Surgery

Second Edition

Surgery
Basic Science and Clinical Evidence

Second Edition

Edited by

Jeffrey A. Norton, MD, FACS
Robert L. and Mary Ellenburg Professor, Department of Surgery; Chief, Divisions of Surgical Oncology and General Surgery, Department of Surgery, Stanford University Medical Center, Stanford, California

Philip S. Barie, MD, MBA, FCCM, FACS
Professor, Departments of Surgery and Public Health; Chief, Division of Critical Care and Trauma, NewYork-Presbyterian Hospital/Weill Cornell Medical College, New York, New York

R. Randal Bollinger, MD, PhD, FACS
Professor, Departments of Surgery and Immunology, Duke University Medical Center, Durham, North Carolina

Alfred E. Chang, MD, FACS
Chief, Division of Surgical Oncology, Hugh Cabot Professor of Surgery, Department of Surgery, University of Michigan, Comprehensive Cancer Center, Ann Arbor, Michigan

Stephen F. Lowry, MD, MBA, FACS
Professor and Chairman, Department of Surgery, University of Medicine and Dentistry of New Jersey, Robert Wood Johnson Medical School, New Brunswick, New Jersey

Sean J. Mulvihill, MD, FACS
Professor and Chair, Department of Surgery; Senior Director of Clinical Affairs, Huntsman Cancer Institute; The University of Utah, Salt Lake City, Utah

Harvey I. Pass, MD, FACS
Professor, Departments of Cardiothoracic Surgery and Surgery, New York University Medical Center, New York, New York

Robert W. Thompson, MD, FACS
Professor of Surgery (Section of Vascular Surgery), Radiology, and Cell Biology and Physiology; Vice-Chairman for Research, Department of Surgery, Washington University School of Medicine, St. Louis, Missouri

Springer

Jeffrey A. Norton, MD, FACS
Robert L. and Mary Ellenburg Professor, Department of Surgery; Chief, Divisions of Surgical Oncology and General Surgery, Department of Surgery, Stanford University Medical Center, Stanford, CA, USA

Philip S. Barie, MD, MBA, FCCM, FACS
Professor, Departments of Surgery and Public Health; Chief, Division of Critical Care and Trauma, NewYork-Presbyterian Hospital/Weill Cornell Medical College, New York, NY, USA

R. Randal Bollinger, MD, PhD, FACS
Professor, Departments of Surgery and Immunology, Duke University Medical Center, Durham, NC, USA

Alfred E. Chang, MD, FACS
Chief, Division of Surgical Oncology, Hugh Cabot Professor of Surgery, Department of Surgery, University of Michigan, Comprehensive Cancer Center, Ann Arbor, MI, USA

Stephen F. Lowry, MD, MBA, FACS
Professor and Chairman, Department of Surgery, University of Medicine and Dentistry of New Jersey, Robert Wood Johnson Medical School, New Brunswick, NJ, USA

Sean J. Mulvihill, MD, FACS
Professor and Chair, Department of Surgery; Senior Director of Clinical Affairs, Huntsman Cancer Institute; The University of Utah, Salt Lake City, UT, USA

Harvey I. Pass, MD, FACS
Professor, Departments of Cardiothoracic Surgery and Surgery, New York University Medical Center, New York, NY, USA

Robert W. Thompson, MD, FACS
Professor of Surgery (Section of Vascular Surgery), Radiology, and Cell Biology and Physiology; Vice-Chairman for Research, Department of Surgery, Washington University School of Medicine, St. Louis, MO, USA

ISBN: 978-0-387-30800-5 e-ISBN: 978-0-387-68113-9
DOI: 10.1007/978-0-387-68113-9

Library of Congress Control Number: 20079218816

Printed on acid-free paper

9 8 7 6 5 4 3 2 1

springer.com

To our families

Preface

When the first edition of *Surgery: Basic Science and Clinical Practice* published, evidence-based medicine principles were just starting to be embraced by the surgery community. Our second edition comes at a critical time in surgical care when surgeons are expected to use the best available evidence to support their every day decisions in patient care, citing critical scientific evidence to support their decisions. No longer is it acceptable to simply say, "We do it this way because we always do it this way." The practice of surgery has evolved from *considering* the principles of evidence-based medicine to actively incorporating those principles into practice. We have taken great care to ensure that *Surgery* meets the needs of both students and clinicians, providing the scientific background, the clinical decision-making skills, and the surgical techniques to provide the best possible patient care.

For this new edition, the editorial board has recruited a new member of the team. In order to provide the necessary emphasis on trauma and critical care, we asked Dr. Philip S. Barie to work with Dr. Stephen F. Lowry to thoroughly expand and improve those topics. The reader will quickly see the added depth and scope of coverage—a marked improvement over the previous edition. We have thoroughly revised every chapter and sharpened the focus on our evidence-based approach, including EBM tables and enhanced figures in every chapter. New chapters discuss transfusion therapy, intraabdominal and nosocomial infections, severe sepsis and shock, mechanical ventilation, imaging in critical care patients, burns and inhalation injury, vascular trauma, traumatic injury of the spine, and surgical rehabilitation. We have identified particular patient populations that require specialized care, including the elderly, neonates, children, and obese patients. We also discuss the needs of pregnant and immunocompromised patients, who require variations in surgical management and care. These chapters are well-illustrated and packed with important evidence to allow enlightened choices.

We have included new chapters on vascular access for dialysis, chemotherapy and nutritional support, thoracic infections, and video-assisted thoracic surgery. The transplant section has been brought up to date and expanded to include transplantation of the intestine. Fundamentals of cancer genomics and proteomics and fundamentals of cancer cell biology and molecular targeting are essential to changes in cancer patient care and treatment, so we have expanded those topics in the oncology section. Finally, there is a new section on biomaterials, energy transfer, and robotics that provide the busy practicing surgeon with new methods and innovative perspectives for modern surgical care. In summary, the book has been thoroughly updated with recent advances in both scientific evidence and clinical practice, including 28 new chapters discussing exciting new areas in surgery. We have focused on current references and evidence to give the reader the most up-to-date information possible.

We hope you will agree that this book, with its consistent and long-established EBM focus, is different from other surgical textbooks. The contributing authors are all clinically active experts who have written comprehensive, current chapters. We believe the chapters on emerging topics strike a balance describing both the current status of practice and the possibilities on the horizon. The chapters have been carefully edited to provide a smooth, readable text. As in previous editions, the evidence-based tables provide information that is consistently formatted and carefully rated, based on the quality of the study design and conduct.

We will soon be embracing the changes in both learning and practice brought on by the ubiquity of computers in medicine. In addition to the print version of this book, we will bring together the timely content of journal articles with the authoritative content of a traditional textbook. At our soon-to-be launched web portal, users will be able to call up topics by book chapter, by general subject, or through a search function. (Similarly, journal readers will be able to access the content of *Surgery* when reading articles in a linked journal.) From this portal, users can navigate easily and seamlessly between book chapters, journal articles, and, where available, videoclips. An online image library, references linked to online databases with full text retrieval (when available), and related clinical and biomedical data will also be available. In addition, an e-book version of *Surgery: Basic Science and Clinical Evidence* is now available, in combination with the print book or as a stand-alone digital resource.

In short, *Surgery: Basic Science and Clinical Evidence* continues to be different and exciting. We have strived to combine the past and present, with an optimistic eye to the future. *Surgery* represents the state of the art and science of the full range of surgical practice as we now know it. We hoped to expand on our past success and create a key reference source for residents and students. We hope readers are as excited about this edition as we are and we invite you to send your comments. Please let us hear from you, as we want to update the book frequently, continuing to improve upon it and make it more reader friendly. We wish you good reading.

Jeffrey A. Norton, MD, FACS
Philip S. Barie, MD, MBA, FCCM, FACS
R. Randal Bollinger, MD, PhD, FACS
Alfred E. Chang, MD, FACS
Stephen F. Lowry, MD, MBA, FACS
Sean J. Mulvihill, MD, FACS
Harvey I. Pass, MD, FACS
Robert W. Thompson, MD, FACS
January 2008

Acknowledgments

The Editorial Board wishes to thank both the editorial and production staff at Springer for their support and encouragement, Mary Shirazi, whose wonderful medical illustrations appear throughout the book, and Barbara Chernow and Kathy Jackson-Cleghorn of Chernow Editorial Services for their outstanding work in coordinating the production of this text.

I personally would also like to thank my family members for their continued help and support, specifically Cathy, John, Meg, Pat, and Tim.

Jeffrey A. Norton, MD

This book is dedicated to all who thirst for knowledge, and strive to improve the care of the surgical patient.

Philip S. Barie, MD, MBA

The untiring support and encouragement of my wife, Monika Bollinger is gratefully acknowledged. I sincerely appreciate the superb work of each author who contributed to the transplantation section and especially the participation of my former colleagues and trainees, Drs. Duane Davis, Douglas Farmer, Bob Harland, Allan Kirk, Stuart Knechtle, Christine Lau, Brian Lima, and Betsy Tuttle-Newhall.

R. Randal Bollinger, MD, PhD

To my wife, Lana, for her support in this effort.

Alfred E. Chang, MD

To Susette, Alex, Lorna, and Kate, who make the "day job" all the more meaningful, and to Debbie, Micki, and Lynn, who help make the "day job" a pleasure. To my mentors, Dick Kraft, Frank Moody, Murray Brennan, and Tom Shires, who instilled a love of surgery and imparted (hopefully) a modicum of their great wisdom.

Stephen F. Lowry, MD

To the surgical trainees who will use this reference for inspiring me with their commitment to excellence, to my own mentor, Haile Debas, MD, for his teaching, advice, and support, and to my wife Kim and sons Michael, Jeffrey, and Timothy for bringing joy to my life.

Sean J. Mulvihill, MD

To my family, Helen, Eric, and Ally Pass, for their constant support.

Harvey I. Pass, MD

To my surgical mentors, Norm Thompson (dad), John Mannick, Ron Stoney, and Greg Sicard, for their inspiration and instruction. To my students, residents, and fellows, who keep me challenged, and to Della for keeping it all in order. To my wonderful wife Michelle and the joy of our lives, Taylor Alexandra, who makes it all worthwhile.

Robert W. Thompson, MD

Contents

[†]Deceased

Section Seven Thoracic Surgery

Section Eight Transplantation Surgery

Section Nine Cancer Surgery

Section Ten Associated Disciplines

Section Eleven Modern Practice of Surgery

Contributors

Craig T. Albanese, MD
Professor, Pediatrics and Obstetrics and Gynecology, Department of Surgery, Stanford University Medical Center; Chief, Division of Pediatric Surgery and Director of Surgical Services, Lucile Packard Children's Hospital, Stanford, CA, USA

David A. August, MD
Associate Professor, Chief, Division of Surgical Oncology, Department of Surgery, University of Medicine and Dentistry of New Jersey, Robert Wood Johnson Medical School, and the Cancer Institute of New Jersey, New Brunswick, NJ, USA

Frank A. Baciewicz, Jr., MD
Associate Professor, Department of Cardio-Thoracic Surgery, Wayne State University/Harper Hospital, Detroit, MI, USA

Carl L. Backer, MD
A. C. Buehler Professor, Division of Cardiovascular-Thoracic Surgery, Department of Surgery, Children's Memorial Hospital, Northwestern University Feinberg School of Medicine, Chicago, IL, USA

Philip S. Barie, MD, MBA
Professor, Departments of Surgery and Public Health; Chief, Division of Critical Care and Trauma, NewYork-Presbyterian Hospital/Weill Cornell Medical College, New York, NY, USA

B. Timothy Baxter, MD
Professor, Department of Surgery, University of Nebraska Medical Center and the Methodist Hospital, Omaha, NE, USA

Gary Binyamin, PhD
Surgical Innovation Fellow, Department of Surgery, Stanford University, James H. Clark Center, Stanford, CA, USA

Mark I. Block, MD
Director, Department of Thoracic Oncology, Memorial Regional Cancer Center, Hollywood, FL, USA

David Bloom, PhD
Postdoctoral Associate, Department of Surgery, University of Florida College of Medicine, Gainesville, FL, USA

Matthew B. Bloom, MD
Resident, Department of Surgery, Stanford University, Stanford, CA, USA

R. Randal Bollinger, MD, PhD
Professor, Departments of Surgery and Immunology, Duke University Medical Center, Durham, NC, USA

Roxana M. Bologa, MD
Assistant Professor, Departments of Clinical Medicine and Surgery, Weill Cornell Medical College; Co-Director, Peritoneal Dialysis, The Rogosin Institute, New York, NY, USA

John Boockvar, MD
Alvina and Willis Murphy Assistant Professor, Departments of Neurological Surgery, and Surgery, Weill Cornell Medical College, New York, NY, USA

Hillary B. Boswell, MD
Staff Physician, The Women's Specialists of Houston, General Obstetrics and Adult Gynecology, Pediatric and Adolescent Gynecology, St. Luke's Medical Tower, Houston, TX, USA

Carol R. Bradford, MD, FACS
Medical Director, Head and Neck Cancer Clinic; Professor, Department of Otolaryngology/Head and Neck Surgery, University of Michigan, UM Comprehensive Cancer Center, Ann Arbor, MI, USA

David Bruce, MD, FACS
Transplant Surgeon, Department of Transplant Surgery, LifeLink Healthcare Institute, Tampa, FL, USA

Steve E. Calvano, PhD
Associate Professor, Department of Surgery, University of Medicine and Dentistry of New Jersey, Robert Wood Johnson Medical School, New Brunswick, NJ, USA

William G. Cance, MD
Professor and Chairman, Department of Surgery, University of Florida College of Medicine, Gainesville, FL, USA

Kathleen King Casey, MD
Chief, Infectious Disease, Department of Medicine, Jersey Shore University Medical Center, Neptune, NJ, USA

George J. Chang, MD
Assistant Professor, Department of Surgical Oncology, The University of Texas M. D. Anderson Cancer Center, Houston, TX, USA

Kyle Chapple, MD
Resident, Department of Neurological Surgery, Weill Cornell Medical College, New York, NY, USA

Edgar Chedrawy, MD
Assistant Professor, Department of Surgery, University of Illinois at Chicago, Chicago, IL, USA

David E. Cohn, MD
Associate Professor, Divisions of Gynecologic Oncology, Departments of Obstetrics and Gynecology, The Ohio State University College of Medicine and Public Health, Columbus, OH, USA

Siobhan A. Corbett, MD
Associate Professor, Department of Surgery, University of Medicine and Dentistry of New Jersey, Robert Wood Johnson Medical School, Clinical Academic Building, New Brunswick, NJ, USA

Raul A. Cortes, MD
Clinical Fellow, Department of Surgery, University of California, San Francisco, San Francisco, CA, USA

Myriam J. Curet, MD, FACS
Associate Professor, Department of Surgery, Stanford University, Stanford, CA, USA

Gail Darling, MD, FACS, FRCSC
Associate Professor, Department of Thoracic Surgery, University Health Network, Toronto, Ontario, Canada

John Mihran Davis, MD
Professor, Department of Surgery, Jersey Shore University Medical Center, Neptune, NJ, USA

R. Duane Davis, MD
Professor, Division of Cardiothoracic Surgery, Department of Surgery, Duke University Medical Center, Durham, NC, USA

Laura A. Dawson, MD
Assistant Professor, Department of Radiation Oncology, University of Toronto/Princess Margaret Hospital, Toronto, Ontario, Canada

Haile T. Debas, MD[†]
Executive Director, UCSF Global Health Sciences; Maurice Galante Distinguished Professor, Dean Emeritus, School of Medicine, Vice Chancellor Emeritus, Medical Affairs, Chancellor Emeritus, Department of Surgery, University of California, San Francisco, San Francisco, CA, USA

William de Bois, MD
Fellow, Department of Surgery, Heart Center at Stony Brook, Stony Brook University, Stony Brook, NY, USA

Ronald P. DeMatteo, MD
Vice Chair, Department of Surgery; Head, Division of General Surgical Oncology; Director, General Surgical Oncology Fellowship Program, Memorial Sloan-Kettering Cancer Center, New York, NY, USA

Frank C. Detterbeck, MD
Professor; Section Chief; Surgical Director, Department Thoracic Oncology; Associate Director, Department for Clinical Affairs, Yale Cancer Center, Yale-New Haven Hospital, New Haven, CT, USA

James P. Dolan, MD
Lieutenant Colonel, USAF, MC, Chief, Department of General Surgery, Keesler Medical Center, Biloxi, MI, USA

Jessica Scott Donington, MD
Assistant Professor, Department of Cardiothoracic Surgery, Stanford University Medical Center, Stanford, CA, USA

John H. Donohue, MD
Professor, Department of Surgery, Mayo Medical School; Consultant, Division of Gastroenterologic and General Surgery, Mayo Clinic, Rochester, MN, USA

David J. Dries, MSE, MD
Assistant Medical Director, Department of Surgical Care, HealthPartners Medical Group; John F. Perry, Jr. Professor, Department of Surgery, University of Minnesota, St. Paul, MN, USA

David L. Dunn, MD, PhD
Vice President for Health Sciences, Professor, Department of Surgery, University at Buffalo/SUNY, Buffalo, NY, USA

Soumitra R. Eachempati, MD
Associate Professor, Departments of Surgery and Public Health, Weill Cornell Medical College; Associate Attending Surgeon, NewYork-Presbyterian Hospital, New York, NY, USA

Eric A. Elster, MD
Assistant Professor, Department of Surgery, Uniformed Services University; Transplantation Branch, National Institutes of Health, Bethesda, MD, USA

Andrew Fang, MD
Attending, Department of Orthopedics, South San Francisco Medical Center, San Francisco, CA, USA

Peter L. Faries, MD
Chief, Departments of Endovascular Surgery and Surgery, Cornell University, Weill Cornell Medical College, Columbia University College of Physicians and Surgeons, New York, NY, USA

Douglas G. Farmer, MD
Associate Professor, Department of Surgery, David Geffen School of Medicine at UCLA; Director, Intestinal Transplant Program, Director, Pediatric Liver Transplant Program, Co-Director, Intestinal Failure Center, Division of Liver and Pancreas Transplantation, Dumont UCLA Transplant Center, Los Angeles, CA, USA

Alison M. Fecher, MD
Fellow, Department of Surgery, Duke University Medical Center, Durham, NC. USA

Hiran C. Fernando, MBBS
Associate Professor, Department of Cardiothoracic Surgery, Boston University, Boston, MA, USA

Mathew I. Foley, MD
Vascular Surgeon, Legacy Columbia Vascular and Endovascular Division, Legacy Emanuel Hospital and Health Center, Portland, OR, USA

Ramsey A. Foty, PhD
Assistant Professor, Department of Surgery, University of Medicine and Dentistry of New Jersey, Robert Wood Johnson Medical School, New Brunswick, NJ, USA

Douglas L. Fraker, MD
Jonathon Rhoads Professor, Department of Surgery; Vice-Chairman, Clinical Affairs, Department of Surgery, University of Pennsylvania, Philadelphia, PA, USA

Justin F. Fraser, MD
Resident, Department of Neurological Surgery, NewYork-Presbyterian Hospital, New York, NY, USA

Joseph S. Friedberg, MD
Associate Professor, Chief, Division of Thoracic Surgery, Department of Surgery, University of Pennsylvania Medical Center at Presbyterian, Philadelphia, PA, USA

Donald E. Fry, MD
Adjunct Professor, Department of Surgery, Northwestern University Feinberg School of Medicine, Chicago, IL, USA

Michael J. Gardner, MD
Senior Clinical Associate, Department of Orthopaedic Surgery, Hospital for Special Surgery, New York, NY, USA

Marc R. Garfinkel, MD
Assistant Professor, Department of Surgery, University of Chicago Medical Center, Center for Advanced Medicine, Chicago, IL, USA

Randolph L. Geary, MD
Professor, Department of General Surgery, Wake Forest University School of Medicine, Winston-Salem, NC, USA

Michael E. Gertner, MD
Consulting Assistant Professor, Department of Surgery, Stanford University, Stanford, CA, USA

Scott N. Gettinger, MD
Assistant Professor, Department of Medicine, Yale Medical Oncology, New Haven, CT, USA

Enrique Ginzberg, MD
Professor, DeWitt Daughtry Family, Department of Surgery, Miller School of Medicine, University of Miami, Miami, FL, USA

Robert E. Glasgow, MD
Assistant Professor, Department of Surgery, University of Utah, Salt Lake City, UT, USA

Claudia E. Goettler, MD
Assistant Professor, Traumatology and Surgical Critical Care, Department of Surgery, Brody School of Medicine, East Carolina University, Greenville, NC, USA

Jason S. Gold, MD
Staff Surgeon, Surgical Service VA Boston Healthcare System, West Roxbury MA; Lecturer, Department of Surgery, Brigham and Women's Hospital, Harvard Medical School, Boston, MA, USA

Michael A. Golden, MD
Chief, Division of Vascular Surgery and Endovascular Therapy, Department of Surgery, Penn Presbyterian Medical Center, Philadelphia, PA, USA

Vita Golubovskaya, PhD
Research Assistant Professor, Department of Surgery, University of Florida College of Medicine, Gainesville, FL, USA

Jeffrey Hammond, MD, MBA, MPH
Professor, Department of Surgery, University of Medicine and Dentistry of New Jersey, Robert Wood Johnson Medical School, New Brunswick, NJ, USA

Douglas W. Hanto, MD, PhD
Lewis Thomas Professor, Department of Surgery, Harvard Medical School; Chief, Division of Transplantation, Beth Israel Deaconess Medical Center, Boston, MA, USA

Robert C. Harland, MD
Associate Professor, Departments of Surgery and Medicine, Director, Kidney and Pancreas Transplantation, Comer Children's Hospital, University of Chicago, Center for Advanced Medicine, Chicago, IL, USA

Hobart W. Harris, MD, MPH
Professor and Chief, Division of General Surgery, Vice-Chair, Department of Surgery, University of California, San Francisco, CA, USA

Roger Hartl, MD
Assistant Professor, Neurological Surgery, Weill Cornell Medical College, New York, NY, USA

David L. Helfet, MD
Professor, Department of Orthopaedic Surgery, Weill Cornell Medical Center, Director, Orthopedic Trauma Service, Hospital for Special Surgery/NewYork-Presbyterian Hospital, New York, NY, USA

Steven N. Hochwald, MD
Assistant Professor, Department of Surgical Oncology, Molecular Genetics and Microbiology, University of Florida College of Medicine, Gainesville, FL, USA

Richard A. Hodin, MD
Associate Professor, Department of Surgery, Massachusetts General Hospital, Harvard Medical School, Boston, MA, USA

Maureen B. Huhmann, MS, RD
Instructor, Department of Primary Care, University of Medicine and Dentistry of New Jersey, New Brunswick, NJ, USA

Danny O. Jacobs, MD, MPH
Professor and Chairman, Department of Surgery, Duke University Medical Center, Durham, NC, USA

Eric H. Jensen, MD
Fellow, Department of Surgical Oncology, H. Lee Moffitt Cancer Center and Research Institute, Tampa, FL, USA

Scott R. Johnson, MD
Instructor, Department of Surgery, Harvard Medical School; Surgical Director of Kidney Transplantation, Beth Deaconess Medical Center, Boston, MA, USA

Daniel B. Jones, MD
Associate Professor, Harvard Medical School; Chief, Minimally Invasive Surgery, Beth Israel Deaconess Medical Center, Boston, MA, USA

Fady M. Kaldas, MD
Surgical Research Fellow, Department of Surgery, University of California, Los Angeles, CA, USA

Seth J. Karp, MD
Assistant Professor, Department of Surgery, Harvard Medical School; Division of Transplantation, Beth Israel Deaconess Medical Center, Boston, MA, USA

K. Craig Kent, MD
Chief, Combined Columbia and Cornell Division of Vascular Surgery, NewYork-Presbyterian Hospital, New York, NY; Professor, Department of Surgery, Columbia University College of Physicians and Surgeons, New York; Greenberg-Starr Professor, Department of Surgery, Weill Cornell Medical College, New York, NY, USA

Khalid Khwaja, MD
Instructor, Department of Surgery, Harvard Medical School; Surgical Director of Pancreas Transplantation, Beth Israel Deaconess Medical Center, Boston, MA, USA

Allan D. Kirk, MD, PhD
Chief, Transplantation Branch, National Institutes of Health, Bethesda, MD, USA

Stuart J. Knechtle, MD
Ray D. Owen Professor, Departments of Transplantation and Surgery, University of Wisconsin Medical School, Madison, WI, USA

Joseph Knight, MS
Biodesign Innovation Fellow, Department of Cardiovascular Medicine, Stanford University, Stanford, CA, USA

Daniel Kreisel, MD, PhD
Assistant Professor, Division of Cardiothoracic Surgery, Department of Surgery, Washington University School of Medicine, St. Louis, MO, USA

Thomas Krummel, MD
Emile Holman Professor and Chair, Department of Surgery, Division of Pediatric Surgery, Stanford University, Stanford, CA, USA

John C. Kucharczuk, MD
Assistant Professor, Department of Cardiothoracic Surgery, Hospital of the University of Pennsylvania, Philadelphia, PA, USA

Kenneth A. Kudsk, MD
Professor, Department of Surgery, Vice Chairman of Surgical Research, University of Wisconsin-Madison, Madison, WI, USA

Terry C. Lairmore, MD
Director, Division of Surgical Oncology, Scott and White Memorial Hospital and Clinic, Texas A&M University System Health Science Center, Temple, TX, USA

Christine L. Lau, MD
Fellow, Division of Cardiothoracic Surgery, Department of Surgery, Washington University School of Medicine, St. Louis, MO, USA

W. Thomas Lawrence, MD, MPH
Professor and Chief, Department of Plastic Surgery, University of Kansas Medical Center, Sutherland Institute, Kansas City, KS, USA

Walter Lawrence, Jr., MD
Professor Emeritus, Division of Surgical Oncology, Department of Surgery, Virginia Commonwealth University College of Medicine, Richmond, VA, USA

David Le, MD
Resident, Department of Surgery, Stanford University Medical Center, Stanford, CA, USA

Alice Y. Lee, MS
Computation Biologist, H. Lee Moffitt Cancer Center and Research Institute, Tampa, FL, USA

Hanmin Lee, MD
Associate Professor, Department of Surgery, Pediatrics, and OB-Gyn and Reproductive Services, University of California, San Francisco, San Francisco, CA, USA

Alan T. Lefor, MD, MPH
Professor, Department of Surgery, Jichi Medical University, Center for Graduate Medical Education, Shimotsuke, Tochigi, Japan

Marcel Levi, MD, PhD
Professor, Department of Medicine, Academic Medical Center, University of Amsterdam, Amsterdam, The Netherlands

Brian Lima, MD
Research Fellow, Department of Cardiothoracic Surgery, Duke University, Durham, NC, USA

Edward Lin, MD
Assistant Professor, Department of Surgery, Emory University School of Medicine, Atlanta, GA, USA

Pamela A. Lipsett, MD
Professor, Department of Surgery, Anesthesiology/Critical Care Medicine, Johns Hopkins University Schools of Medicine and Nursing, Baltimore, MD, USA

Michael T. Longaker, MD, MBA
Deane P. and Louise Mitchell Professor, Department of Surgery (Plastic and Reconstructive); Director, Children's Surgical Research, Lucile Packard Children's Hospital, Stanford University School of Medicine, Stanford, CA, USA

Peter P. Lopez, MD
Assistant Professor, DeWitt Daughtry Family, Department of Surgery, Miller School of Medicine, University of Miami, Ryder Trauma Center, Jackson Memorial Medical Center, Miami, FL, USA

H. Peter Lorenz, MD
Associate Professor, Department of Surgery (Plastic and Reconstructive); Investigator, Children's Surgical Research Program, Stanford University School of Medicine, Stanford, CA, USA

Dean G. Lorich, MD
Assistant Professor, Department of Orthopedic Surgery, Weill Cornell Medical Center; Associate Director, Orthopaedic Trauma Service, Hospital for Special Surgery/NewYork-Presbyterian Hospital, New York, NY, USA

David W. Lowenberg, MD
Chairman, Department of Orthopedic Surgery, California Pacific Medical Center, San Francisco, CA, USA

Adam Lowenstein, MD
Private Practice, Mendacito Center for Aesthetic Plastic Surgery, Santa Barbara, CA, USA

Stephen F. Lowry, MD, MBA
Professor and Chairman, Department of Surgery, University of Medicine and Dentistry of New Jersey, Robert Wood Johnson Medical School, New Brunswick, NJ, USA

Erika J. Lu, MD
Resident, Department of Surgery, Stanford University Medical Center, Stanford, CA, USA

James D. Luketich, MD
Professor, Department of Surgery; Chief, Division of Thoracic and Foregut Surgery, University of Pittsburgh, Pittsburgh, PA, USA

Ronald V. Maier, MD
Jane and Donald D. Trunkey Professor, Vice Chair, Department of Surgery; Surgeon-in-Chief, Department of Surgery, Harborview Medical Center, Seattle, WA, USA

Kim A. Margolin, MD
Associate Director for Clinical Research, Division of Medical Oncology and Therapeutics Research; Professor, Division of Hematology and Hematopoietic Cell Transplantation; Staff Physician, Medical Oncology, City of Hope National Medical Center, Duarte, CA, USA

John C. Marshall, MD
Professor, Department of Surgery, Critical Care Medicine, University of Toronto/St. Michael's Hospital, Toronto, Ontario, Canada

Jeffrey B. Matthews, MD
Christian R. Holmes Professor, Chairman, Department of Surgery, University of Cincinnati College of Medicine, Cincinnati, OH, USA

Constantine Mavroudis, MD
Willis J. Potts Professor, Department of Surgery; Surgeon-in-Chief, Division of Cardiovascular-Thoracic Surgery, Children's Memorial Hospital, Northwestern University Feinberg School of Medicine, Chicago, IL, USA

David A. McClusky, III, MD
Chief Resident, Department of Surgery, Emory University Hospital, Atlanta, GA, USA

Robin S. McLeod, MD, FRCSC
Professor, Department of Surgery, University of Toronto; Head, Division of General Surgery, Mount Sinai Hospital, Toronto, Ontario, Canada

Spencer J. Melby, MD
Senior Resident, Department of General Surgery, Barnes-Jewish Hospital and Washington University School of Medicine, St. Louis, MO, USA

Carlos Mery, MD, MPH
Surgical Innovation Fellow, Department of Surgery, Stanford University, Mountain View, CA, USA

Barbara-Ann Millar, MBChB
Assistant Professor, Department of Radiation Oncology, University of Toronto/Princess Margaret Hospital, Toronto, Ontario, Canada

Edward Miranda, MD
Attending Surgeon, Department of Plastic and Reconstructive Surgery, California-Pacific Medical Center, San Francisco, CA, USA

Jeffrey F. Moley, MD
Professor, Division of General Surgery, Department of Surgery; Chief, Cancer and Endocrine Surgery Section; Associate Director, Siteman Cancer Center, Washington University School of Medicine, St. Louis, MO, USA

Gregory L. Moneta, MD
Professor and Chief, Department of Vascular Surgery, Oregon Health and Science University, Portland, OR, USA

John Morton, MD, MPH
Director, Department of Bariatric Surgery, Stanford School of Medicine, Stanford, CA, USA

Jeffrey S. Moyer, MD
Assistant Professor, Department of Otolaryngology, Director of Medical Student Education, University of Michigan, A. Alfred Taubman Health Care Center, Ann Arbor, MI, USA

Sean J. Mulvihill, MD
Professor and Chair, Department of Surgery; Senior Director of Clinical Affairs, Huntsman Cancer Institute; The University of Utah, Salt Lake City, UT, USA

Lena M. Napolitano, MD
Professor, Department of Surgery; Chief, Surgical Critical Care; Program Director, Surgical Critical Care Fellowship; Associate Chair, Department of Critical Care, University of Michigan School of Medicine, Ann Arbor, MI, USA

Avery B. Nathens, MD, PhD, MPH
Associate Professor, Director, Surgical Critical Care, Department of Surgery, University of Washington/ Harborview Medical Center, Seattle, WA, USA

Tammy Noren, PT, MSPT
Assistant Chief Physical Therapist, Department of Rehabilitation Medicine, NewYork-Presbyterian Hospital, Weill Cornell Medical Center, New York, NY, USA

Jeffrey A. Norton, MD
Robert L. and Mary Ellenburg Professor, Department of Surgery, Chief, Divisions of Surgical Oncology and General Surgery, Department of Surgery, Stanford University Medical Center, Stanford, CA, USA

Michael W. O'Dell, MD
Acting Chief and Professor, Department of Rehabilitation Medicine, New York, NY, USA

Steven M. Opal, MD
Professor, Infectious Disease Division, Department of Medicine, Brown Medical School, Providence, RI, USA

Theodore N. Pappas, MD
Professor and Vice President, Department of Administration and Surgery; Executive Medical Director, Private Diagnostic Clinic, Duke University Medical Center, Durham, NC, USA

Helen A. Pass, MD
Assistant Professor, Department of Clinical Surgery, Columbia University; Assistant Attending Surgeon, NewYork-Presbyterian Hospital/Columbia University Medical Center, New York, NY, USA

Sheela T. Patel, MD
Resident, Department of Surgery, Weill Cornell Medical College, Columbia University College of Physicians and Surgeons, New York, NY, USA

G. Alexander Patterson, MD
Joseph C. Bancroft Professor, Department of Surgery; Chief, Division of Cardiothoracic Surgery, Department of General Thoracic Surgery, Washington University School of Medicine, St. Louis, MO, USA

John F. Perry, Jr., MD
Professor, Department of Surgery, University of Minnesota, Minneapolis, MN, USA

David A. Peterson, MD
Resident, Department of Surgery, Stanford University Medical Center, Stanford, CA, USA

John E. Phay, MD
Assistant Professor, Divisions of Surgical Oncology, Department of Surgery, Vanderbuilt University Medical Center, Nashville, TN, USA

Edward H. Phillips, MD
Director, Center for Minimally Invasive Surgery, Department of Surgery, Cedars-Sinai Medical Center, Los Angeles, CA, USA

Peter W.T. Pisters, MD
Professor, Department of Surgical Oncology, The University of Texas M. D. Anderson Cancer Center, Houston, TX, USA

Joseph C. Presti, Jr., MD
Associate Clinical Professor, Department of Urology, University of California, San Francisco, San Francisco, CA, USA

Janet S. Rader, MD
Professor, Division of Gynecologic Oncology, Department of Obstetrics and Gynecology; Associate Professor, Department of Genetics, Washington University School of Medicine, St. Louis, MO, USA

Michael D. Rollins, MD
Assistant Professor, Department of Surgery, University of Utah, Salt Lake City, UT, USA

Bruce R. Rosengard, MD
Associate Professor, Department of Surgery, Cardiac Surgical Unit, Massachusetts General Hospital, Boston, MA, USA

Todd K. Rosengart, MD
Chief, Cardiothoracic Surgery, Co-Director of the Heart Center at Stony Brook, Stony Brook University, Stony Brook, NY, USA

Michael F. Rotondo, MD
Professor, Chairman, Department of Surgery, Brody School of Medicine, East Carolina University, Greenville, NC, USA

Grace S. Rozycki, MD, MBA
Professor, Department of Surgery; Director, Trauma and Surgical Critical Care, Emory University School of Medicine, Grady Memorial Hospital, Atlanta, GA, USA

Ira M. Rutkow, MD
Clinical Professor, Department of Surgery, University of Medicine and Dentistry of New Jersey, Newark, NJ, USA

Stuart D. Saal, MD
Professor, Departments of Clinical Medicine and Surgery, Weill Cornell Medical College; Vice President for Hospital Affairs; Medical Director, Transplantation Program; Co-Director, Renal Consultation Service; Co-Director, Apheresis, The Rogosin Institute, New York, NY, USA

Courtney Scaife, MD
Assistant Professor, Department of Surgery, University of Utah, Salt Lake City, UT, USA

Thomas M. Scalea, MD
Physician-in-Chief, R Adams Cowley Shock Trauma Center; Director, Program in Trauma, University of Maryland School of Medicine, Baltimore, MD, USA

William P. Schecter, MD
Professor, Department Clinical Surgery, University of California, San Francisco, University of California, San Francisco, San Francisco, CA, USA

Matthew J. Schuchert, MD
Instructor, Department of Surgery, University of Pittsburgh, Pittsburgh, PA, USA

Daniel J. Scott, MD
Associate Professor and William Henderson Chair, Director, Tulane Center for Minimally Invasive Surgery, Tulane University School of Medicine, New Orleans, LA, USA

Bilal Shafi, MD, MSE
Surgical Innovation Fellow, Departments of Surgery and Cardiovascular Medicine, Stanford University, Palo Alto, CA, USA

Michael B. Shapiro, MD
Associate Professor, Department of Surgery, Trauma and Critical Care, Feinberg School of Medicine, Northwestern University, Chicago, IL, USA

Andrew A. Shelton, MD
Assistant Professor, Department of Surgery, Stanford University School of Medicine, Stanford, CA, USA

G. Tom Shires, MD[†]
Professor, Department of Surgery, University of Nevada School of Medicine, Las Vegas, NV, USA

Craig L. Slingluff, Jr., MD
Joseph Helms Farrow Professor, Department of Surgery, University of Virginia, Charlottesville, VA, USA

C. Daniel Smith, MD
Professor and Chair, Department of Surgery, Mayo Clinic Jacksonville, Jacksonville, FL, USA

Mark A. Socinski, MD
Associate Professor, Department of Medicine, Lineberger Comprehensive Cancer Center, University of North Carolina, Chapel Hill, NC, USA

Vernon K. Sondak, MD
Chief, Division of Cutaneous Oncology; Professor, Departments of Surgery and Interdisciplinary Oncology, H. Lee Moffitt Cancer Center and Research Institute, Tampa, FL, USA

David Soybel, MD
Senior Staff Surgeon, Division of General and Gastrointestinal Surgery, Brighams and Women's Hospital, Brigham and Women's Hospital, Division of General and Gastrointestinal Surgery, Boston, MA, USA

Philip Starr, MD, PhD
Associate Professor, Dolores Cakebread Endowed Chair, Co-Director, Functional Neurosurgery Program, Department of Neurological Surgery, University of California, San Francisco; Surgical Director, Parkinson's Disease Research, Education and Care Center (PADRECC) at San Francisco Veteran's Affairs Medical Center, San Francisco, CA, USA

Thomas E. Starzl, MD, PhD
Professor, Department of Surgery, Thomas E. Starzl Transplantation Institute, University of Pittsburgh, Pittsburgh, PA, USA

Deborah M. Stein, MD, MPH
Assistant Professor, Department of Surgery, R Adams Cowley Shock Trauma Center, University of Maryland School of Medicine, Baltimore, MD, USA

Larry W. Stephenson, MD
Ford-Webber Professor, Department of Surgery; Professor and Chief, Cardiothoracic Surgery, Wayne State University, School of Medicine, Detroit, MI, USA

Catherine Sudarshan, FRAS
Attending, Cardiothoracic Division, Papworth Hospital, Cambridge, United Kingdom

Benjamin C. Sun, MD
Associate Professor and Director, Departments of Cardiac Transplantation and Mechanical Support and Surgery, The Ohio State University Medical Center, Columbus, OH, USA

Thoralf M. Sundt, MD
Professor, Department of Surgery, Mayo Clinic, Rochester, MN, USA

Jimmy C. Sung, MD, JD
Senior Resident, Department of Surgery, University of South Florida, Tampa, FL, USA

Jeffrey J. Sussman, MD
Assistant Professor, Department of Surgery, University of Cincinnati/VAMC Cincinnati, Cincinnati, OH, USA

J. Richard Thistlethwaite, MD, PhD
Professor, Department of Surgery; President, Medical Staff, The University of Chicago Medical Center, Chicago, IL, USA

[†]Deceased

Jesse E. Thompson, MD
Professor, Department of Surgery, Baylor University Medical Center, Dallas, TX, USA

Robert W. Thompson, MD
Professor, Departments of Surgery (Section of Vascular Surgery), Radiology, and Cell Biology and Physiology; Vice-Chairman for Research, Department of Surgery; Attending Surgeon, Barnes-Jewish Hospital and Washington University School of Medicine, St. Louis, MO, USA

Bryan W. Tillman, MD, PhD
Assistant Instructor, Department of Surgery, Wake Forest University Medical Center, Winston-Salem, NC, USA

Joseph D. Tobias, MD
Vice-Chairman, Department of Anesthesiology; Russell and Mary Shelden Chair, Department of Pediatric Intensive Care; Chief, Division of Pediatric Anesthesiology; Professor, Department of Pediatrics and Anesthesiology, University of Missouri, Columbia, MO, USA

J.E. Tuttle-Newhall, MD
Assistant Professor, Department of Surgery, Duke University, Durham, NC, USA

Robert Udelsman, MD, MBA
Professor and Chairman, Department of Surgery, Yale University School of Medicine, New Haven, CT, USA

Tom van der Poll, MD, PhD
Professor, Laboratory of Experimental Medicine, Academic Medical Center, University of Amsterdam, Amsterdam, The Netherlands

Madhulika G. Varma, MD
Attending, UCSF Center for Colorectal Surgery, University of California, San Francisco, Medical Center, San Francisco, CA, USA

Malica Vukovic, MD
Instructor, Department of Medicine, Evanston Hospital, Evanston, IL, USA

James Wall, MD
Resident, Department of Surgery, University of California, San Francisco, San Francisco, CA, USA

Russell Wall, MD
Director, Resident Education, Department of Anesthesia, Georgetown University, Washington, DC, USA

Olivia Walton, PA-C
Physicians Assistant, Department of Anesthesiology, University of Utah, Huntsman Cancer Institute, Salt Lake City, UT, USA

John C.L. Wang, MD, PhD
Professor, Departments of Clinical Medicine and Surgery, Weill Cornell Medical College; Vice President for Out-Patient Services; Director, Jack J. Dreyfus Clinic of Rogosin Kidney Center; Director, Adoptive Immunotherapy Program; Director, Nephrology; Co-Director, Renal Consultation Service, The Rogosin Institute, New York, NY, USA

Ronald J. Weigel, MD, PhD
Professor and Head, Department of Surgery, University of Iowa Roy J. and Lucille A. Carver College of Medicine and University of Iowa Hospitals and Clinics, Iowa City, IA, USA

Sharon M. Weinstein, MD
Associate Professor, Department of Anesthesiology, University of Utah, Huntsman Cancer Institute, Salt Lake City, UT, USA

Mark L. Welton, MD
Associate Professor, Department of Surgery, Stanford University Medical Center, Stanford, CA, USA

Michael A. West, MD, PhD
Professor, Department of Surgery, Trauma/Critical Care, Northwestern University, Feinberg School of Medicine, Chicago, IL, USA

Brad A. Winterstein, MD
Assistant Professor, Department of Surgery, University of Nebraska Medical Center and the Methodist Hospital, Omaha, NE, USA

Susannah S. Wise, MD
Instructor, Department of Surgery, University of Medicine and Dentistry of New Jersey, Robert Wood Johnson Medical School, New Brunswick, NJ, USA

Russell K. Woo, MD
General Surgery Resident, Department of Surgery, Stanford University Medical Center, Stanford, CA, USA

Amy D. Wyrzykowski, MD
Assistant Professor, Department of Surgery, Emory University School of Medicine, Grady Memorial Hospital, Atlanta, GA, USA

Marineh Yagubian, MD
Resident, Department of Surgery, Mayo Clinic, Rochester, MN, USA

Timothy J. Yeatman, MD
Associate Center Director, Department of Clinical Investigations; Professor, Department of Interdisciplinary Oncology, H. Lee Moffitt Cancer Center and Research Institute, Tampa, FL, USA

Roger W. Yurt, MD
Johnson and Johnson Distinguished Professor and Vice Chairman, Department of Surgery; Director, William Randolph Hearst Burn Center, Weill Cornell Medical College, NewYork-Presbyterian Hospital, New York, NY, USA

Evidence-Based Tables

All evidence-based tables are indicated in the text by an E.

Surgery

Second Edition

SECTION ONE

Fundamentals of Surgical Care

1

Origins of Modern Surgery

Ira M. Rutkow

It remains a rhetorical question whether an understanding of surgical history is important to the maturation and continued education and training of a surgeon. Conversely, it is hardly necessary to dwell on the heuristic value that an appreciation of history provides in developing adjunctive humanistic, literary, and philosophical tastes. Clearly, medicine is a lifelong learning process that should be an enjoyable and rewarding experience. For a surgeon, the study of surgical history contributes greatly toward making this learning process more pleasurable and is invigorating. To trace the evolution of what one does on a daily basis and to understand it from a historical perspective are enviable goals. It reality, there is no way to separate present-day surgery and one's own practice from the experiences of all the surgeons in all the preceding years.

For the budding surgeon, it is a magnificent adventure to appreciate what he or she is currently learning within the context of past and present cultural, economic, political, and social institutions. The active practitioner will find that the study of the profession, dealing as it rightly must with all aspects of human society, affords an excellent avenue to the appreciation of previous ideas and concepts.

As this chapter is titled "Origins of Modern Surgery," by definition it is concerned primarily with events prior to the 20th century, a time during which surgery evolved into its current status of respected profession.

Ancient Civilizations

Although there is no way of knowing when the earliest surgical operations were performed, it is not unreasonable to assume that frequent attempts at surgery were completed by our most distant prehistorical ancestors. The attempt to remedy day-to-day external discomforts by manual manipulations must have been among the ongoing evolutionary efforts of the human species. Presumably, the earliest attempts at surgery were mainly devoted to the treatment of injuries and included procedures to alleviate nuisances, such as removing splinters, piercing boils or blisters, treating burns, and excising traumatized tissue. Accordingly, surgery by default necessarily preceded internal medicine regarding the rational treatment of human disease.

Speculations by the ancients about bodily "humors," "fluxes," "vital spirits," and other nonsensical doctrines did little to relieve human suffering. Instead, it was the "surgeon," or at least the individual who wielded the knife or treated injuries, who was better equipped to handle diseases and wounds. The clearest example of this is that trephination remains the earliest example of actual major surgery. That prehistorical humans, using the most rudimentary surgical instruments, were able to bore open a human skull—and that the patient survived—is an incredible medical accomplishment. When and how skull boring originated are matters of scientific conjecture. However, skulls from the Mesolithic cultural period have been found with round depressions suggestive of primitive trephination skills, which would date initial efforts at such operations at 10,000 to 5000 BC.

Why would Stone Age humans resort to trephination? There is little archeological or other scientific evidence to suggest that this practice was used for the treatment of diseases such as osteomyelitis or syphilitic lesions of the cranium; most trephinations were performed on intact skulls with no prior signs of violence. It is more likely that trephinations were carried out for spiritual or magical reasons and used in cases of epilepsy, headache, or mental illness.

From the Fertile Crescent in the Middle East, several ancient civilizations have provided some of the earliest known examples of surgical writings. The complex culture of Assyro-Babylonia left the important Code of Hammurabi. Many of the rules in the code concern the outcome of operations (If a physician shall make a severe wound with the bronze operating-knife and kill the patient, or shall open a growth with a bronze operating-knife and destroy his eye, the physician's hands shall be cut off). Thus, despite the lack of archeological evidence regarding surgical tools, it can be assumed that surgical therapies were carried out. Closely connected in spirit and substance with Assyro-Babylonian and Sumerian-Semitic surgery is the surgery of the ancient Jews. A rich collection of surgical lore is found in the Talmud. The text discusses various surgical procedures, including how to suture wounds and clean traumatized edges, methods for dealing with imperforate anus, the advantages of lessening pain during a surgical procedure, reduction of dislocations, amputations and the use of wooden prostheses, cesarean section, and even veterinary procedures.

From ancient Egypt, the Edwin Smith papyrus, written around 1600 BC, addresses strictly surgical problems. Unfortunately, the work, systematically arranged like a textbook of surgery, remains incomplete. The anatomical observations are descriptive, and terms were created to designate structures. This work provides the following information for dealing with the surgical problems: In the case of a skull injury, the pulse is recorded, and a digital exploration of the wound is attempted to ascertain whether there is a depressed fracture of the skull. Feeble pulse and fever are noted in cases of hopeless head injuries. The traumatized skin edges are placed close together, and bandages soaked in a type of glue hold them in position. Fresh meat, perhaps for its hemostyptic value, is the usual dressing for the first day.

The first allusions to surgical subjects in Greek civilization are found in the Homeric poems the *Iliad* and the *Odyssey*, which are generally accepted as dating from 800 to 700 BC. More than 100 passages give realistic descriptions of battle wounds, spearing, sword thrusts, arrow wounds, slingshot injuries, and their treatment. Numerous "schools" of medicine (associations of philosophers, priest-physicians, practitioners, and students) were beginning to develop throughout Greece. The two most important were located at Cnidos and Cos. It was on the latter that the "father of modern medicine," Hippocrates (Fig. 1.1) was said to have been born. He was able to disassociate medicine permanently from the religious mysticism that previously coexisted with it; through his abilities as a teacher, he crystallized the existing knowledge of the Cnidian and Coan schools into a systematic science, and most important, he made physicians understand the high moral inspiration under which they practiced medicine.

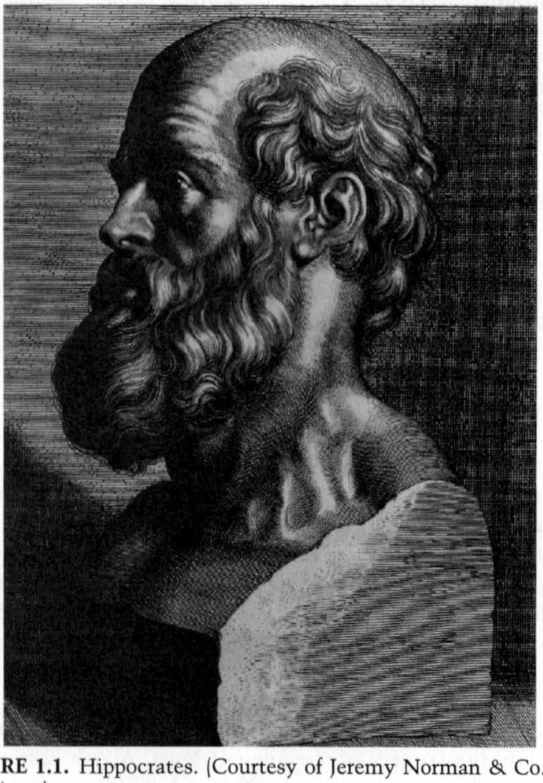

FIGURE 1.1. Hippocrates. (Courtesy of Jeremy Norman & Co., San Francisco.)

A collection of 72 medical works has become known as the *Corpus Hippocraticum*. Undoubtedly, the works of others were included in the *Corpus*, so when the writings of Hippocrates are discussed, it is reasonable to presume more than one author. The surgical texts, including "Wounds and Ulcers," "Hemorrhoids," "Fistulas," "Injuries of the Head," "Fractures," "Articulations," and "Mochlicus" (meaning Bones, Their Injuries and Displacements, and Instruments of Reduction) are the most lucid and brilliant sections of the entire work.

Early Roman surgery is poorly understood because little remains of written information. However, it was believed to have been strongly influenced by Greek medicine and in most aspects reflected the Greek healing traditions. Surgery in Rome was practiced almost entirely by Greek physicians, yet the most erudite accounting of it was written by Cornelius Celsus (25 BC to AD 50), a Roman nobleman. Because he wrote in Latin, not Greek, and because he was not a physician, his works exerted little professional influence during his own time. Even in the handwritten manuscripts of the Middle Ages, his name is mentioned only a few times. When first printed during the Renaissance, however, his books on medicine became highly valued for their purity and precision in style and informative value. Celsus's *De Medicina* is the oldest important medical document after the *Corpus Hippocraticum* and provides a cumulative knowledge of medicine and surgery from the time of Hippocrates to the dawn of the Christian era. This work consists of eight sections or books; the last two discuss diseases considered strictly surgical. In particular, Celsus is best remembered for his description of the characteristics of inflammations: redness, swelling, heat, and pain (rubor, tumor, calor, and dolor, respectively).

The most famous physician of the Roman period is Galen (AD 129–199), who is considered second only to Hippocrates as the most important physician of antiquity. His views dominated European medicine for almost 15 centuries, until the time of the Renaissance. Unlike Hippocrates, about whom little is known, Galen provided much autobiographical information. Born in Pergamum, he later served as chief surgeon to the Roman gladiators. Because human dissection was not permitted, Galen conducted well-publicized anatomical dissections on apes and pigs and drew much human anatomical data from animals rather than *Homo sapiens*. This necessity resulted in the perpetuation of countless errors throughout the medical literature until the 16th century. Despite Galen's overbearing personality and ill-formed misconceptions, the breadth and depth of his writings are staggering. Viewed as a talented technical surgeon, he wrote extensively on the use of various surgical instruments. Most scholars consider his treatise on pathological swellings his foremost contribution to surgery because of its exacting discussion of inflammation and tumors. Due to his pugnacious personality, Galen never acquired any true disciples. However, because the coming Middle Ages were a scientifically and culturally unsettled era, there was a need for certainty and authority in medicine. Galen's answers provided the church and lay leaders with their desire for an absolute truth, regardless of its veracity.

The Middle Ages

The Middle Ages, or the medieval age, is most commonly delineated as beginning with the fall of Rome to the Goths in 476 and concluding with the fall of Constantinople to the Turks in 1453. The early Middle Ages (476–814) is often referred to as the Dark Ages because it is considered a time of widespread ignorance and lack of social progress. The classical thinking of Greco-Roman times, which viewed surgery as an invaluable adjunct to internal medicine, was completely obliterated during the Dark Ages. The clergy carried to the extreme Galen's belief that surgery was "a mode of treatment" by treating surgeons themselves as lackeys and underlings. Through the influence of the Arabian commentators, there was a genuine belief that it was unclean and unholy to touch another human body with one's hands.

It must be understood that the medieval surgeon, whether renowned scholar or roving rogue, stood in jeopardy of life or limb if he operated unsuccessfully on any of the feudal lords. Consequently, the greatest surgeons of the time shrewdly advised their professional brethren to avoid or evade all difficult cases. However, when in the 12th century a number of edicts were issued by the church declaring that the shedding of blood was incompatible with a cleric's holy office, the "educated" class was clearly restricted from performing any type of surgical practice. In so doing, the church totally abandoned the surgical crafts to the secular arm of medieval society.

Because monks were forbidden to perform surgical operations, this skill fell mostly to the "barbers," who had previously assisted the monks in their surgical therapies and in particular had been frequenting monasteries since 1092, when beards were banned. The barbers helped shave the monks and cut their hair in the particular styles of specific religious orders. These barbers soon widened the scope of their professional activities and became specialists. For instance, one operated for hernia, another for bladder calculi, and a third for cataract, with the knowledge handed down from father to son. By the 13th and 14th centuries, surgical techniques were beginning to mature at the hands of barber-surgeons. These faithful and mostly obscure followers of the craft of surgery, although continuously ostracized by clerical bigots, ensured the ultimate survival of surgery.

Despite the church's ban on surgery, via its edict abhorring bloodshed, the craft of surgery steadily advanced. Even more surprising, much of this change was accomplished by surgeons affiliated with religious orders. Prominent among these individuals was Hugh of Lucca (1160–1257) and his major disciple, Theodoric (1205–1296). The *Chirurgia* of Theodoric was completed in 1266 but is most important for providing excellent examples of the overall decline of surgery from its previous Greco-Roman sophistication. Basic surgical precepts had become buried in unintelligible jargon. Yet, despite its many shortcomings, the *Chirurgia* is an important milestone in the history of surgery; it demonstrated the beginnings of independence of thought and observation in surgical therapy. A noteworthy Italian contemporary of Hugh and Theodoric was William of Saliceto (1210–1277). A member of the medical faculty at Bologna, his monumental effort, the *Ciroxia* (1270), stands out as a landmark in the history of surgery because it does not separate surgical diagnosis from internal medicine and even includes a remarkable collection of case histories.

A resurgence of medical and surgical education in western Europe first occurred at the School of Salerno, situated near Naples on the Gulf of Paestum. From this school was authored the most important of early medieval surgical manuscripts, the *Bamberg Surgery*. Covering wounds and fractures of the skull, general wounds of the body, surgical lesions of eye and ear, diseases of the skin, fractures and dislocations, hemorrhoids, herniorrhaphy, bloodletting, and cautery, the work is pragmatic, especially concerning operative surgery. About 20 years after the *Bamberg Surgery* was written, a markedly different type of surgical manuscript appeared at Salerno. Roger of Salerno (circa late 12th century) authored an original, systematic text called the *Surgery of Master Roger*. With topics arranged in sequence from head to lower extremity, it was the preeminent surgical manuscript of the Salernitan school and is the first known independent surgical work in the Western world.

By the end of the 1200s, Italian leadership in surgical education had substantially declined. Among the reasons for this declination was the civil war rampant throughout the country. These difficulties are particularly evident in the career of Lanfranc of Milan (?–1315). Having become involved in the political strife of his native country, Lanfranc resettled in France and became associated with a gathering of surgeons called the Confraternity of Saints Cosmas and Damian. According to popular tradition, Cosmas and his twin, Damian, had been traveling physicians who gave their services freely to those in need. During that earlier era's persecution of Christians, Cosmas and Damian were tortured and beheaded (circa AD 300). They were soon given sainthood for what were regarded as miraculous surgical cures and over the intervening centuries became recognized as the patron saints of surgery.

Little is known about the early organization of the confraternity. However, by the beginning of the 14th century, a guild of Parisian barber-surgeons also existed. In general, these individuals were not permitted to use a knife, and as a result great jealousy existed between them and the confraternity. Noting the chaotic state of affairs, the king of France issued an edict in 1311; only individuals who underwent an examination administered from a royally authorized source should be allowed, according to the edict, to practice surgery in Paris. In this instance, the confraternity assumed the royal order and began academic testing. Those who passed the required examination were to be known as "masters of surgery." By this royal statute, the existence and autonomy of the surgeons were officially recognized.

Paralleling the surgeons' ambitions to attain university status were the barber-surgeons' aspirations to gain entry into the surgeons' ranks. Unwelcome in the confraternity, the barber-surgeons obtained their own special royal charter (1372), legalizing their professional ambitions and the designation *barber-surgeon*. In addition to barbering, they were now entitled to treat carbuncles, bruises, boils, and any other nonmortal open wounds. Into this ever-changing political environment moved Lanfranc, who became one of the founders of modern French surgery. He became a bitter critic of the noncleriсal and essentially uneducated barber-surgeons and soon wrote *Chirurgia Magna* (1296), the foundation of French surgical teaching for many years.

A contemporary of Lanfranc was Henri de Mondeville (1260–1320), considered the first great French master of surgery. Mondeville's prominence lies entirely in his *Chirurgie* and early opposition to surgical quackery and empiricism. He declared that surgery must belong to all of medicine and twitted the church and its hierarchy to explain how its physician-clerks were supposed to learn surgery without permission to touch a human body.

At the same time that Mondeville's career was coming to an end, the university at Montpellier was beginning to rival the university at Paris as the center of European medical and surgical education. The most prominent of its graduates and the individual destined to become the preeminent European surgeon of the late Middle Ages was Guy de Chauliac (1300–1368). His massive Latin manuscript, *Inventorium Seu Collectorium Cyrurgie* (1363), would become the most important medical book then printed in France (*La Grande Chirurgie*, 1478). His methods dominated surgery in France and, to some degree, England for the next 2 centuries.

English surgery during the Middle Ages was not nearly as developed as in France or Italy, but certain individuals did manage to become prominent. The most important was John of Arderne (1306–1390). Settling in London, Arderne joined the Guild of Military Surgeons. In 13th- and 14th-century London, guilds or companies were established to control various types of trades. Initially, barber-surgeons were allowed almost exclusive control over the practice of surgery in the city, which did nothing but political and financial harm to the smaller number of military surgeons. The barber-surgeons fought fierce economic and political battles with the military surgeons for the total right of supervision over anyone who practiced surgery. The London city corporation sided sometimes with one group, sometimes with the other, and indecision was always present.

The Renaissance

The European Renaissance, the great revival of learning via the arts, humanities, and growth of scientific thought, occurred from the late 14th to the 15th century. It began in northern Italy, spread gradually to other countries, and marked the transition from the medieval world to modern civilization. Renaissance society began to hold a worldly rather than a religious point of view, with this new attitude called *humanism*. Humans, not God, became the center of reference. There was a gradual transference of wealth and its attendant political power from the Christian church to various princes. These men assumed an avid interest in learning, and a new age of classicism developed. As a consequence, the all-pervasive religious character of medieval education and governance had become untenable.

The unfettered flowering of surgery during the Renaissance was directly related to fundamental changes in the study of human anatomy. By the end of the Middle Ages, it had become apparent to physicians that further progress in the knowledge of medicine, specifically surgery, could not be attained unless scientific studies of human anatomy were made. By that time, the church's ban on human vivisection was showing some signs of weakness as several popes approved the right to study the human body. Accordingly, by the early 16th century there were no further major hindrances to either dissection or autopsy.

Few individuals have had an influence as overwhelming on the history of surgery as Andreas Vesalius (1514–1564) (Fig. 1.2). Deeply devoted to the study of human anatomy and proficient in human dissection, Vesalius served as professor of anatomy and public prosector at the University of Padua in Italy. The 7 years he spent in Padua left an indelible mark on the evolution of medicine and surgery. His public lectures drew great attendance, and he was in constant demand to provide anatomical discourses and demonstrations in other Italian cities. The indefatigable efforts of Vesalius culminated in the publication of his magnificent *De Humani Corporis Fabrica* (1543). The effect of this work was immediate and self-sustaining, with its many splendid woodcuts demonstrating innumerable peculiarities and minor variations in structures encountered in dissection. Although the *Fabrica* was written in Latin, its impact ultimately extended to individuals who spoke or understood only the vernacular, the everyday language of ordinary people. Galenic errors were boldly swept aside, permitting the emergence of modern medicine and surgery. Among Vesalius's greatest contributions was his research on the vascular system and the question of the circulation of blood. Even more radical than his criticism of past authorities was Vesalius's assertion that anatomical dissection must be completed by the physician/surgeon himself—a direct renunciation of the long-standing doctrine that dissection was a grisly and loathsome task to be performed only by a diener-like individual while from on high the learned physician lectured utilizing orthodox texts. This prin-

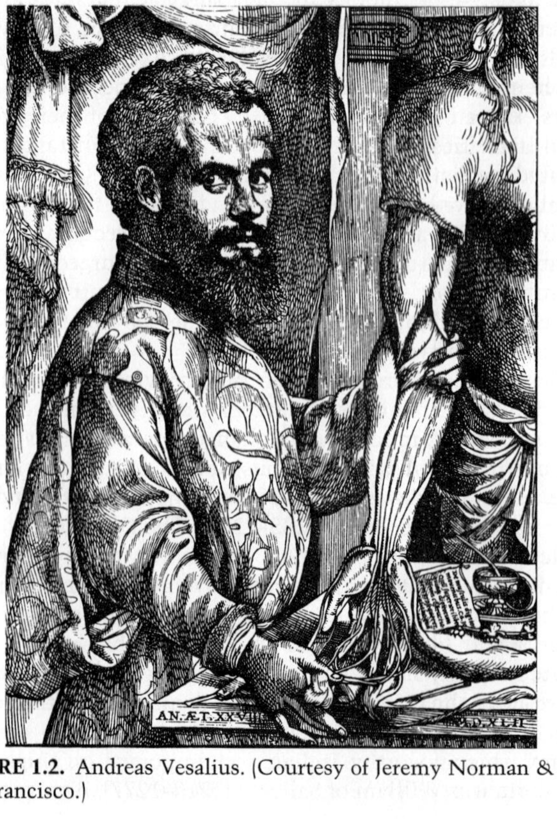

FIGURE 1.2. Andreas Vesalius. (Courtesy of Jeremy Norman & Co., San Francisco.)

ciple of "hands-on" education would remain Vesalius's most important and long-lasting contribution to the teaching of anatomy.

During the Renaissance, each European country began to develop its own recognizable practice of surgery. Both Germany and Switzerland lagged far behind in the awakening of medicine and surgery during the late Middle Ages and in the great surgical renaissance. A number of reasons accounted for this, including the sorry state of university education in central Europe. In the particular case of Germanic surgery, most individuals who practiced the art of surgery were simple craftsmen who, like other artisans, joined together in guilds. It was thought no more suitable for a surgeon to study books than for a carpenter or a blacksmith to do so. Because German surgeons usually had no formal education, they could neither speak nor read Latin. Although not as learned as their foreign colleagues, the German surgeons were well versed in the surgery of war. They were widely experienced in the growing field of military surgery, the subject of their earliest surgical works. These surgical texts were intended as practical handbooks or manuals for the use of their fellow craftsmen. They were written in the vernacular and were concerned almost entirely with the treatment of wounds.

Heinrich von Pfolspeundt was a 15th-century Bavarian army surgeon and the earliest known German surgical writer. He composed his *Buch der Bündth-Ertznei* in 1460, although it remained in manuscript form until 1868, when it was rediscovered, edited, and published. As was typical of the wound surgeon, he had no skill in major operations and did not know how to treat fractures and dislocations. He left minor surgery to the barbers and the larger operative procedures to the cutters. His text was largely limited to discussion of the management of wounds and other injuries. Within a quarter century of Pfolspeundt lived another, more literate German surgeon, Hieronymus Brunschwig (1450–1512). His *Dis ist Das Buch der Cirurgia Hantwirckung der Wundartzney* (1497) is a remarkable publication, the first important printed surgical treatise in German. The last of the famous early German wound surgeons was Hans von Gersdorff (1480–1540). His *Feldtbuch der Wundartzney* (1517), in vernacular German, is particularly valuable for its many important illustrations. Gersdorff is best remembered for his claim to have performed more than 200 amputations for gangrene or erysipelas.

Other renowned Germanic surgeons of this era included Paracelsus (1493–1541), Walter Hermann Ryff (circa first half of the 16th century), Caspar Stromayr (circa 16th century), and Felix Wurtz (1518–1574). The first great book on eye surgery, *Ophthalmolodouleia das ist Augendient* (1583), was written in vernacular German by George Bartisch (1535–1606). Bartisch, considered the founder of modern ophthalmology, was the first to practice the extirpation of the globe in cancer of the eye.

Italian surgeons, unlike their generally illiterate Germanic-speaking counterparts, were often university educated and sometimes attained academic distinction. The vigorous rivalry between the itinerant barber-surgeons and their more sophisticated surgical peers was not readily apparent. Giovanni de Vigo (1460–1525) was the first Italian Renaissance surgeon to write an account of gunshot injuries and their treatment. As an outstanding compiler of surgical works, his *Practica in Arte Chirurgica Copiosa Continens Novem Libros* (1514) provides the most detailed portrait of European surgery as it existed at the end of the 15th century.

Guido Guidi (1508–1569) followed de Vigo as the leading surgeon during the Italian Renaissance. His memory is particularly preserved in the names of several anatomical structures he described, such as the Vidian artery, canal, nerve, and vein. Mariano Santo of Barletta (1490–1550) achieved fame as a lithotomist. Giovanni Andrea della Crose (1514–1575) propagated many concepts of de Vigo and Guidi in his *Chirurgiae Libri Septem* (1573) and *Chirurgiae Universalis Opus Absolutum* (1573). Gaspare Tagliacozzi (1547–1599) has been called the father of plastic surgery. In his *De Curtorum Chirurgia per Institionem* (1597), he described in exacting detail specific operative methods for treating mutilating injuries, especially nasal defects. The last great Italian Renaissance surgeon was Hieronymus Fabricius ab Aquapendente (1533–1620). As professor of anatomy and surgery at Padua, Fabricius had so many pupils that at his own expense he built in Padua the first known permanent anatomical amphitheater.

The most important Spanish surgeon of this era was Francisco Arceo (1493–1573), but little information is available about his schooling and professional life. Dionisio Daza Chacon (1503–1580) wrote the most exhaustive Spanish work on surgery during this period, *Practica y Teorica de Cirurgia* (1600). Bartolome Hidalgo de Aguero (1531–1597) is commonly acknowledged as the father of modern Spanish surgery. He was lecturer on surgery at Seville and gained wide experience in the treatment of battlefield wounds.

European surgery during the Renaissance owed much to France, primarily through the efforts of Pierre Franco (1500–1561) and Ambroise Paré (1510–1590) (Fig. 1.3), whose achievements were especially impressive because both men rose from poverty, and neither was university educated. In the highly stratified society of the time, the lack of university

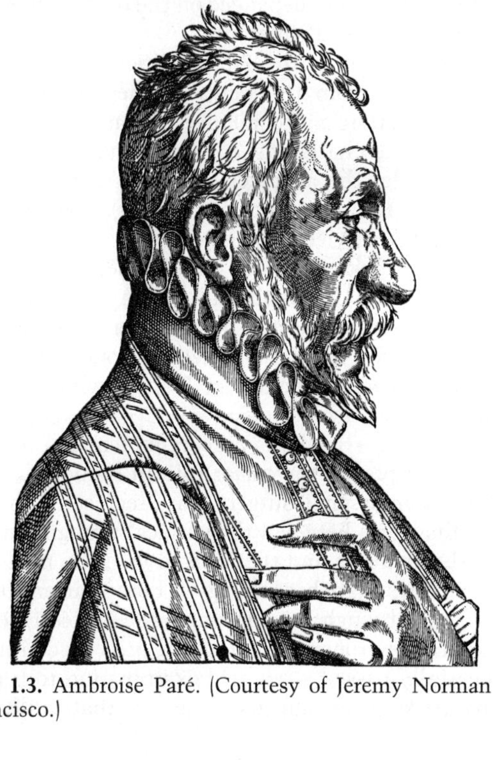

FIGURE 1.3. Ambroise Paré. (Courtesy of Jeremy Norman & Co., San Francisco.)

education usually prevented individuals from obtaining important standing in medicine or surgery. Franco was trained mostly by itinerant lithotomists, cataract couchers, and herniotomists, whereas Paré emerged from the ranks of the barber-surgeons.

During the 16th century, the French barber-surgeons had clearly moved beyond the legal limitations that had earlier been placed on their clinical practice. They came to be known euphemistically as the "surgeons of the short gowns," in contradistinction to the "long-gown" or academic surgeons of the College of St. Côme. The barber-surgeons guild grew much more rapidly than the College of St. Côme, probably because the elitist, exclusive attitude of the college restricted its own membership. For the average Parisian, the barber-surgeon of the short gown was a much more accessible, pleasant, and familiar figure than his academic long-gown counterpart. Eventually, although the barber-surgeons did not have equivalent social status or academic rank, the public recognized their superior skills.

It was during this period that Jean Canappe (1495–1552) translated Guy de Chauliac's works from Latin into French, thus allowing non-Latin-educated barber-surgeons access to printed surgical teachings. Canappe's avowed purpose was to aid the barber-surgeons against the opposition of the more educated university surgeons. Another French academic surgeon who authored a work expressly for the barber-surgeon was Jacques Dalechamps (1513–1588), the *Chirurgie Françoise* (1569).

The controversies in France among itinerant surgeons, barber-surgeons, and university-educated surgeons and between physicians and surgeons were more intense than in any other European country. That Dalechamps could recognize Paré, a barber-surgeon, as the foremost surgeon in France, with Franco, an upstart itinerant, not far behind, was an important step in the eventual decision of the universities to make a university education available to men of the lower classes. It was obvious, at least to Dalechamps, that a positive future for French surgery depended on the outstanding barber-surgeons and occasional itinerant.

The most famous of the French "incisors" was Franco. Although he rose from the ranks of the incisors, he was adamant in his attempts to remove operative surgery from the domain of the charlatans, itinerant quacks, and cutters and place it under the auspices of the regular practitioners (the surgeons of the short and long gowns). Franco accepted the physician's supervision of the surgeon, but he was unrelenting in his attacks on those who abused the true art of surgery. He became especially influential as a result of his writings in the vernacular and the fact that he eagerly operated on patients with hernias and bladder stones, unlike many well-known educated surgeons of France, who shied away from such technical feats.

Paré's position in the history of surgery remains of supreme importance. He played the major role in reinvigorating and modernizing Renaissance surgery. Paré represents the severing of the final link between the surgical thought and techniques of the ancients and the push toward the modern era. His ability to articulate his findings in both written word and clinical practice brought him lasting fame. In 1541, realizing the importance of proper credentials, he presented himself for and successfully passed a required examination to become a master barber-surgeon and a member of that guild. Paré's reputation became so great that he was begrudgingly made a member of the College of St. Côme (1554). Despite at first being refused admission because he had been a barber's apprentice and spoke not in Latin but in the vernacular, Paré gave his inaugural lecture in French and was duly mocked by the envious. However, his membership, championed by Dalechamps, helped bring about a later union of the barber-surgeons and the surgeons of St. Côme. It is a tribute to Paré's remarkable career that he became chief surgeon to four successive kings of France. Most important, he demonstrated true humility in his work with his patients and in the world of healing, a humility most evident in his well-remembered statement, "I treated him. God cured him."

In England, the number of military surgeons had long remained constant, whereas the various barber-surgeons' companies grew more powerful. In 1540, a momentous event in English surgical history occurred. Under the aegis of Henry VIII, Parliament passed a statute uniting the previously chartered Guild or Company of Barber-Surgeons with the small, exclusive Guild of Military Surgeons. This new Royal Commonality of Barber-Surgeons received all the previous powers granted under past British sovereigns and more. The new charter declared that members who practiced surgery should no longer perform barber activities, and that barbers should not undertake any surgery except dental work. As a result of the new royal charter, a vigorous attempt was made to improve educational work. The surgical examiners instituted a series of licensing examinations, which culminated in the student receiving the Grand Diploma as a master in surgery and anatomy. The new company was entitled to receive the bodies of four executed criminals each year for the purpose of dissection. Thus, the Act of 1540 succeeded in creating for London an active educational and licensing body for the practice of surgery. Henry VIII's personal surgeon, Thomas Vicary (1495–1561), was elected first master of the united companies. Vicary was a recognized leader in the profession, although he left behind few memorable written works. Other English surgeons of note were Thomas Gale (1507–1587), William Bullein (?–1576), William Clowes (1540–1604), John Banister (1533–1610), and Peter Lowe (1550–1612).

By the end of the 16th century, the craft of surgery in Europe had attained a tenuous but accepted and respected position within the world of medicine. Although surgeons continued to be viewed askance by their follow physicians, the importance of a surgeon's clinical skills could no longer be blithely dismissed. Admittedly, large areas of medical and surgical practice remained bound with superstition, herb therapy, and quackery. However, the true greatness of the many renowned surgeons during this era is reflected in their increasing scorn for quacks and charlatans and their application of rational empirical observations to daily practices. In essence, the humanism of the Renaissance provided surgeons with their first substantive opportunities to become respected members of the healing profession.

The 17th Century

The scientific revolution of the 17th century represented a turning point in the history of medicine. Emphasis shifted dramatically from speculation to experimentation, with remarkable advances made in the basic sciences. However, the teaching of medicine and surgery was still heavily influenced by ancient philosophies. Initially, supporters of older influences continued to outnumber the more progressive thinkers and scientists, but by the end of the century, the latter group had an overwhelming influence on the craft of surgery. The great centers of medical education in 17th-century Europe were Leyden, Montpellier, Padua, and Paris, but the condition of medicine was vastly improved by the ambitions of royalty to establish small universities and by the formation of scientific societies. Specific advances in anatomy, physiology, and medical instrumentation aided this flowering of medicine.

The most astonishing and influential of these progressive changes was the discovery and fundamental understanding of the anatomy and physiology of the circulation of blood by William Harvey (1578–1657). His *Exercitatio Anatomica De Motu Cordis Et Sanguinis In Animalibus* (1628) has been called the most important book in the history of medicine. Harvey used inductive logic to demonstrate that the heart acts as a muscular pump in propelling the blood along the arteries, and that the blood's motion is continuous and leads back to the heart via veins to form a cycle or circle.

Although from the modern perspective medicine and surgery as practiced during this era hardly appear advanced, it was an era of remarkable innovation. New therapeutic modalities were introduced that would have an enormous impact on the future development of surgical operations. The most important of these were the concept of exhaustive treatment, including bleeding and purging, and the use of intravenous injection of drugs and transfusion of blood. Bloodletting in particular became a source of considerable remuneration for the surgeon. Exactly when the bleeding came into serious vogue remains historical conjecture. However, *Il Barbiere* (1626), the earliest book specifically devoted to barber-surgery, contained engravings detailing bloodletting, including portraits of two female barber-surgeons considered especially adept at the procedure. In Paris, one of the major functions of surgical house officers was to bleed patients. This chore, said to consume an hour's time every afternoon, probably explains why there were more surgical interns than physician interns at the Hôtel Dieu.

The cultural and social aspects of 17th-century medicine and surgery suggest it to have been a time of individual scientific endeavor rather than of concerted advancement of science. Most surgeons were not well compensated, although certain prominent individuals were well off. The medieval custom of paying a lifetime annuity for a successful operation remained somewhat in vogue. Surgery in the 17th century did not keep pace with progress in anatomy and physiology. In comparison to the extensive development of medical literature, the literature of surgery seems meager. Surgeons had not yet achieved the social and academic status of physicians, and bitter antagonisms were still apparent in particular countries.

The 17th century was a time of great political instability in England. As the country became increasingly isolated socially and politically from the rest of western Europe, and consequently from the western European universities, English surgeons had to rely on the teaching organized by various barber-surgeon companies and English universities. The activity of these barber-surgeon companies was reaching its zenith, exemplified by the London barber-surgeon company that obtained an act of Parliament in 1604 and a new charter in 1629, which mandated that no one could practice surgery in that city until the person had passed an examination given in the presence of two or more master barber-surgeons. Still, quarrels continued to arise between surgeons who were not members of the company but instead were attached to hospitals and their medical schools. By the middle of this century, it was becoming evident that an English surgeon, if sufficiently educated and devoted to his craft, could reach a position of equality with the best physicians in the community. In many respects, this changing attitude was brought about by the increasing numbers of well-respected English surgeons and their erudite writings. Included within this group were John Woodall (1556–1643), Alexander Read (1586–1641), and the renowned Richard Wiseman (1620–1676).

In Germany, the overriding societal event was the Thirty Years' War (1618–1648). The barber-surgeons in Germany continued to reign supreme; their various guilds contained men of ability and independent thought. The most prominent 17th-century German surgeon was Wilhelm Fabry von Hilden (1560–1634). Initiated into the art of surgery by a thorough apprenticeship under a succession of skilled and experienced wound surgeons and barber-surgeons, von Hilden authored the first book, *De Combustionibus* (1607), devoted entirely to burns.

Another important German surgeon was Johannes Scultetus (1595–1645). Like increasing numbers of 17th-century surgeons, he was liberal in his indications for surgical intervention, as is evident in his famous *Armamentarium Chirurgicum* (1653), which became the most popular surgical text of that era. Although published posthumously by his nephew, the work was brought out in numerous editions and translations in practically every European country. Among other German surgeons, Matthaeus Purmann (1649–1711) was also well known.

In France, the official status of the guild of barber-surgeons in Paris had greatly improved by the first portion of the 17th century. In 1603, the government of that city authorized the title of the guild to use the words *barber-surgeons* rather than simply *barbers*. Concurrently, master barber-surgeons were given the legal right to treat all kinds of wounds. Three decades later, Louis XIII reaffirmed the enabling statutes of his "dear community of master barber-surgeons" and recognized the community as "the principal source of the knowledge and practice of this art in all our kingdom."

Surprisingly, some master barber-surgeons left the guild to join the ranks of the Confraternity of St. Côme. However, most barber-surgeons did not wish to give up their barber's work in exchange for admission to the more elite organization. In 1613, revolutionary-minded members of both the confraternity and the guild attempted to unite the two companies, and the royal government gave its tacit approval. However, a majority of the academic surgeons of St. Côme disavowed the union, thereby ending the agreement. More than 40 years later, the same plan for unification was proposed and met a far warmer reception from the academic surgeons. In 1655, the surgeons of both the long gown and short gown put aside their centuries-old rivalry and signed a contract of union.

In joining forces with the barber-surgeons, the academic surgeons had an obvious economic incentive. As the membership of the prosperous guild of barber-surgeons increased, the guild threatened the viability of the much smaller confraternity of academic surgeons. The inescapable fact was that it was difficult to make a living by practicing only surgery. Without the mix of barber's work, such as bloodletting and wound care, the economic stability of practicing surgeons was seriously threatened. On a more practical level, barber-surgeons commanded much higher fees than did their academic counterparts.

During the second half of the century, strengthening of the united surgical guild was evident. There was a marked increase in its prestige in the eyes of the public as a new surgical amphitheater was constructed in Paris (1694) to offer public anatomy and operative courses to large audiences. More important, several prominent surgeons, including Pierre Dionis (1643–1718) and Charles-François Felix (1650–1703), were regarded with much favor by Parisian society. Despite this growing prestige, few Paris surgeons actually performed major operations. In the 1690s, of the approximately 400 to 500 master surgeons, perhaps 5% practiced the bold, often-new procedures, such as lithotomy. Most surgeons earned a livelihood by completing minor surgery, which included treating abscesses; applying external medications to various skin ailments, bruises, and cuts; reducing incarcerated hernias; setting fractures; and treating skin tumors, venereal diseases, and ulcers. Realistically, this kind of work was not sufficient to provide a livelihood for the entire surgical community.

By the end of the century, certain surgeons had a growing disdain for what they regarded as socially demeaning work, so surgeons in Paris increasingly began to turn to the practice of "internal medicine." Because French surgery was in confusion, little progress was achieved until the end of the 17th century. More important, by the final years of the era it was evident that Paris barbers and surgeons were going their separate ways. The departure of the barbers reflected tangible alterations in the nature of surgery, which would become more evident in the next century.

The 18th Century

The close relationship that had been established between surgeons and anatomical research continued during most of the 18th century. Thus, many of the period's outstanding anatomical and surgical discoveries were made by so-called surgeon-anatomists. Among the most important of these individuals were William Cheselden (1688–1752); the Monros—father Alexander (*primus*) (1697–1767), son Alexander (*secundus*) (1733–1817), and grandson Alexander (*tertius*) (1773–1859); Percival Pott (1714–1788); William Hunter (1718–1783); the Meckels—father Johann (1724–1774), son Philipp (1756–1803), and two grandsons, Johann (1781–1833) and his younger brother August (1790–1829); Pierre-Joseph Desault (1744–1795); and Antonio Scarpa (1747–1832). Through their combined efforts, the role of surgery in the rise of modern medical thought would be ensured. By the end of the century, surgeons as a group had begun to rise above their traditional social status as technicians or craftsmen to receive acceptance as professionals on a par with physicians. Clearly, surgeons had become scientific as well as technical innovators.

European surgery achieved great prominence in France in the 18th century. At the beginning of the century, new patterns of surgical education and training were apparent. Two kinds of apprenticeships were available. The first was a formal arrangement for a period of 2 years consecutively, during which the apprentice's family and the master surgeon agreed to a legal contract, or *brevet*. The young man would provide certain services and obedience to his mentor; the surgeon agreed to provide education as well as food, shelter, and other basic needs. For families unable to afford a *brevet* apprenticeship, another, known as *garçons chirurgiens* or *serviteurs chirurgiens*, existed. This type of apprentice was in a much more menial position than was the *brevet* apprentice and had less freedom to attend hospital and public lectures. More important, a master surgeon could have only one *brevet* apprentice at a time but was not restricted as to the number of *garçons*.

Regardless of educational tract, neither the *brevet* apprentice nor the *garçon* was likely to learn how to perform major operations from the average Parisian master surgeon. Therefore, several renowned Paris surgeons offered practical training beyond minor surgical operations. These surgeons received fee-paying students, or *pensionnaires*, in addition to the one apprentice permitted them. The *pensionnaire* differed from the apprentice in that he did not enter into a binding agreement with the master surgeon and did not hope to fulfill an entrance requirement of one of the surgical guilds. He was simply allowed to accompany the distinguished master surgeon in his daily routines. The *pensionnaires* tended to be wealthy students from outside Paris and from foreign countries. Most were already graduates of medical school and came to Paris to strengthen their surgical training.

Once a *brevet* apprentice or a *garçon* had completed his service, he began the final stage of surgical training, the journeyman or *compagnon* stage, which usually lasted for 7 years. Most *compagnons* hoped to become eligible for a mastership but were not allowed to practice surgery on their own. Those who chose not to move to the provinces, where a surgical mastership could be acquired with much greater ease, usually left their masters after a few years and commenced independent practices illegally in Paris. None of these individuals could realistically hope to become a Paris master surgeon unless he were a son or son-in-law of such a master or had political connections in the royal court or a hospital.

The actual transformation of French surgeons from practitioners of guild mentality to well-educated professionals can be traced to 1715. In that year, Georges Mareschal (1658–1736), surgeon to Louis XIV, began a formal public campaign to improve the status of the Paris surgical community. Within 15 years, two important events would firmly place the surgeons on an equal social and scientific level with their physician peers. First, in 1731 Mareschal and François La Peyronie (1678–1747) petitioned the king to establish a society that would meet once a week to hear and discuss presentations of papers on surgical topics. This society became known as the Royal Academy or College of Surgery and consisted of the 70 leading master surgeons in Paris. A second major step in the evolutionary process of 18th-century French surgery concerned the Royal Declaration of 1743, which declared that henceforth Paris master surgeons were forbidden to work as barbers. Conversely, barber's work would be considered an inferior profession and would belong solely to the barber-wigmakers. Therefore, when the last few Paris barber-surgeons retired from practice, such an occupation would become extinct.

The transformation of French surgery from a craft guild to a liberal guild profession was complete in 1750, particularly as the French public finally viewed surgeons as on the same societal level as physicians. In the second half of the 18th century, Paris would showcase the talents of its surgeons, and that city became the mecca for surgeons from throughout the civilized world who sought further education and training. The Paris College of Surgery commenced a dissection school with practical instruction in anatomy and surgical operations, and a clinical research and teaching hospital was constructed.

The leading French scientific surgeon of the first half of the 18th century was Jean-Louis Petit (1674–1750). His reputation as a bold, skillful surgeon attracted large numbers of students to his home, where he organized a private school. Petit was the originator of many important surgical methods and invented the screw tourniquet. The most renowned of Petit's pupils was Dominique Anel (1678–1725). Among other prominent French surgeons of this period were Nicolas Andry (1658–1742), Henri Le Dran (1685–1773), and Claude-Nicolas Le Cat (1700–1768).

The French Revolution played such a tremendous part in reshaping the lives of French citizens that, not unexpectedly, surgeons and surgical thinking were also profoundly affected by the upheaval. From 1780 to 1793, politics was thought to hold the key to health. Accordingly, physicians flocked to the side of the revolutionaries. The concept of professional unification as a way to create a new health care delivery system became a subject of lively debate. In late 1790, one of the revolutionary councils decided that physicians and surgeons should be given the same education and undergo the same examinations.

Neither the old guard of Paris surgeons nor the medical faculty had much chance to prevent unification. The surgical institutions of the old regime in Paris were so closely linked to the discredited monarchy that there was no possibility of their remaining in an unaltered state. In 1792, a law passed by the legislative assembly abolished simultaneously the Faculty of Medicine and the College of Surgery. Public instruction at the Paris College of Surgery persisted through 1794, but the college became a shell of its former self. The effect of all these laws would prove to be catastrophic to French surgeons.

With the abolition of degrees in medicine and surgery and the dissolution of all academic colleges, the creation of the Ecole De Santé in 1794 marked the total unification of medicine and surgery in France. Educational requirements for the practice of either medicine or surgery were to be identical, and only one degree, Doctor of Medicine, would be awarded. With the opening of the new school, the destinies of the disciples of St. Côme and the medical faculty of Paris became inextricably intertwined. Pierre-Joseph Desault, a surgeon-anatomist, provided most of the dynamism of late 18th-century French surgery. His greatest impact on the evolution of surgical education and training resulted from his introduction of the clinical surgical lesson. Despite his outstanding reputation, Desault provided little in the way of a written legacy except for his editing of the world's first surgical periodical, the *Journal de Chirurgie* (1791–1794).

In Great Britain, the barber-surgeon companies were in full power at the beginning of the century. In many instances, the surgeons in the various companies were increasingly involved in the financial management, which caused discontentment among the nonsurgical members. As long as the legal monopoly of barber-surgical practice continued, however, both parties were forced to resolve their petty differences in amicable ways. The London Company of Barber-Surgeons had controlled surgery in the metropolis for almost 2 centuries, but changes were taking place within its ranks that would have enormous historical repercussions. Although at the beginning of the century the barbers outnumbered the surgeons 20 to 1, the greater part of the company's income was coming from the surgeons. As the number of British hospitals increased, so did the number, and correspondingly the importance, of surgeons. The two sections of the company had obviously diverged in status and interests, and their separation was inevitable.

At the beginning of the 18th century, little competent surgical instruction was available in England or Scotland; the best was in London. The London Company of Barber-Surgeons acted as the bellwether for most of the country, and its dissolution had an enormous impact on the future of British surgery. The final divorce between the London barbers and surgeons was orchestrated primarily by two men, William Cheselden (1688–1752) and John Ranby (1703–1773). Cheselden was the leading English surgeon during the first half of this era, and his clinical work and administrative expertise ushered that country's surgical education and training into a new period.

In London, the surgical educational system was gradually improving, and the demand for better anatomical teaching had been answered through a system of private schools. Because hospital appointments were difficult to obtain and practices slow to develop, Cheselden began providing a private course in anatomy in 1711. The success of Cheselden's anatomical lectures brought him into direct conflict with the company. He was accused of teaching anatomy in his home at times that conflicted with public dissection at the company hall.

In 1738, Cheselden became a member of the court of assistants of the Company of Barber-Surgeons. Six years later, he became a junior warden, and it was during his tenure in office that the surgeons announced without any prior warning that they wished to separate permanently from the barbers. Parliament appointed a committee to consider the matter; the committee was chaired by Cheselden's son-in-law, with Cheselden himself donating £550 toward payment of the expenses incurred by the proceedings. Not unexpectedly, the committee upheld the petition of the surgeons, and in 1745, Parliament passed a bill forming an independent Company or Corporation of Surgeons. This formal separation was greatly aided by Ranby, who served as sergeant surgeon to the British monarch and was able to perform some persuasive lobbying.

Although the company had a wonderful chance to advance the cause of British surgery, such was not the case. The act of Parliament entitled those who had satisfied a Court of Examiners to practice without hindrance anywhere in Great Britain, and apprenticeship was no longer specifically required. Many foreign nationals who were practicing surgery in London were admitted to the new company without inquiry regarding their training. Thus, it became impossible to ensure that a young surgeon would acquire surgical training in a systematized fashion based on some type of apprenticeship.

The company dragged on in an uninspired existence for almost a half century. Early difficulties led to financial and administrative irregularities that were not readily overcome. The control of the company had gradually passed into the hands of the 10 members of the Court of Assistants, who were also examiners. In most instances, these examiners were appointed for life and were the only regular attendants at meetings. Realistically, during its first 50 years of existence the Company of Surgeons was nothing more than a bloated, inefficient examining body. Clearly, the individualistic attitude of most company surgeons resulted in petty quarrels, tardy publications, and a general lack of cohesiveness and created an untenable educational environment. Nonetheless, the art of surgery, existing outside the company, continued to be consolidated and advanced by careful clinical observations and superb teachers in private settings.

Because the Company of Surgeons failed to adequately organize surgical education, effective licensing was nonexistent. Two types of programs assumed much of the responsibility for education. First were the private schools of anatomical and surgical instruction. In the absence of any great public medical institution, these schools provided excellent instruction but were decidedly transient and had no licensing powers. The many new hospitals and the schools of medicine and surgery that were evolving with them represented the second type of educational institution for surgeons. The surgeons attached to these hospitals had the opportunity to take their apprentices with them while performing surgical operations. In this way, the initial efforts to provide systematic teaching, including bedside instruction, were made. Schools naturally evolved from such individual entrepreneurship, and the emerging surgical educational system was enormously beneficial to the student. The apprentice's physical presence in a hospital also helped increase the overall efficiency of the institution's patient care.

Although there were many teachers of surgery in 18th-century London, the two most outstanding individuals were Percivall Pott (1713–1788) and John Hunter (1728–1793). Hunter particularly stands out because of the volume of his written work and the quality of his research. Considered a dexterous surgeon, he was primarily interested in the pathophysiology of surgical diseases. Ultimately, Hunter's voluminous research and clinical work resulted in a collection of more than 13,000 specimens, which became one of his most important legacies to the world of surgery.

By the last decade of the century, Great Britain, especially London, had displaced Paris as the center for European surgical education and training. Well-known surgeons such as Cheselden, Pott, Hunter, and many others contributed to that success. Among the most prominent of these other surgeons were Samuel Sharp (1700–1780), John Pringle (1707–1782), William Bromfield (1712–1792), William Blizard (1743–1835), Henry Cline (1750–1827), Everard Home (1756–1832), John Abernethy (1764–1831), and William Hey (1736–1819).

In an environment of military and socioeconomic strife, the condition of German surgical practice was decidedly unstable. Formalized surgical education and training were limited. Most individuals obtained surgical treatment from local barbers or itinerant quacks. The populace was overwhelmingly superstitious and ignorant of medical facts. Despite repeated edicts by the kings, nobles, and city authorities to improve conditions for the physicians and surgeons, the unsettled times limited surgical progress. The first surgeon of importance in the 18th century was Lorenz Heister (1683–1758). His *Chirurgie in Welcher Alles was zur Wund-Artzney Gehoret* (1718) became one of the most popular surgical texts of the era and was published in numerous editions and was translated into Latin, English, Spanish, French, Italian, and Dutch. During the last half of the century, the principal German surgeons were Carl Siebold (1736–1807) and August Richter (1742–1812).

In North America, medicine and surgery made few credible advances from 1600 to 1750. There were few actual physicians or surgeons of note, and most of the medical needs of the growing populace were served by three classes of health care providers: governors, clerics, and a wide range of self-educated "physicians," secular preachers, and schoolmasters. By the late 18th century, American medicine began to be distinguished from that of earlier years by the higher regard in which physicians were held by society and the increasing numbers of Americans obtaining medical degrees in Europe and returning to the colonies with valuable clinical acumen and technical skills. Names that recur most commonly in the accounts of surgery in revolutionary times are John Bard (1716–1799); John Jones (1729–1791), who authored the first major surgical work written by an American, *Plain Concise Practical Remarks on the Treatment of Wounds and Fractures* (1775); Samuel Bard (1742–1821); William Baynham (1749–1814); and John Warren (1753–1815).

At the end of the 1700s, the necessary role of surgery within the context of overall medicine had become clearer. There was an increasing interdependence of internal medicine and surgery, which had been cultivated in the common ground of 18th-century pathological anatomy and experimental physiology. At long last, physicians and surgeons had knowledge in areas that were essential to both disciplines. For thousands of years, surgeons had attempted to rely on an objective anatomical diagnosis. With the advent of pathology, physicians were able to regard disease from a perspective that had long been prevalent among surgeons. However, because surgery, to make its most impressive gains, still awaited the advent of anesthesia and antisepsis, 18th-century internal medicine appeared to yield more dramatic results, for example, in diagnosis and treatment.

The 19th Century

During the 19th century, the organized advancement of medical sciences began, and the surgeon emerged as a specialist and a respected medical practitioner. Yet, the era began unobtrusively as a direct continuation of the medical and surgical development of the 18th century. Through the first half of the 19th century, the scope of surgery remained limited. Surgeons, whether university educated or trained in apprenticeships, treated only simple fractures, dislocations, and abscesses and performed amputations with dexterity but high mortality rates. They managed to ligate major arteries for common and accessible aneurysms and made heroic attempts to excise external tumors. Some specialized in the treatment of anal fistulas, hernias, cataracts, and bladder stones. Compound fractures of the limbs with attendant sepsis remained mostly unmanageable, and staggering morbidity and mortality could be anticipated. Although a few bold surgeons endeavored to incise the abdomen in a hope to divide obstructing bands and adhesions, abdominal surgery was virtually unknown.

Within just a few years, the practice of surgery would be altered more abruptly than in all its previous history. Startling new developments rendered the surgery of the 1850s and beyond a scientific profession markedly different from the surgery of the past. Among the most salient of these changes were the discovery and employment of anesthetics; the establishment of antiseptic and aseptic surgery; the improvement on old practices and the advent of radically new operative procedures; the use of roentgen rays; the development of more effective methods of hemostasis; and the evolution of practical blood transfusion. In addition, the total removal of any restrictions on the study of human anatomy and pathology, distinct and far-reaching changes in the methods of educating and training surgeons, the reform of medical care as a result of the rise of nursing as a profession, the formation of national and international surgical societies, and more rapid transfer of information via periodicals and other forms of communication all contributed to this progress. So great were the innovations and so inclusive was the domain of surgery that the foundation of basic operative procedures to be performed throughout the 20th century was laid by the time World War I was concluded (1918).

Numerous efforts had been made throughout history to relieve by various measures the discomfort of surgical operations, and the epoch of ultimate conquest of pain is one of the most important in the evolution of surgery. Soporific, narcotic, and analgesic agents such as hashish, mandrake, and opium had been put to use for thousands of years. Alcoholic beverages also had been used to render a patient sufficiently oblivious to pain to permit the performance of surgical procedures on the surface of the body or on the bones. However, as anatomical knowledge and surgical techniques improved, the search for safer methods to prevent pain became more pressing. By the early 1830s, ether, nitrous oxide, and chloroform had been discovered. In the United States, "laughing gas" parties and "ether frolics" were in vogue. Young people were amusing themselves with the pleasant side effects of these compounds. Throughout the 1830s and 1840s, itinerant "professors" of chemistry traveled to villages, towns, and cities to lecture on these new gases and demonstrate their exhilarating effects. Often, the most important part of such presentations consisted of having young members of the audience inhale ether vapor or nitrous oxide. These individuals lost their sense of equilibrium, felt little pain, and acted with an apparent loss of inhibition.

It became obvious to various American physicians and dentists that the pain-relieving qualities of ether and nitrous oxide could be applicable to surgical operations. By December 1844, Horace Wells (1815–1848), a dentist from Connecticut, had grasped the concept of inhalation anesthesia and shared his findings with another dentist, William Morton (1819–1868). The latter settled in Boston and in October 1846 gave the first public demonstration of the effects of sulfuric ether anesthesia on a surgical patient, from whom John Collins Warren (1778–1856), professor of surgery at Harvard Medical School, removed a vascular tumor of the neck. After the operation, Warren, greatly impressed with the new discovery, uttered his famous words: "Gentlemen, this is no humbug." News of the momentous event spread rapidly throughout the United States and Europe: a new epoch in the history of surgery had begun.

Despite the introduction of general anesthesia, the evolution of surgery could not proceed smoothly until the grave problem of postoperative and hospital-acquired infection was resolved. Without a clear understanding of bacteriology and the sources of infection, however, most surgeons could do little more than provide high standards of surgical cleanliness, adequate hemostasis, and open-wound management. In many respects, the recognition of antisepsis and asepsis was a more important event in the evolution of surgical history than the advent of inhalation anesthesia. There was no arguing that the deadening of pain permitted a surgical operation to be conducted in a more efficacious manner. Haste was no longer of prime concern. However, if anesthesia had never been conceived, a surgical operation could still have been performed, albeit with much difficulty. Such was not the case with listerism. Without antisepsis and asepsis, major surgical procedures more than likely ended in death rather than just pain. Clearly, surgery needed both anesthesia and antisepsis, but in terms of overall importance, antisepsis proved of greater singular impact.

In the long evolution of surgery, the contributions of few individuals are preeminent. Joseph Lister (1827–1912) (Fig. 1.4) can be placed in such an elite list because of his monumental efforts to introduce systematic, scientifically

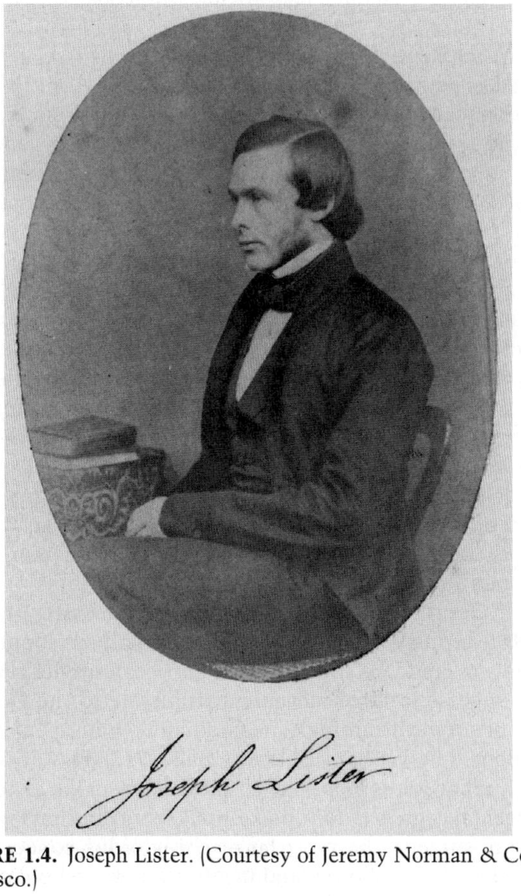

FIGURE 1.4. Joseph Lister. (Courtesy of Jeremy Norman & Co., San Francisco.)

based antisepsis in the treatment of wounds and the performance of surgical operations. Lister pragmatically applied Louis Pasteur's (1822–1895) bacteriological research to human disease. Because infection was now known to be caused by a microscopic living body carried in the air, Lister devised a means of prevention and secured its adoption by a skeptical profession. Although the use of a carbolic acid spray remains his best-remembered detail, it was eventually abandoned in favor of other substances. Lister not only used carbolic acid in the wound but also sprayed it into the atmosphere around the operative field and table. Lister did not emphasize hand scrubbing but merely dipped his fingers into a solution of phenol and corrosive sublimate.

A second important contribution that Lister made to surgical technique was the development of sterile absorbable sutures. He was concerned that much of the deep suppuration found in wounds was created by previously contaminated silk ligatures. Lister evolved a carbolized catgut ligature better than any previously produced (1869). He was able to cut short the ends of his suture, thereby closing the wound tightly and eliminating the necessity of bringing the ends of the suture out through the wound.

Over the years, Lister's principles of antisepsis gave way to those of *asepsis*, the complete elimination of bacteria. Asepsis was especially promulgated by Ernst von Bergmann (1836–1907), who merged the corrosive sublimate method into steam sterilization (1886) and eventually into the elaborate concept of general asepsis (1891). Any lingering doubts about the validity and significance of the momentous concepts Lister had put forth were eliminated on the battlefields of World War I. There, the importance of plain antisepsis became an invaluable lesson for surgeons around the world.

Once antiseptic and aseptic techniques had been finally accepted as part of routine surgical practice, it was inevitable that other elaborate antiseptic rituals would similarly take hold. The use of gloves, face masks, operating gowns, and hats would soon naturally evolve. By the mid-1890s, surgeons were becoming fully satisfied with their antiseptic methods and the attendant results. Wound infection was becoming less of a concern, although difficulties still existed. Equally prominent among the 19th-century discoveries that had an enormous impact on the evolution of surgery was the research conducted by Wilhelm Roentgen (1845–1923) and his elucidation of x-rays in late 1895. Surgeons immediately applied the new discovery to the diagnosis and location of fractures, dislocations, and removal of foreign bodies.

Far-reaching changes in the manner and methods of educating and training surgeons were among the most important organization advances in surgery during this era. The haphazard education of surgeons that had held sway for more than 2000 years became a well-defined system, as first promulgated in Germany, Austria, and the United States. By the mid-19th century, Germany and Austria had supplanted England and France as the centers of European surgical knowledge, a success in large measure attributable to the German system of surgical training. The German "pyramid" plan was soon adopted by William Halsted (1852–1922) (Fig. 1.5) in his program at the Johns Hopkins Hospital. Although Halsted has long been recognized for his original contributions to the science of surgery, the most far-reaching of his concepts lay in the education, training, and inspiration of a school of surgeons imbued with his principles of thought and action. The "Halsted tradition" remains the sine qua non of modern surgical residencies.

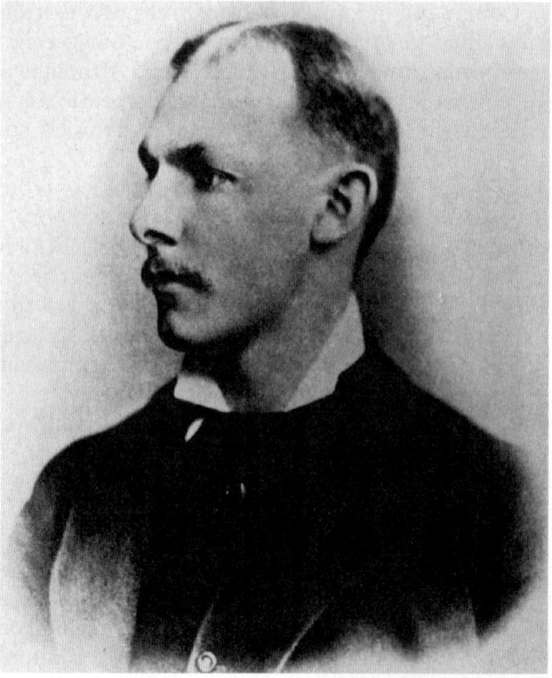

FIGURE 1.5. William Halsted. (Courtesy of Jeremy Norman & Co., San Francisco.)

Although textbooks, monographs, and treatises had always been the foundation of medical writing, the introduction of journals to the surgeon's written armamentarium had a tremendous impact on the development of surgery in the 19th century. Albrecht von Graefe's (1828–1870) *Journal der Chirurgie und Augen-Heilkunde* (1820), Joseph Malgaigne's (1806–1865) *Journal de Chirurgie* (1843), Bernard Langenbeck's (1810–1887) *Archiv für Klinische Chirurgie* (1860), and Lewis Pilcher's (1844–1917) *Annals of Surgery* (1885) were particularly renowned.

London had displaced Paris as the center of international surgical excellence, partially because of the manner in which surgical practice and the education of surgeons had been organized. By 1797, the old Company of Surgeons had ceased to be an effective managerial body, and plans were under way to organize a more responsive institution, the Royal College of Surgeons. In 1800, the Royal College of Physicians, the Royal College of Surgeons, and the Society of Apothecaries controlled the three types of practice, which officially remained mutually exclusive. The members of the Royal College of Physicians were few and had minimal influence outside London. The larger membership of the Royal College of Surgeons included about 400 to 500 individuals trained to practice only surgery. The apothecaries, theoretically under the control of the Royal College of Physicians, were permitted to advise on medical cases but were not allowed to charge for that advice unless they prescribed a medicine. When a surgeon was called in to operate, an apothecary frequently was required to attend the patient afterward or to dress the wound, but he could receive no fee unless he induced the patient to take potions and dressings.

Because there were so few physicians, the requirement for more personnel fell to the apothecaries and members of the Royal College of Surgeons. To better care for patients, the apothecaries, who knew little surgery, joined the college to learn surgery. The typical surgeon, conversely, knew little about pharmaceutical medicine and was forced to obtain an apothecary's license. It became apparent that this new class of general practitioner or surgeon-apothecary needed a comprehensive, regulated form of training.

In 1815, the apothecaries obtained an act of Parliament that enabled them to hold an examination for all who practiced in England and to prosecute unqualified practitioners, the first statute in Great Britain to impose penalties on unlicensed practitioners. Within a few years of the passage of the Act of 1815, the Royal College of Surgeons began to define more clearly its educational requirements and made them complementary to those required by the Society of Apothecaries. Thus, candidates who intended to enter general practice usually obtained both licenses, and a Master of the Royal College of Surgeons, Licentiate of the Society of Apothecaries (MRCS, LSA), became the common qualification.

The Royal College of Surgeons became a licensing body and during the course of the 19th century gradually assumed increasing responsibility for the education of surgeons. Its license, however, was purely optional, and anyone could practice without restriction. In 1843, the college charter was again re-formed: the name was legally changed to the Royal College of Surgeons of England, and the Fellowship of Surgeons was created. During the 19th century, the most prominent English surgeons included Astley Cooper (1768–1841) (Fig. 1.6), Charles Bell (1774–1842), Benjamin Brodie (1783–1862), William Lawrence (1783–1867), Benjamin Travers (1783–1858), George Guthrie (1785–1856), Robert Liston (1794–1847), James Syme (1799–1870), John Hilton (1804–1878), James Paget (1814–1899), John Erichsen (1818–1896), Jonathan Hutchinson (1828–1913), Hugh Owen Thomas (1834–1891), Robert Lawson Tait (1845–1899), and William Macewen (1848–1924).

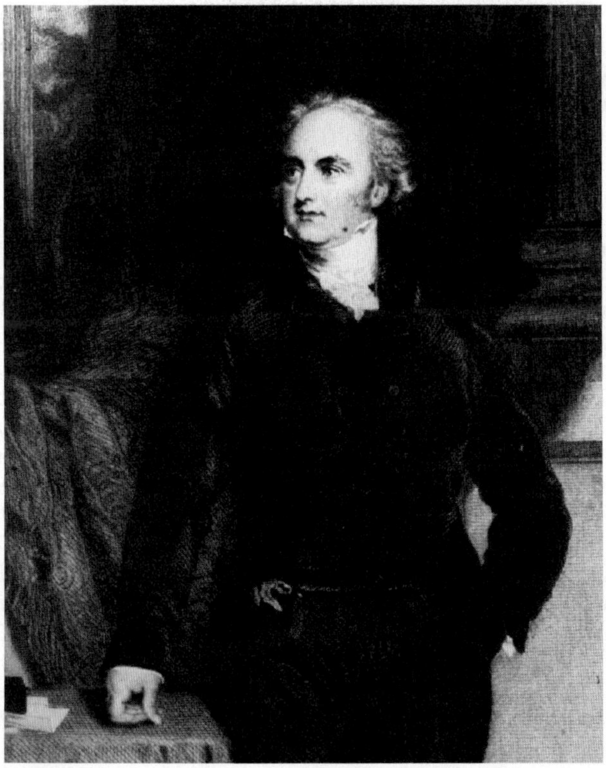

FIGURE 1.6. Astley Cooper. (Courtesy of the New York Academy of Medicine Library.)

The ascendancy of German medicine and surgery did not occur until the latter half of the 19th century. Surgical education and training persisted in an undeveloped state in the German-speaking countries longer than in most other regions in western Europe. Undoubtedly, a major reason for the delay was that at the beginning of the century Germany was a conglomeration of divided, independent political units, with no one central city representing the focus of governmental organization.

The 19th-century German unification process under Prussia presented unlimited opportunities for surgery and its surgeons. As the new Germany began to showcase itself to the international markets, it looked to its universities for image building. In Prussia, a system of medical study had been arranged in 1825. It provided both for physicians who studied at the universities and for surgeons, who were delineated into first and second classes. The surgeons of the first class were required to study at either a university or a "medico-chirurgical school" for 3 years. Unlike the physicians, however, they were not required to know Latin, an indication, perhaps, that surgery was thought of as the more practical craft. Surgeons of the second class were educated only through an apprenticeship with a practicing second-class surgeon. At midcentury, the Prussian government decreed that there should be but a single class of doctors, and that more than a medical degree was necessary before doctors could obtain the right to practice. As the German-speaking empire grew, a great scholastic achievement was coming to fruition in the form of the richly endowed state university—highly organized, academically free, crowded with laboratories, and ever growing.

The national achievements of Germany soon became international, and from the 1860s through World War I, its educational system attracted aspiring students, including physicians and surgeons, from all over the world. In a mighty academic upsurge of less than 40 years, German surgeons wrenched the world surgical stage away from their European neighbors and asserted their own dominance. In 1872, the Deutsche Gesellschaft für Chirurgie was formed. This national organization soon began to hold annual meetings, during which papers were read and criticized. In effect, it acted as a gathering place for the free interchange of new German surgical ideas.

The reasons for the rapid development of surgery in Germany are not easily defined, but it was undoubtedly related to political and economic changes, as well as to the general cultural and scientific climate. The multiplication in the number of chairs of surgery at the universities, the unification of the disparate branches of the healing art, and the organization of learned societies with journals to publicize their proceedings can be counted among the most important factors.

Few surgeons of distinction practiced in Germany during the early part of the century. Franz Hesselbach (1759–1816) and Vincenz von Kern (1760–1829) were among the best known. By the fourth and fifth decades of the 19th century a growing number of German surgeons were achieving prominence. Although their influence would be the catalyst that later propelled Germany toward world prominence, most of them did not live to see the heights to which German surgery rose. Among these individuals were Conrad Langenbeck (1776–1851); Johann Meckel, the younger; Johann Friedrich Dieffenbach (1792–1847); Georg Stromeyer (1804–1876); and Edward Zeis (1807–1868).

During the 1860s, German surgery began its rapid climb to world prominence. In most instances, it fell to the surgeons born during and after the second decade of the century to help showcase the astounding medical and surgical advances and superb technical achievements of German-speaking surgeons. Within this group were Karl Thiersch (1822–1895), Friedrich von Esmarch (1823–1908), Albrech von Graefe (1828–1870), Theodor Billroth (1928–1894), Richard von Volkmann (1830–1889), Ernst von Bergmann (1836–1907), Theodor Kocher (1841–1917) (Fig. 1.7), Vincenz Czerny (1842–1916), and Friedrich Trendelenburg (1844–1924). Following the midpoint of the 19th century, another group of surgeons would lead German domination of the world surgical stage through the tragic lessons of World War I. Included were Johann von Mikulicz-Radecki (1850–1905), Paul Kraske (1851–1930), Anton von Eiselsberg (1860–1939), Hermann Pfannenstiel (1862–1909), Max Wilms (1867–1918), Fritz de Quervain (1868–1940), and George Perthes (1868–1927).

In France, the new Paris medical school was basically the old College of Surgery with the addition of a few physicians. Although surgeons did not literally replace physicians, most physicians of the revolutionary era and the early 19th century had strong surgical backgrounds. In a matter of great symbolism, the new Paris medical school was provided a home within the spacious facilities of the former College of Surgery.

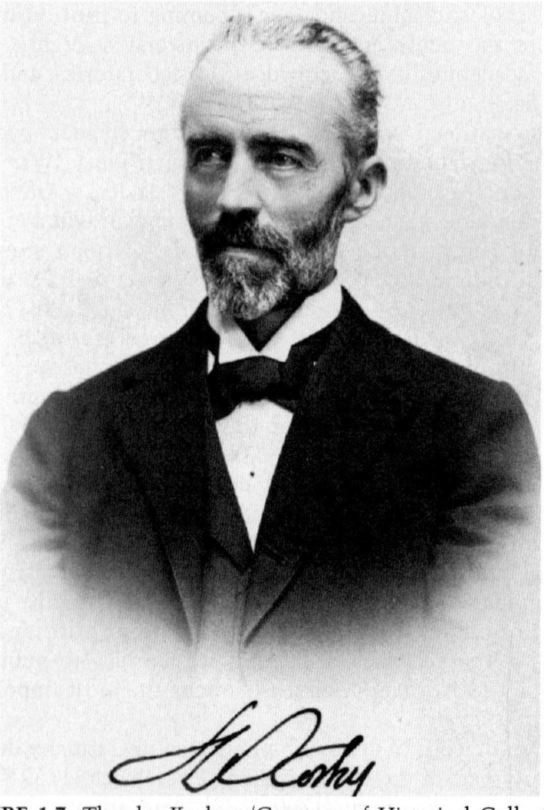

FIGURE 1.7. Theodor Kocher. (Courtesy of Historical Collections, Library of the College of Physicians of Philadelphia.)

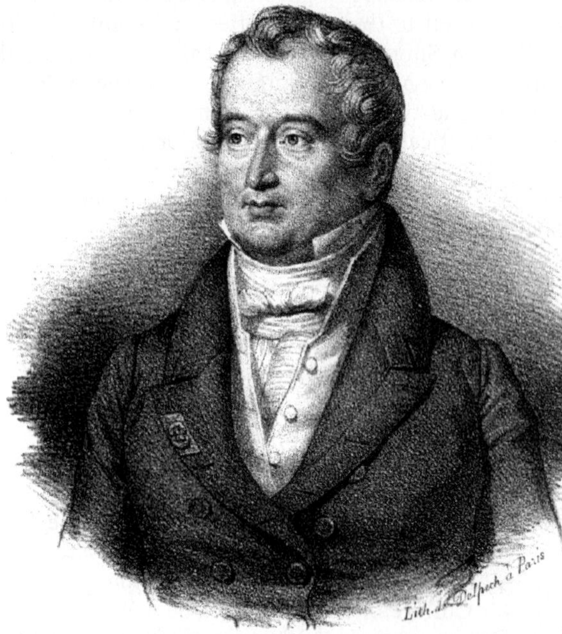

FIGURE 1.8. Guillaume Dupuytren. (Courtesy of Historical Collections, Library of the College of Physicians of Philadelphia.)

The reform of hospital training for young doctors also indicated the strength of Parisian surgeons. In the 19th century, hospital service became an integral aspect of overall medical training. Consequently, such features as the competitive examinations, known as *concours*, and the division of nonresident students (externs) and resident students (interns) were throwbacks to earlier surgical precedents. Many chores that had previously been assigned to young surgeons (wound dressing, phlebotomy, minor surgery) were now undertaken by medical students. Thus, French physicians had a strong surgical inclination, even if they were not actually going to specialize in surgery.

Prelisterian 19th-century French surgery falls into four natural periods: the first, or Napoleonic, era (1800–1814); the second era, from 1815 to 1835, which closely parallels developments in the career of Guillaume Dupuytren (1778–1835) (Fig. 1.8); a preanesthetic period, from Dupuytren's death until 1847; and a fourth period, which lasted until the mid-1870s, when listerian techniques were finally accepted by most French surgeons. Among the well-known French surgeons of the 19th century and the beginning of the 20th century were Dominique Jean Larrey (1766–1842) (Fig. 1.9), Jacques Delpech (1777–1832), Jean Marjolin (1780–1850), Jules Cloquet (1790–1883), Jacques Lisfranc (1790–1847), Alfred Velpeau (1795–1867), Auguste Nélaton (1807–1873), Paul Broca (1824–1880), Jules Péan (1830–1898), Just Lucas-Championière (1843–1913), Henri Hartmann (1860–1952), and Mathieu Jaboulay (1860–1913).

Although the mantle of surgical leadership had been assumed by French and German surgeons during this century, other European surgeons of note dotted the medical landscape. Names that should be mentioned include Antonio Scarpa (1752–1832), Adolf Callisen (1787–1866), Christian

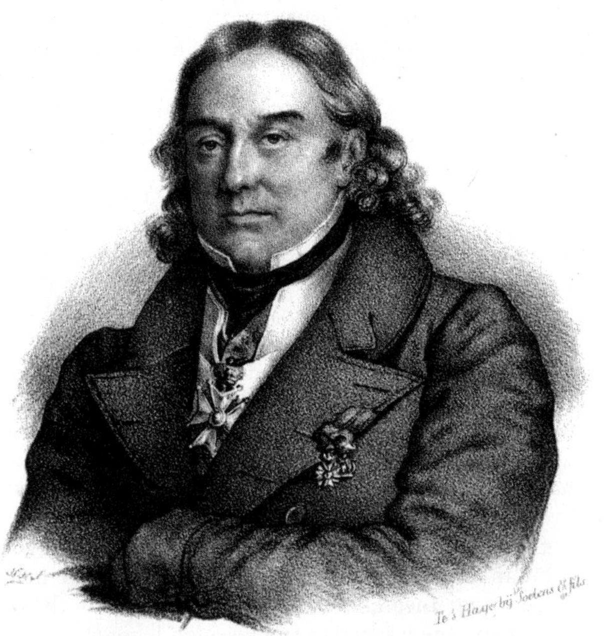

FIGURE 1.9. Dominique Larrey. (Courtesy of Historical Collections, Library of the College of Physicians of Philadelphia.)

Tilanus (1796–1883), Nikolai Pirogoff (1810–1881), Eduardo Bassini (1844–1924), Carl Reyher (1846–1890), Niels Rovsing (1862–1927), and Leonardo Gigli (1863–1908).

The practice of surgery in the United States during the 19th century consisted of several distinct periods, each characterized by conditions sufficiently different to constitute separate surgical eras. The initial decades (1800–1825) were in most respects an extension of medicine as it had developed in the 13 colonies. Few physicians or surgeons in early 19th-century America had become qualified to practice through a systematic course of education because academic facilities in the United States were limited and an extensive medical education generally required attendance at a European medical school. To meet existing conditions, most future practitioners were compelled to become apprentices to practicing physicians in America and to "read medicine and surgery" while working in the physician's office.

During the earliest periods of the century, surgery remained merely a technical mode of medical treatment: there was little to suggest that it had become a branch of scientific medicine. In contrast to Europe, there were virtually no individuals in America who could be considered scientific surgeons. However, several developments during the early part of the century indicated progress toward the professionalizing of American surgery. Increasing numbers of young Americans were beginning to matriculate at leading European medical centers, especially those in Great Britain. Americans who managed to study abroad came to form a considerable proportion of the leading surgeons in sparsely settled America. Among these individuals were Wright Post (1766–1822), Valentine Mott (1785–1865), and J. Kearny Rodgers (1793–1851) of New York City. The Philadelphia surgeons Philip Syng Physick (1768–1837), his nephew John Syng Dorsey (1783–1818), and William Gibson (1788–1868) took lengthy periods of training in London and Edinburgh, and both Ephraim McDowell (1771–1830) and Benjamin Winslow Dudley (1785–1870) returned, after studying in the latter city, to practice in the wilds of Kentucky.

The years from the mid-1820s to 1846, when ether anesthesia was introduced, can also be considered a distinct period in the history of American surgery. During that time, because of the vast proliferation of medical schools throughout the country, nearly every important physician and surgeon in the United States initially studied at an American medical school. From the few scattered 18th-century institutions in Boston, New York City, and Philadelphia to the myriad schools that were opened during the 19th century, medical education became widely available.

From 1847 through 1860, a third era in 19th-century American surgery occurred, a period dominated by the increasing use of surgical anesthesia and tempered by the continued inability to control infection. The surgeon's technical expertise regarding operations also changed markedly. Whereas the trademark of the bold surgeon had always been operative speed (e.g., completing an amputation in less than 60 seconds), the advent of anesthesia enabled the operator to remove his focus from speed alone and to be more precise in his methods. Numbers of surgical operations were beginning to increase, and some surgeons were beginning to pursue scientific investigation. The foremost example of the new type of American surgeons was Samuel Gross (1805–1884). He was adamant in his use of animal models to understand surgical diseases and therapies.

Of unquestioned importance in the development of an American profession of surgery was the tragic experience of the Civil War (1861–1865). This armed struggle produced a huge number of casualties, and the concomitant need for surgical care constituted a unique era in the development of surgery in this country during the 19th century. The contributions to surgical treatment that developed during the Civil War have never been fully appreciated, probably because antiseptic techniques remained unknown, and more deaths and suffering resulted from infectious processes than from battlefield injury. The most important direct effect of the Civil War was the great number of physicians who were introduced to basic principles of surgery. Literally thousands on thousands of the most difficult surgical cases imaginable were handled in a short time; so many cases would not have occurred in many years of peace. These new "surgeons" learned about new ideas and standards of care and became familiar with anesthetic agents. After this on-site surgical education and training, American surgical practice evolved rapidly.

A fifth era of American surgery took place from 1865 through the late 1870s. Rapid advances were made in medical sciences despite the growing presence of various medical sects, including homeopaths, botanics, and eclectics. During the 1870s, for the first time, a substantial number of surgical textbooks and monographs by American surgeons were published. That American surgery had reached a new level of sophistication was evident both in the growth of surgical literature and in the number of well-respected practitioners. However, there still remained no clear delineation between physician and surgeon, and the defining of an American surgeon had become a particularly difficult task.

Clearly, there was a difference between the European concept of a surgeon and his American counterpart. The European medical community had an established history of groups of physicians who performed little but surgical operations, whereas such specialization would not be attained in America until after the 1880s. Therefore, it is likely that most surgeons practicing in the United States through the 1870s practiced more nonsurgical medicine and derived greater income from their medical therapies than their surgical operations. Only toward the end of the 19th century was surgery in the United States increasingly performed by those who considered themselves specialists in surgery. Although most general practitioners continued to perform minor surgical operations (such as those for simple fractures, minor skin trauma, and hernia), the more difficult procedures such as abdominal operations were completed by these new specialists in surgery. This distinction between surgeon and physician was most evident in the large urban areas of the country.

In rural America, the turn toward specialists in surgery would not occur until well into the 20th century. A major part of this delay can be attributed to the large number of rural physicians who received surgical training during the Civil War and to their desire to remain physician/surgeons as a means of augmenting their income. In addition, physicians in rural America were in short supply, and these general practitioner/surgeons were obligated to provide the only surgical expertise available for many miles.

By the conclusion of the 1870s, surgery was practiced with about equal success on both sides of the Atlantic Ocean. The major difference between the two continents was that in most instances any evidence of advanced scientific research was still concentrated in the older, more established European university and hospital centers, not in the United States.

The penultimate evolutionary stage of American surgery in the 19th century, including the existence of well-supported and adequately supplied hospitals and research institutions, occurred during the decades of the 1880s and 1890s. These years brought about a final acceptance of the germ theory in America and with it the introduction of crude antiseptic and aseptic techniques into many of the country's operating rooms. For various reasons, Lister found widespread enthusiastic support for his beliefs among the surgeons of the European continent. In his own country, however, and in the United States, surgeons turned to listerian techniques slowly and, at times, with reluctance. Before the 1880s, there was less infection in America's spacious general hospitals than in the exceptionally crowded charity hospitals of Europe. Consequently, the clinical need for listerian principles was not as great in the United States as in Europe. During the late 1880s, several surgical texts appeared that brought about the final acceptance of Lister's techniques in the United States. The most important of these American publications was Arpad Gerster's (1848–1923) *The Rules of Aseptic and Antiseptic Surgery* (1888) and Nicholas Senn's (1844–1908) *Surgical Bacteriology* (1889).

Two other events during the 1880s were also crucial in the professionalizing of American surgery. In 1880, the American Surgical Association, the country's first surgical organization, was formed. Three years later, the initial volumes of the *Annals of Surgery* were published. For the surgeon, the *Annals* represented the most influential and important of all American medical journals of the 19th century. It was the first American periodical devoted solely to the practice of surgery, and its pages recorded the advancement of American surgery more accurately than did any other written source. By having their own society and journal, American surgeons finally achieved some measure of the social and political organization that European surgeons had experienced for almost a century.

By the beginning of the 1890s, it was evident that both American and European surgery had been affected more profoundly than any other area of 19th-century medical practice by achievements in the medical sciences. The discovery of useful anesthetics and the development of a method to prevent wound infection revolutionized surgical practice. From a crude and dangerous art, surgery rapidly became an influential, prestigious medical specialty in the 19th century. American surgery had finally begun to achieve its status as a distinct medical specialty.

The last developmental era began in 1889, when William Halsted initiated his work in the newly opened Johns Hopkins Hospital in Baltimore. Although other surgeons had more international reputations, it was Halsted who set the tone for the final period of development. His work reveals the beginnings of a new American surgery based as much on physiology as on anatomy. Halsted moved surgery from the heroics of the operating "theater" to the relative sterility of the operating room and the privacy of the research laboratory. American surgery was becoming a true science, and the recognition of surgery's true therapeutic powers would soon follow.

By the end of the 19th century, American surgery had sufficiently matured to acquire a professionalism of its own. Great surgical centers were being constructed in every section of the country, and the practice of surgery was proliferating and progressing. What American surgeons lacked was a cohesiveness brought about by some type of educational organization similar to the Royal Colleges in Great Britain or the Academy of Surgery in France. Although such societies as the American Medical Association (1847), the American Surgical Association, and various surgical specialty groups had begun to be established, they held no overt regulatory powers. They were primarily educational alliances with no control over licensure. Lack of an organized system of surgical education, training, and licensure would plague American surgery well into the 20th century.

Like their European counterparts, 19th-century American surgeons were great individual achievers. Among the most prominent were John Rhea Barton (1794–1871), Nathan Ryno Smith (1797–1877), Willard Parker (1800–1884), Joseph Pancoast (1805–1882), Gurdon Buck (1807–1877), Frank Hamilton (1813–1886), J. Marion Sims (1813–1883), Henry Bigelow (1818–1890), D. Hayes Agnew (1818–1892), Lewis Sayre (1820–1900), Thomas Addis Emmet (1828–1919), William Tod Helmuth (1833–1902), Hunter Holmes McGuire (1835–1900), William W. Keen (1837–1932), Henry Marcy (1837–1924), Charles McBurney (1845–1913), John Wyeth (1845–1922), Roswell Park (1852–1914), Franklin Martin (1857–1935), Howard Kelly (1858–1943), William Mayo (1861–1939), George Crile (1864–1943), Charles Mayo (1865–1939), and Harvey Cushing (1869–1939).

The 20th Century

Three phases of surgical development are noted during the 20th century—from 1900 to 1918, from 1919 to 1945, and from 1946 to the present. Within each period, significant events have transpired that have affected the history of surgery. The first 20 years represent a direct continuation of the tremendous revolution that had occurred within the surgical sciences during the last quarter of the 19th century. Many advances in surgery have been made during armed conflict. Not unexpectedly, therefore, World War I provided a signpost for surgery during the remainder of the 20th century.

At the beginning of this era, a certain sense of social discomfort on the part of surgeons led to continued mockery by "scientific" physicians, who often disqualified surgeons as nonthinkers and surgery as an inferior craft. By 1900, surgeons had basically explored all the cavities of the body. Nonetheless, operative surgery had not yet been accepted by physicians who were not oriented to surgery or, most importantly, by patients and society. Even in the late 1990s, the immediate consequences of surgical operations, such as discomfort and associated complications, often were of more concern to patients than the positive knowledge that surgery can eliminate potentially devastating disease processes.

By the early 20th century, it was becoming evident that research models, theoretical concepts, and valid applications would be necessary to demonstrate the scientific basis of surgery to the public, and that to devise new operative methods, experimental surgery was necessary. Most important, a scientific basis for therapeutic surgical recommendations consisting of empirical data collected and analyzed according to internationally accepted rules and set apart from individual authoritative appreciations would have to be developed. Surgeons needed to allay society's fear of the surgical unknown and present surgery as an accepted part of the established medical armamentarium. The most consequential achievement for 20th-century surgeons was the eventual social acceptability of surgery.

Among the difficulties in studying 20th-century surgery is the abundance of famous names and important written and clinical contributions. It becomes a difficult and invidious task to attempt any selection of representative personalities, particularly after World War I, when the evolution of surgery became affected more than ever before by socioeconomic events and technological advances rather than by unique individual clinical achievements. The vast social transformation of surgery and medicine has begun to control the fate of the individual practitioner in the late 20th and beginning of the 21st century to a much greater extent than the clinicians as a collective force are able to control it by their attempts to direct their own profession.

For American surgeons, the years just before World War I were a time of active coalescence into various social and educational organizations. The most important of these societies was the American College of Surgeons, founded by Franklin Martin in 1914. Patterned after the Royal Colleges of Surgeons of England, Ireland, and Scotland, the American College of Surgeons established professional, ethical, and moral standards for every authorized graduate in medicine who practiced surgery.

From 1919 to 1945, the maturation process for surgical specialties gathered tremendous momentum. This clarion call became a vital stage in the evolution of world surgery and constituted the most significant aspect of surgical history during that period. Ironically, the United States, which had been much slower than European countries to recognize surgeons as a distinct group of clinicians separate from internists and general practitioners, would spearhead the move toward surgical specialization with great alacrity. The course of surgical fragmentation into specialties and subspecialties continues apace today, particularly in the United States.

Bibliography

Bankoff G. The Story of Surgery. London: Arthur Barker; 1947.
Bishop WJ. The Early History of Surgery. London: Robert Hale; 1960.
Cartwright FF. The Development of Modern Surgery. London: Arthur Barker; 1967.
Dally AD. Women Under the Knife: A History of Surgery. London: Hutchinson Radius; 1991.
Glaser H. The Road to Modern Surgery. London: Butterworth; 1960.
Graham H. The Story of Surgery. New York: Doubleday & Doran, 1939.
Haeger K. The Illustrated History of Surgery. New York: Bell; 1988.
Hurwitz A, Degenshein GA. Milestones in Modern Surgery. New York: Hoeber-Harper; 1958.
Leonardo RA. History of Surgery. New York: Froben; 1943.
Meade RH. An Introduction to the History of General Surgery. Philadelphia: Saunders; 1968.
Power D. A Short History of Surgery. London: John Hale; 1933.
Richardson RG. Surgery: Old and New Frontiers. New York: Scribner's; 1968.
Rutkow IM. Surgery: An Illustrated History. St. Louis: Mosby; 1993.
Rutkow IM. American Surgery: An Illustrated History. Philadelphia: Lippincott; 1998.
Thorwald J. The Century of the Surgeon. New York: Pantheon; 1957.
Thorwald J. The Triumph of Surgery. New York: Pantheon; 1960.
Wangensteen OH, Wangensteen SD. The Rise of Surgery From Empiric Craft to Scientific Discipline. Minneapolis: University of Minnesota; 1978.
Zimmerman LM, Veith I. Great Ideas in the History of Surgery. Baltimore: Williams & Wilkins, 1961.

2 Evidence-Based Surgery

Robin S. McLeod

The term *evidence-based medicine* was coined by Sackett and colleagues in the 1980s. They defined it as "the conscientious, explicit, and judicious use of current best evidence in making decisions about the care of individual patients."[1] The practice of evidence-based medicine means integrating individual clinical expertise with the best-available clinical evidence from systematic research. In short, evidence-based medicine means systematically searching for the best evidence rather than relying on expert opinion or anecdotal experience. In addition, Sackett and colleagues recognized the importance of the clinical expertise that most physicians possess and were explicit in stating that the evidence must be integrated with clinical acumen. Finally, the preferences and values of the patient must be considered in the decision making.

Critics of evidence-based medicine have argued that most clinicians already base their decisions on evidence even though, as discussed in this chapter, there is evidence that indicates that may not be true. Others feel that evidence-based medicine does not place a value on the experience of the individual clinician. However, there is a recognition that patients vary in their disease manifestations and response to therapy, so even the best evidence may not be completely generalizable to the individual patient; therefore, the judgment of the clinician is crucial. Similarly, individual patients differ in their expectations and preferences, and management decisions must be guided by them.

There are five linked ideas central to the practice of evidence-based medicine. First, clinical decisions should be based on the best-available scientific evidence; second, the clinical problem, rather than the habits of protocols, should determine the type of evidence to be sought; third, identifying the best evidence means using epidemiological and biostatistical ways of thinking; fourth, conclusions derived from identifying and critically appraising evidence are useful only if put into action in managing patients or making health care decisions; and finally, performance should be constantly evaluated.[2]

Why the necessity for evidence-based medicine? The basis for the traditional practice of surgery has been the understanding of the pathophysiology of a disease, introduction of procedures or maneuvers to alter the process, and close observation of the results of treatment reported through case series.[3] This practice has led to many advances and accepted therapies, including appendectomy for appendicitis, cholecystectomy and common bile duct exploration for cholangitis, and antireflux surgery for gastroesophageal reflux. On the other hand, there are striking examples for which the translation of basic physiological principles has not led to improved clinical outcomes. For example, gastric cooling was found to reduce acid secretion sharply, but when gastric cooling was used clinically to treat bleeding duodenal ulcers, it failed.[4] There has been evidence that inflammatory mediators are elevated in septic shock, but interventions with antagonists have failed to change outcome in these patients.[5,6]

No one would argue that modern medicine is different from that practiced earlier in this or previous centuries. For example, the discovery of penicillin led to a dramatic improvement in outcome in patients with pneumococcal pneumonia. It was obvious that penicillin was effective. Today, rarely do new interventions or technologies lead to such dramatic changes in outcome. More commonly, they lead to a small improvement in survival or possibly no improvement in survival but a change in function or quality of life. Whereas large differences can be readily detected by observation alone, certainty that the small change in outcome is due to the treatment itself and not inherent differences in patients requires more rigorous evaluation. This need for higher-quality evidence has also led to a need for physicians to be able to interpret the evidence.

Since the introduction of the term evidence-based medicine, it has been adopted by a wide range of specialties, including surgery. Many fear that evidence-based medicine is simply an excuse by policymakers to cut costs and curb clinical freedom. It is certainly true that rationing of health care dollars has increased, and with that there is increasing pressure to do more with less. Physicians may be unhappy with that prospect, but it is likely the reality. In the United States, $1.1 trillion were spent on health care in 1997 compared with $700 billion in 1990. Since 1970, the proportion of gross domestic product spent on health care has nearly doubled to 13.6% compared with 7.1%.[7] Thus, with health care costs increasing exponentially, it is understandable that providers have concerns. Clinicians should also be concerned because without judicious use of available funds, there may be inadequate resources for interventions that are effective and thus for the ability to deliver high-quality care.

There are, however, other reasons to practice evidence-based medicine. First, most physicians want to do the best for their patients on an individual basis. To do so, one must be abreast of the current knowledge in the area. Second, patients are better educated and informed and are challenging physicians' views. Patients have access to the medical literature and can often cite it. Not only are individual patients questioning what doctors are doing but also patient advocacy groups are playing a major role in medical care. Finally, if physicians wish to play a role in policy decision making and allocation of resources, they must have the evidence to justify the introduction and maintenance of these programs. Thus, physicians can no longer rely on their anecdotal experience.

Are We Practicing Evidence-Based Medicine?

It has been shown that even high-quality information published in the literature is often not applied by practicing physicians. Antman and colleagues looked at interventions used in the management of acute myocardial infarction.[8] They determined the date when the first randomized controlled trial (RCT) indicated that a treatment was effective or ineffective and the dates of subsequent trials and performed meta-analyses of the individual trials. As a measure of when the treatment became standard practice or conversely was no longer standard practice, they looked at standard medical texts to determine whether the treatment was recommended as standard practice, might be useful, or was experimental. There were discrepancies between the results of meta-analyses and the recommendations of experts. In some cases, over 20 years elapsed between the time a medication was first shown to be effective in an RCT until it was recommended as routine therapy. No similar studies have been performed studying surgical procedures and their adoption or abandonment. However, the marked variations in the rates of some operations observed across small and large areas are likely an indication of the same phenomenon.[9]

Anderson and colleagues[10] reviewed discharge data from 16 hospitals in Massachusetts during an 18-month period between 1985 and 1986. They found that 17% of patients were at high risk for developing a venous thromboembolism. Of these, 50% were surgical patients. Despite evidence from multiple RCTs dating to the 1970s, prophylaxis for venous thromboembolism was administered to only 32% of these high-risk patients. The proportion of patients receiving prophylaxis ranged from 9% to 56% at the study hospitals. Overall, patients at teaching hospitals were more likely to receive prophylaxis.

On the other hand, there is some evidence from two small studies performed at institutions in the United Kingdom suggesting that many of the decisions made by both internists and surgeons are based on high-quality evidence.[11,12] Ellis and colleagues examined the treatments given to 109 patients with a known diagnosis admitted through the emergency room to a general internal medicine ward.[11] They reported that treatment was based on evidence from RCTs in 53% and on convincing nonexperimental evidence in 29%; interventions without substantial evidence were employed in 18%. Those interventions based on RCT evidence included aspirin for transient ischemic attacks, omeprazole for esophagitis, and 100% oxygen for carbon monoxide poisoning. The interventions with convincing nonexperimental evidence included cardiopulmonary resuscitation for cardiac arrest and surgery for complete small bowel obstruction due to a cecal cancer. Treatment of various poisonings, noncardiac chest pain, and presumed food poisoning were classified as having unsubstantial evidence.

A similar study was performed by Howes et al. of 100 patients on a general surgical ward.[12] It is noteworthy that only 24% received treatment based on evidence from RCTs compared with 53% of decisions in the internal medicine study. Treatment based on other convincing evidence was received by 71%. The latter group included the conservative management of adhesive small bowel obstruction, conservative management of splenic hematoma and blunt liver trauma, and endoscopic retrograde cholangiopancreatography and endoscopic management of gallstones and jaundice. The authors concluded that, for the most part, surgical therapy is evidence based. However, it is debatable whether nonsurgeons would be accepting that all of the treatments based on nonexperimental evidence would be based on "convincing" evidence as stated by these surgical authors.

Requirements for Practicing Evidence-Based Surgery

Rosenberg and Donald outlined some of the steps involved in the application of evidence-based practice.[13] First, the clinician must clearly identify and articulate a question that has arisen from clinical practice. External evidence is then sought, usually by performing a focused search of the literature. The information thus retrieved is subjected to critical appraisal; finally, the newly acquired knowledge is implemented in clinical practice. Thus, the necessary elements to practice evidence-based medicine are production and dissemination of high-quality evidence and retrieval and critical appraisal of the evidence. The remainder of this chapter discusses these two major issues.

Providing the Evidence

Various hierarchies have been proposed for classifying study design.[14,15] In simplest terms, studies can be classified as case series, case-control studies, cohort studies, and RCTs. The case series is the weakest and the RCT is the strongest for determining the effectiveness of treatment (Table 2.1).

Case Series

Case reports (arbitrarily defined as involving 10 or fewer subjects) and case series are the typical surgical studies performed. There is no concurrent control group, although there may be a historical control group. Patients may be followed from the same inception point and followed prospectively not

TABLE 2.1. Hierarchy of Study Designs.

	Control group	*Prospective follow-up*	*Random allocation of subjects*
Case series	No	No	No
Case-control study	Yes	No	No
Cohort study	Yes	Yes	No
Randomized controlled trial	Yes	Yes	Yes

for the purpose of the study but in the normal clinical course of the disease. Typically, data from patient charts or clinical databases are reviewed retrospectively. Thus, the outcome of interest is present when the study is initiated.

Despite the limitations of this study design, the importance of results from case series should not be minimized. It is because of careful observation that innovations in surgical practice and techniques have been and continue to be made. However, results from case series should be likened to those observations made in the laboratory. Just as those observations should lead to generation of a hypothesis and performance of an experiment to test it, an RCT should be performed to confirm the observations reported in a case series. Case series are plagued with biases (e.g., selection and referral biases), and because data are not collected specifically for the study, they are often incomplete or even inaccurate. Therefore, incorrect conclusions about the efficacy of a treatment are common, and the mistake that surgeons make is relying solely on evidence from case series.

Case-Control Studies

The case-control study is the design used most frequently by epidemiologists to study risk factors or causation. There are two groups of patients: the case group is composed of subjects in whom the outcome of interest is present, whereas it is not present in subjects in the control group. Controls are selected by the investigator rather than by random allocation, so the likelihood of bias introduction is real; thus, there is a risk of drawing an erroneous conclusion. Generally, the controls are matched to the cases with respect to important prognostic variables other than the factor under study. While it is important to match the subjects to avoid an incorrect conclusion about the significance of the factor studied, it is equally important not to overmatch the controls so that a true difference is not observed.

In case-control studies, as in case series, data are collected retrospectively. Thus, the outcome is present at the start of the study. As an example, Selby and colleagues performed a case-control study to make inferences about the effectiveness of flexible sigmoidoscopy in preventing rectal cancer.[16] The cases were patients who had been receiving regular yearly examinations at a health maintenance organization (HMO) who developed rectal cancer (the outcome of interest). The controls were individuals from the same cohort of patients who had not developed rectal cancer. They were matched to the cases with respect to age, sex, and date of entry into the health plan. Selby and colleagues found that cases were less likely to have had a flexible sigmoidoscopy than controls in the preceding 10 years (8.8% of cases vs. 24.2% of controls).

Cohort Studies

Cohort studies may be performed retrospectively or prospectively. There are two or more groups, but subjects are not randomly allocated to the groups. One group receives the treatment or exposure of interest; the other group of subjects receives another or no treatment or exposure. The inception point may not be defined by the study, and the intervention and follow-up may be ad hoc. However, the outcome is not present at the time that the inception cohort is assembled.

There is less possibility of bias than for a case-control study because cases are not selected and the outcome is not present at the initiation of the study. However, the likelihood of bias is still high because subjects are not randomly allocated to groups. Instead, there is some selection process by either the subject or the clinician that allocates them to groups. For instance, subjects may be allocated to groups according to where they live (when the effect of an environmental toxin is under study), by choice (when a lifestyle factor such as dietary intake is under study), or by physician (when a nonrandomized study of a treatment intervention is performed).

Retrospective cohort studies differ from prospective cohort studies in that data analysis and possibly data collection are performed retrospectively, but there is an identifiable time point that can be used to define the inception cohort. Such a date could be the date of birth, date of first attendance at a hospital, or other selection.

Cohort studies typically are performed by epidemiologists studying risk factors for which randomization of patients is unethical. Although they are more powerful than case-control studies, subjects are not randomized, so the cohorts may potentially be biased. An example of a cohort study would be the use of a database to follow patients who had a mucosectomy versus no mucosectomy in restorative proctocolectomy to determine the long-term outcome.

Randomized Controlled Trials

The RCT is accepted as the best trial design for establishing treatment effectiveness. There are several essential components of the RCT. First, subjects are randomly allocated to two groups: usually a treatment group (in which the new treatment is tested) and a control group (in which the standard therapy or placebo is administered). Thus, the control group is concurrent, and subjects are randomly allocated to the two groups. Second, the interventions and follow-up are standardized and performed prospectively. Thus, it is hoped that both groups are similar in all respects except for the interventions studied. Not only does this guard against differences in factors known to be important, but also it ensures that there are no differences due to unknown or unidentified factors. This latter point is especially important. Statistical techniques such as multivariate analysis can be employed to adjust for known prognostic variables but obviously cannot adjust for unknown prognostic variables. There are multiple examples of studies showing differences between groups that cannot be accounted for by the known prognostic variables.[17]

When differences in treatment effect are small, the RCT may minimize the chance of reaching an incorrect conclusion about the effectiveness of treatment. There are, however, some limitations to RCTs. First, RCTs tend to take a long time to complete because of the time required for planning, accruing and following patients, and finally analyzing results. As a consequence, results may not be available for many years. Second, clinical trials are expensive to perform, although their cost may be recuperated if ineffective treatments are abandoned and only effective treatments are implemented.[18] Third, the results may not be generalizable or applicable to all patients with the disease because of the strict inclusion and exclusion criteria and inherent differences in patients who volunteer for trials. As well, not all patients will respond similarly to treatment. Fourth, when the disease or outcome is rare or only occurs after a long period of follow-up, RCTs are generally not feasible. Finally, the ethics of performing RCTs is controversial, and some clinicians may feel uncomfortable with randomizing their patients when they believe 1 treatment to be superior even if that is based only on anecdotal evidence.

There are elements common to all RCTs as outlined in Table 2.2. The first and perhaps the most important issue in designing an RCT is to enunciate clearly the research question. Most RCTs are based on observations or experimental evidence from the laboratory. Always, RCTs should make biological sense, have clinical relevancy, and be feasible to perform. The research question will determine who will be included, what the intervention will be, and what will be measured.

Frequently, a sequence of RCTs will be performed to evaluate a particular intervention. Initially, a small trial that is highly controlled using a physiological or surrogate endpoint may be performed. This trial would provide evidence that the intervention is effective in the optimal situation (*efficacy trial*). However, it might lack clinical relevance, especially if the endpoint were a physiological measure. However, if it were positive, then it would lead to another trial, with more patients and a more clinically relevant outcome measure. If this were positive, a large trial might be indicated to assess the effectiveness of the intervention in normal practice (*effectiveness trial*). Such an example would be studying the effect of a chemoprevention agent in colon cancer. Initially, the agent might be prescribed to a group of individuals at high risk for polyp formation (e.g., patients with familial polyposis coli) for a short time with the outcome measure a rectal biopsy looking for proliferative changes. A subsequent trial might look at polyp regression in this same cohort of patients, with subsequent trials aimed at the prevention of significant polyps in average-risk individuals followed for several years. As one can see, the selection of subjects, the intervention, the duration of the trial, and the choice of outcome measure may vary depending on the research question. Ultimately, however, investigators wish to generalize the results to clinical practice, so the outcome measures should be clinically relevant. For this reason, quality-of-life measures are often included.

TABLE 2.2. Elements of a Randomized Controlled Trial.

1. Stating the research question
2. Selecting the subjects
3. Allocating the subjects
4. Describing the maneuver
   a. The interventions
   b. Minimizing potential biases
   c. Baseline and follow-up maneuvers
5. Measuring outcome
   a. Assessing treatment effectiveness
   b. Assessing side effects and toxicity
6. Analyzing the data
7. Estimating the sample size
8. Ethical considerations
9. Administrative issues
   a. Feasibility of the trial
   b. Administration of the trial
   c. Data management
   d. Funding issues

While there are elements common to all RCTs, there are issues of special concern in surgical trials.[19] The issue of standardization of the procedure is of major importance in surgical trials. Standardization is difficult because surgeons may vary in their experience with and ability to perform a surgical technique; there may be individual preferences in performing the procedure, and technical modifications may occur as the procedure evolves. Moreover, differences in perioperative and postoperative care may also have an impact on the outcome.

There are two issues related to standardization of the procedure. First, there is the issue of who should perform the procedure: experts only or surgeons of varying ability. Second, there is the issue of standardization of the procedure so it is performed similarly by all surgical participants and can be duplicated by others following publication of the trial results. The implications of these two issues are different, and strategies to address them differ.

The first issue is analogous to assessing compliance in a medical trial. Thus, if the procedure is performed by experts only in a controlled fashion, this is analogous to an efficacy trial. The advantage of such a trial is that if the procedure is truly superior to the other intervention, then this design has the greatest likelihood of detecting a difference. The disadvantage, obviously, is that the results are less generalizable. Like most issues in clinical trials, there is no right or wrong answer. If the procedure is usually performed by experts, then it probably is desirable to have only experts involved in the trial. On the other hand, if a wide spectrum of surgeons performs the procedure usually, then it would be appropriate not to limit surgical participation.

No matter how many surgeons are involved in the trial and that investigators want to mimic routine practice, there must be at least a certain amount of standardization so that readers of the trial results can understand what was done and can duplicate the procedure in their own practice. There are several strategies to ensure a minimum standard. First, all surgeons should agree on the performance of the critical aspects of the procedure. It may not be necessary that there is agreement with all of the technical aspects, but there should be consensus on those that are deemed to be important. Furthermore, if there are aspects of the perioperative and postoperative care that have an impact on outcome (e.g., postoperative adjuvant therapy), then they should be standardized. Teaching sessions may be held preoperatively and feedback given to surgeons on their performance during the trial. As well, obtaining documentation that the procedure has been performed satisfactorily (e.g., through postoperative angiograms to document vessel patency or pathology specimens to document resection margins and lymph node excision) may contribute to ensuring that the surgery is performed adequately. Finally, patients are usually stratified according to surgeon or center to ensure balance in case there are differences in surgical technique between centers or surgeons.

Blinding is often a difficult issue in surgical trials. It may not be an issue if two surgical procedures are compared but is a major issue if a surgical procedure is compared with a medical therapy. There is often a placebo effect of surgery. The classic example was observed in a series of 18 patients in which 13 patients underwent ligation of the internal mammary artery for coronary artery disease, and 5 patients underwent a sham operation.[20] All of the patients in the latter group reported subjective improvement in their symptoms. Currently, it would be difficult ethically to perform a sham operation, so it might be impossible to conceal which treatment the patient received.

The lack of blinding is especially worrisome if the primary outcome is a change in symptoms or quality of life rather than a "hard" outcome measure such as mortality or morbidity. In these situations, if a hard outcome measure is also measured and it correlates with the patient's assessment, then there is less concern about the possibility of bias. Assessments may be performed by an independent assessor who is unaware of the patient's treatment group. Finally, if criteria used to define an outcome (e.g., criteria to diagnose an intraabdominal abscess) are explicitly specified a priori, then it may minimize or eliminate bias. Investigators may also choose in this situation to have a blinded panel review the results of tests to ensure that the tests meet the criteria.

The issue of timing of trials is difficult. Chalmers argued that the first patient who receives a procedure should be randomized.[21] Most surgeons would argue, however, that a learning curve exists in any procedure, and modifications to the technique are made frequently at its inception. By including these early patients, one would almost certainly bias the results against the new procedure. The introduction of laparoscopic cholecystectomy and the initially high rate of common bile duct injuries is a good example of this problem. On the other hand, it may be difficult to initiate a trial when the procedure is widely accepted by both the patient and the surgical community. The paucity of RCTs testing surgical therapies supports this latter contention. This dilemma arises because, unlike the release of medical therapies, there is no regulating body in surgery that restricts performance of a procedure or requires proof of its efficacy. Probably, RCTs should be performed early, before they become accepted into practice, recognizing that future trials may be necessary as the procedure evolves and surgical experience increases. This is analogous to medical oncological trials, in which trials are planned as one is completed. On the other hand, the procedure must be established adequately for one certainly would not want to invest a large amount of money and time into a trial and have the results be of no value at its completion.

Finally, patient issues may be of greater concern in surgical trials. In a medical trial, patients may be randomized to either treatment arm with the possibility that at the conclusion of the trial they can receive the more efficacious treatment if the disease is not progressive and the treatment is reversible. Surgical procedures, however, are almost always permanent. This may be of particular concern if a medical therapy is compared to a surgical procedure or the two surgical procedures differ in their magnitude or invasiveness. Patients may have a preference for one or the other treatments and therefore refuse to participate in the trial. There also tends to be more emotion involved with surgery, and patients may be less willing to leave the decision regarding which procedure will be performed to chance. Surgeons themselves may feel uncomfortable in discussing the uncertainty of randomization with patients requiring surgery.[22] Thus, accruing patients for surgical trials may be more difficult than for medical trials. In a survey of subjects who had already participated in a trial of maintenance therapy for Crohn's disease, Kennedy et al. found that 91% would agree to participate in a trial again if it involved comparison of two medical treatments, but only 44% would agree to participate if it included a surgical arm.[23] While accrual may be more difficult, there are notable examples of important surgical trials that have been performed.[24–26] Thus, they can be performed, though they may require a larger pool of eligible patients for sampling.

Outcome Studies

The outcomes movement probably began in the 1980s in the United States when the Joint Commission on Accreditation of Healthcare Organizations launched a restructuring of its survey and accreditation procedures.[27] Rather than simply measuring processes of care (e.g., number of surgical procedures performed), there was a shift to measuring patient outcomes. The outcomes and health services research movement has continued to gain momentum, and now many countries are employing these techniques to assess health care delivery in their jurisdiction. Health services research, which includes outcomes research, has been defined by the Institute of Medicine as "a multidisciplinary field of inquiry, both basic and applied, that examines the use, costs, quality and accessibility, delivery, organization, financing and outcomes of health care services to increase knowledge and understanding of the structures, processes and effects of health services for individuals and populations."[28]

Health services research includes all types of evaluations, including studies using the RCT design. Outcomes research has been used to describe many different types of research. *Outcomes studies* are usually used to describe those studies for which outcomes are assessed in large cohorts of patients, often using data from administrative databases. These cohorts may include patients registered in an HMO or living in a geographical area or some other defined group. Thus, outcomes studies, using the previously discussed hierarchy of study designs, are cohort studies. The strength and rationale for outcome studies are provided with their focus on populations or large groups of patients to minimize selection and referral biases found in small institutional series. In addition, outcomes studies often use patient-based or patient-derived evaluations of care. The hope for the outcomes movement was that the information derived would inform decision making by clinicians, health care administrators, and patients and thereby lead to a cycle of improved care.

The number of outcomes studies evaluating surgical procedures in all disciplines has increased exponentially in recent years. While they have an important role, they should be viewed as complementary to RCTs. Generally, an RCT is needed to establish the effectiveness of a treatment. The strength of the RCT is that conditions are tightly controlled to minimize bias and the risk of coming to an incorrect conclusion. However, because of this, they also may lack generalizability. Whereas variations in structure and process variables are minimized in RCTs, outcomes studies try to determine what role these factors play in routine care because there is no control over the selection of patients and the practice of physicians.[29]

Optimally, outcome studies can be used to determine whether services work as well in routine practice as they did in trials. For example, NASCET (North American Symptomatic Carotid Endarterectomy Trial) showed that carotid endarterectomy is superior to medical therapy in preventing strokes and reducing mortality in patients with significant carotid stenosis.[30] However, this study was done under controlled conditions by expert surgeons who had to provide evidence, prior to participating in the study, that they could do the operation adequately. Following the trial, experts recommended that carotid endarterectomy should be performed only if perioperative stroke and mortality rates of less than 6% could be achieved. Kucey et al. examined data from the University of Toronto to determine whether the benefits of carotid endarterectomy could be achieved in an academic setting that included surgeons with a range of expertise and potentially including some with resultant higher-than-recommended stroke rates.[31] Overall, the combined stroke and death rate was 6.3% among 27 surgeons at the 8 hospitals, suggesting indeed that the benefit of carotid endarterectomy was realized. Unfortunately, not all surgeons achieved this threshold rate, with hospital complication rates ranging from 4.0% to 30.0%. Information such as this may be useful in determining whether results from RCTs can be generalized to the nontrial situation.[29]

While RCTs are the standard for determining treatment effectiveness, another potential role for outcome studies occurs when RCTs are not feasible (e.g., involving a rare condition) or are not ethical. The availability of large administrative databases and ready access to this information with modern computers and statistical software packages has allowed outcome studies to be performed. These databases have several important limitations. First, the data within a database may be inaccurate or incomplete. Second, the databases have usually been set up for administrative purposes; therefore, clinically relevant data such as comorbid illness may be limited. Occasionally, it may be possible to link the administrative database to a clinical database that contains clinically relevant data. Alternately, additional information can be garnered by abstracting medical records or individual patient records. Finally, like clinical trials, outcome studies tend to be as good as the rigorousness of the methodology of the study. Thus, prior to embarking on the study, a hypothesis should be formulated, outcomes should be specified (e.g., length of stay, reoperative rate, readmission rate, etc.), plus comorbidities or risk factors (e.g., gender, age, hospital or surgeon, etc.) should be explicitly defined. Testing of the database to ensure accuracy is also an important step. Finally, multivariate statistical tests and logistic regression analyses are performed to adjust for possible known confounders (i.e., to control for the case mix).

There are several limitations of outcomes studies. Outcome studies are essentially observational studies, lacking the rigorous control of variables as in an RCT. Thus, there is the risk of bias. If recognized, then adjustments can be made in the analysis. However, there may be unidentifiable factors that bias the results. Thus, inferences must be made cautiously because there may be unmeasured variations in the patients, practitioners, and processes, and these may be the real explanation for differences in outcome. Second, often the available databases used have been set up for another purpose (i.e., to administer health care delivery). Thus, clinically relevant data may be limited. Optimally, patient relevant outcomes such as quality of life should be measured. However, endpoints may be limited to length of hospital stay, operative mortality, reoperation rates, and readmission rates. In addition to the limited number of endpoints, there may be inadequate or inaccurately recorded data on comorbidities. Furthermore, it may be impossible to know whether a comorbidity was present preoperatively or occurred following surgery. This may limit the ability to adjust the data adequately for varying levels of risk or disease severity. Third, outcomes studies can only assess the impact of patient variables and practice patterns on the process of health care delivery. Because patient preferences are not recorded, their impact cannot be assessed. However, certainly these play a major role in both decision making and outcome. Finally, there may be large fluctuations in outcome just due to chance for low-frequency procedures, and rates may not be stable statistically.

The confusion surrounding outcome research includes not only the different design characteristics of outcomes research as described in this section but also because the term has been applied to at least two other kinds of studies: to assess small-area variation and to assess the relationship between volume and outcome.

Small-Area Variation

The term *area variations* describes the phenomenon of differences in the rates of medical and surgical services observed among geographic regions (so-called large areas). These variations have been recorded among countries, states, and provinces and among counties or health services areas (so-called small areas). These findings elicit concern because those in areas of high volume may be receiving too much or inappropriate care (and thereby potentially be exposed to iatrogenic illness and postoperative death), while those in low volume areas may be receiving too little care (and thereby not benefiting from modern medical care).[32] In the Province of Ontario, the rate of breast-conserving operations in females with newly diagnosed breast cancer ranged, by county, from 11% to 84%. Iscoe and colleagues raised concerns that whether a woman had a breast-preserving procedure seemed to be related to factors at the local hospital level and not to patient factors or geography. Indeed, this large variation (15%–76%) was observed even within metropolitan Toronto.[33]

While the 2 main reasons cited for the variations have been differences in physician practice style and access to medical care, Eddy warned that the variations may be due to a multitude of other causes, including difficulties defining or diagnosing the disease, differences in the prevalence and severity of disease, and regional differences in patient preferences in seeking and accepting medical care.[34] Variation in surgical rates is related to variation in physician opinion. For many procedures, there is little variation (including such operations as inguinal hernia, acute myocardial infarction, and hip fractures) when there is general consensus among the medical profession regarding the diagnosis and treatment.[35] However, Wright and colleagues showed that the rates of knee replacement surgery in individual counties was directly related to the opinions of orthopedic surgeons.[36] Where differences in physician opinion do exist, there tends to be large geographic variations. For example, when a panel of experts from the United States and the United Kingdom were asked to review the indications for coronary artery bypass surgery, only 13% of US physicians considered the indications to be inappropriate compared with 35% of British physicians.[37]

The results of such studies are only of value if the causes and consequences of variation can be ascertained so strategies to minimize these variations can be implemented.[38] The conduct of RCTs to improve the quality of evidence available and develop evidence-based practice guidelines may be useful in this regard. An additional problem with the interpretation of area variation studies is knowing what the rate should be.[39] For some procedures, there may be no correct rate if patient preferences are considered.[40]

Volume Outcome Differences

Increasingly, studies have shown that for complex operations (e.g., esophagectomy, Whipple procedure, low anterior resection and abdominoperineal resection, liver resection and sarcoma surgery), surgical volume may have an impact on outcome.[41–44] For instance, Porter and colleagues reported a 2.5-fold increase in local recurrence for patients having curative surgery for rectal cancer when surgery was performed by surgeons who performed at a low volume (defined as fewer than 21 procedures over a 7-year period).[41] Similarly, reports from Canada and the United States have shown a significantly lower postoperative mortality rate in centers performing a high volume of Whipple procedures compared with low-volume centers.[42,43] Birkmeyer et al. reported that the outcomes of low-volume surgeons were equivalent to those of high-volume surgeons if the low-volume surgeon worked at a high-volume hospital,[45] suggesting that the health care team and facilities may be as important or even more important than the individual expertise of the surgeon. This trend has not been consistently observed, particularly in procedures of low or intermediate complexity. Khuri and colleagues studied 30-day outcome information on seven of the most commonly performed operations (e.g., colectomy, total hip arthroplasty, cholecystectomy) at Veterans Affairs hospitals in the United States and found no correlation between mortality and hospital volume.[46]

Halm and colleagues performed a systematic review of the literature pertaining to volume outcome studies.[47] There were 135 studies that covered 27 procedures and clinical conditions. The methodologic rigor of the studies varied, with few using clinical data for risk adjustment. However, 71% of studies of hospital volume and 69% of studies of physician volume reported statistically significant associations between higher volume and better outcomes. The magnitude of the association was variable. Interestingly, studies that performed risk adjustment using clinical data were less likely to report significant associations. Halm et al. concluded that differences in case mix and processes of care might explain part of the observed relationship between volume and outcome.

The implications of such studies are enormous and must be reviewed by policy- and decision makers. There has been a suggestion that there should be regionalization of more complex procedures. Before doing so, however, one must be certain that the results of current studies are not biased, and that observed differences are not due to factors other than volume. Thus, rigorous volume outcome studies with prospective collection of data with risk adjustment and studies addressing patient preferences may be required for each procedure before such decisions can be made. As well, implementation of educational measures may be another strategy to improve outcome.

Levels of Evidence

There are several grading systems for assessing the level of evidence.[14,47–50] The first was developed by the Canadian Task Force on Periodic Health Examination in the 1970s and has been adopted by the US Task Force (Table 2.3). While differing in some respects, most systems consider the a priori design of the study and the actual quality of the study. Studies in which there has been blinded random allocation of subjects are given highest weighting because the risk of bias is minimized. Thus, an RCT will provide level I evidence if it is well executed with respect to the issues discussed in this chapter.

This system is of value because of its simplicity, but difficulties may arise when pooling results from several studies, either informally during reading or when performing systematic reviews or developing guidelines. Decisions must be made on whether studies should be included or excluded depending on the quality of the study. As well, the systems are not sensitive to the relevance of the findings of studies. For instance, the clinical relevance of the outcome measures, the baseline risk of the effect, and the actual results of the studies (e.g., study results that are not consistent with results from other RCTs) are not considered in any system.

In this volume, the quality of the evidence is generally classified according to the system listed in Table 2.3.

The Center for Evidence-Based Medicine (Oxford, UK) has developed[51] the system shown in Table 2.4. It is used for the levels of evidence about prevention, diagnosis, prognosis, therapy, and harm. It differs from that initially proposed by

TABLE 2.3. Levels of Evidence.

I	Evidence obtained from at least one properly randomized controlled trial
II-1	Evidence obtained from well-designed controlled trials without randomization
II-2	Evidence obtained from well-designed cohort or case-control analytic studies, preferably from more than one center or research group
II-3	Evidence obtained from comparisons between times or places with or without the intervention; could also include dramatic results in uncontrolled experiments (e.g., the results of treatment with penicillin in the 1940s)
III	Opinions of respected authorities, based on clinical experience, descriptive studies, or reports of expert committees

Source: From Canadian Task Force on Periodic Health Examination.[14] Used by permission of *Canadian Medical Association Journal.*

TABLE 2.4. Oxford Centre for Evidence Based Medicine Levels of Evidence.

Level	*Therapy/prevention, etiology/harm*	*Prognosis*	*Diagnosis*	*Differential diagnosis/ symptom prevalence study*
1a	Systematic review	Systematic review	Systematic review of Level 1 diagnosis studies	Systematic review of prospective studies
1b	Individual RCT	Individual inception cohort studies	Cohort study with reference standard	Prospective cohort study
1c	All-or-none case series	All-or-none case series		All-or-none case series
2a	Systematic review of cohort studies	Systematic review of either retrospective cohort studies or untreated control groups in RCTs	Systematic review of level <2 diagnostic studies	Systematic review of 2b and better studies
2b	Individual cohort studies	Retrospective cohort study or follow-up of untreated control patients in an RCT	Exploratory cohort study with reference standard	Retrospective cohort study
2c	Outcomes research	Outcomes research		
3a	Systematic review of case-control studies		Systematic review of 3b and better studies	Systematic review of 3b and better studies
3b	Individual case-control study		Nonconsecutive study	Nonconsecutive cohort study
4	Case series	Case series (and poor-quality prognostic cohort studies)	Case-control study	Case series
5	Expert opinion	Expert opinion	Expert opinion	Expert opinion

Source: From Levels of Evidence and Grade Recommendation.[51] Used with permission of the Oxford Centre.

the Canadian Task Force on Periodic Health Examination in that evidence from systematic reviews (discussed in a separate section in this chapter) is given the designation 1a, and evidence from a single RCT is given the designation 1b.

What Is the Quality of Evidence Evaluating Surgical Practice?

There is certainly a perception held by others that surgeons are not adequately assessing surgical procedures. In an editorial in the *Lancet* in 1996, "Surgical Research or Comic Opera: Questions But Few Answers," Richard Horton criticized surgeons for their high reliance on case studies and stated that if surgeons wished to retain their academic reputations, they must find imaginative ways to collaborate with epidemiologists to improve the design of the case series and to plan randomized trials.[52] Furthermore, he quoted a medical statistician, Major Greenwell, who stated, "I should like to shame surgeons out of the comic opera performances which they suppose are statistics of operations."[52] This quotation dated to 1923. In a similar condemnation, Spoddick complained of the "repeated reporting of biased data from uncontrolled or poorly controlled trials, giving an illusion of success due to sheer quantity . . . but that . . . a thousand zeros look impressive on paper, but they still amount to zero."[53]

So, what is the evidence of the evidence? As one would predict, repeated studies have shown that there is a predominance of case studies and a relative paucity of RCTs published. Solomon and I reviewed[15] three surgical journals (*British Journal of Surgery, Surgery,* and *Diseases of the Colon and Rectum*) over two time periods, 1980 and 1990. We found that only 7% of all published clinical articles were RCTs despite the fact that almost half of the articles addressed issues of treatment effectiveness. Furthermore, the proportion did not differ between 1980 and 1990 or among the three journals. Similarly, Barnes noted that only 5% of abstracts accepted at the annual joint meetings of the Society for Vascular Surgery and the International Society for Cardiovascular Surgery dealt with RCTs.[54] Haines reported that only 5% of articles in the *Journal of Neurosurgery* between 1973 and 1977 were controlled clinical trials.[55] In 1996, Horton noted that 7% of articles published in nine surgical journals were reports of RCTs.

What clinical trials are being performed by surgeons? Solomon et al. identified 204 RCTs published in 1990 that were contributed by surgeons, were from a surgical department, or contained at least one surgical arm.[56] Solomon et al. estimated that the search retrieved approximately half of the surgical RCTs published. Of these trials, the majority (75%) compared two medical therapies, whereas trials comparing two surgical therapies comprised only 18%, and trials comparing a medical to a surgical therapy comprised only 5%. Thus, trials comparing antibiotic prophylactic regimens and adjuvant chemotherapy regimens were not uncommon, whereas trials comparing two different operative procedures were infrequent. Furthermore, the published trials tended to be small: almost two-thirds were single-center trials, and in half there was no significant difference detected, probably because the sample size was small and the trial lacked adequate power. Unfortunately, surgeons were the primary author in only a small proportion of studies, even those comparing two surgical procedures and in areas almost exclusively surgical in nature (e.g., trauma). The quality of the trials tended to be poor, especially if they contained one or two surgical arms or were published in surgical journals. Hall and colleagues reviewed the published surgical trials in 10 journals between 1988 and 1994. They also found that the trials tended to be poor quality.[57]

Given the relative paucity of RCTs reported in the literature, our group then wished to determine whether it should be possible to perform RCTs in more instances or whether it is not possible, as has been suggested by some.[58] To address this issue, we identified a sample of 260 questions in the surgical literature relating to the efficacy of general surgical procedures. From this analysis, it was estimated that it should be possible to perform an RCT to answer approximately 40% of questions. In contrast, only 4.6% of the articles reviewed reported results of RCTs, and more than 50% of the articles were case reports or case studies. Although methodological issues unique to surgical trials are commonly cited as the reason for not being able to do an RCT, in fact we felt that methodological issues would preclude doing an RCT only 1% of the time. On the other hand, RCTs would be precluded because of methodological issues. The most common issues to preclude performing an RCT would be strong patient preferences for one or the other treatments or the infrequency of the condition. However, with respect to the former, this was an assessment made by clinicians, and trials (e.g., those comparing mastectomy and lumpectomy and carotid endarterectomy to medical therapy) illustrate that it is possible to do trials even when the alternative treatments differ significantly in magnitude.

While one cannot argue that surgeons do seem to rely on case series rather than RCTs to evaluate new surgical techniques, it is also important to point out that some noteworthy surgical trials that have had a high impact have been performed: mastectomy-versus-lumpectomy trials, carotid endarterectomy and ECIC bypass trials for stroke prevention.[24,25,30] Furthermore, we must not forget the pioneering work of John Goligher, who performed a series of trials assessing the surgical management of peptic ulcer disease long before RCTs were in vogue.[59] On the other hand, while internists may criticize surgeons for not performing more trials, it is also important to realize that perhaps the greatest impetus for medical trials is the requirement by regulating agencies of evidence from clinical trials before release of new medication and therefore the availability of funding from industry to test them.

Assessing the Best Evidence

Practicing evidence-based medicine might be a daunting task for the clinician who has a busy clinical practice, must look after the administrative and financial aspects of his or her practice, and try to keep current with the latest information. It is physically impossible for clinicians to read all published medical journals, even in one's own specialty, much less stay abreast of information that is distributed on the Internet and in non-peer-reviewed sources. Thus, the busy clinician must learn ways to access the best information and be able to appraise it critically to determine its worth and relevance to his or her practice. There may be two scenarios for which clinicians wish to obtain information: for specific patient problems encountered daily and for general maintenance or updating of knowledge. While clinicians will need to have the skills to retrieve information and critically appraise it, there are several information sources that may be of particular help, including systematic reviews and evidence-based practice guidelines.

Systematic Reviews or Meta-analyses

The terms *systematic review* and *meta-analysis* have been used interchangeably. However, systematic reviews or overviews are qualitative reviews, whereas statistical methods are used to combine and summarize the results of several studies in meta-analysis (Table 2.5).[60] In both, there is a specific scientific approach to the identification, critical appraisal, and synthesis of all relevant studies on a specific topic. They differ from the usual clinical review in that there is an explicit, specific question that is addressed. As well, the methodology is explicit, and there is a conscientious effort to retrieve and review all studies on the topic without preconceived prejudice. The value of meta-analysis is that study results are combined, so conclusions can be drawn about therapeutic effectiveness or, if there is not a conclusive answer, to plan new studies.[61] They are especially useful when results from several studies disagree regarding the magnitude or the direction of effect, when individual studies are too small to detect an effect and label it as statistically not significant, or when a large trial is too costly or time consuming to perform. For the clinician, meta-analyses are useful because results of individual trials are combined so the clinician does not have to retrieve, evaluate, and synthesize the results of all studies on the topic. Thus, it may increase the efficiency of the clinician in keeping abreast of recent advances.

Meta-analysis is a relatively new method for synthesizing information from multiple studies. Thus, the methodology is constantly evolving, and like other studies, the quality of individual meta-analysis may be variable. There has been a call for standardization of the methodology used in meta-analysis.[62,63] However, because the rigorousness of the methodology of many published meta-analyses may be variable, the clinician should have some knowledge of meta-analysis methodology and be able to appraise them critically. Published guidelines are available to help (Table 2.6).[64]

There are some basic steps followed in performing a meta-analysis. First, the meta-analysis should address a specific health care question. Second, various strategies should be used to ensure that all relevant studies (RCTs) on the topic are retrieved. These include searching various databases, such as Medline and EMBASE. In addition, proceedings of meetings and reference lists should be checked, and content experts and clinical researchers should be consulted to ensure all published and nonpublished trials are identified. Reliance on Medline searches alone will result in incomplete retrieval of published studies.[58] Third, as in other studies, inclusion criteria regarding which studies will be included should be set a priori. Fourth, data from the individual studies should be extracted by two blinded investigators to ensure that this is

TABLE 2.5. Guidelines for Using a Review.

1. Did the overview address a focused clinical question?
2. Were the criteria used to select articles for inclusion appropriate?
3. Is it unlikely that important, relevant studies were missed?
4. Was the validity of the included studies appraised?
5. Were the assessments of the studies reproducible?
6. Were the results similar from study to study?
7. What are the overall results of the review?
8. How precise were the results?
9. Can the results be applied to my patient care?
10. Were all the clinically important outcomes considered?
11. Are the benefits worth the harms and costs?

Source: Adapted from Oxman et al.[64] Used by permission of the *Journal of the American Medical Association.*

TABLE 2.6. Guidelines for Assessing Practice Guidelines.

1. Were all important options and outcomes clearly specified?
2. Was an explicit and sensible process used to identify, select, and combine evidence?
3. Was an explicit and sensible process used to consider the relative value of different outcomes?
4. Is the guideline likely to account for important recent developments?
5. Has the guideline been subject to peer review and testing?
6. Are practical, clinically important, recommendations made?
7. How strong are the recommendations?
8. What is the impact of uncertainty associated with the evidence and values used in guidelines?
9. Is the primary objective of the guideline consistent with your objective?
10. Are the recommendations applicable to your patients?

Source: Adapted from Hayward et al. for the Evidence Based Medicine Working Group.[77] Used by permission of the *Journal of the American Medical Association.*

done accurately. As well, these investigators should assess the quality of the individual studies. Fifth, the data should be combined using various statistical techniques. Before doing so, statistical tests to determine the "sameness" or "homogeneity" of the individual studies should be performed.

While some have embraced meta-analysis as a systematic approach to synthesizing published information from individual trials, others have cautioned about the results of meta-analysis, and others have been skeptical of the technique completely.[65] LeLorier et al. compared the results of 19 meta-analyses with the results of 12 large trials published subsequently.[66] If the subsequent trials had not been performed, then an ineffective treatment would have been adopted in 32% of cases, and a useful treatment would have been rejected in 33%. Others have pointed out that meta-analyses on the same clinical question have led to different conclusions.[67] Some of these are due to methodological problems. Failure to use broad enough search strategies may result in exclusion of all relevant studies. Most commonly, unpublished studies are excluded, and these are more likely to be negative trials (so-called publication bias).[68] As well, there is evidence that omission of trials not published in English language journals may bias the results.[69] Finally, there is a strong association between statistically positive conclusions of meta-analyses and their quality (i.e., the lower the quality of the studies, the more likely that the meta-analysis reached a positive conclusion).[70]

One of the values of meta-analysis is that the generalizability of the results is increased by combining the results of several trials. However, if there is great variation in studies, including patient inclusion criteria, dosage and mode of administration of medication, and length of follow-up (so-called heterogeneity), then it may be inappropriate to combine results and, if done, doing so may result in invalid results. Other reasons for discrepancies may be the use of different statistical tests and failure to update the meta-analysis. Finally, meta-analysis has generally been restricted to combining the results of RCTs even though there is also a need for combining data from nonrandomized or observational studies.

Dixon and colleagues performed a review of the methodologic quality of published meta-analyses on general surgery topics.[71] Between 1997 and 2002, there were 51 published meta-analyses that pooled the results of primary studies in general surgery on issues of diagnosis, causation, prognosis, or treatment. Of these, 38 were published in general surgery journals. Most studies had major methodological flaws. Those published by individuals without prior meta-analysis publications or by surgeons without the assistance of external collaboration were more likely to be lower quality.

The Cochrane Collaboration is an international organization that prepares, maintains, and disseminates systematic reviews of RCTs of health care interventions.[72] It was named after Archie Cochrane, an eminent statistician in the United Kingdom. The Cochrane Collaboration is a voluntary organization that encourages participation by interested individuals. Cochrane groups are organized by areas of interest (e.g., upper gastrointestinal, inflammatory bowel disease, colorectal cancer, hepatobiliary). In addition to preparing reviews, journals are hand searched, and a database of all published RCTs is maintained. Systematic reviews are constantly updated. The Cochrane Library is available on CD-ROM on a quarterly basis (Cochrane Library, Update Software Inc., 936 La Rueda, Vista, CA 92084 USA). It includes several databases, including the Cochrane Database of Systematic Reviews. This is a valuable source of high-level information for practicing clinicians. Unfortunately, it is of somewhat more limited use to surgeons because of the paucity of published surgical RCTs and meta-analyses.

Practice Guidelines

Practice guidelines have been defined by the Institute of Medicine as "systematically developed statements to assist practitioner and patient decisions about appropriate health care for specific clinical circumstances."[73(p58)] Guidelines are not standards that set rigid rules of care for patients. Rather, guidelines should be flexible so that individual patient characteristics, preferences of surgeons and patients, and local circumstances can be accommodated.[74]

Guideline development has occurred for several reasons.[75] First, as discussed, there is growing evidence of substantial unexplained and inappropriate variation in clinical practice patterns that is probably due in part to physician uncertainty. Second, there is evidence that the traditional methods for delivering continuing medical education are ineffective, and that clinicians have difficulty in assimilating the rapidly evolving scientific evidence. Third, there is concern that, as health care resources become more limited, there will be inadequate funds to deliver high-quality care if current technology and treatments are used inappropriately or ineffectively.

Practice guidelines have been promoted as 1 strategy to assist clinical decision making to increase the effectiveness and decrease unnecessary costs of delivered health care services.[75] Many clinicians are wary of guidelines and believe that they are simply a means to limit resources and inhibit clinical decision making and individual preferences. Guidelines have also been criticized as too idealistic and failing to take into account the realities of day-to-day practice. It is argued that patients differ in their clinical manifestations, associated diseases, and preferences for treatments. Thus, guidelines may be too restrictive or irrelevant. Third, clinicians may be confused because of conflicting guidelines. Finally, guideline development may be inhibited because there is a lack of evidence on which to base guidelines.

Many groups and organizations have begun to develop practice guidelines. Guidelines are developed using different methods.[76] Guidelines can be developed based on informal consensus. The criteria on which decisions are made are often poorly described, and there is no systematic approach to reviewing the evidence. More often, these guidelines are based on the opinion of experts. Readers are unable to judge the validity of the guidelines because, even if a systematic approach was followed, the process is not documented. In many instances, guidelines are self-serving and used to promote a certain specialty or expertise. The National Institutes of Health and others have produced guidelines based on a formal consensus approach. While this approach tends to be more structured than the informal consensus, it suffers from the same potential flaws in that it is less structured and susceptible to the biases of the experts.

Evidence-based guidelines are the most rigorously developed.[49,75,77] There should be a focused clinical question, and a systematic approach to the retrieval, assessment of quality, and synthesis of evidence should be followed. Guideline development should also be a dynamic process with constant updating as more evidence is available. In addition to assessment of the literature, there is usually an interpretation of the evidence by experts, and the evidence may be modulated by current or local circumstances (e.g., cost/availability of technology).

While there has been much attention paid to the preparation of guidelines, there has been much less emphasis on the dissemination of and evaluation of the impact of guidelines. Unfortunately, there is some evidence that evidence-based guidelines may not have as much impact on either changing physician behavior or improving outcome.

Because there are many guidelines available and some with conflicting recommendations, clinicians require some skills to evaluate the guidelines and determine their validity and applicability.[47,77]

Critically Appraising the Literature

Critical appraisal skills must be mastered before evidence-based practice can be implemented successfully.[78] *Critical appraisal skills* are those that enable one to apply certain rules of evidence and laws of logic to clinical, investigative, and published data and information to estimate their validity, reliability, credibility, and utility. Clinicians need critical appraisal skills because of the constant appearance of new knowledge and the short half-life of current knowledge. Thus, clinicians cannot rely on facts learned in medical school. Instead, they must have the necessary skills to assess the validity and relevancy of new knowledge to provide the best care to their patients.

Critical appraisal requires the clinician to have some knowledge of clinical epidemiology, biostatistics, epidemiology, decision analysis, and economics. While this knowledge is helpful, critical appraisal skills improve with practice, and the clinician is encouraged simply to begin using the skills they already have in evaluating the literature and to build on these skills. There are a variety of articles and books written on the topic. The McMaster Evidence Based Medicine Group has published a series of articles in the *Journal of the American Medical Association*.[49,64,77,79–93] Sackett and colleagues consolidated much of this information into a book, *Evidence Based Medicine*.[78] Interested readers are encouraged to seek further information from these and other sources.

To make decisions about a patient, clinicians generally need to know something about the cause of or risk factors for disease, natural history or prognosis of disease, how to quantify aspects of disease (measurement issues), diagnostic tests and the diagnosis of disease, and the effectiveness of treatment. In addition, clinicians now need to have some knowledge of economic analysis, health services research, practice guidelines, systematic reviews, and decision analysis to appreciate the literature fully and make use of all sources of information.

Many clinicians feel that critical appraisal only requires knowledge of statistics. As stated, an array of skills is required. Furthermore, in making decisions about the internal validity of the study (i.e., How good is the study? How confident am I that the results or conclusions are correct?), it is critical that the clinician can assess the study design and how well the study was actually performed. The statistical analysis, while important, is only 1 component of study design.

Generally, clinicians read articles so they can generalize the results of the study and apply them to their own patients. There are two potential sources of error that may lead to incorrect conclusions about the validity of the study results: systematic error (bias) or random error. *Bias* is defined as "any effect at any stage of investigation or inference tending to produce results that depart systematically from the true values."[94] For example, the term *biased sample* is often used to mean that the sample of patients is not typical or representative of patients with that condition.

There are a number of biases that might be present, not just those related to patient selection. It may be difficult to discern whether there is bias and, if there is, the magnitude of it. For instance, suppose two different treatments are compared in two groups of patients from two different hospitals. Although the authors could provide basic demographic information on the patient groups, one could not be certain that there were no differences in the patients, the severity of the disease, ancillary care, and so on at the two different hospitals and that these differences, rather than the treatment, led to an improved outcome.

The risk of an error due to bias decreases as the rigorousness of the trial design increases. Because of the random allocation of patients as well as the other attributes, the RCT is considered the best design for minimizing the risk of bias. In observational studies, including outcomes research (for which patients have not been randomized), various statistical tests (e.g., multivariate analysis) are frequently employed to adjust for differences in prognostic factors between the two groups of patients. However, it is important to realize that it is possible to adjust only for known or measurable factors. In addition to these, there may be other unknown and possibly important prognostic factors that cannot be adjusted. Again, only if patients are randomly allocated can one be certain that the two groups are similar with respect to all known and unknown prognostic variables.

The other type of error is random error. *Random error* occurs due to chance when the result obtained in the sample of patients studied differs from the result that would be

TABLE 2.7. Types of Statistical Tests.

Data type	*Statistical (with no adjustment for prognostic factors)*	*Procedure test (with adjustment for prognostic factors)*
I. Binary (dichotomous)	Fisher exact test or χ^2	Logistic regression Mantel-Haenszel
II. Ordered discrete	Mann-Whitney U	
III. Continuous (normal distribution)	Student *t* test	Analysis of covariance (ANCOVA) (multiple regression)
IV. Time to event (censored data)	Log-rank Wilcoxon	Log-rank (Cox's proportional hazards)

obtained if the entire population were studied.[94] Statistical testing can be performed to determine the likelihood of a random error. The type of statistical test used will vary depending on the type of data. Some of the more common tests are shown in Table 2.7. There are two types of random error, types I and II. The risk of stating that there is a difference between two treatments when really there is not one is known as a type I error. In the theory of testing hypotheses, rejecting a null hypothesis when it is actually true is called a type I error. By convention, if the risk of the result occurring due to chance is less than 5% (a *P* value less than .05), then the difference in the results of treatment is considered statistically significant, and there really is a difference in the effectiveness of the two treatments.

While a result may be statistically significant, the clinician must determine whether it is clinically relevant or important.[78] Typically, treatment effects can be written as absolute or relative risk reductions. The *absolute risk reduction* (ARR) is simply the difference in rates between the control group and the experimental group. whereas the *relative risk reduction* (RRR) is a proportional risk reduction and is calculated by dividing the ARR by the control risk. The advantage of the ARR is that the baseline event rate is considered. For instance, the RRR would be the same in two different studies in which the rates between the control and experimental groups were 50% and 25% and 0.5% and 0.25%, respectively. In other words, while the ARR would be 25% in the first study and 0.25% in the second study, the RRR for both studies would be 50%. Although the RRR is the same in both studies, the treatment benefit in the second scenario may be trivial.

Cook and Sackett coined the term *number needed to treat* (NNT), which may make more intuitive sense to clinicians rather than thinking in terms of ARR and RRR.[95] It is calculated by dividing the ARR into 1. Thus, in the first example, 4 patients would have to be treated to prevent 1 bad outcome (the NNT is 4), whereas 400 would have to be treated to prevent 1 bad outcome (the NNT is 400) in the latter example. Determining whether the treatment benefit is clinically significant requires the judgment of the clinician. The statistician can only determine whether a treatment benefit is statistically significant. Whether the effect is clinically significant will depend on the NNT, the frequency and severity of side effects (sometimes stated as the number needed to harm [NNH]), as well as the cost of treatment and its feasibility and acceptability.

The other random error is the so-called type II error. A type II error occurs when 2 treatments are, in reality, different but one concludes that they are equally effective. In the theory of testing hypotheses, accepting a null hypothesis when it is incorrect is called a type II error. It is not uncommon for clinicians to read about a study in which the results are not statistically significant and to wonder whether the two treatments are equally effective or whether there is a type II error. When investigators plan a trial, they minimize the risk of a type II error by calculating a sample size to ensure that there is adequate power (1- type II error) to show a difference if one really exists. To calculate a sample size, both the type I error and power are specified plus the mean and standard deviation or event rate in the control group and the size of the difference to detect. Not surprisingly, the more variable the subjects, the less frequent the event rate is, or the smaller the difference in the effects of the treatment is, the more subjects that are necessary to be certain a treatment effect has not been missed. Conversely, fewer subjects are necessary if there is less subject variability, the outcome occurs more frequently, or one wishes to detect a large difference in treatment effect.

While a power calculation is performed a priori, a more useful measure for interpreting the study results is the calculation of 95% confidence intervals (CIs).[96] The 95% CI means that there is 95% certainty that the true difference between the two treatments lies within this range of values.[96] Thus, suppose that, in a study comparing stapled to hand-sutured anastomoses, the difference in leak rate was 2% with 95% CIs of 3%. In other words, one can be 95% certain that the true risk of an anastomotic leak is somewhere between 1% lower with a stapled anastomosis and 5% higher. If so, one would be fairly confident that the two different anastomotic techniques are equally effective. On the other hand, if the CIs were 10%, so the true difference in leak rates was somewhere between 8% lower with a stapled anastomosis and 12% higher, one would be less likely to conclude that the two anastomotic techniques were equal. Clinicians can interpret the negative result of a study much better when CIs are calculated than when only a *P* value is given. The wider the CI, the less certain one can be that the two treatments are really similar in effectiveness. Conversely, if the CIs are narrow, then one can be much more certain that the treatments are equally effective.

Conclusion

This chapter is a brief introduction to evidence-based surgery and some of the concepts that it encompasses. Readers are encouraged to learn more about evidence-based surgery by reading some of the sources referenced. While important, the concepts should not be daunting, and practicing evidence-based surgery should lead to improved care for surgical patients as well as more efficient use of health care resources.

References

1. Evidence Based Medicine Working Group. Evidence-based medicine. JAMA 1992;268:2420–2425.
2. Davidoff F, Haynnes B, Sackett D, Smith R. Evidence based medicine. A new journal to help doctors identify the information they need. BMJ 1998;310:1085–1086.
3. Wai E, Wright JG. Evidence-based surgery. 1A. The traditional practice of surgery. Curr Controversies Surg 1999;33:1–15.
4. Ruffin JM, Grizzle JE, Hightower NC, McHardy G, Shull H, Kirsner JB. A co-operative double blind evaluation of gastric "freezing" in the treatment of duodenal ulcer. N Engl J Med 1969;281:16–19.
5. Calandra T, Baumgartner JD, Grau EG, et al. Prognostic values of tumor necrosis factor/cachectin, interleukin-1, interferon-alpha and interferon-gamma in the serum of patients with septic shock. J Infect Dis 1990;161:982–987.
6. Fisher CJ, Dhaniaut JFA, Opal SM, et al. Recombinant human interleukin receptor antagonist in the treatment of patients with sepsis syndrome. JAMA 1994;271:1836–1843.
7. Seward WF. Medical economics. Bull Am Coll Surg 1999;84:12–13.
8. Antman EM, Lau J, Kupelnick B, Mosteller F, Chalmers TC. A comparison of results of meta-analyses of randomized control trials and recommendations of clinical experts. Treatments for myocardial infarction. JAMA 1992;268:240–248.
9. Kreder HJ. Evidence based surgical practice: what is it and do we need it? W J Surg in press.
10. Anderson FA Jr, Wheeler B, Goldberg RJ, Hosmer DW, Forcier A, Patawardhan NA. Physician practices in the prevention of venous thromboembolism. Ann Intern Med 1991;115:591–595.
11. Ellis J, Mulligan I, Rowe J, Sackett D. Inpatient general medicine is evidence based. Lancet 1995;346:407–410.
12. Howes N, Chagla L, Thorpe M, McCulloch P. Surgical practice is evidence based. BJS 1997;84:1220–1223.
13. Rosenberg W, Donald A. Evidence based medicine: an approach to clinical problem-solving. BMJ 1995;310:1126.
14. Canadian Task Force on Periodic Health Examination. The periodic health examination. CMAJ 1979;121:1193–1254.
15. Solomon MJ, McLeod RS. Clinical studies in surgical journals—have we improved? Dis Colon Rectum 1993;36:43–48.
16. Selby JV, Friedman GD, QuesenberryCP, Weiss NS. A case-control study of screening sigmoidoscopy and mortality from colorectal cancer. N Eng J Med 1992;326:653–657.
17. Shapiro S. Evidence of screening for breast cancer from a randomized trial. Cancer 1977;39(suppl):2772.
18. Detsky AS. Are clinical trials a cost effective investment? JAMA 1983;262:1795–1800.
19. McLeod RS, Wright JG, Solomon MJ, Hu X, Walters BC, Lossing A. Randomized controlled trials in surgery; issues and problems. Surgery 1996;119:483–486.
20. Dimond EG, Kittle CF, Crockett JE. Evaluation of internal mamary artery ligation and sham procedure in angina pectoris. Circulation 1958:18:712–713.
21. Chalmers TC. Randomization of the first patient. Med Clin North Am 1975;59:1035–1038.
22. Taylor K, Margolese R, Soskolne CL. Physicians' reasons for not entering eligible patients in a randomized clinical trial of adjuvant surgery for breast cancer. N Engl J Med 1984;310:1363–1367.
23. Kennedy ED, Blair JE, Ready R, et al. Patients' perceptions of their participation in a clinical trial for postoperative Crohn's disease. Can J Gastroenterol 1998;12:287–291.
24. Fisher B, Bauer M, Margolese R, et al. Five year results of a randomized clinical trial comparing total mastectomy and segmental mastectomy with or without radiation in the treatment of breast cancer. N Engl J Med 1985;312:665–673.
25. The EC/IC Bypass Study Group. Failure of extracranial-intracranial arterial bypass to reduce the risk of ischemic stroke. Results of an international randomized trial. N Engl J Med 1985;313:1191–1200.
26. Spechler SJ. Comparison of medical and surgical therapy for complicated gastroesophageal reflux disease in veterans. N Engl J Med 1992;326:786–792.
27. Health Services Research Group. Outcomes and the management of health care. CMAJ 1992;147:1775–1779.
28. Committee to Design a Strategy for Quality Review and Assurance in Medicare, Institute of Medicine. Medicare; a Strategy for Quality Assurance. Washington, DC: National Academy Press; 1990.
29. Greenfield S. The state of outcome research: are we on target? N Engl J Med 1989;320:1142–1143.
30. North American Symptomatic Carotid Endarterectomy Trial collaborators. Beneficial effect of carotid endarterectomy in symptomatic patients with high-grade carotid stenosis. N Engl J Med 1991;325:445–453.
31. Kucey DS, Bowyer B, Iron K, Austin P, Anderson G, Tu JV. Determinants of outcome after carotid endarterectomy. J Vasc Surg 1998;28:1051–1058.
32. Health Services Group. Small-area variations: what are they and what do they mean? CMAJ 1992;146:467–470.
33. Iscoe NA, Goel V, Wu K, Fehringer G, Holowaty EJ, Naylor CD. Variation in breast cancer surgery in Ontario. CMAJ 1994;150:245–352.
34. Eddy DM. Variations in physician practice: the role of uncertainty. Health Aff (Millwood) 1984;3:74–89.
35. Wennberg JE. Dealing with medical practice variations: a proposal for action. Health Aff (Millwood) 1984;3:6–32.
36. Wright JG, Hawker GA, Bombardier C, et al. Physician enthusiasm as an explanation for area variation in the utilization of knee-replacement surgery. Med Care 1999;37:946–956.
37. Brook RH, Kosecoff JB, Park RE, Chassin MR, Winslow CM, Hampton JR. Diagnosis and treatment of coronary disease: comparisons of doctors' attitudes in the USA and UK. Lancet 1988;1:750–753.
38. Blais R. Variations in the use of health care services: why are more studies needed? CMAJ 1994;151:1701–1719.
39. Wennberg JE. Which rate is right? [editorial]. N Engl J Med 1986;314:310–311.
40. Wright JG, Coyte P, Hawker G, et al. Variation in orthopedic surgeon's perceptions of the indications for and outcomes of knee replacement. CMAJ 1995;152:687–697.
41. Porter GA, Soskolne CL, Yakimets WW, Newman SC. Surgeon-related factors and outcome in rectal cancer. Ann Surg 1998;227:157–167.
42. Lieberman MD, Kilburn H, Lindsey M, Brennen MF. Relation of perioperative deaths to hospital volume among patients undergoing pancreatic resection for malignancy. Ann Surg 1995;222:638–645.
43. Simunovic M, To T, Theriault M, Langer B. Relation between hospital surgical volume and outcome for pancreatic resection for neoplasm in a publicly funded health care system. CMAJ 1999;160:643–648.
44. Gordon TA, Burleyson GP, Tielsch JM, Cameron JL. The effects of regionalization on cost and outcome for 1 general high-risk surgical procedure. Ann Surg 1995;221:43–49.
45. Birkmeyer JD, Finlayson SR, Tosteson AN, Sharp SM, Warshaw AL, Fisher ES. Effect of hospital volume on in-hospital mortality with pancreaticoduodenectomy. Surgery 1999;125:250–256.
46. Khuri SF, Henderson WG, Hur K, Hossein M, Daley J. The relationship of surgical volume to outcome in 8 common operations. Paper presented at: the meeting of the American Surgical Association; April 1999; San Diego, CA.
47. Halm EA, Lee C, Chassin MR. Is volume outcome related to outcome in health care? A systematic review and methodo-

logic critique of the literature. Ann Intern Med 2002;137: 511–520.
48. US Preventive Services Task Force. Guide to Clinical Preventive Services. An Assessment of 169 Interventions. Baltimore: Williams & Wilkins; 1989.
49. Guyatt GH, Sackett DL, Sinclair JC, Hayward R, Cook DJ, Cook RJ, for the Evidence Based Medicine Working Group. Users' guides to the medical literature. IX. A method for grading health care recommendations. JAMA 1995;274:1800–1804.
50. Liberati A. Problems in defining hierarchies (levels) of evidence for studies to be included in systematic reviews of effectiveness of interventions. Paper presented at: the Second Symposium on Systematic Reviews: Beyond the Basics; January 1999; Oxford.
51. Levels of evidence and grade recommendation. Available at: http:www.cebm.net/levels_of_evidence.asp.
52. Horton R. Surgical research or comic opera: questions, but few answers. Lancet 1996;347:984–985.
53. Spodick DH. Randomized controlled clinical trials. The behavioral case. JAMA 1982;247:2258–2260.
54. Barnes RW. Understanding investigative clinical trials. J Vasc Surg 1989;9:609–618.
55. Haines SJ. Randomized clinical trials in the evaluation of surgical innovation. Neurosurgery 1979;51:5–11.
56. Solomon MJ, Laxamana A, Devore L, McLeod RS. Randomized controlled trials in surgery. Surgery 1994;115:707–712.
57. Hall JC, Mills B, Nguyen H, Hall JL. Methodological standards in clinical trials. Surgery 1996;119:466–472.
58. Solomon JS, McLeod RS. Should we be performing more randomized controlled trials evaluating surgical operations? Surgery 1995;118:459–467.
59. Goligher JC, Pulvertaft CN, Watkinson G. Controlled trial of vagotomy and gastroenterology, vagotomy and gastroenterostomy, vagotomy and antrectomy and subtotal gastrectomy in elective treatment of duodenal ulcer. BMJ 1964;1455–1460.
60. Cook DJ, Sackett DL, Spitzer WO. Methodologic guidelines for systematic reviews of randomized control trials in health care from the Potsdam consultation on meta-analysis. J Clin Epidemiol 1995;48:167–171.
61. L'Abbee KA, Detsky AS, O'Rourke K. Meta-analysis in clinical research. Ann Intern Med 1987;107:224–233.
62. Spitzer WO, ed. The Potsdam International Consultation on Meta-analysis. J Clin Epidemiol 1995;48:1–171.
63. Chalmers TC, Altman DG, eds. Systematic Reviews. London: British Medical Journal Publishing Group; 1995.
64. Oxman AD, Cook DJ, Guyatt GH. Users' guides to the medical literature. VI. How to use an overview. Evidence-Based Medicine Working Group. JAMA 1994;272:1367–1371.
65. Moher D, Olkin I. Meta-analysis of randomized controlled trials: a concern for standards. JAMA 1995;274:1962–1964.
66. LeLorier J, Gregoire G, Benhaddad A, Lapierre J, Dederian F. Discrepancies between meta-analysis and subsequent large randomized, controlled trials. N Engl J Med 1997;337:536–542.
67. Moher D, Olkin I. Meta-analysis of randomized controlled trials: a concern for standards. JAMA 1995;274:1962–1964.
68. Dickerson K, Scherer R, Lefebvre C. Identifying relevant studies for systematic reviews. BMJ 1994;309:1286–1291.
69. Moher D, Fortin P, Jadad AR, et al. Completeness of reporting of trials published in languages other than English: implications for conduct and reporting of systematic reviews. Lancet 1996;347:363–366.
70. Jadad AR, McQuay HJ. Meta-analyses to evaluate analgesic interventions: a systematic qualitative review of their methodology. J Clin Epidemiol 1996;49:235–243.
71. Dixon E, Hameed M, Sutherland F, Cook DJ, Doig C. Evaluating meta-analyses in the general surgical literature. A critical appraisal. Ann Surg 2005;241:450–459.
72. Cochrane Collaboration. Cochrane Library. Vista, CA: Cochrane Collaboration. (The Cochrane Library is available on CD-ROM on a quarterly basis. The Cochrane Library, Update Software Inc., 936 La Rueda, Vista, CA 92084, USA.)
73. Committee to Advise Public Health Service on Clinical Practice Guidelines (Institute of Medicine) Clinical Practice Guidelines. Directions for a New Program. Washington, DC: National Academy Press; 1990:58.
74. Wright JG, McLeod RS, Mahoney J, Lossing A, Hu X from the Surgical Clinical Epidemiology Group. Surgery 1996;119:706–709.
75. Browman GP, Levine MN, Mohide A, et al. The practice guidelines development cycle: a conceptual tool for practice guidelines development and implementation. J Clin Oncol 1995;13:502–512.
76. Wolff SH. Practice guidelines, a new reality in medicine. II. Methods of developing guidelines. Arch Intern Med 1992;152:946–952.
77. Hayward RSA, Wilson MC, Tunis SR, Bass EB, Guyatt GH, for the Evidence Based Medicine Working Group. Users' guides to the medical literature. VIII. How to use clinical practice guidelines. Are recommendations valid? JAMA 1995;274:570–574.
78. Sackett DL, Richardson WS, Rosenberg W, Haynes RB. Evidence Based Medicine. How to Practice and Teach EBM. Pearson Professional Ltd; 1997.
79. Oxman AD, Sackett DL, Guyatt GH, for the Evidence Based Medicine Working Group. Users' guides to the medical literature. I. How to get started. JAMA 1993;270:2093–2095.
80. Guyatt GH, Sackett DL, Cook DJ. Users' guides to the medical literature. II. How to use an article about therapy or prevention. A. Are the results of the study valid? Evidence-Based Medicine Working Group. JAMA 1993;270:2598–2601.
81. Guyatt GH, Sackett DL, Cook DJ. Users' guides to the medical literature. II. How to use an article about therapy or prevention. B. What were the results and will they help me in caring for my patients? Evidence-Based Medicine Working Group. JAMA 1994;271:59–63.
82. Jaeschke R, Guyatt GH, Sackett DL, for the Evidence Based Medicine Working Group. Users' guides to the medical literature. III. How to use an article about a diagnostic test. A. Are the results of the study valid? JAMA 1994;271:389–391.
83. Jaeschke R, Guyatt GH, Sackett DL, for the Evidence Based Medicine Working Group. Users' guides to the medical literature. III. How to use an article about a diagnostic test. B. What are the results and will they help me in caring for my patients? JAMA 1994;271:703–707.
84. Levine M, Walter S, Lee H, Haines T, Holbrook A, Moyer V, for the Evidence Based Medicine Working Group. Users' guides to the medical literature. IV. How to use an article about harm. JAMA 1994;271:1615–1619.
85. Laupacis A, Wells G, Richardson WS, Tugwell P, for the Evidence Based Medicine Working Group. Users' guides to the medical literature. V. How to use an article about prognosis. JAMA 1994;272:234–237.
86. Richardson WS, Detsky AS, for the Evidence Based Medicine Working Group. Users' guides to the medical literature. VII. How to use a clinical decision analysis. A. Are the results of the study valid? JAMA 1995;273:1292–1295.
87. Richardson WS, Detsky AS, for the Evidence Based Medicine Working Group. Users' guides to the medical literature. VII. How to use a clinical decision analysis. B. What are the results and will they help me in caring for my patients? JAMA 1995;273:1610–1613.
88. Naylor DC, Guyatt GH, for the evidence Based Medicine Working Group. Users' guides to the medical literature. X. How to use an article reporting variations in the outcomes of health services. JAMA 1996;275:554–558.

89. Naylor CD, Guyatt GH, for the Evidence Based Medicine Working Group. Users' guides to the medical literature. XI. How to use an article about a clinical utilization review. JAMA 1996;275:1435–1439.
90. Guyatt GH, Naylor CD, Juniper E, Heyland DK, Jaeschke R, Cook DJ, for the Evidence Based Medicine Working Group. Users' guides to the medical literature. XII. How to use an article about health-related quality of life. JAMA 1997;277:1232–1237.
91. Drummond MF, Richardson WS, O'Brien BJ, Levine M, Heyland D, for the Evidence Based Medicine Working Group. Users' guides to the medical literature. XIII. How to use an article on economic analysis of clinical practice. A. Are the results of the study valid? JAMA 1997;277:1552–1557.
92. O'Brien BJ, Heyland D, Richardson WS, Levine M, Drummond MF, for the Evidence Based Medicine Working Group. Users' guides to the medical literature. XIII. How to use an article on economic analysis of clinical practice. B. What are the results and will they help me in caring for my patients? JAMA 1997;277:1802–1806.
93. Dans AL, Dans LF, Guyatt GH, Richardson S, for the Evidence Based Medicine Working Group. Users' guides to the medical literature. XIV. How to decide on the applicability of clinical trial results to your patient. JAMA 1998;279:545–549.
94. Last JM. A Dictionary of Epidemiology. Oxford Medical Publications; 1983.
95. Cook RJ, Sackett DL. The number needed to treat: a clinically useful measure of treatment effect. BMJ 1995;310:452–454.
96. Guyatt GH, Jaeschke R, Heddle N, Cook D, Shannon H, Walter S. Basic statistics for clinicians: 2. Interpreting study results: confidence intervals. CMAJ 1995;152:169–173.

3 Cell Structure, Function, and Genetics

Siobhan A. Corbett and Ramsey A. Foty

Life arose on Earth about 3.5 billion years ago from the spontaneous assembly of small organic molecules. Over millions of years, these simple molecules acquired the ability to interact and ultimately developed mechanisms of self-replication. These mechanisms became more elaborate as evolutionary forces brought their influence to bear. The first true "cells" arose when DNA, RNA, and proteins became contained within a boundary, the plasma membrane. These first unicellular organisms acquired the ability to interact. Multicellularity endowed these early organisms with the ability to organize into ever more complicated structures, ultimately giving rise to the explosion in biodiversity we see today. Cells, proteins, and genes are so interconnected that it would be impossible to consider only one level of organization. Thus, we begin our chapter with a discussion of the evolution of cell structure. We then consider the structure–function relationships between nucleic acids and proteins. We next describe cellular processes fundamental to cell survival, including gene regulation and cell proliferation. We also explore the process of cell death. We end our chapter by discussing multicellularity and cell communication. This chapter is not intended to be an exhaustive description of cell biology. Rather, it reflects the aim to provide the reader with a solid grasp of basic cell structure and its influence on cell function.

Evolution of Cell Structure

Current thought is that living cells arose on Earth 3.5 billion years ago. Atmospheric conditions on Earth during this time were likely conducive to the spontaneous production and aggregation of simple molecules. Volcanic eruptions, lightning, torrential rains, no free oxygen, and the lack of an ozone layer to absorb ultraviolet radiation led to the spontaneous formation of simple, carbon-based organic molecules. Indeed, laboratory experiments in which mixtures of gases such as CO_2, CH_4, NH_3, and H_2 were heated with water and energized by electrical discharge or ultraviolet radiation generated small organic molecules, such as hydrogen cyanide and formaldehyde. Notably, amino acids, sugars, fatty acids, and nucleotides were also generated, these representing the four major classes of molecules found in cells. Simple organic molecules, such as amino acids and nucleotides, self-assembled to form large polymers. Nucleotides, for example, assembled into long, linear polymers termed *polynucleotides* in the form of RNA and DNA. Similarly, polymers of amino acids formed polypeptides. Polypeptides are the building blocks for the thousands of different kinds of cellular proteins. Polynucleotides and polypeptides are the most important constituents of a cell.[1]

Polymer formation likely occurred in the presence of condensing agents, compounds with free energy that can be used to facilitate macromolecular formation. Polyphosphates were the likely source of free energy during primitive times. The energy released during their breakdown could well have been used to polymerize amino acids and nucleotides. It is interesting to note that present-day cells utilize nucleoside triphosphates, such as adenosine triphosphate (ATP), for this purpose.[2]

Two functions are particularly important to living cells. One is the ability to enhance the rates of chemical reactions, a property referred to as *catalysis*; the other is the ability to store, reproduce, and transmit information. Polypeptides likely served as primitive catalysts. In the same way that organic acids and bases catalyze reactions involving the uptake of protons, simple amino acid polymers containing acidic or basic side chains could readily have served as simple proton catalysts. Indeed, studies have shown that protein polymers spontaneously synthesized in the laboratory have the capacity to catalyze reactions involving hydrolysis, decarboxylation, oxidation–reduction, and amination, all properties typical of present-day enzymatic catalysis. Enzymes likely developed as a result of natural selection, with selection for amino acid polymers with enhanced catalytic activity gradually giving rise to families of enzymes as they exist today.[1]

The instructions for guiding most cellular activities are stored in the base sequence of DNA molecules. This information is reproduced every time a cell divides. Modern cells require a number of highly specific enzyme catalysts to drive this reaction. Primitive cells, not having access to such enzymes, nevertheless developed strategies to accomplish the same reaction. One strategy could have been complementary base pairing. For example, a polyA sequence existing in a soup of free nucleotides could have given rise to a polyU sequence. This in turn would have acted as a template to generate another polyA sequence, in effect duplicating the original template. Moreover, errors in complementary base-pair matching could, in principle, have given rise to stably inherited changes in nucleotide sequences. If these sequence changes in some way imparted a selective advantage to the molecule, through increased function, stability, or the ability to replicate, the altered sequence would have become conserved and replicated. In this way, information transfer could have been accomplished without the need of specific catalysts.[1]

Separately, polynucleotides and polypeptides could not accomplish all the tasks required of a living cell. Polynucleotides are sufficient to store, replicate, and transmit information, but they cannot produce the structural and functional building blocks of the cell. Polypeptides are ideally suited to a large range of structural and chemical tasks but are not self-replicating. Primitive cells must have developed mechanisms that ultimately gave polynucleotides, such as RNA, the ability to direct the synthesis of proteins. This development would have provided RNA with an enormous pool of potential chemical tools, some of them enzymes, that could potentially catalyze the synthesis of more proteins and RNA molecules. Once the evolution of nucleic acids had advanced to the point of specifying enzymes involved in their own synthesis, the proliferation of self-replication would have been substantially accelerated.[1]

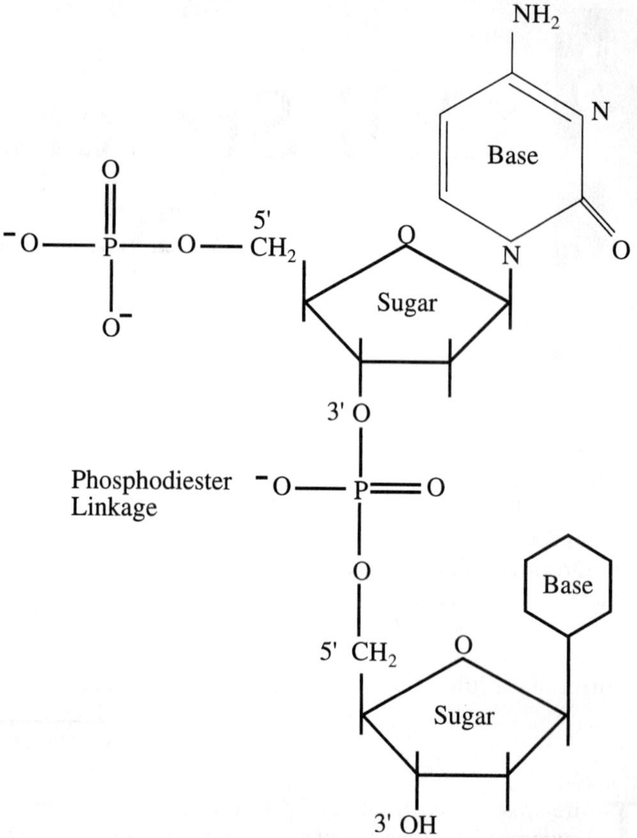

FIGURE 3.1. Nucleic acid structure. Nucleic acids are long polymers of nucleotides. A nucleotide consists of a nitrogen-containing base, a five-carbon pentose sugar, and one or more phosphate groups. Nucleotides are held together by phosphodiester bonds. These covalent bonds between sugars and phosphates form the repeating sugar–phosphate array of the backbone of both DNA and RNA. Phosphodiester bonds link deoxyribose sugars between the 3′ carbon of one sugar and the 5′ carbon of the next sugar.

Nucleic Acid Structure and Function

The Structure of DNA

The primary structure of deoxyribonucleic acid, or DNA, is a linear polymer of four different nucleotides. These nucleotides are composed of a sugar moiety (the pentose deoxyribose), a phosphate group, and a nitrogen-containing base (Fig. 3.1). The phosphate group is a strong acid with a pK_a of about 1; this is why DNA and RNA are called nucleic acids. The nitrogenous bases can either be purines (adenine [A] or guanine [G],) or pyrimidines (cytosine [C] or thymine [T]). Purines are paired fused rings, whereas pyrimidines have only one ring. Both purines and pyrimidines are heterocyclic; the rings are built of more than one kind of atom, in this case nitrogen in addition to carbon (Fig. 3.2). The bases are attached to the 1′ carbon of the deoxyribose sugar, which in turn is attached to the phosphate group through its 3′ and 5′ carbons. The nucleotides are thus linked together to form long polynucleotide chains. Each nucleic acid strand has an orientation: 5′ to 3′ (the 5′ end has a free hydroxyl or phosphate at the 5′ carbon of a sugar) or 3′ to 5′ (the 3′ end has a free hydroxyl group at the 3′ carbon of a sugar).

A DNA molecule is composed of a double helix of two antiparallel chains with complementary nucleotide sequences (Fig. 3.3). The two sugar–phosphate backbones are on the outside of the double helix, and the bases project into the interior. The nitrogenous bases noncovalently connect the two complementary strands of DNA, which are held together principally by hydrogen bonds. Between the two DNA strands, A always pairs with T, and C always pairs with G. This base-pair complementarity is a consequence of the size, shape, and chemical composition of the bases. The adjoining bases in each strand stack on top of one other in parallel planes. Hydrophobic and van der Waals interactions between the stacked adjacent base pairs also contribute significantly to the overall stability of the double helix giving it flexibility along its long axis. This property allows DNA to bend favoring the binding of specific protein molecules functional in

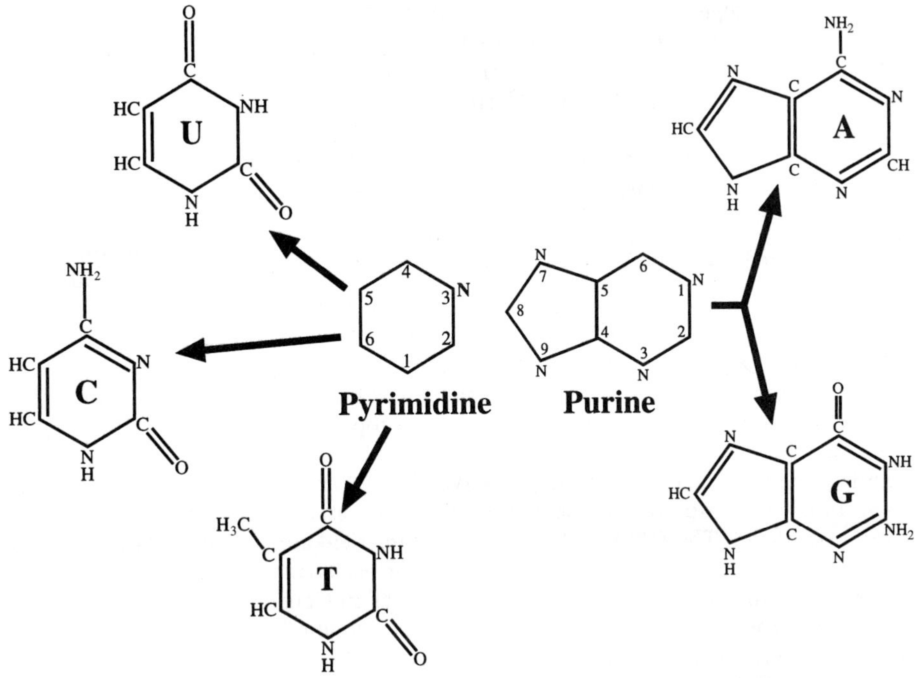

FIGURE 3.2. Nucleotide bases. The bases are N-containing ring compounds known as purines or pyrimidines. Purines are paired, fused rings, whereas pyrimidines have only one ring. In DNA and RNA, the purines are adenine and guanine, abbreviated A and G, respectively. Cytosine (C) is the pyrimidine in DNA and RNA; thymine (T) is the pyrimidine in DNA, and uracyl (U) is the pyrimidine in RNA.

the gene regulation process. Two polynucleotide strands can, in principle, form either a right-handed or a left-handed helix, but natural DNA is right handed. A polynucleotide chain has individuality, which is determined by its nucleotide sequence. This sequence is called the *primary structure*, and it is in this primary structure of DNA that genetic information is stored. Base-pair complementarity is the central principle on which DNA replication, RNA transcription, and protein synthesis are based.[1–4]

The entire cellular DNA consists of approximately 3 billion base pairs. Approximately 1% of the human genome is thought to encode a functional protein or polypeptide (*exons*). These are generally single-copy DNA sequences that appear only once or a few times across the genome. A similar percentage (1%) of the noncoding portion of the genome is under active selection, suggesting that it also has functional significance. These regions may contain the regulatory information that controls the expression of the approximately 25,000 protein-coding genes, in addition to other sequence elements that regulate chromosomal dynamics. About 24% of the human DNA sequence is composed of *introns* (DNA regions interspersed between exons), and the remaining 75% of the genome consists of *intergenic DNA* (DNA regions that flank genes), composed largely of repetitive sequences. These repetitive sequences appear many times in the genome and are found either tightly associated (*tandem repeats*) or scattered about (*interspersed repeats*).[1]

Tandemly repetitive sequences are commonly known as *satellite DNA*, *satellite* referring to any DNA with density in cesium chloride gradient that differs from the bulk of the DNA. Satellite DNAs are classified into three major groups. *Satellites* are highly repetitive long DNA sequences organized into large clusters in the heterochromatin regions of the chromosomes, usually near the centromere. *Minisatellites* are

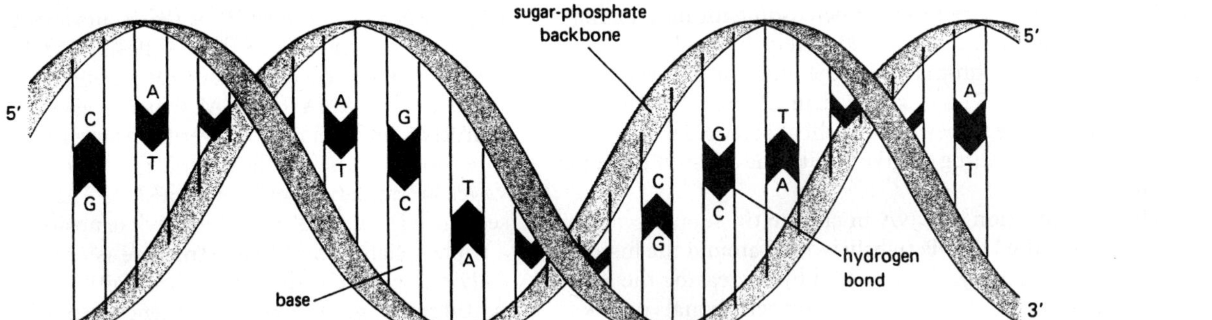

FIGURE 3.3. The DNA double helix. In a DNA molecule, two antiparallel strands that are complementary in their nucleotide sequence are paired in a right-handed double helix with about 10 nucleotide pairs per helical turn. The strands are held together by hydrogen bonds. A schematic representation is illustrated. (From Alberts et al.,[1] with permission of Garland Publishing.)

moderate size, repetitive tandem repeats that are usually organized into smaller clusters located in euchromatin regions. Finally, *microsatellites* are moderately repetitive arrays of short repeats that are also located in euchromatin regions. Due to their high interindividual variability, the polymorphic repeats of monosatellites form the basis for most DNA typing used in forensic medicine.[5]

Packaging of DNA into the Nucleus

The total length of DNA in the nucleus of a human cell is about 10^5 times the diameter of a typical cell. How then is it possible to package such a considerable amount of DNA into such a limited space? Developing mechanisms of coiling DNA into highly compact structures solved this topological problem. Eukaryotic DNA is complexed with a number of specific proteins called *histones*, which serve to compact the DNA into the chromosome structures characteristic of eukaryotic nuclei. The DNA folding is important in eukaryotic cells for two reasons. First, it is essential for packaging the long DNA molecules in an orderly way in the cell nucleus. Second, the exact manner in which a region of the genome is folded in a particular cell can determine the activity of the genes in that region. When eukaryotic chromosomes are isolated and analyzed, there is about twice as much protein as DNA. This mixture of DNA and protein is termed *chromatin*. There are two types of chromatin: euchromatin and heterochromatin. *Heterochromatin* is highly compacted, remains condensed throughout the cell cycle, and is genetically inactive. *Euchromatin* is also compacted during division but decondenses during interphase and is genetically active.

The protein component of chromatin is called *histones*. Histones are relatively small, basic proteins having net positive charge. Histones bind to DNA largely through ionic bonds between the negatively charged phosphate groups of DNA and the positively charged side groups found in the histones. There are five major types of histone proteins: H1, H2A, H2B, H3, and H4. The association of histones with DNA leads to the formation of *nucleosomes*, the unit particles of chromatin. Nucleosomes contain a central core of eight histone proteins, composed of two molecules each of histones H2A, H2B, H3, and H4, around which some 150 base pairs of DNA are bound. Connecting the nucleosome units are short stretches of linker DNA where H1 histone is found. Nucleosomes are arranged as "beads on a string," in which the beads are the nucleosomes and the string connecting the beads is naked DNA. Although nucleosome formation shortens the chromatin strand approximately fivefold, it is clear that much of the chromatin in the nucleus is even more tightly compacted. The next stage in compaction involves wrapping the beaded fiber into a helical solenoidal structure, followed by supercoiling to give rise to the 200-nm diameter chromatin fibers.

The condensation of DNA in chromatin suppresses gene activity. When the DNA is tightly wound around the histone, transcriptional activity is suppressed by decreasing the availability of transcription factors to the transcriptional complex.[6] Histone modifications, including N-terminal phosphorylation, acetylation, methylation, and possibly ubiquitination, can modulate histone interaction with DNA. For example, acetylation of lysine residues on the N-terminal tails of core histone proteins removes the effective positive charge of the residues, resulting in uncoiling of the DNA and increased transcription of a variety of genes.[7] Deacetylation restores the positive charge and condenses the nucleosome structure. Histone acetylation is reversible and is regulated by a group of histone acetyltransferases (HATs), which promote acetylation, and histone deacetylases (HDACs), which promote deacetylation. Histone methylation has been shown to have a similar impact on gene transcriptional events.[6] The availability of pharmacologic agents that modulate histone activity has potential clinical implications. Use of valproic acid (VPA), an agent that can act as an HDAC inhibitor, demonstrated that VPA reduced brain damage and improved functional outcome in a transient focal cerebral ischemia model of rats.[8]

Chromatin fibers become further organized into large units hundreds to thousands of kilobases in length called *chromosomes* (Fig. 3.4). A chromosome is defined as a single, genetically specific DNA molecule to which are attached large numbers of proteins involved in maintaining chromosome structure and regulating gene expression. Each chromosome consists of two sister *chromatids*, which are attached at the centromere. The numbers, sizes, and shapes of chromosomes constitute the *karyotype*, which is distinctive for each species.[1,2,4] Most human DNA is organized into 46 chromosomes. In women, the 46 chromosomes are organized into 23 homologous pairs, one set inherited from the mother and one from the father. Men have 22 pairs of homologous chromosomes. The 23rd pair is partially homologous at the point where it pairs an X chromosome with a Y.

The Structure of RNA

Like DNA, RNA is also a linear polymer of nucleotides. However, the pentose sugar component of RNA is ribose. One other major difference between DNA and RNA is that the pyrimidine thymine in DNA is replaced by uracil in RNA. The RNA also has an additional hydroxyl group at the 2′ position. Consequently, RNA is more chemically labile than DNA. For example, RNA is cleaved into mononucleotides by alkaline solution, whereas DNA is not. Because RNA is also a long phosphodiester chain, it can be double stranded, single stranded, linear, or circular. It can also form DNA–RNA hybrids. RNA binds to specific proteins to form ribonucleoprotein particles.

Three major classes of RNA are found in eukaryotic cells: messenger RNA (mRNA), ribosomal RNA (rRNA), and transfer RNA (tRNA). Messenger RNA represents about 4% of the total cellular RNA and directs the synthesis of proteins in the cytoplasm. It is preceded by a nuclear precursor termed heterogeneous nuclear RNA (hnRNA), which is about 10 times the size of mRNA and has a short lifetime. The mRNA molecule has three main parts. At the 5′ end is a leader sequence, which varies in length from mRNA to mRNA. The 5′ end of this leader sequence is "capped" by a 7-methylguanosine residue linked to a triphosphate. This 5′ cap structure is crucial as it is specifically recognized by ribosomes as an initiation signal for protein synthesis. None of the leader sequence is translated into protein. Following the 5′ leader sequence is the actual coding sequence of the mRNA; this sequence determines the amino acid sequence of a protein during translation. The coding sequence varies in length depending on the length of the protein for

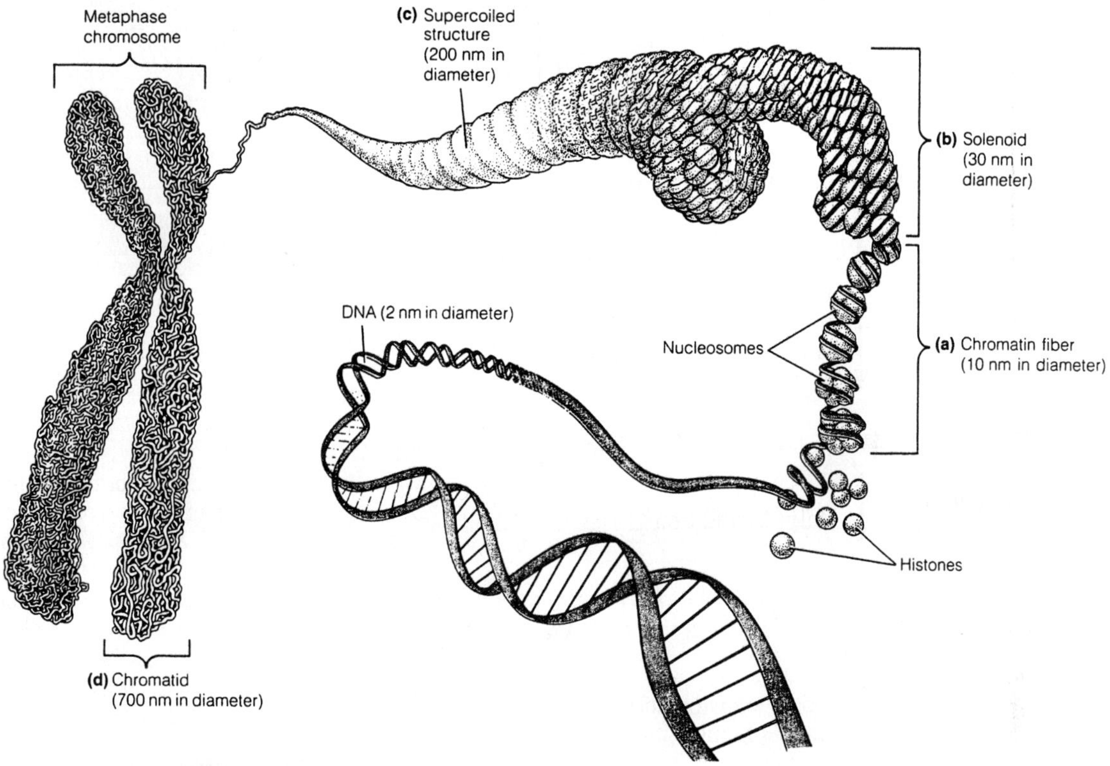

FIGURE 3.4. Levels of chromatin structure. The beaded-string structure is a 10-nm fiber that folds into a solenoidal 30-nm fiber with about six nucleosomes per turn. This fiber can further fold to form fibers 200 nm thick. The chromatin is then further organized into chromosomes. (From Mathews and Van Holde,[74] with permission from Benjamin Cummings.)

which it codes. The mRNA is further modified by the addition of a sequence of 50 to 250 adenine nucleotides on the 3′ end of the mRNA molecule. This sequence is called a *polyA tail* and is found on most of the RNAs of all eukaryotic species. A number of studies have shown that polyA tails help to stabilize the mRNA.[1,2,4]

The primary transcripts of eukaryotic protein-coding genes often contain long insertions of sequences that do not code amino acids. These noncoding sequences, called *introns*, must be excised from each primary transcript (pre-mRNA) to convert the transcript into a mature, functional mRNA molecule. Those parts of the gene that correspond to the mature mRNA molecule are called *exons* (Fig. 3.5).

About 85% of cellular RNA is found in ribosomes. *Ribosomes* are complex cellular particles composed of ribosomal proteins and rRNA molecules. Ribosomes are composed of two subunits of unequal size. Mammalian ribosomes have a sedimentation coefficient (S) of 80S. The sedimentation coefficient is simply the rate at which a molecule sediments as it is spun through a sucrose gradient in an ultracentrifuge. The smaller (40S) subunit contains an 18S RNA molecule and about 30 proteins. The larger (60S) subunit contains three RNA molecules with sedimentation coefficients of 28S, 5S, and 5.8S and about 50 proteins. During the translation of an RNA message into a protein, ribosomes move along the mRNA, successively accepting aminoacyl-tRNAs (aa-TRNAs), selecting them by matching the anticodons to the codon on the mRNA strand. The amino acids are thus transferred to the growing polypeptide chain, and the ribosome moves along to the next codon to repeat the process. This continues until a *stop codon* is read; then, a protein release factor causes both polypeptide and mRNA to be released.[1,2,4]

The tRNA brings amino acids to the ribosome–mRNA complex, where they are polymerized into protein chains in the translation process. The tRNA constitutes between 10% and 15% of total cellular RNA. Each tRNA molecule contains between 73 and 93 nucleotides linked together in a single, covalently bonded chain. The 3′ end always terminates in a CCA sequence, and the 5′ end always contains a 5′-terminal monophosphate group (often guanylic acid). At least one tRNA molecule exists for each amino acid, and for many amino acids more than one occurs. Many tRNAs have been sequenced from a number of organisms, and all the sequences can be arranged into what is called the *cloverleaf model* of tRNA. The cloverleaf itself results from complementary base pairing between different sections of the molecule. Four base-paired stems appear in the molecule, with the number of base pairs in each stem varying from tRNA to tRNA. All tRNAs have three unpaired loops. Loop II contains within it the three-nucleotide sequence called the *anticodon*, which pairs with another three-nucleotide sequence on mRNA called the *codon*. This codon–anticodon pairing is crucial for adding the correct amino acid (as specified by the mRNA) to the growing polypeptide chain. For the 20 different amino acids, a special set of enzymes, called aa-tRNA synthetases, specifically catalyze the linkage of each amino acid to its appropriate tRNA molecule[1,2,4] (Fig. 3.6).

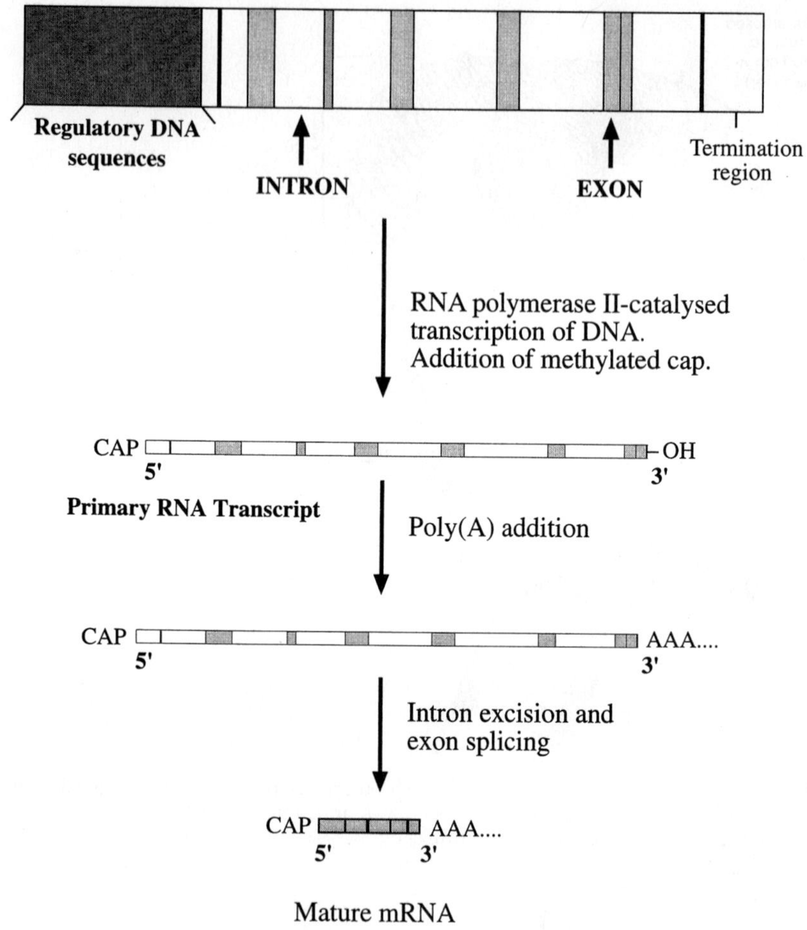

FIGURE 3.5. Processing of mRNA in eukaryotic cells. The primary RNA transcript is transcribed from DNA by RNA polymerase II. This transcript is methylated at the 5′ cap and is polyadenylated at the 3′ tail. Further processing includes excision of introns and the splicing together of exons to produce a mature mRNA molecule.

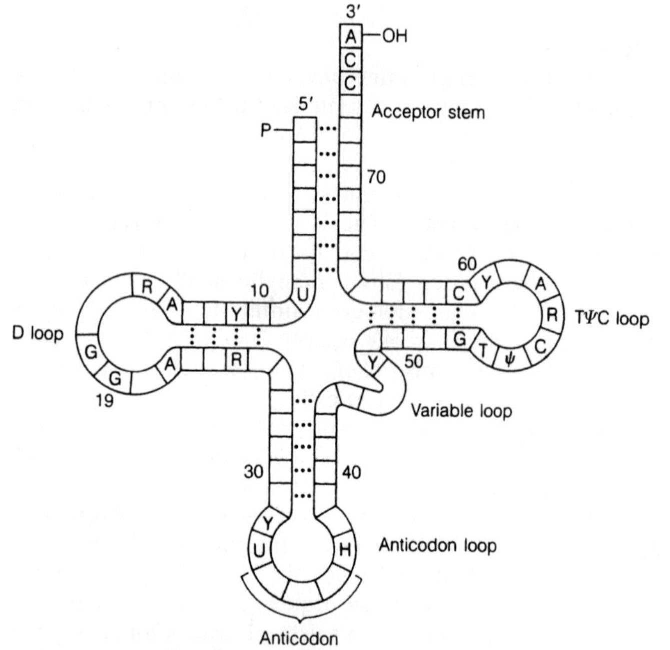

FIGURE 3.6. A schematic representation of the general structure of tRNA. All tRNAs are organized according to the same cloverleaf pattern. Each contains an amino acid attachment site, a dihydrouridine loop, an anticodon region, a variable loop, and a (TCC) loop. Code for bases: *Y*, pyrimidine; *R*, purine; *H*, hypermodified purine; *C*, pseudouridine; *T*, ribothymidine. (From Kleinsmith and Kish,[2] with permission of Pearson Education.)

Protein Structure

Although polynucleotides direct the reproduction and transmission of information in living cells, polypeptides represent the actual building blocks of cells. Proteins have incredibly versatile functions. For example, although most proteins are enzymes that catalyze chemical reactions, they are also essential membrane components that regulate intracellular ion concentration. Further, proteins provide structural support to the cell and, when secreted, form the extracellular matrix (ECM) required for cell attachment. They are also required for cell motility and, perhaps most important, regulate gene function.[1,9,10]

Proteins are polymers composed primarily of amino acids. *Amino acids* are small molecules composed of a central or α-carbon that is linked to four different side groups: an amino group ($-NH_2$), a carboxyl group ($-COOH$), a hydrogen ($-H$), and a variable group ($-R$) (Fig. 3.7A). Although the potential exists for many different side chains, and thus different amino acids, most proteins are made up of the same 20 amino acids that occur over and over again. The specialized properties of amino acids are determined by their R groups, which can be generally categorized by their solubility in water and by whether they are acidic, basic, uncharged but polar, or nonpolar. In addition, a few have distinctive properties. Cysteine, for example, has the capacity to form disulfide bonds.

Amino acids are linked to each other by *peptide bonds.* These bonds are formed by a condensation reaction between

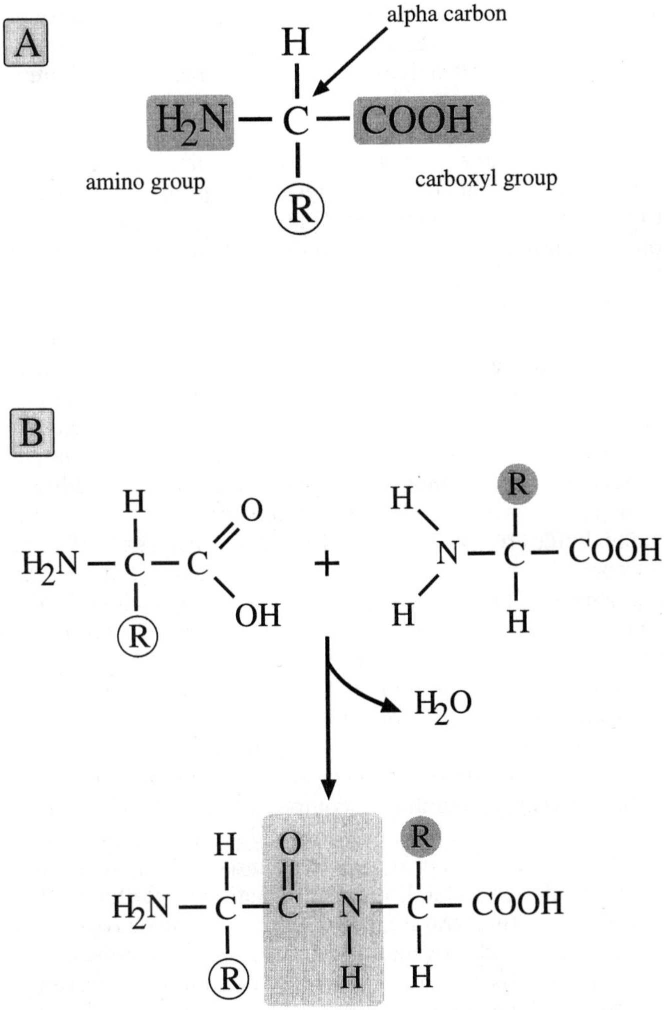

FIGURE 3.7. Proteins are polymers of amino acids that are linked by peptide bonds. **A.** Amino acids have a common general formula. They all contain an amino group and a carboxylic acid group, both linked to a single α-carbon. There are 20 amino acids common to all proteins, each with a different side group designated *R*. At physiological pH, almost all carboxylic acids and amines are in their fully charged forms. **B.** Each amino acid is joined to the next by a covalent amide linkage called a peptide bond (*shaded*). The amino acid sequence determines the primary structure of the protein.

the amino group of one amino acid and the carboxyl group of another (Fig. 3.7B). The specialized characteristics of each protein are determined by its amino acid sequence, which is termed the primary structure of the protein. This sequence dictates the distribution of polar and nonpolar side chains and determines the correct folding of the protein (Fig. 3.8). Although the three-dimensional pattern of folding is unique for each protein, it is apparent that there are recurrent structural motifs in portions of the polypeptide chain. Motifs are regular combinations of secondary structures that are usually in one of two geometric forms: an *α-helix* (two α-helices form a coiled coil) or a *β-sheet* (composed of laterally associated β-strands).

The α-helices are formed when the polypeptide chain turns about itself to create a rigid cylinder. These rodlike elements serve many functions. For example, a bundle of three α-helices is the essential motif of dystrophin, a structural protein required for appropriate muscle function. In addition, α-helices often form the transmembrane portion of receptor proteins. They are also a common secondary structure for DNA-binding proteins because the α-helix fits into the major groove of the double-stranded DNA molecule, thus facilitating DNA–protein interactions.

The β-sheets are composed of short, nearly fully extended polypeptide chains. These β-sheets form when two separate polypeptide chains (or two different regions of the same chain) fold back and forth on themselves, with each section of the chain running in the direction opposite that of its immediate neighbors. The chains then become connected by hydrogen bonds. There are two different forms of β-sheets. In one, the adjacent chains run in the same amino-carboxyl direction, producing a parallel β-sheet; in the other, the adjacent chains run in opposite directions, producing an antiparallel β-sheet. Many globular proteins contain compact regions of β-sheets that support their internal structure, and in some cases the β-sheet will form the floor of a binding pocket. In structural proteins such as silk, layers of β-sheets provide both flexibility and strength.

Combinations of different secondary structures can be organized into a tertiary structure. Often, this tertiary struc-

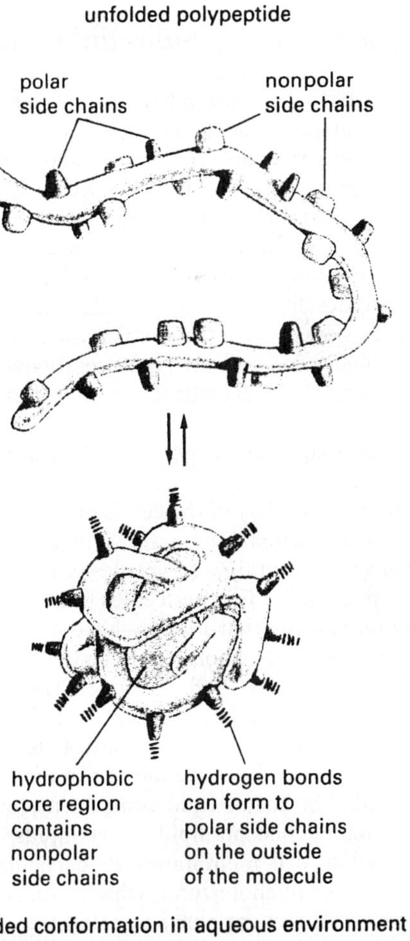

FIGURE 3.8. The amino acid sequence determines correct protein folding. The distribution of the polar and nonpolar R groups determines the folding of a protein. The polar side groups tend to be on the outside of the protein where they can interact with water molecules; the nonpolar groups are hidden on the inside, forming a "hydrophobic core." (From Alberts et al.,[1] with permission.)

ture can be organized into discrete regions called *domains* that are characterized by specific structural or functional features. Tertiary structure domains can be incorporated into proteins as repeating modular units. For example, the ECM protein fibronectin is composed of multiple repeating subunits designated type III repeats. These domains are found in a number of different structural proteins and can provide clues to protein function even if the complete three-dimensional structure of the protein is unknown. The tertiary structure of a protein is stabilized by forces between the molecules and by disulfide bonds between cysteine residues. A protein's tertiary structure can be disrupted in vitro by heat or by chemical agents, leading to unfolding of the protein and loss of function. In many cases, however, the protein will refold spontaneously to form a functionally active molecule. In vivo, proteins become destabilized or damaged through a variety of mechanisms. Misfolded proteins may be induced to refold correctly by the action of molecular chaperones such as heat-shock protein 70 (hsp 70) and hsp 60. If this fails, these and other abnormal proteins are targeted for degradation by coupling to ubiquitin. Ubiquitination targets misfolded proteins to large complexes in the cytosol termed *proteosomes*, where the proteins are degraded to small peptides and released.[1,9]

Cell Organization and Subcellular Structure

Broadly speaking, cells contain four families of small organic molecules: sugars, fatty acids, amino acids, and nucleotides. For primitive cells to evolve, it became important to contain and separate these macromolecules within a boundary. It has been postulated that the first cell was formed when phospholipid molecules in the prebiotic soup spontaneously assembled, enclosing a self-replicating mixture of RNA and protein molecules. All present-day cells are surrounded by a plasma membrane. Over time, eukaryotic cells developed an array of organelles and internal membranes specifically designed to partition specialized cellular function within the cell cytoplasm. Cellular compartmentalization likely evolved as a consequence of the increased complexity of cell function.[11]

The external boundary of the cell is defined by the *plasma membrane*. The plasma membrane is a fluid lipid bilayer composed of a variety of lipid molecules with proteins associated or embedded in it. Lipid molecules that form this defined layer are *amphipathic*; that is, they have polar head regions connected to long hydrophobic side chains, typically composed of fatty acids (Fig. 3.9). In water, the phospholipids orient so that the hydrophobic regions are directed inward, and the polar head groups face outward. It is from this tendency that one can see how the formation of a bilayer structure is favored. The major lipid components of the plasma membrane include phospholipids, glycolipids, and cholesterol. Mammalian cell membranes, in particular, contain a significant amount of cholesterol, which appears to stabilize the membrane and prevent phase transitions.

All membranes contain a large proportion of phospholipids. The four major phospholipids are phosphatidylcholine, phosphatidylserine, phosphatidylethanolamine, and sphingomyelin, a molecule that instead of a glycerol backbone has a sphingosine. The phospholipid composition of different cells varies as different phospholipids have specialized capacity to associate with integral and associated membrane proteins. Moreover, different halves of the lipid bilayer have different lipid compositions. For example, the phospholipids that have choline in their head groups are typically found in the portion of the membrane facing the extracellular compartment, whereas those that contain charged head groups are found in the portion of the membrane facing the intracellular compartment. This asymmetry is important to intracellular signaling events that are dependent on key lipid membrane components such as sphingomyelin and phosphatidylinositol. Glycolipids are a small component of the lipid bilayer and are found exclusively in the noncytoplasmic leaflet. Typically, glycolipids have sugar groups linked to their head regions. These sugar moieties project from the cell surface. The most complex glycolipids, the gangliosides, are important components of the plasma membranes of nerve cells.[1,9,10] In addition to being the structural building blocks of the plasma membrane, lipids are now recognized as the precursors of a diverse number of bioactive molecules that can function as second messengers. The major lipid signaling systems include (1) the glycerophospholipid derivatives diacylglycerol (DAG), inositol 1,4,5-triphosphate (IP_3), arachidonate, the eicosanoids, and the lysophospholipids and (2) the sphingolipids, particularly the sphingomyelinase product ceramide.

Recent data indicate that the cell membrane is organized into lipid-based micro- and macrodomains that are referred to as *lipid rafts*.[12] Lipid rafts are composed principally of cholesterol, sphingolipids, and phospholipids with saturated acyl chains. The conformation of these molecules allows their tight association to facilitate the formation of platforms that organize structural and signaling molecules. Rafts have special biochemical and physical properties when compared to nonraft domains, including resistance to nonionic detergents. Further, as the formation of rafts is dependent on cholesterol content, this process can be disrupted by cholesterol-sequestering agents. One example of lipid raft formation in vivo is the immune synapse that forms in stimulated T cells.[13] Lipid rafts have also been implicated in signaling events in monocytes, where rafts form a microenvironment for CD14-dependent clustering of receptors involved in inflammation and atherogenesis.[14]

The Nucleus

Eukaryotic cells, by definition, have a nucleus (Fig. 3.10). The nucleus is the largest organelle in the cell, ranging in size from 3 to 8 mm in diameter, depending on cell type. All the chromsomal DNA is held in the nucleus, packaged into chromatin fibers by its association with an equal mass of histone proteins. During the process of cell division, the chromatin fibers condense into compact structures known as *chromosomes*. The nucleus is separated from the cytoplasm by the nuclear envelope, a double membrane composed of two lipid bilayers separated by a gap of 20 to 40 nm known as the *perinuclear space*. The nuclear envelope isolates the central genetic processes of DNA replication and RNA synthesis from the cytoplasmic-associated process of protein synthesis. The outer membrane of the nuclear envelope is continuous with the endoplasmic reticulum (ER) and is studded with ribosomes. Specific proteins in the inner membrane interact with a set of proteins that form the underlying nuclear lamina.

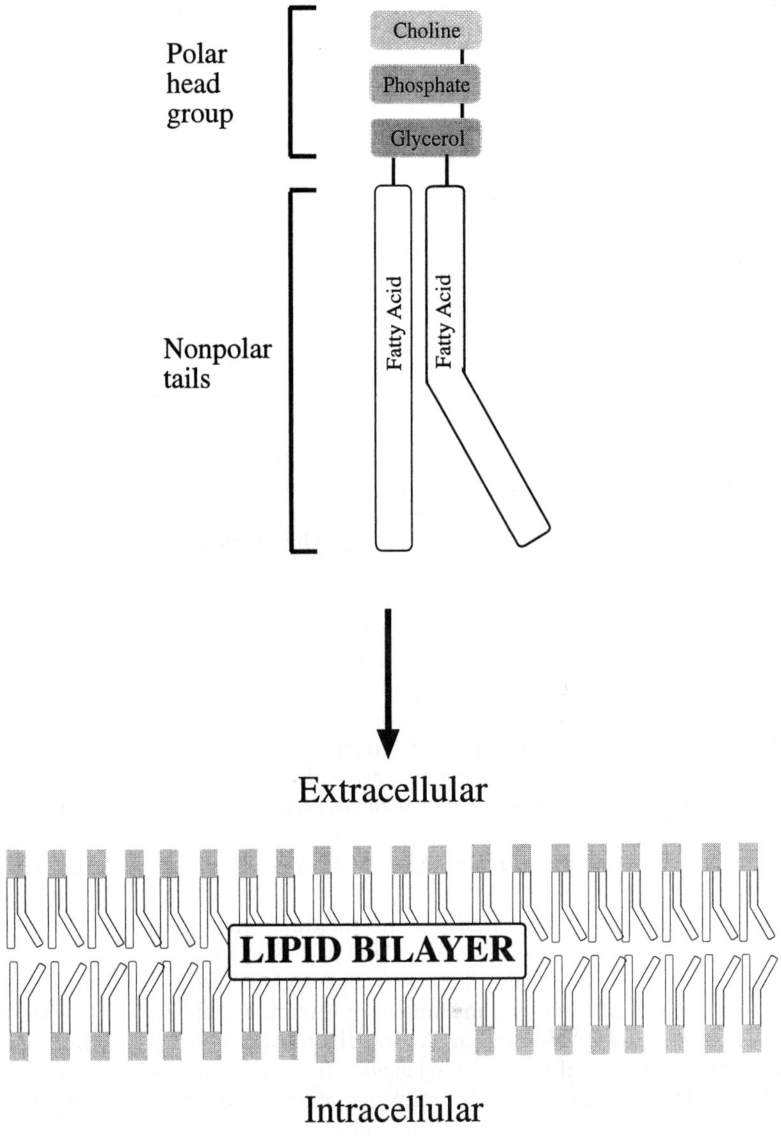

FIGURE 3.9. Eukaryotic cells are enclosed by a phospholipid bilayer membrane. A schematic of a membrane phospholipid, phosphatidylcholine, is shown. Membrane phospholipids are amphipathic; that is, they have a polar head group and a hydrophobic tail that is typically composed of fatty acids. Phospholipid molecules have a tendency to aggregate in water so that their hydrophobic tails are buried. In this fashion, they can form bilayer sheets.

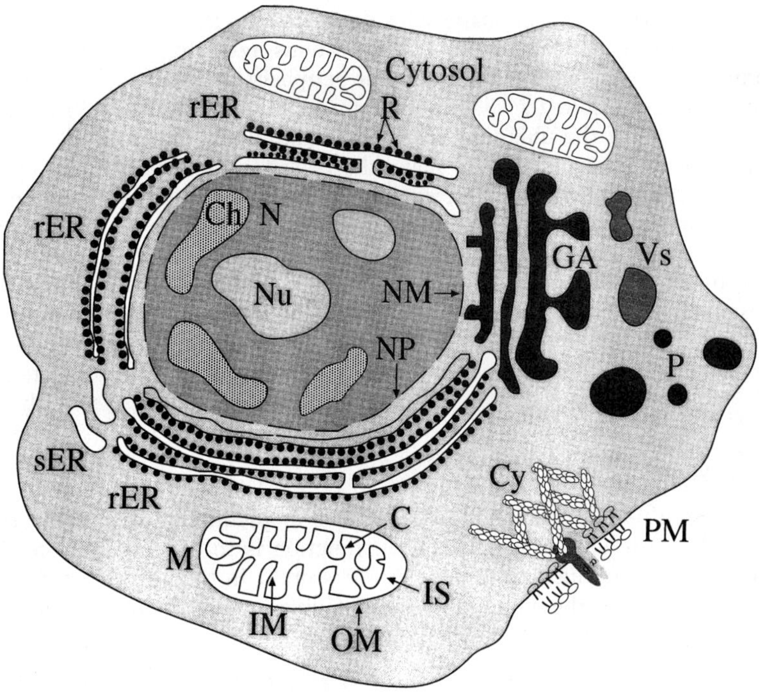

FIGURE 3.10. Schematic of a typical eukaryotic cell: ribosomes (*R*), rough endoplasmic reticulum (*rER*), smooth endoplasmic reticulum (*sER*), nucleus (*N*), nucleolus (*Nu*), nuclear membrane (*NM*), nuclear pore (*NP*), chromatin (*Ch*), mitochondrion (*M*), inner membrane (*IM*), outer membrane (*OM*), intermembrane space (*IS*), cristae (*C*), cytoskeleton (*Cy*), plasma membrane (*PM*), Golgi apparatus (*GA*), lysosome (*LY*), peroxisomes (*P*), transport vesicles (*Vs*).

The nuclear lamina is thought to play a crucial part in organizing both the nuclear envelope and the underlying chromatin. The nuclear lamina is composed of proteins called *lamins*. The nuclear contents communicate with the cytosol by means of openings in the nuclear envelope called *nuclear pores*. The pores are about 50 to 70 nm in diameter, and each is surrounded by a thick, electron-dense ring or annulus known as the *nuclear pore complex*. Each complex is composed of eight large protein granules arranged in an octagonal pattern.

Regions in which the inner and outer nuclear membranes are continuous enable lipid-soluble materials, such as histones, DNA and RNA polymerases, gene regulatory proteins, and RNA processing proteins, to flow from the ER membrane, where they are synthesized into the inner nuclear membrane. The central cavity of the pore provides the main channel by which water-soluble molecules, such as sodium chloride and other ionic compounds, shuttle between the nucleus and the cytoplasm. The central cavity is often plugged by a large central granule believed to represent newly made ribosomes and other particulate matter caught in transit. The nucleus also contains a specialized region, the nucleolus, where ribosomes are assembled (Fig. 3.10). The nucleolus contains large loops of DNA with ribosome RNA genes that are transcribed at a high rate. Such a loop of DNA is called a *nucleolar organizer region*. Unlike the cytoplasmic organelles, the nucleolus has no membrane to keep it contained; rather, it seems to be held together by the binding of unfinished ribosome precursors to each other to form a meshwork. Of the nucleolar mass, 80% is composed of proteins, with the remaining 20% consisting of a mixture of DNA and RNA.[1,11]

The nucleus also contains other distinct subnuclear bodies, including splicing speckles, Cajal bodies, gems, PML (promyelocytic leukemia) bodies, paraspeckle proteins (PSPs), and clastosomes. Many nuclear proteins are able to interact with these structures and markedly influence nuclear activities such as ribosome biogenesis, transcription, and RNA splicing. Paraspeckles, for example, are discrete bodies in the interchromatin nucleoplasmic space and associate with at least three RNA-binding proteins (PSP1, PSP2, and P54/nrb) that interact dynamically with the nucleolus in a transcription-dependent manner. These proteins relocalize to unique cap structures at the nucleolar periphery when transcription is inhibited.[15] Clastosomes are highly enriched in components of the ubiquitin-proteosome pathway. Proteins involved in cell cycle regulation and short-lived transcription factors are specifically targeted for proteosome-mediated degradation by this pathway. Clastosomes disappear when cells are treated by proteosome inhibitors and reappear when the inhibitors are removed, indicating that clastosomes represent sites where proteosome-dependent proteolysis is taking place.[16]

Cytoplasmic Organelles

The Mitochondria

Mitochondria are the major source of energy production in all eukaryotic cells (Fig. 3.10). Their function is to convert energy found in nutrient molecules and store it in the form of ATP, which is the universal energy-yielding commodity in cells, used by enzymes to perform a wide range of cellular functions. To carry out energy conversion, mitochondria require oxygen, which they convert to water. The consumption of oxygen by mitochondria is called *cellular respiration*. Mitochondria contain the enzymes of the citric acid or Krebs cycle, carry out oxidative phosphorylation, and are involved in fatty acid biosynthesis. Mitochondria are among the largest organelles in the cell, measuring approximately 0.5 to 1 mm in diameter. In the liver, they can occupy as much as 20% of the cell volume. They are especially abundant in cells and parts of cells associated with active processes. In cardiac muscle, mitochondria surround the contractile elements.

Mitochondria are cylindrical in shape and are bounded by a double membrane. The outer membrane defines the external boundary of the organelle. The outer membrane is a relatively simple phospholipid bilayer, containing proteins called porins, which render it permeable to molecules of about 10 kDa or less (the size of the smallest proteins). Ions, nutrient molecules, ATP, adenosine diphosphate (ADP), and the like can pass through the outer membrane with ease. The inner membrane exhibits a series of convolutions or invaginations known as *cristae*. The cristae increase the surface area of the inner membrane about fivefold over that of the outer membrane. The inner membrane contains small spherical particles protruding into the matrix space. These inner membrane spheres or knobs are involved with electron transport and oxidative phosphorylation. The inner membrane is almost entirely protein and is freely permeable only to oxygen, carbon dioxide, and water.

The outer and inner mitochondrial membranes divide the mitochondrion into two distinct compartments: the internal matrix space and a narrower intermembrane space. The intermembrane space, as implied, is the region between the inner and outer membranes. It has an important role in the primary function of mitochondria, which is oxidative phosphorylation. The matrix contains a mixture of hundreds of different enzymes and cofactors involved in the final oxidation of sugars and lipids. The intermembrane space also contains several copies of the mitochondrial DNA genome, special mitochondrial ribosomes, and various enzymes required for the expression of mitochondrial genes. The matrix also contains dissolved oxygen, water, carbon dioxide, the recyclable intermediates that serve as energy shuttles, and much more. Because of the folds of the cristae, no part of the matrix is far from the inner membrane. Therefore, matrix components can quickly reach inner membrane complexes and transport proteins.

Mitochondria, like bacteria, have circular DNA genomes that encode for 2 rRNAs, 22 or 23 tRNAs, and 10 to 12 proteins, these being components of the organelle-based translation apparatus. Mitochondrial DNA also codes mRNA for proteins synthesized within the organelle.[1,2,11]

It is thought that mitochondria began as free-living bacteria but were then engulfed by primitive eukaryotes. Once internalized, these symbiotic bacteria flourished within the host eukaryote as *endosymbionts*, supplying the host with the ability to generate energy by oxidative phosphorylation. As protomitochondria became specialized organelles, genes were transferred from the protomitochondria to the host genome. This concept is evident inasmuch as most mitochondrial proteins are now encoded in the nuclear DNA, translated in the cytoplasm, and transported across the outer membrane of the organelle. Only molecules that cannot cross the outer membrane (rRNA, tRNA, mRNA, and proteins coding for mitochondria-related oxidative processes) are encoded by the mitochondrial genome. Mitochondria divide by fission, consistent with the notion that they originated from captive or symbiotic bacteria.[1] Mitochondria are never made de novo but arise by the growth and division of existing mitochondria. Moreover, the number of mitochondria per cell can be regulated according to need. For example, a 5- to 10-fold increase in mitochondria is observed if a resting skeletal muscle is repeatedly stimulated to contract for a prolonged period of time.[1]

The Endoplasmic Reticulum

The ER is a cytoplasmic system of membranes consisting of a series of interconnected flattened disks (cisternae). Two functionally distinct regions can be distinguished in electron photomicrographs. The rough endoplasmic reticulum (rER) is studded with ribosomes on the cytoplasmic side of the membrane and is involved in the synthesis, processing, and transport to the Golgi of proteins destined for the plasma membrane, certain organelles, or secretion (Fig. 3.10). Most proteins synthesized in the rER are glycosylated. The rER is generally arranged as flattened sheets of membrane. The smooth endoplasmic reticulum (sER) lacks any attached ribosomes and typically consists of an interconnected series of convoluted tubules. The sER is primarily involved in the synthesis of fatty acids and lipids.

The most important functions of the ER are to provide surfaces inside the cell for the ribosomes to attach and to transport the substances that the ribosomes need to make proteins from the nucleus to the ribosomes themselves. The relative abundance of rough and smooth ER varies among cell types, with rER predominating in cells actively synthesizing proteins for export, such as pancreatic acinar cells and antibody-secreting plasma cells. Smooth ER is normally associated with cells involved in the metabolism of lipids, steroid hormones, drugs, and toxic substances. Phenobarbital, for instance, is detoxified in the liver; enzymes in the sER convert the toxin into a more water-soluble, conjugated product that is readily secreted from the body.

The ER divides the cytoplasm into two compartments, the cell sap and the ER lumen or cisternal space. The lumen of the ER is separated from the cytosol by a single membrane. Because the ER membrane is continuous with the outer nuclear membrane, the ER lumen and the interior of the nucleus are also only separated by a single membrane, the inner nuclear membrane. The cell sap contains enzymes involved in many metabolic pathways; the cisternal space provides a route for the intracellular movement of materials, especially proteins destined for export.[1,11]

The Golgi Complex and Vesicles

The *Golgi complex* is located near the nucleus and is composed of a series of flattened membrane sacs, or cisternae, surrounded by secretory vesicles (Fig. 3.10). The Golgi complex is structurally and biochemically polarized. That is, it has two distinct faces: a *cis*, or forming face, and a *trans*, or maturing face. The *cis* face normally associates with ribosome-free portions of the rER (termed transitional ER). The *trans* face is closest to the plasma membrane. Small vesicles, called *transport vesicles*, are interposed between the rER and the *cis* face of the Golgi. Large secretory vesicles are found exclusively in association with the *trans* face.

One role of the Golgi complex is to direct macromolecular traffic in the cell. For example, proteins targeted for the plasma membrane are carried from the Golgi complex to the plasma membrane in transport vesicles. Proteins destined for secretion are packaged into secretory vesicles, which form by budding from the Golgi complex. The secretory vesicles migrate to the cell surface, where they fuse with the plasma membrane and release the packaged proteins to the outside of the cell. Proteins are also compartmentalized into large secretory granules in which the contents condense and are stored. The Golgi complex also modifies proteins, most commonly by glycosylation, sulfation, and fatty acid addition. These various modifications follow highly ordered enzymatic pathways. The accurate sorting of proteins to specific intracellular and extracellular destinations is thought to be mediated largely by the coated vesicles that surround the cisternae and to depend on sets of receptors in the Golgi membrane that recognize specific markers of the proteins to be transported.[1,11]

Lysosomes

Lysosomes are cytoplasmic organelles containing hydrolytic enzymes (Fig. 3.10). The enzymes are separated from the cytoplasm by a surrounding membrane. Lysosomes are involved in digesting substances that are brought into the cell by endocytosis. They also participate in the hydrolysis of cellular constituents. Two classes of lysosomes are distinguished: primary and secondary. Primary lysosomes are roughly spherical and contain hydrolytic enzymes but do not contain obvious particulate or membrane debris. Primary lysosomes are formed by budding from the *trans*-most cisternae of the Golgi apparatus. Secondary lysosomes are larger and irregularly shaped. They not only contain hydrolytic enzymes but also membranes and particles undergoing digestion. Secondary lysosomes arise from the fusion of primary lysosomes with engulfed or abnormal organelles or with endocytic vesicles that are bringing extracellular material into the cell for degradation.[1,11]

Most of the hydrolytic enzymes present in lysosomes are glycoproteins synthesized on the rER. Some 40 enzymes are now known to be contained in lysosomes. They are all acid hydrolases, including proteases, nucleases, glycosydases, lipases, phospholipases, phosphatases, and sulfatases. These enzymes are active at acidic pH, so the acidity of lysosomes is maintained at a pH of about 4.8. This control is accomplished by means of the presence of an H^+ ion pump in the membrane of the lysosome. The lysosomal enzymes are inactive at neutral pH; thus, if a lysosome releases its enzymes into the cytosol, where the pH is between 7.0 and 7.3, no degradation will take place.[1,11]

There are at least four pathways by which lysosomes function (Fig. 3.11). These include (1) degradation of foreign matter taken up by *endocytosis*, (2) destruction of nonfunctioning

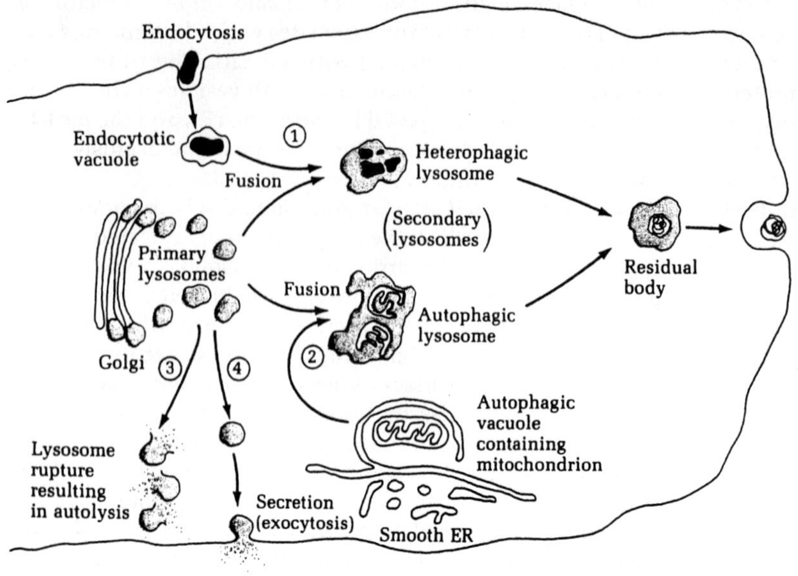

FIGURE 3.11. Schematic representation of the four basic digestive functions of lysosomes: *1*, degradation of material taken up by endocytosis; *2*, autophagy; *3*, autolysis; *4*, exocytosis. (From Kleinsmith and Kish,[2] with permission of Pearson Education.)

organelles (*autophagy*), (3) cell death-associated breakdown of cellular structures (*autolysis*), and (4) *digestion* of extracellular materials.

1. *Endocytosis* refers to the uptake of extracellular materials trapped in membrane vesicles that pinch off from the plasma membrane.[1,11] There are three principal pathways for endocytosis: phagocytosis, receptor-mediated endocytosis, and pinocytosis. *Phagocytosis* is the process by which relatively large particles are internalized. In *receptor-mediated endocytosis*, a specific receptor on the surface of the membrane binds tightly to the extracellular macromolecule, or ligand; the plasma membrane region containing the receptor–ligand complex then undergoes endocytosis, becoming a transport vesicle. This process occurs via clathrin-coated pits and vesicles. Clathrin, a fibrous protein, interacts with several other proteins to form a polyhedral cage around the coated pit. After the receptor–ligand complexes have become clustered within the coated pit, it invaginates and pinches off from the plasma membrane, releasing a coated vesicle into the interior of the cell. This internalized vesicle then sheds its clathrin coat, forming an uncoated vesicle known as an *endosome*. *Pinocytosis* refers to the nonspecific uptake of small droplets of extracellular fluid containing water-soluble macromolecules such as antibodies, enzymes, hormones, and toxins into endocytic vesicles.[1,11]

2. *Autophagy*, the selective destruction of cellular components, is useful to the cell because it removes unwanted organelles and because it permits the chemical building blocks generated during the organelle's destruction to be recycled.

3. *Autolysis*, the digestion of cell structure, plays an important role in the development of certain organ systems and body structures. For example, embryonic formation of fingers or toes from undifferentiated blocks of tissue requires selective destruction of the cells located between the newly forming digits.

4. Extracellular digestion by hydrolytic enzymes is important during fertilization as it facilitates dissolution of the outer layers of the egg membranes, thus allowing sperm to penetrate. Other, less-beneficial effects include a role in posttraumatic or infectious inflammation and the facilitation of invasion and metastasis during carcinogenesis.

Failure of lysosomes to function in their normal capacities can result in several disorders known collectively as *lysosomal storage disease*. One such disorder, Tay-Sachs disease, an inherited recessive disorder, affects nerve cells. It is caused by the absence of a lysosomal enzyme, β-*N*-hexosaminidase A, which ordinarily digests a ganglioside (GM_2) in nerve cell membranes. Normally, GM_2 is continually synthesized and degraded. In Tay-Sachs victims, GM_2 accumulates as concentric lamellae in residual bodies, ultimately filling up the nerve cell and interfering with its function. Tay-Sachs disease causes mental retardation, blindness, muscular weakness, and death, usually by the age of 5 years.[1,11]

Peroxisomes

Peroxisomes are spherical, membrane-limited structures about 0.5 mm in diameter and are found in almost all eukaryotic cells. Peroxisomes contain enzymes that degrade fatty acids to acetyl coenzyme A (CoA); a product of these reactions is hydrogen peroxide (H_2O_2), a corrosive substance. Consequently, peroxisomes also contain the enzyme catalase, which degrades hydrogen peroxide. Catalase utilizes the H_2O_2 to oxidize a variety of substrates, including phenols, formic acid, formaldehyde, and alcohols. Peroxisomes also carry out oxidative reactions using molecular oxygen.[1,11]

The Cytoskeleton

The cytoplasm and organelles of eukaryotic cells exist within a three-dimensional meshwork of cytoplasmic and membrane-associated proteins called the *cytoskeleton*. The cytoskeleton not only provides structural support for cells but also allows cells to perform essential functions such as movement, phagocytosis, and cellular division. This network of protein filaments is rapidly responsive to extracellular cues, assembling and disassembling to facilitate cell shape change. In addition to this structural role, recent data suggest that linkage between cytoskeletal filaments and cell-surface receptors may provide a mechanism for mechanical signal transfer directly to the nucleus. The cytoskeletal scaffolding is dependent on three types of protein filaments: actin microfilaments, intermediate filaments (IFs), and microtubules. It has become clear that alterations in these cytoskeletal proteins can weaken cellular support, thus contributing to a variety of human disorders, ranging from blistering skin disease to Alzheimer's disease.

Intermediate filaments are so named because their 10-nm diameter is intermediate between actin microfilaments (6nm) and microtubules (23nm). In most cells, networks of IFs radiate from the nucleus to the cell periphery, where they are anchored at the plasma membrane at specialized sites. In addition, IFs form a tight mesh that underlies the nuclear membrane. They are differentially expressed in a variety of cells, where their abundance as a percentage of the total protein content of the cell can range from 1% to 85%. The IFs are particularly prominent in cells subject to mechanical stress. For example, epithelial cells contain a large amount of IFs, as do muscle cells. The IFs are distinct from both actin filaments and microtubules in that they are a diverse family of proteins arising from some 50 different genes. However, all IFs share a common structure: a dimer composed of two α-helical chains intertwined to form a coiled-coil rod. The highly conserved ends of the rods allow polymerization of protein monomers in a head-to-tail fashion. Four dimers associate to form a protofibril, and three to four protofibrils intertwine to form a mature filament. The nonhelical head and tail portions of IFs vary greatly, permitting different proteins to associate with them.[1,9,10]

Intermediate filaments in vertebrate cells fall into one of three classes: (1) keratin filaments of hair and epidermal cells, (2) vimentin and related proteins of fibroblasts, and (3) neurofilament proteins. Cells that have abundant IFs, such as epidermal keratinocytes, have provided important clues as to their function. Studies from both human and transgenic mouse models revealed that the normal function of keratin filaments is to provide epidermal cells with structural integrity. The absence or disorganization of the IF network seen with keratin mutations expressed in epidermal cells results in cells that are more fragile when stressed. Subsequently, mutations in keratin genes have been associated with epidermolysis bullosa simplex and other blistering skin disorders. Nerve cells also contain an abundant IF network. Neurofilaments appear to be important for the structuring of axons. Their disorganization is a hallmark of motor neuron diseases, including amyotrophic lateral sclerosis.[4,17]

Microtubules are stiff polymers of tubulin molecules composed of heterodimers of alpha (α) and beta (β) tubulin. They are highly conserved evolutionarily and play an important role in cytoplasmic organization, cell polarity, cell movement, and transport. A microtubule has a cylindrical structure formed from tubulin molecules that are bundled into protofilaments organized around a central core. They are dynamic in nature, with rapid assembly occurring at the plus ("fast-growing") end of the filament. One end of the microtubule is anchored at the *centrosome.* The centrosome is a small, centrally located organelle that is composed of centrioles and serves as the major microtubule-organizing center. Displaying intrinsic polarity, microtubule plus ends face away from the centrosome, while the minus ends face toward the centrosome. Microtubules frequently fluctuate between states of polymerization and depolymerization. This assembly–disassembly behavior, termed *dynamic instability,* facilitates microtubule remodeling required for transitions in the cell cycle, cell shape change, and cell movement.

The energy necessary for polymerization is generated by the hydrolysis of tubulin-bound GTP (guanosine triphosphate) to GDP (guanosine diphosphate) accompanying polymerization. Treatment of tubulin molecules with nonhydrolyzable forms of GTP does not interfere with microtubule assembly but generates stable microtubule protofilaments that are resistant to depolymerization. Delayed hydrolysis of GTP on polymerization facilitates microtubule growth because GTP-tubulin binds other tubulin molecules with higher affinity. Regulation of dynamic instability occurs through a number of cellular factors, including the structural microtubule-associated proteins (MAPs). These proteins bind to and stabilize tubulin molecules, preventing them from depolymerizing. The MAPs are phosphorylated by a novel group of serine-threonine kinases, the microtubule-associated regulatory kinases (MARKs). Phosphorylation of the tubulin-binding domain of MAPs causes their detachment from the microtubules, triggering microtubule disruption.[9,18]

Another group of proteins that associate with microtubules is the microtubule-dependent ATPases kinesin and dynein. These motor proteins and their family members control the direction and velocity of organelle transport and that of other microtubule cargoes, including protein complexes and mRNA. Motor proteins and MAPs both interact with microtubules, suggesting that MAPs may interfere with the movement of motor proteins. Further, there may be a link between overexpression and hyperphosphorylation of MAPs in neurons, the disruption of mitochondrial transport, and the subsequent development of neuronal degeneration typical of Alzheimer's disease. Microtubules are sensitive to drugs that alter the kinetics of assembly–disassembly. One of these is colchicine, an alkaloid that binds tightly to tubulin and prevents its polymerization. Treatment of cells with colchicine causes rapid disappearance of the mitotic spindle. In contrast, the drug taxol binds tightly to microtubules, stabilizing them and thus preventing depolymerization. Taxol-treated cells arrest in the mitotic phase of the cell cycle.[9,19]

Actin is one of the most abundant and evolutionarily highly conserved proteins found in eukaryotic cells. Filamentous, or F, actin, is assembled into 8-nm filaments by the spontaneous polymerization of globular, or G, actin molecules in a process that requires physiological salt concentrations and ATP. The G-actin monomers are assembled in a head-to-tail fashion, creating structurally and functionally polar actin filaments. This polarity is readily visualized by electron microscopy. The preferred end for the addition of G-actin is the barbed or "plus" end; the growth of the "minus" end is much slower. Actin polymerization requires an actin nucleus, consisting of either an actin trimer or a free actin filament end that is generated by the uncapping or severing of an existing actin filament. Similar to tubulin, actin polymerization is a dynamic process that is controlled by proteins that interact with and bind both to monomeric actin and to actin filaments. These actin-associated proteins act through diverse mechanisms to regulate the assembly and disassembly of actin filaments. The assembly of the actin cytoskeleton is both temporally and spatially controlled. For example, actin-dependent cellular processes such as cell locomotion require actin assembly exclusively at the leading edge of the migrating cell. The process through which actin assembly sites are selected is not well understood, but work suggests that the protein zyxin may play an important role.[1,9,20]

The assembly and disassembly of actin filaments in response to extracellular signals is controlled by three Ras-related GTP-binding proteins called Rho, Rac, and Cdc42 (Fig. 3.12). This activity is central to a variety of biological functions, including maintenance of cell shape and polarity and the initiation of cell movement. In response to extracellular signals, Rho activation leads to the formation of bundles of contractile actin-myosin filaments called *stress fibers*. Stress fibers are important for the assembly of focal adhesions, regions of close contact between the cell and the ECM that serve as organizing centers for cytoskeletal and signaling molecules. In contrast, Rac activation leads to the formation of a meshwork of actin filaments proximal to the cell membrane that results in the assembly of lamellopodia and membrane ruffling. The third member of the Rho family, Cdc42, induces actin-rich surface projections called *filopodia*.

Rho GTPases also have the ability to coordinate cell activities other than actin filament assembly. For example, Rho, Rac, and Cdc42 have been reported to regulate members of the mitogen-activated protein kinase (MAPK) signaling

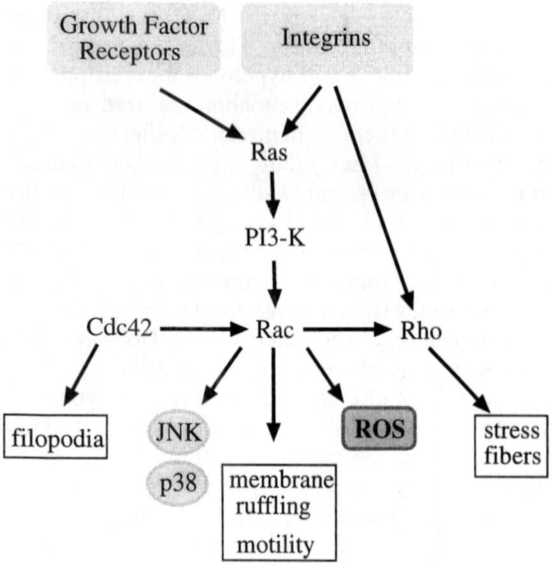

FIGURE 3.12. Rho GTPases and the actin cytoskeleton. Activation of Rho GTPases is responsible for the reorganization of the actin cytoskeleton. Activation of Rho leads to the assembly of actin-myosin stress fibers associated with focal adhesions. Activation of Rac, via growth factors or Ras, causes lamellopodial formation and membrane ruffling. Cdc42 activation leads to the formation of filopodia, small finger-like actin extensions. Both Rac and Cdc42 activity are required for cell spreading. In transfection assays, Rac and Cdc42 activate the *JNK* and p38 MAPK pathways via a mechanism involving the p21-activated kinase (PAK). Rac is known to regulate the NADP (nicotinamide adenine dinucleotide phosphate) oxidase enzyme complex in phagocytes to generate superoxide and reactive oxygen species (*ROS*). Evidence suggests that Rac may accomplish this in other cell types as well.

family, including the c-Jun N-terminal kinase (JNK), and the p38 MAPK. Activity of GTPase is also important for progression through the G_1 phase of the cell cycle, perhaps via a mechanism that involves Rac-regulated generation of reactive oxygen species.[21]

Interestingly, the Rho family proteins are the targets for bacterial protein toxins such as the *Clostridium difficile* toxins A and B and the *Escherichia coli* virulence factor, cytotoxic necrotizing factor. These toxins can either inactivate the GTPases by ADP-ribosylation or glucosylation (toxins A and B) or activate them by deamidation (cytotoxic necrotizing factor). The large clostridial cytotoxins are the major virulence factors for antibiotic-associated diarrhea and are a leading cause of nosocomial diarrhea in the United States. These toxins monoglucosylate Rho proteins, rendering them biologically inactive. This action results in the disorganization of the actin cytoskeleton, cell rounding, and altered cell signaling. In animals, the administration of toxin A leads to epithelial cell disruption and fluid secretion into the intestinal lumen.[22]

Molecular Motors

The cytoskeleton not only provides a structural network for the spatial organization of subcellular organelles but also is the principal means by which proteins and nucleic acids are actively transported within the cell. Key processes such as protein trafficking, cell polarization, and cell division all rely on active transport for distributing macromolecules, organelles, and chromosomes to various parts of the cell. The distribution system is complex and involves a specialized class of cytoskeleton-associated proteins called *motor proteins*: the myosin, kinesin, and dynein motors. Myosin moves along actin filaments, whereas kinesin and dynein utilize the microtubule system. Typically, each protein contains a "tail" region that binds to the element transported and a "head" region that binds to the cytoskeleton. The three motor proteins hydrolyze ATP and utilize the energy released to propel themselves along the cytoskeleton. The direction of transport is determined by both the motor proteins and the cytoskeletal system with which they interact. Microtubules, for example, are polar and are typically organized with their minus ends oriented at a microtubule-organizing center close to the nucleus. The plus ends of the microtubules radiate outward away from the nucleus in a radial manner. Motor proteins are able to recognize this polarity. Most kinesin proteins move toward the plus end and consequently shuttle their "cargo" toward the cell periphery. Dynein, on the other hand, moves toward the minus end and transports cargo toward the nucleus. Actin filaments are more randomly oriented and shorter than microtubules. Actin filaments cluster in areas of low microtubule density such as the cell surface. The filaments orient themselves with their plus ends pointed outward. Myosin-V moves toward the plus end and is therefore able to transport cargo to the very perimeter of the cell. In some cells, the same cargo can be transported on both actin and microtubule filaments and exchanges motor protein to do so. Together, the actin cytoskeleton, microtubules, and motor proteins provide an efficient, rapid means of active transport in the cell and are crucial to all basic cellular processes.[23,24]

Protein Synthesis

As proteins carry out most of the biological activities of the cell, the control of protein synthesis is central to the life of the cell. To understand the control of protein synthesis, it is important to understand the relationship between genes and proteins. Once the double-helical structure of DNA was identified, it became possible to elucidate the relationship between nucleic acid and amino acid sequences. The concept of single gene, single protein was developed based on experiments of mutant proteins with single amino acid replacements. Subsequent experiments with *E. coli* led to the discovery that the position of specific amino acid mutations in the proteins corresponded well to the predicted position of the mutation on the genetic map, suggesting strongly that the gene and its protein product were colinear. It was also apparent, however, that there was no direct correlation between the nucleotide sequence and the amino acid sequence because the number of amino acids (20) exceeded the number of base pairs (4). Therefore, it was postulated that *groups* of bases were required to specify protein sequence. Moreover, it was determined that the DNA sequence could not directly guide polypeptide synthesis inasmuch as the genetic material (DNA) was retained in the nucleus, while protein synthesis occurred in the cytoplasm. The information therefore had to be transferred to an intermediate molecule. The RNA became the ideal candidate for a number of reasons. First, there is significant structural similarity between DNA and RNA, lending support to the idea that DNA could serve as a template for RNA synthesis. Second, cells that expressed large amounts of protein were known to contain large amounts of cytoplasmic RNA.

On the basis of this information, it was postulated that single-stranded DNA directs the synthesis of a complementary strand of either DNA (*replication*) or RNA (*transcription*). In turn, RNA directs the synthesis of proteins (*translation*), and the proteins ultimately regulate further replication and transcriptional events. The enzymes that catalyze the synthesis of DNA from nucleotide triphosphate precursors are termed *DNA polymerases*. They catalyze the formation of DNA in the presence of other single-strand DNA molecules that serve as templates. The DNA polymerases require a primer, a short DNA or RNA sequence that binds to the DNA template. Conversely, RNA polymerases make RNA and, while also requiring an existing DNA template, can initiate nucleic acid synthesis without the need for a primer.

There are three RNA polymerases active in eukaryotic cells. RNA polymerase II transcribes genes that are capable of encoding proteins as well as those encoding small nuclear RNAs. However, genes encoding the 28S (S refers to the rate of sedimentation of RNA in an ultracentrifuge), 18S, and 5.8S rRNAs are transcribed by RNA polymerase I, and those encoding the tRNAs and the 5S rRNA are transcribed by RNA polymerase III. Nucleic acid strand synthesis is unidirectional. All DNA chains and RNA chains grow in the 5′ (phosphate) to 3′ (hydroxyl) direction, as does translation.[1,9]

In 1966, it was determined that the genetic code used by all cells is a triplet code. That is, a sequence of three nucleotides determines a specific amino acid. Each triplet is called a *codon*, and 61 of a possible 64 codons code for specific amino acids, with several amino acids specified by more than 1 codon. The three combinations (UGA, UAG, and UAA) that do not code for amino acids code for *stop* or termination signals. The *start* or initiator codon is AUG; AUG also specifies the amino acid methionine, hence all proteins begin with this amino acid, with few exceptions. To distinguish the start signal from internally coded methionines, the start AUG is usually preceded by a purine-rich sequence. The sequence of nucleotides that runs from a specific start signal to a termination codon is termed a *reading frame*. In general, the majority of RNAs can only be read in one frame.[1,9]

A key element to the understanding of how mRNA is translated into a protein sequence lies in the structure and function of tRNA. The tRNAs have two functions; the first is to link to a particular amino acid, and the second is to recognize a specific triplet codon on the mRNA. This process is facilitated by specific enzymes termed *aa-tRNA synthetases* that recognize only one tRNA and only one amino acid, resulting in the linkage of a specific amino acid to a tRNA with a distinct anticodon. In this manner, once the tRNA is coupled to the correct amino acid, codon–anticodon pairing directs the tRNA to the proper site.

The translation of mRNA to protein requires an RNA–protein complex called the *ribosome*. There are three major RNA-binding sites on the ribosomal complex: the A-site (for aa-tRNA), the P-site (for peptidyl-tRNA), and a separate site for the mRNA (Fig. 3.13). During the translation of an RNA message into a protein, ribosomes move along the mRNA successively accepting aa-tRNAs, selecting them by matching the anticodons to the codon on the mRNA strand. Protein synthesis in eukaryotic cells is initiated by attachment of a free small ribosomal subunit to the 5′ cap of an mRNA (Fig. 3.14). As mentioned, this 5′ "cap" structure consists of a 7-methylguanosine residue linked to a triphosphate. The 5′ cap is followed by a variable-length leader sequence that is not translated into protein. In eukaryotes, the initiator tRNA must be loaded onto the small ribosomal subunit before this subunit can bind to the mRNA. The initiator tRNA is a special tRNA because it must be able to bind to the P-site on the ribosome, the site where normally only peptidyl-tRNA molecules can bind. The initiator tRNA always carries a methionine (met).

After cap recognition, the bound ribosome plus the initiator tRNA slide down the mRNA until the first downstream start signal is located, usually within the regulatory promoter region of the gene. The promoter region corresponds to the nucleotide sequence in the DNA to which the RNA

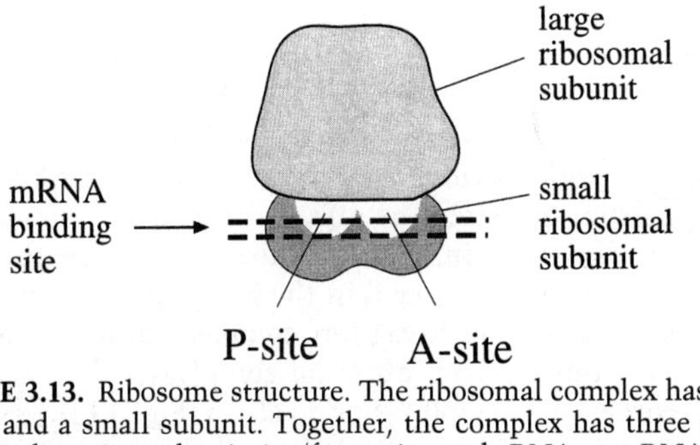

FIGURE 3.13. Ribosome structure. The ribosomal complex has both a large and a small subunit. Together, the complex has three major RNA-binding sites: the *A-site* (for aminoacyl-tRNA, aa-tRNA), the *P-site* (for peptidyl-tRNA), and a separate site for the mRNA.

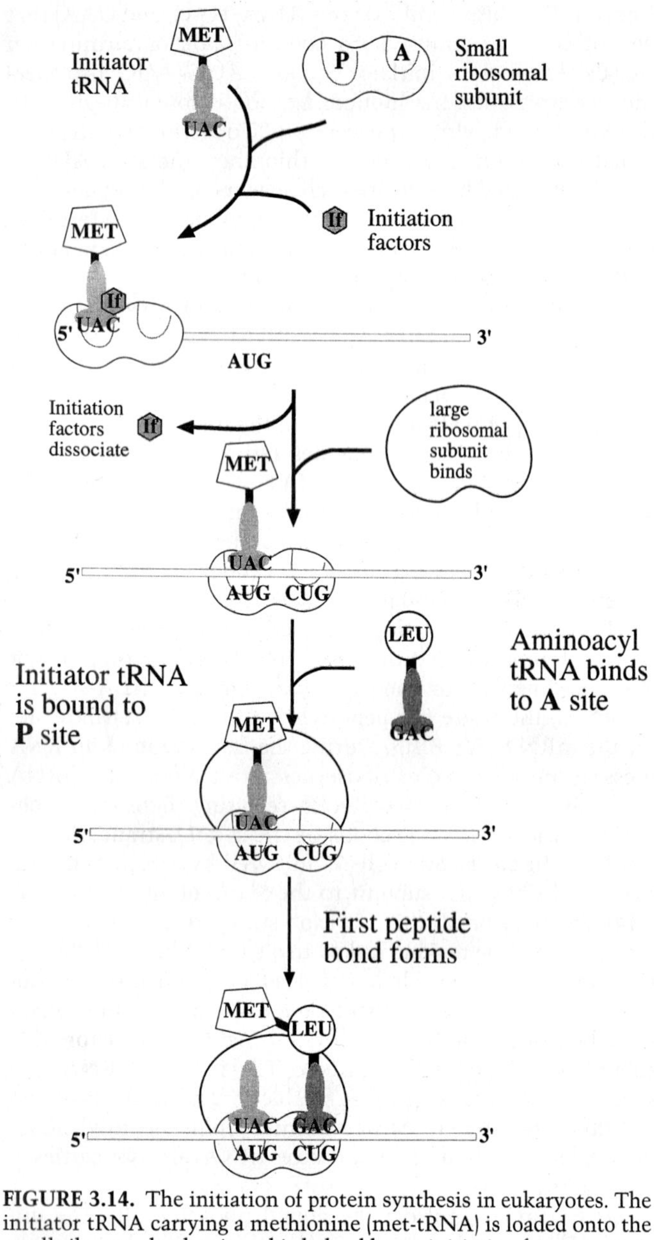

FIGURE 3.14. The initiation of protein synthesis in eukaryotes. The initiator tRNA carrying a methionine (met-tRNA) is loaded onto the small ribosomal subunit and is helped by an initiation factor to position itself correctly in the P-site. The initiator complex then identifies the 5′ cap of the mRNA, binds to it, and scans the mRNA for the start codon, *AUG*. When the initiator tRNA recognizes and binds the AUG, the initiation factors dissociate to make room for the large ribosomal subunit. There is now room in the A-site for the addition of an aminoacyl-tRNA.

polymerase binds to begin transcription. At the start site, the small ribosomal complex associates with a group of proteins called *eukaryotic initiation factors* (eIFs) that help the ribosome find the start site. The eIFs are required for translation initiation, discussed in more detail below. Once the met-tRNA is correctly positioned in the P-site, a large ribosomal complex binds to the initiation complex, forming the 80S initiation complex. The initiation complex is then ready to begin synthesis of the polypeptide chain (Fig. 3.15).

The growing polypeptide chain is always attached to the tRNA that brought in the last amino acid (located in the P-site). A new aa-tRNA binds to the A-site in the ribosome, a process catalyzed by proteins called *eukaryotic elongation factors* (eEFs). The eEFs position the aa-tRNA correctly in the A-site. The peptide chain is then transferred to the amino group of the newly arrived aa-tRNA, generating a peptidyl-tRNA that has acquired a new amino acid and is now bound to the A-site. The 80S ribosomal complex then moves to the next codon, shifting the peptidyl-tRNA to the P-site, vacating the A-site. This translocation is catalyzed by a separate elongation factor, eEF2, and the sequence of events is repeated as each amino acid is added to the peptide chain. Finally, the termination codon, in concert with termination factors, signals the release of the peptidyl-tRNA, which divides into the tRNA molecule and the new polypeptide chain.[1,9,10]

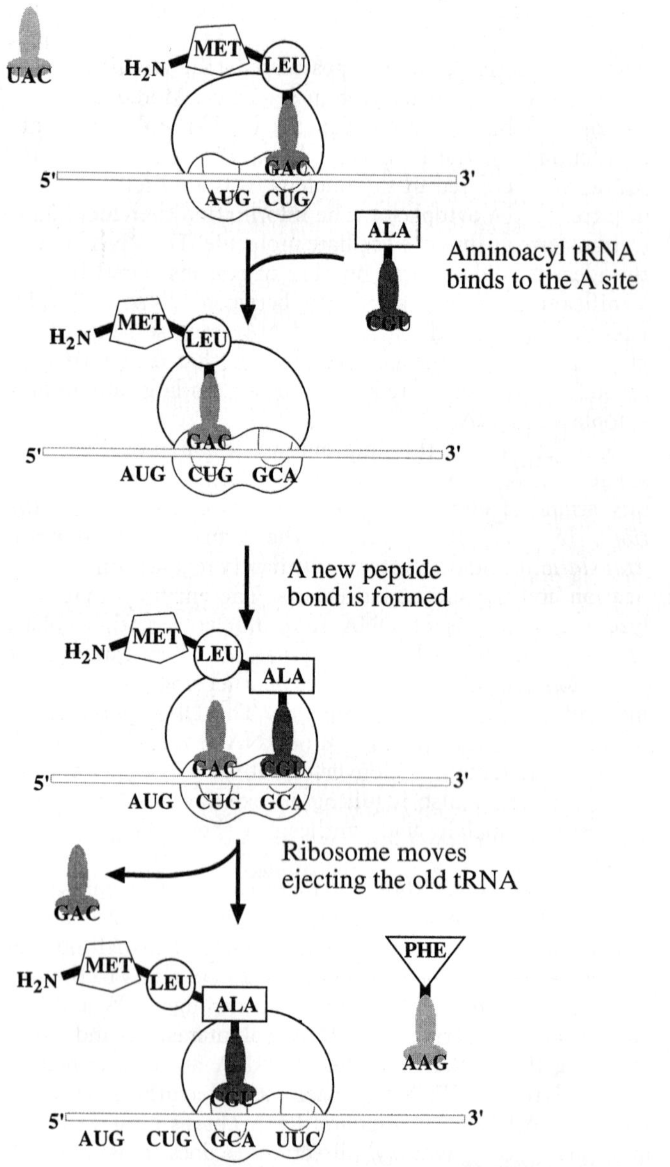

FIGURE 3.15. The elongation phase of protein synthesis in eukaryotes. An aminoacyl-tRNA binds to the A-site on the ribosome. A peptide bond is formed, and the peptide chain is transferred to the aminoacyl-tRNA in that site. The ribosome then shifts its position by three nucleotides, ejecting the old tRNA and resetting the ribosome so that the next aminoacyl-tRNA can bind.

Protein Function

As discussed in this chapter, appropriate folding is essential to proper protein function. However, the three-dimensional structure of a protein is not rigid. Structural modifications coupled to chemical events often result in changes in protein conformation. Depending on the conformational change, proteins may act as catalysts, as signaling machines, or as scaffolds on which multisubunit complexes can be assembled. Protein modification occurs through a number of different mechanisms, each having significantly different effects on protein function.

Perhaps the best described of these are ligand–receptor interactions. For example, the ligation of transmembrane cell-surface receptors known as integrins with their ECM ligands results in a conformational change in the cytoplasmic portion of the integrin receptor, leading to distinct intracellular signaling events. In this instance, the binding of one ligand to the extracellular domain of the receptor affects the binding of a second ligand to the intracellular portion of the receptor. The conformational coupling of two widely separated ligand-binding sites in this fashion is known as *allostery*, and this process can be cooperative or competitive. This type of linkage between ligands is a crucial regulatory mechanism in most cells and is especially prominent in enzymatic cascades.[1,9]

Protein phosphorylation is a common mechanism of controlling allosteric transitions in eukaryotic cells (Fig. 3.16A). The addition of a negatively charged phosphate group to target hydroxyl residues on serine, threonine, or tyrosine residues can lead to a conformational change in the protein that facilitates ligand binding at separate sites. The phosphates are transferred from ATP molecules by protein kinases and removed by protein phosphatases. Stimulation of diverse signaling cascades results in the sequential activation of multiple kinases in pathways that integrate cellular responses to external cues. Often, protein kinases have multiple phosphorylation sites that both positively and negatively regulate their function. Among the best-described protein kinase cascades are the highly conserved mitogen-activated protein kinase (MAPK) family. Another way that eukaryotic cells control protein activity via allosteric shape change is through GTP-binding proteins (Fig. 3.16B). They are also called GTPases because of their intrinsic ability to hydrolyze GTP and thus to convert from an active (GTP-bound) to an inactive (GDP-bound) conformation. Two structurally distinct classes of GTP-binding proteins are recognized: the monomeric GTP-binding proteins (also called monomeric GTPases), which consist of a single polypeptide chain, and the trimeric GTP-binding proteins (also called G proteins), which consist of three different subunits (Table 3.1). The activity of these proteins is controlled by nucleotide exchange. Switching from the inactive to active state is mediated by guanine nucleotide

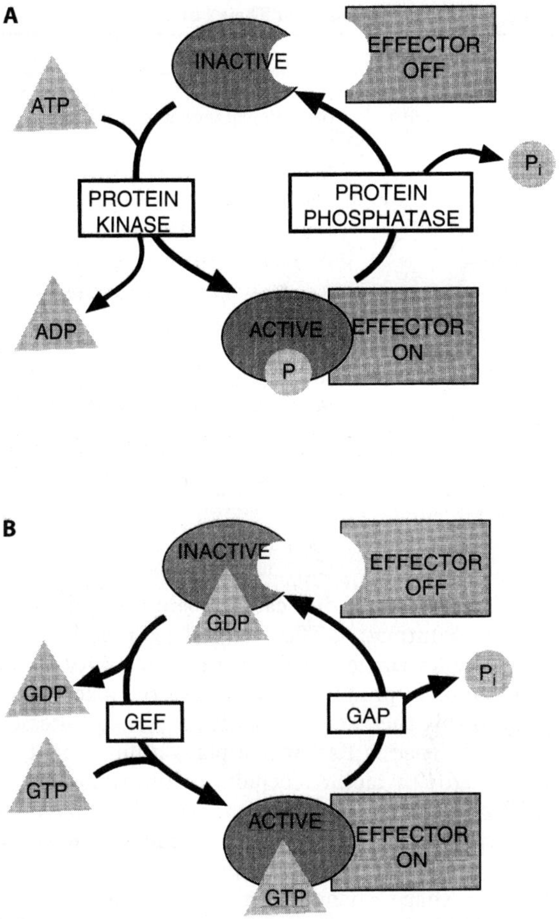

FIGURE 3.16. Allosteric changes in proteins are achieved through protein phosphorylation or by nucleotide exchange. **A.** Protein phosphorylation can control allosteric transitions in eukaryotic cells. The addition of negatively charged phosphate groups to target residues can change the conformation of a protein, leading to effector activation. The phosphates are transferred from ATP molecules by protein kinases and are removed by protein phosphatases. **B.** GTP-binding proteins behave as molecular switches. They cycle between an active (GTP-bound) and inactive (GDP-bound) state, with interconversion occurring by nucleotide exchange or by GTP hydrolysis.

TABLE 3.1. Selected GTP-Binding Proteins and Their Functions.

GTP-binding proteins	*Members*	*Function*
Ras superfamily GTPases	Ras, Ran, Rap, Ral, Rab, Arf, Rho, Rac, Cdc42	Ongogenic transformation, signal transduction, vesicle docking, regulation of cell morphology, actin organization, gene transcription, cell-cycle progression, apoptosis, tumor progression, activation of kinase cascades, membrane trafficking
Trimeric G proteins	G_s, G_{olf}, G_i, G_o, G_t, G_q	Activation/inhibition of adenyl cyclase, activation of Ca^+ and K^+ channels, activation of phospholipase C-β, and activation of cyclic GMP phosphodiesterase in vertebrate rod photoreceptors
Elongation factors	Ef-1, Ef-tu	Kinetic proofreading mechanism for selection of correct tRNA molecule in protein synthesis

TABLE 3.2. Selected ATPases and Their Functions.

ATPase	*Function*
Na^+–K^+ ATPase	Acts as a Na^+/K^+ pump; maintains osmotic balance and stabilizes cell volume
Ca^{2+} ATPase	Maintains cellular calcium gradient and regulates muscle contraction
Kinesin, dynein	Regulate vesicular transport
ATP synthetase	Regulates ATP synthesis
Myosin	Regulates muscle contraction
Uncoating ATPase	Removes the coat from clathrin-coated vesicles
Vacuolar H^+ ATPase	Acidifies all exocytic and endocytic organelles, including phagosomes, lysosomes, selected compartments of the Golgi apparatus, and many transport vesicles

exchange factors (GEFs) that catalyze the exchange of GDP for GTP. In contrast, GTPase-activating proteins (GAPs) accelerate the intrinsic GTP hydrolytic activity of GTP-binding proteins to promote formation of the inactive, GDP-bound form of the protein. Perhaps the quintessential monomeric GTPase is Ras, which plays a fundamental role in coupling growth factor receptors to intracellular signals required for cell growth and differentiation. Data have linked Ras activation in mammalian cells to the MAPK signaling cascade, a primary downstream target.

Allosteric shape changes can also be coupled to ATP hydrolysis (Table 3.2). In this fashion, a series of conformational changes can be made unidirectional, a functional requirement of cellular motor proteins such as myosin, to generate orderly movement. Besides generating mechanical force, allosteric proteins use ATP hydrolysis to do other forms of work, such as acting as ion pumps when membrane bound.

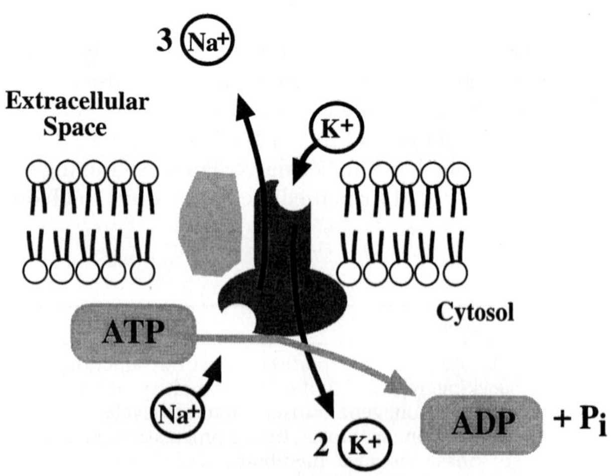

FIGURE 3.17. Hydrolysis of ATP can be used by membrane proteins to establish ion gradients. The Na^+–K^+ ATPase pumps Na^+ out of the cell in exchange for K^+ in a 3:2 ratio for every molecule of ATP that is hydrolyzed. The ion gradient that is established can then be used to drive other membrane-bound transport pumps, such as those that transport glucose and amino acids into the cell in exchange for sodium.

An example of this is Na^+–K^+ ATPase, which pumps Na^+ out of the cell in exchange for K^+ in a 3:2 ratio, thus keeping the Na^+ concentration inside the cell lower than the outside and the K^+ concentration inside the cell higher than the outside (Fig. 3.17). These ion gradients are then used to drive other plasma membrane-bound transport pumps, such as those that exchange glucose and amino acids transported into the cell for sodium transported out of the cell.[1,9]

Control of Cellular Activity

There are about 200 distinct cell types in an adult human being. All these several hundred different cell types share a core of "housekeeping" proteins necessary for metabolism and replication; these include some abundant proteins, such as those of the cytoskeleton, the major histone and nonhistone chromosomal proteins, proteins essential to the ER and Golgi membranes, the proteins of the nuclear lamina, RNA-packaging proteins, ribosomal proteins, and so on. Many of the different enzymes involved in metabolism are also similar in different cell types. Different cell types, however, also express different subsets of the total protein-coding capacity of the genome. For example, hemoglobin is only expressed in red blood cells, although the DNA sequences that code for this protein are present in all mammalian cells. Each of these 200 different cell types contains exactly the same DNA, yet each cell type expresses distinct structural, chemical, and functional characteristics.

How then do cells become specialized? This generation of cellular diversity is known as *differentiation*, a highly programmed, temporal pattern of gene activation and gene repression. A process involving the covert commitment of cells to a particular fate or set of fates precedes this overt change in cellular biochemistry and function. Here, the cell does not appear phenotypically different from its uncommitted state, but somehow its developmental state has been restricted. This control is accomplished by the regulation of gene expression.

Regulation of Gene Expression

As noted, there are many steps in the pathway leading from DNA transcription to polypeptide synthesis. Thus, control of protein synthesis can be achieved at a number of checkpoints (Fig. 3.18). For the vast majority of cells, the primary control of gene expression is at the level of transcription. However, there are a number of posttranscriptional steps at which eukaryotic gene expression can be controlled. For example, variations in RNA processing can modulate *RNA splicing* (alternative splicing), thus allowing the generation of two closely related mRNAs and, in turn, types of proteins from the same primary RNA transcript. Alternatively, RNA stability can be regulated via proteins that bind to the 5′- and 3′-untranslated regions (UTRs) of the mRNA. Cases in which RNA stability is regulated are often those for which rapid and transient availability of the protein is required. Similarly, RNA translational control can select specific mRNAs for transport to the cytoplasm or, once in the cytoplasm, for translation by the ribosomal complex. In general, translational control mechanisms supplement the regulation of gene expression by transcription.[1,9]

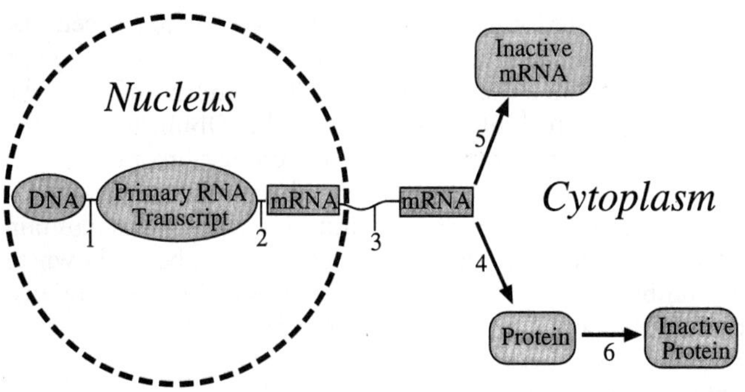

FIGURE 3.18. Eukaryotic gene expression can be controlled at multiple sites. A cell can control the proteins that it makes through a variety of mechanisms. It can control (1) when and how often a gene is transcribed, (2) how the primary RNA transcript is processed, (3) the transport of the mRNA transcripts out of the nucleus, (4) the selection of transcripts for translation, (5) the stability of the mRNA transcript, and (6) the activation of the protein. Transfer time through the cells is quite short, lasting perhaps 20h.

Transcriptional Regulation of Gene Expression

The regulation of gene activity at the transcriptional level has been generally thought to take place through the interaction of gene regulatory proteins called *transcription factors* with specific DNA sequences adjacent to the gene. Eukaryotic RNA polymerase II, for example, requires general transcription factors that must be assembled at the promoter before transcription can occur. These transcription factors must be assembled in a particular order and require binding to a short DNA regulatory sequence, the TATA box, found upstream of almost all RNA polymerase-binding sites. Additional regulatory sequences for the binding of gene regulatory proteins can be found thousands of base pairs away from the start site. Binding sites that activate transcription are termed *enhancer sequences.* Proteins that bind to these sites contain domains that interact with both the enhancer DNA sequence and one of the general transcription factors in the promoter region or with the RNA polymerase itself. Thus, DNA binding, although necessary for transcriptional activation, is not sufficient. A protein that negatively regulates transcription is termed a transcriptional *repressor.* These factors can act either by binding to DNA, thus displacing or preventing the binding of a positive factor, or by directly blocking the transcription machinery. Alternatively, a repressor can bind an activator so that it can no longer enhance transcription.[9,25]

Transcription factors are regulated by distinct mechanisms. For example, factors may be regulated by tissue-specific expression. MyoD is one example of an essential transcriptional activator of muscle-specific genes that is required throughout myogenesis and is found only in muscle tissue. Gene regulatory proteins may also exist in a tissue but be nonfunctioning until a tissue-specific stimulus modifies the protein through conformational change, either through ligand binding or by covalent modification. For example, steroid binding to the glucocorticoid receptor displaces the receptor from heat-shock protein 90, facilitating its movement from the cytosol to the nucleus to activate transcription.

The mammalian CREB (cyclic adenosine 5′-monophosphate [cAMP]-responsive element binding) factor is activated once it is phosphorylated by protein kinase A (PKA), which in turn is activated by binding of cAMP to its regulatory subunit. Phosphorylation also regulates the activation of nuclear factor kappa beta (NF-κB) in response to a variety of stimuli. However, it is the phosphorylation of an associated protein, I-κB (inhibitor of NF-κB), that leads to transcriptional activation. The NF-κB is bound in the cytoplasm to I-κB in an inactive complex. Phosphorylation of I-κB leads to the release of NF-κB from this complex so that NF-κB can translocate to the nucleus to activate gene expression.[25,26] Evidence has indicated that controlling the balance of nuclear import and export of transcription factors may be a common mechanism for regulating transcriptional activation. Examples of transcription factors that may be regulated by nucleocytoplasmic shuttling include signal transducer and activator of transcription 1 (STAT1), adenomatous polyposis coli (APC) protein, and the sry box (SOX) family of developmental transcription factors.[27]

Interactions between DNA and transcription factors are very specific. Typically, DNA-binding proteins contain one of a small set of DNA-binding structural motifs that use either β-sheets or α-helices. The *helix-turn-helix* motif is one of the most common DNA-binding motifs and is characterized by the homeobox proteins in *Drosophila.* It is composed of two α-helices linked by a short amino acid sequence in which the carboxy-terminal α-helix serves as the DNA-binding domain. Other motifs include the *zinc finger motif,* which also uses an α-helix to recognize the major groove of DNA but requires a zinc molecule as a structural element. The DNA-binding proteins that contain the zinc finger motif include TFIIIA, Egr I, and Spl. In addition, the steroid thyroid hormone receptor gene family also encodes proteins with a DNA-binding region that contains a zinc finger motif (Table 3.3).

Most gene regulatory proteins recognize DNA as *dimers.* The ability of selected transcription factors to dimerize provides an additional mechanism of gene regulation by these proteins (see Table 3.3). For example, two identical proteins with identical recognition sequences can form *homodimers,* but proteins with different DNA-binding specificities can also form dimers (*heterodimers*). Often, the homodimers and heterodimers recognize distinct sequences or have different gene

TABLE 3.3. Transcription Factor Domains.

Domain	*Role*	*Factors containing domain*
Cysteine-histidine zinc finger	DNA binding	TFIIIA, SP1, Egr1, MK1, MK2, Evi1
Cysteine-cysteine zinc finger	DNA binding	Nuclear hormone receptor family
Leucine zippers	Protein dimerization	C/EBP, Jun B, Jun, Fos, Fra 1, c-myc, n-myc
Helix-loop-helix	Protein dimerization	c-myc, Myo D

Source: Data from Latchman.[25]

activation properties. For example, c-*fos* and c-*jun* are transcription factors that form dimers. A c-*jun* homodimer binds to the AP-1 transcription site but not a c-*fos* homodimer, whereas a c-*jun*–c-*fos* heterodimer binds to AP-1 with 30-fold greater affinity when compared to the c-*jun* homodimer. Gene regulatory proteins that form dimers contain distinct structural motifs, such as the *leucine zipper motif*, so-called because of the way the α-helices from each monomer interdigitate via leucine-rich regions on the respective helices. The DNA-binding proteins that contain the leucine zipper motif include c/EBP, jun B, c-*jun*, Gcn 4, c-*fos*, Fra 1, c-*myc*, and n-*myc*. The basic *helix-loop-helix* (HLH) motif plays a similar role to the leucine zipper in mediating protein dimerization. These transcription factors are composed of two α-helices connected by a flexible loop. One helix mediates DNA binding; the other interacts with the HLH motif of another protein. The HLH proteins are prevalent in muscle development and include members of the transcription activator family, *MyoD*. Homodimerization of MyoD leads to muscle-specific gene transcription. However, MyoD can also dimerize with a helix-turn-helix protein, Id, which lacks the α-helical extension required for DNA binding. The MyoD–Id heterodimer is unable to bind DNA (Id acts as a transcriptional repressor in this instance). This example illustrates how heterodimerization can be used to both positively and negatively regulate transcription activation.[1,13]

The direct regulation of transcription factor expression or activity is not the sole method of transcriptional regulation. Rather, biological control of transcription may also occur via the modulation of transcriptional coactivators, proteins that dock on transcription factors to allow transcription to take place. Transcriptional coactivators have been shown in some settings to be the primary targets of developmental or biological signals. Coactivators function in a variety of ways but can generally be segregated into three classes. One class of proteins modifies histones to improve the access of other proteins to the DNA. These include p300 and CBP, powerful HATs. A second class of proteins binds to transcription factors and recruits RNA polymerase II to facilitate transcription. Examples of these include members of the TRAP/DRIP/Mediator/ARC complex. The final class of proteins contain DNA unwinding activities that, by improving access of transcription factors to the DNA, create more efficient gene transcription. Transcriptional corepressors have the opposite activity, making the DNA less accessible to transcription factors. These proteins are often associated with HDAC activity.[28]

Silencing of gene transcription can occur through DNA methylation, which is a covalent chemical modification of DNA that results in the addition of a methyl (CH_3) group at the carbon 5 position of the cytosine ring. Most DNA methylation occurs in the sequence context of 5′CG3′, also called the CpG dinucleotide. The DNA methylation is brought about by a group of enzymes known as the *DNA methyltransferases*, of which there are currently eight isoforms identified. Methylation can occur both de novo (when CpG dinucleotides on both DNA strands are unmethylated) and as maintenance (when the CpG dinucleotide on one strand is already methylated). Mice deficient in these enzymes die early in development or shortly after birth. In addition to DNA methyltransferases, the other mechanisms for the regulation of methylation include demethylases, methylation centers that trigger DNA methylation, and methylation protection centers. In the promoter region of target genes, DNA methylation can effectively silence transcription, both by interfering with the binding of transcription factors to the DNA and by the specific binding of transcriptional repressors to methylated regions of the DNA. For example, the transcription factors, AP-1, CREB, and NF-κB recognize sequences that contain CpG sequences, and the binding of each has been shown to be inhibited by methylation. In addition, the methyl-CpG-binding domain (MBD) proteins are transcriptional repressors. Hypermethylation of a number of genes has been associated with oncogenic transformation.[29]

Translational Regulation of Gene Expression

The final step in protein synthesis, the translation of mRNA into protein, is regulated by a variety of biological signals. Two general mechanisms of translational control of protein expression have been described. The first involves the global regulation of translation and usually requires the modification of translation-initiation factors that serve as the rate-limiting step in the translation process. The second method involves the specific regulation of individual mRNAs. This commonly occurs via an interaction between regulatory elements in either the 5′- or 3′-UTRs of the mRNA and specific protein or RNA complexes that target these elements. Plus, there are a variety of structural features of the mRNA that contribute to its translational fate.

Regulation of Translation Initiation

Translation initiation is a complicated event that requires the formation of a large, multiprotein complex. The first step in the process is the binding of a small (40S) ribosomal subunit to the 5′ end of the mRNA, which then scans the mRNA until the initiation codon is identified. This small rRNA is joined by the eIFs to form a 43S preinitiation complex. This complex includes the initiator tRNA attached to methionine. The eIFs that are important to this process include (1) the eIF4E that associates with the 5′ cap structure, (2) the eIF4A that contains RNA helicase activity, and (3) the eIF4G that binds to eIF4E and functions as a scaffold for the recruitment of other eIFs. Together, they form part of the eIF4F translation initiation complex that regulates cap-dependent protein translation. Other eIFs serve important roles by providing the energy source to catalyze the addition of the 60S subunit. For example, eIF2 joins the complex bound to GTP, which is then hydrolyzed to enable the formation of an "elongation-competent" 80S ribosome at the site of the initiation codon.[30]

Global control of mRNA translation usually occurs by changes in the phosphorylation status of the eIFs or their regulators. For example, phosphorylation of the α-subunit of the GTP-donor, eIF2 (eIF2α), blocks GTP-GDP exchange, resulting in the inhibition of translation. Similarly, phosphorylation can modulate the binding of regulatory proteins called 4E-binding proteins (4E-BPs; also called PHAS-1) to the cap complex. These proteins, when hypophosphorylated, disrupt the association between eIF4E and eIF4G, halting translation. The phosphorylation of 4E-BPs frees them from eIF4E, allowing the eIF4E–eIF4G interaction to occur and translation to proceed.[31]

Mammalian Target of Rapamycin and Surgical Disease

One of the key regulators of cell growth and proliferation is the mammalian target of rapamycin (mTOR) pathway. Much of the information regarding mTOR is derived from use of the drug rapamycin (also referred to as sirolimus), a specific inhibitor of mTOR that has significant immunosuppressive properties. Rapamycin inhibits cell growth through its interaction with a cellular receptor called FKBP12. Screens performed in yeast to identify mutants resistant to rapamycin identified two genes, *TOR1* and *TOR2*, which have a single mammalian homologue, mTOR (also known as RAFT, FRAP, and RAPT).[32,33]

The mTOR belongs to a family of phosphoinositide kinase-related kinases that contain a lipid kinase-like domain. However, mTOR functions only as a serine-threonine kinase and does not contain lipid kinase activity. The rapamycin/FKBP12 complex binds to the amino-terminus of mTOR at a site that flanks the mTOR kinase domain and that has been identified as an FKBP12-rapamycin-binding (FRB) domain. As a consequence, mTOR signaling is inhibited. One affected downstream target of mTOR includes 4E-BP1, an important regulator of translation initiation. For example, in times of nutrient sufficiency, mTOR-mediated signaling results in 4E-BP1 becoming highly phosphorylated and dissociating from eIF4E. An additional target of mTOR is the elongation factor eEF2, a GTP-binding protein that mediates the translocation step of peptide-chain elongation. The mTOR signaling regulates a kinase that phosphorylates eEF2 and inhibits the translocation step. In these capacities, mTOR may function as a sensor for nutrient and energy levels in the cell. Dysregulation of mTOR signaling has been implicated in oncogenic transformation, intimal hyperplasia, and cardiac hypertrophy.[32,33]

Control of Translation by RNA Interference

In 1998, initial studies performed in *Caenorhabditis elegans* demonstrated that double-stranded RNA (dsRNA) that was homologous to a specific gene could induce effective post-transcriptional gene-specific silencing. Preliminary attempts to use dsRNA in mammalian systems were initially unsuccessful, primarily because the use of long dsRNA triggered activation of the interferon system. As a consequence, protein translation was inhibited, leading to cellular apoptosis. However, elucidation of the mechanism of action of dsRNA soon revealed the extraordinary potential of small interfering RNA (siRNA).

It is now known that gene silencing occurs via two main steps. The first step in the RNA interference (RNAi) pathway involves the processing of large dsRNA molecules into short (21–23 bp) siRNA molecules. An RNAase III enzyme that recognizes and cleaves the dsRNA is Dicer, a highly conserved enzyme found in diverse species, including yeast, *Drosophila*, mice, and humans. Following the cleavage of dsRNA into siRNAs, the second important stage of mRNA degradation occurs. Hammond et al.[34] demonstrated that RNAi ablates target mRNAs through the generation of a sequence-specific nuclease activity. They termed the enzyme responsible for this activity RISC (RNA-induced silencing complex); RISC is guided to its mRNA target by siRNAs containing homologous sequence. Subsequently, the mechanism of action of RISC has been determined, and it exists in both an active and an inactive form. Although RISC requires double-stranded siRNA, unwinding of the siRNA is required for RISC activation. Then, active RISC associates with the antisense form of the siRNA. These data suggest that the RISC–siRNA complex has ATP-dependent helicase activity or that a helicase enzyme is associated with RISC.[35,36]

To apply RNAi methodology to mammalian cells, gene silencing had to be induced without long dsRNA. Once it was determined that siRNAs targeted mRNA degradation via RISC, small synthetic siRNAs (21–22 bp) were used to bypass the Dicer enzyme. Synthetic siRNAs have now been used successfully to elicit strong suppression of gene expression in mammalian cells both in vitro and in vivo. The short half-life of siRNAs led to the development of short hairpin RNAs (shRNAs). Briefly, shRNAs are generated from expression cassettes composed of the eukaryotic polymerase III promoter followed by the sense strand of the siRNA followed by a spacer and then the antisense strand, which ended in a series of 5 U residues. The spacer sequence permitted the sense and antisense strands to anneal, forming a hairpin RNA molecule that has a longer half-life and can be continuously synthesized. This system has demonstrated potent gene suppression in mammalian cells. The availability of libraries of shRNA expression cassettes has created a powerful tool for the genetic manipulation of mammalian cells.[35]

Small endogenously produced regulatory RNAs have been implicated in the control of translation. Termed microRNAs (miRNAs), these sequences derive from original transcripts. Their features are very close in structure to siRNA but are believed to act by translational repression rather than by inducing RNA degradation. They bind to sequences in the 3′ UTR of the target mRNA. However, the mechanism of translational repression is not known.[37]

The Cell Cycle

The eukaryotic cell cycle is divided into four stages or phases: G_1, S, G_2, and M. The most dramatic of these phases is the *M* or *mitotic phase.* It is during the M phase that the nucleus divides and cytokinesis occurs. The period between successive M phases is known as *interphase.* A nondividing or interphase cell is not a resting cell, as it is sometimes described, because during this period the cell carries out all the normal activities (growth, respiration, protein synthesis, etc.) of the cell with the exception of division. It is thus only "resting" from the actual process of division.

The interphase period may be subdivided into three recognizable stages as follows. In actively dividing cells, the actual division process (M phase) may take 1 or 2 h, the G_1 phase approximately 8 h, the S phase about 6 h, and the G_2 phase about 4 to 5 h. Thus, the total cell cycle (period from one division to the next) in actively dividing cells is quite short, lasting perhaps 20 h.

The significant events that occur within the G_1, S, and G_2 phases are as follows. In the *G_1 phase*, the chromosomes decondense. At this point, the cells become biochemically active, synthesizing proteins needed for the replication and subsequent segregation of DNA. Here, normal cells must decide whether to remain quiescent or to proliferate. Cellular proliferation requires activation of various biomolecular signals, such as the cyclin-dependent kinases (Cdks), transcription factors, and phosphorylation of the retinoblastoma protein. Once a cell becomes committed to proliferation, this biochemical programming becomes irreversible, and the cell progresses into the *S phase*.

Within dividing cells, the S phase is critical because this is the period during which the DNA is replicated in preparation for the next division. Histones and nonhistone proteins are deposited on the daughter DNA molecules to reproduce the chromatin structures. Replication of DNA in eukaryotes is semiconservative. Each DNA strand acts as a template for the synthesis of a new DNA molecule by the sequential addition of complementary base pairs, thereby generating a new DNA strand that is the complementary sequence to the parental DNA. Each daughter DNA molecule ends up with one of the original strands and one newly synthesized strand.[1,2,4,10]

Eukaryotic DNA replication begins with the denaturation of the DNA double helix followed by the assembly of short RNA primer molecules by the action of an enzyme, DNA primase, and the semiconservative replication of the DNA. Initiation of DNA replication occurs at specific sites or origins (mouse chromosomes may contain as many as 25,000 origins) on the chromosome where the double helix denatures into single strands. The precise nature of eukaryotic origins is still somewhat obscure, although sequences have been identified that appear to be essential for replication of plasmid sequences in yeast. They are called autonomously replicating sequences (ARSs).[1,2,4,10]

Topoisomerases and helicases facilitate the unwinding of DNA during replication, the activity of these enzymes increasing as cells enter the S phase of the cell cycle. The DNA helicases move rapidly along single-stranded DNA. When they encounter a region of double helix, they continue to move along their strand, thereby prying apart the helix. Single-stranded DNA-binding (SSB) proteins aid helicases by stabilizing the unwound, single-stranded DNA. The SSB proteins also coat single-stranded regions on the lagging strand, thereby preventing formation of hairpin helices that would otherwise impede synthesis by DNA polymerase. Replication proceeds bidirectionally, and the DNA double helix opens to expose single strands that act as templates for new DNA synthesis. A Y-shaped structure forms when a double-stranded DNA molecule unwinds to expose the two single-stranded templates. This structure is called a *replication fork*.

Replication of DNA is catalyzed by DNA polymerase. Four different polymerases, designated α, β, γ, and δ, have been identified, although only DNA polymerases α and δ are responsible for nuclear DNA replication. Both can use RNA primers for the initiation of DNA replication. The fidelity of "copying" is such that only about 1 error is made in 10^9 base-pair replications. This high fidelity of DNA replication depends on "proofreading" mechanisms that act to remove errors. The exact nature of proofreading proteins in eukaryotes is as yet unclear; however, several eukaryotic proteins have been discovered that are homologous in their amino acid sequence to several bacterial mismatch proofreading enzymes.[1,2,4,10]

Cells that complete the S phase almost always enter the G_2 phase and proceed into cell division. Cells not destined to divide again (e.g., certain epithelial cells, nerve cells, differentiated muscle cells) stop in the G_1 phase and never enter the S phase. It is in the G_1 phase that the cell carries out the normal metabolic processes for that particular cell type. Cells that complete the G_2 phase enter the M (mitotic) phase of the cell cycle.[1,2,4,10]

Mitosis is nuclear division plus *cytokinesis* and produces two identical daughter cells. Mitosis consists of four stages: prophase, metaphase, anaphase, and telophase. During *prophase*, chromatin in the nucleus begins to condense and becomes visible in the light microscope as chromosomes. In *metaphase*, spindle fibers of the developing spindle apparatus penetrate into the region originally occupied by the nucleus and align the chromosomes along the equator of the spindle. During *anaphase*, the paired chromosomes separate at the centromeres, thereby generating two individual chromosomes. The beginning of *telophase* is marked by the arrival of the two sets of chromosomes at opposite poles of the spindle. Cytokinesis, or division of the cytoplasm, also begins during this stage.

Cell-Cycle Regulation

Most molecular mechanisms that control a cell's progress through the cell cycle regulate initiation of the S phase or of mitosis. These regulatory mechanisms operate by using molecular brakes that can stop the cell cycle at one of several checkpoints, effectively keeping the cell cycle from progressing until a stage has been completed. These checkpoints are also points where the control system becomes regulated by signals from other cells. The G_1 checkpoint regulates passage into the S phase and checks for cell size, environment, and DNA damage. Only cells that are competent to progress through the rest of the cell cycle are allowed to proceed. The G_2 checkpoint is the gate for passage into mitosis. Cells here must be of a certain size and must have stockpiled all the necessary components to undergo DNA replication. Both these transitions are regulated by heterodimeric protein kinases composed of a catalytic subunit and a regulatory subunit that contributes to substrate specificity. The regulatory subunits are called *cyclins* because the concentrations of most of them cycle in phase with the cell cycle. The protein kinase activity of the catalytic subunits depends on their association with cyclin, leading to the name *cyclin-dependent kinases*, or Cdks. When activated, these Cdk–cyclin heterodimers phosphorylate multiple different proteins, activating some and inhibiting others, to control the many molecular events associated with DNA replication and mitosis.

Mitosis-promoting factor (MPF) is the cyclin–Cdk complex that controls entry into M phase; it regulates the activity of a large number of other proteins by phosphorylating them. For example, MPF causes chromosomes to condense and the nuclear envelope to break down by phosphorylating lamins. Phosphorylation of MAPs causes reorganization of microtubules to form the mitotic spindle. Two independent processes control Cdk-cyclin activity: (1) phosphorylation of Cdk and (2) proteolysis of cyclins.[1,2,4,10]

How does this system get shut off? Initiation of mitosis results in the activation of a number of genes with protein products that are enzymes that add the ubiquitin peptide to cyclin. This "tags" the cyclin for degradation via the proteosome pathway. The rapid drop in cyclin concentration results in a corresponding drop in Cdk–cyclin enzyme activity.[1,2,4,10]

Cell Death

Programmed cell death, or *apoptosis*, is a process that is important to all multicellular organisms. It regulates cell number and tissue size by balancing cell proliferation with cell death. Cells undergoing apoptosis shrink and condense. Their cytoskeleton collapses, their nuclear envelope disassembles, the nuclear DNA fragments, and the cell surface becomes altered. Apoptotic cells are then rapidly recognized and phagocytosed by neighboring cells, with little residual debris. By contrast, cell death from accidental causes leads to cell swelling and lysis, triggering an inflammatory response in the surrounding tissue. Defects in the apoptotic mechanism have been implicated in a wide variety of disease processes, from the systemic inflammatory response syndrome (SIRS) to cancer, and thus the study of the regulation of this pathway has received enormous attention.

The apoptotic machinery of a cell is produced constitutively. However, survival signals from the cell keep activation of the death program in check. In the event that the cell detaches from its environment or suffers irreversible damage, apoptosis is initiated. For example, DNA damage often leads to the accumulation and activation of the tumor suppressor protein p53. Activation of p53 either leads to growth arrest or directs cells to the apoptotic pathway. Although the mechanisms by which p53 promotes apoptosis are not completely understood, they involve the transcriptional activation or repression of specific target genes that lead to the activation of the apoptotic pathway. For example, p53 controls transcription of proapoptotic members of the Bcl-2 family such as Bax and Bid; p53 may exert transcriptional control on regulatory proteins in the intrinsic apoptotic pathway, including Apaf-1 and caspase-6. Finally, p53 also targets survival signaling by positively regulating the expression of protein tyrosine phosphatase (PTEN), a lipid phosphatase that antagonizes prosurvival signals generated by phosphatidyl inositol 3-kinase (PI 3-kinase).[38]

The morphological appearance of apoptotic cells relies on the activation of a family of proteases. First identified in the nematode *C. elegans*, members of the cell death abnormal (CED) gene family have been found to encode a family of ubiquitously expressed cysteine proteases that cleave their protein target at specific aspartic acid residues and are called *caspases*.[39,40] To date, 14 mammalian caspase family members have been described, of which at least 7 have been implicated in apoptosis (Table 3.4).

TABLE 3.4. Caspases and Their Regulators.

Group	*Caenorhabditis elegans proteins*	*Mammalian proteins*
Initiator caspase	Ced-3	Caspase (2), -8, -9, -10
Effector caspase	?	Caspase (2), -3, -4, -5, -6, -7, -11, -12, -13
Caspase activator	Ced-4	Apaf-1, FADD, RAIDD
Antiapoptotic Bcl-2 homologue	Ced-9	Bcl-2, Bcl-x_L, Bcl-w, Mcl-1

Source: Data from Latchman.[25]

Typically, a caspase molecule is transcribed as a single polypeptide chain that exists as a large inactive precursor in the cytosol and is composed of a large, variable-length, amino-terminal prodomain; a large subunit; and a small subunit. Proapoptotic signals lead to the activation of the procaspase by enzymatic cleavage, often through the action of an associated, initiator caspase. Proteolytic processing separates the three domains, removing the predomain and allowing the two subunits to form a heterodimer. The active caspase is a tetramer composed of two heterodimers. The prodomains are important because they contain regions that regulate the interaction of the caspase with other proteins, targeting them either to the activating death receptor at the cell membrane or to an assembled caspase-activating apparatus in the cytoplasm.

Once activated, caspases cleave other specific proteins in the cell, which serve both to initiate and to directly cause the destruction of the cell (Table 3.5). These so-called death substrates include proteins involved in RNA splicing, DNA repair, and scaffolding of the cytosol and nucleus. Caspases are also known to cleave proteins involved in the maintenance of cell–ECM and cell–cell attachment and to inactivate proteins that function to protect the cell from apoptosis, such as Bcl-2.

TABLE 3.5. Selected Caspase Substrates.

Death substrate	*Function*
Structural proteins Gelsolin Gas-2	Caspase cleavage of the cytoskeletal protein gelsolin and the microfilament protein; Gas-2 induces actin filament disruption
Nuclear lamins	Lamin cleavage induces disassembly of the nucleus
DNA degradation CAD (caspase-activated deoxyribonuclease)	Caspases cleave the inhibitor of CAD, ICAD
Antiapoptotic proteins Bcl-2 Bcl-x_L	Caspase cleavage of Bcl-2 proteins transforms them into proapoptotic molecules
Kinases PAK2 PKC-δ PKC-ν MEKK-1	Caspase cleavage generates a constitutively active kinase resulting in nuclear/cytoplasmic condensation, cellular detachment, and phosphatidyl serine externalization (?? mechanism)

Source: Data from Cryns and Yuan.[39]

The inhibition of caspase function, while preventing the appearance of apoptosis, does not always rescue the cell from the apoptotic pathway and cell death. These data suggest that caspases can be divided into two groups: upstream or "initiator" caspases, which include caspases 2, 8, 9, and 10, and downstream or "effector" caspases, which include caspases 3, 6, and 7 (Fig. 3.19). Initiator caspases contain regions in their prodomains that target them to the plasma membrane, where they are activated as a result of cell-surface-receptor signaling events such as those mediated by the "death receptors" of the tumor necrosis factor-α (TNF-α) superfamily.[41–43] Interestingly, the substrate cleavage preferences for these initiator caspases correspond to the sites of proteolytic activation in several downstream caspases. The activation of effector caspases is carried out by an initiator caspase and is responsible for the cleavage of proteins that leads to cell destruction. The substrate cleavage preferences for these effector caspases correspond to the sites of proteolytic activation in the majority of known apoptotic substrates.

The activation of the apoptotic response occurs through two distinct pathways, designated intrinsic or extrinsic

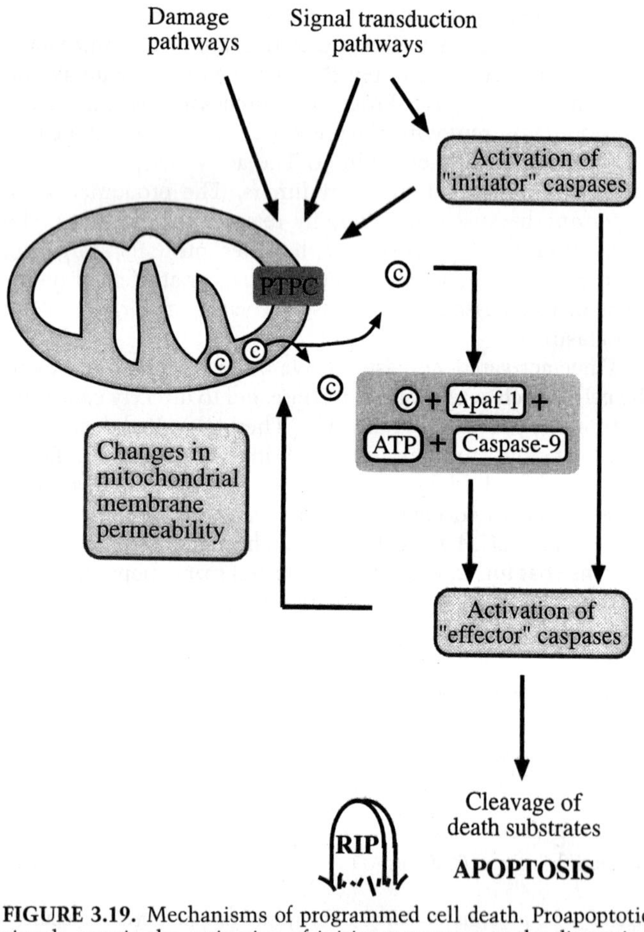

FIGURE 3.19. Mechanisms of programmed cell death. Proapoptotic signals act via the activation of initiator caspases or the disruption of mitochondrial membrane integrity. Mitochondrial membrane collapse leads to the release of cytochrome *c* into the cytoplasm. Once there, cytochrome *c* binds to *Apaf-1* (apoptotic protease-activating factor-1), caspase-9, and ATP to form a complex, referred to as the *vertebrate apoptosome*, that activates pro-caspase-3; this results in the activation of downstream caspases, leading to substrate cleavage. In contrast, the activation of initiator caspases by "death receptors" leads directly to the activation of effector caspases.

depending on the origin of the death stimulus. With the intrinsic pathway, the proapoptotic signal causes the release of proapoptotic proteins from the mitochondria, leading to mitochondrial membrane collapse, membrane depolarization, and the release of proapoptotic proteins from the mitochondria into the cytoplasm. These proteins include cytochrome *c*, SMAC (second mitochondria-derived activator of caspases)/ DIABLO (direct inhibitor of apoptosis [IAP] binding protein with low pI), and AIF (apoptosis-inducing factor), to name a few. In the cytoplasm, cytochrome *c* binds to APAF-1 (apoptotic protease-activating factor-1, a homologue of the worm CED-4), to facilitate the binding of APAF-1 to ATP/dATP, thus forming the vertebrate apoptosome that mediates the activation of caspase-9.[44,45] In fact, caspase-9 is capable of self-processing when bound to APAF-9. This complex results in the activation of procaspase-3 (a downstream caspase) and the processing and activation of other caspases, leading to substrate cleavage. In contrast, SMAC/DIABLO acts by binding to the IAPs in the cytoplasm, relieving the IAP-mediated inhibition of caspase-3 and -9. In this model of the apoptotic pathway, the inhibition of caspases will delay but not prevent cell death. Other caspases, such as caspase-1 and the related caspase-4 and -5, may be able to act as both initiators and effectors.[44,45]

The disruption of mitochondrial membrane integrity leading to mitochondrial membrane permeability (MMP) is often observed before caspase activation is regulated at multiple levels. Induction of MMP can occur by proapoptotic second messengers, including calcium, reactive oxygen species (ROS), cerqamide, and other lipid messengers. In addition, it may involve the activation of the mitochondrial permeability transition pore complex (PTPC), which includes the voltage-dependent anion channels in the outer membrane and the adenine-nucleotide translocase in the inner membrane. This multisubunit complex participates in the regulation of a variety of important mitochondrial membrane functions, and its opening has effects on energy metabolism, the generation of ROS, and the release of cytochrome *c* from the mitochondrial intermembrane space into the cytoplasm. Further, activation of the PTPC has been implicated in the physical disruption of the mitochondrial outer membrane. Although it is not clear which events (i.e., caspase activation or mitochondrial membrane disruption) constitute the "point of no return" in the apoptotic pathway, it is apparent that both are critically interrelated.

A second mechanism exists that enables certain cells to induce other cells to self-destruct. This process is particularly important in the immune system. The receptors that mediate this response are members of the TNF superfamily that contain a conserved cytoplasmic protein–protein interaction module termed the death domain (DD). This cytoplasmic domain, first identified in studies involving the TNF receptor-1 (TNFR-1), is responsible for the generation of cytotoxic death signals and the activation of acid sphingomyelinase.[46] Mammalian death receptors include Fas/APO-1/CD95, TNFR-1, Apo-3/TRAMP, and the TRAIL receptors. The best described of these are CD95 or Fas and TNFR-1 (Fig. 3.20). Clustering of the Fas receptor in response to ligand binding leads to the recruitment of DD-containing adaptor proteins such as FADD (Fas-associated death domain) to the receptor complex. This can occur either directly via FADD DD in the case of the Fas receptor or indirectly via the protein TRADD

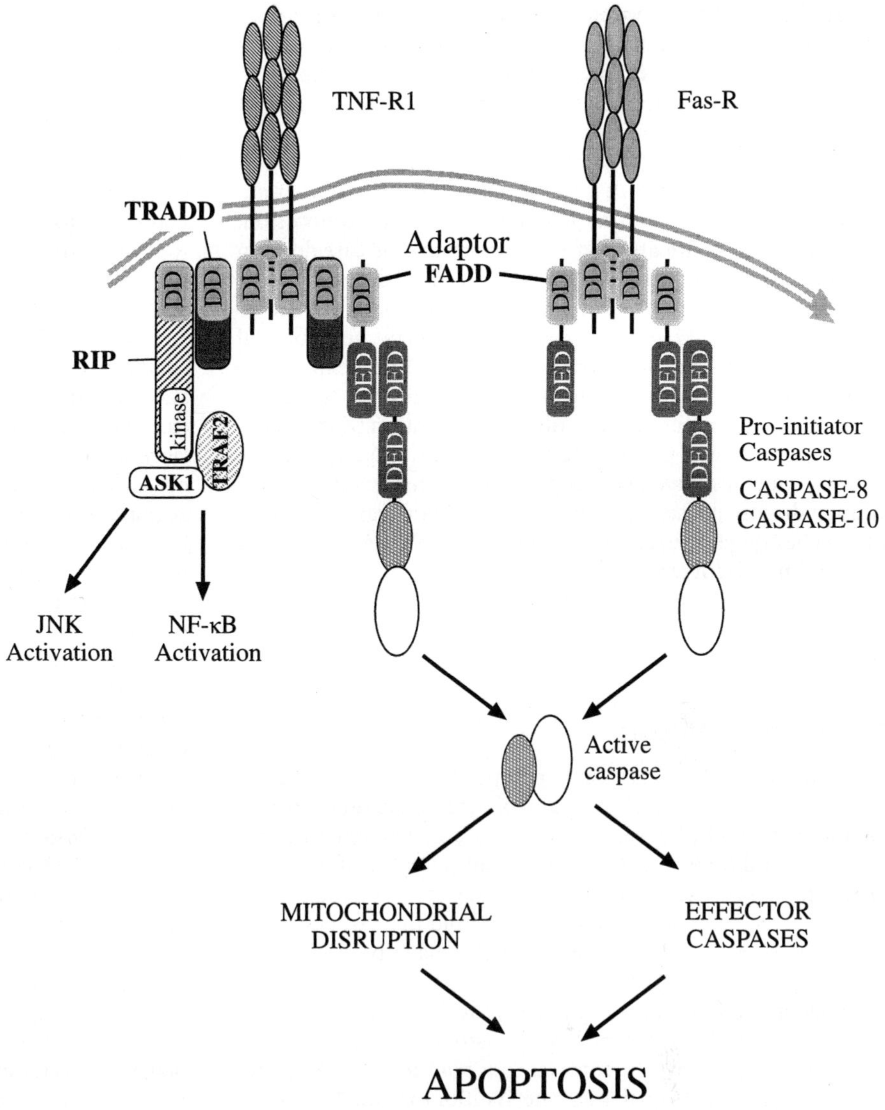

FIGURE 3.20. A schematic of the proposed signaling mechanisms of two members of the tumor necrosis factor receptor (TNFR) superfamily. Ligand binding to *TNFR-1* or to Fas-R leads to receptor oligomerization. Adaptor proteins such as *FADD* (Fas-associated death domain) and *TRADD* (TNFR-1-associated death domain) are recruited to the receptors via their death domains (*DD*). This phase is followed by an interaction between FADD and initiator procaspases (e.g., caspase-8 or -10) via their death effector domains (*DED*). This interaction results in caspase activation, which in turn leads both to activation of downstream caspases and to alterations in mitochondrial membrane permeability. Alternately, ligation of TNFR-1 can recruit *RIP* (receptor interaction protein) to the receptor via an interaction between the DD of TRADD and a DD motif in RIP. The RIP is a serine-threonine kinase with activation that may regulate TNF-mediated activation of NF-κB and c-Jun NH_2-terminal kinase (JNK), possibly resulting in survival signals. An additional mechanism for TNFR-1 signaling is via the recruitment of TRAF-2 (TNF-receptor-associated protein) and ASK-1 (apoptosis signal-regulating kinase-1). ASK-1 is an upstream kinase that leads to the activation of JNK [ASK-1 (JNKK kinase) > JNK kinase (JNKK) > JNK].

(TNFR-1-associated death domain) in the case of TNFR-1. The FADD contains a death effector domain (DED) that interacts with a DED module in procaspase-8 or procaspase-10, leading to their activation. Caspase-2 and -9 also contain DED domains. Caspase-8 then activates, either directly or indirectly, downstream effector caspases (caspase-3 and -7) that cleave key death substrates. The extrinsic pathway can cross-talk to the intrinsic pathway through the caspase-8-mediated cleavage of Bid, a widespread proapoptotic protein of the Bcl-2 pathway.[45,47] Once Bid is cleaved by caspase-8, the C-terminus of Bid moves to the mitochondria, where it induces the dimerization of Bax and Bak to promote the release of cytochrome *c* from the mitochondria. Mammalian inhibitors of the death receptor pathway include FLIP, which may act by displacing caspase-8 or -10 from their interaction with FADD.

The formation of an adaptor protein complex via the DD also initiates important cellular signaling events that are required for the stress response.[46] The TNFR-1-mediated induction of these signals may involve a second receptor-associated protein called RIP (receptor-interacting protein) that is also recruited to the signaling complex via a DD. The RIP is a serine-threonine kinase with activation that may regulate the function of NF-κB and JNK (also called stress-activated protein kinase or SAPK). This action may occur via its association with other receptor-associated signaling molecules such as TRAD-2 (TNF receptor-associated factor-2) and ASK-1 (apoptosis-signal regulating kinase-1). The TNFR engagement also leads to the activation of acid sphingomyelinase. Sphingomyelinase acts on membrane-associated sphingomyelin to generate the lipid second messenger ceramide, which may play an important role in the initiation of apoptosis. Ceramide-induced apoptosis may occur via two separate mechanisms, one involving the transcriptional regulation of the JNK pathway and the other via an alteration in mitochondrial membrane function.[48]

A major class of proteins that are intracellular regulators of apoptosis are the Bcl-2 family members, of which 18 have been identified in mammals thus far (see Table 3.4 for examples). These proteins are characterized by the presence of Bcl-2 homology (BH) domains, designated BH1, BH2, BH3, and BH4, and can be anti- or proapoptotic. In general, the antiapoptotic proteins Bcl-2, BclXL, Mcl-1, and Bcl-w are thought to regulate apoptosis by interacting with the mitochondrial PTPC either to modulate its opening or to preserve mitochondrial ATP synthesis. The proapoptotic Bcl-1 family members Bax, Bak, and Bok exist as monomers in viable cells but oligomerize to form multimers on receipt of a death signal. Also, Bax and Bak are capable of forming heterodimers with the antiapoptotic family members.[47]

Studies have shown that the presence of the BH3 domain among proapoptotic family members is key to their function. Further, the identification of the importance of this domain has led to the discovery of a class of proteins known as the BH3-only proteins. These include Bid, Bad, Bik, and Bim, to list a few. The BH3-only proteins are thought to link cell death signals to the core apoptotic pathway. Their expression is regulated by a variety of mechanisms, including transcriptional regulation, phosphorylation, sequestration by cytoskeletal proteins, and proteolytic cleavage. Increasingly, these small molecules have been implicated in the pathogenesis of human disease processes, including oncogenic transformation and ischemic cell injury, making them important targets for future drug discovery.[47]

Cell Communication

Membrane Transport

The ability of cells to respond appropriately to their environment is dependent on the function of membrane proteins that mediate intercellular signaling. A protein that is embedded in the membrane is referred to as an *integral* or *intrinsic membrane protein.* Virtually all these are transmembrane proteins that span both leaflets of the lipid bilayer. However, some can be anchored only in one leaflet, usually through the presence of a covalently bound hydrocarbon side chain. Classes of these proteins include glycosyl phosphatidylinositol-linked (GPI-linked) proteins, myristosylated proteins, and farnesylated proteins. In contrast, *peripheral* membrane proteins are not integrated into the membrane but rather are bound to the membrane indirectly by an association with an integral membrane protein or with a phospholipid; these include cytoskeletal and signaling molecules such as protein kinase C. In addition, phospholipases such as phospholipase A (PLA) can bind to the fatty acyl groups of phospholipids in the membrane.[1,10]

Integral membrane proteins have common structural motifs. The transmembrane portion of the protein is usually an α-helix composed primarily of hydrophobic amino acids. This portion of the molecule makes a single pass through the membrane. Alternately, proteins may be composed of multiple α-helical regions that pass through the membrane multiple times. It is these multipass proteins that typically serve as transport molecules or as signal transducers. As lipid bilayers are essentially impermeable to even the smallest charged molecules, specialized transport proteins are required to move molecules such as amino acids or ions into and out of the cell.

While membrane proteins can diffuse in the plane of the membrane, some cells can confine specific membrane components to particular regions of the membrane compartmentalizing their function. These cells are termed *polar cells.* The best example of this type of cell is the intestinal epithelial cell, which has an apical surface that is highly specialized for absorption, whereas its basolateral surface mediates the transport of absorbed nutrients out of the cell. Epithelial cell polarity is maintained by tight junctions. Tight junctions are essential structures that segregate specialized regions of the plasma membrane (i.e., fence function) and provide an apical barrier to the paracellular movement of water and solutes. Their structural and functional integrity is based on an intact actin cytoskeleton and requires functional Rho GTPases. Protein components that have been identified in tight junctions include the transmembrane protein occludin and cytosolic plaque proteins ZO-1 and ZO-2.[49]

Membrane proteins that regulate intercellular communication are called *receptors.* When bound to a ligand, receptors serve to transduce signals into the cell through a conformational change, dimerization, enzymatic activation, or association with other molecules; this results in the activation of effector pathways that are specific to individual ligands. Cell-surface receptors have a wide variety of functions. However, they can be divided into two broad categories, transport receptors or signaling receptors; the former ferry required substrates into the cell, whereas the latter link ligand binding to the activation of intracellular signaling pathways.[1,50]

There are two main classes of multipass membrane transport proteins. Carrier proteins bind solutes and undergo conformational change to transfer the solute across the membrane. Channel proteins consist of hydrophilic pores that, when open, allow solutes such as ions to pass through the membrane. All channel proteins and many carrier proteins function by *passive transport.* In this instance, solutes move according to their concentration gradient or to the membrane potential of the cell.

Other carrier proteins have the capacity to move solutes against their concentration gradient by using *active transport,* a process that couples transport to an energy source. One well-described ion pump that is dependent on active transport is the Na^+–K^+ ATPase. The Na^+–K^+ ATPases are found in the plasma membranes of most animal cells and function to transport Na^+ out of the cell in exchange for K^+, thus maintaining low intracellular Na^+ concentration. This process requires the hydrolysis of ATP to ADP. Although the pump is electrogenic, its main function is to regulate cell osmolarity. Cells contain a large concentration of organic solutes in the cytosol, including a high number of negatively charged molecules, thus requiring the retention of positively charged ions for charge balance. This large number of solutes draws water into the cell and must be countered by the extrusion of cations by Na^+–K^+ ATPase, thus contributing to a high extracellular ion concentration (Na^+ and Cl^+). Another membrane-bound ATPase that is homologous to the Na^+–K^+ ATPase is the *calcium pump.* The plasma membrane of most eukaryotic cells contains Ca^{2+} pumps that pump Ca^{2+} out of the cell against its gradient, thus maintaining an extremely low cytosolic Ca^{2+} concentration relative to the outside of the cell. As a result, a small influx of Ca^{2+} can lead to a substantial response within the cell by Ca^{2+}-dependent signaling molecules. Muscle cells also contain a special pump in the sarcoplasmic reticulum. The rapid removal of Ca^{2+} from the cytoplasm following muscle contraction is necessary for muscle relaxation to occur.[1,9]

A separate class of transport proteins that require ATP to function are the ATP-binding cassette (ABC) family of proteins. These include the cystic fibrosis transmembrane regulator (CFTR), P-glycoprotein, the multidrug resistance transporter, and the sulfonylurea receptors. The CFTR receptor is localized predominantly in the apical membrane of epithelial cells, where it functions as an ATP-stimulated Cl^- channel. Evidence has suggested, however, that CFTR may also regulate other Cl^- conductance channels and Na^+ channels, perhaps by facilitating cellular ATP release.

Energy stored in the cell's ion concentration gradients drive active transport. For example, Na^+-driven carrier proteins that are present in the plasma membrane can regulate cytosolic pH by exchanging Na^+ (in) for H^+ (out). The energy stored in the Na^+ gradient is used to drive this transport, which becomes active to decrease acidity when H^+ leaks into or is made in the cell. Alternately, Na^+ can be brought in with bicarbonate (HCO_3^-). The Na^+ concentration gradient can also be used to drive a chloride–bicarbonate exchange, which is also very effective in pH regulation. In addition to ion exchange, the sodium gradient can be coupled to cellular import of glucose and amino acids.

Channel proteins form holes or pores in the plasma membrane, allowing the passage of millions of ions per second when effectively triggered. There are two classes of membrane channel proteins, *gap junctions*, which bridge the cytoplasm between two cells, and *ion channels.* Ion channels, rather than functioning simply as pores, are selective for the ions that pass through (Fig. 3.21). Moreover, they have "gates" that open and close in response to specific stimuli, including (1) a change in voltage across the membrane (voltage-gated channels), (2) a mechanical stimulus, or (3) the binding of a ligand such as a neurotransmitter.

The most common ion channels are those that are permeable to potassium. These channels are important because the potassium gradient across the cell membrane is the primary determinant of the resting membrane potential. Voltage-gated channels are responsible for the generation of action potentials in electrically excitable cells such as neurons and muscle cells and for the recovery of the resting membrane potential once the signal has passed. Ligand-gated channels, such as those activated by neurotransmitters, transfer a chemical signal to an electrical signal. The best-described members of this family are the fast-acting nicotinic acetylcholine receptors of skeletal muscles. These are multisubunit proteins (typically composed of five subunits) that span the plasma membrane multiple times. The subunit architecture forms an array around a central channel that opens in response to acetylcholine binding to the extracellular domain of the receptor, allowing rapid sodium influx and membrane depolarization. In nerve cells, the end result is the initiation of an action potential. In other cells, however, membrane depolarization is linked to voltage-gated calcium channels, leading to increased intracellular Ca^{2+} concentration and triggering of Ca^{2+}-linked signaling events.[1,9]

Cell Signaling

Eukaryotic cells have the capacity to respond to a tremendously diverse array of biological stimuli. How is this information processed in an efficient and effective manner? The ability of cells to respond appropriately to their environment is dependent both on extracellular signaling molecules and on the presence of receptor proteins that bind to signaling molecules and transduce their specific responses. The chemical signaling molecules can be generally categorized by their membrane permeability. Small hydrophilic molecules such as peptide signaling molecules and growth factors require cell-surface receptors to transduce an appropriate signal. Many of these molecules act in a paracrine fashion to signal cells in the immediate environment.

The availability of these signaling molecules is tightly controlled through a variety of mechanisms, including rapid uptake of the molecule and enzymatic degradation. Other molecules are either small enough or lipophilic enough to pass directly across the cell membrane to interact with intracellular targets. One example of this is the gas nitric oxide (NO). It diffuses readily out of the cells where it is produced and passes directly into nearby cells. Its half-life is so short, however, that its effects are kept local. In contrast, lipophilic signaling molecules such as hormones can affect the entire organism and signal in an endocrine fashion. These small hydrophobic molecules are released into the bloodstream and

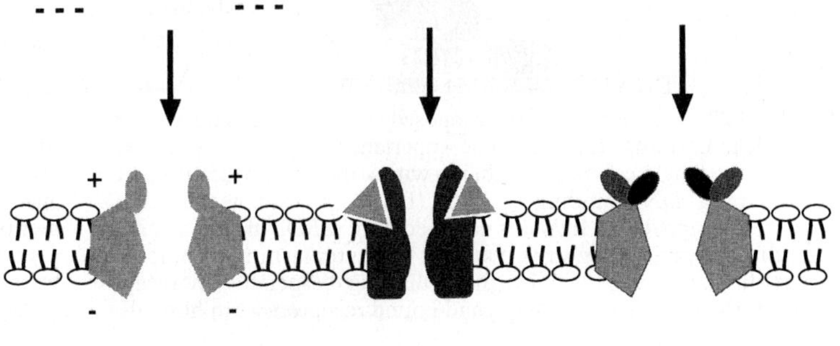

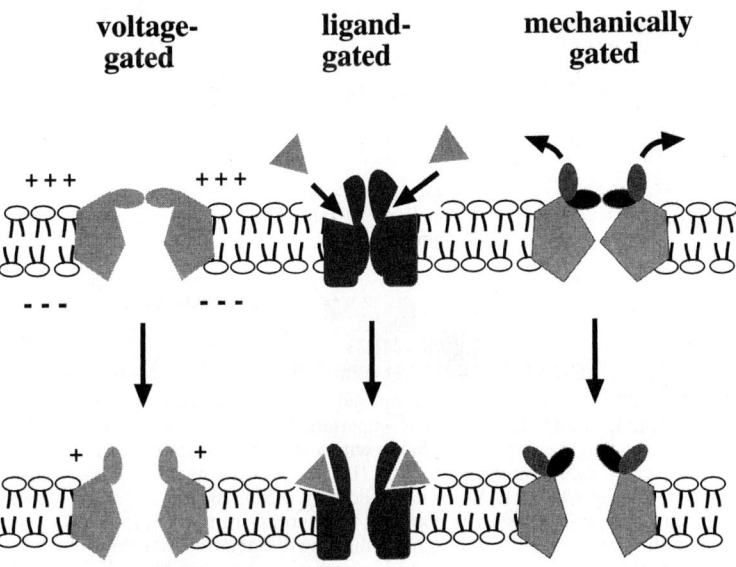

FIGURE 3.21. Ion channels open and close in response to specific stimuli, including (1) a change in the voltage across the membrane, (2) the binding of a ligand, or (3) a mechanical stimulus.

can travel to distant sites, where they permeate target cells and are recognized by specific intracellular receptors that directly regulate gene transcription.

The receptors for these molecules, which include steroid and thyroid hormones, retinoic acid, and vitamin D, are members of the *nuclear hormone receptor* gene superfamily. These proteins are single polypeptide chains with a modular structure that consists of a DNA-binding domain (containing two zinc finger motifs), nuclear localization signals, and a conserved ligand-binding domain (LBD). Unligated steroid receptors are found bound in the cytoplasm to a complex of heat-shock proteins, including hsp 90 and hsp 70. Hormone binding dissociates the receptors from the complex, and the ligand-bound receptors form homodimers via the LBD. The homodimers translocate to the nucleus, where they bind to DNA sequences called hormone response elements in the promoter region of target genes, leading to the activation or repression of gene transcription. In contrast, the nonsteroid family members, which include the vitamin D and retinoic acid receptors, are found bound to their response elements in the nucleus, even in the absence of ligand. In this instance, ligand binding alters the conformation of the receptor protein, increasing the affinity of the receptor for the DNA sequence (Fig. 3.22).

Cells have streamlined the transmission of messages by cell-surface receptors by linking them to a limited number of intracellular signaling pathways. It is apparent that the major currency of signal transduction is through the phosphorylation and dephosphorylation of pivotal regulatory proteins. The membrane receptors involved in signal transduction are grouped on the basis of the mechanism by which they activate downstream effectors. The largest family of signaling receptors is those associated with heterotrimeric GTP-binding proteins (G proteins). These proteins regulate the formation of intracellular second messengers such as calcium and cyclic adenosine 3′,5′-monophosphate (cAMP). A second major family possessing intrinsic or associated enzymatic activity includes receptors with tyrosine kinase, serine-threonine kinase, tyrosine phosphatase, or guanyl cyclase activity. A third class of receptors, already discussed, are those ligand-gated ion channels that initiate cell signaling by allowing rapid flux of ions across the plasma membrane.[1,9]

The G-protein-coupled or serpentine receptors are seven transmembrane-spanning, integral membrane proteins that respond to a variety of stimuli and are linked via one or more G proteins to the activation of specific effector pathways (Fig. 3.23). These stimuli include a diverse variety of factors, including mitogens, vasoactive polypeptides,

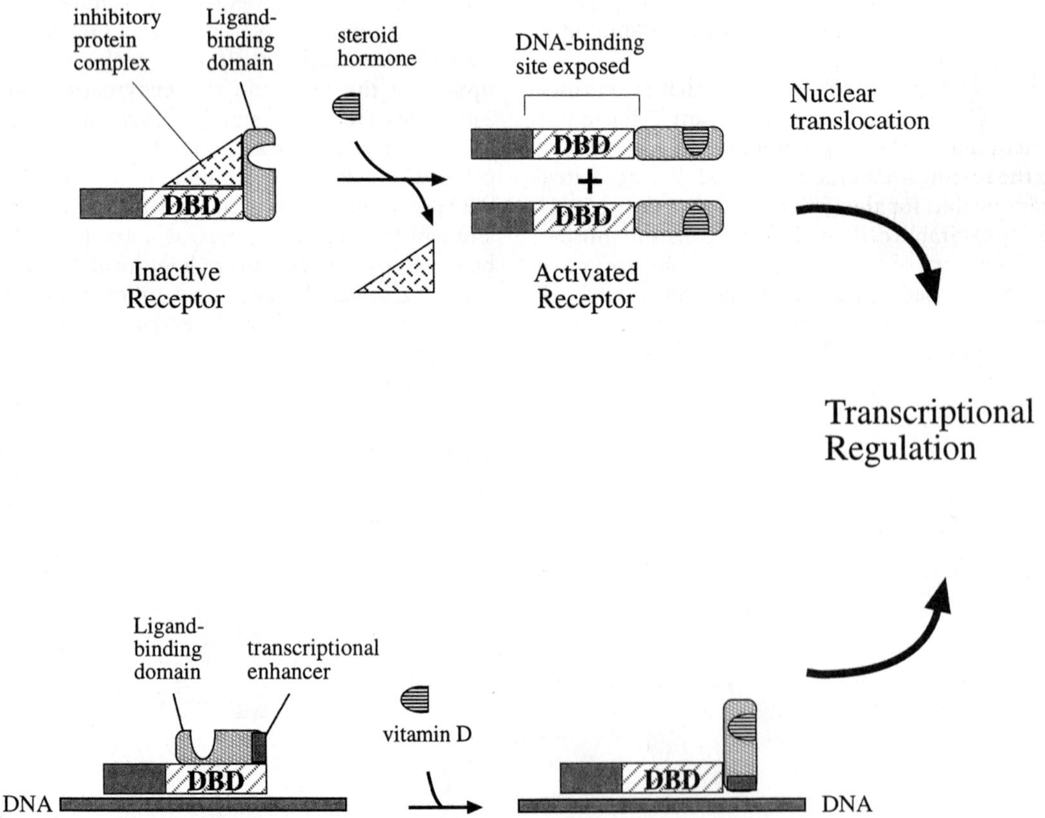

FIGURE 3.22. A schematic of the proposed signaling mechanisms for the nuclear hormone receptor gene superfamily. Nuclear hormone receptors are single polypeptide chains with a modular structure that consists of a DNA-binding domain (*DBD*), nuclear localization signals, and a conserved ligand-binding domain (*LBD*). In the inactive state, the unligated receptor is bound in the cytoplasm to a complex of heat-shock proteins (hsp). Hormone binding dissociates the receptors from the complex, and the ligand-bound receptors form homodimers via the LBD. The homodimers translocate to the nucleus, where they bind to DNA sequences to regulate gene transcription. Other nuclear hormone receptor family members, including the vitamin D and retinoic acid receptors, are found bound to their response elements in the nucleus, even in the absence of ligand. In this instance, ligand binding alters the conformation of the receptor protein, increasing the affinity of the receptor for the DNA sequence, thus activating transcription.

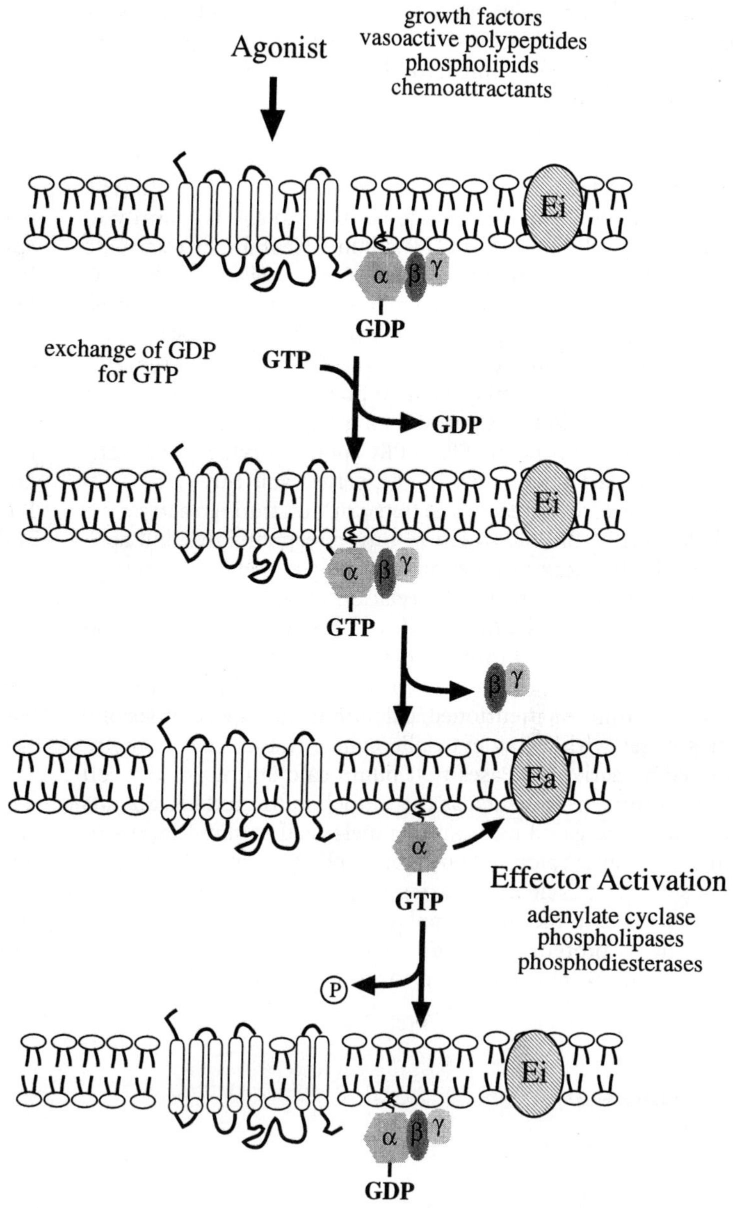

FIGURE 3.23. The G-protein-coupled receptors are integral membrane proteins that are linked via G proteins to a variety of effector pathways. Ligand binding by a G-protein-coupled receptor leads to a conformational change in the receptor that facilitates the exchange of GDP for GTP on the associated Gα subunit. The active GTP-bound Gα subunit then dissociates from the βγ dimer. The free GTP-Gα subunit is then able to associate with inactive membrane-bound effectors (*Ei*) leading to their activation (*Ea*). Specific intracellular effectors that are regulated by G-protein-coupled receptors include adenylate cyclase, phospholipase C, and phospholipase A. The Gαβγ heterotrimer is regenerated by the hydrolysis of GTP-Gα to GDP-Gα, leading to its reassociation with the Gβγ dimer and its inactivation.

neurotransmitters, and phospholipids. The G proteins control the activity of an effector protein, usually an enzyme, and this effector transmits a signal to the downstream target. The G proteins are composed of three subunits: Gα, Gβ, and Gγ. The diversity of function of the G proteins is largely dependent on the Gα subunit, of which there are more than 16. In the absence of activation of the receptor, GDP is bound to the Gα subunit, which together with the βγ dimer forms an inactive heterotrimer. This protein–GDP complex is bound to the unstimulated receptor. Ligation of the serpentine receptor leads to the exchange of GDP for GTP on the Gα subunit, the release of the bound G protein from the receptor, and the dissociation of the heterotrimer into Gα and Gβγ complexes. The free GTP-bound G protein α subunits and βγ subunits are then able to activate specific intracellular effector molecules that include plasma membrane-associated adenylyl cyclases, phospholipases, and phosphodiesterases, in addition to regulators of ion transport and protein kinase activity.[1,9,51]

Perhaps the best-described effector pathway for G-protein-linked receptors regulates the intracellular concentration of cAMP. This control is achieved via the stimulation or inhibition of adenylate cyclase activity by distinct G proteins, the stimulatory G protein G_s (the target of cholera toxin), and the inhibitory G proteins G_{i1} and G_{i2} (both are the targets of pertussis toxin). The effects of cAMP are mediated by a cAMP-dependent protein kinase, PKA. The cAMP binds to the regulatory subunits of PKA so that they dissociate from the catalytic subunit, allowing activation of the enzyme. Activated PKA catalyzes the transfer of a phosphate from ATP to specific serine or threonine residues in selected proteins. An increase in cAMP can also augment gene transcription. The PKA can phosphorylate a gene regulatory protein, CREB, that binds to a short DNA sequence (CRE, cAMP response element) found in the regulatory region of cAMP-responsive genes. The degradation of cAMP is regulated by cAMP phosphodiesterase, which becomes active in response to increases in intracellular calcium. The best-studied examples of receptors coupled to the activation of adenylyl cyclase are the β-adrenergic receptors, which mediate the action of epinephrine and norepinephrine.[10]

A second major effector pathway for serpentine receptors regulates cytoplasmic calcium concentration through G-protein-coupled activation of phospholipase C-β (PLC-β) (Fig. 3.24). The PLC isoenzymes are coupled to the G_Q family of G proteins, which has Gα-GTP subunits that directly activate PLC and are insensitive to cholera or pertussis toxin. The PLC catalyzes the hydrolysis of the membrane phospholipid, phosphatidylinositol 4,5-biphosphate (PIP_2). The hydrolysis of PIP_2 results in the formation of DAG and IP_3. The DAG remains associated with the plasma membrane, where its principal function is to elicit activation of a group of protein kinase C isoenzymes. Similar to PKA, PKC phosphorylates and activates selected target proteins on serine and threonine residues. It can also increase gene transcription through activation of the MAPK ERK-1, which in turn phosphorylates and activates the transcription factor Elk-1. Alternately, PKC activation can lead to the phosphorylation of Iκ-B, which releases the gene regulatory protein NF-κB. In contrast to the action of DAG, IP_3 diffuses into the cytoplasm, where it acts on its intracellular receptor located in the ER to mobilize intracellular calcium. As mentioned, calcium is an important second messenger with a low cytosolic concentration that is maintained by active ATPases that pump calcium out of the cell or into storage sites such as the mitochondria and ER. Signals that activate gated calcium channels lead to rapid increases in cytoplasmic calcium and diverse cellular responses, including smooth muscle cell contraction, secretory vesicle release, and changes in membrane polarization.[1]

The G-protein receptors may also be coupled to the activation of phospholipase A_2 (PLA_2), the enzyme that catalyzes the hydrolysis of membrane phospholipids to free arachidonic acid and lysophospholipids. The principal isoform of PLA_2 that has been linked to G proteins is cytosolic PLA_2.

The largest and best-understood family of receptors with intrinsic enzymatic activity are the receptor tyrosine kinases (RTKs). Examples of these receptors include receptors for platelet-derived growth factor, insulin-like growth factor, and epidermal growth factor, to name a few (Fig. 3.25). Interestingly, the characterization and sequencing of these receptors led to the discovery of an association between RTKs and cellular transformation. For example, the transforming gene of avian erythroblastosis virus, v-*erbB*, encodes a truncated form of the epidermal growth factor receptor with a kinase domain that is constitutively active. The mutation disrupts the regulated activity of the receptor so that it enhances cell growth and survival independent of ligand binding. Other RTK protooncogenes (cancer-causing genes) include *met*, *sis*, and *ret*.

All RTKs share the general structure of an extracellular LBD, a transmembrane domain, a cytoplasmic domain that possesses the catalytic kinase activity, and regulatory sequences. In most cases, the binding of the ligand to these receptors leads to receptor dimerization (Fig. 3.26). This is essential for the activation of the intrinsic kinase activity and the autophosphorylation of the receptor. Receptor phosphorylation has two main functions. First, it allows the receptor to become an effective kinase for other target proteins; second, it creates phosphorylated tyrosine residues that recruit other specialized signaling molecules to the receptor. Two different families of signaling molecules associate with the cytoplasmic domain of the phosphorylated RTK. The first are adaptor proteins that couple the receptor to other signaling molecules but are without intrinsic signaling activity. The second are

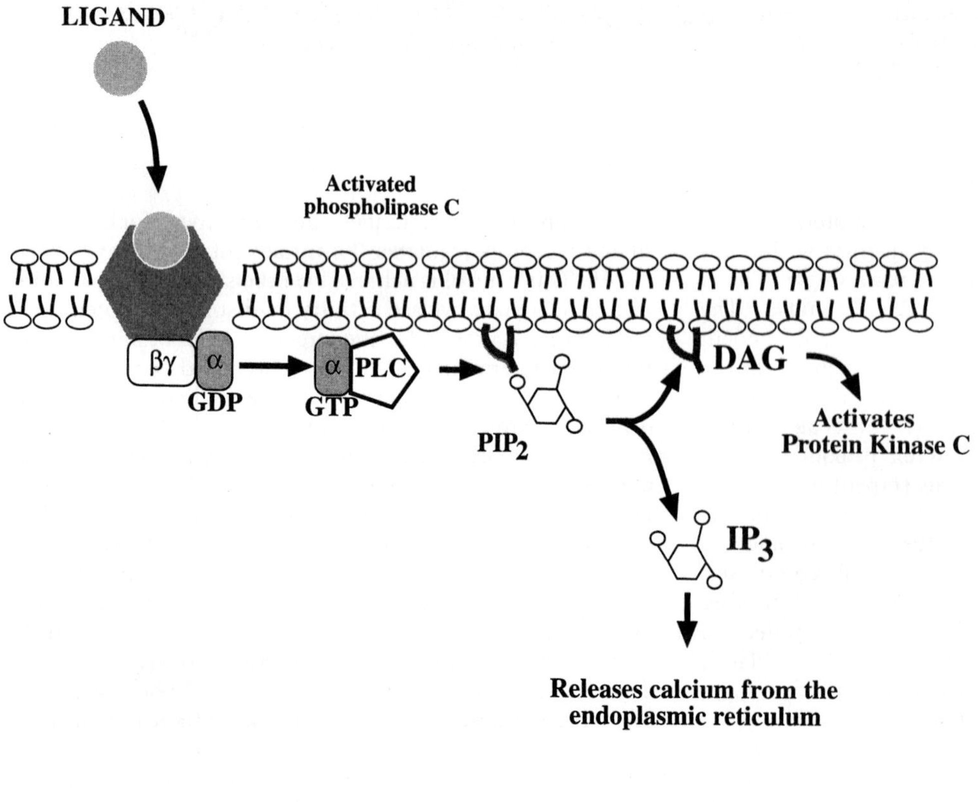

FIGURE 3.24. The G-protein-coupled activation of phospholipase C (*PLC*) leads to the hydrolysis of phosphatidylinositol 4,5-biphosphate (*PIP_2*), yielding diacylglycerol (*DAG*) and inositol 1,4,5-triphosphate (*IP_3*). The activation of PLC isoenzymes is coupled to the G_Q family of G proteins whose Gα-GTP subunits directly activate PLC; PLC catalyzes the hydrolysis of the membrane phospholipid, PIP_2. The hydrolysis of PIP_2 results in the formation of DAG and IP_3, and DAG remains associated with the plasma membrane, where its principal function is to elicit activation of a group of protein kinase C isoenzymes. Similar to PKA, PKC phosphorylates and activates selected target proteins on serine and threonine residues. In contrast to the action of DAG, IP_3 diffuses into the cytoplasm, where it acts on its intracellular receptor located in the endoplasmic reticulum to mobilize intracellular calcium, an important second messenger.

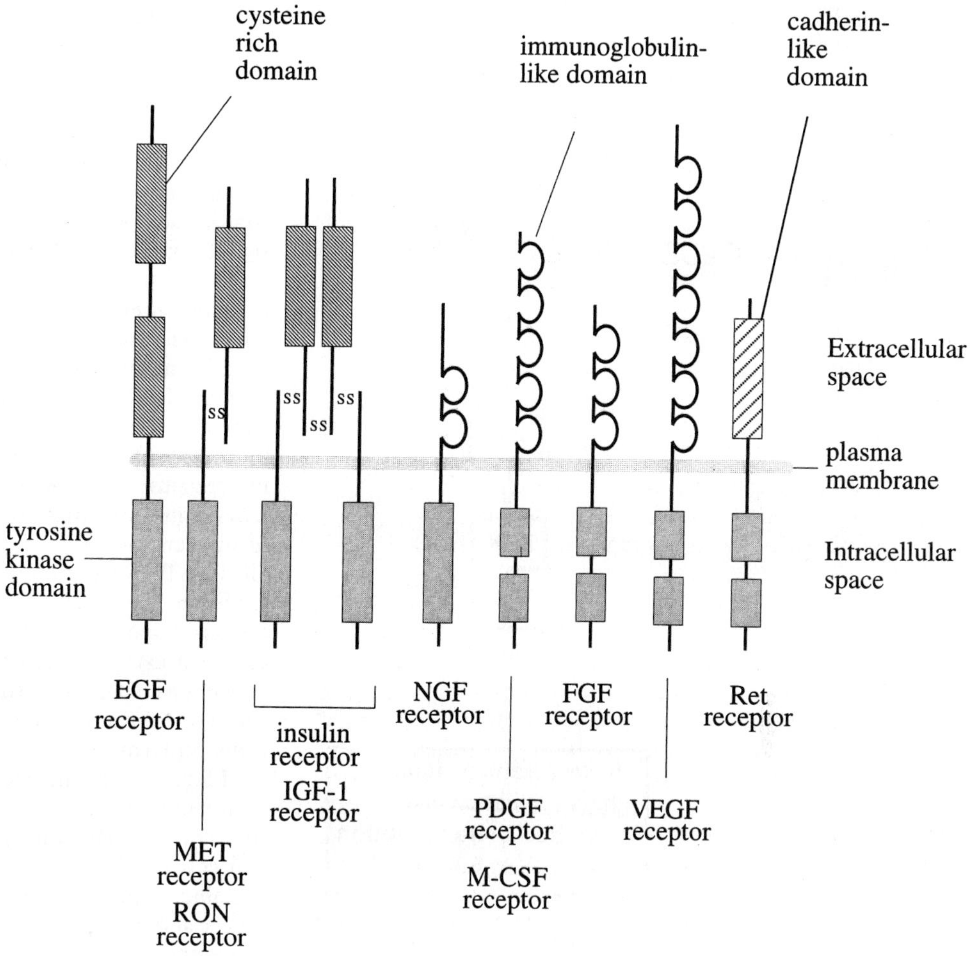

FIGURE 3.25. Eight subfamilies of receptor tyrosine kinases (RTKs). The classification of RTKs is determined by the structural motifs of their extracellular or intracellular domains. Note that in certain receptors the kinase domain is split. Only one or two members of each family are indicated. *EGF*, epidermal growth factor; *IGF-1*, insulin-like growth factor-1; *NGF*, nerve growth factor; *PDGF*, platelet-derived growth factor; *M-CSF*, macrophage-colony-stimulating factor; *FGF*, fibroblast growth factor; *VEGF*, vascular endothelial growth factor.

enzymes involved in the activation of specific effector pathways.[1,10,52]

The RTKs are important regulators of the gene transcription events required for cell proliferation and differentiation.

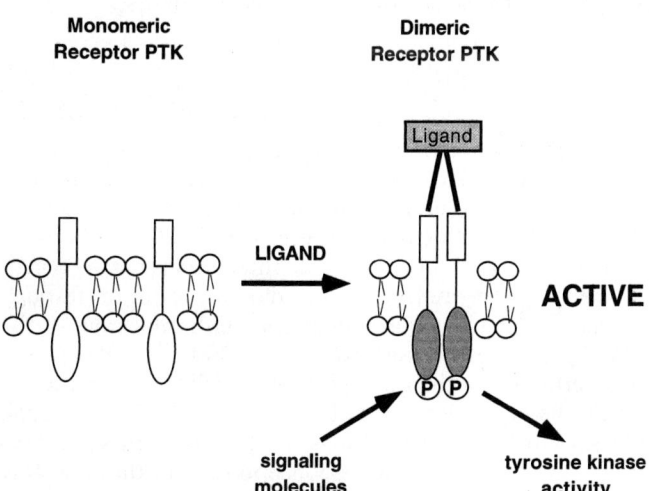

FIGURE 3.26. Dimerization of receptor tyrosine kinases (RTKs) through ligand binding activates the receptor's intrinsic kinase activity and recruits signaling molecules that contain phosphotyrosine-binding motifs to the receptor complex.

Ligand-induced activation of these receptors is essential for biological function, while inappropriate, constitutive activation results in uncontrolled growth and anchorage independence. How are signals transduced from the cell surface to the nucleus? Clues from experiments in yeast and *Drosophila* have identified a major signaling pathway that is highly conserved across diverse species. These important discoveries placed the GTPase *ras* and the serine-threonine kinase *raf* downstream of many RTKs in the signaling pathway mediating cell growth (Fig. 3.27). It is now apparent that the small adaptor protein Grb, which recognizes and binds to the phosphorylated tyrosine residues of the cytoplasmic domain of the RTK, initiates the formation of a multiprotein complex that includes Sos, a GEF that activates ras. The GTP-bound Ras becomes associated with and activates Raf-1, which phosphorylates and activates a downstream kinase known as MAPK or ERK kinase (ME). This step leads to the activation of the mitogen-activated protein kinase ERK, which culminates in the phosphorylation of a variety of substrates including transcription factors. Further characterization of the ras-raf-MEK-ERK signaling cascade has identified related pathways of the same general design that are activated by both environmental stress and cytokines; these include the JNKs or SAPKs and the p38 MAPK families.

The GTP-bound Ras has received much attention because of the high frequency of mutations that occur in the *ras* gene isolated from a variety of tumors. For example, one point

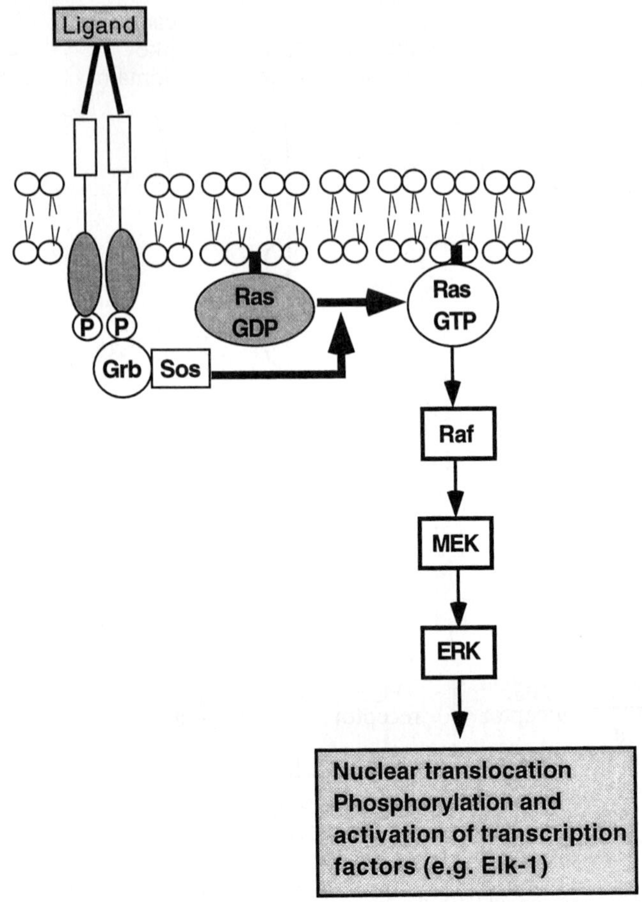

FIGURE 3.27. The RTK dimerization and recruitment of signaling molecules leads to the activation of the Ras-Raf-MEK-ERK signaling cascade that controls cell proliferation.

mutation that is found in the *ras* gene changes the protein sequence by a single amino acid. This mutation reduces the intrinsic GTPase activity of the ras protein, allowing it to remain in the GTP-bound state. As a result, ras signaling bypasses the cell regulatory machinery, causing uncontrolled cell growth and contributing to cellular transformation.[53]

Another molecule recruited to activated RTKs is phosphoinositide-3-OH kinase (PI3K). PI3K is a key regulator of a variety of cellular processes, including cell proliferation, cell shape change, and membrane vesicle trafficking and has been shown to be disturbed in many human cancers. This enzyme is responsible for the phosphorylation of phosphatidylinositols at the D-3 position, creating lipid molecules that are no longer substrates for phospholipases and that rapidly accumulate inside the cell. The primary substrate for PI3K is phosphatidylinositol-4,5-biphosphate ($PI\text{-}4,5\text{-}P_2$) to generate $PI\text{-}3,4,5\text{-}P_3$. The $PI\text{-}3,4,5\text{-}P_3$ accumulates rapidly within the cell following PI3K activation, recruiting signaling molecules to the cell membrane that contain distinct protein–lipid interaction domains called *plekstrin honology* (PH) domains. The PH domains are found in many proteins, including the serine/threonine kinases 3′-phosphoinositide-dependent kinases-1 (PDK1) and Akt/protein kinase B (PKB). The PDK1 phosphorylates and activates Akt at critical residues. Downstream effectors of Akt include kinases involved in cell survival (Bad), cell signaling (CREB and IκB kinase [IKK]), and cell growth (glycogen synthetase kinase3, insulin receptor substrate-1, mTOR). Several studies have also provided evidence that Akt via its action on GSK3 can modulate the activity of the signaling molecule β-catenin to induce the expression of genes involved in cell cycle progression.[54]

There exists a class of signaling receptors that lack intrinsic tyrosine kinase activity but have a mechanism of action that involves tyrosine phosphorylation. Members of this rapidly growing family include the receptors for growth hormone, prolactin, erythropoietin, interferons-α, -β, and -γ, and the interleukins IL-2 to IL-7 and IL-9 to IL-13. These receptors have been found to have an associated partner protein that is activated following ligand binding and receptor oligomerization (Fig. 3.28). The receptors mediate ligand-dependent tyrosine phosphorylation through these partner proteins, which are members of the Janus family (JAK) of nonreceptor tyrosine kinases. The characteristic action of JAKs is the activation by phosphorylation of the STAT family of transcription factors. Tyrosine phosphorylation of STATs allows STAT protein dimerization and nuclear translocation. Once in the nucleus, these transcription factors bind to sequence-specific DNA response elements within the regulatory regions of target genes to promote transcription.[28] Evidence has suggested that constitutive activation of JAKs can contribute to uncontrolled cell growth and cellular transformation.

Members of the transforming growth factor-β (TGF-β) family of signaling molecules regulate the expression of genes that control cell differentiation, cell division, cell motility, and cell death. The TGF-β signals are transduced by transmembrane proteins that possess intrinsic serine-threonine kinase activity. Signaling is initiated via ligand binding to two receptors, type I and type II. The interaction of the growth factor with the type II receptor allows it to serine phosphorylate and activate the type I receptor. The activated type I receptor can then phosphorylate associated molecules that are a subset of the Smad family (receptor Smads [R-Smads]; e.g., Smad-1 or Smad-2). Phosphorylated R-Smads can associate with Smad-4, and this complex translocates to the nucleus, where it can activate the transcription of target genes. The deletion or loss of function of Smad-2 or Smad-4 has been associated with pancreatic and colorectal tumors.[55]

Multicellularity

An early step in the evolution of multicellularity was the association of unicellular organisms to form colonies. Thus, cells must have developed the ability to associate with one another, and this association must have been of selective advantage. In higher eukaryotic organisms, cell association is mediated largely through complex interactions between cell-surface adhesion molecules on adjoining cells or through associations of cell-surface molecules with molecules of the ECM. Specific cells possess particular adhesive functions that are determined by their complement of cell-surface receptors and by the activation state of those receptors. For example, cells such as leukocytes circulate in the vasculature and then extravasate into tissues in response to stimuli that not only upregulate the expression of adhesion receptors but also increase their ligand affinity.

The functional units of cell adhesion are made up of three general classes of proteins: the *cell adhesion molecules/adhe-*

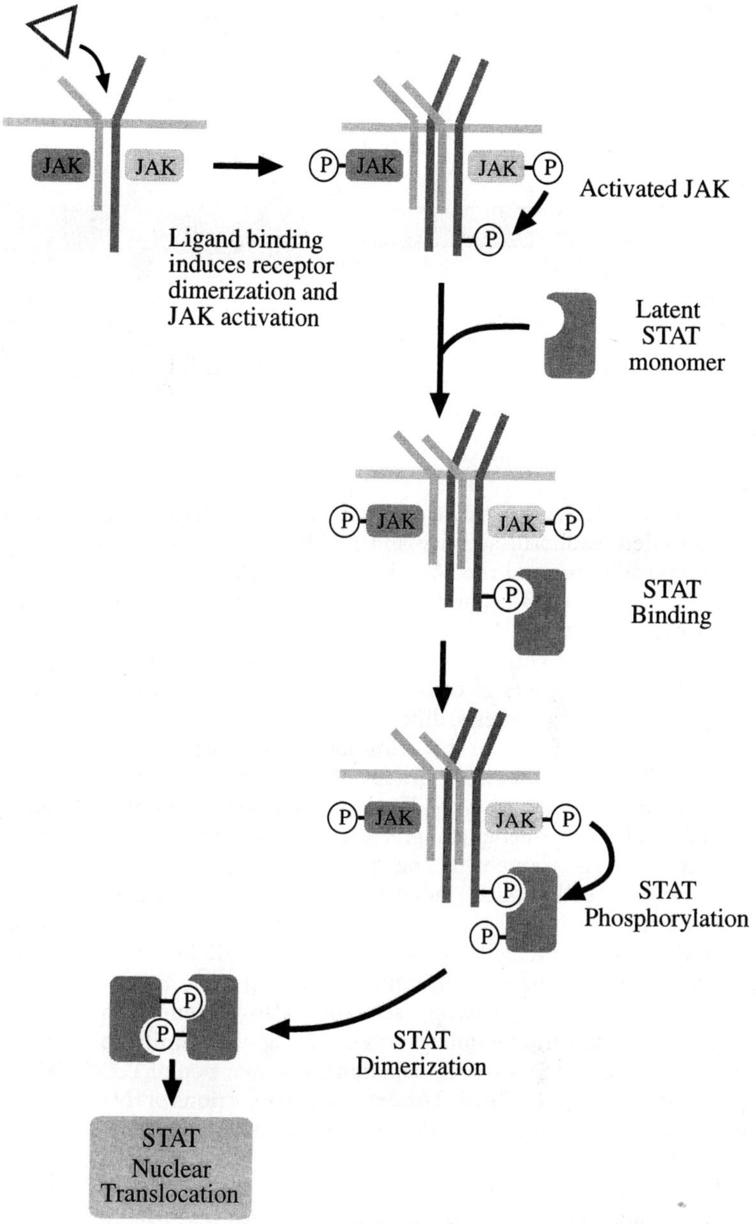

FIGURE 3.28. A schematic for cytokine receptor-mediated activation of the JAK/STAT signaling pathway. Ligand binding to the cytokine receptor induces receptor oligomerization. This process results in the phosphorylation and activation of the associated Janus kinase (*JAK*). The active JAK phosphorylates the cytoplasmic portion of the receptor, creating a docking site for latent *STAT* (*s*ignal *t*ransducer and *a*ctivator of *t*ranscription) molecules. Interaction of the STAT protein with the receptor facilitates its tyrosine phosphorylation by JAKs. Phosphorylated STAT monomers dissociate from the receptor, and subsequently two STATs associate as dimers via reciprocal phosphotyrosine-binding sites. STAT dimers are then able to translocate to the nucleus to bind to DNA response elements in specific target genes to enhance transcription.

sion receptors, ECM proteins, and *cytoplasmic plaque/peripheral membrane proteins.* Cell adhesion molecules or adhesion receptors are cell-surface transmembrane glycoproteins. They serve to mediate either direct cell–cell associations or cell–ECM interactions. These molecules include members of the cadherin, integrin, immunoglobulin, selectin, and proteoglycan superfamilies. The ECM proteins are typically large glycoproteins and include the collagens, fibronectins, and laminins. Cytoplasmic plaque proteins serve to link adhesion receptors to the cytoskeleton, regulate the function of the receptors, and transduce signals from the outside of the cell to the inside of the cell.[1,56] The function of these molecules is largely dependent on the integrity of the cytoskeleton.

Cell–Cell Adhesion

Direct cell–cell associations are largely mediated by *cadherins,* a multifunctional family of Ca^{2+}-dependent, cell–cell adhesion molecules (Fig. 3.29). The cadherin gene superfamily contains more than 40 members. Molecular cloning and sequence comparison have led to the characterization of a highly homologous group of classical cadherins and more distantly related members. The classical cadherins are transmembrane glycoproteins that exhibit, in addition to the structural homologies, a similar overall protein topology. The E-, P-, N-, and R-cadherins, for example, are termed *classical type I* cadherins. Each of these proteins is an integral membrane glycoprotein of 720 to 750 amino acids, and on average, 50% to 60% of the sequence is identical among the various family members. The extracellular domains of two classical cadherin molecules on neighboring cells bind to one another through an His-Ala-Val (HAV) motif in a calcium-dependent fashion, and cells expressing identical cadherins preferentially bind to one another. The cytoplasmic domains of cadherins interact with several cytoplasmic proteins, including α-catenin, β-catenin, γ-catenin (plakoglobin), and the tyrosine kinase

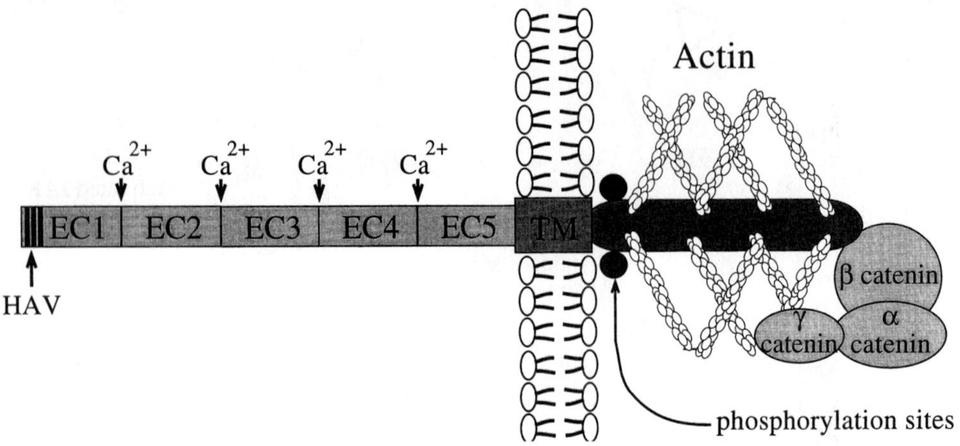

FIGURE 3.29. Classic cadherin structure. Cadherins are transmembrane Ca^{2+}-dependent cell-surface adhesion receptors. The extracytoplasmic fragment of a typical cadherin molecule is composed of five domains (*EC1–EC5*), each containing calcium-binding regions. The EC1 domain contains the putative binding recognition or *HAV* site. Classical cadherins have a short transmembrane segment that serves to anchor the cadherin into the cell membrane. The cytoplasmic domain contains phosphorylation sites and interacts with several proteins, including the *catenins*, and with the *actin* cytoskeleton.

substrate p120cas. Cadherin–catenin interactions are required for complete cadherin activity and regulate the interaction between cadherins and the actin-based cytoskeleton.

Importantly, each cadherin family member has a characteristic tissue distribution. During differentiation, the amount and nature of the cell-surface cadherin expression changes, affecting many aspects of cell–cell adhesion and cell migration. During embryogenesis, differential expression of cadherins drives morphogenesis by stimulating cell aggregation, defining boundaries between groups of cells, and promoting cell migration. Modulation of adhesion systems is also known to play a role in less-beneficial processes. Malignant invasion, for example, is thought to be mediated by modulation of various cell-surface adhesion molecules, notably E-cadherin.[1,56]

Other important cell adhesion molecules fall into two classes, *selectins* and the *immunoglobulin (Ig) superfamily.* Cell–cell adhesion involving selectins also depends on calcium, whereas interactions involving the Ig superfamily do not. The prototype of the Ig superfamily is the neural cell adhesion molecule N-CAM. The extracellular portions of this receptor are characterized by the presence of at least one, and often multiple, immunoglobulin-like domains that are versatile and readily adaptable to different binding functions. Selectins are a family of cell adhesion molecules that adhere to oligosaccharide sequences in glycoproteins or glycolipids of leukocytes. As such, these glycoproteins mediate the adhesion of leukocytes to selectins. Selectins are rapidly upregulated on endothelial cells following an inflammatory stimulus.[1,4]

Cell to Extracellular Matrix Adhesion

Although also mediating cell-to-cell adhesion, *integrins* are the major family of surface receptors that mediate cell adhesion to the ECM. The ECM not only binds cells and tissues together, but also influences the development, polarity, and behavior of the cells that it contacts. The ECM contains various fiber-forming proteins such as collagens, elastin, fibronectin, and laminin, interwoven in a hydrated gel composed of a network of glycosaminoglycan chains.[1] Located on virtually all cell types, integrins are heterodimeric transmembrane glycoproteins composed of one alpha (α) and one beta (β) subunit.[57] Subunit composition determines the ligand-binding specificity of the intact receptor. In mammals, 16 distinct α-subunits and 8 β-subunits combine to form 22 distinct receptors with predictable and often overlapping ligand specificity. Integrins recognize specific sequences present in ECM proteins; the best characterized of these is the RGD (arginine-glycine-aspartate) tripeptide sequence present in the cell-binding domain of fibronectin and other ECM proteins.

Integrins perform an important structural function by linking the ECM to the actin cytoskeleton, thus facilitating cell shape change and movement. However, integrin–ECM interactions also mediate a number of intracellular signaling events.[58–60] One concept suggests that integrins transmit these signals by reorganizing the actin cytoskeleton, thereby regulating cell shape and internal cellular architecture. This process is mediated by direct contact between the integrin cytoplasmic domain and selected cytoskeletal proteins, leading to the accumulation of cytoskeletal and signaling molecules at specialized regions of cell–matrix contact called *focal adhesions* (Fig. 3.30). The recruitment of proteins to these sites is initiated by receptor recognition of a distinct ligand, suggesting a mechanism by which the ECM, through integrins, may modulate cell morphology and in turn regulate cell behavior. Evidence has demonstrated that integrins can also transmit biochemical signals inside the cell. For example, one mode of integrin signal transduction involves the activation of cytoplasmic tyrosine kinases, including focal adhesion kinase and c-*src*. Other signaling events associated with integrin ligation include elevation of intracellular pH and increased synthesis of phosphotidyl inositide second messengers. These signals intersect with a number of important intracellular signaling pathways, including the ERK and JNK members of the MAPK family.

The activation of ERK in response to integrin ligation may require Ras signaling. Evidence has demonstrated that certain integrins are linked to the ras-raf-ERK signaling cascade via the adaptor molecule Shc. Moreover, integrin-mediated signals from the ECM are required both to stimulate the Cdks that mediate progression through the G_1 phase of the cell cycle and to protect normal cells from programmed cell death.[61] Thus, ECM recognition by integrins can be linked to a number of vital biological processes. Cooperative signals from both growth factor receptors and integrins may be required for optimal levels of signaling necessary for appropriate cell behavior, including cell proliferation and differentiation.[58–60]

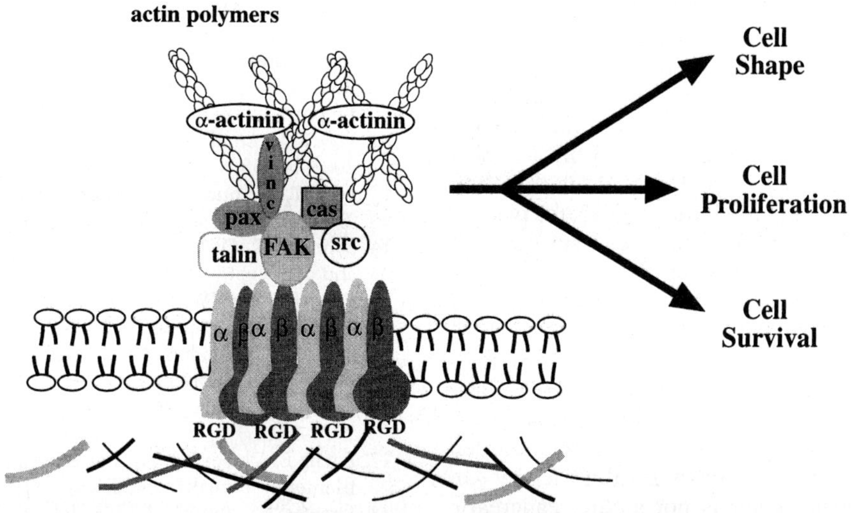

FIGURE 3.30. A schematic of the proposed signaling mechanisms for the integrin receptor superfamily. Integrins are heterodimeric transmembrane glycoproteins composed of one alpha (α) and one beta (β) subunit. Interaction of the integrin receptors with extracellular matrix ligands leads to the clustering of the receptors and the recruitment of both cytoskeletal molecules (e.g., *talin*, α-*actinin*, vinculin) and signaling molecules to specialized regions of cell–matrix contact called *focal adhesions*. Integrin signal transduction involves the activation of cytoplasmic tyrosine kinases, including focal adhesion kinase (*FAK*) and *src* by phosphorylation. Activation of FAK and src leads to the phosphorylation of a number of FAK-associated proteins, including paxillin, tensin, and pp^{130} cas (crk-associated substrate). Cas is a multidomain docking protein that interacts with a number of other adaptor proteins when phosphorylated, thereby regulating signals to the mitogen-activated protein kinase pathways. Integrin-mediated signaling events have been linked to important cellular processes, including cell proliferation, cell motility, and cell survival.

If cells are to function effectively as tissues, then they must form specialized junctions that link the cells both to each other and to the ECM. These junctions include three types of *desmosomes* that impart to cells strength and the ability to resist shear forces: the belt desmosomes, the spot desmosomes, and the hemidesmosomes. Belt desmosomes are points of cell–cell contact where the actin cytoskeleton of adjacent cells is linked via cadherins. Spot desmosomes are found right beneath the belt desmosomes, and are linked through IFs to the plasma membrane at points of cell–cell contact. Hemidesmosomes are stable anchoring structures that mediate the adhesion of stratified and complex epithelia to the ECM. In contrast to focal adhesions, the integrin receptor components of these complexes serve to link the cell's IFs (primarily the keratin filaments) at plasma membrane junctions to the basement membrane.[1]

Stem Cells

We have up to now described some of the molecular and genetic mechanisms employed by cells to differentiate into cell types committed to perform specialized functions. In the 1960s, researchers identified small populations of seemingly unspecialized "stem" cells within adult tissues and organs. These "adult" stem cells possess the capacity for self-renewal and are capable of differentiating into the major specialized cell types found in their organ of origin. The primary role of adult stem cells is to maintain and repair the organ in which they are found. They can remain quiescent for years, then quickly become activated by disease or tissue injury. Adult tissues reported to contain stem cells include brain, bone marrow, peripheral blood, blood vessels, skeletal muscle, skin, liver, and pancreas. Hematopoietic stem cells can trans-differentiate into almost any other type of blood cell, including red blood cells, B and T lymphocytes, natural killer cells, monocytes, and macrophages, among others. Neural stem cells can give rise to both neuronal and nonneuronal cells, including astrocytes and oligodendrocytes. Epithelial stem cells of the digestive tract can trans-differentiate into absorptive cells, goblet cells, Paneth cells, and enteroendocrine cells. Adult stem cells from one tissue also have the ability to trans-differentiate into cell types of other tissues, a phenomenon known as *plasticity*. Stem cells in adult liver, for example, can trans-differentiate into insulin-secreting cells, and hematopoietic stem cells into heart muscle.[3] Various methods have been used to force stem cells to differentiate along specific pathways, including introduction of tissue-specific genes[62] or manipulation of the tissue culture environment in which stem cells are grown.[63]

In the 1980s, scientists developed methods to isolate stem cells from mouse embryos. These were termed embryonic stem (ES) cells and are derived from the inner cell mass (ICM) of the preimplantation mouse or human embryo. The ES cells can proliferate indefinitely in tissue culture in an undifferentiated state as long as they are maintained in the presence of leukemia inhibitory factor (LIF). Once this agent is removed, ES cells differentiate into structures called embryoid bodies (EBs); EBs are composed of all three germ layers: ectoderm, endoderm, and mesoderm. These germ layers have the capacity to differentiate into their respective derivatives, including cardiomyocytes, hematopoietic progenitor cells, smooth muscle cells, adipocytes, hepatocytes, pancreatic islet cells, neurons, glial cells, and so on.[64]

The study of stem cells can lead to important discoveries about embryonic development, carcinogenesis, and intriguingly, how to use stem cells to regenerate, restore, or replace damaged, diseased, or worn-out organs. Stem cells represent a renewable source of cells that can be directed to differentiate into any number of specific cell types to treat diseases such as Parkinson's[65] and Alzheimer's[66] diseases as well as spinal cord injury,[67] heart disease,[68] burns,[69] stroke,[70] and endocrine disorders such as type I diabetes.[71]

The National Institutes of Health estimates that 18.2 million Americans are diabetic. Of these 18.2 million, 206,000 are children under the age of 20. Each year, 1.3 million new cases of diabetes are diagnosed. Type I diabetes is the sixth leading cause of death in the United States. Diabetes is associated with increased risk of heart disease and stroke, high blood pressure, blindness, kidney and nervous system disease, amputation, and complications of pregnancy. It is estimated that $132 billion are spent each year either directly on medical costs associated with diabetes or on costs associated with work loss, disability, and premature mortality (NIH Publication No. 04–3892, April 2004). Diabetes is also becoming a global problem and as such represents an enormous burden on health care systems here and abroad. Insulin therapy can control symptoms of diabetes but is not a cure. Pancreatic islet transplantation is a promising treatment for type I diabetes but is restricted, in part, by limited availability of primary human islets. The in vitro reconstitution of physiologically competent replacement islets using ES or adult stem cells differentiated to produce glucoregulatory factors represents a potential cure for type I diabetes.

Realizing this goal presents several challenges. For instance, once differentiated, the proliferative capacity of the cells must be controllable to avoid the development of insulin-related hypoglycemia.[64] Once transplanted, the differentiated cells must escape immune surveillance and destruction. Interestingly, stem cell-derived islets appear to be less sensitive to recurrent immune destruction than is normally seen in response to islet transplantation.[72] Finally, transplanted islets must become vascularized. Vascularization has been shown to be of paramount importance for islet growth and function.[73] Despite these significant hurdles, stem cell replacement therapy for type I diabetes promises to be a viable and exciting alternative to chronic insulin injections.

References

1. Alberts B, Bray D, Lewis J, Raff F, Roberts K, Watson JD. Molecular Biology of the Cell. New York: Garland Publishing, 1994.
2. Kleinsmith LJ, Kish VM. Principles of Cell Biology. New York: Harper Collins, 1988.
3. Agrawal S, Schaffer DV. In situ stem cell therapy: novel targets, familiar challenges. Trends Biotechnol 2005;23:78–83.
4. Watson JD, Hopkins NH, Roberts JW, Steitz JA, Weiner AM. Molecular Biology of the Gene. Menlo Park: Benjamin/Cummings, 1987.
5. Ugarkovic D, Plohl M. Variation in satellite DNA profiles—causes and effects. EMBO J 2002;21:5955–5959.
6. Peterson CL, Laniel MA. Histones and histone modifications. Curr Biol 2004;14:R546–51.
7. Strahl BD, Allis CD. The language of covalent histone modifications. Nature 2000;403:41–45.
8. Ren M, Leng Y, Jeong M, Leeds PR, Chuang DM. Valproic acid reduces brain damage induced by transient focal cerebral ischemia in rats: potential roles of histone deacetylase inhibition and heat shock protein induction. J Neurochem 2004; 89:1358–1367.
9. Latchman DS. Basic Molecular and Cell Biology. London: Chapman and Hall, 1997.
10. Lodish H, Baltimore D, Berk A, Zipursky S, Matsudaira P, Darnell J. Molecular Cell Biology. New York: W. H. Freeman and Company, 1995.
11. Ross MH, Reith EJ. Histology: A Text and Atlas. New York: Lippincott, 1985.
12. Pike LJ. Lipid rafts: bringing order to chaos. J Lipid Res 2003;44:655–667.
13. He HT, Lellouch A, Marguet D. Lipid rafts and the initiation of T cell receptor signaling. Semin Immunol 2005;17:23–33.
14. Schmitz G, Orso E. CD14 signalling in lipid rafts: new ligands and co-receptors. Curr Opin Lipidol 2002;13:513–521.
15. Fox AH, Lam YW, Leung AK, et al. Paraspeckles: a novel nuclear domain. Curr Biol 2002;12:13–25.
16. Lafarga M, Berciano MT, Pena E, et al. Clastosome: a subtype of nuclear body enriched in 19S and 20S proteasomes, ubiquitin, and protein substrates of proteasome. Mol Biol Cell 2002;13:2771–2782.
17. Fuchs E, Cleveland, D. A structural scaffolding of intermediate filaments in health and disease. Science 1998;279:514–519.
18. Drewes G, Ebneth A, Mandelkow EM. MAPs, MARKs, and microtubule dynamics. Trends Biochem Sci 1998;23:307–311.
19. Hirokawa N. Kinesin and dynein superfamily of proteins and the mechanism of organelle transport. Science 1998;279:519–526.
20. Beckerle MC. Spatial control of actin filament assembly: lessons from *Listeria*. Cell 1998;95:741–748.
21. Hall A. Rho GTPases and the actin cytoskeleton. Science 1998;279:509–514.
22. Aktories K. Rho proteins: targets for bacterial toxins. Trends Microbiol 1997;5:282–288.
23. Mallik R, Gross SP. Molecular motors: strategies to get along. Curr Biol 2004;14:R971–R982.
24. Mountain V, Compton DA. Dissecting the role of molecular motors in the mitotic spindle. Anat Rec 2000;261:14–24.
25. Latchman DS. Gene Regulation: A Eucaryotic Perspective. London: Chapman and Hall, 1995.
26. Bauerle PA, Baltimore D. NF-κB: 10 years after. Cell 1996;87:13–20.
27. Smith JM, Koopman PA. The ins and outs of transcriptional control: nucleocytoplasmic shuttling in development and disease. Trends Genet 2004;20:4–8.
28. Spiegelman BM, Heinrich R. Biological control through regulated transcriptional coactivators. Cell 2004;119:157–167.
29. Das PM, Singal R. DNA methylation and cancer. J Clin Oncol 2004;22:4632–4642.
30. Gebauer F, Hentze MW. Molecular mechanisms of translational control. Nat Rev Mol Cell Biol 2004;5:827–835.
31. Richter JD, Sonenberg N. Regulation of cap-dependent translation by eIF4E inhibitory proteins. Nature 2005;433:477–480.
32. Hay N, Sonenberg N. Upstream and downstream of mTOR. Genes Dev 2004;18:1926–1945.
33. Tee AR, Blenis J. mTOR, translational control and human disease. Semin Cell Dev Biol 2005;16:29–37.
34. Hammond SM, Boettcher S, Caudy AA, Kobayashi R, Hannon GJ. Argonaute2, a link between genetic and biochemical analyses of RNAi. Science. 2001:293(5532):1146–1150.
35. Bantounas I, Phylactou LA, Uney JB. RNA interference and the use of small interfering RNA to study gene function in mammalian systems. J Mol Endocrinol 2004;33:545–557.
36. Silva J, Chang K, Hannon GJ, Rivas FV. RNA-interference-based functional genomics in mammalian cells: reverse genetics coming of age. Oncogene 2004;23:8401–8409.
37. He L, Hannon GJ. MicroRNAs: small RNAs with a big role in gene regulation. Nat Rev Genet 2004;5:522–531.
38. Fridman JS, Lowe SW. Control of apoptosis by p53. Oncogene 2003;22:9030–9040.
39. Cryns V, Yuan J. Proteases to die for. Genes Dev 1998;12:1551–1570.

40. Nunez G, Benedict MA, Hu Y, Inohara N. Caspases: the proteases of the apoptotic pathway. Oncogene 1998;17:3237–3245.
41. Evan G, Littlewood T. A matter of life and cell death. Science 1998;281:1317–1321.
42. Raff M. Cell suicide for beginners. Nature 1998;396:119–122.
43. Thornberry NA, Lazebnik, Y. Caspases: enemies within. Science 1998;281:1312–1316.
44. Riedl SJ, Shi Y. Molecular mechanisms of caspase regulation during apoptosis. Nat Rev Mol Cell Biol 2004;5:897–907.
45. Danial NN, Korsmeyer SJ. Cell death: critical control points. Cell 2004;116:205–219.
46. Baker SJ, Reddy EP. Modulation of life and death by the TNF receptor superfamily. Oncogene 1998;17:3261–3270.
47. Chan SL, Yu VC. Proteins of the bcl-2 family in apoptosis signalling: from mechanistic insights to therapeutic opportunities. Clin Exp Pharmacol Physiol 2004;31:119–128.
48. Mathias S, Pena LA, Kolesnick RN. Signal transduction of stress via ceramide. Biochem J 1998;335:465–480.
49. Balda MS, Matter K. Tight junctions. J Cell Sci 1998;111:541–547.
50. Stone DK. Receptors: structure and function. Am J Med 1998; 105:244–250.
51. Hakonarson H, Grunstein M. Regulation of second messengers associated with airway smooth muscle contraction and relaxation. Am J Respir Crit Care Med 1998;158:S115–S122.
52. Weiss A, Schlessinger J. Switching receptors on or off by receptor dimerization. Cell 1998;94:277–280.
53. Robinson MJ, Cobb MH. Mitogen-activated protein kinase pathways. Curr Opin Cell Biol 1997;9:180–186.
54. Fresno Vara JA, Casado E, de Castro J, Cejas P, Belda-Iniesta C, Gonzalez-Baron M. PI3K/Akt signalling pathway and cancer. Cancer Treat Rev 2004;30:193–204.
55. Hata A, Massague J, Shi Y. TGF-β signalling and cancer: structural and functional consequences of mutations in Smads. Mol Med Today 1998;4:257–262.
56. Gilbert SF. Developmental Biology. Sunderland, MA: Sinauer Associates, 1994.
57. Hynes RO. Integrins: versatility, modulation and signaling in cell adhesion. Cell 1992;69:11–19.
58. Clarke EA, Brugge JS. Integrins and signal transduction pathways: the road taken. Science 1995;268:233–239.
59. Juliano R, Haskill S. Signal transduction from the extracellular matrix. J Cell Biol 1993;120:577–585.
60. Parsons JT. Integrin-mediated signaling: regulation by protein tyrosine kinases and small GTP-binding proteins. Curr Opin Cell Biol 1996;8:146–152.
61. Giancotti FG. Integrin signaling: specificity and control of cell survival and cell cycle progression. Curr Opin Cell Biol 1997;9:691–700.
62. Soria B, Roche E, Berna G, Leon-Quinto T, Reig JA, Martin F. Insulin-secreting cells derived from embryonic stem cells normalize glycemia in streptozotocin-induced diabetic mice. Diabetes 2000;49:157–162.
63. Lumelsky N, Blondel O, Laeng P, Velasco I, Ravin R, McKay R. Differentiation of embryonic stem cells to insulin-secreting structures similar to pancreatic islets. Science 2001;292:1389–1394.
64. Doss MX, Koehler CI, Gissel C, Hescheler J, Sachinidis A. Embryonic stem cells: a promising tool for cell replacement therapy. J Cell Mol Med 2004;8:465–473.
65. Kim SU. Human neural stem cells genetically modified for brain repair in neurological disorders. Neuropathology 2004;24:159–171.
66. Blesch A, Tuszynski MH. Gene therapy and cell transplantation for Alzheimer's disease and spinal cord injury. Yonsei Med J 2004;45(suppl):28–31.
67. Zhou Q, Zhang SZ, Xu RX, Xu K. [Neural stem cell transplantation and postoperative management: report of 70 cases.]. Di Yi Jun Yi Da Xue Xue Bao 2004;24:1207–1209.
68. Lee S, Bick-Forrester J, Makkar RR, Forrester JS. Stem-cell repair of infarcted myocardium: ready for clinical application? Am Heart Hosp J 2004;2:100–106.
69. Shumakov VI, Onishchenko NA, Rasulov MF, Krasheninnikov ME, Zaidenov VA. Mesenchymal bone marrow stem cells more effectively stimulate regeneration of deep burn wounds than embryonic fibroblasts. Bull Exp Biol Med 2003;136:192–195.
70. Haas S, Weidner N, Winkler J. Adult stem cell therapy in stroke. Curr Opin Neurol 2005;18:59–64.
71. Nygaard Jensen J, Jensen J. Cell therapy of diabetes. Adv Exp Med Biol 2004;552:16–38.
72. Petrovsky N, Silva D, Schatz DA. Prospects for the prevention and reversal of type 1 diabetes mellitus. Drugs 2002;62:2617–2635.
73. Beger C, Cirulli V, Vajkoczy P, Halban PA, Menger MD. Vascularization of purified pancreatic islet-like cell aggregates (pseudoislets) after syngeneic transplantation. Diabetes 1998; 47:559–565.
74. Mathews CK, Van Holde KE. Biochemistry. New York: Benjamin/Cummings, 1990.

4 Mediators of Inflammation and Injury

Stephen F. Lowry, Edward Lin, and Steve E. Calvano

The response to injury or infection in the surgical patient is characterized by diverse endocrine, metabolic, and immunological alterations. If the inciting injury is minor and of limited duration, then wound healing and restoration of metabolic and immune homeostasis occur with relatively minimal intervention. By contrast, major insults to the host are associated with greater alterations in endogenous regulatory processes that, without appropriate and timely intervention, impact negatively on survival or full restoration of cellular and organ function. The spectrum of metabolic and immunological dysfunction arising from major injuries or severe infections is complex. Conceptually, it is beneficial to consider the initial response to injury—be it surgical, traumatic, or infectious—as inherently inflammatory, marked by the activation of cellular processes designed to restore or maintain function within tissues while also promoting the eradication of invading microorganisms. The initial proinflammatory processes are followed by anti-inflammatory or counterregulatory processes that are equally important in the restoration of homeostasis to the host (Fig. 4.1).[1]

The mediators that govern the proinflammatory and anti-inflammatory responses to injury represent the collective dynamics of neuroendocrine, immunological, and metabolic activity of the host. Indeed, the concept of integrated systemic and regional inflammatory balance has become a reasonable framework for patient management in virtually every discipline of surgical practice and may serve as the foundation on which interventions and therapeutics are formulated. This chapter addresses the macroendocrine, microendocrine, immunological, and cellular responses to injury. Although issues pertaining to host metabolism and the utilization of fuel substrates during injury are the focus of subsequent chapters, it is important to understand that they are also subject to the influences of hormonal and immunological mediators as discussed in this chapter.

Hormonal Mediators of Injury

Injury sustained by the host is characterized by the release of local bioactive substances, by heightened neural (e.g., pain, tachycardia, hypertension) and systemic responses (e.g., tachycardia and hypertension), and by activation of baroreceptor stimulation from intravascular volume shifts. In a broad sense, the hormones released in response to injury may be divided into those primarily under hypothalamopituitary control and those primarily under autonomic nervous control and composed of a network of signaling and regulatory feedback loops (Fig. 4.2). The hypothalamus may release stimulatory or inhibitory stimuli to the pituitary, which in turn releases tropic hormones to target organs such as the adrenal glands. Target organs may return a feedback signal directly to the pituitary (short loop) or to the hypothalamus (long loop).

Hormone-Signaling Pathways

Hormones may be classified by structure (Fig. 4.3) and by function (Table 4.1). Most membrane-associated hormonal receptors generate signals by one of three major pathways, and these signaling pathways often do overlap (Fig. 4.4). These receptor-signaling pathways are (1) receptor kinases with ligands such as insulin and insulin-like growth factors (IGFs); (2) guanine nucleotide-binding or G-protein-coupled receptors, which are activated by peptide hormones, neurotransmitters, and prostaglandins (PGs); and (3) ligand-gated ion channels that permit ion transport on ligand–receptor binding.

On activation of the membrane receptors, secondary signaling pathways are utilized to amplify the triggering signal. One of the most ubiquitous intracellular second messengers by which hormones exert their effects is the modulation of

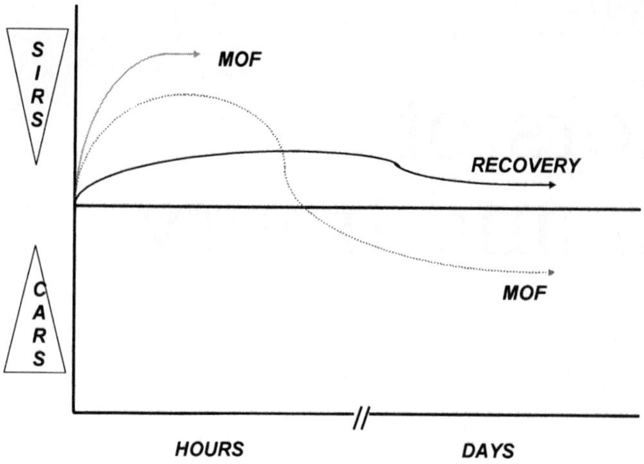

FIGURE 4.1. Schematic representation of the systemic inflammatory response (*SIRS*) to injury, followed by a period of convalescence mediated by counterregulatory antiinflammatory response (*CARS*). Severe inflammation may lead to acute multiple organ failure (*MOF*) and early death following injury (*gray solid arrow*). A lesser inflammatory response followed by excessive CARS may indicate a prolonged immunosuppressed state that can also be deleterious to the host (*dashed arrow*). Normal recovery after injury requires a period of systemic inflammation followed by a return to homeostasis (*black solid arrow*). (Adapted from Guirao and Lowry,[46] with permission from *World Journal of Surgery*.)

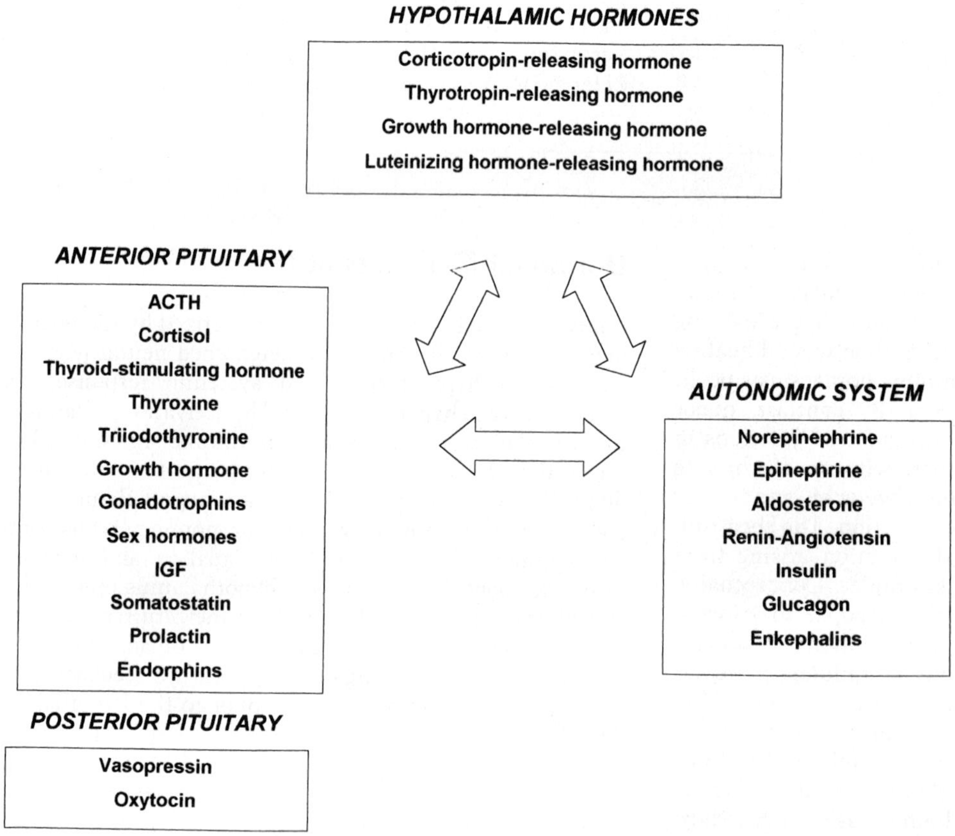

FIGURE 4.2. The hormones regulated by the hypothalamus, pituitary, and autonomic system comprise a complex network of stimulatory and inhibitory signals.

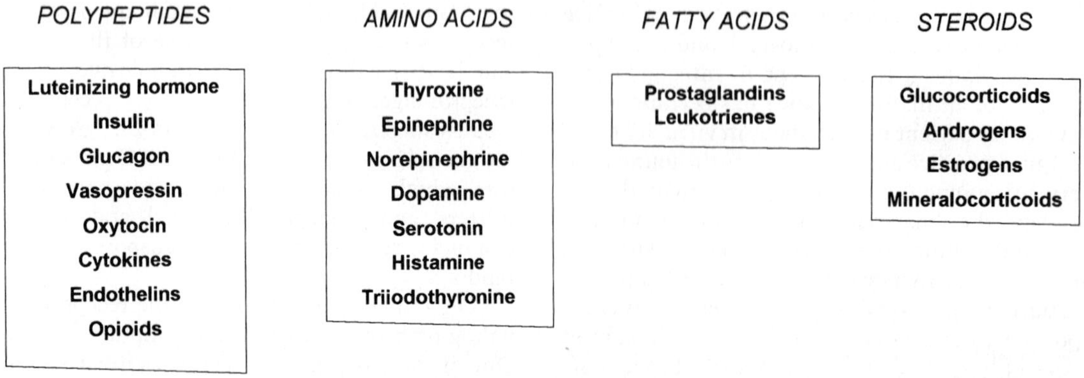

FIGURE 4.3. Hormones as catalogued by chemical structure.

TABLE 4.1. Hormone Classification by Function.

Activation of intracellular receptors	*Activation of surface receptors*	
Androgens	β_2-Adrenergic catecholamines	*cAMP (Second messenger)*
Calcitriol	ACTH	
Estrogens	Antidiuretic hormone	
Glucocorticoids	Calcitonin	
Mineralocorticoids	Chorionic gonadotropin	
Progestins	Corticotropin-releasing hormone	
Retinoic acid	Follicle-stimulating hormone	
Thyroid hormones	Glucagon	
	Lipotropin	
	Luteinizing hormone	
	Melanocyte-stimulating hormone	
	Parathyroid hormone	
	Thyroid-stimulating hormone	
	α_2-Adrenergic catecholamines	
	Angiotensin II	
	Opioids	
	Somatostatin	
	Atrial natriuretic peptide	*cGMP (Second messenger)*
	Nitric oxide	
	α_1-Adrenergic catecholamines	*Calcium/ Phosphatidylinositide (Second messengers)*
	Antidiuretic hormone	
	Epidermal growth factor	
	Gonadotropin-releasing hormone	
	Platelet-derived growth factor	
	Thyrotropin-releasing hormone	
	Acetylcholine (muscarinic)	
	Angiotensin II	
	Chorionic somatomammotropin	*Kinase/phosphatase (Second messengers)*
	Epidermal growth factor	
	Erythropoietin	
	Fibroblast growth factor	
	Growth hormone	
	Insulin	
	Insulin-like growth factor	
	Nerve growth factor	
	Oxytocin	
	Prolactin	

Hormones in the shaded boxes are known to inhibit second messengers.

Source: Adapted with permission from Granner.[187]

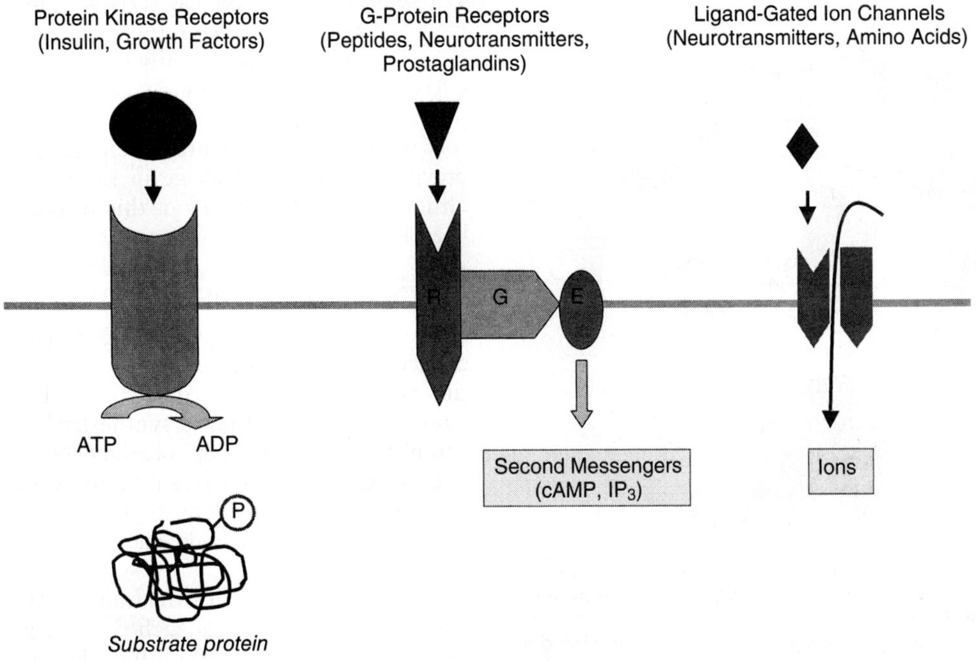

FIGURE 4.4. Three major classes of membrane receptors. The protein kinase receptor phosphorylates various protein kinase pathways. The G-protein receptors respond to ligands such as adrenaline and serotonin. On binding to the receptor (*R*), the *G* protein is activated and in turn activates the effector (*E*) component. The E component subsequently activates second messengers. The ligand-gated ion channel responds to a stimulus such as acetylcholine. On ligand binding, ion influx occurs, and second messengers are activated.

cyclic adenosine monophosphate (cAMP). Hormone–receptor interactions induce cell membrane alterations that activate the enzyme adenylate cyclase. Adenylate cyclase catalyzes the conversion of adenosine triphosphate (ATP) to cAMP, which in turn activates various intracellular protein kinases. Substances that decrease cAMP generally exert an influence opposite to those observed for substances that increase cAMP (see Table 4.1). For instance, increases in intracellular cAMP are associated with functional lymphocyte responses that generally are immunosuppressive.[2] In T lymphocytes, agents that increase cAMP levels diminish proliferation, lymphokine production, cytotoxic functions, and immunoglobulin production. Neutrophils with increased intracellular cAMP manifest decreased chemotaxis as well as reduced production of superoxides, H_2O_2, and lysosomal enzymes.[3] Similarly, basophils or mast cells demonstrate a decreased release of histamine.[4] Many prolonged hormone-mediated responses to injury tend toward increasing intracellular cAMP levels, either through a direct action on membrane receptors or by increasing the sensitivity of leukocytes to substances that directly increase cAMP. Whether this response to hormone stimulation contributes to the immunosuppression following injury is unclear.

Hormonal actions are further mediated by intracellular receptors. These intracellular receptors have binding affinities both for the hormone itself and for the targeted gene sequence on the DNA.[5] These intracellular receptors may be located within the cytosol or may already be localized in the nucleus, bound to the DNA. The classic example of a cytosolic hormonal receptor is a glucocorticoid receptor. Intracellular glucocorticoid receptors are maintained in an active state by linking to the stress-induced protein, heat-shock protein (HSP).[6] When the hormone ligand binds to the receptor, the dissociation of HSP from the receptor activates the receptor–ligand complex and is transported to the nucleus (Fig. 4.5).

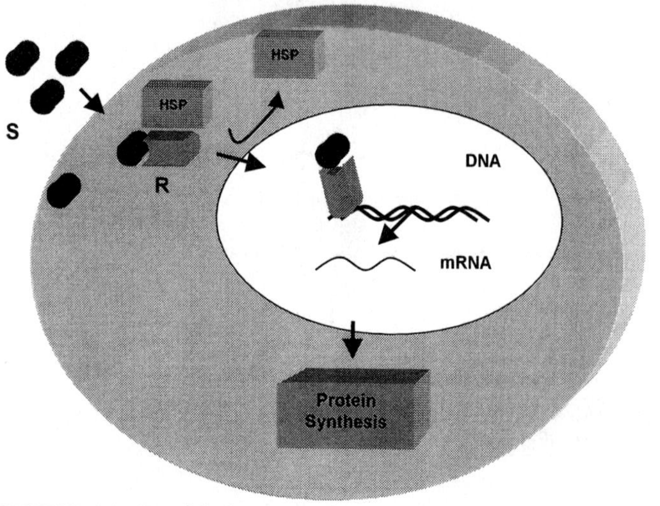

FIGURE 4.5. Simplified schematics of steroid transport into the nucleus. Steroid molecules (*S*) diffuse readily across cytoplasmic membranes. Intracellularly, the receptors (*R*) are rendered inactive by coupling to heat-shock protein (*HSP*). When S and R bind, HSP dissociates, and the S–R complex enters the nucleus, where the S–R complex induces DNA transcription and eventuates in protein synthesis.

Anterior Pituitary Function

Corticotropin-Releasing Hormone

Pain, fear, anxiety, or emotional arousal generate signals to the paraventricular nucleus of the hypothalamus, stimulating the synthesis of corticotrophin-releasing hormone (CRH), which is then delivered by way of the hypothalamic-hypophyseal-portal circulation to the anterior pituitary. Proinflammatory cytokines and vasopressin can also induce CRH synthesis and release. In the anterior pituitary, CRH serves as the major stimulant of corticotropin (ACTH; formerly adrenocorticotropic hormone or adrenocorticotropin) production and release.[7] This effect is accomplished by CRH-mediated activation of adenylate cyclase in the ACTH-producing corticotrophs, which increases intracellular cAMP levels and activates the pathway leading to increased ACTH production.

In laboratory animals, CRH has been demonstrated to induce hyperdynamic cardiovascular responses and catecholamine release characteristic of the sympathetic stress response.[8] The secretion of CRH can be directly activated by[9] angiotensin II (AT-II), neuropeptide Y, serotonin (5-hydroxytryptamine, 5-HT), acetylcholine, interleukin-1 (IL-1), and IL-6. The release of CRH can be inhibited by γ-aminobutyric acid (GABA), substance P, atrial natriuretic peptide (ANP), endogenous opioids, and L-arginine.[10] Aside from the pituitary gland and the central nervous system, receptors for CRH in primates have also been described within the renal medulla, marginal zone, and red pulp of the spleen and within the sympathetic ganglia.

Circulating glucocorticoids serve as potent negative feedback signals to the hypothalamus and have been demonstrated in animal models to reduce CRH messenger RNA (mRNA) transcription. On the other hand, adrenalectomized animals demonstrate elevated CRH mRNA transcriptional activities that are reversed with exogenous administration of dexamethasone or prednisolone. The CRH-binding proteins synthesized by the liver also serve as regulators of CRH activity. These proteins collectively demonstrate endogenous pathways that may potentially regulate or preclude excessive CRH-mediated responses to injury. Injured tissues also produce CRH that may contribute locally to the inflammatory response. Experimental studies suggest a role for CRH in preventing vascular leakage in injured or inflamed tissues, although the implications of this in human injury have not been identified.

Adrenocorticotropic Hormone

Adrenocorticotropic hormone (ACTH; adrenocorticotropin or corticotropin) is synthesized, stored, and released by the anterior pituitary on CRH stimulation. This hormone is a 39-amino-acid peptide that is synthesized as a larger precursor complex known as proopio-melanocortin (POMC).[11] POMC is cleaved within the cytosol to the components β-melanocyte stimulating hormone (β-MSH), lipotropin-stimulating hormone (LSH), the endogenous opiate β-endorphin, and ACTH.

In the nonstressed healthy human, ACTH release is regulated by circadian signals such that the greatest elevation of ACTH occurs late at night until the hours immediately before sunrise. This pattern is dramatically altered or obliterated in injured subjects.[12] Most injury is characterized by elevations

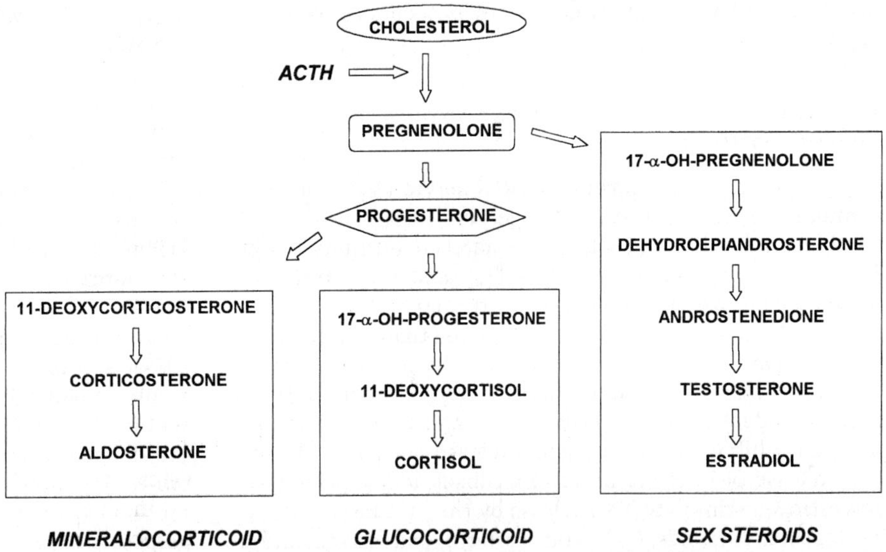

FIGURE 4.6. Steroid synthesis from cholesterol. ACTH is a principal regulator of steroid synthesis. The end products are mineralocorticoids, glucocorticoids, and sex steroids.

in CRH and ACTH that are proportional to the severity of injury. Although pain and anxiety are prominent mediators of ACTH release in the conscious injured patient, other ACTH-promoting mediators may become relatively more active in the injured patient; these include vasopressin, AT-II, cholecystokinin, vasoactive intestinal peptide (VIP), catecholamines, oxytocin, and proinflammatory cytokines.

Within the zona fasiculata of the adrenal gland, ACTH signaling activates intracellular adenylate cyclase, the cAMP-dependent protein kinase pathway, and the mitochondrial cytochrome P-450 system. This chain of activities leads to increased glucocorticoid production via desmolase-catalyzed side-chain cleavage of cholesterol (Fig. 4.6). Conditions of excess ACTH stimulation result in adrenal cortical hypertrophy.

Cortisol/Glucocorticoids

Cortisol is the major glucocorticoid in humans and is essential for survival following significant physiological stress. The cortisol response is altered in injury and may remain persistently elevated depending on the type of systemic stress. Burn patients have demonstrated elevated circulating cortisol levels up to 4 weeks; soft tissue injury and hemorrhage may sustain elevated cortisol levels for as long as a week.[13] Circulating cortisol rapidly returns to normal levels on restoration of blood volume following hemorrhage. Coexisting systemic stress such as infections can also prolong the elevated cortisol levels following injury.

Cortisol is a major effector of host metabolism. It potentiates the actions of glucagon and epinephrine (EPI), leading to hyperglycemia in the host.[14] In the liver, cortisol stimulates the enzymatic activities favoring gluconeogenesis.[15] Peripherally, it decreases insulin binding to insulin receptors in muscles and adipose tissue. In skeletal muscle, cortisol induces proteolysis as well as the release of lactate. The release of available lactate and amino acids has the net effect of shifting substrates for hepatic gluconeogenesis. Cortisol also stimulates lipolysis and inhibits glucose uptake by adipose tissues. It potentiates the lipolytic activities of ACTH, growth hormones (GHs), glucagon, and EPI. The resulting increased plasma free fatty acids, triglycerides, and glycerol from adipose tissue mobilization serve as available energy sources. In plasma, only 10% of cortisol is present in the free, biologically active form. The remaining 90% is bound to corticosteroid-binding globulin (CBG) and albumin. On injury, total plasma cortisol concentrations increase, but CBG and albumin levels decrease by as much as 50%.[16] This alteration can lead to an increase of free cortisol by as much as 10-fold over normal.[17]

Glucocorticoids exert immunosuppressive influences. Administration of glucocorticoids can induce rapid lymphopenia, monocytopenia, eosinopenia, and neutrophilia.[18] Immunological changes include thymic involution, depressed cell-mediated immune responses reflected by decreases in T-killer and natural killer (NK) cell functions, T-lymphocyte blastogenesis, mixed-lymphocyte responsiveness, graft-versus-host reactions, and delayed hypersensitivity responses. With glucocorticoid administration, monocytes lose the capacity for intracellular killing but appear to maintain normal chemotactic and phagocytic properties. Neutrophil function is affected by glucocorticoid treatment in terms of intracellular superoxide reactivity and depressed chemotaxis.[19] However, neutrophil phagocytosis remains unchanged. Finally, glucocorticoids are inhibitors of immunocyte proinflammatory cytokine synthesis and secretion.[20,21] Indeed, glucocorticoid infusion in human endotoxemia downregulates tumor necrosis factor-alpha (TNF-α) production and increases the production of IL-10, the antiinflammatory mediator.[22] This glucocorticoid-induced downregulation of cytokine stimulation serves an important negative regulatory function in the inflammatory response to injury.

Macrophage Inhibitory Factor

Initially identified as a T-lymphocyte-derived inhibitor of macrophage migration, macrophage inhibitory factor (MIF) is a glucocorticoid antagonist produced by the anterior pituitary.[23] This hormone can potentially reverse the immunosuppressive effects of glucocorticoids both systemically via anterior pituitary secretion and at local sites of inflammation where MIF is produced by T lymphocytes. In experiments in which anti-MIF antibodies were administered to endotoxemic mice, survival increased, presumably because glucocorticoid antiinflammatory effects were not counterregulated by MIF.

Thyrotropin-Releasing Hormone and Thyroid-Stimulating Hormone

Thyrotropin-releasing hormone (TRH) serves as the primary stimulant for the synthesis, storage, and release of thyroid-stimulating hormone (TSH) in the anterior pituitary.[24] The TSH in turn stimulates thyroxine (T_4) production from the thyroid gland, which is converted to triiodothyroxine (T_3) by peripheral tissues. The T_3 is more potent than T_4, but both are transported intracellularly by cytosolic receptors, which then bind DNA to mediate the transcription of multiple protein products. Free forms of both T_4 and T_3 in the circulation can inhibit the hypothalamic release of TRH and pituitary release of TSH via negative-feedback loops. Both TRH and estrogen stimulate TSH release by the pituitary, whereas T_3, T_4, corticosteroids, GHs, somatostatin, and fasting inhibit TSH release.

Thyroid hormones (thyronines), when elevated above normal levels, exert diverse influences on cellular metabolism and function. Thyronines enhance membrane transport of glucose and increase glucose oxidation. These hormones increase the formation and storage of fat when carbohydrate intake is excessive, but this process decreases during starvation. The increase in cellular metabolism from excess thyroid hormone production leads to proportional elevations in overall oxygen consumption as well as heat production.

Although T_3 levels are frequently decreased after injury, there is no compensatory rise in TSH release.[25] In fact, following major injury, reduced circulating TSH levels are observed, and peripheral conversion of T_4 to T_3 is impaired concomitant with a reduction in available T_3. This impaired conversion may be explained in part by the inhibitory effects of cortisol and an increased conversion of T_4 to the biologically inactive molecule known as reverse T_3 (rT_3). Elevated rT_3, but reduced T_4 and T_3, is an observation characteristic of acute injury or trauma, referred to as *euthyroid sick syndrome* or *nonthyroidal illness*. Experimentally, mild endotoxemia in otherwise healthy humans has shown that thyroid hormone alteration in systemic inflammation is not mediated by endogenous IL-1. Although total T_4 (protein bound and free) levels may be reduced following injury, free T_4 concentrations remain relatively constant. In severely injured or critically ill patients, a reduced free T_4 concentration has been predictive of high mortality.

Lymphoid cells have high-affinity nuclear and cytoplasmic binding sites for thyronines, and one consequence of exposure to thyronines is an increase in the uptake of amino acids and glucose into the cell. Whether this is a direct effect of thyroid hormones or a secondary effect of increased cellular metabolism is unknown. As with other somatic cells, leukocyte metabolism measured by oxygen consumption is increased in hyperthyroid individuals and subjects receiving thyroid hormones. Functionally, animal studies have demonstrated that surgically or chemically induced thyroid hormone depletion significantly decreases cellular and humoral immunity. By contrast, thyroid hormone repletion is associated with enhancement of both types of immunity. Human monocytes, NK cells, and activated B lymphocytes express receptors for TSH. Exposure of B cells to TSH in vitro induces a moderate increase in immunoglobulin secretion.

Growth Hormones and Insulin-Like Growth Factors

Hypothalamic growth hormone-releasing hormone (GHRH) traverses through the hypothalamo-hypophyseal-portal circulation to the anterior pituitary and stimulates the release of GHs in a pulsatile fashion during the sleeping hours. In addition to GHRH, GH release is influenced by autonomic stimulation, thyroxine, vasopressin, ACTH, β-MSH, glucagon, and sex hormones. Other stimuli for GH release are physical exercise, sleep, stress, hypovolemia, fasting hypoglycemia, decreased circulating fatty acids, and increased amino acid levels. Conditions that inhibit GH release include hyperglycemia, hypertriglyceridemia, somatostatin, α-adrenergic stimulation, and cortisol. During times of stress, GH promotes protein synthesis as well as enhances the mobilization of fat stores. Fat mobilization occurs by direct stimulation in conjunction with potentiation of adrenergic lipolytic effects on adipose stores. In the liver, hepatic ketogenesis is also promoted by GH. Insulin release is inhibited and glucose oxidation is decreased by GH, leading to elevated glucose levels.

The protein synthesis properties of GH following injury are mediated in part by the secondary release of insulin-like growth factor-1 (IGF-1).[26] This hormone, which circulates predominantly in bound form with several binding proteins, promotes amino acid incorporation and cellular proliferation and attenuates proteolysis in skeletal muscle as well as in the liver. The IGFs (formerly referred to as somatomedins) are mediators of hepatic protein synthesis and glycogenesis.[27] In the adipose tissue, IGF increases glucose uptake and lipid synthesis. In skeletal muscles, it increases glucose uptake and protein synthesis. Also, IGF has a role in skeletal growth by promoting the incorporation of sulfate and proteoglycans into cartilage. In vitro studies utilizing proteoglycan synthesis as a marker for IGF-1 activity demonstrated that IL-1α, TNF-α, and IL-6 can inhibit the effects of IGF-1.

There is a rise in circulating GH levels following injury, major surgery, and anesthesia. However, the associated decrease in protein synthesis and observed negative nitrogen balance is attributed to a reduction in IGF-1 levels following injury.[28] Administration of GH has been shown to improve the clinical course of pediatric burn patients, but its use in injured adult patients remains unproven. The liver is the predominant source of IGF-1, and preexisting hepatic dysfunction may further contribute to the negative nitrogen balance following injury. The IGF-binding proteins are also produced within the liver and are necessary for effective binding of IGF to the cell. In sum, IGF has the potential for attenuating the catabolic effects following surgical insults.[29]

Leukocytes express high-affinity surface receptors for GH. In general, GH and IGF-1 are immunostimulatory and promote tissue proliferation. In vitro, GH augments the proliferation of T lymphocytes to mitogens and the cytotoxicity of T killer cells to allogenic stimuli. Macrophages also respond to GH with a modest respiratory burst. Mice deficient in GH manifest immunodeficiencies that can be partially reversed by the administration of GH. However, GH-deficient humans do not display any clinically significant immunological abnormalities. Normal humans given intravenous GH demonstrate no significant immunological changes except for neutrophilia. It is evident that GH has immunomodulating effects, but the clinical relevance of this influence remains to be determined.

SOMATOSTATIN

Somatostatin is a 14-amino-acid polypeptide produced by diverse cell types that include the gastric antrum and pancreatic islet D cells. It is a potent inhibitor of GH, TSH, renin, insulin, and glucagon release.[30] The role of somatostatin during injury is yet unclear, but it may serve to regulate excessive nutrient absorption and the activities of GH and IGF during the convalescence period.

GONADOTROPHINS AND SEX HORMONES

Luteinizing hormone-releasing hormone (LHRH) or gonadotropin-releasing hormone (GnRH or gonadotrophins) is released from the hypothalamus and stimulates follicle-stimulating hormone (FSH) and luteinizing hormone (LH) release from the anterior pituitary. The release of these hormones can be effectively blocked by CRH, prolactin, estrogen, progestins, and androgens. The most relevant clinical correlation is seen following injury, stress, or severe illness when release of LH and FSH is suppressed. The reduction in LH and FSH consequently reduces estrogen and androgen secretion. This change is attributed to the inhibitory activities of CRH on LH and FSH release and accounts for the menstrual irregularity and decreased libido reported following surgical stress and other injuries.

Estrogens inhibit cell-mediated immunity, NK cell activity, and neutrophil function but stimulate antibody-mediated immunity. Androgens appear to be predominantly immunosuppressive. In fact, in animal experiments castration is associated with enhanced immune function that can be reversed by exogenous androgens. Conversely, ovariectomy in the same type of animals results in immunodepression following trauma.[31] Experimental data have shown greater survival rates in female animals following trauma than in male animals.[32] Although a strong experimental basis supports the concept that female animals have improved survival following inflammatory stresses, the documentation of this sexual dimorphism survival bias is far less evident clinically. Studies documented modest differences between young, healthy male and female subjects regarding systemic phenotype responses (temperature, blood pressure) but no differences in cytokine responses after an endotoxin challenge.[33]

PROLACTIN

The role of the hypothalamus is to suppress prolactin secretion from the anterior pituitary; this is achieved by the activities of LHRH/GnRH and dopamine. Stimulants for its release are CRH, TRH, GHRH, serotonin, and VIP.

Elevated prolactin levels following injury have been described in adults; reduced levels are noted in children. The hyperprolactinemia may also account for the amenorrhea frequently seen in women following injury or major surgeries. Like GH, prolactin has immunostimulatory properties. Chemically induced inhibition of prolactin in animals has demonstrated increased susceptibility to infection, decreased lymphocyte proliferation, decreased IL-2 production and receptor expression, decreased interferon-alpha (IFN-α) production, and macrophage dysfunction. Exogenous administration of prolactin reversed these effects. There is increasing evidence that prolactin is also synthesized and secreted by T lymphocytes and may function in an autocrine or paracrine fashion.

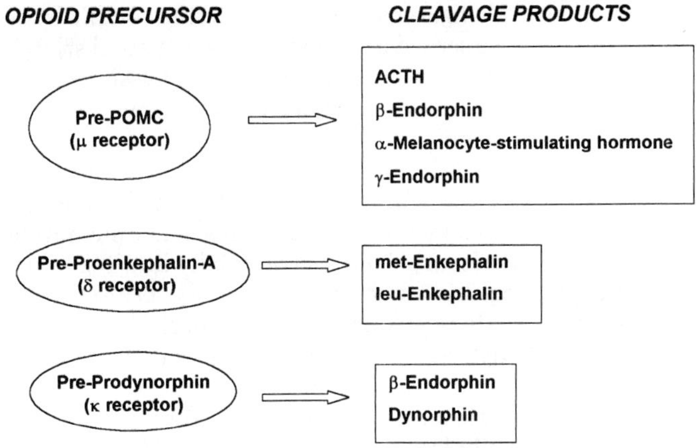

FIGURE 4.7. Precursors of endogenous opioids.

ENDOGENOUS OPIOIDS

Elevated endogenous opioids are measurable after major surgeries or insults to the patient.[34] In addition to their role in attenuating pain perception, β-endorphins are capable of inducing hypotension through a serotonin-mediated pathway. On the other hand, the enkephalins produce hypertension. In the gastrointestinal tract, the occupation of opioid receptors reduces peristaltic activity as well as suppresses fluid secretion. The role of endogenous opioids in glucose metabolism is probably complex.[35] Although endorphins and morphine induce hyperglycemia, they also increase both insulin and glucagon release by the pancreas. In animal models, endogenous opioids such as dynorphins have demonstrated a paracrine role in modulation of vasopressin and oxytocin secretion. Studies demonstrating the presence of opioid receptors in the adrenal medulla also suggest their role in regulating catecholamine release.

Certain immune cells release endorphins that also share an antinociceptive role in modulating the response of local sensory neurons to noxious stimuli. Endorphins also influence the immune system by increasing NK cell cytotoxicity and T-cell blastogenesis.[36] There is evidence that IL-1 stimulates the release of endorphins from the pituitary gland. Both endogenous opioids (endorphin and enkephalin) and exogenous opiates mediate their effects through mammalian delta, kappa, and mu receptors (Fig. 4.7). Opioids appear to compromise both the natural (innate) and specific (adaptive) immune system through dose-dependent inhibition of proliferation and differentiation in lymphocytes and monocytes/macrophages.

Posterior Pituitary Function

VASOPRESSIN

Vasopressin (antidiuretic hormone, ADH) is synthesized in the anterior hypothalamus and transported by axoplasmic flow to the posterior pituitary for storage. The major stimulus for vasopressin release is elevated plasma osmolality as detected by sodium-sensitive hypothalamic osmoreceptors. There is evidence of extracerebral osmoreceptors for vasopressin release in the liver and the portal circulation. Vasopressin release is enhanced by α-adrenergic agonists, AT-II stimulation, opioids, anesthetic agents, pain, and elevated glucose concentrations. Changes in effective circulating volume by as little as 10% can be sensed by baroreceptors, left atrial stretch receptors, and chemoreceptors, leading to vasopressin release. Release of vasopressin is inhibited by β-adrenergic agonists and ANP. There is now substantial evidence documenting a "vasopressin-resistant" condition in many patients suffering from severe injury and sepsis. While efforts to overcome this resistance state have included the exogenous administration of arginine vasoporessin (AVP), the potentially limiting toxicity of the agent requires other support measures. Data confirm that glucocorticoids may improve the vasopressin-resistant condition, although the mechanisms for this interaction remain unclear.[37]

In the kidney, vasopressin promotes reabsorption of water from the distal tubules and collecting ducts. Peripherally, vasopressin mediates vasoconstriction. This effect in the splanchnic circulation may cause the trauma-induced ischemia/reperfusion phenomenon antecedent of gut barrier impairment. Vasopressin, on a molar basis, is more potent than glucagon in stimulating hepatic glycogenolysis and gluconeogenesis. The resulting hyperglycemia increases the osmotic effect, which contributes to the restoration of effective circulating volume. Elevated vasopressin secretion is another characteristic of trauma, hemorrhage, open heart surgery, and other major operations. This elevated level typically persists for 1 week after the insult.

The syndrome of inappropriate antidiuretic hormone release (SIADH) describes the excessive vasopressin release that is manifested by low urine output, highly concentrated urine, and dilutional hyponatremia. Clinically, this diagnosis can only be made if the patient is euvolemic. Once normal volume is established, a plasma osmolality less than 275 mOsm/kg H_2O and a urine osmolality greater than 100 mOsm/kg H_2O are indicative of this diagnosis. SIADH is commonly seen in patients with head trauma and burns.

In the absence of vasopressin, a situation of central diabetes insipidus occurs in which there is voluminous output of dilute urine. Frequently seen in comatose patients, the polyuria in untreated diabetes insipidus can precipitate a state of hypernatremia and hypovolemic shock. Attempts at reversal should include free water and exogenous vasopressin (desmopressin, DDAVP).

Oxytocin

Oxytocin and vasopressin are the only known hormones to be secreted by the posterior pituitary. Although both hormones share structural similarities, the role of oxytocin in the injury response is unknown. In humans, the only consistent stimulus for oxytocin secretion is suckling or other nipple stimulation in lactating women, which stimulates contraction of lactating mammary glands and induces uterine contractions in parturition. There is no recognized stimulus for oxytocin release or any known functions in men.

Autonomic Regulation

A balance of autonomic function is increasingly recognized as important for regulating inflammation at the local and systemic levels.[38] Studies have identified dysfunction of autonomic signaling either via classic neurohumoral mediators, such as catecholamines,[39] or through neurally transmitted signals, such as those elicited by vagus nerve traffic,[40,41] as consequential to the regulation of pro- and antiinflammatory responses. The latter pathway, now termed the *cholinergic antiinflammatory pathway*, appears to regulate the production of TNF-α within tissue macrophages.[42]

Catecholamines

Catecholamines exert significant influence in the physiological response to stress and injury. Indeed, the hypermetabolic state observed following severe injury has been attributed to activation of the adrenergic system. Both norepinephrine (NE) and EPI are increased in plasma immediately following injury, with average elevations of three- to fourfold above baseline. Catecholamines increase immediately after injury and reach their peak in 24 to 48 h before returning to baseline levels. The patterns of both NE and EPI appearance parallel each other following injury. Most of the NE in plasma results from synaptic leakage during sympathetic nervous system activity, whereas virtually all plasma EPI is secreted by adrenal chromaffin cells.

Catecholamines exert metabolic, hormonal, and hemodynamic influences on cells. In the liver, EPI promotes glycogenolysis, gluconeogenesis, lipolysis, and ketogenesis. It also causes decreased insulin secretion but increases glucagon secretion. Peripherally, EPI increases lipolysis in adipose tissues and inhibits insulin-facilitated glucose uptake by skeletal muscle. These effects collectively promote the often-evident stress-induced hyperglycemia, not unlike the effects of cortisol on blood sugar. Catecholamines also increase the secretion of thyroid and parathyroid hormones, T_4 and T_3, and renin but inhibit the release of aldosterone.

Catecholamines elicit discernible influences on immune function. As an example, catecholamine occupation of β-receptors present on leukocytes increases intracellular cAMP, which may decrease immune responsiveness in lymphocytes. Like cortisol, EPI enhances leukocyte demargination with resultant neutrophilia and lymphocytosis. Also, EPI lowers the ratio of $CD4^+$ to $CD8^+$ T lymphocytes. Immunological tissues such as the spleen, thymus, and lymph nodes possess extensive adrenergic innervation. Chemical sympathectomy of peripheral nerves has been demonstrated to augment antibody response following immunization with a specific antigen. It also reverses the depressed mitogenic response of splenocytes preincubated with endotoxin. Normal volunteers infused with EPI exhibited depressed mitogen-induced T-lymphocyte proliferation.

Aldosterone

The mineralocorticoid aldosterone is synthesized, stored, and released in the adrenal zona glomerulosa. Aldosterone release during injury is stimulated by AT-II, hyperkalemia, pituitary aldosterone-stimulating factor, and most potently, ACTH.

The major function of aldosterone is to maintain intravascular volume by conserving sodium and eliminating potassium and hydrogen ions in the early distal convoluted tubules of the nephrons. Although the major effect is exerted in the kidneys, this hormone is also active in the intestines, salivary glands, sweat glands, vascular endothelium, and brain. In the late distal convoluted tubule, further sodium reabsorption takes place while potassium ions are excreted. Vasopressin also acts in concert with aldosterone to increase osmotic water flux into the tubules.

Patients with aldosterone deficiency develop hypotension and hyperkalemia, whereas patients with aldosterone excess develop edema, hypertension, hypokalemia, and metabolic alkalosis. Following injury, ACTH stimulates a brief burst of aldosterone release. Angiotensin II induces a protracted aldosterone release that persists well after ACTH returns to baseline. Like cortisol, normal aldosterone release is also influenced by the circadian cycle, but this effect is lost in the injured patient.

Renin–Angiotensin

Renin is synthesized and stored primarily within the renal juxtaglomerular (JG) apparatus near the afferent arteriole. The JG apparatus is comprised of the JG neurogenic receptor, JG cell, and macula densa. Renin initially exists in an inactive form as prorenin. The activation of renin and its release are mediated by ACTH, vasopressin, glucagon, PGs, potassium, magnesium, and calcium. The JG cells are baroreceptors that respond to a decrease in blood pressure by increasing renin secretion. The macula densa detects changes in chloride concentration within the renal tubules.

Angiotensinogen is a protein primarily synthesized by the liver but also identified in the kidney. Renin catalyzes the conversion of angiotensinogen to angiotensin I (AT-I) within the kidney. Angiotensin I remains physiologically inactive until it is converted in the pulmonary circulation to AT-II by angiotensin-converting enzyme (ACE) present on endothelial surfaces (Fig. 4.8).

The potent vasoconstrictor AT-II also stimulates aldosterone and vasopressin synthesis. It is capable of regulating thirst; AT-II stimulates heart rate and myocardial contractility. It also potentiates the release of EPI by the adrenal medulla, increases CRH release, and activates the sympathetic nervous system. It can induce glycogenolysis and gluconeogenesis. Expectedly, the renin–angiotensin system participates in the response to injury by acting to maintain volume homeostasis.

Insulin

Insulin is derived from pancreatic beta islet cells and released on stimulation by specific substrates, autonomic neural input, and other hormones. In normal metabolism, glucose is the major stimulant of insulin secretion. Other stimulants are amino acids, free fatty acids, and ketone bodies. Hormonal and neural influences during stress alter this response. Insulin release is inhibited by EPI and sympathetic stimulation. Other factors that further diminish insulin release include glucagon, somatostatin, gastrointestinal hormones, endorphins, and IL-1. Peripherally, cortisol, estrogen, and progesterone interfere with glucose uptake. The net result of impaired insulin production and function following injury is stress-induced hyperglycemia. These mechanisms are in keeping with the general catabolic state immediately following major injury. Insulin exerts a global anabolic effect in which it promotes hepatic glycogenesis and glycolysis, glucose transport into cells, adipose tissue lipogenesis, and protein synthesis. In the injured patient, there are two phases to the pattern of insulin release. The first phase occurs within a few hours after injury and manifests as relative suppression of insulin release, reflecting the influence of catecholamines and sympathetic stimulation. The later phase is characterized by a return to normal or excessive insulin production but with persistent hyperglycemia, demonstrating a peripheral resistance to insulin.

Activated lymphocytes express receptors for insulin. Furthermore, insulin has been shown to enhance T-lymphocyte proliferation and cytotoxicity. In fact, mouse spleen cells transiently exposed to a mitogen can continue to proliferate and maintain cytotoxicity if insulin is added to the medium. Clinically, institution of insulin therapy to newly diagnosed diabetics is associated with increased B- and T-lymphocyte populations. The utilization of intensive insulin therapy for control of hyperglycemia has received much attention as this therapy is presumed to exert, at least partial, antiinflammatory influences.[43] Although appealing as an explanation for

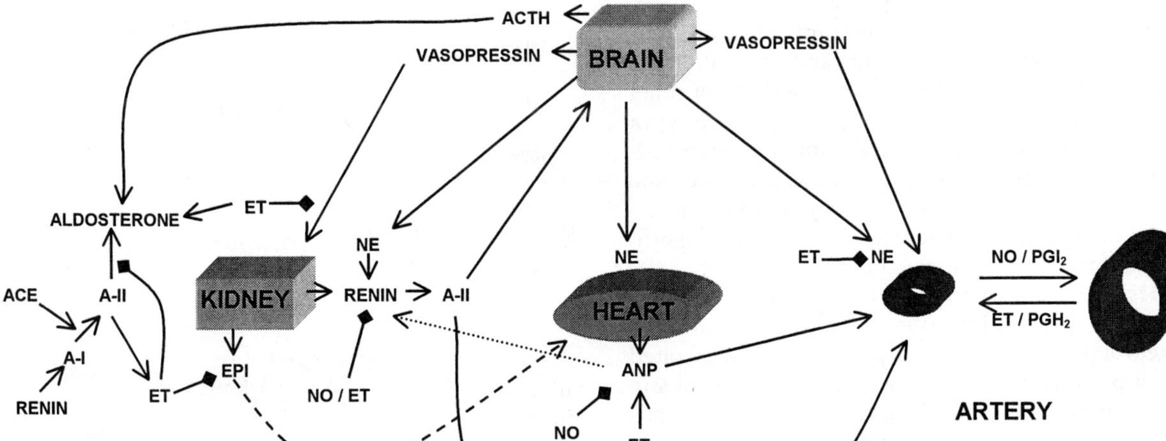

FIGURE 4.8. Endocrine activity of endothelium-derived mediators nitric oxide (*NO*) and endothelin (*ET*). *ANP*, atrial natriuretic peptide; *NE*, norepinephrine; *ACTH*, adrenocorticotropin; *EPI*, epinephrine; *ACE*, angiotensin-converting enzyme; *A-I* and *A-II*, angiotensin I and II, respectively; *PGI_2*, prostacyclin; *PGH_2*, prostaglandin H_2. *Arrows*, stimulatory signal; *lines with diamond symbols*, inhibitory signal. (Adapted from Luscher,[156] with permission.)

the presumed benefit of this therapeutic approach, few, if any, of the several inflammation regulatory mechanisms attributable to insulin have been clearly established.

Glucagon

Glucagon is a product of pancreatic alpha islet cells. Similar to insulin, the release of glucagon is also mediated by its substrates, autonomic neural input, and other hormones. However, whereas insulin is an anabolic hormone, glucagon has catabolic properties. Glucagon has a half-life of approximately 5 min and operates by adenylate cyclase second-messenger activity. The primary stimulants of glucagon secretion are low plasma glucose concentrations and exercise.

Glucagon stimulates hepatic glycogenolysis and gluconeogenesis, which under basal conditions account for approximately 75% of the glucose produced by the liver. In contrast to insulin, glucagon promotes hepatic ketogenesis and lipolysis in adipose tissue. The release of glucagon following injury is initially decreased, but returns to normal 12 h later. By 24 h, glucagon levels are supranormal and can persist for as long as 3 days.

Immune and Cellular Response to Injury

Endogenous mediators of inflammation orchestrate the hemodynamic, metabolic, and immune responses following acute injury and severe infections. Unlike classic hormonal mediators, which are produced by specialized tissues and exert their influence predominantly by endocrine routes, cytokines are polypeptides or glycoproteins produced by diverse cell types at the site of injury as well as by systemic immune cells. Moreover, cytokines are not stored as preformed molecules but rather are produced on demand by active gene transcription and translation by the injured or stimulated cell. Once released into the circulation, cytokines function predominantly via paracrine and autocrine mechanisms.

Cytokines bind to specific cellular receptors that result in activation of intracellular signaling pathways and gene transcription.[44] By this mechanism, cytokines influence immune cell activity, differentiation, proliferation, and survival. These mediators also regulate the production and activity of other cytokines, which may either augment (proinflammatory) or attenuate (antiinflammatory) the inflammatory response. The capacity of cytokines to activate diverse cell types and to incite equally diverse responses underscores the pleiotropism of these inflammatory mediators. There is also significant overlap in bioactivity among different cytokines.

Cytokines are necessary mediators that direct the inflammatory response to sites of infection and injury and are essential promoters of proper wound healing. However, exaggerated production of proinflammatory cytokines from the local site of injury can manifest systemically as hemodynamic instability (e.g., septic shock) or metabolic derangements (e.g., muscle wasting).[45] Following severe injuries or infections, persistently exaggerated proinflammatory cytokine response can contribute to end-organ injury, leading to multiple-organ failure (MOF) and late mortality.[46] The presence of antiinflammatory cytokines may serve to attenuate some of these exaggerated responses. However, it is presently assumed that excessive antiinflammatory cytokine production activity may promote a condition of immunocompromise and enhance susceptibility to infectious morbidity.

Cytokine Response to Injury

The cytokine cascade activated in response to injury is complex. Hence, a proper perspective of the immunobiological functions of cytokines can have important applications in the comprehensive care of the surgical patient (Fig. 4.9).[47] The list of cytokines is rapidly expanding, and the ones described here represent only a partial list of mediators pertinent to injury and the inflammatory response (Table 4.2).

Tumor Necrosis Factor-α

Following acute injury or during infections, TNF-α is among the earliest and most potent mediators of subsequent host responses. The primary sources of TNF-α synthesis include monocytes/macrophages and T cells, which are abundant in the peritoneum and splanchnic tissues.[48] Furthermore, Kupffer cells represent the single largest concentrated population of macrophages in the human body. Therefore, surgical or traumatic injuries to the abdominal viscera undoubtedly have profound influences on the generation of inflammatory mediators and homeostatic responses such as acute-phase protein production.[49,50] Although the half-life of TNF-α is less than 20 min, this brief appearance is sufficient to evoke marked metabolic and hemodynamic changes and activate mediators distally in the cytokine cascade. Also, TNF-α is a major inducer of muscle catabolism and cachexia during stress by shunting available amino acids to the hepatic circulation as fuel substrates. Other functions of TNF-α include coagulation activation, promoting the expression or release of adhesion molecules, PGE_2, platelet-activating factor (PAF), glucocorticoids, and eicosanoids.[51]

Soluble (i.e., circulating) TNF receptors (sTNFRs) are proteolytically cleaved extracellular domains of membrane-

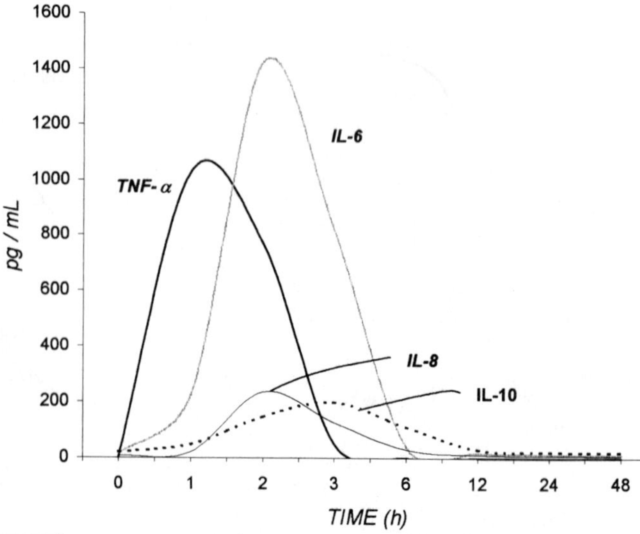

FIGURE 4.9. Sequence of appearance for TNF-α, IL-6, IL-8, and IL-10 following 2 ng/kg intravenous bolus of standardized endotoxin (lot EC-5) administered to five healthy male subjects. Values are mean circulating levels. (Adapted from Lin and Lowry,[47] with permission.)

TABLE 4.2. Sources of Selected Cytokines.

Cytokine	*Source*	*Cytokine*	*Source*
TNF-α	**Macrophages/monocytes** Kupffer cells Neutrophils NK cells Astrocytes Endothelial cells T lymphocytes Adrenal cortical cells Adipocytes Keratinocytes Osteoblasts Mast cells Dendritic cells	IL-6	**T lymphocytes/macrophages** B lymphocytes Neutrophils Basophils Mast cells Fibroblasts Endothelial cells Astrocytes Synovial cells Adipocytes Osteoblasts Megakaryocytes Chromaffin cells Keratinocytes
IL-1	**Macrophages/monocytes** B and T lymphocytes NK cells Endothelial cells Epithelial cells Keratinocytes Fibroblasts Osteoblasts Dendritic cells Astrocytes Adrenal cortical cells Megakaryocytes Platelets Neutrophils Neuronal cells	IL-8	**Macrophages/monocytes** T lymphocytes Basophils Mast cells Epithelial cells Platelets
		IL-10	**T lymphocytes** B lymphocytes Macrophages Basophils Mast cells Keratinocytes
IL-2	**T lymphocytes**	IL-12	**Macrophages/monocytes** Neutrophils Keratinocytes Dendritic cells B lymphocytes
IL-3	**T lymphocytes** Macrophages Eosinophils Mast cells	IL-13	**T lymphocytes**
		IL-15	**Macrophages/monocytes** Epithelial cells
IL-4	**T lymphocytes** Mast cells Basophils Macrophages B lymphocytes Eosinophils Stromal cells	IL-18	**Macrophages** Kupffer cells Keratinocytes Adrenal cortical cells Osteoblasts
IL-5	**T lymphocytes** Eosinophils Mast cells Basophils	IFN-γ	**T lymphocytes** NK cells Macrophages
		GM-CSF	**T lymphocytes** Fibroblasts Endothelial cells Stromal cells

Principal sources are in bold.

Source: Adapted from Lin et al.[184]

associated TNFRs that are elevated and readily detectable in acute inflammation. The sTNFRs retain their affinity for the binding of TNF-α and therefore compete with the cellular receptors for the binding of free TNF-α. This effect potentially represents an endogenous counterregulatory response to excessive systemic TNF-α activity.[52] The functional biology of sTNFR is limited to TNF-α antagonism as these molecules may also serve as a carrier (e.g., transporter) or as a storage pool of bioactive TNF-α in the circulation.

Interleukin-1

Interleukin-1 is primarily released by activated macrophages and endothelial cells. There are two known species of IL-1: IL-1α and IL-1β. The IL-1α is predominantly cell membrane associated and exerts its influence via cellular contacts; IL-1β is more readily detectable in the circulation and is capable of eliciting similar physiological and metabolic alterations as TNF-α.[53] With high doses of either IL-1 or TNF-α, these cytokines independently initiate a state of hemodynamic decompensation. At low doses, they can produce the same response only if administered simultaneously. These observations emphasize the synergistic roles of TNF-α and IL-1 in the inflammatory response.[54] Predominantly, IL-1 is a local mediator with a half-life of approximately 6 min, which makes its detectability in acute injury or illness even less likely than that of TNF-α. Interleukin-1 induces the classic inflammatory febrile response to injury by stimulating local PG activity in the anterior hypothalamus. Attenuated pain perception after surgery can be mediated by IL-1 by promoting the release of β-endorphins from the pituitary gland and increasing the number of central opioid-like receptors.[55]

Endogenous IL-1 receptor antagonists (IL-1ra) are also released during injury and serve as an endogenous autoregulator of IL-1 activity.[56] This molecule effectively competes for binding to IL-1 receptors yet exacts no overt signal transduction.

Interleukin-2

Interleukin-2 is a primary promoter of T-lymphocyte proliferation, immunoglobulin production, and gut barrier integrity. Partly as a result of its circulation half-life, less than 10 min, IL-2 has not been readily detectable following acute injury. Attenuated IL-2 expression associated with major injuries or perioperative blood transfusions potentially contributes to the transient immunocompromised state of the surgical patient.[57] There is evidence to suggest that accelerated lymphocyte apoptosis (i.e., lymphocyte depletion) exacerbates the injury-induced immunocompromise as a result of diminished IL-2 stimulation.[58]

Interleukin-4

Interleukin-4 is produced by activated type 2 T-helper (T_H2) cells and possesses diverse influence on hemopoietic cell proliferation. It is particularly important in antibody-mediated immunity and in antigen presentation.[59] Class switching in differentiating B lymphocytes is induced by IL-4 to produce predominantly immunoglobulin (Ig) G_4 and IgE, which are important immunoglobulins in allergic and antihelminthic responses. Interleukin-4 has potent antiinflammatory properties against activated macrophages by downregulating the effects of IL-1, TNF-α, IL-6, and IL-8, as well as oxygen radical production. Also, IL-4 appears to increase macrophage susceptibility to the antiinflammatory effects of glucocorticoids.[60]

Interleukin-6

Tumor necrosis factor-α and IL-1 are potent inducers of IL-6 production from virtually all cells and tissues, including the gut. After injury, IL-6 levels in the circulation are detectable by 60 min, peak between 4 and 6 h, and can persist for as long as 10 days. Circulating IL-6 levels appear to be proportional to the extent of tissue injury during an operation, more so than the duration of the surgical procedure itself. Evidence has demonstrated both a proinflammatory role and an antiinflammatory role for IL-6.[61] Interleukin-6 is an important mediator of the hepatic acute-phase response during injury and convalescence. Interleukin-6 not only induces neutrophil activation during injury and inflammation but also may delay the disposal of such neutrophils, thereby prolonging the injurious effects mediated by these cells.[62] Also, IL-6 possesses antiinflammatory properties during injury by attenuating TNF-α and IL-1 activity while promoting the release of sTNFRs and IL-1ra.[63]

Interleukin-8

Interleukin-8 is perhaps the best studied of a larger class of proteins (chemokines) that activate and attract leukocytes to sites of inflammation. There are at least four families of chemokines, including the a and b groups, which are defined by the amino acid spacing among cysteine residues. The α chemokines with a glutamic acid–leucine–arginine motif near the N-terminal, such as IL-8, are chemotactic for neutrophils, whereas those without this sequence influence lymphocytes. The β chemokines attract monocytes, eosinophils, basophils, and lymphocytes. There are also several chemokine receptor types that are differentially expressed on leukocytes. The rich diversity of chemokine activities serves in part to orchestrate the specificity and temporal sequencing of inflammatory infiltrates. Those conditions, which are characterized by a predominance of neutrophil infiltration, likely vary considerably in chemokine profile from a site featuring lymphocyte or monocytic infiltrates.[64]

Interleukin-10

Among other activities, IL-10 functions as a modulator of TNF-α activity. Experimental evidence has demonstrated that neutralization of IL-10 during endotoxemia increases monocyte TNF-α production and mortality, but restitution of IL-10 reduces TNF-α levels and the associated deleterious effects.[65] Also, IL-10 is capable of attenuating IL-18 mRNA expression in monocytes.[66] In animal experiments, induction of IL-10 transcription has been shown to attenuate the systemic inflammatory response and reduce mortality during septic peritonitis.[67] However, excessive recombinant IL-10 administration in similar animal models has been associated with increased bacterial load and mortality.

Interleukin-12

Interleukin-12 has a primary role in cell-mediated immunity and promotes the differentiation of T_H1 cells. In mice with fecal peritonitis as well as with burn injury, survival increases with IL-12 administration, while IL-12 neutralization results in high mortality.[68,69] Administration of IL-12 in nonhuman primates is capable of inducing an inflammatory response for up to 48 h, independently of TNF-α and IL-1.[70] Interleukin-12 promotes neutrophil and coagulation activation, as well as the expression of both proinflammatory and antiinflammatory mediators. Furthermore, IL-12 toxicity appears to be synergistic with IL-2.[71] Although IL-12 detection following injury or severe infections is variable, most evidence would suggest that this cytokine contributes to the overall proinflammatory response.

Interleukin-13

Interleukin-13 shares many structural and functional properties of IL-4; both modulate macrophage function, but unlike IL-4, IL-13 has no identifiable effect on T lymphocytes and only has influence on selected B-lymphocyte populations.[72,73] Interleukin-13 can inhibit nitric oxide (NO) production and the expression of proinflammatory cytokines, and it can enhance the production of IL-1ra. Furthermore, IL-13 attenuates leukocyte interaction with activated endothelial surfaces.[74] The net effect of IL-13, along with IL-4 and IL-10, is antiinflammatory.

Interleukin-15

Interleukin-15 is a macrophage-derived cytokine with potent autocrine regulatory properties. As a result of shared receptor signaling components, both IL-15 and IL-2 possess similar bioactivity in promoting lymphocyte activation and proliferation.[75,76] In neutrophils, IL-15 induces IL-8 production and nuclear factor kappa B (NF-κB) activation and enhances phagocytic function against fungal infections.[77,78]

Interleukin-18

Interleukin-18 (formerly IFN-γ-inducing factor) is a proinflammatory cytokine product of activated macrophages. Structurally similar to IL-1β and functionally similar to IL-12, IL-18 promotes early resolution of bacterial infections in mice.[79,80] Bacterial products, IL-4, and IFN-γ can stimulate IL-18 production from monocytes. Interleukin-18 signaling is associated with NF-κB and c-Jun N-terminal kinase (JNK) pathway activation, as well as the expression of functionally active intercellular adhesion molecule-1 (ICAM-1).[81,82] Furthermore, murine endotoxemia models indicate that IL-18 is a downstream mediator of both TNF-α and Fas ligand-induced hepatoxicity.[83] Preliminary data have demonstrated elevations of circulating IL-18 for several weeks during a severe septic episode. This elevation in IL-18 is particularly pronounced in gram-positive sepsis.[84]

Interferon-γ (IFN-γ)

Much of IL-12 and IL-18 biology is mediated via IFN-γ. Human T-helper lymphocytes activated by bacterial antigens, IL-2, IL-12, or IL-18 readily produce IFN-γ. Conversely, IFN-γ can induce the production of IL-2, IL-12, and IL-18.[85,86] When released into the circulation, IFN-γ is detectable in vivo by 6h and may be persistently elevated for as long as 8 days. Injured tissues, such as operative wounds, also demonstrate the presence of IFN-γ production 5 to 7 days after injury.[87] Interferon-γ has important roles in activating circulating and tissue macrophages. Alveolar macrophage activation mediated by IFN-γ may induce acute lung inflammation after major surgery or trauma.

Granulocyte-Macrophage Colony-Stimulating Factor

In vitro studies have demonstrated a prominent role for granulocyte-macrophage colony-stimulating factor (GM-CSF) in delaying apoptosis (programmed cell death) of macrophages and neutrophils.[88–90] This process may contribute to organ injury such as that found in acute respiratory distress syndrome.[91] This growth factor is effective in promoting the maturation and recruitment of functional leukocytes necessary for normal inflammatory cytokine response and potentially in wound healing. Results of perioperative GM-CSF administration in patients undergoing major oncological procedures and in patients with major burns have demonstrated enhanced neutrophil numbers and function.

Immune Cell and Cytokine Interaction

Paradigm of Specific Immunity

Surgery or traumatic injury is associated with acute impairment of the immune response that can potentially manifest as infectious morbidity (Fig. 4.10).[92] This phenomenon, as demonstrated by recent studies, is primarily characterized by impaired cell-mediated immunity and macrophage function.

The T-helper lymphocytes are functionally divided into two subgroups, referred to as T_H1 and T_H2. Both T_H1 and T_H2 cells produce IL-3, TNF-α, and GM-CSF, but T_H1 cell response is further characterized by the production of IFN-γ, IL-2, IL-12, and TNF-β (lymphotoxin); T_H2 cell response is primarily characterized by IL-4, IL-5, IL-6, IL-9, IL-10, and IL-13 production. In severe infections and major injury, there appears to be a reduction in T_H1 (cell-mediated immunity) cytokine production, with a lymphocyte population shift toward the T_H2 response and associated depression in cell-mediated immunity effects. In patients with major burns, a shift to a T_H2 cytokine response has been a predictor of infectious complications.[93] However, studies in patients undergoing major surgery have demonstrated a postoperative reduction in T_H1 cytokine production, but this is not necessarily associated with increased T_H2 response.[94] Nevertheless, depressed T_H1 response and systemic compromise in immune function following major insults to the host may be a useful paradigm in predicting the subset of patients who are prone to infectious complications and poor outcome. It should be noted that an excessive T_H1 response can conceivably lead to overwhelming

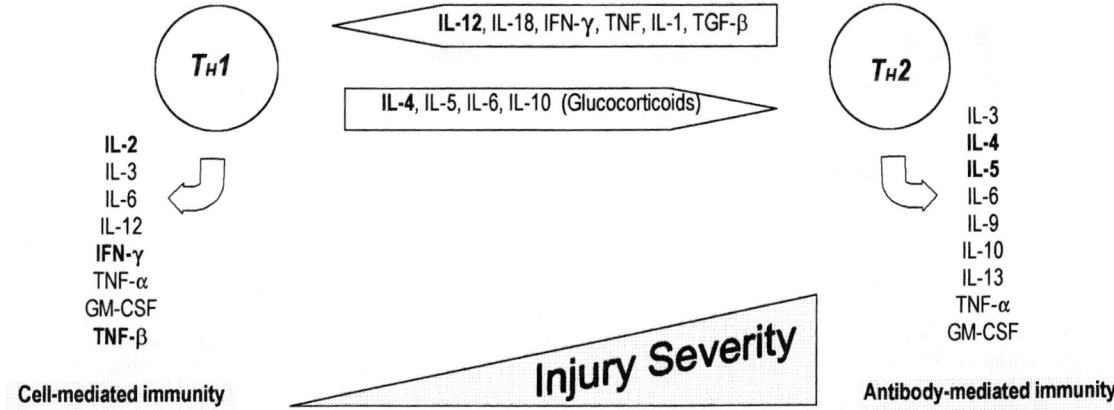

FIGURE 4.10. Specific immunity mediated by type 1 (*T_H1*) and type 2 (*T_H2*) T-helper cells following injury. A T_H1 response is favored in lesser injuries, with intact cell-mediated and opsonizing antibody immunity against microbial infections. This cell-mediated immunity includes activation of monocytes, B lymphocytes, and cytotoxic T lymphocytes. A shift toward the T_H2 response from naive T-helper cells is associated with injuries of greater magnitude and is not as effective against microbial infections. A T_H2 response includes the activation of eosinophils and mast cells and of B lymphocyte IgG_4 and IgE production. Primary stimulants and principal cytokine products of such responses are in **bold** characters. It is known that IL-4 and IL-10 are inhibitors of the T_H1 response, and IFN-γ is a known inhibitor of the T_H2 response. Although not a cytokine, glucocorticoids are potent stimulants of a T_H2 response, which may partly contribute to the immunosuppressive effects of cortisol. (Adapted from Lin et al.[184])

inflammatory response and organ injury, but this phenomenon has not been well documented in surgical or trauma patients.

Immunocyte Apoptosis

In the normal host, apoptosis is the principal mechanism by which senescent or dysfunctional cells, including macrophages and neutrophils, are systematically disposed without activating other immunocytes or the release of proinflammatory contents. The cellular environment created by systemic inflammation is hypothesized to disrupt the normal apoptotic machinery in activated immunocytes, consequently delaying the disposal of these cells. The prolonged survival of inflammatory immunocytes may perpetuate and augment the inflammatory response to injury and infection, precipitating MOF and eventual death in severely injured and critically ill patients.[95] Several proinflammatory cytokines (TNF-α, IL-1, IL-3, IL-6, GM-CSF, granulocyte colony-stimulating factor [G-CSF], IFN-γ) and bacterial products (e.g., endotoxin) have been shown to delay macrophage and neutrophil apoptosis in vitro, while IL-4 and IL-10 accelerate apoptosis in activated monocytes.[96]

In acute inflammation, the response of the immunocyte to TNF-α is perhaps most widely investigated.[97] This cytokine exerts its biological effects by binding to specific cellular receptors TNFR-1 (55 kDa) and TNFR-2 (75 kDa) (Fig. 4.11). Under physiological conditions, TNFR-1 mediates most known biological effects of soluble TNFα, including inflammatory responses, NF-κB activation, and apoptosis.[98] Studies in nonhuman primates also suggest a dominant role for TNFR-1 in TNF-α-mediated toxicity. The administration of mutant TNF-α with exclusive TNFR-1 binding capacity precipitated circulatory shock reminiscent of severe sepsis. However, the administration of mutant TNF-α binding exclusively to TNFR-2 failed to induce any inflammatory responses or shock.[99,100]

Activation of TNFR-2 by soluble TNF-α promotes proliferation of T cells, fibroblasts, and NK cells. Signal transduction experiments and studies employing receptor gene knockout technology have consistently demonstrated intracellular signaling "cross talk" between TNFR-1 and TNFR-2 on receptor activation by TNF-α.[101] TNFR-1 mediates most of the proinflammatory effects of TNF-α, and it has been demonstrated that the early activation of JNK and p38 kinase prevents TNFR-1-mediated apoptosis. The activation of NF-κB and JNK is believed to be the major antiapoptotic, and therefore proinflammatory, signal TNFR-1 and TNFR-2 induces.[102] It is well known that TNF-α-induced NF-κB activation delays cell death and is associated with the activation

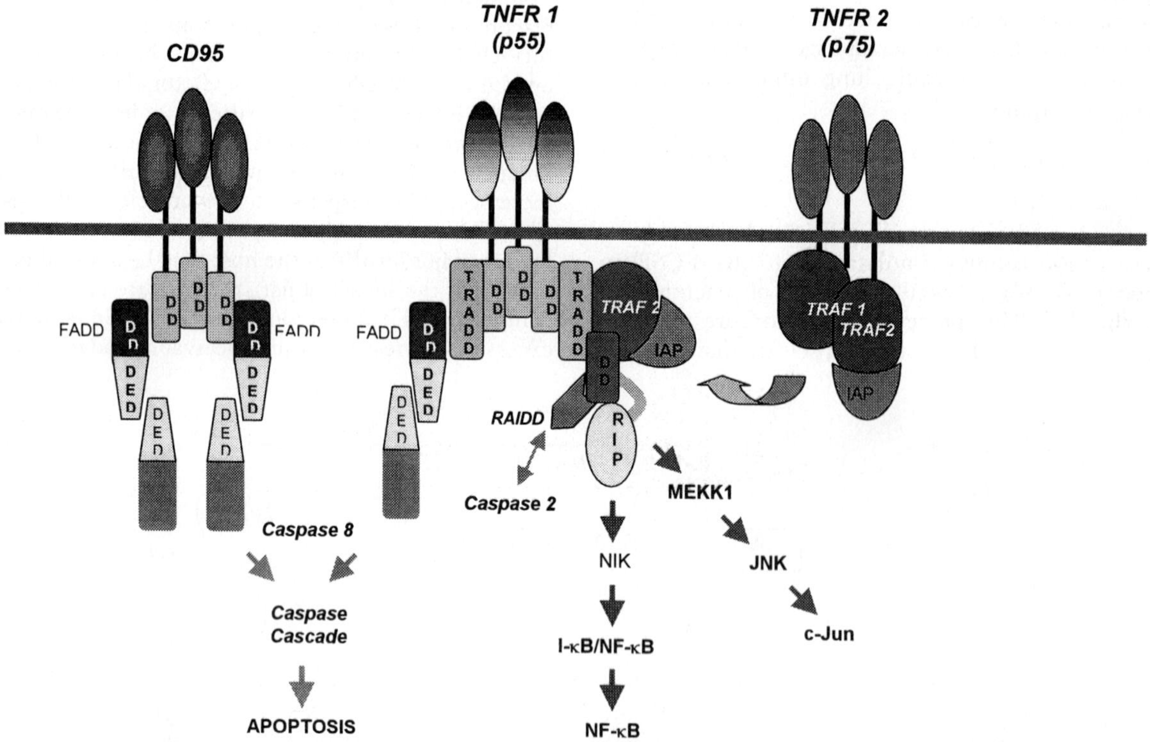

FIGURE 4.11. Signaling pathway for *TNFR-1* (55 kDa) and *TNFR-2* (75 kDa) occurs by the recruitment of several adapter proteins to the intracellular receptor complex. Optimal signaling activity requires receptor trimerization. The TNFR-1 initially recruits *TRADD* (TNFR-associated death domain) and induces apoptosis through the actions of proteolytic enzymes known as caspases, a pathway shared by another receptor known as CD95 (Fas). The CD95 and TNFR-1 possess similar intracellular sequences known as death domains (*DD*), and both recruit the same adapter proteins known as Fas-associated death domain (*FADD*) before activating caspase-8. Also, TNFR-1 induces apoptosis by activating caspase-2 through the recruitment of *RIP* (receptor-interacting protein), which also has a functional component that can initiate NF-κB and c-Jun activation, both favoring cell survival and proinflammatory functions. The TNFR-2 lacks a DD component but recruits adapter proteins known as *TRAF1* and *TRAF2* (TNFR-associated factor) that interact with RIP to mediate NF-κB and c-Jun activation. TRAF2 also recruits additional proteins that are antiapoptotic, known as *IAP* (inhibitors of apoptosis protein). *DED*, death effector domain; *RAIDD*, RIP-associated ICH-1-like protein with death domain, which activates proapoptotic caspases; *MEKK1*, mitogen-activated protein/Erk kinase kinase-1; *JNK*, c-Jun N-terminal kinase; *NIK*, NF-κB-inducing kinase; 1-κB/NF-κB, inactive complex of NF-κB that becomes activated when I-kB portion is cleaved. (Adapted from Lin et al.,[97] with permission.)

of diverse genes that include proinflammatory mediators. Inhibiting NF-κB activation in endothelial cells has been shown to reduce E-selectin, P-selectin, and IL-8 expression.[103] Exaggerated peripheral blood monocyte NF-κB activation has been associated with higher mortality in patients with septic shock.[104]

Members (i.e., homologues) of the intracellular human oncogene product Bcl-2 are also involved in regulating immunocyte survival during systemic inflammation. The intracellular expression of one such member, Bfl-1, is directly dependent on NF-κB activity and capable of suppressing TNF-α-induced apoptosis. Bfl-1 mRNA is inducible in neutrophils stimulated with agonists such as G-CSF, GM-CSF, and lipopolysaccharide (LPS).[105] Inflammatory cytokines can also enhance neutrophil Mcl-1 expression, another antiapoptotic Bcl-2 homologue, suggesting one mechanism by which inflammatory states prolong neutrophil survival.[106] Monocytes activated by inflammatory stimuli such as TNF-α can also have prolonged survival as a result of upregulated Bfl-1 gene expression.

The CD95 (Fas) receptor resembles that of TNFR-1 intracellularly. Unlike TNFR-1, the only known function of CD95 is to initiate programmed cell death. Neutrophils and macrophages express CD95, and this expression may have important implications in the cellular contribution to the inflammatory response. In fact, both clinical sepsis and experimental endotoxemia have demonstrated prolonged survival of neutrophils and diminished responsiveness to CD95 stimuli.[107,108] Although the mechanisms are unclear, CD95 and TNFR activity may participate in organ injury during systemic inflammation.[109–111]

Receptor Alterations

In humans, downregulation in monocyte and neutrophil TNFR expression has been demonstrated experimentally and clinically (Fig. 4.12).[112,113] In clinical sepsis, nonsurviving

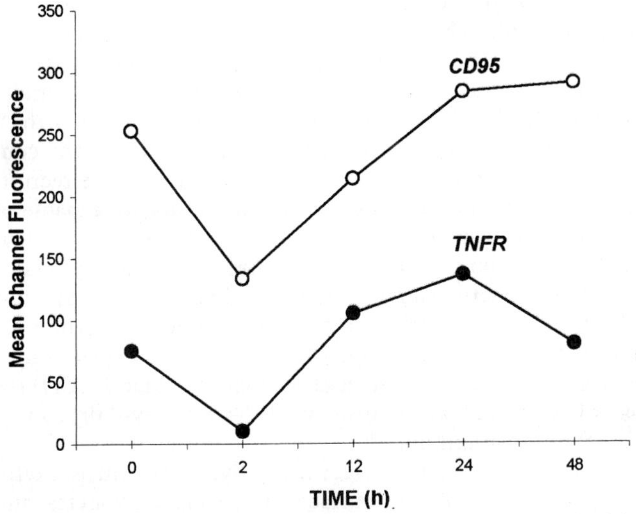

FIGURE 4.12. Monocyte CD95 and TNFR expression in healthy adult subjects following intravenous endotoxin administration at time = 50 h. A reduction in receptor expression is observed at time = 52 h, corresponding to the time of maximal clinical response to the endotoxin. In the absence of further stimulus, receptor expression recovers to normal levels by 48 h. (Adapted from Lin E, Lowry SF.[47])

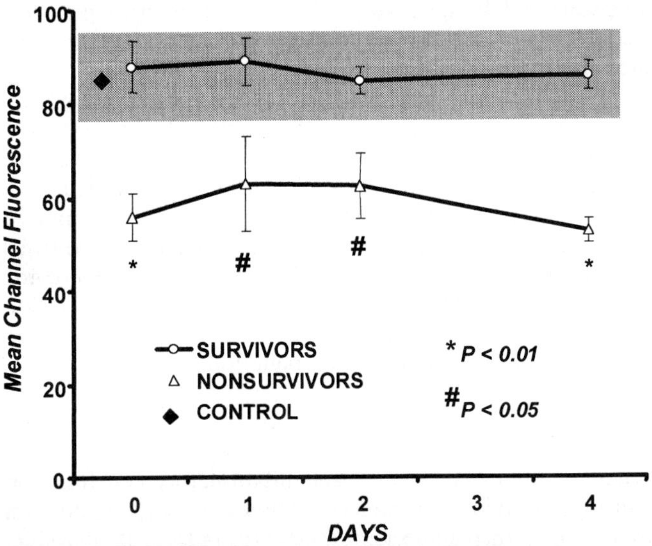

FIGURE 4.13. Monocyte TNFR expression in healthy subjects and in surviving and nonsurviving sepsis patients on days 0 to 4. *Shaded area* encompasses range of monocyte TNFR expression in surviving patients and healthy subjects. (Adapted from Calvano et al.,[113] with permission.)

patients with severe sepsis had an immediate reduction in monocyte surface TNFR expression with failure to recover, while surviving patients had normal or near-normal receptor levels from the outset of clinically defined sepsis (Fig. 4.13). In patients with congestive heart failure, there is also a significant decrease in the amount of monocyte surface TNFR expression when compared with control patients.[114] Thus, TNFR expression can potentially be used as a prognostic indicator of outcome in patients with systemic inflammation.[115] There is also decreased CD95 expression following experimental endotoxemia in humans, which correlates with diminished CD95-mediated apoptosis.[116] Taken together, the reduced receptor expression and delayed apoptosis may be a mechanism for prolonging the inflammatory response during injury or infection.

Hormonal Regulation of Cytokine Activity

Cortisol and Glucocorticoids

The hormonal responses mounted by the injured host or the antecedent hormonal milieu of the cell have considerable influence on the inflammatory cytokine response. The anti-inflammatory effects of glucocorticoids include decreased TNF-α and IL-1 transcription, inducible cyclooxygenase-2 (COX-2) generation, and adhesion molecule expression.[117] In different inflammatory cell types, glucocorticoids increase the intracellular expression of IkBα, which inhibits the activation of NF-κB.[118]

The influences of glucocorticoids on inflammatory cells appear to be cell specific. In vitro and in animal experiments, dexamethasone induces apoptosis in T lymphocytes, with thymocytes the most sensitive, and $CD8^+$ T cells more sensitive than $CD4^+$ cells.[119] Although the mechanisms are unclear, IL-2, IL-4, and IL-10 appear to delay glucocorticoid-induced apoptosis in T lymphocytes.[120] In contrast, in vitro glucocorticoid exposure delays apoptosis in normal neutrophils and prolongs their functional responsiveness.[121]

In healthy human subjects, glucocorticoid administration immediately before or concomitant with endotoxin infusion is able to attenuate the systemic inflammatory response partly by altering cytokine expression.[122,123] Antecedent glucocorticoid administration by 6h or less in experimental human endotoxemia increases IL-10 release, above the IL-10 response mounted to endotoxin alone. In patients undergoing coronary artery bypass, methylprednisolone administration before surgery appears to reduce IL-6 and IL-8 production while leaving IL-10 and IL-1ra production unchanged.[124]

Catecholamines

Catecholamines appear to alter inflammatory cell function and inhibit endotoxin-induced TNF-α and IL-1β production in healthy human subjects.[125] Endotoxin-induced IL-8 production is enhanced by EPI infusion as a function of β-adrenergic receptor signaling. Interestingly, hydrocortisone has been shown to reverse EPI-enhanced IL-8 production.[126] In normal human subjects, short-term preexposure to EPI effectively inhibits endotoxin-induced TNF-α production but increases IL-10 production.[127] This antiinflammatory effect is lost with longer periods of EPI treatment.

Endothelium-Mediated Injury

The activation of endothelial cells represents a fundamental mechanism for the manifestations of local and systemic inflammation that accompany injury and infection. Much of what we consider systemic inflammatory response arises in part from the early and sustained participation of endothelial cell immune functions. In a paracrine fashion, local mediators such as TNF-α, IL-1, endotoxin, thrombin, histamine, and IFN-α are capable of stimulating or activating the endothelial cell during local tissue injury. In response, the endothelial cell releases several mediators, including IL-1, PAF, PGs (PGI_2 [prostacyclin] and PGE_2), GM-CSF, growth factors, endothelin (ET), NO, and small amounts of thromboxane A_2 (TxA_2). Activated endothelial cells also release collagenases capable of autodigesting their basement membranes. This important property permits neovascularization and vascular remodeling at sites of injury for the purposes of facilitating adequate oxygen supply and immunocyte transport. The presence of ACE that converts AT-I to AT-II on the surface of endothelial cells makes it a potent regulator of vascular tone. Systemically, endothelial cell mediators can modulate cardiovascular and renal function as well as influence the HPA (hypothalamic-pituitary-adrenal) axis.

Neutrophil–Endothelium Interaction

The accumulation and infiltration of inflammatory leukocytes, specifically neutrophils, at sites of injury contribute to cytotoxicity of vital tissues and eventuate in organ dysfunction.[128] Injury in the form of ischemia followed by reperfusion (I/R) to a target site organ unleashes a vast array of inflammatory mediators that activate immunocytes as well as promote neutrophil adherence to, and extravasation through, microvascular endothelium.[129] These activated, and localized, neutrophils release reactive oxygen metabolites (e.g., $O_2^{-\cdot}$, $OH^{\cdot}$, H_2O_2) and lysosomal enzymes (e.g., collagenase, elastase, gelatinase) that propagate a chain of injurious events that include, but are not limited to, endothelial injury, microvascular "plugging" and thrombus formation, myeloperoxidase activity, and adjacent tissue injury.[130,131] Indeed, experimental evidence has repeatedly demonstrated that leukocyte depletion by filtration, chemotherapeutic agents, or specific polyclonal antileukocyte serum administration significantly reduces the extent of I/R injury.[132–135] Although I/R-induced leukocyte activation is understood to be an important mechanism for tissue and end-organ injury,[136] specific therapy directed against leukocyte-mediated toxicity is still sought.

In activated states, leukocytes roll along endothelial surfaces (i.e., margination) before firm adhesion at specific sites. The initial action of rolling is predominantly mediated by the selectin family of adhesion molecules present on both endothelial cells and leukocytes. The E- and P-selectins are expressed on the surfaces of activated endothelial cells, with the latter also expressed on the surfaces of activated platelets. The expression of E- and P-selectins has been confirmed on endothelium of vital tissues, including, but certainly not limited to, the lung, heart, small intestine, muscle, and brain.[137] There is evidence to suggest that the expression of P-selectin following injury is biphasic, with an acute but modest peak appearing within 20min and a significant peak by 2 to 4h. The initial expression of P-selectin is attributed to the mobilization of intracellular storage granules followed by rapid internalization and degradation, while the latter appearance is attributed to de novo synthesis. The first phase of P-selectin expression makes it one of the early mediators of leukocyte–endothelial interaction. Furthermore, the presence of P-selectin on platelet surfaces serves to promote microthrombus formation in capillaries and venules of injured tissue.

Expression of E-selectin, as with P-selectins, requires de novo mRNA and protein synthesis, which involves the translocation of intracellular NF-κB onto nuclear promoter sites.[138,139] Following a single stress stimulus such as endotoxin administration in mice, E-selectin expression on stimulated endothelial surfaces is detectable by 2h, is maximally expressed at 3 to 5h, and is rapidly downregulated by 10h.[140] The delay in surface expression virtually precludes the contribution of E-selectin in early rolling and leukocyte recruitment in acute inflammation. The E-selectins are capable of causing significant reductions in the rolling velocity of neutrophils to a point that precedes arrest, suggesting greater adhesion strength than P-selectins.[141] Therefore, the slowest rolling velocity is attributed to E-selectin activity. The ligation of E-selectins also appears to induce the expression of leukocyte β_2-integrin molecules, such as Mac-1 (CD11b/CD18), which are largely responsible for leukocyte firm adhesion and transmigration.[142]

The smallest of the selectin family, L-selectin is exclusively expressed on the surface of normal leukocytes and directly mediates rolling on inflammatory (i.e., activated) endothelium. Furthermore, the initial recognition of endothelium that precipitates leukocyte rolling (i.e., "capture") is attributed to early expression of cell-surface L-selectins.[143]

On activation, L-selectin is readily shed from the leukocyte cell surface, and indeed soluble L-selectin is often detectable in human serum.[144] The precise signaling mechanism governing L-selectin shedding still remains to be elucidated, but it is clear that shedding frees the activated leukocyte to continue its downstream rolling.[145] The fastest rolling is attributed to L-selectin activity by nature of its rapid shedding (Fig. 4.14).

Neutrophil rolling in the first 10 to 20 min following injury is mainly mediated by P-selectin, with minimal L-selectin contribution,[146] which is consistent with the rapid expression of P-selectins from intracellular stores. Beyond 20 min, the influences of P-selectins diminish secondary to internal degradation, and L-selectin becomes the principal mediator of leukocyte rolling. In conjunction with L-selectin, PSGL-1 (P-selectin glycoprotein ligand-1) is responsible for more than 85% of monocyte-to-monocyte and monocyte-to-endothelium adhesion activity.[147] Although there are distinguishable properties among individual selectins in leukocyte rolling, effective rolling most likely involves a significant degree of functional overlap.[148–150] Similarly, L-selectin also initiates neutrophil-to-neutrophil interaction, in part by binding to leukocyte surface PSGL-1.[151]

Endothelium-Derived Nitric Oxide

Endothelium-derived NO is released in response to acetylcholine stimulation, hypoxia, endotoxin, cellular injury, or mechanical shear stress from circulating blood.[152] Induction of vascular smooth muscle relaxation by NO requires the activation of soluble guanylate cyclase and an increase in cytosolic cyclic guanosine monophosphate (cGMP) within the myocytes. Methylene blue inhibits guanylate cyclase, prevents the production of cGMP, and inhibits vascular relaxation. Cyclic GMP is also present in platelets and can be activated by NO. Increased cGMP within platelets is associated with reduced adhesion and aggregation. Therefore, NO induces vasodilation as well as platelet deactivation (Fig. 4.15). Also, NO mediates protein synthesis in hepatocytes and electron transport in hepatocyte mitochondria.[153] It is a readily diffusible substance with a half-life of a few seconds, and it spontaneously decomposes into nitrate and nitrite.

Nitric oxide is formed from oxidation of L-arginine, a process catalyzed by NO synthase. Cofactors of NO synthase activity include calmodulin, ionized calcium, and NADPH (nicotinamide adenine dinucleotide phosphate). In addition to the endothelium, this enzymatic activity is also present in neutrophils, monocytes, renal cells, Kupffer cells, and cerebellar neurons. In normal vasculature, experimental blocking of NO activity induces a state of vasoconstriction readily reversed with L-arginine administration.[154] This result demonstrates that the vasculature is in a constant state of vasodilation because of the continuous basal release of NO. Endogenous inhibitors of NO have also been identified that serve as autoregulators of endothelial tone. Elevations of NO in septic shock and trauma, as measured by its nitrite and nitrate metabolites, are demonstrated in association with low systemic vascular resistance and elevated endotoxin levels.[155]

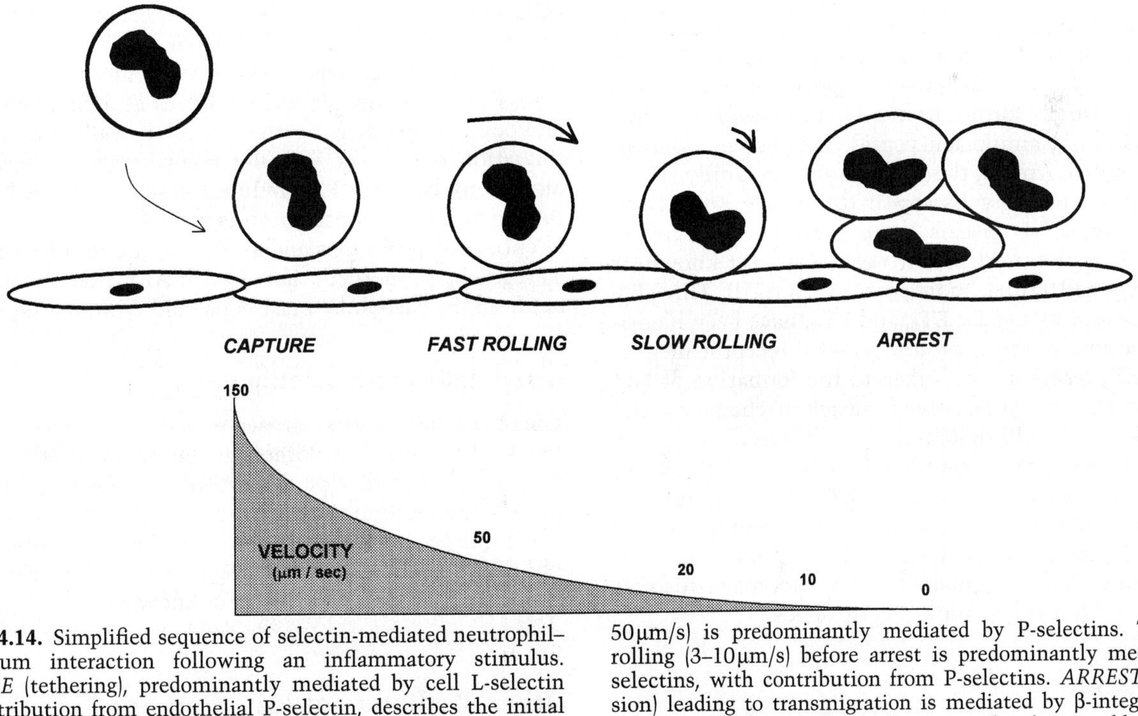

FIGURE 4.14. Simplified sequence of selectin-mediated neutrophil–endothelium interaction following an inflammatory stimulus. *CAPTURE* (tethering), predominantly mediated by cell L-selectin with contribution from endothelial P-selectin, describes the initial recognition between leukocyte and endothelium by which circulating leukocytes marginate toward the endothelial surface. *FAST ROLLING* (50–150 µm/s) is a consequence of rapid L-selectin shedding from cell surfaces and formation of new downstream L-selectin to endothelium bonds, occurring in tandem. *SLOW ROLLING* (20–50 µm/s) is predominantly mediated by P-selectins. The slowest rolling (3–10 µm/s) before arrest is predominantly mediated by E-selectins, with contribution from P-selectins. *ARREST* (firm adhesion) leading to transmigration is mediated by β-integrins and the immunoglobulin family of adhesion molecules. In addition to interactions with the endothelium, activated leukocytes also recruit other leukocytes to the inflammatory site by direct interactions, which are mediated in part by selectins. (Adapted from Lin et al.,[185] with permission.)

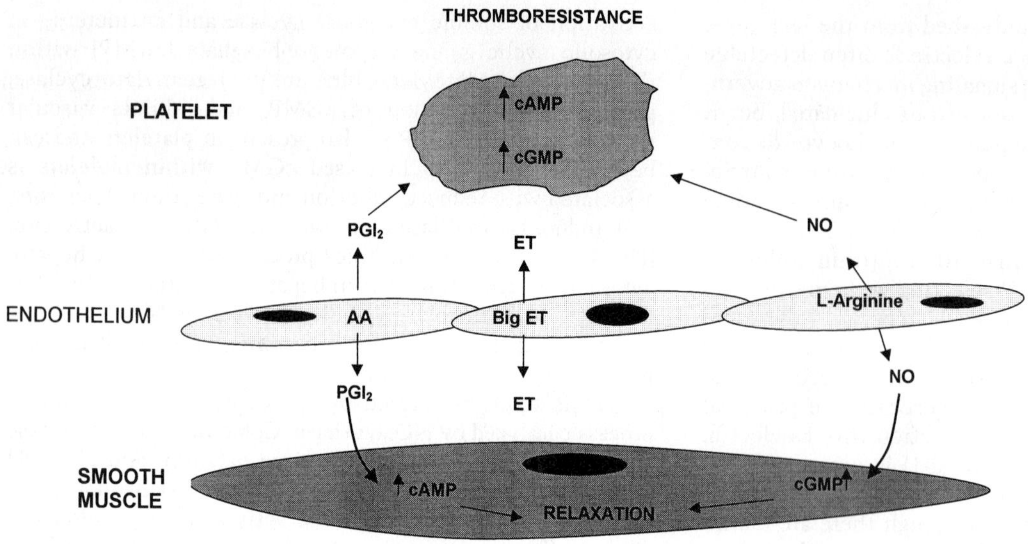

FIGURE 4.15. Endothelium interaction with smooth muscle cells and with intraluminal platelets. Prostacyclin (*PGI₂*) is derived from arachidonic acid, and nitric oxide (*NO*) is derived from L-arginine. The increase in cAMP and cGMP results in smooth muscle relaxation and inhibition of platelet thrombus formation. Endothelins (*ET*) are derived from *"big ET"* and counter the effects of prostacyclin and nitric oxide. (Adapted from Angaard,[186] with permission.)

Prostacyclin

Prostacyclin (PGI_2) is another important endothelium-derived vasodilator synthesized in response to vascular shear stress and hypoxia. It also shares similar functions with NO. While NO is derived from L-arginine and increases cGMP, prostacyclin is derived from arachidonic acid and causes relaxation as well as platelet deactivation by increasing cAMP. Clinically, it has been used to reduce pulmonary hypertension, particularly in the pediatric population.

Endothelins

Endothelins (ETs) are elaborated by vascular endothelial cells in response to injury, thrombin, transforming growth factor-β (TGF-β), IL-1, AT-II, vasopressin, catecholamines, and anoxia.[156] Structurally formed from a 38-amino-acid precursor molecule, ET is a 21-amino-acid peptide with potent vasoconstrictor properties. Among the peptides in this family (ET-1, ET-2, ET-3), endothelial cells appear to produce exclusively ET-1. Moreover, ET-1 appears to be the most biologically active as well as the most potent vasoconstrictor known; it is estimated to be 10 times more potent than AT-II. Three ET receptors, referred to as ET_A, ET_B, and ET_C, have been identified and function by the G-protein-coupled receptor mechanism. The ET_B receptors are linked to the formation of NO and PGI_2, which serve as negative feedback mechanisms, and the maintenance of physiological tone in vascular smooth muscles depends on the balance between NO and ET production. The vasoconstrictor activity of ET can be reversed by the administration of acetylcholine, which stimulates NO production. Increased serum levels of ET correlate with the severity of injury following major trauma, after major surgical procedures, and in cardiogenic or septic shock.[157]

Platelet-Activating Factor

Another endothelial-derived product is PAF, a phospholipid constituent of cell membranes that can be induced by TNF, IL-1, vasopressin, and AT-II.[158] This potent inflammatory mediator can stimulate production of TxA_2 through the cyclooxygenase pathway and promote platelet aggregation; TxA_2 is also a potent vasoconstrictor. PAF has been experimentally demonstrated to increase glucagon and catecholamine activities.[159] It can induce hypotension; enhance vascular permeability, hemoconcentration, pulmonary hypertension, and bronchoconstriction; and prime neutrophil activation, eosinophil chemotaxis/degranulation, and thrombocytopenia. It induces general leukocytopenia by way of margination. Administration of antagonists to PAF in experimental human endotoxemia demonstrates partial attenuation of symptoms such as myalgias and rigors, but these inhibitors are ineffective in reversing any hemodynamic derangements.[160]

Platelet-activating factor alters the shape of endothelial cells, causing them to contract and increase endothelial permeability.[161] In cultured endothelial cells, this cell contraction permits the passage of macromolecules such as albumin across cell junctions. It further serves as a chemotactant for leukocyte adherence to the vascular wall and facilitates migration out of the vascular compartment. The apparent dichotomy between PAF-induced vascular permeability and PAF-induced vasoconstriction is most likely the result of differential receptor types and affinity found in different vascular segments. Other cells that secrete PAF include macrophages, neutrophils, basophils, mast cells, and eosinophils.

Atrial Natriuretic Peptides

The ANPs are peptides released by the central nervous system and by specialized endothelium found in atrial tissues in response to wall tension. The ANPs are potent inhibitors of aldosterone secretion and prevent reabsorption of sodium. In rats, the myocardial NO appears to inhibit the release of ANP, while ET-1 is a potent secretagogue of ANP. The role of ANP in human response to injury is unknown.

Other Mediators of Inflammation

Heat-Shock Proteins

Stimuli such as hypoxia, trauma, heavy metals, local trauma, and hemorrhage all induce the production of intracellular

HSPs.[162] These proteins are presumed to protect cells from the deleterious effects of traumatic stress. The HSPs function intracellularly in the assembly, disassembly, stability, and transport of proteins. The classic example of HSP activity relates to the intracellular transport of steroid molecules.[163] The formation of HSPs requires gene induction by the heat-shock transcription factor (HSF). The expression of HSP may also be ACTH sensitive, and the production may decline with age.[164] Although HSPs are presumed to be important intracellular effectors, their relevance in the human response to injury can only be inferred from animal data.

Reactive Oxygen Metabolites

Reactive oxygen metabolites are short-lived, highly reactive molecular oxygen species with an unpaired outer orbit. They cause tissue injury by peroxidation of cell membrane unsaturated fatty acids.[165]

Oxygen radicals are produced by processes that involve anaerobic glucose oxidation coupled with the reduction of oxygen to superoxide anion. Superoxide anion is also a potent oxygen metabolite, but it can be further metabolized to other reactive species, such as hydrogen peroxide and hydroxyl radicals. Cells are not immune to damage by their own reactive oxygen metabolites but are generally protected by oxygen scavengers that include glutathione (GSH) and catalases. In ischemic tissues, the intracellular mechanisms for production of oxygen metabolites are fully activated but remain nonfunctional because of the lack of oxygen supply. On restoration of blood flow and oxygen supply, large quantities of reactive oxygen metabolites are produced that induce reperfusion injury. The emerging concept of *cytopathic hypoxia* incorporates injury mechanisms related to reactive oxidative and nitrosative species.[166] Several unique compounds designed to neutralize or divert the toxic effects of these mediators have been developed and are in early clinical trials.

Activated leukocytes in response to a stimuli are potent generators of reactive oxygen metabolites. Reactive oxygen metabolites can also induce apoptosis. Studies using T lymphocytes have demonstrated a major apoptotic mechanism mediated by depletion of intracellular GSH or oxygen radical scavenger. The proapoptotic Fas/CD95 receptor activation has been implicated in depleting GSH with resultant intracellular reactive oxygen metabolite accumulation and cell death. Repletion of GSH in these cells can reverse such effects.[167]

Eicosanoids

The eicosanoid class of mediators, which encompasses PGs, Txs, leukotrienes (LTs), hydroxyeicosatetraenoic acids (HETEs), and lipoxins (Lxs), is made up of oxidation derivatives of the membrane phospholipid, arachidonic acid (eicosatetraenoic acid).[168] They are secreted by virtually all nucleated cells except lymphocytes. The synthesis of arachidonic acid from phospholipids requires enzymatic activation of phospholipase A_2 (Fig. 4.16). The cyclooxygenase and the lipoxygenase pathways are two major routes by which arachidonic acid is oxygenated. Most eicosanoids generated from the cyclooxygenase pathway are given the subscript designation of 2 (e.g., TxA_2), whereas products of the lipoxygenase pathway are designated by a subscript 4 (e.g., LTE_4). These subscripts represent the number of carbon double bonds present in the side chains. Products of the cyclooxygenase pathway include all the PGs and Txs. The formation of prostacyclin (PGI_2) requires further enzymatic activity by prostacyclin synthetase, and the formation of TxA_2 requires the activity of thromboxane synthetase. The lipoxygenase pathway generates the LTs and HETE.[169]

Initial phospholipase A_2 activation can be achieved by compounds such as EPI, AT-II, bradykinin, histamine, and thrombin. On the other hand, phospholipase A_2 can be inhibited by lipocortin, which is induced by cortisol. The synthesis of PGs and Txs is also inhibited by nonsteroidal antiinflammatory drugs and salicylates, which are cyclooxygenase inhibitors.[170]

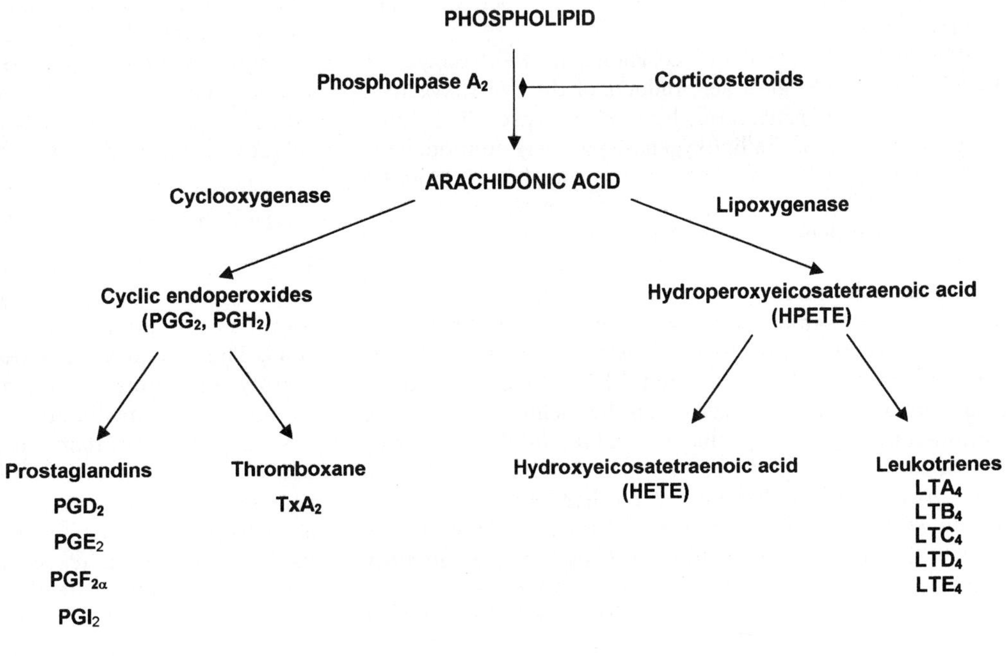

FIGURE 4.16. Schematic of arachidonic acid metabolism.

Eicosanoids are not stored within cells but are rather synthesized rapidly on stimulation by hypoxic and ischemic injury, direct tissue injury, endotoxin, NE, vasopressin, AT-II, bradykinin, serotonin, acetylcholine, and histamine. Many of these stimuli also induce a second cyclooxygenase enzyme referred to as COX-2, which further enhances the production of arachidonic acid metabolites. The activity of COX-2 can be inhibited by glucocorticoids, which provide specific inhibition of cyclooxygenase metabolites as opposed to lipocortin, which inhibits production of arachidonic acid metabolites in general. The products of arachidonic acid metabolism are functionally cell or tissue specific. For instance, vascular endothelium primarily synthesizes PGI_2, which causes vasodilation and platelet deactivation. Thromboxane synthetase converts platelet PGs to TxA_2, a potent vasoconstrictor and platelet aggregator.[171] Monocytes are capable of synthesizing both cyclooxygenase and lipoxygenase products.

Second messengers mediate much of eicosanoid activity. For example, PGE compounds, in a manner similar to ACTH, TSH, and LH, inhibit vasopressin activity and hormone-stimulated lipolysis by activating adenylate cyclase activity, thus generating intracellular cAMP. Thromboxane and LTs have opposite effects from PGE by increasing intracellular free calcium via the phosphatidylinositol pathway.

Eicosanoids have diverse effects systemically on endocrine and immune function, neurotransmission, and vasomotor regulation (Table 4.3). Eicosanoids are major components of the inflammatory response in injured tissue, with the response characterized by vascular permeability, leukocyte migration, and vasodilation. Collectively, their deleterious effects are implicated in acute lung injury, pancreatitis, and renal failure. Leukotrienes are produced by cells of the lung, connective tissue, smooth muscle, monocytes, and mast cells, which mediate the reactions characteristic of anaphylaxis. Leukotrienes are 1000 times more potent than histamines in promoting capillary leakage. They are also effective promoters of leukocyte adherence, neutrophil activation, bronchoconstriction, and vasoconstriction. The role of Lxs is not so well understood, but they are believed to induce neutrophil activation and production of superoxides and degranulation.

The metabolic effects of eicosanoids are well recognized. In the regulation of glucose, products of the cyclooxygenase pathway inhibit pancreatic beta-cell release of insulin, whereas products of the lipoxygenase pathway promote beta-cell activity. Hepatocytes also express specific receptors for PGE_2 that, when activated, inhibit gluconeogenesis. Also, PGE_2 has been demonstrated to inhibit hormone-stimulated lipolysis.

Eicosanoids modulate the immune response in multiple ways. Small amounts of PGE_2 suppress proliferation of human T lymphocytes by mitogens, an effect mediated by downregulation of IL-2 production. Thus, enhanced lymphocyte activation by mitogens can be achieved with the administration of indomethacin, a PGE_2 inhibitor. During phagocytosis, neutrophils release eicosanoids such as LTB_4 that serve as chemoattractants for other leukocytes. Commonly, PGE_2 and LTD_4 are present in local areas of injury and are believed to have direct influences on the inflammatory response.

TABLE 4.3. The Influence of Eicosanoids on Specific Organs.

Organ and function	*Stimulator*	*Inhibitor*
Pancreas		
Glucose-stimulated insulin secretion	12-HPETE	PGE_2
Glucagon secretion	PGD_2, PGE_2	
Liver		
Glucagon-stimulated glucose production	PGE_2	
Fat		
Hormone-stimulated lipolysis	PGE_2	
Bone		
Resorption	PGE_2, PGE-m, 6-K-PGE_1, PGF_{1a}, PGI_2	
Pituitary		
Prolactin	PGE_1	
LH	PGE_1, PGE_2, 5-HETE	
TSH	PGA_1, PGB_1, PGE_1, PGE_{1a}	
GH	PGE_1	
Parathyroid		
PTH	PGE_2	PGF_{2a}
Pulmonary		
Bronchoconstriction	PGF_{2a}, TxA_2, LTC_4, LTD_4, LTE_4	PGE_2
Renal		
Stimulate renin secretion	PGE_2, PGI_2	
Gastrointestinal		
Cytoprotective effect	PGE_2	
Immune response		
Suppress lymphocyte activity	PGE_2	
Hematological		
Platelet aggregation	TxA_2	PGI_2

Source: Adapted from Robertson,[168] with permission.

Resolvins

The rapid injury-induced production of several lipid moieties may serve to attenuate the magnitude and progression of inflammation. Although as yet to be discussed in the context of human systemic inflammation, these unique lipid compounds appear to act effectively as antiinflammatory molecules via attenuation of both immune cell activation and target cell injury.[172,173]

Fatty Acid Metabolites

Fatty acid metabolism potentially has a role in the inflammatory response. Most commercially prepared enteral nutrition formulas contain Ω-6 fatty acids as the primary source of lipid. The Ω-6 fatty acids also serve as precursors of inflammatory mediators associated with injury and the stress response. Such mediators include LTs, PGs, and PAF.[174] By contrast, the antiinflammatory effects of Ω-3 fatty acids on chronic autoimmune diseases such as rheumatoid arthritis, psoriasis, and lupus have been well documented in both animals and humans.[175] Although the mechanisms are yet unclear, animal studies substituting Ω-3 for Ω-6 fatty acids have demonstrated attenuated inflammatory response by hepatic Kupffer cells as measured by TNF and IL-1 release and PGE_2 production.[176] Antiinflammatory properties of Ω-3 have also been demonstrated in injured animals, as manifested by reductions in metabolic rate, normalization of glucose metabolism, and overall weight loss as well as improved nitrogen balance and immune function.[177,178] Feeding supplemented by Ω-3 fatty acid has been variably demonstrated in animals to minimize I/R injury in the myocardium, small intestines, and skeletal muscles, but not following hepatic hypoperfusion.[179] Dietary Ω-3 fatty acids in rats, when compared to Ω-6 fatty acids, have also been shown to ameliorate endotoxin-induced acute lung injury by suppressing the levels of proinflammatory eicosanoids in bronchoalveolar lavage fluid and reducing pulmonary neutrophil accumulation.[180]

In vitro studies coincubating human monocytes with fish oil have demonstrated inhibition of MHC (major histocompatibility complex) class II cell receptors with reduced antigen-presenting capacity. The same study also demonstrated reduced cell-surface adhesion molecule expression that could inhibit cell-to-cell activation and monocyte–endothelial interactions.[181]

Kallikrein–Kinin System

Bradykinins are potent vasodilators produced through kininogen degradation by the serine protease kallikrein.[182] Kallikrein exists in blood and tissues as inactive prekallikrein that is activated by various factors such as Hageman factor, trypsin, plasmin, factor XI, glass surfaces, kaolin, and collagen. Kinins are rapidly metabolized by kinase I and II. Kinase I also degrades the anaphylatoxins C3a, C4a, and C5a. Kinase II is identical to ACE. Of interest is that the use of ACE inhibitors in controlling hypertension may partially block kinin degradation in some patients and enhance the kinin-induced injurious effects on the bronchial tree. Kinins increase capillary permeability and tissue edema, evoke pain, and increase bronchoconstriction. They also increase renal vasodilation and consequently reduce renal perfusion pressure. The resulting increase in renin formation activates sodium and water retention via the renin–angiotensin system.

Bradykinin release is stimulated by hypoxic and ischemic injury. Increased kallikrein activity and bradykinin levels have been detected following hemorrhage, sepsis, endotoxemia, and tissue injury.[183] Furthermore, these observations appear to correlate positively with the magnitude of injury and mortality. Clinical trials utilizing bradykinin antagonists in attempts to reduce the deleterious sequelae of septic shock have demonstrated only modest reversal in gram-negative sepsis but no overall improvement in survival. Metabolically, kinins increase glucose clearance by inhibiting gluconeogenesis. Bradykinin infusion may also increase nitrogen retention.

Serotonin

The neurotransmitter serotonin is a tryptophan derivative found in chromaffin cells of the intestine and in platelets. Patients with midgut carcinoid tumors often secrete 5-HT in excess. This neurotransmitter stimulates vasoconstriction, bronchoconstriction, and platelet aggregation. It is also capable of acting as a myocardial chronotrope and inotrope. Although it is released at sites of injury, its role in the injury response is unclear.

Histamine

Histamine is derived from histidine and stored in neurons, skin, gastric mucosa, mast cells, basophils, and platelets. Its release is activated by increased calcium levels. There are two receptor types for histamine binding. The H_1 binding stimulates bronchoconstriction, intestinal motility, and myocardial contractility; H_2 binding inhibits histamine release. Both H_1 and H_2 receptor activation induce hypotension, peripheral pooling of blood, increased capillary permeability, decreased venous return, and myocardial failure. Histamine release has been demonstrated in hemorrhagic shock, trauma, thermal injury, endotoxemia, and sepsis.

Acknowledgment. This work was supported in part by National Institutes of Health grant GM34695.

References

1. Bone RC. Sir Isaac Newton, sepsis, SIRS, CARS. Crit Care Med 1996;24:1125–1128.
2. Sheth SB, Chaganti K, Bastepe M, et al. Cyclic AMP phosphodiesterases in human lymphocytes. Br J Haematol 1997;99:784–789.
3. Pryzwansky KB, Kidao S, Merricks EP. Compartmentalization of PDE-4 and cAMP-dependent protein kinase in neutrophils and macrophages during phagocytosis. Cell Biochem Biophys 1998;28:251–275.
4. Weston MC, Peachell PT. Regulation of human mast cell and basophil function by cAMP. Gen Pharmacol 1998;31:715–719.
5. Robyr D, Wolffe P. Hormone action and chromatin remodelling. Cell Mol Life Sci 1998;54:113–124.
6. Dao-Phan HP, Formstecher P, Lefebvre P. Disruption of the glucocorticoid receptor assembly with heat shock protein 90 by a peptidic antiglucocorticoid. Mol Endocrinol 1997;11:962–972.
7. Casadevall M, Saperas E, Panes J, et al. Mechanisms underlying the antiinflammatory actions of central corticotropin-releasing factor. Am J Physiol 1999;276:G1016–G1026.
8. Turnbull AV, Rivier C. Corticotropin-releasing factor (CRF) and endocrine responses to stress: CRF receptors, binding protein, and related peptides. Proc Soc Exp Biol Med 1997;215:1–10.
9. Mercer JG, Lawrence CB, Moar KM, Atkinson T, Barrett P. Short-day weight loss and effect of food deprivation on hypothalamic NPY and CRF mRNA in Djungarian hamsters. Am J Physiol 1997;273:R768–R776.
10. Agnello D, Bertini R, Sacco S, Meazza C, Villa P, Ghezzi P. Corticosteroid-independent inhibition of tumor necrosis factor production by the neuropeptide urocortin. Am J Physiol 1998;275:E757–E762.
11. DeBold CR, Menefee JK, et al. Proopiomelanocorticotropin gene is expressed in many normal human tissues and in tumors not associated with ectopic adrenocorticotropin syndrome. Mol Endocrinol 1989;2:862–867.
12. Udelsman R, Holbrook NJ. Endocrine and molecular responses to surgical stress. Curr Probl Surg 1994;31:653–720.
13. Brizio-Molteni L, Molteni A, et al. Prolactin, corticotropin, and gonadotropin concentrations following thermal injury in adults. J Trauma 1984;14:1–9.
14. Kraus-Friedmann N. Hormonal regulation of hepatic gluconeogenesis. Physiol Rev 1984;51:312–322.

15. Rock CS, Coyle SM, Keogh CV, et al. Influence of hypercortisolemia on the acute-phase protein response to endotoxin in humans. Surgery (St. Louis) 1992;112:467–474.
16. Calvano SE, Albert JD, Legaspi A, et al. Comparison of numerical and phenotypic leukocyte changes during constant hydrocortisone infusion in normal humans with those in thermally injured patients. Surgery (St. Louis) 1987;164:509–520.
17. Bessey PQ, Lowe KA. Early hormonal changes affect the catabolic response to trauma. Ann Surg 1993;218:476–491.
18. Newman WH, Zhang LM, Leeper-Woodford SK, Shaker IJ, Erceg SK, Castresana MR. Inhibition of release of tumor necrosis factor-α from human vascular tissue and smooth muscle cells by glucocorticoids. Crit Care Med 1997;25:519–522.
19. Calvano SE, Barber AE, Hawes AS, de Riesthal HF, Coyle SM, Lowry SF. Effect of combined cortisol-endotoxin administration on peripheral blood leukocyte counts and phenotype in normal humans. Arch Surg 1992;127:181–186.
20. Hawes AS, Rock CS, Keogh CV, Lowry SF, Calvano SE. In vivo effects of the antiglucocorticoid RU 486 on glucocorticoid and cytokine responses to *Escherichia coli* endotoxin. Infect Immun 1992;2641–2647.
21. Barber AE, Coyle SM, Marano MA, et al. Glucocorticoid therapy alters hormonal and cytokine responses to endotoxin in man. J Immunol 1993;150:1999–2006.
22. Van der Poll T, Barber AE, Coyle SM, Lowry SF. Hypercortisolemia increases plasma interleukin-10 concentrations during human endotoxemia—a clinical research center study. J Clin Endocrinol Metab 1996;81:3604–3606.
23. Swope MD, Lolis E. Macrophage migration inhibitory factor: cytokine, hormone, or enzyme? Rev Physiol Biochem Pharmacol 1999;139:1–32.
24. Jackson I. Thyrotropin-releasing hormone. N Engl J Med 1982;306:245–250.
25. Calvano SE, Chiao J, et al. Changes in free and total levels of plasma cortisol and thyroxine following thermal injury in man. J Burn Care Rehabil 1984;5:143–149.
26. Ullrich A, Gray A, Tam AW, et al. Insulin-like growth factor I receptor primary structure: comparison with insulin receptor suggests structural determinants that define functional specificity. EMBO J 1986;5:2503–2512.
27. Clemmons DR, Underwood LE. Nutritional regulation of IGF-1 and IGF binding proteins. Annu Rev Nutr 1991;11:393–412.
28. Coates CL, Burwell RG, Carlin SA, et al. Somatomedin activity in plasma from burned patients with observations on plasma cortisol. Burns 1981;7:425–433.
29. Thompson WA, Coyle SM, et al. The metabolic effects of continuous infusion of insulin-like growth factor (IGF-1) in parenterally fed men. Surg Forum 1991;42:23–25.
30. Harris AG. Future medical prospects for sandostatin. Metabolism 1990;39:S180–S185.
31. Knoferl MW, Angele MK, Diodato MD, et al. Surgical ovariectomy produces immunodepression following trauma hemorrhage and increases mortality from subsequent sepsis. Surg Forum 1999;50:235–237.
32. Wichmann MW, Zellweger R, DeMaso CM, et al. Enhanced immune responses in females as opposed to decreased responses in males following hemorrhagic shock. Cytokine 1996;8:853–863.
33. Coyle SM, Calvano SE, Lowry SF. Gender influences in vivo human responses to endotoxin. Shock 2006; 26:538–543.
34. Levy EM, McIntosh T, et al. Elevation of circulatory beta-endorphin levels with concomitant depression of immune parameters after traumatic injury. J Trauma 1986;26:246–251.
35. Shavit Y, Lewis JW, et al. Opioid peptides mediate the suppressive effect of stress on natural killer cell cytotoxicity. Science 1984;223:188–190.
36. Deitch EA, Xo D, et al. Opioids modulate neutrophil lymphocyte function: thermal injury alters plasma beta-endorphin levels. Surgery (St. Louis) 1988;104:41–48.
37. Ertmer C, Bone HG, Morelli A, et al. Methylprednisolone reverses vasopressin hyporesponsiveness in ovine endotoxinemia. Shock 2007;27: in press.
38. Munford RS, Pugin J. Normal responses to injury prevent systemic inflammation and can be immunosuppressive. Am J Respir Crit Care Med 2001;163:316–332.
39. Annane D, Trabold F, Sarshar T, et al. Inappropriate sympathetic activation at the onset of septic shock—a spectral analysis approach. Am J Respir Crit Care Med 1999;160:458–446.
40. Borovikova LV, Ivanova S, Zhang M, et al. Vagus nerve stimulation attenuates the systemic inflammatory response to endotoxin. Nature 2000;405:458–462.
41. van Westerlo DJ, Giebelen IA, Florquin S, et al. The cholinergic anti-inflammatory pathway regulates the host response during septic peritonitis. J Infect Dis 2005;191:2138–2148.
42. Tracey KJ. The inflammatory reflex. Nature 2002;420:853–859.
43. van den Berghe G, Wilmer A, Hermas G, et al. Intensive insulin therapy in the medical ICU. N Engl J Med 2006;354:449–461.
44. Spink J, Cohen J. Synergy and specificity in induction of gene activity by proinflammatory cytokines: potential therapeutic targets. Shock 1997;7:405–412.
45. Tracey KJ, Fong Y, Hesse DG, et al. Anti-cachectin/TNF monoclonal antibodies prevent septic shock during lethal bacteremia. Nature (Lond) 1987;330:662–664.
46. Guirao X, Lowry SF. Biologic control of injury and inflammation: much more than too little or too late. World J Surg 1996;20:437–446.
47. Lin E, Lowry SF. The human response to endotoxin. Sepsis 1998;2:255–262.
48. Van Berge Henegouwen MI, van der Poll T, van Deventer SJH, Gouma DJ. Peritoneal cytokine release after elective gastrointestinal surgery and postoperative complications. Am J Surg 1998;175:311–316.
49. Lin E, Calvano SE, Lowry SF. Cytokine response in abdominal surgery. In: Schein M, Wise L, eds. Cytokines and the Abdominal Surgeon. Austin: Landes, 1998:17–34.
50. Enayati P, Brennan MF, Fong Y. Systemic and liver cytokine activation. Arch Surg 1994;124:1159–1164.
51. Van der Poll, Lowry SF. Tumor necrosis factor in sepsis: mediator of multiple organ failure or essential part of host defense? Shock 1995;3:1–12.
52. Van der Poll, Lowry SF. Endogenous mechanisms regulating TNF and IL-1 during sepsis. In: Vincent JL, ed. Yearbook of Intensive Care and Emergency Medicine. Berlin: Springer-Verlag, 1995:385–397.
53. Dinarello CA. Interleukin-1 and interleukin-1 antagonism. Blood 1991;77:1627–1652.
54. Fong Y, Lowry SF. Cytokines and the cellular response to injury and infection. In: Wilmore DW, Cheung LY, Harken AH, Holcroft JW, Meakins JL, eds. Surgery, Vol. 15. New York: Scientific American, 1996:1–21.
55. Schafer M, Carter L, Stein C. Interleukin-1 beta and corticotropin-releasing factor inhibit pain by releasing opioids from immune cells in immune tissue. Proc Natl Acad Sci USA 1994;91:4219–4223.
56. Ohlsson K, Bjork P, Bergenfeldt M, Hageman R, Thompson RC. Interleukin-1 receptor antagonist reduces mortality from endotoxic shock. Nature (Lond) 1990;348:550–552.
57. Abraham E, Regan RF. The effects of hemorrhage and trauma on interleukin-2 production. Arch Surg 1983;120:1341–1346.
58. Oka M, Hirazawa K, Yamamoto K, et al. Induction of Fas-mediated apoptosis on circulating lymphocytes by surgical stress. Ann Surg 1996;223:434–440.

59. Keegan AD, Ryan JJ, Paul WE. IL-4 regulates growth and differentiation by distinct mechanisms. Immunologist 1996;4:194–198.
60. Mangan DF, Wahl SM. Differential regulation of human monocyte programmed cell death (apoptosis) by chemotactic factors and proinflammatory cytokines. J Immunol 1991;147:3408–3412.
61. Xing Z, Gauldie J, Cox G, et al. IL-6 is an antiinflammatory cytokine required for controlling local or systemic acute inflammatory responses. J Clin Invest 1998;101:311–320.
62. Biffl WL, Moore EE, Moore FA, et al. Interleukin-6 delays neutrophil apoptosis. Arch Surg 1996;131:24–30.
63. Tilg H, Trehu E, Atkins MB. Interleukin-6 (IL-6) as an antiinflammatory cytokine: induction of circulating IL-1 receptor antagonist and soluble tumor necrosis factor receptor p55. Blood 1994;83:113–118.
64. Luster, AD. Chemokines—chemotactic cytokines that mediate inflammation. N Engl J Med 1998;338:436–445.
65. Gerard C, Bruyns C, Marchant A, et al. Interleukin 10 reduces the release of tumor necrosis factor and prevents lethality in experimental endotoxemia. J Exp Med 1993;177:547–550.
66. Marshall JD, Aste-Amezaga M, Chehimi SS, Murphy M, Olsen H, Trinchieri G. Regulation of human IL-18 mRNA expression. Clin Immunol 1999;90:15–21.
67. Van der Poll T, Marchant A, Buurman WA, et al. Endogenous IL-10 protects mice from death during septic peritonitis. J Immunol 1995;155:5397–5401.
68. Steinhauser ML, Hogaboam CM, Lukacs NW, Strieter RM, Kunkel SL. Multiple roles for IL-12 in a model of acute septic peritonitis. J Immunol 1999;162:5437–5443.
69. O'Sulleabhain C, O'Sullivan ST, Kelly JL, et al. Interleukin-12 treatment restores normal resistance to bacterial challenge after burn injury. Surgery (St. Louis) 1996;120:290–296.
70. Lauw FN, Dekkers PE, te Velde AA, et al. Interleukin-12 induces sustained activation of multiple host inflammatory mediator systems in chimpanzees. J Infect Dis 1999;179:646–652.
71. Carson WE, Yu H, Dierksheide J, et al. A fatal cytokine-induced systemic inflammatory response reveals a critical role for NK cells. J Immunol 1999;162:4943–4951.
72. Chomarat P, Banchereau J. Interleukin-4 and interleukin-13: their similarities and discrepancies. Int Rev Immunol 1998;17:1–52.
73. Manna SK, Aggarwal BB. Interleukin-4 down-regulates both forms of tumor necrosis factor receptor and receptor-mediated apoptosis, NF-kappaB, AP-1, and c-Jun N-terminal kinase. Comparison with interleukin-13. J Biol Chem 1998;273:33333–33341.
74. Etter H, Althaus R, Eugster HP, Santamaria-Babi LF, Weber L, Moser R. IL-4 and IL-13 downregulate rolling adhesion of leukocytes to IL-1 or TNF-alpha-activated endothelial cells by limiting the interval of E-selectin expression. Cytokine 1998;10:395–403.
75. Alleva DG, Kaser SB, Monroy MA, Fenton MJ, Beller DI. IL-15 functions as a potent autocrine regulator of macrophage proinflammatory cytokine production: evidence for differential receptor subunit utilization associated with stimulation or inhibition. J Immunol 1997;159:2941–2951.
76. Bulfone-Paus S, Ungureanu D, Pohl T, et al. Interleukin-15 protects from lethal apoptosis in vivo. Nat Med 1997;3:1124–1128.
77. McDonald PP, Russo MP, Ferrini S, Cassatella MA. Interleukin-15 (IL-15) induces NF-kappaB activation and IL-8 production in human neutrophils. Blood 1998;92:4828–4835.
78. Musso T, Calosso L, Zucca M, et al. Interleukin-15 activates proinflammatory and antimicrobial functions in polymorphonuclear cells. Infect Immun 1998;66:2640–2647.
79. Puren AJ, Fantuzzi G, Dinarello CA. Gene expression, synthesis, and secretion of interleukin-18 and interleukin-1b are differentially regulated in human blood mononuclear cells and mouse spleen cells. Proc Natl Acad Sci USA 1999;96:2256–2261.
80. Bohn E, Sing A, Zumbihl R, et al. IL-18 (IFN-γ-inducing factor) regulates early cytokine production in, and promotes resolution of, bacterial infection in mice. J Immunol 1998;160: 299–307.
81. Hoshino K, Tsutsui H, Kawai T, et al. Generation of IL-18 receptor-deficient mice: evidence for IL-1 receptor-related protein as an essential IL-18 binding receptor. J Immunol 1999;162:5041–5044.
82. Kohka H, Yoshino T, Iwagaki H, et al. Interleukin-18/interferon-γ-inducing factor, a novel cytokine, up-regulates ICAM-1 (CD54) expression in KG-1 cells. J Leukocyte Biol 1998;64:519–527.
83. Tsutsui H, Matsui K, Kawada N, et al. IL-18 accounts for both TNF-α- and Fas ligand-mediated hepatotoxic pathways in endotoxin-induced liver injury in mice. J Immunol 1997;159:3961–3967.
84. Oberholzer A, Steckholzer U, Okamura H, Kurimoto M, Trentz O, Ertel W. Increased circulating levels of interleukin-18 during severe sepsis in humans. Surg Forum 1998;49:88–90.
85. Heinzel FP, Rerko DM, Ling P, et al. Interleukin-12 is produced in vivo during endotoxemia and stimulates synthesis of gamma interferon. Infect Immunol 1994;62:4244–4249.
86. Dinarello CA. IL-18: a TH-1 inducing, proinflammatory cytokine and new member of the IL-1 family. J Allergy Clin Immunol 1999;103:11–24.
87. Barbul A, Regan MB. The regulatory role of T lymphocytes in wound healing. J Trauma 1990;30:S97–S102.
88. Keel M, Ungethum U, Steckholzer U, et al. Interleukin-10 counterregulates proinflammatory cytokine-induced inhibition of neutrophil apoptosis during severe sepsis. Blood 1997;90:3356–3363.
89. Ertel W, Keel M, Infanger M, Ungethum U, Steckholzer U, Trentz O. Circulating mediators in serum of injured patients with septic complications inhibit neutrophil apoptosis through upregulation of protein-tyrosine phosphorylation. J Trauma 1998;44:767–775.
90. Fanning NF, Kell MR, Shorten GD, et al. Circulating granulocyte macrophage colony-stimulating factor in plasma of patients with the systemic inflammatory response syndrome delays neutrophil apoptosis through inhibition of spontaneous reactive oxygen species generation. Shock 1999;11:167–174.
91. Goodman ER, Stricker P, Velavicius M, et al. Role of granulocyte-macrophage colony-stimulating factor and its receptor in the genesis of acute respiratory distress syndrome through an effect on neutrophil apoptosis. Arch Surg 1999;134:1049–1054.
92. Decker D, Schondorf M, Bidlingmaier F, Hirner A, von Ruecker AA. Surgical stress induces a shift in the type-1/type-2 T helper cell balance, suggesting down-regulation of cell-mediated and up-regulation of antibody-mediated immunity commensurate to the trauma. Surgery (St. Louis) 1996;119:316–325.
93. Zedler S, Bone RC, Baue AE, Donnersmarck GH, Faist E. T-cell reactivity and its predictive role in immunosuppression after burns. Crit Care Med 1999;27:66–72.
94. Berguer R, Bravo N, Bowyer M, Egan C, Knolmayer T, Ferrick D. Major surgery suppresses maximal production of helper T-cell type 1 cytokines without potentiating the release of helper T-cell type 2 cytokines. Arch Surg 1999;134:540–544.
95. Lin E, Calvano SE, Lowry SF. Disordered apoptosis as a mechanism for adverse outcome in critical illness. In: Vincent JL, ed. Yearbook of Intensive Care and Emergency Medicine. Berlin: Springer-Verlag, 1997:91–99.
96. Lin E, Calvano SE, Lowry SF. The biologic control of systemic inflammatory response. Curr Opin Crit Care 1997;3:299–307.
97. Lin E, Calvano SE, Lowry SF. Tumor necrosis factor receptors in systemic inflammation. In: Vincent JL, ed. Update in Intensive Care and Emergency Medicine: Immune Response in Critical Illness. Berlin: Springer-Verlag, 1999;365–384.

98. Ksontini R, MacKay SLD, Moldawer LL. Revisiting the role of tumor necrosis factor α and the response to surgical injury and inflammation. Arch Surg 1998;133:558–567.
99. Van Zee KJ, Stackpole SA, Montegut WJ, et al. A human tumor necrosis factor (TNF) a mutant that binds exclusively to the p55 TNF receptor produces toxicity in the baboon. J Exp Med 1994;179:1185–1191.
100. Welborn MB, van Zee K, Edwards PD, et al. A human tumor necrosis factor p75 receptor agonist stimulates in vitro T cell proliferation but does not produce inflammation or shock in the baboon. J Exp Med 1996;184:165–171.
101. Weiss T, Grell M, Hessabi S, et al. Enhancement of TNF receptor p60-mediated cytotoxicity by TNF receptor p80. J Immunol 1998;158:2398–2404.
102. Liu ZG, Hsu HL, Goeddel DV, Karin M. Dissection of TNF receptor 1 effector functions: JNK activation is not linked to apoptosis, while NF-κB activation prevents cell death. Cell 1996;87:565–576.
103. Anrather J, Csizmadia V, Brostjan C, Soares JP, Bach FH, Winkler H. Inhibition of bovine endothelial cell activation in vitro by regulated expression of a transdominant inhibitor of NF-κB. J Clin Invest 1997;99:763–772.
104. Bohrer H, Qiu F, Zimmermann T, et al. The role of NF-κB in the mortality of sepsis. J Clin Invest 1997;100:972–985.
105. Zong WX, Edelstein LC, Chen C, Bash J, Gelinas C. The prosurvival Bcl-2 homolog Bfl-1/A1 is a direct transcriptional target of NF-κB that blocks TNF-α-induced apoptosis. Genes Dev 1999;13:382–387.
106. Moulding DA, Quayle JA, Hart CA, Edwards SW. Mcl-1 expression in human neutrophils: regulation by cytokines and correlation with cell survival. Blood 1998;92:2495–2502.
107. Jiminez MF, Watson RW, Parodo J, et al. Dysregulated expression of neutrophil apoptosis in the systemic inflammatory response syndrome. Arch Surg 1997;132:1263–1270.
108. Lin E, Calvano SE, Coyle S, Rumalla V, Kumar A, Lowry SF. Physiologic hypercortisolemia in humans modulates neutrophil CD95 signal transduction. Surg Forum 1999;50:288–290.
109. Ksontini R, Colagiovanni DB, Josephs MD, et al. Disparate roles for TNF-alpha and Fas ligand in convanavalin A-induced hepatitis. J Immunol 1998;160:4082–4089.
110. Kunstel G, Leist M, Uhlig S, et al. ICE-protease inhibitors block murine liver injury and apoptosis caused by CD95 or by TNF-alpha. Immunol Lett 1997;55:5–10.
111. Rodriguez I, Matsuura K, Ody C, Nagata S, Vassalli P. Systemic injection of a tripeptide inhibits the intracellular activation of CPP32-like proteases in vivo and fully protects mice against Fas-mediated fulminant liver destruction and death. J Exp Med 1996;184:2067–2072.
112. Van der Poll T, Calvano SE, Kumar A, et al. Endotoxin induces downregulation of tumor necrosis factor receptors on circulating monocytes and granulocytes in humans. Blood 1995;86:2754–2759.
113. Calvano SE, van der Poll T, Coyle SM, et al. Monocyte tumor necrosis factor receptor levels as a predictor of risk in human sepsis. Arch Surg 1996;131:434–437.
114. Rumalla V, Calvano SE, Spotnitz AJ, Krause TJ, Lin E, Lowry SF. Alterations in immunocyte tumor necrosis factor receptor and apoptosis in preoperative patients with congestive heart failure. Surg Forum 1999;50:120–122.
115. Calvano SE, Coyle S, Barbosa K, et al. Multivariate analysis of nine disease-associated variables for outcome prediction in patients with sepsis. Arch Surg 1998;133:1347–1350.
116. Lin E, Katz JA, Calvano SE, et al. The influence of human endotoxemia on CD95-induced apoptosis. Arch Surg 1998;133:1322–1327.
117. Wissink S, van Heerde EC, van der Burg B, van der Saag PT. A dual mechanism mediates repression of NF-κB activity by glucocorticoids. Mol Endocrinol 1998;12:355–363.
118. Brostjan C, Anrather J, Csizmadia V, Natarajan G, Winkler H. Glucocorticoids inhibit E-selectin expression by targeting NF-κB and not ATF/c-Jun. J Immunol 1997;158:3836–3844.
119. Ayala A, Herson CD, Lehman DL, DeMaso CM, Ayala CA, Chaudry IH. The induction of accelerated thymic programmed cell death during polymicrobial sepsis: control by corticosteroids but not tumor necrosis factor. Shock 1995;3:259–267.
120. Zubiaga AM, Munoz E, Huber BT. IL-4 and IL-2 selectively rescue Th cell subsets from glucocorticoid-induced apoptosis. J Immunol 1992;149:107–112.
121. Liles WC, Dale DC, Klebanoff SJ. Glucocorticoids inhibit apoptosis of human neutrophils. Blood 1995;86:3181–3188.
122. Barber AE, Coyle SM, Marano MA, et al. Glucocorticoid therapy alters hormonal and cytokine responses to endotoxin in man. J Immunol 1993;150:1999–2006.
123. Van der Poll T, Barber AE, Coyle SM, Lowry SF. Hypercortisolemia increases plasma interleukin-10 concentrations during human endotoxemia—a clinical research center study. J Clin Endocrinol Metab 1996;81:3604–3606.
124. Kawamura T, Inada K, Nara N, Wakusawa R, Endo S. Influence of methylprednisolone on cytokine balance during cardiac surgery. Crit Care Med 1999;27:545–548.
125. Van der Poll T, Lowry SF. Epinephrine inhibits endotoxin-induced IL-1b production: roles of tumor necrosis factor-α and IL-10. Am J Physiol 1997;273:R1885–R1890.
126. Van der Poll T, Lowry SF. Lipopolysaccharide-induced interleukin-8 production by human whole blood is enhanced by epinephrine and inhibited by hydrocortisone. Infect Immun 1997;65:2378–2381.
127. Van der Poll T, Coyle SM, Barbosa K, Braxton CC, Lowry SF. Epinephrine inhibits tumor necrosis factor-α and potentiates interleukin-10 production during human endotoxemia. J Clin Invest 1996;97:713–719.
128. Walden DL, McCutchan HJ, Enquist EG, et al. Neutrophils accumulate and contribute to skeletal muscle dysfunction after ischemia-reperfusion. Am J Physiol 1990;259:H1809–H1812.
129. Lin E, Lowry SF, Calvano SE. The systemic response to injury. In: Schwartz SI, ed. Principles of Surgery, 7th ed. New York: McGraw-Hill, 1998:3–51.
130. Barroso-Aranda J, Schmid-Schönbein GW, Zwiefach BW, et al. Granulocytes and no-reflow phenomenon in irreversible hemorrhagic shock. Circ Res 1988;63:437–447.
131. Jerome SN, Smith CW, Korthuis RJ. CD18-dependent adherence reactions play an important role in the development of the no-reflow phenomenon. Am J Physiol 1993;264:H479–H483.
132. Carden EL, Smith JK, Korthuis RJ. Neutrophil-mediated microvascular dysfunction in postischemic canine skeletal muscle: role of granulocyte adherence. Circ Res 1990;66:1436–1444.
133. Klausner JM, Paterson IS, Valeri CR, et al. Limb ischemia-induced increase in permeability is mediated by leukocytes and leukotrienes. Ann Surg 1988;208:755–760.
134. Vedder NB, Winn RK, Rice CL, et al. Inhibition of leukocyte adherence by anti-CD18 monoclonal antibody attenuates reperfusion injury in the rabbit ear. Proc Natl Acad Sci USA 1990;87:2643–2646.
135. Eichacker PQ, Farese A, Hoffman WD, Banks S, Mouginis T, Natanson C. Leukocyte CD11b/CD18 antigen-directed monoclonal antibody improves early survival and decreases hypoxemia in dogs challenged with tumor necrosis factor. Am Rev Respir Dis 1992;145:1023–1029.
136. Patrick DA, Moore FA, Moore EE, Biffl WL, Sauaia A, Barnett CC. The inflammatory profile of interleukin-6, interleukin-8, and soluble intercellular adhesion molecule-1 in postinjury multiple organ failure. Am J Surg 1996;172:425–431.
137. Eppihimer MJ, Wolitzky BA, Anderson DC, Labow MA, Granger DN. Heterogeneity of E- and P-selectin expression in vivo. Circ Res 1996;79:560–569.

138. Read MA, Whitley MZ, Williams AJ, Collins T. NF-κB and IkBa: an inducible regulatory system in endothelial activation. J Exp Med 1994;179:503–512.
139. Anrather J, Csizmadia V, Brostjan C, Soares JP, Bach FH, Winkler H. Inhibition of bovine endothelial cell activation in vitro by regulated expression of a transdominant inhibitor of NF-κB. J Clin Invest 1997;99:763–772.
140. Bevilacqua MP, Pober JS, Mendrick DL, Cotran RS, Gimbrone MA. Identification of an inducible endothelial-leukocyte adhesion molecule. Proc Natl Acad Sci USA 1987;84:9238–9242.
141. Lawrence MB, Springer TA. Neutrophils roll on E-selectin. J Immunol 1993;151:6338–6346.
142. Lo SK, Lee S, Ramos RA, et al. Endothelial-leukocyte adhesion molecule 1 stimulates the adhesive activity of leukocyte integrin CR3 (CD11b/CD18, Mac-1, amb2) on human neutrophils. J Exp Med 1991;173:1493–1500.
143. Butcher EC. Leukocyte-endothelial cell recognition—three (or more) steps to specificity and diversity. Cell 1991;67:1033–1036.
144. Schleiffenbaum BE, Spertini O, Tedder TF. Soluble L-selectin is present in human plasma at high levels and retains functional activity. J Cell Biol 1992;119:229–238.
145. Walcheck B, Kahn J, Fisher JM, et al. Neutrophil rolling altered by inhibition of L-selectin shedding in vitro. Nature (Lond) 1996;380:720–723.
146. Ley K, Bullard D, Arbones ML, et al. Sequential contribution of L- and P-selectin to leukocyte rolling in vivo. J Exp Med 1995;181:669–675.
147. Lim YC, Snapp K, Kansas GS, Camphausen R, Ding H, Luscinskas FW. Important contributions of P-selectin glycoprotein ligand-1-mediated secondary capture to human monocyte adhesion to P-selectin, E-selectin, and TNF-a-activated endothelium under flow in vitro. J Immunol 1998;161:2501–2508.
148. Kanwar S, Steeber DA, Tedder TF, Hickey MJ, Kubes P. Overlapping roles for L-selectin and P-selectin in antigen-induced immune responses in the microvasculature. J Immunol 1999;162:2709–2716.
149. Kansas GS. Selectins and their ligands: current concepts and controversies. Blood 1996;88:3259–3287.
150. Gopalan PK, Smith CW, Lu H, Berg EL, McIntire LV, Simon SI. Neutrophil CD18-dependent arrest on intercellular adhesion molecule 1 (ICAM-1) in shear flow can be activated through L-selectin. J Immunol 1997;158:367–375.
151. Walcheck B, Moore KL, McEver RP, Kishimoto TK. Neutrophil–neutrophil interactions under hydrodynamic shear stress involve L-selectin and PSGL-1. J Clin Invest 1996;98:1081–1087.
152. Nathan C. Nitric oxide as a secretory product of mammalian cells. FASEB J 1992;6:3051–3064.
153. Geller DA, Lowenstein C, Shapiro RA, et al. Molecular cloning and expression of inducible nitric oxide synthase from human hepatocytes. Proc Natl Acad Sci USA 1993;90:3491–3495.
154. Buga GM, Singh R, Pervin S, et al. Arginase activity in endothelial cells: inhibition by *NG*-hydroxy-L-arginine during high-output NO production. Am J Physiol 1996;271:H1988–H1998.
155. Geller DA, Nussler AK, DiSilvio M, et al. Cytokines, endotoxin, and glucocorticoids regulate the expression of inducible nitric oxide synthase in hepatocytes. Proc Natl Acad Sci USA 1993;90:522–526.
156. Luscher TF. The endocrine endothelium. In: Becker KL, et al., eds. Principles and Practice of Endocrinology and Metabolism, 2nd ed. Philadelphia: Lippincott, 1996:1491–1498.
157. Koller J, Mair P, et al. Endothelin and big endothelin concentrations in injured patients. N Engl J Med 1991;325:1518–1524.
158. Diez FL, Nieto ML, Fernandez-Gallardo S, et al. Occupancy of platelet receptors for platelet-activating factor in patients with septicemia. J Clin Invest 1989;83:1733–1740.
159. Thompson WA, Coyle SM, et al. The metabolic effects of PAF antagonism in endotoxemic man. Arch Surg 1994;29:72–76.
160. Moore JM, Earnest MA, DiSimone AG, et al. A PAF receptor antagonist, BN52021, attenuates thromboxane release and improves survival in lethal canine endotoxemia. Circ Shock 1991;35:53–59.
161. Botha AJ, Moore FA, et al. Sequential systemic platelet-activating factor and interleukin 8 primes neutrophils in patients with trauma at risk of multiple organ failure. Br J Surg 1996;83:1407–1415.
162. Jindal S. Heat shock proteins: applications in health and disease. Trends Biotechnol 1996;14:17–25.
163. Udelsman R, Blake MJ, et al. Molecular response to surgical stress: specific and simultaneous heat shock proteins induction in the adrenal cortex, aorta, and vena cava. Surgery (St. Louis) 1991;110:1125–1131.
164. Blake MJ, Udelsman R, et al. Stress-induced heat shock protein 70 expression in adrenal cortex: an adrenocorticotropic hormone-sensitive, age-dependent response. Proc Natl Acad Sci USA 1991;88:9873–9879.
165. Brigham KL, Meyrick B, et al. Antioxidants protect cultured bovine lung endothelial cells from injury from endotoxin. J Appl Physiol 1987;63:840–845.
166. Fink MP. Bench-to-bedside review: cytopathic hypoxia. Crit Care 2002;6:491–499.
167. Chiba T, Takahashi S, et al. Fas-mediated apoptosis is modulated by intracellular glutathione in human T cells. Eur J Immunol 1996;26:1164–1169.
168. Robertson RP. Prostaglandins and other arachidonic acid metabolites. In: Becker KL, et al., eds. Principles and Practice of Endocrinology and Metabolism, 2nd ed. Philadelphia: Lippincott, 1996:1466–1472.
169. Grbic JT, Mannick JA, et al. The role of prostaglandin E_2 in immune suppression following injury. Ann Surg 1991;214:253–260.
170. Lefer AM. Eicosanoids as mediators of ischemia and shock. Fed Proc 1985;44:275–279.
171. Caromona RH, Tsao RC, et al. The role of prostacyclin and thromboxane in sepsis and septic shock. Arch Surg 1984;119:189–194.
172. Sherhan CN, Clish CB, Brannon J. Novel functional sets of lipid derived mediators with antiinflammatory actions derived from omega-3 fatty acids via cyclooxygenase-2 nonsteroidal drugs and transcellular processing. J Exp Med 2000;192:1197–1204.
173. Sherhan CN, Savill J. Resolution of inflammation: the beginning programs the end. Nat Immunol 2005;6:1191–1197.
174. Kinsella JE, Lokesh B. Dietary lipids, eicosanoids and the immune system. Crit Care Med 1990;18:S94–S113.
175. Kremer JM, Jubiz W, Michalek A, et al. Fish oil fatty acid supplementation in active rheumatoid arthritis: a double-blinded, controlled, crossover study. Ann Intern Med 1987;106:497–503.
176. Endres S, Ghorbani R, Kelley VE, et al. The effect of dietary supplementation with *n*-3 polyunsaturated fatty acids on the synthesis of interleukin-1 and tumor necrosis factor by mononuclear cells. N Engl J Med 1989;320:265–271.
177. Trocki O, Heyd TJ, Waymack JP, Alexander JW. Effects of fish oil on postburn metabolism and immunity. J Parenter Enteral Nutr 1987;11:521–528.
178. Sierra P, Ling PR, Istfan NW, Bistrian BR. Fish oil feeding improves muscle glucose uptake in tumor necrosis factor-treated rats. Metabolism 1995;44:1365–1370.
179. Lo CJ, Terasaki M, Garcia R, Helton S. Fish oil-supplemented feeding does not attenuate warm liver ischemia and reperfusion injury in the rat. J Surg Res 1997;71:54–60.
180. Mancuso P, Whelan J, DeMichele SJ, Snider CC, Guszcza JA, Karlstad MD. Dietary fish oil and fish and borage oil suppress intrapulmonary proinflammatory eicosanoid biosynthesis and

attenuate pulmonary neutrophil accumulation in endotoxic rats. Crit Care Med 1997;25:1198–1206.

181. Hughes DA, Pinder AC, Piper Z, Johnson IT, Lund EK. Fish oil supplementation inhibits the expression of major histocompatibility complex class II molecules and adhesion molecules on human monocytes. Am J Clin Nutr 1996;63:267–272.
182. Hartl WH, Herndon DN, Wolfe RR, et al. Kinin/prostaglandin system: its therapeutic value in surgical stress. Crit Care Med 1990;18:1167–1174.
183. Rodell TC. The kallikrein/kinin system and kinin antagonists in trauma. Immunopharmacology 1996;33:279–288.
184. Lin E, Calvano SE, Lowry SF. Inflammatory cytokines and cell response in surgery. Surgery 2000;127:117–126.
185. Lin E, Calvano SE, Lowry SF. Selectin neutralization: does it make biological sense? Crit Care Med 1999;27:2050–2053.
186. Angaard EE. The endothelium: the body's largest endocrine organ? J Endocrinol 1990;127:373–378.
187. Granner DK. Hormonal action. In: Becker KL, et al., eds. Principles and Practice of Endocrinology and Metabolism, 2nd ed. Philadelphia: Lippincott, 1996.

5 Substrate Metabolism

Edward Lin and Stephen F. Lowry

The initial hours following surgical or traumatic injury are associated metabolically with reduced total body energy expenditure and increased urinary nitrogen wasting. This initial phase of injury also demonstrates an augmented release of neuroendocrine hormones, including catecholamines and cortisol. On adequate resuscitation and stabilization of the injured patient, a reprioritization of substrate utilization occurs to preserve vital organ function and for the repair of injured tissue.[1] This phase of recovery is also characterized by augmented metabolic rates and oxygen consumption, enhanced enzymatic pathways for readily oxidizable substrates such as glucose, and stimulation of immune system functions that participate in the restoration of homeostasis.

Substrate Utilization in Fasting

Fuel metabolism during unstressed fasting states has conventionally served as the basis to which metabolic alterations following acute injury and critical illness are compared (Fig. 5.1). To maintain basal metabolic needs (i.e., at rest and fasting), a normal healthy adult requires approximately 25 kcal/kg per day drawn from carbohydrate, lipid, and protein sources. This requirement can be as high as 40 kcal/kg per day in severe stress states, such as seen in burn injury patients.

The metabolic derangements of the postinjury state are often contrasted with unstressed starvation. In the healthy adult, the principal sources of fuel during short-term fasting (<5 days) are derived from muscle protein and body fat, and fat is the most abundant source of energy (Table 5.1).[2] The normal adult body contains 300 to 400 g of carbohydrates in the form of glycogen, of which 75 to 100 g are stored in the liver. Approximately 200 to 250 g of glycogen are stored within skeletal, cardiac, and smooth muscles. The greater glycogen stores within the muscle are not readily available for systemic use because of a deficiency in glucose-6-phosphatase but are available for energy needs of muscle cells.

During fasting, a healthy 70-kg adult utilizes 180 g glucose per day to support the metabolism of obligate glycolytic cells such as neurons, leukocytes, erythrocytes, and the renal medulla. Other tissues that utilize glucose for fuel are skeletal muscle, intestinal mucosa, fetal tissues, and solid tumors. It is obvious that hepatic glycogen stores are rapidly depleted in fasting states, and indeed serum glucose concentration falls within hours (<16 h).

The acute depletion in serum glucose concentration signals for a reduction in insulin release as well as other hormonal responses that promote the production and release of glucose. Glucagon, norepinephrine, vasopressin, and angiotensin II can promote the utilization of glycogen stores (glycogenolysis) through intracellular signaling activity. Glucagon, epinephrine, and cortisol primarily promote gluconeogenesis, whereas epinephrine and cortisol limit the direct utilization of pyruvate as fuel, which allows for pyruvate shuttling to the liver for gluconeogenesis.[3] Precursors for hepatic gluconeogenesis include lactate, glycerol, and amino acids such as alanine and glutamine. Lactate is released by glycolysis within skeletal muscles as well as by erythrocytes and leukocytes. The recycling of lactate and pyruvate for gluconeogenesis, commonly referred to as the *Cori cycle*, can provide up to 40% of plasma glucose during starvation (Fig. 5.2).

Skeletal muscle lactate production is insufficient to maintain systemic glucose levels during short-term fasting. Therefore, significant amounts of protein must be degraded (75 g per day for a 70-kg adult) to provide the amino acids necessary to sustain hepatic gluconeogenesis. Proteolysis, which results primarily from decreased insulin and increased cortisol release, is associated with elevated urinary nitrogen excretion from the normal 7 to 10 g per day up to 30 g or more per day. Proteolysis during starvation occurs mainly within skeletal muscles, but protein degradation in other organs also occurs.

In prolonged starvation, systemic proteolysis is reduced to approximately 20 g/day, and urinary nitrogen excretion

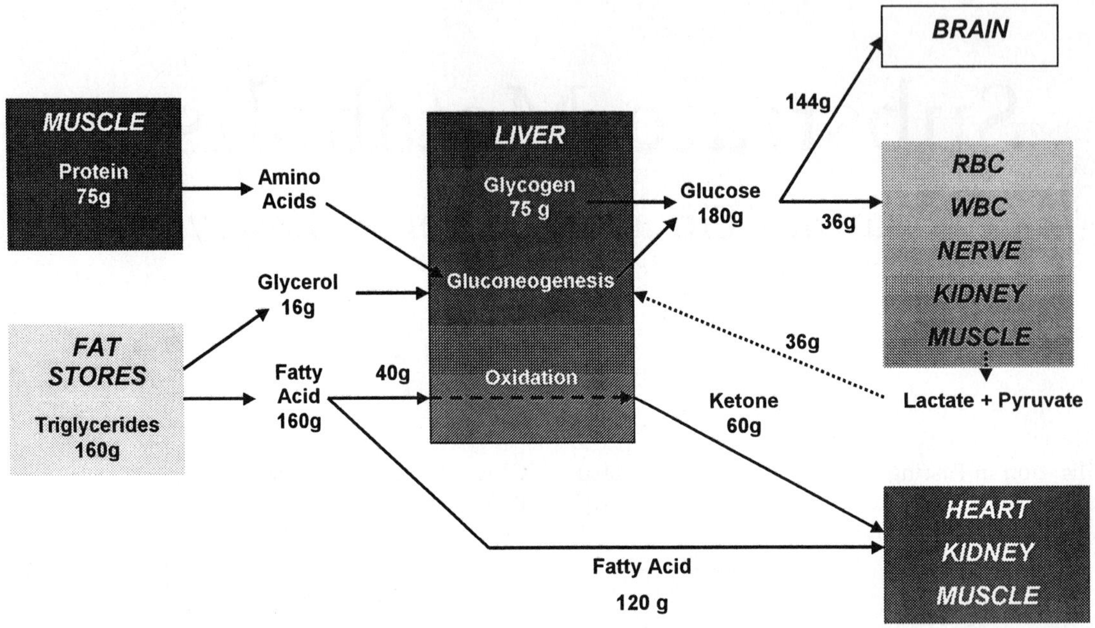

FIGURE 5.1. Fuel utilization in a 70-kg man during short-term fasting with approximate basal energy expenditure of 1800 calories. During starvation, muscle proteins and fat stores provide fuel for the host, with the latter most abundant. *RBC*, red blood cells; *WBC*, white blood cells. (Adapted from Cahill,[2] with permission.)

TABLE 5.1. Body Composition and Energy Reserves in a Normal 70-kg Man at Rest.

Component	*Mass (kg)*	*Energy (kcal)*	*Days available*
Water and minerals	49	0	0
Protein	6	24,000	13
Glycogen	0.2	800	0.4
Fat[a]	15	140,000	78
Total	70	164,800	91.4

[a] Fat remains the primary fuel source.

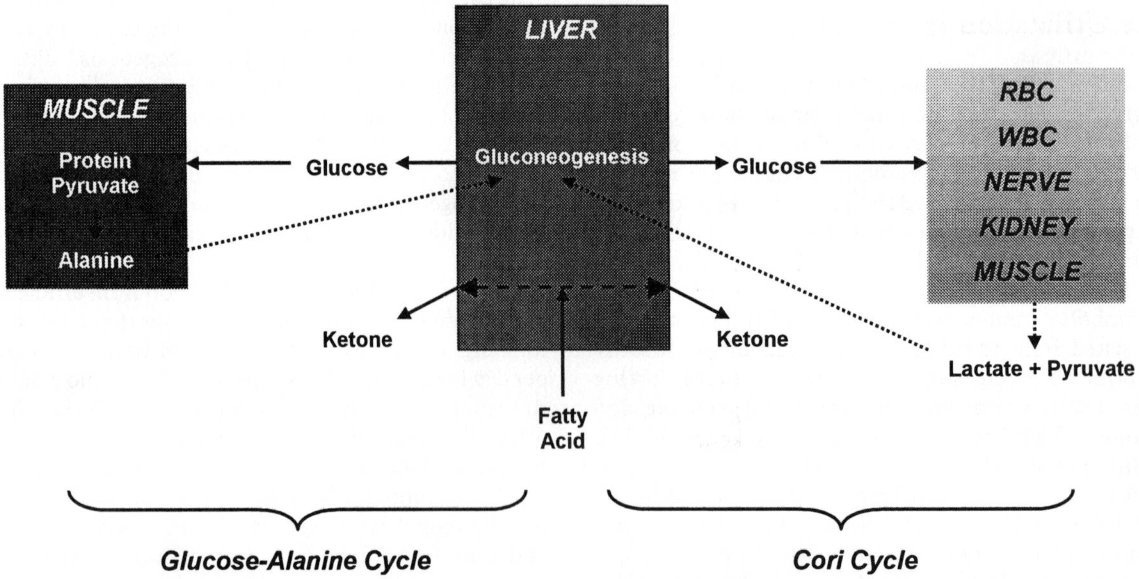

FIGURE 5.2. Recycling of peripheral lactate and pyruvate for hepatic gluconeogenesis in the Cori cycle. Alanine within skeletal muscles can also be utilized as a precursor for hepatic gluconeogenesis. During starvation, such fatty acids provide fuel sources for basal hepatic enzymatic function.

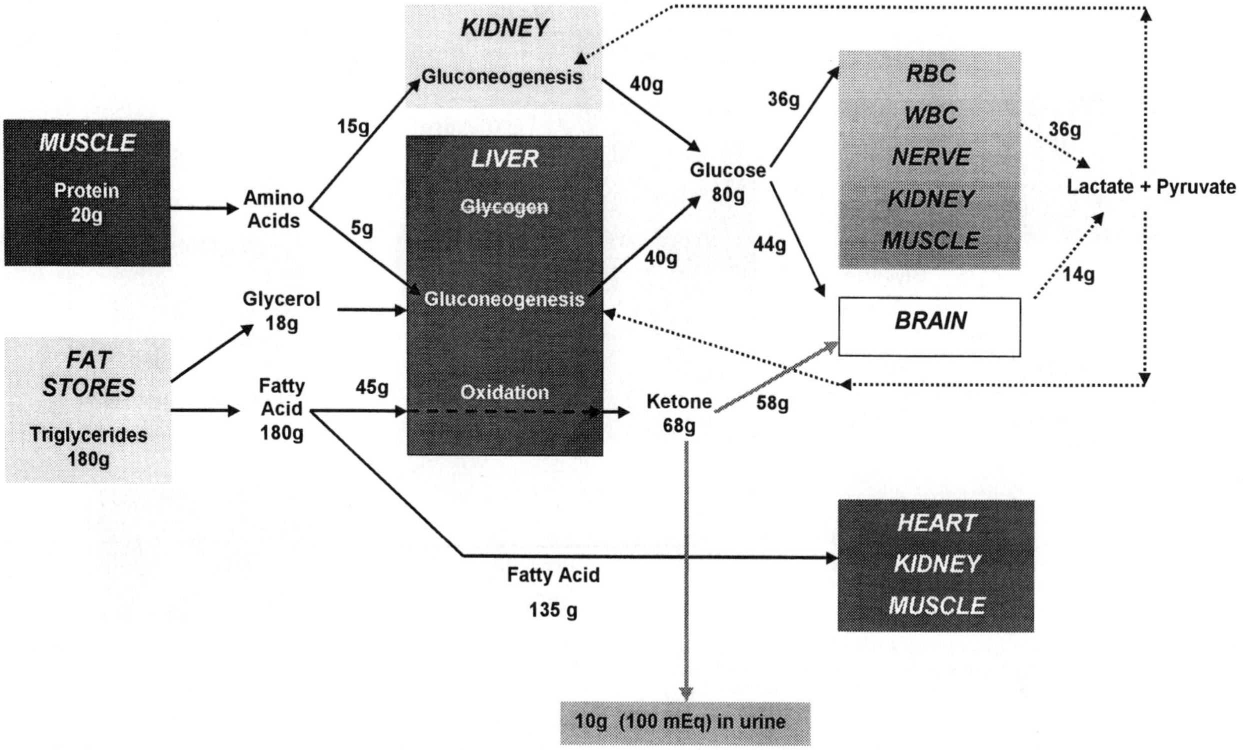

FIGURE 5.3. Fuel utilization in extended starvation. Liver glycogen stores are depleted, and there is adaptive reduction in proteolysis as a source of fuel. The brain utilizes ketones for fuel; the kidneys become important participants in gluconeogenesis. (Adapted from Cahill,[2] with permission.)

stabilizes to 2 to 5 g/day (Fig. 5.3). This reduction in proteolysis reflects the adaptation by vital organs (e.g., myocardium, brain, renal cortex, skeletal muscle, brain) to using ketone bodies as their principal fuel source. In extended fasting, ketone bodies become an important fuel source of the brain after 2 days and gradually become the principal fuel source by 24 days.

Enhanced deamination of amino acids for gluconeogenesis during starvation consequently increases renal excretion of ammonium ions. The kidneys also participate in gluconeogenesis by the utilization of glutamine and glutamate. Indeed, the kidneys can become the primary source of gluconeogenesis during prolonged starvation, accounting for as much as half of systemic glucose production.

Lipid stores within adipose tissue provide up to 40% of caloric expenditure during starvation. Energy requirements for basal enzymatic and muscular functions (e.g., gluconeogenesis, neural transmission, cardiac contraction) are met by the mobilization of triglycerides from adipose tissue. In a resting, fasting 70-kg person, approximately 160 g of free fatty acids and glycerol can be mobilized from adipose tissue. Free fatty acid release is stimulated in part by a reduction in serum insulin levels and in part by the increase in glucagon and catecholamine levels. Such free fatty acids and ketone bodies generated by the liver are used as fuel by tissues such as the heart, kidney (renal cortex), muscle, and liver. The mobilization of lipid stores for energy importantly decreases the rate of glycolysis, gluconeogenesis, proteolysis, and the overall glucose requirement to sustain the host. Furthermore, ketone bodies spare glucose utilization by inhibiting the enzyme pyruvate dehydrogenase.

Substrate Metabolism After Injury

Injuries or infections induce unique neuroendocrine and immunological responses that differentiate injury metabolism from that of unstressed fasting (Fig. 5.4).[4] Such stresses on the patient are accompanied by significant interorgan substrate flux as well as augmented metabolic requirements. Indeed, the magnitude of metabolic expenditure appears to be directly proportional to the severity of insult, with thermal injuries and severe infections exhibiting the highest energy demands (Fig. 5.5).[5] The increase in energy expenditure is mediated in part by sympathetic activation and catecholamine release and has been replicated by the administration of catecholamines to healthy human subjects.

Lipid Metabolism

Adipose stores within the body (triglycerides) are the predominant energy source (50%–80%) during critical illness and following injury, and fat mobilization (lipolysis) occurs mainly in response to catecholamine stimulus on hormone-sensitive triglyceride lipase. Other hormonal influences on lipolysis include adrenocorticotropic hormone (ACTH; corticotropin), catecholamines, thyroid hormone, cortisol, glucagon, growth hormone release, reduction in insulin levels, and increased sympathetic stimulus.

Lipid Absorption

Although the mechanism is poorly understood, during critical illness and injury adipose tissue provides the host fuel in the form of free fatty acids and glycerol. Oxidation of 1 g of fat

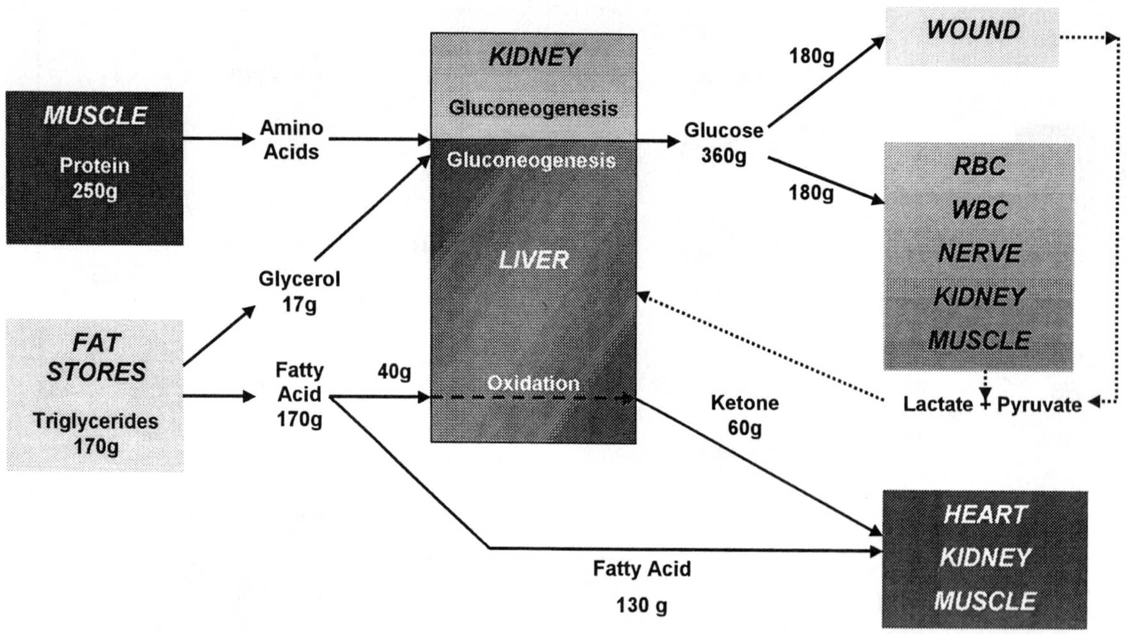

FIGURE 5.4. Acute injury is associated with significant alterations in substrate utilization. There is enhanced nitrogen loss, indicative of catabolism. Fat remains the primary fuel source under these circumstances. (Adapted from Cahill,[2] with permission.)

yields approximately 9 kcal of energy. Although the liver is capable of synthesizing triglycerides from carbohydrates and amino acids, dietary and exogenous sources provide the major source of triglycerides.

Dietary lipids are not readily absorbable in the gut but require pancreatic lipase and phospholipase within the duodenum to hydrolyze the triglycerides into free fatty acids and monoglycerides. The free fatty acids and monoglycerides are then readily absorbed by gut enterocytes, which resynthesize triglycerides by esterification of the monoglycerides with fatty acyl coenzyme A (acyl-CoA) (Fig. 5.6). Long-chain fatty acids (LCFAs), defined as those with 12 carbons or more, generally undergo this process of esterification and enter the circulation through the lymphatic system as chylomicrons. Shorter fatty acid chains directly enter the portal circulation and are transported to the liver by albumin carriers.

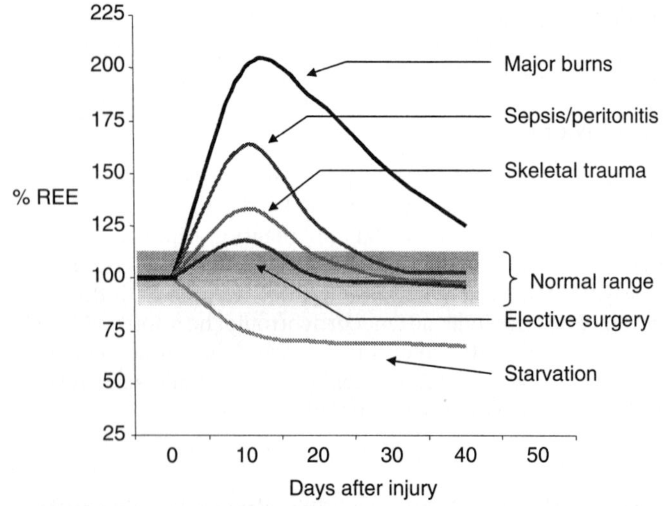

FIGURE 5.5. The influence of injury severity on resting metabolism (resting energy expenditure, *REE*). The *shaded area* indicates normal REE. (Adapted from Long,[5] with permission.)

Hepatocytes utilize free fatty acids as a fuel source during stress states but can also synthesize phospholipids or triglycerides (i.e., lipoproteins with very low density) during fed states. Systemic tissue (e.g., adipose, muscle, heart) can utilize chylomicrons and triglycerides as fuel by hydrolysis with lipoprotein lipase at the luminal surface of capillary endothelium. Starvation or trauma is known to decrease lipoprotein lipase activity in adipose tissue but increase its activity within skeletal muscles. Sepsis, however, suppresses this enzyme activity in both adipose tissue and muscle.[6] Tumor necrosis factor inhibits lipogenesis and decreases lipoprotein lipase activity. During fed states, insulin activity increases lipoprotein lipase activity in adipose tissue but decreases it in muscle. As a negative feedback, unutilized free fatty acids at the luminal surface cause an inhibitory effect on tissue lipoprotein lipase.

Lipolysis and Fatty Acid Oxidation

Periods of energy demand are accompanied by free fatty acid mobilization from adipose stores. This activity is mediated by hormonal influences (e.g., catecholamines, ACTH, thyroid hormones, growth hormone, and glucagon) on triglyceride lipase through a cyclic adenosine monophosphate (cAMP) pathway (Fig. 5.7).[7] In adipose tissues, triglyceride lipase hydrolyzes triglycerides into free fatty acids and glycerol. Free fatty acids enter the capillary circulation and are transported by albumin to tissues requiring this fuel source (e.g., heart and skeletal muscle). Insulin inhibits lipolysis and favors triglyceride synthesis by augmenting lipoprotein lipase activity as well as intracellular levels of glycerol-3-phosphate. The use of glycerol for fuel depends on the availability of tissue glycerokinase, which is abundant in the liver and kidney.

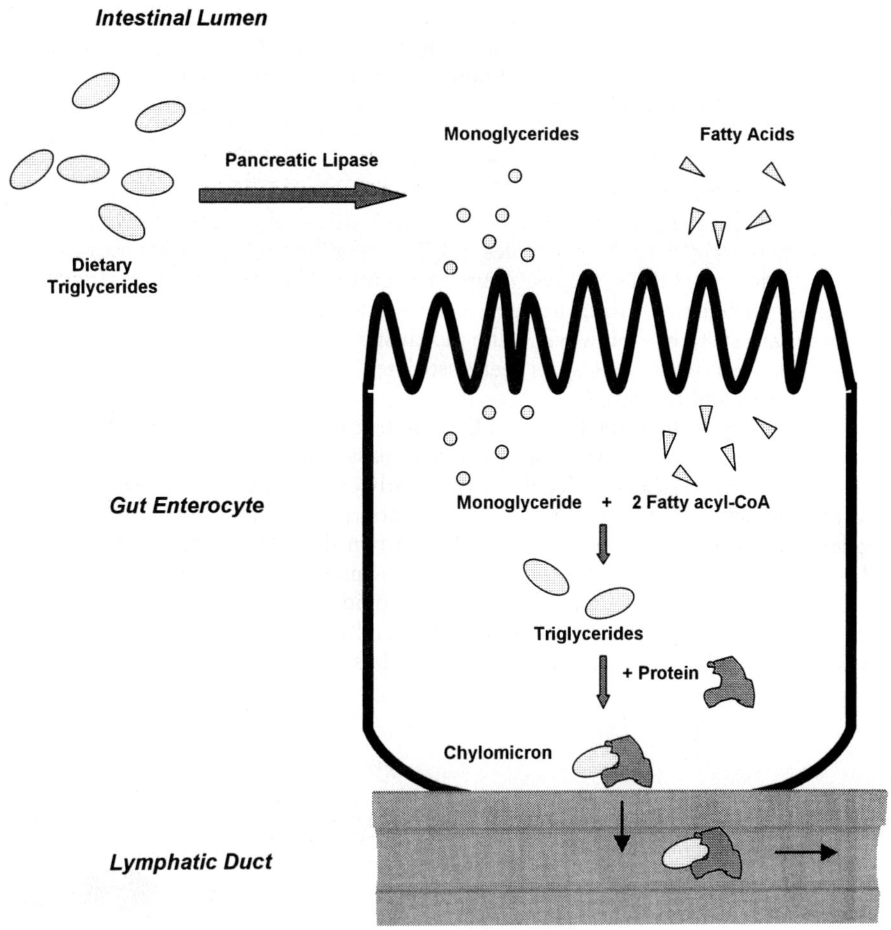

FIGURE 5.6. Pancreatic lipase within the small intestinal brush borders hydrolyzes triglycerides into monoglycerides and fatty acids. These components readily diffuse into the gut enterocytes, where they are reesterified into triglycerides. The resynthesized triglycerides bind carrier proteins to form chyomicrons, which are transported by the lymphatic system. Shorter triglycerides (fewer than 10 carbons) can bypass this process and directly enter the portal circulation for transport to the liver.

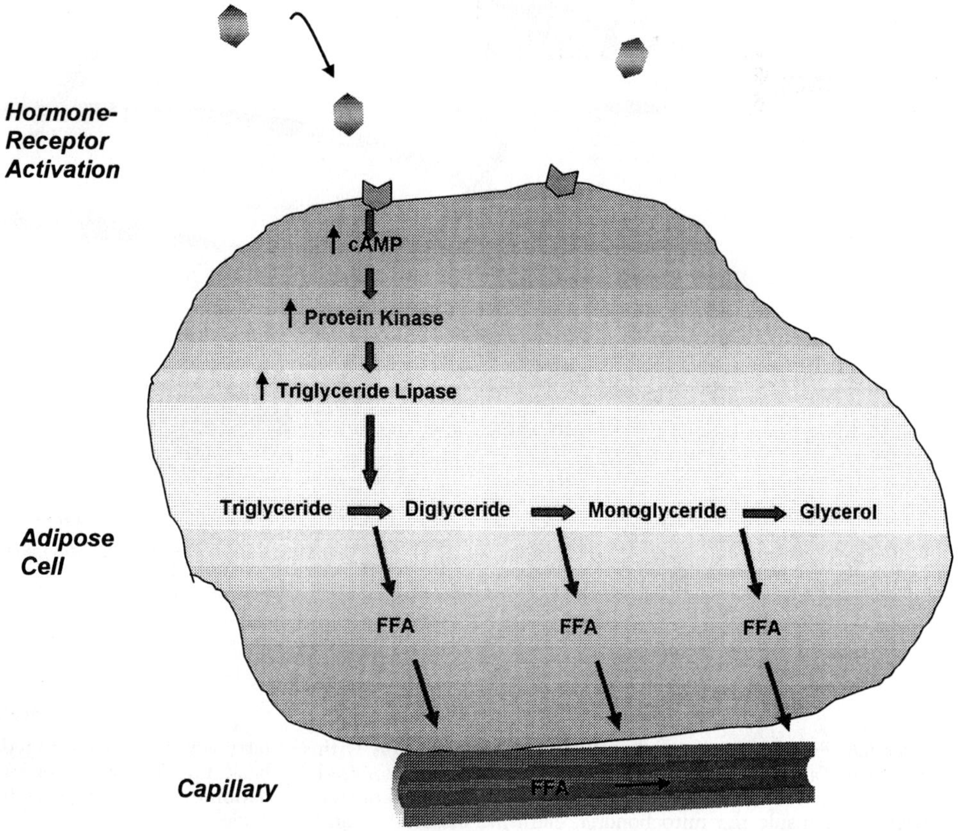

FIGURE 5.7. Fat mobilization in adipose tissue. Triglyceride lipase activation by hormonal stimulation of adipose cells occurs through the cAMP pathway. Triglycerides are serially hydrolyzed with resultant free fatty acid (*FFA*) release at every step. The FFAs diffuse readily into the capillary bed for transport. Tissues with glycerokinase can utilize glycerol for fuel by forming glycerol-3-phosphate. Glycerol-3-phosphate can esterify with FFA to form triglycerides or can be used as a precursor for renal and hepatic gluconeogenesis. Skeletal muscle and adipose cells have little glycerokinase and thus do not use glycerol for fuel.

Free fatty acids absorbed by cells conjugate with acyl-CoA within the cytoplasm. The transport of fatty acyl-CoA from the outer mitochondrial membrane across the inner mitochondrial membrane occurs via the carnitine shuttle (Fig. 5.8). Medium-chain fatty acids, defined as those 6 to 12 carbons in length, bypass the carnitine shuttle and readily cross the mitochondrial membranes. This ability is one reason why medium-chain triglycerides (MCTs) are more efficiently oxidized than long-chain triglycerides (LCTs). Ideally, the rapid oxidation of MCTs makes them less prone to fat deposition, particularly within immune cells and the reticuloendothelial system.[8] However, the exclusive use of MCTs as fuel in animal studies has been associated with high metabolic rates and toxicity.[9]

Within the mitochondria, fatty acyl-CoA undergoes β-oxidation, which produces acetyl-CoA with each pass through the cycle. Each acetyl-CoA molecule subsequently enters the tricarboxylic acid (TCA) cycle for further oxidation to yield 12 adenosine triphosphate (ATP) molecules, carbon dioxide, and water. Excess acetyl-CoA molecules serve as precursors for ketogenesis. Unlike glucose metabolism, oxidation of fatty acids requires proportionally less oxygen and produces less carbon dioxide; this is frequently quantified as the ratio of carbon dioxide produced to oxygen consumed for the reaction, or respiratory quotient (RQ). An RQ of 0.7 would imply greater fatty acid oxidation for fuel, while an RQ of 1 indicates greater carbohydrate oxidation; an RQ of 0.85 suggests the oxidation of equal amounts of fatty acids and glucose.

Ketogenesis

Carbohydrate depletion slows acetyl-CoA entry into the TCA cycle secondary to depleted TCA intermediates and enzyme activity. Increased lipolysis and reduced systemic carbohydrate availability during starvation diverts excess acetyl-CoA toward hepatic ketogenesis. A number of extrahepatic tissues, but not the liver itself, are capable of utilizing ketones for fuel. *Ketosis* represents a state in which hepatic ketone production exceeds extrahepatic ketone utilization.

The rate of ketogenesis appears to be inversely related to the severity of injury.[10] Major trauma, severe shock, and sepsis attenuate ketogenesis by increasing insulin levels and by rapid tissue oxidation of free fatty acids. Minor injuries and infections are associated with modest elevations in plasma free fatty acid concentrations and ketogenesis. However, ketogenesis in minor stress states does not exceed that of nonstressed starvation.

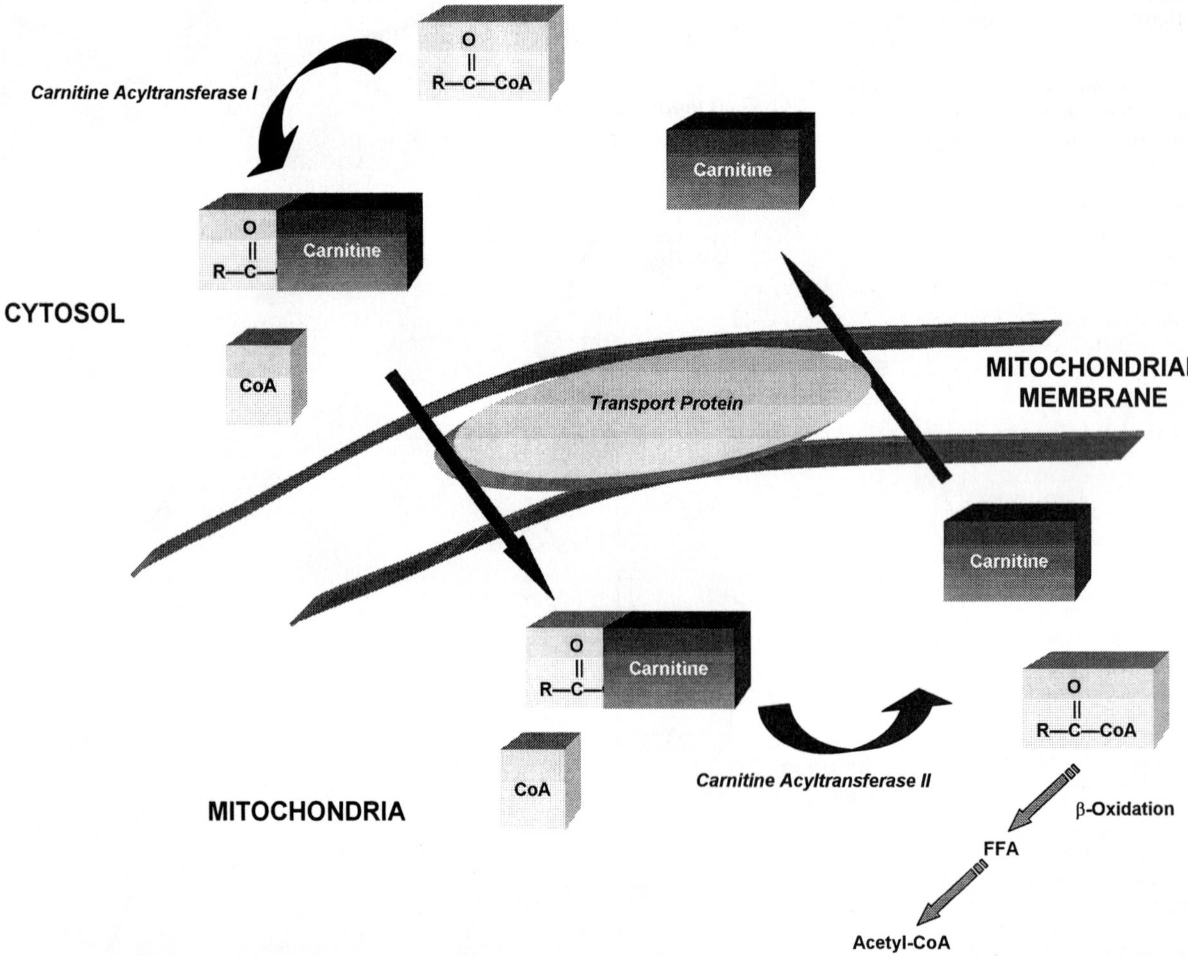

FIGURE 5.8. Free fatty acids in the cells form fatty acyl-CoA with coenzyme A. Fatty acyl-CoA cannot enter the inner mitochondrial membrane and requires carnitine as a carrier protein (carnitine shuttle). Once inside the mitochondria, carnitine dissociates, and fatty acyl-CoA is re-formed. The carnitine molecule is transported back into the cytosol for reuse. The fatty acyl-CoA undergoes β-oxidation to form acetyl-CoA for entry into the tricarboxylic acid (TCA) cycle.

Carbohydrate Metabolism

The oxidation of 1 g of carbohydrate yields 4 kcal, but administered glucose solutions such as those found in intravenous fluids provide only 3.4 kcal per gram of dextrose. In starvation, glucose production occurs at the expense of protein stores (i.e., skeletal muscle). Hence, the primary goal for maintenance glucose administration in surgical patients is to minimize muscle wasting. The exogenous administration of small amounts of glucose (approximately 50 g/day) can also serve to facilitate the oxidation of fat through entry into the TCA cycle and reduce ketosis. Unlike starvation in healthy subjects, studies providing exogenous glucose to septic and trauma patients have never been shown to fully suppress amino acid degradation for gluconeogenesis.[11] This result suggests that, during periods of stress, other hormonal and proinflammatory mediators have profound influences on the rate of protein degradation, and that some degree of muscle wasting is inevitable.[12] The administration of insulin, however, has been shown to reverse protein catabolism during severe stress by stimulating amino acid transport systems and protein synthesis in skeletal muscles and by inhibiting hepatocyte protein degradation.[13] Insulin also stimulates the incorporation of labeled precursors into nucleic acids as well as RNA synthesis in muscle.

In the cells, glucose is phosphorylated to form glucose-6-phosphate (G6P), which can be polymerized during glycogenesis or catabolized in glycogenolysis. Glucose catabolism occurs by cleavage to pyruvate or lactate (pyruvic acid pathway) or by decarboxylation to pentoses, which is a direct oxidative pathway (pentose shunt) (Fig. 5.9). Excess glucose from overfeeding, as reflected by RQs greater than 1.0, can result in conditions such as glucosuria, thermogenesis, and conversion to fat (lipogenesis). Indeed, excessive glucose administration results in elevated carbon dioxide production, which may be deleterious in patients with suboptimal pulmonary functions.

Despite insulin levels severalfold above baseline, injury and severe infections acutely induce a state of peripheral glucose intolerance. This state may occur in part as a result of reduced skeletal muscle pyruvate dehydrogenase activity following injury, which diminishes the conversion of pyruvate to acetyl-CoA and subsequent entry into the TCA cycle. The consequent accumulations of three-carbon structures (pyruvate, lactate) are shunted to the liver as substrate for gluconeogenesis. Furthermore, regional tissue catheterization and isotope dilution studies revealed a 50% to 60% increase in net splanchnic glucose production in septic patients and a 50% to 100% increase in burn patients. The increase in plasma glucose levels was proportional to the severity of injury, and this net hepatic gluconeogenic response is believed to be influenced predominantly by glucagon. Unlike the nonstressed subject, the hepatic gluconeogenic response to injury or sepsis cannot be suppressed by exogenous or excess glucose administration but rather persists in the hypermetabolic critically ill patient.

Hepatic gluconeogenesis, arising primarily from alanine and glutamine precursors, provides a ready fuel source for tissues such as those of the nervous system, wounds, and erythrocytes, which do not require insulin for glucose transport. The elevated glucose concentrations also provide the necessary energy source for leukocytes in inflamed tissues and in sites of microbial invasions. The deprivation of glucose to nonessential organs such as skeletal muscle and adipose tissues is mediated by catecholamines. Experiments infusing catecholamines and glucagon in animals have demonstrated elevated plasma glucose levels as a result of increased hepatic gluconeogenesis and peripheral insulin resistance.[14] While glucocorticoid excess alone does not increase glucose levels, elevated glucocorticoid levels do prolong and augment the hyperglycemic effects of catecholamines and glucagon.

Glycogen stores within skeletal muscles can be mobilized by epinephrine activation of β-adrenergic receptor, a guanosine 5′-triphosphate (GTP)-binding protein (G protein), and subsequent activation of the second-messenger cycle AMP pathway.[15] Cyclic AMP activates phosphorylase kinase, which in turn leads to conversion of glycogen to glucose-1-phosphate. Phosphorylase kinase can also be activated by the second messenger calcium through the breakdown of phosphatidylinositol phosphate, which is the case in vasopressin-mediated hepatic glycogenolysis.

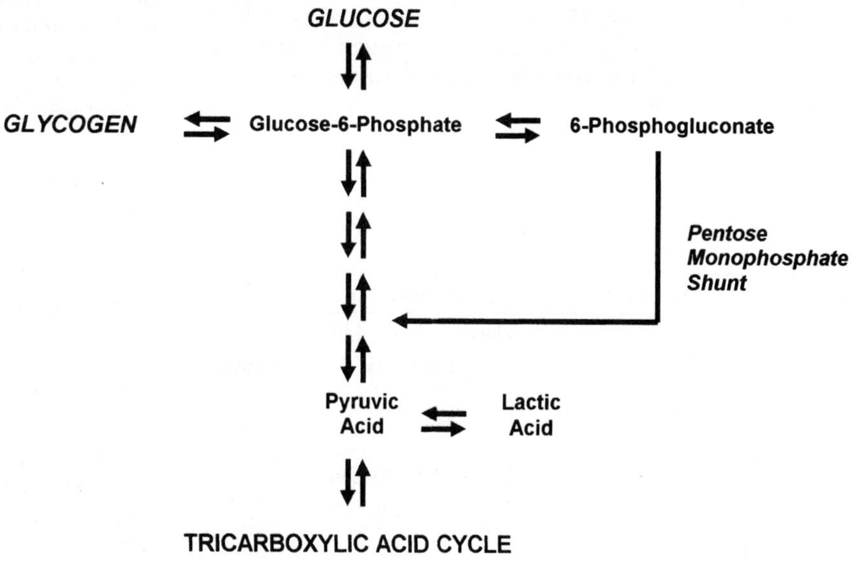

FIGURE 5.9. Simplified schema of glucose catabolism through the pentose monophosphate pathway or by breakdown into pyruvate. Glucose-6-phosphate becomes an important "crossroad" for glucose metabolism. Glycogen stores within skeletal muscles do not directly release glucose systemically because of a deficiency in glucose-6-phosphatase.

Although they may potentially serve as energy sources to minimize protein wasting during injury, the infusion of sorbitol, xylitol, fructose, and possibly mannitol (in neurological injury) does not evoke an increase in plasma insulin levels.

Glucose Transport and Signaling

Hydrophobic cell membranes are relatively impermeable to hydrophilic glucose molecules. There are two distinct classes of membrane glucose transporters in human systems: the facilitated diffusion glucose transporters (GLUTs) that permit the transport of glucose down a concentration gradient (Table 5.2) and the Na^+–glucose transport system, which transports glucose molecules against concentration gradients by active transport.[16] The energy-dependent Na^+–glucose transport system is relatively prevalent on brush borders of small intestine enterocytes and the epithelium of proximal renal tubules.

Mostly through the screening of complementary DNA libraries and transgenic and knockout mice studies, more than five human facilitative-diffusion glucose transporters have been cloned since 1985. In human erythrocytes, *GLUT 1* is the transporter. It is expressed on several other tissues, but little is found in the liver and skeletal muscle. Importantly, it is a constitutive part of the endothelium in the blood–brain barrier. The transporter *GLUT 2* is predominantly expressed in the sinusoidal membranes of liver, renal tubules, enterocytes, and insulin-secreting β-cells of the pancreas; it is important for rapid export of glucose resulting from gluconeogenesis. Although *GLUT 3* is highly expressed in neuronal tissue of the brain, the kidney, and placenta, its messenger RNA has been detected in almost every human tissue. The transporter *GLUT 4* is the primary glucose transporter of the insulin-sensitive tissues, adipose tissue, and skeletal and cardiac muscle. These transporters are usually packaged as intracellular vesicles, but insulin induces rapid translocation of these vesicles to the cell surface. The functions of GLUT 4 and GLUT 5 are less well characterized.

The Na^+–glucose transport systems are distinct glucose transport systems found in the intestinal epithelium and in the proximal renal tubules. This system transports both sodium and glucose intracellularly. In fact, glucose affinity for this transporter increases when sodium ions are attached. In addition, the Na^+–glucose transport system within the intestinal lumen also enhances gut retention of water through osmotic absorption.

TABLE 5.2. Human-Facilitated Diffusion Glucose Transporter Family (GLUT 1–5).

Type	*Amino acids*	*Major expression sites*
GLUT 1	492	Placenta, brain, kidney, colon
GLUT 2	524	Liver, pancreatic β-cells, kidney, small intestine
GLUT 3	496	Brain, testes
GLUT 4	509	Skeletal muscle, heart muscle, brown and white fat
GLUT 5	501	Small intestine, sperm

Source: Adapted from Levin.[16]

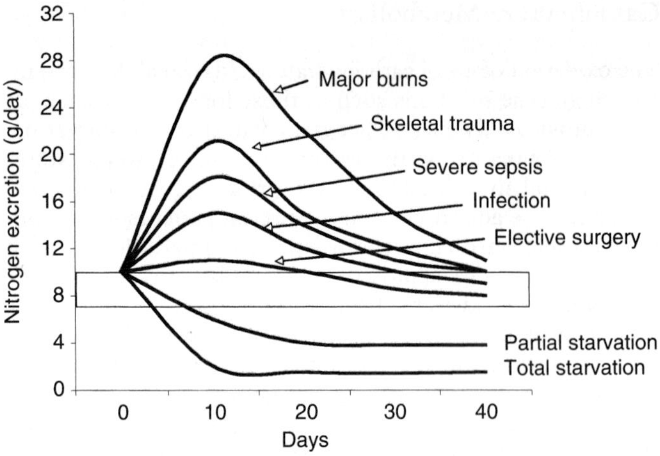

FIGURE 5.10. The effect of injury severity on nitrogen wasting. (Adapted from Long,[5] with permission.)

Protein and Amino Acid Metabolism

The average protein intake in healthy young adults ranges from 80 to 120g per day, and every 6g of protein yields approximately 1g of nitrogen. Following major injury, urinary nitrogen excretion may increase to levels in excess of 30g per day (Fig. 5.10). Protein catabolism following injury can serve to provide substrates for gluconeogenesis and for the synthesis of acute-phase proteins. Radiolabeled amino acid incorporation studies and protein analyses confirmed that skeletal muscles are preferentially depleted following injury, while visceral tissues (liver, kidney) remain relatively preserved. Therefore, amino acids cannot be considered a long-term fuel reserve, and indeed excessive protein depletion (25%–30% of lean body weight) is not compatible with life. The accelerated urea excretion is also associated with the excretion of intracellular elements such as sulfur, phosphorus, potassium, magnesium, and creatinine. Conversely, the rapid uptake of elements such as potassium and magnesium during recovery from major injury may indicate a period of tissue healing.

The net changes in protein catabolism and synthesis correspond to the severity and duration of injury (Fig. 5.10). Elective operations and minor injuries result in lower protein synthesis and normal rates of protein breakdown. Severe trauma, burns, and sepsis are associated with increased protein catabolism. The rise in urinary nitrogen and negative nitrogen balance can be detected early following injury and peak by 7 days. This state of protein catabolism may persist for as long as 3 to 7 weeks. The patient's prior physical status and age appear to influence the degree of proteolysis following injury or sepsis. The degradation of 1g of protein yields approximately 4kcal of energy, almost the same as for carbohydrates.

Glutamine and Arginine

Glutamine is the most abundant amino acid in the human body, comprising nearly two-thirds of the free intracellular amino acid pool. Of this, 75% is found within the skeletal muscles.[17] In healthy individuals, glutamine is considered a nonessential amino acid because it is synthesized within the skeletal muscles and the lungs. Glutamine is a necessary substrate for nucleotide synthesis in most dividing cells and hence provides a major fuel source for enterocytes.[18] It also serves as an important fuel source for immunocytes such as lymphocytes and macrophages, as well as a precursor for glutathione, a major intracellular antioxidant. During stress states such as sepsis or in tumor-bearing hosts, peripheral glutamine stores are rapidly depleted, and this amino acid may be preferentially shunted as a fuel source for visceral organs or tumors, respectively.[19] This creates, at least experimentally, a glutamine-depleted environment, the consequences of which include enterocyte and immunocyte starvation.

However, glutamine metabolism during stress in humans may be more complex than in previously reported animal data. More advanced methods of detecting glutamine traffic in patients with gastrointestinal cancer have not demonstrated more tumor sequestration of glutamine than normal intestine.[20] There are data demonstrating decreased dependency on total parenteral nutrition (TPN) in severe cases of short-bowel syndrome when therapies of glutamine with modified diets and growth hormone are used.[21] However, in patients with milder forms of short-bowel syndrome and better nutritional status, glutamine supplementation did not demonstrate appreciable enhancement in intestinal absorption.[22] In healthy subjects, glutamine-supplemented TPN did not attenuate endotoxin-induced symptoms or proinflammatory cytokine release compared to standard TPN.[23] Although it is hypothesized that provision of glutamine may preserve immune cell and enterocyte function and enhance nitrogen balance during injury or sepsis,[24] the clinical evidence in support of this phenomenon in human subjects remains inconclusive.

Arginine, also a nonessential amino acid in healthy subjects, first attracted attention for its immuno-enhancing properties, wound-healing benefits, and improved survival in animal models of sepsis and injury.[25] As with glutamine, the benefits of experimental arginine supplementation during stress states are diverse. Clinical studies administering arginine enterally have demonstrated net nitrogen retention and protein synthesis compared to isonitrogenous diets in critically ill and injured patients and following surgery for certain malignancies.[26,27] Some of these studies are also associated with in vitro evidence of enhanced immunocyte function.[28,29] The clinical utility of arginine in improving overall patient outcome remains to be established.

Acknowledgment. This work was supported in part by National Institutes of Health grant GM34695.

References

1. Smith MK, Lowry SF. The hypercatabolic state. In: Shils ME, et al., eds. Modern Nutrition in Health and Disease, 9th ed. Baltimore: Williams & Wilkins, 1999:1555–1568.
2. Cahill GF. Starvation in man. N Engl J Med 1970;282:668–675.
3. Brodsky IG. Hormone, cytokine, and nutrient interactions. In: Shils ME, et al., eds. Modern Nutrition in Health and Disease, 9th ed. Baltimore: Williams & Wilkins, 1999:699–724.
4. Bessey PQ, Lowe KA. Early hormonal changes affect the catabolic response to trauma. Ann Surg 1993;218:476–491.
5. Long CL. Metabolic response to injury and illness: estimation of energy and protein needs from indirect calorimetry and nitrogen balance. J Parenter Enteral Nutr 1979;3:452–456.
6. Nordenstrom J, Carpentier YA, Askanazi J, et al. Free fatty acid mobilization and oxidation during total parenteral nutrition in trauma and infection. Ann Surg 1983;198:725–735.
7. Peterson J, Bihain BE. Fatty acid control of lipoprotein lipase: a link between energy metabolism and lipid transport. Proc Natl Acad Sci USA 1990;87:909–913.
8. Rossle C. Medium chain triglycerides induce alterations in carnitine metabolism. Am J Physiol 1990;258:E944–E947.
9. Sailer D, Muller M. Medium chain triglycerides in parenteral nutrition. J Parenter Enteral Nutr 1981;5:115–119.
10. Wiener M, Rothkopf MM, Rothkopf G, et al. Fat metabolism in injury and stress. Crit Care Clin 1987;3:1–25.
11. Long CL, Schiller WR, Geiger JW, et al. Gluconeogenic response during glucose infusions in patients following skeletal trauma or sepsis. J Parenter Enteral Nutr 1978;22:619–625.
12. Elwyn DH, Kinney JM, Jeevanandam M, et al. Influence of increasing carbohydrate intake on glucose kinetics in injured patients. Ann Surg 1979;190:117–127.
13. Long CL, Nelson KM, Akin JM, et al. A physiologic basis for the provision of fuel mixtures in normal and stressed patients. J Trauma 1990;30:1077–1086.
14. Eigler N, Sacca L, Sherwin RS. Synergistic interactions of physiologic increments of glucagon, epinephrine, and cortisol in the dog: a model for stress-induced hyperglycemia. J Clin Invest 1979;63:114–118.
15. Chu CA, Sindelar DK, et al. Comparison of the direct and indirect effects of epinephrine on hepatic glucose production. J Clin Invest 1997;99:1044–1048.
16. Levin RJ. Carbohydrates. In: Shils ME, et al., eds. Modern Nutrition in Health and Disease, 9th ed. Baltimore: Williams & Wilkins, 1999:49–65.
17. Bergstrom J, Furst P, Noree LO, Vinnars E. Intracellular free amino acid concentration in human muscle tissue. J Appl Physiol 1974;36:693–696.
18. Hartmann F, Plauth M. Intestinal glutamine metabolism. Metabolism 1989;38:S18–S24.
19. Souba WW. Cytokine control of nutrition and metabolism in critical illness. Curr Probl Surg 1994;31:577–652.
20. Van der Hulst RRWJ, von Meyenfeldt MF, Deutz NEP, Soeters PB. Glutamine extraction by the gut is reduced in patients with depleted gastrointestinal cancer. Ann Surg 1997;225: 112–121.
21. Byrne TA, Morrissey TB, Nattakom TV, Ziegler TR, Wilmore DW. Growth hormone, glutamine and a modified diet enhance nutrient absorption in patients with severe short bowel syndrome. J Parenter Enteral Nutr 1995;19:296–302.
22. Byrne TA, Persinger RL, Young LS, Ziegler TR, Wilmore DW. A new treatment for patients with short-bowel syndrome. Ann Surg 1995;222:243–255.
23. Braxton CC, Coyle SM, van der Poll T, Roth M, Calvano SE, Lowry SF. Influence of glutamine-supplemented TPN on in vitro and in vivo responses to endotoxin. Surg Forum 1995;46:21–23.
24. Long CL, Nelson KM, DiRienzo DB, et al. Glutamine supplementation of enteral nutrition: impact on whole body protein kinetics and glucose metabolisms in critically ill patients. J Parenter Enteral Nutr 1995;19:470–476.
25. Barbul A. Arginine: biochemistry, physiology, and therapeutic implications. J Parenter Enteral Nutr 1986;10:227–238.
26. Brittenden J, Heys SD, Miller I, et al. Dietary supplementation with L-arginine in patients with breast cancer (>4 cm) receiving multimodality treatment: report of a feasibility study. Br J Cancer 1994;69:918–921.
27. Brittenden J, Heys SD, Ross J, Park KGM, Eremin O. Nutritional pharmacology: effects of L-arginine on host defenses, response to trauma and tumour growth. Clin Sci 1994;86:123–132.
28. Kirk SJ, Barbul A. Role of arginine in trauma, sepsis, and immunity. J Parenter Enteral Nutr 1990;24:S226–S229.
29. Beaumier L, Castillo L, Ajami AM, Young VR. Urea cycle intermediate kinetics and nitrate excretion at normal and therapeutic intakes of arginine in humans. Endocrinol Metab 1995;32: E884–E896.

6

Nutrition

Kenneth A. Kudsk and Danny O. Jacobs

Since the earliest recorded evidence of nutrition support using nutrient enemas some 3500 years ago in Egypt,[1] progressive malnutrition with its negative impact on strength, resistance to infection, and ability to heal have challenged clinicians. With today's highly sophisticated, highly technical procedures to deliver nutrients intravenously or enterally, the field of nutrition support still struggles with the identification and reversal of malnutrition-induced vulnerability in patients. The implications of nutritional intervention—or lack of it—are still being defined despite tremendous growth in nutrition research since the late 1960s, when Dudrick and colleagues supported normal growth and development of beagles by intravenous nutrition alone.[2]

The impact of specialized nutrition support on malnourished or well-nourished patients sustaining, or about to sustain, infectious, operative, or traumatic stress has generated debate concerning the ability to identify nutrition-related risks, the importance of route of nutrition, the effectiveness of administered nutrients, and the appropriate amount and composition of diets for specific clinical conditions. Technological successes generate new complications that warrant consideration as therapy is instituted. Despite clear evidence in randomized, prospective studies of positive effects of nutrition support in defined patient populations, many clinical practices are controversial and highly debated among nutrition support professionals. The institution of any therapy as invasive as nutrition support carries potential costs and benefits defined from studies of a heterogeneous population that may or may not be applicable to an individual patient's condition.

History of Nutrition Support

The modern era dates to the late 1700s, when Hunter used oral gastric feeding with an eel-skin-covered whalebone to administer solutions of eggs, milk, wine, sugar, and jelly.[3] In the late 1800s, rectal feedings were administered, with the most notable case that of U.S. President Garfield's "enteral" support for 79 days using whiskey and beef broth.[4] Small-bore feeding tubes gradually became common practice, as did dilute nutrient solutions, which were soon replaced with "blenderized" foods. Intravenous feeding using feather quills with a pig's bladder as a reservoir dates to the 1600s, when nutrient solutions consisted of milk, sugar, and egg white.

In the 20th century, attempts at infusion of fat, carbohydrate, protein, and alcohol produced thrombosis with hypertonic solutions or pulmonary edema with dilute solutions even if diuretics were given.[5] The subclavian catheter with central access allowed Dudrick, Rhoads, and Wilmore to administer low-volume, hypertonic solutions containing quantities of nutrients necessary to support metabolic needs.[2,6] In the late 1970s, research regenerated interest in the gastrointestinal (GI) tract as a primary route for nutrient administration when Kudsk and Sheldon identified that enteral feeding improved survival of animals after septic peritonitis.[7] Since then, the bias has swung toward provision of nutrients enterally whenever feasible, particularly in malnourished or severely injured trauma patients. The avoidance of immunological and metabolic complications and the preservation of mucosal integrity with enteral feeding has expanded the field of nutrition support and increased insight into malnutrition-related defects.

Implications of Nutrition Support for Clinical Outcome

To critically evaluate a specific therapeutic intervention, three criteria should be satisfied.[8] First, evidence should show that treatment is better than no treatment. Second, beneficial effects should outweigh harmful effects. Third, compared with other alternatives, the treatment should represent wise use of resources. These issues are paramount in nutrition support because comprehensive studies of intravenous nutrition documented a 29% incidence of complications related to catheter placement (5.7%), sepsis (6.5%), metabolic (7.7%) and mechanical (9%) complications, and death (0.2%)[9] caused by fluid and electrolyte problems (e.g., refeeding syndrome with sometimes-lethal drops in potassium, phosphate, and magnesium levels), metabolic complications such as hyperglycemia, and other technical issues. Enteral complications include aspiration, tube dislodgement, and abdominal complications such as diarrhea, nausea, vomiting, and intestinal necrosis.[10] Potential serious and life-threatening complications dictate close inspection of existing clinical data obtained from heterogeneous and homogeneous populations. An evaluation of existing data of nutrition support in medical and surgical patients was published.[10] This review is limited by the failure of the document to judge the quality of individual research studies,[11] but it serves as a guideline for the review of the literature.

Determination of Nutritional Status

The ability to quantify malnutrition, measure metabolic stress, and measure the effectiveness of nutrition is limited. Benefits are clear in some circumstances. Patients with short-gut syndrome from vascular disasters or chronic disease that leave no colon and less than 100 cm of jejunum or less than 50 cm of jejunum or ileum with an intact colon die without parenteral nutrition.[12] Parenteral nutrition restores body composition, allowing a meaningful, productive existence. Without such dramatic GI loss or severely impaired nutritional status, improved clinical outcome with specialized support is less clear.

There is a strong inverse correlation between protein status and complications after patients undergo major GI surgery.[13] Measurement of protein status is inexact because of difficulties quantitating degree of malnutrition and because diseases influence markers of malnutrition and clinical outcome. The continuum of nutritional status ranges from the well-nourished to the cachectic individual.

Weight loss, albumin, prealbumin (PA), and immune competence (measured by delayed cutaneous hypersensitivity or total lymphocyte count) have been used to classify clinical states of malnutrition,[11,14] but individual markers may not accurately represent the status of a patient. Important information is the amount of weight loss or percentage of usual body weight calculated by the following equations:

$$\%\ \text{Body weight loss} = [(\text{Usual body weight} - \text{Current body weight})/\text{Usual body weight}] \times 100$$

or

$$\%\ \text{Usual body weight} = (\text{Current body weight}/\text{Usual body weight}) \times 100$$

In general, a weight loss of 5% to 10% over a month or of 10% to 20% over 6 months is associated with increased complications.[15] Although considered the single best marker of status in stable patients, serum albumin levels are influenced by synthesis rates, degradation rates, and vascular losses into the interstitium or through the gut and kidney. Protein energy malnutrition decreases albumin synthesis, but reduced rates can maintain normal serum levels; for example, marasmus, a severe deficiency of protein and energy, is associated with a normal albumin level, which usually drops precipitously once nutrition is provided. Albumin ($T_{1/2}$ = 21 days), and other transport proteins such as transferrin ($T_{1/2}$ = 8 days) and PA ($T_{1/2}$ = 2–3 days), also drops in inflammatory conditions such as sepsis, peritonitis, trauma, and burns, for which high interleukin (IL) 6 levels stimulate acute-phase protein production, such as C-reactive protein (CRP) and α_1-acid-glycoprotein (AAG), and inhibit transport protein production.[16] Delayed cutaneous hypersensitivity is influenced by injury; hepatic and renal failure; infections; edema; anesthesia; medications such as corticosteroids, coumarin, and cimetidine; and immunosuppressants.

As a predictive tool, combinations of these measurements have been used to quantify the risk of complications. The Prognostic Nutritional Index correlates with poor outcome in the following equation:

$$\text{PNI}\ (\%) = 158 - 16.6\ (\text{ALB}) - 0.78\ (\text{TSF}) - 0.20\ (\text{TFN}) - 5.8\ (\text{DH})$$

where PNI is the risk of complication occurring in an individual patient, ALB is serum albumin (g/dl), TSF is the triceps skinfold thickness (mm), TFN is serum transferrin (mg/dl), and DH is delayed hypersensitivity reaction to one of three recall antigens (0, nonreactive; 1, <5-mm induration; 2, >5-mm induration).[17] Because DH is rarely used in clinical practice, the equation can substitute the lymphocyte score, using a scale of 0 to 2, where 0 is less than 1000 total lymphocytes/mm^3, 1 is 1000 to 2000 total lymphocytes/mm^3, and 2 is more than 2000 total lymphocytes/mm^3.[18] The higher the score using either of these equations, the greater the risk of postoperative complications will be. In acute disease, elevations in acute-phase proteins occur with simultaneous reductions in constitutive proteins.

The Prognostic Inflammatory Nutrition Index (PINI) appears to correlate with recovery from injury as the acute-phase protein response abates in the following equation:

$$\text{PINI} = (\text{CRP})(\text{AAG})/(\text{PA})(\text{ALB})$$

where CRP, AAG, and PA are measured in milligrams per deciliter and albumin in grams per deciliter.[19] The subjective global assessment clinically evaluates nutritional status by determining restriction of nutrient intake, changes in organ function and body composition, and the disease process.[20] There is close interobserver agreement and good prediction of complications in general surgical patients, liver transplant patients,[21] and dialysis patients.[22]

Anthropometry, creatine–height index, and muscle function have been used to assess nutritional status. Anthropometry using TSF and midarm muscle circumference provides an indirect measure of muscle mass and, in general populations, correlates with the degree of malnutrition. Its use is limited by high interobserver variability, influences of hydration and age, and overall response to nutrition therapy. Use of the creatine–height index, requiring complete urinary collection and meat-free diets, has fallen out of favor because of variability in metabolic status. Muscle function assessed by grip strength, respiratory status, and response to electrical stimulation does correlate with postoperative complications and response to nutrition therapy, but correlation with improvement in clinical outcome is unknown.

In summary, there is no "gold standard" for determining nutritional status because of the influence of illness and injury on parameters and difficulty in isolating the individual influences of malnutrition and disease on clinical outcome. This conclusion was supported by nonrandomized prospective, retrospective, or case cohort-controlled studies.[10] Malnutrition is a continuum influenced by the duration of altered nutritional intake, the degree of insult and metabolic stress, and the ability to control or reverse the disease and metabolic perturbations induced by that disease.

Implications of Specialized Nutrition Support in Malnourished Versus Well-Nourished Patients

The effect of nutrition on outcome in patients with midrange degrees of malnutrition is unclear, but significant class I data (class of evidence) describe its impact in nontrauma/noncritically ill general surgical patients at both ends of the nutritional scale, that is, well-nourished and severely malnourished patients (Table 6.1). The six articles on perioperative nutrition that reflect the effect of nutrition support—enteral or parenteral—on well-nourished general surgery patients[23–28] demonstrated no significant impact on patient outcome in five of six studies. In fact, perioperative or postoperative parenteral nutrition was associated with increased septic complications of the respiratory tract[22] or the intra-abdominal cavity.[25]

Severe malnutrition increases complications, the length of stay, and intensive care unit (ICU) days. Under these conditions, perioperative intravenous nutrition reduced postoperative complications without increasing infectious complications.[22] When these data were pooled with nine other older, prospective, randomized, controlled studies of patients with varying degrees of malnutrition, analysis demonstrated approximately a 10% reduction in postoperative complications with perioperative parenteral nutrition.[10]

In patients with a moderate degree of malnutrition, data suggest improved benefit of some nutrition support (Table 6.1). In patients undergoing upper GI tract surgery for malignancy,[29,30] fewer infectious and noninfectious complications and shorter lengths of stay were noted in patients fed enterally with a specialty diet (supplemented with arginine, RNA, and omega-3 fatty acids) compared with patients fed either a nonisonitrogenous[29] or an isonitrogenous isocaloric enteral diet.[30] This result poses a dilemma in some general surgical patients. If immediate postoperative parenteral nutrition is started in general surgical patients considered mildly to moderately malnourished on the basis of weight loss, plasma proteins, or prognostic indicators, then postoperative complications increase by approximately 10% (from a rate of 30% to 40%) compared with unfed patients. However, many of these patients will develop complications (with or without nutrition) restricting or eliminating their ability to take an adequate oral diet within a few days of surgery.

It is probably best to start parenteral (or preferably enteral) nutrition within 5 to 10 days of surgery to avoid starvation-induced malnutrition. One particular population deserves special attention. In a randomized, prospective study, 122 elderly women who were 1 to 2 SD below the average weight of 744 patients sustaining femoral neck fractures were provided a ward diet and randomized to an additional 1000 kcal each night by nasogastric (NG) tube or no supplementation. Patients with the additional nutrition recovered faster, had fewer postoperative complications, and had a reduced hospital stay with a trend toward improved mortality.[31] These results were confirmed in a second study of oral nutrition supplementation after surgical repair of a fractured femoral neck.[32]

Enteral Versus Parenteral Versus No Specialized Nutrition Support

Several class I randomized, prospective studies have investigated the route of nutrient administration in trauma (Table 6.2) and general surgical (Table 6.3) patients. Most of these studies were in patients with blunt and penetrating trauma (Table 6.2, section A) or head injuries (Table 6.2, section B). Most trauma studies showed improved outcome with early enteral feeding.[33–36] The benefits with enteral feeding increase as the severity of injury increases.

The type of injury probably plays an important role. Only one of five studies[37–41] of patients with severe head injury noted benefit with early enteral feeding. Gastroparesis delayed advancement of successful enteral feedings in several of the studies. Grahm et al.[40] compared early nasojejunal feeding with intragastric feeding and noted a significant reduction in bacterial infections with the early nasojejunal feeding, but this study was not replicated by Borzotta et al.,[41] who surgically placed jejunostomies in 27 patients and compared outcome against early parenteral nutrition; no differences in infectious complications were noted. For the most part, patients with closed-head injury given intragastric feeding received insignificant amounts of enteral diet for the first 10 days following injury and were severely underfed. At this point, existing data do not suggest significant benefit or neurological or infectious outcome with enteral or parenteral feeding following severe closed-head injury. The gastroparesis often resolves within 4 to 5 days, allowing institution of early enteral feeding at that point. In patients in whom gastroparesis does not resolve within 6 to 7 days, parenteral nutrition or a transpyloric enteral tube is clinically indicated (level III data) with transition to intragastric feeding when gastroparesis resolves.

In addition to the studies Table 6.2 mentions, 14 investigations[42–55] studied outcome with nutrition in patients sustaining general surgical problems such as surgical resection (Table 6.3, section A), inflammatory bowel disease (Table 6.3, section B), transplantation (Table 6.3, section C), or acute pancreatitis (Table 6.3, section D). Cognizant of the failure of enteral feeding with specialized diets to improve outcome in well-nourished patients following intestinal resection,[26] several

TABLE 6.1.
Perioperative and Early Feeding Studies with Substantial Number of Well-Nourished or Moderately Malnourished Patients.

Author	*Year*	*Class of evidence*	*Conclusions*
Veterans Affair Total Parenteral Nutrition Cooperative Study Group[23]	1991	1	Of 395 malnourished patients requiring laparotomy or noncardiac thoracotomy randomized to 7–15 days preoperative nutrition (n = 192) or no perioperative nutrition support (n = 203) and monitored for 90 days following surgery, the rates of major complications were similar in patients with mild or moderate degrees of malnutrition, with more infectious complications in the TPN group (P = .01) but more noninfectious complications in the control group (P = .02); 90-day mortality rates were also similar. Only in severely malnourished patients did TPN significantly reduce noninfectious complications (5% vs. 43%, P = .03) with no increase in infectious complications.
Fan[24]	1994	I	A randomized prospective study of 124 patients undergoing resection of hepatocellular carcinoma randomized to perioperative intravenous nutrition with 35% branched-chain amino acids, dextrose, and lipid (50% medium-chain triglycerides) for 14 days in addition to oral diet or control group (oral diet alone). Postoperative morbidity rate was reduced in perioperative fed group (34% vs. 55%) because of fewer septic complications (17% vs. 37%) and less deterioration of liver function as measured by indocyanine green. There were no significant differences in deaths, although most of the benefit occurred in cirrhotic patients undergoing major hepatectomy.
Brennan[25]	1994	I	A prospective, randomized trial of 117 moderately malnourished patients randomized to postoperative parenteral nutrition (n = 60, albumin = 3.1, 5.8% preoperative body weight loss) or standard intravenous fluids (n = 57, albumin = 3.3, 6.8% preoperative body weight loss). Complications were significantly greater in TPN-fed patients, with a significant increase in intraabdominal abscess and major complications.
Heslin[26]	1997		Of 195 well-nourished patients undergoing esophageal, gastric, pancreatic, or gastric resection randomized to jejunal feedings (n = 97; albumin 4.08 ± 0.04 g/dl) or intravenous feedings (n = 98; albumin 4.1 ± 0.06 g/dl), no significant differences found in the number of major, minor, or infectious wound complications between groups and no difference in hospital mortality or length of stay. There was one small-bowel necrosis in the enterally fed group.
Doglietto[27]	1996	I	Their 678 patients with normal or mild malnutrition undergoing major elective abdominal surgery randomized to protein-sparing therapy or no specialized nutrition had similar operative mortality rates and postoperative complication rate.
Watters[28]	1997	I	Patients undergoing esophagectomy or pancreatoduodenectomy were randomized to postoperative early jejunal feedings (n = 13; albumin = 4.08 ± 5 g/dl) or no enteral feeding (n = 15; 4.1 ± 4 g/dl) during the first 6 postoperative days. Postoperative vital capacity and fractional expired volume were lower in the fed group, and postoperative mobility was lower in the fed group in this well-nourished group of patients at low risk of nutrition-related complications. This study was confounded by increased epidural anesthesia in the enterally fed group.
Daly[29]	1992		Studied 85 patients randomized to standard (n = 44; albumin = 3.0 ± 1.2 g/dl) versus supplemented (n = 41; albumin = 3.3 g/dl) enteral diets with 77 eligible patients. Infectious and wound complications (P = .02) and length of stay (P = .01) significantly shorter for supplemented group. Diets were not isonitrogenous.
Daly[30]	1995	I	Studied 60 patients with upper GI lesions requiring resection randomized to standard enteral diet (n = 30) or diet supplemented with arginine, omega-3 fatty acids, and nucleotides (n = 30). Patients were moderately malnourished, with albumins less than 3.4. Length of stay and infectious/wound complications significantly reduced (P < .05 for both) in supplemented group. Patients also randomized to jejunal feedings during radiation chemotherapy tolerated chemotherapy significantly better.

TPN, total parenteral nutrition.

authors noted improved outcome in patients receiving enteral feeding following laparotomy compared with parenterally fed patients or patients receiving only intravenous fluids. Most of these included patients undergoing upper GI surgery for carcinoma, and most showed benefit when nutrients were delivered via the GI tract. Enteral feeding is not without complications. Watters et al.[28] noted reduced postoperative mobility and pulmonary status with enteral feeding, although increased use of epidural anesthesia—a factor often associated with prolonged ileus—was more common in the fed group.

A study of ulcerative colitis patients, undergoing resection and randomized to either polymeric enteral nutrition or an isonitrogenous, isocaloric parenteral nutrition solution, noted significant improvement in serum albumin rates with enteral feeding and more postoperative infectious complications with parenteral nutrition.[47] In a study of patients with Crohn's disease, polymeric enteral feeding achieved similar results with steroid treatment in inducing remission.[48]

Following liver transplantation, results have been inconsistent. In 24 patients randomized to nasojejunal feeding or

TABLE 6.2.
Enteral Versus Parenteral or Delayed Feeding in Trauma Patients.

Author	*Year*	*Class of evidence*	*Conclusions*
A. Torso trauma			
Moore[33]	1986	I	Of 63 evaluable of 75 entered patients randomized to jejunostomy feedings ($n = 32$) or no feeding ($n = 31$; TPN started on fifth postoperative day if necessary) and followed for infectious complications, enterally fed patients sustained significantly lower sepsis rate (3/32, 9%) than unfed patients (9/31, 29%, $P < .05$), mainly through reduction in intra-abdominal abscess. In patients with an ATI (abdominal trauma index) of 15–40 (enteral, $n = 26$; unfed, n = 27), sepsis was 4% versus 26% ($P < .05$), respectively.
Moore[34]	1989	I	Of 59 evaluable of 75 patients with ATI > 15 and < 40 randomized to either early enteral feeding ($n = 29$) or immediate TPN ($n = 30$), infectious complications, primarily pneumonia, were significantly lower in enteral than TPN patients (17% vs. 37%, $P < .05$).
Kudsk[35]	1992	I	Of 96 trauma patients randomized to either early jejunal ($n = 51$) or intravenous TPN ($n = 45$), patients in early enteral group sustained significantly fewer pneumonias and intra-abdominal abscesses and line sepsis than parenterally fed patients. Most of the benefit occurred in the most severely injured patients with severe intraabdominal injuries (ATI > 25) or high injury severity scores (ISS > 20).
Kudsk[36]	1996	I	Severely injured trauma patients with high ATI or ISS randomized to standard II (enteral vs. isonitrogenous, isocaloric diet [$n = 18$] or diet supplemented with glutamine, arginine, unfed) omega-3 fatty acids, and nucleotides ($n = 17$). An additional nonfed group was followed prospectively. Supplemented diet group had significantly shorter length of stay and infectious complications compared to standard or unfed group. Unfed group had highest rate of infectious complications, with the standard feeding group midway between. Combined enterally fed groups had significantly fewer infections than unfed patients.
Chuntrasakul[37]	2003	I	Severely injured trauma (ISS 15–30) or burn (body surface area 30%–60% burn) patients were randomized to a standard diet or a diet enriched with arginine, glutamine, and omega-3 fatty acids. The ICU stay was shorter (3.4 vs. 7.8 days) as was days to wean (2.7 vs. 7.4 days) in supplemented group, but neither reached statistical significance.
B. Head injuries			
Rapp[38]	1983	I	There were 38 patients with blunt or penetrating head injuries randomized within 48h to either TPN ($n = 20$, age = 29.4 ± 4.1, GCS [Glasgow Coma Scale] 7.7 ± 0.6) or intragastric feeding (n = 18, age = 34.9 ± 3.8, GCS = 7.2 ± 0.6). Intragastric feeding resulted in caloric intake ≤ 600kcal/day for the first 10 days and less than 900kcal/day over the first 2 weeks due to gastroparesis. Mortality increased in the enterally fed patients (8/18) versus none in the TPN group, and sepsis was approximately 30% in the intragastric group. Sepsis was not reported in the TPN patients. Early intragastric feeding is unsuccessful following severe head injury due to gastroparesis.
Hadley[39]	1986	I	There were 45 patients with GCS ≤ 10 following head injury randomized to intragastric feeding ($n = 21$, GCS = 5.9) or TPN ($n = 24$, GCS = 8). Intragastric feeding resulted in positive caloric balance (140% of basal metabolic rate) in 5% of patients on day 2, 45% by day 3, 70% by day 4, and between 70% and 85% by day 11. Caloric balance was achieved with TPN in 80% of patients by day 5 and 100% by day 9. Complication and infection rates were similar between the two.
Young[40]	1987	I	51 of 58 consented patients with GCS ≤ 4–10 after blunt or penetrating head wounds completed a study following randomization to TPN ($n = 23$, age = 30.3 ± 2.7, GCS = 7.0 ± 0.3) or intragastric feeding ($n = 38$, age = 34.0 ± 2.9, GCS = 6.5 ± 0.4). Intragastric feedings were instituted after bowel sounds returned and NG drainage was below 100ml per shift. Enteral patients received less than 50% of their caloric needs over the first week due to prolonged gastroparesis, but infectious complications were approximately 30% in both groups. There was no difference in neurologic outcome at 1 year. The results failed to reproduce the results of reduced mortality noted in their earlier study.[57]
Grahm[41]	1989	I	22 patients with blunt or penetrating wounds and a GCS < 10 randomized to nasojejunal feeding within 36h of admission (age = 25.5 ± 13.2, GCS = 5.1) or intragastric feeding after day 3 with return of GI function (age = 27.8 ± 9.3, GCS = 7.1). Calculated nutrient needs were achieved by day 3 with jejunal feeding and approached 75% by days 5–7. Early jejunal feeding resulted in significantly fewer respiratory bacterial infections, and goal rates were achieved significantly faster. There was no difference in metabolic rate between the two groups when measured by indirect calorimetry.
Borzotta[42]	1994	I	Head-injured patients (GCS ≤ 8) were randomized to TPN ($n = 21$, age = 28.9 ± 10, ISS = 33.4 ± 9.5, GCS = 5.4 ± 1.9) or surgical jejunostomy ($n = 27$, age = 26.2 ± 10.4, ISS = 32.5 ± 10.1, GCS = 5.2 ± 1.6). Feedings were started within 72h of injury, and all TPN patients had failed intragastric feeding (presumably). Enteral-delivered calories equaled 90.5% of measured resting expenditure by indirect calorimetry by day 3, and there were no differences in infectious complications. Diarrhea was more common with TPN.

TABLE 6.3.
Enteral Versus Parenteral or Other Therapy in General Surgical Patients.

Author	*Year*	*Class of evidence*	*Conclusions*
A. Surgical resections			
Beier-Holgersen[43]	1996	I	After major abdominal surgery, patients were randomized to nutritional supplements (n = 30) or placebo (n = 30) admitted through a nasoduodenal feeding tube; the rate of postoperative infections was significantly lower in the nutrition group (6.6% vs. 46.7%; P = .0009).
Shirabe[44]	1997	I	Of 26 patients undergoing major hepatic resection randomized to early enteral feeding (n = 13) or TPN (n = 13), immunological parameters such as natural killer (NK) activity, lymphocyte number, and PHA response were significantly higher in the enterally fed group (P < .05). Infectious complications were higher in the TPN group (31%) versus the early enteral group (8%), which did not reach statistical significance.
Gianotti[45]	1997	I	Patients undergoing pancreatic or duodenectomy or gastrectomy for cancer were randomized to a standard enteral diet (n = 87), a diet enriched with arginine, omega-3 fatty acids and RNA (n = 87), or parenteral nutrition (n = 86), all of which were isocaloric and isonitrogenous. Postoperative infection rate was 14.9% in the immuno-nutrition group, 22.9% in the standard group, and 27.9% in the parenteral group (P = .06), with length of hospital stay at 16.1 ± 6.2, 19.2 ± 7.9, and 21.6 ± 8.9 days, respectively (immunonutrition, P = .01 vs. standard and P = .004 vs. parenteral group). There was a significantly increased risk of infection with intravenous feeding compared with the supplemental group, with the standard diet midway between.
Sand[46]	1997	I	Of 29 patients undergoing curative total gastrectomy for gastric carcinoma randomized to nasojejunal tube feeding or parenteral nutrition, there were few infective complications in the enteral group versus the parenteral group (23% vs. 31%, NS). The acute-phase protein CRP (C-reactive protein) was lower in the enteral group on day 6 (P = .02).
Hochwald[47]	1997	I	Of 29 patients undergoing resection of upper GI cancer randomized to either enteral feeding (n = 12) via a jejunostomy tube or intravenous fluids (not TPN, n = 17), protein metabolic studies with ^{14}C-leucine documented whole-body protein catabolism significantly less and whole-body net protein balance significantly better in fed group. Free fatty acid values were also significantly lower in the enterally fed group.
Watters[28]	1997	I	Patients undergoing esophagectomy or pancreatoduodenectomy were randomized to postoperative early jejunal feedings (n = 13) or no enteral feeding (n = 15) during the first 6 postoperative days. Postoperative vital capacity and fractional expired volume were lower in the fed group, and postoperative mobility was lower in the fed group in this well-nourished group of patients at low risk of nutrition-related complications. This study was confounded by increased epidural anesthesia.
B. Inflammatory bowel disease			
Gonzalez-Huix[48]	1993	I	Of 42 patients randomized to polymeric enteral nutrition (n = 22; albumin = 3.19 g/dl) or isocaloric, isonitrogenous TPN (n = 20; albumin = 3.3 g/dl), serum albumin significantly increased in the enteral feeding group (P = .019) with fewer adverse advents. Postoperative infections (P = .028) and adverse events (P = .04) were significantly greater with TPN.
Gonzalez-Huix[49]	1993	I	Of 32 patients with active Crohn's disease randomized to polymeric enteral diet (n = 15) or 1 mg/kg/day prednisone (n = 17), incidence of remission was similar at 4 weeks and probability of relapse similar within 1 year. The enteral nutrition was as safe and as effective as steroids in inducing short-term remission in active Crohn's disease.
C. Transplantation			
Wicks[50]	1994	I	The 24 patients received either nasojejunal feeding (n = 514) or TPN (n = 510). No significant differences in outcome between the two groups.
Hasse[51]	1995	I	The 50 transplant patients were randomized to nasojejunal feeding or intravenous fluids until oral diet initiated, with 31 patients completing the study (tube fed, 14; intravenous fluids, 17). Viral infections significantly lower in tube-fed patients (P = .05) with a trend toward reduction in bacterial infections as well (29.4% vs. 14.3%, NS). No significant effect on hospital costs, ventilator days, length of stay in the ICU, or rejection. An enteral feeding tolerated in liver transplant patients.
D. Pancreatitis			
McClave[52]	1997	I	Of 30 patients over 32 admissions randomized to nasojejunal (n = 16) or isocaloric, isonitrogenous TPN (n = 16) admitted for mild, acute pancreatitis, cost and stress-induced hyperglycemia was increased with TPN, and Ranson criteria improved significantly in enterally fed patients.
Windsor[53]	1998	I	Patients with acute pancreatitis stratified according to disease severity were randomized to TPN or enteral nutrition for 7 days. Systemic inflammatory response syndrome, sepsis, organ failure, and ICU stay were improved in enterally fed patients, with improvement in the acute-phase response and disease severity scores. These parameters did not change in parenterally fed patients.

TABLE 6.3. (continued)

Author	*Year*	*Class of evidence*	*Conclusions*
Pupelis[54]	2001	I	60 patients with severe pancreatitis operated on for secondary pancreatitis or failed conservative therapy. Patients randomized to jejunal feeding sustained fewer infections, but this did not reach statistical significance. No difference in length of stay. Reoperative therapy was significantly greater in the control patients than with jejunostomy (26.7% vs. 3.3%, $P = .03$). Mortality higher in control group than with jejunal feedings (23.3% vs. 3.3%, $P = .05$).
Odah[55]	2002	I	Pancreatitis patients randomized to parenteral ($N = 48$) or jejunal feeding ($N = 41$). Septic complications lower in the enteral group ($P = .08$). When early jejunal feeding was combined with antibiotic therapy, septic complications significantly lower ($P = .03$), with trend toward reduced multiple organ failure and mortality.
Abou-Assi[56]	2002	I	Patients with pancreatitis treated initially with bowel rest and intravenous fluids. If not discharged within 4 days, patients randomized to hypocaloric jejunal feeding ($N = 26$) or parenteral feeding ($N = 27$). Enteral feeding was shorter (6.7 vs. 10.8 days, $P < .05$), and nutrition costs were lower, saving approximately $2400 per patient. Enteral feeding was less effective in meeting nutritional requirements (54% vs. 88%, $P < .0001$), but metabolic ($P < .003$) or infectious complications ($P = .01$) were lower.

parenteral nutrition, Wicks et al.[49] demonstrated no difference in outcome, but Hasse et al.[50] noted significantly fewer viral infections and a trend toward reduction in bacterial infections in 50 transplant patients receiving nasojejunal feeding rather than intravenous fluid alone.

During acute pancreatitis, no differences were noted in infectious complications or length of hospital stay between patients randomized to jejunal feeding or parenteral nutrition.[51] Windsor et al.[52] compared enteral with parenteral feeding for 7 days in patients with pancreatitis and noted improvement in systemic inflammatory response parameters, sepsis, organ failure, and ICU stay with enteral feeding, whereas these parameters were unchanged with parenteral feeding. Duodenal feedings are contraindicated in patients with acute pancreatitis because of pancreatic stimulation caused by hormonal responses following intragastric and intraduodenal stimulation. Intravenous feeding and jejunal feedings do not appear to stimulate pancreatic secretions and can be given without fear of aggravating pancreatitis.

Type of Nutrient Diet

Enteral Feeding

While early intragastric feeding *prevents* gastroparesis in burn patients,[57] patients with major head and torso trauma or undergoing major intestinal surgery develop gastroparesis, which precludes successful early intragastric feeding. When delivered beyond the ligament of Treitz via nasojejunal, transgastric, or standard jejunostomy tubes, more complex formulas containing whole proteins, fiber, and the like are usually tolerated with low rates of distension, cramps, or diarrhea. Tolerance decreases as severity of injury increases.[58] Specific substrates may benefit the metabolic and immunological responses following surgery. Specialty enhanced diets have been formulated with various combinations of arginine, omega-3 fatty acids, nucleotides, glutamine, and branched-chain amino acids (BCAAs).

Glutamine, the most abundant free amino acid in the body, becomes "conditionally essential" during stress and sepsis. Free glutamine, unstable in solution particularly during heat sterilization, degrades to pyroglutamic acid and ammonia. While stable in a protein or as a dipeptide (alanyl, glycyl, or glutamine-glutamine), free glutamine must be added to parenteral nutrition solutions prior to infusion. Glutamine production increases during stress and sepsis, while intracellular levels drop. Glutamine is a primary fuel for enterocytes and proliferating immunological cells.[59] Glutamine has been tested in both enteral[60,61] and parenteral[62–67] solutions.

Arginine promotes T-cell proliferation after in vitro stimulation. It is a precursor for nitric oxide, nitrites, and nitrates, putrescine, spermine, and spermidine.[68] Arginine has beneficial effects on cellular immunity, increases fibroblast proliferation in wounds, and improves survival following injury and sepsis.[69] Arginine is a secretagogue for growth hormone, insulin, prolactin, and glucagon.[70]

Polyunsaturated fatty acids (PUFAs) induce immunological effects. Defined by the location of the first double bond from the methylated end, omega-3 and omega-6 fatty acids are metabolized into end products that affect responses to injury. Humans do not synthesize unsaturated fatty acids but can incorporate ingested PUFAs into the cell walls for subsequent metabolism. Once released by phospholipases during stress, the end products of omega-6 fatty acid metabolism produce prostaglandin E_2, thromboxane A_2, and leukotriene B_4 of the 2- and 4-series of prostaglandins and leukotrienes. These products inhibit killer cell activity, antibody formation, and cell-mediated immunity.[71] Omega-3 PUFAs derived from rapeseed (canola oil) or fish oil are metabolized to the 3- and 5-series prostanoids (prostaglandin [PG] I_3, thromboxane A_3, and leukotriene B_5) via the lipoxygenase pathway. In animal studies, omega-3 products are neither proinflammatory nor immunosuppressive. In animal models, they reduce bacterial translocation and mortality after burn injury and increase resistance to infection while promoting cell-mediated immunity.[72]

Nucleotides provide RNA for cell proliferation and immune function, providing structural units for synthesis of DNA and RNA. Deprivation of nucleotides depresses T-helper-cell function and IL-2 production and increases mortality following infection with *Candida albicans* or *Staphylococcus aureus*.[73]

The BCAAs are a primary energy source for muscle protein. Nonbranched-chain amino acids from muscle breakdown are released into the extracellular amino acid pool, but BCAAs are metabolized by the muscle cell itself. The waste nitrogen moieties are transaminated onto pyruvate to produce alanine or onto alpha-keto-glutarate to produce glutamine by the addition of two nitrogen moieties. Although alanine and glutamine compose only 10% to 15% of muscle protein, they comprise approximately 70% of the amino acids released by muscle during stress and sepsis. Clinical data do not substantiate the effectiveness of BCAA supplementation alone in clinical outcome, but they have been incorporated as an element in some formulas.[74]

Many randomized, prospective studies compared the various immune-enhancing diets versus standard enteral diets in trauma, burn, or general surgical patients (Table 6.4). Although there appears to be no benefit of these specialty formulas in well-nourished patients following elective surgery,[74] well-controlled prospective studies showed benefit with specialty formulas in high-risk trauma and, perhaps, some general surgical patients. Although not all studies compared isocaloric and isonitrogenous formulas,[29,61,74,75] there are enough current studies with matched, controlled diets to support their use in severely injured trauma patients. In studies of patients undergoing resection for upper GI tract malignancies,[29,30,45,76–78] studies have suggested that immune-enhancing diets provided reductions in infectious complications, hospital stays, or total complications. Similar results have been found in severely injured trauma patients, with significant reduction in intraabdominal abscess, pneumonia, organ failure, length of stay, and ICU stay.[36,61]

There are conflicting data, however; Saffle et al.[75] studied burn patients given supplemented or standard high-protein enteral diets and noted no differences in outcome. Mendez[80] noted an increase in ventilator days, hospital days, and infectious complications in patients receiving the supplemented diet, although statistical significance was not reached. However, in this study, the patients receiving the immune-enhancing diet had a higher incidence of ARDS (acute respiratory distress syndrome) before entry into the study, and the diets were not routinely started within 24h of injury. Two studies[81,82] of critically ill patients noted benefits when minimum feeding criteria had been met; reductions in length of stay, ICU stay, and systemic inflammatory response parameters were noted.

In a metaanalysis, increased mortality occurred in septic elderly males admitted with pneumonia and given a specialty diet.[83] Although the primary study with these data is not published, established sepsis may prove to be a contraindication to the supplemented diets, possibly due to arginine. In sepsis, arginase is depressed, while arginase levels are increased after trauma.[84] Thus, arginine may become conditionally essential after trauma, but toxic in septic states.

Although the use of enteral formulations supplemented with arginine, glutamine, or other biologically active nutrients or growth factors appears to reduce the length of stay and septic mortality in patients who are severely injured, the dosing levels and durations of treatment needed to improve outcomes have not yet been unequivocally established. In general, the investigations of the immuno-enhancing enteral formulas in the traumatically injured have not studied uniform populations, have used formulas with varying compositions, have initiated and administered enteral feedings for widely varying times during hospitalization, and have used supplementary parenteral nutrition irregularly. Last, many of the published studies have been statistically underpowered. Until large, rigorous, randomized, blinded, and controlled trials are completed, the recommendations for the use of immuno-enhancing dietary formulations should be subject to professional opinion and experience.[85]

Parenteral Feeding

Specialty parenteral formulas for hepatic failure, stress, and sepsis have been tested. Only glutamine-containing formulas have shown potential for clinical benefit. Following bone marrow transplantation, glutamine supplementation increased blood lymphocytes in adult patients[66] and reduced clinical infections and normalized microbial colonization.[61] These results were not confirmed in patients under therapy for bone marrow and solid organ malignancies.[86] In studies of critically ill patients randomized to a glutamine-supplemented or standard parenteral solutions, reduced hospital stay and improved survival with glutamine were noted.[63,64] Intestinal biopsies and lactulose/mannitol tests from patients treated with glutamine should reduce atrophy and less permeability in the intestine,[87] with some changes noted in the cell populations of the mucosa.[65] In the few randomized studies available, there is evidence of benefit with glutamine supplementation, but these studies were limited to small select populations and cannot be generalized to a broader range of general surgical patients.

Nonprotein energy sources have also been studied in parenteral formulas[88–93] (Table 6.5). In patients receiving isocaloric, isonitrogenous parenteral solutions with varying concentrations of glucose and fat, either source of nonprotein calories appeared to produce similar effects on whole-body protein, kinetics, metabolic responses, and muscle protein degradation.[88] Glucose is more effective at suppressing gluconeogenesis than a high-fat diet. Although intravenous omega-3 fatty acid solutions are not available in the United States, they demonstrate no toxicity or other deleterious effects.[92] Intravenous medium-chain triglycerides (MCTs) are well tolerated in mechanically ventilated patients, although administration rates should be reduced because of increased oxygen consumption induced by the MCTs.[90]

A metaanalysis examined the effects of enteral and parenteral glutamine supplementation on length of stay, infectious complications, and mortality in critically ill surgical patients—including those undergoing elective operation.[94] Mortality and new onset infectious complications were the primary outcomes, whereas length of stay was secondary. Studies in which glutamine was only one of several nutrients administered, studies of pediatric patients, and studies of adults undergoing bone marrow transplantation or chemotherapy were excluded.

No adverse effects were identified. Glutamine supplementation was associated with a lower risk of mortality (risk ratio of 0.78, 95% confidence limits 0.58–1.04); a lower rate of infectious complications (risk ratio of 0.81, 95% confidence

TABLE 6.4.
Immune-Enhancing Diets Versus Standard Diet.

Author	*Year*	*Class of evidence*	*Conclusions*
Gottschlich[79]	1990	I	Of 50 acutely burned patients randomized to standard enteral ($n = 14$) diet, supplemented with fish oil and arginine ($n = 17$), or stress formula ($n = 17$), wound infection rates ($P < .03$) and length of stay per percentage body burn ($P < .02$) were significantly lower with the supplemented/fish oil diet.
Daly[29]	1992	I	Of 85 patients randomized to standard versus supplemented enteral diets with 77 eligible patients, infectious and wound complications ($P = .02$) and length of stay ($P = .01$) were significantly shorter for supplemented group. Diets were not isonitrogenous.
Brown[141]	1994	I (human data)	Of 37 patients completing study (of 41 entered) randomized to specialty formula with arginine, α-linolenic acid, beta-carotene, and hydrolyzed protein ($n = 19$) or standard enteral diet ($n = 18$), specialty diet had significantly fewer infections (3/19 vs. 10/18; $P < .05$) and more rapid acute-phase protein reduction. Patients receiving specialty diet had more direct small-bowel access and received more enteral nutrition.
Moore[61]	1994	I	Of 98 evaluable patients randomized to standard diet ($n = 47$) or diet supplemented with glutamine, arginine, omega-3 fatty acids, and nucleotides ($n = 51$), patients receiving supplemented diets had significantly fewer intraabdominal abscesses and less multiple organ failure ($P = .023$ for both) and had improved immunological markers (total lymphocyte count and T-helper-cell numbers). The diets were not isonitrogenous.
Bower[81]	1995	I	Patients with trauma, surgery, or sepsis were randomized to supplemented diet or standard diet. Infectious complications were fewer and lengths of stay were shorter with supplemented diet but not significantly. Immune-enhanced feeding (IMF) decreased length of stay in septic patients ($P < .05$), with possible increase in mortality rate. Patients who met minimum feeding criteria had a reduced length of stay ($P < .05$). Diets were nonisonitrogenous and isocaloric.
Daly[30]	1995	I	Of 60 patients with upper GI lesions requiring resection randomized to standard enteral diet ($n = 30$) or diet supplemented with arginine, omega-3 fatty acids, and nucleotides ($n = 30$), patients were moderately malnourished, with albumin values less than 3.4. Length of stay and infectious/wound complications were significantly reduced ($P < .05$ for both) in supplemented group. Patients also randomized to jejunal feedings during radiation chemotherapy were significantly less chemotherapy intolerant if enterally fed.
Kudsk[60]	1996	I & II	A randomized, prospective study of 35 severely injured patients with enteral access randomized to immune-enhancing diet ($n = 17$) or isonitrogenous, isocaloric diet ($n = 18$). Patients without enteral access and unable to be fed were followed prospectively as unfed controls. There were significantly fewer infectious complications (6%) with immune-enhancing diet than isonitrogenous control group ($P = .02$) or control group ($P = .002$). Infectious complications and use of antibiotics highest in the unfed group, lowest with the immune-enhancing diet, and midway between with the standard diet. Immune-enhancing diet was advantageous in severely injured trauma patients, while fasting was the least desirable.
Schilling[74]	1996	I	Following major abdominal surgery, patients were randomized to supplemented diet ($n = 14$), standard enteral diet ($n = 14$), and a low-calorie/low-fat intravenous solution ($n = 13$). Numerous immunological parameters, including leukocyte counts and reduced CRP levels, significantly better in fed patients than nonfed patients, and infectious complications significantly lower with the supplemented diet versus no feeding.
Mendez[80]	1997	I	Trauma patients were randomized to standard diet ($n = 21$) or diet supplemented with omega-3 fatty acids and arginine ($n = 22$). Ventilator days, hospital days, and infectious complications higher but not significantly so in supplemented diet patients, but this group had more ARDS before entry into the study.
Gianotti[45]	1997	I	Patients undergoing pancreatic or duodenectomy or gastrectomy for cancer were randomized to a standard enteral diet ($n = 87$), a diet enriched with arginine, omega-3 fatty acids and RNA ($n = 87$), or parenteral nutrition ($n = 86$), all of which were isocaloric and isonitrogenous. Postoperative infection rate was 14.9% in the immunonutrition group, 22.9% in the standard group, and 27.9% in the parenteral group ($P = .06$), with length of hospital stay at 16.1 ± 6.2, 19.2 ± 7.9, and 21.6 ± 8.9 days, respectively (immunonutrition $P = .01$ vs. standard and $P = .004$ vs. parenteral group). There was a significantly increased risk of infection with intravenous feeding compared with the supplemental group, with the standard diet midway between.
Senkal[76]	1997		Patients undergoing resection for upper GI malignancy were randomized to diet enhanced with arginine, nucleotides, and omega-3 fatty acids ($n = 77$) or isocaloric, isonitrogenous diet ($n = 77$) after 10 dropouts. Infections after postoperative day 5 were significantly lower with supplemented diet ($P < .05$); length of stay similar, total complications lower with supplemented diet but not statistically significant.
Saffle[75]	1997	I	Of 50 burn patients randomized to a diet supplemented with omega-3 fatty acids, arginine, and RNA ($n = 25$) or standard high-protein diet ($n = 24$) within 48 h of injury, there were no differences between groups in mortality, length of hospital stay, charges, days of ventilator support, or incidence of complications.

(continued)

TABLE 6.4. (continued)

Author	*Year*	*Class of evidence*	*Conclusions*
Atkinson[82]	1998	I	Of 369 ICU patients of 398 enrolled randomized to enteral diet supplemented with arginine, nucleotides, and omega-3 fatty acids or isonitrogenous, isocaloric controlled diet, 101 patients supplemented (n = 50), standard diet (n = 51) received >2.51 within 72h. With successful early enteral feeding, supplemented diet significantly reduced ventilator days, length of stay, ICU stay, and systemic inflammatory response syndrome. No effect on mortality.
Gianotti[142]	2000	I	221 patients undergoing pancreatectomy randomized to a standard diet versus an arginine/omega-3 fatty acid/RNA supplemented diet or parenteral nutrition. Postoperative complications lower in the supplemented (33.8%) than standard diet (43.8%) or parenteral group (58.8%, $P = .005$ vs. supplemented diet). Length of stay shorter in the supplemented group (15.1 days) versus standard (17.0 days, $P < .05$) or parenterally fed groups (18.8 days, $P < .05$).
Galbán[143]	2000	I	176 patients randomized to diet enriched with arginine, RNA, and omega-3 fatty acids or high-protein control diet. Mortality significantly lower (17/89 vs. 28/87, $P < .05$) and bacteremia significantly reduced in the supplemented group (7/89 vs. 19/87, $P = .01$). Significantly reduced nosocomial infections with supplementation (5/89 vs. 17/87, $P = .01$). Reduced mortality rate in supplemented patients with Apache 2 scores between 10 and 15 (1/26 vs. 8/29, $P = .02$).
Caparrós[144]	2001	I	ICU patients randomized to high-protein diet with arginine, fiber, and antioxidants versus a high-protein formula. Infectious complication rates, ICU mortality, and in-hospital mortality similar. Patients receiving the enriched diet had a better survival at 6-month follow-up (76% vs. 67%, $P = .06$) and medical patients had a better survival with the enriched diet (76% vs. 59%, $P < .05$).
deLuis	2002	I	47 patients with oral laryngeal carcinoma randomized to standard diet or isonitrogenous isocaloric diet with arginine and fiber. Total complications similar, but fistula development lower in the enriched nutrient group (0% vs. 20.8%, $P < .05$). Postoperative stay shorter with the enriched diet (22.8 ± 11.8 days vs. 31.2 ± 19.1 days, $P = .07$).
Conejero[145]	2002	I	84 patients with systemic inflammatory response syndrome randomized to glutamine-enriched or standard enteral diet. Infections significantly lower in the enriched group (11 vs. 17, $P < .05$) due primarily to reduced nosocomial pneumonia (6 vs. 11).
Braga[78]	2002	I	196 malnourished patients undergoing elective surgery for GI malignancy randomized to standard postoperative enteral feeding (N = 50), preoperative feeding of a diet enriched with arginine, omega-3 fatty acids and RNA and standard enteral formula postoperatively (N = 50), or enriched diet pre- and postoperatively (N = 50). Baseline demographics, surgical variables, and morbidity factors similar. Complications significantly highest in the group with standard diet alone and lowest in those with the enriched diet pre- and postoperatively. Postoperative length of stay significantly shorter in both groups receiving enriched diet than control group ($P = .01$ for both).
Zhou[146]	2003	I	40 injured patients with body surface burns of 50%–80% and third-degree burns of 20%–40% randomized to groups given glutamine-enriched or a standard enteral formula for 12 days. Hospital stay significantly shorter with glutamine (67 ± 4 days vs. 73 ± 6 days, $P = .026$), and by 30 days wound healing significantly greater (86% ± 2% healed vs. 72% ± 3%, $P = .041$). Cost of hospitalization significantly lower with glutamine ($P = .031$), but cost of nutrition greater.
Hall[147]	2003	I	363 general ICU patients requiring mechanical ventilation randomized to glutamine-supplemented diet or an isonitrogenous isocaloric control. No significant difference in death within 6 months, incidence of severe sepsis or secondary outcomes of infections, duration of febrile episodes, antimicrobial therapy, or use of isotropes. No benefit from enteral glutamine supplementation was noted.
Garrel[148]	2003	I	45 burn patients randomized to either a standard diet or a glutamine-supplemented diet. The length of stay not significantly different (0.9 vs. 1.0 days per % total body surface area burn for glutamine vs. control), but positive blood cultures three times more frequent in control patients (4.3 vs. 1.2 days per patient, $P < .05$). *Pseudomonas aeruginosa* in 6 control versus 0 with glutamine diet ($P < .05$). Mortality rate significantly lower with glutamine (2 deaths vs. 12, $P < .05$).

limits 0.64–1.00); and a shorter hospitalization (risk ratio of −2.6 days, 95% confidence limits −4.5 to −0.7 days). Other subgroup analyses were not statistically different; however, the data suggested that improvements in mortality tended to occur when glutamine was provided parenterally and at high doses compared with enteral or low-dose supplementation. Furthermore, the reduction in length of stay appeared to occur in operated patients relative to those who were critically ill.

Considering the data that are currently available, it would be premature to recommend glutamine supplementation as standard therapy outside its use in new or ongoing clinical trials.[95]

TABLE 6.5.
Carbohydrate Versus Lipid as Primary Nonprotein Calorie Source.

Author	*Year*	*Reference*	*Class of evidence*	*Conclusions*
Smith[88]	1992	The effect on protein and amino acid metabolism of an intravenous nutrition regimen providing seventy percent of nonprotein calories as lipid. Surgery (St. Louis) 111:12–20.	I	20 patients requiring IV nutrition randomized to receive 36 kcal/kg/day with glucose-based solution or 37 kcal/kg/day as a lipid-based solution (70% nonprotein calories as lipid), glucose-based solution increased plasma transferrin and suppressed alanine efflux from peripheral tissues significantly greater than lipid-based formula. Glucose was more effective at suppressing gluconeogenesis.
de Chalain[89]	1992	The effect of fuel source on amino acid metabolism in critically ill patients. J Surg Res 52:167–176.	I	18 evaluable of 50 patients randomized to either glucose or glucose plus lipid-based solution providing 125% of the basal energy expenditure. Whole-body protein synthesis and metabolism correlated with the development of sepsis. The glucose-based solution led to more hyperglycemia, requiring withdrawal of four patients. Both formulas improved whole body protein kinetics.
Chassard[90]	1994	Effects of intravenous medium-chain triglycerides on pulmonary gas exchanges in mechanically ventilated patients. Crit Care Med 22:248–251.	I	Mechanically ventilated patients prospectively randomized in crossover trial to two 8-h infusion periods of either 50% MCTs (50% LCT solution) or 100% LCTs. The MCTs increased oxygen consumption by 28% and minute ventilation by 14%, but CO_2 production, $Pa{O_2}$, and $Pa{CO_2}$ were not different, suggesting slower infusion rate for intravenously administered MCTs.
Kohlhardt[91]	1994	Metabolic response to a high-lipid, high-nitrogen peripheral intravenous nutrition solution after major upper-GI surgery. Nutrition 10:317–326.	I	Of 18 patients status post-upper GI surgery randomized to either peripheral nutrition (75% nonprotein calories as lipid) or central intravenous nutrition with both groups receiving 0.56 g N kg/day and 100:1 calorie:nitrogen ratio, with the central nutrition group receiving only glucose; the metabolic response to major surgery was similar in both groups.
Roulet[92]	1997	Effects of intravenously infused fish oil on platelet fatty acid phospholipid composition and on platelet function in post-operative trauma. J Parenter Enteral Nutr 21:296–301.	I	In 19 postoperative patients randomized to 20% soybean fat emulsion with 10% marine fish oil emulsion or 20% soybean fat emulsion alone, large increases in omega-3 fatty acids in platelet membranes and increase in omega-3/omega-6 ratios and platelets without toxicity or evidence of increased postoperative bleeding were produced.
Tappy[93]	1998	Effects of isoenergetic glucose-based or lipid-based parenteral nutrition on glucose metabolism, de novo lipogenesis, and respiratory gas exchanges in critically ill patients. Crit Care Med 26:813–814.	I	In 16 surgical ICU patients randomized to receive isocaloric isonitrogenous parenteral nutrition with 75% (TPN glucose) or 15% (TPN lipid) glucose over a 5-day period with a metabolic procedure using tracers, TPN glucose increased plasma glucose, plasma insulin, and total CO_2 compared with lipid glucose solution. Both formulas failed to inhibit endogenous glucose production and net protein oxidation, suggesting absence of suppression of gluconeogenesis. Fractional de novo lipogenesis markedly increased by TPN glucose. There was no measured metabolic negative consequence of lipid-based formula.

Potential Mechanism for Reduced Infectious Complications with Enteral Feeding

Intravenous nutrition or lack of enteral feeding is associated with bacterial translocation in animal models of stress.[96] Clinically, bacterial translocation occurs in a few clinical settings, such as bowel obstruction or hemorrhagic shock, but does not appear to correlate with extraintestinal infections.[97]

Within the GI tract, parenteral feeding alters mucosal architecture[98] and increases in permeability.[99] A component of the mucosal barrier defenses is the gut-associated lymphoid tissue (GALT), which composes approximately 50% of the body's total immunity. The GALT is sensitive to route and type of nutrition in the animal model.[100,101] Naïve T cells and B cells produced within the peritoneal cavity and bone marrow circulate through the Peyer's patches. If sensitized by antigens processed by cells within the Peyer's patches, then the cells migrate through mesenteric lymph nodes and into the thoracic duct. The blood carries them to the lamina propria and intraepithelial spaces of the small intestine and to the upper and lower respiratory tract. In these sites, the sensitized B cells become plasma cells that produce immunoglobulin (Ig) A; the sensitized T cells produce cytokines that upregulate or downregulate IgA production.[102] In addition to IgA, defensins, lactoferrin, and other innate defenses as well as mucin provide barriers to prevent attachment of bacteria to the mucosal surfaces.

Parenteral nutrition reduces the size and effectiveness of the GALT.[101] Significant decreases in absolute numbers of T cells and B cells within the small intestine occur in association with decreasing intestinal and respiratory tract IgA levels. These decreases in IgA levels impair resistance against many types of viruses and bacteria.[103] Supplementation of the parenteral nutrition with glutamine partially preserves IgA levels and defenses against IgA-mediated antiviral defenses.[104] Route of nutrient administration also affects peritoneal defenses. With intravenous feeding, the immunological response within the peritoneal cavity is blunted with reduced peritoneal immunological cell numbers and decreased tumor necrosis factor (TNF) response with impaired bacterial killing.[105] Similar cytokine responses to endotoxin have been shown to occur in humans.[106]

Determining Dietary Requirements

Standard equations, such as the Harris–Benedict equation, multiplied by correction factors are used to determine nutrient goals. The use of indirect calorimetry has shown that stress and activity correction factors frequently lead to overestimates of nutrient needs.[107,108] Increased oxygen consumption, increased CO_2 production, hepatic lipogenesis, immunosuppression, and other negative effects occur with overfeeding, and it is important to provide appropriate amounts of each nutrient.

Energy Calculations

Estimated energy requirements must consider organ function, body weight, and the clinical condition. Guidelines are noted in Table 6.6. For calculations using body weight, actual body weight is appropriate for malnourished, euvolemic, or well-nourished patients. Overfeeding results when actual body weight is used in obese patients, and an adjusted form should be used to avoid overfeeding[109]:

$$\text{Adjusted body weight} = \text{Ideal body weight} + 0.25\,(\text{Actual} - \text{Ideal body weight})$$

In cases of significant fluid overload, an estimated dry body weight should be obtained by history.

The Harris–Benedict equation is based on gender, height, weight, and age to generate estimated body energy expenditure (BEE)[110] (Table 6.7, calculation A). Indirect calorimetry has shown these correction factors overestimate energy expenditure,[107,108,111] with a more appropriate correction factor approximately 15% greater than the BEE. Indirect calorimetry by portable metabolic carts uses expired gas analysis to determine overall resting energy expenditure (REE). By measuring carbon dioxide production (VCO_2) and oxygen consumption (VO_2), these values are applied to the Weir equation to determine REE. The metabolic rate in kilocalories as well as protein, carbohydrate, and fat oxidation can be calculated when the VO_2 and VCO_2 are combined with the urine urea nitrogen (UUN)[112] (Table 6.7, calculation B).

TABLE 6.7. Calculations Used to Determine Metabolic and Nutritional Parameters.

A. Male: BEE = $66 + (13.8 \times W) + (5 \times H) - (6.8 \times A)$
Female: BEE = $655 + (9.6 \times W) + (1.85 \times H) - (4.7 \times A)$
where W is the weight in kilograms, H is the height in centimeters, and A is the age in years.

B. Protein oxidation (g/d) = $6.25 \times UUN$
Carbohydrate oxidation (g/d) = $(4.12 \times VCO_2) - (2.91 \times VO_2) - (2.56 \times UUN)$
Fat oxidation (g/d) = $(1.69 \times VO_2) - (1.69 \times VCO_2) - (1.94 \times UUN)$
If UUN is not available, then MEE is calculated by
MEE (kcal/d) = $(3.9 \times VO_2) + (1.1 \times VCO_2)$
If UUN is available, then the MEE is adjusted for protein metabolism in the equation:
Adjusted MEE (kcal/d) = MEE − $(2.17 \times UNN)$

C. Nitrogen balance = Protein intake/6.25 − $[(UUN \times 0.8) + 1]$

MEE, metabolic energy expenditure

Although variations occur in the VO_2 and VCO_2 during a 24h period, intermittent measurements can confirm that the prescription is within a reasonable range of the administered nutrient dose to avoid significant underfeeding or overfeeding. The respiratory quotient (RQ) is the ratio of VCO_2 to VO_2, and a characteristic RQ exists for each fuel metabolized: fat RQ = 0.7, glucose RQ = 1.0, and protein RQ = 0.8; lipogenesis has an RQ of approximately 8. If the RQ of a patient is greater than 1, then it is a strong indicator of overfeeding.

There are limitations to indirect calorimetry. Accuracy is lost in mechanically ventilated patients as the FIO_2 (fraction of inspired oxygen) increases because of measurement errors between inspired and expired oxygen levels. A 1% measurement error in the inspired or expired VO_2 in a patient receiving an FIO_2 of 0.8 produces a 100% error in VO_2 calculation. Air leaks around tracheostomies or through chest tubes must be recognized in measurements. Indirect calorimetry is labor intensive and requires dedicated personnel with defined protocols to provide reliable data.[113]

Because postsurgical patients usually have increases of 10% to 15% over the BEE calculated by the Harris–Benedict equation, the current guidelines in Table 6.6 are adequate for most patients. If 30kcal/kg is provided to most hypermetabolic patients, then approximately 90% of them will attain their energy requirement, with minimal overfeeding in only 15% to 20%.[106]

TABLE 6.6. Energy and Protein Needs for Surgical Patients.

Condition	*kcal/kg/day*	*Protein/kg/day*	*Non-protein calories/gN:N*
Normal-to-moderate malnutrition	25–30 (low stress)	1.0	150:1
Moderate stress	25–30	1.5	120:1
Hypermetabolic, stressed	30–35	1.5–2.0	90–120:1
Burns	35–40	2.0–2.5	90–120:1

Protein Requirements

The recommended daily allowance for protein intake in well-nourished, healthy individuals is approximately 0.8g/kg/day.[114] Each gram provides 4.0kcal/g. The recommended dose of amino acids (or protein with enteral feeding) for stressed or septic patients without renal dysfunction is 1.5 to 2g/kg/

day.[115] Although blood urea nitrogen (BUN) may increase to 40 mg/dl in some patients, this is without adverse consequences.

In nonhypermetabolic patients who have existing malnutrition or who are at risk of developing starvation-induced malnutrition, 1.0 to 1.5 g/kg/day of protein meets nutrient needs. In burn patients, excessive urinary and wound losses generally dictate administration of 2 to 2.5 g/kg/day. These administered doses, however, may need to be reduced in patients with chronic or acute renal failure. Under these conditions, it is prudent to provide 0.6 to 0.8 g of amino acids or protein per kilogram per day before dialysis and increase the dose to 1 to 1.5 g protein/kg/day once dialysis is instituted.

Adequacy of protein administration may be assessed by a determination of nitrogen balance (Table 6.7, calculation C) in a 24 h urine collection. The UUN generally represents approximately 80% of excreted nitrogen, and additional nitrogen losses are estimated at 1 g/day. Accurate urine collection and accurate records of protein intake determine the accuracy of this calculated value.

Glucose

The maximal rate of glucose oxidation is 4 to 5 mg/kg/min or approximately 7.2 g/kg/day. Total glucose administration in intravenous fluids, parenteral nutrition, or enteral nutrition should not exceed these levels.[116] In a 70 kg man, these needs are met by 2l of 25% dextrose solution, providing 500 g of glucose. Blood sugar should ideally be maintained well below 200 mg%. It is suggested that complications are increased with high blood sugars.[117] Administration of the glucose in these doses provides approximately 50% to 60% of total caloric requirements. Hydrated glucose in parenteral nutrition provides 3.4 kcal/g, and oral carbohydrates provide 4.0 kcal/g. Work demonstrated reduced mortality with rigid control of glucose in an ICU setting, although almost all benefit occurred in cardiac patients.[118]

Fat Requirement

Remaining nonprotein caloric needs are met by lipid infusion of approximately 1 g/kg/day. The maximum adult dose of intravenous lipid is 2.5 g/kg/day.[119] Rarely is this higher limit administered except, for example, in the brittle diabetic with uncontrolled hyperglycemia. Enterally, fat provides 9.1 kcal/g. Intravenous lipid provides 10 kcal/g obtained due to emulsifiers and glycerol. If overfeeding is suspected, then total calories should be reduced. In patients with diabetes or receiving corticosteroids, high rates of fat administration may control glucose but induce hyperlipidemia, cholestasis, and perhaps immunosuppression.[120,121] Lipid emulsions available in the United States contain omega-6 PUFAs derived from vegetable oils. There is concern about their immunosuppressive effects.

Intravenous lipid emulsion in the critically ill patient should be limited to 1 g/kg/day if triglyceride levels are less than 300 mg% and withheld in patients with hypertriglyceridemia, particularly if values are greater than 500 mg/dl. There is no evidence that intravenous lipid emulsions aggravate acute pancreatitis if hyperlipidemia is not the cause of the pancreatitis.

Organ System Complications of Overfeeding

Pulmonary Failure

Lipogenesis from overfeeding increases CO_2 production but rarely causes ventilator dependence in patients sustaining multiple trauma or sepsis. Failure to wean is usually the result of the increased metabolic rate, pneumonia, multiple rib fractures, pulmonary contusions, or sepsis. In selected surgical patients—particularly those with chronic pulmonary disease or after prolonged intubation—increasing fat as a percentage of nonprotein calories may assist in reducing CO_2 production and decreasing ventilator demands. These patients usually have GI function, and a high-fat enteral formula may be used with a calorie-to-nitrogen ratio of approximately 120–150:1 with 40% to 50% of the calories as fat. The routine use of these solutions in intubated patients is usually unnecessary.

Hepatic Failure

Hepatic failure generally carries a dismal prognosis, and excessive protein restriction should be avoided. Intravenous amino acid solutions are better tolerated than enteral protein. Typically, these patients should receive 0.5 to 0.8 g of protein and approximately 30 kcal/kg/day. These formulas appear to be of little value in desperate situations of severe hepatic failure in a setting of multiple organ dysfunction secondary to uncontrolled sepsis and metabolic collapse.

Enteral Nutrition

Both clinical and economic considerations support the use of the enteral route for feeding whenever possible. Currently, more than 200 enteral products varying in composition, complexity, and physical characteristics are available to meet restrictions and requirements of most clinical conditions. "Ileus" is often limited to the stomach and colon, whereas the small intestine remains a site capable of absorption of nutrients. Because of the wide array of enteral products and the potential for expensive duplication in a hospital formulary, understanding basic concepts of enteral formulation and techniques of access can produce both clinical and economic benefits.

Enteral Access

Most preoperative and postoperative patients tolerate intragastric feeding. A small-bore NG tube is better tolerated than a large tube. Small-bore tubes reduce the risk of complications such as esophageal stricture, reflux, or necrosis of the nasal alae. Styletted tubes help placement, and their location can be confirmed with aspiration of gastric juice or confirmation via fluoroscopy or x-ray. Simple air insufflation is inadequate to confirm placement because sounds transmitted from the left lung or distal esophagus may be auscultated in the left upper quadrant. In patients at increased risk of aspiration due to reflux, advancement of the tube beyond the ligament of Treitz via endoscopic techniques or fluoroscopy may provide additional protection. A double-lumen tube allows gastric decompression and feeding beyond the pylorus and, ideally, beyond the ligament of Treitz.

Unfortunately, nasojejunal or NG tubes are frequently dislodged, increasing the cost and complexity in providing enteral nutrition. In these situations, if laparotomy is not necessary, an endoscopic gastrostomy with direct intragastric feeding may be preferable because it can be performed with minimal mortality and morbidity (Fig. 6.1). This technique is useful in patients requiring long-term intragastric feeding because of dysphagia or chronic neurological dysfunction. It should be used with caution in patients with a history of esophageal reflux and aspiration. Direct gastric feeding is not recommended in neurologically impaired pediatric patients with recurrent pneumonia secondary to reflux. Access distal in the GI tract or surgical correction of the reflux is advisable.[122]

Laparotomy allows access beyond the ligament of Treitz for direct small-bowel feeding. Jejunostomies with a large-bore (14-, 16-, or 18F) tube or needle catheter jejunostomies (5- and 7F) allow direct administration of tube feedings in patients expected to have prolonged gastroparesis. In critically injured patients with severe intraabdominal or chest, head, bony, or soft tissue injuries, there is a significant reduction in pneumonia and intraabdominal abscess with early small-bowel feeding.[33–35] Needle catheter jejunostomies are useful for 3 to 4 weeks following injury. Jejunostomies should be located at a site with a long mesentery so that abdominal distension does not tear the jejunostomy off the anterior abdominal wall as a result of the tethering effect at the ligament of Treitz. A Witzel tunnel should be constructed for a distance of about 4 cm and the jejunostomy sutured lateral to the rectus sheath with four to five sutures to eliminate volvulus.

Fiber-containing diets can be administered through both small- and large-bore needle catheter jejunostomies,[123] but

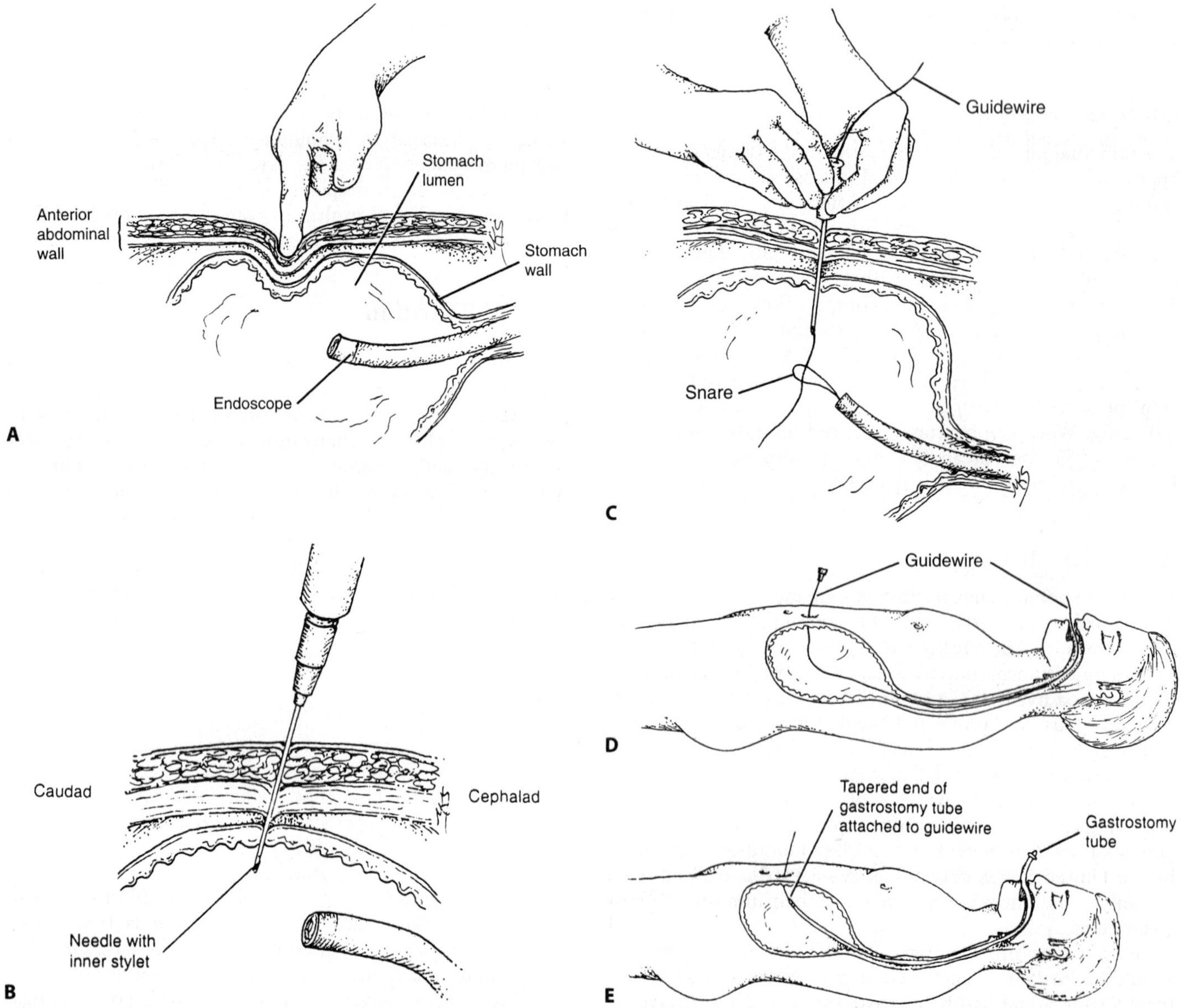

FIGURE 6.1. **A.** The procedure for percutaneous endoscopic gastrostomy includes transillumination of the stomach and identification of the needle insertion site. **B.** A needle is inserted into the stomach across the abdominal wall under direct vision. **C.** A guidewire passed through the lumen of the needle is grasped with a snare. **D.** The ensnared guidewire is removed via the mouth. **E.** The tapered end of the gastrostomy tube is attached to the guidewire and pulled out through the stomach and abdominal wall to seal the button end. The external portion of the gastrostomy tube is then trimmed to fit the patient's body habitus as desired.

protein supplements and immune-enhancing diets clog 5F tubes. Tubes should be flushed at least four times a day. Elixirs in medications coagulate the enteral products and clog the tubes rapidly. Needle catheter jejunostomies usually cannot be replaced once lost. Larger-bore catheters can be replaced after 1 week and are more useful for long-term requirements. Transgastric tubes allow simultaneous decompression of the stomach and feeding into the duodenum (Moss tube) or beyond the ligament of Treitz (transgastric jejunostomy). Location of the distal port in the duodenum stimulates both pancreatic and gastric secretions and may cause fluid and electrolyte problems, but infusion beyond the ligament of Treitz produces little stimulation. Transgastric jejunostomies rarely dislodge back into the stomach, but the size of the jejunal channel dictates product choice similar to 5F needle catheter jejunostomies.

Anastomosis above the site of enteral access or in the mid- or distal small bowel and colon provides no contraindication to direct small-bowel feeding. There is no evidence of increased intraabdominal infection with small-bowel access in patients with no other hollow viscus violation.[124] Enteral feeding is not contraindicated in acute pancreatitis if nutrients are delivered beyond the ligament of Treitz.[51–54] Short-gut syndrome, uncontrollable diarrhea, distal bowel obstruction, or upper GI hemorrhage are relative contraindications.

Initiation of Tube Feeding

Direct intragastric feeding should be attempted in most patients. In burn patients, intragastric feeding soon after admission prevents subsequent gastroparesis with a 95% success rate. The highest success rate occurs when feedings are instituted within 6 to 8h[55]; success drops to less than 50% when feeding is instituted after 18h. Even when pressors are used, intragastric feedings are safe because small-bowel intolerance prompts high gastric residuals, protecting the small intestine from potential necrosis.[125] With direct small-bowel feeding, the low but real rate of intestinal necrosis preempts institution of feeding until resuscitation is complete, tissues are perfused, patients are not receiving pressors, and splanchnic blood flow can increase in response to enteral feeding. Hypertonic or isotonic formulas can be infused into the stomach, but it is preferable to use isotonic solutions with intrajejunal feedings, although more concentrated solutions have been used with success if started as a more dilute solution and then increased in concentration as the volume increases.[33,126]

Gastric feedings can be administered as either bolus or continuous infusions. Jejunostomy feedings should be continuously infused, although some patients adapt to bolus intrajejunal feeding over time. Intragastric and intrajejunal feedings are started at 25 to 30ml/h and advanced over varying times to a goal that meets caloric and nutrient needs. With intragastric feeding, residuals are measured every 4h, and tube feeding is advanced by 25ml/h if residuals remain below 200ml/h. With intrajejunal feedings, signs of intolerance include abdominal distension, diarrhea, and cramping. Most commonly, intrajejunal feedings are increased by 25ml/h over 12 or 24h increments to the goal rate. Direct small-bowel feedings should be discontinued if feedings reflux into the NG tube.

Enteral Formulas

Choice of formula is determined by functional status of the GI tract, patient nutrient requirements, or restrictions imposed by organ failure. A summary of some enteral feeding formulas is presented in Table 6.8. With an intact GI tract and mucosa, formulas with complex proteins, carbohydrates, and fats are well tolerated. Formulas that contain lactose should be avoided in patients who have not been fed via the GI tract for some time because of rapid decreases in disaccharidase production (lactase is the most rapid) in the GI tract.

Critically ill patients have increased protein requirements and may be less tolerant of glucose or lipid. In these conditions, a lower nonprotein calorie-to-nitrogen ratio (range 80–120:1) may better meet these macronutrient needs. In patients with mucosal disease, such as Crohn's disease, chemically defined formulas containing amino acids with di- or tripeptides may improve digestion and absorption. Fiber-containing formulas provide soluble fiber, which can be metabolized by intraluminal bacteria to produce short-chain fatty acids (butyrate, propionate, and acetoacetate), and provide substrate for the colonocyte to maintain water absorption and reduce or prevent diarrhea.[127]

The MCTs may be better tolerated than long-chain triglycerides (LCTs) since they are more easily digested and absorbed. The MCTs do not contain essential fatty acids, and some LCTs must be provided.

Categories of Enteral Feeding Formulations

Standard Isotonic Formulas

Standard isotonic formulas contain an appropriate balance of carbohydrate, protein, and fat (usually with a nonprotein calorie-to-nitrogen ratio of approximately 150:1). The macronutrients require digestion but provide adequate nutrition in a low volume with low osmolality (approximately 300mOsm/l) and a caloric density of 1.0kcal/ml. These diets are considered low residue because they do not contain fiber. In general, these formulas are used in stable patients at risk of starvation-induced malnutrition or those with existing states of malnutrition who are neither stressed nor septic.

Standard Fiber-Containing Formulas

Standard fiber-containing formulas are similar to the standard isotonic products but contain a combination of soluble and insoluble fiber, most often as soy polysaccharide. Fiber prolongs intestinal transit time, stimulates intestinal lipase activity, and provides the substrate for short-chain fatty acid metabolism by intraluminal bacteria.[128] These formulas are tolerated even in critically ill patients fed via needle catheter jejunostomies and appear to reduce the incidence of diarrhea compared with chemically defined diets. They do not occlude small-bore feeding catheters when catheters are properly flushed and often have a high protein content appropriate for critically ill patients.

Specialty, "Immune-Enhancing" Formulas

Several products enriched in nutrients such as BCAAs, glutamine, arginine, omega-3 fatty acids, nucleotides, or beta-

TABLE 6.8. Some Enteral Feeding Formulas.

PRODUCT, Supplier	*kcal/ml*	*Total calorie/ nitrogen*	*Liters to provide 100% RDA vitamins and minerals*	*mOsm*	*Protein*	*Carbohydrate*	*Fat*	*Na*	*K*	*Features*[a]
PRECISION LR, Sandoz	1.1	239	1.7	530	26	248	1.6	30	2.3	P,F
TRAVASORB STD, Baxter	1	184	2	560	30	190	14	40	30	P,U,MCT
REABILAN, O'Brien	1	175	3	350	32	131	39	30	32	L,U,MCT
TRAVASORB, Baxter	1	154	1.9	450	35	136	35	30	31	L,F,MCT
ENSURE, Ross	1	153	1.9	450	37	145	37	37	40	L,F
RESOURCE CRYSTALS, Sandoz	1	154	1.9	450	37	145	37	37	40	F
RESOURCE POWER, Sandoz	1	178	1.9	450	37	145	37	37	40	P,F
ENRICH, Ross	1	148	1.4	480	40	162	37	37	40	L,F, high residue
COMPLEAT, REG, Sandoz	1	131	1.5	405	43	128	43	57	36	L,U
ENSURE HN, Ross	1	125	1.3	470	44	141	35	40	40	L,F
PRECISION HN, Sandoz	1	125	2.8	525	44	216	1.3	43	23	P,F
REABILIAN HN, O'Brien	1.3	125	2.9	490	58	158	52	43	43	L,U,MCT
MERITENE, Doyle	1	104	1.2	550	58	110	32	38	41	L,F
SUSTACAL, Mead Johnson	1	79	1	625	61	140	23	41	53	L,F
MERITENE POWDER, Doyle	1	104	1.2	690	66	113	32	44	68	P,F
SUSTACAL POWDER, M.J.	1.3	80	0.8	899	77	180	34	54	87	Mixed w/whole milk
Isotonic										
PRECISION ISOTONIC, Sandoz	1	183	1.6	300	29	144	30	20	25	P,F
ISOCAL, Mead Johnson	1	167	1.9	300	34	133	44	23	34	L,U,MCT
ENTRITION, Biosearch	1	154	2	300	35	136	35	31	31	L,U
OSMOLITE, Ross	1	153	1.9	300	37	145	39	24	26	L,U,MCT
COMPLEAT MODIFIED, Sandoz	1	131	1.5	300	4.3	141	37	29	36	L,U
PEPTAMEN, Clintec Nutrition	1	131	2	260	40	127	39	22	16	L,U,MCT
OSMOLITE HN, Ross	1	125	1.3	310	44	141	37	40	40	L,U,MCT
ISOTEIN HN, Sandoz	1.2	86	1.8	300	68	156	34	27	27	P,F,MCT
For impaired GI tract and other special situations										
TOLEREX, Eaton	1	284	1.8	550	21	226	1.5	20	30	P,U
VIVONEX T.E.N., Eaton	1	149	2	630	38	206	2.8	20	20	P,U,BCAA
SURGICAL LIQUID, Diet Ross	0.7	117	1.2	545	38	136	0	36	21	P,F
CRITICARE HN, Mead Johnson	1	148	2	650	38	222	3.4	28	34	L,U
VITAL HN, Ross	1	125	1.5	460	42	185	11	20	34	P,F,MCT
TRAUMA-AID HBC, McGaw	1	132	3	640	56	166	7	23	30	P,F,MCT,BCAA
STRESSTEIN, Sandoz	1.2	97	2	910	70	173	27	29	29	P,U,MCT,BCAA
TRAVASORB MCT, Baxter	1.5	100	1.3	450	74	185	49	23	26	L,F,MCT
IMPACT, Novartis	1	91	1.5	375	56	130	28	48	36	L,U,MCT, fish oil
PERATIVE, Ross	1.3	122	1.2	425	67	177	37	45	44	L,U,MCT, arginine
ALITRAQ, Ross	1	120	1.5	480	53	165	16	44	31	F,F, glutamine
SUBDUE, Mead Johnson	1	120	1.2	330	50	127	34	48	41	L,F,MCT

TABLE 6.8. (continued)

PRODUCT, Supplier	*kcal/ml*	*Total calorie/ nitrogen*	*Liters to provide 100% RDA vitamins and minerals*	*mOsm*	*Protein*	*Carbohydrate*	*Fat*	*Na*	*K*	*Features*[a]
For specific pathological entities										
AMINIAID, McGaw	1.9	362	1.95	23	384	25	14	5	For renal failure	
TRAVASORB RENAL, Baxter	Packets of 112 g, 467 cal, 470 mOsm/l	For renal failure								
HEPATIC AID IL, McGaw	1.1	174	1.0	44	158	34	5	6	For liver failure	
TRAVASORB HEPATIC, Baxter	Packets of 96 g, 378 cal, 480 mOsm/l	For liver failure								
PULMOCARE, Ross	1.5	150	1	490	63	106	92	57	49	To decrease CO_2 production
High calorie density										
ENSURE PLUS, Ross	1.5	146	1.6	600	55	200	53	50	54	L,F
SUSTACAL HC, Mead Johnson	1.5	134	1.2	650	61	190	57	37	38	L,F
ENSURE PLUS HN, Ross	1.5	125	0.9	650	62	200	50	51	47	L,F
MAGNACAL, Sherwood	2	154	1	590	70	250	80	44	32	L,F
ISOCAL HCN, Mead Johnson	2	145	1.5	690	75	224	91	35	36	L,F,MCT
TWOCAL HN, Ross	2	126	0.9	700	84	217	90	46	59	L,F,MCT

Protein, carbohydrate, and fat are expressed as gram per liter (g/l) standard dilution, Na and K are expressed as milliequivalents per liter (mEq) standard dilution.
[a]P, powder; L, liquid; F, flavored; U, unflavored; BCAA, branched-chain amino acids; MCT, medium-chain triglycerides.

carotene have been studied in clinical populations. These specialty immune-enhancing formulas are nitrogen rich given the supplementation with arginine or glutamine. The proposed clinical functions of individual nutrients have been previously described.

High-Density Formulas

High-density formulas provide 1.5 to 2 kcal/ml for patients requiring food restriction or very high calorie and protein requirements, but osmolality is higher than that of isotonic formulas. They are most often used as intragastric feedings in patients requiring fluid restriction or those intolerant of large volumes. Potential for diarrhea is greater.

High-Protein Formulas

To meet the high protein needs of severely stressed and injured patients, formulas containing nonprotein calorie-to-nitrogen ratios of less than 125:1 are well suited for critically ill patients. Both isotonic and nonisotonic formulas are available.

Elemental/Peptide-Based Formulas

The products in the elemental/peptide-based formulas have been predigested compared with formulas with intact micronutrients. Protein is provided as mono-, di-, or tripeptides; fat is provided as MCTs and LCTs, and complex carbohydrates are limited. The fat content in some formulas is extremely low (less than 10% of total calories), which limits their long-term usefulness. However, these products are more readily absorbed in patients with maldigestion or malabsorption. In critically ill patients, these formulas should be started at a lower rate (15–20 ml/h) and advanced more slowly or initially diluted with water to produce a more isotonic formula; as the rate increases, the concentration of these formulas can be increased.

Renal Failure Formulas

Renal failure formula products contain only essential amino acids or a high ratio of essential to nonessential amino acids, and they are designed with a high calorie-to-nitrogen ratio to allow endogenous synthesis of nonessential amino acids from urea nitrogen. These formulas also contain moderate to low concentrations of the intracellular electrolytes potassium, phosphorus, and magnesium to control serum levels. They are more expensive, and it is unclear whether there is significant clinical benefit over standard mixes of crystalline amino acids, but the restriction of electrolytes is often beneficial and cannot be achieved with other enteral formulas.

Applications of Enteral Feeding

Complications of tube feeding include diarrhea, aspiration, vomiting, distension, metabolic abnormalities, and tube dislodgment.[128] Avoid intragastric feeding in patients with severe reflux and prior evidence of aspiration. Elevation of the head of the bed by 30°, administration of prokinetic agents, or feedings beyond the ligament of Treitz may minimize aspiration. Diarrhea is frequent in tube-fed patients. Fiber-containing diets may reduce diarrhea by providing substrate for the colonocytes. Administration of medications via the tube or use of antibiotics is often the cause of diarrhea in enterally fed patients.[129] Elixirs in medications are rich in sorbitol, causing diarrhea through osmotic effects. Magnesium-containing antacids, bacterial overgrowth from antibiotics, or the overuse of prokinetic agents also produce diarrhea, which is reversed with discontinuation of these medications. Stools should be cultured for *Clostridium difficile* and medications reviewed for those noted earlier.[128] Diarrhea usually is not caused by the tube feedings but by other therapies.

Metabolic complications include hyperglycemia, hypophosphatemia, hyper- or hypokalemia, and hypomagnesemia in postoperative patients with preexisting nutritional deficiencies, renal failure, or diabetes mellitus. The sodium content in most enteral formulas is 30 to 35 mEq/l, which can lead to hyponatremia, especially when multiple medications are administered in dextrose and water or if the patient has inappropriate antidiuretic hormone secretion. Hypernatremia occurs when medications or intravenous fluids are provided in normal saline or when diabetes insipidus complicates head injuries or neurosurgical procedures. Refeeding syndrome with intracellular mobilization of potassium, phosphate, and magnesium can occur with enteral nutrition, particularly in patients with significant preexisting nutrient deficiencies.[130]

Small-bowel necrosis and pneumatosis intestinalis can occur with direct small-bowel feedings. The cause is unknown, but speculation that inability to increase blood flow to the splanchnic bed may be one etiological factor. It is prudent to delay jejunal feedings until hemodynamic stability is achieved and there is adequate splanchnic perfusion (adequate urine output). Intragastric feedings are safe because high gastric residuals will reflect the small-bowel intolerance.

Parenteral Nutrition

Parenteral Access

Parenteral nutrient solutions with dextrose concentrations greater than 10% are hypertonic and must be administered into a large, centrally located vein to avoid thrombophlebitis and venous sclerosis associated with administration of these hyperosmolar formulas. The superior vena cava is an ideal site in which to administer concentrated parenteral nutrition formulas. Infraclavicular transcutaneous puncture and cannulation of the right subclavian vein usually accomplish access to the superior vena cava (Figs. 6.2 and 6.3). A supraclavicular approach may occasionally be preferred if the infraclavicular approach is contraindicated or inaccessible, as occurs in patients who have suffered chest trauma or burns or have tumor involving this region, have had extensive radiotherapy, or have distorted anatomy. The right side is preferred as this avoids the possibility of injury to the thoracic duct, and the guidewire may be somewhat easier to thread because of a typically more gentle angulation present between the right innominate vein and the superior vena cava as compared to the left side. Access to the superior vena cava can also be obtained by transcutaneous puncture of the external or internal jugular veins, but catheters that exit in the neck are more difficult to care for, more uncomfortable for many patients, and probably more likely to become infected. Multiple-lumen central venous catheters are usually inserted. Catheter infection rates are the lowest when catheters to be used for parenteral nutrition support are inserted under the strictest sterile conditions, including use of a hat, mask, gown, and gloves.[131,132] Currently, safe practice dictates that a chest x-ray should be obtained to verify that the catheter tip is centrally located before concentrated dextrose solutions are administered. Rarely, a lateral chest film will be required to verify that the

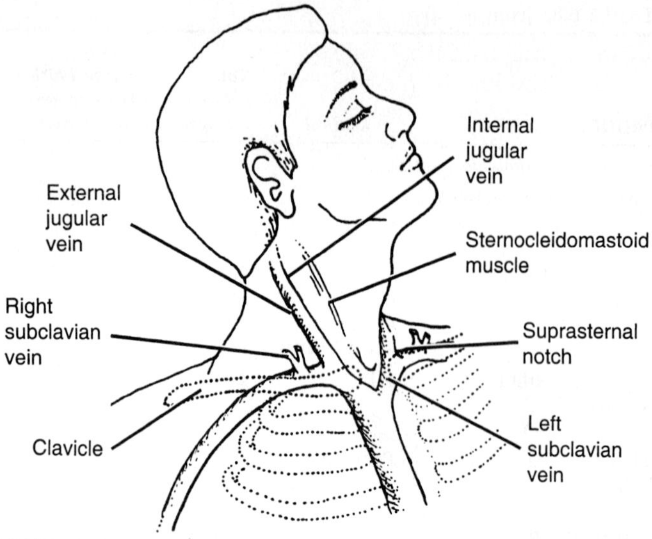

FIGURE 6.2. Anatomic sites and landmarks for central venous access procedures.

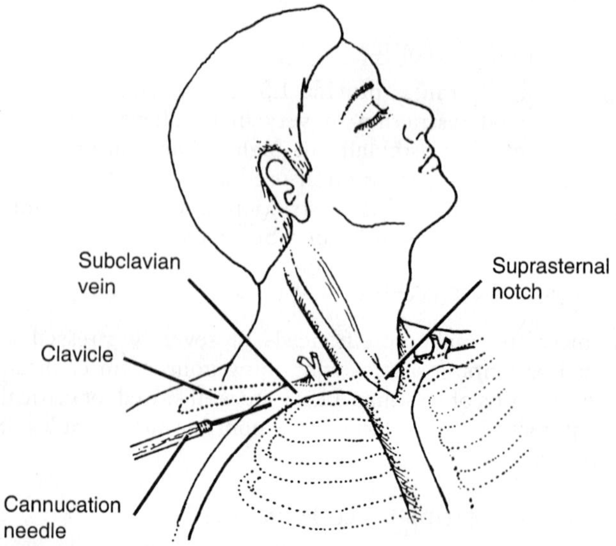

FIGURE 6.3. Cannulation of the subclavian vein by an infraclavicular approach.

catheter tip is located in the superior vena cava rather than in an internal mammary vein.

Once the line is inserted, at least one lumen should be reserved solely for the administration of the parenteral formulation because multiuse catheters appear to have higher infection rates.[132] This precaution makes intuitive sense because of the likely correlation between the number of line breaks and the likelihood of contamination of the nutrient solution. Similarly, although it would be theoretically advantageous to have a single-lumen catheter inserted for the administration of parenteral nutrition, this approach is impractical for most hospitalized patients who require the therapy. Thus, while one lumen of a multiple-lumen catheter should be devoted to the administration of parenteral nutrition, the other lumens may be used for monitoring, for blood drawing, or to administer medications. Regardless of the type of catheter that is inserted, it is critically important that the multilumen catheters be handled carefully and dressing changes be made regularly, typically at least every third day, by a knowledgeable, certified, and trained individual.

Access to the superior vena cava can also be obtained using catheters that are inserted peripherally in the upper extremity and threaded to the appropriate location. Such peripherally inserted central venous catheters, known by the acronym PICC lines, offer the ability to obtain central venous access without the risks associated with subclavian or jugular puncture. As discussed for catheters inserted via other approaches, it is important to dedicate a single lumen for the administration of parenteral nutrition and to manage the catheter carefully. These lines can be used for several months and are often used for hydration or other parenteral therapy for home-bound patients.

Dedicated central venous access via the subclavian or jugular veins may rarely be impossible to obtain, for example, because of preexisting thrombosis or occlusion of the subclavian or innominate veins or superior vena cava or anatomical problems preventing safe puncture, or may be too risky, especially in patients with refractory coagulopathies and pulmonary insufficiency. In these circumstances, most institutions favor a policy by which the dextrose concentration of parenteral nutrition solutions is limited to 15% or less. This measure is recommended in an effort to limit the risk of lower extremity venous thrombosis. It would also appear to be prudent to change these lines every 3 days or more often to minimize the risk of infection associated with the higher number of skin bacteria in the femoral region. Safe parenteral nutritional therapy would also mandate that the dextrose concentration of nondedicated lines, that is, lines that have been used for any purpose other than the administration of nutritional formulas, be limited to 10% or less. This restriction is advised because the risk of infection is probably higher when more concentrated solutions are used.

Composition of Central and Peripheral Venous Solutions

The common macronutrients and their caloric densities and functions are presented in Table 6.9. As mentioned, with central venous nutrition, hypertonic nutrient solutions (>10% dextrose) are infused via a catheter inserted into a large central vein. Access to a large central vein is needed because these formulas usually have osmolarities greater than or equal to 1900 mOsm/kg, and administration of the solutions into peripheral veins causes thrombophlebitis and venous sclerosis (Table 6.10). When infused into the central venous system, the nutrients are rapidly diluted to near isotonicity and then metabolized. These solutions usually contain about 1 kcal/ml. Typically, 2 to 3 l are administered over a 24 h period, thereby providing about 2000 to 3000 kcal/day. Occasionally, as for patients who will require home parenteral nutrition support, it may be advisable and feasible to administer the feeding solution over less than 24 h (a procedure known as *cycling*), if only to provide some time free from intravenous infusion.

Peripheral nutritional alimentation solutions typically have dextrose concentrations of 5%. Between 1000 and 1500 calories can be administered using this method, and the volume of fluid required to administer these calories is usually greater than 2 l/day. In contrast to the case for central venous alimentation solutions, in which the substrate mixture is predominantly composed of carbohydrate, most of the calories from peripheral parenteral nutrition solutions are

TABLE 6.9. Caloric Densities, Sources, and Functions of the Major Macronutrients.

Macronutrient (caloric density)	*Common sources*	*Functions*
Carbohydrates (3.4 kcal/g)	Dextrose	Essential fuels used by glycolytic tissues; normally the major or sole energy source for the central nervous system, peripheral nerves, red blood cells, and some phagocytes. During prolonged starvation, the glucose requirement of the brain decreases as adaptation to ketone oxidation occurs. Are used by tissues that oxidize fat (e.g., muscle) when carbohydrates are administered as the major fuel source. Maintain hepatic glycogen stores, which may protect hepatocytes during hypoxia or exposure to toxins.
Lipids (10 kcal/g)	Polyunsaturated	The most concentrated forms of energy. Long-chain lipids protect vital structures. Complex with fat-soluble molecules like some vitamins are used as structural components in biological triglycerides from soybean oil or a safflower–soybean oil mixture membranes.
Proteins (4 kcal/gm)	Crystalline amino	Major structural component of the body. Some are essential acids (histidine, isoleucine, leucine, valine, methionine, cysteine, phenylalanine, tyrosine, threonine, tryptophan, and lysine) because they cannot be synthesized by the body. Others are nonessential because they can be made from carbon and nitrogen precursors. Act as peptide hormones, enzymes, and antibodies. May join with carbohydrates to form glycoproteins, to serve as plasma proteins and immune globulins, and components of connective tissue cell membranes and mucous secretions.

TABLE 6.10. Central Parenteral Nutrition.

	Central	*Peripheral*
Daily calories	2000–3000	1000–1500
Protein	Variable	56–87 g
Volume of fluid required	1000–3000 ml	2000–3500 ml
Duration of therapy	4–7 days	5–7 days
Route of administration	Dedicated central venous catheter	Peripheral vein or multiuse central catheter
Substrate profile	55%–60% carbohydrate	30% carbohydrate
	15%–20% protein	20% protein
	25% fat	50% fat
Osmolarity	2000 mOsm/l	Approx. 600–900 mOsm/l

derived from fat. Peripheral nutritional prescriptions typically provide approximately 30% of calories as carbohydrate, 20% as protein, and at least 50% of calories as fat.

Peripheral parenteral nutrition is usually undesirable for several reasons. First, there is no evidence that this improves outcomes or significantly decreases nitrogen losses when it does not closely approximate a patient's energy needs. Second, the high-fat content typically administered as part of peripheral parenteral nutrition regimens may impair reticuloendothelial cell function and therefore immune responsiveness.[133]

Parenteral alimentation solutions are prepared by a pharmacist and typically combine 500 ml of 50% dextrose with 500 ml of a 10% to 15% amino acid mixture. Examples of amino acid and intravenous lipid preparations are shown in Tables 6.11 and 6.12, respectively. Vitamins, electrolytes, and

TABLE 6.11. Some Parenteral Amino Acid Solutions.

	Novamine 15%	*Travasol 10%*	*TrophAmine 6%*
Protein equivalent (g/100 ml)	15	10	6
Total nitrogen (g/100 ml)	2.3	1.6	0.93
Osmolarity (mOsm/l)	1300	998	525
pH	5.6	6.0	5.5
Essential amino acids (mg/100 ml)			
Isoleucine	749	600	490
Leucine	1040	730	840
Lysine	1180	580	490
Methionine	749	400	200
Phenylalanine	1040	560	290
Threonine	349	420	260
Tryptophan	250	180	120
Valine	960	580	470
Nonessential amino acids (mg/100 ml)			
Cysteine			14
Arginine	1470	1150	730
Alanine	2170	2070	320
Proline	894	680	410
Glycine	1040	1030	220
Serine	592	500	230
Tyrosine			15

TABLE 6.12. Fatty Acid Content of Intravenous Lipid Preparations.

	Intralipid	*Liposyn II*	*Liposyn III*
Manufacturer	Clintec Nutrition	Abbott	Abbott
Concentration (%)	10	10	10
	20	20	20
Oil (%)			
Safflower		5	
		10	
Soybean	10	5	10
	20	10	20
Fatty acid content (%)			
Linoleic	50	65.8	54.5
	50	65.8	54.5
Oleic	26	17.7	22.4
	26	17.7	22.4
Palmitic	10	8.8	10.5
	10	8.8	10.5
Linoleic	9	4.2	8.3
	9	4.2	8.3
Stearic	3.5	3.4	4.2
	3.5	3.4	4.2
Osmolarity (mOsm/l)	260	276	284
	260	258	292

trace elements are added to the formulation as needed. Central parenteral nutrition solutions usually provide about 55% to 60% of calories as carbohydrate and 15% to 20% of calories as protein. Lipids should contribute no more than 30% of the total calories administered in nearly all circumstances. A typical prescription would administer 2 l of this standard solution each day. Administration of 500 ml of 20% fat emulsion for 1 day each week is sufficient to prevent essential fatty acid deficiency. This method of administration is satisfactory if lipids are needed only as a source of essential fatty acids and are not needed as an additional source of calories, for example, by patients whose caloric requirements would require dextrose infusions at rates greater than 5 mg/kg/min. If additional calories from lipids are needed on a daily basis, then they can be administered as a separate infusion or most commonly as part of a mixture of dextrose and amino acids. These three major nutrients are added together in a 3-l bag in a technique known as *triple mix* or *three-in-one*. In this instance, the entire contents of a single bag are infused during a 24 h period.

With a mixed-fuel system, the rate of infusion of lipid is constant over the infusion period. This method increases the efficiency of fat utilization and may minimize the risk of reticuloendothelial system dysfunction associated with infusion of lipids during the 10 to 12 h period used for intermittent infusion protocols. However, the inclusion of intravenous fat emulsion into a parenteral nutrition admixture changes the conventional nutritional solution into an emulsion. For example, various micronutrients can adversely influence emulsion stability. The higher the cation valence, the greater the destabilizing influence to the emulsifier. Therefore, trivalent cations such as the ferric ion (iron dextran) are more disruptive than divalent cations such as calcium or magnesium ions, which are more disruptive than monovalent cations such as sodium or potassium. Evidence demonstrated that there is no concentration of iron dextran that is safe in triple-mix formulations.[134] In-line filtration is necessary for all parenteral nutrition solutions, including triple-mix solutions, as it is impossible to detect precipitates visually until they are grossly incompatible and unsafe for infusion.

Once the basic solution is created, electrolytes are added as needed (Table 6.13). Sodium or potassium salts are given as chloride or acetate according to the requirements of the individual patient. Normally, equal amounts of chloride and acetate are provided. However, if chloride losses from the body are increased, such as may occur in patients who have NG tubes, then most of the salts should be given as chloride. Similarly, more acetate should be given to patients when additional base is required because acetate generates bicarbonate when it is metabolized. Sodium bicarbonate is incompatible with parenteral nutrition solutions and so cannot be added to the mixture. Phosphate may be given as the sodium or potassium salt. Lipid emulsions contain an additional 15 mmol/l of phosphate.

Commercially available preparations of vitamins, minerals, and trace elements are added to the nutrient mix unless they are contraindicated. Both fat- and water-soluble vitamins should be given. Until recently, a standard 10-ml vial of a multivitamin preparation that contained the recommended doses of vitamins was routinely added to the parenteral nutrition solution[135] (Table 6.14). However, due to a national shortage of this standard preparation, various new vitamin preparations are being introduced into the market. As alluded to, the provision of adequate thiamin is essential for patients receiving parenteral nutrition and can be provided separately. Vitamin K is not a component of any of the vitamin mixtures formulated for adults. Adding vitamin K in the parenteral nutrient solution can satisfy maintenance requirements; 10 mg of vitamin K are given weekly to patients who are not receiving anticoagulants such as warfarin (coumadin).

Trace element preparations that include zinc, copper, manganese, and chromium are added to the parenteral nutrition solution in amounts consistent with the American Medical Association (AMA) guidelines; 60 pg of selenium are also given daily. Because copper and manganese are excreted in the biliary tract, the dosages of these micronutrients should be modified or eliminated in patients with significant liver disease or biliary obstruction. In the absence of clear data in the literature, safe practice would withhold copper and manganese when the patient's serum bilirubin level exceeds 5 mg/dl. Also, 10 to 15 mg/day of zinc are provided to patients whose GI losses are likely to be excessive. Iron is not a part of commercial additive preparations because it is incompatible with triple-mix solutions and may cause anaphylactic reactions when it is given intravenously. Patients who need this trace element should receive it orally or by injection. Iron is not given to the critically ill because hyperferremia can increase bacterial virulence, alter polymorphonuclear cell function, and increase host susceptibility to infection.[134]

TABLE 6.13. Electrolyte Concentrations in Parenteral Nutrition.

Electrolyte	*Recommended central PN doses*	*Recommended peripheral PN doses*	*Usual range of doses*
Potassium (mEq/l)	30	30	0–120 (CVL) 0–80 (PV)
Sodium (mEq/l)	30	30	0–150
Phosphate (mmol/l)	15	5	0–20
Magnesium (mEq/l)	5	5	0–16
Calcium (mEq/l) (as gluconate)	4.7	4.7	0–10
Chloride (mEq/l)	50	50	0–150
Acetate (mEq/l)	40	40	0–100

CVL, central venous line; PN, parenteral nutrition; PV, peripheral vein.

TABLE 6.14. Vitamin and Trace Element Recommendations for Adults.

Vitamin/trace element	*Recommended daily allowance*	*Parenteral requirements*
Vitamin A	4000–5000 IU	3300.0 IU
Vitamin D	400 IU	200.0 IU
Vitamin E	12–15 IU	10.0 IU
Ascorbic acid (C)	60 mg	100.0 mg
Folic acid	400 μg	400.0 μg
Niacin	12–20 mg	40.0 mg
Riboflavin (B_2)	1.1–1.8 mg	3.6 mg
Thiamine (B_1)	1.0–1.5 mg	3.0 mg
Pyridoxine (B_6)	1.6–2.0 mg	4.0 mg
Cyanocobalamin (B_{12})	3 μg	5.0 μg
Pantothenic acid	5–10 mg	15.0 mg
Biotin	150–300 μg	60.0 μg
Zinc	15 mg	2.5–4 mg
Copper	2–3 mg	0.5–1.5 mg
Chromium	0.05–0.2 mg	10–15 μg
Manganese	2.25–5 mg	0.15–1.8 mg
Selenium	0.05–0.2 mg	
Iron	10–15 mg	
Iodine	150 μg	
Fluoride	1.5–4 mg	
Molybdenum	0.15–4 mg	
Cobalt	As part of B_{12} requirements	

Initiation and Maintenance of Infusion: Patient Monitoring

All patients should be metabolically and hemodynamically stable before parenteral nutrition support is begun. Little is known about how vitamin and mineral requirements are changed by disease. In 1979, guidelines for parenteral vitamin and trace element administration were established by the Nutrition Advisory Group of the AMA.[135] The AMA recommendations for daily intravenous intake, as well as the recommended daily allowances, are shown in Table 6.14. It is imperative that patients are provided with adequate vitamins and trace elements while receiving parenteral nutrition.

Patients receiving a carbohydrate load are particularly susceptible to thiamine deficiency. In 1988, several deaths resulted from cardiac failure caused by thiamine deficiency when long-term parenteral nutrition patients did not receive vitamins for a few weeks. Megaloblastic anemia secondary to folate deficiency can occur in parenteral nutrition patients who do not receive folate for several weeks. Selenium is a trace element for which requirements have not been well established, but it nonetheless should be added to solutions for patients receiving prolonged parenteral nutrition. There have been several cases of parenteral nutrition-associated selenium deficiency manifested as cardiomyopathy. Parenteral nutrition-associated deficiencies of copper, zinc, chromium, selenium, and molybdenum have also been reported. There is some evidence to indicate that, in certain disease states, vitamin and mineral requirements are altered because of increased losses, greater utilization, or both.[136] In most instances, vitamin supplementation is accomplished by using single vitamin preparations. For example, higher doses of vitamins A and C are indicated for wound healing, and additional thiamin and folic acid are necessary in patients with alcoholism. As alluded to previously, zinc is required in higher amounts when there are excessive GI losses, as in massive diarrhea from short-bowel syndrome, inflammatory bowel disease, and malabsorption syndromes.

Typically, one initiates parenteral nutrition with up to 2l of the nutrient solution and 500kcal as lipid. However, it may be advisable to start with 1l of parenteral nutrition and then to increase the volume as indicated. Blood glucose concentrations should be less than 200mg/dl, and abnormal electrolyte levels should be corrected, especially for potassium, phosphate, and magnesium, before starting or advancing to the goal nutritional prescription. Obviously, patients with diabetes mellitus may need to be advanced more slowly to prevent severe glucose intolerance. Lipid can be infused as an alternative fuel source to fulfill energy requirements without increasing the glucose infusion rate. The solutions should be administered using a volumetric pump set at a constant rate up to the levels previously specified. It is important not to modify the infusion rate during any given day to try to compensate for excess or inadequate administration of the parenteral nutritional solution. A cyclic schedule (8–16h/day) for patients requiring long-term parenteral nutrition can be initiated once the patient is metabolically stable. Cycling should be done gradually, and the last hour of infusion should be tapered to one-half the maintenance infusion rate to prevent rebound hypoglycemia.

Before central parenteral alimentation is discontinued, the volume of infusion should be decreased by at least half to avoid adverse effects that may occur secondary to relative hyperinsulinemia if the body is not allowed sufficient time to equilibrate. In emergency situations when the central parenteral nutrition solution must be suddenly discontinued, 10% dextrose should be given at the same infusion rate as was used for the parenteral nutrition unless there is severe hyperglycemia. When patients who are receiving parenteral nutrition require a surgical operation, one can continue to administer the solution through the procedure, but decreasing the infusion rate may make circulating glucose and electrolyte levels easier to control, especially in patients with glucose intolerance or other severe organ dysfunction.

During the initiation of central parenteral nutrition, serum chemistries must be monitored frequently. Once the patient has stabilized on his or her individual nutritional prescription, blood samples should be obtained at least twice weekly to measure chloride, CO_2, potassium, sodium, BUN, creatinine, calcium, and phosphate levels and once weekly for liver function tests and albumin, total protein, uric acid, magnesium, and triglyceride levels. Patients should be weighed each day on the same scale. Urine or blood should be tested for sugar and acetone every 6h initially and until blood glucose concentrations are stable. Electrolytes and other medications should be added only by the pharmacist when the parenteral nutrition solution is prepared. Numerous common metabolic abnormalities may arise during the course of parenteral (or enteral) nutrition. Several of these are outlined in Table 6.15.

Parenteral Nutrition for Patients with Abnormal Organ Function

Diabetes Mellitus

Control of blood glucose levels is important for all patients who receive parenteral nutrition. However, regulation may be especially difficult in patients who are known to have diabetes or in patients who develop insulin resistance in response to severe stress or infection. If blood glucose levels are not maintained at less than 200mg/dl, then immune function is likely to be impaired, and patients may be at increased risk for infection.[137–139] In the insulin-dependent patient, the same amount of insulin that would normally be taken is added to the parenteral nutrition solution on the first day. Because as much as one-half of the insulin given binds to the container and intravenous tubing, the insulin given in this manner is almost always an underestimate of actual requirements. For example, if a patient's normal dose of regular insulin is 40U/day for a 2000-kcal diet, then 20U should be added to a parenteral nutrition solution of 1000kcal. Thereafter, blood glucose concentrations obtained by finger-stick or blood sampling are determined every 6h, and a sliding scale for subcutaneous regular insulin is used to provide supplementary insulin doses as needed. For the next day, one-half or all the insulin given on the previous day according to the sliding scale is added to the parenteral nutrition solution, depending on the level of control that is required.

For nondiabetic patients who develop hyperglycemia, a similar procedure is used by which a sliding scale estimates the amount of insulin that is needed to maintain blood glucose levels below 200mg/dl, and one-half this amount is then added to the next day's parenteral nutrition orders.

Acute Renal Failure

In general, most patients with acute renal failure are catabolic with elevated energy requirements. Calories should be provided in sufficient quantities to minimize protein degradation. Energy requirements can generally be met with the provision of 35 to 40kcal/kg dry weight. Protein should be provided in the range of 1.2 to 1.5g/kg/day with a standard solution containing both essential and nonessential amino acids. Traditionally, formulas designed for renal failure contained predominantly essential amino acids. However, there is no conclusive data to show that special formulas containing essential amino acids only are superior to the less-expensive standard formulations containing both nonessential and essential amino acids. Moreover, the provision of nonessential amino acids may enhance protein synthesis and nitrogen retention. A balance of fat and carbohydrate should be provided. Lipid emulsions can be used as a source of concentrated energy in the patients who are fluid restricted. The contribution of fat to the total caloric intake should be no more than

TABLE 6.15. Possible Etiologies and Treatment of Common Complications of Central Parenteral Nutrition.

Problem	*Possible etiology*	*Treatment*
Glucose		
Hyperglycemia, glycosuria, hyperosmolar nonketotic dehydration or coma	Excessive dose or rate of infusion; inadequate insulin production; steroid administration; infection	Decrease the amount of glucose given; increase insulin; administer a portion of calories as fat
Diabetic ketoacidosis	Inadequate endogenous insulin production and/or inadequate insulin therapy	Give insulin; decrease glucose intake
Rebound hypoglycemia	Persistent endogenous insulin production by islet cells after long-term high carbohydrate infusion	Give 5%–10% glucose before total parenteral infusion is discontinued
Hypercarbia	Carbohydrate load exceeds the ability to increase minute ventilation and excrete excess CO_2	Limit glucose dose to 5 mg/kg/min. Give greater percentage of total caloric needs as fat (up to 30%–40%)
Fat		
Hypertriglyceridemia	Rapid infusion; decreased clearance	Decrease rate of infusion; allow clearance (approximately 12 h) before testing blood
Essential fatty acid	Inadequate essential fatty acid administration efficiency	Administer essential fatty acids in doses of 4%–7% of total calories
Amino acids		
Hyperchloremia metabolic acidosis	Excessive chloride content of amino acid solutions	Administer Na^+ and K^+ as acetate salts
Prerenal azotemia	Excessive amino acids with inadequate caloric supplementation calories	Reduce amino acids; increase the amount of glucose
Miscellaneous		
Hypophosphatemia	Inadequate phosphorus administration with redistribution into tissues	Give 15 mm phosphate/1000 i.v. evaluate antacid and Ca^{2+}; administration
Hypomagnesemia	Inadequate administration relative to increased losses (diarrhea, diuresis, medications)	Administer Mg^{2+} (15–20 mEq/1000 kcal)
Hypermagnesemia	Excessive administration; renal failure	Decrease Mg^{2+} supplementation
Hypokalemia	Inadequate intake relative to increased needs for anabolism; diuresis	Increase K^+ supplementation
Hyperkalemia	Excessive administration, especially in metabolic acidosis; renal decompensation	Reduce or stop exogenous K^1; if EKG changes are present, treat with Ca gluconate, insulin, diuretics
Hypocalcemia	Inadequate administration; reciprocal response to phosphorus repletion without simultaneous calcium infusion	Increase Ca^{2+} dose
Hypercalcemia	Excessive administration; excess vitamin D administration	Decrease Ca^{2+} and/or vitamin D administration
Elevated liver transaminases or serum alkaline phosphatase and bilirubin	Enzyme induction secondary to amino acid imbalances or overfeeding	Reevaluate nutritional prescription

30%, while the remainder of the caloric requirements is provided by glucose.

Fluid and electrolyte balances are often impaired in patients with acute renal failure. Potassium, phosphate, and magnesium levels must be monitored carefully, and these should be added to parenteral nutrition if blood levels fall. Acetate salts of potassium or sodium can be administered to help correct a metabolic acidosis. Standard doses of the water-soluble vitamins and additional folic acid (1 mg/day total) should be added to the solution of patients who are undergoing dialysis because these substances are lost from the body in the dialysate bath. The supplementation of fat-soluble vitamins is usually not required, especially in patients who are also eating, because excretion is reduced in renal failure. In anuric patients, trace elements are not added to the nutrient solutions. However, for patients who require prolonged parenteral nutrition support and are dialyzed, trace elements and fat-soluble vitamins should be replaced. The various ultrafiltration techniques are also associated with highly variable but increased amino acid losses in the dialysate. In these instances, additional protein may be required to meet the patient's estimated needs. However, a portion of the patient's nonprotein calorie needs may be met by the dextrose contained in replacement solutions.

Hepatic Dysfunction and Liver Failure

Protein intake for patients with stable chronic liver disease depends on the patient's nutritional status and protein tolerance. Nutritionally depleted patients may require as much as 1.5 g of protein per kilogram estimated dry weight. However, protein intake may need to be decreased in patients with liver failure and encephalopathy. Protein-sensitive encephalopathic patients should be given 0.5 to 0.7 g protein per kilogram per day and increased gradually to 1.0 to 1.5 g/kg/day if possible. These patients have altered plasma amino acid profiles with increased concentrations of aromatic amino acids (phenylalanine, tyrosine, and tryptophan) and methionine and decreased BCAAs (valine, leucine, and isoleucine).

Fluid restriction may be necessary in some patients with ascites and edema. In this instance, the concentration of dextrose can be increased to maintain the number of calories administered as carbohydrate. The amount of sodium given is reduced because these patients excrete nearly sodium-free urine. As mentioned, administration of trace elements is often contraindicated because a major route of excretion for these substances, such as copper and manganese, is via the biliary system. Zinc deficiency is common in cirrhotic patients, and supplementation of this mineral may be necessary, especially if there are excessive GI losses.

Other Conditions and Nutritional Treatments

The catabolism of major surgery, trauma, burns, and sepsis is characterized by a net breakdown of body protein stores to provide substrates for gluconeogenesis and acute-phase protein synthesis. The provision of adequate nutrition can attenuate whole-body catabolism but rarely if ever prevents or reverses loss of lean body mass using conventional management principles during the acute phase of injury. Several new strategies to accomplish this are under investigation; these include the administration of hormones or growth factors and the provision of conditionally essential amino acids, such as glutamine.

Growth hormone administration to patients increases the rate of wound healing and decreases wound infection rates, hospital stays, and perhaps the catabolism and muscle wasting associated with critical illness as well. However, growth hormone is a very expensive therapy. Furthermore, preliminary data suggest that it may be harmful to some critically ill patients.[140] For these reasons, other agents, such as oxandrolone (Oxandrin) are being pursued to induce positive nitrogen balance and enhance wound healing in critically ill patients. The use of growth factors currently remains investigational in acute care settings. The use of adjuvant anabolic agents should be reserved for patients who have not responded to aggressive nutrition support but whose underlying disease processes are controlled.

Common Complications and Their Management

Catheter Sepsis

Catheter sepsis is a very serious complication associated with central venous alimentation. Primary catheter sepsis occurs when there are signs and symptoms of infection, and the indwelling catheter is the only anatomical focus of infection. Secondary catheter infections are associated with another focus or multiple infectious foci that cause bacteremia and seed the catheter.

Management of the patients with catheter infection depends on their clinical condition. If extremely ill patients with high fevers are hypotensive or have local signs of infection around the catheter site, then the catheter should be removed, its tip cultured, and peripheral and central venous blood cultures obtained. In primary catheter sepsis, signs and symptoms should return to normal quickly. The organisms that grow from the catheter tip are the same as the ones that are identified in peripheral blood culture. Usually, more than 1×10^3 organisms are grown from cultures of the catheter tip.

Specific therapy should be initiated against the primary source in patients in whom a source of infection other than the catheter tip is present. Peripheral blood cultures are obtained. One should avoid taking blood cultures from the central venous catheter port dedicated for parenteral nutrition because this increases the risk of contaminating the line. If the infection resolves, then central venous feedings can be continued. If a secondary source is not identified and the symptoms persist, then the catheter should be removed, and its tip should be cultured. If the catheter tip culture returns positive or if the index of suspicion is high, then appropriate antibiotic therapy is initiated. Central venous feeding can be resumed, maintaining blood glucose levels below 200 mg/dl.

Occasionally, the situation arises in which a site of infection other than the catheter is identified, but signs and symptoms persist despite what is assumed to be adequate therapy. As before, if blood cultures are positive, the safest course of action may be to remove the catheter. If peripheral blood cultures are negative, then the catheter may be changed over a guidewire and the catheter tip cultured to determine if it was contaminated. Central venous feedings can be continued during this interval if the patient is stable. If the catheter tip returns a positive culture, then a new catheter should be inserted at a different site. Changing the central venous catheter over a guidewire can also facilitate the diagnosis of primary catheter infections.

Other Complications

Complications of central venous alimentation are usually related to excess administration or underadministration of the energy sources, electrolytes, or trace metals. The etiologies of some common complications and treatment options are outlined in Table 6.15.

Prolonged administration of parenteral nutrition may result in altered hepatic function tests and changes in liver pathological conditions that can lead to liver failure. Initially (1–2 weeks after initiation of parenteral nutrition), serum transaminases may be elevated. These abnormalities frequently resolve without any change in the composition or rate of parenteral nutrition administration. However, in patients receiving long-term (>20 days) parenteral nutrition, serum transaminase levels may remain elevated, even after parenteral nutrition support is discontinued. Serum levels of alkaline phosphatase and bilirubin may also increase in some patients who receive long-term parenteral nutrition. Patients who do not receive some lipid as part of their parenteral nutrition may have more frequent and severe hepatic abnormalities. The provision of excess glucose increases insulin secretion, which stimulates hepatic lipogenesis and results in hepatic fat accumulation. Fatty infiltration is the initial histopathological change; it is readily reversible and may not be accompanied by altered liver function. Longer parenteral nutrition therapy may be associated with cholestasis and nonspecific triaditis and may progress to active chronic hepatitis, fibrosis, and eventual cirrhosis. The management of parenteral nutrition-related liver dysfunction is summarized in Table 6.15.

References

1. McCamish MA, Bounous G, Geraghty ME. History of enteral feeding: past and present perspectives. In: Rombeau JL, Rolandelli RH, eds. Clinical Nutrition: Enteral and Tube Feeding, 3rd ed. Philadelphia: Saunders, 1997:1–11.

2. Dudrick SJ, Wilmore DW, Vars HM, et al. Long-term total parenteral nutrition with growth, development, and positive nitrogen balance. Surgery (St. Louis) 1968;64:134–136.
3. Hunter J. A case of paralysis of the muscles of deglutition cured by an artificial mode of conveying food and medicines into the stomach. Trans Soc Improve Med Chir Know 1793;1:182–186.
4. Bliss DW. Feeding per rectum: as illustrated in the case of the late President Garfield and others. Med Rec 1882;22:64–66.
5. Rhoads JE. Diuretics as an adjuvant in disposing of extra water as a vehicle in parenteral hyperalimentation [abstract]. Fed Proc 1962;21:389–391.
6. Wilmore DW, Dudrick SJ. Growth and development of an infant receiving all nutrients exclusively by vein. JAMA 1968;203:860–863.
7. Kudsk KA, Carpenter G, Petersen S, et al. Effect of enteral and parenteral feeding in malnourished rats with *E. coli*-hemoglobin adjuvant peritonitis. J Surg Res 1981;31:105–110.
8. Wolfe BM, Mathiesen KA. Clinical practice guidelines in nutrition support: can they be based on randomized clinical trials? J Parenter Enteral Nutr 1997;27:1–6.
9. Wolfe BM, Ryder MA, Nishikawa RA, et al. Complications of parenteral nutrition. Am J Surg 1986;152:93–99.
10. Klein S, Kinney J, Jeejeebhoy K, et al. Nutrition support in clinical practice: review of published data and recommendations for future research directions. J Parenter Enteral Nutr 1997;21:133–156.
11. Kudsk KA. Dear Miss Milk Toast [1998 Presidential Address—ASPEN]. J Parenter Enteral Nutr 1998;22:191–198.
12. Nightingale JMD, Lennard-Jones JE, Walter ER, et al. Jejunal efflux in the short bowel syndrome. Lancet 1990;336:765–768.
13. Winsor JA, Hill GL. Risk factors for postoperative pneumonia: the importance of protein depletion. Ann Surg 1988;208:209–214.
14. Jeejeebhoy KN. Assessment of nutritional status. In: Rombeau JL, Caldwell MD, eds. Clinical Nutrition: Enteral and Tube Feeding. Philadelphia: Saunders, 1990:118–126.
15. Blackburn GL, Bistrian BR, Maini BS, et al. Nutritional and metabolic assessment of the hospitalized patient. J Parenter Enteral Nutr 1977;1:11–22.
16. Kudsk KA, Minard G, Wojtysiak SL, et al. Visceral protein response to enteral versus parenteral nutrition and sepsis in trauma patients. Surgery (St. Louis) 1994;116:516–523.
17. Buzby GP, Mullen JL, Mathews DC, et al. Prognostic nutritional index in gastrointestinal surgery. Am J Surg 1980;139:160–167.
18. Niederman MS, Mantivonni R, Schoch P, et al. Patterns and routes of tracheobronchial colonization in mechanically ventilated patients. Chest 1989;95:155–161.
19. Ingenbleek Y, Carpentier YA. A prognostic inflammatory and nutritional index scoring critically ill patients. Int J Vitam Nutr Res 1984;55:91–101.
20. Detsky AS, McLaughlin JR, Baker JP, et al. What is subjective global assessment of nutritional status? J Parenter Enteral Nutr 1987;11:8–13.
21. Pikul J, Sharp MD, Lowndes R, et al. Degree of preoperative malnutrition is predictive of postoperative morbidity and mortality in liver transplant patients. Transplantation (Baltimore) 1994;57:469–471.
22. Enia G, Sicuso C, Alati G, et al. A subjective global assessment of nutrition in dialysis patient. Nephrol Dial Transplant 1993;8:1094–1098.
23. The Veteran Affairs Total Parenteral Nutrition Cooperative Study Group. Perioperative total parenteral nutrition in surgical patients. N Engl J Med 1991;325:525–532.
24. Fan St, Lo CM, Lai EC, et al. Perioperative nutritional support in patients undergoing hepatectomy for hepatocellular carcinoma. N Engl J Med 1994;331:1547–1552.
25. Brennan MF, Pisters PWT, Posner M, et al. A prospective, randomized trial of total parenteral nutrition after major pancreatic resection for malignancy. Ann Surg 1994;220:436–444.
26. Heslin MJ, Latkany L, Leung D, et al. A prospective, randomized trial of early enteral feeding after resection of upper gastrointestinal malignancy. Ann Surg 1997;226:567–577.
27. Doglietto GB, Gallitelli L, Pacelli F, et al. Protein-sparing therapy after major abdominal surgery: lack of clinical effects. Ann Surg 1996;223:357–362.
28. Watters JM, Kirkpatrick SM, Norris SB, et al. Immediate postoperative enteral feeding results in impaired respiratory mechanics and decreased mobility. Ann Surg 1997;226:369–377.
29. Daly JM, Lieberman MD, Goldfine J, et al. Enteral nutrition with supplemental arginine, RNA, and omega-3 fatty acids in patients after operation: immunologic, metabolic, and clinical outcome. Surgery (St. Louis) 1992;112:56–67.
30. Daly JM, Weintraub FN, Shou J, et al. Enteral nutrition during multimodality therapy in upper gastrointestinal cancer patients. Ann Surg 1995;221:327–338.
31. Vascow MD, Rawlings J, Ellison S. Benefits of supplementary tube feeding after fractured neck of femur: a randomized, controlled study. Br Med J 1983;187:1589–1592.
32. Delmi M, Rapin C-H, Bengoa J-M, et al. Dietary supplementation in elderly patients with fractured neck of the femur. Lancet 1990;335:1013–1016.
33. Moore EE, Jones TN. Benefits of immediate jejunostomy feeding after major abdominal trauma—a prospective, randomized study. J Trauma 1986;26:874–879.
34. Moore FA, Moore EE, Jones TN, et al. TEN versus TPN following major abdominal trauma—reduced septic morbidity. J Trauma 1989;29:916–923.
35. Kudsk KA, Croce MA, Fabian TC, et al. Enteral versus parenteral feeding. Effects on septic morbidity after blunt and penetrating abdominal trauma. Ann Surg 1992;215:503–511.
36. Kudsk KA, Minard G, Croce MA, et al. A randomized trial of isonitrogenous enteral diets after severe trauma. An immune-enhancing diet reduces septic complications. Ann Surg 1996;224:531–540.
37. Chuntrasakul C, Siltham S, Sarasombath S, et al. Comparison of a immunonutrition formula enriched arginine, glutamine and omega-3 fatty acid, with a currently high-enriched enteral nutrition for trauma patients. J Med Assoc Thai 2003;86(6):552–561.
38. Rapp RP, Young B, Twym D, et al. The favorable effect of early parenteral feeding on survival in head injured patients. J Neurosurg 1983;58:906–911.
39. Hadley MN, Grahm TW, Harrington T, et al. Nutritional support in neurotrauma: a critical review of early nutrition in 45 acute head injury patients. Neurosurgery (Baltim) 1986;19:367–373.
40. Young B, Ott L, Twyman D, et al. The effect of nutritional support on outcome from severe head injury. Neurosurgery (Baltim) 1987;67:668–676.
41. Grahm TW, Zadrozny DB, Harrington T. The benefits of early jejunal hyperalimentation in the head-injured patient. Neurosurgery (Baltim) 1989;25:729–735.
42. Borzotta AP, Penning S, Papasadero B, et al. Enteral versus parenteral nutrition after severe closed head injury. J Trauma 1994;37:459–468.
43. Beier-Holgersen R, Boesby S. Influence of postoperative enteral nutrition on postsurgical infections. Gut 1996;39:833–835.
44. Shirabe K, Matsumata T, Shimada M, et al. A comparison of parenteral hyperalimentation and early enteral feeding regarding systemic immunity after major hepatic resection—the results of a randomized prospective study. Hepatogastroenterology 1997;44:205–209.
45. Gianotti L, Braga M, Vignali A, et al. Effect of route of delivery and formulation of postoperative nutritional support in patients

undergoing major operations for malignant neoplasms. Arch Surg 1997;132:1222–1229.
46. Sand J, Luostarinen M, Matikainen M. Enteral or parenteral feeding after total gastrectomy: prospective randomized pilot study. Eur J Surg 1997;163:761–766.
47. Hochwald SN, Harrison LE, Heslin MJ, et al. Early postoperative enteral feeding improves whole body protein kinetics in upper gastrointestinal cancer patients. Am J Surg 1997;174:325–330.
48. Gonzalez-Huix F, Fernandez-Banares F, Esteve-Comas M, et al. Enteral versus parenteral nutrition as adjunct therapy in acute ulcerative colitis. Am J Gastroenterol 1993;88:227–232.
49. Gonzalez-Huix F, de Leon R, Fernandez-Banares F, et al. Polymeric enteral diets as primary treatment of active Crohn's disease: a prospective steroid controlled trial. Gut 1993;34:778–782.
50. Wicks C, Somasundaram S, Bjarnason I, et al. Comparison of enteral feeding and total parenteral nutrition after liver transplantation. Lancet 1994;344:837–840.
51. Hasse JM, Blue LS, Liepa GU, et al. Early enteral nutrition support in patients undergoing liver transplantation. J Parenter Enteral Nutr 1995;19:437–443.
52. McClave SA, Greene LM, Snider HL, et al. Comparison of the safety of early enteral nutrition versus parenteral nutrition in mild acute pancreatitis. J Parenter Enteral Nutr 1997;21:14–20.
53. Windsor AC, Kanwar S, Li AG, et al. Compared with parenteral nutrition, enteral feeding attenuates the acute phase response and improves disease severity in acute pancreatitis. Gut 1998;42:431–435.
54. Pupelis G, Selga G, Austrums E, et al. Jejunal feeding, even when instituted late, improves outcomes in patients with severe pancreatitis and peritonitis. Nutrition 2001;17:91–94.
55. Olah A, Pardavi G, Belagyi T, et al. Early nasojejunal feeding in acute pancreatitis is associated with a lower complication rate. Nutrition 2002;18:259–262.
56. Abou-Assi S, Craig K, O'Keefe SJ. Hypocaloric jejunal feeding is better than total parenteral nutrition in acute pancreatitis: results of a randomized comparative study. Am J Gastr 2002;97:2255–2262.
57. McDonald WS, Sharp CW Jr, Deitch EA. Immediate enteral feeding in burn patients is safe and effective. Ann Surg 1991;213:177–183.
58. Jones TN, Moore FA, Moore EE, et al. Gastrointestinal symptoms attributed to jejunostomy feeding after major abdominal trauma—a critical analysis. Crit Care Med 1989;17:1146–1150.
59. Souba WW, Smith RJ, Wilmore DW. Glutamine metabolism by the intestinal tract. J Parenter Enteral Nutr 1985;9:608–617.
60. Kudsk K, Minard G, Croce MA, et al. A randomized trial of isonitrogenous enteral diets after severe trauma. An immune-enhancing diet reduces septic complications. Ann Surg 1996;224:531–540.
61. Moore FA, Moore EE, Kudsk KA, et al. Clinical benefits of an immune-enhancing diet for early postinjury enteral feeding. J Trauma 1994;37:607–615.
62. Ziegler TR, Young LS, Benfell K, et al. Clinical and metabolic efficacy of glutamine-supplemented parenteral nutrition after bone marrow transplantation. A randomized, double-blind, controlled study. Ann Intern Med 1992;116:821–828.
63. MacBurney M, Young LS, Ziegler TR, et al. A cost-evaluation of glutamine-supplemented parenteral nutrition in adult bone marrow transplant patients. J Am Diet Assoc 1994;94:1263–1266.
64. Tremel H, Kienle B, Weilemann LS, et al. Glutamine dipeptide-supplemented parenteral nutrition maintains intestinal function in the critically ill. Gastroenterology 1994;107:1595–1601.
65. Griffiths RD, Jones C, Palmer TE. Six-month outcome of critically ill patients given glutamine-supplemented parenteral nutrition. Nutrition 1997;13:297–302.
66. van der Hulst RR, von Meyenfeldt MF, Tiebosch A, et al. Glutamine and intestinal immune cells in humans. J Parenter Enteral Nutr 1997;21:310–315.
67. Ziegler TR, Bye RL, Persinger RL, et al. Effects of glutamine supplementation on circulating lymphocytes after bone marrow transplantation: a pilot study. Am J Med Sci 1998;315:4–10.
68. Kirk SJ, Barbul A. Role of arginine in trauma, sepsis, and immunity. J Parenter Enter Nutr 1990;14:226S.
69. Gianotti L, Alexander JW, Pyles T, et al. Arginine-supplemented diet improves survival in gut-derived sepsis and peritonitis by modulating bacterial clearance. Ann Surg 1993;217:644–654.
70. Barbul A. Arginine: biochemistry, physiology, and therapeutic implications. J Parenter Enteral Nutr 1986;10:227–238.
71. Kinsella JE, Lokesh B, Broughton S, Whelan J. Dietary polyunsaturated fatty acids and eicosanoids: potential effect on the modulation of inflammatory and immune cells: an overview. Nutrition 1990;6:24–44.
72. Alexander JW, Saito H, Trocki O, et al. The importance of lipid type in the diet after burn injury. Ann Surg 1986;204:1–8.
73. Fanslow WC, Kulkarni AD, Van Buren CT, et al. Effect of nucleotide restriction and supplementation on resistance to supplemental murine candidiasis. J Parenter Enteral Nutr 1988;12:49–52.
74. Schilling J, Vranjes N, Fierz W, et al. Clinical outcome and immunology of postoperative arginine, omega-3 fatty acids, and nucleotide-enriched enteral feeding: a randomized prospective comparison with standard enteral and low calorie/low fat i.v. solutions. Nutrition 1996;12:423–429.
75. Saffle JR, Wiedke G, Jennings K, et al. A randomized trial of immune-enhancing enteral nutrition in burn patients. J Trauma 1997;42:793–802.
76. Senkal M, Mumme A, Eickhoff U, et al. Early postoperative enteral immunonutrition: clinical outcome and cost-comparison analysis in surgical patients. Crit Care Med 1997;25:1489–1496.
77. Gianotti L, Braga M, Gentilini O, et al. Artificial nutrition after pancreaticoduodenectomy. Pancreas 2002;21:344–351
78. Braga M, Gianotti L, Nespoli L, et al. Nutritional approach in malnourished surgical patients: a prospective randomized study. Arch Surg 2002;137:174–180.
79. Gottschlich MM, Jenkins M, Warden G, et al. Differential effects of three enteral dietary regimens on selected outcome variables in burn patients. J Parenter Enteral Nutr 1990;14:225–236.
80. Mendez C. Effects of an immune-enhancing diet in critically injured patients. J Trauma 1997;42:933–941.
81. Bower RH, Cerra FB, Bershadsky B, et al. Early enteral administration of a formula (Impact) supplemented with arginine, nucleotides, and fish oil in intensive care unit patients: results of a multicenter, prospective, randomized, clinical trial. Crit Care Med 1995;23:436–449.
82. Atkinson S, Sieffert E, Bihari D. A prospective randomized, double-blind controlled clinical trial of enteral immunonutrition in the critically ill. Crit Care Med 1998;26:1164–1172.
83. Heyland DK, Novak F. Immunonutrition in the critically ill patient: more harm than good. J Parenter Enteral Nutr 2001 25(2 suppl):S51–S55; discussion S55–S56.
84. Ochoa JB, Makarenkova V, Bansal V. A rational use of immune enhancing diets: when should we use dietary arginine supplementation? Nutr Clin Prac 2004;19:216–225.
85. Jacobs DG, Jacobs DO, Kudsk KA, et al. Practice management guidelines for nutritional support of the trauma patient. J Trauma 2004;57:660–679.
86. Schloerb PR, Amare M. Total parenteral nutrition with glutamine in bone marrow transplantation and other clinical applications (a randomized, double-blind study). J Parenter Enteral Nutr 1993;17:407–413.

87. van der Hulst RRWJ, von Meyenfeldt MF, van Kreel BK, et al. Glutamine and the preservation of gut integrity. Lancet 1993; 334:1363–1365.
88. Smith RC, Mackie W, Kohlhardt SR, Kee AJ. The effect on protein and amino acid metabolism of an intravenous nutrition regimen providing 70% of nonprotein calories as lipid. Surgery (St. Louis) 1992;111:12–20.
89. de Chalain TM, Mitchell WL, O'Keefe SJ, et al. The effect of fuel source on amino acid metabolism in critically ill patients. J Surg Res 1992;52:167–176.
90. Chassard D, Guiraud M, Gauthier J, et al. Effects of intravenous medium-chain triglycerides on pulmonary gas exchanges in mechanically ventilated patients. Crit Care Med 1994;22:248–251.
91. Kohlhardt SR, Smith RC, Kee AJ. Metabolic response to a high-lipid, high-nitrogen peripheral intravenous nutrition solution after major upper-gastrointestinal surgery. Nutrition 1994; 10:317–326.
92. Roulet M, Frascarolo P, Pilet M, et al. Effects of intravenously infused fish oil on platelet fatty acid phospholipid composition and on platelet function in postoperative trauma. J Parenter Enteral Nutr 1997;21:296–301.
93. Tappy L, Schwarz JM, Schneiter P, et al. Effects of isoenergetic glucose-based or lipid-based parenteral nutrition on glucose metabolism, de novo lipogenesis, and respiratory gas exchanges in critically ill patients. Crit Care Med 1998;26:813–814.
94. Novak F, Heyland DK, Avenell A, et al. Glutamine supplementation in serious illness: a systematic review of the evidence. Crit Care Med 2003;30:2022–2029.
95. Miskovitz P. Glutamine supplementation in critically ill and elective surgery patients: does the evidence warrant its use? Crit Care Med 2003;30:2152–2153.
96. Deitch EA. Does the gut protect or injure patients in the ICU? Perspect Crit Care 1988;1:1–31.
97. Moore FA, Moore EE, Poggetti R, et al. Gut bacterial translocation via the portal vein: a clinical perspective with major torso trauma. Trauma 1991;31:629–638.
98. Johnson LR, Copeland EM, Dudrick SJ, et al. Structural and hormonal alterations in the gastrointestinal tract of parenteral fed rats. Gastroenterology 1975;68:1177–1183.
99. Purandare S, Offenbartl K, Westrom B, et al. Increased gut permeability to fluorescein isothiocyanate–dextran after total parenteral nutrition in rat. Scand J Gastroenterol 1989;24:678–682.
100. McGhee JR, Mestecky J, Dertzbaugh MT, et al. The mucosal immune system: from fundamental concepts to vaccine development. Vaccine 1992;10:75–88.
101. Li J, Kudsk KA, Gocinski B, et al. Effects of parenteral nutrition on gut-associated lymphoid tissue. J Trauma 1995;39:44.
102. Tomasi TB Jr. Mechanisms of immune regulation at mucosal surfaces. Rev Infect Dis 1983;5:S784.
103. Kudsk KA, Li J, Renegar KB. Loss of upper respiratory tract immunity with parenteral feeding. Ann Surg 1996;223:629–638.
104. Li J, Kudsk KA, Janu P, Renegar KB. Effect of glutamine-enriched TPN on small intestine gut-associated lymphoid tissue (GALT) and upper respiratory tract immunity. Surgery (St. Louis) 1997; 121:542–549.
105. Lin M-T, Saito H, Fukushima R, et al. Route of nutritional supply influences local, systemic, and remote organ responses to intraperitoneal bacterial challenge. Ann Surg 1996;223:84–93.
106. Fong Y, Marano MA, Barber E, et al. Total parenteral nutrition and bowel rest modify the metabolic response to endotoxin in humans. Ann Surg 1989;210:449–457.
107. Hunter DC, Jaksik T, Lewis D, et al. Resting energy expenditure in the critically ill: estimations versus measurement. Br J Surg 1988;75:875–878.
108. Hwang T-L, Hwang S-L, Chen M-F. The use of indirect colorimetry in critically ill patients—relationship with measured energy expenditure to injury severity score, a septic severity score, and Apache II score. J Trauma 1993;34:247–251.
109. Choban PS, Burge JC, Flancbaum L. Nutrition support of obese hospitalized patients. Nutr Clin Prac 1997;12:149–154.
110. Harris JA, Benedict FG. A Biometric Study of Basal Metabolism in Man. Publication 279. Washington, DC: Carnegie Institution, 1919.
111. Garrel DR, Jobin N, deJonge LHM. Should we still use the Harris and Benedict equations? Nutr Clin Pract 1996;11:99–103.
112. Weir JB de V. New methods for calculating metabolic rate with special reference to protein metabolism. J Physiol (Camb) 1949; 109:1–9.
113. Campbell SM, Kudsk KA. "High tech" metabolic measurements: useful in daily clinical practice? J Parenter Enteral Nutr 1988;12:610–612.
114. Food and Nutrition Board, National Research Council. Recommended Dietary Allowances, 10th ed. Washington, DC: National Academy of Sciences, 1989.
115. Kudsk KA, Teasley-Strausburg KM. Enteral and parenteral nutrition. In: Irwin RS, Cerra FB, Rippe JM, eds. Intensive Care Medicine, 4th ed. New York: Lippincott-Raven, 1998.
116. Wolfe RR, Shaw JHF. Glucose and FFA in kinetics in sepsis: role of glucagon and sympathetic nervous system activity. Am J Physiol 1985;248:E236–E243.
117. Pomposelli JJ, Baxter JK, Babineau TJ, et al. Early postoperative glucose control predicts nosocomial infection rate in diabetic patients. J Parenter Enteral Nutr 1998;22:77–81.
118. van den Berghe G, Wouters P, Weekers F, et al. Intensive insulin therapy in the critically ill patients. N Engl J Med 2001;8;345:1359–1367.
119. Pelham LD. Rational use of intravenous fat emulsions. Am J Hosp Pharm 1981;38:198–208.
120. Kinsella JE, Lokesh B, Broughton S. Dietary polyunsaturated fatty acids and eicosanoids: potential effect on the modulation of inflammatory and immune cells: an overview. Nutrition 1990;6:24–44.
121. Allardyce DB. Cholestasis caused by lipid emulsions. Surg Gynecol Obstet 1982;154:641–647.
122. Fonkalsrud E. Surgical treatment of gastroesophageal reflux (GER) syndrome in infants and children. Am J Surg 1987;154:11–18.
123. Collier P, Kudsk KA, Glezer J, et al. Fiber-containing formula and needle catheter jejunostomies: a clinical evaluation. Nutr Clin Pract 1994;9:101–103.
124. Dent D, Kudsk K, Minard G, et al. Risk of abdominal septic complications following feeding jejunostomy placement in patients undergoing splenectomy for trauma. Am J Surg 1993; 166:686–689.
125. Smith-Choban T, Max MH. Feeding jejunostomy: a small bowel stress test. Am J Surg 1988;155:112–117.
126. Adams S, Dellinger EP, Wertz MJ, et al. Enteral versus parenteral nutritional support following laparotomy for trauma: a randomized prospective trial. J Trauma 1986;26:882–891.
127. Smith CD, Sarr MG. Clinically significant pneumatosis intestinalis with postoperative enteral feeding by needle catheter jejunostomy: an unusual complication. J Parenter Enteral Nutr 1991;15:328–331.
128. Guenter PA, Settle RG, Perlmutter S, et al. Tube feeding-related diarrhea in acutely ill patients. J Parenter Enteral Nutr 1991; 15:277–280.
129. Edes TE, Walk BE, Austin JL. Diarrhea in tube-fed patients: feeding formula not necessarily the cause. Am J Med 1990;88:91–93.
130. Solomon SM, Kirby DF. The refeeding syndrome: a review. J Parenter Enteral Nutr 1990;14:90–97.

131. Pemberton LB, Lyman B, Lander V, et al. Sepsis from triple- versus single-lumen catheters during total parenteral nutrition in surgical or critically ill patients. Arch Surg 1986;121:591.
132. Miller JJ, Venus B, Mathru M. Comparison of the sterility of long-term central venous catheterization using single lumen, triple lumen, and pulmonary artery catheters. Crit Care Med 1984;12:634.
133. Pomposelli JJ, Bistrian BR. Is total parenteral nutrition immunosuppressive? New Horiz (US) 1994;2:224–229.
134. Kumpf VJ. Parenteral iron supplementation. Nutr Clin Pract 1996;11:139–146.
135. American Medical Association Department of Foods and Nutrition, 1975. Multivitamin preparations for parenteral use: a statement by the Nutrition Advisory Group. J Parenter Enteral Nutr 1979;3:258–262.
136. De Biasse MA, Wilmore DW. What is optimal nutritional support? New Horiz 1994;2:122–130.
137. Kwoun MO, Ling PR, Lydon E, et al. Immunologic effects of acute hyperglycemia in nondiabetic rats. J Parenter Enteral Nutr 1997;21:91–95.
138. Delamaire M, Maugendre D, Moreno M, et al. Impaired leucocyte functions in diabetic patients. Diabetes Med 1997;14:29–34.
139. Alexiewicz JM, Kumar D, Smogorzewski M, et al. Polymorphonuclear leukocytes in non-insulin dependent diabetes mellitus: abnormalities in metabolism and function. Ann Intern Med 1995;123:919–924.
140. Pharmacia and Upjohn. Safety Statement From Pharmacia and Upjohn Regarding the Use of Recombinant Somatropin (Genotropin/Genotonorm) for Treatment of Acute Catabolism in Critically Ill Patients. Pharmacia/Upjohn: Kalamazoo, MI, 1997.
141. Brown RO, Hunt H, Mowatt-Larssen CA, et al. Comparison of specialized and standard enteral formulas in trauma patients. Pharmacotherapy 1994;14:314–320.
142. Gianotti L, Gentilini O, Braga M. Nutrition in oncological surgery. Nestle Nutr Workshop Ser Clin Perform Programme 2000;4:239–21; discussion 251–254.
143. Galbán C, Montejo JC, Mesejo A, et al. An immune-enhancing enteral diet reduces mortality rate and episodes of bacteremia in septic intensive care unit patients. Crit Care Med 2000;28:884–885.
144. Caparrós T, Lopez J, Grau T. Early enteral nutrition in critically ill patients with a high-protein diet enriched with arginine, fiber, and antioxidants compared with a standard high-protein diet. The effect on nosocomial infections and outcome. JPEN J Parenter Enteral Nutr 2001;25:299–309.
145. Conejero R, Bonet A, Grau T, et al. Effect of a glutamine-enriched enteral diet on intestinal permeability and infectious morbidity at 28 days in critically ill patients with systemic inflammatory response syndrome: a randomized, single-blind, prospective, multicenter study. Nutrition 2002;18:716–721.
146. Zhou YP, Jiang ZM, Sun YH, Wang XR, Ma EI, Wilmore D. The effect of supplemental enteral glutamine on plasma levels, gut function, and outcome in severe burns: a randomized, double-blind, controlled clinical trial. JPEN J Parenter Enteral Nutr 2003;27:241–245.
147. Hall JC, Dobb G, Hall J, de Sousa R, Brennan L, McCauley R. A prospective randomized trial of enteral glutamine in critical illness. Intensive Care Med 2003;29:1710–1716.
148. Garrel D, Patenaude J, Nedelec B, et al. Decreased mortality and infectious morbidity in adult burn patients given enteral glutamine supplements: a prospective, controlled, randomized clinical trial. Crit Care Med 2003;31:2444–2449.

7 Perioperative Fluids and Electrolytes

Avery B. Nathens and Ronald V. Maier

Surgical patients undergo acute alterations in the volume and composition of fluids in the intracellular and extracellular spaces. To a great extent, these changes occur as a result of the patient's underlying disease. For example, hemorrhage or bowel obstruction may acutely change the volume of fluid in the intravascular or extracellular compartments. However, these alterations are not limited to patients requiring urgent operative intervention as even elective surgery may result in dramatic fluid shifts in the absence of significant blood loss. In addition to changes in fluid volume, surgical patients may develop potentially dangerous fluctuations in concentrations and total body content of important electrolytes. Precise perioperative management of fluids and electrolytes is thus required to minimize perioperative morbidity and mortality.

Physiology

Body Fluid Compartments

Accurate replacement of fluid requires an understanding of the distribution of water, electrolytes, and colloid across the various body fluid compartments. Total body water (TBW) approximates 60% of total body weight, or 42 l in a 70-kg person; TBW is composed of the intracellular and extracellular compartments. The intracellular compartment or intracellular volume (ICV) constitutes 40% of total body weight (28 l in a 70-kg patient), whereas the extracellular volume (ECV) makes up the remaining 20%. The ECV is composed of interstitial fluid (IF) and the intravascular or plasma volume (PV). The PV constitutes 25% of ECV (5% of total body weight or approximately 3.5 l), while the remainder is IF. Red cell volume, approximately 2% to 3% of TBW, is part of the ICV. Thus, total blood volume is approximately 7% to 8% of total body weight, or approximately 5 l in a 70-kg patient (Fig. 7.1). Body water composition differs in obese subjects, with less TBW per unit of weight and a relatively expanded ECV compared to ICV due to the relatively low water content of adipose tissue. This low water content is a reflection of the relative low water content of adipocytes.[1] (Body water composition is also altered in the elderly such that by 80 years of age, TBW contributes only 50% of total body weight.[2])

The solute and colloid compositions of the intracellular and extracellular fluid compartments differ markedly. The ECV contains most of the sodium in the body, with equal sodium concentrations in the PV and IF (140 mEq/l), while the intracellular $[Na^+]$ is only 10 to 12 mEq/l. By contrast, the predominant intracellular cation is potassium, with the intracellular concentration $[K^+]$ approximating 150 mEq/l in contrast to an ECV $[K^+]$ of 4.0 mEq/l. Albumin represents the most important osmotically active constituent of the ECV and is virtually excluded from the ICV. Albumin is unequally distributed within the ECV; the serum concentration of albumin approximates 4.0 g/dl, while the IF concentration averages 1.0 g/dl.

The *distribution volume* of various crystalloid or colloid solutions is that volume in which the administered solution will equilibrate over the short term. For example, TBW is the distribution volume for sodium-free water; ECV is the distribution volume for crystalloid solution in which $[Na^+]$ approximates 140 mEq/l, whereas PV represents the distribution volume for most colloid solutions. To clarify this concept, assume a 70-kg patient has suffered an acute blood loss of 1000 ml, approximately 20% of the predicted 5-l blood volume. Any one of 5% dextrose in water (D5W), lactated Ringer's solution, or 5% albumin may be chosen to replace the lost blood volume. The formula describing the effects of fluid infusion on PV expansion is as follows:

$$\text{Expected PV increment} = \frac{\text{Volume infused} \times \text{Normal PV}}{\text{Distribution volume}}$$

Rearranging the equation would yield the following:

$$\text{Volume infused} = \frac{\text{Expected PV increment} \times \text{Distribution volume}}{\text{Normal plasma volume}}$$

In this example, the expected PV increment is 1 l (to replace shed blood), and the normal PV is approximately 3.5 l. To restore blood volume using D5W, which distributes throughout TBW (42 l), it would be necessary to administer 12 l. By

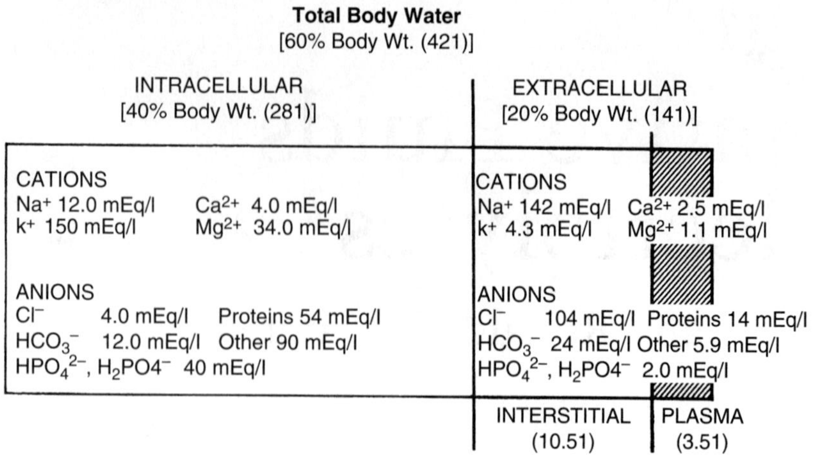

FIGURE 7.1. Distribution of body water and electrolytes in a healthy 70-kg male. (Adapted from Narins and Krishna,[13] with permission.)

contrast, if lactated Ringer's solution (which distributes throughout ECV) were chosen, a 1-l PV increment would require approximately 41 of crystalloid. Colloid solutions with similar oncotic pressures to plasma (e.g., 5% albumin) distribute within the intravascular space and thus have a distribution volume equal to the PV. In this example, 1l of 5% albumin would be required to replace the shed blood.

Maintenance Body Fluid and Electrolyte Requirements

Healthy adults require a minimal amount of fluid and electrolyte intake to maintain systemic homeostasis. Sufficient water is required to replace obligatory urinary losses of approximately 1000ml/day and gastrointestinal (GI) losses of 100 to 200ml/day. Insensible water losses must also be considered in estimating maintenance fluid requirements. Insensible losses amount to 8 to 12ml/kg/day and are equally divided into respiratory and cutaneous water loss. Cutaneous insensitive losses increase by approximately 10% for each degree of temperature greater than 37°C; thus, these losses may become significant in the febrile patient. Respiratory insensitive water losses tend to be greater with inspiration of unhumidified air, as may occur with a tracheostomy. Overall maintenance fluid requirements are dependent on weight and are approximated using either of the approaches in Table 7.1. For example, a 60-kg patient would require approximately 100ml/h of water (4ml/kg × 10kg plus 2ml/kg × 10kg plus 1ml/kg × 40kg) to keep up with obligatory water losses.

Daily sodium intake in normal individuals approaches 100 to 250mEq/day. This intake is balanced by sodium losses in sweat, stool, and urine. However, renal conservation of sodium is extraordinary, and in cases of profound volume depletion, urinary losses of sodium may be less than 1mEq/day. In the perioperative period, adequate maintenance of sodium may be achieved with an intake of 1 to 2mEq/kg/day. Normal potassium intake is approximately 40 to 120mEq/day, approximately 10% to 15% of which is excreted as normal urinary losses. In individuals with normal renal function, body potassium stores can be maintained with an intake of approximately 0.5 to 1.0mEq/kg/day. In the past, glucose-containing fluids have been administered in an effort to prevent hypoglycemia and limit protein catabolism. However, because of the hyperglycemic response associated with surgical stress, only infants and patients receiving insulin or drugs that interfere with glucose synthesis are at high risk for hypoglycemia. The supplementation of other electrolytes (e.g., calcium, magnesium, and phosphate) is usually unnecessary in patients with normal nutritional status.

TABLE 7.1. Maintenance Water Requirements.

Weight	*ml/kg/h*	*ml/kg/day*
First 10kg	4	100
Second 10kg	2	50
Each kilogram above 20kg	1	20

Based on estimated maintenance requirements of Na^+ and K^+, there are several options for maintenance fluid replacement (Table 7.2). A 60-kg patient should receive approximately 60 to 120mEq/day of sodium and 30 to 60mEq/day of potassium. The most commonly used maintenance solutions are D5W 1/2 normal saline (NS) or 2/3 D5W 1/3 NS, which are relatively isotonic and provide the required amount of sodium over a 24h period. Potassium is often added to these solutions at concentrations approximating 20mEq/l to ensure that maintenance requirements are met. Although 0.9% saline is used frequently, the relatively high concentration of chloride results in a hyperchloremic metabolic acidosis because of the inability of the renal tubule to excrete the excess Cl^-.

Perioperative Fluid Requirements

Appropriate management of fluids and electrolytes in the perioperative period requires a flexible yet systematic approach to ensure that fluid administration is appropriately tailored to the patient's changing requirements. The amount of fluids administered in the immediate postoperative period (within the first 12–24h) must take into account the existing deficit, maintenance requirements, and any ongoing losses.

Estimation of the existing deficit must incorporate an approximation of intraoperative blood loss as well as fluid losses from evaporative and third-space (i.e., extravascular) fluid sequestration. It is important to realize that the surgeon's estimated intraoperative blood loss is often 50% less than when calculated using more rigorous methods.[3,4] This discrepancy should be taken into account when estimating postoperative fluid requirements. Due to the shift of crystalloid from the intravascular space to the interstitium, crystalloid should replace blood loss in a ratio of 3–4:1.

TABLE 7.2. Options for Maintenance Fluid Replacement.

	Na^+ (mEq/l)	K^+ (mEq/l)	Cl^- (mEq/l)	Ca^{++} (mEq/l)	Lactate[a] (mEq/l)	Glucose (g/l)
Normal (0.9%) saline (NS)	154	0	154	0	0	0
Dextrose 5% in water (D5W)	0	0	0	0	0	50
D5W 1/2 NS	77	0	77	0	0	50
2/3 D5W, 1/3 NS	50	0	50	0	0	33
Lactated Ringer's	130	4	109	3	28	0

[a]Lactate is used instead of Cl^- to maintain electroneutrality. It is converted to HCO_3^- by hepatic metabolism.

Extravascular fluid sequestration represents another important source of intraoperative fluid loss. Extensive dissection at the operative site induces a localized capillary leak, the result of which is extravasation of intravascular fluid into the interstitium with edema formation. The loss of intravascular volume via this route depends on the extent of exposure and degree of dissection. For example, estimated intravascular fluid losses associated with inguinal herniorrhaphy are approximately 4 ml/kg/h, while losses during aortic aneurysmectomy may be as high as 8 ml/kg/h. This capillary leak may persist as long as 24 h into the postoperative period and should be considered as part of ongoing losses in the immediate postoperative period.

Ongoing fluid requirements usually represent GI losses from stomas, tubes, drains, or fistulae. These losses may be accurately estimated by closely following recorded hourly outputs from any tube or drain. The electrolyte composition of the output depends on the source of effluent[5] (Table 7.3). The replacement fluid should be chosen to best approximate the composition of the ongoing losses. For example, nasogastric losses are typically replaced with NS supplemented with 10 mEq KCl/l, whereas losses from a duodenal fistula may best be replaced using lactated Ringer's solution.

Postoperative fluid orders should take into account the overall fluid balance in the operating room as an estimate of the existing deficit along with maintenance fluid requirements and any ongoing losses. The preferred approach is to reassess the patient frequently to determine intravascular volume status. In this regard, evaluation of heart rate, blood pressure, and most importantly, hourly urine output provides an excellent measure of intravascular volume status. Orders for intravenous fluids should be rewritten frequently to maintain a normal heart rate, a urine output of approximately 1 ml/kg/h, and adequate blood pressure. It has become common practice to avoid potassium supplementation within the first 24 h. The rationale behind this approach is to prevent life-threatening hyperkalemia should oliguria become a significant problem in the early postoperative period. The preferred practice is to administer NS or lactated Ringer's in the first 24 h. The smaller volume of distribution of these solutions compared to dextrose-containing solutions ensures that adequate intravascular volume is maintained despite ongoing extravascular fluid sequestration. On the first postoperative morning, these solutions are switched to dextrose-containing solutions (2/3 D5W 1/3 NS or D5W 1/2 NS) supplemented with KCl, providing that urine output has been adequate.

Disorders of Sodium Homeostasis

Maintenance of a normal serum sodium concentration (135–145 mEq/l) is intimately associated with control of plasma osmolarity (P_{osm}). Plasma osmolarity is determined by the sum of the individual osmotically active substances as described in the following equation:

$$P_{osm} = 2 \times \text{Plasma } [Na^+] + [\text{Glucose}]/20 + [\text{BUN}]/3$$

From this equation, it is evident that plasma $[Na^+]$ is the major determinant of P_{osm} in normal individuals. Further, it is important to realize that plasma $[Na^+]$ alone provides no information about the total content of sodium in the body but simply provides an estimate of the relative amounts of free water and sodium.

Maintenance of the plasma osmolarity within normal limits depends on the ability of the kidneys to excrete water, thus preventing hypoosmolarity, and on a normal thirst mechanism with access to water to prevent hypernatremia. The ability to excrete maximally dilute urine (<100 mOsm/kg) allows the kidneys to excrete in excess of 18 l of water per day. In the presence of normal renal perfusion and intact renal function, antidiuretic hormone (ADH) is the principal regulator of serum osmolarity. A 1% to 2% reduction in P_{osm} maximally inhibits ADH release, leading to a urine osmolarity that is maximally dilute. By contrast, a 1% to 2% increase in P_{osm} above normal or a 5% to 10% decrease in blood volume or blood pressure stimulates ADH release. Importantly, when both a low plasma osmolarity and low blood volume or pressure are present, the latter effect will dominate, resulting in

TABLE 7.3. Volume and Composition of Gastrointestinal Fluid Losses.

Source	Volume (ml)	Na^+ (mEq/l)	Cl^- (mEq/l)	K^+ (mEq/l)	HCO_3^- (mEq/l)	H^+ (mEq/l)
Stomach	1000–4200	20–120	130	10–15	—	30–100
Duodenum	100–2000	110	115	15	10	—
Ileum	1000–3000	80–150	60–100	10	30–50	—
Colon (diarrhea)	500–1700	120	90	25	45	—
Bile	500–1000	140	100	5	25	—
Pancreas	500–1000	140	30	5	115	—

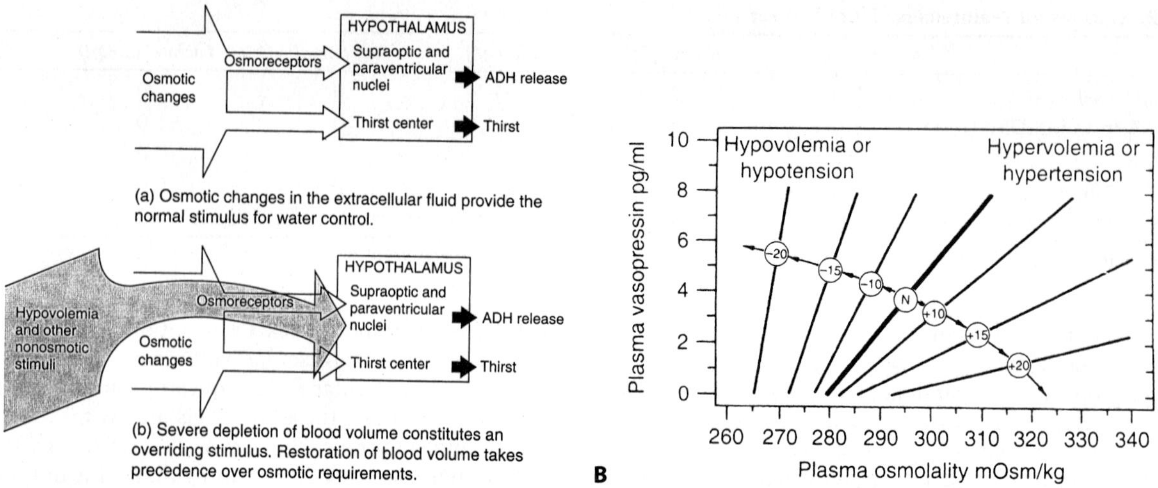

FIGURE 7.2. A. Graphic depiction of the law of circulating volume. In the setting of volume depletion, this stimulus takes precedence over osmotic requirements. *ADH*, antidiuretic hormone. (From Goldberg.[14]) **B.** Effect of intravascular volume on the regulation of osmolality by ADH. Each line represents the relationship of plasma vasopressin to plasma osmolarity in the presence of varying levels of volume status or blood pressure. The hemodynamic influences raise or lower the set point and, to a lesser extent, alter the slope or sensitivity of the osmotic response. (From Robertson,[6] Science and Medicine Publishing.)

an increase in ADH release (Fig. 7.2). This is one of the principal mechanisms leading to the development of hyponatremia in patients with low intravascular volume. In addition, changes in blood pressure or volume status will alter the osmolar set point and, to a lesser extent, the sensitivity of the osmotic response.[6]

The elderly are particularly prone to alterations in sodium homeostasis.[2] The reduction in glomerular filtration rate that occurs with aging limits the ability of the aged to excrete a sodium load, making them more prone to overexpansion of the extracellular fluid compartment. In addition, a combination of impaired thirst mechanism and decreased ability to concentrate the urine predispose them to hypernatremia.

Hyponatremia

The approach to hyponatremia begins with an assessment of the serum osmolarity[5] (Table 7.4). If serum osmolarity is high, then it is important to consider the possibility of other effective plasma osmoles, the most common of which is glucose. Hyperglycemia shifts H_2O from cells, leading to dilutional hyponatremia. As a result, for every 100 mg/dl rise in glucose the $[Na^+]$ falls by 1.3 mEq/l. The treatment requires definitive management of the osmotically active agent, which in the case of glucose, would be insulin. In rare cases, the serum osmolarity may be normal. This phenomenon is referred to as *pseudohyponatremia* and is caused by hyperlipidemia or hyperproteinemia; it is an artifact of the laboratory assay. No treatment is required.

More frequently, a low $[Na^+]$ will be associated with reduced plasma osmolarity. The etiology and treatment of hypoosmolar hyponatremia may be classified into three groups depending on the ECV status of the patient. A reduction in ECV leads to an increase in ADH secretion, impairing the kidney's ability to excrete free water. Either administration of Na^+-free solutions or the ingestion of free water induced by thirst aggravates the resulting hyponatremia. The most common causes of hypovolemic hyponatremia are Na^+ loss. Typically, perioperative isotonic losses (plasma, gastric losses) are replaced with hypotonic solutions in the face of mild hypovolemia. Treatment involves replenishing the extravascular volume with isotonic fluids in concert with restriction of free water.

Hyponatremia in the presence of an increased extravascular volume probably represents the next most common scenario in the perioperative period. Typically, these represent edematous states in which there is a reduction in the effective circulating volume. Low cardiac output states, cirrhosis, and other hypoalbuminemic states are the more common etiologies. Both water restriction and Na^+ restriction are necessary. Depending on the severity of the hyponatremia, a loop diuretic may be required to increase both Na^+ and water loss; in most cases, this induces an excess of urinary water loss over Na^+ loss and should correct the hyponatremia.

Patients with a normal ECV status and hypoosmolar hyponatremia may have the syndrome of inappropriate ADH secretion (SIADH). In the surgical patient, SIADH is not often

TABLE 7.4. Causes of Hyponatremia.

Pseudohyponatremia (normal plasma osmolality)
Hyperlipidemia, hyperproteinemia
Dilutional hyponatremia (increased plasma osmolality)
Hyperglycemia, mannitol
True hyponatremia (reduced plasma osmolality)
Reduction in ECF volume
Plasma, GI, skin, or renal losses (diuretics)
Expanded ECF volume
Congestive heart failure
Hypoproteinemic states (cirrhosis, nephrotic syndrome, malnutrition)
Normal ECF volume
SIADH (syndrome of inappropriate antidiuretic hormone release)
Pulmonary or CNS lesions
Endocrine disorders (hypothyroidism, hypoadrenalism)
Drugs (e.g., morphine, tricyclic antidepressants, clofibrate, antineoplastic agents, chlorpropamide, aminophylline, indomethacin)
Miscellaneous (pain, nausea)

considered as a possible cause of hyponatremia, but nausea, pain, and narcotics, all of which are common in the postoperative period, may result in SIADH and contribute to postoperative hyponatremia. Diagnosis is confirmed by demonstrating a low plasma osmolarity, a less than maximally dilute urine (U_{osm}. > 100 mOsm/l), and renal salt wasting (U_{Na}. > 20 mEq/l).[7] Treatment includes management of the underlying cause and water restriction. Isotonic (0.9%) saline should not be administered to patients with SIADH as it may cause the plasma [Na^+] to fall.

The presence of symptoms in hyponatremia depends on the rate at which hyponatremia occurred. Symptoms of increased intracranial pressure from cerebral edema are the most prominent features and may be present at plasma [Na^+] less than 125 mEq/l if the development of hyponatremia was rapid in onset. If the reduction in [Na^+] occurs slowly, then symptoms may not be evident until plasma [Na^+] drops to as low as 110 mEq/l. Too rapid correction of plasma [Na^+] may result in central pontine myelinosis, a process of demyelination caused by cell shrinkage that may result in irreversible brainstem injury. If the patient is asymptomatic or mildly symptomatic, then the goal should be to raise the [Na^+] by approximately 0.5 mEq/h; if the patient is symptomatic with coma or convulsions, then more rapid correction is necessary. The aim is to give sufficient Na^+ as 3% NaCl until either the symptoms have improved or the plasma [Na^+] has increased by 5 mEq/l, whichever comes first. The following formula may be used to estimate the amount of Na^+ required to raise the [Na^+] to a safe level (approximately 120 mEq/l):

$$Na^+ \text{ deficit} = 0.60 \times \text{Lean body weight (kg)} \times (120 - \text{Measured plasma } Na^+)$$

Hypernatremia

Hypernatremia (plasma [Na^+]. > 150 mEq/l) is far less common than is hyponatremia. Cellular shrinkage caused by fluid shifts from the intracellular space to the extracellular compartment may cause confusion, coma, and intracranial hemorrhage. Symptoms are usually not evident below a plasma [Na^+] of 160 mEq/l.

Elevated plasma [Na^+] occurs as a result of excessive free water loss and is thus frequently associated with hypovolemia. Excessive insensible losses caused by fever, hyperventilation, and burns or hypotonic fluid losses due to perspiration or severe diarrhea are the principal causes. If hypovolemia is sufficiently severe that tissue perfusion is compromised, then initial therapy should be isotonic saline until tissue perfusion is restored. If perfusion is adequate, then 0.5 NS or D5W is sufficient to return plasma [Na^+] to normal.

Polyuria associated with excessive renal free water losses represents another frequent cause of hypernatremia. For example, osmotic diuresis induced by hyperglycemia or mannitol may cause profound hypernatremia if left unchecked. An inability to concentrate urine because of high-output renal failure commonly associated with the recovery phase of acute tubular necrosis may also cause severe hypernatremia. In the context of the clinical scenario, the diagnosis is usually straightforward. Treatment simply involves measuring urinary electrolyte losses and providing adequate free water replacement. Central diabetes insipidus is not uncommon following neurosurgical operations or head injury and may cause profound hypernatremia. Administration of exogenous vasopressin in the form of dDAVP (1-desamino-8d-arginine vasopressin) is both diagnostic and therapeutic.

Rapid correction of severe hypernatremia may cause irreversible neurological deficits. Plasma [Na^+] should not be corrected at a rate faster than 0.5 to 1.0 mEq/l per hour. In the presence of convulsions, sufficient free water should be administered either to return the plasma [Na^+] to the concentration documented before the convulsion or to reduce the [Na^+] by about 6 mmol/l. The following formula may help to guide therapy:

$$\text{Water deficit} = \text{Total body water} \times \{(\text{Plasma } [Na^+] \div \text{Desired plasma } [Na^+]) - 1\}$$

Disorders of Potassium Homeostasis

Potassium is the major intracellular cation. Total intracellular K^+ is approximately 40 to 50 mmol/kg body weight, with only 2% of total body potassium located in the extracellular fluid. Despite the small quantity of K^+ in the extracellular space, slight alterations in plasma [K^+] may have dramatic effects on muscle contraction and nerve conduction as the concentration gradient across the plasma membrane is the main determinant of membrane excitability. For this reason, abnormalities in plasma [K^+] should be treated expeditiously.

Hypokalemia

Hypokalemia in the surgical patient is usually due to losses from the GI tract, kidneys, or skin (Table 7.5). Rarely, transcellular flux of K^+ may cause significant alterations in plasma [K^+], and these causes should be considered in the appropriate context. In the case of diarrhea, stool potassium losses represent the principal reason for hypokalemia. By contrast, the mechanism for hypokalemia in vomiting is more complex. The content of K^+ in gastric secretion is only about 10 mEq/l. As a result, massive vomiting would be necessary to cause hypokalemia. Typically, renal K^+ losses account for potassium depletion associated with vomiting. The ECV contraction leads to elevated levels of aldosterone, which results in enhanced renal Na^+ reabsorption and increased K^+ secretion. Massive burns may also cause hypokalemia because of a combination of tissue breakdown and fluid loss.

TABLE 7.5. Causes of Hypokalemia.

Extrarenal losses
Gastrointestinal (vomiting, nasogastric suction)
Diarrhea
Massive burns
Profuse sweating
Renal losses
Diuretic therapy
Vomiting
Tubular disorders (e.g., type I renal tubular acidosis)
Drugs (cisplatin, amphotericin B)
Transcellular flux of K^+ into the cell
Metabolic alkalosis
Insulin administration
β_2-Adrenergic stimulation
Other
Primary hyperaldosteronism
Renal artery stenosis
Cushing syndrome

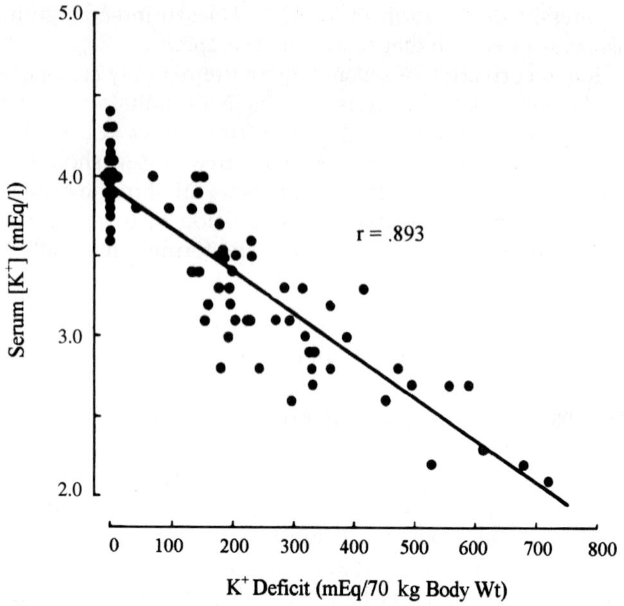

FIGURE 7.3. Effect of potassium depletion on serum potassium. Results are summarized from studies of experimental potassium depletion in normal subjects and in potassium-depleted patients. The relationship between serum potassium and total body potassium appears to be linear when moderate deficits exists. (From Sterns et al.,[15] with permission.)

The major danger associated with hypokalemia is cardiac arrhythmias. The potential for arrhythmias is exacerbated in the presence of a metabolic alkalosis, digoxin, or hypercalcemia. Electrocardiographic (ECG) changes associated with hypokalemia correlate poorly with the plasma [K^+] but typically are not manifest until the plasma [K^+] drops below 3 mmol/l. Early changes include T-wave flattening or inversion and depressed ST segments, followed by the development of U waves and a prolonged QT interval. Hypokalemia may also manifest with weakness once plasma [K^+] drops below 2.5 mmol/l.

Potassium replacement therapy should be geared toward rapid correction of plasma [K^+], followed by slower repletion of the total body K^+ deficit. The potassium deficit may be large. For example, a fall in plasma [K^+] from 4 to 3 reflects a total deficit of 100 to 400 mmol[3] (Fig. 7.3). Too rapid correction may result in inadvertent hyperkalemia because it takes time for the administered K^+ to be transferred into cells. When possible, K^+ supplementation should be administered orally. However, if the plasma [K^+] is less than 3.0 or enteral supplementation is not possible, then parenteral administration is indicated. Potassium can be administered intravenously into peripheral veins in concentrations as high as 40 mmol/l. Higher concentrations may cause phlebitis and thus should be administered into a central vein. The rate of administration in the absence of intractable arrhythmias should be no greater than 20 to 40 mEq/h. At this rate of administration, continuous ECG monitoring is indicated.

Hyperkalemia

Sudden increases in plasma [K^+] are almost always caused by rapid administration or transcellular flux of K^+. By contrast, sustained hyperkalemia implies that there is impairment of renal K^+ excretion. It is important to be aware of pseudohyperkalemia, observed when the serum potassium (as measured by the laboratory) is spuriously elevated by potassium release from red blood cells or platelets after the blood specimen has been obtained. The diagnosis of pseudohyperkalemia can be made by demonstrating that the plasma [K^+] is normal in a nonhemolyzed plasma sample in which clotting is prevented by drawing the blood into a heparinized tube.

Transcellular flux of K^+ from the cell into the extracellular fluid may occur in patients with severe metabolic acidosis, insulin deficiency (e.g., diabetes mellitus), or rhabdomyolysis as the intracellular potassium stores are released. Administration of succinylcholine may also cause a transient rise in plasma [K^+] because of en masse muscle depolarization, particularly following paralysis or prolonged bed rest, such as is seen in severe burn injury. In the surgical patient, hyperkalemia occurs most frequently as a result of impaired renal excretion of K^+ caused by oliguric renal dysfunction. It is for this reason that K^+ should not be added to maintenance intravenous fluid therapy within the first 24 h of surgery. Rarely, hypoaldosterone states may induce hyperkalemia.

The main risks associated with hyperkalemia are similar to those of hypokalemia: weakness and myocardial irritability. Electrocardiographic signs of hyperkalemia proceed from an increase in T-wave amplitude, leading to a narrow, peaked symmetrical T wave, followed by reduced P-wave amplitude and widening of the QRS complexes. If untreated, severe hyperkalemia may eventually cause a sinusoidal ECG complex and ultimately ventricular fibrillation. Signs or symptoms are rare at plasma [K^+] below 6.0 mmol/l; beyond this, there is poor correlation with the serum potassium level and arrhythmias. The rate of rise of plasma [K^+] appears to be extremely important; many patients with chronic renal failure tolerate plasma [K^+] levels in excess of 6 or 6.5 without symptoms. Treatment is dependent on the presence or absence of ECG changes and the plasma [K^+]. Individuals with mild hyperkalemia (<6.0 mmol/l) can usually be treated conservatively by reducing daily intake. Active treatment to lower the plasma [K^+] or to antagonize its effects on the cell membrane should be started if the [K^+] has risen acutely to greater than 6.0 mmol/l or if any ECG manifestations of hyperkalemia are present. These therapeutic modalities should be used in conjunction with other methods to reduce total body potassium stores (Table 7.6).

TABLE 7.6. Treatment of Hyperkalemia.

Treatment	*Mechanism of action*	*Time frame*
Intravenous calcium gluconate	Antagonizes effects of hyperkalemia on the cell membrane	Seconds to minutes
Glucose, insulin, sodium bicarbonate	Translocation of potassium into cells	30–60 min
Rectally or orally administered potassium-binding resins	Binds and hastens excretion of K^+ secreted into colon	1–4 h (rectal); >6 h (oral)
Dialysis	Movement across a concentration gradient and excreted	Immediate

Disorders of Mineral Homeostasis

In most surgical patients, abnormalities in the body fluid composition of calcium (Ca), magnesium (Mg), and phosphate (PO_4) are seldom extreme enough to cause concern. However, in the critically ill patient, these alterations may exacerbate potentially life-threatening situations.

Calcium Abnormalities

Total body calcium stores are approximately 1000 g, with almost 99% apportioned in bone. The remainder is located within the extracellular fluid and is either free (40%) or bound to albumin (50%) or other anions such as citrate, lactate, and sulfate. Only the free or ionized component is biologically active. Acid–base alterations affect the binding of calcium to albumin and account for the symptoms of hypocalcemia associated with hyperventilation. The resultant respiratory alkalosis increases the binding affinity of calcium for albumin, leading to a reduction in the serum ionized calcium levels. Similarly, changes in serum protein levels affect total serum calcium. The ionized calcium level (normal range 4.5–5.5 mg/dl) can be estimated using the following formula:

$$\text{Ionized calcium (mg/dl)} = \text{Total serum calcium (mg/dl)} - 0.83 \times \text{Serum albumin (mg/dl)}$$

Normal daily intake of calcium is between 500 and 1500 mg per day. The GI tract excretes most of this, with the efficiency of intestinal absorption inversely related to the amount ingested. Routine supplementation or assessment in postoperative patients is usually not indicated. However, in patients with major fluid shifts, prolonged immobilization, alterations in GI absorption, or operative procedures on the thyroid or parathyroid, significant alterations in calcium homeostasis may arise.

Hypocalcemia

The most frequent cause of hypocalcemia is low serum albumin. In this case, the ionized fraction remains normal, and no treatment is indicated. Frequent alternate causes to consider include acute pancreatitis, massive soft tissue infection, small-bowel fistulae, and hypoparathyroidism. Massive blood transfusion induces hypocalcemia caused by chelation of calcium with citrate. Each unit of blood contains approximately 3 g of citrate. The normal adult liver metabolizes 3 g of citrate every 5 min, so hypocalcemia may result at blood transfusion rates exceeding 1 unit every 5 min.[7] If the rate of transfusion is less than this, then calcium should only be given if there is biochemical, clinical, or ECG evidence of hypocalcemia.

Manifestations of hypocalcemia may become evident at serum levels less than 8 mg/dl. The earliest symptoms include numbness or tingling in the circumoral region or at the tips of the fingers. Tetany or seizure may arise at more profound levels of hypocalcemia. A positive Trousseau's sign or Chvostek's sign may be suggestive of hypocalcemia. Hypocalcemia alters myocardial repolarization and results in a prolonged QT interval on the ECG. ECG monitoring may be useful to guide calcium supplementation in massive transfusion when rapid assays are unavailable.

The treatment of hypocalcemia depends on its severity. In symptomatic patients with an ionized calcium level less than 3 g/dl, intravenous replacement therapy should be administered: a 10-ml ampule of either 10% calcium gluconate (93 mg elemental calcium) or calcium chloride (232 mg elemental calcium) should be administered in 50 to 100 ml D5W over 10 to 15 min. In less-severe cases, oral supplementation may suffice, and any oral preparation providing 1 to 3 g of elemental calcium per day will be adequate.

Hypercalcemia

There is an extensive differential diagnosis for hypercalcemia (see chapter 55, "Parathyroid"). Primary hyperparathyroidism and malignant disease account for 90% of cases, with the former more common in outpatients and the latter most common among hospitalized patients.[8] Hypercalcemia has protean manifestations, including confusion, lethargy, coma, muscle weakness, anorexia, nausea, vomiting, pancreatitis, and constipation. Renal stones may develop in cases of prolonged hypercalcemia. Hypercalcemia may also induce nephrogenic diabetes insipidus and result in polyuria. Finally, ECG changes include a shortened QT interval. This alteration in cardiac repolarization predisposes the patient to fatal arrhythmias, particularly in the presence of digitalis.

A serum calcium concentration in excess of 15 mg/dl or in association with ECG changes requires urgent treatment. Most patients will respond to vigorous hydration with NS. Dehydration is not uncommon as the result of polyuria, and thus rehydration both dilutes the serum calcium and improves renal calcium excretion. Once the patient is rehydrated, furosemide may be administered to further increase calcium excretion. Rarely, adjunctive measures, including administration of diphosphonates, calcitonin, or mithramycin, may be necessary. These agents may inhibit osteoclast resorption (diphosphonates, calcitonin) or reduce serum calcium levels by forming calcium–phosphate complexes (diphosphonates).[9]

Magnesium Abnormalities

Magnesium is the principal intracellular divalent cation. Approximately 50% of total body magnesium is found in bone and is not readily exchangeable. Serum magnesium concentrations typically range between 1.5 and 2.5 mEq/l. Magnesium absorption occurs throughout the small intestine and is reabsorbed effectively in the renal tubules, with renal excretion as low as 1 mEq/day. Hypomagnesemia may occur because of poor nutritional intake, malabsorption, or increased renal excretion due to diuretics. Hypomagnesemia is common in patients abusing alcohol. In this population, the effect is caused by both dietary deficiency and the diuretic effect of alcohol. The signs and symptoms of hypomagnesemia are characterized by neuromuscular and central nervous system (CNS) irritability and in this respect are similar to those seen with hypocalcemia. Low serum magnesium levels appear to impair parathyroid hormone excretion and may induce hypocalcemia refractory to calcium supplementation unless the hypomagnesemia is corrected.[10]

Hypomagnesemia may be treated with either oral or parenteral magnesium preparations. If the serum magnesium level is less than 1 mEq/l or the patient is symptomatic, then parenteral treatment is indicated. In the presence of normal renal function, up to 2 mEq magnesium per kilogram of body weight may be administered daily. This dosage may be administered as magnesium sulfate diluted in intravenous fluid and administered over 3 to 6 h. If administered in large doses, then vital signs and cardiac rhythm should be monitored as excessively rapid administration may induce hypotension, respiratory or cardiac arrest, or coma. Ongoing oral or parenteral replacement over several days to weeks may be required to correct the total body magnesium deficit.

Hypermagnesemia is extraordinarily rare in the absence of renal failure. Flaccid paralysis, hypotension, confusion, and coma may become evident at serum levels exceeding 6 mEq/l. Electrocardiographic features are similar to those seen in hyperkalemia. Emergency treatment of severe symptomatic hypermagnesemia involves administration of calcium as either calcium gluconate or calcium chloride. Calcium effectively antagonizes the effect of magnesium on neuromuscular function. Definitive treatment requires increasing renal magnesium excretion with a combination of hydration and diuresis. If renal function is impaired, then dialysis will be necessary.

Phosphate Abnormalities

Phosphate is the most abundant intracellular anion, and only 0.1% of total body phosphorus is in the extracellular fluid compartment. As a result, circulating plasma levels do not reflect total body stores. Hypophosphatemia may occur as the result of impaired intestinal absorption or increased renal excretion. Hyperparathyroidism may induce a drop in serum phosphate levels through an increase in renal excretion. Significant hypophosphatemia is common following major liver resection, an effect caused by rapid phosphate utilization in the regenerating hepatocytes.[11] In this clinical setting, serum phosphate should be measured frequently and treated appropriately. Careful monitoring of phosphate should also occur with the administration of parenteral nutrition after prolonged starvation because profound hypophosphatemia may result.[12] The potential adverse effects associated with severe hypophosphatemia include impaired tissue oxygen delivery due to decreased 2,3-diphosphoglycerate levels, muscle weakness, and rhabdomyolysis. Severe hypophosphatemia may be treated parenterally using potassium phosphate. Phosphate (0.08–0.16 mmol/kg body weight) may be diluted in intravenous fluid and administered over 4 to 6 h. Phosphate levels should be reassessed and additional supplementation provided as required.

Hyperphosphatemia is most commonly seen in the setting of impaired renal phosphate excretion and in this scenario is frequently associated with hypocalcemia. Similarly, hypoparathyroidism reduces renal phosphate excretion, leading to an increase in serum phosphate levels. In these cases, treatment should be directed toward the underlying cause.

Acid–Base Abnormalities

The concentration of hydrogen ions in body fluids is maintained within an optimal pH range (7.35–7.45) to ensure adequate function of structural and enzymatic proteins. This narrow range is ensured by the availability of several buffer systems, including intracellular proteins and phosphates and the bicarbonate–carbonic acid system. The former functions primarily as an intracellular buffer and the latter as a buffer in the extracellular fluid. Further, alterations in excretion or retention of CO_2 or HCO_3^- through changes in minute ventilation or renal tubular handling of HCO_3^- provide an additional homeostatic mechanism for maintaining normal pH. By combining information on the various buffering systems, a nomogram can be constructed to describe the normal compensatory responses to acute and chronic acid–base disturbances (Fig. 7.4).

Metabolic Acidosis

Metabolic acidosis arises as a result of retention (or administration) of fixed acids or the loss of bicarbonate. In this way, disorders associated with a metabolic acidosis are categorized by the presence or absence of an anion gap (AG), in that addition of fixed acids results in an AG metabolic acidosis, and bicarbonate loss results in a nonAG metabolic acidosis (Table 7.7). The AG refers to the difference between measured cations (Na^+) and measured anions (Cl^- and HCO_3^-):

$$AG5Na^+ - (Cl^- + HCO_3^-)$$

The normal anion gap ranges from 3 to 11 mM/l. These unmeasured anions consist of proteins (primarily albumin), sulfates, phosphates, and organic acids. A reduction in the plasma albumin concentration will reduce the baseline AG approximately 2.5 mEq for every fall of 1 g/dl in the serum albumin. Thus, a severely hypoalbuminemic patient may have an AG metabolic acidosis with an apparently "normal" AG if this is not considered.

Lactic acidosis represents the most frequent cause of acidosis in hospitalized patients. Most commonly, it arises as a result of impaired tissue oxygenation caused by a reduction in tissue perfusion or hypoxia. Infrequently, it may occur in the presence of severe anemia or carbon monoxide poisoning, both of which impair tissue oxygen delivery, or uncoupling of oxidative phosphorylation as occurs with cyanide poisoning. Finally, hepatic dysfunction may also be associated with the presence of lactic acidosis because of impaired lactate clearance. An AG acidosis is also a feature of renal failure. In uncomplicated renal failure, typically the AG does not exceed 23, and the serum bicarbonate does not drop below 12. If the acidosis extends beyond these parameters, then another cause of acidosis should be considered.

The principal early manifestation of metabolic acidosis is an increase in minute ventilation primarily resulting from an increased tidal volume. The increase in minute ventilation serves to compensate for the metabolic acidosis by eliminating more CO_2. The appropriate ventilatory response should reduce Pa_{CO_2} by 1 mmHg (from 40 mmHg) for every 1 mmol/l drop in HCO_3^-. If the reduction in CO_2 is less than expected, then ventilatory support should be strongly considered because any further aggravation of the acidosis may lead to rapid decompensation. As the pH drops below 7.2, loss of vasomotor tone and a reduction in myocardial contracility may lead to cardiovascular collapse.

Treatment of metabolic acidosis is dependent on the underlying etiology. In the case of lactic acidosis, efforts should be directed toward optimizing tissue perfusion through administration of crystalloid solutions or blood products.

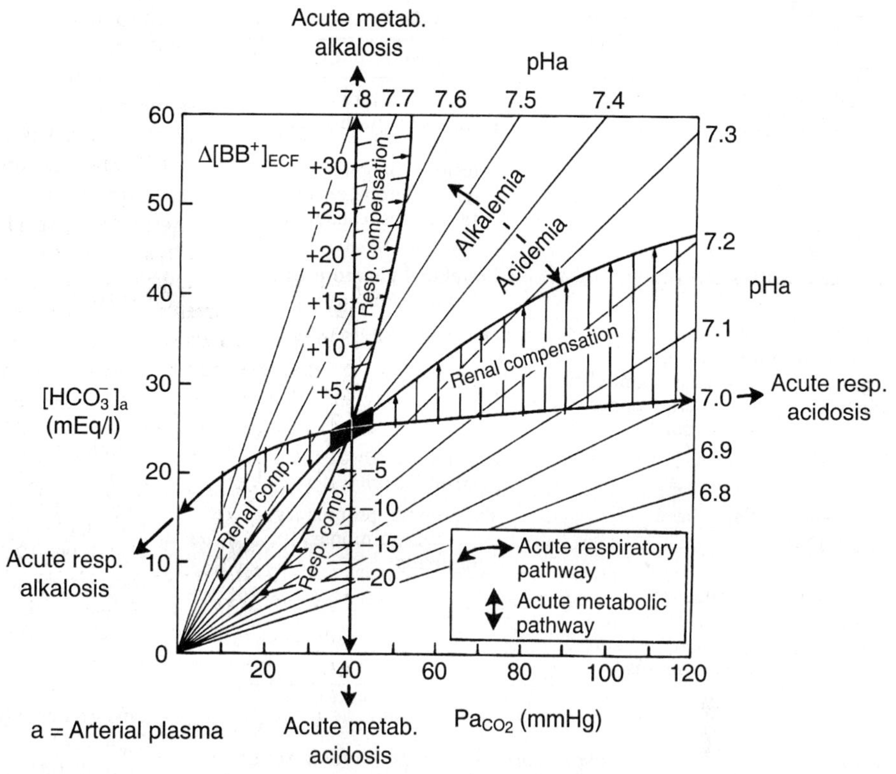

FIGURE 7.4. Compensatory responses to acute and chronic acid base alterations. $[BB^1]_{ECF}$ represents the base deficit. The *black diagonal box in the center* represents the normal range. As an example, if a metabolic acidosis develops such that a base deficit of 215 mEq/l occurs, then the resulting acidosis would lower the pH to 7.1. However, normal respiratory compensation would reduce the Pa_{CO_2} to 27 mmHg and raise the pH to about 7.25. (From Johnson and Ramanathan,[16] with permission.)

Administration of sodium bicarbonate is usually not indicated unless the acidosis is severe (pH < 7.15; HCO_3^- < 12 mmol/l). At this point, the buffering capacity is markedly reduced, and any further reduction in pH can lead to vasomotor collapse. Further, at a pH below 7.2, catecholamine resistance develops such that the myocardium and resistance vessels may not respond to either endogenous or exogenous catecholamines.

Metabolic Alkalosis

Primary metabolic alkalosis is characterized by an elevated plasma HCO_3^- concentration in the presence of an arterial pH greater than 7.4. Manifestations are rare, but when they do occur are chiefly those of excess neuromuscular excitability, including paresthesias, carpopedal spasm, or lightheadedness. Ventricular irritability may also be present at pH greater than 7.55. The expected respiratory response is a reduction in minute ventilation such that for every 1 mmol/l increase in plasma $[HCO_3^-]$ there should be a 0.7 mmHg increase in Pa_{CO_2}.

TABLE 7.7. Metabolic Acidosis.

Anion gap	*Nonanion gap*
Renal failure	GI HCO_3^- loss Diarrhea, ileus, fistula, and ureterosigmoidostomy
Lactic acidosis	Renal HCO_3^- loss Proximal renal tubular acidosis, acetazolamide
Ketoacidosis Diabetic, alcoholic	Failure of renal HCO_3^- production Distal renal tubular acidosis starvation
Toxic ingestions Salicylates, methanol, ethylene glycol, paraldehyde, toluene	

An elevation in plasma $[HCO_3^-]$ may occur as a result of one of three mechanisms: loss of acid from the GI tract or urine; administration of HCO_3^- or a precursor, such as citrate (e.g., as occurs following massive blood transfusions); or loss of fluid with a high chloride/bicarbonate ratio. Metabolic alkaloses are classified as either chloride sensitive or chloride resistant to the extent that they are reversed by the administration of NS.[5] For example, vomiting results in both hypovolemia and loss of both H^+ and chloride. To a great extent, it is the hypovolemia rather than the H^+ loss that contributes to the alkalosis. The hypovolemia associated with vomiting results in increased renal sodium reabsorption. In the presence of chloride depletion, the main anion reabsorbed with sodium is HCO_3^-, which tends to maintain the alkalotic state. Administration of NaCl replenishes depleted Cl^- levels and restores ECV. Chloride-resistant metabolic alkaloses are typically caused by excessive mineralocorticoid activity or renal tubular chloride wasting (Bartter syndrome). In these disorders, the primary abnormality is enhanced renal H^+ excretion and HCO_3^- reabsorption. Treatment should be directed toward the underlying cause.

Respiratory Acid–Base Disorders

Respiratory acid–base disorders are categorized as either acute or chronic. Chronic respiratory acid–base disorders differ from acute disorders because of the time available for renal alterations in either excretion of NH_4^+ or reabsorption of HCO_3^-. This renal compensatory response may occur after several

TABLE 7.8. Respiratory Acid–Base Disorders by Mechanism.

Respiratory acidosis	*Respiratory alkalosis*
Reduced respiratory drive	Increased respiratory drive
Sedatives, hypnotics, narcotics	Pain, fever, gram-negative sepsis, cirrhosis, CNS lesions, pregnancy (progesterone effect), salicylates, theophylline
CNS lesions	
Increased work of breathing	Peripheral chemoreceptor stimulation
Restrictive lung disease: pulmonary fibrosis, pleural effusions, ankylosing spondylitis	Hypoxia, hypotension
Obstructive lung disease: upper air obstruction, asthma	
Myopathies	Pulmonary receptor stimulation
Paralysis, Guillain–Barré syndrome	Pneumonia, pulmonary edema, pulmonary embolus
Increased CO_2 production in concert with a fixed minute ventilation, e.g., fever, seizures, large pulmonary embolus	

hours or days. Chronic respiratory disorders have a renal response that leads to increased serum bicarbonate in respiratory acidosis and a decreased serum bicarbonate in respiratory alkalosis. By contrast, acute changes are characterized by significant changes in $Paco_2$ with minimal alterations in serum HCO_3^-.

In respiratory acidosis, a reduction in effective minute ventilation leads to an increase in $Paco_2$ and a reduction in pH. If the acidosis is acute, then there should be no more than a 3 to 4 mEq/l rise in HCO_3^- as the result of cellular buffering. If chronic, then there should be a 0.3 mEq/l increase in HCO_3^- for each 1 mmHg increment in $Paco_2$. The most common cause of respiratory acidosis in postoperative patients is central respiratory depression due to excessive postoperative sedatives or narcotics (Table 7.8). In a patient with a fixed minute volume (e.g., on a mechanical ventilator), an increase in $Paco_2$ suggests either an increase in alveolar dead space (e.g., pulmonary embolus) or increased CO_2 production. The treatment of respiratory acidosis should be directed toward the underlying cause. If the cause is not easily correctable and the acidosis is severe, then assisted ventilation will be necessary. Administration of exogenous HCO_3^- may lead to a further increase in $Paco_2$ and is therefore not indicated.

Respiratory alkalosis is common in surgical patients. Typically, excessive pain, fever, or gram-negative sepsis leads to an increase in central respiratory drive, causing a reduction in $Paco_2$, and if chronic, a compensatory increase in serum HCO_3^- (Table 7.8). If the alkalosis is acute, then there should be no greater than a 3 to 4 mEq/l reduction in serum HCO_3^-. In chronic respiratory alkalosis, a reduction in HCO_3^- of 0.4 to 0.5 mEq/l for each 1 mmHg reduction in $Paco_2$ is expected. If treatment is indicated, then it should be directed toward the underlying cause.

References

1. Sartorio A, Malavolti M, Agosti F, et al. Body water distribution in severe obesity and its assessment from eight-polar bioelectrical impedance analysis. Eur J Clin Nutr Sept 2004; doi:10.1038/sj.ejcn.1602049.
2. Luckey AE, Parsa CJ. Fluid and electrolytes in the aged. Arch Surg 2003;138:1055–1060.
3. Brecher ME, Monk T, Goodnough LT. A standardized method for calculating blood loss. Transfusion 1997;37:1074.
4. Budny PG, Regan PJ, Roberts AH. The estimation of blood loss during burn surgery. Burns 1993;19:134–137.
5. Halperin ML, Goldstein MB. Fluids, Electrolytes and Acid-Base Physiology, 2nd ed. Philadelphia: Saunders, 1998.
6. Robertson GL. Regulation of vasopressin secretion. In: Seldin DW, Giebisch G, eds. The Kidney: Physiology and Pathophysiology, 2nd ed. New York: Raven Press, 1992.
7. Donaldson MD, Seaman MJ, Park GR. Massive blood transfusion. Br J Anaesth 1992;69:621–630.
8. Lafferty FW. Differential diagnosis of hypercalcemia. J Bone Miner Res 1991;6:S51–S59.
9. Heys SD, Smith IC, Eremin O. Hypercalcaemia in patients with cancer: aetiology and treatment. Eur J Surg Oncol 1998;24:139–142.
10. Fatemi S, Ryzen E, Flores J, Endres DB, Rude RK. Effect of experimental human magnesium depletion on parathyroid hormone secretion and 1,25-dihydroxyvitamin D metabolism. J Clin Endocrinol Metab 1991;73:1067–1072.
11. George R, Shiu MH. Hypophosphatemia after major hepatic resection. Surgery (St. Louis) 1992;111:281–286.
12. Solomon SM, Kirby DF. The refeeding syndrome: a review. J Parenter Enteral Nutr 1990;14:90–97.
13. Narins RG, Krishna GC. Disorders of water balance. In: Stein JH, ed. Internal Medicine, 2nd ed. Philadelphia: Lippincott-Williams & Wilkins, 1987:794–805.
14. Goldberg M. Water control and the dysnatremias. In: Bricker NS, ed. The Sea Within Us. New York: Scientific Medical Publishing, 1975:14–25.
15. Sterns RH, Cox M, Feig PU, Singer I. Internal potassium balance and the control of plasma potassium concentration. Medicine (Baltimore) 1981;60:339–354.
16. Johnson RL, Ramanathan M. Buffer equilibra in the lungs. In: Seldin DW, Giebisch G, eds. The Kidney: Physiology and Pathophysiology, 2nd ed. Philadelphia: Lippincott-Williams & Wilkins, 1992.

8

Hemostasis and Coagulation

Marcel Levi and Tom van der Poll

Basic Considerations

Bleeding is one of the major complications of surgery. Serious intraoperative and postoperative bleeding not only may be caused by a local problem in surgical hemostasis, such as a failed ligature, but also can be caused by a defect in the hemostatic system. Surgical hemostasis and an adequately functioning coagulation system are complementary: In some cases, a patient with a (minor) hemostatic defect may be operated on without any specific perioperative intervention in the coagulation system, whereas in other instances improvement of blood coagulation may be necessary before operation. In this chapter, current insights into the functioning of the coagulation system, and anticoagulant and prohemostatic interventions in this system, are discussed. Subsequently, conditions associated with an enhanced risk of perioperative bleeding (including the preoperative use of anticoagulant agents) and strategies to reduce perioperative blood loss are reviewed. Last, the pathogenesis and clinical management of disseminated intravascular coagulation (DIC) are discussed.

Current Insights into the Function of the Hemostatic System In Vivo

Blood coagulation can be divided into three parts: (1) primary hemostasis, consisting of the formation of a platelet plug and the occurrence of vasoconstriction, as a first line of defense of the body against bleeding; (2) fibrin formation, as a result of the activation of various coagulation proteins, which ultimately results in the generation of thrombin and subsequent fibrinogen-to-fibrin conversion; and (3) removal of fibrin, which is a function of the fibrinolytic system.[1,2]

Primary Hemostasis

After disruption of the integrity of the vessel wall, platelets adhere to the (sub)endothelium by means of their surface membrane glycoprotein receptor Ib. The ligand between this receptor and the vessel wall is the circulating protein named von Willebrand factor. As a consequence, the platelet becomes activated, which results in the expression of the platelet membrane surface receptor glycoprotein IIb/IIIa. Subsequently, platelets may aggregate with each other through this receptor, using circulating fibrinogen as a ligand. Red blood cells appear to play an important role in platelet adhesion and aggregation, potentially because of their physical capability to facilitate platelet transport to the surface (Fig. 8.1). Therefore, adequate function of primary hemostasis is dependent on a sufficiently high hematocrit.[3]

During the activation of the platelets and via a series of enzymatic reactions, arachidonic acid (from the platelet membrane) is converted into several eicosanoids, such as thromboxane A_2 and various prostaglandins (PGs). These mediators may exert a vasoconstricting action and thus promote further activation of primary hemostasis. Another consequence of platelet activation is the release of various proteins from platelet storage granules, including (1) several platelet agonists (such as adenosine diphosphate [ADP] and serotonin); (2) coagulation factors (such as von Willebrand factor and coagulation factor V); (3) heparin-binding proteins (such as platelet factor 4 and β-thromboglobulin); and (4) proteins with activity as a growth factor or chemokine (such as platelet-derived growth factor [PDGF], platelet transforming growth factor-β_1 [platelet TGF-β], epidermal growth factor, or thrombopoietin [TPO]). Last, the phospholipid membrane of the activated platelet provides an excellent surface on which the generation of thrombin and subsequent fibrin formation may take place.[4]

Blood Coagulation

Although the coagulation system has traditionally been divided into an intrinsic and extrinsic pathway, such a division does not exist in vivo.[5] A schematic outline of the activation of coagulation in vivo is provided in Figure 8.2.

The principal route of activation of blood coagulation is via the tissue factor–factor VII pathway (the former "extrinsic

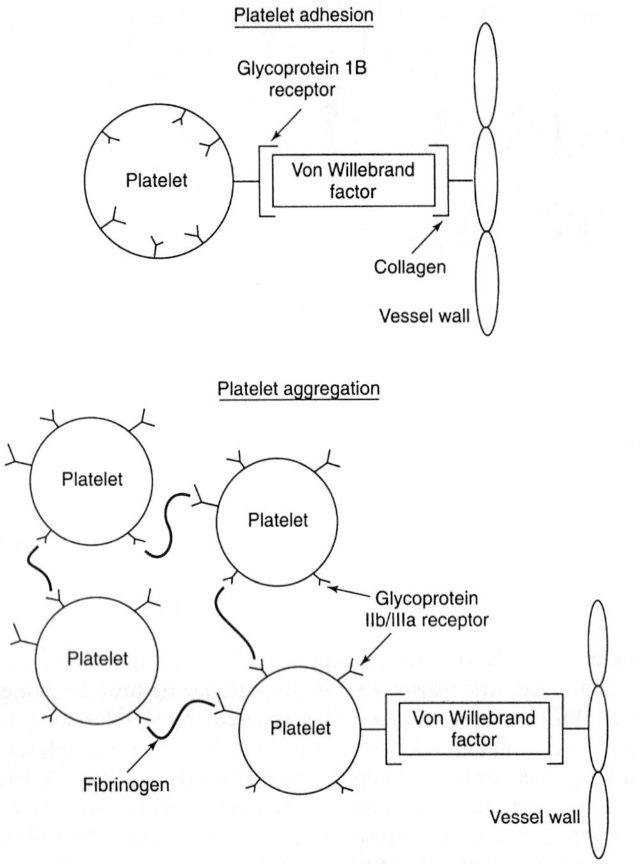

FIGURE 8.1. Platelet adherence to endothelium occurs via interaction of the platelet receptor and von Willebrand factor (*top*). This mechanism results in activation and expression of additional platelet receptors, which may aggregate via fibrinogen to other platelets (*bottom*).

system"). Tissue factor is a membrane-associated glycoprotein that is not in contact with the blood under physiological circumstances. Tissue factor is present at subendothelial sites and becomes exposed to the blood on disruption of the normal architecture of the blood vessel. Alternatively, tissue factor can be expressed by endothelial cells or by mononuclear cells in response to certain stimuli, such as inflammatory mediators. This action may explain the exposition of tissue factor and subsequent activation of coagulation, which may occur under diverse conditions such as traumatic endothelial injury or during systemic infection. After exposition of tissue factor to blood, a complex between tissue factor and factor VII occurs, on which factor VII is converted into its active form (factor VIIa). The tissue factor–factor VIIa complex subsequently binds and activates factor X, resulting in factor Xa. Once factor Xa is formed, it converts prothrombin (factor II) to thrombin (factor IIa). This enzymatic reaction requires the presence of factor V as a cofactor and is most efficient in the presence of a suitable phospholipid surface, such as that provided by the activated platelet.

An alternative route for factor Xa activation by the tissue factor–factor VIIa complex is by the activation of factor IX. The importance of this "secondary" pathway for activation of coagulation is best illustrated by the striking hemorrhagic diathesis of patients with a deficiency of factor VIII or IX (hemophilia A and B, respectively; the incidences of hemophilia A and B are 1:10,000 and 1:70,000, respectively). A third amplifying pathway of the blood coagulation system consists of the activation of factor XI by thrombin. Factor XIa subsequently activates factor IX, resulting in further factor Xa and thrombin generation.

Thrombin is the key enzyme in the activation of coagulation. Thrombin is not only essential for the conversion of fibrinogen into fibrin, but also is able to activate various coagulation factors and cofactors, thereby strongly facilitating its own formation. In addition, thrombin is a very strong activator of platelet aggregation. The formation of cross-linked fibrin is the ultimate step in the coagulation cascade. Thrombin-mediated cleavage of peptides from the fibrinogen molecule results in the formation of fibrin monomers and subsequently polymers. To further stabilize the clot, cross-linking of fibrin takes place by thrombin-activated factor XIII.

Synthesis of most of the coagulation factors takes place in the liver. Some coagulation factors (II, VII, IX, and X) require the presence of vitamin K for proper synthesis; in the absence of vitamin K, inactive precursor molecules are formed.

Natural Anticoagulant Mechanisms

Activation of the coagulation system is regulated at various points (see Fig. 8.2).[6] Inhibition of the tissue factor–factor VIIa complex may occur by the action of tissue factor pathway inhibitor (TFPI), a surface-associated protease inhibitor. Further regulation takes place by the protein C system. Activated protein C, assisted by its essential cofactor (protein S), proteolytically degrades the important cofactors V and VIII. Activated protein C is formed on activation of circulating protein C by the endothelial cell-bound enzyme thrombomodulin in association with thrombin. Hence, thrombin not

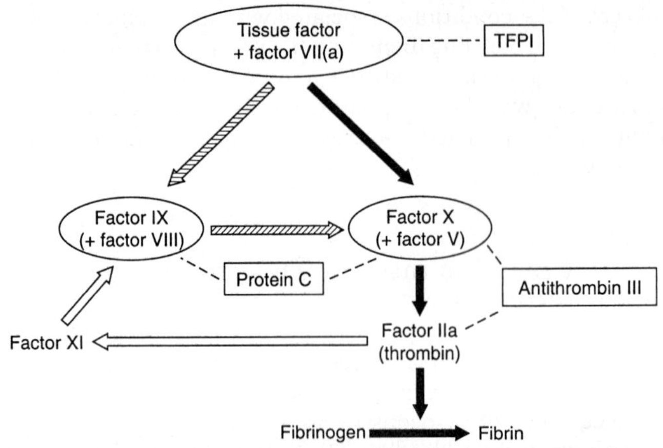

FIGURE 8.2. Schematic representation of the function of blood coagulation in vivo. The principal route of thrombin generation proceeds by the direct activation of factor X by the tissue factor–factor VIIa complex (*black arrows*). An alternative pathway is formed by the activation of factor IX by the tissue factor–factor VIIa complex and the activation of factor X by this activated factor IX (and cofactor VIII) (*shaded arrows*). A third amplifying pathway consists of the thrombin-mediated activation of factor XI, which can subsequently activate factor IX and X (*open arrows*). The point of impact of the three inhibitory systems (antithrombin III, the protein C and S system, and tissue factor pathway inhibitor [*TFPI*], respectively) are indicated with the *dotted lines*.

only plays a pivotal role in coagulation activation but also is involved in the inhibition of blood coagulation. Both protein C and protein S are vitamin K-dependent proteins. A third inhibitory system is formed by antithrombin III; this serine protease inhibitor forms complexes with thrombin and factor Xa, thereby losing their coagulant activity. The inhibitory action of antithrombin III on thrombin and factor Xa is strongly amplified in the presence of heparin.

A (usually hereditary) deficiency of antithrombin III, protein C, or protein S results in a procoagulant state, and patients with these deficiencies are prone to develop thrombosis. This development may occur in particular in situations with an enhanced thrombotic risk, such as the puerperium or postoperatively. A situation in which there is normal functional protein C but an impaired sensitivity of factor V to protein C is called activated protein C resistance (APC resistance) and is caused by a point mutation in factor V (factor V Leiden). The prevalence of this mutation is about 3% to 5% in the general population and may account for about 30% of all idiopathic venous thromboembolism.

Fibrinolysis

Fibrin plays only a temporary role and must be removed to restore normal tissue structure and function. The enzymatic degradation of fibrin is carried out by the fibrinolytic system, which is partly responsible for the unobstructed flow of blood. The fibrinolytic system, resembling the cascade mechanism of blood coagulation, comprises zymogen-to-enzyme conversions, feedback amplification and inhibition, and a finely tuned balance with various inhibitors.[7] The function of the fibrinolytic system is schematically represented in Figure 8.3. The pivotal event in the process of fibrinolysis is the conversion of the inactive zymogen plasminogen into the active protease plasmin, which cleaves cross-linked fibrin, resulting in the dissolution of a clot. Plasminogen activators, of which tissue-type plasminogen activator (tPA) and urokinase-type plasminogen activator (uPA) are most important, mediate the conversion of plasminogen into plasmin. Both activators are present in endothelial cells and may be released by various stimuli, including hypoxia and acidosis, as may occur during thrombotic occlusion. Inhibition of the fibrinolytic system may occur at the level of the plasminogen activators by plasminogen activator inhibitors (PAIs, e.g., PAI-1) or at the level of plasmin by circulating protease inhibitors, of which α_2-antiplasmin is the most important.

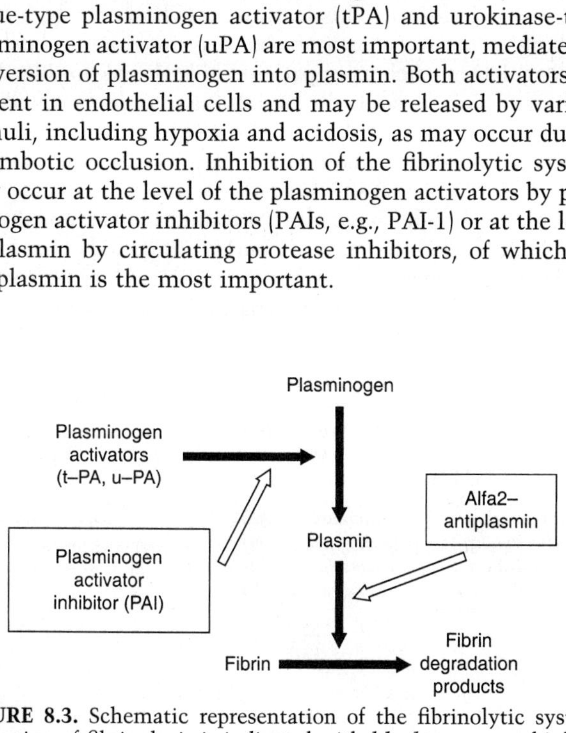

FIGURE 8.3. Schematic representation of the fibrinolytic system. Activation of fibrinolysis is indicated with *black arrows* and inhibition of the system by the *open arrows*.

An imbalance between activators and inhibitors of the fibrinolytic system, resulting in a net antifibrinolytic state, may contribute to the development of thrombosis. After major operations, such a "fibrinolytic shutdown" may be demonstrable. The efficacy of postoperative pneumatic calf compression may be based not only on rheological advantages in the venous circulation but also result from the enhanced release of plasminogen activators from the vessel wall on compression (and venous occlusion), thereby compensating for this fibrinolytic imbalance.

Anticoagulant Agents

Antiplatelet Agents

Platelets play a pivotal role in primary hemostasis and in the initiation of arterial and, to a lesser extent, venous thrombosis. Inhibition of platelet activity has been shown to be an effective strategy in the prevention and treatment of thromboembolic disease. The ability of aspirin (acetylsalicylic acid) to inhibit platelet activity has been known for decades. Despite the fact that several other antiplatelet agents have become available in recent years, aspirin remains the standard regarding efficacy and safety in the management of (arterial) thromboembolic vascular disease.[8]

The antiplatelet effect of *aspirin* is based on the irreversible inhibition of the platelet membrane-associated enzyme cyclooxygenase. Cyclooxygenase is a crucial enzyme in the arachidonic acid metabolic pathway, and inhibition of this enzyme blocks the formation of thromboxane A_2, a potent platelet agonist and mediator of vasoconstriction. Low doses of aspirin preferentially inhibit the formation of platelet thromboxane A_2, whereas interference with the formation of other PGs, such as the platelet antagonist and vasodilator prostacyclin (PGI_2) by endothelial cells seems less prominent. The use of aspirin results in an irreversible (and relatively weak) inhibition of platelet aggregation and may be associated with significant impairment of primary hemostasis and mild enhancement of bleeding as a consequence. Because the antiplatelet effect of aspirin is irreversible, this effect will last for the interval needed to produce a sufficient number of new platelets not affected by aspirin. In view of the life span of platelets (approximately 10 days), 5 to 7 days are usually required after termination of aspirin use to restore adequate platelet function and effective hemostasis. The most important adverse effects of aspirin are bleeding and the occurrence of hemorrhagic gastritis or even gastric ulceration.

Clopidogrel belongs to the class of thienopyridine derivatives, which act by blocking the ADP receptor on the platelet. In a large trial comparing clopidogrel with aspirin as secondary prophylaxis in patients with a myocardial infarction, stroke, or peripheral arterial disease, an equivalent efficacy of these two antiplatelet agents was demonstrated.[9] However, the combination of clopidogrel and aspirin was shown to be superior over aspirin alone in studies of patients after an acute coronary event, percutaneous coronary interventions, and coronary stent placement.[10,11]

Dipyridamole exerts its antiplatelet effect by inhibition of phosphodiesterase, resulting in the intracellular accumulation of cyclic AMP (adenosine monophosphate), which has an antiaggregating effect. Although dipyridamole is a potent inhibitor of platelet aggregation in vitro, it has not shown any significant efficacy on the prevention of thromboembolic disease in large clinical trials.

Inhibitors of the glycoprotein receptor IIb/IIIa are the most potent inhibitors of platelet aggregation by competitively competing for fibrinogen binding to the platelet IIb/IIIa receptor. Although the intravenous form of this medication has been shown to be highly effective in interventional cardiology, oral forms of this class of agents were not effective in the secondary prevention of atherothrombotic events.[12]

Vitamin K Antagonists (Coumarin Derivatives)

Oral anticoagulant agents are *coumarin* derivatives, such as warfarin, acenocoumarol, and phenprocoumon.[13] These compounds block the essential vitamin K-dependent carboxylation of coagulation factors II, VII, IX, and X, resulting in the formation of biologically inactive proteins and a decrease in the coagulant activity of these factors in plasma. The anticoagulant effect of coumarin derivatives is a function of the decay in the concentration of the vitamin K-dependent coagulation factors rather than of the plasma concentration of the drug. The half-life of vitamin K-dependent coagulation factors ranges from 6 (factor VII) to 60h (factor II); hence, the full effect of therapy is delayed for 2 or 3 days. Also, full restoration of normal coagulation after termination of coumarin therapy requires at least 3 to 5 days (see the section, "Consequences of the Preoperative Use"). The dose–effect relationship of oral anticoagulants may vary considerably both between patients (interindividual) and in any patient over time (intraindividual) as the result of changes in binding to plasma albumin, variable vitamin K intake, and variable clearance by the liver. Therefore, close monitoring of the intensity of anticoagulation is required. To do so, the prothrombin time (PT) determination is most often used. To correct for considerable differences in thromboplastin sensitivity, which ultimately result in highly different PT results in patients with an identical intensity of anticoagulation, the International Normalized Ratio (INR) has been established. The INR corrects for the differences of the various thromboplastins used in the PT assays as compared to an international reference thromboplastin preparation. Increasing values of the INR represent higher intensities of anticoagulation, with an INR of 1.0 indicating no anticoagulation.

The most important side effect of coumarin treatment is bleeding. In rare cases, usually associated with a protein C deficiency, coumarin-induced skin necrosis may occur. This is caused by the relatively rapid decay in already low protein C levels at a time when levels of coagulation factors are still normal, resulting in a net procoagulant state.

Heparin, Low Molecular Weight Heparins, and Pentasaccharides

Not all physicians realize that heparin represents a cocktail of more than 100 different molecules.[14] Heparin consists of a large number of glycosaminoglycans of various molecular sizes (4–20kDa), and these are isolated from the intestines or lungs of pig, cow, or other cattle. Heparin binds to antithrombin III, thereby potentiating the inhibitory effect of antithrombin III on coagulation factors IIa (thrombin) and Xa more than 1000-fold. The effect of heparin after intravenous administration is immediate, and heparin has a dose-dependent half-life: After the intravenous administration of a bolus dose of 5000U, the mean half-life is approximately 60 to 90min. Also, the anticoagulant effect of heparin may be highly variable; therefore, frequent laboratory monitoring is required. Usually, the activated partial thromboplastin time (aPTT) is used to tailor heparin treatment. In special conditions, such as extracorporeal cardiopulmonary bypass, the whole blood activated clotting time (ACT) may be applied.

Low molecular weight heparins (LMWHs) have been introduced that have an average molecular weight between 4 and 6kDa.[15] In some situations, these heparin fractions have shown a more favorable antithrombotic effect and induce fewer bleeding complications at therapeutic doses compared to unfractionated heparin. In addition, LMWHs have highly predictable inter- and intraindividual bioavailability and clearance, thereby precluding the need for frequent laboratory monitoring and frequent dose adjustments. The much longer half-life of LMWHs compared to unfractionated heparin is advantageous when stable anticoagulation is required over a longer period of time. This feature may, however, be a complicating factor in situations that require easily adjustable anticoagulation, such as in patients at high risk for bleeding. Large randomized controlled trials have demonstrated the efficacy and safety of LMWH in the postoperative prevention of venous thromboembolism in various surgical patients (Table 8.1).

Pentasaccharides have been introduced into clinical practice. Pentasaccharides are synthetic compounds that exert antithrombin-dependent exclusive inhibition of factor Xa. Pentasaccharides (such as fondaparinux) have been superior

TABLE 8.1.

Summary of Randomized Controlled Trials on the Efficacy and Safety of Low Molecular Weight Heparin in the Prevention of Postoperative Venous Thromboembolism in Patients Undergoing General Surgery, Major Orthopedic Surgery (Total Hip Replacement and Total Knee Replacement), and Trauma Surgery (Level I Evidence).

Type of surgery	*No. of trials*	*No. of patients*	*Incidence of venous thromboembolism (95% CI)*	*Relative risk reduction of postoperative venous thromboembolism (compared with placebo)*	*Increase in total bleeding complications (compared with placebo) (95% CI)*	*Increase in major bleeding complications (compared with placebo) (95% CI)*
General surgery	12	4386	5% (4–6)	80%	16%	3%
Major orthopedic surgery	30	4712	21% (20–22)	71%	7%	−1%
Trauma surgery	5	437	28%	44%	11%	0%

Source: Data from Koch et al.[96] and Palmer et al.[97]

to LMWH in the prophylaxis of venous thromboembolism in patients undergoing hip or knee replacement.[16]

Bleeding is the most frequently encountered adverse effect of heparin or heparin derivative treatment. In addition, heparin-induced thrombocytopenia (HIT) may occur. This entity is an immunological response to heparin characterized by the occurrence of thrombocytopenia and venous and arterial thromboembolism. Usually, HIT occurs at 5 to 7 days after initial exposure to heparin, but it may be an immediate complication if the patient has received heparin previously. It is essential to immediately discontinue heparin in patients with HIT. Alternative anticoagulant therapy may consist of treatment with hirudin or heparinoids but not with coumarin derivatives, which may promote skin necrosis. Last, long-term use of heparin has been associated with the occurrence of osteopenia. These adverse effects appear to have a lower incidence if LMWH is used.

Thrombolytic Agents

Rapid dissolution of clots can be attained by the administration of thrombolytic agents. All thrombolytic agents are plasminogen activators, either recombinant endogenous plasminogen activators (such as recombinant tPA) administered at a dose that is 1000-fold higher than physiological concentration or activators derived from exogenous sources, such as streptokinase. The most important side effect of thrombolytic treatment is bleeding.

Prohemostatic Agents

Platelets, Plasma, and Coagulation Factor Concentrates

Platelet transfusion may be considered in patients with severe thrombocytopenia and bleeding or a risk for bleeding. Platelet concentrates usually contain a mixture of the platelet preparation of the blood donation from six donors (6 units). After platelet transfusion, the platelet count should rise by at least 5×10^9/l per unit of platelets transfused. A lesser response may occur in patients with fever, a consumptive coagulopathy (see "Management of Postoperative Bleeding"), or splenomegaly or may indicate alloimmunization of the patient after repeated transfusion. Platelet transfusion is particularly effective in patients with thrombocytopenia caused by impaired platelet production or increased consumption, whereas in disorders of enhanced platelet destruction (such as immune thrombocytopenia; see the section on immune thrombocytopenia) alternative therapies may provide better results. Guidelines for platelet transfusion are given in Table 8.2.

TABLE 8.2. Suggested Transfusion Guidelines for Platelet Concentrates.

Platelet count $<10 \times 10^9$/l
Platelet count $<50 \times 10^9$/l with demonstrated bleeding or a planned surgical/invasive procedure
Documented platelet dysfunction (e.g., prolonged bleeding time) with (microvascular) bleeding or undergoing a surgical/invasive procedure and (assumed) insufficient efficacy of other interventions (e.g., desmopressin)
Bleeding patients or patients undergoing a surgical procedure who require more than 10U of packed red cells

TABLE 8.3. Suggested Transfusion Guidelines for Fresh Frozen Plasma.

Correction of multiple or specific coagulation factor deficiencies in bleeding patients or if a surgical/invasive procedure is planned
Congenital deficiencies of a specific factor (provided specific factor concentrates are not available, e.g., factor XI)
Acquired deficiencies, such as those related to liver disease, massive transfusion, or disseminated intravascular coagulation
Volume replacement in case of severe bleeding to avoid massive transfusion of gelatin or crystalloid solutions
Thrombocytopenic thrombotic purpura

Fresh or frozen plasma contains all coagulation factors and may be used to replenish congenital or acquired deficiencies in these factors. For more specific therapy, or if the transfusion of large volumes of plasma is not desirable, fractionated plasma of purified coagulation factor concentrate is available.[17] Suggested guidelines for the use of fresh frozen plasma are given in Table 8.3.

Prothrombin complex concentrates (PCCs) contain the vitamin K-dependent coagulation factors II, VII, IX, and X. Hence, these concentrates may be used if immediate reversal of coumarin therapy is required. Also, PCCs may be used if a global replenishment of coagulation factors is necessary and large volumes of plasma are not tolerated. One should realize, however, that only a selected number of coagulation factors are administered, and important deficiencies, such as factor V or fibrinogen, are not treated.

Cryoprecipitate is fractionated plasma that contains mainly von Willebrand factor, factor VIII, and fibrinogen. However, because of problems in the production of cryoprecipitate, particularly regarding standards to prevent the transmission of infectious agents, in most parts of the Western world cryoprecipitate is not readily available.

Purified concentrates containing only that specific factor are available for a selected number of clotting factors. These concentrates are particularly useful in cases of isolated (usually congenital) deficiency of a single clotting factor, such as factor VIII concentrate for the treatment of hemophilia A. Most of these concentrates consist of clotting factors that are purified by affinity chromatography of plasma. Recombinant coagulation factors have become available.

Clotting factor concentrates derived from plasma are of human origin. Potentially, these carry the risk of transmission of blood-borne diseases. Despite all current measures to prevent this complication, these risks are not fully eliminated. Hence, the use of these products should be limited as much as possible, especially if no strict indication is present or an alternative treatment is available.

Desmopressin

Deamino-D-arginine vasopressin (DDAVP, desmopressin) is a vasopressin analogue that induces release of the contents of the endothelial cell-associated Weibel–Palade bodies, including von Willebrand factor.[18] Hence, the administration of DDAVP results in a marked increase in the plasma concentration of von Willebrand factor (and associated coagulation factor VIII) and, by yet unexplained additional mechanisms, a remarkable potentiation of primary hemostasis. Administration of DDAVP can be by different routes (intravenously, subcutaneously, and intranasally) but is usually administered intravenously, resulting in an immediate prohemostatic effect. It is used for the prevention and treatment of bleeding in patients with von Willebrand disease or mild hemophilia A. It is also used in patients with an impaired function of primary hemostasis, such as those with uremia, liver cirrhosis, or aspirin-associated bleeding.

Recombinant Factor VIIa

Given that activation of coagulation in vivo predominantly proceeds by the tissue factor–factor VIIa pathway, recombinant factor VIIa has been developed as a prohemostatic agent and has become available for clinical use. In uncontrolled clinical studies, this compound has been shown to exert potent procoagulant activity and appears to be highly effective in the prevention and treatment of bleeding. Most clinical experience thus far has been obtained in patients with severe and complicated coagulation defects.[19]

In a randomized controlled trial in patients undergoing transabdominal prostatectomy, administration of recombinant factor VIIa resulted in a 50% reduction of blood loss compared with placebo and eliminated the need for blood transfusion, which was required in about 60% of placebo-treated patients.[20]

Subsequent studies have focused on surgery in patients undergoing orthotopic liver transplantation. An initial open-label pilot study in 6 patients showed a strong reduction in transfusion requirements in those who received a single dose of recombinant activated factor VII (80 μg/kg) compared with historic matched controls.[21] However, a subsequent randomized placebo-controlled trial evaluating two different dosages (60 or 120 μg/kg) in 182 patients showed no reduction in transfusion requirements, although a significantly higher proportion of patients treated with recombinant activated factor VII did not need any red blood cell transfusion (8.4% vs. none in the placebo group).[22] Two randomized controlled trials (up to 100 μg/kg at every second hour of surgery) in patients with cirrhosis or normal liver function undergoing major liver resection also showed no significant effect on either the volume of blood products administered or the number of patients transfused.[23,24] Last, recombinant activated factor VII has been evaluated in a small randomized controlled study in 20 patients undergoing noncoronary cardiac surgery requiring cardiopulmonary bypass. Administration of this agent (90 μg/kg after discontinuation of bypass and reversal of heparin) significantly reduced the need for blood transfusion (relative risk of any transfusion 0.26, 95% confidence interval 0.07–0.90).[25]

Trauma is another potential area of interest for the use of recombinant activated factor VII, after several case reports and case series indicated this agent may be effective in reducing major blood loss and transfusion requirements in these patients.[26] A placebo-controlled trial of repeated doses of recombinant activated factor VII (200, 100, and again 100 μg/kg) in 143 patients with severe blunt trauma showed that this schedule significantly reduced red blood cell transfusion (mean reduction 2.6 units) and the need for massive transfusion (defined as more than 20 units of red blood cells) (14% in treated patients vs. 33% in controls). Although there was a trend toward lower mortality and other clinically relevant outcomes (such as organ failure and acute respiratory distress syndrome), statistical significance was not achieved. On the other hand, there were no significant effects in 134 patients with penetrating trauma.[27]

There are several case reports and case series on the use of recombinant factor VIIa in patients with severe postoperative bleeding.[28] There are no randomized controlled clinical trials, which is not surprising in view of the difficulty in performing a meaningful study in these heterogeneous situations. Many reports claim rapid reduction of blood loss or decrease in transfusion requirements after other therapeutic measures had failed. Although many of these reports are compelling, it is difficult to properly assess the utility of recombinant activated factor VII as publication bias may have played a relevant role. Although no thrombotic complications of recombinant factor VIIa treatment have been reported thus far, the safety of this strategy in a general population remains to be established.

Antifibrinolytic Agents

Agents that exert antifibrinolytic activity are aprotinin and the group of lysine analogues.[29] The prohemostatic effect of these agents proceeds both by the inhibition of fibrinolysis (thereby shifting the procoagulant–anticoagulant balance toward a more procoagulant state) and by a protective effect on platelets. The mechanism of this platelet-protective effect has not been fully elucidated. Whether the prohemostatic effect of the antifibrinolytic agents will eventually result in a higher incidence of thromboembolic complications is still a matter of debate (see further), although this has not been shown in initial clinical trials.

Aprotinin is a 58-amino-acid polypeptide, mainly derived from bovine lung, parotid gland, or pancreas. Aprotinin directly inhibits the activity of various serine proteases, including plasmin, coagulation factors or inhibitors, and constituents of the kallikrein–kinin and angiotensin system. This rather nonspecific mode of action of aprotinin is frequently considered a disadvantage, although the interactions of aprotinin with proteases other than plasmin have not been demonstrated to cause clinically important adverse effects. The most important clinical side effect of aprotinin is a rarely occurring, but sometimes serious, allergic or anaphylactic reaction. The use of aprotinin is contraindicated in cases of ongoing systemic intravascular activation of coagulation, as in disseminated intravascular coagulation (DIC) and in patients with renal failure. The safety of aprotinin has been questioned as large clinical practice-based studies showed an increased incidence of renal insufficiency and other adverse outcomes after its use.[30,31] The current Food and Drug Administration advisory recommends the use of aprotinin only when the clinical benefit of reduced blood loss is essential to medical management and outweighs any potential risk.

Lysine analogues (i.e., ε-aminocaproic acid and tranexamic acid) are potent inhibitors of fibrinolysis. The antifibrinolytic action of lysine analogues is based on the competitive binding of these agents to the lysine-binding sites of a fibrin clot, thereby competing with the binding of plasminogen. Impaired plasminogen binding to fibrin delays the conversion of plasminogen to plasmin and subsequent plasmin-mediated fibrinolysis. Subtle molecular variations between different lysine analogues may have important consequences for their fibrinolysis-inhibiting capacity. Indeed, tranexamic acid is at least 10 times more potent than ε-aminocaproic acid. The use of lysine analogues is contraindicated in situations with ongoing systemic activation of coagulation (such as in DIC) and in cases of macroscopic hematuria because the inhibition of fibrinolysis may result in deposition of urinary tract-obstructing clots.

Other Prohemostatic Agents

Conjugated estrogen preparations may also improve primary hemostasis. Currently, there is no sound evidence for the use of these agents to prevent or treat perioperative bleeding although a limited number of mostly uncontrolled studies in patients with uremic thrombocytopathy and preliminary observations in patients who undergo liver transplantation suggest some efficacy.

Fibrin sealant, usually consisting of a combination of human fibrinogen and bovine thrombin, may be used as a topical hemostatic agent. Although a number of controlled studies have shown the efficacy of this treatment in various surgical situations, there is no evidence that application of fibrin sealant results in a reduction of intraoperative or postoperative blood loss or other clinically significant outcome measures. In addition, fibrinogen is usually derived from human donor plasma and may carry the risk of transmission of blood-borne diseases. Further, the bovine origin of the thrombin may result in the formation of anticoagulation factor antibodies cross-reacting with human coagulation factors, resulting in a potentially severe bleeding tendency. Methodologically sound clinical trials that would demonstrate efficacy and safety of fibrin sealants are badly warranted.

Monitoring of Blood Coagulation

The function of the hemostatic system can be monitored using various laboratory tests. For proper function of primary hemostasis, a platelet count of at least 30 to 50 × 10^9 is required. The function of the primary hemostatic system may be tested by performance of the bleeding time. However, clinical studies have shown that there is no correlation between the result of the bleeding time and the occurrence and intensity of perioperative bleeding. More detailed analysis of primary hemostasis may be performed by ex vivo platelet aggregation tests. These tests, however, are labor intensive and may not be widely available.

The most frequently used screening tests for blood coagulation are the PT and the aPTT. Although both PT and aPTT are highly artificial and do not fully reflect coagulation in vivo, these tests are useful to screen for deficiencies of single or multiple coagulation factors. In case of an abnormal test result, assaying the coagulant activity of selected coagulation factors can be performed to more incisively analyze the function of blood coagulation. In addition, the PT is used to monitor coumarin treatment, whereas the aPTT is most frequently used to monitor the intensity of heparin anticoagulation.

Clinical Management of Coagulation Abnormalities and Bleeding

Conditions Associated with an Enhanced Risk of Perioperative Bleeding

Congenital Coagulation Abnormalities

Congenital defects, either in primary hemostasis or in the blood coagulation system, may cause serious intraoperative and postoperative bleeding. Albeit not an absolute rule, a defect in primary hemostasis will cause immediate hemostatic problems, whereas a defective blood coagulation system may cause postoperative bleeding up to 1 week after surgery.

The most frequently occurring congenital defect in primary hemostasis is a deficiency of von Willebrand factor, also called *von Willebrand disease.* (The incidence of severe von Willebrand disease is estimated at 1:25,000, but milder forms of this disorder may be present in 1 to 5 of 1,000 patients.) A deficiency of von Willebrand factor is associated with a bleeding tendency that varies in clinical presentation (partly dependent on the remaining concentration of von Willebrand factor in blood). The von Willebrand factor plays a role as the carrier and stabilizing factor of plasma factor VIII. Low levels of von Willebrand factor are usually associated with low levels of factor VIII and a resulting impairment of blood coagulation. A typical patient with von Willebrand disease has a lifelong bleeding tendency, particularly of mucosal tissues (such as gingival or nose bleeding). Laboratory tests will reveal a prolonged bleeding time and low level of von Willebrand factor (and factor VIII) levels. Treatment of or prevention of bleeding in a patient undergoing an invasive procedure may consist of the administration of desmopressin, which will result in a two- to threefold increase in endogenous von Willebrand factor levels. Prospective studies have shown the efficacy and safety of desmopressin in patients with mild and moderate types of von Willebrand disease undergoing invasive procedures and surgery.[32] If desmopressin has an insufficient effect when retested, then von Willebrand factor concentrate may be administered. Also, adjunctive treatment with lysine analogues has proven to be effective in patients with von Willebrand disease undergoing surgical procedures in small randomized controlled trials.[33]

Other congenital defects in primary hemostasis are *thrombocytopathies*, including the rarely occurring deficiencies of platelet membrane glycoproteins (e.g., deficiency of glycoprotein Ib; syndrome of Bernard Soulier and deficiency of glycoprotein IIb/IIIa; Glanzmann thrombasthenia). (The incidence of inherited thrombocytopathies is actually not known and, due to definition problems, hard to estimate.) The inability of platelets to release their contents on activation (storage pool disease) is another cause of thrombocytopathy. No specific cause can be found in a considerable number of thrombocytopathies. All thrombocytopathies are detected by a prolonged bleeding time. Small uncontrolled trials indicated that a sufficient improvement of primary hemostasis may be achieved by the administration of desmopressin, potentially in combination with lysine analogues.[34] If this is not sufficient, then a platelet transfusion should be considered. The best-known congenital defects in blood coagulation are *hemophilia A* and *hemophilia B*, deficiencies of factor VIII and IX, respectively. Severe hemophilia (factor VIII or IX < 1%) is characterized by a spontaneous bleeding tendency, particularly in muscles and joints. Moderate or mild hemophilia usually presents with bleeding after trauma or an invasive medical intervention. Spontaneous bleeding is rare. A deficiency in factor XI is a relatively frequent disorder and is associated with a bleeding tendency of a variable degree. Deficiencies in all other coagulation proteins do occur but are relatively rare.

Coagulation factor deficiencies may be detected by prolonged clotting times (aPTT or PT), and subsequent analysis reveals a low level of the deficient factor. These screening tests do not detect a deficiency of factor XIII, which is characterized by rebleeding after initial adequate hemostasis. Treatment of coagulation factor deficiencies may be achieved by administration of coagulation factor concentrate. In case of a patient with hemophilia who must undergo a major surgical intervention, coagulation factor administration should continue for at least 7 to 10 days. Prospective trials have shown the safety and efficacy of coagulation factor concentrates in patients with hemophilia who had to undergo major surgery.[35] Hence, the existence of hemophilia should never be a motive to refrain from a necessary surgical intervention.

Liver Failure

Because the liver produces most coagulation factors, insufficient liver function is associated with low levels of coagulation factors.[36] A deficiency of vitamin K, as in cases of biliary tract obstruction (see the section on vitamin K deficiency) or resulting from loss of storage sites in hepatocellular disease, may further lower levels of vitamin K-dependent factors. If liver failure is associated with portal hypertension and associated splenomegaly, then serious thrombocytopenia may also exist. In cirrhotic patients, impaired platelet function is often encountered. Because of these combined coagulation defects, patients with liver failure are at a considerable risk of perioperative bleeding, although no systematic clinical trials have precisely estimated that risk.[37]

Management of such patients includes perioperative assessment of the coagulation status by measuring platelet count, bleeding time, aPTT, and PT (and potentially one or two coagulation factors). A potential vitamin K deficiency should be treated with vitamin K_1. Correction of low levels of coagulation factors may be achieved by the administration of plasma or PCCs. There are some limitations, however, to the use of PCCs in patients with an impaired liver function: These concentrates may contain variable amounts of activated coagulation factors that cannot be adequately neutralized in patients with liver disease because of the reduced plasma concentration of antithrombin III and impaired liver clearance.[37] The effect of plasma on coagulation lasts for a few hours and may require repeated administration of plasma. Large quantities of plasma, however, may precipitate hepatic encephalopathy or cause fluid overload. Patients with severe thrombocytopenia (i.e., platelets < 30–50 × 10^9/l) should receive a transfusion with platelet suspension. However, platelet concentrates may be effective only briefly because of the rapid removal of platelets by the enlarged spleen. In addition, small controlled studies have shown that the administration of desmopressin may result in an improvement of the bleeding time, although it is not clear whether this treatment reduces the risk of perioperative bleeding.[38]

Renal Failure

Patients with renal failure often present with coagulation abnormalities and are at risk for enhanced bleeding. The hemorrhagic tendency in patients with uremia can be attributed to impaired platelet adhesion, aggregation, and release. In addition, a low hematocrit in patients with renal failure may contribute to the impaired function of primary hemostasis, although this is less frequently an important factor because most patients are regularly treated with erythropoietin.[39] The extent of the defect in primary hemostasis may be established by the bleeding time. The administration of desmopressin has been shown to result in a correction of the prolonged bleeding time in patients with uremia.[40] Prospective studies have shown the efficacy and safety of this treatment in uremic patients undergoing invasive procedures such as kidney biopsies and surgery. If an insufficient correction of the bleeding time is achieved, then the administration of platelet concentrates could be added to the desmopressin treatment. Additional measures include the correction of anemia and execution of hemodialysis, which has been shown to (partially) restore the function of primary hemostasis.

Vitamin K Deficiency

Vitamin K is essential for the production of several coagulation factors (factors II, VII, IX, and X), and a deficiency in vitamin K results in low plasma levels of these factors. Dietary vitamin K is a fat-soluble vitamin, which is absorbed in the small intestine. Also, vitamin K is synthesized by endogenous bacterial flora resident in the small intestine and colon. Hence, major causes of vitamin K deficiency are inadequate dietary intake (including patients who are not adequately supplied with vitamin K during parenteral feeding), insufficient adsorption (e.g., in patients with biliary tract obstruction), and loss of storage sites as the result of hepatic disease.[41] A vitamin K deficiency will result in prolongation of global coagulation times, particular for the PT. A final diagnosis may be made by simultaneously measuring vitamin K-dependent and vitamin K-independent coagulation factors. A more practical approach could be to administer vitamin K and to observe the effect on the PT, which should be corrected within 24h. Vitamin K_1 (usually 10mg) can be administered orally and parenterally, but oral treatment is obviously not adequate in case of insufficient adsorption. Intravenous administration is preferred over intramuscular treatment (in view of the risk of muscle bleeds in patients with low levels of coagulation factors) but may be associated with a (small) risk of an adverse response. If immediate correction of deficiency of vitamin K-dependent coagulation factors is required, then the administration of PCC will immediately restore the defect.

Immune Thrombocytopenia and Other Immune Coagulation Disorders

Immune thrombocytopenia (immune thrombocytopenic purpura, ITP) is caused by the presence of autoantibodies, usually directed against platelet glycoproteins. Increased platelet destruction and removal by the reticuloendothelial system may result in splenomegaly. In severe cases, the platelet count may be as low as 10×10^9 platelets/l, and autoantibodies to platelets are almost always detectable in serum. In general, patients with autoimmune thrombocytopenia have an enhanced bleeding risk, and retrospective data indicate that a platelet count of less than 50×10^9/l might predispose for an enhanced risk of perioperative bleeding.[42] Infusion with human immunoglobulin may provide a rapidly occurring but relatively short-lasting increase in the platelet count and thus may be useful in case a nonelective major invasive procedure is necessary. Transfusion of platelets may cause the formation of other antiplatelet antibodies and should be reserved for emergency situations. The incidence of major bleeding complications in patients with autoimmune thrombocytopenia is very low following an appropriate preoperative preparation.

The development of (auto)antibodies to a coagulation factor (most frequently factor VIII) causes a rare but dangerous disorder.[43] These so-called coagulation factor inhibitors may become present in patients treated with coagulation factor concentrates for a congenital coagulation factor deficiency, as well as in patients with a previously normal coagulation system ("acquired hemophilia"). The latter case may arise in the context of a lymphoproliferative or general autoimmune disorder, postpartum, or as a drug reaction. This disorder is characterized by a severe bleeding tendency and is associated with high morbidity and mortality from bleeding. Laboratory tests will reveal a prolongation of the aPTT or PT that is not shortened after addition of normal plasma. A definitive diagnosis can be made by measuring the individual coagulation factors and by quantification of the inhibitor. Treatment may consist of (high doses of) coagulation factor concentrate, activated PCCs, or recombinant factor VIIa. The management of this disorder is complicated and should be carried out in a specialized center.

Other Conditions Associated with Coagulation Abnormalities

Other conditions associated with coagulation abnormalities include myeloproliferative or lymphoproliferative disorders, which may be associated with defective primary hemostasis caused by a combination of thrombocytopenia and impaired platelet function. Patients with malignancies may present with diverse coagulation abnormalities resulting from impaired primary hemostasis, low-grade DIC (see DIC section), or systemic hyperfibrinolysis.

How to Identify Patients at Risk for Bleeding

The cornerstone for recognition of a clinically significant coagulation disorder is the medical history, which should include a specific inquiry about previous surgical procedures, bleeding complicating trauma, and bleeding after tooth extraction. A potential congenital coagulation disorder might be identified on the basis of a history of lifelong bleeding complications after minor trauma or interventions and a bleeding tendency in other members of the family. In addition, the history should particularly focus on the use of drugs that might affect hemostasis. During physical examination, abnormal bruising, petechiae, and splenomegaly are signs that might point to a defect in the coagulation system. Retrospective and prospective studies have shown that routine coagulation tests for most surgical procedures are not useful in patients with a negative medical history and normal physical examination. Possible exceptions may include anticipated extensive surgery or operations that pose a great challenge to hemostatic competence (e.g., neurosurgical procedures). A strategy for preoperative screening in patients with signs or symptoms of a bleeding tendency includes a platelet count, a PTT, and PT.[44] If an abnormality in primary hemostasis is suspected, bleeding time assessment and measurement of von Willebrand factor are performed. If these tests are normal but if a very high suspicion of a bleeding tendency (particularly delayed bleeding after initially adequate hemostasis) persists, then measurement of factor XIII and α_2-antiplasmin should be considered. If screening test results are abnormal, further analysis should be carried out. Table 8.4 summarizes the potential causes of abnormalities in the screening tests and suggests some follow-up tests to further analyze these abnormalities.

Consequences of the Preoperative Use of Anticoagulant Agents for Perioperative Bleeding Complications

Anticoagulant and antiplatelet agents are important in the primary treatment and secondary prevention of atherothrombotic cardiovascular disease and venous thromboembolism. A growing number of patients who must undergo a surgical procedure will be using aspirin, other antiplatelet agents, or oral anticoagulants.

A number of studies have addressed the question whether the preoperative use of aspirin results in an increased risk of perioperative bleeding. For major surgical procedures, most trials indicate that the preoperative use of aspirin resulted in enhanced perioperative bleeding, more transfusion of red blood cells and other blood products, longer operation times, and a higher incidence of reoperation because of excessive bleeding.[45,46] This evidence is provided by retrospective analysis of large clinical trials, determining risk factors for enhanced perioperative bleeding and associated complications. Moreover, a randomized controlled trial of patients using aspirin (500 mg) versus placebo preoperatively showed significantly increased blood loss and an estimated odds ratio for reoperation of 1.82 in comparison with nonusers of aspirin.[47] These observations have been confirmed in other controlled studies.

However, more recent trials showed that the lower doses of aspirin currently in use (100 mg daily), albeit associated with increased perioperative blood loss, do not increase the transfusion need, incidence of reoperation due to bleeding, or duration of hospital stay.[48] Also, published evidence indicates that smaller procedures in patients using aspirin can be performed safely without any specific preoperative intervention. As noted, it has been shown that the results of bleeding time determinations in patients exposed to aspirin shortly before a surgical procedure did not correlate with the amount of surgical bleeding, the number of transfusions, or the duration of the operation. A number of small clinical studies have shown that the administration of DDAVP may effectively reduce the antihemostatic effect of aspirin.[49] Infusion of DDAVP (0.3 μg/kg) in patients who had used aspirin within 7 days before surgery resulted in a reduction of total

TABLE 8.4. Common Causes for Abnormalities in Coagulation Screening Tests and Suggestions for Initial Further Analysis.

Finding	*Potential cause*	*Further test*
Thrombocytopenia	Immune thrombocytopenia (ITP)	Antiplatelet antibodies, thrombopoietin
	Impaired platelet production	Complete blood cell count and bone marrow analysis
	Disseminated intravascular coagulation	aPTT, PT, fibrin degradation products
	Heparin-induced thrombocytopenia	HIT test
Prolonged bleeding time	von Willebrand disease or thrombocytopathy	Platelet aggregation tests and von Willebrand factor
	Uremia, liver failure, myeloproliferative disorder, etc.	—
aPTT prolonged, PT normal	Coagulation factor deficiency (factor VIII, IX, XI, or XII)	Measure coagulation factor
	Use of heparin	—
PT prolonged, aPTT normal	Coagulation factor deficiency (factor VII)	Measure coagulation factor
	Vitamin K deficiency	Measure factor VII (vitamin K dependent) and factor V (vitamin K independent) *or* administer vitamin K and repeat after 1–2 days
	(Mild) Hepatic insufficiency	—
Both aPTT and PT prolonged	Coagulation factor deficiency (factor X, V, II, or fibrinogen)	Measure coagulation factor
	Use of oral anticoagulants	—
	Severe hepatic insufficiency	Measure coagulation factors
	Disseminated intravascular coagulation	Platelets, fibrin degradation products
	Loss/dilution caused by excessive bleeding/massive transfusion	—

blood loss and decreased red cell transfusion compared to placebo. In cardiac surgery, a similar effect may be achieved by the administration of aprotinin (see section on cardiac surgery).

Aspirin treatment should be interrupted at least 5 to 7 days preoperatively in case of elective surgery. For nonelective and emergency situations, minor procedures can be performed without any specific intervention. For major surgery or those procedures for which even minor blood loss is not desirable, transfusion of platelets or administration of desmopressin should be considered.

Prospective studies have shown that the preoperative use of other nonsteroidal antiinflammatory agents is not associated with enhanced perioperative bleeding.[50] As far as the preoperative use of *oral anticoagulants* is concerned, earlier studies showed an unacceptable high incidence of perioperative bleeding, particularly for major surgery. Prospective clinical trials, however, showed that surgery may be safely performed at low levels of anticoagulation (INR < 1.5).[51] The dose of coumarin should be significantly reduced preoperatively to achieve these levels. The indication for coumarin treatment should be taken into account. Interruption of anticoagulant treatment for recent venous thromboembolism may place the patient at high risk for recurrence in the postoperative period. Also, in patients with mechanical heart valves (in particular in combination with heart arrhythmias such as atrial fibrillation), it might not be desirable to interrupt anticoagulant treatment. In such cases, interruption of oral anticoagulation and simultaneous initiation of intravenous heparin should be contemplated. Shortly before the operation, heparin may be discontinued and may be restarted at 6 to 12h postoperatively.[52] A prospective clinical study has shown the safety of this approach regarding perioperative bleeding and prevention of thrombotic complications in patients with mechanical heart valves.[53] In patients with recent venous thromboembolism, interruption of anticoagulation and simultaneous placement of an inferior caval filter to prevent pulmonary embolism could be considered; however, there are no clinical trials to support this approach. In case of nonelective surgery, a rapid (12 to 24h) reversal of coumarin therapy may be achieved by the administration of 10mg of vitamin K. This treatment should be continued for 3 to 5 days, dependent on the half-life of the type of coumarin used. If necessary, immediate and complete correction of coagulation may be achieved by the administration of PCC.

The preoperative use of prophylactic (low molecular weight) *heparin* for the prevention of postoperative venous thromboembolism was not associated with an enhanced risk of intraoperative and postoperative bleeding in a large series of randomized controlled trials.[54] In patients treated with therapeutic doses of heparin, discontinuation of heparin will result in near normalization of coagulation in approximately 3 to 4h. If rapid reversal of heparin treatment is needed (e.g., in case of severe bleeding), then this may be achieved by the administration of protamine.

Reduction of Perioperative Blood Loss by Interventions in the Coagulation System

Perioperative blood loss may result from surgical causes or defective hemostasis. A combination of these causes may be present in some complicated situations. Even if it is not certain that a coagulation disorder is the most important factor in the enhanced blood loss, interventions in the hemostatic system may be beneficial to prevent excessive bleeding and associated complications. This approach has been extensively investigated in cardiac surgery and liver transplantation. In fact, the efficacy and safety of prohemostatic interventions in other types of surgery have not convincingly been shown in clinical trials with appropriate methodology.

Cardiac Surgery

Cardiac surgery may be associated with blood loss resulting from hemostatic imbalances. These mechanisms include (1) the loss of platelets and impairment of platelet function caused by cardiopulmonary bypass, (2) hemodilution with associated decreased plasma concentrations of coagulation factors, (3) incomplete neutralization of heparin given during cardiopulmonary bypass, and (4) an inadequate function of the fibrinolytic system for which no clear explanation is presently available. A number of pharmacological agents have been used in an effort to diminish bleeding associated with cardiopulmonary bypass.

A number of studies have focused on the potential beneficial effect of *aprotinin* on the prevention of excessive bleeding in patients undergoing cardiac surgery. Randomized controlled trials have invariably shown that administration of aprotinin resulted in a reduction of perioperative blood loss, postoperative chest tube drainage, the number of transfused units, and the number of patients receiving any transfusion. Most studies have demonstrated at least a 40% reduction in perioperative blood loss and a 50% reduction in transfusion requirements. These figures do need to be interpreted with caution because of intercenter variations in blood salvage techniques and transfusion practice.

Three meta-analyses summarized the placebo-controlled clinical trials with aprotinin.[55–57] These metaanalyses showed a mean reduction in blood loss of 400ml and a threefold-lower need to give any transfusion in cardiac surgery patients who had received aprotinin. The two most recent metaanalyses suggested that the use of aprotinin results in a threefold reduction in the incidence of reexploration, and the results of one of these studies indicated a twofold reduction in mortality compared with placebo. The dose of aprotinin used in most studies was relatively high, that is, a 280-mg (2×10^6 IU) loading dose over 30min after the induction of anesthesia, followed by a 70mg/h (0.5×10^6 IU) continuous infusion for the duration of the operation, and occasionally a dose of 280mg (2×10^6 IU) added to the priming fluid of the cardiopulmonary bypass circuit. Lower doses of aprotinin have been used as well in a variety of studies. A metaanalysis of studies comparing the higher and the lower dose of aprotinin shows that the higher dose is more effective in reducing blood loss and transfusion requirements but that there is no statistically significant difference in the incidence of rethoracotomy and mortality.

The potential to reduce blood loss by another antifibrinolytic therapy, *lysine analogues*, has also been investigated in a number of clinical trials. Generally, ε-aminocaproic acid showed insufficient efficacy relative to tranexamic acid, and most studies have focused on the latter agent. Tranexamic acid reduced bleeding after cardiac surgery, resulting in reduced transfusion requirements and fewer patients who needed any transfusion. The effects of high-dose tranexamic acid (up to 10g perioperatively) resulted in a 40% reduction in blood loss and a 50% reduction in the number of transfused units in most controlled clinical trials. The above-mentioned metaanalyses of all studies with lysine analogues suggest a 40% reduction in the number of patients who received any blood product and about a 2.5-fold reduction in the incidence of reexploration.

A number of recent studies have directly compared aprotinin and tranexamic acid. A metaanalysis of these trials appeared to indicate higher efficacy of aprotinin compared with lysine analogues, although the differences in the most important clinical endpoints, mortality and rethoracotomy, did not reach statistical significance. Also, it should be noted that the use of aprotinin may result in severe adverse reactions, whereas lysine analogues are devoid of such serious adverse events.[30]

Placebo-controlled trials have provided evidence that the administration of *desmopressin* reduces perioperative blood loss (15%–40%) and decreases transfusion requirements (30%) in patients undergoing coronary artery bypass surgery. However, these favorable findings were not confirmed in other trials, which showed no beneficial effect of desmopressin in the prevention of perioperative blood loss. The differential effects of desmopressin treatment may have been caused by other patient selection criteria in the different clinical trials. Several metaanalyses of controlled clinical trials with desmopressin in cardiac surgery showed a beneficial effect on blood loss and transfusion requirements, whereas the percentage of patients who needed any transfusion, the incidence of reexploration, and mortality were not statistically affected by desmopressin.[58] Subgroup analysis of the various clinical trials suggests that desmopressin might be particularly effective in the preoperative use of aspirin, which is not uncommon in patients undergoing cardiac surgery. The effect of desmopressin, however, appears to be relatively small compared with aprotinin and tranexamic acid.

There is much discussion whether any beneficial effects of therapy for the prevention of excessive perioperative blood loss might be offset by a potentially harmful net procoagulant effect, associated with graft occlusion and thrombotic complications. In one study, patients treated with aprotinin during their coronary artery bypass surgery appeared to have more vein graft occlusions at coronary angiography 1 year postoperatively (20.5% vs. 12.7% in patients who had not received aprotinin). Also, clinical endpoints such as perioperative myocardial infarction did not favor aprotinin treatment.[59] However, all these data were derived from a retrospective analysis of a multicenter trial in which these outcomes may be center dependent. Other, mostly uncontrolled, studies had not demonstrated an increase in clinically important thrombotic events attending the use of aprotinin. At this time, a potential prothrombotic and graft-occluding effect of these interventions has not been clearly established.

Liver Transplantation

Major liver surgery, including orthotopic liver transplantation, may be associated with excessive blood loss. Factors that contribute to this complication are impaired synthesis of coagulation proteins by the diseased liver, preexisting thrombocytopenia and thrombocytopathy, and impaired clearance of activated coagulation and fibrinolytic factors during the anhepatic phase. A few randomized controlled trials showed that the administration of either aprotinin or tranexamic acid results in the reduction of blood loss and transfusion requirements.[60,61] However, studies on the appropriate dose of these agents have yielded conflicting results, and the definitive place of these prohemostatic agents in extensive liver surgery needs to be established.

Management of Postoperative Bleeding

A central issue for a patient who has excessive bleeding during or after surgery is the decision whether the bleeding is a result

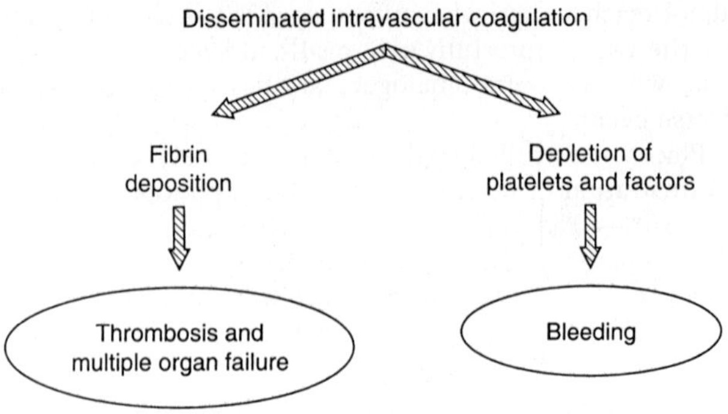

FIGURE 8.4. The clinical picture of disseminated intravascular coagulation (DIC), characterized by simultaneously occurring thrombosis and bleeding.

of a systemic hemostatic defect or a local problem in surgical hemostasis. This distinction may sometimes prove difficult in the absence of clear signs of a generalized bleeding tendency, such as simultaneous bleeding from various locations and sites of intravenous cannulation. In all cases of severe bleeding, a global coagulation screening (i.e., platelet count, aPTT, PT) should be carried out as soon as possible. If these tests show abnormal results, then a brief trial of therapy with replacement of deficient hemostatic factors should be provided. However, unless there is prompt cessation of bleeding, this treatment should not delay the decision to reoperate if even the smallest suspicion of a local surgical problem exists.

Systemic coagulation defects in bleeding patients with a previously normal coagulation system generally arise by two different mechanisms: (1) loss of platelets and coagulation factors due to bleeding and dilution of these elements on massive transfusion of red cells and plasma substitutes and (2) consumption of platelets and coagulation factors in the framework of DIC.

Patients with severe blood loss may require massive fluid replacement therapy with blood substitutes such as crystalloid, colloid, dextran, and starch solutions. The use of these synthetic plasma volume expanders in excess of 1 l/h may in some cases be associated with impairment of primary hemostasis (most probably the result of interference with von Willebrand factor function) and the plasma coagulation system (due to dilution). This association has been established for dextrans and gelatin-based plasma volume expanders.[62] Hence, the disproportionate use of these products may result in a deterioration of hemostatic capability and aggravate bleeding. Therefore, if there is need for massive expansion of circulating volume in bleeding patients or patients at risk for bleeding, then use of these preparations should be accompanied by administration with fresh frozen plasma.

Transfusion with large amounts of packed red cells without concomitant replacement of platelets and coagulation factors may cause generalized dilution coagulopathy,[63] which is readily established by a decrease in platelet count usually to 50 to 100×10^9/l and prolongation of global clotting times (aPTT and PT). Although there is no evidence from clinical studies to support this practice, it is generally recommended that patients who need massive transfusion of red cells receive 1 unit of plasma for every 2 to 3 units of red cells administered. In the absence of other factors that may cause a coagulation defect, this routine will result in a (near) normalization of coagulation times. A more conservative strategy appears to be justified with respect to the low platelet count. A prospective trial demonstrated no benefit of prophylactic transfusion of platelets in patients receiving more than 12 units of red cells in a short period of time.[64] However, retrospective analyses showed that in bleeding patients with a platelet count lower than 50×10^9/l, transfusion of platelets is effective.[65] Hence, the threshold for platelet transfusion in patients with bleeding can be held at 50×10^9/l unless defective platelet function is suspected.

Although there is no evidence from clinical trials to support such treatment, pharmacotherapeutic interventions to improve hemostasis may in some exceptional cases be contemplated. These interventions may consist of antifibrinolytic strategies, such as the administration of ε-aminocaproic acid, tranexamic acid, or aprotinin. The administration of recombinant factor VIIa has given impressive effects in patients with excessive bleeding in a small series of case reports, but the safety and efficacy of this approach requires further study.

Disseminated Intravascular Coagulation

Surgical patients may present with DIC because this is a frequent complication of a variety of disease states common in these patients, such as infection, severe trauma, or malignancies.[66] As a syndrome, DIC is always secondary to an underlying disorder. The syndrome is characterized by systemic activation of the blood coagulation system, the generation and deposition of fibrin, microvascular thrombi in various organs, and in many cases the development of multiorgan failure (Fig. 8.4). Depletion of coagulation proteins and platelets resulting from the ongoing activation of the coagulation system may induce severe bleeding complications, although microclot formation may occur in the absence of severe clotting factor depletion and bleeding.[67] Severe bleeding from DIC poses a particular problem in trauma patients or during the early postoperative phase.

A spectrum of clinical entities has been associated with DIC, and the major conditions are listed in Table 8.5. Infection is the most common cause of DIC, and in patients with septic shock, DIC is a strong predictor of death.[68] Another cause of DIC is malignancy, although in that setting DIC usually is relatively mild. In contrast, the DIC that accompanies obstetrical catastrophes, such as abruptio placentae or

TABLE 8.5. Underlying Surgical Diseases Causing Acute or Chronic Disseminated Intravascular Coagulation (DIC).

Septicemia/infections
Polytrauma
Malignancies
Aortic aneurysm
Brain injury
Extended liver surgery
Extracorporeal circulation
Thermal injury/hypothermia
Fat embolism
Peritoneovenous shunt
Massive transfusion

amniotic fluid embolism, is turbulent but usually self-limiting.

Pathogenesis of DIC

Disseminated intravascular coagulation is characterized by widespread intravascular fibrin deposition resulting from enhanced fibrin formation and impaired fibrin degradation.[69] Enhanced fibrin formation is caused by tissue factor-mediated thrombin generation and simultaneously occurring depression of inhibitory mechanisms (Fig. 8.5). The impairment of endogenous fibrinolysis is caused mainly by high circulating levels of PAI-1, the principal inhibitor of plasminogen activation. These derangements in coagulation and fibrinolysis are probably mediated by several cytokines, as readily demonstrable during DIC associated with infectious disease.

The initiation of the systemic activation of coagulation is dependent on the underlying cause of DIC. The expression of tissue factor to circulating blood appears to be a common pathway for the initiation of blood coagulation activation. The intravenous administration of endotoxin to human subjects or primates results in the activation of coagulation, and this coagulant response could be completely blocked by the simultaneous administration of monoclonal antibodies that inhibit tissue factor or factor VIIa activity.[70,71] A similar important role of the tissue factor–factor VIIa route is also demonstrable for other types of DIC. The expression of tissue factor may be a direct effect, as in the case of trauma when large amounts of subendothelially localized tissue factor become exposed or may be induced by the action of various cytokines produced in response to various pathogenic insults.

In sepsis, the induction of the tissue–factor system and subsequent activation of coagulation seems to be mediated by proinflammatory cytokines such as tumor necrosis factor-α (TNF-α) and interleukins (IL) 1 and 6. Administration of TNF-α to healthy volunteers elicits rapid activation of coagulation.[72] However, the role of TNF in endotoxin-induced activation of coagulation became less clear when subsequent studies showed that monoclonal antibodies directed against TNF activity were able to abolish the endotoxin-stimulated increase in TNF while leaving thrombin generation unchanged.[73] In contrast to this observation, monoclonal antibodies directed against IL-6 were able to completely block the endotoxin-induced activation of coagulation in chimpanzees.[74] In addition, it was shown that IL-6 infusion in baboons and in human cancer patients induced thrombin generation.[75,76] Hence, these data suggest that IL-6 rather than TNF is the primary mediator for the induction of coagulation in sepsis.

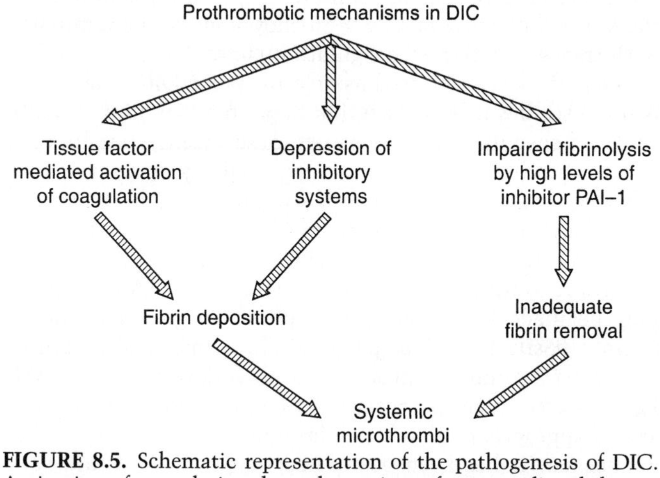

FIGURE 8.5. Schematic representation of the pathogenesis of DIC. Activation of coagulation depends on tissue factor-mediated thrombin generation and a simultaneously occurring depression of the physiological coagulation–inhibitory systems. Impaired function of the fibrinolytic system, caused by high levels of the fibrinolytic inhibitor PAI-1, further contributes to the procoagulant state.

The role of other cytokines, such as IL-1, is less clear. Treatment of septic patients with IL-1 receptor antagonist resulted in lower thrombin generation, as reflected in decreased levels of thrombin–antithrombin complexes.[77] Also, administration of IL-1 to baboons resulted in systemic coagulation activation. It is not clear whether this effect of IL-1 is a direct effect or an effect mediated by other IL-1-induced cytokines.

The thrombin generated by the activated coagulation promotes further activation of coagulation by a number of positive feedback loops. To balance this ongoing activation of coagulation, the human body uses various inhibitory systems. One of the major inhibitors of coagulation is antithrombin III. Antithrombin III is decreased during sepsis in humans due to increased consumption and degradation by elastase released from activated neutrophils. Low antithrombin III levels in DIC are associated with increased mortality.[68,77]

In addition to the decrease in antithrombin III, a significant downregulation of the protein C–protein S system may occur. There are several explanations for an impairment of the protein C–protein S system in DIC. First, protein C and protein S levels are decreased in patients with DIC, probably because of increased consumption. In addition, proinflammatory cytokines can induce downregulation of thrombomodulin on endothelial cells, resulting in decreased activation of protein C.[78] Furthermore the acute-phase protein C4bBP, which can bind protein S, is increased during severe illness, leading to lower levels of the biologically active free protein S.

A third natural anticoagulant pathway consists of TFPI. Most of the TFPI in the body is bound to the endothelium and can be released into the blood. Much of the circulating TFPI is bound to lipoproteins; TFPI is a direct factor Xa inhibitor and, in a factor Xa-dependent manner, produces feedback inhibition of the factor VIIa–tissue factor complex. In a primate model of sepsis, TFPI levels increased 1.2-fold following sublethal and 2-fold following lethal *Escherichia coli* infusion. Evidence for the importance of TFPI in sepsis was provided by a study in baboons that showed that TFPI infusion after the start of a lethal intravenous *E. coli* infusion could prevent the activation of coagulation as well as death in all animals studied.[79]

In patients with DIC, deposition of fibrin in the (micro)vasculature is caused by both the formation and inadequate removal of intravascular fibrin. This inadequate removal is caused by an impaired function of the fibrinolytic system. Following endotoxin exposure, there is rapid but short-lasting activation of fibrinolysis caused by an increase in tissue tPA and uPA. Following this initial activation of fibrinolysis, a complete and sustained inhibition of fibrinolysis can be observed because of an increase in PAI-1. At the time of maximal thrombin generation, fibrinolysis is also markedly inhibited. Thus, a remarkable imbalance between coagulation and fibrinolysis results in a net procoagulant state.[80] Experimental studies have shown that the dysregulation of fibrinolysis in DIC is completely mediated by TNF, whereas other cytokines, such as IL-6, play no major role.[81]

Diagnosis of DIC

No single laboratory test or combination of tests allows a definitive diagnosis of DIC. However, the clinical diagnosis can be made reliable by taking into consideration the underlying disease and a combination of laboratory findings. As the prominent feature of DIC is the occurrence of fibrin in the circulation, measurement of soluble fibrin in blood should theoretically be helpful in confirming the diagnosis. Although some assays for quantitatively measuring soluble fibrin in plasma are being developed, a reliable test has not been available thus far. Assays for the detection of thrombin generation (such as thrombin–antithrombin complexes or prothrombin activation fragment F1 + 2) might be useful but are not available on a routine basis to most hospital laboratories. Hence, the diagnosis of DIC in the normal situation is usually based on markers of advanced consumption of coagulation proteins and platelets, that is, prolonged clotting times (aPTT and PT) and low platelets, in combination with tests that do not detect the generation but rather the degradation of fibrin (fibrin degradation products). It should be realized, however, that a single determination is often not helpful, and repeated measurements may provide more information. The measurement of individual coagulation factors may have some limited value (e.g., to detect a concomitant vitamin K deficiency) but is usually not essential. Measurement of fibrinogen is commonly performed but has been shown to be of no value for the diagnosis of DIC, especially because the acute-phase reactant properties of fibrinogen in many clinical situations may completely obscure ongoing fibrinogen consumption. A simple scoring algorithm for DIC based on routinely available laboratory tests has been introduced and has been validated in consecutive intensive care unit patients[82] (Table 8.6).

Management of DIC

Several issues regarding the proper management of patients with DIC remain controversial.[83] These controversies result from the complexity of the clinical presentation of the syndrome, its variable and unpredictable course, and the (either) subtle or catastrophic clinical consequences of the syndrome. The cornerstone of DIC treatment is the specific and vigorous treatment of the underlying disorder. In some cases, DIC will completely resolve within hours after the resolution of the underlying condition, as, for example, in the case of DIC induced by abruptio placentae and amniotic fluid embolism. However, in other cases, such as in patients with sepsis and a systemic inflammatory response syndrome, DIC may be present for a number of days, even after proper treatment has been initiated. Under such circumstances, supportive measures to manage DIC may be necessary. Administration of coagulation factors or platelets may be useful, particularly in cases of persistent bleeding. In addition, therapeutic interventions aimed at the interruption of ongoing thrombin formation or at the inhibition of thrombin might have a beneficial effect. This effect might be further facilitated by administration of protease inhibitors, such as antithrombin III, levels of which may dramatically decrease in the course of DIC.

Treatment with *plasma or platelet concentrate* is guided by the clinical condition of the patient and should not be instituted on the basis of laboratory findings alone. Replacement may be indicated in patients with active bleeding and in those requiring an invasive procedure or otherwise at risk for bleeding complications. On the other hand, it has been suggested that transfusion of blood components may also be harmful by further stimulating the activated coagulation system. Although this theory has rarely been proven to occur simultaneously, (low-dose) heparin might be useful to prevent this complication.[84] Treatment with plasma is not based on evidence from controlled trials. The only randomized controlled trial in neonates with DIC, comparing administration of fresh frozen plasma and platelets with whole-blood exchange and no specific therapy, failed to show any change in outcome of DIC or survival.[85] Despite the lack of evidence, most authors recommend treatment with fresh frozen plasma, at least when patients are bleeding or are at increased risk for bleeding.[86] To sufficiently correct the coagulation defect, large volumes of plasma may be needed. The use of coagulation factor concentrates may overcome this need. However, these concentrates usually contain only a selected number of the various clotting factors, and they may be contaminated with traces of activated coagulation factors.

Heparin has been used as treatment for DIC since 1959. Animal studies have shown that heparin can inhibit the activation of coagulation in experimental septicemia but does not affect mortality.[87,88] A retrospective analysis of cases of DIC reported in the literature noted similar survival for patients treated and patients not treated with heparin.[89] One can conclude that there is no sound evidence in favor of the use of heparin as routine therapy in patients with DIC. An exception may be made for patients with clinical signs of extensive fibrin deposition, such as purpura fulminans, acral ischemia, or venous thrombosis. In such cases low-dose heparin (5–8 U/kg/h) is advocated, potentially in combination with plasma and, if appropriate, platelet replacement.[90]

Because it has been postulated that *LMWH* would have a decreased bleeding risk while having at least the same antithrombotic potential as unfractionated heparin, these agents might prove useful in patients with DIC. Animal studies showed effective treatment of DIC with LMWH, and

TABLE 8.6. Diagnostic Algorithm for the Diagnosis of Overt DIC.

1. Risk assessment: Does the patient have an underlying disorder known to be associated with overt DIC?
   If yes, proceed. If no, do not use this algorithm.
2. Order global coagulation tests (platelet count, prothrombin time [PT], fibrinogen, soluble fibrin monomers, or fibrin degradation products).
3. Score global coagulation test results.
   Platelet count *(>100 = 0; <100 = 1; <50 = 2)* ________
   Elevated fibrin-related marker (e.g., soluble fibrin monomers/fibrin degradation products) *(no increase: 0; moderate increase: 2; strong increase: 3)* ________
   Prolonged PT *(<3 s = 0; >3 s but <6 s = 1; >6 s = 2)* ________
   Fibrinogen level *(>1.0 g/l = 0; <1.0 g/l = 1)* ________
4. Calculate score. ________
5. If ≥5, compatible with overt DIC. If ≤5, not compatible with overt DIC; repeat next 1–2 days.

successful treatment was suggested in two small uncontrolled studies in humans. A multicenter, double-blind, randomized trial showed that the LMWH dalteparin had superior efficacy compared with unfractionated heparin in reducing bleeding symptoms and in improving subjective organ symptom score.[88] However, there was no influence on mortality by such therapy. The underlying cause of DIC in most of these patients was malignancy, and only 13% of patients suffered from infectious disease. Future studies are needed to definitively indicate a potential role of LMWH in the supportive treatment of DIC patients.

Low levels of *antithrombin III* may play an important role in the pathogenesis of DIC, and it has been shown that low antithrombin III levels are associated with increased mortality.[68,91,92] Mortality caused by gram-negative sepsis could be prevented by the infusion of antithrombin III concentrate in baboons, but only if adequate antithrombin III levels were achieved early in the course of sepsis. Studies compared the administration of supraphysiological doses of antithrombin III (up to plasma levels of 150%–200%) to placebo in patients with septic shock.[93] The antithrombin III-treated patients showed a more rapid recovery from DIC and a reduced blood transfusion requirement. A trend to decreased mortality was found, but statistical significance was not reached. A large-scale, multicenter, randomized controlled trial to address this issue directly showed no significant reduction in mortality of patients with sepsis who were treated with antithrombin concentrate.[94] Interestingly, post hoc subgroup analyses indicated some benefit in patients who did not receive concomitant heparin, but this observation needs prospective validation.

Based on the notion that depression of the protein C system may significantly contribute to the pathophysiology of DIC, supplementation of *activated protein C* might be beneficial. A phase III trial of activated protein C concentrate in patients with sepsis was prematurely stopped because of efficacy in reducing mortality in these patients.[95] All-cause mortality at 28 days after inclusion was 24.7% in the activated protein C group versus 30.8% in the control group (19.4% relative risk reduction). Recombinant human-activated protein C has been licensed in most countries for treatment of patients with severe sepsis and a high APACHE (Acute Physiology and Chronic Health Evaluation) score or two or more organ failures.

Future treatment strategies that are currently being studied are directed against the tissue factor pathway or may consist of the administration of other coagulation inhibitors, such as (activated) protein C.

References

1. Colman RW, Hirsh J, Marder VJ, et al. Hemostasis and Thrombosis. Basic Principles and Clinical Practice. Philadelphia: Lippincott, 1994.
2. Hathaway WE, Goodnight SH. Disorders of Hemostasis and Thrombosis. A Clinical Guide. New York: McGraw-Hill, 1993.
3. Colman RW, Cook JJ, Niewiarowski. Mechanisms of platelet aggregation. In: Colman RW, Hirsh J, Marder VJ, Salzman EW, eds. Hemostasis and Thrombosis: Basic Principles and Clinical Practice. Philadelphia: Lippincott, 1994.
4. Niewiarowski S, Holt JC, Cook JJ. Biochemistry and physiology of secreted platelet proteins. In: Colman RW, Hirsh J, Marder VJ, Salzman EW, eds. Hemostasis and Thrombosis: Basic Principles and Clinical Practice. Philadelphia: Lippincott, 1994.
5. Davie EW. Biochemical and molecular aspects of the coagulation cascade. Thromb Haemost 1995;74:1–7.
6. Davie EW, Fujikawa K, Kisiel W. The coagulation cascade: initiation, maintenance and regulation. Biochemistry 1991;30:10363–10370.
7. Collen D. On the regulation and control of fibrinolysis. Thromb Haemost 1980;43:77.
8. Hirsh J, Dalen JE, Fuster V, et al. Aspirin and other platelet-active drugs. Chest 1995;108:247S–257S.
9. A randomised, blinded, trial of clopidogrel versus aspirin in patients at risk of ischaemic events (CAPRIE). CAPRIE Steering Committee. Lancet 1996;348:1329–1339.
10. Yusuf S, Zhao F, Mehta SR et al. Effects of clopidogrel in addition to aspirin in patients with acute coronary syndromes without ST-segment elevation. N Engl J Med 2001;345:494–502.
11. Steinhubl SR, Berger PB, Mann JT III, et al. Early and sustained dual oral antiplatelet therapy following percutaneous coronary intervention: a randomized controlled trial. JAMA 2002;288:2411–2420.
12. Topol EJ, Easton D, Harrington RA, et al: Randomized, double-blind, placebo-controlled, international trial of the oral IIb/IIIa antagonist lotrafiban in coronary and cerebrovascular disease. Circulation 2003;108:399–406
13. Hirsh J, Dalen JE, Deykin D, et al. Oral anticoagulants. Chest 1995;108:231S–247S.
14. Hirsh J, Raschke R, Warkentin TE, et al. Heparin: mechanism of action, pharmacokinetics, dosing considerations, monitoring, efficacy, and safety. Chest 1995;108:258S–275S.
15. Weitz JI. Low molecular weight heparins. N Engl J Med 1997;337:688–698.
16. Bauer KA, Hawkins DW, Peters PC, et al. Fondaparinux, a synthetic pentasaccharide: the first in a new class of antithrombotic agents—the selective factor Xa inhibitors. Cardiovasc Drug Rev 2002;20:37–52.
17. Edmunds LH, Salzman EW. Hemostatic problems, transfusion therapy, and cardiopulmonary bypass in surgical patients. In: Colman RW, Hirsh J, Marder VJ, Salzman EW, eds. Hemostasis and Thrombosis: Basic Principles and Clinical Practice. Philadelphia: Lippincott, 1994.
18. Mannucci PM. Desmopressin (DDAVP) in the treatment of bleeding disorders: the first 20 years. Blood 1997;90:2515.
19. Limentani SA, Roth DA, Furie BC, Furie B. Recombinant blood clotting proteins for hemophilia therapy. Semin Thromb Hemostasis 1993;19:62–72.
20. Friederich PW, Henny CP, Messelink EJ, et al. Effect of recombinant activated factor VII on perioperative blood loss in patients undergoing retropubic prostatectomy: a double-blind placebo-controlled randomised trial. Lancet 2003;361:201–205.
21. Hendriks HG, Meijer K, de Wolf JT, et al. Reduced transfusion requirements by recombinant factor VIIa in orthotopic liver transplantation: a pilot study. Transplantation 2001;71:402–405.
22. Lodge JP, Jonas S, Jones RM, et al. Efficacy and safety of repeated perioperative doses of recombinant factor VIIa in liver transplantation. Liver Transpl 2005;11:973–979.
23. Lodge JP, Jonas S, Oussoultzoglou E, et al. Recombinant coagulation factor VIIa in major liver resection: a randomized, placebo-controlled, double-blind clinical trial. Anesthesiology 2005;102:269–275.
24. Shao YF, Yang JM, Chau GY, et al. Safety and hemostatic effect of recombinant activated factor VII in cirrhotic patients undergoing partial hepatectomy: a multicenter, randomized, double-blind, placebo-controlled trial. Am J Surg 2006;191:245–249.
25. Diprose P, Herbertson MJ, O'Shaughnessy D, Gill RS. Activated recombinant factor VII after cardiopulmonary bypass reduces

allogeneic transfusion in complex non-coronary cardiac surgery: randomized double-blind placebo-controlled pilot study. Br J Anaesth 2005;95:596–602.
26. Kenet G, Walden R, Eldad A, Martinowitz U. Treatment of traumatic bleeding with recombinant factor VIIa. Lancet 1999;354:1879.
27. Boffard KD, Riou B, Warren B, et al. Recombinant factor VIIa as adjunctive therapy for bleeding control in severely injured trauma patients: two parallel randomized, placebo-controlled, double-blind clinical trials. J Trauma 2005;59:8–15.
28. Levi M. Recombinant factor VIIa: a general hemostatic agent? Not yet. J Thromb Haemost 2004;2:1695–1697.
29. Marder VJ, Butler FO, Barlow GH. Antifibrinolytic therapy. In: Colman RW, Hirsh J, Marder VJ, Salzman EW, eds. Hemostasis and Thrombosis: Basic Principles and Clinical Practice. Philadelphia: Lippincott, 1994.
30. Ferraris VA, Bridges CR, Anderson RP, et al. Aprotinin in cardiac surgery. N Engl J Med 2006;354:1953–1957.
31. Hiatt WR. Observational studies of drug safety—aprotinin and the absence of transparency. N Engl J Med 2006;355:2171–2173.
32. Mannucci PM, Ruggeri ZM, Pareti FI, Capitannio A. DDAVP: A new pharmacological approach to the management of hemophilia and von Willebrand disease. Lancet 1977;1:869–872.
33. Francis JL. The use of drugs to reduce blood loss during surgery. Hematol Rev 1992;7:85–99.
34. Rao AK, Ghosh S, Sum L, et al. Mechanism of platelet dysfunction and response to DDAVP in patients with congenital platelet function defects. A double-blind placebo-controlled trial. Thromb Haemost 1995;74:1071–1078.
35. McIntyre AJ. Blood transfusion and haemostatic management in the perioperative period. Can J Anaesth 1992;39:R101.
36. Levi M, Lensing A, ten Cate JW. Haemostasis, blood coagulation and fibrinolysis in liver disease. In: Tytgat GN, Lygidakis A, et al, eds. Hepatobiliary and Pancreatic Malignancies: Diagnosis, Medical and Surgical Therapy. Stuttgart: Thieme, 1988:173–178.
37. Marassi A, Manzullo V, Di Carlo V, et al. Thromboembolism following prothrombin complex concentrate and major surgery in severe liver disease. Thromb Haemost 1978;39:787.
38. Agnelli G, Parise P, Levi M, Cosmi B, Nenci GG. Effects of desmopressin on hemostasis in patients with liver cirrhosis. Haemostasis 1995;25:241–247.
39. Moia M, Mannucci PM, Vizzotto L, et al. Improvement in the hemostatic defect of uremia after treatment with recombinant human erythropoietin. Lancet 1987;2:1227.
40. Mannucci PM, Remuzzi G, Pusinri F, et al. De-amino-8-D-arginine vasopressin shortens the bleeding time in uremia. N Engl J Med 1983;308:8–12.
41. Hathaway WE. New insights on vitamin K. Hematol Oncol Clin North Am 1987;1:367.
42. Kelton JG, Gibbons S. Autoimmune platelet destruction: idiopathic thrombocytopenic purpura. Semin Thromb Hemostasis 1982;8:83–104.
43. Cohen AJ, Kessler CM. Acquired inhibitors. Baillieres Clin Haematol 1996;9:331–354.
44. Houry S, Georgeac C, Hay JM, Fingerhut A, Boudet MJ. A prospective multicenter evaluation of preoperative hemostatic screening tests. The French Association for Surgical Research. Am J Surg 1995;170:19–23.
45. Watson CJ, Deane AM, Doyle PA, Bullock KN. Identifiable factors in post-prostatectomy haemorrhage: the role of aspirin. Br J Urol 1990;66:85.
46. Billingsley EM, Maloney ME. Intraoperative and postoperative bleeding problems in patients taking warfarin, aspirin, and nonsteroidal antiinflammatory agents. A prospective study. Dermatol Surg 1997;23:381.
47. Kallis P, Tooze JA, Talbot S, Cowans D, Bevan DH, Treasure T. Pre-operative aspirin decreases platelet aggregation and increases post-operative blood loss—a prospective, randomised, placebo controlled, double-blind clinical trial in 100 patients with chronic stable angina. Eur J Cardiovasc Thorac Surg 1994;8:404.
48. Goldman S, Copeland J, Moritz T, et al. Improvement in early saphenous vein graft patency after coronary artery bypass surgery with antiplatelet therapy: results of a Veterans Administration cooperative study. Circulation 1988;77:1324.
49. Flordal PA. Use of desmopressin to prevent bleeding in surgery. Eur J Surg 1998;164:5.
50. Bartley GB, Warndahl RA. Surgical bleeding associated with aspirin and nonsteroidal anti-inflammatory agents. Mayo Clin Proc 1992;67:402.
51. Horskotte D, Schulte HD, Bircks W, et al. Lower intensity anticoagulation therapy results in lower complication rates with the St. Jude medical prosthesis. J Thorac Cardiovasc Surg 1994;107:1136–1145.
52. Kearon C, Hirsh J. Management of anticoagulation before and after elective surgery. N Engl J Med 1997;336:1506–1511.
53. Katholi RE, Nolan SP, McGuire LB. The management of anticoagulation during noncardiac operations in patients with prosthetic heart valves. Am Heart J 1978;96:163–165.
54. Nurmohamed MT, Rosendaal FR, Büller HR, et al. Low molecular weight heparin versus standard heparin in general and orthopedic surgery: a meta-analysis. Lancet 1992;340:152–156.
55. Fremes SE, Wong BI, Lee E, et al. Metaanalysis of prophylactic drug treatment in the prevention of postoperative bleeding. Ann Thorac Surg 1994;58:1580–1588.
56. Laupacis A, Fergusson D. Drugs to minimize perioperative blood loss in cardiac surgery: meta-analyses using perioperative blood loss as the outcome. The International Study of Peri-operative Transfusion (ISPOT) Investigators. Anesth Analg 1997;85:1258–1267.
57. Levi M, Cromheecke ME, de Jonge E, et al. Pharmacological strategies to decrease excessive blood loss in cardiac surgery: a meta-analysis of clinically relevant endpoints. Lancet 1999;354:1940–1947.
58. Cattaneo M, Harris AS, Strömberg U, Mannucci PM. The effect of desmopressin on reducing blood loss in cardiac surgery. A meta-analysis of double-blind placebo-controlled trials. Thromb Haemost 1995;74:1064.
59. van der Meer J, Hillege HL, Kootstra GJ, et al. for the CABADAS Research Group of the Interuniversity Cardiology Institute of the Netherlands. Prevention of one year vein graft occlusion after aortocoronary bypass surgery: a comparison of low dose aspirin, low dose aspirin plus dypiridamole, and oral anticoagulants. Lancet 1993;342:257–264.
60. Garcia Huete L, Domenech P, Sabate A, et al. The prophylactic effect of aprotinin on intraoperative bleeding in liver transplantation: a randomized clinical study. Hepatology 1997;26:1143–1148.
61. Lentschener C, Benhamou D, Mercier FJ, et al. Aprotinin reduces blood loss in patients undergoing elective liver resection. Anesth Analg 1997;84:875–881.
62. de Jonge E, Levi M, Berends F, van der Ende A, ten Cate JW, Stoutenbeek C. Impairment of haemostasis in vivo by intravenous administration of a gelatin-based plasma solution in healthy human subjects. Thromb Haemost 1998;79:286–290.
63. Lim RC, Olcott C, Robinson AJ, et al. Platelet response and coagulation changes following massive blood replacement. J Trauma 1973;18:577.
64. Reed RL, Ciavarella D, Heimbach DM, et al. Prophylactic platelet administration during massive transfusion: a prospective, randomized, double-blind clinical study. Ann Surg 1986;203:40–48.

65. Roy AJ, Jaffe N, Djerassi I. Prophylactic platelet transfusions in children with acute leukemia: a dose-response study. Transfusion (Phila) 1973;13:283–290.
66. Levi M, de Jonge E, van der Poll T, Ten Cate H. Disseminated intravascular coagulation. Thromb Haemost 1999;82:695–705.
67. Baglin T. Disseminated intravascular coagulation: diagnosis and treatment. Br Med J 1996;312:683–687.
68. Fourrier F, Chopin C, Goudemand J, et al. Septic shock, multiple organ failure, and disseminated intravascular coagulation. Compared patterns of antithrombin III, protein C, and protein S deficiencies. Chest 1992;101:816–823.
69. Levi M, ten Cate H, van der Poll T, et al. Pathogenesis of disseminated intravascular coagulation in sepsis. JAMA 1993;270: 975–979.
70. Taylor FB Jr, Chang A, Ruf W, et al. Lethal *E. coli* septic shock is prevented by blocking tissue factor with monoclonal antibody. Circ Shock 1991;33:127–134.
71. Levi M, ten Cate H, Bauer KA, et al. Inhibition of endotoxin-induced activation of coagulation and fibrinolysis by pentoxifylline or by a monoclonal anti-tissue factor antibody in chimpanzees. J Clin Invest 1994;93:114–120.
72. van der Poll T, Buller HR, ten Cate H, et al. Activation of coagulation after administration of tumor necrosis factor to normal subjects. N Engl J Med 1990;322:1622–1627.
73. van der Poll T, Levi M, van Deventer SJ, et al. Differential effects of anti-tumor necrosis factor monoclonal antibodies on systemic inflammatory responses in experimental endotoxemia in chimpanzees. Blood 1994;83:446–451.
74. van der Poll T, Levi M, Hack CE, et al. Elimination of interleukin 6 attenuates coagulation activation in experimental endotoxemia in chimpanzees. J Exp Med 1994;179:1253–1259.
75. Stouthard JM, Levi M, Hack CE, et al. Interleukin-6 stimulates coagulation, not fibrinolysis, in humans. Thromb Haemost 1996;76:738–742.
76. Boermeester MA, van Leeuwen PA, Coyle SM, et al. Interleukin-I blockade attenuates mediator release and dysregulation of the hemostatic mechanism during human sepsis. Arch Surg 1995;130:739–748.
77. Buller HR, ten Cate JW. Acquired antithrombin III deficiency: laboratory diagnosis, incidence, clinical implications, and treatment with antithrombin III concentrate. Am J Med 1989;87:44S–48S.
78. Hesselvik JF, Malm J, Dahlback B, et al. Protein C, protein S and C4b-binding protein in severe infection and septic shock. Thromb Haemost 1991;65:126–129.
79. Creasey AA, Chang AC, Feigen L, et al. Tissue factor pathway inhibitor reduces mortality from *Escherichia coli* septic shock. J Clin Invest 1993;91:2850–2856.
80. Biemond BJ, Levi M, ten Cate H, et al. Endotoxin-induced activation and inhibition of the fibrinolytic system: effects of various interventions in the cytokine and coagulation cascades in experimental endotoxemia in chimpanzees. Clin Sci 1995;88:587–594.
81. Levi M, van der Poll T, ten Cate H, van Deventer SJH. The cytokine-mediated imbalance between coagulant and anticoagulant mechanisms in sepsis and endotoxemia. Eur J Clin Invest 1997;27:3–9.
82. Levi M, de Jonge E, Meijers J. The diagnosis of disseminated intravascular coagulation. Blood Rev 2002; 16:217–223.
83. Corrigan JJ, Colman RW, Robboy SJ. Management of DIC. In: Inglefinger FJ, et al, eds. Controversies in Internal Medicine, Vol. 2. Philadelphia: Saunders, 1974.
84. Wong VK, Hitchock W, Mason WH. Meningococcal infection in children: a review of 100 cases. Pediatr Infect Dis J 1989;8:224–227.
85. Gross SJ, Filston HC. Controlled study of treatment for disseminated intravascular coagulation in the neonate. J Pediatr 1982;100:445–448.
86. Rubin RN, Colman RW. Disseminated intravascular coagulation. Approach to treatment. Drugs 1992;44:963–971.
87. Corrigan JJ Jr, Kiernat JF. Effect of heparin in experimental gram-negative septicemia. J Infect Dis 1975;131:138–143.
88. Corrigan JJ Jr, Jordan CM. Heparin therapy in septicemia with disseminated intravascular coagulation. Effect on mortality and on correction of hemostatic defects. N Engl J Med 1970;283:778–782.
89. Sakuragawa N, Hasegawa H, Maki M, et al. Clinical evaluation of low-molecular-weight heparin (FR-860) on disseminated intravascular coagulation (DIC)—a multicenter co-operative double-blind trial in comparison with heparin. Thromb Res 1993;72:475–500.
90. Feinstein DI. Diagnosis and management of disseminated intravascular coagulation: the role of heparin therapy. Blood 1982;60:284–287.
91. Maki M, Terao T, Ikenoue T, et al. Clinical evaluation of antithrombin III concentrate (BI 6.013) for disseminated intravascular coagulation in obstetrics. Well-controlled multicenter trial. Gynecol Obstet Invest 1987;23:230–240.
92. Blauhut B, Kramar H, Vinazzer H, et al. Substitution of antithrombin III in shock and DIC: a randomized study. Thromb Res 1985;39:81–89.
93. Fourrier F, Chopin C, Huart JJ, et al. Double-blind, placebo-controlled trial of antithrombin III concentrates in septic shock with disseminated intravascular coagulation. Chest 1993;104:882–888.
94. Warren BL, Eid A, Singer P, et al. Caring for the critically ill patient. High-dose antithrombin III in severe sepsis: a randomized controlled trial. JAMA 2001; 286:1869–1878.
95. Bernard GR, Vincent JL, Laterre PF, et al. Efficacy and safety of recombinant human activated protein C for severe sepsis. N Engl J Med 2001; 344:699–709.
96. Koch A, Bouges S, Ziegler S, Dinkel H, Daures JP, Victor N. Low molecular weight heparin and unfractionated heparin in thrombosis prophylaxis after major surgical intervention. Update of previous meta-analyses. Br J Surg 1997;84:750–759.
97. Palmer AJ, Koppenhagen K, Kirchhof B, Weber U, Bergemann R. Efficacy and safety of low molecular weight heparin, unfractionated heparin and warfarin for thrombo-embolism prophylaxis in orthopaedic surgery: a meta-analysis of randomised clinical trials. Haemostasis 1997;27:75–84.

9 Transfusion Therapy

Lena M. Napolitano

In the United States in 2001, approximately 15 million units of blood were collected according to the National Blood Data Resource Center, representing an increase compared to prior years (Fig. 9.1).[1] Approximately 40,000 units of blood are used each day in the United States; every few seconds someone receives a blood transfusion. The majority of the red blood cell (RBC) transfusions in the United States are administered to elective surgical patients (55%) and medical patients with chronic anemia (30%), and only 15% are utilized for trauma and other emergencies. As of November 2000, the American Red Cross (ARC) managed about 45% of the U.S. blood supply, The American Association of Blood Banks (AABB) managed about 45%, and others, such as United Blood Services, managed the remaining 10%.

The use of transfusion therapy (transfusion of RBCs, plasma, platelets) is common in surgical patients. Nearly 20% of blood transfusions in the United States are associated with cardiac surgery. It is therefore important that we have an evidence-based knowledge of the efficacy of specific transfusion therapies in our surgical patients. Blood transfusion is an essential component of health care. Used correctly, it can save life and improve health. However, as with any therapeutic intervention, it may result in acute or delayed complications and is associated with some risk. Transfusion decisions should be based on clinical assessment of the patient and laboratory test results. Guidelines regarding transfusion of blood products are, however, an important aid in decision making.

Components of whole blood available for transfusion include the following: RBCs, plasma, platelets, cryoprecipitate. Whole blood (500 ml) from a donor is collected into an anticoagulant/preservative solution and undergoes no further processing if used as whole blood. The RBCs are prepared from whole blood by the removal of most of the plasma, or they may be obtained by apheresis collection. The RBCs are stored in one of several saline-based anticoagulant/preservative solutions, yielding a hematocrit between 55% and 80%.

All plasma products are prepared by separation from whole blood by centrifugation or by hemapheresis using centrifugation or filtration. The volume of plasma varies and appears on the label. Fresh frozen plasma (FFP) contains all soluble clotting factors and the plasma from one unit of whole blood, approximately 250 ml, separated and frozen within 8 h of collection. Once FFP is thawed, it should be transfused within 24 h. Levels of Factors V and VIII in thawed FFP are reduced, and therefore FFP should not be used to treat patients with deficiencies of these factors.

The appropriate use of blood and blood products (i.e., consistent effective clinical transfusion practices) are essential in the care of surgical and critically ill and injured patients. The World Health Organization (WHO) has published *The Clinical Use of Blood Handbook*[91]; it provides comprehensive information regarding clinical transfusion practices. The WHO principles for the clinical use of blood components are listed in Table 9.1.

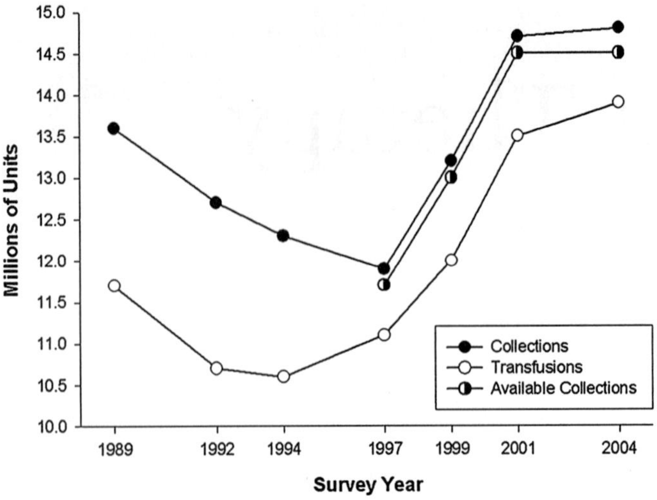

FIGURE 9.1. Blood collection rates in the United States annually from 1989 to 2004. (From the 2005 Nationwide Blood Collection and Utilization Survey Report, with permission, Fig 11-2, p. 52, http://www.aabb.org/apps/docs/05nbcusrpt.pdf.)

Red Blood Cells

Red blood cell transfusion products available include whole blood and packed RBCs. These products can be leukoreduced, washed, irradiated, or frozen/thawed/deglycerolized. The RBCs require compatibility testing and should be ABO and Rh compatible. Indications for RBC transfusion are listed in Table 9.2. One unit of RBCs should increase the hemoglobin of a 70-kg adult by approximately 1 gm/dl and can replace a blood loss of 500 ml in the absence of volume overload or continuing blood loss. Clinical signs and symptoms should be assessed after every unit of RBC transfusion so that the need for additional transfusion and the patient's blood volume status can be assessed. Patients with chronic anemia, who are volume expanded, and other patients susceptible to fluid overload should be transfused slowly. The initial transfusion period should be carefully monitored with a slow transfusion rate to allow the early detection of a transfusion reaction. Transfusion should be completed within 4 h per unit.

The patient should be assessed and have posttransfusion hemoglobin measured to monitor the effectiveness of the RBC transfusion. Lack of clinical benefit may indicate ongoing blood loss or cardiac or pulmonary disease. Causes of a less-than-expected hemoglobin response include increased blood volume due to infusion of crystalloid or colloid solutions; incomplete transfusion of RBCs; ongoing bleeding; a hemolytic transfusion reaction; and transfusion of RBC units near outdate.

TABLE 9.1. World Health Organization Principles for the Clinical Use of Blood Components.

1. Transfusion is only one element of the patient's management.
2. Prescribing decisions should be based on the national guidelines on the clinical use of blood components, taking individual patient needs into account.
3. Blood loss should be minimized to reduce the patient's need for transfusion.
4. The patient with acute blood loss should receive effective resuscitation (intravenous replacement fluids, oxygen, etc.) while the need for transfusion is being assessed.
5. The patient's hemoglobin level, although important, should not be the sole deciding factor in starting transfusion. The decision to transfuse should be supported by the need to relieve clinical signs and symptoms and prevent significant morbidity and mortality.
6. The clinician should be aware of the risks of transfusion-transmissible infection in the blood components that are available for the individual patient.[a]
7. Transfusion should be prescribed only when the benefits to the patient are likely to outweigh the risks.
8. The clinician should record the reason for transfusion clearly.
9. A trained person should monitor the transfused patient and respond immediately if any adverse effects occur.

[a]It should be noted that the rates of noninfective complications are probably higher than those of infective complications.

Source: From WHO,[91] with permission of the World Health Organization.

TABLE 9.2. Indications for Red Blood Cell Transfusion.

Indications: The major indication for red blood cell (RBC) product transfusions is prevention or treatment of symptoms of tissue hypoxia by increasing the oxygen-carrying capacity of blood. The transfusion requirements of each patient should be based on clinical status rather than on predetermined hematocrit or hemoglobin (Hgb) values.

- Symptomatic chronic anemia in normovolemic patients if pharmacologic therapy is not effective or available.
- Patients may become symptomatic from lack of oxygen-carrying capacity when the hgb falls below 8 gm/dl. Younger, healthy patients may tolerate a lower hgb. Few patients will tolerate a hgb less than 6 gm/dl.
- Prophylactic transfusion to prevent morbidity from anemia in patients at greater risk of tissue hypoxia.
- Patients with cardiac, pulmonary, or cerebrovascular disease may become symptomatic with hgb <10 g/dl.
- Active bleeding with signs and symptoms of hypovolemia unresponsive to crystalloid or colloid infusions.
- The clinical assessment of the degree of blood loss is more important than the hgb level or hct since these may not reflect the degree of blood loss. Although patient factors are important in determining the need for red cell transfusion, in healthy individuals blood loss of up to 40%–50% of the blood volume should be replaced with non-red cell resuscitation fluids before red cells are needed.
- Preoperative anemia <9 g/dl with impending major blood loss.
- Sickle cell disease: When general anesthesia is anticipated, when signs and symptoms of anemia are present, or for exchange transfusion when indicated (e.g., pregnancy, stroke, seizures, priapism, or acute chest syndrome).
- Anemia due to renal failure/hemodialysis refractory to erythropoietin therapy.

Red blood cell products should not be transfused for volume expansion only or to enhance wound healing.

References: This table is based on references 39, 101–103.

Plasma

Plasma is provided as FFP. The FFP is plasma within 24 h of thawing. Plasma may be transfused for replacement of any plasma protein deficiency, usually coagulation factor deficiency. Indications for FFP transfusion are listed in Table 9.3. Plasma transfusion should be monitored with specific factor levels or prothrombin time (PT) and activated partial thromboplastin time (aPTT) measurements within 4 h of transfusion. Causes of an inadequate response to plasma transfusion include insufficient dosage, incomplete transfusion, active bleeding or consumptive coagulopathy, coagulation factor inhibitor, heparin administration, and liver disease.

TABLE 9.3. Indications for Plasma Transfusion.

Indications

- Bleeding, preoperative, or massively transfused patients with a deficiency of multiple coagulation factors.
- Patients with bleeding or urgent invasive procedures on warfarin therapy. Vitamin K will reverse the warfarin defect in about 12h.
- Thrombotic thrombocytopenic purpura and related syndromes.
- Congenital or acquired coagulation factor deficiency when no concentrate is available.
- Specific plasma protein deficiencies (i.e., antithrombin III deficiency and C-1 esterase deficiency, hereditary angioedema. Specific treatment protocols for these rare conditions should be referenced.)

Not all Plasma products are suitable for all the above indications. The choice of plasma product should be based on the underlying deficiency and the contents of the available plasma products.

Plasma product transfusion for coagulopathies is not indicated unless the PT or aPTT is >1.5 times the midpoint of the normal values.

Do not transfuse plasma products for volume expansion, for prophylaxis following cardiopulmonary bypass, or as a nutritional supplement.

Dosage and Administration

Plasma product transfusions should be ABO compatible. Crossmatching and Rh compatibility are not required for plasma product transfusions. The usual starting dose is 10–15 ml/kg (i.e., 3–4 units for a 70-kg patient). An assessment of the effect of the product on the bleeding problem should be made before continuing therapy.

Alternative Therapy

For volume expansion, saline, other electrolyte solutions, albumin, or synthetic colloids are safer, cheaper, and more effective. When appropriate, a specific coagulation factor concentrate should be used for treatment. Treatment with vitamin K can avoid the need for plasma transfusion in patients with vitamin K deficiency or on warfarin.

References: This table is based on references. 39, 102, 105, and 106.

Platelets

Platelets are indicated for the prevention or control of bleeding due to thrombocytopenia or platelet dysfunction. Platelets may be provided as pooled whole-blood-derived platelet concentrates ("random-donor" platelets, RDP) and as apheresis platelet concentrates ("single-donor" platelets, SDP). For most patients, these products are equally effective. Apheresis platelets are indicated for patients with immune refractoriness when crossmatched or HLA-matched platelets have better posttransfusion survival. Indications for platelet transfusion are listed in Table 9.4.

TABLE 9.4. Indications for Platelet Transfusion.

Indications:

- Prevention/treatment of nonsurgical bleeding due to thrombocytopenia.

If possible, prior to transfusion the reason for thrombocytopenia should be established. When thrombocytopenia is caused by marrow failure, the following transfusion triggers are considered appropriate:

  - If platelet count is <10,000/μl and no additional abnormalities exist.
  - If platelet count is between 10,000 and 20,000/μl and coagulation abnormalities exist or there are extensive petechiae or ecchymoses.
  - If the patient is bleeding at sites other than skin and platelet count is <40,000–50,000/μl.
- Patients with accelerated platelet destruction with significant bleeding (such as autoimmune thrombocytopenia or drug-induced thrombocytopenia).
  - The endpoint should be cessation of bleeding since an increment in platelet count is not likely to be achieved. Prophylactic transfusion is not indicated in these disorders.
- Prior to surgical and major invasive procedures when the platelet count is <50,000/μl.
  - During neurosurgical and ophthalmologic procedures, some authorities recommend that the platelet count be maintained between 70,000 and 100,000/μl.
- Bleeding with qualitative platelet defect documented by history or laboratory tests.
  - The cause should be identified and corrected, if possible, prior to surgery. Platelet transfusion is indicated only if the defect cannot be otherwise corrected (e.g., a congenital platelet abnormality). Consultation with the blood bank physician is recommended in these situations.
- Diffuse microvascular bleeding after cardiopulmonary bypass or massive transfusion.
  - Platelet count and coagulation studies should be performed prior to the transfusion to guide subsequent therapy. During surgery on patients with quantitative or qualitative platelet defects, the adequacy of hemostasis in patients should be evaluated by the assessment of microvascular bleeding.

Platelet transfusion is contraindicated in thrombotic thrombocytopenic purpura (TTP), heparin-induced thrombocytopenia, and posttransfusion purpura, except in cases of life-threatening hemorrhage. Platelet transfusion is relatively contraindicated in immune thrombocytopenic purpura (ITP).

Dosage and Administration

Compatibility testing is not required. Platelet concentrate products should be ABO identical if possible because platelet increments may be higher. If not possible, then good clinical results are usually obtained with ABO mismatched platelets. In this case, transfusion of large quantities of ABO-incompatible plasma may lead to a positive direct antiglobulin test and, rarely, clinically significant red cell destruction. Although not always possible, Rh compatibility is important. Postexposure prophylaxis with anti-Rh immune globulin should be considered following Rh-positive platelet product transfusions to Rh-negative women who may have children in the future.

A typical platelet transfusion dose is 1 SDP or 4–5 pooled RDP. This should raise the platelet count of a typical 70-kg man approximately 30,000–50,000/μl. Platelet count increments after transfusion may be lower than expected in the presence of certain medications, fever, splenomegaly, infection, or alloimmunization to hLA or specific platelet antigens. Consult the blood bank/transfusion medicine physician or hematologist in such cases.

Alternative Therapy

Desmopressin (DDAVP) may improve the platelet functional defect in uremia. It also raises von Willebrand factor levels in mild-moderate von Willebrand disease, which may improve platelet function. Pharmacologic agents such as aprotinin may reduce major surgical bleeding and thereby avoid the dilutional thrombocytopenia characteristic of massive transfusion. Some of these agents may also have a direct effect on improving platelet function.

References: This table is based on references 106–109.

The RDP are separated from whole blood by differential centrifugation; SDP are harvested from a single donor by hemapheresis. One unit of RDP contains at least 5.5×10^{10} platelets, typically 7.5×10^{10} platelets. Pooled RDP are typically prepared from 4–6 units of RDP. One unit of SDP contains at least 3×10^{11} platelets, typically 4×10^{11} platelets. Platelets are suspended in donor plasma unless washed.

Transfusion of one platelet pool and one unit of apheresis platelets will typically increase the platelet count of an adult by 20,000–40,000/μl. Alternatively, transfusion of one unit per 10kg body weight will typically increase the platelet count by 10,000/μl. Platelets should be transfused immediately before or during an invasive procedure for maximal effectiveness. In a patient with normal splenic function, approximately 40% of transfused platelets will be sequestered in the spleen. This proportion is increased in splenomegaly.

A posttransfusion platelet count should be obtained 10min to 1h after transfusion for best assessment of transfusion effectiveness. Platelet counts obtained later may not allow for differentiation between immune and nonimmune causes of platelet transfusion refractoriness. The corrected count increment (CCI) is usually the best assessment of transfusion effectiveness. A 1-h CCI greater than 5000 is typically considered a satisfactory response.[2] Causes of an inadequate response to platelet transfusion include insufficient dosage, incomplete transfusion, transfusion of platelet concentrates near outdate, immune refractoriness, splenomegaly, and consumption.

Cryoprecipitate

Cryoprecipitate is the cold, insoluble portion of plasma that precipitates when FFP is thawed at 1°C–6°C. The supernatant (cryo-poor plasma) is removed, and the residual volume of cryoprecipitate (approximately 15ml) is refrozen and stored at −18°C. Cryoprecipitate provides therapeutic amounts of factor VIII:C, factor XIII, von Willebrand factor, and fibrinogen. Each bag of cryoprecipitate contains 80–100 units of factor VIII:C and 150–200mg of fibrinogen (factor I). In addition, significant amounts of factor XIII (fibrin-stabilizing factor) and von Willebrand factor (vWF), including the high molecular weight multimers of vWF, are also present. The indications for cryoprecipitate transfusion are listed in Table 9.5. Cryoprecipitate is not a significant source of other coagulation factors and cannot be used as an alternative to plasma.

Clinical response is usually the best assessment of cryoprecipitate transfusion effectiveness. Factor VIII activity, fibrinogen, or von Willebrand factor activity should be measured 1h after transfusion. Lack of expected benefit may be due to inadequate dosage, incomplete transfusion, presence of a factor VIII inhibitor, bleeding, or intravascular coagulation.

Massive Transfusion

Massive transfusion is defined as the replacement of one blood volume within 24h. This is approximately equivalent to transfusion of 10 units of RBCs in an adult. Coagulopathy due to dilutional and consumptive thrombocytopenia and coagulation factor deficiency may occur in massive transfusion. Optimal management should be based on frequent clinical assessment and laboratory monitoring. Consideration should be paid to maintenance of intravascular volume, avoidance of hypothermia, normalization of acid/base status, correction of preexisting hematological or coagulation disorders, maintenance of normal ionized calcium levels, and evaluation of ongoing blood loss.

TABLE 9.5.
Indications for Cryoprecipitate.

Indications

Treatment of bleeding due to hypofibrinogenemia or dysfibrinogenemia.

Cases of disseminated intravascular coagulation for which both fibrinogen and factor VIII may be depleted. Consultation with the blood bank/transfusion medicine physician or hematologist is recommended.

Prophylaxis or treatment of significant factor XIII deficiency.

Historically, patients with von Willebrand disease (vWD) and hemophilia A have been treated with cryoprecipitate. Safer products are now available (see Alternative Therapy). *Cryoprecipitate should not be used in the treatment of hemophilia B (factor IX deficiency, Christmas disease).*

Cryoprecipitate has also been used in the production of "fibrin glue" with the addition of thrombin to form an insoluble clot for application to surgical margins and other surgical applications. Such use is not approved by the Food and Drug Administration, although widespread. The safety of this procedure, including the risk of the thrombin source, has not been established.

Dosage and Administration

For fibrinogen replacement, 10 bags of cryoprecipitate will increase the fibrinogen level of a 70-kg recipient approximately 70mg/dl. Cryoprecipitate is administered after pooling. Compatibility testing is not necessary, but the product should be ABO plasma compatible. The Rh type is not important.

Alternative Therapy

Factor VIII concentrates that are made with recombinant DNA technology or have been pasteurized are safer and are the treatment of choice for patients with hemophilia A and von Willebrand disease. Desmopressin (DDAVP) causes the release of factor VIII and vWF in most patients with mild-moderate hemophilia A and vWD. Therefore, DDAVP may be used instead of cryoprecipitate or factor concentrates in these patients. Consult the blood bank/transfusion medicine physician or hematologist in such cases.

References: This table is based on references 106 and 110.

Patient assessment in massive transfusion should include examination of mucus membranes, intravenous sites, and wounds for microvascular bleeding and laboratory testing to include complete blood count with platelet count, PT, aPTT, and fibrinogen and ionized calcium concentration. Laboratory testing should be repeated frequently (typically after each 5–10 units of red cells transfused). No single transfusion protocol is applicable for all massively transfused patients. The first priority is maintaining intravascular volume and oxygen-carrying capacity. The RBCs, platelets, and plasma should be transfused based on both clinical (i.e., ongoing bleeding) and laboratory (anemia, thrombocytopenia, coagulopathy) criteria. Cryoprecipitate may be useful if the fibrinogen is less than 100 mg/dl. However, cryoprecipitate does not contain other coagulation factors (except factor VIII and von Willebrand factor). Plasma is usually a preferable source of coagulation factors.

Epidemiology

Red Blood Cell Transfusion in Surgery

A significant portion of the entire blood supply is administered in the perioperative setting and to critically ill and injured patients. Previous studies have documented that from 56% to 69% of allogeneic RBCs are transfused to surgical patients.[3,4] A more recent study documented the significant variation of transfusion practice following surgical repair of hip fracture or cardiac surgery, as well as those requiring critical care following a surgical intervention or multiple trauma.[5] Rates of allogeneic red cell transfusion were examined in 41,568 patients admitted to 11 hospitals across Canada between August 1998 and August 2000 as part of a retrospective observational cohort study. The overall rate of red cell transfusion was 38.7%, and it ranged from 23.8% to 51.9% across centers among the 41,568 perioperative and critically ill patients. Women were more likely to be transfused (43.7% vs. 35.3%, $P < .0001$), with higher rates of transfusion in 8 of 11 centers. The median number of transfusions was two units for hip fracture and cardiac surgical patients and three units for intensive care unit (ICU) patients (Fig. 9.2). This study documented the high rate of blood transfusion in surgical and ICU patients and significant interinstitutional variability.

Red Blood Cell Transfusion in Critical Care

The results of a large, multicenter prospective observational study (n = 3534 patients from 146 ICUs) conducted in Western Europe were reported in 2002 and documented the common occurrence of anemia and the high rate of blood transfusion in critically ill patients. The transfusion rate during the ICU period was 37%, with mean transfusion per patient of 4.8 ± 5.2 units per patient. For similar degrees of organ dysfunction, patients who had a transfusion had a higher mortality rate. Furthermore, for matched patients in the propensity analysis, the 28-day mortality was 22.7% among patients with transfusions and 17.1% among those without ($P = .02$); the Kaplan-Meier log-rank test confirmed this difference (Fig. 9.3). This epidemiologic study therefore provided evidence of an association between transfusions and diminished organ function as well as between transfusions and mortality.[6]

This pivotal study and other prior studies (Table 9.6) have clearly confirmed the widespread use of blood transfusion in critically ill patients and a concerning association between blood transfusion and adverse clinical outcome. The data from these studies from diverse locations in Western Europe, Canada, the United Kingdom, and the United States reveal remarkably similar findings. Additional studies have further examined these issues and are summarized next and in much more detail in comprehensive reviews.[7–10]

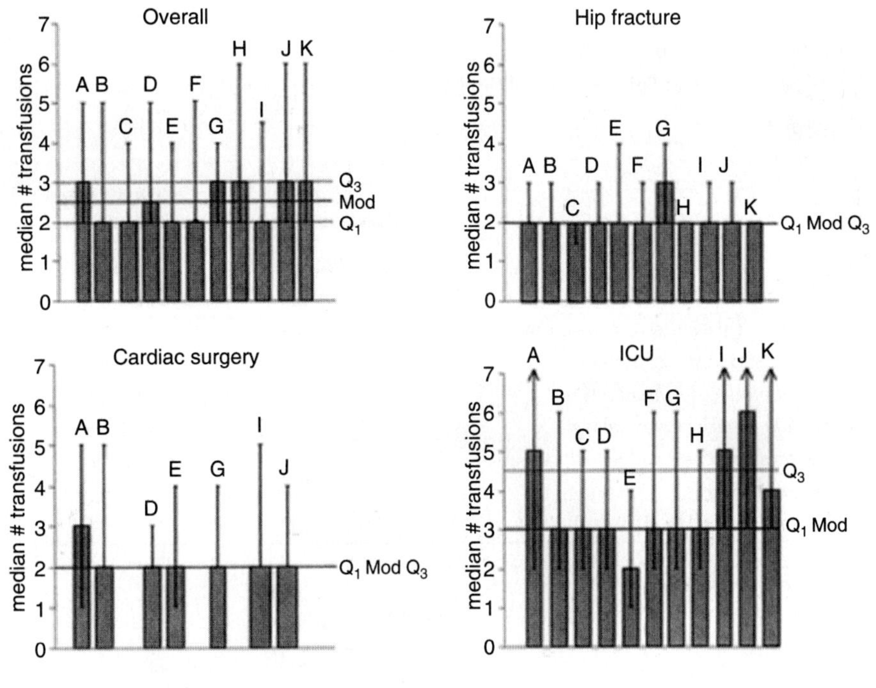

FIGURE 9.2. Median number of RBC transfusions among transfused surgical and ICU patients at 11 participating centers (**A–K**), along with their associated interquartile ranges. ICU, intensive care unit. (From Hutton et al.,[4] by permission of *Canadian Journal of Anaesthesia*.)

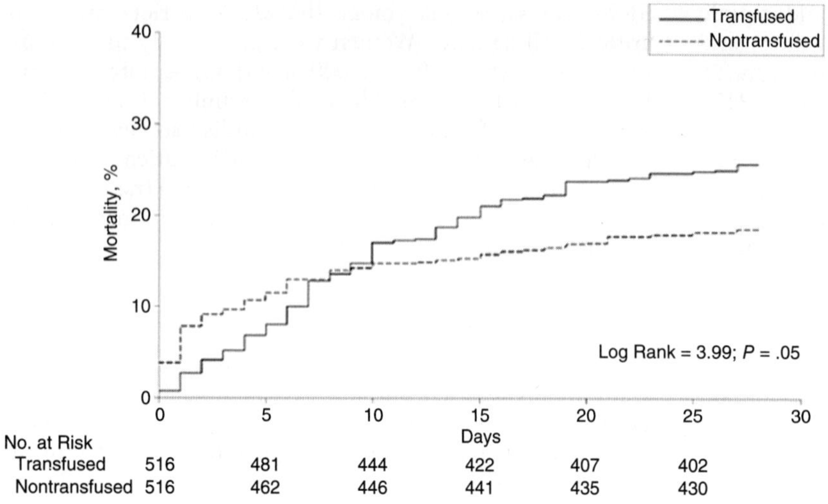

FIGURE 9.3. Survival by transfusion status in propensity-matched critically ill patients in the ABC trial. (From Vincent et al., for the ABC Investigators,[6] by permission of *Journal of the American Medical Association*.)

The CRIT study was a prospective noninterventional study that examined current clinical practice regarding anemia and blood transfusion in the United States.[11] A total of 284 ICUs in 213 hospitals participated in the study, and 4892 critically ill patients from all types of ICUs (including medical, surgical, and medical-surgical) were studied. Patients were enrolled within 48h after ICU admission and followed for up to 30 days or until hospital discharge or death. This study documented that 44% of all patients received one or more RBC transfusions while in the ICU, with a mean RBC transfusion rate of 4.6 ± 4.9 units (Table 9.6). The number of RBC units transfused was an independent predictor of worse clinical outcome and confirmed by a matched propensity analysis (Fig. 9.4). An analysis was performed using matching by propensity score to study mortality rate, and a total of 1059 transfused patients (44.8%) were matched to 1059 patients (41.8%) who did not receive transfusions. After adjusting for the propensity for receiving a blood transfusion, RBC transfusion remained statistically significantly associated with an increased risk for death (adjusted mortality ratio 1.65; 95% confidence interval [CI] 1.35–2.03; log-rank, $P < .001$). The number of RBC transfusions a patient received during the study was independently associated with longer ICU and hospital lengths of stay and an increase in mortality. Patients who received transfusions also had more total complications. Baseline hemoglobin was related to the number of RBC transfusions but was not an independent predictor of length of stay or mortality.

A post hoc analysis of the trauma patient cohort (n = 576) in the CRIT study documented that the majority of trauma patients were anemic (mean baseline hemoglobin 11.1 ± 2.4 g/dl) and remained anemic throughout the study either with or without transfusion.[12] A higher percentage of trauma patients were transfused (55.4%) compared to the entire study cohort, with a mean transfusion rate of 5.8 ± 5.5 units during the ICU stay. Mean pretransfusion hemoglobin in the trauma cohort

TABLE 9.6.
Results of Epidemiological Studies on Anemia and Blood Transfusion in Critical Care.

	ABC Trial (Western Europe)	*CRIT Study (United States)*	*TRICC investigators (Canada)*	*North Thames Blood Interest Group (United Kingdom)*
N	3534	4892	5298	1247
Mean admission hemoglobin (g/dl)	11.2 ± 2.3	11.0 ± 2.4	9.9 ± 2.2	—
Percentage of patients transfused in ICU	37.0%	44.1%	25%	53.4%
Mean transfusions per patient (units)	4.8 ± 5.2	4.6 ± 4.9	4.6 ± 6.7	5.7 ± 5.2
Mean pretransfusion hemoglobin (g/dl)	8.4 ± 1.3	8.6 ± 1.7	8.6 ± 1.3	8.5 ± 1.4
Mean ICU length of stay (days)	4.5	7.4 ± 7.3	4.8 ± 12.6	—
ICU mortality (%)	13.5	13.0	22	21.5
Hospital mortality	20.2	17.6	—	—
Admission APACHE II (mean)	14.8 ± 7.9	19.7 ± 8.2	18 ± 11	18.1 ± 9.1

Data are expressed as mean ± standard deviation; ABC, Anemia and Blood Transfusion in Critical Care; APACHE, Acute Physiology and Chronic Health Evaluation; TRICC, Transfusion Requirements in Critical Care.

Source: From Napolitano,[8] by permission of *Critical Care*.

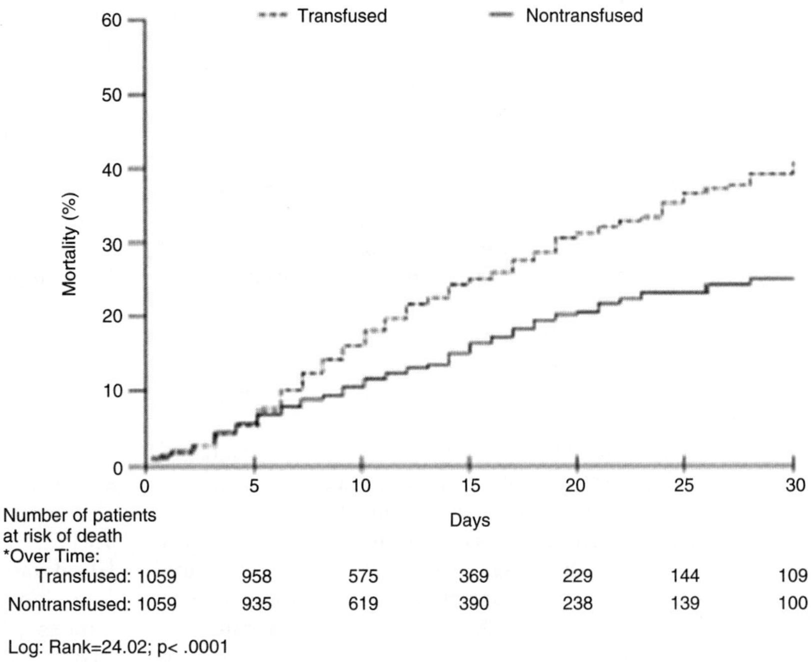

FIGURE 9.4. Mortality by transfusion status for propensity matched patients in the CRIT study. (From Corwin et al.,[11] by permission of *Critical Care Medicine*.)

was 8.9 ± 1.8 g/dl. As compared with the full study population, patients in the trauma subset were more likely to be transfused and received an average of one additional unit of blood. This study confirmed that anemia is common in critically injured trauma patients and persists throughout the duration of critical illness.

Pathophysiology of Anemia in Critical Care

The pathophysiology of ICU-acquired anemia is related to a number of factors, including low endogenous erythropoietin concentrations related to inflammation and increased cytokine concentrations, decreased availability of iron, occult blood loss from the intestine or renal replacement therapies, blood loss related to phlebotomy, and blood loss related to trauma, surgery, or invasive procedures. This is similar to the pathophysiologic mechanism underlying the anemia of chronic disease that is prevalent in patients with cancer and renal failure. Iron deficiency has been reported in 9% of critically ill patients, and others have functional iron deficiency related to the acute-phase response and inflammation. Hepcidin, a liver-derived peptide regulator of iron homeostasis, has been recognized as a key mediator of hypoferremia in inflammation. Using both mice and humans as experimental models, a study documented that interleukin-6 (IL-6) acts directly on hepatocytes to stimulate hepcidin production. Hepcidin in turn acts as a negative regulator of intestinal iron absorption and macrophage iron release, resulting in reduced iron availability.[13]

An animal study documented that bone marrow impairment after shock results not only from altered cell differentiation but also from an increase in the rate of apoptosis (programmed cell death).[14] Apoptosis has a defined role in hematopoiesis regulation, in removal of potentially harmful cells. Increased bone marrow apoptosis, however, may induce compromised bone marrow function, resulting in anemia.

Risks Associated with Red Blood Cell Transfusion

There has been renewed interest in blood transfusion therapy and its associated risks. There are a number of important complications that may occur with transfusion. The most important include volume overload, alloimmunization, iron overload, and exposure to infectious agents. Volume overload is usually caused by too rapid administration of blood. Prevention includes reducing the rate of administration or concurrent administration of loop diuretics in patients with expanded blood volumes or limited cardiac reserve.

Alloimmunization is a common problem occurring in about one-quarter of transfused sickle cell patients. Delayed transfusion reactions, difficulty obtaining blood, and development of autoantibodies are common sequelae. Factors such as racial differences in minor antigen frequency, amount of blood transfused, and previous alloantibodies all predispose to development of new antibodies. Prevention of alloimmunization and delayed transfusion reactions are facilitated by providing a record of previous transfusions, reactions, and alloantibodies to the patient. Identification bracelets should provide alloantibodies and a number to obtain a transfusion history in sensitized individuals. Screening for alloantibodies 6 to 8 weeks after transfusion will document new antibodies that may disappear if there is a prolonged interval without transfusion but may still cause delayed transfusion reactions if further transfusions are required. Limiting the number of units transfused is also important.

Leukocyte depletion prior to storage of red cells prevents febrile reactions. Iron overload can only be effectively prevented by limiting the amount of red cells transfused. Testing for infectious agents markedly reduces but does not eliminate exposure to hepatitis, acquired immunodeficiency syndrome (AIDS), and other viral diseases. All patients receiving transfusion from 1975 through 1985 should be offered counseling about testing for human immunodeficiency virus (HIV) infection. Others given screened blood should be tested for hepatitis or HIV on request or in clinical situations for which infection is likely. Patients who are not immune to hepatitis B should be immunized with the hepatitis B vaccine.

The rates of viral disease transmission have declined substantially with implementation of nucleic acid testing, resulting in a safe U.S. blood supply (Fig. 9.5). Current estimates of risk per unit RBCs transfused are approximately 1/1.9 million for HIV, 1/1.6 million for hepatitis C, and 1/220,000 for hepatitis B.[15] Despite this low risk of viral transmission with blood transfusion, other risks associated with transfusion are increasingly apparent. Current estimates of transfusion-related acute lung injury (TRALI) are 1/8000. Bacterial contamination of platelet concentrates occurs in approximately 1/1000 to 1/2000 units. In 2002, transmission of West Nile virus via blood transfusion was documented.[16]

Substantial advances have been achieved in blood safety during the past 20 years, particularly for transfusion-transmitted viral infections. Currently, the most serious known risks from blood transfusion are administrative error (leading to ABO-incompatible blood transfusion), TRALI, and bacterial contamination in platelet products. Emerging pathogens, such as West Nile virus infection, emphasize the need for implementation of proactive strategies, such as pathogen-inactivation technologies, as well as reactive strategies, such as nucleic acid testing, to ensure continued advances in blood safety.[17]

The risk of transfusion-transmitted infectious diseases has declined dramatically in over the past two decades, primarily because of extraordinary success in preventing HIV and other established transfusion-transmitted viruses from entering the blood supply. Attention is now refocusing on new and emerging pathogens, such as West Nile virus, infectious proteins (the presumed cause of variant Creutzfeldt-Jakob disease), and other transmissible organisms such as bacteria and parasites. It is important to be aware of the individual pathogens and the risks they pose to transfusion recipients and the existing and evolving procedures that are designed to protect the blood supply from this threat.[18]

Studies have also documented a potential increased risk of perioperative bacterial infections associated with blood transfusion. A metaanalysis of 20 peer-reviewed studies, including 13,152 surgical and trauma patients (5215 transfused and 7937 nontransfused), documented the association between allogeneic blood transfusion and postoperative bacterial infection.[19] Multivariate logistic regression analysis documented that blood transfusion was associated with a significantly increased risk of postoperative bacterial infection in the *surgical* patient (odds ratio [OR] 3.45, range 1.43–15.15, $P < .05$) (Fig. 9.6). In the subgroup of *trauma* patients, blood transfusion was associated with higher risk for bacterial infection (OR 5.26, range 5.03–5.43, $P < .05$). Additional studies confirmed these findings in varied patient populations. Multivariate regression analysis confirmed transfusion of allogeneic RBCs as an independent variable predicting postoperative infection (OR 23.65, CI 1.3–422.1, $P = .01$) in orthopedic surgery patients.[20] These data provide additional support for implementation of all strategies to prevent blood transfusion in surgical and trauma patients.

Acute and delayed transfusion reactions occur commonly in surgical patients, and a comprehensive understanding of the diagnosis and management of these reactions is mandatory. Mild and moderate acute transfusion reactions (Table 9.7) are not life threatening. It is extremely important to recognize life-threatening acute transfusion reactions (Table 9.8) and to stop the transfusion immediately and render appropriate life-saving treatment. Furthermore, prompt investigation of the acute transfusion reaction (Table 9.9) is necessary in all patients and warrants a systematic and meticulous approach with collection of data and laboratory samples for diagnosis.

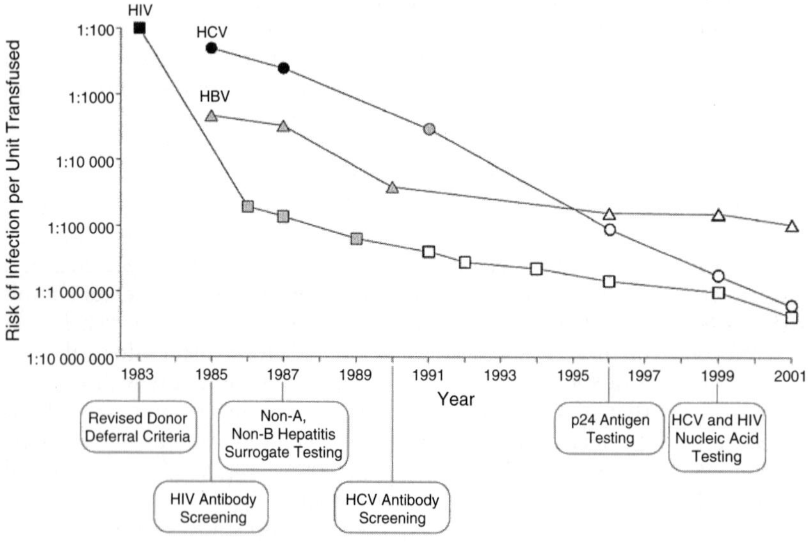

FIGURE 9.5. Risks associated with blood transfusion. (From Busch et al.[92])

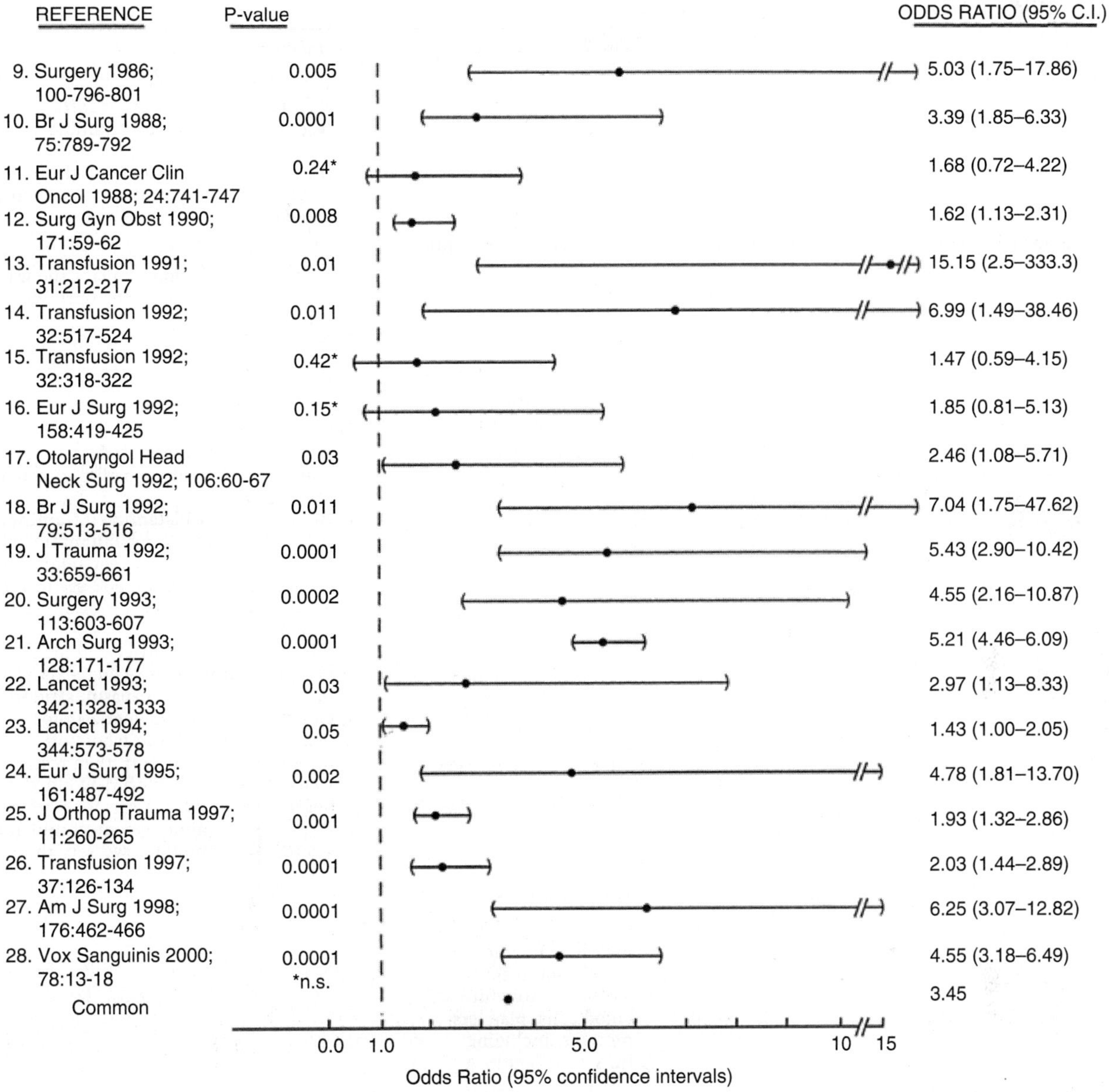

FIGURE 9.6. Blood transfusion association with perioperative bacterial infection. Odds ratios (•) of postoperative bacterial infection (95% confidence intervals) occurring after allogeneic blood transfusion. *Broken vertical line* represents an odds ratio of 1.0 (no increased risk). Values of $P \leq .05$ were considered significant (*n.s., not significant). (From Hill et al.,[19] by permission of *Journal of Trauma*.)

Transfusion-Related Acute Lung Injury

Transfusion-related acute lung injury (TRALI) is a potentially life-threatening complication of allogeneic blood transfusion manifested typically by dyspnea, tachypnea, fever, and hypotension and may result in severe hypoxemia, requirement for mechanical ventilation, and eventual progression to the acute respiratory distress syndrome.[21] It has been estimated to occur in 0.04% to 0.16% of patients transfused, and some studies estimate an incidence as high as 1 in 5000 blood product transfusions. This complication has been identified as the third leading cause of transfusion-related mortality. Despite the increasing recognition that TRALI represents an important clinical syndrome, it remains underreported, and accurate estimates of its incidence are not available.[22] Furthermore, the etiologic factors and pathophysiology of TRALI remain poorly understood.[23]

Now, TRALI is the leading cause of transfusion-related mortality, even though it is probably still underdiagnosed and underreported.[24] Two different etiologies have been proposed: a single antibody-medicated event, involving anti-HLA class I and class II, or antigranulocyte antibodies; and a two-event model, which includes the clinical condition of the patient resulting in pulmonary endothelial activation and neutrophil sequestration. The second event is the transfusion of a biologic response modifier (lipids or antibodies) in the blood component that activates primed neutrophils.

Based on the fact that TRALI is now the leading cause of transfusion-associated mortality, the National Heart, Lung, and Blood Institute convened a working group to identify

TABLE 9.7. Mild and Moderate Blood Transfusion Reactions.

Signs	*Symptoms*	*Possible cause*	*Immediate management*
Category 1: mild reactions			1. Slow the transfusion. 2. Administer antihistamine intramuscularly (e.g., 0.1 mg/kg chlorpeniramine or equivalent). 3. If no clinical improvement within 30 min or if signs and symptoms worsen, then treat as category 2.
Localized cutaneous reactions	Pruritus (itching)	Hypersensitivity (mild)	
Category 2: moderately severe reactions			1. Stop the transfusion. Replace the infusion set and keep intravenous line open with normal saline. 2. Notify the blood bank and the doctor responsible for the patient immediately. 3. Send blood unit with infusion set, freshly collected urine, and new blood samples (one clotted and one anticoagulated) from vein opposite infusion site with appropriate request form to blood bank for laboratory investigations. 4. Administer antihistamine intramuscularly (e.g., 0.1 mg/kg chlorpheniramine or equivalent) and oral or rectal antipyretic (e.g., 10 mg/kg paracetamol, 500 mg to 1 g in adults). Avoid aspirin in thrombocytopenic patients. 5. Give intravenous corticosteroids and bronchodilators if there are anaphylactoid features (e.g., bronchospasm, stridor). 6. Collect urine for the next 24 h for evidence of hemolysis and send to laboratory. 7. If clinical improvement, then restart transfusion slowly with new blood unit and observe carefully. 8. If no clinical improvement within 15 min or if signs and symptoms worsen, then treat as category 3.
Flushing	Anxiety	Hypersensitivity (moderate-severe)	
Urticaria	Pruritus	Febrile nonhemolytic transfusion reactions: antibodies to white blood cells; platelets; proteins, including immunoglobulin A	
Rigors	Palpitations	Possible contamination with pyrogens or bacteria	
Fever	Mild dyspnea		
Restlessness	Headache		
Tachycardia			

Source: From WHO,[91] with the permission of the World Health Organization.

areas of research needed in TRALI.[25] The working group identified the immediate need for a common definition and thus developed the clinical definition of TRALI. The major concept is that TRALI is defined as new acute lung injury occurring during or within 6h after a transfusion, with a clear temporal relationship to the transfusion. Also, another important concept is that acute lung injury temporally associated with multiple transfusions can be TRALI because each unit of blood or blood component can carry one or more of the possible causative agents: antileukocyte antibody, biologically active substances, and other yet-unidentified agents. This group recommended that all future studies utilize the new TRALI definition and proposed that clinicians can diagnose and report TRALI cases to the blood bank. Importantly, researchers can use this TRALI definition to determine accurate incidence, pathophysiology, and strategies to prevent this leading cause of transfusion-associated mortality.

TABLE 9.8. Category 3: Life-Threatening Reactions.

Signs	*Symptoms*	*Possible causes*
Rigors	Anxiety	Acute intravascular hemolysis
Fever	Chest pain	Bacterial contamination and septic shock
Restlessness	Pain near infusion site	Fluid overload
Hypotension (fall of 20% or more in systolic blood pressure)	Respiratory distress/shortness of breath	Anaphylaxis
Tachycardia (rise of 20% or more in heart rate)	Loin/back pain	Transfusion-associated acute lung injury (TRALI)
Hemoglobinuria (red urine)	Headache	
Unexplained bleeding (DIC)	Dyspnea	
Immediate management 1. Stop the transfusion. Replace the infusion set and keep intravenous line open with normal saline. 2. Infuse normal saline (initially 20–30 ml/kg) to maintain systolic pressure. If hypotensive, then give over 5 min and elevate patient's legs. 3. Maintain airway and give high-flow oxygen by mask. 4. Give adrenaline (as 1:1000 solution) 0.01 mg/kg body weight by slow intramuscular injection. 5. Give intravenous corticosteroids and bronchodilators if there are anaphylactoid features (e.g., bronchospasm, stridor). 6. Give diuretic (e.g., 1 mg/kg i.v. frusemide or equivalent). 7. Notify the blood bank and the doctor responsible for patient immediately. 8. Send blood unit with infusion set, fresh urine sample, and new blood samples (one clotted and one anticoagulated) from vein opposite infusion site with appropriate request form to blood bank for investigations. 9. Check a fresh urine specimen visually for signs of hemoglobinuria. 10. Start a 24-h urine collection and fluid balance chart and record all intake and output. Maintain fluid balance. 11. Assess for bleeding from puncture sites or wounds. If there is clinical or laboratory evidence of DIC, give platelets (adult: 5–6 units) and either cryoprecipitate (adult: 12 units) or fresh frozen plasma (adult: 3 units). 12. Reassess. If hypotensive: Give further saline 20–30 ml/kg over 5 min. Give inotrope, if available. 13. If urine output falling or laboratory evidence of acute renal failure (rising K^+, urea, creatinine): Maintain fluid balance accurately. Give further frusemide. Consider dopamine infusion, if available. Seek expert help: The patient may need renal dialysis. 14. If bacteremia is suspected (rigors, fever, collapse, no evidence of a hemolytic reaction), then start broad-spectrum antibiotics intravenously.		

Note: 1. If an acute transfusion reaction occurs, first check the blood pack labels and the patient's identity. If there is any discrepancy, then stop the transfusion immediately and consult the blood bank.
2. In an unconscious or anesthetized patient, hypotension and uncontrolled bleeding may be the only signs of an incompatible transfusion.
3. In a conscious patient undergoing a severe hemolytic transfusion reaction, signs and symptoms may appear quickly—within minutes of infusing only 5–10 ml of blood. Close observation at the start of the infusion of each unit is essential.

Source: From WHO,[91] with permission of the World Health Organization.

TABLE 9.9. Investigation of Acute Transfusion Reactions.

1. Immediately report all acute transfusion reactions, with the exception of mild hypersensitivity (category 1), to the doctor responsible for the patient and to the blood bank that supplied the blood. If you suspect a severe life-threatening reaction, seek help immediately from the duty anesthetist, emergency team, or whoever is available and skilled to assist.
2. Record the following information on the patient's notes:
   Type of transfusion reaction.
   Length of time after the start of transfusion that the reaction occurred.
   Volume, type, and pack numbers of the blood products transfused.
3. Take the following samples and send them to the blood bank for laboratory investigations:
   Immediate posttransfusion blood samples (one clotted and one anticoagulated: EDTA/Sequestrene) from the vein opposite the infusion site for
   - Repeat ABO and RhD group.
   - Repeat antibody screen and crossmatch.
   - Full blood count.
   - Coagulation screen.
   - Direct antiglobulin test.
   - Urea and creatinine.
   - Electrolytes.

   Blood culture in a special blood culture bottle.
   Blood unit and infusion set containing red cell and plasma residues from the transfused donor blood.
   First specimen of the patient's urine following the reaction.
4. Complete a transfusion reaction report form.
5. After the initial investigation of the reaction, send the following to the blood bank for laboratory investigations:
   Blood samples (one clotted and one anticoagulated: EDTA/Sequestrene) taken from the vein opposite the infusion site 12h and 24h after the start of the reaction.
   Patient's 24h urine sample.
6. Record the results of the investigations in the patient's records for future follow-up, if required.

Source: From WHO,[91] with permission of the World Health Organization.

Red Blood Cell Transfusion and Outcome in Surgery

The impact of perioperative RBC transfusion on outcome in surgical patients has come under increased scrutiny. The effect of perioperative RBC transfusion on 30-day and 1-year mortality following coronary artery bypass grafting (CABG) was examined in a retrospective analysis of 3024 consecutive patients (January 1999 to December 2001) in the United Kingdom.[26] Confounding variables were controlled for by constructing a propensity score from core patient characteristics, including the lowest recorded laboratory hemoglobin, for the probability of receiving a transfusion. Of the patients, 940 (31.1%) patients received RBC transfusion during or within 72h of surgery. Predictors of the need for transfusion were low hemoglobin, lower body mass index, use of cardiopulmonary bypass, female sex, number of grafts, renal dysfunction, increased age, extent of disease, and prior CABG. These factors were all included in the propensity score. After 1 year of follow-up, 122 (4.03%) deaths occurred. After adjusting for the propensity score, reoperation for bleeding, perioperative blood loss, and postoperative complications, the adjusted 30-day mortality was 1.9% in transfused patients compared to 1.1% in patients not transfused ($P < .05$). The adjusted HR for 1-year mortality in patients transfused was 1.88 ($P < .01$). The authors concluded that perioperative RBC transfusion after CABG is associated with an increased risk of mortality during a 1-year follow-up period, with a large proportion of deaths occurring within 30 days.

Red Blood Cell Transfusion and Outcome in Critical Care

New evidence has emerged documenting the associated risks and lack of efficacy or improvement in clinical outcome with blood transfusion for the treatment of anemia in critically ill patients who are hemodynamically stable. Emerging data have documented that the use of blood transfusions for the treatment of anemia in hemodynamically stable critically ill patients is not associated with improved outcome. The TRICC (Transfusion Requirements in Critical Care) trial conducted by the Canadian Critical Care Trials group was the only prospective study that randomized patients (n = 838) to a *restrictive* transfusion strategy (red cells transfused if the hemoglobin concentration dropped below 7g/dl and maintained at 7–9g/dl) or a *liberal* strategy (red cells transfused if the hemoglobin concentration fell below 10g/dl and maintained at 10–12g/dl).[27]

Overall, 30-day mortality was similar in the two groups (18.7% vs. 23.3%, $P = .11$). However, mortality rates were significantly lower with the restrictive transfusion strategy among patients who were less acutely ill—those with an Acute Physiology and Chronic Health Evaluation II score below 20 (8.7% in the restrictive-strategy group and 16.1% in the liberal-strategy group, $P = .03$)—and among patients who were less than 55 years of age (5.7% and 13.0%, respectively; $P = .02$). The mortality rate during hospitalization was significantly lower in the restrictive-strategy group (22.2% vs. 28.1%, respectively; $P = .05$). The authors concluded that a restrictive strategy of red cell transfusion is at least as effective as and possibly superior to a liberal transfusion strategy in critically ill patients, with the possible exception of patients with acute myocardial infarction and unstable angina.

Interestingly, in the CRIT study the mean pretransfusion hemoglobin was 8.6 ± 1.7g/dl. This study documented that since the publication in 1999 of the TRICC trial,[28] little has changed in the practice of anemia and blood transfusion in critical care. Critical care practitioners had not yet adopted the restrictive transfusion strategy (transfuse if hemoglobin is <7g/dl) that was recommended by the results of the TRICC trial. In an accompanying editorial, Drs. Shah and Hickey documented that we have had "a decade without change" regarding anemia and blood transfusion practice in the critically ill.[29] They pointed out that 84% of the ICUs in the study had a full-time director, but only 19% of the hospitals had an institutional transfusion protocol. Furthermore, 71% of the ICUs in the study were "open" units, thereby allowing any practitioners to order a blood transfusion.

An interesting secondary analysis of the CRIT study examined the relationship between packed RBC transfusion practice and the development of ventilator-associated pneumonia (VAP).[30] Of 4892 subjects in the original cohort, 1518 received mechanical ventilation of 48 h or longer and did not have preexisting pneumonia. Diagnosis of VAP was made in 311 (20.5%) patients. Multivariate analysis revealed that transfusion independently increased the risk for VAP (OR 1.89, 95% CI 1.33–2.68). The effect of transfusion on late-onset VAP was more pronounced (OR 2.16, 95% CI 1.27–3.66) and demonstrated a positive dose-response relationship (P = .0223 for trend test). This study documented that transfusion of packed RBCs increases the risk of developing VAP. Avoiding the unnecessary use of packed RBC transfusions may decrease the occurrence of VAP.

A study from our research group documented that blood transfusion, independent of shock severity, was associated with worse outcome in trauma. Prospective data were collected on 15,534 patients admitted to a level I trauma center over a 3-year period (1998–2000) and stratified by age, gender, race, Glasgow Coma Scale score, and Injury Severity Score. Admission anemia and blood transfusion were assessed as independent predictors of mortality, ICU admission, ICU length of stay (LOS), and hospital LOS by logistic regression analysis, with base deficit, serum lactate, and shock index as covariates. Blood transfusion was a strong independent predictor of mortality (OR 2.83; 95% CI 1.82–4.40, $P < .001$) after controlling for severity of shock by admission indices of shock (base deficit, serum lactate, shock index, and anemia).[31]

Red Blood Cell Transfusion in Septic Patients

The Surviving Sepsis Campaign guidelines for the management of severe sepsis and septic shock were published in 2004 and are evidence-based guidelines.[32] Recommendations regarding blood product administration in the septic patient are listed in Table 9.10 and recommend a restrictive policy (based on the TRICC trial) of blood transfusion following resolution of tissue hypoperfusion and in the absence of significant coronary artery disease or acute hemorrhage. Guidelines for the use of FFP and platelet component therapy are also listed in Table 9.10.

TABLE 9.10. Blood Product Administration in Severe Sepsis and Septic Shock.

1. Following resolution of tissue hypoperfusion and in the absence of significant coronary artery disease or acute hemorrhage, transfuse red blood cells when hemoglobin decreases to <7.0 g/dl to target a hemoglobin of 7.0 to 9.0 g/dl.
2. Do not use fresh frozen plasma to correct laboratory clotting abnormalities unless there is bleeding or there are planned invasive procedures.
3. Administer platelets when counts are <5000/mm^3 (5 × 10^9/l) regardless of bleeding. Transfuse platelets when counts are 5,000 to 30,000/mm^3 (5–30 × 10^9/l) and there is significant bleeding risk. Higher platelet counts (≥50,000/mm^3 [50 × 10^9/l]) are required for surgery or invasive procedures.

Source: From Dellinger et al.,[32] by permission of *Critical Care Medicine.*

A number of published studies have documented that transfusion of packed RBCs does not consistently improve tissue oxygen consumption, either globally or at the level of the microcirculation, in critically ill patients.[33]

A prospective randomized study in septic patients documented that hemoglobin increase from stored red cell transfusion did not improve either global or regional oxygen utilization in anemic septic patients.[34] Furthermore, RBC transfusion was associated with a significant reduction in right ventricular ejection by increasing the pulmonary vascular resistance index. This effect may, in part, be related to increased concentrations of free hemoglobin in stored blood.[35] Cell-free hemoglobin in the plasma, after transfusion of stored blood, rapidly destroys nitric oxide by oxidation to methemoglobin and nitrate. Nitric oxide reacts at least 1000 times more rapidly with free hemoglobin than with erythrocytes. Subsequently, limited nitric oxide bioavailability promotes regional and systemic vasoconstriction and subsequent organ dysfunction.[36] Lack of efficacy of RBC transfusion in critically ill patients is likely related to a number of factors, including storage time, increased endothelial adherence of stored RBCs, nitric oxide binding by free hemoglobin in stored blood, donor leukocytes, host inflammatory response, and reduced red cell deformability.

Transfusion Protocols and Guidelines

The decision to transfuse a patient must be based on the specifics of each individual case. However, the decision to transfuse any patient for a given indication must balance the risk of not transfusing (influenced, e.g., by disease prognosis) against the risks of transfusion (influenced, e.g., by the probable duration of patient survival and the incubation time of known infective agents). Given the potential risks, however small, each allogeneic transfusion must have a valid, defined, and justifiable indication. The indication for each transfusion should be documented in the patient's record. In a hemodynamically stable patient, one unit of RBCs should be transfused at a time, allowing the benefit of each to be assessed at 24 hourly intervals. The major principle guiding transfusion therapy is to minimize the need for donor blood products (Table 9.11).

The use of transfusion protocols and guidelines, however, has been documented to reduce the use of allogeneic blood transfusion significantly, decrease the total number of patients transfused, and have no adverse effect on patient outcome. Most clinical practice guidelines recommend restrictive red cell transfusion practices with the goal of minimizing exposure to allogeneic blood (Table 9.12).[37–40] A Cochrane systemic review documented that the limited published evidence supports the use of restrictive transfusion triggers in patients who are free of serious cardiac disease.[41] However, most of the data on clinical outcomes were generated by a single trial (TRICC). The effects of conservative transfusion triggers on functional status, morbidity, and mortality, particularly in patients with cardiac disease, need to be tested in further large clinical trials. It is advantageous to have institution- and unit-specific blood transfusion protocols (see, e.g., Fig. 9.7) since physician compliance is improved.

TABLE 9.11. Major Principles of Transfusion Therapy.

Principle: Minimize the need for donor blood products

- Transfusion carries risks; some of these are specifically due to the use of allogeneic blood (i.e., blood from another person). Autologous blood also has some risks.
- Good clinical practice demands that any blood product should only be given when the patient is judged likely to benefit (i.e., the transfusion will do more good than harm).
- Prescribing decisions should be based on the best available clinical guidelines, modified according to individual patient needs. The reasons for giving blood should be written in the notes.
- The need for transfusion can in some cases be reduced by stimulating red cell production with erythropoietin or by using drugs such as aprotinin to reduce surgical bleeding. In some situations, the need for donor blood can be reduced by retransfusing the patient's own shed blood (blood salvage).
- For some patients in some clinical situations, it is preferable to use the patient's own blood that has been collected in advance of planned surgery (autologous transfusion).
- Modifications of routine practice can minimize the need to transfuse red cells, for example:
  Checking for and correcting anemia before planned surgery.
  Stopping anticoagulants and antiplatelet drugs before planned surgery.
  Minimizing the amount of blood taken for laboratory samples.
  Using a simple protocol to guide when hemoglobin should be checked and when red cells should be transfused.

Source: Reproduced with permission from Handbook of Transfusion Medicine.[112]

TABLE 9.12. Perioperative Blood Transfusion for Elective Surgery: A National Clinical Guideline, Scottish Intercollegiate Guidelines Network.

Hemoglobin Transfusion Thresholds

The transfusion threshold is the hemoglobin value at which transfusion will normally be indicated, under stable conditions, and in the absence of other clinical signs or symptoms of anemia.

- A transfusion threshold should be defined as part of an overall strategy to provide optimal patient management.
- The transfusion threshold should be viewed as the hemoglobin value below which the patient should not fall during the perioperative period, particularly in the context of ongoing or anticipated blood loss.

Preoperative Thresholds

All patients undergoing major elective surgery should have a full blood count performed prior to surgery to avoid short-term cancellation and to allow those patients presenting with anemia to be investigated and treated appropriately (e.g., iron therapy).

When possible, anemia should be corrected prior to major surgery to reduce exposure to allogeneic transfusion.

Intraoperative Thresholds

There is no indication that thresholds should differ during this period, but the use of intraoperative transfusion must reflect the ongoing rate of surgical blood loss, continued hemodynamic instability, and anticipated postoperative bleeding.

Postoperative Thresholds

Transfusion is unjustified at hemoglobin levels >10 g/dl.

Transfusion is required at hemoglobin levels <7 g/dl.

Patients with cardiovascular disease, or those expected to have covert cardiovascular disease (e.g., elderly patients or those with peripheral vascular disease), are likely to benefit from transfusion when their hemoglobin level falls below 9 g/dl.

Source: Based on the Scottish Intercollegiate Guidelines Network. Perioperative blood transfusion for elective surgery: a national clinical guideline. Edinburgh; SIGN: 2001. (SIGN guideline 54) pp 7–8, with permission.[113,114]

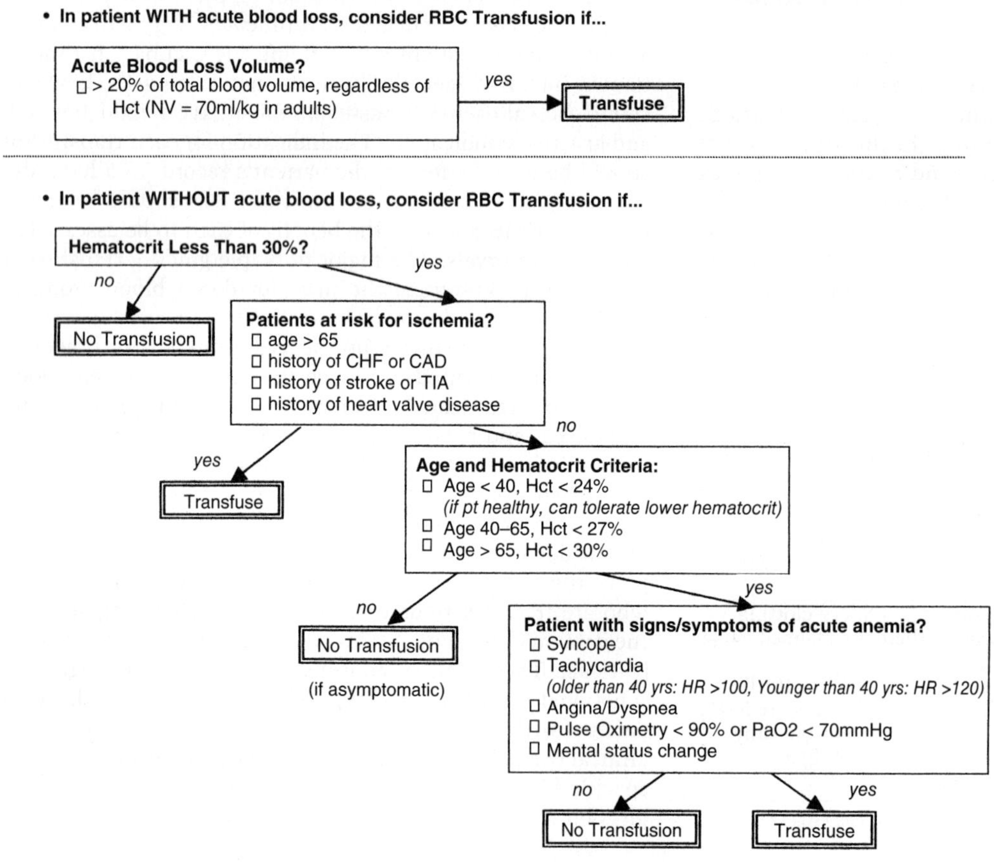

FIGURE 9.7. Blood transfusion protocol at Stanford Surgery ICU. Background: There are divergent views on the risks of anemia and the benefits of blood transfusion in critically ill patients. Blood products are not without risk, and unnecessary blood transfusion contributes to increased morbidity, costs, and in some studies, mortality. In an effort to promote decision consistency and reduce the number of inappropriate blood transfusions, an evidenced-based transfusion guideline should be employed. Indications: The major indication for RBC product transfusion is to prevent or treat symptoms of tissue hypoxia by augmenting the oxygen-carrying capacity in blood. Principles: Patients should be informed of transfusion when possible. In the setting of acute blood loss, transfusion should not be used to expand vascular volume when oxygen-carrying capacity is adequate. (This figure was based on references 37 and 93–100. : From http://scalpel.stanford.edu/articles/Stanford%20Blood%20Txf%20Guidelines.pdf, with permission of Stanford University, 2003–2004.)

Patient Safety and Blood Transfusion

Current risk from transfusion is largely because of noninfectious hazards and defects in the overall process of delivering safe transfusion therapy. Significant among these risks is the potential for human error and the subsequent transfusion of the incorrect blood component. In the first annual report of the Serious Hazards of Transfusion (SHOT) initiative from the United Kingdom and Ireland, 366 cases were reported over 24 months, of which 191 (52%) were episodes of "wrong blood to patient."[42] Analysis of these revealed multiple errors of identification, often beginning when blood was collected from the blood bank. The second annual report of the SHOT initiative reported a 36% increase in these cases that may be related partly to improved reporting.[43] With progress in prevention of viral disease transmission, human error is associated with 100- to 1000-fold greater hazard of severe adverse effects than getting HIV or hepatitis from blood transfusion.

New technology is becoming increasingly available to improve the performance of sample labeling and the bedside clerical check. Several technology solutions are in various stages of development and include wireless, handheld, portable digital assistants; advanced bar coding; radio-frequency identification; and embedded chip technology.[44] Bar code technology for blood transfusion has been adopted by the Veterans Affairs hospitals in the United States and by the National Blood Service in the United Kingdom.[45] In the United Kingdom, significant improvements were found in the procedure for the administration of blood following the introduction of bar code patient identification, including an improvement from 11.8% to 100% in the correct verbal identification of patients ($P < .001$). Technology-based solutions for transfusion safety will depend on the larger issue of the technology for patient identification. Devices for transfusion safety hold exciting promise but need to undergo clinical trials to show effectiveness and ease of use.[46]

Strategies to Reduce Allogeneic Blood Transfusion in Surgery

The transfusion of allogeneic RBCs and allogeneic coagulation products is associated with risk to the patient and the depletion of an increasingly scarce resource. A number of factors have an impact on the need for allogeneic blood transfusion in surgery, including surgical technique, degree of intraoperative bleeding, presence of preoperative anemia, hemodilution with crystalloid resuscitation, and postoperative bleeding complications. A number of strategies are currently available to address each of these issues in efforts to reduce blood transfusion.

Diagnosis and Treatment of Preoperative Anemia

Preoperative anemia is common in surgical patients, yet diagnosis and treatment of preoperative anemia is not commonly practiced. Using prospective data from the National Veterans Administration Surgical Quality Improvement Program from 1995 to 2000, we previously identified that preoperative anemia (hematocrit < 36%) was present in 33.9% of all noncardiac surgical patients (n = 6301). Postoperative anemia was more common, identified in 84.1% of the study cohort. Multiple logistic regression analysis documented that low preoperative hematocrit, low postoperative hematocrit, and increased blood transfusion rates were associated with increased mortality ($P < .01$), increased postoperative pneumonia ($P \leq .05$), and increased hospital length of stay ($P < .05$). This study confirmed that there is a high incidence of preoperative and postoperative anemia in surgical patients, with a coincident increase in blood utilization.[47]

Certain surgical patient populations are at higher risk for preoperative anemia, including patients with a diagnosis of cancer. We identified that the incidence of preoperative anemia was 46.1% in a prospective cohort study of 311 surgical patients with colorectal carcinoma.[48] Furthermore, preoperative anemia was most common in patients with right colon cancer, with an incidence of 57.6%, followed by left colon cancer (42.2%) and rectal cancer (29.8%). The European Cancer Anemia Survey confirmed a high (53.7%) incidence of anemia in cancer patients (n = 15,367) and documented that anemia was treated in only 38.9% of patients who were diagnosed with anemia. Treatment included erythropoietin (17.4%), blood transfusion (14.9%), and iron (6.5%). Mean hemoglobin to initiate anemia treatment was 9.7 g/dl.[49]

Consideration should be given to preoperative diagnosis and correction of anemia with iron, vitamin B_{12}, folate supplementation, or administration of recombinant human erythropoietin (rHuEpo). The EORTC guidelines for the use of erythropoietic proteins in anemia patients with cancer provide an evidence-based review and confirm level I evidence that supports the effectiveness of erythropoietic proteins in the prevention and treatment of anemia in cancer patients receiving chemotherapy or radiotherapy or in those undergoing cancer surgery.[50]

A prospective randomized study (n = 93) documented that the preoperative use of erythropoietin was effective in increasing hematocrit in surgical patients with preoperative anemia. This study also confirmed that two injections of erythropoietin were sufficient to reach a hematocrit of 40% in the majority of patients. Furthermore, the use of preoperative erythropoietin was associated with a higher hematocrit on postoperative days 1 and 3 and at discharge and improved cost-effectiveness compared to preoperative autologous blood donation (PABD) in elective orthopedic surgical patients.[51]

Preoperative anemia has also been associated with a higher risk of intraoperative and postoperative complications. A prospective analysis of elective total hip replacements performed over a 10-month period (n = 225) documented that patients with preclinical anemia on admission had a higher incidence of postoperative infection and transfusion ($P < .001$) and a longer postoperative inpatient stay.[52] Preoperative iron supplementation in patients with preclinical iron deficiency anemia resulted in a significant reduction in transfusion requirements ($P = .00125$). These data suggest that identification and treatment of patients with preclinical anemia preoperatively may reduce postoperative infection and transfusion needs and result in a shorter inpatient stay. Future efforts should be focused on such simple strategies for optimization of preoperative hematocrit.

Surgical Technique and Intraoperative Blood Loss

A number of studies have documented that specific surgical techniques may significantly reduce intraoperative blood loss and result in reduced need for transfusion. Total mesorectal excision (TME) for rectal cancer is associated with decreased local recurrence rate and improved survival compared with conventional surgery. Furthermore, TME was associated with less intraoperative bleeding and transfusion compared with conventional surgery.[53] Comparison of transfusion history in rectal cancer resections in two different multicenter studies confirmed that TME resulted in a significant reduction in intraoperative blood loss (median 100 ml vs. 550 ml, $P < .001$) and reduction in perioperative blood transfusion, from 73% to 43% ($P < .001$).[54] Importantly, this study also identified that factors other than blood loss seemed to influence the decision of blood transfusion in these surgical patients.

Similarly, minimally invasive surgery with the use of laparoscopy can assist in reducing intraoperative blood loss. A case-matched study (n = 147) documented that a laparoscopic approach for colorectal surgery led to significantly less intraoperative blood loss and perioperative blood transfusions than matched open colectomy cases.[55] A similar study in 384 patients with colorectal diseases randomized patients to laparoscopic or open resection.[56] Patients who underwent laparoscopic resection had faster recovery of bowel function ($P = .0001$) and a shorter length of stay ($P = .0001$). In the whole cohort of patients, multivariate analysis identified open surgery ($P = .003$), duration of surgery ($P = .01$), and homologous blood transfusion ($P = .01$) as risk factors for postoperative morbidity. This study confirmed that laparoscopic surgery was associated with significant reduction in allogeneic blood transfusion.

Several techniques and devices have been developed in an effort to reduce or avoid intraoperative blood loss. One such device is a new water-cooled, saline-enhanced, high-density, monopolar radio-frequency device (Tissuelink Monopolar Floating Ball, Tissuelink Medical, Inc., Dover, NH) that can be used in solid organ resections. A study in hepatic resections documented that the mean blood loss was 150 ml (range 50 to 300 ml). No vascular clamping was used with the exception of one patient. This study confirmed that the Tissuelink Monopolar Floating Ball permitted excellent coagulation of the cut liver surface, thus avoiding bleeding and vascular clamping, with a resultant significant decrease in the need for allogeneic blood transfusion.[57] Similarly, the use of the Tissuelink device was associated with a significant reduction in intraoperative blood loss in patients undergoing open partial nephrectomy compared to needlepoint electrocautery.[58]

Other adjuncts to local surgical hemostasis, including fibrin sealants, have been associated with reduced incidence of both intraoperative and postoperative bleeding, resulting in decreased need for allogeneic blood transfusions.[59] A Cochrane Database Systematic Review of fibrin sealant use for minimizing perioperative allogeneic blood transfusion concluded that overall the results suggest that fibrin sealants are efficacious in reducing both postoperative blood loss and perioperative exposure to allogeneic RBC transfusions.[60] Seven trials, including a total of 388 patients, reported data on perioperative exposure to allogeneic RBC transfusion. Fibrin sealant treatment, on average, reduced the rate of exposure to allogeneic red cell transfusion by a relative 54% (relative risk [RR] = 0.46, 95% CI = 0.32 to 0.68). Eight trials, including a total of 442 patients, provided data for postoperative blood loss. Fibrin sealant treatment reduced blood loss on average by approximately 134 ml per patient (95% CI = 51 to 217 ml). However, the trials reviewed were small and of poor methodological quality (91% unblinded). Overall, the results suggest that fibrin sealants are efficacious in reducing both postoperative blood loss and perioperative exposure to allogeneic RBC transfusion. However, due to the lack of blinding, transfusion practices may have been influenced by knowledge of the patient's treatment status. This raises concerns about the use of blood transfusion practice as an outcome variable in trials of fibrin sealant. In the case of blood loss, the results must be interpreted with caution in view of the statistically significant heterogeneity in treatment effect observed. Large, methodologically rigorous, randomized controlled trials of fibrin sealants are needed. It is also clear that some specific complex surgical procedures result in significant intraoperative blood loss, and all efforts to minimize the need for blood transfusion in these procedures should be considered.[61]

Acute Normovolemic Hemodilution

The efficacy of acute normovolemic hemodilution (ANH) remains uncertain. A study assessed the effects of ANH on allogeneic transfusion and postoperative complications in major gastrointestinal surgery (n = 160).[62] Consecutive patients undergoing major gastrointestinal surgery were randomized to a planned three-unit ANH or no ANH. Both groups underwent identical management, including adherence to a transfusion protocol after surgery. There was no significant difference between groups in the number of patients receiving allogeneic blood (28% vs. 30%), the total number of allogeneic units transfused (90 vs. 93), complication rate, or duration of stay. The ANH significantly increased anesthetic time, and significantly fewer patients in the ANH group experienced oliguria in the immediate postoperative period (47% vs. 67%, $P = .012$). The most significant factors affecting transfusion were blood loss, starting hemoglobin, and age. When compared with matched historical controls, the introduction of a transfusion protocol reduced the transfusion rate in colorectal patients from 136/333 (41%) to 37/138 (27%) ($P = .004$). This study documented that ANH did not affect the allogeneic transfusion rate in major gastrointestinal surgery. Instead, reduced preoperative hemoglobin (preoperative anemia), blood loss, and transfusion protocol were the key factors influencing allogeneic blood transfusion.

The efficacy of ANH and intraoperative cell salvage (ICS) in blood-conservation strategies for infrarenal aortic surgery was also examined. This multicenter, prospective, randomized trial compared standard transfusion practice with autologous transfusion combining ANH with ICS in 145 patients undergoing elective aortic surgery. The primary outcome measures were the proportion of patients requiring allogeneic blood and the volume of allogeneic transfusion. The secondary outcome measures were the frequency of complications, including postoperative infection, and postoperative hospital stay. The combination of ANH and ICS reduced the volume of allogeneic blood transfused from a median of two units to zero units. The proportion of patients transfused was 56% in allogeneic and 43% in autologous groups. There were no significant differences in complications or length of hospital stay. Therefore, both ANH and ICS were safe and reduced the allogeneic blood transfusion requirement in patients undergoing elective infrarenal aortic surgery.[63]

In cardiac surgical patients who require cardiopulmonary bypass, a simple strategy of autotransfusion of the residual blood from the cardiopulmonary bypass circuit is considered one of the methods enabling reduction in the need for blood transfusion in the postoperative period. A study assessed the efficacy of autologous autotransfusion of centrifuged RBCs from the residual blood of the cardiopulmonary bypass circuit after cardiac surgery.[64] This study compared three groups of patients: Group 1 received all residual blood in the bypass circuit, group 2 did not receive residual blood, group 3 received *centrifuged* RBCs from the residual blood in the bypass circuit. Group 3 patients had a significant reduction in blood transfusions, postoperative infections, and hospital length of stay. Therefore, autotransfusion of centrifuged RBCs from the residual blood in the bypass circuit should be considered in all cardiac surgery patients requiring cardiopulmonary bypass.

Intraoperative Blood Salvage and Autotransfusion

One strategy for reducing perioperative allogeneic blood transfusion is the use of intraoperative blood salvage and autotransfusion. A single-center prospective clinical trial documented that fewer patients randomized to intraoperative autotransfusion required perioperative blood transfusion (21 vs. 31, $P = .038$), and the median blood requirement per patient was two units lower ($P = .012$). There was a higher incidence of pulmonary infection (12 vs. 4 patients, $P = .049$) and systemic inflammatory response syndrome (SIRS) (20 vs. 9 patients, $P = .020$) in the control group. This study confirmed that the use of autotransfusion effectively reduced the need for allogeneic blood transfusion and was associated with a reduced incidence of postoperative SIRS and infectious complications.[65]

A previous retrospective review documented that routine use of red cell salvage and autotransfusion was an effective means for reducing transfusion requirements in elective abdominal aortic aneurysm repair.[66] Interestingly, a prior prospective randomized study of intraoperative autotransfusion during elective infrarenal aortic surgery (n = 100) found no net benefit.[67] There were no significant differences identified between patients randomized to intraoperative autotransfusion and control groups in estimated blood loss; allogeneic blood transfusion (units administered intraoperatively, postoperatively, and total); proportion of patients not receiving allogeneic blood (34% vs. 28% of control patients); postoperative hemoglobin/hematocrit levels; and complications.

A Cochrane Database Systematic Review in 2003 examined the evidence for the efficacy of cell salvage in reducing allogeneic blood transfusion and the evidence for any effect on clinical outcomes.[68] Overall, the use of cell salvage reduced the rate of exposure to allogeneic RBC transfusion by a relative 40% (RR = 0.60, 95% CI = 0.51 to 0.70). The absolute risk reduction (ARR) of receiving an allogeneic RBC transfusion was 23% (95% CI = 16% to 30%). In orthopedic procedures, the relative risk of exposure to RBC transfusion was 0.42 (95% CI = 0.32 to 0.54) compared to 0.78 (95% CI = 0.68 to 0.88) for cardiac procedures. The use of cell salvage resulted in an average saving of 0.64 units of allogeneic RBCs per patient (weighted mean difference [WMD] = −0.64, 95% CI = −0.86 to −0.46). Cell salvage did not appear to have an adverse impact on clinical outcomes. The results suggest cell salvage is efficacious in reducing the need for allogeneic red cell transfusion in adult elective surgery. However, the methodological quality of trials was poor. As the trials were unblinded and lacked adequate concealment of treatment allocation, transfusion practices may have been influenced by knowledge of the patient's treatment status biasing the results in favor of cell salvage.

Preoperative Autologous Blood Donation

Preoperative autologous blood donation (PABD) is an additional strategy to consider in attempts to reduce perioperative allogeneic blood transfusion. A study of 100 consecutive patients undergoing hepatectomy for biliary hilar malignancies documented that PABD was possible in 73 patients (3.4 ± 1.2 units). Intraoperative blood loss was high in these procedures (1850 ± 1000 ml, range 677–5900 ml). Intraoperatively, only 10% (7 of 73) of patients who underwent PABD received allogeneic blood transfusion compared to 67% (18 of 23) of those patients who did not. The incidence of postoperative complications was higher in the 35 patients who received perioperative allogeneic transfusion than in 65 patients who did not (94% vs. 52%, $P < .0001$). This study documented that approximately two-thirds of hepatectomies can be performed in an experienced center without perioperative allogeneic blood transfusion using PABD.[69]

Similarly, a study of autologous blood transfusion during total hip arthroplasty (n = 253) documented that the mean total volume of intraoperative blood loss was 2039 (standard deviation 992) ml in revision surgery and 1673 (717.3) ml in primary surgery ($P < .05$). The rate of avoidance of homologous blood transfusion was 75% among patients who underwent primary surgery and 61% among those who underwent revision surgery. The rate was 95% in cases in which a combination of preoperative autologous donation and intraoperative recovery was used, 49% in cases in which the preoperative autologous donation alone was used, and 42% in those in which the intraoperative recovery system alone was employed. The autologous blood had to be disposed of in 3 (1%) cases, all of which were revision procedures with replacement of the polyethylene liner alone. This study documented that the combined use of the PABD and intraoperative recovery systems is effective for avoiding homologous blood transfusion.[70]

In contrast, a prospective study of patients undergoing breast reconstruction with TRAM flaps documented that patients who did not donate autologous blood had statistically significantly higher preoperative and postoperative day 3 hemoglobin levels than patients in the groups that did predonate. No difference in blood transfusion rates was identified. The authors concluded that preoperative autologous donation of blood does not confer any clinical advantage to patients undergoing autologous breast reconstruction using pedicled TRAM flaps.[71]

A Cochrane Database Systematic Review in 2002 examined the evidence for the efficacy of PABD in reducing the need for perioperative allogeneic RBC transfusion.[72] Overall, PABD reduced the risk of receiving an allogeneic blood transfusion by a relative 63% (RR = 0.37, 95% CI 0.26–0.54). The absolute reduction in risk of allogeneic transfusion was 43.8% (RD = −0.438, 95% CI −0.607–0.268). In contrast, the results showed that the risk of receiving any blood transfusion (allogeneic or autologous) is actually increased by PABD (RR = 1.29, 95% CI 1.12–1.48). Trials were unblinded, and allocation concealment was not described in 87.5% of the trials. Although the trials of PABD showed a reduction in the need for allogeneic blood, the methodological quality of the trials was poor, and the overall transfusion rates (allogeneic or autologous) in these trials were high and were increased by recruitment into the PABD arms of the trials. This raises questions about the true benefit of PABD.

We should be aware that there are significant risks associated with autologous transfusion, and that many of these are the same risks as with allogeneic blood transfusion. These include transfusion reaction, laboratory error resulting in an unmatched transfusion, and bacterial contamination of autologous blood. In the hematology literature, data suggest that even autologous transfusion can result in significant immune suppression, which may be associated with poorer prognosis. Furthermore, approximately 50% of all autologous blood transfusions are not utilized. Costs associated with autologous donation and transfusion are difficult to quantify but must include costs of collection, storage, and transfusion and clerical costs. The costs increase dramatically if preoperative recombinant erythropoietin is part of an autologous donation protocol. Objective assessments of these costs have led a number of authors to question the widespread use of presurgical autologous donation. In fact, there has been a significant reduction in the use of autologous blood transfusion in surgical patients. In the absence of large, high-quality trials using clinical endpoints, it is not possible to say whether the benefits of PABD outweigh the risks.

Pharmacologic Strategies for Reduction of Allogeneic Blood Transfusion

A number of pharmacologic strategies have been investigated to reduce allogeneic blood transfusion in surgery, including aprotinin, desmopressin, tranexamic acid (TXA), and ε-aminocaproic acid (EACA). The vast majority of these studies have been performed in cardiac surgery.

In 1997, a metaanalysis of randomized trials evaluating the efficacy and safety of aprotinin, desmopressin, TXA, and EACA in cardiac surgery was published.[73] All identified randomized trials (n = 60) in cardiac surgery were included in the metaanalysis. The primary outcome was the proportion of patients who received at least one perioperative allogeneic red cell transfusion. The largest number of patients (5808) was available for the metaanalysis of aprotinin, which significantly decreased exposure to allogeneic blood (OR 0.31, 95% CI 0.25–0.39, $P < .0001$). The efficacy of aprotinin was not significantly different regardless of the type of surgery (primary or reoperation), aspirin use, or reported transfusion threshold. The use of aprotinin was associated with a significant decrease in the need for reoperation because of bleeding (OR 0.44, 95% CI 0.27–0.73, $P = .001$). The TXA significantly decreased the proportion of patients transfused (OR 0.50, 95% CI 0.34–0.76, $P = .0009$). The authors concluded that aprotinin and TXA, but not desmopressin, decreased the exposure of cardiac surgery patients to allogeneic blood transfusion perioperatively.

Subsequently in 2001, a Cochrane Database Systematic Review was performed to assess the effects of the antifibrinolytic drugs aprotinin, TXA, and EACA on perioperative RBC transfusion (Table 9.13).[74] All randomized controlled trials of antifibrinolytic drugs in adults scheduled for nonurgent surgery were included. Aprotinin reduced the rate of RBC transfusion by a relative 30% and saved 1.1 units of RBCs in those patients requiring transfusion. Aprotinin also significantly reduced the need for reoperation due to bleeding (RR = 0.40, 95% C: 0.25 to 0.66). The TXA reduced the rate of RBC transfusion by a relative 34% and resulted in a saving of 1.03 units of RBCs in those requiring transfusion. Use of EACA resulted in a statistically nonsignificant reduction in RBC transfusion. There was no significant difference between aprotinin and TXA in the rate of RBC transfusion: RR = 1.21 (95% CI 0.83 to 1.76). Aprotinin did not seem to be associated with an excess risk of adverse effects, including thromboembolic events (thrombosis RR = 0.64, 95% CI 0.31 to 1.31) and renal failure (RR = 1.19, 95% CI 0.79 to 1.79). Aprotinin reduced the need for red cell transfusion and the need for reoperation due to bleeding without serious adverse effects. However, there was significant heterogeneity in trial outcomes and some evidence of publication bias. Similar trends were seen with TXA and EACA, although the data were sparse. The poor evaluation of these last drugs is unfortunate as results suggest they may be equally as effective as aprotinin but are significantly less expensive. The evidence from this review supports the use of aprotinin in cardiac surgery. Future trials should be large enough to compare the efficacy and cost-effectiveness of aprotinin with that of TXA and EACA. An additional prospective, randomized, double-blind, placebo-controlled trial confirmed that low-dose postoperative aprotinin use in patients taking aspirin until just before primary CABG surgery not only significantly reduced the rate and total amount of postoperative mediastinal blood loss but also lowered postoperative blood product use.[75]

In 2004, the evidence for the efficacy of desmopressin acetate (1-deamino-8-D-arginine-vasopressin; DDAVP) in reducing perioperative blood loss and the need for red cell transfusion in patients who do not have congenital bleeding disorders was examined.[76] Eighteen trials of DDAVP (n = 1295) reported data on the number of patients receiving allogeneic RBC transfusion. In subjects treated with DDAVP, the

TABLE 9.13. Comparison of Pharmacologic Strategies for Transfusion Avoidance in Surgery.

Drug	*Trials (n)*	*Patients (n)*	*Red blood cell transfusion relative risk reduction (RR) (95% CI)*	*Red blood cell transfusion absolute risk reduction (ARR) (95% CI)*	*Saved units RBCs (95% CI)*
Aprotinin	61	7027	RR 0.70 (0.64 to 0.76)	ARR 20.4% (15.6% to 25.3%)	1.1 units (0.69 to 1.47)
Tranexamic acid	18	1342	RR 0.66 (0.54 to 0.81)	ARR 17.2% (8.7% to 25.7%).	1.03 units (0.67 to 1.39)
ε-Aminocaproic acid	4	208	RR 0.48 (0.19 to 1.19)	NA	NA

Source: Adapted from Henry,[74] by permission of Cochrane Database System Review.

pooled relative risk of exposure to perioperative allogeneic RBC transfusion was 0.95 (95% CI = 0.86 to 1.06). The use of DDAVP did not significantly reduce blood loss (WMD = −114.3 ml, 95% CI = −258.8 to 30.2 ml per patient) or the volume of RBC transfused (WMD = −0.35 units, 95% CI = −0.70 to 0.01 units). In DDAVP-treated patients, the relative risk of requiring reoperation due to bleeding was 0.69 (95% CI = 0.26 to 1.83). There was no statistically significant effect overall for mortality and nonfatal myocardial infarction in DDAVP-treated patients compared with control (RR = 1.72, 95% CI = 0.68 to 4.33 and RR = 1.38, 95% CI = 0.77 to 2.50, respectively). There is no convincing evidence that desmopressin minimizes perioperative allogeneic RBC transfusion in patients who do not have congenital bleeding disorders. These data suggest that there is no benefit from using DDAVP as a means of minimizing perioperative allogeneic RBC transfusion.

A metaanalysis of randomized head-to-head trials of these drugs compared the efficacy of aprotinin to the less-expensive lysine analogues TXA and EACA.[77] The available data are conflicting regarding the equivalence of lysine analogues and aprotinin in reducing perioperative bleeding, transfusion, and the need for reoperation. Decisions are sensitive to the choice of clinical outcome and noninferiority boundary. The data are an uncertain basis for replacing aprotinin with the cheaper lysine analogues in clinical practice. Progress has been hampered by small trials and failure to study clinically relevant outcomes.

Selective and Combination Therapies

Donation of autologous blood before elective surgery is inconvenient and costly, causes phlebotomy-induced anemia, and may be wasteful and unnecessary in the nonanemic patient. In fact, approximately 50% of autologous units of blood are wasted. Based on these findings, there has been a national decline in PABD by approximately 50%.[78]

The development of a blood-conservation algorithm that (1) does not require predonation of autologous blood, (2) utilizes selective recombinant erythropoietin, and (3) advocates evidence-based transfusion criteria has been documented as successful in reduction of perioperative allogeneic blood transfusion in total joint arthroplasty.[79] Some centers have advocated policies that include the use of recombinant erythropoietin when baseline hematocrit is 37% or less and avoidance of PABD in nonanemics (baseline hematocrit >37%). The application of this policy in patients undergoing primary total hip or knee arthroplasty was associated with a marked decrease in blood transfusion rates (from 43% to 12%, $P < .0001$), with no change in discharge hematocrit and a 39% financial savings.[80] Although erythropoietin is expensive, it can be used with cost savings in selected patients because the overall cost of blood transfusion is reduced.

A prospective, randomized, double-blind, placebo-controlled trial investigated combination practices to avoid transfusion in patients undergoing first-time cardiac surgery.[81] Patients were randomized to one of three pharmacologic treatment groups: aprotinin, TXA, and saline control. Intraoperative cell salvage was used for all patients. Patients were 2.5 times more likely to receive any allogeneic transfusion in the tranexamic group than in the aprotinin group (21 patients of 60 compared with 9 out of 60, respectively). The relative risk of any allogeneic transfusion comparing aprotinin with TXA was 0.43 (95% CI 0.21–0.86, $P = .019$). Patients in the control group were four times more likely to receive any allogeneic transfusion when compared with the aprotinin group (37 patients of 60 compared with 9 out of 60, respectively). The relative risk of any allogeneic transfusion comparing aprotinin with control was 0.24 (95% CI 0.13–0.46, $P < .001$). This study confirmed that, when used in addition to intraoperative cell salvage, aprotinin is the most efficacious pharmacologic therapy for reducing patient exposure to any allogeneic transfusion during first-time cardiac surgery.

Blood transfusion rates in cardiac surgery remain high despite major advances in perioperative blood conservation, with large variations among individual centers. A review documented that the adoption of available blood-conservation techniques we discussed that are available, safe, and efficacious in patients undergoing cardiac surgery could result in an estimated 75% reduction of unnecessary blood transfusions. The success of previously reported blood-conservation programs in cardiac surgery should call for a reevaluation of allogeneic transfusion practices in patients undergoing cardiac surgery. By applying the numerous reported blood-conservation strategies for the management of patients presenting for cardiac surgery, we can preserve our dwindling blood resources and help alleviate some of the direct costs of blood as well as the indirect costs of treating noninfectious and infectious complications of transfusion.[82]

Patients at Increased Risk for Red Blood Cell Transfusion

Nine risk factors have been identified that predict the need for allogeneic transfusion:

- Low preoperative hemoglobin, either before intervention or on day of surgery
- Low weight
- Short height
- Female sex
- Age over 65 years
- Availability of PABD
- Estimated surgical blood loss
- Type of surgery
- Primary or revision surgery

In addition, the administration of antiplatelet drugs before surgery is associated with increased risk of major hemorrhage and increased need for perioperative blood transfusion. Clopidogrel has become the standard of care to prevent thrombotic complications following cardiological interventions, in particular intracoronary stenting. In addition, patients with aspirin intolerance and those with carotid and peripheral vascular disease are also increasingly treated with clopidogrel. Platelet inhibition may become a concern for hemostasis in patients treated with clopidogrel who need emergency and undelayed surgery.

A retrospective cohort study (n = 659) of CABG patients documented that a greater mean number of units of RBCs were transfused among those who received clopidogrel alone (2.9) or in combination with aspirin (2.4) compared to those on aspirin alone (1.9) or neither antiplatelet drug (1.4) ($P = .001$). A similar trend was seen for the respective mean number of transfused units of platelets (3.6, 3.7, 1.3, and 1.0, respectively; $P < .001$) and FFP (2.5, 3.1, 2.3, and 1.6, respectively; $P = .01$). Compared to nonusers, the associated risk of excessive blood product transfusion was highest among recipients of aspirin and clopidogrel together (adjusted OR 2.2, 95% CI 1.1–4.3).[83]

Another study examined the outcome of 505 consecutive patients who underwent isolated CABG and compared two groups: those with clopidogrel exposure until 72h prior to surgery (n = 136) and those without exposition to clopidogrel (n = 369).[84] Clopidogrel exposure 3 days or less prior to CABG surgery significantly increased the risk of postoperative bleeding, the need for perioperative transfusion, and the incidence of reexploration for bleeding. This study suggests that aggressive correction of platelet dysfunction is required before chest closure in patients with clopidogrel exposure preoperatively.

Similar findings were reported in a study of 45 patients receiving clopidogrel within 6 days of surgery and 45 control subjects undergoing CABG. Compared with control subjects, clopidogrel recipients required significantly more transfusions of platelets (9.0 ± 1.7 vs. 1.2 ± 0.5 units; $P < .0001$) and packed RBCs (4.3 ± 0.6 vs. 2.3 ± 0.5 units; $P = .01$) and required longer periods of controlled ventilation (12.4 ± 1.3 vs. 8.6 ± 0.8h; $P = .02$). This study also documented that the measurement of preoperative platelet dysfunction before heparin administration for cardiopulmonary bypass, by using adenosine diphosphate aggregometry (response < 40%), identified patients at highest risk for perioperative bleeding and transfusions and could be used to implement strategies to reduce the perioperative transfusion requirement in these high-risk patients.[85]

Perioperative management of patients treated with antiplatelet therapy or chronically anticoagulated patients is a complex medical problem. It is clear that all measures should be implemented to avoid perioperative bleeding in patients receiving antiplatelet or anticoagulant therapy.[86] Decision making will depend on whether the surgery is elective or urgent and whether cardiopulmonary bypass is required. Temporary discontinuation of these drugs, reversal of the drug effects, judicious use of replacement blood products (platelets/plasma), or delay of surgery may all need to be considered in these patients.

Strategies for Prevention of Blood Transfusion in Critical Care

Phlebotomy for diagnostic testing is a contributing cause of anemia in critical care. Multiple studies have documented daily phlebotomy volumes from 40 to 70ml/day. A number of strategies to reduce blood loss related to phlebotomy are available, including the use of blood-conservation devices, pediatric or low-volume adult blood sampling tubes, and reduction in laboratory testing by elimination of automatic daily laboratory orders.[87] The use of blood-conservation devices to minimize phlebotomy blood loss is effective since it eliminates discarded blood volume and instead reinfuses blood to the patient.[88] Similarly, changing from the standard large-volume adult tubes to tubes with smaller volume is a simple, effective strategy to reduce blood loss in the ICU. Despite documented efficacy, these preventive strategies are not used frequently in critical care units.[89]

Two prospective randomized studies have examined the use of rHuEpo for the treatment of anemia in critically ill patients in an effort to reduce blood transfusion rates.[90] In the first study (n = 160), therapy with rHuEpo was associated with an almost 50% reduction in blood transfusions compared with placebo; a loading dose strategy (300 U/kg daily for 5 days, then every other day until ICU discharge) was used. In the second study (n = 1302), treatment with rHuEpo resulted in a 10% reduction in the number of patients receiving any blood transfusion and a 20% reduction in the total number of units transfused; an rHuEpo dosing strategy of 40,000 U weekly was used. The third prospective randomized trial of rHuEpo in critical care is under way and results will form the basis for the final application to the Food and Drug Administration for approval of the use of rHuEpo in critical care.

Conclusion

Blood transfusion is commonly utilized in surgical and ICU patients. Anemia is also common in surgical and ICU patients. Blood and blood products are scarce resources and should be reserved for treatment of patients with acute hemorrhage. Surgical and critically ill patients with anemia who are hemodynamically stable can tolerate hemoglobin concentrations of 7g/dl. Reduction of blood transfusion in surgery and critical care requires a multidisciplinary effort, including the use of institutional or unit-based transfusion protocols, educational efforts, and preventive strategies to reduce blood loss.

References

1. http://www.aabb.org/About_the_AABB/Nbdrc/index.htm.
2. Butch SH, Davenport RD, Cooling L. Blood transfusion policies and standard practices of the University of Michigan, July 2004. Available at: http://www.pathology.med.umich.edu/bloodbank/manual/.
3. Brien WF, Butler RJ, Inwood MJ. An audit of blood component therapy in a Canadian general teaching hospital. CMAJ 1989;140:812–815.
4. Ghali WA, Palepu A, Paterson WG. Evaluation of red blood cell transfusion practices with the use of preset criteria. CMAJ 1994;150:1449–1454.
5. Hutton B, Fergusson D, Tinmouth A, McIntyre L, Kmetic A, Hebert PC. Transfusion rates vary significantly amongst Canadian medical centres. Can J Anaesth 2005 52:581–590.
6. Vincent JL, Baron JF, Reinhart K, et al., and the ABC (Anemia and Blood Transfusion in Critical Care) Investigators. Anemia and blood transfusion in critically ill patients. JAMA 2002;288:1499–1507.
7. Napolitano LM, Corwin HL, Fink MP, eds. Anemia in critical care: etiology, treatment and prevention. Crit Care 2004;8(suppl 2):S1–S64.
8. Napolitano LM. Review: scope of the problem: epidemiology of anemia and use of blood transfusions in critical care. Crit Care 2004;8(suppl 2):S1–S8.
9. Hebert PC, Corwin HL. Blood transfusion in the critically ill. Crit Care Clin 2004;20:159–328.
10. Pearl RG, Wibbald WJ. Anemia and blood management in critical care. Crit Care Med 2003;31(12 suppl):S649–S715.
11. Corwin HL, Gettinger A, Pearl RG, et al. The CRIT Study: anemia and blood transfusion in the critically ill—current clinical practice in the United States. Crit Care Med 2004;32:39–52.

12. Shapiro MJ, Gettinger A, Corwin HL, et al. Anemia and blood transfusion in trauma patients admitted to the intensive care unit. J Trauma 2003;55:269–273; discussion 273–274.
13. Nemeth E, Rivera S, Gabayan V, et al. IL-6 mediates hypoferremia of inflammation by inducing the synthesis of the iron regulatory hormone hepcidin. J Clin Invest 2004;113:1271–1276.
14. Parreira JG, Rasslan S, Poli de Figueiredo LF, et al. Impact of shock and fluid resuscitation on the morphology and apopotosis of bone marrow: an experimental study. J Trauma 2004;56:1001–1008.
15. Goodnough LT. Risks of blood transfusion. Crit Care Med 2003;31(12 suppl):S678–S686.
16. Pealer LN, Marfin AA, Petersen LR, and West Nile Virus Transmission Investigation Team. Transmission of West Nile virus through blood transfusion in the United States in 2002. N Engl J Med 2003;349:1236–1245.
17. Goodnough LT. Risks of blood transfusion. Crit Care Med 2003;31(12 suppl):S678–S686.
18. Fiebig EW, Busch MP. Emerging infections in transfusion medicine. Clin Lab Med 2004;24:797–823, viii.
19. Hill GE, Frawley WH, Griffith KE, Forestner JE, Minei JP. Allogeneic blood transfusion increases the risk of postoperative bacterial infection: a meta-analysis. J Trauma 2003;54:908–914.
20. Innerhofer P, Klingler A, Klimmer C, Fries D, Nussbaumer W. Risk for postoperative infection after transfusion of white blood cell-filtered allogeneic or autologous blood components in orthopedic patients undergoing primary arthroplasty. Transfusion 2005;45:103–110.
21. Webert KE, Blajchman MA. Transfusion-related acute lung injury. Transfus Med Rev 2003;17:252–262.
22. Kopko PM, Marshall CS, MacKenzie MR, Holland PV, Popovsky MA. Transfusion-related acute lung injury: report of a clinical look-back investigation. JAMA 2002;287:1968–1971.
23. Silliman CC, Boshkov LK, Mehdizadehkashi Z, et al. Transfusion-related acute lung injury: epidemiology and a prospective analysis of etiologic factors. Blood 2003;101:454–462.
24. Goodnough LT, Hewitt PE, Silliman CC. Transfusion medicine: joint ASH and AABB educational session. Hematology (Am Soc Hematol Educ Program) 2004:457–72.
25. Toy P, Popovsky MA, Abraham E, et al., and the National Heart, Lung and Blood Institute Working Group on TRALI. Transfusion-related acute lung injury: definition and review. Crit Care Med 2005;33:721–726.
26. Kuduvalli M, Oo AY, Newall N, et al. Effect of peri-operative red blood cell transfusion on 30-day and 1-year mortality following coronary artery bypass surgery. Eur J Cardiothorac Surg 2005;27:592–598.
27. Hebert PC, Wells G, Blajchman MA, et al. A multicenter, randomized, controlled clinical trial of transfusion requirements in critical care. Transfusion Requirements in Critical Care Investigators, Canadian Critical Care Trials Group. N Engl J Med 1999;340:409–417.
28. Hebert PC, Wells G, Blajchman MA, et al. A multicenter, randomized, controlled clinical trial of transfusion requirements in critical care. N Engl J Med 1999;340:409–417.
29. Shah JS, Hickey R. Anemia and blood transfusion in the critically ill: a decade without change. Crit Care Med 2004;32:290–291.
30. Shorr AF, Duh MS, Kelly KM, Kollef MH, and the CRIT Study Group. Red blood cell transfusion and ventilator-associated pneumonia: a potential link? Crit Care Med 2004;32:666–674.
31. Malone DL, Dunne J, Tracy JK, Putnam AT, Scalea TM, Napolitano LM. Blood transfusion, independent of shock severity, is associated with worse outcome in trauma. J Trauma 2003;54:898–905; discussion 905–907.
32. Dellinger RP, Carlet JM, Masur H, et al., and the Surviving Sepsis Campaign Management Guidelines Committee. Surviving sepsis campaign guidelines for management of severe sepsis and septic shock. Crit Care Med 2004;32:858–873.
33. Napolitano LM, Corwin HL. Efficacy of red blood cell transfusion in the critically ill. Crit Care Clin 2004;20:255–268.
34. Fernandes CJ Jr, Akamine N, De Marco FV, De Souza JA, Lagudis S, Knobel E. Red blood cell transfusion does not increase oxygen consumption in critically ill septic patients. Crit Care 2001;5:362–367.
35. Nishiyama T, Hanaoka K. Hemolysis in stored red blood cell concentrates: modulation by haptoglobin or ulinastatin, a protease inhibitor. Crit Care Med 2001;29:1979–1982.
36. Schechter AN, Gladwin MT. Hemoglobin and the paracrine and endocrine functions of nitric oxide. N Engl J Med 2003;348:1483–1485.
37. Expert Working Group. Guidelines for red blood cell and plasma transfusion for adults and children. CMAJ 1997;156(11 suppl): S1–S24.
38. Murphy MF, Wallington TB, Kelsey P, et al., and the British Committee for Standards in Haematology, Blood Transfusion Task Force. Guidelines for the clinical use of red cell transfusions. Br J Haematol 2001;113:24–31.
39. Practice guidelines for blood component therapy: a report by the American Society of Anesthesiologists Task Force on Blood Component Therapy. Anesthesiology 1996;84:732–747.
40. Eindhoven GB, Diercks RL, Richardson FJ, et al. Adjusted transfusion triggers improve transfusion practice in orthopaedic surgery. Transfus Med 2005;15:13–18.
41. Hill SR, Carless PA, Henry DA, et al. Transfusion thresholds and other strategies for guiding allogeneic red blood cell transfusion. Cochrane Database Syst Rev 2002;2:CD002042.
42. Williamson LM, Lowe S, Love EM, et al. Serious Hazards of Transfusion (SHOT) initiative: analysis of the first two annual reports. BMJ 1999;319:16–19.
43. Williamson L, Cohen H, Love E, Jones H, Todd A, Soldan K. The Serious Hazards of Transfusion (SHOT) initiative: the UK approach to haemovigilance. Vox Sang 2000;78(suppl 2):291–295.
44. Dzik WH, Corwin H, Goodnough LT, et al. Patient safety and blood transfusion: new solutions. Transfus Med Rev 2003;17:169–180.
45. Turner CL, Casbard AC, Murphy MF. Barcode technology: its role in increasing the safety of blood transfusion. Transfusion 2003;43:1200–1209.
46. Dzik WH, Corwin H, Goodnough LT, et al. Patient safety and blood transfusion: new solutions. In: Manuel BM, Nora PF, eds. American College of Surgeons Surgical Patient Safety: Essential Information for Surgeons in Today's Environment. Amer Coll Surgeons, Chicago, Ill 2004:119–132.
47. Dunne JR, Malone D, Tracy JK, Gannon C, Napolitano LM. Perioperative anemia: an independent risk factor for infection, mortality, and resource utilization in surgery. J Surg Res 2002;102:237–244.
48. Dunne JR, Gannon CJ, Osborn TM, Taylor MD, Malone DL, Napolitano LM. Preoperative anemia in colon cancer: assessment of risk factors. Am Surg 2002;68:582–587.
49. Ludwig H, VanBelle S, Barrett-Lee P, et al. The European Cancer Anemia Survey (ECAS): a large, multinational prospective survey defining the prevalence, incidence, and treatment of anemia in cancer patients. Eur J Cancer 2004;40:2293–2306.
50. Bokemeyer C, Aapro MS, Courdi A, et al. EORTC guidelines for the use of erythropoietic proteins in anaemic patients with cancer. Eur J Cancer 2004;40:2201–2216.
51. Rosencher N, Poisson D, Albi A, Aperce M, Barre J, Samama CM. Two injections of erythropoietin correct moderate anemia in most patients awaiting orthopedic surgery. Can J Anaesth 2005;52:160–165.
52. Myers E, Grady PO, Dolan AM. The influence of preclinical anaemia on outcome following total hip replacement. Arch

Orthop Trauma Surg 2004;124:699–701. Epub October 29, 2004.
53. Bulow S, Christensen IJ, Harling H, et al.; Danish TME Study Group; RANX05 Colorectal Cancer Study Group. Recurrence and survival after mesorectal excision for rectal cancer. Br J Surg 2003;90:974–980.
54. Mynster T, Nielsen HJ, Harling H, Bulow S, the Danish TME-group, and the RANX05-group. Blood loss and transfusion after total mesorectal excision and conventional rectal cancer surgery. Colorectal Dis 2004;6:452–457.
55. Kiran RP, Delaney CP, Senagore AJ, Millward BL, Fazio VW. Operative blood loss and use of blood products after laparoscopic and conventional open colorectal operations. Arch Surg 2004;139:39–42.
56. Vignali A, Braga M, Zuliani W, Frasson M, Radaelli G, Di Carlo V. Laparoscopic colorectal surgery modifies risk factors for postoperative morbidity. Dis Colon Rectum 2004;47:1686–1693.
57. DiCarlo J, Barbagallo F, Toro A, Sofia M, Guastella T, Latteri F. Hepatic resections using a water-cooled, high-density, monopolar device: a new technology for safer surgery. J Gastrointest Surg 2004;8:596–600.
58. Ilbeigi P, Ahmed M, Szobota J, Munver R, Sawczuk IS. Open partial nephrectomy using saline-enhanced monopolar radiofrequency device: evaluation of novel surgical technique with TissueLink DS3.0 Dissecting Sealer. Urology 2005;65:578–582.
59. Schwartz M, Madariaga J, Hirose R, et al. Comparison of a new fibrin sealant with standard topical hemostatic agents. Arch Surg 2004;139:1148–1154.
60. Carless PA, Henry RA, Anthony DM. Fibrin sealant use for minimizing perioperative allogeneic blood transfusion. Cochrane Database Syst Rev 2003;2:CD004171.
61. Tuncbilek G, Vargel I, Erdem A, Mavili ME, Benli K, Erk Y. Blood loss and transfusion rates during repair of craniofacial deformities. J Craniofac Surg 2005;16:59–62.
62. Sanders G, Mellor N, Rickards K, et al. Prospective randomized controlled trial of acute normovolaemic haemodilution in major gastrointestinal surgery. Br J Anaesth 2004;93:775–781. Epub October 1, 2004.
63. Wong JC, Torella F, Haynes SL, et al., and the ATIS Investigators. Autologous versus allogeneic transfusion in aortic surgery: a multicenter randomized clinical trial. Ann Surg 2002;235:145–151.
64. Sirvinskas E, Lenkutis T, Raliene L, Veikutiene A, Vaskelyte J, Marchertiene I. Influence of residual blood autotransfused from cardiopulmonary bypass circuit on clinical outcome after cardiac surgery. Perfusion 2005;20:71–75.
65. Mercer KG, Spark JI, Berridge DC, Kent PJ, Scott DJ. Randomized clinical trial of intraoperative autotransfusion in surgery for abdominal aortic aneurysm. Br J Surg 2004;91:1443–1448.
66. Szalay D, Wong D, Lindsay T. Impact of red cell salvage on transfusion requirements during elective abdominal aortic aneurysm repair. Ann Vasc Surg 1999;13:576–581.
67. Clagett GP, Valentine RJ, Jackson MR, Mathison C, Kakish HB, Bengtson TD. A randomized trial of intraoperative autotransfusion during aortic surgery. J Vasc Surg 1999;29:22–30; discussion 30–31.
68. Carless PA, Henry DA, Moxey AJ, O'Connell Dl, Fergusson DA. Cell salvage for minimising perioperative allogeneic blood transfusion. Cochrane Database Syst Rev 2003;4:CD001888.
69. Nagino M, Kamiya J, Arai T, Nishio H, Ebata T, Nimura Y. One hundred consecutive hepatobiliary resections for biliary hilar malignancy: preoperative blood donation, blood loss, transfusion, and outcome. Surgery 2005;137:148–155.
70. Yamamoto K, Imakiire A, Masaoka T, Shinmura K. Autologous blood transfusion in total hip arthroplasty. J Orthop Surg 2004;12:145–152.
71. Lennox PA, Clugston PA, Beasley ME, Bostwick J 3rd. Autologous blood transfusion in TRAM breast reconstruction: is it necessary? Ann Plast Surg 2004;53:532–535.
72. Henry DA, Carless PA, Moxey AJ, et al. Pre-operative autologous donation for minimising perioperative allogeneic blood transfusion. Cochrane Database Syst Rev 2002;2:CD003602.
73. Laupacis A, Fergusson D. Drugs to minimize perioperative blood loss in cardiac surgery: meta-analyses using perioperative blood transfusion as the outcome. The International Study of Perioperative Transfusion (ISPOT) Investigators. Anesth Analg 1997;85:1258–1267.
74. Henry DA, Moxey AJ, Carless PA, et al. Anti-fibrinolytic use for minimising perioperative allogeneic blood transfusion. Cochrane Database Syst Rev 2001;1:CD001886.
75. Alvarez JM, Jackson LR, Chatwin C, Smolich JJ. Low-dose postoperative aprotinin reduces mediastinal drainage and blood product use in patients undergoing primary coronary artery bypass grafting who are taking aspirin: a prospective, randomized, double-blind, placebo-controlled trial. J Thorac Cardiovasc Surg 2001;122:457–463.
76. Carless PA, Henry DA, Moxey AJ, et al. Desmopressin for minimising perioperative allogeneic blood transfusion. Cochrane Database Syst Rev 2004;1:CD001884.
77. Carless PA, Moxey AJ, Stokes BJ, Henry DA. Are antifibrinolytic drugs equivalent in reducing blood loss and transfusion in cardiac surgery? A meta-analysis of randomised head-to-head trials. BMC Cardiovasc Disord 2005;5:19.
78. Goodnough LT. Autologous blood donation. Anesthesiol Clin North Am 2005;23:263–270.
79. Pierson JL, Hannon TJ, Earles DR. A blood-conservation algorithm to reduce blood transfusions after total hip and knee arthroplasty. J Bone Joint Surg Am 2004;86-A:1512–1518.
80. Couvret C, Laffon M, Baud A, Payen V, Burdin P, Fusciardi J. A restrictive use of both autologous donation and recombinant human erythropoietin is an efficient policy for primary total hip or knee arthroplasty. Anesth Analg 2004;99:262–271.
81. Diprose P, Herbertson MJ, O'Shaughnessy D, Deakin CD, Gill RS. Reducing allogeneic transfusion in cardiac surgery: a randomized double-blind placebo-controlled trial of antifibrinolytic therapies used in addition to intra-operative cell salvage. Br J Anaesth 2005;94:271–278. Epub December 10, 2004.
82. Shander A, Moskowitz D, Rijhwani TS. The safety and efficacy of "bloodless" cardiac surgery. Semin Cardiothorac Vasc Anesth 2005;9:53–63.
83. Ray JG, Deniz S, Olivieri A, et al. Increased blood product use among coronary artery bypass patients prescribed preoperative aspirin and clopidogrel. BMC Cardiovasc Disord 2003; 3:3.
84. Englberger L, Faeh B, Berdat PA, Eberli F, Meier B, Carrel T. Impact of clopidogrel in coronary artery bypass grafting. Eur J Cardiothorac Surg 2004;26:96–101.
85. Chen L, Bracey AW, Radovancevic R, et al. Clopidogrel and bleeding in patients undergoing elective coronary artery bypass grafting. J Thorac Cardiovasc Surg 2004;128:425–431.
86. Harder S, Klinkhardt U, Alvarez JM. Avoidance of bleeding during surgery in patients receiving anticoagulant and/or antiplatelet therapy: pharmacokinetic and pharmacodynamic considerations. Clin Pharmacokinet 2004;43:963–981.
87. Barie PS. Phlebotomy in the intensive care unit: strategies for blood conservation. Crit Care 2004;8(suppl 2):S34–S36.
88. Peruzzi WT, Parker MA, Lichtenthal PR, Cochran-Zull C, Toth B, Blake M. A clinical evaluation of a blood conservation device in medical intensive care unit patients. Crit Care Med 1993;21:501–506.
89. O'Hare D, Chilvers RJ. Arterial blood sampling practices in intensive care units in England and Wales. Anaesthesia 2001;56: 568–571.

90. Corwin HL. Anemia and blood transfusion in the critically ill patient: role of erythropoietin. Crit Care 2004;8(suppl 2):S42–S44.
91. The Clinical Use of Blood Handbook. Geneva, Switzerland: World Health Organization.
92. Busch MP, Kleinman SH, Nemo GJ. Current and emerging infectious risks of blood transfusions. JAMA 2003;289:959–962.
93. Guidelines for Canadian Clinical Practice Guidelines. Ottawa: Canadian Medical Association, 1994.
94. Hebert PC. A multicenter, randomized, controlled clinical trial of transfusion requirements in clinical care. N Engl J Med 1999;340:439–447.
95. Goodnough LT. Transfusion medicine, first of two parts. N Engl J Med 1999;340:438–447.
96. Consensus Conference: perioperative red blood cell transfusion. JAMA 1988;260:2700–2703
97. American College of Physicians. Practice strategies for elective red blood cell transfusion. Ann Intern Med 1992;116:403–406
98. Guidelines for Blood Transfusion Services at MGH.
99. The University of Iowa Hospitals and Clinics. Transfusion Guidelines.
100. Brundage S, Curet M, Dicker R, et al, and the Blood Transfusion Guidelines Committee. Blood Transfusion Guidelines, University of Michigan Medical Center.
101. Triulzi DJ (ed.) Blood Transfusion Therapy; A Physician's Handbook, 6th ed. American Association of Blood Banks. Bethesda, MD, 1999.
102. Guidelines for Blood Utilization Review. American Association of Blood Banks. Bethesda, MD, 2001.
103. Simon TL, Alverson DC, AuBuchon J, et al. Practice parameter for the use of red blood cell transfusions. Arch Pathol Lab Med 1998;122:130–8.
104. American Red Cross—New England Region. Red cell transfusion guidelines. Available at: http://www.newenglandblood.org/professional/redcellguide.htm.
105. National Institutes of Health. Fresh Frozen Plasma: Indication and Risks. NIH Consensus Statement. Bethesda, MD; National Institutes of Health, 1984.
106. Task Force of the American College of American Pathologists. Practice parameter for the use of FFP, cryoprecipitate, and platelets. JAMA 1994;271:777–781.
107. Practice guidelines for blood component therapy: Task Force of the American Society of Anesthesiologists. Anesthesiology 1996;84:498–501.
108. Rebulla P, Finazzi G, Marangoni F, et al. The threshold for prophylactic platelet transfusions in patients with acute myeloid leukemia. New Engl J Med 1997;337:1870–1875.
109. Schiffer CA, Anderson KC, Bennett CL, et al. Platelet transfusion for patients with cancer: clinical practice guidelines of the American Society of Clinical Oncology. J Clin Oncol 2001;19:1519–1538.
110. Pool JG, Shannon AE. Production of high potency concentrates of antihemophilic globulin in a closed bag system; assay in vitro and in vivo. N Engl J Med 1965;273:1443–1447.
111. American Red Cross Blood Services—New England Region. Cryoprecipitate transfusion guidelines. Available at: http://www.newenglandblood.org/professional/cryoguide.htm.
112. Handbook of transfusion medicine. Available at: http://www.transfusionguidelines.org.uk/.
113. Scottish Intercollegiate Guidelines Network (SIGN). Perioperative blood transfusion for elective surgery. Edinburgh: Scottish Intercollegiate Guidelines Network (SIGN), October 2001. SIGN Publication no. 54.
114. Scottish Intercollegiate Guidelines Network (SIGN). Perioperative blood transfusion for elective surgery. Update to printed guideline. Edinburgh: Scottish Intercollegiate Guidelines Network (SIGN), August 31, 2004. Available at: http://www.sign.ac.uk/new.html.

10

Wounds: Biology, Pathology, and Management

H. Peter Lorenz and Michael T. Longaker

Wound healing is an orchestrated biological process initiated by tissue injury and culminating in restoration of tissue integrity. The end result of the repair process is fibrosis and scar in all organ systems except bone and except for specialized conditions of liver injury. Because surgeons induce tissue injury, a thorough understanding of the wound repair process is fundamental to the practice of surgery; thus, surgeons and wound repair have enjoyed a close relationship from the beginning of surgery.

Surgeons can now actively influence the healing of wounds through pharmacologic treatments. Armed with a more detailed understanding of the repair processes and their regulation, investigators have modulated experimental wounds to heal faster than normal. In addition, reversal of the healing impairment that occurs in several pathologic states (e.g., diabetes and steroid immunosuppression) has been demonstrated experimentally, which is translating to clinical use.

Wound Biology

The overlapping segments of the repair process are conceptually defined as inflammation, proliferation, and remodeling. During the inflammatory phase, hemostasis occurs, and an acute inflammatory infiltrate ensues. The proliferative phase is characterized by fibroplasia, granulation, contraction, and epithelialization. The final phase is remodeling, which is commonly described as *scar maturation* (Fig. 10.1).

Inflammation

Inflammation is the first stage of wound healing. After tissue injury, the lacerated vessels immediately constrict, and thromboplastic tissue products, predominantly from the subendothelium, are exposed. Platelets aggregate and form the initial hemostatic plug. The coagulation and complement cascades are initiated. The intrinsic and extrinsic coagulation pathways lead to activation of prothrombin to thrombin, which converts fibrinogen to fibrin, which is subsequently polymerized into a stable clot.

As thrombus is formed, hemostasis in the wound is achieved (Fig. 10.2). The aggregated platelets degranulate, releasing potent chemoattractants for inflammatory cells, activation factors for local fibroblasts and endothelial cells, and vasoconstrictors (Table 10.1). Platelet adhesiveness is mediated by integrin receptors such as GPIIb/IIIa (αIIbβ3 integrin).[1,2]

Within minutes, the repair processes are initiated. After the transient vasoconstriction induced by platelet factors, local small vessels dilate secondary to the effects of the coagulation and complement cascades. Bradykinin is a potent vasodilator and vascular permeability factor that is generated by activation of Hageman factor in the coagulation cascade.[2] The complement cascade generates the C3a and C5a anaphylatoxins, which directly increase blood vessel permeability and attract neutrophils and monocytes to the wound. These complement components also stimulate the release of histamine and leukotrienes C4 and D4 from mast cells. The local endothelial cells then break cell-to-cell contact, which enhances the margination of inflammatory cells into the wound site.[2]

An efflux of bone marrow-derived white blood cells (first neutrophils, later monocytes) and plasma proteins enter the wound site (Fig. 10.3). The early neutrophil infiltrate scavenges cellular debris, foreign bodies, and bacteria. Activated complement fragments aid in bacterial killing through opsonization. The primary role of the neutrophil is to sterilize the wound. Accordingly, the initial neutrophil infiltrate is decreased in clean surgical wounds when compared to contaminated or infected wounds.

Within 2 to 3 days, the inflammatory cell population begins to shift to one of monocyte predominance (Fig. 10.4). Circulating monocytes are attracted and infiltrate the wound site.[3] These elicited monocytes differentiate into macrophages

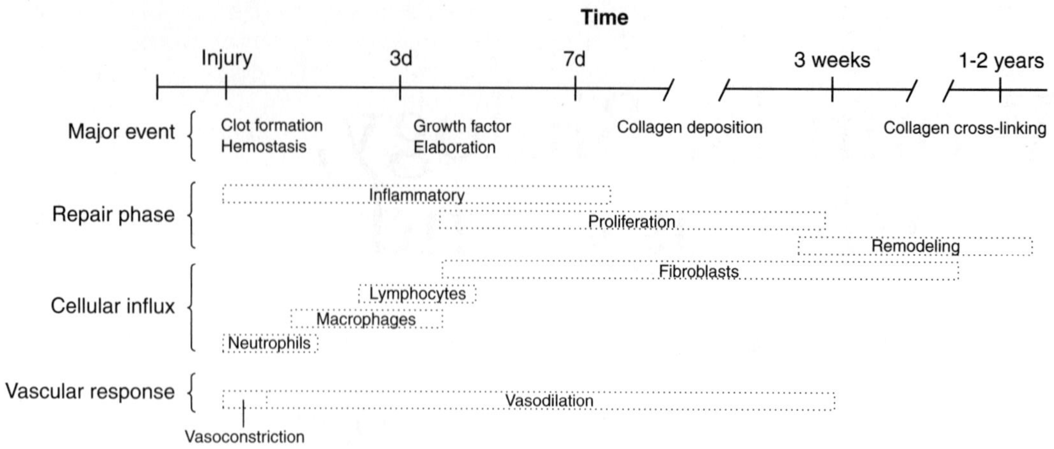

FIGURE 10.1. The temporal relationship of repair stages and cellular infiltrates into the wound. Overlap occurs between the stages, and the beginning and endpoints are approximate.

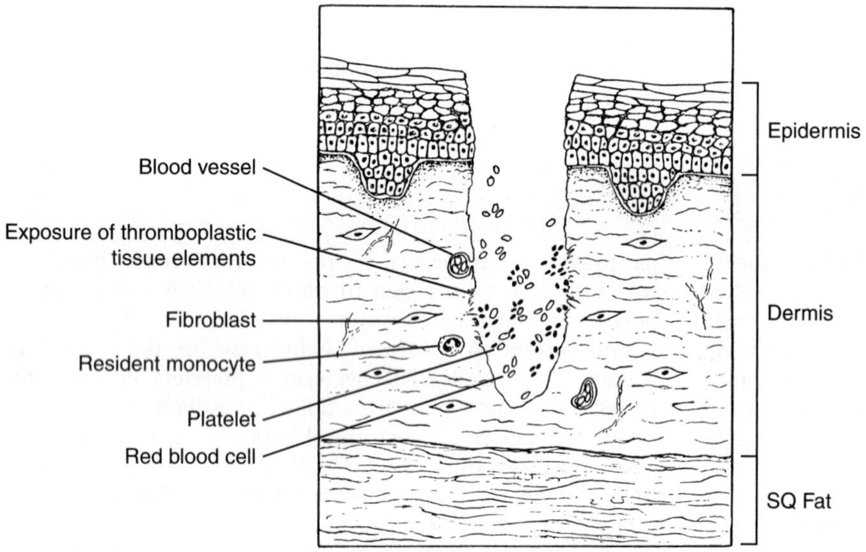

FIGURE 10.2. Immediately after tissue injury, hemostasis is stimulated by platelet degranulation and exposure of tissue thromboplastic agents. SQ, subcutaneous.

TABLE 10.1. Platelets Contain Both Alpha and Dense Granules, Which Are Released at the Wound Site.

	Biologic effect
Alpha Granules	
Platelet-derived growth factor	Matrix deposition
Transforming growth factor-β	Matrix deposition
Transforming growth factor-α	Epithelialization
Insulin-like growth factor binding protein-3	Matrix deposition
Platelet factor 4	Activation of growth factors
β-Thromboglobulin	Activation of growth factors
Dense granules	
Adenosine diphosphate	Platelet aggregation
Calcium	Platelet aggregation
Serotonin	Vasoconstriction
Cytosol	
Von Willebrand factor VIII	Mediator of platelet adhesion
Fibronectin	Ligand for platelet aggregation
Fibrinogen	Ligand for platelet aggregation
Thrombospondin	Ligand for platelet aggregation
Factor V	Hemostasis
Platelet-activating factor	Platelet activation
Thromboxane A_2	Vasoconstriction
12-Hydroxyeicosatetranoic acid (12-HETE)	Vasoconstriction

In addition, multiple activators and mediators of the hemostatic cascades are present on the platelet surface membrane. The substances released have myriad effects on the repair process. Vascular endothelial growth factor is present within platelets but its exact intracellular location is unknown.[28]

Source: Data compiled from several sources (reviewed in references 1–3).

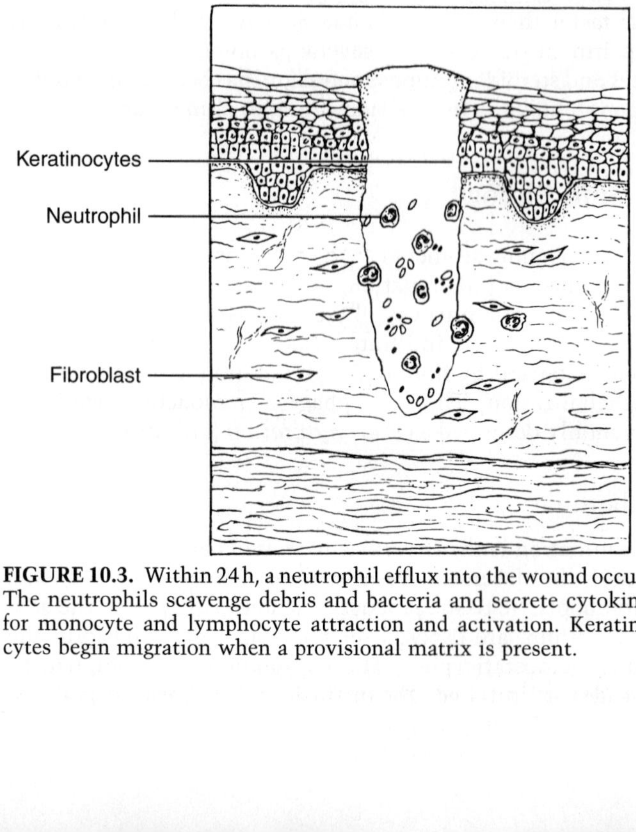

FIGURE 10.3. Within 24 h, a neutrophil efflux into the wound occurs. The neutrophils scavenge debris and bacteria and secrete cytokines for monocyte and lymphocyte attraction and activation. Keratinocytes begin migration when a provisional matrix is present.

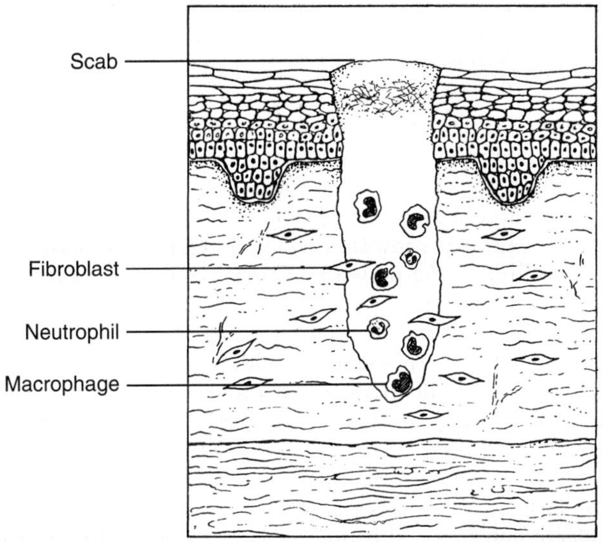

FIGURE 10.4. At 2–3 days after injury, the macrophage becomes the predominant inflammatory cell type in clean, noninfected wounds. These cells then regulate the repair process by secretion of myriad growth factors, including types that induce fibroblast and endothelial cell migration and proliferation. Bone marrow-derived mesenchymal progenitor cells are also present in the wound.

and, in conjunction with resident macrophages, orchestrate the repair process. Macrophages not only continue to phagocytose tissue and bacterial debris but also secrete multiple growth factors. These peptide growth factors activate and attract local endothelial cells, fibroblasts, and keratinocytes to begin their respective repair functions. Over 20 different cytokines and growth factors are known to be secreted by macrophages (Table 10.2).[4] Depletion of monocytes and macrophages causes a severe alteration in wound healing, with poor debridement, delayed fibroblast proliferation, and inadequate angiogenesis.[5] The macrophage is an inflammatory cell type that is requisite for repair, indicating a primary responsibility for regulation of the healing processes.

Besides contributing to the inflammatory processes, bone marrow-derived cells have been shown to actively deposit collagen during repair. Subpopulations of these circulating cells, termed *fibrocytes*, migrate to the wound site, express collagen, and ultimately become resident antigen-presenting dendritic cells.[6] Other subpopulations, without inflammatory markers, termed *mesenchymal progenitor cells*, regulate the proliferation and migration of dermal and epidermal cells at the wound site. These mesenchymal progenitor cells express collagens and integrate into the resident dermal fibroblast population after repair is complete.[7,8]

Proliferation

Fibroplasia

Deposition of the collagen scar matrix and the activation and proliferation of local fibroblasts marks the proliferative phase. The initial fibrin–fibrinogen matrix is populated with platelets and macrophages and other bone marrow-derived cells. These cells and the local extracellular matrix (ECM) release growth factors that initiate fibroblast activation. Fibroblasts migrate into the wound using the newly deposited fibrin and fibronectin matrix as a scaffold. They become activated and increase protein synthesis in preparation for cell division. As fibroblasts proliferate, they become the prominent cell type by 3–5 days in clean, noninfected wounds (Fig. 10.5). After cell division and proliferation, fibroblasts begin synthesis and secretion of ECM products. The control of ECM deposition is

TABLE 10.2. Partial List of Growth Factors Present at the Wound Site.

Growth factor	*Cellular source*	*Target cells*	*Biologic activity*
TGF-β1 and -β2	Macrophages, platelets, fibroblasts, keratinocytes	Inflammatory cells, keratinocytes, fibroblasts	Chemotaxis, proliferation, matrix production (fibrosis)
TGF-β3	Macrophages	Fibroblasts	Antiscarring?
TGF-α	Macrophages, platelets, keratinocytes	Keratinocytes, fibroblasts, endothelial cells	Proliferation
TNF-α	Neutrophils	Macrophages, keratinocytes, fibroblasts	Activation of growth factor expression
PDGF	Macrophage, platelets, fibroblasts, endothelial cells, vascular smooth muscle cells	Neutrophils, macrophages, fibroblasts, endothelial cells, vascular smooth muscle cells	Chemotaxis, proliferation, matrix production
FGF-1, FGF-2, FGF-4	Macrophage, fibroblasts, endothelial cells	Keratinocytes, fibroblasts, endothelial cells, chondrocytes	Angiogenesis, proliferation, chemotaxis
FGF-7 (KGF-1), FGF-10 (KGF-2)	Fibroblasts	Keratinocytes	Proliferation, chemotaxis
EGF	Platelets, macrophages, keratinocytes	Keratinocytes, fibroblasts, endothelial cells	Proliferation, chemotaxis
IGF-1/Sm-C	Fibroblasts, macrophages, serum	Fibroblasts, endothelial cells	Proliferation, collagen synthesis
IL-1α and IL-1β	Macrophages, neutrophils	Macrophages, fibroblasts, keratinocytes	Proliferation, collagenase synthesis, chemotaxis
CTGF	Fibroblasts, endothelial cells	Fibroblasts	Downstream of TGF-β1
VEGF	Macrophages, keratinocytes	Endothelial cells	Angiogenesis

Redundant biologic effects through both autocrine and paracrine mechanisms are apparent. CTGF, connective tissue growth factor; EGF, epidermal growth factor; FGF, fibroblast growth factor; IGF-1, insulin-like growth factor-1; IL-1, interleukin-1; KGF, keratinocyte growth factor; PDGF, platelet-derived growth factor; Sm-C, somatostatin-C; TGF-α, transforming growth factor-α; TGF-β, transforming growth factor-α; TNF-α, tumor necrosis factor-α; VEGF, vascular endothelial cell growth factor.

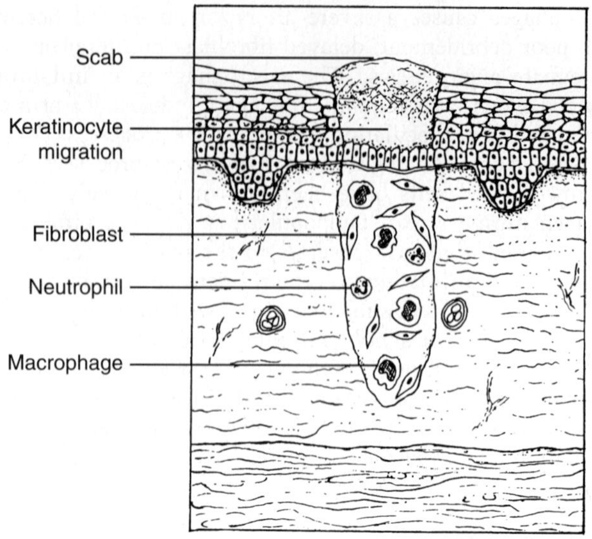

FIGURE 10.5. Local fibroblasts and elicited progenitor cells are activated and present at the wound by 3–5 days after injury. These cells secrete matrix components and growth factors that continue to stimulate healing. Keratinocyte migration (epiboly) begins over the new matrix. Migration starts from the wound edges as well as from epidermal cell nests at sweat glands and hair follicles in the center of the wound.

complex and thought to be regulated not only by growth factors but also by interactions between integrins and other cell membrane receptors with the ECM.

Integrins are transmembrane proteins with extracellular, membrane, and intracellular domains. They are heterodimeric and composed of alpha and beta subunits that interact to form the active protein receptor. Ligands include growth factors, ECM structural components such as collagen, elastin, and other cells. After ligands bind, a structural change occurs in the cytoplasmic domain of the integrin receptor, and phosphorylation occurs. This typically starts a signal transduction cascade that ultimately results in transcription factor synthesis and new gene expression. Subsequently, new cellular function ensues. Thus, the cell has been regulated to change its behavior (Fig. 10.6).

The initial wound matrix is provisional and is composed of fibrin and the glycosaminoglycan (GAG) hyaluronic acid.[3] Because of its large water of hydration, hyaluronic acid provides a matrix that enhances cell migration. Adhesion glycoproteins, including fibronectin, laminin, and tenascin, are present throughout the early matrix and facilitate cell attachment and migration. Integrin receptors on cell surfaces bind to the matrix GAGs and glycoproteins. As fibroblasts enter and populate the wound, they utilize hyaluronidase to digest the provisional hyaluronic acid-rich matrix, and larger, sulfated GAGs are subsequently deposited. Concomitantly, collagens are deposited by fibroblasts onto the fibronectin and GAG scaffold in a disorganized array.

Collagen types I and III are the major fibrillar collagens comprising the ECM and are the major structural proteins in both unwounded and wounded skin. The ratio of collagens type I:III is 4:1 in skin and wound scar. Type III collagen is initially present in relatively greater amounts in wounds but always is less than type I collagen in mature scar.[9]

There are now at least 27 different types of collagens described.[9–12] Most collagen types are synthesized by fibroblasts; however, it is now known that some types are synthesized by epidermal cells.[13] The collagens share common characteristics: The basic structural unit is a right-handed triple helix. Unique structural properties that distinguish the different collagen types include segments that interrupt the triple helix and fold it into other kinds of structures, conferring unique properties to that type.

Dermal collagen, the major structural component of wound repair, is synthesized and secreted by fibroblasts into an extracellular fiber network. This is accomplished through a complex intra- and extracellular process. Coordinated transcription of genes on different chromosomes (2, 6, 7, 12, 13, 17, and 21) has been found. In addition, several intra- and extracellular modifications are required to form the new collagen fiber.[9] In the nucleus, messenger RNA splicing modifications occur after transcription. In the rough endoplasmic reticulum, five major modifications occur to form the triple helix. The signal peptide is cleaved, followed by hydroxylation of selected proline and lysine residues. Next, addition of N-linked oligosaccharides and addition of galactose to hydroxylysine residues occurs. The three single-protein chains, called *pro-alpha chains*, align with disulfide bond formation and form a right-handed triple-helical procollagen. Each of the pro-alpha chains that forms the triple helix is coded for by a single gene. Most collagen types have three identical chains (e.g., types II, III, VII, X, and XII). However, some types have two different pro-alpha chains coded for by two different genes that form the triple helix with two chains of one pro-alpha type and one chain of the other type without variation (e.g., types I, IV, V). Collagen types VI, IX, and XI each have three different pro-alpha chains.[9]

After triple-helix formation in the endoplasmic reticulum, the procollagens are transported to the Golgi apparatus. There, further hydroxylation occurs prior to exocytosis. In the ECM, N- and C-terminal propeptides are removed, and tropocollagen is formed. Tropocollagen molecules laterally aggregate and are covalently cross-linked by the enzyme lysyl oxidase to form collagen fibrils.[14] The fibrils interact with other fibril types, which then aggregate into fibers. For example, in skin, collagen types I and VI fibrils interact to form the collagen fibers that are imaged with electron microscopy.[10]

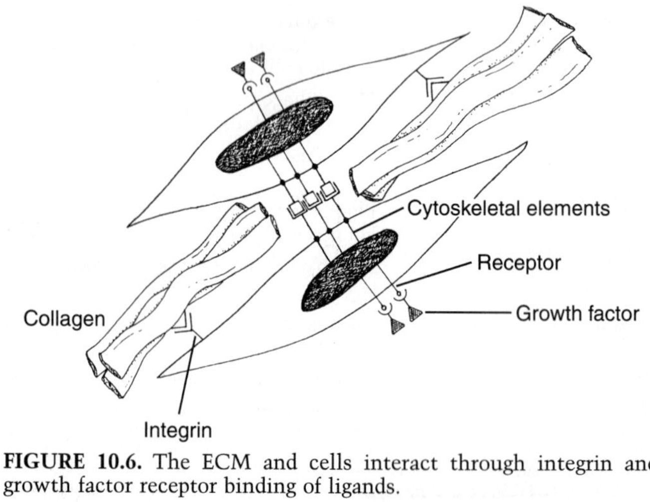

FIGURE 10.6. The ECM and cells interact through integrin and growth factor receptor binding of ligands.

Granulation

Granulation tissue is present in wounds healing by secondary intention. This tissue is clinically characterized by its beefy-red appearance (i.e. "proud flesh"), which is a consequence of the rich bed of new capillary networks (neoangiogenesis) that have formed due to endothelial cell division and migration. The directed growth of vascular endothelial cells is stimulated by platelet and activated macrophage and fibroblast products. One example is vascular endothelial growth factor, which is secreted by macrophages and acts to induce migration and proliferation of endothelial cells. Granulation tissue is a dense population of blood vessels, macrophages, and fibroblasts embedded within a loose provisional matrix of fibronectin, hyaluronic acid, and collagen.

The presence of granulation tissue is used as a clinical indicator that the wound is ready for skin graft treatment. Wounds that benefit are from skin grafts and are of sufficient size that the healing time would be decreased. Granulation tissue has a high level of vascularity due to the abundance of new capillary formation. This degree of vascularity enables granulation tissue to readily accept and support skin grafts.

Contraction

Open wounds are characterized by *contraction*, a phenomenon not present in closed surgical incisions. Open wounds occur after trauma and burns and when previously closed wounds are secondarily opened due to infection. Contraction is the process in which the surrounding skin is pulled circumferentially toward the wound (Fig. 10.7). Wound contraction decreases the size of the wound dramatically without new tissue formation. This repair component allows the wound to close and thus heal much more rapidly than by epithelialization alone. In addition, the area of insensate scar is smaller.

Mammalian animals have much greater capacity for wound contraction than do humans. Most mammalian animals (e.g., rodents, cats, dogs, sheep, and rabbits) have a panniculus carnosus, which is a myofascial layer between the subcutaneous fat and musculoskeletal layers. The resultant anatomy is a plane of low resistance between two fascial layers, which allows for enhanced skin mobility and contraction. The amount of contraction is related to the size of the wound and mobility of the skin. In humans, contraction is greatest in the trunk and perineum, least on the extremities, and intermediate on the head and neck. Up to 80% of wound closure can be due to contraction in the trunk and perineum. These regional differences are thought to be due to the relative differences in skin laxity in those areas.

The wound contraction mechanism is not completely understood. The contractile forces are likely generated by myofibroblasts.[15,16] These are fibroblast-like cells that contain alpha smooth muscle actin and microfilaments. It is not known whether these cells act to pull the surrounding skin by their movement through the matrix scaffold or by intrinsic cellular forces.

Clinically, wound contraction can lead to *contracture*, which distorts tissue and leads to decreased function. For example, wound contraction across a joint can lead to a contracture in that joint. The range of motion, and thus function, of the joint is diminished. Contractures can develop in the extremities, eyelids, neck, spine, and fingers.

Open wounds invariably become colonized by bacteria. The wound has no protective barrier to prevent bacterial adherence in the exposed dermis or subcutaneous fat/muscle. Colonization does not preclude healing. However, if bacterial infection occurs, then healing not only can be delayed but also can stop. Clinical infection implies bacterial invasion into the deeper layers of the surrounding tissue. It is treated by debridement of necrotic tissue, which is a nutrient source for bacteria, and by appropriate antibiotic therapy.

Epithelialization

Within hours after injury, morphologic changes in keratinocytes at the wound margin are evident. In skin wounds, the epidermis thickens, and marginal basal cells enlarge and migrate over the wound defect (see Fig. 10.5). Once these epithelial cells begin migrating, they do not divide until epidermal continuity is restored. New epithelial cells for wound closure are provided by fixed basal cells in a zone near the edge of the wound.[17] Their daughter cells flatten and migrate over the wound matrix as a sheet (epiboly). Cell adhesion glycoproteins, such as tenascin and fibronectin, provide the "railroad tracks" to facilitate epithelial cell migration over the wound matrix. Following the reestablishment of the epithelial layer, keratinocytes and fibroblasts secrete laminin and type IV collagen to form the basement membrane.[13] The keratinocytes then become columnar and divide as the layering of the epidermis is established, thus re-forming a barrier to further contamination and moisture loss.

Interestingly, keratinocytes can respond to foreign body stimulation with migration as well. Sutures in skin wounds provide tracts along which these cells can migrate. Subsequent epithelial thickening and keratinization produce fibrotic reactions, cysts, or sterile abscesses centered on the suture. These are treated by removal of the inciting suture and epithelial cell sinus tract or cyst.

Remodeling Phase

The ECM is the scaffold that supports cells both in the unwounded and wounded states. The ECM is dynamic and during repair is constantly undergoing remodeling. The regulation of the remodeling is poorly understood but simplistically can be conceptualized as the balance among synthesis, deposition, and degradation. Lysyl oxidase is the major intermolecular collagen cross-linking enzyme.[14] Collagen

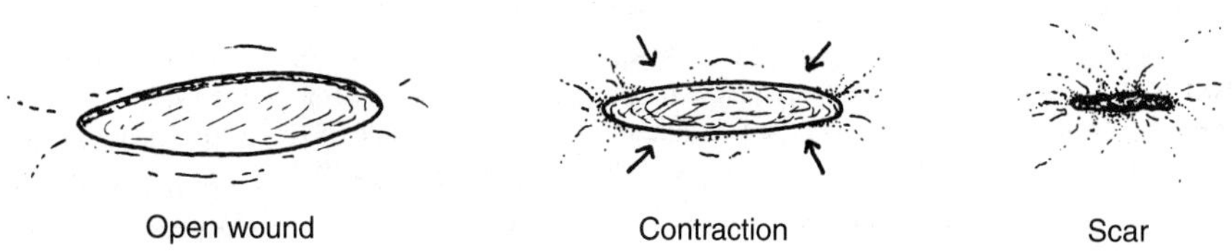

FIGURE 10.7. Wound contraction is the process by which the surrounding tissue is pulled radially toward the wound. The wound size is decreased, which shortens the healing time.

cross-linking improves wound tensile strength. Collagenases, gelatinases, and stromelysins are matrix metalloproteinases (MMPs) that degrade ECM components. These proteinases also are active in local carcinoma invasion into the ECM and therefore have gained attention in recent years.[18] The balance of collagen deposition and degradation is in part determined by the regulation of MMP activity. Proteins called tissue inhibitor of matrix metalloproteinases (TIMPs) specifically inactivate the MMPs.[19] Current investigation is examining the regulation of MMP/TIMP balance during wound ECM remodeling.[18,20]

Ultimately, the outcome of mammalian wound healing is scar formation (Fig. 10.8). Scar is defined morphologically as the lack of tissue organization compared to surrounding normal tissue architecture and is characterized by disorganized collagen deposition. New collagen fibers secreted by fibroblasts are present as early as 3 days after wounding. As the collagenous matrix forms, densely packed fibers fill the wound site. The ultimate pattern of collagen in scar is one of densely packed fibers and not the reticular pattern found in unwounded dermis.

The scar remodels slowly over months to years to form a "mature" scar. The early scar is red due to its dense capillary network. Over a period of months, the capillaries regress until relatively few remain, and the appearance of the scar is no longer red. Scars are usually hypopigmented and appear lighter than the surrounding skin after full maturation. However, scars can be hyperpigmented and darker than the surrounding skin in some darkly pigmented patients or those lighter-pigmented patients whose scars receive excess sun exposure. For this reason, surgeons recommend sun protective measures for patients with early scars on sun-exposed areas such as the scalp, face, and neck.

During remodeling, wounds gradually become stronger with time. Wound tensile strength increases rapidly from 1 to 8 weeks postwounding. Thereafter, tensile strength increases at a slower pace and has been documented to increase up to 1 year after wounding in animal studies (Fig. 10.9). However, the tensile strength of wounded skin at best only reaches approximately 80% that of unwounded skin.[21] The final result of tissue repair is scar, which is brittle, less elastic than normal skin, and does not contain any skin appendages such as hair follicles or sweat glands. The major benefit of repair by scar is the relatively rapid reformation of tissue integrity.

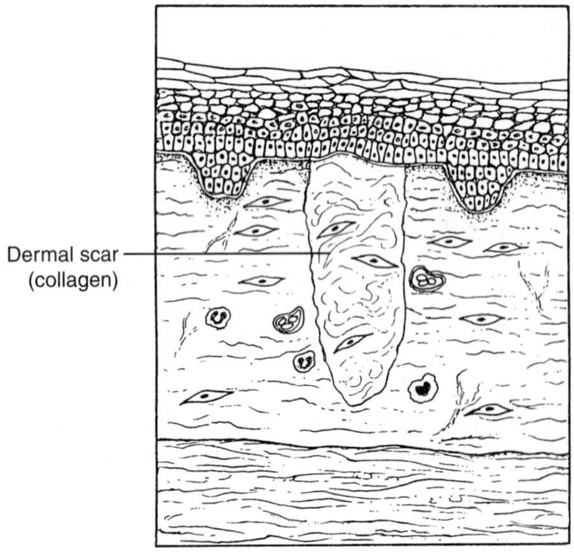

FIGURE 10.8. Scar formation is the outcome of healing in postnatal skin. Scar is composed of densely packed, disorganized collagen fiber bundles. Remodeling occurs up to 1–2 years after injury and consists of further collagen cross-linking and regression of capillaries, which account for the softening of scar and its color change from red to white.

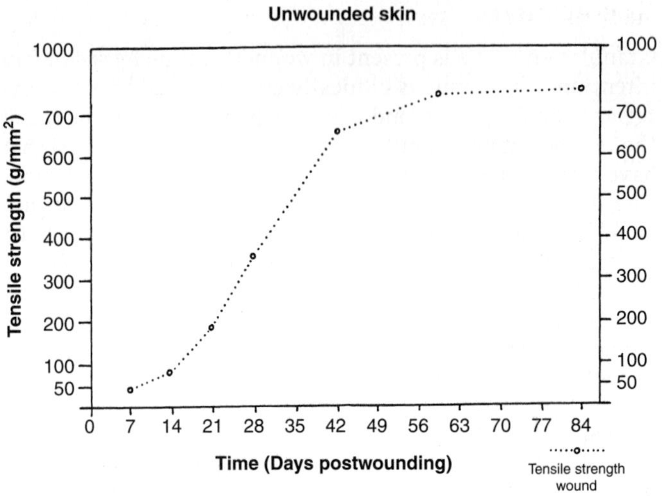

FIGURE 10.9. Wound tensile strength as a function of time. Maximal wound tensile strength is 75%–80% of unwounded skin. (From Levenson et al.[21])

Regulation of Wound Repair

Growth Factors

Growth factors play a prominent role in the regulation of wound healing. These polypeptides are released by a variety of activated cells at the wound site (Table 10.2). They act in either paracrine or autocrine fashion to stimulate or inhibit protein synthesis by cells in the wound. Growth factors also chemoattract new cells to the wound. Myriad growth factors are present in wounds, and many have overlapping functions. The biologic effects of growth factors are only beginning to be unraveled.

In addition to the growth factors themselves, their signaling receptors are another locus for regulation of repair. Growth factors do not have an effect on target cells without a functioning signaling receptor present. The best-studied growth factors have multiple different receptor types to which they can bind and induce cell signaling. Scientists are now beginning to understand some of the differences between receptor binding affinity, growth factor isoforms, and target cell effect. In the future, treatment of wound healing deficiency states may be possible by stimulating or neutralizing specific receptors via pharmacologic ligands.

Platelet-Derived Growth Factor

Platelet-derived growth factor (PDGF) is released from platelet alpha granules immediately after injury. The PDGF attracts neutrophils, macrophages, and fibroblasts to the wound and serves as a powerful mitogen. Macrophages, endothelial cells, and fibroblasts also synthesize and secrete PDGF. The PDGF stimulates fibroblasts to synthesize new ECM, predominantly noncollagenous components such as GAGs and adhesion proteins. Also, PDGF increases the amount of fibroblast-secreted collagenase, indicating a role for this cytokine in tissue remodeling.[22,23]

Transforming Growth Factor-β

Transforming growth factor-β (TGF-β) directly stimulates collagen synthesis and decreases ECM degradation by fibroblasts.[15,24] It is released from platelets and macrophages at the wound. In addition, TGF-β is released from fibroblasts and keratinocytes. The TGF-β acts in an autocrine fashion to further stimulate its own synthesis and secretion. Also, TGF-β chemoattracts fibroblasts and macrophages to the wound.

Transforming growth factor-β is a profibrotic growth factor and accelerates wound repair when applied experimentally to otherwise normal wounds. However, the increase in repair rate is at the expense of increased fibrosis. In addition, increased TGF-β activity is associated with pathologic fibrosis in multiple different organ systems, including heart, lung, brain, liver, and kidney. It is also thought to be a factor in the formation of intestinal adhesions. Synthesis of ECM is stimulated by TGF-β by increasing collagen, elastin, and GAG synthesis. It increases integrin expression and therefore enhances cell–matrix interactions. The TGF-β increases ECM accumulation by decreasing MMP and increasing TIMP expression. Through these mechanisms, TGF-β augments fibrosis at the wound site.[25,26]

Fibroblast Growth Factors

Angiogenesis is stimulated by acidic and basic fibroblast growth factors (FGF-1 [or aFGF] and FGF-2 [or bFGF], respectively).[27] Endothelial cells, fibroblasts, and macrophages produce FGF-1 and FGF-2. These growth factors are bound by heparin and the GAG heparan sulfate in the ECM. Basement membrane serves as a storage depot for FGF-2, which is released on degradation of the heparin components of the basement membrane. The FGFs stimulate endothelial cells to divide and form new capillaries. They also chemoattract endothelial cells and fibroblasts.

Vascular Endothelial Growth Factor

Vascular endothelial growth factor is also a potent angiogenic stimulus.[28] It acts in a paracrine manner to stimulate proliferation by endothelial cells after release from platelets, macrophages, fibroblasts, and keratinocytes.[29] Its expression is also increased in hypoxic conditions, such as those found at the wound site.[30]

Other Growth Factors

Epithelialization is directly stimulated by at least three growth factors: epidermal growth factor (EGF) and keratinocyte growth factor-1 and -2 (KGF-1 [or FGF-7] and KGF-2 [or FGF-10], respectively).[27,31,32] The EGF is released by keratinocytes to act in an autocrine fashion, whereas the KGFs are released by fibroblasts to act in a paracrine fashion to stimulate keratinocyte division and differentiation.

Multiple other growth factors affect wound repair. For example, insulin-like growth factor-1 (IGF-1) stimulates collagen synthesis by fibroblasts, and IGF-1 functions synergistically with PDGF and bFGF to facilitate fibroblast proliferation.[33] Interferon-γ has been shown to downregulate collagen synthesis. The various interleukins mediate inflammatory cell functions at the wound site.[34]

Surgeons may soon have the ability to enhance repair by adding or deleting growth factors to wounds. Investigators have accelerated healing rates in normal wounds by adding exogenous TGF-β, PDGF, IGF-1, or FGF-2.[27,35,36] Addition of these same growth factors has also augmented repair in animal models of impaired wound-healing conditions such as diabetes and chronic steroid use.[24,37–43] Further studies are needed to determine the precise growth factor combination that is optimal for specific wound types before clinical application is appropriate.

The Extracellular Matrix

The ECM is a depository of growth factors in latent forms under normal, unwounded conditions. With injury and matrix destruction, the previously bound and inactive growth factors are released from the ECM in active form and thereby assist in initiating and regulating the repair process. For example, TGF-β is bound in the ECM to the proteoglycan decorin and is inactive when bound. At sites of injury, TGF-β, with its binding protein, latency-associated protein (LAP), is released. Under acidic conditions, such as those at sites of hypoxia and tissue injury, LAP disassociates, and active TGF-β is formed.[44] Also, LAP can be proteolytically cleaved and released by MMPs and other proteases at the wound site. Active TGF-β immediately binds to one of its two serine-threonine kinase receptors (TGF-β-RI and -RII), which are present on fibroblasts, macrophages, and endothelial cells.[45,46] The TGF-β-RI and -RII receptors then form heterodimeric complexes with each other, and TGF-β biologic activity is initiated in the target cell.

Another example of growth factors bound by the ECM are the FGFs, which are bound to the GAG heparan sulfate. Also, PDGF has been shown to bind to ECM proteins. Thus, by binding growth factors and releasing them during injury, the ECM participates in wound repair by release of growth factors thought to regulate the biology of repair.

Scarless Repair: The Fetal Paradigm

Unlike the adult, the fetus in early gestation can heal skin wounds with regenerative-type repair and not with scar formation.[47,48] The epidermis and dermis are restored to a normal architecture in which the collagen matrix pattern is reticular and unchanged from unwounded dermis. The wound hair follicle and sweat gland patterns are normal.

The ability of the fetus to heal a wound without scar is a function of both gestational age and wound size.[49,50] As gestation progresses, a transition from scarless to healing with scar formation occurs prior to birth. In large-animal models, such as the fetal lamb and monkey, this transition occurs during the early part of the third trimester for incisional, closed wounds. In addition, wound size affects the temporal occurrence of this transition. The larger the excisional wound size is, the earlier in gestation it must be made for it to heal without scar.[49] The transition in repair outcome is not abrupt but instead occurs gradually, with an intermediate repair outcome that is neither regeneration nor scar: a *transition wound*. The transition wound has a normal reticular collagen and connective tissue matrix pattern but without restoration of epidermal appendages.[51]

Scarless healing by the fetus is not dependent on the fetal environment. Fetal skin grafts heal wounds without scar after transplantation to a postnatal environment. Thus, amniotic fluid, the intrauterine environment, and fetal serum factors are not required for scarless healing. Scarless repair appears to be inherent to the fetal tissue.[52,53] For example, the TGF-β ligand profile is different with greater TGF-β3 and less -β1 in scarless wounds compared to scarring wounds.[54] Scarless fetal repair occurs during a period with high levels of morphogen expression, which have an impact on the regenerative repair outcome.

Inflammation plays a prominent role in postnatal repair, but it is not present in significant amounts in fetal skin wounds. There is little or no acute inflammatory cell infiltrate in the sterile fetal skin wound. Prompted by fetal wound-healing observations, investigators have now decreased the inflammatory response in experimental postnatal wounds and noted less scar formation.[55,56] However, due to redundancy of action among growth factors, TGF-β will likely not be the only target with neutralization that reduces human scar and fibrosis.

In contrast to the fetus, adult tissue injury, whether due to trauma or disease, results in scar and fibrosis. Examples of fibrotic disease include pulmonary fibrosis, hepatic fibrosis, keloids, intraperitoneal adhesions, and burn wound contractures. Other conditions, such as a myocardial infarction, represent a tissue response to injury resulting in a scar. Thus, fetal repair is the blueprint for ideal repair. To unravel the genes regulating scarless fetal versus adult repair, investigators are using noncandidate gene approaches, such as microarray analysis. An understanding of the biology of scarless fetal wound repair will help surgeons develop therapeutic strategies to minimize scar and fibrosis.

Wound Pathology

Nonhealing Wounds

Chronic or nonhealing wounds are open wounds that fail to epithelialize and close in a reasonable amount of time. These wounds are clinically stagnant and without evidence of further closure. There are likely many reasons why these wounds do not heal, but no broad, unifying theory exists. Simply put, chronic wounds may be thought of as lacking appropriate "start" signals. These wounds can be broadly categorized into three groups: pressure sores, lower extremity ulcers, and radiation skin injury.

Pressure Sores

Pressure sores develop over a bony prominence, usually in the immobile patient. There are mistakenly called decubitus ulcers or bed sores. The sacrum, ischium, and greater trochanter are the most common locations affected.[57] However, the metatarsal heads, ankles, heels, knees, and occiput are susceptible under the right conditions. A not-uncommon problem is malleolar skin pressure necrosis due to constricting cast placement.

Pressure necrosis is a function of the amount of pressure on the tissue and duration of pressure. Microcirculation is compromised when the tissue pressure is greater than 25–30 mmHg, which blocks capillary perfusion pressure. Necrosis can occur with as little as 2 h of sustained pressures at this level.[58] Skin is more resistant to pressure necrosis than the underlying fat and muscle, which explains the common finding of a small area of skin ulceration overlying a large area of subcutaneous fat and muscle necrosis.

To begin treatment of these patients, efforts should be made to control the factors leading to increased pressure. Paralyzed patients require periodic rotation and air mattress or other types of low-pressure beds. In addition, behavior and contractures may need to be addressed. Tight-fitting casts should be removed and replaced by those with no excess pressure. Other contributing factors should be identified and controlled, such as malnutrition, infection, and diabetes control. Necrotic tissue requires debridement.

With avoidance of pressure over the involved area, most pressure sores will heal. However, they heal with scar formation, which is less resistant to trauma than intact skin. Thus, a higher incidence of recurrence exists after spontaneous closure of these wounds than if they are closed surgically with flaps of normal skin and muscle over the bony prominence.[59,60]

Lower Extremity Ulcers

Leg ulcers generally arise from one of two different vascular diseases: arterial or venous insufficiency. Most (80%–90%) result from venous valvular disease (venous insufficiency).[57,61,62] Increased venous pressure in the dependent lower extremity leads to localized edema and tissue necrosis. Tissue edema is thought to be a major inhibitor of repair at the ulcer site, but the exact mechanism is not known. Oxygen delivery and diffusion are likely impaired. Postcapillary obstruction leads to increased perfusion pressure and hypoxia. Protein and red blood cell extravasation occurs, which further limit diffusion and oxygen delivery.

Arterial insufficiency to the lower extremity greatly impairs healing. Minor trauma, resulting from scratches and abrasions that would otherwise heal quickly in a normal patient, can progress into large wounds and ultimately necrotizing infection that is not only limb but also life threatening. A reliable clinical sign of adequate arterial inflow is the simple presence of an arterial pulse. If a single palpable pulse is present in the foot, then most wounds will heal. Transcutaneous oxygen ($TCPo_2$) measurements have been shown to have 83% accuracy in predictability of wound closure in an ischemic extremity.[63] A $TCPo_2$ of 30 at the wound edge denotes a wound that is more likely than not to heal. A nonhealing wound in an ischemic extremity is generally regarded as an indication for revascularization of that extremity.

Radiation Injury

External beam radiation through skin to treat deep pathology has both acute and chronic effects on skin. Acutely, a self-limiting erythema may develop that spontaneously resolves. Its late effect can be a more significant injury to fibroblasts, keratinocytes, and endothelial cells. Cell DNA damage propagates over time and impairs the ability of these cells to divide successfully. Ultimately, a skin ulcer may appear

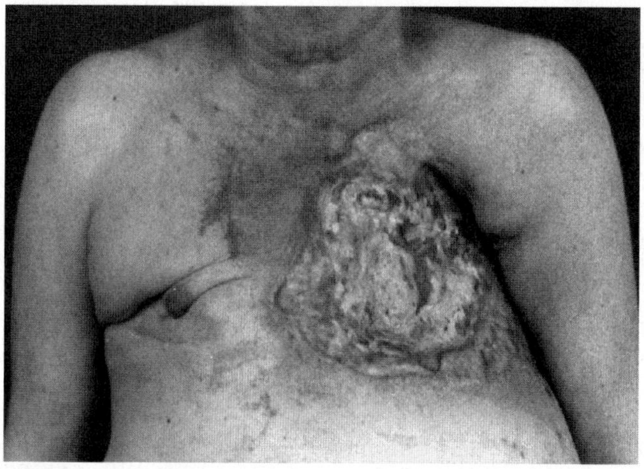

FIGURE 10.10. Chest wound due to radiation injury for breast cancer treatment after modified radical mastectomy. The wound was treated with debridement and subsequent reconstruction with microsurgical transfer of a free transverse rectus myocutaneous flap. (Photograph courtesy of Andrew Da Lio, MD.)

spontaneously, but usually it occurs after repeated mild trauma such as abrasions (Fig. 10.10).[64] If a surgical incision needs to be placed through an area of irradiated skin, then that incision is not likely to heal. Currently, the only treatment modalities for these wounds are hyperbaric oxygen therapy or coverage with vascularized tissue flaps.

Clinical Factors Affecting Repair

Infection

Wound infection is an imbalance between host resistance and bacterial growth.[65] Bacterial infection impairs healing through several mechanisms.[66] At the wound site, acute and chronic inflammatory infiltrates slow fibroblast proliferation and thus slow ECM synthesis and deposition. Although the exact mechanisms are not known, sepsis causes systemic effects that can impede the repair processes.

A threshold number of bacteria in the wound appears to be necessary to overcome host resistance and cause clinical wound infection. Bacterial contamination results in clinical infection and delays healing if greater than 10^5 organisms/gram tissue are present in the wound.[66,67] Skin grafts on open wounds are likely to fail if quantitative culture shows greater than 10^5 organisms/gram tissue, which provides further evidence that bacterial load has an impact on repair.[68] Similarly, well-vascularized muscle flaps heal open wounds successfully if bacterial loads are not greater than 10^5 organisms/gram tissue.[69] These studies demonstrate that high levels of bacteria inhibit the normal healing processes.

Treatment of the closed, infected wound depends on whether fluid or necrotic tissue is present. If no fluid is draining or loculated, then the cellulitis can be successfully treated with appropriate antibiotics. The wound should be opened, sutures removed, irrigated, and debrided if pus or necrotic tissue are present. Appropriate antibiotic administration following wound cultures treats surrounding cellulitis. Signs of wound infection include fever, tenderness, erythema, edema, and drainage.

Nutrition

Wound healing is an anabolic event that requires additional caloric intake.[70] However, the precise calorie requirements for optimal wound healing have not been determined. Large injuries such as burns greatly increase metabolic rate and nutritional requirements.[71] Severely malnourished and catabolic patients clinically appear to have diminished healing; however, no studies have definitely proved this finding.[72] Experimentally in dogs, chronic protein depletion impairs wound healing.[73] Wound dehiscence risk is increased in protein-depleted rats; however, this can be reversed with protein repletion immediately after wounding.[74]

Vitamin C (ascorbic acid) deficiency results in scurvy. In these patients, wound healing is arrested during fibroplasia. Normal quantities of fibroblasts are present in the wound, but they produce an inadequate amount of collagen.[75] Vitamin C is necessary for hydroxylation of proline and lysine residues.[76] Without hydroxyproline, newly synthesized collagen is not transported out of cells. Without hydroxylysine, collagen fibrils are not cross-linked.

Vitamin A (retinoic acid) is involved in multiple facets of repair: fibroplasia, collagen synthesis and cross-linking, and epithelialization processes.[75] Vitamin A requirements increase following injury. Severely injured patients require supplemental vitamin A to maintain normal serum levels. Animal studies show that vitamin A also reverses the impaired healing that occurs with chronic steroid treatment.[77,78] While not proved conclusively in human studies, most surgeons administer vitamin A postoperatively to their patients on steroid therapy. Vitamin A is fat soluble and can be taken in toxic doses, so careful administration is essential. The oral dose is 25,000 U/day.[75]

Vitamin B_6 (pyridoxine) deficiency impairs collagen cross-linking.[79] Vitamin B_1 (thiamine) and vitamin B_2 (riboflavin) deficiencies cause syndromes associated with poor wound repair. Supplementation with these vitamins does not improve healing unless a preexisting deficiency condition is present.

Trace metal deficiencies (e.g., of zinc and copper) have been implicated with poor wound repair since these divalent cations are cofactors in many important enzymatic reactions.[75] Zinc deficiency is associated with poor epithelialization and chronic, nonhealing wounds. Trace metal deficiency is now extremely rare in both enterally and parenterally fed patients.

Vitamin and mineral excess administration can be detrimental and cause toxicity, especially by the fat-soluble vitamins. Adequate amounts are present in today's enteral feeding solutions and as supplemental additives to parenteral solutions. Supplemental administration is necessary only in deficiency states and certain unique clinical situations as described.

Oxygen and Perfusion

Wounds require adequate oxygen delivery to heal. Ischemic wounds heal poorly and have a much greater risk of infection.[80,81] Wound ischemia occurs secondary to a variety of factors: occlusive vascular disease, vasoconstriction, and hypovolemia. Excessive suture tension during wound closure will cause local wound ischemia and result in wound-healing complications. Conversely, increased oxygen delivery at the wound improves wound healing.[80,82] Experimentally, collagen synthesis by fibroblasts is increased with supplemental oxygen.[83,84]

Anemia in the normovolemic patient is not detrimental to wound repair as long as the hematocrit is greater than 15% because oxygen content in blood does not affect wound collagen synthesis.[83] However, increasing the pO_2 in blood to high levels with hyperbaric oxygen therapy allows more oxygen to diffuse to the relatively poorly vascularized wound edge. This mechanism is hypothesized to account for the repair improvement that occurs in nonhealing, radiation injury wounds during hyperbaric oxygen therapy.[85]

Tissue perfusion is the ultimate determinate of wound oxygenation and nutrition. To optimize wound repair, those factors leading to wound ischemia should be prevented. Sutures should not be placed too tightly. The patient should be kept warm, pain should be well controlled to prevent vasoconstriction, and hypovolemia should be corrected.

Diabetes Mellitus and Obesity

Wound healing is impaired by unknown mechanisms in diabetic patients, although studies have implicated a lack of KGF and PDGF function in the wound.[86,87] Many of these patients have microvascular occlusive disease that may cause ischemia and impaired repair. Healing is enhanced if glucose levels are well controlled.[88] Obesity interferes with repair independently of diabetes.[89] Obese patients with diabetes have impaired wound healing independent of glucose control and insulin therapy. Poor wound perfusion and necrotic adipose tissue probably contribute to impaired healing in both diabetic and nondiabetic obese patients.

Corticosteroids

Both topically applied and pharmacologic steroid use impairs healing, especially when given in the first 3 days after wounding.[90,91] Steroids reduce wound inflammation, collagen synthesis, and contraction.[75] The exact mechanisms underlying how steroids impair healing are not fully understood. Glucocorticoids have been shown to decrease PDGF and KGF expression in experimental wounds.[87,92] Steroids stabilize lysosomal membranes and thereby decrease the release of lysosomes at the repair site, which may slow repair processes. Because steroids decrease inflammation, they may decrease host bacterial resistance and thus increase wound infection complications. The entire repair process is slowed, and risk of dehiscence and infection is increased. As stated in the discussion of nutrition, vitamin A administration can reverse this effect.[78]

Radiation Therapy

Both radiation and chemotherapeutic agents have their greatest effects on dividing cells. The division of endothelial cells, fibroblasts, and keratinocytes is impaired in irradiated tissue, which retards wound healing. Irradiated tissue usually has some degree of residual endothelial cell injury and progressive endarteritis, which results in atrophy, fibrosis, and poor tissue repair.[64] Improvement in repair can be achieved with hyperbaric oxygen therapy.[93,94] Surgical reconstruction involves wide resection of the wound back to normal, nonirradiated tissue and coverage with well-vascularized flaps.

Chemotherapy

During the proliferative phase of repair, numerous cell types are active at the wound site. Antiproliferative chemotherapeutic agents act to slow this process and thus retard healing.[95] Following oncologic surgical procedures, in most institutions, chemotherapeutic agents are not administered until at least 5 to 7 days postoperatively to prevent impairment of the initial healing events.

Excessive Healing

Normal wounds have stop signals that halt the repair process when the dermal defect is closed and epithelialization is complete. When these signals are absent or ineffective, then the repair process may continue and result in a condition of excessive scar. The underlying regulatory mechanisms leading to excessive repair are not yet known. Profibrotic cytokine overexpression has been implicated.[96,97] A lack of programmed cell death, apoptosis, at the conclusion of repair with continued presence of activated fibroblasts secreting ECM components has also been implicated.[98]

Notwithstanding the molecular regulation of excessive scar formation, there are clinical factors that affect scar formation. Some of these factors can be addressed by the surgeon. To minimize visible scar on skin, elective incisions are least noticeable when placed parallel to the natural lines of skin tension (Langer's lines). This placement location has two advantages: The scar is parallel or within a natural skin crease, which camouflages the scar, and this location places the least amount of tension on the wound. Wound tension prevents thin scar formation. Sharply defined and aligned wound edges approximated without tension heal with the least amount of scar. Infection or separation of the wound edges with subsequent secondary intention repair also results in more scar formation.

Hypertrophic Scar

Hypertrophic scars and keloids are unique to humans and do not occur in other animals for unknown reasons. These pathologic scar types are distinguished based on their clinical characteristics. *Hypertrophic scars* are defined as scars that have not overgrown the original wound boundaries but are instead raised (Fig. 10.11). They usually form secondary to excessive tensile forces across the wound and are most common in wounds across flexion surfaces, the extremities, breasts, sternum, and neck. Physical therapy with range of motion exercises is helpful in minimizing hypertrophic scar as well as joint contracture in the extremities.

Hypertrophic scar is a self-limited type of overhealing after tissue injury and usually regresses with time. These scars generally fade in color as well as flatten to the surrounding skin level. There has never been a clear histologic difference between hypertrophic scar and keloid. Early studies found that keloids contained bundles of collagen around focal nodules of proliferation.[99] However, later studies refuted this distinction.[100] Because of similar histologic findings in both hypertrophic scar and keloid, they are more easily differentiated by their clinical characteristics.

Hypertrophic scars and keloids are both fibroproliferative disorders of wound repair with excess healing.[96] However, because there are no animal models of either disease

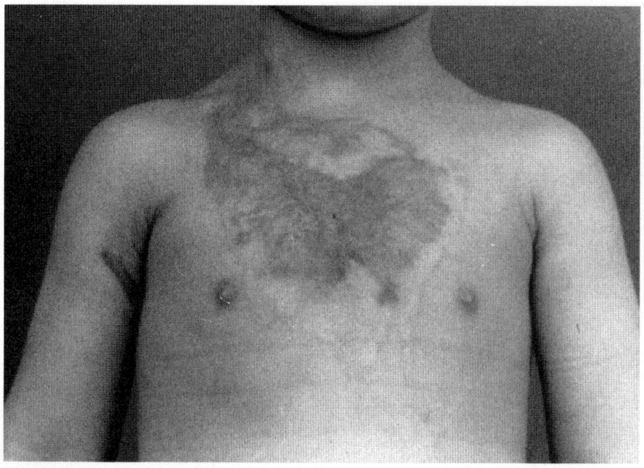

FIGURE 10.11. Chest hypertrophic scar after a hot water burn in a child. The scar is raised and erythematous yet has not grown beyond the borders of the original injury. (Photograph courtesy of Andrew Da Lio, MD.)

condition, there is little biochemical and molecular data that distinguish the two entities well in direct comparison. In addition, most studies analyze either one or the other, but not both. For example, one study found that fibroblasts isolated from hypertrophic scars synthesize less decorin than normal dermal fibroblasts.[101] No comparison with keloid fibroblasts was performed. In general, both keloid and hypertrophic scar fibroblasts have an upregulation of collagen synthesis, deposition, and accumulation.[102] It may be that keloid fibroblasts respond to a greater degree than do hypertrophic scar fibroblasts to the signals stimulating scar formation. For example, keloid fibroblasts respond to exogenous TGF-β with a much greater increase in collagen production than do hypertrophic scar fibroblasts.[103]

Treatment options for hypertrophic scars include the application of pressure garments or topical silicone sheets, laser therapy, and reexcision with primary closure.[104,105] The last option is most useful in cases of excess scar due to infection or dehiscence. If the original wound was closed following the basic tenets described, then reexcision with primary closure is not likely to result in an improved scar compared to the initial procedure. Recurrence of hypertrophic scar is high in these circumstances, and therefore most surgeons do not treat hypertrophic scar with excision and primary closure unless they plan adjuvant therapy.

Keloid

Scars that overgrow the original wound edges are called *keloids*. This clinical characteristic distinguishes keloid from hypertrophic scar. True keloid scar is not common and occurs mainly in darkly pigmented individuals, with an incidence of 6% to 16% in African populations.[106] It has a genetic predisposition with autosomal dominant features. The keloid scar continues to enlarge past the original wound boundaries and behaves like a benign skin tumor with continued slow growth. However, complete excision and primary closure of the defect result in recurrence in the majority of cases.

A skin field defect affecting the repair process may result in excessive stimuli or lack the appropriate "stop" signals for healing. In the latter instance, the lack of stop signals in the wound results in continued and unchecked repair. Studies have looked at apoptotic cell numbers in keloids and found that there are similar amounts of apoptotic cells at the advancing wound edge in both normal wound scar and hypertrophic scar.[107] However, apoptotic gene expression was decreased in keloids.[108] A possible mechanism of keloid formation may be the presence of persistent signals pushing fibroblasts to keep "healing" the wound site despite complete coverage of the original wound.

Keloids consist mainly of collagen. They are relatively acellular in their central portions, with fibroblasts present along their enlarging borders. They do not contain a significant excess number of fibroblasts. Collagen scar deposition outpaces degradation, and the lesion continues to enlarge. Keloid fibroblasts respond differently from normal wound fibroblasts to growth factors found at the repair site.[102,109,110] For example, TGF-β treatment causes a greater degree of collagen gene expression in keloid compared to normal wound fibroblasts in in vitro studies.[102]In addition, there is a greater degree of profibrotic growth factor expression in keloids than in normal wounds.[109] Moreover, keloid keratinocytes also are phenotypically different compared to normal scar keratinocytes. Keloid keratinocytes secrete greater profibrotic factors.[111] These and other studies suggest that keloid formation occurs due to an increased expression and activity of proliferative and fibrotic growth factors at the wound site.

No uniformly successful treatment of keloid scar exists. Excision and primary closure invariably results in recurrence. Therefore, some form of additional therapy is necessary. The type of treatment also depends on the time point when the patient presents. Steroid injection directly into the keloid has the most benefit early in the course.[112] It has been shown to decrease collagen gene expression.[113] Mixed with 2% plain lidocaine in a 50:50 ratio, 10mg/ml triamcinolone acetonide should be used initially; if no response occurs, then a concentration of 40mg/ml should be attempted.

Patients presenting with mature lesions they have had for months to years and that are slowly changing respond poorly to steroid injection. The only viable treatment options for mature keloids are to monitor and do nothing or to excise and administer adjuvant therapy. A short course of low-dose radiation therapy to the keloid excision wound immediately after excision has been shown to reduce the rate of recurrence.[114] Steroid injection intra- and postoperatively also has been performed.[115,116] Benefit with topical silicone sheeting placement has been found.[117,118] Topical antiinflammatory creams (e.g., Aldara) have been used with some success.[119,120] Experimentally, tamoxifen has been shown to decrease collagen synthesis by keloid fibroblasts in vitro.[121,122] However, resection of keloid with adjuvant therapy still has a high rate of recurrence, with the risk that the next keloid will be larger and more difficult to control.

Clinical Management of Wounds

Primary Intention

Primary intention healing occurs in *closed wounds*, which are wounds with the edges approximated (Fig. 10.12A). These wounds are usually closed in layers along tissue planes.

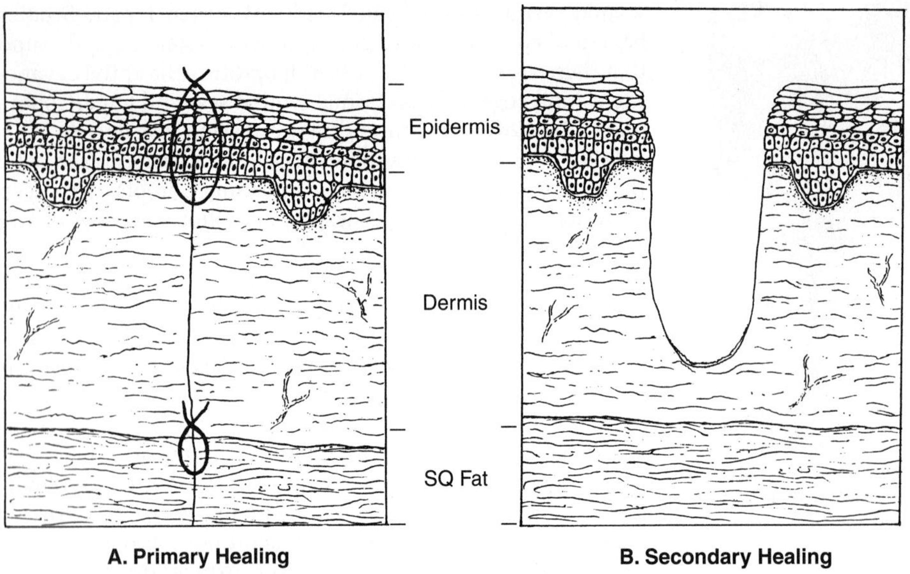

FIGURE 10.12. **A**. Wound healing by primary intention. The edges are approximated. **B**. Wound healing with secondary intention. The wound is open, and the edges are not approximated. These wounds heal by contraction and epithelialization.

Deep sutures are placed in collagen-rich layers such as fascia and dermis. These layers are strong and can hold sutures with a high degree of tension. Fatty tissue layers, such as subcutaneous fat, do not have significant collagen and cannot hold sutures under tension. For this reason, most surgeons do not close the subcutaneous fat layer, even in the morbidly obese patient. Dead space here is better obliterated with a short course of closed suction drainage postoperatively rather than by placing sutures that serve as bacterial culture sources.

The amount of tissue injury and degree of contamination influence the length and quality of healing. Small, clean closed wounds heal quickly with little scar formation, whereas large, open, dirty wounds heal slowly with significant scar. To decrease scar formation and risk of infection, meticulous hemostasis should be performed. This limits the amount of hematoma to be cleared and thus decreases the inflammatory phase and likely decreases scar. Because hematoma is a culture medium for bacteria, less bleeding also decreases the risk of infection. By limiting inflammation with sterile technique and tight hemostatic control, repair by activated fibroblasts can begin earlier and shorten the healing period.

Smaller surgical scars are achieved with no skin edge trauma and less resultant inflammation. Forceps crush injury of the epidermis and dermis should be avoided by using fine forceps and skin hooks to retract and assist in dermal closure. This decreases the amount of necrotic tissue at the wound edge and thereby reduces inflammation. Because suture material is a foreign body, it generates an immune response and is susceptible to infection. Some surgeons therefore close the epidermis with Steri-strips. There is no suture to leave a railroad track scar or serve as an infection locus in the skin. Fibrin and other biologic glues and sealants are now being developed for use during wound closure with the potential benefit of less scar formation.[123,124]

Uncomplicated wounds healing with primary intention epithelialize within 24–48 h. At this point, water barrier function has been restored, and patients can be allowed to shower or wash. This has a psychological benefit during the postoperative recovery period. In addition, gentle cleansing removes old serum and blood, which reduces potential bacterial accumulation and infection risk.

Secondary Intention

Open wounds heal with the same basic processes of inflammation, proliferation, and remodeling as closed wounds. The major difference is that each sequence is much longer, especially the proliferative phase. There is much more granulation tissue formation and contraction. This type of healing process is referred to as *secondary intention* (Fig. 10.12B).

Open wound edges are not approximated but are instead separated, which necessitates epithelial cell migration across a longer distance. Before epiboly can occur, a provisional matrix must be present. Granulation tissue must form. There are variable amounts of bacteria, tissue debris, and inflammation present depending on wound location and etiology. Infection, with high protein exudative losses and acute and chronic inflammation, can disregulate repair and transform the healing wound into a clinically nonhealing wound. The exact molecular mechanisms causing this shift from a healing to a nonhealing wound with infection remain unknown.

During the proliferative phase of an uncomplicated course of secondary intention healing, a bed of granulation tissue will be present. If no infection is present and the area is of sufficient size that healing will not be complete for at least 2–3 weeks, then placement of a partial- or full-thickness skin graft should be considered. Grafts readily adhere to granulation tissue and will quickly speed the repair process. Partial-thickness skin graft donor sites can heal in as little as 2 weeks, depending on graft thickness.

When an open wound heals, which is generally defined as *complete epithelialization*, the dermal defect has been filled with collagen scar covered by epithelium. This scar has less tensile strength and is more susceptible to trauma than normal skin. Thus, after healing these scars more easily break down due to local trauma such as pressure.

Topical Wound Treatment

Local Care

Closed Wounds

Closed wounds healing by primary intention require much less care than open wounds. Closed wounds should be kept sterile for 24–48h until epithelialization is complete. Tensile strength is only 20% of normal skin at 3 weeks when collagen cross-linking is becoming significant. At 6 weeks, wounds are at 70% of the tensile strength of normal skin, which is nearly the maximal tensile strength achieved by scar (75%–80% of normal; Fig. 10.9).[21] Therefore, if absorbable suture is used to close deep structures that are under significant tension, such as abdominal fascia, then the suture should retain significant tensile strength for at least 6 weeks before absorption severely weakens the suture. In addition, heavy activity should be limited for a minimum of 6 weeks while healing of deep fascial structures occurs.

Open Wounds

Necrotic material should be removed from open wounds on initial presentation and subsequently as it accumulates. Necrotic tissue serves only as a culture source for bacteria and does not aid healing. The only exception to immediate debridement is a dry, chronic, arterial insufficiency eschar without evidence of infection. These types of wounds may be best treated by revascularization prior to debridement.

Open wounds heal optimally in a moist, sterile environment. Although sterility is not possible to achieve clinically, numerous experimental and clinical studies have demonstrated that a moist environment speeds healing.[125] This is thought to occur by preventing desiccation at the base of the wound. Desiccation causes necrosis at the base of the wound until an eschar forms, which may take several days. During this time, the wound is enlarging and initiation of the healing process is delayed. By keeping the wound covered and moist without infection, desiccation necrosis and healing delay are prevented.[126]

Wound Dressings

A plethora of wound dressings are available for all types of wounds. No type has conclusively been shown to accelerate healing above the others despite several claims. Substantial improvements have been gained in convenience and comfort with a new class of engineered skin replacements that show great promise in affecting chronic wound care.

The optimal open wound dressing maintains a moist, clean environment that prevents pressure and mechanical trauma, reduces edema, stimulates repair, and is inexpensive. Less-frequent dressing changes and prevention of skin irritation are also beneficial. At this time, no ideal dressing exists.

Plain gauze and saline with or without antibiotic ointment remain the simplest and least-expensive dressing. Its major disadvantages are frequent need for changes, painful changes, and difficulty with desiccation and tape irritation to adjacent skin. Types of dressings listed by class are shown in Table 10.3. The films are gas permeable, maintain a moist environment, and are useful for partial-dermal thickness wounds such as skin graft donor sites. For highly exudative wounds, the absorptive dressings are useful to create a moist environment without excess fluid and proteinaceous material accumulation.

Hydrocolloid dressings are useful for locations where adhesion is necessary, such as the extremities and over bony prominences. They are relatively thick and can stay in place for 2–3 days. As the absorptive capacity is reached, they lose adhesiveness, and gentle atraumatic removal is facilitated. Hydrogels are similar to hydrocolloid dressings except that they have little adhesiveness and are especially useful for facial wound dressings.

The vacuum-assisted closure (VAC) device is now commonly used to treat large wounds, including those with exposed fascia, tendon, or bone. The apparatus consists of sponge, vacuum, and transparent film.[127] The device aids the healing of pressure sores, skin graft donor sites, venous stasis ulcers, and infected surgical wounds.[127,128] It also provides wound coverage and care until definitive reconstructive surgery is performed for large scalp, trunk, and extremity wounds. The vulnerary mechanisms are hypothesized to relate to reduction of surrounding edema and increased blood flow to the wound site.

Engineered Skin Replacements

With the biotechnology revolution, several dermal and skin replacements are now available through tissue engineering technology (Table 10.3). These products have the additional potential benefit of accelerating or augmenting repair due to their biocomponents. Growth factors are present in products with acellular dermal matrices. Some products contain living fibroblast and keratinocyte layers that secrete matrix components and active growth factors. This unique biology of skin replacement dressings shows great promise to aid impaired healing conditions.

Pharmacologic Treatment

Antibiotic Ointments

Antibiotic ointments are commonly used in burn wound care as well as deep partial-thickness injuries. They remain controversial in the nonburn patient because the risk of developing an invasive infection by resistant bacteria may be too high to justify their use. Open wounds are colonized by bacteria, and systemic antibiotics are indicated only if invasive infection is present. Nonburn wounds without infection will likely heal without topical antibiotic treatment as long as local care is adequate.

In burn patients, silver sulfadiazine is commonly used. It is inexpensive, has few side effects, and rarely induces bacterial resistance. It can be useful in chronic wound dressings as well. It is inexpensive and is well tolerated by pediatric and geriatric patients alike.

Collagenases

The collagenases are useful for treating wounds that require fine debridement of necrotic tissue not amenable to surgical debridement. This could be a thin layer of adherent exudate or small amounts of necrotic tissue remaining after a bedside wound debridement. Theoretically, collagenase would be detrimental to a clean wound in the proliferative phase when

TABLE 10.3. Classes of Wound Dressings and Skin Replacements Currently Available.

Class	*Composition*	*Characteristics/function*	*Commercial examples*
Gauze	Woven cotton fibers	Permeable with desiccation; debridement; painful removal	Curity
Calcium alginates	Seaweed polymer that forms a gel when absorbs fluid	Absorbs exudate; nonadherent; nonirritating; requires a cover dressing (permeable)	Algisorb, Sorbsan
Impregnated gauzes	Fine mesh fabric (silicone, nylon) with dermal porcine collagens	Nonadherent; semipermeable	Biobrane II
Films	Plastic (polyurethane); semipermeable	Allows water vapor permeation; adhesive	Opsite, Tegaderm
Foams	Hydrophilic (wound side) and hydrophobic (outer side); semipermeable	Necrotic/exudative wounds	Lyofoam, Allevyn
Hydrogels	Water (96%) and polymer (polyethylene oxide)	Aqueous environment; requires secondary dressing; no adherence; not recommended if infection is present; semipermeable	Vigilon, Aquasorb
Hydrocolloids	Hydrophilic colloidal particles and adhesive	Absorbs fluid; necrotic tissue autolysis; little adherence; occlusive	Duoderm, Intrasite
Absorptive powders and pastes	Starch copolymers, hydrocolloidal particles	Absorbs exudate; used as a filler; good for deep wounds	Geliperm, Duoderm granules
Silicone	Silicone sheets	Sheet induces a localized electromagnetic field; decreases scar formation	Sil-K
Mechanical vacuum	Vacuum, sponge, plastic film	Sponge conforms to wound; vacuum removes edema fluid, increases blood flow; stimulation of repair	VAC device
Dermal matrix replacements	Acellular matrix	Permeable; increased stimulation of repair	Alloderm (human, dermis), SIS (porcine, small bowel submucosa), Integra (bovine collagen, GAG, and silicone epidermal-type layer)
Dermal living replacements	Absorbable matrix populated with fibroblasts	Permeable; increased stimulation of repair	Dermagraft
Skin living replacement	Bovine collagen matrix populated with human fibroblasts with an outer layer of human keratinocytes	Impermeable; increased stimulation of repair	Apligraf (FDA approved)

A multitude of brands within each class is available, and only a few examples are listed. Skin replacements have become available. Although expensive, they have great potential clinical usefulness. No particular brands are recommended in any class.

Source: Data partially taken from Feedar.[135]

ECM synthesis and deposition favors accumulation rather than degradation.

Growth Factors

Experimentally, exogenous application of several growth factors has been shown to accelerate normal healing as well as improve healing rates and efficacy in impaired models of healing.[27,40,42,129–133] The best-studied growth factors with the most promise to improve healing are PDGF, TFG-β, and members of the FGF family (Table 10.2). Several obstacles must be overcome prior to widespread use, including efficacious application, vehicle development, and cost. For example, nonhealing human wound fluid has increased protease activity, which would likely rapidly degrade exogenously applied peptide growth factors.[134] Random, double-blind studies demonstrating clinical efficacy in the human patient are necessary. These studies are particularly difficult to design and perform due to the great degree of variability between patients in terms of wound types, local wound care, and concomitant control of active medical diseases.

In 1998, the first growth factor for treatment of wounds was approved by the Food and Drug Administration (FDA). Recombinant human PDGF-BB was shown to improve healing of lower extremity diabetic neuropathic ulcers in a double-blind, placebo-controlled, multicenter study. This 20-week trial included only patients with ulcers free of necrotic tissue and with adequate oxygenation documented by transcutaneous oxygen tensions of 30 mmHg or greater.[130] Complete wound healing occurred in 48% of the treated group compared to 25% of the control group.[130] On the basis of this and other studies, human recombinant PDGF-BB is approved for the treatment of diabetic neuropathic wounds. Other growth factors no doubt will be approved for wound treatment.

Extreme redundancy exists in the function of growth factors at the wound site. In addition, multiple simultaneous processes are occurring during repair. Thus, it is likely that multiple growth factors may need to be added, in combination, on impaired and even otherwise normal wounds to effect a clinically significant improvement in repair quality and rate. Different growth factor combinations may be needed to treat impaired wounds due to different underlying diseases, such as diabetes versus arterial insufficiency. To further complicate matters, neutralization of certain growth factors may be necessary as well as augmentation of other factors in the same wound. Our understanding of the molecular basis of repair regulation is still primitive but is rapidly expanding. With further knowledge, we will beneficially manipulate the repair outcome in different types of both wounds and tissue.

References

1. Ginsberg MH, Du X, Plow EF. Inside-out integrin signalling. Curr Opin Cell Biol 1992;4:766–771.
2. Roberts HR, Tabares AH. Overview of the coagulation reactions. In: High KA, Roberts HR, eds. Molecular Basis of Thrombosis and Hemostasis. New York: Marcel Dekker, 1995:35–50.
3. Clark RAF. Wound repair. Overview and general considerations. In: Clark RAF, ed. The Molecular and Cellular Biology of Wound Repair, 2nd ed. New York: Plenum Press, 1996:3–50.
4. DiPietro LA. Wound healing: the role of the macrophage and other immune cells. Shock 1995;4:233–240.
5. Leibovich SJ, Ross R. The role of the macrophage in wound repair. A study with hydrocortisone and antimacrophage serum. Am J Pathol 1975;78:71–100.
6. Chesney J, Bucala R. Peripheral blood fibrocytes: mesenchymal precursor cells and the pathogenesis of fibrosis. Curr Rheumatol Rep 2000;2:501–505.
7. Fathke C, Wilson L, Hutter J, et al. Contribution of bone marrow-derived cells to skin: collagen deposition and wound repair. Stem Cells 2004;22:812–822.
8. Kataoka K, Medina RJ, Kageyama T, et al. Participation of adult mouse bone marrow cells in reconstitution of skin. Am J Pathol 2003;163:1227–1231.
9. Miller EJ, Gay S. Collagen structure and function. In: Cohen IK, Diegelmann RF, Lindblad WJ, eds. Wound Healing. Biochemical and Clinical Aspects. Philadelphia: W. B. Saunders Company, 1992:130–151.
10. Lodish H, Baltimore D, Berk A, Zipursky SL, Matsudaira P, Darnell J. Multicellularity: cell–cell and cell–matrix interactions. In: Molecular Cell Biology, 4th ed. New York: Scientific American Books, Inc., 1995:1123–1200.
11. Koch M, Schulze J, Hansen U, et al. A novel marker of tissue junctions, collagen XXII. J Biol Chem 2004;279:22514–22521.
12. Boot-Handford RP, Tuckwell DS, Plumb DA, Rock CF, Poulsom R. A novel and highly conserved collagen (pro(alpha)1(XXVII)) with a unique expression pattern and unusual molecular characteristics establishes a new clade within the vertebrate fibrillar collagen family. J Biol Chem 2003;278:31067–31077.
13. Marinkovich MP, Keene DR, Rimberg CS, Burgeson RE. Cellular origin of the dermal-epidermal basement membrane. Dev Dyn 1993;197:255–267.
14. Kobayashi H, Ishii M, Chanoki M, et al. Immunohistochemical localization of lysyl oxidase in normal human skin. Br J Dermatol 1994;131:325–330.
15. Pierce GF, Vande Berg J, Rudolph R, Tarpley J, Mustoe TA. Platelet-derived growth factor-BB and transforming growth factor beta 1 selectively modulate glycosaminoglycans, collagen, and myofibroblasts in excisional wounds. Am J Pathol 1991; 138:629–646.
16. Gabbiani G. Evolution and clinical implications of the myofibroblast concept. Cardiovasc Res 1998;38:545–548.
17. Woodley DT. Reepithelialization. In: Clark RAF, ed. The Molecular and Cellular Biology of Wound Repair. New York: Plenum Press, 1996:339–350.
18. Moses MA, Marikovsky M, Harper JW, et al. Temporal study of the activity of matrix metalloproteinases and their endogenous inhibitors during wound healing. J Cell Biochem 1996;60:379–386.
19. Talhouk RS, Bissell MJ, Werb Z. Coordinated expression of extracellular matrix-degrading proteinases and their inhibitors regulates mammary epithelial function during involution. J Cell Biol 1992;118:1271–1282.
20. Witte MB, Thornton FJ, Kiyama T, et al. Metalloproteinase inhibitors and wound healing: a novel enhancer of wound strength. Surgery 1998;124:464–470.
21. Levenson SM, Geever EF, Crowley LV, Oates JF, Berard CW, Rosen H. The healing of rat skin wounds. Ann Surg 1965;161:293–308.
22. Pierce GF, Brown D, Mustoe TA. Quantitative analysis of inflammatory cell influx, procollagen type I synthesis, and collagen cross-linking in incisional wounds: influence of PDGF-BB and TGF-beta 1 therapy. J Lab Clin Med 1991;117:373–382.
23. Pierce GF, Mustoe TA, Altrock BW, Deuel TF, Thomason A. Role of platelet-derived growth factor in wound healing. J Cell Biochem 1991;45:319–326.
24. Cromack DT, Pierce GF, Mustoe TA. TGF-beta and PDGF mediated tissue repair: identifying mechanisms of action using impaired and normal models of wound healing. Prog Clin Biol Res 1991;365:359–373.
25. Roberts AB. Molecular and cell biology of TGF-beta. Miner Electrolyte Metab 1998;24:111–119.
26. Roberts AB, Sporn MB. Transforming growth factor-β. In: Clark RAF, ed. The Molecular and Cellular Biology of Wound Repair. New York: Plenum Press, 1996:275–308.
27. Mustoe TA, Pierce GF, Morishima C, Deuel TF. Growth factor-induced acceleration of tissue repair through direct and inductive activities in a rabbit dermal ulcer model. J Clin Invest 1991;87:694–703.
28. Nissen NN, Polverini PJ, Koch AE, Volin MV, Gamelli RL, DiPietro LA. Vascular endothelial growth factor mediates angiogenic activity during the proliferative phase of wound healing. Am J Pathol 1998;152:1445–1452.
29. Banks RE, Forbes MA, Kinsey SE, et al. Release of the angiogenic cytokine vascular endothelial growth factor (VEGF) from platelets: significance for VEGF measurements and cancer biology. Br J Cancer 1998;77:956–964.
30. Frank S, Hubner G, Breier G, Longaker MT, Greenhalgh DG, Werner S. Regulation of vascular endothelial growth factor expression in cultured keratinocytes. Implications for normal and impaired wound healing. J Biol Chem 1995;270:12607–12613.
31. Werner S, Smola H, Liao X, et al. The function of KGF in morphogenesis of epithelium and reepithelialization of wounds. Science 1994;266:819–822.
32. Han DS, Li F, Holt L, et al. Keratinocyte growth factor-2 (FGF-10) promotes healing of experimental small intestinal ulceration in rats. Am J Physiol Gastrointest Liver Physiol 2000;279: G1011–G1022.
33. Robertson JG, Pickering KJ, Belford DA. Insulin-like growth factor I (IGF-I) and IGF-binding proteins in rat wound fluid. Endocrinology 1996;137:2774–2781.
34. Heino J, Heinonen T. Interleukin-1 beta prevents the stimulatory effect of transforming growth factor-beta on collagen gene expression in human skin fibroblasts. Biochem J 1990;271:827–830.
35. Cromack DT, Porras-Reyes B, Purdy JA, Pierce GF, Mustoe TA. Acceleration of tissue repair by transforming growth factor beta

1: identification of in vivo mechanism of action with radiotherapy-induced specific healing deficits. Surgery 1993;113:36–42.
36. Giannobile WV, Hernandez RA, Finkelman RD, et al. Comparative effects of platelet-derived growth factor-BB and insulin-like growth factor-I, individually and in combination, on periodontal regeneration in *Macaca fascicularis*. J Periodont Res 1996;31:301–312.
37. Suh DY, Hunt TK, Spencer EM. Insulin-like growth factor-I reverses the impairment of wound healing induced by corticosteroids in rats. Endocrinology 1992;131:2399–2403.
38. Tanaka E, Ase K, Okuda T, Okumura M, Nogimori K. Mechanism of acceleration of wound healing by basic fibroblast growth factor in genetically diabetic mice. Biol Pharm Bull 1996;19:1141–1148.
39. Bitar MS. Insulin-like growth factor-1 reverses diabetes-induced wound healing impairment in rats. Horm Metab Res 1997;29:383–386.
40. Greenhalgh DG, Sprugel KH, Murray MJ, Ross R. PDGF and FGF stimulate wound healing in the genetically diabetic mouse. Am J Pathol 1990;136:1235–1246.
41. Wu L, Brucker M, Gruskin E, Roth SI, Mustoe TA. Differential effects of platelet-derived growth factor BB in accelerating wound healing in aged versus young animals: the impact of tissue hypoxia. Plast Reconstr Surg 1997;99:815–822; discussion 823–824.
42. Slavin J, Nash JR, Kingsnorth AN. Effect of transforming growth factor beta and basic fibroblast growth factor on steroid-impaired healing intestinal wounds. Br J Surg 1992;79:69–72.
43. Albertson S, Hummel RPD, Breeden M, Greenhalgh DG. PDGF and FGF reverse the healing impairment in protein-malnourished diabetic mice. Surgery 1993;114:368–372; discussion 372–373.
44. Abe M, Oda N, Sato Y. Cell-associated activation of latent transforming growth factor-beta by calpain. J Cell Physiol 1998;174:186–193.
45. Burmester JK, Qian SW, Ohlsen D, Phan S, Sporn MB, Roberts AB. Mutational analysis of a transforming growth factor-beta receptor binding site. Growth Factors 1998;15:231–242.
46. Gold LI, Sung JJ, Siebert JW, Longaker MT. Type I (RI) and type II (RII) receptors for transforming growth factor-beta isoforms are expressed subsequent to transforming growth factor-beta ligands during excisional wound repair. Am J Pathol 1997;150:209–222.
47. Ferguson MW, Whitby DJ, Shah M, Armstrong J, Siebert JW, Longaker MT. Scar formation: the spectral nature of fetal and adult wound repair. Plast Reconstr Surg 1996;97:854–860.
48. Beanes SR, Hu FY, Soo C, et al. Confocal microscopic analysis of scarless repair in the fetal rat: defining the transition. Plast Reconstr Surg 2002;109:160–170.
49. Cass DL, Bullard KM, Sylvester KG, Yang EY, Longaker MT, Adzick NS. Wound size and gestational age modulate scar formation in fetal wound repair. J Pediatr Surg 1997;32:411–415.
50. Longaker MT, Whitby DJ, Adzick NS, et al. Studies in fetal wound healing, VI. Second and early third trimester fetal wounds demonstrate rapid collagen deposition without scar formation. J Pediatr Surg 1990;25:63–68; discussion 68–69.
51. Lorenz HP, Whitby DJ, Longaker MT, Adzick NS. Fetal wound healing. The ontogeny of scar formation in the non-human primate. Ann Surg 1993;217:391–396.
52. Lorenz HP, Lin RY, Longaker MT, Whitby DJ, Adzick NS. The fetal fibroblast: the effector cell of scarless fetal skin repair. Plast Reconstr Surg 1995;96:1251–1259; discussion 1260–1261.
53. Lorenz HP, Longaker MT, Perkocha LA, Jennings RW, Harrison MR, Adzick NS. Scarless wound repair: a human fetal skin model. Development 1992;114:253–259.
54. Soo C, Beanes SR, Hu FY, et al. Ontogenetic transition in fetal wound transforming growth factor-beta regulation correlates with collagen organization. Am J Pathol 2003;163:2459–2476.
55. Shah M, Foreman DM, Ferguson MW. Neutralising antibody to TGF-beta 1,2 reduces cutaneous scarring in adult rodents. J Cell Sci 1994;107:1137–1157.
56. Ashcroft GS, Yang X, Glick AB, et al. Mice lacking Smad3 show accelerated wound healing and an impaired local inflammatory response [see comments]. Nature Cell Biol 1999;1:260–266.
57. Young T. Pressure sores: incidence, risk assessment and prevention. Br J Nurs 1997;6:319–322.
58. Schubert V, Perbeck L, Schubert PA. Skin microcirculatory and thermal changes in elderly subjects with early stage of pressure sores. Clin Physiol 1994;14:1–13.
59. Relander M, Palmer B. Recurrence of surgically treated pressure sores. Scan J Plast Reconstr Surg Hand Surg 1988;22:89–92.
60. Kierney PC, Engrav LH, Isik FF, Esselman PC, Cardenas DD, Rand RP. Results of 268 pressure sores in 158 patients managed jointly by plastic surgery and rehabilitation medicine. Plast Reconstr Surg 1998;102:765–772.
61. Burton CS. Venous ulcers. Am J Surg 1994;167:37S–40S; discussion 40S–41S.
62. Margolis DJ, Cohen JH. Management of chronic venous leg ulcers: a literature-guided approach. Clin Dermatol 1994;12:19–26.
63. Padberg FT, Back TL, Thompson PN, Hobson RW 2nd. Transcutaneous oxygen ($TcPo_2$) estimates probability of healing in the ischemic extremity. J Surg Res 1996;60:365–369.
64. Bernstein EF, Harisiadis L, Salomon GD, et al. Healing impairment of open wounds by skin irradiation. J Derm Surg Oncol 1994;20:757–760.
65. Robson MC. Infection in the surgical patient: an imbalance in the normal equilibrium. Clin Plast Surg 1979;6:493–503.
66. Robson MC. Wound infection. A failure of wound healing caused by an imbalance of bacteria. Surg Clin North Am 1997;77:637–650.
67. Robson MC, Stenberg BD, Heggers JP. Wound healing alterations caused by infection. Clin Plast Surg 1990;17:485–492.
68. Robson MC, Krizek TJ. Predicting skin graft survival. J Trauma 1973;13:213–217.
69. Murphy RC, Robson MC, Heggers JP, Kadowaki M. The effect of microbial contamination on musculocutaneous and random flaps. J Surg Res 1986;41:75–80.
70. Barbul A, Purtill WA. Nutrition in wound healing. Clin Dermatol 1994;12:133–140.
71. Muller MJ, Herndon DN. The challenge of burns. Lancet 1994;343:216–220.
72. Albina JE. Nutrition and wound healing. J Parenter Enteral Nutr 1994;18:367–376.
73. Thompson WD, Ravdin IS, Frank IL. Effect of hypoproteinemia on wound disruption. Arch Surg 1938;26:500–508.
74. Modolin M, Bevilacqua RG, Margarido NF, Lima-Goncalves E. Effects of protein depletion and repletion on experimental open wound contraction. Ann Plast Surg 1985;15:123–126.
75. Levenson SM, Demetriou AA. Metabolic factors. In: Cohen IK, Diegelmann RF, Lindblad WJ, eds. Wound Healing, Biochemical and Clinical Aspects. Philadelphia: W. B. Saunders Company, 1992:248–273.
76. Alcain FJ, Buron MI. Ascorbate on cell growth and differentiation. J Bioenerg Biomembr 1994;26:393–398.
77. Ehrlich HP, Hunt TK. Effects of cortisone and vitamin A on wound healing. Ann Surg 1968;167:324–328.
78. Ehrlich HP, Tarver H, Hunt TK. Effects of vitamin A and glucocorticoids upon inflammation and collagen synthesis. Ann Surg 1973;177:222–227.
79. Masse PG, Pritzker KP, Mendes MG, Boskey AL, Weiser H. Vitamin B_6 deficiency experimentally-induced bone and joint

disorder: microscopic, radiographic and biochemical evidence. Br J Nutr 1994;71:919–932.
80. LaVan FB, Hunt TK. Oxygen and wound healing. Clin Plast Surg 1990;17:463–472.
81. Allen DB, Maguire JJ, Mahdavian M, et al. Wound hypoxia and acidosis limit neutrophil bacterial killing mechanisms. Arch Surg 1997;132:991–996.
82. Hopf HW, Hunt TK, West JM, et al. Wound tissue oxygen tension predicts the risk of wound infection in surgical patients. Arch Surg 1997;132:997–1004; discussion 1005.
83. Jonsson K, Jensen JA, Goodson WH, et al. Tissue oxygenation, anemia, and perfusion in relation to wound healing in surgical patients. Ann Surg 1991;214:605–613.
84. Hunt TK, Pai MP. The effect of varying ambient oxygen tensions on wound metabolism and collagen synthesis. Surg Gynecol Obstet 1972;135:561–567.
85. Uhl E, Sirsjo A, Haapaniemi T, Nilsson G, Nylander G. Hyperbaric oxygen improves wound healing in normal and ischemic skin tissue. Plast Reconstr Surg 1994;93:835–841.
86. Werner S, Breeden M, Hubner G, Greenhalgh DG, Longaker MT. Induction of keratinocyte growth factor expression is reduced and delayed during wound healing in the genetically diabetic mouse. J Invest Dermatol 1994;103:469–473.
87. Beer HD, Longaker MT, Werner S. Reduced expression of PDGF and PDGF receptors during impaired wound healing. J Invest Dermatol 1997;109:132–138.
88. Goodson WH, Hunt TK. Wound healing in experimental diabetes mellitus: importance of early insulin therapy. Surg Forum 1978;29:95–98.
89. Goodson WH, Hunt TK. Deficient collagen formation by obese mice in a standard wound model. Am J Surg 1979;138:692–694.
90. Ehrlich HP, Hunt TK. The effects of cortisone and anabolic steroids on the tensile strength of healing wounds. Ann Surg 1969;170:203–206.
91. Marks JG Jr, Cano C, Leitzel K, Lipton A. Inhibition of wound healing by topical steroids. J Derm Surg Oncol 1983;9:819–821.
92. Brauchle M, Fassler R, Werner S. Suppression of keratinocyte growth factor expression by glucocorticoids in vitro and during wound healing. J Invest Dermatol 1995;105:579–584.
93. Schwentker A, Evans SM, Partington M, Johnson BL, Koch CJ, Thom SR. A model of wound healing in chronically radiation-damaged rat skin. Cancer Lett 1998;128:71–78.
94. Zhao LL, Davidson JD, Wee SC, Roth SI, Mustoe TA. Effect of hyperbaric oxygen and growth factors on rabbit ear ischemic ulcers. Arch Surg 1994;129:1043–1049.
95. Drake DB, Oishi SN. Wound healing considerations in chemotherapy and radiation therapy. Clin Plast Surg 1995;22:31–37.
96. Tredget EE, Nedelec B, Scott PG, Ghahary A. Hypertrophic scars, keloids, and contractures. The cellular and molecular basis for therapy. Surg Clin North Am 1997;77:701–730.
97. Yang GP, Lim IJ, Phan TT, Lorenz HP, Longaker MT. From scarless fetal wounds to keloids: molecular studies in wound healing. Wound Repair Regen 2003;11:411–418.
98. Wassermann RJ, Polo M, Smith P, Wang X, Ko F, Robson MC. Differential production of apoptosis-modulating proteins in patients with hypertrophic burn scar. J Surg Res 1998;75:74–80.
99. Blackburn WR, Cosman B. Histologic basis of keloid and hypertrophic scar differentiation. Clinicopathologic correlation. Arch Pathol 1966;82:65–71.
100. Kischer CW, Shetlar MR, Chvapil M. Hypertrophic scars and keloids: a review and new concept concerning their origin. Scan Electron Microsc 1982(pt 4):1699–1713.
101. Scott PG, Dodd CM, Ghahary A, Shen YJ, Tredget EE. Fibroblasts from post-burn hypertrophic scar tissue synthesize less decorin than normal dermal fibroblasts. Clin Sci 1998;94:541–547.
102. Bettinger DA, Yager DR, Diegelmann RF, Cohen IK. The effect of TGF-beta on keloid fibroblast proliferation and collagen synthesis. Plast Reconstr Surg 1996;98:827–833.
103. Younai S, Nichter LS, Wellisz T, Reinisch J, Nimni ME, Tuan TL. Modulation of collagen synthesis by transforming growth factor-beta in keloid and hypertrophic scar fibroblasts. Ann Plast Surg 1994;33:148–151.
104. Mustoe TA, Cooter RD, Gold MH, et al. International clinical recommendations on scar management. Plast Reconstr Surg 2002;110:560–571.
105. Alster T. Laser scar revision: comparison study of 585-nm pulsed dye laser with and without intralesional corticosteroids. Dermatol Surg 2003;29:25–29.
106. Murray JC. Keloids and hypertrophic scars. Clin Dermatol 1994;12:27–37.
107. Appleton I, Brown NJ, Willoughby DA. Apoptosis, necrosis, and proliferation: possible implications in the etiology of keloids. Am J Pathol 1996;149:1441–1447.
108. Sayah DN, Shaw WW, Holmes EC, et al. Downregulation of apoptosis genes accounts for aberrant cellular growth in keloid tissue. Surg Forum 1998;49:596–598.
109. Tuan TL, Nichter LS. The molecular basis of keloid and hypertrophic scar formation. Mol Med Today 1998;4:19–24.
110. Kikuchi K, Kadono T, Takehara K. Effects of various growth factors and histamine on cultured keloid fibroblasts. Dermatology 1995;190:4–8.
111. Lim IJ, Phan TT, Song C, Tan WT, Longaker MT. Investigation of the influence of keloid-derived keratinocytes of fibroblast growth and proliferation in vitro. Plast Reconstr Surg 2001;107:797–808.
112. Maguire HC. Treatment of keloids with triamcinolone acetonide injected intralesionally. JAMA 1965;192:325–327.
113. Kauh YC, Rouda S, Mondragon G, et al. Major suppression of pro-alpha1(I) type I collagen gene expression in the dermis after keloid excision and immediate intrawound injection of triamcinolone acetonide. J Am Acad Dermatol 1997;37:586–589.
114. Klumpar DI, Murray JC, Anscher M. Keloids treated with excision followed by radiation therapy. J Am Acad Dermatol 1994;31(2 pt 1):225–231.
115. Minkowitz F. Regression of massive keloid following partial excision and post-operative intralesional administration of triamcinolone. Br J Plast Surg 1967;20:432–435.
116. Griffith BH, Monroe CW, McKinney P. A follow-up study on the treatment of keloids with triamcinolone acetonide. Plast Reconstr Surg 1970;46:145–150.
117. Lee SM, Ngim CK, Chan YY, Ho MJ. A comparison of Sil-K and Epiderm in scar management. Burns 1996;22:483–487.
118. Palmieri B, Gozzi G, Palmieri G. Vitamin E added silicone gel sheets for treatment of hypertrophic scars and keloids. Int J Dermatol 1995;34:506–509.
119. Kelly AP. Medical and surgical therapies for keloids. Dermatol Ther 2004;17:212–218.
120. Berman B, Villa A. Imiquimod 5% cream for keloid management. Dermatol Surg 2003;29:1050–1051.
121. Chau D, Mancoll JS, Lee S, et al. Tamoxifen downregulates TGF-beta production in keloid fibroblasts. Ann Plast Surg 1998;40:490–493.
122. Mancoll JS, Chau D, Munger J, et al. Tamoxifen downregulates TGF-β production by keloid fibroblasts. Surg Forum 1997;48:133–137.
123. Otani Y, Tabata Y, Ikada Y. A new biological glue from gelatin and poly (L-glutamic acid). J Biomed Mater Res 1996;31:158–166.
124. DeBono R. A simple, inexpensive method for precise application of cyanoacrylate tissue adhesive. Plast Reconstr Surg 1997;100:447–450.

125. Breuing K, Eriksson E, Liu P, Miller DR. Healing of partial thickness porcine skin wounds in a liquid environment. J Surg Res 1992;52:50–58.
126. Svensjo T, Pomahac B, Yao F, Slama J, Eriksson E. Accelerated healing of full-thickness skin wounds in a wet environment. Plast Reconstr Surg 2000;106:602–612; discussion 613–614.
127. Argenta LC, Morykwas MJ. Vacuum-assisted closure: a new method for wound control and treatment: clinical experience. Ann Plast Surg 1997;38:563–576; discussion 577.
128. Genecov DG, Schneider AM, Morykwas MJ, Parker D, White WL, Argenta LC. A controlled subatmospheric pressure dressing increases the rate of skin graft donor site reepithelialization. Ann Plast Surg 1998;40:219–225.
129. Richard JL, Parer RC, Daures JP, et al. Effect of topical basic fibroblast growth factor on the healing of chronic diabetic neuropathic ulcer of the foot. A pilot, randomized, double-blind, placebo-controlled study. Diabetes Care 1995;18:64–69.
130. Steed DL. Clinical evaluation of recombinant human platelet-derived growth factor for the treatment of lower extremity diabetic ulcers. Diabetic Ulcer Study Group. J Vasc Surg 1995;21:71–78; discussion 79–81.
131. Steed DL, Donohoe D, Webster MW, Lindsley L. Effect of extensive debridement and treatment on the healing of diabetic foot ulcers. Diabetic Ulcer Study Group. J Am Coll Surg 1996;183:61–64.
132. Pierce GF, Tarpley JE, Allman RM, et al. Tissue repair processes in healing chronic pressure ulcers treated with recombinant platelet-derived growth factor BB. Am J Pathol 1994;145:1399–1410.
133. Jones SC, Curtsinger LJ, Whalen JD, et al. Effect of topical recombinant TGF-beta on healing of partial thickness injuries. J Surg Res 1991;51:344–352.
134. Bullen EC, Longaker MT, Updike DL, et al. Tissue inhibitor of metalloproteinases-1 is decreased and activated gelatinases are increased in chronic wounds. J Invest Dermatol 1995;104:236–240.
135. Feedar JA. Clinical management of chronic wounds. In: McCulloch JM, Kloth LC, Feedar JA, eds. Wound Healing Alternatives in Management. Philadelphia: F. A. Davis Company, 1995:137–185.

11

Diagnosis and Treatment of Infection

David L. Dunn

Over the span of recorded history, the occurrence of serious infection after injury has been the rule rather than the exception, with such sequelae of our interaction with the microbial world often resulting in death. For centuries, infection after traumatic wounding was considered a desirable outcome, as evidenced by the epithet "laudable pus," which, once drained, was associated with wound healing in those patients who were able to survive both the inciting event and the ensuing infection. During the past century, the development and use of anesthesia, fluid resuscitation, blood transfusion, and hemodynamic monitoring were key advances that allowed surgical practitioners to carry out increasingly complex procedures. However, before the widespread application of aseptic surgical technique and the subsequent discovery and therapeutic use of antimicrobial agents, the evolution and performance of even routine surgical procedures was hindered by the frequent association with serious, often life-threatening infections.

Considering the large numbers of microbes that individuals encounter and the magnitude, complexity, and frequency with which many surgical procedures are now performed, it is noteworthy that more infections do not occur. Today, we have the ability to prevent many, albeit not all, infections from developing after operative procedures and subsequent to trauma, as well as the capacity to effectively diagnose and treat most that do arise. However, despite considerable progress in the areas of prevention, diagnosis, and therapy, postoperative nosocomial infection as well as those types of infection that require surgical intervention as a component of treatment continue to be associated with considerable morbidity and mortality. It is of paramount importance, therefore, that the surgical practitioner be familiar with the precepts of diagnosis and management of infectious diseases and the appropriate use of antimicrobial agents for prophylaxis and therapy.

Microbes and Host Defenses

The development of infection, whether it remains contained at a specific site or spreads to adjacent or distant sites via the bloodstream and whether it exerts deleterious effects on the host, is highly dependent on the outcome of the interaction of invading microbes with innate host defenses. The complex process of host–microbe interactions can be conceptualized as an equation in which the risk of infection is directly proportional to a number of microbial factors and inversely proportional to the presence and vigor of various facets of host defenses. Microbial factors of importance include (1) number (inoculum size) and types of microbes, (2) rate of microbial proliferation, and (3) microbial virulence factors. These aspects are counterbalanced by host factors that include (1) strength of resident host defenses in the local environment at the site of microbial invasion, (2) magnitude and rate of recruitment of host defenses to the site of infection, and (3) potency of systemic host defenses should either local containment of microbes fail or microbes are directly introduced into the bloodstream. Each component of the following infection risk equation is discussed in turn, although it should be noted that precise characterization and quantitation of each element rarely is possible even in experimental animal models, let alone the clinical setting. However, it is useful to consider when determining whether intervention such as surgery, administration of antibiotics, or both should be undertaken.

$$\begin{aligned}\text{Infection} &= \text{Microbial Invasion/Host defenses}\\ &= (\text{Inoculum size} \times \text{Species} \times \text{Division rate}\\ &\quad \times \text{Virulence factors})/[\text{Potency}\\ &\quad (\text{Resident/Recruited/Systemic})\\ &\quad \times \text{Recruitment rate/Magnitude}]\end{aligned}$$

Classification and Identification of Microbes

Microbes capable of causing infection may be encountered in the external environment or as part of the host microflora. The scope of potential pathogens that the surgeon may be called on to diagnose and treat is enormous and includes many different bacteria, fungi, viruses, and parasites. These microbes are classified on the basis of a variety of characteristics that range from colonial morphology directly visualized without magnification to sophisticated genetic analysis. Microbiological diagnostic techniques of importance fall into several general categories: (1) differential staining; (2) isolation via colonial selection; (3) differential growth under various conditions; (4) observation of specific growth characteristics or traits; (5) direct identification of microbial antigens via immunological assays or demonstration of the presence of a host antibody response or, less commonly, a cellular immune response directed against them; and (6) identification of microbial genetic material.

Preliminary identification of bacteria and fungi within a sample of body fluid or tissue suspected of harboring infection is undertaken via microscopic observation using a number of different stains. Thereafter, in vitro growth in various types of media that facilitate isolation of the organism in pure culture takes place using standard techniques. For example, streaking onto an agar plate of a sample from an initial culture into which the specimen has been inoculated facilitates selection of a single bacterial colony for further growth in routine media. Use of selective enrichment media to facilitate isolation of a particular type of organism also can be undertaken. A pure culture can then be grown and examined for colonial morphology, the presence of motility, metabolic by-products (e.g., gas formation), or toxin formation (e.g., hemolysins). Concurrently, differential growth characteristics in aerobic or anaerobic environments, at different temperatures, with or without the presence of certain nutrients or exogenous compounds (e.g., antibiotics), as well as specific staining characteristics are observed; in composite, these steps allow precise identification.

Those microbes that do not readily replicate in vitro are identified by antibody-based tests that serve to detect specific microbial antigens, the host immune response to them, or both. These tests are of particular use for identifying the presence of bacteria and fungi that exhibit fastidious nutritional requirements or that replicate slowly, many viruses that do not readily replicate in mammalian cell lines, and most parasites because they possess complex life cycles that require a host for growth. Sophisticated techniques such as phase contrast and transmission or scanning electron microscopy for distinguishing characteristic microbial particles or pathological effects and for identification and analysis of genetic sequences unique to microbial ribosomal RNA or DNA increasingly are employed as detection tools. Automated analysis in which vast arrays of characteristic genetic sequences of potential pathogens are embedded on microchips to facilitate rapid, precise identification of microbes from minuscule tissue or body fluid samples may be realized in the near future.

Bacteria are responsible for the majority of surgical infectious diseases, and particular species are identified according to their Gram stain and growth characteristics subsequent to isolation from a site of suspected or overt infection. The Gram stain is a simple but important assay that can be performed rapidly by first fixing the specimen on a microscope slide using heat, staining it with crystal violet dye, fixing it with iodine-KI solution as a mordant, then washing the specimen with either acetone or alcohol and counterstaining with a red dye such as safranin. Microscopic characteristics related to initial dye retention due to the structure of the bacterial cell wall serve to define bacteria according to color—gram positive (blue) or gram negative (red). Other parameters such as shape (round cocci, rodlike bacilli); patterns of division (single organisms, groups of organisms in pairs [diplococci], clusters [staphylococci], or chains [streptococci]); and presence and location of spores (e.g., terminal, central) facilitate initial identification.

Gram-positive bacteria of importance to surgeons include aerobes such as staphylococci (*Staphylococcus aureus* and *Staphylococcus epidermidis*), enterococci (*Enterococcus faecalis* and *Enterococcus faecium*), streptococci that are classified according to their hemolytic and antigenic properties (e.g., β-hemolytic *Streptococcus pyogenes*, α-hemolytic [also termed viridans] such as *Streptococcus salivarius*, as well as *Streptococcus pneumoniae*) or anaerobic growth requirements (peptostreptococci and peptidostreptococci). Relevant aerobic gram-negative bacteria are numerous, but common pathogenic types include those belonging to the family Enterobacteriaceae such as *Escherichia coli*, *Klebsiella pneumonia*, *Serratia marcescens*, *Enterobacter* spp., *Acinetobacter* spp., and *Citrobacter* spp. as well as pseudomonads such as *Pseudomonas aeruginosa*, *Pseudomonas cepacia*, and *Pseudomonas fluorescens*. Anaerobic bacteria are numerous as well, encompassing genera including *Bacteroides*, *Fusobacterium*, and *Clostridia*. Less common bacterial organisms such as *Nocardia asteroides*, *Mycobacterium tuberculosis*, *Mycobacterium avium-intracellulare*, *Mycobacterium chelonei*, *Mycobacterium kansasii*, and other species can be identified initially by use of the Ziehl–Neelsen stain; in this test, only such organisms remain stained after exposure to acetic acid, hence the term *acid-fast* bacilli. Observation of growth characteristics in vitro on different types of media also allows identification, although many of these organisms grow slowly, necessitating observation for several weeks or even months. Organisms such as *Legionella pneumophila* and *Legionella micdadei* are not grown readily in vitro and are identified by immunofluorescence staining techniques and the presence of a host antibody response.

Similar principles are applied for identification of fungi, although many of these microbes are dimorphic, replicating as single, separate cells (yeast) under certain nutrient and temperature conditions and as colonies in which the cells form long filaments (hyphae) under others. Occasionally, the presence of these pathogens can be deduced from the observation of characteristic large gram-positive microbes on Gram staining, but more commonly they are identified by use of special stains (e.g., KOH, India ink, Giemsa, methanamine silver). The manner in which cell division (septation) and chain branching (ramification) occurs in stained specimens or after growth in vitro and staining facilitates initial identification. Subsequently, observation of differential growth characteristics in vitro similar to that described for bacteria as well as at different temperatures (25°C and 37°C) leads to the identification of a specific microbe. Fungi of importance in surgery include *Candida albicans*, *Candida glabrata*, *Candida krusei*, *Candida parapsilosis*, *Candida tropicalis*, and other species; *Aspergillis fumigatus*, *Aspergillis niger*, *Aspergillis terreus*, and other species; *Cryptococcus neoformans*; *Histoplasma capsulatum*; *Blastomyces dermatitidis*; and *Mucor* and *Rhizopus* spp.

Viruses of importance to surgeons include those belonging to the class Herpesviridae, such as cytomegalovirus (CMV), herpes simplex virus (HSV); those that, albeit unrelated, cause hepatitis (primarily hepatitis B virus [HBV] and hepatitis C virus [HCV]); as well as so-called retroviruses such as human immunodeficiency virus (HIV) and a number of other agents. Although growth in cell culture is possible for some pathogens, the presence of many viruses must be inferred by identification of the host immune (e.g., antibody) response. Use of a monoclonal antibody that is directed against a specific viral antigen and labeled with a marker (enzyme or immunofluorescent compound) can be useful for rapid microscopic identification of the presence of viral pathogens in body fluids or tissues. The presence of certain viral pathogens can be ascertained by use of routine light microscopy for identification of characteristic cytopathic abnormalities (e.g., CMV inclusion bodies) or via observation of characteristic viral particles via electron microscopy. Increasingly, viruses are identified based on the presence of viral genetic material using a test based on the polymerase chain reaction (PCR). As mentioned, the presence of parasites generally is confirmed by direct microscopic identification, by identification of a host antibody response to parasitic antigens, or the presence of these antigens by use of antibody-based tests, or by a combination of these assays.

Table 11.1 provides a list of those pathogens of importance that is by no means exhaustive. The infectious diseases that they cause in surgical patients are discussed in greater detail next.

TABLE 11.1. Common Microbial Pathogens Capable of Causing Infection in Surgical Patients.

Gram-positive bacterial aerobes
Enterococcus faecium, faecalis
Staphylococcus aureus, epidermidis
Streptococcus pyogenes
Streptococcus pneumoniae
Streptococcus salivarius
Gram-negative bacterial aerobes
Acinetobacter calcoaceticus
Aeromonas hydrophila
Citrobacter freundii
Enterobacter cloacae, aerogenes
Escherichia coli
Hemophilus influenza
Klebsiella pneumoniae
Morganella morgagnii
Proteus mirabilis
Providencia stuartii
Pseudomonas aeruginosa
Pseudomonas cepacia, fluorescens
Serratia marcescens
Xanthomonas maltophilia
Fungi
Absidia
Aspergillus fumigatus
Aspergillus niger, terreus, flavus
Blastomyces dermatiditis
Candida albicans
Candida glabrata, torulopsis, parapsilopsis, krusei
Coccidioides imitis
Cryptococcus neoformans
Fusarium
Histoplasma capsulatum
Mucor
Pneumocystis carinii
Rhizopus
Gram-positive bacterial anaerobes
Clostridium perfringens, tetani, septicum
Clostridium difficile
Peptidostreptococcus
Peptostreptococcus
Gram-negative bacterial anaerobes
Bacteroides fragilis
Bacteroides distasonis, thetaiotaomicron
Fusobacterium
Acid-fast bacteria
Mycobacterium avium-intracellulare
Mycobacterium kansasii, chelonei
Mycobacterium tuberculosis
Nocardia asteroides and brasiliensis
Other bacteria
Legionella pneumophila, micdadii
Listeria monocytogenes
Viruses
Cytomegalovirus
Epstein–Barr virus
Hepatitis B, C, and D viruses
Herpes simplex virus
Herpesvirus 6
Human immunodeficiency virus
Varicella zoster virus

Microbial Factors of Importance in the Development of Infection

One of the primary determinants of whether infection develops is the size of the initial microbial inoculum, which for bacteria is expressed in terms of colony-forming units (CFU). Even large numbers of low-virulence microbes can overwhelm resident and recruited host defenses by direct toxicity or via subsequent division and proliferation, with the end result morbidity in the form of established infection, which can in turn be lethal. Two major reservoirs of microbes exist that can form the initial inoculum leading to infection in surgical patients: (1) host endogenous microflora and (2) microbes within the external milieu, which often represents the nosocomial environment for hospitalized individuals. As discussed, the presence of host microflora is normal in healthy individuals; these microbes as well as microbes in the environment are precluded from invading and proliferating within the body by a number of potent host defense mechanisms.

The rate at which microbes proliferate in a specific environment represents a critical factor in the development of infection. Particularly in relation to bacteria and fungi, microbial division depends on ambient temperature and oxygen concentration, sources of nutrients, and inherent properties that determine the maximal division rate under optimal conditions. After provided with ideal growth conditions in vitro, microbes experience a lag phase, following which they enter log-phase growth, during which exponential cell division occurs. Limitation of growth occurs thereafter as nutrients are expended and microbial by-products accumulate, followed by microbial death. In vivo, however, conditions are much more complex, as evidenced by our incomplete understanding of the manner in which specific microbes cause infection only in certain tissues and only in particular patients. In addition, microbial growth is dependent on the above-mentioned factors as well as the capacity of one type of microbe to inhibit or promote the growth of another, the latter process being termed microbial synergy if associated with adverse effects greater than those caused by either organism alone during clinical infection. Finally, microbes may secrete toxins only under certain growth conditions, and some possess virulence mechanisms such as large polysaccharide capsules or leukocyte toxins that render them capable of evading or inhibiting host defenses.

The terms *pathogenicity* and *virulence* are relative designations and must be considered in relation to both host defenses and microbial virulence mechanisms (e.g., toxin secretion). Pathogenic microbes are those that are capable of causing disease; those that cause severe infection consistently are termed virulent. Low-virulence microbes are those that inconsistently cause infectious diseases in normal individuals. However, the host exists in a state of equilibrium with resident microflora and microbes within the environment that possess pathogenic potential but are interdicted from causing disease by host defenses. Disruption or suppression of host defenses may allow invasion of microbes. Intriguingly, only some species proliferate and cause infection, although even low-virulence organisms that rarely cause infection in an individual with intact host defense mechanisms can become pathogens in an immunosuppressed patient.

Host Defenses

Once a portal of entry for microbes is established (e.g., surgical wound, indwelling catheter, gut perforation), resident host defenses act to attempt to eliminate microbes that are present, and additional host defenses are recruited to the site of entry as microbes proliferate. The mammalian host possesses many different types of endogenous defense mechanisms that serve to prevent microbial invasion, limit proliferation of microbes within the host, and sequester or eradicate invading microbes. These defenses consist of (1) physical barriers, (2) sequestration mechanisms, and (3) humoral and cellular host defenses in association with cytokines. All host defenses are tightly integrated such that the various components function as a complex, highly regulated system that is extremely effective in coping with microbial invaders. In addition, some elements of host defenses are redundant; however, despite this redundancy, perturbation of one or more components may have a substantial negative impact on resistance to infection.

Physical Barriers and Host Microflora

The first line of host defense against both exogenous and endogenous microbes consists of physical, anatomical barriers. The hallmark of all barriers is that they possess either an epithelial (integument) or endothelial (respiratory, gut, urogenital) surface. These barriers serve to interdict the ingress of microbes into areas of the host that are sterile under normal circumstances. Microbes normally are associated with some but not all barriers, and in composite they are termed resident, endogenous, or autochthonous microflora. For example, the urogenital, biliary, pancreatic ductal, and distal respiratory endothelia do not possess resident microflora in healthy individuals, although microbes may be present if these barriers are affected by disease (e.g., malignancy, inflammation, calculi, foreign body) or if microorganisms are introduced from an external source (e.g., urinary catheter, pulmonary aspiration). In contradistinction, significant numbers of microbes are associated with the skin and skin appendages as well as the oropharynx and the distal gastrointestinal tract. Common autochthonous microbes in various parts of the body are delineated in Table 11.2.

TABLE 11.2. Common Autochthonous Microbes in Various Parts of the Body.

Region	*Microbes*[a]	*Quantity*[b]
Skin (all areas)	*Acinetobacter* *Brevibacterium* *Corynebacterium* *Micrococcus* *Pityrosporum* *Proprionibacterium* ***Staphylococcus aureus*** *and* ***epidermidis*** ***Streptococcus*** (nonenterococcal)	102–103
Skin (infraumbilical)	*Candida* *Corynebacterium* ***Streptococcus faecalis*** *and* ***faecium*** ***Escherichia coli*** *Proprionibacterium* ***Staphylococcus aureus*** *and* ***epidermidis*** ***Streptococcus*** (nonenterococcal)	102–105
Oropharynx	*Actinomyces* ***Bacteroides*** (non-*fragilis*) *Bifidobacterium* *Eubacterium* ***Fusobacterium*** ***Haemophilus*** *Moraxella* ***Peptostreptoccus*** *Porphyromonas* *Prevotella* ***Staphylococcus aureus*** *and* ***epidermidis*** ***Streptococcus*** (nonenterococcal) *Veillonella*	109–1011
Stomach	***Candida*** ***Streptococcus*** (nonenterococcal)	102–103
Proximal small intestine	***Bacteroides fragilis*** and other spp. *Bifidobacterium* *Clostridium* ***Escherichia coli*** and other *Enterobacteriaceae* *Eubacterium* *Lactobacillus* ***Peptostreptococcus*** *Proprionibacterium*	103–107
Distal ileum	***Streptococcus faecalis, faecium***	105–108
Colorectum	*Veillonella*	1011–1012

[a]Potentially pathogenic organisms are designated in **bold type**.

[b]Colony-forming units (CFU)/ml or per gram feces.

While barrier function remains intact, resident microflora are saprophytes, commensals, or symbionts; however, these same microbes often represent the initial inoculum of pathogens when damage to or breach of a barrier occurs. This information is of considerable importance to surgeons because prevention of infection is predicated on reducing the number of resident microbes before barrier disruption using topical microbicides or intraluminal antiseptics or antibiotics plus systemic antibiotics to reduce the threat of microbial invasion and proliferation once wounding—either planned or traumatic—occurs.

First and foremost among the physical barriers is the integument. This extensive structure possesses the largest interface for contact with the external microbial milieu, acting to prevent ingress of pathogens. In addition, the skin possesses its own resident microflora that may interdict the attachment and invasion of noncommensal microbes. Under normal conditions, the predominant organisms are gram-positive aerobic microbes belonging to the genera *Staphylococcus* and *Streptococcus*, as well as *Corynebacterium* and anaerobic *Proprionibacterium* species. These organisms plus *E. faecalis*, *E. faecium*, *E. coli* and yeast such as *C. albicans* can be isolated in the inguinal, perineal, and gluteal infraumbilical regions. Ancillary host defenses also exist as part of the integumentary barrier. For example, sebaceous glands secrete a variety of compounds that exhibit antimicrobial activity, which most likely both limits the number of resident microflora and prevents extensive colonization by virulent pathogens including *S. aureus* and *S. pyogenes.*

The respiratory tract possesses a number of host defense mechanisms, of which mucous secretion and ciliary action of specialized epithelial cells are the most critical. Mucus traps particles, including microbes, that are swept into the upper airways and oropharynx by ciliary action of specialized respiratory epithelial cells; coughing and expectoration follow. Any process that diminishes these host defenses can lead to microbial proliferation and invasion, usually eventuating in the presence of increasing numbers of microbes such that these organisms enter the distal branches of the respiratory tract, causing bronchitis or pneumonia.

The number of endogenous microbes varies throughout the gastrointestinal tract. Large numbers ($\sim 10^{11}$ CFU/ml) of aerobic and anaerobic bacteria are present at both ends of the gut, that is, oropharynx and colorectum, although the typical species differ somewhat among these two sites.[1] Few microbes (10^{2}–10^{3} CFU/ml) are present within the normal stomach because of the low pH and initial slow transit, which serve to promote microbial killing of ingested microbes in this highly acidic environment. Disease processes and drugs that inhibit gastric acidity may allow overgrowth of microbes in the stomach and thereby the small intestine, although in the absence of obstruction the relatively rapid transit time in the latter portion of the gut moves fluid, particles, and microbes aborally, counteracting overgrowth.

Normally, the upper portion of the small-bowel lumen contains few microbes, but the number of resident microbes gradually increases aborally such that about 10^{5}–10^{8} CFU/ml are present in the terminal ileum. The number of gut microbes present distal to the ileocecal valve increases exponentially such that within the sigmoid colon and rectum about 10^{11}–10^{12} CFU/g feces are present. The predominant forms are gram-negative and gram-positive aerobes such as *E. coli*, *E. faecalis*, and *E. faecium*, as well as facultative and strict anaerobes such as *Bacteroides fragilis*, *Bacteroides distasonis*, *Bacteroides thetaiotomicron*, *Peptostreptococcus* and *Fusobacterium* species, and many other anaerobic microbes. Anaerobes represent the predominant type of microbe, outnumbering aerobes by about 100 to 1.

Large numbers of microbes exist within a dense layer of mucus that covers gut endothelial cells. Microbes adhere to gut endothelial cells, mucus, and each other; although these complex adherence interactions are not understood entirely, the autochthonous microflora create a highly anaerobic environment and act to prevent adherence, proliferation, overgrowth, and invasion of pathogens. This phenomenon is associated with the physical barrier and is termed *colonization resistance*. It probably occurs at all barriers that possess microflora, but it has been best characterized in the gut.

Sequestration Mechanisms

The mammalian host possesses a number of primitive host defenses that serve to sequester microbes at the site of infection, thereby preventing dissemination. In any tissue, resident and recruited host defenses attempt to kill and eradicate all microbes, and the influx of inflammatory fluid contains fibrinogen, which during polymerization to fibrin traps bacteria in the extracellular milieu.[2,3] Also, within the abdomen, the omentum moves to a site of viscus perforation or inflammatory disease; this process, in conjunction with ileus and intestinal distension, serves to wall off infection. However, sequestration also partitions microbes from resident and recruited host defenses, with the end result invariably an abscess. The purulent material within the abscess represents the by-product of the death of both microbes and local and recruited humoral and cellular host defense components, and it is relatively impermeable to recruitment of additional host defenses or penetration of antibiotics. In addition, the presence of viable microbes within the abscess renders it a nidus for intermittent bacteremic episodes and complications related to its presence such as fever, pain, and bowel obstruction within the abdomen. Most likely, sequestration host defenses serve to convert serious, immediately life-threatening infections into more indolent, albeit chronic, types of infection. Invariably, an abscess requires some form of drainage, although on occasion spontaneous discharge occurs. Rarely, if ever, can treatment be accomplished with antibiotics alone.

Finally, a number of proteins are present within the plasma and extracellular milieu that act to sequester nutrients that microbes require to divide. For example, transferrin and lactoferrin bind iron and thus limit the amount of this critical microbial growth factor. Low or high oxygen tension in certain parts of the body limits growth of aerobes or anaerobes, respectively.

Humoral and Cellular Immunity

Humoral immunity, so named because the components circulate within blood and body fluids as proteins, consists of two components: (1) antibodies (immunoglobulin, Ig) and (2) complement.[4] Antibodies are composed of a basic structure, two similar heavy (α, δ, ε, γ, or μ) and two similar light (κ or λ) chains. Disulfide bonds bind each heavy chain to one another, and a light chain is bound to each heavy chain in the Ig molecule in a similar fashion. Several distinct hypervariable regions within the terminal portion of the heavy and light chains spatially fold to form the region that for each heavy–light chain pair binds a specific antigen. Different antibodies may be capable of binding to different portions of an antigen, particularly if the antigen is a large, complex structure such as a microbe. The most limited antigenic region to which an antibody binds is termed an *epitope*, typically defined by competitive inhibition of binding of two or more distinct monoclonal antibodies. In humans, there are five different classes of antibodies: IgG, IgM, IgD, IgE, and IgA. There are four subclasses of IgG (IgG_{1-4}) and two of IgA ($IgA_{1,2}$). In addition, certain portions of the heavy chain of IgM and IgG possess the capacity to activate the complement cascade (IgM >> IgG) once antigen binding occurs, and the terminal Fc portion of some subclasses of IgG is capable of binding to leukocyte receptors, markedly enhancing phagocytosis.

Antibodies are produced by B lymphocytes in response to the presence of substances, including microbes, that the mammalian host recognizes as a foreign antigen and not part of itself. In composite, B cells possess the ability to make a huge number of different Ig molecules ($>10^8$) via recombination and somatic mutation of genes that encode for the constant, variable, and hypervariable regions of each heavy and light chain; each B cell is capable of secreting Ig that binds to a specific antigen. The B-cell-bound IgD is capable of binding antigen directly, which triggers proliferation of a clone of B cells that secretes antibody; some of these cells circulate for long periods of time (memory cells). It has become clear, however, that T-helper lymphocytes and macrophages interact with B cells, acting as accessory cells that facilitate the antibody response. Some antigens are capable of directly stimulating B cells to produce antibody absent accessory cell interactions, although in general this type of response is less vigorous.

The humoral immune response serves to target multiantigenic pathogens for complement-mediated lysis and augmented phagocytosis that occurs via the Fc portion of the Ig molecule. Eventually, antigens are cleared from the body sites or the systemic circulation if they are present in the circulation. Most types of antigens engender production of antibody of the pentameric IgM class initially, but within about 2 to 3 weeks antibody of similar binding specificity but of the IgG class is secreted. Thereafter, if antigen persists or reexposure occurs after initial clearance, IgG of greater binding affinity is produced in ever-larger amounts. Two subclasses of dimeric IgA (IgA_1, IgA_2) are secreted at mucosal surfaces by submucosal resident B lymphocytes, which act to prevent the ingress of antigens, including pathogenic microbes, while IgE is present in small amounts in the circulation and is secreted into the respiratory tract. Although natural antibodies exist in low levels to many pathogens, initial contact followed by subsequent exposure to a particular pathogen triggers a more intense response because of the presence of memory cells. This phenomenon is the basis for vaccination against specific pathogens or toxins.

Complement consists of a large number of inactive proteins that circulate within the bloodstream; these proteins are activated and thereby modified in a specific sequence, several steps of which serve to trigger the production of large amounts of bioactive compounds. Activation of this cascade of proteins occurs by means of the binding of certain types of Ig to microbial antigens (IgM is extremely efficient) and via direct activation by specific components of the microbial cell wall, such as gram-negative bacterial lipopolysaccharide (endotoxin, LPS) or yeast saccharides such as *Candida* mannan. Two different complement activation pathways (classical, alternate [Properdin]) lead to a single common pathway in which complement protein fragments play key roles in the host defense response. For example, C3b and C4b enhance Ig adherence, while C3bi and C1q serve as opsonins, leading to enhanced phagocytosis of microbes by leukocytes. The fragments C5a, C3a, and C4a are anaphylatoxins (listed in order of potency) acting to increase vascular permeability and concurrent influx of additional proteins; C5a also is a chemoattractant that causes phagocytic cell chemotaxis. Finally, C5b6–9 form what is termed a membrane attack complex that creates a hole in microbes, leading to osmotic cell disruption and death.

Monocytes and polymorphonuclear leukocytes (PMNs) are capable of engulfing microbes via the process of phagocytosis. Once internalized, the portion of the leukocyte membrane that has enveloped the pathogen (phagocytic vacuole) fuses with an intracellular structure termed the *lysosome*, which contains a variety of enzymes (e.g., lysozyme, cathepsin) and reactive oxygen metabolites (O_2–, OH) that serve to kill and degrade the invading microorganism. The body contains large numbers of resident macrophages within various tissues that serve as one of the first lines of host defense against microbial invasion. For example, pulmonary alveolar macrophages within the lung, Kupffer cells within the liver, and peritoneal macrophages act in this capacity.

Microbial invasion also triggers the recruitment of PMNs to the site of infection via the aforementioned activity of the complement cascade and because of the presence of peptide sequences in which *N*-formyl methionine is present. The latter compounds are found in microbes and mammalian mitochondria and are potent chemoattractants for PMNs. This characteristic leads to an influx of large numbers of these highly active phagocytic cells within 2 to 4 h of invasion, with the magnitude and duration of this response proportional to the size of the inoculum and ability of the microbes to proliferate and remain at the site of infection or spread. Both macrophages and PMNs secrete a number of highly bioactive substances into the internal milieu during cellular activation. Unfortunately, many of these compounds also exert deleterious effects on the host. For example, the contents of lysosomes and reactive oxygen metabolites are extremely toxic to mammalian cells, and release of copious amounts of cytokines secreted by macrophages in response to bacterial cell wall products is thought to be responsible in large part for sepsis syndrome.

Cytokines function as regulatory molecules that play an important role during infection as follows: (1) coordination of cellular immunity with other aspects of host defense and (2) regulation of host defense via augmentation and suppression of specific defense components, including their own activity. Bacteria and fungal cell wall compounds trigger macrophages to synthesize and secrete large amounts of what are termed *proinflammatory cytokines*: tumor necrosis factor-α (TNF-α), interleukin-1β (IL-1β), interleukin-6 (IL-6), and interferon-γ (IFN-γ). Presumably because cytokines exert such potent effects within the local tissue environment and systematically, counterregulatory compounds are secreted in response to the release of proinflammatory cytokines. This process has been precisely delineated in response to endotoxin challenge in animals and humans as this gram-negative microbial cell wall component represents an extremely potent macrophage activator provoking cytokine secretion. Similar effects occur in response to challenge with intact gram-negative bacteria, as well as gram-positive bacteria and yeast. It should be noted, however, that the sequence of events that occurs during clinical infection has been difficult to elucidate, probably because the magnitude, temporal onset, and duration of the infectious insult as well as the ensuing host response varies from patient to patient.

Subsequent to endotoxin challenge, it is well established that peak serum levels of TNF-α occur within 1.5 to 2h and rapidly decline thereafter in animals and humans.[5] Maximal secretion of IL-1β occurs slightly later, although it has been more difficult to measure, and elevated levels are observed inconsistently, particularly during clinical infection. The IL-6 levels rise even later (~4h) after endotoxin injection in animals and humans, as do IL-8 levels in humans.[6] Peak TNF-α levels can occur much later (10–16h) after bacterial challenge in experimental models of infection, in contrast to the early peak evidenced after endotoxin injection.[7] This difference is most probably related to the fact that host defense initially may be able to contain infection, after which such containment fails and unchecked microbial proliferation occurs. Cytokines, acting in concert with the cellular and humoral branches of the immune system, are an important host defense mechanism against infection, acting to activate other cells within the local tissue milieu in the presence of invading microbes. However, widespread activation of tissue macrophages at many sites can lead to the presence of high systemic levels of cytokines such as TNF-α that provoke deleterious effects on the host. This process may represent one of the inciting events that lead to sepsis syndrome, septic shock, and multiple system organ failure (MSOF), although many other mediators may play significant roles in these processes.

Effects of TNF-α and IL-1β are mediated by binding to and interacting with their specific cellular receptors; TNF-α has two receptors, TNF RI (p55) and TNF RII (p75). The effects of TNF-α appear to be manifested primarily by signal transduction through TNF RI, while TNF RII plays an integral role in T-cell proliferation.[8] There are two IL-1 receptors, IL-1 RI (p80) and IL-1 RII (p68). However, only IL-RI appears to be functional because no cellular signaling has yet been identified for IL-1 RII.[9] These cytokine receptors exist in both membrane-associated and soluble forms, which appear to serve regulatory functions as well.

Coordination of Host Defenses

Complex regulatory events occur in relation to the humoral, cellular, and cytokine components of host defense (Fig. 11.1). As noted, repeated antigenic stimulation leads to refinement of the antibody response such that high levels of increasingly high-affinity IgG are produced. Intriguingly, it is not solely Ig clearance of antigen that serves to regulate this response as antiidiotypic Ig directed against the antigen-binding site of the initial Ig is produced in small amounts as well. In addition, it has become clear that the host cellular response to infection is not confined to phagocytic cells. The T lymphocytes have been thought to be an important defense mainly against intracellular pathogens such as *M. tuberculosis*, but their role in defense against common bacterial infections has been elucidated as well. A paradigm in which a subset of T-helper lymphocytes (Th_1) is associated with proinflammatory cytokines including IL-2, IFN-γ, and TNF-α has emerged, and this system is regulated by a separate subset of similar cells (Th_2) that are associated with antiinflammatory cytokines such as IL-4 and IL-10.

Concurrent with the secretion of IL-1β and TNF-α during gram-negative bacterial infection and endotoxemia, a complex network of endogenous cytokine antagonists for these cytokines functions to damp the host cytokine response. Interleukin-1 receptor antagonist (IL-1ra) is secreted, tumor necrosis factor-binding protein (TNF-BP) is shed from the cell surface (representing TNF RI), and other agents tightly regulate cytokine elaboration under normal circumstances, although during severe infection an exaggerated, dysregulated

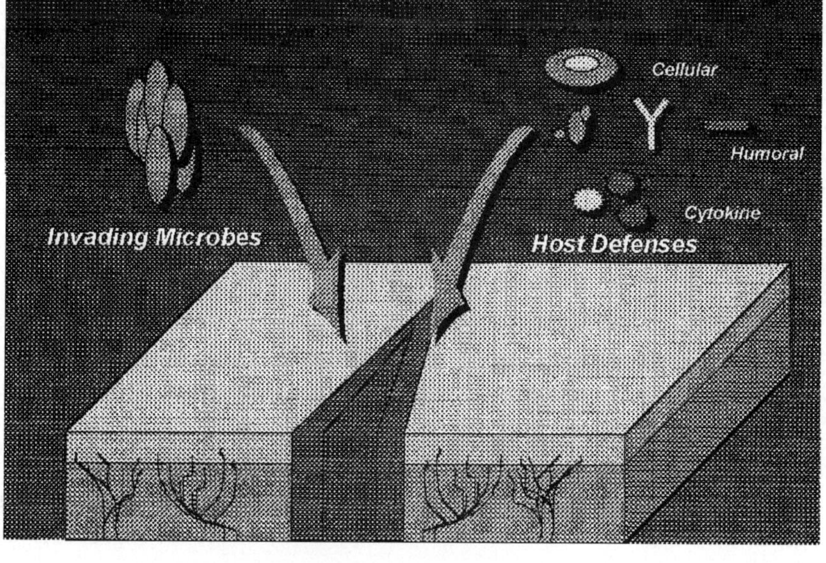

FIGURE 11.1. Complex regulatory events occur in relation to the humoral, cellular, and cytokine components of host defense in the surgical wound.

cytokine response can occur.[10–12] In addition, there is increasing evidence that those cytokine receptors that bind a particular cytokine but do not transduce an intracellular signal serve to damp the initial response as well. Recent data indicate that elevated levels of both a specific cytokine and its cellular receptor may not lead to adverse effects early in sepsis, while exaggerated cytokine secretion concurrent with secretion of the endogenous antagonist for several days may most closely correlate with deleterious consequences.[13] Most likely, this response represents a surrogate marker for uncontrolled infection at the primary site of disease.

Finally, certain parts of the body possess unique host defense mechanisms. For example, specialized areas on the peritoneal mesothelial surface of the diaphragm form stomata that lead into lymphatic channels, which in turn coalesce into large channels within the thoracic cavity that eventually drain into the thoracic duct.[14] Via this pathway, large volumes of fluid containing phagocytic cells, erythrocytes, or microbes can be pumped from the peritoneal cavity. However, if a large inoculum of microbes enters the bloodstream via this mechanism, sepsis syndrome can occur.

Antimicrobial Agents

Subsequent to the discovery and successful clinical use of penicillin and sulfonamides, a profuse number of antibiotics have been developed. New agents appear each year; many are suitable for use in surgical patients. The precepts of antimicrobial agent usage entail familiarity with the following: (1) microbes commonly encountered during the prevention or treatment of specific types of infections; (2) antibiotic class, mechanism of action, and spectrum of activity of index agents; (3) spectrum of activity of specific agents within a class; (4) prophylactic, empiric (preemptive), or therapeutic use coupled with duration of administration; (5) global, institutional, and unique patient care unit microbial antibiotic resistance patterns; (6) culture and antibiotic sensitivity patterns of organisms cultured from a specific site; and (7) clinical course of the patient. Types of antimicrobial agents are discussed first, then specific types of infection and the manner in which they are diagnosed and treated are described. A representative, but by no means exhaustive, list of antimicrobial agents and their spectrum of activity is provided in Table 11.3.

β-Lactam Agents

Four subclasses of β-lactam drugs have been developed; all are bactericidal: penicillins, cephalosporins, monobactams, and carbapenems. These drugs act to inhibit bacterial cell wall synthesis, with the β-lactam ring competitively inhibiting transpeptidation of the D-alanyl group of *N*-acteylmuramic acid residues. This step in microbial cell wall peptidoglycan synthesis and cross-linking is critical to microbial cell wall integrity. Numerous agents have been developed within each class, and although general rules regarding their spectrum of activity can be stated, numerous exceptions exist that must be considered carefully when the surgeon selects a particular agent.

Penicillin G is the index drug for this class; it possesses activity against many common gram-positive organisms, such as most streptococci, including anaerobic species, and against less commonly encountered microbes such as *Clostridium perfringens* and *Treponema pallidum.* However, today it exhibits activity to only a limited number of strains of *S. aureus* and enterococci, and resistant isolates of *S. pneumoniae* now are common. Depot forms of the drug (procaine and benzathine penicillin) remain extremely useful agents, and penicillin V is available as an oral formulation. Ampicillin and amoxicillin exhibit activity against some enterococci and streptococci and a limited number of strains of gram-negative aerobes, such as *E. coli.* So-called semisynthetic penicillins such as methicillin exhibit substantial gram-positive activity, similar to penicillin G for streptococci, plus activity against *S. aureus,* although the prevalence of methicillin-resistant *S. aureus* (MRSA) strains has increased substantially. Carboxypenicillins (carbenicillin, ticarcillin) and ureidopenicillins (acylampicillins [piperacillin, azlocillin]) exhibit substantial activity against gram-negative aerobes, including many strains of *P. aeruginosa,* and the latter agents also are active against some strains of enterococci based on their derivation from ampicillin.

Many microbes secrete enzymes that cleave the β-lactam ring of these agents, and several inhibitors of these virulence factors have been developed (clavulanate, sulbactam, tazobactam). These compounds have been combined with β-lactam antibiotics, and the combined drugs (ticarcillin-clavulanate, amoxicillin-clavulanate, ampicillin-sulbactam, piperacillin-tazobactam) possess an extended spectrum of activity that generally includes more strains of gram-positive and gram-negative aerobes than the parent antibiotic alone plus potent anaerobic activity.

A large number of cephalosporins have been developed as well, and these agents are grouped into first-, second-, third-, and more recently, fourth- (cefipime) and fifth-generation (ceptobiprole) drugs. A simple way to remember the spectrum of activity of the agents in each generation is that first-generation drugs exhibit considerable gram-positive aerobic activity, including activity against methicillin-sensitive *S. aureus* (MSSA), but little gram-negative aerobic activity. Gram-positive activity decreases progressively with second- and third-generation agents, whereas the gram-negative activity increases; selected second- and third-generation agents (ceftriaxone, cefoxitin, cefotetan) possess considerable activity against anaerobes. This activity occurs because bacterial enzymes located at the cell wall division plate to which different types of β-lactam antibiotics bind are distinct among gram-positive and gram-negative bacteria. Finally, most cephalosporin agents do not possess any degree of enterococcal activity, with the exception of recently developed novel agents currently under investigation.

A single monobactam agent has been developed (aztreonam), and this drug has activity against only gram-negative aerobes such as *E. coli* and some strains of *P. aeruginosa.* Finally, an increasing number of carbapenem agents derived from a parent thienamycin compound are available for use; all exhibit potent activity against many gram-negative aerobes, including *P. aeruginosa* and most anaerobes, and varying degrees of activity against gram-positive aerobes. Imipenem-cilastatin is a combination drug in which cilastatin prevents degradation of the β-lactam component by renal

TABLE 11.3. Activity of Selected Antimocrobial Agents.[a]

	Streptococcus pyrogenes	*Staphylococcus aureus*	*Staphylococcus epidermidis*	*Enterococcus faecalis*	*Enterococcus faecium*	*Escherichia coli*	*Pseudomonas aeruginosa*	*Anaerobes*
β-Lactam agents								
Penicillins								
Penicillin G	+++++	+	+	+	+	—	—	—
Methicillin	+++++	++	+	+	+	—	—	—
Ticarcillin	+++	++	+	++	++	++	++	—
Ampicillin	++	+	+	+++	+++	+	—	—
Penicillin agent1β-lactamase inhibitors								
Piperacillin	+	+	—	+++	+++	+++	++++	+
Ampicillin-sulbactam	++	++	+	+++	+++	++	++	++++
Ticarcillin-clavulanate	+++	++	+	++	++	++	++	++++
Piperacillin-tazobactam	+	+	—	+++	+++	++++	++++	++++
First-generation cephalosporins	+++	++++	++	—	—	—	—	—
Second-generation cephalosporins[b]	++	++	++	—	—	+++	++	V
Cefoxitin	++	++	++	—	—	+++	++	+++
Cefaperazone	++	++	++	—	—	+++	++	—
Third-generation cephalosporins[b]	6	6	—	—	—	+++++	V	V
Cefotaxime	+	6	—	—	—	+++++	++	—
Cefotetan	+	+	—	—	—	++++	+	+++
Ceftazadime	+	+	—	—	—	+++++	+++++	—
Ceftriaxone	+	+	—	—	—	+++++	++	++++
Fourth-generation cephalosporins								
Cefapime	6	6	—	—	—	+++++	++++	—
Aztreonam								
Carbapenems	++	+	+	+	+	+++++	++++	++++
Vancomycin	+++++	+++++	+++++	++++	++++	—	—	—
Quinupristine-dalfopristine	++++	++++	++++	—	++++	—	—	—
Erythromycin	++++	++	++	+	+	—	—	++
Aminoglycosides	+	+	+	++	+	+++++	++++	—
Quinolones[b]	V	V	V	V	V	V	V	V
Naladixic acid	—	—	—	—	—	++	+	—
Norfloxacin	—	—	—	—	—	+++	++	
Ciprofloxacin	+	—	—	++	++	++++	++++	
Moxifloxacin	+	+	+	++	++	++++	++++	+++
Trimethoprim-sulfamethoxazole	—	—	—	—	—	++++	++	—
Clindamycin	+++	++	+	++	++	—	—	++++
Metronidazole	—	—	—	—	—	—	—	+++++

[a]+++++ indicates maximal activity; — indicates none.

[b]V indicates variability within the group, as denoted by the difference in activity among specific agents for certain types of organisms.

tubular epithelial brush border dihydropeptidases. Meropenem, ertapenem, and doripenem are not degraded in this fashion.

Glycopeptides

Vancomycin and teicoplanin are glycopeptides that act to kill bacteria by inhibiting bacterial cell wall synthesis in a fashion distinct from that of β-lactam drugs. These agents demonstrate potent activity against most strains of gram-positive pathogens, including streptococci, many enterococci, MSSA, and MRSA. Bacteria resistant to one agent are generally resistant to the other. Vancomycin exhibits nephrotoxicity, and drug-level and serum creatinine monitoring generally is required. Potential advantages of teicoplanin include reduced nephrotoxicity and less-frequent dosing, although it is not available for use in the United States. Vancomycin-resistant enterococci increasingly are encountered, and strains of *S. aureus* with intermediate or high levels of resistance to vancomycin have been isolated, albeit infrequently.

Aminoglycosides

The aminoglycosides are available only in parenteral formulation and are bactericidal, acting to inhibit microbial ribosomal protein synthesis plus a second poorly defined microbicidal mechanism, both of which lead to bacterial killing. Their spectrum of activity is primarily gram-negative aerobes, including Enterobacteriaceae and pseudomonads, and they exhibit some degree of activity against some strains of gram-positive microbes, such as *E. faecalis* and *E. faecium* as well, although they rarely are used alone for treatment of the latter organisms. Their use is associated with nephrotoxicity, and for that reason many clinicians believe that drug levels and serum creatinine values should be monitored to avoid high peaks and troughs of drug levels if more than 3 days of therapy are needed or if the patient exhibits renal dysfunction before initial administration.

Quinolones

The quinolones act to inhibit bacterial replication by binding to one of several DNA topoisomerases. Naladixic acid is the index agent, and this drug possesses activity primarily against gram-negative aerobic microbes, such as *E. coli.* Derivatives of this drug have been developed (e.g., norfloxacin) that demonstrated superior activity to a broader array of these types of bacteria. More recently, a number of fluoroquinolones have become available; all possess greater activity against gram-negative aerobes and some degree of gram-positive activity compared to the aforementioned agents in this class. For example, ciprofloxacin demonstrates suitable activity against gram-negative aerobes, including *P. aeruginosa,* while levofloxacin, ofloxacin, gatifloxacin, and moxifloxacin exhibit activity against select gram-positive bacteria as well.

Sulfonamides

Sulfonamide agents act by inhibition of microbial folic acid production, blocking the synthesis of tetrahydropteroid acid. A number of agents are available, and one of the most useful is sulfamethoxazole. When combined with trimethoprim, which inhibits the enzyme dihydrofolate reductase that catalyzes a later step in the same biosynthetic pathway, these drugs are extremely active against a wide spectrum of pathogens, including gram-negative aerobes such as *E. coli*, as well as organisms such as *N. asteroides, Listeria monocytogenes, Pneumocystis carinii*, and *L. pneumophila.* This agent commonly is used to treat urinary tract infections (UTIs) and to prevent and treat infection caused by these last pathogens in immunosuppressed patients.

Other Antibacterial Agents

Erythromycin is a macrolide antibiotic that acts to inhibit bacterial protein synthesis by binding to the 50S ribosomal subunit. It possesses activity against a number of gram-positive organisms and some degree of anaerobic activity. Azithromycin and clarithromycin also are macrolides and possess greater anaerobic activity. None of these drugs should be considered "first-line" agents for either staphylococci or streptococci, although they often are administered to patients who are allergic to β-lactam drugs.

Streptogramins are a class of agents that act to prevent bacterial growth by inhibition of ribosomal synthesis. Streptogramins A and B act via two separate mechanisms, both of which are distinct from that of other protein synthesis inhibitors. Quinupristine-dalfopristine combines these two types of streptogramins and is active against many gram-positive pathogens, including streptococci, *S. aureus* (including many MRSA strains) and *S. epidermidis*, and *E. faecium* but not *E. faecalis.* At present, only an intravenous formulation is available.

Linezolid, an oxazolidinone antibiotic, also inhibits ribosomal synthesis by binding to the 23S subunit. It possesses activity against many gram-positive aerobes, including many vancomycin-sensitive and resistant *E. faecium* and *E. faecalis.*

Clindamycin, chloramphenicol, and various tetracyclines are structurally unrelated but act to inhibit various steps in bacterial protein synthesis; they possess considerable activity against anaerobes as well as many gram-positive pathogens. Metronidazole is a drug that is available in oral and intravenous formulations; it possesses potent activity against virtually all anaerobic bacteria as well as gut parasites such as *Giardia lamblia* and *Entamoeba histolytica.* It is often used to treat the anaerobic component of a polymicrobial infection; it is also effective against *Clostridium difficile*, and its oral formulation is used to treat colonic infection caused by this pathogen.

Antifungal Agents

A more limited number of agents are available to treat fungal pathogens; these consist of amphotericin B azole drugs and echinocandins. Amphotericin B acts to prevent fungal growth and kills fungi by binding to fungal cell wall sterols and causing cell death via lysis. However, this agent causes nephrotoxicity, the occurrence of which is related to the cumulative dose of drug administered. Several different liposomal preparations of this agent have been developed that allow administration of much higher (three- to fivefold) doses with less associated nephrotoxicity and equivalent or perhaps superior efficacy, albeit at higher cost, compared to the routine preparation. Azole agents inhibit fungal sterol synthesis that is critical to cell wall growth and therefore division. Agents such as ketaconazole are active against many commonly encountered fungi, such as *Candida,* as well as specific agents such as *Blastomyces dermatiditis*. Triazole drugs (fluconazole, itraconazole, voriconazole) are active against a wider array of fungi. For example, fluconazole possesses greater activity than ketaconazole against *C. albicans*, although *C. krusei*, *C. tropicalis*, and *C. glabrata* are routinely resistant. Itraconazole demonstrates efficacy against some strains of *Aspergillus*, although it is not as active as amphotericin B and is available only as a parenteral formulation. A single echinocandin (caspofungin) has been developed, and it possesses activity against *Candida* spp., including azole-resistant strains as well as many *Aspergillus* spp.; it acts by inhibiting fungal cell wall synthesis.

Antiviral Agents

Only a limited number of viral agents are available, although the number has increased. Acyclovir, ganciclovir, and their derivatives valacyclovir and valganciclovir exhibit activity primarily directed against herpesviruses. Acyclovir and valacyclovir possess activity against HSV, herpes zoster, Epstein–Barr viruses (EBVs), and, to a lesser extent, CMV. Ganciclovir and foscarnet possess activity against CMV, although the latter agent is nephrotoxic, which represents a concern in renal transplant patients or patients with renal dysfunction. Amantadine is effective against influenza virus A (but not B), a pathogen that causes disease rarely even in immunosuppressed patients. Ribavarin is used to treat respiratory syncytial virus, and although it has been used to treat infection caused by adenovirus, its efficacy for this and other pathogens is limited.

The hepatitides are diseases caused by a diverse group of pathogens considered together because of their propensity to cause hepatocellular cytotoxicity, eventual cirrhosis and hepatic failure, and hepatocellular carcinoma. The most common pathogens among surgical patients are HBV and HCV, both of which can be transmitted via blood or body fluid exposure. Disease caused by HBV can be prevented by vaccination, and individuals at high risk for exposure (hemodialysis patients and all surgeons and health care workers who participate in invasive procedures) should receive three doses of the recombinant vaccine.[15] Disease caused by HBV can range from asymptomatic infection identified solely by serological studies to fulminant hepatic failure. Postexposure prophylaxis of nonimmunized individuals consists of administration of hepatitis B immune globulin (0.06 ml/kg i.m. immediately and at 1 month), following which standard vaccination should take place. There is some evidence that progression of hepatitis can be ameliorated by use of lamivudine, and patients undergoing liver transplantation whose underlying disease is caused by this virus can receive this agent plus HBIg to attempt to reduce the high incidence of recurrent disease in the allograft.

Transmission of HCV occurs in a fashion similar to HBV and also is identified via serological studies as well as RNA-based assays. Interferon-α_{2b} is used to treat chronic hepatitis caused by HCV (3×10^6 U s.c. 3 × a week × 12 months), and a vaccine is under development.[16] Various other hepatitis viruses (D and E) have been identified; most appear to be associated and to require HBV coinfection to cause disease. Five classes of drugs have been developed against HIV, including three types of agents that act to prevent viral growth by inhibiting retroviral reverse transcriptase (nucleoside, nucleotide, and nonnucleoside reverse transciptase inhibitors), as well as protease inhibitors and a fusion inhibitor. Current recommendations for postexposure prophylaxis in health care workers consist of administration of zidovidine plus lamivudine for 1 month or in combination with other retroviral agents for serious or massive exposure, including deep percutaneous injury.[17]

Appropriate Use of Antimicrobial Agents

Antibiotic usage in surgical patients can be categorized as prophylaxis, empiric (referred to as preemptive by some authors), and treatment. For surgical patients, antibiotics generally are used to prevent infection (prophylaxis) when the risk of wound infection is high, that is, the likelihood of presence of microbes is substantial. In this situation, one or more agents that possess activity against the most likely pathogens should be administered. For example, if only skin microbes are likely to be present and prosthetic material is to be implanted, then a single dose of a parenteral first-generation cephalosporin agent (or vancomycin if MRSA commonly is encountered) should be administered 5 to 10 min before creating the incision to allow ample time for the antibiotic to be present in the wound tissue fluid. Similarly, patients undergoing procedures in which substantial numbers of aerobic and anaerobic microbes may be present, such as elective colonic resection, should receive mechanical bowel preparation using a polyethylene glycol-based agent, oral antibiotics such as erythromycin and neomycin, and a single dose of an agent that exhibits activity against skin and colonic microflora. In general, second-generation cephalosporin agents such as cefoxitin, cefotetan, or penicillin drugs with a β-lactamase inhibitor (e.g., ampicillin-sulbactam) are chosen for this purpose. So-called preemptive therapy entails the use of preoperative prophylaxis, following which postoperative doses are administered as well in a situation in which a large inoculum is likely to be present such as penetrating gastrointestinal tract trauma. Although antibiotics routinely are used to treat infection, it should be noted that for many disease processes the precise duration of therapy has not been established.

Basic tenets regarding antibiotic therapy in surgical patients are as follows: (1) define the disease process treated and its severity and set duration of antibiotic therapy from the outset; (2) reevaluate the patient's clinical course on an ongoing basis in relation to the need for antibiotic administration; (3) use antibiotics in conjunction with other treatment modalities such as drainage and debridement; (4) use stains, cultures, and sensitivity studies and other laboratory tests to guide therapy but do not change agents or extend the antibiotic treatment course in a patient who is faring well solely on the basis of this information; (5) review the patient's drug allergy history carefully; (6) choose the least toxic drug appropriate for the infection; and (7) consider cost and, if equivalent agents are available, select the least expensive.[18]

Antibiotic Allergy

It is important to ascertain whether a patient has had any type of allergic reaction in association with administration of a particular antibiotic. However, one should take care to ensure that the purported reaction consists of true allergic symptoms and signs such as urticaria, bronchospasm, or other similar manifestations rather than indigestion or nausea. Penicillin allergy is common, occurring in 7 to 40 of 1000 treatment courses. The incidence of cross-reactivity to other β-lactam drugs is difficult to ascertain because some initial cephalosporin preparations contained penicillin drugs as well. Although avoiding the use of any β-lactam drug is appropriate in patients who manifest significant allergic reactions to penicillins, the incidence of cross-reactivity appears highest for carbapenems, much lower for cephalosporins (~5%–7%), and extremely small for monobactams.

Severe allergic manifestations to a specific class of agents, such as anaphylaxis, generally preclude the use of any agents in that class except when use of an agent represents a life-saving measure. In some centers, patients also can undergo intradermal testing of a dilute solution of a particular antibiotic to determine whether a severe allergic reaction would be elicited after parenteral administration, although this type of testing is rarely employed because it is simpler to select alternative classes of agents.

Endocarditis Prophylaxis

Patients with valvular heart disease, prosthetic heart valves, or other cardiac defects should receive prophylactic antibiotics before undergoing dental, upper respiratory, and gastrointestinal or genitourinary procedures to prevent the occurrence of microbial endocarditis. Suggested regimens are listed in Table 11.4.

TABLE 11.4. Recommendations for Endocarditis Prophylaxis in Adult Surgical Patients.

Procedure	*Routine oral*	*Routine parenteral*	*β-Lactam allergy*
Oropharyngeal/ dental	Amoxicillin[a]	Ampicillin[b]	Clindamycin[c]
Clean	Amoxicillin	Cetazolin[d]	Clindamycin
Gastrointestinal/ genitourinary[e]	Amoxicillin	Ampicillin[d]	Vancomycin[d]
Gentamicin[f]	Gentamicin[g]		

[a]2g p.o. 1h before procedure.

[b]2g i.m. or i.v. 30min before procedure.

[c]600mg 1h before procedure; cephalosporins such as cephalexin or cefradroxil or macrolides such as azithromycin or clarithromycin also are suitable alternatives.

[d]1g i.m. or i.v. 1h before procedure.

[e]Consideration should be given to use of amoxicillin-clavulanate as an oral agent instead of amoxicillin or the addition of clindamycin or use of an agent such as ampicillin-sulbactam in place of gentamicin to provide wound infection prophylaxis in selected patients, particularly those undergoing colonic procedures.

[f]1.5mg/kg (120mg maximum dose) i.m. or i.v. 30min before procedure.

[g]1g i.v. administered slowly 1h before procedure.

Antibiotic Resistance

The widespread use of antibiotics for the treatment of infectious diseases has led to significant improvements in morbidity and mortality rates but has concomitantly heralded the appearance of microbes resistant to many different agents. Resistance patterns parallel the duration and extent of usage both of classes of agents and of a particular agent, particularly within an institution. Currently, MRSA continues to plague patients in many hospitals, yet this has been superseded by the appearance of multidrug-resistant gram-negative aerobes belonging to the genera *Pseudomonas*, *Serratia*, *Aeromonas*, *Acinetobacter*, and *Citrobacter*. Moreover, both vancomycin-resistant *Enterococcus faecalis* and *E. faecium* (VRE or VREF) exhibiting either low- or high-level resistance to this drug have become prevalent, with their appearance temporally associated with third-generation cephalosporin and vancomycin use. A small number of strains of vancomycin-resistant *S. aureus* have been identified, which has caused great consternation for practitioners because there are few, if any, alternative agents that are capable of treating infection caused by such organisms. Resistance of fungal and viral pathogens to fluconazole and to acyclovir and ganciclovir, respectively, has been reported as well. It is imperative that the practitioner become familiar with global, institutional, and patient care unit resistance patterns, which are of particular importance in surgical patients, for whom prophylactic and preemptive therapy frequently is employed, the latter before culture and sensitivity results are available.

A number of maneuvers serve to decrease resistance rates, most of which have not been subjected to rigorous examination in the clinical setting. These include (1) precluding patient-to-patient spread by routine procedures such as handwashing by health care personnel after each patient contact; (2) limiting extent of use of antimicrobial agents such that patients receive then under highly constrained circumstances and for a defined course of therapy; (3) using appropriate bactericidal doses and only sufficient duration of therapy because a prolonged course of suboptimal doses of any agent foments resistance; and (4) switching global usage within a unit to a distinct class of antibiotics after a defined period of usage of a particular antibiotic class. It is by no means clear that antibiotic restriction programs do anything more than serve as a surrogate for attempting to employ these principles, and such programs should never be coupled with a mandated consultative process by infectious disease experts.

Surgical Infectious Diseases

Surgical infectious disease states encompass both infections occurring in surgical patients and infections that require surgical intervention as part of the treatment regimen. Ancient physicians diagnosed and treated many infections that occurred after traumatic wounding in battle, and it is intriguing to note that many advances in surgery were principally related to human conflict. Early physician-surgeons described a series of symptoms and signs that occur during infection and that remain useful today, and it is intriguing that they speculated about the existence of the microbial world. These signs are calor (warmth), rubor (redness), tumor (swelling), dolor (pain), and *functio laessa* (loss of function). The hallmark of infection is the development of purulent material, part of the body's attempt to limit infection to a local site. From a teleological standpoint, this makes sense because local infections generally are less morbid, may resolve, and may not be associated with mortality compared to systemic infection. However, in many surgical patients these external manifestations do not occur, and for that reason the importance of clinical acumen regarding epidemiology and causative pathogens in the diagnosis of surgical infections cannot be overemphasized.

Nosocomial Infections in Surgical Patients

Evaluation of postoperative fever in surgical patients represents an important diagnostic undertaking in which the onus is on the surgeon to exclude the presence of a serious infection that may have profound detrimental effects on the patient.[19] Potential sites of such nosocomial infections in surgical patients include UTIs, pneumonia, surgical site (wound) infections (SSIs), and bloodstream infection bacteremia; the last may occur with or without infection identified at a specific site, including that of an intravascular device. Extensive survey data have been collected regarding the epidemiology of nosocomial infections, including (1) site-specific rates, (2) causative pathogens, and (3) associated morbidity and mortality (Table 11.5).[20] This information is useful in identifying and monitoring high-risk patients, implementing preventive strategies, and diagnosing and treating those infections that occur.

Urinary Tract Infection and Pneumonia

The most common type of nosocomial infection, UTIs can occur in surgical patients as the result of underlying genitourinary disease or prolonged indwelling catheter drainage.[21] For that reason, every attempt should be made to remove this type of device after the initial operation. In general, this can be accomplished within 1 to 3 days even for major procedures. However, many patients in surgical intensive care units (SICUs) require prolonged urinary and tracheal intubation. Although urinary catheters do become colonized and elicit diapedesis of PMNs into the urine, significant infection can be diagnosed based on the presence of more than 100,000 CFU/ml. Initial therapy should be directed against common gram-negative aerobic organisms such as *E. coli*, although UTIs caused by gram-positive bacteria such as *E. faecalis* and *E. faecium* are common as well. Meticulous aseptic technique during catheter insertion and tubing changes and daily meatal care diminish the risk of such infections. If a UTI occurs during the postoperative period, then it should be treated for 10 to 14 days with an antibiotic demonstrated to have efficacy based on sensitivity testing, and a urine sample should be obtained for culture 3 to 5 days after completion of therapy. Identification of recurrent infection mandates a search for an underlying anatomical abnormality.

The occurrence of postoperative pneumonia in a surgical patient is a grave, potentially highly morbid event. In some patients, the diagnosis is readily established based on the presence of a discrete area of pulmonary consolidation on chest roentgenogram and a single organism identified on Gram stain and culture from a sample of sputum. In most hospitals, initial empiric therapy should be directed against gram-negative aerobic pathogens, although gram-positive microbes such as *S. aureus* also cause such infections. In some SICUs, highly antibiotic-resistant gram-negative bacteria such as *P. aeruginosa*, *Acinetobacter calcoaceticus*, and *Citrobacter freundii* are common, and in those settings initial single- or dual-drug therapy should be instituted on the basis of the institutional and unit sensitivity patterns for these microbes. Patients who undergo prolonged tracheal intubation who develop fever and infiltrates on chest roentgenogram should undergo diagnostic bronchoscopy if routine sputum sampling does not reveal the presence of more than 25 PMNs per low-power field (100×) via microscopic examination and a single causative organism using the former technique or routine culture. Use of the so-called covered-brush technique to obtain satisfactory specimens has not been unequivocably demonstrated as beneficial in establishing the diagnosis. Postoperative pneumonia should be treated with a 14- to 21-day course of an appropriate parenteral antibiotic; it is associated with a mortality rate of more than 50% among patients requiring mechanical ventilation.[22,23]

TABLE 11.5. Epidemiology of Nosocomial Infections in Patients in Surgical Intensive Care Units.

Nosocomial infection	*Rate*	*Distribution*[a] *(%)*
Urinary tract	5.3[b]	20.7
Surgical site	0.14–5.28[c]	13.2
Pneumonia	14.5[d]	31.4
Central line-associated bacteremia	4.9[e]	15.1
Other	19.6	

[a]Percentage that each type of infection contributes to 100% of infections among surgical patients.

[b]Number of urinary catheter days/number of patient days.

[c]Number of infections per 100 cases.

[d]Number of ventilator days/number of patient days.

[e]Number of central line days/number of patient days.

Source: From National Nosocomial Infections Surveillance (NNIS) System report.[20]

Surgical Site Infections

The SSIs are categorized according to whether they involve the superficial wound that constitutes the skin and subcutaneous tissue above the fascia, the deep wound that is the body cavity in which the procedure is performed, or both regions concurrently. Rigorous definitions of wound infection have been established (Table 11.6), and wound infection surveillance is mandated in the United States at all major inpatient facilities.

Because of the importance of administering prophylactic antibiotics in reducing wound infection rates for certain types of procedures, surgical wounds are classified into three strata according to the potential risk of microbial contamination. Class I or clean wounds are those in which only skin microflora are likely to contaminate the operative field; because no hollow viscus that possesses endogenous microflora is entered, the risk of infection is low (~1%–4%). A subset of class I wounds (ID) are those in which prosthetic material such as mesh, a vascular graft, a cardiac valve, or a medical device is implanted; although the risk of infection is similar to other

TABLE 11.6. Criteria for Diagnosis of Superficial and Deep (Organ Space) Surgical Site Infections Within 30 Days of All Procedures (1 Year If Prosthetic Material Is Implanted).

Purulent drainage from superficial wound is seen
Surgeon declares the presence of a wound infection (cellulitis, fever, and suspected infection) and opens superficial wound
Superficial or deep wound exudes fluid that demonstrates bacteria on Gram stain or culture from specimens obtained under aseptic conditions
Presence of an abscess in the deep wound
Deep wound (organ space) reexplored because of dehiscence in the presence of infection

class I wounds, the consequences of wound infection can be dire, often defeating the purpose of the procedure. Class II clean contaminated wounds are those in which a hollow viscus likely to harbor microbes is entered (gut, biliary tract), such that both skin microflora plus resident microbes may be present in the wound, producing a slightly higher risk of infection (~3%–6%). Class III wounds are those in which substantial microbial contamination (e.g., fecal soilage; traumatic heavily contaminated wound) may be present, and the overall wound infection risk is substantial (~4%–20%), particularly if the skin edges of the superficial wound are apposed.

Note that some degree of overlapping risk occurs among the various wound classes. For this reason, survey data using a separate wound infection risk index have been accumulated using additional variables, including patient American Society of Anesthesiology score and duration of procedure. Examples of operative procedures and ranges of wound infection rates are provided in Table 11.7. Wound classification systems are used by the surgeon to decide whether to administer prophylactic antibiotics, whether to select agents with activity against pathogens that are likely to contaminate the wound and cause infection, and whether to close the skin edges of the wound per primum.

A series of maneuvers appear, in composite, to reduce the rate of infection of either the superficial or deep portions of the wound or both sites. These include (1) preoperative patient skin preparation in the form of scrubbing the prospective wound area and showering using a topical microbicide; (2) clipping of hair, but avoidance of shaving the skin of the prospective wound site, particularly in advance of the procedure because microbial proliferation can occur in areas of epidermal damage; (3) surgeon hand scrubbing and patient skin preparation using a topical microbicide immediately before the procedure; (4) instrument sterilization and avoidance of breaks in aseptic technique; (5) use of mechanical preparation, intraluminal antibiotics, or antiseptics for selected procedures to reduce the microbial inoculum within a hollow viscus that will be entered as part of the procedure; and (6) administration of prophylactic antibiotics that possess activity against numerically common, albeit not all, potential pathogens that may contaminate the wound during the operation. It should be noted that not all these modalities have been examined in rigorous fashion as independent variables in randomized, prospective clinical trials, although they represent the standard of care for most patients. The effect of prophylactic antibiotics, however, has been carefully examined experimentally and in the clinical setting.

Although they are in routine use today, less than three decades ago the importance of prophylactic antibiotics in reducing the incidence of wound infections had not been determined. Using an experimental animal model, Burke demonstrated that there was a "golden period" 2 to 4h after inoculation of microbes into a wound during which prophylactic antibiotics were effective.[24] Subsequent clinical trials demonstrated the efficacy of antibiotics in reducing wound infection rates that in some institutions were as high as 50% to 70%.[25,26] In current clinical practice, prophylactic usage of antibiotics consists of administration of an agent with activity against pathogens that could be present in substantial numbers and in which the statistical likelihood of these microbes causing infection is low but measurable. For practi-

TABLE 11.7. Surgical Site Infection Risk Stratification and Rates of Infection.

Class	*Definition*	*Examples*	*Rate (%)*
I: Clean	Atraumatic wound No inflammation No break in aseptic technique No entry of biliary, respiratory, GI, or GU tracts	Herniorraphy Excision of skin lesion Thyroidectomy	1–4
ID: Clean; prosthetic	Same as I, clean Cardiac valve replacement	Vascular surgery with graft material implanted	1–4
II: Clean contaminated	Atraumatic wound No inflammation Minor break in aseptic technique Biliary, respiratory, GI, or GU tracts entered with either minimal spillage or prior preparation	Appendectomy without perforation Elective colectomy after bowel preparation Cholecystectomy	3–6
III: Contaminated	Traumatic wound with delay in therapy or exogenous contamination Inflammation or purulence Major break in aseptic technique Entry of biliary, respiratory, GI, or GU tract with gross spillage of contents	Colectomy for colonic perforation Open drainage of intraabdominal abscess	4–20

GI, gastrointestinal; GU, genitourinary.

cal purposes, this amounts to a risk of infection of more than 2% to 4%. Thus, standard practice entails administration of a prophylactic antibiotic 5 to 10min before creating the skin incision for class ID, II, and selected class III procedures (Table 11.8).[27–30] In addition, the agent should be readministered during those procedures in which the duration of the operation exceeds the serum $t_{1/2}$ of the agent to ensure that microbial levels are continually present. For many commonly administered prophylactic antibiotics, this occurs between 4 and 5h.[31]

In general, the risk–benefit analysis demonstrates that administering antibiotics to 100 patients to prevent as few as 2 to 4 wound infections is reasonable, and that few adverse events occur. Because the risk of infection for many, if not most, types of clean surgery falls below this value, whether systemic antibiotics should be administered to patients undergoing clean surgery continues to be debated. Several clinical trials have attempted to resolve this issue, but none has provided definitive evidence of the value of prophylactic antibiotics in reducing wound infection rates.[32,33] The subset of patients undergoing clean surgery in whom a prosthetic device is implanted into a tissue space (e.g., pacemaker, vascular graft) should receive an agent directed against skin microflora because in most cases wound infection is associated with considerable morbidity and occasional mortality. Frequently, the device must be removed to cure the infection, obviating the purpose of the initial procedure.

The effect of prophylactic antibiotics has been most carefully examined in patients undergoing elective colonic resection. Initial studies provided evidence of the efficacy of mechanical preparation of the bowel using cathartics and enemas plus oral antibiotics administered on three occasions before the operation. Poorly absorbed agents directed against gram-negative aerobes (neomycin) and absorbable agents with activity against anaerobes (erythromycin, tetracycline, metronidazole) were examined, and clear benefits in reducing both superficial and deep wound infection rates were observed.[34] Statistical analysis demonstrated that entry of about 1500 patients is required to determine the added benefits of a single dose of a parenteral agent over and above that of mechanical preparation of the large bowel and administration of neomycin and erythromycin in reducing the rate of superficial and deep wound infection.[35] Current standard of care based on survey results conducted during the past decade is the use of mechanical bowel preparation, two separate oral agents, plus a single dose of a parenteral agent with a spectrum of activity against aerobes and anaerobes.[36]

Primary closure of class III wounds remains controversial because of the high rate of infection. However, the controversy revolves around the attendant morbidity and cost associated with the occurrence of wound infection. Few studies have demonstrated the efficacy of use of topical antimicrobial powder, wicks, or open or closed wound irrigation systems to achieve primary closure without infection. Rarely, closure of a contaminated wound is associated with the occurrence of necrotizing fasciitis, sepsis syndrome, or death. Many clinicians employ delayed primary closure techniques in this setting, although this approach does not entirely obviate the occurrence of wound infection.

Superficial surgical wound infection must be treated by opening the wound, draining purulent material, debriding devitalized tissue, and instituting dressing changes that include packing the wound with gauze. Obtaining cultures and using an antimicrobial agent should be reserved for patients who exhibit extensive cellulitis (>2cm from incision margin) and immunosuppressed patients in whom unusual pathogens may be causative, although the added benefit of antibiotics has not been rigorously studied. Cultures may serve to direct therapy for the rare serious soft tissue infection that ensues and may provide important epidemiological and microbiological data, but routinely obtaining cultures is hard to justify in relation to cost-containment measures. Deep wound infections require percutaneous drainage if no ongoing source of infection, such as a leaking anastomosis, is present, although in some patients reexploration is required.

Finally, although wound infection surveillance is required in the United States for a minimum of 30 days in all patients undergoing major operative procedures (1 year for any ID procedures), it has not been established that this process itself serves to alter wound infection rates. However, it seems clear that surveillance retrospectively serves to carefully monitor adherence to standards of clinical practice and to direct atten-

TABLE 11.8. Indications for Use of Prophylactic Antibiotics in Surgical Patients.

Procedure	*Standard*	*Alternatives*	*β-Lactam allergy*
Class I and ID			
Cardiac	Cefazolin	Cefuroxime	Vancomycin
Vascular	Cefazolin	Cefuroxime	Vancomycin
Orthopedic	Cefazolin	Cefuroxime	Vancomycin
Class II			
Upper gastrointestinal	Cefazolin		Vancomycin
Biliary	Cefazolin		Vancomycin
Lower gastrointestinal	Oral neomycin + erythromycin plus intravenous cefoxitin	Same oral plus intravenous cefotetan or ampicillin-sulbactam or cefazolin + metronidazole	Clindamycin + gentamicin
Thoracic	Cefazolin	Cefuroxime	Vancomycin
Genitourinary	Ciprofloxacin		
Gynecological	Cefoxitin	Cefotetan	Gentamicin + clindamycin
Head and neck	Gentamicin + clindamycin		
Class III			
Perforated viscus	Cefoxitin	Cefotetan or ampicillin-sulbactam or cefazolin + metronidazole	Gentamicin + clindamycin
Traumatic wound	Cefazolin		

tion to any deviations that could be subsequently avoided. In addition, variance in intensity of surveillance among institutions may confound direct comparisons of outcome measures.

Bloodstream Infections and Sepsis Syndrome

Bloodstream infections occur frequently in the nosocomial environment; currently, the incidence of nosocomial bloodstream infection is about 250,000 to 300,000 per annum in the United States.[20,37] Gram-positive microbes account for about 50% to 60% of events and gram-negative bacteria about 30%; fungemia, mainly caused by *Candida* spp., accounts for the remainder. Sepsis syndrome occurs in a subset of patients who manifest the systemic inflammatory response syndrome (SIRS) on the basis of infection. Currently, SIRS describes patients with two or more of the following: temperature above 38°C, heart rate greater than 90 beats/min, respiratory rate above 20 breaths/min, white blood cell count above 12,000 cells/mm^3, and the presence of more than 10% immature band forms of neutrophils on the peripheral blood smear.[38] It is highly likely, however, that most episodes of bacteremia and fungemia are both intermittent and transient, precluding isolation of the offending pathogens during every clinical event. The term *severe sepsis syndrome* refers to the added presence of organ dysfunction. *Septic shock* is defined as the sepsis syndrome in association with hypotension that persists despite adequate fluid resuscitation.

Clinical studies indicated that about 45% of patients who develop SIRS harbor infection such that they are classified as having sepsis syndrome.[39] Bacteremic episodes are causally most closely linked to sepsis syndrome, although the latter process can occur without identification of bloodstream infection. Clinical trials have provided evidence that fewer than 50% of patients who develop sepsis syndrome have a microbial pathogen cultured from their bloodstream. Sepsis syndrome can progress to MSOF and is the 13th most common cause of death among patients in the United States, with as many as 400,000 cases occurring annually, and surgical patients account for about 30% of these cases.[40,41] Despite improvements in antimicrobial therapy and intensive care (e.g., aggressive fluid resuscitation, hemodynamic monitoring, and metabolic support), mortality associated with sepsis syndrome remains at about 40%, a statistic that has changed but little over the past several decades. Even more distressing, bacteremia and sepsis syndrome caused by antibiotic-resistant gram-positive or gram-negative microbes are associated with higher mortality rates.

Staphylococcus epidermidis has become a major causative pathogen of bacteremic episodes and intravascular catheter infections; it is now the most common gram-positive organism isolated from blood (~30% of isolates) and accounts for the majority of infections that are associated with an intravascular catheter. Formerly thought to possess minimal virulence, this organism increasingly has become recognized as a significant pathogen. *Staphylococcus aureus* and *Enterococcus* spp. also have become prevalent as etiological agents. Of particular concern is the increasing identification of bacterial strains that are resistant to multiple antimicrobial agents (MRSA, VRE) as pathogens causing bacteremic episodes.

Because staphylococci are responsible for the majority of gram-positive bacteremic events, initial antibiotic therapy should target these organisms. Because of the appearance and rapid spread of VRE that has been associated with widespread vancomycin use, consideration should be given to the use of semisynthetic penicillins such as nafcillin or methicillin or a first-generation cephalosporin as initial empiric therapy. For the patient allergic to β-lactams or a patient who has developed a life-threatening infection, a short course (at most 3 days) of vancomycin should be administered, after which empiric therapy with this drug should be halted if no gram-positive organism is isolated either from blood or from a specific site of infection. In critically ill surgical patients such as those with extensive burns or traumatic injuries, antimicrobial coverage should also be directed against *E. faecalis* and *E. faecium* (ampicillin or an acylampicillin aminoglycoside, or vancomycin alone for patients allergic to β-lactam drugs or those who develop infection associated with sepsis syndrome or aggressive local infection with bacteremia). Empiric therapy subsequently can be tailored based on culture and sensitivity data. The VRE isolates that cause infection require use of agents such as quinupristine-dalfopristine, tetracycline, rifampin, chloramphenicol, or other drugs alone or in combination according to the sensitivity pattern of the particular organism. In VRE isolates that demonstrate low-level vancomycin resistance, teicoplanin can be considered an alternative agent.

Bacteremia caused by gram-negative bacterial infections remains common, accounting for about 30% to 35% of cases. The mortality associated with gram-negative bacteremia in normal individuals is 10% and may exceed 50% in immunocompromised patients. A wide variety of gram-negative bacteria are capable of causing infection in the clinical setting. Commonly isolated microbes include *E. coli*, *Klebsiella pneumoniae*, *Pseudomonas aeruginosa*, and *Enterobacter aerogenes* and *Enterobacter cloacae*. Although infections caused by *Pseudomonas* and *Klebsiella* species appear to be more virulent, these infections occur more commonly in patients with serious underlying diseases (e.g., extensive trauma, burns, or malignancy), such that it has not been possible to ascertain the relative contributions of bacterial virulence and the underlying disease process to overall outcome.

Antibiotic therapy should be initiated if evidence of sepsis syndrome and a potential source of gram-negative bacterial infection are identified; therapy should not be delayed for culture documentation of bacteremia. The initial choice of antimicrobial agent should be based on the institutional or care unit antibiotic resistance patterns. Aminoglycosides remain potent agents but have fallen into disfavor because of their associated nephro- and ototoxicity and the perceived need for drug-level monitoring. In general, many β-lactam drugs such as third-generation cephalosporins, acylampicillins, monobactams, and carbapenems exhibit satisfactory activity against gram-negative bacteria. Quinolones and trimethoprim-sulfamethoxazole may be useful for specific organisms. After a specific organism has been identified and antibiotic sensitivity testing performed, refinements in antimicrobial agent therapy can be made.

Clinical trials in which febrile neutropenic patients were treated with either single agents or two agents in combination, usually a β-lactam drug plus an aminoglycoside, have provided evidence that the dual-agent therapy is more effective than single-agent therapy in this particular heavily immunosuppressed patient population. Currently, a single broad-spectrum β-lactam agent is used with or without vancomycin.[42,43] Although use of dual-agent therapy frequently is extended to other patient groups, no clinical trials have been performed to provide evidence of similar efficacy in the general patient population. Thus, the added benefit of two agents has not been demonstrated in patients who are not neutropenic, and single-agent therapy targeting the infecting organism should be utilized in most circumstances. When a microbe is identified that is typically highly resistant to many agents (e.g., *Pseudomonas* or *Xanthomonas* species), dual-agent therapy should be considered.[44]

Prolonged treatment of high-risk patient populations such as immunosuppressed diabetics with broad-spectrum antibacterial agents coupled with the widespread use of intravascular devices represent some of the factors that have led to an increase in the incidence of fungemia. *Candida* species are the most common isolates, and *C. albicans* accounts for more than half the fungi cultured from clinical infections. Isolation of *Candida* from the bloodstream should prompt immediate initiation of antifungal treatment and a search for the source of infection. In nonneutropenic patients, either intravenous fluconazole or amphotericin B can be used initially unless the isolate is known to be resistant to triazole drugs.[45] Fluconazole is efficacious against many strains of *Candida*, particularly the commonly encountered *C. albicans*, although some isolates of *C. krusei*, *C. tropicalis*, *C. glabrata*, and *Candida guilliermondii* are resistant and may emerge during fluconazole prophylaxis in immunosuppressed patients.[46] If the infection is unresponsive to such therapy based on clinical parameters or if an organism resistant to fluconazole is identified, then amphotericin B therapy should be instituted. Fungemic patients who exhibit hemodynamic instability or neutropenia should receive amphotericin B as the initial therapeutic agent. Therapy for bacteremia or fungemia should be continued for 10 to 21 days, although the precise duration of therapy is unknown and has not been examined in clinical trials.

Endotoxin and a number of different endogenous mediators (TNF-α, IL-1, platelet-activating factor [PAF]) have been implicated in the development of sepsis syndrome, and for that reason clinical trials have been performed in an attempt to diminish lethality from this disease process. Two different antiendotoxin monoclonal antibodies were developed (E5, HA-1A), and their efficacy was examined in several randomized, placebo-controlled trials. Unfortunately, the target patient population with sepsis syndrome caused by gram-negative microbes represented only about one-third of the patients, and in composite these trials did not demonstrate a decrease in mortality in either the overall group of patients or the subgroup of patients with presumed endotoxemia.[47–50] Clinical trials in which large numbers of patients who had developed sepsis syndrome received either one of a number of anti-TNF-α agents (TNF-BP, TNFR:Fc, anti-TNF-α monoclonal antibodies), IL-1ra, anti-IFN-γ, or a PAF receptor antagonist (PAFra BN 52021) were subsequently conducted.[51–55] However, data obtained from these trials did not provide evidence of efficacy in any of these agents in decreasing mortality during sepsis syndrome. Currently, clinical trials using more potent antiendotoxin agents such as bactericidal permeability-increasing protein (BPI) and cytokines that appear to exert antiinflammatory effects on the host defense response (e.g., IL-10) are under way or in consideration.

Intravascular Catheter Infections

Within the nosocomial environment, many bacteremic episodes are associated with intravascular catheters and other devices. These devices serve a variety of functions: drug administration, parenteral nutrition, hemodynamic monitoring, hemodialysis, or plasmapheresis. Many patients undergo intravascular catheter placement at some time during their hospitalization, and epidemiological data indicate that among about 3 million central venous catheters inserted per annum in the United States, approximately 25% will become colonized, and about 5% (150,000) will become colonized and be associated with bacteremia. Similar events are 10-fold less common when peripheral catheters are considered, probably because of their short duration of use.[56]

Prevention of catheter infections requires adherence to strict aseptic technique and subsequent meticulous insertion site care. The risk of catheter infection is increased if inserted through infected or contaminated skin (e.g., burns), so these areas should be avoided if at all possible. Femoral vein catheters are more likely to become infected than subclavian or internal jugular vein catheters, probably related to both degree of skin contamination and catheter movement in and out of the exit site. Multilumen catheters may also have a higher rate of infection than single-lumen catheters, but this may not be clinically significant because multilumen catheters are typically used for short periods of time. Although tunneled or cuffed catheters initially were thought to decrease infection, several prospective studies have shown that these devices offer no advantage over noncuffed catheters.[57] In composite, the risk of infection increases significantly with the length of time a catheter is in place, although this is most probably a surrogate marker for catheter use and manipulation.

The use of routine catheter changes either via guidewire exchange or insertion at a separate site has been rigorously examined. The former increased infection rates; the latter increased the incidence of mechanical complications.[58] Administration of prophylactic antibiotics before catheter insertion or during the period of time that the catheter is in place in the patient is not indicated as only data from small-scale clinical trials among patients with hematological malignancies have provided evidence supporting their use, and this form of prophylaxis is expensive and assuredly promotes antibiotic resistance.[59] Clinical trials have examined the capacity of intravascular catheters in which antibiotic is bonded to the prosthetic material to reduce the incidence of colonization and infection. Two types of catheters have been studied: (1) chlorhexidine-silver sulfadiazine bonded on the extraluminal surface and (2) minocycline-rifampin bonded on both the intra- and extraluminal surfaces.[60–62] On balance, it would appear that colonization and infection rates indeed are reduced, but it remains to be determined whether the cost of these devices is justified. In particular, it may be that many catheter infections can be prevented by applying sound surgical judgment such that no catheter is inserted or, if one is inserted, it is left in place for only a short period of time.

Identification of infection of intravascular catheters can prove vexing; this process can involve solely the exit site, the intravascular portion of the catheter itself, or both regions. If the intravascular portion of the catheter is involved, then bacteremia can occur. Several key principles should be considered when attempting to diagnose intravascular catheter infections: (1) infections extending along the track of a tunneled catheter or subcutaneous port pocket are potentially serious and do not invariably manifest either locally or systemically, and (2) catheter infection should be suspected in any patient with an intravascular catheter who exhibits bacteremia and no other obvious source of infection.

Superficial, limited intravascular catheter-related infections are diagnosed by the presence of redness, swelling, pain, and occasionally purulent exudate in proximity to the peripheral or central venous catheter exit or subcutaneous port site. Infection of a peripheral intravenous line site in general can be cured by removal of the catheter, and culture of the catheter tip or insertion site is unnecessary. Antibiotics directed against gram-positive microbes should be used to treat accompanying cellulitis or ascending lymphangitis, and the appearance of a doughy vein proximal to a peripheral catheter site is cause for concern because suppurative thrombophlebitis may be present. Under these circumstances, the catheter should be removed and the site examined; if more than 1 ml of purulent material is encountered, then the patient should be taken to the operating room and this area explored. The presence of purulent material and infected clot extending proximally in the vein mandates removal of the infected vein and treatment with a 14- to 21-day course of a parenteral antibiotic selected on the basis of initial Gram stain and subsequent culture and sensitivity data.

Purulent material at the catheter exit site should be cultured, and ultrasonography can be used to identify and percutaneously sample fluid within a subcutaneous port pocket. Demonstrably infected wounds should be locally explored and drained, and in most cases catheter removal is required. In the absence of obvious infection, however, blood cultures should be obtained peripherally and through the catheter, but the diagnosis is established unequivocally only by removing the device, demonstrating large numbers of microbes on the device itself, and observing resolution of the patient's signs and symptoms. Increasingly, however, potentially infected catheters are allowed to remain in situ; identification, via blood culture obtained through the catheter itself and from peripheral blood samples, of the same microbe with the identical antibiotic sensitivity pattern at the exit site establishes the diagnosis. Rarely, however, can the same organism be isolated from all three sites. More commonly, the same organism is isolated from peripheral blood cultures and from blood withdrawn via the catheter or from the catheter tip after guidewire exchange, either of which supports but does not establish the diagnosis. Therefore, additional microbiological techniques have been employed.

In the most commonly used semiquantitative method, the distal 2 cm of the catheter is rolled across an agar plate and growth of more than 15 colonies per plate is considered diagnostic of catheter infection. However, a number of studies have shown that as few as 5 colonies may be associated with bacteremia.[63] Because the most serious event with catheter infection is bacteremia, a positive blood culture is probably of the most practical importance. Blood cultures drawn through the catheter growing 5- to 10-fold more colonies than peripheral cultures obtained simultaneously verify the catheter as the source of bacteremia. In general, patients with signs of infection and a positive blood culture drawn through the catheter or a positive catheter tip culture (>15 colonies per plate) should be treated for catheter infection.

Patients should undergo catheter removal if catheter infection is suspected and the device can be readily removed without altering the patient's treatment course. However, if the catheter is required for ongoing treatment, then the potentially infected line can be removed, the tip cultured, and a new catheter inserted over a guidewire. If the catheter tip culture shows that the original catheter was infected, then a new catheter can be placed at a fresh site. Neither the need for delaying catheter reinsertion to prevent catheter seeding nor the need for antimicrobial therapy or specific duration of therapy to treat vascular catheter infections, particularly after catheter removal or exchange, has been determined in clinical trials. Antibiotic therapy should be adjusted on the basis of culture data, including halting therapy among patients in whom neither bacteremia nor catheter colonization is identified, particularly in those individuals in whom systemic manifestations resolve rapidly.

Approximately 80% of catheter infections are caused by increasingly common gram-positive microbes, and about 75% to 85% can be successfully treated with a 14- to 21-day course of a parenteral antibiotic without catheter removal.[64,65] A small number of trials also have provided data indicating that instilling an antibiotic such as teicoplanin and allowing it to dwell for 12h before removal may eradicate some catheter infections.[66] Because of the high incidence of *S. epidermidis* that is resistant to most β-lactam drugs as well as MRSA, vancomycin usually is selected for initial therapy among patients who exhibit systemic manifestations such as fever or an elevated serum white blood cell count. Initial empiric antibiotic therapy should not be extended more than 3 to 5 days without confirming the presence of a gram-positive microbe in blood or catheter exchange cultures. If a gram-positive microbe sensitive to β-lactam agents is isolated, then therapy can be refined to obviate the use of vancomycin. In addition, serious enterococcal infections often are treated by combining ampicillin with an aminoglycoside because this combination appears to be synergistic. Antibiotic therapy should not be continued if the patient's clinical course fails to improve after 24 to 48h. Under those conditions, the catheter should be removed.

Patients who exhibit sepsis syndrome initially; those who harbor catheters infected with gram-negative bacterial pathogens or fungi, whether or not sepsis syndrome is manifest; and those who exhibit recrudescence soon after completion of an initial treatment for gram-positive catheter infections do not respond solely to antibiotic therapy. Under any of these conditions, the catheter should be removed without a trial of antimicrobial agent administration in the presence of an infected device. In immunocompromised patients, gram-negative infections are likely, and antibiotic coverage should be broadened to cover these microbes (usually by adding a second- or third-generation cephalosporin or, less commonly, an aminoglycoside) before establishing the diagnosis.

Vascular and Cardiovascular Infections

Infections involving the vascular system are rare and probably occur subsequent to hematogenous seeding of either a pathological abnormality or one created by operative intervention. *Salmonella* and staphylococcal infection can involve the great vessels on rare occasions, leading to "mycotic" aneurysm formation. This type of aneurysm can rapidly expand, and the risk of rupture is high.

Acute and chronic infection of prosthetic vascular grafts are more common, occurring after about 2% to 6% of vascular procedures in which such material is implanted.[67] Complications associated with these infections include rupture, thrombosis, distal embolization, bacteremia, and sepsis syndrome. Standard care consists of removal of the infected portion of the graft and any surrounding infected tissue, concurrent vascular bypass to avoid recontamination (often extraanatomical), and administration of a 6- to 12-week course of an antimicrobial agent. The microbiology of these infections is similar to that of intravascular catheter infections in that gram-positive microbes (i.e., *S. aureus* and *S. epidermidis*) predominate. Anecdotal clinical studies have examined the effect of antibiotic impregnation of prosthetic grafts in reducing the incidence of these types of infection, but added benefit has not been clearly demonstrated.

It remains controversial regarding whether extraanatomical bypass invariably needs to be performed if removal of the entire graft is required; some surgeons advocate the use of in situ reconstruction, favoring the use of autogenous graft over prosthetic material. The results of several retrospective series have demonstrated satisfactory results using this technique, although no prospective clinical trials have been performed.[68,69] In general, more prolonged antibiotic treatment courses are selected when in situ reconstruction is performed or highly virulent microbes are present. If multidrug antibiotic-resistant, virulent organisms are encountered, then a second antimicrobial agent with a separate mechanism of action often is added to the regimen. Treatment of recurrent infection generally requires graft removal.

Native or prosthetic cardiac valvular infection initially is treated with a 6- to 12-week course of one or more antibiotics, but significant cardiac dysfunction, recurrent infection, particularly that associated with sepsis syndrome unresponsive to initial antimicrobial agent therapy, or fungal infection warrants valvular removal and replacement.[70] Every attempt should be made to reduce the inoculum size via administration of perioperative antibiotics, and the resected valve tissue should be examined microscopically for the presence of microbes and cultured. Generally, implantation of autogenous valves is preferred over use of prosthetic valves in this situation, and parenteral antibiotics should be continued for about 6 to 12 weeks after replacement of an infected cardiac valve in an attempt to reduce the likelihood of recurrent infection.

Skin and Soft Tissue Infections

Many eponyms have been used historically that often describe the same disease process (e.g., Fornier's gangrene, scrotum; Meleney's synergistic gangrene, abdominal wall). Currently, these infections are classified according to (1) tissue plane affected and extent of invasion, (2) anatomical site, and (3) causative pathogen(s) (Table 11.9).[71] Parameters such as rapidity of progression and clinical manifestations (e.g., septic shock) are important to consider as well. The most common of these diseases are superficial infections (cellulitis, erysipelas, lymphangitis, and furunculosis) caused by gram-positive aerobic skin microflora, although gram-negative bacteria and yeast also are capable of causing these infections, particularly in immunocompromised patients. Most commonly, erythema and mild cellulitis are associated with mild abrasive or penetrating trauma to the surrounding skin, the presence of dermatological disease, or a superficial surgical wound infection. These infections rarely progress to more serious infection and can be treated by a 3- to 5-day course of an oral first-generation cephalosporin or a semisynthetic penicillin. Superficial surgical wound infection must be treated by opening the wound, as mentioned.

TABLE 11.9. Classification of Soft Tissue Infections.

Superficial soft tissue infections	*Deep soft tissue infections*
Cellulitis	Necrotizing fasciitis
Erysipelas	Necrotizing myositis
Furuncles	Parasitic muscle infections
Lymphangitis	Pyomyositis

More extensive cellulitis in which spread of erythema occurs is referred to as *erysipelas*. A life-threatening form of this disease occurs as the result of β-hemolytic streptococci; rapid progression of disease from a single site occurs, and systemic toxicity is severe because of bacterial exotoxin secretion.[72] Treatment consists of administration of 16 to 20MU/day of penicillin G i.v. and debridement of necrotic tissue. Spread of infection via lymphatic drainage channels manifests as "streaks" and is termed *lymphangitis*. Either of these types of infection should be treated with a parenteral antibiotic with gram-positive activity until resolution occurs. An involved extremity should be elevated and mobility restricted until the infection is effectively treated. *Furuncuolosis* represents more extensive disease in which superficial subcutaneous abscesses form; treatment generally requires antimicrobial agent therapy and surgical incision and drainage if spontaneous drainage does not occur. In all patients with what appears to be superficial infection, a careful search for the presence of a more aggressive underlying soft tissue infection should be undertaken.

Aggressive infections involving the deep soft tissues can occur with or without the presence of a superficial infection, and the most difficult to diagnose and treat are those that involve only the deep tissue because few external manifestations occur. Deep soft tissue infections are classified as follows: (1) necrotizing fasciitis, (2) necrotizing myositis, (3) pyomyositis, and (4) parasitic muscle infections.[73,74] These infections are rare and difficult to diagnose, and it remains difficult to predict their occurrence. For that reason, few if any rigorous clinical trials have been performed examining the impact of various therapeutic modalities on outcome. The body of literature in this area provides evidence that several factors must coincide in the same patient to facilitate the occurrence of these infections: (1) impairment of some aspect of the immune system and host defenses, (2) compromise of fascial blood supply, and (3) presence of microbes capable of proliferating in this area.

The most common types of deep soft tissue infections are necrotizing fasciitis and necrotizing myositis. The former is a necrotizing infection of the fascia deep to the panniculus adiposus. Invariably, there is rapid, extensive spread in the deep soft tissues that may secondarily involve the surrounding muscles. Necrotizing myositis primarily involves the muscles and will rapidly involve and impair muscle bed and spread to adjacent soft tissues. Either of these types of infection can be caused by a single organism, most commonly *S. pyogenes* or *C. perfringens*, and rarely gram-negative aerobes such as *P. aeruginosa* or *Vibrio vulnificans*. More commonly, however, polymicrobial infections occur. These infections involve gram-positive aerobes such as *S. pyogenes*, *S. aureus*, or *E. faecalis* plus gram-negative aerobes (*E. coli*, *P. aeruginosa*) as well as anaerobes, including *C. perfringens*, *B. fragilis*, and *Peptostreptococcus*, and occasionally fungi.

The clinical presentation of such infections often is indolent. Fever and confusion may be the first signs, and there may be pain out of proportion to any findings on physical examination, particularly if an extremity is involved. Drainage of watery, grayish fluid from the wound or an open sore, an odd coppery hue of the skin, brawny induration, and skin blebs or crepitus are pathognomonic of these infections, and rapid extension to adjacent sites can occur. Patients often exhibit high fever, tachycardia, hypotension, shock, incipient MSOF with disseminated intravascular coagulation (most probably related to bacterial exotoxin secretion and bacterial synergistic interactions that occur during polymicrobial infections), and occasionally renal failure secondary to rhabdomyolysis.

Ascertaining the presence of a deep soft tissue infection can be difficult. Initially, the patient's history should be reviewed for the presence of any risk factors, and the patient should be thoroughly examined to determine whether possible entry sites, skin changes, or crepitus are present. Plain roentgenograms looking for gas in the soft tissue should be performed, and computerized tomography or magnetic resonance imaging can occasionally be helpful in establishing the diagnosis. However, radiological studies, particularly time-consuming scans, should not be performed if it seems highly likely that a deep soft tissue infection is present, particularly if the patient exhibits hemodynamic instability. Under those circumstances, rapid fluid resuscitation should take place, and an incisional biopsy should be performed in the operating room, obtaining direct visualization of both the soft tissue and muscle. Fluid can be obtained for performance of Gram stain and cultures.

The presence of a deep soft tissue infection mandates radical debridement of all infected tissue, and the surgeon must be prepared to proceed with such intervention at the time of initial diagnostic exploration. For the most part, the surgeon must use personal judgment to debride tissue to the point at which all devitalized tissue has been removed. Some clinicians have advocated frozen section analysis, but it remains unclear whether this definitively provides information to assist with determining the extent of resection.[75] This type of surgery often is cosmetically disfiguring and may involve amputation of an extremity to save the patient's life. Planned reexploration and debridement must occur in almost all cases until the infection has been eradicated.

Antibiotic therapy initially should be directed against gram-positive aerobes, gram-negative aerobes, anaerobes, and *C. perfringens* until Gram stain and culture results are available. Antifungal therapy is often administered as well to immunosuppressed patients. Initial antimicrobial agent therapy consists of aqueous penicillin G (approximately 16–20×10^6U every 24h) plus vancomycin plus an aminoglycoside or a third-generation cephalosporin plus clindamycin or metronidazole. Alternative regimens include vancomycin plus a single broad-spectrum agent such as imipenem-cilastatin, ampicillin-sulbactam, ticarcillin-clavulanate, or piperacillin-tazobactam. Amphotericin B therapy should be instituted if fungi are identified. Alterations and refinements in antibiotic therapy can be made within 1 to 2 days based on microbiological data.

Deep soft tissue infections are associated with a mortality rate of about 50%, even with rapid diagnosis, radical debridement, and administration of appropriate antibiotics. Minimal debridement, incision and drainage plus antibiotics, or use of antibiotics alone is associated with approximately 80% to 100% mortality.[76] Higher rates of morbidity and mortality are associated with delay of diagnosis, less than radical debridement, initial selection of antibiotics that in retrospect prove to be ineffective against the pathogens encountered, and the occurrence of these infections in elderly, diabetic, or immunosuppressed patients. Several studies have been performed in an attempt to determine whether added benefit is achieved by use of hyperbaric oxygen (HBO) therapy in addition to the aforementioned treatment regimen.[77–79] Although there is some experimental evidence to support the use of HBO, no prospective clinical trials have been performed that unequivocally demonstrated efficacy, and several trials have used historical controls or have not carefully stratified patients regarding each aspect of multimodality therapy. The HBO therapy is expensive and seems to be used at centers that possess such equipment. At best, it most likely represents adjunctive therapy that provides a modicum of benefit in selected patients. The referral of patients who develop deep soft tissue infection solely to centers that possess HBO equipment is not invariably indicated for use of that modality alone, although many such institutions possess considerable expertise in the management of these patients.

Pyomyositis consists of abscesses deep within the muscle compartment. Patients develop fever and localized swelling. The surrounding muscle initially is not involved but may become infected subsequently. Causative organisms include *S. aureus* and *E. coli*.[80] Treatment consists of open drainage and debridement and antibiotics. Parasitic myositis is similar, but occurs as the result of *Trichinella* or *Toxocara* among patients in tropical environments or those infected with HIV. The presentation is more indolent, and treatment also consists of open-drainage administration of an antiparasitic agent.

Intraabdominal Infections

Infection within the abdominal cavity is termed *microbial peritonitis* and is classified according to etiology into primary, secondary, and tertiary forms. During any type of microbial challenge, resident (peritoneal macrophages, translymphatic clearance) and recruited (PMNs) host defenses act efficiently, and sequestration mechanisms become active. However, effective treatment of this type of closed-space infection requires use of antimicrobial agents, operative intervention particularly if a potential ongoing source of peritoneal soilage (perforated viscus, abscess) is present, or both modalities.

Primary microbial peritonitis occurs without the presence of perforation of a hollow viscus and probably is caused by seeding of microorganisms, directly or perhaps via bacterial translocation from the gut or via hematogenous dissemination, into the peritoneal cavity. This process is caused by a single type of organism (monomicrobial), and common causative pathogens include *E. coli* or other aerobic gram-negative bacilli, *S. aureus*, *E. faecalis*, *E. faecium*, and less frequently *C. albicans*. This disease process is associated with the presence of abnormal amounts of fluid within the peritoneal cavity, which normally contains only 50ml or less. Thus, patients who develop hepatic cirrhosis and ascites and individuals undergoing peritoneal dialysis are prone to this type of infection. Patients who harbor these conditions and subsequently develop primary microbial peritonitis generally present complaining of diffuse abdominal pain without localization. The presence of any of the disease processes just mentioned should lead the surgeon to suspect this diagnosis and perform abdominal paracentesis. Confirmatory evidence includes the presence of numerous PMNs and a single type of microbe on Gram stain. If polymicrobial flora are observed on Gram stain, then the diagnosis of primary microbial peritonitis is incorrect, and secondary microbial peritonitis most likely is present. Treatment of primary microbial peritonitis consists of administration of parenteral antimicrobial agents directed against the causative pathogen for 14 to 21 days. Removal of prosthetic material such as a peritoneal dialysis catheter generally is necessary, although it may be possible to treat some patients solely with antibiotics. Resolution of symptoms is the best indicator of successful therapy, although posttreatment paracentesis can be considered for severe or recurrent cases.

Secondary microbial peritonitis occurs subsequent to perforation of a hollow viscus in which endogenous microbes spill out into the peritoneal cavity, forming the initial inoculum. Intriguingly, despite the huge number of microbes that form the initial inoculum during gastrointestinal tract perforation, only a limited number are capable of causing infection. Clinical observations and experimental studies have made clear that microbial simplification occurs among the hundreds of microbes initially present by means of a variety of mechanisms such that only a limited number of species (~3–12) survive the initial stages of infection during the first 2 to 7 days after contamination.[81] These mechanisms include (1) microbial numerical contribution to the initial inoculum; (2) additive, inhibitory, and synergistic effects of one microbe on the growth of others; and (3) inhibition of specific host defenses.

Not surprisingly, perforation of the colon is associated with higher infection rates compared to other types of perforation because of the large inoculum size, consisting of both aerobes and anaerobes. After such contamination, the clinical manifestations of infection include severe abdominal pain associated with distension, ileus, and fever and evidence of free intraperitoneal air or leakage from the gut on routine radiographic studies or those using contrast material, respectively.

At the time of abdominal exploration, fibrinopurulent peritonitis is encountered that may be localized or diffuse. Aerobic microbes (e.g., *E. coli* and other gram-negative bacilli such as *Enterobacter*, gram-positive microbes including *E. faecalis* and *E. faecium*), and anaerobic isolates (*B. fragilis* and other species; *Peptidostreptococcus*, *Peptostreptococcus*, and *Clostridium* species) are encountered in about 80% to 90% of specimens; rarely are only aerobes or anaerobes isolated. *Candida albicans* is isolated in about 10% to 20% of cases.

Subsequent to expeditious fluid resuscitation, patients who develop secondary microbial peritonitis should undergo surgery to alleviate the source of ongoing peritoneal soilage.

The optimal duration of therapy has proved difficult to ascertain among all patients who develop intraabdominal infection, although it has been determined for certain types of patients. For example, those patients who suffer penetrating gastrointestinal tract trauma clearly benefit from a short course (12–24h) of an antibiotic that exhibits both aerobic and anaerobic activity, whereas massive blood loss and colon perforation and performance of a colostomy are associated with higher rates such that 3 to 5 days of therapy have been demonstrated to be more effective.[82,83]

Several major trauma centers have developed algorithms based on these data to use during the operative procedure that allow selection of high-risk patients for more prolonged treatment courses. Also, gangrenous or perforated appendicitis without diffuse fibrinopurulent peritonitis can be treated with 3 to 5 days of therapy after operative intervention. In general, after appropriate surgical intervention, patients with any type of localized peritoneal contamination can be treated with a 3- to 5-day course of an antimicrobial agent, whereas longer courses are indicated for immunosuppressed patients and patients with more extensive contamination. Severe fibrinopurulent peritonitis in immunosuppressed patients generally is treated for longer periods (10–14 days), although the efficacy of such prolonged therapy has not been rigorously compared to shorter treatment course.

Formerly, the mortality rate attributed to secondary microbial peritonitis was greater than 30% to 50%.[84] Currently, 10% or fewer patients die if the initial therapy cures the disease; however, the mortality rate remains about 30% to 50% among those individuals with unsuccessful initial therapy that is not successful.

Even after timely surgical intervention and preemptive antibiotic therapy, about 15% to 30% of patients demonstrate ongoing infection consisting of recurrent secondary microbial peritonitis, intraabdominal abscess, or tertiary microbial peritonitis. This problem has been studied in a large number of both retrospective and prospective randomized clinical trials. Concurrently, because aerobes and anaerobes are present in most cases, antimicrobial agent therapy directed against both these types of pathogens should be administered. Initially, it was demonstrated in a series of trials that the efficacy of two agents in combination was superior to that of single agents that demonstrated efficacy against either type of pathogen. It also was demonstrated that anaerobic coverage could be achieved with similar results using either clindamycin or metronidazole, and the specific aminoglycoside selected was of little consequence.[35,85]

Such therapy can be achieved by using two agents, one directed against gram-negative aerobes (e.g., third-generation cephalosporin, aminoglycoside) plus an antianaerobic agent (e.g., clindamycin, metranidazole) or by use of a single broad-spectrum agent that encompasses a similar spectrum of activity. The latter type of therapy is simple and increasingly common, and a large number of suitable agents are available. Commonly selected antibiotics include cefoxitin, cefotetan, ampicillin-sulbactam, ticarcillin-clavulanate, imipenem-cilastatin, and piperacillin-tazobactam. The last two agents are extremely potent and often are used for patients who develop more severe infections, such as hospitalized individuals who develop peritonitis after an initial surgical procedure, immunosuppressed patients, or patients with severe disease.

An extensive review of clinical trials performed in this patient population determined that a success rate of 70% to 85% can be expected, but only when initial surgical intervention is appropriate and suitable agents with concurrent aerobic and anaerobic activity are selected.[86–90] In addition, it has been rigorously demonstrated that it is possible to switch from a parenteral to an oral drug regimen without detrimental effects at the juncture in the postoperative period at which the patient regains gut function.[91] Parameters that should alert the surgeon to the presence of ongoing intraabdominal infection, particularly at the conclusion of antibiotic therapy, include fever (temperature above 37.6°C), more than 10,000 peripheral white blood cells/ml, and band forms on peripheral smear.[92,93] Note, however, that the presence of these indicators does not necessarily warrant continuance of antibiotics or alteration of agents to cure recrudescent infection; rather, it mandates an intensive search for a problem (e.g., intraabdominal abscess, leaking anastomosis, UTI, catheter infection) that may be rectified by further intervention.

Although, historically, culture data have provided the basis of our understanding of the microbiology of intraabdominal infection, currently their associated cost precludes their extensive use for all patients. Increasingly, it has become apparent that initial culture information serves to direct subsequent therapy only in a small subgroup of patients. This issue has been examined retrospectively in about 450 patients; the conclusion reached was that antibiotic changes were not helpful and were in some cases detrimental.[94] Unfortunately, some patients underwent alterations in therapy that were discordant with culture and sensitivity data. Thus, selection of a highly efficacious agent with activity against aerobes and anaerobes from the outset is appropriate, and alterations in antibiotic therapy should not be made for patients who exhibit resolution of infection.

A subset of patients who develop secondary microbial peritonitis and who are unable to either eradicate or sequester intraabdominal infection develop what has been termed *persistent* or *tertiary microbial peritonitis*.[95] Many of these patients are immunosuppressed and require reexploration to ensure that a source of ongoing contamination is not present. Generally, cloudy infected peritoneal fluid is encountered, and cultures reveal the presence of microbes that frequently are resistant to the antibiotics used to treat the initial episode of secondary microbial peritonitis. These microbes include low-virulence pathogens such as *S. epidermidis*, *E. faecalis*, and *E. faecium* as well as more virulent organisms such as *C. albicans* and *P. aeruginosa*. It seems highly likely that the combination of diminished peritoneal host defenses plus initial use of potent antibiotics directed against gram-negative aerobes and anaerobes facilitates the selection of such organisms. Treatment is directed against pathogens isolated at the time of reexploration, and frequent abdominal reexploration to perform lavage and debridement may be required. The mortality of this disease process remains above 50% despite use of potent antibacterial and antifungal agents and reexploration.

The subgroup of patients who develop intraabdominal infection due to appendicitis bears mention. Many studies have been performed examining the effect of antimicrobial agents on the incidence of superficial and deep (intraabdominal abscess) wound infection. A series of studies demonstrated that (1) either dual-agent or single-agent therapy was effective as long as the spectrum of activity encompassed gram-negative aerobes and anaerobes, and (2) under such circumstances the wound edges could be closed with an infection rate of about 2% to 3%.[96–98] Other studies have examined the effect of antimicrobial agents in reducing the wound infection rate with severity of inflammatory disease of the appendix at the time of surgery, with a clear correlation demonstrated. In particular, only minimal impact of preemptive antibiotics could be demonstrated in patients who exhibited minimal disease, whereas a substantial decrease in wound infection rate was evidenced among patients who suffered more serious disease such as perforation or gangrene with surrounding fibrinopurulent peritonitis.[99]

The efficacy of routine use of antifungal or antienterococcal agents for the treatment of intraabdominal infection has not been subjected to rigorous scrutiny in the clinical setting, and any additive beneficial effects of such agents have not been substantiated. The number of patients in whom enterococcus is encountered has not been carefully studied in relation to outcome. Similarly, only retrospective data support the use of antifungal agent therapy when *Candida* is cultured during intraabdominal infection.[100] Patients who suffer gastroduodenal perforation and in whom *Candida* is isolated probably do not require antifungal therapy if surgical intervention is prompt. However, based on retrospective analysis of patients in whom yeast was isolated from established intraabdominal infection, seriously ill immunocompromised patients probably benefit from such therapy with either amphotericin B (300–500 mg total dose) or a triazole drug. In selected patients who suffer less-severe disease, amphotericin B can be used initially and then switched to an oral triazole to allow earlier discharge. Both these organisms are less virulent, present in smaller numbers than more commonly encountered pathogens, and therefore probably contribute to a lesser extent to serious intraabdominal infection in a subset of patients. Because large numbers of patients were required to establish the efficacy of the combination of antiaerobic and antianerobic agents, it is doubtful that controlled trials will be conducted to determine whether coverage of additional antienterococcal or antifungal agents will provide added benefit.

Other Bacterial Infections

Mediastinal infection after cardiothoracic surgery requires exploration, drainage, and debridement. Watery gray purulent material with lack of culture of microbes may be indicative of the presence of *Mycoplasma hominis* infection, a rare cause of mediastinal infection after cardiac surgery. This infection should be treated by administration of a tetracycline antibiotic. Gram-positive microbes cause most of these types of infection. Extensive infection may require open packing and eventual coverage using vascularized muscle flaps.

Large (>3–5 cm) hepatic, splenic, and pulmonary abscesses can be percutaneously drained. Concurrent antibiotic therapy against aerobes and anaerobes should be administered. Abscess drainage catheters should be left in place until such time as the output falls below about 30 to 50 ml/day, although some surgeons have noted that removal within 5 days is associated with recurrence, probably because collapse of the cavity has not occurred. However, the appropriate duration of catheter drainage treatment has not been rigorously examined.

Clostridium difficile colonization and infection can occur in hospitalized patients, and colonic and intestinal inflammatory disease caused by this pathogen is closely linked to antimicrobial agent usage, immunosuppression, and spread within the hospital environment. Treatment consists of oral metronidazole for 10 to 14 days. Recrudescence occurs in 10% to 15% of patients and should be treated with a 10- to 14-day course of oral vancomycin. Rarely, severe disease leads to severe colitis with sepsis syndrome, colonic necrosis, or perforation, any of which require subtotal or total colectomy.

Fungal Infections

The incidence of fungal infections has increased markedly over the past decade, in large part because of the increase in HIV infection as well as the ability to treat cancer and perform bone marrow and solid organ transplantation. Fungi are identified as a component of a polymicrobial infection or as sole pathogens. These types of infections can be classified according to (1) site of infection and (2) pathogenic and invasive potential of the causative microbe. *Candida* represent fungi that generally possess low pathogenic potential when present in superficial sites such as the intertrigonous folds of the skin, although they are capable of invasive behavior, as is *C. neoformans.* More highly pathogenic fungi include *Aspergillus, Histoplasma,* and *Blastomyces,* while those organisms belonging to the order *Mucorales* (*Mucor, Rhizopus,* and *Absidia*) are highly invasive and resistant to antifungal agents.

Common fungal infections encountered by surgeons include those caused by *Candida* and *Aspergillus,* and although other organisms bear mention they are less commonly cultured. Urinary tract infections, esophagitis, and fungemic events caused by *C. albicans* can be treated with a 14- to 21-day course of fluconazole or amphotericin B. Azole-resistant *Candida* should be treated with amphotericin B. *Cryptococcus neoformans* can cause cerebromeningitis in immunosuppressed patients and can be treated with either amphotericin B or fluconazole, although there is some indication that the latter form of therapy is associated with slightly higher recurrence rates in HIV-infected patients.[101] More aggressive fungal infections caused by *Aspergillus* may manifest as pulmonary nodules or infiltrates in immunosuppressed individuals, although diffuse bronchoalveolar infection caused by this organism is common in this patient population. Although infections limited to a single site have been treated with itraconazole, most such infections require prolonged amphotericin B therapy (1.5–2.0 g total dose) concurrent with a reduction in immunosuppressive drug therapy in transplant patients.

Lack of complete resolution within 3 to 4 weeks mandates consideration of surgical extirpative therapy. Fungi belonging to the *Mucor–Rhizopus* group are highly invasive and can cause aggressive rhinocerebral or wound infection in immunosuppressed patients and diabetics who suffer poor glucose control. Aggressive surgical intervention is required from the outset, plus high-dose amphotericin B therapy (2.0–3.0 g). On occasion, dual therapy using amphotericin B and either fluconazole or itraconazole has been employed with success for the treatment of highly drug-resistant fungi, although whether additive or synergistic effects of two drugs together occur remains to be established. Also, some patients who develop invasive infection from minimally pathogenic organisms probably can receive initial amphotericin B followed by oral triazole therapy, the latter in the outpatient setting.

Pulmonary infection caused by *P. carinii* occurs in immunosuppressed patients and produces cough, tachypnea, mild fever, and bilateral diffuse alveolar infiltrates or interstitial pneumonia on the chest roentgenogram. Bronchoscopy should be performed in patients who develop these manifestations; treatment consists of parenteral trimethoprim-sulfamethoxazole, trimethoprim-dapsone, or pentamidine even if the diagnosis is presumptive.

Viral Infections

Viral infections that come to the attention of surgeons include herpesviruses, HBV, HCV, HIV, and many other pathogens. Many of these types of infections occur in immunosuppressed solid organ and bone marrow transplant patients or in patients who have developed AIDS due to HIV. Generally, HSV and varicella zoster virus (VZV) cause mucocutaneous lesions that are self-limited, while VZV can present as shingles. Either can be effectively treated with a 14- to 21-day course of acyclovir. Therapy often is initiated using a parenteral formulation, following which oral drug is administered. On occasion, either virus can cause severe disease (encephalitis, pneumonitis, and endophthalmitis) in immunocompromised patients. Such manifestations should be treated with high-dose parenteral acyclovir (~10–12.5 mg/kg every 6 h in patients with normal renal function) and a concurrent reduction in exogenous immunosuppression in solid organ transplant patients. Infrequently, EBV causes a primary mononucleosis syndrome that should be treated with high-dose acyclovir, but more commonly it is closely associated with posttransplant lymphoproliferative disorders (PTLDs) in immunosuppressed patients. The incidence among solid organ transplant patients ranges from about 1% to 5% and appears to be correlated with the extent of exogenous immunosuppression. The optimal treatment of PTLD remains controversial; reduction in immunosuppression, surgical extirpation, acyclovir, ganciclovir, IFN-α2b, and multidrug cancer chemotherapy regimens all have been employed alone or in combination with anecdotal success. Mortality rates in limited series remain at about 40% to 70%.[102]

In solid organ transplant patients, CMV remains a common problem, with 50% to 75% reported rates of infection; clinical disease is somewhat less frequent (~15%–25%).[103] Infection with CMV occurs in temporal association with maximal host immunosuppression and thus is frequent during the first several months after transplantation; after antirejection therapy, particularly with potent agents such as antilymphocyte antibody (polyclonal or monoclonal); after repeated courses of antirejection therapy; and after cadaver transplantation because of the higher doses of immunosuppressive agents generally administered to this last group of patients. In addition, several experimental and clinical studies have indicated that CMV exerts a direct immunosuppressive effect on the host, acting to diminish T-helper lymphocyte function.

Infection with CMV can occur via several distinct mechanisms. Primary CMV infection occurs when an individual who has not been previously infected with CMV becomes infected by viral transmission from an organ or a blood donor who harbors latent CMV infection. Secondary infection occurs as the result of reactivation of a strain of virus that caused an initial infection in the recipient and entered the latent state, only to again become active during suppression of host defenses. Superinfection with a second strain of CMV also can occur after a patient has experienced CMV infection from one strain of virus and is inoculated with a second strain. If this second strain is sufficiently different from the first or host defenses are diminished to the point that the second strain can produce an infection, then CMV disease may occur because of reactivation, superinfection, or both. Any of these types of infection can lead to clinical manifestations of CMV disease.

Several studies have provided information indicating that CMV disease caused by primary infections is the most severe, that caused by superinfection is less severe, and reactivation disease is most frequently mild. Infection with CMV often presents as a mild disease syndrome consisting of fever, myalgias, malaise, lethargy, leukopenia, and mild dyspnea. More serious illness may present initially as severe retinitis, interstitial pneumonia, gastrointestinal hemorrhage, hepatitis, or pancreatitis and may evolve into a lethal CMV syndrome consisting of severe hypoxia and respiratory failure caused by progressive pneumonitis, as well as hypotension, disseminated intravascular coagulation, massive gastrointestinal hemorrhage, MSOF, and death. Superinfections due to other viral, bacterial, and fungal agents are often present as well, and it is often difficult to determine whether CMV is a primary infecting pathogen.

With the advent of new immunosuppressive drugs that can be used in combination with reduced toxicity plus potent agents that exhibit efficacy against CMV, the impact of this pathogen has diminished such that mortality is rare, and morbidity in terms of allograft loss and intercurrent superinfections has diminished.[103,104] A series of randomized, prospective clinical trials has demonstrated that prophylactic administration of acyclovir, anti-CMV Ig, ganciclovir, and valacyclovir during the first 3 months after solid organ transplantation can reduce the incidence of CMV disease.[104–107] Many centers use initial parenteral ganciclovir, following which oral drug is administered. Patients who develop CMV disease should receive 14 to 21 days of parenteral ganciclovir, following which an additional 9 to 10 weeks of oral therapy is administered to prevent recurrent disease, which occurs in 10% to 25% of patients. Foscarnet is rarely used because of its nephrotoxicity, and few ganciclovir-resistant strains of CMV have been identified among patients receiving this drug for initial prophylaxis. Reduced efficacy of prophylaxis and recurrent disease occur more commonly among patients who suffer primary CMV infection and disease.

Parasitic Infections

Entamoeba histolytica, *Echinococcus multilocularis*, and *Echinococcus granulosus* can cause hepatic abscesses.[108] Generally, such abscesses are large and can become secondarily infected with bacterial pathogens. The diagnosis of infection caused by these pathogens should be established by examination of the stool, serological studies, and abdominal computerized tomography for amoebic disease; only the last two approaches are helpful in identifying echinococcal infection as humans are not definitive hosts. Treatment of amoebic abscesses consists of antiparasitic drugs such as metronidazole or tinidazole, although a number of alternative agents are available. Percutaneous drainage is not undertaken unless rupture seems imminent or there is no response to therapy within 72h.

Echinococcal liver disease generally requires cyst excision via pericystectomy and placement of omentum within the liver defect; hepatectomy is associated with higher rates of morbidity and mortality.[109] Initial sterilization of the cyst(s) can occur either preoperatively or intraoperatively using a scolicidal agent such as 3N saline or formalin, and antiparasitic agent therapy should be administered thereafter. Care must be taken to avoid cyst rupture and spillage, which can lead to widespread intraabdominal dissemination of daughter cysts containing viable scolices capable of peritoneal implantation and growth.

Occasionally, surgeons encounter biliary tract disease caused by the liver fluke *Chlonorchis senesis* or patients who develop acute abdominal pain from visceral larval migrans or bowel obstruction caused by helminths. Operative intervention invariably is required under these circumstances to treat the underlying disease in addition to therapy with antiparasitic agents. *Toxoplasma gondii* can cause necrotizing encephalitis, myocarditis, pneumonitis, and death in immunosuppressed patients, and a higher incidence of infection occurs among cardiac transplant patients. Treatment consists of administration of pyrimethamine and sulfadiazine.

References

1. Dunn DL. Autochthonous microflora of the gastrointestinal tract. Perspect Colon Rectal Surg 1990;2:105–119.
2. Dunn DL, Barke RA, Knight NB, Humphrey EW, Simmons RL. Role of resident macrophages, peripheral neutrophils, and translymphatic absorption in bacterial clearance from the peritoneal cavity. Infect Immun 1985;49:257–264.
3. Dunn DL, Simmons RL. Fibrin in peritonitis. III. The mechanism of bacterial trapping by polymerizing fibrin. Surgery (St. Louis) 1982;92:513–519.
4. Dunn DL, Meakins JL. Humoral immunity to infection and the complement system. In: Howard RJ, Simmons RL, eds. Surgical Infectious Diseases, 3rd ed. Norwalk: Appleton and Lange, 1995:295–312.
5. Fong Y, Moldawer LL, Shires GT, Lowry SF. The biologic characteristics of cytokines and their implication in surgical injury. Surg Gynecol Obstet 1990;170:363–378.
6. Hack C, Aarden LA, Thijs LG. Role of cytokines in sepsis. Adv Immunol 1997;66:101–195.
7. Battafarano RJ, Burd RS, Kurrelmeyer KM, Ratz CA, Dunn DL. Inhibition of splenic macrophage tumor necrosis factor-α secretion in vivo by antilipopolysaccharide monoclonal antibodies. Arch Surg 1994;129:179–186.
8. Banner DW, D'Arcy A, Janes W, et al. Crystal structure of the soluble human 55 kDa TNF receptor-human TNF beta complex: implications for TNF receptor activation. Cell 1993;73:431–445.

9. Giri JG, Wells J, Dower SK, et al. Elevated levels of shed type II IL-1 receptor in sepsis: potential role for type II receptor in regulation of IL-1 responses. J Immunol 1994;153:5802–5809.
10. Porteu F, Nathan CF. Shedding of tumor necrosis factor receptors by activated human neutrophils. J Exp Med 1990;172:599–607.
11. Pruitt J, Copeland E, Moldawer L. Interleukin-1 and interleukin-1 antagonism in sepsis systemic inflammatory response syndrome and septic shock. Shock 1995;3:235–251.
12. Aderka D. The potential biological and clinical significance of the soluble tumor necrosis factor receptors. Cytokine Growth Factor Rev 1996;7:231–240.
13. Goldie AS, Fearon KC, Ross JA, et al. Natural cytokine antagonists and endogenous antiendotoxin core antibodies in sepsis syndrome. The Sepsis Intervention Group. JAMA 1995;274:172–177.
14. Dunn DL, Barke RA, Ewald DC, Simmons RL. Macrophages and translymphatic absorption represent the first line of host defense of the peritoneal cavity. Arch Surg 1987;122:105–110.
15. Barie PS, Dellinger EP, Dougherty SH, Fink MP. Assessment of hepatitis B virus immunization status among North American surgeons. Arch Surg 1994;129:27–31.
16. Updated U.S. public health service guidelines for management of occupational exposure to HBV, HCV, and HIV and recommendations for postexposure prophylaxis. Recommendations for prevention and control of hepatitis C virus (HCV) infection and HCV-related chronic disease. Centers for Disease Control and Prevention. MMWR Morb Mortal Wkly Rep 2001;50:1–42.
17. Panlilio AL, Cardo DM, Grohskopf LA, et al. Updated U.S. public health service guidelines for the management of occupational exposure to HIV and recommendations for postexposure prophylaxis: provisional public health service recommendation for chemoprophylaxis after occupational exposure to HIV. MMWR Morb Mortal Wkly Rep 2005;54:1–17.
18. Sawyer MS, Dunn DL. Appropriate use of antimicrobial agents. Nine principles. Postgrad Med 1991;90:115–122.
19. O'Grady NP, Barie PS, Bartlett JG, et al. Practice guidelines for evaluating new fever in critically ill adult patients. Task Force of the Society of Critical Care Medicine and the Infectious Diseases Society of America. Clin Infect Diseases 1998;26:1042–1059.
20. National Nosocomial Infections Surveillance (NNIS) System report, data summary from October 1986–April 1998, issued June 1998. Am J Infect Control 1998;26:522–533.
21. Tambyah PA, Halvorson KT, Maki DG. A prospective study of pathogenesis of catheter-associated urinary tract infections. Mayo Clin Proc 1999;74:131–136.
22. Heyland D, Cook DJ, Griffith L, Keenan SP, Brun-Buisson C. The attributable morbidity and mortality of ventilator-associated pneumonia in the critically ill patient. The Canadian Critical Trials Group. Am J Respir Crit Care Med 1999;159:1249–1256.
23. Bowton DL. Nosocomial pneumonia in the ICU—year 2000 and beyond. Chest 1999;115:28S–33S.
24. Burke JF. Preventing bacterial infection by coordinating antibiotic and host activity: a time dependent activity. South Med J 1977;1:24–29.
25. Polk HC Jr, Lopez-Mayor JF. Postoperative wound infection: a prospective study of determinant factors and prevention. Surgery (St. Louis) 1969;66:97–103.
26. Nichols RL, Webb WR, Jones JW, Smith JW, LoCicero J III. Efficacy of antibiotic prophylaxis in high risk gastroduodenal operations. Am J Surg 1982;143:94–98.
27. Bold RJ, Mansfield PF, Berger DH, et al. Prospective, randomized, double-blind study of prophylactic antibiotics in axillary lymph node dissection. Am J Surg 1998;176:239–243.
28. Gonzalez RP, Holevar MR. Role of prophylactic antibiotics for tube thoracostomy in chest trauma. Am Surg 1998;64:617–621.
29. Midtvedt K, Hartmann A, Midtvedt T, Brekke IB. Routine perioperative antibiotic prophylaxis in renal transplantation. Nephrol Dial Transplant 1998;13:1637–1641.
30. Dobay KJ, Freier DT, Albear P. The absent role of prophylactic antibiotics in low-risk patients undergoing laparoscopic cholecystectomy. Am Surg 1999;65:226–228.
31. Dellinger EP, Gross PA, Barrett TL, et al. Quality standard for antimicrobial prophylaxis in surgical procedures. The Infectious Diseases Society of America. Infect Control Hosp Epidemiol 1994;15:182–188.
32. Platt R, Zaleznik DF, Hopkins CC, et al. Perioperative antibiotic prophylaxis for herniorrhaphy and breast surgery. N Engl J Med 1990;322:153–160.
33. Classen DC, Evans RS, Pestonik SL, Horn SD, Menlove RL, Burke JP. The timing of prophylactic administration of antibiotics and the risk of surgical-wound infection. N Engl J Med 1992;326:281–286.
34. Bartlett JG, Condon RE, Gorbach SL, Clarke JS, Nichols RL, Ochi S. Veterans Administration Cooperative Study on Bowel Preparation for Elective Colorectal Operations: impact of oral antibiotic regimen on colonic flora, wound irrigation cultures and bacteriology of septic complications. Ann Surg 1978;188:249–254.
35. Sawyer MD, Dunn DL. Antimicrobial therapy of intra-abdominal sepsis. Infect Dis Clin North Am 1992;6:545–570.
36. Nichols RL, Smith JW, Garcia RY, Waterman RS, Holmes JW. Current practices of preoperative bowel preparation among North American colorectal surgeons. Clin Infect Dis 1997;24:609–619.
37. Dunn DL. Gram-negative bacterial sepsis and sepsis syndrome. Surg Clin North Am 1994;74:621–635.
38. Bone RC, Balk RA, Cerra FB, et al. Definitions for sepsis and organ failure and guidelines for the use of innovative therapies in sepsis. The ACCP/SCCM Consensus Conference Committee. American College of Chest Physicians/Society of Critical Care Medicine. Chest 1992;101:1644–1655.
39. Bossink AW, Groeneveld J, Hack CE, Thijs LG. Prediction of mortality in febrile medical patients: how useful are systemic inflammatory response syndrome and sepsis criteria? Chest 1998;113:1533–1541.
40. Burd RS, Cody CS, Dunn DL. Immunotherapy of Gram-Negative Bacterial Sepsis. Austin, TX: Landes, 1992.
41. Dunn DL. Endotoxin antagonism. In: Baue AE, Faist E, Fry DE, eds. Multiple Organ Failure: Pathophysiology, Prevention, and Therapy. New York: Springer-Verlag, 2000.
42. Bodey G, Abi-Said D, Rolston K, Raad I, Whimbey E. Imipenem or cefoperazone-sulbactam combined with vancomycin for therapy of presumed or proven infection in neutropenic cancer patients. Eur J Clin Microbiol Infect Dis 1996;15:625–634.
43. Hathorn JW, Lyke K. Empirical treatment of febrile neutropenia: evolution of current therapeutic approaches. Clin Infect Dis 1997;24:S256–S265.
44. Gross PA, Barrett TL, Dellinger EP, et al. Quality standard for the treatment of bacteremia. The Infectious Diseases Society of America. Infect Control Hosp Epidemiol 1994;15:189–192.
45. Rex JH, Bennett JE, Sugar AM, et al. A randomized trial comparing fluconazole with amphotericin B for the treatment of candidemia in patients without neutropenia. Candidemia Study Group and the National Institute. N Engl J Med 1994;331:1325–1330.
46. Goodman JL, Winston DJ, Greenfield RA, et al. A controlled trial of fluconazole to prevent fungal infections in patients undergoing bone marrow transplantation. N Engl J Med 1992;326:845–851.
47. Ziegler EJ, Fisher CJ Jr, Sprung CL, et al. Treatment of gram-negative bacteremia and septic shock with HA-1A human monoclonal antibody against endotoxin. A randomized, double-

blind, placebo-controlled trial. The HA-1A Sepsis Study Group. N Engl J Med 1991;324:429–436.
48. Greenman RL, Schein RM, Martin MA, et al. A controlled clinical trial of E5 murine monoclonal IgM antibody to endotoxin in the treatment of gram-negative sepsis. JAMA 1991;266:1097–1102.
49. McCloskey RV, Straube RC, Sanders C, Smith SM, Smith CR. Treatment of septic shock with human monoclonal antibody HA-1A. A randomized, double-blind, placebo-controlled trial. CHESS Trial Study Group. Ann Intern Med 1994;121:1–5.
50. Bone RC, Balk RA, Fein AM, et al. A second large controlled clinical study of E5, a monoclonal antibody to endotoxin: results of a prospective, multicenter, randomized, controlled trial. The E5 Sepsis Study Group. Crit Care Med 1995;23:994–1005.
51. Abraham E, Wunderink R, Silverman H, et al. Efficacy and safety of monoclonal antibody to human tumor necrosis factor-α in patients with sepsis syndrome. JAMA 1995;273:934–941.
52. Fisher CJ Jr, Slotman GJ, Opal SM, et al. Initial evaluation of human recombinant interleukin-1 receptor antagonist in the treatment of sepsis syndrome: a randomized, open-label, placebo-controlled multicenter trial. The IL-1RA Sepsis Syndrome Study Group. Crit Care Med 1994;22:12–21.
53. Fisher CJ Jr, Dhainaut JF, Opal SM, et al. Recombinant human interleukin 1 receptor antagonist in the treatment of patients with sepsis syndrome. Results from a randomized, double-blind, placebo-controlled trial. Phase III rhIL-1ra Sepsis Syndrome Study Group. JAMA 1994;271:1836–1843.
54. Fisher CJ Jr, Agosti JM, Opal SM, et al. Treatment of septic shock with the tumor necrosis factor receptor:Fc fusion protein. The Soluble TNF Receptor Sepsis Study Group. N Engl J Med 1996;334:1697–1702.
55. Abraham E, Glauser MP, Butler T, et al. A p55 tumor necrosis factor receptor fusion protein in the treatment of patients with severe sepsis and septic shock. A randomized controlled multicenter trial. Ro 45-2081 Study Group. JAMA 1997;277:1531–1538.
56. Bullard KM, Dunn DL. Diagnosis and treatment of bacteremia and intravascular catheter infections. Am J Surg 1996;172:S13–S19.
57. Andrivet P, Bacquer A, Ngoc CV, et al. Lack of clinical benefit from subcutaneous tunnel insertion of central venous catheters in immunocompromised patients. Clin Infect Dis 1994;18:34–36.
58. Cobb D, High KP, Sawyer RG, et al. A controlled trial of scheduled replacement of central venous and pulmonary-artery catheters. N Engl J Med 1992;327:1062–1068.
59. Lim SH, Smith MP, Machin SJ, Goldstone AH. A prospective randomized study of prophylactic teicoplanin to prevent early Hickman-catheter-related sepsis in patients receiving intensive chemotherapy for haematological malignancies. Eur J Haematol 1993;54:10–13.
60. Maki DG, Stolz SM, Wheeler S, Mermel LA. Prevention of central venous catheter-related bloodstream infection by use of an antiseptic-impregnated catheter. A randomized, controlled trial. Ann Intern Med 1997;127:257–266.
61. Raad I, Darouiche R, Dupuis J, et al. Central venous catheters coated with minocycline and rifampin for the prevention of catheter-related colonization and bloodstream infections. A randomized, double-blind trial. The Texas Medical Center Catheter Study Group. Ann Intern Med 1997;127:267–274.
62. Darouiche RO, Raad II, Heard SO, et al. A comparison of two antimicrobial-impregnated central venous catheters. Catheter Study Group. N Engl J Med 1999;340:1–8.
63. Collignon PJ. Intravascular catheter associated sepsis: a common problem. The Australian Study on Intravascular Catheter Associated Sepsis. Med J Aust 1994;161:374–378.
64. Martinez E, Mensa J, Rovira M, et al. Central venous catheter exchange by guidewire for treatment of catheter-related bacteraemia in patients undergoing BMT or intensive chemotherapy. Bone Marrow Transplant 1999;23:41–44.
65. Raad I, Bompart F, Hachem R. Prospective, randomized dose-ranging open phase II pilot study of quinupristin/dalfopristin versus vancomycin in the treatment of catheter-related staphylococcal bacteremia. Eur J Clin Microbiol Infect Dis 1999;18:199–202.
66. Johnson DC, Johnson FL, Goldman S. Preliminary results treating persistent venous catheter infections with the antibiotic lock technique in pediatric patients. Pediatr Infect Dis 1994;13:930–931.
67. Henke PK, Bergamini TM, Rose SM, Richardson JD. Current options in prosthetic vascular graft infection. Am Surg 1998;64:39–45.
68. Sladen JG, Chen JC, Reid JD. An aggressive local approach to vascular graft infection. Am J Surg 1998;176:222–225.
69. O'Brien T, Collin J. Prosthetic vascular graft infection. Br J Surg 1992;79:1262–1267.
70. Reardon MJ, Vinnerkvist A, LeMaire SA. Mitral valve homograft for mitral valve replacement in acute bacterial endocarditis. J Heart Valve Dis 1999;8:71–73.
71. Dunn DL, Sawyer MD. Deep soft tissue infections. Curr Opin Infect Dis 1990;3:691–696.
72. Bilton BD, Zibari GB, McMillan RW, Aultman DF, Dunn G, McDonald JC. Aggressive surgical management of necrotizing fasciitis serves to decrease mortality: a retrospective study. Am Surg 1998;64:397–400.
73. Sawyer MD, Dunn DL. Deep soft tissue infections. Curr Opin Infect Dis 1991;4:649–654.
74. Sawyer MD, Dunn DL. Serious bacterial infections of the skin and soft tissues. Curr Opin Infect Dis 1995;8:293–297.
75. Stamenkovic I, Lew DP. Early recognition of potentially fatal necrotizing fasciitis. The use of frozen-section biopsy. N Engl J Med 1984;310:1689–1696.
76. Stone HH, Martin JD. Synergistic necrotizing cellulitis. Ann Surg 1972;175:702–711.
77. Riseman JA, Zamboni WA, Curtis A, Graham DR, Konrad HR, Ross DS. Hyperbaric oxygen therapy for necrotizing fasciitis reduces mortality and the need for debridements. Surgery (St. Louis) 1990;108:847–850.
78. Brown DR, Davis NL, Lepawsky M, Cunningham J, Kortbeek J. A multicenter review of the treatment of major truncal necrotizing infections with and without hyperbaric oxygen therapy. Am J Surg 1994;167:485–489.
79. Topper SM, Plaga BR, Burner WL. Necrotizing myonecrosis and polymicrobial sepsis. The role of adjunctive hyperbaric oxygen. Orthop Rev 1990;14:895–900.
80. Hall RL, Callaghan JJ, Moloney E, Martinez S, Harrelson JM. Pyomyositis in a temperate climate. Presentation, diagnosis, and treatment. J Bone Joint Surg 1990;72:1240–1244.
81. Dunn DL, Simmons RL. The role of anaerobic bacteria in intraabdominal infections. Rev Infect Dis 1984;6:S139–S146.
82. Nichols RL, Smith JW, Klein DB, et al. Risk of infection after penetrating abdominal trauma. N Engl J Med 1984;311:1065–1070.
83. Dellinger EP, Wertz MJ, Lennard ES, Oreskovich MR. Efficacy of short-course antibiotic prophylaxis after penetrating intestinal injury. A prospective randomized trial. Arch Surg 1986;121:23–30.
84. Bohnen J, Boulanger M, Meakins JL, McLean AP. Prognosis in generalized peritonitis. Relation to cause and risk factors. Arch Surg 1983;118:285–290.
85. Dunn DL, Simmons RL. Anaerobic microorganisms in intraabdominal infection: significance and treatment. In: Simmons RL, ed. Topics in Intraabdominal Surgical Infection, Vol. 2. New York: Appleton Century Crofts, 1984:1–16.
86. Solomkin JS, Dellinger EP, Christou NV, Busuttil RW. Results of a multicenter trial comparing imipenem/cilastatin to tobra-

mycin/clindamycin for intra-abdominal infections. Ann Surg 1990;212:581–591.
87. Bohnen JM, Solomkin JS, Dellinger EP, Bjornson HS, Page CP. Guidelines for clinical care: anti-infective agents for intra-abdominal infection. A Surgical Infection Society policy statement. Arch Surg 1992;127:83–89.
88. Christou NV, Barie PS, Dellinger EP, Waymack JP, Stone HH. Surgical Infection Society intra-abdominal infection study. Prospective evaluation of management techniques and outcome. Arch Surg 1993;128:193–198.
89. Condon RE, Walker AP, Sirinek KR, et al. Meropenem versus tobramycin plus clindamycin for treatment of intraabdominal infections: results of a prospective, randomized, double-blind clinical trial. Clin Infect Dis 1995;21:544–550.
90. Barie PS, Vogel SB, Dellinger EP, et al. A randomized, double-blind clinical trial comparing cefepime plus metronidazole with imipenem-cilastatin in the treatment of complicated intra-abdominal infections. Cefepime Intra-abdominal Infection Study Group. Arch Surg 1997;132:1294–1302.
91. Solomkin JS, Reinhart HH, Dellinger EP, et al. Results of a randomized trial comparing sequential intravenous/oral treatment with ciprofloxacin plus metronidazole to imipenem/cilastatin for intra-abdominal infections. The Intra-Abdominal Infection Study Group. Ann Surg 1996;223:303–315.
92. Stone HH, Bourneuf AA, Stinson LD. Reliability of criteria for predicting persistent or recurrent sepsis. Arch Surg 1985;120:17.
93. Lennard ES, Dellinger EP, Wertz MJ, et al. Implications of leukocytosis and fever at conclusion of antibiotic therapy for intra-abdominal sepsis. Ann Surg 1982;195:19.
94. Mosdell DM, Morris DM, Voltura A, et al. Antibiotic treatment for surgical peritonitis. Ann Surg 1991;214:543–549.
95. Rotstein OD, Pruett TL, Simmons RL. Microbiologic features and treatment of persistent peritonitis in patients in the intensive care unit. Can J Surg 1986;29:247.
96. Berne TV, Yellin AW, Appleman MD, Heseltine PNR. Antibiotic management of surgically treated gangrenous or perforated appendicitis. Comparison of gentamicin and clindamycin versus cefamandole versus cefoperazone. Am J Surg 1982;144:8–13.
97. Heseltine PNR, Yellin AE, Appleman MD, et al. Imipenem therapy for perforated and gangrenous appendicitis. Surg Gynecol Obstet 1986;162:43–48.
98. Berne TV, Yellin A, Appleman MD, Gill MA, Chenella FC, Heseltine PNR. Surgically treated gangrenous or perforated appendicitis. A comparison of aztreonam and clindamycin versus gentamicin and clindamycin. Ann Surg 1987;205:133–137.
99. Bauer R, Vennits B, Holm B, et al. Antibiotic prophylaxis in acute nonperforated appendicitis. The Danish multicenter study group 111. Ann Surg 1989;209:307–311.
100. Solomkin JS, Flohr AB, Quie PG, Simmons RL. The role of *Candida* in intraperitoneal infections. Surgery (St. Louis) 1980;88:524–530.
101. Powderly WG, Saag MS, Cloud GA, et al. A controlled trial of fluconazole or amphotericin B to prevent relapse of cryptococcal meningitis in patients with the acquired immunodeficiency syndrome. The NIAID AIDS Clinical Trials Group and Mycoses Study Group. N Engl J Med 1992;326:793–798.
102. Morrison VA, Peterson BA, Dunn DL. Post-transplant lymphoproliferative disorders: pathogenesis, presentation, and approaches to therapy. In: Faist E, Baue AE, Schildber FW, eds. The Immune Consequences of Trauma, Shock and Sepsis—Mechanisms and Therapeutic Approaches. Berlin: Pabst, 1996:592–602.
103. Dunn DL, Mayoral JL, Gillingham KJ, et al. Treatment of invasive cytomegalovirus disease in solid organ transplant patients with ganciclovir. Transplantation 1991;51:98–106.
104. Dunn DL, Gillingham KJ, Kramer MA, et al. A prospective randomized study of acyclovir versus ganciclovir plus human immune globulin prophylaxis of cytomegalovirus infection after solid organ transplantation. Transplantation 1994;57:876–884.
105. Snydman DR, Werner BG, Heinze-Lacey B. Use of cytomegalovirus immune globulin to prevent cytomegalovirus disease in renal-transplant recipients. N Engl J Med 1987;317:1049–1054.
106. Balfour HH, Chace BA, Stapleton JT. A randomized, placebo-controlled trial of oral acyclovir for the prevention of cytomegalovirus disease in recipients of renal allografts. N Engl J Med 1989;320:1381–1385.
107. Lowance D, Neumayer HH, Legendre CM, et al. Valacyclovir for the prevention of cytomegalovirus disease after renal transplantation. International Valacyclovir Cytomegalovirus Prophylaxis Transplantation Study Group. N Engl J Med 1999;340:1462–1470.
108. Sharma MP, Dasarathy S. Amoebic liver abscess. Trop Gastroenterol 1993;14:3–9.
109. Di Matteo G, Bove A, Chiarini S, et al. Hepatic echinococcus disease: our experience over 22 years. Hepato-Gastroenterology 1996;43:1562–1565.

12

Infections of Skin and Soft Tissue

Philip S. Barie and Soumitra R. Eachempati

Infections of skin and soft tissue (SSTIs) encompass a diverse set of conditions, but there are commonalities that justify their consideration as a group. Some SSTIs are not dangerous to the patient, whereas others are life threatening and require radical surgical debridement as well as broad-spectrum antibiotic therapy. The U.S. Food and Drug Administration (FDA) classified SSTIs as uncomplicated or complicated infections for the purposes of clinical trial design and enrollment. This framework is also useful for clinical description.[1]

Uncomplicated SSTIs are those that are superficial or self-limited. They may require only incision and drainage (without antibiotics) or oral antibiotics (without drainage). Hospitalization is rarely necessary. Examples of uncomplicated infections include cellulitis, impetigo, erysipelas, furunculosis, carbunculosis, and small abscesses. Cellulitis may coexist with the last three entities. Uncomplicated infections are excluded from trials of antibiotic therapy for complicated SSTI (cSSTI) and vice versa.

Complicated SSTIs involve deeper tissues or require major surgical intervention. An infection is also considered complicated if the patient has medical comorbidities, specifically renal insufficiency, diabetes mellitus, or peripheral arterial disease. Examples of cSSTIs include major abscesses, deep-space infections, diabetic foot infections (DFIs), some postoperative surgical site infections (SSIs; those with systemic signs of infection), infected decubitus ulcers, and necrotizing soft tissue infections (NSTIs). Clinical trials of drug therapy for cSSTI exclude NSTIs because the mortality rate is high, and the timeliness and extent of surgical debridement are crucial in determining the outcome.

Uncomplicated Skin and Soft Tissue

Cellulitis

Cellulitis is an acute, pyogenic infection of the dermis and subcutaneous tissues, usually complicating a breach of skin integrity.[2] The infected tissue is warm, erythematous, edematous, and tender; the lower extremity is the most common site of infection. The differential diagnosis of cellulitis includes both infectious and noninfectious entities. Early manifestations of NSTIs may be modest and can be confused initially for cellulitis. Inflammatory conditions that can mimic cellulitis include insect bites, acute gout, deep venous thrombosis, drug reactions, pyoderma gangrenosum (characteristic of inflammatory bowel disease or collagen vascular disease), and metastatic carcinoma.

Identification of the source of cellulitis can provide important clues to help define therapy. The most common cause of cellulitis is trauma to the skin. Edema predisposes to cellulitis (e.g., ipsilateral arm edema after mastectomy).[3] Other important clues include physical activity, water contact, and human or animal bites. Cellulitis may also manifest a deeper infection, (e.g., spread of subjacent osteomyelitis, cellulitis of the thigh following colon perforation into the retroperitoneum). Bloodstream infection is a rare cause of SSTI, but cases have been reported after meningococcal, pneumococcal, or staphylococcal bacteremia. *Pseudomonas* bacteremia can cause skin lesions in neutropenic patients. Bacteremic SSTI (usually an NSTI) caused by *Vibrio vulnificus* has been associated with ingestion of raw shellfish, and NSTI caused by *Bacillus cereus* has been associated with ingestion of a wide variety of foodstuffs.

The diagnosis of cellulitis is made clinically based on the circumstances and the appearance of the lesion; neither imaging studies nor cultures of the lesion have a high diagnostic yield. Needle aspiration yields an organism only about 30% of the time. Punch biopsies of skin have a higher yield, but the invasiveness is seldom justified as empiric therapy is usually successful in uncomplicated cases. Bloodstream infection is uncommon in cellulitis; the incidence of positive blood cultures is less than 5%, and therefore they are not cost-effective except perhaps for cellulitis complicating lymphedema, for which the incidence of bloodstream infection may be higher. Radiologic studies are unnecessary in most patients unless a complicated,

TABLE 12.1. Summary of Recommendations from Practice Guideline for Diagnosis and Treatment of Skin and Soft Tissue Infections (SSTIs), Infectious Diseases Society of America.

Level I	
Impetigo	Mupirocin is the best topical agent, and is equivalent to oral systemic antimicrobials when lesions are limited in number. Patients with numerous lesions or who do not respond to topical therapy should receive an oral antimicrobial agent. PCN or penicillinase-resistant PCN are TOCs for nonbullous lesions. PCN or 1-G cephalosporin is recommended for bullous lesions.
Erysipelas	PCN is TOC for streptococcal infection. Penicillinase-resistant PCN or 1-G cephalosporin is recommended if staphylococci are suspected.
Cellulitis	Penicillinase-resistant PCN or 1-G cephalosporin are the TOCs unless resistant organisms are common in the community. Use clindamycin or vancomycin for PCN-allergic patients.
Cutaneous abscess	Incision and drainage is the TOC.
Furunculosis	Recurrent furunculosis may be treated with mupirocin to the anterior nares (for chronic staphylococcal carriers) or clindamycin 150 mg/day for 3 months.
MRSA	Linezolid, daptomycin, and vancomycin have excellent efficacy in SSTI in general and in particular those caused by MRSA.
NSTI	Surgical intervention is the major therapeutic intervention.
Type I NSTI	Ampicillin-sulbactam plus ciprofloxacin plus clindamycin is TOC for community-acquired infection.
Type II NSTI	Clindamycin/PCN combination therapy is TOC.
Level II	
Furunculosis	Attempt to eradicate the staphylococcal carrier state among colonized persons.
Type I NSTI	A variety of antimicrobials directed against aerobic gram-positive and -negative bacteria and anaerobes may be used in mixed necrotizing infection.
Type II NSTI	Consider intravenous gamma globulin (IVIG) therapy. PCN/clindamycin combination therapy is the TOC for infections caused by *Clostridium perfringens.*
Animal bites	Oral amoxicillin-clavulanic acid or intravenous ampicillin-sulbactam or ertapenem should be administered to non-PCN-allergic patients because of suitable activity against *Pasturella multocida*. Acceptable alternative regimens include piperacillin-tazobactam, imipenem-cilastatin, and meropenem.
Level III	
Cutaneous abscess	Gram stain, culture, and systemic antibiotics are rarely necessary.
Furuncle	Systemic antibiotics are usually unnecessary, absent fever or extensive surrounding cellulitis.
Animal bites	1-G cephalosporins, penicillinase-resistant PCN, macrolides, and clindamycin should be avoided as therapy because of poor activity against *P. multocida.*
Human bites	Intravenous ampicillin-sulbactam or cefoxitin are the TOCs for non-PCN-allergic patients. A hand surgeon should evaluate clenched-fist injuries for penetration into synovium, joint capsule, or bone.

1-G, First-generation cephalosporin; MRSA; methicillin-resistant *Staphylococcus aureus*; NSTI, necrotizing soft tissue infection; PCN, penicillin; SSI: surgical site infection; TOC, treatment of choice.

Suspicion of possible SSI does not justify use of antibiotics without a definitive diagnosis and the initiation of other therapies, such as opening the incision. All infected surgical incisions should be opened.

Source: From Stevens,[1] by permission of *Clinical Infectious Diseases*.

deep-seated SSTI or NSTI cannot be excluded by examination of the patient.

Most cases of cellulitis are caused by gram-positive cocci, either streptococci or *Staphylococcus aureus*.[4] Diffuse or poorly circumscribed lesions are more likely to be caused by streptococci. The β-lactam antibiotics with activity against penicillinase-producing *S. aureus* (methicillin-sensitive *S. aureus*, MSSA) are the treatment of choice for most cases of cellulitis. Oral therapy is appropriate unless the patient has systemic signs (e.g., fever, chills); medical comorbidity; or a rapidly spreading lesion, any of which indicate initial intravenous therapy. Choices for initial parenteral therapy include penicillin G (for erysipelas; see below); cefazolin; nafcillin (or oxacillin or methicillin); or ceftriaxone (Table 12.1). If methicillin-resistant *S. aureus* (MRSA) is suspected or the patient is highly allergic to penicillin (i.e., anaphylactoid reaction), then vancomycin or linezolid may be chosen. Appropriate oral agents include dicloxacillin, cephalexin, cephradine, or cefadroxil. Minocycline or linezolid may be appropriate for oral therapy of MRSA.

Methicillin-Resistant *Staphylococcus Aureus* in Surgical Site Infection

Methicillin-resistant *S. aureus* in SSTI requires particular mention. Approximately 60% of hospital isolates of *S. aureus* are MRSA;[5] hospitalized or recently hospitalized patients who develop an SSTI must be considered for empiric therapy against MRSA. Increasingly, MRSA SSTIs are observed among patients who have had no contact with the health care system. Community-onset or community-acquired MRSA (CA-MRSA) has emerged since 2001 as a major pathogen.[6] Molecular epidemiologic studies show clearly that CA-MRSA is not a feral, escaped clone of the hospital-associated MRSA, but is a unique pathogen that has a unique antibiotic susceptibility pattern. The CA-MRSA clone probably arose from antibiotic selection pressure on a commensal, saprophytic *Staphylococcus* sp. that is part of normal skin flora. Community-associated MRSA may cause pneumonia as well as SSTI; either manifestation may be associated with tissue necrosis; a handful of cases of NSTI have been reported as well.[7] However, about 75% of infections caused by CA-MRSA are SSTIs. In many areas of the United States, CA-MRSA is now the predominant cause of SSTIs that present to emergency departments.[8]

The antimicrobial susceptibilities of CA-MRSA differ from the hospital clones. Although CA-MRSA is similarly susceptible to vancomycin and linezolid, CA-MRSA may be susceptible in vitro to macrolides, clindamycin, and co-trimoxazole; the last drug is most reliable for oral therapy. Clindamycin resistance that is inducible by macrolides has been associated with treatment failures; therefore, caution is advised if using clindamycin for therapy,[9] especially if the organism is macrolide resistant.

Outbreaks of CA-MRSA have been associated with groups of people who are in close contact, including prison inmates, amateur and professional sports teams, military recruits, and clients of day care centers.[6] Direct contact with skin is a definite risk factor, as are shared personal hygiene items such as towels or bars of soap. Other patient groups at risk are young children and people of lower socioeconomic status. Infections (SSTIs) caused by CA-MRSA have a characteristic appearance that may raise suspicion of the diagnosis. The lesions are usually superficial and well demarcated, often with a necrotic center (Fig. 12.1). If the lesions are uncomplicated, then incision and drainage alone or topical mupirocin ointment or chlorhexidine solution may be sufficient therapy. If antibiotic therapy is required, then co-trimoxazole should be considered.

Erysipelas

Erysipelas, a form of cellulitis, is distinguished from other uncomplicated SSTIs by two factors.[10,11] Lesions of erysipelas are raised above the level of surrounding skin, and there is sharp demarcation between infected and normal skin. Most infections remain superficial, but deep extension is reported. Erysipelas is most common among young children and older adults. The etiologic agent is almost always group A streptococci, sometimes group C or G streptococci, or rarely group B streptococci or *S. aureus*. Because of the streptococcal predominance, penicillin is the treatment of choice unless staphylococci are suspected[1] (Table 12.1).

Impetigo

Impetigo is a common SSTI that consists of discrete purulent lesions that are nearly always caused by β-hemolytic streptococci or *S. aureus*[12] (Fig. 12.2). Impetigo is most common among economically disadvantaged children in warm climates (during the summer in temperate climates). Organisms probably initially colonize unbroken skin as a prelude to impetigo, emphasizing personal hygiene in the pathogenesis. Inoculation into skin by minor trauma occurs subsequently.

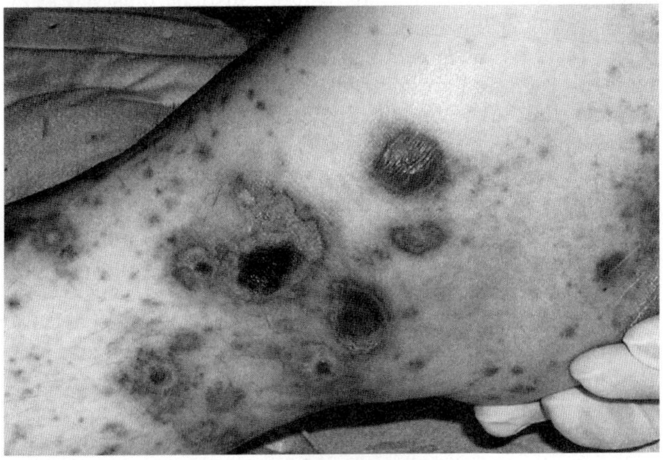

FIGURE 12.1. Necrotizing skin lesion characteristic of community-associated methicillin-resistant *S. aureus* infection.

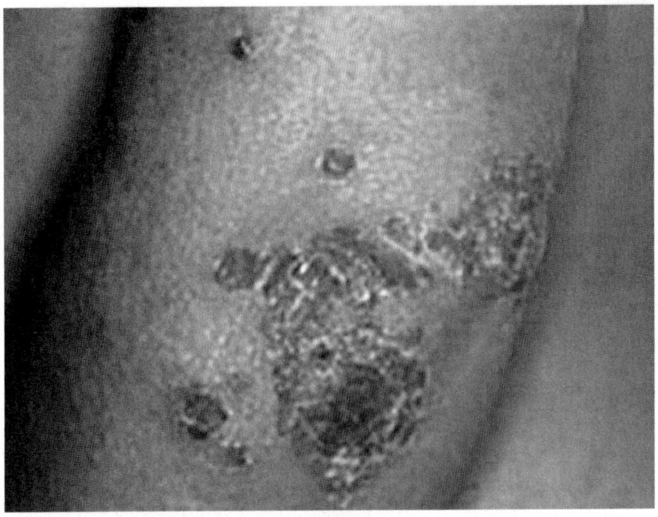

FIGURE 12.2. Staphylococcal impetigo.

Nasal carriage of staphylococci is a risk factor for impetigo caused by those organisms. Impetigo usually invades exposed skin, primarily of the face and extremities. The lesions are usually multiple and may be bullous (*S. aureus*) or nonbullous. A deeply ulcerated form of impetigo is known as ecthyma. A penicillinase-resistant penicillin or first-generation cephalosporin is preferred for therapy, but cases caused by MRSA are on the increase. Topical therapy with mupirocin is equivalent to therapy with oral antibiotics[1] (Table 12.1).

Cutaneous Abscess

Cutaneous abscesses may infect the dermis and subcutaneous tissue. These lesions are usually painful, tender, and fluctuant, with a central pustule and surrounding erythema and edema. These infections are typically polymicrobial, with pure culture of *S. aureus* isolated in only one-quarter of cases. Epidermoid cysts (erroneously called sebaceous cysts) may contain skin flora in the soft, keratinous, "cheesy" center, even when not inflamed. Inflammation usually results from cyst rupture with extrusion of cyst contents into surrounding tissue rather than infection per se. Organisms, when identified, are usually skin flora. Treatment of cutaneous abscesses is incision and drainage, with mechanical destruction of intracavitary loculations (Table 12.1).[1] Gram stain, culture, or systemic antibiotics are rarely necessary unless a patient has systemic signs or severe immunocompromise.

Furuncles ("boils") are infected hair follicles, usually caused by *S. aureus*.[1] Suppuration extends through the dermis to subcutaneous tissue, forming a small abscess. This contrasts with *folliculitis*, which is also an infection arising in hair follicles, but the inflammation is more superficial, and pus is present in the epidermis. Furuncles can appear anywhere on hair-bearing skin. Infection of several adjacent follicles can cause coalescence, with multiple draining sites, which is called a *carbuncle* (Fig. 12.3). Carbuncles have a strong predilection to form on the dorsum of the neck in patients with diabetes mellitus. Small furuncles may be treated with moist heat, which promotes spontaneous drainage. Systemic antibiotics again are rarely necessary. Outbreaks of staphylococcal furunculosis (either MSSA or MRSA)

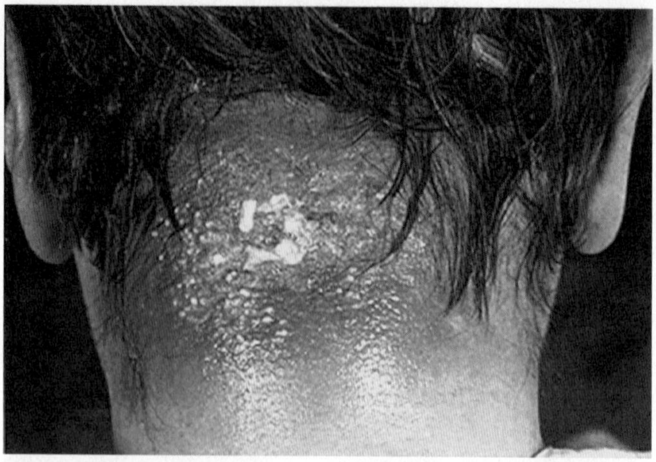

FIGURE 12.3. Several furuncles have coalesced to form a spontaneously draining carbuncle on the nape of the neck. Formal incision and drainage is necessary.

among persons in close personal contact (e.g., prisoners, families, team sports participants) may require institution of infection control measures, such as bathing with antibacterial soaps, careful laundering, no sharing of personal hygiene items, and eradication of the staphylococcal carrier state if present. Some patients are also subject to recurrent episodes of furunculosis, for which nasal carriage of staphylococci is a strong predisposing factor. Intranasal 2% mupirocin ointment twice daily for 5 days each month can reduce the incidence of recurrence by one-half.[13] Oral clindamycin 150 mg/day for 3 months is even more successful, reducing recurrences by 80%.[14]

Hidradenitis Suppurativa

Hidradenitis suppurativa is a chronic acneiform infection of the cutaneous apocrine glands that also can involve adjacent subcutaneous tissue and fascia of the axillae, groin, or wherever apocrine glands are concentrated.[15–18] In addition to common manifestations in the axilla or groin, the areola, the intramammary cleft, gluteal folds, perineum, circumanal area, or infraumbilical skin may be affected. Ingrown hairs are a predisposing factor; thus, the incidence is increased in patients with curly hair. The incidence of hidradenitis suppurativa is greater in females. Hidradenitis suppurativa does not present in prepubescent patients because apocrine secretion is hormone sensitive. The condition may be observed in patients of any age after puberty, and symptoms may be affected by the menstrual cycle. Hot weather, excessive perspiration, and obesity may be aggravating factors. A genetic predisposition to hidradenitis suppurativa exists, including Down syndrome. Disease activity may be related to stress or in association with other chronic conditions such as inflammatory bowel disease, irritable bowel syndrome, or autoimmune disorders such as arthritis, Hashimoto thyroiditis, or Sjögren syndrome.

Hidradenitis suppurativa occurs when apocrine gland secretion becomes obstructed by perspiration or glands are unable to drain normally because of structural abnormality. Trapped secretions and bacteria extravasate bacteria into surrounding tissue, causing subcutaneous inflammation and infection. As suppuration progresses, surrounding cellulitis may be present. The condition presents most commonly as painful, tender, firm, nodular lesions in one or both axillae. When infection is active, hidradenitis suppurativa may resemble bacterial folliculitis or furunculosis. The differential diagnosis also includes granuloma inguinale, lymphogranuloma venereum, pilonidal cyst, and tuberculosis of the skin. The nodules may open and drain pus spontaneously, then heal slowly, with or without drainage, over a 2- to 4-week period. Remissions may last months or years, but recurrences are frequent, and some patients are afflicted continuously. Patients with chronic affliction may present with multiple nodules that have coalesced and are associated with a fibrotic reaction that results in scarring and an unsightly appearance.

Most nodules will resolve without surgical drainage. Incision and drainage may be helpful for fluctuant nodules that have not opened spontaneously. Antibiotics are indicated if cellulitis or fever is present, and hospitalization should be considered if the patient has systemic toxicity. In severe or intractable cases, excision of the pathologic tissue with split-thickness skin grafting offers the best chance for cure. Radiation and laser treatments are investigational but have shown some promise for patients with severe hidradenitis suppurativa.

Complications or intractable disease include lymphedema due to inflammation and scarring of lymphatic channels, restricted limb mobility from scarring and contracture, or arthritis secondary to inflammatory injury of synoval tissue or cartilage. Disseminated infection is rare. Squamous cell carcinoma may develop in indolent sinus tracts.

Prevention includes minimized heat exposure and consequent perspiration. Patients should lose weight if overweight. Constrictive clothing and frictional trauma to affected skin should be avoided, as should underarm antiperspirants and deodorants. Affected hair-bearing areas should be kept shaved to prevent re-ingrowth of hair.

Complicated Skin and Soft Tissue

Complicated SSTIs involve deeper tissues or require major surgical intervention. Infection in the presence of medical comorbidities, particularly renal insufficiency, diabetes mellitus, or peripheral arterial disease, also defines a cSSTI. Examples of cSSTIs include major abscesses, deep-space infections, DFIs, some postoperative SSIs (those with systemic signs of infection), infected decubitus ulcers, and NSTIs. Clinical trials of drug therapy for cSSTI exclude NSTIs because the mortality rate is high, and the timeliness and extent of surgical debridement are crucial in determining the outcome. Table 12.2 presents an evidence-based summary of recent clinical trials of antibiotic therapy.[19–27] Most trials are designed to demonstrate "noninferiority" of the tested regimen against the comparator regimen, so numerous regimens appear comparable despite widely divergent spectra of activity. Notably, comparable outcomes are achieved by agents that treat only gram-positive cocci (e.g., vancomycin, linezolid, daptomycin, dalbavancin), but the many options available to investigators (e.g., choice of comparator in "standard therapy" regimens, addition of aztreonam) makes the literature a challenge to interpret.

TABLE 12.2.
Recent Prospective Trials of Antibiotic Therapy for Complicated Skin and Skin Structure Infections.

Study	*Drug*	*Comparator*	*Result*	*Notes*
Stevens[19]	Linezolid 600 mg i.v. daily	Vancomycin 1 g i.v. every 12 h	73% vs. 73% cure, E population 95% CI (−16.6 to 16.8)	MRSA only; open label; 7 days of therapy; underpowered
Seltzer[20]	Dalbavancin 1 g i.v. day 1 and 500 mg day 8	Standard therapy	94% vs. 76%, E population; only result for 2 doses of dalbavancin shown	Open-label, dose-ranging, phase 2 trial
Arbeit[21]	Daptomycin 4 mg/kg i.v. daily	Standard therapy or vancomycin 1 g i.v. every 12 h, oral switch to synthetic penicillin OK if MSSA	83% vs. 84% cure, E population; 95% CI (−4.0 to 5.6)	Combined report of two phase 3 trials; noninferior treatment for 7–14 days
Wilcox[22]	Linezolid 600 mg i.v./p.o. every 12 h	Teicoplanin dose determined by investigator	96% vs. 88% cure, ITT population; 95% CI (2.5 to 13.2)	Linezolid superior to teicoplanin, but dose of teicoplanin questionable
Giordano[23]	Moxifloxacin 400 mg i.v./p.o. every 12 h	Piperacillin-tazobactam 3.375 g i.v. every 6 h; amoxicillin-clavulanate 800 mg p.o. every 12 h	79% vs. 82% cure, E population; 95% CI (−12.04 to 3.29)	Noninferior treatment for 7–14 days
Ellis-Grosse[24]	Tigecycline 100 mg load, then 50 mg i.v. every 12 h	Vancomycin 1 g every 12 h plus aztreonam 2 g i.v. every 12 h	80% vs. 82% cure, mITT population; 95% CI (−7.1 to 2.8)	Combined report of two phase 3 trials; noninferior treatment
Jauregui[25]	Dalbavancin 1 g day 1, 500 mg day 8	Linezolid 600 mg i.v./p.o. every 12 h	89% vs. 91% cure, E population; 97.5% CI calculated, only lower limit of −7.28 reported	Randomized; D:L 2:1; treatment for 14 days
Weigelt[26]	Linezolid 600 mg every 12 h i.v./p.o., aztreonam permitted	Vancomycin 1 g i.v. every 12 h; switch to semisynthetic penicillin if MSSA, aztreonam permitted	92% vs. 89% cure, ITT population; 95% CI (−0.11 to 7.47)	Open-label, phase 4; treatment up to 14 days; linezolid superior in MRSA subset; 95% CI (6.08 to 25.70)
Fabian[27]	Meropenem 500 mg i.v.	Imipenem-cliastatin 500 mg i.v. every 8 h	73% vs. 75% cure, mITT group; 95% CI (−2.8 to 9.3)	mitt population: eligible, randomized, and received at least one dose of drug

E, evaluable patient group; ITT, intention-to-treat patient group; i.v., intravenous; mITT, modified intention-to-treat patient group; p.o., oral administration.

Standard therapy means that selection of the comparator agent was at the discretion of the investigator. Noninferiority is defined statistically when the lower limit of the 95% confidence interval is greater than −15, and the confidence interval contains zero. A trial with a relatively narrow confidence interval is likely to have greater statistical power (or more homogeneous results) than one with a wider interval.

Diabetic Foot Infection

Foot infections in patients with diabetes mellitus cause considerable morbidity, including limb loss.[28,29] Diabetic foot infections usually begin in skin ulcerated from either abrasions or ischemia. One-third of patients presenting with a DFI have had a foot lesion for more than 1 month prior to presentation. Skin ulcers are common in diabetic patients not only because of vascular insufficiency, but also because of peripheral sensory neuropathy, which may render the foot insensate. Two-thirds of patients with DFI will present with peripheral arterial disease, and the prevalence of sensory neuropathy is about 80%. Although most DFIs remain superficial, as many as 25% of such infections will spread contiguously to involve subcutaneous tissue or bone (osteomyelitis). The compartmentalized anatomy of the foot, with its various spaces, tendon sheaths, and neurovascular bundles, may create conditions that favor ischemic necrosis of tissues within a compartment or spread along anatomic tissue planes. Recurrent infections are common as 10%–30% of affected patients may come to amputation eventually.[30]

Diabetic patients are predisposed to foot infections not only because of the portal of entry, but also because of defects in humoral immunity, including impaired neutrophil chemotaxis, phagocytosis, and intracellular killing;[31] and impaired monocyte/macrophage function, which appear to correlate with the adequacy of glycemic control.[32] Cell-mediated immunity and complement function may be impaired as well. Diabetic patients have a higher prevalence of nasal carriage of *S. aureus*, which also predisposes to SSTIs.

Acute infections in untreated patients are usually caused by gram-positive cocci, most commonly *S. aureus*, often as monomicrobial infections[33,34] (Table 12.3). *Staphylococcus aureus* is the most important pathogen in DFI; even when it is not the only isolate, it is usually part of the flora of mixed infections. Chronic wounds or recurrent infections may harbor complex flora. Serious infections in hospitalized patients are more likely to be mixed infections, including

TABLE 12.3. Pathogens Isolated in a Clinical Trial of Antibiotic Therapy of Diabetic Foot Infection.

Organisms	*Isolates*
Staphylococci	
Staphylococcus aureus (total)	158
Methicillin-sensitive *S. aureus*	127
Methicillin-resistant *S. aureus*	31
Coagulase-negative staphylococci	65
Streptococci	
Streptococcus agalactiae	52
β-hemolytic streptococci	6
Streptococcus species	14
Enterococci	60
Pseudomonas species	27
Enterobacteriaceae	88

Of cases, 50% had only gram-positive cocci isolated.

Source: Data from Lipsky et al.[34]

both aerobic and anaerobic flora.[35] Among gram-negative bacilli, bacteria of the family Enterobacteriaceae are common, and *Pseudomonas aeruginosa* may be isolated from wounds that have been treated with hydrotherapy or wet dressings. Enterococci may be recovered from patients treated previously with a cephalosporin. Anaerobic bacteria seldom cause DFIs as the sole pathogen, but they may be isolated from deep infections or necrotic tissue. Antibiotic-resistant bacteria, especially MRSA, may be isolated from patients who have received antibiotics previously or who have been hospitalized or reside in long-term care facilities.

Infections affect the forefoot most commonly, especially the toes and the metatarsal heads on the plantar surface. Infection must be diagnosed clinically because all skin wounds contain microorganisms, many of which are commensal. The presence of systemic signs (e.g., fever, chills, leukocytosis); purulent drainage; or at least two local signs of inflammation (e.g., calor [warmth], rubor [redness], dolor [pain or tenderness], and tumor [induration]) are suggestive. Deep-space infections may have few surface signs. Chronic wounds may manifest discoloration, friability, delayed healing, or malodor. Signs of systemic toxicity are uncommon in DFI, even with limb-threatening infection, but metabolic abnormalities (e.g., poorly controlled blood sugar, ketoacidosis, hyperosmolar state) may provide a clue. Many patients do not complain of pain on presentation, and more than one-half of patients do not have fever, leukocytosis, or an elevated erythrocyte sedimentation rate (ESR). Whenever the diagnosis of DFI is considered, aggressive management is indicated because these infections sometimes progress rapidly.

Several severity scores have been proposed for DFI,[36] but none has achieved universal acceptance. Severity may be assessed clinically by determining the depth of the wound and whether tissue ischemia is present. Local wound exploration with a sterile surgical instrument is important to identify necrotic tissue or the presence of a foreign body (e.g., a needle that the patient stepped on but did not feel at the time) and the possibility of osteomyelitis.[37,38] An assessment of severity is essential to select an antibiotic regimen (including route of administration) and determine the need for hospitalization and the potential necessity and timing of surgical debridement or level of amputation. Systemic signs, when present, should raise suspicion of a deep-space infection. Indications for hospitalization include fluid resuscitation, correction of metabolic abnormalities, parenteral antibiotic therapy, or the need for surgical intervention. Other reasons to hospitalize a patient with a DFI include an inability or unwillingness of the patient to provide local wound care or to maintain non-weight-bearing status or likely noncompliance with an outpatient antibiotic regimen. Antibiotic therapy alone will not overcome suboptimal wound care and glycemic control.

Antibiotic Therapy

Of diabetic patients who are treated for a foot ulcer, 40% to 60% receive antibiotics, but antibiotic therapy does not improve the outcome of uninfected foot lesions in diabetic patients.[29,39] Successful antibiotic therapy requires achievement of a therapeutic drug concentration at the site of infection. Intravenous antibiotics are indicated for patients with systemic illness, severe infection, intolerance of oral antibiotics, or pathogens that are not susceptible to oral agents. After the patient is stabilized and shows signs of improvement, a switch to oral antibiotic therapy may be appropriate. The slower delivery of antibiotic with an initial oral dose is inconsequential for noncritically ill patients, so the main issue with oral antibiotic therapy is the bioavailability of the chosen agent. Among the potential choices of oral antibiotics for DFIs, clindamycin and fluoroquinolones have good oral bioavailability. Even parenteral antibiotics may not penetrate tissue adequately in the presence of peripheral arterial disease, even when serum concentrations are adequate.[40]

Most initial therapy is empiric, directed at common pathogens.[34,39,41,42] Severity of infection may influence antibiotic choice in that mild infections may be treated more narrowly because disease progression is unlikely to interfere with the opportunity to modify the regimen when microbiology data become available. Regimens for severe infections should utilize broad-spectrum intravenous antibiotics. Any regimen must also account for allergy, renal function, recent antibiotic therapy and the possibility of antibiotic-resistant pathogens, and local susceptibility patterns. Empiric coverage for gram-positive bacteria (staphylococci and streptococci) is almost always required, so the usual question is whether to broaden the regimen to cover gram-negative bacteria (Table 12.4).[34,41,42] Anaerobic coverage should be considered for necrotic or foul-smelling wounds. If the patient responds to the empiric therapy, then the regimen may be narrowed when microbiology data become available. If the patient does not respond, then the possibility of fastidious organisms missed by culture should be reconsidered, or surgery may be needed.

Agents that have been effective for therapy of DFIs in clinical trials include cephalosporins, β-lactamase inhibitor combination antibiotics, fluoroquinolones, clindamycin, carbapenems, vancomycin, and linezolid. Select results from clinical trials are shown in Table 12.4. The optimal duration of therapy for DFI has not been determined. A 1-week course of therapy is sufficient for most mild infections, whereas up to 2 weeks may be necessary for serious infections. Adequate debridement, resection, or amputation can shorten the necessary duration of therapy. Bloodstream infection is a rare complication for which many experts recommend 2 weeks of therapy. Therapy may be discontinued when

TABLE 12.4.

Recent Prospective Trials of Antibiotic Therapy for Complicated Skin and Skin Structure Infections of the Foot in Patients with Diabetes Mellitus.

Study	*Drug*	*Comparator*	*Result*	*Notes*
Lipsky[34]	Linezolid 600 mg i.v./p.o.	Ampicillin-sulbactam 3 g i.v. every 6 h, then amoxicillin-clavulanate 875 mg every 12 h	Clinical cure 81% vs. 71% (*P* = n.s.); linezolid superior in post hoc foot ulcer and nonosteomyelitis groups	Open label; randomized; L:A-S 2:1; treatment for 7–28 days
Harkless[41]	Piperacillin-tazobactam 4.5 g every 8 h i.v.	Ampicillin-sulbactam 3 g i.v. every 6 h	Clinical cure 81% vs. 83%; confidence interval not reported	Open label; vancomycin 1 g i.v. every 12 h optional for both groups
Lipsky[42]	Ertapenem 1 g daily	Piperacillin-tazobactam 3.375 g every 6 h for 5 days, amoxicillin-clavulanate 1 g p.o. every 12 h for up to 23 days	94% vs. 92% cure, E population; 95% CI (−2.9 to 6.9)	Noninferior; treatment for up to 28 days

all signs and symptoms of infection have resolved; incomplete wound healing is not an indication to prolong antibiotic therapy.

Adjuncts to Antibiotic Therapy

Hyperbaric oxygen may improve wound healing and decrease the rate of amputation of DFI according to one double-blind randomized trial.[43] However, most evidence of hyperbaric oxygen effect in DFI is anecdotal.[44] The hyperbaric oxygen literature is difficult to interpret because of poor controlling for multiple patient comorbidities, small sample sizes, and poor documentation of wound size and severity. Potential candidates for hyperbaric oxygen therapy include those patients with deep infections who are unresponsive to therapy, making amputation a definite possibility. Objectively, hyperbaric oxygen may be most beneficial when the transcutaneous oxygen tension is less than 40 mmHg before therapy and increases to above 200 mmHg after therapy.[44]

Surgical revascularization may also be considered.[45] Improving blood flow to the ischemic, infected foot may be a crucial determinant of outcome. Initial debridement is undertaken in the presence of infection; revascularization is generally postponed until sepsis is controlled, but should not be postponed more than a few days lest there be additional tissue loss. Successful revascularization of an ischemic, infected foot can result in 3-year limb salvage rates of up to 98%.[46]

A good outcome may be expected in 80%–90% of mild cases treated appropriately and 50%–60% for more advanced DFIs. Aggressive surgical debridement is often needed for infections of deep tissue or bone. Partial amputations (e.g., toe amputation, "ray" amputation of a metatarsal) may be foot sparing and lead to effective control of infection in more than 80% of cases. Healing is facilitated when there is no exposed bone, absent tissue edema, a palpable popliteal pulse, ankle systolic blood pressure above 80 mmHg, and a white blood cell (WBC) count below 12,000/mm^3. Infection recurs in 20%–30% of cases and should increase the suspicion of underlying osteomyelitis.

Osteomyelitis

Osteomyelitis is a feared complication of DFI (incidence, 50%–60% in serious DFIs and 10%–20% in mild infections),[38] but diabetic patients may have destructive bone lesions that are caused by peripheral neuropathy (e.g., Charcot joint). Distinguishing between neuropathic and infectious destruction of bone can be difficult. The likelihood of osteomyelitis is increased with foot ulcers that are chronic (>4 weeks), large (>2 cm diameter), deep (>3 mm), or associated with a marked elevation of ESR (>70 mm/h).[38] Wound exploration that "probes to bone" has a positive predictive value of more than 90% for the diagnosis of osteomyelitis.

The initial diagnostic test should be plain radiographs of the foot. It may take 2 weeks for radiographic changes to become manifest, so repeating an initially negative study in a stable patient may be a better strategy than proceeding immediately to more sophisticated imaging. If clinical and plain radiographic findings are nondiagnostic, then various types of scans may be useful. Technetium 99m bone scans are 85% sensitive but only 45% specific. Leukocyte scans (e.g., ^{111}In) are comparably sensitive but more specific (~75%). However, magnetic resonance imaging (MRI) is usually the diagnostic test of choice despite its expense because of high sensitivity (>90%) and specificity (>80%). A definitive diagnosis of osteomyelitis requires a bone biopsy for culture and histology, obtained without traversing an open wound to avoid contamination by colonizing organisms. Surgical biopsy is indicated if the diagnosis remains in doubt after imaging studies are obtained or if the etiologic agent(s) cannot be ascertained because of previous antibiotic therapy or confusing culture results. Most cases of osteomyelitis are polymicrobial; *S. aureus* is isolated most commonly (~40%), but *S. epidermidis*, streptococci, and Enterobacteriaceae are also isolated commonly.

Antibiotic therapy of osteomyelitis should be based on results of bone culture because soft tissue culture results do not predict bone pathogens accurately.[38] Empiric therapy should always cover *S. aureus*; broader coverage should be administered based on history or results of soft tissue cultures. Most antibiotics penetrate bone poorly, and leukocyte function is impaired, so long-term (at least 6 weeks) parenteral (at least initially) therapy is required. Osteomyelitis complicating DFI can be arrested by antibiotic therapy alone in about two-thirds of cases, so resection of infected bone is not always necessary. Oral antibiotics with good bioavailability (e.g., fluoroquinolones, clindamycin) may be useful for most of the therapeutic course. If all infected bone is removed, then a shorter course of therapy (e.g., 2 weeks) may be appropriate. Clinical resolution may be documented by a decrease to normal of the ESR or loss of increased uptake on a leukocyte scan.

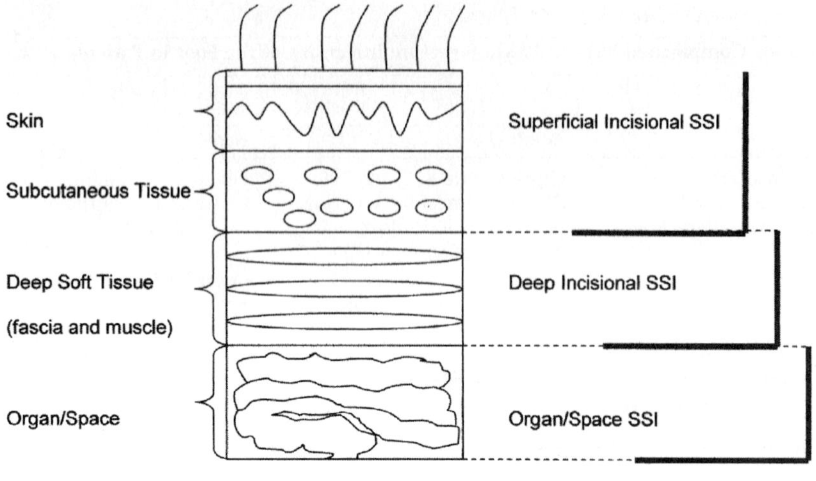

FIGURE 12.4. Cross section of the abdominal wall depicting U.S. Centers for Disease Control and Prevention (CDC) classifications of surgical site infection. (*Source:* Adapted from Mangram et al.,[16] by permission of *Infection Control Hospital Epidemiology.*)

Surgical Site Infection

Infections of surgical incisions are now referred to as surgical site infections (SSIs),[47] a common surgical complication that occurs after about 3% of all surgical procedures.[48] Potential complications of SSIs include tissue destruction, failure or prolongation of wound healing, incisional hernias, and occasionally bloodstream infection. Recurrent pain and disfiguring scars may also result. The SSIs result in substantial morbidity, prolonged hospital stays, and increased direct patient costs, creating a huge economic burden on health care systems.[49]

Infection may occur within the surgical site at any depth, from the skin to the intracavitary operative field. Superficial incisional SSI involves tissues down to the fascia (Fig. 12.4), whereas deep incisional SSI extends beneath the fascia but not intracavitary. Organ/space infections are intracavitary, but if related directly to an operation, are considered to be SSIs.

TABLE 12.5. Risk Factors for the Development of Surgical Site Infections.

Patient factors	
	Ascites
	Chronic inflammation
	Corticosteroid therapy (controversial)
	Obesity
	Diabetes
	Extremes of age
	Hypocholsterolemia
	Hypoxemia
	Peripheral vascular disease (especially for lower extremity surgery)
	Postoperative anemia
	Prior site irradiation
	Recent operation
	Remote infection
	Skin carriage of staphylococci
	Skin disease in the area of infection (e.g., psoriasis)
	Undernutrition
Environmental factors	
	Contaminated medications
	Inadequate disinfection/sterilization
	Inadequate skin antisepsis
	Inadequate ventilation
Treatment factors	
	Drains
	Emergency procedure
	Hypothermia
	Inadequate antibiotic prophylaxis
	Oxygenation (controversial)
	Prolonged preoperative hospitalization
	Prolonged operative time

Source: Adapted from National Nosocomial Infections Surveillance System (NNIS) System Report,[50] by permission of the *American Journal of Infection Control.*

Epidemiology

Numerous factors determine whether a patient will develop an SSI, including factors contributed by the patient, the environment, and the treatment (Table 12.5).[50] As described by the National Nosocomial Infections Surveillance System (NNIS)[50–52] of the U.S. Centers for Disease Control and Prevention (Table 12.6), the most recognized factors are the wound classification (contaminated or dirty; see below and Table 12.7), American Society of Anesthesiologists (ASA) designation above class 3 (chronic active medical illness; Table 12.8), and prolonged operative time, with time longer than the 75th percentile for each such procedure. Clean surgical procedures (class I) (Table 12.7) involve only integumentary and musculoskeletal soft tissues (e.g., groin hernia, breast, thyroid). Clean-contaminated procedures (class II) open a hollow viscus (e.g., alimentary, biliary, genitourinary, respiratory tract) under controlled circumstances (e.g., elective colon surgery). Contaminated procedures (class III) involve extensive introduction of bacteria into a normally sterile body cavity but too briefly to allow infection to become established (e.g., penetrating abdominal trauma, enterotomy during adhesiolysis for mechanical bowel obstruction). Dirty procedures (class IV) are those when the surgery is performed to control

TABLE 12.6. National Nosocomial Infections Surveillance System (NNIS) Risk Index for Surgical Site Infections.

Traditional class	*0*	*1*	*2*	*3*	*All*
Clean	1.0%	2.3%	5.4%	NA	2.1%
Clean/contaminated	2.1%	4.9%	9.5%	NA	3.3%
Contaminated	NA	3.4%	6.6%	13.2%	6.4%
Dirty	NA	3.1%	8.1%	12.8%	7.1%
All	1.5%	2.9%	6.8%	13.0%	2.8%

NA, not applicable.

Source: Adapted from National Nosocomial Infections Surveillance System (NNIS) System Report,[50] by permission of the *American Journal of Infection Control.*

TABLE 12.7. Surgical Site Infection Wound Classification and Approximate Rates of Infection.

Class	*Definition*	*Examples*	*Rate (%)*
I: Clean	Atraumatic wound No inflammation No break in aseptic technique No entry of biliary, respiratory, GI, or GU tracts If drained, by closed drainage	Herniorraphy Excision of skin lesion Thyroidectomy	1–5
I_D: Clean; prosthetic material implanted	Same as I, clean Cardiac valve replacement	Vascular surgery with graft	1–5
II: Clean-contaminated	Atraumatic wound No inflammation Minor break in aseptic technique Biliary, respiratory, GI, or GU tract entered under controlled conditions with minimal contamination	Appendectomy without perforation Elective colectomy after bowel preparation Cholecystectomy	2–9
III: Contaminated	Traumatic wound with delay in therapy or exogenous contamination Acute nonpurulent inflammation Major break in aseptic technique Entry of biliary, respiratory, GI, or GU tract with gross spillage of contents	Penetrating abdominal with hollow viscus injury Inadvertent enterotomy during adhesiolysis for mechanical small intestinal obstruction	3–13

GI, gastrointestinal; GU, genitourinary.

established infection (e.g., colon resection for complicated diverticulitis).

According to the NNIS classification, the risk of SSI increases with an increasing number of risk factors present, irrespective of the wound class and almost without regard for the type of operation. Laparoscopic abdominal surgery is associated with a decreased incidence of SSI under certain circumstances, which has required a modification of the NNIS risk classification.[47] For laparoscopic biliary, gastric, and colon surgery, one risk factor is subtracted if the operation is performed via the laparoscope—a new category has been created specifically for the circumstance, representing essentially minus one risk factor. Laparoscopy decreases the risk of SSI for several reasons, including decreased wound size, limited use of cautery, and a diminished stress response to tissue injury. Laparoscopic appendectomy, on the other hand, is a unique circumstance in that the risk of SSI is reduced by laparoscopy only if no risk factors are present (i.e., the patient is otherwise healthy, the appendix is not perforated, and the operation does not take more than 1 h).

Outpatient surgery poses problems for surveillance of SSI.[53] Although many SSIs will develop in the first 5–10 days after surgery, an SSI may develop up to 30 days after surgery. Estimates of the incidence of SSI after ambulatory surgery thus depend on inherently unreliable voluntary self-reporting by surgeons. Therefore, the incidence of SSI in NNIS is almost certainly an underestimate. Organ/space SSIs also are not identifiable separately in the data reported by NNIS.

Host-derived factors are important contributors to the risk of SSI, which the ASA score may not capture. Increased age,[54] obesity, malnutrition, diabetes mellitus,[55,56] hypocholesterolemia,[57] and other factors are not accounted for specifically by NNIS. In a study of 2345 patients undergoing cardiac surgery, the incidence of SSI was 8.5% (199/2345).[58] The relative risk (RR) of SSI among diabetic patients was 2.29 (95% confidence interval [CI] 1.15–4.54), and the RR among obese patients (body mass index >30) was 1.78 (95% CI, 1.24–2.55). Malone et al. found an incidence of SSI of 3.2% among 5031 noncardiac surgery patients at a Veterans Affairs hospital. Independent risk factors for the development of SSI included ascites, diabetes mellitus, postoperative anemia, and recent weight loss but not chronic obstructive pulmonary disease, tobacco use, or corticosteroid use.[58] Other studies have linked low serum albumin concentration and increased serum creatinine concentration to an increased risk of SSI.[59]

TABLE 12.8. American Society of Anesthesiologists (ASA) Physical Status Score.

ASA 1	A normal healthy patient.
ASA 2	A patient with mild-to-moderate systemic disturbance that results in no functional limitations. Examples: hypertension, diabetes mellitus, chronic bronchitis, morbid obesity, extremes of age.
ASA 3	A patient with severe systemic disturbance that results in functional limitations. Examples: poorly controlled hypertension, diabetes mellitus with vascular complications, angina pectoris, prior myocardial infarction, pulmonary disease that limits activity.
ASA 4	A patient with a severe systemic disturbance that is life threatening with or without the planned procedure. Examples: congestive heart failure; unstable angina pectoris; advanced pulmonary, renal, or hepatic dysfunction.
ASA 5	A morbid patient not expected to survive with or without the operative procedure. Examples: ruptured abdominal aortic aneurysm, pulmonary embolism, traumatic brain injury with increased intracranial pressure.
ASA 6	Any patient for whom the procedure is an emergency.

Source: From Cohen and Duncan.[130]

Microbiology

Inoculation of the surgical site occurs during surgery, either inward from the skin or outward from the tissues operated on. The microbiology of SSI depends on the type of operation,

TABLE 12.9. Incidence of Pathogen Isolation in Surgical Site Infection (Collected Series).

Organism	*Percentage*
Staphylococcus aureus	20
Coagulase-negative staphylococci	14
Enterococci	12
Pseudomonas aeruginosa	8
Escherichia coli	8
Enterobacter spp.	7
Proteus mirabilis	3
Streptococcus spp.	3
Klebsiella pneumoniae	3
Candida albicans	2

with an increased likelihood of gram-negative bacilli after gastrointestinal surgery or infrainguinal vascular surgery. However, most SSIs are caused by gram-positive cocci that are commensal skin flora (Table 12.9),[60] including *S. aureus*, coagulase-negative staphylococci (usually *S. epidermidis*), and *Enterococcus* spp. Head and neck surgery (if pharyngo-esophageal structures are entered) and intestinal surgery may be associated with SSI caused by enteric facultative (e.g., *Escherichia coli*) and anaerobic (e.g., *Bacteroides fragilis*) bacteria.

Preoperative Preparation

The patient should be assessed before elective surgery for correctable risk factors. Open skin lesions should heal beforehand if possible. The patient should be free of bacterial infections of any kind and should quit smoking if possible, preferably 1 month before surgery. The patient should shower with an antibacterial soap the night before the operation. The patient must not be shaved the night before, considering that the risk of SSI is increased by bacteria that colonize the inevitable small cuts and abrasions.[60] Particular attention should be paid to the patient's nutritional status. Obese patients should lose as much weight as is safely possible. Malnourished patients can reduce the risk of SSI significantly with as few as 5 days of enteral nutritional supplementation.[61,62]

Antibiotic Prophylaxis and the Risk of SSI

Preoperative administration of prophylactic antibiotics to reduce the risk of postoperative SSI is of proven benefit in many circumstances (Table 12.10). However, only the

TABLE 12.10. Appropriate Cephalosporin Prophylaxis for Selected Operations.[a]

Operation	*Alternative prophylaxis in serious penicillin allergy*
First-generation cephalosporin (i.e., cefazolin,cefuroxime)	
Cardiovascular and thoracic	Clindamycin (for all cases herein except amputation)[b]
Median sternotomy	Vancomycin
Pacemaker insertion	
Vascular reconstruction involving the abdominal aorta, insertion of a prosthesis, or a groin incision (except carotid endarterectomy, which requires no prophylaxis)	
Implantable defibrillator	
Pulmonary resection	
Lower limb amputation	Gentamicin and metronidazole
General	
Cholecystectomy (high risk only: age >60, jaundice, acute, prior biliary procedure)	Gentamicin
Gastrectomy (high risk only: not uncomplicated chronic duodenal ulcer)	Gentamicin and metronidazole
Hepatobiliary	Gentamicin and metronidazole
Major debridement of traumatic wound	Gentamicin
Genitourinary (ampicillin plus gentamicin is a reasonable alternative)	Ciprofloxacin
Gynecological	
Cesarean section (STAT)	Metronidazole (after cord clamping)
Hysterectomy (cefoxitin is a reasonable alternative)	Doxycycline
Head and neck/oral cavity	
Major procedures entering oral cavity or pharynx	Gentamicin and clindamycin or metronidazole
Neurosurgery	
Craniotomy	Clindamycin, vancomycin
Orthopedics	
Major joint arthroplasty	Vancomycin[b]
Open reduction of closed fracture	Vancomycin[b]
Second-generation (i.e., cefoxitin)[c]	
Appendectomy	Metronidazole with or without gentamicin (for all cases herein)
Colon surgery[d]	
Surgery for penetrating abdominal trauma	

[a]Should be given as a single intravenous dose just before the operation. Consider an additional dose if the operation is longer than 3–4 h.

[b]Primary prophylaxis with vancomycin (i.e., for the non-penicillin-allergic patient) may be appropriate for cardiac valve replacement, placement of a nontissue peripheral vascular prosthesis, or total joint replacement in institutions where a high rate of infections with methicillin-resistant *Staphylococcus aureus* or *Staphylococcus epidermidis* has occurred. The precise definition of *high rate* is debated. A single dose administered immediately before surgery is sufficient unless operation lasts for more than 6 h, in which case the dose should be repeated. Prophylaxis should be discontinued after a maximum of two doses but may be continued for up to 48 h.

[c]An intraoperative dose should be given if cefoxitin is used and the duration of surgery exceeds 3–4 h because of the short half-life of the drug. A postoperative dose is not necessary but is permissible for up to 24 h.

[d]Benefit beyond that provided by bowel preparation with mechanical cleansing and oral neomycin and erythromycin base is debatable.

TABLE 12.11.
Systemic Antimicrobial Prophylaxis in Colorectal Surgery: Systematic Review of Randomized Controlled Trials.

Analysis	*No. of trials*	*OR*	*95% CI*
Cefuroxime + metronidazole			
vs. metronidazole alone	4	0.32	0.15–0.68
vs. mezlocillin	3	0.55	0.32–0.93
vs. all comparators overall	16	No difference (not reported)	
First*-generation cephalosporins			
vs. later-generation cephalosporins	6	1.07	0.54–2.12
Single-dose prophylaxis			
vs. multiple-dose prophylaxis	17	1.17	0.90–1.53
Parenteral antibiotics			
vs. parenteral plus oral antibiotics	4	1.13	0.60–2.14

*With or without metronidazole.
Source: Data from Song and Glenny.[66]

incision itself is protected, and antibiotics are not a panacea. If not administered properly, then antibiotic prophylaxis will not be effective and may be harmful.

Antibiotic prophylaxis is indicated for most clean-contaminated and contaminated (or potentially contaminated) operations. An example of a clean-contaminated operation for which antibiotic prophylaxis is not always indicated is elective cholecystectomy.[63] Antibiotic prophylaxis is indicated only for high-risk biliary surgery; patients at high risk include those over age 70 or who have diabetes mellitus and patients whose biliary tract has been instrumented recently (e.g., biliary stent).[63] The vast majority of patients who undergo laparoscopic cholecystectomy do not require antibiotic prophylaxis.[64] An example of a potentially contaminated operation is adhesiolysis for mechanical small bowel obstruction; intestinal ischemia cannot be predicted accurately before surgery, and an enterotomy during adhesiolysis increases the risk of SSI twofold. Antibiotics for dirty operations represent treatment for an infection, not prophylaxis.

Elective colon surgery is a clean-contaminated procedure for which preparatory practices are in evolution.[65] Historically, mechanical bowel preparation to reduce bulk feces made colon surgery safe, but trauma surgeons have demonstrated that the injured, unprepared colon can be operated on safely. Antibiotic bowel preparation, standardized in the 1970s by the oral administration of nonabsorbable neomycin and erythromycin base, reduced the risk of SSI further to its present rate of approximately 4%–8%, depending on the number of risk factors. However, preoperative oral antibiotics are omitted increasingly because there may be no additive benefit beyond parenteral antibiotic prophylaxis with cefoxitin or ampicillin-sulbactam (or a quinolone or monobactam plus metronidazole for the penicillin-allergic patient) given within 1h prior to the skin incision.[65] Parenteral antibiotic prophylaxis is undeniably effective (Table 12.11).[66] Compliance with the performance standards of the Surgical Care Improvement Program (SCIP),[67] which is mandatory for U.S. health care facilities, will be achieved by oral or parenteral prophylaxis or both (Table 12.12).

Antibiotic prophylaxis of clean surgery has been controversial. If bone is incised (e.g., craniotomy, sternotomy) or a prosthesis is inserted, then antibiotic prophylaxis is generally indicated. Some controversy persists with clean surgery of soft tissues (e.g., breast, hernia). Meta-analysis of randomized controlled trials shows some benefit of antibiotic prophylaxis of breast cancer surgery without immediate reconstruction[68,69] (Table 12.13), but no decrease of SSI rate for groin hernia surgery,[70,71] even when a nonabsorbable mesh prosthesis is implanted (Table 12.13).

Arterial reconstruction with prosthetic graft material of vein is an example of clean surgery for which the susceptibility to infection is high owing to the presence of ischemic tissue and the infrainguinal location of many such operations. Several aforementioned strategies have been studied in an attempt to reduce the risk of SSI. A meta-analysis[72] identified 35 randomized, controlled trials for prevention of infection after peripheral arterial reconstruction, with 23 of these pro-

TABLE 12.12. Surgical Care Improvement Program: Approved Antibiotic Prophylactic Regimens for Elective Surgery.

Type of operation	*Antibiotic(s)*
Cardiac (including coronary artery bypass grafting [CABG]),[a] Vascular[b]	Cefazolin or cefuroxime or vancomycin[c]
Hip/knee arthroplasty[b]	Cefazolin or cefuroxime or vancomycin[c]
Colon[d,e]	Oral: neomycin sulfate plus either erythromycin base or metronidazole administered for 18h before surgery Parenteral: cefoxitin or cefotetan or cefazolin plus metronidazole or ampicillin-sulbactam
Hysterectomy[e]	Cefazolin or cefoxitin or cefotetan or cefuroxime or ampicillin-sulbactam

[a]Prophylaxis may be administered for up to 48h for cardiac surgery; for all other cases, the limit is 24h.

[b]For β-lactam allergy, clindamycin or vancomycin are acceptable substitutes for cardiac, vascular, and orthopedic surgery.

[c]Vancomycin is acceptable with a physician-documented justification for use in the patient's medical record.

[d]For β-lactam allergy, clindamycin plus gentamicin, a fluoroquinolone, or aztreonam; or metronidazole plus gentamicin or a fluoroquinolone are acceptable choices.

[e]For colon surgery, either oral or parenteral prophylaxis alone or both combined are acceptable.

TABLE 12.13.
Antibiotic Prophylaxis for Reduction of Surgical Site Infection Following Clean Surgery: Two Meta-Analyses.

Analysis	*No. of trials*	*OR*	*95% CI*
Breast surgery[a]			
Overall	5/1307	0.60	0.45–0.81
Breast cancer surgery[b,c]			
No immediate reconstruction	5/1254	0.66	0.48–0.89
Immediate reconstruction	Insufficient data for analysis		
Abdominal wall hernia surgery			
Overall results[d]	8/2907	0.65	0.35–1.21
Inguinal herniorraphy (no prosthetic material)		0.84	0.53–1.34
Inguinal hernioplasty (prosthetic material used)		0.28	0.02–3.14
Overall results[e] (groin, mesh repairs only)	6/2507	0.54	0.24–1.21
Deep incisional SSI (groin, mesh)	5/1987	0.50	0.12–2.09
Other abdominal wall hernias, mesh	Insufficient data for analysis		

[a]Data from Tejirian et al.[68]
[b]Data from Cunningham et al.[69]
[c]Analysis of the same five trials.
[d]Data from Sanchez-Manuel and Seco-Gil.[71]
[e]Data from Aufenacker et al.[70]

phylactic systemic antibiotics trials (Table 12.14). Prophylactic systemic antibiotics reduced the risk of SSI by approximately 75% and early graft infection by about 69%. There was no benefit to prophylaxis for more than 24h, of antibiotic bonding to the graft material itself, or preoperative bathing with an antiseptic agent compared with unmedicated bathing.

Four principles should guide selection of the appropriate antimicrobial agent for prophylaxis: The agent should be safe; the agent should have an appropriately narrow spectrum of coverage of relevant pathogens; the agent should not be one that is relied on for therapy of infection (owing to the possible induction of resistance with heavy usage); and the agent must be administered for a defined, brief period of time (ideally, a single dose; certainly for no more than 24h). According to these principles, third-generation cephalosporins or quinolones should never be used for surgical prophylaxis. Given that most SSIs are caused by gram-positive cocci, the antibiotic chosen should be directed primarily against staphylococci for clean cases and high-risk, clean-contaminated elective biliary and gastric surgery. A first-generation cephalosporin is preferred (Table 12.10), with clindamycin used for penicillin-allergic patients.[73] Vancomycin prophylaxis is appropriate only in institutions where the incidence of MRSA infection is high (>20% of all SSIs caused by MRSA).

TABLE 12.14.
Meta-Analysis of Measures to Prevent Infection Following Arterial Reconstruction.

Intervention	*No. of trials*	*Odds ratio*	*95% CI*
Systemic antibiotic prophylaxis			
Surgical site infection	10	0.25	0.17–0.38
>24h prophylaxis	3	1.28	0.82–1.98
Early graft infection	5	0.31	0.11–0.85
Rifampicin bonding of polyester grafts			
Graft infection, 1 month	3	0.63	0.27–1.49
Graft infection, 2 years	2	1.05	0.46–2.40
Suction wound drainage, groin			
Surgical site infection	2	0.96	0.50–1.86
Preoperative antiseptic bath			
Surgical site infection	3	0.97	0.70–1.36
In situ surgical technique			
Surgical site infection	2	0.48	0.31–0.74

Source: Data from Stewart et al.[72]

The optimal time to give parenteral antibiotic prophylaxis is within 1h prior to the time of incision.[74] Antibiotics given sooner are ineffective, as are agents that are given after the incision is closed. Antibiotics with short half-lives (<2h, e.g., cefazolin or cefoxitin) should be redosed every 3–4h during surgery if the operation is prolonged or bloody.[75] Choice, timing, and duration of prophylactic antibiotic administration have been standardized as part of SCIP[67] (Tables 12.12 and 12.15), and institutional compliance (eventually, possibly compliance by individual surgeons) will be required.

Preoperative topical antiseptics or antibiotics may also help prevent SSI. A preoperative shower with an antiseptic soap (e.g., chlorhexidine) should be a standard part of preoperative preparation but is omitted often. Topical 2% mupirocin ointment applied to the nares of patients who are chronic carriers of *S. aureus* may reduce the increased incidence of SSI that is characteristic of chronic staphylococcal carriage.[76,77]

Unfortunately, excessively prolonged antibiotic prophylaxis is both pervasive and potentially harmful. Recent U.S. data showed that only 40% of patients who receive antibiotic prophylaxis do so for less than 24h.[78] Antibiotic penetration into the incision immediately after surgery is questionable as a result of ischemia caused by surgical hemostasis. Single-dose preoperative prophylaxis is often sufficient, with intraoperative dosing as noted above, but 24- to 48-h regimens (the latter for cardiac surgery) have become standardized. Antibi-

TABLE 12.15. Surgical Care Improvement Project: Performance Measures Relevant to Prevention of Surgical Site Infection.

Antibiotic prophylaxis
- Proportion of patients who have their antibiotic dose initiated within 1 h before surgical incision (2 h for vancomycin or fluoroquinolones)
- Proportion of patients who receive prophylactic antibiotics consistent with current recommendations (published guidelines)
- Proportion of patients whose prophylactic antibiotics were discontinued within 24 h of surgery end time (48 h for cardiac surgery)

Clindamycin use is preferred for patients allergic to β-lactam antibiotics. Vancomycin is allowed for prophylaxis of cardiac, vascular, and orthopedic surgery if there is a physician-documented reason in the medical record or documented β-lactam allergy.

Glucose control (cardiac surgery patients)
- Blood glucose concentration must be maintained <200 mg/dl for the first 2 days after surgery

Blood glucose determination closest to 6:00 a.m. on postoperative days 1 and 2 (surgery end date is postoperative day 0) will be monitored.

Proper hair removal
- No hair removal should be performed

If hair is removed, clippers or a depilatory agent should be used immediately prior to surgery. Razors are not to be used.

Normothermia (colorectal surgery patients)
- Core body temperature should be between 96.8°F and 100.4°F within the first hour after leaving the operating room.

otics should not be given to "cover" indwelling drains or catheters, in lavage/irrigation fluid, or as a substitute for poor surgical technique.

Prolongation of antibiotic prophylaxis beyond 24 h not only provides no benefit but also is associated with complications. *Clostridium difficile*-associated disease (CDAD) follows disruption of the normal balance of gut flora, resulting in overgrowth of the enterotoxin-producing *C. difficile*.[79] Although virtually any antibiotic may cause CDAD (even after a single dose) prolonged antibiotic prophylaxis increases the risk. Prolonged prophylaxis also increases the risk of nosocomial infections unrelated to the surgical site and the emergence of multidrug-resistant pathogens. Both pneumonia and catheter-related infections have been associated with prolonged prophylaxis,[79,80] as has the emergence of SSI caused by MRSA.[81]

Antibiotic Prophylaxis of Trauma-Related Infections

Trauma is profoundly immunosuppressive, and injured patients are at high risk for infection. An overall infection incidence of approximately 25% occurs after trauma,[33] with infection of a wound (or an incision made as treatment) and nosocomial infection equally likely. Certain patterns of injury are independently associated with infectious morbidity, including hemorrhagic shock, the need for blood transfusion, heavy wound contamination, central nervous system injury, colon injury, combined thoraco-abdominal injuries, four or more organs injured, and increasing injury severity.[82]

Certain characteristics of trauma add complexity. By definition, antibiotics are administered after injury, but injured tissues are vulnerable beforehand. Patients in shock have vasoconstriction, which may decrease tissue penetration of antibiotics. Ongoing blood loss may result in antibiotic loss in shed blood if the agent is highly protein bound (i.e., not well distributed to tissues) or administered before bleeding is controlled. Postinjury fluid shifts and hypoalbuminemia can cause fluctuations in volume of distribution.

Despite the higher risk, basic principles of antibiotic prophylaxis still apply after injury: use a safe, narrow-spectrum agent for a defined brief period (certainly no more than 24 h), preferably one that has a limited role as therapy (i.e., a first- or second-generation cephalosporin).[76] Multiple studies indicate unequivocally that 24 h of prophylaxis with a second-generation cephalosporin is sufficient following penetrating abdominal trauma, even with colon injury or shock.[82] Although injury severity increases infection risk, severe injury does not justify prolonged prophylaxis.[83]

Operating Room Environment

Lapses in the operating room can result in increased rates of SSI. The elements of proper operating room design, management, and comportment have been reviewed in an evidence-based manner.[60] Although such factors as proper sterilization technique and ventilation should not be the everyday concern of the surgeon, operating room personnel must remain vigilant. The surgeon must be attentive to personal hygiene (e.g., hand scrubbing, hair) and that of the entire team. Data indicate that a brief rinse with soap and water followed by use of an alcohol gel hand rub is equivalent to a prolonged (and ritualized) session with soap and water at the scrub sink.[84]

Careful preparation of the skin with an appropriate antiseptic is essential. Chlorhexidine-based skin preparation solutions have superior microbicidal activity and are supplanting povidone-iodine-based solutions. No data show that adhesive plastic drapes (iodophor impregnated or not) reduce the risk of SSI, so routine usage may be foregone.

Surgical gloves are punctured or torn during an operation about 20% of the time, increasing the chance of contamination of the operative field (as well as contact between surgeon and the patient's body fluids). Therefore, gloves must be inspected regularly during a procedure. Likewise, most surgical gowns in use offer limited protection (1.5–2 h at most) against strikethrough of fluids. It may be prudent to change gowns and gloves regularly (every 2 h or so) during long procedures and certainly if there is any breach of integrity of barrier materials.

Although most flora that cause SSIs are skin derived and inoculated during the procedure, airborne bacteria, especially staphylococci, do pose some risk. Surgeons who are chronic nasal carriers of *S. aureus* have higher rates of SSI than do their noncolonized brethren. Surgical masks should cover the nose and mouth at all times, and unnecessary foot traffic and conversation in the operating room should be minimized.

Patients may become hypothermic during surgery owing to exposure, evaporative water losses, administration of room temperature fluids, and other factors. Maintenance of normal core body temperature is crucial for decreasing the incidence of SSI and is mandatory for colorectal surgery patients under SCIP (Table 12.15). Mild intraoperative hypothermia is associated with an increased rate of SSI following various types of operations.[85,86] In one randomized study, 30 min of active preoperative warming reduced the rate of SSI following minor clean operations.[87]

Management of the Incision

Cosmesis is important to patients. On the other hand, closure of a contaminated or dirty wound is widely believed to increase the risk of SSI. Few good studies exist to help resolve the issue. Tissues should be handled gently, and electrocautery for hemostasis should be minimized.[88] Traditionally, high-risk incisions for SSI are left open after surgery, with delayed primary closure performed with sutures or adhesives approximately 4 days after surgery if the incision "looks okay." Incisions that are "not ready" or that fail delayed primary closure are left to heal by secondary intention, which takes weeks and consumes precious home care resources.

Can contaminated incisions be closed primarily? The data are mixed, and the type of incision may be a determinant. It appears that muscle-splitting appendectomy incisions can be closed primarily; decision analysis indicates that primary closure is cost-effective if the rate of SSI is less than 27%.[89] However, wound management techniques that are appropriate after open appendectomy may not be suitable elsewhere. A prospective study demonstrated that primary closure of contaminated midline abdominal incisions led to more wound failures and greater cost than did delayed primary closure.[90]

Drains placed in incisions probably cause more infections than they prevent. Sealing of the wound by epithelialization is prevented, and the drain becomes a conduit, holding open a portal for invasion of the wound by pathogens colonizing the skin. Drains placed into clean or clean-contaminated incisions do not decrease the rate of SSI[91,92]; in fact, the rate is increased.[93,94] Considering that drains pose a risk and accomplish little, they should be used as seldom and removed as soon as possible.[95] Prolonged antibiotic prophylaxis should never be administered to "cover" indwelling drains.

Wound irrigation is controversial as a means to reduce the risk of SSI. Routine low-pressure washing of an incision with saline has no effect,[96] but high pressure (e.g., pulse irrigation) may be beneficial.[97] Topical antibiotics placed into the incision during surgery may minimize the risk of SSI,[98,99] but use of topical antiseptics rather than antibiotics may minimize the possibility of the development of resistance.

Postoperative Period

Blood Transfusion

In hemorrhage and trauma, blood transfusions may be lifesaving; alternatives to transfusion in the acute setting are few, but hemoglobin concentrations of more than 7 g/dl are well tolerated for hemodynamically stable postoperative patients.[100] Blood transfusion should be avoided, if possible, because it has been associated with immunosuppression, disruption of the microcirculation, and an increased incidence of nosocomial infection. Even a single-unit transfusion carries demonstrable risk.[101] The risk of infection increases as the total transfusion volume increases, especially when older units are transfused (>14 days of storage).[102] A recent meta-analysis estimated that transfusion of any volume of red blood cell (RBC) concentrates more than triples the risk of nosocomial infection compared with no transfusion.[103] Observational studies suggested that transfusion of critically ill patients not only increases the risk of infection[104] but also may worsen organ dysfunction and increase mortality.[105]

Hyperglycemia, Nutrition, and Control of Blood Sugar

Hyperglycemia is deleterious to host immune function, most notably impairing function of neutrophils and mononuclear phagocytes. Hyperglycemia may also be a marker of the catabolism and insulin resistance associated with the surgical stress response.

Poor control of blood glucose during surgery and in the perioperative period increases the risk of infection and worsens outcome from sepsis. Diabetic patients undergoing cardiopulmonary bypass surgery have a higher risk of infection of both the sternal incision and the vein harvest incisions on the lower extremities.[106] Tight control of blood glucose by the anesthesiologist during surgery and during the early postoperative period decreases the risk. Control of blood glucose for cardiac surgery patients is mandatory under SCIP (Table 12.15). Moderate hyperglycemia (>200 mg/dl) at any time on the first postoperative day increases the risk of SSI fourfold after noncardiac surgery.[56] In a large randomized trial of critically ill postoperative patients, exogenous insulin administration to keep blood glucose concentrations below 110 mg/dl was associated with a 40% decrease of mortality, fewer nosocomial infections, and less organ dysfunction.[107] Meta-analysis of the approximately 35 existing trials indicates that the risk of mortality is decreased significantly (relative risk [RR] 0.85, 95% CI 0.75–0.97] by tight glucose control, especially so for critically ill surgical patients (RR 0.58, 95% CI 0.22–0.62), regardless of whether the patients had diabetes mellitus (RR 0.71, 95% CI 0.54–0.93) or stress-induced hyperglycemia (RR 0.73, 95% CI 0.58–0.90).[108]

The need to manage carbohydrate metabolism carefully has important implications for the nutritional management of surgical patients. Gastrointestinal surgery may render the gastrointestinal tract unusable for feeding, sometimes for prolonged periods. Ileus is common in surgical intensive care units (ICUs), whether from traumatic brain injury, narcotic analgesia, prolonged bed rest, inflammation in proximity to the peritoneal envelope (e.g., lower lobe pneumonia, retroperitoneal hematoma, fractures of the thoraco-lumbar spine, pelvis, or hip), or other causes. Parenteral nutrition is used frequently for feeding, despite evidence of a lack of efficacy[109] and the possibility of hepatic dysfunction; hyperglycemia may be an important complication as well. Every effort should be made to provide enteral feedings, including the use of promotility agents such as erythromycin to improve tolerance.[110] Early enteral feeding (within 36 h) reduces the risk of nosocomial infection by more than one-half among critically ill and injured patients.[111]

Oxygenation

It is somewhat intuitive that the administration of oxygen in the postoperative period would be beneficial for wound healing and the prevention of infection.[112] The fresh surgical incision is ischemic; maintenance of normothermia may promote vasodilation of local tissue beds to improve nutrient blood flow to the incision. Moreover, oxygen has been postulated to have a direct antibacterial effect. However, clinical trials have had conflicting results.[113,114] In a study of 500 patients undergoing elective colorectal surgery, administration of 80% oxygen (vs. 30% oxygen) during surgery and for 2h thereafter decreased the incidence of SSI by more than 50% (5.2% vs. 11.2%),[113] whereas another prospective trial of the utility of 80% versus 35% oxygen administered to 165 patients undergoing major intraabdominal procedures showed that the infection rate was twice as high (25.0% vs. 11.3%) after 80% oxygen.[114] Although the latter trial can be criticized for the high overall rate of SSI (18.1%) and possible underpowering, supplemental oxygenation administration specifically to reduce the incidence of SSI is now controversial.

Diagnosis and Treatment of Surgical Site Infection

Specific criteria have been established by the Centers for Disease Control and Prevention for the diagnosis of SSI (Table 12.16). Adherence to these diagnostic guidelines is important because SSI can be misdiagnosed otherwise. Not all draining or erythematous incisions are infected. A superficial swab culture will likely become contaminated during specimen collection and be overinterpreted. Proper surveillance requires the prospective involvement of specifically trained personnel, adhering to the aforementioned criteria, who inspect incisions directly. Retrospective studies are nearly certain to be plagued by diagnostic inaccuracy and therefore are inherently dubious. Likewise, voluntary self-reporting by surgeons produces notorious underestimates of incidence because reporting does not occur and because the plethora of ambulatory surgical procedures escape hospital-based surveillance programs. Therefore, published data from the NNIS (Table 12.6) probably are at or near the lower end of the confidence interval.

TABLE 12.16. Criteria for Diagnosis of Superficial and Deep (Organ Space) Surgical Site Infections (SSIs) Within 30 Days of All Procedures (1 Year If Prosthetic Material Is Implanted).

Incisional SSI

Superficial: Infection involves skin or subcutaneous tissue of the incision *and* at least one of the following:

1. Purulent drainage from the superficial incision.
2. Organisms isolated from an aseptically obtained culture from the superficial incision.
3. One or more of the following: pain, localized swelling, erythema, or heat, and incision is opened deliberately by surgeon unless incision is culture negative.
4. Diagnosis of superficial incisional SSI by surgeon.

Deep: Infection involves fascial or muscle layer of the incision *and* at least one of the following:

1. Purulent drainage from the deep incision, excluding organ/space.[a]
2. Incision that dehisces spontaneously or is opened deliberately by a surgeon in the presence of fever (>38°C) or pain, unless site is culture negative.
3. Evidence of infection is found on direct examination, during repeat surgery, or by histopathologic or radiologic examination.[b]
4. Diagnosis of deep incisional SSI by surgeon.

Organ/space SSI

Infection of any part of the anatomy (e.g., organs or surgically created spaces) opened or manipulated during an operation *and* at least one of the following:

1. Purulent drainage from a drain that is placed into the organ/space.
2. Organisms isolated from an aseptically obtained culture from the organ/space.
3. Evidence of infection is found on direct examination, during repeat surgery, or by histopathologic or radiologic examination.[b]
4. Diagnosis of an organ/space SSI by surgeon.

For all classifications, infection is defined as occurring within 30 days after the operation if no implant is placed or within 1 year if an implant is in place and the infection is related to the incision.

[a]Report infection that involves both superficial and deep incision sites as a deep incisional SSI.

[b]Report an organ/space SSI that drains spontaneously through the incision as a deep incisional SSI.

Source: Adapted from Mangram et al.,[60] by permission of *Infection Control Hospital Epidemiology.*

There is only one constant in the management of established SSI: incise and drain the incision. Often, opening the incision and applying basic wound care (e.g., topical saline-soaked wet-to-dry cotton gauze dressings) is sufficient, provided that the incision is opened wide enough to facilitate wound care and the diagnosis of associated conditions. Making an incision that is too small may fail to bring the infection under control. Most nostrums other than physiologic saline applied to gauze dressings (e.g., modified Dakin's solution, 0.25% acetic acid solution) actually suppress fibroblast proliferation and may delay secondary wound healing.

Opening the incision adequately is essential not only to gain control of the infection but also to diagnose and treat any associated conditions, such as skin, subcutaneous tissue, or fascial necrosis that requires debridement; fascial dehiscence or evisceration that requires formal abdominal wall reconstruction; or drainage from beneath the fascia that could signal an organ/space infection or an enteric fistula. Without control of complicating factors, a SSI will be difficult to control, if not impossible.

Antibiotic therapy is not required for uncomplicated SSIs that are opened and drained adequately and that receive appropriate local care. Likewise, if antibiotic therapy is unwarranted, then culture and susceptibility testing of wound drainage are of no value and can be omitted. Even if cultures are taken, routine swabs of drainage are not recommended because the risk of contamination by commensal skin flora is high. Rather, tissue specimens or an aliquot of pus collected aseptically and anaerobically into a syringe are recommended for analysis.

Antibiotics may be indicated if there is systemic evidence of toxicity (e.g., fever, leukocytosis) or cellulitis that extends more than 2cm beyond the incision. Antibiotics are also indicated as adjunctive management of several of the complications mentioned. The choice of antibiotic is defined by the operation performed through the incision and the likely infecting organism, as discussed. Coverage against gram-positive cocci is indicated in most circumstances.

Wound closure by secondary intention can be protracted and disfiguring. Reports of vacuum-assisted wound closure (VAC) are proliferating. Putative benefits of VAC dressings include reduced inflammation, increased fibroblast activity, improved wound hygiene as fluid is aspirated continuously from the field, and more rapid wound contraction and closure.[115] However, these benefits remain conjectural in the absence of definitive class I data.

Necrotizing Soft Tissue Infection

Necrotizing soft tissue infections (NSTIs) are dangerous but fortunately also uncommon.[116] There is danger because of rapid progression and much systemic toxicity. Bacterial proteases cleave tissue planes, facilitating the rapid spread of infection. Host defenses are rapidly overwhelmed, leading to hemodynamic instability and hypoperfusion. Ischemic tissue in turn is susceptible to progression of the infection, and organ dysfunction may also result. Necrotizing STIs are also dangerous because they are uncommon, and their initial manifestations can be subtle, increasing the possibility of a delay in diagnosis. Although most presentations are obvious, an NSTI must always be considered whenever a patient presents with severe pain, particularly of the perineum or an extremity, that is out of proportion to any physical findings. There may be no obvious portal. The presence of gas in the soft tissues on examination (crepitus) or by imaging study is helpful but unreliable if absent.

Delayed definitive therapy (i.e., surgical debridement) is the major risk factor for mortality in cases of NSTI; therefore, familiarity is crucial for anyone (e.g., surgeon, emergency physician, primary care physician) who might encounter an early presentation. True NSTIs cannot be treated successfully with antibiotics alone (although broad-spectrum antibiotics are an essential adjunct to surgery), so timely surgical consultation is mandatory. Even with optimal therapy, mortality is approximately 25%–30%, and the hospitalization will be protracted, complicated, and expensive regardless of the outcome.

Although many names have been applied to these serious infections, such as synergistic gangrene and the eponymous Fournier gangrene (of the scrotum), it is most useful to characterize NSTIs based on the deepest tissue layer involved by necrosis. Involvement of the skin and subcutaneous tissue only is *necrotizing cellulitis*, whereas involvement of the fascia (most common) is referred to as *necrotizing fasciitis*, and involvement of underlying muscle is referred to as *necrotizing myositis* or sometimes *myonecrosis*. Some experts classify NSTIs further by the causative pathogen (e.g., clostridial myositis) or whether the infection is polymicrobial (type I) or caused by a single organism (type II). It is important to distinguish NSTIs from their nonnecrotizing SSTIs because the latter may be treated effectively with intravenous antibiotics alone. However, only operative debridement can classify accurately the anatomic extent of NSTI; therefore, attempts to classify NSTIs preoperatively can only engender dangerous, even life-threatening, delay.

Etiology

Necrotizing STIs can be primary or secondary events. Primary, or idiopathic, infections are less common and lack a portal of entry. Whether the source of bacteria in primary NSTIs is the bloodstream or epithelial disruptions too small to be apparent is debated; either mechanism is possible. One well-known example, the halophilic marine bacteria of the genus *Vibrio* (especially *V. vulnificus*),[117] can cause NSTIs after ingestion of raw seafood or skin trauma while wading in seawater. Another example is an NSTI caused by *Clostridium septicum*, which is specifically associated with occult carcinoma of the colon (and likely arises after a bacteremia). Much more common are the secondary infections, which may arise after burns or trauma, in recent surgical incisions, or as a consequence of unrecognized, neglected, or inadequately treated SSTIs. Other potential portals of entry include human, animal, or insect bites and parenteral drug abuse.[118]

Secondary NSTIs often have associated conditions that can predispose to tissue necrosis or impede containment by local host defenses. Inadequate treatment of SSTIs, such as decubitus ulcers,[119] ischemic leg ulcers, Bartholin cyst abscess, or perirectal or ischiorectal abscess pose a high risk of progression to NSTI. However, for reasons unclear, SSTIs of the face, neck, or chest[120–123] progress less often to NSTI than infections of the perineum and lower extremity.

Microbiology

Approximately 80% of NSTIs are polymicrobial (type I NSTI), with bacteria acting synergistically to promote dissemination and increase toxicity. Monomicrobial NSTIs are most commonly caused by *Streptococcus pyogenes*, with *Clostridium perfringens* also a relatively common pathogen. Rare causes of monomicrobial NSTI include *V. vulnificus*, community-associated MRSA,[7] and *B. cereus.*[124] *Pseudomonas aeruginosa* rarely is a pathogen of NSTI; rarer still are the infections caused by *C. septicum* and *V. vulnificus.* Phycomycotic NSTI (mucormycosis) caused by *Rhizopus*, *Mucor*, or *Absidia* spp. may occur in profoundly immunosuppressed patients or after accidental burial by a landslide. In contrast, polymicrobial NSTI is the norm, with aerobic gram-positive and -negative bacteria and anaerobes usually all present in tissue. *Escherichia coli* and *B. fragilis* are the most common anaerobic and aerobic isolates, respectively. The most likely gram-positive coccus to be isolated depends on the clinical context. For example, enterococci are more likely to be isolated when the NSTI complicates a recent abdominal incision.

Pathogenesis

After inoculation of susceptible tissue, several factors determine the extent of infection, including the size of the inoculum, the invasiveness of the organism,[125,126] the presence of a foreign body or ischemic tissue, and impaired host responses. Inoculation can occur from delayed or inadequate treatment of an initially localized process, inappropriate closure of a contaminated surgical incision that should have been left open, or in the presence of an enterostomy or retention sutures. Inoculation may also be occult; for example, NSTI of the thigh can be the initial manifestation of a colon perforation into the retroperitoneum.

The hallmark of NSTI is rapid progression and a fulminant clinical course, especially for monomicrobial infections, but polymicrobial NSTIs are also bona fide emergencies that require rapid diagnosis and definitive treatment. Several bacterial enzymes cause tissue damage and promote bacterial invasiveness, including hemolysin, fibrinolysin, hyaluronidase, and streptokinase elaborated by *S. pyogenes*, collagenase elaborated by *P. aeruginosa*, and lecithinase elaborated by *C. perfringens*. Polymicrobial NSTIs are characterized by synergistic activity of facultative aerobes and anaerobes. Tissue hypoxia and impaired neutrophil function create conditions favorable for the proliferation of facultative bacteria, which

TABLE 12.17. Objective Criteria to Distinguish Necrotizing Soft Tissue Infections from Nonnecrotizing Infections.

A. Diagnostic Accuracy

	Sensitivity (%)	*Specificity (%)*	*Positive predictive value (%)*	*Negative predictive value (%)*
Tense edema	38	100	100	62
Gas on x-ray	39	95	88	62
Bullae	24	100	100	57
WBC > 14 × 10^9/l	81	76	77	80
Sodium < 135 mg/dl	75	100	100	77
Chloride < 95 mg/dl	30	100	100	55
BUN > 15 mg/dl	70	88	88	71

B. Incidence of Positive Laboratory Parameters (Univariate Analysis)

	Necrotizing fasciitis	*Other infection*	*P value*
WBC > 14 × 10^9/l	17/21 (81%)	5/21 (24%)	.0002
Sodium < 135 mEq/l	15/20 (75%)	0/17 (0%)	.0001
Chloride < 95 mEq/l	6/20 (30%)	0/17 (0%)	.02
Serum urea nitrogen > 15 mg/dl	14/20 (70%)	2/17 (12%)	.0007

Source: Data from Hohlweg-Majert et al.[121] and Toran et al.[122]

consume oxygen in the microenvironment and lower the tissue redox state, thereby creating conditions favorable for the growth of anaerobes.

Extensive tissue necrosis develops from direct tissue injury caused by bacterial toxins, inflammation and tissue edema, and vascular thrombosis. The subcutaneous fat and fascia are more likely than the overlying skin to develop necrosis. Thus, there may be little or no early cutaneous evidence of underlying infection. However, as the infection progresses, thrombosis of the cutaneous microcirculation leads to the characteristic erythema, edema, bullae, and overt gangrene of advanced NSTI.

Soft tissue gas may or may not be present, depending on the pathogens involved, but develops as a result of anaerobic wound conditions that allow proliferation of gas-forming organisms, including *C. perfringens, B. fragilis, E. coli, Klebsiella pneumoniae, P. aeruginosa,* and *Proteus* spp. These bacteria produce insoluble gases such as hydrogen, nitrogen, and methane, which remain in the tissue to a variable degree. Gas in the tissue tends to be a late finding in nonclostridial polymicrobial infections and to be absent in NSTI caused by *S. pyogenes.*

Diagnosis

The diagnosis of NSTI is based primarily on the history and physical examination. One notable early characteristic is a complaint of severe pain that is disproportionate to local physical findings. Inspection of the overlying skin may yield few early clues. Characteristic features to elicit include edema and tenderness that extend beyond the margin of erythema, skin vesicles or bullae, crepitus, and the absence of lymphangitis and lymphadenitis. As infection progresses, cutaneous anesthesia and necrosis develop along with clinical manifestations of sepsis (fever, tachycardia, hypotension, encephalopathy). Occasionally, patients with clostridial sepsis will present with anemia and jaundice secondary to hemolysis, and patients with myonecrosis will present with myoglobinuria, rhabdomyolysis, and acute renal failure.

Some common laboratory tests may point the clinician toward the diagnosis of NSTI in the appropriate clinical context. Wall et al. showed that hyponatremia ($[Na]_{serum}$ < 135 mEq/dl) and leukocytosis (WBC count > 14 × 10^9/l) have good diagnostic accuracy[127,128] (Table 12.17). Wong et al. described the Laboratory Risk Indicator for Necrotizing Fasciitis (LRINEC) score (Table 12.18),[129] which may be even more accurate. Although these observation have not been subjected to independent validation, they may be valuable to the extent that it *heightens* the suspicion of a clinician confronted with a possible NSTI who has seen one previously only rarely, if at all.

If the diagnosis is not obvious by physical examination and laboratory testing, then radiographic studies may be obtained provided surgical exploration, which is the definitive diagnostic test as well as therapeutic intervention, is not unduly delayed. Plain radiographs can demonstrate gas in the soft tissues in the absence of crepitus, but the absence of gas does not exclude the presence of NSTI as it is usually a late finding when it does develop. Computed tomography (CT) is sensitive for the presence of soft tissue gas, and it may also demonstrate asymmetric edema of tissue planes (a nonspecific finding). A CT scan may be helpful in the evaluation of the obese patient with a deep-seated infection, for whom the physical examination can be unreliable. However, to the extent that obtaining any imaging study will delay the operative management of the patient, they should be avoided. The use of imaging studies as "confirmatory" tests cannot be

TABLE 12.18. Laboratory Risk Indicator for Necrotizing Fasciitis (LRINEC) Score.

Parameter	*Point value*
C-Reactive protein, mg/l	
<150	0
≥150	4
White blood cell count, mm³	
<15	0
15–25	1
>25	2
Hemoglobin, g/dl	
>13.5	0
11–13.5	1
<11	2
Sodium, mEq/l	
>135	0
≤135	2
Creatinine, mg/dl	
≤1.6	0
>1.6	2
Glucose, mg/dl	
≤180	0
>180	1

The maximum LRINEC score is 13 points. A score greater than 6 points should raise the suspicion of a necrotizing soft tissue infection, whereas a score of more than 8 points is strongly predictive. The model was constructed retrospectively but has a positive predictive value of 92% at a cutoff score of 6 points and a negative predictive value of 96%.

Source: Adapted from Wong et al.,[129] by permission of *Critical Care Medicine.*

condoned. Clinical diagnosis alone is sufficient to begin broad-spectrum antimicrobial therapy and to undertake surgical exploration and debridement.

Both fine-needle aspiration and incision biopsy of questionably affected areas have been recommended. Gram stain of the biopsy material can demonstrate causative organisms and an inflammatory cell infiltrate, and frozen section demonstration of necrosis, thrombosis, or pathogens in tissue are diagnostic. However, clinical suspicion is sufficient to explore the patient with suspected NSTI; therefore, these less-invasive approaches to diagnosis are usually superfluous and must not engender delay.

Treatment

The management of NSTI is a true emergency. The elapsed time between the onset of symptoms and the initial operative treatment is the single most important factor influencing morbidity and mortality. Delay in diagnosis must be avoided at all costs as the success of management depends on prompt recognition and operative debridement. Once the diagnosis of NSTI is made, tissue salvage and patient survival can only be achieved by prompt, widespread debridement. Identification of the causative organism(s) and underlying pathology can wait. Antibiotics are a necessary adjunct and must be started immediately (see below), but they are only an adjunct; the mortality of true NSTI managed nonoperatively is 100%.

The first surgical objective is a thorough wound exploration to confirm the presence and extent of NSTI. Debridement of all infected, devitalized tissue must be aggressive. The underlying tissue necrosis usually extends far beyond the boundary of the skin involvement; therefore, exposure must be wide, and dissection must extend beyond the boundary of tissue viability. Considering that these infections spread rapidly, resection of a margin of viable tissue is prudent even at the cost of additional deformity or disability. When the margin of viability is indistinct, frozen section examination of the limits of resection can occasionally be helpful. Wound drainage must be submitted for comprehensive microbiologic testing. Fasciotomies should be performed if compartment syndrome is suspected. A temporary prosthesis may be necessary to reconstruct the abdominal wall to prevent evisceration in some cases. All open wounds are irrigated before loose packing with saline-moistened gauze.

Reexploration in the operating room is routine at 24h to ensure that all necrotic tissue has been debrided. Patients with NSTIs are often unstable, so ICU management must also be aggressive with mechanical ventilation, fluids, blood and blood products, and inotrope/vasopressor agents as appropriate so that the crucial return trip to the operating room can occur on schedule. Operative debridement is continued daily until the infection is controlled. Extremity amputation or colostomy may be necessary to manage severe infections of the extremity or perineum, respectively.

Empiric antibiotics must be effective against a broad range of potential pathogens (gram-positive cocci; gram-negative bacilli, including *Pseudomonas*; and anaerobes) because the infecting organism usually cannot be discerned from inspection alone. Empiric antifungal therapy is unnecessary in most cases of NSTI. Antibacterial monotherapy can be achieved with a carbapenem, either imipenem-cilastatin (2–3g daily) or meropenem (1g every 8h). Piperacillin-tazobactam is an effective, less-costly alternative (13.5g daily). Current guidelines recommend ampicillin-sulbactam, but activity may be inadequate against *E. coli* and *K. pneumoniae*. Clindamycin in high dosage may be preferable to penicillin G for streptococcal infections because of good evidence that clindamycin inhibits toxin production. Clindamycin is also effective against MSSA. Metronidazole can be substituted for clindamycin for therapy of type I NSTI because of better anaerobic coverage. Gentamicin is best avoided because of the additive risk of acute renal failure in patients who may be hypovolemic or hypotensive. However, gentamicin is an efficient microbicide when given in adequate dosage; single daily dose administration provides an adequate peak serum concentration while minimizing the development of toxicity. Combination therapy that includes vancomycin is now popular, especially considering that nearly 60% of *S. aureus* strains are now MRSA. Vancomycin can be added to piperacillin-tazobactam or a carbapenem if MRSA is suspected.

All identified pathogens should be treated. The duration of therapy must be individualized, but most NSTIs will require a minimum of 10 days of therapy. Once culture and sensitivity data are available, the empiric antibiotic regimen should be adjusted accordingly. Adjustment can be challenging when multiple pathogens are isolated from a polymicrobial infection, but an attempt must be made to decrease the chance of superinfection by multidrug-resistant pathogens. Clostridial infections are best treated with penicillin alone, but many clinicians prefer high-dose clindamycin to penicillin for NSTIs caused by *S. pyogenes* alone because of its antitoxin properties. Anaerobic infections of the head, neck, and upper extremity tend to be caused by penicillin-susceptible anaerobes, whereas those of the trunk and lower extremity tend to include *B. fragilis*, against which penicillin is ineffective. Rare phycomycotic infections may require amphotericin B; fluconazole is ineffective.

Patients with traumatic wounds should receive tetanus toxoid or immune globulin, depending on their immunization status. Other therapy is supportive, including early nutritional support and prophylaxis against venous thromboembolic disease. Hyperbaric oxygen therapy has been advocated, especially for clostridial infections. Among the putative benefits of hyperbaric oxygen are inhibition of exotoxin production, increased tissue oxygen tension, and improved neutrophil function. However, there has never been evidence of benefit from a randomized trial of hyperbaric oxygen therapy of NSTI. A "dive" takes a minimum of 2h to arrange and complete. Most clinicians consider that time better spent in the operating room.

References

1. Stevens DL, Bisno AL, Chambers HF, et al. Practice guidelines for the diagnosis and management of skin and soft-tissue infections. Clin Infect Dis 2005;41:1373–1406.
2. Swartz MN. Cellulitis. N Engl J Med 2004;350:904–912.
3. Miller SR, Mondry T, Reed JS, et al. Delayed cellulitis associated with conservative therapy for breast cancer. J Surg Oncol 1998;242–245.
4. Brook I, Frazier EH. Aerobic and anaerobic bacteriology of wounds and cutaneous abscesses. Arch Surg 1990;125:1445–1451.
5. National Nosocomial Infections Surveillance (NNIS) System report, data summary from January 1992 through June 2004,

issued October 2004. Am J Infect Control 2004;232:5470–485.

6. Fridkin SK, Hageman JC, Morrison M, et al. Active Bacterial Core Surveillance Program of the Emerging Infections Program Network. Methicillin-resistant *Staphylococcus aureus* disease in three communities. N Engl J Med 2005;352:1436–1444.
7. Miller LG, Perdreau-Remington F, Rieg G, et al. Necrotizing fasciitis caused by community-associated methicillin-resistant *Staphylococcus aureus* in Los Angeles. N Engl J Med 2005;352:1445–1453.
8. Frazee BW, Lynn J, Charlebois ED, et al. High prevalence of methicillin-resistant *Staphylococcus aureus* in emergency department skin and soft tissue infections. Ann Emerg Med 2005;45:311–320.
9. Lewis JS 2nd, Jorgensen JH. Inducible clindamycin resistance in staphylococci: should clinicians and microbiologists be concerned? Clin Infect Dis 2005;40:280–285.
10. Dupuy A, Benchikhi H, Roujeau JC, et al. Risk factors for erysipelas of the leg (cellulitis): case-control study. BMJ 1999;318:1591–1594.
11. Bisno AL, Stevens DL. Streptococcal infections in skin and soft tissues. N Engl J Med 1996;334:240–245.
12. Hirshmann JV. Impetigo: etiology and therapy. Curr Clin Top Infect Dis 2002;22:42–51.
13. Raz R, Miron D, Colodner R, et al. A 1-year trial of nasal mupirocin in the prevention of recurrent staphylococcal nasal colonization and skin infection. Arch Intern Med 1996;156: 1109–1112.
14. Klempner MS, Styrt B. Prevention of recurrent staphylococcal skin infections with low-dose clindamycin therapy. JAMA 1988;260:2682–2685.
15. Attanoos RL, Appleton MA, Douglas-Jones AG. The pathogenesis of hidradenitis suppurativa: a closer look at apocrine and apoeccrine glands. Br J Dermatol 1995;133:254–258.
16. Deroo H, Aelbrecht M, t'Kindt J. Hidradenitis suppurativa. Dermatologica 1990;180:193–194.
17. Edlich RF, Silloway KA, Rodeheaver GT. Epidemiology, pathology, and treatment of axillary hidradenitis suppurativa. J Emerg Med 1986;4:369–378.
18. Jemec GB, Heidenheim M, Nielsen NH. Hidradenitis suppurativa—characteristics and consequences. Clin Exp Dermatol 1996;21:419–423.
19. Stevens DL, Herr D, Lampiris H, Hunt JL, Batts DH, Hafkin B. Linezolid versus vancomycin for the treatment of methicillin-resistant Staphylococcus aureus infections. Clin Infect Dis 2002;34:1481–1490.
20. Seltzer E, Dorr MB, Goldstein BP, et al., and the Dalbavancin Skin and Soft-Tissue Study Group. Once-weekly dalbavancin versus standard of care antimicrobial regimens for treatment of skin and soft-tissue infections. Clin Infect Dis 2003;37:1298–1303.
21. Arbeit RD, Maki D, Tally FP, et al., and the Daptomycin 98-01 and 99-01 Investigators. The safety and efficacy of daptomycin for the treatment of complicated skin and skin-structure infections. Clin Infect Dis 2004;38:1673–1681.
22. Wilcox M, Nathwani D, Dryden M. Linezolid compared with teicoplanin for the treatment of suspected or proven gram-positive infections. J Antimicrob Chemother 2004;53:335–344.
23. Giordano P, Song J, Pertel P, et al. Sequential intravenous/oral moxifloxacin versus intravenous piperacillin-tazobactam followed by oral amoxicillin-clavulanate for the treatment of complicated skin and skin structure infections. Int J Antimicrob Agents 2005;26:357–365.
24. Ellis-Grosse EJ, Babinchak T, Dartois N, et al., for the Tigecycline 300 and 305 cSSSI Study Groups. The efficacy and safety of tigecycline in the treatment of skin and skin-structure infection: results of two double-blind phase 3 comparison studies with vancomycin-aztreonam. Clin Infect Dis 2005;41(suppl 5): S341–S353.
25. Jauregui LE, Babazadeh S, Seltzer E, et al. Randomized, double-blind comparison of once-weekly dalbavancin versus twice-daily linezolid therapy for the treatment of complicated skin and skin structure infections. Clin Infect Dis 2005;41:1407–1412.
26. Weigelt J, Itani K, Stevens D, et al. Linezolid versus vancomycin in treatment of complicated skin and soft tissue infections. Antimicrob Agents Chemother 2005;49:2260–2266.
27. Fabian TC, File TM, Embil JM, et al. Meropenem versus imipenem-cilastatin for the treatment of hospitalized patients with complicated skin and skin structure infections: results of a multicenter, randomized, double-blind comparative study. Surg Infect 2005;6:269–282.
28. Lipsky BA. Medical treatment of diabetic foot infections. Clin Infect Dis 2004;39(suppl 2):S104–S114.
29. Lipsky BA, Berendt AR, Deery HG, et al. Diagnosis and treatment of diabetic foot infections. Clin Infect Dis 2004;39:885–910.
30. Reiber GE, Pecoraro RE, Knepsell TD. Risk factors for amputation in patients with diabetes mellitus: a case control study. Ann Intern Med 1992;117:97–105.
31. Wilson RM. Neutrophil function in diabetes. Diabet Med 1986;3:509–512.
32. McMahon MM, Bistrian BR. Host defenses and susceptibility to infection in patients with diabetes mellitus. Infect Dis Clin North Am 1005;9:1–10.
33. Wheat LJ, Allen SD, Henry M, et al. Diabetic foot infections: bacteriologic analysis. Arch Intern Med 1986:146:1935–1940.
34. Lipsky BA, Itani K, Norden C, et al., and the Linezolid Diabetic Foot Infections Study Group. Treating foot infections in diabetic patients: a randomized, multicenter, open-label trial of linezolid versus ampicillin-sulbactam/amoxicillin-clavulanate. Clin Infect Dis 2004;38:17–24.
35. Gerding DN. Foot infections in diabetic patients: the role of anaerobes. Clin Infect Dis 1995;20(suppl 2):S283–S288.
36. Armstrong DG, Lavery GA, Harkless LB. Validation of a diabetic wound classification system: the contribution of depth, infection, and ischemia to risk of amputation. Diabetes Care 1998;21:855–859.
37. Jeffcoate WJ, Lipsky BA. Controversies in diagnosing and managing osteomyelitis of the foot in diabetes. Clin Infect Dis 2004;39(suppl 2):S115–S122.
38. Lipsky BA. Osteomyelitis of the foot in diabetic patients. Clin Infect Dis 1997;25:1318–1326.
39. Lipsky BA. Evidence-based antibiotic therapy of diabetic foot infections. FEMS Immunol Med Microbiol 1999;26:267–276.
40. Raymakers JT, Houben AJ, van de Hayden JJ, et al. The effect of diabetes and severe ischemia in the penetration of ceftazidime into tissues of the limb. Diabetes Med 2001;18:229–234.
41. Harkless L, Boghossian J, Pollak R, et al. An open-label, randomized study comparing efficacy and safety of intravenous piperacillin/tazobactam and ampicillin/sulbactam for infected diabetic foot ulcers. Surg Infect 2005;6:27–40.
42. Lipsky BA, Armstrong DG, Citron DM, et al. Ertapenem versus piperacillin/tazobactam for diabetic foot infections (SIDESTEP): prospective, randomised, controlled, double-blinded, multicentre trial. Lancet 2005;366:1695–1703.
43. Stone JA, Cianci P. The adjunctive role of hyperbaric oxygen in the treatment of lower extremity wounds in patients with diabetes. Diabetes Spectrum 1997;10:118–123.
44. Wunderlich RP, Peters EJG, Lavery L. Systemic hyperbaric oxygen therapy, lower extremity wound healing, and the diabetic foot. Diabetes Care 2000;23:1551–1555.
45. Estes JM, Pomposelli FB Jr. Lower extremity arterial reconstruction in patients with diabetes mellitus. Diabet Med 1996;13: S43–S50.

46. Tannenbaum GA, Pomposelli FB Jr, Marcaccio EJ, et al. Safety of vein bypass grafting to the dorsal pedal artery in diabetic patients with foot infections. J Vasc Surg 1992;15:982–990.
47. Horan TC, Gaynes RP, Martone WJ, Jarvis WR, Emori TG. CDC definitions of nosocomial surgical site infections, 1992: a modification of CDC definitions of surgical wound infections. Infect Control Hosp Epidemiol 1992;13:606–608.
48. Barie PS. Surgical site infections: epidemiology and prevention. Surg Infect 2002;3(suppl 1):S9–S21.
49. Fry DE. The economic costs of surgical site infection. Surg Infect 2002;3(suppl 1):S37–S43.
50. National Nosocomial Infections Surveillance System (NNIS) System Report: data summary from January 1992–June 2001, issued August 2001. Am J Infect Control 2001;29:404–421.
51. Garibaldi RA, Cushing D, Lerer T. Risk factors for postoperative infection. Am J Med 1991;91(suppl 3B):158S–163S.
52. Dellinger EP, Hausmann SM, Bratzler DW, et al. Hospitals collaborate to decrease surgical site infections. Am J Surg 2005;190:9–15.
53. Emori TG, Gaynes RP. An overview of nosocomial infections, including the role of the microbiology laboratory. Clin Microbiol Rev 1993;6:428–442.
54. Raymond DP, Pelletier SJ, Crabtree TD, et al. Surgical infection and the ageing population. Am Surg 2001;67:827–832.
55. Latham R, Lancaster AD, Covington JF, et al. The association of diabetes and glucose control with surgical-site infections among cardiothoracic surgery patients. Infect Control Hosp Epidemiol 2001;22:607–612.
56. Pomposelli JJ, Baxter JK III, Babineau TJ, et al. Early postoperative glucose control predicts nosocomial infection rate in diabetic patients. JPEN J Parenter Enteral Nutr 1998;22:77–81.
57. Delgado-Rodriguez M, Medina-Cuadros M, Martinez-Gallego G, et al. Total cholesterol, HDL cholesterol, and risk of nosocomial infection: a prospective study in surgical patients. Infect Control Hosp Epidemiol 1997;18:9–18.
58. Malone DL, Genuit T, Tracy JK, et al. Surgical site infections: reanalysis of risk factors. J Surg Res 2002;103:89–95.
59. Scott JD, Forrest A, Feuerstein S, et al. Factors associated with postoperative infection. Infect Control Hosp Epidemiol 2001;22:347–351.
60. Mangram AJ, Horan TC, Pearson ML, et al. Guideline for prevention of surgical site infection, 1999. Hospital Infection Control Practices Advisory Committee. Infect Control Hosp Epidemiol 1999;20:250–278.
61. Tepaske R, Velthuis H, Oudemans-van Straatan HM, et al. Effect of preoperative oral immune-enhancing nutritional supplement on patients at high risk of infection after cardiac surgery: a randomized placebo-controlled trial. Lancet 2001;358:696–701.
62. Gianotti L, Braga M, Nespoli L, et al. A randomized controlled trial of preoperative oral supplementation with a specialized diet in patients with gastrointestinal cancer. Gastroenterology 2002;122:1763–1770.
63. Higgins A, London J, Charland S, et al. Prophylactic antibiotics for elective laparoscopic cholecystectomy: are they necessary? Arch Surg 1999;134:611–613.
64. Harling R, Moorjani N, Perry C, MacGowan AP, Thompson MH. A prospective, randomised trial of prophylactic antibiotics versus bag extraction in the prophylaxis of wound infection in laparoscopic cholecystectomy. Ann R Coll Surg Engl 2000;82:408–410.
65. Lewis RT. Oral versus systemic antibiotic prophylaxis in elective colon surgery: a randomized study and meta-analysis send a message from the 1990s. Can J Surg 2002;45:173–180.
66. Song F, Glenny A-M. Antimicrobial prophylaxis in colorectal surgery: a systematic review of randomized controlled trials. Br J Surg 1998;85:1232–1241.
67. http://www.medqic.org/dcs/ContentServer?cid=1089815967030&pagename=Medqic%2FContent%2FParentShellTemplate&parentName=Topic&c=MQParents. Accessed January 2, 2007.
68. Tejirian T, DiFrtonzo LA, Haigh PI. Antibiotic prophylaxis for preventing wound infection after breast surgery: a systematic review and metaanalysis. J Am Coll Surg 2006;203:729–734.
69. Cunningham M, Bunn F, Handscomb K. Prophylactic antibiotics to prevent surgical site infection after breast cancer surgery (review). Cochrane Database Syst Rev 2006;2:CD005360.
70. Aufenacker TJ, Koelemay JW, Gouma DJ, Simons MP. Systematic review and meta-analysis if the effectiveness of antibiotic prophylaxis in prevention of wound infection after mesh repair of abdominal wall hernia. Br J Surg 2006;93:5–10.
71. Sanchez-Manuel FJ, Seco-Gil JL. Antibiotic prophylaxis for hernia repair. Cochrane Database Syst Rev 2004;4:CD003769.
72. Stewart A, Evers PS, Earnshaw JJ. Prevention of infection in arterial reconstruction. Cochrane Database Syst Rev 2006;3:CD003073.
73. Bratzler DW, Houck PM, and the Surgical Infection Prevention Guideline Writers Workgroup. Antimicrobial prophylaxis for surgery: an advisory statement from the National Surgical Infection Prevention Project. Am J Surg 2005;189:395–404.
74. Classen DC, Evans RS, Pestotnik SL, et al. The timing of prophylactic administration of antibiotics and the risk of surgical-wound infection. N Engl J Med 1992;326:281–286.
75. Zaneti G, Giardina R, Platt R. Intraoperative redosing of cefazolin and risk for surgical site infection in cardiac surgery. Emerg Infect Dis 2001;7:828–831.
76. Mest DR, Wong DH, Shimoda KJ, et al. Nasal colonization with methicillin-resistant *Staphylococcus aureus* on admission to the surgical intensive care unit increases the risk of infection. Anesth Analg 1994;78:644–650.
77. Perl TM, Cullen JJ, Wenzel RP, et al., and the Mupirocin and the Risk of *Staphylococcus aureus* Study Team. Intranasal mupirocin to prevent postoperative *Staphylococcus aureus* infections. N Engl J Med 2002;346:1871–1877.
78. Bratzler DW, Houck PM, Richards C, et al. Use of antimicrobial prophylaxis for major surgery. Baseline results from the National Surgical Infection Prevention Project. Arch Surg 2005;140:174–182.
79. Morris AM, Jobe BA, Stoney M, et al. *Clostridium difficile* colitis: an increasingly aggressive iatrogenic disease? Arch Surg 2002;137:1096–1100.
80. Namias N, Harvill S, Ball S, et al. Cost and morbidity associated with antibiotic prophylaxis in the ICU. J Am Coll Surg 1999;188:225–230.
81. Fukatsu K, Saito H, Matsuda T, et al. Influences of type and duration of antimicrobial prophylaxis on an outbreak of methicillin-resistant *Staphylococcus aureus* and on the incidence of wound infection. Arch Surg 1997;132:1320–1325.
82. Bozorgzadeh A, Pizzi WF, Barie PS, et al. The duration of antibiotic administration for penetrating abdominal trauma. Am J Surg 1999;177:125–131.
83. Velmahos GC, Toutouzas KG, Sarkysian G, et al. Severe trauma is not an excuse for prolonged antibiotic prophylaxis. Arch Surg 2002;137:537–541.
84. Parienti JJ, Thibon P, Heller R, et al. Hand-rubbing with an aqueous alcoholic versus traditional surgical hand-scrubbing and 30-day surgical site infection rates: a randomized equivalence study. JAMA 2002;288:722–727.
85. Kurz A, Sessler DI, Lenhardt R. Perioperative normothermia to reduce the incidence of surgical-wound infection and shorten hospitalization, Study of Wound Infection and Temperature Group. N Engl J Med 1996;334:1209–1215.
86. Flores-Maldonado A, Medina-Escobedo CE, Rios-Rodriguez HM, et al. Mild hypothermia and the risk of wound infection. Arch Med Res 2001;32:227–231.

87. Melling AC, Ali B, Scott EM, et al. Effects of preoperative warming on the incidence of wound infection and clean surgery: a randomized controlled trial. Lancet 2001;358:876–880.
88. Janik J. Electric cautery lowers contamination threshold for infection by laparotomies. Am J Surg 1998;175:263–266.
89. Brasel KJ, Borgstrom DC, Weigelt JA. Cost-utility analysis of contaminated appendectomy wounds. J Am Coll Surg 1997;184:23–30.
90. Cohn SM, Giannotti G, Ong AW, et al. Prospective randomized trial of two wound management strategies for dirty abdominal wounds. Ann Surg 2001;233:409–413.
91. Al-Inany H, Youssef G, Abd ELMaguid A, et al. Value of subcutaneous drainage system in obese females undergoing cesarean section using Pfannenstiel incision. Gynecol Obstet Invest 2002;53:75–78.
92. Magann EF, Chauhan SP, Rodts-Palenik D, et al. Subcutaneous stitch closure versus subcutaneous drain to prevent wound disruption after cesarean delivery: a randomized clinical trial. Am J Obstet Gynecol 2002;186:1119–1123.
93. Noyes LD, Doyle DJ, McSwain NE. Septic complications associated with the use of peritoneal drains in liver trauma. J Trauma 1998;28:337–346.
94. Magee C, Rodeheaver GT, Golden GT, et al. Potentiation of wound infection by surgical drains. Am J Surg 1976;131;28:14–20.
95. Barie PS. Are we draining the life from our patients? Surg Infect 2002;3:159–160.
96. Platell C, Papadimitriou JM, Hall JC. The influence of lavage on peritonitis. J Am Coll Surg 2000;191:672–680.
97. Cervantes-Sanchez CR, Gutierrez-Vega R, Vasquez-Carpizio JA, et al. Syringe pressure irritation of subdermic tissue after appendectomy to decrease the incidence of postoperative wound infection. World J Surg 2000;24:38–41.
98. Yoshii S, Hosaka S, Suzuki S, et al. Prevention of surgical site infection by antibiotic spraying in the operating field during cardiac surgery. Jpn J Thorac Cardiovasc Surg 2001;49:279–281.
99. O'Connor LT Jr, Goldstein M. Topical perioperative antibiotic prophylaxis for minor clean inguinal surgery. J Am Coll Surg 2002;194:407–410.
100. Hebert PC, Wells G, Blajchman MA, et al. A multi-center, randomized, controlled clinical trial of transfusion requirements in critical care. Transfusion Requirements in Critical Care Investigators, Canadian Critical Care Trials Group. N Engl J Med 1999;340:409–417.
101. Claridge JA, Sawyer RG, Schulman AM, et al. Blood transfusions correlate with infections in trauma patients in a dose-dependent manner. Am Surg 2002;68:566–572.
102. Offner PJ, Moore EE, Biffl WL, et al. Increased rate of infection associated with transfusion of old blood after severe injury. Arch Surg 2002;137:711–717.
103. Hill GE, Frawley WH, Griffith KE, et al. Allogeneic blood transfusion increases the risk of postoperative bacterial infection: a meta-analysis. J Trauma 2003;54:908–914.
104. Taylor RW, Manganaro L, O' Brian J, et al. Impact of allogenic packed red blood cells transfusion on nosocomial infection rates in the critically ill patient. Crit Care Med 2002;30:2249–2254.
105. Vincent JL, Baron J-F, Reinhart K, et al. Anemia and blood transfusion in critically ill patients. JAMA 2002;288:1499–1507.
106. Latham R, Lancaster AD, Covington JF, et al. The association of diabetes and glucose control with surgical-site infections among cardiothoracic surgery patients. Infect Control Hosp Epidemiol 2001;22:607–612.
107. van den Berghe G, Wouters P, Weekers F, et al. Intensive insulin therapy in the critically ill patients. N Engl J Med 2001;345:1359–1367.
108. Pittas AG, Siegel RD, Lau J. Insulin therapy for critically ill hospitalized patients: a meta-analysis of randomized controlled trials. Arch Intern Med 2004;164:2005–2011.
109. Heyland DK, MacDonald S, Keefe L, et al. Total parenteral nutrition in the critically ill patient: a meta-analysis. JAMA 1998;280:2013–2019.
110. Berne JD, Norwood SH, McAuley CE, et al. Erythromycin reduces delayed gastric emptying in critically ill trauma patients: a randomized, controlled trial. J Trauma 2002;53:422–425.
111. Marik PE, Zaloga GP. Early enteral nutrition in acutely ill patients: a systematic review. Crit Care Med 2001;29:2264–2270.
112. Gottrupp F. Oxygen in wound healing and infection. World J Surg 2004;28:312–315.
113. Greif R, Akca O, Horn EP, et al. Supplemental perioperative oxygen to reduce the incidence of surgical-wound infection. Outcomes Research Group. N Engl J Med 2000;342:161–167.
114. Pryor KO, Fahey TJ 3rd, Lien CA, Goldstein PA. Surgical site infection and the routine use of perioperative hyperoxia in a general surgical population: a randomized controlled trial. JAMA 2004;291:79–87.
115. Fuchs U, Zittermann A, Stuettgen B, et al. Clinical outcome of patients with deep sternal wound infection managed by vacuum-assisted closure compared to conventional therapy with open packing: a retrospective analysis. Ann Thorac Surg 2005;79:526–531.
116. File TM. Necrotizing soft tissue infections. Curr Infect Dis Rep 2003;5:407–415.
117. Oliver JD. Wound infections caused by *Vibrio vulnificus* and other marine bacteria. Epidemiol Infect 2005;133:383–391.
118. Ebright JR, Pieper B. Skin and soft tissue infections in injection drug users. Infect Dis Clin North Am 2002;16:697–712.
119. Cunningham SC, Napolitano LM. Necrotizing soft tissue infection from decubitus ulcer after spinal cord injury. Spine 2004;29: E172–E174.
120. Skitarelic N, Mladina R, Morovic M, Skitarelic N. Cervical necrotizing fasciitis: sources and outcomes. Infection 2003;31:39–44.
121. Hohlweg-Majert B, Weyer N, Metzger MC, Schon R. Cervicofacial necrotizing fasciitis. Diabetes Res Clin Pract 2006;72:206–208.
122. Toran KC, Nath S, Shrestha S, Rana BB. Odontogenic origin of necrotizing fasciitis of head and neck—a case report. Kathmandu Univ Med J 2004;2:361–363.
123. Praba-Egge AD, Lanning D, Broderick TJ, Yelon JA. Necrotizing fasciitis of the chest and abdominal wall arising from an empyema. J Trauma 2004;56:1356–1361.
124. Darbar A, Harris IA, Gosbell IB. Necrotizing infection due to *Bacillus cereus* mimicking gas gangrene following penetrating trauma. J Orthop Trauma 2005;19:353–355.
125. Chhatwal GS, McMillan DJ. Uncovering the mysteries of invasive streptococcal diseases. Trends Mol Med 2005;11:152–155.
126. Gillespie SH. New tricks from an old dog: streptococcal necrotising soft-tissue infections. Lancet 2004;363:672–673.
127. Wall DB, Klein SR, Black S, de Virgilio C. A simple model to help distinguish necrotizing fasciitis from nonnecrotizing soft tissue infection. J Am Coll Surg 2000;191:227–231.
128. Wall DB, de Virgilio C, Black S, Klein SR. Objective criteria may assist in distinguishing necrotizing fasciitis from nonnecrotizing soft tissue infection. Am J Surg 2000;179:17–21.
129. Wong CH, Khin LW, Heng KS, et al. The LRINEC (Laboratory Risk Indicator for Necrotizing Fasciitis) score: a tool for distinguishing necrotizing fasciitis from other soft tissue infections. Crit Care Med 2004;32:1535–1541.
130. Cohen MM, Duncan PG. Physical status score and trends in anesthetic complications. J Clin Epidemiol 1988;41:83–90.

13

Intraabdominal Infections

Michael A. West and Michael B. Shapiro

A century ago, infectious complications severely limited the capacity of surgeons to care for abdominal pathology. Advances in medical care over the past 100 years have made abdominal surgery remarkably safe. There is a sense that even extensive procedures are "routine," particularly in patients who do not have major comorbidities. Although we often think that progress has limited infectious complications, the reality is that in 2006 infections are the most frequent cause of morbidity and mortality in surgical patients.[1–3]

Factors that Prevent Intraabdominal Infection

Intraabdominal infections are encountered frequently by physicians and surgeons.[1–7] If not managed properly, they result in significant mortality and morbidity[2,5,8]; therefore, it is important to understand how to recognize and treat these infections. At the most fundamental level, three things must be understood to manage these infections: (1) how infections arise, (2) factors that normally prevent development of abdominal infections, and (3) the treatment priorities that apply when infections do arise. Under normal circumstances, there is balance among bacterial factors, host defenses, and environmental factors.[2,5,8] This balance prevents development of clinically evident infection. To understand the pathogenesis of intraabdominal infection, each of these three factors is considered.

Bacteria

There are huge numbers of bacteria on the surface of the skin and within the gastrointestinal (GI) tract. The vast majority of bacteria in the colon are anaerobic species that contribute little to clinical intraabdominal infection. In point of fact, the bacteria isolated from clinical infection make up less than 0.1% of the normal colonic flora.[9,10] Table 13.1 shows the most common aerobic and anaerobic species isolated from clinical intraabdominal infection.[9,11,12]. It is clear in both recent series that *Escherichia coli* and *Bacteroides fragilis* were isolated most frequently, and bacteria such as *Pseudomonas aeruginosa* are infrequent primary pathogenic isolates. It is also important to note that most intraabdominal infections are polymicrobial. *Escherichia coli* is often described as the "prototypic" aerobic organism, and *Bacteroides* species are representative of anaerobic bacteria.[13,14] Even the most common anaerobic pathogen, *B. fragilis*, accounts for only about 1% of colonic flora (Fig. 13.1).

It is important to recognize that the bacteria that cause peritonitis or intraabdominal abscesses possess virulence factors that separate them from other types of bacteria that do not cause clinical infection. For example, in the case of *B. fragilis*, only strains possessing a polysaccharide capsule cause abscesses.[15,16] Injections of purified polysaccharide capsule, in the absence of viable organisms, can substitute for the presence of *B. fragilis* in generation of abscesses.[17]

The experimental results shown in Figure 13.2 illustrate the relative pathogenic contributions of aerobic and anaerobic bacteria in intraabdominal sepsis. Using an experimental model it was shown that injection of *E. coli* alone resulted in significant mortality but a low incidence of abscess formation in survivors.[18] In contrast, injection of pure *B. fragilis* into the peritoneal cavity resulted in low mortality, but 95% of animals developed abscesses. When a combination of *E. coli* and *B. fragilis* was injected, the typical clinical condition was seen, with significant mortality and bacteremia and with most survivors developing abscesses. Thus, gram-negative aerobes are largely responsible for mortality and bacteremia, whereas the anaerobic bacteria contribute to the development of intraabdominal abscesses. These observations form the basis for the use of antimicrobial therapy for intraabdominal infection.

In the case of clinical infection, the organisms do not exist in isolation. Rather, aerobic and anaerobic bacteria are present at the same time, and the property known as *microbial synergy* is such that the sum of the effects of the combined infection is greater than the individual components of each type of bacteria. In experimental models, simultaneous injec-

TABLE 13.1.
Bacteria Isolated from Clinical Intraabdominal Infection (% of Patients in Whom a Particular Organism Was Recovered).

Organism	*Solomkin*[10]	*Mosdell*[12]
Gram-negative aerobes		
Escherichia coli	58%	69%
Enterobacter/Klebsiella	39%	23%
Pseudomonas aeruginosa	15%	19%
Gram-positive. ND, not detected		
Staphylococci	11%	11%
Proteus spp.	6%	3%
Anaerobes		
Bacteroides fragilis	23%	45%
Enterococcus	23%	11%
Other bacteroides	21%	N.D.
Fusobacterium spp.	6%	5%
Peptostreptococci	7%	16%

tion of *B. fragilis* along with *E. coli* significantly augments the lethality of the *E. coli* even though *B. fragilis* by itself results in no mortality.[19,20] The bowel flora are also influenced significantly by prior antibiotic treatment. As mentioned, most of the anaerobic bacterial species in the colon are nonpathogenic; however, under the influence of broad-spectrum antibiotics the susceptible organisms are killed, leaving an altered flora of resistant organisms and pathogenic fungi.[21–24]

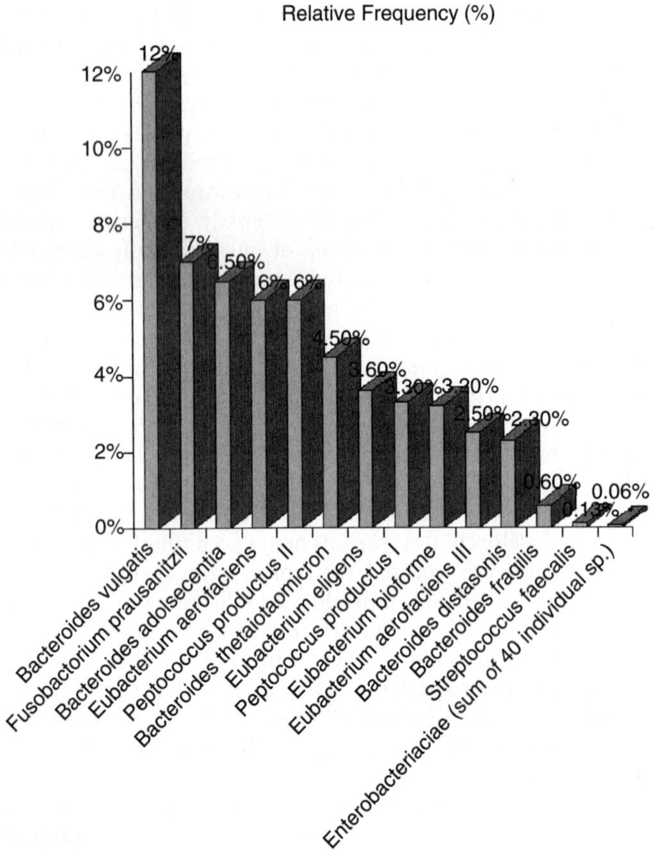

FIGURE 13.1. Relative frequency of pathogen isolation from intraabdominal infections. (*Source:* Adapted from Howard and Simmons,[173] with permission.)

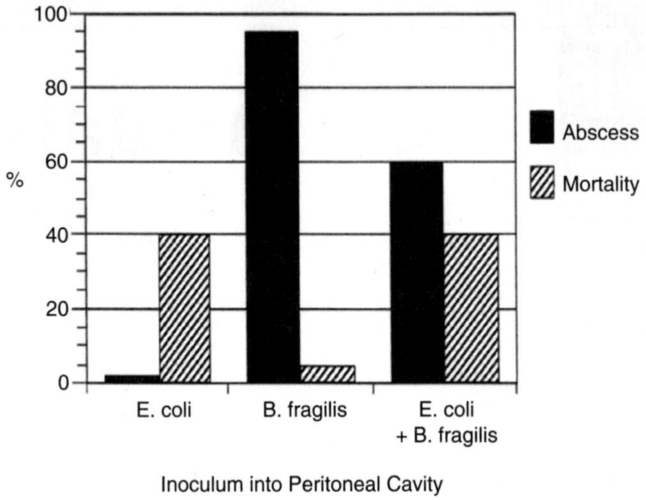

FIGURE 13.2. Contribution of aerobic and anaerobic bacteria to the pathogenesis and mortality of polymicrobial intraabdominal infection. Experimental inoculation of *E. coli* alone, *B. fragilis* alone, or a combination of *E. coli* and *B. fragilis* into the rat peritoneal cavity was performed. The mortality and incidence of abscesses in survivors were measured. With *E. coli* alone, there was significant (40%) mortality, but abscesses were rare in survivors. When *B. fragilis* alone was inoculated, there was little mortality, but essentially all survivors had abscesses. If both bacteria were inoculated, then a situation similar to untreated human intraabdominal infection was observed. That is, there was a significant mortality, associated with gram-negative bacteremia, and survivors had a high incidence of intraabdominal abscesses. (*Source:* Adapted from Weinstein,[172] by permission of *Infection and Immunity*.)

Host Defenses

The first line of host defense in the peritoneal cavity is the presence of soluble factors such as complement and preformed antibodies.[9,25] Cellular host defense consists primarily of the monocytes and macrophages normally present in the peritoneal cavity. These cells coordinate the inflammatory response and have the capacity to ingest and kill invading bacteria. They also function importantly as antigen-presenting cells. Macrophages recruit additional host defense cells in the form of neutrophils (PMNs, polymorphonuclear leukocytes). Neutrophils are one of the key effector cells in the inflammatory response; however, neutrophils are also responsible for much of the parenchymal destruction associated with inflammation.[26] These cells are able to produce large quantities of reactive oxygen intermediates (ROIs) with generation of hydrogen peroxide and superoxide.[27,28]

Following the inoculation of bacterial components into the peritoneal cavity, there is subsequent release of proinflammatory cytokines into the systemic circulation.[29] Peak levels of tumor necrosis factor (TNF) are seen at 60 to 90 min, whereas interleukin-1 and interleukin-6 (IL-1 and IL-6) lag behind. Appearance of these cytokines in the bloodstream coincides with the development of clinical signs and symptoms, including fever, chills, and leukocytosis.

Environmental Factors

Under normal circumstances, the integrity of the skin and the GI tract ensures that bacteria on the surface do not gain access to the sterile portions of the body. Bacteria are usually

TABLE 13.2. Characteristics that Determine Surgical Options in the Gastrointestinal Tract.

Characteristic	*Stomach*	*Duodenum*	*Small bowel*	*Large bowel*
Blood supply	Excellent	Very good	Very good	Very good
Bacterial counts	$<10^2$ CFU/ml (10^5–10^6 if achlorrhydic)	~10^3–10^4 CFU/ml	~10^3–10^4 CFU/ml	10^3–10^6 CFU/ml
Redundancy	Good	Little/none	Excellent	Excellent
Mobility	Very good	Slight	Excellent	Excellent
Serosa	Yes	Partial	Yes	Yes
Intraperitoneal	Yes	Partial	No	Mostly

present on all surfaces of the skin, and there are enormous numbers of bacteria within the lumen of the GI tract.[1,7,8,15,30,31] A number of factors may upset this balance, ranging from elective surgery to severe traumatic injury. It is also good to keep in mind that the number, as well as the type, of bacteria vary significantly with progression down the GI tract from mouth to colon (Table 13.2). The upper GI tract is normally inhabited by lactobacilli in relatively low numbers. In contrast, the distal GI tract normally contains 10^{10-12} pathogenic aerobic and anaerobic bacteria.[32,33]

Pathogenesis of Intraabdominal Infection

Intraabdominal infections present in a wide variety of forms and at numerous locations. In the broadest terms, classification schemes have distinguished between localized and diffuse infections.[5,7,30,31,34,35] For most practical purposes, *localized infections* represent an infected fluid collection or an intraabdominal abscess. *Diffuse infections* present clinically as generalized peritonitis and reflect the absence or failure of an effective local immune response.[26,36] By definition, diffuse infections encompass all or most of the peritoneal cavity. Localized infections or abscesses can be located anywhere in the subphrenic, subhepatic, or pelvic recesses, as well as between loops of intestine, within the lesser sac, and even within the substance of solid organs (e.g., liver, spleen, kidney).[31,34,35,37–39] Most surgical intraabdominal infections arise as a result of a break in the integrity of the GI tract.[31,39,40] This realization clarifies the need for a "surgical intervention" (although such an intervention may be a radiological or minimally invasive procedure) to obtain primary control of the source of the leak (see Table 13.2).[41,42] It is axiomatic that antimicrobial agents alone are seldom sufficient to eradicate serious intraabdominal infections.

If the bacterial inoculum is contained by the host defense, then a localized inflammatory process results, recognized clinically as an abscess. With a larger inoculum or in the absence of adequate host defenses, the bacteria can disseminate more widely, resulting in a diffuse inflammatory response, recognized clinically as peritonitis.[31,35,43] Uncontrolled peritonitis will frequently result in death. Bacteria within the peritoneal cavity can rapidly gain access to the systemic circulation via subdiaphragmatic lymphatic channels.[9,10] In fact, bacteria can be isolated from the bloodstream within 5–10min after inoculation into the peritoneal cavity.[44]

The process described above underscores the importance of the balance between bacterial inoculum and host defense. The ultimate outcome is, in many respects, a "race" between bacterial multiplication and bacterial destruction mediated by the host defenses. Miles and Burke suggested the concept of a "decisive period" that was important for determining the development of bacterial infection.[45] This concept refers to the time required for bacterial numbers in fluid or tissue to exceed $10^5/cm^3$. Once these levels are achieved, an infection is established. On the other hand, if the host defenses are able to keep the bacterial numbers below this threshold, then infection is averted. When this is examined experimentally, bacteria counts drop rapidly following inoculation due to the influence of complement and preformed antibody. Complement attracts PMNs into the tissue, with a further rapid decrease in the number of surviving bacteria. Vascular permeability is altered by complement and is further increased as a result of the ROI released by PMNs. With altered vascular permeability, the redness and swelling that are typically associated with infection is seen. For PMNs to kill bacteria, molecular oxygen is a key cofactor. Oxygen delivery to the tissues is optimized by adequate resuscitation as well as vigorous debridement to ensure that any nonviable tissue is removed.

So-called adjuvant substances are also important for the development of infection.[43,46,47] The inoculum of bacteria required for infection is significantly decreased in the presence of adjuvant substances. These substances serve both to increase bacterial virulence and to interfere with host defenses. The most important adjuvant substance in clinical infection is blood. Other adjuvants that frequently contribute to the pathogenesis of intraabdominal infection include bile salts, gastric mucin, pancreatic secretions, urine, and chyle. Foreign bodies also increase the likelihood of clinical infection. Microorganisms adhere to foreign materials, making it far more difficult for phagocytes to ingest or kill them. In addition, the foreign body itself may induce an inflammatory reaction.

If the bacterial inoculum is contained within an abscess to a large extent, then the bacteria have been "removed" from the host.[30,34,48] A well-defined abscess is usually contained within a collagen capsule, with an inner rim of white blood cells that keep the bacteria from further invading the host. Although bacteria may be contained within abscesses, the characteristics of the abscess center are inhospitable to host leukocytes, impairing the ability of these cells to clear the abscess of bacteria and resolve the infection. Characteristics of the abscess center include a low pH, low po_2, huge numbers of bacteria, opsonin-deficient fluid, and the presence of necrotic material and proteolytic enzymes.[10]

TABLE 13.3.
Adjunctive (Nonantibiotic) Measures to Prevent Infection.

Author	*Year*	*N*	*Study type*	*Condition*	*Conclusion*
Perioperative Glucose Control					
Furnay[61]	2004	4864	PNRCT	Diabetic patients undergoing open heart surgery/ sternotomy	Glucose below 150 associated with decreased risk of deep sternal wound infection, lower mortality and decreased length of stay
Effect of oxygen					
Grief[158]	2000	500	PRCT	Elective colon resection	High FIO_2 during operation decreased incidence of postop SSI
Pryor[159]	2004	165	PRCT	General surgery patients undergoing elective operation	High FIO_2 did not reduce incidence of SSI
Preoperative mechanical bowel preparation					
Wille-Jorgensen[160]	2003	?	Rev: PRCT	Elective colorectal surgery	No evidence for beneficial effects from bowel preparation; cleansing may be associated with an increased risk of anastomotic dehiscence.
Zmora[161]	2003	380	PRCT	Colonic diseases/elective colectomy requiring anastomosis	Preoperative mechanical bowel preparation (polyethylene glycol) made no difference in wound infection, anastomotic leak, or intra-abdominal abscess
Bucher[162]	2004	1144	Rev; PRCT	Colonic diseases/elective colectomy requiring anastomosis	Preoperative mechanical bowel preparation did not reduce postoperative infections and may increase anastomotic leak rate
Selective digestive decontamination					
Nathens[163]	1999	—	Meta-analysis of PRCT	Critically ill patients with intraabdominal infection	Selective decontamination of the digestive tract notably reduces mortality in critically ill surgical patients, while critically ill medical patients derive no such benefit
Source control					
Marshall[42]	2003	—	EB review	Modified Delphi method, systematic review	Source control (drain infected fluid, debride infected tissue, remove infected device, or correct anatomic derangement abnormality producing ongoing microbial contamination) considered crucial to success of intra-abdominal infection control, although scant grade A or B evidence
Prophylactic drainage					
Petrowsky[108]	2004	—	EB review	Patients undergoing abdominal surgery entered into study that randomized drains or none	Many GI operations can be performed safely without prophylactic drainage; drains should be omitted after hepatic, colonic, or rectal resection with primary anastomosis and appendectomy for any stage of appendicitis (recommendation grade A), whereas prophylactic drainage remains indicated after esophageal resection and total gastrectomy (recommendation grade D)
Jesus[164]	2004	1140	Rev; PRCT	Colorectal surgery with anastomosis	No evidence showing that routine drainage after colorectal surgery alters anastomotic or infectious complications
Wound management in face of gross peritonitis					
Cohn[165]	2001	51	PRCT	Patients with gross contamination secondary to perforated appendicitis, trauma or intraabdominal abscess/laparotomy	Delayed primary wound closure at 4 days was associated with a lower incidence of SSI

SSI, surgical site infection; PNRCT, prospective, non-randomized clinical trial; PRCT, prospective, randomized clinical trial; Rev, review; EB, evidenced-based.

Prevention of Intraabdominal Infection

Information about how intraabdominal infections arise and how to treat these serious infections also provides important information about an even more effective strategy: prevention.[49–52] There is now abundant evidence pertaining to a variety of readily achievable measures that can be employed to prevent infection during routine abdominal surgical procedures. These measures include clipping hair rather than shaving,[52] preoperative bowel preparation,[49,53] antibiotic prophylaxis initiated before the skin incision,[51,54] discontinuing prophylactic antibiotics within 24h after the procedure,[51,54] administration of adequate intraoperative fluid to avoid "relative hypovolemia,"[55] maintaining normothermia,[56,57] administration of supplemental oxygen,[58,59] and "tight" perioperative glucose control.[60,61] In addition, the very nature of abdominal surgery has qualitatively changed with the widespread application of "minimally invasive," frequently laparoscopic surgical techniques.[62] Table 13.3 summarizes evidence-based measures that have been shown to be effective in decreasing the incidence of infection.

Principles of Treatment

Most clinically important surgical intraabdominal infections arise as a result of so-called secondary peritonitis.[10,30,31,34] Primary peritonitis is usually seen in immunocompromised patients or in children.[63] The bacteria arise from an exogenous source, and surgery is seldom required. Most of these infections are also due to a single species of bacteria. In contrast, secondary peritonitis arises in relatively normal patients. The bacteria arise from the patients themselves, and isolation of multiple bacteria species is the rule. Surgery is generally required. A third form of intraabdominal infection, so-called tertiary peritonitis,[64–66] develops in intensive care unit (ICU) patients with multiple-organ dysfunction syndrome (MODS). The source of bacteria is again endogenous, and multiple bacteria are isolated from these types of infections. The role of surgery in tertiary peritonitis, however, is less clear-cut.

Surgical intervention has a key role in treating typical secondary peritonitis. The most important factor is to correct the primary pathology. In many cases, this may require exploratory surgery.[39,67] Once the defect in the GI tract or source of infection is identified, resection, patching, repairing, debriding, or draining the underlying cause is the mainstay of treatment. At the same time, it is important to recognize that the inflammatory response results in enormous "third-space" fluid losses that require aggressive fluid resuscitation and concurrent monitoring. Finally, there is clearly an important role for appropriate antibiotics.[51,54,68] Choice of antibiotics should be based on knowledge of the underlying pathogens likely to be involved in the infection. This can be determined (in part) based on knowledge of where in the GI tract the perforation or inoculation occurred (see Table 13.2).

If surgical intervention is required, then the timing of that intervention may dramatically influence the outcome. For example, there is little morbidity if gastric or proximal small bowel perforations are closed within the first 24h or colon perforations are repaired within 12h.[50,54,69] With a longer delay, these infections become more established, widespread, and associated with more complications. In some cases, the morbidity may include development of severe sepsis or even MODS.[70–72] Finally, the timing of the intervention may determine what is treated (i.e., peritonitis vs. an abscess).

When a surgical intervention is performed, it is important to adhere to general principles of abdominal source control[3,39,73]: (1) prompt control of ongoing contamination, (2) removal of all necrotic tissue, and (3) ensuring an excellent blood supply. If a repair is performed, then it should be tension free. The mainstay of treatment for intraabdominal abscess is drainage, which can be performed either surgically or radiologically.[74,75] Drainage results in resolution of the abscess because it tips the standoff between bacterial invasion and host defense back in favor of the host.[76] Drainage results in more favorable conditions for host inflammatory cells within the abscess center, including an increase in pH and po_2, removal of large numbers of bacteria, obliteration of dead space, and collapse of abscess walls due to removal of the infected fluid. Drainage should be continued until the cavity is completely obliterated.

The goal of antimicrobial therapy in intraabdominal infection is to hasten elimination of the infecting microorganism. Appropriate antimicrobial therapy should shorten clinical manifestations of infection and minimize the risk of recurrent infection. Antimicrobial therapy should be initiated when the diagnosis is suspected based on the anticipated pathogens that will be encountered at the site of presumed infection/proliferations.[51,77–79] In many new intraabdominal infections, the initial antibiotic choice needs to be empiric. This choice depends on the site of presumed infection, patient risk factors, and the recognition of whether the infection is arising from the community or within the hospital environment. Subsequently, it is appropriate to adjust therapy based on culture results in the context of the anticipated pathogens.

Appropriate choices for antimicrobial therapy for intraabdominal infection have been reviewed.[51,79] Many guidelines for antibiotic choices divide therapy into single agents or combination therapy and further subdivide the therapeutic choices based on whether the infection is community acquired of mild to moderate intensity or a severe community or a nosocomial infection. Evidence-based guidelines for appropriate choices for single or combination therapy are summarized in Table 13.4, based on the Surgical Infection Society (SIS) and Infections Disease Society of America (IDSA) guidelines.[51,79]

Antibiotic resistance is becoming a more serious problem in surgical patients with infection. Analogous to the distinction between community-acquired and hospital-acquired pneumonia is the concern of whether intraabdominal infection arises in the community or in the hospital. For example, although gram-positive bacteria (e.g., *Enterococcus*, *Staphylococcus aureus*) *may* be cultured, they are seldom important pathogens for community-acquired infections.[80,81] However, the epidemiology is altered under the selection pressure of systemic antimicrobial therapy within medical centers.[21–24,82] Microorganisms isolated from in-hospital abdominal infection include *Enterococcus*, *Pseudomonas*, methicillin-resistant *S. aureus* (MRSA), *Staphylococcus epidermidis*, and *Candida* spp., reflecting the alterations in the GI flora from prior antibiotic exposure.[5,24,64] Such infections are much more difficult to treat, and this is reflected in the higher mortality with in-hospital intraabdominal infection.

TABLE 13.4.
Use of Perioperative Antibiotic Prophylaxis.

Author	*Year*	*N*	*Study type*	*Condition*	*Conclusion*
Antibiotic prophylaxis versus none					
Andersen[92]	2003	9,757	Rev: PRCT, PCCT	Acute appendicitis/ appendectomy	Antibiotic prophylaxis was superior to placebo for reducing infectious complications in acute appendicitis; benefit was present in both children and adults irrespective of appendiceal pathology
Mazuski[51]	2002	—	EB review	PRCT evaluating antibiotic use in intraabdominal infection 1990–2000	Strong evidence supporting antibiotic use, choice, spectrum, and timing of administration; paucity of good data on duration and treatment of high-risk patients
Duration					
Mazuski[51]	2002	—	EB review	PRCT evaluating antibiotic use in intraabdominal infection 1990–2000	Strong evidence supporting antibiotic use, choice, spectrum, and timing of administration; paucity of good data on duration and treatment of high-risk patients
Wong[166]	2005	5,094	Review: RCT and "quasi-randomized" clinical trial	Adults requiring antimicrobial treatment of secondary peritonitis	No specific recommendations for first-line antibiotic treatment of secondary peritonitis in adults; all regimens showed equivocal efficacy; factors such as local guidelines and preferences, ease of administration, costs, and availability should be considered in determining antibiotic regimen of choice
Single versus multiple antibiotics					
Sims[167]	1997	291	PRCT	Penetrating abdominal trauma/laparotomy	No difference in outcome with single vs. multiple antibiotics
Bratzler[168]	2005	34,133	Random sample of Medicare records	Patients undergoing surgery for a wide variety of conditions	An antibiotic dose was administered to 55.7% within 1 h before incision; antimicrobial agents consistent with guidelines were administered to 92.6% of patients; antimicrobial prophylaxis was discontinued within 24 h of surgery in 40.7% of patients; substantial opportunities exist to improve use of prophylactic antimicrobials for patients undergoing major surgery

PNRCT, prospective, non-randomized clinical trial; PRCT, prospective, randomized clinical trial; EB, evidenced-based; PCCT, prospective, controlled clinical trial.

Specific Surgical Conditions

In the sections that follow, some specific aspects of the most common intraabdominal surgical infectious conditions encountered by practicing surgeons are reviewed. The conditions discussed certainly do not comprise an exhaustive list, yet many of the principles that pertain to these specific, common conditions could be applied, alone or in combination, to address treatment of almost every variety of intraabdominal infection.

Acute Appendicitis

Acute appendicitis is a common problem encountered by the majority of surgeons. The peak incidence of appendicitis extends from childhood into early adulthood, although the condition can be encountered at all ages. For nonperforated acute appendicitis, the current standard of care is surgical removal, although debate is ongoing regarding whether an open or laparoscopic approach is preferable (see below).

Acute appendicitis arises when there is an obstruction to the lumen of the appendix. Initially, this results in crampy abdominal pain, nausea, anorexia, or emesis with discomfort localized to the epigastrium. Subsequently, as pressure builds within the appendix, there is invasion of the mucosa with inflammatory changes, resulting in development of localized peritoneal signs over McBurney's point in the right lower quadrant. Classically, the diagnosis is made on the basis of a characteristic history and the presence of localized peritoneal irritation in the right lower quadrant. More recently, there has been increased use of diagnostic adjuncts, including ultrasound and abdominal computed tomographic (CT) scans. Ultrasound is used more frequently in the pediatric population, and abdominal CT is used with increasing frequency in both pediatric and adult populations. On CT scan, the characteristics of acute appendicitis include the presence of a dilated appendix with wall enhancement, which is frequently associated with periappendiceal inflammatory changes (fat stranding). Prior to the use of these diagnostic adjuncts, clinical judgment resulted in a 90%–95% accurate diagnosis in males and an 80%–90% accurate diagnosis in females of child-bearing age. With the increasing use of these other modalities, the accuracy rate has increased to 95%–97% in both genders.[83]

Debate continues regarding whether an open or laparoscopic approach is the ideal modality for removal of the

TABLE 13.5.
Open Appendectomy (OA) Versus Laparoscopic Appendectomy (LA) for Acute Appendicitis.

Author	*Year*	*N*	*Study type*	*Condition*	*Conclusion*
Eysach[86]	2002	—	Review of randomized controlled studies comparing LA to OA	Patients undergoing surgery for acute appendicitis	LA was associated with lower incidence of SSI (OR 0.5) but a higher rate of intraabdominal abscess (OR 3); diagnostic accuracy was superior to OA
Katkhouda[84]	2005	247	PRDBCT	Patients undergoing surgery for acute appendicitis	No advantage of LA over OA in all studied parameters except quality-of-life scores at 2 weeks; choice of procedure should be based on surgeon or patient preference
Sauerland[169]	2004	—	Cochrane review of 45 studies	Patients undergoing surgery for acute appendicitis	In clinical settings where surgical expertise and equipment are available and affordable, *diagnostic laparoscopy* and LA seem to have various advantages over OA; clinical effects of LA are small and of limited clinical relevance

PRDBCT, prospective, randomized, double-blind clinical trial.

inflamed appendix. Several prospective, randomized clinical trials have been performed; in most cases, there was no major advantage to one approach or the other.[84–86] Data from several of these studies are included in Table 13.5. A potential advantage of the laparoscopic approach is the ability to rule out other conditions, particularly in women of child-bearing age. This advantage is largely negated if an abdominal CT scan is used for preoperative diagnosis. With either modality, the acute condition can be readily treated with hospitalizations ranging from 1 to 3 days for uncomplicated appendicitis.[84,85,87] The presence of perforation, frequently associated with greater than 24- to 48-h history of symptoms, complicates therapy by either approach. Most series of laparoscopic appendectomy report a 5% to 10% conversion to open operation,[84,88] and this is more frequent in the case of advanced clinical disease with peritonitis.[89,90] Laparoscopic appendectomy is also associated with slightly greater cost, although this may be surgeon dependent and reflects the use of disposable instrumentation.[87,91]

There is clear evidence that perioperative antibiotic prophylaxis represents the standard of care for acute appendicitis.[92] In uncomplicated acute appendicitis, there is no advantage to continuing the antibiotics longer than 24h.[93,94] Most clinicians will treat perforated appendicitis with a more prolonged course of antibiotics, although the exact duration remains a point of contention.[94,95] Many authors recommend 5–7 days of antibiotics. In the setting of a prolonged duration of symptoms or CT-documented perforation (e.g., abscess or a large phlegmon), percutaneous drainage may be the preferred option in conjunction with prolonged antibiotics.[96,97] The choice of antibiotics reflects the general choices for infections arising in the distal GI tract, with coverage for both aerobic and anaerobic bacteria (see Table 13.4).

Acute Cholecystitis

Acute cholecystitis represents another common intraabdominal surgical infection. Acute cholecystitis arises when the cystic duct is obstructed; the gallbladder becomes increasingly distended, resulting in a cycle of progressive distention and gallbladder wall ischemia.[98,99] Infections usually arise secondary to bile stasis and represent proliferation of the bacteria already present. With progressive ischemia or necrosis of the mucosa and gallbladder wall, these bacteria add an infectious component to the ischemia-induced inflammatory changes. The clinical diagnosis is made on the basis of ultrasound findings of marked gallbladder wall thickening with or without pericholecystic fluid. Patients frequently have a significant elevation of the white blood cell count with a left shift. On physical examination, most patients have right upper quadrant peritoneal signs in addition to a positive Murphy's sign. The presence of a positive Murphy's sign in and of itself does not indicate a clinical diagnosis of acute cholecystitis because pressure alone elicits discomfort with a distended gallbladder. Acute pancreatitis and ascending cholangitis need to be ruled out in the setting of localized severe right upper quadrant pain with fever.[99] Patients presenting with acute cholecystitis frequently receive parenteral antibiotics, although the evidence supporting this is largely based on expert opinion.[100]

In most cases, operative removal of the gallbladder is appropriate for patients with acute cholecystitis,[101–103] but the timing of surgical intervention has been a matter of ongoing debate. Most investigators recommend early operative intervention (within 1–4 days) following the onset of symptoms.[104] With more prolonged duration of symptoms, the severe inflammatory changes make removal of the gallbladder exceedingly difficult, increasing risk of injury to the common bile duct. Experienced surgeons are often able to remove even markedly inflamed gallbladders via the laparoscopic route; however, the incidence of complications or conversion to open operation remains as high as 40%.[105] Open cholecystectomy can be an appropriate modality for patients with acute cholecystitis and is still used preferentially by many surgeons.[102,103] Finally, percutaneous drainage of the gallbladder is an option for patients with multiple comorbidities or with evidence of severe inflammatory changes or prolonged duration of the condition.[101] Percutaneous drainage of the gallbladder is most often performed by interventional radiologists using a transhepatic route. The precise role of interval cholecystectomy remains undefined, although this is probably indicated in the absence of severe comorbid conditions.

Antibiotics chosen for acute cholecystitis should provide coverage for aerobic gram-negative bacteria (see Table 13.4). Enterococcus is commonly isolated from bile,[106] although empiric antibiotics that include antienterococal coverage are probably unnecessary.[51,107] Even with severe inflammatory changes, if gallbladder removal takes away the primary focus of infection, then 24h of antibiotics are sufficient. If there is evidence of significant systemic disease (e.g., rigors, bacteremia, acidosis), then antibiotics are often continued for 5–7 days or more, although evidence supporting this practice is lacking.[100] There is little or no evidence supporting routine prophylactic closed-suction drainage after cholecystectomy,[108] although this is still frequently employed (see Table 13.3).

Acute Diverticulitis

Acute, uncomplicated diverticulitis is seldom seen by surgeons. Most reviews of acute diverticulitis show that an uncomplicated first attack is appropriately treated medically, with antibiotics the mainstay of treatment.[109–111] Antibiotics in this setting should include coverage for aerobic and anaerobic bacteria (see Table 13.4). After a second episode of acute diverticulitis or with complication arising secondary to diverticulitis (e.g., fistula, perforation), surgical resection of the involved colon is indicated.[111,112]

Perforated acute diverticulitis frequently presents as a surgical emergency with signs and symptoms of generalized peritonitis. Radiographic evaluation often shows free intra-abdominal air on plain films or CT scans. On physical examination, most patients have localized peritoneal signs in the left lower quadrant. If peritoneal signs are localized, then a course of antibiotics or percutaneous drainage of abscesses may facilitate one-stage surgery at the time of exploration. Appropriate broad-spectrum antibiotics should be initiated as soon as the diagnosis is confirmed. The presence of generalized peritonitis is usually an indication for exploratory laparotomy. Patients with generalized peritonitis often require aggressive fluid resuscitation, and this should be performed prior to bringing these patients to the operating room.

A variety of surgical options for treatment of acute diverticulitis have been delineated.[112–116] In the recent past, a three-stage approach was considered the standard of care. This entailed construction of a diverting stoma at the first operation, followed days or weeks later by resection of the diseased colon (second stage). The third stage with this approach involved colostomy takedown with reestablishment of colorectal continuity. More recently, a two-stage approach with resection, proximal colostomy, and distal Hartman's pouch construction at the initial operation has been used. Subsequently, these patients need colostomy takedown, generally after 2–4 months.

Currently, there is considerable evidence (see Table 13.6) supporting one-stage operations in appropriately selected patients.[112,116] Performance of a one-stage operation is facilitated by preoperative control of the acute infection and in some cases even preoperative bowel preparation. The general principles regarding construction of a safe anastomosis apply (tension-free repair, excellent blood supply, minimal bowel wall edema, and the absence of peritonitis). If these conditions can be achieved with resection of the diseased segment and the patient is hemodynamically stable, then primary resection and anastomosis can be considered. Although the incidence of infectious complications is higher than that seen after elective operations, the combined incidence of intra-abdominal infection associated with the two-stage operation is higher still (see Table 13.6).

Bowel Infarction/Ischemia

Intestinal ischemia can arise secondary to strangulation (e.g., internal hernia, adhesions) or low-flow states (e.g., shock, vascular insufficiency).[117] Overall, the small intestine has a better blood supply than the colon, but both organs are susceptible to infarction/ischemia. Vasopressor therapy may make a patient particularly susceptible to decreased intestinal blood flow inasmuch as intestinal perfusion is often the "first

TABLE 13.6.
Single-Stage Versus Two-Stage Operation for Complicated Acute Diverticulitis.

Author	*Year*	*N*	*Study type*	*Condition*	*Conclusion*
Salem[113]	2004	1620	Retrospective review	Patients undergoing Hartman procedure (1051) vs. primary resection and anastomosis (569) for acute perforated diverticulitis	Reported mortality and morbidity in patients with diverticular peritonitis who underwent primary anastomosis were *not* higher than those in patients undergoing Hartmann's procedure; this suggests that primary anastomosis is a safe operative alternative in certain patients with peritonitis
Gooszen[112]	2002	60	Retrospective	Patients undergoing surgery for complicated acute diverticulitis	No statistically significant difference in complication rate between one- and two-stage operations
Zeitoun[170]	2000	105	PRCT	Complicated diverticulitis with peritonitis	Single-stage resection is superior for treatment of generalized peritonitis complicating sigmoid diverticulitis; this approach associated with less postoperative peritonitis, fewer reoperations, and shorter LOS

PRCT, prospective, randomized clinical trial; LOS, length of stay.

to go" and the "last to return" in systemic low-flow states. This fact underscores the importance of aggressive resuscitation and adequate patient monitoring.

The metabolic rate of the intestinal mucosa is significantly higher than that of the muscularis or serosa; thus, the mucosa is more vulnerable to ischemic conditions.[118–120] Indeed, significant mucosal ischemia may be visualized endoscopically at the same time that the intestinal musculature remains viable and the external appearance is normal. On the other hand, the fact that the mucosa is more vulnerable provides the clinician with a high degree of assurance with respect to intestinal viability if the mucosa looks viable in the setting of suspected low-flow states. Low blood flow to the intestine, with varying degrees of mucosal ischemia, results in enhanced bacterial translocation or even progression to frank ulceration.[121–123]

A variety of methods has been used to identify intestinal ischemia pre- or intraoperatively.[117,124] Preoperatively, angiography is the mainstay of diagnosis; however, with improved software packages and bolus contrast infusion, CT scanning is providing increasingly reliable information regarding intestinal blood flow. From a practical standpoint, magnetic resonance imaging (MRI) is seldom used to evaluate acute ischemia, but this modality has a significant role in the evaluation of chronic intestinal ischemic conditions (e.g., artherosclerotic mesenteric occlusive disease). Intraoperatively, clinical judgment and visual inspection of the bowel are the primary assessments used to determine intestinal viability.[125–127] Segmental full-thickness necrosis needs to be resected to avoid perforation and generalized peritonitis. In select circumstances, areas of marginal viability may be revascularlized (with segmental bypass, angioplasty, or thrombolytics). In some instances, intestinal perfusion can be assessed using a sterile Doppler probe and evaluating the blood flow in the peripheral aspects of the mesenteric circulation. Historically, intravenous administration of fluorescine along with ultraviolet illumination (Wood's lamp) was used to assess intestinal viability, although this is rarely used today.

As noted above, all areas of frankly necrotic bowel should be resected at the initial operation.[41] In addition, there is a large body of evidence that supports a planned second-look operation 24 to 48 h after the initial procedure.[128,129] This approach is a variation on the so-called damage control laparotomy (see below) that has been incorporated into the algorithm for operative management of acute trauma.[129–132] Using this approach, bowel resections are performed at the initial operation, but no anastomoses or stomas are constructed. During the planned reexploration, the remaining bowel can be carefully assessed for viability. Areas with progression of necrosis should be resected, and if there are no residual ischemic segments, then it is generally safe to perform an anastomosis at the second or subsequent operation.[133,134]

An additional benefit of the damage control approach is the ability to delay fascial closure. In severe bowel ischemia, there is frequently tremendous third-space losses into the bowel wall or lumen. This often results in significant swelling within the peritoneal cavity, which could further compromise blood flow and set in motion a cycle of increasing pressure with progressive ischemic necrosis of the bowel. Performance of a temporary abdominal closure aids in the appropriate aggressive perioperative fluid resuscitation and avoids development of abdominal compartment syndrome.[131,135]

Anastomotic Breakdown/Intraabdominal Abscess

Intraabdominal abscesses arise secondary to localized infection within the peritoneal cavity. While generally considered to be an adverse outcome, in a sense abscess development represents a "victory" for the host defenses since the generalized infection has become localized. Material contaminating the peritoneal cavity generally occurs from a break in the integrity of the GI tract. If surgical source control and antibiotics are unable to completely eradicate the infection, then abscesses ensue. The best means to minimize the development of an intraabdominal abscess is appropriate primary surgical source control.[39,41,136,137] Table 13.2 discusses some of the anatomic factors that need to be considered with respect to source control of GI perforations.

Intraabdominal abscesses or infected fluid collections are frequently encountered in the postoperative period.[36,136,138] Primary healing of an intestinal anastomosis requires excellent blood supply to both ends of the bowel, no tension on the anastomosis, absence of peritonitis or localized inflammatory changes, and technically optimal performance of the anastomosis. If any of these factors are deficient, then anastomotic breakdown with intraperitoneal leakage of intestinal contents occurs. Interloop abscesses are frequently encountered with postoperative anastomotic breakdown or intestinal perforation, and these can be much more difficult to treat.

At this time, the preferred approach to management of intraabdominal fluid collections/abscesses is percutaneous drainage.[37,75] Anatomic localization of the abscess can generally be accomplished using abdominal CT scan or ultrasound.[139] Once the abscess or fluid collection is identified, a safe anatomic trajectory is determined, and the fluid collection is aspirated or drained. It is important to obtain postprocedural radiologic verification that the fluid collections in question have been adequately drained.[75] An additional benefit of the percutaneous approach is the ability to obtain "clean" specimens for culture. Broad-spectrum antibiotics (see Table 13.4) directed against the pathogens to be encountered at the level of the GI tract where the perforation occurred are administered preprocedure and generally are continued for 7 to 10 days.[39,51,54] Data to support this arbitrary duration of treatment are scant.

If more generalized infection arises secondary to anastomotic breakdown, then reexploration may be needed. Such patients should be resuscitated, receive invasive monitoring, and be prepared for emergent surgery. It is generally unwise to perform an anastomosis in the setting of acute peritonitis, and therefore preoperative discussion regarding construction of a diverting stoma is appropriate.[39]

If percutaneous drainage is able to control the acute infection, development of an enterocutaneous fistula is frequent.[3,37,140,141] In the absence of distal obstruction, most enterocutaneous fistulae heal spontaneously.[140] There are numerous anecdotal reports of decreased output from proximal fistulae or healing of fistulae using somatostatin[142]; however, there are no good prospective randomized trials addressing the role of this agent. Aggressive nutritional support is also an important component of the management of an enterocutaneous fistula.[141] In general, low-residue or

TABLE 13.7.
Antibiotics for Abdominal Trauma.

Author	*Year*	*N*	*Study type*	*Condition*	*Conclusion*
Cornwell[153]	1999	63	PRCT	Colonic trauma in high-risk patients (multiple blood transfusions, more than 4h from injury to operation, penetrating abdominal trauma index more than 25)	No benefit of duration of antibiotic administration longer than 24h
Velamhos[171]	2002	250	PNRCT	Trauma patients requiring operation *and* ICU stay longer than 3 days	No benefit to multiple antibiotics or antibiotic duration longer than 24h
Kirton[152]	2000	317	PRCT	Penetrating abdominal trauma with ≥ 1 hollow viscus injury/laparotomy	No difference in incidence of postoperative infection with 1 day vs. 5 days of antibiotics
Bozorgzadeh[154]	1999	314	PRCT	Penetrating abdominal trauma/laparotomy	No difference in incidence of postoperative infection with 1 day vs. 5 days of antibiotics

PRCT, prospective, randomized clinical trial; PNRCT, prospective, non-randomized clinical trial.

elemental enteric formulation can be useful if it does not adversely affect the fistula output. Alternatively, total parenteral nutrition (TPN) may be employed, but it may take 4–8 weeks for complete resolution of a fistula; therefore, this will likely need to be continued after discharge from the hospital.

Surgery for Trauma

It is not surprising that intraabdominal infections arise frequently after traumatic injuries, particularly following penetrating trauma.[30,130,143] Penetrating trauma has the potential for significant bacterial contamination secondary to holes in the intestinal tract and simultaneous low-flow or shock states that interfere with delivery of host defenses or antibiotics to the intestinal cavity.[144] With penetrating abdominal trauma, broad-spectrum antibiotics, directed at aerobic and anaerobic gram-negative bacteria, should be administered as presumptive treatment.[50,51] Most experienced clinicians adopt an approach of assuming that there is a hole in the intestine and beginning empiric treatment to address the "worst-case scenario" of massive contamination and peritonitis. Antibiotics are initiated in the trauma resuscitation area as soon as penetrating abdominal injuries are identified, recognizing that it may be some time before source control can be accomplished because of other diagnostic or treatment priorities in the injured patient. Surgical exploration and source control are performed as soon as possible. At the time of abdominal exploration, the first priority in the trauma patient is control of bleeding, even in the face of massive fecal or enteric contamination. Once hemorrhage control is achieved, the GI tract injuries must be addressed.

Damage control laparotomy has assumed an increasingly important role in the armamentarium of general/trauma surgeons.[132,145] In this approach, the immediately life-threatening injuries are identified and controlled. With respect to injuries to the GI tract, immediate control may simply involve tying off or resecting a segment for temporary closure of GI perforations, thereby minimize ongoing contamination. Not infrequently, packing materials are utilized for hemorrhage control (the primary goal), but as foreign bodies these have a propensity to increase the likelihood of late infection.[30,146]

Overall, there is abundant evidence that survival is improved and long-term outcome is not impaired with the damage control approach.[145] A mainstay of this approach is avoidance of primary anastomoses or stoma construction at the time of the initial operation along with temporary abdominal closure. Gross enteric/fecal contamination should be removed using crystalloid lavage of the peritoneal cavity. There is no compelling evidence to suggest that massive peritoneal lavage decreases the likelihood of late infectious complications.[147–150] Theoretically, massive lavage has the potential to remove more of the host defense cells while at the same time having a minimal impact on the number of bacteria that may be left behind.[151]

The duration of antibiotic administration after traumatic injuries has been subjected to several well-controlled, prospective, randomized, multicenter trials[152–154] (Table 13.7). These data show that in the absence of established infection (recognized clinically by the presence of massive bowel wall edema, erythema, and fibrinopurulent exudates) removal of gross contamination, 24h of broad spectrum antibiotic coverage is sufficient. There is *no* benefit to continuing antibiotics beyond 24h if primary source control is achieved.[152,154] Recent experiences call into question the traditional 12-h time frame for acute source control of colonic injuries.[155] Posttraumatic intraabdominal infectious complications (abscess, anastomotic leak, infected fluid collections) are still encountered, even if antibiotics are administered for a prolonged interval.[152,154] The reasons that prolonged antibiotics do not decrease late infections relate more to the severity of initial injury, residual necrotic debris, or posttraumatic immunosuppression.[50,152,156] Prolonged administration of antibiotics will not eliminate these late complications but has been shown to increase the likelihood that late infections have decreased antimicrobial sensitivity.[24,157]

Conclusion

With each new technological advance, surgeons identify new challenges and new opportunities for improved care and results. Bacterial infection remains a factor that must be prevented or controlled for optimal patient care. Remaining controversial issues include the scope of empiric antibiotic regimens in high-risk patients, the appropriate duration of antibiotic therapy, and minimizing the emergence of microbial resistance. Immunomodulatory strategies currently continue as largely experimental.

References

1. Cheadle WG, Spain DA. The continuing challenge of intra-abdominal infection. Am J Surg 2003;186(5A):15S–22S; discussion 31S–34S.
2. Raymond DP, Pelletier SJ, Crabtree TD, et al. Surgical infection and the aging population. Am Surg 2001;67:827–832; discussion 832–833.
3. Barie PS. Serious intra-abdominal infections. Curr Opin Crit Care 2001;7:263–267.
4. Uggeri FR, Perego E, Franciosi C, Uggeri FA. Surgical approach to the intraabdominal infections. Minerva Anestesiol 2004;70:175–179.
5. Marshall JC, Innes M. Intensive care unit management of intra-abdominal infection. Crit Care Med 2003;31:2228–2237.
6. Brook I. Microbiology and management of intra-abdominal infections in children. Pediatr Int 2003;45:123–129.
7. van Goor H. Surgical treatment of severe intra-abdominal infection. Hepatogastroenterology 1997;44:975–981.
8. Barie PS. Management of complicated intra-abdominal infections. J Chemother 1999;11:464–477.
9. Hau T. Management of peritonitis. Curr Surg 1984;41:165–167.
10. Solomkin JS, Wittman DW, West MA, Barie PS. Intraabdominal Infections. In: Schwartz SI, Shires GT, Spencer FC, et al., eds. Principles of Surgery, 7th ed. New York: McGraw-Hill, 1999:1515–1550.
11. Solomkin JS, Dellinger EP, Christou NV, Busuttil RW. Results of a multicenter trial comparing imipenem/cilastatin to tobramycin/clindamycin for intra-abdominal infections. Ann Surg 1990;212:581–591.
12. Mosdell DM, Morris DM, Voltura A, et al. Antibiotic treatment for surgical peritonitis. Ann Surg 1991;214:543–549.
13. Onderdonk AB, Weinstein WM, Sullivan NM, et al. Experimental intra-abdominal abscesses in rats: quantitative bacteriology of infected animals. Infect Immun 1974;10:1256–1259.
14. Onderdonk AB, Kasper DL, Mansheim BJ, Louie TG, Gorbach SL, Bartlett JG. Experimental animal models for anaerobic infections. Rev Infect Dis 1979;1:291–301.
15. Polk BF, Kasper DL. Bacteroides fragilis subspecies in clinical isolates. Ann Intern Med 1977;86:569–571.
16. Zaleznik DF, Kasper DL. The role of anaerobic bacteria in abscess formation. Annu Rev Med 1982;33:217–229.
17. Onderdonk AB, Kasper DL, Cisneros RL, Bartlett JG. The capsular polysaccharide of *Bacteroides fragilis* as a virulence factor: comparison of the pathogenic potential of encapsulated and unencapsulated strains. J Infect Dis 1977;136:82–89.
18. Bartlett JG, Onderdonk AB, Louie T, et al. A review. Lessons from an animal model of intra-abdominal sepsis. Arch Surg 1978;113:853–857.
19. Rotstein OD, Kao J. The spectrum of *Escherichia coli–Bacteroides fragilis* pathogenic synergy in an intraabdominal infection model. Can J Microbiol 1988;34:352–357.
20. Dunn DL, Rotstein OD, Simmons RL. Fibrin in peritonitis. IV. Synergistic intraperitoneal infection caused by *Escherichia coli* and *Bacteroides fragilis* within fibrin clots. Arch Surg 1984;119:139–144.
21. Evans HL, Sawyer RG. Cycling chemotherapy: a promising approach to reducing the morbidity and mortality of nosocomial infections. Drugs Today (Barc) 2003;39:733–738.
22. Noskin GA. Vancomycin-resistant enterococci: clinical, microbiologic, and epidemiologic features. J Lab Clin Med 1997;130:14–20.
23. Mylotte JM, Goodnough S, Tayara A. Antibiotic-resistant organisms among long-term care facility residents on admission to an inpatient geriatrics unit: retrospective and prospective surveillance. Am J Infect Control 2001;29:139–144.
24. Raymond DP, Kuehnert MJ, Sawyer RG. Preventing antimicrobial-resistant bacterial infections in surgical patients. Surg Infect (Larchmt) 2002;3:375–385.
25. Heemken R, Gandawidjaja L, Hau T. Peritonitis: pathophysiology and local defense mechanisms. Hepatogastroenterology 1997;44:927–936.
26. Hau T, Ahrenholz DH, Simmons RL. Secondary bacterial peritonitis: the biologic basis of treatment. Curr Probl Surg 1979;16:1–65.
27. Dallegri F, Ottonello L. Tissue injury in neutrophilic inflammation. Inflamm Res 1997;46:382–391.
28. Suntres ZE, Omri A, Shek PN. *Pseudomonas aeruginosa*-induced lung injury: role of oxidative stress. Microb Pathog 2002;32:27–34.
29. Hesse DG, Tracey KJ, Fong Y, et al. Cytokine appearance in human endotoxemia and primate bacteremia. Surg Gynecol Obstet 1988;166:147–153.
30. Malangoni MA. Pathogenesis and treatment of intra-abdominal infection. Surg Gynecol Obstet 1990;171(suppl):31–34.
31. Wittmann DH, Schein M, Condon RE. Management of secondary peritonitis. Ann Surg 1996;224:10–18.
32. Schwan A, Ryden AC, Laurell G. Fecal bacterial flora of four nordic population groups with diverse incidence of large bowel cancer. Nutr Cancer 1982;4:74–79.
33. Mai V, Morris JG Jr. Colonic bacterial flora: changing understandings in the molecular age. J Nutr 2004;134:459–464.
34. Farthmann EH, Schoffel U. Epidemiology and pathophysiology of intraabdominal infections (IAI). Infection 1998;26:329–334.
35. Dellinger EP, Wertz MJ, Meakins JL, et al. Surgical infection stratification system for intra-abdominal infection. Multicenter trial. Arch Surg 1985;120:21–29.
36. Davis JL. Treatment of peritonitis. Vet Clin North Am Equine Pract 2003;19:765–778.
37. Kirkpatrick AW, Baxter KA, Simons RK, et al. Intra-abdominal complications after surgical repair of small bowel injuries: an international review. J Trauma 2003;55:399–406.
38. Dobremez E, Lavrand F, Lefevre Y, et al. Treatment of post-appendectomy intra-abdominal deep abscesses. Eur J Pediatr Surg 2003;13:393–397.
39. Schein M. Surgical management of intra-abdominal infection: is there any evidence? Langenbecks Arch Surg 2002;387:1–7.
40. Evans HL, Raymond DP, Pelletier SJ, et al. Diagnosis of intra-abdominal infection in the critically ill patient. Curr Opin Crit Care 2001;7:117–121.
41. Jimenez MF, Marshall JC. Source control in the management of sepsis. Intensive Care Med 2001;27(suppl 1):S49–S62.
42. Marshall JC, Maier RV, Jimenez M, Dellinger EP. Source control in the management of severe sepsis and septic shock: an evidence-based review. Crit Care Med 2004;32(11 suppl):S513–S526.
43. Berger D, Buttenschoen K. Management of abdominal sepsis. Langenbecks Arch Surg 1998;383:35–43.
44. Dunn DL, Barke RA, Knight NB, et al. Role of resident macrophages, peripheral neutrophils, and translymphatic absorption in bacterial clearance from the peritoneal cavity. Infect Immun 1985;49:257–264.
45. Burke JF, Miles AA. The sequence of vascular events in early infective inflammation. J Pathol Bacteriol 1958;76:1–19.
46. Pruett TL, Rotstein OD, Wells CL, et al. Mechanism of the adjuvant effect of hemoglobin in experimental peritonitis. IX:

The infection-potentiating effect of hemoglobin in *Escherichia coli* peritonitis is strain specific. Surgery 1985;98:371–377.
47. Hau T, Lee JT Jr, Simmons RL. Mechanisms of the adjuvant effect of hemoglobin in experimental peritonitis. IV. The adjuvant effect of hemoglobin in granulocytopenic rats. Surgery 1981;89:187–191.
48. Rotstein OD. Role of fibrin deposition in the pathogenesis of intraabdominal infection. Eur J Clin Microbiol Infect Dis 1992;11:1064–1068.
49. Sganga G. New perspectives in antibiotic prophylaxis for intra-abdominal surgery. J Hosp Infect 2002;50(suppl A):S17–S21.
50. Fabian TC. Infection in penetrating abdominal trauma: risk factors and preventive antibiotics. Am Surg 2002;68:29–35.
51. Mazuski JE, Sawyer RG, Nathens AB, et al. The Surgical Infection Society Guidelines on antimicrobial therapy for intra-abdominal infections: an executive summary. Surg Infect (Larchmt) 2002;3:161–173.
52. Mangram AJ. A brief overview of the 1999 CDC Guideline for the Prevention of Surgical Site Infection. Centers for Disease Control and Prevention. J Chemother 2001;13(spec no 1):35–39.
53. Guenaga KF, Matos D, Castro AA, et al. Mechanical bowel preparation for elective colorectal surgery. Cochrane Database Syst Rev 2003:CD001544.
54. Solomkin JS, Mazuski JE, Baron EJ, et al. Guidelines for the selection of anti-infective agents for complicated intra-abdominal infections. Clin Infect Dis 2003;37:997–1005.
55. Arkilic CF, Taguchi A, Sharma N, et al. Supplemental perioperative fluid administration increases tissue oxygen pressure. Surgery 2003;133:49–55.
56. Mathieson A. Pre-op warming reduces infections. Br J Perioper Nurs 2000;10:541.
57. Saadat D, Lowenfels AB. Effect of preoperative warming on wound infection. Lancet 2002;359:445–446.
58. Greif R, Sessler DI. Supplemental oxygen and risk of surgical site infection. JAMA 2004;291:1957; author reply 1958–1959.
59. Akca O, Sessler DI. Supplemental oxygen and risk of surgical site infection. JAMA 2004;291:1956–1957; author reply 1958–1959.
60. Guvener M, Pasaoglu I, Demircin M, Oc M. Perioperative hyperglycemia is a strong correlate of postoperative infection in type II diabetic patients after coronary artery bypass grafting. Endocr J 2002;49:531–537.
61. Furnary AP, Wu Y, Bookin SO. Effect of hyperglycemia and continuous intravenous insulin infusions on outcomes of cardiac surgical procedures: the Portland Diabetic Project. Endocr Pract 2004;10(suppl 2):21–33.
62. Balague Ponz C, Trias M. Laparoscopic surgery and surgical infection. J Chemother 2001;13(spec no 1):17–22.
63. Mowat C, Stanley AJ. Review article: spontaneous bacterial peritonitis—diagnosis, treatment and prevention. Aliment Pharmacol Ther 2001;15:1851–1859.
64. Malangoni MA. Evaluation and management of tertiary peritonitis. Am Surg 2000;66:157–161.
65. Nathens AB, Rotstein OD, Marshall JC. Tertiary peritonitis: clinical features of a complex nosocomial infection. World J Surg 1998;22:158–163.
66. Evans HL, Raymond DP, Pelletier SJ, et al. Tertiary peritonitis (recurrent diffuse or localized disease) is not an independent predictor of mortality in surgical patients with intraabdominal infection. Surg Infect (Larchmt) 2001;2:255–263; discussion 264–265.
67. Bosscha K, van Vroonhoven TJ, van der Werken C. Surgical management of severe secondary peritonitis. Br J Surg 1999;86:1371–1377.
68. Holzheimer RG, Dralle H. Antibiotic therapy in intra-abdominal infections—a review on randomised clinical trials. Eur J Med Res 2001;6:277–291.
69. Fabian TC, Croce MA, Payne LW, et al. Duration of antibiotic therapy for penetrating abdominal trauma: a prospective trial. Surgery 1992;112:788–794; discussion 794–795.
70. Marshall JC, Cook DJ, Christou NV, et al. Multiple organ dysfunction score: a reliable descriptor of a complex clinical outcome. Crit Care Med 1995;23:1638–1652.
71. Livingston DH, Mosenthal AC, Deitch EA. Sepsis and multiple organ dysfunction syndrome: a clinical-mechanistic overview. New Horiz 1995;3:257–266.
72. Rotstein OD. Pathogenesis of multiple organ dysfunction syndrome: gut origin, protection, and decontamination. Surg Infect (Larchmt) 2000;1:217–223; discussion 223–225.
73. Bohnen JM, Marshall JC, Fry DE, et al. Clinical and scientific importance of source control in abdominal infections: summary of a symposium. Can J Surg 1999;42:122–126.
74. Jaffe TA, Nelson RC, Delong DM, Paulson EK. Practice patterns in percutaneous image-guided intraabdominal abscess drainage: survey of academic and private practice centers. Radiology 2004;233:750–756.
75. Sirinek KR. Diagnosis and treatment of intra-abdominal abscesses. Surg Infect (Larchmt) 2000;1:31–38.
76. Dougherty SH, Simmons RL. The biology and practice of surgical drains. Part 1. Curr Probl Surg 1992;29:559–623.
77. Nathens AB, Rotstein OD. Antimicrobial therapy for intra-abdominal infection. Am J Surg 1996;172(6A):1S–6S.
78. Farber MS, Abrams JH. Antibiotics for the acute abdomen. Surg Clin North Am 1997;77:1395–1417.
79. Solomkin JS, Umanskiy K. Intraabdominal sepsis: newer interventional and antimicrobial therapies for infected necrotizing pancreatitis. Curr Opin Crit Care 2003;9:424–427.
80. Burnett RJ, Haverstock DC, Dellinger EP, et al. Definition of the role of enterococcus in intraabdominal infection: analysis of a prospective randomized trial. Surgery 1995;118:716–271; discussion 721–723.
81. Wacha H, Hau T, Dittmer R, Ohmann C. Risk factors associated with intraabdominal infections: a prospective multicenter study. Peritonitis Study Group. Langenbecks Arch Surg 1999;384:24–32.
82. Smith RL 2nd, Sawyer RG, Pruett TL. Hospital-acquired infections in the surgical intensive care: epidemiology and prevention. Zentralbl Chir 2003;128:1047–1061.
83. Rosengren D, Brown AF, Chu K. Radiological imaging to improve the emergency department diagnosis of acute appendicitis. Emerg Med Australas 2004;16:410–416.
84. Katkhouda N, Mason RJ, Towfigh S, et al. Laparoscopic versus open appendectomy: a prospective randomized double-blind study. Ann Surg 2005;242:439–448; discussion 448–450.
85. Guller U, Hervey S, Purves H, et al. Laparoscopic versus open appendectomy: outcomes comparison based on a large administrative database. Ann Surg 2004;239:43–52.
86. Eypasch E, Sauerland S, Lefering R, Neugebauer EA. Laparoscopic versus open appendectomy: between evidence and common sense. Dig Surg 2002;19:518–522.
87. Ignacio RC, Burke R, Spencer D, et al. Laparoscopic versus open appendectomy: what is the real difference? Results of a prospective randomized double-blinded trial. Surg Endosc 2004;18:334–337.
88. Carbonell AM, Burns JM, Lincourt AE, Harold KL. Outcomes of laparoscopic versus open appendectomy. Am Surg 2004;70:759–765; discussion 765–766.
89. Mancini GJ, Mancini ML, Nelson HS Jr. Efficacy of laparoscopic appendectomy in appendicitis with peritonitis. Am Surg 2005;71:1–4; discussion 4–5.
90. Ball CG, Kortbeek JB, Kirkpatrick AW, Mitchell P. Laparoscopic appendectomy for complicated appendicitis: an evaluation of postoperative factors. Surg Endosc 2004;18:969–973.

91. Sauerland S, Lefering R, Neugebauer EA. Laparoscopic versus open surgery for suspected appendicitis. Cochrane Database Syst Rev 2002:CD001546.
92. Andersen BR, Kallehave FL, Andersen HK. Antibiotics versus placebo for prevention of postoperative infection after appendicectomy. Cochrane Database Syst Rev 2003:CD001439.
93. Wittmann DH, Schein M. Let us shorten antibiotic prophylaxis and therapy in surgery. Am J Surg 1996;172(6A):26S–32S.
94. Mui LM, Ng CS, Wong SK, et al. Optimum duration of prophylactic antibiotics in acute non-perforated appendicitis. ANZ J Surg 2005;75:425–428.
95. Gorecki P, Schein M, Rucinski JC, Wise L. Antibiotic administration in patients undergoing common surgical procedures in a community teaching hospital: the chaos continues. World J Surg 1999;23:429–432; discussion 433.
96. Brown CV, Abrishami M, Muller M, Velmahos GC. Appendiceal abscess: immediate operation or percutaneous drainage? Am Surg 2003;69:829–832.
97. Yamini D, Vargas H, Bongard F, et al. Perforated appendicitis: is it truly a surgical urgency? Am Surg 1998;64:970–975.
98. Barie PS, Eachempati SR. Acute acalculous cholecystitis. Curr Gastroenterol Rep 2003;5:302–309.
99. Trowbridge RL, Rutkowski NK, Shojania KG. Does this patient have acute cholecystitis? JAMA 2003;289:80–86.
100. Kanafani ZA, Khalife N, Kanj SS, et al. Antibiotic use in acute cholecystitis: practice patterns in the absence of evidence-based guidelines. J Infect 2005;51:128–134.
101. Ito K, Fujita N, Noda Y, et al. Percutaneous cholecystostomy versus gallbladder aspiration for acute cholecystitis: a prospective randomized controlled trial. AJR Am J Roentgenol 2004;183:193–196.
102. Glavic Z, Begic L, Simlesa D, Rukavina A. Treatment of acute cholecystitis. A comparison of open versus laparoscopic cholecystectomy. Surg Endosc 2001;15:398–401.
103. Koperna T, Kisser M, Schulz F. Laparoscopic versus open treatment of patients with acute cholecystitis. Hepatogastroenterology 1999;46:753–757.
104. Chandler CF, Lane JS, Ferguson P, et al. Prospective evaluation of early versus delayed laparoscopic cholecystectomy for treatment of acute cholecystitis. Am Surg 2000;66:896–900.
105. Kanaan SA, Murayama KM, Merriam LT, et al. Risk factors for conversion of laparoscopic to open cholecystectomy. J Surg Res 2002;106:20–24.
106. Lee WJ, Chang KJ, Lee CS, Chen KM. Surgery in cholangitis: bacteriology and choice of antibiotic. Hepatogastroenterology 1992;39:347–349.
107. Teppler H, McCarroll K, Gesser RM, Woods GL. Surgical infections with enterococcus: outcome in patients treated with ertapenem versus piperacillin-tazobactam. Surg Infect (Larchmt) 2002;3:337–349.
108. Petrowsky H, Demartines N, Rousson V, Clavien PA. Evidence-based value of prophylactic drainage in gastrointestinal surgery: a systematic review and meta-analyses. Ann Surg 2004;240:1074–1084; discussion 1084–1085.
109. Floch MH, Bina I. The natural history of diverticulitis: fact and theory. J Clin Gastroenterol 2004;38(5 suppl):S2–S7.
110. Acosta JA, Grebenc ML, Doberneck RC, et al. Colonic diverticular disease in patients 40 years old or younger. Am Surg 1992;58:605–607.
111. Buchanan GN, Kenefick NJ, Cohen CR. Diverticulitis. Best Pract Res Clin Gastroenterol 2002;16:635–647.
112. Gooszen AW, Gooszen HG, Veerman W, et al. Operative treatment of acute complications of diverticular disease: primary or secondary anastomosis after sigmoid resection. Eur J Surg 2001;167:35–39.
113. Salem L, Flum DR. Primary anastomosis or Hartman's procedure for patients with diverticular peritonitis? A systematic review. Dis Colon Rectum 2004;47:1953–1964.
114. Pessaux P, Muscari F, Ouellet JF, et al. Risk factors for mortality and morbidity after elective sigmoid resection for diverticulitis: prospective multicenter multivariate analysis of 582 patients. World J Surg 2004;28:92–96.
115. Tursi A. Acute diverticulitis of the colon—current medical therapeutic management. Expert Opin Pharmacother 2004;5:55–59.
116. Schilling MK, Maurer CA, Kollmar O, Buchler MW. Primary versus secondary anastomosis after sigmoid colon resection for perforated diverticulitis (Hinchey stage III and IV): a prospective outcome and cost analysis. Dis Colon Rectum 2001;44:699–703; discussion 703–705.
117. Yasuhara H. Acute mesenteric ischemia: the challenge of gastroenterology. Surg Today 2005;35:185–195.
118. Revelly JP, Ayuse T, Brienza N, et al. Endotoxic shock alters distribution of blood flow within the intestinal wall. Crit Care Med 1996;24:1345–1351.
119. Hiltebrand LB, Krejci V, Banic A, et al. Dynamic study of the distribution of microcirculatory blood flow in multiple splanchnic organs in septic shock. Crit Care Med 2000;28:3233–3241.
120. Hiltebrand LB, Krejci V, tenHoevel ME, et al. Redistribution of microcirculatory blood flow within the intestinal wall during sepsis and general anesthesia. Anesthesiology 2003;98:658–669.
121. Tsunooka N, Hamada Y, Imagawa H, et al. Ischemia of the intestinal mucosa during cardiopulmonary bypass. J Artif Organs 2003;6:149–151.
122. Tsunooka N, Maeyama K, Hamada Y, et al. Bacterial translocation secondary to small intestinal mucosal ischemia during cardiopulmonary bypass. Measurement by diamine oxidase and peptidoglycan. Eur J Cardiothorac Surg 2004;25:275–280.
123. Meddah AT, Leke L, Romond MB, et al. The effects of mesenteric ischemia on ileal colonization, intestinal integrity, and bacterial translocation in newborn piglets. Pediatr Surg Int 2001;17:515–520.
124. Wiesner W, Khurana B, Ji H, Ros PR. CT of acute bowel ischemia. Radiology 2003;226:635–650.
125. Park WM, Gloviczki P, Cherry KJ Jr, et al. Contemporary management of acute mesenteric ischemia: factors associated with survival. J Vasc Surg 2002;35:445–452.
126. Bulkley GB, Zuidema GD, Hamilton SR, et al. Intraoperative determination of small intestinal viability following ischemic injury: a prospective, controlled trial of two adjuvant methods (Doppler and fluorescein) compared with standard clinical judgment. Ann Surg 1981;193:628–637.
127. Johansson K, Ahn H, Lindhagen J. Intraoperative assessment of blood flow and tissue viability in small-bowel ischemia by laser Doppler flowmetry. Acta Chir Scand 1989;155:341–346.
128. Anadol AZ, Ersoy E, Taneri F, Tekin EH. Laparoscopic "second-look" in the management of mesenteric ischemia. Surg Laparosc Endosc Percutan Tech 2004;14:191–193.
129. Moore EE, Burch JM, Franciose RJ, et al. Staged physiologic restoration and damage control surgery. World J Surg 1998;22:1184–1190; discussion 1190–1191.
130. Nicholas JM, Rix EP, Easley KA, et al. Changing patterns in the management of penetrating abdominal trauma: the more things change, the more they stay the same. J Trauma 2003;55:1095–1108; discussion 1108–1110.
131. Johnson JW, Gracias VH, Schwab CW, et al. Evolution in damage control for exsanguinating penetrating abdominal injury. J Trauma 2001;51:261–269; discussion 269–271.
132. Finlay IG, Edwards TJ, Lambert AW. Damage control laparotomy. Br J Surg 2004;91:83–85.
133. Sharp KW, Locicero RJ. Abdominal packing for surgically uncontrollable hemorrhage. Ann Surg 1992;215:467–474; discussion 474–475.
134. Hau T, Ohmann C, Wolmershauser A, et al. Planned relaparotomy versus relaparotomy on demand in the treatment of

intra-abdominal infections. The Peritonitis Study Group of the Surgical Infection Society-Europe. Arch Surg 1995;130:1193–1196; discussion 1196–1197.
135. Sherck J, Seiver A, Shatney C, et al. Covering the "open abdomen": a better technique. Am Surg 1998;64:854–857.
136. Wittmann DH. Operative and nonoperative therapy of intraabdominal infections. Infection 1998;26:335–341.
137. McGilvray ID, Rotstein OD. Management of infection in the surgical patient: an update. Surg Technol Int 2003;11:39–43.
138. Chambers WM, Mortensen NJ. Postoperative leakage and abscess formation after colorectal surgery. Best Pract Res Clin Gastroenterol 2004;18:865–880.
139. Fry DE. Noninvasive imaging tests in the diagnosis and treatment of intra-abdominal abscesses in the postoperative patient. Surg Clin North Am 1994;74:693–709.
140. Danielson D, West MA. Recent developments in clinical management of surgical sepsis. Curr Opin Crit Care 2001;7:367–370.
141. Falconi M, Pederzoli P. The relevance of gastrointestinal fistulae in clinical practice: a review. Gut 2001;49(suppl 4):iv2–iv10.
142. Curtin JP, Burt LL. Successful treatment of small intestine fistula with somatostatin analog. Gynecol Oncol 1990;39:225–227.
143. Freeark RJ. Penetrating wounds of the abdomen. N Engl J Med 1974;291:185–188.
144. Morales CH, Villegas MI, Villavicencio R, et al. Intra-abdominal infection in patients with abdominal trauma. Arch Surg 2004;139:1278–1285; discussion 1285.
145. Shapiro MB, Jenkins DH, Schwab CW, Rotondo MF. Damage control: collective review. J Trauma 2000;49:969–978.
146. Granchi TS, Abikhaled JA, Hirshberg A, et al. Patterns of microbiology in intra-abdominal packing for trauma. J Trauma 2004;56:45–51.
147. Schein M, Saadia R. To wash or not to wash? Intra-operative peritoneal lavage in the contaminated peritoneal cavity. S Afr J Surg 1989;27:22–23.
148. Kimmelstiel F, Anaise D, Waltzer WC, Rapaport FT. Continuous postoperative peritoneal lavage for the management of intra-abdominal sepsis in renal allograft recipients. Transplant Proc 1988;20:101–104.
149. Schein M, Gecelter G, Freinkel W, et al. Peritoneal lavage in abdominal sepsis. A controlled clinical study. Arch Surg 1990;125:1132–1135.
150. Whiteside OJ, Tytherleigh MG, Thrush S, et al. Intra-operative peritoneal lavage—who does it and why? Ann R Coll Surg Engl 2005;87:255–258.
151. Dunn DL, Barke RA, Ahrenholz DH, et al. The adjuvant effect of peritoneal fluid in experimental peritonitis. Mechanism and clinical implications. Ann Surg 1984;199:37–43.
152. Kirton OC, O'Neill PA, Kestner M, Tortella BJ. Perioperative antibiotic use in high-risk penetrating hollow viscus injury: a prospective randomized, double-blind, placebo-control trial of 24h versus 5 days. J Trauma 2000;49:822–832.
153. Cornwell EE 3rd, Dougherty WR, Berne TV, et al. Duration of antibiotic prophylaxis in high-risk patients with penetrating abdominal trauma: a prospective randomized trial. J Gastrointest Surg 1999;3:648–653.
154. Bozorgzadeh A, Pizzi WF, Barie PS, et al. The duration of antibiotic administration in penetrating abdominal trauma. Am J Surg 1999;177:125–131.
155. Kamwendo NY, Modiba MC, Matlala NS, Becker PJ. Randomized clinical trial to determine if delay from time of penetrating colonic injury precludes primary repair. Br J Surg 2002;89:993–998.
156. Griswold JA, Muakkassa FF, Betcher E, Poole GV. Injury severity dictates individualized antibiotic therapy in penetrating abdominal trauma. Am Surg 1993;59:34–39.
157. Solomkin JS. Antibiotic resistance in postoperative infections. Crit Care Med 2001;29(4 suppl):N97–N99.
158. Greif R, Akça O, Horn EP, Kurz A, Sessler DI. Supplemental perioperative oxygen to reduce the incidence of surgical-wound infection. Outcomes Research Group. N Engl J Med 2000;342:161–167.
159. Pryor KO, Fahey TJ 3rd, Lien CA, Goldstein PA. Surgical site infection and the routine use of perioperative hyperoxia in a general surgical population: a randomized controlled trial. Jama 2004;291:79–87.
160. Wille-Jorgensen P, Guenaga KF, Castro AA, Matos D. Clinical value of preoperative mechanical bowel cleansing in elective colorectal surgery: a systematic review. Dis Colon Rectum 2003;46:1013–1020.
161. Zmora O, Mahajna A, Bar-Zakai B, et al. Colon and rectal surgery without mechanical bowel preparation: a randomized prospective trial. Ann Surg 2003;237:363–367.
162. Bucher P, Mermillod B, Morel P, Soravia C. Does mechanical bowel preparation have a role in preventing postoperative complications in elective colorectal surgery? Swiss Med Wkly 2004;134:69–74.
163. Nathens AB, Marshall JC. Selective decontamination of the digestive tract in surgical patients: a systematic review of the evidence. Arch Surg 1999;134:170–176.
164. Jesus EC, Karliczek A, Matos D, et al. Prophylactic anastomotic drainage for colorectal surgery. Cochrane Database Syst Rev 2004:CD002100.
165. Cohn SM, Giannotti G, Ong AW, et al. Prospective randomized trial of two wound management strategies for dirty abdominal wounds. Ann Surg 2001;233:409–413.
166. Wong PF, Gilliam AD, Kumar S, et al. Antibiotic regimens for secondary peritonitis of gastrointestinal origin in adults. Cochrane Database Syst Rev 2005:CD004539.
167. Sims EH, Thadepalli H, Ganesan K, Mandal AK. How many antibiotics are necessary to treat abdominal trauma victims? Am Surg 1997;63:525–535.
168. Bratzler DW, Houck PM, Richards C, et al. Use of antimicrobial prophylaxis for major surgery: baseline results from the National Surgical Infection Prevention Project. Arch Surg 2005;140:174–182.
169. Sauerland S, Lefering R, Neugebauer EA. Laparoscopic versus open surgery for suspected appendicitis. Cochrane Database Syst Rev 2004:CD001546.
170. Zeitoun G, Laurent A, Rouffet F, et al. Multicentre, randomized clinical trial of primary versus secondary sigmoid resection in generalized peritonitis complicating sigmoid diverticulitis. Br J Surg 2000;87:1366–1374.
171. Velmahos GC, Toutouzas KG, Sarkisyan G, et al. Severe trauma is not an excuse for prolonged antibiotic prophylaxis. Arch Surg 2002;137:537–541; discussion 541–542.
172. Weinstein WM, Onderdonk AB, Bartlett JG, Gorbach SL. Experimental intra-abdominal abscesses in rats: development of an experimental model. Infect Immun 1974;10:1250–1265.
173. Howard R, Simmons R. Surgical Infectious Diseases, 3rd ed. Norwalk, CT: Appleton and Lange, 1995.

14

Nosocomial Infections

Pamela A. Lipsett

A *nosocomial infection* (NI) is defined as an infection that is not present or incubating when the patient is admitted to a hospital or other health care facility.[1] Generally, an infection that is discovered 48–72 h after admission is indicative of nosocomial, rather than community-acquired, infection. Although usually associated with hospital admission (hence the term hospital-acquired infection), NIs can arise after admission to any health care facility, and the term *health care-associated infection* is now preferred. Nosocomial infections are increasingly considered as a measure of quality of care and are the focus of safety and quality improvements efforts in many hospitals today.[2–8] To date, the extent these NIs are avoidable under real-life hospital conditions and what represents the irreducible minimum remain unclear.[9–11] A number of observational studies implementing multimodality strategies and standardized policies and practices have demonstrated a 10% to 70% reduction in infection rates depending on the setting, study design, type of infection, and baseline infection rates.[9–15]

Among hospitalized patients, NIs are a leading cause of morbidity and mortality.[16–18] Infections acquired in the hospital occur in 5%–15% of patients and can lead to complications in 25%–50% of those admitted to intensive care units (ICUs).[7,8,16] Although fewer patients were admitted to U.S. hospitals in 1995 compared with 1975 (36 million vs. 38 million) and the average duration of stay decreased (7.9 to 5.3 days), the national NI rate has risen. In 1975, there were 7.2 NIs per 1000 patient-days compared with 9.8 per 1000 in 1995, an increase of 36%.[19] In addition, it has been estimated that there are approximately 90,000 deaths attributed to NIs annually, ranking it as the fifth leading cause of death in acute care hospitals.[20,21] However, the total cost of NIs to society is not clear. Among the directives of *Healthy People 2010* is the reduction of NIs in ICUs by 10% (objectives 14–20).[19] To meet this goal, it is essential that the effectiveness and efficiency of prevention and control strategies be carefully evaluated so that interventions with demonstrated value can be implemented.[21] Interventions that are the best candidates for widespread implementation not[3] only must work (i.e., be associated with reduced infections) but also must be feasible.

Globally, urinary tract and surgical site infections are the most frequent infections, followed by respiratory and bloodstream infections.[7] However, in ICUs, respiratory tract infections are the most frequent infections, followed by central-line infections, urinary tract infections (UTIs), and surgical site infections (Table 14.1).[3,16] In addition to their association with increased morbidity and mortality, NIs are frequently associated with drug-resistant microorganisms, including methicillin-resistant *Staphylococcus aureus* (MRSA), resistant gram negatives such as *Acinetobacter* and *Candida* species.[16,22] In this chapter, I briefly describe (1) the pathophysiology and epidemiology of NI in general; (2) specific NIs (nosocomial pneumonia, bacteremia, UTIs, miscellaneous infections); (3) strategies for diagnosis and treatment of these specific infections; and (4) the evidence of effective preventive therapies.

Pathophysiology

The two key features contributing to the development of NI are a reduction in the patient's normal immune or defense systems and colonization by pathogenic or potentially pathogenic pathogens.[3] While these factors may develop independently, for infection to occur both must be present to some extent. The postoperative state, especially when associated with critical illness, is characterized by alterations in the immune response, in T cells and B-cell activation, and in cytokine production. Antiinflammatory mediators such as interleukin-10, interleukin-1 receptor antagonist, and tumor necrosis factor receptors create an immunosuppressed postoperative state that some refer to as *immunoparalysis*.[23–26] Normal bodily functions impaired in the postoperative state include coughing, sneezing, and mucociliary clearance, to name a few. Each of these functions is an important host defense mechanism in the prevention of respiratory infection. In addition, the use of invasive devices such as endotracheal intubation and central lines can reduce these local defenses,

TABLE 14.1. Incidence of Infections in Surgical Intensive Care Units in the United States.

Infection	*Incidence (pooled mean)*
Ventilator-associated pneumonia	9.3[a]
Catheter-related bloodstream infection	4.6[b]
Urinary tract	4.4[c]

[a]Number of ventilator days/number of patient days.
[b]Number of central line days/number of patient days.
[c]Number of urinary catheter days/number of patient days.
Source: Data modified from NNIS System.[16]

predisposing to respiratory infection and bacteremia, especially in mechanically ventilated patients.[3,27–31]

Invasive devices are also implicated in contributing to colonization by serving as a nidus for bacterial and fungus attachment and biofilm growth. Because these invasive devices cause infection, repeated courses of antibiotics are often administered. Administration of antibiotics can then cause local colonic bacteria to be altered; thus, the defenses provided by the native colon flora are altered.[32]

Microbial Flora

Microbial pathogens can be divided into those endogenous to the host or those exogenously transmitted. Bacteria and fungi are located throughout the body on epithelial and mucosal surfaces. For example, the colon contains as many as 10^{12} bacteria per gram of tissue and more than 100 species.[33] These bacteria are an important source of local host defenses by occupying many of the mucosal attachment sites, thus protecting the patient from invasion of "foreign" pathogens. This defense mechanism is called *colonization resistance* and can be applied to prevention of colonization of exogenously introduced organisms and to prevention of overgrowth by potential pathogens such as *Escherichia coli*.[33]

A variety of factors can affect the overgrowth of intestinal pathogens and subsequent transmission of NI. While much of this work has focused on *Clostridium difficile* and antibiotic-resistant microbes, similar principles apply to antibiotic-sensitive pathogens. Nosocomial pathogens can be present in the indigenous microflora at admission or can originate from an exogenous source. *Clostridium difficile* and vancomycin-resistant enterococcus (VRE) are usually acquired in health care settings, while *Enterobacter* species and *Candida albicans* often emerge from the indigenous microflora.[34,35] The oropharynx, gastrointestinal tract, and urinary tract appear to be the sites of greatest colonization of nosocomial pathogens.

The normal acidic pH of the stomach reduces the number of ingested microorganisms that enter the intestinal tract, with more than 99.9% of ingested coliform bacteria killed within 30min by normal gastric acidity.[32] Medications that inhibit production of stomach acid (e.g., proton pump inhibitors and H_2 blockers) have been associated with several pathogens, including *C. difficile, S. aureus*, VRE, and gram-negative bacilli.[32,36,37]

The ability of microbes to adhere to the host tissue is dependent on microbial adhesion factors that interact with mucosal surfaces to bind bacteria and appear to be pathogen and tissue specific.[38] Either changes in adhesion molecules or complementary attachment to epithelial cells may be seen with resistant organisms.[39] Pathogens may be inhibited by blocking attachment sites of pathogenic bacteria, depletion of nutrients, or production of inhibitory substances (e.g., volatile fatty acids and anaerobic conditions).[32]

Pathogens from an exogenous source can colonize or infect patients via direct contact, droplet, or aerosolized spread. For direct contact, spread occurs principally by contamination from the hands of health care workers and visitors.[34,40] However, the environment and medical devices can also contribute to direct contamination. Some pathogens are typically spread by airborne contamination and include *Mycobacterium tuberculosis* and some viral pathogens, most notably the recent outbreak of severe acute respiratory syndrome (SARS). Environmental surface contamination can occur with pathogens that survive for lengthy periods (VRE) and where spores may not be killed with commonly used cleaning solutions (*C. difficile*).[34]

Hand hygiene, whether by traditional washing with soap and water or with an alcohol-based gel or foam, is one of the single most important and infrequently practiced opportunities for infection control.[41] Numerous studies documented low compliance with hand hygiene, especially in high-risk individuals in the ICU where many interactions with staff occur.[41–46] Multiprofessional, multimodality approaches to improving hand hygiene can effectively reduce infection rates when the interventions are focused on system and behavioral changes.[42,44,46] Since NIs occur at a specific site, each is discussed separately, as well as specific evidenced-based preventive therapy, where available. Since alternative chapters are devoted to soft tissue infections and intraabdominal infections, these specific infections are not discussed here.

Epidemiology

The quoted incidence of NI depends on the type of hospital (size, teaching vs. nonteaching); the specific hospital location (ward, ICU, surgical unit, medical unit); the patient population; and the definitions of infection utilized.[3,22,47] The Centers for Disease Control and Prevention (CDC) established definitions for hospitals participating in the National Nosocomial Infection Surveillance System (NNIS). The NNIS was established in the 1970s when selected hospitals in the United States began presenting aggregated infection surveillance data to a national database. Today, more than 300 U.S. hospitals collect and report data that can be used to benchmark a hospital's or unit's performance regarding specific infections or pathogens.[6,16,48,49]

In a study from France with more than 110,000 patients, among the 1945 patients who died during the study, 26.6% had an NI.[50] The authors stated that NI contributed to the deaths of 284 (14.6%) patients, thereby ranking NI as the fourth most frequent cause of death. Lower respiratory tract, bloodstream, and surgical site infections were responsible for 39%, 20%, and 14%, respectively, of all NIs in these patients. Thus, the focus here is on specific infections. Surgical site infections are covered elsewhere.

Specific Diseases

Nosocomial Pneumonia

Nosocomial pneumonia is the most frequent hospital-acquired infection in the ICU (second overall) and the leading cause of death from hospital-acquired infections, with an associated crude mortality of approximately 30%.[7,51] Although the incubation period varies among specific infections, by definition hospital-acquired pneumonia (HAP) includes any case of pneumonia that has developed in this ≥48- to 72-h time frame after admission.[48,51] Ventilator-associated pneumonia (VAP) occurs in patients intubated and mechanically ventilated for more than 48h. There are approximately 300,000 cases of HAP annually in the United States, representing roughly 5 to 10 cases per 1000 hospital admissions.[52] Based on NNIS data from 14,000 ICU patients, HAP is the second most common NI after UTI, affecting approximately 27% of all critically ill patients.[6]

The two main access routes for bacteria to reach the tracheobronchial tree are aspiration, which is of major clinical relevance, and inhalation.[52] Hematogenous and contiguous dissemination of infection are only occasional mechanisms. The lower respiratory tract is normally sterile, and the presence of bacteria is usually the result of the aspiration of secretions. While the exact contribution of each site is uncertain, the potential sources of contaminating bacteria include the oral cavity, upper airway, nasal sinuses, mechanical circuits, and the stomach.[53–56] Several randomized trials have found a relation between lowering gastric pH with stress ulcer prophylaxis and higher rates of nosocomial pneumonia.[57–60] Nasogastric tubes may also facilitate colonization of the oropharynx by gram-negative pathogens, such as *Pseudomonas aeruginosa*; the ability of these pathogens to adhere to plastic surfaces and form biofilm may contribute to colonization of this site.[61,62] However, using transpyloric feeding tubes to avoid large gastric volumes does not reduce the incidence of nosocomial pneumonia.[54,63,64] More than one-half of healthy adults aspirate oropharyngeal contents during sleep. Therefore, a large inoculum (reported risk ratio of 3.25), virulent bacteria, or a compromised immune status is required to develop aspiration pneumonia. Surgeons should be aware that patients who are critically ill, are intubated, have a head injury, had neurosurgery, or have a need for reintubation all appear to bear significant risk for the development of nosocomial pneumonia.[51,53,56,61–66] Additional risk factors are listed in Table 14.2.

TABLE 14.2. Risk Factors for the Development of Ventilator-Associated Pneumonia.

Risk factor class, type	*OR (95% CI)*
Nonmodifiable risk factors	
Patient-related risk factor	
Chronic obstructive pulmonary disease (COPD)	1.9 (1.4–2.6) 18.3 (3.8–89.8)
Organ System Failure Index > 2	10.2 (4.5–23)
Age > 60 years	5.1 (1.9–14.1)
Coma	40.3 (3.3–423.1)
Acute respiratory distress syndrome (ARDS)	9.7 (1.6–59.2)
Head trauma	5.2 (0.9–30.3)
Male sex	2 (1.5–2.7)
Intervention-related risk factor	
Neurosurgery	10 (1.6–64.9)[a]
Thoracic surgery	2.16
ICP monitor	4.2 (1.7–10.5)
Transportation out of ICU	3.8 (2.8–5.5)
Reintubation	5.94 (1.27–22.71)
Modifiable risk factor	
Intervention-related risk factor	
Use of H_2 antagonist	2.5 (1.2–5)
	2.33
Use of antacids	20
Use of sucralfate	3.44
24-h circuit changes, compared with 48-h circuit changes	2.3 (1.2–5)
Use of antibiotics	3.1 (1.4–6.9)
	2.3
	0.1 (0.01–0.7)
Supine position	2.9 (1.3–6.6)
Receipt of enteral nutrition	31.2 (3.3–294.8)
Failed subglottic aspiration	5.3(1.2–22.6)
Intracuff pressure of <20cm H_2O	4.2 (1.1–15.9)
Tracheostomy	3.1 (2.2–4.5)

Source: Bonten et al.[27]

Pathogens

The microbiology of HAP typically differs from that of community-acquired pneumonia. Gram-negative organisms comprise the majority of infecting pathogens in HAP/VAP; individual pathogens include *P. aeruginosa*, *Enterobacter* species, *Klebsiella pneumonia*, *Acinetobacter* species, and *S. aureus*.[51,67] While anaerobes appear to play a role in aspiration pneumonia in nonintubated patients, they have a limited role in HAP/VAP.[68] While these are the general pathogens involved in VAP, there can be vast differences within and between hospitals and countries. Thus, each unit should be aware of their local microbiology and should appropriately choose antibiotics on this basis.

Diagnostic Strategies

Pneumonia is commonly clinically defined as the presence of a new, persistent pulmonary infiltrate not otherwise explained on chest radiographs in combination with at least two criteria, including (1) temperature of greater than 38.3°C, (2) leukocytosis of greater than 10,000 cells/mm, and (3) purulent respiratory secretions.[69] Numerous studies have evaluated the performance of bronchoscopic techniques and nonbronchoscopic procedures for the diagnosis of VAP.[51,64,67] However, the precise manner of diagnosis of VAP remains highly controversial, and no true diagnostic gold standard is both accepted and utilized today.[69–81] A consensus opinion of international experts was gathered to guide the selection of patients for the study of VAP, and they formed the working definition of VAP from which different diagnostic methods could be compared.[82] In addition, they recommended the injection of at least 140 ml when performing bronchoalveolar lavage (BAL).[83]

Michaud and colleagues reviewed the studies of diagnostic methods for VAP and examined the effect of study design bias on the outcome of the different diagnostic strategies.[70] In particular, the authors wanted to examine how both the study design and previous antibiotic exposure affected the reported accuracy of the protected specimen brush (PSB), BAL, endotracheal aspirates (EAs), and intracellular organism count (IOC) in mechanically ventilated, nonimmunocompromised adults with suspected VAP. After constructing

TABLE 14.3. Analysis of Varied Diagnostic Tests for Ventilator-Associated Pneumonia.

	PSB (10^3 CFU/ml or more)		*BAL (10^4 CFU/ml or more)*		*IOC (5% or more)*		*EA (10^5 CFU/ml or more)*	
	Studies (n)	*P values*	*Studies (n)*	*P values*	*Studies (n)*	*P values*	*Studies (n)*	*P values*
Crude analysis	21	—	17	—	10	—	7	—
Agreement with patient selection consensus criteria								
Yes	13	.005	9	10	6	.11	5	NA
No	8		8		4		2	
Agreement with diagnostic consensus criteria								
Yes	5	.016	5	.19	4	.10	1	NA
No	16	—	12	—	6		6	
BAL volume								
≥140 ml	—	—	6	.023	2	NA	—	—
<140 ml			11		8			
Antibiotic exposure[a]								
No antibiotics	14	—	10	—	6	—	4	—
Former antibiotics	4		3		4		—	
Recent antibiotics	9		9		3		4	

[a]Considered adequate.
Source: From Michaud et al.[70]

receiver operating curves (ROCs) for each study and as a summary value, the authors utilized a Q value to determine the discriminate ability of a test. The Q value is a summary measure of the test's discriminative ability and represents the intersection between the summary ROCs and the line where sensitivity equals specificity. The greater the Q value, the more discriminative the test is; a value of 1 indicates a perfect test, and a value of 0.5 indicates a nondiscriminative test. Table 14.3 indicates the values seen for the various tests.[70] These tests appear to have variable results depending on patient selection criteria, volume infused, and previous antibiotic exposure. Thus, consideration of which diagnostic strategy to use depends on additional factors. A meta-analysis also confirmed that there are few studies that examine the impact of diagnostic strategies on the outcome of suspected VAP. Moreover, these authors found that invasive strategies do not alter mortality but may affect antibiotic use and prescribing.[84]

While many individuals claim superiority of one method over another, in fact none of the strategies has proven benefit over the others.[77] Only six trials have assessed the effect of diagnostic strategy on outcome and antibiotic use (Table 14.4). In comparing strategy 1 versus 2, Singh et al.[85] used the modified Clinical Pulmonary Infections Score (CPIS) by Pugin et al.[78] to guide antibiotic therapy. Based on the earlier work by Pugin suggesting that a score greater than 6 was likely to indicate pulmonary infection, Singh et al. enrolled patients with a CPIS less than or equal to 6 to limited antibiotic therapy of 3 days (ciprofloxacin) in the experimental group, while standard patients continued to have routine antibiotics for 10–21 days. In the group with a CPIS of less than or equal to 6, antibiotics were continued beyond 3 days in 96% of the standard therapy group and in none of the experimental group. Hospital length of stay and mortality did not differ between the groups. Antimicrobial resistance developed in 35% of the standard therapy group and in 15% in the short-therapy group.

In a multicenter prospective cohort study comparing 92 patients managed with bronchoscopic diagnostic testing versus 42 patients managed with clinical evaluation alone, Heyland et al. determined that BAL patients received fewer antibiotics (31 of 92 vs. 9 of 49, $P = .05$), with more frequent discontinuation of antibiotics in the group that had invasive testing.[79] While neither duration of mechanical ventilation nor ICU stay differed between the groups, mortality was lower in the group that underwent bronchoscopy (18.5% vs. 34.7%, $P = .03$).[79] Unfortunately, decisions about discontinuation of antibiotics based on microbiology were not part of the study by Sole-Violan et al., which examined strategy 3 versus 5 or 6.[86]

TABLE 14.4. Clinical Studies and Practices Can Be Placed into One of Six Strategies for Ventilator Pneumonia.

Diagnostic plan (studies of outcome and antibiotics)	*Evaluation*
Strategy 1 (one RCT trial, 1 vs. 2; one cohort, 1 vs. 6)	Clinical evaluation alone; no bacteriologic samples
Strategy 2	Clinical evaluation alone; short-course antibiotic therapy
Strategy 3 (two RCTs, 3 vs. 6)	Clinical evaluation alone; qualitative bacteriologic samples from trachea
Strategy 4 (two RCTs, 4 vs. 6)	Clinical evaluation alone; quantitative bacteriologic samples from trachea
Strategy 5	Clinical or microbiologic techniques associated with nonbronchoscopic techniques for sampling the lower respiratory tract
Strategy 6	Clinical and microbiologic techniques with bronchoscopic techniques of either protected brush specimen (PBS) or bronchoalveolar lavage (BAL) for sampling the lower respiratory tract

RCT, random controlled trial.
Source: From Fagon.[77]

In the largest study to date on this topic, Fagon et al. examined strategy 3 (clinical qualitative cultures) versus strategy 6 in 413 patients suspected as having VAP.[73] Antibiotics were not initiated or discontinued in the invasive diagnostic group (strategy 6) unless there was a positive direct examination of the PSB or BAL samples or positive quantitative cultures (PSB > 10^3 CFU/ml, BAL > 10^4 CFU/ml).[73] Empirical antibiotics were started in 91% of the clinical group (strategy 3) versus 52% in the BAL/PSB group (strategy 6). In addition, the invasive diagnostic group (strategy 6) had less antibiotic use (mean number of antibiotic-free days at day 14, 2 ± 3 vs. 5 ± 5, $P < .001$); lower mortality rate on day 14 (25% vs. 16%, $P = .02$); and lower sepsis-related organ failure assessment scores on days 3 and 7 ($P = .04$).

Thus, based on evidence from limited trials, if and only if physicians are willing to begin or discontinue antibiotics, the invasive strategy may be advantageous.

The invasive strategies (6) have also been compared with quantitative cultures in two studies involving 127 patients,[80,81] with antibiotic management duration determined by either the quantitative tracheal aspirates versus the invasive BAL/PSB. No significant differences were seen between the groups in length of stay, duration of mechanical ventilation, and mortality. However, the studies did not manage empiric antibiotic use or duration.

Therapy

Therapy for HAP is usually started empirically based on clinical and radiological features, previous antibiotic use, day of onset of infection after intubation, specific patient risk factors, and local pathogens. Microbiological direct assessment of respiratory tract secretions (lower) for the presence of intracellular bacteria and Gram stain (or similar direct tests) can help in selecting the initial antimicrobial agent but do not help in defining which patient does or does not have pneumonia.[77,87]

The American Thoracic Society (ATS) has published a series of guidelines for the treatment of HAP, with that in 2005 the most recent.[51] Several factors are considered: (1) severity of illness, (2) presence of risk factors for specific organisms, and (3) time of onset from hospital admission. According to the ATS criteria, severe pneumonia is associated with the need for ICU admission, respiratory failure, swift radiological presentation or cavitation, or the presence of severe sepsis or septic shock.

Based on the former ATS recommendations for antibiotic use, an international consensus panel did not favor the risk stratification named by the ATS and believed that the previous use of antibiotics, local pathogens, and resistance patterns should be primary considerations in the selection of therapy.[87] Luna et al.[88] and Ibrahim et al.[89] have shown a lower mortality when antibiotics were administered quickly and were appropriately selected.

Antibiotic-resistant bacteria are important pathogens in VAP, making selection of appropriate antibiotics difficult. Thus, clinicians are faced with the dilemma of using broad-spectrum agents initially while trying to minimize the further acquisition of resistant pathogens. Micek and colleagues performed a randomized controlled trial of an antibiotic discontinuation policy for clinically suspected VAP.[90] Previously, this group had demonstrated that a local clinical guideline for VAP improved the number of appropriate antibiotics and reduced overall duration of antibiotic administration.[89] Given the need for initial broad coverage of both *S. aureus* and *Pseudomonas* in their unit, the authors used a combination of either vancomycin or linezolid for suspected gram positives and cefipime and either ciprofloxacin or gentamicin for gram negatives. By outlining criteria for stopping antibiotics, duration of treatment was 2 days shorter in the guideline versus the conventional group (6.0 ± 4.9 vs. 8.0 ± 5.6 days) without altering secondary VAP, length of stay, or mortality.[89] These authors have also successfully used a similar strategy for gram positives and a carbapenam with either an aminoglycoside or fluroquinolone.

A national trend of an increasing incidence of MRSA has been reported.[16] With this trend, there has been an interest in whether to use vancomycin or linezolid when pneumonia is suspected or proven to be caused by MRSA.[91,92] Because vancomycin is poorly concentrated in lung tissue, some experts have advocated for the use of linezolid.[51] However, reports of linezolid-resistant organisms have already surfaced, and prolonged use (>2 weeks) is often associated with reversible thrombocytopenia.

Prevention

The risk of VAP ranges from 1% to 3% per day a patient is intubated in the ICU, with an overall incidence in some studies of 40%–60%.[66] In a prospective, matched cohort study, patients with VAP remained in the ICU 4.3 days (95% CI, 1.5 to 7.0 days) longer than patients who did not have VAP and had a trend toward an increased risk for death (absolute risk increase 5.8%; CI –2.4% to 14.0%).[93]

Since HAP/VAP is at least a morbid, costly, if not mortal complication,[94–99] the focus should not be on diagnosis or therapy but on methods to prevent the disease from occurring. To this end, the Canadian Critical Care Society and Canadian Critical Care Trials Group collaborated to publish a formal evidence-based analysis of the literature of physical, pharmacologic, and positional interventions for effective prevention of VAP with strict analysis of the quality of the data.[64] This article should be read in its entirety by those caring for critically ill patients. The authors found evidence to recommend the following: the orotracheal route of intubation, changes of ventilator circuits only for each new patient and if the circuits are soiled, use of closed endotracheal suction systems that are changed for each new patient and as clinically indicated, the use of heat and moisture exchangers in the absence of contraindications, weekly changes of heat and moisture exchangers, and semirecumbent positioning in the absence of contraindications.[64] While widespread implementation and costs have not been formally measured, the authors believed that practitioners should also consider endotracheal tubes with subglottic secretion drainage and the use of kinetic beds. The authors could not recommend sucralfate as an agent to prevent VAP in patients at high risk for gastrointestinal bleeding or topical antibiotics to prevent VAP. Because of insufficient or conflicting evidence, the panel could not make recommendations about systematically searching for maxillary sinusitis, chest physiotherapy, the timing of tracheostomy, prone positioning, prophylactic intravenous antibiotics, or intravenous plus topical antibiotics.[64]

Bloodstream Infections

Nosocomial (hospital-acquired) bloodstream infections (BSIs) are an important cause of morbidity and mortality, with an estimated 250,000 cases occurring each year in the United States.[49] The BSIs comprise about 15% of all infections, with an incidence of about 5 per 1000 catheter days.[6,16] The impact of BSI on outcome is tremendous: BSIs are associated with a crude mortality rate of 35%–53% in ICU patients,[100–102] prolonged ICU (7.5–25 days) and hospital length of stay (4.5–32), and increased costs by as much as $77,000.[102] Inappropriate initial antibiotic therapy is an important predictor of death in patients with bacteremia.[103]

Bloodstream infections are primarily catheter associated, with intravascular catheters more commonly involved than urinary catheters.[7,8] Bloodstream infections may be either primary (i.e., direct infection) or secondary.[104] Secondary infections are related to infections at other sites, such as the urinary tract, lung, postoperative wounds, and skin.

Primary BSIs comprise the majority (64%) of NIs reported to the CDC's NNIS.[6,16] Primary BSI has traditionally been classified as community or nosocomially acquired. However, a group from Duke has proposed adding the category of health care-associated BSI to this classification. A large number of patients that present with bacteremia have health care-associated infection, defined as BSI in patients residing in long-term care facilities; in those receiving home health care, intravascular therapy at home, or in an outpatient facility; and in those hospitalized within 90 days. Clinicians should reconsider therapy for patients with community-acquired BSIs if their recent care falls into the health care-associated category. The choice of empirical antibiotics should cover the commonly isolated staphylococci (often with oxacillin resistance) rather than simply organisms such as *E. coli* or *Streptococcus pneumoniae*, which are more characteristic of community-acquired BSI. In addition, the provider should be increasingly aware of community-acquired MRSA.[104]

Definitions

A primary BSI occurs when the recognized pathogen is isolated from blood culture *and* the pathogen is not related to infection at another site.[105] In situations in which common skin organisms could be contaminants or actual infecting organisms are isolated such as coagulase-negative staphylococcus (CoNS), diphtheroids, *Bacillus* spp., *Propionibacterium* spp., and micrococcus, patients must have clinical signs of infection (fever > 38°C, chills, or hypotension) *and* meet one of the following criteria: (1) the common skin contaminant is isolated from two blood cultures drawn on separate occasions *and* the organism is not related to infection at another site; or (2) the common skin contaminant is isolated from a single blood culture in a patient with an intravascular access device *and* the physician institutes appropriate antimicrobial therapy.

Infections associated with the use of catheters include both catheter-associated infections and catheter-related infections. While perhaps an overestimate of the incidence of infection, catheter-associated infections include primary BSI and clinical sepsis events that are epidemiologically associated with the use of an intravascular device. Catheter-related infections include catheter colonization, skin exit site infection, and microbiologically proven device-related BSI. Central line-related bloodstream infection (CR-BSI) is a primary BSI in a patient with a central venous catheter with at least one positive blood culture obtained from a peripheral vein *and* at least one of the following: (1) a positive semiquantitative (>CFU/catheter segment) or quantitative (>10^3 CFU/catheter segment) culture with the same organism (species and antibiogram) isolated from the catheter segment and peripheral blood; (2) simultaneous quantitative blood cultures with a 5:1 or higher ratio (CVC vs. peripheral), or (3) if central venous catheter blood turns positive 2h sooner than simultaneously drawn peripheral blood. Patient risk factors and best practices for the placement and maintenance of the catheters have been well described.[106]

Epidemiology, Pathogenesis, Pathogens

Catheters may become infected through one of four common pathways. First, the skin and therefore the external surface of the catheter may become colonized, and the bacteria may move along the catheter into the bloodstream.[8] Skin colonization is a strong predictor of infection. The internal surface of the catheter may become colonized or infected by contaminating the hub and intraluminal surface of the catheter.[106] Frequent opening of the hub is an important source of contamination. These two processes are believed to account for the majority of infections. In addition, it is possible for the catheter to become contaminated by infusing infected fluids or by hematogenous spread of bacteria from a distant site.[106]

A biofilm is rapidly formed on catheters and can contribute to enhanced attachment to foreign material of some pathogens, such as *S. aureus* and CoNS. In addition, some pathogens (CoNS) produce a substance called slime that can allow additional attachment of pathogens and protection from antimicrobial penetration.[106]

The Surveillance and Control of Pathogen of Epidemiological Importance (SCOPE) project is a compilation of data from 49 hospitals dispersed throughout the United States.[107] The data from SCOPE have been highly correlated with the data from NNIS and are similar to that reported from large epidemiological studies in other countries. Data from the SCOPE project on 24,179 cases of nosocomial BSI over a 7-year period ending in 2002 demonstrated a BSI incidence of 60 cases per 10,000 hospital admissions.[107] Of BSIs, 87% were monomicrobial. Gram-positive organisms caused 65% of these BSIs, gram-negative organisms caused 25%, and fungi caused 9.5%. The crude mortality rate in that series was 27%. The most common organisms causing BSIs were CoNS (31% of isolates), *S. aureus* (20%), enterococci (9%), and *Candida* species (9%). Interestingly, there were differences in time between presentation and certain pathogens. The mean interval between admission and infection was 13 days for infection with *E. coli*,16 days for *S. aureus*, 22 days for *Candida* species and *Klebsiella* species, 23 days for enterococci, and 26 days for *Acinetobacter* species. In ICU patients, CoNS, *Pseudomonas* species, *Enterobacter* species, *Serratia* species, and *Acinetobacter* species were more likely to cause infections.[107] Of significant concern was the report that the proportion of *S. aureus* isolates with methicillin resistance increased from 22% in 1995 to 57% in 2001, and in some reports it is even greater today.[104] In addition, vancomycin resistance was seen in 2% of *Enterococcus faecalis* isolates and in 60% of *Enterococcus faecium* isolates.

Treatment

In patients with primary bacteremia, clinicians should consider the catheter as a potential source for infection and should examine exit sites and tunnels closely.[108] If there are local signs of infection at the exit site or in the tunnel, then the catheter should be removed. The likelihood of the catheter acting as a source of infection is related to many of the processes, procedures, and decisions made about the insertion and care of the catheter.

If the catheter is suspected to be the source of infection, then a guidewire exchange rather than simple removal of the catheter is appropriate.[7,8,108] Guidewire exchange decreases the likelihood of technical complications associated with reinsertion but increases the likelihood of catheter colonization. Thus, neither guidewire exchange nor routine reinsertion of catheters should be performed without a clinical suspicion of a catheter infection.[109] If an exchanged catheter is colonized (>15 colonies by semiquantitative roll plate or > 10^3 colonies by sonication), then the catheter should be removed. In this setting, a course of antibiotics is not recommended.

If a catheter and blood are positive (CR-BSI) and the catheter is a short-term catheter, then it should be removed. While some authors advocate that catheters can be treated through the catheter with an antibiotic lock, this cannot be generally recommended except in patients for whom venous access is a significant concern.[110] For patients with a long-term catheter and CR-BSI, the risks and benefits of keeping the catheter in situ should be balanced. For many pathogens, success can be obtained by treating through the catheter. However, some authors would argue that for catheter-related infection and certain microorganisms such as *S. aureus* and *Candida* species, the time until microbial clearance is shortened, the possibility of metastatic infection decreased, and perhaps survival is improved by earlier catheter removal.

Antibiotics should be directed toward the likely pathogens.[103,104] Since more than two-thirds of all patients will have a gram-positive CR-BSI, antibiotics should be selected with this in mind. Risk factors considering the likelihood of MRSA should be carefully examined, including duration of hospital stay, known colonization with MRSA or location near a patient who is colonized with MRSA, antibiotic therapy, and an open wound. If risk factors are present, then therapy with an agent that covers MRSA (vancomycin or linezolid) should be considered. If not, then therapy with a staphylococcus direct penicillin such as oxacillin or nafcillin would be appropriate. Duration of therapy depends on the pathogen isolated. If the patient has *S. aureus* bacteremia, then therapy should be at least 10–14 days due to the high rate of relapse if duration is 7 days or less, and an echocardiogram may be required to determine which patients should have prolonged therapy. If the patient has relapse, continuous fever, or bacteremia despite catheter removal, then a search for complications such as endocarditis or metastatic infection should be undertaken.

Prevention

The majority of infections associated with the use of intravascular devices in critically ill patients requiring short-term catheterization are preventable.[9] Prevention relies first on strict observation of the basic rules of hygiene, of which hand hygiene represents the first and most important. More specific measures, including the use of maximal sterile barriers during insertion,[110] optimal insertion site preparation,[111] detailed guidelines for catheter replacement, and defining particular situations in which the use of antiseptic- or antibiotic-coated devices may be used have been examined in detail in hundreds of clinical studies.[112–116] Detailed recommendations based on education were updated[106] and should now be systematically included in the process of improving the overall quality of patient care. Table 14.5 details accepted processes of care.

Intensive care units should be aware of the ongoing incidence of CR-BSI and should have in place a quality improvement process to drive the infection rate as close to zero as possible. A multimodality multidisciplinary approach to the process is most likely to succeed. Education about best practices has been successful in decreasing rates of infections,[117–119] as have several simple interventions, including the

TABLE 14.5. A Practical Approach to Prevention of Catheter-Related Bloodstream Infection.

Topic	*Manner*
Indication	Assessment of need, development of complications, daily goals sheet
Hand hygiene	Hand disinfection with alcohol or soap and water, checklist compliance
Preparation	Collect all necessary equipment, including gowns, gloves, hat, mask, full-barrier precautions; line cart facilitates placement in one area
Patient	Proper positioning, site selection (subclavian unless it is a dialysis catheter or contraindication), skin preparation (chlorhexidine 2%); maximal sterile technique (gown, gloves, mask, hat, full-barrier drape); checklist ensures compliance
Dressing	Gauze or transparent dressing; change when soiled or loose
Maintenance	Stopcocks should be avoided; new caps on all hubs after opening; aseptic technique for blood drawing, drug infusion; intravenous infusion set changed every 3 days
Replacement	Intravenous infusion set changed every 3 days, as well as dressing if not as above; lipid and transfusion sets should be changed every 24h; routine central line replacement not recommended

Source: Adapted from Berenholtz.[9]

use of checklists to ask every day if a catheter or tube can be removed.[9]

Urinary Tract Infections

Urinary tract infections are the most common NIs, accounting for up to 40% of all NIs; most are associated with the use of a urinary catheter.[120,121] Approximately 24 million urinary catheters are used annually in the United States, and nearly 25% of hospitalized patients have a urinary catheter during their hospitalization.[122] Some studies have indicated that attending and resident physicians are unaware that patients have a urinary catheter in place in as many as 38% of patients, and that the catheter is frequently not indicated.[123]

Catheter use can be divided into short- and long-term use by time, with fewer than 30 days defining short-term use and the difference between common and universal colonization with bacteria or fungi.[124] For short-term use, the risk of developing bacteriuria in catheterized patients has been reported to be between 3% and 5% per day of catheterization, with an estimated probability of bacteriuria in patients not receiving antibiotics and having a catheter in place for 2–10 days is at 26% (95% CI 23%–29%).[125] After the development of bacteriuria the development of symptomatic UTI without bacteremia has been estimated at 25% (16%–32%) and for the development of bacteremia at 3.6% (95% CI 3.4%–3.8%).[126]

In the United States, it is estimated that 9 million episodes of nosocomial UTI occur annually, increasing the cost of health care by more than $500 million annually (estimated minimum of $676 per episode without bacteremia, $2836 for those with UTI and bacteremia).[126] In addition to the direct effect of treating complicated UTIs, many catheter cultures represent colonization and do not require antibiotic therapy. Although the costs of catheter-associated UTIs are not as high as, for example, those for a deep surgical site infection or a nosocomial pneumonia, UTIs are a major reservoir of resistant pathogens.[127,128]

Pathogenesis

Much like other NIs, a UTI is caused by the combination of an invasion of local defenses and the easy transmission of pathogens through the uretheal meatus into the bladder.[120,121,129] In addition, the presence of a foreign body allows for the formation of a biofilm and the development of a protected site for the growth of bacteria and accounts for the difficulty in penetration of antibiotics into the biofilm. Extraluminal contamination of the urinary tract can occur via breaks in sterile technique during insertion of the catheter or from colonization of the meatus and ascent of pathogens along the catheter into the bladder.[129] Intraluminal contamination occurs from breaks in the drainage system during irrigation of the bladder or because of improper technique and lack of hand hygiene when draining the closed drainage system. Pathogens can then ascend from the collection bag into the bladder, where they can easily multiply.

In a large study of more than 1000 patients, more than two-thirds of infections were attributed to extraluminal contamination, and one-third were intraluminal.[130] Interestingly, there was a difference in the type of organism by mode of acquisition. *Candida*, enterococci, and staphylococci more commonly ascended along the catheter from the perineum. On the other hand, the water-borne gram negatives such as *Pseudomonas, Enterobacter*, and *Acinetobacter* were more commonly associated with the intraluminal route from the collection bag.

Risk Factors

Several studies[131–133] have examined the risk factors for the development of a UTI in hospitalized patients. The two most important risk factors are the duration of catheterization and female gender. Other risk factors that have been identified include having the catheter placed in an environment outside the operating room, having the patient on a urology service (which may be a proxy for structural abnormalities of the urinary tract), other infections, malnutrition, diabetes, and renal failure. In improvement efforts, only efforts to keep the drainage bag below the patient have consistently been helpful in decreasing the infection rate.[124]

Diagnosis

While the diagnosis of a UTI may seem straightforward, in fact there is controversy and lack of consistency about the exact classification, diagnosis, and management of a UTI.[134,135] General classification and considerations include site of infection (bladder vs. kidney), the presence or absence of symptoms (asymptomatic vs. symptomatic), origin of infection (community vs. hospital), and the severity of infection (uncomplicated vs. complicated). While these broad aspects of classification may help determine pathogens and need for treatment, they are not clearly defined or universally accepted. For instance, a complicated UTI can be found in at-risk patient populations or those with specific conditions, such as the elderly, pregnant, critically ill, those with structural abnormalities of the urinary tract, or catheterized patients.[124]

The presence of pyuria is used as a general criterion for a UTI in noncatheterized patients. However, a study of more than 750 patients demonstrated that pyuria was a better predictor of the presence of gram-negative infection; the presence of large numbers of yeast, staphylococci, and enterococci was not as frequently associated with pyuria.[136] This difference is postulated to be due to the lower levels of inflammation elicited by these pathogens. Thus, pyuria should not be used as the sole criterion in determining the need for a urine culture or treatment. Unfortunately, symptoms cannot be used to determine who should have therapy. In a large prospective study, no differences were seen in the presence or absence of fever or symptoms such as dysuria or suprapubic pain in patients with and without catheter-associated UTI. This is likely secondary to the fact that the catheter itself may cause symptoms, and that the catheter prevents bladder distention and thereby bladder symptoms. However, when the catheter becomes obstructed, symptoms develop, and infection is also much more likely.[129]

Pathogens

In contrast to uncomplicated UTIs, for which *E. coli* is the predominant pathogen, catheter-associated UTIs have additional pathogens, including the enterococci (including VRE) and *C. albicans*.[124,129,137] In complicated UTIs, polymicrobial infections are not uncommon.

Treatment

As is true in any infection, knowledge of the likely pathogens is essential in selecting the appropriate antimicrobial agent. A urinary culture must be obtained in suspected cases of UTI, and antibiotic therapy should be molded to isolated pathogens. There are many available oral and intravenous agents that are appropriate for UTIs (Table 14.6), and no state-of-the art guidelines exist to suggest preferred agents.

In seriously ill or critically ill patients with a suspected UTI, empirical coverage with an antipseudomonal agent is recommended until cultures have returned (Table 14.7).[124,129,131] Empiric coverage of the gram-positive agents is usually reserved for proven serious infection based on cultures, known colonizers, or a Gram stain with gram-positive agents alone. These gram-positive infections can be treated with vancomycin, quinpristin/dalfopristin, or linezolid following identification.[138–140] Uncomplicated UTIs can be treated for 3 days, while complicated UTIs should be treated for 7–14 days.

While *E. coli* remains the most common pathogen if the UTI is an initial infection, resistance to the sulfa (trimethoprim/sulfamethoxazole) agents commonly suggested as first-line therapy may be seen in as many as 10%–22% of isolates. Recurrent *E. coli* and the remaining gram-negative isolates tend to be more resistant. These resistant *E. coli* strains are often susceptible to the fluroquinolones, nitrofurantoin, carbapenems, and the aminoglycosides. Agents that were cffective for *Klebsiella* include the third- and fourth-generation cephalosporins, pipercillin-tazobactam, the carbapenems, aminoglycosides, and fluroquinolones. The most active fluroquinolones against *Pseudomonas* in vitro studies was ciprofloxacin (75% susceptible), followed by levofloxacin (71%) and gatifloxacin (66%).[136] A randomized controlled trial demonstrated that a single dose of ciprofloxacin (1000mg) was as effective as ciprofloxacin given twice daily for the treatment of complicated UTIs for 7–14 days.[140]

TABLE 14.6. Distribution of Infecting Urinary Pathogens in Two Large Study Populations.

Pathogen	*Percentage of isolates*[a]	*Percentage of isolates*[b]
Escherichia coli	13	46.9
Enterococcus spp.	21	12.8
Klebsiella spp.	Other gram negatives	11.0
Pseudomonas. aeruginosa	25	7.5
Staphylococcus aureus	11	
Proteus mirabilis	Other gram negatives	5.0
Coagulase-negative staphylococci	5.0	3.4
Streptococcus spp.	8	
Miscellaneous	See below	3.4
Other gram negatives	13	Listed above
Other gram positives	1	Not listed
Yeast	3	Not listed

[a]Data from Merle et al.[161]

[b]Data from Jones et al.[162]

TABLE 14.7. Empiric Antibiotic Selection for Catheter-Associated Urinary Tract Infection.

Empirical agents for UTI, *Pseudomonas* not suspected
Fluroquinolones: Ciprofloxacin, gatifloxacin, levofloxacin
Cephalosporins: Second generation (cefuroxime, cefotiam), third generation (cefotaxime, ceftriaxone)
Penicillins: Amoxicillin/clavulanic acid; ampicillin/sulbactam
Aminoglycosides: Gentamicin, tobramycin, amikacin
Carbapenem: Ertapenam
Severe infections or *Pseudomonas* suspected
Fluroquinolone: Ciprofloxacin
Penicillin: Pipercillin/tazobactam
Cephalosporin: Cetazadome, cefipime ± aminoglycoside
Carbapenem: Imipenem, meropenem

The goals of antimicrobial therapy are to rapidly resolve symptoms, eradicate pathogens, minimize recurrence and resistance, and reduce morbidity and mortality. Correction of underlying risk factors such as catheter removal or correction of an underlying abnormality should be performed as able.

Prevention

One of the primary areas for prevention of UTIs involves the decision whether to use a urinary catheter.[120,141] In men, an alternative to the indwelling catheter is the condom catheter.[142] While there have not been any properly designed studies directly comparing these two modes, repeat studies from the same institutions suggest a substantially lower incidence of bacteriuria. However, it should be noted that urine inside the condom catheters may contain a large number of bacteria, skin breakdown may occur, the meatus may become colonized, and bacteriuria may develop. Intermittent catheterization is a reasonable alternative to indwelling catheters, with an incidence of bacteriuria of about 1%–3% per catheterization. No well-designed studies have compared long-term indwelling catheters with intermittent catheterization for overall or specific outcomes.

Catheters should not be placed indiscriminately, for convenience, or as "routine" postoperative care if a patient can urinate spontaneously. Use of indwelling catheters should be limited to patients with anatomic or physiologic urinary obstruction; patients undergoing surgery of the genitourinary tract; patients requiring accurate monitoring of urine output (i.e., critically ill or postoperative patients); and debilitated, comatose, or paralyzed patients.

If a catheter has been placed, then two clear practices should be used to decrease infection risk. First, the catheter should be removed as soon as possible. In our ICUs, we use a daily goals sheet that specifically ask if any lines or catheters can be discontinued.[9] This tool has helped eliminate unnecessary devices. Second, the drainage system must remain closed except at the bag-tube drain, and care should be made to avoid the emptying port from touching contaminated containers.[143–145]

While logical to decrease urethral colonization, topical application of microbial agents has not effectively decreased infection. In fact, in some series the incidence of bacteriuria increased. Similarly, bladder irrigation had not been effective.[125]

Antiinfective agents applied to catheters have been a subject of significant interest, especially with silver as an antimicrobial.[146–154] Thirteen trials of silver-coated catheters generally supported the use of these devices, but few had patients in an ICU setting or demonstrated a homogeneous benefit of prevention, and there is no consensus about whether these catheters should be widely used.

Miscellaneous

With the exception of surgical site infections, this chapter has covered the most common NIs. Postoperative fever is not always indicative of infection, and risk factors such as operation performed, time from operation, patient risk factors, and signs and symptoms should be defined. A thorough search for localizing signs and symptoms should thus be undertaken. While not all infectious causes can be discussed, two additional diseases should be considered, infections with *C. difficile* and sinusitis.

Clostridium difficile-associated disease (CDAD) is the major hospital-acquired gastrointestinal infection, with an estimated 3 million cases annually in the United States.[155] The annual estimated cost of CDAD has been estimated at $1.1 billion, with an increase in length of stay of 3.6 days and hospital costs of $3669 per case, 54% more than for patients without CDAD. Several reports have suggested an increase in the incidence of this disease, which has been confirmed by NNIS ICU data in hospitals with more than 500 beds.[156]

For a hospitalized patient with diarrhea, *C. difficile* will be responsible for 30% of cases; for patients with colitis and antibiotics, the number is 50%–70%, and if pseudomembranes are present, nearly 100% are due to *C. difficile*.[157] Risk factors associated with hospital-acquired CDAD include antimicrobial use, advanced age, laxative use, antineoplastic chemotherapeutic agent use, bowel colonization with *C. difficile*, production of toxin A, renal insufficiency, or gastrointestinal surgery or procedures. The three antibiotics most closely linked to CDAD include ampicillin (amoxicillin), clindamycin, and the cephalosporins, especially the third-generation agents.

Clostridium difficile produces two toxins: toxin A, which is both enteropathic and cytotoxic, and toxin B, which is only cytotoxic. The enteropathic toxin A effects induce fluid flux into the bowel, as potent as cholera toxin. However, the range of presentation of disease is wide and varies from asymptomatic, culture positive in 20% to an overwhelming life-threatening toxic presentation. Diarrhea is not always present; leukocytosis is often present and can be marked. Diagnosis is established based on immunoassay on fructose agar as the most sensitive test; culture has a 20%–25% false-positive rate. The immunoassay is rapid but a bit less sensitive (70%–75%) for a single stool specimen; additional specimens may increase sensitivity by 10%. Serial studies should not be performed to assess treatment effectiveness or test of cure since the stool may be positive for 3 to 6 weeks after successful treatment and does not predict relapse.[157] Endoscopy should not be performed routinely but may be indicated when a rapid diagnosis is needed, where immunoassay is not available, when the assay is negative but CDAD is strongly suspected, or when alternative colon diseases may be present.[157]

Treatment of CDAD depends somewhat on symptoms. Antibiotics should be stopped or changed to those with a lower propensity for causing disease. Asymptomatic patients should not be treated as well as some patients with mild disease because spontaneous resolution is not associated with relapse. Metronidazole (either 250mg every 6h or 500mg every 8h) should be the first-line agent of choice and can be administered orally in those who can tolerate it or intravenously in those who cannot. Cure rates are in the range of 95%, with relapse rates of 5%–15%. If patients are not improving after 3–5 days, then 125mg vancomycin p.o. every 6h is recommended, as well as in those patients pregnant or lactating. A vancomycin retention enema can be used as an adjunct to intravenous metronidazole in patients with an ileus. Additional agents with some efficacy against CDAD include bacitracin, rafixamine, and an agent not available in the United States, tecoplanin. In their recent Cochrane review, authors concluded that vancomycin is the only agent compared to and better than placebo, but this was a small trial. They did not support a clear choice of the available agents based on current information.[158]

Acute purulent sinusitis is a well-known cause of fever of unknown origin in the ICU. The disease has a wide spectrum of presentation and can be a life-threatening problem requiring urgent diagnosis. The problem with diagnosis of this disease in postoperative patients is that radiographic findings in patients with nasogastric tubes are almost uniformly found after 48h, and microbiologic cultures may indicate contamination or colonization. Moreover, purulent secretions may be sterile. A study of antral puncture versus rhinoscopy demonstrated that 25 of 53 patients had mucopurulent effusions, most commonly polymicrobial (40%). *Staphylococcus aureus* and gram negatives were the most common isolates. While antral puncture was safe and effective, with anterior rhinoscopy showing a normal examination, only 8% of cultures would be positive.[159] In a study specifically designed to examine anaerobic cultures, 18/30 patients with nosocomial sinusitis had anaerobes isolated.[160] Thus, anaerobic coverage should be strongly considered. As stated earlier, while sinusitis and VAP are linked, there is no clear evidence that a systematic search for sinusitis should be undertaken in all patients.

Conclusion

This chapter has covered the common NIs, risk factors, methods of diagnosis, treatment, and effective methods for prevention. Nosocomial infections are among the most important causes of postoperative morbidity, prolonged hospital and ICU stay, increased costs, and mortality. Every effort should be made to employ the proven preventive strategies.

References

1. Garner J, Jarvis W, Emori T, et al. CDC definitions for nosocomial infections, 1988. Am J Infect Control 1988;16:128–140.
2. CDC. Public health focus: surveillance, prevention and control of nosocomial infections. MMWR Morb Mortal Wkly Rep 1992;41:783–787.
3. Vincent J. Nosocomial infections in the adult intensive care unit. Lancet 2003;361:2068–2077.
4. Kohn L, Corrigan J, Donaldson M. To Err Is Human: Building a Safer Health System. Washington, DC: Institute of Medicine, National Academy Press, 1999.
5. Gaynes R, Solomon S. Improving hospital-acquired infection rates: the CDC experience. JCAHO J Quality Improvement 1996;22:457–467.

6. CDC. National Nosocomial Infections Surveillance (NNIS) system report, data summary from January 1990–May 1999. Am J Infect Control 1999;27:520–532.
7. Eggimann P, Pittet D. Infection control in the ICU. Chest 2001;120:2059–2093.
8. Eggimann P, Sax H, Pittet D. Catheter-related infection. Microbes Infect 2004;6:1033–1042.
9. Berenholtz S, Pronovost P, Lipsett P, et al. Eliminating catheter-related bloodstream infections in the intensive care unit. Crit Care Med 2004;32:2014–2020.
10. National Center for Health Statistics. Healthy People 2000 Review 1998–1999. Hyattsville, MD: U.S. Department of Health and Human Services, CDC, 2000.
11. Culver D, White J, Morgan W, et al. The efficacy of infection surveillance and control programs in preventing nosocomial infections in U.S. hospitals. Am J Epidemiol 1985;121:182–205.
12. Eggimann P, Harbarth S, Constantin M, et al. Impact of a prevention strategy targeted at vascular access care on incidence of infections acquired in intensive care. Lancet 2000;355:1864–1868.
13. Hacek D, Suriano T, Noskin G, et al. Medical and economic benefit of a comprehensive infection control program that includes routine determination of microbial clonality. Am J Clin Pathol 1999;111:647–654.
14. Dumigan D, Kohan C, Reed C, et al. Utilizing national nosocomial infection surveillance system data to improve urinary tract infection rates in three intensive-care units. Clin Perform Qual Health Care 1998;6:172–178.
15. McConkey S, L'Ecuyer P, Murphy D, et al. Results of a comprehensive infection control program for reducing surgical-site infections in coronary artery bypass surgery. Infect Control Hosp Epidemiol 1999;8:533–538.
16. NNIS System. National Nosocomial Infections Surveillance (NNIS) System report, data summary from January 1992 through June 2004, issued October 2004. Am J Infect Control 2004;32:470–485.
17. Saint S, Savel R, Matthay M. Enhancing the safety of critically ill patients by reducing urinary and central venous catheter-related infections. Am J Respir Crit Care Med 2002;165:1475–1479.
18. Wenzel R, Edmond M. The impact of hospital-acquired bloodstream infections. Emerg Infect Dis 2001;7:174–177.
19. U.S. Department of Health and Human Services. Healthy People 2010, U.S. Department of Health and Human Services, conference ed. Washington, DC: U.S. Department of Health and Human Services, 2000.
20. Monitoring hospital-acquired infections to promote patient safety—United States, 1990–1999. MMWR Morb Mortal Wkly Rep 2000;49:149–153.
21. Stone P, Larson E, Nijab Kawar L. A systematic audit of economic evidence linking nosocomial infections and infection control interventions: 1990–2000. Am J Infect Control 2002; 30:145–152.
22. Vincent J, Bihari D, Suter P, et al. The prevalence of nosocomial infection in intensive care units in Europe. Results of the European Prevalence of Infection in Intensive Care (EPIC) study. JAMA 1995;274:639–644.
23. Döcke W, Randow F, Syrbe H, et al. Monocyte deactivation in septic patients: restoration by IFN-γ treatment. Nat Med 1997; 3:678–681.
24. Asadullah K, Woiciechowsky C, Docke W, et al. Immunodepression following neurosurgical procedures. Crit Care Med 1995; 23:1976–1983.
25. Schinkel C, Sendtner R, Zimmer S, et al. Functional analysis of monocyte subsets in surgical sepsis. J Trauma 1998;44:743–748.
26. Peters M, Petros A, Dixon G, et al. Acquired immunoparalysis in paediatric intensive care: prospective observational study. BMJ 1999;319:609–610.
27. Bonten M, Kollef M, Hall J. Risk factors for ventilator-associated pneumonia: from epidemiology to patient management. Clin Infect Dis 2004;38:1141–1149.
28. Beck-Sague C, Sinkowitz R, Chinn R, et al. Risk factors for ventilator-associated pneumonia in surgical intensive care-unit patients. Infect Control Hosp Epidemiol 1994;17:374–376.
29. Craven D, Kunches L, Kilinsky V, et al. Risk factors for pneumonia and fatality in patients receiving continuous mechanical ventilation. Am Rev Respir Dis 1986;133:792–796.
30. Torres A, Gatell J, Aznar E, et al. Re-intubation increases the risk of nosocomial pneumonia in patients needing mechanical ventilation. Am J Respir Crit Care Med 1995;152:137–141.
31. Rello J, Sonora R, Jubert P, et al. Pneumonia in intubated patients: role of respiratory airway care. Am J Respir Crit Care Med 1996;154:111–115.
32. Donskey C. The role of the intestinal tract as a reservoir and source for transmission of nosocomial pathogens. Clin Infect Dis 2004;39:219–226.
33. Vollaard E, Clasener H. Colonization resistance. Antimicrob Agents Chemother 1994;38:409–414.
34. Hendrix C, Hammond J, Swoboda S, et al. Surveillance strategies and impact of vancomycin-resistant enterococcal (VRE) colonization and infection in critically ill patients. Ann Surg 2001;233:259–265.
35. Pelz R, Lipsett P, Swoboda SM, et al. The diagnostic value of fungal surveillance cultures in critically ill patients. Surg Infect 2000;1:273–281.
36. Ray A, Pultz N, Bhalla A, et al. Coexistence of vancomycin-resistant *Enterococcus* and *Staphylococcus aureus* in the intestinal tracts of hospitalized patients. Clin Infect Dis 2003; 37:875–881.
37. Cunningham R, Dale B, Undy B, Gaunt N. Proton pump inhibitors as a risk factor for *Clostridium difficile* diarrhoea. J Hosp Infect 2003;54:243–245.
38. Estes R, Meduri G. The pathogenesis of ventilator-associated pneumonia, 1: mechanisms of bacterial transcolonization and airway inoculation. Intensive Care Med 1995;21:365–383.
39. Livrelli V, De Champs C, Di Martino P, et al. Adhesive properties and antibiotic resistance of *Klebsiella*, *Enterobacter*, and *Serratia* clinical isolates involved in nosocomial infections. J Clin Microbiol 1996;34:1963–1969.
40. Wang J, Chang S, Ko W, et al. A hospital-acquired outbreak of methicillin-resistant *Staphylococcus aureus* infection initiated by a surgeon carrier. J Hosp Infect 2001;47:104–109.
41. Pettinger A, Nettleman M. Epidemiology of isolation precautions. Infect Control Hosp Epidemiol 1991;12:303–307.
42. Pittet D. Improving adherence to hand hygiene practice: a multidisciplinary approach. Emerg Infect Dis 2001;7:225–240.
43. Lipsett P, Swoboda S. Handwashing compliance depends on professional status. Surg Infect 2001;2:241–245.
44. Pittet D, Hugonnet S, Harbarth S, et al. Effectiveness of a hospital-wide programme to improve compliance with hand hygiene. Lancet 2000;356:1307–1290.
45. Pittet D, Mourouga P, Perneger T, et al. Compliance with handwashing in a teaching hospital. Ann Intern Med 1999;130:126–130.
46. Swoboda S, Earsing K, Strauss K, et al. Electronic monitoring and voice prompts improve hand hygiene and decrease nosocomial infections in an intermediate care unit. Crit Care Med 2004;32:358–363.
47. Streit J, Jones R, Sader H, et al. Assessment of pathogen occurrences and resistance profiles among infected patients in the intensive care unit: report from the SENTRY Antimicrobial Surveillance Program (North America, 2001). Int J Antimicrob Agents 2004;24:111–118.
48. Emori T, Edwards J, Culver D, et al. Accuracy of reporting nosocomial infections in intensive care unit patients to the

National Nosocomial Infections Surveillance (NNIS) system: a pilot study. Infect Control Hosp Epidemiol 1998;19:308–316.
49. Jarvis W. Benchmarking for prevention: the Centers for Disease Control and Prevention's National Nosocomial Infections Surveillance (NNIS) system experience. Infection 2003;suppl 2:44–48.
50. Kaoutar B, Joly C, L'Heriteau F, et al. Nosocomial infections and hospital mortality: a multicenter epidemiological study. J Hosp Infect 2003;58:269–272.
51. The American Thoracic Society and Infectious Disease Society of America. Guidelines for the management of adults with hospital-acquired, ventilator-associated, and healthcare-associated pneumonia. Am J Respir Crit Care Med 2005;171:388–416.
52. Kollef M. Prevention of hospital-associated pneumonia and ventilator-associated pneumonia. Crit Care Med 2004;32:1396–1405.
53. Kollef M. Epidemiology and risk factors for nosocomial pneumonia. Emphasis on prevention. Clin Chest Med 1999;20:653–670.
54. Kollef M. The prevention of ventilator-associated pneumonia. N Engl J Med 1999;340:627–634.
55. Zack J, Garrison T, Trovillion E, et al. Effect of an education program aimed at reducing the occurrence of ventilator-associated pneumonia. Crit Care Med 2002;30:2407–2412.
56. Cook D, Kollef M. Risk factors for ICU-acquired pneumonia. JAMA 1998;279:1605–1606.
57. Messori A, Trippoli S, Vaiani M, et al. Bleeding and pneumonia in intensive care patients given ranitidine and sucralfate for prevention of stress ulcer: meta-analysis of randomised controlled trials. BMJ 2000;321:1103–1106.
58. Ben-Menachem T, Fogel R, Patel R, et al. Prophylaxis for stress-related gastric hemorrhage in the medical intensive care unit. A randomized, controlled, single-blind study. Ann Intern Med 1994;121:568–575.
59. Eddleston J, Pearson R, Holland J, et al. Prospective endoscopic study of stress erosions and ulcers in critically ill adult patients treated with either sucralfate or placebo. Crit Care Med 1994;22:1949–1954.
60. Cook D, Guyatt G, Marshall J, et al. A comparison of sucralfate and ranitidine for the prevention of upper gastrointestinal bleeding in patients requiring mechanical ventilation. N Engl J Med 1998;338:791–797.
61. Bonten M, Bergmans D, Ambergen A, et al. Risk factors for pneumonia, and colonization of respiratory tract and stomach in mechanically ventilated ICU patients. Am J Respir Crit Care Med 1996;154:1339–1346.
62. Garrouste-Oregas M, Chevret S, Arlet G, et al. Oropharyngeal or gastric colonization and nosocomial pneumonia in adult intensive care unit patients: a prospective study based on genomic DNA analysis. Am J Respir Crit Care Med 1997;156:1647–1655.
63. Heyland D, Drover J, Dhaliwal R, Greenwood J. Optimizing the benefits and minimizing the risks of enteral nutrition in the critically ill: role of small bowel feeding. JPEN J Parenter Enteral Nutr 2002;26:S51–S55.
64. Dodek P, Keenan S, Cook D, et al. Evidenced-based clinical practice guideline for the prevention of ventilator-associated pneumonia. Ann Intern Med 2004;141:305–313.
65. Drakulovic M, Torres A, Bauer T, et al. Supine body position as a risk factor for nosocomial pneumonia in mechanically ventilated patients: a randomised trial. Lancet 1999;354:1851–1858.
66. Cook D, Walter S, Cook R, et al. Incidence of and risk factors for ventilator-associated pneumonia in critically ill patients. Ann Intern Med 1998;129:433–440.
67. Hernandez G, Rico P, Diaz E, et al. Nosocomial lung infections in adult intensive care units. Microbes Infect 2004;6:1004–1014.
68. Marik P, Careau P. The role of anaerobes in patients with ventilator-associated pneumonia, and aspiration pneumonia: a prospective study. Chest 1999;115:178–183.
69. Hubmair. R. Statement of the Fourth International Consensus Conference in Critical Care on ICU-Acquired Pneumonia, Chicago, IL, May 2002. Intensive Care Med 2002;28:1521–1536.
70. Michaud S, Suzuki S, Harbath S. Effect of design-related bias in studies of diagnostic tests for ventilator-associated pneumonia. Am J Respir Crit Care Med 2002;166:1320–1325.
71. Waterer G, Wunderink R. Controversies in the diagnosis of ventilator-associated pneumonia. Med Clin North Am 2001;85:1565–1581.
72. Mehta R, Niederman M. Nosocomial pneumonia in the intensive care unit: controversies and dilemmas. J Intensive Care Med 2003;18:175–188.
73. Fagon J, Chastre J, Wolff M, et al. Invasive and noninvasive strategies for management of suspected ventilator-associated pneumonia: a randomized trial. Ann Intern Med 2000;132:621–630.
74. Sole Violan J, Fernandez J, Benitez A, et al. Impact of quantitative invasive diagnostic techniques in the management and outcome of mechanically ventilated patients with suspected pneumonia. Crit Care Med 2000;28:2737–2741.
75. Baughman R, Thorpe J, Staneck J, et al. Use of the protected specimen brush in patients with endotracheal or tracheostomy tubes. Chest 1987;91:233–236.
76. Chastre J, Fagon J, Soler P, et al. Diagnosis of nosocomial bacterial pneumonia in intubated patients undergoing ventilation: comparison of the usefulness of bronchoalveolar lavage and the protected specimen brush. Am J Med 1988;85:499–450.
77. Fagon J. Hospital-acquired pneumonia: diagnostic strategies: lessons from clinical trials. Infect Dis Clin N Am 2003:17;717–726.
78. Pugin J, Auckenthaler R, Mili N, et al. Diagnosis of ventilator associated pneumonia by bacteriologic analysis of bronchoscopic and nonbronchoscopic "blind" bronchoalveolar lavage fluid. Am Rev Respir Dis 1991;143:1121–1129.
79. Heyland D, Cook D, Marshall J, et al. The clinical utility of invasive diagnostic techniques in the setting of ventilator-associated pneumonia. Canadian Critical Care Trials Group. Chest 1999;115:1076–1084.
80. Sanchez-Nieto J, Torres A, Garcia-Cordoba F, et al. Impact of invasive and noninvasive quantitative culture sampling on outcome of ventilator-associated pneumonia: a pilot study. Am J Respir Crit Care Med 1998;157:371–376.
81. Ruiz M, Torres A, Ewig S, et al. Noninvasive versus invasive microbial investigation in ventilator-associated pneumonia: evaluation of outcome. Am J Respir Crit Care Med 2000;162:119–125.
82. Pingleton S, Fagon J, Leeper K Jr. Patient selection for clinical investigation of ventilator-associated pneumonia: criteria for evaluating diagnostic techniques. Chest 1992;102:553S–556S.
83. Meduri G, Chastre J. The standardization of bronchoscopic techniques for ventilator-associated pneumonia. Chest 1992; 102:557S–564S.
84. Shorr A, Sherner J, Jackson W, et al. Invasive approaches to the diagnosis of ventilator-associated pneumonia: a meta-analysis. Crit Care Med 2005;33:46–53.
85. Singh N, Rogers P, Atwood C, et al. Short-course empiric antibiotic therapy for patients with pulmonary infiltrates in the intensive care unit: a proposed solution for indiscriminate antibiotic prescription. Am J Respir Crit Care Med 2000;162:505–511.
86. Sole-Violan J, Fernandez J, Benitez A, et al. Impact of quantitative invasive diagnostic techniques in the management and outcome of mechanically ventilated patients with suspected pneumonia. Crit Care Med 2000;28:2737–2741.

87. Rello J, Paiva J, Baraibar K, et al. International Conference for the Development of the Consensus on the Diagnosis and Treatment of Ventilator-Associated Pneumonia. Chest 2001;120:955–970.
88. Luna C, Vujacich P, Niederman M, et al. Impact of BAL data on the therapy and outcome of ventilator-associated pneumonia. Chest 1997;111:676–685.
89. Ibrahim E, Ward S, Sherman G, et al. Experience with a clinical guideline for the treatment of ventilator-associated pneumonia. Crit Care Med 2001;29:1109–1115.
90. Micek S, Ward S, Fraser V, et al. A randomized controlled trial of an antibiotic discontinuation policy for clinically suspected ventilator-associated pneumonia. Chest 2004;125:1791–1799.
91. Wunderink R, Cammarata S, Oliphant T, et al. Continuation of a randomized, double-blind, multicenter study of linezolid versus vancomycin in the treatment of patients with nosocomial pneumonia. Clin Ther 2003;25:980–992.
92. Rubinstein E, Cammarata S, Oliphant T, et al. Linezolid (PNU-100766) versus vancomycin in the treatment of hospitalized patients with nosocomial pneumonia: a randomized, double-blind, multicenter study. Clin Infect Dis 2001;32:402–412.
93. Heyland D, Cook D, Griffith L, et al. The attributable morbidity and mortality of ventilator-associated pneumonia in the critically ill patient. The Canadian Critical Trials Group. Am J Respir Crit Care Med 1999;159:1249–1256.
94. Fagon J, Chastre J, Hance A, et al. Nosocomial pneumonia in ventilated patients: a cohort study evaluating attributable mortality and hospital stay. Am J Med 1993;94:281–288.
95. Baker A, Meredith J, Haponik E. Pneumonia in intubated trauma patients. Microbiology and outcomes. Am J Respir Crit Care Med 1996;153:343–349.
96. Cunnion K, Weber D, Broadhead W, et al. Risk factors for nosocomial pneumonia: comparing adult critical-care populations. Am J Respir Crit Care Med 1996;153:158–162.
97. Craig C, Connelly S. Effect of intensive care unit nosocomial pneumonia on duration of stay and mortality. Am J Infect Control 1984;12:233–238.
98. Kappstein I, Schulgen G, Beyer U, et al. Prolongation of hospital stay and extra costs due to ventilator-associated pneumonia in an intensive care unit. Eur J Clin Microbiol Infect Dis 1992; 11:504–508.
99. Papazian L, Bregeon F, Thirion X, et al. Effect of ventilator-associated pneumonia on mortality and morbidity. Am J Respir Crit Care Med 1996;154:91–97.
100. Pittet D, Tarara D, Wenzel R. Nosocomial bloodstream infection in critically ill patients. Excess length of stay, extra costs, and attributable mortality. JAMA 1994;271:1598–1601.
101. Heyland D, Cook D, Griffith L, et al. The attributable morbidity and mortality of ventilator-associated pneumonia in the critically ill patient. The Canadian Critical Trials Group. Am J Respir Crit Care Med 1999;159:1249–1256.
102. Dimick J, Pelz R, Consunji R, et al. Increased resource use associated with catheter-related bloodstream infection in the surgical intensive care unit. Arch Surg 2001;136:229–234.
103. Harbath S, Garbino J, Pugin J, et al. Inappropriate initial antibiotic therapy and its effect on survival in a clinical trial of immunomodulating therapy for severe sepsis. Am J Med 2003; 115:529–535.
104. Farr B. Prevention and control of methicillin-resistant *Staphylococcus aureus* infections. Curr Opin Infect Dis 2004;17:317–322.
105. Garner J, Jarvis W, Emori T, et al. CDC definitions for nosocomial infections. Am J Infect Control 1988;16:128–140.
106. O'Grady N, Alexander M, Dellinger E, et al. Guidelines for the prevention of intravascular catheter-related infections. Centers for Disease Control and Prevention. MMWR Morb Mortal Wkly Rep 2002;51:1–29.
107. Wisplinghoff H, Bischoff T, Tallent S, et al. Nosocomial bloodstream infections in U.S. hospitals: analysis of 24,179 cases from a prospective nationwide surveillance study. Clin Infect Dis 2004;39:309–317.
108. Mermel L, Farr B, Sherertz R, et al. Infectious Diseases Society of America, American College of Critical Care Medicine, and Society for Healthcare Epidemiology of America. Guidelines for the management of intravascular catheter related infections. Clin Infect Dis 2001;32:1249–1272.
109. Cobb D, High K, Sawyer R, et al. A controlled trial of scheduled replacement of central venous and pulmonary-artery catheters. N Engl J Med 1992;327:1062–1068.
110. Raad I, Hohn D, Gilbreath B, et al. Prevention of central venous catheter-related infections by using maximal sterile barrier precautions during insertion. Infect Control Hosp Epidemiol 1994;15:231–238.
111. Maki D, Ringer M, Alvarado C. Prospective randomised trial of povidone-iodine, alcohol, and chlorhexidine for prevention of infection associated with central venous and arterial catheters. Lancet 1991;338:339–343.
112. Darouiche R, Raad I, Heard S, et al. A comparison of two antimicrobial-impregnated central venous catheters. N Engl J Med 1999;340:1–8.
113. Veenstra D, Saint S, Sullivan S. Cost-effectiveness of antiseptic-impregnated central venous catheter for the prevention of catheter-related bloodstream infection. JAMA 1999;282:554–560.
114. Veenstra D, Saint S, Saha S, et al. Efficacy of antiseptic-impregnated central venous catheters in preventing catheter-related bloodstream infection. A meta-analysis. JAMA 1999; 281:261–267.
115. Maki D, Stolz, S, Wheeler S, et al. Prevention of central venous catheter-related bloodstream infection by use of an antiseptic-impregnated catheter. A randomized, controlled trial. Ann Intern Med 1997;127:257–266.
116. Raad I, Darouiche R, Dupuis J, et al. A central venous catheter coated with minocycline and rifampin for the prevention of catheter-related colonization and bloodstream infections. A randomized, double-blind trial. Ann Intern Med 1997;127:267–274.
117. Sherertz R, Ely E, Westbrook D, et al. Education of physicians-in-training can decrease the risk for vascular catheter infection. Ann Intern Med 2000;132:641–648.
118. Coopersmith C, Rebmann T, Zack J, et al. Effect of an education program on decreasing catheter-related bloodstream infections in the surgical intensive care unit. Crit Care Med 2002;30:59–64.
119. Warren D, Zack J, Cox M, et al. An educational intervention to prevent catheter-associated bloodstream infections in a non-teaching, community medical center. Crit Care Med 2003;31: 1959–1963.
120. Warren J. Catheter-associated urinary tract infections. Int J Antimicrob Agents 2001;17:299–303.
121. Stamm W. Catheter-associated urinary tract infections: epidemiology, pathogenesis, and prevention. Am J Med 1991;91:65S–71S.
122. Haley R, Hooton T, Culver D, et al. Nosocomial infections in U.S. hospitals, 1975–1976: estimated frequency by selected characteristics of patients. Am J Med 1981;70:947–59.
123. Saint S, Wiese J, Amory J, et al. Are physicians aware of which of their patients have indwelling urinary catheters? Am J Med 2000;109:476–480.
124. Warren J. Catheter-associated urinary tract infections. Infect Dis Clin North Am 1997;11:609–622.
125. Warren J, Platt R, Thomas R, et al. Antibiotic irrigation and catheter-associated urinary-tract infections. N Engl J Med 1978; 299:570–573.
126. Saint S. Clinical and economic consequences of nosocomial catheter related bacteriuria. Am J Infect Control 2000;28:68–75.

127. Silveira F, Fujitani S, Paterson D. Antibiotic-resistant infections in the critically ill adult. Clin Lab Med 2004;24:329–341.
128. Wagenlehner F, Naber, K. Hospital-acquired urinary tract infections. J Hosp Infect 2000;46:171–181.
129. Tambyah P. Catheter-associated urinary tract infections: diagnosis and prophylaxis. Int J Antimicrob Agents 2004;24S;S44–S48.
130. Tambyah P, Halvorson K, Maki D. A prospective study of the pathogenesis of catheter-associated urinary tract infection. Mayo Clin Proc 1999;74:131–136.
131. Platt R, Polk B, Murdock B, et al. Risk factors for nosocomial urinary tract infection. Am J Epidemiol 1986;124:977–985.
132. Johnson J, Roberts P, Olsen R, et al. Prevention of catheter-associated urinary tract infection with a silver oxide-coated urinary catheter: clinical and microbiologic correlates. J Infect Dis 1990;162:1145–1150.
133. Riley D, Classen D, Stevens L, et al. A large randomized clinical trial of a silver-impregnated urinary catheter: lack of efficacy and staphylococcal superinfection. Am J Med 1995;98:349–356.
134. Stark R, Maki D. Bacteriuria in the catheterized patient. What quantitative level of bacteriuria is relevant? N Engl J Med 1984; 311:560–564.
135. Urinary Tract Infection (UTI) Working Group: Naber K, Bergman B, et al. EAU guidelines for the management of urinary and male genital tract infections. Eur Urol 2001;40:576–588.
136. Tambyah P, Maki D. Catheter-associated urinary tract infection is rarely symptomatic: a prospective study of 1497 catheterized patients. Arch Intern Med 2000;160:678–682.
137. Ronald A. The etiology of urinary tract infection: traditional and emerging pathogens. Am J Med 2002;113:14S–19S.
138. Wagenlehner F, Naber K. New drugs for gram-positive uropathogens. Int J Antimicrob Agents 2004;24S:S39–S43.
139. Carson C, Naber K. Role of fluroquinolones in the treatment of serious bacterial urinary infections. Drugs 2004;64:1359–1373.
140. Talan D, Klimberg I, Nicolle L, et al. Once daily extended release ciprofloxacin for complicated urinary tract infections and acute uncomplicated pyelonephritis. J Urol 2004;171:734–739.
141. Maki D, Tambyah P. Engineering out the risk for infection with urinary catheters. Emerg Infect Dis 2001;7:342–347.
142. Ouslander J, Greengold B, Chen S. External catheter use and urinary tract infections among incontinent male nursing home patients. J Am Geriatr Soc 1987;35:1063–1070.
143. Huth T, Burke J, Larsen R, et al. Clinical trial of junction seals for the prevention of urinary catheter-associated bacteriuria. Arch Intern Med 1992;152:807–812.
144. Kunin C, McCormack R. Prevention of catheter-induced urinary-tract infections by a new sterile closed drainage system. Antimicrobial Agents Chemother 1965;5:631–638.
145. Classen D, Larsen R, Burke J, et al. Prevention of catheter-associated bacteriuria: clinical trial of methods to block three known pathways of infection. Am J Infect Control 1991;19:136–142.
146. Darouiche R, Smith J, Hanna H, et al. Efficacy of antimicrobial-impregnated bladder catheters in reducing catheter-associated bacteriuria: a prospective, randomized, multicenter clinical trial. Urology 1999;54:976–981.
147. Karchmer T, Giannetta E, Muto C, et al. A randomized crossover study of silver-coated urinary catheters in hospitalized patients. Arch Intern Med 2000;160:3294–3298.
148. Johnson J, Roberts P, Olsen R, et al. Prevention of catheter-associated urinary tract infection with a silver oxide-coated urinary catheter: clinical and microbiologic correlates. J Infect Dis 1990;162:1145–1150.
149. Saint S, Elmore J, Sullivan S, et al. The efficacy of silver alloy-coated urinary catheters in preventing urinary tract infection: a meta-analysis. Am J Med 1998;105:236–241.
150. Karchmer T, Giannetta E, Muto C, et al. A randomized crossover study of silver-coated urinary catheters in hospitalized patients. Arch Intern Med 2000;160:3294–3298.
151. Maki D, Knasinski V, Halvorson K, et al. A novel silver hydrogel-impregnated indwelling urinary catheter reduces catheter related urinary tract infections: a prospective double-blind trial [abstract]. Infect Control Hosp Epidemiol 1998;19:682.
152. Thibon P, Le Coutour X, Leroyer R, et al. Randomized multicentre trial of the effects of a catheter coated with hydrogel and silver salts on the incidence of hospital-acquired urinary tract infections. J Hosp Infect 2000;45:117–124.
153. Verleyen P, De Ridder D, Van Poppel H, et al. Clinical application of the Bardex IC Foley catheter. Eur Urol 1999;36:240–246.
154. Bologna R, Tu L, Polansky M, et al. Hydrogel/silver ion-coated urinary catheter reduces nosocomial urinary tract infection rates in intensive care unit patients: a multicenter study. Urology 1999;54:982–987.
155. Gerding D, Johnson S, Peterson LR, et al. *Clostridium difficile*-associated diarrhea and colitis. Infect Control Hosp Epidemiol 1995;16:459–477.
156. Archibald L, Banerjee S, Jarvis W. Secular trends in hospital-acquired *C. difficile* disease in the United States 1897–2001. J Infect Dis 2004;189:1585–1589.
157. Oldfield E. *Clostridium difficile*-associated diarrhea: risk factors, diagnostic methods, and treatment. Rev Gastroenterol Disord 2004;4:186–195.
158. Bricker E, Garg R, Nelson R. Antibiotic treatment of *Clostridium difficile*-associated diarrhea in adults. Cochrane Database Syst Rev 2005;1CD 004610, pub2.
159. Vandenbussche T, De Moor S, Bachert C, et al. Value of antral puncture in the intensive care patient with fever of unknown origin. Laryngoscope 2000;110:1702–1706.
160. LeMoal G, Lemerre D, Grollier G, et al. Nosocomial sinusitis with isolation of anaerobic bacteria in ICU patients. Intensive Care Med 1999;25:1066–1071.
161. Merle V, Germain JM, Bugel H, et al. Nosocomial urinary tract infections in urologic patients: assessment of a prospective surveillance program including 10,000 patients. Eur Urol 2002;41: 48–49.
161. Jones RN, Kugler KC, Pfaller MA, et al. Characteristics of pathogens causing urinary tract infections in hospitals in North America: results from the SENTRY Antimicrobial Surveillance Program 1997. Diagn Microbiol Infect Dis 1999;35:55–63.

15

Severe Sepsis and Septic Shock

Steven M. Opal

This chapter reviews the remarkable recent advances in the understanding of the molecular basis that underlies the pathophysiology of sepsis. This knowledge has improved diagnostic techniques and introduced new therapeutic agents into the standard management of patients with severe sepsis/septic shock. The current treatment regimens for sepsis are discussed, and the evidence to support each major treatment strategy is outlined in detail. Research priorities to further the optimal management of septic shock in the future are highlighted.

Sepsis: Definitions and Epidemiology

Definitions

The terminology used to describe the septic process is, by necessity, imprecise and lacking in analytical clarity since there is no single, universally accepted, diagnostic or confirmatory test for sepsis. This has plagued the field of sepsis research as the majority of intensive care specialists in a recent survey[1] felt that the current definitions are inadequate and frequently miss the correct diagnosis. The loosely applied term *sepsis* is used to connote a syndrome when a patient develops a deleterious systemic host response to an infectious process. In its early stages, sepsis can be difficult to distinguish from an appropriate and localized inflammatory reaction to an uncomplicated infection. The innate immune response and coagulation networks evolved to defend the host from blood loss and generalized infection following minor injury. These same inflammatory and clotting systems can be detrimental when they become excessive or dysfunctional, as they often become following major injury or systemic infection.

The clinical syndrome of sepsis becomes more readily recognizable and distinguishable for controlled inflammation when overt signs of systemic inflammatory responses, tissue hypoperfusion, and organ dysfunction develop. According to current consensus definitions,[2] sepsis accompanied by objective signs of organ dysfunction is classified as *severe sepsis.* It is often apparent only in retrospect that the patient was "becoming septic," and that subtle, telltale signs were progressing to a potentially devastating pathologic state such as severe sepsis. *Septic shock* is defined as sepsis complicated by organ dysfunction and systemic hypotension refractory to an adequate fluid challenge. These definitions are independent of the nature of the infecting microorganism, and they correctly acknowledge the central role of the host inflammatory and coagulation response rather than microbial factors in the pathogenesis of sepsis. A brief summary of the recommended terminology of sepsis definitions is listed in Table 15.1. While these consensus definitions are imperfect and have limitations,[1] they have stood the test of time, and the sepsis definitions in common parlance today are still useful as working definitions for clinical use and for comparative clinical trials.[2]

Epidemiology and Secular Trends

Sepsis, and the associated multiorgan failure that often accompanies this systemic inflammatory process, remains a leading cause of mortality in the intensive care units (ICUs) worldwide.[3] It is currently estimated that as many as 700,000 patients develop severe sepsis each year in the United States,[4,5] with similar incidence rates in several European countries.[6,7] The incidence of severe sepsis/septic shock has continuously increased over the past three decades, and the occurrence of sepsis likely will further increase over the next several decades as the population of elderly and vulnerable patients continues to expand. The mortality rate for fully developed septic shock remains between 35% and 45% despite recent improvements in treatment options and outcome.[2,7–9] The outcome in sepsis is highly variable and dependent on a large number of preexisting and physiological elements; nonetheless, it is clear that this process alone accounts for hundreds of thousands of deaths per year.[4,5]

The incidence of sepsis is increasing for several reasons, but primary among them is the fact that sepsis largely has become a disease of medical progress. While sepsis certainly

TABLE 15.1. Classification and Working Definitions of Sepsis.

Term	*Definition*	*Comments*
Bacteremia (or fungemia)	Presence of viable bacteria (or fungi) in the bloodstream	Bacteremia or fungemia is not necessary or sufficient for the diagnosis of sepsis. Microorganisms may transit the bloodstream briefly and without clinical consequences; fatal septic shock may occur in the absence of documented bacteremia or fungemia.
Sepsis	A clinical syndrome manifested as a deleterious host response to an infectious process	Infection (local or systemic) accompanied by a systemic inflammatory response (e.g., fever, leukocytosis, tachycardia, tachypnea). It may be difficult to distinguish a physiologic host response to infection from a deleterious (septic) response.
Severe sepsis	Sepsis complicated by one or more major organ dysfunction(s)	Sepsis-induced organ dysfunction (central nervous system dysfunction, acute lung injury, renal failure, hepatic dysfunction, coagulopathy, metabolic acidosis, cardiovascular dysfunction) remote from the site of active infection; this should be distinguished from preexisting organ dysfunction.
Septic shock	Severe sepsis with systemic hypotension refractory to early fluid therapy	This is clinically defined as failure to maintain a systolic blood pressure above 90 mmHg (or mean arterial pressure >65 mmHg) following an adequate fluid challenge (>40 ml/kg over 6 h).

Source: From Levy et al.,[2] by permission of *Critical Care Medicine.*

occurs in previously healthy persons (e.g., meningococcal sepsis, toxic shock syndrome, and severe community-acquired pneumonia), the majority of septic patients have significant underlying diseases that place them at risk for sepsis.[10] Successful management of a variety of severe trauma situations and medical illnesses and advances in surgical interventions are salvaging patients who only a few generations ago would have rapidly succumbed. This has produced a large susceptible population of patients with prolonged critical illness and impaired host defenses.[11] These patients have a greatly increased risk of developing sepsis. Innovations in organ transplantation, implanted prosthetic devices, and long-term vascular access devices continue to expand in this patient population. The gradual aging of the population in many developed countries and the increasing prevalence of antibiotic-resistant microbial pathogens also conspire to increase the incidence of severe sepsis/septic shock.

In a study by Martin et al., over 10 million cases of sepsis from the National Hospital Discharge Survey were reviewed over a 21-year time period throughout the United States.[5] They found that the incidence of sepsis increased by an average of 8.7% per year from 1979 to 2000, from 82.7 to 240/100,000 population. Sepsis was consistently and significantly more common in men than women and more common in non-white populations compared to white populations. The mean age of patients with severe sepsis was 60 years,[5] but the incidence of sepsis by age was heavily splayed to the extremes of age, with a small peak in the neonatal period and a marked and progressive rise in sepsis in the elderly after age 65.[4]

Gram-positive bacterial pathogens now outnumber gram-negative pathogens as a cause of sepsis, and the incidence of fungal sepsis has increased by over 200% in the past two decades. While the incidence has progressively increased, the overall crude mortality rate has steadily decreased to less than 18% from 27.9% average 20 years earlier.[5] Similar findings have been reported in a large French study, with significant improvements in management outcomes from sepsis noted over the past decade.[10]

The human resource losses attributable to sepsis for affected patients, family members, and society in terms of years of life lost, long-term disability, and diminished quality-of-life indices are enormous and incalculable. Recent evidence indicates that the long-term disability suffered by survivors of sepsis and other critical illnesses is considerable.[12] The financial implications in health care expenditures for the management of sepsis are daunting as well. Each episode of severe sepsis extends the average hospital length of stay by 11 additional days and costs approximately $40,000/episode. The added costs accrued from sepsis that develops in patients while hospitalized for other medical or surgical indications may be even higher.[13] Angus and colleagues estimated that expenditures in the United States for sepsis alone account for an incremental annual cost of nearly $17 billion.[4]

Sepsis Pathogenesis

Predisposing Factors

Severe sepsis and septic shock usually arise in an unexpected fashion in patients who have another primary illness,[10] and the severity of the underlying illness is a principal determinant of the mortality rate attributable to sepsis. This relationship was first noted by Jackson and McCabe several decades ago,[14] and it remains true today despite numerous advances and innovations in supportive care and in medical and surgical management.[15] The source of the septic focus has repeatedly been shown to have a major impact on the risk of adverse outcome from sepsis. Catheter-related sepsis and urinary tract infections have the most favorable prognosis, while intraabdominal sites of sepsis and pulmonary sources of sepsis are associated with the worst outcome.[16,17]

The risk of disseminated infection and sepsis following the onset of tissue invasion by pathogens from an initial site of injury varies markedly depending on the type of infection, location and degree of tissue invasion, and the intrinsic virulence of the causative pathogen. The likelihood of developing multiorgan dysfunction, hemodynamic compromise, and lethal septic shock after infection begins is heavily dependent on the antimicrobial defense capacity and fundamental nature of the individual host response to the microbial challenge. Many hereditary and acquired factors contribute to the risk of severe sepsis following similar types of microbial challenge. While it is widely appreciated that the elderly patient,[18] the neutropenic patient,[19] and the asplenic patient[20] all have readily measurable differences in outcome when compared with the same type of systemic infection in an otherwise healthy young adult, it is increasingly apparent that much of the mortality risk from sepsis is actually determined by our genomic background.[21]

An expanding array of polymorphisms in immune response and regulatory genes are known to potentially affect the risk of sepsis and its outcome.[22–33] A major research priority in clinical research at present is the development of an information system that can rapidly and correctly identify and balance the influence of all the relevant genes and gene products that ultimately determine the fate of patients with systemic inflammatory states. The magnitude, dynamics, and complexity of interacting networks that contribute to acute inflammatory states such as sepsis indicate that deciphering this process in real-time patient care settings will be a challenge indeed. An entirely different conceptual framework on which to formulate a greater understanding of sepsis pathophysiology may be required to adequately integrate this information.

An initial attempt at accomplishing the goal of reanalyzing sepsis in the genomic era has been proposed as the PIRO system,[2] which stands for predisposing factors, infection, response, and organ dysfunction. This classification system is depicted in Table 15.2 and is fashioned after the TNM (tumor, nodes, metastases) system in codifying malignant diseases. It is predicated on the hypothesis that breaking down sepsis into its component parts (the reductionist approach to complexity) will lead to an improved understanding of the mechanisms that underlie sepsis itself. Intuitively, a classification scheme that adequately separates a number of important and easily recognizable subgroups of patients with very different risk factors for the development of sepsis, and risk of death from sepsis, is an appealing strategy in better understanding sepsis in general.

Microbial Factors

Microbial Mediators

The microbiology of sepsis (or the I in the PIRO system) has changed over the past 50 years from what was once a primarily gram-negative bacterial infection in the 1950s through the 1980s (previously termed *gram-negative sepsis* or *endotoxic shock*) to what is now principally a gram-positive bacterial process.[5] The ubiquitous use of vascular catheters, other implantable devices, progressive antibiotic resistance among gram-positive bacteria, and improved antimicrobial agents against gram-negative bacterial pathogens have all contributed to the progressive emergence of gram-positive bacterial pathogens as the major causative microorganisms of sepsis by the beginning of the 21st century.[34]

Fungal organisms are increasingly recognized as important pathogens as a cause of sepsis in ICU patients, and these infections are associated with a markedly increased mortality rate compared to bacterial sepsis.[4,16] Polymicrobial infections account for up to 30% of severe sepsis and are primarily related to complex infections such as a contaminated wound, perforated viscus, or intraabdominal abscess.[16] No clear microbial agent is recognized in approximately 15% of septic patients, and this is most often attributable to the widespread use of empiric antibiotic therapy that obscures culture documentation of infection. Translocation and circulation of microbial mediators in the absence of viable and cultivatable

TABLE 15.2. The PIRO Conceptual Framework for the Study of Sepsis.

Category	*Specific element*	*Comments*
P: Predisposing factors	Recognition of preexisting conditions in sepsis pathogenesis (immunodeficiency, diabetes, cancer, chronic disease states, medications); genetic factors; nutritional, age, and gender differences	The use of genomics and proteomics may define genetic polymorphisms of the immune response to systemic infection; need to recognize important patient subgroups based on baseline predisposing factors.
I: Infection	Accounts for differences in the site of infection, quantity, and intrinsic virulence of each type of infecting microorganism; different causative organisms induce different signaling networks within the innate immune and coagulation systems	Outcomes differ in sepsis depending on the site of infection and number and type of pathogen. Rapid microbial detection systems (LPS, lipopeptides, fungal elements, bacterial DNA or RNA) may direct sepsis therapies according to the nature of the pathogen.
R: Response	Mortality risk primarily determined by the patient's response to sepsis; optimal host mediator-targeted therapy predicated on ability to rapidly assess individual host responses	Markers of inflammation (PCT or IL-6); status of host responsiveness (e.g., HLA-DR, TNF receptor, or TLR density); or gene transcript profiles by genomics and proteomics may guide individualized therapy in the future.
O: Organ dysfunction	Preexisting organ damage and variations in the pattern of organ dysfunction affect outcome in sepsis; organ damage caused by microbial pathogen or its toxins requires different approach than remote organ injury from host immune response	Dynamic measures of organ-specific cellular and microcirculatory responses to infection or insult (apoptosis, cytopathic hypoxia, cell stress, and energy depletion) may provide a system to guide therapy for individual patient needs.

HLA, human leukocyte antigen; IL, interleukin; LPS, lipopolysaccharide; PCT, procalcitonin; TLR, Toll-like receptor; TNF, tumor necrosis factor.

Source: Adapted from Levy et al.,[2] by permission of *Critical Care Medicine*.

microorganisms may also account for some cases of "culture-negative" sepsis.[35]

Role of Endotoxin

Bacterial endotoxin, which is composed of lipopolysaccharide (LPS), is an intrinsic component of the outer membrane of gram-negative bacteria and is essential for the viability of enteric bacteria.[36] An endotoxin-deficient strain of *Neisseria meningitidis* has been isolated that is viable and is 10- to 100-fold less potent an inducer of cytokine production than wild-type bacteria.[37] Lipopolysaccharide is a phosphorylated, polar macromolecule that contains hydrophobic elements in the fatty acids of its lipid A core structure and hydrophilic elements in its repeating polysaccharide surface components.

Humans are one of the most susceptible species to the profound immunostimulant properties of endotoxin, which may be lethal following intravenous challenge in minute doses. Whether endotoxin is released into the human circulatory system in its free form (released from dead organisms or shed from the membrane of viable organisms as microparticles) or bound to the cell wall of intact bacteria, an intense systemic inflammatory response results. Endotoxin in the prototypic pathogen-associated molecular pattern (PAMP) that functions to alert the host's innate immune defenses to the presence of invading gram-negative bacteria.[38] It is the host response to the systemic release of endotoxin (or other PAMPs), rather than the endotoxin itself, that accounts for its potentially lethal consequences.[2]

In human plasma, endotoxin immediately comes in contact with endotoxin-binding proteins, the most important of which is LPS-binding protein (LBP).[39] This protein facilitates the transfer of LPS to the surface of immune effector cells expressing the anchoring receptor molecule CD14.[40] Another endogenous LBP in plasma is bactericidal permeability-increasing protein (BPI),[41] which is principally expressed on neutrophil membranes and primary granules. Bactericidal permeability-increasing protein binds with high affinity to LPS and is a potent inhibitor of endotoxin activity. The concentration of LBP in the plasma is two to three orders of magnitude higher than that of BPI, and therefore, most of the LPS released in the plasma binds to LBP and is efficiently carried to myeloid cells in its active form. The BPI functions as an endogenous antiendotoxin molecule, and systemic infusions of high levels of BPI may become a treatment strategy for endotoxin-induced injury.[42]

The long-sought-after primary cellular receptor for endotoxin on immune cells has been identified.[43–45] The Toll-like receptors (TLRs) are type 1 transmembrane receptors and are now known to be the receptors for multiple microbial structures such as endotoxin, peptidoglycan, bacterial lipopeptides, viral and bacterial nucleic acids, flagella, and lipoteichoic acid. The TLRs belong to a network of pattern recognition receptors of the innate immune system that alert effectors cells to the presence of a microbial pathogen.[38] This system includes up to 11 TLRs, CD14, and components of the alternate complement system and mannose-binding lectin system (Table 15.3).[46–50]

TABLE 15.3. Human Toll-like Receptors, Their Ligands, and Other Pattern Recognition Receptors.

Receptor	*Major cell type*	*Known actions and recognized ligands*
TLR1	Myeloid cells, T and B lymphocytes, NK cells	Forms heterodimers with TLR2 for bacterial lipopeptide, outer surface proteins of *Borrelia* spp., and possibly other microbial ligands
TLR2	Myeloid cells, T cells	Bacterial and *Mycoplasma* lipopeptide, ? peptidoglycan; lipoarabinomannan from *Mycobacteria*, lipoteichoic acid, fungal cell wall components, LPS of spirochetes
TLR3	Dendritic cells, epithelial cells	Double-stranded viral RNA probably signals from inside endosomal vacuoles
TLR4	Myeloid cells	LPS, respiratory syncytial virus proteins, HSP60, fibrinogen, heparan sulfate
TLR5	Myeloid cells, epithelial cells	Flagellin from gram-positive or gram-negative bacteria
TLR6	Myeloid cells, dendritic cells	Forms heterodimers with TLR2 in recognition of *Mycoplasma* lipopeptides and fungal elements (zymosan)
TLR7	B cells, plasmacytoid dendritic cells	Binds to single-strand (ss) RNA in mice (? humans); binds to antiviral compounds, imidazoquinolines[47]
TLR8	Myeloid cells, dendritic cells	Recognizes ssRNA in humans inside intracellular endosomes; binds imidazoquinolines[47]
TLR9	B cells, plasmacytoid dendritic cells, epithelial cells	Unmethylated CpG motifs in microbial DNA; signaling occurs inside endosomal vacuoles
TLR10	B cells, myeloid cells	Unknown, may interact with TLR2 to form heterodimers
TLR11	Macrophages, uroepithelial cells	Recognizes uropathogenic bacteria in the urogenital tract in mice (? humans)[48]
CD14	Myeloid cells	Recognizes LPS, peptidoglycan, lipoarabinomannan, fungal antigens; binds with TLRs for cell signaling
Alternate C pathway	Plasma proteins	Pathogen-associated molecular patterns that are exposed to the C3 thioester bond[49]
MBL	Plasma protein	Recognizes mannosides expressed on bacterial, fungal, viral surfaces and activates C4 and C2[50]

C′, complement; HSP, heat-shock protein; LPS, lipopolysaccharide; MBL, mannose-binding lectin; TLR, Toll-like receptor.

Source: Adapted from Cristofaro and Opal,[46] by permission of *Expert Opinion on Therapeutic Targets*.

The principal endotoxin transmembrane receptor is TLR4.[43] It functions along with an extracellular adaptor protein known as MD2 and a critically important pattern recognition receptor CD14 that anchors microbial antigens to the surface of myeloid cells.[39,51] These surface receptor molecules aggregate on membrane regions known as *lipid rafts* where the intracellular signaling process begins. The precise mechanisms by which TLR4 activates gene transcription of cytokines, acute-phase proteins, coagulation, and nitric oxide synthase (NOS) are known in considerable detail (Fig. 15.1),[46] although other regulatory and accessory pathways of gene induction and control have not yet been fully characterized.[23] A well-characterized series of tyrosine and theonine/serine kinases is activated by TLR4 engagement with LPS, and this intracellular signaling leads to phosphorylation of IκB (inhibitor of nuclear factor kappa B [NF-κB]). This releases the transcriptional activator NFκB from the cytoplasm and allows it to translocate into the nucleus. The NFκB and a number of other of transcriptional activators are transferred to the nucleus, where hundreds of genes are activated or suppressed in response to the presence of endotoxin.[52,53] Details of these events and interactions are important as they form the molecular basis for novel therapeutic agents to treat sepsis.

The receptor TLR2 recognizes a large number of bacterial, fungal, mycobacterial, and mycoplasma surface structures in heterodimeric combination with either TLR1 or TLR6.[54] Toll-like receptor 9 is the cellular receptor for unmethylated CpG motifs found in bacterial DNA,[55] while TLR3 recognizes double-strain viral RNA,[56] and TLR8 detects single-strand RNA.[47] Also, TLR5 recognizes bacterial flagellin found on motile gram-positive and gram-negative bacteria.[57]

The TLRs belong to the pattern recognition molecules' innate immune system and initiate this rather nonspecific, antimicrobial defense system. It lacks the precision of the highly specific and clonal acquired immune system (B cells and T cells), yet its rapid reaction time in phagocytosis and clearance of pathogens in the early phases of microbial invasion makes the innate immune response a critical host defense mechanism. Excessive activation and disordered regulation of the innate immune system and its cellular components (neutrophils, monocytes, macrophages, natural killer [NK] cells) are primarily responsible for the pathogenesis of early septic shock.[23,38] Elements of the acquired immune system and defects in adaptive immunity may play a pivotal role in toxic shock syndromes[58] and in the later stages of sepsis (the late immune-suppressive phase of sepsis).[59]

Bacterial Superantigens

Another important microbial mediator in some forms of septic shock from gram-positive bacterial pathogens is bacterial superantigen. Superantigens are a unique group of microbially derived protein antigens found in some streptococci,

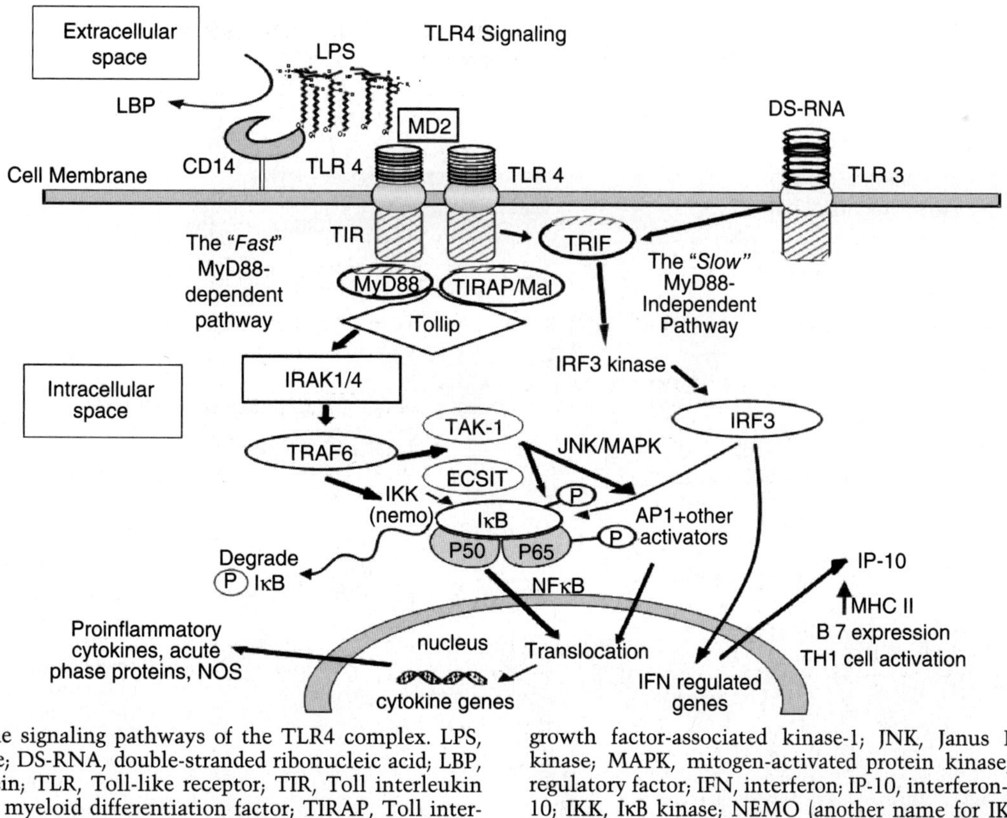

FIGURE 15.1. The signaling pathways of the TLR4 complex. LPS, lipopolysaccharide; DS-RNA, double-stranded ribonucleic acid; LBP, LPS-binding protein; TLR, Toll-like receptor; TIR, Toll interleukin receptor; MyD88, myeloid differentiation factor; TIRAP, Toll interleukin receptor adapter protein; Mal, MyD88 adapter like; Tollip, Toll interactive protein; TRIF, TIR domain adapter inducing interferon-γ; IRAK, interleukin 1 receptor-associated kinase; TRAF6, tumor necrosis factor receptor associated factor 6; ECSIT, evolutionarily conserved signaling intermediate of Toll; TAK-1, transforming growth factor-associated kinase-1; JNK, Janus N-terminal-linked kinase; MAPK, mitogen-activated protein kinase; IRF3, interferon regulatory factor; IFN, interferon; IP-10, interferon-inducible protein-10; IKK, IκB kinase; NEMO (another name for IKK-NFκB essential modulator); IκB, inhibitory subunit κB; NFκB, nuclear factor κB; MHC, major histocompatibility complex; NOS, nitric oxide synthase; TH_1, type 1 thymic-derived $CD4^+$ lymphocyte helper cells. (*Source:* Modified from Cristofaro and Opal,[46] by permission of Expert Opinion on Therapeutic Targets.)

staphylococci, and perhaps other pathogens; each possesses an unusual immunologic property. These superantigens have the capacity to rapidly activate large numbers of $CD4^+$ T cells by circumventing the conventional antigen-processing and presentation system of adaptive immunity.[58]

Conventional protein antigens are internalized by antigen-presenting cells (APCs) and undergo limited proteolysis. They are then processed within the endosomal component of macrophages or dendritic cells. Appropriate size peptide sequences of these antigens (epitopes) are then processed and inserted into the central groove of major histocompatibility (MHC) class II molecules on the membrane surface of APCs. Specific, clonotypic $CD4^+$ T cells that recognize each unique epitope are then activated. Clonal expansion of this small subset of T cells results in a physiologic immune response to the neoantigen.[60]

Superantigens, by contrast, do not undergo processing by APCs and bind directly to class II molecules outside the epitope-specific peptide groove on APCs. Superantigens then bind to the Vβ region of the T-cell receptor (TCR) on $CD4^+$ T cells. This binding brings $CD4^+$ T cells, and APC forms a bridge that then activates both the APC and T-cell populations expressing the appropriate Vβ region of the TCR. Conventional peptide antigens specifically stimulate about 1 in 10^5 circulating lymphocytes that can recognize its unique epitope. Superantigens such as the toxic shock syndrome toxin-1 from *Staphylococcus aureus* binds to the Vβ2 region of T cells that is found in up to 10%–20% of human lymphocyte populations.[58] This activates large numbers of both lymphocytes and macrophages, and the synthesis and release of proinflammatory cytokines proceeds in an uncontrolled fashion. Staphylococcal and streptococcal strains can produce a variety of different superantigenic exotoxins capable of widespread immune activation if introduced into the circulation.[58,60,61]

Superantigen-induced immune activation may terminate in a form of septic shock known as toxic shock syndrome if the source of the superantigen is not expeditiously removed. Polymicrobial infections that release both bacterial superantigens and endotoxin may be particularly injurious to the host. The systemic toxicity of bacterial endotoxin is magnified by immune activation by superantigens that prime the immune system to overreact to endotoxin signaling (Fig. 15.2).[62]

Peptidoglycan from the cell wall of bacteria, capsular antigens, lipoteichoic acid, lipopeptides, microbial DNA, viral RNA, fungal elements, microbial toxins, and procoagulant substances produced by microbial pathogens may all contribute to the pathogenesis of sepsis. Peptidoglycan and lipopeptides from gram-positive bacteria interact with CD14 molecules and activate inflammatory cells via TLR2 in a manner comparable to that observed by bacterial endotoxin.[54] Moreover, gram-positive bacterial and fungal pathogens may induce hypotension with redistribution of blood flow and splanchnic vasoconstriction. The ischemia and reperfusion of blood vessels that supply the mucosal surfaces of the gastrointestinal (GI) tract may disrupt the permeability barrier to bacterial products. Translocation of microbial antigens, including bacterial endotoxin, may occur during periods of hypoperfusion of the GI mucosa.[63] This injurious process has prompted interest in efforts to boost the GI mucosal barrier through immunonutrition, epithelial growth factors, and selective decontamination of the GI tract in critical illness.

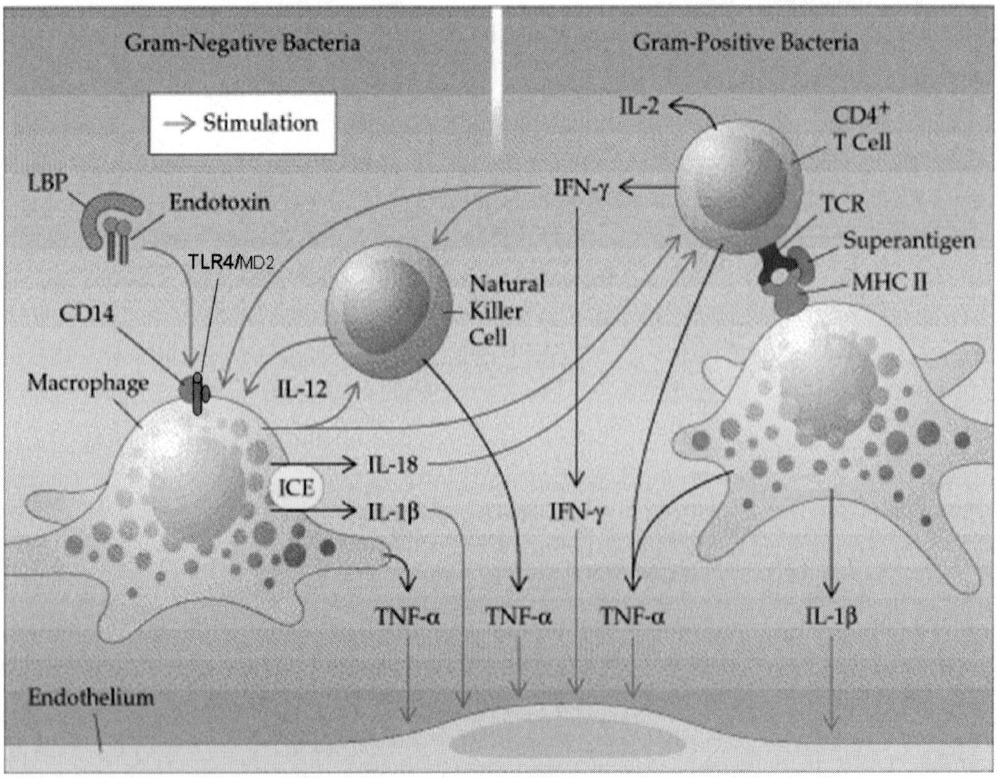

FIGURE 15.2. Interactions between bacterial endotoxin and bacterial superantigen. Interactions between bacterial endotoxin and bacterial superantigens. CD4, $CD4^+$ T cell; TLR2/4, Toll-like receptor 2/4; ICE, interleukin-1β converting enzyme (also known as caspase 1); IFN-γ, interferon-γ; IL, interleukin; LBP, LPS-binding protein; TNF-α, tumor necrosis factor-α. (*Source:* Modified from Opal and Huber,[62] with permission from *Scientific American Medicine.*)

Host Response

Cytokine Networks

Proinflammatory cytokines play a pivotal role in the pathogenesis of sepsis. In animal studies, the administration of human tumor necrosis factor-α (TNF-α), an endogenous monocyte-macrophage-derived protein, is potentially lethal,[64] and pronounced hemodynamic, metabolic, and hematologic changes occurred when TNF-α was administered to human volunteers.[65] Hypotension induced by even minute amounts of interleukin-1α (IL-1α) when given as an infusion to humans is a graphic demonstration of the pathologic potential of proinflammatory cytokines.[66]

The major proinflammatory cytokines, TNF-α and IL-1β, function in concert with an expanding group of host-derived proinflammatory mediators and an equally impressive array of antiinflammatory mediators that work in a coordinated fashion to produce the systemic inflammatory response (see Table 15.4). Cytokines and chemokines function as a network of communication signals among neutrophils, monocytes, macrophages, lymphocytes, and endothelial cells. Autocrine and paracrine activation amplifies cytokine signaling of the inflammatory response within the microenvironment once it is activated by a systemic microbial challenge (e.g., endotoxemia). Much of the proinflammatory response is compartmentalized within the proximal region of initial injury (e.g., lung tissue or peritoneum). If local control is not achieved, then the inflammatory response spills over into the systemic circulation, resulting in a generalized reaction with endothelial injury, coagulation activation, and remote organ injury. The endocrine-like effects of the circulating cytokines and chemokines maintain the generalized inflammatory process that typifies the septic state.[67,68]

The proinflammatory mediators are activated in the early phases of sepsis (the first 12 to 24 h) and are rapidly countered by the endogenous antiinflammatory components of the systemic immune response. Cytokine antagonists, decoy receptors, soluble receptors, antiinflammatory cytokines, and downregulation of tissue receptors prevail in the later phases of sepsis.[59] Mice deficient in T cells and B cells respond to endotoxin challenge in the same manner as normal mice,[69] indicating that neutrophils and monocyte-macrophage generated cytokines are sufficient to induce the early septic process. Lymphocyte activity and their cytokines and interferons become important in the regulation of later phases of sepsis and may ultimately determine the outcome in septic shock.

Immune-Refractory State of Sepsis

Important functional differences exist within $CD4^+$ T cells. Activated, yet uncommitted, $CD4^+$ T cells (TH_0 cells) have two major pathways of functional differentiation. The T cells exposed to IL-12 in the presence of IL-2 are driven toward a TH_1-type functional development. These cells produce large quantities of interferon-γ (IFN-γ), TNF-α, and IL-2 and promote a proinflammatory, cell-mediated immune response. Uncommitted $CD4^+$ T cells exposed to IL-4 will preferentially develop into a TH_2-type phenotype; TH_2 cells secrete IL-4, IL-10, and IL-13. These cytokines promote humoral immune responses and attenuate macrophage and neutrophil activity.[70]

The TH_1-type cytokines suppress the expression of TH_2-type cytokines. Interferon-γ inhibits the synthesis of IL-10; conversely, the TH_2-cell-derived cytokine IL-10 is a potent inhibitor of TNF-α and IFN-γ synthesis by TH_1 cells. The nature of the initial lymphocyte response is critical because the system tends to polarize over time into either a TH_2- or

TABLE 15.4. Host-Derived Inflammatory Mediators in Septic Shock.

Proinflammatory mediators	***Antiinflammatory mediators***
Proinflammatory cytokines: TNF-α, interleukins-1, -2, -12, -18, lymphotoxin-α Fas ligand	Antiinflammatory cytokines: Interleukins-4, -6, -10, -11, -13 Interleukin-1 receptor antagonist
Proinflammatory chemokines: IL-8, MCP-1	Soluble cytokine receptors: sTNF receptor, sIL-1 receptor, sIL-6R
Interferon-γ	Type 1 interferons (IFN-αβ)
Complement activators and components: C3a, C5a, MBL, C reactive protein	Complement inhibitors: C1 inhibitor, factor H
Lipid mediators: Leukotriene B_4, platelet-activating factor, oxidized phospholipids, phospholipase A_2	Stress hormones: Glucocorticoids, epinephrine, norepinephrine
Bradykinin, histamine	Prostaglandin E_2, prostacyclin
Prooxidants Reactive oxygen and nitrogen species	Antioxidants Glutathione, selenium, uric acid
Granulocyte-macrophage colony-stimulating factor	Granulocyte colony-stimulating factor
Macrophage migration inhibitory factor	Decoy cytokine receptors (IL-1 type 2 R)
Upregulation of receptors: TLR4, TLR2, CD14	Downregulation of receptors: TLR4, MHC II, TNF R, glucocorticoid receptors
Coagulation factors: Thrombin, factor Xa, tissue factor: FVIIa, fibrinogen, heparan sulfate, uPAR	Anticoagulants: Antithrombin, tissue factor pathway inhibitor, activated protein C
High-mobility group box-1	Transforming growth factor-β Vagal cholinergic antiinflammatory reflex

MBL, mannose-binding lectin; MCP, monocyte chemoattractant protein; R, receptor; TLR, Toll-like receptor; uPAR, urokinase plasminogen activator receptor.

TH_1-type response.[71] Functional differentiation of CD8 cells has also been detected ($CD8^+$ type 1 and type 2 cells).[70] Cytotoxic T cells can induce apoptosis by surface expression of Fas ligand, which fixes to cell membrane Fas on target cells and via the release of perforins and granzymes. Regulation of T-cell activity in sepsis is clinically relevant. A generalized TH_2-type response characteristically occurs after an initial septic insult. The stress hormone response in septic shock, with expression of adrenocorticotropic hormone, corticosteroids, prostaglandins, and catecholamines, promotes a TH_2 response after systemic injury.

Hotchkiss et al.[59,72] have provided another potential explanation for the relative immune suppression (or immune paralysis) that often accompanies sepsis. Selective apoptosis of $CD4^+$ T cells and B cells along with follicular dendritic cells is highly characteristic of severe sepsis. This selective loss of immune effector cells may contribute to the increased risk for secondary bacterial or fungal infection in the later phases of sepsis. Neutrophils are naturally apoptotic cells, and inflammatory cytokines and growth factors actually cause delayed apoptosis of neutrophils in sepsis.[73] Accelerated caspase function and excess apoptosis also occur in intestinal epithelial cells, compromising mucosal permeability barrier function of the gut.[59] This pathophysiologic state is further aggravated by sepsis-induced endotoxin tolerance (or reprogramming)[74] and deactivation of monocytes, macrophages, and neutrophils by cytokine inhibitors such as IL-1 receptor antagonist and antiinflammatory cytokines such as IL-10.[75] Depressed expression of MHC class II antigens (HLA-DR), TNF receptors, TLRs, and perhaps other cell surface activation signals may contribute to this functionally immunosuppressed state.[59]

Role of Nitric Oxide

Nitric oxide (NO) is a freely diffusible gas and highly reactive free radical with a short half-life (1–3 s).[76] It has an essential role in the pathophysiology of septic shock. Nitric oxide is generated by one of three isoforms of NOS (endothelial, neuronal, and inducible NOS).[77] Regulation of the human NOSs is complex. Full expression of the inducible form of NOS requires TNF-α, IL-1, LPS, and probably other regulatory elements. Nitric oxide is the major endothelial-derived relaxing factor that initiates the systemic hypotension observed in septic shock. Nitric oxide activates guanylate cyclase, which increases cyclic guanosine monophosphate levels inside vascular smooth muscle cells. The resultant smooth muscle relaxation in precapillary arterioles lowers peripheral vascular resistance.[76]

The other major physiologic effects of NO in septic shock are increased intracellular killing and regulation of platelet and neutrophil adherence. In the presence of reactive oxygen intermediates such as superoxide anion, NO leads to the formation of peroxynitrite. Peroxynitrite decays intracellularly into highly cytotoxic molecules, including hydroxyl radicals and nitrosyl chloride. These reactive nitrogen intermediates (RNI) activate an intracellular enzyme known as PARP (poly ADP-ribose polymerase). This enzyme rapidly depletes the cellular contents of adenosine triphosphate (ATP), resulting in cellular energy starvation.[78] These RNIs also induce lipid peroxidation and cause loss of cell viability.[76] Nitric oxide also inhibits a variety of metalloenzymes and essential enzymes in the tricarboxylic acid cycle, the glycolytic pathway, DNA repair systems, and electron transport pathways.

As with many other elements of the host inflammatory response, NO may have both advantageous and disadvantageous properties in sepsis. Nitric oxide regulates microcirculation to vital organs and contributes to intracellular killing of microbial pathogens. Excess and prolonged release of NO, however, results in systemic hypotension and contributes to septic shock. Regulation of NO synthesis remains an experimental target in the treatment of sepsis, but preservation of the favorable attributes of NO in the microcirculation while limiting its toxic effects remains a major therapeutic challenge.[77]

Role of the Coagulation System

Activation of the coagulation system, generation of a consumptive coagulopathy, systemic fibrinolysis, and diffuse microthrombi are potentially life-threatening complications of severe sepsis.[79] The innate immune system and the coagulation system coevolved as early defense systems against microbial invasion and tissue injury and remain highly integrated and coregulated. The tissue factor pathway (formerly known as the extrinsic pathway) is the principal mechanism by which the coagulation system is activated in human sepsis.[80] The contact factors (also known as the intrinsic pathway) play an accessory role as amplifiers of clotting once thrombin is generated (Fig. 15.3). Intravascular fibrin deposition impairs blood flow, promotes neutrophil and platelet adherence, and may contribute to at least some forms of multiorgan failure in sepsis.[81] Depletion of coagulation factors and activation of plasmin, antithrombin, and activated protein C may result in a hemorrhagic diathesis in some septic patients. Depletion of endogenous anticoagulants and impaired fibrinolysis may generate a procoagulant state and portend a poor prognosis.[82]

Inflammatory signals generated by intravascular thrombin generation and fibrin deposition contribute to microvascular injury as neutrophils and monocytes are drawn into areas of clot formation. Specialized receptors known as the protease-activated receptors (PAR 1–4) recognize thrombin, tissue factor:factor VII complex, factor X, and activated protein C.[83] These receptors are present on endothelial surfaces, neutrophils, and platelets and initiate the release of inflammatory cytokines, chemokines, platelet-activating factor, and P-selectin, among other mediators. The clotting system works in concert with the inflammatory networks in an attempt to localize the site of injury or infection from the rest of the host tissues. Extensive injury or failure of the early local control mechanism leads to generalized coagulation activation, inflammation, and the pathologic process of severe sepsis and septic shock.[84]

Clinical trials with recombinant tissue factor pathway inhibitor,[85] activated protein C,[86] and plasma-derived antithrombin[87] for treatment of sepsis resulted in disappointing results except for recombinant human activated protein C (drotrecogin alfa activated). This treatment strategy yielded a statistically significant survival benefit in a multicenter clinical trial with 1690 patients. The 28-day all-cause mortality in the recombinant human activated protein C group was 24.7%, while the mortality rate in the placebo group was

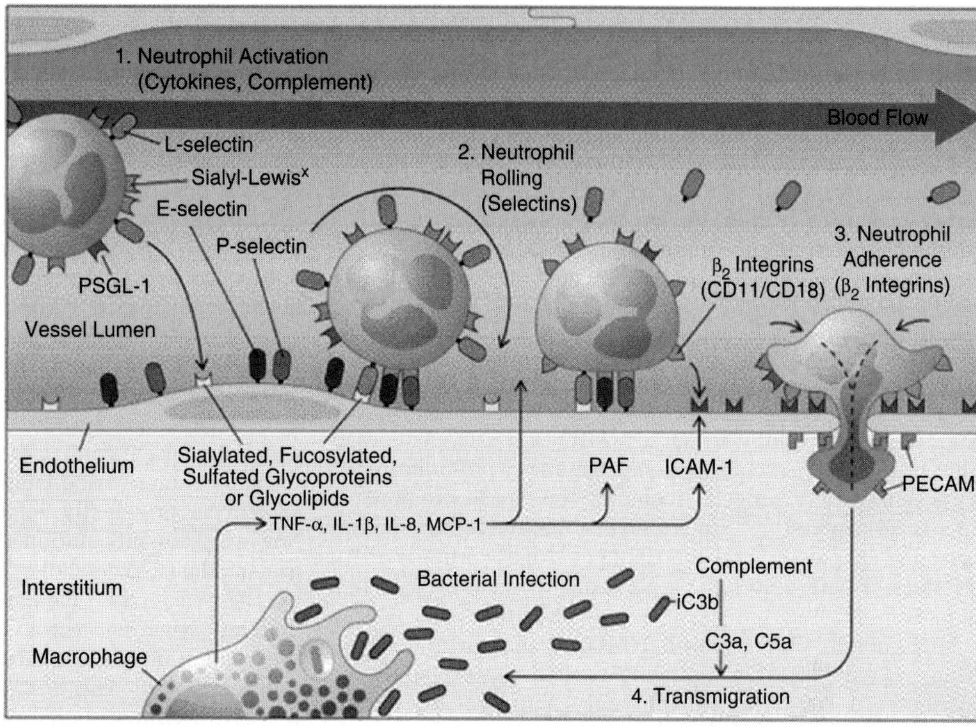

FIGURE 15.3. The interactions between coagulation and inflammation in sepsis. Solid bold arrows, major coagulation pathways; thin solid arrows, accessory and amplification clotting pathways; open arrows, inflammation and clotting interactions; dashed open arrows, inhibitory pathways; TF, tissue factor; uPA, urokinase plasminogen activator; tPA, tissue plasminogen activator; PAI-1, plasminogen activator inhibitor-1; Fbg, fibrinogen; PAR, protease-activated receptor; IL, interleukin; TNF, tumor necrosis factor; MIF, macrophage migration inhibitory factor; MCP-1, monocyte chemoattractant protein-1.

30.9% ($P < .005$, with a 6.1% absolute reduction in mortality).[86] This drug received regulatory approval in 2002 for the use of drotrecogin alfa activated in severe sepsis/septic shock at high risk of mortality (e.g., multisystem failure or an APACHE [Acute Physiology and Chronic Health Evaluation] II score of 25 or greater). The precise mechanism of action of recombinant human activated protein C that accounts for its beneficial effects is not entirely clear, but it is not likely to be its direct anticoagulant activity.[88] Heparin alone and other anticoagulants such as hirudin have not been shown to improve outcome in clinical settings or experimental models of sepsis,[89,90] and all of these endogenous anticoagulants have antiinflammatory properties.[91] Activated protein C also has profibrinolytic activity and antiapoptotic activities on endothelial cells in experimental systems,[88] which may spare the endothelial surface for the injurious effects of systemic inflammation and disordered coagulation.[81,91] Clinical investigations with antithrombin, tissue factor pathway inhibitor, and other coagulation inhibitors continue as possible treatment regimens for specific subgroups of septic patients.

Monocyte, Platelet, Neutrophil, and Endothelial Cell Interactions in Sepsis

The recruitment of neutrophils, platelets, and other inflammatory cells to an area of localized infection or clot formation is an essential component of the host innate immune response. Localization and eradication of invasive microorganisms at the initial site of injury is the primary defense strategy against microbial pathogens. This physiologic process may become deleterious if diffuse neutrophil–endothelial cell interactions occur throughout the circulation in response to systemic inflammation.[84,91,92]

The mechanisms responsible for the migration of neutrophils from the intravascular space into the interstitium, where invasive microorganisms are found, are depicted in Figure 15.4.[62] Activated neutrophils degranulate and expose endothelial surfaces and surrounding structures to reactive oxygen and nitrogen intermediates, and a number of lytic proteases, including elastase. This process involves ongoing communication between endothelial surfaces and inflammatory cells. The process is initiated by the selectins and culminated by engagement of neutrophil β-2 integrins (CD11/CD18) and adhesion molecules on endothelial cells such as

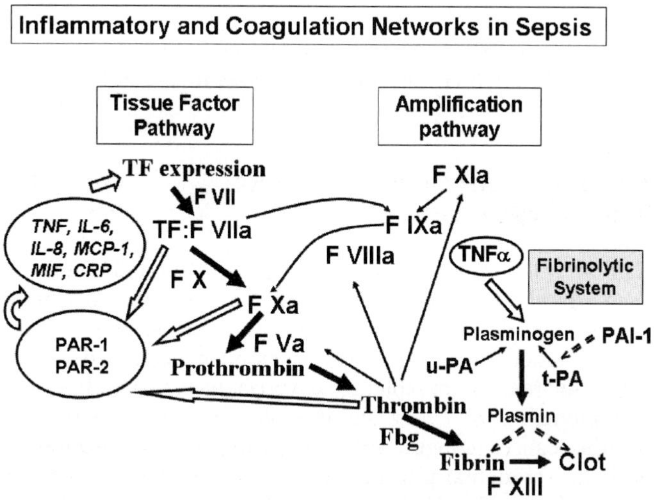

FIGURE 15.4. Neutrophil–endothelial cell interactions in sepsis. Ls, L-selectin; PSGL-1, P-selectin glycoprotein ligand-1; Ps, P-selectin; Es, E-selectin; sLe^x, sialylated-Lewis^x; ICAM-1, intercellular adhesion molecule-1; PAF, platelet-activating factor; TNF-α, tumor necrosis factor-α; IL-1β, interleukin-1β; MCP-1, monocyte chemoattractant protein-1; C, complement; PECAM, platelet endothelial cell adhesion molecule. (*Source:* From Opal and Huber,[62] with permission from *Scientific American Medicine.*)

intercellular adhesion molecule-1 and -2. Neutrophil egress commences and chemotactic factors direct phagocytic cells to the site of microbial infection. Platelet and monocyte infiltration follow and provide additional inflammatory signals, adherence molecules, and procoagulant surfaces for clot formation and cell migration. This process may lead to diffuse endothelial injury in the face of generalized systemic inflammatory responses. Regulation of events at the neutrophil–endothelial interface is an important area for therapeutic intervention in the management of sepsis.[79,81,84,88,91]

Other Mediators of Sepsis

It has been discovered that several host-derived mediators may contribute to the pathogenesis of septic shock. Macrophage migration inhibitory factor (MIF) is a late mediator induced by glucocorticoid excess; it has many proinflammatory actions on effector cells, including the capacity to upregulate TLR4 expression,[93] impair myocardial function,[94] delay neutrophil apoptosis,[95] and contribute to lethal septic shock.[96] Inhibitors of MIF may have a potential therapeutic role in human sepsis.[93,96]

High-mobility group box-1 (HMGB-1) protein is a late-acting cytokine-like DNA-binding protein that appears to contribute to late-onset inflammatory activities in septic shock.[97,98] Inhibitors of HMGB-1 demonstrate some therapeutic benefit in experimental sepsis.[99] Complement components, particularly the chemoattractant factor C5a,[100] and loss of the regulatory element C1 esterase inhibitor[91] can produce vasodilatation and may participate in the pathogenesis of septic shock. The triggering receptor expressed on myeloid cells TREM-1[101] and NOD1/NOD2 (nucleotide-binding oligomerization domain protein)[102] are additional, recently identified, signaling systems that mediate inflammatory signals independent of the TLRs and may play a pathogenic role in the initiation of the septic process. The cholinergic antiinflammatory system is a well-characterized vagally transmitted mechanism by which the nervous system is able to directly modulate host macrophage inflammatory signals via a nicotinic receptor-mediated process.[103] This neuronal–immune communication system may also prove to be amenable to therapeutic modulation in the care of septic patients.

Diagnostic Methods for Severe Sepsis/Septic Shock

Fully developed septic shock is obvious to the clinician, yet the early phases of severe sepsis and even septic shock may be quite subtle even to experienced clinicians. Early symptoms include confusion, apprehension, or decreased sensorium. Sudden and unexplained dyspnea (respiratory alkalosis) is a frequent early event, and it is often missed or attributed to other causes (congestive heart failure, anemia, pulmonary embolus, bronchial plugging, etc.). Fever is usually, but not invariably, present. Hypothermia in fact is a more specific and reliable finding; its presence portends an unfavorable prognosis. An unexplained decrease in urinary output, sudden onset of cholestatic jaundice, unexplained metabolic acidosis, excessive bleeding at venipuncture sites, or even sudden unexplained hypotension may be the presenting finding in septic shock. Clinicians need to recognize these early signs and symptoms since successful outcomes from severe sepsis/septic shock depend on early recognition and rapid intervention.[2]

Myriad clinical, laboratory, and hemodynamic abnormalities are recognized in septic shock (Table 15.5). There is no single clinical or laboratory test that is pathognomonic of septic shock; therefore, the clinical diagnosis of sepsis remains a challenging problem.[1] Blood cultures need not be positive (and reveal no pathogen in about two-thirds of septic patients); leukocytosis or neutropenia may occur; hyperglycemia, euglycemia, or hypoglycemia may be observed; and a variety of acid–base abnormalities may occur. It is the progressive evolution of a constellation of signs and symptoms that leads to a clinical diagnosis of septic shock.

The most common hemodynamic findings in early septic shock are a high cardiac output and a low systemic vascular resistance state. Vasodilatation within the peripheral vascular system is principally related to increased NO synthesis; however, downregulation of adrenergic receptors with progressive loss of catecholamine sensitivity; excess production of the vasoactive mediators histamine, adrenomedullin, platelet-activating factor, and bradykinin; and deficiency of vasopressin all contribute to reduced vascular tone in sepsis.[84,100,104–106] The heart attempts to compensate for the loss of systemic vascular tone despite diminished myocardial performance even in the early phases of septic shock.[100] Without adequate intervention, circulating blood volume is continually lost into the interstitial spaces and intracellular locations. The heart cannot compensate indefinitely as myocardial depressant factors (NO, MIF, IL-6, TNF, other factors) are released, and cardiac performance deteriorates. Late septic shock is marked by systolic hypotension despite intense peripheral vasoconstriction and reduced cardiac index.[91,94,100]

Septic shock may be associated with a loss of normal autoregulation within the microcirculation, with an imbalance between oxygen delivery and oxygen consumption.[107] A supply-dependent dysoxia may occur, and cytopathic hypoxia[108] from diminished oxygen utilization may develop as well. Attempts to enhance oxygen delivery in sepsis to supranormal levels have not improved outcomes,[3,109] but a controlled clinical trial of early goal-directed resuscitation found rapid restoration of tissue perfusion and oxygen delivery remains a critically important target in sepsis therapy.[110]

Experimental Diagnostic Methods and Biomarkers for Sepsis

Since timely intervention is essential for successful outcomes in severe sepsis/septic shock, a concerted effort has been undertaken to improve the early diagnostic tools available to detect sepsis. Improved blood culture methods or measurement of plasma endotoxin levels may have diagnostic utility.[111] Circulating levels of bacterial superantigens can be detected in selected patients with toxic shock syndrome.[112]

Interleukin-6 has been considered an indicator of cytokine activation as its synthesis is induced by TNF-α and IL-1β. Patients with elevated IL-6 levels appear to respond favorably to anticytokine therapies.[113] In several studies,[113–115] elevations of IL-6 or failure of IL-6 levels to decline over time have been associated with poor outcome. Unfortunately, the variability and lack of specificity or IL-6 measurement limits its reliability as a diagnostic method for septic shock.

TABLE 15.5. Characteristic Hemodynamic and Laboratory Findings in Severe Sepsis.

Parameter	*Common findings*	*Clinical interpretation and implications*
Mixed venous O_2 saturation	<70%	Low mixed venous O_2 indicates inadequate O_2 delivery to tissues in sepsis
Cardiac index (cardiac output/m_2 [surface area])	>4 l/min/m^2	Cardiac index elevated in early septic shock; may be depressed in late septic shock
Pulmonary arterial wedge pressure (PAWP)	4–10 mmHg	Volume resuscitation should continue until return of normal MAP or PAWP reaches 12–15 mmHg
Systemic vascular resistance (SVR)	<800 dyne/s/cm^{-5}	SVR characteristically low in early septic shock secondary to peripheral vasodilation
Oxygen delivery (DO_2)		
CI × Arterial O_2 content	<550 ml/min/m^2	Goal of treatment is to provide sufficient DO_2 to maintain adequate mixed venous O_2 saturation
Platelet count	<100,000/µl	Poor prognostic factor in sepsis; increased bleeding risk; thrombocytopenia may be accompanied by DIC
Glucose	Hyperglycemia or hypoglycemia	Acute stress response (hyperglycemia), inhibition of hepatic gluconeogenesis (hypoglycemia)
Clotting measurements	Elevated PT, aPPT, d-dimer, FDPs, low fibrinogen, AT, PC	Coagulopathy often seen with systemic endotoxin release; coagulation activation is almost uniform in sepsis but clinically overt DIC is uncommon
Plasma lactate	(>2.2 mmol/l)	Hypermetabolism, hypoperfusion of tissues, inhibition of pyruvate dehydrogenase
C-reactive protein, procalcitonin, IL-6	Elevated	Acute-phase proteins and products of immune cells, variable levels, sensitive but not specific indicators
Arterial blood gases	Respiratory alkalosis (early); metabolic acidosis (late)	Measurements of O_2 content and mixed venous O_2 saturation useful in management to ensure adequate tissue oxygenation and fluid resuscitation

aPTT, activated partial thromboplastin time; AT, antithrombin; DIC, disseminated intravascular coagulation; FDP, fibrin degradation products; IL, interleukin; PC, protein C; PT, prothrombin time.

Procalcitonin (PCT) is the propeptide of calcitonin, and under pathological conditions of systemic inflammation PCT is produced in abundant amounts by a variety of tissues. A specific protease cleaves procalcitonin into calcitonin, katacalcin, and an amino-terminal peptide.[116] Procalcitonin has many favorable attributes as a potential marker for sepsis. It has a long half-life (approximately 24 h) and will increase from undetectable levels to greater than 100 ng/ml in severe sepsis/septic shock. Higher levels are associated with more severe systemic infection.[117] The diagnostic and therapeutic value of PCT measurement needs to be tested in large clinical trials to determine its ultimate clinical applicability.[118] The usefulness of plasma C-reactive protein, clotting factors, platelet counts, and plasma lactate levels are listed in Table 15.5.[62] It is anticipated that progress in real-time functional genomics and proteomics in the near future will greatly aid the early recognition of incipient sepsis in patients, although the level of complexity and heterogeneity in host responses remain major, unsolved challenges in this field of medical informatics.[52,53]

Organ Dysfunction in Sepsis

One of the most remarkable and characteristic findings in sepsis is the development of organ injury remote from the initial site of infection. The development of one or more organ dysfunctions at the onset of severe sepsis, or over the course of sepsis, is a poor prognostic factor and major determinant of outcome (Table 15.6).[3,15] The diffuse endothelial injury, proapoptotic signals, immune dysregulation, and coagulopathy induced from septic shock conspire in concert to produce organ dysfunction distant from the original site of infection. It is generally assumed that the activation signals in the pathogenesis of multiorgan injury derive from plasma factors (e.g., proinflammatory cytokines, complement, phospholipid mediators),[67] but cellular signals from circulating blood components[72] or neuroendocrine signals may also contribute to remote organ injury.[103]

Inadequate blood supply to vital tissues likely contributes to organ dysfunction. The failure of the microcirculation to maintain tissue viability is related to hypoperfusion, redistribution of blood flow within vascular beds, functional arteriovenous shunting, obstruction of blood flow from microthrombi, platelet or white blood cell aggregates, or abnormal deformability of red blood cells. Direct endothelial injury from NO, reactive oxygen and nitrogen intermediates, proinflammatory cytokines, activated cytotoxic T cells and NK cells, and inducers of apoptosis may directly damage endothelial surfaces.[59,72,105]

Acute lung injury occurs as a result of damage to the pulmonary vascular circulation and the alveolar-capillary membranes. The acute respiratory distress syndrome (ARDS) remains a major cause of morbidity and mortality in septic shock.[3] Avoidance of barotrauma and volutrauma, avoidance of oxidant injury, maintenance of functional alveolar capillary units through position change (prone position), judicious

TABLE 15.6. Organ Dysfunction Syndromes that May Accompany Severe Sepsis.

Organ system	*Clinical-metabolic abnormalities*	*Histopathologic findings*
Immune system	Initial activation of innate immunity and late depression of innate and adaptive responses	Adherence and extravasation and delayed apoptosis of neutrophils, selective loss of B cells, $CD4^+$ T cells, and follicular dendritic cells
Musculoskeletal system	Muscle tenderness, loss of muscle mass and power	Increased muscle catabolism, progressive loss of somatic muscle tissue
Central nervous system	Encephalopathy, decreased sensorium	Cerebral edema, microthrombi
Cardiovascular	Decreased myocardial performance; myocardial depressant factors (TNF, IL-1, IL-6, nitric oxide)	Altered calcium influx, interstitial edema, myocardial hibernation
Lung	Acute respiratory distress syndrome	Exudation of fluid into the alveolar spaces, neutrophil plugging, hyaline membrane formation
Kidney	Acute tubular necrosis	Hypoperfusion, focal ischemia, microthrombi
Endocrine	Relative adrenal insufficiency, adrenal hemorrhage, decreased vasopressin output, thyroid abnormalities	Focal or diffuse hemorrhage, ischemic necrosis of adrenals, increased vascular sensitivity to vasopressin
Hepatobiliary system	Cholestatic jaundice, acute phase protein response, decreased clotting factors, hepatic metabolism of drugs	Zonal necrosis, acalculous cholecystitis
Gut	Translocation of endotoxin and microorganisms, decreased motility, increased permeability	Diffuse interstitial edema, breaks in the epithelial membrane integrity, mucosal necrosis

fluid management, and semirecumbent body positioning all reduce progressive lung damage in ventilated patients.[119] The ARDS clinical trials network study confirmed the value of low stretch tidal volume settings (6 ml/kg) over more conventional high tidal volume settings (12 ml/kg).[120] Low tidal volume ventilation should be utilized whenever feasible to minimize further acute lung injury in a ventilated patient. Epidemiologic studies have conclusively demonstrated that even multiple organ dysfunction from sepsis is potentially amenable to treatment if instituted rapidly and skillfully in ICUs.[3,5]

Management of Septic Shock

Priorities in the Management of Sepsis

There are four immediate objectives in the initial management of septic shock: (1) early recognition; (2) reestablishment of tissue perfusion and arterial blood pressure by early resuscitation; (3) optimal supportive care of organ dysfunction; and (4) appropriate intervention to eradicate the causative septic focus. The 2004 surviving sepsis campaign treatment guidelines provide a useful, up-to-date, and evidence-based review of the standard treatment of sepsis.[3] They rank the level of evidence to support treatment decisions as follows: grade A, supported by at least two large, randomized trials; grade B, one large randomized trial; grade C, supported by smaller randomized or nonrandomized trials; grade D, supported by nonrandomized trials; or grade E, nonrandomized clinical data and expert opinion. There is considerable agreement regarding basic resuscitation strategies and organ support maneuvers. There is general consensus about the need to remove the septic focus as soon as possible and initiate appropriate antimicrobial agents against the causative pathogens. Treatment options vary considerably with respect to the timing of interventions, amount and type of fluid administration, value of specific vasopressor therapies, and advisability of treatment interventions of unclear or experimental clinical utility. Areas of general agreement and options lacking uniform consensus are addressed in this section.

Initial Resuscitation

Fluid resuscitation is an essential first step in the management of septic shock. The loss of vasomotor tone and increased vascular permeability necessitate immediate correction to maintain tissue perfusion and provide adequate circulating blood volume. Debate has raged for decades over the relative merits of colloids versus crystalloid fluids. The lack of clear evidence of benefit of colloid agents (e.g., albumin, dextran, and plasma expanders) and their high cost have favored the use of saline solutions for volume expansion.[121,122] A large, controlled clinical trial was undertaken recently in Australia and New Zealand in an effort to finally settle this debate.[123] In a comparative study of nearly 7000 critically ill patients randomized to saline versus 4% albumin, the 28 day all-cause mortality was virtually identical (relative risk 0.99, P = n.s.). This would seem to have settled the debate except that a subgroup analysis of over 1200 septic patients suggested an improved outcome in the albumin group (30.7% vs. 35.3% saline group, $P = .06$). Current consensus opinion still favors cystalloid solutions.[3]

The optimal amount of fluid therapy for patients in septic shock remains unclear, but a study by Rivers and colleagues[110] supported the notion that early, aggressive, and goal-directed resuscitation fluids should be widely adopted as the standard approach to early fluid administration. They recommended a treatment regimen aimed at resolving lactic acidemia, recovery of mean arterial blood pressure over 65 mmHg, and return of central venous pressure above 8 mmHg and mixed venous oxygen saturation above 70% within 6 h of initial presentation (grade B evidence).

A delicate balance is required between maintenance of tissue perfusion and prevention of fluid overload, with its attendant risk of lung injury. Decreased myocardial performance in sepsis may necessitate a higher filling pressure for adequate cardiac output; however, exudation of fluids into the alveolar space in lung tissue and into the interstitium in other vital organs continues to be a major problem. Maintenance of a pulmonary arterial occlusion pressure of approximately 12 mmHg is considered a reasonable starting point for those patients with a hemodynamic monitor in place (grade B).[3]

Use of Vasopressors for Blood Pressure Support

When patients fail to recover hemodynamic stability with fluid resuscitation alone, vasopressor agents are indicated to reestablish systemic arterial blood pressure. Dopamine has been the vasopressor agent of choice for several decades based on its presumed salutary effects on renal vasodilatation and its modest inotropic effects.[124] The actual clinical value of dopamine compared with other vasopressor agents has been brought into question. Dopamine has complex effects as this catecholamine has its own receptors (D1 and D2 dopaminergic receptors) and variable affinities for α- and β-adrenergic receptors. The net effect of dopamine depends on many variables, including the receptor density in specific vascular beds, blood volume, and the rate of administration of drug dose used. Higher doses of dopamine increase the systemic vascular resistance by its effects on α-adrenergic receptors in the peripheral circulation. Dopamine may have adverse effects on splanchnic blood flow,[3,124] and there is no evidence in controlled trials that dopamine has any meaningful renal perfusion benefits.[3] The use of dopamine as a "renal-sparing" agent is no longer justified (grade B).[3,125]

Norepinephrine is a potent vasoconstrictor that is used more frequently to treat the hemodynamic effects of septic shock. Earlier concerns regarding adverse consequences of norepinephrine on renal blood flow may have been overstated; studies suggested that norepinephrine may actually increase urine output and creatinine clearance in septic patients.[126] Norepinephrine may rapidly restore perfusion pressure within the glomerulus and result in improved glomerular filtration in patients with adequate fluid resuscitation. Current consensus opinion recommends either dopamine or norepinephrine as the initial vasopressor to correct hypotension in septic shock (grade D).[3]

Vasopressin is a potent vasopressor in refractory sepsis. Endogenous vasopressin levels rapidly fall in sepsis, and vasopressin has its own vascular receptors that are distinct from adrenergic receptors and often upregulated in sepsis.[127] There is concern about diminished splanchnic blood flow with higher doses of vasopressin, and myocardial ischemia may occur at infusion rates above 0.04 unit/min. Vasopressin may be considered in refractory shock, but it has not replaced dopamine or norepinephrine for first-line vasopressors in septic shock (grade E).[3]

Dobutamine, a β-agonist, may improve cardiac output and oxygen delivery in some patients in septic shock with persistently low cardiac output. Dobutamine may cause peripheral vasodilatation in septic patients, and it increases myocardial oxygen consumption by its inotropic effects.[3]

Another approach to improved tissue oxygen delivery is by use of vasodilators to open up poorly perfused capillary beds in patients with septic shock. Spronk et al.[128] reported the use of nitroglycerin therapy in patients following intravascular volume resuscitation. Using an optical device to measure microcirculatory flow (orthogonal polarization spectral imaging), they were able to show improved microvascular flow rates in septic patients who received adequate fluid repletion. This is an appealing strategy but must be considered experimental at present until further clinical trials are completed using this approach.

Numerous techniques are under study to clinically measure tissue oxygenation by gastric tonometry, hepatic venous oxygen measurements, direct tissue oxygen probes, and microcirculatory units for visualized capillary blood flow.[3] The practical value of these measurements in the clinical management of sepsis has yet to be demonstrated.

Blood Product Support and Nutritional Support

The relative merits of blood transfusion or erythropoietin necessity to improve the oxygen-carrying capacity of blood remains a subject of considerable debate.[129,130] It has been demonstrated that humans are remarkably resistant to adverse effects from isovolumetric anemia.[131] Banked, stored red blood cells are less deformable, less efficient at releasing their oxygen from 2,3-biphosphoglycerate-depleted hemoglobin stores, and may have immunosuppressive effects.[129] Efforts to promote endogenous erythrocyte production with erythropoietin treatments have yet to be proven superior to blood transfusions.[130] Further clinical trials are warranted with this treatment approach. The lower limit of transfusion threshold in septic shock has not been defined, but it appears to be considerably lower than the traditional transfusion threshold of less than 10 g/dl. Studies of patients in the ICU setting indicated that a conservative transfusion policy at 7–9 g/dl may be preferable[132] (grade B recommendation).

Expert management of acute renal failure, renal replacement therapy, ARDS treatment, hepatic decompensation, acid–base disturbances, and disordered hemodynamics are of critical importance in the management of sepsis. These topics have been addressed in recent treatment guidelines[3] and are dealt with extensively in other chapters in this book. Nutritional support in the critically ill patient has changed radically over the past two decades. Reliance on total parenteral nutrition has given way to early and extensive use of enteral hyperalimentation. Enteral feeding of septic patients has been shown to benefit enterocyte function, help maintain the intestinal permeability barrier, and prevent gut-derived endotoxin and cytokine generation.[133] Nutritional supplementation with glutamine, arginine, and omega-3 fatty acids has experimental support and remains an active area of research, yet convincing clinical efficacy studies are not yet available.[134]

Fever is frequently concomitant to severe infection and is generally considered advantageous to the host.[135] Experimental animals with peritonitis clear infection and recover more rapidly when allowed to develop fever compared to a control group with externally controlled normothermia.[136] Heat-shock proteins function as molecular chaperones and prevent protein denaturation during cellular stress. Heat-shock protein induction may actually improve outcomes in experimental endotoxin challenge.[137] Cooling blankets to lower body temperature should be avoided as they are uncomfortable for patients and generally ineffective unless true hyperthermia is present.[138]

Antibiotics are considered an adjuvant therapy to source control with drainage, relief of obstruction, or removal of the

TABLE 15.7. **Suggested Initial Empirical Antibiotic Choices for Severe Sepsis.**

Suspected source of infection	*Primary pathogens*	*Antimicrobial choice*[a]
Intraabdominal infections	Enteric aerobic gram-negative bacilli, enterococci, bowel anaerobes	Third- or fourth-generation cephalosporins or extended-spectrum penicillins or β-lactam-β-lactamase inhibitor with metronidazole or clindamycin; or carbapenem ± an aminoglycoside (alternative: fluoroquinolone)
Soft tissue infections	Staphylococci, streptococci, mixed aerobes/anaerobes	Extended-spectrum penicillin or third- or fourth-generation cephalosporin or carbapenem or β-lactam-β-lactamase inhibitor; add clindamycin if streptococcal or staphylococcal toxic shock suspected
Community-acquired pneumonia	*Streptococcus pneumoniae*, *S. aureus*, Legionella, oral anaerobes	Third-generation cephalosporin with a macrolide (alternative: fluoroquinolones)
Hospital-acquired pneumonia	*S. aureus*, *Pseudomonas aeruginosa*, gram-negative bacilli	Third-/fourth-generation cephalosporins, extended-spectrum penicillins ± an aminoglycoside (alternatives: fluoroquinolones, carbapenems, β-lactam-β-lactamase inhibitor)
Urinary tract infections	Gram-negative aerobic bacilli, enterococci	Extended-spectrum β-lactam agent (third-generation cephalosporin or extended-spectrum penicillin); or a fluoroquinolone (add ampicillin or vancomycin if enterococci are present, linezolid if vancomycin-resistant enterococci)
Biliary tract infections	*Klebsiella* spp., *Escherichia coli*, *Clostridia*	Extended-spectrum penicillin ± an aminoglycoside or fluoroquinolone (add metronidazole if hepatic abscess present)
Neutropenic patients	*P. aeruginosa*, aerobic gram-negative bacilli	Extended-spectrum β-lactam agent ± an aminoglycoside or quinolone (add vancomycin if evidence of gram-positive infection)

[a]Assuming no drug allergies an empiric choice should be based on local antibiotic resistance patterns.

offending focus of infection when possible (grade E recommendation[3]). Suggested empiric choices of antimicrobial agents are listed in Table 15.7. In septic shock, combinations of bactericidal antimicrobial agents are generally given on an empirical basis, yet monotherapy with an effective broad-spectrum β-lactam or fluoroquinolone is usually sufficient (grade D[3]). Ineffective empiric antibiotic choices for initial therapy for sepsis have adverse consequences,[139,140] and therefore it is preferable to ensure adequate initial therapy and then deescalate to single narrow-spectrum agents after the causative organism is identified.[140]

Euglycemia, Steroids, and Recombinant Human Activated Protein C

Other important supportive management techniques in sepsis are tight regulation of blood glucose levels and use of stress dose glucocorticoids in the presence of relative adrenal insufficiency. Hyperglycemia can increase procoagulant activity on endothelial surfaces and may induce excess apoptosis.[141] Van den Berghe et al.[142] demonstrated improved survival, shorter ICU stays, and less bacteremia in some surgical population with strict control over blood sugar (target was continuous euglycemia) versus conventional care in a cardiovascular ICU setting. It is recommended that blood sugar levels be kept under 150mg/dl if at all feasible in septic patients (grade D[3]).

Annane and coworkers[143] reported significant survival benefits in a study of 299 patients with vasopressor-dependent septic shock; the study used hydrocortisone (50mg every 6h for 7 days) and fludrocortisone (50μg/day for 7 days). This treatment strategy is based on the frequent occurrence of relative adrenal insufficiency in patients with septic shock.[144,145] The low-dose corticosteroid therapy was only effective in those patients with evidence of inadequate adrenal responses to a short corticotropin test.[143] Stress dose steroids should be discontinued if normal cortisol levels and corticotropin responses are found (grade C).

The results of the recombinant human activated protein C trial (drotrecogin alfa activated) represent the first successful phase III international trial in severe sepsis.[86] It is given as a continuous infusion at 24μg/kg/h for 4 days. Since the molecule is an endogenous anticoagulant, the major side effect of treatment is bleeding. Carefully selected patients benefit from this treatment regardless of the type of infecting microorganism that caused sepsis[16] (grade B recommendation[3]).

Experimental Therapies for Sepsis

The wealth of new discoveries into the central molecular events that underlie sepsis and the unmet medical need for improved therapies for sepsis have created an ongoing impetus to develop innovative treatments for sepsis. Some of those experimental strategies that are in clinical trials or nearing clinical investigation are listed in Table 15.8 along with their presumed mechanism of action. Translational research has already brought novel treatments such as stress dose steroids, low stretch mechanical ventilation, enteral nutrition, and activated protein C into clinical use. It is anticipated that the genomic era will speed the development of innovations into clinical practice. Much-needed research continues on preventive strategies, improved diagnostics, and more effective treatment interventions to improve the outlook for this ever-growing population of septic patients.

TABLE 15.8. Experimental Therapies in the Treatment of Septic Shock.

Treatment target	*Experimental agents*	*Possible mechanisms*
Endotoxin	Bactericidal/permeability-increasing protein	Endotoxin-neutralizing human protein
Endotoxin	Phospholipid emulsions	Complexes and clears LPS
Endotoxin	E5564	Toll-like receptor 4 antagonist
Endotoxin	Polymyxin B–binding columns	Endotoxin-binding antibiotic
Poly ADP ribosyl polymerase-1 (PARP-1)	Small molecule PARP inhibitor	Inhibits cellular depletion of ATP and limits cellular necrosis
High-mobility group box-1 (HMGB-1)	Antibody or small molecule inhibitors of HMGB-1 or its receptor	Blocks the lethal effects of this late-acting cytokine-like molecule
Macrophage migration inhibitory factor (MIF)	Antibody to MIF	Blocks the lethal effects of this late-acting cytokine
Adrenal function	Low-dose corticosteroids[a]	Treat adrenal hypofunction of sepsis
Coagulation system	Tissue factor pathway inhibitor, recombinant human antithrombin, tissue factor or factor X inhibitors	Inhibitors of DIC, microthrombi; decreases thrombin-induced inflammatory actions
Cytokines and endotoxin	Hemoperfusion systems, small molecule signal transduction inhibitors	Removes inflammatory mediators and endotoxin during hemoperfusion, inhibition of cytokine gene induction
Disordered microcirculation	Nitroglycerin infusion	Opens up poorly perfused capillary beds along with intravenous fluids
Immunonutrition	Arginine, glutamine, nucleic acids, micronutrients	Improves immune function and provides antioxidants
Cellular apoptosis	Caspase inhibitors	Block excess apoptosis of immune cells and endothelial cells

[a]One clinical trial demonstrated benefit[143]; other studies are ongoing (recent unpublished report of no benefit for one trial).

References

1. Poeze M, Ramsay G, Gerlach H, et al. International sepsis survey: A study of doctor's knowledge and perception about sepsis. Crit Care 2004;8:409–413.
2. Levy M, Ramsey G, Fink M, et al. The 2001 SCCM/ESICM/ACCP/ATS/SIS International Sepsis Definitions Conference. Crit Care Med 2003;31:1250–1256.
3. Dellinger RP, Carlet JM, Masur H, et al. Surviving sepsis campaign guidelines for the management of severe sepsis and septic shock. Crit Care Med 2004;32:858–871.
4. Angus DC, Linde-Zwirble WT, Lidicker J, Clermont G, Carcillo J, Pinsky MR. Epidemiology of severe sepsis in the United States: analysis of incidence, outcome, and associated costs of care. Crit Care Med 2001;29:1303–1310.
5. Martin GS, Mannino DM, Eaton S, et al. Epidemiology of sepsis in the United States from 1979–2000. N Engl J Med 2003;348:1546–1554.
6. Alberti C, Brun-Buisson C, Burchardi H, et al. Epidemiology of sepsis and infection in ICU patients from international multicenter cohort study. Intensive Care Med 2002;28:108–121.
7. Valles J, Leon C, Alvarez-Lerma F. Nosocomial bacteremia in critically ill patients: a multicenter study evaluating epidemiology and prognosis. Spanish Collaborative Group for Infections in Intensive Care Units of the Sociedad Espanola de Medicina Intensiva Unidades Coronarias (SEMIUC). Clin Infect Dis 1997; 24:387–395.
8. Friedman G, Silva E, Vincent J-L. Has the mortality of septic shock changed with time? Crit Care Med 1998;26:2078–2086.
9. Sands KE, Bates DW, Lanken PN, et al. Epidemiology of sepsis syndrome in eight academic medical centers. JAMA 1997; 278:234–240.
10. Brun-Buisson C, Meshaka P, Pinton P, et al. EPISEPSIS: a reappraisal of the epidemiology and outcome of severe sepsis in French intensive care units. Intensive Care Med 2004;30:580–588.
11. Opal SM, Esmon C. Functional relationships between coagulation and the innate immune response and their respective roles in the pathogenesis of sepsis. Crit Care 2003;7:23–38.
12. Hund E. Neurological complications of sepsis: critical illness polyneuropathy and myopathy. J Neurol 2001;248:929–934.
13. Brun-Buisson C, Roudot-Thoraval F, Girou E, et al. The costs of septic syndromes in the intensive care unit and the influence of hospital-acquired sepsis. Intensive Care Med 2003;29:1464–1471.
14. Kreger BE, Craven DE, Carling PC, McCabe WR. Gram-negative bacteremia. III. Reassessment of etiology, epidemiology and ecology in 612 patients. Am J Med 1980;68:332–343.
15. Pittet D, Thiívent B, Wenzel RP, et al. Importance of pre-existing co-morbidities for prognosis of septicemia in critically ill patients. Intensive Care Med 1993;19:265–272.
16. Opal SM, Maki D, Larosa S, et al. Systemic host response to sepsis based upon the infectious microorganism and effects of drotrecogin alfa activated. Clin Infect Dis 2003;37:50–58.
17. Cohen J, Brun-Buisson C, Torres A, et al. Diagnosis of infection in sepsis: an evidence-based review. Crit Care Med 2004;32: S466–S494.
18. Ely EW, Wheeler AP, Thompson BT, et al. Recovery rate and prognosis in older persons who develop acute lung injury and the acute respiratory distress syndrome. Ann Intern Med 2002; 136:25–29.
19. Hughes WT, Armstrong D, Bodey GP, et al. 2002 guidelines for the use of antimicrobial agents in neutropenic patients with cancer. Clin Infect Dis 2002;34;730–751.
20. Styrt B. Infection associated with asplenia: risks, mechanisms and prevention. Am J Med 1990;88:33N–42N.
21. Sorensen TIA, Nielsen GG, Andersen PK, Teasdale TW. Genetic and environmental influences on premature death in adult adoptees. N Engl J Med 1988;318:727–732.
22. Newport MJ, Huxley CM, Huston S, et al. A mutation in the interferon-γ receptor gene and susceptibility to mycobacterial infection. N Engl J Med 1996;335:1941–1949.

23. Beutler B. Science review: key inflammatory and stress pathways in critical illness. Crit Care 2003;7:39–46.
24. Lorenz E, Mira J-P, Frees KG, Schwartz DA. Relevance of mutations in the TLR4-receptor in patients with gram-negative septic shock. Arch Intern Med 2002;162:1028–1031.
25. Gibot S, Cariou A, Drouet L, Rossignol M, Ripoll L. Association between a genomic polymorphism with the CD14 locus and septic shock susceptibility and mortality rate. Crit Care Med 2002;30:969–973.
26. Agnese DM, Calvano JE, Hahm SJ, et al. Human toll-like receptor 4 mutations but not CD 14 polymorphisms are associated with increased risk of gram-negative infections J Infect Dis 2002;185:1522–1525.
27. Mira JP, Cariou A, Grall F et al. Association of *TNF2*, a TNFα promoter polymorphism, with septic shock susceptibility and mortality. JAMA 1999;282:561–568.
28. Read RC, Camp NJ, Di Giovine FS, et al. An interleukin-1 genotype is associated with fatal outcome of meningococcal disease. J Infect Dis 2000;182:1557–1560.
29. Nadel S, Newport MJ, Booy R, et al. Variation in the tumor necrosis factor-α gene promoter region may be associated with death from meningococcal disease. J Infect Dis 1996;174:878–880.
30. Smirnova I, Mann N, Dols A, et al. Assay of locus-specific genetic load implicates rare Toll-like receptor 4 mutations in meningococcal susceptibility. Proc Natl Acad Sci U S A 2003;100:6075–6080.
31. O'Keefe G, Hybki DL, Munford RS. The G→ a single nucleotide polymorphism at the –308 position in the tumor necrosis factor-alpha promoter increases the risk for severe sepsis. J Trauma 2002;52:817–826.
32. Stuber F, Petersen M, Bokelmann F, et al. A genomic polymorphism within the tumor necrosis factor locus influences plasma tumor necrosis factor-alpha concentrations and outcome patients with severe sepsis. Crit Care Med 1996;24:381–384.
33. Schlüter B, Raufhake C, Erren M, et al. Effect of the interleukin-6 promoter polymorphism (–174G/C) on the incidence and outcome of sepsis. Crit Care Med 1002;30:32–37.
34. Bone RC: Gram-positive organisms in sepsis. Arch Intern Med 1994;154:26–31.
35. Danner RL, Elin RJ, Hosseini JM, et al. Endotoxemia in human septic shock. Chest 1991;99:169–175.
36. Rietschel ET, Kirikae T, Schade FU, et al. Bacterial endotoxin: molecular mechanisms of structure to activity and function. FASEB J 1994;218: 217–225.
37. Pridmore AC, Wyllie DH, Abdillahi F, et al. A lipopolysaccharide-deficient mutant of *Neisseria meningitidis* elicits attenuated cytokine release by human macrophages and signals via toll-like receptor (TLR)2 but not via TLR4/MD2. J Infect Dis 2001;183:89–96.
38. Medzhitov R, Janeway, C. Innate immunity. N Engl J Med 2000;343:338–344.
39. Fenton MJ, Golenbock DT.LPS-binding proteins and receptors. J Leukoc Biol 1998;64:25–32.
40. Pugin J, Heumann ID, Tomasz A, et al. CD14 is a pattern recognition receptor. Immunity 1994;1:509–516.
41. Lin Y, Leach WJ, Ammons WS. Synergistic effect of a recombinant N-terminal fragment of bactericidal/permeability increasing protein and cefamandole in treatment of rabbit gram-negative sepsis. Antimicrobial Agents Chemother 1996;40:65–69.
42. Levin M, Qunit PA, Goldstein B, et al. Recombinant bactericidal/permeability-increasing protein ($rBPI_{21}$) as adjunctive treatment for children with severe meningococcal sepsis: a randomised trial. Lancet 200;356:961–967.
43. Poltorak A, He X, Smirnova I, et al. Defective signaling in C3H/HeJ and C57BL/10ScCr mice: mutations in *Tlr4* gene. Science 1998;282:2085–2088.
44. Takeuchi O, Hoshino K, Kawai T, et al. Differential roles of TLR2 and TLR4 in recognition of gram-negative and gram-positive bacterial cell wall components. Immunity 1999; 11:443.
45. Brightbill HD, Libraty DH, Krutzik SR, et al. Host defense mechanisms triggered by microbial lipoproteins through toll-like receptors. Science 1999;285:732–735.
46. Cristofaro P, Opal S. The human toll-like receptors as a therapeutic target. Expert Opin Therapeutic Targets. 2003;7:603–612.
47. Heil F, Hemmi H, Hochrein H, et al. Species-specific recognition of single-stranded RNA via toll-like receptor 7 and 8. Science 2004;303:1526–1529.
48. Zhang D, Zhang G, Hayden MS, et al. A toll-like receptor that prevents infection by uropathogenic bacteria. Science 2004;303:1522–1526.
49. Wolbink GJ, Bossink AW, Groeneveld AB, et al. Complement activation in patients with sepsis is in part mediated by C-reactive protein. J Infect Dis 1998;177:81–87.
50. Roy S, Knox K, Griffiths D, et al. MBL genotype and risk of invasive pneumococcal disease: a case-control study. Lancet 2002;359:1569–1573.
51. Landmann R, Müller B, Zimmerli W. CD14, new aspects of ligand and signal diversity. Microb Infect 2000;2:295–304.
52. Nau GJ, Richmond JF, Schlesinger A, et al. Human macrophage activation programs induced by bacterial pathogens. Proc Natl Acad Sci U S A 2002;99:1503–1508.
53. Boldrick JC, Alizadeh AA, Diehn M, et al. Stereotyped and specific gene expression programs in human innate immune responses to bacteria. Proc Natl Acad Sci U S A 2002;99:972–977.
54. Means TK, Golenbock DT, Fenton MJ. The biology of toll-like receptors. Cytokine Growth Factor Rev 2000;11:219–232.
55. Hemmi H, Osamu T, Kawai T, et al. A toll-like receptor recognizes bacterial DNA. Nature 2000;408:740–744.
56. Alexopoulou L, Holt AC, Medzhitov R, et al. Recognition of double stranded RNA and activation of NFκB by Toll-like receptor 3. Nature 2001;413:732–738.
57. Hayayashi F, Smith KD, Ozinski A, et al. The innate immune response to bacterial flagellin is mediated by Toll-like receptor 5. Nature 2001;420:1099–1103.
58. Choi Y, Lafferty JA, Clements JRL. Selective expansion of T cells expressing Vb2 in toxic shock syndrome. J Exp Med 1990;172:981.
59. Hotchkiss RS, Karl IE. The pathology and treatment of sepsis. N Engl J Med 2003;348:138–150.
60. Florquine S, Goldman M: Immunoregulatory mechanisms of T-cell-dependent shock induced by bacterial superantigen in mice. Infect Immun 1996;64:3443.
61. Kusunoki T, Hailman E, Juan TS-C, et al. Molecules from *Staphylococcus aureus* that bind CD14 and stimulate innate immune responses. J Exp Med 995;182:1673.
62. Opal SM, Huber CE. Sepsis. Sci Am Med. 2001;30:1–17.
63. Opal SM, Scannon PJ, Vincent JL, et al. Relationship between plasma levels of lipopolysaccharide (LPS) and LPS-binding protein in patients with severe sepsis and septic shock. J Infect Dis 1999;180:1584–1589.
64. Tracey KJ, Beutler B, Lowry SF, et al. Shock and tissue injury induced by recombinant human cachectin. Science 1998;234:470–474.
65. Bauer KA, ten Cate H, Barzegar S, et al. Tumor necrosis factor infusions have a procoagulant effect on the hemostatic mechanism of humans. Blood 1989;74:165.
66. Fisher CJ, Slotman GJ, Opal SM, et al. Initial evaluation of human recombinant interleukin-1 receptor antagonist in the treatment of sepsis syndrome: a randomized, open-label, placebo-controlled multicenter trial. Crit Care Med 1994;22:12–21.

67. Dinarello CA, Gelfand JA, Wolff SM. Anticytokine strategies in the treatment of the systemic inflammatory response syndrome. JAMA 1993;269:1825–1832.
68. Luster AD. Chemokines: chemotactic cytokines that mediate inflammation. N Engl J Med 1998;338:436–442.
69. Falk LA, McNally R, Perera PY, et al. LPS-inducible responses in severe combined immunodeficiency (SCID) mice. J Endotoxin Res 1995;2:273.
70. Szabo SJ, Dinghe AS, Gubler U, et al. Regulation of the interleukin (IL)-12Rb2 subunit expression in developing T helper 1 (Th1) and Th2 cells. J Exp Med 1997;185:817.
71. Schneider C, von Aulock S, Siegfried Z, et al. Perioperative recombinant human granulocyte colony-stimulating factor (filgrastim) treatment prevents immunoinflammatory dysfunction associated with major surgery. Ann Surg 2004;239:75–81.
72. Hotchkiss RS, Swanson PE, Freeman BD, et al. Apototic cell death in patients with sepsis, shock and multiple organ dysfunction. Crit Care Med 1999;27:1230–1251.
73. Kell M, Ungethüm U, Steckholzer U, et al. Interleukin-10 counterregulates proinflammatory cytokine-induced inhibition of neutrophil apoptosis during severe sepsis. Blood 1997;90:3356–3363.
74. van Deventer SJH, Buller HR, ten Cate JW, et al. Experimental endotoxemia in humans: analysis of cytokine release and coagulation, fibrinolytic and complement pathways. Blood 1990;76: 2520–2526.
75. Greenberger MJ, Strieter RM, Kunkel SL, et al. Neutralization of IL-10 increases survival in a murine model of *Klebsiella pneumonia*. J Immunol 1995;155:722–729.
76. MacMicking J, Xie QM, Nathan C. Nitric oxide and macrophage function. Annu Rev Microbiol 1997;15:323–350.
77. Shenep JL, Toumanen E. Prospective: targeting nitric oxide in the adjuvant therapy of sepsis in meningitis. J Infect Dis 1998;177:766–771.
78. Liaudet L Poly (adenosine 5′phosphate) ribose polymerase activation as a cause of metabolic dysfunction in critical illness. Curr Opin Clin Nutr Metab Care 2002;5:175–184.
79. Vervloet MG, Thijs LG, Hack CE. Derangements of coagulation and fibrinolysis in critically ill patients with sepsis and septic shock. Semin Thromb Hemost 1998;24:33–44.
80. McGilvray ID, Rotstein OD. Role of the coagulation system in the local and systemic inflammatory response. World J Surg 1998;22:179–86.
81. Aird W. The role of the endothelium in severe sepsis and multiple organ dysfunction syndrome. Blood 2003;101:3765–3777.
82. Lorente JA, Garcia-Frade LJ, Landin L, et al. Time course of hemostatic abnormalities in sepsis and its relation to outcome. Chest 1993;103:1536–1542.
83. Coughlin SR. Thrombin receptor function and cardiovascular disease. Trends Cardiovasc Med 1994;4:77–83.
84. Levi M, ten Cate H. Disseminated intravascular coagulation. N Engl J Med 1999;341:586–592.
85. Abraham E, Reinhart K, Opal SM, et al. Efficacy and safety of tifacogin (recombinant tissue factor pathway inhibitor) in severe sepsis: a randomized controlled trial. JAMA 2003;290:238–251.
86. Bernard GR, Vincent JL, Laterre PF, et al. Safety and efficacy of activated protein C for severe sepsis. N Engl J Med 2001;344:699–709.
87. Warren BL, Eid A, Singer P, et al. High-dose antithrombin III in severe sepsis. A randomized controlled trial. JAMA 2001;286: 1869–1878.
88. Joyce DE, Gelbert L, Ciaccia A, et al. Gene expression profile of antithrombotic protein C defines new mechanisms modulating inflammation and apoptosis. J Biol Chem 2001;276:11199–11203.
89. Corrigan JJ Jr. Heparin therapy in bacterial septicemia. J Pediatr 1977;91:695–700.
90. Hoffmann JN, Vollmar B, Inthorn D et al. The thrombin antagonist hirudin fails to inhibit endotoxin-induced leukocyte/endothelial cell interaction and microvascular perfusion failure. Shock 2000;14:528–534.
91. Wheeler AP, Bernard GR. Treating patients with severe sepsis. N Engl J Med 1999;340:207–214.
92. Esmon CT. Why do animal models (sometimes) fail to mimic human sepsis? Crit Care Med 2004;32:S219–S22.
93. Roger T, Froidevaux C, Martin C, et al. Macrophage migration inhibitory factor (MIF) regulates host responses to endotoxin through modulation of Toll-like receptor 4 (TLR4). J Endotoxin Res 2003;9:119–123.
94. Garner LB, Willis MS, Carlson DL, et al. Macrophage migration inhibitory factor is a cardiac-derived myocardial depressant factor. Am J Physiol Heart Circ Physiol 2003;285:H2500–H2509.
95. Baumann R, Casaulta C, Simon D, et al. Macrophage migration inhibitory factor delays apoptosis in neutrophils by inhibiting the mitochondria-dependent death pathway. FASEB J 2003;17: 2221–2230.
96. Bozza FA, Gomes RN, Japiassu AM, et al. Macrophage migration inhibitory factor levels correlate with fatal outcome in sepsis. Shock 2004;22:309–313.
97. Eriandsson Harris H, Andersson U. Mini-review: the nuclear protein HMGB1 as a proinflammatory mediator. Eur J Immunol 2004;34:1503–1512.
98. Wang H, Yang H. Tracey KJ. Extracellular role of HMGB1 in inflammation and sepsis. J Intern Med 2004;255:320–331.
99. Yang H, Ochani M, Li J, et al. Reversing established sepsis with antagonists of endogenous high-mobility group box 1. Proc Natl Acad Sci U S A 2004;101:296–301.
100. Riedermann NC, Guo RF, Ward PA. Novel strategies for the treatment of septic shock. Nat Med 2003;9:517–524.
101. Bouchon A, Facchetti F, Weigand MA, et al. TREM-1 amplifies inflammation and is crucial mediator of septic shock. Nature 2001;410:1103–1107.
102. Chamaillard M, Hashimoto M, Horie Y, et al. An essential role for NOD-1 in host recognition of peptidoglycan containing diaminopimelic acid. Nat Immunol 2003;4:702–707.
103. Borovikova LV, Ivanov S, Zhang M, et al. Vagus nerve stimulation attenuates the systemic inflammatory response to endotoxin. Nature 2000;405:458–462.
104. Nishio K, Akai Y, Murao Y, et al. Increased plasma concentrations of adrenomedullin correlate with relaxation of vascular tone in patients with septic shock. Crit Care Med 1997;25:953–957.
105. Landry DW, Oliver JA. The pathogenesis of vasodilatory shock. N Engl J Med 2001;345:588–595.
106. Zimmermann GA, McIntyre TM, Prescott SM, et al. The platelet-activating factor signaling system and its regulators in syndromes of inflammation and thrombosis. Crit Care Med 2002; 30(suppl):S294–S301.
107. Shoemaker WC, Montgomery ES, Kaplan E, et al. Physiologic patterns in surviving and non-surviving shock patients. Arch Surg 1973;106:630.
108. Fink M. Cytotoxic hypoxia in sepsis. Acta Anaesthesiol Scand 1997;110:87–95.
109. Hayes MA, Timmins AC, Yau EHS, et al. Elevation of systemic oxygen delivery in the treatment of critically ill patients. N Engl J Med 1994;330:1717.
110. Rivers E, Nguyen B, Havstadt S, et al. Early goal-directed therapy in the treatment of severe sepsis and septic shock. N Engl J Med 2001;345:1368–1377.
111. Marshall JC, Foster D, Vincent JL, et al. Diagnostic and prognostic implications of endotoxemia in critical illness: results of the Medic trial. J Infect Dis 2004;190:527–534.
112. Sriskandan S, Moyes D, Cohen J. Detection of circulating bacterial superantigen and lymphotoxin alpha in patients with streptococcal toxic-shock syndrome. Lancet 1986;348:1315.

113. Reinhart K, Wiegand-Lohnert C, Grimminger F, et al. Assessment of the safety and efficacy of the monoclonal anti-tumor necrosis factor antibody-fragment, MAK 195F, in patients with sepsis and septic shock: a multicenter, randomized, placebo-controlled, dose-ranging study. Crit Care Med 1996;24:733–740.
114. Damas P, Ledoux D, Nys M, et al. Cytokine serum levels during severe sepsis in humans: IL-6 as a marker of severity. Ann Surg 1992;215:356.
115. Fisher CJ, Dhainaut JF, Opal SM, et al. Recombinant human interleukin 1 receptor antagonist in the treatment of patients with sepsis syndrome. Results from a randomized, double blind, placebo-controlled trial. JAMA 1994;271:1836–1843.
116. Karzai W, Oberhoffer M, Meier-Helmann A, et al. Procalcitonin: a new indicator of systemic response to severe infections. Infection 1997;6:629–634.
117. Gendrel D, Assicot M, Raymond J, et al. Procalcitonin as a marker for the early diagnosis of neonatal infection. J Pediatr 1996;128:570–573.
118. deWerra I, Jacchard C, Corradin SB, et al. Cytokines, nitrite/nitrate, soluble tumor necrosis factor receptors, and procalcitonin concentration: comparisons in patients with septic shock, cardiogenic shock, and bacterial pneumonia. Crit Care Med 1997;25:607–615.
119. Drakulovic MB, Torres A, Bauer TT, et al. Supine body position as a risk factor for nosocominal pneumonia in mechanically ventilated patients: a randomised trial. Lancet 1999;354:1851–1858.
120. ARDS-Network. Ventilation with lower tidal volumes as compared with traditional tidal volumes for acute lung injury and the acute respiratory distress syndrome. N Engl J Med 2000;342:1301.
121. Cochrane Injuries Group Albumin Reviewers. Human albumin administration in critically ill patients: systematic review of randomized controlled trials. BMJ 1998;317:235–240.
122. Wilkes MM, Navickis RJ. Patient survival after human albumin administration. Ann Intern Med 2001;135:149–164.
123. Finfers, Bellomo R, Boyce N, et al. A comparison of albumin and saline for fluid resuscitation in the intensive care unit. N Engl J Med 2004;350:2247–2256.
124. Martin C, Papazian L, Perrin G, et al. Norepinephrine or dopamine for the treatment of hyperdynamic septic shock? Chest 1993;103:1826.
125. Kellum J, Decker J. Use of dopamine in acute renal failure: a meta-analysis. Crit Care Med 2001;29:1752–1758.
126. Marin C, Eon B, Saux P, et al. Renal effects of norepinephrine used to treat septic shock patients. Crit Care Med 1990;18: 282.
127. Holmes CL, Patel BM, Russell JA, et al. Physiology of vasopressin relevant to management of septic shock. Chest 2001;120:989–1002.
128. Spronk PF, Ince C, Gardien MJ et al. Nitroglycerin in septic shock after intravascular fluid resuscitation. Lancet 2002;360: 1395–1396.
129. Wu W, Rathore SS, Wang Y, et al. Blood transfusion in elderly patients with acute myocardial infarction. N Engl J Med 2001;345:1230–1236.
130. Corwin HL, Gettinger A, Rodriguez RM, et al. Efficacy of recombinant human erythropoietin in the critically ill patient: a randomized, double-blind, placebo-controlled trial. Crit Care Med 1999;27:2346–2350.
131. Weiskopf RB, Viely MK, Feiner J, et al. Human cardiovascular and metabolic response to acute, severe isovolemic anemia. JAMA 1998;279:217–221.
132. Hebert PC, Wells G, Blajchman M, et al. A multicenter, randomized, controlled clinical trial of transfusion requirements in critical care. N Engl J Med 1999;340:409–417.
133. Kudsk KA, Croce MA, Fabian TC, et al. Enteral versus parenteral feeding: effects on septic morbidity after blunt and penetrating abdominal trauma. Ann Surg 1992;15:503–508.
134. Bower RH, Cerra FB, Bershadshy B, et al. Early enteral administration of a formula (Impact) supplemented with arginine, nucleotides, and fish oil in intensive care unit patients: results of a multicenter prospective, randomized, clinical trial. Crit Care Med 1995;23:436–442.
135. Kluger MJ, Kozak W, Conn C, et al. The adaptive value of fever. Infect Dis Clin North Am 1996;10:1–22.
136. Jiang Q, Cross AS, Singh IS, et al. Febrile core temperature is essential for optimal host defense in bacterial peritonitis. Infect Immun 2000;68:1265–1270.
137. Ribeiro SP, Chu E, Slutsky AS. Heat stress after injection of LPS in rats decreases mortality. Am J Respir Crit Care Med 1996;153: A252.
138. O'Donnell J, Axelrod R, Fisher C, et al. Use and effectiveness of hypothermia blankets for febrile patients in the intensive care unit. Clin Infect Dis 1997;24:1208–1211.
139. Kollef MH. Optimizing antibiotic therapy in the intensive care unit setting. Critical Care 2001;5:189–195.
140. Ibrahim EM, Sherman G, Ward S, et al. The influence of inadequate antimicrobial treatment of blood stream infection on patient outcomes in the ICU setting. Chest 2000;118:146–155.
141. Rao AK, Chouhan V, Chen X, et al. Activation of the tissue factor pathway of blood coagulation during prolonged hyperglycemia in young healthy men. Diabetes 2002;48:1156–1161.
142. van den Berghe G, Wouters P, Weekers F, et al. Intensive insulin therapy in critically ill patients. N Engl J Med 2001;345:1349–1346.
143. Annane D, Sebille V, Charpentier C, et al. Effects of treatment with low doses of hydrocortisone and fludrocortisone on mortality in patients with septic shock. JAMA 2002;288:862–871.
144. Schroeder S, Wichers M, Klingmüller D, et al. The hypothalamic-pituitary-adrenal axis of patients with severe sepsis: altered response to corticotropin-releasing hormone. Crit Care Med 2001;29:310–316.
145. Keh D, Boehnke T, Weber-Cartens S, et al. Immunologic and hemodynamic effects of "low dose" hydrocortisone in septic shock. A double-blind, randomized, placebo-controlled crossover study. Am J Respir Crit Care Med 2003;167:512–520.

16

Shock and Resuscitation

Avery B. Nathens and Ronald V. Maier

In 1872, Gross referred to shock as the "manifestation of the rude unhinging of the machinery of life."[1] We now know that shock, at its most fundamental level, represents the clinical syndrome arising as a result of inadequate tissue perfusion. The discrepancy between substrate delivery and the cellular substrate requirement leads to cellular metabolic dysfunction. Inadequate oxygen delivery is implicated as the principal defect in shock states. The clinical manifestations of shock are caused by end-organ dysfunction secondary to impaired perfusion *and* the body's sympathetic and neuroendocrine response to an insufficient cellular supply/demand ratio for oxygen.

Timely restoration of perfusion and oxygen delivery usually reverses the shock state. However, the persistence or progression of shock may occur as a result of an ongoing occult perfusion defect, irreversible cellular injury, or a combination of the two phenomena. In addition, there is substantial clinical and laboratory evidence suggesting that cellular injury leads to the elaboration of proinflammatory mediators that may further compromise perfusion through functional and structural changes in the microvasculature. This form of secondary injury further impairs perfusion, creating a vicious cycle by which cellular injury leads to impaired perfusion, which further exacerbates cellular injury. Last, following recovery from the clinical shock state (i.e., total body hypoperfusion), there is diffuse activation of potent inflammatory cells that may lead to the systemic inflammatory response syndrome (SIRS). It is postulated that persistence of SIRS, through the secondary induction of global cellular dysfunction, may be causative in the development of the multiple-organ dysfunction syndrome (MODS).[2–4]

Several classification schemes based on the underlying cause of shock have been proposed, but none is ideal. The classic scheme, proposed by Blalock in 1930, recognized hypovolemic, cardiogenic, neurogenic, and vasogenic shock as separate entities, but a somewhat more elaborate classification better takes into account the pathophysiological mechanisms leading to the shock state (Table 16.1). It is critical to appreciate that strict adherence to a classification scheme can be difficult because clinical shock syndromes often involve a combination of processes. For example, hypovolemia is often a component of shock caused by trauma or sepsis, while relative adrenal insufficiency might contribute to hemodynamic alterations in all shock states.

Hypovolemic Shock

Hypovolemic shock is the most common cause of shock. It may arise as a result of one of two processes: (1) hemorrhage, representing intravascular volume depletion through the loss of red blood cell mass; or (2) loss of plasma volume only through extravascular fluid sequestration *or* gastrointestinal, urinary, and insensible losses. Hemorrhage is the form of volume loss that can be most readily quantified and reproduced and thus represents the best-understood form of shock, whereas extravascular fluid sequestration, also referred to as *third-space fluid losses*, is frequently underappreciated as a cause of shock. Third-space fluid losses are the principal cause of hypovolemia in the early postoperative period and in local inflammatory processes, such as pancreatitis, in which local changes in capillary permeability result in fluid extravasation from the intravascular space into the interstitium. Fluid sequestration is the principal cause of shock in patients with small-bowel obstruction. In this case, hypovolemia results from fluid loss into the interstitium and bowel lumen and exudation of fluid into the peritoneal cavity. The clinical manifestations of nonhemorrhagic forms of hypovolemic shock are the same as with hemorrhage, although onset can be more insidious.

The physiological responses to hypovolemic shock are geared toward maintenance of cerebral and coronary perfusion and the restoration of effective circulating blood volume. The major compensatory mechanisms include an increase in sympathetic activity, release of stress hormones and expansion of intravascular volume through resorption of interstitial

TABLE 16.1. Classification of Shock States.

Hypovolemic
Traumatic
Cardiogenic
Intrinsic
Compressive
Septic
Neurogenic
Hypoadrenal

fluid, mobilization of intracellular fluid, and conservation of fluids and electrolytes by the kidney. The clinical manifestations are simply a reflection of the intense adrenosympathetic response and renal conservation of fluid. Microvascular hypoperfusion of selected vascular beds results from the combination of low intravascular blood volume, diminished cardiac output from a reduction in preload, and compensatory peripheral vasoconstriction.

A clinical staging system of hemorrhagic shock based on the percentage of acute blood volume loss has been described (Table 16.2). Mild volume loss can be tolerated with relatively few external signs, particularly in the supine, resting patient. Loss of 10% to 15% of the blood volume or class I hemorrhage (500–750 ml in a 70-kg patient) causes minimal change in the patient's clinical condition. Class I hemorrhage is exemplified by the status of a patient following the donation of a single unit of blood. Slight tachycardia with a drop in pulse pressure may be the only manifestation.

With class II hemorrhage, consisting of a 15% to 30% blood volume loss (750–1500 ml), the patient becomes anxious and mildly tachycardic with a clear drop in pulse pressure. Systolic blood pressure is still maintained by virtue of peripheral vasoconstriction, manifested as pallor and delayed capillary refill. Elevated levels of vasopressin and aldosterone coupled with adrenergic-mediated renal arteriolar constriction induce a mild oliguria.

Blood volume loss of 30% to 40% (1500–2000 ml), or class III hemorrhage, leads to the classic findings of hemorrhagic shock. Patients almost always present with marked tachycardia, tachypnea, significant alterations in mental status, and a measurable fall in blood pressure. In normal individuals, this is the least amount of blood loss that consistently causes a drop in systolic blood pressure.

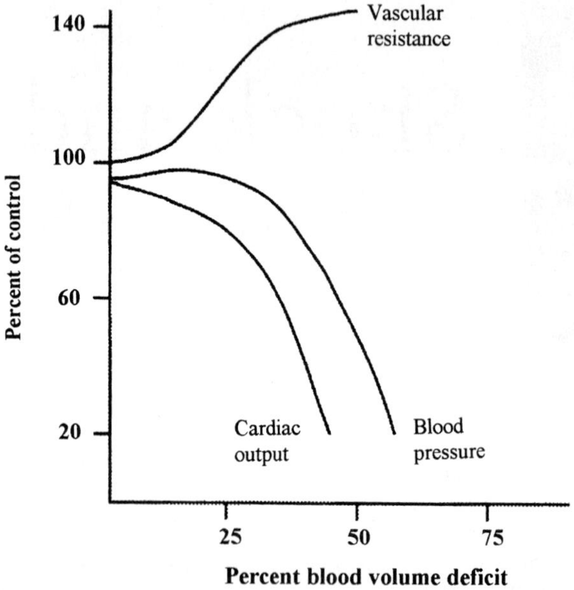

FIGURE 16.1. The compensatory neuroendocrine response to hemorrhage maintains an adequate blood pressure until blood loss exceeds 30%–40% of total blood volume. The relatively early increase in systemic vascular resistance and reduction in cardiac output implies that tissue perfusion is impaired far sooner than the development of hypotension would suggest. (*Source:* Adapted from Schwaitzberg et al.,[111] with permission.)

Severe blood loss, or class IV hemorrhage, with 40% or more blood volume loss (>2000 ml), represents a severe physiological insult. Systolic hypotension may be profound, and the diastolic blood pressure may be unobtainable. Mental status changes progress from restlessness and agitation to listlessness and obtundation, producing a moribund condition because cerebral blood flow is insufficient to maintain neurological function. Loss of more than 50% of circulating blood volume results in loss of consciousness, pulse, and blood pressure.

Typically, classes I and II are referred to as compensated shock states in which the adrenergic response maintains a normal blood pressure (Fig. 16.1). Passage from an initially compensated state of shock to class IV shock may occur rapidly, particularly in children and young adults. It is crucial to recognize compensated shock and intervene as early as possible. Decompensation of homeostatic mechanisms and

TABLE 16.2. Estimated Fluid and Blood Losses Based on Patient's Initial Presentation.*

	Class I	*Class II*	*Class III*	*Class IV*
Blood loss (mL)	Up to 750	750–1500	1500–2000	>2000
Blood loss (% blood volume)	Up to 15%	15%–30%	30%–40%	>40%
Pulse rate	<100	≥100	>120	>140
Blood pressure (mm Hg)	Normal or increased	Decreased	Decreased	Decreased
Pulse pressure (mm Hg)	Normal or increased	Decreased	Decreased	Decreased
Respiratory rate	14–20	20–30	30–40	>35
Urine output (mL/h)	>30	20–30	5–15	Negligible
CNS/mental status	Slightly anxious	Mildly anxious	Anxious, confused	Confused, lethargic
Fluid replacement (3:1 rule)	Crystalloid	Crystalloid	Crystalloid and blood	Crystalloid and blood

*For a 70-kg man. The guidelines are based on the 3-for-1 rule. This rule derives from the empiric observation that most patients in hemorrhagic shock require as much as 300 mL of electrolyte solution for each 100 mL of blood loss. Applied blindly, these guidelines can result in excessive or inadequate fluid administration. For example, a patient with a crush injury to the extremity may have hypotension out of proportion to his or her blood loss and require fluids in excess of the 3:1 guidelines. In contrast, a patient whose ongoing blood loss is being replaced by blood transfusion requires less than 3:1. The use of bolus therapy with careful monitoring of the patient's response can moderate these extremes.

Source: Reprinted with permission from Advanced Trauma Life Support for Doctors, Committee on Trauma, American College of Surgeons. Chicago: 2004.

inability to maintain systolic blood pressure above 90 mmHg after trauma-induced hypovolemia are associated with a mortality of more than 50%.[5] However, rapid and adequate restoration of circulating blood volume simultaneous with control of bleeding can reverse even severe hemorrhagic shock. If shock is prolonged, then hypoperfusion of the various microvascular beds may lead to cellular injury and the elaboration of inflammatory mediators, setting up the vicious self-propagation of ongoing tissue injury and organ dysfunction.[6,7]

Hypovolemic shock is easily diagnosed when there is an obvious source of volume loss and when overt signs of hemodynamic instability and increased adrenergic output are present. However, assessment is more difficult with lesser degrees of hypovolemia. Table 16.3 demonstrates the diagnostic utility of changes in heart rate and systolic blood pressure.[8] Most evident is the lack of sensitivity of these measures in patients with moderate acute blood loss. The most helpful physical findings are severe postural dizziness (preventing measurement of upright vital signs) or a postural pulse increment of 30 beats/min or more. Supine hypotension and tachycardia are frequently absent, even with more than 1000 ml blood loss. In addition, capillary refill time, once considered a valuable physical sign of hypovolemia, has a sensitivity for moderate blood loss of only 11% and specificity of 89%[8] The diagnosis is even more challenging when there is an occult source or a slower rate of volume loss, such as might occur with excessive gastrointestinal, urinary, or insensible loss.

Laboratory evaluation may provide some diagnostic information. Nonhemorrhagic forms of hypovolemic shock tend to cause hemoconcentration. If the principal abnormality is caused by loss of free water, then hemoconcentration will be accompanied by hyponatremia. Acutely following hemorrhage, there may be no alteration in the hemoglobin or hematocrit values until compensatory fluid shifts have occurred or exogenous red cell-free resuscitation fluid is administered. In the absence of exogenous resuscitation, these values decrease secondary to transcapillary refill or osmotic-induced shifts, a process that may take several hours to achieve.

The diagnosis of hypovolemic shock is usually made on the basis of the complete clinical picture. However, when the underlying shock state is not clear, the most critical distinction is to ensure that one is not treating cardiogenic shock as the appropriate therapy differs dramatically. The findings of jugular venous distension, rales, and the presence of an S_3 gallop in cardiogenic shock may assist in their differentiation. Both forms of shock, however, are associated with a reduction in cardiac output and a compensatory sympathetic-mediated response. Further, both types of shock may be treated with, and respond to, volume resuscitation. If the diagnosis is in doubt or the clinical situation suggests both as a possibility, then invasive monitoring using a pulmonary artery catheter (PAC) might be helpful.

Treatment of hypovolemic shock involves achieving two primary goals concurrently: reexpanding the circulating blood volume and proceeding with any necessary interventions to control ongoing volume loss. The rate at which volume expansion is achieved should take into account the clinical status of the patient. In patients with hemorrhagic shock, there is increasing evidence to suggest that limiting volume until bleeding is controlled is not harmful and might in fact be beneficial.[9] However, in patients with clear evidence of shock in whom ongoing blood loss is not a concern, vigorous volume resuscitation is paramount. Adequate repletion of the circulating volume reexpands capacitance vessels, restores venous return, and reestablishes ventricular filling. As a result of improved left ventricular end-diastolic volume, contractile function, stroke volume, and cardiac output respond positively; as cardiac output improves, the systemic vascular resistance returns to normal, and tissue perfusion is restored. Even after adequate resuscitation, diastolic compliance may remain abnormal for some time because of increased myocardial interstitial fluid. This reduced compliance may necessitate higher left ventricular end-diastolic pressures to optimize ventricular performance.

Intravenous Access

Resuscitation of hemorrhagic shock or severe hypovolemia irrespective of the cause requires two large-bore (16-gauge or larger) intravenous lines for rapid volume restoration. Access may be achieved by peripheral vein catheterization; cutdowns on the basilic, greater saphenous, or cephalic veins; or percutaneous central venous access via subclavian, internal jugular,

TABLE 16.3. Systematic Review of the Diagnostic Utility of Changes in Heart and Blood Pressure in the Assessment of Hemorrhagic Shock.

	Sensitivity (95% confidence interval)		*Specificity (95% confidence interval)*
	Moderate blood loss (450–630 ml)	Large blood loss (630–1150 ml)	Specificity
Postural[a] pulse increment ≥30/min or severe postural dizziness	22 (6%–48%)	97 (91%–100%)	98 (97–99)
Postural hypotension (≥20 mmHg decrease in systolic blood pressure) Age ≤65	9 (6–12)	NA	94 (84–99)
Age ≥65	27 (14–40)	NA	86 (76–97)
Supine tachycardia (pulse >100/min)	0 (0–42)	12 (5–24)	96 (88–99)
Supine hypotension (systolic blood pressure ≤95 mmHg)	13 (0–50)	33 (21–47)	97 (90–100)

NA, not applicable in this setting.

[a]Supine to standing position.

Source: From McGee et al.,[8] by permission of the *Journal of the American Medical Association.*

or femoral venous puncture. In a large, randomized controlled trial, femoral venous catheterization was associated with a 4-fold increase in rates of catheter-related infection and over a 10-fold increased risk of thrombotic complications,[10] suggesting that this approach should be used only when other sites are inaccessible. If absolutely required, then the catheter should be removed at the earliest possible time.

For the purposes of resuscitation, the most important consideration for vascular access is the choice of catheter and tubing. The rate of flow is proportional to the fourth power of the radius of the cannula and is inversely related to its length (Poiseuille's law). Thus, a short, large-bore catheter connected to the widest administration tubing possible or direct insertion of beveled tubing via a cutdown venotomy provides the most rapid flow rates. There is a 10-fold increase in flow rates when a large-bore introducer catheter (8.5 French) is used in conjunction with trauma administration tubing (0.22 inch internal diameter) compared to a typical 18-gauge catheter with regular intravenous tubing (0.10 inch internal diameter).[11] Flow rates are also dependent on the viscosity of the administered fluid. Finally, accurate placement with avoidance of catheter kinking is critical to maximize flow rates (Fig. 16.2).

Choice of Fluid for Volume Resuscitation

The optimal fluid for volume resuscitation has been a subject of controversy for decades. The most efficacious and cost-effective approach is to restore intravascular volume with rapid infusion of isotonic saline or a balanced salt solution. Infusion of 2 to 3l of crystalloid over 10 to 30min should restore adequate intravascular volume in most cases as the result of its large volume of distribution. In patients with hemorrhagic shock, final restoration of blood volume with crystalloid usually requires at least three times the estimated blood loss. However, if blood pressure does not improve after rapid administration of 2l of crystalloid, this suggests that blood loss is in excess of 1500ml, there is ongoing active bleeding, or another cause of shock must be considered. Further volume resuscitation should therefore include simultaneous blood transfusion, either as fully cross-matched blood, type-specific blood, or in dire circumstances, O-positive or O-negative packed cells.

Although administration of isotonic crystalloid and blood products remains the conventional approach to patients with hemorrhagic or hypovolemic shock, several other products have been considered and promoted as possible alternatives. These options include hypertonic saline (HS), a variety of colloids, and blood substitutes.

Hypertonic Saline

Hypertonic (7.5%) saline has been considered an alternative to isotonic solutions for several reasons. First, it achieves a similar increase in intravascular volume with the administration of smaller infusion volumes by drawing water out of the intracellular space and thus replenishes the depleted extracellular space; in effect, it is a form of autotransfusion from the relatively large intracellular compartment to the smaller interstitial and intravascular compartments. The relative cellular dehydration induced by HS might also play a role in reducing cerebral edema (and thus lower intracranial pressure) in patients with head injury. In addition, there are experimental data suggesting that hypertonic solutions might lessen the inflammatory response following shock and resuscitation.[12–14] To increase the intravascular oncotic pressure, hyperonic saline is often administered in 6% dextran. The colloid component transiently partitions the recruited fluid to the intravascular space and thus, in theory, should prolong

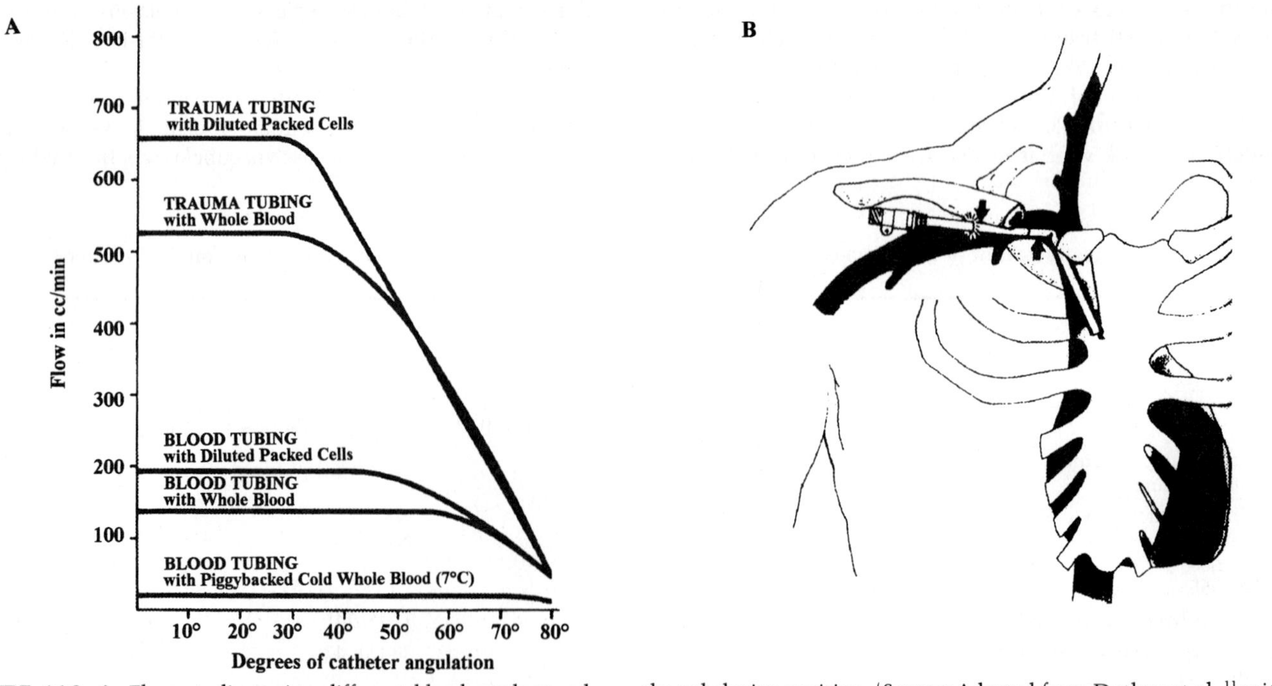

FIGURE 16.2. **A**. Flow studies using different blood products administered through an 8.5-French catheter. **B**. Kinking is a frequent problem and significantly reduces maximal flow rates, particularly in the subclavian position. (*Source:* Adapted from Dutkey et al.,[11] with permission.)

the beneficial hemodynamic effects of the solutions. In addition, HS induces a poorly defined pressor response following its administration.

In most clinical trials, outcomes of patients receiving HS with or without dextran (HSD) are compared to those receiving standard crystalloid solutions of either lactated Ringer's or 0.9% saline. The solution is administered as a 250-ml bolus either in the prehospital setting or as the first resuscitation fluid in the emergency department. When dextran is administered with HS, it persists in the circulation with a half-life of 7 to 10h; thus, some effect should persist beyond the acute resuscitation phase.[15]

In a large American multicenter study trial consisting of 359 evaluable patients with hypotension caused by trauma, patients were randomized to receive either HSD (250ml) or standard isotonic resuscitation during prehospital transport.[16] Mortality was 83% in patients receiving HSD compared to 80% in those receiving standard crystalloid solutions, an insignificant difference. Post hoc subset analysis demonstrated a significant survival benefit in those patients requiring operation for penetrating trauma. However, when this group of patients was studied prospectively, there was only a trend toward improved survival in the patients receiving HSD.[17] Unfortunately, the small sample size (48 patients) precludes any definitive interpretation of the effect of HS as a resuscitation fluid in this subset of patients.

In the highest-quality randomized controlled trial to date, 229 patients in coma with shock following injury were randomized to receive either a single 250-ml bolus of 7.5% saline or Ringer's lactate in the field. In-hospital survival and long-term (6-month) neurological outcomes were equivalent across groups.[18]

To specifically evaluate the importance of dextran, a large multicenter trial was performed to evaluate the effects of isotonic saline and HS with or without dextran during the prehospital resuscitation of trauma patients with hemorrhagic shock.[19] This study suggested only a trend toward improved survival in the entire cohort of patients receiving HS solutions. There was no significant benefit with the addition of dextran. However, post hoc subset analysis demonstrated a significantly improved survival in patients with severe head injury in combination with hemorrhagic shock. Unfortunately, this effect did not persist in a subsequent trial in which this subset of patients was specifically evaluated prospectively.[20]

Most, but not all, of the studies to date do not have sufficient statistical power to detect a difference in outcome between patients treated with HSD and isotonic crystalloid solutions. To circumvent this problem, two meta-analyses have been published.[21,22] In one evaluation, individual patient data were collated from all randomized controlled trials of HSD or HS in patients with hemorrhagic shock due to trauma.[21] The overall study population consisted of more than 600 patients. When the entire population of patients was considered, there was a definite suggestion of an improvement in survival associated with HSD, with the greatest effect demonstrable in patients requiring surgery for penetrating injuries. In a separate publication, these data were analyzed specifically to determine the effectiveness of HS resuscitation in patients with severe head injury.[23] In an analysis of 233 patients with combined shock and severe head injury from six different trials, patients receiving HSD were twice as likely to survive until discharge. However, these results do not include data from the more recent, negative, large randomized controlled trial.[18]

In a second meta-analysis, the effects of HS, HSD, and isotonic crystalloid in patients with traumatic hemorrhagic shock were evaluated.[22] This study differs because of the use of intent-to-treat analysis; that is, patients were evaluated according to treatment assignment rather than actual treatment received. After an analysis of more than 1200 patients in a total of 14 studies, there was no difference in survival. Patients treated with HS generally exhibited larger blood pressure increases and had reduced early and 24-h total fluid and blood requirements than observed in patients treated with isotonic solutions.

Based on published data, HS with or without dextran probably offers little benefit to standard resuscitation regimens. Hypertonic saline as a method of small-volume resuscitation may also offer certain advantages in less-controlled medical environments where prolonged transport or evacuation times require longer periods of resuscitation with limited supplies. In addition, the low weights and small volumes of HS required for resuscitation may prove advantageous in the battlefield.

Fluid Resuscitation Using Colloid

Much of the controversy regarding the optimal fluid for shock resuscitation has centered on the use of crystalloid solutions versus colloid solutions. In addition, there is controversy regarding which colloid offers the greatest benefit. In a meta-analysis of 31 randomized controlled trials in which albumin was compared to crystalloid solutions, mortality was 50% higher in patients receiving albumin.[24] For every 20 patients treated with albumin, it is estimated that there is 1 additional death. Another meta-analysis suggested neither harm nor benefit with albumin infusion.[25] Taken together, the absence of benefit and potential for harm coupled with the certain increase in costs, albumin cannot be recommended for shock resuscitation.

The putative mechanisms by which administration of albumin may exert any adverse effects are unclear. Potentially, increased transcapillary flux of albumin from increased microvascular permeability might reduce the oncotic pressure difference across the capillary wall, making edema more likely and more resistant to subsequent mobilization. An increase in interstitial edema may globally worsen tissue oxygenation while impairing alveolar gas exchange in the lungs.[26] There is also some evidence to suggest that albumin may impair sodium and water excretion and worsen renal failure.[27]

There are several forms of synthetic colloid in use. Most are derived from a 6% hydroxyethyl starch solution and differ in the molecular weights of the hydroxyethyl moiety. These large molecules provide superb oncotic properties while maintaining the agent in the intravascular space. As a result of these properties, these agents have a volume-expanding effect that lasts as long as 24h (Fig. 16.3).

Potential disadvantages with the use of hydroxyethyl starch solutions include rare anaphylactic reactions and a coagulopathy when given in large volumes. The development of coagulopathy depends on the specific colloid and is frequent in some with larger molecular weights (e.g., hetastarch)

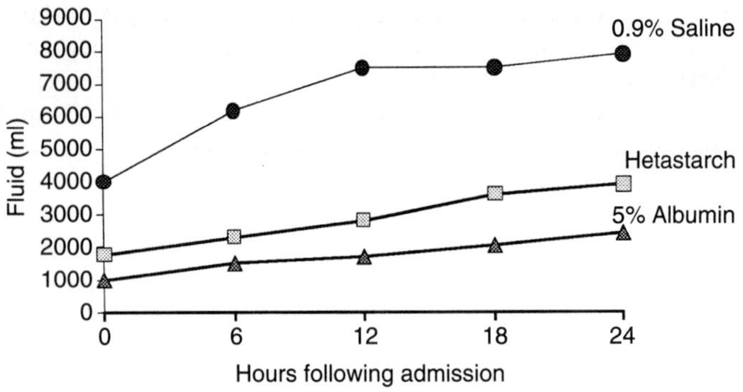

FIGURE 16.3. Total fluid requirements in patients with hypovolemic shock receiving a synthetic colloid (hetastarch), 5% albumin, or 0.9% saline. Synthetic colloids have a far greater volume-expanding effect than crystalloid solutions, roughly equal to that of 5% albumin. (*Source:* Adapted from Rackow et al.[112])

compared to others with relatively small molecular weights (e.g., pentastarch).[27,28] Randomized controlled trials in a variety of clinical settings suggested that these solutions do provide volume expansion superior to crystalloid solutions[29,30] and, along with this, some improvement in microcirculatory blood flow.[31] There is a suggestion that these synthetic colloids might increase the risk of acute renal failure, an effect dependent on the in vitro molecular weight of the compound, the degree of substitution (the proportion of hydroxyethylated glucose molecules), and the volume administered as these characteristics affect the time to elimination from the intravascular space and the degree of macromolecule accumulation.[32]

Alternatives to Blood Transfusion

Although the current blood supply is safer than ever owing to improved donor screening and testing, it is likely, because of the inevitable appearance of new viruses and the potential for false-negative screening tests, that disease transmission will never be completely eradicated. In addition, there is some evidence to suggest that blood transfusion is an independent risk factor for posttraumatic organ dysfunction, an effect putatively mediated by priming of recipient neutrophils by inflammatory mediators within stored blood.[33,34] In this regard, a randomized controlled trial of a restrictive (maintaining hemoglobin between 7 and 9 g/dl) versus a liberal (maintaining hemoglobin between 10 and 12 g/dl) transfusion policy demonstrated a reduced risk of death and organ dysfunction in the restrictive group. This effect was significant in patients less than 55 years of age and in those with scores below 20 on the APACHE (Acute Physiology and Chronic Health Evaluation) II.[35] Finally, blood transfusion involves the need for compatibility testing, which increases the time required for its availability. To circumvent the problems associated with the transfusion of allogeneic blood, two alternatives exist to standard blood transfusion: autotransfusion and red blood cell substitutes.

Autotransfusion

Autotransfusion of shed blood is a valuable adjunct to elective cardiothoracic, abdominal, orthopedic, and vascular surgery, although its use in the resuscitation of trauma patients was first reported more than 50 years ago.[36] Transfusion of shed blood has several advantages over homologous blood. In the acutely injured patient in need of immediate blood, autotransfusion is readily available. Autotransfusion is safe without risk of hemolytic, febrile, or allergic reactions or transmissible disease. Further, salvaged blood is already warm and has better oxygen-transport properties because of preservation of normal levels of 2,3-diphosphoglycerol. Despite reductions in platelet count and function, labile clotting factors are present in greater concentration than in banked blood, although fibrinogen levels drop significantly in salvaged blood.[37] Although enteric contamination was at one point considered a contraindication to the use of autotransfusion devices, there is evidence to suggest that even moderate amounts of contamination pose little risk if perioperative antimicrobial therapy is used.[38,39]

Despite the potential advantages of autotransfusion, its contribution to blood replacement in the patient with hemorrhagic shock is variable. In several studies, autologous blood met from 11% to 45% of the total blood requirement.[37,40–42] In the exsanguinating patient, two limitations preclude its greater use. First, there is usually insufficient time available to organize the necessary personnel and equipment. In addition, by design the suction apparatus is less efficient at aspirating blood to minimize hemolysis, and this feature makes it less useful in patients with massive hemoperitoneum. Regardless, the use of autotransfusion devices is cost-effective and reduces the use of banked blood.[42] Its use should be considered in any operative patient with hemorrhagic shock who does not immediately respond to crystalloid resuscitation in the emergency room.[40]

Red Blood Cell Substitutes

There are several potential benefits to using a red blood cell substitute, including immediate availability, no need for compatibility testing, freedom from disease transmission, and long-term storage. Diaspirin cross-linked hemoglobin (DCLH) is the most well studied of the currently available blood substitutes. It has been evaluated in two clinical trials in patients with hemorrhagic shock following injury. In the first study, there was a significantly increased risk of organ failure and death in patients receiving DCLH.[43] Another study in a similar group of patients in whom the DCLH was administered in the prehospital phase of care demonstrated no benefit in the treatment group.[44] In other studies in patients undergoing major surgery, DCLH spared the transfusion of allogeneic red blood cells but frequently resulted in decreases in cardiac index and jaundice, hemoglobinuria, pancreatitis, and abnormalities in liver function tests.[45–47]

Preliminary data on other blood substitutes do not suggest an increase in adverse events. For example, an open-label prospective trial of human polymerized hemoglobin (Polyheme) in 39 patients with acute blood loss due to either trauma or emergency surgery demonstrated a relatively good safety profile.[48,49] In a subsequent randomized, prospective evaluation of polymerized human hemoglobin versus allogeneic blood in a series of trauma patients, there were no significant adverse effects except for a small rise in bilirubin evident by day 3, representing the clearance and metabolism of acellular hemoglobin.[50] Large randomized controlled trials are under way with both Polyheme and Hemopure, a form of bovine polymerized hemoglobin.

Traumatic Shock

The major contributor to shock following trauma is hypovolemia, and acute hemorrhage is a frequent cause of death after injury.[5] Once hemorrhage ceases or is controlled, patients can continue to suffer loss of plasma volume into the interstitium of injured tissues and develop progressive hypovolemic shock. In addition, hypovolemia coupled with tissue injury evokes a greater systemic inflammatory response and a potentially more devastating degree of shock than hypovolemia alone. Specific injuries can also produce superimposed cardiogenic or neurogenic shock. Pericardial tamponade or tension pneumothorax can produce hemodynamically significant compression of the heart, and myocardial contusion can cause cardiogenic shock. Neurogenic shock can accompany spinal cord injury.

The degree to which direct tissue injury and an inflammatory response participate in the development and progression of traumatic shock distinguishes it from hypovolemic shock. Cellular injury, devitalized tissues, ischemia-reperfusion injury, bacterial contamination, and accumulations of blood or other body fluids contribute to the development of SIRS. It is the inflammatory response to these various stimuli that evokes the functional and metabolic disturbances that follow and place the trauma patient at high risk for postinjury organ dysfunction and death.

The management of traumatic shock is similar to that of hypovolemic shock. Apart from prompt reversal of perfusion defects, efforts must be focused on limiting the inflammatory response to other stimuli. For example, maneuvers directed toward aggressive early reestablishment of the circulation to ischemic tissues, prompt debridement of devitalized or necrotic tissues, and early fracture fixation[51,52] might all play a role in limiting the inflammatory response.

Cardiogenic Shock

The syndrome of *cardiogenic shock* has been defined as the inability of the heart—as a result of impairment of its pumping function—to deliver sufficient blood flow to the tissues to meet resting metabolic demands.[53] Thus, the purest clinical definition of cardiogenic shock requires a low cardiac output and evidence of tissue hypoxia in the presence of an adequate intravascular volume. If hemodynamic monitoring is available, then the diagnosis is confirmed by the combination of a low systolic blood pressure and a depressed cardiac index ($<2.2\,l/min/m^2$) in the presence of an elevated pulmonary capillary wedge pressure (>15 mmHg).

Intrinsic causes of cardiogenic shock include myocardial infarction, contusion from direct chest trauma, cardiomyopathy, valvular heart disease, and rhythm disturbances. In the context of myocardial infarction, autopsy studies show that cardiogenic shock is generally associated with loss of more than 40% of left ventricular myocardium.[54] The cumulative nature of myocardial damage should be taken into account. In a patient in whom compensation for previous myocardial damage is marginal, even a small additional amount of infarction or direct contusion from blunt trauma can result in cardiogenic shock. In addition, the loss of a functional component of the heart, including a valve or valvular support, free wall, or ventricular septum, because of acute ischemic necrosis or direct trauma can result in shock either in isolation or in conjunction with loss of left ventricular function. Finally, a variety of other causes may result in acute deterioration leading to cardiogenic shock; these include acute myocarditis, sustained arrhythmias, acute primary valvular catastrophes, and decompensation in patients with previous end-stage cardiomyopathies.

In a large prospective cohort study assessing outcomes of cardiogenic shock following acute myocardial infarction, left ventricular failure was the most frequent etiology leading to shock (78%); isolated right ventricular failure was causal in only 2.8%. Only 1.4% of patients in cardiogenic shock had evidence of tamponade due to rupture of the ventricular wall, 6% had severe mitral regurgitation as a result of papillary muscle dysfunction or rupture, and 4% had ventricular septal rupture.[55] Although these mechanical complications leading to cardiogenic shock following myocardial infarction account for the etiology in only 12% of patients, they require prompt recognition and treatment to ensure survival.

The mechanisms leading to the development of cardiogenic shock reflect a complex interplay between the heart, the peripheral circulation, and maladaptive compensatory responses. The progressive deterioration that occurs in the absence of intervention can be seen as a vicious cycle in which normal physiological compensatory mechanisms in response to reduced cardiac output tend to propagate in a downward spiral, ultimately leading to death (Fig. 16.4). A reduction in blood pressure activates the sympathetic nervous system through the stimulation of baroreceptors. The adrenergic response leads to an increase in heart rate, myocardial contractility, and arterial and venous vasoconstriction. The renin–angiotensin system is activated by inadequate renal perfusion and sympathetic stimulation, leading to additional vasoconstriction and salt and water retention. Finally, hypotension potentiates the secretion of antidiuretic hormone, which further increases water retention. The reduction in

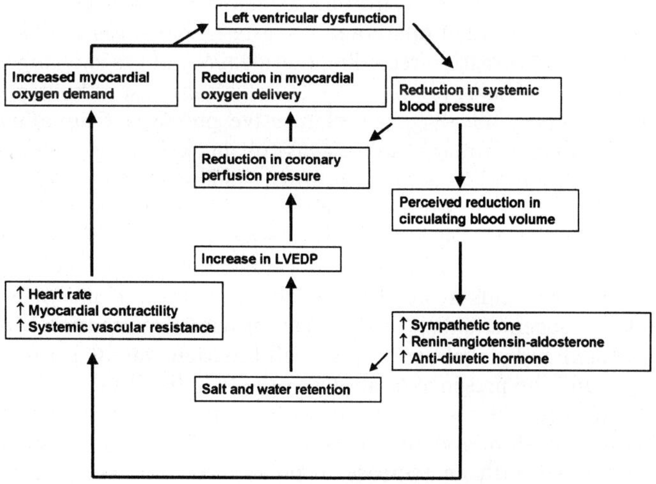

FIGURE 16.4. The reduction in cardiac output associated with left ventricular dysfunction results in a series of compensatory responses that function to maintain blood pressure at the expense of aggravating any disparity in myocardial oxygen demand and supply. This imbalance increases left ventricular dysfunction and sets up a vicious cycle.

blood pressure in conjunction with an elevated left ventricular end-diastolic pressure resulting from fluid retention and impaired left ventricular function reduces coronary perfusion pressure and thus myocardial oxygen delivery. Meanwhile, the increase in heart rate, systemic vascular resistance, and contractility all increase myocardial oxygen consumption and demand. The discrepancy between myocardial oxygen demand and oxygen delivery further impairs left ventricular function and will lead to circulatory collapse unless appropriate and timely intervention interrupts the cycle.

The manifestations of cardiogenic shock develop as a consequence of a reduction in peripheral perfusion, the associated adrenergic response, and the inability of the heart to accommodate pulmonary venous return. Except for the last, the clinical features of cardiogenic shock are remarkably similar to those of hypovolemic shock. If right-sided failure predominates, then the predominant clinical features are those of accumulation of blood in the systemic veins and capacitance vessels. If this is severe or chronic, then peripheral edema, hepatomegaly, and hepatojugular reflux may develop. By contrast, the principal features of left-sided failure are related to an increase in extravascular lung water. The large capacitance pulmonary vasculature initially accommodates the increase in pulmonary venous pressures and blood volume. With normal pulmonary capillary permeability, pulmonary interstitial fluid flow overwhelms the capacity of pulmonary lymphatics, and edema develops at capillary pressures higher than 20 mmHg. Overt pulmonary edema develops at pressures of more than 24 mmHg.

In making the diagnosis of cardiogenic shock, any history of cardiac disease may be of diagnostic value. Physical exam may demonstrate evidence of inadequate tissue perfusion in conjunction with an elevated jugular venous pressure, an S_3 gallop, and pulmonary edema. An electrocardiogram should be obtained immediately because evidence of serious abnormalities should direct the investigation toward the myocardium. A chest radiograph provides valuable diagnostic information regarding the presence of pulmonary edema, pleural effusion, or cardiac chamber enlargement. Laboratory data are supportive and may offer critical information for optimal management. Cardiac enzymes may provide evidence of acute myocardial infarction, and arterial blood gas analysis provides information regarding the adequacy of gas exchange. Severe hypoxia in the presence of a normal chest radiograph may support the diagnosis of massive pulmonary embolus rather than a primary cardiac cause of shock. Urinary indices may demonstrate decreased urinary sodium and elevated urine osmolarity, a function of renal conservation of sodium and water in response to a drop in renal perfusion. Transthoracic and transesophageal echocardiography are excellent noninvasive aids in sorting through the differential diagnosis of cardiogenic shock; they may provide information on regional and global ventricular wall function, valvular integrity, and the presence or absence of pericardial fluid.

In selected cases, it is difficult to ascertain the role of cardiac dysfunction in the shock state. Pulmonary edema associated with an increase in pulmonary capillary permeability may arise from noncardiac causes. Mechanical ventilation or underlying pulmonary disease may obscure the role of cardiogenic failure. Occasionally, a sudden cardiac event may lead to a fall or motor vehicle crash, making the differential diagnosis of shock particularly difficult. In these situations, use of a PAC may provide additional diagnostic information.

Management of cardiogenic shock is geared toward therapeutic interventions that interrupt the vicious cycle leading to progressive myocardial dysfunction. General supportive measures should be initiated immediately concurrent with the diagnostic evaluation. Critical elements include ensuring adequate oxygenation and ventilation, correction of electrolyte and acid–base abnormalities, and restoration of sinus rhythm. In the case of supraventricular tachycardia associated with hypotension, synchronized cardioversion will rapidly establish a normal sinus rhythm. Administration of crystalloid may improve perfusion if inadequate intravascular volume is contributing to the shock state. In patients with inadequate tissue perfusion and adequate intravascular volume, infusion of inotropic or vasopressor drugs should be begun immediately. However, it is important to be cognizant that pharmacological therapy, through an increase in heart rate, contractility, or systemic vascular resistance, tends to increase myocardial oxygen requirements. Dobutamine, because of its beneficial effect on afterload reduction, is preferable to other sympathomimetics unless substantial hypotension is present. Through its vasodilatory and inotropic effects, it increases left ventricular emptying while augmenting diastolic coronary blood flow. In the presence of moderate hypotension, dopamine is the preferred agent, whereas norepinephrine is reserved for cases of profound hypotension while other resuscitative measures are undertaken.[56] Inotropic support should be considered only a temporizing measure; it has never been demonstrated to improve survival in patients with cardiogenic shock.[57]

Afterload reduction through the use of vasodilators may be beneficial for patients in cardiogenic shock, but caution must be exercised because of the risk of exacerbating hypotension. Either intravenous nitroglycerin or sodium nitroprusside may be used. Although nitroprusside is a more potent arterial vasodilator, nitroglycerin is preferred as it has the advantage of not producing coronary steal (preferential coronary blood flow to nonischemic vascular beds).[58]

Patients with right ventricular infarction leading to cardiogenic shock deserve special mention. The marked reduction in right ventricular compliance causes these patients to be extremely sensitive to volume depletion. The focus of therapy in such patients should be the immediate restoration of adequate left ventricular filling pressure while accepting significantly elevated central venous pressures. If volume resuscitation fails to resolve hypotension, then dobutamine should be used in an attempt to improve the contractility of the dysfunctional right ventricle.[53]

One adjunctive approach to patients with severe cardiac dysfunction is the use of intraaortic balloon counterpulsation (IABC), which is achieved by placing a counterpulsation balloon catheter in the descending thoracic aorta via the femoral artery.[59] Inflation of the balloon during diastole augments diastolic pressure at the aortic root and thus improves coronary blood flow; deflation during systole then provides some degree of afterload reduction. The reduction in afterload in concert with improved coronary perfusion is reflected by favorable changes in myocardial oxygen metabolism, with a decrease in oxygen extraction and a shift from lactate production to lactate extraction.[60] Thus, unlike inotropic support, use of the intraaortic balloon pump reduces rather than increases myocardial oxygen requirements. Objective findings include immediate and significant increases in cardiac index, stroke volume, and stroke work index, while reduction in pulmonary capillary wedge pressure and systemic vascular resistance are noted within hours.[61]

Generally, IABC is used as a means of temporary support for patients in cardiogenic shock, either with the hope of recovering myocardial function or while preparations are made for other interventions, whether they are percutaneous or operative attempts at myocardial revascularization, correction of other anatomical defects, or cardiac transplantation. There is some evidence that use of the IABC in patients subsequently undergoing revascularization may offer a significant survival benefit.[62] However, a randomized controlled trial comparing early revascularization (within 6h) to initial medical stabilization (thrombolysis or IABC) in patients with cardiogenic shock following acute myocardial infarction showed a significant benefit in functional status and mortality at 1 year, suggesting that prolonged attempts at medical stabilization are unwarranted if facilities for revascularization are available.[63]

Compressive (or obstructive) cardiogenic shock is a discrete entity that occurs as a result of extrinsic compression of the heart. The extrinsic compression limits diastolic filling, effectively reducing preload, which adversely affects stroke volume and cardiac output. Blood or fluid within the poorly distensible pericardial sac may cause pericardial tamponade, which is the most frequently cited cause of extrinsic cardiogenic shock. However, any cause of increased intrathoracic pressure—such as tension pneumothorax, herniation of abdominal viscera through a diaphragmatic hernia, mediastinal hematomas (rarely pneumomediastinum), and in some instances excessive positive pressure ventilation or intraabdominal compartment pressure—can cause cardiogenic shock.

The classic clinical findings of pericardial tamponade include jugular venous distension, muffled heart sounds, and hypotension (Beck's triad). A drop in blood pressure of more than 10mmHg with inspiration, known as *pulsus paradoxus*, may be demonstrated. Placement of a central venous catheter confirms the elevation in right-sided filling pressures despite persistent hypotension. In the patient at risk, echocardiography is the most sensitive and specific modality to demonstrate pericardial fluid and need for operation. Pericardiocentesis as a diagnostic maneuver is not ideal because of the likelihood of inadvertent ventricular puncture causing a false-positive diagnosis, risk of significant iatrogenic injury, and the inability to withdraw clotted blood that has not yet lysed. These pitfalls limit the technique to only acute lifesaving situations.

Septic Shock

Septic shock is the second most frequent cause of shock in the surgical patient. Invasive bacterial infection represents the most common cause of septic shock, with the most likely sites of infection the lungs, abdomen, and urinary tract. Bacteremia occurs in 40% to 60% of such patients. In the remainder, causative organisms may not be isolated because of previous exposure to antibiotics, episodic patterns of seeding, or fastidiousness of the organisms. In the past, gram-negative aerobic organisms were thought to be the primary organisms responsible for septic shock. It is now clear that the same clinical features may be evident in patients with gram-positive, fungal, viral, and protozoal infections.

The pathophysiological alterations in septic shock are a result of the local and systemic response to bacteria and their products. Although endotoxin from gram-negative bacilli is the best studied of these bacterial toxins, other bacterial products may initiate a similar response. These agents derived from infectious organisms include formyl peptides, exotoxins, and proteases from gram-negative organisms as well as exotoxins, enterotoxins, peptidoglycans, and lipoteichoic acid from gram-positive organisms. Bacterial products stimulate the release of endothelial and macrophage-derived proinflammatory cytokines, the most potent of which are tumor necrosis factor-α (TNF-α) and interleukin-1 (IL-1). The TNF-α and IL-1 may stimulate the release of IL-6, IL-8, and other mediators, including thromboxanes, leukotrienes, platelet-activating factor, prostaglandins, complement, and nitric oxide (NO).

The inflammatory milieu induces several circulatory changes that impair tissue perfusion. First, myocardial depression is often evident despite an increase in cardiac index. Several factors contribute to cardiac dysfunction, including biventricular dilation,[64] myocardial hyporesponsiveness to catecholamines,[65] and diastolic dysfunction.[66] Together, these phenomena result in a significant reduction in ejection fraction and a suboptimal response to volume infusion that persists for as long as 10 days. Possibly in conjunction with NO, TNF-α and IL-1 are thought to be responsible for these alterations.[67]

The increase in cardiac index despite a reduction in myocardial contractility occurs as a result of a profound reduction in vasomotor tone, the principal cause of hypotension in septic shock. Decreases in vascular tone affect both arterial and venous circuits. The reduction in venous tone leads to pooling in large capacitance vessels, effectively reducing circulating blood volume. Dilation of the small arterioles in skeletal muscle beds contributes to the decreased systemic vascular resistance and hypotension on the basis of the large microvascular surface area and volume, respectively, of skeletal muscle.[68] Based on several clinical and experimental studies, NO appears to be the principal mediator responsible for the changes.[69,70] Pharmacologic blockade of nitric oxide synthase reverses the septic shock state more readily than conventional catecholamine-based inotropes and vasopressors in phase II studies.[71] However, a phase III study was discontinued at interim analysis due to higher mortality in patients receiving the nitric oxide synthase inhibitor. Presumably, the vasopressor effects of NO blockade increased systemic vascular resistance (to achieve an increase in blood pressure) and thus reduced cardiac output, leading to greater impairment of tissue oxygenation.[72]

Several microcirculatory changes distinct from changes in vasomotor tone also play a role in the manifestations of septic shock. The mediator environment of sepsis results in activation of the coagulation cascade, leading to microthrombus formation and marked decreases in deformability of neutrophils and erythrocytes, leading to capillary plugging.[73] This microvascular occlusive phenomenon induces the opening of arteriovenous shunts, effectively depriving tissues of adequate perfusion. Several proinflammatory mediators also increase neutrophil–endothelial adherence and subsequent extravasation of activated inflammatory cells into the interstitium, where they induce tissue injury. This same process also significantly increases endothelial permeability. The combination of increased capillary pressure secondary to capillary plugs in concert with an increase in vascular permeability results in loss of intravascular volume into the interstitium, further exacerbating hypotension and edema. Edema effectively increases the diffusion distance required for cellular oxygen delivery and may, in concert with opening of arteriovenous shunts, induce cellular hypoxia. In addition to shunting, there also appears to be a direct or indirect toxic effect on mitochondrial utilization of oxygen. Thus, even in the face of normally adequate delivery of oxygen, the ability to utilize O_2 leads to a relative intracellular hypoxia and anaerobic metabolic shift.

Early manifestations of severe sepsis include tachypnea, tachycardia, oliguria, and changes in mental status. These clinical features may precede the onset of fever and leukocytosis, particularly in immunocompromised patients. Thus, these simple clinical features should be considered evidence of impending shock in those at risk.

Early, aggressive management is critical for minimizing the morbidity and mortality of septic shock. Patients often require intubation and ventilatory support, particularly if there is evidence of acute respiratory distress syndrome (ARDS). Because of the systemic vasodilation and increase in microvascular permeability, it is not unusual for patients to require large amounts of intravenous fluid to restore a normal blood pressure. Vasopressor support with dopamine, epinephrine, or norepinephrine may be necessary if there is an inadequate blood pressure response to fluid resuscitation. As a result of the increase in microvascular permeability within the pulmonary capillary network, administration of large amounts of intravenous fluid may reduce lung compliance and impair alveolar gas exchange. Although early use of vasopressors may minimize the possibility of pulmonary edema, it is not often possible or wise to limit volume resuscitation to prevent this clinical scenario; thus, close monitoring in an intensive care unit setting is essential to optimize resuscitation. In patients not responding to fluid infusion or those with underlying cardiac or renal disease, the use of a PAC might guide therapy. Relative adrenal insufficiency might contribute to the manifestations of septic shock and should be considered and treated (see below).

During the resuscitation process, it is imperative that all measures be taken to reverse the infectious process as expediently as possible. If the organism or site is unknown, then treatment may require empiric broad-spectrum antimicrobial agents, based in part on known bacterial patterns in the institution, until further information is available. The correct choice of antibiotic or antibiotic combination is critical as there is a significantly higher case-fatality rate if inappropriate antimicrobials are administered (see Chapter 11).[74] If the infection source is an abscess or there is ongoing soiling of the pleural or peritoneal cavities, then either drainage or control of contamination is mandatory. Similarly, necrotic, infected tissue requires aggressive debridement.

In patients with sepsis, tissue injury occurs as a result of the host inflammatory response rather than the organism per se. As a result, a variety of therapies directed toward modulating the inflammatory response have been attempted with discouraging results. These approaches and their limitations are more fully discussed in Chapters 4 and 15.

Neurogenic Shock

Hypotension and bradycardia may occur following acute cervical or high thoracic spinal cord injury as a result of disruption of sympathetic outflow in conjunction with unopposed vagal tone. This constellation of clinical features is referred to as *neurogenic shock*, a syndrome that must be considered separately from the inappropriate term *spinal shock*, which refers to loss of spinal cord reflexes below the level of spinal cord injury.

Following acute spinal cord transection, there is a marked systemic pressor response from acute activation of the sympathetic nervous system and adrenal medulla. This response, manifested as hypertension and tachycardia, lasts for several minutes and because of its short duration is usually not appreciated.[75] As the pressor response abates, the interruption of descending supraspinal fibers in the intermediolateral cell column that activate the preganglionic sympathetic nervous system results in the loss of sympathetic activity. As the sympathetic nerves generally exit from the first thoracic to the first lumbar segment, any patient with a spinal cord injury above the level of L1 is potentially at risk. The loss of sympathetic tone results in hypotension secondary to arterial vasodilation and venodilation. Hypotension is frequently accompanied by marked bradycardia due to loss of the sympathetic cardioaccelator fibers and persistent, unopposed vagal tone.

Neurogenic shock typically manifests in patients with cervical spinal cord injuries, particularly when there is complete loss of motor function below the level of injury. In this group of patients, bradycardia is a universal feature with hypotension an accompaniment in approximately two-thirds of patients.[76] Partial cervical spinal cord injuries may cause bradycardia but only rarely is hypotension problematic. Finally, patients with injuries to thoracolumbar segments rarely demonstrate features of neurogenic shock. The cardiovascular abnormalities are only transient and tend to resolve spontaneously in 2 to 6 weeks.

The diagnosis should be suspected in any patient with hypotension and bradycardia following injury. In some cases, these findings may represent the first suggestion of a spinal cord injury in a comatose patient. The patient with neurogenic shock is typically warm and well perfused. If a PAC is in situ, the cardiac index may be elevated while the systemic vascular resistance is markedly reduced.[77] It is critical to remember that hemorrhage remains the most common cause of shock in patients with spinal cord injury. Thus, occult hemorrhage should be ruled out before attributing spinal cord injury as the exclusive cause of hypotension.

Hypoadrenal Shock

Shock secondary to adrenal insufficiency occurs infrequently and usually within the context of a concomitant critical illness. As a result, the diagnosis of adrenal insufficiency as a cause of the shock state is rarely suspected until late in the disease process. Unfortunately, if the diagnosis is missed, the patient will likely succumb to refractory shock. In North America, adrenal insufficiency most commonly arises as a consequence of the chronic therapeutic administration of high-dose exogenous corticosteroids with resultant suppression of the hypothalamic-pituitary-adrenal axis. If adrenal insufficiency is slow in onset, then there may be adequate cortisol production to maintain homeostasis in the unstressed state. By contrast, once the patient is severely stressed, typically following major infection, operation, or trauma, adrenocortical function may be insufficient to support the necessary physiological response, and the clinical picture of shock due to adrenal insufficiency will become manifest. In a small proportion of patients, adrenal insufficiency onset is abrupt and occurs directly as a result of the acute underlying illness. For example, overwhelming sepsis may cause adrenal insufficiency because of adrenal infarction secondary to hypotension or adrenal hemorrhage caused by coagulopathy.

Diagnosis of shock secondary to hypocortisolism requires a high level of suspicion. Findings associated with adrenal insufficiency include weakness, fatigue, anorexia, abdominal pain, fever, nausea, vomiting, and weight loss. If longstanding (i.e., Addison's disease), then there may be hyperpigmentation of the skin and mucous membranes. Hyponatremia, hypochloremia, and hyperkalemia are consistent with decreased mineralocorticoid activity. Adrenal insufficiency may also present acutely with fever, shock, and an acute abdomen. More typically, surgical patients with adrenal insufficiency present with refractory shock in the course of injury or illness. There may be no findings other than the failure to respond to standard shock therapy. Hypotension may be marked despite massive fluid resuscitation and inotropic support.

The hemodynamic changes associated with acute adrenal insufficiency tend to occur in two predictable patterns. In the relatively hypovolemic patient, the appearance is one of cardiogenic shock with decreased preload, depressed myocardial contractility, and high systemic vascular resistance. By contrast, if the patient had been adequately volume resuscitated, the cardiac output is usually high with a low systemic vascular resistance, suggesting that there are no classic hemodynamic features of hypoadrenalism. In this regard, evidence suggests that adrenal insufficiency has been underrecognized, and there is a large proportion of critically ill patients who have relative adrenal insufficiency. These patients do not present in fulminant shock but typically have persistent inotropic requirements or prolonged ventilator dependence. It is important to identify these patients as corticosteroid replacement leads to significantly improved outcomes (see below).

In patients in whom the diagnosis is suspected, a blood sample for measurement of plasma cortisol and corticotrophin should be obtained and a cosyntropin (synthetic corticotrophin) stimulation test performed. Although several methods for cosyntropin stimulation testing have been suggested, a standard test involves an intravenous bolus of 250 μg of cosyntropin and repeat cortisol levels 30 and 60 min later. Relative adrenal insufficiency is defined as an increase in serum cortisol of 9 μg/dl or less.[78,79] In a large, double-blind, randomized controlled trial, approximately 75% of patients presenting with septic shock met the criteria for relative adrenal insufficiency.[78] In this study, there was a significant reduction in mortality among nonresponders receiving 50 mg hydrocortisone every 6 h in concert with 50 μg fludricortisone daily for 7 days. Several other randomized controlled trials have confirmed the benefits of corticosteroid replacement (i.e., stress dose) in patients with septic shock. A meta-analysis of these and other trials using higher doses of corticosteroids suggests a 20% reduction in mortality in patients with septic shock receiving steroids at low dose (<300 mg/day) for at least 5 days.[80] By contrast, patients receiving high dose (>300 mg/day) for shorter periods of time demonstrated no benefit.

Together, these data suggest that low-dose corticosteroid replacement should be administered to all patients with septic shock while waiting for the results of a cosyntropin stimulation test. If the test is negative (i.e., an increase in serum cortisol of >9 μg/dl), then the corticosteroids can be discontinued. The number needed to treat (irrespective of responder status) to prevent a single death is only 8, indicating that this intervention might have tremendous benefit to critically ill patients with shock due to sepsis.

Diagnostic and Therapeutic Adjuncts in the Management of Shock

Pulmonary Artery Catheter

The differential diagnosis of the shock state is usually relatively straightforward. The clinical setting in conjunction with physical examination is often sufficient to guide diagnosis and therapy. However, occasionally the cause of the shock state is unclear. Typically, this occurs when the cause of the shock state may be multifactorial. For example, a trauma patient with persistent hypotension may have a combination of spinal shock and hemorrhagic shock. Alternatively, an elderly patient with septic shock may have significant myocardial dysfunction that often will confuse the clinical picture. In these scenarios, hemodynamic parameters derived from a PAC may provide valuable insight into the principal mechanism underlying the shock state (Table 16.4).

Despite its conceptual appeal, there are no data supporting an improvement in outcome among patients whose resuscitation is guided by a PAC. In one randomized controlled trial of 201 patients with shock or acute respiratory failure, patients with a PAC had more fluid administration, a higher incidence of renal failure, and a greater incidence of thrombocytopenia.[81] In another such study involving almost 700 patients with shock or ARDS, patients receiving a PAC had equivalent outcomes to those without.[82]

TABLE 16.4. Differential Diagnosis of Shock States Based on Hemodynamic Parameters.

Type of shock	*CVP or PCWP*	*Cardiac output*	*Systemic vascular resistance*	*Venous O_2 saturation*
Hypovolemic	↓↓	↓	↑	↓
Cardiogenic	↑	↓	↑	↓
Septic	↓↑	↑	↓	↑
Traumatic	↓	↓↑	↓↑	↓
Neurogenic	↓	↓	↓	↓
Hypoadrenal	↓↑	↓↑	↑↓	↓

CVP, central venous pressure; PCWP, pulmonary capillary wedge pressure.

Resuscitative Thoracotomy

Resuscitative thoracotomy (also referred to as emergency room thoracotomy) represents an adjunctive measure to manage patients in extremis or profound shock following trauma. This approach involves performing a left anterolateral thoracotomy in the emergency room while the rest of the resuscitation team continues with managing the airway, intravenous access, and fluid resuscitation. After entry into the left chest, the pericardium is inspected for evidence of tamponade, and a pericardiotomy is performed to decompress the pericardial space or allow for open cardiac massage. Major pulmonary hemorrhage or hilar injury can be managed by cross-clamping the pulmonary hilum. The descending thoracic aorta can be occluded, thus optimizing perfusion to the coronary and cerebral circulation while limiting intraabdominal hemorrhage.

The results of resuscitative thoracotomy have been reported in the form of retrospective studies from individual institutions. Despite the heterogeneity of patients, the effectiveness of this approach appears to depend on both the site and mechanism of injury and the physiological status of the patient. Although the survival in unselected patients ranges from 1.8% to 13%,[83–85] survival in patients with penetrating cardiac injury may be as high as 22%.[85,86] By contrast, patients undergoing resuscitative thoracotomy following hypovolemic arrest caused by blunt trauma have 0% to 2% chance of survival.[84–86] The principal reason for this differential survival benefit is that a resuscitative thoracotomy with pericardiotomy may prove to be the definitive management for patients in cardiogenic shock due to tamponade, while an easily remediable problem is rarely evident in blunt trauma patients. Several reports have attempted to prognosticate survival based on the presence or absence of respiratory attempts, brainstem reflexes, movement, or vital signs (blood pressure, pulse, or viable cardiac rhythms). It is clear that survival is negligible in patients without signs of life in the prehospital phase of care.[86] Based on these data, the American College of Surgeons Committee on Trauma and the National Association of EMS Physicians have come out with a joint position statement indicating that a resuscitative thoracotomy in blunt trauma patients found apneic, pulseless, and without organized electrocardiogram (ECG) activity on the arrival of emergency medical services (EMS) at the scene is unwarranted.[87] Similarly, a resuscitative thoractomy is not warranted in victims of penetrating trauma found by EMS to be apneic and pulseless and who have no signs of life (pupillary reflexes, spontaneous movement, or organized ECG activity) at the scene.

Inotropes and Vasopressors

Management of shock requires manipulation of intravascular volume (preload), systemic vascular resistance (afterload), and myocardial contractility. Optimal volume resuscitation should precede pharmacological intervention. The use of inotropic agents should be considered when tissue perfusion remains inadequate despite adequate fluid administration. Both catecholamine and noncatecholamine agents are used clinically, and the agents differ in their degree of α- and β-activity, chronotropic effects, and influence on myocardial oxygen consumption.

Dopamine

Dopamine is an endogenous sympathetic amine that is a biosynthetic precursor of epinephrine and also functions as a central and peripheral neurotransmitter. At low doses (1–3 mg/kg/min), dopamine may increase renal blood flow and maintain diuresis via effects mediated through DA1 and DA2 receptors in the renal vasculature.[88,89] At moderate doses (5 mg/kg/min), stimulation of cardiac β-receptors produces increases in contractility and cardiac output with little effect on heart rate or blood pressure. With increasing doses (5–10 mg/kg/min), β-adrenergic effects still predominate, but further increases in cardiac output are accompanied by increases in heart rate and blood pressure. At higher doses (more than 10 mg/kg/min), peripheral vasoconstriction from increasing α-activity becomes more prominent, resulting in elevation of systemic vascular resistance, blood pressure, and myocardial oxygen consumption.

Dobutamine

Dobutamine is a synthetic catecholamine that has been used for its β-adrenergic effects and the absence of significant α-activity. The predominant effect is an increase in cardiac contractility with little increase in heart rate. Dobutamine also has a peripheral vasodilating effect resulting from β_2-receptor activation that is independent of any increase in cardiac output. The combination of increased contractility and reduction in afterload contribute to improved left ventricular emptying and a reduction in pulmonary capillary wedge pressure. Blood pressure may drop slightly. As a result of these properties, dobutamine is an ideal agent when the therapeutic goal is to improve cardiac output rather than to improve blood pressure. This improvement in cardiac output frequently occurs without a significant increase in myocardial oxygen requirement due to the reduction in afterload and little, if any, chronotropic effect.

Norepinephrine

The sympathetic neurotransmitter norepinephrine exerts both α- and β-adrenergic effects. The β-adrenergic effects are most prominent at lower infusion rates, leading to increases in heart rate and contractility. With increasing doses, the α-mediated effects become evident and are responsible for increases in systemic vascular resistance and blood pressure. Due to favorable effects on the splanchnic circulation, either norepinephrine or dopamine are the recommended vasopressors in patients with septic shock.[90]

Epinephrine

Epinephrine has a broad spectrum of systemic actions. At lower rates of infusion, β-adrenergic responses predominate, leading to an increase in heart rate and contractility (β_1-effect) in conjunction with peripheral vasodilation (β_2-effect). These effects result in an increase in stroke volume and cardiac output with a variable effect on blood pressure. At a higher rate of infusion, α-effects predominate, leading to an increase in systemic vascular resistance and blood pressure. Limitations in the use of epinephrine arise from its renal vasoconstrictive activity, its arrhythmogenic potential, and its substantial contribution to increasing myocardial oxygen demand. However, epinephrine remains the drug of choice for anaphylactic reactions, primarily because of extensive experience with this agent for this indication. In septic shock, it is considered a second-line agent for patients not responding to dopamine or norepinephrine.

Amrinone

Amrinone (or milrinone) is a synthetic bipyridine with inotropic and vasodilator effects. Its principal mechanism of action involves phosphodiesterase inhibition, through which it raises the intracellular concentration of cyclic adenosine monophosphate (AMP). It appears to be a useful agent in cardiogenic shock complicating myocardial infarction as it may significantly increase cardiac contractility and cardiac output without increasing myocardial oxygen requirement due to concomitant vasodilation and afterload reduction. Drawbacks to the use of amrinone are the variability of the individual response, its relatively long half-life (3.6h), and the potential for acute significant hypotension if intravascular volume is inadequate. In addition, its use is not infrequently accompanied by the development of thrombocytopenia.

Vasopressin

Vasopressin is a peptide hormone synthesized in the hypothalamus and then transported to and stored in the pituitary gland, where it is released in response to decreases in intravascular volume and increased plasma osmolarity. There is evidence to suggest that vasopressin secretion might be impaired in patients with shock, and several case series have demonstrated the effectiveness of exogenous vasopressin administration in patients with catecholamine-resistant septic shock. It is typically administered at a rate of 0.04u/min (ranging from 0.01u/min to as high as 0.08u/min). Vasopressin acts as a vasopressor and might reduce cardiac index and tissue oxygen delivery. Relatively small randomized controlled trials suggest that it spares the use of norepinephrine and improves creatinine clearance.[91,92] There are no studies comparing outcomes in patients treated with vasopressin compared to conventional catecholamine-based vasopressors. Currently, it is recommended for use as second-line therapy after norepinephrine or dopamine.[90]

Complications of Shock and Resuscitation

Multiple Organ Dysfunction Syndrome

The syndrome associated with multiple organ dysfunction (MODS) has evolved only recently as a result of advances in our ability to salvage patients who would have otherwise died as a result of their shock state. Shock in all its forms represents the most common predisposing factor leading to the development of MODS. Although the mechanisms leading to the development of organ dysfunction following shock are unclear, it appears that an unbridled systemic inflammatory response is in part responsible.

There is no specific treatment for MODS. Efforts should be directed toward minimizing the duration of shock and rapidly ensuring adequate organ perfusion. Infection should either be prevented if possible or treated early and aggressively. Fracture fixation and debridement of necrotic tissue should be performed early to reduce the systemic inflammatory response associated with tissue injury.[51,52,93] Novel approaches to modulating the aberrant host response are currently under evaluation to determine their effectiveness in minimizing reperfusion injury.

Hypothermia

A potential adverse consequence of massive volume resuscitation to reverse shock is hypothermia. Prolonged extrication or examination in a cold environment following trauma and evaporative heat losses in the operating room also may contribute to this condition. Iatrogenic paralysis may prevent endogenous heat production through shivering. Nearly one-half of patients develop incidental hypothermia between the time of injury and completion of surgery.[94]

Hypothermia invokes a variety of systemic responses, including a reduction in heart rate and cardiac output, while temperatures below 32°C may induce supraventricular or ventricular arrhythmias.[95] Most importantly, at temperatures less than 35°C, hypothermia induces coagulopathy due to effects on both coagulation factors and platelet function. Because coagulation assays are routinely performed after warming blood samples to 37°C, the clinical impact of the patient's hypothermia is often underestimated. In fact, coagulation assays that appear normal at 37°C are significantly prolonged and clinically important when performed at the core body temperature of the hypothermic patient.[96] The combination of coagulopathy and hypothermia produces a vicious cycle; the coagulopathy leads to more blood loss, requiring more replacement with cool fluids or blood products, leading to further hypothermia and aggravation of the coagulopathy.

Prevention of hypothermia should be considered in all patients with shock. Fluid warmers utilizing a countercurrent heating technique allow for rapid administration of warm fluids or blood products. Warming blankets and warmed ventilator circuits should be used routinely. Rewarming techniques, including pleural or peritoneal lavage with warm crystalloid solutions may be useful. Continuous arteriovenous rewarming may be the most efficacious method because it allows for rapid rewarming using an extracorporeal countercurrent mechanism through percutaneously placed catheters in the femoral artery and vein[97] (Fig. 16.5). This process does not require a pump and rapidly rewarms from 30°C to 36°C in less than 30min. In a randomized prospective study of this rapid rewarming technique, patients undergoing rapid rewarming required less fluid resuscitation, were more likely to rewarm, and demonstrated improved survival compared to those receiving standard rewarming techniques.[98]

Abdominal Compartment Syndrome

The abdominal compartment syndrome (ACS) is a sequela of massive resuscitation following shock or visceral ischemia. The most common clinical scenarios giving rise to ACS are emergent repair of an abdominal aortic aneurysm, abdominal trauma, pancreatitis, severe intraabdominal infection, and burns. Aggressive fluid resuscitation in concert with alterations in microvascular permeability result in marked visceral edema. Similarly, increasing soft tissue edema results in a reduction in abdominal wall compliance. The combination of an increase in the volume of intraabdominal contents in

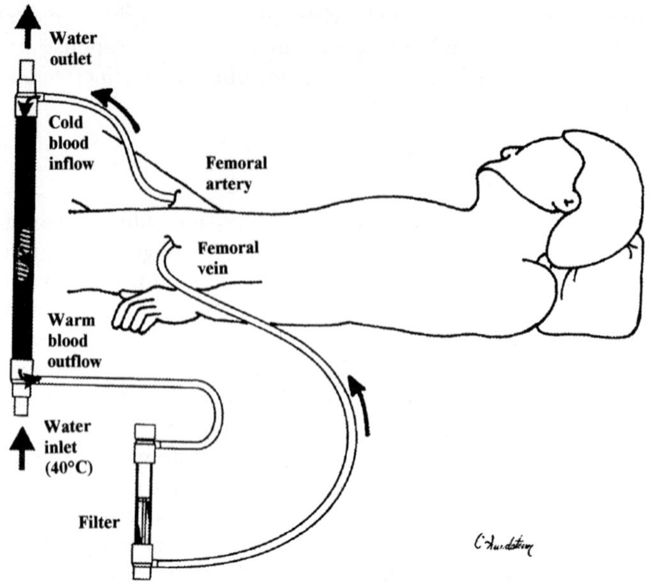

FIGURE 16.5. Continuous arteriovenous rewarming is achieved by cannulating the femoral artery and vein using an 8.5- or 10-French catheter and creating a circulatory fistula through a countercurrent heating mechanism. (*Source:* Adapted from Gentillelo et al.,[97] with permission.

concert with a stiff abdominal wall significantly increases the pressure in the abdominal cavity, a phenomenon that may be exacerbated by intraabdominal packing to control bleeding or hematoma.

A progressive increase in intraabdominal pressure (IAP) produces a graded decrease in cardiac output, an effect mediated by a reduction in venous return and an increase in systemic vascular resistance due to caval compression and mechanical compression of capillary beds, respectively.[99] Left and right atrial filling pressures obtained using a pulmonary artery catheter may be spuriously elevated because of the increase in intrathoracic pressure.[100]

Passive elevation of the diaphragm allows the transmission of high IAP into the pleural cavity, reducing both static and dynamic lung compliance.[101,102] This reduction in compliance results in the need for high inspiratory airway pressures to maintain effective ventilation. Intraabdominal hypertension may also result in significant increases in intracranial pressure due to impaired cerebral venous outflow secondary to an increase in intrathoracic pressure.[103,104]

Oliguria is the most overt clinical manifestation of sustained intraabdominal hypertension. The etiology of renal dysfunction in ACS is multifactorial. A reduction in cardiac output and hence renal blood flow is in part responsible; however, the most plausible explanation for the renal effects of elevated IAP is renal vein compression, leading to increased venous pressure within the renal parenchyma. The combined effect of increased renal parenchymal pressure and a reduction in renal blood flow decrease the pressure gradient across the glomerular membrane and thus the glomerular filtration rate.[104] The local effects of intraabdominal hypertension are not limited to the kidney as even moderate increases in IAP may result in visceral mucosal ischemia and acidosis.[105,106]

Diagnosis of the ACS requires recognizing the clinical syndrome and, ultimately, some objective measurement of IAP. The classic clinical clues to the presence of ACS are (1) a tense or distended abdomen, (2) massive intravenous fluid requirements, (3) elevated central venous and pulmonary capillary wedge pressures, (4) decreased cardiac output, (5) elevated peak airway pressures, and (6) oliguria. In a prospective study, Rapanos et al. compared physical exam to objective evaluation of IAP in a series of critically ill blunt trauma patients. Physical exam was notoriously unreliable in detecting clinically significant elevations in IAP (>15 mmHg), suggesting that an objective evaluation of IAP may be necessary for the patient with a clinical presentation suggestive of ACS.[107]

The most widely used method of measuring IAP involves transurethral measurement of urinary bladder pressure using a Foley catheter.[106,108] In the supine position, the normal IAP is less than 10 mmHg. Following abdominal surgery, pressures are typically in the range of 3 to 15 mmHg.[106] Treatment should be considered if IAPs exceed 25 to 30 mmHg.[109,110] Optimally, management involves either reopening a prior laparotomy incision or, in patients without a recent laparotomy, opening the peritoneal cavity via a midline incision. Some form of temporary abdominal closure is then necessary to bridge the fascial defect and prevent evisceration. The morbidity associated with an "open abdomen" is significant, with fluid, electrolyte, and nutritional implications, and should not be undertaken unless clear benefit is expected. There are no studies demonstrating a survival benefit with decompressive celiotomy.

References

1. Gross SG. A System of Surgery: Pathological, Diagnostic, Therapeutic, and Operative. Philadelphia: Lea and Febiger, 1872.
2. Rangel-Frausto MS, Pittet D, Costigan M, Hwang T, Davis CS, Wenzel RP. The natural history of the systemic inflammatory response syndrome. JAMA 1995;273:117–123.
3. Muckart DJJ, Bhagwanjee S. American College of Chest Physicians/Society of Critical Care Medicine consensus conference definitions of the systemic inflammatory response syndrome and allied disorders in relation to critically injured patients. Crit Care Med 1997;25:1789–1795.
4. American College of Chest Physicians—Society of Critical Care Medicine Consensus Conference. Definitions for sepsis and organ failure and guidelines for the use of innovative therapies in sepsis. Crit Care Med 1992;20:864–875.
5. Heckbert SR, Vedder NB, Hoffman W, et al. Outcome after hemorrhagic shock in trauma patients. J Trauma 1998;45:545–549.
6. Abramson D, Scalea TM, Hitchcock R, et al. Lactate clearance and survival following injury. J Trauma 1993;35:584–589.
7. Davis JW, Kaups KL, Parks SN. Base deficit is superior to pH in evaluating clearance of acidosis after traumatic shock. J Trauma 1998;1998:114–118.
8. McGee S, Abernethy WB, III, Simel DL. The rational clinical examination. Is this patient hypovolemic? JAMA 1999;281:1022–1029.
9. Dutton RP, Mackenzie CF, Scalea TM. Hypotensive resuscitation during active hemorrhage: impact on in-hospital mortality. J.Trauma 2002;52:1141–1146.
10. Merrer J, De Jonghe B, Golliot F, et al. Complications of femoral and subclavian venous catheterization in critically ill patients: a randomized controlled trial. JAMA 2001;286:700–707.
11. Dutkey PA, Stevens SL, Maull KI. Factors affecting rapid fluid resuscitation with large-bore introducer catheters. J Trauma 1989;29:856–860.

12. Junger WG, Coimbra R, Liu FC, et al. Hypertonic saline resuscitation: a tool to modulate immune function in trauma patients. Shock 1998;8:235–241.
13. Hartl R, Medary MB, Ruge M, Arfors KE, Ghahremani F, Ghajar J. Hypertonic/hyperoncotic saline attenuates microcirculatory disturbances after traumatic brain injury. J Trauma 1997;42(suppl 5):S41–S47.
14. Rizoli SB, Kapus A, Fan J, Li YH, Marshall JC, Rotstein OD. Immunomodulatory effects of hypertonic resuscitation on the development of lung inflammation following hemorrhagic shock. J Immunol 1998;161:6288–6296.
15. Wade CE, Dubick MA, Vassar MJ, Perry CA, Holcroft JW. Plasma dextran concentrations in trauma patients administered hypertonic saline-dextran 70. Clin Chem 1996;42:779–780.
16. Mattox KL, Maningas PA, Moore EE, et al. Prehospital hypertonic saline/dextran infusion for post-traumatic hypotension: the USA multicenter trial. Ann Surg 1991;213:482–491.
17. Maningas PA, Mattox KL, Pepe PE, Jones RL, Feliciano DV, Burch JM. Hypertonic saline-dextran solutions for the prehospital management of traumatic hypotension. Am J Surg 1989; 157:528–534.
18. Cooper DJ, Myles PS, McDermott FT, et al. Prehospital hypertonic saline resuscitation of patients with hypotension and severe traumatic brain injury: a randomized controlled trial. JAMA 2004;291:1350–1357.
19. Vassar MJ, Fischer RP, O'Brien PE, et al. A multicenter trial for resuscitation of injured patients with 7.5% sodium chloride: the effect of added dextran 70. Arch Surg 1993;128:1003–1013.
20. Vassar MJ, Perry CA, Holcroft JW. Prehospital resuscitation of hypotensive trauma patients with 7.5% NaCl with added dextran: a controlled trial. J Trauma 1993;34:622–632.
21. Wade C. Efficacy of hypertonic saline (HSD) in patients with traumatic hypotension: meta analysis of individual patient data. Acta Anaesthesiol Scand Suppl 1997;110:77–79.
22. Wade CE, Kramer GC, Grady JJ, Fabian TC, Younes RN. Efficacy of hypertonic 7.5% saline and 6% dextran in treating trauma: a meta-analysis of controlled clinical studies. Surgery (St. Louis) 1997;122:609–616.
23. Wade CE, Grady JJ, Kramer GC, Younes RN, Gehlsen K, Holcroft JW. Individual patient cohort analysis of the efficacy of hypertonic saline/dextran in patients with traumatic brain injury and hypotension. J Trauma 1997;42:S61–S65.
24. Alderson P, Bunn F, Lefebvre C, et al. Human albumin solution for resuscitation and volume expansion in critically ill patients. Cochrane Database Syst Rev 2002(1):CD001208.
25. Wilkes MM, Navickis RJ. Patient survival after human albumin administration. A meta-analysis of randomized, controlled trials. Ann Intern Med 2001;135:149–164.
26. Fleck A, Raines G, Hawker F, et al. Increased vascular permeability: a major cause of hypoalbuminemia in disease and injury. Lancet 1985;1:781–784.
27. Moon MR, Lucas CE, Ledgerwood AM, Kosinski JP. Free water clearance after supplemental albumin resuscitation for shock. Circ Shock 1989;28:1–8.
28. Strauss RG, Pennell BJ, Stump DC. A randomized, blinded trial comparing the hemostatic effects of pentastarch versus hetastarch. Transfusion 2002;42:27–36.
29. Langeron O, Doelberg M, Ang ET, Bonnet F, Capdevila X, Coriat P. Voluven, a lower substituted novel hydroxyethyl starch (HES 130/0.4), causes fewer effects on coagulation in major orthopedic surgery than HES 200/0.5. Anesth Analg 2001;92:855–862.
30. Nagy KK, Davis J, Duda J, Fildes J, Roberts R, Barrett J. A comparison of pentastarch and lactated Ringer's solution in the resuscitation of patients with hemorrhagic shock. Circ Shock 1993;40:289–294.
31. Younes RN, Yin KC, Amino CJ, Itinoshe M, Rocha e Silva M, Birolini D. Use of pentastarch solution in the treatment of patients with hemorrhagic hypovolemia: randomized phase II study in the emergency room. World J Surg 1998;22:2–5.
32. Schortgen F, Lacherade JC, Bruneel F, et al. Effects of hydroxyethyl starch and gelatin on renal function in severe sepsis: a multicentre randomised study. Lancet 2001;357:911–916.
33. Moore FA, Moore EE, Sauaia A. Blood transfusion: an independent risk factor for postinjury multiple organ failure. Arch Surg 1997;132:620–625.
34. Patrick DA, Moore EE, Barnett CC, Silliman CC. Human polymerized hemoglobin as a blood substitute avoids transfusion induced neutrophil priming. Surg Forum 1996;47:36–38.
35. Hebert PC, Wells G, Blajchman MA, et al. A multicenter, randomized controlled clinical trial of transfusion requirements in critical care. N Engl J Med 1999;340:409–417.
36. Griswold RA, Ortner AB. The use of autotransfusion in surgery of the serous cavities. Surg Gynecol Obstet 1943;77: 167.
37. Jacobs LM, Hsieh JW. A clinical review of autotransfusion and its role in trauma. JAMA 1984;251:3283.
38. Tiimberlake GA, McSwain NE. Autotransfusion of blood contaminated by enteric contents: a potentially life saving measure in the massively hemorrhaging trauma patient. J Trauma 1988;28:855–857.
39. Ozmen V, McSwain NE, Nichols RL, Smith J, Flint LM. Autotransfusion of potentially culture-positive blood (CPB) in abdominal trauma: preliminary data from a prospective study. J Trauma 1992;32:36–39.
40. Jurkovich GJ, Moore EE, Mediana G. Autotransfusion in trauma: a pragmatic analysis. Am J Surg 1984;148:782.
41. Smith LA, Barker DE, Burns RP. Autotransfusion utilization in abdominal trauma. Am Surg 1997;63:47–49.
42. Huth JF, Maier RV, Pavlin EG, et al. Utilization of blood recycling in nonelective surgery. Arch Surg 1983;118:626–629.
43. Sloan EP, Koenigsberg M, Gens D, et al. Diaspirin cross-linked hemoglobin (DCLHb) in the treatment of severe traumatic hemorrhagic shock: a randomized controlled efficacy trial. JAMA 1999;282:1857–1864.
44. Kerner T, Ahlers O, Veit S, Riou B, Saunders M, Pison U. DCL-Hb for trauma patients with severe hemorrhagic shock: the European "On-Scene" multicenter study. Intensive Care Med 2003;29:378–385.
45. Bloomfield EL, Rady MY, Esfandiari S. A prospective trial of diaspirin cross-linked hemoglobin solution in patients after elective repair of abdominal aortic aneurysm. Mil Med 2004; 169:546–550.
46. Schubert A, O'Hara JF Jr, Przybelski RJ, et al. Effect of diaspirin cross-linked hemoglobin (DCLHb HemAssist) during high blood loss surgery on selected indices of organ function. Artif Cells Blood Substit Immobil Biotechnol 2002;30:259–283.
47. Lamy ML, Daily EK, Brichant JF, et al. Randomized trial of diaspirin cross-linked hemoglobin solution as an alternative to blood transfusion after cardiac surgery. The DCLHb Cardiac Surgery Trial Collaborative Group. Anesthesiology 2000;92:646–656.
48. Gould SA, Moore EE, Moore FA, et al. Clinical utility of human polymerized hemoglobin as a blood substitute after acute trauma and urgent surgery. J Trauma 1997;43:325–332.
49. Gould SA, Moss GS. Clinical development of human polymerized hemoglobin as a blood substitute. World J Surg 1996;20:1200–1207.
50. Gould SA, Moore EE, Hoyt DB, et al. The first randomized trial of human polymerized hemoglobin as a blood substitute in acute trauma and emergent surgery. J Am Coll Surg 1998;187:113–122.

51. Broos PL, Stappaerts KH, Luite EJ, Gruwez JA. The importance of early internal fixation in multiply injured patients to prevent late deaths and sepsis. Injury 1987;18:235–237.
52. Lozman J, Deno DC, Feustel PJ, et al. Pulmonary and cardiovascular consequences of immediate fixation or conservative management of long-bone fractures. Arch Surg 1986;121:992–999.
53. Kinch JW, Ryan TJ. Right ventricular infarction. N Engl J Med 1994;330:1211–1217.
54. Alonso Dr, Scheidt S, Post M, Killip T. Pathophysiology of cardiogenic shock: quantification of myocardial necrosis, clinical, pathologic and electrocardiographic correlations. Circulation 1973;48:588–596.
55. Hochman JS, Buller CE, Sleeper LA, et al. Cardiogenic shock complicating acute myocardial infarction—etiologies, management and outcome: a report from the SHOCK Trial Registry. SHould we emergently revascularize Occluded Coronaries for cardiogenic shocK? J Am Coll Cardiol 2000;36(3 suppl A):1063–1070.
56. Califf RM, Bengston JR. Cardiogenic shock. N Engl J Med 1994; 330:1724–1730.
57. Moscucci M, Bates ER. Cardiogenic shock. Cardiol Clin 1995; 13:391–406.
58. Becker LC, Fortuin NJ, Pitt B. Effect of ischemia and antianginal drugs on the distribution of radioactive microspheres in the canine left ventricle. Circ Res 1971;28:263–269.
59. Freed PS, Wasfre T, Zado B, Kentrowitz A. Intraaortic balloon pumping for prolonged circulatory support. Am J Cardiol 1988;61:554.
60. Muller H, Ayres SM, Giannelli S, et al. Effect of isoproterenol, L-norepinephrine, and intraaortic counterpulsation on hemodynamics and myocardial metabolism in shock following acute myocardial infarction. Circulation 1972;45:335.
61. Bardet J, Mesquet C, Kahn JC, Gourgon R, Bourdarics JP. Clinical and hemodynamic results of intraaortic balloon counterpulsation and surgery for cardiogenic shock. Am J Heart 1977;93:280.
62. Sanborn TA, Sleeper LA, Bates ER, et al. Impact of thrombolysis, intra-aortic balloon pump counterpulsation, and their combination in cardiogenic shock complicating acute myocardial infarction: a report from the SHOCK Trial Registry. SHould we emergently revascularize Occluded Coronaries for cardiogenic shocK? J Am Coll Cardiol 2000;36(3 suppl A):1123–1129.
63. Hochman JS, Sleeper LA, White HD, et al. One-year survival following early revascularization for cardiogenic shock. JAMA 2001;285:190–192.
64. Parker MM, Shelhamer JH, Bacharach SL, et al. Profound but reversible myocardial depression in patients with septic shock. Ann Intern Med 1984;100:483–490.
65. Silverman HJ, Penaranda R, Orens JB, Lee NH. Impaired beta-adrenergic receptor stimulation of cyclic adenosine monophosphate in human septic shock: association with myocardial hyporesponsiveness to catecholamines. Crit Care Med 1993; 21:31–39.
66. Jafri SM, Lavine S, Field BE, Bahorozian MT, Carlson RW. Left ventricular diastolic function in sepsis. Crit Care Med 1990; 18:709–713.
67. Parker MM. Pathophysiology of cardiovascular dysfunction in septic shock. New Horizons 1998;6:130–138.
68. Garrison RN, Cryer HM. Role of the microcirculation to skeletal muscle during shock. Prospect Shock Res 1989;1:43–52.
69. Avontuur JAM, Nolthenius T, van Bodegom JW, Bruining HA. Prolonged inhibition of nitric oxide synthesis in severe septic shock: a clinical study. Crit Care Med 1998;26:660–667.
70. Palmer RMJ. The discovery of nitric oxide in the vessel wall: a unifying concept in the pathogenesis of sepsis. Arch Surg 1993;128:396–401.
71. Bakker J, Grover R, McLuckie A, et al. Administration of the nitric oxide synthase inhibitor NG-methyl-L-arginine hydrochloride (546C88) by intravenous infusion for up to 72h can promote the resolution of shock in patients with severe sepsis: results of a randomized, double-blind, placebo-controlled multicenter study (study no. 144–002). Crit Care Med 2004;32: 1–12.
72. Lopez A, Lorente JA, Steingrub J, et al. Multiple-center, randomized, placebo-controlled, double-blind study of the nitric oxide synthase inhibitor 546C88: effect on survival in patients with septic shock. Crit Care Med 2004;32:21–30.
73. Hinshaw LB. Sepsis/septic shock: participation of the microcirculation: an abbreviated review. Crit Care Med 1996;24:1072–1078.
74. Leibovici L, Drucker M, Konigsberger H, et al. Septic shock in bacteremic patients: risk factors, features and prognosis. Scand J Infect Dis 1997;29:71–75.
75. Piepmeier JM, Kenneth LB, John LG. Cardiovascular instability following acute cervical spinal cord trauma. Cent Nerv Syst Trauma 1985;2:153.
76. Lehmann KG, Lane JG, Piepmeier JM, Batsford WP. Cardiovascular abnormalities accompanying acute spinal cord injury in humans: incidence, time course and severity. J Am Coll Cardiol 1987;10:46–52.
77. Levi L, Wolf A, Belzberg H. Hemodynamic parameters in patients with acute cervical cord trauma: description, intervention, and prediction of outcome. Neurosurgery (Baltim) 1993;33:1007–1017.
78. Annane D, Sebille V, Charpentier C, et al. Effect of treatment with low doses of hydrocortisone and fludrocortisone on mortality in patients with septic shock. JAMA 2002;288:862–871.
79. Annane D, Sebille V, Troche G, Raphael JC, Gajdos P, Bellissant E. A 3-level prognostic classification in septic shock based on cortisol levels and cortisol response to corticotropin. JAMA 2000;283:1038–1045.
80. Annane D, Bellissant E, Bollaert PE, Briegel J, Keh D, Kupfer Y. Corticosteroids for severe sepsis and septic shock: a systematic review and meta-analysis. BMJ 2004;329:480.
81. Rhodes A, Cusack RJ, Newman PJ, Grounds RM, Bennett ED. A randomised, controlled trial of the pulmonary artery catheter in critically ill patients. Intensive Care Med 2002;28:256–264.
82. Richard C, Warszawski J, Anguel N, et al. Early use of the pulmonary artery catheter and outcomes in patients with shock and acute respiratory distress syndrome: a randomized controlled trial. JAMA 2003;290:2713–2720.
83. Esposito TJ, Jurkovich GJ, Rice CL, Maier RV, Copass MK, Ashbaugh DG. Reappraisal of emergency room thoracotomy in a changing environment. J Trauma 1991;31:881–885.
84. Branney SW, Moore EE, Feldhaus KM, Wolfe RE. Critical analysis of two decades of experience with postinjury emergency department thoracotomy in a regional trauma center. J Trauma 1998;45:87–94.
85. Lorenz HP, Steinmetz B, Lieberman J, Schecoter WP, Macho JR. Emergency thoracotomy: survival correlates with physiologic status. J Trauma 1992;32:780–785.
86. Ivatury RR, Kazigo J, Rohman M, Gaudino J, Simon R, Stahl WM. "Directed" emergency room thoracotomy: a prognostic prerequisite for survival. J Trauma 1991;31:1076–1081.
87. Hopson LR, Hirsh E, Delgado J, Domeier RM, McSwain NE, Krohmer J. Guidelines for withholding or termination of resuscitation in prehospital traumatic cardiopulmonary arrest: joint position statement of the National Association of EMS Physicians and the American College of Surgeons Committee on Trauma. J Am Coll Surg 2003;196:106–112.
88. Stevens PE, Gwyther SJ, Hanson ME. Noninvasive monitoring of renal blood flow characteristics during acute renal failure in man. Intensive Care Med 1990;16:153–158.
89. McDonald RH, Goldberg LI, McNay JL, et al. Effects of dopamine in man: augmentation of sodium excretion, glomerular

filtration rate, and renal plasma flow. J Clin Invest 1973;45:733–742.

90. Hollenberg SM, Ahrens TS, Annane D, et al. Practice parameters for hemodynamic support of sepsis in adult patients: 2004 update. Crit Care Med. 2004;32:1928–1948.
91. Dunser MW, Mayr AJ, Ulmer H, et al. Arginine vasopressin in advanced vasodilatory shock: a prospective, randomized, controlled study. Circulation 2003;107:2313–2319.
92. Patel BM, Chittock DR, Russell JA, Walley KR. Beneficial effects of short-term vasopressin infusion during severe septic shock. Anesthesiology 2002;96:576–582.
93. Goris RJA. Prevention of ARDS and MOF by prophylactic mechanical ventilation and early fracture stabilization. Prog Clin Biol Res 1987;236B:163.
94. Gregory JS, Flancbaum L, Townsend MC, Cloutier CT, Jonasson O. Incidence and timing of hypothermia in trauma patients undergoing operations. J Trauma 1991;31:795–798.
95. Paton BC. Cardiac function during accidental hypothermia. In: Pozos RE, Wittmer LE, eds. The Nature and Treatment of Hypothermia. Minneapolis: University of Minnesota Press, 1983:133–142.
96. Gubler KD, Gentilello LM, Hassantash SA, Maier RV. The impact of hypothermia on dilutional coagulopathy. J Trauma 1994;36:847–851.
97. Gentilello LM, Cobean RA, Offner PJ, Soderberg RW, Jurkovich GJ. Continuous arteriovenous rewarming: rapid reversal of hypothermia in critically ill trauma patients. J Trauma 1992;32:316–327.
98. Gentilello LM, Jurkovich GJ, Stark MS, Hassantash SA, O'Keefe GE. Is hypothermia in the victim of major trauma protective or harmful? A randomized, prospective study. Ann Surg 1997; 226:439–447.
99. Ivatury RR, Diebel L, Porter JM, Simon RJ. Intra-abdominal hypertension and the abdominal compartment syndrome. Surg Clin North Am 1997;77:783–800.
100. Cullen DJ, Coyle JP, Teplick R, Long MC. Cardiovascular, pulmonary, and renal effects of massively increased intra-abdominal pressure in critically ill patients. Crit Care Med 1989;17:118–121.
101. Meldrum DR, Moore FA, Moore EE, Haenel JB, Cosgriff N, Burch JM. Cardiopulmonary hazards of perihepatic packing for major liver injuries. Am J Surg 1995;170:537–542.
102. Bloomfield GL, Ridings PC, Blocher CR, Marmarou A, Sugerman HJ. A proposed relationship between increased intra-abdominal, intrathoracic and intracranial pressure. Crit Care Med 1997;25:496–503.
103. Bloomfield GL, Ridings PC, Blocher CR, Marmarou A, Sugerman H. Effects of increased intra-abdominal pressure upon intracranial and cerebral perfusion pressure before and after volume expansion. J Trauma 1996;40:936–943.
104. Caldwell CB, Ricotta JJ. Evaluation of intra-abdominal pressure and renal hemodynamics. Curr Surg 1986;43:495–498.
105. Bongard F, Pianim N, Dubecz S, Klein SR. Adverse consequences of increased intraabdominal pressure on bowel tissue oxygen. J Trauma 1995;39:519–525.
106. Kron IL, Harman PK, Nolan SP. The measurement of intra-abdominal pressure as a criterion for abdominal re-exploration. Ann Surg 1984;199:28–30.
107. Kirkpatrick AW, Brenneman FD, McLean RF, Rapanos T, Boulanger BR. Is clinical examination an accurate indicator of raised intra-abdominal pressure in critically injured patients? Can J Surg 2000;43:207–211.
108. Iberti TJ, Kelly KM, Gentili DR, Hirsch S, Benjamin E. A simple technique to accurately determine intra-abdominal pressure. Crit Care Med 1987;15:1140–1142.
109. Burch JM, Moore EE, Moore FA, Franciose R. The abdominal compartment syndrome. Surg Clin North Am 1996;76:833–842.
110. Meldrum DR, Moore FA, Moore EE, Franciose RJ, Sauia A, Burch JM. Prospective characterization and selective management of the abdominal compartment syndrome. Am J Surg 1997;174: 667–672.
111. Schwaitzberg SD, Bergman KS, Harris BH. A pediatric trauma model of continuous hemorrhage. J Pediatr Surg 1988;23:605–609.
112. Rackow EC, Falk JL, Fein IA, et al. Fluid resuscitation in circulatory shock: a comparison of albumin, hetastarch and saline solutions in patients with hypovolemic and septic shock. Crit Care Med 1983;11:839–850.
113. American College of Surgeons. Shock. In: Advanced Trauma Life Support Manual. Chicago: American College of Surgeons, 1997:87–107.

17

Perioperative Management

Philip S. Barie

Perioperative care, put simply, is the medical care provided to prepare a patient for surgery and to hasten recovery thereafter. Perioperative patient care is as integral to the outcome of the patient as the operation itself. In many cases, quality care may be more important to the achievement of a good outcome than the operation (e.g., when a major complication occurs after minor surgery or when a patient with complex medical problems must be managed for a straightforward operation). The simplicity of these statements belies the complexity of the issues because numerous fundamental questions must be addressed before considering the specifics involved. What is the duration of the perioperative period, and what marks its beginning and end? What constitutes a good outcome, and from the perspective of whom—the physician, the patient, or some external agency? What constitutes quality care, how can quality be measured, and are there characteristics of high-quality providers or units that are worthy of emulation? What standards of evidence should be applied for the evaluation of efficacy and effectiveness, and what are their flaws? Even the question of who should provide perioperative care is debated, especially for the hospitalized and seriously ill patient. By addressing these questions, it is intended that the reader create a framework for independent analysis rather than an expectation of "right" or "wrong" answers that sometimes do not exist.

Defining the Perioperative Period

The concept that the perioperative period can be defined temporally is arbitrary but necessary despite obvious flaws. The necessity has derived from the impetus to describe the incidence of "postoperative complications"; the flaws include the compartmentalization that results when an event occurs subsequent to a defined point in time or from speculation that a complication is "unrelated" to a procedure. Surgical literature relating to the preoperative period is scant compared to that relating to intraoperative management and postoperative care, perhaps because the definition of the preoperative period is nebulous, or perhaps because so much of the care in the prehospital setting is provided by nonsurgeons. Regardless, it is crucial for surgeons to be involved in all phases of perioperative care because many stand ready to provide care if surgeons are not involved.

The preoperative period begins when it is decided that a patient needs surgery. This period may extend for the few minutes that it takes to get a trauma patient to the operating room or for several weeks if comorbid factors must be addressed in preparation. The postoperative period is more defined, albeit arbitrarily, as 30 days after surgery; operative mortality and complication rates are generally reported using that criterion. Other models use the length of hospital stay to define the period, but that is increasingly irrelevant in modern practice considering that many surgical patients are never hospitalized. A model that has financial underpinnings is the use of the Center for Medicare and Medicaid Services (CMS) concept of the "aftercare" period, which varies depending on the magnitude of the procedure and constitutes the postoperative care portion of the global surgical fee. Set at 90 days for most procedures, even minor operations, it is 10 days for some procedures (e.g., tube gastrostomy), 0 days for others (e.g., central venous catheter insertion, tube thoracostomy), and is therefore unusable for clinical results reporting. It is increasingly apparent that long-term outcome data (extending well past the 90-day period) are important. To continue to justify the expensive, high-complexity treatments that are offered to increasingly older, high-risk patients, long-term benefit must be demonstrable.

Who Should Provide Perioperative Care?

Fundamental questions are being asked about the evidence of efficacy for even "standard" interventions. Millions of patients undergo ambulatory surgery annually without the "benefit" of hospitalization. Minimal-access surgery is reducing the metabolic stress response to surgery and challenging conventional widsom regarding wound care, pain management, recovery of gut function, and whether hospitalization is necessary in the immediate postoperative period. Traditionally, perioperative care was provided by the surgeon with consultative assistance by the primary care physician. In that reversal of roles (consultant as primary caregiver, primary physician as consultant), the primacy of the surgeon in directing perioperative care was perpetuated. Now, there is nothing simple about perioperative care, and traditions are becoming anachronisms. The diagnosis of surgical illness is often made before the patient sees a surgeon; patients now often present to the surgeon for management of acute appendicitis after a diagnostic computed tomographic (CT) scan.[1]

Even as postoperative care is provided increasingly in the outpatient setting, conceptions are changing regarding who should be providing perioperative care. Nonphysicians (e.g., advanced practice nurses) increasingly practice without direct medical supervision, can be primary care providers, or may provide care in acute inpatient settings such as the intensive care unit (ICU). Physician assistants require supervision but can be credentialed to provide sophisticated, invasive care such as placement of catheters for hemodynamic monitoring.[2] Even primary care physicians sometimes limit their practices to the outpatient setting, just as some surgeons now do. The medical care of hospital inpatients is increasingly transferred to hospital-based physicians, known as *hospitalists*. Hospitalist physicians are willing and increasingly able to provide perioperative care and have the time to devote to the patient that the surgeon, performing more operations for less reimbursement, decides to spend in the operating room. That decision is also a factor in the rising phenomenon of closed ICUs,[3] where care is provided to patients by dedicated multiprofessional critical care teams, while the operating surgeon is a consultant.

Traditionally, the operating surgeon has had primary responsibility for perioperative care for reasons that are several and substantial.[4] *Critical care* is defined as one of the core components of general surgery by the American Board of Surgery, and sufficient experience with the management of critically ill patients must be gained for the surgeon to be proficient in providing critical care in practice. Primary responsibility for the care of critically ill surgical patients may rest with a surgeon, pulmonary-critical care physician, or anesthesiologist. The individual who provides perioperative critical care must have an intimate knowledge of surgical physiology.

In a true open ICU model, all patient care decisions are made by the primary team. Continuity of care is ensured, and surgical residents receive the experience requisite to their training. In a true closed ICU model, decisions regarding triage and therapy become the responsibility of the ICU service. In academic centers, the ICU team is most often led by surgeons and sometimes anesthesiologists, but in other circumstances a nonsurgical team is in charge. In effect, the operating surgeon becomes a consultant on his or her own patient, but other involved subspecialty consultants are fewer. This model is effective for cost containment[5,6] and highly concentrated educational activities. Communication is often facilitated, which is a positive attribute of high-quality units.[7,8] Data indicate that the closed ICU model may provide superior and cost-effective patient care.[3,9,10]

Several comparisons between open and closed ICU care models are available.[3,9,10] One study examined a before–after cohort comparison in which the cohorts were well matched for age and admission severity of illness (Acute Physiology and Chronic Health Evaluation [APACHE] III).[3] There were no differences in the duration of invasive hemodynamic monitoring, antibiotic use, the route of feeding, or the administration of vasopressors. Length of stay in the ICU was not decreased, but the overall rate of morbidity was significantly reduced by 20%, and mortality was reduced by 57% (14.4% vs. 6.0%; $P < .05$).

The status of perioperative care is in flux, as is the even-thornier issue of whether complex or rarely performed operations should be undertaken outside specialized centers.[11,12] For surgeons to maintain a central role in perioperative care, they are well advised to exert leadership rather than to assert ownership.

What Sort of Evidence Should Be Accepted?

Much of perioperative care is empirical, meaning that interventions have more of a basis than simply a hypothesis. However, empirical evidence may derive from observation, experience, or experiment, and much patient care is not based firmly on the last. Evidence-based medicine emphasizes consideration of the quantity and quality of the evidence as part of the evaluation process. There is a paucity of top-quality studies on which to base day-to-day decisions. In one prospective evaluation,[13] each of 281 pediatric surgical patients was allotted a primary diagnosis and intervention, and each intervention was recorded and over a 1-month period categorized according to its level of scientific support. Only 31 interventions (11%) were based on randomized controlled trials; 66% of the interventions could be traced to "convincing nonexperimental evidence," such that the conduct of a randomized controlled trial might be considered unethical or unjustified. However, 23% of interventions were not supported by evidence. This result has many implications, not all of them negative. Literature searches may be flawed, and all evidence may not be identified. Targets for focused research projects can be identified for which expense is high, alternative therapies carry morbidity, and complexity can be reduced. On the other hand, beliefs can be held strongly, and the literature is replete with examples of clinical trials that failed because of low patient accrual and a lack of cooperation from practitioners.[14]

Although surgical procedures and devices should be evaluated by randomized clinical trials in the same manner as medical therapy,[15] such an inherently desirable outcome has many obstacles. Despite the desire and even the wherewithal to conduct more trials, many aspects of surgical care may not be amenable to a rigorous prospective evaluation. Considering that randomized prospective clinical trials (class I data) are few, what other types of evidence can be relied on? Prospective nonrandomized trials or case-control studies with a clearly defined comparison cohort constitute class II data, whereas class III evidence is composed of retrospective studies, small case series, or case reports. Within classes, the quality of the study can be defined by blinding, the methods of treatment allocation, protocol violations, whether the data set was clinical (patient derived) or administrative (e.g., statewide trauma database),[16] and whether the data analysis was on an intention-to-treat basis. After the evidence has been compiled and classified, recommendations are made by a panel of experts.

Classification systems abound, but they share the characteristic of providing recommendations based on the strength of the evidence. I have taken some license here to convert these to standardized terminology so that a level I recommendation is one that is based on sufficient class I data. Level II recommendations represent strong recommendations but indicate the data are not quite as solid scientifically, are equivocal, or depend to a degree on expert opinion. Level III recommendations are by definition weakest, depending on retrospective data, scant prospective but nonrandomized studies, or expert opinion in large part. In every case, the reader is encouraged to consult the original document for answers to questions or the resolution of detail.

It would be virtually impossible to assemble evidentiary tables for an independent review of the evidence for the many aspects of perioperative care in a chapter of this scope, and therefore I chose to rely on published analyses, if available. Many such publications exist, and they also are of uneven quality. Hundreds of clinical practice guidelines have been published on a multitude of topics. Many of those are evidence based, which ideally have been accompanied by publication of evidentiary tables. Evidence-based guidelines (EBGs) generally are thoughtful documents of high quality. These must be distinguished from consensus-based guidelines (CBGs), which although often produced by a panel of experts and crafted with great care, do not disclose the quality of the evidence on which they are based and therefore are of lesser value.

Meta-analysis is a statistical method by which the results of several trials may be pooled for an aggregate analysis.[17] There is disagreement regarding the strength of evidence represented by meta-analysis. Is it class I data or class III? Meta-analysis is unique in that underpowered trials (with possible type II errors); negative trials (to the extent they can be identified, as many are not published); data in abstract form only (and therefore not peer reviewed); and non-English publications are all eligible for review and inclusion, making the assessment of methodological quality a crucial issue. The inclusion of poor-quality studies, small studies, or other flawed data sets can lead a meta-analysis to an erroneous conclusion[18] or two analyses to disparate conclusions from a largely similar primary data set.[19] Sometimes, a pivotal clinical trial reaches a conclusion opposite to that of a previous meta-analysis. In such a circumstance, was the meta-analysis flawed by a lack of quality data, the exclusion of important studies, or some other methodological error? Would the conclusion hold up if the analysis were redone to incorporate the additional data? Considering that this chapter incorporates the results of meta-analysis in several important areas, the reader must be aware of the limitations of the technique.[20–22] Because of the limitations and potential error, some consider meta-analysis to be class III data, with less persuasive force than recommendations made in the context of an EBG.

What Constitutes Quality of Care?

Quality patient care has been defined variously as maximized patient welfare, consistent contributions to the improvement or maintenance of quality and duration of life, or the degree to which health services increase the likelihood of desired health outcomes consistent with current health knowledge.[23] The complexity and variability of terminology can be confusing, especially when the endpoints are vague or the ideal means to achieve a defined outcome are unknown.

From the perspective of the caregiver, quality consists of appropriate care provided with skill. In other words, both the decision making and the performance must be of high quality. Intangibles that help define quality include communication (between providers and with patient and family), proper distribution of workload (so that the right person is performing the correct task), trust, and compassion. Quality of care can also be evaluated in terms of structure or outcome in addition to process. Quality-of-care criteria based on structure or process data must demonstrate that variations lead to differences in outcome. Conversely, it must be demonstrated that different outcomes can be attributed to changes in structure or process. For individual encounters, the implicit criteria are three: Was the process adequate? Could better care have improved the outcome? Considering the process and outcome, was the overall quality acceptable[24]?

Two other methods examine explicit process criteria: Was a cholesterol concentration checked in the past 12 months in this patient with heart disease? What percentage of the population was checked (against some benchmark value) in the past 12 months? Increasingly, the latter, more strict, process-type criteria are examined, which has important implications. In a given population, the percentage of patients who receive adequate care will be lower than if implicit criteria are used. However, not every patient needs every possible intervention to improve, and costs may escalate to achieve explicit process targets with only a marginal benefit in outcome.

Error in Medicine

The need to describe and evaluate quality through the use of systematic evidence reviews, EBGs, analysis of resource utilization, and outcomes assessments has been heightened by developing evidence that serious errors are commonplace in medical care. There has been much recent emphasis on errors in health care, which are prevalent and for the most part preventable. The proportion of hospitalizations in which some sort of adverse event occurs exceeds 3%, and more than 50% are associated with errors that are preventable.[25,26] Adverse events are associated with mortality in 9% to 14% of episodes, resulting in as many as 98,000 deaths annually in the United States that are attributable to preventable medical errors.[25,26] Deaths from medication errors alone exceed the number of workplace deaths each year. In ICUs, where patients are seriously ill and treated with invasive procedures, the chance of an adverse event has been reported to be 46%, with 18% producing either disability or death. The likelihood of an adverse event increases about 6% for each day of hospitalization.[27] Medication-related complications tend to be most common, followed by surgical site infections (SSIs; but many are not errors) and technical complications.[28]

Errors can also be described as "active" or "latent" errors.[29] Active medical errors are usually made by direct caregivers, and their effects are recognizable almost immediately. Latent errors, sometimes called system errors, tend to be out of the direct control of individuals (e.g., poor design, inadequate installation, faulty maintenance, and poor organizational structure). Latent errors have more potential to cause harm in complex systems because they often go unrecognized and may result in many types of active errors. Administrative responses to errors tend to focus on punitive measures directed at the individual causing the active error. However, such a focus is an ineffective way to prevent recurrence because the latent failures remain in the system. Elimination of latent failures is more likely to increase safety than minimizing active errors.

Outcomes Assessment

Increasingly, a good surgical outcome is defined by the quality of life enjoyed by the patient after surgery.[30] Surgical results reporting must extend beyond the hospital portal. These types of quality endpoints will be incorporated increasingly into clinical research and quality audits, and therefore clinicians must be familiar with the administration and interpretation of these types of studies.

Quality-of-life assessment tools have five essential characteristics[31]: reliability, validity, responsiveness (sensitivity to change), appropriateness, and practicality. Many published tools have not been evaluated carefully for all these characteristics,[32] so the researcher must be careful in the choice of an instrument. Validated instruments can be divided into three types.[30] Generic instruments are applicable across a wide variety of diseases and breadth of illness severity, making them especially valuable for long-term follow-up of ICU care. Disease-specific instruments are especially sensitive for the measurement of changes of clinical importance over time for a discrete entity. Symptom-severity instruments focus solely on symptoms without measuring the impact of the symptoms on other aspects of the quality of life. No one instrument can fit all situations, but general guidance for the choice is available.[33]

Preoperative Cardiovascular Assessment

More than 3 million patients with coronary artery disease (CAD) undergo surgery each year in the United States. Among them, 50,000 patients sustain a perioperative myocardial infarction (MI). The incidence may be increasing because of an aging population. Overall mortality for perioperative MI remains nearly 40%. Aortic and peripheral vascular surgery, orthopedic surgery, and major intrathoracic and intraperitoneal procedures are more frequently associated with perioperative cardiac mortality than are other types of surgery. Absent a history of heart disease, men are at increased risk above 35 years of age, whereas women are at increased risk after age 40. Cardiac mortality risk increases markedly in patients over age 70. Cigarette smoking also confers increased risk.

Crucial to the task of risk–benefit analysis is the prospective identification of the patient at risk for a perioperative cardiac complication. Unfortunately, although the presence of CAD is not difficult to demonstrate by screening techniques, there is little evidence that prophylactic coronary revascularization, whether by open surgery or angioplasty, can reduce risk before noncardiac surgery. Routine noninvasive testing is expensive, and clinical criteria may be nearly as good for the identification of patients at high risk. Until recently, it has been unclear whether medical management in preparation for surgery accomplishes much unless the patient has decompensated disease (e.g., congestive heart failure, recent MI),[34] but new evidence indicates that perioperative β-blockade can reduce cardiovascular mortality even when started immediately preoperatively.[35,36]

In addition to the presence of CAD, the perioperative history and physical examination must ascertain the presence of valvular heart disease (particularly asymptomatic aortic stenosis [AS]), congestive heart failure (CHF), or arrhythmias. Congestive heart failure is strongly predictive of perioperative pulmonary edema and other complications. A prospective study of 254 predominantly hypertensive diabetic patients who underwent elective general surgery operations revealed a 17% incidence of perioperative CHF among patients with cardiac disease (previous MI, valvular disease, or CHF).[37] Patients with both diabetes and heart disease were at especially high risk. In contrast, CHF developed in fewer than 1% of patients without prior cardiac disease.

Severe AS (defined as a pressure gradient >50 mmHg) must be detected preoperatively because the risk of perioperative mortality has been estimated at 13%. The increased mortality results from a limited capacity to increase cardiac output in response to stress, vasodilation, or hypovolemia. Patients with AS tolerate poorly the development of hypovolemia, tachycardia, or new-onset atrial fibrillation. Moreover, left ventricular hypertrophy decreases ventricular compliance and leads to decreased diastolic filling. Elective aortic valve replacement before noncardiac surgery may be indicated in severe AS, even in the absence of symptoms. Patients with less-critical AS require invasive hemodynamic monitoring in the perioperative period and caution with the use of afterload-reducing agents.

Aortic and mitral insufficiency subject the left ventricle to high-volume loads that may impair contractility, but the risk is comparatively small compared to that conferred by AS. Occult ventricular dysfunction may be present in the asymptomatic patient, and therefore close monitoring is required, but patients can be expected to tolerate surgery well if they are not in CHF. Patients with mitral stenosis or hypertrophic cardiomyopathy are at intermediate risk of perioperative pulmonary edema, especially with tachycardia and decreased left atrial emptying. Perioperative fluid shifts of little consequence to the healthy patient may wreak havoc in the setting of mitral stenosis. Hypovolemia and a resultant low-flow state may occur despite relatively high pulmonary vascular pressures, but overzealous volume or blood administration may cause pulmonary edema rapidly.

Atypical or unstable chest pain requires careful evaluation. Stable chest pain does not increase perioperative risk, but unstable disease (e.g., new-onset or crescendo angina, a recent MI, or recent or current CHF) certainly warrants both evaluation and stabilization. The preoperative evaluation of

TABLE 17.1. Risk Stratification Parameters and Criteria for Cardiac Events Following Noncardiac Surgery.

Parameter	*Low risk*	*Intermediate risk*	*High risk*
Clinical characteristic	Advanced age	Mild angina	Myocardial infarction within previous 7–30 days
	Abnormal ECG (LVH, LBBB, ST-T abnormalities)	Prior myocardial infarction	Unstable or severe angina
	Atrial fibrillation or other nonsinus rhythm	Previous or compensated congestive heart failure	
	Low functional capacity (climb <1 flight of stairs with bag of groceries)	Diabetes mellitus	
	Hypertension		
	History of stroke		
Type of operation (partial list): Low, <1% cardiac risk; high, >5% cardiac risk	Endoscopic procedures	Carotid endarterectomy	Emergent major surgery
	Skin or skin structure operation (i.e., groin hernia, breast procedure)	Head and neck procedure	Aortic and other major vascular procedures, including peripheral procedures
	Cataract excision	Intraabdominal procedures	Long procedures/major fluid shifts or blood loss
		Intrathoracic procedures	
		Orthopedic surgery	
		Prostate surgery	
Characteristics of ECG stress test (i.e., treadmill)	No ischemia	Ischemia at moderate-level exercise (heart rate 100–130)	Ischemia at low-level exercise (heart rate <100)
	Ischemia only at high level exercise (heart rate >130)		
	ST depression >0.1 mV	ST depression >0.1 mV	ST depression >0.1 mV
	Typical angina	Typical angina	Typical angina
	One or two abnormal leads	Three or four abnormal leads	Five or more abnormal leads
		Persistent ischemia 1–3 min after exercise	Persistent ischemia >0.3 min after exercise

a patient with angina should determine whether the patient's disease and symptoms are truly stable. If so, surgery may proceed with the maintenance of an effective antianginal regimen during and after operation. Similarly, asymptomatic or only minimally symptomatic patients who have previously undergone coronary bypass grafting tolerate surgery well.

A recent MI is the single most important risk factor for perioperative infarction (Table 17.1). The risk is greatest within the early aftermath following an infarction, probably the first 30 days. Estimates of the risk of anesthesia following an MI range as high as a 27% reinfarction rate within 3 months, 11% between 3 and 6 months, and 5% after a 6-month interval. Patients who suffer nontransmural (non-Q-wave) infarctions appear to be at identical risk. However, cardiac risk management strategies may be succeeding. With intraoperative hemodynamic monitoring, the risk may be reduced to as low as 6% within 3 months of the first MI and only 2% incidence within 3 to 6 months. Elective surgery should be postponed for 6 months following an acute MI. When major emergency surgery is necessary, it should be performed with intraoperative hemodynamic monitoring. When operation is urgent, as for a potentially resectable malignant tumor, it can be undertaken from 4 to 6 weeks after infarction if the patient has had an uncomplicated recent course and the results of noninvasive stress testing are favorable.

The Cardiac Risk Index System (CRIS) is an accepted system that was developed from a cohort of patients aged 40 years or more who underwent noncardiac surgery.[38] Risk classes (I–IV) are assigned on the basis of accumulated points (Table 17.2). According to CRIS, any elective operation is

TABLE 17.2. Cardiac Risk Index System (CRIS).

Factors	*Points*
History	
Age >70 years	5
Myocardial infarction ≤6 months ago	10
Aortic stenosis	3
Physical examination	
S_3 gallop, jugular venous distension or congestive heart failure	11
Bedridden	3
Laboratory	
PO_2 <60 mmHg	3
PCO_2 >50 mmHg	3
Potassium <3 mEq/dl	3
Blood urine nitrogen >50 mg/dl	3
Creatinine >3 mg/dl	3
Operation	
Emergency	4
Intrathoracic	3
Intraabdominal	3
Aortic	3

Approximate cardiac risk (percentage incidence of major complications)

Class[a] baseline	*I*	*II*	*III*	*IV*	
Minor surgery	1	0.3	1	3	19
Major noncardiac surgery, age >40 years	4	1	4	12	48
Abdominal aortic surgery or age >40 with other characteristics	10	3	10	30	75

[a]CRIS class I, 0–5 points; class II, 6–12 points; class III, 13–25 points; class IV, ≥26 points.

Source: Adapted from Goldman et al.,[38] by permission of *New England Journal of Medicine.*

contraindicated if the patient falls within class IV. One benefit of CRIS is that more than one-half of the total points are potentially controllable (e.g., treating CHF reduces the score by 11 points, delaying surgery for a recent MI decreases it by 10 points), thereby reducing risk. Further study of CAD serves primarily to quantify risk in patients with identified risk factors. Whether patients with no cardiac risk factors should undergo additional preoperative testing is still debated. Algorithms from the American College of Cardiology/American Heart Association (ACC/AHA) Task Force on Practice Guidelines can be used to guide the evaluation (Table 17.3; Figs. 17.1–17.3).[39]

The routine resting electrocardiogram (ECG) remains the primary screening modality for virtually all patients over age 40 who are to undergo general anesthesia. It is undeniably cost-effective but may be normal in many patients with CAD. However, evidence of a prior MI (Q-wave 0.04 s or wider and at least one-third the height of the R-wave) is nearly indisputable evidence of CAD. A wide array of other tests have been employed for the preoperative assessment of cardiac risk, including ambulatory ECG, exercise ECG, stress echocardiography, radionuclide imaging, and coronary angiography. Noninvasive tests are sufficiently sensitive to identify most patients at increased risk. Exercise ECG (exercise stress testing) is the historical standard to unmask myocardial ischemia. The sensitivity for detection of CAD ranges up to 81%, whereas specificity varies up to 96%, depending on the testing protocol. Testing has important prognostic value when ST segment depression of 1.5 mm or greater occurs early during testing, is sustained into the recovery period, is associated with a submaximal increase in heart rate or blood pressure, or is accompanied by angina or an arrhythmia. However, false-negative studies are problematic. Moreover, the test has limited value as a screening procedure for healthy, asymptomatic individuals.

Radionuclide cardiac imaging is popular for preoperative evaluation of cardiac disease, most commonly with thallium perfusion scanning, which can be performed at rest, during

TABLE 17.3. Evaluation Steps Corresponding to ACC/AHA Guideline Algorithms for Perioperative Cardiovascular Evaluation of Noncardiac Surgery.[a]

Step 1.	What is the urgency of the proposed surgery? If emergent, detailed risk assessment must be deferred to the postoperative period.
Step 2.	Has the patient had myocardial revascularization within the past 5 years? If so, further testing is generally unnecessary if the patient is stable/asymptomatic.
Step 3.	Has the patient had a cardiologic evaluation within the past 2 years? If so, further testing is generally unnecessary if the patient is stable/asymptomatic.
Step 4.	Does the patient have unstable symptoms or a major predictor of risk? Unstable chest pain, decompensated congestive heart failure, symptomatic arrhythmias, and severe valvular heart disease require evaluation and treatment before elective surgery.
Step 5.	Does the patient have intermediate clinical predictors of risk, such as prior myocardial infarction, angina pectoris, prior or compensated heart failure, or diabetes? Consideration of the patient's capacity to function and the level of risk inherent in the proposed surgery can help identify patients who will benefit most from perioperative noninvasive testing.
Step 6.	Patients with intermediate risk and good-to-excellent functional capacity can undergo intermediate-risk surgery with very little risk. Consider additional testing for patients with multiple predictors about to undergo higher-risk surgery.
Step 7.	Further testing can be performed on patients with poor functional capacity in the absence of clinical predictors of risk, especially if vascular surgery is planned.
Step 8.	For high-risk patients about to go to high-risk surgery, coronary angiography or even cardiac surgery may be less risky than the noncardiac operation. Clinical, surgery-specific, and functional parameters are taken into account to make the decision. Indications for coronary revascularization are identical whether or not considered in preparation for noncardiac surgery.

[a]See Figs. 17.1–17.3.

Source: Adapted from Eagle et al.,[39] by permission of the *Journal of the American College of Cardiology*.

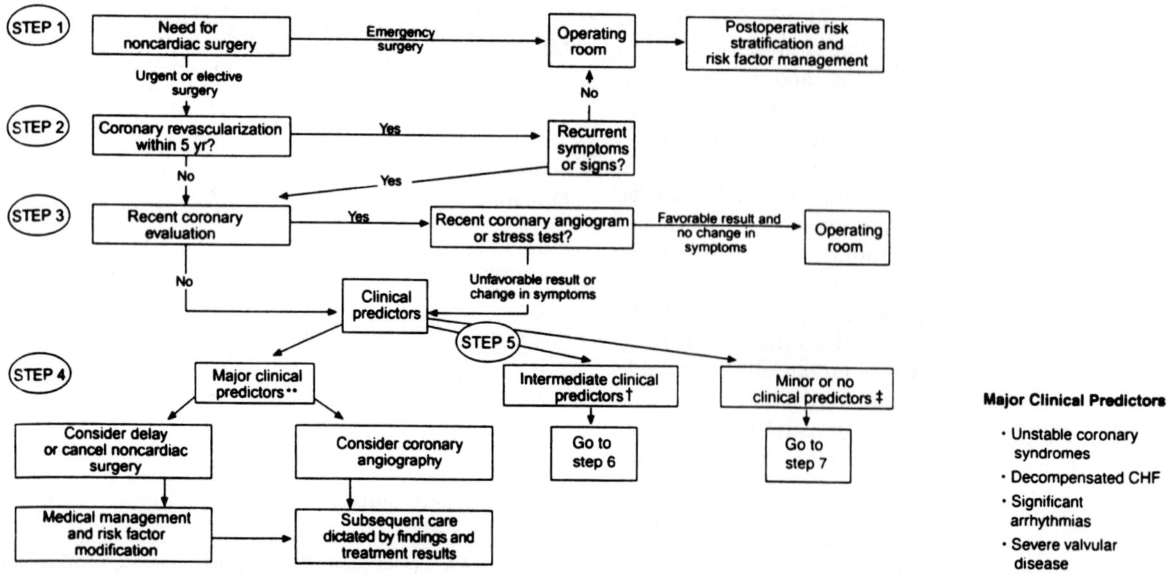

FIGURE 17.1. American College of Cardiology/American Heart Association guideline algorithm for evaluation of cardiac risk before noncardiac surgery. Patients with major clinical predictors of risk may have to have surgery postponed or cancelled or undergo an invasive evaluation. See Table 17.5 for additional information. (Reprinted from Eagle et al.,[39] with permission.)

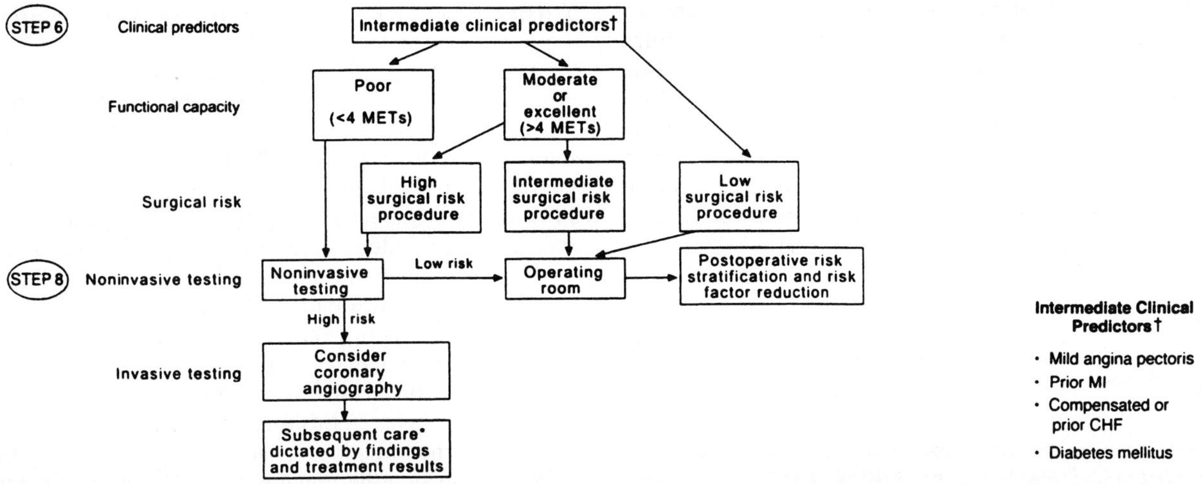

FIGURE 17.2. American College of Cardiology/American Heart Association guideline algorithm for evaluation of cardiac risk before noncardiac surgery. Patients with intermediate clinical predictors of risk or who are about to undergo high-risk surgery may have to have noninvasive testing before surgery. See Tables 17.3 and 17.5 for additional information. Four metabolic equivalents (METs) are equivalent to climbing one flight of stairs with a bag of groceries. (Reprinted from Eagle et al.,[39] with permission.)

exercise, or during a pharmacological exercise equivalent (e.g., dipyridamole) for patients who cannot exercise (e.g., those with peripheral vascular disease, lower-extremity orthopedic problems). Myocardial perfusion imaging using intravenous ^{201}Th analyzes the extent and localization of CAD, the reversibility of the lesions, and the stress response of ^{201}Th in the coronary circulation. The isotope is taken up by myocytes in a manner analogous to potassium. Rapid uptake allows visualization of ischemic or unperfused myocardium. Normal coronary blood flow is relatively homogeneous, such that perfusion deficits cannot be detected in the resting state unless severe (90% or greater) coronary artery stenosis is present. Heterogeneity can therefore be enhanced by superimposed myocardial stress, which reflects ischemia. Because myocardial clearance of ^{201}Th is rapid, redistribution during reperfusion of ischemic myocardium can also be observed. The accuracy of ^{201}Th perfusion scans is limited by lower sensitivity with lesser degrees of coronary stenosis. Single-vessel disease involving the circumflex or right coronary circulations may not be detected, and disease in the left anterior descending artery may go unrecognized if redistribution occurs in other segmental circulations. Although the negative predictive value is high (90%), the presence of redistribution during reperfusion is identified so often, particularly in vascular surgical patients, that its positive predictive value is low (30%). It is also possible to estimate the left ventricular ejection fraction (LVEF), which portends increased risk when below 35% however it is measured (e.g., echocardiography).

Stress echocardiography (usually with infusion of dobutamine) may be even more accurate than ^{201}Th scanning according to a meta-analysis of the recent literature.[40] Dobutamine echocardiography is less expensive than a ^{201}Th perfusion scan and has the advantage of additional imaging possibilities. Valvular function can be assessed, wall motion and wall thickening can be quantified, and an estimate of LVEF can be made from measurements of end-systolic and end-diastolic areas. Dobutamine echocardiography should probably be

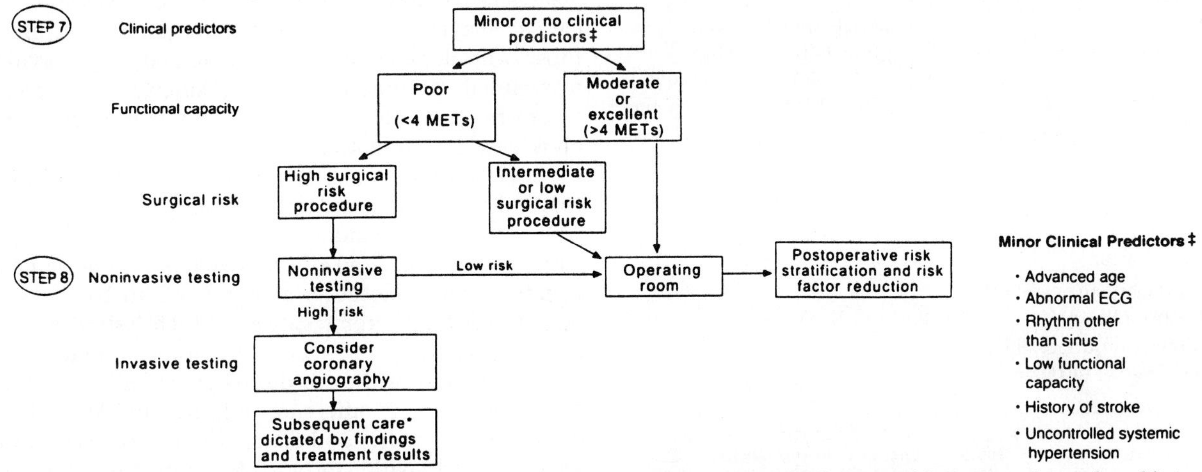

FIGURE 17.3. American College of Cardiology/American Heart Association guideline algorithm for evaluation of cardiac risk before noncardiac surgery. Patients with minor or no clinical predictors who are about to undergo high-risk surgery may have to have noninvasive testing before surgery. See Tables 17.3 and 17.5 for additional information. Four metabolic equivalents (METs) are equivalent to climbing one flight of stairs with a bag of groceries. (Reprinted from Eagle et al.,[39] with permission.)

considered the provocative test of choice for moderate- to high-risk patients. Echocardiographic estimates of ventricular function correlate well with angiographic and radionuclide data. Such information can be of great value as reduced LVEF (<35%) correlates strongly with perioperative myocardial events. Some patients may be evaluated more safely at rest than under pharmacological stress. An equivocal or positive result from noninvasive testing is an indication for cardiac catheterization (Table 17.4; see Figs. 17.1–17.3).

TABLE 17.4.
Guidelines to Perioperative Cardiovascular Evaluation of Noncardiac Surgery.

Indications for assessment of left ventricular function at rest (radionuclide angiography, echocardiography, contrast ventriculography)	
Level I (helpful):	Patients with current or poorly controlled congestive heart failure
Level II (possibly helpful):	Patients with prior congestive heart failure or dyspnea of unknown etiology
Level III (not helpful):	Routine testing of ventricular function in patients without prior congestive heart failure
Indications for cardiac catheterization	
Level I:	High-risk results during noninvasive testing
Unstable chest pain syndrome	
Nondiagnostic or equivocal noninvasive testing result in high-risk patient before high-risk procedure	
Level II:	Intermediate results from noninvasive testing
Nondiagnostic or equivocal noninvasive testing result in low-risk patient before high-risk procedure	
Urgent noncardiac surgery after a recent acute myocardial infarction	
Perioperative myocardial infarction	
Level III:	Low-risk noninvasive testing result in patient with known CAD before a low-risk procedure
Screening before a noninvasive test	
Asymptomatic patient with normal exercise tolerance after coronary revascularization	
Normal coronary angiography in previous 5 years	
Revascularization impossible, contraindicated, or refused a priori	

Summary of evidence-based recommendations for supplemental evaluation of the American College of Cardiology/American Heart Association Task Force on Practice Guidelines, Committee on Perioperative Cardiovascular Evaluation for Noncardiac Surgery, 1996.

Source: Adapted from Eagle et al.,[39] by permission of the *Journal of the American College of Cardiology*.

Adjustment of Cardiovascular Medications

To minimize risk, the patient must be in optimal medical condition. Such optimization is ultimately the responsibility of the operating surgeon but may often be undertaken by the referring physician or a consultant. Congestive heart failure, poorly controlled hypertension (diastolic blood pressure >110mmHg), and diabetes mellitus must be stabilized before an elective procedure is undertaken. In general, cardiovascular medications should be continued through the perioperative period. Continuation of antihypertensive therapy throughout the perioperative period does not contribute to hemodynamic instability, although the data are conflicting regarding whether continuation of antihypertensive therapy actually decreases morbidity. Discontinuation of antihypertensive therapy does pose potential hazards. Rebound hypertension may be precipitated when centrally acting α_2-adrenergic agonists (e.g., clonidine) are withheld abruptly. Congestive heart failure may recur if angiotensin-converting enzyme inhibitors or angiotensin receptor blockers are withheld. Diuretic therapy may cause hypovolemia or hypokalemia, but neither problem poses major difficulties if recognized and treated. There is widespread agreement that β-adrenergic blockade should not be discontinued abruptly. Abrupt discontinuation may be associated with a hyperadrenergic withdrawal syndrome characterized by unstable angina, tachyarrhythmias, MI, or sudden death.

Tachycardia is common in the perioperative period, whether from pain, discomfort from positioning or an indwelling catheter, hypovolemia, or many other reasons. Less evident but equally important is ECG evidence of myocardial ischemia, which may be inapparent unless it is specifically sought by ST-segment trend analysis.[41] The diagnosis of perioperative MI can be elusive because most are silent clinically, many are nontransmural (non-Q-wave) and therefore have minimal accompanying ECG changes, and the incision of muscle may elaborate creatine phosphokinase and confound enzymatic diagnosis. Current ACC/AHA recommendations are to screen for MI in patients without evidence of CAD only if signs of cardiovascular dysfunction develop. For patients with CAD undergoing high-risk operations, an ECG at baseline, immediately postoperatively, and daily for the first 2 postoperative days should be obtained. Measurements of cardiac enzymes are best reserved for patients at high risk or those who demonstrate ECG or hemodynamic evidence of myocardial dysfunction.[39] Increasingly, measurement of serum troponin concentration is supplanting creatine phosphokinase determination.

Several studies suggested that both short- and long-term survival can be improved by β-adrenergic blockade for patients who undergo noncardiac surgery.[35,36] In one study,[35] 200 patients with CAD and at least two risk factors were randomized to receive placebo or atenolol at 5 to 10mg i.v. 30min before major noncardiac surgery, which lasted an average of 6h. Atenolol at 5 to 10mg every 12h i.v. or 50 to 100mg p.o. daily was continued until discharge or for a maximum of 7 days. There was no difference in in-hospital MI or death rate, but overall mortality and deaths from cardiovascular disease were reduced significantly at 6 months and 2 years. At 2 years, reduction of the relative risk for death was 48%, and there was a 15% absolute increase in event-free survival at 2 years, from 68% to 83%. In another study,[36] a randomized multicenter trial of bisoprolol versus standard perioperative care was conducted in high-risk patients (clinical indicators and the results of dobutamine echocardiography) not already taking β-blockers and about to undergo major vascular surgery. The medication was started 1 week before surgery and continued for 30 days thereafter. Those who received β-blockers had statistically lower rates of perioperative (30-day) MI and death.

On the other hand, continuation of calcium channel antagonists in the perioperative period is controversial. Rebound phenomena associated with abrupt drug discontinuance are less common than with β-blockers, but patients receiving combined therapy with β-adrenergic and calcium channel blockers are at increased risk of conduction abnormalities and depressed ventricular function. Digoxin therapy for chronic CHF, particularly with complicating supraventricular tachyarrhythmias, should be continued.

Preoperative Preparation in the Intensive Care Unit

Preoperative admission to the ICU for final preparation for surgery has fallen out of favor. Preoperative "optimization" is no longer utilized routinely because of the chronic shortage of ICU beds and nurses and a lack of supporting data. Only patients who need active therapy, such as aggressive fluid resuscitation, should be considered candidates for preoperative ICU admission. Patients likely to benefit from preoperative evaluation in the ICU include those with unstable angina, severe valvular heart disease or decompensated CHF, shock, or perhaps severe renal disease.

TABLE 17.5.
Evidence-Based Pulmonary Risk Stratification for Noncardiothoracic Surgery.

Factor	*Grade of evidence*	*Odds ratio*
Patient-related factors		
Congestive heart failure	A	2.93
ASA score ≥2	A	2.55
Advanced age	A	2.09
COPD	A	1.79
Functional dependence	A	1.65
Weight loss	B	1.62
Impaired sensorium	B	1.39
Cigarette use	B	1.26
Alcohol use	B	1.21
Laboratory test-related factors		
Serum albumin <3.5 g/dl	A	2.53
Abnormal chest radiograph	B	4.81
Procedure-related factors		
Aortic aneurysm repair, open	A	6.31
Thoracic surgery	A	4.24
Upper abdominal surgery	A	2.91
Neurosurgery	A	2.53
Surgery >2.5–4 h	A	2.26
Head and neck surgery	A	2.21
Emergency surgery	A	2.21
Vascular surgery, open	A	2.10
General anesthesia	A	1.83
Perioperative transfusion	B	1.47

ASA, American Society of Anesthesiologists; COPD, chronic obstructive pulmonary disease; grade A, good evidence that pulmonary complications are reduced and that benefit outweighs risk; grade B, fair evidence that pulmonary complications are reduced and that benefit outweighs risk.

Preoperative Pulmonary Evaluation

Patients with a history of lung disease or those for whom a pulmonary resection is planned may benefit from preoperative assessment and optimization of pulmonary function. Late postoperative pulmonary complications are leading causes of morbidity and mortality, second only to cardiac complications as causes of death after surgery. Prolonged postoperative decreases in functional residual capacity (FRC) and forced vital capacity (FVC) are associated with atelectasis, decreased pulmonary compliance, increased work of breathing, and tachypnea at low tidal volumes. Poor cough effort and impaired airway reflexes increase susceptibility to retained secretions, bacterial invasion, and pneumonia. Older age, upper abdominal and thoracic incisions, neurosurgical procedures, emergency operations, prolonged operative time, increased severity of underlying pulmonary disease (chronic obstructive pulmonary disease [COPD] or chronic bronchitis), alcohol abuse, cigarette smoking, poor preoperative nutrition, and preoperative blood transfusion are independent risk factors for major pulmonary morbidity[42] (Table 17.5).

Pulmonary morbidity may be anticipated after thoracotomy. Resection of a lung tumor requires removal of functional, albeit abnormal, tissue from patients who have limited pulmonary reserve. Operability is assessed by evaluation of baseline pulmonary function, including the contribution to overall pulmonary function of the tissue proposed for resection (by split-function studies). In contrast, preoperative assessment before nonthoracic surgery should focus on identification of chronic airway obstruction, possible preoperative intervention to minimize risk, and the choice of surgical incision in the case of celiotomy and laparoscopic surgery as an alternative. However, few data suggest that outcome is improved by optimization of pulmonary function before elective procedures. There is no doubt, however, that prophylaxis of venous thromboembolic complications is important for patients at risk.

Preoperative chest radiography, of no value routinely, may be of value for dyspneic patients with underlying lung disease or to serve as a basis for comparison. Radiographic indicators of possible airflow obstruction include depression of the right hemidiaphragm at or below the seventh rib anteriorly on a conventional posteroanterior view, a cardiac silhouette with a transverse dimension less than 11.5 cm, and a retrosternal air space greater than 4.4 cm on a lateral view. Substantive airflow obstruction may be associated with a normal X-ray.

Most laboratory studies, other than the serum albumin concentration, are of little benefit for prediction of pulmonary morbidity (Table 17.5). An elevated serum bicarbonate concentration suggests chronic respiratory acidosis, whereas polycythemia may suggest chronic hypoxemia. A room air arterial oxygen tension (Pa_{O_2}) less than 60 mmHg correlates

TABLE 17.6.
Evidence-Based Strategies to Reduce Pulmonary Risk for Noncardiothoracic Surgery.

Factor	*Grade of evidence*
Demonstrated benefit	
Lung expansion modalities[a]	A
Probable benefit	
Selective nasogastric tube decompression[b]	B
Shorter-acting neuromuscular blockade[c]	B
Possible benefit	
Laparoscopic vs. open operation	C
Uncertain benefit	
Smoking cessation	I
Intraoperative neuraxial blockade (epidural or spinal)	I
Postoperative epidural analgesia	I
Immunonutrition	I
No benefit	
Pulmonary artery catheterization	D
Routine enteral or parenteral nutritional support	D

Grade A, good evidence that pulmonary complications are reduced and that benefit outweighs risk; grade B, fair evidence that pulmonary complications are reduced and that benefit outweighs risk; grade C, limited evidence that pulmonary complications are reduced and that benefit outweighs risk; grade D, at least fair evidence that pulmonary complications are not reduced or that risk outweighs benefit; grade I, evidence of effectiveness is conflicting, of poor quality, insufficient, or lacking or the balance between benefit and risk cannot be determined.

[a]Incentive spirometry, chest physiotherapy, continuous positive airway pressure.

[b]Use only for postoperative nausea/vomiting, intolerance of oral intake, abdominal distention.

[c]Atracurium or vecuronium as opposed to pancuronium.

Source: Data from Lawrence et al.[43]

with pulmonary hypertension, whereas a Pa_{CO_2} greater than 45 mmHg is associated with increased perioperative morbidity. Spirometry before and after bronchodilators is simple and safe to obtain. Analysis of forced expiratory volume in 1 s (FEV_1) and FVC usually provides sufficient information for clinical decision making. Dyspnea is assumed to occur when FEV_1 is less than 2 l, whereas an FEV_1 less than 50% of the predicted value correlates with exertional dyspnea. In COPD, the FVC decreases less than the FEV_1, resulting in an FEV_1/FVC ratio less than 0.8. Spirometry correlates with the development of postoperative atelectasis and pneumonia, particularly if FEV_1 is less than 1.2 l or less than 70% of predicted, if FVC is less than 1.7 l or less than 70% of predicted, or if FEV_1/FVC is less than 0.65. If spirometric parameters improve by 15% or more after bronchodilator therapy, then such therapy should be continued. If pulmonary resection is planned, then split-lung function can be determined. An FEV_1 of approximately 800 ml from the contralateral lung is required to proceed with pneumonectomy. For abdominal surgery, there is no indication for evaluation beyond spirometry and arterial blood gas analysis.

Preoperative pulmonary toilet is of unproven benefit and probably accomplishes more by patient education than by actually improving gas exchange. However, lung expansion exercises (e.g., spirometry) are of proven benefit in the postoperative period (Table 17.6).[43] Chronic bronchodilator therapy should be continued perioperatively. A short course of oral antibiotics can treat acute bronchitis before surgery if the sputum is purulent or tenacious, but expectorants and mucolytic agents are of no value and may actually promote bronchospasm. Cessation of cigarette smoking has been advocated for those who smoke more than 10 cigarettes per day, but the benefit is uncertain (Table 17.6). Short-term abstinence (48 h) decreases the carboxyhemoglobin concentration to that of a nonsmoker, abolishes the effects of nicotine on the cardiovascular system, and improves mucosal ciliary function. Sputum volume decreases after 1 to 2 weeks of abstinence, and spirometry improves after about 6 weeks.

Prophylaxis of Venous Thromboembolism

The morbidity and mortality of venous thromboembolism make consideration of prophylaxis mandatory for every major operation. Several risk factors have been identified (Table 17.7), including increasing age, obesity, previous thromboembolic disease, varicose veins, cigarette smoking, major surgery (especially pelvic, urological, orthopedic, and cancer surgery), and several hematologic disorders; risk is increased further by the presence of several risk factors (Table 17.8).[44] The lowest-risk patients are those who are undergoing only minor surgery and who have no risk factors; prophylaxis is not usually needed. However, risk is increased somewhat for any patient over the age of 40 who undergoes general anesthesia for more than 30 min. Many prophylactic regimens have proven efficacy for patients at moderate to high risk, and the morbidity is acceptable[45]; therefore, standard regimens are employed increasingly for virtually all patients (Tables 17.8 and 17.9).

TABLE 17.7. Risk Factors[a] for the Development of Venous Thromboembolism in the Perioperative Period.

General	*Hematological*
Age	Activated protein C resistance (factor V Leiden mutation)
Cancer	Antiphospholipid antibody
Congestive heart failure	Antithrombin III deficiency
Estrogen therapy	Disorders of plasminogen/ plasminogen activation
Fracture of pelvis, hip, or leg	Dysfibrinogenemia
Indwelling femoral vein catheter	Heparin-associated thrombocytopenia
Inflammatory bowel disease	Hyperviscosity syndromes
Major surgery (abdomen, pelvis, lower extremity)	Homocysteinemia
Myocardial infarction	Lupus anticoagulant
Nephrotic syndrome	Myeloproliferative disorders
Obesity	Protein C deficiency
Prior venous thromboembolic disease	Thrombocytosis
Prolonged immobility; paralysis	
Stroke	
Varicose veins	

[a]Patients may have multiple risk factors. If multiple factors are present, then the risk is cumulative.

Source: Adapted from Clagett et al.,[44] by permission of *Chest*.

TABLE 17.8. Risk Stratification Scheme and Incidence of Venous Thromboembolic Events.

Level of risk (% incidence)	*Low (no risk factors)*	*Moderate (any surgery, age 40–60; major surgery age <40; no other risks)*	*High (major surgery, age >60, no risk factors; major surgery age >40 with risk)*	*Very high (Major surgery at age >40 with major risk factors [VTE, cancer, coagulopathy, elective lower-extremity surgery, hip fracture, stroke, multiple trauma, spinal cord injury])*
Event				
Calf vein thrombosis	2	10–20	20–40	40–80
Proximal deep venous thrombosis	0.4	2–4	4–8	10–20
Clinical pulmonary embolism	0.2	1–2	2–4	4–10
Fatal pulmonary embolism	0.002	0.1–0.4	0.4–1.0	1–5
Prevention strategies	None needed	LDUH every 12h LMWH IPC	LDUH every 8h LMWH IPC	LMWH Warfarin IPC plus a heparinoid Intravenous adjusted-dose heparin Vena cava interruption

IPC, intermittent pneumatic compression device; LDUH, low-dose unfractionated heparin; LMWH, low molecular weight heparin; VTE, venous thromboembolism.

Source: Data from Clagett et al.[44] and Palmer et al.[45]

TABLE 17.9.
Summary of Evidence-Based Guidelines for Prevention of Venous Thromboembolic Disease in Surgical Patients from Fifth American College of Chest Physicians Consensus Conference on Antithrombotic Therapy, 1998.

General Surgery	
Level I:	In moderate-risk patients, it is recommended that low-dose unfractionated heparin, low molecular weight heparin, an intermittent pneumatic compression device, or graded-compression elastic stockings be used. In high-risk patients, it is recommended that low-dose unfractionated heparin in higher dosage or low molecular weight heparin be used for prophylaxis. For patients at high risk for wound complications such as hematoma or infection, an intermittent pneumatic compression device is a good alternative. Aspirin is not recommended for prophylaxis because other measures are more efficacious.
Level II:	In very high risk patients, it is recommended that low-dose unfractionated heparin or low molecular weight heparin be combined with an intermittent pneumatic compression device. For selected patients, warfarin (international normalized ratio 2.0–3.0) may be used.
Level III:	For low-risk patients, no specific prophylaxis is recommended other than early ambulation.
Total Hip Replacement	
Level I:	In patients undergoing hip replacement surgery, prophylaxis with low molecular weight heparin should begin 12–24h before surgery, or warfarin (international normalized ratio 2.0–3.0) should be started preoperatively or immediately after surgery, or adjusted-dose heparin should be started preoperatively. Adjuvant prophylaxis with intermittent pneumatic compression or graded-compression elastic stockings may provide additional protection. Low-dose unfractionated heparin, aspirin, dextran, and intermittent pneumatic compression alone are less effective and are not recommended. In patients undergoing elective knee replacement surgery, low molecular weight heparin, warfarin, or intermittent pneumatic compression should be used for prophylaxis. The optimal duration of prophylaxis is uncertain. Abundant data suggest that a 7- to 10-day duration of prophylaxis is appropriate. Emerging data suggest that a 29- to 35-day duration of prophylaxis may confer additional protection, but additional data are needed. Routine screening with duplex ultrasonography is not recommended after hip or knee replacement surgery in asymptomatic patients.

Source: Adapted from Clagett et al.[44]

TABLE 17.10. Effectiveness of Various Modalities for Risk Reduction in Prophylaxis of Perioperative Deep Venous Thrombosis.

General surgery	*Total hip replacement* *n*	*Modality* *(%)*	*Incidence*[a] *(%)*	*Risk reduction* *n*	*Incidence*[a] *(%)*	*Risk reduction* *(%)*
Controls		54	25		13	51
LDUH	53	8	–68	10	31	–39
LMWH	17	7	–72	20	11	–78
Warfarin	2	10	–60	7	22	–57
Dextran	11	18	–28	5	30	–41
Aspirin	5	10	–60	7	52	None
IPC device	5	10	–64	4	22	–57

IPC, intermittent pneumatic compression device; LDUH, low-dose unfractionated heparin; LMWH, low molecular weight heparin; n, number of studies reviewed.

[a]95% confidence intervals for the incidence.

Source: Data extracted from Claggett et al.[44]

For general surgery patients, prophylaxis options of proven benefit in prospective trials include low-dose unfractionated heparin (LDUH), low molecular weight heparin (LMWH), intermittent pneumatic compression, and oral warfarin (Table 17.10). Subcutaneous heparinoids must be administered 2h before induction to be maximally effective, making them somewhat inconvenient for use in ambulatory or same-day admission settings. Moreover, it is recommended that LMWH should be administered for 1 week postoperatively in orthopedic surgery patients, but it is unknown whether this applies to general surgery patients as well (Table 17.9). Meta-analysis of more than 30 randomized controlled trials comparing LMWH to LDUH in general surgery patients demonstrated comparable efficacy for the prevention of thromboembolic phenomena but at a consequence of a slightly higher incidence of minor wound bleeding.[45] Low molecular weight heparin is inadvisable for a patient with recent neurosurgery, gastrointestinal bleeding, or renal insufficiency and has been reported to cause spinal or epidural hematomas in patients with epidural catheters. It is recommended that an epidural catheter should be removed at least 12h before instituting LMWH for any indication. Concomitant LMWH and epidural catheterization are contraindicated.

Patients at high risk require aggressive prophylaxis; multimodality therapy (e.g., anticoagulation plus intermittent pneumatic compression) is common (see Table 17.9), although supporting data are scant. The increased cost and risks of combined-modality prophylaxis are offset by the potential devastation of a pulmonary embolism. Although expensive and lacking any randomized prospective trials, prophylactic placement of vena cava filters is popular. In longitudinal outcome studies, filters are more than 96% effective, and the incidence of complications is low. High-risk patients undergoing high-risk surgery may be appropriate candidates, such as those who have a history of deep venous thrombosis or pulmonary embolism or certain patients with multiple trauma. Newer, potentially retrievable filters may expand the indications by reducing long-term complications further, but experience remains limited.

Evaluation of the Risk of Bleeding

Evaluation of the patient's risk of bleeding requires a careful history and physical assessment to be cost-effective because the routine screening tests of hemostasis have a low yield. Important historical data include whether the patient or a relative has had a prior episode of bleeding or a thromboembolic event and whether the patient reports prior transfusions, prior surgery, heavy menstrual bleeding, easy bruising, frequent nosebleeds, or bleeding gums after brushing the teeth. Coexistent liver or kidney disease, poor diet, excessive alcohol use, ingestion of aspirin, other nonsteroidal antiinflammatory drugs, lipid-lowering drugs (possible vitamin K deficiency), and anticoagulant therapy (usually warfarin) must be ascertained. Answers to these questions should uncover most potential problems with hemostasis. If the history is completely negative and the patient has had a previous hemostatic challenge from surgery or trauma, then an important hemostatic defect is extremely unlikely. A mild coagulopathy in the previously unchallenged patient is not excluded; however, the consequences once such a mild defect is unmasked can be managed readily.

Many hematologic tests can be omitted safely from the preparation protocol if there is no clinical suspicion of a coagulopathy, even before major surgery. Notable exceptions are those operations known to affect coagulation, including cardiopulmonary bypass procedures, prostatectomy, and possibly peripheral vascular surgery. Laboratory testing is overutilized and almost never yields a finding of importance in patients with a negative history and physical examination.[46] Many screening coagulation tests can generate false-positive results that do not translate into increased surgical bleeding. Minor problems, such as oozing from the subcutaneous portion of the incision, can be managed readily by a number of techniques. In the absence of clinical suggestion of a bleeding disorder, the chance that a patient will have a major clotting disorder during surgery has been estimated to be less than 0.01%. Even when indicated, the usual screening tests (prothrombin time [PT], activated partial thromboplastin time [aPTT], and platelet count) identify abnormalities of importance in only 0.2% of patients. False-positive results are especially common with the aPTT; one study found the test to be abnormal 14% of the time but consequential in only 16% of positives (2.2% overall). Similarly, prolongation of the template bleeding time (e.g., after aspirin ingestion) does not correlate with increased operative blood loss. If a clinically important coagulopathy is identified, therapeutic strategies for management of various coagulation disorders in preparation for surgery are listed in Table 17.11.

TABLE 17.11. Preoperative Management of Selected Coagulation Disorders.

Diagnosis Treatment
Factor deficiencies
Hemophilia A
Mild Factor VIII > .10%; desmopressin 0.3 mg/kg i.v. every 12–24 h for 5–7 days for minor surgery
Severe Factor VIII concentrate (level 50%–75% for mild–moderate injury, 75%–100% for severe insults)
Dose: 1 U will increase factor VIII level by 2% in a 70-kg patient; give one-half i.v. every 12 h or 1/24 dose i.v. every 1 h by infusion after the initial bolus
Levels should be maintained for 5–7 (moderate injury) or 7–14 days (severe injury) as delayed bleeding is typical; levels of 25%–30% are adequate for a minor operation
Hemophilia B
Mild Desmopressin 0.3 mg/kg i.v. every 12–24 h
Severe Factor IX concentrate (level 50%–75% for mild–moderate injury, 75%–100% for severe insults)
Dose: 1 U will increase factor IX level by 2% in a 70-kg patient; give one-half i.v. every 18–24 h after the initial bolus; levels should be maintained for 5–7 (moderate injury) or 7–14 days (severe injury) as delayed bleeding is typical; levels of 10%–25% are adequate for a minor operation von Willebrand's disease
Type 1 Desmopressin 0.3 mg/kg i.v. every 12–24 h for 5–7 days; tachyphylaxis can be restored by a 24-h drug holiday to allow repletion of endothelial stores; Keep VIII:vWF 60% for 24–72 h for minor surgery, 80% for 5–7 days for major surgery
Type 2 Trial of desmopressin (unpredictable effect)
Cryoprecipitate (contains 80–100 U vWF/10 U)
Liver disease (multifactorial) Based on specific defect; fresh-frozen plasma to keep PT/aPTT < 1.3 × control (difficult to correct factor VII deficiency)
Vitamin K 10 mg i.m. if vitamin K deficiency suspected
Platelet count > 50,000–100,000
Cryoprecipitate if low fibrinogen (<100–150 mg/dl), factor VIII
Warfarin (vitamin K deficiency, factors II, VII, IX, X)
Fresh-frozen plasma to keep PT < 1.33 control; vitamin K 10 mg i.m. if the patient does not require immediate correction (<12–48 h) or short-term anticoagulation
Platelet abnormalities
Thrombocytopenia Transfuse platelets < 50,000 if bleeding or invasive procedure is anticipated; > 20,000 otherwise
Idiopathic thrombocytopenic purpura Intravenous immunoglobulin 2 g/kg over 2–4 days (*very* expensive)
Platelet infusion after ligation of the splenic artery during splenectomy if the response to immune globulin is poor
Drug induced Discontinue all noncritical medications
Transfuse platelets only if surgery cannot be delayed to allow spontaneous recovery
Uremia Aggressive hemodialysis?
Transfuse to hematocrit ~30% to allow improved adhesion?
Desmopressin 0.3 mg/kg i.v. every 12–24 h (rapid effect of short duration)
Cryoprecipitate, 10 U (rapid effect but short duration)
Conjugated estrogens 25 mg i.v./day for 3 days (slow onset of action but effective for up to 2 weeks)

Management of the Therapeutically Anticoagulated Patient

It is often necessary to operate on an anticoagulated patient. In such circumstances, it is desirable to reverse the patient's anticoagulation temporarily so that hemostasis can be optimized. Procoagulant therapy may sometimes obviate the need for surgery by stopping the bleeding (e.g., gastrointestinal hemorrhage). Previously, perioperative anticoagulant management was needed for patients with a metal prosthetic heart valve, but now chronic atrial fibrillation is the most common indication for long-term warfarin. The approach can be individualized, based on the urgency and magnitude of the surgery to be performed and the strength of the indication for anticoagulation.

Most patients who take warfarin and who are to undergo ambulatory or same-day admission elective surgery can be managed simply by discontinuing the warfarin several days before surgery. Most such patients are on a stable dose of warfarin and are sophisticated regarding their medication and diet because of the need for frequent monitoring of their anticoagulation. The timing of the medication adjustment depends on the degree of anticoagulation determined by preoperative testing, which in turn depends on the indication for the anticoagulation. For example, a patient with a valve prosthesis can be maintained chronically at an international normalized ratio (INR) of 2.5 to 3.0. If there is concern that the patient should not be without anticoagulation, then the patient can be heparinized systemically with an infusion of unfractionated heparin or placed on LMWH. The heparin infusion is discontinued approximately 4 h preoperatively (the half-life of heparin is about 90 min), and surgery proceeds with good hemostasis. However, data are insufficient for a definitive recommendation regarding LMWH.

Clopidogrel, a potent selective inhibitor of adenosine diphosphate-mediated platelet aggregation, is prescribed increasingly for prophylaxis of thrombosis of drug-coated stents placed for management of coronary artery occlusive disease. The effect of clopidogrel on platelets is immediate and irreversible, so optimally the drug should be withheld for 5 to 7 days prior to elective surgery. However, there is increased risk of stent occlusion without clopidogrel for at least 6 months after stent placement, so benefit and risk must be considered, including referral of elective surgery for the 6-month period.

In most circumstances, there is less urgency for reanticoagulation than is generally appreciated. Protection of a cardiac valve prosthesis is the most urgent indication, but a metallic valve can be left without anticoagulation for at least 72 h and perhaps as long as 1 week (especially in the aortic position), although such a long interval is seldom necessary. High-risk patients or those unable to take warfarin by mouth can be heparinized safely as early as 12 h after almost any operation with secure hemostasis, except neurosurgical procedures and some operations for major trauma. Patients who take clopidogrel appear to be at risk for postoperative bleeding for up to 2 weeks even if clopidogrel is withheld for several days after surgery, so the drug should be reintroduced with particular caution.

Steroid Prophylaxis

It is traditional that patients who are on a maintenance glucocorticoid regimen, or who have received corticosteroids within the past 6 months, should receive supplemental "stress dose" steroid prophylaxis owing to concern that a hypophysis–pituitary–adrenal axis suppressed by exogenous steroids may not respond to surgical stress. Large doses (100mg hydrocortisone i.v. every 8h or equivalent) were given for undefined periods without any monitoring, despite the fact that normal adrenal glands, stimulated maximally, increase their output from about 35 to 150mg cortisol/day on average, and that exogenous high-dose steroids have deleterious effects on wound healing, host defenses, carbohydrate metabolism, and other systems. Moreover, there has been no accounting for variability in the stress response (i.e., that a hernia repair causes less stress than an esophagogastrectomy or that laparoscopic procedures appear to be less stressful than their open counterparts). A CBG (there are virtually no class I data) has suggested that such doses are far too high and are given for too long.[47] A minor surgical stress (e.g., inguinal herniorraphy) may not need steroid supplementation at all, whereas a major stress (e.g., esophagogastrectomy) may need only 150 to 200mg hydrocortisone/day for 1 to 2 days.

Of course, there must be a high index of suspicion for adrenal insufficiency in such patients, which can be precipitated by postoperative events, such as infection. The diagnosis is best made by a stimulation test using cosyntropin. A baseline cortisol concentration is drawn, and 0.01 or 0.25mg cosyntropin is administered intravenously; the merits of the two doses are under debate. The serum cortisol concentration is repeated 30 to 60min after the challenge. Glucocorticoids can be given immediately thereafter as indicated, pending the results. The diagnosis is confirmed if neither of the values exceeds 15ng/ml or the stimulated cortisol concentration does not increase by at least 9ng/ml. Patients respond hemodynamically within 12 to 24h of starting glucocorticoid (50 to 75mg hydrocortisone every 8h or equivalent), but it may take several days to correct the electrolyte abnormalities or for fever to dissipate.

Resuscitation: The Interface Between Preoperative and Postoperative Care

Fluid resuscitation is an ubiquitous issue in the perioperative period, one that is multifaceted and context sensitive. Among the many facets are the choice of fluid, the monitoring modalities, and the choice of endpoint. Whether to use isotonic crystalloid or colloid solutions for resuscitation has been a matter of debate for more than three decades. However, one meta-analysis of fluid resuscitation for shock indicated that albumin administration is associated with excess mortality.[48] Considering that human albumin solutions are nearly 100-fold more expensive than equivalent volumes of crystalloid, there no longer seems to be any justification for the administration of colloids for fluid resuscitation unless the patient is markedly hypoalbuminemic (<2g/dl).

Among the many considerations in addition to the volume status are whether shock is present and vasopressor/inotropic therapy is needed in addition to fluid,[49] whether the patient is bleeding, whether relevant preexisting disease is present (e.g., CHF, chronic renal insufficiency, diabetes mellitus), or if there has been an acute decompensation of vital organ function (e.g., acute MI, acute respiratory distress syndrome [ARDS], or acute tubular necrosis [ATN]). The patient may require resuscitation to prepare for surgery (e.g., small bowel obstruction, penetrating trauma to the torso), or resuscitation may be the primary therapeutic modality (e.g., acute alcoholic pancreatitis, anatomically stable pelvic fracture with no associated injuries). Postoperative patients often require fluid resuscitation, especially if intraoperative fluid requirements have been underestimated, evaporative losses are high because a body cavity (especially both chest and abdomen) is open for a prolonged period, the patient is hypothermic, or there has been osmotic diuresis from hyperglycemia or the administration of mannitol.

The goal of fluid resuscitation is to support the circulation to provide sufficient oxygen and metabolic fuel for cellular function, thereby facilitating the resolution of the inflammatory response[50] and preventing or ameliorating the development of the multiple-organ dysfunction syndrome.[51]

Blood Tests and Monitoring Technology as Guides to Resuscitation

Several blood tests are available to guide resuscitation, but not all can be obtained without invasive sampling. A lactate concentration can be measured, or the base deficit can be calculated. Either, in the absence of another cause of metabolic acidosis, can be used to estimate the adequacy of global tissue perfusion. There is no convincing evidence that one is superior, but a persistent base deficit and hyperlactatemia during resuscitation have each been associated with increased mortality in several models. Simple measurement of the serum bicarbonate concentration correlates well with the base deficit.[52] The two indicators do not always correlate because they are not assessing exactly the same parameter. A misconception surrounding resuscitation is that an increased lactate concentration reflects anaerobic metabolism. In actuality, recent metabolic studies have found no correlation between hyperlactatemia and anaerobic conditions.[53] Rather, lactate is generated by deranged amino acid metabolism in the pyruvate kinase pathway. Regardless, the clinical utility of lactate measurements is not diminished by this revelation.

Hemodynamic monitoring is usually instituted at some point if the clinician is disconcerted by the volume of fluid required by a high-risk patient, or if there is persistent acidosis or hemodynamic instability. Vascular access is usually obtained via percutaneous cannulation of a subclavian or internal jugular vein (see chapters 8 and 9). Central venous pressure (CVP) can be measured from the superior vena cava; the access is more reliable than that provided by peripheral vein cannulas, and prodigious volumes of fluid (several liters/hour) can be administered through a multilumen catheter. Central venous pressure provides an estimate of intravascular volume or myocardial function; it can provide an estimate of right ventricular preload, but right ventricular function is more a function of right ventricular end-diastolic volume than any right-sided pressure. Only in the setting of left ventricular function that is known to be normal can a strong inference be drawn from CVP data. Valvular heart disease (especially mitral stenosis and tricuspid insufficiency) and pulmonary hypertension can make CVP readings difficult to interpret.

Even more invasive is placement of a balloon-tipped pulmonary artery (PA) flotation catheter. Data that are of use in resuscitation can be obtained but at a commensurate increase in risk. A meta-analysis of 13 randomized controlled trials of

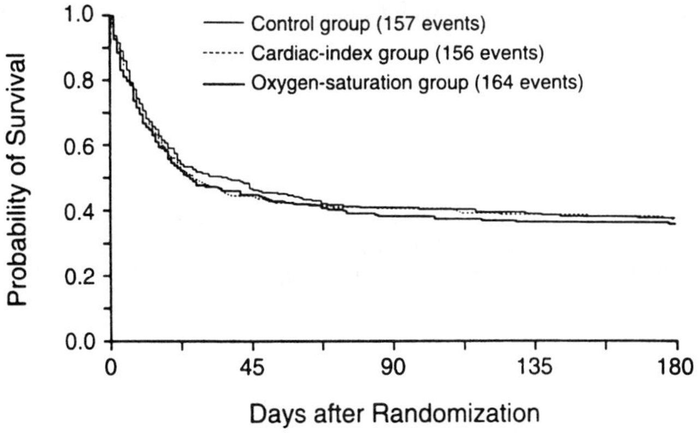

PATIENTS AT RISK (NO. OF EVENTS)

Control group	252 (129)	108 (13)	94 (4)	90 (3)	87
Cardiac-index group	253 (133)	102 (8)	90 (4)	86 (3)	83
Oxygen-saturation group	257 (133)	106 (16)	89 (4)	85 (1)	84

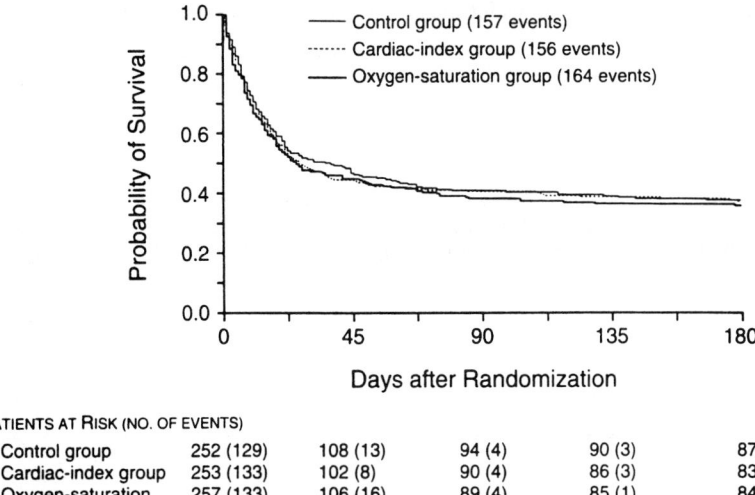

FIGURE 17.4. Kaplan–Meier plot of 180-day survival for three resuscitation strategy groups. There was no significant difference among the groups. (Reprinted from Gattinoni et al.,[55] with permission.)

5051 patients estimated the odds ratio (OR) for death associated with the use of the PA catheter. Overall, the OR for death was 1.04 (95% confidence interval [CI] 0.90–1.20, $P = .59$). Use of a PA catheter was associated with greater use of inotropic agents (OR 1.58; 95% CI 1.19–2.12, $P = .02$) and intravenous vasodilators (OR 2.35; 95% CI 1.75–3.15, $P < .001$). However, use of a PA catheter in selected patients (e.g., for shock, CHF, acute renal failure) may still be justified (see Chapter 16)[54].

Oxygen delivery ($\dot{D}O_2$) and consumption ($\dot{V}O_2$) may also be calculated if actual O_2 context is measured separately. In contrast to directly measured $\dot{V}O_2$ (e.g., by indirect calorimetry), calculated $\dot{V}O_2$ data can be misinterpreted because of a bias called *shared measurement error* that is introduced because calculated $\dot{D}O_2$ and $\dot{V}O_2$ are not independent variables. This bias misinformed the resuscitation of critically ill patients for many years, based on a strategy of enforced supraphysiological $\dot{D}O_2$ rather than mere restoration to physiological levels (see chapter 16).

Gattinoni et al. tested this hypothesis directly in a multicenter trial performed in 56 ICUs.[55] A total of 10,726 patients were screened to identity 762 patients in predefined diagnostic categories (Simplified Acute Physiology Score above 11 and one of the following: high surgical risk, massive blood loss, severe sepsis or septic shock, acute respiratory failure, or multiple trauma). The patients were randomized to therapy consisting of resuscitation via increasing the cardiac index to a predetermined level (>4.5 l/min/m^2), increasing the mixed venous oxygen saturation to normal (70%), or a control group. Mortality was not different among the groups (Fig. 17.4) and ranged from 48% to 52% at the time of ICU discharge to 62% to 64% at 6-month follow-up. Among survivors, there were no differences among groups in terms of organ dysfunction or the length of ICU stay. There were no differences in mortality when stratified by diagnostic subgroup (Fig. 17.5) or among the subsets of patients in which the resuscitation goal was met. Velmahos et al.[56] found in a randomized prospective trial of normal versus supranormal oxygenation that those who achieved supranormal oxygen transport had better outcomes, but they did so spontaneously; therapy had no effect on whether the endpoint was achieved. Younger patients were much more likely to achieve supranormal oxygenation; elderly patients rarely did so. These studies may be considered definitive, and the enforced oxygen transport hypothesis to be therefore disproved.

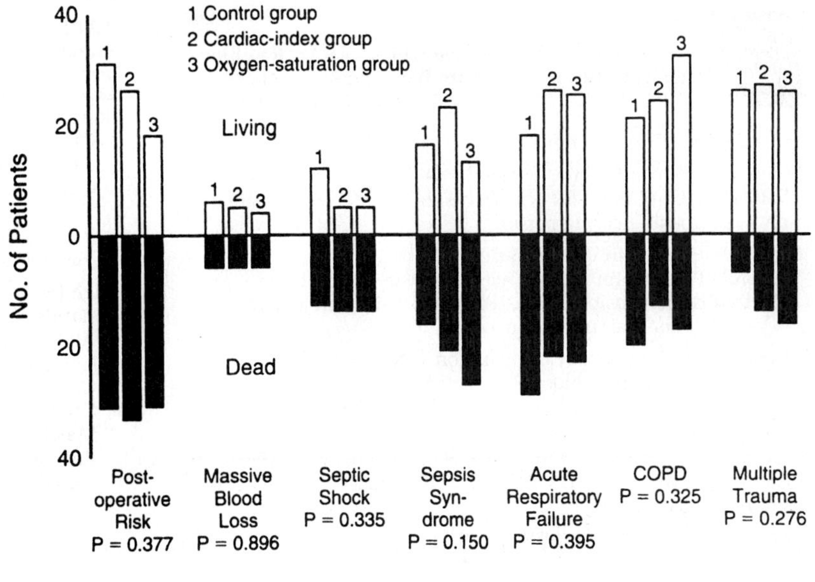

FIGURE 17.5. Overall survival for three resuscitation strategy groups, stratified by study inclusion criteria. There was no significant difference within or among the groups. (Reprinted from Gattinoni et al.,[55] with permission.)

TABLE 17.12. Indications for Blood and Blood Component Therapies.

Leukocyte-reduced red blood cell units
Congenital hemolytic anemias
Hypoproliferative anemias likely to need multiple transfusions
Recurrent severe febrile hemolytic transfusion reactions
Known HLA alloimmunization
Irradiated cellular blood components
Bone marrow/stem cell transplants
Intrauterine/postuterine transfusions
Directed donations (HLA-matched or blood-relative donors)
Hodgkin disease
Acute lymphocytic leukemia
Solid-organ transplant recipients
Antineoplastic chemo- or radiotherapy
Exchange transfusion/extracorporeal membrane oxygenation
HIV opportunistic infections

Transfusion of Blood and Blood Products

The issue of blood transfusion is of great concern to patients and physicians because of real and perceived risks of infectious disease transmission, increased risk of nosocomial infections, and other consequential complications (also see chapter 9). The decision to transfuse a patient with blood or blood products must be predicated on several factors, such as the underlying diagnosis (Tables 17.11–17.15),[57,58] the availability of blood, the "optimal" hematocrit for oxygen transport, and alternatives to transfusion itself. Options for blood transfusion therapy currently include no transfusions whatsoever (which may be dictated for religious reasons), a lowering of the transfusion "trigger" such that a lower hematocrit is tolerated, or possibly therapy with recombinant human erythropoietin (rHuEPO). Alternatives to allogeneic (anonymous volunteer donor) transfusion include blood from a designated donor, autologous transfusion of blood predonated by the patient, and intraoperative isovolemic hemodilution with autotransfusion of reserved blood at the end of the case.

Several studies indicated that higher transfusion targets (hemoglobin 8–10 g/dl) may lead to higher mortality than the more parsimonious strategy of transfusion for a hemoglobin concentration of about 7 g/dl.[59,60] Spiess et al. observed 2202 patients prospectively who underwent coronary artery bypass grafting.[59] The hematocrit value on admission to the ICU after surgery was classified as high (>34%), medium (25%–33%), or low (<24%). Predefined adverse events included Q-wave MI, death, dialysis-dependent acute renal failure, a neurological event, or the need for aortic balloon counterpulsation. A high hematocrit was statistically associated with a higher incidence of MI and more left ventricular dysfunction. By multivariable analysis, the ICU admission hematocrit was the most significant predictor of any adverse event (relative risk (RR) 2.2; 95% CI 1.04–4.76). Hebert et al. randomly assigned 838 critically ill patients (stratified by an APACHE II score cutoff point of 15 points) who had hemoglobin con-

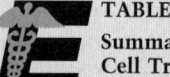

TABLE 17.13.
Summary of Evidence-Based Guidelines for Red Blood Cell Transfusions for Acute Blood Loss.[a]

Evaluate for risk of ischemia
Estimate/anticipate degree of blood loss
<30% rapid volume loss probably does not require transfusion in a previously healthy person
Measure hemoglobin concentration
<6 g/dl: Transfusion usually needed
6–10 g/dl: Transfusion dictated by clinical circumstance
>10 g/dl: Transfusion rarely needed
Measure vital signs/tissue oxygenation when hemoglobin 6–10 g/dl and extent of blood loss is unknown
Tachycardia hypotension refractory to volume: Transfusion needed
Pvo_2, O_2 extraction ratio >.50%, Vo_2,50% of baseline: Transfusion usually needed

[a]Practice Parameter of the College of American Pathologists, 1997.

TABLE 17.14.
Summary of Evidence-Based Guidelines for Red Blood Cell and Plasma Transfusions.[a]

Red blood cell transfusions	
Level I:	No recommendations.
Level II:	Transfusions should be given to alleviate symptoms or mortality.
	No single transfusion trigger is appropriate for all patients or situations.
	Red blood cell concentrates should not be used to expand intravascular volume when oxygen-carrying capacity is adequate.
	Red blood cell concentrates should not be used to treat anemia if less-risky alternatives are available.
Fresh-frozen plasma transfusions	
Level I:	FFP is indicated for adult thrombotic thrombocytopenic purpura, followed by plasmapheresis.
Level II:	FFP is indicated for bleeding in patients with abnormal PT, aPTT, or INR. FFP is not indicated prophylactically for INR <2.0.
	FFP is indicated for therapy of disseminated intravascular coagulation provided the precipitant can be treated effectively.
	FFP is indicated for massive transfusion with microvascular bleeding and abnormal tests of coagulation.

[a]Canadian Medical Association Expert Working Group; level III guidelines excluded.

Source: Adapted from Innes.[58]

TABLE 17.15. Selected Surgical Procedures and Likelihood of Blood Transfusion.

Low (<15%) risk: No likely benefit from preoperative autologous donation
Childbirth
Cesarean section
Cholecystectomy
Transurethral prostatectomy
Vaginal delivery
Vaginal hysterectomy
High (>5%) risk: Likely benefit from preoperative autologous donation
Abdominal hysterectomy
Cardiac surgery
Colorectal surgery
Craniotomy
Mastectomy
Radical prostatectomy
Spinal surgery
Total joint replacement
Vascular graft surgery

centrations below 9 g/dl to two different protocols for transfusion of red blood cell concentrates.[60] One group was transfused only if the hemoglobin concentration dropped below 7 g/dl; the other group received blood to maintain the hemoglobin concentration at 10 to 12 g/dl. Thirty-day mortality was similar overall but was higher for the hospitalization in patients who were transfused at the higher hemoglobin trigger ($P < .05$). Mortality was also higher among less severely ill patients (APACHE II < 20) who were transfused liberally ($P < .05$) and among those over the age of 55 ($P < .05$). There was no difference in mortality in patients with "clinically significant" coronary disease, although patients transfused liberally had a higher incidence of MI and acute pulmonary edema. Overall, no difference in the pattern of development of multiple-organ dysfunction syndrome was apparent.

Predonation Strategies

Acute preoperative hemodilution with reinfusion and perioperative autologous blood salvage ("cell-saver") techniques are essentially autologous transfusion practices. However, from the standpoint of preparation for elective surgery, preoperative autologous blood donation is the popular approach. Directed-donor transfusions are no safer than transfusions from anonymous volunteer donors because clerical error or contamination during processing is still possible, but these transfusions are encouraged when the likelihood of transfusion is high. Such a strategy can decrease the likelihood of allogeneic transfusion by up to 80% in elective surgery. Successful predonation of blood requires attention to the mechanics of the donation process (see Table 17.14). Patients who are not anemic (hematocrit > 40%) can donate approximately one unit of blood per week, although the final donation can be as few as 3 days before surgery. Anemic patients are less likely to complete the scheduled donations and to receive allogeneic blood and therefore may benefit from aggressive and innovative blood procurement strategies.

The physiological benefit of autologous predonation is a function of the degree to which erythropoiesis is stimulated. Typical autologous donation protocols produce a submaximal response. Administration of rHuEPO may facilitate collection, but the optimal dose, route, and timing of administration have yet to be established in the surgical setting. Published guidelines suggest the same criteria for autologous and allogeneic transfusions (see Table 17.13) because the leading causes of acute transfusion reactions are administrative error and bacterial contamination. Neither is eliminated as a potential problem by an autologous transfusion. A unit of autologous blood should not be infused simply because it is available.

Gastrointestinal Prophylaxis

Most prophylaxis of the gastrointestinal tract begins in the postoperative period. Most prophylactic efforts are directed against stress-related gastric mucosal hemorrhage, which has decreased in incidence and importance in the aftermath of the introduction of effective prophylactic methods and improved nutritional support. Historically, "stress gastritis," as it is known popularly but inaccurately, affected about 20% of critically ill patients, but the incidence has been reduced by about 90%.

The incidence began to decrease in the early 1980s with the introduction of antacid prophylaxis, and the decline accelerated as parenteral H_2-histamine receptor antagonists became available. As effective as prophylaxis was, epidemiological studies suggested that gastric acid suppression might lead to overgrowth of gram-negative bacteria in the stomach and that, if aspiration occurred, could result in nosocomial pneumonia. Sucralfate became popular as an alternative method of prophylaxis, but depending on the chosen definition of gastric mucosal injury, sucralfate was not as effective a method as H_2-histamine receptor antagonists.[19] Sucralfate is now seldom used, in that a parenteral proton pump inhibitor (PPI) is available, although class I data regarding PPI use for prophylaxis are scant.[61–63] A prospective but nonrandomized study suggested that only patients who are coagulopathic or who require mechanical ventilation for more than 48 h require prophylaxis, but that adequate prophylaxis in high-risk patients reduces the risk of clinically important bleeding by only one-half.[64] Acid reduction does not in fact increase the risk of nosocomial pneumonia.[19]

Nutritional Support

Total Parenteral Nutrition

Total parenteral nutrition (TPN) is standard therapy for many hospitalized patients when clinical conditions preclude enteral or oral feeding. Long-term nutritional support is possible by administration of vitamins and minerals along with amino acids and dextrose and the periodic supplementation of 10% lipid emulsion. The concentration of amino acids and dextrose can be modified to tailor therapy to specific conditions (e.g., 40% dextrose rather than 25% for patients whose fluid intake must be minimized).

Parenteral nutrition has numerous complications that limit its use. Although dilute solutions are sometimes administered peripherally, TPN therapy requires administration into a central vein. Complications associated with central vein administration include those related to catheter placement or the indwelling state (e.g., infection, especially bloodstream infection), central vein thrombosis, and the rare complications of air embolism or erosion of the catheter tip into the mediastinum.

Potential metabolic complications include fluid overload, electrolyte abnormalities, hyperglycemia or hypoglycemia, and overfeeding. Hyperglycemia is common because of the large number of diabetic patients who require major surgery and because of the insulin resistance that is characteristic of sepsis and surgical stress (see following). Regular insulin not only can be added to the solution directly but also can be administered by supplemental infusion. Absorption after subcutaneous administration can be erratic in hemodynamically unstable patients or those with large volumes of tissue edema.

Hypoglycemia may occur for several reasons. The least likely scenario should be overestimation of the insulin requirement if appropriate caution is exercised. More likely is the failure to adjust the insulin dose downward as the patient's condition improves. Completely avoidable is hypoglycemia associated with the need to interrupt the TPN infusion abruptly. In the event of an abrupt cessation of TPN therapy, the infusion of even a 5% dextrose solution should be sufficient to prevent hypoglycemia. In unusual cases, hepatic dysfunction (usually resulting from ischemia–reperfusion injury or cholestasis, but to which TPN may contribute) may become so severe that gluconeogenesis is impaired.

Patients who are fed intravenously with TPN sustain small-bowel mucosal atrophy and may have impaired immune function. Whether this translates into a clinically important injury in most patients remains a matter of speculation. Patients fed with TPN may develop cholestasis with or without the formation of sludge or stones in the gallbladder. Unfortunately, neither the administration of cholecystokinin nor enteral feeding prevent the development of acute acalculous cholecystitis (ACC) because it is primarily an ischemic injury.[65] It has been hypothesized that the administration of even small amounts of enteral feedings to TPN-dependent patients may protect the gut, but proof is lacking.

Patients fed with TPN are often seriously ill and therefore vulnerable to the myriad potential complications of TPN. The substantial morbidity associated with TPN may negate any beneficial aspects of intravenous nutrition. A meta-analysis of 26 randomized trials of TPN selected from 210 publications from 1980 to 1998 that evaluated TPN versus standard care (i.e., no nutritional supplementation other than intravenous dextrose and an oral diet; comparisons of TPN and enteral supplementation were not examined).[66] Surgical or trauma patients were studied in all but two of the trials selected for inclusion, but the authors considered only six of the studies to contain patients who would normally require ICU care. Trauma patients were relatively few, and medical ICU patients almost nonexistent. When the trials were aggregated, TPN had no effect on mortality (RR 1.03; 95% CI 0.81–1.31) or the complication rate (RR 0.84; 95% CI 0.64–1.09).

Enteral Nutrition

At least 18 randomized, controlled prospective trials have examined the effects of early enteral feedings (usually defined as feedings within 24h vs. 3–5 days), mostly after trauma, burns, or major elective abdominal surgery (Jacobs/Kudsk).[67] The principal endpoints involved have been mortality, length of stay, and the incidence of infection. Significant benefit was demonstrated in five of seven studies of major abdominal surgery, without a predominant type of benefit. In contrast, an improved outcome was demonstrated in six of seven studies of trauma patients, manifested notably by a reduced length of hospital stay of patients with a femur fracture. An improved outcome was also noted in all three studies of burn patients.

All patients who undergo abdominal surgery may have a catheter placed directly into the jejunum, whether by a nasoenteric or transabdominal approach. Aside from the nasoenteric tube, percutaneous endoscopic gastrostomy is performed most commonly. Common complications of nasoenteric tubes include difficulty with insertion, aspiration, intubation of the lower respiratory tract with pneumothorax (even in patients with an endotracheal tube and the cuff inflated), difficulty in negotiating the catheter tip through the pylorus, and intolerance of feedings. Positioning may be assisted endoscopically or with videofluoroscopy, but it is not clear that the catheter tip must be in the duodenum before the initiation of feedings. Many clinicians now have few reservations about feeding into the stomach as long as caution is exercised (head of bed up 30°, frequent checks for residuals that may reflect ileus or intolerance, meticulous pulmonary toilet, and use of promotility agents [e.g., erythromycin]).

The most common complication of enteral nutrition is diarrhea, which causes loss of nutrients as well as fluid and electrolyte abnormalities. Diarrhea can occur even when feeding with an iso-osmotic solution. Evaluation of the stool for parasites or aerobic gram-negative bacteria is almost never of value, but the differential diagnosis does include antibiotic-associated colitis (AAC) caused by *Clostridium difficile*, even if the patient has received only routine perioperative antibiotic prophylaxis and the patient does not have fever, abdominal signs, or leukocytosis. Treatment of diarrhea due to AAC may exacerbate symptoms because of the retention of toxin in the colon; therefore, it is often necessary to exclude the diagnosis with an assay for *C. difficile* enterotoxin performed on a fresh stool sample in any patient whose diarrhea persists for more than 24h. False negatives are few, so a single test will usually suffice. Once excluded, diarrhea may be controlled by the addition of opioids (e.g., dilute tincture of opium), fiber, or discontinuance of any promotility agents. Hyperglycemia is less of a problem than with TPN but is managed similarly. The clinician must also be alert to the possibility of the late complications of sinusitis and tracheoesophageal fistula, especially in patients with endotracheal or tracheostomy tubes.

Management of Blood Glucose

Carbohydrate metabolism is inherently unstable surrounding periods of surgical stress. The perceived need for patients to receive nothing by mouth for several hours before elective endotracheal intubation will decrease caloric intake, as will mechanical bowel preparation before colon surgery. For those patients who require insulin and inject small amounts frequently according to current recommended protocols, fluctuations in blood glucose can be smoothed. For these patients who take long-acting insulin or oral hypoglycemic agents, the potential danger of hypoglycemia before surgery often leads to a recommendation to reduce the drug dosages. In the case of metformin, cessation of therapy 48h before surgery is mandatory to preclude the rare development of severe lactic acidosis.

Historically, there has been little concern about the need to moderate perioperative hyperglycemia. In fact, such hyperglycemia is common in the immediate postoperative period owing to metabolic stress and counterregulatory hormone responses. Emergency surgery for infections and elective surgery for morbid obesity or involving cardiopulmonary bypass pose particular risk for hyperglycemia. Patients with liver disease or on steroid therapy are also at increased risk. Tissue insulin resistance, catabolism of lean tissue for fuel substrate, and catecholamine-mediated glycogenolysis and gluconeogenesis contribute to the propensity of the surgical patient for hyperglycemia. Increased protein catabolism may be mediated by complex interactions between insulin-like growth factors (IGFs) and their binding proteins (IGFBPs). Concentrations of IGF-1 and IGF-2 decrease rapidly with surgery, in concert with a decrease in IGFBP-3, and take up to 6 weeks to recover.[68] In seriously ill or injured patients, resting energy expenditure may exceed the patient's normal daily caloric intake, and "excess" calories must be provided. Concentrated feeding, especially parenterally, can aggravate hyperglycemia. Hyperglycemia begets glycosuria, which in turn is associated with osmotic diuresis. Impaired wound healing and impaired leukocyte function are additional consequences of hyperglycemia.

Exogenous insulin can reverse or overcome many of the metabolic disturbances, but blood glucose is not always checked during surgery, and insulin is not always administered, despite the widespread availability of accurate handheld glucometers. It may take 3 to 5 days after major surgery to restore metabolic homeostasis.[69,70]

Data indicate clearly that hyperglycemia is in fact deleterious and must be controlled. *Tight glucose control*, as it has come to be called, reduces mortality, organ dysfunction, and the incidence of nosocomial infection among critically ill surgical patients. In a landmark study, Van den Berghe et al. randomized 1548 surgical patients (70% postcardiac surgery) to tight glucose control (blood glucose concentration 80–100 mg/dl) with a continuous infusion of insulin versus maintenance of the blood glucose concentration between 180 and 200 mg/dl.[71] Intensive insulin therapy reduced mortality from 8.0% to 4.6% ($P < .05$); the benefit was concentrated among patients who remained in the ICU for more than 5 days (20.2% vs. 10.6%, $P < .01$). Intensive insulin therapy also reduced overall in-hospital mortality by 34%, bloodstream infections by 46%, and the median number of transfusions of red blood cell concentrates by 50%. Insulin is an anabolic hormone with antiinflammatory properties, so the putative mechanism of benefit is still being defined. However, acute control of glucose concentration is more important than the amount of insulin administered,[72] and the benefit accrues to both diabetic and nondiabetic patients.

Pittas et al.[73] performed a meta-analysis of 35 trials of critically ill patients who were treated with insulin. Combining data from all trials using a random effects model showed that insulin reduced short-term mortality by 15% (RR 0.85; 95% CI 0.75–0.97). Insulin therapy reduced mortality markedly in the surgical ICU (RR 0.58; 95% CI 0.22–0.62). The benefit was observed when the aim was glucose control (RR 0.71; 95% CI 0.54–0.93) and in patients with diabetes mellitus (RR 0.73; 95% CI 0.58–0.90).

Van den Berghe et al. were unable to demonstrate an overall reduction of mortality in a randomized trial of 1200 critically ill medical patients treated with intensive insulin therapy.[74] In the intention-to-treat analysis, intensive insulin therapy reduced blood glucose concentrations but did not reduce hospital mortality (40.0% vs. 37.3% in the intensive treatment group, $P = .33$). However, morbidity was significantly reduced by the prevention of acute renal failure, shorter duration of mechanical ventilation, and accelerated discharge from the ICU and the hospital.

The literature is mixed with respect to attributable morbidity and mortality from diabetes mellitus. Mackenzie and Charlson found that complications were rare (4% incidence) in patients who did not already have end-organ dysfunction from their diabetes,[75] and a retrospective case-control study in cardiac surgical patients found no differences in the rates of MI, renal failure, neurological sequelae, leg infections, or thromboembolic events.[76] However, Pomposelli et al. found a relationship between perioperative glucose control and the incidence of postoperative nosocomial infection rates in a prospective study of patients undergoing elective surgery.[77] One hundred consecutive patients were stratified into groups with "poor" (any blood glucose value > 220 mg/dl) and "good" (all values <220 mg/dl) glucose management. Poor glucose control on the first postoperative day was sensitive (87.5%) but not specific (33.3%) as a predictor of later nosocomial infection. Patients with hyperglycemia on postoperative day 1 were 2.7 times more likely to develop any infection (31% vs. 12%) and 5.7 times more likely to develop nonurinary tract infections. Only 18% of the variance could be explained by differences in severity of illness.

Anesthesia induces many of the perioperative changes in carbohydrate metabolism.[78] Serial intravenous glucose tolerance tests during prolonged sevoflurane anesthesia show deranged carbohydrate metabolism within 35 min of the induction of anesthesia, characterized by a depressed disappearance rate for glucose and diminished maximum insulin responsiveness.[79] These effects were accentuated when reexamined at the 6-h period. In another study, insulin resistance was evaluated after elective upper abdominal surgery of moderate severity using a euglycemic insulin clamp technique.[80] Patients were randomized to receive either general anesthesia followed by parenteral opioids or epidural anesthesia followed by epidural opioids. Paired insulin clamp studies were performed preoperatively. Glucose disappearance was depressed on postoperative day 1 in both groups, but the response was attenuated in the epidural catheter group.

Several characteristics of cardiopulmonary bypass in diabetic patients deserve mention. Infusion of a glucose-insulin-potassium solution during surgery may stabilize myocardial metabolism and improve myocardial function.[81] In a randomized study conducted 6 h after coronary artery bypass grafting[82] of patients who received an insulin (7.1 U/kg) plus dopamine (7 mg/kg/min) infusion, cardiac output was increased significantly more by the insulin–dopamine combination, whereas heart rate and myocardial oxygen consumption remained equivalent. This effect may be caused by reduced left ventricular afterload because insulin is known to have a vasodilatory effect that persists for several hours postoperatively after intravenous administration during cardiopulmonary bypass.[83] This effect may result in improved lower-extremity perfusion, but glucose uptake into both skeletal muscle and myocardium is enhanced.[84]

Diabetic Ketoacidosis

Insulin deficiency and a synergistic increase in "stress" hormone (i.e., epinephrine, cortisol, glucagon) secretion produce a volume-depleted, acidemic, hyperglycemic, and ketonemic state with severe electrolyte abnormalities. Acutely decompensated type I diabetes mellitus is the most common underlying problem, and the cause of the destabilization is usually infection. Frequently, diabetic ketoacidosis (DKA) is the presenting manifestation of previously undiagnosed diabetes. Other precipitants may include pregnancy, acute MI, trauma, acute psychiatric illness, or major surgery. Endocrine precipitants include thyrotoxicosis and pheochromocytoma.

The massive hyperglycemia is caused primarily by accelerated gluconeogenesis in the face of reduced peripheral glucose utilization and catabolism of lean tissue and lipid stores. Serum hyperosmolarity precipitates an osmotic diuresis with subsequent volume depletion and paradoxical dilutional hyponatremia. Ketonemia results from the inability to metabolize mobilized long-chain fatty acids via lipogenic pathways. A high index of suspicion for DKA is indicated in patients with dehydration, vomiting, tachypnea, severe abdominal pain, obtundation, or a combination of those findings. Diagnostic criteria for DKA include blood glucose above 300 mg/dl, serum osmolarity above 340 mOsm/l, arterial pH below 7.30 with Pa_{CO_2} 40 mmHg or less, ketonemia, and ketonuria. The differential diagnosis includes lactic acidosis, uremia, various intoxicants (including ethanol), sepsis syndrome, cerebrovascular accident, and intraabdominal catastrophe. Patients with hyperosmolar nonketotic coma (HHNC; see following) by definition do not have ketonemia, although HHNC and DKA may coexist.

Effective treatment for DKA requires simultaneous metabolic management and a search for the precipitant. An ECG must always be obtained to rule out the "silent" MI typical of diabetic patients. Patients with DKA may have a volume deficit as great as 10 l, and therefore vigorous fluid replacement is essential. Hypotonic saline is the treatment of choice. In the first 30 min, 1 l is given, followed by 500 to 1000 ml/h. Shock or hyponatremia is an indication for isotonic saline. When the blood glucose decreases below 250 mg/dl, resuscitation continues with 5% dextrose in water (D_5W) to prevent hypoglycemia and cerebral edema. Central hemodynamic monitoring is used as indicated.

All patients in DKA require prompt insulin treatment. After a bolus dose of 10 to 30 U, a continuous infusion of short-acting (regular) insulin, 5 to 10 U/h, is effective and safe if monitored closely. Higher doses carry a greater risk of hypokalemia and hypoglycemia. If close monitoring of blood glucose shows that glucose has not decreased by 30% or more within 4 h or by at least 50% within 8 h, then the insulin dosage should be doubled. Once blood glucose decreases to 250 mg/dl, the continuous infusion is discontinued, and subcutaneous doses of short-acting insulin are substituted, provided the patient is no longer ketotic. Longer-acting insulin preparations should not be used until the patient's condition has stabilized and oral intake is possible.

Bicarbonate therapy in DKA is seldom necessary because metabolism of acetoacetate and β-hydroxybutyrate generate bicarbonate. Indications for bicarbonate therapy in DKA include arterial pH below 7.1 or HCO_3 concentration below 10 mEq/dl or relief of the discomfort of Kussmaul respirations. If indicated, then 100 to 150 mEq $NaHCO_3$ can be added to the first liter of saline. In contrast, potassium supplementation is invariably required. Ketonuria, diuresis, and frequent vomiting can produce marked potassium depletion, which may be masked initially as intracellular stores shift to the extracellular space in response to acidosis. Correction of acidosis will unmask marked hypokalemia. Potassium chloride, 20 to 40 mEq, is added to the second liter of resuscitation fluid and supplemented further as appropriate. If the patient is hypokalemic and acidemic at presentation, then potassium depletion is profound, and replacement (40–60 mEq/l) should begin with the first liter of resuscitation fluid.

Hyperglycemic Hyperosmolar Nonketotic Coma

Patients with HHNC present with very high blood glucose concentrations (sometimes >1000 mg/dl), depressed sensorium, marked dehydration, and prerenal azotemia. By definition, acidosis, ketonemia, and ketonuria are absent unless there is coexistent DKA. Precipitants include many stresses typical of the surgical patient, including burns, severe infections, pancreatitis, and major surgery. Mortality appears to be higher in cases associated with sepsis or pancreatitis. Therapy with β-blockers, diazoxide, furosemide, glucocorticoids, TPN, or thiazides may precipitate HHNC, as may renal replacement therapy.

Diabetic ketoacidosis and HHNC share two similarities: relative insulin deficiency and marked volume depletion. The diagnosis of HHNC should be suspected in the setting of marked hyperglycemia (>700 mg/dl) and azotemia without ketonemia. The serum sodium concentration may be factitiously normal in the setting of elevated blood glucose (decreased 3 mEq/dl per 100 mg glucose elevation). Ketosis is absent because sufficient insulin is present to suppress lipolysis. Hyperglycemia itself suppresses lipolysis, and the stress hormone response in HHNC is modest compared to that in DKA. Changes in mental status can be related directly to the degree of hyperosmolarity. Neurological abnormalities include lethargy, focal or generalized seizures, or coma.

As with DKA, therapy consists of rehydration, intravenous insulin, electrolyte replacement, and correction of the precipitant. Isotonic saline is the fluid of choice except for the hypernatremic patient. As much as 10 l may be required in the first 24 h. Potassium supplementation up to 20 mEq/h may be necessary. Fluid administration is then adjusted based on the response to resuscitation. Intravenous insulin is given as an infusion of 6–10 U/h until blood glucose is below 250 mg/dl, when a change is also made to dextrose-containing fluid to prevent hypoglycemia and cerebral edema.

Approach to the Febrile Surgical Patient

Fever is common in surgical patients. The list of potential causes of fever is long and includes many noninfectious etiologies (Table 17.16). Any fever in a surgical patient is a potential cause for concern. A tendency to equate fever with infection is understandable, but approximately one-half of febrile episodes in surgical patients are noninfectious in origin. Unfortunately, there are few comprehensive epidemiological studies of fever in surgical patients. The workup and therapy for the individual patient will vary depending on the patient's underlying diagnosis, clinical appearance, and the clinician's suspicion of infection. Current guidelines for the evaluation of fever in critically ill adults suggest that fever mandates a history and physical examination (Table 17.17).[85] Subsequent testing should be based on the findings of the clinical evaluation; in some instances, no further evaluation will be necessary.

What Constitutes a Fever?

The magnitude of temperature elevation necessary to constitute a fever may simply be the particular temperature at which the clinician believes that investigation is necessary, most commonly in the range of 38.0°C to 38.5°C. Elevated body temperature increases basal metabolic rate 7%–15%/°C, but aside from increased insensible fluid losses and some

TABLE 17.16. Noninfectious Causes of Fever of Importance in Surgical Patients.

Cardiovascular	Inflammatory
Myocardial infarction	Gout/pseudogout
Aortic dissection	Intramuscular injections
Pericarditis	Transplant rejection
	Vasculitis
Central nervous system disease	Endocrine/metabolic
Cavernous sinus thrombosis	Adrenal insufficiency
Hypothalamic dysfunction	Alcohol/drug withdrawal
Nonhemorrhagic infarction/stroke	Hyperthyroidism
Seizures	Miscellaneous
Subarachnoid hemorrhage	Allergic drug reaction
Traumatic brain injury	Drug fever
Gastroenterological	Tissue ischemia/infarction
Acalculous cholecystitis	Neoplastic
Gastrointestinal hemorrhage	Febrile neutropenia
Hepatitis (toxic/ischemic)	Metastatic disease
Inflammatory bowel disease	Primary tumors
Ischemic colitis	Pulmonary/airway
Pancreatitis (early)	Acute respiratory distress syndrome (fibroproliferative phase)
Hematological	Atelectasis
Venous thrombosis (superficial or deep)	Aspiration pneumonitis
Retroperitoneal/pelvic hemorrhage/hematoma	Pulmonary embolism/infarction
Transfusion reaction	

discomfort, fever is usually not the primary source of morbidity. Tachycardia or increased oxygen demand may make it desirable to suppress fever in select patients with coronary ischemia or critical acute respiratory failure. However, most adults without a neurologic diagnosis do not specifically require antipyresis unless temperature exceeds 40°C; in fact, to do so may be harmful because of the salutory effects of fever on host defenses (e.g., enhanced neutrophil function, suppressed bacterial growth). If antipyretic therapy is chosen, then cyclooxygenase (COX) inhibition is most effective, bearing in mind that deleterious effects on renal function and the gastric mucosa are possible with COX inhibitors. Topical cooling is generally ineffective (cutaneous vascoconstriction causes core retention of heat), although core cooling (e.g., iced fluid lavage of the stomach) can be effective.

The site where the temperature is determined may also influence the observed temperature value. The accepted standard for measuring an accurate core body temperature is the thermistor reading of a PA catheter, now seldom increasingly used. Rectal temperatures may be several tenths of a degree higher than the core temperature, and axillary values generally are lower and poorly reproducible. Infrared tympanic membrane devices have been popularized and do represent the core temperature, but there may be problems with reproducibility.

Noninfectious Causes of Fever

A nosocomial infection is a less likely cause of postoperative fever than a noninfectious cause in the first 72h after surgery. The problem of postoperative fever is a useful paradigm for consideration of the priorities in the workup. Perhaps more money is wasted in evaluation of early postoperative fever than in any other aspect of postoperative care. Although common, fever in the early postoperative period can be the result of a few things, provided pulmonary aspiration and gross breaks in surgical technique or for insertion of intravascular catheters are avoided.

The most common cause of early postoperative fever is atelectasis. If atelectasis is present, then pulmonary physiotherapy and early ambulation (if possible) should be undertaken immediately; cultures are generally not useful in the immediate postoperative period. It is unusual for a fresh postoperative patient to have been admitted with a community-acquired pneumonia, but the clinician must remain alert to the possibility. After the third postoperative day, nosocomial pneumonia is possible. In addition to atelectasis, aspiration pneumonitis (which is usually noninfectious), tissue ischemia or infarction, acute vasculitis, gout or pseudogout, intracerebral hemorrhage, retroperitoneal hematoma, pericarditis, and transfusion reactions can cause fever. There are several miscellaneous causes of fever that are not caused by infection. Withdrawal from alcohol, benzodiazepines, or opioids can all cause fever.

Endocrine emergencies, including acute adrenal insufficiency or thyroid storm, can be challenging to diagnose because they can be precipitated by infection. Adrenal insufficiency and thyrotoxicosis can create high fevers with a constellation of systemic signs. Two types of patients are at high risk for adrenal insufficiency: those with a history of corticosteroid use and those with an acute condition that ablates adrenal function. It is debatable whether stress can otherwise unmask latent adrenal insufficiency in previously asymptomatic patients. Both conditions are rare (thyrotoxicosis, especially) and therefore treacherous because the diagnosis can be overlooked. Patients with adrenal insufficiency present with variable degrees of temperature elevation, hypotension, hyponatremia, hyperkalemia, or hypoglycemia. Severe thyrotoxicosis or thyroid storm can cause fevers above 39.0°C with a variety of other systemic signs, including tachyarrhythmias; atrial fibrillation; diaphoresis; palpitations; CHF; gastrointestinal symptoms (abdominal pain, nausea, vomiting, and diarrhea); neurological symptoms (tremors, seizures, anxiety); and heat intolerance. Treatment is supportive and includes propranolol, fluids, iodine, and possibly antithyroidal agents such as methimazole or propylthiouracil.

TABLE 17.17.

Evidence-Based Practice Management Guideline for the Evaluation of Fever in Critically Ill Adult Patients.[a]

Temperature measurement	
Level I:	Record the temperature and the site of measurement in the patient's medical record.
	The nosocomial spread of pathogens must be avoided when using temperature measurement devices.
Level II:	Temperature is measured most accurately by indwelling vascular or bladder thermistors, but most other sites are acceptable. Axillary measurements should not be used.
	Laboratory testing for the evaluation of fever should be individualized for each patient.
Blood cultures	
Level I:	For skin preparation, povidone-iodine should be allowed to dry for 2 min or tincture of iodine for 30 s. Alcohol skin preparation, an acceptable alternative for iodine-allergic patients, need not be allowed to dry.
Level II:	Obtain a single pair of blood cultures after appropriate skin disinfection after the initial temperature elevation and another pair within 24 h thereafter from a second peripheral site. Additional cultures should be based on high clinical suspicion of bacteremia or fungemia and not instituted automatically for each temperature elevation.
	If two peripheral sites are not available, then one pair of cultures may be drawn through the most recently inserted catheter, but the diagnostic accuracy is reduced.
	Draw at least 10–15 ml blood/culture.
Suspected intravascular catheter infection	
Level II:	Examine the catheter insertion site for purulence and distally on the extremity for signs of vascular compromise or embolization.
	Any expressed purulence from an insertion site should be collected for culture and Gram stain.
	The catheter should be removed and cultured for evidence of a tunnel infection, embolic phenomena, vascular compromise, or sepsis.
	Two blood cultures should be drawn peripherally, or one may be drawn from the most proximal port (if a multilumen catheter).
	Both the introducer and the catheter itself should be cultured for suspected pulmonary artery catheter infection.
	It is not routinely necessary to culture the intravenous fluid infusate.
Suspected ICU-acquired pneumonia	
Level I:	A chest x-ray should be obtained to evaluate for suspected pneumonia. Posteroanterior and lateral films or computed tomography of the chest can offer more information.
Level II:	Lower respiratory tract secretions should be sampled for direct examination and culture. Bronchoscopy may be considered.
	Respiratory secretions should be transported to the laboratory within 2 h of collection.
	Pleural fluid should be obtained for culture and Gram stain if there is an adjacent infiltrate or another reason to suspect infection.
Evaluation of the febrile patient with diarrhea	
Level II:	If more than two diarrheal stools occur, then a single stool sample should be sent for *Clostridium difficile* evaluation. A second sample should be sent if the first is negative and suspicion remains high.
	If illness is severe and rapid testing is unavailable or nondiagnostic, then consider flexible sigmoidoscopy.
	If illness is severe, then consider empiric therapy with metronidazole until the results of studies are available. Empiric therapy (especially with vancomycin) is not recommended if two stool evaluations have been negative for *C. difficile* and is discouraged because of the risk of producing resistant pathogens.
	Stool cultures are rarely indicated for other enteric pathogens if the patient is HIV negative or did not present to the hospital with diarrhea.
Suspected urinary tract infection	
Level II:	Obtain urine for culture and to evaluate for pyuria. If the patient has an indwelling Foley catheter, urine should be collected from the urine port and not the drainage bag.
	The specimen should be transported rapidly to the laboratory or refrigerated if transport will exceed 1 h.
Suspected sinusitis	
Level I:	Aspirate should be Gram stained and cultured.
Level II:	Computed tomography of the facial sinuses is the imaging modality of choice for the diagnosis of sinusitis.
	Puncture and aspiration of the sinuses should be performed using sterile technique if mucosal thickening or an air–fluid level is present in the sinus.
Postoperative fever	
Level II:	Examine the surgical wound for erythema, fluctuance, tenderness, or purulent drainage.
	Open the wound for suspicion of infection.
	Culture and Gram stain should be obtained from purulent material if from deep within the wound.
Suspected central nervous system infection	
Level II:	Gram stain and culture of cerebrospinal fluid should be performed in cases of suspected infection. Other tests should be predicated on the clinical situation.
	A computed tomographic study is usually required before lumbar puncture, which may need to be deferred if a mass lesion is present.
	Consider lumbar puncture for new fever with unexplained alteration of consciousness or focal neurological signs.
	In febrile patients with an intracranial device, cerebrospinal fluid should be sent for culture and Gram stain.
Noninfectious causes of fever	
Level II	Reevaluate all recent medications and blood products the patient has received.
	Stop all nonessential medications or substitute medications for treatments that cannot be stopped.

[a]Summary of clinical recommendations, Society of Critical Care Medicine, 1998; level III guidelines excluded.

Source: Adapted from O'Grady et al.[85]

Drug Fever

Fever coincident with administration of a drug that disappears after discontinuance, when no other cause of fever is apparent, characterizes the disorder. The diagnosis is therefore one of exclusion, and skepticism is always in order lest another treatable cause of fever is overlooked. True drug-related fever probably accounts for no more than 2% to 3% of episodes of fever in hospitalized patients. Most are hypersensitivity reactions; therefore, malignant hyperthermia and the neuroleptic malignant syndrome (NMS; see following) are generally not classified as drug fever. Other potential mechanisms associated with drug administration include chemical phlebitis or sterile abscesses, pyrogenic contaminants, or generation of endogenous pyrogens. Some drugs, notably thyroxine, atropine, and epinephrine, may affect thermoregulation directly. Most classes of drugs require long latent administration periods, but antibiotics, phenytoin, and antineoplastic agents are capable of producing fever within a few days. As a group, antimicrobial agents are the most common cause of fever. Penicillins, cephalosporins, tetracyclines, and vancomycin are commonly prescribed culprits. Fever usually abates within 72h of discontinuance of the offending drug unless its half-life is prolonged (e.g., phenytoin), so additional therapy is usually unwarranted.

Hyperthermia occurs when heat production exceeds heat loss in the presence of a normal set point. Work or exercise in hot environments may precipitate hyperthermia (heat stroke), as may an inability to dissipate heat (such as in a high-humidity environment where evaporation cannot occur). In some patients, set-point temperature is increased by trauma, hemorrhage, or tumors of the hypothalamus. However, such "central" or "hypothalamic" fevers are unusual, except in neurosurgical patients.

Malignant hyperthermia syndrome can occur when certain anesthetics and adjuncts (e.g., succinylcholine, volatile hydrocarbons) produce in susceptible patients a rapid uncoupling of oxidative phosphorylation, which is often fatal (30%–70% mortality). Rare causes of malignant hyperthermia include anoxia, lymphoma, and viral infections. Most cases occur in the operating room but may develop up to 24h after the offending agent has been given. Patients are predisposed genetically to this disorder, which can be suspected by a family history of anesthesia complications and confirmed by genetic testing. Medication for both prophylaxis and the overt syndrome includes the administration of freshly prepared dantrolene (1–2mg/kg every 10min) along with supportive care. Malignant hyperthermia usually does not respond to antipyretic therapy.

Another form of hyperthermia, NMS, occurs in patients taking neuroleptic drugs, typically phenothiazines or butyrophenones, although metoclopramide therapy has been implicated. All such drugs decrease hypothalamic dopaminergic tone. Despite the different etiology, both malignant hyperthermia and NMS present with similar symptoms and have similar therapies, except that the magnitude of the core temperature response is somewhat lower, and signs of muscle damage (e.g., tenderness, immobility, and elevated serum creatinine phosphokinase) are absent in NMS.

Hematologic Causes of Fever

Several hematologic causes of fever exist (see Table 17.16). One of the most common causes of fever in the inpatient setting is a transfusion reaction. Passenger leukocytes are the chief cause of alloimmunization to leukocyte-specific antigens in transfusion recipients. Alloimmunization may result in febrile transfusion reactions, platelet refractoriness, or acute lung injury.[86] Leukocytes are also the vector for transfusion-associated cytomegalovirus infection. Technological advances have made it possible to reduce the number of leukocytes to fewer than 10^7 per transfusion. The use of leukocyte-reduced cellular blood components may minimize or prevent recurrent febrile reactions and alloimmunizations to leukocyte antigens and minimize the risk of cytomegalovirus transmission (see Table 17.12), but the data are mixed. The presence of a coexisting hematologic dyscrasia may also increase the likelihood of a transfusion reaction. Almost any neoplasm itself may manifest fever. The postchemotherapeutic state may lead to the *tumor lysis syndrome,* which is a common source of fever in hospitalized cancer patients. Febrile neutropenia is common on oncology wards and bone marrow transplant units, and the initiation of therapy with any of the colony-stimulating factors or cytokines (e.g., interleukin-2 therapy) may also cause fever.

Almost any intracranial pathology can lead to centrally mediated fevers. Any traumatic or infectious condition of the brain can stimulate a hyperpyrexic response, but most common is subarachnoid hemorrhage. In actuality, a blood clot anywhere in the body can cause fever. Hematomas can occur in the soft tissue from trauma or in the retroperitoneum or abdominal wall spontaneously in the anticoagulated patient. A clot in the vasculature may be either an arterial or a venous thrombosis. Suspicion of deep venous thrombosis and pulmonary embolism must be high because these problems are often occult. High fever can certainly be caused by uncomplicated superficial phlebitis of a subcutaneous vein of an extremity. Fine-needle aspiration with Gram stain and culture may be necessary to exclude suppuration. Uncomplicated superficial phlebitis responds promptly to warm soaks, elevation, and ibuprofen (if not contraindicated), but the vein must be explored and excised to bleeding tissue for suppurative phlebitis. For lower-extremity deep venous thrombosis, the diagnostic approach includes lower extremity duplex ultrasound studies or, in some institutions, magnetic resonance imaging of the pelvic veins.[87] Although ICU patients are at high risk for venous thromboembolism, routine screening does not appear to be cost-effective. Many authorities believe that helical CT has now supplanted venography/pulmonary angiography for the diagnosis of venous thromboembolism.[88]

If a central catheter-related venous thrombosis occurs, then the therapy includes the removal of the catheter and the possible institution of anticoagulant or thrombolytic therapy. If thrombolysis is chosen, then it must be accomplished before the catheter is removed to avoid the possibility of hemorrhage. With arterial thrombosis, it is often the resulting tissue ischemia that causes fever.

Infectious Causes of Fever: Nosocomial Infection

Many emergency operations are performed for control of an infection. Even under optimal circumstances (definitive surgical source control, timely administration of appropriate broad-spectrum antibiotics), it may take 72h or more for the patient to defervesce. New or persistent fever more than 3 days after surgery should raise a strong suspicion of persistent illness or a new complication.

Device-Related Infections, Catheter-Related Infections, and Ventilator-Associated Pneumonia

Health care-associated (nosocomial) infections are potentially devastating complications. Therefore, every effort must be made to prevent them (Table 17.18).[89,90] Nosocomial infections often arise in association with indwelling devices, such as intravascular catheters, endotracheal or tracheostomy tubes, or other devices that breach or degrade a natural epithelial barrier to infection.[91]

The patients most at risk for pneumonia are those who require prolonged mechanical ventilation (ventilator-associated pneumonia, VAP). Pneumonia is a particular problem for surgical patients, with cardiothoracic, neurosurgical, and trauma patients and those who have undergone major head and neck or gastrointestinal operations at high risk (Table 17.19). Although the presence of (1) purulent sputum, (2) fever, (3) leukocytosis, and (4) a new or changed radiographic infiltrate (i.e., the definition of the U.S. Centers for Disease Control and Prevention) may suggest pneumonia, only about 40% of patients with these four typical findings are found to have pneumonia when evaluated with a consistent and systematic protocol that includes noncontaminated sputum collection[92] and microbiology. Bronchoalveolar lavage or protected specimen-brush sampling increases the specificity and therefore the accuracy of the diagnosis of pneumonia.[93]

TABLE 17.19. Device-Related Nosocomial Infection Rates 1992–1998.[a]

	Type of infection		
Type of ICU	*Urinary catheter*	*Central line bacteremia*	*Ventilator-associated pneumonia*
Burn	10.0 (N/A)	12.8 (N/A)	21.1 (N/A)
Cardiothoracic	3.3 (2.1)	2.8 (1.8)	11.7 (11.3)
Medical	7.8 (7.0)	6.1 (5.3)	8.5 (7.6)
Neurosurgical	8.5 (7.8)	5.4 (4.4)	17.3 (13.8)
Surgical	5.7 (4.9)	5.7 (4.9)	14.9 (12.7)
Trauma	7.9 (N/A)	7.0 (N/A)	17.0 (N/A)

N/A, not available.

Data are expressed as mean (median), and as Number of occurrences/Number of patient-days with device indwelling x 1000.

[a]National Nosocomial Infection Surveillance System, Centers for Disease Control and Prevention. Data are available in the public domain at www.cdc.gov/ncidod/hip/nnis/sar98net.pdf.

TABLE 17.18.
Summary of Evidence-Based Clinical Guidelines for the Prevention of Nosocomial Bacterial Pneumonia.[a]

Surveillance

Level I: Conduct surveillance of bacterial pneumonia among ICU patients at high risk.
Routine surveillance cultures of patients, equipment, or devices is unnecessary.

Interrupting person-to-person transmission of bacteria

Level I: Regardless of whether gloves are worn, wash hands after contact with mucous membranes, respiratory secretions, or objects contaminated with respiratory secretions.
Regardless of whether gloves are worn, wash hands both before and after contact with a patient who has an endotracheal or tracheostomy tube in place, or for handling respiratory secretions.
Change gloves and wash hands after handling respiratory secretions or objects before contact with another patient, object, or environmental surface.
Change gloves and wash hands between contacts with a contaminated body site and the respiratory tract or device on the same patient.

Level II: Use aseptic techniques when changing a tracheostomy tube.

Modifying host risk for infection

Level I: Do not routinely administer systemic antimicrobial agents to prevent nosocomial pneumonia.

Level II: Discontinue enteral tube feeding and remove devices as soon as the clinical indications are resolved.
If not contraindicated, elevate the head at an angle of 30°–45° of the bed of a patient at high risk for aspiration.
Routinely assess the patient's intestinal motility and adjust the rate and volume of enteral feeding to avoid regurgitation.
Before deflating the cuff of an endotracheal tube, ensure that secretions are cleared from above the tube cuff.
Instruct preoperative patients, especially those at high risk for contracting pneumonia, regarding frequent coughing, taking deep breaths, and ambulating.
Encourage postoperative patients to cough frequently, take deep breaths, move about the bed, and ambulate unless medically contraindicated.
Control pain that interferes with coughing and deep breathing during the immediate postoperative period.

Source: Adapted from Centers for Disease Control and Prevention.[90]

Any oropharyngeal or nasopharyngeal apparatus can promote the development of sinusitis.[91] Patients with maxillofacial or skull fractures, traumatic brain injury, or nasotracheal intubation are at high risk. The optimal diagnostic test for sinusitis is a CT scan with thin cuts of the facial bones, followed by sinus aspiration and lavage for culture of any patient with mucosal thickening or an air–fluid level. Although the diagnostic yield is low and the evaluation is laborious, the incidence of sinusitis is increasing. For prevention and treatment, early removal of transpharyngeal devices is important, especially nasotracheal tubes, which are associated with sinusitis approximately one-third of the time after nasotracheal intubation.[89]

Peripheral or central venous catheters may become infected and then cause a bloodstream infection. The complication is serious but largely preventable with rigid adherence to infection control practice and meticulous technique for catheter insertion and maintenance. Central venous catheters impregnated with antimicrobial agents may decrease the risk of infection in high-incidence units.[94]

Urinary tract infection is commonplace because of the ubiquitous use of urinary catheters but is seldom destabilizing. Nosocomial upper urinary tract infections are rare in nonneurological patients. Most of these infections are caused by instrumentation of the urinary bladder. The duration of catheterization is the most important risk factor for the development of nosocomial bacterial cystitis. Most episodes of bacteriuria are asymptomatic, but symptoms, including fever and leukocytosis, can develop in 10% to 30% of patients. The indications for catheterization should be reviewed daily. The best prevention and therapy is removal of the catheter at the earliest opportunity. The closed drainage system should be handled as little as possible and only with meticulous attention to good infection control practice.

Nosocomial Infections Not Related to Devices

Surgical site infection (SSI) or infection of a traumatic wound is rare in the first few days after operation because effective methods of prevention are recognized. The only important exceptions to this rule are the development of erysipelas, a necrotizing soft tissue infection caused by pyogenic streptococci, and clostridial fasciitis or myonecrosis. Thus, it is important to take down the surgical dressing to inspect the incision for a fever in the early postoperative period, but the diagnosis of these serious infections can be made by inspection alone, and such patients are usually "toxic" appearing. Crush injury syndrome and tetanus are two rare complications of traumatic wounds that may cause fever. Other SSIs, either of the incision or intracavitary for surgery of the torso, generally manifest themselves after the fourth postoperative day in the absence of a gross break in technique.

Antibiotic-Associated Colitis

One complication to which every surgical patient who receives antibiotics is potentially subject is AAC. The most distinguishable of these syndromes, *Clostridium difficile*-associated disease (CDAD), results from overgrowth and toxin production after antibiotic use, even a single dose of a cephalosporin used appropriately for surgical incision prophylaxis. Practically every antibiotic has been implicated in the pathogenesis. The symptoms are nonspecific because the spectrum of disease is broad, ranging from asymptomatic disease to fulminant colonic ischemia. The proportion of severe cases is increasing because of a mutation of a suppressor gene for toxin production.[95–97] The diagnosis of AAC usually depends on isolation of exotoxin A or B from a fresh stool sample. Sigmoidoscopic visualization of colonic pseudomembranes may assist in the diagnosis when the exotoxins are not detected, but the pseudomembranes are present less than 50% of the time, and endoscopy is therefore seldom performed.

Treatment for AAC includes supportive care, the exclusion of peritonitis or an indication for laparotomy, and metronidazole (intravenous or oral), which is comparable to oral vancomycin at about 80% effectiveness, even for clinically severe cases. Oral vancomycin can be used for patients who are intolerant of metronidazole or who fail therapy with metronidazole, but vancomycin use is discouraged for infection control reasons. Vancomycin can be administered by gavage or enema if necessary because intravenous vancomycin is ineffective. Increasingly, severe cases require a total abdominal colectomy for cure, with attendant operative mortality of up to 50%.[97]

Acute Acalculous Cholecystitis

Acute acalculous cholecystitis (AAC) may complicate surgery or critical illness or injury.[65] Diabetes mellitus, abdominal vasculitis, CHF, cholesterol embolization, and resuscitation from major trauma or burns, hemorrhagic shock, or cardiac arrest have been associated with AAC. The unifying theme is that the pathogenesis of AAC is ischemia–reperfusion injury of the gallbadder.

The diagnosis of AAC can be difficult to make. These patients almost invariably are jaundiced and often unable to communicate. The differential diagnosis of jaundice in the critically ill patient is complex, including intrahepatic cholestasis from sepsis or drug toxicity and "fatty liver" induced by TPN, in addition to cholecystitis. The diagnosis of ACC should be considered in every critically ill or injured patient with a clinical picture of sepsis and no other obvious source. Fever is generally present, but other physical findings are less reliable. Leukocytosis and hyperbilirubinemia are nonspecific, and biochemical assays of hepatic enzymes are of little help. The diagnosis of ACC thus often rests on radiologic studies. Ultrasound of the gallbladder is the preferred modality to diagnose ACC because of low cost and the ability to image the patient at the bedside. Thickening of the gallbladder wall of 3.5 mm or more is the most accurate criterion. Radionuclide hepatobiliary imaging is unreliable in critically ill or injured patients because of false-positive scans due to fasting, alcoholism or other forms of liver disease, or TPN feeding. Computed tomography is as accurate as ultrasound in the diagnosis of ACC, and the diagnostic criteria for ACC are similar.

The mainstay of therapy for ACC is percutaneous cholecystectomy.[65] The advantages of percutaneous cholecystostomy are bedside applicability, local anesthesia, and avoidance of an open procedure. The technique controls the acute syndrome in about 85% of patients.

Diagnostic Approach to Fever

The likelihood of infection as a cause and the potential for destabilization of a tenuous patient create a sense of urgency surrounding the workup of many febrile episodes. However, some fevers are not destabilizing and do not require either workup or treatment. An individual approach is essential, both for evaluation and for therapy. Unlikely diagnoses should not be pursued initially until more common problems have been considered and excluded. However, it is costly as well as nonbeneficial to make diagnoses that are unlikely to have an important effect on the patient's overall diagnosis or treatment.

Two major problems to resolve are distinguishing sterile systemic inflammation from systemic infection and distinguishing bacterial colonization from tissue invasion. Many patients with sterile inflammation (e.g., early pancreatitis, major trauma, burns) develop an inflammatory host response characterized by elaboration of the very cytokines implicated in the febrile response. The picture may be indistinguishable from clinical infection. The distinction is crucial because these patients are at high risk to develop antibiotic-resistant infections if unnecessary antibiotics are administered.[98]

A careful history and physical examination should direct further diagnostic tests, recognizing that individual tests may yield equivocal or even misleading results. Severe sepsis can occur with a normal or even low white blood cell (WBC) count. A very low WBC count from transient bone marrow suppression in a nonimmunocompromised patient may be highly suggestive of sepsis. Also, any stressed state such as the postoperative or posttraumatic state can cause leukocytosis via epinephrine- and cortisol-mediated demargination, as can administration of either as a drug in the absence of infection.

Other diagnostic tests may be helpful in certain patients. The most commonly ordered initial tests are cultures of blood, sputum, and urine, although the yield of blood cultures is low in the early postoperative period (<72 h) and in patients already on broad-spectrum antibiotics.[99] Other possible culture sites include stool (the yield is extremely low in surgical patients), cerebrospinal fluid (central nervous system infection is rare except in neurosurgical patients), sinus fluid, or vascular catheters and depends on the individual patient's circumstances. Importantly, after positive cultures are reported, the astute clinician must determine whether the culture represents infection that may require treatment or colonization that does not require specific therapy.

The most commonly performed imaging study to evaluate fever is chest radiography. However, a CT scan can often be helpful, especially after abdominal surgery. Because of the earlier presence of various nonspecific changes, the best yield for CT scan for suspected intraabdominal abscess is for scans obtained at least 7 days after operation. Chest CT scans may be useful in some patients to help rule out an empyema or to rule out pneumonia in a patient with ARDS (itself an increasingly recognized noninfectious cause of fever) or to exclude venous thromboembolic disease.

Empiric Antibiotic Therapy

The decision to administer empiric antibiotic therapy is not considered with sufficient care in many circumstances. The result is that many courses of antibiotic therapy are inappropriate because infection is not present, therapy is delayed, the chosen drug is not effective against the likely pathogens, or the duration of treatment is too long.

Several questions are worth asking each time empiric antibiotic therapy is considered. First, are antibiotics indicated at all? The answer is ultimately often no, but the decision to start treatment must often be made before definitive information becomes available if the patient is unstable. In the absence of definitive data, the decision to start antibiotics is based on the likelihood of infection, its likely source and the likely pathogens, and whether the patient's condition is sufficiently precarious that a delay will be detrimental. Outcome is improved if antibiotics are started promptly, but on the other hand, only about 50% of fever episodes in hospitalized patients are caused by infection. Many causes of the systemic inflammatory response syndrome (SIRS) (e.g., aspiration pneumonitis, burns, trauma, pancreatitis) are not due to infection, although they may be complicated later by infection. Multiple-organ dysfunction syndrome may progress as the result of a dysregulated host response even after an infectious precipitant has been controlled.

Must antibiotics be started immediately? If the patient is stable hemodynamically, then the decision also depends on the overall status of the patient, considering such host factors as age, debility, renal and hepatic function, and immunosuppression. Culture yields are highest when collected before antibiotics are administered. However, for many infections (e.g., bacteremia, intraabdominal infection, pneumonia), data indicate that early therapy with an appropriate antibiotic in adequate dosage improves outcome.

Which organisms are the likely pathogens, and are they likely to be antibiotic resistant? This assessment requires rapid formulation of the differential diagnosis, for which there may not be time to perform diagnostic testing other than blood testing and obtaining specimens for culture. The clinical setting must be considered (e.g., nosocomial vs. community-acquired infection, recent antimicrobial therapy), as must the patient's environment (e.g., proximity to other infected patients, the presence of resistant organisms in the unit) and any recent microbiology obtained from the patient.

Will a single antimicrobial agent suffice? This answer depends on the answers to the questions regarding the likely diagnosis and the nature of the probable pathogens. Under certain circumstances, it is desirable to use more than one antibiotic to treat an infection. This approach is most common with empiric therapy, for which the pathogen (or even the source of the infection) is assumed (or guessed at) and the potentialities are so broad and the consequences of inaccurate initial therapy so deleterious that more than one drug must be chosen. Two-drug empiric therapy is commonplace for presumed polymicrobial infections such as nosocomial pneumonia or recurrent or persistent intraabdominal infection or for sepsis of unknown origin. If there is reason to suspect a nosocomial gram-positive pathogen (e.g., SSI, catheter-related infection, infection of an implanted prosthetic device, pneumonia) and methicillin-resistant staphylococci are endemic, then empiric vancomycin is appropriate. Serious *Pseudomonas* infections may require dual-agent therapy with agents that act in a dissimilar manner (e.g., an antipseudomonal β-lactam drug to disrupt the bacterial cell wall along with an aminoglycoside to disrupt protein synthesis). Infections that involve anaerobic pathogens are usually mixed anaerobic–aerobic infections, the only common exceptions being community-acquired aspiration pneumonia and clostridial soft tissue infections. Nosocomial mixed anaerobic infections can be treated effectively by a single agent if a β-lactam/β-lactamase inhibitor combination drug or a carbapenem is chosen; for community-acquired infections, a second-generation cephalosporin may be appropriate, whereas carbapenem therapy is not. If the aerobic component is treated with a fluoroquinolone, monobactam, or a late-generation cephalosporin, then metronidazole is the preferred antianaerobic agent. Whatever is chosen, it is recommended strongly that triple-antibiotic regimens (e.g., ampicillin *or* vancomycin *plus* gram-negative coverage *plus* metronidazole) should be avoided because administration costs are high, and there is no added benefit.

Duration of Therapy

The endpoint of antibiotic therapy is difficult to define. Unfortunately, duration of therapy is not well established in the literature, and new studies are seldom designed with duration of therapy as a primary endpoint. Much depends on expertise and clinical judgment, which is accumulating in favor of shorter courses of therapy. If bona fide evidence of infection is evident, then treatment is continued as indicated clinically. Careful culture techniques and specimen handling, combined with modern microbiology laboratory support, make it unlikely that substantive pathogens will be missed. Therefore, continuing empiric antibiotic therapy beyond 48 h becomes difficult to justify. There are two possible exceptions. One occurs when fungal infection is suspected because the organisms can be difficult to culture, and the other occurs when deep cultures are needed from areas that are inaccessible until a drainage procedure is performed.

There is a clear trend toward shorter courses of antibiotics for established infections. Many infections can be treated with therapy lasting 5 days or less. Infections that require 24 h of therapy or less (sometimes just a single dose) include uncomplicated acute appendicitis or cholecystitis, uncomplicated bacterial cystitis (with some agents), and intestinal infarction without perforation. Most cases of intraabdominal infection require no more than 5 days of treatment. Every decision to start antibiotics must be accompanied by a decision regarding the duration of therapy. A reason to continue therapy beyond the predetermined endpoint must be compelling. Bacterial killing is rapid in response to effective agents, but the host response may not subside immediately. Therefore, the clinical response of the patient should not be the sole determinant for continuation of therapy. If a patient still has sepsis syndrome at the end of a defined course of therapy, then it is more useful to stop therapy and obtain a new set of cultures to look for new sites of infection, resistant pathogens, and noninfectious causes of inflammation. There is seldom justification to continue antibacterial therapy for more than 10 days. Examples of bacterial infections that require more than 14 days of therapy include tuberculosis of any site, endocarditis, osteomyelitis, brain abscess, liver abscess, lung abscess, postoperative meningitis, and endophthalmitis.

Among the many reasons to limit therapy is that antibiotic therapy has adverse consequences. Adverse consequences of antibiotics include allergic reactions; development of nosocomial superinfections, including fungal infections, enterococcal infections, and CDAD; organ toxicity; promotion of antibiotic resistance; reduced yield from subsequent cultures; and vitamin K deficiency. The worldwide emergence of multidrug-resistant bacteria, superinfections in immunosuppressed patients, and the increased mortality associated with nosocomial infections in general make it important that adequate therapy is provided rapidly and for the shortest possible duration.

References

1. Rao PM, Rhea JT, Novelline RA, et al. Effect of computed tomography of the appendix on treatment of patients and use of hospital resources. N Engl J Med 1998;338:141–146.
2. Miller W, Riehl E, Napier M, et al. Use of physician assistants as surgery/trauma housestaff at an American College of Surgeons-verified level II trauma center. J Trauma 1998;44:372–376.
3. Ghorra S, Reinert SE, Cioffi W, et al. Analysis of the effect of conversion from open to closed surgical invensive care unit. Ann Surg 1999;229:163–171.
4. Trunkey DD. An unacceptable concept. Ann Surg 1999;229:172–173.
5. Barie PS, Hydo LJ. Learning to not know: results of a program for ancillary cost reduction in surgical critical care. J Trauma 1996;41:714–720.
6. Barie PS, Hydo LJ. Lessons learned: durability and progress of a program for ancillary cost reduction in surgical critical care. J Trauma 1997;43:590–596.
7. Knaus WA, Draper EA, Wagner DP, Zimmerman JE. An evaluation of outcome from intensive care in major medical centers. Ann Intern Med 1986;104:410–418.
8. Daley J, Forbes MG, Young GJ, et al. Validating risk-adjusted surgical outcomes: site visit assessment of process and structure. J Am Coll Surg 1997;185:341–351.
9. Hanson CW III, Deutschman CS, Anderson HL III, et al. Effects of an organized critical care service on outcomes and resource utilization: a cohort study. Crit Care Med 1999;27:270–274.
10. Pronovost PJ, Jenckes MW, Durman T, et al. Organizational characteristics of intensive care units related to outcomes of abdominal aortic surgery. JAMA 1999;281:1310–1317.
11. Gordon TA, Burleyson GP, Tielsch JM, Cameron JL. The effects of regionalization on cost and outcome for one general high-risk surgical procedure. Ann Surg 1995;221:43–49.
12. Glasgow RE, Showstack JA, Katz PP, et al. The relationship between hospital volume and outcomes of hepatic resection for hepatocellular carcinoma. Arch Surg 1999;134:30–35.
13. Kenny SE, Shankar KR, Rintala R, et al. Evidence-based surgery: interventions in a regional paediatric surgical unit. Arch Dis Child 1997;76:50–53.
14. Sugerman HJ, Wolfe L, Pasquale MD, et al. Multicenter, randomized, prospective trial of early tracheostomy. J Trauma 1997;43:741–747.
15. Solomon MJ, McLeod RS. Should we be performing more randomized controlled trials evaluating surgical operations? Surgery 1995;118:459–467.
16. Romano PS, Roos LL, Luft HS, et al. A comparison of administrative versus clinical data: coronary artery bypass surgery as an example. Ischemic Heart Disease Patient Outcomes Research Team. J Clin Epidemiol 1994;47:249–260.
17. Egger M, Snith GD, Phillips AN. Meta-analysis: principles and procedures. Br Med J 1997;315:1533–1537.
18. Moher D, Pham B, Jones A, et al. Does quality of reports of randomised trials affect estimates of intervention efficacy reported in meta-analyses? Lancet 1998;352:609–613.
19. Cook DJ, Reeve BK, Guyatt GH, et al. Stress ulcer prophylaxis in critically ill patients: resolving discordant meta-analyses. JAMA 1996;275:308–314.
20. Hardy RJ, Thompson SG. Detecting and describing heterogeneity in meta-analysis. Stat Med 1998;17:841–856.
21. Davey Smith G, Egger M. Meta-analysis. Unresolved issues and future developments. Br Med J 1998;316:221–225.
22. Flather MD, Farkouh ME, Pogue JM, Yusuf S. Strengths and limitations of meta-analysis: larger studies may be more reliable. Controlled Clin Trials 1997;18:568–579.
23. Blumenthal D. Quality of health care. Part 1. Quality of care—what is it? N Engl J Med 1996;335:891–894.
24. Brook RH, Cleary PD. Quality of health care. Part 2. Measuring quality of care. N Engl J Med 1996;335:966–970.
25. Brennan TA, Leape LL, Laird NM, et al. Incidence of adverse events and negligence in hospitalized patients: results of the Harvard Medical Practice Study. II. N Engl J Med 1991;324:377–384.
26. Leape LL, Brennan TA, Laird NM, et al. Incidence of adverse events and negligence in hospitalized patients: results of the Harvard Medical Practice Study. N Engl J Med 1991;324:370–376.
27. Andrews LB, Stocking C, Krizek T, et al. An alternative strategy for studying adverse events in medical care. Lancet 1997;349:309–313.
28. Bates DW, Leape LL, Petrycki S. Incidence and preventability of adverse drug events and potential adverse drug events: Implications for prevention. JAMA 1995;274:29–34.
29. Leape LL. Error in medicine. JAMA 1994;272:1851–1857.
30. Velanovich V. Using quality-of-life instruments to assess surgical outcomes. Surgery 1999;126:1–4.

31. Fitzpatrick R, Fletcher A, Gore S, et al. Quality-of-life measures in healthcare. Applications and issues in assessment. Br Med J 1992;305:1074–1077.
32. Gill TM, Feinstein AR. A critical appraisal of quality of life measurements. JAMA 1994;272:619–626.
33. Fletcher A, Gore S, Jones O, et al. Quality of life measures in healthcare. II. Design, analysis, and interpretation. Br Med J 1992;305:1145–1148.
34. Goldman L. Cardiac risk for vascular surgery. J Am Coll Cardiol 1996;27:799–802.
35. Mangano DT, Layug EL, Wallace A, Tateo I. Effect of atenolol on mortality and cardiovascular morbidity after noncardiac surgery. Multicenter Study of Perioperative Ischemia Research Group. N Engl J Med 1996;335:1713–1720.
36. Poldermans D, Boersma E, Bax JJ, et al. The effect of bisoprolol on perioperative mortality and myocardial infarction in high-risk patients undergoing vascular surgery. N Engl J Med 1999; 341:1789–1794.
37. Charlson ME, MacKenzie CR, Gold JP, et al. Risk for postoperative congestive heart failure. Surg Gynecol Obstet 1991; 172:95–104.
38. Goldman L, Caldera DL, Nussbaum SR, et al. Multifactorial index of cardiac risk in noncardiac surgical procedures. N Engl J Med 1977;297:845–850.
39. Eagle KA, Brundage BH, Chaitman BR, et al. Guidelines for perioperative cardiovascular evaluation for noncardiac surgery. Report of the American College of Cardiology/American Heart Association Task Force on Practice Guidelines (Committee on Perioperative Cardiovascular Evaluation for Noncardiac Surgery). J Am Coll Cardiol 1996;27:910–948.
40. Fleischmann KE, Hunink MG, Kuntz KM, Douglas PS. Exercise echocardiography or exercise SPECT imaging? A meta-analysis of diagnostic test performance. JAMA 1998;280:913–920.
41. Mangano DT, Hollenberg M, Fegert G, et al. Perioperative myocardial ischemia in patients undergoing noncardiac surgery. I. Incidence and severity during the 4 day perioperative period. The Study of Perioperative Ischemia (SPI) Research Group. J Am Coll Cardiol 1991;17:843–850.
42. Smetana GW, Lawrence VA, Cornell JE. Preoperative pulmonary risk statification for noncardiothoracic surgery: systematic review for the American College of Physicians. Ann Intern Med 2006;144:581–595.
43. Lawrence VA, Cornell JE, Smetana GW. Strategies to reduce postoperative pulmonary complications after noncardiothoracic surgery: systematic review for the American College of Physicians. Ann Intern Med 2006;144:596–608.
44. Clagett GP, Anderson FA Jr, Geerts W, et al. Prevention of venous thromboembolism. Chest 1998;114(suppl 5):531S–560S.
45. Palmer AJ, Schramm W, Kirchhof B, Bergemann R. Low molecular weight heparin and unfractionated heparin for prevention of thrombo-embolism in general surgery: a meta-analysis of randomised clinical trials. Haemostasis 1997;27:65–74.
46. Wattsman TA, Davies RS. The utility of preoperative laboratory testing in general surgery patients for outpatient procedures. Am Surg 1997;63:81–90.
47. Salem M, Tainsh RE Jr, Bromberg J, et al. Perioperative glucocorticoid coverage. A reassessment 42 years after emergence of a problem. Ann Surg 1994;219:416–425.
48. Schierhout G, Roberts I. Fluid resuscitation with colloid or crystalloid solutions in critically ill patients: a systematic review of randomised trials. Br Med J 1998;316:961–964.
49. Task Force of the American College of Critical Care Medicine, Society of Critical Care Medicine. Practice parameters for hemodynamic support of sepsis in adult patients in sepsis. Crit Care Med 1999;27:639–660.
50. Talmor M, Hydo L, Barie PS. Relationship of systemic inflammatory response syndrome (SIRS) to organ dysfunction, length of stay, and mortality in critical surgical illness: effect of intensive care unit resuscitation. Arch Surg 1999;134:81–87.
51. Barie PS, Jones WG. Multiple organ failure. In: Barie PS, Shires GT, eds. Surgical Intensive Care. Boston: Little Brown, 1993;147–207.
52. Eachempati SR, Reed RL II, Barie PS. Serum bicarbonate concentration correlates with arterial base deficit in critically ill patients. Surg Infect 2003:4:193–198.
53. Gore DC, Jahoor F, Hibbert JM, De Maria EJ. Lactic acidosis during sepsis is related to increased pyruvate production, not deficits in tissue oxygen availability. Ann Surg 1996;224:97–102.
54. Shah MR, Hasselblad V, Stevenson LW, et al. Impact of the pulmonary artery catheter in critically ill patients. Meta-analysis of randomized clinical trials. JAMA 2005;294:1664–1670.
55. Gattinoni L, Brazzi L, Pelosi P, et al. A trial of goal-oriented hemodynamic therapy in critically ill patients. SvO_2 collaborative group. N Engl J Med 1995;333:1025–1032.
56. Velmahos GC, Oemetriades O, Shoemaker WC, et al. Endpoints of resuscitation of critically injured patients: normal or supranormal? A prospective randomized trial. Ann Surg 2000;232:409–418.
57. Simon TL, Alverson DC, Au Buchon J, et al. Practice parameter for the use of red blood cell transfusions: developed by the Red Blood Cell Administration Practice Guideline Development Task Force of the College of American Pathologists. Arch Pathol Lab Med 1998;122:130–138.
58. Innes G. Guidelines for red blood cells and plasma transfusion for adults and children: an emergency physician's overview of the 1997 Canadian blood transfusion guidelines. Part 1: red blood cell transfusion. Canadian Medical Association Expert Working Group. J Emerg Med 1998;16:129–131.
59. Spiess BD, Let C, Body SC, et al. Hematocrit value on intensive care unit entry influences the frequency of Q-wave myocardial infarction after coronary artery bypass grafting. J Thorac Cardiovasc Surg 1998;116:460–467.
60. Hebert PC, Wells G, Blajchman MA, et al. A multicenter, randomized, controlled clinical trial of transfusion requirements in critical care. N Engl J Med 1999;340:409–417.
61. Devlin JW, Welage LS, Olsen KM. Proton pump inhibitor formulary considerations in the acutely ill. Part 1: pharmacology, pharmacodynamics, and available formulations. Ann Pharmacother 2005;39:1667–1677.
62. Devlin JW, Welage LS, Olsen KM. Proton pump inhibitor formulary considerations in the acutely ill. Part 2: clinical efficacy, safety, and economics. Ann Pharmacother 2005;39:1844–1851.
63. Daley RJ, Rebuck JA, Welage LS, Rogers FB. Prevention of stress ulceration: current trends in critical care. Crit Care Med 2004; 32:2008–2013.
64. Cook DJ, Fuller HD, Guyatt GH, et al. Risk factors for gastrointestinal bleeding in critically ill patients. Canadian Critical Care Trials Group. N Engl J Med 1994;330:377–381.
65. Barie PS, Eachempati SR. Acute acalculous cholecystitis. Curr Opin Gastorenterol 2003;5:302–309.
66. Heyland DK, MacDonald S, Keefe L, Drover JW. Total parenteral nutrition in the critically ill patient: a meta-analysis. JAMA 1998;280:2013–2019.
67. Zaloga GP. Early enteral nutritional support improves outcome: fact or fancy? Crit Care Med 1999;27:259–261.
68. Cotterill AM, Mendel P, Holly JM, et al. The differential regulation of the circulating levels of the insulin-like growth factors and their binding proteins (IGFBP) 1, 2, and 3 after elective abdominal surgery. Clin Endocrinol 1996;44:91–101.
69. Kaufman FR, Devgan S, Roe TF, Costin G. Perioperative management with prolonged intravenous insulin infusion versus subcutaneous insulin in children with type I diabetes mellitus. J Diabetes Complications 1996;10:6–11.

70. Thorell A, Efendic S, Gutmak M, et al. Insulin resistance after abdominal surgery. Br J Surg 1994;81:59–63.
71. Van den Berghe G, Wouters P, Weekers F, et al. Intensive insulin therapy in the critically ill patients. N Engl J Med 2001;345:1359–1367.
72. Van den Berghe G, Wouters PJ, Bouillon R, et al. Outcome benefit of intensive insulin therapy in the critically ill: insulin dose versus glycemic control. Crit Care Med 2003;31:359–366.
73. Pittas AG, Siegel RD, Lau J. Insulin therapy for critically ill hospitalized patients: a meta-analysis of randomized controlled trials. Arch Intern Med 2004;164:2005–2011.
74. Van den Berghe G, Wilmer A, Hermans G, et al. Intensive insulin therapy in the medical ICU. N Engl J Med 2006;354:449–461.
75. Mackenzie CR, Charlson ME. Assessment of perioperative risk in the patient with diabetes mellitus. Surg Gynecol Obstet 1988; 167:293–299.
76. Clement R, Ronson JA, Engelman RU, Breyer RH. Perioperative morbidity in diabetics requiring coronary artery bypass surgery. Ann Thorac Surg 1988;46:321–323.
77. Pomposelli JJ, Baxter JK III, Bakineau TJ, et al. Early postoperative glucose control predicts nosocomial infection rate in diabetic patients. JPEN J Parenter Enteral Nutr 1998;22:77–81.
78. Jwasaka H, Itoh K, Myakawa H, et al. Glucose intolerance during prolonged sevoflurane anaesthesia. Can J Anaesth 1996;43: 1059–1061.
79. Uchida I, Asoh T, Shirasaka C, Tsuji H. Effect of epidural analgesia on postoperative insulin resistance as evaluated by insulin clamp technique. Br J Surg 1988;75:557–562.
80. Svedjeholu R, Hakanson E, Vanhaneu I. Rationale for metabolic support with amino acids and glucose-insulin-potassium (GIP) in cardiac surgery. Ann Thorac Surg 1995;59(suppl 2):515–522.
81. Svedjeholu R, Ekroth R, Joachinersson PO, Tyden H. High-dose insulin improves the efficacy of dopamine early after cardiac surgery. A study of myocardial performance and oxygen consumption. Scand J Thorac Cardovasc Surg 1991;25:215–221.
82. Svensson S, Ekroth R, Nilsson F, et al. Insulin as a vasodilating agent in the first hour after cardiopulmonary bypass. Scand J Thorac Cardiovasc Surg 1989;23:139–143.
83. Svensson S, Ekroth R, Milocco I, et al. Glucose and lactate balances in heart and leg after coronary surgery: influence of insulin infusion. Scand J Thorac Cardiovasc Surg 1989;23:145–150.
84. Brandi LS, Fredian M, Oleggini M, et al. Insulin resistance after surgery: normalization by insulin treatment. Clin Sci 1990;79: 443–450.
85. O'Grady NP, Barie PS, Bartlett JG, et al. Practice guidelines for evaluating new fever in critically ill adult patients. Task Force of the Society of Critical Care Medicine and the Infectious Diseases Society of America. Clin Infect Dis 1998;26:1042–1059.
86. Muylle L, Joos M, Wouters E, et al. Increased tumor necrosis factor alpha (TNF-α), interleukin-1, amid interleukin-6 (IL-6) levels in the plasma of stored platelet concentrates: relationship between TNF-α and IL-6 levels and febrile transfusion reaction. Transfusion 1993;33:195–199.
87. Montgomery KD, Potter HG, Helfet DL. Magnetic resonance venography to evaluate the deep venous system of the pelvis in patients who have an acetabular fracture. J Bone Joint Surg [Am] 1995;77:1639–1649.
88. Ferretti GR, Bosson JL, Buffaz PD, et al. Acute pulmonary embolism: role of helical CT in 164 patients with intermediate probability at ventilation-perfusion scintigraphy and normal results at duplex US of the legs. Radiology 1997;205:453–458.
89. Pearson ML. Guideline for prevention of intravascular device-related infections. Hospital Infection Control Practices Advisory Committee. Infect Control Hosp Epidemiol 1996;17:438–473.
90. Centers for Disease Control and Prevention. Guidelines for prevention of nosocomial pneumonia. MMWR Morb Mortal Wkly Rep 1997;46(RR-1):1–79.
91. Talmor M, Li P, Barie PS. Acute paranasal sinusitis in critically ill patients: guidelines for prevention, diagnosis and treatment. Clin Infect Dis 1997;25:1441–1446.
92. Meduri GU, Mauldin GL, Wunderink RG, et al. Causes of fever and pulmonary densities in patients with clinical manifestations of ventilator-associated pneumonia. Chest 1994;106:221–235.
93. Croce MA, Fabian TC, Waddle-Smith L, et al. Utility of Gram's stain and efficacy of quantitative cultures for posttraumatic pneumonia: a prospective study. Ann Surg 1998;227:743–751.
94. Veenstra DL, Saint S, Saha S, et al. Efficacy of antiseptic-impregnated central venous catheters in preventing catheter-related bloodstream infection: a meta-analysis. JAMA 1999;281:261–267.
95. Bartlett JG, Perl TM. The new *Clostridium difficile*—what does it mean? N Engl J Med 2005;353:2503–2505.
96. McDonald LC, Killgore GE, Thompson A, et al. An epidemic, toxin gene-variant strain of *Clostridium difficile*. N Engl J Med 2005;353:2433–2441.
97. Loo VG, Poirier L, Miller MA, et al. A predominantly clonal multiinstitutional outbreak of *Clostridium difficile*-associated diarrhea with high morbidity and mortality. N Engl J Med 2005; 353:2442–2449.
98. Kollef MH. Antibiotic use and antibiotic resistance in the intensive care unit: are we curing or creating disease? Heart Lung 1994;23:363–367.
99. Darby JM, Linden P, Pasculle W, Saul M. Utilization and diagnostic yield of blood cultures in a surgical intensive care unit. Crit Care Med 1997;25:989–994.

18

Anesthesia

Joseph D. Tobias and Russell Wall

There are five basic methods for the administration of anesthesia: local; monitored anesthesia care; peripheral nerve blockade; and neuraxial anesthesia, including spinal or epidural anesthesia; and general anesthesia. Peripheral nerve blockade and neuraxial anesthesia are frequently considered together under the title of regional anesthesia. Local anesthesia involves the infiltration of a surgical site with a local anesthetic agent to render the site insensitive to pain.

Monitored anesthesia care involves monitoring a patient with standard noninvasive monitors (see below for a description of standard American Society of Anesthesiologists [ASA] monitors), administering a sedative or analgesic agent intravenously to make the patient comfortable, and frequently infiltrating the surgical site with a local anesthetic agent. It frequently is provided using a combination of a drug with amnestic properties (midazolam or propofol) with a drug that provides analgesia (an opioid such as fentanyl). With monitored anesthesia care, the goal is to have the patient maintain spontaneous ventilation during the procedure. The depth of sedation may range from minimal, in which the patient is in an awake, relaxed state and able to respond to verbal stimuli, to deep, in which a painful stimulus is required to elicit a response.

A peripheral nerve block involves the injection of a local anesthetic agent around a nerve or group of nerves (plexus) to render a specific dermatome or dermatomes insensitive to pain. Examples of plexus blockade include cervical plexus blockade for carotid endarterectomy, brachial plexus blockade for upper-extremity or shoulder procedures, or lumbar plexus blockade for hip or leg surgery. Alternatively, a single nerve or select number of nerves can be blocked if the surgical procedure is confined to the distribution of that nerve or those nerves, for example, median nerve and ulnar nerve blockade for carpal tunnel surgery or femoral and sciatic nerve blockade for procedures on the lower extremity distal to the knee. Intravenous regional anesthesia (Bier block), may be considered another example of a peripheral nerve block. A Bier block is produced by injecting a specific volume of a dilute local anesthetic intravenously into an extremity after that extremity has been exsanguinated by wrapping it with a bandage and then occluded with a tourniquet.

Neuraxial anesthesia involves injecting a local anesthetic into the subarachnoid or epidural space to block an area of the spinal cord and its accompanying nerve roots to render an entire region of the body (lower abdomen, pelvis, perineum, or lower extremities) insensitive to pain. Examples of neuraxial anesthesia include spinal, epidural, and caudal anesthesia.

During regional anesthesia (peripheral nerve block, Bier block, or neuraxial anesthesia), patients are monitored and generally receive intravenous sedatives or analgesics for comfort. A regional anesthetic technique such as a peripheral nerve block or epidural anesthesia is frequently combined with a general anesthetic (see below) as part of a balanced anesthetic technique. In many cases, the regional anesthetic technique can be continued into the postoperative period by use of a continuous infusion via catheter and thereby provide ongoing postoperative analgesia.

General anesthesia includes four requisites: amnesia, analgesia, muscle relaxation, and the attenuation of the sympathetic nervous system's response to surgical trauma. General anesthesia can be broken down into induction, maintenance, and emergence phases. The induction of anesthesia can be provided by the administration of an intravenous anesthetic agent (a barbiturate such as thiopental, propofol, or etomidate) or by the inhalation of an inhalational anesthetic agent such as halothane or sevoflurane. The advantages of intravenous induction include rapid onset of anesthesia and avoidance of the pungent odor of the inhalational anesthetic agents.

In pediatric patients, the inhalation induction of anesthesia is frequently chosen to avoid the need for obtaining intravenous access on an awake child. The downside of such a technique is the lack of intravenous access during a time when airway and cardiovascular problems may occur with the administration of an inhalational anesthetic agent. Hemodynamic compromise was more common with the use of halothane given its negative inotropic and chronotropic properties. Such issues are less of a concern with the introduction of the newer inhalational anesthetic agent sevoflurane, which is now widely used in the practice of pediatric anesthesia for inhalation induction. However, laryngospasm and glottic closure may still occur, resulting in an inability to ventilate the patient. In such instances, the intramuscular administration of succinylcholine may be used to break laryngospasm and prevent hypoxia if intravenous access is immediately attainable. The inhalation induction of anesthesia also allows the maintenance of spontaneous ventilation even during deep planes of anesthesia (deep enough to allow for direct laryngoscopy and endotracheal intubation). Such a technique may be used if there is any question regarding the ability to bag-valve-mask ventilate the patient, such as patients with airways compromised by infection, tumor, or anatomic abnormalities.

Maintenance of general anesthesia can be accomplished by balanced, inhalation, or combination techniques. The balanced technique includes nitrous oxide or a continuous infusion of an intravenous anesthetic, a nondepolarizing muscle relaxant, and an opioid. The inhalation technique includes a potent inhalation anesthetic such as halothane, enflurane, isoflurane, desflurane, or sevoflurane in nitrous oxide and oxygen or air and oxygen. The combination technique is the balanced technique plus the addition of a small concentration of a potent inhalation agent. In most circumstances, the choice of maintenance anesthesia is based on the presence of comorbid features and the preferences of the attending anesthesiologists.

Preoperative Evaluation

Regardless of the type of procedure, a preoperative evaluation is recommended. In many hospitals, the preoperative evaluation is performed in a specialized clinic and frequently accomplished the same day that the patient sees the surgeon. Alternatively, in low-risk patients without accompanying comorbid diseases, the preoperative evaluation can be performed the day of surgery. The preoperative evaluation of the patient for anesthesia and surgery includes obtaining a history of present illness, past medical problems, past surgical and anesthetic history, and reviewing the patient's current and possibly prior medical record and medication list. Current medical problems should receive optimal therapy before surgery.

The physical examination is directed primarily at the central nervous, cardiovascular, and respiratory systems, including an examination of the airway. An ASA physical status classification is assigned to the patient based on their comorbid features and associated medical conditions (Table 18.1).[1] The physical classification is based on the physical condition of the patient and does not include the planned surgical procedure. In addition to the history and physical examination, a review of current drug therapy, a history of allergies, and an interpretation of laboratory data are essential. Laboratory tests should be ordered on the basis of positive findings obtained during the history and physical examination and on the complexity of the surgical procedure.[2]

TABLE 18.1. American Society of Anesthesiologists (ASA) Physical Status Classification.

Classification	*Description*
1	Normal healthy patient
2	Mild systemic disease with no functional limitation
3	Severe systemic disease with functional limitation
4	Severe systemic disease that is a constant threat to life
5	Moribund patient not expected to survive without operation
6	Brain-dead patient; organs are being removed for donor purposes
E	Emergency operation

Source: From American Society of Anesthesiologists,[1] with permission of *Anesthesiology*.

Preoperative testing of all patients for elective surgery is unjustified and expensive. However, state, local, and accrediting body regulations may necessitate policies requiring certain tests. In general, in males who are 40 years of age or younger without identified comorbid conditions, no laboratory or radiologic evaluation is necessary; a hemoglobin is all that is generally recommended for women who are 40 years of age or younger. A 12-lead electrocardiogram (ECG) is generally recommended in patients who are 40 years of age or older; a chest radiograph may be obtained in patients who are 50 years of age or above. In addition, an ECG or chest radiograph should be obtained in patients with a history or symptoms suggestive of respiratory or cardiovascular disease. Although commonly performed, routine testing of coagulation function has been shown to be of limited value without an antecedent history of bleeding problems.[3]

Another area of ongoing controversy is the role of routine preoperative pregnancy testing. Given the theoretical potential for anesthetic agents to be teratogenic and the risks of spontaneous abortion, the history should include specific questioning about the potential for pregnancy, including information about the patient's last menstrual cycle. In addition, some centers routinely obtain urinary pregnancy tests.

The planned management of anesthesia is discussed with each patient, and risks and possible complications are reviewed. Options and plans for postoperative pain management are discussed. Answering questions and obtaining an informed consent completes the preoperative evaluation.

Patients with preexisting heart disease who are to have noncardiac surgery may present a significant perioperative challenge.[4,5] The goals of the preoperative evaluation in the patient with the potential for underlying cardiac disease are to identify patients with ischemic heart disease who may require specific perioperative monitoring for ischemia detection; evaluate the patient's cardiac function (generally by means of echocardiography or occasionally cardiac catheterization); identify patients with ischemic heart disease that requires intervention (stenting or coronary artery bypass grafting) prior to elective surgical procedures; ensure that maximal pharmacologic therapy has been obtained to optimize the patient's cardiovascular performance; and identify those patients who may benefit from perioperative therapy, including the use of β-adrenergic blockade to decrease the risk of perioperative cardiac events (see below).[4,5]

The evaluation of patients for the presence of ischemic heart disease starts with a thorough history and physical examination with an evaluation of the patient's symptomatology and exercise tolerance. This is supplemented by a standard 12-lead ECG. As the ECG may be a relatively insensitive marker of ischemic heart disease in the absence of a pervious myocardial infarction or some type of ongoing acute ischemic event, additional evaluation may include exercise testing ("stress test") or a pharmacologic stress test using dobutamine in patients who cannot actively exercise; this increases their heart rate to the specific threshold necessary to provide diagnostic information. The last group includes patients with various conditions, including orthopedic issues which limit activity.

Clinical markers may be major, intermediate, or minor predictors of increased perioperative cardiovascular risk. Major predictors include unstable coronary syndromes (myocardial infarction within the past 6 months, unstable or severe angina), decompensated congestive heart failure (CHF), significant dysrhythmias, and severe valvular disease. Intermediate predictors include minor angina, prior myocardial infarction, compensated CHF, and diabetes mellitus. Minor predictors include advanced age, an abnormal ECG, rhythms other than sinus, low functional capacity, history of stroke, and uncontrolled hypertension. Although a preoperative cardiology evaluation is frequently performed to assess such patients, the use of the cardiologist or internist to "clear patients for surgery" should no longer be practiced. Consultant physicians are asked to assess the patient's cardiovascular status, perform diagnostic evaluations such as echocardiography or stress testing, and determine if additional preoperative evaluations (cardiac catheterization to evaluate for coronary artery disease) or changes in the patient's pharmacologic regimens are needed. In addition to continuing the patient's current pharmacologic regimen, perioperative morbidity and mortality may be reduced by preoperative preparation with β-adrenergic antagonists or α-adrenergic agonists (clonidine).[6–8]

In addition to patient-specific issues, there may also be surgery-related factors that have an impact on perioperative outcome. Surgery-specific risks are determined by the type of surgery and the degree of hemodynamic stress created by the surgery. High-risk surgeries include major emergency surgery, especially for the elderly, major vascular (aortic) and peripheral vascular surgery, and prolonged procedures with large fluid shifts or blood loss. Intermediate-risk surgeries include carotid endarterectomy, head and neck surgery, intraperitoneal and intrathoracic procedures, orthopedic surgery, and prostatic surgery. Low-risk procedures include endoscopic procedures, superficial procedures, cataract extractions, and surgeries on the breast.

Is regional anesthesia safer than general anesthesia? Although some studies suggest that regional anesthesia and regional anesthesia in combination with general anesthesia result in less cardiac morbidity than general anesthesia alone, studies examining this question in patients undergoing peripheral vascular surgery have reported no significant difference in cardiac morbidity and mortality among general, spinal, and epidural anesthesia.[9–12]

Guidelines for Patients Receiving Nothing by Mouth

Although the pulmonary aspiration of gastric contents is an uncommon event, the consequences may be severe (pneumonitis, respiratory failure, death), and other than supportive therapy, there is no specific therapy. Classical teaching relates that the severity of the aspiration injury relates to the volume aspirated as well as its pH, with severe complications occurring with the aspiration of greater than 0.4 ml/kg or with aspirates with a pH less than 2.5. Although aspiration may occur in any setting, patients at risk include parturients; obese patients; diabetics; patients who have received opioids; patients with gastrointestinal (GI) disease (reflux, obstruction); patients with altered mental status; patients with intra-abdominal pathology (acute abdominal emergencies, including appendicitis); and patients in whom difficult airway management is anticipated. These factors may predispose to aspiration by limiting the patient's ability to protect his or her airway, decreasing the normal barrier to aspiration (lower esophageal sphincter tone), increasing gastric volume, or delaying gastric emptying.[13,14] Patients at greatest risk are those with high ASA physical status classifications and those having emergency surgery. The majority of aspirations occur during the induction of anesthesia or following tracheal extubation when the patient has blunted or lost protective airway reflexes.

Classically, keeping patients *nil per os* (NPO) has been the mainstay of therapy to prevent acid aspiration. In the past, adult patients were fasted 8 to 12 h before surgery to reduce the volume of gastric contents at the time of induction of anesthesia and to decrease the risk of aspiration pneumonitis. This preoperative fast does not take into account differences in gastric emptying of clear liquids and solids. Clear liquids have a gastric emptying time of 1 to 2 h. Solids have an unpredictable gastric emptying time greater than 6 h. There is no scientific evidence confirming the benefit of a fluid fast.[15–18] The ingestion of clear liquids up to 2 h before surgery does not increase gastric fluid volume or acidity. As a result, the liberalization of guidelines for ingestion of clear liquids for elective surgery of otherwise healthy patients has been recommended.[19,20] A national survey of anesthesiologists in the United States has shown that 69% have either changed their NPO policy or are flexible in their practice in allowing clear liquids before elective operations in children and in 41% of adults.[21] Suggested guidelines for patients with no known risk factors include no solid food for at least 8 h before surgery and unrestricted clear liquids until 2 h before surgery. Oral medications may be given 1 to 2 h before surgery with as much as 150 ml of water. Some centers even allow the ingestion of one cup of coffee prior to elective outpatient surgical procedures as a common complaint of outpatients is a postoperative headache related to caffeine withdrawal.

What should be done with patients with risk factors for acid aspiration? Although no definitive studies have demonstrated its efficacy, many centers routinely use preoperative medications to decrease the acidity of the gastric fluid (H_2-antagonists or proton pump inhibitors) and speed gastric emptying (metoclopramide). However, to be effective, it is recommended that these medications be administered 60–90 min prior to anesthetic induction. Alternatively, a nonparticulate antacid (sodium bicitrate) can be given immediately prior to anesthetic induction, which is a common practice in obstetrical anesthesia. In addition, in patients at risk for acid aspiration, rapid sequence induction is practiced. This involves the use of a rapidly acting neuromuscular blocking agent (NMBA; see below) with an anesthetic induction agent and the application of cricoid pressure. As the cricoid is the only complete ring of the trachea, it can be gently pushed posteriorly to effectively occlude the esophagus and prevent passive regurgitation of gastric contents.

Preoperative Medication

There are several categories and uses of preoperative medications (Table 18.2). The most common use of a preoperative medication is to provide sedation and anxiolysis prior to transport to the operating room. Preparing the patient for surgery includes psychological preparation and frequently pharmacological premedication. Psychological preparation includes the preoperative visit and an interview by the anesthesiologist. Pharmacological premedication may be given orally or rarely intramuscularly 1 to 2h before the induction of anesthesia or intravenously in the immediate preoperative period. Popular choices include benzodiazepines such as midazolam or occasionally α_2-adrenergic agonists such as clonidine. Analgesia for placement of invasive lines such as arterial cannulae or central venous lines can be provided by incremental intravenous doses of fentanyl while the patient is in the preoperative holding area, where appropriate monitoring of hemodynamic and respiratory status can be provided.

Additional preoperative medications may be used in patients with certain comorbid features. This includes the use of H_2-antagonists or proton pump inhibitors or motility agents to increase gastric pH and decrease gastric volume in patients at risk for acid aspiration, while inhaled β-adrenergic agonists (albuterol) or anticholinergic agents (ipratropium) may be administered to patients with reactive airway diseases (asthma, recent upper respiratory infection, or chronic obstructive pulmonary diseases). Anticholinergic agents may be used to dry airway secretions in patients requiring fiber-optic intubation.

TABLE 18.2. Types and Uses of Premedications.

Type of medication	*Purpose*
Benzodiazepines	Sedation, anxiolysis, amnesia
Opioids	Analgesia during invasive procedures
Anticholinergic agents (atropine, glycopyrrolate)	Prevent bradycardia, blunt airway reflexes, dry secretions
Inhaled β-adrenergic agonists (albuterol), inhaled anticholinergic agents (ipratroprium)	Prevention or relief of bronchospasm
H_2-antagonists, proton pump inhibitors	Decrease pH of stomach contents
Promotility agents	Decrease volume of gastric secretions

Monitoring

The standards for basic anesthetic monitoring have been developed by the ASA and apply to all general anesthetics, regional anesthetics, peripheral nerve blocks, and monitored anesthesia care. Similar monitoring guidelines have also been suggested for nonanesthesiologists who are providing procedural sedation. The standards for intraoperative monitoring include the presence of qualified anesthesia personnel throughout all anesthetics and the ongoing evaluation of a patient's oxygenation, ventilation, circulation, and temperature. To fulfill these criteria, the following monitors are used: oxygen analyzer, blood pressure cuff, continuous ECG, pulse oximeter, end-tidal carbon dioxide analyzer, precordial or esophageal stethoscope, temperature probe, and a ventilator disconnect alarm. Based on the medical condition of the patient and the surgical procedure, more elaborate, invasive monitoring may be added. These additional monitors may include a urinary catheter; catheters for measuring intraarterial, central venous, and pulmonary artery (PA) pressures; and transesophageal echocardiography (TEE).

Few studies have compared outcomes in patients managed perioperatively with or without PA catheters.[22,23] The ASA recommends considering three variables when assessing benefit versus risk of PA catheters: disease severity, magnitude of the surgical procedure, and practice setting.[24] The American College of Cardiology/American Heart Association (ACC/AHA) guidelines indicate that the patients most likely to benefit from PA catheters in the perioperative period are those with recent myocardial infarctions complicated by CHF, those with significant coronary artery disease undergoing surgery associated with significant hemodynamic stress, and those with systolic or diastolic left ventricular dysfunction, cardiomyopathy, or valvular disease undergoing high-risk operations.[5]

Additional information regarding structural and functional issues of the myocardium may be obtained by the use of TEE. The strongest indications for perioperative TEE that are supported by evidence-based medicine include cardiac surgery procedures such as repair of valvular lesions (insufficiency or stenosis) or congenital lesions, assessments and repairs of thoracic aortic aneurysms and dissections, pericardial window procedures, and the repair of hypertrophic obstructive cardiomyopathy.[25] For noncardiac surgery, intraoperative TEE is indicated to evaluate acute, persistent, and life-threatening hemodynamic disturbances in which ventricular function and its determinants are uncertain and have not responded to treatment, especially when placement of a PA catheter is not feasible.

In addition to routine ASA monitors and invasive hemodynamic monitoring, there is continued interest in the development and potential use of "consciousness" or "awareness" monitors. The importance of such monitors is highlighted by the results of several different studies, which demonstrated that intraoperative awareness may occur in anywhere from 0.1% to 0.2% of all patients, with even higher incidences in specific procedures, including trauma, cardiac, obstetrical, and emergency surgery. Of even more concern is the fact that as many as one-third of patients who have intraoperative awareness will have long-term consequences, such as a post-traumatic stress disorder.[26–28] To avoid such issues, several manufacturers have marketed or are developing monitors that provide the anesthesia provider with a numerical value against which anesthetic agents are titrated. There are currently five such monitors: the Bispectral Index (BIS monitor, Aspect Medical, Newton, MA); the Narcotrend (MonitorTechnik, Bad Bramstedt, Germany), which is currently available only in Europe; Patient State Analyzer (PSA 4000, Baxter Healthcare, Deerfield, IL); SNAP (Everest Medical, Minneapolis, MN); and Auditory Evoked Potential Monitor (AEP Monitor, Danmetter Medical). To date, the one that has received the most clinical use is the BIS monitor.

The BIS is a modified electroencephalographic (EEG) monitor that uses a preset algorithm based on intraoperative data obtained from adults to evaluate the EEG. The BIS number is determined from three primary factors: the frequency of the EEG waves, the synchronization of low- and high-frequency information, and the percentage of time in burst suppression. Part of the simplicity and attraction of the BIS monitor is that the depth of sedation/anesthesia is displayed numerically, ranging from 0 to 100, with 40–60 a suitable level of anesthesia to ensure amnesia and lack of recall. With the use of BIS monitoring, a decreased incidence of awareness has been demonstrated as well as a decrease in the total amount of anesthetic agent used.[29–31] Additional studies have suggested faster recovery times and faster discharge times from the postanesthesia care unit, all of which may translate into reduced perioperative costs.[31,32]

Although not yet considered the standard of care for intraoperative anesthesia care, the ASA does recommend the availability of such monitors whenever general anesthesia is provided. Given the success of such monitors in the perioperative arena, there is ongoing interest in the application of such technology in the ICU and the procedural sedation arena.[33,34]

Airway Management

Tracheal intubation is performed on many patients receiving general anesthesia for surgery. The ASA Closed Claims Project has demonstrated that airway misadventures such as inadequate ventilation, difficult intubation, and esophageal intubation are the leading causes of complications involving the respiratory system and are responsible for the most serious injuries (death, brain injury, airway trauma). Guidelines have been developed by the ASA to facilitate management of the difficult airway and decrease the likelihood of adverse outcomes.[35]

A *difficult airway* is defined as a clinical situation in which a conventionally trained anesthesiologist experiences difficulty with mask ventilation, difficulty with tracheal intubation (more than three attempts or more than 10 min required for completion), or both. The preoperative evaluation can identify many patients with a difficult airway. An airway history should be obtained seeking medical, surgical, and anesthetic factors that may indicate a difficult airway. Examination of previous anesthesia records is helpful, although a patient's airway may change with changes in weight or the development of comorbid conditions. A physical examination of the airway is performed to detect physical characteristics associated with a difficult airway such as a large tongue, small mouth, short neck (shortened thyromental distance), recessed mandible, limited extension or flexion of the neck, limited mouth opening, and difficulty visualizing the uvula and tonsillar pillars when the patient opens his or her mouth. The last is assessed with the Mallampati grading system so that visualization of the entire uvula and tonsillar pillars (Mallampati grade) suggests that endotracheal intubation will be uncomplicated, while failure to visualize the tonsillar pillars and the soft palate (Mallampati class IV) is suggestive that endotracheal intubation will be difficult.

When a difficult intubation is suspected, preparation to manage the airway includes having the following readily available: laryngoscope blades of various sizes and designs; endotracheal tubes of different sizes; stylets/guides/wands; fiber-optic intubation equipment; retrograde intubation equipment; equipment for emergency nonsurgical ventilation (transtracheal jet ventilator, hollow jet ventilation stylet, laryngeal mask airway [LMA], esophageal-tracheal Combitube); equipment for emergency surgical airway; and an end-tidal carbon dioxide detector. This equipment should be available on a separate cart (difficult airway cart) so that it can be immediately moved into the operating room when needed for dealing with the unsuspected difficult airway. In addition to the appropriate equipment, every anesthesiologist should have a preformulated strategy for managing the difficult airway.[35,36]

When securing the airway in any setting, there are three basic management options: (1) awake endotracheal intubation versus endotracheal intubation after the induction of general anesthesia, (2) nonsurgical versus surgical approaches (cricothyrotomy or tracheostomy), and (3) maintenance of spontaneous ventilation versus ablation of spontaneous ventilation. In most anesthetic scenarios, the assessment of the airway is such that the decision is made to proceed with the intravenous induction of anesthesia and routine oral endotracheal intubation with a standard laryngoscopic approach. In this scenario, the patient is brought into the operating room and routine ASA monitors are placed. The patient is then allowed to breathe 100% oxygen via the anesthesia circuit and a tight-fitting anesthesia mask. This "denitrogenates" the patient's lungs so that there is little nitrogen left (less than 5%), and the lungs are filled with 100% oxygen.

When anesthesia is induced and an NMBA administered, the lung volume will fall to its functional residual capacity (FRC). In an otherwise healthy patient without alveolar space disease (pneumonia or adult respiratory distress syndrome), the FRC is approximately 25–30 ml/kg or 2 l in a 70-kg adult. Given that the normal oxygen consumption is approximately 200–250 ml/minute, this will provide the patient with an oxygen reserve to maintain an acceptable oxygen saturation during up to 6–8 minutes of apnea. This provides a significant margin of safety if there are problems with bag-valve-mask ventilation or endotracheal intubation. After preoxygenation, anesthesia is induced with a rapid-acting intravenous anesthetic agent (see below) such as thiopental, propofol, or etomidate, and once apnea occurs, effective bag-valve-mask ventilation is demonstrated. Once this has been accomplished, endotracheal intubation is facilitated by the use of an NMBA (see below).

Techniques for managing an unconscious patient who is difficult to ventilate include the insertion of oral or nasopharyngeal airways; two-person bag-valve-mask ventilation; and use of an LMA (Fig. 18.1), an esophageal-tracheal Combitube (Fig. 18.2), an intratracheal jet stylet, a rigid ventilating bronchoscope; transtracheal jet ventilation; and surgical airway access.[36,37] Techniques for managing the unconscious patient who can be ventilated but is difficult to intubate include using alternative laryngoscope blades, a light wand, an intubation stylet/tube changer, blind intubation (oral or nasal), fiber-optic intubation, retrograde intubation, and surgical airway access. Multiple attempts at endotracheal intubation should be avoided since this may result in progressive airway trauma, thereby turning the "cannot intubate/can ventilate" scenario into the "cannot intubate/cannot ventilate" scenario (see below). In elective or urgent cases, the most prudent measure may be to continue bag-valve-mask ventilation and allow the effects of the intravenous induction agent and NMBA to dissipate.

In a small percentage of patients, an airway emergency occurs in that the patient cannot be bag-valve-mask ventilated and endotracheal intubation cannot be accomplished. This is known as the cannot intubate/cannot ventilate scenario. When this occurs, there are four appropriate choices after a second attempt has been made at endotracheal intubation: (1) insertion of an LMA, (2) insertion of a Combitube; (3) institution of transtracheal jet ventilation, or (4) establishing a surgical airway.[37] Given the emergency nature of this scenario, an organized, prerehearsed approach to such problems is mandatory. In many instances, the patient can be rescued with the placement of an LMA and ventilation provided. When placing the LMA, cricoid pressure (see below) should be released as it has been shown to be more difficult to obtain correct LMA placement with the application of cricoid pressure. Although the LMA does not protect against acid aspiration, it may provide effective ventilation and oxygenation when bag-valve-mask ventilation fails. The LMA can also be used as a conduit for blind endotracheal intubation or fiber-optic assisted intubation.

The same preformulated strategy is also necessary to extubate a patient with a difficult airway. Follow-up care includes documenting and informing the patient of the difficult airway management and observing for potential complications such as airway edema or bleeding, tracheal or esophageal perforation, a pneumothorax, and aspiration. The development of the ASA difficult airway algorithm has resulted in a dramatic decrease in the number of respiratory-related anesthetic adverse outcomes.

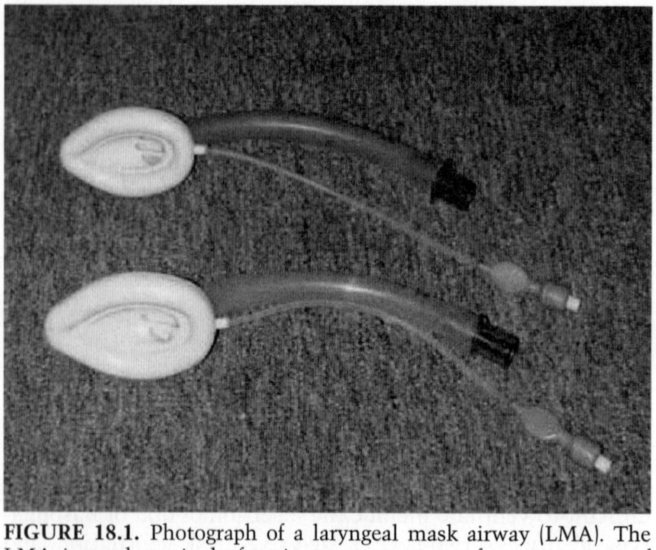

FIGURE 18.1. Photograph of a laryngeal mask airway (LMA). The LMA is used routinely for airway management for many types of surgical procedures and is a key element in the American Society of Anesthesiologists' difficult airway algorithm.

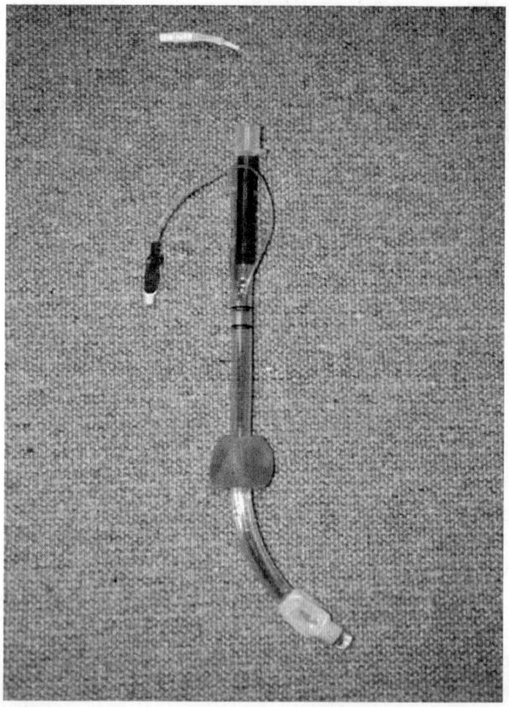

FIGURE 18.2. Photograph of a Combitube. The Combitube is a modification of the esophageal obturator airway that is a suggested means of managing the airway in the American Society of Anesthesiologists' difficult airway algorithm.

Pharmacology of Anesthetic Practice

Local Anesthetic Agents

There are two chemically distinct classes of local anesthetics: amino esters and amino amides. Amino esters used in anesthetic practice include procaine, chloroprocaine, and tetracaine. Amino amides used clinically include lidocaine, mepivacaine, prilocaine, bupivacaine, levobupivacaine, and ropivacaine. These two classes of local anesthetic agents differ in their site of metabolism, plasma half-lives, adverse effect profile, and allergic potential. Amino esters are metabolized in the plasma by cholinesterases, while amino amides are metabolized in the liver. Para-aminobenzoic acid (PABA) is a metabolite of amino ester breakdown and rarely may result in allergic reactions, whereas amino amides rarely cause allergic reactions. Regardless of their chemical structure (ester vs. amide), the mechanism of action for the majority of local anesthetic agents involves blockade of sodium channels in the nerve membrane, thereby preventing depolarization. The nonionized portion of the local anesthetic agent penetrates the lipid membrane, while the ionized portion reversibly blocks the inner aspect of the sodium channel.

Local anesthetic agents differ in intrinsic potency, onset of action, duration of action, and their ability to produce differential sensory and motor blockade (Table 18.3). Potency is determined primarily by lipid solubility. The higher the lipid

TABLE 18.3. Local Anesthetic Agents.

Agent	*Onset*	*Relative potency*	*pK_a*	*Duration*	*% Protein binding*	*Maximum dose range (mg/kg)*[a]
Esters						
Procaine	Slow	1	8.9	Short	6	7–10
Chloroprocaine	Fast	1	9.1	Short	—	7–10
Tetracaine	Slow	8	8.5	Long	76	—
Amides						
Mepivacaine	Fast	2	7.6	Moderate	78	5–7
Prilocaine	Fast	2	7.7	Moderate	55	8–10
Lidocaine	Fast	2	8.1	Moderate	64	5–7
Bupivacaine	Moderate	8	8.1	Long	96	2–3
Ropivacaine	Moderate	6	8.2	Long	94	2–4
Etidocaine	Fast	6	8.1	Long	94	3–4

[a]Upper dose range is for drug combined with epinephrine.

solubility partition coefficient, the more potent the local anesthetic agent is.[38] Bupivacaine and tetracaine are examples of potent local anesthetic agents. The onset of action of a local anesthetic agent is determined primarily by the pK_a.[39,40] The pK_a of local anesthetic agents ranges from 7.6 to 9.1. The closer the pK_a is to the physiological pH of 7.4, the more rapid the onset of action because the percentage of local anesthetic in the nonionized form is greater, promoting penetration of the nerve membrane. Lidocaine has a pK_a of 7.7, and at a pH of 7.4, 35% exists in the nonionized base form, yielding a relatively rapid onset of blockade. In contrast, tetracaine has a pK_a of 8.6, with only 5% in the nonionized form at a tissue pH of 7.4, resulting in a slower onset of blockade than lidocaine. Duration of action is determined primarily by the degree of protein binding.[41]

Local anesthetic agents bind to protein receptors in the sodium channels. A greater degree of protein binding produces a longer-lasting blockade of sodium channels and a longer duration of action. Bupivacaine, levobupivacaine, tetracaine, and ropivacaine are long-acting local anesthetic agents. Duration of action is also influenced by the degree of vasodilation produced by the local anesthetic.[42] Lidocaine and mepivacaine have similar degrees of protein binding, but mepivacaine creates less vasodilation and therefore remains at the site of action longer. A desirable feature of several local anesthetic agents is their ability to produce significant sensory anesthesia while creating minimal inhibition of motor activity.[43] Bupivacaine and ropivacaine demonstrate this property, which is beneficial for postoperative analgesia administered through an epidural catheter so that patients are able to ambulate with minimal discomfort.

When performing regional anesthesia, the practitioner's experience, knowledge of anatomy, and manual dexterity are important. Knowledge about the appropriate dose of the local anesthetic, the use of a vasoconstrictor, and the impact of the site of administration are necessary to increase the rate of success and limit potential complications. Increasing the dose of a local anesthetic yields a faster onset of effect, a longer duration of action, and a greater depth of blockade.[43,44] Dosage can be increased by increasing the concentration or the volume of the local anesthetic. However, higher plasma concentrations of the local anesthetic agent will also be achieved, thereby increasing the risks of toxicity (see below).

Epinephrine (0.5 µg/ml or a concentration of 1:200,000) may be added to the local anesthetic solution during performance of a regional anesthetic technique (epidural or peripheral nerve blockade) to decrease the vascular absorption of the drug, thereby increasing the number of anesthetic molecules available to diffuse to the nerve membrane.[45] This results in an increase in duration of action and an increase in the density of the blockade. However, the ability of epinephrine to prolong duration of action depends on the local anesthetic used and the site of administration. For peripheral nerve blocks and skin infiltration, epinephrine prolongs the duration of action of all local anesthetics.[46] For epidural anesthesia, epinephrine added to lidocaine increases the duration of action, but epinephrine added to bupivacaine does not.[47,48] This relates to the fact that lidocaine causes more vasodilation than bupivaine. Therefore, the addition of epinephrine to lidocaine counteracts its vasodilatory effects, which would normally hasten the resolution of the block. Since less vasodilation occurs with bupivacaine, the effect of epinephrine is less pronounced. For spinal anesthesia, epinephrine added to a local anesthetic will prolong duration of action through decreased vascular absorption and possibly through a direct antinociceptive effect on the spinal cord.[49]

Epinephrine is also used as a marker for inadvertent intravascular injection. This is especially important when large doses of local anesthetic agents (epidural or plexus blockade) are administered. For such procedures, gentle aspiration is recommended prior to injection and intermittently while the dose of local anesthetic agent is administered. However, even with negative aspiration for blood, there is the potential for inadvertent intravascular administration. In attempt to identify such a problem, a "test dose" is frequently used. This test dose entails the administration of 3 ml of the 5 µg/ml epinephrine solution or a total epinephrine dose of 15 µg. If this amount of epinephrine is injected intravascularly, then it generally can be detected by changes in heart rate, blood pressure, or the ST-T wave segments of the ECG and thereby alert the practitioner that inadvertent intravascular injection is occurring.[50]

The site of injection of the local anesthetic agent also has a significant impact on its clinical effects. The shortest durations of action are seen with intrathecal (i.e., spinal anesthesia) and subcutaneous administration, whereas the longest durations of action (and slowest onsets) are seen with major peripheral nerve blocks (i.e., brachial plexus blockade). Spinal anesthesia with bupivacaine has an onset of 5 min and a duration of 3 to 4 h, while a brachial plexus block with bupivacaine will take effect in 20 to 30 min and last 6 to 8 h.[51,52] The site of administration also determines the vascular absorption of the drug and hence the plasma concentration. The highest venous plasma concentration of local anesthetic agents occurs following an intercostal nerve block or interpleural analgesia, followed by a paracervical block, caudal epidural, lumbar/thoracic epidural, brachial plexus, peripheral nerve blockade, subarachnoid anesthesia, and last, subcutaneous infiltration.[53] For example, 400mg of lidocaine for a brachial plexus block yields a peak venous plasma concentration of 3mg/ml, whereas 400mg of lidocaine for an intercostal nerve block yields a plasma concentration of 7mg/ml.

With the use of local anesthetic agents, the greatest risk of morbidity is the potential for the achievement of toxic plasma concentrations of the drug. Local anesthetic-induced systemic toxicity affects the central nervous system (CNS) and the cardiovascular system. With most local anesthetic agents, CNS toxicity occurs at doses and blood levels below those that produce cardiovascular toxicity. This provides some degree of safety as the CNS symptoms (seizures) are generally more amenable to treatment than the cardiovascular effects (arrhythmias and conduction blockade). Toxicity with lidocaine occurs in the CNS at 8 to 10mg/ml, whereas cardiovascular toxicity occurs at 20mg/ml.[54] The signs and symptoms of CNS toxicity include lightheadedness, dizziness, circumoral numbness, tinnitus, twitching, tremors, and ultimately tonic–clonic seizures. With higher doses, CNS excitation, including seizure activity, is followed by CNS depression, unconsciousness, and respiratory arrest. Seizures result from the blockade of inhibitory pathways in the cerebral cortex yielding unopposed activity of facilitatory neurons.[55] Depression of the CNS and unconsciousness result from inhibition of inhibitory and facilitatory pathways. Hypercarbia and acidosis decrease the convulsive threshold of local anesthetic agents as well as potentiating their cardiotoxicity.[56]

Death from local anesthetic toxicity is most commonly the result of the cardiovascular effects of these agents. Local anesthetic toxicity can adversely affect cardiac electrical and mechanical activity.[57] Bupivacaine may produce severe cardiac dysrhythmias by inhibiting the fast sodium channels and the slow calcium channels in the cardiac membrane. Local anesthetic agents depress myocardial contractility, with the most potent drugs (bupivacaine, tetracaine) causing the greatest dose-dependent myocardial depression.[58] At toxic plasma concentrations, bupivacaine can cause profound myocardial depression and intractable cardiac arrest. These effects are so profound that resuscitative measures for ventricular tachycardia/fibrillation, including standard advanced candiac life support (ACLS) protocols, may be ineffective. Anecdotal case reports have suggested the potential role of various agents such as amiodarone for refractory ventricular arrhythmias or lipid emulsions, which bind the local anesthetic agent and decrease its free fraction. It is only the free fraction and not the local anesthetic that is bound to plasma proteins that has the potential to cause toxicity. In some cases, resuscitation has included the use of extracorporeal circulation. The toxic effects of bupivacaine on the CNS and cardiovascular system occur at the same plasma level of 3 to 5μg/ml. Ropivacaine and levobupivacaine have pharmacological properties similar to bupivacaine but demonstrate fewer cardiodepressant and arrhythmogenic effects.[59]

The signs of local anesthetic cardiovascular toxicity include hypertension and tachycardia during the CNS excitation phase, followed by myocardial depression and mild-to-moderate hypotension, then sinus bradycardia, profound hypotension, ventricular dysrhythmias, and finally circulatory collapse. Hypercarbia, acidosis, and hypoxia potentiate the negative chronotropic and inotropic effects of high plasma concentrations of local anesthetic agents. On vascular smooth muscle, most local anesthetics have a biphasic effect, producing vasoconstriction at low concentrations and vasodilation at high concentrations. When considering the subject of local anesthetic toxicity, the primary method of treating the toxicity should be avoidance by careful calculation of the dose, use of the lowest necessary dose (concentration and volume), use of a test dose with epinephrine to identify inadvertent intravascular injection, intermittent aspiration to identify vascular penetration, and slow incremental injection of the dose.

Local anesthetic agents in recommended concentrations and doses are relatively free of localized tissue effects or irritation. However, additives can cause tissue damage. Prolonged sensorimotor blockade with the epidural and subarachnoid administration of large doses of chloroprocaine was attributed to the low pH of the solution and sodium bisulfite, the antioxidant.[60,61] As a result, the pH was raised, and sodium bisulfate was replaced with EDTA, thereby eliminating the potential neurotoxic effects. However, EDTA may result in back pain from spasms by chelating calcium in paraspinous muscles following epidural anesthesia.[62] Although the addition of epinephrine is recommended to aid in the identification of inadvertent intravascular administration, it should not be added when the local anesthetic will be injected into the area around end arteries (digits, nose, ear, penis) as intense vasoconstriction and tissue necrosis may occur.

Intravenous Anesthetic Agents

Anesthetic agents are administered intravenously to induce general anesthesia or in lower doses to provide sedation. The ideal intravenous anesthetic would have a rapid, smooth onset of action following a nonirritating and painless injection. The drug would demonstrate a steep dose–response relationship, allowing a rapid change in anesthetic depth, and would be rapidly metabolized to inactive metabolites. It would cause minimal cardiovascular and respiratory depression and reduce cerebral blood flow (CBF), cerebral metabolism, and intracranial pressure (ICP). It would allow a rapid and smooth return of consciousness even after prolonged administration and a rapid recovery without postoperative side effects. It would have a low potential to cause histamine release or precipitate hypersensitivity reactions.

Commonly used intravenous anesthetic agents include the barbiturates thiopental and thiamylal; propofol, an alkylphenol; etomidate, an imidazole; ketamine, an arylcyclohexylamine; and midazolam, a benzodiazepine. Sodium thiopental, although far from ideal, remains the most commonly used intravenous induction agent (along with propofol) and is the gold standard against which all other intravenous anesthetics are compared. Although any of these agents can be used to induce anesthesia and begin the anesthetic process, the specific choice of the agent and its dose are based on the clinical scenario, the anticipated duration of the surgical procedure, and the patient's underlyng hemodynamic status.

The intravenous induction agents produce their effects by enhancing inhibitory or inhibiting excitatory neurotransmission. Thiopental, midazolam, propofol, and etomidate interact with different components of the $GABA_A$ receptor complex to enhance the function of the inhibitory neurotransmitter system, γ-aminobutyric acid (GABA).[63–66] When the $GABA_A$ receptors are activated, transmembrane chloride conductance increases to create a hyperpolarization of the postsynaptic cell membranes and a functional inhibition of postsynaptic neurons. Ketamine acts differently by blocking open channels of *N*-methyl-D-aspartate (NMDA) receptors that have been activated by glutamate, an excitatory transmitter, and interacting with brain acetylcholine to create a dissociation between the thalamocortical and limbic systems.[67–69]

The intravenous anesthetic agents demonstrate different pharmacodynamic effects in the CNS and respiratory and cardiovascular systems. The barbiturates propofol and etomidate reduce cerebral metabolism cerebral metabolic rate O_2 ($CMRO_2$), CBF, and ICP and therefore are valuable induction agents for neuroanesthesia or in critically ill patients with increased ICP. Etomidate may be preferred in the latter setting because it provides greater hemodynamic stability, and as a result, cerebral perfusion pressure (CPP = MAP – ICP) is maintained, whereas propofol and thiopental may decrease mean arterial pressure (MAP) through effects on systemic vascular resistance (vasodilation) and negative inotropic effects. Thiopental and perhaps etomidate and propofol may also possess "neuroprotective" properties secondary to reducing $CMRO_2$, which improves the ability of the brain to tolerate incomplete ischemia during procedures such as carotid endarterectomy or the temporary occlusion of cerebral arteries during an aneurysm repair.[70,71] Ketamine's direct effects on ICP remain somewhat controversial, with the older literature suggesting that ketamine may directly increase CBF and ICP. However, it is apparent from recent studies that ketamine has limited effects on CBF and ICP when given in combination with other anesthetic agents, including midazolam.[72–74]

Propofol, midazolam, and the barbiturates have similar EEG effects, causing a transient period of high-frequency activity at low brain concentrations, followed by lower-frequency, higher-amplitude waveforms at high brain concentrations, and finally by burst suppression. Most intravenous anesthetics are anticonvulsants, with both the barbiturates and propofol used in algorithms for the treatment of refractory status epilepticus.[75,76] Etomidate can produce involuntary myoclonic movements from an imbalance of inhibitory and excitatory influences in the thalamocortical tract and can stimulate the EEG pattern, increasing amplitude and frequency.[76] Myoclonic movements and opisthotonic posturing have also been reported following the administration of propofol. These movements are attributed to propofol's antagonism at glycine receptors in subcortical structures.

Thiopental, propofol, etomidate, and midazolam cause dose-dependent respiratory depression with a decrease in tidal volume and minute ventilation and a rightward shift in the CO_2 response curve. The potential for respiratory depression is increased in patients with specific comorbid conditions, including chronic respiratory or cardiovascular disease, and in patients receiving opioids. Following an induction dose of any of these agents, a transient period of apnea occurs. In contrast, ketamine causes minimal respiratory depression in clinically relevant doses and may preserve protective airway reflexes, although aspiration has been reported.[77,78]

Ketamine is the only intravenous anesthetic with bronchodilating properties from the release of endogenous catecholamines.[79] Although it lacks inherent bronchodilating properties, propofol has been shown to be an effective induction agent for patients with reactive airway disease, resulting in limited risk of a wheezing postintubation.

In a prospective trial, 77 patients were randomized to receive propofol (2.5 mg/kg), etomidate (0.4 mg/kg), or thiopental (5 mg/kg) for anesthetic induction and tracheal intubation.[80] Following placement of the endotracheal tube, respiratory resistance was significantly lower with propofol when compared to either etomidate or thiopental. In a second study, asthmatic or nonasthmatic patients were randomized to anesthetic induction with thiopental/thiamylal (5 mg/kg), methohexital (1.5 mg/kg), or propofol (2.5 mg).[81] In asthmatic patients, the incidence of wheezing was 45% with thiopental/thiamylal, 26% with methohexital, and 0% with propofol. In nonasthmatic patients, the incidence of wheezing was 16% with thiopental/thiamylal and 3% with propofol.

The potential beneficial effects of propofol on airway reactivity are further supported by animal studies. Propofol attenuates carbachol-induced airway constriction in canine tracheal smooth muscle.[82] The reported mechanism involves a decrease of intracellular inositol phosphate, resulting in a decrease of intracellular calcium availability. Propofol has also been shown to be more effective in preventing bronchoconstriction following provocative agents in an isolated guinea pig tracheal smooth muscle model.[83]

Intravenous anesthetic agents can depress the cardiovascular system by various mechanisms, including a reduction of central or peripheral autonomic nervous system activity, blunting compensatory baroreceptor reflexes, decreasing preload or afterload, or directly depressing myocardial contractility. Hemodynamic function during the induction of anesthesia may also be affected by preexisting cardiovascular disease, volume status, resting sympathetic nervous system tone, residual effects of chronically administered drugs (angiotensin-converting enzyme inhibitors, β-adrenergic antagonists), and the administration of preinduction drugs, including opioids and benzodiazepines. An induction dose of thiopental causes a variable decrease in cardiac output, systemic vascular resistance, and MAP.[84] The decrease in cardiac output is the result of venodilation and direct myocardial depression. This effect is generally well tolerated in patients with adequate cardiovascular function but is exaggerated with preexisting cardiovascular disease, necessitating the use of a lower dose of thiopental or preferably the use of alternative agents in patients with compromised cardiovascular function.

Likewise, propofol demonstrates cardiovascular depressant effects similar to or greater than those of thiopental. Propofol is a direct myocardial depressant and reduces systemic vascular resistance. Significant cardiovascular responses following propofol administration are more common with high doses, in hypovolemic patients, in elderly patients, and in patients with significant cardiovascular disease.[85,86] The administration of calcium chloride (10 mg/kg) has been shown to prevent the deleterious cardiovascular effects of propofol.[87] In addition to its effects on systemic vascular resistance and myocardial function, propofol may augment central vagal tone, leading to bradycardia, conduction disturbances, and asystole.[88,89] Bradycardia may be more likely when propofol is combined with other medications known to alter cardiac chronotropic function (fentanyl or succinylcholine). Although the relative bradycardia is generally considered a beneficial effect in patients at risk for myocardial ischemia, it may be detrimental in patients with a fixed stroke volume in whom cardiac output is heart rate dependent.

In contrast, etomidate causes minimal cardiovascular depression and is frequently the induction agent of choice in patients with significant cardiovascular disease.[90,91] Ketamine stimulates the cardiovascular system by central and peripheral activation of the sympathetic nervous system and release of endogenous catecholamines.[92] Induction doses of ketamine (1–2 mg/kg) generally increase heart rate and MAP. Therefore, ketamine is not recommended in patients with significant coronary artery disease in whom the balance of myocardial oxygen supply and demand is critical. Aside from its indirect effects with the release of endogenous catecholamines and stimulation of the sympathetic nervous system, ketamine is a direct myocardial depressant, but this effect is seen only when catecholamine reserves are depleted. Midazolam demonstrates relative hemodynamic stability, causing a mild decrease in MAP secondary to a decrease in systemic vascular resistance.

A number of other significant pharmacodynamic and physiologic effects may occur with each of the specific intravenous anesthetic agents. Etomidate inhibits the activity of 17-α-hydroxylase and 11-β-hydroxylase, which are necessary for the production of adrenal corticosteroids.[93,94] This effect occurs even after the use of a single dose for anesthetic induction, with adrenal suppression lasting 5 to 8 h. There is no evidence to suggest that the adrenal suppression from a single induction dose of etomidate has clinical sequelae, although increased mortality has been reported in critically ill patients in the intensive care unit (ICU) when receiving continuous infusions of etomidate for days.[95]

Etomidate and ketamine can also cause significant postoperative nausea and vomiting (PONV). In contrast, propofol is the only intravenous anesthetic with antiemetic properties.[96,97]

Ketamine is unique in producing profound analgesia, while the other anesthetic induction agents do not have analgesic properties. Thiopental, midazolam, and etomidate can precipitate acute intermittent porphyria and are therefore contraindicated in patients with this comorbidity.[98] Although all intravenous anesthetics except etomidate cause some histamine release, the incidence of severe anaphylactic reactions is low.

Additional problems with propofol relate to its delivery in a lipid emulsion (the same lipid preparation used in parenteral hyperalimentation solutions, otherwise known as intralipid). These problems include rare reports of anaphylactoid reactions (more likely in patients with a history of egg allergy[99]), pain on injection, and elevated triglyceride levels with prolonged infusions. Variable success in decreasing the incidence of pain has been reported with various maneuvers, including the preadministration of lidocaine, mixing the lidocaine and propofol in a single solution, mixing the propofol with thiopental,[100] diluting the concentration of the propofol, or cooling the propofol prior to bolus administration. Another alternative is the administration of a small dose of ketamine (0.5 mg/kg) prior to the administration of propofol.[101] Since propofol has limited analgesic properties, ketamine and propofol can be administered together to take advantage of the analgesia provided by ketamine and the rapid recovery with propofol.

Additional problems related to the lipid content of propofol may occur when propofol is used for continuous sedation in the ICU setting. High doses and prolonged infusions may result in hypertriglyceridemia and its associated effects. A propofol infusion of 2 mg/kg/h provides approximately 0.5 gm/kg/day of fat. In an attempt to eliminate or lessen such problems, a 2% solution of propofol (twice the amount of propofol with the same amount of lipid per milliliter as the 1% solution) is undergoing clinical evaluations.[102,103] Although the issues related to increased triglycerides may be eliminated with the 2% solution, there may be an alteration in propofol's bioavailability as there seems to be an increased dose requirement when the 2% solution is used compared with the 1% solution.

The pharmacokinetic profile of intravenous anesthetic agents is characterized by a rapid onset of CNS effects secondary to their high lipid solubility and the high percentage of cardiac output perfusing the brain. The termination of the central effect occurs from redistribution of the drug from the central to the peripheral compartment and is not dependent on primary metabolism and elimination of the drug from the body. Most intravenous anesthetics are metabolized in the liver and excreted in the kidney. Some metabolites are active, such as desmethyldiazepam (diazepam) and norketamine (ketamine), and may result in prolonged effects. There is a wide variation in the elimination half-lives of intravenous anesthetic agents because of differences in clearance. Drugs with short elimination half-lives include propofol, etomidate, ketamine, and midazolam, whereas thiopental has a long elimination half-life. Propofol is widely used, especially in ambulatory surgery centers, because of its short duration of action, fast recovery time, and early discharge potential.[104,105] Drugs with short elimination half-lives are suitable for continuous infusions that yield less fluctuation in plasma drug levels and fewer side effects, thereby making the use of a propofol infusion a popular choice for brief, outpatient surgical procedures in which a rapid recovery from anesthesia and discharge from the hospital are desirable.[106]

Each intravenous anesthetic has unique features that affect its clinical use (Table 18.4). Thiopental is highly alkaline (pH 10) and very irritating to tissues if extravasation into soft tissues occurs. Inadvertent intraarterial injection of thiopental can cause intense vasoconstriction, thrombosis, and tissue necrosis. Seventy-five percent to 85% of thiopental is bound to plasma albumin and therefore is inactive. Drug interactions and pathological states (renal or liver dysfunction) that affect plasma albumin levels can alter the amount of unbound, active thiopental and have an impact on the dose required. Although thiopental is classified as an ultrashort-acting barbiturate with return of consciousness occurring 5 to 10 min after an induction dose, the return to recovery can be significantly delayed because of its long elimination half-life.

Propofol is widely used, especially in ambulatory surgery centers, because of its rapid recovery time and limited residual postoperative sedation and psychomotor impairment. Propofol is solubilized in a solution of soybean oil, glycerol, and egg phosphatide that can support bacterial growth. Bacterially contaminated propofol has been reported to cause sepsis and death, and strict guidelines have been developed for its safe use.[106,107] Pain may be experienced with the injection of pro-

TABLE 18.4. Clinical Characteristics of Commonly Used Intravenous Induction Agents.

Agent	*Onset*	*Induction*	*Cardiovascular effects*	*Respiratory effects*	*Analgesia*	*Emergence*	*Additional notes*
Thiopental	Rapid	Smooth	Depression	Depression	None	Rapid to intermediate with some hangover effect with residual lethargy	Cardiovascular effects make it a poor choice for patients with compromised hemodynamic function
Etomidate	Rapid	Pain on injection, myoclonic activity	Minimal	Minimal	None	Rapid	Adrenal suppression even with single induction dose; not recommended for continuous infusion; may lead to postoperative nausea and vomiting
Midazolam	Intermediate	Smooth	Minimal	Depression	None	Intermediate	Rarely used alone for anesthetic induction; frequently combined with opioids
Ketamine	Rapid	Excitatory	Increased heart rate and blood pressure	Limited	Yes	Intermediate	May elevate ICP when used alone; emergence phenomena or hallucinations without coadministration of benzodiazepine or other anesthetic agent
Propofol	Rapid	Pain on injection	Depression	Depression	No	Rapid	Popular drug for anesthetic induction given rapid awakening and antiemetic effect

pofol, especially through smaller-gauge intravenous cannulae placed on the dorsum of the hand. The incidence and severity of pain can be attenuated by pretreatment with intravenous lidocaine or fentanyl. Etomidate also produces pain on injection secondary to the solubilizing additive propylene glycol. This also can be reduced by pretreatment with intravenous lidocaine or fentanyl.

Ketamine is structurally related to the hallucinogen phencyclidine and is a dissociative anesthetic, creating a functional and electrophysiological dissociation between the thalamoneocortical system and the limbic system. It produces a state known as *dissociative anesthesia* in which the eyes remain open with a slow nystagmic gaze, and corneal and light reflexes remain intact, making it difficult to judge the anesthetic depth of the patient. Emergence phenomena (hallucinations) can occur when ketamine is used as a sole agent. These can be limited or prevented by pretreatment with benzodiazepines. There is also ongoing work with the isolated enantiomere, s(+) ketamine, which is more potent when compared with the racemic mixture of ketamine but it may lack the psychomimetic effects. Unlike the other intravenous anesthetic induction agents, ketamine can be administered intramuscularly as well as intravenously and is occasionally used in combative patients (mentally retarded adults) in whom intravenous access cannot be achieved. Ketamine is a recommended induction agent for patients in hypovolemic shock from trauma or patients with cardiac tamponade because it supports hemodynamic function and systemic vascular resistance better than other induction agents. Ketamine also remains an acceptable choice for the intravenous induction of patients with asthma because of its bronchodilating properties.

Midazolam is not a popular intravenous anesthetic induction agent because of its slower onset of action, limited potency, and prolonged recovery time. However, it is versatile and can be used for premedication or sedation during **monitored anesthesia care**, peripheral nerve blocks, or regional anesthesia. It is an anxiolytic, sedative, hypnotic, and amnestic. It can also be administered intramuscularly or by nonparenteral routes (orally mixed in a flavored syrup, intranasally, rectally, or sublingually) as a premedication in children prior to inhalation induction. Its effects can be reversed with the antagonist flumazenil, although initial therapy when adverse hemodynamic effects occur with its use are directed at airway management and hemodynamic support as the onset time of flumazenil may be prolonged (minutes). In addition, flumazenil is meant only to reverse the effects of the acute administration of benzodiazepines. When used in other settings, such as for patients chronically receiving benzodiazepines, those with underlying seizure disorders, or when other medications have been administered (tricyclic antidepressants), adverse effects, including seizures and ventricular arrhythmias, have been reported.

Opioids

Opioids can be classified as natural, semisynthetic, or synthetic compounds with morphine-like properties. The naturally occurring opioid, morphine, and especially the synthetic compounds of the fentanyl family (fentanyl, sufentanil, remifentanil, and alfentanil) are commonly used in anesthesia practice. Opioids are used as premedicants, sedatives, intravenous anesthetics, components of general anesthetics, postoperative analgesics, and intraspinal analgesics. The commonly used opioids are pure agonists that are selective for μ (mu) opioid receptors located at discrete sites throughout the spinal cord and the CNS.[108] With increasing plasma concentrations, opioids produce analgesia, sedation, and ultimately hypnosis (sleep). Even in doses sufficient to produce profound analgesia and apnea, the opioids do not consistently produce amnesia in healthy patients, and therefore other agents are required for intraoperative anesthetic care to ensure amnesia.[109] Opioids produce analgesia that attenuates or abolishes autonomic and somatic responses to surgical stimuli (stress response).

Respiratory depression is the major toxicity of opioids. They produce a dose-related depression of the ventilatory response to CO_2 through a direct effect on the respiratory centers in the medulla.[110] The opioids also blunt the ventilatory response to hypoxia. As the dose is increased, the respiratory rate slows. The slowing of the respiratory rate is initially offset by an increase in tidal volume. Analgesic doses rarely cause significant respiratory depression unless the patient has significant preexisting pathology or prior sedative/analgesic administration. Equianalgesic doses of all opioids (fentanyl, morphine, meperidine, etc.) produce equivalent degrees of respiratory depression. The myth that using one opioid versus another provides some safety regarding respiratory depression is false (Table 18.5). Opioid-induced respiratory depression is antagonized by pain, movement, and opioid antagonists such as naloxone. When used properly (small incremental doses of 1 μg/kg every 2 to 3 min), it is generally possible to reverse opioid-induced respiratory depression without reversing analgesia.

When confronted with the patient with opioid-induced respiratory depression, treatment begins with addressing airway and breathing by the administration of supplementation oxygen or assisted ventilation using bag-valve-mask ventilation as needed. Opioid administration should be discontinued and incremental doses of naloxone administered as needed to provide an acceptable respiratory rate. Given the short half-life of naloxone (20–30 min), repeated doses may be needed if longer-acting opioids (morphine, meperidine, or hydromorphone) have been administered. Longer-acting opioid antagonists (nalmefene) are now clinically available but have had little clinical use in the practice of anesthesia. Opioid reversal using naloxone and similar agents can result in undesirable or dangerous hemodynamic responses, such as hypertension, tachycardia, and myocardial infarction. The potential for such effects must be weighed against the anticipated benefits of opioid reversal.

TABLE 18.5. Potency and Half-life of Opioids.

Agent	*Potency*	*Half-life (h)*	*Active metabolites*
Morphine	1	2 to 3	Yes
Meperidine	0.1	2 to 3	Yes
Hydromorphone	5	2 to 4	No
Oxymorphone	10	2 to 4	No
Methadone	1	12 to 24	No
Fentanyl	100	20 to 30 min	No
Sufentanil	1000	20 to 30 min	No
Alfentanil	20	10 to 15 min	No
Reminfentanil	100	5 to 8 min	No

Opioids generally produce minimal cardiovascular effects at usual analgesic doses. With higher doses, when combined with other anesthetic drugs, or in patients with comorbid features, opioids may produce bradycardia and vasodilation, resulting in hypotension and decreased cardiac output. Bradycardia results from stimulation of the central nuclei of the vagus nerve leading to prolonged atrioventricular (AV) conduction and direct depression of the sinoatrial (SA) node.[111] Peripheral vasodilation is the result of depression of the vasomotor centers in the medulla.[112] Patients with elevated levels of sympathetic tone (hypovolemia, CHF) are more likely to become hypotensive after opioids. Anesthetic techniques with high doses of opioids may result in bradycardia and peripheral vasodilation. However, given that minimal direct myocardial effects occur, these techniques are effective for patients with myocardial pathology, including patients undergoing cardiovascular surgery in whom administration of high doses of fentanyl (25–75 μg/kg) is a frequently chosen anesthetic technique. Decreases in blood pressure with such techniques result from a direct decrease in systemic vascular resistance and can be treated with direct-acting α-adrenergic agonists such as phenylephrine. Given their relatively short half-lives, longer-acting agents (morphine, hydromorphone) are required during the perioperative period to provide effective analgesia. There may be minor differences in the cardiovascular effects noted with the other opioids. Morphine may result in more profound venodilation, leading to decreased venous return, decreased cardiac output, and hypotension. Meperidine, given its structural similarity to atropine, may result in mild tachycardia.

Large intravenous doses of fentanyl, sufentanil, remifentanil, or alfentanil can produce a generalized hypertonus of skeletal muscle.[113] The synthetic opioids bind to receptors in extrapyramidal nuclei, increasing dopamine biosynthesis and inhibiting the release of the inhibitory neurotransmittor GABA.[114] This problem usually occurs during the induction of anesthesia when large doses of synthetic opioids are administered rapidly. The rigidity may involve the abdominal, thoracic, neck, or extremity muscles. In its most severe form, the rigidity can prevent spontaneous or mechanical ventilation because of contraction of the laryngeal and pharyngeal muscles and a loss of chest wall compliance. Positive pressure ventilation and small doses of NMBAs are required for treatment.

In the GI tract, opioids decrease the propulsive activity of the small and large bowel, delay gastric emptying, and cause smooth muscle contraction of the biliary tree and spasm of the sphincter of Oddi.[100] The biliary effects can be antagonized by naloxone, glucagon, nitroglycerine, or atropine.[115] The GI effects of opioids can be particularly bothersome during the postoperative period, leading to constipation, impaction, and delayed enteral feeding. Although tolerance develops to many of the other adverse effects of opioids, tolerance to the GI effects does not develop, making GI issues particularly bothersome when using long-term opioid therapy in patients with chronic pain.

In an effort to deal with the GI effects of both the acute and chronic use of opioids, current research is directed at the use of oral opioid antagonists that are not absorbed and do not cross the blood–brain barrier. These agents may be able to block the GI effects without affecting the analgesic potency of opioids.

In the genitourinary tract, opioids increase the tone of the detrusor muscle of the bladder and urinary sphincter, thereby causing urinary retention. Other opioid effects include the suppression of cough centers in the medulla; stimulation of the chemoreceptor trigger zone (CTZ), causing nausea and vomiting; and stimulation of the Edinger–Westphal nucleus of the oculomotor nerve to produce miosis. Pinpoint pupils are a pathognomonic sign of opioid use as well as overdose.

True allergic reactions to opioids are rare. Morphine produces a nonimmunological release of histamine from tissue mast cells, while opioids of the fentanyl family do not release histamine.[116] Tolerance and physical dependence occur with chronic opioid use, and withdrawal symptoms may be seen with the abrupt discontinuation of therapy. However, psychological dependence and addiction are rare when opioids are used in the management of acute pain, and fears of such problems should not prevent the appropriate use of opioids and dose escalations in the treatment of acute pain issues.

The main reasons for selecting a particular opioid for anesthesia is based on the time of onset and the duration of action of the drug.[117,118] Morphine is the least lipophilic of the commonly used opioids and has a slow onset of action and a long duration of analgesia. Morphine is biotransformed in the liver, and the metabolites of hepatic metabolism are excreted in the urine. In part, morphine is converted to morphine-6-glucoronide (M6G), a metabolite with a potency far greater than that of the parent compound. However, given that it is water soluble, there is limited penetration of M6G into the CNS through the blood–brain barrier and therefore limited clinical effects. In patients with renal insufficiency or failure, a significant amount of M6G can accumulate and result in respiratory depression.

Alternatives to morphine include meperidine and hydromorphone. Meperidine has a potency a tenth that of morphine with a similar half-life (2–3 h). It undergoes hepatic metabolism to normeperidine, a metabolite that may accumulate in certain clinical scenarios, including renal insufficiency. High plasma concentrations of normeperidine may cause seizures. Given these concerns and a higher incidence of psychomimetic effects with meperidine, our current clinical practice does not include its use in low doses (10 mg) to treat postanesthesia shivering.

Hydromorphone has a potency that is six to eight times that of morphine with a half-life of 2–3 h. As there are no active metabolites of hydromorphone, it may be an effective alternative to morphine in patients with renal insufficiency. In addition, hydromorphone causes less histamine release than morphine and may be an effective agent when adverse effects such as pruritus occur with morphine use.

Fentanyl, sufentanil, and alfentanil are potent, highly lipid-soluble drugs with rapid onsets and short durations of action. They are biotransformed in the liver, excreted by the kidney, and do not have active metabolites. Although sufentanil has 10 times the potency of fentanyl, the pharmacokinetics are similar, with both drugs short acting at low doses and longer acting at higher doses. The termination of their effect is dependent on redistribution, and because both drugs have long elimination half-lives, accumulation and prolonged duration of action occur after multiple doses or with infusions. Alfentanil is less potent than sufentanil and fentanyl and has very rapid onset and short duration of action. Because its elimination half-life is substantially less than that of sufentanil and fentanyl, it is suitable for multiple dosing and continuous infusions and is popular for ambulatory surgery in many centers.

Remifentanil is the newest of the synthetic opioids. It is the first true ultrashort-acting opioid.[119] It is structurally unique, having ester linkages that are hydrolyzed by blood and tissue nonspecific esterases to inactive metabolites. It has a rapid onset of activity and a short, predictable duration of action. Its elimination half-life is 8 to 10 min, and its potency is comparable to fentanyl. It is administered as a continuous infusion and remains short acting regardless of the duration of the infusion. Unlike the other opioids, which have longer half-lives and a variable duration of effect in neonates and infants, the duration of action and half-life of remifentanil are constant across all age ranges, thereby making it a suitable agent in neonatal anesthesia.

The opioids play a key role in anesthesia practice. Fentanyl, sufentanil, and alfentanil are common components of various anesthetic techniques. They have replaced their predecessors (morphine, meperidine) because of their faster onsets of action, shorter and more predictable duration of action, and minimal hemodynamic side effects. For general anesthesia, they reduce the surgical stress response and the associated cardiovascular responses to endotracheal intubation and surgical stimulation. They potentiate the hypnotic effects of barbiturates and benzodiazepines. They produce a dose-related decrease in the need for potent inhalational anesthetic agents. High-dose opioid techniques are commonly used in cardiac surgery because the synthetic opioids produce a smooth induction process, provide hemodynamic stability, suppress the hemodynamic responses to various surgical stimulations, reduce the production of stress hormones, and provide a smooth transition to mechanical ventilation at the end of the case.

Inhalational Anesthetic Agents

The inhalational anesthetic agents include nitrous oxide (N_2O) and five potent inhalational agents (halothane, enflurane, isoflurane, sevoflurane, and desflurane). The potent agents are two chemically distinct classes (alkanes and ethers) with similar hypnotic properties. Halothane is an alkane (a two-carbon chain), while the other four agents (enflurane, isoflurane, desflurane, and sevoflurane) are ethers. The potent inhalational anesthetic agents are volatile liquids and are administered to the patient via a vaporizer that is situated on the anesthesia machine. The vaporizer allows the anesthesia provider to increase or decrease the inspired concentration of the agent by turning the dial on the device. As the concentration is increased, more of the fresh gas flow from the anesthesia machine is diverted into the vaporizer, thereby increasing the output of the agent and thereby its inspired concentration. As the vapor pressures of the potent inhalational anesthetic agents vary, in modern anesthetic practice each vaporizer is specific for the individual potent inhalational anesthetic agent.

The onset and duration of action of an inhalational agent are determined by its blood–gas solubility coefficient. This coefficient describes how the anesthetic partitions itself between the arterial blood and alveolar gas when equilibrium is reached. The goal is to achieve a specific partial pressure of the inhalation anesthetic in the brain to create the desired effect. An agent with a high blood–gas solubility (partition) coefficient has a slower onset of action and a longer duration of action on discontinuation than an agent with a low blood–gas solubility coefficient. In addition, the depth of anesthesia can be adjusted more quickly with an agent that has a lower blood–gas solubility coefficient. Of the potent inhalation agents, desflurane has the lowest blood–gas solubility coefficient and therefore the most rapid onset and offset of activity, followed in order by sevoflurane, isoflurane, enflurane, and halothane. The lower solubility in blood allows the alveolar concentration of the agent and hence the blood and brain concentrations of the agent to increase more rapidly than agents with a higher solubility in blood. Nitrous oxide has a low blood–gas solubility coefficient, comparable to desflurane.

The potency of inhalational anesthetic agents is measured by MAC (minimum alveolar concentration). The MAC is defined as the percentage of the inhalational agent in 1 atmosphere that is required to prevent 50% of patients from moving in response to a surgical stimulus. Since it is not acceptable to have 50% of patients moving, 1.5 to 2.5 MAC of an agent are required to maintain anesthesia solely with a potent inhalation agent. However, in most clinical scenarios, 1.0–1.5 MAC of an inhalational anesthetic agent is combined with N_2O, opioids, or intravenous anesthetic agents to provide maintenance anesthesia during a surgical procedure.

The lower the MAC value for an inhalation agent, the more potent the gas. Halothane is the most potent inhalational anesthetic agent, followed in order by isoflurane, enflurane, sevoflurane, and desflurane. Nitrous oxide has a very low potency (MAC of 110%) and must be combined with other intravenous sedatives/analgesics/anesthetics or a potent inhalational anesthetic agent to fulfill the prerequisites (unconsciousness, analgesia, muscle relaxation, decrease in sympathetic nervous system activity) of a general anesthetic (Table 18.6).

Nitrous oxide is the oldest of the commonly used inhalational anesthetic agents, and although there has been a decline in its use with the introduction of newer inhalational anesthetic agents with low blood–gas solubility coefficients (desflurane, sevoflurane), it remains a common component of many general anesthetics. Depending on the concentration administered, N_2O can be a sedative/analgesic or a weak anesthetic. In concentrations of 70%, N_2O (with 30% O_2) will render the majority of patients amnestic and provide moderate-to-significant analgesia. However, only minor surgical procedures can be performed with N_2O and O_2 alone.

TABLE 18.6. Characteristics of the Inhalational Anesthetic Agents.

Agent	*Blood–gas partition coefficient*	*Minimum alveolar concentration*	*Percentage metabolized*
Nitrous oxide	0.47	105	0
Halothane	2.4	0.75	15–20
Enflurane	1.9	1.68	2–3
Isoflurane	1.4	1.15	0.2
Desflurane	0.42	6.0	<0.1
Sevoflurane	0.6	2.0	5–10

Nitrous oxide causes minimal respiratory and cardiac depression.[120] Recovery from N_2O is rapid given its low blood-gas solubility coefficient. During recovery, high concentrations of O_2 are needed to avoid diffusion hypoxia.[121] As N_2O diffuses from the blood into the alveoli, its concentration rises, thereby decreasing the effective concentration of oxygen, which can lead to diffusion hypoxia. Chronic exposure to N_2O can lead to impairment of bone marrow function and anemia by inactivation of methionine synthetase, an enzyme necessary for vitamin B_{12} metabolism.[122,123] This same effect on vitamin B_{12} metabolism can, with repeated or prolonged exposure, lead to neurological signs and symptoms with deterioration of the posterior columns of the spinal cord. Nitrous oxide diffuses into and expands gas-containing closed spaces in the body (obstructed bowel, pneumothorax, middle ear, pneumocephalus, and air embolus) because it is significantly more soluble in blood than nitrogen.[124] With time, the pressure in the closed cavity and size of the cavity can increase to dangerous levels, with resultant physiologic changes based on the site of accumulation.

The potent inhalational agents provide all of the necessary prerequisites of a general anesthetic. How potent inhalational anesthetic agents work has not been fully determined, although recent work suggests that they stabilize critical proteins, possibly receptors of neurotransmitters.[125] All of the potent inhalational anesthetic agents are nonflammable and nonexplosive in clinical concentrations. Halothane and sevoflurane are less pungent to the airway than the other agents and are preferred for the inhalation induction of anesthesia. Given its limited potential for causing myocardial depression when compared with halothane, sevoflurane has become the preferred agent for inhalation induction in pediatric patients. Surveys of the etiology of cardiac arrest during general anesthesia in infants and children have implicated inadvertent overdosing of halothane as the primary factor responsible for many of these events.

All of the potent agents cause a dose-related depression of cardiovascular and respiratory function. With increasing anesthetic depth, the inhalational anesthetic agents result in a progressive decrease in alveolar ventilation characterized by a significant reduction in tidal volume in spontaneously breathing patients and an increase in Pa_{CO_2}. The potent agents also interfere with the normal ventilatory responses to hypercarbia and hypoxia and inhibit mucociliary function. Beneficial effects on the airways include a direct effect on bronchial smooth muscle with bronchodilation, making them an effective agent outside the OR for the treatment of patients with refractory status asthmaticus.

The inhalational anesthetic agents decrease mean arterial pressure, myocardial contractility, and myocardial oxygen consumption. The decrease in mean arterial pressure reduces renal blood flow and hepatic blood flow. Changes in cardiac output, systemic vascular resistance, and heart rate vary from agent to agent. Isoflurane and desflurane result primarily in vasodilation with reflex tachycardia, while a decrease in heart rate is commonly seen with sevoflurane and halothane. Halothane, because of its alkane structure, sensitizes the myocardium to catecholamines and can cause dysrhythmias, especially when there is associated hypercarbia or high circulating catecholamines. The latter may occur when anesthetized patients receive large doses of epinephrine-containing local anesthetic agents.

The potent inhalational agents cause a dose-related decrease in CNS activity, reducing cerebral metabolic oxygen consumption and depressing EEG activity. Enflurane and sevoflurane can activate the EEG and produce clinical and EEG evidence of seizure activity at high concentrations. Such problems are more common during hyperventilation and the development of hypocarbia. Cerebral blood flow increases via a reduction in cerebral vascular resistance, which can lead to an elevation in ICP in patients with compromised intracranial compliance. The effect on ICP is least with isoflurane and can be blunted by hyperventilation and hypocarbia. These effects make isoflurane a common choice for neurosurgical anesthesia. The potent inhalational anesthetic agents depress neuromuscular activity and enhance the effect of the NMBAs. The potent inhalational anesthetic agents are potential triggering agents for malignant hyperthermia (MH), an inherited disorder of muscle metabolism.

The chemical structure of the potent agent determines its stability and its eventual metabolic fate. In addition to the parent compound, metabolic products may be responsible for the toxicity of these agents. For halothane, 15% to 20% is recovered as metabolites compared to 5% to 10% for sevoflurane, 2% to 3% for enflurane, 0.2% for isoflurane, and less than 0.1% for desflurane. Hepatotoxicity can occur by an immune-mediated reaction following exposure to halothane, enflurane, isoflurane, or desflurane.[126–129] The metabolic product trifluoroacetic acid (TFA) can act as a hapten, binding to hepatocytes and inducing an immune-mediated hepatitis. Although described primarily with halothane, there have been rare anecdotal reports of hepatitis with all of the other potent inhalational agents except for sevoflurane. The metabolic pathway of sevoflurane is different and does not result in the production of TFA.

Two types of halothane hepatotoxicity, mild and fulminant, have been described. The mild injury affects 20% of adults who receive halothane, while the fulminant form (halothane hepatitis) occurs in 1 of every 10,000 adult patients who receive halothane. Patients with the fulminant form develop massive hepatic necrosis with a mortality rate of 50% to 75%. Most of the these patients (up to 95%) have had a prior exposure to halothane.

The most important predictive factor for anesthesia-induced hepatotoxicity is prior anesthetic exposure. Other risk factors include female gender, middle age, and obesity. Chronic ethanol ingestion and isoniazid use increase enzyme levels responsible for the metabolism of the potent inhalational anesthetic agents and increase the risk. Given these concerns, halothane is not recommended for adult use but remains popular in pediatric anesthesia because halothane hepatitis is rare in children (1/200,000).[130,131] Because cross-sensitization may occur, all of the potent inhalational anesthetic agents should be avoided in patients who have an unexplained postoperative hepatic injury following a prior exposure to a potent agent.

Several of the potent inhalational anesthetic agents have demonstrated toxic potential to the kidney related either to release of fluoride during metabolism or the production of potentially toxic metabolic by-products. Prolonged enflurane anesthesia has been shown to significantly diminish renal concentrating ability because of the metabolism of enflurane with the release of fluoride. Prolonged sevoflurane anesthesia may also produce transient renal injury. Sevoflurane reacts with the CO_2 absorbent in the carbon dioxide absorber of the anesthesia machine to produce a vinyl ether, compound A.[132–134] The safe concentration of compound A is unknown in humans, as is the mechanism of renal injury. Because of the concerns of the potential nephrotoxicity of sevoflurane, higher fresh gas flows (2l/min) are recommended during its use. An additional possible toxicity with potent inhalational agents results from degradation of the agent by strong bases in the carbon dioxide absorbent to produce carbon monoxide.[135,136] Although all of the potent inhalational anesthetic agents can produce carbon monoxide, desflurane yields the highest levels, followed in order by enflurane, isoflurane, sevoflurane, and halothane. Production of clinically significant levels of carbon monoxide is rare and has only been reported with desiccated soda lime.

The potent inhalational anesthetic agents are unique in providing all four requirements of a general anesthetic. The addition of nitrous oxide enables a reduction in the concentration of the potent agent required and therefore a decrease in the undesirable features caused by the agent. The dose required of the potent inhalational anesthetic agent varies from patient to patient and is continuously adjusted to match surgical stimulation. The alveolar concentration, a close approximation of brain concentration, of a potent inhalational anesthetic agent is continuously monitored during the course of a case by sampling the exhaled gases from the anesthesia circuit. The increase in outpatient surgery has necessitated the development of potent inhalational anesthetic agents with low blood–gas solubilities, which provide rapid awakening and hospital discharge. These needs have resulted in the addition to anesthesia practice of desflurane and sevoflurane.[137]

Neuromuscular Blocking Agents

Skeletal muscle relaxation can be achieved by potent inhalational anesthetic agents, regional anesthesia, or NMBAs. The NMBAs are used to facilitate endotracheal intubation, decrease muscle tone during general anesthesia, and assist with mechanical ventilation in the ICU. Their site of action is the neuromuscular junction. They have no effect on the level of consciousness and provide neither amnesia nor analgesia. When NMBAs are used, the patient requires an adequate level of general anesthesia and in the ICU an adequate level of sedation. This is especially important since clinical signs of inadequate anesthesia (movement) are abolished. It is also important to recognize that the airway must be controlled when NMBAs are used These agents are contraindicated if there is any concern regarding one's ability to control ventilation.

The NMBAs are classified by their mechanism of action (depolarizing vs. nondepolarizing); duration of action (ultrashort, short, intermediate, and long acting); and chemical structure (steroidal, benzylisoquinoline, ester). The choice of NMBA is influenced by the required speed of onset, duration of action, route of elimination, and associated side effects (Table 18.7).

The NMBAs inhibit the activation of the nicotinic receptor–ion channel complex at the muscle's motor end plate by acetylcholine. The postjunctional receptor is composed of five subunits (two α-chains and one each of the β-, γ-, and δ-chains). The two α-subunits are binding sites for

TABLE 18.7. Characteristics of Neuromuscular Blocking Agents.

Agent	*Classification*	*Onset*	*Clinical duration (min) following standard intubating dose*	*Recovery time (min)*	*Standard intubating dose (mg/kg)*
Succinylcholine	Ultrashort	Very rapid	6–8	15	1–2
Mivacurium	Short	Intermediate	10–20	20–30	0.2
Atracurium	Intermediate	Intermediate	30–50	50–70	0.6
Vecuronium	Intermediate	Intermediate	30–50	50–70	0.1
Rocuronium	Intermediate	Rapid	30–50	50–70	0.6
cis-Atracurium	Intermediate	Intermediate	30–50	50–70	0.2
Pancuronium	Long	Slow	60–90	90–180	0.1

acetylcholine and are the sites occupied by NMBAs. The nondepolarizing NMBAs act as competitive antagonists for acetylcholine at the end plate, competitively blocking its binding with the receptor and preventing depolarization of the sarcolemma or muscle membrane. Depolarizing agents activate the acetylcholine receptor, causing depolarization. However, the depolarizing agents are resistant to degradation by acetylcholinesterase and therefore occupy the receptor for much longer than acetylcholine and thereby prevent repolarization. Without repolarization, subsequent depolarization cannot occur, leading to neuromuscular blockade.

Succinylcholine is an ultrashort-acting NMBA with the most rapid onset of action. It is the only depolarizing NMBA in clinical use. It consists of two acetylcholine molecules linked together and reacts with the two α-subunits of the nicotinic receptors at the neuromuscular junction to keep the receptor–ion channel open. Prolonged depolarization and paralysis occur. After succinylcholine diffuses away from the receptors, the membrane repolarizes and will then respond to neuromuscular transmission.

The greatest advantage of succinylcholine is its rapid onset (30–60 s) and brief duration of action (5–10 min). Succinylcholine is resistant to acetylcholinesterase, and its effect is terminated by diffusion away from the site and subsequent metabolism by plasma cholinesterase (pseudocholinesterase). Occasionally, patients are unable to metabolize succinylcholine because of either a low quantity (liver disease; effects of medications, including various chemotherapeutic agents; pregnancy) or abnormal quality (atypical cholinesterase) of plasma cholinesterase. The latter can be inherited as a Mendelian trait; therefore, part of the normal preoperative workup is to question the patient regarding a family history of the need for postoperative mechanical ventilation. Such patients can be identified by measuring the level of pseudocholinesterase when a quantitative deficit is suspected or by assaying the quality of the enzyme. The latter assay is generally performed only in specialized reference laboratories by obtaining a dibucaine number, which determines the functional effects of the enzyme. When prolonged neuromuscular blockade occurs following the administration of succinylcholine due to issues with pseudocholinesterase levels or function, postoperative mechanical ventilation may be required for up to 4–6 h. During this time, adequate amnesia must be ensured. Although the enzyme is present in fresh frozen plasma, the most prudent action is generally to provide mechanical ventilation and amnesia and avoid the use of blood products.

Succinylcholine is commonly used for endotracheal intubation in emergency situations, when there is a concern regarding a potentially difficult airway, or in patients with a "full stomach" as part of a rapid sequence induction. In the past, prior to the development and marketing of short-acting NMBAs, succinylcholine was administered as a continuous infusion to provide a longer period of neuromuscular blockade while allowing rapid recovery once the procedure was completed.

Succinylcholine also binds to nicotinic receptors in autonomic ganglia and muscarinic cholinergic receptors in the heart and can have hemodynamic consequences, including hypertension, dysrhythmias, or bradycardia. The last is particularly prevalent in infants and children or in patients experiencing hypoxemia. In these situations, atropine is recommended prior to the administration of succinylcholine. The most lethal adverse effect of succinylcholine is hyperkalemia. Although a modest increase in the serum potassium level (0.5 mEq/l) occurs in most patients following the administration of succinylcholine, more profound hyperkalemia may occur in various comorbid features, including patients with burns, massive tissue trauma, upper and lower motor neuron lesions, and extensive skeletal muscle denervation. Extrajunctional receptors are synthesized in these states, and plasma levels of potassium can increase significantly following the administration of succinylcholine as activation of these receptors results in the opening of ion channels and the release of intracellular potassium. Succinylcholine is generally avoided in infants and children except in emergency situations when rapid securing of the airway is necessary, when the potential exists for a difficult airway, or when intravenous access is not present. In addition to its rapid onset of action when administered intravenously, succinylcholine can also be used intramuscularly when airway emergencies (laryngospasm) occur during the inhalation induction of anesthesia prior to securing intravenous access.

However, succinylcholine is no longer recommended for routine use in pediatric patients given the potential for hyperkalemia in patients with a previously undiagnosed myopathy.[138] In these cases, sudden death has occurred within minutes after succinylcholine administration due to massive rhabdomyolysis and severe hyperkalemia. Other potential adverse effects of succinylcholine include muscle fasciculations, which may result in severe postoperative pain; myalgias, masseter spasm (trismus); increases in intraocular pressure (IOP), intragastric pressure, and ICP; myoglobinemia; anaphylaxis; and MH. The increases in IOP that occur with succinylcholine relatively contraindicate its use in patients with an open globe injury. Large doses of succinylcholine may create a prolonged block (phase II block) that resembles the type of neuromuscular blockade that is seen with the use of nondepolarizing NMBAs.

Nondepolarizing NMBAs competitively inhibit acetylcholine at the motor end plate by occupying one or two of the α-subunits of the nicotinic receptor–channel complex close to the ion channel and thereby preventing depolarization. Nondepolarizing NMBAs are highly ionized at physiological pH, and their duration of action depends on redistribution to inactive tissue sites with subsequent metabolism and clearance from the body. Clinically, they are classified into short-, intermediate-, and long-acting drugs.

The ideal nondepolarizing NMBA would have a rapid onset of action, no hemodynamic side effects (histamine release, ganglionic blockade), and alternate pathways of elimination.[139,140] A fast-onset, ultrashort-acting nondepolarizer to replace succinylcholine has not been developed. Currently available alternatives (see below) to succinylcholine have a longer onset to optimal intubating conditions (60 s vs. 30–45 s with succinylcholine) and have a prolonged duration (60 min) of action following the doses needed to provide a rapid onset. The latest addition to the NMBA family, rapacurium, which was thought to rival the onset and offset of succinylcholine, was withdrawn from clinical use because of its effects on respiratory function and reports of profound bronchospasm and death with its use for emergency airway management.[141–144] Subsequent laboratory research has demonstrated that rapacuronium preferentially blocks the M_2-muscarinic receptor (receptor on the presynaptic side of the neuromuscular junction) in addition to the M_3 receptor (acetylcholine receptor on the sarcolemma). The M_2-muscarinic receptor regulates ongoing acetylcholine release and its blockade inhibits the normal negative feedback process, thereby augmenting acetylcholine release.

Mivacurium, a benzylisoquinoline, is the only nondepolarizing NMBA with a short duration of action.[145] Like succinylcholine, it is metabolized by plasma cholinesterase. Its onset of action following the recommended intubating dose of 0.2 mg/kg is slower than that of succinylcholine. Rapid administration of higher doses will increase the speed of onset; however, time to optimal intubating conditions remains at 1.5–2 min. Histamine release is seen commonly with routine intubating doses of 0.2 mg/kg and may lead to hypotension in patients with poor cardiovascular function. In the majority of patients, histamine release results in clinically insignificant cardiovascular changes but may result in total body erythema. Increasing the dose to achieve a more rapid onset results in increased histamine release and a greater potential for a decrease in MAP. Mivacurium can be administered in a continuous infusion to provide a prolonged effect with a predictable offset with discontinuation of the infusion. When this is done, the infusion rate is titrated using train-of-four (TOF) monitoring (see below). As with succinylcholine, a prolonged duration of action occurs in patients with decreased or atypical plasma cholinesterase.

Atracurium, a benzylisoquinoline, has an intermediate onset of activity and an intermediate duration of action.[146] It is not dependent on hepatic or renal function for elimination as it is metabolized by ester hydrolysis and Hoffman elimination (a nonenzymatic breakdown of the drug). High doses administered rapidly cause histamine release and a decrease in MAP. The principal metabolite of Hoffman degradation is laudanosine, which may be epileptogenic in high concentrations. When used for the usual duration of cases in the operating room, this is not a concern; however, a continuous infusion for several days in the ICU can result in high plasma concentrations of laudanosine, especially in the elderly and in patients with combined renal and hepatic failure. Hoffman degradation is affected by changes in body temperature, resulting in decreased dose requirements during hypothermia.

Like atracurium, *cis*-atracurium has an intermediate onset of activity and an intermediate duration of action that is independent of hepatic or renal function. As an isomer of atracurium, *cis*-atracurium is more potent, does not cause histamine release, and yields lower plasma levels of laudanosine following prolonged use. It would be an ideal intermediate-acting relaxant except that it has a slower onset time than atracurium.[147]

Vecuronium, a steroidal analogue of pancuronium, is an intermediate-acting NMBA with no direct cardiovascular effects.[148] It undergoes hepatic metabolism with active metabolites excreted primarily not only in the bile, but also in the kidney. The 3-OH metabolite has neuromuscular-blocking properties and is eliminated by the kidneys. Persistent plasma levels and extended blockade can occur following prolonged infusions in the ICU, especially in patients with renal insufficiency or failure. Patients with liver disease or renal disease may experience a prolonged effect following intraoperative use. To increase the speed of onset, larger doses of vecuronium (0.3 mg/kg) can be administered. These result in acceptable conditions for endotracheal intubation in approximately 60 s. Although the higher doses have no cardiovascular effects, a prolonged duration of action occurs (60–90 min).

Rocuronium, an analogue of vecuronium, is an intermediate-acting NMBA with a pharmacokinetic profile similar to vecuronium.[149] Unlike other nondepolarizing NMBAs, it has a rapid onset of action, producing good-to-excellent conditions for endotracheal intubation within 60 s, although its effect will also be prolonged (60 min) following intubating doses of 1 mg/kg. Rocuronium undergoes primarily hepatic metabolism, with some degree of renal excretion. Hence, its duration of action increases in patients with liver or kidney disease. Especially at higher doses, a mild vagolytic effect is seen, with a resultant increase in heart rate.

Pancuronium, pipecuronium, and doxacurium are long-acting (60–90 min) NMBAs with slow onset times (3–5 min). Given their duration of action, they are reserved for cases that last more than 2 h. Pancuronium, the oldest and most popular long-acting NMBA, is a steroidal molecule primarily eliminated by the kidneys. Hence, it has a prolonged duration of action in patients with renal disease. Pancuronium has a vagolytic effect through blockade of muscarinic receptors in the SA node. It increases transmission through sympathetic ganglia and inhibits norepinephrine reuptake in sympathetic terminals, resulting in tachycardia, elevations in MAP and cardiac output, and dysrhythmias. Pipecuronium and doxacurium demonstrate no cardiovascular side effects.[150] Their durations of action are prolonged in patients with renal failure.

The duration of action of any of the nondepolarizing NMBAs can be prolonged by neuromuscular diseases, potent inhalational anesthetic agents, aminoglycoside antibiotics, magnesium, local anesthetics (lidocaine), cardiac antidysrhythmics (quinidine), calcium channel blockers (verapamil), hypothermia, acidosis, and hypokalemia. Although allergic reactions are rare, NMBAs are high on the list of agents responsible for intraoperative anaphylactoid reactions second only to antibiotics.

Neuromuscular blockade may be used only to facilitate endotracheal intubation or may be continued throughout the surgical procedure to provide surgical relaxation. When ongoing neuromuscular blockade is required, incremental doses that are approximately a fourth to a fifth of the initial intubating dose are administered based on the response obtained using neuromuscular blockade monitoring. Neuromuscular blockade monitoring is used to predict optimal conditions for endotracheal intubation, adequacy of surgical muscle relaxation, effectiveness of reversal of neuromuscular blockade, and appropriate use of NMBAs in the ICU. The goal of such monitoring is to allow incremental titration of NMBAs to maintain the desired level of blockade while maintaining sufficient neuromuscular function to allow reversal of residual neuromuscular blockade at the completion of the surgical procedure. To accomplish monitoring of neuromuscular blockade, a supramaximal electrical stimulation from a peripheral nerve stimulator is delivered to electrodes placed over the distribution of the ulnar nerve at the wrist or elbow, the common peroneal nerve as it passes over the head of the fibula, or the facial nerve. When placed over the ulnar nerve, which innervates the adductor pollicis muscle, movement will be noted by adduction of the thumb. Electrical stimulation can be delivered as a single twitch, TOF, double-burst suppression, tetanus, and posttetanic stimulation. As any of these involve electrical stimulation, they are painful and should be performed only in an appropriately anesthetized patient. Each stimulation stresses the neuromuscular junction differently, and accurate interpretation enables the observer to determine the degree of neuromuscular blockade present. In most clinical scenarios, the anesthesiologist uses the TOF, by which two electrical stimuli are delivered each second for 2 s to give four twitches or a TOF.

Although used in common clinical practice, TOF monitoring is relatively nonspecific in that up to 70%–80% of the acetylcholine receptors must be blocked to achieve any visible decrement in the TOF. The goal of monitoring is to ensure that some residual neuromuscular function is present at the completion of the surgical procedure so that the effects can be reversed. The goal of reversal is for the patient to sustain minute ventilation and maintain a patent airway to allow for tracheal extubation.[147,151] In most clinical circumstances, one or two twitches of the TOF must be present to allow for effective pharmacologic reversal. A TOF of 0.7 or greater, in which the fourth twitch is 70% or more of the height of the first twitch, is evidence of adequate reversal.

Other tests of adequacy of reversal include a sustained response to tetanus, a sustained head lift for 5 to 10 s, and strong grip strength. In infants, sustained hip flexion is a useful clinical sign. Patients demonstrating profound blockade (no response to electrical stimulation) should not be reversed until some evidence of return of neuromuscular function has occurred. Despite adequate reversal, recurrence of partial paralysis resulting in respiratory insufficiency or upper airway obstruction may occur while the patient is in the postanesthesia care unit.

At the completion of the surgical procedure, reversal of residual neuromuscular blockade is accomplished using a drug that inhibits acetylcholinesterase, such as edrophonium, neostigmine, or pyridostigmine. By inhibiting acetylcholinesterase, these medications result in the accumulation of acetylcholine at the nicotinic (neuromuscular junction) and muscarinic sites, thereby increasing the competition between acetylcholine and the NMBA for the α-subunits of the nicotinic cholinergic receptor. Anticholinesterases have quaternary ammonium structures that limit their penetration into the CNS. However, as these medications also inhibit acetylcholinesterase at muscarinic sites, they must be coadministered with an anticholinergic agent such as atropine or glycopyrrolate to prevent bradycardia or asystole. An inadequate response to the anticholinesterase medication with residual weakness may be secondary to excessive blockade at the time of reversal, allowing inadequate time since the administration of the reversal drug, an altered acid–base or electrolyte status, hypothermia, effects of other medications, or impaired clearance of NMBAs from the plasma secondary to renal or hepatic dysfunction.

Intraoperative Anesthetic Care

Maintenance Anesthesia

This chapter has discussed the sequence of events from the time the patient presents for the preoperative evaluation through premedication, monitoring, and induction of general anesthesia. Once the airway has been secured and ventilation/oxygenation established, it becomes necessary to provide maintenance anesthesia. As is evident from the discussion of the various inhalational anesthetic agents, intravenous anesthetic agents, and opioids, there are several pharmacologic agents that can be used to provide the various prerequisites of general anesthesia. The choice of agent varies widely and is determined by the personal preferences and experiences of the anesthesia provider; the patient's comorbid features, most importantly the underlying cardiovascular function; the anticipated duration of the surgical procedure; the postoperative requirements (Will the patient's trachea be extubated at the completion of the procedure? Is ongoing postoperative analgesia required?); and the operative setting (Is rapid turnover of cases desirable, and are rapid awakening and hospital discharge needed?).

In most scenarios, the baseline level of anesthesia is provided by either a potent inhalational anesthetic agent or propofol and supplemented with intermittent dosing or a continuous infusion of an opioid. If ongoing neuromuscular blockade is required, a continuous infusion of a short-acting agent or intermittent dosing of an intermediate-to-long-acting agent can be used. Although controlled ventilation is most commonly practiced, there are many surgical procedures for which spontaneous ventilation is acceptable. The use of spontaneous ventilation is more common in the outpatient setting, where endotracheal intubation is less common, and general anesthesia is provided using a mask or an LMA.

In addition to commonly monitored hemodynamic parameters, spontaneous ventilation provides an effective means of assessing the depth of anesthesia and respiratory rate and provides the optimal parameter for dosing of opioids. When spontaneous ventilation is used, opioids can be dosed based on the patient's respiratory rate to ensure that an appropriate amount is administered to provide postoperative analgesia while avoiding overdosing and postoperative respiratory depression.

Intraoperative Fluid Management

In addition to monitoring hemodynamic and respiratory function, the anesthesiologist must maintain fluid, electrolyte, and glucose homeostasis during anesthetic care. Intraoperative fluid management uses isotonic crystalloid solutions such as lactated Ringer's (LR), normal saline (NS), or Plasmalyte to provide ongoing maintenance fluids and replace preoperative deficits, intraoperative third-space losses, and blood losses when blood therapy is not necessary. Third-space losses may be relatively trivial during superficial procedures (2–3 ml/kg/h) or significant (10–15 ml/kg/h) for intraabdominal procedures.

Although generally considered an isotonic fluid, LR has only 130 mEq of sodium per liter and therefore is relatively contraindicated in patients at risk for cerebral edema, including the multiple trauma patient. Large volumes of NS, although effective in supporting the serum sodium, can result in a dilutional acidosis. These issues have led to the consideration of using a combination of NS and LR or the use of a more balanced solution such as Plasmalyte, which contains 140 mEq/l of sodium, physiologic amounts of chloride, and gluconate/acetate as buffers.

Given the distribution between the intravascular and extravascular space, if blood therapy is not administered, blood loss is routinely replaced as 3 ml of crystalloid for each 1 ml of blood loss. Alternatives to isotonic crystalloid solutions include synthetic and natural colloids such as hydroxyethyl starch, albumin, or gelatins (these are not currently available in the United States). As with resuscitation in other areas, there are currently no studies demonstrating the superiority of any of these solutions over standard isotonic crystalloids, and it is likely that the crystalloid-colloid debate will continue for many years. Potential drawbacks to the use of hydroxyethyl starch solutions, including hetastarch solutions (Hespan or Hexted), include the potential for platelet dysfunction when amounts greater than 15–20 ml/kg are administered. This reversible platelet dysfunction results from alterations in the efficacy of von Willebrand factor by the hydroxyethyl starch solutions.

During the postoperative period, especially in pediatric patients, given the potential for the development of postoperative hyponatremia, fluids more hypotonic than half-normal saline are rarely indicated. For short surgical procedures when a Foley catheter is not inserted, aggressive fluid therapy with replacement of the preoperative deficit is not necessarily required since bladder distention during emergence from anesthesia may be uncomfortable for the patient. In addition, specific surgical procedures such as intracranial neurosurgical procedures and thoracic procedures or underlying cardiovascular dysfunction may mandate that the patient "be kept dry" to improve the intraoperative and postoperative course. However, in many other surgical procedures, especially intraabdominal cases, burn debridement, or other cases with significant third-space losses, the administration of significant amounts of isotonic crystalloids may be required to maintain intravascular volume status. Except for the neonatal population or patients chronically receiving parenteral nutrition fluids, dextrose-containing fluids are rarely administered. In high-risk patients, those receiving glucose-containing fluids, and diabetics, intermittent monitoring of blood glucose may be indicated. Although a review of the perioperative care of the diabetic patient is beyond the scope of this chapter, recent evidence has demonstrated that the postoperative outcome of such patients may be improved by tight perioperative glucose control. With the availability of rapid bedside testing, the rapid and intermittent determination of blood glucose concentrations is feasible.

Specific Perioperative Issues

Postoperative Analgesia

Inadequate pain relief following surgery has been attributed to inappropriate methods of administration more than to ineffective analgesic agents. The inadequacy of traditional intramuscular opioid regimens results from variable absorption and unpredictable plasma opioid concentrations in addition to patients' reluctance to ask for pain medications due to the pain associated with intramuscular injections.[152] Fortunately, the area of acute and postoperative analgesia has been of intense research, which has resulted in the development of new techniques and refinement of treatment strategies.[153] Current modalities to provide better postoperative analgesia include intravenous patient-controlled analgesia (PCA) and the use of epidural and spinal local anesthetics or opioids.

With PCA, patients self-administer opioids to obtain analgesia. Analgesia occurs when the plasma opioid concentration reaches the minimum effective analgesic concentration (MEAC). There is considerable interpatient variability of MEAC and therefore significant interpatient variability in analgesic requirements.[154] With PCA, patients titrate the opioid-to-plasma concentrations close to the MEAC and can maintain consistent analgesia.[155,156] Numerous studies have demonstrated improved analgesia, fewer adverse effects, and decreased opioid consumption with the use of PCA. Prior to the initiation of PCA, the patient receives multiple small doses of an opioid to achieve the MEAC and provide effective analgesia. Once this is accomplished, the PCA is started, and a dose of opioid (morphine 1 mg) is self-administered at a specific interval or lockout period (generally 5–10 min) as needed by the patient. In addition, a continuous infusion can be added to the PCA regimen, although it has been suggested that this negates the safety feature of PCA in which no opioid is delivered if the patient is too sleepy to push the button. With the continuous infusion, opioid is infused regardless of the patient's demand, which may increase the incidence of adverse effects, including respiratory depression.

In addition to the use of opioids, acetaminophen and nonsteroidal antiinflammatory agents play a significant role in the control of postoperative pain. Nonsteroidal antiinflammatory drugs (NSAIDs), acetaminophen, and salicylates act through the inhibition of the enzyme cyclooxygenase, thereby blocking the synthesis of prostaglandins that stimulate the free nerve endings of the peripheral nervous system. In distinction to opioids, these agents demonstrate a ceiling effect, so that once a specific plasma concentration is achieved, no further analgesia is provided by increasing the dose.

Although available as over-the-counter medications, these agents represent an effective means to control mild-to-moderate pain. They are classified according to their chemical structure as (1) para-amino phenol derivatives (acetaminophen), (2) NSAIDs (ibuprofen), and (3) salicylates (acetylsalicylic acid, choline magnesium trisalicilate).[157] When considering the para-aminol phenol derivatives, acetaminophen has a significant role in the management of acute pain, while phenacetin is no longer used given its potential toxicity profile (renal papillary necrosis). Although currently available only as an oral or rectal medication in the United States, acetaminophen or its prodrug propacetamol is available in Europe and elsewhere throughout the world. Although generally effective, there are issues with pain on administration, which has led to the development of an intravenous acetaminophen preparation that is currently undergoing clinical trials. Issues regarding Reye's syndrome in children and adolescents and its effects on platelet function have markedly decreased the use of salicylates during the past 20–30 years. Choline magnesium trisalicilate offers the analgesic advantages of an aspirin product while having limited effects on platelet function, making it an effective option in patients with qualitative and quantitative platelet issues. Commonly used NSAIDs include either ibuprofen for oral administration or ketorolac for intravenous administration. The reader is referred to reference 161 for a more in-depth discussion of the prostaglandin synthesis inhibitors.

The role of the prostaglandin synthesis inhibitors to treat acute pain includes their use as the sole agent for minor pain, their combination with weak opioids for oral administration to control moderate pain, and their addition to parenteral opioids and regional anesthetic techniques for severe pain. In the last situation, their use does not replace opioids or neuraxial techniques but rather provides adjunctive analgesia, thereby lowering the total amount of opioid required. As the majority of opioid-related adverse effects are dose related, modalities that decrease total opioid consumption play a significant role in decreasing or preventing opioid-associated adverse effects. When used for this purpose, the prostaglandin synthesis inhibitor is administered around the clock and not on an as-needed basis.

Decisions regarding prostaglandin synthesis inhibitors include the agent to be used and the route of administration. In most cases, oral administration is an effective and cost-beneficial alternative to intravenous administration. However, with oral administration, obstacles may arise that interfere with effective analgesia, including a delay in the onset, decreased bioavailability when compared with parenteral administration, refusal to take the medication, vomiting, and an inability to give enteral medications due to ileus or abdominal complaints.

Regional anesthetic techniques, including either neuraxial blockade (epidural or spinal analgesia) or peripheral nerve blockade can be continued into the postoperative period to provide effective analgesia while avoiding the potential adverse effects associated with parenteral opioid therapy. Epidural and spinal local anesthetics provide profound analgesia; however, undesirable side effects of the use of high concentrations of local anesthetics include blockade of the sympathetic nervous system with hypotension, urinary retention, and blockade of motor function. Epidural and spinal opioids can provide intense, segmental, localized analgesia without sensory, motor, or sympathetic nervous system effects. However, adverse effects of neuraxial opioids may include respiratory depression, nausea, pruritus, sedation, and urinary retention. As a result, combinations of low-dose epidural local anesthetics and opioids are commonly used to take advantage of their synergistic effects and limit the side effects of each.

Fentanyl and morphine are commonly used opioids, and bupivacaine is the usual local anesthetic of choice. The lipid solubility of the opioid predicts its clinical behavior. Fentanyl is a very lipid soluble, penetrating the dura and rapidly binding to spinal cord opioid receptors, producing a fast onset of action but a short duration of action. Significant vascular absorption of fentanyl also occurs, decreasing its epidural effect and reducing its advantage over parenteral administration. Morphine is lipid insoluble and has a slower onset of action but a much longer duration of action. However, given its hydrophilic nature, morphine remains in the cerebrospinal fluid for a longer period of time with cephalad spread and the risks of delayed respiratory depression for up to 24 h after neuraxial administration, thereby mandating ongoing monitoring of respiratory function during this time.

Other methods of postoperative analgesia include the use of long-acting local anesthetic agents for either wound infiltration or peripheral nerve blockade. Examples of peripheral nerve blockade include brachial plexus blocks for upper extremity pain, femoral nerve blocks for femur and knee surgeries, sciatic nerve blocks for analgesia below the knee, and intercostal nerve blocks for thoracic and abdominal surgeries. Options include the placement of a catheter to allow for a continuous infusion during the postoperative period and to provide long-term analgesia for up to 3–5 days.

Epidural analgesia with a local anesthetic agent or a combination of a local anesthetic agent and opioids can provide significant postoperative pain relief for many surgical procedures. Epidural analgesia also effectively blunts the surgical stress response. Although it theoretically appears that epidural analgesia should reduce postoperative morbidity, no studies have demonstrated a significant improvement in patient outcome.[158] Epidural analgesia has been shown to have beneficial effects during the postoperative period by blunting the adverse physiologic effects of surgical stress response on the cardiovascular system, the coagulation cascade, pulmonary dysfunction, the GI system, and immune function.[159] The greatest decrease in stress response occurs when epidural local anesthetics are initiated preoperatively (preemptive analgesia), maintained intraoperatively, and continued into the postoperative period.[160] Activation of the sympathetic nervous system can increase cardiac morbidity by increasing myocardial oxygen demand or decreasing oxygen supply. Neuraxial anesthesia blunts the stress response and maintains the concentrations of stress mediators (epinephrine, norepinephrine, cortisol) at preoperative levels. Epidural local anesthetics can completely block the stress response to procedures below the umbilicus and partially block the response to surgeries above the umbilicus.[161]

Although neuraxial analgesia may provide superior analgesia when compared to parenteral opioids, additional beneficial effects may be seen in patients with comorbid features, including ischemic heart disease. Thoracic epidural anesthesia by selectively blocking the cardiac accelerator fibers T_{1-4} may improve the balance in supply and demand in patients with ischemic heart disease by increasing coronary blood flow to ischemic regions while reducing heart rate, afterload, and contractility.[162] Lumbar epidural anesthesia may reduce myocardial morbidity for operations on the lower abdomen and lower extremities by reducing pain and the stress response.[163,164] However, randomized, prospective trials are still needed to confirm the clinical impression that postoperative epidural analgesia is associated with a significant decrease in cardiac morbidity and mortality.

Additional benefits of neuraxial analgesia during the perioperative period include improvements in coagulation and GI, respiratory, and immune function. Neuraxial anesthesia and analgesia can significantly decrease or eliminate postoperative hypercoagulability. In patients at high risk for vasoocclusive events (lower extremity revascularization procedures), lumbar epidural anesthesia and postoperative analgesia can decrease the incidence of thrombosis of vascular grafts.[165] Mechanisms responsible include an increase in blood flow secondary to the sympathectomy, an increase in fibrinolytic activity and an inhibition in platelet aggregation from the impaired stress response, and a decrease in platelet aggregation from systemically absorbed local anesthetics.

In patients undergoing total hip replacement, intraoperative epidural anesthesia and postoperative analgesia have been shown to decrease the risk of deep venous thrombosis and pulmonary embolism.[165,166] Clinical studies have demonstrated that postoperative epidural local anesthetics can reduce the duration of an ileus.[166,167] A thoracic epidural anesthetic can block nociceptive afferents and sympathetic efferents while sparing parasympathetic innervation, thereby increasing propulsive activity of the colon. Patients at high risk for postoperative pulmonary dysfunction may benefit from the intraoperative administration of epidural local anesthetics.

In addition to analgesia, epidural local anesthetics can decrease the degree of diaphragmatic dysfunction and improve abdominal and chest wall compliance, decreasing the number of episodes of hypoxemia.[168] Epidural anesthesia followed by epidural analgesia with local anesthetics may aid in preserving perioperative immune function by decreasing the release of stress mediators, which are potent immunosuppressants.[169] In addition, epidural analgesia with local anesthetics alone or in combination with opioids provides better analgesia than systemic opioids for many surgeries. By affecting the surgical stress response, epidural local anesthetics appear to reduce the incidence and severity of many perioperative physiological perturbations. The effect of this mode of analgesic therapy on patient outcome remains to be clarified. Patients in high-risk groups undergoing major operations appear to benefit most from epidural anesthesia and analgesia.

Postoperative Nausea and Vomiting

Nausea and vomiting are among the most common and bothersome postoperative complaints.[170,171] These problems may occur after local anesthesia only, **monitored anesthesia care**, a peripheral nerve block, or neuraxial or general anesthesia. The incidence of postoperative nausea and vomiting (PONV) is in the range of 20% to 30%, although with the increased use of propofol as the induction agent, elimination or provocative intraoperative factors (see below), and the use of preemptive therapy, the incidence is decreasing. Severe nausea and vomiting occur in 0.1% of patients, with the risk of its antecedent consequences including dehydration and electrolyte imbalance. Also, PONV may result in an increased risk of aspiration, delayed discharge from the recovery room or hospital, venous hypertension, increased bleeding from surgical sites, and tension on suture lines. Severe PONV is one of the more common factors, along with uncontrollable pain, which mandates unplanned admission to the hospital after outpatient surgical procedures.

Vomiting is controlled by the emetic center (parvicellular reticular formation) located in the lateral reticular formation close to the tractus solitarius in the brainstem. Stimuli to the emetic center are conveyed by afferent fibers from the pharynx, GI tract, mediastinum, visual center, vestibular portion of cranial nerve VIII, and the CTZ in the area postrema. The CTZ can be activated by chemical stimuli from blood and cerebrospinal fluid. Dopamine, opioid, and serotonin receptors in the area postrema of the brainstem and enkephalin, histamine, and muscarinic cholinergic receptors in the nucleus tractus solitarius play important roles in transmitting impulses to the emetic center. The emetic center sends motor output from the dorsal nucleus of the vagus nerve and the nucleus ambiguous to initiate the act of vomiting.

Nonanesthetic and anesthetic factors are associated with PONV. Nonanesthetic risk factors include patient-related predispositions, such as young age, with the peak incidence in the 11- to 14-year-old age group; gender, with a higher incidence in women; obesity; history of motion sickness or previous PONV; anxiety; and gastroparesis. Other nonanesthetic factors include the operative procedure with the highest incidence of PONV occurring with gynecologic laparoscopies, dental extractions, dilation and curettage of the uterus, knee arthroscopies, lithotripsies, head and neck surgeries, and gastric, duodenum, and gallbladder operations. In addition, PONV has been shown to be higher in nonsmokers when compared with smokers. Surgeries in children that may have a high incidence of PONV include orchiopexies, otoplasties, tonsilloadenoidectomy, middle ear surgeries, and strabismus repairs. The duration of surgery is also a factor, with longer procedures associated with a higher incidence.

Anesthesia-related factors include preoperative medications, various anesthetic drugs or techniques, and postoperative issues. Gastric distension from intraoperative positive pressure ventilation via a mask is a possible cause. Components of general anesthesia such as opioids, etomidate, ketamine, nitrous oxide, halothane, enflurance, isoflurane, desflurane, and sevoflurane can all increase the incidence of PONV. There is no significant difference in incidence among the potent inhalation agents. The balanced technique of nitrous oxide, an opioid, and an NMBA is associated with a higher incidence of PONV than the inhalation technique. Reversal of neuromuscular blockade with the use of an anticholinesterase agent is also a risk factor for PONV.

Opioids are a common cause of PONV; however, postoperative pain can also result in PONV as numerous studies have shown that patients with higher pain scores also have a higher incidence of PONV. There is no consistent or significant difference between opioids or their route of administration on the incidence of emesis. Opioids vary in their ability to cause nausea and vomiting in individual patients, and substitutes such as peripheral or neuraxial blockade should be considered when appropriate for analgesia if PONV is a problem. Opioids directly stimulate the CTZ, which activates the vomiting center. Apomorphine, a morphine derivative, is commonly used as an emetogenic agent in Europe for patients with toxic ingestions. Ironically, high doses of opioids can have antiemetic effects by depressing the vomiting center proper. The dose required for antiemesis has not been determined. Nonsteroidal antiinflammatory drugs have a lower incidence of emesis and may be a valuable option for analgesia.

Regional anesthesia is associated with less nausea and vomiting than general anesthesia, but emesis following a central neuroaxial block (spinal, epidural) can occur from significant hypotension secondary to the sympathetic nervous system blockade. Epidural opioids, especially morphine, can cause nausea and vomiting by spreading rostrally in the cerebral spinal fluid to reach the CTZ.

Postoperative factors that can cause PONV include pain, dizziness, ambulation, oral intake, and opioids. Patients may have their first bout of PONV when riding home from the hospital after outpatient surgery when the car makes the first turn, which causes stimulation of the middle ear vestibular apparatus. Ambulation with sudden motion or change in position are common causes and can be exacerbated by opioids, which sensitize the vestibular system to motion.

Although practiced in many centers, routine prophylaxis against PONV may not be mandatory because fewer than 30% of patients are affected and many of those only transiently, not requiring antiemetic therapy. In addition, antiemetics of the phenothiazine and butyrophenone class may produce significant side effects, including sedation, potentiation of opioid-induced respiratory depression, dysphoria, and extrapyramidal signs and symptoms. More recently, concern has been expressed regarding the use of the butyrophenone droperidol and its potential link with prolongation of the QT interval and fatal ventricular arrhythmias. Given these concerns, droperidol has been removed from most hospital formularies and is no longer used perioperatively.

Prophylactic antiemetic therapy is justified in high-risk populations. Unfortunately, no single drug is universally effective. There are at least four sites of action in the CTZ for antiemetic drugs: dopamine, histamine, cholinergic muscarinic, and serotonin receptors. Antiemetic drugs may have effects at more than one receptor site but tend to act predominantly at one or two receptors. As a result, combinations of drugs usually are more effective than a single drug.[172,173] Minimally effective doses should be used to reduce side effects. Antiemetic drugs include the phenothiazines (chlorpromazine, promethazine); butyrophenones (droperidol, haloperidol); antihistamines (hydroxyzine, diphenhydramine); anticholinergics (atropine, scopolamine); benzamides (metoclopramide); and serotonin antagonists (ondansetron, dolasetron). Phenothiazines, butyrophenones, and benzamides antagonize dopamine receptors and can produce sedation, ventricular repolarization delays, and extrapyramidal side effects. An additional action of metoclopramide is to increase the tone of the lower esophageal sphincter and increase gastric and small-bowel motility. Antihistamines act on the vestibular pathways to attenuate motion sickness and PONV following middle ear surgery. In addition to the pharmacological treatment of PONV, maintaining adequate hydration and providing effective pain relief are effective means of limiting PONV.

Malignant Hyperthermia

Malignant hyperthermia (MH) is a rare, potentially lethal inherited disorder of skeletal muscle. This hypermetabolic syndrome is triggered in susceptible patients by exposure to a potent inhalation anesthetic or succinylcholine. The incidence is reported to range from 1 in 4500 (when succinylcholine is used) to 1 in 60,000 anesthesias in adults and slightly more frequently in the pediatric populations. Most cases occur in children and young adults. Most families demonstrate an autosomal dominant pattern of inheritance with variable expression. Intense interest in identifying a gene for MH has demonstrated a linkage between MH and genes on chromosomes 1, 3, 7, 17, and 19 in individual families. Because MH is heterogenetic, a simple DNA-based diagnostic test appears remote.

Malignant hyperthermia is caused by an uncontrolled elevation of intracellular calcium in skeletal muscle. Normally, intracellular calcium is controlled primarily by the sarcoplasmic reticulum. In MH, there is an uninhibited release of free, unbound, ionized calcium from the sarcoplasmic reticulum. The mechanism responsible for this reaction is unclear. Most studies are focusing on the calcium channel, which links muscle membrane depolarization to the signal for calcium release, the ryanodine receptor.[174] The role of second messengers and modulators of calcium release are also under exploration. The anesthetic agents that trigger MU include the potent inhalational agents (halothane, enflurane, isoflurane, desflurane, and sevoflurane) and the depolarizing NMBA succinylcholine.

The clinical presentation of MH is variable in onset and severity. Some reactions are acute and severe, whereas others are delayed and subtle. Malignant hyperthermia may manifest only during the postoperative period, and although an extremely uncommon event, it should be considered important in the evaluation of patients who manifest postoperative fevers. The hypermetabolic response is characterized by increased carbon dioxide production, increased oxygen consumption, acid–base imbalance, and skeletal muscle breakdown. The earliest signs of MH include an elevation in the end-tidal CO_2 level, tachycardia, and tachypnea. Other common signs include acidosis, muscle rigidity, rhabdomyolysis, hyperkalemia, and dysrhythmias. Hyperthermia is frequently a late sign. Without therapy, the mortality of MH approaches 100%. Conditions that can mimic MH include a pheochromocytoma, hyperthryoidism, cocaine intoxication, and sepsis.

Treatment for MH includes immediately discontinuing the triggering agent, hyperventilation with 100% oxygen, and administering dantrolene at 2.5 mg/kg until signs of MH abate, up to a total dose of 10 mg/kg. With effective supportive therapy and dantrolene, mortality is less than 10%.[175] Other therapeutic measures include volume resuscitation, surface and central cooling, sodium bicarbonate for metabolic acidosis, diuresis and maintenance of urine output for renal protection from rhabdomyolysis and myoglobinuria, and treatment of hyperkalemia with insulin and glucose. Following successful treatment, dantrolene is continued at 1 mg/kg intravenously every 6 h for 24 h. Potassium salts, digoxin, and calcium channel blockers should not be administered during the treatment of MH as they have been associated with increased mortality.

The time-honored diagnostic test for MH is the halothane-caffeine contracture test.[176] Skeletal muscle from patients with MH demonstrates larger contractures to halothane and caffeine than normal muscle. A piece of vastus lateralis muscle is used for testing. This test has a sensitivity greater than 95% and a specificity of 80% to 85%. There are a limited number of biopsy centers in North America, which requires appropriate handling and shipping of the specimen to these centers. Patients with a family history of MH or a suspicious clinical history of MH such as masseter muscle rigidity (MMR) should be tested. Succinylcholine-induced MMR occurs in 1 in 100 children induced with halothane and given succinylcholine. The clinical incidence of MH following MMR is 15%. Muscle biopsy with contracture testing reveals that 50% of patients with MMR are MH susceptible.[177] Creatinine kinase (CK) levels exceeding 20,000 IU/l have a high correlation with a positive muscle-contracture testing. The peak CK level usually occurs 12 to 18 h after MMR.

The MH-susceptible patients may present with past medical histories that include an unexplained intraoperative death of a family member; an unexpected adverse event under anesthesia; exercise-induced rhabdomyolysis; muscle abnormalities such as ptosis, strabismus, or scoliosis; a history of heat stroke or heat intolerance; or a myopathy. Certain myopathic disorders such as central core disease and King–Denborough syndrome are associated with MH. For MH-susceptible patients, no pretreatment with dantrolene is necessary, and an anesthetic without triggering agents should be used. The Malignant Hyperthermia Association of the United States (MHAUS) has a 24-h hotline to assist physicians treating acute MH episodes (1-800-98-MHAUS).

References

1. American Society of Anesthesiologists. New classification of physical status. Anesthesiology 1963;24:111.
2. Kaplan EB, Sheiner LB, Boeckmann AI, et al. The usefulness of preoperative laboratory screening. JAMA 1985;253:3576–3581.
3. Burk CD, Miller L, Hander SD, Cohen AR. Preoperative history and coagulation screening in children undergoing tonsillectomy. Pediatrics 1992;89:691–695.
4. American College of Physicians. Guidelines for assessing and managing the perioperative risk from coronary artery disease associated with major noncardiac surgery. Ann Intern Med 1997;127:313–328.
5. Eagle K, Brundage B, Chaitman B, et al. Guidelines for perioperative cardiovascular evaluation of the noncardiac surgery. A report of the AHA/ACC Task Force on Assessment of Diagnostic and Therapeutic Cardiovascular Procedures. Circulation 1996;93:1278–1317.
6. Selzman CH, Miler SA, Zimmerman MA, Harken AH. The case for beta-adrenergic blockade as prophylaxis against perioperative cardiovascular morbidity and mortality. Arch Surg 2001;136:286–290.
7. Lindenhauer PK, Pekow P, Wang K, et al. Perioperative beta-blocker therapy and mortality after major noncardiac surgery. New Engl J Med 2005;353:349–361.
8. Nishina K, Mikawa K, Uesugi T, et al. Efficacy of clonidine for prevention of perioperative myocardial ischemia: a critical appraisal and meta-analysis of the literature. Anesthesiology 2002;96:323–329.
9. Go AS, Browner WS. Cardiac outcomes after regional or general anesthsia. Anesthesiology 1996;84:1–2.
10. Bode RH Jr, Lewis KP, Zarich SW, et al. Cardiac outcome after peripheral vascular surgery: comparison of general and regional anesthesia. Anesthesiolgy 1996;84:3–13.
11. Cook PT, Davies MJ, Cronin KD, et al. A prospective randomized trial comparing spinal anesthesia using hyperbaric cinchocaine with general anesthesia for lower limb surgery. Anaesth Intensive Care 1986;14:373–380.
12. Christopherson R, Beattie C, Frank SM, et al. Perioperative morbidity in patients randomized to epidural or general anesthesia for lower extremity vascular surgery. Perioperative Ischemia Randomized Anesthesia Trial Study Group. Anesthesiology 1993;79:422–434.
13. Warner MA, Warner ME, Weber JG. Clinical significance of pulmonary aspiration during the perioperative period. Anesthesiology 1993;78:56–62.
14. Kallar SK, Everett LL. Potential risk and preventive measure for pulmonary aspiration: new concepts in preoperative fasting guidelines. Anesth Analg 1993;77:171–182.
15. Crawford M, Lerman J, Christensen S, et al. Effects of duration of fasting on gastric fluid pH and volume in healthy children. Anesth Analg 1990;71:400–403.
16. Shevde K, Trivedi N. Effects of clear liquids on gastric volume and pH in healthy volunteers. Anesth Analg 1991;72:528–531.
17. Phillips S, Hutchinson S, Davidson T. Preoperative drinking does not affect gastric contents. Br J Anaesth 1993;70:6–9.
18. Read MS, Vaughn RS. Allowing pre-operative patients to drink: effects on patients' safety and comfort of unlimited oral water until 2 hours before anaesthesia. Acta Anaesthesiol Scand 1991;35:591–595.
19. Goresky GV, Maltby JR. Fasting guidelines for elective surgical patients. Can J Anaesth 1990;37:493–495.
20. Strunin L. How long should patients fast before surgery? Time for new guidelines. Br J Anaesth 1993;70:1–2.
21. Green CR, Pandit SK, Schork MA. Preoperative fasting time: is the traditional policy changing? Results of a national survey. Anesth Analg 1996;83:123–128.
22. Tuman KJ, Roizen MF. Outcome assessment and pulmonary artery catheterization: why does the debate continue? Anesth Analg 1997;84:1–4.
23. Connors AF, Speroff T, Dawson NV, et al. The effectiveness of right heart catheterization in the initial care of critically ill patients. JAMA 1996;276:889–897.
24. American Society of Anesthesiologists. Practice guidelines for pulmonary artery catheterization. Anesthesiology 1993;78:380–392.
25. American Society of Anesthesiologists. Practice guidelines for preoperative transesophageal echocardiography. Anesthesiology 1996;84:986–1006.
26. Gan TJ, Glass PS, Windsor A, et al. Bispectral index monitoring allows faster emergence and improved recovery from propofol, alfentanil, and nitrous oxide anesthesia. BIS Utility Study Group. Anesthesiology 1997;87:808–815.
27. Sandin RH, Enlund G, Samuelsson P, et al. Awareness during anaesthesia: a prospective case study. Lancet 2000;355:707–711.
28. Ekman A, Lindholm ML, Lennmarken C, et al. Reduction in the incidence of awareness using BIS monitoring. Acta Anaesthesiol Scand 2004;48:20–26.
29. Myles PS, Lelie K, McNeil J, et al. Bispectral index monitoring to prevent awareness during anaesthesia: the B-aware randomized control trial. Lancet 2004;363:1757–1763.

30. Gan TJ, Glass PS, Windsor A, et al. Bispectral index monitoring allows faster emergence and improved recovery from propofol, alfentanil and nitrous oxide anesthesia. Anesthesiology 1997; 87:808–815.
31. Guignard B, Coste D, Menigaux C, et al. Reduced isoflurane consumption with bispectral index monitoring. Acta Anaesthesiol Scand 2001;45:308–314.
32. Courtman SP, Wardurgh A, Petros AJ: Comparison of the bispectral index monitor with the COMFORT score in assessing level of sedation of critically ill children. Intensive Care Med 2003; 29:2239–2246.
33. Berkenbosch JW, Fichter CR, Tobias JD: The correlation of the bispectral index monitor with clinical sedation scores during mechanical ventilation in the pediatric intensive care unit. Anesth Analg 2002;94:506–511.
34. Grindstaff R, Tobias JD. Applications of bispectral index monitoring in the pediatric intensive care unit. J Intensive Care Med 2004;19:111–116.
35. American Society of Anesthesiologists. Practice guidelines for management of the difficult airway. Anesthesiology 1993;78:597–602.
36. Benumof JL. Management of the difficult airway. Anesthesiology 1991;75:1085–1110.
37. Benumof JL. The LMA and the ASA difficult airway algorithm. Anesthesiology 1996;84:686–699.
38. Wildsmith JA, Brown DT, Paul D, et al. Structure–activity relationships in differential nerve block at high and low frequency stimulation. Br J Anaesth 1989;63:444–452.
39. Covino BG. Pharmacology of local anaesthetic agents. Br J Anaesth 1986;58:701–716.
40. Wildsmith JA, Gissen AJ, Takman B, et al. Differential nerve blockade: esters versus amides and the influence of pK_a. Br J Anaesth 1987;59:379–384.
41. Butterworth JF, Strichartz GR: Molecular mechanisms of local anesthesia: a review. Anesthesiology 1990;72:711–734.
42. Johns RA, DiFazio CA, Longnecker DE. Lidocaine constricts or dilates rat arterioles in a dose-dependent manner. Anesthesiology 1985;62:141–144.
43. Scott DB, McClure JH, Giasi RM, et al. Effects of concentration of local anesthetic drugs in extradural block. Br J Anaesth 1980;52:1033–1037.
44. Crawford OB. Comparative evaluation in epidural anesthesia of lidocaine, mepivacaine, and L-67, a new local anesthetic agent. Anesthesiology 1964;25:321–329.
45. Braid DP, Scott DB. The systemic absorption of local analgesic drugs. Br J Anaesth 1965;37:394–404.
46. Swerdlow M, Jones R. The duration of action of bupivacaine, prilocaine, and lignocaine. Br J Anaesth 1970;42:335–339.
47. Bromage PR. A comparison of the hydrochloride salts of lignocaine and prilocaine for epidural analgesia. Br J Anaesth 1965; 37:753–761.
48. Sinclair CJ, Scott DB. Comparison of bupivacaine and etidocaine in extradural blockade. Br J Anaesth 1984;56:147–152.
49. Eisenach JC, Dewan DM, Rose JC, et al. Epidural clonidine produces antinociception, but not hypotension, in sheep. Anesthesiology 1987;66:496–501.
50. Tobias JD. Caudal epidural block: a review of test dosing and recognition of systemic injection in children. Anesth Analg 2001;93:1156–1161.
51. Sheskey MC, Rocco AG, Bizzarri-Schmid M, et al. A dose-response study of bupivacaine for spinal anesthesia. Anesth Analg 1983;62:931–935.
52. Bromage PR, Gretal M. Improved brachial plexus blockade with bupivacaine hydrochloride and carbonated lidocaine. Anesthesiology 1972;36:479–487.
53. Tucker GT, Mather LE. Clinical pharmacokinetics of local anesthetics. Clin Pharmacokinet 1979;4:241–278.
54. Scott DB. Toxic effects of local anaesthetic agents on the central nervous system. Br J Anaesth 1986;58:732–735.
55. Wagman IH, DeJong RH, Prince DA. Effects of lidocaine on the central nervous system. Anesthesiology 1967;28:155–172.
56. Englesson S. The influence of acid–base changes on central nervous system toxicity of local anesthetic agents. Acta Anaesthesiol Scand 1974;18:79–87.
57. Moller RA, Covino BG. Cardiac electrophysiologic effects of lidocaine and bupivacaine. Anesth Analg 1988;67:107–114.
58. Block A, Covino BG. Effect of local anesthetic agents on cardiac conduction and contractility. Reg Anesth 1982;6:55.
59. Pitkanen M, Feldman HS, Arthur GR, et al. Chronotropic and inotropic effects of ropivacaine, bupivacaine, and lidocaine in the spontaneously beating and electrically paced isolated, perfused rabbit heart. Reg Anesth 1992;17:183–192.
60. Ravindran RS, Bond VK, Tasch MD, et al. Prolonged neural blockade following regional analgesia with 2-chloroprocaine. Anesth Analg 1980;59:447–451.
61. Reisner LS, Hochman BN, Plumer MH. Persistent neurologic deficit and adhesive arachnoiditis following intrathecal 2-chloroprocaine injection. Anesth Analg 1980;59:452–454.
62. Fibuch EE, Opper SE. Back pain following epidurally administered Nesacaine–MPF. Anesth Analg 1989;69:113–115.
63. Concas A, Santoro G, Mascia MP, et al. The general anesthetic propofol enhances the function of alpha aminobutyric acid-coupled chloride channel in the rat cerebral cortex. J Neurochem 1990;55:2135.
64. Ho IK, Harris RA. Mechanism of action of barbiturates. Annu Rev Pharmacol Toxicol 1981;21:83–111.
65. Johnston GA, Willow M. GABA and barbiturate receptors. Trends Pharmacol Sci 1982;3:328–330.
66. Olsen RW. Drug interactions at the GABA receptor-ionophore complex. Annu Rev Pharmacol Toxicol 1982;22:245–277.
67. MacDonald JF, Miljkovic Z, Pennefather P. Use-dependent block of excitatory amino acid currents in cultured neurons by ketamine. J Neurophysiol 1987;58:251–266.
68. Mayer ML, Westbrook GL, Vyklicky L. Sites of antagonist action on N-methyl-D-aspartatic acid receptors studied using fluctuation analysis and a rapid perfusion technique. J Neurophysiol 1988;60:645–663.
69. Vincent JP, Cavey D, Kamenka JM, et al. Interaction of phencyclinidines with the muscarinic and opiate receptors in the central nervous system. Brain Res 1978;152:176–182.
70. Michenfelder JD, Theye RA. Cerebral protection by thiopental during hypoxia. Anesthesiology 1973;39:510–517.
71. Michenfelder JD, Milde JH, Sundt TM Jr. Cerebral protection by barbiturate anesthesia. Arch Neurol 1976;33:345–350.
72. Langsjo JW, Maksimow A, Salmi E, et al. S-Ketamine anesthesia increases cerebral blood flow in excess of the metabolic needs in humans. Anesthesiology 2005;103:258–268.
73. Bourgoin A, Albanese J, Wereszczynski N, et al. Safety of sedation with ketamine in severe head injury patients: comparison with sufentanil. Crit Care Med 2003;31:711–717.
74. Mayberg TS, Lam AM, Matta BF. Ketamine does not increase cerebral blood flow velocity or intracranial pressure during isoflurane/nitrous oxide anesthesia in patients undergoing craniotomy. Anesth Analg 1995;81:84–89.
75. Modica PA, Tempelhoff R, White PF. Pro and anticonvulsant effects of anesthetics. Part I. Anesth Analg 1990;70:303–315.
76. Modica PA, Tempelhoff R, White PF. Pro and anticonvulsant effects of anesthetics. Part II. Anesth Analg 1990;70:433–444.
77. Carson IW, Moore J, Balmer JR, et al. Laryngeal competence with ketamine and other drugs. Anesthesiology 1973;38:128–133.
78. Bourke DL, Malit LA, Smith TC. Respiratory interactions of ketamine and morphine. Anesthesiology 1987;66:153–156.

79. Hirshman CA, Downes H, Farbood A, Bergman NA. Ketamine block of bronchospasm in experimental canine asthma. Br J Anaesth 1979;51:713–718.
80. Eames WO, Rooke GA, Sai-Chuen R, Bishop M. Comparison of the effects of etomidate, propofol, and thiopental on respiratory resistance after tracheal intubation. Anesthesiology 1996;84: 1307–1311.
81. Pizov R, Brown RH, Weiss YS, et al. Wheezing during induction of general anesthesia in patients with and without asthma. A randomized, blinded trial. Anesthesiology 1995;82:1111–1116.
82. Chih-Chung L, Ming-Hwang S, Tan PPC, et al. Mechanisms underlying the inhibitory effect of propofol on the contraction of canine airway smooth muscle. Anesthesiology 1999;91:750–759.
83. Pedersen CM, Thirstrup S, Nielsen-Kudsk JE. Smooth muscle relaxant effects of propofol and ketamine in isolated guinea-pig tracheas. Eur J Pharm 1993;238:75–80.
84. Chamberlain JH, Sede RG, Chung DC. Effect of thiopentone on myocardial function. Br J Anaesth 1977;49:865–870.
85. Claeys MA, Gepts E, Camu F. Hemodynamic changes during anaesthesia induced and maintained with propofol. Br J Anaesth 1988;60:3–9.
86. Cullen PM, Turtle M, Prys-Roberts C, et al. Effects of propofol anesthesia on baroreflex activity in humans. Anesth Analg 1987;66:1115–1120.
87. Tritapepe L, Voci P, Marino P, et al. Calcium chloride minimizes the hemodynamic effects of propofol in patients undergoing coronary artery bypass grafting. J Cardiothoras Vasc Anesth 1999;13:150–153.
88. Sochala C, Van Deenen D, De Ville A, Govaerts MJM. Heart block following propofol in a child. Paediatr Anaes 1999;9:349–351.
89. Egan TD, Brock-Utne JG. Asystole and anesthesia induction with a fentanyl, propofol, and succinylcholine sequence. Anesth Analg 1991;73:818–820.
90. Gooding JM, Weng JT, Smith RA, et al. Cardiovascular and pulmonary response following etomidate induction of anesthesia in patients with demonstrated cardiac disease. Anesth Analg 1979;58:40–41.
91. Tarnow J, Hess W, Kline W. Etomidate, althesin and thiopentone as induction agents for coronary artery surgery. Can Anaesth Soc J 1980;27:338–344.
92. White PF, Way WL, Trevor AJ. Ketamine—its pharmacology and therapeutic uses. Anesthesiology 1982;56:119–136.
93. Wagner RL, White PF. Etomidate inhibits adrenocortical function in surgical patients. Anesthesiology 1984;61:647–651.
94. Wagner RL, White PF, Kan PB, et al. Inhibition of adrenal steroidogenesis by the anesthetic etomidate. N Engl J Med 1984;310:1415–1421.
95. Wagner RL, White PF, Kan PB, et al. Inhibition of adrenal steroidogenesis by the anesthetic etomidate. New Engl J Med 1984;310:1415–1421.
96. McCollum JS, Milligan KR, Dundee JW. The antiemetic action of propofol. Anaesthesia 1988;43:239–240.
97. Borgeat A, Wilder-Smith O, Forni M, et al. Adjuvant propofol enables better control of nausea and emesis secondary to chemotherapy for breast cancer. Can J Anaesth 1994;41:1117–1119.
98. Harrison PG, Moore MR, Meissner TM. Porphyrogenicity of etomidate and ketamine as continuous infusions: screening in the DDC-primed rat model. Br J Anaesth 1985;57:420–423.
99. Laxenaire MC, Mata-Bermejo E, Moneret-Vautrin DA, Gueant JL. Life-threatening anaphylactoid reactions to propofol. Anesthesiology 1992;77:275–280.
100. Griffin J, Ray T, Gray B, et al. Pain on injection of propofol: a thiopental/propofol mixture versus a lidocaine/propofol mixture. Am J Pain Manage 2002;12:45–49.
101. Tobias JD. Prevention of pain associated with the administration of propofol in children: lidocaine versus ketamine. Am J Anesthesiol 1996;23:231–232.
102. Camps AS, Sanchez-Izquierdo Riera JA, Vazquez DT, et al. Midazolam and 2% propofol in long-term sedation of traumatized, critically ill patients: efficacy and safety comparison. Crit Care Med 2000;28:3612–3619.
103. Barrientos-Vega R, Sanchez-Soria M, Morales-Garcia C, et al. Pharmacoeconomic assessment of propofol 2% used for prolonged sedation. Crit Care Med 2001;29:317–322.
104. Smith I, White PF, Nathanson M, et al. Propofol: an update on its clinical use. Anesthesiology 1994;81:1005–1043.
105. Crawford M, Pollock J, Anderson K, et al. Comparison of midazolam with propofol for sedation in outpatient bronchoscopy. Br J Anaesth 1993;70:419–422.
106. Veber B, Gachot B, Bedos JP, et al. Severe sepsis after intravenous injection of contaminated propofol. Anesthesiology 1994;80: 712–713.
107. Bennett SN, McNeil MM, Bland LA, et al. Postoperative infections traced to contamination of an intravenous anesthetic, propofol. N Engl J Med 1995;333:147–154.
108. Fine PG, Hare BD. The pathways and mechanisms of pain and analgesia: a review and clinical perspective. Hosp Formul 1985; 20:972–985.
109. Bailey PL, Wilbrink J, Zwanikken P, et al. Anesthetic induction with fentanyl. Anesth Analg 1985;64:48–53.
110. Keats AS. The effects of drugs on respiration in man. Annu Rev Pharmacol Toxicol 1985;25:41–65.
111. Urthaler F, Isobe JH, James T. Direct and vagally mediated chronotropic effects of morphine studied by selective perfusion of the sinus node of awake dogs. Chest 1975;68:222–228.
112. Zelis R, Mansour EJ, Capone RJ, et al. The cardiovascular effects of morphine. The peripheral capacitance and resistance vessels in human subjects. J Clin Invest 1974;54:1247–1258.
113. Benthuysen JL, Ty Smith N, Sanford TJ, et al. Physiology of alfentanil-induced rigidity. Anesthesiology 1986;64:440–446.
114. Costall B, Fortune DH, Naylor RJ. Involvement of mesolimbic and extrapyramidal nuclei in the motor depressant action of narcotic drugs. J Pharm Pharmacol 1978;30:566–572.
115. Radnay PA, Duncalf D, Novakovic M, et al. Common bile duct pressure changes after fentanyl, morphine, meperidine, butorphanol, and naloxone. Anesth Analg 1984;63:441–444.
116. Flacke JW, Flacke WE, Bloor BC, et al. Histamine release by four narcotics: a double-blind study in humans. Anesth Analg 1987;66:723–730.
117. Shafer SL, Varvel JR. Pharmacokinetics, pharmacodynamics and rational opioid selection. Anesthesiology 1991;74:53–63.
118. Mather LE. Pharmacokinetic and pharmacodynamic profiles of opioid analgesics: a sameness amongst equals? Pain 1990;43:3–6.
119. Burkle H, Dunbar S, Van Aken H: Remifentanil: a novel, short-acting, μ opioid. Anesth Analg 1996;83:646–651.
120. Smith NT, Eger EJ II, Stoelting RK, et al. The cardiovascular and sympathomimetic responses to the addition of nitrous oxide to halothane in man. Anesthesiology 1970;32:410–421.
121. Fink BR. Diffusion anoxia. Anesthesiology 1955;16:511–519.
122. Deacon R, Lumb M, Perry J, et al. Selective inactivation of vitamin B_{12} in rats by nitrous oxide. Lancet 1978;2:1023–1024.
123. Hadzic A, Glab K, Sanborn KV, et al. Severe neurologic deficit after nitrous oxide anesthesia. Anesthesiology 1995;83:863–866.
124. Eger EI II, Saidman LJ. Hazards of nitrous oxide anesthesia in bowel obstruction and pneumothorax. Anesthesiology 1965; 26:61–66.
125. Eckenhoff R. Do specific or nonspecific interactions with proteins underlie inhalational anesthetic action? Mol Pharmacol 1998;54:610–615.

126. Subcommittee on the National Halothane Study of the Committee on Anesthesia. Possible association between halothane anesthesia and postoperative hepatic necrosis. JAMA 1966;197:775–788.
127. Kenna JG, Jones RM. The organ toxicity of inhaled anesthetics. Anesth Analg 1995;81(suppl):S51–S66.
128. Brown BR Jr, Gandolfi AJ. Adverse effects of volatile anesthetics. Br J Anaesth 1987;59:14–23.
129. Pohl LR, Satoh H, Christ DD, et al. The immunologic and metabolic basis of drug hypersensitivities. Annu Rev Pharmacol 1988;28:367–387.
130. Wark HJ. Postoperative jaundice in children—the influence of halothane. Anaesthesia 1983;38:237–242.
131. Warner LO, Beach TP, Garvin JP, et al. Halothane and children: the first quarter century. Anesth Analg 1984;63:838–840.
132. Morio M, Fujii K, Satoh N, et al. Reaction of sevoflurane and its degradation products with soda lime. Toxicity of the byproducts. Anesthesiology 1992;77:1155–1164.
133. Frink EJ Jr, Malan TP, Morgan SE, et al. Quantification of the degradation products of sevoflurane in two CO_2 absorbents during low-flow anesthesia in surgical patients. Anesthesiology 1992;77:1064–1069.
134. Mazze RI. The safety of sevoflurane in humans. Anesthesiology 1992;77:1062–1063.
135. Fang ZX, Eger EI II, Laster MJ, et al. Carbon monoxide production from degradation of desflurane, enflurane, isoflurane, halothane, and sevoflurane by soda lime and Baralyme®. Anesth Analg 1995;80:1187–1193.
136. Baum J, Sachs G, Driesch C, et al. Carbon monoxide generation in carbon dioxide absorbents. Anesth Analg 1995;81:144–146.
137. Eger EI II. New inhaled anesthetics. Anesthesiology 1994;80:906–922.
138. Rosenberg H, Gronert GA. Intractable cardiac arrest in children given succinylcholine. Anesthesiology 1992;77:1054.
139. Miller RD, Rupp SM, Fisher DM, et al. Clinical pharmacology of vecuronium and atracurium. Anesthesiology 1984;61:444–453.
140. Brull SJ, Silverman DG. Intraoperative use of muscle relaxants. Anesth Clin North Am 1993;11:325–344.
141. Abouleish EI, Abboud TS, Bikhazi G, et al. Rapacuronium for modified rapid sequence induction in elective Cesarean section: neuromuscular blocking effects and safety compared with succinylcholine and placental transfer. Br J Anaesth 1999;83:862–867.
142. Tobias JD, Johnson JO, Sprague K, et al. Effects of rapacuronium on respiratory function during general anesthesia. Anesthesiology 2001;95:908–912.
143. Jooste E, Zhang Y, Emala CW. Rapacuronium preferentially antagonizes the function of M2 versus M3 muscarinic receptors in guinea pig airway smooth muscle. Anesthesiology 2005;102:117–124.
144. Rajchert DM, Pasquariello CA, Watcha MG, et al. Rapacuronium and the risk of bronchospasm in pediatric patients. Anesth Anagl 2002;94:488–493.
145. Savarese JJ, Ali HH, Basta SJ, et al. The clinical neuromuscular pharmacology of mivacurium chloride: a short-acting nondepolarizing ester neuromuscular blocking drug. Anesthesiology 1988;68:723–732.
146. Hughes R, Chapple DJ. The pharmacology of atracurium: a new competitive neuromuscular blocking agent. Br J Anaesth 1981;53:31–44.
147. Kopman AF, Ng J, Zank LM, et al. Residual postoperative paralysis: pancuronium versus mivacurium; does it matter? Anesthesiology 1996;85:1253–1259.
148. Savage DS, Sleigh T, Carlyle I. The emergence of ORG NC 45 from the pancuronium series. Br J Anaesth 1980;52(suppl 1):3S–9S.
149. Van den Broek L, Wierda JM, Smeulers NJ. Clinical pharmacology of rocuronium: study of the time course of action, dose requirement, reversibility, and pharmacokinetics. J Clin Anesth 1994;6:288–296.
150. Larijani GE, Bartkowski RR, Azad SS, et al. Clinical pharmacology of pipecuronium bromide. Anesth Analg 1989;68:734–739.
151. Kopman AF, Yee PS, Neuman GG. Correlation of the train-of-four fade ratio with clinical signs and symptoms of residual curarization in awake volunteers. Anesthesiology 1997;86:765–771.
152. Austin KL, Stapleton JV, Mather LE. Multiple intramuscular injections: a major source of variability in analgesic response to meperidine. Pain 1980;8:47–62.
153. American Society of Anesthesiologists. Practice guidelines for acute pain management in the perioperative setting. Anesthesiology 1995;82:1071–1081.
154. Austin KL, Stapleton JV, Mather LE. Relationship between blood meperidine concentrations and analgesic response: a preliminary report. Anesthesiology 1980;53:460–466.
155. Dahlstrom B, Tamsen A, Paalzow L, et al. Patient-controlled analgesic therapy. Part IV. Pharmacokinetics and analgesic plasma concentration of morphine. Clin Pharmacokinet 1982;7:266–279.
156. Tamsen A, Hartvig P, Fagerlund C, et al. Patient-controlled analgesic therapy. Part II. Individual analgesic demand and analgesic plasma concentrations of pethidine in postoperative pain. Clin Pharmacokinet 1982;7:164–175.
157. Tobias JD. Weak analgesics and nonsteroidal anti-inflammatory agents in the management of children with acute pain. Pediatr Clin North Am 2000;47:527–543.
158. Liu S, Carpenter RL, Neal JM. Epidural anesthesia and analgesia—their role in postoperative outcome. Anesthesiology 1995;82:1474–1506.
159. Breslow MJ, Parker SD, Fran SM, et al. Determinants of catecholamine and cortisol responses to lower extremity revascularization. Anesthesiology 1993;79:1202–1209.
160. Kissin I. Preemptive analgesia—why its effect is not always obvious. Anesthesiology 1996;84:1015–1019.
161. Salo M. Cytokines and attenuation of responses to surgery. Acta Anaesthesiol Scand 1996;40:141–142.
162. Blomberg S, Emanuelsson H, Kvist H, et al. Effects of thoracic epidural anesthesia on coronary arteries and arterioles in patients with coronary artery disease. Anesthesiology 1990;73:840–847.
163. Yeager MP, Glass DD, Neff RK, et al. Epidural anesthesia and analgesia in high-risk surgical patients. Anesthesiology 1987;66:729–736.
164. Tuman KJ, McCarthy RJ, March RJ, et al. Effects on epidural anesthesia and analgesia on coagulation and outcome after major vascular surgery. Anesth Analg 1991;73:696–704.
165. Sharrock N, Ranawat C, Urquhart B, et al. Factors influencing deep vein thrombosis following total hip arthroplasty under epidural anesthesia. Anesth Analg 1993;76:756–771.
166. Modig J, Maripuu E, Sahlstedt B. Thromboembolism following total hip replacement: a prospective investigation of 94 patients with emphasis on the efficacy of lumbar epidural anesthesia in prophylaxis. Reg Anesth 1986;11:72–79.
167. Scheinen B, Asantila R, Orko R. The effect of bupivacaine and morphine on pain and bowel function after colonic surgery. Acta Anaesthesiol Scand 1987;31:161–164.
168. Pansard JL, Mankikian B, Bertrand M, et al. Effects of thoracic extradural block on diaphragmatic electrical activity and contractility after upper abdominal surgery. Anesthesiology 1993;78:63–71.
169. Tonnesen E, Wahlgreen C. Influence of extradural and general anesthesia on natural killer cell activity and lymphocyte subpopulations in patients undergoing hysterectomy. Br J Anaesth 1988;60:500–507.

170. Watcha MF, White PF. Postoperative nausea and vomiting—its etiology, treatment, and prevention. Anesthesiology 1992;77: 162–184.
171. Forrest JB, Cahalan MK, Rehder K, et al. Multicenter study of general anesthesia. II. Results. Anesthesiology 1990;72:262–268.
172. Naguib M, el Bakry AK, Khoshim MH, et al. Prophylactic antiemetic therapy with ondansetron, tropisetron, granisetron, and metoclopramide in patients undergoing laparoscopic cholecystectomy: a randomized, double blind comparison with placebo. Can J Anaesth 1996;43:226–231.
173. Davis PJ, McGowan FX Jr, Landsman I, et al. Effect of antiemetic therapy on recovery and hospital discharge time: a double-blind assessment of ondansetron, droperidol, and placebo in pediatric patients undergoing ambulatory surgery. Anesthesiology 1995; 83:956–960.
174. Pessah IN. Complex pharmacology of malignant hyperthermia. Anesthesiology 1996;84:1275–1279.
175. Wedel DJ, Quinlan JG, Iazzio P. Clinical effects of intravenous dantrolene. Mayo Clin Proc 1995;70:241–246.
176. Larach MG. Standardization of the caffeine halothane muscle contracture test. Anesth Analg 1989;69:511–515.
177. Schwartz L, Rockoff MA, Koka BV. Masseter spasm with anesthesia: incidence and implications. Anesthesiology 1984;61:772–775.

19

Management of Perioperative Pain

Susannah S. Wise

Pain has always been linked with surgical intervention. Pain may occur because of the preexisting disease that led to the need for an operation, the surgical procedure itself (with the associated tissue trauma, instrumentation, or complications), or a combination of both the disease process and the intervention. Optimal management of acute pain during the perioperative period is increasingly recognized as reducing the risk of adverse perioperative events, in addition to providing comfort, relieving suffering, and aiding in return to normal function.

Public perception is changing, as evidenced by the popular press and medical journals. The public feels that they have a "right" to adequate pain control. Pain is no longer seen as an inevitable consequence of surgery. Increasingly, the media have focused on pain management concerns. In addition, there have been cases of elder abuse brought to court with judgments rendered against docters and nursing homes for not providing adequate pain control to their patients.

Government agencies, such as the Joint Commission of Accreditation of Health Care Organizations, now mandate that pain is monitored and requires that hospitals collect data and measure performance on pain control issues.[1] The Veterans Administration enacted a program that has received widespread acceptance; it is to monitor pain as a "fifth vital sign." Assessing pain has become a mandatory practice. Treating pain effectively therefore follows as the next step. Optimal pain control should help to improve patient care and surgical outcomes. Acute pain management services are becoming more accessible and have been found to be a cost-effective adjunct.[2]

The American Society of Anesthesiologists Task Force on Acute Pain Management has outlined reasons why understanding and utilizing adequate pain management techniques is important.[3] The purposes of these guidelines are to facilitate the safety and effectiveness of acute pain management in the perioperative setting, reduce the risk of adverse outcomes, maintain the patient's functional abilities and physical and psychological well-being, and enhance the quality of life for patients with acute pain during the perioperative period.[3]

Adverse outcomes that may result from the undertreatment of perioperative pain include (but are not limited to) thromboembolic and pulmonary complications, additional time spent in an intensive care unit or hospital setting, hospital readmission for further pain management, needless suffering, impairment of health-related quality of life, and development of chronic pain.

Adverse outcomes associated with the management of perioperative pain include (but are not limited to) respiratory depression, brain or other neurologic injury, sedation, circulatory depression, nausea, vomiting, pruritus, urinary retention, impairment of bowel function, and sleep disruption. Health-related quality of life includes (but is not limited to) physical, emotional, social, and spiritual well-being.[3]

Types of Pain

Somatic pain is the typical postoperative pain that is caused by activation of peripheral nociceptors due to tissue injury. This nociceptive input is transmitted via A delta and C fibers. Visceral pain is due to compression or distention of the viscera. Visceral nociceptors may also be stimulated by inflammation or ischemia. This nociceptive input is transmitted via afferent sympathetic pathways. Neuropathic pain is related to compression or infiltration of peripheral nerves.

Pain may also be classified by its duration and its physiologic response. *Acute pain* is of recent onset, often due to tissue trauma or an active disease process. Nociceptive impulses cause autonomic and somatic reflex response to acute pain. Postoperative pain is most often acute and will resolve as tissue trauma heals and the noxious stimuli resolve, although poorly treated acute pain may lead to chronic pain.

Chronic pain by definition must be present for over 3 months. Unlike acute postoperative pain, chronic pain does not lead to an autonomic response. Chronic pain is especially prevalent in the older patient. Of patients in nursing homes, 45% to 80% have chronic pain issues related to osteoarthritis, osteoporosis, neuropathy, vascular disease, and cancer.[4–6]

Mechanism of Pain Perception

Acute pain is caused by direct injury and activation of free nerve terminals as well as release of inflammatory mediators such as prostaglandins, bradykinin, serotonin, histamine, and hydrogen ions. Nociception causes peripheral nerve transmission to the dorsal horn via A delta or C fibers or afferent sympathetic nerves. From the dorsal horn, the stimuli travel to the spinothalamic tracts and to the hypothalamus (Fig. 19.1).

Surgeons may be able to reduce pain by changing this pathway by reduction of tissue damage and the ensuing inflammatory response, increasing the release of endogenous opioids, and providing enough exogenous medication to bind to peripheral and central pain receptors.

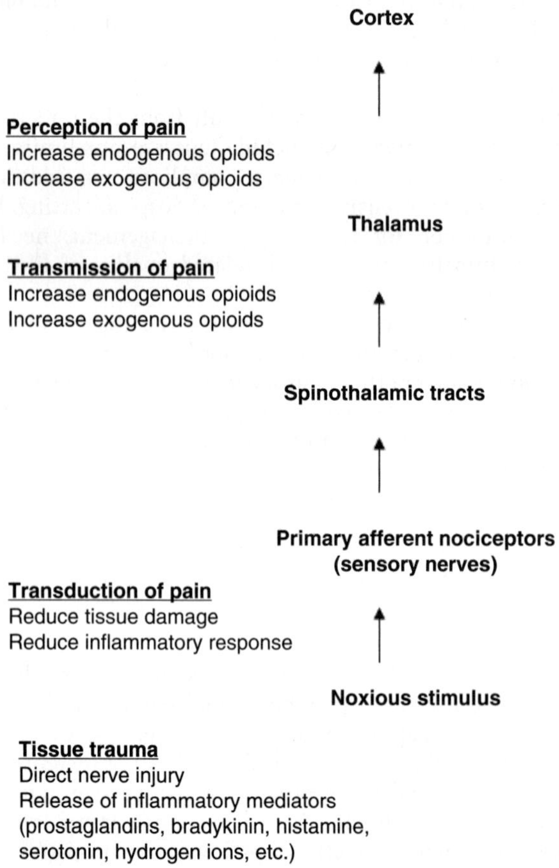

FIGURE 19.1. Mechanism of pain perception, nociceptive pathway. Tissue trauma starts the process of causing pain by inducing direct nerve injury and release of inflammatory mediators. The stimulus is transmitted from the peripheral nerve to the dorsal horn via A delta or C fibers or afferent sympathetic nerves. From the dorsal horn, the stimuli travels to the spinothalamic tracts and to the hypothalamus.

TABLE 19.1. Functional Pain Scale.

0 = No pain
1 = Tolerable (does not prevent activities)
2 = Tolerable (does prevent some activities)
3 = Intolerable (can use phone, watch TV, or read)
4 = Intolerable (cannot use phone, watch TV, or read)
5 = Intolerable (unable to verbally communicate)
There are a number of ways to assess pain. The visual analogue scale is a method to give a pain score based on a numerical score. This functional pain scale incorporates the patient's activity.

Source: From Gloth,[7] by permission of *Clinical Geriatric Medicine.*

Assessing Pain

Inadequate pain control is linked with underrecognition. Assessing pain is the first step in recognizing and treating pain. There are a host of pain scales available to assess pain and response to its treatment. Verbal, numerical, and visual scales are in current common usage. The newer pain scales incorporate a verbal as well as a functional component and may prove to be even more useful in assessing pain[7] (Table 19.1).

Pain recognition may be harder to assess in noncommunicative patients. Assessing facial expression (Is the face relaxed or tight?); upper limb position (Is the arm relaxed or contracted?); and ventilation (Is the patient breathing comfortably or fighting?) can gauge pain in those who cannot speak on their own behalf.[8]

Physiology of Pain in the Postoperative Period

The physiologic changes and comorbidities that lead to reduced functional reserve and reduced ability to compensate for physiologic stress may be significantly affected after an operative procedure. Pain can add to the stress. Adequate pain control may help reduce the consequences of postoperative pain, but each medication also can have detrimental effects. The careful balance of the right pain regimen is necessary.

Endocrine and Metabolic Stress Response

The metabolic—endocrine stress response to pain includes tachycardia, hyperglycemia, and increased protein breakdown. Overall, there is an increase in sympathetic tone and therefore metabolic rate. In theory, treating pain can help control this response.

Blocking the autonomic effects on pain may extend the duration of anesthetic protection. For example, administering atenolol for 7 days during the postoperative period in patients with a high risk of myocardial ischemia helped to reduce postoperative mortality by 50% over 2 years postoperatively.[9]

Pulmonary Function

Pulmonary dysfunction is commonly seen when patients are in pain. There is a reduced vital capacity, reduced diaphragmatic shortening, and hypoxemia. This, coupled with the physiologic decompensation that naturally occurs with age, makes respiratory complications especially common in the older surgical patient.[10] With age, there is a decrease in lung elasticity, leading to an increased alveolar–arterial oxygen gradient. Decreased upper airway reflexes lead to an increased risk of aspiration.[11] Over 10% of patients over the age of 80 years old have pulmonary complications postoperatively.[12] These complications include aspiration, bronchospasm, hypoxemia, pneumonia, pneumothorax, and respiratory failure. Major abdominal or thoracic procedures will increase the restrictive pulmonary deficit because of splinting. Functional residual capacity may be reduced by 70% during the immediate postoperative period and up to 1 week after the operation.[13] Optimizing pain control is clearly important for pulmonary function.

Cardiac Function

Cardiovascular complications are a major concern, especially in the older surgical patient. Of people over the age of 80 years old, 80% have coronary artery disease,[14] and 10% have congestive heart failure.[15] Octogenarians have a 17% incidence of cardiovascular mortality versus 2.6% in patients younger than 50 years of age who undergo similar noncardiac operations.[12] There is a linear increase in systolic blood pressure with age.[16] In addition, there is an increase in systemic vascular resistance and ventricular hypertrophy.[17] Pain control in painful hip fractures has been reviewed. In patients over the age of 70, those with epidural analgesia had a 50% reduction in cardiac events compared to those receiving intramuscular narcotics.[18] Further investigation regarding pain control and reduction a catecholamine release and cardiac events needs to be made.

Gastrointestinal Function

Whether adequate pain control can help accelerate gastrointestinal function is still unclear. Pain causes reduced motility of the gastrointestinal tract and leads to nausea, vomiting, ileus, and constipation. However, opioids also decrease gastrointestinal motility. Inhibiting the nociceptive stimulus may help improve function. Local analgesia via epidural catheter has been shown to slightly decrease time to gastrointestinal function.[19]

Coagulation System

Pain control is thought to play a role in reducing thromboembolic complications after surgery. Hypercoagulability after surgery is related to an activation of the coagulation cascade, an increase in platelet activity, and decreased fibrinolytic activity. Epidural anesthesia in the perioperative period has shown a reduction in rate of thrombotic complications.[20] Studies revealed less platelet activation, better fibrinolytic function, and fewer thromboembolic complications.[21] The local analgesia in epidural anesthesia may be the reason. Early ambulation is also more frequent if pain is well controlled, and this may play a role in reduction of thromboembolic complications.

Cognitive Function

Preservation of cognitive function is more of a critical issue in the elderly surgical patient than in the younger surgical patient. Cognitive dysfunction usually presents initially on the second postoperative day. Usually, this dysfunction recovers in a week, but in the elderly it may take as long as 3 months to recover. Increased morbidity and increased hospital stay are often related to cognitive dysfunction. Delirium affects 15%–25% of older patients who have undergone a major operation.[22] Delirium is the decreased ability to maintain attention to external stimuli and appropriately shift attention to new stimuli. Mortality related to delirium is quoted at between 10% and 65%.[22,23] Higher postoperative pain scores have been shown in prospective studies to be associated with an increased risk for delirium.[24] The quality of pain relief may be more important than the method of pain relief. A postoperative "geriatric" consult focusing on pain control and drug interactions reduced the risk of delirium by one-third in one study.[25] Certain drugs, including meperidine, have been implicated in causing delirium.[19,26]

Timing of Analgesia

Preemptive

Preoperative, preemptive analgesia, although intuitively sensible, is controversial. A 2002 meta-analysis from the Cochrane library did not show any decrease in postoperative pain or pain medication requirements. This qualitative and quantitative systematic review of preemptive analgesia did not provide any evidence that timing of single-dose or continuous postoperative pain treatment was important for postoperative analgesia[27] (Table 19.2). Although there are single studies demonstrating a decrease in postoperative opioid requirement with preemptive analgesia, this review of multiple studies did not support any benefit. This topic still draws heated debate. Other studies suggested that preoperative epidural analgesia minimizes central sensitization and consequently lessens the intensity of the postoperative pain experience.[28]

Intraoperative

The benefit of intraoperative pain control is also controversial. Current data show no difference in mortality or morbidity related to use of regional versus general anesthesia. Studies from the 1970s and 1980s showed a reduction in morbidity and mortality with regional anesthesia.[29,30] More recent studies do not demonstrate a difference.[31] Although clinical perception and theoretic considerations suggest that regional anesthesia should be safer than general anesthesia, there appears to be no difference in mortality or major morbidity as long as perioperative hemodynamics are well controlled and postoperative analgesia is provided. Many of the perceived benefits of regional anesthesia may actually be that the benefits of regional analgesia get extended into the postoperative period.[31] Perioperative local analgesia by wound infiltration does have benefits.[3] Preincisional injection does not show any difference compared with postincisional injection. Nonetheless, local anesthetic by wound injection or infusion pump does lead to improved postoperative pain reduction.[3]

Postoperative

With the above concepts in mind, postoperative pain control seems to be the first place to focus. Accurate assessment of

TABLE 19.2.
Preoperative Versus Postoperative Analgesia.

Presurgical versus postsurgical NSAIDs[69–87]
- Some aspects of postoperative pain control were improved by preemptive treatment in 4 of 20 trials. Overall, the data demonstrated preemptive NSAIDs to be of no analgesic benefit when compared with postincisional administration of these drugs.

Presurgical versus postsurgical intravenous opioids[88–95]
- No improvement in postoperative pain control was observed after preemptive administration of systemic opioids.

Presurgical versus postsurgical intravenous and intramuscular NMDA receptor antagonists[96–103]
- No improvement in postoperative pain control was observed after preemptive administration of systemic ketamine. Both studies on dextromethorphan were positive, but data are too sparse to reach a definitive conclusion.

Presurgical versus postsurgical single-dose epidural analgesic regimens[104–112]
- The quantitative analysis of mean visual analog pain scores showed no significant reduction by preemptive single-dose epidural analgesia with opioid, local anesthetic, or a mixture. However, significant reductions in analgesic demand were demonstrated in 7 of 11 treatment arms.

Presurgical versus postsurgical continuous epidural analgesic regimens[113–120]
- No improvement in postoperative pain control was observed after preemptive versus postincisional continuous epidural analgesia.

Presurgical versus postsurgical caudal analgesia in children and presurgical versus postsurgical intrathecal anesthesia and analgesia[121–126]
- Preemptive treatment was ineffective in four of five studies of caudal block and in the one study of intrathecal block.

Presurgical versus postsurgical wound infiltration, peripheral nerve block, and intraperitoneal instillation with local anesthetics[127–145]
- There is no evidence for improved pain relief with preemptive local anesthetic wound infiltration compared with similar postincisional administration.
- The limited data available do not allow conclusions regarding a positive effect of preemptive analgesia with peripheral nerve blocks or intraperitoneal local anesthetic.

Source: A summary of Møiniche's qualitative and quantitative systematic review of preemptive analgesia for postoperative pain relief.[27]

pain may be as critical as treatment. Nurses' and physicians' assessment of pain is routinely found to be less than the patients' own assessment.[32] Adequate treatment of pain may help reduce postoperative complications by minimizing the autonomic response to pain. Most surgical morbidity and mortality occur postoperatively. Mortality in the first 24h is twice that of intraoperative mortality, and over the next 6 days it is 10 times that of intraoperative mortality.[33]

Strategies for Treating Acute Postoperative Pain

Medications are the mainstay of pain control in surgical patients. These medications are categorized as acetaminophen, nonsteroidal antiinflammatory drugs (NSAIDs), opioids, and experimental medications. Local anesthetics can also play a substantial role. There are a host of other medications and nonpharmacological modalities for more chronic and neuropathic pain syndromes not discussed here. Current drugs such as antidepressants and neuroleptics are in use for chronic pain syndromes but have little role in acute pain management in the postoperative period.

Pharmacological Agents

Acetaminophen

Acetaminophen is an analgesic and antipyretic with no antiinflammatory effect. Acetaminophen is the basis of pain control for mild postoperative pain. There is a ceiling dose past which there is no further effect. In addition, there is known hepatic toxicity that limits dosing. In patients with liver disease, dosing is limited to 2g/day. In patients without liver disease, 4g/day is the maximum dose.

Nonsteroidal Antiinflammatory Drugs

The NSAID group blocks prostaglandin production and release by inhibiting the cyclooxygenase (COX) enzymes. The physiologic effects of prostaglandin-mediated inflammation are therefore inhibited (Fig. 19.2). However, there are adverse consequences to this interaction. Most notably, gastric mucosa protection is compromised, and platelet dysfunction occurs.

Dyspepsia and upper gastrointestinal bleeding increases in a linear fashion with age in patients using NSAIDs.[34,35] Antacids, H_2 blockers, and proton pump inhibitors may decrease this risk.[36] An additional side effect of NSAIDs is platelet dysfunction, which occurs irreversibly for the life of the platelet. Platelet aggregation is inhibited, and there may be an increased risk of bleeding. Renal injury may also occur.[37] The risk of fluid retention is a concern, especially in patients with underlying renal disease, congestive heart failure, hepatic disease, or those patients on diuretics. Like acetaminophen, there is a ceiling dose above which there is no increase in analgesia.

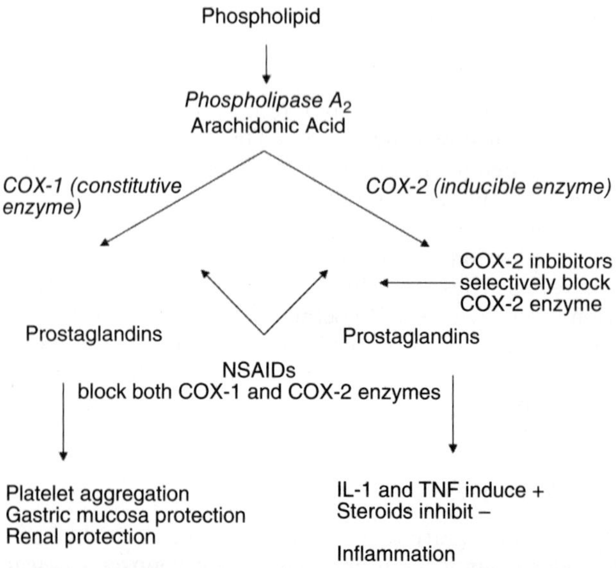

FIGURE 19.2. Prostaglandin biosynthesis. The NSAIDs act by blocking prostaglandin synthesis and block both COX-1 and COX-2 enzymes. The COX-2 inhibitory class of medication only blocks the COX-2 enzyme.

Ketoralac is an NSAID that can be given parenterally. It has the same side-effect profile as most conventional oral NSAIDs. Some studies have shown decreased opioid requirement when ketoralac is given postoperatively.[38,39] There are no cardiopulmonary side effects known. Use is limited to 5 days only.[40] Dosing in the elderly patient must be reduced. Typically, a 30-mg dose is thought to be equivalent to 12 mg of morphine. In the older individual, the dose should be reduced to no more than 15 mg i.v. every 6 h.[41,42]

The COX-2 inhibitors are a new generation of NSAID that block only the COX-2 enzyme and not the COX-1 enzyme; COX-1 is a constitutive enzyme found in most tissues in the body, whereas COX-2 is undetectable in most tissue but is expressed in response to painful stimuli.[34,43,44] The COX-2 inhibitors are 200–300 times more selective for COX-2 compared to COX-1. Renal side effects are similar to other NSAIDs, but there is no antiplatelet effect and less gastrointestinal risk. There also is a mild anticoagulation effect, and these drugs interact with warfarin, causing an increase in the international normalized ratio (INR) by as much as 10%. Celecoxib, one of the current COX-2 inhibitors, has a sulfonamide moiety that may cause an allergic reaction in patients with a sulfa allergy. Vioxx, one of the three current COX-2 inhibitors, has been withdrawn from the market because of concerns about increased cardiac events in patients taking the medication over an 18-month period. Current concerns regarding the safety of this class of drug are under investigation.

Opioids

Opioid medication was originally derived form the poppy plant but now is primarily produced from synthetic sources. Opioid drugs mimic the naturally occurring opioid peptides. Opioid receptors include the Mu_1 receptor found in the brain (periaquiductal gray matter, locus ceruleus, nucleus raphe magnum) and the Mu_2 receptor found in the dorsal horn of the spinal cord as well as the kappa and delta fibers.

Opioids have no ceiling effect. There is no known long-term toxicity. Most opioids are metabolized by the liver. Morphine undergoes glucuronidation to morphine-6-glucuronide, which is an active metabolite that has the same affinity for opioid receptors as morphine. Tolerance develops over time. Tolerance to the side effects of most opioids actually develops more readily than tolerance to the analgesic effect.[45] Side effects include respiratory depression, which is dose dependent. Opioids blunt the response to hypoxic and hypercarbic stimuli mediated by the Mu_2 receptor in the brainstem. This can lead to shallow breaths and even apnea. Hypotension may occur in patients as opioids lower sympathetic tone. This is more apt to occur in the hypovolemic patient.

Nausea is common, with 10% to 40% of patients experiencing nausea related to opioid receptor triggers. Vomiting may occur as well. Opioids reduce lower esophageal sphincter tone, increase gastric secretions, and reduce gastric secretion transit. Ileus is common. Ileus is mediated by Mu_2 receptors in the brain and intestinal plexus.[46] Constipation is a common problem, especially in the older adult. Urinary retention can also occur. Urinary retention is more common when opioids are administered by the epidural route. Renal effects occur with some opioids.

All opioids can cause sedation. Delirium, which is especially concerning in the elderly patient, has been closely linked with meperidine administration. Fear of addiction keeps many older patients from asking for opioid-based medication. These fears are unfounded. In one chart review of 12,000 patients, there were only 4 who developed an addiction.[47] Other studies mentioned a 1 in 1000 risk of addiction when opioids are used for acute pain treatment.[48] Dosing should begin with short-acting opioids initially. A switch to a longer-acting, controlled-release medication can occur after good pain control has been established. Dosing should be patient controlled whenever possible as opposed to scheduled or as needed (prn), especially in the immediate postoperative period.

Weak Opioids

Codeine has a mild-to-moderate analgesic effect; it does have a ceiling for its analgesic effect but no ceiling for its adverse effects. Codeine has an antitussive effect as well. Oxycodone is an analgesic with a short half-life. It is combined with either acetaminophen or aspirin, and dosing is based on these medications' limits. There is a low potential for metabolite accumulation. Propoxyphene has been found in studies to have no greater analgesic effect than aspirin or acetaminophen. There is, however, a substantial risk of addiction and renal injury with this medication.[49] Pentazocine can cause delirium and agitation in the elderly and should be avoided in these patients.[50] It works as a mixed opioid agonist/antagonist. Tramadol is a nonopioid that binds to the opiate receptor. It causes minimal sedation and minimal respiratory depression. Nausea is the main side effect.[51]

Strong Opioids

Morphine is the mainstay of postoperative pain management. Morphine is available in almost every conceivable form (oral, intravenous, intramuscular, rectal, sublingual, liquid, spinal, epidural, topical). Prospective studies compared postoperative morphine consumption in the younger and the older postoperative patient and found that the two groups had equal intravenous morphine requirements.[52,53]

Hydromorphone is eight times more potent than morphine.[54] It has a short half-life and a low potential for metabolite accumulation, although it may accumulate in renal failure.[55] Hydromorphone is well tolerated in the elderly.[54]

Fentanyl is 100 times more potent than morphine and has a faster onset of action. Fentanyl has a short duration of action, but it may have a prolonged effect in the older patient; therefore, dosing should be reduced in the elderly. Fentanyl has a cardiac-stabilizing effect.[54] Fentanyl also comes in a patch form. This should be used with caution in the elderly patient because dosing fluctuates in older people as body temperature and percentage body fat affect transdermal dosing. Dosing of fentanyl should never start over 25 μg/h in an opioid-naïve older patient.

Methadone is typically used in the maintenance of heroin addicts undergoing treatment. It has a long half-life and may accumulate, especially in the older patient. It is not recommended for the elderly patient.

Meperidine is 1/10 as potent as morphine. Meperidine is metabolized into normeperidine, which is a toxic metabolite that causes central nervous system excitability. The half-life of this metabolite is 40h. It may lead to myoclonus and seizures. These effects are more pronounced in the elderly and in patients with renal failure.[56,57] Meperidine may lead to delirium.[24] Meperidine is more apt to lead to respiratory depression than morphine. For these reasons, this drug should not be used in the older patient.

Experimental

Investigation of other approaches to block the pain response is an exciting research topic. Ion channel blockers are the most talked about up-and-coming analgesic class. They target pain at the peripheral neuron in hope of avoiding central effects. Ziconotide (the prototype of this class of drugs) is 1000 times more potent than morphine. It is derived form the venom of a Pacific Ocean marine snail and blocks the electrical impulses that generate pain by blocking the calcium ion channel. Theoretically, by targeting the synapse of the peripheral nerve, there will be fewer side effects. However, ziconotide currently has prohibitive side effects, such as confusion, memory loss, dizziness, and tremors.[58] This drug is still in the experimental stage and is not recommended.

Others

The postoperative period is associated with an increased production of cytokines, which increase pain sensitivity. The investigation of medications such as clonidine and atenolol, which are thought to blunt the release of proinflammatory cytokines by blocking the autonomic effect of acute pain, is of current interest. A double-blind, placebo-controlled study looked at the use of epidural clonidine. Patients in the clonidine group exhibited longer patient-controlled analgesia (PCEA) trigger times, lower pain scores at rest and while coughing, less morphine consumption, and a faster return of bowel function throughout the 72-h postoperative observation period compared with patients in the control group. For patients in the clonidine group, production of interleukin-1 receptor antagonist (IL-1RA), interleukin-6 (IL-6), and IL-8 was significantly less at the end of the surgical procedure and at 12 and 24h after surgery. However, the concentrations of IL-1β and tumor necrosis factor-α (TNF-α) were not significantly increased.[59]

Local/Regional Block/Infusion Pumps

Local anesthetics work by blocking conduction in nerve fibers. Local anesthetics may be used by local infiltration, topical application, local wound infusion by continuous postoperative pump, epidural infusion, and peripheral nerve infusion. Topical application of local anesthetic is obtained using agents such as EMLA cream, which contains prilocaine and lidocaine. This agent can be used for superficial procedures and can be placed 40 to 60min before surgical incision. The development of disposable and lightweight infusion pumps is leading to the increasing use of peripheral nerve infusion in the ambulatory setting (Table 19.3). Complications encoun-

TABLE 19.3.
Local Infusion Pump Versus Systemic Opioids.

Trial	*Year*	*Level*	*Group*	*Design*	*Median follow-up*	*Major endpoint*	*Interpretations*
146	2003	I	N = 36 NS 0.25% bupivacaine 0.5% bupivacaine	Prospective, randomized, placebo-controlled, double-blind (postcardiac surgery sternal infusion pump)	Postop inpatient stay	Pain score and opioid requirement	Compared with the control group, there was a statistically significant reduction in verbal rating scale pain scores and patient-controlled analgesia morphine use in the bupivacaine 0.5% group.
147	1998	II-1	N = 72 Pump containing bupivacaine; pump containing normal saline control group without a pump	Randomized controlled (patient undergoing Lichtenstein hernia repair)	5 days postop	Pain scores	Patients who had a local anesthetic infusion had significantly less pain than either the placebo or control groups. This was greatest during the first 48h (day 1, $P = .028$ and .011, respectively; day 2, $P = .012$ and .037, respectively).
148	2000	II-1	N = 62 NS, 31 0.25% bupivacaine, 31	Prospective, randomized (consecutive patients undergoing arthroscopic subacromial decompression had an indwelling pain control infusion catheter)	7 days postop	Pain score and narcotic and nonnarcotic use	There was a statistically significant difference in pain in all parameters tested in the bupivacaine group as compared with the saline control group ($P < .05$).

NS, normal saline.

References: From a review of the literature regarding local infusion pump use.[146–148] tered with these infusion pump systems include tissue necrosis, surgical wound infection, and cellulitis.[60]

Nonpharmacological Agents

Transcutaneous Electrical Nerve Stimulation

Transcutaneous electrical nerve stimulation (TENS) is used clinically by a variety of health care professionals for the reduction of pain. Clinical effectiveness of TENS is controversial, with some studies supporting and others refuting its clinical use. Although used by health professionals for decades, the mechanisms by which TENS produces analgesia or reduces pain are still being elucidated. It is a noninvasive modality that is easy to apply with relatively few contraindications. However, the clinical efficacy of TENS will remain equivocal until the publication of sufficient numbers of high-quality, randomized controlled clinical trials.[61]

Audiovisual Distraction

Using audiovisual distraction (i.e., playing a movie of the patient's choice through a special headset) may reduce pain, reduce patient movement during the procedure, decease autonomic stimulation, and therefore perhaps decrease cardiac risk. This technique was presented at the 2004 American College of Surgeons Clinical Congress but the Food and Drug Administration has not cleared this technique for use.[62]

Minimally Invasive Surgery

Surgeons can help reduce postoperative pain by employing less-traumatic operative methods. Minimally invasive techniques tend to limit tissue trauma and therefore may have less associated postoperative pain (Table 19.4).

TABLE 19.4.
Minimally Invasive Surgery Versus Open Surgery.

Trial	*Year*	*Level*	*Group*	*Design*	*Median follow-up*	*Major endpoint*	*Interpretations*
149	2003	II-2	N = 481 L = 53 O = 428	Retrospective review (all patients undergoing colectomy)	Postop inpatient stay	Morphine use in milligrams	The laparoscopic colectomy group used a mean of 89.7 mg MSO_4 versus 170.6 mg MSO_4. $P = .0001$
150	2000	II-1	N = 49 L = 27 O = 22	Prospective randomized (laparoscopic vs. open cholecystectomy)	Postop period until return to work	Length of hospital stay and the duration of the sick leave	The median (range) hospital stay was significantly shorter after LC than OC. The duration of sick leave was also significantly shorter after LC than OC. Patients had significantly less postoperative pain after LC than OC as reflected by the need for opioids.
151	2001	II-1	N = 198 L = 93 O = 105	Prospective randomized (laparoscopic vs. open appendectomy)	Postop period until return to work	Operating time, return to regular diet, need for parenteral analgesia, length of hospital stay, total cost	The laparoscopic group had a shorter duration of parenteral analgesia (mean 1.6 vs. 2.2 days; $P < .01$), fewer morphine-equivalent milligrams of parenteral narcotic (median 14 mg vs. 34 mg; $P = .001$), a shorter postoperative hospital stay (mean 2.6 vs. 3.4 days; $P < .01$), and earlier return to full activity (median 14 vs. 21 days; $P < .02$).
152	2000	II-2	N = 60 L = 30 O = 30	Prospective randomized (laparoscopic vs. open Nissen fundoplication)	Postop period until return to work	Operating time, need for parenteral analgesia, length of hospital stay, pulmonary function, time to return to work	The laparoscopic group used less morphine (33.9 mg vs. 67.5 mg morphine, respectively) per total hospital stay ($P < .001$). There was no significant difference in postoperative nausea and vomiting. On the first day after operation, patients in the laparoscopy group had better respiratory function. Postoperative hospital stay was shorter in the laparoscopic group, median (range) 3 (2–6) versus 3 (2–10) days ($P = .021$). No difference was found in the duration of sick leave.

L, laparoscopic approach; O, open approach.

References: From a review of the literature looking at pain after minimally invasive surgery.[149–152]

Special Patient Populations

Pediatrics

Children often do not receive adequate pain control because of inadequate knowledge, poor assessment of the patient's pain, and concerns about addiction. Children are usually reluctant to report pain and may be concerned that pain correlates with worse disease.

There are some special considerations in treating children. Drug equilibration and clearance is slower in young children (less than 6 months). Morphine should be dosed at 0.1 mg/kg (half that dose if less than 6 months). Patient-controlled analgesia (PCA) is appropriate at age 7 years in general. Use of EMLA cream may help by providing topical analgesia, but a 30- to 60-min wait after application is necessary.

Pregnancy

While pregnant, 2% of women need nonobstetric operations. The physiologic changes associated with pregnancy may complicate their management (Table 19.5).

During pregnancy, NSAIDs are contraindicated. These drugs can cause premature closure of the ductus in the third trimester, which leads to decreased fetal urine output and oligohydramnios.

Tylenol and narcotics are not contraindicated. Patient-controlled analgesia is appropriate, but basal dosing may have an increased risk of respiratory depression. Fentanyl has a short duration and is becoming the drug of choice in pregnancy. Epidural PCA with the local anesthetic bupivacaine is protein bound and limits transplacental transfer, making this a safe method as well.

Sleep Apnea

Obstructive sleep apnea (OSA) in the adult obese patient may be due in part to an increased amount of pharyngeal tissue; therefore, there is an increased risk of intubation and extubation difficulties, and pain management can be complicated by narcotic/sedative-induced pharyngeal collapse.[63] It is estimated that 18 million Americans have OSA.

Obese OSA patients have an increased risk of opioid-induced upper airway obstruction (even epidural analgesia and PCA may be problematic), and this is a reason why these patients may need a monitored care environment. Factors to be considered in this risk-benefit analysis are the body mass index of the patient, the severity of the OSA, the degree of associated cardiopulmonary disease, and the postoperative narcotic requirement. Based on these factors, a plan for adequate monitoring should be made.[63]

TABLE 19.5. Physiologic Changes with Pregnancy.[a]

Mild chronic respiratory alkalosis
Increased oxygen consumption
Decreased functional residual capacity
Increased risk for hypoxia and acidosis
Increased difficulty in masking and intubating
Increased blood volume
Hypercoagulable state
Thromboembolic events common
Hypotension common
Decrease LES pressure
Decreased epidural space

LES, lower esophageal sphincter.

[a]The physiologic changes seen with pregnancy may affect pain management choices.

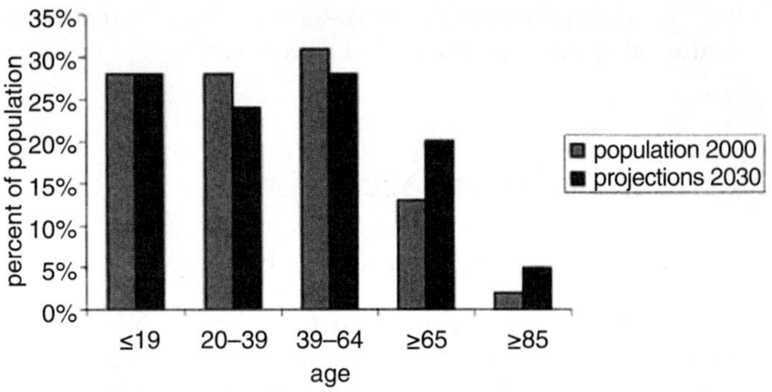

FIGURE 19.3. Population projections, U.S. Census. The older group (those over 65 years of age) of patients is the fastest-growing population in the United States. (From U.S. Census.[68])

Geriatric

Patients over the age of 65 currently comprise 12% of the U.S. population. One-third of the 25 million operations performed annually are on patients in this segment of the population, which is continuing to grow (Fig. 19.3). Unfortunately, the rate of inadequate pain control seems to be highest in this group of patients. Physiology changes that come with aging make adequate pain control even more important in the elderly patient (Table 19.6).

There are some considerations when dosing medications in this group of patients. Drug elimination half-life changes. For example, the normal 250-min half-life of fentanyl may increase to 925 min in an older patient. When using NSAIDs in the older patient, use those with a short half-life. Parenteral forms require reduced dosing. Be wary of the renal and antiplatelet effects in older patients. Opioids may be administered. The PCA dosing is usually appropriate. Meperidine should not be used. Propoxipene should not be used. Intramuscular injection should be avoided as this population usually has less muscle mass.

Regional and local anesthetics offer decreased postoperative negative nitrogen balance, endocrine stress, thromboembolic events, blood loss, and mental status changes. However,

TABLE 19.6. Physiologic Changes with Aging.

Decreased vascular compliance
Increased vascular resistance, therefore increased blood pressure
Decreased parasympathetic response
Decreased β-receptor response, therefore less ability to increase heart rate
Decreased pulmonary compliance
Decreased glomerular filtration rate
Decreased drug affinity to serum proteins
Increase in percentage body fat
Decreased liver and renal function
Decreased functioning central nervous system mass

TABLE 19.7.
Epidural Versus Intravenous Opioid Postoperative Analgesia.

Trial	*Year*	*Level*	*Group*	*Design*	*Median follow-up*	*Major endpoint*	*Interpretations*
153	2003	II-3	N = 2696 E = 1670 IV = 1026	Prospective review (review of all patients undergoing major surgery over a 5-year period)	Postop inpatient stay	Pain score	Overall patients in the epidural group had less pain. Insufficient dosing, leg weakness, pruritus were more common in the epidural group. Respiratory depression, sedation, hallucinations, nightmares, confusion more common in intravenous group.
154	2003	I	N = 36 E = 18 IV = 20	Prospective randomized, not blinded (patients undergoing laparoscopic colectomy)	Postop inpatient stay	Pain score	The epidural group had better early postoperative pain scores but equivalent length of stay
65	2000	I	N = 70 E = 35 IV = 35	Prospective randomized, not blinded (patients over the age of 70 undergoing colectomy)	Postop inpatient stay	Pain score	Epidural group had better pain relief at rest and with coughing. No difference in incidence of delirium. Equivalent length of stay.

E, epidural catheter; IV, intravenous opioids.

References: From a review of the literature looking at pain control using epidural versus intravenous opioids.[65,153,154]

spinal anesthetic is more likely to lead to hypotensive events.

Methods of Administration

After major surgical procedures, in the immediate postoperative period, the current guidelines are for intravenous opioids, epidural opioids with or without local anesthetic, or regional blockade.[3] In general, patient-controlled dosing has proven to be superior to continuous or as-needed dosing. Intramuscular injection should not be used since intravenous administration has been found to be superior, with more consistent systemic absorption.[64]

Studies have shown that patients (including older patients) get better titration of pain medication when they control dosing. Baseline cognitive function is required. Overall, studies of PCA use revealed improved analgesia, fewer pulmonary complications, and less confusion. In a study comparing a younger population to an older group using intravenous PCA after major surgery, the same amount of intravenous opioid was given in the first 24 h to both groups. Both groups took PCA morphine for "adequate" relief but not for "complete" relief of pain.[52] In conclusion, both younger and older patients attained comparable levels of analgesia; they were equally satisfied, and the total dose of narcotic administered was equivalent.

Epidural catheters allow administration of opioid analgesia as well as a local analgesic. The placement of such a catheter is costly, and there are contraindications, such as coagulopathy, local infection, and spinal abnormalities (Table 19.7).

A prospective, randomized trial compared PCA with intravenous morphine versus PCA with epidural 0.125% bupivacaine and sufentanil.[65] Seventy patients over the age of 70 who had undergone laparotomy for cancer were randomized to intravenous PCA or epidural PCA. Pain intensity, mental status, cardiopulmonary function, gastrointestinal function, and patient satisfaction were assessed. In the epidural PCA group, there was a significant improvement in pain relief and satisfaction and a quicker return to gastrointestinal function; mental status improved more rapidly. The duration of hospitalization was equivalent. The episodes of delirium were equivalent, as were cardiopulmonary complications.

In a different study, not limited to an older patient population, epidural with bupivacaine alone or bupivacaine with morphine reduced length of gastrointestinal dysfunction by 1.5 days compared to intravenous narcotics.[19] This is significant because currently ileus is estimated to cost $750 million.[66,67]

Recommendations

After major laparotomy or thoracotomy, patients who have the ability to use PCA should be given the opportunity. The epidural route with opioid and local anesthetic seems to provide some benefit if an epidural can be placed safely. For patients who are unable to control their own pain relief, a well-monitored continuous epidural or intravenous dosing is most likely to provide the best pain control (Table 19.8). Two agents that work in alternate ways via the same or a different route are recommended to optimize pain management.[3]

TABLE 19.8. Recommended Analgesia for More Painful Procedures: Thoracotomy/Laparotomy.

Cognitively intact	*Cognitively impaired*
Epidural	Epidural
Lipophilic opioid and local analgesic	Lipophilic opioid and local analgesic
Continuous or PCA	Continuous
Intravenous	Intravenous
Strong opioid	Strong opioid
Continuous or PCA	Continuous

Local and regional analgesia should be used when appropriate. Additional treatment with a second agent with different mechanism of action should also be considered.

TABLE 19.9. Cost of Pain Control to the Hospital.

Oral narcotics	$0.16
Sustained-release narcotics	$2
Fentanyl patch	$41
PCA morphine 50mg/ml	$10
Epidural	$1000

Source: Data from American College of Surgeons 89th Clinical Congress.[154]

Cost

How to assess the cost benefit of pain control is still a question that does not have clear answers. Oral narcotics have a small cost per dose to the health care system. A single dose costs the hospital about 16 cents. Patient-controlled devices using intravenous morphine are more expensive to the system at about $10 for 50mg of morphine. Epidural catheters are 100 times the cost of 50mg of PCA morphine (Table 19.9).

Conclusion

Providing adequate pain control in the perioperative period should be a routine part of the procedure. A new focus on the importance of adequate pain control has led to the development of pain management services in many facilities. Surgeons, anesthesiologists, and nursing staff all should be involved in assessing and addressing pain issues. Patient comfort and recovery is closely linked with pain control. There are well-established recommendations for addressing perioperative pain; there is also a burgeoning body of literature on new techniques that will require further review, but it is becoming clearer that patients have physiologic improvement with optimal pain management.

References

1. Joint Commission on Accreditation of Healthcare Organizations Pain Management Standard. Available at: www.jcaho.org/accredited=organizations/hospitals/standards/revisions/2001/pain=managment1.htm.
2. Stadler M, Schlander M, Braeckman M, et al. A cost-utility and cost-effectiveness analysis of an acute pain service. J Clin Anesth 2004;16:159–167.
3. Ashburn M, Caplan R, Carr D, et al. Practice guidelines for acute pain management in the perioperative setting. Anesthesiology 2004;100:1573–1584.
4. Roy R, Michael T. A survey of chronic pain in an elderly population. Can Fam Physician 1986;32:513.
5. Sengstaken EA, King SA. The problem of pain and its detection among geriatric nursing home residents. J Am Geriatr Soc 1993;41:541.
6. Ferrell BA. Pain management in elderly people. J Am Geriatr Soc 1991;39:64–73.
7. Gloth FM. Principles of perioperative pain management in older adults. Clin Geriatr Med 2001;17:553–573.
8. Gloth FM. Pain management in older adults. Prevention and treatment. J Am Geriatr Soc 2001;49:188–199.
9. Wallace A. Prophylactic atenolol reduces postoperative myocardial ischemia. McSPI Research Group. Anesthesiology 1998;88:7–17.
10. Khuri SF, Daley J, Hendeson W, et al. The National Veterans Administration Surgical Risk Study: risk adjustment for the comparative assessment of the quality of surgical care. J Am Coll Surg 1995;180:519–531.
11. Erskine RJ, Murphy PJ, Langton JA, et al. Effects of age on the sensitivity of upper airway reflexes. Br J Anaesth 1993;70:574–575.
12. Pedersen T, Eliasen K, Henriksen E. A prospective study of risk factors and cardiopulmonary complications associated with anesthesia and surgery: risk indicators of cardiopulmonary morbidity. Acta Anaesthesiol Scand 1990;34:144–155.
13. Schwieger I, Gamuliln Z, Suter PM. Lung function during anesthesia and respiratory insufficiency in the postoperative period: physiological and clinical implications. Acta Anaesthesiol Scand 1989;33:527–534.
14. Mangano DT. Perioperative cardiac morbidity. Anesthesiology 1990;12:153–184.
15. Kannel WB, Belanger AJ. Epidemiology of heart failure. Am Heart J 2991;121:951–957.
16. Franklon SS, Gustin WT, Wong ND, et al. Hemodynamic patterns of age-related changes in blood pressure: the Framingham Heart Study. Circulation 1997;96:308–315.
17. Landahl S, Bengtsson C, Sigurdsson JA, et al. Age-related changes in blood pressure. Hypertension 1986;8:1004–1009.
18. Matot I, Oppemheim-Eden A, Ratrot R. Preoperative cardiac events in elderly patients with hip fracture randomized to epidural or conventional analgesia. Anesthesiology 2003;98:156–163.
19. Liu SS, Carpenter RL, Mackey DC. Effects of perioperative analgesic techniques on rate of recovery after colon surgery. Anesthesiology 1995;83:757–765.
20. Kehlet H. Modification of responses to surgery by neural blockade: clinical implications. In: Cousins MJ, Bridenbaugh PO, eds. Clinical Anesthesia and Management of Pain, 3rd ed. New York: Lippincott-Raven, 1998:129–175.
21. Rodgers A, Walker N, Schug S, et al. Reduction of postoperative mortality and morbidity with epidural or spinal anaesthesia: results from overview of randomised trials. BMJ 2000;321:1493.
22. Inouye S. The dilemma of delirium; clinical and research controversies regarding diagnosis and evaluation of delirium in hospitalized elderly medical patients. Am J Med 1994;97:278–288.
23. Lipowski Z. Delirium in the elderly patient. N Engl J Med 1989;320:278–288.
24. Lynch EP, Lazor MA, Gellis JE, Orav J, Goldman L, Marcantonio ER. The impact of postoperative pain on the development of postoperative delirium. Anesth Analg 1998;86:781–785.
25. Marcantonio ER, Flacker JM, Wright RJ, et al. Reducing delirium after hip fracture: a randomized trial. J Am Geriatr Soc 2001;49:516–522.
26. Meador K. Cognitive side effects of medication. Neurol Clin North Am 1998;16:141–155.
27. Møiniche S. A qualitative and quantitative systematic review of preemptive analgesia for postoperative pain relief. Anesthesiology 2002;96:725–742.
28. Katz J, Cohen L, Schmidt R, et al. Postoperative morphine use and hyperalgesia are reduced by preoperative but not intraoperative epidural analgesia. Anesthesiology 2003;98:1449–1460.
29. McLaren AD. Mortality studies. Reg Anesth 1982;7(suppl):172.
30. Yeager MP, Glass DD, Neff RK, et al. Epidural anesthesia and analgesia in high-risk surgical patients. Anesthesiology 1987;66:729.
31. Roy RC. Choosing general versus regional anesthesia for the elderly. Anesthesiol Clin North Am 2000;18:90–104.
32. Abrahm JL. Advances in pain management for older adult patients. Clin Geriatr Med 2000;16:269–311.
33. Pedersen T, Eliasen K, Henriksen E. A prospective study of mortality associated with anaesthesia and surgery: risk indica-

tors of mortality in hospital. Acta Anaesthesiol Scand 1990;34: 176–182.
34. Bell GM, Schnitzer TJ. COX-2 inhibitors and other nonsteroidal anti-inflammatory drugs in the treatment of pain in the elderly. Clin Geriatr Med 2001;17:489–502.
35. Bjorkman D. Current status of nonsteroidal anti-inflammatory drug use in the United States: risk factors and frequent complications. Am J Med 1999;107(suppl 6A):3S.
36. Hawkey C. Progress in prophylaxis against nonsteroidal anti-inflammatory drug-associated ulcers and erosions. Am J Med 1998;104:67S.
37. Whelton A. Nephrotoxicity of nonsteroidal anti-inflammatory drugs: physiologic foundations and clinical implications. Am J Med 1999;106(suppl 5B):13S.
38. Etches DC, Warriner CB, Badner N, et al. Continuous intravenous administration of ketorolac reduces pain and morphine consumption after total hip replacement or knee arthroplasty. Anesth Analg 1995;81:1175–1180.
39. Stouten E, Armbuster S, Houmes R, et al. Comparison of ketorolac and morphine for postoperative pain after major surgery. Acta Anesthesiol Scand 1992;336:716–721.
40. Strom DL, Berlin JA, Kinman JL, et al. Parenteral ketorolac and risk of gastrointestinal and operative site bleeding: a postmarketing surveillance study. JAMA 1996;275:376–382.
41. Camu F, Lauwers MH, Vandersberghe C. Side effects of NSAIDs and dosing recommendations for ketorolac. Acta Anaesthesiol Belg 1996;47:143–149.
42. Malieka J, Elboim CM. Gastrointestinal complications associated with intramuscular ketorolac therapy in the elderly. Ann Pharmacother 1995;29:698–701.
43. Noor MG. Cycolooxygenase-2 inhibitors. Anesth Analg 2003; 96:1720–1738.
44. Furst D. Pharmacology and efficacy or cyclooxygenase (COX) inhibitors. Am J Med 1999;107(suppl 6A):18S.
45. Melzack R. The tragedy of needless pain. Sci Am 1990;262(2): 27–33.
46. Evans C, Hammond D, Frederickson R. The opioid peptides. In: Pasternak G, ed. The Opiate Receptors. Clifton Park, NJ: Humana Press, 1988:23–71.
47. Porter J, Jick H. Addiction is rare in patients treated with narcotics [letter]. N Engl J Med 1980;302:123.
48. Fishbain D, Rosomoff H, Rosomoff R. Drug abuse, dependence, and addiction in chronic pain patients. Clin J Pain 1992;8: 77–850.
49. Beaver WT. Impact of non-narcotic oral analgesics on pain management. Am J Med 1988;84:3–15.
50. Morrison RS, Carney MT, Manfredi LM. Pain Management, Principles and Practice of Geriatric Surgery. New York: Springer, 2001:160–171.
51. Moore R, McQuay H. Single-patient data meta-analysis of 3453 postoperative patients: oral tramadol versus placebo, codeine, and combination analgesics. Pain 1997;69:287–294.
52. Gagliese L, Jackson M, Ritvo P. Age is not an impediment to effective use of patient-controlled analgesia by surgical patients. Anesthesiology 2000;93:597–598.
53. Aubrun F, Bunge D, Langeron O. Postoperative morphine consumption in the elderly patient. Anesthesiology 2003;99: 160–174.
54. Austrup ML, Korean G. Analgesic agents for the postoperative period. Surg Clin North Am 1999;79:253–273.
55. Babul N, Darke A, Hagen N. Hydromorphone metabolite accumulation in renal failure. J Pain Symptom Manage 1995;10: 184–186.
56. Szeto H, Inturrisi C, Houde R, et al. Accumulation of normeperidine, an active metabolite of meperidine, in patients with renal failure and cancer. Ann Intern Med 1977;86:738–740.
57. Kaiko R, Foley K, Grabinski P, et al. Central nervous system excitatory effects of meperidine in cancer patients. Ann Neurol 1983;13:180–185.
58. Garber K. Stopping pain. Technol Rev 2003;11:48–57.
59. Wu CT, Jao SW, Borel CO, et al. The effect of epidural clonidine on perioperative cytokine response, postoperative pain, and bowel function in patients undergoing colorectal surgery. Anesth Analg 2004;99:502–509.
60. Brown SL, Morrison AE. Local anesthetic infusion pump systems adverse events reported to the Food and Drug Administration. Anesthesiology 2004;100:1305–1307.
61. Sluka KA. Transcutaneous electrical nerve stimulation: basic science mechanisms and clinical effectiveness. J Pain 2003;4(3): 109–121.
62. Wallace A. American College of Surgeons 90th Clinical Congress 10/2004. Selected Topics in Perioperative Pain Management; p. 29.
63. Benumof J. Sleep apnea. Anesthesiol Clin North Am 2002;20: 789–811.
64. Forrest J. Pharmacology of opioids. In: Forest J, ed. Acute Pain: Pathophysiology and Treatment. Grimsby, Ontario, Canada: Manticore, 1998:75–98.
65. Mann C, Pouzeratte Y, Boccara G. Comparison of intravenous or epidural patient-controlled analgesia in the elderly after major abdominal surgery. Anesthesiology 2000;92:433–441.
66. Livingston E, Passaro E. Postoperative ileus. Dig Dis Sci 1990;35:121–132.
67. Steinbrook RA. Epidural anesthesia and gastrointestinal motility. Anesth Analg 1998;86:837–844.
68. U.S. Census. Available at: http://www.census.gov/population/nation/intfile2–1.txt.
69. Gustafsson I, Nyström E, Quiding H. Effect of preoperative paracetamol on pain after oral surgery. Eur J Clin Pharmacol 1983;24:63–65.
70. Bridgman JB, Gillgrass TG, Zacharias M. The absence of any pre-emptive analgesic effect for non-steroidal anti-inflammatory drugs. Br J Oral Maxillofac Surg 1996;34:428–431.
71. Sisk AL, Grover BJ. A comparison of preoperative and postoperative naproxen sodium for suppression of postoperative pain. J Oral Maxillofac Surg 1990;48:674–678.
72. Sisk AL, Mosley RO, Martin RP. Comparison of preoperative and postoperative diflunisal for suppression of postoperative pain. J Oral Maxillofac Surg 1989;47:464–468.
73. Buggy DJ, Wall C, Carton EG. Preoperative or postoperative diclofenac for laparoscopic tubal ligation. Br J Anaesth 1994;73: 767–770.
74. Nordbladh I, Ohlander B, Björkman R. Analgesia in tonsillectomy: a double-blind study on pre- and post-operative treatment with diclofenac. Clin Otolaryngol 1991;16:554–558.
75. Nelson WE, Henderson RC, Almekinders LC, et al. An evaluation of pre- and postoperative nonsteroidal antiinflammatory drugs in patients undergoing knee arthroscopy: a prospective, randomized, double-blind study. Am J Sport Med 1993;21: 510–516.
76. Bünemann L, Thorshauge H, Herlevsen P, et al. Analgesia for outpatient surgery: placebo versus naproxen sodium (a non-steroidal anti-inflammatory drug) given before or after surgery. Eur J Anaesth 1994;11:461–464.
77. Flath RK, Hicks ML, Dionne RA, et al. Pain suppression after pulpectomy with preoperative flurbiprofen. J Endodontics 1987; 13:339–347.
78. Fletcher D, Zetlaoui P, Monin S, et al. Influence of timing on the analgesic effect of intravenous ketorolac after orthopedic surgery. Pain 1995;61:291–297.
79. Rogers JE, Fleming BG, Macintoch KC, et al. Effect of timing of ketorolac administration on patient-controlled opioid use. Br J Anaesth 1995;75:15–18.

80. Rømsing J, Østergaard D, Walther-Larsen S, et al. Analgesic efficacy and safety of preoperative versus postoperative ketorolac in pediatric tonsillectomy. Acta Anaesthesiol Scand 1998;42:770–775.
81. Parke TJ, Lowson SM, Uncles DR, et al. Pre-emptive versus post-surgical administration of ketorolac for hysterectomy. Eur J Anaesthesiol 1995;12:549–553.
82. Vanlersberghe C, Lauwers, Camu F. Preoperative ketorolac administration has no preemptive analgesic effect for minor orthopaedic surgery. Acta Anaesthesiol Scand 1996;40:948–952.
83. Peduto VA, Toscano A, D'Uva R, et al. Profilassi con ketorolac del dolore acuto postoperatorio. Minerva Anestesiol 1995;61: 367–372.
84. Cabell CA. Does ketorolac produce preemptive analgesic effect in laparoscopic ambulatory surgery patients. AANA J 2000;68:343–349.
84A. Likar R, Krumpholz R, Mathiaschitz K, et al. The preemptive action of ketoprofen: randomized, double-blind study with gynecologic operation. Anaesthesist 1997;46:186–190.
85. Likar R, Krumpholz, Pipam W, et al. Randomized, double-blind study with ketoprofen in gynecologic patients: preemptive analgesia study following the Breivik-Stubhaug design. Anaesthesist 1998;47:303–310.
86. Vogel RI, Desjardins PJ, Major KV. Comparison of presurgical and immediate postsurgical ibuprofen on postoperative periodontal pain. J Periodontol 1992;63:914–918.
87. Richmond CE, Bromley LM, Woolf CJ. Preoperative morphine pre-empts postoperative pain. Lancet 1993;342:73–75.
88. Mansfield MD, James KS, Kinsella J. Influence of dose and timing of administration of morphine on postoperative pain and analgesic requirements. Br J Anaesth 1996;76:358–361.
89. Millar AY, Mansfield MD, Kinsella J. Influence of timing of morphine administration on postoperative pain and analgesic consumption. Br J Anaesth 1998;81:373–376.
90. Fassoulaki A, Sarantopoulos C, Zotou M, et al. Preemptive opioid analgesia does not influence pain after hysterectomy. Can J Anaesth 1995;42:109–113.
91. Griffin MJ, Hughes D, Knaggs A, et al. Late-onset preemptive analgesia associated with preincisional large-dose alfentanil. Anesth Analg 1999;85:1317–1321.
92. Wilson RJ, Leith S, Jackson IJ, et al. Pre-emptive analgesia from intravenous administration of opioids. Anaesthesia 1994;49: 591–593.
93. Sarantopoulos C, Fassoulaki A. Sufentanil does not preempt pain after abdominal hysterectomy. Pain 1996;65:273–276.
94. Nagasaka H, Taguchi M, Mizumoto Y, et al. Pre-emptive analgesia from intravenous administration of opioid: no effect with pentazocine. Masui 1996;45:750–755.
95. Fu ES, Miguel R, Scharf JE. Preemptive ketamine decreases postoperative narcotic requirements in patients undergoing abdominal surgery. Anesth Analg 1997;84:1086–1090.
96. Adam F, Libier M, Oszustowicz T, et al. Preoperative small-dose ketamine has no preemptive analgesic effect in patients undergoing total mastectomy. Anesth Analg 1999;89:444–447.
97. Heinke VW, Grimm D. Präemptive effekte durch ko-analgesie mit ketamin bei gynäkologischen laparotomien? Anesthesiol Reanim 1999;24:60–64.
98. Menigaux C, Fletcher D, Dupont X, et al. The benefit of intraoperative small-dose ketamine on postoperative pain after anterior cruciate ligament repair. Anesth Analg 2000;90:129–135.
99. Dahl V, Ernoe PE, Steen T, et al. Does ketamine have preemptive effects in women undergoing abdominal hysterectomy procedures? Anesth Analg 2000;90:1419–1422.
100. Mathisen LC, Aasbø, Ræder J. Lack of pre-emptive analgesic effect of (R)-ketamine in laparoscopic cholecystectomy. Acta Anaesthesiol Scand 1999;43:220–224.
101. Chia Y, Liu K, Chow L, et al. The preoperative administration of intravenous dextromethorphan reduces postoperative morphine consumption. Anesth Analg 1999;89:748–752.
102. Wu CT, Yu JC, Yeh CC, et al. Preincisional dextromethorphan treatment decreases postoperative pain and opioid requirement after laparoscopic cholecystectomy. Anesth Analg 1999;88: 1331–1334.
103. Rockemann MG, Seeling W, Bischof C, et al. Prophylactic use of epidural mepivacaine/morphine, systemic diclofenac and metamizole reduces postoperative morphine consumption after major abdominal surgery. Anesthesiology 1996;84:1027–1034.
104. Katz J, Kavanagh BP, Sandler AN, et al. Preemptive analgesia: clinical evidence of neuroplasticity contributing to postoperative pain. Anesthesiology 1992;77:439–446.
105. Katz J, Clairoux M, Kavanagh BP, et al. Pre-emptive lumbar epidural anaesthesia reduces postoperative pain and patient-controlled morphine consumption after lower abdominal surgery. Pain 1994;59:395–403.
106. Kundra P, Gurnani A, Bhattacharya A. Preemptive epidural morphine for postoperative pain relief after lumbar laminectomy. Anesth Analg 1997;85:135–138.
107. Espinet A, Henderson DJ, Faccenda KA, et al. Does pre-incisional thoracic extradural block combined with diclofenac reduce postoperative pain after abdominal hysterectomy. Br J Anaesth 1996;76:209–213.
108. Gil GM, Aguado RG, Rosso MT, et al. Estudio comparativo entre morfina epidural lumbar preventiva o postincisional en cirugía resectiva pulmonar: informe preliminar. Rev Esp Anesthesiol Reanim 1998;45:384–388.
109. Richards JT, Read JRM, Chambers WA. Epidural anaesthesia as a method of pre-emptive analgesia for abdominal hysterectomy. Anaesthesia 1998;53:296–298.
110. Choe H, Choi YS, Kim YH, et al. Epidural morphine plus ketamine for upper abdominal surgery: improved analgesia from preincisional administration. Anesth Analg 1997;84:560–563.
111. Subramaniam B, Pawar DK, Kashyap L. Pre-emptive analgesia with epidural morphine or morphine and bupivacaine. Anaesth Intensive Care 2000;28:392–398.
112. Wong CS, Lu CC, Cherng CH, et al. Pre-emptive analgesia with ketamine, morphine and epidural lidocaine prior to total knee replacement. Can J Anaesth 1997;44:31–37.
113. Aguilar JL, Rincón R, Domingo V, et al. Absence of an early pre-emptive effect after thoracic extradural bupivacaine in thoracic surgery. Br J Anaesth 1996;76:72–76.
114. Dahl JB, Hansen BL, Hjortsø NC, et al. Influence of timing on the effect of continuous extradural analgesia with bupivacaine and morphine after major abdominal surgery. Br J Anaesth 1992;69:4–8.
115. Dahl JB, Daugaard JJ, Rasmussen B, et al. Immediate and prolonged effects of pre- versus postoperative epidural analgesia with bupivacaine and morphine on pain at rest and during mobilisation after total knee arthroplasty. Acta Anaesthesiol Scand 1994;38:557–561.
116. Nonaka A, Kashimoto S. Does pre-operative epidural buprenorphine improve postoperative pain? Pain Clin 1996;9:41–48.
117. Obata H, Saito S, Fujita N, et al. Epidural block with mepivacaine before surgery reduces long-term post-thoracoctomy pain. Can J Anaesth 1999;46:1127–1132.
118. Flisberg P, Törnebrandt K, Walther B. A comparison of the effects on postoperative pain relief of epidural analgesia started before or after surgery. Eur J Anaesthesiol 2000;17:627–633.
119. Nakamura T, Yokoo H, Hamakawa T. Preemptive analgesia produced with epidural analgesia administered prior to surgery. Masui 1994;43:1024–1028.
120. Rice LJ, Pudimat MA, Hannallah RS. Timing of caudal block placement in relation to surgery does not affect duration of postoperative analgesia in paediatric ambulatory patients. Can J Anaesth 1990;37:429–431.

121. Holthausen H, Eichwede F, Stevens M, et al. Preemptive analgesia: comparison of preoperative with postoperative caudal block on postoperative pain in children. Br J Anaesth 1994;73: 440–442.
122. Ho JW, Khambatta HJ, Pang LM, et al. Preemptive analgesia in children: does it exist? Reg Anesth 1997;22:125–130.
123. Kundra P, Deepalakshmi K, Ravishankar M. Preemptive caudal bupivacaine and morphine for postoperative analgesia in children. Anesth Analg 1998;87:52–56.
124. Goodarzi M. The effect of perioperative and postoperative caudal block on pain control in children. Paediatr Anaesth 1996;6: 475–477.
125. Dakin MJ, Osinubi OYO, Carli F. Preoperative spinal bupivacaine does not reduce postoperative morphine requirement in women undergoing total abdominal hysterectomy. Reg Anesth 1996;21:99–102.
126. Ejlersen E, Andersen H, Eliasen K, et al. A comparison between pre- and postincisional lidocaine infiltration on postoperative pain. Anesth Analg 1992;74:495–498.
127. Dierking G, Dahl J, Kanstrup J, et al. The effect of pre- versus postoperative inguinal field block on postoperative pain after herniotomy. Br J Anaesth 1992;68:344–348.
128. Turner GA, Chalkiadis G. Comparison of preoperative with postoperative lignocaine infiltration on postoperative analgesic requirements. Br J Anaesth 1994;72:541–543.
129. Ørntoft S, Løngren A, Møiniche S. A comparison of pre- and postoperative tonsillar infiltration with bupivacaine on pain after tonsillectomy: a pre-emptive effect? Anaesthesia 1994;94: 151–154.
130. Victory RA, Gajraj NM, Van Elstraete A, et al. Effect of preincision versus postincision infiltration with bupivacaine on postoperative pain. J Clin Anesth 1995;7:192–196.
131. Dahl V, Ræder JC, Ernø PE, et al. Pre-emptive effect of preincisional infiltration of local anaesthesia on children undergoing hernioplasty. Acta Anaesthesiol Scand 1996;40:847–851.
132. Badner NH, Bourne RB, Rorabeck CH, et al. Intra-articular injection of bupivacaine in knee-replacement operations: results of use for analgesia and for preemptive blockade. J Bone Joint Surg 1996;78:734–738.
133. Bourget JL, Clark J, Joy N. Comparing preincisional with postincisional bupivacaine infiltration in the management of postoperative pain. Arch Surg 1997;132:766–769.
134. Campbell WI, Kendrick RW. Pre-emptive analgesia using local anaesthesia: a study in bilaterally symmetrical surgery. Br J Anaesth 1997;79:657–659.
135. Campbell WI, Kendrick RW, Ramsay-Baggs P, et al. The effect of pre-operative administration of bupivacaine compared with its postoperative use. Anaesthesia 1997;52:1212–1216.
136. O'Hanlon DM, Colbert ST, Keane PW. Preemptive bupivacaine offers no advantage to postoperative wound infiltration in analgesia for outpatient breast biopsy. Am J Surg 2000;180:29–32.
137. Molliex S, Haond P, Baylot D, et al. Effect of pre- versus postoperative tonsillar infiltration with local anesthetics on postoperative pain after tonsillectomy. Acta Anaesthesiol Scand 1996;40:1210–1215.
138. Likar R, Morianz U, Wieser S, et al. Präemptive analgesie mit ropivacain bei tonsillektomien im erwachsenealter. Anaesthesist 1999;48:373–378.
139. Elhakim M, Abdel Hay H. Comparison of preoperative with postoperative topical lidocaine spray on pain after tonsillectomy. Acta Anaesthesiol Scand 1995;39:1032–1035.
140. Ke RW, Portera SG, Bagous W, et al. A randomized, double-blinded trial of preemptive analgesia in laparoscopy. Obstet Gynecol 1998;92:972–975.
141. Huffnagle HJ, Norris MC, Leighton BL, Arkoosh VA. Ilioinguinal iliohypogastric nerve blocks: before or after cesarean delivery under spinal anesthesia? Anesth Analg 1996;82:8–12.
142. Altintas F, Bozkurt P, Ipek N, et al. The efficacy of pre- versus postsurgically axillary block on postoperative pain in paediatric patients. Paediatr Anaesth 2000;10:23–28.
143. Doyle E, Bowler GMR. Pre-emptive effect of multimodal analgesia in thoracic surgery. Br J Anaesth 1998;80:147–151.
144. Pasqualucci A, De Angelis V, Contardo R. Preemptive analgesia: intraperitoneal local anesthetic in laparoscopic cholecystectomy. Anesthesiology 1996;85:11–20.
145. White PF, Rawal S, Latham P, et al. Use of a continuous local anesthetic infusion for pain management after median sternotomy. Anesthesiology 2003;99:918–923.
146. Oakley MJ, Smith JS, Anderson JR, et al. Randomized placebo-controlled trial of local anaesthetic infusion in day-case inguinal hernia repair. Br J Surg 1998;85:797–799.
147. Savoie FH, Field LD, Jenkins RN, et al. The pain control infusion pump for postoperative pain control in shoulder surgery. Arthroscopy 2000;16:339–342.
148. Joels CS, Mostafa G, Matthews BD, et al. Factors affecting intravenous analgesic requirements after colectomy. J Am Coll Surg 2003;197:780–785.
149. Hendolin HI, Paakonen ME, Alhava EM, et al. Laparoscopic or open cholecystectomy: a prospective randomised trial to compare postoperative pain, pulmonary function, and stress response. Eur J Surg 2000;166:394–399.
150. Long KH, Bannon MP, Zietlow SP, et al. A prospective randomized comparison of laparoscopic appendectomy with open appendectomy: clinical and economic analyses. Surgery 2001; 129:390–400.
151. Nilsson G, Larsson S, Johnsson F. Randomized clinical trial of laparoscopic versus open fundoplication: blind evaluation of recovery and discharge period. Br J Surg 2000;87:873–878.
152. Flisberg P. Pain relief and safety after major surgery. A prospective study of epidural and intravenous analgesia in 2696 patients. Acta Anaesthesiol Scand 2003;47:457–465.
153. Senagore AJ. Randomized clinical trial comparing epidural anaesthesia and patient-controlled analgesia after laparoscopic segmental colectomy. Br J Surg 2003;90:1195–1199.
154. American College of Surgeons 89th Clinical Congress 10/2003. Acute pain Management in Patients with Chronic Nonmalignant Pain; p. 45.

Suggested Reading

Karanikolas M. Current trends in perioperative pain management. Anesthesiol Clin North Am 2000;18:575–599.

Schecter WP, Bongard FS, Gainor BJ. Pain control in outpatient surgery. J Am Coll Surg 2002;195:95–104.

SECTION TWO

Biology and Practice of Trauma and Critical Care

20 Development of Trauma and Critical Care

G. Tom Shires

The contemporary historian, Meade,[1] states "It is hardly surprising that surgery of a number of parts of the human body had its origin in the treatment of wounds, for in many respects man's environment is a hostile one, threatening him on all sides with insults to the body that is ill-adapted to resist force." Aside from the mute testimony of the remains of our forebears, however, the first actual account of the treatment of wounds is to be found in the Edwin Smith Papyrus. According to Breasted, it was written about 1700 BC, but composed of texts dating back as far as 3000 BC The fascinating Smith Papyrus, which is now translated and in print,[2] includes the records of 48 cases with discussions of diagnosis, treatment, and prognosis (Figure 20.1).

The first really great surgical renaissance occurred about the fifth century BC when the school of Hippocrates (460–377 BC) brought the state of the healing art to a position of scientific medicine. This great renaissance was so profound that the history of medicine and surgery for the ensuing 2000 years was largely a struggle to retain those peaks of excellence that were attained during this golden age of Greece, 400 years before the Christian era.[3]

The second surgical renaissance coincided with what is generally known throughout the world as the Renaissance, which came in about the fifteenth century following the Dark Ages. This is not to say that significant contributions were not made with the dawning of the Christian era. Certainly the work of Celsus, when he produced his remarkable book, *De Re Medica*, is truly a milestone of description. Subsequently, however, monumental work by Harvey, Malpighi, the great Ambroise Paré, and others, aided by the discovery of the microscope, produced a true rebirth of medical and surgical knowledge.

The last half of the nineteenth century was clearly the third surgical renaissance, which truly formed the foundation for all modern surgery. This renaissance began with the discovery of ether and chloroform in 1848 and, subsequently, the work of Pasteur and the great Lister with antisepsis and asepsis, which laid the foundations for modern surgery. The pace of progress since this third renaissance has truly been staggering. Many reasons exist for the rapidity and extent of this progress, not the least of which are the coincident advances in scientific knowledge, such as chemistry and physiology, that have taken place.

However, the greatest American contribution to surgery was clearly the development of anesthesia. All those participating in this discovery were Americans. This story is well known to all of us, from the use of ether inhalation anesthesia by Crawford Long, who did not report his experiences until 1849; the development of nitrous oxide for painless tooth extraction in 1884 by Horace Wells, a dentist from Hartford; and in 1846 the use by William Morton, also a dentist and pupil of Wells, of ether anesthesia inhalation in an operation performed by John Collins Warren at the Massachusetts General Hospital. This contribution clearly was a milestone and the beginning of modern surgery. Shortly following the adoption of Joseph Lister's precepts of surgical antisepsis, which were first published in 1867, surgeons in America began to change a totally undisciplined and empirical art into surgical practice with a basis in science. A veritable flood of new hospitals appeared around the country. In addition, innumerable medical schools and universities developed medical education almost overnight. The proprietary schools were finally dealt a death blow by legislation following the historic Abraham Flexner report on medical education in 1910. In parallel fashion, the formal postgraduate training of surgeons was developed. The great William Stuart Halsted designed the unique school of surgical training in American surgery. His structuring of the residency program has, with some modifications, persisted since his establishment of this school in the late 1890s.

If one compares the treatment of wounds as described in the Smith Papyrus, it is clear that the only treatment available initially was the body's natural defenses. If we consider the same injuries in a patient today, the advances and successes are truly remarkable. One sees a patient who has been transported quickly, resuscitated early, given physiological support in the form of blood, fluid, and electrolytes, and had a detailed surgical approach to correct the injury. In addition, one sees biological monitoring in its fullest form and organ support in a variety of forms, whether cardiac, pulmonary, renal, nutritional, or others—this, in a patient who had the surgical procedure under painless anesthesia, with strict aseptic technique and the benefit of antibiotic prophylaxis.[4]

A number of developments occurred in the twentieth century that were absolutely essential to the development of the care of the injured patient and the critically ill patient.[5] Some of the necessary procedures include the following:

1900: Blood typing—Landsteiner
1901: Imaging—Roentgen
1923: Intensive care unit (ICU) (neuro), first ICU

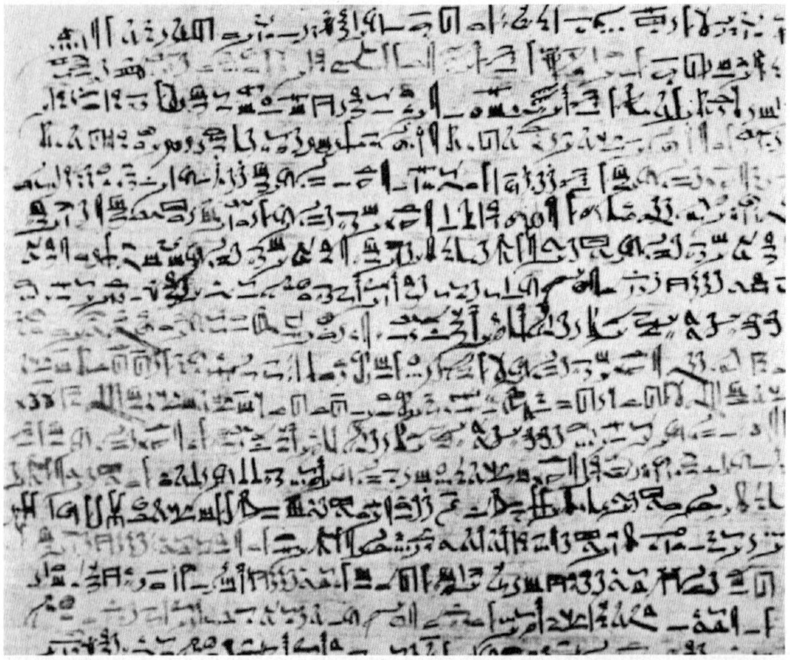

FIGURE 20.1. The Edwin Smith Surgical Papyrus, published in facsimile and hieroglyphic transliteration with translation and commentary. (Courtesy of The Oriental Institute of The University of Chicago.)

1940: Ventilation (Denmark), developed originally to manage the polio epidemic
1940: Dialysis—Kolff
1940: Antibiotics
1953: Open heart surgery
1956: Defibrillator—Zoll
1960: Cardiopulmonary resuscitation (CPR)—Kouivenhoven
1960: Adult ICU and CCU
1965: 95% hospital ICU prevalence
1970: Triage, resuscitation, fluids, acute respiratory distress syndrome (ARDS)
1971: Ultrasound
1972: Computer-assisted tomography (CAT) scan
1973: Magnetic resonance imaging (MRI)
1975: Multiple organ failure described
1980: Thrombolytic therapy
1981: Organ transplantation-effective immunosuppression

As technological and biological advances occur in many fields, success becomes more difficult to measure. In a milestone report published in *Science* in 1976, Comroe and the late Dr. Robert Dripps reported the scientific basis of the support of biomedical research.[6] These respected investigators examined clinical advances since the early 1940s, specifically in the field of cardiovascular and pulmonary diseases. The top 10 clinical advances in cardiovascular and pulmonary medicine and surgery in the past 30 years were elucidated by asking 40 physicians to list the advances they considered the most important for their patients. These selections were then tabulated and sent to another 50 specialists in each field, asking each to vote on the list and add additional advances they believed belonged on the list. Their votes selected the top 10 advances. With the help of 140 consultants, Comroe and Dripps identified the essential bodies of knowledge that had to be developed before each of the 10 clinical advances could reach its current state of achievement. As their study pointed out, general anesthesia was first put to use in 1846, and it was not until 107 years later that John Gibbon performed the first successful operation on an open heart with complete cardiopulmonary bypass. For all 10 advances they identified 137 essential bodies of knowledge. To arrive at these conclusions they examined 4000 published articles; 2500 specific scientific reports were particularly important to the development of one or more of the 137 essential bodies of knowledge. From this, 529 key articles were selected as a prerequisite background to this one major clinical advance.

Another major reason for success in research by the surgical biologist relates to funding of biomedical research. Before World War II, research played a relatively minor role in the nation at large and certainly in academic institutions. The total national expenditure for medical research in 1940 was $45 million, of which more than half was expended by and within industry, mainly for privately-oriented research. The federal government's investment in biomedical research then amounted to only $3 million; today that figure is more than $15 billion. Although a number of important advances resulted from medical research during the pre-World War II era, particularly in regard to control of infectious diseases by immunizations, the rate of discovery was slow by recent standards. The 25-year period between 1945 and 1970 was a golden era in biomedical research during which substantial financial support was available and enormous advances in the prevention and treatment of disease were accomplished. Dr. James A. Shannon,[7] the remarkable director of the NIH (National Institutes of Health) at that time, developed the support and the peer review system that persists today (Figure 20.2).

Similarly, in the Comroe and Dripps report in *Science* (1976) mentioned previously, it was stated, "it is easy to select examples in which basic undirected nonclinical research led to dramatic advances in clinical medicine and equally easy to give examples in which either clinically oriented research or development was all-important." In that

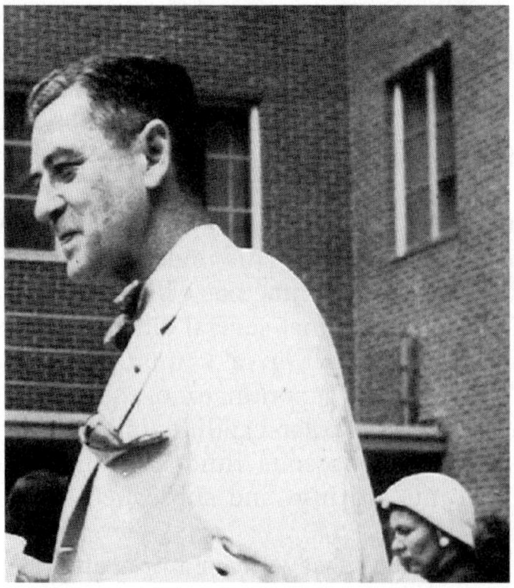

FIGURE 20.2. Dr. James A. Shannon.

study, 41% of all work to be judged essential for later clinical advancment was not clinically oriented at the time that it was done. Consequently, it seems clear that patient care-initiated basic or applied research will be the future cutting edge for advances in surgery because 60% of all such work was clinically related. We are now experiencing the fourth great surgical renaissance.

When turning to specific injuries in specific patients, there are obviously an enormous number of factors that have led to improvement in survival. One could list things such as improvement in early diagnosis, the early restoration of body fluids with blood and electrolyte solutions, the early presumptive use of antibiotics, intensive care support of visceral organ function, and improvements in operative techniques themselves. Some examples of specific improvements that resulted from research can be cited.

The concept of a constant internal environment was first articulated by the great French physiologist Claude Bernard. Bernard stated "the stability of the milieu intérieur is the primary condition for freedom and independence of existence: The mechanism which allows of this is that which insures in the milieu intérieur the maintenance of all the conditions necessary to the life of the elements." The constancy of the internal environment is protected by multiple intrinsic mechanisms, including renal, pulmonary, hepatic, and even cell membrane function.[8] Walter Cannon, a professor of physiology at Harvard, subsequently evolved the term homeostasis, which led to the concept that fitness for survival is directly related to the capacity of an organism to maintain physiological stability.[9] From this concept evolved the biological precept that the extracellular fluid, including the circulation, is the true milieu of life because it enables the cells of the body to function. One of the earliest attempts at resuscitation was carried out by the administration of large volumes of salt solutions intravenously. Latta[10] and O'Shaughnessy[11] treated cholera victims by the administration of large volumes of salt solutions intravenously in 1831. This was one of the first documented attempts to replace and maintain the extracellular internal environment.

During World War I, a variety of theories existed concerning the cause of vascular collapse in injured patients. It was assumed that this vascular collapse was caused primarily by toxins. In a unique set of experiments beginning with Blalock,[12] it was determined that almost all acute injuries are associated with changes in fluid and electrolyte metabolism. These studies showed that the alterations were primarily the result of reductions in the effective circulating blood volume. However, reduction in the effective circulating volume following injury may be the result of loss of blood as in hemorrhage; but also as a loss of vascular tone, as in sepsis or neurogenic shock; pump failure as in cardiac tamponade or myocardial infarction; or loss of large volumes of extracellular fluid, as occurs in patients with diarrhea, vomiting, and fistula drainage. Blalock's studies clearly showed that fluid loss in injured tissues was loss of extracellular fluid that was unavailable to the intravascular space for maintenance of circulation. The original concept of a "third space" in which fluid would be sequestered, and therefore unavailable to the intravascular space, evolved from those studies. As a consequence, by the time World War II occurred, plasma became the favored resuscitative solution in addition to whole-blood replacement. However, the concept that a limited amount of salt and water should be given to a patient after surgical or other injuries prevailed through the Korean War, largely due to the work of Coller and Moyer in experiments done at the University of Michigan (Figure 20.3).[13] These capable surgical investigators showed what was called "salt intolerance in response to operative trauma." These data are still reproducible; however, these patients had developed extracellular fluid volume deficits incident to the trauma, and consequently the renal retention of sodium and water was physiologically a desirable response to surgery. The mechanism of this response was later shown to be mediated via aldosterone for sodium retention and vasopressin (ADH, antidiuretic hormone) for water retention. The exact mechanism for the production of electrolyte changes, as well as the marked diminution in extracellular water that occurs following hemorrhagic shock, is not

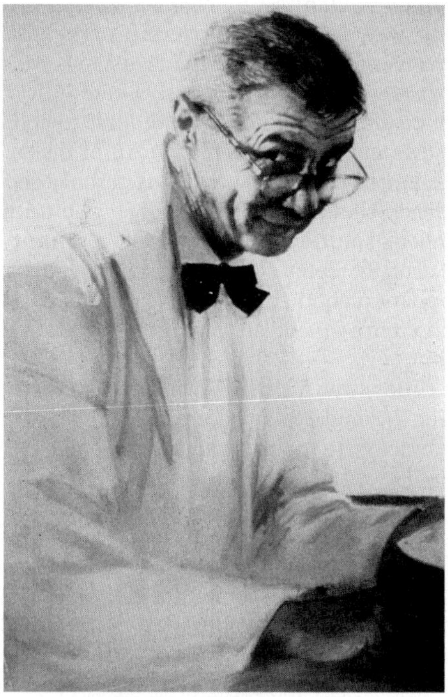

FIGURE 20.3. Dr. Carl A. Moyer.

known. It appears that these may well represent a reduction in the efficiency of an active ionic pump mechanism, or a selective increase in muscle cell membrane permeability to sodium, or both.[14]

In this modern day of instant travel and instant communication, research data are often transformed into therapeutic regimens very quickly. Responses to this kind of research have led to different forms of resuscitation for injured patients. Detailed reviews of resuscitation in thousands of civilian injuries have been reported with excellent results. Similarly, large numbers of battle casualties have been resuscitated, using newer forms of resuscitation. A review of Vietnam battle casualty resuscitations led Hardaway to write, "Intravenous blood and fluid administration is the single important factor in the treatment of shock." Additional statistics on the mortality rate of seriously injured patients in Vietnam tended to approximate those in Korea (2.5%). However, the ratio of wounded to killed was 6:1 in Vietnam whereas in Korea it was 3:1. This change dramatically indicates that more patients than ever before were surviving combat injuries. Further battlefield experience has shown reduced mortality from injury in Gulf War I compared with Vietnam, and even further reduced mortality in the Iraq/Afghanistan theaters. Posttraumatic renal failure in Vietnam occurred in approximately 1 in 1867 combat casualties, whereas in Korea the incidence of posttraumatic renal failure was approximately 1 per 200 casualties. Consequently, it is obvious that a number of factors, including rapid transportation, better resuscitation, and more appropriate definitive care, have reduced substantially the mortality from serious injury in the past 50 years.[14]

Most of the fluid resuscitation regimens used in recent years have been either normal saline or lactated Ringer's solution. The primary ion responsible for volume repletion has been and continues to be sodium. Most studies concerning fluid resuscitation in hemorrhagic shock indicate that cellular damage is induced by hemorrhage with or without resuscitation, which is manifest by changes in resting membrane potential as well as cytokine overproduction. In addition, apoptosis is very sensitive to fluid therapy. Many studies conclude that certain fluids are associated with a decreased level of apoptosis and thus contribute least to cellular death. Recent studies indicate that replacement of the DL isomer of lactate in lactated Ringer's solution with only the L isomer, and in addition the use of ketone Ringer's solution or bicarbonate Ringer's solution, may well have a salutory effect on the production of apoptotic cells. Whether apoptosis is a necessary phenomenon to remove dead cells as a benefit or detriment in terms of organ damage or failure is yet to be delineated.[15]

By the time of the Vietnam War, the provision of volume resuscitation beyond replacement of shed blood became an acceptable practice to maintain adequate homeostasis. During World War II, acute tubular necrosis was a common consequence of hypovolemic shock. However, because of the liberal use of fluid resuscitation during the Vietnam War, the incidence of acute tubular necrosis decreased dramatically.[16] With advances in the management of hemorrhagic shock and support of circulatory and renal function in injured patients, more patients survived, and 1% to 2% of significantly injured patients (with previously normal lungs) developed acute respiratory failure in the postinjury period. Initially this lung injury was believed to be related specifically to the shock state and resuscitation. This idea was implied by names such as "shock lung" and "traumatic wet lung," which have been applied to acute respiratory insufficiency following injury. It is now recognized that there are many similarities in the pathophysiology and clinical presentation of acute lung injury/acute respiratory distress syndrome (ALI/ARDS) following a variety of insults. This understanding has resulted in the realization that the lung has a limited number of ways of reacting to injury and that several different causes of acute diffuse lung injury result in a similar pathophysiological response. The common denominator of this response appears to be damage at the alveolar–capillary interface, with resulting leakage or proteinaceous fluid from the intravascular space into the interstitium and subsequently into alveolar spaces.

A variety of factors have been implicated as capable of producing ARDS or pulmonary failure following injury and resuscitation: these include (1) sepsis syndrome (80%); (2) aspiration (5%); (3) pulmonary contusion (5%); and (4) multiple fractures, (5) multiple transfusions, and (6) drowning or near-drowning (4, 5, and 6, combined, 10%).[17] In burn injuries many specific factors can be reasonably assessed. Pruitt[18] reviewed the mortality percentage by percent of body surface burn before and after the use of topical chemotherapy. In the salvageable burn category, the mortality rate, which was as great as 50%, was essentially halved by the introduction of topical chemotherapy. The development of the Parkland formula, by Baxter and Shires,[19] has clearly resulted in a reduction in mortality with adequate fluid replacement from the initial shock phase of burn injury.

As Donald Trunkey has pointed out, the fact remains that one-half of all trauma deaths occur before hospitalization and many of these are from fatal multiple injuries, including traumatic brain injury. The remaining half of trauma deaths occur in the hospital, and of these 62% occur within the first four hours of hospitalization, emphasizing the crucial necessity for early and adequate correction of fluid and electrolyte balances as well as supportive care and prompt surgical intervention. The third death peak in trauma occurs late, in approximately 20% of all trauma deaths. The majority of these deaths are caused by sepsis and multiple organ dysfunction syndrome (formerly, multiple organ failure). Consequently, it is clear that the need to prevent and control sepsis is a major issue in the improvement of survival following injury.

The isolation and characterization of bacterial endotoxin/lipopolysaccharide (LPS) led to the subsequent delineation of pathophysiological responses attributable to LPS. Wide derangements of organ function and cellular homeostasis characterized by acute inflammatory responses, altered energy metabolism, and lethal tissue injury are observed after LPS administration. It is now known that many (if not all) of these effects are mediated by humoral factors released in response to endotoxemia.[20] The role of the macrophage-secreted protein tumor necrosis factor-alpha (TNF-α) as an early or proximal mediator of the deleterious event induced by LPS was the first of the cytokines to be incriminated when in excess. Subsequently, many proinflammatory cytokine mediators and receptors have been described. Recently, antiinflammatory cytokines have also been identified, but the putative balance of pro- and antiinflammatory effects in the pathogenesis of tissue injury, host responses, and organ dysfunction is still debated.

In summary, the development of intensive care and modern trauma care has occurred primarily since 1960. These advances in patient care have been brought about by a number of different disciplines during the past 40 to 50 years, and progress is still being made by many specialities in medicine.

References

1. Meade RH. An Introduction to the History of General Surgery. Philadelphia: Saunders, 1968.
2. Breasted JH. The Edwin Smith Surgical Papyrus. [Published in facsimile and hieroglyphic transliteration with translation and commentary.] Chicago: University of Chicago Press, 1930.
3. Zimmerman LM. Great Ideas in the History of Surgery. Baltimore: Williams & Wilkins, 1961.
4. Shires GT. Presidential Address: The fourth surgical renaissance? Ann Surg 1980;192:269–281.
5. Calvin JE, Habert K, Parrillo JE. Critical care in the United States. Who are we and how did we get there? Crit Care Clin 1997;13(2):363–376.
6. Comroe JH, Dripps RD. Scientific basis for the support of biomedical science. Science 1976;192:105.
7. Shannon JA. Research in the service of man: biomedical knowledge, development and use. Document 55, U.S. Senate, 90th Congress, 1st Session; 1967:72.
8. Bernard C. An Introduction to the Study of Experimental Medicine (Green HC, transl.). New York: Macmillan, 1927.
9. Cannon WB. The Wisdom of the Body. New York: Norton, 1937.
10. Latta R (quoted by Weatherhill I). Case of malignant cholera in which 480 ounces of fluid were injected into the vein with success. Lancet 1831–1832;2:688.
11. O'Shaughnessy WB. Experiments on the blood in cholera. Lancet 1831–1832;1:490.
12. Blalock A. Experimental shock: the cause of low blood pressure caused by muscle injury. Arch Surg 1930;20:959.
13. Coller FA, Iob V, Vaughn HH, et al. Translocation of fluid produced by intravenous administration of isotonic salt solutions in man postoperatively. Ann Surg 1945;122:663.
14. Shires GT. Current status of resuscitation: solutions including hypertonic saline. Adv Surg 1995;28:133–170.
15. Shires GT, Browder LK, Steljes TP, Williams SJ, Browder TD, Barber AE. The effect of shock resuscitation fluids on apoptosis. Am J Surg 2005;1989:85–91.
16. Whelton A, Donadiq JV Jr. Post-traumatic acute renal failure in Vietnam. Johns Hopkins Med J 1969;124:95–105.
17. Shires GT III, Canizaro P,Carrico CJ. Shock. In: Schwartz SI, Shires GT, Spencer FC, eds. Principles of Surgery, 5th ed. New York: McGraw-Hill, 1989:171–177.
18. Pruitt B Jr. Host–opportunist interactions in surgical infection. Arch Surg 1986;121:13–22.
19. Baxter CR, Shires GT. Physiological response to crystalloid resuscitation of severe burns. Ann N Y Acad Sci 1968;150:875–894.
20. Tracey KJ, Beutler B, Lowry SF, et al. Shock and tissue injury induced by recombinant human cachectin. Science 1986;234:470.

21

Trauma Systems, Triage, and Disaster Management

Jeffrey Hammond

Appreciation of the magnitude of the health burden posed by traumatic injury, in terms of lives lost, disabilities, and economic cost, dates to the landmark publication *Accidental Death and Disability: The Neglected Disease of Modern Society*, published by the National Academy of Sciences in 1966.[1] The concept of a network of trauma centers is an extension of a larger trauma system approach to what has been termed a public health epidemic.[2] Such efforts culminated in the passage by the U.S. Congress of the Trauma Care Systems and Development Act (PL 101-590) in 1990, which, although not renewed in 1995, provided public funds to spur planning and development of model trauma systems. The development of such regional systems has provided substantially the most significant improvement in the care of the injured during the past two decades.[3]

To be successful, the trauma system must encompass an approach to trauma care broader than merely the designation of tertiary receiving hospitals. The spectrum of trauma care extends from the moment of injury through the pre-hospital and hospital phases to the patient's optimal recovery and return to work, school, or society. The necessary elements of a trauma system must therefore address four primary patient needs: access to care, pre-hospital care, hospital care, and rehabilitation. The trauma system concept revolves around the basic tenet of getting the right person to the right place at the right time along that continuum of care.

The essential components of a trauma system in the United States were derived from 20th-century military experience.[4] These components include rapid triage and timely evacuation through progressive echelons of care, planned "surge" capacity to manage a mass casualty incident, attention to resuscitation science, expertise in definitive management of injury, and aggressive rehabilitation. Characteristics of a trauma system include delivery of a full range of care to all injured patients in a defined geographic area, coordination with pre-hospital services, efficient use of resources through regionalization, population-based planning, and integration with the public health system to include an emphasis on injury prevention.

Within the civilian arena, "accident hospitals," devoted exclusively to the care of accident victims, have been in existence since 1882.[5] Nearly a century later, the seminal study of West et al., published in 1979, compared Orange County, California, with San Francisco, and demonstrated that delayed or inadequate care in the county without a trauma system was associated with preventable or possibly preventable deaths in up to two-thirds of the cases. A substantial reduction in preventable deaths was documented after implementation of a trauma center-based system involving one Level I and four Level II centers.[6] This mechanism of needs assessment and documentation, regional and governmental support for system implementation, and reporting and dissemination of systems results follows the Public Health Model and has become a template for change.

Through the efforts of the American College of Surgeons and the American College of Emergency Physicians, principally through the Advanced Trauma Life Support (ATLS) course and its companion Pre-Hospital Trauma Life Support (PHTLS) course, the management approach and principles of trauma care have been codified and standardized. The system does not depend upon individual expertise, but on a standardized multidisciplinary approach. Trauma system development in Europe has great country-by-country variation and tends to lag behind the United States and Canada.[7]

Epidemiology

Trauma is the fourth leading cause of death overall in the United States and the leading cause of death during the first four decades of life. It is the fifth most common cause of death overall in Canada. Because it tends to be a disease of the young, trauma is the leading cause of years of potential life lost (YPLL) in both the United States and Canada.[8] Trauma accounts for 7% of all hospital admissions in the United States. Major trauma constitutes 11% of these 412 hospitalizations per 100,000 person-years,[9] but this volume is sufficient in trauma system development.

Trauma-related mortality exhibits a trimodal distribution. The first cohort, approximately 50% of trauma deaths, occurs in the immediate postinjury period, and represents death from overwhelming injury such as spinal cord transection, aortic disruption, or massive intraabdominal injuries. These patients die at the scene or during transport before hospital arrival. Despite modern emergency medical systems (EMS) networks, there is little that sophisticated treatment systems can do to salvage these patients; thus, efforts should be directed at prevention.

It is in the second peak in the trimodal distribution, however, that trauma systems and trauma centers can perhaps make their greatest contributions. Deaths in this group, usually caused by severe traumatic brain injury or uncontrolled hemorrhage, occur within hours of the injury, and represent perhaps one-third of all trauma deaths. Preventable death studies report reduction in preventable death rates of 20% to 50% to less than 10% and as low as 2% upon institution of trauma system or trauma center development.[10]

The third peak occurs 1 day to 1 month postinjury and comprises approximately 10% to 20% of deaths. These "late" deaths are most often caused by refractory increased intracranial pressure subsequent to closed head injury or pulmonary complications. With aggressive critical care, nonpulmonary sources of sepsis, renal failure, and multiple organ dysfunction syndrome as causes of death are decreasing.

Trauma Center Evaluation

The modern civilian trauma center in the United States dates to 1966 with the establishment of identifiable trauma care units at San Francisco General Hospital and Cook County Hospital in Chicago.[11] Systems of trauma care originally developed and improved based on expert opinion and informed consensus. Use of evidence-based medicine and the establishment of a research agenda resulted in a more scientific approach to trauma system evaluation and adaptation.[12] Since 1979, more than two dozen studies have demonstrated as much as a 50% reduction in preventable deaths after implementation of regionalized and dedicated trauma care.[13] Unfortunately, these studies almost uniformly rely on mortality as the primary indicator of effectiveness. Nevertheless, as demonstrated in evidence tables from a comprehensive literature review, the consistency of the data does support the supposition that organized systems of trauma care are good health policy even if cost-effectiveness has not been studied.[14]

Pediatric trauma systems have developed "by necessity" within adult systems.[15] Pediatric injury-focused content was first introduced into the ATLS course in 1983. The federally supported Emergency Medical Services for Children program was launched in 1984. Outcomes at "adult" trauma centers that are committed to pediatric care and obtain added qualifications appear to be equal to those in pediatric trauma centers,[16] although there are some conflicting data to imply that more procedures are performed.[17]

Trauma care in rural areas is one of the great challenges for a trauma system. Death rates for comparable injuries are greater in rural compared to urban areas. The needs and capabilities of the local hospitals that take on the trauma burden differ greatly from metropolitan areas. Pre-hospital and transport times are longer, providers may have less training or exposure to trauma, and subspecialty services may be limited. One solution has been the development of inclusive trauma systems in which virtually all hospitals participate in the trauma system, designated as Level III–V trauma centers as their resources permit.[18] Results as to reduction of mortality are conflicting, although preventable death rates can be reduced in this setting,[19] and processes of care can be improved.[20]

One of the salient features of the Trauma Center concept is the emphasis on quality improvement and objective evaluation. This emphasis has taken the form of self-monitoring complemented by external review and audit by subject matter experts, either through the verification process of American College of Surgeons Committee on Trauma (ACSCOT) or by state agencies.

The core concept for the ACSCOT verification process has changed little since initiated in 1987 as codified by West et al. On-site hospital visits by impartial out-of-area survey teams assess compliance with defined standards.[21] Established standards are reviewed periodically by ACSCOT, updating essential and desirable components linked to level of hospital designation. The lack of a robust and effective performance improvement program is the most common deficiency.[22] Other important common deficiencies include lack of a defined trauma service, absence of the trauma surgeon in the emergency department at time of patient arrival, inadequate trauma registry, lack of 24-h operating room capability, inadequate evidence of continuing medical education, and lack of adequate authority or job description for the trauma director. Adherence to these rigorous standards does have a positive impact on patient survival, however, and can alleviate some of the cost burden of maintaining a trauma center, principally through reduced length of stay.[23,24]

Essential Components and System Characteristics

The hospital is just one component of a trauma system. The goal of the system is to create a network of community resources that meet adequately the needs of injured patients in a rapid, efficient, and consistent manner.[25] Moreover, systematized trauma care involves not only the medical components, but also social, political, and economic solutions addressing injury prevention, patient education, research, financial planning, and disaster preparedness.

At its core, a trauma system is *inclusive*, incorporating a variety of sectors, including nontrauma centers. The template was originally described in the 1992 Health Resources Services Administration (HRSA) document, The Model Trauma Care System Plan. This inclusive philosophy implies that all injured patients are cared for within the system and that a tiered approach establishes a role for all to play.

In addition to the trauma center(s), which might be thought of as the hub of a hub-and-spoke wheel configuration, the trauma system requires administrative and legislative leadership, financial support, robust pre-hospital emergency medical systems (EMS) including communications and operational guidelines, information systems, rehabilitation capabilities, and an evaluative process. Additional components must address the needs of public education and injury prevention.

By its very nature, a trauma system will centralize components of trauma care into specialized or designated facilities. This process may present political or economic challenges for a community and demands that all stakeholders be part of the development process. These challenges can best be met if the system is rooted in legal authority conferred by legislation. This mode permits creation of an oversight agency to regulate the system, allocation, and designation of trauma centers based on a needs assessment, management of a system trauma registry, and enforcement of performance standards.

Three states, Maryland, Florida, and Illinois, pioneered the trauma system concept in the United States.[4] In 1969, the Maryland Institute for Emergency Medicine, under the direction of R. Adams Cowley, initiated helicopter transport of injured patients in cooperation with the Maryland State Police.[26] This "shock-trauma" approach included interhospital transfer from regional hospitals. Efforts in Florida during the 1970s focused on the development of trained and professional pre-hospital providers, coupled with improved communications. Development of advanced EMS led to a 38% reduction in motor vehicle crash deaths in Jacksonville, Florida.[27] Efforts in Illinois incorporated both urban and rural hospitals in a regionalized approach and introduced a ranking scheme based on criteria for equipment, resources, and personnel. Also integral to the Illinois system, described in a series of articles by Boyd et al.,[28] was the introduction of a trauma registry as a cornerstone for a "medical audit" system of quality improvement.[29]

A 1987 telephone survey of state health departments and directors of emergency medical services identified only two states, Maryland and Virginia, that had in place all eight of what were deemed essential components of a trauma system (Table 21.1).[30] Nineteen other states were in various stages of system development. The failure to control the number and distribution of trauma centers based on a needs-based methodology was the most common failing.

By 1995, with an expanded inventory of essential components, 5 states were identified as meeting all essential components. As trauma system evolution continued, 35 states were actively working to develop comprehensive programs in 1998.[31] Financial constraints imposed by the labor- and resource-intensive requirements to start and maintain a trauma center,[32] and the difficulty in retention in personnel, have been cited as reasons for the waxing and waning of trauma system development.[33]

A 2002 national inventory by MacKenzie et al., using the American Trauma Society's Trauma Information Exchange Program (TIEP), documented a doubling of the number of trauma centers in the United States since 1991.[34] Fewer than one-half of these 1154 facilities were designated as Level I or II centers using the ACSCOT classification.[35] Moreover, the distribution was not uniform. Nevertheless, in every state there was at least one hospital that demonstrated a substantial commitment to the care of patients. Still, an analysis of more than one-half million injury-related hospital discharges from 18 states documented that 56% of all trauma patients, and more than one-third of patients with major trauma, are cared for in nondesignated trauma centers or those at a lower level of designation.[36]

Trauma Triage

A cornerstone of trauma care is the timely identification and transport to a trauma center of those patients most likely to benefit; that is, the principle of triage. Triage, adapted from a French military concept, is at its simplest the sorting of patients based on need for treatment and an inventory of available resources to meet those needs, which may take place in the field or within the institution. Indeed, effective systems incorporate triage principles sequentially at different points in the patient's transit through the trauma system: the field emergency department, the intensive care unit, and the operating room, for example.

Trauma triage is founded upon the recognition that the nearest emergency department may not be the most appropriate destination. On a more complex level, it involves the development of an algorithm that seeks to balance avoiding under-triage (and possible adverse outcomes) while minimizing over-triage (and overloading the system).

Multiple pre-hospital scoring mechanisms have been suggested to assist in the triage decision. It has been hoped that some scoring technique would facilitate identification of the 5% to 10% of trauma patients estimated to require the sophisticated trauma center. Current triage schemas tend to assess the potential for life- or limb-threatening injury utilizing physiological, anatomic, and/or mechanism of injury criteria.[37] In general, physiological criteria offer the greatest yield, whereas anatomic criteria are intermediate and mechanism-based criteria have a low yield.[38] Highest yield criteria include prolonged pre-hospital time, a pedestrian struck at greater than 20 mph, associated death of another vehicular occupant, and the physiological criteria of systolic blood pressure less than 90 mmHg, respiratory rate less than 10 or more

TABLE 21.1. Essential Components of a Regional Trauma System.

1.	A legal authority responsible for trauma center designation
2.	Formal process for designating trauma centers
3.	Trauma center distribution based on patient volume or population density
4.	Use of American College of Surgeons standards
5.	Use of independent survey teams from other areas for on-site verification visits
6.	Written trauma triage criteria including transfer agreements with specialty centers and bypass or diversion protocols
7.	Ongoing monitoring systems
8.	Statewide coverage by the trauma center system

than 29 breaths per minute, or Glasgow Coma Scale score of less than 13 points.

Variation within trauma systems is a common occurrence, and rigid adherence to guidelines is often offset by expert opinion. Even within a mature trauma system such as that of Pennsylvania, a large proportion of seriously injured trauma patients are not transported to trauma centers.[27] Older patients, women, people who have fallen, and rural patients are more likely to be mis-triaged or under-triaged. However, logistic regression analysis of more than 72,000 patient admissions over 5 years in a regionalized system in Quebec, Canada, identified only pre-hospital notification and protocols, and the use of performance improvement programs, as having a positive effect on adjusted mortality.[39] A multiple tier system of trauma triage and alert can reduce over- and under-triage, leading to reduced emergency department time.[40]

Role in Disaster Management

Failure to prepare is preparation to fail. Although the task may seem daunting, or even hopeless, planning for disasters or mass casualty events is essential. It may be true that disasters defy planning and that the best one might hope for is controlled chaos, but the success of a well-crafted and rehearsed disaster plan is measured by its ability to facilitate the restoration of order from the chaos.

Although disasters are unpredictable and sudden, they are not necessarily random, and they can be anticipated. In certain geographic areas, the form of disaster (e.g., tornado, wildfire, earthquake, nuclear power plant event) can be anticipated. Disasters, even from terrorism, may follow a pattern from which we can learn strategies to mitigate the damage.

Disasters and mass casualty events, intentional or unintentional, are likely to require surgical management to some extent, whereas the volume of traumatic injuries may be small in some instances, such as flooding, and injuries and trauma may appear during subsequent phases, for example, as homeowners attempt to repair roofs. In other scenarios, such as after a terrorist bombing, traumatic injuries will predominate, with 10% to 20% being classified as severe.[41]

Recent experience utilizing a statewide trauma system model has demonstrated the importance of trauma centers, trauma systems, and trauma surgeons in disaster preparedness and response in an all-hazard approach.[42] The initial response to a disaster will be chaotic. The second phase of the sequence leading to recovery is site clearing and reorganization, followed by search and rescue. From the vantage point of the hospital or trauma center, the better the planning and training, the more likely that organization can be reestablished in a timely fashion.

The first step in preparing a disaster plan is conducting an institutional Hazard Vulnerability Analysis (HVA). This exercise in risk assessment and communication guides an organization to focus on threats that are most likely and which pose the highest risk. The steps in development of an HVA start with identification of all internal and external threats, followed by an estimation of the probability of a hazard occurring. For each hazard listed, a level of preparedness should be defined, thus identifying areas needing improvement. Such an all-hazards approach builds upon the common elements of potential hazards while still permitting flexibility and adaptability to meet unique demands.[43]

TABLE 21.2. The DISASTER Paradigm.

<u>D</u>etect
<u>I</u>ncident command
<u>S</u>cene security and safety
<u>A</u>ssess hazards
<u>S</u>upport
<u>T</u>riage and treatment
<u>E</u>vacuation
<u>R</u>ecovery

Core parts of a disaster response are generic regardless of the type of incident, consistent with the "all-hazards" approach to emergency planning. These core concepts include confirmation of the information available, data gathering, activating a control station, evacuation of the emergency department of noncritical patients, alert and recall of extra medical and paramedical staff, and designating a triage officer/team. The DISASTER paradigm has been advanced as a framework to address systematically the administrative and clinical issues necessary to disaster management (Table 21.2).[44]

Impediments to success include poor planning, poor drilling, communication breakdowns, security lapses, and unclear command and control.[45] The Hospital Emergency Incident Command System (HEICS) is an effective organization model that addresses these potential lapses. The HEICS model, which is being incorporated into the Federal Emergency Management Agency's (FEMA) National Incident Management System (NIMS), comprises a hierarchical system with five major domains: command, operations, logistics, planning, and finance/adminstrative.[46]

The HEICS recognizes the need for a medical facility or system to continue to function in an orderly fashion despite a mass casualty incident or disaster. Indeed, the facility or network plan should take into account the possibility that one is in the middle of the disaster.[46] To react to the community needs, maintain continuity of services, and protect the facility, HEICS provides a comprehensive resource management strategy. In essence, it does on a larger scale what trauma teams do on a day-to-day basis.

Key principles in any incident command system or organized response include a common terminology, modular organization, integrated communications, consolidated action plans, manageable span of control and predesignated areas, and a unified command structure. An example of the HEICS domains and division of functions is shown in Figure 21.1.

The trauma center often serves as the hospital of "last resort" in a disaster. Trauma surgeons and trauma centers are ideally suited to deal with disaster and mass casualty events. They have experience in multiple casualty events, linked and redundant communications, practice disaster responses as part of their core mission and to comply with designation requirements, perform triage in some fashion in a practical fashion on a daily basis, and are integrated with the local and regional public health, EMS system, and surrounding hospitals.

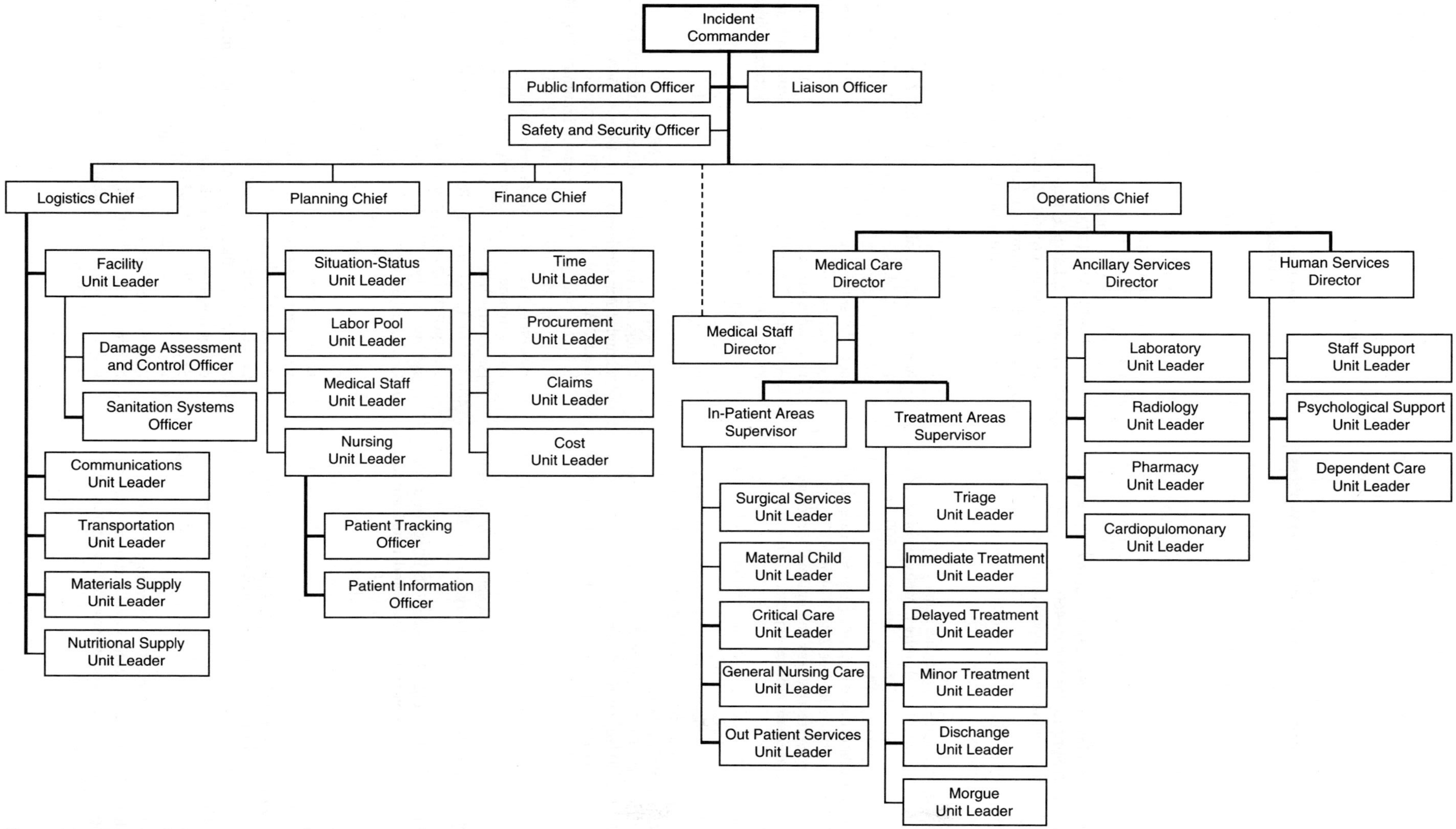

Figure 21.1. Hospital Emergency Incident Command System organization chart. (From the Hospital Emergency Incident Command System, Third Edition, by permission of The San Mateo County Health Services Agency, Emergency Medical Services, June 1998.)

References

1. National Academy of Sciences/National Research Council. Accidental Death and Disability: The Neglected Disease of Modern Society. Washington, DC: National Academy of Sciences, 1966.
2. National Research Council and the Institute of Medicine. Injury in America. Washington, DC: National Academy Press, 1985.
3. Mann NC, Mullins RJ, MacKenzie EJ, et al. A systematic review of published evidence regarding trauma system effectiveness. J Trauma 1999;47:S15–S21.
4. Mullins RJ. A historical perspective of trauma system development in the United States. J Trauma 1999;47(suppl):S8–S14.
5. Freeark RJ. Accident hospitals. Bull Am Coll Surg 1986;71:24–30.
6. West JG, Trunkey DD, Lim RC. Systems of trauma care: a study of two counties. Arch Surg 1979;114:455–460.
7. Leppaniemi A. Trauma systems in Europe. Curr Opin Crit Care 2005;11:576–579.
8. Liberman M, Mulder DS, Lavoie A, Sampalis J. Implementation of a trauma care system: evolution through evaluation. J Trauma 2004;56:1330–1335.
9. http://www.ahrq.gov/data/his96/clinclas.htm.
10. Cayten CG, Stahl W, Agarwal N, Murphy J. Analyses of preventable deaths by mechanism of injury among 13,500 trauma admissions. Ann Surg 1992;21:510–520.
11. Trunkey DD. History and development of trauma care in the United States. Clin Orthop Relat Res 2000;374:36–46.
12. Mann NC. Assessing the effectiveness and optimal structure of trauma systems: a consensus among experts. J Trauma 1999; 47(suppl):S69–S73.
13. Eastman B. Blood in our streets: status and evolution of trauma care systems. Arch Surg 1992;127:677–681.
14. Mann NC, Mullins R, MacKenzie EJ, et al. Systematic review of published evidence regarding trauma system effectiveness. J Trauma 1999;47(suppl):S25–S33.
15. Morrison W, Wright JL, Paidas CN. Pediatric trauma systems. Crit Care Med 2002; 30 (suppl): S448–S456.
16. Hulka F. Pediatric trauma systems: critical distinctions. J Trauma 1999;47(suppl):S85–S89.
17. Keller MS, Vane D. Management of pediatric blunt splenic injury: comparison of pediatric and adult trauma surgeons. J Pediatr Surg 1995;30:221–224.
18. Nathens AB, Brunet F, Maier RV. Development of trauma systems and effect on outcomes after injury. Lancet 2004;363: 1794–1801.
19. Esposito TJ, Danddal T, Reynolds S, Sandall N. Effect of a voluntary trauma system on preventable death and inappropriate care in a rural state. J Trauma 2003;54:663–670.
20. Olson CJ, Arthur M, Mullins RJ, et al. Influence of trauma system implementation on process of care delivered to seriously injured patients in rural trauma centers. Surgery (St. Louis) 2001;130:273–279.
21. West JG, Williams M, Trunkey DD, Wolferth CC. Trauma systems: current status—future challenges. JAMA 1988;259:3597–3600.
22. Mitchell FL, Thal ER, Wolferth CC. Analysis of American College of Surgeons trauma consultation program. Arch Surg 1995;130:578–584.
23. DiRusso S, Holly C, Kamath R, et al. Preparation and achievement of American College of Surgeons Level 1 trauma verification raises hospital performance and improves patient outcome. J Trauma 2001;51:294–300.
24. Piontek FA, Coscia R, Marselle CS, et al. Impact of American College of Surgeons verification on trauma outcomes. J Trauma 2003;54:1041–1047.
25. Hammond JS, Gomez G, Eckes J. Trauma systems: economic and political considerations. J Fla Med Assoc 1990;77:603–605.
26. Cowley RA, Hudson R, Scanlon E, et al. An economical and proved helicopter program for transporting the emergency critically ill and injured patient in Maryland. J Trauma 1973;13:1029–1038.
27. Waters J, Wells C. The effects of a modern emergency medical care system in reducing automobile crash deaths. J Trauma 1973;13:645–647.
28. Boyd DR, Dunea MM, Flasher BA. The Illinois plan for a statewide system of trauma centers. J Trauma 1973;13:24–31.
29. Boyd DR, Lowe R, Baker R, Nyhus L. Trauma registry: new computer method for multifactorial evaluation of a major health problem. JAMA 1973;223:422–428.
30. Eastman AB, Lewis F, Champion H, Mattox K. Regional trauma system design: critical concepts. Am J Surg 1987;154:79–87.
31. Bazzoli GJ. Community based trauma system development: key barriers and facilitating factors. J Trauma 1999;47(suppl):S22–S29.
32. Hammond JS, Breckinridge MB. Longitudinal analysis of the impact of a level 1 trauma center designation at a university hospital. J Am Coll Surg 1999;188:217–224.
33. Mann NC, MacKenzie E, Teitelbaum SD, et al. Trauma system structure and viability in the current healthcare environment: a state-by-state assessment. J Trauma 2005;58:136–147.
34. MacKenzie EJ, Hoyt D, Sacra J, et al. National inventory of hospital trauma centers. JAMA 2003;289:1515–1522.
35. American College of Surgeons Committee on Trauma. Resources for the Optimal Care of the Injured Patient. Chicago: American College of Surgeons, 2003.
36. Nathens AB, Jurkovich GJ, MacKenzie EJ, Rivara F. A resource-based assessment of trauma care in the United States. J Trauma 2004;56:173–178.
37. Norcross E, Ford D, Cooper M, et al. Application of American College of Surgeons field triage guidelines by pre-hospital personnel. J Am Coll Surg 1995;181:539–544.
38. Baez AA, Lane P, Sorondo B. System compliance with out-of-hospital trauma triage criteria. J Trauma 2003; 54:344–351.
39. Liberman M, Mulder DS, Jurkovich GJ, Sampalis JS. The association between trauma system and trauma center components and outcome in a mature regionalized trauma system. Surgery (St. Louis) 2005;137:647–658.
40. Kaplan L, Santora T, Blank-Reid C, Trooskin SZ. Improved emergency department efficiency with a three tier trauma triage system. Injury 1997;28:449–453.
41. Gutierrez de Ceballos JP, Turegano Fuentes F, Perez Diaz D, et al. Casualties treated at the closest hospital in the Madrid, March 11, terrorist bombings. Crit Care Med 2005;33(1 suppl): S107–S112.
42. Jacobs L, Burns K, Gross R. Terrorism: a public health threat with a trauma system response. J Trauma 2003;55:1014–1021.
43. American Medical Association. Advanced Disaster Life Support, provider manual, version 2.0. Chicago: AMA, 2004.
44. Avitzour M, Libergal M, Assaf J, et al. A multicasualty event: out-of-hospital and in-hospital organizational aspects. Acad Emerg Med 2004;11:1102–1104.
45. Klein J, Weigelt JA. Disaster management: lessons learned. Surg Clin N Am 1991;71:257–266.
46. Norcross ED, Elliott BE, Adams D, Crawford F. Impact of a major hurricane on surgical services in a university hospital. Am Surg 1993;59:28–33.

22 Monitoring of Cardiovascular and Respiratory Function

Philip S. Barie and Soumitra R. Eachempati

Patient acuity is increasing in the intensive care unit (ICU), requiring more sophisticated methods to monitor, support, and evaluate critically ill patients.[1–3] Mechanical ventilation is a mainstay of modern ICU care. Monitoring of blood flow, acid–base status, oxygen transport, coagulation, pulmonary and other visceral organ function, and the development of nosocomial infection are a few of several aspects of patient surveillance.

Blood Testing

Blood testing is essential for patient monitoring, but such testing can be excessive. Cost and quality are linked; expenditure of additional resources decreases quality if there is no benefit to the patient. Blood removed for testing can average more than 70 mL/day[4]; an indwelling arterial catheter may increase blood testing by one-third.[5] Waste of blood occurs each time a catheter is aspirated and flushed,[6] and the risk of nosocomial infection is increased by catheter manipulation[7] and transfusion of red blood cell concentrates.[8] Strategies to reduce blood testing while preserving optimal patient care include noninvasive hemodynamic monitoring, adoption of practice parameters for diagnostic evaluation, and point-of-care testing.

Point-of-Care Testing

Point-of-care (POC) testing of blood occurs at or near the bedside and is recognized to be accurate and to confer numerous advantages. Turnaround time is reduced, enhancing clinical care and reducing repetitive testing. Very small (i.e., microliter) blood samples are required, and in some cases samples are not even removed from the patient if indwelling sensors or a closed-circuit extracorporeal sampling device is employed.

Perhaps the most prevalent example of POC testing is glucose monitoring,[9] which is performed frequently now that the benefits of "tight" glucose control (i.e., serum glucose concentration 80–110 mg/dL) by use of a continuous infusion of insulin are recognized to reduce the risk of nosocomial infection, duration of mechanical ventilation, organ dysfunction, and death among critically ill surgical patients.[10] Expected error tolerances for bedside glucose monitoring are ± 15%. Blood gases and electrolyte concentrations can also be analyzed accurately at the bedside with good precision across a range of concentrations for each analyte. In a recent comparison trial,[11] precision studies performed at three different concentrations for each analyte demonstrated an intraassay coefficient of variation of 2.5% or less and interassay precision of 4% or less in all tests.

Blood Gas Monitoring

Blood gas analyzers report several results, but the parameters measured directly are the partial pressures of oxygen (pO_2) and carbon dioxide (pCO_2) and blood pH. Hemoglobin saturation (SaO_2) is calculated from the pO_2 using the oxyhemoglobin dissociation curve, assuming a normal P_{50} (the pO_2 at which SaO_2 is 50%, normally 26.6 mmHg), and normal hemoglobin structure. Blood gas analyzers with a co-oximeter measure the various forms of hemoglobin directly, including oxyhemoglobin, total hemoglobin, carboxyhemoglobin, and

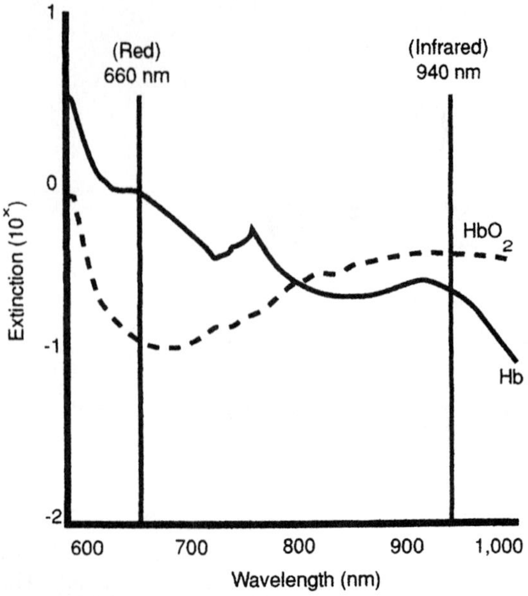

FIGURE 22.1. Modern pulse oximetry uses two wavelengths of light, red (660nm) and infrared (940nm), to differentiate oxyhemoglobin (HbO_2) from deoxyhemoglobin (Hb). (Adapted with permission from J Crit Illness 1989;4:23–31.)

methemoglobin. The actual bicarbonate, standard bicarbonate, and base excess are calculated from the pH and pCO_2.

A fresh, heparinized, bubble-free arterial blood sample is required. Heparin is acidic; if present to excess, pCO_2 and HCO_3 are reduced spuriously. Delay in measurement allows continued metabolism by erythrocytes, reducing pH and pO_2 and increasing pCO_2. An iced specimen can be assayed accurately for up to 1 h. Air bubbles decrease pCO_2 and increase pO_2.

The solubility of all gases in blood increases with a decrease in temperature; thus, hypothermia causes pO_2 and pCO_2 to decrease and pH to increase. Analysis at 37°C of a sample taken from a hypothermic patient will cause a spurious increase in pO_2 and pCO_2, but the error is usually too small to be meaningful.

Electrocardiography

Electrocardiographic (ECG) monitoring is standard in many clinical settings.[12] Four or five limb and chest leads are used for routine monitoring, which provides instantaneous information regarding cardiac rhythm and rate. Tachycardia is underappreciated as a source of serious morbidity, especially in older patients, and may be a manifestation of hypovolemia, hemorrhage, inadequate analgesia, or other causes. Because tachycardia may precipitate myocardial ischemia, it is inherently dangerous. However, routine ECG monitoring is insensitive for detection of acute ST-T wave changes,[13] which may portend ischemia[14] detectable by 12-lead ECG.[15] Continuous 12-lead ECG monitoring is a sensitive indicator of myocardial ischemia, but it is prone to lead displacement and is not used widely.

Continuous ECG monitoring is invaluable in assuring ongoing control of heart rate in patients at risk for myocardial ischemia[16] Perioperative mortality is decreased among patients who receive beta-adrenergic blockade preoperatively, and continued for 1 week after surgery.[17] Even if beta-blockade cannot be started before an emergency operation (e.g., uncorrected hypovolemia), it should be started as soon as possible thereafter.[18]

Pulse Oximetry

Pulse oximetry has revolutionized perioperative monitoring in that even slight decreases in SaO_2 are detectable with only about a 60-s delay.[19] So successful has been pulse oximetry that deaths attributable to general anesthesia have decreased dramatically. The device calculates SaO_2 by estimating the difference in signal intensity between oxygenated and deoxygenated blood from red (660nm) and near-infrared (940nm) light. Pulse oximetry must detect pulsatile blood flow to be accurate (Figure 22.1; Table 22.1), but all things being equal, data can be obtained from a detector on the finger, the earlobe, or the forehead.[20] Pulse oximetry is generally accurate (±2%) over the range of SaO_2 70% to 100%, but it is less accurate below 70%.

Interestingly, a recent Cochrane systematic review was unable to identify any demonstrable benefit of pulse oximetry.[21] Several aspects of the technology and patient physiology limit the accuracy of pulse oximetry.[22] If the device cannot detect pulsatile flow, the waveform will be damped. Consequently, patients with hypothermia, hypotension, hypovolemia, or peripheral vascular disease, or who are treated with vasoconstrictor medications (e.g., norepinephrine), may have inaccurate pulse oximetry readings. Additionally, an elevated carboxyhemoglobin concentration will lead to falsely elevated SaO_2 because reflected light from these entities is absorbed at the same wavelength as oxyhemoglobin (Figure 22.2). Other

Table 22.1. Sources of Error in Pulse Oximetry.

False depression of SaO_2
Methemoglobinemia (reads at 85%)
Methylene blue dye
Indocyanine green dye
Nonpulsatile blood flow (no reading may be appreciable at all)
Vasoconstriction
Hypotension
Hypothermia
Hypovolemia
Venous congestion with exaggerated venous pulsation
Peripheral edema
Nail polish
Fluorescent lighting
Use of electrocautery (electrical interference)
Severe anemia (hemoglobin concentration 3–4g/dL)
Shivering (may cause mechanical loss of signal)
False elevation of SaO_2
Carboxyhemoglobin
No effect
Fetal hemoglobin
Hyperbilirubinemia

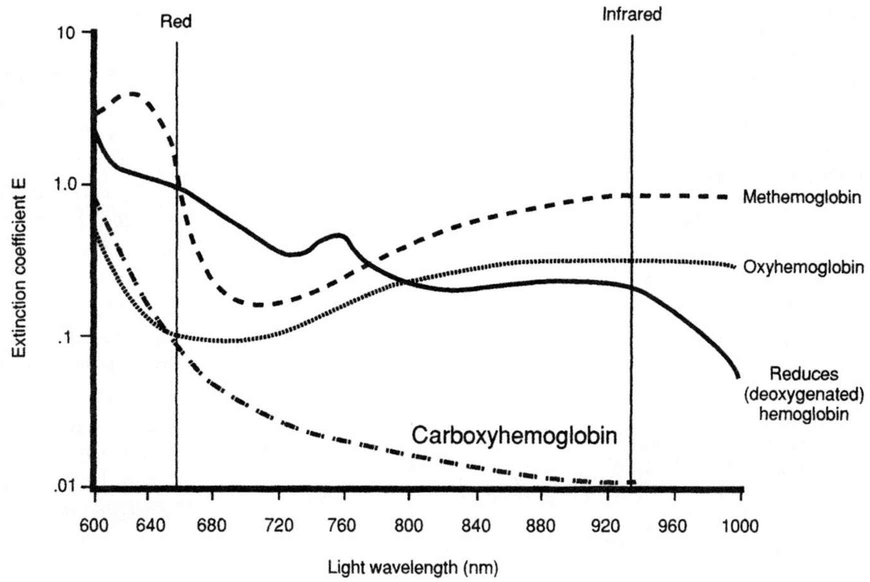

FIGURE 22.2. Different forms of dyshemoglobinemia, in particular methermoglobinemia and carboxyhemoglobin, mimic the light absorbance characteristics of oxyhemoglobin, resulting in false pulse oximetry reading of the true oxyhemoglobin saturation. (Adapted with permission from J Crit Illness 1988;3:103–107.)

causes of inaccurate pulse oximetry include ambient light and motion artifact.

Temperature

Measurement of core body temperature is an essential part of routine monitoring. Hypothermia may contribute to metabolic acidosis, vasoconstriction, myocardial dysfunction, arrhythmias, electrolyte imbalances, altered pharmacokinetics and metabolism, platelet dysfunction, and an increased risk of surgical site infection. Hypothermia may develop under anesthesia for many reasons, including exposure, evaporative water loss, and rapid infusion of ambient temperature fluid or cold blood, and must be avoided by the use of fluid warmers and warming blankets. On the other hand, hyperthermia results in an increased metabolic rate that will increase a patient's heart rate, oxygen consumption, insensible fluid losses, and maintenance fluid requirement.[23] The most reliable method of temperature monitoring is to obtain a core temperature, whether by transoral esophageal probe, bladder catheter thermistor, or the thermistor tip of a pulmonary artery catheter (PAC).

Capnography

Capnography measures changes in the concentration of CO_2 in expired gas during the ventilatory cycle. This technique is most reliable in ventilated patients and employs either mass spectroscopy or infrared light absorption to detect the presence of CO_2. The gas sample may be collected by either sidestream or mainstream sampling; the former is more common and has the advantage that the analyzer is light in weight. However, sidestream sampling is susceptible to accumulation of water vapor in the sampling line. In the ICU, where respiratory gases are humidified, mainstream sampling may be preferable.

The peak CO_2 concentration occurs at end-exhalation and is regarded as the patient's "end-tidal CO_2" ($ETCO_2$), at which time $ETCO_2$ is in close approximation to the alveolar gas concentration (Figure 22.3). Capnography is useful in the assessment of successful tracheostomy or endotracheal tube placement, to monitor weaning from mechanical ventilation, and as a monitor of resuscitation (Table 22.2).[24] The ability to detect hypercarbia during ventilator weaning of intubated patients can diminish the need for serial determinations of blood gases. In conjunction with pulse oximetry, many patients can be weaned successfully from mechanical ventilation altogether, without reliance upon arterial blood gases or invasive hemodynamic monitoring.

Other information is acquired from capnography as well. Prognostically, an $ETCO_2$–$PaCO_2$ gradient of 13 mmHg or more after resuscitation has been associated with increased mortality in trauma patients. A sudden decrease or even dis-

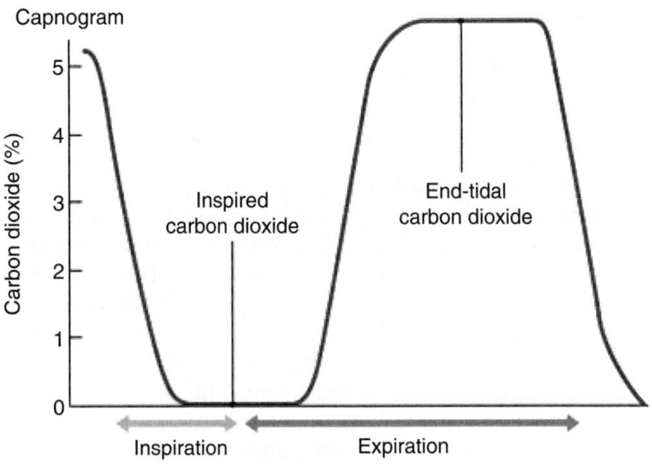

FIGURE 22.3. A normal capnograph tracing.

TABLE 22.2. Changes in End-Tidal CO_2 ($ETCO_2$).

Increased $ETCO_2$	
Decreased alveolar ventilation	
	Reduced respiratory rate
	Reduced tidal volume
	Increased equipment dead space
Increased CO_2 production	
	Fever
	Hypercatabolic state
	Excess feeding with carbohydrate
Increased inspired CO_2 concentration	
	CO_2 absorber exhausted
	Increased CO_2 in inspired gas
	Rebreathing of expired gas
Decreased $ETCO_2$	
Increased alveolar ventilation	
	Increased respiratory rate
	Increased tidal volume
Decreased CO_2 production	
	Hypothermia
	Hypocatabolic state
Increased alveolar dead space	
	Decreased cardiac output
	Pulmonary embolism (clot, air, fat)
	High positive end-expiratory pressure (PEEP)
Sampling error	
	Air in sample line (no or diminished signal)
	Water in sample line (no or diminished signal)
	Inadequate tidal volume (no or diminished signal)
	Disconnection of monitor from tubing (no signal)
	Artificial airway not in trachea (e.g., esophageal intubation) (no signal)

appearance of $ETCO_2$ can be correlated with potentially serious pathology or events, such as a low cardiac output state, disconnection from the ventilator, or pulmonary thromboembolism (see Table 22.2).[25] A gradual increase of $ETCO_2$ can be seen with hypoventilation; the converse is also true. Another cause of gradually decreasing $ETCO_2$ is hypovolemia. The characteristics of the waveform can indicate information about the patient's pulmonary status and in particular whether obstructive disease or inadequate ventilation is present.[26] Recently, some investigators have studied sublingual capnography and its utility as a marker of tissue perfusion, but this technology is still awaiting clinical substantiation as a useful technique.[27]

Invasive Hemodynamic Monitoring

Arterial Catheterization

Measurement of a patient's arterial blood pressure is one of the simplest and most reproducible methods of evaluating hemodynamic status. For most operations, automated noninvasive blood pressure cuff devices, in conjunction with continuous ECG monitoring, can assess the anesthetized patient's volume status adequately (error, ± 2%). These automated blood pressure devices can be set to measure the patient's blood pressure as often as every 5 min. In some patients in whom blood pressure fluctuations occur more frequently than these intermittent measurements can capture, continuous monitoring is needed via an indwelling arterial catheter.[28] These catheters may be placed either preoperatively or intraoperatively in patients undergoing major operations such as cardiac bypass procedures, surgery for multiple trauma, or major chest or abdominal surgery. Blood pressure will be overestimated if the cuff is too small and if actual systolic blood pressure is less than 60 mmHg. Arrhythmias such as atrial fibrillation affect accuracy adversely.

Alternatively, an arterial monitoring catheter may be placed for monitoring of potentially or actually unstable patients in the ICU. Candidates for intraoperative invasive arterial monitoring include patients whose operations are anticipated to be longer than 4 h in duration, those who are already unstable hemodynamically (e.g., intraabdominal infection complicated by septic shock) or who may lose substantial amounts of blood, those who need frequent monitoring of blood samples, or those who may need precise blood pressure control (e.g., neurosurgical patients, patients on cardiopulmonary bypass). Patients with an anticipated postoperative need for continuous blood pressure monitoring, ventilator support, or inotropic support often benefit from intraoperative arterial catheterization. Arterial monitoring catheters are often placed in the ICU for monitoring of hemodynamic instability or mechanical ventilation, among other indications. Although there is morbidity from insertion and from indwelling catheters, there is also morbidity from repetitive arterial punctures; the risk:benefit analysis is a matter of clinical judgment for "less unstable" patients.

Arterial catheters may be placed in any of several locations. The catheter should be a special-purpose thin-walled catheter to maintain fidelity of the waveform and also to obstruct minimally the lumen of the vessel. A standard intravenous cannula should not be used for arterial catheterization. The radial artery at the wrist is the most commonly used site; although the ulnar artery is usually of larger diameter, it is relatively inaccessible to percutaneous access compared with the radial artery. Careful assessment to ensure patency of the collateral circulation to the hand is mandatory before cannulation of an artery at the wrist, to minimize the possibility of tissue loss from arterial occlusion or embolization of debris or clot from the catheter tip. Alternative sites are many. In neonates, the umbilical artery may be catheterized; intestinal ischemia is a rare complication. The axillary artery is relatively spared by atheromatous plaque, supported by good collaterals at the shoulder, and easy to cannulate percutaneously, making it a suitable choice. The superficial femoral artery may also be used, but this is not a location of choice because the burden of plaque (and therefore the risk of distal embolization) is higher, as is the infection rate because skin bacterial counts in the inguinal crease are among the highest anywhere on the body. The superficial temporal artery is difficult to cannulate because of small caliber and tortuosity. The dorsalis pedis artery is accessible but should be avoided in patients with peripheral vascular disease. The brachial artery should be strictly avoided because the collateral circulation around the elbow is poor and the risk of ischemia of the hand or forearm is high. The waveform may be damped by severe peripheral vasoconstriction in patients who are being treated with vasopressors, and it may be necessary to use a longer catheter at a more central location (e.g., axillary, femoral) to get the catheter tip into an artery in the torso that would be less affected. Nosocomial infection of arterial monitoring is unusual provided basic tenets of infection control are honored and femoral artery catheterization is avoided.[29]

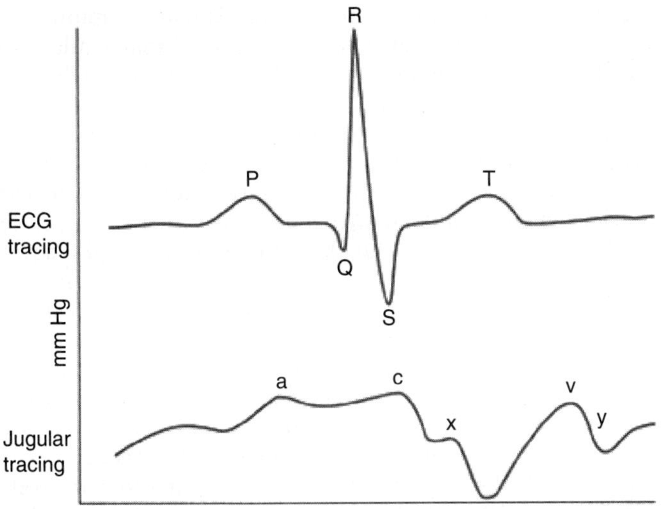

FIGURE 22.4. The central venous pressure waveform. See text for explanation.

Other complications from arterial catheterization include bleeding, hematoma, and pseudoaneurysm.

Central Venous Pressure Monitoring

The central venous pressure (CVP) is an interplay of the circulating blood volume, venous tone, and right ventricular function. The CVP measures the filling pressure of the right ventricle, providing an estimate of intravascular volume status. The normal CVP waveform (Figure 22.4) consists of three upward deflections (a, c, and v waves) and two downward deflections (x and y descents). These waves are produced as follows: The "a" wave is produced by right atrial contraction and occurs just after the P wave on the ECG. The "c" wave occurs as a consequence of isovolumic ventricular contraction, forcing the tricuspid valve to bulge upward into the right atrium. The pressure within the right atrium then decreases as the tricuspid valve is pulled away from the atrium during right ventricular ejection, forming the "x" descent. The right atrium continues to fill during late ventricular systole, forming the "v" wave. The "y" descent occurs when the tricuspid valve opens and blood from the right atrium empties rapidly into the right ventricle during early diastole.

The indications for cannulation of a central vein are numerous and the contraindications are relatively few (Table 22.3). Strict adherence to asepsis, full barrier precautions, and the principles of infection control are crucial if the serious, potentially life-threatening complication of catheter-related bacteremia is to be avoided.[30] Central venous access can be obtained at several body sites, including the basilic vein, femoral vein, external jugular vein, internal jugular vein, or subclavian vein. The basilic vein is used only for placement of a peripherally inserted central catheter (PICC), which is generally used only for long-term venous access (e.g., antibiotics, chemotherapy, parenteral nutrition). The external jugular vein is used rarely outside the operating room. In the ICU, the internal jugular, subclavian, and femoral veins are used, listed in decreasing frequency. Each has advantages and disadvantages. The internal jugular vein site is most popular because of ease of accessibility, a high technical success rate of cannulation, and a low rate of complications. However, it is difficult to keep an adherent dressing in place, and the infection rate is higher than for subclavian vein catheters.

TABLE 22.3. Indications and Contraindications for Central Venous Pressure Monitoring and Pulmonary Artery Catheterization.

Central venous catheter placement
Indications
Major operative procedures involving large fluid shifts or blood loss
Hypovolemia or shock
Intravascular volume assessment when urine output is not reliable or unavailable (e.g.: renal failure)
Major trauma
Surgical procedures with a high risk of air embolism, such as sitting-position craniotomy or major liver resection
Frequent venous blood sampling
Venous access for vasoactive or irritating drugs
Chronic drug administration
Inadequate peripheral IV access
Rapid infusion of IV fluids (using large cannulae)
Parenteral nutrition
Insertion of other devices
PA catheters
Transvenous pacing wires
Access for renal replacement therapy
Absolute contraindications
Infection at the site of insertion
Large tricuspid valve vegetations
Superior vena cava syndrome
Tumor or thrombus in the right atrium
Relative contraindications
Anticoagulant therapy
Coagulopathy
Contralateral diaphragm dysfunction (risk of recurrent nerve injury with internal jugular cannulation)
Newly inserted pacemaker wires
Presence of carotid disease
Recent cannulation of the internal jugular vein
Thyromegaly or prior neck surgery (especially ipsilateral carotid endarterectomy)
Pulmonary artery catheterization:
Indications
Cardiac surgery:
Poor left ventricular function (ejection fraction <0.4; end-diastolic pressure >18 mmHg)
Recent myocardial infarction
Complications of myocardial infarction (e.g., mitral insufficiency, ventricular septal defect, ventricular aneurysm)
Combined lesions, e.g., coronary artery disease with mitral insufficiency or aortic stenosis
Asymmetrical septal hypertrophy
Intraaortic balloon pump
Noncardiac indications
Shock of any cause
Severe pulmonary disease
Complicated surgical procedures
Multiple trauma
Hepatic transplantation
Aortic surgery
Contraindications
The same contraindications for central venous catheterization apply here. Additionally:
Absolute
Tricuspid or pulmonary valvular stenosis
Right ventricular masses (tumor or thrombus)
Tetralogy of Fallot
Relative
Ventricular arrhythmia

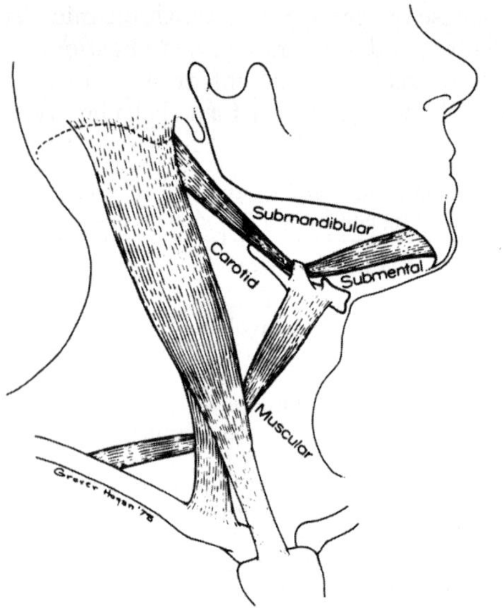

FIGURE 22.5. The subdivision of the anterior triangle of the neck. (By permission of JE Skandalakis, SW Gray, and JR Rowe, *Am Surg* 45(9):590–596, 1979.)

The subclavian site is the most technically demanding for placement and has the highest rate of pneumothorax (1.5%–3%),[30] but the infection rate is the lowest of the three because catheter care is facilitated by the relatively flat surface of the upper chest. The femoral vein site is least preferred, despite the relative ease of catheter placement. It is accessible during cardiopulmonary resuscitation or emergency intubation, so procedures can occur concurrently. However, the site is particularly prone to infection, and the risks of arterial puncture (9%–15%) and venous thromboembolic complications are much higher than for jugular or subclavian venipuncture. Overall complications are comparable for internal jugular and subclavian vein cannulation (6%–12%) and much higher for femoral vein cannulation (13%–19%).[30]

The internal jugular vein begins just medial to the mastoid process at the base of the skull and runs directly inferior from the mastoid process, passing under the sternal end of the clavicle where it joins the subclavian vein. In terms of surface landmarks, the internal jugular vein courses straight down from the mastoid process to the medial side of the insertion point of the clavicular head of the sternocleidomastoid muscle. For purposes of internal jugular vein access, an important anatomic triangle is formed by the two heads of the sternocleidomastoid muscle and the medial one-third of the clavicle (Figure 22.5). Within the triangle, the internal jugular vein is most safely and readily cannulated (Figures 22.6, 22.7) (on the left, the thoracic duct may be punctured inadvertently; Figure 22.8). Within the triangle, the carotid artery lies medial and slightly posterior to the internal jugular vein; the incidence of carotid artery puncture during internal jugular vein cannulation (6%–9%) is somewhat higher than that of puncture of the subclavian artery during subclavian vein catheterization (3%–5%) (Figure 22.9).[30]

Pulmonary Artery Catheterization

A pulmonary artery catheter (PAC) is a balloon-tipped, flow-directed catheter that is usually inserted percutaneously via a central vein and transits the right side of the heart into the pulmonary artery. This catheter can provide a variety of clinical information and typically contains several ports that can monitor pressure or be used for administration of fluids. Some PACs also include a sensor to measure central (mixed) venous oxygen saturation ($S_{mv}O_2$) or right ventricular volume. Data from PACs are used mainly to determine cardiac output (Q) and preload, which is most commonly estimated in the clinical setting by the pulmonary artery occlusion pressure (PAOP).

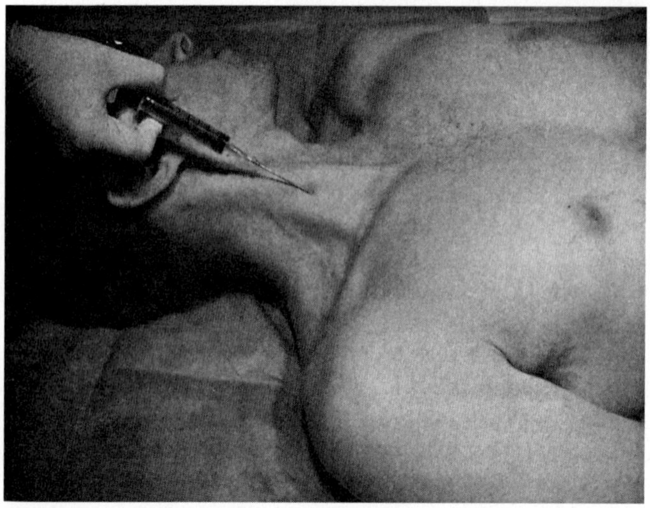

FIGURE 22.6. Internal jugular vein cannulation. When using the middle approach, the apex of a triangle formed by the medial and lateral heads of the sternocleidomastoid muscle (SCM) with the clavicle is localized. The vein runs parallel to and below the lateral head of the SCM. Applying gentle pressure (to avoid collapsing the vein that lies in the same sheath), the operator locates the carotid artery pulse with the index finger of the nondominant hand. The needle is inserted at the apex of the triangle and directed toward the ipsllateral nipple.

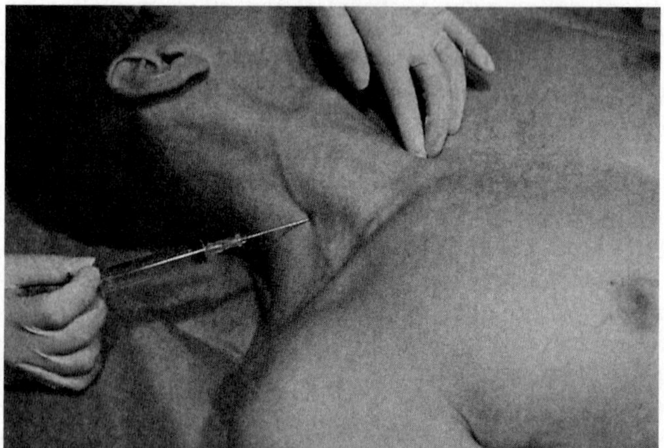

FIGURE 22.7. Internal jugular vein cannulation. When using the posterior approach, the operator locates the posterior aspect of the lateral belly of the sternocleidomastoid muscle. The needle is inserted above the point where the external jugular vein traverses the lateral belly of the sternocleidomastoid muscle and is directed (underneath the muscle) toward the suprasternal notch.

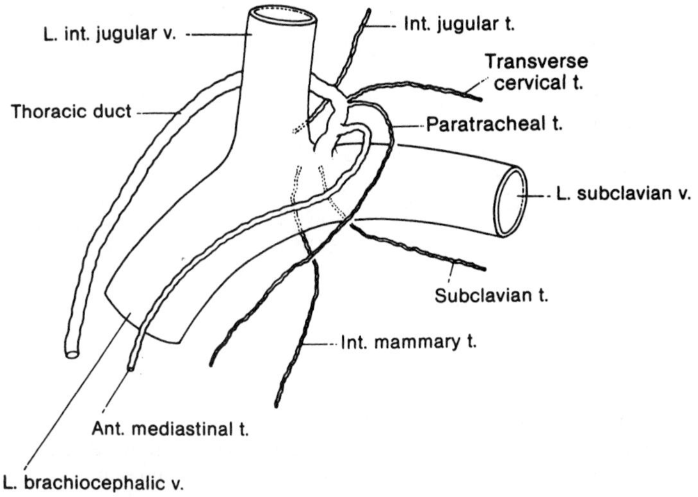

FIGURE 22.8. The thoracic duct and main left lymphatic trunks. Trunks are variable and may enter the veins with the thoracic duct or separately. (By permission of JE Skandalakis, SW Gray, and JR Rowe, *Anatomical Complications in General Surgery*, New York: McGraw-Hill, 1983.)

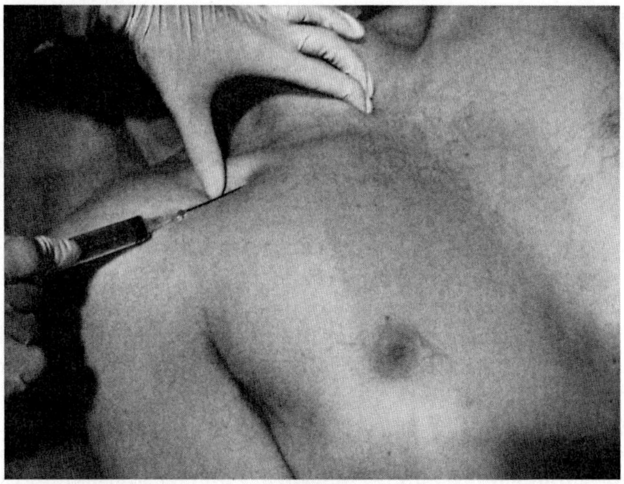

FIGURE 22.9. Subclavian vein cannulation. The operator locates the junction of the middle and medial thirds of the clavicle. The needle is inserted 1 cm below this point and directed toward the suprasternal notch, which is marked by the operator's nondominant hand's index finger. The needle is maintained as parallel to the skin as possible.

Insertion and Monitoring

The insertion of the PAC (as well as a central venous catheter) is performed in the following manner. The operator dons cap, mask, eye protection, and a sterile gown and gloves before preparing the patient's skin (2% chlorhexidine gluconate is associated with a lower incidence of catheter-related infection than 10% povidine-iodine solution) and draping the patient completely with a full-bed drape. After infiltration of a local anesthetic, an introducer sheath is placed into the subclavian or internal jugular vein, and the catheter is inserted through the introducer with the balloon deflated. Once the catheter tip reaches the superior vena cava (after approximately 20 cm), partial inflation of the balloon (generally 0.5 mL) permits blood flow to advance the catheter. The position of the catheter tip is usually determined by pressure monitoring or occasionally by fluoroscopy. Entry into the right ventricle is indicated by a sudden increase in systolic pressure to at least 30 mmHg (Figure 22.10), while the diastolic pressure remains unchanged from right atrial or vena caval pressure. When the catheter enters the pulmonary artery, the systolic pressure does not change, but diastolic pressure increases above right ventricular end-diastolic pressure or central venous pressure (CVP), and consequently, the pulse pressure narrows. Advancement of the catheter with periodic inflation of the catheter wedges the balloon, usually in a lobar pulmonary artery. A chest X-ray confirms proper placement and rules out complications such as hemothorax or pneumothorax. As a general rule, if the tip of the catheter extends beyond the hilum, it has advanced too far and must be withdrawn partially and repositioned.

The pulmonary artery systolic pressure (normal, 15–30 mmHg) and diastolic pressure (normal, 5–13 mmHg) are recorded with the catheter balloon deflated. The diastolic pressure corresponds well to the PAOP. Diastolic pressure can exceed the PAOP when pulmonary vascular resistance is high secondary to primary pulmonary disease (e.g., pulmonary fibrosis, pulmonary hypertension).

The PAOP is measured in the following manner.[31] With the balloon inflated, the tip of the catheter records the static

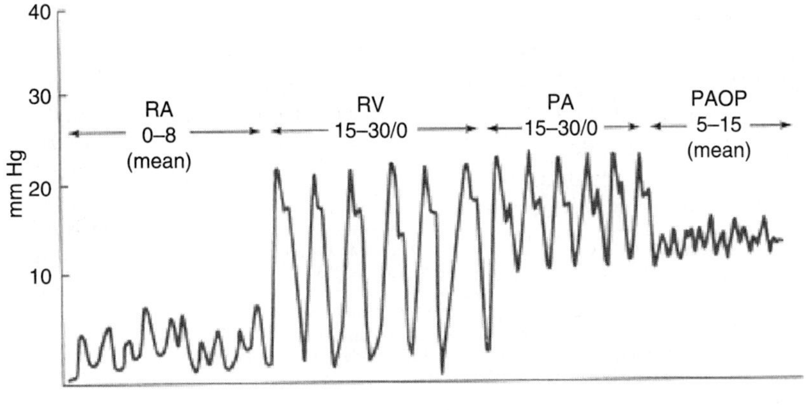

FIGURE 22.10. Waveform for insertion of a pulmonary artery catheter. See text for explanation.

back-pressure of the pulmonary veins. The balloon must not remain inflated for longer than 30s to prevent pulmonary artery rupture or pulmonary infarction. Normally, PAOP approximates left atrial pressure, which in turn approximates left ventricular end-diastolic pressure (LVEDP), itself a reflection of left ventricular end-diastolic volume (LVEDV). The LVEDV represents preload, which is the actual target parameter. Many factors cause PAOP to reflect LVEDV inaccurately: these factors include mitral stenosis, high levels of positive end-expiratory pressure (PEEP > 10 cm H_2O), and changes in left ventricular compliance (e.g., because of myocardial infarction, pericardial effusion, or increased afterload). Inaccurate readings may result from balloon overinflation, improper catheter position, alveolar pressure exceeding pulmonary venous pressure (as with ventilation with PEEP), or severe pulmonary hypertension (which may make PAOP measurement difficult or, indeed, hazardous). Elevated PAOP occurs in left-sided heart failure. Decreased PAOP occurs with hypovolemia or decreased preload.

A desirable feature of PA catheterization is the ability to measure $S_{mv}O_2$, although controversially, sampling from the superior vena cava via a central venous catheter may provide data of comparable utility. True mixed venous blood is composed of blood from both the superior and inferior vena cava that has admixed in the right atrium. The blood may be sampled for blood gas analysis from the distal port of the PAC, but some catheters have embedded fiberoptic sensors that measure $S_{mv}O_2$ saturation directly. Causes of low $S_{mv}O_2$ include anemia, pulmonary disease, carboxyhemoglobinemia, low Q, and increased tissue oxygen demand. The SaO_2:(SaO_2 – $S_{mv}O_2$) ratio determines the adequacy of O_2 delivery (DO_2). Ideally the $P_{mv}O_2$ should be 35–40 mmHg, with a $S_{mv}O_2$ of about 70%. Values of $P_{mv}O_2$ less than 30 mmHg are critically low.

Another monitoring feature of the PAC includes the ability to measure Q. With these catheters, Q is measured either by intermittent bolus injection of ice water or, in new catheters, continuous warm thermodilution.[32] Other parameters can be calculated from the Q, including systemic and pulmonary vascular resistance (SVR, PVR) and right and left ventricular stroke work (RVSW, LVSW) (Table 22.4).

TABLE 22.4. Derived Hemodynamic Parameters from Pulmonary Artery Catheter Data.

Formula	*Normal value*
CI = CO (L/min)/BSA	2.8–4.2 L/min/m^2
SV = (L/min) CO·1000/HR	50–110 mL/beat
SI = SV/BSA	30–65 mL/beat/m^2
LVSWI = 1.36·(MAP – PAOP)·SVI/100	45–60 g.m/beat/m^2
RVSWI = 1.36·(PAP – CVP)·SVI/100	5–10 g.m/beat/m^2
SVR = (MAP – CVP)·80/CO	900–1400 dyne.s.cm^{-5}
SVRI = (MAP – CVP)·80/CI	1500–2400 dyne.s.cm^{-5}
PVR = (PAP – PAOP)·80/CO	150–250 dyne.s.cm^{-5}
PVRI = (PAP – PAOP)·80/CI	250–400 dyne.s.cm^{-5}

BSA, body surface area; CI, cardiac index; CO, cardiac output; CVP, central venous pressure; g.m, gram.meter; HR, heart rate; LVSWI, left ventricular stroke work index; MAP, mean arterial blood pressure; PAOP, pulmonary artery occlusion pressure; PAP, pulmonary artery pressure; PVR, pulmonary vascular resistance; PVRI, pulmonary vascular resistance index; RVSWI, right ventricular stroke work index; SI, stroke volume index; SV, stroke volume; SVR, systemic vascular resistance; SVRI, systemic vascular resistance index.

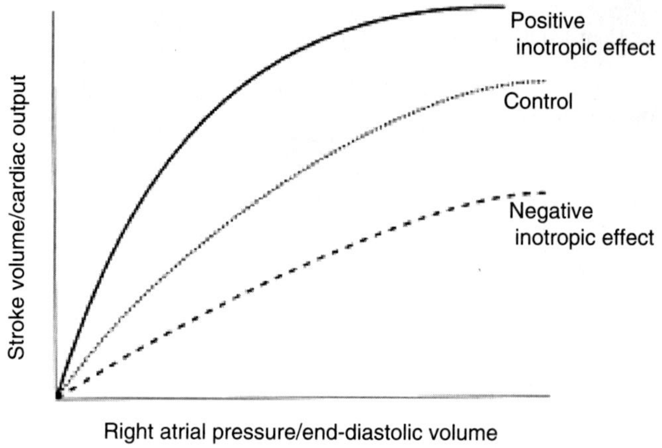

FIGURE 22.11. A stylized Frank–Starling curve. A wide range of cardiac output values is possible for a given filling pressure.

Clinical Use of the Pulmonary Artery Catheter

Many indications have been championed for the PAC,[24] despite a lack of convincing evidence. One suggested indication is perioperative monitoring of patients with coronary artery disease or congestive heart failure undergoing noncardiac surgery (see Table 22.3).[33–35] A specific population that has been studied frequently is perioperative vascular surgery patients.[36–38] A purported benefit to the preoperative placement of a PAC is that it allows the "optimization" of cardiac function. By this technique, the incremental manipulation of fluids, blood products, inotropes, and possibly diuretics is undertaken to define the Frank–Starling curve for the individual patient before surgical stress (Figure 22.11).[39–41] Additionally, the patient would be prepositioned to undergo aggressive resuscitation intraoperatively if it were necessary,[42] theoretically reducing the risk of organ dysfunction in the perioperative period. Despite this rationale, no studies have demonstrated unequivocally that PAC use decreases morbidity or mortality (Table 22.5).

However attractive the concept may be of perioperative cardiac optimization to decrease morbidity (the lack of data notwithstanding), certain features of the practice make it undesirable for routine use in surgical patients.[43] First, monitoring by a less invasive method such as central venous monitoring or even by physical examination and clinical judgment may be equally useful in determining volume status in many patients.[44,45] Second, PAC-derived data can be difficult to interpret, and inexperienced practitioners misinterpret frequently the data derived, oftentimes with deleterious consequences. Cardiac pathology that may confound even experienced clinicians includes valvular disease, pulmonary hypertension, cardiomyopathy, or fluctuations in core temperature. Imprecise "optimization" of a patient's cardiac function may augment myocardial work excessively and contribute to myocardial ischemia. The lack of demonstrable benefit, coupled with the trend to same-day admission for elective surgery, have decreased PAC placement in substantially in the perioperative period.[46,47]

Pulmonary artery catheters may still be useful in selected circumstances, such as cardiomyopathy, shock of various etiologies, or an unpredicted or poor response to conventional fluid therapy. The PAC may be useful during aortic surgery; proximal aortic cross-clamping/declamping may cause

TABLE 22.5.
Evidence for Utility of Pulmonary Artery Catheter in Perioperative Patients.

Author	*Class of data*	*Population*	*Numbers of patients: protocol/control*	*Findings*
Bonazzi et al.[40]	I	Elective infrarenal abdominal aortic aneurysm optimized to CI > 3.0 L/min/m^2, DO_2 > 600 mL/min/m^2	50/50	No differences in in-hospital mortality, cardiovascular morbidity, renal failure, hospital length of stay
Bender et al.[34]	I	Mandatory PA catheter monitoring vs. conventional treatment in elective vascular surgery	51/53	No mortality, morbidity difference, or change in ICU or hospital length
Isaacson et al.[35]	I	PA catheter vs. CVP monitoring in elective abdominal aortic aneurysm surgery	51/51	No morbidity or mortality difference
Boyd et al.[47]	I	High-risk elective surgery patients randomized to PA catheter optimization to DO_2 > 600 mL/min/m^2	54/53	Decreased mortality and morbidity in protocol group
Berlauk et al.[36]	I	Elective vascular surgery patients randomized to CI > 2.8	68/21	Decreased mortality in PA catheter group
Valentine et al.[38]	I	Elective vascular patients receiving aortic surgery randomized to CI > 2.8, SVR < 1100	60/60	No differences in mortality or adverse postoperative events
Ziegler et al.[37]	I	Elective vascular surgery patients randomized to PCWP > 12, SVO_2 > 65%	32/40	No differences in mortality or complications between groups

CI, cardiac index; CVP, central venous pressure; DO_2, oxygen delivery; ICU, intensive care unit; PA, pulmonary artery; PAOP, pulmonary artery occlusion pressure; SvO_2, venous oxygen saturation; SVR, systemic vascular resistance.

marked, instantaneous hemodynamic changes. Intraoperative transesophageal echocardiography has its advocates for intraoperative monitoring, but it is not widely available outside cardiac surgery operating rooms, and requires considerable expertise for data interpretation. Critically ill patients receiving one or more inotropic agents despite resuscitation with large volumes of fluid may also benefit from monitoring by PAC, both in the operating room and in the ICU.[48] A summary of the data regarding the use of pulmonary artery catheters for monitoring of critically ill patients is provided in Table 22.6.[41,42,48]

Shoemaker et al. achieved superior outcomes in a small number of critically ill patients who were resuscitated to "supranormal" (i.e., oxygenation in excess of metabolic need) oxygen transport endpoints, but the hypothesis that more rapid "repayment" of the "oxygen debt" incurred in shock/hypoperfusion is beneficial has been disproved by multiple recent studies.[50] Another study suggested that use of a PAC may be associated with decreased mortality after acute renal failure.[51] However, the preponderance of data has failed to demonstrate benefit, as shown in Table 22.6.[52–54] Some retrospective data even suggest that PAC use is associated with excess mortality.[55,56]

Several theories may explain why PAC use has not improved outcomes. In observational studies, mortality may be higher with PAC use because they are more likely to be placed in sicker patients,[57] leading to a higher incidence of complications as well as misinterpretation of the data.[58] Other clinicians have noted that goal-directed therapy guided by a PAC may lead to increased fluid administration and resultant abdominal compartment syndrome.[59] Nevertheless, clinicians continue to believe that PACs do aid in the management of certain critically ill patients when combined with other objective and clinical data.[60] As with many physiological measurements, a changing trend in measurable parameters may be more informative than a single abnormal value.

In the past 15 years, innovative new PACs have become available, including catheters that allow continuous monitoring of Q and continuous oximetric monitoring of $S_{mv}O_2$. Continuous availability of data may be useful in certain circumstances where oxygen transport is marginal, such as patients with acute respiratory distress syndrome (ARDS) on high levels of positive end-expiratory pressure (PEEP). The application of PEEP can decrease venous return markedly, and therefore Q, in a short time period; maintenance of Q is important to maintain ventilation-perfusion matching.

Pulmonary artery catheters that measure right heart function by estimating right ventricular volume have also been championed in recent years. Proponents of this technology claim that a more accurate assessment of right ventricular preload can be obtained.[61] This contention is arguable; there is a paucity of Class I data from patients managed by these "right ventricular" catheters.

Complications specific or common to PACs include difficulty with insertion, infection (2%–5%), hemopneumothorax (2%–5%), migration (5%–10%), patient discomfort, arrhythmia (10%–15%), and hemorrhage (0.2%). Other more rare complications have been reported, including catheter knotting resulting from redundancy of the catheter within the right ventricle (especially in patients with heart failure, cardiomyopathy, or increased pulmonary pressure); pulmonary

TABLE 22.6.
Evidence for Utility of Pulmonary Artery Catheter in Monitoring Critically Ill Patients.

Author	*Class of data*	*Population*	*Numbers of patients: protocol/control*	*Findings*
Richard et al.[49]	I	ICU patients with shock, sepsis, ARDS randomized with or without PA catheter	335/341	No significant differences in mortality with or without catheter at day 14
Sandham et al.[42]	I	High-risk surgical patients randomized with or without PA catheter	78/77	No survival difference for in-hospital stay, 6 months or 12 months; PA catheter group with more pulmonary embolism
Rhodes et al.[41]	I	ICU patients randomized with or without a PA catheter	90/105	No survival difference; PA group had more fluids and more renal failure by ICU day 3
Yu et al.[48]	I	ICU patients with shock, sepsis, ARDS randomized to DO_2 > 600 or 450 mL/min/m^2	27/21 (89 originally enrolled patients)	No mortality or myocardial infarction difference
Balogh et al.[59]	II	Severely ill trauma patients resuscitated to 600 mL/min/m^2 (supranormal) vs. 500 mL/min/m^2 (normal) before and after ICU protocol change	85/71	Supranormal group with more organ failure, mortality, abdominal compartment syndrome
Tuchschmidt et al.[53]	I	ICU patients with septic shock randomized to CI > 6.0 or CI 3.0	26/25	No significant mortality difference
Fleming et al.[52]	I	Severely ill trauma patients randomized to CI > 4.5 L/min/m^2 or DO_2 > 670 mL/min/m^2	33/34	Decreased mortality in protocol patients compared to control patients
Hayes et al.[54]	I	ICU patient randomized to supranormal goals of CI > 4.5 L/min/m^2, DO_2 > 600 mL/min/m^2, CO_2 > 170 mL/min/m^2	50/50	Decreased mortality in control group compared to protocol group

ARDS, acute respiratory distress syndrome; CI, cardiac index; DO_2, oxygen delivery; ICU, intensive care unit; PA, pulmonary artery; VO_2, oxygen consumption.

infarction secondary to an overinflated or "permanently wedged" balloon; pulmonary artery perforation; intracardiac perforation; valvular injury; and endocarditis. A devastating complication is pulmonary artery rupture, which occurs in less than 0.1% of cases of PAC usage. This catastrophic complication is generally fatal and occurs upon wedging the catheter during insertion or during routine determination of PAOP. Distal migration of the PAC within the pulmonary artery increases the risk dramatically of pulmonary artery rupture and argues for routine daily bedside chest radiography for all patients with an indwelling PAC.[62]

Noninvasive Cardiac Output

Thoracic bioimpedance systems to monitor Q are being developed for clinical use. Thoracic bioimpedance derives information from topical electrodes placed onto the anterior chest and neck to estimate Q by incorporating a modified form of the Kubicek equation and by estimating the left ventricular systolic time interval from time 1/μ derivative bioimpedance signals. The lag time for the system to provide data is approximately 2 to 5 min from initial lead placement and activation. The main drawback of thoracic bioimpedance is that the technique is very sensitive to any alteration of the electrode contact or positioning on the patient.

The esophageal Doppler monitor (EDM) device is a soft, 6-mm catheter that is placed noninvasively into the esophagus. A Doppler flow probe at its tip allows continuous monitoring of Q and stroke volume. A 4-MHz continuous wave ultrasound frequency is reflected to produce a waveform, representing the change in blood flow in the descending aorta (about 80% of Q) with each pulsation. In contrast to the invasive PA catheter, the EDM does not require percutaneous insertion.[63] The EDM also avoids the risk of infection. An EDM may yield more accurate hemodynamic data than a PA catheter in patients with cardiac valvular lesions, septal defects, arrhythmias, or pulmonary hypertension. The primary disadvantage of the EDM is that the device may sometimes lose its waveform with only a slight positional change and render damped, inaccurate readings.[64]

Consequently, although both thoracic bioimpedance and esophageal Doppler monitoring represent potentially useful techniques for monitoring of Q, neither device has proved to be as consistently reliable as the invasive method of Q measurement via PAC. Currently, no data exist to demonstrate superior outcomes between invasive and noninvasive hemodynamic monitoring techniques. However, a prospective study comparing patients monitored simultaneously with PAC and bioimpedance techniques concluded that the methods gave comparable estimates of Q.[65] Similarly, a trial comparing measurements between esophageal echo-Doppler and pulmonary artery catheters did demonstrate comparable values.[66] The noninvasive modalities may still supplant the use of the PAC if equivalent results can be obtained with greater safety.

Intracranial Pressure Monitoring

Monitoring of intracranial pressure (ICP) has become a standard method of evaluating patients with severe traumatic brain injury (TBI).[67] Several different types of ICP monitors have been described. In TBI, these devices can be used to "optimize" the cerebral perfusion pressure (CPP) (mean arterial pressure minus ICP). Typically, the CPP should be kept above 60 mmHg in these cases. Importantly, although ICP monitoring and calculation of CPP have become standard, no Class I data in human beings show an outcome benefit for ICP monitoring in patients with traumatic encephalopathy.[68]

Perhaps the most useful method of ICP monitoring involves the use of the intraventricular or "ventriculostomy" catheter. This device is the preferred method of ICP monitoring because the catheter can also drain cerebrospinal fluid and consequently decrease elevated ICP. In this way, the ventriculostomy can be both diagnostic and therapeutic. However, ventriculostomy is also the most invasive method of ICP monitoring and poses the highest infection risk (~8%). Occasionally, the ventriculostomy may be impossible to place or may become occluded because of severe brain edema or extruding brain matter. Other types of intracranial devices include an intraparenchymal monitor or the epidural bolt; no consensus has developed as to how to choose among these devices. Despite the high risk of infection with ventriculostomy, neither prolonged antibiotic prophylaxis nor, controversially, regular replacement of the catheter at 5- to 7-day intervals serves to reduce the risk.

Gastric Tonometry

Tonometry is used to determine the gut intramucosal pH (pH_i) of the patient. Tonometer catheters are available for placement via the stomach or sigmoid colon. The tonometry catheter contains a port that leads to a chamber with a semipermeable membrane into which saline is instilled and allowed to equilibrate with the intragastric (or intracolonic) milieu. Investigators have focused on both the absolute pH_i and the tissue CO_2 to arterial CO_2 gradient as being surrogates of splanchnic perfusion and consequently markers of resuscitation. Proponents of the device believe it to be a valuable tool because gastric mucosal ischemia is an early sign of impaired splanchnic perfusion, which in turn is believed to be more sensitive as an indicator of hypoperfusion than global indicators such as Q or acidosis.[69] Optimal splanchnic perfusion during surgery has been suggested to decrease complications postoperatively after abdominal surgery, cardiac surgery, and aortic aneurysm repair.[70,71] A recent multicenter, observational study in elective general surgery patients revealed that patients monitored with semicontinuous gastric tonometry could be predicted accurately to have postoperative complications based on the gastric : $ETCO_2$ ratio.[72]

Questions persist as to the utility of gastric tonometry. Prospective trials demonstrating superior outcomes with the device have yet to be published, despite more than a decade of use. Tonometry has fallen into disfavor as well because the device is expensive, difficult to use, and prone to dislodgment and errors of calibration. Consequently, most clinicians currently use acidosis, base deficit, hyperlactatemia, creatinine clearance, or $S_{mv}O_2$ to guide resuscitation. Newer tonometers that utilize air rather than saline, or which use fiberoptic infrared technology to measure mucosal blood flow directly, may revitalize this approach to monitoring.

Near-Infrared Spectroscopy

Near-infrared (NIR) technology relies on the principle that mitochondrial cytochrome a, a redox shifts can be determined by near-infrared wavelength reflection, which can penetrate skin and bone. In animal studies, significant correlations were detected between certain NIR waveform attributes and oxygen delivery during shock, with NIR probes placed directly on the stomach, small bowel, and other viscera. Consequently, NIR technology appears to be useful for assessing tissue perfusion.[73] Also, NIR monitoring of small bowel pH may be used to gauge the adequacy of resuscitation. However, the technique is still being adapted, especially for indications other than hemorrhagic shock.

Near-infrared spectroscopy may also develop a variety of other clinical uses including detection of compartment syndrome, neonatal perfusion, vascular graft patency, and microvascular flap perfusion.[74] This technology is useful for the early detection of ischemia by external placement of the probe after free tissue transfer. The technology may prove useful for postoperative monitoring of the patency of lower extremity vascular bypass grafts, onset of extremity compartment syndrome, or the risk of wound failure or surgical site infection after surgery.

References

1. Ahrens T. Utilization of intensive care unit technology. New Horiz 1998;6:41–51.
2. Eachempati SR, Barie PS. Minimally invasive and noninvasive diagnosis and therapy in critically ill and injured patients. Arch Surg 1999;134:1189–1196.
3. Barie PS. Advances in critical care monitoring. Arch Surg 1997;132:734–739.
4. Corwin HL, Parsonnet KC, Gettinger A. RBC transfusion in the ICU. Is there a reason? Chest 1995;108:767–771.
5. Low LL, Harrington GR, Stoltzfus DP. The effect of arterial lines on blood-drawing practices and costs in intensive care units. Chest 1995;108:216–219.
6. Lin JC, Strauss RG, Kulhavy JC, Johnson KJ. Phlebotomy overdraw in the neonatal intensive care nursery. Pediatrics 2000;106: E19.
7. Adal KA, Farr BM. Central venous catheter-related infections: a review. Nutrition 1996;12:208–213.
8. Ottino G, De Paulis R, Pansini S, et al. Major sternal wound infection after open-heart surgery: a multivariate analysis of risk factors in 2,579 consecutive operative procedures. Ann Thorac Surg 1987;44:173–179.

9. Louie RF, Tang Z, Sutton DV, et al. Point-of-care glucose testing: effects of critical care variables, influence of reference instruments, and a modular glucose meter design. Arch Pathol Lab Med 2000;124:257–266.
10. van den Berghe G, Wouters P, Weekers F, et al. Intensive insulin therapy in the critically ill patients. N Engl J Med 2001;345:1359–1367.
11. Chance JJ, Li DJ, Sokoll LJ, et al. Multiple site analytical evaluation of a portable blood gas/electrolyte analyzer for point of care testing. Crit Care Med 2000;28:2081–2085.
12. Drew BJ, Califf RM, Funk M, et al. American Heart Association. Practice standards for electrocardiographic monitoring in hospital settings: an American Heart Association scientific statement from the Councils on Cardiovascular Nursing, Clinical Cardiology, and Cardiovascular Disease in the Young: endorsed by the International Society of Computerized Electrocardiology and the American Association of Critical-Care Nurses. Circulation 2004;110:2721–2146.
13. Sejersten M, Pahlm O, Pettersson J, et al. The relative accuracies of ECG precordial lead waveforms derived from EASI leads and those acquired from paramedic applied standard leads. J Electrocardiol 2003;36:179–188.
14. Chun AA. McGee SR. Bedside diagnosis of coronary artery disease: a systematic review. Am J Med 2004;117:334–343.
15. Salerno SM, Alguire PC, Waxman HS. Competency in interpretation of 12-lead electrocardiograms: a summary and appraisal of published evidence. Ann Intern Med 2003;138:751–760.
16. Giles JW, Sear JW, Foex P. Effect of chronic beta-blockade on peri-operative outcome in patients undergoing non-cardiac surgery: an analysis of observational and case control studies. Anaesthesia 2004;59: 574–578.
17. Mangano DT, Layug EL, Wallace A, et al. Effect of atenolol on mortality and cardiovascular morbidity after noncardiac surgery. N Engl J Med 1996;335:1713–1720.
18. Auerbach AD, Goldman L. Beta-blockers and reduction of cardiac events in noncardiac surgery: scientific review. JAMA 2002;287:1435–1444.
19. Reuss JL. Factors influencing fetal pulse oximetry performance. J Clin Monit Comp 2004;18:13–24.
20. Branson RD, Mannheimer PD. Forehead oximetry in critically ill patients: the case for a new monitoring site. Respir Care Clin N Am 2004;10:359–367.
21. Pedersen T, Dyrlund A, Pedersen B, et al. Pulse oximetry for perioperative monitoring. Cochrane Database Syst Rev 2003;3: CD002013.
22. Aoyagi T. Pulse oximetry: its invention, theory, and future. J Anesth 2003;17:259–266.
23. Barie PS, Eachempati. SR. Fever in the ICU. In: Read RC, ed. Managing Difficult Infections. London: SP Science Press, 1999:63–76.
24. Soubani AO. Noninvasive monitoring of oxygen and carbon dioxide. Am J Emerg Med 2001;19:141–146.
25. Hatlestad D. Capnography as a predictor of the return of spontaneous circulation. Emerg Med Serv 2004;33:75–80.
26. Thompson JE, Jaffe MB. Capnographic waveforms in the mechanically ventilated patient. Respir Care 2005;50:100–109.
27. Maciel AT, Creteur J, Vincent JL. Tissue capnometry: does the answer lie under the tongue? Intensive Care Med 2004;30:2157–2165.
28. Pinsky MR. Hemodynamic monitoring in the intensive care unit. Clin Chest Med 2003;24:549–560.
29. Bowdle TA. Complications of invasive monitoring. Anesth Clin N Am 2002;20:571–588.
30. McGee DC, Gould MK. Preventing complications of central venous catheterization. N Engl J Med 2003;348:1123–1133.
31. O'Quin R, Marini JJ. Pulmonary artery occlusion pressure; clinical physiology, measurement and interpretation. Am Rev Respir Dis 1983;128:319–326.
32. Stetz CW, Miller RG, Kelly GE, et al. Reliability of the thermodilution method in the determination of cardiac output in clinical practice. Am Rev Respir Dis 1982;126:1001–1010.
33. Barie PS. Perioperative management. In: Norton JA, Lowry SF, Pass H, et al., eds. Surgery: Scientific Basis and Current Practice. New York: Springer-Verlag, 2000:363–395.
34. Bender JS, Smith-Meek MA, Jones CE. Routine pulmonary artery catheterization does not reduce morbidity and mortality of elective vascular surgery: results of a prospective, randomized trial. Ann Surg 1997;226:229–236.
35. Isaacson IJ, Lowdon JD, Berry AJ, et al. The value of pulmonary artery and central venous monitoring in patients undergoing abdominal aortic reconstructive surgery: a comparative study of two selected, randomized groups. J Vasc Surg 1990;12:754–760.
36. Berlauk JF, Abrams JH, Gilmour IJ, et al. Perioperative optimization of cardiovascular hemodynamics improves outcome in peripheral vascular surgery. Ann Surg 1991;214:290–299.
37. Ziegler DW, Wright JG, Choban PS, et al. A prospective randomized trial of preoperative optimization of cardiac function in patients undergoing elective peripheral vascular surgery. Surgery (St. Louis) 1997;22:584–592.
38. Valentine RF, Duke ML, Inman MH, et al. Effectiveness of pulmonary artery catheters in aortic surgery. A randomized trial. J Vasc Surg 1998;27:203–212.
39. Fischer SP. Cost-effective preoperative evaluation and testing. Chest 1997;115(suppl):96S–100S.
40. Bonazzi M, Gentile F, Biasi GM, et al. Impact of perioperative haemodynamic monitoring on cardiac morbidity after major vascular surgery in low risk patients. A randomised pilot trial. Eur J Vasc Endovasc Surg 2002;23:445–451.
41. Rhodes A, Cusack RJ, Newman PJ, et al. A randomised, controlled trial of the pulmonary artery catheter in critically ill patients. Intensive Care Med 2002;28:256–264.
42. Sandham JD, Hull RD, Brant RF, et al. A randomized, controlled trial of the use of pulmonary-artery catheters in high-risk surgical patients. N Engl J Med 2003;348:5–14.
43. Morris AH, Chapman RH, Gardner RM. Frequency of technical problems encountered in the measurement of pulmonary artery wedge pressure. Crit Care Med 1984;12:164–170.
44. Trottier SJ, Taylor RW. Physicians attitudes toward and knowledge of the pulmonary artery catheter: Society of Critical Care Medicine membership survey. New Horiz 1997;5:201–206.
45. Shippy CR, Appel PL, Shoemaker WC. Reliability of clinical monitoring to assess blood volume in critically ill patients. Crit Care Med 1984;12:107–112.
46. Connors AF, Speroff T, Dawson NV, et al. The effectiveness of right heart catheterization in the initial care of critically ill patients. JAMA 1996;276:889–897.
47. Boyd O, Grounds RM, Bennett ED. A randomized clinical trial of the effect of deliberate perioperative increase of oxygen delivery on mortality in high-risk surgical patients. JAMA 1993;270:2699–2707.
48. Yu M, Takanishi D, Myers SA, et al. Frequency of mortality and myocardial infarction during maximizing oxygen delivery: a prospective, randomized trial. Crit Care Med 1995;23:1025–1032.
49. Richard C, Warzawski J, Anguel N, et al. French Pulmonary Artery Catheter Study Group. Early use of the pulmonary artery catheter and outcome in patients with shock and acute respiratory distress syndrome: a randomized controlled trial. JAMA 2003;290:2713–2720.
50. Shoemaker WC, Appel PL, Kram HB, et al. Prospective trial of supranormal values of oxygenation as therapeutic goals in high-risk surgical patients. Chest 1988;94:1176–1186.

51. Uchino S, Doidg GS, Beloomo R, et al. Diuretics and mortality in acute renal failure. Crit Care Med 2004;32:1669–1677.
52. Fleming A, Shop M, Shoemaker W, et al. Prospective trial of supranormal values as goals of resuscitation in severe trauma. Arch Surg 1992;7:1175–1179.
53. Tuchschmidt J, Fried J, Astiz M, et al. Elevation of cardiac output and oxygen delivery improves outcome in septic shock. Chest 1992;102:216–220.
54. Hayes MA, Timmins AC, Yau EH, et al. Elevation of systemic oxygen delivery in the treatment of critically ill patients. N Engl J Med 1994;330:1717–1722.
55. Marik PE. Pulmonary artery catheterization and esophageal Doppler monitoring in the ICU. Chest 1999;116:1085–1091.
56. Connors AFJ, Speroff T, Dawson NV, et al. The effectiveness of right heart catheterization in the initial care of critically ill patients. SUPPORT Investigators. JAMA 1996;276:889–897.
57. Zion MM, Balkin J, Rosenmann D, et al. Use of pulmonary artery catheters in patients with acute myocardial infarction. Analysis of experience with 5,841 patients in the SPRINT registry. Chest 1990;98:1331–1335.
58. Iberti TJ, Fischer EP, Leibowitz AB, et al. A multicenter study of physician's knowledge of the pulmonary artery catheter: Pulmonary Artery Catheter Study Group. JAMA 1990;264:2928–2932.
59. Balogh Z, McKinley BA, Cocanour CS, et al. Supranormal trauma resuscitation causes more cases of abdominal compartment syndrome. Arch Surg 2003;138:637–643.
60. Shoemaker WC. Use and abuse of the balloon tipped pulmonary artery (Swan–Ganz) catheter: are patients getting their money's worth? Crit Care Med 1990;18:1294–1296.
61. Diebel L, Wilson R, Tagett MG, et al. End diastolic volume: a better indicator of preload in the critically ill. Arch Surg 1992;127:817–822.
62. Fong Y, Whalen GF, Hariri RH, Barie PS. Utility of daily chest radiographs in the surgical intensive care unit: a prospective study. Arch Surg 1995;130:764–768.
63. Eachempati SR, Young C, Alexander J, et al. The clinical use of an esophageal Doppler monitor for hemodynamic monitoring in sepsis. J Clin Monit Comput 1999;15:223–225.
64. Lefrant JY, Bruelle P, Aya AG, et al. Training is required to improve the reliability of esophageal Doppler to measure cardiac output in critically ill patients. Intensive Care Med 1998;24:347–352.
65. Shoemaker WC, Belzberg H, Wo CC, et al. Multicenter study of noninvasive monitoring systems as alternatives to invasive monitoring of acutely ill emergency patients. Chest 1998;114:1643–1652.
66. Su NY, Huang CJ, Tsai P, et al. Cardiac output measurement during cardiac surgery: esophageal Doppler versus pulmonary artery catheter. Acta Anaesthiol Sin 2002;40:127–133.
67. Rincon F, Mayer SA. Novel therapies for intracerebral hemorrhage. Curr Opin Crit Care 2004;10:94–100.
68. Forsyth R, Baxter P, Elliott T. Routine intracranial pressure monitoring in acute coma. Cochrane Database Syst Rev 2001;3: CD002043.
69. Hameed SM, Cohn SM. Gastric tonometry: the role of mucosal pH measurement in the management of trauma. Chest 2003;123(5 suppl):475S–481S.
70. Gardeback M, Settergren G, Brodin LA, et al. Splanchnic blood flow and oxygen uptake during cardiopulmonary bypass. J Cardiothorac Vasc Anesth 2002;16:308–315.
71. Frumento RJ, Mongero L, Naka Y, Bennett-Guerrero E. Preserved gastric tonometric variables in cardiac surgical patients administered intravenous perflubron emulsion. Anesth Analg 2002;94:809–814.
72. Lebuffe G, Vallet B, Takala J, et al. A European, multicenter, observational study to assess the value of gastric-to-end tidal PCO_2 difference in predicting postoperative complications. Anesth Analg 2004;99:166–172.
73. Cohn SM, Crookes BA, Proctor KG. Near-infrared spectroscopy in resuscitation. J Trauma 2003;54(5 suppl):S199–S202.
74. Gentilello LM, Sanzone A, Wang L, et al. Near-infrared spectroscopy versus compartment pressure for the diagnosis of lower extremity compartmental syndrome using electromyography-determined measurements of neuromuscular function. J Trauma 2001;51:1–9.

23

Imaging of the Critically Ill Patient

Amy D. Wyrzykowski and Grace S. Rozycki

For reasons of cost-effectiveness, time savings, and, most importantly, patient safety, diagnostic and therapeutic procedures are being performed more frequently in the intensive care unit (ICU) at the patient's bedside. This development is not surprising, because the transport of patients to other areas of the hospital, the "road trip," may be associated with risks that should not be undertaken without a judicious assessment of the risk:benefit ratio of the test. Some of the adverse events that have occurred during these transports include delays in the administration of medication, equipment malfunction, malposition of the patient's endotracheal tube, and cardiopulmonary arrest.[1,2] Although the implementation of a specially trained ICU transport team has been shown to reduce these complications, there is a trend to avoid the risks altogether by doing as much imaging in the ICU as possible.[1,3,4] To that end, the following includes a discussion of the most commonly performed imaging procedures in the intensive care environment.

Chest Radiographs

The portable chest radiograph (pCXR) is one of the most common radiologic tests performed on the critically ill patient. In a recent study, it was estimated that about 12,000 pCXRs were performed annually in one academic medical center.[5] Table 23.1 lists the common indications for the performance of a portable CXR in the ICU. Frequently, the film is both ordered and interpreted by the surgeon who knows the patient's history, performs the physical examination or invasive procedure, and understands the patient's clinical picture. With this comprehensive knowledge of the patient and a systematic method for reading the film (Table 23.2), the surgeon can make rapid and accurate decisions about the patient's management.

The clinical utility and the cost-effectiveness of performing routine daily pCXRs on patients in the ICU have been questioned and, therefore, the frequency with which they should be performed has yet to be clearly established. Although some authors suggest that daily pCXRs should be performed on almost all patients in the ICU, others recommend that the decision to perform a pCXR be based on the patient's clinical picture.[5,6] The latter practice is supported by a study that showed no decrease in either length of stay or mortality of critically ill patients who had daily pCXRs.[5] In contrast, however, there are data to support that the routine performance of these films is beneficial when unanticipated pathology or the malposition of a life support device is detected and addressed before a complication ensues.[7] Figures 23.1, 23.2, and 23.3 provide examples of unanticipated findings from daily pCXRs that required intervention. Although both sides of the argument are reasonable, clinical judgment and patient acuity should be taken into consideration when deciding if a daily, routine pCXR is needed. Furthermore, as the patient's clinical condition changes, this issue should be reassessed frequently.

In addition to cost, another concern raised regarding the use of a daily pCXR is the cumulative radiation exposure to which the patient is subjected. In reality, the amount of radiation exposure with a CXR is minimal compared with other radiographic studies. Even in the most critically ill patients with prolonged ICU stays, the cumulative radiation exposure from daily pCXRs is only two to three times that of the background radiation in the United States and well within safe limits.[8,9] Regardless, it is recommended that appropriate lead shields be utilized, particularly for children and gravid patients, to protect the neck and pelvis as appropriate. Of note, so long as standard radiation precaution protocols are adhered to, it has also been documented that these studies do not pose a radiation hazard to the healthcare provider in the intensive care unit.[10]

Ultrasound

The surgeon's use of ultrasound is particularly applicable to the evaluation of critically ill patients for several reasons: (1) many patients have a depressed mental status, making it dif-

TABLE 23.1. Common Indications for pCXR in the ICU.

Indication for pCXR	*What to look for*
Change in clinical status	
Hypoxia	• Atelectasis • Poor placement of endotracheal tube • Lobar collapse • Effusion • Hemothorax • Pneumothorax • Infiltrate • Contusion • ARDS
Fever	• Infiltrate • Loculated effusion
Purulent sputum	• Infiltrate
Postprocedure monitoring	
Intubation	• Appropriate tube position
Central line placement	• Ensure tip is in SVC • Evaluate for pneumothorax
Pulmonary artery catheter (PAC)	• Ensure PAC tip is in appropriate position • Evaluate for pneumothorax
Thoracentesis	• Evaluate adequacy of procedure • Evaluate for pneumothorax
Chest tube placement	• Evaluate position of tip of tube • Evaluate position of sentinel hole • Assess resolution of pneumothorax, hemothorax, or effusion

pCXR, portable chest X-ray; PAC, pulmonary artery catheter; SVC, superior vena cava; ARDS, acute respiratory distress syndrome.

ficult to elicit pertinent signs by physical examination; (2) physical examination is further hampered by tubes, drains, and monitoring devices; (3) the clinical picture often changes, necessitating frequent reassessments; (4) transportation to other regions of the hospital is not without risk; and (5) these patients frequently develop complications, which if diagnosed and treated expediently may lessen their morbidity, length of stay in the ICU, and mortality.[11]

Both diagnostic and therapeutic ultrasound examinations can be performed by the surgeon while on rounds in the ICU. These focused examinations should be done with a specific purpose and as an extension of the physical examination, <u>not</u> as its replacement. Several retrospective studies have documented the utility of portable ultrasound examinations performed in diverse groups of critically ill patients.[12–14] In these studies, evaluation for sepsis of unknown origin, suspected gallbladder pathology, and renal dysfunction were the most common indications for the examinations. Slasky et al. reported their findings on the ultrasound evaluations of 107 patients in the ICU.[14] The sonographic results of their examinations supported the suspected diagnosis in 29 (27%) patients and excluded the initial diagnosis in 78 (73%) patients. There were no false-negative studies in this series. Additionally, 22 of the ultrasound examinations showed unsuspected abnormalities, but the management of only 5 patients was altered on the basis of these findings.

Lichtenstein and Axler performed ultrasound examinations prospectively on 150 consecutive patients admitted to the medical ICU.[13] The purpose of their study was to determine which patients had their clinical management altered as a result of routine ultrasound examinations performed within 48h of admission. Examinations of both pleural cavities, the abdomen, and the femoral veins were performed and interpreted by members of the ICU team. They found that information derived from their sonographic examinations contributed directly to a change in the management of 33 (22%) patients. There was one missed diagnosis in this series in which the ultrasound examination was initially believed to be consistent with peptic ulcer disease; however, the patient was diagnosed subsequently with and treated for renal pathology. They concluded that ultrasound examinations of critically ill patients should be performed frequently because of their diagnostic accuracy and positive effect on patient care.

Lerch et al. performed and interpreted 690 ultrasound examinations on patients admitted to a medical ICU.[12] A total of 71 patients during the study required emergency abdominal surgery. The bedside sonographic examination provided the definitive diagnosis in 18 (25%) of the 71 patients, thereby

TABLE 23.2. A Suggested Systematic Method for Reading a Chest X-Ray.

Area or part visualized	*What to look for*
Label	• Correct patient • Correct day
Penetration and position	• CXR should not be under- or overpenetrated • The symmetrical view of the clavicles is a good indicator of the patient's position.
Bones and soft tissues	• Examine all the bone fractures, including the clavicles and scapula • Examine the soft tissue for signs of subcutaneous emphysema
Tubes and lines	• Note the position of the endotracheal tube, central lines, and foreign bodies
Hemidiaphragm	• Nonvisualization of the hemidiaphragm should prompt consideration of the following: 1. Diaphragm rupture 2. Pulmonary contusion 3. Infiltrate 4. Effusion 5. Atelectasis • An abnormally high diaphragm may be indicative of: 1. A paralyzed diaphragm 2. An intraabdominal process (especially with pneumoperitoneum without recent (<7 days) abdominal surgery) • An abnormally low costophrenic angle may be indicative of a pneumothorax (deep sulcus sign)
Lung parenchyma	• Examine for: 1. Pneumothorax 2. Hemothorax/effusion 3. Infiltrate 4. Contusion 5. Atelectasis
Comparison with previous film	• Subtle changes, new lesions

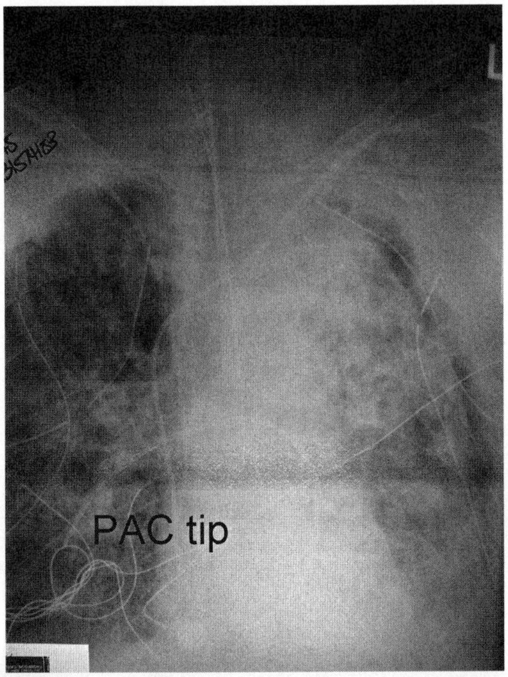

FIGURE 23.1. Pulmonary artery catheter (PAC) advanced too far. Note the position of the tip of the PAC. Attempting to wedge the PAC in this position by inflating the balloon could result in the lethal complication of pulmonary artery rupture.

obviating the need for further diagnostic studies. Operative findings at exploration confirmed the initial clinical diagnosis in all 18 cases. The authors suggested that the patients most likely to benefit from a bedside ultrasound examination are those with occult hemorrhage and sepsis of unknown origin.

In the surgical intensive care unit (SICU) at Grady Memorial Hospital, surgeons routinely perform bedside ultrasound on patients to examine for intraabdominal fluid collections, hemoperitoneum, pleural effusions, and femoral vein thrombosis, and as a guide for the cannulation of central veins in patients with difficult access.

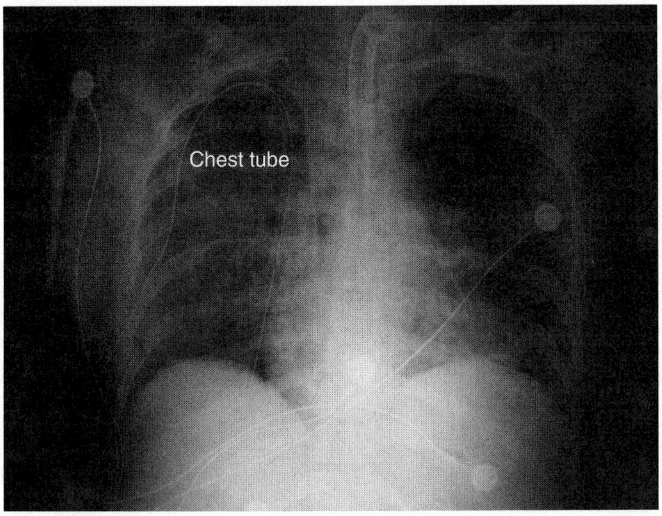

FIGURE 23.2. Inappropriately placed right thoracostomy (chest) tube.

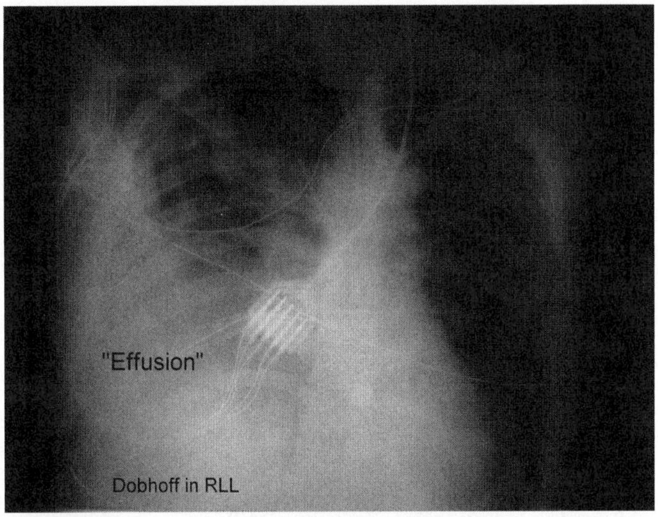

FIGURE 23.3. Film taken approximately 12h following the initiation of tube (enteral) feeding. The feeding tube labeled *Dobhoff* was placed at the bedside the previous day, and position was confirmed by auscultation. As it was believed the feeding tube was placed appropriately in the stomach, feedings were initiated. This portable chest X-ray (pCXR) taken the following morning clearly shows that the feeding tube is actually in the right lower lobe (RLL) bronchus. The *"effusion"* is actually feeding solution.

Intraperitoneal Fluid/Blood

Developed for the evaluation of injured patients, the Focused Assessment for the Sonography of Trauma (FAST) is a rapid diagnostic examination to assess patients with potential truncal injuries.[15–17] The test surveys sequentially for the presence or absence of blood in the pericardial sac and dependent abdominal regions, including the right upper quadrant, left upper quadrant, and pelvis. Ultrasound transmission gel is applied on four areas of the thoracoabdomen, and the examination is conducted in the following sequence: the pericardial area, right upper quadrant, left upper quadrant, and the pelvis (Figure 23.4) The pericardial area is visualized first so that blood within the heart can be used as a standard to set the gain and ensure that hemoperitoneum will appear anechoic.

A 3.5-MHz convex transducer is oriented for sagittal sections and positioned in the subxiphoid region to identify the heart and to examine for blood in the pericardial sac. Normal and abnormal views of the heart are shown in Figure 23.5. Occasionally, this view is unobtainable in a patient who has a narrow subxiphoid area, and a parasternal or apical view is needed.

The transducer is then placed in the right midaxillary line between the 11th and 12th ribs to identify the liver, kidney, and diaphragm. The presence or absence of fluid is sought in Morison's pouch and in the subphrenic space (Figure 23.6) Next, with the transducer positioned in the left posterior axillary line between the 10th and 11th ribs, the spleen and kidney are visualized. The presence or absence of blood is sought in between the two organs and in the subphrenic space (Figure 23.7). Finally, the transducer is directed for a transverse view and placed about 4cm superior to the symphysis pubis. It is swept inferiorly to obtain a coronal view of the

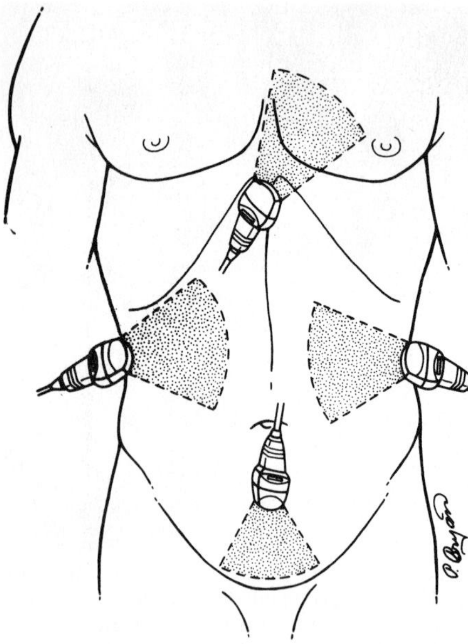

FIGURE 23.4. Transducer positions for the Focused Assessment for the Sonography of Trauma (FAST) examination of the abdomen: pericardial, right upper quadrant, left upper quadrant, and pelvis.

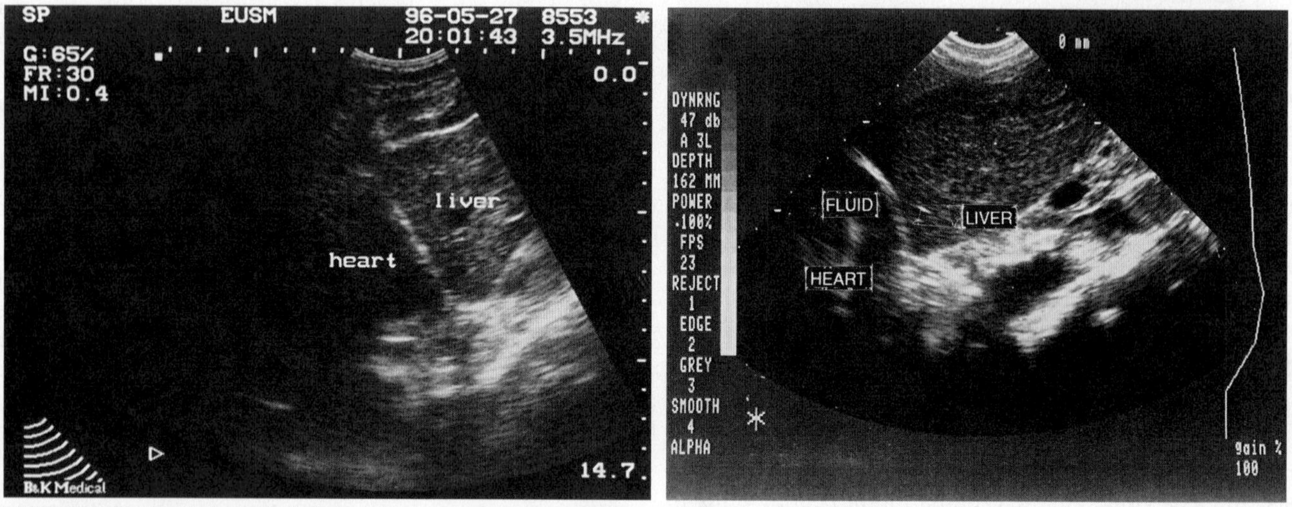

FIGURE 23.5. Pericardial view of the FAST. **A.** Normal pericardial window. Note that the heart and liver appear contiguous, separated only by the pericardium. **B.** Abnormal pericardial view with fluid appearing as an anechoic band between the heart and the pericardium.

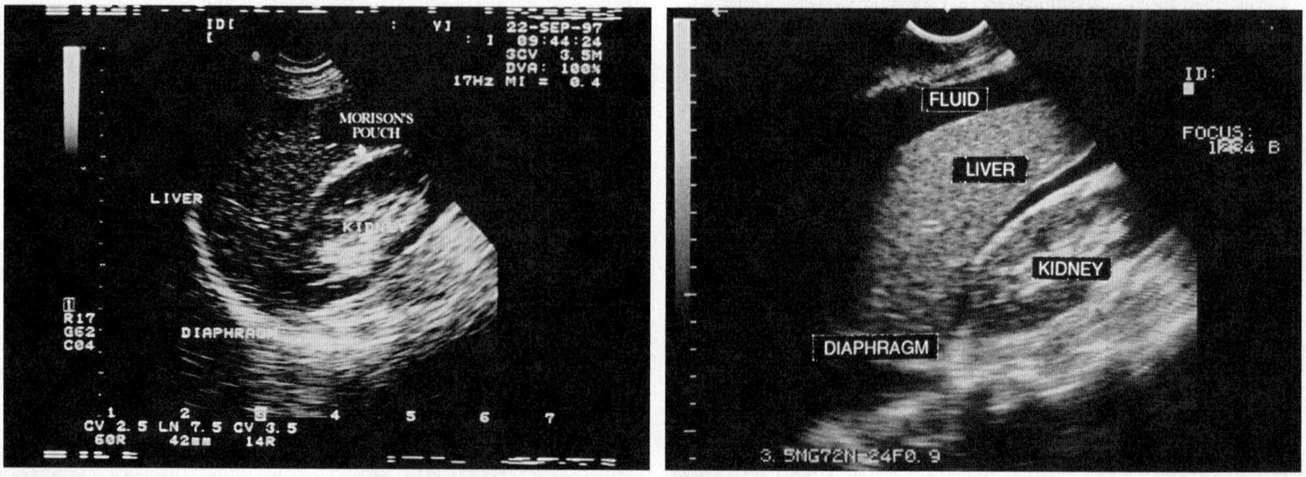

FIGURE 23.6. Right upper quadrant FAST. **A.** Normal ultrasound examination of the right upper quadrant or Morison's pouch. Note the diaphragm abuts the liver, which rests directly on the right kidney. **B.** A copious amount of fluid appears between the diaphragm and the liver as well as between the liver and the right kidney.

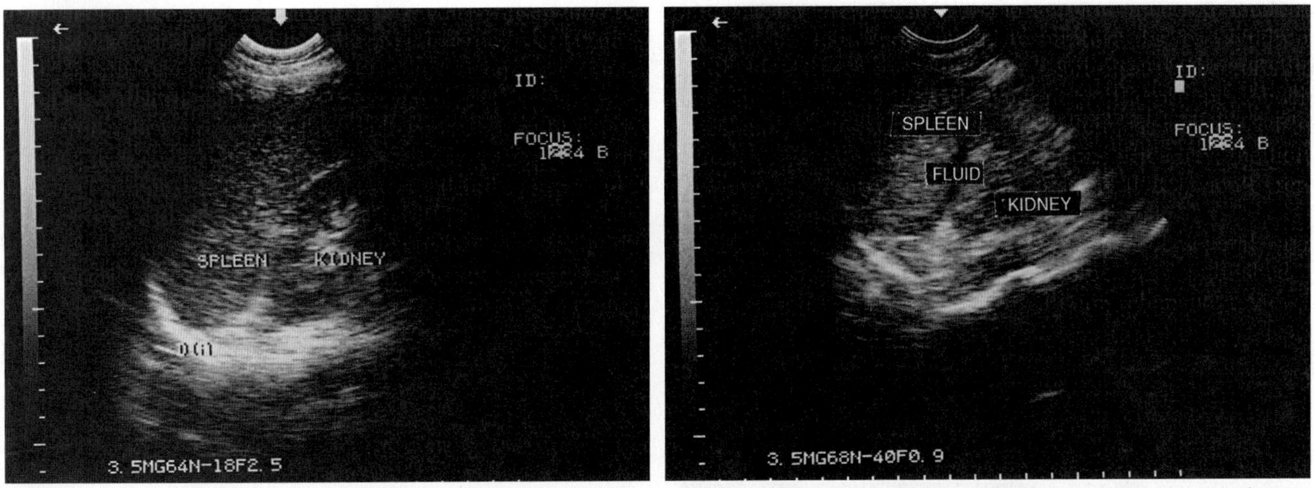

A B

FIGURE 23.7. Left upper quadrant FAST. **A.** Normal left upper quadrant FAST or splenorenal window. Note that the spleen appears to be in direct contact with the kidney. **B.** Fluid is clearly present between the spleen and kidney, making this an abnormal examination.

full bladder and the pelvis, examining for the presence or absence of blood (Figure 23.8a,b). In our experience, an indirect sign of a pelvic hematoma is elongation of the bladder, as shown in Figure 23.8c.

A sudden decrease in a patient's blood pressure or persistent metabolic acidosis despite continued resuscitation are common indications to reassess the peritoneal cavity as the source of hemorrhage. The FAST examination can be performed as needed at the patient's bedside to exclude hemoperitoneum as a potential source of hypotension. This examination may be applied to the patient with multisystem injuries or the patient receiving anticoagulant therapy. In these cases, ultrasound can detect hemoperitoneum rapidly, or, occasionally, retroperitoneal hemorrhage. Ultrasound can also be used to evaluate a patient who has ascites and to perform an ultrasound-guided aspiration of the fluid without injury to the bowel.

Technique

The ultrasound study used to detect or exclude hemoperitoneum is the FAST examination that was described earlier. Examination of the peritoneal cavity with ultrasound should be performed in a systematic fashion to ensure that abnormal findings are not missed. As described by Miner and Sly, the patient is placed in the supine position, and the right upper quadrant is imaged with the transducer oriented for longitudinal sections.[18] The gallbladder, liver, and kidney are identified with special attention focused on the subhepatic space. The mobility of the diaphragm is also confirmed as the patient breathes, and the right subdiaphragmatic region and right pleural cavity are inspected for fluid collections. The left upper quadrant is imaged in a similar fashion with the transducer oriented in the longitudinal direction. The diaphragm, spleen, and left kidney are identified, and the pleural cavity, subphrenic space, and splenorenal recess are examined for fluid. Parys et al. conducted their own study of surgeon-performed ultrasound examinations for the evaluation of patients with acute abdominal pain.[19] These studies demonstrated that surgeons can perform ultrasound examinations successfully for patients with acute abdominal pain and use the information to assist with management.

Pleural Effusions

One of the earliest reports on the use of ultrasound for the evaluation of fluid collections in the pleural space was written by Joyner et al. in 1967.[20] Gryminski et al.[21] were the first to document the superiority of ultrasound over standard radiography for the detection of pleural fluid. Using A-mode ultrasonography, they found that ultrasonography detected pleural fluid in 74 (93%) of 80 patients, whereas plain radiography detected pleural fluid in only 66 (83%) of these patients. In addition, ultrasonography established the absence of fluid in 32 (89%) of 36 patients compared to only 26 (61%) for standard X-rays. Adams and Galati used M-mode ultrasound to identify fluid in 34 of 50 patients whose physical and radiographic examinations were nondiagnostic for pleural cavity disease.[22] In this series, 30 of 34 (88%) patients had a successful ultrasound-guided thoracentesis with the aspirates ranging from 10 mL to 1 L.

Using a slight modification of the FAST and applying basic ultrasound physics principles, a focused thoracic ultrasound examination was developed that can be used for the detection of a traumatic or nontraumatic pleural effusion.[23] The ultrasound examination of the thorax is performed using a 3.5-MHz convex transducer while the patient is supine. Ultrasound transmission gel is applied to the right and left lower thoracic areas in the mid- to posterior axillary lines (Figure 23.9). The transducer is slowly advanced cephalad to interrogate the supradiaphragmatic space for the presence or absence of an effusion (Figure 23.10).

In our institution, we recently examined the utility of ultrasound in the SICU and its value in teaching physical examination to a medical student. Serial focused thoracic ultrasound examinations were performed by a surgeon-sonographer and medical student for the early detection of pleural effusions in critically ill patients.[24] Ultrasound images were

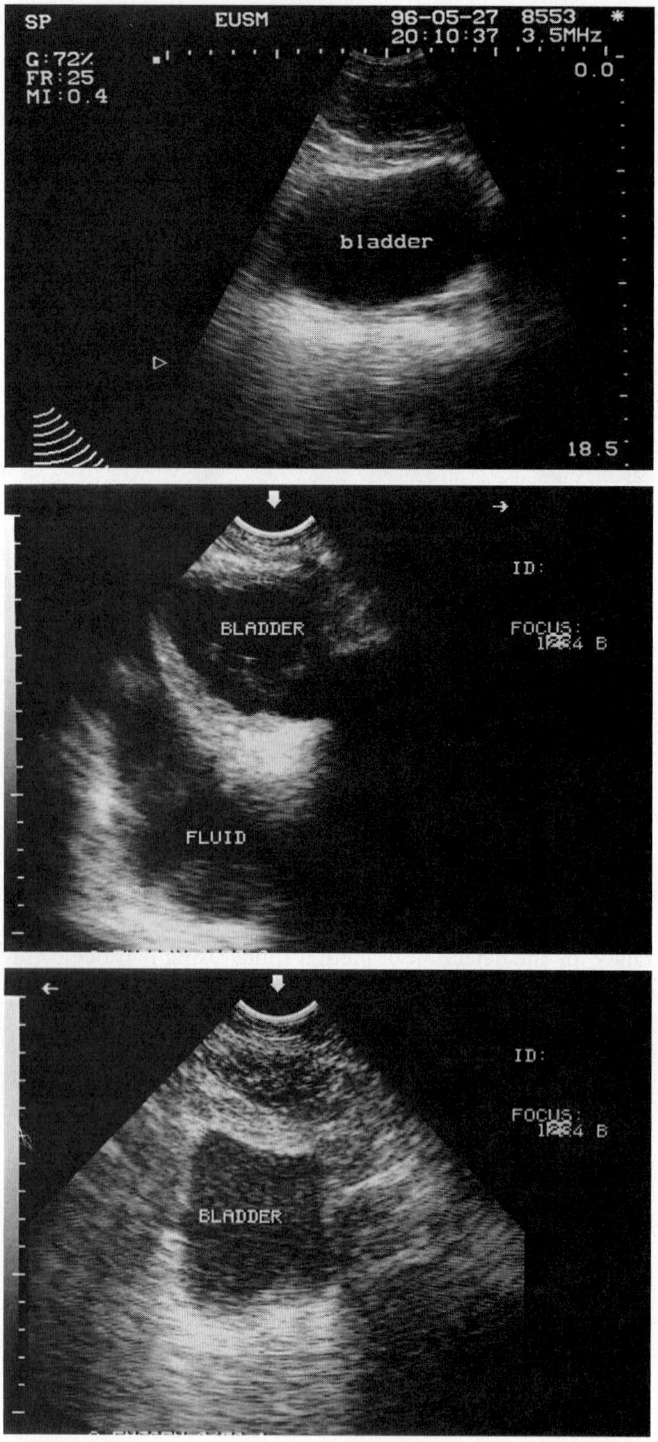

FIGURE 23.8. **A.** Normal ultrasound view of the pelvis. **B.** Fluid is seen to surround the bladder. **C.** Deformation of the normal contour of the bladder suggests the presence of a pelvic hematoma that compresses the bladder extrinsically.

recorded on hard copy and videotape and then compared with the chest X-ray readings, yielding an 83.6% sensitivity, 100% specificity, and 94% accuracy for the detection of pleural effusion with ultrasound. Based on these findings, some patients underwent an early thoracentesis or insertion of a thoracostomy tube. We concluded that a focused thoracic ultrasound examination detects pleural effusions reliably in critically ill patients and that the results can be used successfully in the decision matrix for patient care.

Technique

In the SICU at Grady Memorial Hospital, ultrasound-directed thoracentesis procedures are performed at the bedside by the Surgery/ICU Team. The head of the bed is elevated to a 45°–60° angle if the patient's spine is not injured; if spine precautions are needed, the patient is kept flat but the bed is placed in the reverse Trendelenburg position. A 3.5- or 5.0-MHz transducer is oriented for sagittal sections and placed on the chest wall in the region of the midaxillary line at the sixth or seventh intercostal region. The liver (or spleen) and diaphragm are identified. Normally, the lung is seen poorly as a result of the presence of air within the alveoli, which produces weak transmission of the ultrasound waves. In contrast, in the presence of pleural fluid, the lung can be seen moving freely with respirations during real-time imaging. After the fluid is localized, the area adjacent to the transducer is marked using a felt-tipped pen, and the chest is prepared and draped for this procedure using sterile technique. Local anesthesia is injected into the skin near the mark and extended to the underlying subcutaneous tissue and parietal pleura with a 22- or 25-gauge needle. The pleural space is entered with an 18-gauge needle obtained from a commercial central line kit and then the pleural fluid is aspirated in its entirety. For large effusions, a guidewire is passed through the needle into the pleural cavity using the Seldinger technique. A small skin incision is made around the guidewire and, if necessary, a dilator is passed just through the dermis, but not into the pleural cavity, to facilitate passage of the catheter. A standard central venous catheter is placed into the pleural space, and a three-way stopcock is connected to one of the ports so that the fluid can be aspirated entirely and collected for analysis. The catheter is removed from the pleural space while applying constant suction with a syringe, and then an occlusive

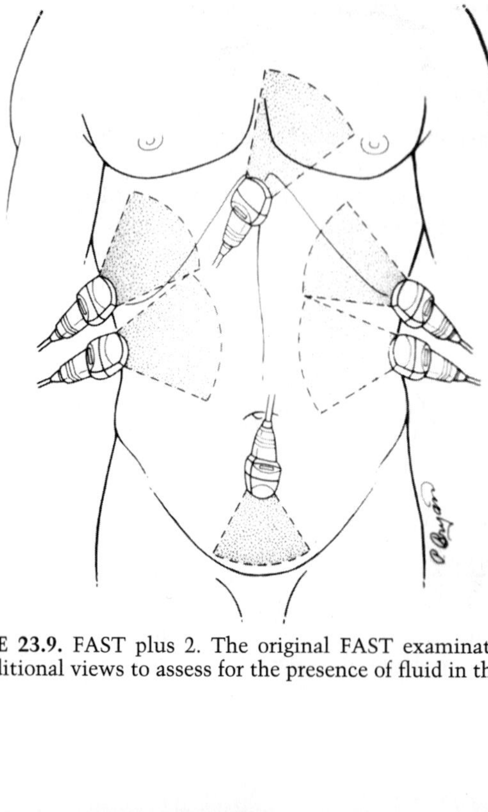

FIGURE 23.9. FAST plus 2. The original FAST examination with two additional views to assess for the presence of fluid in the pleural cavity.

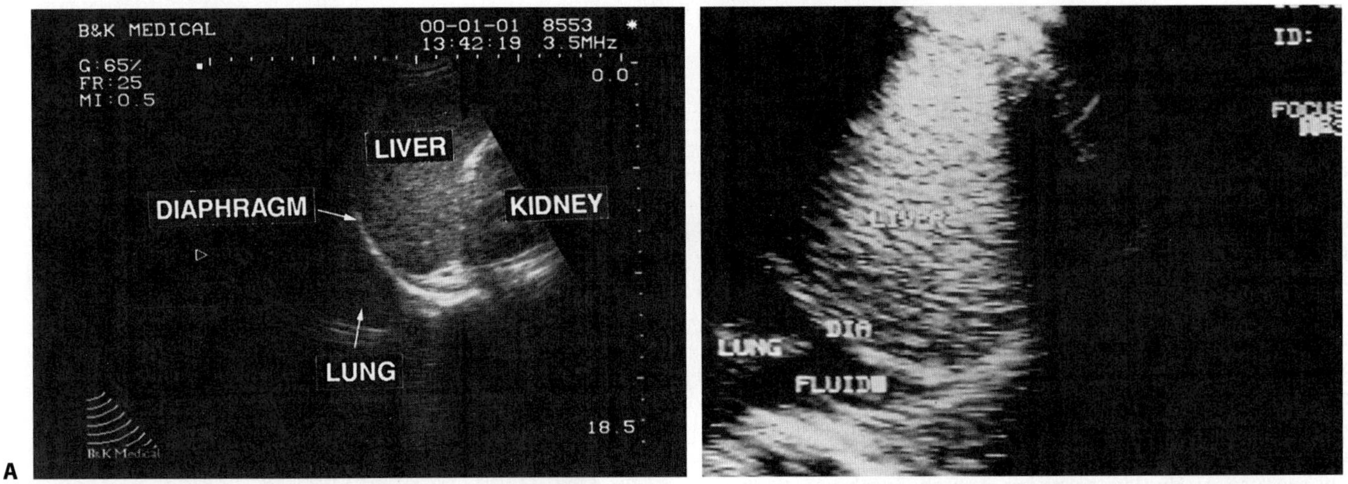

FIGURE 23.10. Ultrasound examination of the pleural cavity. **A.** Normal view of the pleural cavity on ultrasound examination. The normal lung is difficult to discern as the alveoli are filled with air, which is not a good medium for ultrasound transmission. **B.** Lung is clearly seen "floating" in fluid within the pleural cavity.

dressing is placed over the small incision. Real-time ultrasound imaging can also be used for the detection and aspiration of small or loculated fluid collections because the needle is observed as it enters the collection and collapse of the space confirms that the fluid is removed entirely.

Central Venous Catheter Insertion

Placement of a central venous catheter is a commonly performed procedure for critically ill patients. Complication rates range from 0.3% to 12% and include failure to cannulate the vessel, hemothorax, pneumothorax, dysrhythmia, venous thrombosis, and misplacement of the catheter.[25,26] As expected, adverse events occur more frequently when cannulation is performed by inexperienced physicians. In the past decade, several studies have evaluated the use of ultrasound as an aid for central venous catheter placement to reduce the incidence of complications.[26–31] Fry et al. used ultrasound guidance to obtain central venous access successfully in 52 patients who had relative contraindications to the procedure. With the exception of a single pneumothorax, no other complications were noted.[31] These studies suggest that the use of real-time audio Doppler or duplex ultrasound results in a decreased number of cannulation attempts and complications for subclavian and internal jugular venous catheter procedures. This result was especially notable when the procedures were performed by junior housestaff.[29] On the other hand, Mansfield et al. reported a large experience of 821 cannulations of the subclavian vein in a prospective, randomized trial using duplex imaging.[25] The authors found no difference in the rate of successful cannulations or complications using this localization technique. Although surgical residents are generally adept at the insertion of central venous catheters, ultrasound-guided procedures may be helpful when the resident is learning the technique initially, or when the patency of a vessel is uncertain.

Technique

The central veins in the cervical and upper thoracic region can be imaged easily with a 7.5-MHz linear transducer and an ultrasound machine that has color flow duplex and Doppler capabilities. We have found that ultrasound-guided central venous catheter insertions are especially useful in patients with anasarca or morbid obesity and for the immobilized patient with a potential cervical spine injury.

The internal jugular vein is easily visualized with ultrasound. With a 7.5-MHz transducer, the internal jugular vein and common carotid artery are identified using B-mode imaging. Although color flow duplex and Doppler imaging can be used to localize the vein, such technology is generally not necessary. The skin insertion site may be marked before creating a sterile field, or the cannulation can be performed with real-time imaging.

Cannulation of the subclavian vein is slightly more difficult because of its location beneath the clavicle and, therefore, color flow duplex and Doppler ultrasound may be beneficial in identifying the vein before cannulation. We suggest a technique similar to that described by Gualtieri et al.[29] The axillary vein and artery are identified caudal to the lateral aspect of the clavicle. Patency of the vein is determined by its ability to be compressed easily with the ultrasound transducer. The vein is then imaged about 2 to 3 cm medially to the point of the planned insertion site. The transducer should be held in the nondominant hand, and the cannulating needle is followed during real-time imaging as it traverses the soft tissue toward the vein. Once the vein is cannulated, the remainder of the procedure is completed using the standard Seldinger technique.

Common Femoral Vein Thrombosis

Important risk factors associated with deep vein thrombosis (DVT) after major trauma include head and spinal cord injuries, prolonged immobilization, pelvic fractures, major venous injury, and advanced age.[32–35] Depending on the methods of detection and the index of suspicion, the incidence of DVT varies from 4.7% to 60% in these patients.[34,36–38] Many thromboses, however, remain silent clinically or present as sudden death from a pulmonary embolism, making the actual incidence of DVT higher. Despite DVT prophylaxis with low-dose unfractionated heparin, low molecular weight heparin, and sequential pneumatic compression devices to the lower extremities, DVT still occurs in high-risk injured patients, emphasizing the inadequacy of prophylaxis alone.[33,37,39]

In our SICU, select high-risk patients receive DVT prophylaxis and a weekly screening formal duplex study. The characteristics of venous thrombosis as seen on the duplex imaging study include the following: dilation, incompressibility, echogenic material within the lumen, absent or decreased spontaneous flow, loss of phasic flow with respiration, and absent or decreased augmentation of flow with compression of the veins.[40,41] In the diagnosis of acute DVT, incompressibility and visualization of the thrombus are the major diagnostic criteria.[40,42,43] The other ultrasound characteristics of DVT, such as absent or decreased spontaneous flow, loss of phasic flow with respiration, and absent or decreased augmentation of flow with compression, are evident with the use of duplex scanning, which combines B and Doppler flow modes. Although each ultrasound characteristic of a thrombosed vein is important in making the diagnosis of DVT, loss of compressibility of a thrombus-filled vein is the most useful with the other criteria considered supportive of the diagnosis.[41,43–45]

In an effort to detect DVT as early as possible and to define further those patients who develop DVT despite prophylaxis, we developed a focused ultrasound examination of the femoral veins for the detection of intraluminal thrombus.[46] Our focused ultrasound examination is based on the following principles: (1) most lethal pulmonary emboli originate from the iliofemoral veins; (2) the common femoral artery is identified as a pulsatile vessel lateral to the common femoral vein on B-mode ultrasound, therefore providing a consistent anatomic landmark; (3) B-mode ultrasound can be used to evaluate for vein incompressibility, echogenic material (thrombus) within the lumen of the vein, and dilation of the vein; and (4) surgeons are familiar with B-mode ultrasound because it is used frequently by them to detect hemopericardium, hemoperitoneum, and pleural effusion/traumatic hemothorax in critically ill patients, hence enhancing its practical applicability in this setting.[17,23,47–50]

In addition to its role as a diagnostic modality for DVT, ultrasound is increasingly being utilized in the prevention of pulmonary embolism. Using real-time intravascular ultrasound to assess the diameter of the inferior vena cava and location of the renal veins, inferior vena cava filters can be placed at the bedside in the critically ill patient safely and accurately.[51,52] In addition to avoiding the need for transportation of the critically ill patient to the radiology suite or operating room for filter placement, the bedside ultrasound-guided procedure also eliminates the need for potentially nephrotoxic intravenous contrast.

Technique

The focused ultrasound examination of the common femoral veins is performed with the patient in the supine position as an extension of the physical examination. A 7.5-MHz transducer is used to examine the common femoral veins according to the following protocol, as described by Lensing et al.[41]

1. The transducer is oriented for transverse imaging and the right common femoral vein and artery are visualized (Figure 23.11a).

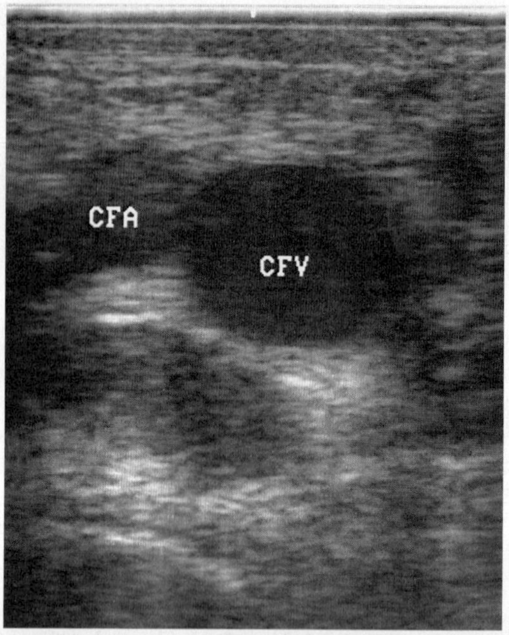

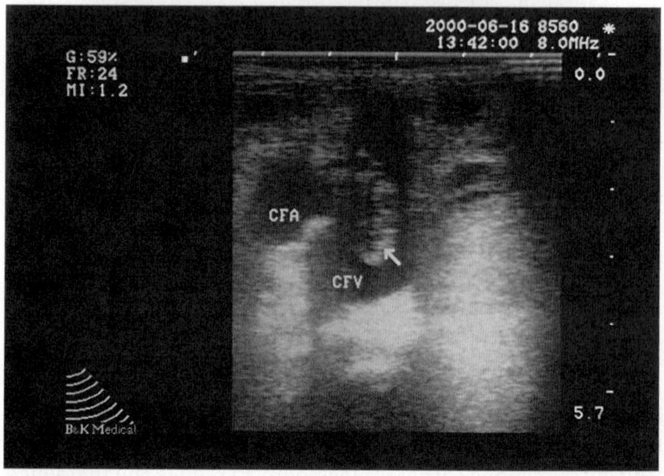

FIGURE 23.11. Ultrasound examination of the femoral vasculature. **A.** Normal transverse view of the common femoral artery (CFA) and common femoral vein (CFV). **B.** Attempt to compress the common femoral vein unmasks the presence of thrombus within the lumen of the CFV.

2. The vein is examined for the presence or absence of intraluminal echogenicity (consistent with thrombus) (Figure 23.11b) and for ease of compressibility.
3. The transducer is positioned for sagittal images and a view of the common femoral vein is identified. The vein is inspected for intraluminal thrombus and adequate compressibility. The diameter of the vein is measured just distal to the saphenofemoral junction.
4. The same examination (steps 1 through 3) is then conducted on the left lower extremity.[41,46]

A positive study is defined as dilation of the common femoral vein (more than 10% increase) when compared to the opposite extremity, incompressibility of the vein, or the presence of echogenic foci consistent with an thrombus.[53] A negative study is the presence of a normal caliber vein with good compressibility and the absence of an echogenic intraluminal thrombus.

Although this focused examination is not equivalent to the duplex imaging study, it can provide valuable clinical information as a routine screening tool or for the rapid assessment of a patient in acute distress in whom pulmonary embolism is in the differential diagnosis. For example, a 68-year-old man with a history of prostate cancer and a recent subtotal colectomy for lower gastrointestinal bleeding underwent a focused routine ultrasound screening of the common femoral veins while in the SICU. He was asymptomatic with adequate DVT prophylaxis, but a thrombus was noted in the right femoral vein on focused examination, later confirmed by duplex imaging; the patient underwent placement of an inferior vena cava filter. Another example is that of a 74-year-old man who underwent a colectomy for cancer and in the postanesthesia care unit suddenly developed cardiopulmonary collapse. The pCXR and electrocardiogram were unremarkable, but the arterial blood gas showed a markedly abnormal D[A–a]O_2. Ultrasound of the right femoral vein demonstrated a thrombus. In contrast, evaluation of the left femoral vein was normal. Such findings supported the diagnosis of a pulmonary embolism and facilitated early treatment.

Developing Portable Technologies

Portable Computed Tomography

Computed axial tomography (CT) scans have become integral in the management of the critically ill patient. CT scans are used to follow up on known injuries such as traumatic brain injury and blunt solid organ injuries that are being managed nonoperatively. These scans provide valuable diagnostic information for a wide range of maladies from sinusitis to intraabdominal abscesses to tumors. Interventions such as the drainage of abscesses, bilomas, loculated pleural effusions, and empyemas performed with CT guidance have also become invaluable. Unfortunately, it is often the most critically ill patients, patients with decompensated septic shock or worsening neurological examinations, who need CT scans, and physicians are often reticent to transport these tenuous patients even with appropriate resources.

To address these issues, portable CT scanners have been developed and are in use in a handful of centers worldwide. Although the data on portable CT scans are limited, initial reviews have been favorable, with portable CT offering a potentially safer alternative to conventional CT scan.[54–56]

Conclusion

Theoretically, any imaging modality that exists within the hospital is available to the critically ill patient in the ICU. However, the risks of road trips required to accomplish this imaging should not be underestimated in these often tenuous patients. To minimize these risks, we recommend that as much imaging as possible be conducted within the ICU, which is arguably the safest environment for the patient. To that end, the use of pCXR and ultrasound should be optimized.

References

1. Stearley HE. Patients' outcomes: intrahospital transportation and monitoring of critically ill patients by a specially trained ICU nursing staff. Am J Crit Care 1998;7(4):282–287.
2. Lovell MA, Mudaliar MY, Klienberg PL. Intrahospital transport of critically ill patients: complications and difficulties. Anaesth Intensive Care 2001;29(4):400–405.
3. Waydhas C. Intrahospital transport of critically ill patients. Crit Care 1999;3:R83–R89.
4. Warren J, Fromm R, Orr R, et al. Guidelines for the inter- and intrahospital transport of critically ill patients. Crit Care Med 2004;32:256–262.
5. Krivopal M, Shoblin O, Schwartzstein R. Utility of daily routine portable chest radiographs in mechanically ventilated patients in the medical ICU. Chest 2003;123(5):1607–1614.
6. Hall J, White S, Karrison T. Efficacy of daily routine chest radiographs in intubated, mechanically ventilated patients. Crit Care Med 1991;19:689–693.
7. Brainsky A, Fletcher R, Glick H, et al. Routine portable chest radiographs in the medical intensive care unit: effects and costs. Crit Care Med 1997;25(5):801–805.
8. Pandit-Bhalla M, Diethelm L, Espenan G. Portable chest radiographs in the intensive care units: referral patterns and estimated cumulative radiation exposures. J Thorac Imaging 2002;17:211–213.
9. Kim P, Gracias V, Maidment A, et al. Cumulative radiation dose caused by radiologic studies in critically ill trauma patients. J Trauma 2004;57:510–514.
10. Mostafa G, Sing R, McKeown R, et al. The hazard of scattered radiation in a trauma intensive care unit. Crit Care Med 2002;30(3):574–576.
11. Braxton C, Reilly P, Schwab C. The traveling intensive care unit patient: road trips. In: Schwab C, Reilly P, eds. Critical Care of the Trauma Patients. Philadelphia: Saunders, 2000:949–956.
12. Lerch M, Riehl J, Buechsel R, et al. Bedside ultrasound in decision making for emergency surgery: its role in medical intensive care patients. Am J Emerg Med 1992;10:35–38.
13. Lichtenstein D, Axler O. Intensive use of general ultrasound in the intensive care unit: prospective study of 150 consecutive patients. Intensive Care Med 1993;19:353–355.
14. Slasky B, Auerbach D, Skolnick M. Value of portable real-time ultrasound in the ICU. Crit Care Med 1983;11:160–164.
15. Rozycki G, Ochsner M, Jaffin J, et al. Prospective evaluation of surgeons' use of ultrasound in the evaluation of trauma patients. J Trauma 1993;34:516–527.
16. Rozycki G, Ochsner M, Schmidt J, et al. A prospective study of surgeon-performed ultrasound as the primary adjuvant modality for injured patient assessment. J Trauma 1995;39:492–500.
17. Rozycki G, Ballard R, Feliciano D, et al. Surgeon-performed ultrasound for the assessment of truncal injuries: lessons learned from 1,540 patients. Ann Surg 1998;228:557–567.
18. Miner N, Sly F. Fever of unknown origin. In: Sanders RC, ed. Clinical Sonography: A Practical Guide. Boston: Little, Brown, 1991:255–264.
19. Parys B, Barr H, Chantarasak N, et al. Use of ultrasound scan as a bedside diagnostic aid. Br J Surg 1987;74:611–612.
20. Joyner C Jr, Herman R, Reid J. Reflected ultrasound in the detection and localization of pleural effusion. JAMA 1967;200:399–402.
21. Gryminski J, Krakowka P, Lypacewicz G. The diagnosis of pleural effusion by ultrasonic and radiologic techniques. Chest 1976;70:33–37.
22. Adams F, Galati V. M-mode ultrasonic localization of pleural effusion. JAMA 1978;239:1761–1764.
23. Sisley A, Rozycki G, Ballard R, et al. Rapid detection of traumatic effusion using surgeon-performed ultrasound. J Trauma 1998;44:291–297.

24. Rozycki G, Pennington S. Surgeon-performed ultrasound in the critical care setting: its use as an extension of the physical examination to detect pleural effusion. J Trauma 2001,50:636–642.
25. Mansfield P, Hohn D, Fornage B, et al. Complications and failures of subclavian-vein catheterization. N Engl J Med 1994:331:1735–1738.
26. Mallory D, McGee W, Shawker T, et al. Ultrasound guidance improves the success rate of internal jugular vein cannulation: a prospective, randomized trial. Chest 1990;98:157–160.
27. Gilbert T, Seneff M, Becker R. Facilitation of internal jugular venous cannulation using an audio-guided Doppler ultrasound vascular access device: results from a prospective, dual-center, randomized, crossover clinical study. Crit Care Med 1995;23:60–65.
28. Gratz I, Ashfar M, Kidwell P, et al. Doppler guided cannulation of the internal jugular vein: a prospective, randomized trial. J Clin Monit 1994;10:185–188.
29. Gualtieri E, Deppe S, Sipperly M, et al. Subclavian venous catheterization: greater success rate for less experienced operators using ultrasound guidance. Crit Care Med 1995;23:692–697.
30. Leger D, Nugent M. Doppler localization of the internal jugular vein facilitates central venous cannulation. Anesthesiology 1984;60:481–482.
31. Fry W, Clagett G, O'Rourke P, et al. Ultrasound-guided central venous access. Arch Surg 1999;134:738–741.
32. Knudson M, Collins J, Goodman S, et al. Thromboembolism following multiple trauma. J Trauma 1992;32:2–11.
33. Knudson M, Lewis F, Clinton A, et al. Prevention of venous thromboembolism in trauma patients. J Trauma 1994;37:480–487.
34. Geerts W, Code K, Jay R, et al. A prospective study of venous thromboembolism after major trauma. N Engl J Med 1994;331:1601–1606.
35. Shackford S, Davis J, Hollingsworth-Fridlund P. Venous thromboembolism in patients with major trauma. Am J Surg 1990;159:365–369.
36. Kudsk K, Fabian T, Baum S, et al. Silent deep vein thrombosis in immobilized multiple trauma patients. Am J Surg 1989;158:515–9.
37. Burns G, Cohn S, Frumento B, et al. Prospective ultrasound evaluation of venous thrombosis in high-risk trauma patients. J Trauma 1993;35:405–408.
38. Flinn W, Sandager G, Cerullo L, et al. Duplex venous scanning for the prospective surveillance of perioperative venous thrombosis. Arch Surg 1989;124:901–905.
39. Knudson M, Morabito D, Paiement G, et al. Use of low molecular weight heparin in preventing thromboembolism in trauma patients. J Trauma 1996;41:446–459.
40. Langsfeld M, Hershey F, Thorpe L, et al. Duplex B-mode imaging for the diagnosis of deep venous thrombosis. Arch Surg 1987;122:587–591.
41. Lensing A, Prandoni P, Brandjes D, et al. Detection of deep-vein thrombosis by real-time B-mode ultrasonography. N Eng J Med 1989;320:342–345.
42. Sullivan E, Peter D, Cranley J. Real-time B-mode venous ultrasound. J Vasc Surg 1984;1:546–571.
43. Appleton P, De Jong T, Lampmann L. Deep venous thrombosis of the leg: US findings. Radiology 1987;163:743–746.
44. Polak J, Culter S, O'Leary D. Deep veins of the calf: assessment with color Doppler flow imaging. Radiology 1989;171:481–485.
45. Vogel P, Laing F, Jeffrey R Jr, et al. Deep venous thrombosis of the lower extremity: US evaluation. Radiology 1987;163:747–751.
46. Rozycki G, Tchorz K, Riehle K, et al. A prospective study of a focused surgeon-performed ultrasound examination for the detection of occult common femoral vein thrombosis in critically ill patients. Arch Surg 2004;139:275–280.
47. Wheeler H, Anderson F Jr. Can noninvasive tests be used as the basis for treatment of deep vein thrombosis? In: Bernstein E, ed. Noninvasive Diagnostic Techniques in Vascular Disease. St. Louis: Mosby, 1985:805–818.
48. Rozycki G, Feliciano D, Schmidt J, et al. The role of surgeon-performed ultrasound in patients with possible cardiac wounds. Ann Surg 1996;223:737–746.
49. Rozycki G, Feliciano D, Ochsner M, et al. The role of ultrasound in patients with possible penetrating cardiac wounds: a prospective multicenter study. J Trauma 1999;46:543–552.
50. Boulanger B, Brenneman F, McClellan B, et al. A prospective study of emergent abdominal sonography after blunt trauma. J Trauma 1995;39:325–330.
51. Ashley D, Gamblin T, McCampbell B, et al. Bedside use of vena cava filters in the intensive care unit using intravascular ultrasound to locate renal veins. J Trauma 2004;57:26–31.
52. Wellons E, Rosenthal D, Shuler F, et al. Real-time intravascular ultrasound-guided placement of a removable inferior vena cava filter. J Trauma 2004;57:20–25.
53. Effeney D, Friedman M, Goading G. Iliofemoral venous thrombosis: real-time ultrasound diagnosis, normal criteria, and clinical application. Radiology 1984;150:787–792.
54. Teichgräber U, Pinkernell J, Jürgensen J, et al. Portable computed tomography performed on the intensive care unit. Intensive Care Med 2003;29:491–495.
55. McCunn M, Mirvis S, Reynolds M, et al. Physician utilization of a portable computed tomography scanner in the intensive care unit. Crit Care Med 2000;28(12):3808–3812.
56. Maher M, Hahn P, Gervais D, et al. Portable abdominal CT: analysis of quality and clinical impact in more than 100 consecutive cases. AJR 2004;183:663–670.

24 Risk Prediction, Disease Stratification, and Outcome Description in Critical Surgical Illness

John C. Marshall

The first half of the 20th century saw a number of important advances in the ability of the surgeon to care for the critically ill or multiply injured patient. An understanding of fluid resuscitation, the development of blood transfusion, and the development of positive-pressure mechanical ventilation and hemodialysis all served to reduce the mortality for wartime trauma from close to 100% at the turn of the century to less than 5% by the time of the Vietnam War.[1] Rapid death from acute physiological insufficiency gave way to uncomplicated recovery for some; for others, it opened the door to an unprecedented series of clinical challenges—the sequelae of life-threatening physiological instability and of the deleterious consequences of the interventions employed to sustain life during a period of otherwise lethal organ system insufficiency. Known as the multiple organ dysfunction syndrome (MODS),[2] this complex disorder has emerged as the leading unsolved problem in the management of the critically ill patient.

Acute physiological instability is the antecedent of MODS, a disorder of chronic physiological instability. It is self-evident that the patients who are most likely to die during their intensive care unit (ICU) stay are those who are the sickest. A corollary of this concept is that the risk of death in critical illness can be quantified through accurate evaluation of how sick the patient is.[3] This awareness has given rise to a number of scoring systems that use measures of acute physiological severity determined early during the course of illness to estimate the probability of survival and so to provide an objective estimate of illness severity at the onset of care,[4–6] or that use measures of chronic physiological instability to describe the outcome of such care, using the construct of the MODS.[7–10]

Historical Background

Remote organ dysfunction as a consequence of, but not pathologically related to, an acute life-threatening disorder was first recognized in the first half of the 19th century, when Curling published his classic description of gastrointestinal hemorrhage in burn patients.[11] During the Second World War, syndromes of hepatic[12] and renal[13] dysfunction were recognized in the survivors of battlefield injuries. However, in the absence of technologies to support patients with life-threatening organ system insufficiency, these syndromes were uncommon and generally lethal.

Techniques for endotracheal intubation and mechanical ventilation, central venous access and monitoring, and renal dialysis were all developed in the decade following the Second World War and provided the impetus for the first dedicated ICU, established in Baltimore in 1958.[14] During the next decade, ICUs became a standard fixture in tertiary care hospitals. The evolution of the MODS parallels the development of the ICU. Acute respiratory insufficiency in association with severe peritonitis was described by Burke et al. in 1963,[15] and 4 years later, Ashbaugh and Petty defined the phenomenon as the adult (now *acute*) respiratory distress syndrome (ARDS).[16] Descriptive studies of gram-negative bacteremia[17] and the characteristic hemodynamic profile of septic shock[18] appeared during this period, and their association with a number of syndromes of acute organ insufficiency, including disseminated intravascular coagulation (DIC), acute renal failure, and stress ulceration, was recognized.

The first suggestion that the failure of several organ systems might comprise a syndrome was published in 1969,[19] followed 4 years later by a comprehensive review of sequential organ failure following repair of ruptured aneurysms.[20] Baue, in an editorial published in 1975, commented on the remarkable similarities in autopsy findings of patients dying of diverse diseases in the ICU, and suggested that multiple organ failure, rather than the isolated failure of a single system, was the most important unsolved problem in critical care.[21] His ideas opened the door to a number of investigators who proceeded to characterize the clinical course of organ failure[22,23] and to emphasize the important role played by uncontrolled infection in the pathogenesis of the syndrome.[23–25]

The MODS has gone by various names, including multiple organ failure[22] and multiple system organ failure.[23] The terminology *multiple organ dysfunction syndrome* was proposed by a consensus conference in 1991, in recognition of the fact that the syndrome is characterized by graded degrees of potentially reversible dysfunction, rather than by the absolute failure of vital organ function.[2] It is generally accepted that MODS develops in approximately 80% of all patients dying in a surgical ICU[7,26,27] and that the syndrome is the leading cause of ICU morbidity. Indeed, critically ill patients in a contemporary ICU rarely die as a direct consequence of the disease process that led to admission, but rather of a complex pattern of physiological derangements that arise from the host response to the underlying disease and its treatment in the ICU.

Defining Risk in the Intensive Care Unit

ICUs provide supportive physiological care for a heterogeneous group of patients with organ system dysfunction, rather than curative therapy for a group of patients with a particular disease. As a consequence, physiological derangements alone, rather than the distinctive manifestations of a unique disease process, provide the best measure of illness severity. Acute, preresuscitation physiological derangements are crucial early determinants of the probability of survival and the focus of scales that have been developed to predict outcome. Chronic, stable, and postresuscitation physiological abnormalities comprise the syndrome of MODS and so are the focus of organ dysfunction scales whose purpose is to measure outcome. The distinction between scores designed as predictive tools and those designed as measurement tools is subtle but important (Table 24.1).

Clinical intervention in a disease serves to increase the probability of survival (to reduce mortality) or to reduce pain and suffering and to improve the quality of life (to reduce morbidity). Measurement tools, therefore, are developed on the basis of their ability to predict mortality or to measure morbidity. Death is a relatively common outcome for patients who are ill enough to be admitted to an ICU; thus, the prediction of survival is the basis for the most widely used prognostic scoring systems, and parameters are selected and calibrated on the basis of their ability to maximize the prediction of death. Hospital mortality is generally used as the criterion against which such scales are developed, because hospital survival usually implies a return to an independent existence.

However, the role of the contemporary ICU is not simply to sustain life at any cost. Indeed, as surgeons increasingly care for sicker patients with significant underlying comorbid conditions, the therapeutic focus is shifting from mere survival to improved quality of life. And as the limitations of ICU supportive care become better understood, it is apparent that the majority of patients who die in an ICU do so not because of unsupportable organ failure, but because a conscious decision is made by the patient's family and the clinical caregivers that continued support is inappropriate and that supportive measures should be discontinued.[28] The need for objective measures of ICU quality of life, therefore, is increasing. Organ dysfunction scales represent a response to this need. They emanate from the assumption that improved quality of life within the ICU is reflected in reduced dependence on ICU technology. Although predictive scores are calibrated to hospital mortality, organ dysfunction scores are generally calibrated with reference to ICU mortality, because survival outside the ICU can be equated to survival without the need for technological intervention, even if the consequence is imminent death. Similarly, in an environment where the majority of deaths follow the withdrawal of support, death in the ICU reflects the ongoing need for physiological supportive measures.

ICUs generate volumes of data that, taken in isolation, often provide contradictory impressions of patient status. Is the patient with an elevated white blood cell count and vasopressor dependence, but relatively intact neurological function, sicker than another patient who is hemodynamically stable but unresponsive to all but painful stimuli? The calculation of a severity score allows the intensivist to evaluate the potential impact of these divergent parameters by transforming them into a single numeric result that itself is known to correlate with outcome. In essence, a score permits the physician to compare apples and oranges by converting them to fruit. However, the score does not provide the clinician with new information: it simply integrates existing information.

TABLE 24.1. Scoring Systems in the ICU: Methodological Considerations.

	Prognostic scales: severity of illness scores	*Outcome measures: organ dysfunction scales*
Uses	Prognostication; risk stratification	Outcome measurement; evaluation of clinical course over time
Timing of ascertainment	Early during ICU stay	Following resuscitation; at any time during ICU stay
Selection of variables	Physiological measures Worst values Selected to maximize predictive capability	Measures of physiology or therapeutic response Stable, representative values Selected to reflect clinical construct
Calibration	Maximize prediction	Maximize description

ICU, intensive care unit.

Scoring Systems: Methodological Principles

A scoring system relates two or more predictor variables (the independent variables) to a single outcome variable (the dependent variable). That outcome is commonly, although not necessarily, death.

Prognostic Scores

Three models for the early evaluation of illness severity in the ICU have found widespread use: the APACHE (Acute Physiology, Age, and Chronic Health Evaluation) score,[29] the SAPS (Simplified Acute Physiology Score),[30] and the MPM (Mortality Prediction Model).[31] Each of these models has undergone several revisions since its initial iteration.

Prognostic scores are developed so that their predictive capacity is optimized, which is accomplished by evaluating the ability of a panel of candidate parameters to predict mortality (or any other outcome of interest) independently using logistic regression analysis, a statistical technique that relates continuous or binary independent (predictor) parameters to a binary (yes or no) dependent (outcome) variable. Analyses are performed in a stepwise fashion to produce a model that maximizes predictive capacity; during this process, parameters that do not contribute independently to the predictive capability of the model are eliminated. The weight that each parameter contributes to the predictive model can be determined by its coefficient in the logistic regression equation; parameters are then weighted to reflect their differing predictive influence.

The performance of a predictive model is evaluated in two ways. *Discrimination* is the ability of the score to predict survival and nonsurvival correctly at differing levels of the score; it can be determined by calculating the area under a receiver operating characteristic (ROC) curve that plots sensitivity against 1—specificity (Figure 24.1). In general, values greater than 0.80 indicate good discrimination.[32] *Calibration* is the agreement between the observed and expected numbers of deaths at differing levels of the score; it is evaluated using the Hosmer–Lemeshow goodness of fit chi-square statistic. Probability values greater than 0.10 (i.e., the absence of a significant difference between groups) indicate good calibration.[33] The validity and reproducibility of the score are determined by evaluating the performance of the score in different groups of patients from the original one in which it was developed.

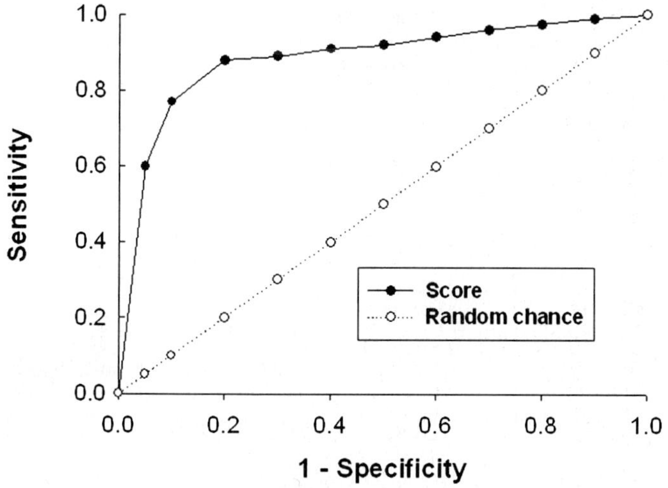

FIGURE 24.1. A receiver operating characteristic (ROC) curve plots sensitivity against 1—specificity; discrimination is evaluated as the area under the curve. (From Hanley J, McNeil B,[32] by permission of Radiology.)

Outcome Scores

A number of scales have been developed to measure the severity of organ dysfunction, including the Multiple Organ Failure score,[34] the Multiple Organ Dysfunction (MOD) score,[7] the Sequential Organ Failure Assessment (SOFA) score,[8] the Brussels score,[9] and the Logistic Organ Dysfunction (LOD) score.[10] Pediatric versions have also appeared.[35,36] The intent of these measures is not to predict an outcome but rather to describe it. Thus, although it is generally accepted that the MODS is the leading cause of death in critical illness, an organ dysfunction scale is not developed primarily on the basis of its ability to predict death, but rather on its ability to reflect organ dysfunction as the clinician sees it. Such a scale should give a low score to a patient who dies of a process other than MODS (for example, an acute myocardial infarction or an exsanguinating hemorrhage) and a high score to a patient who survives with the syndrome.

An outcome measure must be reliable, reproducible, and valid.[37] *Validity*, in turn, entails a variety of domains. *Construct validity* reflects the ability of the score to measure the outcome of interest as the clinician views it. *Content validity* reflects the ability of the score to embody the entire spectrum of the outcome of interest, whereas *criterion validity* refers to the ability of the score to measure an outcome when evaluated against an independent gold standard. For the MOD score,[7] construct validity of the variables was maximized through the use of a systematic review of previously published systems for quantifying organ dysfunction; the SOFA score[8] used a process of expert consensus. Because there is no independent biochemical measure of MODS, both scores use ICU mortality for the establishment of criterion validity.

There are, therefore, two classes of measurement tools available to the intensivist. Predictive scores integrate data available early during the course of care to provide an objective estimate of the probability that a patient will survive. They maximize predictive capacity at the cost of construct validity (the ability to mirror a process as the clinician sees it). Organ dysfunction scales combine stable physiological data to provide an objective measure of the extent of morbidity at a single point in time, or over a defined time interval: they emphasize construct validity over predictive power. The uses and limitations of these are explored next in greater detail.

Risk Prediction: Prognostic Scores

Generic Prognostic Scores

APACHE (Acute Physiology, Age, and Chronic Health Evaluation)

The first scale that measured acute severity of illness in the ICU by predicting the risk of nonsurvival using data available at the time of ICU admission was the APACHE system, developed by Knaus et al. at George Washington University[29] (Table 24.2). The APACHE score incorporates a panel of common physiological variables measured within the first 24h following ICU admission to provide a numeric estimate of illness severity that predicts the likelihood of survival to hospital discharge. The initial variables of APACHE were selected through a process of expert consensus. The 34 variables of APACHE were subsequently reduced to 12 physiological variables by eliminating those that were measured infrequently or which provided less predictive power, giving rise to the widely used APACHE II score.[4] The score yields a number between 0 and 71 that correlates in a graded fashion with the predicted risk of hospital mortality (Figure 24.2). Estimates of the risk of death are further refined using an equation that integrates the physiological data with the patient's underlying diagnosis: for a given APACHE II score, for example, the risk of death is higher for patients with a diagnosis of sepsis than for those with a diagnosis of diabetes mellitus, reflecting in part the fact that diabetes mellitus can be readily controlled with insulin.

More recently, additional variables have been incorporated into the APACHE III score.[38] The APACHE III score incorporates revised diagnostic codes and parameters that correct for potential lead time bias through consideration of the patient's location before ICU admission. However, its use is less intuitive than the APACHE II system, and the extent to which it represents an improvement in predictive power is uncertain. Moreover, unlike its predecessors, APACHE III is a proprietary system, and its additional costs and complexity have limited its acceptance outside the United States.

Simplified Acute Physiology Score

The Simplified Acute Physiology Score (SAPS) was developed in Europe and first published in 1984.[30] A revised version, SAPS II, was published in 1993.[5] The score incorporates 17

TABLE 24.2. The APACHE II Score Sheet: Use Worst Physiological Values Within First 24h of ICU Care.

	Low abnormal range					*High abnormal range*			
PHYSIOLOGICAL VARIABLE	4	3	2	1	0	1	2	3	4
Temperature (Celsius)	<30	30–31.9	32–33.9	34–35.9	36–38.4	38.5–38.9		39–40.9	>40.9
Mean arterial pressure	<50		50–69		70–109		110–129	130–159	>159
Heart rate	<40	40–54	55–69		70–109		110–139	140–179	>179
Respiratory rate (patient + ventilator)	<6		6–9	10–11	12–24	25–34		35–49	>49
Oxygenation:									
a. FIO_2 >= 0.5 record $A\text{-}aDO_2$	$AaDO_2 = (710 \times FIO_2) \times (PCO_2 \times 1.25) - PO_2$				<200		200–349	350–499	≥500
b. FIO_2 < 0.5 record only PO_2	<55	55–60		61–70	>70				
Arterial pH	<7.15	7.15–7.24	7.25–7.32		7.33–7.49	7.5–7.59		7.6–7.69	>7.69
Serum sodium (mMol/L)	<111	111–119	120–129		130–149	150–154	155–159	160–179	>179
Serum potassium (mMol/L)	<2.5		2.5–2.9	3–3.4	3.5–5.4	5.5–5.9		6–6.9	>6.9
Serum creatinine (mMol/L)* →	*Acute Renal Failure: score 2×		<53		53–129		130–169	170–304	>305
Hemoglobin (g/L)	<67		67–99		100–153	154–166	167–200		>200
White blood count (total/mm³)	<1		1–2.9		3–14.9	15–19.9	20–39.9		>39.9
Glasgow Coma Scale score (GCS)	Actual points 15 GCS *(use best GCS for postop/sedated pts)*								
Acute Physiology Score (APS)	Total points from 12 variables above =								

Chronic Health Score = ______

Score:
0—No organ insufficiency
2—Organ insufficiency + elective postop
5-Organ insufficiency + emergency postop OR nonoperative
—Organ TX

Definitions for Organ Insufficiency:
As defined below AND occurred before ICU admission:

RESP: 1. Severe COPD or restrictive lung disease i.e., Unable to climb stairs/perform household duties

Documented chronic hypoxia, hypercapnia, or systolic pulmonary pressure >40mm Hg

CVS: SOB or angina on minimal activities

LIVER: 1. Cirrhosis

Past hepatic encephalopathy or variceal bleeding

RENAL: Dialysis/ESRD
IMMUNOCOMPROMISED/Tumor:
Due to treatment: recent chemotherapy, radiation, high-dose steroids

Due to disease: e.g., leukemia, lymphoma, AIDS

Age Score = ______

Age (years)	*Score*
<45	0
45–54	2
55–64	3
65–74	5
>75	6

APACHE II Score =

APS Score + Chronic Health Score + Age Score

APACHE II Score = ______

APACHE, Acute physiology and chronic health evaluation; TX, transplantation; POSTOP, postoperative; PTS, patients; COPD, chronic obstructive pulmonary disease; ICU, intensive care unit; SOB, shortness of breath; CVS, cardiovascular system; ESRD, end-stage renal disease; AIDS, acquired immune deficiency syndrome.

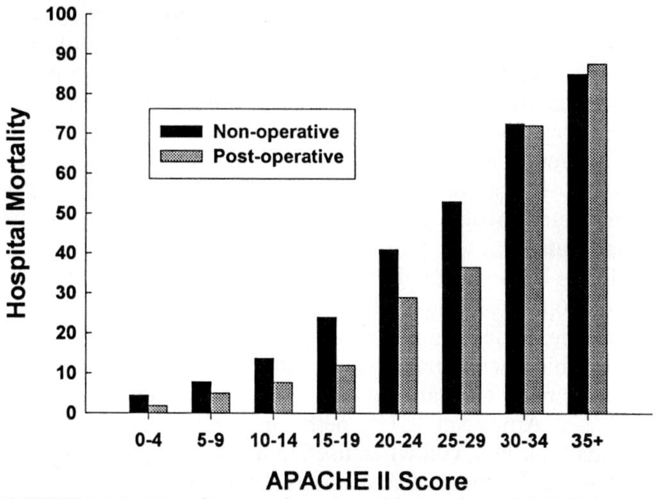

FIGURE 24.2. Mortality as a function of increasing APACHE (Acute Physiology, Age, and Chronic Health Evaluation) II score. Although mortality is slightly lower for postoperative patients at comparable score levels, for both, an APACHE II score of 25–29 is associated with approximately 50% mortality. (From Knaus et al.,[4] with permission.)

parameters: 12 physiological parameters, age, type of admission, and 3 parameters reflecting concomitant disease, specifically acquired immunodeficiency syndrome (AIDS), metastatic cancer, and hematological malignancy. Risk of mortality can be calculated independent of the patient's diagnosis, although customization for particular pathological processes such as sepsis has been reported.[39]

Mortality Prediction Model

The Mortality Prediction Model (MPM), and its updated version, MPM II,[31] employ a somewhat different approach to prognostication. Its parameters are less physiology-based than are those of APACHE and SAPS, and they are recorded as binary (yes or no) states. In contrast to APACHE and SAPS, which were developed and validated based on abnormalities present during the first 24h of ICU admission, MPM permits recalculation of the risk of mortality at 24 and 48h and so incorporates an evaluation of the response to therapy.

Sources of Error in Prognostic Scores

There are multiple potential sources of random or systematic error (bias) that may render inaccurate the estimates derived from a prognostic scale. First, the individual calculating the score must be fully versed in the basics of score calculation. Common errors in the calculation of APACHE II, for example, include assignment of maximal neurological points for the patient who returns from the operating room still anesthetized and paralyzed,[40] or the inappropriate assignment of chronic health points. Similarly, because the score records the worst value for a given parameter, a higher score is more likely to be recorded when parameters are measured more frequently. Thus, the use of an automated data collection system that records data continuously results in higher mortality predictions, with the result that the performance of an ICU with such a system appears to be better than one in which data are measured less frequently.[41] Similarly, because most scores assign a value of 0 to missing data, a score is likely to be recorded as higher when more comprehensive data collection occurs. The impact of these sources of error can be considerable.[42]

Although prognostic scores generally consider the worst values for a parameter during the first 24h of care, there is considerable variability in how this time is measured.[43] Parameters may be recorded from the flowsheets for the first ICU day and thus reflect a time interval ranging from several hours to an entire day. Data collected at the time the patient presented initially may not be available. In addition, scores may be artifactually low for patients who have received their initial resuscitation and treatment in another ward or hospital,[44,45] a phenomenon termed *lead-time bias*.

Scores developed in large heterogeneous databases may not reflect adequately the clinical prognosis of more homogeneous patient populations; the incorporation of diagnosis to generate a probability of mortality does not eliminate this problem entirely.[46–48] Similarly, regional variability in clinical approaches to care or changing practices over time may render prognostic estimates inaccurate. Mortality predictions with a given model are most reliable when the population under study reflects the population from which the model was derived. In contrast, in a specialized ICU, a preponderance of patients with a particular diagnosis may affect model performance adversely.[49]

Keeping Score: A Comparison of Prognostic Scales

Although subtle differences in performance can be demonstrated when differing scales are compared in distinct patient populations, there is no convincing evidence that any one is superior to another, and considerations of familiarity, ease of use, and specific needs generally guide the choice of a given score.[50] The performance of APACHE II and III, SAPS I and II, and MPM I and II was studied in a cohort of nearly 15,000 patients admitted to 137 ICUs in Europe and North America.[51] The performance of the newer versions of the scores was considered superior, based on larger areas under the ROC curve, and better fit; all showed good discrimination and calibration.

The APACHE II and APACHE III scores were compared in a British study.[52] The APACHE III score did not show superior performance characteristics; in fact, for surgical admissions, the risk estimations of APACHE II were superior. The APACHE III score has also been evaluated in a cohort of more than 37,000 patients from 285 American ICUs; discrimination was good (area under the ROC curve, 0.89); however the goodness of fit of the model was suboptimal, particularly for trauma patients.[53] Similarly, a European comparison of SAPS I and SAPS II showed better discrimination for SAPS II, but less than ideal calibration.[54]

Prognostic scores have also been compared to clinical judgment, with parameter results. Marks et al. found that the subjective prediction of an experienced ICU doctor and nurse was superior to APACHE II in identifying patients who were likely to die.[55] In reality, small but statistically significant differences in discrimination or calibration that are reported when scores are compared head to head in large databases are probably not meaningful clinically. A prognostic score is not a diagnostic test and cannot be used reliably to make clinical decisions regarding the management of individual patients.[56] Indeed, if a score could predict the outcome for an individual patient reliably, one would be forced to conclude that care provided following ICU admission is irrelevant to the final outcome.

Uses of Prognostic Scores

Severity scores have found a number of uses in the management of complex critically ill patients. However, it is important to emphasize two key points. First, a score does not provide new information but simply provides a method of integrating information that is already available. Second, despite the increasing sophistication of the methodologies used to develop prognostic scores, their power derives from their application across groups of patients, and they cannot, therefore, be expected to provide definitive prognostic information for an individual patient.[57]

Optimizing the Process of ICU Care

Scoring systems can provide insight into the impact of administrative measures on ICU performance. For example, analysis of the reasons that survival varied for similar predicted outcomes among different ICUs in the APACHE II database revealed that better than expected survival rates could be attributed to processes of care such as the presence of dedicated full-time intensivists and a team approach to patient care that involved both nurses and physicians.[58] Using the MPM to stratify patients, Multz et al. found that the transition of an ICU from an "open" to a "closed" unit was associated with a significant reduction in length of ICU stay, days on mechanical ventilation, and mortality.[59] An Israeli study found that hospital mortality was significantly lower for patients admitted to the ICU than for those to whom admission was denied, particularly for patients with APACHE II scores between 11 and 20, the population for which intensive care has the most to offer.[60]

Scoring systems have also been used to evaluate the acuity of illness in a unit so that appropriate staffing and resources can be provided. Similarly, variability in illness acuity has been used by regional health administrators to rationalize the distribution of critical care resources among healthcare institutions, or to provide "report cards" on quality of care in differing units.

Audit and Quality Assurance Activities

Severity scales can play an important role in quality assurance activities. Clinical outcomes that differ strikingly from predicted outcomes—either death when survival was predicted, or survival when death was predicted—can be audited for quality assurance purposes. Such an approach has proved to be superior to the performance of a random audit of cases in identifying potentially correctable problems with the delivery of care.[61] Severity scores also provide an objective basis for comparing the performance of similar types of ICUs in a given region[62] and, perhaps, for stratifying ICUs on the basis of performance characteristics.[63]

Evaluation of Regional, National, and International Differences in ICU Care

Prognostic scoring systems have been used to compare patient demographics and outcome of care between ICUs in different regions or countries. Because of the many unrecognized sources of error already discussed, the comparison of different ICUs can be misleading,[64,65] especially if data collection is not standardized and lead-time bias is not recognized.[42] Moreover, differences in case mix between ICUs can exert a significant, but unmeasured, effect on mortality prediction.[66] Nonetheless, as qualitative measures of variability in the process of providing critical care services, such comparisons can be enlightening.

It has been observed that when prognostic scores derived in one population are applied to a new and unrelated patient group, the models show good discrimination but poor calibration.[67] This discordance is least evident when the two populations are most similar. The APACHE system, developed in a cohort of American ICUs, performs well when applied in Canada[68] but less well when used in Britain,[69] Japan,[70] Brazil,[71] or Tunisia.[72] These differences may reflect differences in available resources, personnel training, or quality of care; however, the complex interplay of these factors makes it risky to attempt to draw simplistic inferences regarding ICU performance. A comparison of Canadian and American ICUs, for example, found ICU use to be more frequent in the United States and clinical acuity of illness to be lower. There was no evidence that increased ICU utilization resulted in a more favorable clinical outcome.[73]

Severity Stratification for Clinical Research

One of the most important applications of severity scores has been as an instrument in clinical research, to provide an objective measure of the severity of illness in a particular study population and to ensure that mortality risk is equally distributed among study arms at baseline. Scores can be used as an inclusion criterion to define a minimum severity of illness or as an exclusion criterion to define a maximum severity of illness. Moreover, severity scores can be used to stratify patients into differing risk groups; it is a common finding that the benefit or harm resulting from a particular study intervention is not homogeneous but may vary in subgroups with low or high severity scores. In a randomized trial comparing a liberal with a restrictive transfusion strategy in critically ill patients, the greatest benefit associated with limiting blood exposure was seen in the stratum of patients with a lower APACHE II score.[74]

Clinical Decision Making

Although severity scores are not sufficiently reliable to be used in isolation for decision making in individual patients, they can provide the clinician with objective data to support discussions of prognosis and limiting of support.[75] For a predicted mortality of 90%, the therapeutic decision reached in the management of a 24-year-old trauma victim may well differ from that made for a 78-year-old patient with disseminated malignant disease. Moreover, awareness that survival is improbable when the patient first presents for care provides some consolation to the family and caregivers when a decision is made to terminate support in the face of a failure to respond.

Quantification of risk early in the course of a disease process also allows the surgeon to implement measures that might reduce that risk. An elevated SAPS or APACHE score in a patient with acute pancreatitis identifies a patient who is likely to benefit from admission to an ICU for more intensive management,[76] whereas the risk of developing nosocomial infection in the ICU increases with increasing admission SAP scores.[77]

Implicit in the ability to prognosticate outcome for a population of patients is the recognition that the ultimate outcome is determined to an important degree by events that have occurred before the patient received medical attention and that are, therefore, not amenable to any therapeutic intervention. The magnitude of the contribution of severity of illness is unknown but may be as high as 75%.

Organ Dysfunction Scores as Outcome Measures

The severity of acute physiological derangement, independent of its cause, is the predominant determinant of survival for patients admitted to an ICU. However, the mortality of critical illness does not occur precipitously because of an inability to reverse the acute physiological abnormalities. Rather, their correction sets the stage for the development of a more chronic form of physiological derangement whose evolution mirrors both the initial injury and the consequences of resuscitation and ongoing supportive care. This process—the leading unsolved problem in acute care—has been termed MODS.[2]

A disorder characterized by the development of acute but potentially reversible physiological dysfunction involving two or more organ systems, MODS arises in the wake of a potent threat to normal homeostasis. There is considerable clinical variability in the particular systems that are involved in a given patient, in the temporal sequence in which organ dysfunction occurs, and in the severity of the syndrome. Moreover, it is uncertain whether the particular patterns of organ dysfunction that develop in an individual patient represent a single pathophysiological process with variable expression, or multiple discrete disorders with a common phenotypic presentation; that is, whether MODS denotes a disease, or a single syndrome, or simply the limited repertoire of manifestations of a common final pathway to death. Nonetheless, it is apparent that prognosis is a function of both the number of failing systems and of the degree of dysfunction within a given system.

Description of MODS as a clinically relevant process denotes more than the self-evident truism that the sickest patients are those who are most likely to die. First, the concept of MODS emphasizes the fact that morbidity and mortality in the ICU are multifactorial and that the clinician can rarely point to a single disease or event as being responsible for the patient's demise. Second, because organ dysfunction is generally supportable, and often reversible (at lesser degrees), death from the syndrome sometimes reflects a conscious decision by the ICU staff and the family of the patient to discontinue active supportive care in the face of a lack of response to therapy (or a relapse).[28] Finally, MODS almost invariably arises following the activation of a systemic inflammatory response. Just as *functio laesa*, or loss of function, is a cardinal manifestation of local inflammation, MODS is a manifestation of systemic inflammation. A number of descriptive systems have been developed to quantify the severity of MODS.[7–10,34,78,79]

The Multiple Organ Failure Score

The initial reports establishing the concept of multiple organ failure quantified its severity as the number of failing organ systems. Goris et al. were the first to extend the quantification of organ failure to consider not only the number of failing systems but also the degree of failure within each system.[34] The MOF score evaluates the dysfunction of each of seven organ systems on a scale from 0 (normal function) to 2 (failure); the maximum number of organ failure points, therefore, is 14.

The Multiple Organ Dysfunction Score

The Multiple Organ Dysfunction Score[7] evaluates organ dysfunction in six organ systems, using physiological parameters that are measured without reference to therapy (Tables 24.3, 24.4). Parameters were selected to maximize construct, content, and criterion validity. Intervals for each of the variables were established so that a score of 0 in a given system reflects normal function and an ICU mortality rate of less than 5%, whereas a score of 4 reflects markedly deranged function and an ICU mortality rate in excess of 50%; intervening values are established to reflect equal increments, with sensible cutoffs.

The MOD score employs a novel variable to quantify cardiovascular dysfunction: the pressure-adjusted heart rate (PAR). Developed by analogy to the PaO_2:F_IO_2 ratio, the PAR is calculated as the product of the heart rate (HR) and the central venous pressure (CVP) divided by the mean arterial pressure (MAP):

$$\text{Pressure-adjusted rate (PAR)} = \text{HR} \times \text{CVP/MAP}$$

In the absence of a central line, the CVP is assumed to be normal and is assigned a value of 8.

An increase in the heart rate or a decrease in blood pressure increases the value of the PAR, as does fluid administration resulting in increased right atrial pressure. The value, therefore, increases with increasing cardiovascular dysfunction, and high values reflect hemodynamic instability that is refractory to volume challenge.

Sequential Organ Failure Assessment Score

The sequential organ failure assessment (SOFA) score was developed in Europe as an alternate method of quantifying organ dysfunction.[8] It also evaluates organ dysfunction in six systems, but uses as its cardiovascular component the amcount of inotropic support provided. It differs from the MOD score in that it employs the worst daily values for its variables.

Other Organ Failure Scores

Hebert et al. reported an organ failure score that counts the number of failing organs using seven readily measured clinical variables.[78] Bernard developed a scale that is similar to the MOD and SOFA scores, differing in the parameter used to quantify cardiovascular dysfunction.[9] The originators of the SAPS score have developed a score called the Logistic Organ Dysfunction (LOD) score.[10] Differing from other organ

TABLE 24.3. Multiple Organ Dysfunction (MOD) and Sequential Organ Failure Assessment (SOFA) Scores.

Number of Points *System*	*0*	*1*	*2*	*3*	*4*
Respiratory					
PaO_2/F_IO_2	>300	226–300	151–225	76–150	≤75
PaO_2/F_IO_2	>400	301–400	201–300	101–200 (with support)	≤100 (with support)
Renal					
Creatinine (mmol/L)	≤100	101–200	201–350	351–500	>500
Creatinine or Urine output	<110	110–170	171–299	300–440; or urine output <500 mL/day	>440; or urine output <200 mL/day
Cardiovascular					
Pressure-adjusted rate[a]	≤10.0	10.1–15.0	15.1–20.0	20.1–30.0	>30.0
Use of vasoactive agents[b]	No hypotension	MAP <70 mmHg	Dopamine <5 μg	Dopamine >5 μg, or norepinephrine ≤0.1	Dopamine >15 or norepinephrine >0.1
Hematological					
Platelets (/mL × 10^{-3})	>120,000	80–120,000	50–80,000	20–50,000	<20,000
Platelets (/mL × 10^{-3})	>150,000	101–150,000	51–100,000	21–50,000	≤20,000
Hepatic					
Bilirubin (μmol/L)	≤20	21–60	61–120	121–240	>240
Bilirubin (μmol/L)	<20	21–32	33–101	102–204	>204
Neurological					
Glasgow Coma Score	15	13–14	10–12	7–9	≤6
Glasgow Coma Score	15	13–14	10–12	6–9	<6

Bold-face type represents SOFA score; no bold, the MOD score.

The worst daily value is used in the calculation of the SOFA score, a representative value (usually the first of the day) is used for the calculation of the MOD score.

[a]The pressure-adjusted rate (PAR) is the product of the heart rate and the central venous pressure, divided by the mean arterial pressure; in the absence of a central line, the CVP is imputed normal, and assigned a value of 8.

[b]Doses of adrenergic agents are given in μg/kg/min, and must have been administered for at least 1 h.

To convert bilirubin mg/dL to μmol/L, multiply by 17.1. To convert creatinine mg/dL to μmol/L, multiply by 88.4.

TABLE 24.4. Calculating the MOD Score: An Example.

A 78-year-old man is admitted to the ICU following a laparotomy and omental patch for a large perforated duodenal ulcer. He is mechanically ventilated on an F_IO_2 of 0.4; his PaO_2 is 80 mmHg. He is receiving fluids and vasopressors. His heart rate is 90 beats per minute and his blood pressure is 110/65 mmHg; the central venous pressure is 15 cm H_2O. He remains anesthetized and sedated. His creatinine is mildly elevated at 135 μmol/L, and his total bilirubin concentration is normal; the platelet count is 150,000 mm^3. He shows initial clinical improvement: Although he remains intubated, he is liberated from vasopressors by the second ICU day, and opens his eyes to voice. However, he deteriorates over the next 2 days, with worsening arterial blood gases, thrombocytopenia, and a rising bilirubin concentration. Bile leaks from the wound, and he is returned to the OR for a tube duodenostomy to control the leak. Over the next week he develops anuric renal failure requiring renal replacement therapy. A ventilator-associated pneumonia is diagnosed and treated with antibiotics. His ICU course is prolonged, but after 71 days he is discharged to the floor. Clinical data at selected time points are shown below.

ICU day	F_IO_2	PO_2	*Heart rate*	*MAP*	*CVP*	*GCS*	*Platelets*	*Creatinine*	*Bilirubin*
1	0.4	80	90	80	15	—	210,000	135	16
2	0.4	110	80	85	14	11	220,000	130	14
3	0.3	80	84	85	10	13	180,000	128	—
4	0.4	75	120	64	18	11	120,000	165	—
5	0.5	80	110	70	16	10	87,000	215	58
6	0.5	70	120	65	15	10	82,000	290	72
7	0.5	75	110	65	14	10	81,000	370	—
11	0.4	80	105	75	13	12	110,000	420	114
15	0.4	90	105	80	14	12	130,000	560	70
30	0.3	85	96	80	—	14	220,000	245	—

Day 1. His admission MOD score is 5, calculated as follows. His $PaO_2:F_IO_2$ ratio is 200 (2 points), and his PAR is 17 (90 × 15/80), also 2 points. He receives no points for his platelet count (210,000) or bilirubin (16), and 1 point for a creatinine concentration of 135. Because his GCS cannot be measured (the effects of anesthesia are still present), and because it has not previously been abnormal, he receives 0 points for this parameter.

Day 3. Consistent with early clinical improvement, his score is now 3 (1 point each for the respiratory, neurological, and renal systems).

Day 5. Worsening cardiovascular function, and evolving hematological, renal, and hepatic dysfunction combine to produce a day 5 score of 12.

Day 7. A bilirubin concentration is not recorded on this day; however, since the previous value was abnormal, this value is brought forward; his daily score is 15 on this day, the worst of his ICU stay.

Day 30. He is improving gradually; absent values for the cardiovascular and hepatic parameters are scored 0, as there is no reason to expect that they are abnormal. His aggregate MOD score is 17, calculated by summing the worst values for the respiratory system (Day 6), cardiovascular system (Day 4), CNS (Day 5), hematological system (Day 7), renal system (Day 15), and hepatic system (Day 11). His delta MOD score (aggregate – admission) is 12, reflecting two life-threatening complications that developed while he was in the ICU. Overall clinical improvement or deterioration is reflected in the change in score from one day to the next, whereas the rate of such change is reflected in serial scores observed over time (see Figure 24.5).

FIO_2, fraction of inspired oxygen; PaO_2, arterial oxygen tension; MAP, mean arterial pressure; CVP, central venous pressure; GCS, Glasgow Coma Scale; MOD, multiple organ dysfunction.

To convert bilirubin from mg/dL to μmol, multiply by 17.1.

To convert creatinine from mg/dL to μmol, multiply by 88.4.

dysfunction scores, it uses the methodology of a prognostic score to define and weight its variables, emphasizing the quantification of organ dysfunction early during the ICU stay as a predictor of subsequent outcome. Pediatric organ dysfunction scores have also been developed.[35,36]

Therapeutic Intervention Scoring System

The Therapeutic Intervention Scoring System (TISS) measures the need for ICU services and has been used widely to quantify illness severity and resource utilization over time (Table 24.5).[80] One to four points are assigned by TISS to each of a large number of common ICU interventions to create an aggregate score that reflects the intensity of care, a direct measure of nursing acuity, and an indirect measure of illness severity at a given time point which correlates well with ultimate outcome.[81] Scores generated by TISS also correlate well with aggregate ICU costs in populations of patients, although the relationship is less reliable for the individual patient.[82]

Uses of Organ Dysfunction Scores

In contrast to prognostic scores, organ dysfunction scores have found relatively limited use in contemporary ICU practice. Their potential uses are many.[83]

Quantification of Baseline Severity of Illness

Calculation of an organ dysfunction score on the day of ICU admission provides a global measure of the severity of illness, using the construct of organ dysfunction. Not surprisingly, the degree of global organ dysfunction is strongly correlated with the ultimate risk of ICU mortality.[84,85]

Evaluation of the degree of organ dysfunction present at the time of ICU admission can serve several purposes. It provides a measure of the degree of ICU support that a given patient will require and establishes a baseline measure of illness severity against which subsequent improvement or deterioration can be measured. In ICU clinical research, baseline scores provide a measure of illness severity and an estimate of the comparability of the study populations.

TABLE 24.5. The Therapeutic Intervention Scoring System.

Four points	
(a)	Cardiac arrest and/or countershock within past 48 h
	Score for 2 days after most recent cardiac arrest
	Full controlled ventilation (excluding intermittent mandatory ventilation or pressure support)
(c)	Controlled ventilation with intermittent or continuous muscle relaxants
(d)	Balloon tamponade of varices
(e)	Continuous arterial infusion
(f)	Pulmonary artery catheter
(g)	Atrial and/or ventricular pacing (includes active pacing with a chronic pacemaker)
(h)	Hemodialysis in unstable patient (first two rounds of acute dialysis or chronic dialysis in unstable patient)
(i)	Peritoneal dialysis
(j)	Induced hypothermia (to achieve core temperature less than 33°C)
(k)	Pressure-active blood infusion with blood pump or manually
(l)	G-suit (pneumatic pressure garment)
(m)	Intracranial pressure monitoring
(n)	Platelet transfusion
(o)	Intraaortic balloon assist
(p)	Emergency operative procedures (within past 24 h)
(q)	Lavage of acute gastrointestinal bleeding
(r)	Emergency endoscopy or bronchoscopy
(s)	Vasoactive drug infusion (>1 drug)
Three points	
(a)	Central intravenous parenteral nutrition
(b)	Pacemaker on standby
(c)	Chest tubes
(d)	Intermittent mandatory ventilation or pressure support ventilation
(e)	Continuous positive airways pressure (CPAP)
(f)	Concentrated K^+ infusion via central catheter
(g)	Nasotracheal or orotracheal intubation
(h)	Blind intratracheal suctioning
(i)	Complex metabolic balance (frequent intake and output)
(j)	Multiple blood gas, bleeding, and/or stat studies (>4 per shift)
(k)	Frequent infusions of blood products (>5 units/24 h)
(l)	Bolus intravenous medication (nonscheduled)
(m)	Vasoactive drug infusion (1 drug)
(n)	Continuous infusion of antiarrhythmic agents
(o)	Cardioversion for arrhythmia (not defibrillation)
(p)	Hypothermia blanket
(q)	Arterial line
(r)	Acute digoxin administration (within 48 h)
(s)	Measurement of cardiac output
(t)	Active diuresis for fluid overload or cerebral edema
(u)	Active therapy for metabolic alkalosis
(v)	Active therapy for metabolic acidosis
(w)	Emergency thora-, para-, and pericardiocentesis
(x)	Acute anticoagulation (initial 48 h)
(y)	Phlebotomy for volume overload
(z)	Administration of more than 2 intravenous antibiotics
(aa)	Therapy of seizures or metabolic encephalopathy (within 48 h of onset)
(bb)	Complicated orthopedic traction
Two points	
(a)	Central venous pressure monitoring
(b)	Two peripheral intravenous catheters
(c)	Hemodialysis (stable patient)
(d)	Fresh tracheostomy (less than 48 h)
(e)	Spontaneous respiration via endotracheal tube or tracheostomy
(f)	Enteral feedings
(g)	Replacement of excess fluid loss
(h)	Parenteral chemotherapy
(i)	Hourly neurological vital signs
(j)	Multiple dressing changes
(k)	Pitressin infusion
One point	
(a)	ECG monitoring
(b)	Hourly vital signs
(c)	One peripheral intravenous catheter
(d)	Chronic anticoagulation
(e)	Standard intake and output (every 24 h)
(f)	Stat blood tests
(g)	Intermittent scheduled intravenous medications
(h)	Routine dressing changes
(i)	Standard orthopedic traction
(j)	Tracheostomy care
(k)	Decubitus ulcer (preventive therapy)

Source: From Keene AR, Cullen DJ.,[80] by permission of *Critical Care Medicine*.

Daily Quantification of Illness Severity

Organ dysfunction scores calculated on a daily basis provide a composite picture of clinical course over time.[86] Barie and Hydo demonstrated that although surviving and nonsurviving patients admitted to a surgical ICU have comparable degrees of organ dysfunction at baseline, they can be differentiated by the second day on the basis of the resolution of organ dysfunction in survivors and its persistence in nonsurvivors[87] (Figure 24.3). Moreover, resolution of organ dysfunction, reflected in serial reduction in score values in patients with postoperative peritonitis, suggests satisfactory control, whereas prolonged elevation suggests persistence of infection.[88] Because physiological derangement implies the need for therapeutic intervention, daily scores also provide a point measure of the intensity of resource utilization, analogous to the TISS score (see following). Serial scores can be compared between two or more populations in a randomized controlled clinical trial to measure treatment effect over time: Staubach et al., for example, showed that pentoxifylline can attenuate organ dysfunction in severe sepsis.[89]

Quantification of Global Physiological Derangement: Aggregate Scores

Summing the worst daily scores for each of the component variables of an organ dysfunction score provides a composite picture of the severity of organ dysfunction over a defined time period. This time period may be the ICU stay but can also be any arbitrarily defined interval (for example, over 28 days following an experimental intervention) (Figure 24.4).

Delta MOD Scores

The difference between the aggregate score and the score recorded at the time of ICU admission provides a measure of organ dysfunction arising following ICU admission and therefore attributable to events occurring within the ICU (and potentially amenable to therapeutic intervention). Jacobs et al., for example, found that although survivors and nonsurvivors of septic shock had similar admission MOD scores, nonsurvivors had significantly higher delta scores.[90] Delta scores can be calculated over any defined time interval, such as during the administration of an experimental therapy, over the ICU stay, or over any defined time period. In addition, analysis of changes in individual organ system function has shown that mortality risk varies by system over time with the result, for example, that respiratory or hepatic dysfunction are associated only with increased mortality when they arise later during the ICU stay.[91]

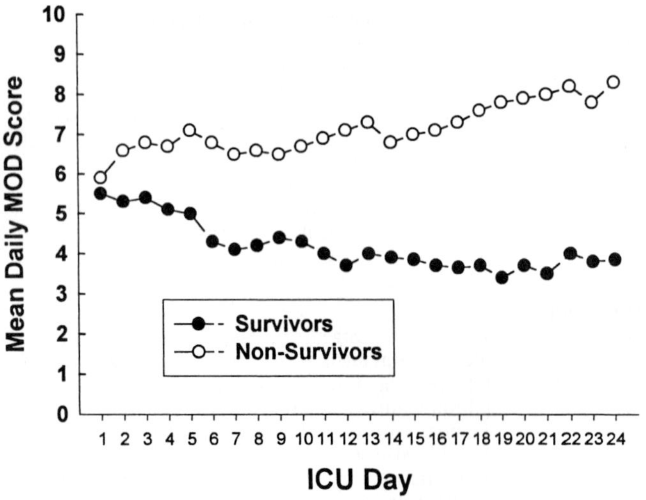

FIGURE 24.3. Daily multiple organ dysfunction (MOD) scores for 115 patients remaining in a surgical intensive care unit (ICU) for more than 3 weeks. Daily scores of nonsurvivors (*open circles*) are significantly higher than those of survivors (*closed circles*) after the first ICU day. (From Barie et al.,[87] with permission.)

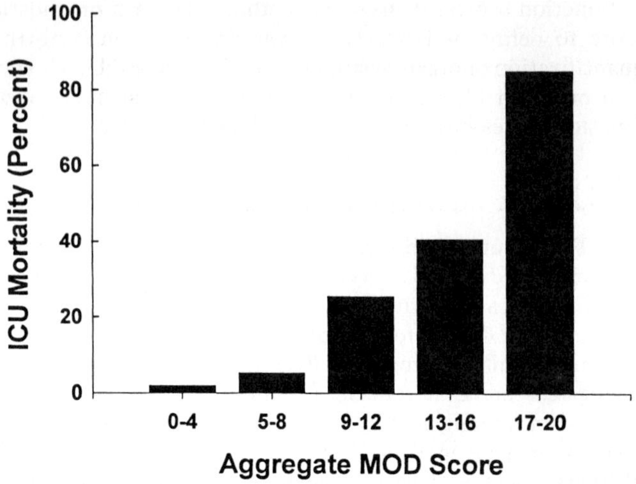

FIGURE 24.4. ICU survival as a function of the aggregate MOD score in a cohort of 851 critically ill surgical patients. (From Marshall et al.,[99] with permission.)

Mortality-Adjusted MOD Scores

A single combined measure of morbidity and mortality can be derived through the calculation of mortality-adjusted MOD scores: The aggregate score is recorded for patients who survive, whereas those who die are assigned a maximal number of points plus one. In a randomized multicenter controlled trial evaluating transfusion needs in critical illness, Hebert et al. showed significant benefit for patients who were not transfused until the hemoglobin level dropped below 7, in comparison to patients who were transfused at a threshold of 10 g/dL. Measured as mortality or organ dysfunction alone, evidence of benefit just failed to attain statistical significance; mortality-adjusted MOD scores, however, were significantly different between the two groups.[74]

From Scores to Staging Systems

Scores such as those described here provide prognostic information but are of relatively limited use in making therapeutic decisions because they stratify patients by risk of adverse outcome but not by their potential to respond to a particular therapy. Although some interventions appear to be more efficacious in certain populations stratified on the basis of acute physiological derangements or degree of organ dysfunction,[74,92] staging based on potential to respond to treatment is a relatively new concept in the ICU setting.

On the other hand, staging has been a fixture of cancer therapy for a full century,[93] and it would be unthinkable for a surgeon treating a patient with carcinoma of the colon to make a definitive decision in the absence of information regarding the clinical and pathologic stage of the tumor. Staging in oncology stratifies patients on their risk of developing recurrent disease, but even more importantly, on their potential to benefit from specific treatments. A localized colon cancer without nodal spread may be cured by surgical resection alone, whereas nodal spread identifies a population that is more likely to benefit from chemotherapy, and the presence of distant metastases shifts the treatment program toward palliation and symptom control.

By analogy to the TNM (tumor, nodes, metastasis) staging system used in oncology, a template for a staging system for critical illness has recently been proposed.[93,94] The PIRO model proposes the stratification of patients with sepsis on the basis of their Predisposition, the nature of the Insult, the Response of the patient, and the degree of Organ dysfunction present. Ample evidence exists to support the concept that each factor can individually influence both prognosis and the potential to respond to treatment. Genetic factors are potent determinants of outcome for patients with infection,[95] and genetic variability or polymorphisms in key innate immune response genes are strongly associated with the risk of mortality in sepsis,[96,97] whereas the response to therapies that target the inflammatory response (for example, corticosteroids or activated protein C) is affected by the nature of that response, whether measured as a response to corticotropin (ACTH) stimulation[98] or the degree of organ dysfunction at the time of intervention.[92] However, development of the PIRO model awaits more extensive epidemiological study.

Conclusion

Scoring systems have become a standard fixture of ICU practice because they facilitate the integration of large amounts of disparate and often contradictory clinical data into a single number that correlates with a recognizable outcome. Just as an experienced clinician relies on a clinical gestalt ("she is getting better" or "I am worried about him") to provide a context for the results of investigations, the intensivist can use the data provided by a score to interpret the status or prognosis of an individual patient, and the investigator can use these data as reliable population descriptors. But neither a gestalt nor a score can predict what will happen to the individual patient: they simply suggest a probable trajectory. So long as clinical intervention retains the capacity to alter clinical outcome, mathematically derived scores will remain a decision tool, rather than a divining rod.

References

1. Root HD. The way we were: 1989 presidential address, American Association for the surgery of trauma. J Trauma 1990;30:1309–1315.
2. Bone RC, Balk RA, Cerra FB, et al. ACCP/SCCM Consensus Conference. Definitions for sepsis and organ failure and guidelines for the use of innovative therapies in sepsis. Chest 1992;101:1644–1655.
3. Knaus WA, Wagner DP, Lynn J. Short-term mortality predictions for critically ill hospitalized adults: science and ethics. Science 1991;254:389–394.
4. Knaus WA, Draper EA, Wagner DP, Zimmerman JE. APACHE II: a severity of disease classification system. Crit Care Med 1985;13:818–829.
5. Le Gall J-R, Lemeshow S, Saulnier F. A new simplified acute physiology score (SAPS II) based on a European/North American multicenter study. JAMA 1993;270:2957–2963.
6. Lemeshow S, Klar J, Teres D, et al. Mortality probability models for patients in the intensive care unit for 48 or 72 hours: a prospective, multicenter study. Crit Care Med 1994;22:1351–1358.
7. Marshall JC, Cook DJ, Christou NV, Bernard GR, Sprung CL, Sibbald WJ. Multiple organ dysfunction score: a reliable descriptor of a complex clinical outcome. Crit Care Med 1995;23:1638–1652.
8. Vincent JL, Moreno R, Takala J, et al. The sepsis-related organ failure assessment (SOFA) score to describe organ dysfunction/failure. Intensive Care Med 1996;22:707–710.
9. Bernard G. The Brussels score. Sepsis 1997;1:43–44.
10. Le Gall JR, Klar J, Lemeshow S, et al. The logistic organ dysfunction system: a new way to assess organ dysfunction in the intensive care unit. JAMA 1996;276:802–810.
11. Curling TB. On acute ulceration of the duodenum in cases of burns. Med-Chir Tr Lond 1842;25:260–281.
12. Bywaters EGL. Anatomical changes in the liver after trauma. Clin Sci 1946;6:19.
13. Bywaters EGL, Beall O. Crush injuries with impairment of renal function. Br Med J 1941;1:427–432.
14. Safar P, DeKornfeld T, Pearson J, et al. Intensive care unit. Anesthesia 1961;16:275.
15. Burke JF, Pontoppidan H, Welch CE. High output respiratory failure: an important cause of death ascribed to peritonitis or ileus. Ann Surg 1963;158:581–595.
16. Ashbaugh DG, Bigelow DB, Petty TL, Levine BE. Acute respiratory distress in adults. Lancet 1967;2:319–323.
17. McCabe WR, Jackson GG. Gram negative bacteremia. Etiology and ecology. Arch Intern Med 1962;110:83–91.
18. Maclean LD, Mulligan WG, Mclean APH, Duff JH. Patterns of septic shock in man: a detailed study of 56 patients. Ann Surg 1967;166:543–562.
19. Skillman JJ, Bushnell LS, Goldman H, Silen W. Respiratory failure, hypotension, sepsis, and jaundice. A clinical syndrome associated with lethal hemorrhage and acute stress ulceration in the stomach. Am J Surg 1969;117:523–530.
20. Tilney NL, Bailey GL, Morgan AP. Sequential system failure after rupture of abdominal aortic aneurysms: an unsolved problem in postoperative care. Ann Surg 1973;178:117–122.
21. Baue AE. Multiple, progressive, or sequential systems failure. A syndrome of the 1970s. Arch Surg 1975;110:779–781.
22. Eiseman B, Beart R, Norton L. Multiple organ failure. Surg Gynecol Obstet 1977;144:323–326.
23. Fry DE, Pearlstein L, Fulton RL, Polk HC. Multiple system organ failure. The role of uncontrolled infection. Arch Surg 1980;115:136–140.
24. Polk HC, Shields CL. Remote organ failure: a valid sign of occult intraabdominal infection. Surgery 1977;81:310–313.
25. Bell RC, Coalson JJ, Smith JD, Johanson WG. Multiple organ system failure and infection in adult respiratory distress syndrome. Ann Intern Med 1983;99:293–298.
26. Deitch EA. Multiple organ failure. Pathophysiology and potential future therapy. Ann Surg 1992;216:117–134.
27. Beal AL, Cerra FB. Multiple organ failure syndrome in the 1990s. Systemic inflammatory response and organ dysfunction. JAMA 1994;271:226–233.
28. Cook D, Rocker G, Marshall J, et al. Withdrawal of mechanical ventilation in anticipation of death in the intensive care unit. N Engl J Med 2003;349:1123–1132.
29. Knaus WA, Zimmerman JE, Wagner DP, Draper EA, Lawrence DE. APACHE, acute physiology and chronic health evaluation:

a physiologically based classification system. Crit Care Med 1981;9:591–597.
30. Le Gall JR, Loirat P, Alperovitch A, et al. A simplified acute physiology score for ICU patients. Crit Care Med 1984;12:975–977.
31. Lemeshow S, Teres D, Klar J, Avrunin JS, Gehlbach SH, Rapoport J. Mortality probability models (MPM 11) based on an international cohort of intensive care unit patients. JAMA 1993;270:2478–2486.
32. Hanley J, McNeil B. The meaning and use of the area under a receiver operating characteristic (ROC) curve. Radiology 1982;143:29–36.
33. Lemeshow S, Hosmer DW. A review of goodness of fit statistics for use in the development of logistic regression models. Am J Epidemiol 1982;115:92–106.
34. Goris RJA, te Boekhorst TPA, Nuytinck JKS, Gimbrere JSF. Multiple organ failure. Generalized autodestructive inflammation? Arch Surg 1985;120:1109–1115.
35. Leteurtre S, Martinot A, Duhamel A, et al. Validation of the paediatric logistic organ dysfunction (PELOD) score: prospective, observational, multicentre study. Lancet 2003;362: 192–197.
36. Graciano AL, Balko JA, Rahn DS, Ahmad N, Giroir BP. The Pediatric Multiple Organ Dysfunction Score (P-MODS): development and validation of an objective scale to measure the severity of multiple organ dysfunction in critically ill children. Crit Care Med 2005;33:1484–1491.
37. Guyatt GH, Veldhuyzen van Zanten SJO, Feeney DH, Patrick DL. Measuring quality of life in clinical trials: a taxonomy and review. Can Med Assoc J 1989;140:1441–1448.
38. Knaus WA, Wagner DP, Draper EA, et al. The APACHE III prognostic system. Risk prediction of hospital mortality and critically ill hospitalized adults. Chest 1991;100:1619–1636.
39. Le Gall J-R, Lemeshow S, Leleu G, et al. Customized probability models for early severe sepsis in adult intensive care patients. JAMA 1995;273:644–650.
40. Bastos PG, Sun X, Wagner DP, Wu AW, Knaus WA. Glasgow Coma Scale score in the evaluation of outcome in the intensive care unit: findings from the acute physiology and chronic health evaluation III study. Crit Care Med 1993;21:1459–1465.
41. Bosman RJ, Oudemane van Straaten HM, Zandstra DF. The use of intensive care information systems alters outcome prediction. Intensive Care Med 1998;24:953–958.
42. Goldhill DR, Withington PS. Mortality predicted by APACHE II. The effect of changes in physiological values and post-ICU hospital mortality. Anaesthesia 1996;51:719–723.
43. Rowan K. The reliability of case mix measurement in intensive care. Curr Opin Crit Care 1996;2:209–213.
44. Dragsted L, Jorgensen J, Jensen NH, et al. Interhospital comparisons of patient outcome from intensive care: importance of lead-time bias. Crit Care Med 1989;17:418–422.
45. Escarce JJ, Kelley MA. Admission source to the medical intensive care unit predicts hospital death independent of APACHE II score. JAMA 1990;264:2389–2394.
46. Goldhill DR, Withington PS. The effect of case mix adjustment on mortality as predicted by APACHE II. Intensive Care Med 1996;22:415–419.
47. Osler TM, Rogers FB, Glance LG, Cohen M, Rutledge R, Shackford SR. Predicting survival, length of stay, and cost in the surgical intensive care unit: APACHE II versus ICISS. J Trauma 1999;45:234–238.
48. Cerra FB, Negro F, Abrams J. APACHE II score does not predict multiple organ failure or mortality in postoperative surgical patients. Arch Surg 1990;125:519–522.
49. Murphy-Filkins RL, Teres D, Lemeshow S, Hosmer DW. Effect of changing patient mix on the performance of an intensive care unit severity-of-illness model: how to distinguish a general from a specialty intensive care unit. Crit Care Med 1996;24:1968–1973.
50. Lemeshow S, Le Gall JR. Modeling the severity of illness of ICU patients. A systems update. JAMA 1994;272:1049–1055.
51. Castella X, Artigas A, Bion J, Kari A. A comparison of severity of illness scoring systems for intensive care unit patients: results of a multicenter, multinational study. The European/North American Severity Study Group. Crit Care Med 1995;23:1327–1335.
52. Beck DH, Taylor BL, Millar B, Smith GB. Prediction of outcome from intensive care: a prospective cohort study comparing Acute Physiology and Chronic Health Evaluation II and III prognostic systems in a United Kingdom intensive care unit. Crit Care Med 1997;25:9–15.
53. Zimmerman JE, Wagner DP, Draper EA, Wright L, Alzola C, Knaus WA. Evaluation of acute physiology and chronic health evaluation III predictions of hospital mortality in an independent database. Crit Care Med 1998;26:1317–1326.
54. Bertolini G, D'Amico R, Apolone G, et al. Predicting outcome in the intensive care unit using scoring systems: is new better? A comparison of SAPS and SAPS II in a cohort of 1393 patients. Med Care 1998;36:1371–1382.
55. Marks RJ, Simons RS, Blizzard RA, Browne DR. Predicting outcome in intensive therapy units: a comparison of APACHE II with subjective assessments. Intensive Care Med 1991;17: 159–163.
56. Teres D, Lemeshow S. Why severity models should be used with caution. Crit Care Clin 1994;19:93–110.
57. Lemeshow S, Klar J, Teres D. Outcome prediction for individual intensive care patients: useful, misused, or abused? Intensive Care Med 1995;21:770–776.
58. Knaus WA, Draper EA, Wagner DP, Zimmerman JE. An evaluation of outcome from intensive care in major medical centers. Ann Intern Med 1986;104:410–418.
59. Multz AS, Chalfin DB, Samson IM, et al. A "closed" medical intensive care unit (MICU) improves resource utilization when compared with an "open" MICU. Am J Respir Crit Care Med 1998;157(5 pt 1):1468–1473.
60. Sprung CL, Geber D, Eidelman LA, et al. Evaluation of triage decisions for intensive care admission. Crit Care Med 1999;27:1073–1079.
61. Mackenzie TA, Greenaway-Coates A, Djurfeldt MS, Hopman WM. Use of severity of illness to evaluate quality of care. Int J Qual Health Care 1996;8:125–130.
62. Teres D, Lemeshow S. Using severity measures to describe high performance intensive care units. Crit Care Clin 1993;9:543–554.
63. Teres D, Higgins T, Steingrub J. Defining a high-performance ICU system for the 21st century: a position paper. J Intensive Care Med 1998;13:195–205.
64. Randolph AG, Guyatt GH, Carlet J, for the Evidence Based Medicine in Critical Care Group. Understanding articles comparing outcomes among intensive care units to rate quality of care. Crit Care Med 1998;26:773–781.
65. Boyd O, Grounds RM. Physiological scoring systems and audit. Lancet 1993;341:1573–1574.
66. Rowan KM, Kerr JH, Major E, McPherson K, Short A, Vessey MP. Intensive Care Society's APACHE II study in Britain and Ireland. I: Variations in case mix of adult admissions to general intensive care units and impact on outcome. BMJ 1993;307:972–977.
67. Teres D, Pekow P. A night in Tunisia. Crit Care Med 1998;26: 812–813.
68. Wong DT, Crofts SL, Gomez M, McGuire GP, Byrick RJ. Evaluation of predictive ability of APACHE II system and hospital outcome in Canadian intensive care unit patients. Crit Care Med 1995;23:1177–1183.

69. Rowan KM, Kerr JH, Major E, McPherson K, Short A, Vessey MP. Intensive Care Society's APACHE II study in Britain and Ireland. II: Outcome comparisons of intensive care units after adjustment for case mix by the American APACHE II method. BMJ 1993;307:977–981.
70. Sirio CA, Tajimi DT, Tase C. An initial comparison of intensive care in Japan and the United States. Crit Care Med 1992;20:1207–1215.
71. Bastos PG, Sun X, Wagner DP, Knaus WA, Zimmerman JE. Application of the APACHE III prognostic system in Brazilian intensive care units: a prospective multicenter study. Intensive Care Med 1996;22:564–570.
72. Nouira S, Belghith M, Elatrous S, et al. Predictive value of severity scoring systems: comparison of four models in Tunisian adult intensive care units. Crit Care Med 1998;26:852–859.
73. Rapoport J, Teres D, Barnett R, et al. A comparison of intensive care unit utilization in Alberta and western Massachusetts. Crit Care Med 1995;23:1336–1346.
74. Hebert PC, Wells G, Blajchman MA, et al. A multicenter randomized controlled clinical trial of transfusion requirements in critical care. N Engl J Med 1999;340:409–417.
75. Halevy A. Severity of illness scales and medical futility. Curr Opin Crit Care 1999;5:173–175.
76. Nathens AB, Curtis JR, Beale RJ, et al. Management of the critically ill patient with severe acute pancreatitis. Crit Care Med 2004;32:2524–2536.
77. Girou E, Pinsard M, Auriant I, Canone M. Influence of severity of illness measured by the amplified Acute Physiology Score (SAPS) on occurrence of nosocomial infections in ICU patients. J Hosp Infect 1996;34:131–137.
78. Hebert PC, Drummond AJ, Singer J, Bernard GR, Russell JA. A simple multiple system organ failure scoring system predicts mortality of patients who have sepsis syndrome. Chest 1993;104:230–235.
79. Moore FA, Moore EE, Poggetti R, et al. Gut bacterial translocation via the portal vein: a clinical perspective with major torso trauma. J Trauma 1991;31:629–638.
80. Keene AR, Cullen DJ. Therapeutic intervention scoring system: update 1983. Crit Care Med 1983;11:1–3.
81. Cullen DJ, Ferrara LC, Briggs BA, Walker PF, Gilbert J. Survival, hospitalization charges and follow-up results in critically ill patients. N Engl J Med 1976;294:982–987.
82. Dickie H, Vedio A, Dundas R, Treacher DF, Leach RM. Relationship between TISS and ICU costs. Intensive Care Med 1998;24:1009–1017.
83. Marshall JC, Vincent JL, Guyatt G, et al. Outcome measures for clinical research in sepsis: a report of the 2nd Cambridge Colloquium of the International Sepsis Forum. Crit Care Med 2005;33:1708–1716.
84. Pettila V, Ppetilla M, Sarna S, Voutilainen P, Takkunen O. Comparison of multiple organ dysfunction scores in the prediction of hospital mortality in the critically ill. Crit Care Med 2002;30:1705–1711.
85. Peres Bota D, Melot C, Lopes Ferreira F, Nguyen Ba V, Vincent J-L. The Multiple Organ Dysfunction Score (MODS) versus the Sequential Organ Failure Assessment (SOFA) score in outcome prediction. Intensive Care Med 2002;28:1619–1624.
86. Ferreira FL, Bota DP, Bross A, Vincent J-L. Serial evaluation of the SOFA score to predict outcome in critically ill patients. JAMA 2001;286:1754–1758.
87. Barie PS, Hydo LJ. Influence of multiple organ dysfunction syndrome on duration of critical illness and hospitalization. Arch Surg 1996;131:1318–1323.
88. Paugam-Burtz C, Dupont H, Marmuse JP, et al. Daily organ-system failure for diagnosis of persistent intra-abdominal sepsis after postoperative peritonitis. Intensive Care Med 2002;28: 594–598.
89. Staubach KH, Schröder J, Stüber F, Gehrke K, Traumann E, Zabel P. Effect of pentoxifylline in severe sepsis. Results of a randomized, double-blind, placebo-controlled study. Arch Surg 1998;133:94–100.
90. Jacobs S, Zuleika M, Mphansa T. The multiple organ dysfunction score as a descriptor of patient outcome in septic shock compared with two other scoring systems. Crit Care Med 1999; 27:741–744.
91. Cook RJ, Cook DJ, Tilley J, Lee KA, Marshall JC. Multiple organ dysfunction: baseline and serial component scores. Crit Care Med 2001;29:2046–2050.
92. Bernard GR, Vincent J-L, Laterre PF, et al. Efficacy and safety of recombinant human activated protein C for severe sepsis. N Engl J Med 2001;344:699–709.
93. Marshall JC, Vincent J-L, Fink MP, et al. Measures, markers, and mediators: towards a staging system for clinical sepsis. Crit Care Med 2003;31:1560–1567.
94. Levy MM, Fink MP, Marshall JC, et al. 2001 SCCM/ESICM/ACCP/ATS/SIS International Sepsis Definitions Conference. Intensive Care Med 2003;29:530–538.
95. Sorenson TI, Nielsen GG, Andersen PK, Teasdale PW. Genetic and environmental influences on premature death in adult adoptees. N Engl J Med 1988;318:727–732.
96. Mira J-P, Cariou A, Grall F, et al. Association of *TNF2*, a TNF-α promoter polymorphism, with septic shock susceptibility and mortality. JAMA 1999;282:561–568.
97. Gibot S, Cariou A, Drouet L, Rossignol M, Ripoll L. Association between a genomic polymorphism within the CD14 locus and septic shock susceptibility and mortality rate. Crit Care Med 2002;30:969–973.
98. Annane D, Sebille V, Charpentier C, et al. Effect of treatment with low doses of hydrocortisone and fludrocortisone on mortality in patients with septic shock. JAMA 2002;288:862–871.
99. Marshall J, Foster D, McKenna C, et al. Quantification of the multiple organ dysfunction syndrome (MODS) as a risk factor, outcome descriptor, and surrogate measure of morbidity in the ICU. Crit Care Med 1996;24:A53.

25

Burns and Inhalation Injury

Roger W. Yurt

The disruption of homeostasis caused by a major burn injury provides one of the greatest challenges in clinical patient care. The loss of integrity of the skin destroys the barrier between the balanced inner environment and that of the external world, leading to loss of body temperature, fluids, proteins, and electrolytes, and at the same time allowing ingress of foreign material and invasion by microbes. However, the local tissue damage and the response to it is only the external sign of what quickly becomes a massive systemic response leading to fluid loss in uninjured tissues and dysfunction of distant tissues and organs. From a teleological perspective, the injured human being has not evolved to survive such a massive insult, and therefore it is only in recent years that advances in resuscitation, infection control, and wound care have allowed survival to the point that the full expression of the body to such an injury can be recognized. Success in caring for these patients has come in a stepwise fashion and provides demonstrable support for the value of continuing investigation and the advantages of integrated multidisciplinary care of seriously ill patients.

Evaluation of the Patient

The initial evaluation of the patient with burn injury is the same as with all victims of trauma. Initially, attention is turned to maintenance of the airway, breathing, and circulation. Although some aspects of the evaluation are specific with regard to burns, for example, inhalation injury, it should always be remembered that a burn-injured patient may have multiple system injuries. Only the aspects of evaluation that are peculiar to the burn-injured patient are emphasized in this chapter.

Extent of Burn Injury

The extent of injury sustained from tissue damage by burning is more easily quantified than in most other types of trauma. A knowledge of the surface area involved and the depth of injury assists in determining a prognosis for the patient and is used to guide fluid resuscitation and to develop a plan of care. The area of the total body surface that has been injured can be estimated in adults by using the rule of nines, which divides the surface area into sections or multiples of 9% (Figure 25.1). Although the use of this estimate is helpful in initial assessment and triage of patients, a more exact measurement should be made using a Lund & Browder chart or Berkow's formula.[1] A section taken from the patient chart used at the Burn Center of NewYork-Presbyterian Hospital (Figure 25.1) shows the distribution of surface area at several different ages. It is essential that such a chart be used when children are evaluated because the distribution of body surface area varies with age.

The determination of the depth of injury presents a greater challenge because the clinical findings are not exact except in the extremes and the wound is dynamic. A partial-thickness burn involves the outer layer of the skin and may extend into the dermis. This wound, commonly termed a second-degree burn, is characterized by blistering of the skin and is red, moist, and painful; sensation is intact. This depth of injury is further subdivided into superficial and deep partial-thickness injury. The clinical differentiation of these different depths of injury is challenging, as evidenced by the fact that even experienced burn surgeons are able to accurately determine depth of injury only 64% of the time.[2] Although some believe that the depth of injury can be assessed by identifying the fact that a pinprick is appreciated as sharp in superficial injury and as a pressure sensation in deeper injury, the only absolute way to confirm the depth of injury is by the length of time it takes these injuries to heal. A superficial partial-thickness burn should heal within 2 weeks, whereas a deep partial-thickness wound takes 3 weeks to reepithelialize. Figure 25.2 depicts a cross section of skin with indication of the various depths of injury. As shown, the superficial burn wound involves the epidermis but spares islands of epidermis that provide the source of epidermal regeneration. The deep partial-thickness injury can only resurface from residual epidermis from the organelles of the skin.

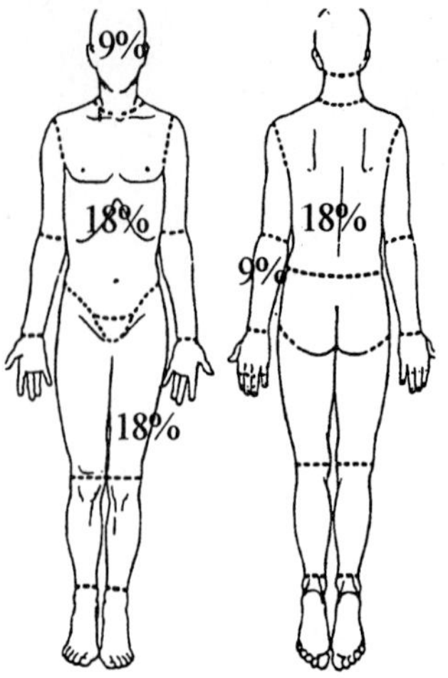

AREA	0-1 YEAR	5-9 YEARS	ADULT
Head	19	11	7
Neck	2	2	2
Ant. Trunk	13	13	13
Post. Trunk	13	13	13
R. Buttock	2 ½	2 ½	2 ½
L. Buttock	2 ½	2 ½	2 ½
Genitalia	1	1	1
R.U. Arm	4	4	4
L.U. Arm	4	4	4
R.L. Arm	3	3	3
L.L. Arm	3	3	3
R. Hand	2 ½	2 ½	2 ½
L. Hand	2 ½	2 ½	2 ½
R. Thigh	5 ½	8	9 ½
L. Thigh	5 ½	8	9 ½
R. Leg	5	5 ½	7
L. Leg	5	5 ½	7
R. Foot	3 ½	3 ½	3 ½
L. Foot	3 ½	3 ½	3 ½

FIGURE 25.1. Distribution of body surface area at different ages.

The clinical importance of differentiating the depth of injury lies in the recognition that a superficial wound heals with minimal cosmetic or functional consequence. The deep partial-thickness wound, although it will heal given enough time, results in both cosmetic deformity and disturbance of function. Skin grafting of deep partial-thickness burns will improve the outcome and is the preferred approach. Because wound care is directed by the depth of injury, numerous attempts have been made to improve diagnostic accuracy in assessing the depth of partial-thickness wounds.

More recent studies have applied laser Doppler-based techniques to evaluate wounds. Schiller et al.[3] were able to differentiate between hand burns that would heal within 15 days and those that required a mean of 42 days to heal; however, they were unable to correlate these findings with cosmetic or functional results. Other studies[4] have shown that this technique works well when low blood flow is detected but is less helpful when high flow is observed in partial-thickness burns. That this approach may be of assistance in evaluating the depth of injury is supported by studies in which measurements with a heated laser Doppler flowmeter could predict whether burn wounds would heal within 3 weeks of injury.[5]

An additional complicating factor in evaluating depth of injury is the fact that the wound evolves over a 3-day period and that external influences such as adequacy of resuscitation, exposure of the wound to noxious agents, and infection modify the progression of the wound. Thus, complications or even inexpert care may deepen the depth of injury or convert a partial-thickness burn to a full-thickness injury. Furthermore, wounds often are of mixed depth such that evaluation of discrete areas may not reflect the depth of the overall wound.

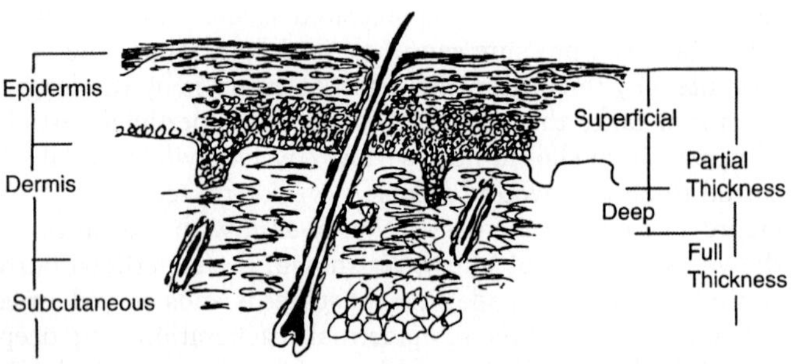

FIGURE 25.2. Cross section of skin showing tissue levels and depth of injury.

Full-thickness wounds are leathery, white or charred, dry, and insensate. Because all the epidermis is destroyed (see Figure 25.2), these wounds can heal only by migration of epidermis from the margins of the wound. During the process of healing, contraction occurs; this decreases the area that must be epithelialized but leads to a poor cosmetic result and a wound that is less resistant to trauma. Further, if the wound is adjacent to or involves a joint, the function of the joint will be impaired. Except for small surface area wounds, full-thickness wounds should be either excised and closed primarily or grafted with the patient's skin.

Types of Injury

The pathophysiology involved in the wounds of a patient with a burn injury is basically the same regardless of the cause. In the superficial area of injury, coagulative necrosis occurs. In this zone protein is denatured irreversibly and cellular integrity is lost.[6] Adjacent to this zone is the zone of stasis in which tissue is viable but subject to further necrosis as the wound evolves. A third zone has been recognized below the zone of stasis and is characterized as a zone of hyperemia. The zones of stasis and hyperemia are the areas where the inflammatory response of the patient is initiated.

The depth of the coagulative necrosis that occurs in burns that are caused by scalding, flame, or contact with a hot object is related directly to the temperature, duration of exposure, thickness of the tissue, and state of the blood supply in the tissue. For example, with the same temperature and duration of exposure, wounds on the inner aspect of the arm or thigh will be deeper than wounds on the lateral aspect. Injury of the back or sole of the foot is less likely to be deep because the epidermis is thicker in those areas. The skin of the face is more protected than other areas because the rich blood supply dissipates heat and provides for rapid recovery of injured tissues.

TABLE 25.1. Common Agents that Cause Burn Injury to the Skin by Category.

Agent	*Site of injury*	*Treatment*
Acids		
Hydrochloric nitric, sulfuric	Superficial	Irrigate with water
Hydrofluoric	Deep	Initial irrigation with water, then calcium gluconate
Phenol	Deep	Irrigate with 50:50 water and polyethylene glycol
Alkali		
Ammonia, sodium hydroxide	Deep	Irrigate with water
Cement	Superficial	Irrigate with water
Tar	Superficial/deep	Cool, then Vaseline

Chemical burns cause denaturation of protein and disruption of cellular integrity. The degree of injury is dependent on the time of exposure, the strength of the agent, and the solubility of the agent in tissue. Alkali tends to penetrate deeper into tissues than does an acid. One exception to this is hydrofluoric acid, which penetrates lipid membranes readily. Table 25.1 provides a list of common agents that cause burn injury.[7]

The major concern in evaluating patients who sustain electrical injuries is that the surface injury, which may appear similar to other burn injuries, is often not indicative of the extent of injury. In the local area of injury subcutaneous tissue, muscle, and bone may be injured. Electrical current follows the path of least resistance and therefore will pass through nerves and blood vessels preferentially[8] and cause injury to these tissues. If the current passes through the torso of the patient, organ injury may result. Injury of the heart is primarily associated with arrhythmia.[9] Injury of other viscera including the pancreas and gastrointestinal tract has been reported.[11] Late sequelae of electrical injury include the development of cataracts and transverse myelitis of the spinal cord. These sequelae have been reported to occur months or even years after electrical injury.[11]

Injury caused by exposure to ionizing radiation may be limited to the skin but often is deeper. Because these wounds do not heal well, care must be taken to avoid additional damage of the tissue. The vasculitis that is associated with these injuries is usually a lifelong problem.[12]

Inhalation Injury

Inhalation injury is often attributed inappropriately to heat-related damage to the airway or lung. Thermal injury to the airway is rare because the upper airway can dissipate heat effectively, but upper airway injury may occasionally be associated with a direct inhalation of superheated steam.[13] The majority of injuries to the lung are caused by inhalation of toxic chemical products of combustion. The deleterious components of smoke are primarily aldehydes.[14] In addition, carbon monoxide and cyanide may be inhaled. Similar to a chemical burn of the skin, these agents cause erythema and edema of the airway and can lead to blistering, ulceration, erosions, and sloughing of airway mucosa, possibly resulting in airway obstruction. The local edema, infiltration of the tissue with polymorphonuclear leukocytes, and sloughing of bronchial mucosa lead to the formation of an endobronchial cast and obstruction of terminal bronchioles. Pulmonary edema occurs from damage to the alveolar-capillary membrane, microvascular injury, and increased pulmonary lymph flow and microvascular permeability.[15] The debris in the airway cannot be cleared because injury to the mucosa disrupts airway host defenses, including mucociliary transport. Small airway obstruction and accumulation of carbonaceous material and necrotic debris, and impaired local host defenses provide a fertile ground for the development of infection. Some authors have reported that the incidence of pneumonia in these patients is as high as 70%[16] within a week of injury.

Because the diagnosis of inhalation injury is difficult to make, a presumptive diagnosis is made based on a history that is consistent and signs and symptoms that are associated with injury to the airway. Any patient who sustains injury in a closed space and has burns above the clavicle, singeing of nasal vibrissae, hoarseness, or carbonaceous sputum should be assumed to have sustained an inhalation injury. Elevated carboxyhemoglobin concentrations confirm exposure to carbon monoxide but are not diagnostic for lung injury. Because the primary concern early after inhalation injury is airway obstruction, the upper airway should be evaluated immediately, usually in the emergency department. Flexible bronchoscopy provides the opportunity to confirm the diagnosis and initiate therapy. An endotracheal tube is passed over the bronchoscope before the endoscopy, and if injury is identified in the airway the tube is passed over the scope into the trachea.

Injury to the parenchyma of the lung is subtle in presentation in the early period after injury except in the most severe injuries such as those found in patients who sustained cardiac or respiratory arrest in the field. Findings on chest X-ray, arterial blood gases, and physical examination are frequently not helpful in the first 48 to 72h post injury.[17] Xenon ventilation/perfusion scans are of value in detecting parenchymal injury to the lung; however, the extent of injury cannot be determined with this test. The results of multiple evaluations with pulmonary function testing and xenon scanning improve diagnostic accuracy.[18] Nevertheless, because the therapy for lung injury is not specific and the injury is not quantified by testing, most patients are treated presumptively. Therapy consists of aggressive pulmonary toilet, use of mucolytics, and early identification and treatment of infection. Prophylaxis with antibiotics is not used, and glucocorticoids are of no benefit and are potentially harmful.[19]

Table 25.2 provides evidence for management of inhalation injury. The practice guidelines for burn care, developed by the American Burn Association, indicate that there are insufficient data to support a standard treatment guideline.[20]

Decision to Transfer to Specialized Care

The resources required to care for patients with major burn injury are not available at many medical centers. For this reason, a regionalized system for care of the burn-injured patient has been developed. Although travel time and distance to a burn center are of concern, transfer of burn-injured patients after initial evaluation has been shown to be safe especially if initiated early after injury.[21] Patients with burns over more than 30% of their body surface area, those at the

TABLE 25.2.
Management of Inhalation Injury.

Trial	*Year*	*Class of evidence*	*Groups*	*Intervention/design*	*Comments*
19	1978	II	Steroids/gentamicin	Prospective	No benefit with either
20	1982	III	± Steroids	Two cohorts	No difference in outcome
21	1991	III	Volumetric Diffusive Respiration	Prospective	Outcome improved
22	1995	III	Permissive Hypercarbia	Prospective (historical control)	Decreased mortality

extremes of age, with injury of crucial body parts such as genitalia, and those with substantial preexisting disease should be cared for in a burn center. Specific guidelines have been published by the American Burn Association.[22]

Resuscitation

General Principles

Because intravascular fluid loss begins to occur immediately after burn injury, initial resuscitative efforts are oriented toward volume replacement. If transport of the patient to an emergency care facility can be accomplished within 30min of injury, intravenous access can be delayed until arrival at the receiving institution. Peripheral venous cannulation is preferred over central venous access and may be performed through burn-injured tissue if access through noninjured sites is not available. Patients with greater than 20% total body surface area (TBSA) injury (15% in children) require intravenous fluid resuscitation and should have a urinary bladder catheter placed. In addition, patients who have sustained a major injury should have a nasogastric tube placed to decompress the dilated stomach. During transport and resuscitation, every effort should be made to maintain body temperature. Patients are wrapped in clean sheets or blankets and the room is warmed in the initial phase in the emergency care area. Recirculating forced-air warming blankets are also of use. Resuscitation fluids should be warmed when fluids are given at rates of greater than 200mL/h. Burn-injured extremities should be elevated above the level of the heart.

Fluid Resuscitation

During the first 24h after injury, there is fluid loss into and through the burn injury. In addition, there is a shift of intravascular fluid into noninjured tissues. There is general agreement that during this period crystalloid solutions should be used.[23–25] As the fluid losses are large, formulae have been developed to provide an estimate of the fluid requirements. Every guideline that has been developed carries with it the mandate that the patient's response to resuscitation be used as the actual determinant of fluid administration, not the formula! The goal of resuscitation is to maintain adequate tissue perfusion and therefore preserve organ function. The traditional assessment of adequacy of resuscitation in burn injury has been based on observation of blood pressure, heart rate, and urine output.[26] In this approach the patient is "titrated" with fluid to maintain a normal blood pressure and heart rate and a urine output of 1mL/kg/h or 30 to 50mL/h in an adult patient. That this is the best method to resuscitate these patients has been challenged by reports suggesting that hyperdynamic resuscitation[27] yields improved outcome. Furthermore, controversy has arisen regarding the best endpoint to use in assessing adequacy of resuscitation from shock in general (reviewed by Elliott[28]). Elliot reports that a variety of studies of resuscitation from shock suggests that mean arterial pressure should be maintained at 60mmHg and that measurement of blood lactate concentrations may be a useful adjunct in assessing response to resuscitation.

The Parkland formula[29] is the crystalloid-based formula that provided the foundation for current methods of resuscitation. This formula calls for the initiation of resuscitation with Ringer's lactate solution at a rate based on the TBSA of burn

TABLE 25.3. Fluid Resuscitation in Patients with Thermal Injury.

Regimen	*Fluid required* *% of Parkland*	 *mL/kg/% burn*	*Serum Sodium*	*Weight gain*[a] *(%)*	*Reference*
Hypertonic	75		141.6[b]	7.3	36
Hypertonic + colloid	57		143.8	7.3	36
Ringer's lactate		4.8		13.9	37
Hypertonic		3.16		11.99	37
Fresh-frozen plasma		2.68		4.37	37
Ringer's lactate		5.3	135[c]		35
Hypertonic		3.9	153[c]		35

[a]At 48h compared to initial.
[b]Mean value, first 24h. [c]At 3 days after injury.

TABLE 25.4.
Burn Shock Resuscitation.

Trial	*Year*	*Class of Evidence*	*Intervention/Design*	*Minor*	*Major*	*Comments*
37	1981	II	Retrospective		Resuscitation	4 mL/kg/% burn
38	1981	III			Resuscitation	2 mL/kg/% burn
39	1985	III	Retrospective	Inhalation injury	Resuscitation	3.9 mL/kg/% burn 5.7 mL/kg/% burn
40	2003	II	Prospective	Fluid required	Base deficit	Greater deficit = 8.5 mL/kg/% burn Lesser deficit = 6.3 mL/kg/% burn
41	2000	III	Retrospective		Fluid required	58% required >4.3 mL/kg/% burn
36	2001	III	Review		Fluid required	No standard, most 2–4 mL/kg/% burn

injury and the patient's body mass. The calculated resuscitation volume for the first 24 h is 4 mL times mass in kilograms times the percent of the TBSA that is burned. One-half of this volume is given in the first 8 h after injury and the other half is given in the following 16 h. Resuscitation of children is based on this volume plus a volume equal to the estimated daily maintenance fluid requirements. Graves et al.,[30] at the U.S. Army Institute of Surgical Research, suggested that the same success can be obtained by using a formula that estimates requirements as 3 mL/kg per percent of the TBSA that is burned. To minimize the volume of fluid used during resuscitation, Monafo et al.[31] recommended the use of higher concentrations of sodium in the resuscitation fluid. Others have not had success with hypertonic saline resuscitation regimens and in fact have reported higher complication and mortality rates compared to historical controls who were resuscitated with Ringer's lactate solution.[32] A comparison of various regimens of fluid resuscitation (Table 25.3) indicates that various regimens lead to differences in weight gain and serum sodium concentration. Evidence is not sufficient to develop a guideline at this time.[33] The current evidence, summarized in Table 25.4, supports a crystalloid-based regimen in the range of 2–4 mL/kg/% burn in the first 24 h. However, it should be noted that more recent data indicate that patients who have sustained inhalation injury and all patients in general are receiving more than estimated needs. Delay in the initiation of resuscitation may result in higher than anticipated fluid requirements.

Most authors continue to suggest that administration of colloid-containing solutions be reserved for the second 24 h after injury when the capillary leak is assumed to have resolved. Thereafter, daily maintenance fluids are given with a recognition of ongoing evaporative losses and the knowledge that total body sodium content is high. Evaporative fluid loss from the burn-injured tissue has been estimated to occur at an hourly rate equal to the sum of 25 and the percent of the TBSA that is injured multiplied by the TBSA.

Wound Care

General Principles

Small (2-cm diameter or less) blisters are often left intact whereas larger blisters and full-thickness wounds should be debrided and covered with a topical agent. Inpatient wound care is provided in a warm environment at the bedside or more often in an area reserved for wound care in a burn center. The objective of wound care is to avoid infection and protect the wound from further injury. Agents that may cause additional tissue damage are avoided, and the perfusion of the wound is protected by avoiding hypotension and excluding the use of alpha-adrenergic agents (e.g., norepinephrine, phenylephrine), which will lead to additional tissue ischemia. Sterile gloves should be worn at all times when a wound is manipulated. Chemical injury of tissue is treated with irrigation with copious amounts of either normal saline or tap water for as long as 6 h. Neutralizing agents are not used because they can lead to additional tissue damage caused by heat generated in an exothermic reaction between the chemicals. Hydrofluoric acid injuries can lead to systemic hypocalcemia, and therefore brief irrigation should be followed by topical application of calcium gluconate gel. If pain persists, clysis (subeschar infusion) of the wound with calcium gluconate is used, except in digits. For injury to distal extremities, intraarterial infusion of calcium gluconate has been recommended.[34]

Prophylaxis Against Wound Infection

Because there is concern for inducing microbial resistance to antibiotics, systemic antimicrobial prophylaxis is not used in burned patients admitted to the hospital. The wounds are observed closely for infection, and treatment is initiated if this occurs. There are differences in how antibiotics are used in the outpatient setting.[35] Some have advocated the use of systemic antibiotics in outpatients whereas others have not.[36] If it is anticipated that compliance with a topical therapy regimen will be poor, systemic prophylaxis should be provided.

The advent of effective topical antimicrobial agents has substantially reduced the mortality associated with burn wound infection.[37] The commonly used agents and their advantages and disadvantages are listed in Table 25.5. The ideal topical regimen includes the use of an agent with good antimicrobial activity that also provides an opportunity to evaluate the wound easily and to perform regular physical therapy. According to a recent international survey,[38] 1% silver sulfadiazine is the topical agent used most commonly for partial-thickness (32% use), mixed partial- and full-

TABLE 25.5. Commonly Used Topical Antimicrobial Agents.

Agent	*Wound dressing*	*Advantages*	*Disadvantages*
Silver sulfadiazine (1%)	Open or light gauze	Soothing, optimal physical therapy, good antimicrobial activity	Does not penetrate eschar possible neutropenia
Mafenide acetate cream (5%)	Open or light gauze	Penerates eschar, optimal physical therapy, good antimicrobial activity	Painful, metabolic acidosis caused by inhibition of carbonic anhydrase
Mafenide acetate (5% solution)	Continuous moist bulky dressing	Good antimicrobial, use over skin grafts	Restricts physical therapy, stains wound
Aqueous silver nitrate (0.5%)	Continuous moist bulky dressing	Good antimicrobial	Hyponatremia, does not penetrate

thickness (34% use), and full-thickness (30% use) burn wounds. Because this agent and most others do not penetrate burn wounds well, they are indicated for prophylaxis against infection but not for therapy. An aqueous solution of 0.5% silver nitrate has been used for years for its topical antimicrobial activity; however, only 4% of centers employ this agent currently for primary topical use. Mafenide acetate does penetrate the wound and is the first-line agent used for therapy of burn wound infection, either as a cream or topical solution. More recent approaches include the use of silver as an antimicrobial; preliminary reports[39] suggest that Acticoat (Smith & Nephew, Hull, UK), a silver-coated polyethylene mesh dressing, provides antimicrobial activity in a dressing that may be left on a partial-thickness wound for 2 to 3 days.

Surgical Care

Excision and closure of wounds has the advantage of reducing the extent of injury and eliminating the risk of wound infection. Tangential excision, which is the sequential removal of layers of necrotic tissue until viable tissue is identified, is the most commonly used method of excision of burn-injured tissue. The advantage of this method is that it yields the best cosmetic and functional result; however, it also is associated with considerable blood loss. Tourniquets have been shown to minimize blood loss when they are applied during excision of extremities.[40] This approach presents a challenge to even the experienced burn surgeon because the identification of the depth to excise to viable tissue is difficult to ascertain in the absence of capillary bleeding. Excision of the wound to the level of the fascia is associated with minimal blood loss and is used when wounds are deep full thickness, are infected, or when large areas are excised. The cosmetic results are poor, and lymphatic drainage is impaired after this type of excision.

Early excision of burn wounds has led to a decrease in length of hospital stay and a decrease in complications,[41,42] but there are no randomized prospective data to indicate that outcome is affected. Excision has been initiated by some within the first 24h after injury[43]; however, many authors suggest that excision is best done when the patient with a large burn has been stabilized and within 3 to 4 days after injury.[44,45] In addition to the stability of the patient, coexistent factors such as inhalation injury affect the timing of operative intervention. When a patient has wounds that will require grafting, that is, deep partial- and full-thickness wounds over more than 40% of the TBSA, the strategy for surgical intervention must take into account the skin donor sites available and a goal of reducing the amount of open wound as soon as possible. In such cases, closure of the wound takes precedence over cosmetic and functional considerations.

At the present time, the ultimate closure of the excised wound requires the use of autograft. If sufficient donor sites are available, the preferred skin graft is a split-thickness autograft (0.008–0.01 inch in thickness). A thicker, full-thickness graft is preferred for cosmetic reconstruction and in areas where scarring would lead to functional compromise. However, this thickness of donor skin requires grafting in turn of the donor site. When donor sites are limited, autograft can be expanded by passing it through a mechanical meshing device to enlarge the skin graft up to six times the surface area of the intact donor skin, but not usually more than threefold for practical purposes.

Closure of the excised wound may be staged by temporary coverage with biological or manufactured dressings. Allograft (skin harvested from a human cadaver) provides for closure of the wound and also may be used as a test graft in areas where there is a concern for infection or when the adequacy of the excised wound bed is suspect. If an allograft is left in place for longer than 10 to 14 days, it becomes incorporated into the wound to the extent that the wound must be excised to remove it. In recent years, a number of skin substitutes have been developed that replace the function of some or all layers of the skin. Integra provides a temporary epidermis as an outer layer of silastic and an inner layer matrix for the growth of a neodermis. Success with use of this product has been reported by a number of authors,[46,47] all of whom noted improved cosmetic and functional results. However, there is concern regarding increased rates of infection when the wound bed is subject to contamination. A thin layer of epidermis must ultimately be grafted onto the neodermis. Alloderm is human dermis that has been processed to provide an acellular nonantigenic matrix that provides a scaffold upon which a thin epidermal graft may be placed, which may improve cosmesis.[48] The advantage of these products for patients with large burns is that donor sites are available sooner for reharvesting of epidermis for further grafting. Immediate application of other products such as pigskin or Biobrane (a synthetic membrane composed of silastic and a chondroitin sulfate-coated surface) on partial-thickness wounds moderates pain and eliminates the need to change dressings, but these products will slough off from deep partial-thickness wounds. A new dressing called TransCyte (Smith & Nephew) derived from human fibroblasts is reported to increase the rate of epidermal healing in partial-thickness wounds.[49] These products are only temporary skin substitutes.

Circumferential Burns

A full-thickness circumferential burn injury carries with it the risk of compression of structures underneath the wound. In the extremities, the combination of increased extravascular fluid in the wound and underlying tissues and the lack of elasticity of the burn wound can lead to subeschar pressures that compromise blood flow to viable tissue. All extremities with circumferential full-thickness burns should be elevated to minimize edema formation and should be evaluated hourly for signs of vascular compromise. The classic signs of ischemia—pallor, pain, parasthesia, paralysis, and poikilothermia—should be assessed. Because these signs are often difficult to evaluate in a burn-injured extremity, blood flow, measured by Doppler, should be assessed. However, loss of Doppler signals may not occur until after tissue becomes damaged,[50] and therefore one should have a low threshold for performing an escharotomy to release subeschar pressure. An escharotomy is performed by making an incision through the eschar on the lateral surface of the extremity. An additional escharotomy may need to be performed on the medial surface as well. The preferred sites for escharotomy are indicated in Figure 25.3. A multicenter study has suggested that delay in decompression of extremities may be associated with occult intracompartmental infection.[51] Decompression of the hand should be performed when full-thickness burn injury of the hand leads to ischemia and dysfunction. Escharotomies are performed on fingers in the midaxial line on the ulnar side and on the radial side of the thumb so as to preserve tactile sensation of the surfaces of opposition of the fingers and thumb. A recent review[52] emphasizes the importance of timely escharotomy of the fingers and the dorsum of the hand that has sustained full-thickness burn injury.

A circumferential full-thickness burn of the chest can compromise chest wall motion and cause a decrease in total pulmonary compliance. When this occurs, escharotomy of the chest in the anterior axillary line will often decrease the inspiratory pressures required to maintain tidal volume. If in addition there are circumferential full-thickness burns of the abdomen and back, an escharotomy following the costal margin may be necessary. Incision of the eschar may be performed with a scalpel but is often done with electrocautery so that minor bleeding can be controlled. Because full-thickness wounds are insensate and avascular, anesthesia is not necessary, and these procedures may be performed under sterile conditions at the bedside. Circumferential full-thickness burns on the abdominal wall can contribute to the development of increased intraabdominal pressure during resuscitation. If abdominal compartment syndrome develops, it may be relieved by escharotomy, drainage of intraabdominal fluid, or decompressive laparotomy.[53]

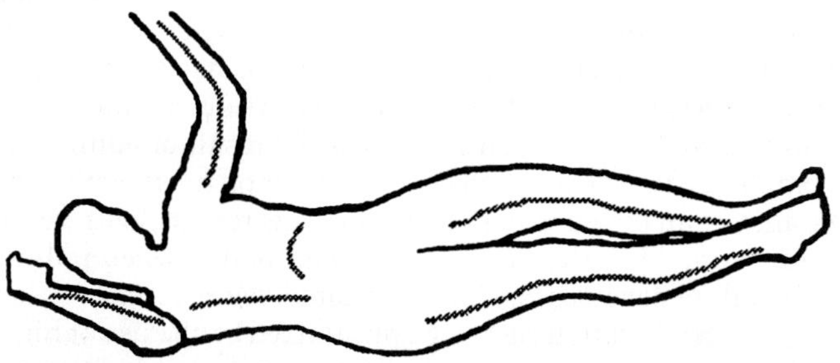

FIGURE 25.3. Preferred sites for escharotomy incisions. The patient should be in the anatomical position as depicted. The incisions are made in the lateral or medial aspect of the extremities.

Infection

General Aspects in Burn Injury

The systemic inflammatory response that is associated with a major burn ignites a cascade of events that presents a clinical syndrome that is difficult to distinguish from infection. These patients often have core body temperatures of 39° to 39.5°C, often develop an intestinal ileus, become disoriented, develop hyperglycemia, and develop positive fluid balance. The burn wound has been seen as a "black box" in which a local inflammatory process occurs that leads to leakage of mediators of inflammation into the systemic circulation and causes activation of cells as they pass through the milieu of the wound.[54] These events compound the responses to injury and are described here only to the extent that they distinguish the burn-injured patient from patients with other injuries. Artunson has summarized the pathophysiology that occurs in the burn wound.[55] Locally produced prostanoids may not only cause local injury[56] but may lead to effects elsewhere.

An increased susceptibility to infection related to the extent of burn injury that has been noted clinically has been confirmed in animal models.[57] Those studies indicated that polymorphonuclear leukocytes (PMNs, neutrophils, granulocytes) were activated. Others have confirmed that granulocytes from burn patients have a baseline increase in cytosolic oxidase activity,[58] suggesting that in vivo activation has occurred. In addition, PMN surface receptors are altered following thermal injury[59,60]; this may lead to increased adhesion of PMNs, causing neutrophil aggregation and sequestration.[59,61] The decrease in bactericidal activity that has been noted may also be the result of in vivo stimulation of the PMN, which leads to a decrease in oxidase activity.[58,62] Decreases in oxidase activity were shown to decrease production of superoxide anion and decrease oxygen consumption[63] by PMNs from burn-injured patients. That there are other mechanisms that modulate the overall activity of PMN is supported by the report that apoptosis in PMNs is inhibited after a burn, possibly by exposure of the cells to granulocyte-macrophage colony-stimulating factor (GM-CSF) or by other mediators in plasma.[64] A randomized prospective study has shown that a monoclonal antibody to intercellular adhesion molecule-1 diminishes progression of tissue injury in partial-thickness burns.[65] These data suggest that leukocyte adherence is involved in the pathogenesis of burn injury.

Cytokines are elevated following a burn injury, and plasma levels of interleukin-1-beta (IL-1β), interleukin-6 (IL-6), and tumor necrosis factor-alpha (TNF-α) have been found to be elevated in severely burned patients.[66–69] IL-6 and TNF concentrations were reported to be higher in patients with severe infection,[68] and TNF concentrations have been noted to be elevated early after burn injury in as many as 80% of patients. It has been suggested that IL-10 production by CD41 T-helper cells is increased following severe burn injury[70] and that this cytokine may increase susceptibility to infection. The net result of activation of cells and mediator pathways appears to be indiscriminant recruitment of the normal pathways that maintain homeostasis, which leads to increased susceptibility of infection and distant organ and further local tissue injury.

Burn Wound Infection

In an attempt to standardize the evaluation and classification of infection in the wounds of the burn-injured patient, a subcommittee of the American Burn Association has provided a proposal for categorization of these infections,[71] providing a foundation for describing the four categories of wound-related infection that occur in the patient with burn injury.

Impetigo

Impetigo "involves the loss of epithelium from a previously reepitheialized surface such as a grafted burn, a partial thickness burn allowed to heal by secondary intention, or a healed donor site."[71] This definition assumes that no other cause for epithelial loss is present such as mechanical damage, hematoma formation, or ischemia. This infection, which has also been termed melting graft syndrome,[72] is not necessarily associated with systemic signs of fever or elevated white blood cell count. Although it is often caused by streptococcal or staphylococcal species, it may be caused by other organisms as well. In distinction to burn wound surface cultures, which give no insight into what is occurring in the wound, surface cultures are helpful in determining the organism that is the agent of these infections. Treatment consists of local care of the wound and systemic antibiotics.

Open Surgical Site Infection

These infections occur in wounds associated with surgical intervention that are not healed. As defined by the committee, they may occur in an ungrafted excised burn or donor sites that have not healed and are associated with culture-positive purulent exudate. In addition, at least one of the following conditions is present:

1. Loss of synthetic or biological covering of the wound
2. Changes in wound appearance, such as hyperemia
3. Erythema in the uninjured skin surrounding the wound
4. Systemic signs, such as fever or leukocytosis

These infections require a change in local wound care, usually the addition of a topical antimicrobial agent, more frequent dressing changes, and the administration of systemic antibiotics.

Cellulitis

The local inflammatory response to a burn injury is manifest at the wound margin as erythema. This finding is differentiated from cellulitis by its localized nature, usually less than 1 to 2 cm from the margin of the wound, and by its lack of extension beyond that zone. The guidelines suggest that in addition to a requirement for antibiotic treatment the definition of cellulitis requires at least one of the following:

1. Localized pain, tenderness, swelling, or heat at the affected site
2. Systemic signs of infection, such as hyperemia, leukocytosis, or sepsis
3. Progression of erythema and swelling
4. Signs of lymphangitis, lymphadenitis, or both

Invasive Infection

The diagnosis of invasive burn wound infection rests on the recognition of changes in the wound, which include discoloration, maceration, or early separation of eschar and systemic manifestations of infection. In addition to the clinical assessment of the wound, biopsy may be performed for quantitative culture or histological evaluation. When more than 10^5 organisms per gram are cultured, it has been held that invasive wound infection is present.[73] However, considerable variability in results with the use of this technique[74] and its lack of correlation with histological findings[75] have limited its application to use for identification of organisms in wounds. Histological evaluation, although not readily available at most institutions, is diagnostic for invasive infection when organisms are identified in viable tissue.[76] Invasive wound infection requires surgical excision of the wound to the level of viable tissue and administration of systemic antibiotics. Topical antimicrobials are not used for therapy for invasive burn wound infection because they do not penetrate eschar, with the exception of mafenide acetate, which may be used in preparation for excision.

The criteria for definition of invasive infection as outlined in the guidelines may be associated with these conditions:

1. Inflammation of the surrounding uninjured skin
2. Histological examination that shows invasion of the organism into adjacent viable tissue
3. Bacteremia in the absence of other infection
4. Systemic signs of infection such as hyperthermia, hypothermia, leukocytosis, tachypnea, hypotension, oliguria, hyperglycemia at a previously tolerated level of dietary carbohydrate, or mental confusion

Pneumonia

Effective topical antimicrobial agents for prevention and therapy of wound infection along with earlier surgical intervention in wound care has decreased the incidence of wound infection. Respiratory failure is now the leading cause of death in the patient with thermal injury.[77] Although inhalation injury is a prominent cause of respiratory complications in these patients, there is a high incidence of pneumonia and acute respiratory distress syndrome even when direct lung injury is not present.[78] Up to 40% of deaths have been attributed to respiratory failure,[79] and even a higher number of children succumb to their injuries as the result of pulmonary complications.[80] Early detection of pulmonary infection by Gram's stain of sputum and culture of secretions, with respiratory support with volume-cycled ventilators when pulmonary failure develops, are standard care.[81] More recent studies suggest that barotrauma can be minimized by the use of high-frequency ventilation in these patients, particularly those with inhalation injury.[82] The presence of white blood cells and bacteria in the sputum associated with other signs of infection should prompt the initiation of systemic antimicrobials that will address the organisms which predominate in the flora of the unit at the time. Specific antimicrobials are then selected when culture reports are available.

Suppurative Thrombophlebitis

Bacterial colonization of venous catheters in patients in intensive care units[83] and in particular of central catheters in the burn-injured patient has been reported to be as high as 25%.[84] Many centers have a policy, such as that at the Hearst Burn Center at NewYork-Presbyterian Hospital, that requires that all peripheral, central venous, and arterial lines are changed over a wire on day 3 and a new site is used on day 6. Others have suggested that a once-a-week catheter change is sufficient to maintain a rate of catheter-related sepsis at 3.2%.[85]

The reason for concern, especially in burn-injured individuals, is that suppurative thrombophlebitis can be an insidious and life-threatening infection.[86] The only findings may be persistent fever and bacteremia that continues despite appropriate antibiotic treatment. Peripheral veins are affected. The classic findings that are associated with phlebitis of edema—erythema, pain, and a palpable cord at an intravenous site—may not be identifiable. Diagnosis is confirmed by aspiration of purulent material from the affected vein, and treatment consists of excision of the involved vein to the point that the vessel is normal where bleeding is encountered.[87]

Suppurative Chondritis

Infection of the external ear that has sustained a partial- or full-thickness injury can lead to loss of integrity of the entire ear.[88] The cartilage of the ear has minimal protection and blood supply and is highly susceptible to infection when the overlying tissue is damaged. Dressings should not be applied to the ear, and pillows should not be used. Auricular burns should be treated with twice-daily open wound care and debrided gently. The topical agent of choice is mafenide acetate because it penetrates eschar and avascular cartilage. When suppurative chondritis occurs, systemic antibiotics are of little value because cartilage is avascular,[89] and the ear must be surgically drained under anesthesia by bivalving of the cartilage with excision of devitalized tissue.

Bacteremia Associated with Wound Manipulation

It may be anticipated that debridement and surgical excision of the burn wound will cause bacteremia; however, the data are not consistent. Bacteremia has been observed transiently in 21% of procedures related to burn care,[90] and 46%[91] of burn patients have bacteremia following burn excision. That the incidence of bacteremia in wound manipulation is related to the extent of injury is supported by the finding of an 8% incidence of bacteremia in patients with 31% to 60% TBSA burns compared to an incidence of 75% in those with more than 60% TBSA burns. More recent studies have suggested that the incidence of bacteremia is low in the early period after injury, and the authors have questioned the need for perioperative antibiotics.[92] Nevertheless, bacteremia related to burn care, especially in patients with a large burn injury who have colonized or infected wounds, may seed distant sites such as cardiac valves or the brain,[93] making perioperative administration of antibiotics of likely benefit.

Other Infections

Just as in any seriously injured patient, host immunosuppression may set the stage for infection at any site. These patients have a high incidence of urinary tract infections and pneumonia.[94] They also develop other infections such as appendicitis and diverticulitis but often do not present with classic features because of the lack of the normal inflammatory response. A high index of suspicion is necessary to detect these infections. Additional infections of concern in the burn-injured patient are listed next.

Sinusitis

One source of sepsis that is frequently overlooked in the burn patient is nosocomial sinusitis.[95] Factors that predispose to sinusitis are indwelling catheters for nasogastric or nasoduodenal feeding and nasotracheal intubation, especially in patients with inhalation injury. The clinical diagnosis of nosocomial sinusitis is difficult because purulent nasal discharge is present in only 27% of cases.[96] The diagnosis is made by computerized tomography of the sinuses, followed by maxillary sinus aspiration and culture. If diagnosed, treatment of sinusitis consists of removal of all tubes and catheters and appropriate antibiotic therapy. If a nasotracheal tube is responsible, it may be necessary to perform a tracheostomy. Persistent or recurrent infection may require formal surgical drainage of the sinuses.

Bacterial Endocardiditis

Immunocompromise, recurrent bacteremia, and the frequent presence of central venous catheters in the patient with burn injury provide a basis for the development of endocarditis.[97] That central venous and pulmonary artery catheters are associated with the development of bacterial endocarditis in these patients is well documented.[98,99] Similar to suppurative thrombophlebitis, this infection is insidious and should be suspected after any bacteremia without an obvious source, especially because the incidence of bacterial endocarditis is 14 to 70 times higher than in other intensive care unit patients. The presence of a new cardiac murmur supports the diagnosis, which should be confirmed by echocardiography. Bacterial endocarditis was associated previously with nearly 100% mortality with burn injury,[97] but early diagnosis and valve replacement have led to improved survival in recent years.

Hypermetabolism and Nutrition

The classic description of the metabolic response to injury includes an early ebb phase that is characterized by low cardiac output and a decreased metabolic rate followed by a hypermetabolic phase that starts at 24 to 36h after injury. After burn injury, the increase in metabolic rate may often exceed the resting energy expenditure (REE) by twofold,[100] but this is variable among patients. Various prior estimates of the caloric needs of these patients often overestimated the needs of current patients; this has been attributed to improved care

TABLE 25.6. Comparison of Metabolic Rate in Thermally Injured Patients: Estimates by Various Formulae Compared to Rate Based on Measurement of Resting Energy Expenditure (REE).

Formula	*Calculation*	*kcal/day*	*% of HBEE*
HBEE[103]	66.5113.75 (kg) + 15.0 (cm) + 26.76 (years)	1837	—
Actual[103]	Based on measured REE	3260	178
Curreri et al.[112]	25 (kg) + 40 (%TBSA burn)	4097	223
Wilmore et al.[100]	2000 (BSA)	3928	214
Long[116]	2.1 (HBEE) (1.2 or 1.3)[a]	4629	252
Molnar et al.[117]	2 (HBEE)	3674	200
Xie and Wang[118]	1000 (BSA) + 125 (% TBSA burn)	3240	176

HBEE, Harris–Benedict energy expenditure; TBSA, total body surface area.

[a]Dependent on level of activity.

Source: Data from Kohrram-Sefat et al.[103]

of the thermally injured patient.[101,102] That the metabolic rate of these patients is substantially increased has recently been reconfirmed by measurement of the REE of patients during the first 20 days after injury.[103] These data confirm those of others[104] and that of the summary of the 28 studies that had been performed before 1990.[105] A comparison of the calculated caloric requirements of various formulae is shown in Table 25.6. These data, taken from the report of Khorram-Sefat et al.,[103] are listed by year of publication from the 1974 study of Curreri et al. to the 1993 report by Xie and Wang and support the suggestion that the metabolic requirements of patients cared for in the modern era are not as high as those of the past. Nevertheless, even the more recent studies indicate that there is a wide variation in metabolic rate among patients and that the hypermetabolism associated with thermal injury may persist well beyond wound closure. Patients with large burns often do not return to a normal metabolic rate until weeks or months after the burn wound is closed.[106] Most clinicians advocate the use of a formula such as that of Curreri or the Harris–Benedict equation adjusted with a stress factor, but in patients with a large injury or those who sustain complications, the metabolic rate should be measured by indirect calorimetry.

Because of losses in the wound, muscle breakdown, and increased demands for healing of the wound, the patient with thermal injury has a requirement for protein replacement that is proportionately greater than that for calories. Protein administration should be two to three times greater than the normal requirement of 0.8 g/kg/day or 2.0 to 2.5 g/kg/day. This amount can be provided in relationship to the estimated or measured calorie needs by providing a nonprotein calorie to nitrogen ratio of 100 to 150:1.[107]

Prognosis

Survival after burn injury has improved significantly during the past 20 years[108] and appears to have reached a plateau over the past 10 years in some studies.[109] Because mortality rates have changed, the suggestion of two decades ago[110] that mortality could be estimated as the addition of age and percent of the body surface area that sustained thermal injury no longer holds true. However, multiple studies have confirmed that patient age and extent of injury are the two most powerful predictors of outcome.[108,111,112] Studies from the past 10 years (summarized in Table 25.7) suggest that the overall mortality rate in burn centers is approximately 4%.[113] These data also confirm the significant contribution of inhalation injury in that the mortality rate was 25% to 35% in the presence of this injury and only 0.5% to 4% in its absence. The high mortality rate when thermal injury is associated with inhalation injury[114,115] is well recognized in other reports of an increase in mortality as high as 20% with inhalation injury.[13] A comparative study of patients matched for burn size and age[16] reported an observed mortality rate of 9.6% in patients without inhalation injury compared to 46.6% in those with inhalation injury.

The report of outcome in multiple centers[116] indicates that 50% of young adults survive a burn injury that involves 81% of their TBSA. To specifically prognosticate the outcome

TABLE 25.7.
Reports on Mortality in Patients with Thermal Injury in the Past Decade.

						Mortality (%)	
Trial	*Year*	*Class of Evidence*	*Design*	*%TBSA*	*Incidence of inhalation (%)*	*Overall*	*Inhalation (with/without)*
126	1990	III	Retrospective	15.1	7.3	4.1	34.7/1.7
127	1994	III	Retrospective	18.0	19.6	9.5	31.0/4.3
128	1995	III	Retrospective	14.1	10.9	4.1	29.4/2.2
122	1998	III	Retrospective	15.0	14	4.0	24.6/0.49
11,234 (total patients)				14.9	11.9	4.8	29.4/2.0

of the thermally injured patient, most authors have suggested that multivariate statistical techniques, such as probit[110,117] or regression[41,111] analysis, be applied. A recent report[109] suggests that mortality can be predicted by a risk scoring system in which one point is given for each of burn size greater than 40% of the TBSA, age greater than 60 years, and presence of inhalation injury. This analysis suggests that mortality rates are 0.3% with no risk factors, 3% with one factor, and 33% and 90% for two or three risk factors, respectively. Although this approach provides a quick estimate, it does not include other variables such as preexisting medical conditions and also does not allow for a continuous stratification of patients by age and extent of injury.[118]

Rehabilitation

Advances in medical care leading to increased survival from thermal injury have led to a renewed emphasis on quality of life after these injuries. Rehabilitation of the patient with a burn injury begins from the time of initial medical care, requires intense care in the first year after injury, and often is lifelong. Splinting of injured extremities begins as soon as the patient is stabilized, and range-of-motion exercises begin within the first day. The team approach is important to coordinate therapy, surgical intervention, and medical care. As soon as wounds have a stable epidermal closure, usually within 2 weeks after grafting or primary healing has occurred, attention is turned to wound and scar management. Garments that apply pressure to the wounds are tailor made for the patient and worn 24h per day. The opportunity to modulate the development of cicatrix is restricted to the time when the wound is immature and actively remodeling. This period may extend up to a year postinjury, but mechanical intervention is of little benefit beyond that time. Surgical intervention for cosmetic deformity is usually delayed until the wound is mature, as is intervention for functional restriction, unless a surgical procedure is necessary to allow for physical therapy.

References

1. Miller SF, Finley RK, Waltman M, et al. Burn size estimate reliability: a study. J Burn Care Rehabil 1991;12:546–559.
2. Heimbach DM, Afromowitz MA, Engrav LH, et al. Burn depth estimation—man or machine. J Trauma 1984;24:373–377.
3. Schiller WR, Garren RL, Bay RC, et al. Laser doppler evaluation of burned hands predicts need for surgical grafting. J Trauma 1997;43:35–40.
4. Yeong EK, Mann R, Goldberg M, et al. Improving accuracy of burn wound assessment using laser Doppler. J Trauma 1996;40:956–962.
5. Atiles L, Mileski W, Purdue G, et al. Laser Doppler flowmetry in burn wounds. J Burn Care Rehabil 1995;16:388–393.
6. Jackson D. The diagnosis of the depth of burning. Br J Surg 1953;40:588–596.
7. Goodwin CW, Finkelstein JL, Madden MR. Burns. In: Schwartz SI, Shires GT, Spencer FC, et al., eds. Principles of Surgery. New York: McGraw-Hill, 1994:265–268.
8. Lee RC. Injury by electrical forces: pathophysiology, manifestations, and therapy. Curr Probl Surg 1997;34:677–764.
9. Arrowsmith J, Usgaocar RP, Dickson WA. Electrical injury and the frequency of cardiac complications. Burns 1997;23:576–578.
10. Haberal M, Bayraktar U, Oner Z, et al. Visceral injuries, wound infection and sepsis following electrical injuries. Burns 1996;22:158–161.
11. Ratnayake B, Emmanuel ER, Walker CC. Neurologic sequelae following a high voltage electrical burn. Burns 1996;22:574–577.
12. Mathes SJ, Alexander J. Radiation injury. Surg Oncol Clin N Am 1996;5:809–824.
13. Pruitt BA Jr, Cioffi WG, Shimazu T, et al. Evaluation and management of patients with inhalation injury. J Trauma 1990;30:S63–S68.
14. Zikria BA, Ferrer JM, Floch HF. The chemical factors contributing to pulmonary damage in "smoke poisoning." Surgery (St. Louis) 1972;71:704–709.
15. Kramer GC, Herndon DN, Linares HA, et al. Effects of inhalation injury on airway blood flow and edema. J Burn Care Rehabil 1989;10:45–51.
16. Shirani KZ, Pruitt BA Jr, Mason AD. The influence of inhalation injury and pneumonia on burn mortality. Ann Surg 1986;205:82–87.
17. Agee RN, Long JM III, Hunt JL, et al. Use of 133 xenon in early diagnosis of inhalation injury. J Trauma 1976;16:218–224.
18. Brown DL, Archer SB, Greenhalgh DG, et al. Inhalation injury severity scoring system: a quantitative method. J Burn Care Rehabil 1996;17:552–557.
19. Levine BA, Petroff PA, Slade CL, et al. Prospective trials of dexamethasone and aerosolized gentamycin in the treatment of inhalation injury in the burned patient. J Trauma 1978;18:188–193.
20. Ahrenholz DH, Cope N, Dimick AR et al. Inhalation injury: initial management in practice guidelines for burn care. J Burn Care Rehabil 2001(suppl):23S–26S.
21. Treat RC, Sirinek KR, Levine BA, et al. Air evacuation of thermally injured patients: principles of treatment and results. J Trauma 1980;20:275–279.
22. Committee on Trauma. Guidelines for the operations of burn units. In: Resources for Optimal Care of the Injured Patient. Chicago: American College of Surgeons, 1999:55–62.
23. Goodwin CW, Dorethy J, Lam V, et al. Randomized trial of efficacy of crystalloid and colloid resuscitation on hemodynamic response and lung water following thermal injury. Ann Surg 1983;197:520–531.
24. Shirani KZ, Vaughan GM, Mason AD, et al. Update on current therapeutic approaches in burns. Shock 1996;5:4–16.
25. Morehouse JD, Finkelstein JL, Marano MA, et al. Resuscitation of the thermally injured patient. Crit Care Clin1992;8:355–365.
26. Baxter CR. Fluid volume and electrolyte changes in the early postburn period. Clin Plast Surg 1974;1:693–703.
27. Schiller WR, Bay RC, Garren RL, et al. Hyperdynamic resuscitation improves survival in patients with life-threatening burns. J Burn Care Rehabil 1997;18:10–16.
28. Elliot DC. An evaluation of the endpoints of resuscitation. J Am Coll Surg 1998;187:536–547.
29. Baxter CR, Shires T. Physiologic response to crystalloid resuscitation of severe burns. Ann NY Acad Sci 1968;150:874–894.
30. Graves TA, Cioffi WG, McManus WF, et al. Fluid resuscitation of infants and children with massive thermal injury. J Trauma 1988;28:1656–1659.
31. Monafo WW, Halverson JD, Schechtman K. The role of concentrated sodium solutions in the resuscitation of patients with severe burns. Surgery (St. Louis) 1984;95:129–135.
32. Huang PP, Stucky FS, Dimick AR. Hypertonic sodium resuscitation is associated with renal failure and death. Ann Surg 1995;221:543–557.
33. Griswold JA, Anglin BL, Love RT. Hypertonic saline resuscitation: efficacy in a community-based burn unit. South Med J 1991;84:692–696.

34. Graudins A, Burns MJ, Aaron CK. Regional intravenous infusion of calcium gluconate for hydrofluoric acid burns of the upper extremity. Ann Emerg Med 1997;30:604–607.
35. Fakhry SM, Alexander J, Smoth D, et al. Regional and institutional variation in burn care. J Burn Care Rehabil 1995;16:86–90.
36. Boss WK, Brand DA, Acampora D, et al. Effectiveness of prophylactic antibiotics in the outpatient treatment of burns. J Trauma 1985;25:224–227.
37. Pruitt BA Jr, McManus AT. The changing epidemiology of infections in burn patients. World J Surg 1992;16:57–67.
38. Hermans MHE. Results of a survey on the use of different treatment options for partial and full thickness burns. Burns 1998; 24:539–551.
39. Tredget EE, Shankowski HA, Groeneveld A, et al. A matched-pair, randomized study evaluating the efficacy and safety of Acticoat silver-coated dressing for the treatment of burn wounds. J Burn Care Rehabil 1998;19:531–537.
40. Marano MA, O'Sullivan G, Madden M, et al. Tourniquet technique for reduced blood loss and wound assessment during excisions of burn wounds of the extremity. Surg Gynecol Obstet 1990;171:249–250.
41. Tompkins RG, Remensnyder JP, Burke JF, et al. Significant reductions in mortality for children with burn injuries through the use of prompt eschar excision. Ann Surg 1988;208:577–585.
42. Pruitt BA Jr, McManus AT, Kim SH, et al. Burn wound infections: current status. World J Surg 1998;22:135–145.
43. Still JM, Law EJ, Craft-Coffman B. An evaluation of excision with application of autografts or porcine xenografts within 24 hours of injury. Ann Plast Surg 1996;36:176–179.
44. Marano MA, Madden MR, Finkelstein JL, et al. Early excision in burn therapy: selection, technique, results. Adv Trauma Crit Care 1991;6:73–78.
45. McManus WF, Mason AD, Pruitt BA Jr. Excision of the burn wound in patients with large burns. Arch Surg 1989;124:718–720.
46. Heimbach D, Luterman A, Burke J, et al. Artificial dermis for major burns. A multicenter randomized clinical trial. Ann Surg 1988;208:313–320.
47. Clayton MC, Bishop JF. Perioperative and postoperative dressing techniques for Integra Artificial Skin: views from two medical centers. J Burn Care Rehabil 1998;19:358–363.
48. Wainwright DJ. Use of an acellular allograft dermal matrix (Alloderm) in the management of full thickness burns. Burns 1995;21:243–248.
49. Purdue GF, Hunt JL, Still JM. A multicenter clinical trial of a biosynthetic skin replacement, Dermagraft-TC, compared to cryopreserved human cadaver skin for temporary coverage of excised burn wounds. J Burn Care Rehabil 1997;18:52–57.
50. Clayton JM, Russell HE, Hartford CE, et al. Sequential circulatory changes in the circumferentially burned limb. Ann Surg 1977;185:391–396.
51. Sheridan RL, Tompkins RG, McManus WF, et al. Intracompartmental sepsis in burn patients. J Trauma 1994;36:301–305.
52. Smith MA, Munster AM, Spence RJ. Burns of the hand and upper limb—a review. Burns 1998;24:493–505.
53. Sheridan RL, Tompkins RG. What's new in burns and metabolism. J Am Coll Surg 2004;198:243–263.
54. Yurt RW. Tissue hormones. In: Dolecek R, Brizio-Molteni L, Molteni A, Traber D, eds. Endocrinology of Thermal Trauma. Philadelphia: Lea & Febiger, 1990.
55. Arturson G. Pathophysiology of the burn wound and pharmacological treatment. The Rudi Hermans Lecture, 1995. Burns 1996; 22:255–274.
56. Liu XS, Luo ZH, Yang ZC, Li AN. Clinical significance of the alterations of plasma prostaglandins E_2 (PGE_2) in severely burned patients. Burns 1996;22:298–302.
57. Yurt RW, McManus AT, Mason AD Jr, et al. Increased susceptibility to infection related to extent of injury. Arch Surg 1984;119:183–188.
58. Cioffi WG Jr, Burleson DG, Jordan BS, et al. Granulocyte oxidative activity after thermal injury. Surgery (St. Louis) 1992;112(5): 860–865.
59. Bjerknes R, Vindenes H, Laerum OD. Altered neutrophil function in patients with large burns. Blood Cells 1990;16:127–143.
60. Rodeberg DA, Bass RC, Alexander JW, et al. Neutrophils from burn patients are unable to increase the expression of CD11b/CD18 in response to inflammatory stimuli. J Leukocyte Biol 1997;61(5):575–582.
61. Mileski W, Borgstrom D, Lightfoot E, et al. Inhibition of leukocyte endothelial adherence following thermal injury. J Surg Res 1992;52:334–339.
62. Sparkes BG. Immunological responses to thermal injury. Burns 1997;23:106–113.
63. Rosenthal J, Thurman GW, Cusack N, et al. Neutrophils from patients after burn injury express a deficiency of the oxidase components p47-phox and p67-phox. Blood 1996;88:4321–4329.
64. Chitnis D, Dickerson C, Munster AM, et al. Inhibition of apoptosis in polymorphonuclear neutrophils from burn patients. J Leukocyte Biol 1996;59(6):835–839.
65. Mileski WJ, Burkhart D, Hunt JL, et al. Clinical effects of inhibiting leukocyte adhesion with monoclonal antibody to intercellular adhesion molecule-1 (enlimomab) in the treatment of partial-thickness burn injury. J Trauma 2003;54:950–958.
66. Drost AC, Burleson DG, Cioffi WG Jr, et al. Plasma cytokines following thermal injury and their relationship to mortality, burn size, and time post burn. J Trauma 1993;35:335–339.
67. Drost AC, Larsen B, Aulick LH. The effects of thermal injury on serum interleukin 1 activity in rats. Lymphokine Cytokine Res 1993;12(3):181–185.
68. Drost AC, Burleson DG, Cioffi WG Jr, et al. Plasma cytokines after thermal injury and their relationship to infection. Ann Surg 1993;218(1):74–78.
69. Colewell Vanni HE, Gordon BR, Levine DM, et al. Cholesterol and IL-6 concentrations relate to outcomes in burn injured patients. J Burn Care Rehabil 2003;24(3):133–141.
70. Burleson DG, Mason AD Jr, Pruitt BA Jr. Lymphoid subpopulation changes after thermal injury and thermal injury with infection in an experimental model. Ann Surg 1987;207(2):208–212.
71. Peck MD, Weber J, McManus A, et al. Surveillance of burn wound infections: a proposal for definitions. J Burn Care Rehabil 1998;19:386–389.
72. Matsumura H, Meyer NA, Mann R, et al. Melting graft-wound syndrome. J Burn Care Rehabil 1998;19:292–295.
73. Teplitz C. The pathology of burns and the fundamentals of burn wound sepsis. In: Artz CP, Moncrief JA, Pruitt BA Jr, eds. Burns: A Team Approach. Philadelphia: Saunders, 1979.
74. Woolfrey BF, Fox JM, Quall CO. An evaluation of burn wound quantitative microbiology. Am Soc Clin Pathol 1980;75:532–537.
75. McManus AL, Kim SH, McManus WF, et al. Comparison of quantitative microbiology and histopathology in divided burn-wound biopsy specimens. Arch Surg 1997;122:74–76.
76. Pruitt BA Jr, Foley DF. The use of biopsies in burn patient care. Surgery (St. Louis) 1973;73:887–897.
77. Pruitt BA Jr, Flemma RJ, DiVencenti FC, et al. Pulmonary complications in burn patients. J Thorac Cardiovasc Surg 1970;59:7–20.
78. Achauer BM, Allyn PA, Furnas DW, et al. Pulmonary complications in burns: the major threat to the burn patient. Ann Surg 1973;177:311–319.
79. Benmeir P, Sagi A, Greber B, et al. An analysis of mortality in patients with burns covering 40 percent BSA or more: a retrospective review covering 24 years (1964–88). Burns 1991;17: 402–405.

80. Reynolds EM, Ryan DP, Doody DP. Mortality and respiratory failure in a pediatric burn population. J Pediatr Surg 1993;28:1326–1330.
81. Nguyen TT, Gilpen DA, Meyer NA, et al. Current treatment of severely burned patients. Ann Surg 1996;223:14–25.
82. 82. Cioffi WG, Graves TA, McManus WE, et al. High-frequency percussive ventilation in patients with inhalation injury. J Trauma 1989;29:350–354.
83. Samsoondar W, Freeman JB, Coultish I, et al. Colonization of intravascular catheters in the intensive care unit. Am J Surg 1985;149:730–732.
84. Still JM, Law E, Thiruvaiyaru D, Belcher K, et al. Central line-related sepsis in acute burn patients. Am Surg 1998;64(2):165–170.
85. Sheridan RL, Weber JM, Peterson HF, et al. Central venous catheter sepsis with weekly catheter change in paediatric burn patients: an analysis of 221 catheters. Burns 1995;21(2):127–129.
86. Pruitt BA Jr, McManus WF, Kim SH, et al. Diagnosis and treatment of cannula-related intravenous sepsis in burn patients. Ann Surg 1980;191:546–554.
87. Khan EA, Correa AG, Baker CJ. Suppurative thrombophlebitis in children: a ten-year experience. Pediatr Infect Dis J 1997; 16(1):63–67.
88. Bentrem DJ, Bill TJ, Himel HN, et al. Chondritis of the ear: a late sequelae of deep partial thickness burns of the face. J Emerg Med 1996;14:469–471.
89. Mills DC II, Roberts LW, Mason AD Jr, et al. Suppurative chondritis: its incidence, prevention, and treatment in burn patients. Plast Reconstr Surg 1988;82(2):267–276.
90. Sasaki TM, Welch GW, Herndon DN, et al. Burn wound manipulation-induced bacteremia. J Trauma 1979;19(1):46–48.
91. Beard CH, Ribiero CD, Jones DM. The bacteraemia associated with burns surgery. Br J Surg 1975;62:638–641.
92. Mozingo DW, McManus AT, Kim SH, et al. Incidence of bacteremia after burn wound manipulation in the early postburn period. J Trauma 1997;42:1006–1010.
93. Suzuki T, Ueki I, Isago T, et al. Multiple brain abscesses complicating treatment of a severe burn injury: an unusual case report. J Burn Care Rehabil 1992;13(4):446–450.
94. Weber JM, Sheridan RL, Pasternack MS, et al. Nosocomial infections in pediatric patients with burns. Am J Infect Control 1997;25:195–201.
95. Browers BL, Purdue GF, Hunt JL. Paranasal sinusitis in burn patients following nasal tracheal intubation. Arch Surg 1991;126: 1411–1412.
96. Lum Cheong RS, Cornwell EE. Suppurative sinusitis in critically ill patients: a case report and review of the literature. J Natl Med Assoc 1992;84(12):1057–1059.
97. Baskin TW, Rosenthal A, Pruitt BA Jr. Acute bacterial endocarditis: a silent source of sepsis in the burn patient. Ann Surg 1974;184:618–621.
98. Sasaki TM, Panke TW, Dorethy JF, et al. The relationship of central venous and pulmonary artery catheter position to acute right-sided endocarditis in severe thermal injury. J Trauma 1979;19:740–743.
99. Ehrie M, Morgan AP, Moore FD, et al. Endocarditis with the indwelling balloon-tipped pulmonary artery catheter in burn patients. J Trauma 1978;18(9):664–666.
100. Wilmore DW. Nutrition and metabolism following thermal injury. Clin Plast Surg 1974;1:603–619.
101. Carlson DE, Cioffi WG, Mason AD Jr, et al. Resting energy expenditure in patients with thermal injuries. Surg Gynecol Obstet 1992;174:270–276
102. Milner EA, Cioffi WG, Mason AD, et al. A longitudinal study of resting energy expenditure in thermally injured patients. J Trauma 1994;37:167–170.
103. Khorram-Sefat R, Behrendt W, Heiden A, et al. Long-term measurements of energy expenditure in severe burn injury. World J Surg 1999;23:115–122.
104. Cunningham JJ, Hegarty MT, Meara PA, et al. Measured and predicted calorie requirements of adults during recovery from severe burn trauma. Am J Clin Nutr 1989;49:404–408.
105. Cunningham JJ. Factors contributing to increased energy expenditure in thermal injury: a review of studies employing indirect calorimetry. J Parenter Enteral Nutr 1990;14:449–456.
106. Saffle JR, Medina E, Raymond J, et al. Use of indirect calorimetry in the nutritional management of burned patients. J Trauma 1985;25:32–39.
107. Rodriguez DJ. Nutrition in major burn patients: state of the art. J Burn Care Rehabil 1996;17:62–70.
108. Tompkins RG, Burke JF, Schoenfeld DA, et al. Prompt eschar excision: a treatment system contributing to reduced burn mortality: a statistical evaluation of burn care at the Massachusetts General Hospital (1974–1984). Ann Surg 1986;204:272–281.
109. Ryan CM, Schoenfeld DA, Thorpe WP, et al. Objective estimates of the probability of death from burn injuries. N Engl J Med 1998;338:362–366.
110. Zawacki BE, Azen SP, Imbus SH, et al. Multifactorial probit analysis of mortality in burned patients. Ann Surg 1979;189:1–5.
111. Pruitt BA Jr, Tumbusch WT, Mason AD Jr, et al. Mortality in 1,100 consecutive burns treated at a burns unit. Ann Surg 1964;159:396–401.
112. Curreri PW, Richmond D, Marvin J, Baxter CR. Dietary requirements of patients with major burns. J Am Diet Assoc 1974; 65:415–417.
113. Monafo WW. Initial management of burns. N Engl J Med 1996;335:1581–1586.
114. Sobel JB, Goldfarb IW, Slater H, et al. Inhalation injury: a decade without progress. J Burn Care Rehabil 1992;13:573–575.
115. Head JM. Inhalation injury in burns. Am J Surg 1980;139:508–512.
116. Long C. Energy expenditure of major burns. J Trauma 1979; 19(Suppl 11):904–906.
117. Molnar J, Wolfe R, Burke F. Metabolism and nutritional therapy in thermal injury. In: Schneider I, Howard A, Anderson CE, Coursin OB, eds. Nutritional Support of Medical Practice, 2nd ed. Philadelphia: Harper & Row; 1983:260–281.
118. Xie WG, Li A, Wang SL. Estimation of the calorie requirements of burned Chinese adults. Burns 1993;19:146–149.

26

Traumatic Brain Injury

Kyle Chapple and Roger Hartl

Traumatic brain injury (TBI) is graded as mild, moderate, or severe based on the level of consciousness or the Glasgow Coma Scale (GCS) score after resuscitation (Table 26.1). Mild TBI is defined with a GCS score between 13 and 15. In most cases it represents a concussion, and there is full neurological recovery, although many patients reveal short-term memory and concentration deficits. Patients with moderate TBI are typically stuporous and lethargic with a GCS score between 9 and 13. A comatose patient who is unable to open his or her eyes or follow commands has a GCS score of less than 9 and by definition has a severe TBI.

During the past two decades, it has become increasingly clear that patients with TBI are susceptible to posttraumatic arterial hypotension, hypoxia, and brain swelling, or so-called secondary brain injury. All major advances in the care of these patients have been achieved by reducing the occurrence and severity of these secondary insults on the already injured central nervous system. Initial resuscitation and rapid transport of trauma patients in the field and direct transport to a major trauma center, and improved critical care management with intracranial pressure monitoring, have decreased the rate of mortality from as much as 50% in the 1970s and 1980s to between 15% and 25% in most recent series.[1,2] The development of scientifically based management protocols for the treatment of patients with TBI holds considerable promise for further improvement in outcome. The goal of this chapter is to familiarize the reader with the basic principles of TBI management. Herein, reference is made to recently published evidence-based guidelines for the pre-hospital and in-hospital surgical and medical management of patients with severe TBI.[3–5] These guidelines have been endorsed by the American Association of Neurological Surgeons (AANS) and the Congress of Neurological Surgeons and can be accessed via the Internet at http://www.braintrauma.org.

Epidemiology

About 1.6 million people sustain a TBI each year in the United States, and 270,000 require hospitalization. With about 52,000 deaths per year, TBI is the most common cause of death and disability in young people and accounts for about one-third of all trauma deaths.[6] The costs of TBI to society are enormous; neurotrauma is a serious public health problem requiring continuing improvement in the care of injured patients. Motor vehicle crashes are the major cause of TBI, particularly for young people. Falls are the leading cause of death and disability from TBI for people older than 65 years of age.

Pathophysiology: Secondary Brain Injury

Neurological injury not only occurs during the impact (primary injury) but also evolves over the following hours and days (secondary brain injury). Within the first days and weeks after TBI, the brain is extremely vulnerable to decreases in blood pressure and oxygenation that are well tolerated by the noninjured central nervous system (Figure 26.1).[7] Secondary brain damage is the most dominant cause of TBI in-hospital death. The most important insults that may lead to secondary brain damage and poor outcome are listed in Table 26.2. Many of these insults are preventable. In the pre-hospital phase, hypoxia and arterial hypotension have been shown to be the most important secondary insults. Studies have reported that 27% to 55% of TBI patients are hypoxemic (SaO_2 <90%) at the scene, in the ambulance, or on arrival in the emergency department. Arterial hypotension is defined as a single systolic blood pressure reading of less than 90 mmHg. Hypotensive episodes were observed in 16% and 32% of patients with severe TBI at the time of hospital arrival and during surgical

TABLE 26.1. Glasgow Coma Scale.

Points	*Eyes open*	*Best verbal response*	*Best motor response*
6	—	—	Obeys commands
5	—	Oriented and converses	Localizes painful stimuli
4	Spontaneously	Disoriented and converses	Flexion withdrawal
3	To verbal command	Inappropriate words	Flexion-abnormal
2	To painful stimuli	Incomprehensible sounds	Extension
1	No response	No response	No response

The Glasgow Coma Scale (GCS) scoring system is routinely used as part of the neurological examination in severe traumatic brain injury. Note that the GCS represents the best response elicited from the patient. The lowest score is 3 and the highest is 15. GCS scores less than 9 indicate coma and portend a worse outcome from traumatic brain injury (TBI).

procedures, respectively.[8] A single hypotensive episode has been shown to be associated with increased morbidity rate and a doubling of the mortality rate. Therefore, the recommendation based on the CNS/AANS guidelines is that the mean arterial blood pressure in patients with severe TBI should always be maintained above 90 mmHg to keep the cerebral perfusion pressure at least 60 mmHg.

Soon after the primary injury, brain swelling occurs. Brain swelling can be caused by vascular engorgement or an increase in brain water content, called brain edema. Depending on the underlying mechanism, it is possible to distinguish several types of brain swelling: swelling caused by hyperemia or venous congestion, which both lead to increased cerebral blood volume, vasogenic brain edema, and cytotoxic brain edema.[9]

Disruption of the blood–brain barrier, within minutes after TBI, leads to accumulation of fluid in the extravascular compartment and vasogenic edema. Vasogenic edema can also develop later within or around areas of contused brain tissue and hemorrhage. Despite the effectiveness of corticosteroids to treat vasogenic edema in patients with brain tumors, they have not proven to be of benefit in patients with TBI. The most common type of brain swelling after TBI probably results from cytotoxic edema. This type of edema is characterized by a failure of sodium/potassium pumps to maintain intracellular homeostasis; this leads to an influx of ions and water into the cells and initiates a self-destructive cascade culminating in progressive ischemia and intracranial hypertension.

The reason for the ischemic cascade is that the brain is contained inside a rigid closed space, the skull. The skull is noncompliant, providing a fixed amount of space for the brain to occupy. As intracranial space is taken up by edema, blood, or any other mass-occupying lesion, the pressure inside the skull (ICP) increases (Figure 26.2). As the ICP elevates, it becomes increasingly difficult for oxygen- and nutrient-rich blood to be pumped into the brain and perfuse viable tissue. As already described, the tissue becomes ischemic, further perpetuating the problem (see Figure 26.1). This downward pathological spiral causes substantial damage, even death, if untreated.

Several pharmacological agents that interfere with this cascade, such as calcium antagonists, free-radical scavengers, and *N*-methyl-D-aspartate antagonists, have been tested, but none has been proven effective.[10] The lack of available pharmacological agents to treat patients with TBI reinforces the importance of optimal critical care management and monitoring and treatment of brain pressure, blood pressure, and oxygenation to maintain and improve cerebral perfusion.

Management of Patients with Severe Traumatic Brain Injury

Pre-Hospital Management

The pre-hospital management of patients with severe TBI is outlined in Table 26.3.[3] Rapid and physiological resuscitation is the first priority in these patients. Following stabilization of airway, breathing, and circulation, the GCS score should be determined by direct verbal or physical interaction with the patient. Patients with a GCS score less than 9 should be brought to a trauma center with the following TBI capabilities: 24-h availability of computed tomography (CT) scans; 24-h availability of an operating room and prompt neurosurgical care; and the ability to monitor intracranial pressure and treat intracranial hypertension.

Comatose patients with a GCS score less than 9 should be intubated for airway stability and protection regardless of their ability to oxygenate and ventilate at the time. All patients should have their oxygenation and blood pressure assessed at least every 5 min. Arterial oxygen saturation should be maintained above 90%, and systolic blood pressure should be kept above 90 mmHg during the initial assessment.

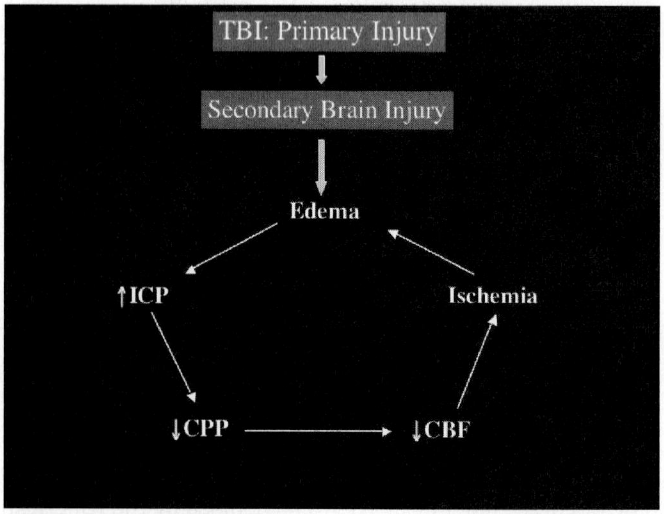

FIGURE 26.1. The relationship of secondary brain injury causing edema and eventually cerebral ischemia. The circular cascade follows as elevated intracranial pressure (*ICP*) causes decreased cerebral perfusion pressure (*CPP*) and cerebral blood flow (*CBF*). Cerebral ischemia then ensues, leading to more edema.

TABLE 26.2. Causes of Secondary Brain Injury.

Secondary insult	*Critical values in TBI*	*Main cause*
Arterial hypotension	Systolic blood pressure <90 mmHg	Blood loss, sepsis, cardiac failure, spinal cord injury, brain stem injury
Hypoxemia	Arterial O_2 saturation <90%, PaO_2 <60 mmHg, apnea, canosis	Hypoventilation, thoracic injury, aspiration
Hypocapnia	Sustained $PaCO_2$ <25 mmHg	Induced or spontaneous hyperventilation
Intracranial hypertension	ICP >20–25 mmHg	Mass lesion, cerebral swelling caused by vasodilation or increased water content

TBI, traumatic brain injury; ICP, intracranial pressure.

In-Hospital Management

Initial Management in the Emergency Department

Maintaining brain perfusion is the overarching priority in managing comatose patients with severe TBI. The cornerstones of the resuscitation of the severely head-injured patient include resuscitation according to Advanced Cardiac Life Support (ACLS)/Advanced Trauma Life Support (ATLS) protocol (airway, breathing, circulation); primary survey with cervical spine control and brief neurological assessment; and secondary survey with complete neurological examination and determination of the GCS score (see Table 26.1). All patients who have had a loss of consciousness, however brief, should undergo an initial head CT scan even if then conscious, lucid, and with a normal neurological examination.

Emergency room patients with mild or moderate TBI or suspected TBI need to be observed closely for neurological deterioration, ideally with "neurochecks" every 15 min in the acute period. A complete trauma evaluation following the ATLS protocol should be initiated if there is any suspicion of associated injuries. Nausea or vomiting, new-onset or progressive headaches, restlessness, pupillary asymmetry, seizures, and increasing lethargy should be interpreted as signs of neurological deterioration, and a head CT scan should be obtained immediately or repeated if the symptoms and signs reflect a change in condition. It is important to remember that with expanding intracranial mass lesions, pupillary changes can precede a significant change in mental status. Blood alcohol concentration and a urine toxicology screen should be considered in all patients presenting with TBI. Routine blood tests, including arterial blood gases and coagulation parameters, should be obtained in patients with moderate and severe TBI and in patients with associated injuries. Tetanus toxoid must be administered if there are any associated open wounds. Immobilization of the cervical spine using a hard collar is mandatory in all patients with head injury. All patients with severe TBI need radiographic evaluation of the cervical spine from the craniocervical junction down to T1. Any complaint of neck pain in patients with mild or moderate TBI should also lead to a radiographic assessment of the cervical spine. A list of typical admission orders for a patient with severe TBI is provided in Table 26.4.

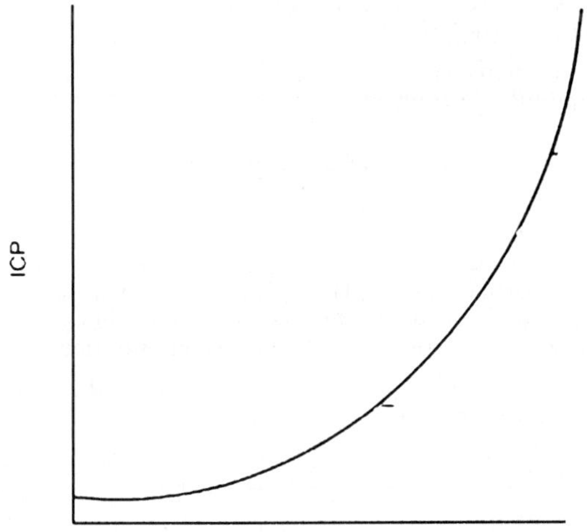

FIGURE 26.2. A simple curve representing the relationship of cerebral volume and intracranial pressure (*ICP*). ICP elevates as the cerebral volume increases.

General principles of the diagnostic evaluation of TBI workup are summarized here. Normocapnia should be maintained. Unless there are signs of cerebral herniation (pupillary asymmetry, dilated/fixed pupils, and/or extensor posturing or flaccidity to noxious stimuli), patients should not be hyperventilated and the arterial $PaCO_2$ should be maintained around 35 mmHg. Isotonic fluids should be used for resuscitation to avoid free water overload. CT is the imaging study of choice to detect skull fractures and intracranial injury with hemorrhage and to assess the necessity of surgical evacuation of a mass lesion. A head CT scan can also demonstrate findings that are closely associated with intracranial hypertension, such as obliterated basal cisterns, compressed cerebral ventricles, and midline shift. All comatose patients with an abnormal CT scan and a GCS score less than 9 should undergo intracranial pressure (ICP) monitoring. Plain radiographs of the cervical spine should be obtained as soon as possible, and a CT scan of suspicious areas should be obtained. Once the patient has been stabilized, a careful physical examination should be repeated.

Computed Tomography Scan Assessment

After resuscitation, all stable patients with severe TBI should undergo a CT scan of the head as soon as possible to identify a life-threatening mass lesion that requires surgical evacuation, evidence of raised ICP, and the degree of intracranial injury to determine prognostic indicators of outcome.

Approximately 10% of initial head CT scans in patients with severe TBI show no abnormalities. The absence of abnormalities on CT scan at admission does not preclude increased ICP. Important new lesions and increased ICP may develop in 40% of patients with an initially normal head CT scan. In addition, patients with normal CT findings, systolic blood pressure lower than 90 mmHg, age greater than 40 years, or motor posturing are at the same risk for intracranial hypertension as those with abnormal head CT findings.[11]

TABLE 26.3. Immediate Assessment and Treatment of Patients with Traumatic Brain Injury.

Parameter	*Critical findings*	*Immediate intervention*
1. Resuscitation		
Oxygenation/ventilation	Apnea, cyanosis, oxygen saturation <90%	Intubation if hypoxemic despite supplemental O_2, no hyperventilation
Blood pressure	Systolic blood pressure <90 mmHg	Resuscitation, consider vasopressor therapy
2. Primary survey/postresuscitation		
Spinal stability	Pain, step-off, external signs of trauma to neck, mechanism	Immobilization, radiographs
Postresuscitation GCS score	<9	Intubation, normoventilation, head CT
Motor examination, papillary diameter, light reflex, direct orbital trauma	Suspect cerebral herniation: flaccidity or motor posturing and asymmetrical or fixed and dilated pupils	Short-term hyperventilation ± mannitol, if herniation suspected
3. Placement of vascular, urinary, and gastric catheters, and cervical spine, chest, and pelvic radiographs		
4. Secondary survey/detailed neurological examination		

TABLE 26.4. Typical Order Set for Admission of Patient with Severe TBI.

Admit to intensive care unit

Monitoring and notifications
- Check vital signs and neurostatus q 1 h, call for neurological change
- Check temperature q4h, call for T > 38.3°C; If T > 38.3°C, remove sheets, use cooling blankets, ice packs to decrease temperature
- Monitor end-tidal CO_2; call for $PaCO_2$ <30 mmHg
- Notify for SBP > 180 or SBP <90 mmHg
- Specify ventriculostomy settings (height, open or clamped, drain above 15–20 mmHg)
- Monitor CPP, call for CPP < 70 mmHg
- Monitor CVP, call for CVP < 5 or CVP >10 mmHg
- If pulmonary artery catheter in place, measure cardiac parameters q 4 h, call for pulmonary artery occlusion pressure <8 or >15 mmHg
- Strict recording of intake/output; call for urine output >200 mL/h × 2 h

Activity
- Bed rest with head of bed up 30°
- Log roll, spine precautions
- Cervical collar

Nursing
- Foley catheter
- Pneumatic compression devices
- Daily weights
- 2–4 L O_2 per nasal cannula if not intubated/mechanically ventilated
- Orogastric tube, nasogastric tube if no basilar skull fracture

Diet
- Start tube feedings within 24–36 h

Maintenance IV fluids
- D5 Normal saline ± 20 mEq/L KCl at 1–2 mL/h, typically 80–120 mL

Medication
- Stool softener
- Docusate sodium 100 mg PO tid

Antiemetic
- Trimethobenzamide 200 mg IM q 8 h prn or
- Prochlorperazine 5–10 mg IM q 6 h prn

Analgesia
- Codeine 30–60 mg IM/PO q 3 h prn moderate pain
- Morphine 1–6 mg IV/IM q 4–6 h prn severe pain or IV drip up to 5–10 mg/h for severe pain or
- Fentanyl 50–150 μg bolus, then 30–100 μg/h maintenance by continuous infusion

Antipyretics
- Acetaminophen 650–1000 mg PO/PR q 6 h prn if T > 38.3°C or
- Ibuprofen 400 mg NG/PR q 8 h prn if T > 38.3°C

Sedation
- Propofol drip, titrate dose to level of sedation and to maintain SBP (preferred) or
- Lorazepam drip, titrate dose to level of sedation

GI prophylaxis
- Famotidine (Pepcid) 20 mg PO/IV bid or proton pump inhibitor IV/PO

Seizure prophylaxis
- Phenytoin 1 g IV loading dose over 1 h
- Phenytoin 300 mg IV qd

Arterial hypertension
- Call for SBP > 180 mmHg

Others
- Lidocaine 2% IV infusion 5 mL down endotracheal tube before suctioning or bronchoscopy

Laboratory studies
- Complete blood count, platelet count, prothrombin time, activated partial thromboplastin time, type and crossmatch for possible blood transfusion, biochemical profile, blood and urine for toxicology screening, blood alcohol concentration

Ventilator settings to maintain SaO_2 above 90% and $PaCO_2$ approximately 35 mmHg

Intracranial Pressure Monitoring and Treatment of Increased Intracranial Pressure

Comatose head injury patients (GCS score, 3 to 8) with abnormal CT scans should undergo ICP monitoring. ICP monitoring helps in the earlier detection of intracranial mass lesions, can limit the indiscriminate use of therapies to control ICP, which themselves can be potentially harmful, can reduce ICP by cerebrospinal fluid drainage and thus improve cerebral perfusion, helps in determining prognosis, and may improve outcome.[11]

Elevated ICP is present in the majority of TBI patients. Cerebral perfusion pressure is defined as the mean arterial blood pressure minus ICP. This physiological variable defines the pressure gradient driving cerebral blood flow and metabolite delivery and is therefore closely related to cerebral ischemia. A threshold for cerebral perfusion pressure of approximately 60 mmHg for adults is recommended currently.[12]

The CNS/AANS Guidelines recommend that ICP monitoring is appropriate in severe head injury patients (GCS score, 3 to 8) with an abnormal CT scan, or a normal CT scan if two or more of the following are noted upon admission: systolic blood pressure less than 90 mmHg, age greater than 40 years, and unilateral or bilateral motor posturing.[11]

Treatment of increased intracranial pressure should be initiated at an upper threshold of 20 or 25 mmHg. Cerebral perfusion pressure (mean arterial pressure minus ICP) should be maintained at approximately 60 mmHg. In the absence of cerebral ischemia, aggressive attempts to maintain cerebral perfusion pressure (CPP) about 70 mmHg with fluids and pressors should be avoided because of the risk of acute respiratory distress syndrome.[13] Increased ICP should be treated vigorously. The management of the typical severe TBI patient with ICP monitoring at our institution is outlined in Table 26.5.

Mannitol

Mannitol is effective for control of raised ICP after severe TBI. Limited data suggest that intermittent bolus doses may be more effective than continuous infusion. Effective doses range from 0.25 to 1 g/kg body weight. Hypovolemia should be avoided by fluid replacement. Serum osmolarity should be kept below 320 mOsm to avoid renal failure. Euvolemia should be maintained by adequate fluid replacement. A Foley catheter must be placed to monitor urine output whenever mannitol is administered. Reduction of ICP reaches a maximum approximately 30 to 60 min after bolus infusion and persists between 90 min and 6 h or longer. Mannitol together with furosemide may cause rapid diuresis and depletion of intravascular volume and electrolytes and is therefore not recommended. Effective doses range from 0.25 to 1 g/kg body weight.

Hyperventilation

Hyperventilation should not be used routinely in patients with TBI because of the risk of further compromising cerebral perfusion.[14] Hyperventilation should be used only for brief periods when there is acute neurological deterioration or if intracranial hypertension is refractory to other treatment interventions. Under these circumstances, we use intraparenchymal brain tissue oxygen monitoring to titrate the degree of hyperventilation and to avoid cerebral ischemia (see Table 26.5). The use of prophylactic hyperventilation ($PaCO_2$

TABLE 26.5. Management of Elevated Intracranial Pressure (ICP) in the Patient with Severe TBI.

In all patients with GCS score below 9	*Add if ICP >20 mmHg*	*Add if ICP >25 mmHg*	*Add for persistent ICP >25 mmHg*	*Add for persistent ICP >25 mmHg or pupillary abnormalities*
ICP monitoring				
Elevate head of bed 30°	Ventricular CSF drainage	Neuromuscular blockade: vecuronium, atracurium	Moderate hypothermia, core temperature 34°–36°C	High-dose propofol infusion
Maintain euvolemia and hemodynamic stability, keep CVP 5–10 mmHg	Sedation: midazolam or lorazepam	Mannitol 0.25–1 g/kg IV over 5–10 min q 4–6 h PRN; serum osmolarity 300–320 mOsm/L, serum sodium 150–155 mEq/L	Hyperventilation to $PaCO_2$ 30–35 mmHg	Hyperventilation to $PaCO_2$ 25–30 mmHg
PaO_2 > 90 mmHg	Analgesia: fentanyl or morphine			Consider hypertonic saline bolus infusion; consider decompressive craniectomy
$PaCO_2$ 35–40 mmHg				
Systolic blood pressure >90 mmHg	"CPP management": inotropic and pressor support to maintain CPP (dopamine, 5–20 μg/kg/min, norepinephrine, 0.05–0.5 μg/kg/min			
CPP approximately 70 mmHg	Repeat head CT to exclude operable mass lesion			

CSF, cerebrospinal fluid; CVP, central venous pressure; CPP, cerebral perfusion pressure; CT, computed tomography.

<35 mmHg) therapy during the first 24 h after severe TBI should be avoided because hypocarbia causes a cerebral vasoconstriction response and can compromise cerebral perfusion.

Hypertonic Saline

Hypertonic saline is now being used as a second-tier therapy in the treatment of intracranial hypertension resistant to conventional treatment maneuvers. Hypertonic saline has been used both as a bolus infusion for treatment of acutely elevated ICP (up to concentrations of 23.4% NaCl) and as a continuous infusion of 1.8% to 3% saline (or sodium acetate, if saline-induced or (potentiated metabolic acidosis is problematic) to increase serum osmolarity.[15–23] Hypertonic saline decreases ICP by reducing brain water content. Clinical data demonstrate that bolus infusion decreases ICP reliably in patients in whom mannitol has lost its effectiveness. A hyperosmolar state with serum osmolarities well above 320 mOsm/L may develop, but this state seems to be tolerated well so long as euvolemia and arterial normotension are maintained.

Glucocorticoids

Glucocorticoids have been shown to not improve outcome after severe TBI.[4] A recent international trial has shown that corticosteroids are associated with increased rates of severe disability and death when used in the treatment of patients with significant TBI.[24]

Propofol

Propofol at low doses is used commonly for baseline sedation in patients requiring mechanical ventilation. Propofol is a useful sedative for many reasons, including its short half-life, metabolism, and elimination that depends on neither hepatic nor renal function, and the induction of 10 to 15 min of retrograde amnesia because short-term memory is impaired. Propofol infusion can be stopped on as little as 10 to 15 min advance notice for the performance of a reliable neurological examination. In recent years, high-dose propofol has gained popularity as an alternative to barbiturates in patients with intracranial hypertension refractory to maximal medical and surgical ICP-lowering therapy.[25] The main advantage of propofol is that it is short acting, but it can cause hypotension, and, even though ICP decreases, overall cerebral perfusion pressure may drop. Prolonged use of propofol can cause hyperlipidemia. Propofol should not be used in pediatric patients.

Nutritional Support

Studies have shown that not feeding severely head-injured patients by the first week increases mortality. Enteral feedings should be administered, ideally nasoduodenally, within the first 2 days after TBI. However, intestinal ileus is common after TBI, and this condition may preclude early use of the gut for nutritional support.

Prophylaxis and Treatment of Seizures

Posttraumatic seizures (PTS) are divided into early (less than 7 days after TBI) and late seizures. In recent TBI studies that followed high-risk patients up to 36 months, the incidence of early PTS varied between 4% and 25%, and the incidence of late PTS varied between 9% to 42% without prophylaxis. Prophylaxis with phenytoin, carbamazepine, or phenobarbital is not recommended for preventing late PTS.[4] Anticonvulsant prophylaxis with either phenytoin or carbamazepine is effective for prevention of early PTS in patients at high risk for seizures following head injury. However, the available evidence does not indicate that prevention of early PTS improves outcome following head injury. Prophylaxis for longer than 1 week following head injury is therefore not recommended. If late PTS occurs, patients should be managed in accordance with standard approaches to patients with new-onset seizures. A common confounder of the administration of anticonvulsants is the development of fever. Drug fever is a diagnosis of exclusion after infectious and other noninfectious causes of fever. Fever may develop 1 to 8 weeks after exposure to phenytoin, phenobarbital, or carbamazepine.

Barbiturate Coma

High-dose barbiturate therapy may be considered in hemodynamically stable, salvageable, severe TBI patients with intracranial hypertension refractory to maximal medical and surgical ICP-lowering therapy. Barbiturates appear to exert their cerebral protective and ICP-lowering effects through several distinct mechanisms: alterations in vascular tone, suppression of metabolism, and inhibition of free radical-mediated lipid peroxidation. The most important effect may relate to coupling of cerebral blood flow to regional metabolic demands, such that the lower the metabolic requirements, the less the cerebral blood flow and related cerebral blood volume with subsequent beneficial effects on ICP and global cerebral perfusion. However, serum concentration, therapeutic benefit, and systemic complications correlate poorly. The risk of arterial hypotension induced by peripheral vasodilation is high. A reliable form of monitoring is the electroencephalographic pattern of burst suppression. Near-maximal reductions in cerebral metabolism and cerebral blood flow occur when burst suppression is induced. To conduct a reliable brain death examination, pentobarbital concentration should be 1 mg/dL (10 μg/mL) or less.

Surgical Management

The decision as to whether an intracranial lesion requires surgical evacuation can be difficult to make and is based on the patient's GCS score, pupillary examination findings, comorbidities, CT findings, age, and, in delayed decisions, the ICP. Neurological deterioration over time is also an important factor influencing the decision to operate. Trauma patients presenting to the emergency department with altered mental status, pupillary asymmetry, and abnormal flexion or extension are at high risk for an intracranial mass lesion, and it is prudent to notify the operating room that an emergency craniotomy will most likely be necessary even before obtaining a CT scan.

Epidural Hematoma

The incidence of surgical and nonsurgical epidural hematoma (EDH) among TBI patients is around 3%. Among patients in coma, up to 9% harbor an EDH requiring craniotomy. The peak incidence of EDH is in the second decade of life, and the mean age of patients with EDH is between 20 and 30 years.

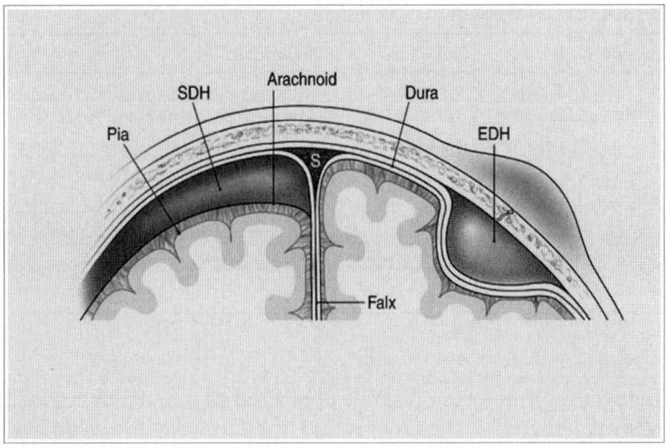

FIGURE 26.3. A subdural hematoma (*SDH*) below the dura mater on the patient's right side. An epidural hematoma (*EDH*), above the dura mater, is shown on the patient's left with a skull fracture and scalp hematoma overlying.

Traffic-related incidents, falls, and assaults account for the majority of all cases of EDH, which usually results from injury to the middle meningeal artery that is related to an overlying parietal skull fracture. However, EDH can also be caused by bleeding from the middle meningeal vein, the diploic veins, or the venous sinuses (Fig. 26.3). Among patients with EDH, one-third to one-half are comatose on admission or immediately before surgery. The classically described "lucid interval," which describes a patient who is initially unconscious, but who then awakens, only to deteriorate soon after, is observed in approximately one-half of patients who undergo surgery for EDH. Increased magnitude of clot thickness, hematoma volume, and midline shift (MLS) on the preoperative CT scan are all related to an adverse outcome.

Noncomatose patients without focal neurological deficits who harbor an acute EDH of less than 15 mm thickness, a MLS less than 5 mm, and a hematoma volume less than 30 mL can be managed nonoperatively with serial CT scanning and close neurosurgical evaluation (Fig. 26.4). The first follow-up CT scan in stable patients managed nonoperatively should be obtained within 6 to 8 h after TBI. Epidural hematoma overlying the temporal lobe is associated with a higher likelihood of successful nonoperative management and should lower the threshold for surgery. Patients with a GCS score less than 9 and an EDH larger than 30 mL should undergo immediate surgical evacuation of the lesion,[5] but all patients should be considered for surgery if the volume of their EDH exceeds 30 mL, regardless of GCS scores. Patients with an EDH volume less than 30 mL should be considered for surgery but may be managed successfully without surgery in selected cases. Patients who deteriorate during evaluation must undergo surgical evaluation as soon as possible. Prolongation of the time from neurological deterioration to surgery correlates inversely with outcome; every hour of delay in surgery is associated with progressively worsened outcome.[26–28]

Acute Subdural Hematoma

A subdural hematoma (SDH) is diagnosed by CT scan as an extracerebral, hyperdense, crescentic collection between the dura and the brain parenchyma (see Figure 26.3); these can be divided into acute and chronic lesions. The incidence of acute SDH is between 12% and 29% in patients admitted with severe TBI. The mean age of affected patients is between 31 and 47 years, with most patients being male. Most SDHs are caused by motor vehicle-related accidents, falls, and assaults. Falls have been identified as the main cause of traumatic SDH in patients older than 75 years of age. Between 37% and 80% of patients with acute SDH present with initial GCS scores of 8 or below. Clot thickness or volume and MLS on the preoperative CT scan also correlate inversely with outcome of acute SDH. Patients with SDH presenting with a clot thickness of greater than 10 mm or MLS greater than 5 mm should undergo surgical evacuation, regardless of the GCS score (Figure 26.5).[5] Patients who present with SDH in coma (GCS score less than 9) but with a clot thickness of less than 10 mm and MLS less than 5 mm can be treated nonoperatively, providing that they undergo ICP monitoring, are neurologically stable since injury, have no pupillary abnormalities, and do not have intracranial hypertension (ICP >20 mmHg). For comatose patients or patients with progressive neurological deterioration, urgent evacuation is necessary.[27,29,30]

Traumatic Parenchymal Lesions

Traumatic parenchymal mass lesions occur in up to 10% of all patients with TBI and 13% to 35% of patients with severe

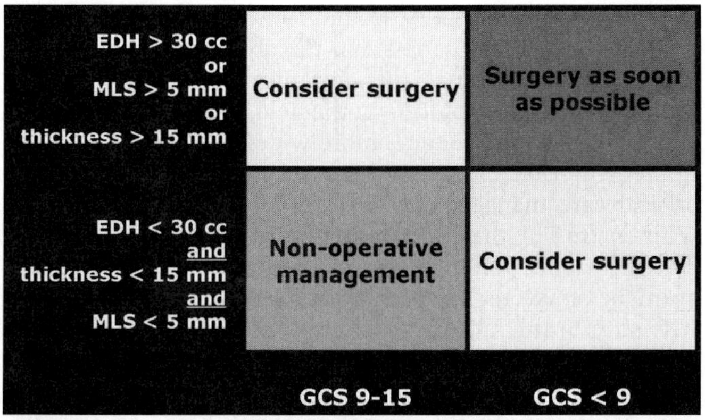

FIGURE 26.4. Considerations for nonoperative versus operative management of epidural hematomas (*EDH*). *MLS*, midline shift; *GCS*, Glasgow Coma Scale.

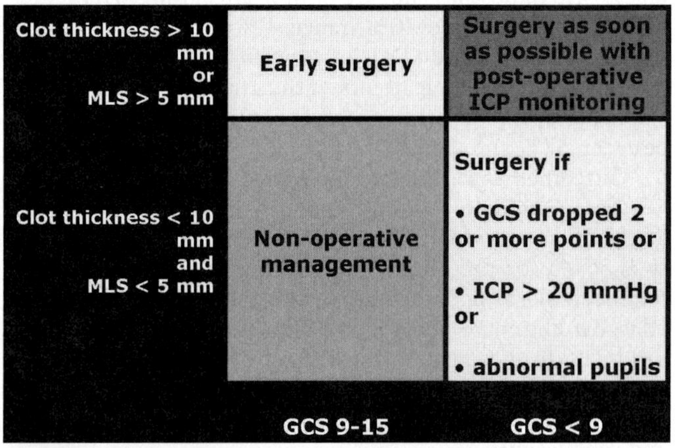

FIGURE 26.5. Considerations for nonoperative versus operative management of subdural hematomas (SDH). *MLS*, midline shift; *GCS*, Glasgow Coma Scale.

TBI. Most small parenchymal lesions do not require surgical evacuation. However, the development of mass effect from larger lesions may result in secondary brain injury, placing the patient at risk of further neurological deterioration, herniation, and death. Parenchymal lesions tend to evolve, and the timing of the surgery affects the outcome. Patients with parenchymal mass lesions and signs of progressive neurological deterioration referable to the lesion, medically refractory intracranial hypertension, or signs of mass effect on CT scan should be treated operatively.[5] Comatose patients with frontal or temporal contusions greater than 20 mL in volume and with MLS of 5 mm or cisternal compression on CT scan, or both, and patients with any lesion greater than 50 mL in volume should be treated surgically. Patients with parenchymal mass lesions who do not show evidence for neurological compromise, have controlled ICP, and have no signs of substantial mass effect on CT scan can be managed nonoperatively.

Depressed Skull Fractures

Depressed skull fractures complicate up to 6% of head injuries, and the presence of skull fracture is associated with a higher incidence of intracranial lesions, neurological deficit, and poorer outcome. Patients with open skull fractures depressed more than the thickness of the skull should undergo surgical intervention to prevent infection. Patients with open depressed skull fractures should receive antibiotic prophylaxis for 24 h.[5]

Decompressive Craniectomy for Control of Intracranial Hypertension

Decompressive procedures, such as subtemporal decompression, temporal lobectomy, and hemispheric decompressive craniectomy, are surgical procedures that are used to treat patients with refractory intracranial hypertension and diffuse parenchymal injury. Decompressive craniectomy can be very effective if it is done early after TBI in young patients who are expected to develop postoperative brain swelling and intracranial hypertension.[5]

Early Prognostic Indicators of Severe TBI

Following admission, ICP greater than 20 mmHg is a poor prognostic indicator. The rate of mortality from EDH requiring surgery is around 10% (range, 7%–12.5%). The rate of mortality from acute SDH is between 40% and 60%.[5] The mortality rate among patients with acute SDH presenting to the hospital in coma with subsequent surgical evacuation is between 57% and 68%.[5]

Outcome from TBI is frequently described using the Glasgow Outcome Scale at 6 months following TBI (Table 26.6). This is a widely accepted and standardized scale that is of value for the clinical description of patients and also for medicolegal documentation and research purposes. The Glasgow Outcome Scale is poor for assessing patients with mild TBI. In these patients, more refined outcome measures are used that describe functional status based on neuropsychological testing, cognitive function, return-to-work data, and productivity.

The most important early presenting factors influencing outcome from severe TBI are age, GCS score, pupillary examination findings, the presence of arterial hypotension, and CT scan findings.[31]

TABLE 26.6. Glasgow Outcome Scale.

Score	*Rating*	*Definition*
5	Good	Recovery: resumption of normal life despite minor deficits.
4	Moderate disability	Disabled but independent. Can work in sheltered setting.
3	Severe disability	Conscious but severely disabled. Dependent for daily support.
2	Persistent vegetative	No conscious behavior.
1	Death	

The probability of poor outcome increases with decreasing admission GCS score in a continuous, stepwise manner below a GCS score of 9. Patients with very low GCS scores have a mortality rate between 70% and 90%, but up to 10% may survive with Glasgow Outcome Scale scores of 4 or 5. Increasing age is a strong independent factor in prognosis from severe TBI, with a significant increase in poor outcome in patients older than 60 years of age; this is not explained by the increased frequency of systemic complications in older patients. Several studies confirm that comatose patients with acute herniation made a good recovery. The pupillary diameter and the pupilloconstrictor light reflex can also prognosticate outcome from severe TBI. Bilaterally unreactive pupils following resuscitation on admission are associated with a greater than 90% chance of poor outcome. A systolic blood pressure less than 90 mmHg measured en route to the hospital after severe TBI or while hospitalized has been associated with a nearly 70% likelihood of a poor outcome. Combined with hypoxia, this likelihood increases to 79%. Even a single recording of arterial hypotension doubles the rate of mortality from severe TBI. Among these early prognostic indicators of outcome, arterial hypotension is the only factor that can be significantly affected by therapeutic intervention.

The CT scan findings associated with poor outcome from severe TBI are compressed or absent basal cisterns, traumatic subarachnoid hemorrhage, and MLS greater than 5 mm.[31]

Conclusion

Overall, the mortality from severe TBI has been reduced from as much as 50% in the 1970s and 1980s to between 15% and 25% in most recent series.[1,2] In the absence of any pharmacological breakthrough, this improvement is attributed to more effective resuscitation in the field, rapid transport of TBI patients to trauma centers, more widespread acceptance and implementation of ICP monitoring, and improvements in critical care management. In a recent study of 93 patients with severe TBI, the 6-month mortality rate was reduced 50% by the introduction of evidence-based protocols for the management of severe TBI.[2] The treatment guidelines supported ICP monitoring, adequate volume resuscitation, aggressive treatment of low blood pressure and oxygenation, avoidance of extreme hyperventilation, and early nutritional intervention. Multidisciplinary clinical pathways based on scientifically sound, evidence-based treatment guidelines for TBI streamline patient care, standardize critical care management, and hold the potential for substantial improvements in patient outcome and reduced costs. Early recognition and treatment of cerebral hypoperfusion and intracranial hypertension are key to managing these patients. Medical personnel in the prehospital and trauma center settings should be aware of and trained in these principles of TBI care.

References

1. Fakhry SM, Trask AL, Waller MA, et al. Management of brain-injured patients by an evidence-based medicine protocol improves outcomes and decreases hospital charges. J Trauma 2004;56:492–499.
2. Palmer S, Bader M, Qureshi A, et al. The impact on outcomes in a community hospital setting of using the AANS traumatic brain injury guidelines. American Association for Neurologic Surgeons. J Trauma 2001;50:657–664.
3. Guidelines for Prehospital Mangement of Traumatic Brain Injury. New York: Brain Trauma Foundation, 2000.
4. Guidelines for the Management of Severe Traumatic Brain Injury. J Neurotrauma 2000;17:449–554.
5. Langlois JA, Rutland-Brown W, Wald MM. The epidemiology and impact of traumatic brain injury: a brief overview. J Head Trauma Rehabil 2006;21:375–378.
6. Sosin D, Sniezek J, Waxweiler R. Trends in death associated with traumatic brain injury. JAMA 1995;273:1778–1780.
7. Stocchetti N, Furlan A, Volta F. Hypoxemia and arterial hypotension at the accident scene in head injury. J Trauma 1996;40: 764–767.
8. Chesnut R, Marshall L, Klauber M, et al. The role of secondary brain injury in determining outcome from severe head injury. J Trauma 1993;34:216–222.
9. Unterberg AW, Stover J, Kress B, et al. Edema and brain trauma. Neuroscience 2004;129:1021–1029.
10. Narayan RK, Michel ME, Ansell B, et al. Clinical trials in head injury. J Neurotrauma 2002;19:503–557.
11. The Brain Trauma Foundation. The American Association of Neurological Surgeons. The Joint Section on Neurotrauma and Critical Care. Indications for intracranial pressure monitoring. J Neurotrauma 2000;17:479–491.
12. Update Notice. Guidelines for the management of severe traumatic brain injury: cerebral perfusion pressure. Neurotrauma Crit Care News 2004;7:3.
13. Robertson CS, Valadka AB, Hannay HJ, et al. Prevention of secondary ischemic insults after severe head injury. Crit Care Med 1999;27:2086–2095.
14. The Brain Trauma Foundation. The American Association of Neurological Surgeons. The Joint Section on Neurotrauma and Critical Care. Hyperventilation. J Neurotrauma 2000;17:513–520.
15. Battison C, Andrews PJ, Graham C, et al. Randomized, controlled trial on the effect of a 20% mannitol solution and a 7.5% saline/6% dextran solution on increased intracranial pressure after brain injury. Crit Care Med 2005;33:196–202.
16. Hartl R, Ghajar J, Hochleuthner H, et al. Hypertonic/hyperoncotic saline reliably reduces ICP in severely head-injured patients with intracranial hypertension. Acta Neurochir Suppl (Wien) 1997;70:126–129.
17. Horn P, Munch E, Vajkoczy P, et al. Hypertonic saline solution for control of elevated intracranial pressure in patients with exhausted response to mannitol and barbiturates. Neurol Res 1999;21:758–764.
18. Munar F, Ferrer AM, de Nadal M, et al. Cerebral hemodynamic effects of 7.2% hypertonic saline in patients with head injury and raised intracranial pressure. J Neurotrauma 2000;17:41–51.
19. Qureshi AI, Suarez JI, Bhardwaj A, et al. Use of hypertonic (3%) saline/acetate infusion in the treatment of cerebral edema: effect on intracranial pressure and lateral displacement of the brain. Crit Care Med 1998;26:440–446.
20. Qureshi AI, Suarez JI, Castro A, et al. Use of hypertonic saline/acetate infusion in treatment of cerebral edema in patients with head trauma: experience at a single center. J Trauma 1999;47:659–665.
21. Schatzmann C, Heissler HE, Konig K, et al. Treatment of elevated intracranial pressure by infusions of 10% saline in severely head injured patients. Acta Neurochir Suppl (Wien) 1998;71:31–33.
22. Shackford SR, Bourguignon PR, Wald SL, et al. Hypertonic saline resuscitation of patients with head injury: a prospective, randomized clinical trial. J Trauma 1998;44:50–58.
23. Vialet R, Albanese J, Thomachot L, et al. Isovolume hypertonic solutes (sodium chloride or mannitol) in the treatment of refractory posttraumatic intracranial hypertension: 2 mL/kg 7.5% saline is more effective than 2 mL/kg 20% mannitol. Crit Care Med 2004;31:1683–1687.
24. Edwards P, Arango M, Balica L, et al. Final results of MRC CRASH, a randomised placebo-controlled trial of intravenous corticosteroid in adults with head injury-outcomes at 6 months. Lancet 2005;365:1957–1959.
25. Oertel M, Kelly DF, Lee JH, et al. Efficacy of hyperventilation, blood pressure elevation, and metabolic suppression therapy in controlling intracranial pressure after head injury. J Neurosurg 2002;97:1045–1053.
26. Cohen J, Montero A, Israel Z. Prognosis and clinical relevance of anisocoria-craniotomy latency for epidural hematoma in comatose patients. J Trauma 1996;41:120–122.
27. Haselsberger K, Pucher R, Auer L. Prognosis after acute subdural or epidural haemorrhage. Acta Neurochir (Wien) 1988;90:111–116.
28. Lee E, Hung Y, Wang L, et al. Factors influencing the functional outcome of patients with acute epidural hematomas: analysis of 200 patients undergoing surgery. J Trauma 1998;45:B946–B952.
29. Sakas D, Bullock M, Teasdale G. One-year outcome following craniotomy for traumatic hematoma in patients with fixed dilated pupils. J Neurosurg 1995;82:961–965.
30. Wilberger JJ, Harris M, Diamond D. Acute subdural hematoma: morbidity and mortality related to timing of operative intervention. J Trauma 1990;30:F733–F736.
31. Jiang JY, Gao GY, Li WP, et al. Early indicators of the prognosis in 846 cases of severe traumatic brain injury. J Neurotrauma 2002;19:869–874.

27

Trauma to the Torso

Deborah M. Stein and Thomas M. Scalea

Injuries to the torso account for a large portion of deaths from trauma. Second only to death from central nervous system injury, hemorrhage accounts for 30%–40% of traumatic deaths.[1,2] Most commonly, bleeding is secondary to injury to the chest or abdomen.[3] Thoracic injury alone accounts for 20% to 25% of all trauma deaths,[4] most commonly caused by injury to the heart or great vessels. Minor injury to the thorax is common, including rib fracture, pneumothorax, and pulmonary contusion. Major abdominal injuries occur in approximately 25% of severely injured patients and are often associated with multiple system injuries.[5]

The incidences of abdominal and chest injuries vary depending on the mechanism of injury. Mechanisms are generally divided into two categories: blunt and penetrating. The percentage of patients injured by these mechanisms varies widely, depending on the location and environment in which the injury occurs. For example, urban settings tend to have a higher percentage of penetrating injuries as compared to rural settings. The injury patterns, and therefore diagnosis and treatment algorithms, vary considerably depending on the mechanism.

Diagnosis

Penetrating Trauma

Penetrating trauma to the torso can present a complex diagnostic and therapeutic challenge. Injuries can occur to the precordium, the thoracoabdominal region, abdomen, flank, back, or pelvis (Figure 27.1). Often these injuries occur to several body regions from either single or multiple missiles. Each of these body regions may require a different approach for both diagnosis and treatment. Penetration from the nipple line to the inguinal ligaments anteriorly and from the tip of the scapula to the inferior gluteal folds posteriorly should prompt suspicion of intraabdominal injury. The degree of hemodynamic stability dictates the initial approach to these patients. Figure 27.2 depicts an algorithm for the diagnostic workup of patients with penetrating injury to the torso.

Physical Examination

For penetrating injuries, often a rapid evaluation of the sites of entry of missiles or stab wounds allows for determination of the need for further evaluation or operation. For instance, transaxial gunshot wounds are associated with a much higher mortality and higher incidence of cardiac, vascular, and spinal injuries. Incorrect initial incisions, missed injuries, and the need for early operation are more frequent in the transaxial group as compared to patients with unilateral injury.[6] In addition, a palpable bullet and determination of bullet tracts helps set priorities and determine the plan of care.[7]

Although auscultation of the chest may sometimes reveal a pneumothorax or hemothorax, several authors have described the potential inaccuracies of physical examination alone in penetrating injuries to the chest.[8–10] However, the high positive predictive value of physical examination for detection of abnormal breath sounds in penetrating chest trauma does not require radiographic confirmation before treatment of hemo- or pneumothorax.[8,10,11]

The physical examination of the patient who has sustained penetrating trauma to the abdomen can be useful in determining the need for operative intervention versus further diagnostic workup. Serial physical examinations alone, in the hemodynamically stable patient, can identify the need for operative intervention.[12–16] Penetrating injuries to the flank

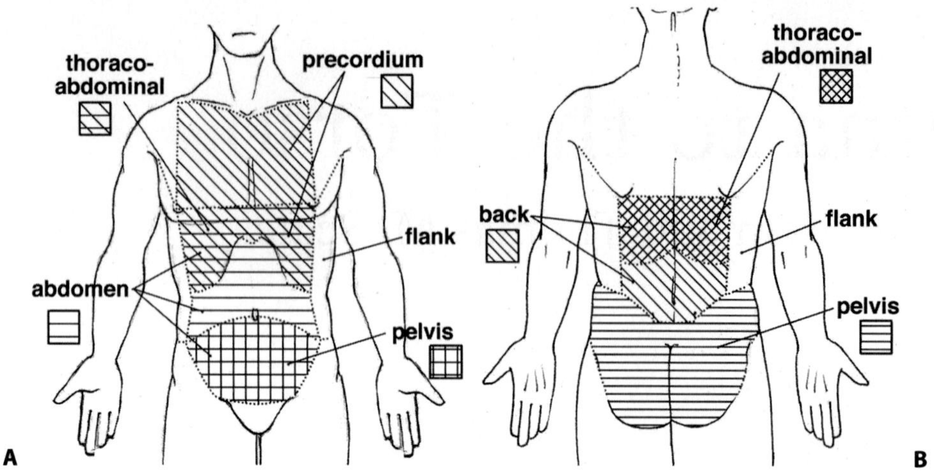

FIGURE 27.1. **A.** Anterior view. **B.** Posterior view. Penetrating trauma can occur to the precordium, thoracoabdominal region, abdomen, flank, back, or pelvis.

and back are somewhat more problematic, with physical examination being less reliable.[16,17] In the patient with stable vital signs, the presence of peritonitis or evisceration is the clearest indication for celiotomy.

Radiographs

The accuracy of detection of hemo- or pneumothorax is increased greatly with the addition of chest radiography.[8–10] Additionally, a normal chest X-ray and physical examination are sufficient to evaluate for thoracic vascular injury with 100% sensitivity and negative predictive value.[18] A normal chest X-ray following penetrating chest trauma with one 3-h follow-up film is sufficient to rule out hemo- or pneumothorax and allow for safe hospital discharge.[19] Few published data are available to evaluate the efficacy of plain radiographs in the setting of penetrating injury to the abdomen or flank, but, clearly, meaningful information can be gained from radiographs that demonstrate bullet fragments or pneumoperitoneum.

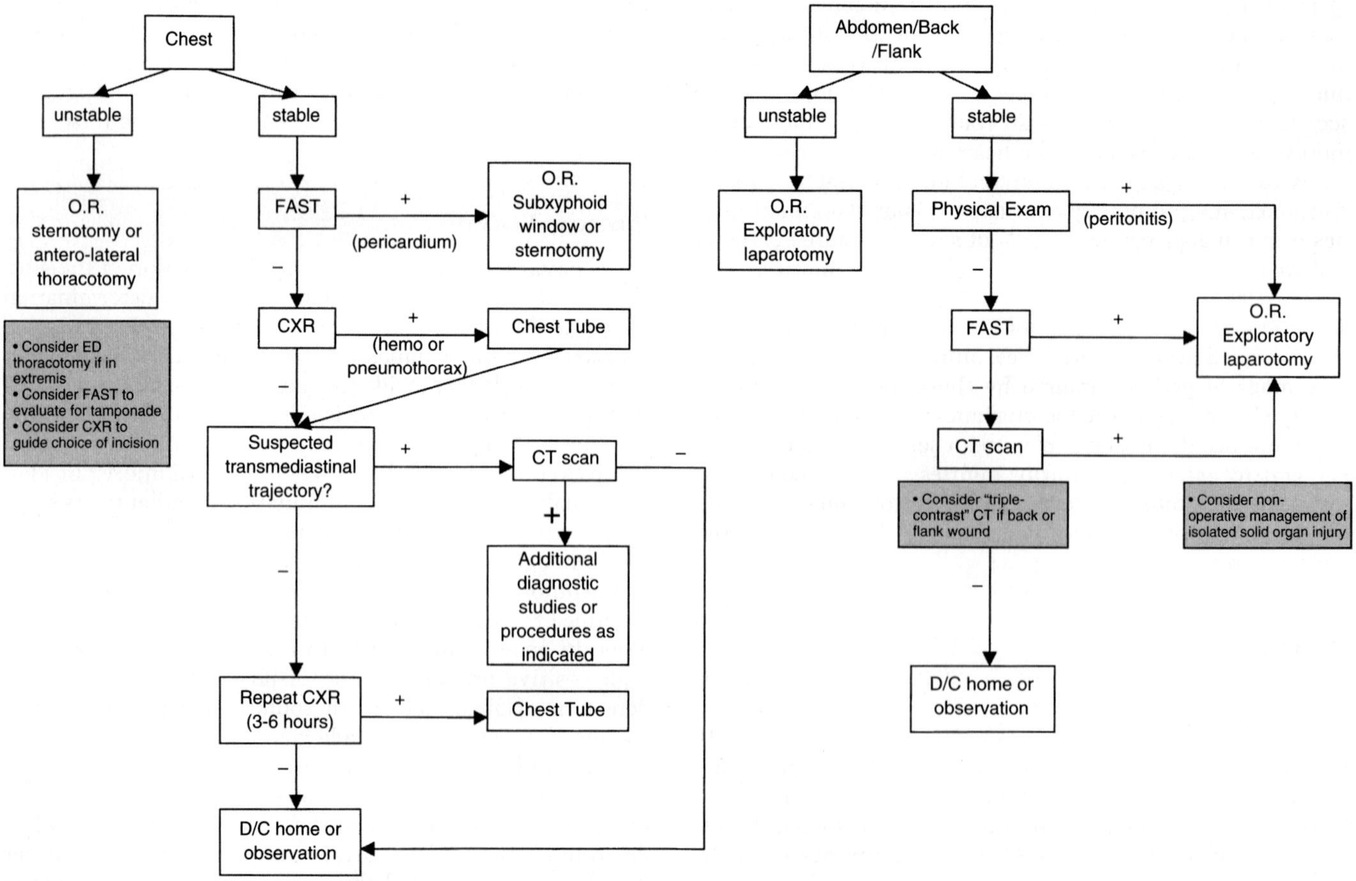

FIGURE 27.2. Algorithm for the evaluation of penetrating torso trauma. *CXR*, chest radiograph; *FAST*, focused assessment for sonography in trauma; *O.R.*, operating room; *ED*, emergency department; *DPL*, diagnostic peritoneal lavage; *D/C*, discharge; *CT*, computed tomography.

Local Wound Exploration

In the setting of stab wounds to the anterior abdomen, local wound exploration can diagnose fascial penetration. The exploration can be performed in the emergency department with the use of local anesthetic. If the wound has not caused fascial penetration, it is safe to treat the wound locally and discharge the patient. Penetrating injuries to the chest, back, and flank should never be explored locally; other diagnostic modalities should be employed to determine the depth of penetration and underlying injury.

Diagnostic Peritoneal Lavage

Root et al. first described diagnostic peritoneal lavage (DPL) in 1965 for the evaluation of blunt abdominal trauma.[20] Since that time, a number of investigators have extended its use for evaluation of penetrating trauma, either alone or in combination with local wound exploration for stab wounds.[21–25] Three techniques have been described: the "open" technique, the "semiopen" technique, and the Seldinger technique. Despite the invasive nature of this test, each of these techniques is associated with relatively low complication rates (0.5%–1%).[26–30] The red blood cell count criterion for a positive lavage in penetrating trauma has varied widely in the literature from 1,000 to 50,000 cells/mm^3; this uncertainty has caused a significant variation in reported sensitivity (85%–99%) and specificity (43%–99%) for detection of intraabdominal injury.[22–24] The presence of enteric material or bile in the setting of penetrating trauma should prompt surgical exploration. Many have questioned the sensitivity of DPL for penetrating injuries to the back and flank because of the incidence of missed retroperitoneal injuries.[31,32] A positive DPL in the setting of a back or flank injury should prompt exploration. Limitations of this technique include its relative contraindication in patients with previous laparotomies. With the advent of better technology and increasing availability of ultrasound and computed tomography scans, the use of DPL in penetrating trauma has decreased substantially.

Computed Tomographic Scanning

The computed tomography (CT) scan has value in the diagnosis of penetrating injuries to the torso. Although it is rare to have major thoracic injury with a normal plain radiograph, CT scan of the chest can often detect occult pneumo- or hemothorax and fractures. Hemodynamically stable patients with transmediastinal gunshot wounds were classically evaluated with angiography, esophagoscopy, or esophagography, and possibly, bronchoscopy. Recent work by Hanpeter et al. has described the accuracy of helical CT scan in the detection of mediastinal injury.[33] This work was later validated by other authors.[34] The use of CT scan for these types of injuries is now widely accepted as standard.

The use of CT scans to diagnose penetrating injuries to the flank and back has also become standard in hemodynamically stable patients. First described by Meyer et al. for selective management of patients with stab wounds to the back, the use of CT has become widely accepted for the diagnosis of intra- and retroperitoneal injuries from penetrating wounds of the back and flank.[35,36] The addition of rectal contrast instillation with colonic opacification plus intravenous and oral contrast has been advocated to improve sensitivity and specificity to nearly 100%.[37–39]

Despite early concerns about the low sensitivity of CT scan for the diagnosis of hollow viscus injury,[26,27,40,41] improvements in technology and the use of helical CT have largely alleviated these concerns. Several large series have described the usefulness of CT scan in stable patients for penetrating injuries to the anterior, as well as posterior, torso.[36,42–49] CT is useful in this context not only to determine whether peritoneal or retroperitoneal violation has occurred but also to evaluate injuries that may be managed nonoperatively, such as isolated solid organ injury. Table 27.1 presents representative clinical experiences with the use of CT scan for the diagnosis of penetrating torso injury.

Ultrasound

The use of ultrasound in the setting of torso trauma has been described and evaluated widely. In both prospective and retrospective reviews, focused assessment for sonography in trauma (FAST) has been found to be highly reliable in the detection of hemoperitoneum, hemopericardium, and hemothorax in trauma patients.[50–58] The technique includes placing a 3.5-MHz tranducer in the pericardial, right upper quadrant, left upper quadrant, and pelvic regions to evaluate for the presence of free fluid. This method has been extended to include an evaluation of the right and left subdiaphragmatic regions to determine the presence of pleural fluid.[54] The EFAST, or extended FAST, has also been used to detect pneumothorax with a higher sensitivity than chest radiograph (49% vs. 21%), and equivalent specificity (99%).[59] One recent study demonstrated 100% sensitivity, specificity, positive predictive value, and negative predictive value for the detection of pneumothorax following penetrating thoracic trauma.[60] Large studies of the use of FAST in combined groups of penetrating and blunt trauma patients have demonstrated overall sensitivity of 81% to 90%, specificity of 99% to 100%, and accuracy of 99% for the detection of pleural fluid.[50–54] In the presence of hemoperitoneum, the FAST exam is most commonly positive in the right upper quadrant of the abdomen, even in the presence of isolated splenic injuries.[61]

Several studies have looked specifically at the use of the FAST in penetrating torso trauma.[55–58] One multicenter trial demonstrated a sensitivity of 100% and specificity of 97% for the detection of hemopericardium in penetrating precordial injuries, resulting in minimal delay to operation.[62] Another study demonstrated 100% sensitivity and 99.3% specificity in patients with penetrating precordial or transthoracic trauma.[52] However, other studies have reported lower sensitivities of 46% to 67% and specificities of 94% to 100% for the presence of intraperitoneal or intrapericardial fluid. A negative FAST examination after penetrating abdominal trauma does not exclude intraperitoneal injury, and further evaluation is always warranted.[55,57,58] In patients with positive examinations, operative intervention is usually indicated. Additionally, the EFAST exam can be valuable in determining the correct operative site in hemodynamically unstable patients with multicavitary penetration.

Laparoscopy

The use of laparoscopy in trauma was first described by Gazzaniga et al. in 1976.[63] Since that time numerous reports

TABLE 27.1.
Representative Clinical Experience with CT Scan for the Diagnosis of Penetrating Torso Trauma.

Trial	*Year*	*Level of evidence*	*Number of patients*	*Intervention/design*	*Median follow-up*	*Minor endpoint*	*Major endpoint*	*Interpretations/comments*
33	2000	II	24	All patients with suspected transmediastinal trajectory underwent CT scan, followed by angiography or esophageal evaluation as indicated	N/A	N/A	Identification of mediastinal injury on CT scan	Demonstrated that CT scan was a reliable and safe screening test to evaluate missile trajectory in hemodynamically stable patients with suspected transmediastinal gunshot wounds and to identify patients who would benefit from additional studies.
34	2002	III	22	Chart review of patients who had CT scans of the chest to evaluate transmediastinal gunshot wounds	N/A	N/A	Identification of mediastinal trajectory with CT scan	CT scan of the chest can be used to screen for patients with a transmediastinal trajectory to evaluate who would benefit from additional imaging
42	1998	III	50	Review of patients with gunshot wounds to the torso who underwent CT scan for diagnosis of trajectory and injury	4.3 days	N/A	Identification of transthoracic, transperitoneal, or transmediastinal trajectory and identification of injuries	CT of the chest and abdomen are useful in identifying patients who require laparotomy or further diagnostic testing and may identify injuries that can be safely observed.
36	1998	III	83	Chart review of patients with CT scan performed for evaluation of flank and abdominal gunshot wounds.	N/A	N/A	Identification of peritoneal violation and intraperitoneal injuries with CT scan	In hemodynamically stable patients with gunshot wounds to the flank or abdomen, CT scan can safely and effectively evaluate for injuries that necessitate laparotomy and those that may be observed. With equivocal studies, laparoscopy may be helpful in determining if peritoneal penetration had occurred. Overall accuracy for anterior abdominal wounds was 71% and 98% for flank wounds.
48	1999	III	16	Review of patients selected for nonoperative management of gunshot wounds to the liver diagnosed by CT scan	11.7 days	N/A	Failure of nonoperative management	CT scan can identify hemodynamically stable patients who may be managed non-operatively. Patients must be monitored closely as the failure rate in this series was more than 30%.
44	2001	II	75	Prospective study of patients who underwent CT scan of the abdomen for penetrating abdominal, back, flank, lower chest, or pelvis wounds	N/A	N/A	Identification of peritoneal violation and intraperitoneal injuries with CT scan	CT scan of patients with penetrating torso trauma accurately predicts the need for laparotomy, excludes peritoneal violation, and can identify patients who may be managed nonoperatively. The use of rectal contrast is helpful in identifying rectal or colonic injuries.
45*	2001	II	104	Prospective study of patients who underwent CT scan of the abdomen for penetrating abdominal, back, flank, lower chest, or pelvis wounds	N/A	N/A	Identification of peritoneal violation and intraperitoneal injuries with CT scan	CT scan of patients with penetrating torso trauma accurately predicts the need for laparotomy, excludes peritoneal violation, and can identify patients who may be managed nonoperatively. A 97% accuracy was reported in predicting the need for laparotomy.
46**	2004	II	242	Prospective study of patients who underwent CT scan of the abdomen for penetrating abdominal, back, flank, lower chest, or pelvis wounds	N/A	N/A	Identification of peritoneal violation and intraperitoneal injuries with CT scan	Penetrating injuries of the torso can be safely evaluated with CT scan in the absence of specific indications for laparotomy. Sensitivity of 97% and specificity of 98% are reported.
32	2004	II	47	Prospective evaluation of hemodynamically stable patients who underwent CT scan for gunshot wounds to the torso	N/A	N/A	Determination of intraabdominal injury by CT scan	Patients with gunshot wounds to the abdomen, back, and flank can safely and accurately be evaluated with CT scan for the presence of intraabdominal injury. Overall accuracy rate was 96% in this study.

CT, computed tomography; N/A, not available.

*Includes patients from Reference 44.

**Includes patients from Reference 45.

and series have described the use of laparoscopy for diagnostic purposes in penetrating torso trauma.[64–76] Laparoscopy is generally used for identification of peritoneal violation in the setting of penetrating trauma. Additionally, evaluation of diaphragmatic injury, a notoriously difficult injury to evaluate, is easily accomplished laparoscopically.[72] However, as technology and experience with laparoscopy increase, formal explorations and treatment of specific injuries have been described.[71,75,77] Studies have shown that the rates of nontherapeutic laparotomies can be decreased with the utilization of diagnostic laparoscopy.[65–68,70,72–76,78] Additionally, the identification of minor isolated solid organ injury from peritoneal penetration with laparoscopy can avoid nontherapeutic laparotomies. However, the sensitivity and specificity for the detection of hollow organ injuries may be poor.[66,70] Thoracoscopy has also been described for diagnosis and treatment of diaphragm injuries in the setting of penetrating trauma.[67,78]

Blunt Trauma

Blunt trauma, most commonly as a result of motor vehicle collisions or falls, accounts for the majority of injuries and deaths from trauma. Severe blunt injuries to the torso often occur in concert with other system injuries, such as major orthopedic, brain, fascial, or spinal cord injury. Several modalities are available to evaluate and diagnose torso injuries, each with inherent strengths and weaknesses. Often multiple modalities play complementary roles. Patients with an abnormal physical examination of either the chest or abdomen require either imaging or operative evaluation. The presence of associated injuries should also prompt further investigation as a consequence of the known association of thoracic and lumbar spine, lower rib, and pelvic fractures with intraperitoneal injury. Hematuria and acute anemia or decreasing hematocrit should prompt investigation as well. Patients with major distracting injuries, severe brain or spinal cord injuries, or drug/alcohol intoxication should also undergo diagnostic evaluation. Figure 27.3 depicts an algorithm for the evaluation of blunt torso trauma.

Physical Examination

Physical examination is the essential first step after blunt trauma. In the hemodynamically unstable patient, auscultation of the lungs or palpation of subcutaneous gas (crepitus)

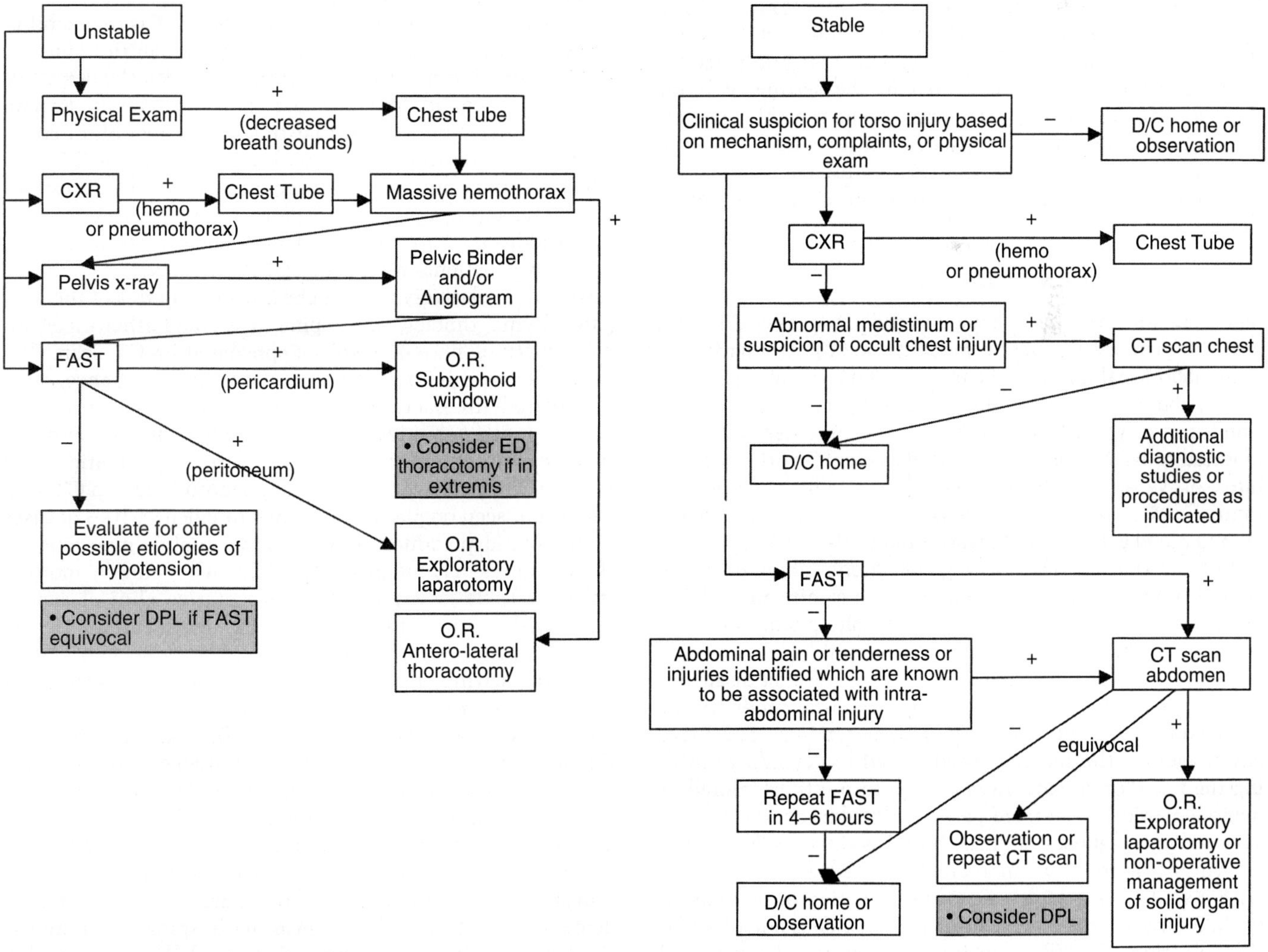

FIGURE 27.3. Algorithm for the evaluation of blunt torso trauma. *CXR*, chest radiograph; *FAST*, focused assessment for sonograph in trauma; *O.R.*, operating room; *ED*, emergency department; *DPL*, diagnostic peritoneal lavage; *D/C*, discharge; *CT*, computed tomography.

may reveal a pneumothorax that may be treated promptly with tube thoracostomy. Some evidence suggests that physical examination of the chest alone may be adequate for the detection of these injuries in blunt trauma patients, and in the presence of abnormal physical examination of the chest, intervention before confirmation with radiography is certainly indicated.[8,9]

In the unstable patient, the presence of abdominal distension or peritonitis on physical examination may be enough to prompt laparotomy. The presence of a "seatbelt sign," noted on physical examination, is associated with a high incidence of intraabdominal injuries.[79–81] There are several situations in which physical examination in the blunt trauma patient has been historically considered inaccurate, including intoxication, multiple injuries, or head injury.[82–84] However, recent data demonstrated that a normal physical examination of the awake and alert patient, even in the presence of mild intoxication, can exclude intraabdominal injury safely and accurately.[85–88]

Radiography

Considering the high incidence of chest injury following blunt injury, plain radiographs offer high-yield information with low risk. Injuries of the bony structures, lungs, heart, or great vessels may be suggested by radiographic abnormalities. A chest X-ray has a high sensitivity but low specificity for the presence of intrathoracic injury. There is little place for plain radiographs of the abdomen in the setting of blunt trauma. However, pelvic radiographs can be valuable in determining and excluding extraperitoneal causes of hemodynamic stability. Abnormal pelvic, thoracic, or lumbar radiographs should also prompt further investigation of intraabdominal injury.[89]

Diagnostic Peritoneal Lavage

Before the routine use of ultrasound and advances in CT, DPL was the primary diagnostic modality for the evaluation of blunt abdominal trauma. The utility of DPL in the evaluation of intraabdominal injuries not detected by physical examination is unequivocal.[90] Sensitivities and specificities have been reported to be 97% and 99%, respectively,[22,91] with accuracy rates of 92% to 98% for detection of blunt abdominal injury.[28,92–96] A positive DPL is generally considered to have 10^5 red blood cells/mm^3 of lavage fluid in the setting of blunt abdominal trauma. The presence of enteric material or bile should prompt surgical exploration. The significance of the presence of elevated amylase or alkaline phosphatase concentrations or white blood cells is controversial.[97–102]

There are a number of discrete advantages and disadvantages to using DPL as the primary diagnostic modality for intraabdominal injury in blunt trauma patients. The main advantages are the superior speed and efficiency in determining the need for surgical intervention in multiply injured or hemodynamically unstable patients.[103] Additionally, DPL is superior for diagnoses of small bowel perforation[91,104,105] and mesenteric injury.[106] Its main disadvantage is its invasiveness with a small, but real, incidence of laceration or perforation of abdominal organs.[26–30] Additionally, DPL does not allow for the detection of solid organ injuries that may be managed nonoperatively. The sensitivity and specificity may be decreased in the presence of peritoneal adhesions from previous surgery or if pelvic fracture with retroperitoneal hematoma is present. For patients with pelvic hematomas, a supraumbilical approach is recommended.[107]

Despite the suggestion that DPL is best used as a screening modality to determine who should undergo further evaluation with CT,[108] this role has largely been supplanted by the FAST. Given that DPL has similar sensitivity to both US and CT,[91] DPL is a good diagnostic tool if FAST is unavailable or the examiner is inexperienced, especially in the presence of hemodynamic instability. In unstable patients with a nondiagnostic FAST exam, DPL can also be useful.

Computed Topography

The CT scan has become the diagnostic modality of choice to evaluate the hemodynamically stable blunt torso trauma patient. Rarely should an unstable patient be brought to CT scan. In the unstable patient, CT scan should only be attempted after preliminary studies (e.g., chest radiograph, EFAST, DPL) have ruled out intrathoracic or intraabdominal bleeding. The specific clinical situation, staff, and resources available should dictate other situations in which a CT scan is obtained on an unstable patient, weighing the benefit against the considerable risk of managing and monitoring an unstable patient in the scanner.

The most common indication for chest CT is the inability to "clear" the mediastinum and exclude an aortic injury by chest X-ray. Historically, angiography has been the definitive diagnostic modality for the detection of aortic injury. Several studies have demonstrated that the diagnosis of blunt aortic rupture can be made reliably with the use of chest CT.[109–122] The sensitivity and negative predictive value of CT scan for traumatic aortic rupture is 100% in many series.

In addition, there are some data to support the use of chest CT even in patients with a normal chest X-ray.[109,123–125] In the setting of a relatively normal chest X-ray, injuries of the lung parenchyma, thoracic cage, spine, heart, and other mediastinal structures may be readily appreciated by CT scan.[124–126] Many of these injuries may be of minor importance, such as isolated rib fractures or minor pulmonary contusions. However, other injuries such as pericardial effusions or pneumomediastinum may necessitate further evaluation and therapy. The presence of an occult pneumothorax on CT scan that is not seen on plain radiography (incidence, 10% of cases of traumatic pneumothorax) may be vitally important, as these injuries may progress to produce major clinical morbidity.[127–129] Table 27.2 presents representative clinical experiences with the use of CT scan for the identification of chest injuries in the setting of blunt trauma.

In the setting of blunt abdominal trauma, CT scan plays an important role in the hemodynamically stable patient. Despite early work that failed to demonstrate superiority of CT over DPL,[130] improvements in technology and the use of helical CT scan have allowed CT scanning to become the diagnostic test of choice in hemodynamically stable patients suspected of having intraabdominal injury.[131] CT scan of the abdomen is beneficial, even in the absence of discrete clinical indicators, in patients with traumatic brain injury, or depressed level of consciousness with spinal cord injury, resulting in an unreliable physical exam.[123,132,133] Additionally, any patient with an abnormal physical examination such as abdominal tenderness or hematuria should undergo abdominal CT.[85,134,135] Detection of an elevated aspartate aminotransferase concentration may also be an indication for CT scan to evaluate for liver injury.[136] Other studies have demonstrated the efficacy of routine CT scans in hemodynamically stable patients with possible intraabdominal injury.[135]

Computed tomography scans have a number of advantages over other diagnostic tests. Sensitivities of 92% to 97% and specificities of 99% have been reported for the presence of intraabdominal injury.[132,134] Although historically CT scan was not considered a good diagnostic modality for the detection of mesenteric or bowel injury,[40,104,137–139] improvements in technology and the use of helical CT have achieved increased accuracy. Reported sensitivities are 94% to 98% for bowel injury and 96% for mesenteric injury,[133,139,140] whereas specificity is as high as 99.6%.[133,140] Recent studies have questioned the need for enteral contrast even for the detection of bowel injury.[140,141] Accuracy rates in predicting the need for operative intervention for bowel injury have ranged from 75% to 94%.[139,142,143]

Abdominal CT scan is efficacious for the detection of occult pneumothorax[144] and provides the best evaluation of the retroperitoneum injuries that may be underappreciated by DPL or ultrasound.[135,145,146] CT also provides for excellent evaluation of solid organ injury[132] and identifies patients who may have nonoperative management.[147,148] The routine use of CT scan in suspected intraabdominal injury reduces nontherapeutic laparotomy rates.[132] Many believe that the negative predictive value of abdominal CT is sufficiently high to permit safe discharge from the emergency department following a negative CT scan.[85,149] Table 27.3 presents representative clinical experiences with the use of CT scan in the setting of blunt trauma.

The main disadvantage of routine CT scanning is the requirement for moving the patient to a separate area, sometimes remote from trauma personnel, which can potentially be dangerous in the event of clinical deterioration. Additionally, there are risks of intravenous contrast allergies, renal failure from contrast injection, and exposure to radiation. As the technology improves, the literature has become replete with papers expressing concern over the routine use of CT scan in low-risk patients.[85,131,134,136,150]

Ultrasound

The use of ultrasound in the setting of blunt trauma has become common. Surgeon-performed ultrasound (FAST) is noninvasive, rapid, and can be performed at the bedside while resuscitation is ongoing. Other practitioners can also conduct the FAST examination reliably with minimal training, including emergency medicine physicians, radiologists, and technicians.[50–52,151–157] Ultrasound may be more cost-effective as a screening test than DPL or CT scanning.[158–160]

Ultrasound (FAST) is useful also for evaluation of blunt thoracic trauma.[53,54,59,161,162] Ultrasonography can reliably detect traumatic effusion or hemothorax with a sensitivity greater than 96% and specificity of 99% to 100%. Additionally, the EFAST may be more accurate than chest radiographs for the detection of pneumothorax.[59,161] Ultrasound evaluation of the pericardium can be invaluable in detection of pericardial tamponade or effusion. Ultrasound has also been used in detection of rib and sternal fractures, with results that demonstrate superior accuracy over both plain radiography and clinical impression,[162] yet adoption has not been widespread.

In the setting of blunt abdominal trauma, FAST has reported sensitivities of 73% to 92% and specificities of 95% to 100%,[51,52,91,151–153,155,163–165] being considered positive when free fluid is visualized in one of four areas of the abdomen or pericardium. At least 200 mL fluid must be present to be detectable with ultrasound.[154] Thus, injuries to the bowel or injuries not associated with hemoperitoneum may be missed by ultrasound alone.[61,135,165] Additionally, solid organ injuries cannot be graded by ultrasound and therefore may still require CT scanning for therapeutic decision making. The use of higher-frequency linear ultrasound probes may identify splenic injuries without relying on surrogate markers, such as hemoperitoneum, but this technique is not commonly in practice.[166] Retroperitoneal injuries may similarly be underappreciated with the use of ultrasound.[135,167] The FAST examination, however, can be repeated for serial evaluation of intraabdominal injuries. It is invaluable in the multiply injured or unstable patient to evaluate rapidly the potential sources of hemorrhage.[51,52,87,165,168] A positive examination of an unstable patient should prompt immediate surgical intervention.[52]

Selected groups of patients may benefit from CT scan in addition to FAST, as ultrasound alone misses injuries in specific high-risk groups of patients.[135,148,167,169] Patients with abdominal tenderness or pain, pelvic ring fractures, hematuria, lumbar fractures, or lower rib fractures should be further evaluated with CT scan even in the setting of a negative ultrasound.[52,167,169,170] Indeterminate or equivocal ultrasound studies, most often secondary to patient factors such as body habitus, should be followed by CT scan to evaluate properly for intraabdominal injury.[171] CT can be useful with a positive FAST in hemodynamically stable patients for further characterization of injuries.[52] Table 27.4 presents representative clinical experiences with the use of ultrasound for diagnosis of injuries following blunt torso trauma.

Laparoscopy

Diagnostic thoracoscopy and laparoscopy have been described for use in blunt torso trauma. Initial reports demonstrated limited benefit in blunt trauma patients,[64,172] but accumulating data have demonstrated better results.[75,173–175] In small selected groups of patients, diagnostic laparoscopy can be quite sensitive and specific[67] and may avoid nontherapeutic laparotomies.[63,67,75,175] Although there may be a role for these procedures in blunt trauma, use remains sporadic.

Other Modalities

Depending on the particular clinical presentation and resources available, thorough evaluation of the patient with torso trauma may require a multidisciplinary approach with utilization of multiple diagnostic modalities. In the setting of both blunt and penetrating torso trauma, there are numerous other diagnostic modalities that can be utilized to identify injuries. These techniques include, but are not limited to, echocardiography for evaluation of aortic or cardiac injury, angiography for detection of vascular injury of the great vessels or visceral arteries, bronchoscopy for evaluation of tracheobronchial injuries, esophagoscopy or contrast esophagography for identification of esophageal injuries, and cystography for

TABLE 27.2.
Representative Clinical Experience with CT Scan for the Diagnosis of Blunt Chest Trauma

Trial	*Year*	*Level of evidence*	*Number of patients*	*Intervention/design*	*Median follow-up*	*Minor endpoint*	*Major endpoint*	*Interpretations/comments*
124	2000	II	375	Prospective cohort study of trauma patients admitted to an ICU who had chest CT on admission compared with those who did not	11.4 days	Detection of chest injuries with chest CT that result in altered management	Improvement in clinical outcomes in patients who had chest CT on admission over those who were studied with plain radiograph	Chest CT detects more injuries than chest X-ray and may lead to altered management; this does not correlate in a difference in clinical outcome, however.
109	2001	II	71	Prospective study of consecutive blunt trauma patients who underwent chest X-ray and chest CT scan	N/A	N/A	Detection of chest injuries with chest CT scan not appreciated on chest radiograph	In the setting of a normal chest X-ray, 50% of chest CT scans demonstrated abnormalities, including two aortic injuries. Routine chest CT should be performed on all patients with major chest trauma.
125	2001	II	169	Prospective study of hemodynamically stable blunt patients who underwent chest CT in addition to chest X-ray to evaluate for intrathoracic injury	N/A	N/A	Identification of patients who benefit from the addition of chest CT scan to plain radiographs	Thoracic CT is most beneficial when there is radiographic suspicion of chest injury. Changes in management occur 20% of the time. CT identifies occult injuries in 5% of patients with a significant mechanism of injury and normal radiograph.
119	1996	III	677	Retrospective review of the use of chest CT for the identification of traumatic aortic rupture	N/A	N/A	Successful identification of aortic injury with chest CT in blunt trauma patients	The finding of mediastinal hemorrhage alone was 87% sensitive and 90% specific for traumatic aortic rupture, while the identification of an aortic injury on chest CT was 99% sensitive and 100% specific.
120	1998	II	494	Prospective study comparing helical chest CT to aortography in the diagnosis of traumatic aortic rupture (TAR)	N/A	N/A	Identification of TAR with chest CT in blunt trauma patients	Sensitivity of thoracic CT for the detection of TAR was 100% with specificity of 83% and 86% accuracy. A normal chest CT safely excludes a traumatic aortic rupture and requires no further evaluation. Aortography was only performed regardless of CT findings during the first year of the 4-year study.
122	1998	II	1104	Prospective study of consecutive blunt trauma patients who underwent chest CT to evaluate for the presence of TAR	N/A	N/A	Identification of TAR with chest CT in blunt trauma patients	Spiral chest CT was 100% sensitive and 99.7% specific for the detection of TAR in blunt trauma patients with an abnormal chest radiograph. Overall accuracy was 99.7%

TABLE 27.2. (continued)

Trial	Year	Level of evidence	Number of patients	Intervention/design	Median follow-up	Minor endpoint	Major endpoint	Interpretations/comments
110	2000	II	1561	Prospective study of the use of thoracic CT scan to evaluate for TAR	N/A	Successful prediction of TAR based on a scoring system by mechanism of injury	Successful identification of aortic injury with chest CT in blunt trauma patients	CT was found to be 100% sensitive with a negative predictive value of 100% for the detection of aortic injury in blunt trauma patients. Patients with unequivocal CT scans should proceed directly to operative intervention without aortography.
121	2001	III	54	Retrospective review of patients undergoing aortic repair following blunt trauma with helical CT scan as the initial diagnostic study	N/A	N/A	Accurate identification of aortic injuries on chest CT allowing for operative repair without aortography	Direct operative repair of TAR is indicated in patients with an unequivocal chest CT. Aortography should be reserved for patients with equivocal chest CT.
112	2001	II	142	Prospective evaluation of chest CT versus aortography for the detection of TAR in blunt trauma patients	N/A	Cost of CT scan versus aortography in patients suspected of having TAR	Accurate detection of TAR by helical CT scan in blunt trauma patients	Helical CT, like aortography, has a 100% sensitivity and negative predictive value for the detection of TAR. Using CT scan as the diagnostic modality of choice decreases costs.

CT, computed tomography; N/A, not available.

diagnosis of bladder injury. These additional modalities should be used in conjunction with standard diagnostic tools.

Indications for Thoracotomy

Between 10% and 15% of patients with thoracic injury will require operative treatment.[176] Most thoracic trauma can be treated with pain medication, supportive care, or bedside procedures. After both blunt and penetrating injuries, indications for emergency thoracotomy include exsanguinating hemorrhage, massive hemothorax (>1500mL or >200mL/h over 4h), cardiac tamponade, evidence of major vascular or cardiac injury, massive air leak, or evidence of esophageal or tracheal injury. Nonacute, or delayed, thoracotomy may be performed days to years following the injury in the setting of retained hemothorax, persistent air leaks, empyema, missed esophageal or tracheal injuries, diaphragmatic hernias, or posttraumatic major vessel injury such as arteriovenous fistula. Thoracoscopy is also useful in the nonemergent setting for evacuation of retained hemothorax, repair of diaphragmatic injuries, control of chest wall bleeding, and repair of minor lung injuries.[67,177–179]

Transmediastinal gunshot wounds have historically been considered an indication for intervention. Recent work has demonstrated that patients can safely undergo diagnostic workup, and up to 50% of patients can be managed nonoperatively.[180] Some authors believe the indications for thoracotomy should be different for blunt and penetrating trauma secondary to the higher likelihood of nontherapeutic thoracotomy after blunt trauma.[181,182]

The incision chosen for operative intervention for of thoracic trauma must be individualized. Median sternotomy, anterolateral thoracotomy with or without extension into the contralateral chest (the "clam-shell" thoracotomy), and posterolateral thoracotomy each provide access to certain intrathoracic and mediastinal structures. A median sternotomy generally provides the best access to the heart and proximal great vessels. It can be easily extended superiorly or laterally to obtain control of the more distal great vessels. Likewise, it can be extended inferiorly to the abdomen if laparotomy is necessary. It is the incision of choice in the setting of cardiac tamponade or penetrating cardiac trauma. Anterolateral thoracotomy provides the quickest access to the lung and hilum and can be performed without special positioning of the patient. If a concomitant laparotomy is necessary, supine or 30° partial decubitus positioning of the patient allows access to the abdomen. Extending an anterolateral thoracotomy across the sternum to the contralateral chest provides excellent access to the heart and proximal great vessels. Posterolateral thoracotomy is usually reserved for isolated injury to one hemithorax (e.g., the descending aorta) and provides excellent exposure to the entire hemithorax, but unstable patients may not tolerate lateral positioning.

TABLE 27.3.
Representative Clinical Experience with CT Scan for the Diagnosis of Blunt Abdominal Trauma.

Trial	*Year*	*Level of evidence*	*Number of patients*	*Intervention/design*	*Median follow-up*	*Minor endpoint*	*Major endpoint*	*Interpretations/comments*
132	1986	II	128	Prospective evaluation of the use of abdominal CT scan in stable blunt trauma patients with an equivocal abdominal exam, closed head injury, spinal cord injury, hematuria, or pelvic fracture	N/A	N/A	Detection of abdominal injuries in stable blunt trauma patients	Accuracy for the detection of intraabdominal injuries with CT scan was 98.3%. Solid organ injuries were reliably detected as were minor injuries requiring no specific therapy.
143	1994	III	26	Retrospective review of blunt trauma patients with small bowel injuries who underwent abdominal CT scan	N/A	N/A	Identification of blunt small bowel injuries by abdominal CT scan	Overall accuracy of CT scan for the detection of small bowel injury was 94%. Sensitivity was 92% and specificity was 94%. Subtly abnormal findings on CT scan warrant further evaluation or observation.
147	1996	III	256	Retrospective review of blunt trauma patients who underwent CT of the abdomen	N/A	N/A	Identification of intraabdominal injury by CT scan in hemodynamically stable blunt trauma patients	Abdominal CT detected 83.7% of injuries. It is safe and noninvasive. Sensitivity of pancreatic and intestinal injuries was low in this study. The use of CT in this setting can avoid nontherapeutic laparotomies.
139	2001	III	74	Retrospective review of patients with blunt bowel and mesenteric injuries who underwent laparotomy and helical CT scan	N/A	N/A	Detection of small bowel injuries by CT scan in blunt trauma patients	Helical CT scan had an overall sensitivity of 94% for bowel injury and 96% for mesenteric injury. The need for operative intervention was correctly established in 86% of patients with bowel injuries but only 75% of mesenteric injuries.
133	2002	III	87	Retrospective review of hollow viscus injuries identified by abdominal CT scan in blunt trauma patients	9 days	N/A	Accurate detection of small bowel injuries by CT scan in blunt trauma patients	CT was 97.7% sensitive, 98.5% specific, and 99.4% accurate for the diagnosis of blunt small bowel injury. CT is useful in patients with an unreliable physical exam secondary to depressed level of consciousness.
123	2003	III	457	Retrospective chart review of patients who underwent CT of the torso in conjunction with cranial CT scan	6.6 days	N/A	Identification of torso injury in patients with suspected brain injury who underwent routine body CT when cranial CT was performed	Torso CT scan when performed routinely in patients undergoing head CT is beneficial. Thirty-eight percent of patients had an unexpected finding of the torso. Management was altered in 10%.
140	2004	II	500	Prospective evaluation of the use of abdominal CT without oral contrast administration	N/A	N/A	Accurate identification of blunt intestinal and mesenteric injuries	The sensitivity and specificity of abdominal CT without oral contrast for the detection of blunt bowel and mesenteric injuries was 95% and 99.6% respectively. Oral contrast is not necessary for the detection of these injuries.

Emergency Department Thoracotomy

Emergency department (ED) or resuscitative thoracotomy should be performed only in a limited set of circumstances for patients in extremis. Patients with penetrating thoracic trauma who have lost vital signs or with severe hypotension may benefit from ED thoracotomy, although the survival rates vary widely in the literature. Survival was 46% in one series in patients with no vital signs and 75% when ED thoracotomy was performed in patients with penetrating injury in shock.[183,184] In patients without "signs of life," defined as absence of blood pressure, cardiac activity, respiratory effort, or pupillary response, survival is 0% to 4% in the setting of penetrating injury, although one series reported a survival of 24% in patients with cardiac injuries.[185–188] Patients with cardiac injuries from stab wounds are the most likely to benefit from resuscitative thoracotomy.[184,189,190] In blunt trauma, the reported success rates in the larger series are typically less than 2%.[186,187,189,191–193] ED thoracotomy is generally not recommended in the setting of cardiac arrest or profound shock secondary to blunt trauma except in extraordinary circumstances.[193,194]

Emergency department thoracotomy begins with a rapid left anterolateral thoracotomy at the fourth or fifth interspace. The incision can be extended across the sternum for wider access and better exposure of the heart. If the sternum is transected, the internal mammary arteries must be identified and ligated if resuscitation is successful. Once the thorax is entered, the pericardium is elevated and entered. Care should be exercised to avoid injury to the phrenic nerves. Opening the pericardium releases tamponade and provides the best access for open cardiac massage and internal defibrillation. To improve coronary perfusion or if there is suspicion of infradiaphragmatic hemorrhage, aortic cross-clamping can be performed inferior to the hilum of the lung. Clamping the pulmonary hilum can control bleeding from the lung parenchyma. Cardiac injuries can be temporized with clamping, manual occlusion, a skin stapler, or a Foley catheter with the balloon inflated. If vital signs are regained, the patient should be transported rapidly to the operating room for definitive management.

Indications for Laparotomy

The most clear-cut indication for laparotomy in the setting of torso trauma is hemodynamic instability with evidence of intraabdominal injury. Whether secondary to blunt or penetrating abdominal trauma, hemorrhagic shock is an absolute indication for surgical exploration. Regardless of the diagnostic modality used, other clear indications include peritonitis, evidence of hollow organ or pancreatic injury, intraperitoneal bladder rupture, evisceration, diaphragmatic injury, and impalement of objects in the abdominal wall.[195,196] In the absence of these clear indications, laparotomy may also be used as a diagnostic modality when clinical suspicion warrants further evaluation unobtainable by radiographic studies or DPL. Laparoscopy may provide an alternative to diagnostic laparotomy in the hemodynamically stable patient.[63,67,75,175]

Gunshot wounds with a possibility of transperitoneal trajectory have been considered an indication for mandatory laparotomy. Work done in several centers has demonstrated that a subset of these patients (i.e., tangential injury) may be safely managed nonoperatively with careful serial physical examinations and additional diagnostic studies such as CT or DPL.[13,36,42–49,197–199] Stab wounds to the abdomen with evidence of fascial penetration were also previously considered an indication for laparotomy. Recently, it has been demonstrated that a subset of these patients can similarly be managed safely with observation and serial physical examinations[14] or with further diagnostic workup to determine whether intra- or retroperitoneal injury has occurred.[44,45] Diagnostic laparoscopy may also be helpful in identifying intraabdominal injury in some patients with penetrating abdominal injury.[36,78,198] Other more controversial indications for operative intervention for blunt abdominal trauma include the presence of free intraperitoneal fluid without evidence of solid organ injury.[200–203]

Laparotomy for trauma is performed via a midline incision from xiphoid to pubis. The skin should be prepared from neck to midthigh in case entry into the thorax or vein harvest for revascularization is needed. The room should be warm and, ideally, rapid infusion and reinfusion systems should be available. Upon entry into the abdomen, depending on the degree of hemoperitoneum, the abdomen should be packed sequentially with laparotomy pads and evaluated systematically. Priorities include control of bleeding, identification of injuries, control of contamination, and prioritization and performance of definitive repair. The surgeon must be cognizant of the development of hypothermia, coagulopathy, and acidosis in assigning priorities.

Damage Control

The abbreviated laparotomy was first described by Stone et al. in 1983.[204] The concept emerged with recognition that the development of coagulopathy, acidosis, and hypothermia (the "lethal triad") secondary to hemorrhagic shock was an almost uniformly lethal event.[205–210] Rotondo et al. then coined the term "damage control" for use in the setting of profound shock secondary to penetrating trauma.[211] The technique of "damage control" includes three steps: rapid control of bleeding and contamination followed by abdominal packing and temporary closure, active warming and resuscitation in an intensive care unit (ICU), and return to the operating room for definitive repair of injuries once the patient is stabilized and the acidosis and coagulopathy have been reversed. In their original report, Rotondo et al. noted that survival was greater when damage control was used in the subset of patients with major vascular injury and two or more visceral injuries. Subsequent work has demonstrated a discrete survival advantage in patients with penetrating abdominal trauma.[212,213]

Damage control has now become standard for patients with severe hemorrhagic shock from both penetrating and blunt trauma. The techniques for damage control in the abdomen include hepatic packing, balloon tamponade of bleeding, temporary enteric closures, placement of vascular shunts, rapid splenectomy, nephrectomy or distal pancreatectomy, use of topical hemostatic agents, the use of systemic hemostatic agents (Factor VIIa), and intraperitoneal packing. Major morbidity of damage control, if successful in preventing early death, includes abdominal compartment syndrome,

TABLE 27.4.
Representative Clinical Experience with Ultrasound for the Diagnosis of Torso Trauma.

Trial	*Year*	*Level of evidence*	*Number of patients*	*Intervention/design*	*Median follow-up*	*Minor endpoint*	*Major endpoint*	*Interpretations/comments*
50	1995	II	245	Prospective evaluation of US for the detection of free intrathoracic and intraperitoneal fluid by emergency department physicians in patients with blunt trauma	N/A	N/A	Accurate detection of pleural, pericardial, retroperitoneal, and intraperitoneal fluid	US was accurate in detecting fluid in blunt trauma patients. Sensitivity was 90%, specificity was 99%, and accuracy was 99%. Emergency department physicians can perform and interpret this diagnostic test.
163	1995	II	206	Prospective evaluation of US compared to CT or DPL in patients with blunt trauma	N/A	N/A	Evaluation of US to detect intraperitoneal fluid	US is an effective method of determining the presence of intraabdominal fluid in patients with blunt abdominal trauma. Accuracy was 96% and could be performed rapidly.
51	1995	II	371	Prospective study of surgeon-performed ultrasound in patients with both blunt and penetrating trauma	N/A	N/A	Identification of hemoperitoneum or pericardial effusion	US can be used reliably as a primary diagnostic modality in patients with traumatic injuries. Sensitivity was 81.5% and specificity was 99.7%. Initial evaluation of injured I5 patients with ultrasound may be cost-effective.
164	1996	III	1,000	Evaluation of an institutional algorithm to evaluate patients with BAT utilizing US as the preliminary diagnostic modality	N/A	N/A	Accurate identification of intraabdominal injuries necessitating further diagnostics or intervention	US accurately detected injuries in 97% of patients. Sensitivity and specificity were 88% and 99%, respectively. US is an effective primary modality to evaluate patients with BAT.
153	1996	II	800	Prospective evaluation of the diagnostic accuracy of US in selected patients with BAT	N/A	N/A	Identification of intraabdominal injuries using US	US can be performed rapidly and in conjunction with resuscitation to evaluate patients with BAT. Overall accuracy for the detection of abdominal injury was 97%.
168	1996	II	69	Blinded prospective evaluation of the accuracy of US in detecting the need for urgent laparotomy in hypotensive BAT patients	N/A	N/A	Accuracy of detection of hemoperitoneum in hypotensive patients	US is a rapid method of detecting hemoperitoneum in unstable patients after BAT. Sensitivity of 100%, specificity of 94%, and accuracy of 96% were reported for predicting the need for laparotomy.
54	1998	II	360	Prospective evaluation of the ability of US to detect traumatic effusions in injured patients	6.4 days	N/A	Accuracy of detection of traumatic pleural effusions by US	Surgeon-performed US can accurately detect traumatic pleural effusions. Accuracy is equivalent to radiographs and can be performed faster.
165	1998	III	1,239	Retrospective evaluation of the use of US to detect intraabdominal injuries	N/A	N/A	Identification of intraabdominal injuries following trauma with US	Sensitivity of US was 94.6% with a specificity of 95.1%. Overall accuracy was 94.9%.

TABLE 27.4. (continued)

Trial	*Year*	*Level of evidence*	*Number of patients*	*Intervention/design*	*Median follow-up*	*Minor endpoint*	*Major endpoint*	*Interpretations/comments*
52	1998	II	1,540	Prospective study of the accuracy of FAST by trauma team members	N/A	N/A	Determination of the accuracy of FAST in detection of injuries following precordial or thoracic penetrating trauma or blunt abdominal trauma	US is rapid and accurate. Sensitivity of 83.3% and specificity of 99.7% are reported. Sensitivity of 100% is reported for hypotensive patients with BAT and precordial penetrating injuries. US should be the initial test of choice in hemodynamically unstable patients or in the setting of penetrating precordial trauma. A positive FAST in this setting warrants immediate surgical intervention.
58	2001	II	75	Prospective study of the use of FAST in hemodynamically stable patients with penetrating abdominal injury	N/A	N/A	Identification of intraabdominal injury in hemodynamically stable patients with penetrating abdominal trauma with ultrasound	In patients with penetrating abdominal injury, a positive FAST is predictive of the need for laparotomy. Negative studies should be followed by additional testing due to the low negative predictive value (60%).
55	2001	II	72	Prospective evaluation of clinical protocols to determine the efficacy of the FAST exam in the setting of penetrating trauma	5.2 days	N/A	Detection of intraabdominal or intrapericardial fluid in patients with penetrating torso trauma	The use of FAST in the setting of penetrating torso trauma is beneficial. Negative exams, however, do not exclude abdominal injury.
57	2004	II	177	Prospective study of the use of US in the setting of penetrating abdominal trauma	N/A	N/A	Correlation of US results with patient outcome and the need for therapeutic laparotomy and thoracotomy	Routine use of FAST does not change the management in a significant number of patients with penetrating torso injury. Sensitivity of 48%, specificity of 98%, and accuracy of 85% were reported.

US, ultrasound; FAST, focused assessment for sonography in trauma; DPL, diagnostic peritoneal lavage; BAT, blunt abdominal trauma.

multiple organ dysfunction syndrome, and complications associated with an open abdomen, such as enteric fistulas.[213–218] One of the tenets of damage control is that patients who manifest clinical signs of ongoing bleeding or abdominal compartment syndrome following damage control laparotomy should be reexplored or undergo adjunctive procedures, such as angiography.[215,219]

There are many unresolved issues surrounding damage control for trauma. There are no defined selection criteria that are clearly predictive of who would benefit from damage control or who should have a definitive procedure on presentation, although several authors have suggested such algorithms.[210,214,215,220–224] Generally, patients with multisystem trauma, multiple abdominal injuries, or a large transfusion requirement, coagulopathy, acidosis, or hypothermia benefit from damage control. Clearly, the earlier damage control is instituted, the better the outcome.[215] Issues concerning the timing of reoperation have also been discussed extensively in the literature.[214,215,219,225–228] In general, the patient should be returned to the operating room once coagulopathy and acidosis have been corrected and the patient has been stabilized, usually within 24 to 48 h. Caution must be taken as excessive time to reoperation increases the risk of infection, and tissue inflammation and friability makes definitive repair technically difficult. Also unresolved are the optimal temporary abdominal closure and how to provide definitive abdominal wall reconstruction.[214]

The principles of damage control have also been extended to areas of the body other than the abdomen. Damage control thoracotomy has been well described.[215,229–233] The general principles are the same as for damage control laparotomy. Several techniques have been described for rapid operative management in unstable patients with thoracic injury. These include thoracic packing, pulmonary tractotomy, nonanatomic pulmonary resection, intravascular shunting, esophageal diversion and drainage, placement of double-lumen endotracheal tubes for tracheal or bronchial injuries, and temporary chest closure.[215,229–231,233–235]

Cardiac Injury

Cardiac injuries can occur from either penetrating or blunt mechanisms. Penetrating injuries are frequently fatal, with widely varying survival rates from 25% to 89%.[232–239] Survival from stab wounds is markedly better than from gunshot wounds.[232–239] Stab wounds to the heart tend to present with evidence of pericardial tamponade. Gunshot wounds often cause profound hemorrhage and shock from hypovolemia secondary to the large cardiac defects caused by bullets. The right ventricle is most frequently injured secondary to its anterior location.[232,239,240] Multichamber injuries are most likely to be fatal.[237,238]

In the setting of hemodynamic instability, immediate operation is indicated. With cardiac arrest or profound hypotension, ED thoracotomy may be performed. In centers in which there is not a surgeon immediately available, pericardiocentesis may be used as a temporizing measure. In the hemodynamically stable patient, diagnosis is typically made by ultrasound. Sensitivity has been reported to be as high as 100% in this setting.[52,62] Echocardiography can also be useful, as can the performance of a diagnostic subxiphoid window.

All penetrating injuries to the heart require operative intervention. Median sternotomy or left anterolateral thoracotomy can be used. Simple lacerations are typically repaired with pledgeted sutures, avoiding injury to the coronary arteries, valves, and septum. If a distal coronary artery is lacerated as a result of the primary injury, it may be ligated. Injuries to proximal or midcoronary arteries will likely require repair or bypass. Typically, patients are followed with echocardiography to identify delayed complications.[239,241–243] Recent data suggest that only symptomatic patients require echocardiography and that asymptomatic patients can be followed with physical examination, chest radiography, and electrocardiography.[240,244]

Blunt trauma can result in a spectrum of injury from mild "contusion" to free cardiac rupture. The reported incidence of blunt myocardial injury varies widely in the literature secondary to discrepancies in diagnostic criteria.[245–248] Typically, these patients have sustained major chest trauma and are usually injured in motor vehicle collisions or falls from a great height.[249,250] The cardiac injury is secondary to a direct force to the precordium, which compresses the heart between the sternum and vertebral bodies.[245] Blunt cardiac injury (BCI) may be associated with sternal or rib fractures. The incidence of associated traumatic brain, abdominal, and aortic injuries in these patients is high.[251] The principles of treatment are the same for blunt cardiac injury with rupture as for penetrating injuries.

The less dramatic forms of BCI, previously named cardiac "contusion," are seen much more frequently. Presentation of BCI varies widely from minor electrocardiogram (ECG) changes and hemodynamically insignificant arrhythmias to cardiogenic shock and cardiac arrest.[245] The diagnosis can be difficult and requires a high index of suspicion. There is good evidence that in the hemodynamically stable patient with clinical suspicion of BCI, a normal ECG effectively excludes a BCI. If these patients have no other comorbidities, they may be discharged home safely from the emergency department.[252–260] If abnormalities are found, or if the patient is symptomatic, admission to a telemetry unit for 24 to 48h is indicated for observation.[252,253,258,261] The role of cardiac isoenzymes and serum troponin concentrations in the diagnosis of BCI is controversial, with some studies supporting their use,[245,248,262–265] whereas others demonstrate no clinical benefit.[252,254,255,257,261,266–270] Additional testing such as echocardiography should be reserved for patients with symptoms, dysrhythmias, or underlying cardiac disease[253,259,260,269,271]; transesophageal echocardiography may be more useful than transthoracic echocardiography in this setting.[272,273] Arrhythmias and cardiac dysfunction resulting from BCI are usually self-limited and treated with supportive care. Even if BCI is diagnosed, the risk of cardiac complications requiring emergency surgery is not increased if the patient is stable hemodynamically, and necessary interventions need not be delayed. Although rare, long-term complications of BCI can occur, including wall motion abnormalities, pericardial effusions, valvular dysfunction, ventricular aneurysms, and ventricular thrombi.[274,275]

Injury to the Chest Wall, Lung, and Trachea

Injuries to the chest account for 25% of all trauma deaths in the United States.[275] Chest wall injuries are most commonly caused by blunt mechanisms, but occasionally high-velocity penetrating injuries can cause extensive destruction of the bony thorax. Fractures of the ribs, sternum, clavicles, or scapula are often associated with underlying pulmonary injury with resultant pulmonary complications.[276–280] The identification of chest wall injuries should prompt a search for other injuries as these injuries rarely occur in isolation.[281] Injuries of the chest wall caused by major mechanisms include traumatic asphyxia (which usually affects children), open chest wall defects, flail chest, and scapulothoracic dissociation. These injuries carry high mortality and severe long-term morbidity in survivors.[282,283] Treatment is primarily supportive, but major chest wall disruption may require operative stabilization or closure.[284–286] The morbidity of more minor injuries, including rib, sternal, or clavicle fractures, is commonly the result of associated injuries. Elderly patients are particularly at risk for morbidity from these types of injuries.[276,287–289] Pain control and early mobilization are the mainstays of therapy.[278–280]

Injuries to the lung and pleura occur after both blunt and penetrating trauma. Penetrating injuries tend to manifest early, whereas blunt injuries may not become apparent for hours or days. Some of these injuries can be immediately life threatening, such as tension pneumothorax or massive hemothorax, whereas others, such as simple pneumothorax, may progress if left untreated. One very common disorder of the lung secondary to trauma is pulmonary contusion, which can range from minor and clinically insignificant to profound acute respiratory failure. The diagnosis of pulmonary injury is typically made by physical examination and chest radiography, but CT scans can also be useful in detecting small contusions, hemothorax, or occult pneumothorax and for differentiating between pleural and parenchymal disease.

Most lung trauma can be treated appropriately with supportive care. Pneumothorax and hemothorax are treated with tube thoracostomy. Chest tubes placed for trauma indications should have a large bore (at least 32–36 Fr.) and be placed in a superior and posterior position. Once the acute process has resolved, chest tubes should be removed expeditiously. Management of chest tubes according to an institutional protocol improves efficiency and possibly decreases complication rates.[290,291] Although tube thoracostomy is usually a relatively straightforward bedside procedure, complication rates approach 20% to 25%.[292,293] Prophylactic antibiotics to decrease infectious complications of bedside tube thoracostomy are controversial.[294–297] There is also controversy as to whether patients with "occult" pneumothorax, seen on CT scan but not chest X-ray, require chest tubes.[298–302] This decision is particularly an issue for patients on mechanical ventilation, as there is concern of progression of these pneumothoraces with positive-pressure ventilation.[302] Pulmonary contusions are treated with supportive care, sometimes requiring mechanical ventilation. Judicious fluid administration is advised, but this must be weighed against the need to provide adequate resuscitation of these often multiply injured patients.

Emergency thoracotomy for lung injury is reserved for patients with hemodynamic instability, massive hemothorax, or massive air leaks. Operative techniques for lung trauma include anatomic and nonanatomic resections, tractotomy, stapling of peripheral injuries, and repair of major pulmonary vasculature. The morbidity and mortality in these patients is quite high, with survival rates of less than 50% following pneumonectomy and less than 70% after lobectomy.[303–308] Thoracotomy for injury to the lung in patients with blunt injury carries a higher mortality than in penetrating trauma victims.[303] Delayed thoracotomy or thoracoscopy may be necessary for retained hemothorax, empyema, or persistent air leak.

Intrathoracic tracheal and major bronchial injuries are relatively rare and require a high index of suspicion for diagnosis. When secondary to penetrating trauma, these injuries often coexist with major lung, great vessel, or cardiac trauma; consequently, the morbidity and mortality are high. When secondary to blunt trauma, these injuries typically occur within 2 cm of the carina. The clinical presentation varies widely; approximately 60% of the more minor injuries in the thorax will not be diagnosed for more than 24 h.[309,310] The diagnosis is typically made with the discovery of pneumomediastinum or persistent pneumothorax following tube thoracostomy, usually with a large air leak. Bronchoscopy is the test of choice for diagnosis.[311] Most of these injuries will require operative repair. Operative management consists of debridement of devitalized tissue and primary repair in most instances. Studies have demonstrated that outcome is improved when the repair is done early after injury.[312–314]

Injury to the Esophagus

Injuries to the thoracic esophagus are fortunately quite rare, as they are difficult to diagnose and morbidity and mortality are high. Most esophageal injuries are secondary to penetrating injury, but the incidence is still relatively low, even with gunshot wounds.[315] There is a high rate of injuries to surrounding structures secondary to the anatomic position of the thoracic esophagus in the posterior mediastinum.[316] Most patients demonstrate some abnormality on chest radiograph, although these are likely to be nonspecific.[317,318] Esophagoscopy can be used for diagnosis, but there may be a small risk of worsening the injury with endoscopy.[319] Esophagography is also used for diagnosis. The treatment of thoracic esophageal injuries is always surgical. Early intervention is paramount.

Operative strategies for the treatment of thoracic esophageal injuries include debridement of devitalized tissue, primary repair, muscle flap coverage, and wide drainage. Injuries less than 24 h old can usually be repaired primarily.[317,320] If operation is delayed more than 24 h, or if there is substantial inflammation or contamination, esophageal diversion and wide drainage are prudent. Complications, such as leaks and subsequent mediastinitis, are common, extremely morbid, and often fatal.

Injury to the Diaphragm

Diaphragm injuries are common, particularly in centers with a large proportion of penetrating injuries. Penetrating injuries tend to cause smaller, more discrete injuries, whereas blunt trauma often causes larger avulsion-type injuries. Diaphragm injuries secondary to both blunt and penetrating causes are often associated with injuries to the lungs and abdominal viscera. The diagnosis of a diaphragm injury can be difficult.[321–323] In any penetrating injury in the thoracoabdominal region, a diaphragm injury should be suspected.[78] In blunt injuries, physical examination is notoriously unreliable. If thoracotomy or laparotomy is performed secondary to associated injuries, the diaphragm should be inspected thoroughly for evidence of injury and repaired at that time. In patients in whom operative intervention is not needed, the diagnosis can easily be missed by plain radiographs, as the findings are often misinterpreted as pulmonary pathology.[322–324] CT scans have low sensitivity for esophageal injury.[323,325,326] Other possible diagnostic modalities include magnetic resonance imaging (MRI), contrast studies, and ultrasonography.[327–330] Diagnostic laparoscopy or thoracoscopy can be extremely valuable, but requires a high index of suspicion to select patients in whom to perform the procedure.[72,78] Some authors suggest that all thoracoabdominal penetrating injuries should be evaluated with laparoscopy or thoracoscopy to determine diaphragm injury in the absence of other indications for surgical intervention.[78]

Once identified, all diaphragm injuries should be repaired secondary to the risk of visceral herniation days to years after injury. This morbid complication of untreated diaphragmatic injuries is associated with substantial morbidity and mortality.[323,331] Most diaphragm injuries are repaired via laparotomy. The edges of the injury should be debrided and closed primarily if possible. Large defects may require prosthetic mesh placement, and a thoracoabdominal approach may be needed. Concomitant bowel injuries with local contamination by enteric contents necessitate irrigation or drainage of the thorax secondary to the high risk of empyema. Chronic diaphragmatic hernias secondary to missed injuries have traditionally been approached via thoracotomy secondary to abdominal adhesion formation. However, there are numerous reports of successful laparoscopic repair of diaphragm injuries, which may prove to be the optimal approach to a relatively isolated injury.[75,77]

Injury to the Liver

The liver is the most frequently injured organ in blunt abdominal trauma and, because of its size and location, is often injured in penetrating trauma as well. The Organ Injury Scaling Committee of the American Association for the Surgery of Trauma (AAST) has outlined a classification scheme that can be used to describe the degree of injury.[332] Injuries range from minor lacerations and capsular hematomas, which have little clinical importance, to hepatic avulsion, which is a uniformly fatal injury. The mortality rises substantially with each grade, as the incidence decreases.[333]

The first step in operative treatment of hepatic injuries is the division of the ligamentous attachments to facilitate inspection. Thoracotomy or a thoracoabdominal incision may be needed to fully access the injury. Many techniques for control of hepatic hemorrhage have been described. The Pringle maneuver controls vascular inflow at the porta hepatis.[334] Failure to control major bleeding with the Pringle maneuver should call attention to the possibility of a retrohepatic vena cava or other major venous injury. Retrohepatic vena cava injuries are often fatal, and these patients are typically profoundly unstable.[333] Several techniques must often be used in concert for severe injuries (Grades III–V). These patients are frequently acidotic and coagulopathic and often require a damage control approach. Hepatic packing is the most effective temporizing measure for massive hemorrhage. Damage control measures may include atriocaval shunting, venovenous bypass, or hepatic vascular isolation.[335–340] If a damage control approach is used for hemorrhage not attributable to major venous injury, packing and deep liver sutures can be used as a temporizing measure. Other damage control techniques for massive hepatic trauma include balloon tamponade and hepatic resection. These patients may benefit from angiographic embolization as an adjunctive measure.[341–343]

If the patient stabilizes, definitive repair is attempted, which can be accomplished with a finger fracture technique.[344–346] This technique allows direct visualization and ligation of blood vessels and bile ducts. Devascularized tissue is then debrided, and omental packs can be used to tamponade minor bleeding.[347] Other techniques such as topical hemostatic agent or argon beam coagulation may be helpful as well. Closed-suction drains are routinely placed to prevent abscess or biloma formation.[333,348] Some patients may benefit from hepatic resection in the case of major hepatic vascular injury or tissue destruction. Hepatorrhaphy with absorbable mesh has also been described.[349,350] Minor hepatic injuries, when discovered at laparotomy, rarely require treatment beyond simple electrocautery coagulation, argon beam coagulation, or topical hemostatic agents. Indications for operative management in the setting of hemodynamic stability include treatment of associated injuries and management of complications such as abscesses, bilomas, biliary injury, or failure of nonoperative therapy.[351] Postoperative complications include biliary and infectious complications.[352]

As many as 50% to 80% of patients with liver injuries may be managed nonoperatively.[353,354] Selection of patients is determined by the degree of hemodynamic stability, as opposed to injury grade or CT findings.[355,356] The failure rate of nonoperative management is generally attributable to associated injuries,[357] but a few failures are secondary to hemorrhage from the liver itself.[353,358] Nonoperative management may result in fewer abdominal complications, and there is good evidence that patients treated nonoperatively have lower transfusion requirements than with operative intervention.[353,355] Length of stay for these patients may also be lower.[353,354,359] High-grade injuries can often be safely managed nonoperatively, but need to be observed closely secondary to the higher rate of failure.[353] Table 27.5 presents representative clinical experiences with nonoperative management of hepatic injuries.

Findings on CT scan may identify patients who will benefit from angiographic embolization.[353,360] Patients with a "blush" on CT or active extravasation of contrast, regardless of the grade of injury, should undergo hepatic artery angiography and embolization.[353,356] Angiography and embolization may also be a useful adjunctive therapy in patients with high-grade lesions even in the absence of pseudoaneurysm or extravasation.[342] Follow-up CT scans are useful in identifying patients at risk for infectious and biliary complications.[361] The timing of routine follow-up CT scan is controversial, with some advocating early imaging (48–72 h) and others advocating for later routine follow-up, or sequential examinations.[353,359]

Nonoperative management of hepatic injuries is usually successful, but potential complications are numerous. In the largest reported series, bleeding was the most common complication of nonoperative management.[353] Biliary complications also occur; bilomas can often be treated successfully with percutaneous drainage, although occasionally operative intervention is required.[351–353] Endoscopic retrograde cholangiopancreatography (ERCP) can be a valuable adjunct in the identification and treatment of biliary complications, and allows therapy with sphincterotomy and biliary stenting.[356,362] Infectious complications, such as hepatic and intraabdominal abscesses, have also been reported.[358] One of the most morbid complications of nonoperative management of hepatic injuries is the development of the abdominal compartment syndrome.[48,351,357,362,363] Routine intraabdominal pressure monitoring in these patients has been advocated by some centers.[363] There are also numerous reports of missed abdominal injuries when nonoperative management of hepatic trauma is undertaken.[353,355,364] Fortunately, the incidence of missed associated injuries is small, but clinicians must be vigilant about careful observation of all these patients.

Injury to the Spleen

The spleen is also commonly injured following blunt trauma, albeit not as often as the liver. Penetrating injury to the left thoracoabdominal region also can injure the spleen. The AAST has outlined a classification scheme that describes the degree of splenic injury.[332] As with the liver, Grade I spleen injuries are the most minor, often simple lacerations or

TABLE 27.5.
Representative Clinical Experience with Nonoperative Management of Blunt Hepatic Injuries.

Trial	*Year*	*Level of evidence*	*Number of patients*	*Intervention/design*	*Median follow-up*	*Minor endpoint*	*Major endpoint*	*Interpretations/comments*
354	1994	III	72	Retrospective review of all patients with blunt hepatic injuries admitted to a single institution	N/A	Transfusion requirements	Successful nonoperative management of blunt hepatic injuries	Ninety-seven percent of patients in whom nonoperative management was attempted were safely managed without surgery. The nonoperative groups had lower transfusion requirements and shorter length of stay.
359	1994	II	30	Prospective study of nonoperative vs. operative management of blunt hepatic injuries	N/A	Complications of nonoperative management	Successful nonoperative management of blunt hepatic injuries	Nonoperative management of blunt hepatic injuries is safe and efficacious in hemodynamically stable patients. Transfusion requirements were lower in the nonoperative group.
355	1995	II	112	Prospective study of nonoperative management of blunt hepatic injuries of all severities compared to operative management in a matched cohort	N/A	Transfusion requirements, length of stay, abdominal complications	Successful nonoperative management of blunt hepatic injuries	Nonoperative management of blunt hepatic injuries is safe even for high-grade injuries. Transfusion requirement, were less in the nonoperative groups as were abdominal complications, although there was no difference in length of stay.
353	1996	III	404	Retrospective multicenter study of nonoperative management of blunt hepatic injuries	N/A	Transfusion requirements, length of stay, complications	Mortality from nonoperative management of blunt hepatic injuries	Nonoperative management of blunt hepatic injuries is safe and efficacious. There were 27 deaths (7%), but only 2 were attributable to the liver injury. Hemorrhage occurred in 3.5% with 0.7% requiring operative intervention. Higher-grade injuries were more likely to fail.
358	2003	II	63	Prospective evaluation of a protocol for the nonoperative management of blunt hepatic injury in hemodynamically stable patients	N/A	Complications of nonoperative management	Failure of nonoperative management in patients with blunt hepatic trauma	Failure of nonoperative management occurred in 17.5% of patients. ICU length of stay and transfusion requirements were higher in the group who failed. Complication rates of nonoperative management was 9.5%.
357	2003	II	55	Prospective evaluation of a protocol for the nonoperative management of blunt hepatic injury in hemodynamically stable patients	N/A	Factors associated with nonoperative failure	Failure of nonoperative management in patients with blunt hepatic trauma	Failure of nonoperative management was 15%. None of these failures was attributable to the liver itself. Nonoperative management is safe regardless of the grade of liver injury. Failure may be predicted by fluid and blood requirements and the presence of associated intraabdominal injuries.

ICU, intensive care unit; N/A, not available.

subcapsular hematomas. Grade V injuries are splenic avulsion or complete devascularization.

In the early 1980s, operative exploration and splenectomy was believed to be necessary for every splenic injury. However, concerns about the incidence of overwhelming postsplenectomy infection (OPSI) led pediatric surgeons to begin to observe selected splenic injuries. Their success prompted use of the same strategy in adults. However, early results were not as good. Simple observation failed approximately 15% to 20% of the time.[365]

Few objective data are available to guide nonoperative therapy. Observation generally involves keeping the patient at bed rest for several days, maintaining the patient on nothing by mouth and utilizing serial abdominal examinations and hematocrits to gauge the efficacy of nonoperative management. Triggers to abandon nonoperative treatment are not clearly defined and vary among institutions and individual clinicians.

The evolution of CT scanning has allowed clinicians to reliably exclude associated injuries, estimate the severity of splenic injury, and plan nonoperative management. However, CT grading does not correlate with operative findings. Early on, observation was restricted to those under the age of 55 years secondary to evidence that failure rates were higher in older patients.[366] Early recommendations were that observation should only be attempted with splenic injury grades of less than 3.[367] However, it became clear that some higher-grade injuries could also be treated nonoperatively as well.[368,369] Additionally, studies have demonstrated that older patients may also be safely managed with observation of splenic injuries.[370,371]

Hemodynamic instability mandates operative management of blunt splenic injuries; this may occur at the time of patient presentation or if patients bleed while being observed. Any patient who presents with hemodynamic stability and does not have another indication for laparotomy is a candidate for nonoperative management. There would be great utility in knowing which patients are more likely to fail observation. In the Eastern Association for the Surgery of Trauma (EAST) multi-institutional retrospective trial, Peitzman et al. demonstrated that splenic injury grade, degree of hemoperitoneum, and hemodynamic stability at the time of patient presentation most accurately predicted who would fail.[367] Approximately 40% of these nearly 1500 patients over 15 years of age were managed primarily with laparotomy. Seventy percent of patients who failed observation did so within 24 h of admission. In addition, the presence of a contrast "blush" on CT scan predicts failure of simple observation, as does the presence of pseudoaneurysm on helical CT scan.[372,373] Pseudoaneurysms are often not visible at the time of initial CT but may appear on repeat CT scan several days later. Complications of simple observation of splenic injuries include hemorrhage, development of pseudoaneurysms, and splenic abscesses.[367,372,374]

Angiographic embolization may improve splenic salvage during nonoperative management. First described in 1995 by Sclafani et al., the splenic artery is embolized proximal to the pancreatic branches.[375] Splenic viability is maintained via collateral blood flow. The first series demonstrated a 98.5% splenic salvage rate, the highest reported in the literature. Several recent series have demonstrated statistically significantly better results in higher-grade splenic injuries when compared against the EAST trial.[369,371,372,376,377] Selective use of angiography also reduces hospital charges and length of stay.[378] Complications following embolization, other than failure of hemostasis, are relatively uncommon but include technical errors, splenic infarctions, and splenic abscess.[376,378] Table 27.6 presents representative clinical experiences with nonoperative management of splenic injuries.

Operative management of splenic injury includes either splenorrhaphy or splenectomy. As 90% of patients with blunt splenic injury are now treated nonoperatively, the need for splenectomy is higher in those undergoing operative management. Splenic salvage is a reasonable option in stable patients without other life-threatening injuries who have injury architecture amenable to splenorrhaphy. Unstable patients or those with other priorities should undergo splenectomy. Patients who have a splenectomy should be vaccinated against pneumococcus to prevent OPSI. Whether vaccination is necessary against meningococci or *Hemophilus influenzae* is debatable. Those who will be exposed to large groups of people (i.e., students or those in the military) should be considered for immunization against *Hemophilus* and meningococcus. Autotransplantation of pieces of the spleen into the omentum after splenectomy may offer some immunological benefit. Options for operative splenic salvage include simple topical hemostasis, fibrin sealants, or use of the argon beam coagulator. Deeper lacerations can be treated by suture repair with Teflon or absorbable pledgets. Multiple lacerations or capsular avulsions may be treated by utilizing a wrap of polyglycolic acid mesh. Proximal splenic artery ligation works similarly to proximal coil embolization.

Injury to the Pancreas and Duodenum

Injuries to the duodenum and pancreas can occur as result of either blunt or penetrating trauma. The mortality of duodenal injuries ranges from 12% to 25% for penetrating injuries and from 10% to 35% for blunt injuries.[379–384] Similarly, for pancreatic injuries the mortality ranges from 3% to 36% in the setting of penetrating injury and is about 20% for blunt injuries.[385–388] Fatalities in these patients are often secondary to associated injuries to the surrounding major vasculature.[389] Isolated injuries to the pancreas or duodenum are rare.[390,391] The retroperitoneal location of these structures protects the duodenum and pancreas from frequent injury, but also makes their diagnosis and treatment extremely challenging. Delay in the diagnosis and treatment of these injuries results in significantly increased morbidity and mortality.[380,385,386]

In the setting of penetrating trauma, the diagnosis typically is made by laparotomy. With blunt trauma, in the absence of indications for exploration, the diagnosis is often made by CT. A high index of suspicion must be maintained for these patients, as findings on physical examination or CT scan may be equivocal or delayed. Once recognized, the degree of hemodynamic stability, associated injuries, and the grade of the injuries determine the treatment. Organ injury scales exist for both duodenal and pancreatic injury and can be helpful in guiding treatment.[392] As a general rule, all these injuries require formal operative evaluation. Full mobilization of the overlying viscera is essential for proper identification and management of these injuries.

Minor duodenal injuries, such as mural hematomas or serosal tears, can be managed with careful inspection and close observation. Intermediate-grade injuries can often be treated with primary repair and drainage.[393] In a large multicenter review of duodenal injuries, primary repair was performed in 71% of cases.[382] The most severe injuries may require resection and diversion or enteric bypass. These repairs and anastomoses should generally be protected with omental or serosal patches, pyloric exclusion, or retrograde duodenostomy tubes.[379–381] Placement of enteral feeding access distal to the duodenum is advisable. Care must always be exercised in evaluating the ampulla of Vater and common bile duct in the setting of a proximal duodenal injury. Concomitant injuries to these structures require alternative techniques, such as choledochojejunostomy or pancreaticoduodentomy. Complications from duodenal injuries include dehiscence and duodenal fistula. The incidence is higher in the setting of a concomitant pancreatic injury.[394] Mortality from these complications alone may be as high as 20%.[380–382]

Pancreatic injuries are similarly treated based on organ injury scaling and often occur in concert with duodenal injuries secondary to their close anatomic relationship. The principles of treatment of pancreatic injuries are to control exocrine secretion while preserving endocrine function. Pancreatic injuries must be evaluated in two ways: whether the injury is to the head or tail, and whether the main pancreatic duct is involved. Determination of the duct's integrity is essential in the management of these injuries.

Minor injuries without duct disruption require no more than closed-suction drainage.[395] If the duct is involved, and the injury is to the tail of the pancreas, distal pancreatectomy is prudent. The most morbid injuries are with major duct disruption in the head of the pancreas. If relatively isolated, these injuries may be managed with wide drainage and postoperative ERCP and stenting.[396] Often these pancreatic head injuries are associated with severe duodenal and major vascular injuries. Damage control may be needed with a staged reconstruction once the patient is stabilized. Very rarely (e.g., combined pancreatic/duodenal injury) is a pancreaticoduodenectomy indicated in the acute setting.[397] All pancreatic injuries should be drained widely, and distal enteral access should be achieved for postoperative nutrition.[398] Complications of pancreatic injuries include fistula, abscess, pseudocyst, late hemorrhage, pancreatitis, pancreatic enzyme deficiency, and diabetes mellitus.[388,395,396] Complications may be seen in more than one-third of patients with pancreatic injuries who survive at least 48 h.[395]

Injury to the Gastrointestinal Tract

Injuries to the stomach and small intestine occur infrequently from blunt injury, but are quite common in the setting of penetrating trauma,[399,400] particularly gunshot wounds. Diagnosis is typically made at laparotomy in the setting of penetrating injury, as these injuries frequently cause peritonitis on physical examination. Pneumoperitoneum, seen on plain radiograph or CT scan, always necessitates laparotomy. The treatment is relatively straightforward and consists of debridement of devitalized tissue and primary repair or resection with anastomosis. If damage control is being utilized, both stomach and small bowel can be readily stapled closed, with definitive repair or resection performed later.

In the setting of blunt trauma, small bowel and stomach injuries can be more difficult to identify.[400] If secondary to motor vehicle collisions, a "seat-belt sign" may be present.[80,81,400,401] CT may be helpful in diagnosis, as is DPL. Findings on CT may include only free peritoneal fluid or bowel wall edema.[200] Delayed presentations can occur with blunt injuries. Often these injuries are associated with other major injuries as substantial force is needed to cause blunt perforation. Mesenteric tears or hematomas can also be seen that may cause small bowel devascularization, which must be addressed operatively. The principles of treatment are the same as in penetrating trauma, with resection of devitalized tissue and repair or resection and anastomosis.

Colon injuries are also common after penetrating trauma. Blunt injuries are relatively rare, but occur secondary to the same mechanisms that cause small bowel injury.[402–404] Blunt injuries may be frank perforations, serosal tears, or devascularizations from mesenteric injury. Diagnosis is often made by physical examination, but DPL and CT scan may be useful as well. At laparotomy these injuries can be subtle, especially when caused by stab wounds or small-caliber bullets. All colonic hematomas should be inspected carefully and opened to confirm the integrity of the bowel wall.

The management of these injuries has been extensively debated in the literature. Three basic options exist: primary repair, resection and reanastomosis, or resection with diversion. Historically, all colonic injuries were treated with diversion. In 1979, Stone and Fabian challenged the notion of diversion for all colonic injuries and demonstrated that primary repair or anastomosis was safe in a select group of patients.[405] Work by others reached similar conclusions and demonstrated that more than 50% of patients may be treated safely with primary repair or anastomosis.[406–418] One study demonstrated an increased failure rate in left-sided anastomoses when compared to ileo-colostomies.[419] Certain conditions must be met to perform primary repair and anastomosis safely,[405,407,408,419] including hemodynamic stability, modest blood loss, no associated abdominal injuries, minimal degree of fecal contamination, and short time interval from injury to laparotomy. These factors may be predictive of anastomotic failure and abscess formation. The risk of these complications must be weighed against the morbidity of colostomy and additional surgery. Several studies have demonstrated increased morbidity in patients treated with diversion, but this may be secondary to the clinical scenario that led the surgeon to choose diversion, rather than the morbidity of colostomy per se.[412,414,415,417,418] All these patients should be given perioperative antibiotics directed against bowel flora[416,418] for 24 h, but longer antibiotic prophylaxis is not beneficial.

Rectal injuries usually occur secondary to penetrating injuries, usually from transpelvic gunshot wounds. Other injuries may occur through transanal insertion of objects or from pelvic fractures with bony penetration. In any patient with a suspected rectal injury, digital rectal examination should be performed, which may demonstrate gross blood. Rigid proctoscopy or sigmoidoscopy should be performed as well if the patient is hemodynamically stable. However, these exams may be nondiagnostic, with nonspecific findings such as intraluminal blood.[420] Attempts to identify rectal injuries

TABLE 27.6.
Representative Clinical Experience with Nonoperative Management of Blunt Splenic Injuries

Trial	*Year*	*Level of evidence*	*Number of patients*	*Intervention/design*	*Median follow-up*	*Minor endpoint*	*Major endpoint*	*Interpretations/comments*
365	1989	III	112	Review of blunt splenic injuries managed nonoperatively	N/A	N/A	Outcome following observation of blunt splenic injuries	Failure rates of 11.6%. Of the patients who failed observation, 58% had splenic salvage at laparotomy. No deaths were attributable to splenic injury. Recommends that low-grade (I–III) splenic injuries can safely be observed in hemodynamically stable patients.
373	1995	III	99	Review of CT findings in patients with blunt splenic injuries	N/A	N/A	Identification of factors predictive of failure of nonoperative management of blunt splenic injuries	Failure rate of 13% is reported. Contrast blush on CT scan predicted failure with nonoperative management and was present in 67% of failures vs. only 6% of patients successfully managed with observation alone.
375	1995	III	150	Review of an algorithm for management of blunt splenic injury to determine the efficacy of angiography and embolization	N/A	Determination of the efficacy of coil embolization in nonoperative management	Determination of the angiographic findings that predict successful nonoperative management of blunt splenic injuries	Overall success rate was 88%. Splenic salvage rate was 97%. Hemodynamically stable patients with splenic injuries can be safely managed nonoperatively regardless of grade. The absence of contrast extravasation on angiography is predictive of success of nonoperative management. Proximal coil embolization is effective and increases the number of patients who can be managed nonoperatively.
374	1998	III	87	Retrospective review of patients with blunt splenic injury managed nonoperatively	N/A	Number of units transfused, ICULOS, LOS, and outcome	Identification of delayed complications following nonoperative management of blunt splenic injuries	Failure rate for patients managed nonoperatively was 6%. Complications occurred in 8% of those observed. Complications included bleeding, pseudoaneurysm formation, and splenic abscess.
372	1998	III	344	Retrospective review of patients with blunt splenic injury managed nonoperatively	N/A	N/A	Identification of factors predictive of failure of nonoperative management of blunt splenic injuries	Nonoperative management was successful in 94% of patients in whom it was attempted. Presence of a pseudoaneurysm on CT scan is strongly predictive of failure of observation alone. Splenic artery pseudoaneurysms may not be apparent on the initial CT scan.

TABLE 27.6. (continued)

Trial	*Year*	*Level of evidence*	*Number of patients*	*Intervention/design*	*Median follow-up*	*Minor endpoint*	*Major endpoint*	*Interpretations/comments*
367	2000	III	913	Multi-institutional retrospective review of patients managed with observation following blunt splenic trauma	N/A	N/A	Identification of factors predictive of failure of nonoperative management of blunt splenic injuries	Failure rate was 10.8% in those patients in whom nonoperative management was attempted. Sixty-one percent of failures occurred in the first 24 h following injury. Failure rates increased significantly with increased grade and an increased degree of hemoperitoneum on CT.
369	2001	III	126	Retrospective review of patients with blunt splenic injury who underwent angiography as an adjunct to nonoperative management	N/A	N/A	Nonoperative salvage rates for patients with blunt splenic injuries managed with angiography and embolization as indicated	Vascular injury is more frequent with higher-grade injuries. Nonoperative salvage rates of 92% are reported with the addition of angiography. Ten percent of patients who initially had negative angiograms required laparotomy or a second angiogram.
371	2004	III	140	Multi-institutional retrospective review of patients managed with splenic embolization following blunt splenic trauma	N/A	Complications of splenic embolization, factors predictive of failure	Failure of nonoperative management of splenic trauma with splenic artery embolization	Failure rate following embolization was 10%. This rate was not different whether proximal coil embolization or selective techniques were applied. Failure was not predicted by degree of hemoperitoneum. Higher-grade injuries demonstrated better results when compared with other studies using simple observation. Complications occurred in 32%.
376	2005	III	368	Retrospective review of patients treated nonoperatively for blunt splenic injuries	N/A	N/A	Splenic salvage rates for patients treated nonoperatively for blunt splenic injuries	Failure of nonoperative management occurred in 0% of patients observed, 6% with a negative angiogram, and 10% who were treated with splenic embolization. Salvage rates decreased with increasing grade of injury. Nonoperative salvage rate was 80% in grade IV and V injuries. Arteriovenous fistulas predict failure of nonoperative therapy.

CT, computed tomagraphy; ICULOS, intensive care unit length of stay; N/A, not available.

at laparotomy can be difficult secondary to the deep extraperitoneal pelvic location of most of the rectum. The safest course of action is to treat the patient as if a rectal injury is present rather than risk the high morbidity of a missed injury. The treatment of rectal injuries consists of diversion, repair, and drainage. The Hartmann procedure (coletomy, end colostomy, and closure of the distal rectal stump) is performed for extensive injuries, rather than attempting a primary repair. Repair with a proximal loop colostomy is advocated for more minor injuries.[420–423] The necessity of drainage for all extraperitoneal injuries has recently been challenged.[420,422–424] There is conflicting literature on whether distal irrigation of the rectum is needed as well.[422,425–427] There is some evidence that small distal injuries may be treated safely with drainage and antibiotics alone, or transanal repair without diversion.[428] In the setting of associated open pelvic fractures, drainage and diversion are essential to prevent pelvic sepsis.[421]

Injuries to the Kidney, Ureter, and Bladder

Hematuria is the hallmark of renal injury, although it is not invariably present. Although the diagnosis is made at laparotomy when performed to treat other injuries, CT scan and contrast studies are the diagnostic modalities that often identify these injuries. Minor injuries rarely require specific treatment, whereas a Grade V renal injury (shattered or avulsed kidney) typically necessitates nephrectomy. Documentation of contralateral renal function is important before nephrectomy. The moderate-grade injuries can be treated by a variety of algorithms. Intraoperative options include nephrectomy, partial nephrectomy, or nephrorrhaphy. Nonoperative management of the stable patient can be accomplished safely for both penetrating and blunt injuries.[341,429–432] Kidney salvage rates are typically greater than 95%.[429,431] Angiographic embolization plays an important role in the management of these injuries. Urine leaks can typically be managed with external drainage with or without ureteral stenting.[431]

Ureter injuries are almost entirely secondary to penetrating trauma. Associated injuries are common. Hematuria in these patients is typically microscopic or may be absent.[433,434] Contrast studies or CT scan may help to identify injuries.[430,433] Missed injuries are not uncommon, especially when major associated injuries are present, and may cause substantial morbidity.[435,436] The management of ureteral injuries includes debridement and primary repair, typically over a stent. Psoas hitch and the Boari flaps are techniques that can be used if blast injury resection results in loss of a segment more than 2 to 3 cm in length.[433]

Bladder injuries are quite common in the setting of blunt trauma, especially in association with pelvic fractures.[437] Hematuria in the presence of a pelvic fracture should prompt evaluation of the bladder with cystography.[438] Often, these injuries are extraperitoneal and require only simple transurethral catheter drainage.[439] Repeat cystography after 7 to 10 days usually demonstrates healing of the injury, but occasionally direct repair may be needed. Intraperitoneal bladder injury from either blunt or penetrating trauma requires operative repair. Direct two-layer closure is recommended. Transurethral bladder drainage is advisable when possible, as suprapubic tubes may lead to higher complication rates.[440]

Complications

Complications of torso trauma are quite frequent and are the leading cause of death among patients who survive the initial insult.[1] Most commonly, death is secondary to the development of multiple organ dysfunction syndrome. Infectious complications and missed injuries contribute dramatically to postinjury morbidity and mortality.[441–443] Strategies to reduce the incidence of missed injuries include the tertiary survey of the patient, "24-h" observation, routine reimaging, and maintenance of a high level of suspicion in the event of clinical deterioration.[443–448] One of the major pitfalls of nonoperative management of solid organ injury is the potential for missed injuries.[364] The risk of missed injuries must be weighed against the risk of complication of negative laparotomy, however, which was reported to be 12% in one recent series.[449] In all patients with traumatic injury, the surgeon must remain vigilant and flexible and utilize sound clinical judgment to guide therapy.

Abdominal Compartment Syndrome

One of the most morbid sequelae of major trauma is the development of the abdominal compartment syndrome (ACS). This complication occurs most frequently in the setting of severe abdominal injury,[450] commonly the result of ongoing intraabdominal or retroperitoneal hemorrhage. Secondary compartment syndrome has been well described, in which massive volume resuscitation and transfusions lead to increased abdominal pressure.[450–453] Abdominal compartment syndrome can occur after damage control procedures, secondary to abdominal packing and massive resuscitation.[216–218,450,454] For this reason, fascial closure following damage control is ill advised.[217] Additionally, ACS may occur following nonoperative management of liver injuries.[351,362,363] Third-spacing of fluid, blood, and severe bowel edema contribute to increased intraabdominal pressure, which can adversely effect the cardiovascular, pulmonary, and renal systems. The gastrointestinal tract may be particularly sensitive to elevated abdominal pressure; some work has focused on measurement of gastric mucosal pH as a harbinger of the development of ACS.[454–456]

If left untreated, ACS is fatal.[450] Physical examination is notoriously unreliable.[457] Monitoring is performed most commonly with the measurement of urinary bladder pressure, first described by Kron et al. in 1984.[458] Treatment usually consists of decompressive laparotomy. A grading system has been developed as a guide for decompression.[450] Grades III (bladder pressure 25–35 mmHg) and IV (bladder pressure >35 mmHg) almost invariably require decompression. The authors stress, however, that the specific clinical picture must dictate treatment, as some patients will manifest symptoms at lower bladder pressures. Some authors have suggesting using an "abdominal perfusion pressure" as a guide for the decision to perform decompression.[459]

Early decompression improves survival.[451,460] The development of both primary and secondary ACS may predict multiple organ dysfunction syndrome in severely injured patients.[455,456,461] Secondary compartment syndrome is a particularly morbid scenario. The mortality rate of secondary ACS is between 38% and 54% in reported series, despite early decompression.[452,462] Even in the setting of an open abdomen, compartment syndrome may develop with associated organ dysfunction. Termed the "open abdomen ACS" or, at our institution, "tertiary" compartment syndrome,[463] this is a highly lethal event.

References

1. Sauaia A, Moore FA, Moore EE, et al. Epidemiology of trauma deaths: a reassessment. J Trauma 1995;38:185–193.
2. MacKenzie EJ, Fowler CF. Epidemiology. In: Mattox KL, Feliciano DV, Moore EE, eds. Trauma, 4th ed. New York: McGraw-Hill, 2000:21–40.
3. Shackford SR, Mackersie RC, Holbrook TL, et al. The epidemiology of traumatic death: a population-based analysis. Arch Surg 1993;128:571–575.
4. Wall MJ, Storey JH, Mattox KL. Indications for thoracotomy. In: Mattox KL, Feliciano DV, Moore EE, eds. Trauma, 4th ed. New York: McGraw-Hill, 2000:473–482.
5. Fabian TC, Croce MA. Abdominal trauma, including indication for celiotomy. In: Mattox KL, Moore EE, Feliciano DV, eds. Trauma, 3rd ed. Stamford: Appleton and Lange, 1996.
6. Hirshberg A, Or J, Stein M, Walden R. Transfix gunshot wounds. J Trauma 1996;41:460–461.
7. Kennedy F, Sullivan J, Arellano D, Roulier R. Evaluating the role of physical and radiographic examinations in assessing bullet tract termination for gunshot victims. Am Surg 2000;66:296–301.
8. Chen SC, Chang KJ, Hsu CY. Accuracy of auscultation in the detection of haemopneumothorax. Eur J Surg 1998;164:643–645.
9. Bokhari F, Brakenridge S, Nagy K, et al. Prospective evaluation of the sensitivity of physical examination in chest trauma. J Trauma 2002;53:1135–1138.
10. Chen SC, Markmann JF, Kauder DR, Schwab CW. Hemopneumothorax missed by ascultation in penetrating chest injury. J Trauma 1997;42:86–89.
11. Hirshberg A, Thomson SR, Huizinga WK. Reliability of physical examination in penetrating chest injuries. Injury 1998;19:407–409.
12. Demetriades D, Rabinowitz B, Sofianos C, et al. The management of penetrating injuries of the back. A prospective study of 230 patients. Ann Surg 1988;207:72–74.
13. Demetriades D, Charalambides D, Lakhoo M, Pantanowitz D. Gunshot wound of the abdomen: role of conservative management. Br J Surg 1991;78:220–222.
14. van Haarst E, van Bezooijen BPJ, Coene PPLO, Luitse JSK. The efficacy of serial physical examination in penetrating abdominal trauma. Injury 1999;30:599–604.
15. Demetriades D, Rabinowitz B, Sofianos C, et al. The management of penetrating injuries of the back. Ann Surg 1988;207:72–74.
16. Jackson G, Thal E. Management of stab wounds to the back and flank. J Trauma 1979;19:660–664.
17. Coppa G, Davalle M, Pachter H, et al. Management of penetrating wounds of the back and flank. Surg Gynecol Obstet 1984;159:514–518.
18. Gasparri MG, Lorelli DR, Kralovich KA, Patton JH. Physical examination plus chest radiography in penetrating periclavicular trauma: the appropriate trigger for angiography. J Trauma 2000;49:1029–1033.
19. Shatz DV, de la Pedraja J, Erbella J, et al. Efficacy of follow-up evaluation in penetrating thoracic injuries: 3- vs. 6-hour radiographs of the chest. J Emerg Med 2001;20:281–284.
20. Root HD, Hauser CW, McKinley CR, et al. Diagnostic peritoneal lavage. Surgery (St. Louis) 1965;57:633–637.
21. Thal ER. Evaluation of peritoneal lavage and local exploration in lower chest and abdominal stab wounds. J Trauma 1977;17:642–649.
22. Alyono D, Morrow CE, Perry JF. Reappraisal of diagnostic peritoneal lavage criteria for operation in penetrating and blunt trauma. Surgery (St. Louis) 1982;92:751–757.
23. Oreskovich MR, Carrico CJ. Stab wounds of the anterior abdomen: analysis of a management plan using local wound exploration and quantitative peritoneal lavage. Ann Surg 1983;198:411–418.
24. Merlotti GJ, Marcet E, Sheaff CM, et al. Use of peritoneal lavage to evaluate abdominal penetration. J Trauma 1985;25:228–231.
25. Nagy KK, Krosner SM, Joseph KT, et al. A method of determining peritoneal penetration in gunshot wounds to the abdomen. J Trauma 1997;43:242–246.
26. Marx JA, Moore EE, Jorden RC, et al. Limitations of computed tomography in the evaluation of acute abdominal trauma: a prospective comparison with diagnostic peritoneal lavage. J Trauma 1985;25:933–937.
27. Davis JW, Hoyt DB, Mackersie RC, McArdle MS. Complications in evaluating abdominal trauma: diagnostic peritoneal lavage versus computerized axial tomography. J Trauma 1990;30:1506–1509.
28. Fischer RP, Beverlin BC, Engrav LH. Diagnostic peritoneal lavage: fourteen years and 2586 patients later. Am J Surg 1978;136:701–704.
29. Powell DL, Bivens BA, Bell RM. Diagnostic peritoneal lavage. Surg Gynecol Obstet 1982;155:257–264.
30. Soderstrom CA, DuPriest RW, Cowley RA. Pitfalls of peritoneal lavage in blunt abdominal trauma. Surg Gynecol Obstet 1980;151:513–518.
31. Goldstein AS, Sclafani SJA, Kupferstein NH, et al. The diagnostic superiority of computerized tomography. J Trauma 1985;25:938–946.
32. Thal ER, May RA, Beesinger D. Peritoneal lavage: its unreliability in gunshot wounds of the lower chest and abdomen. Arch Surg 1980;115:430–433.
33. Hanpeter DE, Demetriades D, Asensio JA, et al. Helical computed tomographic scan in the evaluation of mediastinal gunshot wounds. J Trauma 2000;49:689–695.
34. Stassen NA, Lukan JK, Spain DA, et al. Reevaluation of diagnostic procedures for transmediastinal gunshot wounds. J Trauma 2002;53:635–638.
35. Meyer DM, Thal ER, Weigelt JA, Redman HC. The role of abdominal CT in the evaluation of stab wounds to the back. J Trauma 1989;29:1226–1230.
36. Ginzburg E, Carrillo EH, Kopelman T, et al. The role of computed tomography in selective management of gunshot wounds to the abdomen and flank. J Trauma 1998;45:1005–1009.
37. McAllister E, Perez M, Albrink MH, et al. Is triple contrast computed tomographic scanning useful in the selective management of stab wounds to the back? J Trauma 1994;37:401–403.
38. Kirton OC, Wint D, Thrasher B, et al. Stab wounds to the back and flank in the hemodynamically stable patient: a decision algorithm based on contrast-enhanced computed tomography with colonic opacification. Am J Surg 1997;173:189–193.
39. Phillips T, Sclafani SJA, Goldstein A, et al. Use of the contrast CT enema in the management of penetrating trauma to the flank and back. J Trauma 1986;26:593–601.
40. Sherck JP, Oakes DD. Intestinal injuries missed by computed tomography. J Trauma 1990;30:1–7.
41. Butela ST, Federle MP, Chang PJ, et al. Performance of CT in detection of bowel injury. AJR 2001;176:129–135.
42. Grossman MD, May AK, Schwab CW, et al. Determining anatomic injury with computed tomography in selected torso gunshot wounds. J Trauma 1998;45:446–456.
43. Ginzburg E, Carrillo EH, Kopelman T, et al. The role of computed tomography in selective management of gunshot wounds to the abdomen and flank. J Trauma 1998;45:1005–1009.
44. Chiu WC, Shanmuganathan K, Mirvis SE, Scalea TM. Determining the need for laparotomy in penetrating torso trauma: a pro-

spective study using triple-contrast enhanced abdominopelvic computed tomography. J Trauma 2001:51:860–869.
45. Shanmuganathan K, Mirvis SE, Chiu WC, et al. Triple-contrast helical CT in penetrating torso trauma: a prospective study to determine peritoneal violation and the need for laparotomy. AJR 2001;177:1247–1256.
46. Shanmuganathan K, Mirvis SE, Chiu WC, et al. Penetrating torso trauma: triple-contrast helical CT in peritoneal violation and organ injury: a prospective study in 200 patients. Radiology 2004;231:775–784.
47. Munera F, Morales C, Soto JA, et al. Gunshot wounds of abdomen: evaluation of stable patients with triple-contrast helical CT. Radiology 2004;231:399–405.
48. Demetriades D, Gomez H, Chahwan S, et al. Gunshot wounds to the liver: the role of selective nonoperative management. J Am Coll Surg 1999;188:343–348.
49. Demetraides D, Velmahos G, Cornwell EE, et al. Selective nonoperative management of gunshot wounds of the anterior abdomen. Arch Surg 1997;132:178–183.
50. Ma OJ, Mateer JR, Ogata M, et al. Prospective analysis of a rapid trauma ultrasound examination performed by emergency physicians. J Trauma 1995;38:879–885.
51. Rozycki GS, Ochsner MG, Schmidt JA, et al. Prospective study of surgeon-performed ultrasound as the primary adjuvant modality for injured patient assessment. J Trauma 1995;39:492–500.
52. Rozycki GS, Ballard RB, Feliciano DV, et al. Surgeon-performed ultrasound for the assessment of truncal injuries: lessons learned from 1540 patients. J Trauma 1998;228:557–567.
53. Ma OJ, Mateer JR. Trauma ultrasound examination versus chest radiography in the detection of hemothorax. Ann Emerg Med 1997;29:312–316.
54. Sisley AC, Rozycki GS, Ballard RB, et al. Rapid detection of traumatic effusion using surgeon-performed ultrasonography. J Trauma 1998;44:291–297.
55. Boulanger BR, Kearney PA, Tsuei B, Ochoa JB. The routine use of sonography in penetrating torso injury is beneficial. J Trauma 2001;51:320–325.
56. Kirkpatrick AW, Sirois M, Ball CG, et al. The hand-held ultrasound for penetrating abdominal trauma. Am J Surg 2004;187:660–665.
57. Soffer D, McKenney MG, Cohn S, et al. A prospective evaluation of ultrasonography for the diagnosis of penetrating torso trauma. J Trauma 2004;56:953–959.
58. Udobi KF, Rodriguez A, Chiu WC, Scalea TM. Role of ultrasonography in penetrating abdominal trauma: a prospective clinical study. J Trauma 2001;50:475–479.
59. Kirkpatrick AW, Sirois M, Laupland KB, et al. Hand-held sonography for detecting post-traumatic pneumothoraces: the extended focused assessment with sonography for trauma (EFAST). J Trauma 2004;57:288–295.
60. Knudtson JL, Dort JM, Helmer SD, Smith RS. Surgeon-performed ultrasound for pneumothorax in the trauma suite. J Trauma 2004;56:527–530.
61. Rozycki GS, Ochsner MG, Feliciano DV, et al. Early detection of hemoperitoneum by ultrasound examination of the right upper quadrant: a multicenter study. J Trauma 1998;45:878–883.
62. Rozycki GS, Feliciano DV, Ochsner MG, et al. The role of ultrasound in patients with penetrating cardiac wounds: a prospective multicenter study. J Trauma 1999;46:543–552.
63. Gazzaniga AB, Stanton WW, Bartlett RH. Laparoscopy in the diagnosis of blunt and penetrating injuries to the abdomen. Am J Surg 1976;131:315–318.
64. Salvino CK, Esposito TJ, Marshall WJ, et al. The role of diagnostic laparoscopy in the management of trauma patients: a preliminary assessment. J Trauma 1993;34:506–515.
65. Sosa JL, Markley M, Sleemen D, et al. Laparoscopy in abdominal gunshot wounds. Surg Laparosc Endosc 1993;3:417–419.
66. Ivatury RR, Simon RJ, Stahl WM. A critical evaluation of laparoscopy in penetrating abdominal trauma. J Trauma 1993;34:822–828.
67. Carey JE, Koo R, Stein M, Miller R. Laparoscopy and thoracoscopy in evaluation of abdominal trauma. Am Surg 1995;61:92–95.
68. Sosa JL, Arrillaga A, Puente I, et al. Laparoscopy in 121 consecutive patients with abdominal gunshot wounds. J Trauma 1995;39:501–506.
69. Guth AA, Pachter HL. Laparoscopy for penetrating thoracoabdominal trauma: pitfalls and promises. J Surg Laparosc Surg 1998;2:123–127.
70. Ortega AE, Tang E, Froes ET, et al. Laparoscopic evaluation of penetrating thoracoabdominal traumatic injuries. Surg Endosc 1996;10:19–22.
71. Gorecki PJ, Cottam D, Angus LD, Shaftan GW. Diagnostic and therapeutic laparoscopy for trauma: a technique of safe and systematic exploration. Surg Laparosc Endosc Percutan Tech 2002;12:195–198.
72. McQuay N, Britt LD. Laparoscopy in the evaluation of penetrating thoracoabdominal trauma. Am Surg 2003;69:788–791.
73. Chelly MR, Major K, Spivak J, et al. The value of laparoscopy in management of abdominal trauma. Am Surg 2003;69:957–960.
74. Miles EJ, Dunn E, Howard D, Mangram A. The role of laparoscopy in penetrating abdominal trauma. J Surg Laparosc Surg 2004;8:304–309.
75. Choi YB, Lim KS. Therapeutic laparoscopy for abdominal trauma. Surg Endosc 2003;17:421–427.
76. Zantut LF, Ivatury RR, Smith RS, et al. Diagnostic and therapeutic laparoscopy for penetrating abdominal trauma: a multicenter experience. J Trauma 1997;42:825–831.
77. Matthews BD, Bui H, Harold KL, et al. Laparoscopic repair of traumatic diaphragm injuries. Surg Endosc 2003;17:254–258.
78. Conrad MF, Patton JH, Parikshak M, Kralovich KA. Selective management of penetrating truncal injuries: is emergency department discharge a reasonable goal. Am Surg 2003;69:266–273.
79. Chandler CF, Lane JS. Seatbelt sign following blunt trauma is associated with increased incidence of abdominal injury. Am Surg 1997;63:88–89.
80. Chandler CF, Lane JS. Seatbelt sign following blunt trauma is associated with increased incidence of abdominal injury. Am Surg 1997;63:885–888.
81. Velmahos GC, Tatevossian R, Demetriades D. The "seat belt mark" sign: a call for increased vigilance among physicians treating victims of motor vehicle accidents. Am Surg 1999;65:181–185.
82. Peitzman AB, Makaroun MS, Slasky BS, et al. Prospective study of computed tomography in initial management of blunt abdominal trauma. J Trauma 1986;26:585–591.
83. Rodriguez A, DuPriest RW, Shatney CH. Recognition on intra-abdominal injury in blunt trauma victims. Am Surg 1982;48:456–459.
84. Mackersie RC, Tiwary AD, Shackford SR, Hoyt DB. Intraabdominal injury following blunt trauma. Arch Surg 1989;124:809–813.
85. Richards JR, Derlet RW. Computed tomography for blunt abdominal trauma in the ED: a prospective study. Am J Emerg Med 1998;16:338–342.
86. Gonzalez RP, Dziurzynski K, Maunu M. Emergent extra-abdominal trauma surgery: is abdominal screening necessary? J Trauma 2000;49:195–204.
87. Schurink GWH, Bode PJ, van Luijt PA, van Vugt AB. The value of physical examination in the diagnosis of patients with blunt abdominal trauma: a retrospective study. Injury 1997;28:261–265.

88. Mavridis SP, Firilas AM. Blunt trauma in intoxicated patients: is computed tomography of the abdomen always necessary. S Med J 2000;93:403–405.
89. Sturm JT, Perry JF. Injuries associated with fractures of the transverse processes of the thoracic and lumbar vertebrae. J Trauma 1984;24:597–599.
90. Bivins BA, Sachatello CR, Daughtery ME, et al. Diagnostic peritoneal lavage is superior to clinical evaluation in blunt abdominal trauma. Am Surg 1978;44:637–641.
91. Liu M, Lee CH, P'eng FK. Prospective comparison of diagnostic peritoneal lavage, computed tomographic scanning, and ultrasonography for the diagnosis of blunt abdominal trauma. J Trauma 1993;35:267–270.
92. Smith SB, Andersen CA. Abdominal trauma: the limited role of peritoneal lavage. Am Surg 1982;48:514–517.
93. Henneman PL, Marx JA, Moore EE, et al. Diagnostic peritoneal lavage: accuracy in predicting necessary laparotomy following blunt and penetrating trauma. J Trauma 1990;30:1345–1355.
94. Krausz MM, Manny J, Austin E, et al. Peritoneal lavage in blunt abdominal trauma. Surg Gynecol Obstet 1981;152:327–330.
95. Moore JB, Moore EE, Markivchick VJ, et al. Diagnostic peritoneal lavage for abdominal trauma: superiority of the open technique at the infraumbilical ring. J Trauma 1981;21:570–572.
96. Jacob ET, Cantor E. Discriminate diagnostic peritoneal lavage in blunt abdominal injuries: accuracy and hazards. Am Surg 1979;45:11–14.
97. McAnena OJ, Marx JA, Moore EE. Peritoneal lavage enzyme determinations following blunt and penetrating abdominal trauma. J Trauma 1991;31:1161–1164.
98. McAnena OJ, Marx JA, Moore EE. Contributions of peritoneal lavage enzyme determinations to the management of isolated hollow visceral abdominal injuries. Ann Emerg Med 1991;20:834–837.
99. Megison SM, Weigelt JA. The value of alkaline phosphatase in peritoneal lavage. Ann Emerg Med 1990;19:503–505.
100. D'Amelio LF, Rhodes M. A reassessment of peritoneal lavage leukocyte count in blunt abdominal trauma. J Trauma 1990;30:1291–1293.
101. Soyka JM, Martin M, Sloan EP, et al. Diagnostic peritoneal lavage: is an isolated WBC count greater than or equal to 500/mm^3 predictive of intra-abdominal injury requiring celiotomy in blunt trauma patients? J Trauma 1990;30:874–879.
102. Jacobs DG, Angus L, Rodriguez A, et al. Peritoneal lavage white count: a reassessment. J Trauma 1990;30:607–612.
103. Blow O, Bassam D, Butler K, et al. Speed and efficiency in the resuscitation of blunt trauma patients with multiple injuries: the advantage of diagnostic peritoneal lavage over abdominal computerized tomography. J Trauma 1998;44:287–290.
104. Meyer DM, Thal ER, Weigelt JA, et al. Evaluation of computed tomography and diagnostic peritoneal lavage in blunt abdominal trauma. J Trauma 1989;29:1168–1170.
105. Burney RE, Mueller GL, Coon WW, et al. Diagnosis of isolated small bowel injury following blunt abdominal trauma. Ann Emerg Med 1983;12:71–74.
106. Ceraldi CM, Waxman K. Computerized tomography as an indicator of isolated mesenteric injury. A comparison with peritoneal lavage. Am Surg 1990;56:806–810.
107. Cochran W, Sobat WS. Open versus closed diagnostic peritoneal lavage. A multiphasic prospective randomized comparison. Ann Surg 1984;200:24–28.
108. Gonzalez RP, Ickler J, Gachassin P. Complementary roles of diagnostic peritoneal lavage and computed tomography in the evaluation of blunt abdominal trauma. J Trauma 2001;51:1128–1136.
109. Exadakktylos AK, Sclabas G, Schmid SW, et al. Do we really need routine computed tomographic scanning in the primary evaluation of blunt chest trauma in patients with "normal" chest radiograph. J Trauma 2001;51:1173–1176.
110. Dyer DS, Moore EE, Ilke DN, et al. Thoracic aortic injury: how predictive is mechanism and is chest computed tomography a reliable screening tool? A prospective study of 1,561 patients. J Trauma 2000;48:673–682.
111. Melton SM, Kerby JD, McGiffin D, et al. The evolution of chest computed tomography for the definitive diagnosis of blunt aortic injury: a single-center experience. J Trauma 2004;56:243–250.
112. Parker MS, Matheson TL, Rao AV, et al. Making the transition: the role of helical CT in the evaluation of potentially acute thoracic aortic injuries. AJR 2001;176:1267–1272.
113. Mirvis SE, Kostrubiak I, Whitley NO, et al. Role of CT in excluding major arterial injury after blunt thoracic trauma. AJR 1987;149:601–605.
114. Ishikawa T, Nakajima Y, Kaji T. The role of CT in traumatic rupture of the thoracic aorta and its proximal branches. Semin Roentgenol 1989;24:38–46.
115. Richardson P, Mirvis SE, Scorpio R, Duham CM. Value of CT in determining the need for angiography when findings of mediastinal hemorrhage on chest radiographs are equivocal. AJR 1991;156:273–279.
116. Madayag MA, Kirshenbaum KJ, Nadimpalli SR, et al. Thoracic aortic trauma: role of dynamic CT. Radiology 1991;179:853–855.
117. Raptopoulos V, Sheiman RG, Phillips DA, Davidoff A. Traumatic aortic tear: screening with chest CT. Radiology 1992;182:667–673.
118. Gavant ML, Menke PG, Fabian T, et al. Blunt traumatic aortic rupture: detection with helical CT of the chest. Radiology 1995;197:125–133.
119. Mirvis SE, Shanmuganathan K, Miller BH, et al. Traumatic aortic injury: diagnosis with contrast-enhanced thoracic CT: five year experience at a major trauma center. Radiology 1996;200:413–422.
120. Fabian TC, Davis KA, Gavant ML, et al. Prospective study of blunt aortic injury: helical CT is diagnostic and antihypertensive therapy reduces rupture. Ann Surg 1998;227:666–677.
121. Downing SW, Sperling JS, Mirvis SE, et al. Experience with spiral computed tomography as the sole diagnostic method for traumatic aortic rupture. Ann Thorac Surg 2001;72:495–502.
122. Mirvis SE, Shanmuganathan K, Buell J, Rodriguez A. Use of spiral computed tomography for the assessment of blunt trauma patients with potential aortic injury. J Trauma 1998;45:922–930.
123. Self ML, Blake AM, Whitley M, et al. The benefit of routine thoracic, abdominal, and pelvic computed tomography to evaluate trauma patients with closed head injuries. Am J Surg 2003;186:609–614.
124. Guerrero-Lopez F, Vazquez-Mata G, Alcazar-Romero PP, et al. Evaluation of the utility of computed tomography in the initial assessment of the critical care patient with chest trauma. Crit Care Med 2000;28:1370–1375.
125. Omert L, Yeaney WW, Protetch J. Efficacy of thoracic computerized tomography in blunt chest trauma. Am Surg 2001;67:660–664.
126. Shanmuganathan K, Mirvis SE. Advances in emergency radiology: imaging diagnosis of nonaortic thoracic injury. Radiol Clin N Am 1999;37:533–551.
127. Rhea JT, Novelline RA, Lawrason J, et al. The frequency and significance of thoracic injuries detected on abdominal CT scans in multiple trauma patients. J Trauma 1989;29:502–509.
128. Tocino IM, Miller MH, Fairfax WR. Distribution of pneumothorax in supine and semi-recumbent critically ill patients. AJR 1985;144:901–905.
129. Wall SD, Federle MP, Jeffrey RB, et al. CT diagnosis of unsuspected pneumothorax after blunt trauma. AJR 1983;141:919–921.
130. Fabian TC, Mangiante EC, White TJ, et al. A prospective study of 91 patients undergoing both computed tomography and peri-

toneal lavage following blunt abdominal trauma. J Trauma 1986;26:602–607.
131. Poletti PA, Mirvis SE, Shanmuganathan K, et al. Blunt abdominal trauma patients: can organ injury be excluded without performing computed tomography. J Trauma 2004;57:1072–1081.
132. Peitzman AB, Makaroun MS, Slasky BS, et al. Prospective study of computed tomography in initial management of blunt abdominal trauma. J Trauma 1986;26:585–592.
133. Pal JD, Victorino GP. Defining the role of computed tomography in blunt abdominal trauma: use in the hemodynamically stable patient with a depressed level of consciousness. Arch Surg 2002;137:1029–1033.
134. Webster VJ: Abdominal trauma: pre-operative assessment and postoperative problems in intensive care. Anaesth Intensive Care 1985;13:258–262.
135. Miller MT, Pasquale MD, Bromberg WJ, et al. Not so fast. J Trauma 2003;54:52–60.
136. Stassen NA, Lukan JK, Carrillo EH, et al. Examination of the role of abdominal computed tomography in the evaluation of victims of trauma with increased aspartate aminotransferase in the era of focused abdominal sonography for trauma. Surgery (St. Louis) 2002;132:642–647.
137. Ceraldi CM, Waxman K. Computerized tomography as an indicator of isolated mesenteric injury. A comparison with peritoneal lavage. Am Surg 1990;56:806–810.
138. Nolan BW, Gabram SG, Schwartz RJ, et al. Mesenteric injury from blunt abdominal trauma. Am Surg 1995;61:501–506.
139. Kearney PA, Vahey T, Burney RE, Glazer G. Computed tomography and diagnostic peritoneal lavage in blunt abdominal trauma. Arch Surg 1989;124:344–347.
140. Allen TL, Mueller MT, Bonk T, et al. Computed tomography scanning without oral contrast solution for blunt bowel and mesenteric injuries in abdominal trauma. J Trauma 2004;56:314–322.
141. Stafford RE, McGonigal MD, Weigelt JA, Johnson TJ. Oral contrast solution and computed tomography for blunt abdominal trauma: a randomized study. Arch Surg 1999;134:622–627.
142. Janzen DL, Zwirewich CV, Breen DJ, Nagy A. Diagnostic accuracy of helical CT for detection of blunt bowel and mesenteric injuries. Clin Radiol 1998;53:193–197.
143. Sherck J, Shatney C, Sensaki K, Selivanov V. The accuracy of computed tomography in the diagnosis of blunt small bowel perforation. Am J Surg 1994;168:670–675.
144. Neff MA, Monk JS, Peters K, Nikhilesh A. Detection of occult pneumothoraces on abdominal computed tomographic scans in trauma patients. J Trauma 2000;49:281–285.
145. Lang EK. Intra-abdominal and retroperitoneal organ injuries diagnosed on dynamic computed tomograms obtained for assessment of renal trauma. J Trauma 1990;30:1161–1168.
146. Kane NM, Dorfman GS, Cronan JJ. Efficacy of CT following peritoneal lavage in abdominal trauma. J Comp Assist Tomogr 1987;11:998–1002.
147. Udekwu PO, Gurkin B. The use of computed tomography in blunt abdominal injuries. Am Surg 1996;62:56–60.
148. Ochsner MG, Knudson MM, Pachter HL, et al. Significance of minimal or no intraperitoneal fluid visible on CT scan associated with blunt liver and splenic injuries: a multicenter analysis. J Trauma 2000;49:505–510.
149. Livingston DH, Lavery RF, Passannante MR, et al. Admission or observation is not necessary after a negative abdominal computed tomographic scan in patients with suspected blunt abdominal trauma: results of a prospective, multi-institutional trial. J Trauma 1998;44:272–282.
150. Garber BG, Bigelow E, Yelle JD, Pagliarello G. Use of abdominal computed tomography in blunt trauma: do we scan too much? Can J Surg 2000;43:16–22.
151. McKenney M, Lentz K, Nunez D, et al. Can ultrasound replace diagnostic peritoneal lavage in the assessment of blunt trauma? J Trauma 1994;37:439–441.
152. Smith SR, Kern SJ, Fry WR, et al. Institutional learning curve of surgeon-performed trauma ultrasound. Arch Surg 1998;133:530–536.
153. Healey MA, Simons RK, Winchell RJ, et al. A prospective evaluation of abdominal ultrasound in blunt trauma: is it useful? J Trauma 1996;40:875–883.
154. Branney SW, Wolfe RE, Moore EE, et al. Quantitative sensitivity of ultrasound in detecting free intraperitoneal fluid. J Trauma 1995;39:375–380.
155. Kern SJ, Smith RS, Fry WR, et al. Sonographic examination of abdominal trauma by senior surgical residents. Am Surg 1997; 63:669–674.
156. Thomas B, Falcone RE, Vasquez D, et al. Ultrasound evaluation of blunt abdominal trauma: program implementation, initial experience, and learning curve. J Trauma 1997;42:384–390.
157. Gracias VH, Frankel H, Gupta R, et al. Defining the learning curve for the focused abdominal sonogram for trauma (FAST) examination: implications for credentialing. Am Surg 2001;67: 364–368.
158. Branney SW, Moore EE, Cantrill SV, et al. Ultrasound based key clinical pathway reduces the use of hospital resources for the evaluation of blunt abdominal trauma. J Trauma 1997;42:1086–1090.
159. Glaser K, Tschmelitsch J, Klingler P, et al. Ultrasonography in the management of blunt abdominal and thoracic trauma. Arch Surg 1994;129:743–747.
160. McKenney KL, McKenney MG, Nunez DB, et al. Cost reduction using ultrasound in blunt abdominal trauma. Emerg Radiol 1997;4:3–6.
161. Rowan KR, Kirkpatrick AW, Liu D, et al. Traumatic pneumothorax detection with thoracic US: correlation with chest radiography and CT: initial experience. Radiology 2002;225: 210–214.
162. Rainer TH, Griffith JF, Lam E, et al. Comparison of thoracic ultrasound, clinical acumen, and radiography in patients with minor chest injury. J Trauma 2004;56:1211–1213.
163. Boulanger BR, Brenneman FD, McLellan BA, et al. A prospective study of emergent abdominal sonography after blunt trauma. J Trauma 1995;39:325–330.
164. McKenney MG, Martin L, Lentz K, et al. 1000 consecutive ultrasounds for blunt abdominal trauma. J Trauma 1996;40:607–612.
165. Yoshii H, Sato M, Yamamoto S, et al. Usefulness and limitations of ultrasonography in the initial evaluation of blunt abdominal trauma. J Trauma 1998;45:45–51.
166. Stengel D, Bauwens K, Sehouli J, et al. Discriminatory power of 3.5 MHz convex and 7.5 MHz linear ultrasound probes for the imaging of traumatic splenic lesions. J Trauma 2001;51:37–43.
167. Sirlin CB, Brown MA, Deutsch R, et al. Screening US for blunt abdominal trauma: objective predictors of false-negative findings and missed injuries. Radiology 2003;229:766–774.
168. Wherrett LJ, Boulanger BR, McLellan BA, et al. Hypotension after blunt abdominal trauma: the role of emergent abdominal sonography in surgical triage. J Trauma 1996;41:815–820.
169. Chiu WC, Cushing BM, Rodriguez A, et al. Abdominal injuries without hemoperitoneum: a potential limitation of focused abdominal sonography for trauma (FAST). J Trauma 1997;617–625.
170. Ballard RB, Rozycki GS, Newman PG, et al. An algorithm to reduce the incidence of false-negative FAST examinations in patients at high risk for occult injury. J AM Coll Surg 1999;189:145–151.

171. Boulanger BR, Brenneman FD, Kirkpatrick AW, et al. The indeterminate abdominal sonogram in multisystem blunt trauma. J Trauma 1998;45:52–56.
172. Elliott DC, Rodriguez A, Moncure M, et al. The accuracy of diagnostic laparoscopy in trauma patients: a prospective, controlled study. Int Surg 1998;83:294–298.
173. Mathonnet M, Peyrou P, Gainant A, et al. Role of laparoscopy in blunt perforations of the small bowel. Surg Endosc 2003;17: 641–645.
174. Iannelli A, Fabiani P, Karimdjee BS, et al. Therapeutic laparoscopy for blunt abdominal trauma with bowel injuries. J Laparoendosc Adv Surg Tech 2003;13:189–191.
175. Taner AS Topgul K, Kucukel F, et al. Diagnostic laparoscopy decreases the rate of unnecessary laparotomies and reduces hospital costs in trauma patients. J Laparoendosc Adv Surg Tech 2001;11:207–211.
176. Mattox KL. Indications for thoracotomy: deciding to operate. Surg Clin N Am 1989;69:47–58.
177. Mineo T, Ambrogi A, Benedetto C, et al. Changing indications for thoracotomy in blunt chest trauma after the advent of videothoracoscopy. J Trauma 1999;47:1088–1091.
178. Lang-Lazdunski L, Mouroux J, Pons, et al. Role of videothoracoscopy in chest trauma. Ann Thorac Surg 1997;63:327–333.
179. Ahmed N, Jones D. Video-assisted thoracic surgery: state of the art in trauma care. Injury, Int J Care Injured 2004;35:479–489.
180. Renz BM, Cava RA, Feliciano DV, Rozycki GS. Transmediastinal gunshot wounds: a prospective study. J Trauma 2000;48:416–422.
181. Hoth JJ, Scott MJ, Bullock TK, et al. Thoracotomy for blunt trauma: traditional indications may not apply. Am Surg 2003;69: 1108–1111.
182. Mansour MA, Moore EE, Moore FA, Read RR. Exigent postinjury thoracotomy analysis of blunt versus penetrating trauma. Surg Gynecol Obstet 1992;175:97–101.
183. Mattox KL, Beall AC, Jordan GL, et al. Cardiorrhaphy in the emergency center. J Thorac Cardiovasc Surg 1974;68:886–895.
184. Tavares S, Hankins JR, Moulton AL, et al. Management of penetrating cardiac injuries: the role of emergency room thoracotomy. Ann Thorac Surg 1984;38:183–187.
185. Rohman M, Ivatury RR, Streicher FM, et al. Emergency room thoracotomy for penetrating cardiac injuries. J Trauma 1983;23: 570–576.
186. Lorenz HP, Steinmetz B, Leiberman J, et al. Emergency department thoracotomy: survival correlates with physiologic status. J Trauma 1992;32:780–788.
187. Mazzorana V, Smith RS, Morabito DJ, et al. Limited utility of emergency department thoracotomy. Am Surg 1994;60:516–520.
188. Washington B, Wilson RF, Steiger Z. Emergency department thoracotomy: a four-year review. Ann Thorac Surg 1985;40:188–191.
189. Branney SW, Moore EE, Feldhaus KM, Wolfe RE. Critical analysis of two decades of experience with postinjury emergency department thoracotomy in a regional trauma center. J Trauma 1998;45:87–94.
190. Rhee PM, Acosta J, Bridgeman A, et al. Survival after emergency department thoracotomy: review of published data from the past 25 years. J Am Coll Surg 2000;190:288–298.
191. Velhamos GC, Degiannis E, Souter I, et al. Outcome of a strict policy on emergency department thoracotomies. Arch Surg 1995;130:774–777.
192. Shimazu S, Shatney CH. Outcomes of trauma patients with no vital signs on hospital admission. J Trauma 1983;23:213–216.
193. Brown SE, Gomez GA. Penetrating chest trauma: should indications for emergency room thoracotomy be limited? Am Surg 1996;62:530–534.
194. Kennedy F, Sharif S. Emergency room thoracotomy: a single surgeon's thirteen-year experience. Am Surg 2000;66:56–60.
195. Leppaniemi AK, Voutilainen PE, Haapiainen RK. Indications for early mandatory laparotomy in abdominal stab wounds. Br J Surg 1999;86:76–80.
196. Nagy K, Roberts R, Jospeh K, et al. Evisceration after abdominal stab wounds: is laparotomy required? J Trauma 1999;47:622–626.
197. Chmielewski GW, Nicholas JM. Nonoperative management of gunshot wounds of the abdomen. Am Surg 1995;61:665–669.
198. Pryor JP, Reilly PM, Dabrowski GP, et al. Nonoperative management of abdominal gunshot wounds. Ann Emerg Med 2004;43: 344–353.
199. Velmahos GC, Demetriades D, Cornwell EE. Transpelvic gunshot wounds: routine laparotomy or selective management? World J Surg 1998;22:1034–1038.
200. Ng AKI, Simons RK, Torreggiani WC, et al. Intra-abdominal free fluid without solid organ injury in blunt abdominal trauma: an indication for laparotomy. J Trauma 2002;52:1134–1140.
201. Livingston DH, Lavery RF, Passannante MR, et al. Free fluid on abdominal computed tomography without solid organ injury in blunt abdominal trauma does not mandate celiotomy. Am J Surg 2001;182:6–9.
202. Cunningham MA, Tyroch AH, Kaups KL, Davis JW. Does free fluid on abdominal computed tomographic scan after blunt trauma require laparotomy? J Trauma 1998;44:599–602.
203. Brasel KJ, Olson CJ, Stafford RE, Johnson TJ. Incidence and significance of free fluid on abdominal computed tomographic scan in blunt trauma. J Trauma 1998;44:889–892.
204. Stone HH, Strom PR, Mullins RJ. Management of major coagulopathy with onset during laparotomy. Ann Surg 1983;197:532–535.
205. Ferrara A, MacArthur JD, Wright HK, et al. Hypothermia and acidosis worsen coagulopathy in the patient requiring massive transfusion. Am J Surg 1990;160:515–518.
206. Wudel JH, Morris JA, Yates K, et al. Massive transfusion: outcome in blunt trauma patients. J Trauma 1991;31:1–7.
207. Phillips TF, Soulier G, Wilson RF. Outcome of massive transfusion exceeding two blood volumes in trauma and emergency surgery. J Trauma 1987;27:903–910.
208. Luna GV, Maier RV, Pavlin EG, et al. Incidence and effect of hypothermia in seriously injured patients. J Trauma 1987; 27:1014–1018.
209. Jurkovich GJ, Greiser WB, Luterman A, et al. Hypothermia in trauma victim: an ominous predictor of survival. J Trauma 1987;27:1019–1024.
210. Moore EE. Staged laparotomy for the hypothermia, acidosis and coagulopathy syndrome. Am J Surg 1996;172:405–410.
211. Rotondo MF, Schwab CW, McGonigal MD, et al. "Damage control": an approach for improved survival in exsanguinating penetrating abdominal trauma. J Trauma 1993;35:375–383.
212. Johnson JW, Gracias VH, Schwab CW, et al. Evolution in damage control for exsanguinating penetrating abdominal injury. J Trauma 2001;51:561–571.
213. Nicholas JM, Rix EP, Easley A, et al. Changing patterns in the management of penetrating abdominal trauma: the more things change, the more they stay the same. J Trauma 2003;55:1095–1110.
214. Moore EE, Burch JM, Franciose RJ, et al. Staged physiologic restoration and damage control surgery. World J Surg 1998;22: 1184–1191.
215. Loveland JA, Boffard KD. Damage control in the abdomen and beyond. Br J Surg 2004;91:1095–1101.
216. Raeburn CD, Moore EE, Biffl WL, et al. The abdominal compartment syndrome is a morbid complication of postinjury damage control surgery. Am J Surg 2001;182:542–546.

217. Offner PJ, deSouza AL, Moore EE, et al. Avoidance of abdominal compartment syndrome in damage-control laparotomy after trauma. Arch Surg 2001;136:676–681.
218. Ertel W, Oberholzer A, Platz A, et al. Incidence and clinical pattern of the abdominal compartment syndrome after "damage-control" laparotomy in 311 patients with severe abdominal and/or pelvic trauma. Crit Care Med 2000;28:1747–1753.
219. Hirshberg A, Stein M, Adar R. Damage control surgery. Surg Clin N Am 1997;77:897–907.
220. Sugrue M, D'Amours SK, Joshipura M. Damage control surgery and the abdomen. Injury, Int J Care Injured 2004;35:642–648.
221. Garrison JR, Richardson JD, Hilakos AS, et al. Predicting the need to pack early for severe intra-abdominal hemorrhage. J Trauma 1996;40:923–929.
222. Hirshberg A, Wall MJ, Mattox KL. Planned reoperation for trauma: a two year experience with 124 consecutive patients. J Trauma 1994;37:365–369.
223. Hirshberg A, Mattox KL. Planned reoperation for severe trauma. Ann Surg 1995;222:3–8.
224. Asensio JA, Petrone P, Roldan G, et al. Has evolution in awareness of guidelines for institution of damage control improved outcome in the management of the posttraumatic acute abdomen. Arch Surg 2004;139:209–214.
225. Burch JM, Ortiz VB, Richardson RJ, et al. Abbreviated laparotomy and planned reoperation for critically injured patients. Ann Surg 1992;215:476–482.
226. Carrillo C, Fogler RJ, Shaftan GW. Delayed gastrointestinal reconstruction following massive abdominal trauma. J Trauma 1993;34:233–235.
227. Sharp KW, Locicero RJ. Abdominal packing for surgically uncontrolled hemorrhage. Ann Surg 1992;215:467–474.
228. Talbert S, Trooskin SZ, Scalea T, et al. Packing and reexploration for patients with nonhepatic injuries. J Trauma 1992;33:121–125.
229. Wall MJ, Soltero E. Damage control for thoracic injuries. Surg Clin N Am 1997;77:863–878.
230. Rotondo MF, Bard MR. Damage control surgery for thoracic injuries. Injury Int J Care Injured 2004;35:649–654.
231. Vargo DJ, Battistella FD. Abbreviated thoracotomy and temporary chest closure: an application of damage control after thoracic trauma. Arch Surg 2001;136:21–24.
232. Wilson A, Wall MJ, Maxson R, Mattox K. The pulmonary hilum twist as a thoracic damage control procedure. Am J Surg 2003;186:49–52.
233. Caceres M, Buechter KJ, Tillou A, et al. Thoracic packing for uncontrolled bleeding in penetrating thoracic injuries. South Med J 97;2004:637–641.
234. Wall MJ, Villavicencio RT, Miller CC, et al. Pulmonary tractotomy as an abbreviated thoracotomy technique. J Trauma 1998;45:1015–1023.
235. Asensio JA, Demetriades D, Berne JD, et al. Stapled pulmonary tractotomy: a rapid way to control hemorrhage in penetrating pulmonary injuries. J Am Coll Surg 1997;185:486–487.
236. Thourani VH, Feliciano DV, Cooper WA, et al. Penetrating cardiac trauma at an urban trauma center: a 22-year perspective. Am Surg 1999;65:811–818.
237. Tyburski JG, Astra L, Wilson RF, et al. Factors affecting prognosis with penetrating wounds of the heart. J Trauma 2000;48:587–591.
238. Asensio JA, Berne JD, Demetriades D, et al. One hundred five penetrating cardiac injuries: a 2-year prospective evaluation. J Trauma 1998;44:1073–1082.
239. Mittal V, McAleese P, Young S, Cohen M. Penetrating cardiac injuries. Am Surg 1999;65:444–448.
240. Wall MJ, Mattox KL, Baldwin JC. Acute management of complex cardiac injuries. J Trauma 1997;42:905–912.
241. Symbas PN, DiOrio DA, Tyras DH, et al. Penetrating cardiac wounds: significant residual and delayed sequelae. J Thorac Cardiovasc Surg 1973;66:526–532.
242. Fallah-Nejad M, Wallace HW, Su CC, et al. Unusual manifestations of penetrating cardiac injuries. Arch Surg 1975;191:1357–1362.
243. Fallah-Nejad M, Kutty ACK, Wallace HW. Secondary lesions of penetrating cardiac injuries: a frequent complication. Ann Surg 1980;191:228–233.
244. Mattox KL, Limacher MC, Feliciano DV, et al. Cardiac evaluation following heart injury. J Trauma 1985;25:758–765.
245. Sybrandy KC, Cramer MJM, Burgersdijk C. Diagnosing cardiac contusion: old wisdom and new insights. Heart 2003;89:485–489.
246. Vougiouklakis T, Peschos D, Doulis A, et al. Sudden death from contusion of the right atrium after blunt chest trauma: case report and review of the literature. Injury Int J Care Injured 2005;36:213–217.
247. Frazee RC, Mucha P, Farnell MB, Miller FA. Objective evaluation of blunt cardial trauma. J Trauma 1986;26:510–520.
248. Collins JN, Cole FJ, Weireter LJ, et al. The usefulness of serum troponin levels in evaluating cardiac injury. Am Surg 2001;67:821–826.
249. Kato K, Kushimoto S, Mashiko K, et al. Blunt traumatic rupture of the heart: an experience in Tokyo. J Trauma 1994;36:859–863.
250. Turk EE, Tsokos M. Blunt cardiac trauma caused by fatal fall from height: an autopsy-based assessment in the injury pattern. J Trauma 2004;57:30–304.
251. Fulda G, Braithwaite CEM, Rodriguez A, et al. Blunt traumatic rupture of the heart and pericardium: a ten-year experience (1979–1989). J Trauma 1991;31:167–172.
252. Wisner DH, Reed WH, Riddick RS. Suspected myocardial contusion. Triage and indications for monitoring. Ann Surg 1990;212:82–86.
253. Dowd MD, Krug S. Pediatric blunt cardiac injury: epidemiology, clinical features, and diagnosis. Pediatric Emergency Medicine Collaborative Research Committee: Working Group on Blunt Cardiac Injury. J Trauma 1996;40:61–67.
254. Schick EC. Nonpenetrating cardiac trauma. Cardiol Clin 1995;13:241–247.
255. Miller FB, Shumate CR, Richardson JD. Myocardial contusion: when can the diagnosis be eliminated? Arch Surg 1989;124:805–808.
256. Foil MB, Mackersie RC, Furst SR, et al. The asymptomatic patient with suspected myocardial contusion. Am J Surg 1990;160:638–643.
257. Illig KA, Swierzewski MJ, Feliciano DV, et al. A rational screening and treatment strategy based on the electrocardiogram alone for suspected cardiac contusion. Am J Surg 1991;162:537–544.
258. Fildes JJ, Betlej TM, Manglano R, et al. Limiting cardiac evaluation in patients with suspected myocardial contusion. Am Surg 1995;61:832–835.
259. Cachecho R, Grindlinger GA, Lee VW. The clinical significance of myocardial contusion. J Trauma 1992;33:68–73.
260. Malangoni MA, McHenry CR, Jacobs DG. Outcome of serious blunt cardiac injury. Surgery (St. Louis) 1994;116:628–633.
261. McLean RF, Devitt JH, McLellan BA, et al. Significance of myocardial contusion following blunt chest trauma. J Trauma 1992;33:240–243.
262. Rajan G, Zellweger R. Cardiac troponin I as a predictor of arrhythmia and ventricular dysfunction in trauma patients with myocardial contusion. J Trauma 2004;57:801–808.
263. Helling TS, Duke P, Beggs CW, et al. A prospective evaluation of 68 patients suffering blunt chest trauma for evidence of cardiac injury. J Trauma 1989;29:961–966.
264. Feghali NT, Prisant LM. Blunt myocardial injury. Chest 1995;108:1673–1677.

265. Adams JE, Davila-Roman VG, Bessey PQ, et al. Improved detection of cardiac contusion with cardiac troponin I. Am Heart J 1996;13:308–312.
266. Fabian TC, Cicala RS, Croce MA, et al. A prospective evaluation of myocardial contusion: correlation of significant arrhythmias and cardiac output with CPK-MB measurements. J Trauma 1991;31:653–660.
267. Biffl WL, Moore FA, Moore EE, et al. Cardiac enzymes are irrelevant in the patient with suspected myocardial contusion. Am J Surg 1994;168:523–528.
268. Ferjani M, Droc G, Dreux S, et al. Circulating cardiac troponin T in myocardial contusion. Chest 1997;111:427–433.
269. Fabian TC, Mangiante EC, Patterson CR, et al. Myocardial contusion in blunt trauma: clinical characteristics, means of diagnosis, and implications for patient management. J Trauma 1988;28:50–57.
270. Keller KD, Shatney CH. Creatine phosphokinase-MB assays in patients with suspected myocardial contusion: diagnostic test or test of diagnosis? J Trauma 1988;28:58–63.
271. Karalis DG, Victor MF, Davis GA, et al. The role of echocardiography in blunt chest trauma: a transthoracic and transesophageal echocardiographic study. J Trauma 1994;36:53–58.
272. Brooks SW, Young JC, Cmolik B, et al. The use of transesophageal echocardiography in the evaluation of chest trauma. J Trauma 1992;32:761–768.
273. Weiss RL, Brier JA, O'Connor W, et al. The usefulness of transesophageal echocardiography in diagnosing cardiac contusions. Chest 1996;109:73–77.
274. Lindstaedt M, Germing A, Lawo T, et al. Acute and long-term clinical significance of myocardial contusion following blunt thoracic trauma: results of a prospective study. J Trauma 2002;52:479–485.
275. LoCicero J, Mattox KL. Epidemiology of chest trauma. Surg Clin N Am 1989;69:15–19.
276. Ziegler AW, Agarwal NN. Morbidity and mortality of rib fractures. J Trauma 1994;37:975–979.
277. Bolliger CT, Van Eeden SF. Treatment of multiple rib fracture: randomized controlled trial comparing ventilatory with nonventilatory management. Chest 1990;97:943–948.
278. Bulger EM, Arneson MA, Mock CN, Jurkovich GJ. Rib fractures in the elderly. J Trauma 2000;48:1040–1047.
279. Barnea Y, Kashtan H, Shornick Y, Werbin N. Isolated rib fractures in elderly patients: mortality and morbidity. Can J Surg 2002;45:43–46.
280. Richardson JD, Adams L, Flint LM. Selective management of flail chest and pulmonary contusion. Ann Surg 1982;196:481–487.
281. Shorr RM, Crittenden M, Indeck M, et al. Blunt thoracic trauma: analysis of 515 patients. Ann Surg 1987;206:200–205.
282. Damschen DD, Cogbill TH, Siegel MJ. Scapulothoracic dissociation caused by blunt trauma. J Trauma 1997;42:537–540.
283. Landercasper J, Cogbill TH. Long-term follow-up after traumatic asphyxia. J Trauma 1985;25:838–841.
284. Ahmed Z, Moyhuddin Z. Management of flail chest injury: internal fixation versus endotracheal intubation and ventilation. J Thorac Cardiovasc Surg 1995;110:1676–1680.
285. Thomas AN, Blaisdell FW, Lewis FR Jr, Schlobohm RM. Operative stabilization for flail chest after blunt trauma. J Thorac Cardiovasc Surg 1978;75:793–801.
286. Hassler GB. Open fixation of flail chest after blunt trauma. Ann Thorac Surg 1990;49:993–995.
287. Svennevig JL, Bugge-Asperheim B, Geiran OR, et al. Prognostic factors in blunt chest trauma: analysis of 652 cases. Ann Chir Gynaecol 1986;75:8–14.
288. Shorr RM, Rodriguez A, Indeck MC, et al. Blunt chest trauma in the elderly. J Trauma 1989;29:234–237.
289. Cameron P, Dziukas L, Hadj A, et al. Rib fractures in major trauma. Aust N Z J Surg 1996;66:530–534.
290. Adrales G, Huynh T, Broering B, et al. A thoracostomy tube guideline improves management efficiency in trauma patients. J Trauma 2002;52:210–216.
291. Martino S, Merrit S, Boyakye K, et al. Prospective randomized trial of thoracostomy tube removal guidelines. J Trauma 1999;46:369–373.
292. Deneuville M. Morbidity of percutaneous tube thoracostomy in trauma patients. Eur J Cardiothorac Surg 2002;22:673–678.
293. Etoch SW, Bar-Natan MF, Miller FB, Richardson JD. Tube thoracostomy: factors related to complications. Arch Surg 1995;130:521–526.
294. Cant PJ, Smyth S, Smart DO. Antibiotic prophylaxis is indicated for chest stab wounds requiring closed tube thoracostomy. Br J Surg 1993;80:464–466.
295. Grover FL, Richardson JD, Fewel JG, et al. Prophylactic antibiotics in the treatment of penetrating chest wounds. A prospective double-blind study. J Thorac Cardiovasc Surg 1977;74:528–536.
296. Mandal AK, Montano J, Thadepalli H. Prophylactic antibiotics and no antibiotics compared in penetrating chest trauma. J Trauma 1985;25:639–643.
297. Demetriades D, Breckon V, Breckon C, et al. Antibiotic prophylaxis in penetrating injuries of the chest. Ann R Coll Surg Engl 1991;73:348–351.
298. Rhea JT, Novelline RA, Lawrason J, et al. The frequency and significance of thoracic injuries detected on abdominal CT scans of multiple trauma patients. J Trauma 1989;29:502–505.
299. Bridges KG, Welch G, Silver M, et al. CT diagnosis of occult pneumothoraces in multiple trauma patients. J Emerg Med 1993;11:179–186.
300. Garramone RR, Jacobs LM, Sahdev P. An objective method to measure and manage occult pneumothorax. Surg Gynecol Obstet 1991;173:257–261.
301. Brasel KJ, Staffors RE, Weigelt JA, et al. Treatment of occult pneumothoraces from blunt trauma. J Trauma 1999;46:987–991.
302. Enderson BL, Abdalla R, Frame SB, et al. Tube thoracostomy for occult pneumothorax: a prospective randomized study of its use. J Trauma 1993;35:726–730.
303. Stewart KC, Uyrschel JD, Nakai SS, et al. Pulmonary resection for lung trauma. Ann Thorac Surg 1997;63:1587–1588.
304. Gasparri M, Karmy-Jones, Kralovich KA, et al. Pulmonary tractotomy versus lung resection: viable options in penetrating lung injury. J Trauma 2001;51:1092–1097.
305. Hankins JR, McAslan TC, Shin B, et al. Extensive pulmonary laceration caused by blunt trauma. J Thorac Cardiovasc Surg 1977;74:519–527.
306. Bowling R, Mavroudis C, Richardson JD, Flint LM, et al. Emergency pneumonectomy for penetrating and blunt trauma. Am Surg 1985;51:136–139.
307. Thompson DA, Rowlands BJ, Walker WE, et al. Urgent thoracotomy for pulmonary or tracheobronchial injury. J Trauma 1988;28:276–280.
308. Tominaga GT, Waxman K, Scannell G, et al. Emergency thoracotomy with lung resection following trauma. Am Surg 1993;59:834–837.
309. Dowd NP, Clarkson K, Walsh MA, Cunningham AJ. Delayed bronchial stenosis after blunt chest trauma. Anesth Analg 1996;82:1078–1081.
310. Barmada H, Gibbons JR. Tracheobronchial injury in blunt and penetrating chest trauma. Chest 1994;106:74–78.
311. Hancock BJ, Wiseman NE. Tracheobronchial injuries in children. J Pediatr Surg 1991;26:1316–1319.
312. Hood RM, Sloan HE. Injuries of the trachea and major bronchi. J Thorac Cardiovasc Surg 1959;38:458–480.
313. Reece GP, Shatney CH. Blunt injuries of the cervical trachea: review of 51 patients. South Med J 1988;81:1542–1548.
314. Balci AE, Eren N, Eren S, Ulku R. Surgical experience of post-traumatic tracheo-bronchial injuries: a 14-year experience. Eur J Cardiothorac Surg 2002;22:984–989.

315. Cornwell EE, Kennedy F, Ayad IA, et al. Transmediastinal gunshot wounds. A reconsideration of the role of aortography. Arch Surg 1996;131:949–953.
316. Weiman DS, Walker WA, Brosnan KM, et al. Noniatrogenic esophageal trauma. Ann Thorac Surg 1995;59:845–850.
317. White RK, Morris DM. Diagnosis and management of esophageal perforations. Am Surg 1992;58:112–119.
318. Glatterer MS, Toon RS, Ellestad C, et al. Management of blunt and penetrating external esophageal trauma. J Trauma 1985;25: 784–792.
319. Nesbitt JC, Sawyers JL. Surgical management of esophageal perforation. Am Surg 1987;53:183–191.
320. Sung SW, Park JJ, Kim YT, Kim JH. Surgery in thoracic esophageal perforation. Dis Esophagus 2002;15:204–209.
321. Gelman R, Mirvis SE, Gens D. Diaphragmatic rupture due to blunt trauma: sensitivity of plain chest radiograph. AJR Am J Roentgenol 1991;156:51–57.
322. Guth AA, Pachter HL, Kim U. Pitfalls in the diagnosis of blunt diaphragmatic injury. Am J Surg 1995;170:5–9.
323. Patselas TN, Gallagher EG. The diagnostic dilemma of diaphragm injury. Am Surg 2002;68:633–639.
324. Miller L, Bennett EV, Root HD, et al. Management of penetrating and blunt diaphragmatic injury. J Trauma 1984;24:403–409.
325. Haciibrahimoglu G, Solak O, Olcmen A, et al. Management of traumatic diaphragm rupture. Surg Today 2004;34:111–114.
326. Flancbaum L, Dauber M, Demas C, et al. Early diagnosis and treatment of blunt diaphragmatic injury. Am Surg 1988;54:195–199.
327. Kuligowska E, Mueller PR, Simeone JF, et al. Ultrasound in upper abdominal trauma. Semin Roentgenol 1984;19:281–295.
328. Chen JC, Wilson SE. Diaphragmatic injuries: recognition and management in sixty-two patients. Am Surg 1991;57:810–815.
329. Heiberg E, Wolverson MK, Hurd RN, et al. CT recognition of traumatic rupture of the diaphragm. Am J Roentgenol 1980;135:369–372.
330. Boulanger BR, Mirvis SE, Rodriguez A. Magnetic resonance imaging in traumatic diaphragmatic rupture: case reports. J Trauma 1992;32:89–93.
331. Gourin A, Garzon AA. Diagnostic problems in traumatic diaphragmatic hernia. J Trauma 1974;14:20–31.
332. Moore EE, Cogbill TH, Jurkovich GJ, et al. Organ injury scaling: spleen and liver (1994 revision). J Trauma 1995;38:323–324.
333. Cogbill TH, Moore EE, Jurkovich GJ, et al. Severe hepatic trauma: a multi-center experience with 1,335 liver injuries. J Trauma 1988;28:1433–1438.
334. Pringle JH. Notes on the arrest of hepatic hemorrhage due to trauma. Ann Surg 1908;48:541.
335. Pachter HL, Spencer FC, Hofstetter SR, et al. The management of juxtahepatic venous injuries without an atriocaval shunt: preliminary clinical observations. Surgery (St. Louis) 1986;99: 569–575.
336. Baumgartner F, Milliken J, Scudamore C, et al. Extracorporeal methods of vascular control for difficult IVC procedures. Am Surg 1996;62:246–248.
337. Baumgartner F, Scudamore C, Nair C, et al. Venovenous bypass for major hepatic and caval trauma. J Trauma 1995;39:671–673.
338. Rogers FB, Reese J, Shackford SR, Osler TM. The use of venovenous bypass and total vascular isolation of the liver in the surgical management of juxtahepatic venous injuries in blunt hepatic trauma. J Trauma 1997;43:530–533.
339. Horowitz JR, Black T, Lally KP, Andrassy RJ. Venovenous bypass as an adjunct for the management of a retrohepatic venous injury in a child. J Trauma 1995;39:584–585.
340. Yellin AE, Chaffee CB, Donovan AJ. Vascular isolation in treatment of juxtahepatic venous injuries. Arch Surg 1971;102:566–573.
341. Velmahos GC, Demetriades D, Chahwan S, et al. Angiographic embolization for arrest of bleeding after penetrating trauma to the abdomen. Am J Surg 1999;178:367–373.
342. Duane TM, Como JJ, Bochicchio GV, Scalea TM. Reevaluating the management and outcomes of severe blunt liver injury. J Trauma 2004;57:494–500.
343. Asensio JA, Roldan G, Petrone P, et al. Operative management and outcomes in 103 AAST-OIS grades IV and V complex hepatic injuries: trauma surgeons still need to operate, but angioembolization helps. J Trauma 2003;54:647–654.
344. Feliciano DV, Mattox KL, Jordan GL, et al. Management of 1000 consecutive cases of hepatic trauma (1979–1984). Ann Surg 1986;204:438–445
345. Pachter HL, Spencer FC, Hofstetter SR. Experience with the finger fracture technique to achieve intra-hepatic hemostasis in 75 patients with severe injuries to the liver. Ann Surg 1983;197:771–778.
346. Pachter HL, Spencer FC, Hofstetter SR, et al. Significant trends in the treatment of hepatic trauma: experience with 411 injuries. Ann Surg 1992;215:492–502.
347. Stone HH, Lamb JM. Use of pedicled omentum as an autogenous pack for control of hemorrhage in major injuries of the liver. Surg Gynecol Obstet 1975;141:92–94.
348. Fabian TC, Croce MA, Stanford GG, et al. Factors affecting morbidity following a prospective analysis of 482 liver injuries. Ann Surg 1991;213:540–548.
349. Stevens Sl, Maull KI, Enderson BL, et al. Total mesh wrapping for parenchymal liver injuries: a combined experience and clinical study. J Trauma 1991;31:1103–1109.
350. Jacobson LE, Kirton OC, Gomez GA. The use of absorbable mesh wrap in the management of major liver injuries. Surgery (St. Louis) 1992;111:455–461.
351. Goldman R, Zilkoski M, Mullins R, et al. Delayed celiotomy for the treatment of bile leak, compartment syndrome, and other hazards of nonoperative management of blunt liver injury. Am J Surg 2003;185:492–497.
352. Knudson MM, Lin RC, Olcott EW. Morbidity and mortality following major penetrating liver injuries. Arch Surg 1994;129:256–261.
353. Pachter HL, Knudson MM, Esrig B, et al. Status of nonoperative management of blunt hepatic injuries in 1995: a multicenter experience with 404 patients. J Trauma 1996;40:31–38.
354. Meredith JW, Young JS, Bowling J, et al. Nonoperative management of blunt hepatic trauma: the exception or the rule. J Trauma 1994;36:529–535.
355. Croce MA, Fabian TC, Menke PG, et al. Nonoperative management of blunt hepatic trauma is the treatment of choice for hemodynamically stable patients: results of a prospective trial. Ann Surg 1995;221:744–755.
356. Delgado Millan MA, Deballon PO. Computed tomography, angiography, and endoscopic retrograde cholangiopancreatography in the nonoperative management of hepatic and splenic trauma. World J Surg 2001;25:1397–1402.
357. Velmahos GC, Toutouzas K, Radin R, et al. High success with nonoperative management of blunt hepatic trauma. Arch Surg 2003;138:475–481.
358. Al-Mulhim AS, Mohammad HA. Non-operative management of blunt hepatic injury in multiply injured adult patients. Surgeon 2003;1:81–85.
359. Sherman HF, Savage BA, Jones MA, et al. Nonoperative management of blunt hepatic injuries: safe at any grade? J Trauma 1994;37:616–621.
360. Fang JF, Chen RJ, Wong YC, et al. Classification and treatment of pooling of contrast material on computed tomographic scan of blunt hepatic trauma. J Trauma 2000;49:1083–1088.
361. Knudson MM, Lim RC, Oakes DD, Jeffrey RB. Nonoperative management of blunt liver injuries in adults: the need for continued surveillance. J Trauma 1990;30:1494–1450.

362. Yang EY, Marder SR, Hastings G, Knudson MM. The abdominal compartment syndrome complicating nonoperative management of major blunt liver injuries: recognition and treatment using multimodality therapy. J Trauma 2002;52:982–986.
363. Chen RJ, Fang JF, Chen MF. Intra-abdominal pressure monitoring as a guideline in the nonoperative management of blunt hepatic trauma. J Trauma 2001;51:44–50.
364. Miller PR, Croce MA, Bee TK, et al. Associated injuries in blunt solid organ trauma: implications for missed injury in nonoperative management. J Trauma 2002;53:238–244.
365. Cogbill TH, Moore EE, Jurkovich GJ, et al. Nonoperative management of blunt splenic trauma: a multicenter experience. J Trauma 1989;29:1312–1317.
366. Harbrecht BG, Peitzman AB, Rivera L, et al. Contribution of age and gender to outcome of blunt splenic injury in adults: multicenter study of the Eastern Association for the Surgery of Trauma. J Trauma 2001;51:887–895.
367. Peitzman AB, Heil B, Rivera L, et al. Blunt splenic injury in adults: multi-institutional study of the Eastern Association for the Surgery of Trauma. J Trauma 2000;49:177–189.
368. Ruess L, Sivit CJ, Eichelberger MR, et al. Blunt hepatic and splenic trauma in children: correlation of a CT injury severity scale with outcome. Pediatr Radiol 1995;25:321–325.
369. Haan J, Scott J, Boyd-Kranis RL, et al. Admission angiography for blunt splenic injury: advantages and pitfalls. J Trauma 2001;51:1161–1165.
370. Albrecht RM, Schermer CR, Morris A. Nonoperative management of blunt splenic injuries: factors influencing success in age >55 years. Am Surg 2002;68:227–231.
371. Haan JM, Biffl W, Knudson MM, et al. Splenic embolization revisited: a multicenter review. J Trauma 2004;56:542–547.
372. Davis KA, Fabian TC, Croce MA, et al. Improved success in nonoperative management of blunt splenic injuries: embolization of splenic artery pseudoaneurysms. J Trauma 1998;44:1008–1015.
373. Schurr MJ, Fabian TC, Gavant M, et al. Management of blunt splenic trauma: computed tomographic contrast blush predicts failure of nonoperative management. J Trauma 1995;39:507–513.
374. Cocanour CS, Moore FA, Ware DN, et al. Delayed complications of nonoperative management of blunt adult splenic trauma. Arch Surg 1998;133:619–625.
375. Sclafani SJ, Shaftan GW, Scalea TM, et al. Nonoperative salvage of computed tomography-diagnosed splenic injuries: utilization of angiography for triage and embolization for hemostasis. J Trauma 1995;39:818–827.
376. Haan JM, Bochicchio GV, Kramer N, Scalea TM. Nonoperative management of blunt splenic injury: a 5-year experience. J Trauma 2005;58:492–498.
377. Liu PP, Lee WC, Cheng YF, et al. Use of splenic artery embolization as an adjunct to nonsurgical management of blunt splenic injury. J Trauma 2004;56:768–773.
378. Haan JM, Ilahi ON, Kramer M, Scalea TM. Protocol-driven nonoperative management in patients with blunt splenic trauma and minimal associated injury decreases length of stay. J Trauma 2003;55:317–322.
379. Vaughn G, Grazier O, Graham D, et al. The use of pyloric exclusion in the management of severe duodenal injuries. Am J Surg 1977;134:785–790.
380. Ivatury R, Nallathambi M, Gaudino J, et al. Penetrating duodenal injuries: an analysis of 100 consecutive cases. Ann Surg 1985;202:153–158.
381. Stone H, Fabian T. Management of duodenal wounds. J Trauma 1979;19:334–339.
382. Cogbill T, Moore E, Felician D, et al. Conservative management of duodenal trauma: a multicenter perspective. J Trauma 1990; 30:1469–1475.
383. Corley RD, Norcross WJ, Shoemaker WCZ. Traumatic injuries to the duodenum: a report of 98 patients. Ann Surg 1975;181:92–98.
384. Lucas C, Ledgerwood A. Factors influencing outcome after blunt duodenal injury. J Trauma 1975;15:839–846.
385. Cogbill T, Moore E, Morris JJ, et al. Distal pancreatectomy for trauma: a multicenter experience. J Trauma 1991;31:1600–1606.
386. Ivatury R, Nallathambi M, Rao P, Stahl WM. Penetrating pancreatic injuries: analysis of 103 consecutive cases. Am Surg 1990;56:90–95.
387. Stone H, Fabian T, Satiani B, Turkleson ML. Experiences in the management of pancreatic trauma. J Trauma 1981;21:257–262.
388. Graham J, Mattox K, Jordan G. Traumatic injuries of the pancreas. Am J Surg 1978;136:744–748.
389. Young PR, Meredith JW, Baker CC, et al. Pancreatic injuries resulting from penetrating trauma: a multi-institution review. Am Surg 1988;64:838–844.
390. Jones RC. Management of pancreatic trauma. Am J Surg 1985; 150:698–704.
391. Craig MH, Talton DS. Pancreatic injuries from blunt trauma. Am Surg 1995;61:125–129.
392. Moore EE, Cogbill T, Malangoni M, et al. Organ injury scaling II: pancreas, duodenum, small bowel, colon, and rectum. J Trauma 1990;30:1427–1429.
393. McInnis W, Aust J, Cruz A, et al. Traumatic injuries of the duodenum: a comparison of primary closure and the jejunal patch. J Trauma 1975;15:847–853.
394. Behrman SW, Bertken KA, Stefanacci HA, Parks SN. Breakdown of intestinal repair after laparotomy: incidence, risk factors, and strategies for prevention. J Trauma 1998;45:227–233.
395. Vasquez JC, Coimbra R, Hoyt DB, Fortlage D. Management of penetrating pancreatic trauma: an 11-year experience of a level-1 trauma center. Injury Int J Care Injured 2001;32:753–759.
396. Patton J, Lyden S, Croce M, et al. Pancreatic trauma: a simplified management guideline. J Trauma 1997;43:234–241.
397. Asensio JA, Petrone P, Roldan G, et al. Pancreaticoduodenectomy: a rare procedure for the management of complex pancreaticoduodenal injuries. J Am Coll Surg 2003;197:937–942.
398. Kudsk K, Croce M, Fabian T, et al. Enteral versus parenteral feeding: effects on septic morbidity after blunt and penetrating abdominal trauma. Ann Surg 1991;215:503–513.
399. Brunsting LA, Morton JH. Gastric rupture from blunt abdominal trauma. J Trauma 1987;27:887–891.
400. Wisner DH, Chun Y, Blaisdell FW. Blunt intestinal injury: keys to diagnosis and management. Arch Surg 1990;125:1319–1322.
401. Shuck JM, Lowe RJ. Intestinal disruption due to blunt abdominal trauma. Am J Surg 1978, 136:668–673.
402. McKenzie AD, Bell GA. Nonpenetrating injuries of the colon and rectum. Surg Clin N Am 1972;52:735–746.
403. Howell HS, Bartizal JF, Freeark RJ. Blunt trauma involving the colon and rectum. J Trauma 1976;16:624–632.
404. Duaterive AH, Flancbaum L, Cox EF. Blunt intestinal trauma: a modern-day review. Ann Surg 1985;201:198–203.
405. Stone HH, Fabian TC. Management of perforating colon trauma: randomization between primary closure and exteriorization. Ann Surg 1979;190:430–433.
406. Taheri PA, Ferrara JJ, Johnson CE, et al. A convincing case for primary repair of penetrating colon injuries. Am J Surg 1993; 166:39–44.
407. Flint LM, Vitale GC, Richardson JD, et al. The injured colon: relationships of management to complications. Ann Surg 1981;193:619–623.
408. Shannon FL, Moore EE. Primary repair of the colon: when is it a safe alternative? Surgery (St. Louis) 1985;98:851–860.
409. Burch JM, Brock JC, Gevirtzman L, et al. The injured colon. Ann Surg 1986;203:701–711.

410. Adkins RB, Zirkle PK, Waterhouse G. Penetrating colon trauma. J Trauma 1984;24:491–499.
411. George SM, Fabian TC, Voeller GR, et al. Primary repair of colon wounds: a prospective trial in nonselected patients. Ann Surg 1989;209:728–734.
412. Chappius CW, Frey DJ, Dietzen CD, et al. Management of penetrating colon injuries: a prospective randomized trial. Ann Surg 1991;213:492–498.
413. Falcone RE, Wanamaker SR, Santanelo SA, Carey LC. Colorectal trauma: primary repair or anastomosis with intracolonic bypass vs. ostomy. Dis Colon Rectum 1992;35:957–963.
414. Sasaki LS, Allaben RD, Golwala R, Mittal VK. Primary repair of colon injuries: a prospective randomized study. J Trauma 1995;39:895–901.
415. Gonzalez RP, Merlotti GJ, Holevar MR. Colostomy in penetrating colon injury: is it necessary? J Trauma 1996;41:271–275.
416. Fealk M, Osipov R, Foster K, et al. The conundrum of traumatic colon injury. Am J Surg 2004;188:663–670.
417. Curran TJ, Borzotta AP. Complications of primary repair of colon injury: literature review of 2,964 cases. Am J Surg 1999; 177:42–47.
418. Demetriades D, Murray JA, Chan L, et al. Penetrating colon injuries requiring resection: diversion or primary anastomosis? An AAST prospective multicenter study. J Trauma 2001;50:765–775.
419. Burch JM, Martin RR, Richardson RJ, et al. Evolution of the treatment of injured colon in the 1980s. Arch Surg 1991;126:979–984.
420. Burch JM, Feliciano DV, Mattox KL. Colostomy and drainage of civilian rectal injuries: is that all? Ann Surg 1989;209:600–611.
421. Maull KI, Sachatello CR, Ernst CB. The deep perineal laceration—an injury frequently associated with open pelvic fractures: a need for aggressive surgical management. A report of 12 cases and review of the literature. J Trauma 1988;17:989–696.
422. Levy RD, Strauss P, Aladgem D, et al. Extraperitoneal rectal gunshot injuries. J Trauma 1995;38:273–277.
423. Velmahos GC, Gomez H, Falabella A, Demetriades D. Operative management of civilian rectal gunshot wounds: simpler is better. World J Surg 2000;24:114–118.
424. Vitale GC, Richardson JD, Flint LM. Successful management of injuries to the extraperitoneal rectum. Am J Surg 1983;49:159–162.
425. Shannon FL, Moore EE, Moore FA, McCroskey BL. Value of distal colon washout in civilian rectal trauma: reducing bacterial gut translocation. J Trauma 1988;28:989–994.
426. Thomas DD, Levison MA, Dysktra B, Bender JS. Management of rectal injuries: dogma versus practice. Am Surg 1990;56:507–510.
427. Tuggle D, Huber PJ. Management of rectal trauma. Am J Surg 1984;148:806–808.
428. Levine JH, Longo WE, Pruitt C, et al. Management of selected rectal injuries by primary repair. Am J Surg 1996;172:575–579.
429. Armenakas NA, Duckett CP, McAninch JW. Indications for nonoperative management of renal stab wounds. J Urol 1999;161: 768–771.
430. Hagiwara A, Sakaki S, Goto H, et al. The role of interventional radiology in the management of blunt renal injury: a practical protocol. J Trauma 2001;51:526–531.
431. Nance ML, Lutz N, Carr MC, et al. Blunt renal injuries in children can be managed nonoperatively: outcome in a consecutive series of patients. J Trauma 2004;57:474–478.
432. Wessells H, Suh D, Porter JR, et al. Renal injury and operative management in the United States: results of a population-based study. J Trauma 2003;54:423–430.
433. Carver BS, Bozeman CB, Venable DD. Ureteral injury due to penetrating trauma. South Med J 2004;97:462–464.
434. Brandes SB, Chelsky MJ, Buckman RF, et al. Ureteral injuries form penetrating trauma. J Trauma 1994;36:766–769.
435. Campbell EW, Filderman PS, Jacobs SC. Ureteral injury due to blunt and penetrating trauma. Urology 1992;40:216–220.
436. Presti JC, Carroll PR, McAninch LW. Ureteral and renal pelvic injuries form external trauma. J Trauma 1989;29:370–374
437. Spirnak JP. Pelvic fracture and injury to the lower urinary tract. Surg Clin N Am 1988;68:1057–1069.
438. Carroll PR, McAninch JW. Bladder trauma: mechanisms of injury and a unified method of diagnosis and repair. J Urol 1984; 132:254–257.
439. Bodner DR, Selzman AA, Spirnak JP. Evaluation and treatment of bladder rupture. Semin Urol 1995;13:62–65.
440. Margolin DJ, Gonzalez RP. Retrospective analysis of traumatic bladder injury: does suprapubic catheterization alter outcome of healing? Am Surg 2004;70:1057–1060.
441. Davis JW, Hoyt DB, McArdle MS, et al. An analysis of errors causing morbidity and mortality in a trauma system: a guide for quality improvement. J Trauma 1992;32:660–666.
442. Ong AW, Cohn SM, Cohn KA, et al. Unexpected findings in trauma patients dying in the intensive care unit: results of 153 consecutive autopsies. J Am Coll Surg 2002;194:401–406.
443. Brooks A, Holroyd B, Riley B. Missed injury in major trauma patients. Injury Int J Care Injured 2004;35:407–410.
444. Biffl WL, Harrington DT, Cioffi WG. Implementation of a tertiary trauma survey decreases missed injuries. J Trauma 2003;54:38–44.
445. Buduhan G, McRitchie DI. Missed injuries in patients with multiple trauma. J Trauma 2000;49:600–605.
446. Houshian A, Larsen MS, Holm C. Missed injuries in a level I trauma center. J Trauma 2002;52:715–719.
447. Cowell VL, Ciraulo D, Gabram S, et al. Trauma 24-hour observation critical path. J Trauma 1998;45:147–150.
448. Henneman PL, Marx JA, Cantrill SC, Mitchell M. The use of an emergency department observation unit in the management of abdominal trauma. Ann Emerg Med 1989;18:647–660.
449. Haan J, Kole K, Brunetti A, et al. Nontherapeutic laparotomies revisited. Am Surg 2003;69:562–565.
450. Burch JM, Moore EE, Moore FA, Francoise R. The abdominal compartment syndrome. Surg Clin N Am 1996;76:833–842.
451. Maxwell RA, Fabian TC, Croce MA, Davis KA. Secondary abdominal compartment syndrome: an underappreciated manifestation of severe hemorrhagic shock. J Trauma 1999;47:995–999.
452. Balogh Z, McKinley BA, Cocanour CS, et al. Secondary abdominal compartment syndrome is an elusive early complication of traumatic shock resuscitation. Am J Surg 2002;184:538–544.
453. Balogh Z, McKinley BA, Cocanour CS, et al. Supranormal trauma resuscitation causes more cases of abdominal compartment syndrome. Arch Surg 2003;138:637–643.
454. Ivatury RR, Porter JM, Simon RJ, et al. Intra-abdominal hypertension after life-threatening penetrating abdominal trauma: prophylaxis, incidence, and clinical relevance to gastric mucosal pH and abdominal compartment syndrome. J Trauma 1998;44: 1016–1023.
455. Saggi BH, Sugerman HJ, Ivatury RR, Bloomfield GL. Abdominal compartment syndrome. J Trauma 1998;45:597–609.
456. Balogh Z, McKinley BA, Cox CS, et al. Abdominal compartment syndrome: the cause or effect of postinjury multiple organ failure. Shock 2003;20:483–492.
457. Kirkpatrick AW, Brenneman FD, McLean RF, et al. Is clinical examination an accurate indicator of raised intra-abdominal pressure in critically injured patients? Can J Surg 2000;43:207–211.
458. Kron IL, Harman PK, Nolan SP. The measurement of intra-abdominal pressure as a criterion for abdominal re-exploration. Ann Surg 1984;199:28–30.

459. Cheatham ML, White MW, Sagraves SG, et al. Abdominal perfusion pressure: a superior parameter in the assessment of intra-abdominal hypertension. J Trauma 2000;49:621–627.
460. Meldrum DR, Moore FA, Moore EE, et al. Prospective characterization and selective management of the abdominal compartment syndrome. Am J Surg 1997;174:667–673.
461. Balogh Z, McKinley BA, Holcomb JB, et al. Both primary and secondary abdominal compartment syndrome can be predicted early and are harbingers of multiple organ failure. J Trauma 2003;54:848–861.
462. Biffl WL, Moore EE, Burch JM, et al. Secondary abdominal compartment syndrome is a highly lethal event. Am J Surg 2001; 182:645–648.
463. Gracias VH, Braslow B, Johnson J, et al. Abdominal compartment syndrome in the open abdomen. Arch Surg 2002;137:1298–1300.

28

Trauma to the Pelvis and Extremities

Dean G. Lorich, Michael J. Gardner, and David L. Helfet

Pelvic Trauma

Pelvic fractures account for 3% to 8% of all skeletal injuries.[1–3] Two distinct patient populations sustain pelvic fractures: those involved in high-energy trauma, frequently motor vehicle or pedestrian versus motor vehicle collisions, and those who sustain a low-energy event, commonly an elderly patient with osteoporosis who sustains a fall resulting in a pelvic fracture with a stable pelvic ring and minimal concomitant injuries. High-energy mechanisms are involved in 13% to 18% of all pelvic fractures[1,4] and are often accompanied by bony pelvic instability and severe soft tissue injuries, both locally and in remote systems. Injuries to the genitourinary and gastrointestinal system as a direct result of a pelvic fracture are frequent.[5–7] Despite advances in organized trauma systems and intensive care, these fractures continue to present treatment dilemmas acutely and are a major source of morbidity and of mortality, which ranges from 7% to 50%.[4,5,8–13] Appropriate assessment and management by a multidisciplinary team are crucial to maximize the chance of survival of these patients and their return to preinjury function.

Biomechanics of the Pelvic Ring

High-energy fractures of the pelvic ring following blunt trauma can be classified broadly as either stable or unstable.[14] The former group has minimal damage to the supporting ligaments of the pelvis, and the fracture will withstand physiological forces without displacement.[15] The latter group has a grossly displaced pelvic ring and often requires emergent control of hemorrhage and pelvic stabilization. Pelvic stability is assessed initially by physical examination and confirmed by X-ray. Radiographic signs of instability include displacement and deformity, avulsion of the ischial spine, and fractures of the transverse processes of the L5 vertebra.[1]

Sequential sectioning studies have demonstrated that pubic symphysis diastasis of greater than 2.5 cm requires an application of force sufficient to also cause a destabilizing ligamentous injury.[16] When the strong posterior structures remain intact, the pelvis is rendered rotationally unstable.[14,16] If the posterior ligament complex or sacroiliac joint is disrupted, a markedly unstable hemipelvis results, leading to both rotational and vertical displacement.[17] Knowledge of the structural injuries that produce characteristic radiographic and clinical findings has important implications for resuscitation requirements, concomitant injuries, and prognosis.[11,18–20] In addition, the abdominal fascial attachments have an important stabilizing effect on the pelvic ring,[21] which underscores the importance of ensuring pelvic stability before or during a laparotomy procedure.[21–23]

Classification

Several pelvic fracture classification systems, based on different parameters, have been proposed in the past. The most commonly used system is that of Young and Burgess, which accounts for mechanism of injury.[24] Injury patterns are divided into lateral compression (LC), anteroposterior compression (APC), vertical shear (VS), and combined mechanisms (Figure 28.1). The value of this system is that it is readily applied from information provided by a single anteroposterior pelvic X-ray and it is predictive of concomitant injuries, resuscitative requirements, and outcomes.[18] Lateral compression patterns have a high incidence of vascular injury and shock as severity increases, but the characteristic feature of this group

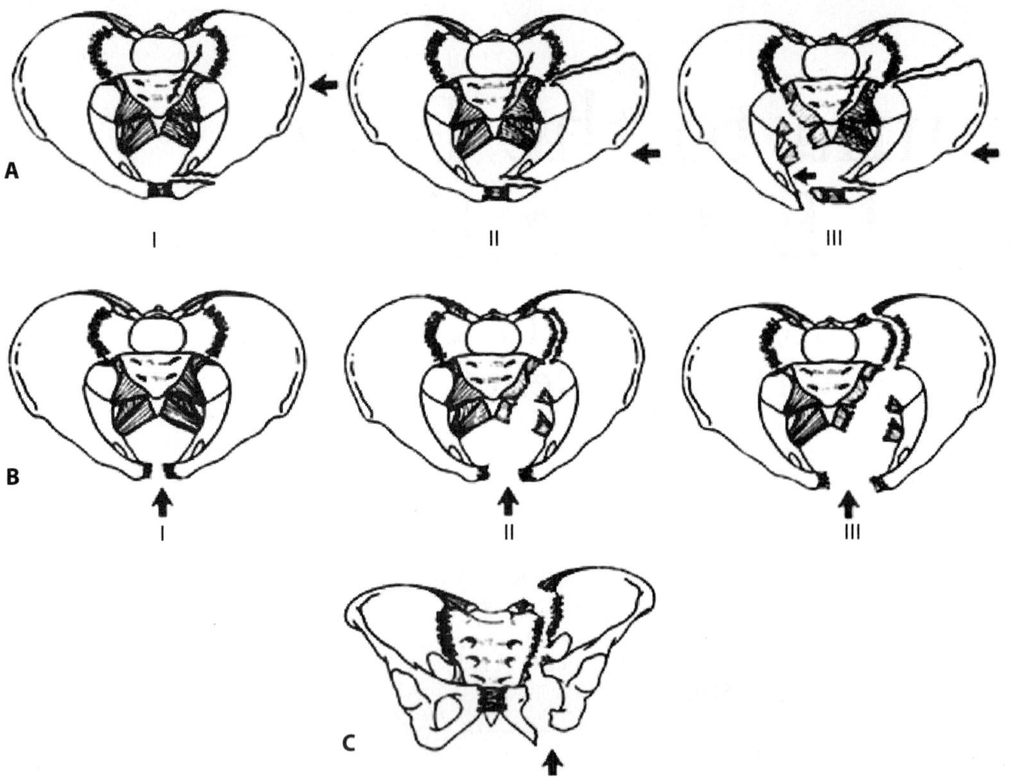

FIGURE 28.1. Schematic of the Young and Burgess classification of pelvic fractures, which includes (**A**) lateral compression (LC), (**B**) anteroposterior compression (APC), and (**C**) vertical shear (VS). (Reprinted from Browner BD, Jupiter J, Levine A, Trafton P, eds. Skeletal Trauma: Basic Science, Management, and Reconstruction, 3rd ed., Philadelphia. Elsevier, 2003, with permission.)

is the concomitant head, lung, and abdominal injuries that are contributory causes of death. Anteroposterior patterns, on the other hand, are associated more frequently with a high incidence of hemorrhage, volume loss, shock, sepsis, and acute respiratory distress syndrome (ARDS). High-grade APC injuries have the largest fluid requirements and the highest mortality.[11,18] Regardless of the propensity of some fracture patterns to lead to greater hemorrhage, it is important to consider that all pelvic fractures, regardless of radiographic classification, may be associated with hemorrhage and hemodynamic instability.[20,25]

Hemorrhage in Pelvic Fractures

One of the most common causes of early death following high-energy pelvic fracture is exsanguinating hemorrhage, which occurs in 10% to 20% of pelvic fractures.[13,18,19,26–28] Fractures that exit into the greater sciatic notch, or those which cause an increased pelvic volume, are more likely to lead to hemorrhage.[18,20,29] A negative chest X-ray, abdominal ultrasound or peritoneal lavage, and physical examination for lacerations and long bone fractures help rule out other sources of major blood loss, making it likely the pelvic fracture is the source of bleeding. More than 90% of pelvic bleeding is believed to arise from the presacral venous plexus and cancellous bone surfaces, and disruption of ligamentous checkreins and soft tissue envelopes allows for uncontrolled bleeding into the retroperitoneum.[1,21,30–2] In an autopsy study of 147 cadavers with pelvic fractures, Huittinen and Slatis reported that the fracture site was the major source of bleeding in 84% to 88% of cases.[33] Thus, stabilization of these surfaces to minimize clot dislodgment during transport is crucial. A third, less common, source of blood loss is from arterial injury, which may result from vessel laceration from a fracture spike, direct traumatic external forces, or shearing of vessels at their site of origin.[25,34] Vascular injury has been reported to occur in 2% and 10% of fractures.[5,34–36] Depending on fracture anatomy, laceration or transaction of the superior gluteal artery or branches of the hypogastric artery can cause life-threatening hemorrhage.

Early diagnosis of pelvic hemorrhage is important to maximize the chance of successful therapeutic intervention. Contrast-enhanced computed tomography (CT) scan, which may be performed in stable or borderline patients, can detect brisk bleeding accurately from the pelvic vasculature.[37,38] The sensitivity of CT for identification of pelvic bleeding has been reported to be as high as 90%, and the specificity is as high as 98%.[37,39,40]

Initial Treatment

Mortality caused by pelvic fractures is generally bimodal, resulting from either uncontrolled bleeding in the acute phase, or secondary to ARDS, multiple organ dysfunction syndrome (MODS), or other posttraumatic complications in the late phase.[23] Alterations in inflammatory mediators shortly after injury contribute to the development of these late conditions and have been termed the "first hit phenomenon."[3,27,41] Surgical intervention (the "second hit") exacerbates the traumatic physiological disturbances and should be minimized to the least invasive or shortest procedure necessary to control hemorrhage and contamination, allowing intensive care unit (ICU) resuscitation to continue relatively unabated.[42,43] "Damage control" surgery, which was applied initially to abdominal trauma,[42] is a fundamental principle in the management of unstable patients with pelvic fractures as well (Table 28.1). Late infection after nonoperative management of a pelvic fracture may also constitute a second hit.

Stabilization of the pelvic ring early in the treatment algorithm is of major importance (Figure 28.2). In patients with unstable pelvic fractures, multiple transfers allow for clot dislodgment, persistent blood loss, and ongoing soft tissue injury. Many methods for stabilization have been recommended, ranging from noninvasive to maximally invasive techniques, some of which may be applied in the prehospitalization phase and some of which require an operating room.

Pneumatic Antishock Garment

The pneumatic antishock garment (PASG) applies circumferential compression to the lower extremities, immobilizing

TABLE 28.1. Damage Control Principles for the Initial Management of High-Energy Pelvic Fractures.

Closed reduction of the pelvis at admission:
External fixation
Wrapping pelvis with sheets with inner rotation and slight flexion of knees
External fixator
Pelvic C-clamp
Pneumatic antishock garment
Control of hemorrhage
Pelvic packing
Angiography
Control of contamination
Repair of genitourinary and rectal injuries
Debridement of necrotic tissue in the case of open injury

From Ertel WK.[23] General assessment and management of the polytrauma patient. In: Tile M, Helfet DL, Kellam JK, eds. Fractures of the Pelvis and Acetabulum. Philadelphia: Lippincott Williams & Wilkins, 2003, with permission.

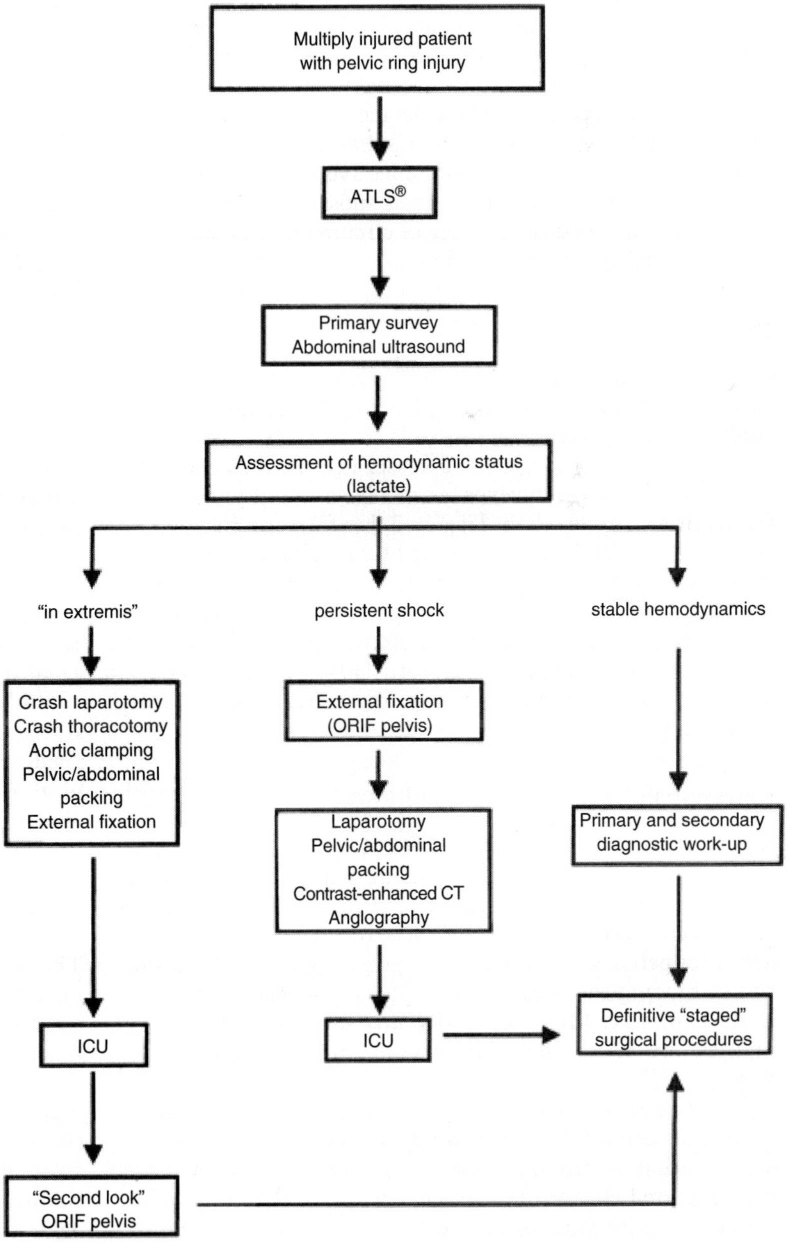

FIGURE 28.2. Algorithm for management of pelvic fracture in the multiply-injured patient. ATLS, Advanced Trauma Life Support; CT, computed tomography; ICU, intensive care unit; ORIF, open reduction and internal fixation.

the pelvis and theoretically increasing venous return from the lower extremities to the systemic circulation.[1] Several smaller series have shown potential benefits in hemodynamically unstable patients.[26,44] However, these devices block access to the patient's abdomen and genitourinary system, restrict diaphragmatic excursion, and may lead to compartment syndromes.[1,32] Evers et al.[28] found that PASG did not control hemorrhage from pelvic fracture as well as did external fixation in their series of 245 patients. A meta-analysis reported no benefit from use of PASGs and that in fact their use may increase morbidity and mortality.[45,46] Consequently, PASGs are no longer used as an adjunct to the resuscitation of trauma patients.

Pelvic Sheeting

Noninvasive circumferential compression with a sheet or sling has recently been advocated as a technique that is effective, inexpensive, and readily available.[47,48] A sheet is folded, wrapped around the greater trochanters, and clamped or knotted, allowing abdominal access if necessary. Prefabricated slings have recently become available specifically for this purpose. Special training or imaging modalities are not required for application of these devices, which may be done in the trauma bay. A small series has used CT scans to demonstrate that this technique effectively decreases pelvic volume in open-book injuries,[49] and a subsequent biomechanical study confirmed the efficacy of circumferential compression in reducing open-book injuries.[50]

Pelvic Packing

Open pelvic packing has been recommended by several authors for treatment of pelvic bleeding.[4,27] The arterial vasculature of the pelvis consists of a large network of collateral vessels; rarely, is a single large vessel identified as the only source of bleeding. However, as has been noted previously, the peritoneum is often lacerated by fracture fragments, causing difficulty in tamponading bleeding by packing anteriorly, and posterior application of a C-clamp is also recommended with open packing.[4,51] Open packing is typically performed concurrently with laparotomy, and cross-clamping of the aorta is possible as a last resort. This technique is rarely indicated and is used only in the most critically unstable patients.[1,47]

External Fixation

Anterior external fixators have become a mainstay in the resuscitation of the unstable patient with pelvic fracture. External fixation provides provisional immobilization, reapproximates and splints cancellous fracture surfaces, and decreases pelvic volume, likely tamponading venous bleeding and stabilizing the initial clot.[21,30–32,52] Rotationally unstable (APC II or LPC III) or vertically unstable (APC III or VS) injuries are most likely to benefit from early external fixation.[1,11,16]

Controversy persists over whether external fixation should be applied before or after angiography for possible embolization of bleeding vessels. No conclusive data have been reported supporting one approach over the other. The major reason for differing protocols among centers is a practical one, in that some have an in-house interventional radiologist available and angiography is obtainable immediately, whereas in other institutions initial application of external fixation in the operating room is more feasible. Although external fixation is believed to be ineffective in controlling arterial bleeding, the low incidence of arterial injury, combined with the ability of external fixation to stabilize the initial hematoma, has led most authors to advocate early pelvic stabilization before angiography.[9,27,28,34,36]

Riemer et al.[9] evaluated outcomes of pelvic fracture patients treated before and after the institution of a new management protocol. The new protocol consisted of a newly formed multidisciplinary team, but the authors attributed a significant decrease in mortality (26%–6% overall; 41%–21% in hemodynamically unstable patients) partly to the increased use of early external fixation (0% vs. 31% in the later time period). When no other source of bleeding could be identified by cystogram, CT scan, or peritoneal lavage, an external fixator was placed empirically. These authors stressed that external fixation controlled bleeding and pain, allowing effective resuscitation and earlier mobilization of the patient to an upright position.[9]

Angiography

In most pelvic fractures, early intravascular volume replacement and pelvic stabilization are sufficient to control pelvic hemorrhage.[34,53–57] In a subset of patients, however, hemodynamic instability persists despite these measures, often because of arterial bleeding. Therapeutic angiographic embolization has been advocated in these cases. Embolization acts to slow or stop bleeding at sites of arterial injury, augmenting the tamponade effect of the hematoma to control venous bleeding.[34] A retrospective review by Agolini et al.[36] revealed that only 1.9% of all pelvic fractures required embolization to control hemorrhage, but that the technique was effective when used. Success rates of identifying and treating sites of bleeding angiographically have been reported to be between 50% and 100%, with most reports greater than 90%.[5,34,36,58] The mortality following embolization still ranges from 18% to 47%,[34] but patients requiring embolization clearly have more severe injuries (Table 28.2). Predictive factors of survival following angiography include identification and successful embolization of bleeding, time to embolization, and initial hemodynamic instability.[59] In an analysis of 507 pelvic fractures, of whom 17 (3.4%) underwent embolization, Wong et al. found that for each 1 unit/h increase in blood transfusion required, the risk of death increased 62%.[34]

Extremity Trauma

The optimal timing and technique of long bone fracture stabilization in the multiply injured patient has been a topic of debate and controversy. Over the past few decades, the importance of early definitive fracture fixation of long bones to minimize morbidity in the multitrauma patient has been emphasized by many authors.[60–69] Femoral shaft fractures are the long bone injury with the most at stake when deciding on treatment, both because of their high incidence in multitrauma patients and because of the associated soft tissue damage and blood loss consequent to its large soft tissue

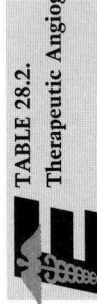

TABLE 28.2.
Therapeutic Angiographic Embolization.

Trial	*Year*	*Level of evidence*	*Groups (n)*	*Intervention/ design*	*Median follow-up*	*Minor endpoints*	*Major endpoints*	*Number of patients who required angiography (%)*	*Number of these patients who required embolization (%)*	*Number of these with successful embolization (%)*	*Comments*
Kimbrell et al.[54]	2004	II-2	2 (n = 17, 75)	Prospective cohort	Hospitalization	Success	Mortality	92 (9%)	55 (60%)	55 (100%)	Patients over 60 years had higher risk of requiring angiography for hemorrhage following pelvic fx
Cook et al.[55]	2002	II-2	2 (n = 23, 127)	Retrospective cohort	Hospitalization	Injury pattern	Embolization, mortality	23 (15%)	18 (78%)	18 (100%)	43% mortality after angiography when it occurred before ex-fix placement; recommended ex-fix before angiography
Velmahos et al.[56]	2002	II-3	1 (n = 100)	Prospective cohort	Hospitalization	Success, complications	Mortality	N/S	57 (57%)	53 (93%)	Angiography and embolization are highly effective and safe in pelvic fx
Demetriades et al.[5]	2002	II-3	1 (n = 1545)	Case Series	Hospitalization	Need for angiography	Incidence of concomitant injury, mortality	72 (4.7%)	36 (50%)	N/S	ISS = 25 predictive for need for angiography
Wong et al.[34]	2000	II-3	1 (n = 507)	Case Series	Hospitalization	Mortality	Success of embolization	22 (3.4%)	17 (77%)	17 (100%)	Mortality 18% after successful embolization
Perez et al.[57]	1998	II-3	1 (n = 721)	Case series	Hospitalization	Mortality	Complications	8 (1.1%)	5 (63%)	5 (100%)	Concluded limited applications for pelvic angiography
Agolini et al.[36]	1997	II-3	1 (n = 806)	Case Series	Hospitalization	Complications	Success, Mortality	35 (4.3%)	15 (60%)	15 (100%)	Very effective technique, but only in carefully selected patients
Evers et al.[28]	1989	II-3	1 (n = 245)	Case series, retrospective protocol evaluation	Hospitalization	Transfusion requirement	Mortality	16 (1.1%)	9 (56%)	8 (89%)	Recommended external fixation before angiography

ISS, Injury Severity Score; fx, fracture; ex-fix, external fixator; N/S not stated.

envelope. Patients treated with early fixation are able to be mobilized to an upright position to allow for pulmonary toilet, and are at less risk for ARDS, fat embolism syndrome (FES), pneumonia, and deep venous thromboembolism.[65,68,69] Early stabilization also minimizes ongoing soft tissue damage and pain at the fracture site. In contrast, unstabilized long bone fractures may exacerbate soft tissue injury and ongoing bleeding and lead to fat embolization, autonomic disturbances, and respiratory insufficiency.[61–64,70] Riska et al., in some of the earliest reports proposing early long bone fixation, reported significantly fewer complications in patients so treated.[63,64]

Only two prospective trials addressing the question of early versus delayed femoral fixation have been conducted. Lozman et al.[71] randomized 18 patients to early or delayed treatment and found that the early group had less pulmonary dysfunction and a higher cardiac index, suggesting a clinical benefit to early fixation. In 1989, Bone et al.[65] conducted a seminal study, analyzing 178 patients prospectively with acute femoral shaft fractures. In the subset of patients who were injured severely [Injury Severity Score (ISS) > 18], delaying fixation markedly increased the incidence of ARDS, fat embolism syndrome, and pneumonia, and the length of hospital stay.[65] Many retrospective series subsequently corroborated these findings, and early definitive fixation became the gold standard in trauma patients, shifting the paradigm from "too sick to operate" to "too sick *not* to operate."[59–64,66–69,72]

Damage Control Orthopedics

During the past decade, several authors noted poor outcomes with early definitive fracture fixation in patients with severe injuries and challenged the dogma that immediate intramedullary nailing of femoral shaft fractures was ideal for all trauma patients.[70,73–77] Several reports of an increased incidence of ARDS and MODS following reamed nailing of femoral fractures in the most severely injured patients caused investigators to reexamine the pathophysiology of this situation.[70,78,79] Inflammatory mediators came under scrutiny both for their possible role in the pathogenesis of systemic complications and for their potential use in monitoring and prognostication.[80] Concomitantly, several centers defined new high-risk patient groups[81] and proposed modified treatment algorithms to minimize inflammatory response in these patients.[76,77,82]

Basic Science of Long Bone Fractures

Long bone fractures are associated with a variety of local and systemic cellular events and microvascular changes, the pathogenesis of which are complex and have not been elucidated fully. Fat-laden bone marrow contents extravasate into the venous circulation and embolize the lung, directly stimulating an inflammatory response and lung microvascular injury.[83,84] However, although fat emboli to the lungs following long bone fracture almost always occur, clinically apparent respiratory changes occur rarely.[83] Additionally, "fat embolism syndrome," which classically involves the triad of refractory hypoxia, neurological changes, and petechiae, may in fact not be a unique syndrome at all but rather one of several precipitants of ARDS. Therefore, actual mechanical lodging of fat globules in the pulmonary microcirculation may be irrelevant to the pathogenesis of respiratory failure after long bone fracture.[85]

A local inflammatory response is elicited at the fracture site as well.[86] Cytokine concentrations, both locally and systemically, correlate with the severity of soft tissue injury. Persistently increased cytokine concentrations in the circulation following local trauma, particularly interleukin (IL)-6 and IL-8, have been demonstrated to be an "overspill" of local immune mediators from the fracture site.[87] This upregulated systemic inflammatory response results in neutrophil activation and adhesion to endothelial cells, with subsequent extravasation.[88] Proteases and reactive oxygen species are released, increasing capillary permeability and causing interstitial edema, ultimately leading to organ dysfunction.[85]

Basic Science of Long Bone Fracture Treatment

Intramedullary nailing of femoral shaft fractures is a reliable procedure that facilitates early mobilization and predictable bony union. Compared to traditional plate fixation, intramedullary fixation leads to less soft tissue disruption and a decreased rate of infection.[89,90] However, instrumentation of the femoral canal causes local pressure in the marrow cavity to increase up to 600 mmHg,[91] leading to further embolization of marrow contents and an inflammatory burst, both of which may be deleterious to the trauma patient (Figure 28.3).[92–94] En route to the lung, the fat globules aggregate with platelets and other mediators and increase in size.[95] Once in the lung, these particles may induce the coagulation and fibrinolytic systems.[93,96–98] Barie et al.[99] reported a dose-related increase in endothelial permeability when bone marrow was injected experimentally into the pulmonary circulation. Mechanical occlusion may be responsible for transitory pulmonary hypertension as well, although this appears to play a lesser role.[93,100] Overall, a complex proinflammatory response occurs, involving both local mechanisms (e.g., vasoactive mediators) and systemic factors such as shock and coagulopathy.[94,101,102]

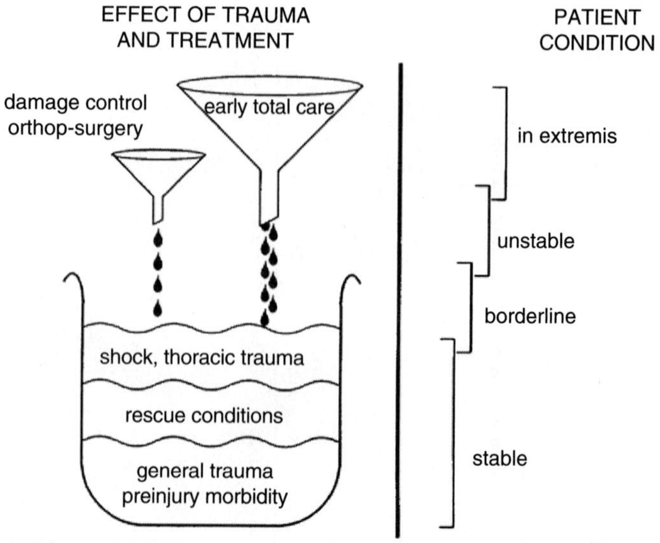

FIGURE 28.3. Schematic of the cumulative physiological effects of the preinjury morbidity, traumatic incident, and subsequent treatment. (Reprinted from Pape HC, Giannoudis P, Krettek C,[77] by permission of American Journal of Surgery, Excerpta Medica.)

Although many physical and biochemical effects of femoral reaming and nailing have been investigated in animal and human studies, their clinical significance is still being determined. Kropfl et al.[103] evaluated 39 patients with femur fractures prospectively who underwent intramedullary nailing and, despite a correlation between the pressure generated and the amount of fat extravasated into the circulation, neither could be related to the development of FES or ARDS, even in patients with thoracic injury.[103] Robinson et al.[93] found several changes in cardiopulmonary parameters between patients who underwent reamed versus unreamed nailing, but there was no clinical difference in the traumatic femur fracture group. Other studies have also indicated that the inflow of fat into the pulmonary vasculature may be a necessary prerequisite for development of ARDS following nailing, but insufficient to cause ARDS alone, and that other pathophysiological events must also occur.[98,104–109]

The numerous combinations of possible injuries, as well as the various biological responses to trauma in individual patients, makes quantifying the systemic physiological burden of the trauma and surgery difficult by clinical parameters. Advances in molecular medicine have allowed the analysis of systemic inflammatory mediators to quantify the trauma-induced burden and the subsequent effects of treatment.[110,111] Initial reports of the responses of interleukin-1β (IL-1β) and tumor necrosis factor-alpha (TNF-α) showed promise in this role, but their clinical utility was subsequently found to be limited.[76,112–114] More recently, IL-6 and IL-8 concentrations have been shown to correlate well with the ISS after trauma.[73,115] Changes in IL-6 are also reliable in quantifying the immunological burden following femoral nailing,[92] as well as other physiological secondary insults,[116] and predict which patients are at a higher risk for postoperative complications.[117–119]

Clinical Aspects of Damage Control

It has been suggested in several series that a subgroup of patients exists, the so-called "borderline patients" (Table 28.3),[81] whose clinical status is neither stable nor hemodynamically unstable, and in whom a greater risk of deterioration exists following invasive procedures.[70,120] These patients have a limited biological reserve following the initial insult of the trauma and are particularly susceptible to a "second hit" superimposed by a physiologically demanding surgical procedure.[121] Subclinical inflammatory responses and subsequent surgical procedures are compounded and may lead to MODS.[102] Several authors have stressed the importance of taking a "damage control" approach to patients who fall into this category.[76,81,82,121]

TABLE 28.3. Clinical Parameters in "Borderline" Patients, Which May Indicate a Patient May Not Tolerate the Physiological Stress of Primary Intramedullary Nailing.

Polytrauma + ISS >20 and additional thoracic trauma (AIS > 2)
Polytrauma with abdominal/pelvic trauma (>Moore 3) and hemodynamic shock (initial BP <90 mmHg)
ISS 40 or above in the absence of additional thoracic injury
Radiographic findings of bilateral lung contusion
Initial mean pulmonary arterial pressure >24 mmHg
Pulmonary artery pressure increase during intramedullary nailing >6 mmHg

ISS, Injury Severity Scale score; AIS, abbreviated injury scale; BP, blood pressure.

Source: Reprinted from Pape HC, Giannoudis P, Krettek C,[81] by permission of American Journal of Surgery, Excerpta Medica.

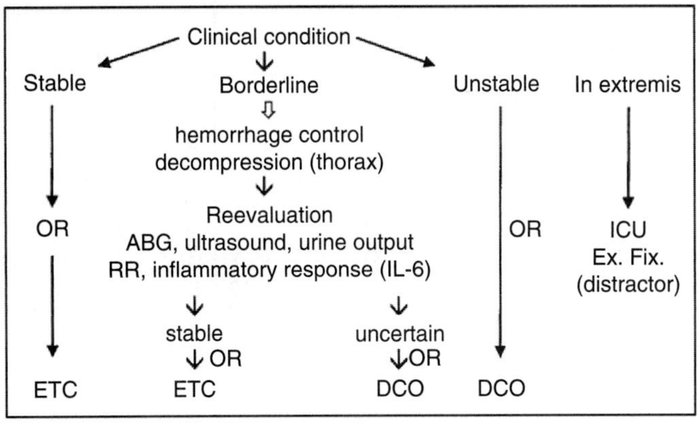

OR = operating room; ICU = intensive care unit;
ETC = early total care; DCO = damage control orthopedic;
Ex.Fix. = external fixation; ABG = arterial blood gas; RR = respiratory rate.

FIGURE 28.4. Suggested flow diagram for managing femur fractures in multitrauma patients, incorporating damage control orthopedics, and focusing on borderline patients. (Reprinted from Pape HC, Giannoudis P, Krettek C,[81] by permission of American Journal of Surgery, Excerpta Medica.)

Principles of damage control include immediate debridement of open fractures, control of hemorrhage, decompression of fascial compartments and intracranial lesions, and stabilization of femoral fractures in an attempt to minimize soft tissue injury, fat embolism, and the inflammatory response. In unstable or borderline patients, external fixation of the femur is an expedient and minimally invasive technique that stabilizes the fracture effectively but avoids a prolonged procedure.[121] In the next phase of treatment, resuscitation in the ICU continues until any coagulopathy, hypothermia, acidosis, or hemodynamic instability is reversed (Figure 28.4). This procedure is akin to the management of the multitrauma patient with an unstable pelvic fracture, which has been the standard of practice for many years.

Fakhry et al.[75] conducted a large database review of 2805 femoral shaft fractures and found the highest mortality in patients treated nonoperatively. Among those treated surgically, patients with an ISS of 15 or more who underwent nailing within 24 h had a higher mortality. Reynolds et al.[74] identified 105 consecutive patients with an ISS of 18 or more who underwent intramedullary nailing of a long bone at different time points following injury. In their series, outcomes were related to severity of injury, not time to fixation, and they hypothesized that fluid shifts associated with surgery may compound the first hit of the trauma.[74] Scalea et al.,[76] who first coined the term "damage control orthopedics," also reported on the usefulness of external fixation of femoral shaft fractures in the severely injured patient to allow ongoing resuscitation and to avoid the physiological insult of intramedullary nailing.

To evaluate prospectively the effect of a damage control approach versus early intramedullary nailing, a randomized multicenter study was conducted in Europe.[73] These investigators found greater increases in inflammatory mediators,

TABLE 28.4.
Prospective Evaluation of the Effect of a Damage Control Approach Versus Early Intramedullary Nailing.

Trial	*Year*	*Level of evidence*	*Groups (n)*	*Intervention/ design*	*Median follow-up*	*Minor endpoints*	*Major endpoints*	*Time cutoff for early fixation*	*Comments*
Pape et al.[73]	2003	I	2 (n = 17, 18)	Prospective, randomized, multicenter	Hospitalization	Inflammatory markers	Complications, mortality	24h	Immediate IMN has higher inflammatory response (IL-6 & IL-8) than ex-fix, but no clinical differences
Pape et al.[102]	2002	II-3	3 (n = 235, 88, 191)	Retrospective cohort over different time periods	3 weeks	Demographics	Mortality, complications	24h	DCO era had fewer complications, compared to earlier time group
Scalea et al.[76]	2000	II-2	2 (n = 43, 284)	Retrospective cohort	Hospitalization	Blood loss, OR time	Mortality, ARDS	24h	Ex-fix took avg 35min (vs. 130) and blood loss was 90mL (vs. 400) with IM nails, good alternative
Nowotarksi et al.[77]	1997	II-3	1 (n = 54)	Case series	12 months	Fracture healing	Mortality, complications	N/A	Safe treatment, no comparison group
Reynolds et al.[74]	1995	II-2	3 (n = 35, 13, 57)	Retrospective cohort	Hospitalization	ICU stay, ventilator days	Pulmonary complications	24h, 24–48h, >48h	Outcome related to severity of injuries, not timing of femoral nailing
Fakhry et al.[75]	1994	II-2	8 (n = 665, 965, 387, 256, 200, 212, 55, 65)	Retrospective cohort	Hospitalization	Length of stay	Mortality	24h, 24 days, >4 days	Higher mortality in patients with femoral nailing within 24h of injury
Pape et al.[70]	1993	II-2	4 (n = 24, 26, 33, 23)	Retrospective cohort	Hospitalization	Pneumonia	ARDS, mortality	24h	Higher incidence of mortality, ARDS, and pneumonia following early nailing with chest trauma

IMN, intramedullary nailing; DCO, damage control orthopedics; ARDS, acute respiratory distress syndrome; Ex-fix, extenal fixation; ICU, intensive care unit; IL, interleukin; OR, operating room.

most notably IL-6 and IL-8, in patients treated with initial nailing compared to those who underwent external fixation. Additionally, this substantial increase in cytokine concentration did not occur when patients underwent conversion from external fixation to a femoral nail at an average of 2.9 days. Most notably, there were no differences in complications, including ARDS or mortality, between the groups (Table 28.4).[73]

To address the most appropriate timing for secondary definitive skeletal fixation, a large retrospective study concluded that procedures requiring more than 3h should be undertaken after postinjury day 4 to minimize the risk of developing MODS.[122] A prospective study confirmed these recommendations, reporting greater concentrations of IL-6 and a threefold greater incidence of postoperative organ dysfunction in patients who underwent definitive surgery between days 2 and 4.[115] In this time period following severe trauma, fluid balance and immunological disturbances are often still normalizing, and it may not be an ideal time for definitive procedures.[43]

Femoral Fractures and Concomitant Chest Trauma

A multitude of animal and echocardiographic studies demonstrating embolization of fat and debris to the lung following intramedullary nailing have raised concern about the effects of femoral nailing in patients with chest injury.[94–101,103–105,107–109,123] Patients with trauma to the pulmonary parenchyma may be particularly susceptible to the deleterious effects of early intramedullary fixation as a consequence of the priming of the immune system and the subclinical effects of the initial pulmonary injury.[124,125] Pape et al.[70] reported retrospectively on 106 patients treated from 1982 to 1991 with a femoral shaft fracture and an ISS greater than 18 points. Patients with chest trauma who underwent femoral nailing within 24h had a higher incidence of ARDS (33% vs. 7.7%) and mortality (21% vs. 4%).[70] This report spurned controversy and led to much research into the harmful effects of early femoral nailing following chest trauma.

Several multicenter retrospective studies subsequently contradicted these data (Table 28.5). Bosse et al.[126] compared plate fixation to reamed intramedullary nailing in femur fractures in more than 200 patients with lung injury, finding no differences in the development of ARDS or mortality. They concluded that postoperative complications in patients with multiple trauma and lung injury were unrelated to reamed nailing. Further investigations into the pulmonary dysfunction caused by intramedullary nailing concluded that a preoperative increase in alveolar dead space was predictive of pulmonary dysfunction but that increased dead space was not the consequence of femoral nailing.[109] Similarly, Weresh et al.[127] concluded that intramedullary nailing did not produce enough embolization of the pulmonary microcirculation to affect the physiological dead space or alveolar-arterial oxygen gradient.[127] Bone et al.[128] reported that the lowest rates of ARDS occurred with early femoral fixation in patients with pulmonary injury. Several other authors have reported that early reamed femoral nailing in patients with a coexistent thoracic injury causes no harmful effect.[67,129,130] Of note, Charash et al.[68] duplicated the study by Pape et al.[70] at their institution and were unable to demonstrate similar detrimental effects of early intramedullary nailing on the outcomes of patients with pulmonary injury. Likewise, van der Made et al. could demonstrate no ill effect of reamed intramedullay nailing on coexistent pulmony injury.[131]

The majority of data refutes the notion that lung injury is exacerbated by reamed intramedullary nailing, despite the biochemical and animal studies. However, it is important to keep in mind that these data largely compare early to delayed nailing. Early external fixation has few drawbacks; the infection rate has been reported to be only 2% and 3% following intramedullary fixation,[76,77] it is less likely to cause intraoperative hypotension (which itself may exacerbate lung injury),[98] and it allows immediate stabilization of the fracture. Because of minimal disadvantages and theoretical benefits, it may be the preferable technique when any doubt exists about the patient's pulmonary status, although no prospective data are available.

Femoral Fractures in Patients with Traumatic Brain Injury

Traumatic brain injuries (TBIs) occur in up to 20% of multitrauma patients and are the most common cause of death.[132] Similarly, femur fractures occur in up to 22% of severely traumatized patients.[133] The timing of skeletal stabilization after TBI, particularly of the femur, has been much debated. Despite the many apparent advantages associated with early skeletal stabilization in multiply injured patients in general,[60,65] other associated risks may outweigh these benefits, in the subset of patients with TBI, as protection of the central nervous system is the first priority. Several mechanisms of secondary brain injury have been postulated following trauma, with hypotension and resulting cerebral hypoxia being key components.[134–137] A hypoxic episode, even as brief as 5min, can have profound negative effects on patient outcome,[138–140] and early hypotension doubles the mortality.[141] It has been suggested that early, prolonged operations may cause intraoperative hypotension, hypoxia, coagulopathy, and blood loss that compromise cerebral perfusion, exacerbating the traumatic event.[127] Specifically, reaming of the femoral canal carries the risk of extravasation of marrow contents with fat microembolization to the brain, with a subsequent increase in edema and intracranial pressure.[83,142,143]

Jaicks et al.[144] reviewed 33 patients with TBI and long bone fractures over a 4-year period and reported that the 19 patients who underwent fracture fixation within 24h required greater intraoperative fluid and blood administration, had a higher incidence of hypoxic episodes (16% vs. 7%), and had slightly worse neurological outcomes. The authors suggested that secondary brain injury from the procedures contributed to the neurological complications. However, their groups were small and heterogeneous with respect to orthopedic injuries, which were treated with unspecified techniques.[144] Martens and Ectors[145] reported on 77 patients, 22 of whom had fractures. Early fracture stabilization led to worse neurological outcomes, and these authors recommended delayed fixation (Table 28.6).

Several more recent series have reported that early fixation of fractures may not be deleterious in the brain-injured patient.[142,143,146–152] Kotwica et al.[148] evaluated 100 patients retrospectively, and those patients who received fracture care within 12h of presentation, simultaneously with

TABLE 28.5.
Plate Fixation to Reamed Intramedullary Nailing in Chest Injury.

Trial	*Year*	*Level of evidence*	*Groups (n)*	*Intervention/design*	*Median follow-up*	*Minor endpoints*	*Major endpoints*	*Comments*
Carlson et al.[130]	1998	II-2	4 (n = 532, 43, 18, 64)	Retrospective cohort	Hospitalization	ARDS, pneumonia	Mortality	No detrimental effect of reamed nailing in patients with chest injury
Bosse et al.[126]	1997	II-2	3 (n = 221, 232, 254)	Retrospective cohort	Hospitalization	Complications	Mortality	No difference in outcomes in patients with both thoracaic and femur fx vs. patients with one or the other
Boulanger et al.[129]	1997	II-3	4 (n = 68, 57, 15, 9)	Retrospective cohort	Hospitalization	ICU stay, ventilation time	Mortality	No effect on mortality or complications with reamed nailing with coexistent chest injury
van der Made et al.[131]	1996	II-2	3 (n = 21, 17, 22)	Retrospective cohort	Hospitalization	ARDS, MODS	Mortality	No effect on mortality or ARDS with reamed nailing with coexistent chest injury
Bone et al.[128]	1995	II-2	3 (n = 24, 18, 55)	Retrospective cohort	Hospitalization	ICU Stay	Mortality, ARDS	Only severity of chest injury was predictive of pulmonary dysfunction, not reamed nailing
Charash et al.[68]	1994	II-2	4 (n = 49, 8, 56, 25)	Retrospective cohort	Hospitalization	ICU stay, intubation time	Mortality, ARDS	Duplicated Pape et al. study; only surgical delay was predictive of pulmonary compromise, particularly in high ISS patients
van Os et al.[67]	1994	II-2	2 (n = 30, 27)	Retrospective cohort	Hospitalization	Mortality	Pulmonary function	Concluded thoracic injury not a contraindication for early surgical stabilization of femur fractures
Pape et al.[70]	1993	II-2	4 (n = 24, 26, 33, 23)	Retrospective cohort	Hospitalization	ICU stay, intubation time	Mortality, ARDS	Group with chest trauma treated early had higher ARDS and mortality

ARDS, acute respiratory distress syndrome; fx, fracture; ICU, intensive care unit; ISS, injury severity score; MODS, multiple organ dysfunction syndrome.

TABLE 28.6.
Early Fracture Stabilization and Worse Neurological Outcomes.

Trial	*Year*	*Level of evidence*	*Groups (n)*	*Intervention/ design*	*Median follow-up*	*Minor endpoints*	*Major endpoints*	*Time cutoff for early fixation*	*Comments*
Townsend et al.[153]	1998	II-2	4 (n = 22, 24, 3, 12)	Retrospective cohort	Hospitalization	Hypotensive episodes	Neurological outcomes	<2h, 2–12h, 12–24h, >24h	Eightfold increase in hypotension if stabilized 0–2h, twofold increase if 2–24h
Jaicks et al.[144]	1997	II-2	2 (n = 19, 14)	Retrospective cohort	Hospitalization	Intraoperative hypotension/ hypoxia; fluid administration	Neurological complications	24h	Early fixation led to greater fluid administration and more hypoxic episodes (16% vs. 7%)
Martens and Ectors[145]	1988	II-3	2 (n = 55, 22)	Retrospective cohort	Hospitalization	Neurological outcomes	Mortality	24h	Patients with early fixation had worse neurological outcomes

neurosurgical treatment, had decreased incidences of fat embolism and mortality. In another review of 58 patients, the 15 patients treated with early fixation had a lower mortality and better neurological outcomes despite more severe injuries.[149] Poole et al.[142] evaluated 114 patients retrospectively with early, delayed, or no fixation, and demonstrated that early fixation had no negative effects on cerebral events, which were related only to the severity of the TBI. Poole et al. stressed that early stabilization facilitated nursing care.[142] In a retrospective review of 171 patients with TBI and lower extremity fractures, Scalea et al.[146] found that surgical fixation within 24h, which included intramedullary nailing, plating, and external fixation, did not lead to more neurological events or an increased risk of mortality. Kalb et al.[150] reported that early fixation required vigilant intraoperative monitoring and administration of larger amounts of blood and fluids but was not associated with more hypotensive episodes or neurological events. In a large trauma registry review, Brundage et al.[72] reported no increase in mortality or adverse neurological outcomes associated with early femoral fracture fixation in patients with TBI (Table 28.7).

No prospective studies with Class I evidence exist to evaluate the timing of fracture fixation in patients with TBI. Several retrospective reviews suggest that the risk of secondary brain injury from intraoperative hypotension and hypoxemia may not justify early fixation.[144,145,153] Most series, however, have reported no increased risk of neurological events with early fracture stabilization in patients with TBI, provided vigilant monitoring is maintained.[142,148,149,154] In general, these retrospective cohort studies rarely describe the criteria used to determine which patients underwent early fixation. Although injury severity is often compared, some studies are skewed toward sicker patients, who tended to have their fixation delayed,[143,144] whereas in other studies there is a strong bias toward early fixation.[146]

These conflicting data have precluded the generation of stringent guidelines, rather suggesting that the surgeon individualize management when treating TBI patients with long bone fractures. Important to consider is the mobilization allowed by early stabilization; and a valuable option may be immediate external fixation, which avoids reaming and instrumentation of the intramedullary canal while still allowing fracture splinting and hematoma consolidation.[127] Retrospective data are available, and although studies are often conflicting and poorly controlled, there does not appear to be a significant disadvantage with early fracture fixation after TBI, provided necessary precautions and monitoring are utilized.[134] Neurological prognosis is likely most closely related to the severity of the brain injury,[133,142] and any surgical procedure must be undertaken with invasive monitoring of both hemodynamics and intracranial pressure, with aggressive resuscitation to avoid hypoxic episodes.[134,140,146,153]

Conclusion

Patients who sustain high-energy pelvic fractures are often difficult to treat, and the associated soft tissue injuries and hemorrhage continue to be a substantial source of morbidity and mortality. Evidence exists that in the setting of hemodynamic instability and unstable pelvic fracture patterns, mechanical stabilization is crucial. In the case of refractory hemodynamic instability when other sources have been excluded, emergent angiography is often successful in treating arterial bleeding, although this applies only to a small group of patients. Several large series have demonstrated improved outcomes with formal clinical trauma pathways and pelvic fracture management algorithms, and adherence to a multidisciplinary approach is essential.

TABLE 28.7.
Early Fixation of Fractures in the Brain-Injured Patient with Good Outcomes.

Trial	*Year*	*Level of evidence*	*Groups (n)*	*Intervention/design*	*Median follow-up*	*Minor endpoints*	*Major endpoints*	*Time cutoff for early fixation*	*Comments*
Nau et al.[154]	2003	II-2	2 (*n* = 28, 120)	Retrospective case-control	Discharge	Hospital/ICU stay, neurological outcomes	Mortality	24 h	Early fixation had no impact on mortality or neurological complications
Brundage et al.[72]	2002	II-2	2 (*n* = 238, 95)	Retrospective cohort	Discharge	Hospital/ICU stay, neurological outcomes	Mortality, pulmonary complications	24 h	Early femoral fixation was associated with lowest mortality and morbidity
Scalea et al.[146]	1999	II-2	2 (*n* = 147, 24)	Retrospective cohort	Discharge	ICU/hospital stay, fluid/blood requirements	Mortality, discharge GCS, neurological complications	24 h	No evidence that early fixation led to neurological compromise
Kalb et al.[150]	1998	II-2	2 (*n* = 84, 39)	Retrospective cohort	8–34 months	Fluid/blood administration	Hypoperfusion, mortality, cardial hypotension	24 h	Early fixation group had more blood and fluid requirements, but no increase in hypoperfusion or adverse outcomes
Velmahos et al.[151]	1998	II-2	2 (*n* = 22, 25)	Retrospective cohort	Discharge	Neurological complications, ventilation day, LOS	Intraoperative hypoxia, mortality	24 h	Early fixation had no impact on neurological complications
Starr et al.[143]	1998	II-2	2 (*n* = 14, 18)	Retrospective cohort	Discharge	CNS complication	Mortality, pulmonary complication	24 h	Fracture stabilization delay increased pulmonary risk, early stabilization had no increased CNS events
McKee et al.[147]	1997	II-2	2 (*n* = 46, 99)	Retrospective case-control	Discharge	Hospital/ICU stay	Mortality, neurological outcomes	24 h	Early intramedullary of femur fractures in head-injured patients had no deleterious effects
Malisano et al.[152]	1994	II-2	2 (n = 88, 20)	Retrospective cohort	18 months to 4 years	Union, sepsis	Mortality, pulmonary complication, neurological complication	N/S	Aggressive operative intervention produced no additional attributable neurological sequelae
Poole et al.[142]	1992	II-2	3 (*n* = 46, 26, 42)	Retrospective cohort	Discharge	Neurological outcome	Pulmonary outcomes	24 h	Cerebral events related only to severity of head injury, not timing of fixation; no deleterious effects
Hofman and Goris[149]	1991	II-2	58 (*n* = 15, 43)	Retrospective cohort	Discharge	Neurological outcome	Mortality	24 h	Early fixation group had higher ISS but lower mortality and better neurological outcomes
Kotwica et al.[148]	1990	II-2	2	Retrospective cohort	—	—	Mortality	12 h	Early fixation had less fat embolism and lower mortality than delayed
Lozman et al.[71]	1986	I	2 (*n* = 9)	Prospective, randomized	Discharge	Cardiac index, pulmonary indices	Mortality, ARDS	N/S	Minor differences in indices, no difference clinically, recommend early fixation

ARDS, acute respiratory distress syndrome; CNS, central nervous system; ICU, intensive care unit; LOS, length of stay; N/S, not stated.

The issue of technique and timing in the treatment of multiply injured patients with femoral fractures has not been resolved fully. The benefits of early fixation in the less severely injured patient are clear. Patients with a multitude of severe injuries (ISS > 18) are likely to benefit from a damage control approach to fixation, which centers on initial external fixation of long bone fractures to minimize the overall physiological insult, followed by continued aggressive resuscitation. Direct measurement of inflammatory mediators has recently become available in some centers and may become commonplace in quantifying the physiological insult of trauma and the risk of subsequent interventions. Prospective evidence exists that early definitive fixation leads to an increased inflammatory response, but this response has not coincided with poorer outcomes.

In patients with concurrent chest or brain injury, there is no clinical evidence that early reamed nailing exacerbates either injury. A plethora of in vitro and animal data have demonstrated the pulmonary fat microembolization following reaming, as well as the potentially detrimental consequences of fat microembolization in pulmonary or cerebral tissue. No prospective data are available to address this question, but the available retrospective clinical data, which include several large multicenter studies, have failed to show any harmful effects in these circumstances.

References

1. Wolinsky PR. Assessment and management of pelvic fracture in the hemodynamically unstable patient. Orthop Clin N Am 1997;28:321–329.
2. Gansslen A, Pohlemann T, Paul C, et al. Epidemiology of pelvic ring injuries. Injury 1996;27(suppl 1):S-A13–S-A20.
3. Giannoudis PV, Pape HC. Damage control orthopaedics in unstable pelvic ring injuries. Injury 2004;35:671–677.
4. Pohlemann T, Bosch U, Gansslen A, Tscherne H. The Hannover experience in management of pelvic fractures. Clin Orthop 1994;305:69–80.
5. Demetriades D, Karaiskakis M, Toutouzas K, et al. Pelvic fractures: epidemiology and predictors of associated abdominal injuries and outcomes. J Am Coll Surg 2002;195:1–10.
6. Taffet R. Management of pelvic fractures with concomitant urologic injuries. Orthop Clin N Am 1997;28:389–396.
7. Brandes S, Borrelli J Jr. Pelvic fracture and associated urologic injuries. World J Surg 2001;25:1578–1587.
8. Allen CF, Goslar PW, Barry M, Christiansen T. Management guidelines for hypotensive pelvic fracture patients. Am Surg 2000;66:735–738.
9. Riemer BL, Butterfield SL, Diamond DL, et al. Acute mortality associated with injuries to the pelvic ring: the role of early patient mobilization and external fixation. J Trauma 1993;35: 671–675; discussion 676–677.
10. Rittmeister M, Lindsey RW, Kohl HW III. Pelvic fracture among polytrauma decedents. Trauma-based mortality with pelvic fracture: a case series of 74 patients. Arch Orthop Trauma Surg 2001;121:43–49.
11. Burgess AR, Eastridge BJ, Young JW, et al. Pelvic ring disruptions: effective classification system and treatment protocols. J Trauma 1990;30:848–856.
12. Eastridge BJ, Burgess AR. Pedestrian pelvic fractures: 5-year experience of a major urban trauma center. J Trauma 1997;42: 695–700.
13. Naam NH, Brown WH, Hurd R, et al. Major pelvic fractures. Arch Surg 1983;118:610–616.
14. Olson SA, Pollak AN. Assessment of pelvic ring stability after injury. Indications for surgical stabilization. Clin Orthop 1996;329:15–27.
15. Kellam JF, McMurtry RY, Paley D, Tile M. The unstable pelvic fracture. Operative treatment. Orthop Clin N Am 1987;18:25–41.
16. Tile M. Pelvic ring fractures: should they be fixed? J Bone Joint Surg Br 1988;70:1–12.
17. Stocks GW, Gabel GT, Noble PC, et al. Anterior and posterior internal fixation of vertical shear fractures of the pelvis. J Orthop Res 1991;9:237–245.
18. Dalal SA, Burgess AR, Siegel JH, et al. Pelvic fracture in multiple trauma: classification by mechanism is key to pattern of organ injury, resuscitative requirements, and outcome. J Trauma 1989;29:981–1000; discussion 1000–1002.
19. Cryer HM, Miller FB, Evers BM, et al. Pelvic fracture classification: correlation with hemorrhage. J Trauma 1988;28:973–980.
20. Hamill J, Holden A, Paice R, Civil I. Pelvic fracture pattern predicts pelvic arterial haemorrhage. Aust N Z J Surg 2000;70: 338–343.
21. Ghanayem AJ, Wilber JH, Lieberman JM, Motta AO. The effect of laparotomy and external fixator stabilization on pelvic volume in an unstable pelvic injury. J Trauma 1995;38:396–400; discussion 400–401.
22. Latenser BA, Gentilello LM, Tarver AA, et al. Improved outcome with early fixation of skeletally unstable pelvic fractures. J Trauma 1991;31:28–31.
23. Ertel WK. General assessment and management of the polytrauma patient. In: Tile M, Helfet DL, Kellam JK, eds. Fractures of the Pelvis and Acetabulum. Philadelphia: Lippincott Williams & Wilkins, 2003.
24. Young JW, Burgess AR, Brumback RJ, Poka A. Pelvic fractures: value of plain radiography in early assessment and management. Radiology 1986;160:445–451.
25. Biffl WL, Smith WR, Moore EE, et al. Evolution of a multidisciplinary clinical pathway for the management of unstable patients with pelvic fractures. Ann Surg 2001;233:843–850.
26. Moreno C, Moore EE, Rosenberger A, Cleveland HC. Hemorrhage associated with major pelvic fracture: a multispecialty challenge. J Trauma 1986;26:987–994.
27. Tscherne H, Pohlemann T, Gansslen A, et al. Crush injuries of the pelvis. Eur J Surg 2000;166:276–282.
28. Evers BM, Cryer HM, Miller FB. Pelvic fracture hemorrhage. Priorities in management. Arch Surg 1989;124:422–424.
29. Blackmore CC, Jurkovich GJ, Linnau KF, et al. Assessment of volume of hemorrhage and outcome from pelvic fracture. Arch Surg 2003;138:504–508; discussion 508–509.
30. Ganz R, Krushell RJ, Jakob RP, Kuffer J. The antishock pelvic clamp. Clin Orthop 1991;267:71–78.
31. Flint L, Babikian G, Anders M, et al. Definitive control of mortality from severe pelvic fracture. Ann Surg 1990;211:703–706; discussion 706–907.
32. Failinger MS, McGanity PL. Unstable fractures of the pelvic ring. J Bone Joint Surg Am 1992;74:781–791.
33. Huittinen VM, Slatis P. Postmortem angiography and dissection of the hypogastric artery in pelvic fractures. Surgery (St. Louis) 1973;73:454–462.
34. Wong YC, Wang LJ, Ng CJ, et al. Mortality after successful transcatheter arterial embolization in patients with unstable pelvic fractures: rate of blood transfusion as a predictive factor. J Trauma 2000;49:71–75.
35. Agnew SG. Hemodynamically unstable pelvic fractures. Orthop Clin N Am 1994;25:715–721.
36. Agolini SF, Shah K, Jaffe J, et al. Arterial embolization is a rapid and effective technique for controlling pelvic fracture hemorrhage. J Trauma 1997;43:395–399.
37. Stephen DJ, Kreder HJ, Day AC, et al. Early detection of arterial bleeding in acute pelvic trauma. J Trauma 1999;47:638–642.

38. Shanmuganathan K, Mirvis SE, Sover ER. Value of contrast-enhanced CT in detecting active hemorrhage in patients with blunt abdominal or pelvic trauma. AJR Am J Roentgenol 1993;161:65–69.
39. Cerva DS Jr, Mirvis SE, Shanmuganathan K, et al. Detection of bleeding in patients with major pelvic fractures: value of contrast-enhanced CT. AJR Am J Roentgenol 1996;166:131–135.
40. Pereira SJ, O'Brien DP, Luchette FA, et al. Dynamic helical computed tomography scan accurately detects hemorrhage in patients with pelvic fracture. Surgery (St. Louis) 2000;128:678–685.
41. Moore FA, Moore EE. Evolving concepts in the pathogenesis of postinjury multiple organ failure. Surg Clin N Am 1995;75:257–277.
42. Rotondo MF, Schwab CW, McGonigal MD, et al. "Damage control": an approach for improved survival in exsanguinating penetrating abdominal injury. J Trauma 1993;35:375–382; discussion 382–383.
43. Waydhas C, Nast-Kolb D, Trupka A, et al. Posttraumatic inflammatory response, secondary operations, and late multiple organ failure. J Trauma 1996;40:624–630; discussion 630–631.
44. Flint LM Jr, Brown A, Richardson JD, Polk HC. Definitive control of bleeding from severe pelvic fractures. Ann Surg 1979;189:709–716.
45. Dickinson K, Roberts I. Medical anti-shock trousers (pneumatic anti-shock garments) for circulatory support in patients with trauma (Cochrane Review). Cochrane Database Syst Rev 2004;2: CD001856.
46. Mattox KL, Bickell W, Pepe PE, et al. Prospective MAST study in 911 patients. J Trauma 1989;29:1104–1111; discussion 1111–1112.
47. Kregor PJ, Routt ML Jr. Unstable pelvic ring disruptions in unstable patients. Injury 1999;30(suppl 2):B19–B28.
48. Routt ML Jr, Falicov A, Woodhouse E, Schildhauer TA. Circumferential pelvic antishock sheeting: a temporary resuscitation aid. J Orthop Trauma 2002;16:45–48.
49. Simpson T, Krieg JC, Heuer F, Bottlang M. Stabilization of pelvic ring disruptions with a circumferential sheet. J Trauma 2002;52:158–161.
50. Bottlang M, Simpson T, Sigg J, et al. Noninvasive reduction of open-book pelvic fractures by circumferential compression. J Orthop Trauma 2002;16:367–373.
51. Ertel W, Keel M, Eid K, et al. Control of severe hemorrhage using C-clamp and pelvic packing in multiply injured patients with pelvic ring disruption. J Orthop Trauma 2001;15:468–474.
52. Grimm MR, Vrahas MS, Thomas KA. Pressure-volume characteristics of the intact and disrupted pelvic retroperitoneum. J Trauma 1998;44:454–459.
53. Ben-Menachem Y, Coldwell DM, et al. Hemorrhage associated with pelvic fractures: causes, diagnosis, and emergent management. AJR Am J Roentgenol 1991;157:1005–1014.
54. Kimbrell BJ, Velmahos GC, Chan LS, Demetriades D. Angiographic embolization for pelvic fractures in older patients. Arch Surg 2004;139:728–732.
55. Cook RE, Keating JF, Gillespie I. The role of angiography in the management of haemorrhage from major fractures of the pelvis. J Bone Joint Surg (Br) 2002;84:178–182.
56. Velmahos GC, Toutouzas KG, Vassiliu P, et al. A prospective study on the safety and efficacy of angiographic embolization for pelvic and visceral injuries. J Trauma 2002;53:303–308.
57. Perez JV, Hughes TM, Bowers K. Angiographic embolisation in pelvic fracture. Injury 1998;29:187–191.
58. Mucha P Jr, Welch TJ. Hemorrhage in major pelvic fractures. Surg Clin N Am 1988;68:757–773.
59. Mucha P Jr, Farnell MB. Analysis of pelvic fracture management. J Trauma 1984;24:379–386.
60. Johnson KD, Cadambi A, Seibert GB. Incidence of adult respiratory distress syndrome in patients with multiple musculoskeletal injuries: effect of early operative stabilization of fractures. J Trauma 1985;25:375–384.
61. Goris RJ, Gimbrere JS, van Niekerk JL, et al. Early osteosynthesis and prophylactic mechanical ventilation in the multitrauma patient. J Trauma 1982;22:895–903.
62. Seibel R, LaDuca J, Hassett JM, et al. Blunt multiple trauma (ISS 36), femur traction, and the pulmonary failure-septic state. Ann Surg 1985;202:283–295.
63. Riska EB, Myllynen P. Fat embolism in patients with multiple injuries. J Trauma 1982;22:891–894.
64. Riska EB, von Bonsdorff H, Hakkinen S, et al. Prevention of fat embolism by early internal fixation of fractures in patients with multiple injuries. Injury 1976;8:110–116.
65. Bone LB, Johnson KD, Weigelt J, Scheinberg R. Early versus delayed stabilization of femoral fractures. A prospective randomized study. J Bone Joint Surg Am 1989;71:336–340.
66. Bone LB, McNamara K, Shine B, Border J. Mortality in multiple trauma patients with fractures. J Trauma 1994;37:262–264; discussion 264–265.
67. van Os JP, Roumen RM, Schoots FJ, et al. Is early osteosynthesis safe in multiple trauma patients with severe thoracic trauma and pulmonary contusion? J Trauma 1994;36:495–498.
68. Charash WE, Fabian TC, Croce MA. Delayed surgical fixation of femur fractures is a risk factor for pulmonary failure independent of thoracic trauma. J Trauma 1994;37:667–672.
69. Behrman SW, Fabian TC, Kudsk KA, Taylor JC. Improved outcome with femur fractures: early vs. delayed fixation. J Trauma 1990;30:792–797; discussion 797–798.
70. Pape HC, Auf'm'Kolk M, Paffrath T, et al. Primary intramedullary femur fixation in multiple trauma patients with associated lung contusion—a cause of posttraumatic ARDS? J Trauma 1993;34:540–547; discussion 547–548.
71. Lozman J, Deno DC, Feustel PJ, et al. Pulmonary and cardiovascular consequences of immediate fixation or conservative management of long-bone fractures. Arch Surg 1986;121:992–999.
72. Brundage SI, McGhan R, Jurkovich GJ, et al. Timing of femur fracture fixation: effect on outcome in patients with thoracic and head injuries. J Trauma 2002;52:299–307.
73. Pape HC, Grimme K, Van Griensven M, et al. Impact of intramedullary instrumentation versus damage control for femoral fractures on immunoinflammatory parameters: prospective randomized analysis by the EPOFF Study Group. J Trauma 2003;55:7–13.
74. Reynolds MA, Richardson JD, Spain DA, et al. Is the timing of fracture fixation important for the patient with multiple trauma? Ann Surg 1995;222:470–478; discussion 478–481.
75. Fakhry SM, Rutledge R, Dahners LE, Kessler D. Incidence, management, and outcome of femoral shaft fracture: a statewide population-based analysis of 2805 adult patients in a rural state. J Trauma 1994;37:255–260; discussion 260–261.
76. Scalea TM, Boswell SA, Scott JD, et al. External fixation as a bridge to intramedullary nailing for patients with multiple injuries and with femur fractures: damage control orthopedics. J Trauma 2000;48:613–621; discussion 621–623.
77. Nowotarski PJ, Turen CH, Brumback RJ, Scarboro JM. Conversion of external fixation to intramedullary nailing for fractures of the shaft of the femur in multiply injured patients. J Bone Joint Surg Am 2000;82:781–788.
78. Giannoudis PV, Abbott C, Stone M, et al. Fatal systemic inflammatory response syndrome following early bilateral femoral nailing. Intensive Care Med 1998;24:641–642.
79. Giannoudis PV, Cohen A, Hinsche A, et al. Simultaneous bilateral femoral fractures: systemic complications in 14 cases. Int Orthop 2000;24:264–267.
80. Smith RM, Giannoudis PV. Trauma and the immune response. J R Soc Med 1998;91:417–420.

81. Pape HC, Giannoudis P, Krettek C. The timing of fracture treatment in polytrauma patients: relevance of damage control orthopedic surgery. Am J Surg 2002;183:622–629.
82. Pape HC, Hildebrand F, Pertschy S, et al. Changes in the management of femoral shaft fractures in polytrauma patients: from early total care to damage control orthopedic surgery. J Trauma 2002;53:452–461; discussion 461–462.
83. Levy D. The fat embolism syndrome. A review. Clin Orthop 1990:281–286.
84. Hulman G. The pathogenesis of fat embolism. J Pathol 1995;176:3–9.
85. Robinson CM. Current concepts of respiratory insufficiency syndromes after fracture. J Bone Joint Surg Br 2001;83:781–791.
86. Hauser CJ, Zhou X, Joshi P, et al. The immune microenvironment of human fracture/soft-tissue hematomas and its relationship to systemic immunity. J Trauma 1997;42:895–903; discussion 903–904.
87. Perl M, Gebhard F, Knoferl MW, et al. The pattern of preformed cytokines in tissues frequently affected by blunt trauma. Shock 2003;19:299–304.
88. Eppihimer MJ, Granger DN. Ischemia/reperfusion-induced leukocyte-endothelial interactions in postcapillary venules. Shock 1997;8:16–25.
89. Bhandari M, Guyatt GH, Khera V, et al. Operative management of lower extremity fractures in patients with head injuries. Clin Orthop 2003;407:187–198.
90. Winquist RA, Hansen ST, Jr., Clawson DK. Closed intramedullary nailing of femoral fractures. A report of five hundred and twenty cases. J Bone Joint Surg Am 1984;66:529–539.
91. Wenda K, Runkel M, Degreif J, Ritter G. Pathogenesis and clinical relevance of bone marrow embolism in medullary nailing—demonstrated by intraoperative echocardiography. Injury 1993;24(suppl 3):S73–S81.
92. Giannoudis PV, Smith RM, Bellamy MC, et al. Stimulation of the inflammatory system by reamed and unreamed nailing of femoral fractures. An analysis of the second hit. J Bone Joint Surg Br 1999;81:356–361.
93. Robinson CM, Ludlam CA, Ray DC, et al. The coagulative and cardiorespiratory responses to reamed intramedullary nailing of isolated fractures. J Bone Joint Surg Br 2001;83:963–973.
94. Strecker W, Gonschorek O, Fleischmann W, et al. Thromboxane: co-factor of pulmonary disturbances in intramedullary nailing. Injury 1993;24(suppl 3):S68–S72.
95. Pape HC, Bartels M, Pohlemann T, et al. Coagulatory response after femoral instrumentation after severe trauma in sheep. J Trauma 1998;45:720–728.
96. Christie J, Robinson CM, Pell AC, et al. Transcardiac echocardiography during invasive intramedullary procedures. J Bone Joint Surg Br 1995;77:450–455.
97. Saldeen T. Intravascular coagulation in the lungs in experimental fat embolism. Acta Chir Scand 1969;135:653–662.
98. Wozasek GE, Thurnher M, Redl H, Schlag G. Pulmonary reaction during intramedullary fracture management in traumatic shock: an experimental study. J Trauma 1994;37:249–254.
99. Barie PS, Minnear FL, Malik AB. Increased pulmonary vascular permeability after bone marrow injection in sheep. Am Rev Respir Dis 1981;123:648–653.
100. Gossling HR, Pellegrini VD Jr. Fat embolism syndrome: a review of the pathophysiology and physiological basis of treatment. Clin Orthop 1982;165:68–82.
101. Pape HC, Giannoudis PV, Grimme K, et al. Effects of intramedullary femoral fracture fixation: what is the impact of experimental studies in regards to the clinical knowledge? Shock 2002;18:291–300.
102. Giannoudis PV, Pape HC, Cohen AP, et al. Review: systemic effects of femoral nailing: from Kuntscher to the immune reactivity era. Clin Orthop Relat Res 2002:404:378–386.
103. Kropfl A, Berger U, Neureiter H, et al. Intramedullary pressure and bone marrow fat intravasation in unreamed femoral nailing. J Trauma 1997;42:946–954.
104. Schemitsch EH, Jain R, Turchin DC, et al. Pulmonary effects of fixation of a fracture with a plate compared with intramedullary nailing. A canine model of fat embolism and fracture fixation. J Bone Joint Surg Am 1997;79:984–996.
105. Aoki N, Soma K, Shindo M, et al. Evaluation of potential fat emboli during placement of intramedullary nails after orthopedic fractures. Chest 1998;113:178–181.
106. Pell AC, Christie J, Keating JF, Sutherland GR. The detection of fat embolism by transoesophageal echocardiography during reamed intramedullary nailing. A study of 24 patients with femoral and tibial fractures. J Bone Joint Surg Br 1993;75:921–925.
107. Duwelius PJ, Huckfeldt R, Mullins RJ, et al. The effects of femoral intramedullary reaming on pulmonary function in a sheep lung model. J Bone Joint Surg Am 1997;79:194–202.
108. Willis BH, Carden DL, Sadasivan KK. Effect of femoral fracture and intramedullary fixation on lung capillary leak. J Trauma 1999;46:687–692.
109. Norris BL, Patton WC, Rudd JN Jr, et al. Pulmonary dysfunction in patients with femoral shaft fracture treated with intramedullary nailing. J Bone Joint Surg Am 2001;83A:1162–1168.
110. Smith RM, Giannoudis PV, Bellamy MC, et al. Interleukin-10 release and monocyte human leukocyte antigen-DR expression during femoral nailing. Clin Orthop 2000;16:233–240.
111. Giannoudis PV, Hildebrand F, Pape HC. Inflammatory serum markers in patients with multiple trauma. Can they predict outcome? J Bone Joint Surg Br 2004;86:313–323.
112. Roumen RM, Redl H, Schlag G, et al. Inflammatory mediators in relation to the development of multiple organ failure in patients after severe blunt trauma. Crit Care Med 1995;23:474–480.
113. Riche F, Panis Y, Laisne MJ, et al. High tumor necrosis factor serum level is associated with increased survival in patients with abdominal septic shock: a prospective study in 59 patients. Surgery (St. Louis) 1996;120:801–807.
114. Casey LC, Balk RA, Bone RC. Plasma cytokine and endotoxin levels correlate with survival in patients with the sepsis syndrome. Ann Intern Med 1993;119:771–778.
115. Pape HC, van Griensven M, Rice J, et al. Major secondary surgery in blunt trauma patients and perioperative cytokine liberation: determination of the clinical relevance of biochemical markers. J Trauma 2001;50:989–1000.
116. Ogura H, Tanaka H, Koh T, et al. Priming, second-hit priming, and apoptosis in leukocytes from trauma patients. J Trauma 1999;46:774–781; discussion 781–783.
117. Partrick DA, Moore FA, Moore EE, et al. Jack A. Barney Resident Research Award winner. The inflammatory profile of interleukin-6, interleukin-8, and soluble intercellular adhesion molecule-1 in postinjury multiple organ failure. Am J Surg 1996;172:425–429; discussed 429–431.
118. Pape HC, Schmidt RE, Rice J, et al. Biochemical changes after trauma and skeletal surgery of the lower extremity: quantification of the operative burden. Crit Care Med 2000;28:3441–448.
119. Pape HC, Remmers D, Grotz M, et al. Reticuloendothelial system activity and organ failure in patients with multiple injuries. Arch Surg 1999;134:421–427.
120. Nast-Kolb D, Waydhas C, Jochum M, et al. [Is there a favorable time for the management of femoral shaft fractures in polytrauma?] Chirurg 1990;61:259–265.
121. Giannoudis PV. Surgical priorities in damage control in polytrauma. J Bone Joint Surg Br 2003;85:478–483.
122. Pape H, Stalp M, von Griensven M, et al. [Optimal timing for secondary surgery in polytrauma patients: an evaluation of 4,314 serious-injury cases.] Chirurg 1999;70:1287–1293.

123. Wozasek GE, Simon P, Redl H, Schlag G. Intramedullary pressure changes and fat intravasation during intramedullary nailing: an experimental study in sheep. J Trauma 1994;36:202–207.
124. Pape HC, Regel G, Dwenger A, et al. Influences of different methods of intramedullary femoral nailing on lung function in patients with multiple trauma. J Trauma 1993;35:709–716.
125. Talucci RC, Manning J, Lampard S, et al. Early intramedullary nailing of femoral shaft fractures: a cause of fat embolism syndrome. Am J Surg 1983;146:107–111.
126. Bosse MJ, MacKenzie EJ, Riemer BL, et al. Adult respiratory distress syndrome, pneumonia, and mortality following thoracic injury and a femoral fracture treated either with intramedullary nailing with reaming or with a plate. A comparative study. J Bone Joint Surg Am 1997;79:799–809.
127. Weresh MJ, Stover MD, Bosse MJ, et al. Pulmonary gas exchange during intramedullary fixation of femoral shaft fractures. J Trauma 1999;46:863–868.
128. Bone LB, Babikian G, Stegemann PM. Femoral canal reaming in the polytrauma patient with chest injury. A clinical perspective. Clin Orthop 1995;347:91–94.
129. Boulanger BR, Stephen D, Brenneman FD. Thoracic trauma and early intramedullary nailing of femur fractures: are we doing harm? J Trauma 1997;43:24–28.
130. Carlson DW, Rodman GH Jr, Kaehr D, et al. Femur fractures in chest-injured patients: is reaming contraindicated? J Orthop Trauma 1998;12:164–168.
131. van der Made WJ, Smit EJ, van Luyt PA, van Vugt AB. Intramedullary femoral osteosynthesis: an additional cause of ARDS in multiply injured patients? Injury 1996;27:391–393.
132. Grotz MR, Giannoudis PV, Pape HC, et al. Traumatic brain injury and stabilisation of long bone fractures: an update. Injury 2004;35:1077–1086.
133. Kushwaha VP, Garland DG. Extremity fractures in the patient with a traumatic brain injury. J Am Acad Orthop Surg 1998;6: 298–307.
134. Schmeling GJ, Schwab JP. Polytrauma care. The effect of head injuries and timing of skeletal fixation. Clin Orthop 1995;318: 106–116.
135. Sarrafzadeh AS, Peltonen EE, Kaisers U, et al. Secondary insults in severe head injury: do multiply injured patients do worse? Crit Care Med 2001;29:1116–1123.
136. Schoettle RJ, Kochanek PM, Magargee MJ, et al. Early polymorphonuclear leukocyte accumulation correlates with the development of posttraumatic cerebral edema in rats. J Neurotrauma 1990;7:207–217.
137. Schmoker JD, Zhuang J, Shackford SR. Hemorrhagic hypotension after brain injury causes an early and sustained reduction in cerebral oxygen delivery despite normalization of systemic oxygen delivery. J Trauma 1992;32:714–720; discussion 721–722.
138. Chesnut RM, Marshall LF, Klauber MR, et al. The role of secondary brain injury in determining outcome from severe head injury. J Trauma 1993;34:216–222.
139. Pietropaoli JA, Rogers FB, Shackford SR, et al. The deleterious effects of intraoperative hypotension on outcome in patients with severe head injuries. J Trauma 1992;33:403–407.
140. Wald SL, Shackford SR, Fenwick J. The effect of secondary insults on mortality and long-term disability after severe head injury in a rural region without a trauma system. J Trauma 1993;34:377–381; discussion 381–382.
141. Chesnut RM. Secondary brain insults after head injury: clinical perspectives. New Horiz 1995;3:366–375.
142. Poole GV, Miller JD, Agnew SG, Griswold JA. Lower extremity fracture fixation in head-injured patients. J Trauma 1992;32:654–659.
143. Starr AJ, Hunt JL, Chason DP, et al. Treatment of femur fracture with associated head injury. J Orthop Trauma 1998; 12:38–45.
144. Jaicks RR, Cohn SM, Moller BA. Early fracture fixation may be deleterious after head injury. J Trauma 1997;42:1–5; discussion 5–6.
145. Martens F, Ectors P. Priorities in the management of polytraumatised patients with head injury: partially resolved problems. Acta Neurochir (Wien) 1988;94:70–73.
146. Scalea TM, Scott JD, Brumback RJ, et al. Early fracture fixation may be "just fine" after head injury: no difference in central nervous system outcomes. J Trauma 1999;46:839–846.
147. McKee MD, Schemitsch EH, Vincent LO, et al. The effect of a femoral fracture on concomitant closed head injury in patients with multiple injuries. J Trauma 1997;42:1041–1045.
148. Kotwica Z, Balcewicz L, Jagodzinski Z. Head injuries coexistent with pelvic or lower extremity fractures early or delayed osteosynthesis. Acta Neurochir (Wien) 1990;102:19–21.
149. Hofman PA, Goris RJ. Timing of osteosynthesis of major fractures in patients with severe brain injury. J Trauma 1991;31:261–263.
150. Kalb DC, Ney AL, Rodriguez JL, et al. Assessment of the relationship between timing of fixation of the fracture and secondary brain injury in patients with multiple trauma. Surgery (St. Louis) 1998;124:739–744; discussion 744–745.
151. Velmahos GC, Arroyo H, Ramicone E, et al. Timing of fracture fixation in blunt trauma patients with severe head injuries. Am J Surg 1998;176:324–329.
152. Malisano LP, Stevens D, Hunter GA. The management of long bone fractures in the head-injured polytrauma patient. J Orthop Trauma 1994;8:1–5.
153. Townsend RN, Lheureau T, Protech J, et al. Timing fracture repair in patients with severe brain injury (Glasgow Coma Scale score <9). J Trauma 1998;44:977–982; discussion 982–983.
154. Nau T, Aldrian S, Koenig F, Vecsei V. Fixation of femoral fractures in multiple-injury patients with combined chest and head injuries. ANZ J Surg 2003;73:1018–1021.

29

Vascular Trauma

Peter P. Lopez and Enrique Ginzberg

Identification and management of vascular injuries is challenging. The surgeon must have a good understanding of the arteries and veins that are likely to be injured, and which diagnostic modalities are needed to identify the injury, as well as the surgical techniques necessary to repair these injuries. It is imperative that one knows how to diagnose a patient who is stable but who may have an unsuspected vascular injury as well as to manage the patient who is hemorrhaging from an obvious injury. Most patients with vascular injuries require a multidisciplinary approach to care, possibly including treatment from an interventional radiologist for diagnosis and endovascular management, an orthopedic surgeon for concurrent fracture management, cardiac surgeons or neurosurgeons for selected types of vascular injuries, and plastic surgeons for wound coverage.[1] The trauma surgeon must remain in charge of the care of the trauma patient while simultaneously orchestrating all consultant services in a timely fashion to save both life and limb. This chapter presents an evidence-based approach to the evaluation and management of trauma patients with vascular injuries.

Historical Perspective

The historical approach to treatment of vascular trauma has been, first, to control hemorrhage and, second, to repair the damaged vessels. The initial control of hemorrhage at the time of injury is by direct compression: this simple principle remains valid today. Other methods used in the past to compress the wound and coagulate the bleeding included simple bandaging along with animal and vegetable tissues, hot irons, cold instruments, or boiling pitch or oils. In the Middle Ages, copper sulfate was used for hemostasis. Today, compression dressings with fibrin or poly-*n*-acetylglucosamine modified Rapid Deployment Hemostat dressing (mRDH) have been shown to stop hemorrhage when applied to vessels or solid organs.[2] Following compression, it was soon recognized that ligation of the bleeding vessel was effective at stopping the hemorrhage. Rufus of Ephesus noted in the first century that an artery that was partly severed continued to bleed, whereas bleeding stopped from an artery that was completely transected and contracted.[3] Ligation was not universally accepted until Ambrose Paré in the 1500s firmly established the use of ligature for control of hemorrhage from injured actively bleeding vessels. In 1674, Morel introduced a stick into the bandage and twisted it until blood flow ceased, creating the first modern tourniquet.[4] In 1873, von Esmarch introduced his elastic rubber tourniquet bandage for first aid on the battlefield.[5] Tourniquets now allow surgeons to operate electively in a dry, bloodless field.

Surgical repair of vessels began in 1759. Hallowell, at the suggestion of Lambert, repaired a brachial artery injury by placing a pin through the arterial walls and holding the edges in position by applying a suture in a figure-of-eight fashion about a pin (farrier's or veterinarian's stitch).[6] In Chicago in 1896, John B. Murphy repaired a transected femoral artery with an end-to-end anastomosis.[7] In 1906, Goyanes resected a popliteal artery aneurysm and used the popliteal vein to reconstruct the artery.[8] This was the first report of the clinical use of an autogenous vein arterial repair. A list of important contributions to vascular trauma surgery that paved the way to repair of damaged vessels is given in Table 29.1.

However, it was not until the Korean War that these principles could be applied to large numbers of battle casualties. During World War I and World War II, the transport time from injury to aid stations and the high incidence of infection led to the policy of ligation and amputation rather than vessel repair. During the Korean and Vietnam conflicts, amputation rates decreased from 49% (WW II) to 13%. This decrease resulted from rapid evacuation of the wounded by helicopter; the advancements of early debridement, delayed primary closure, and antibiotics led to a decrease in traumatic wound infections and surgical site infections, increasing the overall success rate of vascular repair. The Vietnam conflict yielded

TABLE 29.1. Contributions to Vascular Trauma Surgery.

Surgeon	*Year*	*Contribution*
Hallowell-Lambert	1759	Lateral repair with pin and thread
Broca	1762	Suture of a longitudinal incision in artery
Schede	1882	First lateral suture repair of femoral vein
Heidenhain	1894	Catgut suture to repair iatrogenic injury of axillary artery
Murphy	1896	End-to-end anastomosis using invagination technique
Carrel and Guthrie	1902	Triangulation technique of arterial anastomosis
Goyanes	1906	Vein graft repair, popliteal vein for popliteal artery
Lexer	1907	Saphenous vein graft to replace artery

Source: Modified from Rich NM. Vascular trauma. Surg Clin N Am 1973;53:1367–1392.

understanding of the importance of concomitant repair of venous injuries and also stimulated the establishment of a vascular registry. The repair of venous injuries not only contributed to successful arterial repairs but also substantially decreased long-term morbidity from venous insufficiency. The registry allowed outcome analysis including descriptions of the injury, the repair, and the return to activities of daily living for these patients.

Epidemiology

The true incidence of vascular trauma is unknown because incidence is reported for repaired injuries but excludes those with vascular injuries who die before arriving at the hospital. Most war-related vascular injuries affected the extremities as a result of fragments from exploding devices or bullets. Table 29.2 summarizes the anatomic distributions of vascular injuries during World War II and the Korean and Vietnam wars. In contrast to war-related vascular trauma, the civilian experience has been to have more torso-penetrating vascular injuries than extremity injuries. Mattox et al. reported their experience with vascular trauma in the Houston area over a 30-year period.[9] The incidence of vascular trauma from penetrating, blunt, and iatrogenic causes increased over the three decades of this study. This trend will probably continue as the numbers of assaults, high-speed motor vehicle crashes, falls from heights, and invasive medical procedures continue to increase. In 1992, Oller et al. presented a review of North Carolina's vascular trauma experience from the statewide trauma registry,[10] demonstrating that patients in rural settings who sustained vascular trauma were older, more often victims of blunt trauma, more often white, and less often male than urban trauma patients. Also, patients with vascular injuries were more severely injured than those without vascular injury, presenting with higher injury severity scores and having higher mortality, longer hospital stays, and higher hospital charges when compared to those patients without vascular trauma.

Penetrating injuries remain the dominant cause of vascular trauma in both urban and rural civilian settings, accounting for more than 80% of such injuries. Penetrating injuries caused by gunshot wounds cause about 50% of vascular injuries whereas stab wounds and shotgun injuries account for 30% and 5%, respectively. Blunt trauma represents the cause of the remaining 15% of vascular injuries. The anatomic distribution of penetrating injuries is related to the mechanism of injury. Gunshot wounds are most likely to involve abdominal vessels, followed by the lower extremities.[9] Stab wounds are more likely to involve the upper extremities, neck and trunk.

Blunt trauma associated with vascular injuries is caused commonly by high-speed motor vehicle crashes, pedestrians hit by motor vehicles, falls from heights, and crush injuries. Because of the high-energy transfer of force during the accident, blunt trauma victims with vascular injuries usually have other associated injuries to the brain, lung, liver, or pelvis.[11,12] Blunt thoracic vascular injuries are more common in persons with first-rib, scapular, or sternal fractures.[13] Hyperextension of the neck following blunt trauma can lead to carotid and vertebral vascular injuries. Pelvic arterial and venous injuries are associated with severe pelvic fractures. The association of popliteal artery injuries with posterior knee dislocations and supracondylar femur fracture has been well described. The association of brachial artery injuries with mid- and distal humerus fractures is well known, especially in children.[14]

Pathophysiology

Arteries and veins are injured in several ways, each with different clinical consequences (Fig. 29.1). Lacerations and transections are the two most common types of injuries, accounting for 80% to 85% of all injuries. Partial transection leads to greater hemorrhage than complete transection because the vessel cannot develop spasm and contract to reduce blood flow. Pseudoaneurysms, arteriovenous fistulae, and intimal disruption or flaps may result from either blunt or penetrating trauma. The clinical manifestations of these injuries include exsanguination and shock, complete thrombosis and distal ischemia, partial thrombosis and distal embolization, swelling with compression of adjacent structures

TABLE 29.2. Trends in Anatomic Distribution of Vascular Injuries in Military and Urban Warfare.

Site of injury	*World War II (n = 2471)*[137]	*Korean War (n = 304)*[138]	*Vietnam War (n = 1000)*[142]	*Houston (n = 5760)*[9]	*Urban (n = 1526)*[163]
Neck	1%	4%	5%	12%	10%
Trunk	2%	2%	4%	54%	52%
Extremity	97%	94%	91%	34%	38%

Source: Modified from Caps MT. The epidemiology of vascular trauma (table 58.1). In: Rutherford R, ed. Vascular Surgery. New York: Lippincott, Williams & Wilkins, 2001.

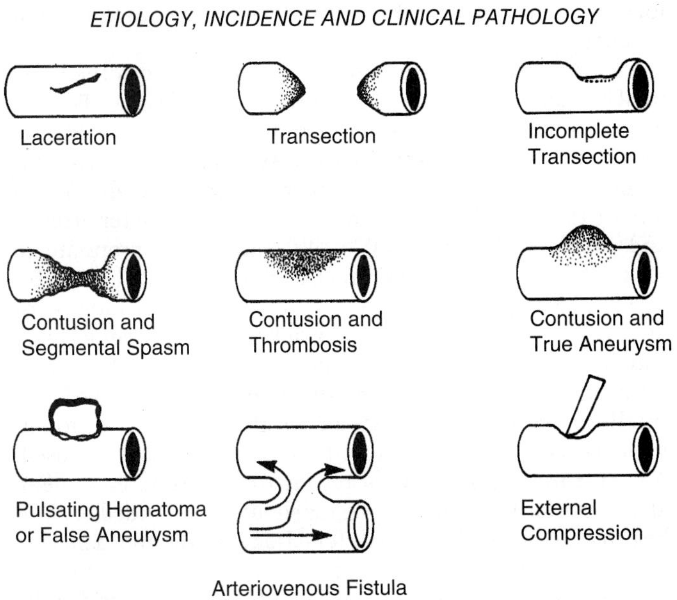

FIGURE 29.1. Common types of arterial injury. (From Rich NM. Vascular trauma. Surg Clin North Am 1973;53:1367–1392, with permission.)

and development of compartment syndrome, or, infrequently, the development of arterial and venous insufficiency.

Pseudoaneurysms develop when the extravasated blood is contained in the surrounding tissue. Pseudoaneurysms usually enlarge over time and produce local symptoms of pain, nerve compression, or thrombosis or embolization. Small pseudoaneurysms (less than 2 cm) usually resolve or improve without treatment.

An arteriovenous fistula results when adjacent lacerations occur to both an artery and a vein. These fistulas usually enlarge over time and cause local edema in the extremity and chronic venous stasis changes. If the arteriovenous fistula becomes larger, congestive heart failure may ensue.

Acute arterial occlusion results in profound ischemia to the involved organ and extremity if collateral circulation is inadequate or absent, or an ipsilateral stroke if the occlusion occurred in a neck vessel. Acutely ischemic extremities manifest the five "P's" of ischemia on physical examination: these signs are pulselessness, pallor, pain, paresthesias (or paralysis), and poikilothermia (Table 29.3). Interruption of arterial flow produces ischemia to the organs and tissues distal to the injury. Nerves are extremely sensitive to ischemia whereas skeletal muscle can tolerate up to 4 to 6 h with no blood flow. However, with restoration of flow a reperfusion injury can occur. This ischemia-reperfusion injury can exacerbate local injury to tissues as well as cause a systemic inflammatory state mediated by reactive oxygen species as well as cytokines, with acute lung injury and acute renal failure.

Prolonged skeletal muscle ischemia without collateral blood flow causes muscle necrosis or rhabdomyolysis with release of potassium and myoglobin into the circulation. Reperfusion exacerbates muscle injury.[15] Myoglobinuria may result. The diagnosis is confirmed with elevated creatinine phosphokinase concentrations, usually greater than 50,000 units/L, and red- or brown-tinged urine without red blood cells present by microscopy. Myoglobin is filtered in the kidney and can precipitate in the tubules, causing acute renal failure. Treatment includes maintaining a high urine output (more than 100 mL/h) and alkalizing the urine (pH $\geq$ 6.0) to prevent precipitation of myoglobin in the tubules.

General Principles

The priorities of managing trauma patients with vascular injuries are to treat life-threatening injuries immediately by maintaining a patent airway, supporting ventilation and oxygenation, restoring circulation, and evaluating neurological function. This systematic approach to the care of the trauma patient is well established and is espoused by the Advanced Trauma Life Support (ATLS) course offered by the American College of Surgeons.[16] The key to the management of all vascular injuries remains a thorough physical examination. Physical findings indicating vascular injury have been categorized into hard signs or soft signs[17] (Table 29.3).

In the past, all patients with injuries in proximity to major vessels were explored to rule out vascular injury. Sirinek et al. reported on their experience with exploration of the neck and extremities based on proximity of a wound.[18] In their series of 390 patients, the incidence of positive explorations was 36% (139 patients). They concluded that routine exploration resulted in an unacceptably high negative exploration rate. Today, the decision regarding further observation, immediate exploration, or additional diagnostic tests is influenced by the history, mechanism of injury, and physical findings. In general, patients who present with any hard signs of a vascular injury do not require preoperative arteriography but rather should be explored immediately. Exceptions to this rule include those patients who are hemodynamically stable, where performance of arteriogram may provide a diagnosis that will lead to improved operative planning (e.g., a more appropriate incision), or where treatment of the injury may be possible by endovascular techniques. Frykberg et al. evaluated 310 patients with 366 penetrating extremity wounds by physical examination.[19] All 21 extremity wounds with hard signs had vascular trauma that required surgical repair, yielding a positive predictive value of 100% for physical examination alone.

TABLE 29.3. Physical Findings Indicating Vascular Injury.

Hard signs	*Soft signs*
Absent distal pulses	Proximity of injury to artery
Active arterial bleeding	History of arterial bleeding at the scene
Expanding or pulsatile hematoma	Diminished distal pulse
Bruit or thrill at injury site	Small nonpulsatile hematoma
Five "P's" of vascular injury Pulselessness Pallor Pain Paresthesia or paralysis Poikilothermia	Questionable neurological deficit Fracture Knee dislocation

Source: Modified from Mattox K. Vascular trauma. In: Haimovici H, ed. Vascular Surgery. Norwalk: Appleton & Lange, 1989.

The optimal way to evaluate a patient with soft signs of a vascular injury continues to evolve and be debated. However, based on studies wherein mandatory surgical exploration or arteriography was performed for patients with soft signs, the incidence of vascular injury was low, yielding positive results from 1% to 25%.[20,21]

Interventional radiologists will continue to play a role in the diagnosis and treatment of vascular injuries in the future. Interventional angiography can be both diagnostic and therapeutic for certain vascular injuries. Angiography remains the preferred procedure for pelvic and retroperitoneal bleeding after pelvic fractures. It also remains helpful in the diagnosis and treatment of injuries to the distal internal carotid artery and vertebral arteries.[22] Interventional radiology can place coils or stents to stop bleeding or treat intimal flaps or dissections causing arterial occlusion or stenosis.[23] Patients who present with a delayed pseudoaneurysm or arteriovenous fistula of a large artery have been treated successfully with stented grafts.

General Principles of Management of Traumatic Vascular Injuries

The general principles of resuscitation should follow the guidelines set forth by the ATLS course, including to secure an airway, control breathing, and control hemorrhage. Patients with penetrating neck trauma may present with airway obstruction or develop it suddenly from increased swelling of soft tissues and hematoma expansion. Patients should be intubated early to prevent airway compromise. Fiberoptic endotracheal intubation by an experienced team member may be required. If fiberoptic and orotracheal attempts are unsuccessful, then emergency cricothyroidotomy may be necessary. A firm compression bandage over the site of injury can temporarily control bleeding. Penetrating wounds should not be probed so as not to dislodge a clot and cause or reinstate bleeding, except for formal local exploration of the abdominal wall to ascertain penetration by stab wounds to the abdomen. The temptation to blindly place clamps into a wound to stop bleeding should be avoided. The operative management of vascular trauma requires proximal and distal control of the bleeding vessel. The patient must be prepared and draped widely to allow rapid exposure of the neck, chest, abdomen, and extremities for resuscitation and control of inflow. A large operative field allows for the ability to perform arteriography for diagnosis and assessment of repair, to harvest autologous vein from an uninjured leg, to perform fasciotomies if needed, and to access directly the distal pulses of an extremity under repair. Ideally, proximal and distal control of the injured vessel is achieved before exposing the injury; this may not be possible with active hemorrhage in an unstable patient. During these times an expedient and direct approach to expose the injury is necessary. A generous incision should be made to expose the vessels. If possible shed blood should be collected and autotransfused back into the patient, although autotransfusion remains controversial for patients with vascular injuries of the abdomen and concomitant gastrointestinal injuries. Vascular clamps or vessel loops are used to obtain control of inflow and outflow to the vascular injury (proximal and distal control). Heparin at 100 units/mL can be injected locally into the proximal and distal vessels before the vascular clamps are applied.

Thrombosis is common of injured vessels; both the proximal and distal vessel should be cleared of clot using a Fogarty embolectomy catheter of appropriate size. Vascular anastomosis should be performed with a synthetic, monofilament suture, usually polypropylene. Suture size is usually 5-0 to 6-0 for the femoral and brachial or similar diameter arteries and smaller, whereas a 3-0 or 4-0 suture is appropriate to repair the aorta, vena cava, and thoracic vessels. The anastomosis is usually performed in a continuous fashion with double-armed suture. The full thickness of the vessel wall should be approximated. The sutures are placed about 1 to 2 mm apart and 1 to 2 mm from the edge of the vessel. For small vessel reconstruction, or in children where growth must be accommodated, interrupted sutures may be used. The best method for arterial reconstruction is an end-to-end anastomosis. The damaged vessel should be debrided back to healthy tissue, including stretched adventitia and damaged intima. The anastomosis must be tension-free, so either an autologous or synthetic conduit may be needed to bridge the gap when performing an end-to-end anastomosis. Lateral arteriorrhaphy or venorrhaphy is appropriate for small punctures or lacerations. Occasionally, a vein patch is required. Lateral arteriorrhaphy will cause iatrogenic stenosis.

Autologous greater saphenous vein from an uninjured extremity is the conduit of choice for extremity trauma and for vessels 6 mm or less in diameter,[24] and is also preferred for patch angioplasty. If autologous vein is not available or unsatisfactory, synthetic conduits made from polyester or polytetrafluroethylene (PTFE) have been used successfully.[25] For larger vessels, these synthetic conduits are the only choice. Feliciano et al. reported on 236 PTFE grafts placed for traumatic vascular injuries to the femoral, brachial, carotid, popliteal, axillary, iliac, or subclavian arteries and mesenteric vessels.[26] Only 7 (3%) grafts became infected, 5 of which had inadequate soft tissue coverage because of the severity of the injuries. For vessels less than 6 mm in diameter, the long-term patency rate of PTFE grafts is less than that reported for vein grafts, but the infection rate is comparable. For vessels with a diameter greater than 6 mm, the long-term patency rates and infection rates of PTFE grafts are acceptable.[27] The use of PTFE grafts is preferable when time is crucial, especially for patients with multiple injuries and shock who require rapid revascularization. The completion arteriogram should include the area of the anastomosis, area of the clamp application, and the distal circulation to identify spasm, narrowing, clot, or additional injury. All vascular repairs need soft tissue coverage to minimize infection, thrombosis, and anastomotic dehiscence. Devitalized tissue in the wound must be debrided before closure. Drains should not be placed near a vascular anastomosis as they may erode into or cause infection of the graft.

Clinical Presentation, Diagnosis, and Management

Cervical Vascular Injuries

Penetrating and blunt injuries to the neck are difficult to assess and manage because of the dense concentration of vital vascular, aerodigestive, and neurological structures. The neck is commonly divided into three zones as described by Monson et al.[28] Zone I extends from the sternal notch to 1 cm above the clavicular head; zone II, from 1 cm above the clavicular head to the angle of the mandible; and zone III, from the angle of the mandible to the base of the skull. Each zone has a corresponding algorithm dictating the management of penetrating trauma; however, an injury to one zone does not preclude a concomitant injury to another zone.

Penetrating Carotid Injury

Most penetrating carotid injuries are caused by stab wounds or low-velocity missiles. Carotid artery injuries occur in 6% of penetrating injuries and account for 22% of all cervical vascular injuries.[29] Common carotid injuries are more common than internal carotid artery injuries. Associated injuries to the esophagus, trachea, or larynx are present in 30% of these patients. Management of penetrating neck trauma depends on two factors: the patient's clinical status and the anatomic zone of injury. Patients who present with obvious signs and symptoms of major vascular or aerodigestive tract injuries should undergo immediate operative exploration and repair. Patients with soft signs should undergo an evaluation to rule out vascular injuries. Three options are currently available to rule out vascular injuries to the neck: surgical exploration, angiography, and observation. Proponents for routine neck exploration suggest that physical examination alone is not reliable and that potentially devastating injuries could be missed.[30] Apffelstaedt and Muller[31] performed a prospective study of mandatory neck explorations in 393 patients with stab wounds and penetration of the platysma. Clinical signs of injury were absent in 30% of patients with positive explorations and in 58% of patients who had negative explorations. Five patients (2.2%) had minor complications after surgery, and the average hospital stay was 1.5 days. The authors concluded that mandatory neck exploration requires no further specialized diagnostic testing and that nontherapeutic operations are safe and do not prolong hospital stay. Some authors advocate observing patients with a normal physical examination. Menawat et al. reported on a retrospective series of patients with penetrating zone II injuries.[32] In their series of 110 patients, 45 underwent angiography and 65 patients were evaluated by physical examination alone. One patient had a small pseudoaneurysm that required surgical repair. Physical examination resulted in a 0.9% missed injury rate, similar to angiography; however, there were three carotid artery intimal defects, three asymptomatic occlusions, and six vertebral artery injuries identified in the patients who received no intervention. Demetriades et al.[33] performed angiography in only 7 of 335 patients with penetrating neck injuries; 269 patients (80%) were selected for nonoperative management, and only 2 of those patients required subsequent operations during the same hospitalization. Some vascular injuries not requiring treatment may not have been identified. Early (16 days) and late (48 days) follow-up on 192 patients showed no complications in the nonoperative group.

Clinical evaluation is highly accurate in determining which patients with zone II penetrating injuries need surgical treatment; nevertheless, there is an appreciable incidence of occult asymptomatic vascular injuries.[34,35] In hemodynamically stable patients with penetrating neck injury, the selective workup of possible injury has gained acceptance as it is safe and cost-effective.[36] Management by observation of occult segmental narrowing, intimal flap, or pseudoaneurysm is safe provided the patients have close follow-up until complete resolution. A small percentage of patients with occult injuries will become symptomatic, even several years later.[37] Alternatively, Kuehne et al.[38] recommended that all stable patients undergo arteriography. Kuehne et al. opined that an occlusion of the internal carotid artery in a neurologically intact patient, anticoagulant therapy should be started if possible. If there is a neurological deficit, if the carotid artery is patent, the injury should be repaired regardless of the neurological status. However, routine use of angiography for all penetrating neck injuries would subject large numbers of patients to an invasive procedure with known complications. Currently, routine angiography is performed for penetrating zone I and zone III injuries and for confirming injuries in zone II detected by duplex ultrasound. Several studies have emphasized the accuracy of duplex sonography in the diagnosis and follow-up of cervical vascular injuries,[39,40] with 100% sensitivity and 85% specificity in one series.[41] The accuracy of a duplex ultrasound evaluation relies heavily on the skill and experience of a trained technologist. If such resources are not available, then angiographic examination is necessary. The role of computed tomography (CT) with contrast in the evaluation of penetrating neck trauma is being determined.[42,43] Inaba et al. showed that CT angiography is a sensitive initial screening examination for 62 patients with penetrating neck trauma.[44] In the future, CT will likely play a dominant role in the workup of penetrating neck trauma. A clinical algorithm for evaluating penetrating neck injuries is presented in Figure 29.2.

Neck Exploration for Penetrating Trauma

Surgical neck exploration for diagnosis and repair of penetrating injuries to the neck is usually started by making an incision along the anterior border of the sternocleidomastoid muscle. The incision can be extended into a median sternotomy for proximal lesions. Exposure for high (distal) internal carotid artery injuries is a major challenge. Anterior subluxation of the mandible may improve exposure. Alternatively, an oromaxillofacial surgeon can perform a vertical mandibular ramus osteotomy to help expose these distal internal carotid arteries.[45] Carotid lesions should be repaired[46,47] unless the artery is completely occluded or possibly if the patient is comatose. Surgical techniques include lateral arteriorraphy, patch graft, or excision with an end-to-end anastomosis or interposition graft repair. If a graft is required, saphenous vein is preferred but prosthetic grafts are acceptable. Isolated external carotid artery injuries may be repaired or ligated, but more complex injuries should be ligated. For internal carotid artery injury, transposition of the external carotid artery is an option. Ligation is recommended only for distal, thrombosed, or nonreconstructable internal carotid artery injuries. Following ligation, anticoagulation therapy is necessary for 3 months to prevent propagation of thrombus.[48,49] In the presence of associated aerodigestive tract injury or repair, the sternocleidomastoid muscle can be transposed between the vascular repair and the aerodigestive repair. This procedure provides protection from salivary enzymes and

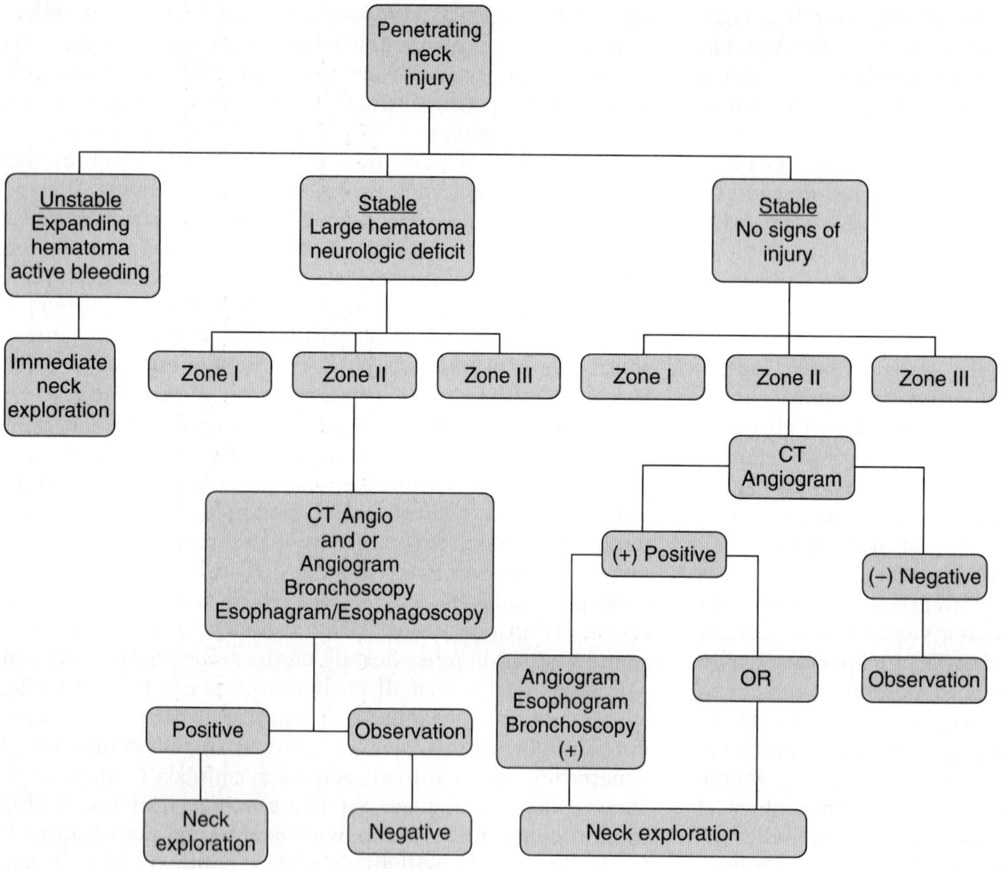

FIGURE 29.2. Algorithm for evaluating penetrating neck injuries.

bacterial contamination, which can lead to anastomotic failure and hemorrhage. Patients who die after carotid revascularization usually die of cerebral edema and transtentorial brain herniation, not of a hemorrhagic infarct.[34,41] Patients who present in coma have a poor prognosis; some have argued that the best chance for improvement in neurological outcome is immediate revascularization.[50]

Blunt Carotid Injury

Blunt carotid injuries are uncommon and differ in their clinical presentation, management, and anticipated outcomes from penetrating injuries. Blunt injury accounts for about 3% to 30% of all carotid injuries.[51] The internal carotid artery is affected more commonly than the common carotid. The most common causes of blunt carotid artery injury are cervical hyperextension/rotation and direct contusion. The incidence of bilaterality is 30%.[52] Blunt carotid artery injury can result in dissection, thrombosis, pseudoaneurysm formation, or transection.[53] Fabian et al. noted an incidence of carotid artery injury of 0.33% after blunt trauma and 0.067% after blunt trauma caused by motor vehicle collision.[54] A high index of suspicion is required to diagnose blunt carotid artery injuries. Most have no immediate neurological sequelae; only about one-third present with a focal neurological deficit. Most injuries are identified after a neurological event. Neurological deficits unexplained by CT of the brain should raise the suspicion of a blunt carotid injury. The gold standard for diagnosing blunt carotid injuries remains cerebral arteriogram. More data are needed with duplex ultrasound, helical CT, and magnetic resonance angiography to validate their efficacy in diagnosing zone III blunt carotid injuries.

Most blunt carotid artery injuries result in intimal disruption with dissection or thrombosis.[55] Treatment of these lesions is systemic anticoagulation with unfractionated heparin, which limits the propagation of thrombus and distal embolization. Outcomes after blunt carotid artery depend on the presence or absence of an initial neurological deficit. Heparin therapy is associated with improved survival,[54] and, if started before the onset of symptoms, heparin therapy can prevent neurological deterioration.[42] Anticoagulation therapy should continue with warfarin for 3 months.[56] Endovascular stent therapy is being used successfully for blunt carotid injury, especially for patients who cannot be anticoagulated, but the precise indications and outcomes of this technology are still evolving.[57,58] With conservative treatment most lesions heal in 3 months. It is important that these patients have follow-up to document healing. Pseudoaneurysms may occur in up to 30% of patients treated with anticoagulation and can be managed with endovascular techniques.

Vertebral Artery Injuries

Trauma to the vertebral artery is relatively rare when compared to other structures in the neck, but the frequency of injury is increasing with the advent of routine angiography in the workup of neck injuries as well as the more common use of helical CT angiography. The overall incidence of vertebral artery injuries in neck injuries is 1.2% or 10% of all major vascular injuries of the neck.[29] The vertebral artery is divided into four segments. The first segment includes the origin from the subclavian artery to the sixth cervical foramen. On the left side, the thoracic duct crosses over the vertebral artery anteriorly. The second segment ascends vertically through the cervical foramina and is encased in a dense network of veins and sympathetic nerve fibers. The third segment begins as the artery exits the foramen of the atlas and ends as it passes under the atlanto-occipital membrane. The fourth segment is within the dura mater, ending as both vertebral arteries culminate in the basilar artery. This anatomy allows proximal ligation of the artery without devastating neurological complications.

The clinical presentation after vertebral artery injury depends on the presence of other associated injuries. A high index of suspicion should prompt cerebral angiography for patients who present with severe oral or maxillofacial trauma, basilar skull fractures, or cervical spine injury. Cerebral angiogram is the only reliable method to evaluate for vertebral artery injuries, as color flow Doppler ultrasonography does not evaluate segments 2–4 well. Most patients with vertebral artery lesions such as active bleeding, false aneurysms, or arteriovenous fistula should be treated with proximal and distal embolization. About 10% to 15% of patients with vertebral artery injury present with shock and will need emergent operative control of the bleeding.[59]

Exposure of the vertebral artery is a technical challenge. The standard incision is made along the anterior border of the sternocleidomastoid muscle. After retracting the carotid sheath laterally, the prevertebral space is exposed and the longus coli muscle is retracted medially off the bone. Then the anterior rim of the vertebral foramen costotransverse bar is removed with a bone rongeur to expose the vertebral artery and ligate it.[60] Given the difficulty of the operative approach, most lesions of the vertebral artery should be managed nonoperatively by angiographic embolization. Surgical ligation should be reserved for patients with severe active bleeding or when embolization fails.

Venous Injuries

Jugular venous injuries are caused most commonly by penetrating neck trauma. Most such injuries are unrecognized because low venous pressure allows tamponade before major hemorrhage or a large hematoma develops. Internal jugular venous injuries should be repaired, if possible, especially if bilateral, when at least one should be repaired either by lateral venorrhaphy, patch venoplasty, resection with end-to-end anastomosis, or resection with graft reconstruction to prevent severe cerebral or cervicofacial edema. Thrombosis is a risk after any major venous repair. External jugular veins may be ligated without consequence.[61] Air embolism is a major complication after a venous injury that can be prevented if the patient is placed in the Trendelenburg position when an internal jugular venous injury is discovered at the time of neck exploration.

Thoracic Vascular Trauma

Injuries to the thoracic great vessels occur after both penetrating and blunt trauma. Because of the usually complex surgical exposure of these vessels, a detailed anatomic understanding of this area is crucial. Vessels at risk in this area include the aortic arch, innominate artery, subclavian arteries, proximal carotid arteries, superior vena cava, innominate vein, and azygos vein. Uncontrolled hemorrhage, air embolism, and associated injuries can cause death.

Subclavian and Axillary Artery Injuries

Injuries to the subclavian and axillary arteries are uncommon, and most trauma surgeons have limited experience with them. Most subclavian and axillary artery injuries are caused by penetrating trauma. About 3% of all penetrating neck and chest injuries are associated with these vascular injuries.[62] Blunt trauma to these vessels is rare. Richardson et al. reported three subclavian artery injuries (5.5%) in 55 patients with first-rib fractures after blunt trauma.[63] Subclavian artery injuries are commonly associated with venous and brachial plexus injuries; subclavian or axillary vascular injuries are associated with high mortality, and many afflicted patients die before reaching the hospital. In a study of 228 patients by Demetriades et al.,[60] 61% (139/228) of the patients were dead before arrival at a medical facility. The operative mortality was 15.5%. The overall mortality of this study was as high for subclavian venous injuries as arterial injuries (21% vs. 18%).

All patients who present with periclavicular trauma should be evaluated for vascular trauma. Severe bleeding, unexplained shock or anemia, large expanding or pulsatile hematomas, and absent or diminished peripheral pulses remain hard diagnostic signs for vascular injury. Suspicious (soft) signs of vascular trauma include proximity of entrance wounds to vessels, continuous oozing from the wound, mild transient hypotension or anemia, or a nonexpanding hematoma. A distal pulse does not exclude a proximal arterial injury because of collateral blood flow around the injury; Cox et al. reported a radial pulse deficit in only 12 of 56 (21%) subclavian artery injuries.[64]

All patients presenting with severe hypotension or a threatened limb should undergo emergency surgery. Specific investigations in stable patients for suspected subclavian or axillary artery injury should start after a complete physical examination. A plain X-ray of the chest or neck may show hematoma, missile fragments, associated fractures, or hemothorax. The ankle-brachial index (ABI; the ratio of the systolic blood pressure at the two sites) should be obtained in all patients with suspected subclavian or axillary artery injury. An ABI less than 0.9 is usually diagnostic for an arterial injury; for upper extremity evaluation, the brachial blood pressure is divided by that of the ankle, but an injury that does not disrupt blood flow could be present with a normal ABI.[65] Helical CT scan with intravenous contrast is replacing the arteriogram in the initial workup of patients with proximity injuries to vessels in the chest and shoulder area. The main objectives are to identify the missile tract and associated injuries. If the projectile path is close to the artery but no injury is identified by CT, an arteriogram should be performed. Helical CT may identify the vascular injury and avoid the need for angiography. However, angiography can be both diagnostic and therapeutic. False aneurysm, arteriovenous fistula, arterial stenosis, and active bleeding from a main artery or tributary can be managed angiographically.[66]

Patients who present in extremis should have vascular access placed on the opposite side (e.g., left vs. right), and also

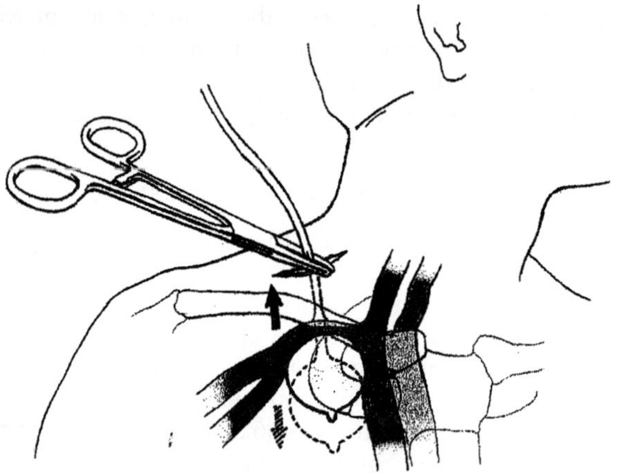

FIGURE 29.3. Balloon tamponade of subclavian vascular bleeding. A Foley catheter is inserted in the supraclavicular wound and is advanced as far as it can go. The balloon is inflated and firm traction is applied to the catheter. The balloon compresses the subclavian vessels against the clavicle and first rib. If persistent external bleeding occurs, a second catheter is inserted and the balloon is inflated inside the wound tract, superficial to the first balloon. (Modified with permission from Demetriades D. Penetrating injuries to the thoracic great vessels. J Cardiac Surg 1997;12:173–180.)

the side of the diaphragm (e.g., above vs. below) opposite the injury. Ipsilateral fluid administration may cause loss of fluid through a major venous injury. An emergent thoracotomy should be done on the side of the injury with the incision extended to the opposite side if necessary. External bleeding can be controlled by applying direct pressure or applying the balloon tamponade technique (Fig. 29.3).[67] A standard clavicular incision for mid- and distal subclavian and proximal axillary vessels starts at the sternoclavicular junction, extends over the medial half of the clavicle and then curves downward toward the deltopectoral groove. The medial half of the clavicle is removed, or the sternoclavicular joint is dislocated and the clavicle is retracted up and laterally (Fig. 29.4). Injuries of the right proximal subclavian artery, proximal left carotid artery, and innominate artery all require a median sternotomy for proper exposure with or without a standard clavicular incision. A proximal left subclavian artery injury requires a median sternotomy with a left clavicular extension or creation of a "trap door" incision, which includes the addition of an anterior, left thoracotomy (see Figure 29.4). However, the trap door incision is not preferred because of intraoperative chest wall bleeding, substantial postoperative pain, and postoperative pulmonary complications. For distal axillary artery injuries, the incision should start below the middle of the clavicle and extend into the deltopectoral groove. Repair of the injured artery should be done in all cases. In critical (unstable) patients, temporary shunting with a definitive repair at a later time may prevent ligation of the subclavian and axillary artery, which causes ischemia of the upper limb in a substantial proportion of patients. Definitive repair can be with debridement and suture, resection with end-to-end anastomosis, or resection with an interposition graft. The choice of autologous vein or prosthetic graft is a matter of personal preference, availability of a suitable vein, and the overall condition of the patient. A completion angiogram is

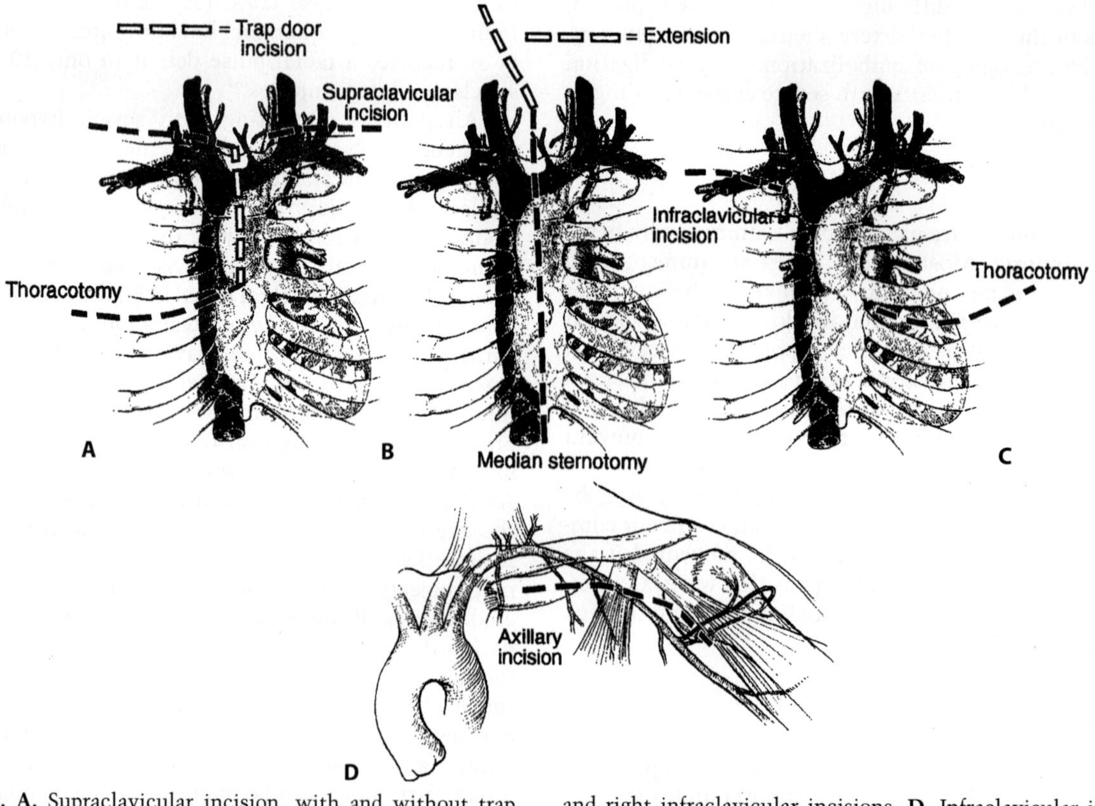

FIGURE 29.4. A. Supraclavicular incision, with and without trap door incision. B. Median sternotomy with extension to the neck for exposure of more distal lesions. C. Left posterolateral thoracotomy and right infraclavicular incisions. D. Infraclavicular incision with extension to the deltopectoral groove and division of the pectoralis minor muscle.

performed, especially if the anastomosis is suboptimal or a pulse deficit remains. Repair of associated venous injuries should be done only if a simple suture repair of the vein can be performed without stenosis; otherwise, ligation of the axillary/subclavian vein is well tolerated, and arm swelling usually resolves over time. Brachial plexus injuries should be repaired at the first operation if the patient remains stable, but if not possible, the branches of the plexus should be tagged for later identification and repair. Thoracic duct injury should be sought when there is an injury near the junction of the left jugular and left subclavian vein, and the duct ligated if found. Fibrin glue can be applied topically after thoracic duct ligation to prevent a lymphocutaneous fistula.

Intrathoracic Vascular Injuries

Injuries to the intrathoracic aorta and great vessels have the highest mortality of all arterial wounds because of exsanguination.[68] Penetrating external and iatrogenic trauma causes more than 90% of all thoracic great vessel injuries.[69] These injuries are challenging due to the difficulty in establishing the diagnosis and the need for wide surgical exposure to control bleeding. Combined arterial and venous injuries are common with penetrating injuries to the upper chest. Venous injuries to the mediastinum are more lethal than isolated arterial injuries because of bleeding and the risk of air embolism. Thirty percent of patients with thoracic vascular trauma present initially with no clinical signs of vascular injury.[70] Diminutive wounds to the upper chest may be associated with serious vascular injuries to the aortic arch and great vessels.

Unstable patients should proceed quickly to the operating room. An urgent left anterior thoracotomy should be done with the incision extended across the sternum to provide immediate exposure of most vessels. Some surgeons prefer a median sternotomy for these injuries with cervical extension. Stable patients should undergo a helical CT scan after a plain chest X-ray and physical examination have been performed. Several findings on chest X-ray are associated with blunt injuries to the intrathoracic great vessels of the thoracic cavity (Table 29.4). The most reliable of these signs for blunt aortic injury is loss of the aortic knob contour.[71] The use of transesophageal echocardiography (TEE) in the evaluation of patients with suspected blunt aortic injury has a sensitivity of 87.5% and a specificity of 92%.[72] The limited accuracy of TEE has limited its use as a screening tool for blunt aortic trauma. Helical CT scan of the chest has become the primary screening test for blunt aortic injury.[73,74] An arteriogram after a positive CT scan preceding repair of the aortic injury may be helpful but is not always necessary. If the CT scan is negative and suspicion for vascular injury is low, no further studies need be done. Arteriography is commonly necessary to identify the injury and plan an appropriate incision. The aortic arch, pulmonary vessels, proximal carotids, arteries, proximal right subclavian artery, and major thoracic veins are best approached through a median sternotomy. The descending aorta and proximal left subclavian artery are best approached through a left posterolateral or left anterolateral thoracotomy. Occasionally, endovascular techniques for management of vascular injuries can be used to avoid major surgery.[75]

Blunt injury to the great vessels may involve not only the aorta but also the innominate artery, pulmonary veins, or vena cava. About 8000 blunt aortic injuries occur per year in the United States.[76] Blunt aortic injuries occur most commonly to the proximal descending thoracic aorta (54%–64%), just below the ligametum arteriosum; other sites include the ascending aorta (10%–14%), mid- or distal descending thoracic aorta (12%), or at multiple sites along the thoracic aorta (13%–18%).[77,78] The second most commonly injured artery by blunt trauma is the innominate artery. Prehospital mortality is 85% for patients who sustain blunt injury to the proximal descending aorta.[79] Of those who reach the trauma center, 30% die within 6h, 40% within 24h, and 72% within the first week. Mortality is greater than 90% among patients who receive no treatment.[80]

Blunt aortic injuries are caused by vehicular deceleration, falls from heights, crush injuries, auto–pedestrian accidents, blast injuries, and equestrian accidents.[81] Although head-on collisions are considered the typical mechanism of injury, up to 50% of blunt aortic tears are from motor vehicle crashes with side impact.[82]

Once the diagnosis is suspected or made of a blunt aortic injury (using the same algorithmic approach described for penetrating aortic injury), pharmacological reduction of the patient's blood pressure and contractility (dP/dT) with beta-blockers and sometimes vasodilators should begin and continue until definitive repair is performed or follow-up studies document complete healing of the arterial defect.[83,84] A reasonable goal is to maintain a heart rate of 60 beats/min and a systolic blood pressure of 100 to 110mmHg. Labetalol given by continuous infusion may achieve these goals with a single agent. Alternatively, a beta-blocker (e.g., esmolol, metoprolol, or propranolol) may be combined with a vasodilator (e.g., nicardipine or nitroprusside).

Patients who have no contraindications to repair should proceed to surgery immediately. Patients with a stable thoracic aortic hematoma and concomitant, head, thoracic, abdominal, or pelvic injuries who remain stable but who would not tolerate a thoracotomy, with or without cardiopulmonary bypass, should have their aortic surgery delayed. Another appropriate reason to delay aortic reconstruction for a few hours for the stable patient is to assemble the most experienced surgical team, which may or may not be intact during off-hours. These patients should be treated medically to decrease their pulse pressure and blood pressure.[85] Patients with stable thoracic hematomas but who are unstable from abdominal or pelvic bleeding should undergo emergency laparotomy, with or without external pelvic fixation, and then a pelvic arteriogram for embolization of persistent sites of bleeding. Repair of the descending thoracic aorta is by posterolateral thoracotomy through the fourth intercostal space.

TABLE 29.4. Findings on Chest X-Ray Associated with Blunt Aortic Injury.

Presence of widened mediastinum (>8cm at the aortic knob in adults)
Deviation of the trachea, nasogastric tube, or endotracheal tube to the right
Presence of an apical cap of pleural fluid
Depression of the left mainstem bronchus >140° from trachea
Obliteration of aortic knob contour
"Funny"-looking mediastinum

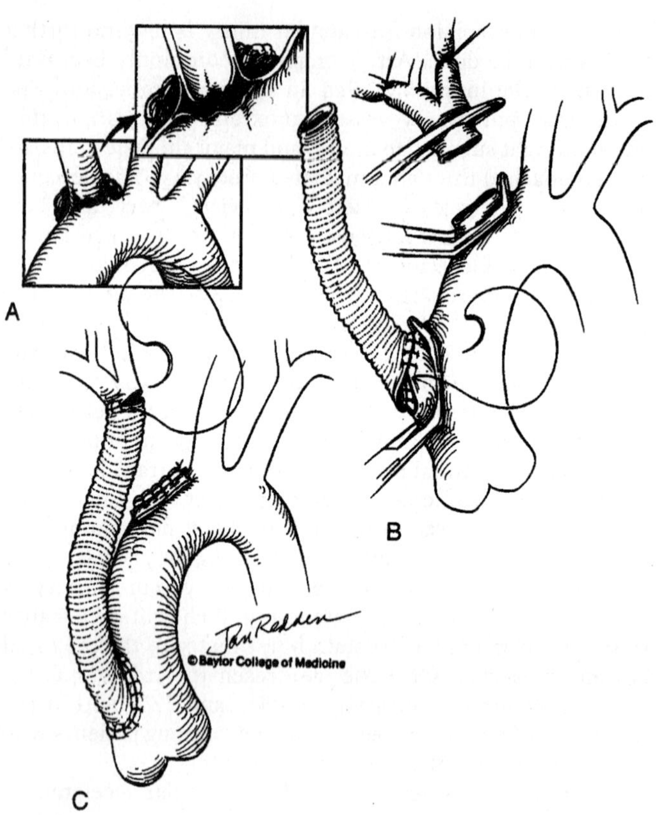

FIGURE 29.5. Bypass exclusion principle for management for innominate artery injuries. The chest is opened by way of a median sternotomy. **A.** A 10-mm Dacron graft is sewn end to side to the aorta with a partial occluding clamp avoiding the hematoma. **B.** The innominate artery is isolated just proximal to its bifurcation, divided, and sewn end to end to the graft without heparin, shunts, or cardiopulmonary bypass. **C.** After restoration of flow, the aortic arch is controlled with a large partial occluding clamp and oversewn. (Courtesy of Baylor College of Medicine, with permission.)

The injury is usually located on the descending aorta just below the origin of the left subclavian artery at the ligamentum arteriosum. The current standard technique of repair involves vascular clamping and direct reconstruction with an interposition graft, whether by the "clamp and sew" technique, use of a temporary shunt, or pump-assisted left heart bypass, which may be either by traditional pump bypass (heparin) or the use of a centrifugal pump (no heparin).[86] Anatomy, the risk of heparin administration, and the experience of the surgeon all affect the choice of technique. Operative mortality after repair ranges from 5% to 25% but mortality is related to associated injuries.[87] The most feared complication after repair of the descending aorta is paraplegia caused by decreased blood flow while the aorta is clamped. In a multicenter trial reported by Fabian et al.,[88] the clamp and sew technique without bypass and cross-clamp time greater than 30 min were associated with higher rates of paraplegia. In more recent series,[89–91] each author has reported low or no postoperative paraplegia after each of these three techniques, but no prospective, randomized trial has identified the superiority of any single method of repair.

Blunt injuries to the innominate artery are approached through a median sternotomy and commonly involve the proximal innominate/aortic arch. These injuries commonly require repair by the bypass exclusion technique[92] (Fig. 29.5).

Internal mammary artery injuries can occur with penetrating trauma but are commonly injured iatrogenically during anterior lateral thoracotomy and with extension of this incision to the right chest. Both the artery and vein must be ligated. Intercostal arteries may be injured from either blunt or penetrating trauma. Precise ligation of these injured vessels may be difficult and only is achieved with circumferential ligatures around the rib on either side of the intercostal vessel injury. Some patients have had intercostal hemorrhage controlled by embolization.

Venous injuries are commonly associated with penetrating arterial injuries. Lateral venorrhaphy should be done if possible. Ligation of the subclavian vein is acceptable and usually well tolerated. Injury to the azygos vein is best managed by suture ligation.

Abdominal Vascular Trauma

Abdominal vascular injuries are among the most lethal and challenging injuries sustained by trauma patients. Abdominal vascular injury may occur to any vessel located in the midline retroperitoneum (zone I), upper lateral retroperitoneum (zone II), pelvic retroperitoneum (zone III), and portal hepatic area (Fig. 29.6; Table 29.5). Asensio et al.[93] reported 302 abdominal vascular injuries accrued over a 6-year period. The incidence of abdominal vascular injuries after stab wounds was 10%, whereas the incidence was 20% to 25% after gunshot wounds (GSW).[94] The incidence of abdominal vascular injury

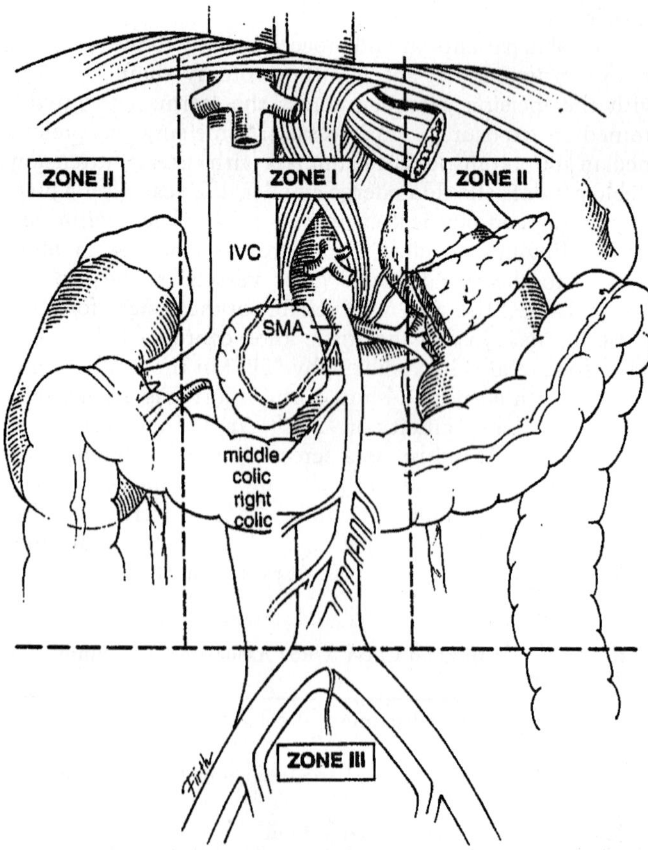

FIGURE 29.6. Zones of the retroperitoneum. *SMA*, superior mesenteric artery; *IVC*, inferior vena cava. (From Asensio J, Demetriades D, eds. Atlas and Textbook of Techniques in Complex Trauma Surgery. Philadelphia: Saunders, 2000.)

TABLE 29.5. Zones of Retroperitoneum.

Zone I: Midline Retroperitoneum
Supramesocolic area:
Suprarenal aorta
Celiac axis
Proximal superior mesenteric artery
Proximal renal artery
Superior mesenteric vein
Inframesocolic area:
Infrarenal aorta
Infrahepatic inferior vena cava
Zone II: Upper lateral retroperitoneum (right and left)
Renal arteries
Renal veins
Zone III: Pelvic retroperitoneum
Iliac arteries
Iliac veins
Portal-retrohepatic area
Portal vein
Hepatic artery
Retrohepatic vena cava

after blunt injury is 5% to 10%.[95] Penetrating injuries account for 90% to 95% of abdominal vascular injuries. Abdominal blood vessels are rarely injured in isolation, with two to four concomitant intraabdominal injuries being typical.[96] Blunt abdominal vascular injuries are caused by either deceleration or direct blows; either mechanism may lead to avulsuion with free bleeding, false aneurysm formation, or intimal flaps with thrombosis.[97] Penetrating trauma can cause abdominal vascular injury by several mechanisms, including blast effect with intimal flap and secondary thrombosis, lateral wall defects with free bleeding or pulsatile hematomas (early false aneurysms), or complete transection with free bleeding or thrombosis.[98] Any penetrating injury occurring between the nipples and the groin poses a risk for abdominal vascular injury. Regardless of mechanism, the clinical presentation of patients with abdominal vascular injuries depends on whether free intraperitoneal hemorrhage or contained retroperitoneal hematoma has developed. Patients presenting in shock should undergo an emergency laparotomy. It may be necessary, for a patient in extremis, to perform an emergency department thoracotomy and aortic cross-clamping or internal cardiac massage before laparotomy; however, the survival rate is a dismal 5% or less.[99] Prompt attention to the airway, venous access, and early aggressive volume replacement with cystalloids and blood are required for successful resuscitation. These patients suffer from shock, tissue hypoperfusion, and massive blood loss, and from generalized edema and reperfusion injury if resuscitation and repair are successful. Gross intestinal contamination by enteric contents from intestinal injuries contribute to the high morbidity and mortality. Patients with blunt injury who present with hypotension but who respond to fluid, and those who remain stable, can proceed with the usual workup for abdominal trauma. Patients with transient hypotension, who have a positive surgeon-performed ultrasound (focused assessment by sonography for trauma [FAST]) examination should go to the operating room promptly, whereas those same patients with a negative FAST examination should go for an abdominal/pelvic CT with contrast to rule out active retroperitoneal or pelvic bleeding.

Abdominal injuries should be explored through a midline incision extending from the xyphoid to the pubis. Immediate control of life-threatening hemorrhage is essential, whether by direct compression of the abdominal aorta at the diaphragm or by aortic crossclamp. Control of intestinal injury is of secondary importance. The abdominal cavity is then explored fully. The surgeon needs to classify the hemorrhage or hematomas by anatomic zones (see Fig. 29.6). Zone I (the midline) extends from the aortic hiatus to the sacral promontory and is divided into supramesocolic and inframesocolic zones. Zone II extends on either side from the renal hila to the pericolic gutters. Zone III begins at the sacral promontory and encompasses the pelvis.[100] Each zone requires complex techniques for exposure. The supramesocolic area of zone I is approached by a left-sided medial viscera rotation that rotates the left colon, spleen, body and tail of the pancreas, and stomach medially to expose the aorta at the aortic hiatus, celiac artery, superior mesenteric artery (SMA), and left renal vascular pedicle. Aortic exposure in the inframesocolic area of zone I is obtained by elevating the transverse colon and mesentery cephalad, eviscerating the small bowel to the right, and incising the peritoneum at the ligament of Treitz down along the left side of the aorta. The inferior vena cava (IVC) in this zone is exposed by performing a right-sided medial viscera rotation, sweeping the right colon, duodenum, and head of the pancreas to the left. Zone II on the right is exposed by mobilizing the right colon and hepatic flexure, performing a Kocher maneuver to expose the IVC infrarenally, and continuing the dissection superiorly until the right renal vein is encountered anterior and inferior to the right renal artery. Exposure of zone II on the left is by exposure of the infrarenal aorta (see above) and continuing the dissection cephalad along the aorta until the left renal vein crosses over the aorta. The left renal artery is also found inferior and superior to the left renal artery. Exposure of zone III vessels is obtained by displacing the right and left colons cephalad, isolating each ureter as it crosses over the common iliac artery, and then dissecting the iliac vessels caudad. Regardless of location, all identified injuries should be graded according to the American Association for the Surgery of Trauma–Organ Injury Scale (AAST-OIS) for vascular injuries[101] (Table 29.6).

Injuries to Zone I: Midline Supramesocolic Area

Injury to the suprarenal aorta should be repaired by primary aortorrhaphy when feasible. When primary repair results in narrowing, or if a large portion of the aortic wall is missing, repair may require the use of a synthetic vascular conduit after debridement of the injured portion.[102] Many of these patients have gastrointestinal injuries as well. Repairs of these intestinal injuries should not be done simultaneously with the aortic repair. The perforated bowel should be packed away and the area irrigated copiously; afterward, the surgical team should change gloves. Repair of the aorta proceeds with sewing the aortic graft in place with 3-0 or 4-0 polypropylene suture. The retroperitoneum is then closed in a watertight fashion with an absorbable suture. The intestinal injuries are then addressed definitively if the operation is not in damage control mode. Historically, survival rates of patients with injuries to the suprarenal aorta have been 8% to 35%.[97,98] Injuries to the celiac axis should be ligated. These vessels are difficult to expose and repair because of the dense neural and lymphatic plexuses surrounding these vessels. The common hepatic artery can be ligated proximal to the gastroduodenal

TABLE 29.6. American Association for the Surgery of Trauma-Organ Injury Scale for Abdominal Vascular Injury (AAST-OIS).

Grade I:	No named superior mesenteric artery or vein No named branches of inferior mesenteric artery or vein Phrenic artery/vein Lumbar artery/vein Gonadal artery/vein Ovarian artery/vein Other no named small arterial or venous structures requiring ligation
Grade II:	Right, left, or common hepatic artery Splenic artery/vein Right and left gastric artery/vein Gastroduodenal artery Inferior mesenteric artery, trunk or inferior mesenteric vein, trunk Primary named branches of the mesenteric artery (ileocolic artery) or mesenteric vein Other named abdominal vessels requiring ligation/repair
Grade III:	Superior mesenteric vein, trunk Renal artery/vein Iliac artery/vein Hypogastric artery/vein Vena cava, infrarenal
Grade IV:	Superior mesenteric artery, trunk Celiac axis proper Vena cava, suprarenal and infrahepatic Aorta, infrarenal
Grade V:	Portal vein Extraparenchymal hepatic vein Vena cava, retrohepatic or suprahepatic Aorta, suprarenal and subdiaphragmatic

This classification system is applicable for extraparenchymal vascular injuries. If the vessel injury is within 2 cm of the organ parenchyma, refer to specific organ injury scale. Increase one grade for multiple grade III or IV injuries involving >50% vessel circumference. Downgrade one grade if <25% laceration for grades IV or V.

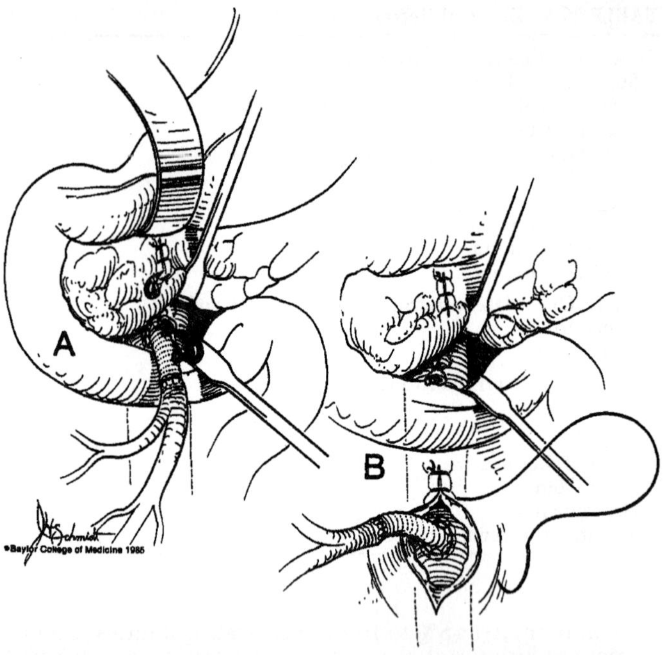

FIGURE 29.7. It may be dangerous to place the proximal suture line of a graft in Fullen zone I or II of the superior mesenteric artery near an associated pancreatic injury (**A**). The proximal suture line should be on the lower aorta (**B**), away from the upper abdominal injuries, and covered with retroperitoneal tissue. (Courtesy of Baylor College of Medicine, 1985, with permission.)

artery without sequelae because collateral flow will perfuse the liver. Necrosis to the gallbladder usually follows ligation of the celiac axis; cholecystectomy is indicated. The SMA may be injured anywhere along its course. Fullen et al.[103] described an anatomic classification of injuries to the SMA (Table 29.7). Management of SMA injuries in Fullen zones I and II should be by primary repair when possible, but these injuries may also be repaired with autogenous or prosthetic grafts, usually from the infrarenal aorta[103] (Fig. 29.7). Injuries in zone I may require division of the pancreas at the neck to repair the injury. Temporary shunting to allow time for damage control before definitive repair of the SMA has also been described.[104] Overall survival was 58% in 116 patients with SMA injuries but was substantially less if an interposition graft was necessary.[105] Injuries to the more distal SMA (zones III and IV) should also be repaired, because ligation may lead to segmental bowel ischemia.[106] The superior mesenteric vein (SMV) lies to the right of the SMA and may also be injured. For injuries to the SMV at the portal vein confluence, division of the pancreas may also be necessary. Ideally, the SMV should be repaired, but it may be ligated if necessary. Survival in 27 patients treated with SMV ligation was 81%.[107] The mean survival rate of patients who sustain an injury to the SMV is 58.3%.[108]

Injuries to Zone I: Midline Inframesocolic Area

Injuries to the infrahepatic suprearenal and infrarenal IVC are repaired by primary venorraphy. If both anterior and posterior injuries are found (through-and-through) the anterior wound can be extended to permit repair of the posterior injury from within the vein, followed by anterior venorrhaphy. If necessary, the infrarenal IVC may be ligated, but a large fluid requirement and a need for bilateral four-compartment infrarenal fasciotomies must be anticipated. The infrahepatic suprarenal IVC should be reconstructed because, if ligated, renal insufficiency will develop with resultant high mortal-

TABLE 29.7. Fullen's Anatomic Classification of Superior Mesenteric Artery (SMA) Injury by Zone.

Zone	*Segment of SMA*	*Ischemic category*	*Bowel segments affected*
I	Trunk proximal to first major collateral	Maximal	Jejunum, ileum, right colon branch (inferior pancreaticoduodenal)
II	Trunk between inferior pancreaticoduodenal and middle colic arteries	Moderate	Major segment, small bowel, or right colon
III	Trunk distal to middle colic artery	Minimal	Minor segment or segments, small bowel, or right colon
IV	Segmental branches; jejunal, ileal, or colic	None	No ischemic bowel

ity. Innovative procedures to reconstruct the IVC have included the use of paneled saphenous vein or interposition grafts of polyester or PTFE.[109] Another useful technique for controlling hemorrhage from the IVC in all locations is Foley balloon catheter tamponade.[110] Porter et al. documented a short-term patency rate of 86% (24/28) for lateral venorrhaphy of the IVC.[111] Survival of infrarenal IVC injuries is 76.1%.[112]

Blunt or penetrating injuries to the infrarenal aorta may be repaired by primary repair with sutures, patch aortoplasty, or performance of an end-to-end anastomosis by woven polyester or PTFE interposition graft. It may be necessary to place omentum over the graft repair to prevent infection and to prevent the development of aortoenteric fistula. The survival rate of an infrarenal aortic injury is 34%.[113] Injuries to the inferior mesenteric artery can be repaired if possible; otherwise, ligation is well tolerated secondary to good collateral blood flow.

Injuries in Zone II: Upper Lateral Retroperitoneum

If an expanding hematoma or active hemorrhage is present in the lateral perirenal area, injury to the renal artery, renal vein, or the kidney itself should be suspected. Blunt trauma injuries are usually identified by CT scan. All patients found to have a perirenal hematoma or pulsatile mass in zone II at the time of exploration for a penetrating abdominal wound should have the hematoma explored. Gonzalez et al. reported that gaining control of the renal vessels at the hilum before opening the hematoma had no effect on rate of nephrectomy, transfusion requirement, or blood loss.[114] Renovascular injuries are difficult to expose and manage because these vessels are relatively inaccessible deep in the retroperitoneum. Injuries to the renal artery may be repaired primarily or grafted with an autologous or prosthetic graft. Small injuries to the renal vein may be repaired by lateral venorrhaphy. If the right renal vein requires ligation, a right nephrectomy should be performed. The left renal vein may be ligated without nephrectomy if the gonadal and adrenal veins remain intact. Penetrating injuries to renal hilar vessels usually lead to nephrectomy because of the other multiple intraabdominal injuries these patients often sustain. Before a nephrectomy, normal function of the contralateral kidney should be confirmed intraoperatively by excretory urography, if stability allows. On occasion, if the patient has only one kidney, a renal vascular injury can be managed by autotransplantation of the injured kidney into the pelvis.[115] The survival rate of patients who have renal artery injuries is 65%, and that from renal vein injuries is 60%.[116]

Blunt injuries to the renal arteries are usually intimal tears that lead to thrombosis. A CT scan of the abdomen with intravenous contrast usually shows abnormal flow to the affected kidney with no parenchymal enhancement or excretion, but the outer edge of the kidney may light up, leading to the pathognomonic cortical rim sign. The time interval from the accident until revascularization of the affected kidney (warm ischemia time) is the most crucial factor in saving the affected kidney.[117] Controversy exists about the exact length of warm ischemia time that is tolerated by the kidney, but revascularization of the kidney should be performed as quickly as possible, with the best results for renal salvage within 6h.[118] If there is kidney function, and a zone II hematoma from blunt trauma is neither expanding nor pulsatile, the hematoma should not be entered.

Injuries to Zone III: Pelvic Retroperitoneum

A hematoma or hemorrhage in the pelvic retroperitoneum may be from an injured iliac artery, iliac vein, or both. The prevention of death from exsanguination is the greatest problem in the management of patients with iliac vascular injuries. Large pelvic hematomas after blunt trauma to the pelvis are often caused by bleeding from iliac vessels in association with a major (often unstable) pelvic fracture.[119] Nonexpanding pelvic hematomas after blunt trauma can be left alone. CT may show a blush from a small bleeding vessel in the pelvis that can be treated by embolization in the interventional radiology suite. Pelvic hematomas from penetrating injuries must be explored. Proximal control of the iliac arteries should be obtained at the aortic bifurcation. Distal control of the external iliac artery is obtained proximal to the inguinal ligament. The internal iliac artery is controlled by pulling up on the common iliac and external iliac arteries.

Injuries to the common and external iliac arteries should be repaired. Ligation of these vessels leads to ischemia of the lower extremity. Options for repair include lateral arteriorrhaphy, end-to-end anastomosis, or insertion of a saphenous vein or PTFE bypass graft.[120] For patients in extremis, damage control principles should be followed by placement of a temporary intraluminal shunt. In contrast, the internal iliac artery can be ligated without sequela. Late postoperative complications such as pseudoaneurysms and suture line dehiscence caused by infection have been described after repair of the common and external iliac arteries, especially if the repair was conducted in the presence of enteric or fecal contamination. If contamination precludes repair, ligation of the artery and closure of the abdomen followed by a femorofemoral crossover graft can be performed.[121]

Injuries to the iliac veins are repaired primarily if possible. Exposure of the right common iliac vein may be difficult and may require the division of the right common iliac artery to expose the vein.[122] Exposure of the internal iliac vein may require ipsilateral transection and ligation of the internal iliac artery.[123] Lateral venorraphy of injured iliac veins is optimal. In desperate conditions, ligation of an iliac vein may be lifesaving and well tolerated so long as the ipsilateral lower extremity is elevated and watched for the development of compartment syndrome. If the vein is narrowed after repair, postoperative anticoagulation should be considered to prevent thromboembolism. In a series by Burch et al., the in-hospital mortality was 28% for iliac vessel injuries.[124]

Injuries of the Porta Hepatis

Injuries in the region of the portal triad in the right upper quadrant may involve the portal vein, hepatic artery or common bile duct. To obtain initial control of bleeding in this area, a Pringle maneuver is performed with a noncrushing vascular clamp or an umbilical tape placed around the proximal hepatoduodenal ligament. Before placing any sutures to repair the hepatic artery or portal vein, the structures must be identified precisely because of the proximity of the common bile duct. Injuries to the common hepatic artery, particularly if proximal to the gastroduodenal artery, are usually treated by ligation, which is well tolerated because of extensive collateral flow.[125,126] Ligation of the right proper hepatic artery requires a cholecystectomy. Injuries to the hepatic artery are rare, and mortality from these injuries is usually dependent on the number and magnitude of associated injuries.

Injuries to the portal vein are difficult to expose given its dorsal location relative to the bile duct and hepatic artery. After performing an extensive Kocher maneuver, mobilization of the common bile duct to the left usually allows for visualization of a suprapancreatic portal vein injury. As with SMA and SMV injuries, it may be necessary to divide the pancreas at its neck to expose the injured proximal portal vein. The preferred technique of portal venorraphy is lateral suture with 4-0 or 5-0 polypropylene. Other options include resection with end-to-end anastomosis, ligation with an end-to-side portocaval shunt, interposition graft, or venous vein patch graft. In damage control mode, the portal vein can be ligated.[127] Stone et al. reported a survival rate of 50% (9/18) after portal vein ligation, similar to the 42% survival rate (15 of 36) reported by Ivatury et al.[128] Portal vein ligation will induce a large fluid requirement to compensate for marked but transient splanchnic hypervolemia.[129] The overall survival rate from injuries to the portal vein may be as high as 61%.[130]

The retrohepatic IVC is perhaps the most difficult area to control surgically. Three common approaches to the retrohepatic IVC include hepatic vascular isolation with clamps, placement of an atriocaval shunt, and endovascular balloon occlusion.[131] Mortality remains high in patients treated with atriocaval shunts because this rarely employed technique is resorted to too late in the course of the operation. Khaneja et al.[132] reported 10 patients of whom 7 survived, using the technique of total vascular isolation. Total hepatic vascular isolation is performed by doing a Pringle maneuver, clamping the aorta at the diaphragm, and clamping the suprarenal and suprahepatic vena cava. In patients with vascular isolation, the use of venovenous bypass is crucial to maintain venous return and to avoid hypotension and arrhythmias.[133]

Extremity Vascular Trauma

Vascular trauma to the extremities is common in both the civilian and military arenas. Successful treatment of these highly morbid extremity vascular injuries is dependent upon early recognition and prompt management. Two major determinants of clinical outcome are the severity of the injury (to vessel and surrounding tissues) and the length of ischemia time before reperfusion.

Historical Perspective

Before the 1950s, the common treatment of vascular injuries to the extremities was ligation of both venous and arterial injuries followed commonly by amputation. Debakey and Simeone stated, in their classic work about vascular injuries to American troops in WW II, "Ligation with or without amputation is not a procedure of choice. It is a procedure of stern necessity, for the purpose of controlling hemorrhage."[134]

Before WW II, long evacuation times, lack of antibiotics, and lack of fluid and blood for resuscitation dictated that ligation be performed to prevent death from exsanguination or sepsis. Debakey and Simeone reported an amputation rate of 49%.[134] The amputation rate during the Korean War was decreased to 13.6% among 227 patients who underwent acute suture repair.[135,136] Ferguson et al. reported a 10-fold increase in the percentage of peripheral vascular injuries repaired rather than ligated in Atlanta, Georgia, in the 1950s.[137] Building on the military surgical principles of early diagnosis and treatment, resection of grossly damaged arterial segments, intimal approximation, and maintenance of palpable pulses after repair, the amputation rates following extremity vascular injury currently are less than 5%.[138]

Epidemiology

Vascular injuries to the extremities occur from both blunt and penetrating trauma. Rich et al. reported a 2% incidence of peripheral vascular injuries during the Vietnam War.[139] Oller et al.[140] reported a 3.7% incidence of civilian peripheral vascular trauma. More than 80% of arterial injuries of the extremity are caused by penetrating trauma, which can affect both the upper and lower extremities. The most common artery injured in the upper extremity is the brachial artery, whereas the most common artery injured in the lower extremity is the superficial femoral artery. Associated injuries to major veins, nerves, and soft tissue usually accompany arterial injuries, most commonly of a major vein. Neurological injury is a primary determinant of outcome. Thus, it is important to perform and document a good physical examination of the injured extremity, including a neurological examination.

Diagnostic Evaluation

All patients with injured extremities must be evaluated for a vascular injury to maximize limb function. Patients with extremity arterial injuries have varied clinical presentations. Few patients present with obvious "hard signs" of arterial injury such as pulsatile bleeding, an enlarging hematoma, absent distal pulses, or an ischemic limb. These patients require immediate surgical exploration without further workup. In most cases where an arteriogram is needed, an intraoperative arteriogram usually suffices to identify the location and extent of the injury and guide surgical treatment. Most cases of injury to the extremities from either blunt or penetrating trauma present without hard signs. It is more common for arterial injuries to present insidiously, posing a diagnostic challenge. In military conflicts, the severity of associated soft tissue injuries prompted the recommendation that all penetrating extremity wounds in proximity to a neurovascular bundle be explored routinely.

When this policy was applied in civilian trauma centers, a large number of nontherapeutic explorations were performed. Once trauma surgeons were able to obtain arteriograms for these injuries, screening or exclusion arteriograms became routine, which also led to a high number of negative arteriograms with their own morbidity, not to mention the cost (normal vessels in up to 90%).[141] Weaver et al.[142] reported 373 patients with penetrating extremity trauma who had an arteriogram for proximity alone or for signs suggestive of an arterial injury. Arteriograms were obtained for a distal pulse or neurological deficit, hematoma, history of large amount of blood loss or hypotension, fracture, major soft tissue injury, delayed capillary refill, or in the absence of these signs when the path of the penetrating object passed in proximity to the neurovascular bundle. An arterial injury was present in 65 of 216 (30%) patients who presented with one or more abnormal physical signs. When proximity was the sole indication for arteriography, an arterial injury was found in only 11% of the patients (17 of 157). In this study, significant predictors for arterial injury were a pulse deficit, neurological deficit, or a shotgun injury. A prospective study of routine arteriography to rule out arterial injury after blunt lower extremity trauma was reported by Applebaum et al.[143] Fifty-three patients had arteriograms performed, 31 of whom had physical findings suggestive of an arterial injury and 22 of whom had no signs of injury. Fifteen arterial injuries were identified with physical findings (48.4%), but only 3 minor injuries that did not require treatment were found in the absence of physical findings (13.6%).

In a study of 37 blunt traumatic knee dislocations, popliteal arterial injury was identified by arteriography in only 6 patients (16%).[144] Miranda and Dennis confirmed these findings subsequently.[145] Following blunt lower extremity, arteriography may be unnecessary when the physical examination is negative. Johansen and Lynch[146] advocated the use of physical examination and noninvasive pressure measurements of the extremity [ankle-arm (brachial) index, ABI] after both blunt and penetrating injuries to the extremities. In their series, 100 patients had arteriograms and ABIs. With arteriography being the gold standard, arterial injuries that required treatment were identified in 14 patients, whereas an ABI less than 0.90 predicted arterial injury with 87% sensitivity and 97% specificity. In this study, there were two false-positive arteriogram results; thus, the sensitivity and specificity of the ABI test with a value of 0.90 or less were even higher, 95% and 97%, respectively.[146]

Today, a patient who sustains either a penetrating or blunt injury to an extremity and who has a normal extremity pulse examination and an ABI greater than 0.90 does not require an arteriogram. All clinically important arterial injuries are found in extremities with a pulse deficit or an ABI less than 0.90. Arteriography may be useful to locate the injury and to plan operative treatment. Even with careful physical examination and blood pressure measurements, occasional injuries are missed. In most cases, these missed injuries are minor and either need no treatment (occlusion of minor branch vessels) or heal without intervention (a major vessel with a minor intimal injury).[147] Intimal irregularities, focal spasm with narrowing, and small pseudoaneurysms that are asymptomatic and found only on arteriography can be treated nonoperatively so long as these injuries are followed up carefully. If a patient needs surgical intervention, hard signs will usually be present on physical examination within 2 weeks of the initial injury. As noninvasive vascular imaging has improved, color flow ultrasonography has become readily available and reliable and has been suggested as a substitute for or a complement to arteriography.[148] However, color flow ultrasonography is highly operator-dependent, and the sensitivity, specificity, and accuracy have been reported to vary widely.[149,150] Color flow Doppler studies can be used to document healing of minor intimal injuries treated nonoperatively. With these principles in mind, a diagnostic algorithm is presented in Figure 29.8.

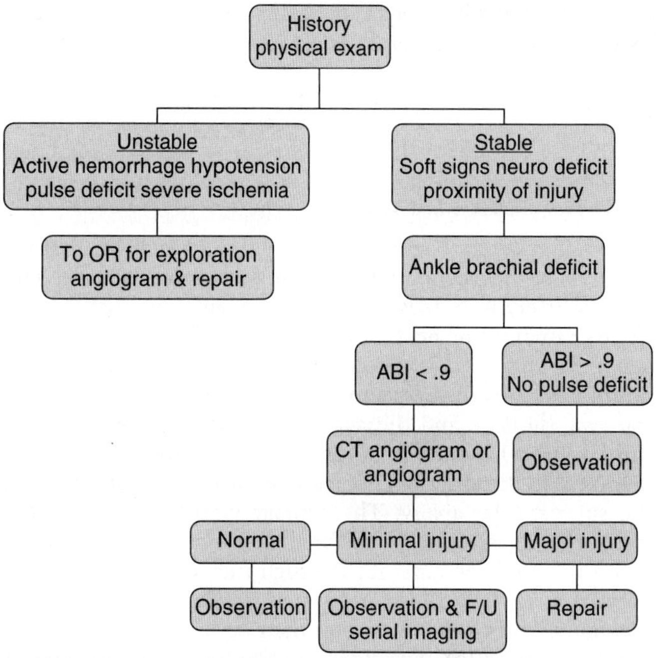

FIGURE 29.8. Algorithm for the management of penetrating extremity trauma. ABI, ankle–brachial index; CT, computed tomography; F/U, followup; OR, operating room.

Operative Management of Extremity Vascular Injury

Patients with extremity trauma must be assessed for other injuries. Antibiotic prophylaxis should be administered as soon as possible after injury. Tetanus prophylaxis should be given for all open wounds. Systemic heparin should be considered for all patients who do not have a contraindication, especially those with isolated extremity injuries. Both extremities, as well as the chest or abdomen in proximal injuries, should be prepared in the surgical field to allow for harvest of the cephalic or saphenous vein from the uninjured extremity. The first priority is to obtain proximal and distal control of the injured vessel through incisions placed over the area of injury, with extension of the incision parallel to the course of the injured vessel. When control of the injured vessel is obtained, proximal and distal thrombus should be extracted by careful passage of embolectomy catheters. Heparinized saline (30 mL normal saline containing 100 units heparin) should be flushed into the proximal and distal vessels for regional anticoagulation during repair. Damaged vessels should be debrided back to normal tissue. A tension-free end-to-end anastomosis should be preformed whenever possible. Autogenous vein or prosthetic interposition grafting may be necessary when primary repair cannot be performed. An intraoperative completion angiogram should be performed after all repairs to document patency of the repair and adequacy of distal runoff. Adequate, well-vascularized, healthy soft tissue coverage must be available to cover all vascular repairs. Early fracture stabilization helps to protect the vascular repair during its construction.

Surgical repair is desirable whenever possible, but ligation of arteries may be necessary when patients have hemodynamic instability, acidosis, hypothermia, and coagulopathy. The use of an arterial shunt can be temporizing as part of a damage control operation before staged definitive repair.[151,152]

Injuries to the radial, ulnar, or tibial arteries can be ligated so long as adequate collateral distal perfusion is documented.

Upper Extremity Injuries

Axillary Arterial Injury

The axillary artery begins at the lateral margin of the first rib and ends at the lateral margin of the teres major muscle. The axillary artery is divided into three sections: The first section lies proximal to the pectoralis minor muscle and gives off the superior thoracic artery. The second section of the axillary artery lies beneath the pectoralis minor muscle and gives off the long thoracic and thoracoacromial arteries, whereas the third section lies lateral to the pectoralis minor muscle and gives rise to the anterior and posterior circumflex arteries and the subscapsular artery. The axillary vein lies anterior and inferior to the artery. The brachial plexus surrounds the axillary artery and accounts for the high incidence of associated nerve injuries in axillary artery trauma. Axillary artery injuries are slightly more common than subclavian artery injuries, accounting for approximately 5% to 10% of all arterial injuries[153]; penetrating injuries account for the majority. Blunt trauma to the axillary artery can follow fracture of the proximal humerus or anterior dislocation of the shoulder. Thrombosis of the axillary artery may occur from chronic recurrent impingement of the artery by the misuse of crutches. Patients present commonly with a pulse deficit, advanced ischemia, pulsatile bleeding, or an expanding hematoma. However, as with subclavian arterial injury, some patients present with a palpable pulse because of excellent collateral circulation. Common associated injuries include the axillary vein, followed by injury to the cords or branches of the brachial plexus. Occasionally, patients with a history of penetrating axillary trauma present with a palpable radial pulse and a thrill or bruit, indicating an arteriogram to rule out an arteriovenous fistula.

Surgical treatment starts with wide preparation of the neck, shoulder, and arm including the fingertips as well as the contralateral leg to harvest a vein graft if needed. Exposure of the proximal axillary artery is best obtained by an infraclavicular incision, which can be extended into the axilla and down onto the upper arm if necessary to obtain distal control. Proximal and distal control of the artery should be obtained with vascular clamps after full exposure of the artery is completed to avoid iatrogenic venous or brachial plexus injuries. Debridement of the injured artery, proximal and distal catheter thrombectomy, and the use of local heparinization are done before vascular repair. Primary repair or resection of the injured vessel with end-to-end anastomosis is the preferred method of repair. Sacrifice of collateral vessels should not be performed to mobilize the injured segments into position for primary repair. If the vascular deficit is large or if any tension is placed on an end-to-end anastomosis, an interposition graft should be inserted. Ligation of the axillary artery is acceptable in patients who are unstable because of the rich collateral circulation of the upper extremities. An option for moribund patients is temporary shunting and wound packing until the patient is stabilized and a proper vascular repair can be performed.[154] Excellent patency rates reported after axillary artery repair are reflected in low mortality and amputation rates. Axillary venous injuries should be repaired when possible. Except for arm swelling, there has been little morbidity associated with ligation of an isolated axillary vein injury. However, long-term functional outcomes following axillary vascular injury (as determined by complete resolution of swelling, pain, and neurological deficit) are suboptimal because of associated neurological injury, which may result in long-term neuralgia or reflex sympathetic dystrophy (causalgia).[155]

Brachial Artery Injury

The brachial artery is a continuation of the axillary artery, beginning at the teres major muscle and terminating 1 inch below the antecubital fossa at the bifurcation into the radial and ulnar arteries. The brachial artery has three main braches, the most proximal and important of which is the profunda brachii. If the brachial artery is injured proximal to the profunda brachii, the amputation rate is 50%; if below, the amputation rate is only 25%.[134] The median nerve courses along with the brachial artery throughout its course, and the radial and ulnar nerves also parallel portions of the brachial artery. Thus, brachial artery injury is associated with peripheral nerve injury. Nerve injury is the most important prognostic factor of long-term extremity function.[156] The brachial artery is one of the most commonly injured peripheral arteries, penetrating injury being most common. Blunt trauma can cause a brachial artery injury, especially after anterior elbow dislocation or supracondylar fracture of the humerus. Patients present commonly with a pulse deficit, active hemorrhage, or a palpable mass. Ocrutt et al.[157] noted that 25% of patients with brachial artery injuries had an arterial occlusion, an intimal tear, or partial transection with no pulse deficit; furthermore, 14% of patients with a radial artery injury had a palpable radial pulse. Thus, for proximity injuries in the upper extremity with soft signs or a neurological deficit, an arteriogram should be performed. In the future, CT angiography may become the diagnostic modality of choice.[158]

After a careful physical examination and comprehensive documentation of the vascular and neurological findings, the patient may undergo operative exploration. Brachial arterial injuries require expedient repair, usually within 4h.[159] Exposure of the brachial artery is obtained by a longitudinal incision in the palpable groove between the triceps and biceps muscle along the medial aspect of the arm (Fig. 29.9). The extent of repair is determined by the type and extent of injury to the artery. Lateral arteriorraphy should attempted only be for small needle or puncture wounds. Vein patch repair is usually unsuccessful because of the high frequency of thrombosis. Adequate debridement of the injured segment is important for successful repair. Spasm is common when repairing small vessels and is usually treated with the topical application of lidocaine. Primary repair of brachial artery injuries is usually possible with an end-to-end anastomosis; if not, a reversed saphenous vein autogenous graft is preferred. If associated orthopedic injuries are present, a temporary shunt allows fracture stabilization before definitive vascular repair. Nonoperative treatment of brachial arterial injuries has been suggested for low-velocity injuries with minimal artery wall disruption (<5 mm intimal defect, pseudoaneurysm, or downstream intimal flap), intact distal circulation, and no active

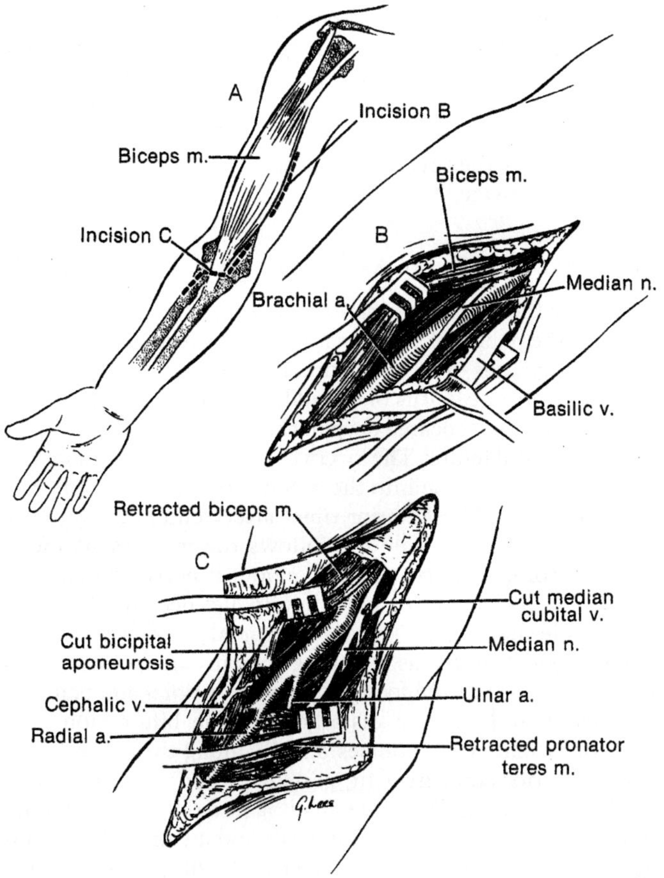

FIGURE 29.9. Surgical exposure of the brachial artery is rapidly obtained by a longitudinal incision along the course of the artery, with an extension as an S-curve either across the axilla proximally or across the antecubital fossa distally as needed. The median nerve and basilic veins are in close proximity to the artery.

hemorrhage.[161] Associated venous injuries should be repaired if not complicated, or they can be ligated.

After the brachial artery transits the antecubital fossa, the ulnar artery is the larger of the two tributaries. The radial artery travels to the wrist and terminates in the deep palmar arch. The ulnar artery travels to the wrist and terminates in the superficial palmar arch. Ulnar and radial arterial injuries often occur with penetrating trauma to the forearm. Complete interruption of either the radial or ulnar artery often has no adverse affect on the circulation of the forearm or hand because of the vast collateral circulation. Occasionally, a patient presents with a swollen forearm and parathesias, which is consistent with a compartment syndrome; fasciotomies are needed as well as revascularization. With injuries to either the radial or ulnar artery alone, the injured artery can be ligated without adverse sequelae.[160] If both arteries are injured, the ulnar artery should be repaired preferentially, as it is the larger of the two vessels. Exposure of the proximal radial and ulnar arteries is through an S-shaped incision in the antecubital fossa (Fig. 29.10). The distal segments of the arteries are exposed through longitudinal incisions over the course of the artery just proximal to the hand. Surgical repair usually follows debridement of the injured segment with either an end-to-end anastomosis or interposition vein grafting. Venous injuries are ligated.

Lower Extremity Injuries

Femoral Arterial Injury

The common femoral artery arises from the external iliac artery as it passes under the inguinal ligament. Approximately 5 cm below the inguinal ligament, the common femoral artery divides into the superficial femoral and the profunda femoris arteries. The profunda femoris artery exists most commonly as a single posterolateral branch of the common femoral artery. The superficial femoral artery originates in the femoral triangle and travels posteromedially to the adductor canal, where it becomes the popliteal artery. The superficial femoral vein travels posteromedial to the artery. The saphenous nerve lies anterior to the artery.

Femoral vessels are one of the more commonly injured extremity vessels, with greater than 90% of these injuries being caused by penetrating trauma, mostly by GSW.[161] Most patients who sustain a femoral arterial injury present with hard signs, such as active bleeding, shock, or a pulseless extremity. These patients should be taken to the operating room expeditiously. Arteriography is indicated in a hemodynamically stable patient with an equivocal examination, in whom the exact location of the injury or the possibility of more than one injury would modify operative management. Injuries to the femoral vessels are not commonly associated

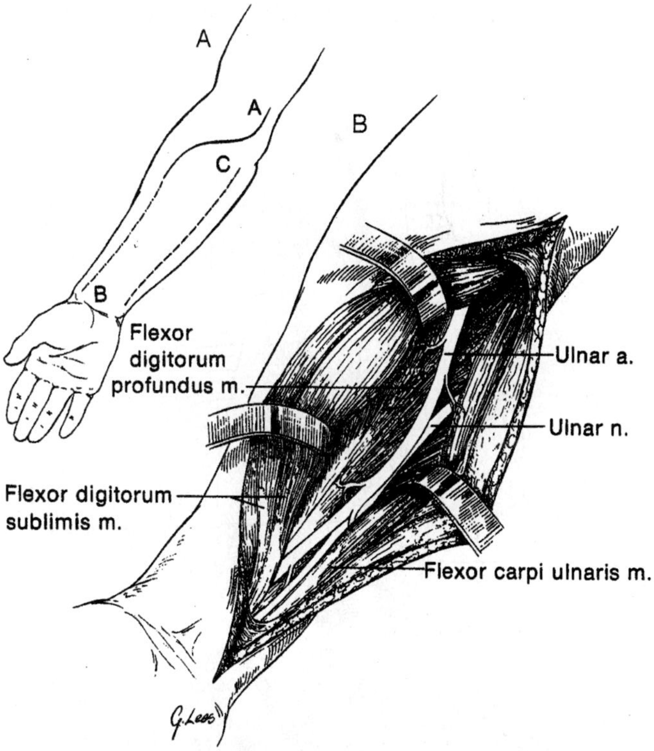

FIGURE 29.10. Elective incisions that can be used to approach the radial and ulnar arteries. **A.** An S-type incision starting along the course of the distal brachial artery, carried through the antecubital fossa and continued down on the forearm, gives excellent exposure of the proximal ulnar and radial arteries, as well as the origin of the common interosseous artery (*A*). An extension off this incision (*B*) along the course of the radial artery can be used for exposure to the wrist level. A separate incision can be used over the course of the ulnar artery (*C*). **B.** This drawing demonstrates exposure of the ulnar neurovascular bundle within the deep muscle layers, which have been split proximally.

with fractures of the femoral shaft, although there is an association with more proximal and especially distal femur fractures.

The common femoral artery, proximal superficial femoral artery, and profunda femoris artery are best exposed through a longitudinal incision overlying its course from the inguinal ligament inferiorly for 8 to 12 cm (Fig. 29.11). Occasionally, the external iliac artery may have to be isolated to gain proximal control, which can be accomplished through an oblique incision above the inguinal ligament carried down into the retroperitoneum, where the artery and vein can be controlled without entering the peritoneal cavity. The profunda femoris artery is found after dissecting distal on the proximal superficial femoral artery and then posterolaterally. The lateral circumflex femoral vein should be identified and ligated as it crosses over the profunda femoral artery about 3 cm from its origin. The middle and distal superficial femoral arteries are exposed through an oblique incision in the thigh over the course of the sartorius muscle. The muscle is retracted medially, and the artery is first found at the adductor canal and followed proximally.

Once proximal and distal control has been obtained, direct repair of the arterial injury is preferred. If the injury is extensive, an interposition graft should be placed to create a tension-free anastomosis. For femoral artery injuries, the reversed saphenous vein graft remains the first choice for interposition grafting when available. A PTFE interposition graft is an acceptable alternative.[162] The profunda femoris artery should be repaired if possible, but the vessel can be ligated in unstable patients as long as the superficial femoral artery is patent. Long-term patency rates after successful primary repair or short segment interposition grafts are excellent. Lower extremity function following vascular repair is determined by the severity of the associated soft tissue, bone, and nerve damage.[163]

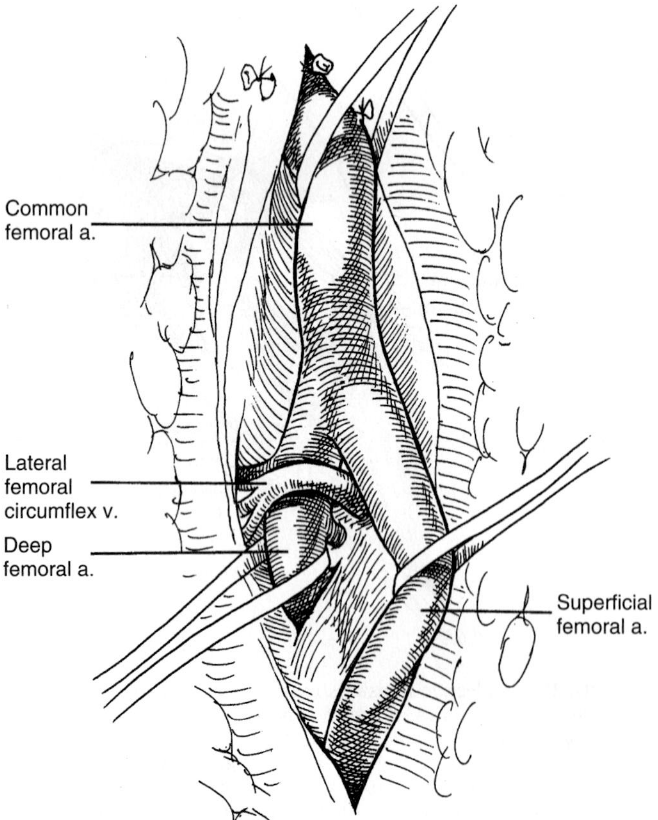

FIGURE 29.11. The deep femoral artery normally arises laterally off the common femoral trunk between 3 and 5 cm distal to the inguinal ligament. Its origin is crossed by the lateral femoral circumflex vein.

Popliteal and Tibial Artery Injuries

Injury to the popliteal artery is a limb-threatening injury because the popliteal artery is a true end artery. The popliteal artery originates from the superficial femoral artery as it emerges from the hiatus of the adductor magnus muscle. The popliteal artery is located deep in the posterior fossa along the posterior distal femur. The artery continues distally and bifurcates 90% of the time into the anterior tibial artery and tibial perineal trunk. The anterior tibial artery enters the anterior compartment of the calf and follows the interosseus membrane, accompanied by the deep peroneal nerve and anterior tibial vein. This neurovascular bundle lies deep to the extensor muscles of the calf. The anterior tibial artery becomes the dorsalis pedis artery as it emerges from the extensor retinaculum on top of the foot. The posterior tibial and peroneal arteries arise 3 to 6 cm distally from the bifurcation. The posterior tibial artery courses distally along the fascia in the deep posterior compartment, passing posterior to the medial malleolus at the ankle before dividing into the plantar arteries of the foot. The deep peroneal nerve and a pair of deep veins accompany the posterior tibial artery. The peroneal artery travels down the middle of the leg. It branches into the anterior and posterior calcaneal arteries above the ankle and has no direct connection to the arterial arches of the foot. It travels with a pair of deep veins but no nerves.

Most popliteal and tibial artery injuries are caused by blunt trauma to the lower extremity. Fracture or dislocation at the knee (popliteal) or ankle are the predominant mechanisms. Penetrating injuries also occur to these vessels but are rare in civilian practice. Most injuries to the popliteal artery present with distal ischemia from arterial thrombosis. A thorough peripheral vascular and neurological examination is the key to recognizing and treating these injuries promptly. The physical examination and the use of the ABI are all that is usually necessary to make the diagnosis of a lower extremity arterial injury. Arteriography should be reserved for patients with equivocal physical findings. Associated venous and neurological injuries are extremely morbid. Factors that clearly affect outcome are the time interval between injury and treatment and associated injuries and mechanism of injury. Blunt trauma has a worse prognosis than penetrating trauma. A history of chronic vascular occlusive disease and presentation with ischemia, shock, or active hemorrhage portend a worse outcome.[164] Occlusion of a single tibial vessel is well tolerated if no other injuries or disease affects the other two distal arteries.

Popliteal injuries are best approached through a medial incision. However, either the medial or posterior approach to the popliteal artery can be used (Fig. 29.12). During medial exposure, care must be taken to avoid injury to the saphenous vein, as this may become the only venous drainage of the lower extremity. The proximal popliteal artery is controlled as it emerges from the adductor canal. Detachment of the

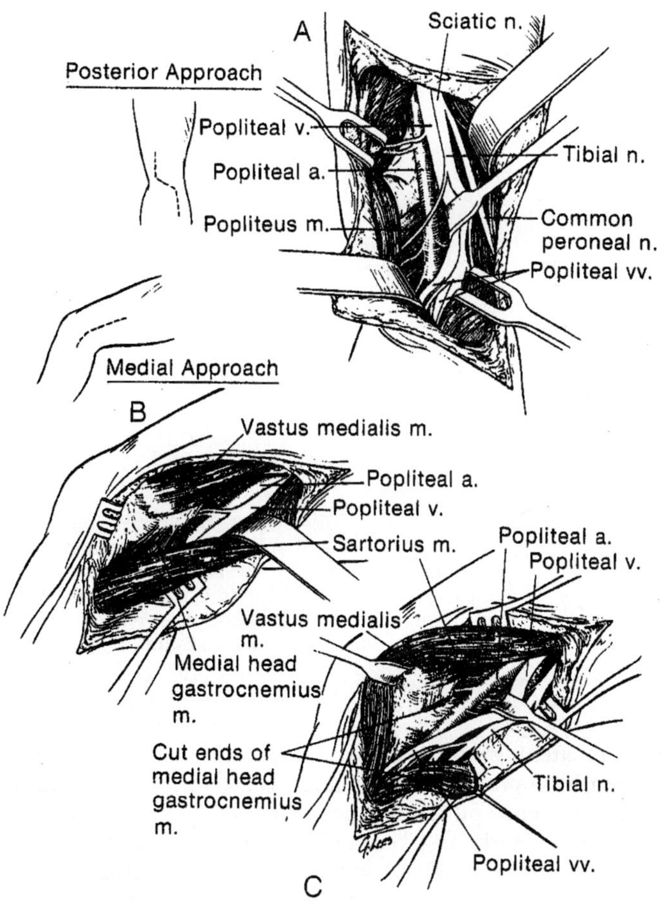

FIGURE 29.12. The posterior and medial approaches to the popliteal artery. **A.** A modified S-shaped incision is used in the posterior approach to avoid contracture across the knee joint. **B.** The medial approach requires a more extensive dissection but provides better access to proximal and distal vessels. **C.** Both approaches can be used successfully in the exposure and repair of the popliteal vessels.

gastrocnemius, semimembranosus, and semitendinosus muscles is required to expose the artery behind the knee. The distal popliteal artery is exposed after making an incision along the posterior tibia and then dividing the soleus muscle longitudinally to expose the neurovascular bundle.

Tibial vessel exposure requires cautious dissection in the upper medial calf. The origin of the vessels can be found by continuing distal dissection of the distal popliteal artery through the area of the triceps surae. The anterior tibial artery is exposed by retracting the popliteal vein posteriorly. Because the anterior tibial vein is injured easily, it should be ligated to prevent iatrogenic hemorrhage. After ligation of this vein the proximal anterior tibial artery and tibial peroneal trunk are exposed. Distal exposure of the posterior tibial artery is obtained through a medial incision along the posterior margin of the tibia down to and posterior to the medial malleolus. The distal anterior tibial artery is exposed through an incision along the middle of the anterior compartment.

Popliteal and tibial arterial injuries usually require repair with interposition grafting. The contralateral reversed saphenous vein remains the interposition graft of choice. An intraoperative completion arteriogram should be performed after all arterial repairs of the popliteal or tibial arteries. Early occlusion should be investigated to rule out a technical problem with the repair. Soft tissue coverage of arterial repairs is required to prevent postoperative infection, thrombosis, or hemorrhage.

Venous Injury of the Lower Extremities

Venous injuries of the lower extremity pose major challenges for the trauma surgeon. Venous injuries are associated with arterial injuries, especially after penetrating trauma. Because of low venous pressures, major hemorrhage is uncommon except after large lacerations to the popliteal or femoral veins. Controversy exists over the best treatment of venous injuries. Most experts prefer to ligate injuries to minor veins and to repair major veins if the patient is stable and without other life-threatening injuries.[165,166] Life-threatening associated injuries and hemodynamic instability mandate ligation of all venous injuries, whereas extensive soft tissue injury with loss of collateral venous outflow mandates venous reconstruction. If possible, a venous injury should be repaired before an arterial injury, using a temporary arterial shunt while the venous repair is constructed using a contralateral reversed saphenous venous interposition graft. These grafts can thrombose early, and the use of aspirin, low molecular weight dextran, can limit platelet adhesion. Systemic heparinization should be reserved for proved deep venous thrombosis. If thrombosis occurs, recannulation is possible in some patients. Pulmonary or clopidogrel embolism is uncommon following venous repairs.[167] Postinjury lower extremity swelling and edema after ligation should be treated by lower extremity elevation and compression dressings.

Extremity Compartment Syndrome

Extremity compartment syndrome results from increased pressure within a closed anatomic space. The upper and lower extremities are comprised of muscles, nerves, and vessels enclosed in a rigid fascial membrane. After either penetrating or blunt injury, pressure in these rigid compartments increases as tissue edema develops. As the pressure in the compartment rises, perfusion to the compartment is compromised at some level. If the high pressure in the compartment is not diagnosed, severe dysfunction of the extremity can result, with a high risk of limb loss. Early signs and symptoms of compartment syndrome are swelling, loss of sensation or movement, and pain out of proportion to the injury. The pressure in the compartment can be measured directly with introduction of a needle connected to a pressure transducer. Pressures less than 20 mmHg are acceptable. Pressures greater than 30 mmHg indicate compartment syndrome. Pressures between 20 and 30 mmHg are worrisome for compartment syndrome, and one must rely on the clinical examination and mechanism of injury to make a decision regarding fasciotomy. Serum creatinine phosphokinase (CPK) concentration and myoglobinuria have been used as markers of compartment syndrome because both are released with muscle necrosis, but as such are late findings. Acute compartment syndrome raises CPK concentration to more than 5000 U within 4 to 6 h.[168] Myoglobin is toxic to the renal tubules and may precipitate acute renal failure if the compartment syndrome remains untreated.[169]

Treatment of established or suspected extremity compartment syndrome is surgical decompression of the affected

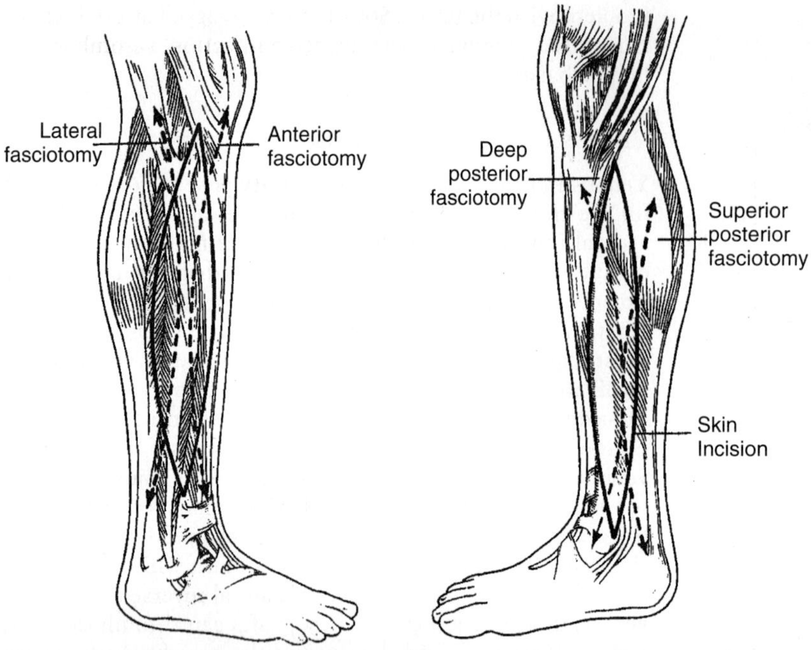

FIGURE 29.13. Lateral and medial leg incisions for a four-compartment faciotomy. The lateral and anterior compartments are decompressed through the lateral incision and the superficial and deep posterior compartments through the medial incision.

extremity by fasciotomies.[170,171] Fasciotomy along the length of the entire compartment is necessary to release pressure and restore microperfusion to the compromised compartment. In the lower extremity, a two-incision, four-compartment fasciotomy is performed (Fig. 29.13). A medial incision is placed 5 cm posterior to the tibia; through this incision, the superficial and deep posterior compartments are decompressed. A lateral incision is made anterior to the fibula, and both the lateral and anterior compartments are decompressed in this incision. The thigh compartments are decompressed through both medial and lateral incisions. The anterior and posterior compartments are decompressed through the lateral incision and the medial compartment is decompressed through the medial incision. In the upper arm, longitudinal lateral and medial incisions are made to decompress the anterior and posterior compartments. In the forearm, a straight dorsal and a "lazy S" incision are made on the volar surface (Fig. 29.14).

Fasciotomies should be closed as soon as possible. The decision for closure is made individually for each case, because there is no ideal time for closure. If possible, wounds should be closed primarily, but skin grafts can be used to close large defects, or they may be allowed to close by secondary intention.

Mangled Extremity

Patients who suffer severe soft tissue, bone, vascular, and neurological injury to the extremity after trauma are considered to have a mangled extremity. Many times these injuries lead to a difficult decision for the trauma team, regarding when to operate and salvage these mangled extremities or just to proceed with amputation. The Mangled Extremity Severity Score (MESS) has been used by some to help guide decision making (Table 29.8).

Patients with severe neurological dysfunction should probably undergo primary amputation. If the patient has other life-threatening injuries, early amputation of the mangled extremity is prudent. If the mangled extremity is not a threat to the patient and neurological function is intact, the best treatment is early irrigation and debridement of the soft tissue and bone injuries, along with vascular reconstruction and fracture stabilization. However, an insensate, functionless extremity will only impede the progress of rehabilitation. These patients take a lot of time, resources, and dedication to have success in regaining function. Many patients suffer from depression and chronic pain, which makes these patients a challenge to manage.

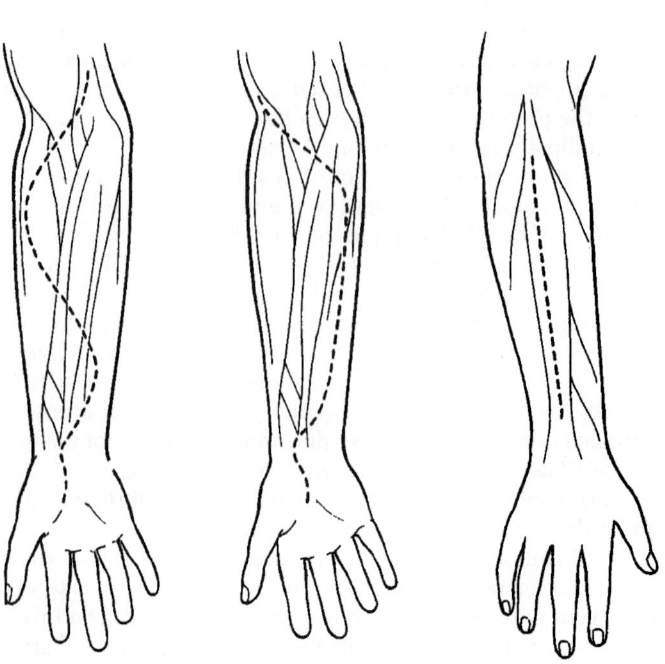

FIGURE 29.14. Volar (S-type or straight) and dorsal (straight) incisions for forearm fasciotomies.

TABLE 29.8. Mangled Extremity Severity Score (MESS).

Diagnosis	*Points*
Skeletal/soft tissue injury	
Low energy (stab, simple fracture)	1
Medium energy (open/multiple fracture)	2
High energy (shotgun or crush)	3
Limb ischemia	
Reduced pulse but normal perfusion	1[a]
Pulseless, paresthesias	2[a]
Cool, paralyzed, insensate	3[a]
Shock	
Blood pressure always >90 mmHg	0
Hypotensive transiently	1
Persistent hypotension	2
Age (years)	
More than 30	0
More than 30 but less than 50	1
More than 50	2

Sum individual diagnoses from MESS; MESS greater than 7 suggests amputation.

[a]Score is doubled for ischemia >6 h.

Source: From Johansen K, Daines M, Howey T, et al. Objective criteria accurately predict amputation following lower extremity trauma. J Trauma 1990;30:568–572.

References

1. Bankey PE. Vascular trauma. In: Norton JA, Bollinger RR, Chang AE, Lowry SF, Mulvihill SJ, Pass HI, Thompson RW, eds. Surgery: Basic Science and Clinical Evidence. New York: Springer, 2001:1111–1134.
2. King DR, Cohn SM, Proctor KG. Modified rapid deployment hemostat bandage terminates bleeding in coagulopathic patients with severe visceral injuries. J Trauma 2004;57:756–759.
3. Schwartz AM. The historical development of methods of hemostasis. Surgery 1958;44:604.
4. Rich NM, Rhee P. An historical tour of vascular injury management. Surg Clin N Am 2001;81:1199.
5. Esmarch F. The Surgeons Handbook of the Treatment of the Wounded in War. New York: Schmidt, 1878.
6. Lambert. Med Observ Inq 1762;2:360.
7. Murphy JB. Resection of arteries and veins injured in continuity—end to end suture: experimental and clinical research. Med Rec 1897;51:73–104.
8. Baird RN, Abbott WM. Vein grafts. An historical prospective. Am J Surg 1977;134:293.
9. Mattox KL, Feliciano DV, Burch J, et al. Five thousand seven hundred sixty cardiovascular injuries in 4459 patients: epidemiologic evolution 1958 to 1987. Ann Surg 1989;209:698–705.
10. Oller DW, Rutledge R, Clancy T, et al. Vascular injuries in a rural state: a review of 978 patients from a state trauma registry. J Trauma 1992;32:740–745.
11. Sirinek KR, Gaskill HV III, Root HD, et al. Truncal vascular injury: factors influencing survival. J Trauma 1983;23:372–377.
12. Brown MF, Graham JM, Feliciano DV, et al. Carotid artery injuries. Am J Surg 1982;144:748–753.
13. Hardy JD, Rau S, Neely WA, et al. Aortic and other arterial injuries. Ann Surg 1975;181:640–653.
14. Treiman GS, Yellin AE, Weaver FA, et al. Examination of the patient with a knee dislocation. The case for selective arteriography. Arch Surg 1992;127:1056–1062.
15. Haimovici H. Metabolic complications of acute arterial occlusions and related conditions: role of free radicals. In: Haimovici H, ed. Vascular Surgery. Norwalk: Appleton & Lange, 1989:386–408.
16. Advanced Trauma Life Support, 7th ed. Chicago: American College of Surgeons, 2004.
17. Mattox K. Vascular trauma. In: Haimovici H, ed. Vascular Surgery. Norwalk: Appleton & Lange, 1989:370–385.
18. Sirinek K, Levine B, Gaskill H, et al. Reassessment of the role of routine operative exploration in vascular trauma. J Trauma 1981;21:339–344.
19. Frykberg ER, Dennis JW, Bishop K, et al. The reliability of the physical examination in the evaluation of penetrating extremity trauma for vascular injury: results at 1 year. J Trauma 1991;31: 502–511.
20. Feliciano D, Cruse P Burch J, et al. Delayed diagnosis of arterial injuries. Am J Surg 1987;154:579–584.
21. Martin L, McKenney M, Sosa JL, et al. Management of lower extremity arterial injury. J Trauma 1994;37:591–599.
22. Higashida RT, Halbach VV, Tsai FY, et al. Interventional neurovascular treatment of traumatic carotid and vertebral artery lesions: results in 234 cases. Am J Radiol 1989;153:577–584.
23. Becker GJ, Beenati JF, Zemel G, et al. Percutaneous placement of a balloon expandable intraluminal stent graft for life-threatening subclavian arterial hemorrhage. J Vasc Interv Radiol 1991;2:225–229.
24. Mitchell FL III, Thal ER. Results of venous interposition grafts in arterial injury. J Trauma 1990;30:336–339.
25. Stone KS, Walshaw R, Sugilyama GT, et al. Polytetrafluroethylene versus autologous vein grafts for vascular reconstruction in contaminated wounds. Am J Surg 1984;147:692–695.
26. Feliciano D, Mattox KL, Graham J, et al. Five-year experience with PTFE grafts in vascular wounds. J Trauma 1985;25:71–82.
27. Shah D, Leather RP, Corson JD, et al. Polytetrafluoropropylene grafts in the rapid reconstruction of acute contaminated peripheral vascular injuries. Am J Surg 1984;148:229–233.
28. Monson DO, Saletta JD, Freeark RJ. Carotid vertebral trauma. J Trauma 1969;9:987–999.
29. Demetriades D, Theodorouu D, Cromwell E, et al. Evaluation of penetrating injuries to the neck: a prospective study of 223 patients. World J Surg 1997;21:41–47.
30. Timberlake GA, Rice JC, Kerstein MD, et al. Penetrating injury to the carotid artery. A reappraisal of management. Am Surg 1989;55:154–157.
31. Apffelstaedt JP, Muller R. Results of mandatory exploration for penetrating neck trauma. World J Surg 1994;18:917–920.
32. Menawat S, Dennis J, Laneve L, et al. Are arteriograms necessary in penetrating zone II neck injuries? J Vasc Surg 1992;16:397–401.
33. Demetriades D, Charalambides D, Lakhoo M, et al. Physical examination and selective conservative management in patients with penetrating injuries to the neck. Br J Surg 1993;80:1534–1536.
34. Beitsch P, Weigelt J, Flynn E, et al. Physical examination and arteriography in patients with penetrating zone II neck wounds. Arch Surg 1994;129:577–581.
35. Biffl W, Moore E, Rehse D, et al. Selective management of penetrating neck trauma based on cervical level of injury. Am J Surg 1997;174:678–682.
36. Wood J, Fabian TC, Mangiante EC. Penetrating neck injuries: recommendations for selective management. J Trauma 1989;29: 602–605.
37. Stain S, Yellin A, Weaver F, et al. Selective management of nonocclusive arterial injuries. Arch Surg 1989;124:1136–1140.
38. Kuehne JP, Weaver FA, Papanicolaou G, et al. Penetrating trauma of the internal carotid artery. Arch Surg 1996;131:942–948.
39. Fry WR, Dort JA, Smith RS, et al. Duplex scanning replaces arteriography and operative exploration in the diagnosis of potential cervical vascular injury. Am J Surg 1994;168:693–695.
40. Demetriades D, Thoudorou D, Cromwell E, et al. Penetrating injuries of the neck in stable patients: physical examination,

arteriography, or color flow doppler. Arch Surg 1995;130:971–979.
41. Ginzberg E, Montalvo B, Leblang S, et al. The use of duplex ultrasonography in penetrating neck injury. Arch Surg 1996;131:691–693.
42. LeBlang SD, Nunez DB, Rivas LA, et al. Helical computed tomographic angiography in penetrating neck trauma. Emerg Radiol 1997;4:200–206.
43. Munera F, Soto J, Palacio D, et al. Diagnosis of arterial injuries caused by penetrating trauma to the neck: comparison of helical CT angiography and conventional angiography. Radiology 2000;216:556–562.
44. Inaba K, Munera F, McKenney M, et al. Prospective evaluation of screening multislice helical computed tomographic angiography in the initial evaluation of penetrating neck injuries. J Trauma 2006;61:144–149.
45. Yellin AE, Weaver FA. Vascular system. In: Donovan AJ, ed. Trauma Surgery. St. Louis: Mosby, 1994:209–264.
46. Ledgerwood AM, Mullins RJ, Lucas CE.: Primary repair versus ligation for carotid artery injuries. Arch Surg 1980;115:488–493.
47. Ramadan F, Rutledge R, Oller D, et al. Carotid artery trauma: a review of cotemporary trauma center experience. J Vasc Surg 1995;21:46–55.
48. Ledgerwood AM, Mullins RJ, Lucas CE. Primary repair versus ligation for carotid artery injuries. Arch Surg 1980;115:488–493.
49. Ramadan F, Rutledge R, Oller D, et al. Carotid artery trauma: a review of contemporary trauma center experience. J Vasc Surg 1995;21:46–55.
50. Weaver FA, Yellin AE, Wagner WH, et al. The role of arterial reconstruction in carotid injuries. Arch Surg 1988;123:1106–1111.
51. Cogbill TH, Moore EE, Meissner M, et al. The spectrum of blunt injury to the carotid artery: a multicenter perspective. J Trauma 1994;37:473–479.
52. Zelenock G, Kazmers A, Whitehouse W, et al. Extracranial internal carotid artery dissections. Arch Surg 1982;117:425–432.
53. Zelenock GB. Penetrating and blunt injuries to the carotid artery. In: Ernest CB, Stanley JC, eds. Current Therapy of Vascular Surgery. St. Louis: Mosby, 2001.
54. Fabian TC, Patton JH, Croce MA, et al. Blunt carotid injury: importance of early diagnosis and anticoagulant therapy. Ann Surg 1996;223:513–522.
55. Kumar SR, Weaver FA, Yellin AE. Cervical vascular injuries. Surg Clin North Am 2001;81:1331–1344.
56. Carillo EH, Osburne DL, Spain DA, et al. Blunt carotid artery injuries: Difficulties with the diagnosis prior to neurologic event. J Trauma 1999;46:1120–1125.
57. Amirjamshidi A, Abbossaioun K, Rahmat H. Traumatic aneurysms and arteriovenous fistulas of the extracranial vessels in war injuries. Surg Neurol 2000;53:136–145.
58. Duke BJ, Ryu RK, Coldwell DM, et al. Treatment of blunt carotid artery by using endovascular stents: an early experience. J Neurosurg 1997;6:825–829.
59. Reid JD, Weigelt JA. Forty-three cases of vertebral trauma. J Trauma 1988;28:1007–1012.
60. Demetriades D, Rabinowitz B, Pezkis A, et al. Subclavian vascular injuries. Br J Surg 1987;74:1001–1003.
61. Nair R, Robbs JV, Muckart DJ. Management of penetrating cervicomediastinal venous trauma. J Vasc Endovasc Surg 2000;19:65–69.
62. Demetriades D, Chahwan S, Gomez H, et al. Penetrating injuries to the subclavian and axillary vessels. J Am Coll Surg 1999;188:290–295.
63. Richardson JD, McElvein RB, Trinkle JF. First rib fracture: a hallmark of severe trauma. Ann Surg 1975;181:251–254.
64. Cox CS Jr, Allen GS, Fischer RP, et al. Blunt versus penetrating subclavian artery injury: presentation, injury pattern, and outcome. J Trauma 1999;46:445–449.
65. Demetriades D, Asensio JA. Subclavian and axillary vascular injuries. Surg Clin N Am 2001;81:1357–1373.
66. Dutort DF, Strauss DC, Blaszczyk M, et al. Endovascular treatment of penetrating thoracic outlet arterial injuries. Eur J Vasc Endovasc Surg 2000;19:489–495.
67. Gilroy D, Lakhoo M, Charalambides D, et al. Control of life threatening hemorrhage from the neck. A new indication for balloon tamponade. Injury 2000;23:557–559.
68. Perry MO. Penetrating injuries to the aortic arch and innominate and subclavian arteries. In: Ernst CB, Stanley JC, eds. Current Therapy in Vascular Surgery, 4th ed. New York: Dekker, 2001.
69. Conroy C, Hoyt DB, Eastman AB, et al. Motor vehicle-related cardiac and aortic injuries differ from other thoracic injuries. J Trauma 2007;62:1462–1467.
70. Flint LM, Snyder WH, Perry MO, et al. Management of major vascular injuries in the base of the neck: an 11-year experience with 146 cases. Arch Surg 1973;106:407–413.
71. Miller FB, Richardson JD, Thomas HA. Role of CT in the diagnosis of major arterial injury artery blunt thoracic trauma. Surgery (St. Louis) 1989;106:596.
72. Ben-Menachem Y. Assessment of blunt aortic-brachiocephalic trauma: should angiography be supplemented by transesophageal echocardiography? J Trauma 1997;42:969.
73. Fabian TC, Davis KA, Gavant M, et al. Prospective study of blunt aortic injury: helico-CT is diagnostic and antihypertensive therapy reduces rupture. Ann Surg 1998;227:666–677.
74. Dyer DS, Moore EE, Ilke DN, et al. Thoracic aortic injury: how predictive is mechanism and is chest computed tomography a reliable screening tool? A prospective study of 1561 patients. J Trauma 2000;48:673–682.
75. Marin ML, Veith FJ, Panetta TF et al. Transluminally placed endovascular stented graft repair of arterial trauma. J Vasc Surg 1994;20:466–473.
76. Mattox KL. Fact and fiction about management of aortic transection. Ann Thorac Surg 1989;48:1.
77. Williams JS, Graff JA, Uku JM, et al. Aortic injury in vehicular trauma. Ann Thorac Surg 1994;57:726.
78. Feczko JD, Lynch L, Pless JE, et al. An autopsy case review: 142 non-penetrating (blunt) injuries of the aorta. J Trauma 1992;33:846.
79. Parmley LF, Mattingly TW, Marian WC, et al. Nonpenetrating traumatic injury of the aorta. Circulation 1958;17:1086.
80. Avery JE, Hail DP, Adams JE. Traumatic rupture of the thoracic aorta. South Med J 1979;75:653.
81. McCollum CH, Graham JM, Noon GP, et al. Chronic traumatic aneurysms of the thoracic aorta: an analysis of 50 patients. J Trauma 1979;19:248.
82. Katyal D, McLellan BA, Brenneman FD, et al. Lateral impact motor vehicle collisions: significant cause of blunt traumatic rupture of the thoracic aorta. J Trauma 1997;42:769.
83. Warren RL, Akins CW, Conn AKT, et al. Acute traumatic disruption of the thoracic aorta: emergency department management. Ann Emerg Med 1992;21:391.
84. Pate JW, Fabian TC, Walker WA. Traumatic rupture of the aortic isthmus: an emergency? World J Surg 1995;19:119.
85. Pate JW, Galvant ML, Weiman DS, et al. Traumatic rupture of the aortic isthmus: program of selective management. World J Surg 1999;23:59–63.
86. Wall MJ Jr, Hirshberg A, Lemaire SA, et al. Thoracic aortic and thoracic vascular injuries. Surg Clin North Am 2001;81:1375–1393.
87. Von Oppell UO, Dunne TT, Degroot MK, et al. Traumatic aortic rupture: twenty-year meta-analysis of mortality and risk of paraplegia. Ann Thorac Surg 1994;58:585.

88. Fabian TC, Richardson JD, Croce MA, et al. Prospective study of blunt aortic trauma: multicenter trail of the American Association for the Surgery of Trauma. J Trauma 1997;42:374–383.
89. Cowley RA, Turney SZ, Hankins JR, et al. Rupture of thoracic aorta due to blunt trauma: a 15 year experience. J Thorac Cardiovasc Surg 1990;100:652.
90. Mattox KL, Holtzman M, Pickard LR, et al. Clamp/repair: a safe technique for the treatment of blunt injury to the descending thoracic aorta. Ann Thorac Surg 1985;40:456.
91. Hilgenberg AD, Logan KL, Akins CW, et al. Blunt injuries of the thoracic aorta. Ann Thorac Surg 1992;53:233.
92. Johnson RH Jr, Wall MJ, Mattox KL. Innominate artery injury: a thirty year experience. J Vasc Surg 1993;17:134.
93. Asensio JA, Chahwan S, Hanpeter D, et al. Operative management and outcome of 302 abdominal vascular injuries. AAST-OIS correlates well with mortality. Southwestern Surgical Congress. Am J Surg 2000;180:528–534.
94. Carrillo EH, Bergamini TM, Richardson JD. Abdominal vascular injuries. J Trauma 1997;43:164.
95. Cox CF. Blunt abdominal trauma. A 5-year analysis of 870 patients requiring celiotomy. Ann Surg 1984;199:467.
96. Feliciano DV, Bitondo CG, Mattox KL, et al. Civilian trauma in the 1980s. A 1-year experience with 456 vascular and cardiac injuries. Ann Surg 1984;199:717.
97. Roth SM, Wheeler JR, Gregory RT, et al. Blunt injury of the abdominal aorta. J Trauma 1997;42:748.
98. Feliciano DV. Pitfalls in the management of peripheral vascular injuries. Probl Gen Surg 1986;3:101.
99. Richardson JD, Bergimini TM, Spain DA, et al. Operative strategies for the management of abdominal aortic gunshot wounds. Surgery (St. Louis) 1996;120:667.
100. Feliciano DV. Abdominal vascular injury. In: Moore EE, Feliciano DV, Mattox KL, eds. Trauma, 5th ed. New York: McGraw-Hill, 2004.
101. Moore EE, Cogbill TH, Jurkovich GJ, et al. Organ injury scaling. III: Chest wall, abdominal vascular, ureter, bladder, and urethra. J Trauma 1992;33:337–339.
102. Acola KD, Feliciano DV, Mattox KL, et al. Management of injuries to the suprarenal aorta. Am J Surg 1987;154:613.
103. Fullen WD, Hunt J, Altemeier WA. The clinical spectrum of penetrate injury to the superior mesenteric arterial circulation. J Trauma 1972;12:656.
104. Reilly PM, Rotondo MF, Carpenter JP, et al. Temporary vascular continuity during damage control: intraluminal shunting for proximal superior mesenteric artery injury. J Trauma 1995;39:757.
105. Acola KD, Feliciano DV, Mattox KL, et al. Management of injuries to the superior mesenteric artery. J Trauma 1986;26:313.
106. Pennington CJ, Gwaltney N, Sweitzer D. Microvascular repair of jejunal and ileal vessels for near complete mesenteric avulsion after seat-belt injury. J Trauma 2000;48:327.
107. Stone HH, Fabian TC, Turkelson ML. Wounds to the portal venous system. World J Surg 1992;6:335.
108. Davis TP, Feliciano DV, Rozycki GS, et al. Results with abdominal vascular trauma in the modern era. Am Surg 2001;67:565.
109. Oldhafer KJ, Freker M Winkler M, et al. Complex inferior vena cava and renal vein reconstruction after abdominal gunshot injury. J Trauma 1999;46:721.
110. Ravikumar S, Stahl WM. Intraluminal balloon catheter occlusion for major vena cava injuries. J Trauma 1985;25:458.
111. Porter JM, Ivatury RR, Islam SZ, et al. Inferior vena cava injuries: noninvasive follow-up of venorrhaphy. J Trauma 1997;42:913.
112. Klein SR, Baumgartner FJ, Bongard FS. Contemporary management strategy for major inferior vena caval injuries. J Trauma 1994;37:35.
113. Tyburski JG, Wilson RF, Dente C, et al. Factors affecting mortality rates in patients with abdominal vascular injuries. J Trauma 2001;50:1020.
114. Gonzalez RP, Falimirski M, Holevar MR, et al. Surgical management of renal trauma: Is vascular control necessary? J Trauma 1999;47:1039.
115. Murphy J, Borman K, Dawidson I. Renal autotransplantation after horseshoe kidney injury: a case report and literature review. J Trauma 1996;40:840–844.
116. Feliciano DV. Abdominal vascular injury. In: Moore EE, Feliciano DV, Mattox KL, eds. Trauma, 5th ed. New York: McGraw-Hill, 2004.
117. Carrol PR, McAnninch JW, Klosterman P, Greenblatt M. Renovascular trauma: risk assessment, surgical management, and outcome. J Trauma 1990;30:547.
118. Haas CA, Dinchman KH, Nasrallah PF, et al. Traumatic renal artery occlusion: a 15-year review. J Trauma 1998;45:557.
119. Rothenberger DA, Fischer RP, Perry JF Jr. Major vascular injuries secondary to pelvic fractures: an unsolved problem. Am J Surg 1978;136:660.
120. Landerscasper RJ, Lewis DM, Synder WH. Complex iliac arterial trauma: autologous or prosthetic vascular repair. Surgery (St. Louis) 1993;114:9.
121. Feliciano DV. Approach to major abdominal vascular injury. J Vasc Surg 1988;7:730.
122. Salam AA, Stewart MT. New approach to wounds of the aortic bifurcation and inferior vena cava. Surgery 1985;98:105.
123. Vitelli CE, Scalea TM, Phillips TF, et al. A technique for controlling injuries to the iliac vein in a patient with trauma. Surg Gynecol Obstet 1988;166:551.
124. Burch JM, Richardson RJ, Martin RR, Mattox KL. Penetrating iliac vascular injuries: experience with 233 consecutive patients. J Trauma 1990;30:1450.
125. Mays ET, Wheeler CS. Demonstration of collateral arterial flow after interruption of hepatic arteries in man. N Engl J Med 1974;290:993.
126. Flint LM Jr, Polk HC Jr. Selective hepatic artery ligation: limitations and failures. J Trauma 1979;19:319.
127. Patcher HL, Drager S, Godfrey N, et al. Traumatic injuries of the portal vein. Ann Surg 1979;189:383.
128. Ivatury RR, Nallathambi M, Lankin DH, et al. Portal vein injuries. Noninvasive follow-up of venorrhaphy. Ann Surg 1987;206:733.
129. Stone HH, Fabian TC, Turkleson ML: Wounds of the portal venous system. World J Surg 6:335,1982.
130. Peterson SR, Sheldon GF, Lim RC Jr. Management of portal vein injuries. J Trauma 1979;19:616.
131. Feliciano DV. Management of traumatic retroperitoneal hematoma. Ann Surg 1990;211:109.
132. Khaneja SC, Pizzi WF, Barie PS, et al. Management of penetrating juxtahepatic inferior vena cava injuries under total vascular occlusion. J Am Coll Surg 1997;184:469.
133. Biffl W, Moore EE, Franciose R. Venovenous bypass and hepatic vascular isolation as adjuncts in the repair of destructive wounds to the retrohepatic vena cava. J Trauma 1998;45:400.
134. DeBakey ME, Simeone FA. Battle injuries of the arteries in World War II: an analysis of 2,471 cases. Ann Surg 1946;123:534.
135. Hughes CW. Arterial repair during the Korean War. Ann Surg 1958;147:555.
136. Jahnke EJ, Seeley SF. Acute vascular injuries in the Korean War: an analysis of 77 consecutive cases. Ann Surg 1953;138:158.
137. Ferguson IA, Byrd WM, McAfee K. Experiences in the management of arterial injuries. Ann Surg 1961;153:980.

138. Fryberg ER, Schinco MA. Peripheral vascular injury. In: Mattox KL, Moore EE, Feliciano DV, eds. Trauma. New York: McGraw Hill, 2005.
139. Rich NM, Baugh JH, Hughes CW. Acute arterial injuries in Vietnam: 1000 cases. J Trauma 1970;10:359.
140. Oller DW, Rutledge R, Clancy T, et al. Vascular injuries in a rural state: a review of 978 patients from a state trauma registry. J Trauma 1992;32:740–745.
141. Guede JW, Hobson RW, Padberg FT, et al. The role of contrast arteriography in suspected arterial injuries of the extremities. Am Surg 1985;51:89.
142. Weaver FA, Yellin AE, Bauer M, et al. Is arterial proximity a valid indication for arteriography in penetrating extremity trauma? A prospective analysis. Arch Surg 1990;125:1256.
143. Applebaum R, Yellin AE, Weaver FA, et al. The role of routine arteriography in blunt lower extremity trauma. Am J Surg 1990;160:221.
144. Kendall RW, Taylor DC, Salvian AJ, O'Brien PJ. The role of arteriography in assessing vascular injuries associated with dislocations of the knee. J Trauma 1993;35:875.
145. Miranda FE, Dennis JW, Veldenz HC, Dovgan PS, Frykberg ER. Confirmation of the safety and accuracy of physical examination in the evaluation of knee dislocation for injury of the popliteal artery: a prospective study. J Trauma 2002;52:247.
146. Johansen K, Lynch K, Paun M, Copass M. Non-invasive vascular tests reliably exclude occult arterial trauma in injured extremities. J Trauma 1991;31:515.
147. Dennis JW, Frykberg ER, Veldenz HC, et al. Validation of non-operative management of occult vascular injuries and accuracy of physical examination alone in penetrating extremity trauma: 5 to 10 year follow-up. J Trauma 1998;44:243.
148. Meissner M, Paun M, Johansen K. Duplex scanning for arterial trauma. Am J Surg 1991;161:552.
149. Schwartz M, Weaver FA, Yellin AE, Ralls P. The utility of color flow Doppler examination in penetrating extremity arterial trauma. Am Surg 1993;59:375.
150. Gagne PJ, Cone JB, McFarland D, et al. Proximity penetrating extremity trauma: the role of duplex ultrasound in the detection of occult venous injuries. J Trauma 1995;39:1157.
151. Reber PU, Patel AG, Sapio NLD, et al. Selective use of temporary intravascular shunts in coincident vascular and orthopedic upper and lower limb trauma. J Trauma 1999;47:72.
152. Pasch AR, Bishara RA, Lim LT, et al. Optimal limb salvage in penetrating civilian trauma. J Vasc Surg 1986;3:189.
153. Perry MO, Thal ER, Shires GT. Management of arterial injuries. Ann Surg 1971;173:403.
154. Granchi T, Schimittling Z, Vasquez J, et al. Prolonged use of intraluminal arterial shunts without systemic anticoagulation. Am J Surg 2000;180:493.
155. Sise MJ, Shackford SR. Extremity vascular trauma. In: Rich NM, Mattox KL, Hirshberg A, eds. Vascular Trauma, 2nd ed. Philadelphia: Elsevier Saunders, 2004.
156. Ballard JL, Bunt TJ, Malone JM. Management of small artery vascular trauma. Am J Surg 1992;164:316.
157. Ocrutt MB, Levine BA, Gaskill HV, et al. Civilian vascular trauma of the upper extremity. J Trauma 1986;26:63.
158. Soto JA, Munera F, Morales C, et al. Focal arterial injuries of the proximal extremities: helical CT arteriography as the initial method of diagnosis. Radiology 2001;218:188.
159. Shackford S, Rich N. Peripheral vascular injury. In: Feliciano DV, Moore EE, Mattox KL, eds. Trauma, 3rd ed. Norwalk: Appleton & Lange, 1996:819.
160. Sitzmann JV, Ernst CB: Management of arm arterial injuries. Surgery 1984;96:896.
161. Feliciano DV, Bitondo CG, Mattox KL, et al. Civilian trauma in the 1980s: a one year experience with 456 vascular and cardiac injuries. Ann Surg 1984;199:717.
162. Feliciano DV, Herskowitz K, O'Gorman RB, et al. Management of vascular injuries in the lower extremity. J Trauma 1988; 28:319.
163. Hafez HM, Woolgar J, Robbs JV. Lower extremity injury: results of 550 cases and review of risk factors associated with limb loss. J Vasc Surg 2001;33:11212.
164. Frykberg ER. Popliteal vascular injuries. Surg Clin N Am 2002;82:67.
165. Zamir G, Berlatzky Y, Rivkind A, et al. Results of reconstruction in major pelvic and extremity venous injuries. J Vasc Surg 1998;28:901.
166. Timberlake GA, Kerstein MD. Venous injury: to repair or ligate, the dilemma revisited. Am Surg 1995;61:139.
167. Nypaver TJ, Schuler JJ, McDonnell P, et al. Long-term results of venous reconstruction after vascular trauma in civilian practice. J Vasc Surg 1992;16:762.
168. Velmahos GC, Toutouzas KG. Vascular trauma and compartment syndromes. Surg Clin N Am 2002;82:125.
169. Ward MM. Factors predictive of acute renal failure in rhabdomyolysis. Arch Intern Med 1988;148:153.
170. Shah PM, Wapnir I, Babu S, et al. Compartment syndrome in combined arterial and venous injury of the lower extremity. Am J Surg 1989;158:136.
171. Lagerstorm CF, Reed LR, Rowlands BJ, et al. Early fasciotomy for acute clinically evident post-traumatic compartment syndrome. Am J Surg 1989;158:36.

30

Traumatic Injury of the Spine

Justin F. Fraser, John Boockvar, and Roger Hartl

Acute injury to the spine is a major cause of morbidity in trauma patients. Of 39.15 million reported injury-related emergency department visits in 2002, 5.1% (1.997 million) were related to the spine.[1] The incidence of traumatic spinal cord injury (SCI) alone is estimated to be 11,000 to 14,000 cases per year in the United States, with an estimated annual cost of medical and supportive care exceeding $9.7 billion.[2–7] SCI are particularly debilitating; more than 50% of patients with SCI are between 16 and 30 years old.[2] In the acute trauma setting, SCI may be missed if appropriate clinical and radiographic tests are not performed. For example, in a 10-year retrospective study, Poonnoose et al. found that among 569 patients with SCI, 9.1% of the diagnoses were missed initially; in 50% of missed cases, mismanagement resulted in worsened neurological status.[8,9] The medical and fiscal costs of caring for spine injuries are high, and spinal pathology, especially if undiagnosed, may complicate the prognosis and treatment of the trauma patient. Outcome depends highly on appropriate management, skilled surgical intervention, and management of comorbid conditions. As such, it is important to approach the patient with a potential traumatic injury of the spine with an accurate understanding of potential pathology and stability, to manage the patient appropriately.

Epidemiology

Of the types of spinal trauma, injuries to the cervical spine are the most common, can be the most debilitating, and also can be missed if effective diagnostic modalities are not used. Cervical spine injuries occur in 2% to 3% of all trauma patients, accounting for approximately 60% (1.2 million) of spine-related injury emergency department visits in 2002 (inclusive of SCI and bony/ligamentous injuries).[1,10] Although the most common site of cervical injury is C5, approximately 20% of cervical spine injuries involve the axis (C2), with odontoid fracture representing the most common type of C2 injury.[7,11–16] Careful diagnosis of suspected cervical injuries is important in patients with traumatic brain injury (TBI), as several investigators have demonstrated an approximate 5% incidence rate of spine injury in patients with concurrent head injury.[17,18] In overall blunt polytrauma, the rate of cervical spine injury is reported to be 2% to 12%.[19–26] In a survey of all members of the Orthopedic Trauma Association (OTA) and of 1000 members of the North American Spine Society (NASS), Harris et al. found 48% of OTA and 40% of NASS respondents admitted having missed an occult neck injury, mostly located from C2 to C6.[10] Therefore, effective and appropriate diagnosis of cervical spine injury in the trauma patient is crucial.

Spine Trauma, Spinal Cord Injury, and Outcome

In considering spine trauma diagnosis and treatment, understanding the functional outcome for patients suffering acute spinal injuries is important. In a retrospective series of 1500 trauma patients, Akmal et al. found that 263 patients (17.5%) had sustained injuries to the spinal column.[27] Mortality was significantly higher in patients with spinal injury (27% versus 20%, respectively).[27] Functional recovery can be quantified by the Functional Independence Measure (FIM): FIM of 126 implies total independence, whereas 18 implies total dependence.[27] Akmal et al. found that functional scores were poor using the FIM in spine trauma patients who survived, but mean FIM scores at 12-month follow-up were significantly improved from initial presentation (124 versus 86, respectively).

Other factors contribute to outcome, such as age and comorbid conditions. Age plays an important epidemiological role in stratifying pathological risk profile for different injuries of the spine. In a study of adult versus geriatric (more than 65 years old) patients with spinal fractures, Irwin et al. found that geriatric patients had fewer cervical injuries, lower-force injuries, less severe injuries, and decreased paralysis, but greater pre-existing morbidity; decreased probability of surgical intervention resulted in significantly higher 60-day mortality (9.7% versus 1.6%).[6] Although the presence of comorbidities and paralysis significantly worsened mortality in both adult and geriatric populations, surgical intervention

TABLE 30.1. Summary of Evidence-Based Guidelines for the Management of Acute Spine and Spinal Cord Injury.

Preadmission Spine Immobilization
Level III
- All patients with actual or potential cervical spine injury should be immobilized at the scene and during transport
- A combination of a rigid cervical collar and supportive blocks or a backboard with straps is recommended for limiting motion of the cervical spine

Transportation of Patients with Acute, Traumatic Spinal Cord Injury
Level III
- Expeditious and careful transport is recommended to the nearest capable definitive care medical facility

Clinical Assessment-Neurological Examination
Level III
- American Spine Injury Association standards for neurological and functional classification of spinal cord injury are preferred as the examination tool for evaluation of acute spinal cord injury.

Clinical Assessment-Functional Outcome Assessment
Level II
- Use the Functional Independence Measure (FIM) score for functional outcome assessment

Level III
- Use the modified Barthel Index for functional outcome assessment

Radiographic Assessment of the Cervical Spine in Asymptomatic Trauma Patients
Level I
- Radiographic assessment of the cervical spine is not recommended in trauma patients who are awake, alert, and not intoxicated, who are without neck pain or tenderness, and who do not have distracting associated injuries

Radiographic Assessment of the Cervical Spine in Symptomatic Trauma Patients
Level I
- Three-view [anteroposterior, lateral, odontoid (open-mouth)] plain radiographs are recommended. Supplement the plain films with computed tomography (CT) to define areas that are suspicious or not well visualized on the plain cervical X-rays

Level III
- Discontinue spine immobilization in awake patients with neck pain or tenderness and normal radiographic studies after dynamic flexion/extension radiographs or a magnetic resonance imaging (MRI) study is obtained within 48h of injury
- Discontinue spine immobilization in obtunded patients after dynamic flexion/extension radiographs under fluoroscopic guidance, or after MRI, or at the discretion of the treating physician

Pharmacological Therapy After Acute Spinal Cord Injury
Level III
- Treatment with methylprednisolone for either 24 or 48h is recommended, but should be undertaken only with the knowledge that evidence of harmful side effects is more consistent than evidence of clinical benefit
- Treatment with GM1 ganglioside is recommended as an option without demonstrated clinical benefit

Prophylaxis of Venous Thromboembolic Disease
Level I
- Prophylaxis of venous thromboembolic disease is recommended
- Low molecular weight heparin, rotating beds, adjusted-dose heparin, or a combination are recommended as prophylaxis
- Low-dose unfractionated heparin with pneumatic compression stockings or electrical stimulation is recommended as prophylaxis

Level II
- Low-dose unfractionated heparin alone is not recommended
- Oral anticoagulation alone is not recommended

Level III
- Duplex Doppler ultrasound, impedance plethysmography, or venography is recommended for diagnostic use
- A 3-month duration of prophylaxis is recommended

Inferior vena cava filter placement is recommended for patients who do not respond to anticoagulant prophylaxis, or when anticoagulants or mechanical devices are contraindicated

Initial Closed Reduction of Cervical Spine Fracture-Dislocation Injuries
Level III
- Early closed reduction with craniocervical traction is recommended in awake patients
- Closed reduction is not recommended in patients with an additional rostral injury
- Patients with cervical spine fracture-dislocation injuries who cannot be examined should undergo MRI before attempted reduction
- Evaluate with MRI those patients who fail closed reduction
- The value of pre-reduction MRI in patients with facet subluxation is unclear

Management of Acute Spinal Cord Injury in the Intensive Care Unit (ICU) or Monitored Setting
Level III
- Management of patients with acute spinal cord injury in an ICU or similar monitored setting is recommended, particularly with severe cervical level injury
- Use of cardiac, hemodynamic, and respiratory monitoring devices is recommended after acute spinal cord injury

was associated with a significantly decreased 60-day mortality rate in both groups.[6] Surgical candidates must be selected appropriately, and initial trauma management should include appropriate neurological monitoring, effective care of comorbid conditions, and skillful surgical intervention when appropriate.

Initial Assessment and Intervention

Initial assessment and intervention are vitally important elements in the treatment of traumatic injuries to the spine. All patients with blunt trauma should be assessed, but clinical suspicion of spinal injury should be especially high in patients presenting after motor vehicle collisions and falls, two of the most common causes. As with any trauma patient, clinicians should assess and treat according to the "ABC" algorithm: stabilization of airway, breathing, and circulation are integral to the primary trauma survey. In particular, continuous blood pressure monitoring is essential as hemodynamic instability may result from high cervical injury and loss of sympathetic adrenergic tone. Although only Class III data exist regarding blood pressure maintenance after SCI, the American Association of Neurological Surgery/Congress of Neurological Surgeons (AANS/CNS) recommend a mean arterial pressure of 85–90mmHg for at least 7 days postinjury as a treatment option.[28] Proper immobilization of the spine in the field, during transport, and in the trauma bay is vital. Up to 25% of SCIs may occur during the process of transport and assessment after the initial trauma.[29–32] Although no Class I or Class II data exist to validate strict restriction of spinal movement for trauma patients, the Section on Disorders of the Spine and Peripheral Nerves of the American Association of Neurological Surgeons and the Congress of Neurological Surgeons (AANS/CNS) guidelines recommends that all trauma patients with cervical spine injury or a mechanism for spine injury be immobilized both in the field and at the care center before investigation of possible spine pathology[29] (Table 30.1). Given

TABLE 30.1. (continued)

Blood Pressure Management after Acute Spinal Cord Injury
Level III
- Hypotension (systolic blood pressure <90 mmHg) should be avoided if possible, or corrected as soon as possible
- Maintain mean arterial blood pressure 85–90 mmHg for the first 7 days after acute spinal cord injury

Nutritional Support
Level III
- Nutritional support is recommended. Energy expenditure is best determined by indirect calorimetry

Spinal Cord Injury Without Radiographic Abnormality (SCIWORA)
Diagnosis

Level III
- Plain X-rays and CT are recommended with attention to the suspected level of neurological injury
- MRI may be useful with attention to the suspected level of neurological injury
- Consider plain X-rays of the entire spinal column; neither spinal angiography nor myelography is recommended

Treatment

Level III
- Immobilize the spine until stability is confirmed by flexion-extension views
- Consider empiric spine immobilization for up to 12 weeks
- Avoid "high-risk" activities for up to 6 months

Prognosis

Level III
- MRI may be useful for prognostication

Atlanto-Occipital Dislocation
Diagnosis

Level III
- Lateral cervical spine plain film is recommended for diagnosis
- Upper cervical prevertebral swelling on an otherwise nondiagnostic plain X-ray should prompt additional testing
- CT may be useful if there is clinical suspicion and plain films are nondiagnostic

Treatment

Level III
- Use of internal fixation and arthrodesis is recommended. Traction may be used but causes a 10% risk of neurological deterioration

Isolated Fracture of the Atlas
Level III
- Base treatment on the specific fracture type. Fractures without disruption of the transverse atlantal ligament may be treated with immobilization alone. With ligament injury, surgical fixation and fusion is an option

Isolated Fracture of the Axis
Odontoid

Level II
- Fractures in patients over the age of 50 years should be considered for surgical fixation

Level III
- Treat types I, II, and III with cervical immobilization
- Type II and III fractures may be treated surgically with dens displacement >5 mm, comminuted type II fracture (type IIa), or failure of external immobilization

"Hangman's"

Level III
- This fracture may be managed initially with cervical immobilization in most cases. Consider surgical fixation with severe angulation of C2 on C3, disruption of the C2–C3 disk space, or failure of external immobilization

Management of Combined Fractures of Atlas and Axis
Level III
- Base management on the specific characteristics of the axis fracture. External immobilization is possible for most fracture combinations (see original guideline document for detailed consideration of specific fracture combinations)

Treatment of Subaxial Cervical Spine Fracture
Facet dislocation

Level III
- Closed or open reduction is recommended
- Rigid external immobilization, anterior arthrodesis with plate fixation, or posterior arthrodesis is recommended
- Prolonged bed rest in traction is recommended if more contemporary treatment methods are not available

Injuries without facet dislocation

Level III
- Closed or open reduction is recommended
- Rigid external immobilization, anterior arthrodesis with plate fixation, or posterior arthrodesis is recommended

Management of Acute Central Cervical Spinal Cord Injury
Level III
- ICU monitoring is recommended, especially with neurological deficits
- Maintain mean arterial blood pressure 85–90 mmHg for the first 7 days after injury
- Early reduction is recommended
- Spinal decompression is recommended, particularly if cord compression is focal and anterior

Vertebral Artery Injury
Diagnosis

Level III
- Angiography or MR angiography is recommended after blunt cervical trauma in the setting of complete cord injuries, fracture through the transverse foramen, facet dislocation, or vertebral subluxation

Treatment

Level III
- Anticoagulate with intravenous adjusted-dose heparin if there is evidence of posterior circulation stroke
- Observe or anticoagulate with intravenous adjusted-dose heparin if there is evidence of posterior circulation ischemia
- Observe patients with injury if there is no evidence of posterior circulation ischemia

Source: American Spinal Injury Association: International Standards for Neurological Classification of Spinal Cord Injury, revised 2002; Chicago, IL. American Association of Neurological Surgery/Congress of Neurological Surgeons (AANS/CNS): the primary source document is published as a supplement to Neurosurgery 2002;50:S1–S199. Level I in the source document is called a "standard." Level II in the source document is called a "guideline." Level III in the source document is called an "option." Some statements are paraphrased for clarity. If the level of evidence is omitted under a subject heading, no statement was made. Consult the source document for clarifications, review of the primary data sources, or recommendations for pediatric patients.

the risk of further injury, such a protocol is necessary to protect the spine and spinal cord.

Frequent, reproducible neurological examinations are necessary. A basic neurological examination assesses mental status, cranial nerves, motor strength and tone, sensation, reflexes (including Babinski and bulbocavernosus), and coordination. Additionally, tenderness over the spine can be an important sign of blunt trauma and biomechanical injury. There are several functional scales for assessment and prognostication. Frankel et al. provided one of the first grading scales for patients with neurological lesions.[33] Currently, the AANS/CNS guidelines recommend the American Spinal Injury Association (ASIA) rating system for neurological examination and the FIM for functional outcome assessment based upon studies demonstrating interrater reliability and prognostic significance.[34–40] An abbreviated form of the ASIA scale is often employed clinically to determine prognosis from acute SCI (Figs. 30.1, 30.2). This condensed scale permits rapid understanding of disease severity, potential morbidity, and prognosis (Table 30.2). In addition, it is important to assess sacral sparing, as it portends a better prognosis. Data from the Model Spinal Cord Injury Systems (a 10-year follow-up of 3585 patients with SCI) demonstrated that, in patients with motor-complete lesions with some sensory preservation (ASIA B), sacral sparing increased the chance of recovery to motor-incomplete status from 13.3% to 53.6%.[16] For this reason, assessment of the bulbocavernosus and anal *wink* reflexes is especially important.

Acute Medical Intervention

Several acute medical interventions have been explored as adjuncts to spine immobilization. Stability of the airway and hemodynamics must be underscored. Cervical spine injury may induce changes in regulation of sympathetic tone, resulting in hemodynamic instability. For this reason, SCI patients should be observed in an ICU setting for at least 48 to 72h, with particular attention to blood pressure management [mean arterial pressure (MAP) >85–90mmHg].

An intervention studied in randomized prospective trials is high-dose methylprednisolone. The National Acute Spinal Cord Injury Study (NASCIS) was established in 1975, and was followed by NASCIS II (1992).[41,42] Analysis of NASCIS II data supported early administration of methylprednisolone (MP) for complete and partial SCI.[43] In 1997, NASCIS III was published, representing the most current large-scale prospective randomized trial studying MP in acute SCI. In NASCIS III, 499 patients with acute SCI received either MP (initial bolus of 30mg/kg), followed by an infusion (5.4mg/kg/h) for either 24h (24MP) or 48h (48MP), or tirilazad, a 21-aminosteroid (2.5mg/kg bolus every 6h) for 48h (48T).[44] The study found significant neurological improvement for the 48MP group at 6 weeks ($P = 0.04$) and 6 months ($P = 0.01$) if therapy was initiated within 3 to 8h posttrauma, by post hoc subgroup analyses. However, the 48MP group also demonstrated significantly higher rates of pneumonia (48MP 5.8%, 24MP 2.6%, 48T 0.6%; $P = 0.02$) and possibly severe sepsis (48MP 2.6%, 24MP 0.6%, 48T 0%; $P = 0.07$).[44] As such, the study group recommended methylprednisolone bolus (30mg/kg) followed by 24-h infusion (5.4mg/kg/h) for therapy initiated less than 3h posttrauma, and methylprednisolone bolus (30mg/kg) followed by 48-h infusion (5.4mg/kg/h) for therapy initiated 3 to 8h posttrauma,[44] without strong underlying support from the data. There are several detrimental effects of high-dose MP, as demonstrated by other retrospective and small prospective studies.[45,46] Additionally, McCutcheon et al. found in a random retrospective analysis of 1227 patients with acute SCI that MP administration among patients surviving to discharge was associated with significantly higher hospital charges ($41,831 vs. $24,258; $P < 0.01$) and longer length of stay (17.7 versus 13.8 days; $P < 0.01$).[47] However, patients who received MP were significantly younger (mean, 39.5 versus 44.2 years; $P < 0.05$) and injured more severely ($P < 0.05$).[47] That the MP data are not compelling is reflected by the controversy surrounding its use. In a survey of 41 trauma medical directors, only 48.7% believed that the data regarding MP treatment of SCI supported its use.[48] Such contradicting opinion is reflected in the AANS/CNS guidelines and in the Canadian Neurosurgical Society recommendations, which declared MP administration to be a treatment option, rather than as a guideline or standard of care, in the management of acute SCI.[45,49,50]

The naturally occurring GM1 ganglioside has also been studied in clinical trials for SCI. Early studies in the 1990s culminated in the Sygen Multicenter Acute Spinal Cord Injury Study to evaluate GM1 ganglioside as a neuroprotective agent in SCI. Seven hundred sixty eligible patients were randomized to three groups (placebo, low-dose GM1, high-dose GM1); all groups received the NASCIS II protocol for MP before starting the treatment intervention, which was given daily for 56 days.[51] Primary functional and neurological outcome endpoints showed no differences among groups, but GM1 ganglioside-treated patients showed earlier marked recovery ($P = 0.01$ for all treated versus placebo)[51] as a secondary endpoint despite the fact that patients in the study could

ASIA IMPAIRMENT SCALE

- ☐ **A = Complete:** No motor or sensory function is preserved in the sacral segments S4-S5.
- ☐ **B = Incomplete:** Sensory but not motor function is preserved below the neurological level and includes the sacral segments S4-S5.
- ☐ **C = Incomplete:** Motor function is preserved below the neurological level, and more than half of key muscles below the neurological level have a muscle grade less than 3.
- ☐ **D = Incomplete:** Motor function is preserved below the neurological level, and at least half of key muscles below the neurological level have a muscle grade of 3 or more.
- ☐ **E = Normal:** Motor and sensory function are normal

CLINICAL SYNDROMES

- ☐ Central Cord
- ☐ Brown-Sequard
- ☐ Anterior Cord
- ☐ Conus Medullaris
- ☐ Cauda Equina

FIGURE 30.1. An abbreviated version of the American Spinal Injury Association (ASIA) Impairment Scale for spinal cord injury. (From Standard Neurological Classification of Spinal Cord Injury, American Spinal Injury Association, 2000, by permission. Available at: http://www.asia-spinalinjury.org/publications/2001_Classif_worksheet.pdf.)

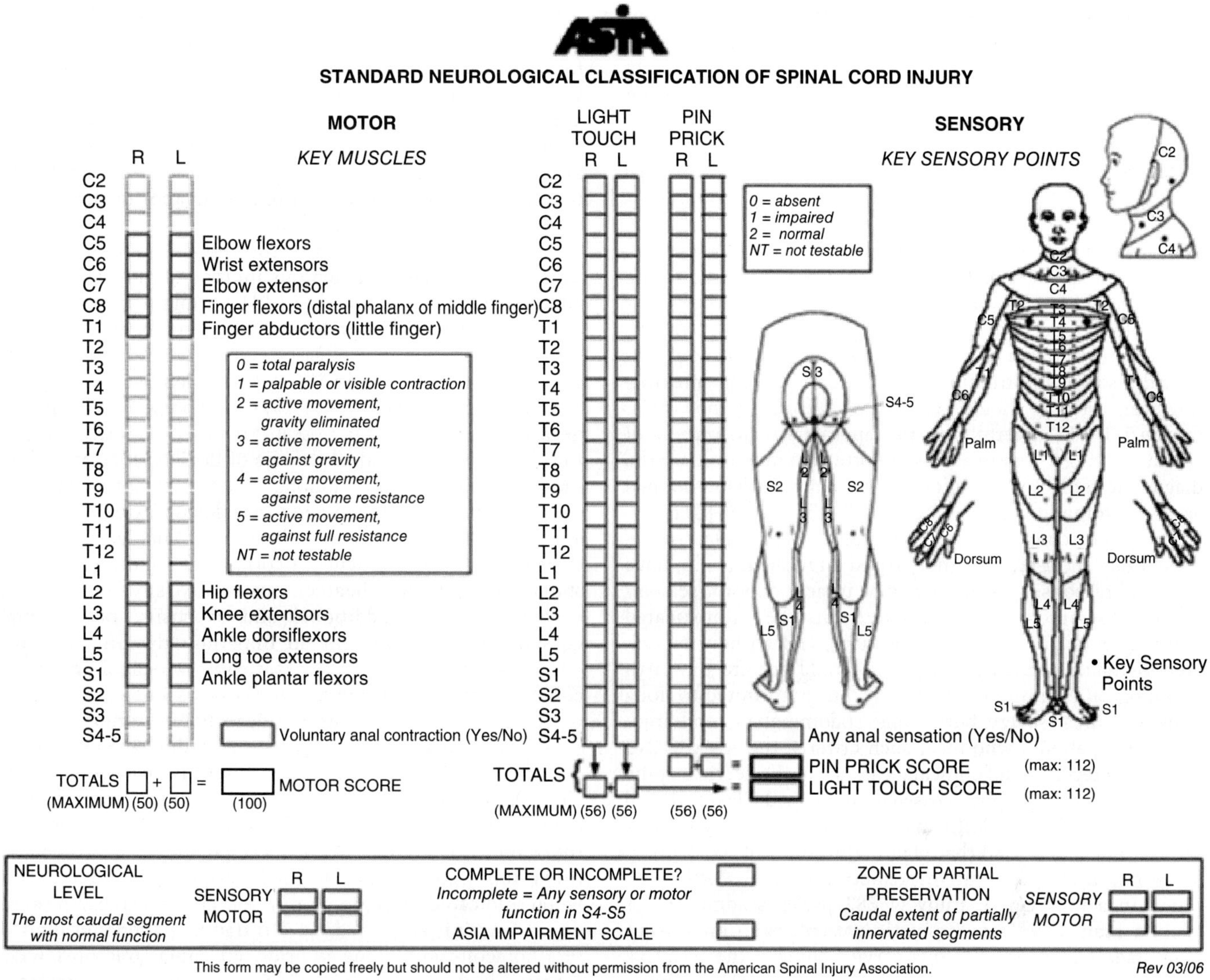

FIGURE 30.2. The ASIA grading scale and classification of spinal cord injury. (From Standard Neurological Classification of Spinal Cord Injury [American Spinal Injury Association], 2000, by permission. Available at: http://www.asia-spinalinjury.org/publications/2001_Classif_worksheet.pdf.)

not receive GM1 ganglioside until 24 to 48h postinjury. Although not the primary endpoint, the data suggest that the utilization of GM1 ganglioside (300-mg loading dose followed by 100mg/day × 56 days) may be useful for SCI. Given the lack of major adverse effects (other than a modest, transient increase in serum total cholesterol and triglyceride concentration), the AANS/CNS guidelines recommend GM1 ganglioside administration after MP administration as an additional treatment option for SCI.[45]

TABLE 30.2. Morbidity of Spinal Injury Based on American Spinal Injury Association (ASIA) Grade.

ASIA grade at admission	*ASIA grade at 1 year (%)*					*Duration to readmission for medical morbidity (months ± SE)*
	A	*B*	*C*	*D*	*E*	
A	84.6	7.3	5.8	2.3	0	35.9 ± 3.1
B	7.8	19.4	38.0	33.3	1.5	25.9 ± 5.0
C	3.1	1.3	25.1	66.7	3.8	36.3 ± 4.1
D	0	0	1.4	94.4	4.2	59.6 ± 3.6

Source: From Middleton JW, Lim K, Taylor L, et al. Spinal Cord 2004;42:359–367, with permission.

Finally, in the acute setting, cervical traction is a useful tool for cervical injuries. Traction provides not only a method for stabilizing the cervical spine from further dislocation but also a tool for closed reduction of fractures. Data regarding cervical traction lack Class I or II evidence, limiting the AANS/CNS Guidelines to list it as a treatment option for early closed reduction of cervical spine fracture-dislocation injuries in awake patients.[52] Class III evidence from case series has demonstrated that early (<5–8h postinjury) closed reduction can improve overall outcome and ASIA scores (by 24h postinjury).[53,54] However, because of reported cases of worsened injury in patients with disk herniation, the AANS/CNS Guidelines have recommended prereduction magnetic resonance imaging (MRI) in patients who cannot be examined to evaluate for disk trauma; the presence of significant disk herniation is a relative indication for decompression before reduction of a cervical injury.[52] Although Class I data are needed to further evaluate the appropriate protocol for cervical traction, it represents an important tool for neurosurgeons in the initial management of cervical trauma. As such, early neurosurgical involvement in cervical trauma is vital if such tools are to be applied to aid in patient care.

Radiographic Assessment of Spine Trauma

Radiography is an essential tool for the diagnosis and management of spinal trauma. The armamentarium available to the clinician includes plain films of the spine [anteroposterior (AP), lateral, odontoid views, and flexion/extension views], CT, CT myelogram, and MRI. Each radiographic tool can provide some information for clinical decision making; however, imaging should be obtained selectively, not indiscriminately. In determining the appropriate utilization of spinal imaging for trauma, it is important to first evaluate the diagnostic tools for asymptomatic patients. Patients defined as asymptomatic must be neurologically normal (Glasgow Coma Scale score, GCS) 15, oriented to person/place/time, have intact short-term memory based on recall at 5 min, have a normal response to stimuli, and be intact on motor/sensory testing. Asymptomatic patients must also be unintoxicated (without evidence of drug/alcohol use), and without associated distracting injury (injuries that could prevent thorough neurological examination including, but not limited to, long bone fractures, severe burns, and abdominal visceral injuries).[55] For patients who meet such criteria, the AANS/CNS guidelines recommend clinical clearance of the cervical spine without any radiography,[56] based on published Class I, II, and III evidence. Of note, Hoffman et al. studied 4309 asymptomatic patients and found that plain radiographs of the cervical spine had a 99.9% negative predictive value.[55] Roth et al. found in a prospective study of 682 patients admitted for trauma that, of 96 asymptomatic patients who underwent plain radiography to rule out cervical injury, the negative predictive value in asymptomatic patients was 100%.[57] Therefore, in patients defined strictly as asymptomatic, spine imaging studies have a relatively low yield and are not recommended.

For patients not classifiable as asymptomatic, and for patients with suspicious presentations, radiographic assessment of the spine is recommended. The standard of care includes three-view cervical spine series (AP, lateral, odontoid) for initial evaluation, with cervical spine CT as a supplement for suspicious pathology or poorly defined anatomy,[58] supported by Class I, II, and III evidence. MacDonald et al., in a study of 775 motor vehicle injury victims, of whom 92 (12%) had cervical injuries, found that standard plain radiographs (including odontoid and swimmer's view) had a sensitivity of 83% and a specificity of 97%.[23] In a Class I prospective study of multiply injured patients, Berne et al. found that, among 58 patients who underwent three-view plain films and helical CT of the spine, the sensitivity of the plain films was 60% with a positive predictive value of 100%,[59] whereas for helical CT alone, the sensitivity was 90%, specificity 100%, and the positive predictive value 100%.[59] As such, although properly performed cervical plain films can be used to evaluate the cervical spine reliably in trauma patients, CT does have a demonstrated superiority in injury detection. Thin-cut (1-mm slice interval or less) spinal CT with coronal and sagittal reconstructions provides a more complete view of the anatomy.[59,60,61] In 360 trauma patients for whom plain radiographs could not adequately evaluate C7–T1, CT demonstrated fractures in 11 patients.[62] The authors of the study concluded through Medicare reimbursement data analysis that such a tool was cost-effective in averting sequelae of underdiagnosed injury.[62] As such, CT of the cervical spine provides an important tool in the evaluation of the symptomatic patient.

Flexion-extension views of the cervical spine have been utilized to evaluate ligamentous injury and movement-associated instability. In a study of 141 trauma patients studied with plain cervical films followed by flexion-extension views, Lewis et al. reported a negative predictive value of greater than 99%.[58,63] Flexion-extension views demonstrated spinal instability in 11 patients (of 141), of whom 4 had initially negative plain films.[63] Of those 4, 3 required surgical stabilization.[63] Brady et al. studied the use of flexion-extension films in 451 trauma patients; among 79 patients with abnormal initial plain films, 16 had abnormal flexion-extension films, and 4 required surgical stabilization.[64] Therefore, flexion-extension films can provide important information regarding spinal stability and ligamentous injury similar to MRI, without requiring additional and expensive radiographic equipment; they represent an important dynamic tool for clinicians evaluating trauma patients for spinal injury to complement static imaging.

There is little consensus regarding thoracolumbar imaging for blunt trauma. Thoracolumbar plain radiographs should be used in cases where lower spinal injury is suspected; suspicion should depend on mechanism of injury, neurological history and examination, and the presence of cervical or thoracolumbar injuries. AP and lateral thoracolumbar plain films, followed by more detailed imaging (CT and/or MRI) when indicated, can be useful for conscious patients in whom injury is suspected. Of 110 trauma patients evaluated for thoracolumbar spine injuries, all spinal fractures were detected in 94 patients with GCS greater than 11, whereas 4 of 9 injuries were missed initially in 16 patients with GCS less than 10 who sustained thoracolumbar injuries.[65] The risk of missed injury is increased with high-velocity injury, decreased level of consciousness, associated TBI, and pelvis/lower extremity injury.[65] Further, Samuels and Kerstein conducted a retrospective study of 756 blunt trauma patients, of whom 106 received thoracolumbar plain films.[66] Among the 55 patients with no clinical evidence of thoracolumbar injury, none had radiographic evidence of injury; however, among the 24 patients with clinical evidence of injury, 14 (58%) had abnormal findings on plain films.[66] Furthermore, in 20 patients whose clinical examinations were equivocal, 1 patient had radiographic evidence of injury.[66] Therefore, there is little evidence to support radiographic screening of the thoracolumbar spine in trauma patients without clinical evidence of injury. However, for patients with clinical findings or cervical spine fractures, or for patients who cannot be examined reliably because of distracting injury or poor mental status, plain radiographic interrogation of the thoracolumbar spine may identify injuries that otherwise might be missed.

CT myelography and MRI represent two other important tools in the evaluation of spinal injury. Detailed information about bony and ligamentous structures is provided by MRI, as well as defining injury and compression to the spinal cord and nerve roots. However, the high sensitivity of MRI raises the possibility of *overcall* of spinal injury (false-positive interpretation of MRI).[58] Benzel et al. studied with 174 MRI patients with symptomatic spinal trauma within 48 h of injury; of 62 patients with demonstrated MRI abnormalities, only 2 had unstable injuries, both of which were also demonstrated with plain films and CT.[67] As such, MRI is not recommended for routine screening for spinal injury. Rather, MRI is helpful for high-resolution definition of spinal anatomy and for detailed evaluation of known spinal injuries. The role of CT myelogram has been largely supplanted by MRI. In a 1988 comparison study of lesions of the cervical and thoracic spinal cord, MRI was equal or superior to CT myelography in depicting cord compression, cord atrophy, cord enlargement, and tissue characterization, and did not suffer limitations of artifact and cerebrospinal fluid (CSF) blockage. Additionally, MRI resolution and imaging have improved substantially since the late 1980s.[68] Despite such advantages, CT myelography can be used in patients unable to undergo MRI (e.g., implants of ferrous metals, permanent pacemakers) and can provide accurate information about spinal cord compression in cases of spinal injury.[69]

Injury detection requires appropriate selection of radiographic studies. However, once injury is identified, each type of study can play a role in understanding the severity, pathophysiology, and stability of the injury. Whereas plain films can assess sagittal and coronal balance of the spine, CT aids in determining the extent of bony injury, providing high-resolution visualization of bony collapse, comminution, and canal compromise. For assessment of spinal cord, ligamentous, and other soft tissue injuries, MRI is superior.

The severely injured or obtunded patient represents a particular dilemma for radiographic diagnosis of spinal injury. In such cases, especially for patients in whom no clinical examination can be obtained reliably for the first 48 to 72 h after injury, a clear methodology for ruling out spinal injury is lacking, with much variation in clinical practice.[22,70] Conservatively, some practitioners do not consider the cervical spine "cleared" despite adequate plain films and CT. As a result, multiple trauma patients without a reliable clinical examination may develop complications from prolonged immobilization including decubitus wounds and skin breakdown (especially of the occiput) from rigid (hard) cervical collars (resulting in substantial morbidity), or prolonged traction or immobilization without a therapeutic endpoint. Furthermore, hard collars provide a false sense of security; for example, Philadelphia collars have allowed 89° of passive flexion/extension, 142° of passive axial rotation, and 92° of passive lateral bending (compared to 141°, 190°, and 102°, respectively, without a collar).[71–74] Three-view cervical plain films are often stated to miss up to 10% of injuries in this patient population, but combining adequate three-view plain films with CT is estimated to reduce the false-negative rate to less than 1%.[24] Widder et al. conducted a 3-year prospective cohort study of obtunded, severely injured trauma patients (GCS < 9) in which patients had three-view plain films and CT scans.[74] Among 102 eligible patients with a mean GCS of 7.8, CT had sensitivity of 100% for detecting injury, whereas plain films had sensitivity and specificity (compared to CT) of 39% and 98%, respectively.[74] In a prospective study of 1006 patients with altered mental status or distracting injury, CT from occiput to T1 with sagittal/coronal reconstruction was compared to plain films; 116 patients had 172 cervical spine injuries. Plain films had sensitivity and specificity of 44% and 100%, whereas CT had sensitivity and specificity of 97.4% and 100%.[75] CT scan outperformed plain radiography as a screening tool for cervical spine injury. Therefore, cervical spine evaluation in the obtunded patient should include high-resolution cervical CT (occiput to T1) with sagittal/coronal reconstructions to rule out cervical injury, as well as thoracolumbar and AP/lateral films.

Cervical plain films and CT are well documented as static studies in obtunded trauma patients. A dynamic assessment of injury is also important, as it aids in identifying patients with instability. In patients without reliable clinical examinations, who cannot report pain with movement, standard radiographic flexion-extension films should be avoided, as the spine is not visualized during forced movement. Another modality advocated previously for obtunded patients is bedside fluoroscopy. Bolinger et al. evaluated bedside fluoroscopic flexion-extension evaluation in 56 comatose trauma patients. All patients had previously normal plain films, and some had normal CT scans; fluoroscopic flexion-extension views identified 1 type II odontoid fracture and missed important instability (C6–C7 dislocation) in 1 patient.[76] Furthermore, visualization to the C7–T1 motion segment was achieved in only 4% of patients.[76] Therefore, bedside fluoroscopy provides a dynamic study that may identify fractures not seen on static studies, but, more importantly, evaluates ligamentous injury and associated instability. However, such a study must entail adequate visualization from the occiput to the C7–T1 junction; without proper visualization, important injuries may be missed. Therefore, in trauma patients without a clinical examination, an adequate static study must be followed by an adequate dynamic study to rule out ligamentous injury or instability under motion. By combining static and dynamic imaging, one can effectively minimize missed cervical injuries.

Traumatic Injuries to the Spine

Atlanto-Occipital Dislocation

Atlanto-occipital dislocation (AOD) is an uncommon, yet devastating, spine injury. Biomechanically, there is a disruption of the normal anatomical relationship between the altas (C1) and the occiput, an abnormality that frequently results in death. It has been estimated that traumatic AOD accounts for 6% to 8% of all traffic fatalities.[77–81] Traynelis et al. classified AOD into three types: type I, anterior displacement of the occiput relative to the atlas; type II, a longitudinal distraction injury without subluxation (Fig. 30.3); and type III, a posterior displacement of the occiput on the atlas.[82] A number of measurements of anatomic relationships exist to assess AOD on sagittal cervical films, including methods by Dublin et al., Powers et al., and Wholey et al.[83–85] The Powers ratio, probably the best known, represents the ratio of the basion-posterior atlas arch distance to the opistheion-anterior atlas arch distance. A Powers ratio greater than 1 is considered abnormal.[84] However, in later studies of reliability, the Powers ratio, along with the other aforementioned measurements, was found to be a poor screening tool for AOD, as its tested

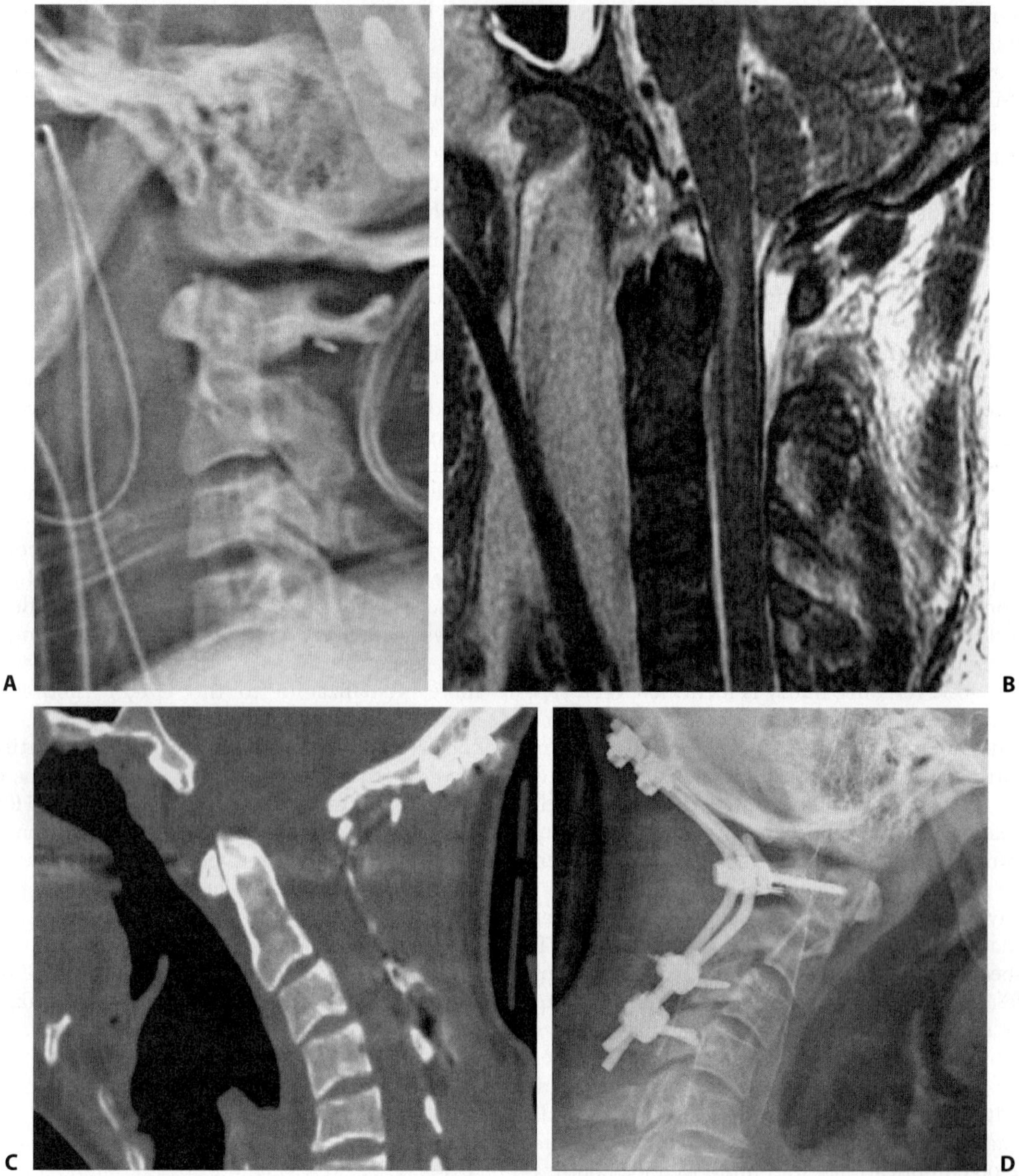

FIGURE 30.3. A 33-year-old firefighter forced to jump several stories from a building presented after becoming acutely quadriplegic. Type II atlanto-occipital dislocation was noted (**A**), with a hematoma anterior to the cord (**B**), causing neurological deficits; the patient was an ASIA B with intact sensorium. The distraction of the occipital-dental interval is notable on computed tomography (CT) (**C**), and the patient underwent occipital-cervical fusion (**D**). After rehabilitation, the patient ambulates with assistance.

sensitivity ranged from 33% to 60%.[86,87] The most recent method of diagnosis, and the most reliable in published literature, is the basion-axial interval–basion-dental interval (BAI-BDI) method.[88] This method, described by Harris et al., involves measurement of the basion to the posterior axial line (rostral extension of posterior cortex of the axis body) and the basion to rostral tip of the dens (basion–dental interval).[89] In both cases, the interval should be less than 12 mm in adults, and the BAI should be less than 12 mm in children under 13 years of age (BDI is not reliable in children).[86] Even through the use of such measurements, AOD can be missed easily; as such, prevertebral soft tissue swelling noted on plain film, lower cranial nerve findings, or craniocervical subarachnoid hemorrhage (SAH) should raise suspicion for AOD and prompt more specific radiographic investigation with CT or MRI.[88,90,91]

Once diagnosed, atlanto-occipital dislocation should be approached with caution, as there is a risk of further neurological deterioration with manipulation. As there are reported cases of deterioration as a result of manipulation, traction is generally not recommended.[88] No Class I evidence exists evaluating the treatment of AOD; the recommended treatment is surgical internal fixation and arthrodesis, typically with an occipital-cervical fusion.[88] Although a case of vagus nerve (CN X) damage as an operative complication has been reported, the majority of reported cases of AOD treated with surgical fixation resulted in neurological improvement at follow-up.[88,91]

Atlanto-Axial Dislocation

Atlanto-axial dislocation (AAD) generally carries less morbidity than AOD, and can involve either rotatory or anterior-posterior subluxation. These injuries should be suspected in patients who have suffered flexion-extension injuries with or without a rotatory component.[81] In cases with an intact transverse ligament, the dislocation is often rotatory. In the case of rotatory subluxation, patients may be treated with cervical traction, starting with 7 to 8 lb in children and 15 lb in adults.[92] Nonsurgical immobilization (typically by halo vest) may also be used to treat rotatory subluxation, although patients with long-standing subluxation refractory to halo immobilization should be treated with arthrodesis after traction. More ominous than rotatory subluxation is anterior atlanto-axial dislocation, which results in neurological deficit or death in approximately one-third of patients. Altanto-dental interval (ADI; the distance between the anterior margin of the dens and the closest point of the C1 anterior arch) provides a useful measurement on lateral cervical plain film for assessing anteroposterior atlanto-axial dislocation. An ADI greater than 3 mm in males, greater than 2.5 mm in females, and greater than 4 mm in children 15 years or younger suggests disruption of the transverse ligament and should prompt further radiographic investigation by CT or MRI. To underscore the severity of this injury relative to isolated rotational subluxation, Fielding and Hawkins published a classification system for atlanto-axial fixation: type I indicates rotatory fixation with less than 3 mm of anterior displacement of C1 on C2; type II indicates the presence of transverse ligament injury with less than 5 mm of displacement; type III indicates complete disruption of the transverse ligament with greater than 5 mm of displacement; and type IV indicates posterior displacement, and can be associated with odontoid injuries.[81,93] Such classification systems underscore the importance of the transverse ligament in maintaining C1–C2 stability. For patients with atlanto-axial dislocation, fusion is the treatment of choice for patients with disruption of the transverse ligament or with irreducible subluxation. As such, CT and MRI are essential diagnostic tools for therapeutic planning.

Fractures of C1: The Jefferson Fracture

The Jefferson fracture represents a burst fracture of the anterior and posterior arches with or without rupture of the transverse atlantal ligament. First described by Cooper in 1822, it is named for Jefferson, who reviewed cases of C1 fractures in 1920.[94,95] The Jefferson fracture is typically the result of impact trauma, including motor vehicle crashes, falls from a height, equestrian accidents, and falling down stairs.[96] It may result in additional abnormalities of the atlanto-occipital and atlanto-axial joints, including subluxation and dislocation. Jefferson fractures comprise approximately 2% of all injuries to the cervical spine, although some publications quote the incidence to be as high as 13% of cervical spine fractures.[97–101] The diagnosis of the Jefferson fracture was made without the aid of CT or MRI, using only plain radiographs of the cervical spine after Spence et al. published cadaveric anatomic data measuring the relationship between the C1 lateral masses and C2.[102] The current "Rule of Spence" reflects the original C1–C2 relationships, confirmed by studies of anteroposterior radiographs, and adjusted for the magnification factor appreciated on open-mouth odontoid radiographic views (the view of choice for applying the "Rule of Spence"). Current publications suggest that, if the sum of the C1 lateral mass (summation of right and left) displacements on C2 is greater than 8.1 mm on open-mouth odontoid view radiographs, then a fracture of C1 should be suspected.[102–104] Should suspicion for injury to C1 be raised by a positive Rule of Spence, MRI represents the best test to assess the injury fully. Vital information about the transverse atlantal ligament is provided by MRI, the disruption of which defines a true unstable Jefferson fracture (as described by Jefferson). No Class I evidence exists to provide guidelines for treatment modalities, but it is generally accepted to treat C1 fractures with a hard collar or halo immobilization unless there is evidence of transverse atlantal ligament disruption. In such cases, most clinicians would consider the fracture unstable, and would treat with either halo immobilization or, more likely, with C1–C2 stabilization, internal fixation, and arthrodesis.[96,97] New techniques of transoral reduction and fixation provide some preservation of rotatory function to the atlanto-axial joint, although some controversy exists because these interventions do not address the disrupted transverse ligament.[100]

The Odontoid Fracture

One of the most common isolated bony injuries to the cervical spine is the odontoid fracture. Odontoid fractures represent up to 60% of all axis fractures and up to 18% of all cervical spine fractures (range, 5%–18%).[105–109] Odontoid fractures are classified into three types—I, II (may include a IIa subtype), and III—based on the system devised by Anderson and D'Alonzo.[11] Type I represents an oblique avulsion fracture at the superior third of the odontoid above the transverse ligament, and the avulsed fragment remains attached to the alar ligament. Rare (1%–5% of odontoid fractures) and considered stable in isolation, these fractures can be associated with atlanto-occipital dislocation, and their diagnosis of a type I odontoid fracture should raise suspicion of AOD.[110] Type II represents the most common type of odontoid fracture, and is defined as a fracture between the dens and C2 body crossing the base of the odontoid body (Fig. 30.4). Hadley et al. added the IIa subtype, defined as a type II fracture with comminution at the base, usually with associated free fragments; they considered this subtype to be extremely unstable, with an inability to obtain reduction and realignment, and requiring surgical fixation.[111] Type III represents a fracture of the odontoid extending into the C2 body. These fractures are often considered simple fractures of the body of the axis. Utilizing such a classification system, much has been published on therapeutic approaches to the odontoid fracture.

Treatment recommendations for odontoid fractures depend upon their classification. Cervical hard collar and halo immobilization both are demonstrably successful in treating type I fractures.[27,110,112–114] Similarly, there has been some reported success in treating type III fractures with cervical hard collar therapy or halo immobilization. Published fusion rates for cervical hard collar therapy vary from 50% to 65%, whereas those for halo immobilization vary from 84% to 100%.[7,113–116] It is recommended to consider each patient's anatomy individually in approaching type III fractures. In cases of dens displacement greater than 5 mm, or if the frac-

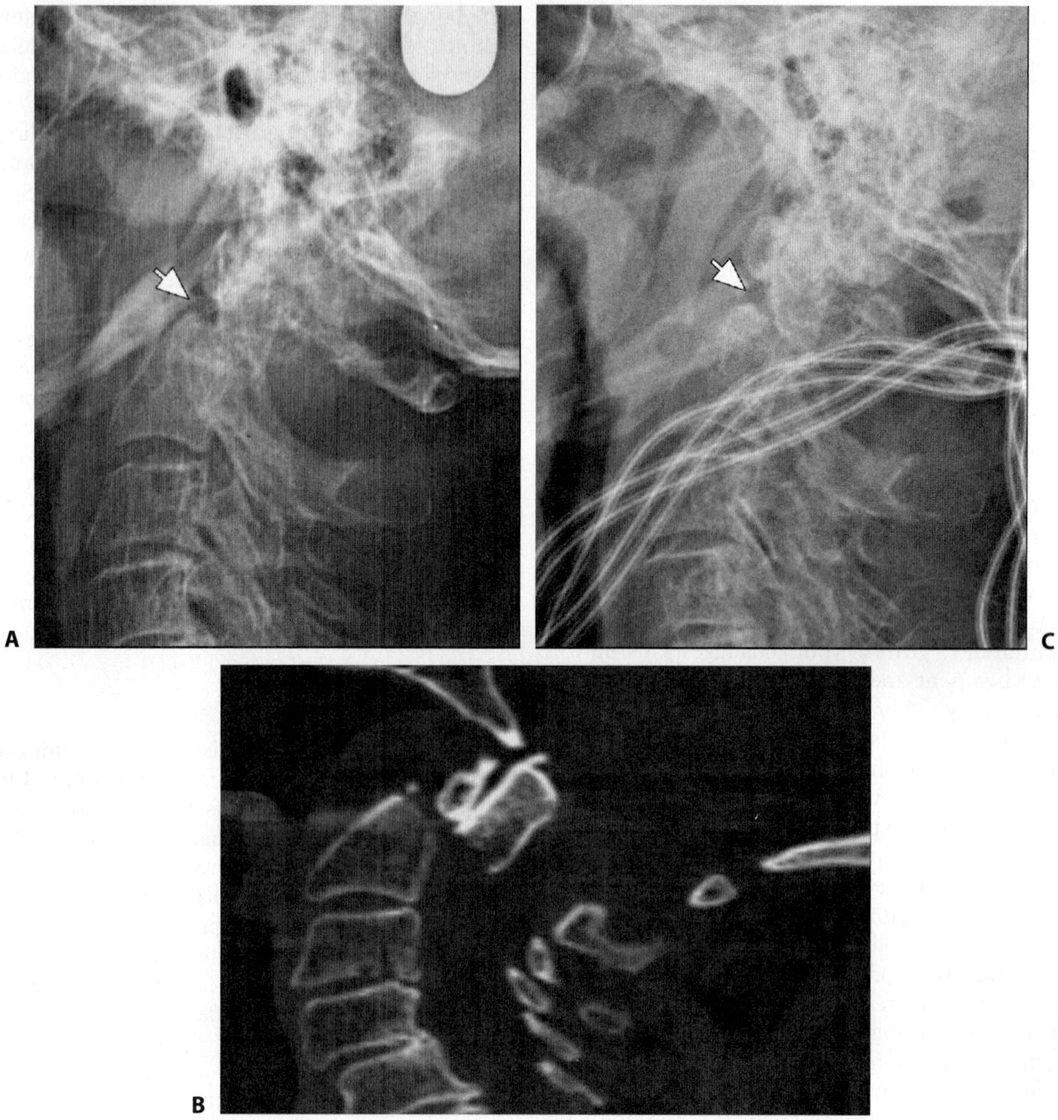

FIGURE 30.4. A 70-year-old man presented with neck pain after a fall related to a syncopal episode; he was neurologically intact on examination. CT demonstrated a type II dens fracture with significant angulation (**A**). A magnetic resonance image (MRI) demonstrated soft tissue swelling into the canal without compromise to the spinal cord (**B**). The patient underwent surgical fixation with an odontoid screw and remained without neurological deficit (**C**).

ture is close to the neck of the odontoid, the probability of nonunion from external immobilization is higher; such fractures may require internal fixation.[108,113,117] Type II fractures, as compared to types I and III, have a poor fusion rate with external immobilization, ranging in the literature from 35% to 85%.[105,108,113,115,118] Predictors of poor fusion include initial displacement greater than 6 mm, age greater than 40 years, posterior displacement of the odontoid, delay in diagnosis, and marked fracture angulation (>10°).[108,114] Of particular note, there is Class II evidence suggesting that patients older than 50 years with type II fractures are at 21-fold-higher risk of nonunion than those under age 50; based on this evidence, the AANS/CNS Guidelines recommend surgical stabilization and fusion as a treatment guideline for type II fractures.[117,119] Furthermore, Hadley et al. recommend surgical stabilization and fixation for type IIa fractures for reasons of instability and the tendency toward nonunion.[111] Surgical treatment options for odontoid fractures include posterior atlanto-axial arthrodesis and direct anterior odontoid screw fixation. Anterior screw fixation preserves atlanto-axial joint mobility, has a published fusion rate of 90% to 100%, and is also indicated for elderly patients.[7,120–123] However, contraindications to anterior screw fixation include an established nonunion, irreducible fracture, osteoporosis or osteopenia preventing solid screw purchase, and known unstable injury to the transverse ligament.[81,124] More research is necessary to elucidate the absolute indications and contraindications for different methods of surgical fixation in odontoid fractures, but it is clear that a precise diagnosis is necessary so that appropriate treatment modalities may be planned.

Traumatic Spondylolisthesis of the Axis: The Hangman's Fracture

Traumatic spondylolisthesis of the axis is aptly named "the Hangman's Fracture," as it represents a hyperextension injury in which the isthmus of C2 is broken bilaterally as the occipital base provides shear forces on the posterior structures of C2.[125,126] Additional injury may occur in the soft tissue structures (ligaments and disks) of C2 and C3.[126] In addition to being hanged, motor vehicle crashes, falls, and cranial angled impact injuries such as diving may cause a hangman's fracture.[117,127] A number of classification systems have been used to define traumatic spondylolisthesis injuries to C2, but the most recognized is that published by Levine and Edwards, which represents a modification of the Effendi classification.[128,129] Type I injuries typically result from a hyperextension-axial loading force and represent a fracture of the C2 pars interarticularis with less than 3 mm of displacement and no angulation. Type II injuries typically result from the same mechanism, but are followed by severe flexion; they represent fractures of the pars interarticularis with more than 3 mm of displacement and with substantial angulation. Type IIa injuries result from flexion-distraction and involve a fracture of the pars interarticularis with minimal or no displacement but substantial angulation, and with C2–C3 unilateral or bilateral facet dislocation. Type III injuries result from flexion-compression with rebound extension and involve a displacement of an anterior fragment with angulation, C2–C3 facet dislocation, and C2–C3 disk space disruption.[128,129] According to Levine and Edwards, type I injuries are stable and require only hard collar immobilization, whereas type II injuries require more rigid halo immobilization (type II injuries benefit from initial traction, whereas type IIa injuries worsen with traction but reduce with mild extension); type III injuries are unstable and require surgical fixation.[129] Vaccaro et al. also found halo immobilization to be effective in treating type II and IIa fractures, especially in patients with angulation less than 12°.[130] Few data exist to support one treatment over another, but it is generally recognized that type I fractures, the most common type (approximately 65%), can be treated with immobilization via halo or hard collar.[114,117,128] Absent any Class I evidence to support surgical management of hangman's fractures, the AANS/CNS guidelines support surgical stabilization and fixation in cases of severe angulation (some type II and type IIa fractures) and in cases of disk space disruption (type III).[117] Additionally, for patients with combination fractures of C1 and C2, the prevailing standard is to treat according to the type of C2 injury.[131,132]

Lower Cervical Spine Fractures

Fractures from C3 to C7 are classified using several different systems, but the most recognized is based upon the mechanism of injury. This system, developed by Allen et al., divides lower cervical injuries into mechanistic categories: compression flexion (resulting in anterior vertebral body fractures with kyphosis and teardrop fractures), distraction flexion (resulting in locked facets and ligamentous injury; Fig. 30.5), vertical compression (burst fracture with or without retropulsion), compression extension (facet fracture), distraction extension (anterior longitudinal ligament disruption with superior retrolisthesis), flexion alone (facet dislocation), and extension alone (spinous process fractures with or without lamina fractures).[133] Such a system provides distinct diagnostic categories for each fracture, but the management of lower cervical injuries requires an assessment of spinal stability. White and Panjabi categorized clinical criteria for stability assessment; some important elements include spinal cord or nerve root damage, change in radiographic or clinical examination with traction, abnormal disk anatomy, congenital canal stenosis, anterior-posterior displacement greater than 3.5 mm, sagittal plane angulation greater than 11°, and sagittal plane rotation.[134] The presence of such factors should prompt further radiographic investigation with CT and MRI. Particular fracture types that are recognized easily on plain cervical films are the teardrop fracture (a compression flexion injury) and locked facets (a distraction flexion injury). A teardrop fracture is an oblique fracture through the vertebral body with resulting posterior displacement of the inferior fracture margin into the spinal canal.[135] Radiographic findings can include a "teardrop" shape of bone displaced anteriorly from the vertebral body (may be confused with an avulsion fracture), a large triangular portion of the vertebral body representing the inferior fracture margin, disrupted facet joints, soft tissue swelling (soft tissue shadow greater than 5–7 mm from C2–C4 and 22 mm from C5–C7 in adults).[92,136] If a teardrop fracture is suspected, it should be evaluated fully and ruled out definitively, as teardrop fractures are generally considered unstable and require fusion in most cases because of retropulsion of the inferior fragment into the central canal. Locked facets occur from distraction flexion injury and involve unilateral or bilateral dislocation of the facets with reversal of the normal relationship. Typical radiographic signs of unilateral locked facets include ipsilateral rotation of the spinous processes superior to the locked facet on AP plain films and a "bow-tie" sign on lateral plain film (visualization of the left and right facets at the level of the injury that are normally superimposed). Treatment choices for locked facets include traction and surgical reduction/stabilization; the employment of one over the other depends upon factors affecting stability in each patient.

Thoracic and Lumbar Spine Fractures: A Three-Column Injury Model

In assessing injury to the thoracolumbar spine, the biomechanical relationships inherent in the anatomy must be understood. Denis developed a biomechanically based system for classifying thoracolumbar injuries known as the three-column model (Fig. 30.6).[137] The anterior column is defined as the anterior half of the vertebral body and intervertebral disk and includes the anterior longitudinal ligament and the anterior annulus fibrosus. The middle column is defined as the posterior half of the vertebral body and disk and includes the posterior longitudinal ligament. The posterior column is defined as the posterior spinal bony complex, including the facet joints, the ligamentum flavum, the spinous processes, and supraspinous and interspinous ligaments. Injuries to just one part of one column are generally considered stable and include isolated transverse process fractures (posterior column), isolated pars interarticularis fractures, and spinous process fractures.[92] Similarly, evidence of injury to multiple columns should prompt the consideration of instability until further diagnostic studies can elucidate clearly the extent of injury. Current classification of thoracolumbar fracture injuries is based upon the column model, the classification system developed by McAfee, and more recent systems that account for mechanism of injury as well as factors affecting instability.[138–141] Major thoracolumbar injuries are divided

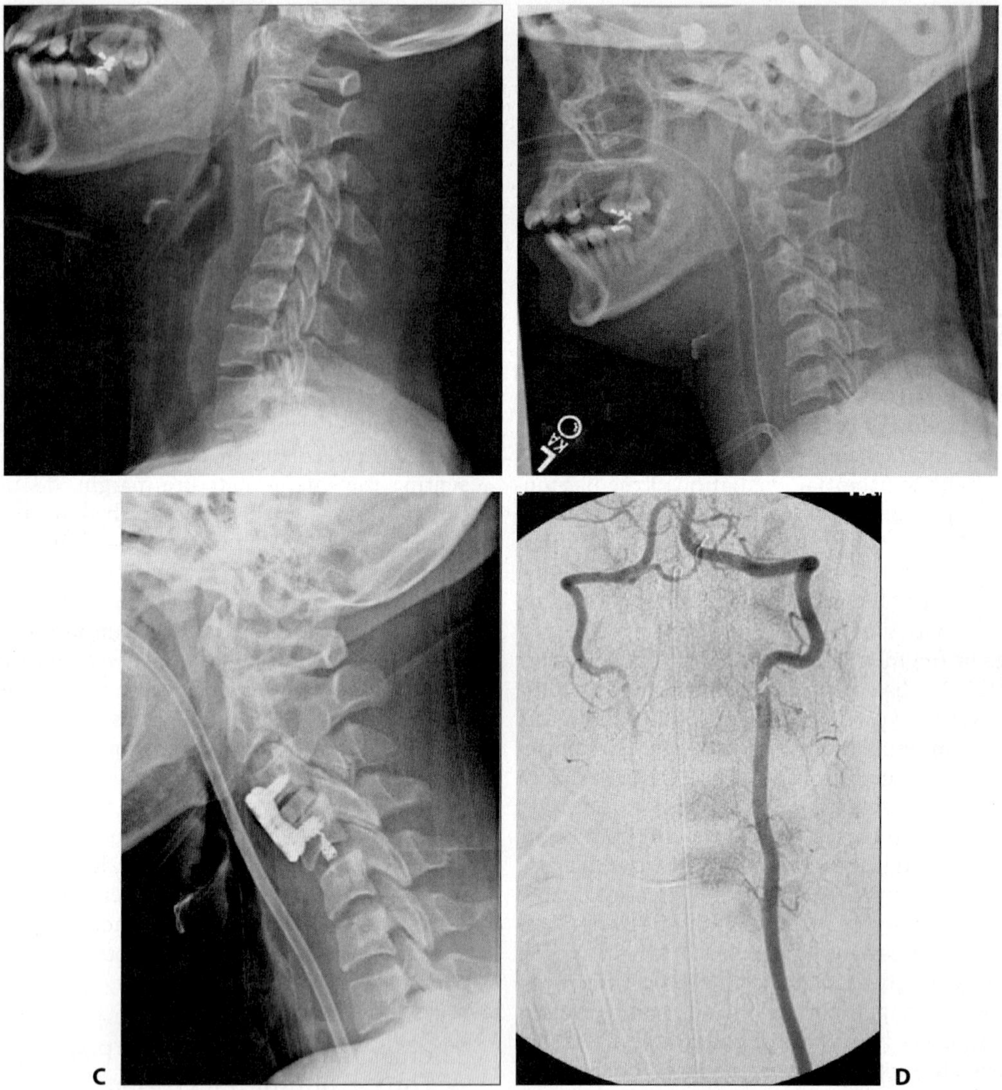

FIGURE 30.5. A 26-year-old woman was pushed down a flight of stairs and presented neurologically intact with a C3–C4 acute fracture and subluxation (**A**). After 15 lb traction, her alignment corrected (**B**), and she was fused anteriorly (**C**). In addition, the patient underwent an angiogram that found a right vertebral dissection (**D**); the vessel was occluded intentionally after collateral cross-filling was noted.

into four categories: compression fractures, burst fractures, flexion-distraction fractures (also called Chance or seat-belt-type fractures), and fracture-dislocations. A compression fracture reflects a failure of the anterior column, with an intact middle column, possibly resulting in a wedge kyphotic deformity. These fractures involve no significant loss of height of the vertebral body, no subluxation, and no neurological deficit, but do disrupt the vertebral body anterior endplate. Most occur from T11 to L2 and are the result of a motor vehicle crash or fall.[142] In assessing the resulting kyphosis for these and other types of fractures, the Cobb angle (angle measured between the superior endplate of the next cephalad vertebral body and the inferior endplate of the next caudal vertebral body) may be helpful both to monitor preoperative kyphotic progression and to assess postoperative reduction and fixation. Although generally considered stable, worsening kyphosis by measurement may result in refractory pain and instability, necessitating more aggressive therapy. As such, patients with compression fractures should be followed clinically and radiographically.

Burst fractures result from an axial load on the spine and cause failure of the anterior and middle columns (see Figure 30.6). These fractures result from falls from height and motor vehicle crashes. Typical radiographic findings include loss of vertebral body height both anteriorly and posteriorly, retropulsion of bone fragments from the endplates into the spinal canal, and widening interpedicular distance (on AP radiograph). Once diagnosed, stability must be assessed; there are no strict criteria, but the categorical standards of White and Panjabi apply.[134] Of note, loss of vertebral body height greater than 50% of normal is associated with progressive kyphosis and spinal stenosis and represents one factor favoring surgical intervention.[142,143] A prospective, randomized study comparing operative versus nonoperative treatment of thoracolumbar burst fractures without neurological deficit or disruption of the posterior ligamentous complex in 53 patients demonstrated no benefit in follow-up kyphosis, canal compromise, return to work, or postinjury pain for surgically treated patients.[144] Although this represents Class I evidence for nonoperative management, debate continues regarding the limi-

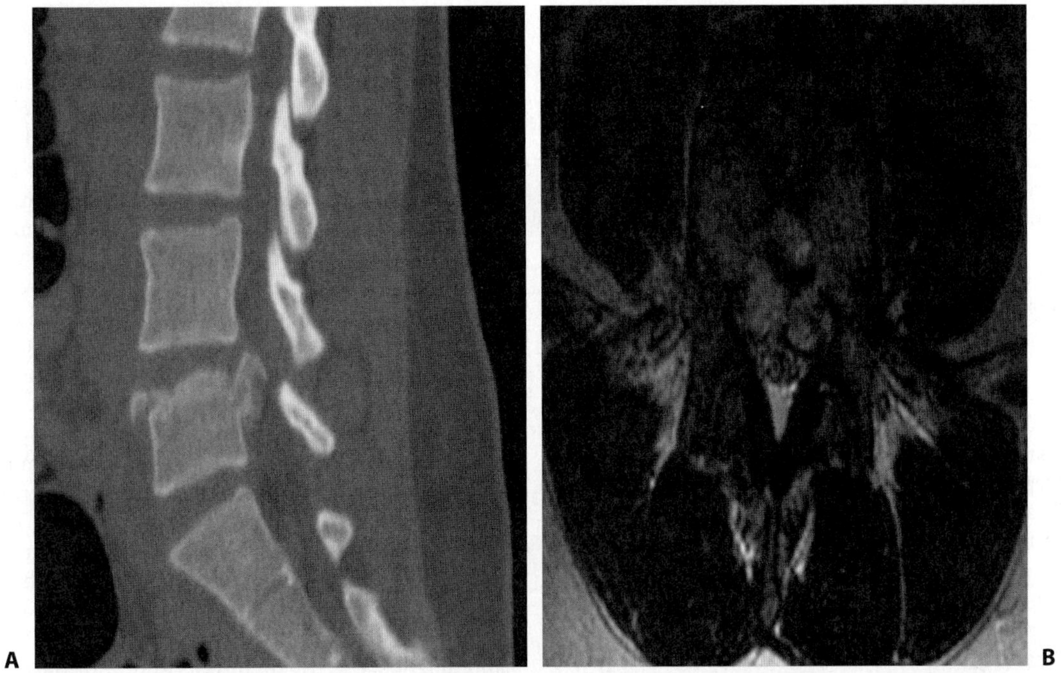

FIGURE 30.6. An 18-year-old female patient presented neurologically intact with an L5 burst fracture and canal stenosis. CT demonstrated bony retropulsion into the spinal canal (**A**), with approximately 50% canal compromise on MRI (**B**).

tations of this study (including the small sample size and integrity of the posterior ligamentous complex (PLC) as an exclusion criterion) and its clinical implications.[145,146] Thus, in evaluating burst fractures for appropriate treatment it is important to note neurological status and to obtain CT and MRI to evaluate the extent of retropulsion, kyphotic deformity, and PLC disruption.

Flexion-distraction injuries, commonly called Chance fractures (see Fig. 30.6), can result from high-speed motor vehicle crashes with a waist seatbelt but without shoulder belt (hence the "seat-belt-type" injury). Distraction of the middle and posterior columns (with possible mild compression injury to the anterior column) is the mechanism. Both CT and MRI are useful for full definition of anatomical abnormalities and assessment of the neural elements (cord and nerve roots). Typical plain radiographic findings include increased interspinous distances, fractures of the pars interarticularis, and pedicle/transverse process fractures. Patients may present frequently without neurological deficit, these fractures are typically considered unstable, and require some surgical intervention (usually posterior fixation).[138] Of note, Chance fractures are associated with a high rate of intra-abdominal injury (45%), and their diagnosis should prompt suspicion of visceral trauma.[142,147]

Finally, fracture-dislocations represent an injury to all three columns by shear, distraction, and rotational forces (Fig. 30.7). As they involve all columns, the rate of total neurological deficit is highest in this group.[143] Usually recognized

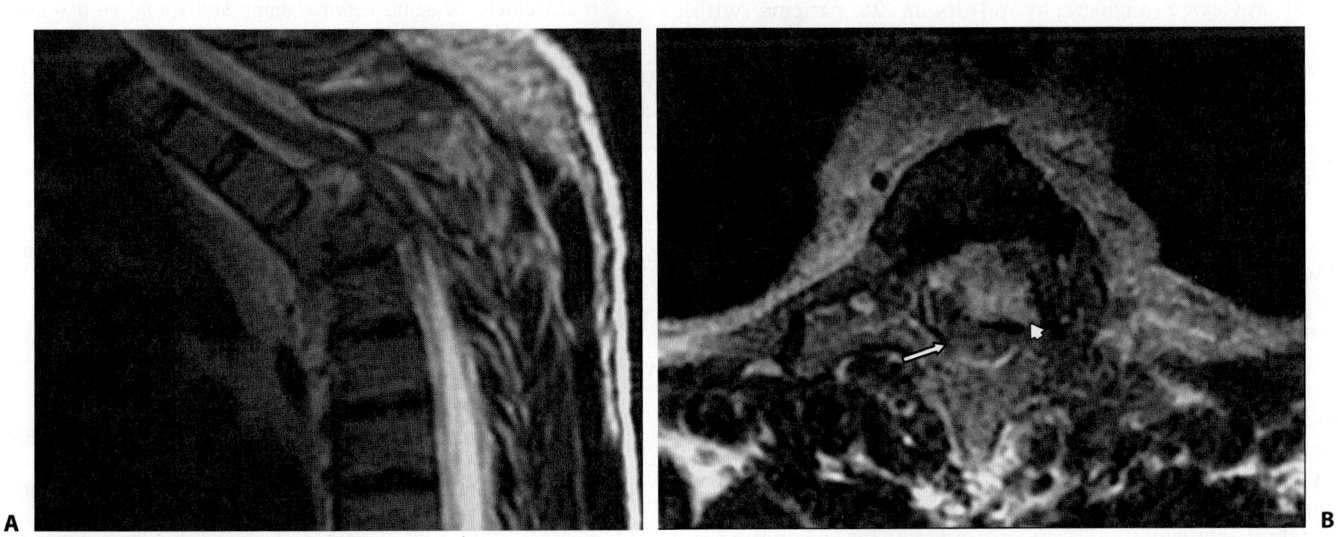

FIGURE 30.7. A 31-year-old man presented after a motorcycle crash and multiple trauma, an ASIA B with a fracture-dislocation. The fracture was demonstrated by MRI on sagittal (**A**) and axial (**B**) sequences, with retropulsing fragments, ruptured disk, hematoma (*thick arrow*), and compression of the spinal cord (*thin arrow*).

easily on plain radiograph by horizontal translation of spinal elements, they may sometimes be self-reduced at the time of imaging. As such, multiple rib fractures, spinous process fractures, and unilateral fractures through articular processes should raise suspicion for a fracture-dislocation.[92] In such cases, further imaging with CT and MRI is necessary as these fractures are considered unstable by definition; surgical reduction and fixation is the standard for such injuries.[138]

A system of classification by Vaccaro et al. adds additional elements to classification in an attempt to define a treatment algorithm. This system classifies injuries based upon morphometry (e.g., compression, translation/rotation, distraction), integrity of the posterior ligamentous complex (PLC), and neurological status.[140] Based loosely on the three-column model, this system incorporates clinical status into the calculation for treatment algorithm. Whereas a patient with a compression fracture, intact PLC, and intact neurological exam could be treated nonoperatively, a patient with a fracture dislocation and disrupted PLC requires stabilization. Debate still exists regarding the most appropriate treatment algorithms for management of thoracolumbar fractures, but clearly not all fractures are the same, and each patient requires an individualized approach that combines radiographic findings with clinical status.

Vascular Injury Associated with Spine Trauma

Cervical spine trauma may lead to an occult pathology that could result in thromboembolic events in the posterior circulation (see Figure 30.3D). Although vertebrobasilar stroke is a relatively rare cause of cerebral ischemia, it may be particularly devastating, as ischemic stroke of supplied structures, particularly the brainstem, results in substantial morbidity and mortality.[148,149] Typical injury mechanisms include motor vehicle crashes and pedestrians struck by motor vehicles, and have been reported to involve hyperflexion, hyperextension, and fracture-dislocations.[149] Willis et al. reviewed angiography results in 26 patients with blunt cervical injury (with locked facets, fractured facet joints, or fractures through the foramen transversarium); the incidence of vertebral artery injury was 46%.[150] Thus, the presence of such injuries should prompt suspicion of a vertebral artery injury. Workup should include CT angiogram (CTA), MR angiogram (MRA), or conventional angiography.[151] However, in a prospective examination of 216 patients with suspicions of blunt cerebrovascular injury (including patients with cervical spine fractures, LeFort II or III facial fractures, Horner's syndrome, skull base fractures involving the foramen lacerum, or neck soft tissue injury), Miller et al. found that CTA and MRA had sensitivities for vertebral artery injury of 53% and 47% respectively when compared with conventional angiography.[152] Debate continues regarding appropriate diagnostic workup for vertebral artery injury. As MR and CT technology improves, patients with traumatic injuries involving the vertebral course should be considered for angiographic workup to rule out injury.

Conclusion

It is vital to consider the possibility of spinal injury, particularly after blunt trauma, and to diagnose such injuries early. Spine injuries cause major morbidity, and can be missed easily on initial evaluation without proper and appropriate assessment. Clinical history (including a history of injury mechanism), neurological examination, and radiographic findings represent crucial components in the workup of spinal injury. Initial immobilization is key for prevention of further injury. Although requiring judicious use and consideration of risk/benefit, early utilization of steroids and possibly GM1 ganglioside may improve outcome. The most vital part of early care, however, is appropriate diagnosis. Suspicious findings on clinical examination and plain radiographs should be followed with more specific testing and imaging. Of equal importance is the need to ensure that screening radiographs are adequate; for example, a lateral cervical spine film must provide adequate visualization from the occiput to the C7–T1 joint complex. Finally, an understanding of the most common diagnoses, their causes, and their clinical and radiographic presentations provides a framework for prompt evaluation and diagnosis. With such tools and information, the clinician can evaluate the spine of the trauma patient with confidence and provide the early diagnosis that can improve profoundly the prognosis for the unstable spine.

References

1. McCaig LF, Burt CW. National Hospital Ambulatory Medical Care Survey: 2002 emergency department summary. Adv Data 2004;340:1–34.
2. Baker SP, O'Neill B, Ginsburg M, Li G. The Injury Fact Book. 2nd ed. New York. Oxford University Press, 1992.
3. Bracken MB, Freeman DH Jr, Hellenbrand K. Incidence of acute traumatic hospitalized spinal cord injury in the United States, 1970–1977. Am J Epidemiol 1981;113:615–622.
4. Fehlings MG, Tator CH. An evidence-based review of decompressive surgery in acute spinal cord injury: rationale, indications, and timing based on experimental and clinical studies. J Neurosurg Spine 1999;91:1–11.
5. Hadley MN, Walters BC, Grabb PA, et al. Guidelines for the management of acute cervical spine and spinal cord injuries. Clin Neurosurg 2002;49:407–498.
6. Irwin ZN, Arthur M, Mullins RJ, et al. Variations in injury patterns, treatment, and outcome for spinal fracture and paralysis in adult versus geriatric patients. Spine 2004;29:796–802.
7. Julien TD, Frankel B, Traynelis VC, Ryken TC. Evidence-based analysis of odontoid fracture management. Neurosurg Focus 2000;8: article 1.
8. Gunnarsson T, Fehlings MG. Acute neurosurgical management of traumatic brain injury and spinal cord injury. Curr Opin Neurol 2003;16:717–723.
9. Poonnoose PM, Ravichandran G, McClelland MR. Missed and mismanaged injuries of the spinal cord. J Trauma 2002;53:314–320.
10. Harris MB, Kronlage SC, Carboni PA, et al. Evaluation of the cervical spine in the polytrauma patient. Spine 2000;25:2884–2891; discussion 2892.
11. Anderson LD, D'Alonzo RT. Fractures of the odontoid process of the axis. J Bone Joint Surg Am 1974;56:1663–1674.
12. Anderson LD, D'Alonzo RT. Fractures of the odontoid process of the axis. 1974. J Bone Joint Surg Am 2004;86A:2081.

13. Benzel EC, Hart BL, Ball PA, et al. Fractures of the C-2 vertebral body. J Neurosurg 1994;81:206–212.
14. Hadley MN, Dickman CA, Browner CM, et al. Acute axis fractures: a review of 229 cases. J Neurosurg 1989;71:642–647.
15. Huelke DF, O'Day J, Mendelsohn RA. Cervical injuries suffered in automobile crashes. J Neurosurg 1981;54:316–322.
16. Marino RJ, Ditunno JF Jr, Donovan WH, et al. Neurologic recovery after traumatic spinal cord injury: data from the Model Spinal Cord Injury Systems. Arch Phys Med Rehabil 1999;80: 1391–1396.
17. Drainer EK, Graham CA, Munro PT. Blunt cervical spine injuries in Scotland 1995–2000. Injury 2003;34:330–333.
18. Hills MW, Deane SA. Head injury and facial injury: is there an increased risk of cervical spine injury? J Trauma 1993;34:549–553; discussion 553–554.
19. Chiu WC, Haan JM, Cushing BM, et al. Ligamentous injuries of the cervical spine in unreliable blunt trauma patients: incidence, evaluation, and outcome. J Trauma 2001;50:457–463; discussion 464.
20. Davis JW, Phreaner DL, Hoyt DB, et al. The etiology of missed cervical spine injuries. J Trauma 1993;34:342–346.
21. Demetriades D, Charalambides K, Chahwan S, et al. Nonskeletal cervical spine injuries: epidemiology and diagnostic pitfalls. J Trauma 2000;48:724–727.
22. Grossman MD, Reilly PM, Gillett T, et al. National survey of the incidence of cervical spine injury and approach to cervical spine clearance in U.S. trauma centers. J Trauma 1999;47:684–690.
23. MacDonald RL, Schwartz ML, Mirich D, et al. Diagnosis of cervical spine injury in motor vehicle crash victims: how many X-rays are enough? J Trauma 1990;30:392–397.
24. Morris CG, McCoy E. Clearing the cervical spine in unconscious polytrauma victims, balancing risks and effective screening. Anaesthesia 2004;59:464–482.
25. Morris CG, Mullan B. Clearing the cervical spine after polytrauma: implementing unified management for unconscious victims in the intensive care unit. Anaesthesia 2004;59:755–761.
26. Schenarts PJ, Diaz J, Kaiser C, et al. Prospective comparison of admission computed tomographic scan and plain films of the upper cervical spine in trauma patients with altered mental status. J Trauma 2001;51:663–668; discussion 668–669.
27. Akmal M, Trivedi R, Sutcliffe J. Functional outcome in trauma patients with spinal injury. Spine 2003;28:180–185.
28. Blood pressure management after acute spinal cord injury. Neurosurgery 2002;50:S58–S62.
29. Cervical spine immobilization before admission to the hospital. Neurosurgery 2002;50:S7–S17.
30. Brunette DD, Rockswold GL. Neurologic recovery following rapid spinal realignment for complete cervical spinal cord injury. J Trauma 1987;27:445–447.
31. Burney RE, Waggoner R, Maynard FM. Stabilization of spinal injury for early transfer. J Trauma 1989;29:1497–1499.
32. Prasad VS, Schwartz A, Bhutani R, et al. Characteristics of injuries to the cervical spine and spinal cord in polytrauma patient population: experience from a regional trauma unit. Spinal Cord 1999;37:560–568.
33. Frankel HL, Hancock DO, Hyslop G, et al. The value of postural reduction in the initial management of closed injuries of the spine with paraplegia and tetraplegia. I. Paraplegia 1969;7:179–192.
34. Clinical assessment after acute cervical spinal cord injury. Neurosurgery 2002;50:S21–S29.
35. Cohen ME, Ditunno JF Jr, Donovan WH, et al. A test of the 1992 International Standards for Neurological and Functional Classification of Spinal Cord Injury. Spinal Cord 1998;36:554–560.
36. El Masry WS, Tsubo M, Katoh S, et al. Validation of the American Spinal Injury Association (ASIA) motor score and the National Acute Spinal Cord Injury Study (NASCIS) motor score. Spine 1996;21:614–619.
37. Hamilton BB, Laughlin JA, Fiedler RC, et al. Interrater reliability of the 7-level functional independence measure (FIM). Scand J Rehabil Med 1994;26:115–119.
38. Jonsson M, Tollback A, Gonzales H, et al. Inter-rater reliability of the 1992 international standards for neurological and functional classification of incomplete spinal cord injury. Spinal Cord 2000;38:675–679.
39. Maynard FM Jr, Bracken MB, Creasey G, et al. International Standards for Neurological and Functional Classification of Spinal Cord Injury. American Spinal Injury Association. Spinal Cord 1997;35:266–274.
40. Stineman MG, Marino RJ, Deutsch A, et al. A functional strategy for classifying patients after traumatic spinal cord injury. Spinal Cord 1999;37:717–725.
41. Bracken MB, Collins WF, Freeman DF, et al. Efficacy of methylprednisolone in acute spinal cord injury. JAMA 1984;251:45–52.
42. Bracken MB, Shepard MJ, Collins WF, et al. A randomized, controlled trial of methylprednisolone or naloxone in the treatment of acute spinal-cord injury. Results of the Second National Acute Spinal Cord Injury Study. N Engl J Med 1990;322:1405–1411.
43. Bracken MB, Holford TR. Effects of timing of methylprednisolone or naloxone administration on recovery of segmental and long-tract neurological function in NASCIS. J Neurosurg 1993;79:500–507.
44. Bracken MB, Shepard MJ, Holford TR, et al. Administration of methylprednisolone for 24 or 48 hours or tirilazad mesylate for 48 hours in the treatment of acute spinal cord injury. Results of the Third National Acute Spinal Cord Injury Randomized Controlled Trial. National Acute Spinal Cord Injury Study. JAMA 1997;277:1597–1604.
45. Pharmacological therapy after acute cervical spinal cord injury. Neurosurgery 2002;50:S63–S72.
46. Matsumoto T, Tamaki T, Kawakami M, et al. Early complications of high-dose methylprednisolone sodium succinate treatment in the follow-up of acute cervical spinal cord injury. Spine 2001;26:426–430.
47. McCutcheon EP, Selassie AW, Gu JK, et al. Acute traumatic spinal cord injury, 1993–2000. A population-based assessment of methylprednisolone administration and hospitalization. J Trauma 2004;56:1076–1083.
48. Peter Vellman W, Hawkes AP, Lammertse DP. Administration of corticosteroids for acute spinal cord injury: the current practice of trauma medical directors and emergency medical system physician advisors. Spine 2003;28:941–947; discussion 947.
49. Hugenholtz H. Methylprednisolone for acute spinal cord injury: not a standard of care. C Med Assoc J 2003;168:1145–1146.
50. Hugenholtz H, Cass DE, Dvorak MF, et al. High-dose methylprednisolone for acute closed spinal cord injury: only a treatment option. Can J Neurol Sci 2002;29:227–35.
51. Geisler FH, Coleman WP, Grieco G, et al. The Sygen multicenter acute spinal cord injury study. Spine 2001;26:S87–S98.
52. Initial closed reduction of cervical spine fracture-dislocation injuries. Neurosurgery 2002;50:S44–S50.
53. Grant GA, Mirza SK, Chapman JR, et al. Risk of early closed reduction in cervical spine subluxation injuries. J Neurosurg 1999;90:13–18.
54. Hadley MN, Fitzpatrick BC, Sonntag VK, et al. Facet fracture-dislocation injuries of the cervical spine. Neurosurgery 1992;30: 661–666.

55. Hoffman JR, Mower WR, Wolfson AB, et al. Validity of a set of clinical criteria to rule out injury to the cervical spine in patients with blunt trauma. National Emergency X-Radiography Utilization Study Group. N Engl J Med 2000;343:94–99.
56. Radiographic assessment of the cervical spine in asymptomatic trauma patients. Neurosurgery 2002;50:S30–S35.
57. Roth BJ, Martin RR, Foley K, et al. Roentgenographic evaluation of the cervical spine. A selective approach. Arch Surg 1994;129: 643–645.
58. Radiographic assessment of the cervical spine in symptomatic trauma patients. Neurosurgery 2002;50:S36–S43.
59. Berne JD, Velmahos GC, El-Tawil Q, et al. Value of complete cervical helical computed tomographic scanning in identifying cervical spine injury in the unevaluable blunt trauma patient with multiple injuries: a prospective study. J Trauma 1999;47: 896–902; discussion 903.
60. Borock EC, Gabram SG, Jacobs LM, et al. A prospective analysis of a two-year experience using computed tomography as an adjunct for cervical spine clearance. J Trauma 1991;31:1001–1005; discussion 1005–1006.
61. Mace SE. Emergency evaluation of cervical spine injuries: CT versus plain radiographs. Ann Emerg Med 1985;14:973–975.
62. Tan E, Schweitzer ME, Vaccaro L, et al. Is computed tomography of nonvisualized C7–T1 cost-effective? J Spinal Disord 1999;12: 472–476.
63. Lewis LM, Docherty M, Ruoff BE, et al. Flexion-extension views in the evaluation of cervical-spine injuries. Ann Emerg Med 1991;20:117–121.
64. Brady WJ, Moghtader J, Cutcher D, et al. ED use of flexion-extension cervical spine radiography in the evaluation of blunt trauma. Am J Emerg Med 1999;17:504–508.
65. Stanislas MJ, Latham JM, Porter KM, et al. A high risk group for thoracolumbar fractures. Injury 1998;29:15–18.
66. Samuels LE, Kerstein MD. 'Routine' radiologic evaluation of the thoracolumbar spine in blunt trauma patients: a reappraisal. J Trauma 1993;34:85–89.
67. Benzel EC, Hart BL, Ball PA, et al. Magnetic resonance imaging for the evaluation of patients with occult cervical spine injury. J Neurosurg 1996;85:824–829.
68. Karnaze MG, Gado MH, Sartor KJ, et al. Comparison of MR and CT myelography in imaging the cervical and thoracic spine. AJR Am J Roentgenol 1988;150:397–403.
69. Jelsma RK, Rice JF, Jelsma LF, et al. The demonstration and significance of neural compression after spinal injury. Surg Neurol 1982;18:79–92.
70. Pasquale M, Fabian TC. Practice management guidelines for trauma from the Eastern Association for the Surgery of Trauma. J Trauma 1998;44:941–956; discussion 956–957.
71. Davis JW, Parks SN, Detlefs CL, et al. Clearing the cervical spine in obtunded patients: the use of dynamic fluoroscopy. J Trauma 1995;39:435–438.
72. Sandler AJ, Dvorak J, Humke T, et al. The effectiveness of various cervical orthoses. An in vivo comparison of the mechanical stability provided by several widely used models. Spine 1996;21:1624–1629.
73. Sees DW, Rodriguez Cruz LR, Flaherty SF, et al. The use of bedside fluoroscopy to evaluate the cervical spine in obtunded trauma patients. J Trauma 1998;45:768–771.
74. Widder S, Doig C, Burrowes P, et al. Prospective evaluation of computed tomographic scanning for the spinal clearance of obtunded trauma patients: preliminary results. J Trauma 2004;56:1179–1184.
75. Diaz JJ Jr, Gillman C, Morris JA Jr, et al. Are five-view plain films of the cervical spine unreliable? A prospective evaluation in blunt trauma patients with altered mental status. J Trauma 2003;55:658–663; discussion 663–664.
76. Bolinger B, Shartz M, Marion D. Bedside fluoroscopic flexion and extension cervical spine radiographs for clearance of the cervical spine in comatose trauma patients. J Trauma 2004;56:132–136.
77. Adams VI. Neck injuries: I. Occipitoatlantal dislocation: a pathologic study of twelve traffic fatalities. J Forensic Sci 1992;37:556–564.
78. Alker GJ Jr, Oh YS, Leslie EV. High cervical spine and craniocervical junction injuries in fatal traffic accidents: a radiological study. Orthop Clin N Am 1978;9:1003–1010.
79. Bucholz RW, Burkhead WZ. The pathological anatomy of fatal atlanto-occipital dislocations. J Bone Joint Surg Am 1979;61:248–250.
80. Saeheng S, Phuenpathom N. Traumatic occipitoatlantal dislocation. Surg Neurol 2001;55:35–40.
81. Vaccaro AR, Cook CM, McCullen G, et al. Cervical trauma: rationale for selecting the appropriate fusion technique. Orthop Clin N Am 1998;29:745–754.
82. Traynelis VC, Marano GD, Dunker RO, et al. Traumatic atlanto-occipital dislocation. Case report. J Neurosurg 1986;65:863–870.
83. Dublin AB, Marks WM, Weinstock D, et al. Traumatic dislocation of the atlanto-occipital articulation (AOA) with short-term survival. With a radiographic method of measuring the AOA. J Neurosurg 1980;52:541–546.
84. Powers B, Miller MD, Kramer RS, et al. Traumatic anterior atlanto-occipital dislocation. Neurosurgery 1979;4:12–17.
85. Wholey MH, Bruwer AJ, Baker HL Jr. The lateral roentgenogram of the neck; with comments on the atlanto-odontoid-basion relationship. Radiology 1958;71:350–356.
86. Harris JH Jr, Carson GC, Wagner LK, et al. Radiologic diagnosis of traumatic occipitovertebral dissociation: 2. Comparison of three methods of detecting occipitovertebral relationships on lateral radiographs of supine subjects. AJR Am J Roentgenol 1994;162:887–892.
87. Lee C, Woodring JH, Goldstein SJ, et al. Evaluation of traumatic atlantooccipital dislocations. AJNR Am J Neuroradiol 1987;8:19–26.
88. Diagnosis and management of traumatic atlanto-occipital dislocation injuries. Neurosurgery 2002;50:S105–S113.
89. Harris JH, Carson GC, Wagner LK. Radiologic diagnosis of traumatic occipitovertebral dissociation: 1. Normal occipitovertebral relationships on lateral radiographs of supine subjects. AJR Am J Roentgenol 1994;162:881–886.
90. Bulas DI, Fitz CR, Johnson DL. Traumatic atlanto-occipital dislocation in children. Radiology 1993;188:155–158.
91. Przybylski GJ, Clyde BL, Fitz CR. Craniocervical junction subarachnoid hemorrhage associated with atlanto-occipital dislocation. Spine 1996;21:1761–1768.
92. Greenberg MS. Handbook of Neurosurgery. New York: Thieme, 2001.
93. Fielding JW, Hawkins RJ. Atlanto-axial rotatory fixation. Fixed rotatory subluxation of the atlanto-axial joint. J Bone Joint Surg Am 1977;59:37–44.
94. Jefferson G. Fractures of the atlas vertebra: report of four cases and review of those previously reported. Br J Surg 1920;7:407–422.
95. Segal LS, Grimm JO, Stauffer ES. Non-union of fractures of the atlas. J Bone Joint Surg Am 1987;69:1423–1434.
96. Hein C, Richter HP, Rath SA. Atlantoaxial screw fixation for the treatment of isolated and combined unstable Jefferson fractures: experiences with 8 patients. Acta Neurochir (Wien) 2002;144:1187–1192.
97. Isolated fractures of the atlas in adults. Neurosurgery 2002;50: S120–S124.
98. Hadley MN, Dickman CA, Browner CM, et al. Acute traumatic atlas fractures: management and long-term outcome. Neurosurgery 1988;23:31–35.
99. Levine AM, Edwards CC. Fractures of the atlas. J Bone Joint Surg Am 1991;73:680–691.

100. Ruf M, Melcher R, Harms J. Transoral reduction and osteosynthesis C1 as a function-preserving option in the treatment of unstable Jefferson fractures. Spine 2004;29:823–827.
101. Sherk HH, Nicholson JT. Fractures of the atlas. J Bone Joint Surg Am 1970;52:1017–1024.
102. Spence KF Jr, Decker S, Sell KW. Bursting atlantal fracture associated with rupture of the transverse ligament. J Bone Joint Surg Am 1970;52:543–549.
103. Fielding JW, Cochran GB, Lawsing JF III, et al. Tears of the transverse ligament of the atlas. A clinical and biomechanical study. J Bone Joint Surg Am 1974;56:1683–1691.
104. Heller JG, Viroslav S, Hudson T. Jefferson fractures: the role of magnification artifact in assessing transverse ligament integrity. J Spinal Disord 1993;6:392–396.
105. Apuzzo ML, Heiden JS, Weiss MH, et al. Acute fractures of the odontoid process. An analysis of 45 cases. J Neurosurg 1978;48:85–91.
106. Hadley MN, Browner C, Sonntag VK. Axis fractures: a comprehensive review of management and treatment in 107 cases. Neurosurgery 1985;17:281–290.
107. Marchesi DG. Management of odontoid fractures. Orthopedics 1997;20:911–916.
108. Sasso RC. C2 dens fractures: treatment options. J Spinal Disord 2001;14:455–463.
109. Vaccaro AR, Cotler JM. Traumatic injuries of the upper cervical spine. In: An HS, Simpson JM, eds. Surgery of the Cervical Spine. London: Martin Dunitz, 1994:227–265.
110. Scott EW, Haid RW Jr, Peace D. Type I fractures of the odontoid process: implications for atlanto-occipital instability. Case report. J Neurosurg 1990;72:488–492.
111. Hadley MN, Browner CM, Liu SS, et al. New subtype of acute odontoid fractures (type IIA). Neurosurgery 1988;22:67–71.
112. Chutkan NB, King AG, Harris MB. Odontoid fractures: evaluation and management. J Am Acad Orthop Surg 1997;5:199–204.
113. Clark CR, White AA III. Fractures of the dens. A multicenter study. J Bone Joint Surg Am 1985;67:1340–1348.
114. Greene KA, Dickman CA, Marciano FF, et al. Acute axis fractures. Analysis of management and outcome in 340 consecutive cases. Spine 1997;22:1843–1852.
115. Bucholz RD, Cheung KC. Halo vest versus spinal fusion for cervical injury: evidence from an outcome study. J Neurosurg 1989;70:884–892.
116. Wang GJ, Mabie KN, Whitehill R, et al. The nonsurgical management of odontoid fractures in adults. Spine 1984;9:229–230.
117. Isolated fractures of the axis in adults. Neurosurgery 2002;50: S125–S139.
118. Seybold EA, Bayley JC. Functional outcome of surgically and conservatively managed dens fractures. Spine 1998;23:1837–1845; discussion 1845–1846.
119. Lennarson PJ, Mostafavi H, Traynelis VC, et al. Management of type II dens fractures: a case-control study. Spine 2000;25:1234–1237.
120. Borm W, Kast E, Richter HP, et al. Anterior screw fixation in type II odontoid fractures: is there a difference in outcome between age groups? Neurosurgery 2003;52:1089–1092; discussion 1092–1094.
121. ElSaghir H, Bohm H. Anderson type II fracture of the odontoid process: results of anterior screw fixation. J Spinal Disord 2000;13:527–530; discussion 531.
122. Graziano G, Jaggers C, Lee M, et al. A comparative study of fixation techniques for type II fractures of the odontoid process. Spine 1993;18:2383–2387.
123. Harrop JS, Przybylski GJ, Vaccaro AR, et al. Efficacy of anterior odontoid screw fixation in elderly patients with type II odontoid fractures. Neurosurg Focus 2000;6: article 6.
124. Greene KA, Dickman CA, Marciano FF, et al. Transverse atlantal ligament disruption associated with odontoid fractures. Spine 1994;19:2307–2314.
125. Arand M, Neller S, Kinzl L, et al. The traumatic spondylolisthesis of the axis. A biomechanical in vitro evaluation of an instability model and clinical relevant constructs for stabilization. Clin Biomech (Bristol, Avon) 2002;17:432–438.
126. Cornish BL. Traumatic spondylolisthesis of the axis. J Bone Joint Surg Br 1968;50:31–43.
127. Schneider RC, Livingston KE, Cave AJ, et al. "Hangman's fracture" of the cervical spine. J Neurosurg 1965;22:141–154.
128. Effendi B, Roy D, Cornish B, et al. Fractures of the ring of the axis. A classification based on the analysis of 131 cases. J Bone Joint Surg Br 1981;63B:319–327.
129. Levine AM, Edwards CC. The management of traumatic spondylolisthesis of the axis. J Bone Joint Surg Am 1985;67:217–226.
130. Vaccaro AR, Madigan L, Bauerle WB, et al. Early halo immobilization of displaced traumatic spondylolisthesis of the axis. Spine 2002;27:2229–2233.
131. Management of combination fractures of the atlas and axis in adults. Neurosurgery 2002;50:S140–S147.
132. Dickman CA, Hadley MN, Browner C, et al. Neurosurgical management of acute atlas-axis combination fractures. A review of 25 cases. J Neurosurg 1989;70:45–49.
133. Allen BL Jr, Ferguson RL, Lehmann TR, et al. A mechanistic classification of closed, indirect fractures and dislocations of the lower cervical spine. Spine 1982;7:1–27.
134. White AA, Panjabi MM. The Problem of Clinical Instability in the Human Spine: A Systematic Approach. Clinical Biomechanics of the Spine, 2nd ed. Philadelphia: Lippincott, 1990:277–378.
135. Kahn EA, Schneider RC. Chronic neurological sequelae of acute trauma to the spine and spinal cord. I. The significance of the acute-flexion or tear-drop fracture-dislocation of the cervical spine. J Bone Joint Surg Am 1956;38A:985–997.
136. Harris JH Jr, Edeiken-Monroe B, Kopaniky DR. A practical classification of acute cervical spine injuries. Orthop Clin N Am 1986;17:15–30.
137. Denis F. Spinal instability as defined by the three-column spine concept in acute spinal trauma. Clin Orthop 1984:65–76.
138. Chedid MK, Green C. A review of the management of lumbar fractures with focus on surgical decision-making and techniques. Contemp Neurosurg 1999;21:1–5.
139. McAfee PC, Levine AM, Anderson PA. Surgical management of thoracolumbar fractures. Instr Course Lect 1995;44:47–55.
140. Vaccaro AR, Lehman RA Jr, Hurlbert RJ, et al. A new classification of thoracolumbar injuries: the importance of injury morphology, the integrity of the posterior ligamentous complex, and neurologic status. Spine 2005;30:2325–2333.
141. Vaccaro AR, Zeiller SC, Hulbert RJ, et al. The thoracolumbar injury severity score: a proposed treatment algorithm. J Spinal Disord Tech 2005;18:209–215.
142. McAfee PC, Yuan HA, Lasda NA. The unstable burst fracture. Spine 1982;7:365–373.
143. Vaccaro AR, Kim DH, Brodke DS, et al. Diagnosis and management of thoracolumbar spine fractures. Instr Course Lect 2004;53:359–373.
144. Wood K, Buttermann G, Mehbod A, et al. Operative compared with nonoperative treatment of a thoracolumbar burst fracture without neurological deficit. A prospective, randomized study. J Bone Joint Surg Am 2003;85A:773–781.
145. Verlaan JJ, Oner FC. Operative compared with nonoperative treatment of a thoracolumbar burst fracture without neurological deficit. J Bone Joint Surg Am 2004;86A:649–650; author reply 650–651.

146. Wettstein M, Mouhsine E. Operative compared with nonoperative treatment of a thoracolumbar burst fracture without neurological deficit. J Bone Joint Surg Am 2004;86A:651–652; author reply 652.
147. Anderson PA, Rivara FP, Maier RV, et al. The epidemiology of seatbelt-associated injuries. J Trauma 1991;31:60–67.
148. Biller J, Hingtgen WL, Adams HP Jr, et al. Cervicocephalic arterial dissections. A ten-year experience. Arch Neurol 1986;43:1234–1238.
149. Haldeman S, Kohlbeck FJ, McGregor M. Risk factors and precipitating neck movements causing vertebrobasilar artery dissection after cervical trauma and spinal manipulation. Spine 1999;24:785–794.
150. Willis BK, Greiner F, Orrison WW, et al. The incidence of vertebral artery injury after midcervical spine fracture or subluxation. Neurosurgery 1994;34:435–441; discussion 441–442.
151. Management of vertebral artery injuries after nonpenetrating cervical trauma. Neurosurgery 2002;50:S173–S178.
152. Miller PR, Fabian TC, Croce MA, et al. Prospective screening for blunt cerebrovascular injuries: analysis of diagnostic modalities and outcomes. Ann Surg 2002;236:386–393.

31

Multiple Organ Dysfunction Syndrome

Donald E. Fry

Death following severe injury or infection assumed a different clinical presentation beginning with the evolution of the intensive care unit (ICU) in acute care hospitals. An improved understanding of hypovolemic shock and techniques of resuscitation during the 1960s led to survival of patients with severe injuries beyond the initial 24 to 48h. The evolution of ventilator support in combination with other organ support measures in the ICU permitted longer survival of the critically ill patient and the emergence of a new clinical syndrome—multiple organ dysfunction syndrome (MODS).[1]

A seminal observation in the evolution of the concept of MODS began with the description of adult (now acute) respiratory distress syndrome (ARDS) by Ashbaugh et al. in 1967.[2] In 1969, Skillman et al.[3] made the clinical association of pulmonary failure with jaundice, stress-related gastrointestinal bleeding, and sepsis. Tilney et al.[4] identified multiple sequential organ failure among surgical patients managed following ruptured aortic aneurysms. Eiseman et al.[5] and Polk and Shields[6] associated MODS with uncontrolled intraabdominal infection and observed that surgical control of abdominal infection was the treatment. Baue[7] offered an organizational premise to MODS as the failure of lung, liver, kidney, gastrointestinal tract, coagulation cascade, and the central nervous system as clinically associated events. Noting that the components of MODS were associated with many different clinical scenarios, Baue proposed that a common pathophysiological pathway was potentially responsible.

In the early 1980s, the Louisville group studied multiple different cohorts of patients and identified clinical sepsis as the most important associated clinical parameter of MODS, noting the progressive increase in the probability of death as the number of organs involved increased.[8–11] Infection from any anatomic site, when associated with clinical sepsis (i.e., a proinflammatory response to infection), was the dominant association with MODS. Deutschman et al.[12] identified that the septic response had a common pathophysiological pathway regardless of the bacterial, fungal, or viral pathogen responsible for the infection. It became apparent that the sepsis response was a nonspecific response of the host that was not associated with a specific anatomic site of infection, or with a specific pathogen.[13]

The "septic" response was soon recognized to not be specific to infection at all. Goris et al.[14] noted a sepsis-like response in patients without infection. It became apparent that nonspecific activation of the systemic proinflammatory response led to MODS. Hypovolemic shock, ischemia-reperfusion injury, extensive soft tissue injury, and other systemic perturbations, in addition to invasive infection, could lead to a "sepsis syndrome" that is now called the systemic inflammatory response syndrome (SIRS).[15] The sustained clinical state of SIRS is associated with the evolution of MODS. Thus, MODS is the auto-destructive consequence of the uncontrolled systemic activation of human inflammation. It is the premise of this chapter that MODS is the consequence of unregulated SIRS and that new treatments in the management of severe sepsis, septic shock, SIRS, and MODS require efforts to control or modulate the systemic activation of inflammation.

Pathophysiology of Multiple Organ Dysfunction Syndrome

An understanding of MODS and the treatment of MODS requires a basic understanding of the human inflammatory cascade.

Local Inflammation

A simple cutaneous wound is a suitable prototype to understand the local inflammatory response and, similarly, to understand the effects of systemic activation of the same mechanisms. With a cut, crush, or burn injury, the initiator events of local inflammation are activated (Figure 31.1). Local injury disrupts cells and releases adenosine diphosphate (ADP)

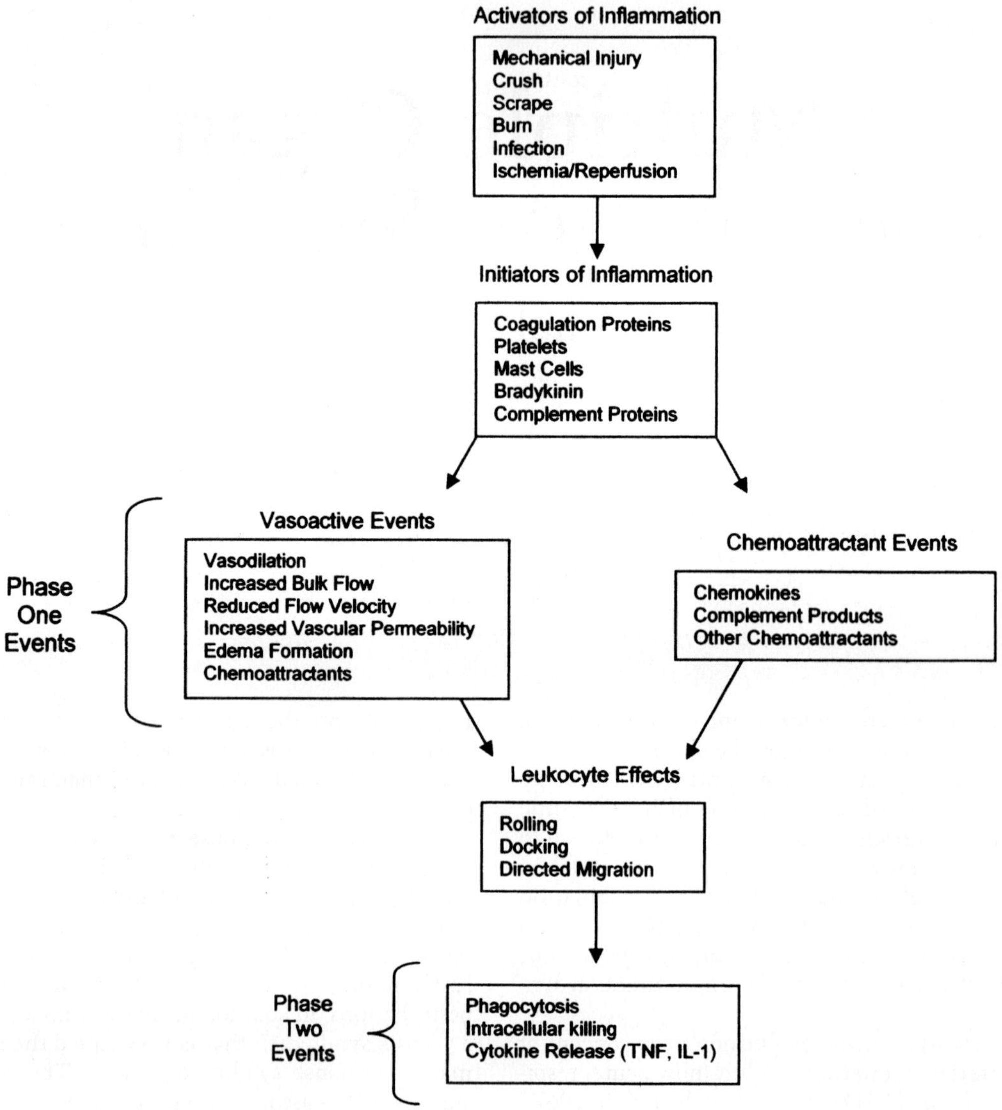

FIGURE 31.1. Normal pathway of events in localized human inflammation. The end products of inflammation are the vasoactive changes herein referred to as phase 1 and the phagocytic events as phase 2.

and other cellular products, injures vascular endothelium, exposes interstitial collagen, and activates tissue factor. The immediate consequence of tissue injury is the activation of coagulation proteins and platelets, which not only serve their role for hemostasis but become the foundation events for local activation of inflammation. Activated coagulation proteins and released platelet enzymes become the proinflammatory stimuli for mast cell degranulation, bradykinin synthesis, and activation of the complement cascade. Full local activation of inflammation results in activation of all five initiator events. Activation of one activates all. This duplicative and redundant feature of inflammation assumes paramount importance as consideration turns subsequently to methods for control of the process.

The consequences of the initiator events are changes within the local microcirculation. Relaxation of vascular smooth muscle results in vasodilation, increased local blood flow, and enhanced oxygen delivery, but reduction of flow velocity and induction of shear forces on the surface of the endothelium. Vasodilation and cytoskeletal changes within the endothelial cell increase vascular permeability. Enhanced permeability provides the exit routes for phagocytic cells to invade the subendothelial interstitial matrix and permits circulating opsonins and other proteins access to injured tissues. Edema formation produces aqueous conduits to permit migration of phagocytic cells through the normally condensed extracellular matrix. The microvascular changes of inflammation are herein referred to as phase I (see Figure 31.1), and serve to prepare the local environment for phase II of inflammation, or the phagocytic phase.

The epicenter of soft tissue injury within a cut, bruise, or abrasion becomes the source of specific and nonspecific chemoattractants that functionally become "beacons" to direct the movement of phagocytic cells into the site. Chemokines are clearly the most important of these chemoattractant signals.[16,17] There are some 50 different chemokines of similar protein structure, which target 18 receptor sites and provide for specificity of the cell types that penetrate the inflammatory environment.[18,19] Chemoattractant signals diffuse from the injury site to adjacent microcirculatory units where they bind to endothelial receptors, which changes the expression of selectin and integrin adhesion molecules. The upregulation of selectins and selectin counterreceptors initiates the rolling of the neutrophil on the endothelial surface, and this is followed by the stable binding of the integrin–intercellular adhesion molecule (CAM) complex, with resultant "margination" of phagocytes as they adhere firmly to the endothelium. Platelet-activating factor (PAF) is an important signal in facilitating the migration of the neutrophil out of the intravascular space, through gap junctions between endothelial cells, and into the extracellular matrix. Orderly phagocytosis of pathogens, contaminants, and nonviable host cells and cellular debris then proceeds after the activated neutrophil enters the area of injury.

The monocyte follows the same general mechanisms and pathways as are characteristic of neutrophil migration, although presence in the tissue of the monocyte is delayed by several hours. Monocyte migration is slower because of the selective effects of the different chemokine signals, but potentially also because of the less efficient movement of the large nucleus rather than the spindly neutrophil nucleus out of the intravascular compartment through the narrow interstices between endothelial cells. Activated monocytes transform in tissue into macrophages, which are efficient phagocytes and active producers of cytokines and other regulators of inflammation.

Chemoattractants provide both directional signals but also powerful signals to stimulate proinflammatory cytokine production. Minimal injury produces a mild chemoattractant signal, slower monocyte chemotaxis, and a milder stimulus of proinflammatory signaling. Severe injury or extensive contamination provokes an abundant chemoattractant signal, a vigorous chemotactic response, and a robust proinflammatory response. Tumor necrosis factor-alpha (TNF-α), interleukin 1 (IL-1), IL-6, and many other proinflammatory cytokines are released. Among its many functions, TNF-α is a potent stimulus of neutrophil phagocytosis.[20] The intense paracrine effects of TNF-α provoke a frenzy of phagocytic activity that even leads to fusion of the lysosomal bodies with the plasma membrane and external release of acid hydrolases and reactive oxygen species. Lipid peroxidation and extracellular enzymatic digestion lead to neutrophil death and further enhancement of the inflammatory milieu. The intense local inflammatory environment leads to local tissue necrosis and liquefaction, dead neutrophils, and a richly proteinaceous extracellular edema fluid that collectively is referred to as pus. The perimeter about the inflammatory focus becomes a fibrinous barricade to sequester the host from the intense activation of inflammation. Egress of bacteria, bacterial cell products (e.g., endotoxin), and proinflammatory signals to the systemic microcirculation is occluded by the brisk response of the coagulation system, causing thrombosis within the microcirculation at the perimeter. When the local responses are fully manifest, a prototypical abscess is the result. Containment in an abscess means that the local inflammatory process has served its principal function, initially, eradication of microbes, and secondarily, the containment of microbial cells, cell products, and inflammatory signals from gaining systemic access to the host. However, local containment often fails, for reasons that are not completely understood.

Systemic Inflammatory Response

The local human inflammatory response of eradication and containment is beneficial to the host. However, escape of bacteria, bacterial endotoxins or exotoxins, or proinflammatory signals to the systemic circulation causes a generalized activation of inflammation that is deleterious to the host. Systemic activation of coagulation, platelets, mast cells, bradykinin, and complement triggers phase I and II of inflammation systemically, with the clinical sequelae being the SIRS. Systemic vasodilation results in loss of peripheral vascular resistance, increased vascular capacitance, and diffuse tissue edema. The pathophysiological consequence of severe phase I systemic inflammation is, if induced by infection, septic shock. The shock state may be accompanied by normal or even elevated cardiac output, but the loss of afterload caused by vasodilation results in hypotension. Afterload reduction when combined with adequate volume preload (as is achieved with fluid resuscitation) results in the typical hyperdynamic circulation of human sepsis. Inadequate cardiac reserve, from underlying cardiac disease or as the result of depressed cardiomyocyte contraction caused by cytokines, may provoke a low cardiac output syndrome as another clinical scenario. Before the development of the ICU, the lack of supportive care of the hemodynamic instability of phase I systemic inflammation resulted in death. Improved supportive care now often allows patients to persevere through phase I of systemic inflammation, but then to develop clinical organ dysfunction as the systemic expression of uncontrolled phase II inflammation.

The systemic phase II of inflammation, or MODS, is illustrated in Figure 31.2. The systemic release of chemoattractants results in systemic changes of adhesion proteins on the endothelium. Margination of neutrophils occurs systemically. However, in contrast to the events of local inflammation, the systemic inflammatory response does not provide a gradient or direction for neutrophil migration. Directionless margination and movement results in random distribution of neutrophils into the perivascular spaces, while other phagocytic cells remain marginated on the endothelial surface. The diffuse release of chemoattractant signals results in stimulation of neutrophils; moreover, the monocyte/macrophage response occurs systemically as well, amplifying the inflammation response. Tumor necrosis factor-alpha, IL-1, and other proinflammatory signals are released systemically, with the result being amplification of the activated neutrophil and monocyte/macrophage responses and neutrophil-mediated endothelial and perivascular injury. Microcirculatory injury leads to disruption or cessation of nutrient blood flows from complete thrombosis of specific vascular units. Local tissue inflammation and necrosis leads to tissue-level restimulation of the initiator events. The consequence is progressive damage and functional impairment of the organ. Furthermore, even when the activator event that triggered the initial cascade is eliminated clinically, the self-stimulatory and self-energizing cycle of inflammation proceeds with progressive organ impairment and eventually the death of the host. The need to disrupt this cycle of self-recycling inflammation characterizes the search for biomodulation therapy in the treatment of MODS.

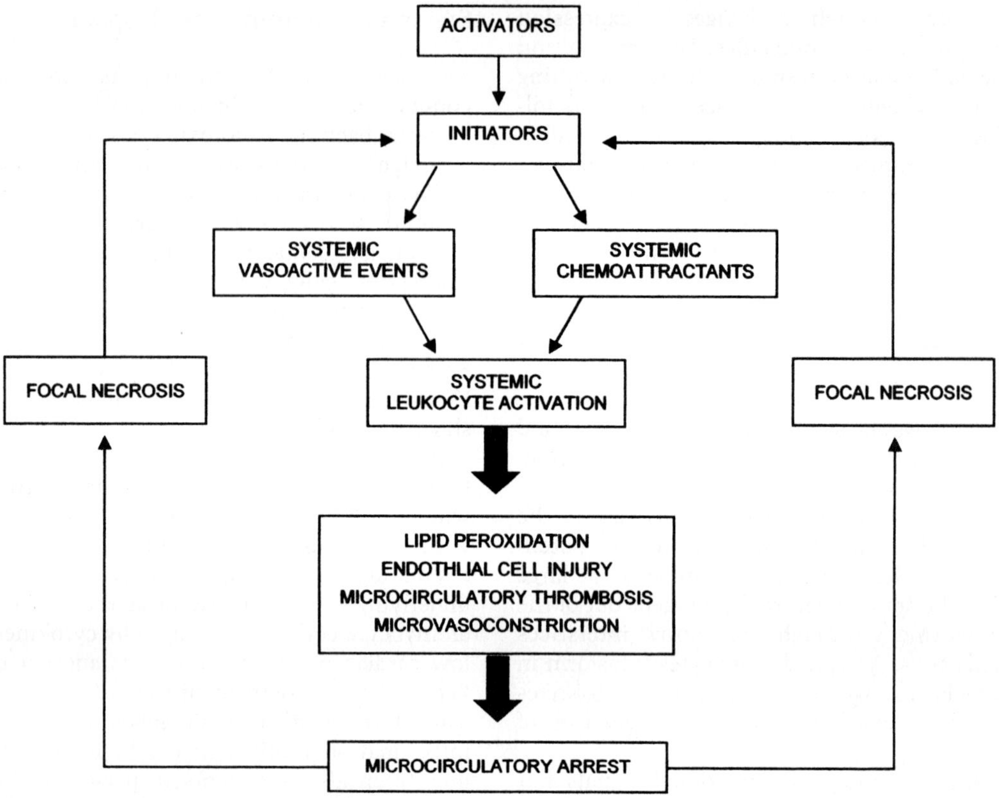

FIGURE 31.2. Schematic illustrating systemic activation of the inflammatory cascade in Figure 31.1 leading to microcirculatory inflammatory damage, microcirculatory arrest, and focal necrosis. Focal necrosis within the tissue then serves as an activator to reenergize the systemic inflammatory response.

Treatment of the Patient with Multiple Organ Dysfunction Syndrome

The foregoing discussion has been a hypothetical construct of the mechanisms that are responsible for the evolution of SIRS and MODS. Systemic inflammation that is activated by invasive infection begets a clinical diagnosis of sepsis. Severe sepsis is defined by sepsis with dysfunction of at least one organ, whereas hypotension that is refractory to fluid administration in association with sepsis-mediated SIRS defines septic shock. The management of severe sepsis or septic shock become the clinical scenarios in which SIRS and MODS are treated most commonly.

Management begins with diagnosis. The diagnosis of failure of the individual organ systems has been defined in multiple different ways and with different grading scales by different authors over a 30-year period.[21–25] Reasonable definitions are presented in Table 31.1. The cascade of organ failure usually begins with pulmonary dysfunction, with other organ systems following in a sequential or synchronous fashion. The sequence and magnitude of organ failures is dependent upon the underlying physiological reserve of each organ system within the host, and no longer is characterized by the stereotypical, all-or-nothing response described initially. Rapidly evolving SIRS or sepsis may produce a clinical picture of synchronously failing systems.

Rapid, accurate diagnosis of the activating event becomes essential in formulating an effective treatment strategy. Microbiological identification of the site of a putative infection or positive blood culture is important to document sepsis and to direct antibiotic therapy. However, neither SIRS nor MODS requires positive blood cultures or circulating endotoxins, but rather may be the consequence of a "mediator shower" from a large, intense focus of infection such as peritonitis. Other activating events such as hemorrhagic shock, or massive tissue injury, may also initiate the inflammatory cascade. Whether SIRS and MODS are caused by infection, shock, soft tissue injury, or a combination of any of these events, the subsequent management of the patients (except for antibiotic therapy) remains largely the same.

When sepsis is the activating event in SIRS/MODS, mechanical control of the infectious focus and appropriate antibiotic therapy are crucially important components of management. Sources of infection needing mechanical control (source control) include gastrointestinal perforations, leaking surgical anastomoses, abscess in the abdominal cavity, empyema of the pleural space, and infected devices (e.g., intravascular catheters or prosthetic implants). Drainage, debridement, exteriorization, resection, repair, percutaneous drainage, and device/prosthesis removal all become important measures that may be necessary for blunting the activation of the inflammatory cascade.[26]

Antimicrobial chemotherapy is an important part of the management of the infected patient with SIRS/MODS. Organ dysfunction arising from community-acquired intraabdominal infection requires antibiotic coverage for enteric aerobic-gram negative bacilli (e.g., *Escherichia coli*) and enteric anaerobic species (e.g., *Bacteroides fragilis*).[27] Community-

TABLE 31.1. Practical and Applicable Definitions of the Commonly Recognized Elements of Multiple Organ Dysfunction Syndrome.

Organ system	*Definition*
Pulmonary failure	Ventilatory support 72h or more; F_IO_2 0.4 or more; requirement for positive end-expiratory pressure
Cardiac failure	High filling pressures; low cardiac output; cardiac arrhythmias; inotropic/vasopressor support
Hepatic failure	Total bilirubin >2mg/dL; AST or ALT more than twice normal; elevated serum ammonia concentration
Renal failure	Sustained oliguria (more than 8h) <20mL/h; creatinine >2mg/dL; requirement for dialysis
Gastrointestinal failure	Endoscopically confirmed gastric mucosal erosions with bleeding; gastroduodenal perforation; sustained (more than 5 days) intestinal ileus
Coagulation failure	Thrombocytopenia (<60,000/μL); white blood cell count <1000/μL; clinical bleeding diathesis; disseminated intravascular coagulation
Neurological failure	Glasgow Coma Scale score 6 or less; suppressed neurological responsiveness; coma

F_IO_2, fraction of inspired oxygen; ALT, alanine aminotransferase; AST, aspartate aminotransferase.

Several validated MODS scores use these definitions to a greater or lesser degree. Quantification of a standardized score is encouraged.

acquired soft tissue infection may occur from multiple different pathogens (Table 31.2) and requires both precise microbiological diagnosis and antibiotic therapy tailored to susceptibility testing. Postoperative MODS from sepsis arises from where "the hands of man" have been and requires evaluation of the surgical site. Healthcare-associated (nosocomial) infections include pneumonia, urinary tract infection, intravascular device infection, and bloodstream infection. The pathogens of healthcare-associated infection include methicillin-resistant *Staphylococcus aureus*, *Staphylococcus epidermidis*, *Pseudomonas aeruginosa*, extended-spectrum beta-lactamase-producing gram-negative bacilli, *Enterococcus* spp., and *Candida albicans*. Tertiary peritonitis is another uncommon but difficult infection in MODS patients that characteristically has resistant nosocomial pathogens which are different from the pathogens isolated during the secondary phase of the infection.[28]

The patient with SIRS exhibits all the features of a septic response, but infection is not identified. Fever, leukocytosis, tachycardia, tachypnea, and the evolution of MODS become a tempting scenario for starting antibiotics. However, antibiotic administration without infection leads to the colonization of the patient with resistant bacteria and creates an adverse situation when nosocomial infection caused by multidrug-resistant bacteria emerges in the wake of the antibiotic treatment.

Circulatory Failure

Vasodilation and increased vascular permeability from the phase I effects of inflammation mean that vascular capacitance is vastly increased, and "third spacing" of intravascular fluid into the interstitial space creates intravascular hypovolemia.[29–31] Thus, maintenance of cardiac preload is essential for maintaining arterial blood pressure and tissue perfusion. In the patient with MODS, preload is maintained preferentially with crystalloid solutions, given the permeability changes of the inflammatory state, and studies show no advantage to resuscitation of sepsis with colloids. Volume targets should generally be (1) mean arterial pressure ≥60mmHg, (2) urine output ≥0.5mL/kg/h, (3) central venous pressure 8–12mmHg, and (4) mixed venous oxygen saturation

TABLE 31.2. Types of Infection, Pathogens, and Antibiotic Therapy for the Different Clinical Types of Aggressive Soft Tissue Infections Associated with MODS.

Organism	*Recommended antibiotic choices*	*Comments*
Clostridium perfringens	Penicillin and Clindamycin	An uncommon clinical infection with a fulminate course that requires prompt recognition and surgical intervention.
Streptococcus pyogenes	Penicillin and Clindamycin	An uncommon but rapidly progressing necrotizing infection associated with a toxic shock-like syndrome. Clindamycin is recommended because it presumably reduces toxin production.
Methicillin-sensitive *Staphylococcus aureus*	Beta-lactam antibiotics	A common pyogenic infection. Cultures are required to determine antibiotic susceptibility because of increasing methicillin resistance.
Community-associated *Staphylococcus aureus*	Clindamycin Trimethoprim/Sulfamethoxazole Vancomycin Linezolid Daptomycin Tigecycline	A new variant of methicillin-resistant staphylococci that commonly has 70%–90% susceptibility to non-beta lactam antibiotics. Presents as a necrotizing skin infection, or rarely pneumonia.
Hospital-associated	Vancomycin Linezolid Daptomycin Tigecycline	Resistant to most antibiotics. It now represents 60% of hospital-cultured staphylococci.
Polymicrobial infections (e.g., ulcers, diabetic foot, necrotizing soft tissue infection)	Double- or triple-drug therapy	Cultures are essential. Usually a mixed infection with gram-negative bacilli, enterococci, or staphylococci, and anaerobes.

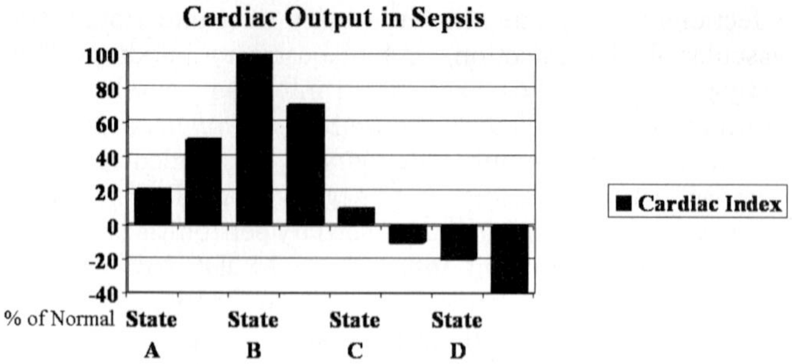

FIGURE 31.3. Changes in cardiac output between the stress response of *state A*, the systemic inflammatory response of *state B*, and the decompensated *state C* and *state D* where septic shock is clinically identified.

≥70%.[32,33] Improvement in the metabolic acidosis that is associated with hypovolemia can be expected if these therapeutic endpoints are achieved, realizing that inflammatory injury of the microcirculation may not fully restore tissue perfusion, and that metabolic acidosis may persist for reasons other than hypovolemia.

When volume expansion has been optimized, shock will still be present in selected patients and either vasoactive or inotropic therapy is necessary. Shock in the SIRS and MODS patient is fundamentally a disjointed relationship between cardiac output and systemic vascular resistance.[13] The relationships between cardiac output and vascular resistance are illustrated in Figures 31.3 and 31.4. State A is the normal stress response seen with severe injury or major surgical procedures. There is a modest reduction in peripheral vascular resistance and a modest increase in cardiac output. In state B, there is an exaggerated stress response characterized by a marked reduction of systemic vascular resistance and a dramatic increase in cardiac output, assuming adequate preload and an appropriate physiological reserve of the left ventricle. State B is the typical SIRS response with acceptable mean arterial pressure. State C represents shock from systemic loss of vascular resistance (i.e., "warm shock"), although cardiac output is normal or even somewhat elevated. State D represents "cold shock" when cardiac output is inadequate and vascular resistance is increased. Management of shock in the patient with SIRS/MODS requires therapy to increase vascular resistance or increase cardiac output, or a combination of both.

Vasoconstrictive therapy may be used to increase vascular resistance and improve arterial blood pressure, but perhaps with negative consequences for splanchnic perfusion. Norepinenephrine or dopamine are used commonly as treatments for this purpose;[33–35] the former is generally considered superior for therapy of septic shock. Epinephrine is generally not recommended because of associated tachycardia and splanchnic vasoconstriction. Vasopressin therapy is controversial. Although vasopressin concentrations are decreased in septic shock, it is unclear whether vasopressin should be administered in fixed dosage for a hormone deficiency state or titrated to achieve a blood pressure endpoint. Vasopressin is a potent vasoconstrictor and is associated with reduction in cardiac output and with coronary and visceral ischemia.[36] Inotropic support may be necessary in patients where cardiac output is inadequate. Dobutamine is the preferred inotropic agent, but it may reduce peripheral vascular resistance and may be associated with marked tachycardia if hypovolemia persists.[33] Use of any vasopressors or inotropes requires invasive hemodynamic monitoring.

The use of corticosteroid therapy in patients with sepsis, SIRS, and MODS has been evaluated for decades (Table 31.3). Pharmacological doses of corticosteroids are not of value in septic shock, SIRS, or MODS patients.[37,38] For shock associated with SIRS/MODS, daily administration of 200–300 mg/day of hydrocortisone (for 7 days) reduces mortality,[39–41] but this is not recommended in the absence of shock.

Pulmonary Failure

The SIRS and sepsis processes have major influences upon pulmonary function. The microcirculation of the lung is affected profoundly by systemic inflammatory processes, as are airway host defenses. The pathophysiological consequences are increased resistance to lung perfusion, ventilation/perfusion mismatching with areas of shunt (perfused, nonventilated lung), and dead space ventilation (nonperfused lung), increased interstitial water, decreased pulmonary compliance, increased airway resistance, and impaired alveolar gas exchange. The lung is the most common organ to become dysfunctional in SIRS/MODS patients: only rarely is it the sole organ system to fail.

Oxygenation is vitally important and almost inevitably requires mechanical ventilator support in severe MODS. Treatment strategies for maintaining oxygenation and ventilation have changed dramatically during the past two to three decades. Ideal objectives in treatment are to keep arterial oxygen saturation ≥90%, arterial pO_2 ≥60 mmHg, and arterial pCO_2 ~40 mmHg. However, current management employs smaller tidal volumes to avoid barotrauma than had been used traditionally (6 mL/kg),[42–46] which may require permissive hypercapnea ($PaCO_2 \leq 80$, pH ≥ 7.20),[47] along with positive end-expiratory pressure[48] (Table 31.4). Elevation of the head of the bed[49] and rapid weaning strategies are also standard. Either bolus or continuous infusion of sedatives is necessary for the ventilated patient with ARDS.[50] Although neuromuscular blockade may occasionally be necessary, an attempt to avoid paralysis is desirable.[51] Prone positioning improves oxygenation by transient restoration of ventilation/perfusion mismatching but does not improve survival.[52]

Renal Failure

Renal function is challenging to maintain during the cascade of events in the SIRS/MODS patient. Preservation of renal function in the patient at risk is best achieved by maintenance of renal perfusion with volume support, systemic oxy-

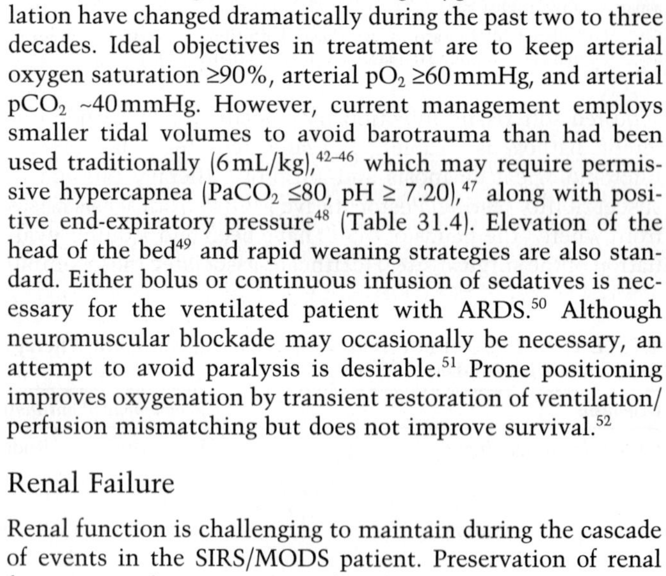

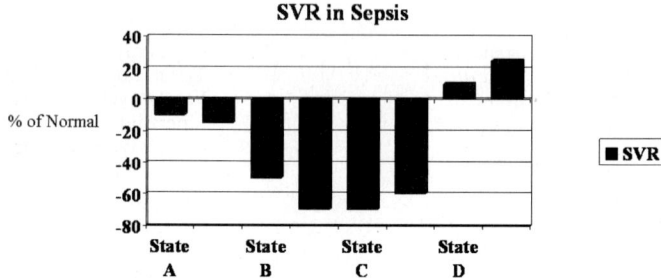

FIGURE 31.4. Changes in systemic vascular resistance (SVR) that occur in the different states of sepsis. In *state C*, there is a profound loss of vascular resistance. In the low cardiac output *state D*, SVR increases above normal.

TABLE 31.3.

Published Reports of Studies of Corticosteroids in the Management of Patients with Sepsis/Systemic Inflammatory Response Syndrome (SIRS)/MODS. All Studies Were Prospective, Randomized Trials (Class 1 Evidence).

Trial (year)	*Total randomized patients*	*Intervention*	*Endpoint*
Bone (1987)[37]	382	30 mg/kg methylprednisolone	Survival
Comment: No difference in survival with corticosteroid treatment. Increased mortality rate in steroid-treated group with renal failure ($P < 0.01$).			
Veterans Administration (1987)[38]	223	30 mg/kg methylprednisolone + 5 mg/kg/h for 9 h more.	Survival
Comment: Demonstrated no difference in survival at 14 days ($P = 0.97$) and no difference in any subgroup of gram-negative bacteremia or gram-positive bacteremia.			
Bollaert (1998)[39]	41	300 mg hydrocortisone daily × 5 days	Shock reversal, survival
Comment: Demonstrated significant reversal of septic shock ($P = 0.007$). No significant difference in survival ($P = 0.09$), but study was inadequately powered to demonstrate a survival difference.			
Briegel (1999)[40]	40	100 mg hydrocortisone × 1; then 18 mg/kg/h	Shock reversal, survival
Comment: No difference in reversal of shock or survival. Treated patients had reduced time to cessation of vasopressors. Study inadequately powered.			
Annane (2002)[41]	299	50 mg hydrocortisone Q 6 h and 50 mg oral fludrocortisone daily	Survival
Comment: Patients who were nonresponders ($n = 229$) to corticotrophin test demonstrated improved survival ($P = 0.02$). There were high death rates in both treated (53%) and untreated (63%) patients.			

genation, cardiac output/blood pressure management, and avoidance of nephrotoxic drugs insofar as possible. Nonoliguric (>400 mL urine/day) renal failure is easier to manage from the perspective of fluid/electrolyte, and nutrition management, but diuretic therapy does not influence the natural history of acute renal failure. When renal failure develops in the setting of MODS and renal replacement therapy is required, either continuous venovenous hemofiltration (CVVH) or intermittent hemodialysis may be employed.[53,54] Fluid and electrolyte balance are the objectives with renal

TABLE 31.4.

Five Randomized, Prospective Trials that Studied Lower Tidal Volumes Versus Conventional Tidal Volumes in Patients Requiring Ventilator Support.

Trial (year)	*Total randomized patients*	*Intervention*	*Endpoint*
Amato(1998)[42]	52	$V_T = 12$ mL/kg vs. $V_T = 6$ mL/kg	Mortality, total ventilator days, barotrauma
Comment: The 28-day survival($P < 0.001$), fewer ventilator days ($P = 0.005$), and less clinical barotrauma ($P = 0.02$) were statistically favorable in the low tidal volume group. The study population was small, interval analysis had been previously undertaken, and survival to discharge from the hospital was not different ($P = 0.37$).			
Stewart(1998)[43]	120	$V_T = 8$ mL/kg; PP ≤ 30 mmHg vs. $V_T = 10$–15 mL/kg; PP ≤ 50 mmHg	Mortality, barotrauma, MODS
Comment: Mortality rates, barotraumas, and episodes of organ failure were not different between the two groups. Lower tidal volume was associated with greater use of paralytics ($P = 0.05$) and a greater need for renal dialysis ($P = 0.04$).			
Brochard (1998)[44]	116	$V_T = 7$ mL/kg; PP = 26 mmHg vs. $V_T = 10$ mL/kg; PP = 32 mmHg	Mortality, ventilator days, pneumothorax, MODS
Comment: Lower tidal volume did not improve outcome in any of the study parameters in a well-stratified population of patients.			
Brower (1999)[45]	52	$V_T = 7$ mL/kg; PP = 25 mmHg vs. $V_T = 10$ mL/kg; PP = 31 mmHg	Mortality, ventilator days, sedation
Comment: No differences were observed between the two groups in any of the study parameters.			
ARDS Network (2000)[46]	861	$V_T = 6$ mL/kg; PP ≤ 30 mmHg vs. $V_T = 12$ mL/kg; PP ≤ 50 mmHg	Mortality, ventilator days
Comment: The mortality rate was 31% in the low tidal volume group vs. 40% in the high tidal volume group ($P = 0.007$). Ventilator-free days were 12 vs. 10 days ($P = 0.007$). The large number of randomized patients allowed a statistically significant outcome.			

V_T, tidal volume; PP, peak inspiratory pressure.

replacement therapy. CVVH may be more safely undertaken when hemodynamic instability is present. Metabolic acidosis from renal failure adds to the fundamental lactic acidosis of SIRS and sepsis. However, bicarbonate therapy has not been demonstrated to improve outcomes[55] and should be used only when the arterial pH is below 7.2.[31] Although some have advocated hemofiltration for elimination of microbial toxins or proinflammatory signals, no clinical evidence supports this indication.[56–59]

Hepatic/Metabolic Failure

The SIRS/MODS patient often has elevation of hepatic enzymes and may occasionally have clinical jaundice. All such patients have the characteristic features of hypermetabolism, increased hepatic gluconeogenesis, increased hepatic ureagenesis, and increased urinary nitrogen loss. Maintenance of splanchnic perfusion and effective nutritional support become the management strategies for hepatic and metabolic failure.

Strategies in nutritional support have evolved over the past 30 years from "hyperalimentation," in which calories were given in excess of metabolic need, to current strategies of more selective nutritional replacement, especially with proteins. Slight underfeeding (basal nonprotein calories of 25 kCal/kg/day) is preferred under nonstressed conditions; questions regarding resting energy expenditure can be resolved by indirect calorimetry. Currently, enteral feeding is preferred over parenteral feeding if the gut is accessible and functioning. The basic goal of nutritional support is 1.5 to 2.0 g protein/kg with a calorie to nitrogen ratio of about 80–100:1. Lipid calories are provided two to three times per week. Enriched enteral formulations with ω-3 fatty acids, arginine, and nucleotides have been associated with reduced risk of nosocomial infections in several ICU studies, but these have not been documented to be beneficial in decreasing mortality in the setting of established MODS.[60] An important consideration in the nutritional management of the MODS patient is glucose control. A prospective, randomized trial has demonstrated a reduction in mortality, infections, and the need for renal replacement therapy if blood sugar was maintained between 80 and 110 mg/dL rather than between 180 and 200 mg/dL.[61]

Gastrointestinal Failure

A frequent issue in the MODS patient in the 1970s and 1980s was stress-related gastric mucosal hemorrhage, which has largely disappeared in recent years as a consequence of improved resuscitation, better nutritional support, and the general use of H_2 histamine receptor blockade for prevention. The effectiveness of H_2 blockade has been generally accepted over antacids or sucralfate.[62] Proton pump inhibitors have not been examined systematically as prophylaxis but are used increasingly.

Another component of gastrointestinal failure may be microbial translocation. This hypothetical event consists of failure of the normal gut barrier from sustained illness, shock, malnutrition, or sepsis. Failure of the complex intestinal mucosal barrier is hypothesized to permit microbes and microbial cell products to gain access to the regional lymph nodes or into the portal circulation. Microbes believed to be "translocators" include *Candida albicans*, *Enterococcus* spp., and some gram-negative bacilli (e.g., *Pseudomonas aeruginosa*). The translocation phenomenon, which has been well documented experimentally, may be a driver of the sepsis syndrome when infection cannot be documented. Treatment would require enhancement of the gut barrier; enteral nutrition to supply glutamine to the small bowel enterocytes and short-chain fatty acids (from fermentable fiber) to the colonocytes has been advocated but not adopted in practice. The strategy of probiotic therapy by the delivery of specific microbes to recolonize the gut is under preliminary investigation as a new treatment.[63]

Coagulation Failure

Laboratory evidence of coagulation failure is a consistent finding in MODS, although overt bleeding or the formal diagnosis of disseminated intravascular coagulation (DIC) is identified less frequently.[64] The clinical syndrome of DIC poses formidable treatment problems in that the use of heparin in the face of clinical bleeding, although often appropriate, is counterintuitive.

Although decreased coagulation is an issue, thromboembolic complications from hypercoagubility continue to be a source of morbidity and mortality for critically ill patients. Both unfractionated and low molecular weight heparin (LMWH) preparations are used for prophylaxis and therapy, but LMWH must be used with extreme caution for patients with renal insufficiency (serum creatinine ≥2.0 mg/dL) as it can accumulate dangerously and cause hemorrhage if the dosage is not reduced.[65] Prophylactic administration of a heparinoid has been demonstrated to prevent deep venous thrombophlebitis and, by inference, pulmonary thromboembolism. When contraindications to anticoagulation exist, an intermittent pneumatic device may be used. Prophylactic vena cava filters have been advocated for selected high-risk patients, but technology and techniques are still being refined.

Innovative Therapy of Systemic Inflammatory Response/Syndrome/Multiple Organ Dysfunction Syndrome

Management of patients at risk for MODS has focused upon improved resuscitation, maintenance of oxygenation, and support or cardiac function to attempt to prevent the syndrome. When organ dysfunction emerges, organ-specific supportive strategies have been used to manage the pathophysiological aftermath of generalized inflammation. Aggressive source control and antibiotic therapy strategies have been used but do not help when infection has not been the precipitant. Moreover, a theoretical point is reached in the pathophysiological cascade of systemic inflammation where eradication of the infection, even when this is the inciting etiology, may not disrupt the domino effects of systemic inflammation. Simplistically, once turned "on," inflammation (or its damaging effects) may reach a point where no therapy, no matter how well targeted, can turn the response "off." Appreciation of the need for new therapies has led to clinical trials of numerous experimental therapies to disrupt or modulate the cascade of events that results in MODS.

Blockade/Neutralization of Activators of Inflammation

Blockade of the initial activating stimulus of inflammation has been proposed, but what is that stimulus? In fact, the precipitant is likely to vary among patients. Endotoxin has been the most studied activator, not only because it has been viewed as a major effector of the virulence of gram-negative infection but also because of its presumed secondary role in the pathogenesis of hypovolemic shock, gut barrier dysfunction, and microbial translocation. Several polyclonal or monoclonal antibodies against the lipid A moiety of the endotoxin molecule have been evaluated in blinded placebo-controlled clinical trials. Initial enthusiasm for results of the early polyclonal antibody trials and from subgroup analysis of the HA-1A monoclonal antibody trials has waned because clinical efficacy was not validated in rigorous prospective trials (Table 31.5).[66–72] Hemofiltration[57] and binding[59] of endotoxin have been studied in human sepsis but remain unproved, as are neutralization with bactericidal/permeability-inducing protein[73] and soluble CD-14 receptor.[74] Given that endotoxin is not a ubiquitous participant in SIRS/MODS, methodologies for combating endotoxin (or any other specific single mediator, for that matter) appear to be of limited value until better bedside diagnostics permit identification of the appropriate patient for treatment.

Inhibition of Phase I of Inflammation

Considerable experimental and some clinical investigations have been performed on blockade or modulation of phase I (vasoactive phase) inflammation. These efforts have been directed principally at inhibiting the activation process of the effectors of the initiators of inflammation (Table 31.6).

Inhibition of the coagulation cascade and platelet activation has been pursued experimentally with studies of antithrombin III and heparin in animal models and human trials of sepsis. Inhibition of Factor XII has been explored experimentally. A clinical trial of antithrombin III failed to achieve endpoints.[75] The use of recombinant human activated protein C (APC) has been the most promising clinical investigation to date in mechanism-directed therapy for the MODS patient with sepsis. A large clinical trial has demonstrated a statistically significant reduction in survival from 31% to 25% in a heterogeneous population of septic patients with Acute Physiology and Chronic Health Evaluation (APACHE) II scores of 25 or more and severe sepsis or septic shock.[76] Patients at high risk for bleeding were excluded from the trial because APC has anticoagulant and profibrinolytic properties. The reduced mortality rate in the treated patients, albeit modest, raises hope that mechanism-based therapies will be identified in the future. In a trial of patients with APACHE II scores less than 25, no difference in survival was identified.[77]

Other efforts at modulation of the initiator events have been unsuccessful. Bradykinin inhibition,[78] tissue factor pathway inhibitor,[79] and nitric oxide synthase inhibition[80] have failed to improve survival in clinical trials of patients with sepsis (see Table 31.6).

Inhibition of Phase II of Inflammation

Experimental efforts to modify phase II of inflammation have been directed variously toward inhibition of leukocyte migration, inhibition of proinflammatory signaling, and inhibition of effector events after neutrophil/monocyte activation. Anti-CD 18 antibodies and other antagonists to adhesion molecules have shown an effect in experimental models, but not

TABLE 31.5.
Studies Designed to Neutralize or Bind Endotoxin in the Management of Patients with Sepsis, Septic Shock, and Organ Failure.

Trial (year)	*Total randomized patients*	*Intervention*	*Endpoint*
Ziegler (1982)[66]	212	Polyclonal anti-endotoxin antibody	Survival
Comment: Significant ($P = 0.011$) increase in survival with treatment. Considered a foundation study for the development of monoclonal antibody against lipid A component of endotoxin.			
Ziegler (1991)[67]	197	Human monoclonal anti-endotoxin antibody (HA-1A)	Survival
Comment: Significant ($P = 0.017$) increased survival for treated patients with gram-negative bacteremia. This study was a subset analysis from 543 randomized patients with sepsis. There was no difference between treated and placebo groups without substratification.			
McCloskey (1994)[68]	621	Human monoclonal anti-endotoxin antibody (HA-1A)	Survival
Comment: Treatment was not significant for patients with gram-negative bacteremia ($P = 0.864$) or for those without gram-negative bacteremia ($P = 0.073$) (placebo, 37% vs. HA-1A, 41% survival).			
Greenman (1991)[69]	316	Mouse monoclonal anti-endotoxin antibody (E5)	Survival
Comment: No difference among all 316 patients with confirmed gram-negative sepsis, but improved survival was seen in those not in shock ($n = 137$) at study entry ($P = 0.01$).			
Bone (1995)[70]	530	Mouse monoclonal anti-endotoxin antibody (E5)	Survival
Comment: No difference in survival among gram-negative sepsis patients ($P = 0.21$). Among 139 patients with organ failure, treated patients had greater resolution of organ failure ($P = 0.005$).			
Angus (2000)[71]	915	Mouse monoclonal anti-endotoxin antibody (E5)	Survival
Comment: A very large trial of gram-negative sepsis demonstrated no difference in survival at 14 days ($P = 0.67$) and 28 days ($P = 0.56$) in survival.			
Albertson (2003)[72]	826	Human monoclonal IgM anti-endotoxin antibody (MAB-T88)	Survival
Comment: There was no difference in 28-day survival between the randomized groups ($P = 0.44$).			

IgM, immunoglobulin M.

TABLE 31.6.
Clinical Trials that Have Attempted to Block or Modulate the Vasoactive Phase (Phase I) of the Systemic Inflammatory Response. All Interventions Were Prospective and Placebo-Controlled.

Trial (year)	*Total randomized patients*	*Intervention*	*Endpoint*
Warren (2001)[75]	2314	Antithrombin III	28-day mortality
Comment: The treated patients had a mortality rate of 38.9% versus 38.7% in the placebo group ($P = 0.94$). An increased rate of bleeding complications was seen in the antithrombin III group when heparin was added.			
Bernard (2001)[76]	1690	Human activated protein C (drotrecogin alfa)	28-day mortality
Comment: The study was conducted in patients with severe sepsis. The mortality rate was 30.8% in the control group and 24.7% in the treated group ($P = 0.005$). This study is the only appropriately powered and statistically significant study showing improvement in outcome with a novel treatment for human sepsis.			
Abraham (2005)[77]	2613	Human activated protein C (drotrecogin alfa)	28-day mortality
Comment: This study was in septic patients with an APACHE score <25. The 28-day mortality was 18.5% in the treated group and 17% in the placebo controls ($P = 0.34$). Therapy with human activated protein C should be reserved for patients with APACHE scores of 25 or less.			
Fein (1997)[78]	504	Bradykinin antagonist	28-day mortality
Comment: No difference was observed in mortality rates in the treated versus placebo groups.			
Abraham (2003)[79]	1754	Tifacogin (tissue factor pathway inhibitor)	28-day mortality
Comment: All-cause mortality was 34.2% in the treated group versus 33.9% in the placebo group. Subgroup analysis showed a significantly better survival ($P < 0.001$) in the patients with a normal prothrombin time.			
Lopez (2004)[80]	797	Nitric oxide synthase inhibitor	28-day mortality
Comment: The 28-day mortality rate was 59% in the treated group and 49% in the placebo group ($P < 0.001$). Adverse hemodynamic events in the treated group were considered causes for the increased mortality rate with nitric oxide synthase inhibitor.			

uniformly so; therefore, large-scale clinical trials have not been undertaken. Platelet-activating factor (PAF) is an inflammatory signal that assumes significance of importance. Inhibition of PAF with several antagonists has failed uniformly in clinical trials (Table 31.7).[81–83]

Inhibition of TNF-α and IL-1 has received the greatest attention because of encouraging results identified in animal models of sepsis.[84–94] However, clinical trials with anti-TNF-α antibodies and IL-1 receptor antagonists have demonstrated no clinical improvement (Table 31.8). In one study, MODS patients treated with anti-TNF-α antibodies actually had poorer outcomes than nontreated patients.

Neutralization of the toxic products released by activated leukocytes has also shown promise in the experimental laboratory. Neutralization of reactive oxygen species with superoxide dismutase and catalase has been effective in experimental endotoxemia and acute bacterial infection, but these agents are untried for sepsis/SIRS/MODS in the clinic. Nitrones are scavengers of both reactive oxygen and reactive nitrogen species but have not been employed clinically. Lazaroids reduce lipid peroxidation and have undergone some limited human investigation (e.g., in traumatic brain injury) but not in SIRS/MODS.

Counterinflammatory Cytokine Therapy

Another overriding concept about the pathophysiology and treatment of SIRS/MODS is excessive systemic activation of the inflammatory cascade. Counterinflammatory signals such as IL-4, IL-10, IL-13, and transforming growth factor-beta

TABLE 31.7.
Platelet-Activating Factor (PAF).

Trial (year)	*Total randomized patients*	*Intervention*	*Endpoint*
Dhainaut (1998)[81]	609	PAF receptor antagonist	28-day mortality
Comment: The 28-day mortality rate was 50% in the placebo group and 44% in the PAF antagonist-treated group ($P = 0.50$). Subgroup analysis confirmed no indications of favorable variables for this treatment.			
Poeze (2000)[82]	98	PAF receptor antagonist (TCV-309)	56-day mortality
Comment: The 56-day mortality rate for control patients was 41.7% and was 51% for treated patients ($P = 0.47$). The authors reported significantly fewer failed organs in the antagonist treated group ($P = 0.04$). The study was not powered correctly for a survival study of patients with severe sepsis and septic shock.			
Opal (2004)[83]	1261	PAF acetylhydrolase	28-day mortality
Comment: The 28-day mortality was 25% in the treated group compared to 24% in the placebo group of patients with severe sepsis. No differences were seen at secondary endpoints nor in subgroup analysis.			

All studies were prospective, randomized, and double-blinded (Class I evidence). The aggregate results have failed to demonstrate any survival benefit for patients with this form of treatment.

TABLE 31.8.

Clinical Trials that Have Attempted to Modulate the Cytokine Response of Phase 2 of the Inflammatory Response. All Trials Were Prospective and Placebo Controlled (Class 1 Evidence) in Patients with the Clinical Diagnosis of Sepsis.

Trial (year)	*Total randomized patients*	*Intervention*	*Endpoint*
Abraham (1995)[84]	971	Anti-TNF monoclonal antibody	28-day mortality
Comments: This was a three-arm study, with one-third of the patients receiving 15 mg/kg antibody, one-third receiving 7.5 mg/kg, and one-third receiving the placebo. For only the patients with septic shock, the 28-day mortality was 38% for both doses of the monoclonal antibody and 46% for the placebo patients, which was not statistically significant. For all treated patients, no significance in reduction of mortality was seen.			
Reinhart (1996)[85]	122	Anti-TNF monoclonal antibody fragment (MAK 195F)	28-day mortality
Comments: There was no difference in survival between the treated and placebo patients in this underpowered study.			
Cohen (1996)[86]	553	Anti-TNF monoclonal antibody	28-day mortality
Comments: The 28-day mortality was 42.9% in the placebo group, 36.7% in the 3 mg/kg treatment arm, and 44.6% in the 15 mg/kg treatment arm for patients with septic shock, which was not significant. Analysis of all patients showed no difference. Shock was reversed faster in treated patients, and treated patients had a delay in onset of first organ failure.			
Fisher (1996)[87]	141	TNF receptor:Fc fusion protein	28-day mortality
Comments: The study was of septic shock patients with a single placebo group and three groups of gradually increased doses of the fusion protein. There was a 30% mortality rate in the placebo group, but a 53% mortality rate in the high-dose fusion protein treatment group ($P = 0.02$).			
Abraham (1997)[88]	498	p55 TNF fusion protein	28-day mortality
Comments: There was no difference between placebo and treated patients ($P = 0.30$) A subset analysis of patients with early septic shock identified suggested potential benefit in the treated patients.			
Abraham (1998)[89]	1879	Murine anti-TNF monoclonal antibody	28-day mortality
Comments: The 28-day mortality of septic shock patients was 42.8% in placebo treatment and 40.3% in those receiving the monoclonal antibody ($P = 0.27$).			
Abraham (2001)[90]	1342	p55 TNF fusion protein	28-day mortality
Comments: The 28-day mortality in these severe sepsis patients with and without shock was 28% in the placebo patients and 27% in the fusion protein-treated patients.			
Reinhart (2001)[91]	446	Anti-TNF monoclonal antibody fragment (afelimomab)	28-day mortality
Comments: Only IL-6-positive sepsis patients were studied. The 28-day mortality rate was 57.7% for placebo treatment and 54% for antibody fragment-treated patients.			
Panacek (2004)[92]	2634	Anti-TNF monoclonal antibody fragment (afelimomab)	28-day mortality
Comments: Patients were segregated into IL-6-positive and -negative patients. Using logistic regression analysis, IL-6-positive patients had a reported 5.8% adjusted improvement in survival ($P = 0.041$). Analysis of IL-6-negative patients and analysis of all patients together demonstrated no significant difference between groups.			
Fisher (1994)[93]	893	Human IL-1 receptor antagonist	28-day mortality
Comments: A study of sepsis syndrome patients; there was no difference in 28-day survival between placebo and treated patients, but some evidence of an increase in survival time in the treated patients.			
Opal (1997)[94]	696	Human IL-1 receptor antagonist	28-day mortality
Comments: The 28-day mortality rate was 36.4% for the placebo-treated patients and 33.1% in the receptor antagonist-treated group ($P = 0.36$). Subgroup analysis failed to identify subpopulations that might benefit from treatment.			

TNF, tumor necrosis factor; IL-1, interleukin-1.

(TNF-β) counteract the proinflammatory signals (e.g., TNF-α, IL-1). Thus, a treatment strategy that has been explored experimentally is to administer counterinflammatory cytokines as therapy to counteract excessive inflammation.[95] Unfortunately, the antiinflammatory response is not as recognizable clinically as the proinflammatory response; accurate recognition and quantification would be a prerequisite to antiinflammatory therapy. Although not used clinically to this point, identification of counterinflammatory signals in the MODS suggests that an inadequate counterinflammatory response may be an important issue.

Alternatively, ICU patients may in fact have a dominant counterinflammatory response, known as the compensatory antiinflammatory response syndrome (CARS).[96] These patients demonstrate profound immunosuppression and have a clinical course of repeated nosocomial infections. The facilitating concept in these patients is the lack of proinflammatory signaling. Thus, future therapeutic efforts likely need to focus upon the balanced relationship of proinflammatory and counterinflammatory signals and understanding under what conditions one or the other predominates.

Conclusion

Only limited success has been achieved thus far to modulate the destructive effects of human inflammation as the fundamental driving force in the development of MODS. Key issues need to be kept in mind as the effort to treat MODS continues.

Inflammation is a redundant and complex process. It may be naïve to believe that blocking a single pathway will result in improved outcomes. Inflammation evolved for the benefit of the host. As has been seen in some clinical trials, blocking steps in the inflammatory pathway may have an adverse impact upon outcomes. Better diagnostics and better staging of the SIRS/MODS patient are needed. When is endotoxemia of clinical significance? Are all MODS patients pathophysiologically the same? It is unlikely that one treatment will fit all. Bedside phenotyping or the use of microarray (gene chip) technology may be one approach to improved diagnostics. Better animal models are needed for study. Not surprisingly, good results in animal models have not been validated in patients. We remain ignorant about the variability of host responses among different populations of patients. Host augmentation (or therapeutic immunosuppression) as a strategy requires that we have better measures of the host response. Specifically, a better understanding of the human counterinflammatory response is needed. The ultimately successful treatment of SIRS and of MODS may lie in a better understanding of normal counterinflammatory mechanisms and how they may be amplified selectively.

References

1. American College of Chest Physicians/Society of Critical Care Medicine Consensus Conference. Definition for sepsis and organ failure and guidelines for the use of innovative therapies in sepsis. Crit Care Med 1992;20:864.
2. Ashbaugh DG, Bigelow DB, Petty TL, Levine BE. Acute respiratory distress in adults. Lancet 1967;2:319–323.
3. Skillman JJ, Bushnell LS, Goldman H, Silen W. Respiratory failure, hypotension, sepsis, and jaundice. Am J Surg 1969;117: 523–530.
4. Tilney NL, Bailey GL, Morgan AP. Sequential system failure after rupture of abdominal aortic aneurysms: an unsolved problem in postoperative care. Ann Surg 1973;178:117–122.
5. Eiseman B, Beart R, Norton L. Multiple organ failure. Surg Gynecol Obstet 1977;144:323–326.
6. Polk HC Jr, Shields CL. Remote organ failure: a valid sign of occult intra-abdominal infection. Surgery (St. Louis) 1977;81:310–313.
7. Baue AE. Multiple, progressive, or sequential systems failure. Arch Surg 1975;110:779–781.
8. Fry DE, Pearlstein L, Fulton RL, Polk HC Jr. Multiple system organ failure: the role of uncontrolled infection. Arch Surg 1980;115:136–140.
9. Fry DE, Garrison RN, Heitch RC, et al. Determinants of death in patients with intraabdominal abscess. Surgery (St. Louis) 1980;89:517–523.
10. Fry DE, Garrison RN, Polk HC Jr. Clinical implications in *Bacteroides* bacteremia. Surg Gynecol Obstet 1979;149:189–192.
11. Fry DE, Garrison RN, Williams HC. Patterns of morbidity and mortality in splenectomy for trauma. Am Surg 1980;46:28–32.
12. Deutschman CS, Konstantinides FN, Tsai M, et al. Physiology and metabolism in isolated viral septicemia: further evidence of an organism-independent, host-dependent response. Arch Surg 1987;122:21–25.
13. Siegel JH, Cerra FB, Coleman B, et al. Physiologic and metabolic correlations in human sepsis. Surgery (St. Louis) 1979;86:163–193.
14. Goris RJ, Beokhorst PA, Nuytinck KS. Multiple organ failure: generalized autodestructive inflammation. Arch Surg 1985;120: 1109–1115.
15. Fry DE. Sepsis syndrome. Am Surg 2000;66:126–132.
16. Luster AD. Chemokines: chemotactic cytokines that mediate inflammation. N Engl J Med 1998;338:436–445.
17. Baggiolini M. Chemokines in pathology and medicine. J Intern Med 2001;250:91–104.
18. Olson TS, Ley K. Chemokines and chemokine receptors in leukocyte trafficking. Am J Physiol Regul Integr Comp Physiol 2002;283:R7–R28.
19. Dianqing WU. Signaling mechanisms for regulation of chemotaxis. Cell Res 2005;15:52–56.
20. Klebanoff SJ, Vedes MA, Harlan JM, et al. Stimulation of neutrophils by tumor necrosis factor. J Immunol 1986;136:4220–4225.
21. Fry DE, Pearlstein L, Fulton RL, Polk HC Jr. Multiple system organ failure. Arch Surg 1980;115:136–140.
22. Knaus WA, Draper EA, Wagner DP, et al. Prognosis in acute organ-system failure. Ann Surg 1985;202:685–693.
23. Goris RJA, te Bockhorst TPA, Nuytinck JKS, Gimbrere JSF. Multiple organ failure. Arch Surg 1985;120:1109–1110.
24. Marshall JC, Christou NV, Horn R, Meakins JL. The microbiology of multiple organ failure. Arch Surg 1988;123:309–315.
25. Vincent JL. Organ dysfunction as an outcome measure: the SOFA score. Sepsis 1997;1:53–54.
26. Bohnen JM, Marshall JC, Fry DE, et al. Clinical and scientific importance of source control in abdominal infections: summary of a symposium. Can J Surg 1999;42:122–126.
27. Mosdell DM, Morris DM, Voltura A, et al. Antibiotic treatment for surgical peritonitis. Ann Surg 1991;214:543–549.
28. Nathens AB, Rotstein OD, Marshall JC. Tertiary peritonitis: clinical features of a complex nosocomial infection. World J Surg 1998;22:158–163.
29. Rackow EC, Falk JL, Fein IA, et al. Fluid resuscitation in circulatory shock: a comparison of the cardiorespiratory effects of albumin, hetastarch, and saline solutions in patients with hypovolemic and septic shock. Crit Care Med 1983;11:839–850.
30. Newman M, Demling RH. Colloid vs. crystalloid during septic shock. Int Crit Care Dig 1990;9:3–8.
31. Wheeler AP, Bernard GR. Current concepts: treating patients with severe sepsis. N Engl J Med 1999;340:207–214.
32. Rivers E, Nguyen B, Havstad S, et al. Early goal-directed therapy in the treatment of severe sepsis and septic shock. N Engl J Med 2001;345:1368–1377.
33. Dellinger RP, Carlet JM, Masur H, et al. Surviving sepsis campaign guidelines for management of severe sepsis and septic shock. Crit Care Med 2004;32:858–873.
34. Denton MD, Chertow GM, Brady HR. "Renal dose" dopamine for the treatment of acute renal failure: scientific rationale, experimental studies and clinical trials. Kidney Int 1996;50:4–14.
35. Meadows D, Edwards JD, Wilkins RG, Nightingale P. Reversal of intractable septic shock with norepinephrine therapy. Crit Care Med 1988;16:663–666.
36. Holmes CL, Walley KR, Chittock DR, et al. The effects of vasopressin on hemodynamics and renal function in severe septic shock: a case series. Intensive Care Med 2001;27:1416–1421.
37. Bone RC, Fisher CJ, Clemmer TP. A controlled clinical trial of high-dose methylprednisolone in the treatment of severe sepsis and septic shock. N Engl J Med 1987;317:653–658.
38. The Veterans Administration Systemic Sepsis Cooperative Study Group: Effect of high-dose glucocorticoid therapy on mortality in patients with clinical signs of sepsis. N Engl J Med 1987;317:659–665.
39. Bollaert PE, Charpentier C, Levy B, et al. Reversal of late septic shock with supraphysiologic doses of hydrocortisone. Crit Care Med 1998;26:645–650.
40. Briegel J, Forst H, Haller M, et al. Stress doses of hydrocortisone reverse hyperdynamic septic shock: a prospective, randomized double-blind, single-center trial. Crit Care Med 1999;27:723–732.
41. Annane D, Sebille V, Charpentier C, et al. Effect of treatment with low doses of hydrocortisone and fludrocortisone on mortal-

ity in patients with septic shock. JAMA 2002;21:288:862–871.
42. Amato MB, Barbas CS, Medeiros DM, et al. Effect of a protective-ventilation strategy on mortality in the acute respiratory distress syndrome. N Engl J Med 1998;338:347–354.
43. Stewart TE, Meade MO, Cook DJ, et al. Evaluation of a ventilation strategy to prevent barotraumas in patients at high risk for acute respiratory distress syndrome. Pressure and volume-limited ventilation strategy group. N Engl J Med 1998;338:355–361.
44. Brochard L, Roudat-Thoraval F, Roupie E, et al. Tidal volume reduction for prevention of ventilator-induced lung injury in acute respiratory distress syndrome. The multicenter trial group on tidal volume reduction in ARDS. Am J Respir Crit Care Med 1998;158:1831–1838.
45. Brower RG, Fessler HE. Mechanical ventilation in acute lung injury and acute respiratory distress syndrome. Clin Chest Med 2000;21:491–510.
46. The Acute Respiratory Distress Syndrome Network. Ventilation with lower tidal volumes as compared with traditional tidal volumes for acute lung injury and the acute respiratory distress syndrome. N Engl J Med 2000;342:1301–1308.
47. Bidani A, Tzouanakis AE, Cardenas VJ, et al. Permissive hypercapnia in acute respiratory failure. JAMA 1994;272:957–962.
48. Pesenti A, Marcolin R, Prato P, et al. Mean airway pressure vs. positive end-expiratory pressure during mechanical ventilation. Crit Care Med 1985;13:34–37.
49. Drakulovic M, Torres A, Bauer T, et al. Supine body position as a risk factor for nosocomial pneumonia in mechanically ventilated patients: a randomized trial. Lancet 1999;354:1851–1858.
50. Brook AD, Ahrens TS, Schaiff R, et al. Effect of a nursing-implemented sedation protocol on the duration of mechanical ventilation. Crit Care Med 1999;27:2609–2615.
51. Manthous CA, Chatila W. Prolonged weakness after withdrawal of atracurium. Am J Respir Crit Care Med 1994;150:1441–1443.
52. Gattinoni L, Tognoni G, Pesenti A, et al. Effect of prone positioning on the survival of patients with acute respiratory failure. N Engl J Med 2001;345:568–573.
53. Mehta RL, McDonald B, Gabbai FB, et al. A randomized clinical trial of continuous versus intermittent dialysis for acute renal failure. Kidney Int 2001;60:1154–1163.
54. Kellum J, Angus DC, Johnson JP, et al. Continuous versus intermittent renal replacement therapy: a meta-analysis. Intensive Care Med 2002;28:29–37.
55. Cooper DJ, Walley KR, Wiggs BR, Russell JA. Bicarbonate does not improve hemodynamics in critically ill patients who have lactic acidosis: a prospective, controlled clinical study. Ann Intern Med 1990;112:492–498.
56. Morgera S, Haase M, Rocktaschel J, et al. Intermittent high-permeability hemofiltration modulates inflammatory response in septic patients with multiorgan failure. Nephron Clin Pract 2003;94:c75–c80.
57. Bengsch S, Boos KS, Nagel D, et al. Extracorporeal plasma treatment for the removal of endotoxin in patients with sepsis: clinical results of a pilot study. Shock 2005;23:494–500.
58. Reinhart K, Meier-Hellmann A, Beale R, et al. Open randomized phase II trial of an extracorporeal endotoxin adsorber in suspected gram-negative sepsis. Crit Care Med 2004;32:1662–1668.
59. Vincent JL, Laterre PF, Cohen J, et al. A pilot-controlled study of a polymixin B-immobilized hemoperfusion cartridge in patients with severe sepsis secondary to intra-abdominal infection. Shock 2005;23:400–405.
60. Heyland DK, Novak F, Drover JW, et al. Should immunonutrition become routine in critically ill patients? A systematic review of the evidence. JAMA 2001;286:944–953.
61. van den Berghe G, Wouters P, Weekers F, et al. Intensive insulin therapy in the surgical intensive care unit. N Engl J Med 2001;345:1359–1367.
62. Cook D, Guyatt G, Marshall J, et al. A comparison of sucralfate and ranitidine for the prevention of upper gastrointestinal bleeding in patients requiring mechanical ventilation. Canadian Critical Care Trials Group. N Engl J Med 1998;338:791–797.
63. McNaught CE, Woodcock NP, Anderson AD, MacFie J. A prospective randomized trial of probiotics in critically ill patients. Clin Nutr 2005;24:211–219.
64. Kinasewitz GT, Yan SB, Basson B, et al. Universal changes in biomarkers of coagulation and inflammation occur in patients with severe sepsis, regardless of causative micro-organism. Crit Care 2004;8:R82–R90.
65. Samama MM, Cohen AT, Darmon JY, et al. A comparison of enoxaparin with placebo for the prevention of venous thromboembolism in acutely ill medical patients. Prophylaxis in medical patients with enoxaparin study group. N Engl J Med 1999;341:793–800.
66. Ziegler EJ, McCutchan JA, Fierer J, et al. Treatment of gram-negative bacteremia and shock with human antiserum to a mutant *Escherichia coli.* N Engl J Med 1982;307:1225.
67. Ziegler EJ, Fischer CJ, Sprung CL Jr, et al. Treatment of gram-negative bacteremia and septic shock with HA-1A human monoclonal antibody against endotoxin: a randomized, double-blind, placebo-controlled trial. N Engl J Med 1991;324:429.
68. McCloskey RV, Straube RC, Sanders C, et al. Treatment of septic shock with human monoclonal antibody HA-1A. A randomized, double-blind, placebo-controlled trial. CHESS Trial Study Group. Ann Intern Med 1994;121:1–5.
69. Greenman RL, Schein RMH, Martin MA, et al. A controlled clinical trial of E5 murine monoclonal IgM antibody to endotoxin in the treatment of gram-negative sepsis. JAMA 1991;266:1097.
70. Bone RC, Balk RA, Fein AM, et al. A second large controlled study of E5, a monoclonal antibody to endotoxin: results of a prospective, multicenter, randomized, controlled trial. The E5 Sepsis Study Group. Crit Care Med 1995;23:994–1006.
71. Angus DC, Birmingham MC, Balk RA, et al. E5 murine monoclonal antiendotoxin antibody in gram-negative sepsis: a randomized controlled trial. E5 study investigators. JAMA 2000;283:1723–1730.
72. Albertson TE, Panacek EA, MacArthur RD, et al. Multicenter evaluation of a human monoclonal antibody to *Enterobacteriaceae* common antigen in patients with gram-negative sepsis. Crit Care Med 2003;31:419–427.
73. Levin M, Quint PA, Goldstein B, et al. Recombinant bactericidal/permeability-increasing protein (rBPI 21) as adjunctive treatment for children with severe meningococcal sepsis: a randomized trial. rBPI 21 meningococcal sepsis study group. Lancet 2000;356:961–967.
74. Reinhart K, Gluck T, Ligtenberg J, et al. CD14 receptor occupancy in severe sepsis: results of a phase I clinical trial with a recombinant chimeric CD14 antibody. Crit Care Med 2004;32:1223–1224.
75. Warren BL, Eid A, Singer P, et al. Caring for the critically ill patient. High-dose antithrombin III in severe sepsis: a randomized controlled trial. JAMA 2001;286:1869–1878.
76. Bernard GR, Vincent JL, Laterre PF, et al. Efficacy and safety of recombinant human activated protein C for severe sepsis. N Engl J Med 2001;344:699–709.
77. Abraham E, Laterre PF, Garg R, et al. Drotrecogin alfa(activated) for adults with severe sepsis and a low risk of death. N Engl J Med 2005;353:1332–1341.
78. Fein AM, Bernard GR, Criner GJ, et al. Treatment of severe systemic inflammatory response syndromes and sepsis with a novel bradykinin antagonist, deltibant (CP-0127). Results of a

randomized, double-blind, placebo-controlled trial. CP-1027 SIRS and Sepsis Study Group. JAMA 1997;277:482–487.

79. Abraham E, Reinhart K, Opal S, et al. Efficacy and safety of tifacogin (recombinant tissue factor pathway inhibitor) in severe sepsis: a randomized controlled trial. JAMA 2003;290:238–247.
80. Lopez A, Lorente JA Steingrub J, et al. Multiple-center, randomized, placebo-controlled, double-blind study of the nitric oxide synthase inhibitor 546C88: effect on survival in patients with septic shock. Crit Care Med 2004;32:21–30.
81. Dhainaut JF, Tenaillon A, Hemmer M, et al. Confirmatory platelet-activating factor receptor antagonist trial in patients with severe gram-negative bacterial sepsis: a phase III, randomized, double-blind, placebo controlled, multicenter trial. BN 52021 Sepsis Investigator Group. Crit Care Med 1998;26:1963–1971.
82. Poeze M, Froon AH, Ramsay G, et al. Decreased organ failure in patients with severe SIRS and septic shock treated with the platelet-activating factor antagonist TCV-309: a prospective, multicenter, double-blind, randomized phase II trial. TCV-309 septic shock study group. Shock 2000;14:421–428.
83. Opal S, Laterre PF, Abraham E, et al. Recombinant human platelet-activating factor acetylhydrolase for treatment of severe sepsis: results of a phase III, multicenter, randomized, double-blind, placebo-controlled, clinical trial. Crit Care Med 2004; 32:332–341.
84. Abraham E, Wunderink R, Silverman H, et al. Efficacy and safety of monoclonal antibody to human tumor necrosis factor alpha in patients with sepsis syndrome. A randomized, controlled, double-blind, multicenter clinical trial. JAMA 1995;273:934–941.
85. Reinhart K, Wiegard-Lohnert C, Grimminger F, et al. Assessment of the safety and efficacy of the monoclonal anti-tumor necrosis factor antibody-fragment, MAK 195F, in patients with sepsis and septic shock: a multicenter, randomized, placebo-controlled, dose-ranging study. Crit Care Med 1996;24:733–742.
86. Cohen J, Carlet J. Intersept: an international, multicenter, placebo-controlled trial of monoclonal antibody to human tumor necrosis factor-alpha in patients with sepsis. International Sepsis Trial Study Group. Crit Care Med 1996;24:1431–1440.
87. Fisher CJ Jr, Agosti JM, Opal SM, et al. Treatment of septic shock with the tumor necrosis factor receptor: Fc fusion protein. The soluble TNF Receptor Sepsis Study Group. N Engl J Med 1996;334:1697–1702.
88. Abraham E, Glauser MP, Butler T, et al. p55 tumor necrosis factor receptor fusion protein in the treatment of patients with severe sepsis and septic shock. A randomized controlled multicenter trial. Ro 45-2081 study group. JAMA 1997;277:1531–1538.
89. Abraham E, Anzueto A, Gutierrez G, et al. Double-blind randomized controlled trial of monoclonal antibody to human tumour necrosis factor in treatment of septic shock. NORASEPT Group. Lancet 1998;351:929–933.
90. Abraham E, Laterre PF, Garbino J, et al. Lenercept (p55 tumor necrosis factor receptor fusion protein) in severe sepsis and early septic shock: a randomized, double-blind, placebo-controlled, multicenter phase III trial with 1,342 patients. Crit Care Med 2001;29:503–510.
91. Reinhart K, Menges T, Gardlund B, et al. Randomized, placebo-controlled trial of the anti-tumor necrosis factor antibody fragment afelimomab in hyperinflammatory response during severe sepsis: the RAMSES study. Crit Care Med 2001;29:765–769.
92. Panacek EA, Marshall JC, Albertson TE, et al. Efficacy and safety of the monoclonal anti-tumor necrosis factor antibody (ab')2 fragment afelimomab in patients with severe sepsis and elevated interleukin-6 levels. Crit Care Med 2004;32:2173–2182.
93. Fisher CJ Jr, Dhainaut JF, Opal SM, et al. Recombinant human interleukin 1 receptor antagonist in the treatment of patients with sepsis syndrome. Results from a randomized, double-blind, placebo-controlled trial. Phase III rhIL-1ra Sepsis Syndrome Study Group. JAMA 1994;271:1836–1843.
94. Opal SM, Fisher CJ Jr, Dhainaut JF, et al. Confirming interleukin-1 receptor antagonist trial in severe sepsis. A phase III, randomized, double-blind, placebo-controlled, multicenter trial. The Interleukin-1 Receptor Antagonist Sepsis Investigation Group. Crit Care Med 1997;25:1115–1124.
95. Kumar A, Zanotti S, Bunnell G, et al. Interleukin-10 blunts the human inflammatory response to lipopolysaccharide without affecting the cardiovascular response. Crit Care Med 2005;33: 331–340.
96. Bone RC, Grodzin CJ, Bulk RA. Sepsis: a new hypothesis for pathogenesis of the disease process. Chest 1997;112:235–243.

32

Mechanical Ventilation

David J. Dries and John F. Perry, Jr.

Positive-pressure ventilation as we know it came into its own during the polio epidemics of the 1950s.[1] Since that time, the use of mechanical ventilatory support has been synonymous with the growth of critical care medicine. Early ventilation used neuromuscular blocking agents to suppress spontaneous respiratory effort. Today, patient–ventilator interaction is understood to be crucial, and there is a growing awareness of complications associated with neuromuscular blockade.[2] Finally, there is increasing recognition that ventilators can induce various forms of lung injury, which has led to reappraisal of the goals of ventilatory support.[3] Although it seems that each manufacturer of mechanical ventilators has introduced differing modes of mechanical ventilation, fundamental principles of ventilator management of critically ill patients remain unchanged.

Positive-pressure ventilation can be lifesaving in patients with hypoxemia or respiratory acidosis refractory to simpler measures. In patients with severe cardiopulmonary distress with excessive work of breathing, mechanical ventilation substitutes for the action of respiratory muscles.[4] In the setting of respiratory distress, respiratory muscles may account for as much as 40% of total oxygen consumption (VO_2).[5,6] In these circumstances, mechanical ventilation allows reallocation of oxygen to other tissue beds, which may be otherwise vulnerable to hypoxia. In addition, reversal of respiratory muscle fatigue, which may contribute to respiratory failure, depends on respiratory muscle rest. Positive-pressure ventilation can reverse or prevent atelectasis by allowing inspiration at a more favorable region of the pressure–volume curve describing pulmonary function. With improved gas exchange and relief from excessive respiratory muscle work, an opportunity is provided for the lungs and airways to heal.

Mechanical ventilation is not therapeutic in itself. Positive-pressure ventilation may aggravate or initiate alveolar damage. These recognized dangers of ventilator-induced lung injury (VILI) have led to reappraisal of the objectives of mechanical ventilation. Rather than seeking normal arterial blood gas values, it is often better to accept a degree of respiratory acidosis and possibly relative hypoxemia to avoid large tidal volumes (V_T) and high inflation pressures.[4]

Mechanical ventilation may have hemodynamic effects as well. Positive-pressure ventilation decreases cardiac output (Q) frequently, primarily as a result of decreased venous return.[7] In other circumstances, mechanical ventilation may paradoxically increase Q in the setting of impaired myocardial contractility because left ventricular afterload decreases with increased intrathoracic pressure.[8] Alveolar distension compresses alveolar vessels and the resulting increase in pulmonary vascular resistance and right ventricular afterload produce a leftward shift in the interventricular septum. Left ventricular compliance is decreased both by the bulging interventricular septum and increased juxtacardiac pressure from distended lungs. There seems little doubt that either adding mechanical ventilation or removing this support from critically ill patients can be a substantial imposed stress (Fig. 32.1).

Mechanical ventilation strategies are clearly affected by underlying pulmonary disease. For example, in patients with acute respiratory failure (ARF), chronic obstructive pulmonary disorder (COPD), asthma, or other conditions associated with a high minute ventilation$_E$ (V_E), gas trapping develops in alveoli as patients have inadequate expiratory time available for exhalation before the next breath begins.[9] Patients experiencing this, termed *breath stacking*, have an alveolar peripheral positive end-expiratory pressure (PEEP). Also termed *auto-PEEP*, this retained alveolar gas makes triggering the ventilator more difficult, because the patient needs to generate a negative pressure equal in magnitude to the level of auto-PEEP in addition to the trigger threshold of the machine. This is one factor that may contribute to inability to trigger the ventilator despite obvious respiratory effort.[10] Auto-PEEP may be undetected because it is not registered routinely on the pressure manometer of the ventilator. Newer machines have software to detect auto-PEEP. In older machines, occluding the expiratory port of the circuit at the end of expiration in a relaxed patient causes pressure in the lungs and ventilator circuit to equilibrate, displaying the level of auto-PEEP on

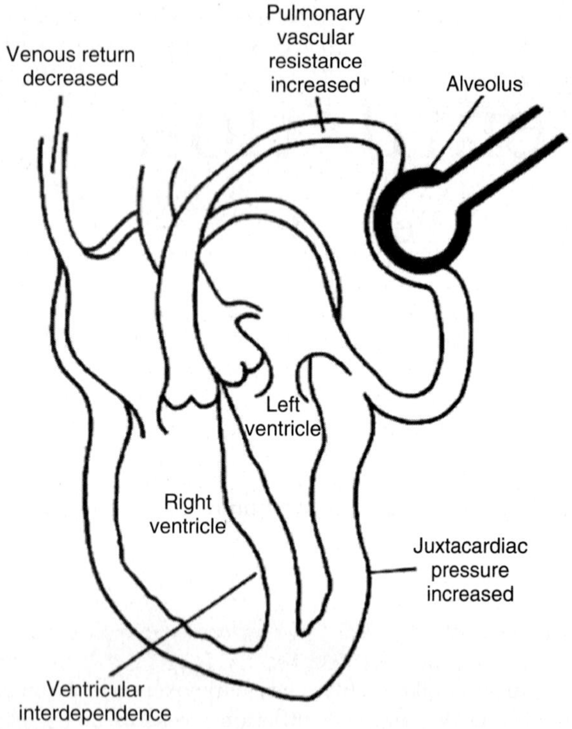

FIGURE 32.1. Factors responsible for the decrease in cardiac output during positive-pressure ventilation. An increase in intrathoracic pressure compresses the vena cava and thus decreases venous return. Alveolar distension compresses the alveolar vessels, and the resulting increases in pulmonary vascular resistance and right ventricular afterload produce a leftward shift in the interventricular septum. Left ventricular compliance is decreased by both the bulging septum and the increased juxtacardiac pressure resulting from distended lungs. (From Tobin,[4] by permission of New England Journal of Medicine.)

the manometer.[11] Fortunately, in most patients, auto-PEEP does not become a problem until the respiratory rate reaches 30 breaths/min.[12] If auto-PEEP or breath stacking is detected, respiratory rate and V_T should be reduced to permit breath stacking and auto-PEEP to resolve.

Mechanical Ventilator Modes and Settings

Technological developments have provided a wide variety of modes by which a patient may be ventilated mechanically,[13] with the hope of improving gas exchange, patient comfort, or promoting a rapid return to spontaneous ventilation. Nearly all modes allow full rest of the patient, on the one hand, and periods of exercise on the other. Thus, in the great majority of patients, choice of mode is merely a matter of physician or patient preference. Because controlled ventilation with abolition of spontaneous breathing rapidly leads to atrophy of respiratory muscles, various assisted modes that are triggered by patients' inspiratory efforts are preferred.[2] The most common triggered modes are assist-control ventilation (ACV), intermittent mandatory ventilation (IMV), and pressure support ventilation (PSV).[14] On some ventilators, V_T can be selected by the physician or respiratory therapist, whereas on others V_E and respiratory rate are chosen secondary to determining the V_T. Similarly, on some machines an inspiratory gas flow rate is selected, while on other ventilators inspiratory gas flow depends on the ratio of inspiratory time to total respiratory cycle time and respiratory rate or an inspiratory to expiratory time ratio and respiratory rate.[15]

Assist Control Ventilation

Set parameters in the ACV mode are inspiratory flow rate, frequency, and V_T.[16] The ventilator delivers a set number of equal breaths per minute each of a given V_T. Tidal volume and flow determine inspiratory and expiratory time as well as the ratio of inspiratory to expiratory time. Plateau or alveolar pressure is related to V_T and the compliance of the respiratory system. The difference between peak and plateau pressures includes contributions from flow and inspiratory resistance. The patient has the ability to trigger extra breaths by exerting an inspiratory effort exceeding a preset trigger pressure difference. Typically, each patient will display a preferred rate for a given V_T and will trigger all breaths when the ventilator frequency is set a few breaths per minute below the patient's rate. In this setting, the control rate serves as underlying support should the patient stop initiating breaths (become apneic). When high inspiratory effort continues during a ventilator-delivered breath, the patient may trigger a second superimposed breath. Patient effort can be increased, if increased exercise is desired, by increasing the magnitude of the required trigger threshold or lowering V_T. In a multi-institutional survey of medical and medical/surgical intensive care units, the ACV mode is used most commonly.[14]

Synchronized Intermittent Mandatory Ventilation

In a passive patient, synchronized intermittent mandatory ventilation (SIMV) cannot be distinguished from controlled ventilation in the ACV mode.[17] Ventilation is determined by the mandatory frequency and V_T. However, if the patient is not truly passive, he or she may perform respiratory work during mandatory breaths.[18] In addition, the patient may trigger additional breaths by lowering the airway opening pressure below a preset trigger threshold.[19] If this triggering effort comes in a brief, defined interval before the next mandatory breath is due, the ventilator will deliver the mandatory breath ahead of schedule to synchronize with the patient's inspiratory effort. If a breath is initiated outside the synchronization window, V_T, flow, and inspiratory to expiratory time ratio are determined by patient effort and respiratory system mechanics, not by ventilator settings.[20] These spontaneous breaths tend to be of small volume and are highly variable from breath to breath. The SIMV mode is often used to gradually augment the patient's work of breathing by lowering the mandatory breath frequency or V_T, driving the patient to breathe more rapidly to maintain adequate V_E. This approach appears to prolong separation from mechanical ventilation. SIMV is used widely but there is relatively little rationale for it.

Pressure Control Ventilation

In the passive patient, ventilation is determined by respiratory rate, inspiratory pressure increment, the inspiratory to expiratory time ratio, and the time constant of the patient respiratory system.[21] In patients without severe airway obstruction, given a sufficiently long inspiratory time, there is equilibration between ventilator-determined inspiratory pressure and alveolar pressure so that inspiratory flow ceases. In this situation, V_T is highly predictable based on equality between inspiratory and alveolar pressure and mechanical properties of the respiratory system. In essence, the driving pressure of the source of inspired gas, which can be set, determines the exhaled V_T. In the presence of airflow obstruction or short inspiratory time, V_T is less predictable and may be less than intended if the breath is terminated by reaching a limiting airway pressure before the desired V_T is delivered.

The active patient can trigger additional breaths by reducing airway opening pressure below a triggering threshold. In this mode, inspiratory time is generally set by the physician, and care must be taken to assess the patient's inspiratory effort from waveforms or physical examination and adjust the ventilator accordingly; otherwise, additional sedation may be required.

Pressure Support Ventilation

The patient must trigger the ventilator to activate this mode; thus, pressure support ventilation (PSV) is not applied in passive, paralyzed, or heavily sedated patients. Ventilation is determined by preset inspiratory pressure, patient-determined rate, and patient effort. Once a breath is triggered, the ventilator attempts to maintain inspiratory pressure at the physician-determined level using whatever flow is necessary to accomplish this.[22,23] Eventually, flow begins to fall as a result of either cessation of patient inspiratory effort or increasing elastic recoil of the respiratory system as V_T rises. The ventilator will maintain inspiratory pressure until inspiratory flow falls an arbitrary amount (for example, to 25% of initial flow) or below an absolute flow rate. Patient work of breathing can be increased by lower inspiratory pressure or making the trigger less sensitive and can inadvertently increase if respiratory system mechanics change with no change in ventilator settings. A potential advantage of PSV is improved patient comfort and, for some patients with very high respiratory drive, reduced work of breathing compared with volume preset modes.[24]

Some ventilators allow combinations of modes. Most commonly used is SIMV plus PSV. Some physicians use SIMV as a means to add "sighs" to PSV and decrease atelectasis. Because SIMV plus PSV guarantees some minimum backup minute ventilation, which PSV alone does not, this mode combination may have value in patients at high risk for deteriorating central respiratory drive.[15]

Ventilator Triggering

In the ACV, SIMV, and PSV modes, the patient must lower airway pressure below a preset threshold to trigger the ventilator. In most situations, this is straightforward; the more negative the sensitivity, the greater the effort demanded of the patient. When breath stacking or auto-PEEP is present, the patient must lower alveolar pressure by the amount of auto-PEEP then further by the trigger amount to initiate a breath; this can dramatically increase the effort required to initiate a breath.[15,25]

Flow triggering systems have been used to reduce the work of triggering the ventilator. In contrast to the usual approach in which the patient must open a demand valve to receive assistance, continuous flow systems maintain a high continuous flow, then further augment flow when the patient initiates a breath. These systems reduce the work of breathing slightly below that present using conventional demand valves, but do not solve the triggering problem when breath stacking occurs.

Unconventional Ventilatory Modes

Inverse ratio ventilation (IRV) is defined as a mode in which the ratio of inspiratory to expiratory time is greater than one.[26,27] IRV is done in one of two ways: pressure-controlled inverse ratio ventilation has a preset airway pressure delivered for a fixed period of time at an inspiratory to expiratory time ratio greater than one; in volume-controlled inverse ratio ventilation, a fixed V_T is delivered at a slow inspiratory flow rate to yield an inspiratory to expiratory time ratio greater than one. The physician must specify the inspiratory airway pressure, rate, and inspiratory to expiratory time ratio while V_T and flow are determined by respiratory system impedance. Compared to conventional modes of ventilation, oxygenation is often improved with IRV owing to increased mean alveolar pressure and volume consequent to longer time above functional residual capacity or by creation of auto-PEEP. Because auto-PEEP is a common consequence of IRV, serial determination of auto-PEEP is important for safe use of this mode. Heavy sedation is frequently required.

Airway pressure release ventilation consists of continuous positive airway pressure, which is intermittently released to allow a brief expiratory interval.[28] A potential advantage of airway pressure release ventilation is that mean alveolar pressure is lower that it would be during positive-pressure ventilation from the same amount of continuous positive airway pressure, possibly reducing the risks of hemodynamic compromise and alveolar injury. The clinical benefit of this mode remains to be demonstrated.

Some modes attempt to combine the benefits of volume and pressure preset modes. For example, the pressure-regulated volume control mode allows a time-limited pressure and adjusts the pressure of subsequent breaths, as needed, to assure a set V_T.[29] Proposed advantages of this mode are prevention of alveolar overdistension by limiting pressure and high initial inspiratory flows while guaranteeing a V_T. However, as patient effort increases, the ventilator actually reduces support. In volume-assured pressure support mode, volume is monitored during each pressure support breath and, if a preset V_T is not achieved, additional volume is given at a constant flow to augment that breath.[30] With this mode comes a risk of alveolar overdistension and injury.

Proportional assist ventilation is intended for patients who are breathing spontaneously. The goal of this mode is to normalize the relationship between patient effort and resulting ventilatory consequences. The ventilator adjusts inspiratory pressure in proportion to patient effort throughout any given breath and from breath to breath,[31] which allows the patient to modulate breathing pattern and total ventilation. Instantaneous flow and the volume of gas moving from ventilator to patient are monitored. Potential advantages of this method are greater patient comfort, lower peak airway pressure, and enhancement of the patient's reflexive and behavioral respiratory control.

High Frequency Ventilation

By definition, high frequency ventilation uses a V_T smaller than dead space volume and respiratory rates outside physiological limits. Gas exchange does not occur through convection as during conventional ventilation but through bulk flow, tailored effusion, molecular diffusion, nonconvective mixing, and possibly other mechanisms.[32] These modes include high frequency oscillatory ventilation and high frequency jet ventilation. The theoretical benefit of high frequency ventilation is a lower risk of barotrauma as a result of smaller tidal excursion with improved gas exchange through more uniform distribution of ventilation and improved healing of wounds such as bronchopleural fistulas.[33,34] Split-lung ventilation for complex pulmonary operations can be facilitated by high frequency ventilation. Clear risks are that auto-PEEP is invariably present and that alveolar pressure is underestimated by monitoring pressure at the airway opening. This is not a new ventilatory strategy, and controlled trials have failed to demonstrate clinically relevant benefit. Complications stemming from alveolar and tracheal injury are common. Nonetheless, high frequency ventilation is the logical extension of lowering V_T as a means to prevent alveolar overdistension.

Routine Ventilator Settings

Ventilator settings are based on the patient's size and condition. The risk of pulmonary oxygen toxicity is minimized by using the lowest fraction of inspired oxygen that can satisfactorily oxygenate arterial blood. The usual goal is an arterial oxygen tension (PaO_2) of 60 mmHg or an oxygen saturation of 90% because higher values do not substantially enhance tissue oxygenation.[4]

Historical practice has included V_T of 10 to 15 mL/kg of body weight, which is two to three times normal.[4] This approach is now considered inappropriate because of convincing data indicating that alveolar overdistension can produce endothelial, epithelial, and basement membrane injuries associated with increased microvascular permeability and lung injury (ventilator-induced lung injury, VILI).[3,35,36] To reduce this risk, one would ideally prefer to monitor alveolar volume, but this is not feasible with current technology. A reasonable substitute is to monitor peak alveolar pressure as obtained from the plateau pressure measured in a relaxed patient by occluding the ventilatory circuit briefly at end-inspiration.[37] The incidence of VILI increases markedly when plateau pressure is high. Particularly in patients with significant underlying pulmonary dysfunction, there is a growing tendency to reduce the V_T delivered to 4–7 mL/kg to achieve a plateau (alveolar) pressure no higher than 30–35 cmH_2O; this may lead to an increase in arterial carbon dioxide ($PaCO_2$) tension. Acceptance of elevated carbon dioxide tension in exchange for controlled alveolar pressure is termed permissive hypercapnia.[4,38,39] It is important to focus on pH rather than $PaCO_2$ if this approach is employed. If the pH falls below 7.20, some physicians will increase V_E or administer sodium bicarbonate.

The rate of ventilation that is set depends on the mode. With ACV, a backup rate should be about 4 breaths/min less than the patient's spontaneous rate; this ensures that the ventilator will continue to supply an adequate minute ventilation should the patient have a sudden decrease in respiratory effort. With SIMV, the rate is typically high at first and then gradually decreased in accordance with patient tolerance.[4]

An inspiratory flow rate of 60 L/min is used with most patients during ACV and SIMV.[40] In patients with chronic obstructive pulmonary disease, better gas exchange may be achieved at a flow rate of 100 L/min, probably because the resulting increase in expiratory time allows for more complete emptying of gas-trapped regions. If the flow rate is insufficient to meet the patient's ventilatory requirements, the patient will strain against his or her own pulmonary impedance and that of the ventilator with a consequent increase in the work of breathing.[41] Examination of the monitoring waveform for airway pressure may be helpful when flow rate and ventilator trigger sensitivity are adjusted.

Positive End-Expiratory Pressure

Few aspects of ventilator management are more controversial than the use of positive end-expiratory pressure (PEEP). In patients with acute respiratory distress syndrome (ARDS), PEEP produces a substantial increase in oxygenation; this is probably caused by reduction in intrapulmonary shunting (Q_S/Q_T) as a result of redistribution of lung water from alveoli to the perivascular interstitial space.[42] Total extravascular lung water is not decreased by PEEP. Provided the improvement in PaO_2 is not decreased cardiac output, F_IO_2 can be decreased, which is the principal therapeutic benefit of PEEP. The application of PEEP influences lung mechanics. Patients with acute lung injury (ALI) commonly have decreased end-expiratory lung volumes and thus, tidal breathing occurs on the low flat portion of the pressure volume curve. By shifting tidal breathing to a more compliant portion of the curve, PEEP can reduce the work of breathing.[43] In patients having air flow limitation or auto-PEEP with difficulty triggering the ventilator, the addition of external PEEP (to a level not exceeding the level of auto-PEEP) can help counteract this problem, because to trigger the ventilator the alveolar pressure needs only be decreased below the level of external PEEP rather than below zero.[44,45] Typical PEEP settings range from 3 to 5 cmH_2O in adults without coexisting pulmonary problems and can range to 15–20 cmH_2O or more in the setting of ARDS or ALI.[46]

Patient Management

Initial Ventilator Settings

Initial ventilator settings depend on the goals of ventilation such as full respiratory muscle rest versus partial exercise, the patient's respiratory system mechanics, and V_E needs. In all patients, the initial F_IO_2 should usually be 0.5 to 1.0 to assure adequate oxygenation, although it can usually be lowered within minutes when guided by pulse oximetry and, in the appropriate setting, the application of PEEP.[47] In the first minutes after institution of mechanical ventilation, the physician should be alert for several common problems, including most notably airway malposition, aspiration of gastric contents, and hypotension. Positive-pressure ventilation may reduce venous return, and thus Q, especially in patients with low mean systemic pressure (e.g., hypovolemia, vasodilating drugs, decreased sympathetic tone) or a high ventilation-related pleural pressure (e.g., chest wall restriction, high PEEP, high auto-PEEP). If hypotension occurs, intravascular volume should be expanded and pleural pressure reduced by decreasing V_T and/or V_E. Although uncommon, tension pneumothorax may be catastrophic in this setting.

For patients with relatively normal respiratory mechanics and gas exchange, initial ventilator orders should include a F_IO_2 of 0.5 to 1.0, V_T of 8–12 mL/kg, rate of 8 to 12 breaths/min, and inspiratory flow rate of 40–60 L/min. Alternatively, if the patient has sufficient drive and is not profoundly weak, PSV may be used.[47,48] The level of pressure support is adjusted (frequently in the range of 10–20 cmH_2O above PEEP) to bring respiratory rate down to the low twenties, corresponding to a V_T of approximately 400 mL in the adult. If gas exchange is normal, F_IO_2 may be further reduced based on pulse oximetry or arterial blood gas determinations.

Optimal care of the mechanically ventilated patient is not limited to management of the ventilator. Evidence-based medicine has led to the development of the *ventilator bundle* (Table 32.1), several strategies that reduce the incidence of ventilator-associated pneumonia and other pulmonary complications. Keeping the head of the bed up 30° at all times has been proved to decrease the risk of aspiration and pneumonia (A–C). Prophylaxis of stress-related gastric mucosal hemorrhage, believed previously to increase the risk of pneumonia, particularly if gastric acid production was suppressed, in fact does not, and is an integral part of the ventilator bundle (D–F).

TABLE 32.1. Ventilator Bundle.

- Head of Bed Elevation (30°–45°)
  - A. Drakulovic MB, Torres A, Bauer TT, et al. Supine body position as a risk factor for nosocomial pneumonia in mechanically ventilated patients: a randomised trial. Lancet 1999; 354:1851–1858
  - B. Torres A, Serra-Batlles J, Ros E, et al. Pulmonary aspiration of gastric contents in patients receiving mechanical ventilation: the effect of body position. Ann Intern Med 1992; 116:540–543.
  - C. Collard HR, Saint S, Matthay MA. Prevention of ventilator-associated pneumonia: an evidence-based systematic review. Ann Intern Med 2003; 138:494–501.
- Stress Ulcer Prophylaxis
  - D. Cook D, Guyatt G, Marshall J, et al. A comparison of sucralfate and ranitidine for the prevention of upper gastrointestinal bleeding in patients requiring mechanical ventilation. Canadian Critical Care Trials Group. N Engl J Med 1998; 338:791–797.
  - E. Saint S, Matthay MA. Risk reduction in the intensive care unit. Am J Med 1998; 105:515–523.
  - F. Dodek P, Keenan S, Cook D, et al. Evidence-based clinical practice guideline for the prevention of ventilator-associated pneumonia. Ann Intern Med 2004; 141:305.313
- Sedation Holiday
  - G. Kress JP, Pohlman AS, O'Connor MF, et al. Daily interruption of sedative infusions in critically ill patients undergoing mechanical ventilation. N Engl J Med 2000; 342:1471–1477.
- DVT Prophylaxis
  - H. Geerts WH, Pineo GF, Heit JA, et al. Prevention of venous thromboembolism: the Seventh ACCP Conference on antithrombotic and thrombolytic therapy. Chest 2004; 126:338S–400S.

The benefit of prophylaxis of *stress gastritis* may be the avoidance of blood loss that requires transfusion of red blood cell concentrates, because transfusion increases the risk of pneumonia and other nosocomial infections substantially. Most patients under mechanical ventilation require sedation for comfort or to prevent patient–ventilator dyssynchrony, which in turn begets even higher sedation requirements. Among possible sedatives given intravenously, propofol is useful because of its short half-life and enzymatic degradation that is independent of hepatic or renal function. Among the benzodiazepines, alprazolam is relatively short acting and does not have active metabolites that prolong the half-life. Midazolam is not generally recommended for sedation during mechanical ventilation because, although its half-life is short with bolus administration, active metabolites do accumulate during continuous infusion of midazolam, increasing the duration of sedation dramatically. The duration of sedative effect is of crucial importance, because a daily "sedation holiday" with assessment of prospects for liberation from mechanical ventilation shortens the duration of ventilation significantly (G). The fourth part of the ventilator bundle is prophylaxis against venous thromboembolic disease (H); pulmonary embolism is morbid, often lethal, a major cause of prolonged mechanical ventilation, and preventable for the most part.

Severe airflow obstruction is often observed in patients with asthma, but also may be encountered in individuals sustaining inhalation injury or those with central airway lesions such as a tumor or foreign body that is distal to the tip of the endotracheal tube. These patients are frequently anxious and distressed. Deep sedation should be provided in such instances, supplemented in the occasional individual by therapeutic administration of muscle relaxants. Notably, the use of such agents may cause long-lasting weakness.[2] These interventions help to reduce oxygen consumption and carbon dioxide production, to lower airway pressures, and to reduce the risk of self-extubation. Because gas-exchange abnormalities in patients with severe airflow obstruction are generally limited to ventilation–perfusion mismatch, a F_IO_2 of 0.5 will be adequate in the majority of cases.[49] Ventilation is most commonly initiated using the ACV mode (or SIMV); the V_T should be small (5–7 mL/kg), and a respiratory rate of 12–15 breaths/min is chosen. A peak flow of 60 L/min is recommended, and higher flow rates do little to increase expiratory time.[47] These patients are at high risk for development of auto-PEEP, and the minimum acceptable V_E is frequently employed. If the patient is triggering the ventilator, PEEP may be added to reduce the work of breathing (triggering). In general, auto-PEEP is not increased by PEEP so long as PEEP is not set higher than about 85% of auto-PEEP.[50,51] Goals in this setting are to minimize alveolar over-distension (plateau pressure <30 cm H_2O) and to minimize dynamic hyperinflation (auto-PEEP <15 cm H_2O). Reducing minute ventilation to achieve these goals may cause arterial PCO_2 to rise above 40 mmHg, often to 50–70 mmHg or higher. Although this requires sedation, such permissive hypercapnia is tolerated well, except in patients with increased intracranial pressure and perhaps those with critical pulmonary hypertension or ventricular dysfunction.[47]

A third group of patients of particular importance to the surgeon are those experiencing acute hypoxemic respiratory failure. This situation is created by alveolar flooding with blood, pus, or edema fluid, leading to alveolar collapse and *derecruitment*. The end result is impaired lung mechanics and gas exchange. Gas-exchange impairment results from intrapulmonary shunt largely refractory to oxygen therapy. In acute respiratory distress syndrome (ARDS), the reduced functional residual capacity arising from alveolar flooding and collapse leaves many fewer alveoli to accommodate the V_T, overdistending the remaining functional alveoli, decreasing lung compliance, and dramatically increasing the work of breathing.[52,53] The ARDS lung should be viewed as a small lung, however, rather than a stiff lung. Consistent with this current concept of ARDS, it is clearly established that overdistension of functioning alveoli of the ARDS lung compounds lung injury and may induce systemic inflammation.[54] The goals of mechanical ventilation are to reduce the work of breathing, avoid oxygen toxicity, and avoid ventilator settings that amplify lung damage. The initial F_IO_2 should be high to counteract hypoxemia rapidly, which is typical. Ventilation with PEEP is indicated in patients with diffuse lung lesions but may not be helpful in patients with focal infiltrates such as lobar pneumonia. In patients with ARDS, PEEP should be instituted immediately and adjusted to the lowest PEEP necessary to maintain SaO_2 above 90% at an F_IO_2 below 0.6. V_T should be 6mL/kg on assist–control ventilation; a higher V_T is associated with higher mortality. Pressure control ventilation can be used as well, but parameters that assure lung protective ventilation have not been rigorously examined in that mode. Inspiratory pressure targets proposed are 30–35 cmH_2O (PEEP plus pressure increment). In either mode, respiratory rate may be set as high as 24–28 breaths/min in the absence of auto-PEEP.[47] An occasional consequence of lung protective ventilation is hypercapnia; preferring hypercapnia to alveolar overdistension is well tolerated and appropriate. Management of ARDS is discussed at length later in this chapter.

A final group of patients of interest to surgeons is that with restriction of pulmonary excursion frequently associated with chest wall edema (massive resuscitation) or morbid obesity. A small V_T (5–7mL/kg) and relatively rapid rate (18–24 breaths/min) are valuable in this patient group to minimize hemodynamic consequences of positive-pressure ventilation and reduce the likelihood of iatrogenic injury to the lung.[47] The degree of alveolar filling or collapse determines the necessary F_IO_2. When the restrictive abnormality involves the chest wall (which may also include the abdomen), a large ventilation-induced increase in pleural pressure has the potential to compromise cardiac output, which will in turn reduce mixed venous PO_2 and, in the setting of ventilation–perfusion mismatch or shunt, the arterial PO_2 as well. If the physician response to this falling arterial PaO_2 is augmenting PEEP or increasing minute ventilation, further circulatory compromise ensues, and a potentially catastrophic cycle begins of worsening gas exchange, increasing ventilator settings, and progressive shock. This situation must be recognized and treated by reduction in V_E and increased intravascular volume.

Monitoring

Selecting the mode and settings on the ventilator is a dynamic process based on the patient's physiological response rather than a fixed set of numbers. Ventilator settings require repeated adjustment over the period of dependency on the ventilator, and iterative interaction requires careful monitoring. Most key parameters in monitoring can be measured at the bedside (Table 32.2).[55] In complex situations, such as the patient with ARDS requiring high levels of positive airway pressure, a pulmonary artery catheter may be valuable to permit titration of fluid or vasoactive drug therapy. Ventilator monitors allow evaluation of patient effort and timing of response to ventilation. Patients with extreme effort may develop respiratory muscle fatigue even with a ventilator strategy designed to minimize the work of breathing. One can also follow changes in gas flow to appreciate earlier inappropriate ventilator triggering, with which auto-PEEP is likely to occur.

TABLE 32.2. Parameters Used in the Monitoring of Patients Receiving Mechanical Ventilation.

GAS EXCHANGE
Arterial oxygen tension or saturation
Arterial carbon dioxide tension and pH
AIRWAY PRESSURE
Peak inspiratory pressure
Plateau (end-inspiratory occlusion) pressure
PEEP, external and auto-waveform of pressure
BREATHING PATTERN
Minute ventilation
Tidal volume
Respiratory frequency
HEMODYNAMIC FUNCTION
Blood pressure
Urinary output
Cardiac output
Pulmonary artery occlusion pressure
CHEST FILM
Endotracheal tube position
Signs of barotrauma
Signs of pneumonia

Source: From Tobin,[4] by permission of New England Journal of Medicine.

Weaning

Discontinuation of mechanical ventilation can be easy for patients requiring short-term support. However, discontinuation can be difficult for patients recovering from a major episode of acute respiratory failure, a complicated operative procedure, or major torso trauma. Weaning such patients from the ventilator is a major clinical challenge and constitutes a major portion of the workload in an intensive care unit.[4] Timing is important in separation of patients from mechanical ventilation. If weaning is delayed unnecessarily, the patient remains at risk for ventilator-associated complications. If weaning is performed prematurely, cardiopulmonary decompensation may delay extubation, or if followed by extubation, may require reintubation and replacement of the ventilator.[15,56,57] In general, discontinuation of mechanical ventilation is not attempted in a patient with cardiopulmonary instability or arterial PO_2 less than 60mmHg with a F_IO_2 of 0.40 or higher. However, satisfactory oxygenation does not reliably predict successful weaning. A more important determinant of weaning outcome is the ability of respiratory muscles to assume increased respiratory work. Similarly,

TABLE 32.3.
Major Contemporary Trials Comparing Ventilator Weaning Modes.

	Brochard[59]	*Esteban*[60]
Description	Single center Prospective Randomized	Multicenter Prospective Randomized
Modes	T-piece PSV SIMV	T-piece PSV SIMV
Population	100 med/surg Patients failed conventional weaning	130 med/surg Patients failed conventional weaning
Results	PSV fastest, most effective weaning. T-piece also better than SIMV	T-piece fastest, most effective weaning. PSV also better than SIMV
Comment	Operator-dependent, favors uniform support for each breath. SIMV weaning least effective.	Operator dependent, favors uniform support for each breath. SIMV weaning least effective.

See text for abbreviations.

parameters traditionally gathered by respiratory care practitioners including maximal inspiratory pressure, vital capacity, and V_E have been used to evaluate a patient's readiness for weaning, but these parameters have a limited predictive accuracy. The dividend of respiratory frequency to V_T (expressed as a decimal fraction) during 1 min of spontaneous breathing (rapid shallow breathing index) may be a more accurate predictor. A value less than 105 indicates that weaning is more likely to be successful.[58] Two recent trials compared ventilator modes used in weaning the patient who does not immediately separate from mechanical ventilation (Table 32.3). T-piece trial (e.g., spontaneous breathing through the endotracheal tube with flow-by of fresh gas), SIMV, and PSV were compared. These trials demonstrated that the weaning mode used does affect outcome in the complex patient. Modes providing equal treatment of each breath (T-piece trials and PSV) gave better results than SIMV.[59,60]

The process of weaning begins by determining patient readiness. In addition to the recommendations from the Task Force for Evidence-Based Guidelines for Weaning and Discontinuing Ventilatory Support (Table 32.4), surgical patients should be carefully screened for mental status, respiratory muscle strength, consistent and adequate wakefulness, ability to manage secretions, nutritional repletion, and normalization of acid–base and electrolyte status.[61] Particular attention should be given to acceptance of hypercapnia if chronically present and avoidance of new metabolic alkalosis. Finally, normality of electrolytes affecting muscle function (calcium, phosphate, and potassium) must be assured. If the aforementioned conditions are addressed, weaning may be attempted. A protocol utilizing the rapid shallow breathing index in separation of patients from mechanical ventilation has been successful in our intensive care unit (Fig. 32.2).[62,63]

Noninvasive Ventilation

When ventilatory support is delivered without establishing an artificial endotracheal airway, it is termed noninvasive ventilation. Historically, noninvasive ventilation has been given with the use of devices that apply intermittent negative pressure. With the advent of positive-pressure ventilation, noninvasive ventilation is delivered through a nasal or face mask. Recent technical advances have greatly expanded the use of noninvasive ventilation. Noninvasive ventilation may be administered as continuous positive airway pressure (CPAP) (for hypoxic, normocarbic respiratory failure) or bilevel positive airway pressure (BiPAP, for hypoxic, hypercarbic respiratory failure). Noninvasive ventilation has a role in the management of acute and chronic respiratory failure and may have a role for some patients with heart failure. Noninvasive approaches preserve swallowing, feeding, and speech. Cough and physiological air warming and humidification are also preserved. Noninvasive ventilation can eliminate the need for intubation or tracheostomy, preventing problems such as injury to the vocal cords or trachea and lower respiratory tract infections.[64,65] However, for noninvasive ventilation the mask must achieve a snug, occlusive, gas-tight seal, which can be uncomfortable for some patients.

Benefits of Noninvasive Ventilation

Reported benefits of noninvasive ventilation are numerous, most prominently the avoidance of endotracheal intubation and its associated complications (Fig. 32.3).[66] Nonintubated patients communicate more effectively, require less sedation, and are often more comfortable than intubated patients. In addition, patients are often able to maintain standard oral nutritional intake. Ventilation without tracheal intubation eliminates complications such as trauma with tube insertion and mucosal ulceration, and decreases the risks of aspiration, infection (pneumonia and sinusitis), and impaired swallowing after extubation. The most obvious benefit of noninvasive ventilation is avoidance of ventilator-associated pneumonia.[67,68] Some authors propose that noninvasive ventilation reduces total days of intubation and mechanical ventilation. Antonelli and coworkers showed a significant decrease in infections in a prospective, randomized trial that directly compared noninvasive ventilation to intubation and mechanical ventilation.[69] A case-controlled study from a medical intensive care unit demonstrated a reduction in nosocomial infections including pneumonia. In another study of 52 immunocompromised patients that compared noninvasive versus conventional mechanical ventilation for acute respiratory failure, patients who received noninvasive ventilation had significantly lower rates of intubation, complications, and mortality.[70,71]

Contraindications to Noninvasive Ventilation

Crucial to the success of noninvasive ventilation in studies to date has been enrollment of awake, cooperative, spontaneously breathing patients who have intact airway reflexes.[67] Hemodynamic instability, an unstable airway, or acute cardiac rhythm disturbances argue against the use of noninvasive ventilation; thus, the unconscious trauma patient with multiple injuries including maxillofacial fractures is not a

TABLE 32.4. Recommendations from the Task Force for Evidence-Based Guidelines for Weaning and Discontinuing Ventilatory Support.

Recommendation 1: In patients requiring mechanical ventilation for >24 h, a search for all the causes that may be contributing to ventilatory dependence should be undertaken. This is particularly true in the patient who has failed attempts at withdrawing the mechanical ventilator. Reversing all possible ventilatory and nonventilatory issues should be an integral part of the ventilator discontinuation process.

Recommendation 2: Patients receiving mechanical ventilation for respiratory failure should undergo a formal assessment of discontinuation potential if the following criteria are satisfied:

1. Evidence for some reversal of the underlying cause for respiratory failure.
2. Adequate oxygenation (e.g., PaO_2/F_IO_2 ratio > 150 to 200; requiring positive end-expiratory pressure (PEEP) ≤ 5 to 8 cmH_2O; F_IO_2 ≤ 0.4 to 0.5); and pH (e.g., ≥7.25).
3. Hemodynamic stability, as defined by the absence of active myocardial ischemia and the absence of clinically significant hypotension (i.e., a condition requiring no vasopressor therapy or therapy with only low-dose vasopressors such as dopamine or dobutamine, <5 µg/kg/min); and
4. The capability to initiate an inspiratory effort.

The decision to use these criteria must be individualized. Some patients who do not satisfy all the above criteria (e.g., patients with chronic hypoxemia values below the thresholds cited) may be ready for attempts at the discontinuation of mechanical ventilation.

Recommendation 3: Formal discontinuation assessments for patients receiving mechanical ventilation for respiratory failure should be performed during spontaneous breathing rather than while the patient is still receiving substantial ventilatory support. An initial brief period of spontaneous breathing can be used to assess the capability of continuing on to a formal spontaneous breathing trial (SBT). The criteria with which to assess patient tolerance during SBTs are the respiratory pattern, the adequacy of gas exchange, hemodynamic stability, and subjective comfort. The tolerance of SBTs lasting 30 to 120 min should prompt consideration for permanent ventilator discontinuation.

Recommendation 4: The removal of the artificial airway from a patient who has successfully been discontinued from ventilatory support should be based on assessments of airway patency and the ability of the patient to protect the airway.

Recommendation 5: Patients receiving mechanical ventilation for respiratory failure who fail an SBT should have the cause for the failed SBT determined. Once reversible causes for failure are corrected, and if the patient still meets weaning criteria, subsequent SBTs should be performed every 24 h.

Recommendation 6: Patients receiving mechanical ventilation for respiratory failure who fail a SBT should receive a stable, nonfatiguing, comfortable form of ventilatory support.

Recommendation 7: Anesthesia/sedation strategies and ventilator management aimed at early extubation should be used in postoperative patients.

Recommendation 8: Weaning/discontinuation protocols that are designed for nonphysician healthcare professionals (HCPs) should be developed and implemented by ICUs. Protocols aimed at optimizing sedation also should be developed and implemented.

Recommendation 9: Tracheostomy should be considered after an initial period of stabilization on the ventilator when it becomes apparent that the patient will require prolonged ventilator assistance. Tracheostomy then should be performed when the patient appears likely to gain one or more of the benefits ascribed to the procedure. Patients who may derive particular benefit from early tracheostomy are the following:

1. Those requiring high levels of sedation to tolerate translaryngeal tubes
2. Those with marginal respiratory mechanics (often manifested as tachypnea) in whom a tracheostomy tube having lower resistance might reduce the risk of muscle overload
3. Those who may derive psychological benefit from the ability to eat orally, communicate by articulated speech, and experience enhanced mobility
4. Those in whom enhanced mobility may assist physical therapy efforts

Recommendation 10: Unless there is evidence for clearly irreversible disease (e.g., high spinal cord injury or advanced amyotrophic lateral sclerosis), a patient requiring prolonged mechanical ventilatory support for respiratory failure should not be considered permanently ventilator dependent until 3 months of weaning attempts have failed.

Recommendation 11: Critical care practitioners should familiarize themselves with facilities in their communities, or units in hospitals they staff, that specialize in managing patients who require prolonged dependence on mechanical ventilation. Such familiarization should include reviewing published peer-reviewed data from those units, if available. When medically stable for transfer, patients who have failed ventilator discontinuation attempts in the ICU should be transferred to those facilities that have demonstrated success and safety in accomplishing ventilator discontinuation.

Recommendation 12: Weaning strategies in prolonged mechanical ventilation patients should be slow-paced and should include gradually lengthening self-breathing trials.

Source: From Weaning Guidelines, with permission from Chest 2001;120(suppl):375S–395S.

candidate for noninvasive ventilation.[64] Additional contraindications include compromised cough and secretion clearance. A common reason for failure of noninvasive ventilation is copious airway secretions (see Figure 32.3). Relative contraindications include the inability to adequately fit and seal the mask, inability to cough, or difficulty or inability to remove the mask in the event of emesis.

Cardiogenic pulmonary edema is controversial. Many workers now believe that noninvasive ventilation helps to unload respiratory muscles and decrease the work of breathing. Other investigators suggest that noninvasive ventilation for cardiogenic pulmonary edema is associated with an increased risk of myocardial infarction, perhaps because of the hemodynamic effects of noninvasive ventilation.[72,73]

Of more concern to the general surgeon is the hypothetical contraindication resulting from aerophagia and gut distension following gastrointestinal surgery. If pressures used to ventilate the patient are maintained below 30 cmH_2O, the closing pressure at the lower esophageal sphincter should not be overcome and aerophagia should be uncommon. The respiratory care literature reports a 1% to 2% risk of gastric distension with noninvasive ventilation, but this point has not been reviewed in postoperative patients. Similarly, morbid obesity is a relative contraindication secondary to increased ventilatory pressure requirements arising from body habitus and the weight of the chest wall and abdominal viscera while the patient is supine.[74–76]

In a randomized, prospective trial, standard postoperative therapy including invasive mechanical ventilation was compared with nasal mask noninvasive ventilation of 48 patients with acute hypoxemic respiratory insufficiency after pulmonary resection.[77] Most patients underwent single lobe resections, although seven patients in each group underwent pneumonectomy. The primary outcome parameter was the need for invasive mechanical ventilation; the secondary outcome parameters were in-hospital and 120-day mortality, duration of intensive care unit (ICU) stay, and duration of hospital stay. The need for postoperative intubation was significantly reduced in patients receiving noninvasive ventilation as a part of respiratory support. Nine patients treated with invasive ventilation died during the trial, whereas only three deaths occurred in the group whose postoperative management included noninvasive ventilation.

Complications of Noninvasive Ventilation

The primary complication of noninvasive ventilation is focal skin necrosis secondary to prolonged pressure from the mask on the underlying skin (see Fig. 32.3).[64,78] The incidence is 7% to 10% with full facemask (as opposed to the nasal mask) noninvasive ventilation. Necrosis usually occurs over the bridge of the nose, but may also occur over the zygoma, and is prevented by avoiding excessive pressure when affixing the mask to the face. The mask should be just tight enough to seal any large air leaks. Skin necrosis can also be prevented by the prophylactic placement of DuoDERM (Convatec,

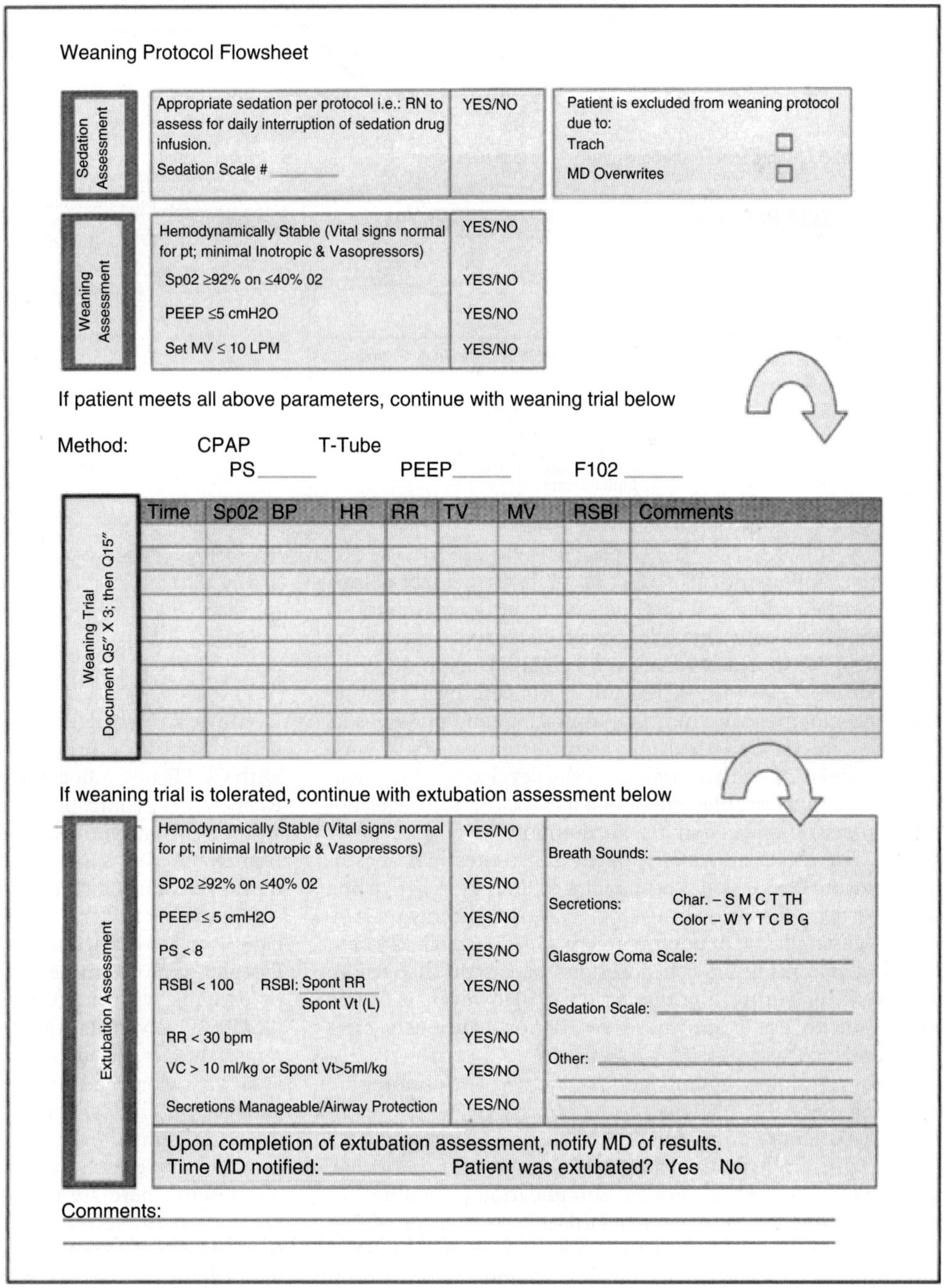
Weaning Protocol Flowsheet

Sedation Assessment

Appropriate sedation per protocol i.e.: RN to assess for daily interruption of sedation drug infusion. Sedation Scale # ______	YES/NO

Patient is excluded from weaning protocol due to:
Trach ☐
MD Overwrites ☐

Weaning Assessment

Hemodynamically Stable (Vital signs normal for pt; minimal Inotropic & Vasopressors)	YES/NO
Sp02 ≥92% on ≤40% 02	YES/NO
PEEP ≤5 cmH2O	YES/NO
Set MV ≤ 10 LPM	YES/NO

If patient meets all above parameters, continue with weaning trial below

Method: CPAP T-Tube
PS______ PEEP______ F102 ______

Weaning Trial — Document Q5″ X 3; then Q15″

Time	Sp02	BP	HR	RR	TV	MV	RSBI	Comments

If weaning trial is tolerated, continue with extubation assessment below

Extubation Assessment

Hemodynamically Stable (Vital signs normal for pt; minimal Inotropic & Vasopressors)	YES/NO
SP02 ≥92% on ≤40% 02	YES/NO
PEEP ≤ 5 cmH2O	YES/NO
PS < 8	YES/NO
RSBI < 100 RSBI: Spont RR / Spont Vt (L)	YES/NO
RR < 30 bpm	YES/NO
VC > 10 ml/kg or Spont Vt>5ml/kg	YES/NO
Secretions Manageable/Airway Protection	YES/NO

Breath Sounds: ______
Secretions: Char. – S M C T TH; Color – W Y T C B G
Glasgrow Coma Scale: ______
Sedation Scale: ______
Other: ______

Upon completion of extubation assessment, notify MD of results.
Time MD notified: ______ Patient was extubated? Yes No

Comments: ______

FIGURE 32.2. Weaning protocol flow sheet. (From Dries DJ, McGonigal MD, Malian MS, et al.,[63] by permission of Journal of Trauma.)

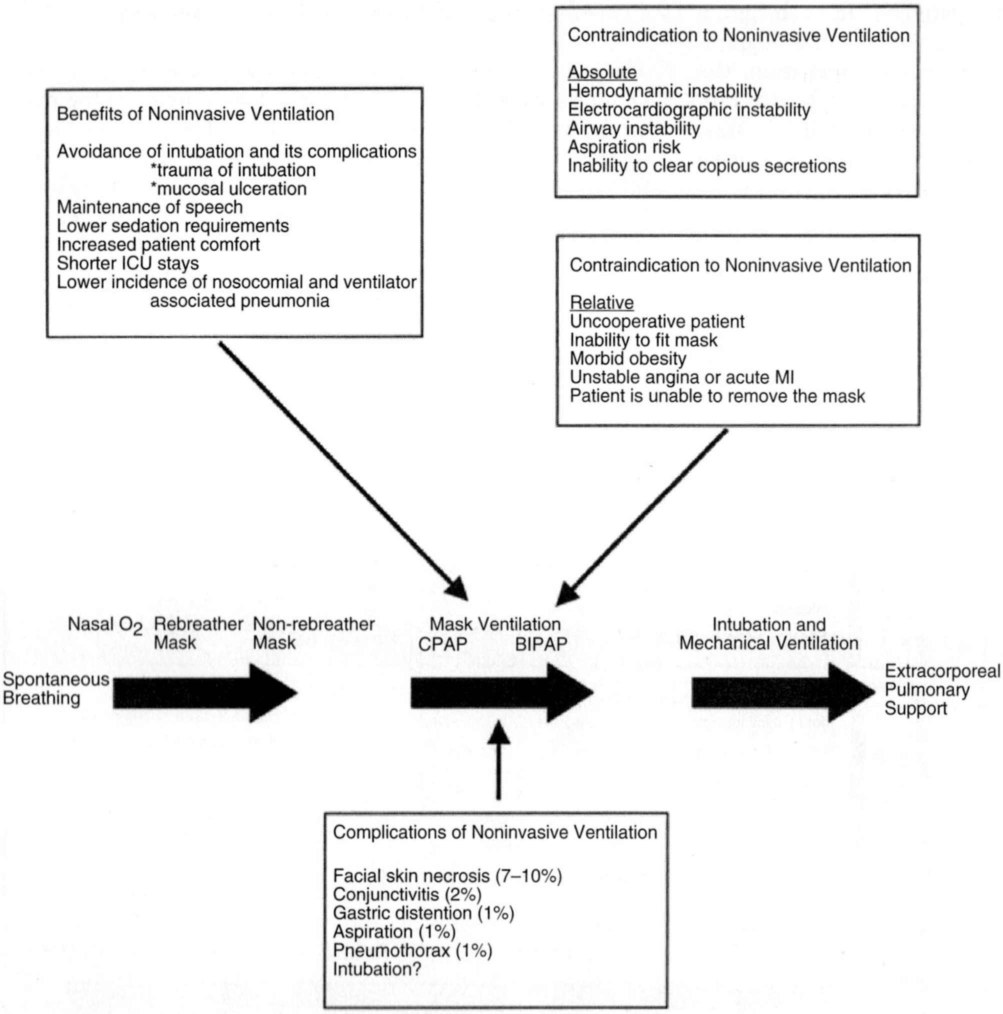

Contraindication to Noninvasive Ventilation
Absolute
Hemodynamic instability
Electrocardiographic instability
Airway instability
Aspiration risk
Inability to clear copious secretions
Benefits of Noninvasive Ventilation
Avoidance of intubation and its complications
*trauma of intubation
*mucosal ulceration
Maintenance of speech
Lower sedation requirements
Increased patient comfort
Shorter ICU stays
Lower incidence of nosocomial and ventilator associated pneumonia
Contraindication to Noninvasive Ventilation
Relative
Uncooperative patient
Inability to fit mask
Morbid obesity
Unstable angina or acute MI
Patient is unable to remove the mask
Nasal O2
Rebreather Mask
Non-rebreather Mask
Mask Ventilation
CPAP
BIPAP
Intubation and Mechanical Ventilation
Spontaneous Breathing
Extracorporeal Pulmonary Support
Complications of Noninvasive Ventilation
Facial skin necrosis (7–10%)
Conjunctivitis (2%)
Gastric distention (1%)
Aspiration (1%)
Pneumothorax (1%)
Intubation?

FIGURE 32.3. The spectrum of respiratory support. See text for abbreviations. (From Acton RD, Hotchkiss JR, Dries DJ,[64] by permission of Journal of Trauma.)

Princeton, NJ) or similar product on the bony contact points. Other complications, all of which occur at approximately a 1% to 2% incidence, include gastric distension (avoided by ventilating with pressures below 30 cmH_2O), aspiration, and pneumothorax. Gastric distension is concerning for subsequent development of vomiting, aspiration, and pneumonia. However, in studies addressing gastric distension, there is no direct correlation with aspiration or the development of pneumonia. Prophylactic placement of a nasogastric tube does not prevent gastric distension.[79,80] Furthermore, hypothetical air swallowing and disruption of upper gastrointestinal anastomotic suture lines has not been reported. In two studies using CPAP in patients recovering from cholecystectomy, gastric bypass, gastroplasty, or bowel surgery, CPAP as high as 12 cm H_2O did not result in complications of gastric distension, aspiration, or suture line disruption.[81,82] However, it seems reasonable to use noninvasive ventilation cautiously after esophageal or gastric surgery.

Less common complications include pneumothorax and conjunctivitis, secondary to air leakage near the eyes in 2% of patients.[76] Treatment of conjunctivitis includes sealing the air leak and administration of synthetic eye lubricants. The most serious complication is failure to recognize when noninvasive ventilation is not providing adequate ventilation, oxygenation, or airway support. Delayed intubation may cause continued dangerous deterioration of the patient; a patient should never be lost for failure to intubate.

Where Does Noninvasive Ventilation Fit?

Noninvasive ventilation can be used as an adjunctive therapy before intubation or after extubation. Outcomes in patients with COPD or cardiogenic pulmonary edema should be good. Randomized, controlled trials also support the use of noninvasive ventilation to reduce the need for endotracheal intubation in immunosuppressed patients with infiltrates and in individuals during recovery from lung resection.[64,65]

Noninvasive ventilation has also been used to avoid intubation or reintubation. A prospective, randomized trial by Esteban et al. examined the role of noninvasive ventilation in patients with acute respiratory failure after extubation. Noninvasive ventilation did not result in reduced intubation rates.[83] In fact, delays in reintubation were noted and associated with worsened survival. When noninvasive ventilation is effective, clinical status generally improves within hours, including reduction of respiratory rate and use of accessory muscles, along with improvement in pH, $PaCO_2$, and PaO_2.[64] At present, there are no data supporting use of noninvasive ventilation to facilitate discontinuation of assisted ventilation other than in patients with COPD or cardiogenic pulmonary edema.[84]

Acute Respiratory Distress Syndrome

Acute respiratory distress syndrome and the acute lung injury (ALI) syndrome are examples of acute hypoxemic respiratory failure. Pulmonary dysfunction in this setting arises from collapse or flooding of alveoli, with resulting increased dead space ventilation and shunt. Beyond hypoxemia, interstitial and alveolar fluid accumulation causes decreased lung compliance, imposing a mechanical load and resulting in increased work of breathing.[52,53] Work of breathing may also be increased by bronchospasm induced by mediators of the inflammatory response.

Low-pressure pulmonary edema [pulmonary wedge pressure (P_{PW}) <18 mmHg] in ARDS results from injury to the pulmonary microcirculation sustained from direct insults (e.g., aspiration, inhalation injury, or infection) or indirectly by systemic processes (sepsis, massive resuscitation following trauma). The former is termed pulmonary ARDS and the latter extrapulmonary ARDS.[85] Some investigators hypothesize that these entities are associated with different lung mechanical properties and a different response to ventilator maneuvers designed to reopen dysfunctional alveoli, but this idea is unproved.[86]

It is also useful to distinguish between early ARDS and ALI and events that occur subsequently. Early ARDS/ALI is characterized by flooding of the lung with proteinaceous fluid and minimal cellular injury.[52,53] By electron microscopy, endothelial cell swelling is seen with widening of intracellular junctions, increased pinocytotic vesicles, and disruption and denudation of basement membranes. This early phase of diffuse alveolar damage has been termed *exudative*, during which pulmonary edema and its effects are pronounced. Over subsequent days, patients with ALI/ARDS demonstrate alveolar hyaline membrane formation and inflammatory cells become more numerous. This later phase is dominated by disordered healing. This second or later phase can occur as early as 7 to 10 days after the initial pulmonary injury and often includes pulmonary fibrosis.[87–89] This second or later phase has been termed the *proliferative* phase of ALI/ARDS. Pulmonary edema may not be as prominent in this later phase of lung injury, and the clinician managing the patient is challenged by a large dead space fraction and V_E. These patients may also exhibit progressive pulmonary hypertension, reduced responsiveness to PEEP, and further reduction in lung compliance. In 1994, an American/European consensus conference published specific definitions of ARDS/ALI (Table 32.5).[90]

Ventilator Management of ARDS

Over the past several years, both clinical and preclinical data have led to reconsideration of the ventilation of patients with ARDS. Prior clinical practice was based on early observations that mechanical ventilation of ARDS required use of large V_T and high inflation pressures, in part, because newer modes of ventilation were impossible before the advent of microprocessor-controlled ventilators. The simple bellows ventilators with set volume or pressure limits were all that were available. Recognition that high-V_T, positive-pressure ventilators could cause lung injury in animals with normal lungs or worsen preexisting lung injury has led to the reconsideration.[3] Laboratory studies suggest that VILI may induce lung inflammation that resembles ARDS. However, although the experimental data are compelling, the clinician cannot be sure in any particular case whether and to what extent pulmonary injury is caused by the ventilator strategy as opposed to the underlying pulmonary insult.

Animal work investigating support of ALI suggests that VILI is related to the distending volume to which the lung is subjected, rather than distending pressure as measured at the mouth. Elegant experiments in which the chest is banded (simulating restrictive disease) and mechanical ventilation is conducted with high airway pressures but low V_T resulting from the restricted chest wall do not produce lung injury, whereas higher V_T at comparable pressures creates widespread pulmonary injury.[91–93] In addition to the detrimental effects of overdistension, numerous investigators have suggested a protective effect of PEEP in patients with ALI/ARDS[94] via avoidance of repetitive alveolar collapse and reopening. In the aggregate, these studies offer a strategy to ventilate patients with ALI/ARDS and avoid VILI.[86] During the respiratory cycle, PEEP acts to avoid cyclic alveolar opening and collapse at end-expiration, whereas V_T is controlled to avoid alveolar overdistension. In ARDS, the respiratory system inflation pressure–volume curve exhibits a sigmoidal shape with lower and upper inflection points (Fig. 32.4). The lower inflection point is consistent with edematous lung behaving as a two-compartment structure, with a population of alveoli exhibiting near-normal compliance and another recruitable population of alveoli distensible only at higher transpulmonary pressures. As transpulmonary pressure is increased above the lower inflection point, lung compliance improves, as reflected by the increase in the slope of the pressure-volume curve. Volume tends to increase in a linear fashion as pressure is increased until the upper inflection point is reached, where flattening of the curve is interpreted as alveolar overdistension.[95,96] Ventilator management strategies for patients with ARDS, therefore, are designed to avoid alveolar collapse near the lower inflection point by titration of PEEP and overdistension near the upper inflection point by limitation of V_T.[86]

TABLE 32.5. The 1994 American-European Consensus Conference Definitions of Acute Lung Injury (ALI) and the Acute Respiratory Distress Syndrome (ARDS).

	Timing	*Oxygenation*	*CXR*	*Ppw*
ALI Criteria	Acute onset	PaO_2: F_IO_2 < 300 (regardless of PEEP level)	Bilateral infiltrates	<18 mmHg or no clinical evidence right atrial hypertension
ARDS Criteria	Acute onset	PaO_2: F_IO_2 < 200 (regardless of PEEP level)	Bilateral infiltrates	<18 mmHg or no clinical evidence right atrial hypertension

See text for abbreviations.

Source: From Bernard GR, Artigas A, Brigham KL, et al.,[90] by permission of American Journal of Respiratory and Critical Care Medicine.

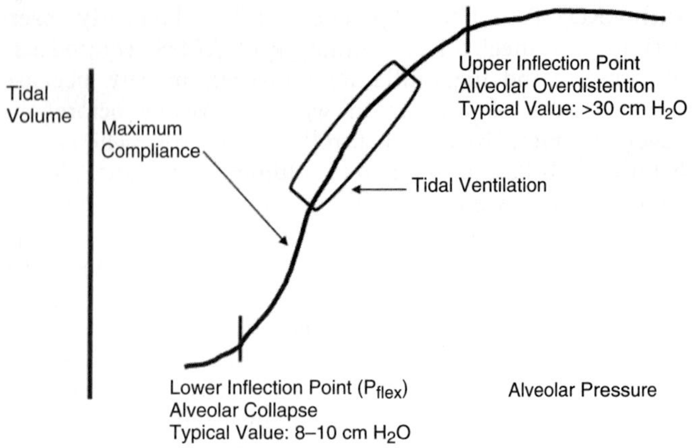

FIGURE 32.4. This simple description of changes in pulmonary volume with applied airway pressure allows theoretical description of contemporary dosing of mechanical ventilation. In patients at risk for airway closure, positive end-expiratory pressure (PEEP) is applied to avoid cyclic alveolar opening and collapse. Typically, the amount of PEEP required is 10–15 cmH_2O. Alveolar overdistension occurs with alveolar pressures of 30 cmH_2O or more. Thus, regardless of tidal volume, tidal ventilation is dosed to keep pulmonary performance on the point in this pressure–volume relationship where maximum compliance is observed. To increase the population of alveoli open for gas exchange, recruitment maneuvers, discussed later, may be employed. (Data from Weaning Guidelines, Chest 2001;120(suppl): 375S–395S.)

Clinical Studies of Ventilator Management in ALI/ARDS

Hickling et al. reported a favorable impact on survival of reduced V_T and permissive hypercapnia in the management of patients with ARDS, comparing outcome to historical controls. Lack of a randomized, prospective control group made interpretation difficult in light of data showing that survival of patients with ARDS is improving apart from details of mechanical ventilatory support.[97,98] Since that time, numerous clinical trials of ventilatory strategies for ALI/ARDS have been undertaken (Table 32.6).

The first contemporary prospective, randomized trial testing a strategy of limiting V_T and utilizing PEEP to avoid alveolar collapse was conducted by Amato et al.[99] (Table 32.7), who randomized patients with ARDS to two treatments: ACV with V_T of 12 mL/kg PEEP sufficient to maintain adequate SaO_2, F_IO_2 below 0.6, and respiratory rate to maintain $PaCO_2$ of 25–38 mmHg. No efforts were made to control peak inspiratory or plateau airway pressures. Comparison was made to pressure-control, inverse-ratio ventilation (PC-IRV), PSV, or pressure support (VC-PSV) with V_T less than 6 mL/kg, recruitment maneuvers, peak airway pressures less than 40 cmH_2O, and PEEP titrated to maintain lung inflation above the lower inflection point. Patients managed with the latter approach demonstrated more rapid recovery of pulmonary compliance, a decreased requirement for oxygen, a lower rate of lung injury, and a higher rate of liberation from the ventilator. These individuals also demonstrated a decreased 28-day mortality, although not at hospital discharge. Concerns regarding this study are that the sample size was small, and that there were multiple treatment differences between groups, including PEEP strategy, V_T utilization, $PaCO_2$ target, V_E, and mode of ventilation. Moreover, mortality was high (71%) in the conventional ventilation group.

The controversy over proper V_T for management of patients with ARDS has been largely resolved by the NIH-funded ARDSNet trial of 861 patients[100–103] randomized to ventilation with V_T of either 12 mL/kg or 6 mL/kg based on ideal body weight. If plateau airway pressure, used as a surrogate of end-inspiratory lung stretch, exceeded 30 cmH_2O in the low V_T group, V_T was reduced further to reduce plateau pressure to that level. The ARDSNet trial was stopped prematurely because of a striking difference in outcome in favor of the lower V_T group. Notably, the low V_T group had a modest increase in $PaCO_2$ and a modestly decreased pH. The potential for greater degrees of respiratory acidosis between groups was minimized by use of higher respiratory rates in the low V_T group. The primary study endpoint, 28-day mortality, was significantly decreased (31.0% versus 39.8%, P = 0.007) with low V_T ventilation. In addition, the number of ventilator-free days during the study was greater in the low V_T group. This trial confirmed earlier basic and clinical studies suggesting that low V_T can improve outcomes after ARDS. Perhaps the best evidence-based recommendation for routine management of patients with ARDS undergoing mechanical ventilation is to implement the ARDSNet protocol (Table 32.8).

Some have called the ARDSNet trial results into question[104]; V_T was not tested between 6 and 12 mL/kg. Survival was better for patients with lower V_T, perhaps because of detrimental effects of high V_T ventilation and not superiority of lower V_T. Additionally, the proper use of PEEP is not defined.[105] Some investigators use PEEP only as necessary to achieve adequate PaO_2 and avoid oxygen toxicity (these thresholds are not established). Others recommend higher PEEP levels with the goals of achieving maximal alveolar recruitment and avoiding mechanical events such as collapse and reinflation, which occur near the lower inflection point of the pressure volume curve. Data do not support either strategy strongly.

Current options in ARDS/ALI management have been summarized by Marini and Gattinoni.[86] Ventilator parameters are adjusted empirically rather than by formula-driven rules. Prevention of mechanical trauma to the lung takes precedence over maintenance of normocapnia and avoidance of oxygen toxicity. No exact upper limits for acceptable plateau pressure or F_IO_2 can be specified, but very high F_IO_2 risks absorption atelectasis and oxygen toxicity. Therefore, maintenance of F_IO_2 below 0.7 is recommended. Similarly, it is desired to use the least PEEP and V_T necessary to achieve acceptable gas exchange while avoiding tidal collapse and reopening of unstable alveoli. Knowing that moderate hypercapnia is well tolerated, therapeutic priorities are lung protection and maintenance of appropriate hemodynamics and oxygen delivery (DO_2). A contemporary surrogate for invasive hemodynamic monitoring is measurement of central venous oxygen saturation. A value of more than 70% and a difference of 25% or less between SaO_2 and S_VO_2 is generally associated with adequate Q.

Patients should be assessed for severity of disease and for the potential of mechanical ventilation to recruit alveoli. One strategy is as follows. After hypovolemia is corrected, recruitment potential is gauged by application of high-level PCV: PEEP of 15–20 cmH_2O, driving pressure of 30 cmH_2O, and plateau pressure of 50 cmH_2O for 1 to 2 min as tolerated. Even higher pressures may be appropriate for a patient with low total lung compliance (e.g., patients with chest wall circum-

TABLE 32.6.
Overview of Ventilatory Strategies for Acute Lung Injury and the Acute Respiratory Distress Syndrome

Strategy Type	*Year*	*Type of Study*	*Patients*	*Findings*	*Study*
PEEP					
High levels of PEEP	1975	Observational	28	High incidence of pneumothorax	Kirby et al.[118]
Prophylactic PEEP (8 cm of water)	1984	Phase 3 single center trial	92	No benefit	Pepe et al.[119]
High versus low PEEP	2004	Phase 3	549	No difference	NIH[105]
Prone Ventilation					
	1997	Observational	13	Inconclusive	Mure et al.[120]
	2000	Observational	39	Inconclusive	Nakos et al.[121]
	2001	Multicenter Randomized	304	Improved oxygenation Survival unchanged	Gattinoni et al.[128]
Combined Modes					
"Open-lung" approach	1998	Phase 3 single center trial	53	Decreased 28-day mortality but not in-hospital mortality (as compared with conventional ventilation)	Amato et al.[99]
Prone plus PEEP	2003	Prospective Randomized Single center	25	Prone ventilation and PEEP offer additive effects	Gainnier et al.[129]
Tidal Volume					
Low tidal volume	1998	Phase 3	120	No benefit in patients at risk for the acute respiratory distress syndrome	Stewart et al.[102]
Low tidal volume	1998	Phase 3	116	No benefit	Brochard et al.[100]
Low tidal volume	1999	Prospective	52	No difference in mortality	Brower et al.[101]
Low tidal volume	2000	Phase 3	861	Decreased mortality by 22% (as compared with traditional tidal volumes)	NIH[103]
Alternative Strategies					
Extracorporeal membrane oxygenation	1979	Phase 3 multi-center trial	90	No benefit	Zapol et al.[122]
High frequency jet ventilation	1983	Phase 3 single center trial	309	No benefit	Carlon et al.[123]
Pressure-controlled inverse ratio ventilation	1994	Observational	9	Inconclusive	Lessard et al.[124]
Extracorporeal removal of carbon dioxide	1994	Phase 3 single center trial	40	No benefit	Morris et al.[125]
Liquid ventilation	1996	Observational	10	Probably safe, needs further study	Hirshl et al.[126]
High-frequency oscillation	1997	Observational	17	Probably safe, needs further study	Fort et al.[127]
High-frequency oscillation	2002	Randomized Controlled	148	High-frequency oscillation is safe and offers comparable outcomes to conventional ventilation	Derdak et al.[33]

Source: Modified from Ware LB, Matthay MA,[52] by permission of N Engl J Med.

TABLE 32.7.
Summary of Randomized Trials of Low Tidal Volume Ventilatory Strategies in Treatment of Adult Patients with ALI/ARDS.

	Study (reference no.)				
	Amato and coworkers (99)	*Brochard and coworkers (100)*	*Brower and coworkers (101)*	*Stewart and coworkers (102)*	*NIH (103)*
Population					
Entry criteria	LIS > 2.5, Ppa, we < 16, MV < 7 d	LIS > 2.5, MV < 3 d	$PaO_2/F_IO_2 < 200$, MV < 1 d	$PaO_2/F_IO_2 < 250$, MV < 1 d	$PaO_2/F_IO_2 < 300$, MV < 36 h
Exclusion criteria	Coronary insufficiency, prior lung disease, barotrauma, uncontrolled acidosis, intracranial hypertension terminal disease	Left heart failure, acute or chronic organ failure, chest wall abnormality, intracranial hypertension, head injury, terminal disease	Ave < 18, left heart failure, acute neurologic disease, chronic lung disease, thoracic surgery	Age < 18, left heart failure, myocardial ischemia, acute or chronic neurologic disease, PIP > 30 for 2 h, terminal disease	Age < 18, left heart failure, acute neurologic disease, life expectancy <6 mo, hepatic failure
Characteristics at Inclusion					
APACHE II	28 versus 27	18 versus 17	90 versus 85 (APACHE III)	22 versus 21	
PaO_2/F_IO_2	112 versus 134	144 versus 155	129 versus 150	123 versus 145	
LIS	3.4 versus 3.2	3.0 versus 3.0	2.7 versus 2.8	—	
Targeted Settings					
Intervention	$V_T < 6$ mL/kg, PIP < 40 cm H_2O, Pdriving <20 cm H_2O, CPAP recruiting	Pplateau ≤ 25–30 cm H_2O V_T = 6–10 ml/kg	Pplateau ≤ 30 cm H_2O V_T ≤ 8 ml/kg IBW	PIP < 30 cm H_2O V_T ≤ 8 ml/kg IBW	V_T ≤ 6 ml/kg IBW, reduce VT if Pplateau > 30 cm H_2O
Control	V_T = 12 mL/kg, Pa_{CO_2} 35–38 mmHg, PIP unlimited	V_T = 10–15 mL/kg, PIP < 60 cm H_2O	Pplateau ≤ 45–55 cm H_2O, V_T = 10–12 mL/kg IBW	PIP < 50 cm H_2O V_T = 10–15 mL/kg IBW	V_T = 12 mL/kg IBW, reduce V_T if Pplateau > 50 cm H_2O
PEEP, cm H_2O					
Intervention	2 above Pflex	0–15, titrated to best P:F ratio	5–20 titrated to best P:F ratio	5–20 titrated to best P:F ratio	Titrated to gas exchange
Control	Titrated to P:F ratio	Same	Same	Same	Titrated to gas exchange
Resulting Settings					
Pplateau, cm H_2O	30 versus 37	26 versus 32	25 versus 32	22 versus 28	25 versus 32–34
PEEP, cmH_2O	16 versus 7	11 versus 11	10 versus 9	9 versus 7	8–9, both groups
V_T ml or ml/kg	350 versus 770 mL	7 versus 10 mL/kg	7 versus 10 mL/kg	7 versus 11 mL/kg	6.2 versus 11.8 mL/kg
Pa_{CO_2}, mmHg	55 versus 32	60 versus 41	50 versus 40	54 versus 46	
Outcomes					
Mortality	13/29 (45%) versus 17/24 (71%)	47% versus 38%	13/26 (50%) versus 12/26 (46%)	30/60 (50%) versus 28/60 (47%)	31% versus 39%
Barotrauma	2 (7%) versus 10 (42%)	8 (14%) versus 7 (12%)	1 (4%) versus 2 (8%)	6 (10%) versus 4 (7%)	No difference

Definitions of abbreviations: CPAP = continuous airway pressure; IBW = ideal body weight (note: the formulas used for calculation of IBW were not uniform across studies; Brochard and coworkers used "dry weight" to determine tidal volume); LIS = lung injury score; MV = mechanical ventilation; Pdriving = driving pressure; Pflex = pressure at lower inflection point of pressure-column curve; P:F = PaO_2: F_IO_2 ratio; PIP = peak inspiratory pressure; Ppa.we = pulmonary artery wedge pressure; Pplateau = plateau pressure; VT = tidal volume.

Source: From International consensus conferences in intensive care medicine: ventilator-associated lung injury in ARDS. Am J Respir Crit Care Med 1999;160: 2118–2124.

ferential burns). Although sustained inflation with high pressure has been used traditionally, it is less well tolerated hemodynamically than recruitment by PCV, which achieves lower average airway pressure but similar peak airway pressure during inspiration.[106,107] If oxygenation and lung mechanics do not improve thus, the patient is considered to have low recruitment potential. Management goals in the recruitable group emphasize maintenance of high-level PEEP to maintain inflation of opened gas-exchange units. In poorly recruitable patients, PEEP may be maintained as low as feasible, generally in the range of 5–10 cmH_2O. In both groups, end-expiratory plateau pressure is kept below 30 cmH_2O except when chest wall compliance is low. Patients with recruitable lung units should respond to increased PEEP in recruiting

TABLE 32.8. ARDSNet Ventilator Management.

- Assist control mode—volume ventilation
- Reduce V_T to 6 mL/kg lean body weight
- Keep Pplat <30 cm H_2O
  - ○ Reduce V_T as low as 4 mL/kg lean body weight to limit Pplat
- Maintain SaO_2 88%–95%

F_IO_2	0.3	0.4	0.4	0.5	0.5	0.6	0.7	0.7	0.7	0.8	0.9	0.9	0.9	1.0
PEEP	5	5	8	8	10	10	10	12	14	14	14	16	18	20–24

Lean Body Weight:
- ○ Male—50 + 2.3 (height [inches] – 60) or 50 + 0.91 (height [cm] – 152.4)
- ○ Female—45.5 + 2.3 (height [inches] – 60) or 45.5 + 0.91 (height [cm] – 152.4)

Pplat, plateau airway pressure during exhalation.

Source: From The Acute Respiratory Distress Syndrome Network,[46] by permission of New England Journal of Medicine.

maneuvers by demonstrating improved PaO_2 and normalized $PaCO_2$ (Figure 32.5).[86]

Prone positioning may be considered for patients with severe gas-exchange impairment that has not responded to other strategies. Prone positioning may be employed in patients requiring more than 10 cmH$_2$O PEEP and F_IO_2 of 0.6 or more to maintain SaO_2 above 90% absent a contraindication. Prone positioning will improve gas exchange by restoration of ventilation-perfusion matching from redistributed lung water, but the benefit lasts only until gravitational force returns the water to dependent portions of lung. The preferred angle for head elevation in supine patients is 30° to horizontal, with turning at least every 2 to 4 h. Similar rules apply in the prone position; reverse Trendelenburg at 15° to 30° is preferred to flat. V_T is the same value as in the supine position. No improvement in mortality was demonstrated in a randomized prospective trial.

Management of Proliferative ARDS

Recovery from ALI/ARDS is recognized by improving P:F and decreasing V_E. Radiographic opacity of the lung fields will also diminish but can lag clinical improvement substantially. Adjustments are then made to sedation and ventilating pressures; spontaneous breathing may be encouraged by conversion to PSV or PCV. Reductions in F_IO_2 are undertaken before cutbacks of PEEP, and PEEP is weaned slowly when F_IO_2 is 0.5 or less and P:F is more than 200.

A subset of patients with ARDS will progress to disordered healing and pulmonary fibrosis, typically after the first week of mechanical ventilation. This state is characterized by increasing airway pressures or decreasing V_T and a further reduction in lung compliance, less responsiveness to PEEP, and a honeycomb appearance on chest X-ray.[52] Progressive pulmonary hypertension and rising V_E are also characteristic. Pulmonary edema is less prominent as the microvascular injury is repaired. Strategies to reduce intravascular volume and edema actually result in increased V_D, pulmonary hypoperfusion, and further compromised gas exchange.

Interventions to influence the course of pulmonary fibrosis directly are not well established, but administration of high-dose corticosteroids to these patients has been advocated. One small, prospective trial has shown improved survival with the use of corticosteroids in late ARDS. Patients with advanced ARDS are at high risk not only for pulmonary dysfunction but also dysfunction of other organs, and

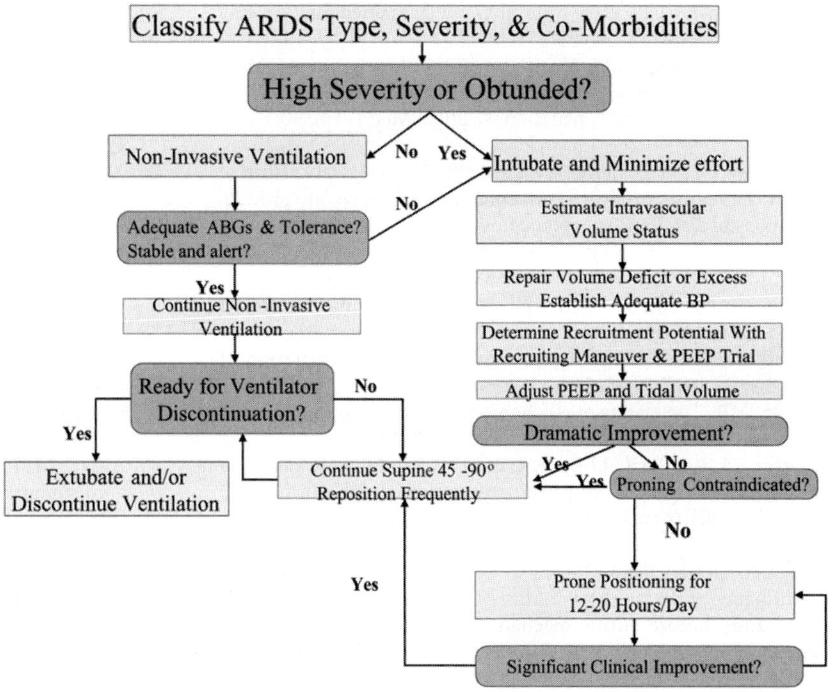

FIGURE 32.5. Management for ventilator management of acute lung injury (ALI)/acute respiratory distress syndrome (ARDS). (From Marini JJ, Gattinoni L,[86] by permission of Critical Care Medicine.)

consideration of corticosteroids in this setting may be reasonable. If corticosteroids are used, aggressive measures are essential to monitor for ventilator-associated pneumonia, which has a high incidence (up to 60%) and high mortality (up to 80%) in patients with ARDS. Patients should be evaluated carefully for the presence of pneumonia before initiation of steroid therapy, including sputum collection assisted by bronchoscopy and quantitative microbiological analysis.[87–89]

Outcomes of ARDS

A limited body of literature is available to describe the long-term sequelae of ARDS.[108] Patients may recover with minimal or no abnormalities by routine pulmonary function testing, or they may remain substantially impaired for a year or longer, if not permanently. Approximately one-quarter of patients show no impairment at 1 year whereas one-half of patients have mild impairment. Only a small proportion of recovering ARDS patients have severe impairment in pulmonary function. Exertional dyspnea is the most common respiratory symptom, although cough and wheezing may be manifest. Spirometry reveals mixed restrictive and obstructive abnormalities. Determining prognosis of ARDS may be facilitated by pulmonary function studies at the time of hospital discharge. Patients with substantial pulmonary dysfunction should be referred for appropriate specialist follow-up. Although pulmonary dysfunction may be relatively inconsequential in many patients, weight loss, muscular weakness, and neuropsychiatric dysfunction related to critical illness may be more symptomatic than pulmonary dysfunction.[109–117]

References

1. Ibsen B. The anesthetist's viewpoint on the treatment of respiratory complications in poliomyelitis during the epidemic in Copenhagen, 1952. Proc R Soc Med 1954;47:72–74.
2. Hansen-Flaschen J, Cowen J, Raps EC. Neuromuscular blockade in the intensive care unit. More than we bargained for. Am Rev Respir Dis 1993;147:234–236.
3. Dreyfuss D, Saumon G. Ventilator-induced lung injury. Am J Respir Crit Care Med 1998;157:294–323.
4. Tobin MJ. Mechanical ventilation. N Engl J Med 1994;330:1056–1061.
5. Robertson CH Jr, Foster GH, Johnson RL Jr. The relationship of respiratory failure to the oxygen consumption of, lactate production by, and distribution of blood flow among respiratory muscles during increasing inspiratory resistance. J Clin Invest 1977;59:31–42.
6. Robertson CH Jr, Pagel MA, Johnson RL Jr. The distribution of blood flow, oxygen consumption, and work output among the respiratory muscles during unobstructed hyperventilation. J Clin Invest 1977;59:43–50.
7. Pinsky MR. The effects of mechanical ventilation on the cardiovascular system. Crit Care Clin 1990;6:663–678.
8. Mathru M, Rao TLK, El-Etr AA, et al. Hemodynamic response to changes in ventilatory patterns in patients with normal and poor left ventricular reserve. Crit Care Med 1982;10:423–426.
9. Rossi A, Gottfried SB, Zocchi L, et al. Measurement of static compliance of the total respiratory system in patients with acute respiratory failure during mechanical ventilation: the effect of intrinsic positive end-expiratory pressure. Am Rev Respir Dis 1985;131:672–677.
10. Gurevitch MJ, Gelmont D. Importance of trigger sensitivity to ventilator response delay in advanced chronic obstructive pulmonary disease with respiratory failure. Crit Care Med 1989;17:354–359.
11. Pepe PE, Marini JJ. Occult positive end-expiratory pressure in mechanically ventilated patients with airflow obstruction: the auto-PEEP effect. Am Rev Respir Dis 1982;126:166–170.
12. Richecoeur J, Lu Q, Vieira SR, et al. Expiratory washout versus optimization of mechanical ventilation during permissive hypercapnia in patients with severe acute respiratory distress syndrome. Am J Respir Crit Care Med 1999;160:77–85.
13. Slutsky AS. Mechanical ventilation. Chest 1993;104:1833–1859.
14. Esteban A, Anzueto A, Alia I, et al. How is mechanical ventilation employed in the intensive care unit? An international utilization review. Am J Respir Crit Care Med 2000;161:1450–1458.
15. Tobin MJ. Advances in mechanical ventilation. N Engl J Med 2001;344:1986–1996.
16. Mador MJ. Assist-control ventilation. In: Tobin JM, ed. Principles and Practice of Mechanical Ventilation. New York: McGraw-Hill, 1994:207–219.
17. Groeger JS, Levinson MR, Carlon GC. Assist control versus synchronized intermittent mandatory ventilation during acute respiratory failure. Crit Care Med 1989;17:607–612.
18. Sassoon CSH. Intermittent mandatory ventilation. In: Tobin JM, ed. Principles and Practice of Mechanical Ventilation. New York: McGraw-Hill, 1994:221–237.
19. Downs JB, Perkins HM, Modell JH. Intermittent mandatory ventilation. Arch Surg 1974;109:519–523.
20. Marini JJ, Smith TC, Lamb VJ. External work output and force generation during synchronized intermittent mechanical ventilation: effect of machine assistance on breathing effort. Am Rev Respir 1988;138:1169–1179.
21. Marini JJ. Pressure-controlled ventilation. In: Tobin JM, ed. Principles and Practice of Mechanical Ventilation. New York: McGraw-Hill, 1994:305–317.
22. MacIntyre NR. Respiratory function during pressure support ventilation. Chest 1986;89:677–683.
23. Brochard L, Pluskwa F, Lemaire F. Improved efficacy of spontaneous breathing with inspiratory pressure support. Am Rev Respir Dis 1987;136:411–415.
24. Brochard L. Pressure support ventilation. In: Tobin JM, ed. Principles and Practice of Mechanical Ventilation. New York: McGraw-Hill, 1994:239–257.
25. Leung P, Jubran A, Tobin MJ. Comparison of assisted ventilator modes on triggering, patient effort, and dyspnea. Am J Respir Crit Care Med 1997;155:1940–1948.
26. Marcy T, Marini J. Inverse ratio ventilation: rationale and implementation. Chest 1991;100:494–504.
27. East T, Böhm S, Wallace C, et al. A successful computerized protocol for clinical management of pressure control inverse ratio ventilation in ARDS patients. Chest 1992;101:697–710.
28. Stock M, Downs J, Frolicher D. Airway pressure release ventilation. Crit Care Med 1987;15:462–466.
29. Product literature. Siemens Servo 300 ventilator, reference manual, ventilation modes no. 60–26–608-E313E. Solna, Sweden: Siemens Corp., 1992.
30. Amato MBP, Barbas CSV, Bonassa J, et al. Volume-assured pressure support ventilation (VAPSV). A new approach for reducing muscle workload during acute respiratory failure. Chest 1992;102:1225–1234.
31. Younes M, Puddy A, Roberts D, et al. Proportional assist ventilation: results of an initial clinical trial. Am Rev Respir Dis 1992;145:121–129.
32. Drazen JM, Kamm RD, Slutsky AS, et al. High-frequency ventilation. Physiol Rev 1984;64:505–543.

33. Derdak S, Mehta S, Stewart TE, et al. High-frequency oscillatory ventilation for acute respiratory distress syndrome in adults: a randomized, controlled trial. Am J Respir Crit Care Med 2002;166:801–808.
34. Mehta S, Granton J, MacDonald RJ, et al. High-frequency oscillatory ventilation in adults: the Toronto experience. Chest 2004;126:518–527.
35. Kolobow T, Moretti MP, Fumagalli R, et al. Severe impairment in lung function induced by high peak airway pressure during mechanical ventilation: an experimental study. Am Rev Respir Dis 1987;135:312–315.
36. Hernandez LA, Coker PJ, May S, et al. Mechanical ventilation increases microvascular permeability in oleic acid-injured lungs. J Appl Physiol 1990;69:2057–2061.
37. Tobin MJ. Respiratory monitoring in the intensive care unit. Am Rev Respir Dis 1988;138:1625–1642.
38. Tuxen DV. Permissive hypercapnia. In: Tobin MJ, ed. Principles and Practice of Mechanical Ventilation. New York: McGraw-Hill, 1994:371–392.
39. Darioli R, Perret C. Mechanical controlled hypoventilation in status asthmaticus. Am Rev Respir Dis 1984;129:385–387.
40. Connors AF Jr., McCaffree DR, Gray BA. Effect of inspiratory flow rate on gas exchange during mechanical ventilation. Am Rev Respir Dis 1981;124:537–543.
41. Marini JJ, Capps JS, Culver BH. The inspiratory work of breathing during assisted mechanical ventilation. Chest 1985;87:612–618.
42. Malo J, Ali J, Wood LDH. How does positive end-expiratory pressure reduce intrapulmonary shunt in canine pulmonary edema? J Appl Physiol 1984;57:1002–1010.
43. Katz JA, Marks JD. Inspiratory work with and without continuous positive airway pressure in patients with acute respiratory failure. Anesthesiology 1985;63:598–607.
44. Smith TC, Marini JJ. Impact of PEEP on lung mechanics and work of breathing in severe airflow obstruction. J Appl Physiol 1988;65:1488–1499.
45. Tobin MJ, Lodato RF. PEEP, auto-PEEP, and waterfalls. Chest 1989;96:449–451.
46. The Acute Respiratory Distress Syndrome Network. Ventilation with lower tidal volumes as compared with traditional tidal volumes for acute lung injury and the acute respiratory distress syndrome. N Engl J Med 2000;342:1301–1308.
47. Schmidt GA, Hall JB. Management of the ventilated patient. In: Hall JB, Schmidt GA, Wood LDH, eds. Principles of Critical Care, 2nd ed. New York: McGraw-Hill, 1998.
48. Aubier M, Trippenbach T, Roussos C. Respiratory muscle fatigue during cardiogenic shock. J Appl Physiol 1981;51:499–508.
49. Rodriguez-Roisin R, Ballester E, Roca J, et al. Mechanisms of hypoxemia in patients with status asthmaticus requiring mechanical ventilation. Am Rev Respir Dis 1989;139:732–739.
50. Gay PC, Rodarte JR, Hubmayr RD. The effects of positive expiratory pressure on isovolume flow and dynamic hyperinflation in patients receiving mechanical ventilation. Am Rev Respir Dis 1989;139:621–626.
51. Tuxen DV. Detrimental effects of positive end-expiratory pressure during controlled mechanical ventilation of patients with severe airflow obstruction. Am Rev Respir Dis 1989;140:5–9.
52. Ware LB, Matthay MA. The acute respiratory distress syndrome. N Engl J Med 2000;342:1334–1349.
53. Brower RG, Ware LB, Berthiaume Y, et al. Treatment of ARDS. Chest 2001;120:1347–1367.
54. Ranieri VM, Suter PM, Tortorella C, et al. Effect of mechanical ventilation on inflammatory mediators in patients with acute respiratory distress syndrome: a randomized controlled trial. JAMA 1999;282:54–61.
55. Respiratory monitoring. In: Tobin MJ, ed. Principles and Practice of Intensive Care Monitoring. New York: McGraw-Hill, 1998:187–718.
56. Tobin MJ, Perez W, Guenther SM, et al. The pattern of breathing during successful and unsuccessful trials of weaning from mechanical ventilation. Am Rev Respir Dis 1986;134:1111–1118.
57. Jubran A, Mathru M, Dries D, et al. Continuous recordings of mixed venous oxygen saturation during weaning from mechanical ventilation and the ramifications thereof. Am J Respir Crit Care Med 1998;158:1763–1769.
58. Yang KL, Tobin MJ. A prospective study of indexes predicting the outcome of trials of weaning from mechanical ventilation. N Engl J Med 1991;324:1445–1450.
59. Brochard L, Rauss A, Benito S, et al. Comparison of three methods of gradual withdrawal from ventilatory support during weaning from mechanical ventilation. Am J Respir Crit Care Med 1994;150:896–903.
60. Esteban A, Frutos F, Tobin MJ, et al. A comparison of four methods of weaning patients from mechanical ventilation. N Engl J Med 1995;332:345–350.
61. Stoller JK. Establishing clinical unweanability. Respir Care 1991;36:186–198.
62. Tobin MJ, Alex CH. Discontinuation of mechanical ventilation. In: Tobin MJ, ed. Principles and Practice of Mechanical Ventilation. New York: McGraw-Hill, 1994:1177–1206.
63. Dries DJ, McGonigal MD, Malian MS, et al. Protocol-driven ventilator weaning reduces use of mechanical ventilation, rate of early reintubation, and ventilator-associated pneumonia. J Trauma 2004;56:943–952.
64. Acton RD, Hotchkiss JR, Dries DJ. Noninvasive ventilation. J Trauma 2002;53:593–601.
65. Liesching T, Kwok H, Hill NS. Acute applications of noninvasive positive pressure ventilation. Chest 2003;124:699–713.
66. McCulloch TM, Bishop MJ. Complications of translaryngeal intubation. Clin Chest Med 1991;12:507–521.
67. Meduri GU. Noninvasive positive-pressure ventilation in patients with acute respiratory failure. Clin Chest Med 1996;17:513–553.
68. Guerin C, Girard R, Chemorin C, et al. Facial mask noninvasive ventilation reduces the incidence of nosocomial pneumonia: a prospective epidemiological study from a single ICU. Intensive Care Med 1997;23:1024–1032.
69. Antonelli M, Conti G, Rocco M, et al. A comparison of noninvasive positive-pressure ventilation and conventional mechanical ventilation in patients with acute respiratory failure. N Engl J Med 1998;339:429–435.
70. Girou E, Schortgen F, Deldaux C, et al. Association of noninvasive ventilation with nosocomial infections and survival in critically ill patients. JAMA 2000;284:2361–2367.
71. Hilbert G, Gruson D, Vargas F, et al. Noninvasive ventilation in immunosuppressed patients with pulmonary infiltrates, fever and acute respiratory failure. N Engl J Med 2001;344:481–487.
72. Hotchkiss JR, Marini JJ. Noninvasive ventilation: an emerging supportive technique for the emergency department. Ann Emerg Med 1998;32:470–478.
73. Rusterholtz T, Kempf J, Berton C, et al. Noninvasive pressure support ventilation (NIPSV) with face mask in patients with acute cardiogenic pulmonary edema (ACPE). Intensive Care Med 1999;25:21–28.
74. Pennock BE, Kaplan PD. Noninvasive ventilation for postoperative support and facilitation of weaning. Respir Care Clin N Am 1996;2:293–311.
75. Abir F, Bell R. Assessment and management of the obese patient. Crit Care Med 2004;32(sppl):S87–S91.
76. Abou-Shala N, Meduri GU. Noninvasive mechanical ventilation in patients with acute respiratory failure. Crit Care Med 1996;24:705–715.

77. Auriant I, Jallot A, Hervé P, et al. Noninvasive ventilation reduces mortality in acute respiratory failure following lung resection. Am J Respir Crit Care Med 2001;164:1231–1235.
78. Mehta S, Hill N. Noninvasive ventilation in acute respiratory failure. Respir Care Clin N Am 1996;2:267–292.
79. Meduri GU, Turner RE, Abou-Shala N, et al. Noninvasive positive pressure ventilation via face mask: first-line intervention in patients with hypercapnic and hypoxemic respiratory failure. Chest 1996;109:179–193.
80. Meduri GU, Abou-Shala N, Fox RC, et al. Noninvasive face mask mechanical ventilation in patients with acute hypercapnic respiratory failure. Chest 1991;100:445–454.
81. Stock MC, Downs JB, Gauer PK, et al. Prevention of postoperative pulmonary complications with CPAP, incentive spirometry, and conservative therapy. Chest 1985;87:151–157.
82. Lindner KH, Lotz P, Ahnefeld FW. Continuous positive airway pressure effect on functional residual capacity, vital capacity and its subdivisions. Chest 1987;2:66–70.
83. Esteban A, Frutos-Vivar F, Niall D, et al. Noninvasive positive-pressure ventilation for respiratory failure after extubation. N Engl J Med 2004;350:2452–2460.
84. Truwit JD, Bernard GR. Noninvasive ventilation—don't push too hard. N Engl J Med 2004;350:2512–2515.
85. Gattinoni L, Pelosi P, Suter PM, et al. Acute respiratory distress syndrome due to pulmonary and extra-pulmonary disease: different syndromes? Am J Respir Crit Care Med 1998;158:3–11.
86. Marini JJ, Gattinoni L. Ventilatory management of acute respiratory distress syndrome: a consensus of two. Crit Care Med 2004;32:250–255.
87. Meduri GU, Belenchia JM, Estes RJ, et al. Fibroproliferative phase of ARDS: clinical findings and effects of corticosteroids. Chest 1991;100:943–952.
88. Meduri GU, Chinn AJ, Leeper KV. Corticosteroid rescue treatment of progressive fibroproliferation in late ARDS: patterns of response and outcome. Chest 1994;105:1516–1527.
89. Meduri GU, Headley AS, Golden E, et al. Effect of prolonged methylprednisolone therapy in unresolving acute respiratory distress syndrome: a randomized controlled trial. JAMA 1998; 280:159–165.
90. Bernard GR, Artigas A, Brigham KL, et al. The American European Consensus Conference on ARDS: definitions, mechanisms, relevant outcomes, and clinical trial coordination. Am J Respir Crit Care Med 1994;149:818–824.
91. Dreyfuss D, Basset G, Soler P, et al. Intermittent positive-pressure hyperventilation with high inflation pressures produces pulmonary microvascular injury in rats. Am Rev Respir Dis 1985;132:880–884.
92. Dreyfuss D, Soler P, Basset G, et al. High inflation pressure pulmonary edema: respective effects of high airway pressure, high tidal volume, and positive end-expiratory pressure. Am Rev Respir Dis 1988;137:1159–1164.
93. Dreyfuss D, Soler P, Saumon G. Spontaneous resolution of pulmonary edema caused by short periods of cyclic overinflation. J Appl Physiol 1992;72:2081–2089.
94. Amato MBP, Barbas CSV, Medeiros DM, et al. Beneficial effects of the "open lung approach" with low distending pressures in acute respiratory distress syndrome. Am J Respir Crit Care Med 1995;152:1835–1846.
95. Marini JJ. Lung mechanics in the adult respiratory distress syndrome: recent conceptual advances and implications for management. Clin Chest Med 1990;11:673–690.
96. Benito S, LeMaire F. Pulmonary pressure-volume relationship in acute respiratory distress syndrome in adults: role of positive end-expiratory pressure. J Crit Care 1990;5:27–34.
97. Hickling KG, Henderson SJ, Jackson R. Low mortality associated with low volume pressure limited ventilation with permissive hypercapnia in severe adult respiratory distress syndrome. Intensive Care Med 1990;16:372–377.
98. Hickling KG, Walsh J, Henderson S, et al. Low mortality rate in adult respiratory distress syndrome using low-volume, pressure-limited ventilation with permissive hypercapnia: a prospective study. Crit Care Med 1994;22:1568–1578.
99. Amato MB, Barbas CS, Medeiros DM, et al. Effect of a protective-ventilation strategy on mortality in the acute respiratory distress syndrome. N Engl J Med 1998;338:347–354.
100. Brochard L, Roudot-Thoraval F, Roupie E, et al. Tidal volume reduction for prevention of ventilator-induced lung injury in acute respiratory distress syndrome: the Multicenter Trial Group on Tidal Volume Reduction in ARDS. Am J Respir Crit Care Med 1998;158:1831–1838.
101. Brower RG, Shanholtz CB, Fessler HE, et al. Prospective, randomized, controlled clinical trial comparing traditional versus reduced tidal volume ventilation in acute respiratory distress syndrome patients. Crit Care Med 1999;27:1492–1498.
102. Stewart TE, Meade MO, Cook DJ, et al. Evaluation of a ventilation strategy to prevent barotrauma in patients at high risk for acute respiratory distress syndrome. N Engl J Med 1998;338:355–361.
103. The Acute Respiratory Distress Syndrome Network. Ventilation with lower tidal volumes as compared with traditional tidal volumes for acute lung injury and the acute respiratory distress syndrome. N Engl J Med 2000;342:1301–1308.
104. Eichacker PQ, Gerstenberger EP, Banks SM, et al. Meta-analysis of acute lung injury and acute respiratory distress syndrome trials testing low tidal volumes. Am J Respir Crit Care Med 2002;166:1510–1514.
105. Brower RG, Lanken PN, MacIntyre N, et al. Higher versus lower positive end-expiratory pressures in patients with the acute respiratory distress syndrome. N Engl J Med 2004;351:327–336.
106. Lim SC, Adams AB, Simonson DA, et al. Intercomparison of recruitment maneuver efficacy in three models of acute lung injury. Crit Care Med 2004;32:2371–2377.
107. Lim SC, Adams AB, Simonson DA, et al. Transient hemodynamic effects of recruitment maneuvers in three experimental models of acute lung injury. Crit Care Med 2004;32:2378–2384.
108. O'Connor M, Hall JB, Schmidt GA, et al. Acute hypoxemic respiratory failure. In: Hall JB, Schmidt GA, Wood LDH, eds. Principles of Critical Care. New York: McGraw-Hill, 1998:537–559.
109. Milbert JA, Davis DR, Steinberg KP, et al. Improved survival of patients with acute respiratory distress syndrome (ARDS): 1983–1993. JAMA 1995;273:306–309.
110. Abel SJC, Finney SJ, Brett SJ, et al. Reduced mortality in association with the acute respiratory distress syndrome (ARDS). Thorax 1998;53:292–294.
111. McHugh LG, Milberg JA, Whitcomb ME, et al. Recovery of function in survivors of the acute respiratory distress syndrome. Am J Respir Crit Care Med 1994;150:90–94.
112. Ghio AJ, Elliott CG, Crapo RO. Impairment after adult respiratory distress syndrome: an evaluation based on American Thoracic Society recommendations. Am Rev Respir Dis 1989;139:1158–1162.
113. Elliott CG, Rasmusson BY, Crapo RO, et al. Prediction of pulmonary function abnormalities after adult respiratory distress syndrome (ARDS). Am Rev Respir Dis 1987;135:634–638.
114. Suchyta MR, Elliott CG, Jensen RL, et al. Predicting the presence of pulmonary function impairment in adult respiratory distress syndrome survivors. Respiration 1993;60:103–108.
115. Weinert CR, Gross CR, Kangas JR, et al. Health-related quality of life after acute lung injury. Am J Respir Crit Care Med 1997;156:1120–1128.
116. Davidson TA, Caldwell ES, Curtis JR, et al. Reduced quality of life in survivors of acute respiratory distress syndrome compared with critically ill control patients. JAMA 1999;281:354–360.

117. Herridge MS, Cheung AM, Tansey CM, et al. One-year outcomes in survivors of the acute respiratory distress syndrome. N Engl J Med 2003;348:683–693.
118. Kirby RR, Downs JB, Civetta JM, et al. High level positive end expiratory pressure (PEEP) in acute respiratory insufficiency. Chest 1975;67:156–163.
119. Pepe PE, Hudson LD, Carrico CJ. Early application of positive end-expiratory pressure in patients at risk for adult respiratory-distress syndrome. N Engl J Med 1984;311:281–286.
120. Mure M, Martling C-R, Lindahl SGE. Dramatic effect on oxygenation in patients with severe acute lung insufficiency treated in the prone position. Crit Care Med 1997;25:1539–1544.
121. Nakos G, Tsangaris I, Kostanti E, et al. Effect of the prone position on patients with hydrostatic pulmonary edema compared with patients with acute respiratory distress syndrome and pulmonary fibrosis. Am J Respir Crit Care Med 2000;161:360–368.
122. Zapol WM, Snider MT, Hill JD, et al. Extracorporeal membrane oxygenation in severe acute respiratory failure: a randomized prospective study. JAMA 1979;242:2193–2196.
123. Carlon GC, Howland WS, Ray C, et al. High-frequency jet ventilation: a prospective randomized evaluation. Chest 1983;84: 551–559.
124. Lessard MR, Guerot E, Lorino H, et al. Effects of pressure-controlled with different I:E ratios versus volume-controlled ventilation on respiratory mechanics, gas exchange, and hemodynamics in patients with adult respiratory distress syndrome. Anesthesiology 1994;80:983–991.
125. Morris AH, Wallace CJ, Menlove RL, et al. Randomized clinical trial of pressure-controlled inverse ratio ventilation and extracorporeal CO_2 removal for adult respiratory distress syndrome. Am J Respir Crit Care Med 1994;149:295–305.
126. Hirschl RB, Pranikoff T, Wise C, et al. Initial experience with partial liquid ventilation in adult patients with the acute respiratory distress syndrome. JAMA 1996;275:383–389.
127. Fort P, Farmer C, Westerman J, et al. High-frequency oscillatory ventilation for adult respiratory distress syndrome: pilot study. Crit Care Med 1997;25:937–947.
128. Gattinoni L, Tognoni G, Pesenti A, et al. Effect of prone positioning on the survival of patients with acute respiratory failure. N Engl J Med 2001;345:568–573.
129. Gainnier M, Michelet P, Thirion X, et al. Prone position and positive end-expiratory pressure in acute respiratory distress syndrome. Crit Care Med 2003;31:2719–2726.

33

Renal Replacement Therapy

John C.L. Wang, Roxana M. Bologa, and Stuart D. Saal

Acute renal failure (ARF) is a commonly anticipated diagnosis in critically ill patients in the intensive care unit (ICU). Its actual frequency varies from less than 10% to approximately 25% in different series including different patient demographics and definitions of ARF.[1–5] The elevations in serum creatinine and urea nitrogen concentrations observed in a majority of these patients (more than 90%) are caused by renal hypoperfusion and related parenchymal dysfunction, the latter referred to as acute tubular necrosis (ATN)[3,6] (Tables 33.1, 33.2). Between one-third and one-half of the observed ATN occurs during infection/sepsis, with the rest related to medical-surgical conditions, including hypotension and toxin exposure.[3,6] ARF is typically accompanied by a number of comorbidities [i.e., respiratory failure (67%), heart failure (48%), and liver failure (31%)].[7] In many series, more than one-half of the patients who develop ARF in the ICU require some form of renal replacement therapy (RRT).[3,6,7]

Considering the foregoing, including frequent comorbidities, it is not surprising that patients with ARF seen in an ICU continue to have extremely high mortality. In the critical care setting, the mortality for patients who undergo RRT may exceed 50%,[3,5,6] and mortality is also increased among patients whose ARF does not progress to the point of needing RRT. Measurements for dialysis delivery and adequacy have been developed and applied to patients receiving chronic RRT. However, in the complicated scenario that accompanies ARF in critical illness, it may be difficult to truly characterize and quantify the dialysis-related outcome.

It is becoming evident that the impact of ARF extends beyond the obvious observations of "renal" dysfunction (e.g., volume overload, metabolic acidosis, hyperkalemia, and azotemia). For example, volume overload may aggravate hypertension and congestive heart failure, whereas acidosis may depress cardiac output and contribute to hypotension.[7–10] Although some of these examples of dysregulation may contribute to a broad inflammatory response,[7,11] the actual ARF pathophysiology may itself exacerbate multiple organ dysfunction.[12] For example, in a renal ischemia model, it takes approximately 48h for elevated systemic tumor necrosis factor-alpha (TNF-α) concentrations to return to baseline after successful reperfusion. Even after systemic concentrations of proinflammatory mediators have returned to normal, local paracrine effects may persist; for example, cardiac muscle may demonstrate increased staining for interleukin-1 (IL-1) and TNF-α. This effect is accompanied by intercellular adhesion molecule (ICAM-1) messenger RNA expression, evidence of neutrophil infiltration, and myocardial apoptosis (programmed cell death). In these models, the latter can be demonstrated in the absence of azotemia. Myocardial dysfunction resulting from decreased myocardial muscle fractional shortening is the observed clinical correlate. Similar results are not observed in animals simply undergoing sham surgery or nephrectomy. Neutrophil infiltration is also evident in other organs (e.g., lung and liver).[12] Downregulation of pulmonary epithelial sodium channels, Na-K-ATPase, and aquaporin 5, as demonstrated after ischemic ARF, may contribute to observed pulmonary dysfunction.[11]

This systemic pathophysiology provides an understanding for the increased morbidity and mortality observed in patients with ARF when they are compared to a matched cohort that does not develop ARF.[13] Renal failure appears to increase the risk of developing severe nonrenal complications.[13] Writing a prescription for optimal RRT is important for managing fluid and electrolyte balance and treating some extrarenal manifestations of uremia (e.g., mental status changes, bleeding, or pericarditis). In fact, there are limited examples to suggest that more intensive treatment of ARF improves overall outcome.[14] However, based on the recognition and understanding of this extensive pathophysiology (i.e., ARF is a "systemic condition"), there may be a limit to what can be achieved to improve organ dysfunction, and therefore ARF-related morbidity and mortality, by even optimized RRT.

TABLE 33.1. Differential Diagnosis of Acute Renal Failure.

Types of acute renal failure and underlying problem	*Possible disorders*
Prerenal acute renal failure:	
Intravascular volume depletion	Sepsis, hemorrhage, overdiuresis, inadequate fluid intake, vomiting, diarrhea
Decreased effective circulating volume	Congestive heart failure, cirrhosis, nephrotic syndrome
Impaired renal blood flow (drug-induced)	Angiotensin-converting enzyme inhibitors, angiotensin II receptor blockers, nonsteroidal antiinflammatory drugs
Intrinsic acute renal failure:	
Acute tubular necrosis	Ischemia
	Toxins: drugs (e.g., aminoglycosides), contrast agents, pigments (e.g., myoglobin, hemoglobin)
Glomerular disease	Rapidly progressive glomerulonephritis: systemic lupus erythematosus, small vessel vasculitis, endocarditis, poststreptococcal or postpneumococcal infection, endocarditis, cryoglobulinemia, antiglomerular basement membrane disease
Vascular disease	Microvascular disease: cholesterol plaque microembolism, thrombotic thrombocytopenic purpura, hemolytic uremic syndrome, HELLP syndrome
	Macrovascular disease: renal artery occlusion, severe abdominal aortic disease
Interstitial disease	Allergic reaction to drugs (antibiotics most common), systemic lupus erythematosus or mixed connective tissue disease, pyelonephritis, infiltrative disease (lymphoma or leukemia)
Postrenal acute renal failure	Benign prostatic hypertrophy or prostate cancer, cervical cancer, retroperitoneal fibrosis, tubular obstruction (crystals or myeloma light chains), ureteral or bladder calculus, pelvic mass or invasive pelvic tumor, intraluminal bladder mass (clot, tumor), iatrogenic injury to ureter, occluded ureteral catheter, neurogenic bladder, urethral stricture, unrecognized intraperitoneal bladder laceration or leak with systemic reabsorption of urine

HELLP, Hemolysis, Elevated Liver enzymes, Low Platelets.

TABLE 33.3. Indications for Initiation of Dialysis.

Fluid and electrolyte abnormalities
- Fluid overload
- Hyperkalemia
- Hypernatremia
- Hyponatremia
- Hypercalcemia
- Hyperphosphatemia
- Hyperuricemia
- Metabolic acidosis
- Metabolic alkalosis

Uremic symptoms
- Pericarditis
- Uremic bleeding
- Encephalopathy
- Nausea/vomiting

Indications for Renal Replacement Therapy in the Critical Care Setting

RRT (i.e., dialysis) is a standard treatment for end-stage renal disease (ESRD) and used commonly for the treatment of ARF. Although there is a growing consensus that supports use of the National Kidney Foundation (NKF) Kidney Disease Outcomes Quality Initiative (K/DOQI) guidelines to guide the treatment of ESRD,[15] no unified approach has been accepted for ARF. There is variation in the indications for RRT and choice of available modalities. The first international consensus conference on continuous RRT developed evidence-based practice recommendations for the management of ARF.[7] However, these Acute Dialysis Quality Initiative (ADQI) guidelines expressed uncertainty on issues of timing (when to begin/stop RRT), dose, and technique.

Optimal management of the critically ill patient who requires RRT includes an understanding of the types of problems that can be corrected effectively by RRT, and the issues or complications that may arise as a consequence of RRT.

Indications for initiating RRT in critical illness should be based on renal and nonrenal considerations. For patients with ARF, when fluid and electrolyte abnormalities are uncontrollable and no longer responding to conservative medical management, and when development of uremia is expected, RRT should be initiated. The established uses for dialysis as therapy are listed in Table 33.3. RRT can be utilized to remove or add solutes and fluid, regulate plasma composition and volume, correct acid–base abnormalities, and treat uremic symptoms.

TABLE 33.2. Blood and Urine Studies to Distinguish Prerenal from Intrinsic Acute Renal Failure.

Type of renal failure	*BUN: creatinine*	*Urine osmolality*	*Urine sediment*	*Urine sodium*	*FeNa*[a]
Prerenal acute renal failure	>20:1	>500 mOsm/L	Scant	<10 mEq/L	<1%
Intrinsic acute renal failure	<20:1	250–300 mOsm/L	Variable[b]	>20 mEq/L	>3%

BUN, blood urea nitrogen (mg/dL).

[a]The fractional excretion of sodium (FeNa) is calculated using the formula: 100 × (urine sodium/serum sodium) ÷ (urine creatinine/serum creatinine). FeNa is most useful in the setting of oliguric acute renal failure.

[b]Acute tubular necrosis: epithelial cells; muddy-brown, coarsely granular casts; white blood cells; low-grade proteinuria.

[b]Allergic interstitial nephritis: white blood cells and possible WBC casts; red blood cells with dysmorphic cells; epithelial cells; eosinophils; low to moderate proteinuria.

[b]Glomerulonephritis: red blood cell casts, dysmorphic red cells, moderate to severe proteinuria.

The decision to begin dialysis is based on clinical judgment. Fluid overload and electrolyte abnormalities may require correction by RRT despite a lack of uremic symptoms. On the other hand, "uremia" manifested by related signs or symptoms may affect a patient's condition adversely, regardless of a specific creatinine or blood urea nitrogen concentration, and warrant initiation of RRT. In addition, so-called prophylactic dialysis has been employed to prevent the complications of ARF. In general, it is reasonable to initiate early dialysis in a patient with persistent oliguria, suggesting that resolution of ARF is not imminent. In comparison, RRT can be withheld from a patient with ARF if there are no symptoms and if the urine output has begun to increase, indicating the onset of recovery.

The nonrenal indications for dialysis have been expanded. In the setting of normal renal function, some drug overdoses may benefit from dialysis or hemoperfusion. Critical serum concentrations for several drugs are listed in Table 33.4. The decision to institute hemodialysis or hemoperfusion must be made on an individual basis.[16] Dialysis can also be effective in raising core body temperature and can be utilized as therapy for hypothermic patients.[17] Peritoneal dialysis in particular has been used in the treatment of profound hypothermia.[18] Peritoneal dialysis has also been advocated by some investigators to treat severe acute pancreatitis,[19] and a few anecdotal reports of success have been published.[20,21] However, a large prospective, randomized study failed to substantiate these reports.[22]

Other indications that have been offered for considering and implementing RRT in the critical care setting include removal of inflammatory mediators,[23,24] treatment of congestive heart failure,[25] and prevention of contrast-induced nephropathy (CIN).[10]

High-volume hemofiltration has been used to remove cytokines in sepsis.[23,24] However, a closer look at the data (Figure 33.1), including the filtration barrier provided by typical hemofiltration membranes, the molecular weight of a number of inflammatory mediators, and the observed sieving coefficients for these mediators, reveals that the actual clearance of a variety of inflammatory mediators may be much less than what would be predicted based on the size barrier provided by a dialyzer and the molecular weights of the mediators in question. Two possible explanations contributing to this discrepant observation are spontaneous aggregation and variable protein binding of the mediators in question. In fact, continuous venovenous hemofiltration (CVVH), including

TABLE 33.4. Serum Concentrations at Which Hemodialysis (HD) or Hemoperfusion (HP) Is Indicated.

Drug	*Serum concentration (mg/dL)*	*Treatment choice*
Phenobarbital	10	HD or HP
Glutethimide	4	HP
Methaqualone	4	HP
Salicylates	80	HD
Theophylline	30–40	HP
Lithium	2.5 (mEq/L)	HD
Methanol	100	HD

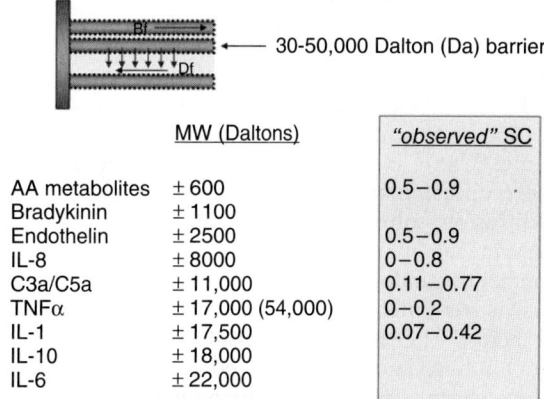

CRRT – cytokines clearance – sieving coefficients (SC)

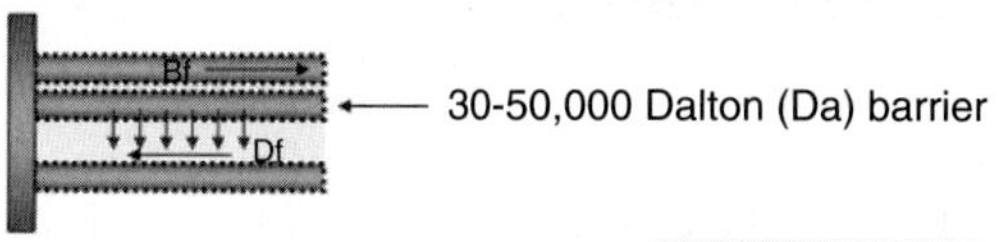

	MW (Daltons)	"observed" SC
AA metabolites	± 600	0.5–0.9
Bradykinin	± 1100	
Endothelin	± 2500	0.5–0.9
IL-8	± 8000	0–0.8
C3a/C5a	± 11,000	0.11–0.77
TNFα	± 17,000 (54,000)	0–0.2
IL-1	± 17,500	0.07–0.42
IL-10	± 18,000	
IL-6	± 22,000	

FIGURE 33.1. Molecular weight of molecules participating in the inflammatory response and their observed sieving coefficients in relation to a high-flux dialyzer barrier. *AA*, amino acid; *IL*, interleukin; *C*, complement fragment; *TNF-α*, tumor necrosis factor-alpha.

2 L/h fluid exchange in critically ill patients, did not produce a predictable decrease in inflammatory mediators, including complement fragments (C3a, C5a), IL-6, -8, and -10, and TNF-α after 48 h treatment.[26] Much of the observed clearance may be the result of these mediators adhering to the dialysis membrane. Thus, even in the absence of production, current RRT technologies and applications probably do not remove circulating inflammatory mediators effectively in patients with sepsis and ARF.

Various ultrafiltration prescriptions have been used to treat patients with diuretic-resistant, refractory congestive heart failure.[27,28] During ultrafiltration, the intravascular plasma compartment is able to refill (mobilize fluid from the interstitial space) at a rate of approximately 700 mL/h. Treatments that provide ultrafiltration at hourly rates less than this (i.e., slow continuous ultrafiltration using hemodialysis or a variant of the continuous therapies to be described) are able to relieve related symptoms. The claims that these treatments may restore diuretic responsiveness have not been examined in a controlled evaluation.

Patients with preexisting renal failure are at particularly high risk for contrast-induced nephropathy (CIN). The strategy of performing hemodialysis immediately after the administration of a contrast agent did not diminish the rate of complications, including CIN.[29] However, Marenzi et al. compared periprocedural hemofiltration given in an ICU setting to normal saline hydration alone in patients with chronic renal failure who were undergoing percutaneous coronary intervention.[10] Hemofiltration was effective in preventing deterioration of renal function and was associated with improved in-hospital and long-term outcomes. However, the use of a bicarbonate-based replacement fluid (which itself may be effective in preventing CIN) and the actual magnitude of contrast removal based on the continuous renal replacement therapy (CRRT) prescription raise questions about the study conclusion. Based on the unanswered questions and the cost, CRRT cannot be recommended to prevent CIN at present.

Overview of Available Modalities for Renal Replacement Therapy

In general, RRT can be rendered either intermittently or continuously. Commonly available dialysis modalities are listed in Table 33.5. Each modality has clinical advantages and disadvantages, although their physiological principles remain the same. There are two mechanisms involved for solute transport: diffusion and convection.

In diffusion, solutes and toxins can pass (diffuse) through a semipermeable membrane (i.e., the peritoneum or a dialysis membrane) by random molecular motion. Equilibration (i.e., dialysis) is dependent on the concentration gradient established across the membrane. Molecular weight, charge, protein binding, and membrane pore size affect diffusion. Clearance during intermittent hemodialysis treatments is largely based on diffusion. In convection, ultrafiltration (i.e., convective transport) occurs when water is driven by either a hydrostatic or osmotic pressure gradient across a semipermeable membrane. In forming an ultrafiltrate, the water brings with it (i.e., a "drag effect") dissolved solutes based on their molecular weight, charge, protein binding, and membrane pore size. The convective clearance that results is an important contribution to overall clearance in both peritoneal dialysis and continuous RRTs.

Although intermittent hemodialysis (IHD) and peritoneal dialysis (PD) were the main renal replacement techniques used in the past, longer duration treatments such as sustained low efficiency dialysis (SLED) and CRRT are now utilized increasingly in the critical care setting. These newer therapies provide for the slow removal of water and solutes over a prolonged period of time. As a result, they create less drastic changes and instability and are more suitable for critically ill patients.

Peritoneal Dialysis

Peritoneal dialysis (PD) is a currently available RRT for patients who develop ARF in the critical care setting.[30] Despite being technically simple, very inexpensive, and not requiring sophisticated equipment, PD has lost its popularity to other forms of slow dialysis.[31]

PD remains a preferred RRT for patients who are hemodynamically unstable.[32] It is particularly suitable for patients with bleeding abnormalities or heparin allergy and for patients in whom vascular access is difficult to obtain. Patients with recent abdominal surgery, abdominal adhesions, abdominal hernia, diaphragmatic pleuroperitoneal defects, or severe liver failure are not candidates for PD.

TABLE 33.5. Renal Replacement Therapy Modalities.

Intermittent renal replacement therapy (IRRT)
Hemodialysis (HD)
Sustained low efficiency dialysis (SLED)
Intermittent peritoneal dialysis (IPD)
Continuous renal replacement therapy (CRRT)
Slow continuous ultrafiltration (SCUF)
Continuous venovenous hemofiltration (CVVH)
Continuous venovenous hemodialysis (CVVHD)
Continuous venovenous hemodiafiltration (CVVHDF)
Continuous peritoneal dialysis (CPD)

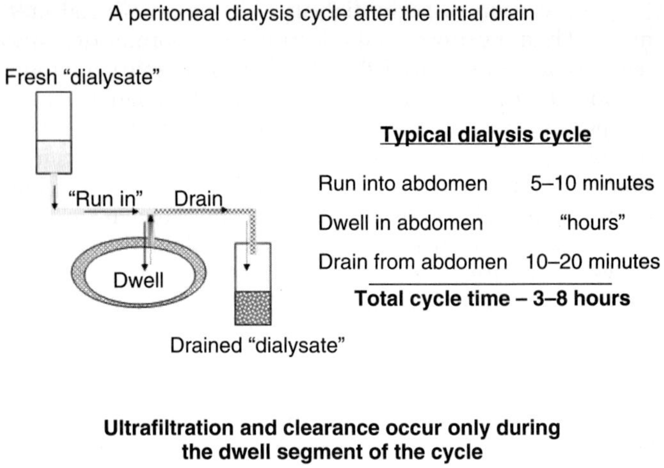

FIGURE 33.2. A typical peritoneal dialysis exchange cycle.

To perform PD, specifically designed catheters are inserted into the lower part of the abdominal cavity. The PD solution (dialysate) is introduced into the abdominal cavity and after a prescribed "dwell" period is drained and discarded. A regular PD exchange actually starts with the drainage of fluid already in the abdominal cavity followed by the infusion of fresh dialysate (Figure 33.2). The dialysate inflow should take an average of 5 to 10 min. Drainage lasts twice as long. In between, the fluid remains (dwells) in the abdomen for the prescribed dwell time in hours.

The passage of uremic toxins and electrolytes[33] across the peritoneal membrane from peritoneal capillaries[34] into the abdominal cavity occurs only during the dwell part of the cycle and is driven by the concentration gradient established between the blood and the infused dialysate for the various dialyzable substances (e.g., urea, creatinine, phosphorus). Passage is relatively slow, avoiding undesired disequilibrium and related side effects. Acid–base status is corrected by the absorption of dialysate lactate that is metabolized by the liver to bicarbonate. Ultrafiltration and subsequent water removal are achieved by an osmotic gradient created by the high glucose content of the PD dialysate relative to the serum glucose concentration. The maximum gradient is present within the first 2 h of any PD exchange. Over time, glucose from the dialysate is absorbed into the circulation, the concentration gradient decreases, and ultrafiltration diminishes. PD dialysis may thus make accomplishment of tight glucose control more difficult to achieve. PD can be performed continuously or intermittently (i.e., every day for a fixed time period). It may be performed "manually" by the nursing staff or "automatically" using an automated cycler.

The dialysis membrane used for PD is the patient's own peritoneal membrane,[35] which excludes any concerns about bio-incompatibility[36] with the potential for stimulating the production of inflammatory cytokines and triggering an inflammatory reaction. The peritoneal membrane is multilayered and allows bidirectional transfer between capillaries and dialysate of almost all sizes of molecules, including proteins and various protein-bound drugs. The peritoneal membrane of each individual has specific characteristics for transferring urea, creatinine, and glucose. Whether a patient is a slow or "low transporter" or a fast or "high transporter" is extremely important in deciding the frequency of the dialysis exchanges.[37]

Preparing the Patient for Peritoneal Dialysis: Access Selection

Semirigid catheters are available for percutaneous, trocar-guided, bedside placement under local anesthesia. They are sutured to the skin and have no physical barrier to outside infection. Although these catheters can be used immediately, they have to be removed after a short period of time. Percutaneous, acute catheter insertion may result in malposition, bowel perforation, infection, or dialysate leakage around the catheter. These complications make this type of PD catheter less desirable. Placement of soft-coiled, tunneled catheters[38] (single- or double-cuffed) has gained popularity, especially in cases when severe ARF requiring dialysis is anticipated. Placement typically occurs in the operating room and may be completed during a primary surgical procedure. Soft-coiled catheters may also be inserted at the bedside by a skilled team. Laparoscopic placement is preferable to ensure pelvic position and to avoid damaging surrounding tissues and organs. Soft-coiled catheters are tunneled into the subcutaneous tissue, allowing for the use of dialysate volumes larger than 1 L with lower chances of pericatheter dialysate leakage or infection. Both types of catheters can be used immediately if the patient is kept supine. They should be removed as soon as PD is no longer necessary.

Preparing the Patient for Peritoneal Dialysis: Dialysate Selection

The PD dialysate contains dextrose (D) in various concentrations (1.5% D, 2.5% D, or 4.25% D) to provide an osmotic gradient for ultrafiltration (i.e., higher concentrations stimulate more ultrafiltration). The amount of glucose absorbed during the dwell time may provide a patient with at least 1000 kcal /day and contribute to overall nutritional status, as well as a requirement for insulin therapy. Also included are several electrolytes: sodium, chloride, calcium, magnesium, and lactate. Lactate (35–40 mEq/L) is absorbed and metabolized to bicarbonate to compensate for metabolic acidosis. Patients with severe liver failure may not be able to complete this conversion. PD solutions do not contain potassium; thus, PD can be used to treat hyperkalemia. However, even using a dialysate potassium concentration of zero provides relatively low potassium clearance; therefore, PD is not the preferred RRT for severely hyperkalemic patients. On the other hand, if hypokalemia develops, it can be corrected by adding 2–3 mEq KCl to each liter of dialysate.

Writing the Peritoneal Dialysis Prescription

The PD prescription[39] should take into account that solute clearance and ultrafiltration occur only during the dwell period of the cycle. Maximum ultrafiltration[40] can be achieved with short dwell times, whereas appropriate uremic toxin clearance, especially for midsized or large uremic molecules, requires longer dwell times. Dialysis adequacy[41] can be estimated by using a specific formula that takes into account urea and creatinine concentration in the serum and the effluent. Hypercatabolic states require prescriptions for higher urea and creatinine clearances.

The PD prescription should include as many exchanges per day, typically between 5 and 12, as are necessary to obtain the desired ultrafiltration and clearance. Extremely short cycles (i.e., less than 1–2 h) are unlikely to achieve either goal. Short exchanges increase the opportunity for a break in sterile technique and are more likely to be complicated by peritonitis.

More "fine-tuning" of the PD prescription to match the ongoing changes in a patient's condition is possible when treatments are performed manually. However, in comparison to treatments performed using an automated cycler, manual exchange requires more nursing intervention. Depending on the patient's clinical condition, fluid status, blood pressure, and laboratory parameters, PD prescriptions (i.e., number of exchanges per 24 h, dialysate electrolyte and dextrose concentrations, and volume of fluid infused per exchange) should be evaluated every 24 h or more frequently if necessary.

The nursing staff should be instructed to analyze each aliquot of effluent (e.g., for clarity, volume, blood-tinged or bloody appearance, the presence of fibrin clots, or vegetable or fecal matter) and report any abnormalities immediately. PD effluent should be sent for cell count and bacterial and fungal cultures at the earliest suspicion of infection.

Medications Commonly Added to the Peritoneal Dialysis Solution

Heparin

Heparin can be added to the dialysate (200–500 IU/L) when intraperitoneal infection or PD-related or other intraperitoneal bleeding (not resulting from surgery) complicates treatments. Although it may seem counterintuitive to add heparin to a bloody dialysate, the heparin is added to prevent fibrin or blood clot formation, partial or total obstruction, and malfunction of the catheter. Even in cases of prolonged heparin administration, there is no need for monitoring the activated partial thromboplastin time (aPTT) because heparin is not absorbed systemically.

Regular Insulin

Regular insulin can be added to the PD solution for better blood glucose control, especially for the diabetic patient. The recommended starting dose of regular insulin is 4–5 units/L for a 1.5% dextrose dialysate, 5–6 units/L for a 2.5% dextrose dialysate, and 7–10 units/L for a 4.25% dextrose dialysate. Ideally, just enough insulin is administered to "cover" the amount of dextrose presumed to be absorbed from the PD solution. Because glucose control is very important in the overall care of critically ill patients, serum glucose concentration may need to be monitored at the start of each exchange.

Antibiotics

A wide spectrum of antibiotics with activity against gram-positive and gram-negative bacteria can be added to the PD dialysate. However, systemic absorption after intraperitoneal administration is unpredictable, and this route of administration should not be used to treat a systemic infection. On the other hand, PD peritonitis may not have a prompt response to systemic antibiotics and should be treated with intraperitoneal antibiotics. Antibiotics should be added to each PD exchange, but once-daily administration may be considered if a single dwell time of at least 6 to 8h is prescribed.

Peritoneal Dialysis-Related Complications

The most common complications related to PD are a result of the abdominal distension caused by the volume of infused dialysate. Some patients can experience abdominal pain or discomfort or mild respiratory distress secondary to diaphragm elevation or poor inspiratory excursion, leading to atelectasis. Infusing smaller dialysate volumes or maintaining the patient in a supine position may improve symptoms.

Another important PD-related complication is dialysate leakage around the PD catheter or into the abdominal wall or perineum; this usually occurs when catheters, especially nontunneled catheters, are used immediately. Management includes discontinuing the dialysis to allow fluid reabsorption, tissue healing, and sealing the pericatheter area.

Other potential complications include abdominal pain or hypothermia related to infusion of PD fluid that has not been warmed properly, inadequate drainage of the PD fluid as a consequence of decreased bowel motility, adhesion of bowel to the catheter, or migration of the PD catheter from the normal position in the pelvis. Rarely, intraabdominal organ perforation may occur related to the placement of a semirigid PD catheter.

PD-related infectious complications[42] (i.e., PD-related peritonitis or exit site infection of the PD catheter) may be avoided by following the proper exchange technique including catheter exit site cleansing[43] with an antiseptic solution or adding mupirocin ointment[44] to the daily local care. Peritonitis secondary to PD can be diagnosed clinically by identifying cloudy fluid in a patient complaining of abdominal pain, nausea, or anorexia. Fever is uncommon. Examination of the PD fluid reveals more than 100 white blood cells per high-power field, including more than 50% polymorphonuclear leukocytes, and the presence of bacteria on Gram stain of the fluid. Dialysate cultures are used to identify organisms and specific antibiotic susceptibility. Coagulase-negative *Staphylococcus* sp. or *Staphylococcus aureus* are responsible for the majority of PD catheter-related infections in the ICU. As already mentioned, PD peritonitis can be treated with intraperitoneal antibiotics. First-generation cephalosporins or vancomycin are used for treatment of gram-positive infections, whereas gentamicin or third-generation cephalosporins can be administered in the dialysate for treatment of gram-negative infections. When microbiology data are available, the antibiotic regimen should be tailored accordingly. During PD peritonitis, there may be a decrease in ultrafiltration, so the PD regimen may need to be adjusted. If there is no response to antibiotic treatment, the PD catheter should be removed, systemic antibiotics are administered, and the patient is converted to hemodialysis.

Intermittent Hemodialysis

The successful use of intermittent hemodialysis (IHD) to treat ARF dates back to World War II. With the exception of PD, all other forms of RRT are simply a variation on the traditional HD model. Figure 33.3 illustrates a generic extracorporeal circuit common to all forms of extracorporeal RRT.

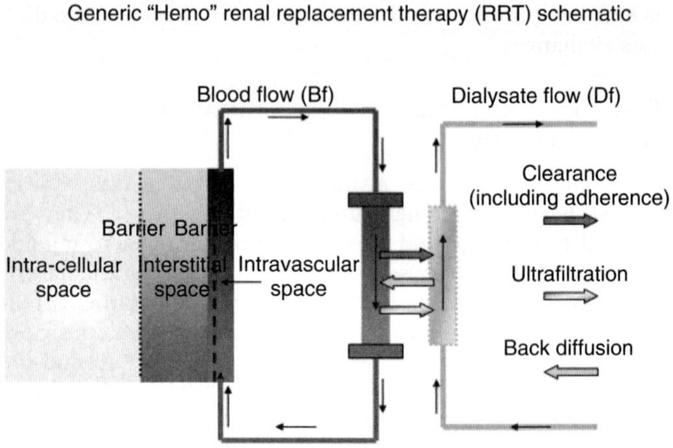

FIGURE 33.3. The generic extracorporeal circuit for providing renal replacement therapy (RRT).

Figure 33.3 includes arrows indicating blood flow, dialysate flow (they are in opposite directions) and dialyzer "events" [i.e., dialysis, ultrafiltration (UF), and the passage of solute from dialysate into blood (back-diffusion)]. Although clearance is usually thought of in terms of a substance passing from the blood compartment through the dialyzer and into the dialysate, the diagram also illustrates that some substances (e.g., inflammatory mediators) may be "cleared" by passing from the blood compartment and adhering to the dialyzer itself.[45]

Essentially, HD involves dialyzing the intravascular or blood compartment. During a treatment, intravascular refilling from the extravascular compartments (interstitial and intracellular space) provides the solutes (e.g., urea, creatinine, and water for continuous clearance and ultrafiltration). This is an important concept, because a dialysis prescription that attempts to ultrafiltrate a patient (i.e., remove fluid) more rapidly than the volume that can be mobilized from the extravascular compartment is likely to result in a decrease in blood pressure[46]; this is obviously a common problem and limitation to RRT in the ICU. A stable, chronic renal failure patient[47] may mobilize extravascular fluid at approximately 1 L/h; the critically ill patient receiving dialysis often cannot.

Selecting Hemodialysis

A typical outpatient chronic renal failure patient may have three hemodialysis sessions for 3 to 4.5h per week; this may not be appropriate or sufficient for a critically ill patient. Intermittent HD treatments should be individualized and prescribed on the basis of the patient's clinical condition and specific needs (e.g., fluid, electrolyte, and metabolic requirements); this may mean five or six treatments per week, if necessary. Generally, hemodynamic stability (i.e., the patient's ability to maintain blood pressure in the absence of pressor use) is the first consideration for selecting IHD.

Peritoneal dialysis or a variant of continuous renal replacement therapy (CRRT) (e.g., CVVH, CVVHHD) may be more suited for hemodynamically "unstable" patients. Table 33.6 includes selected parameters for some IHD variants.[48–51] Few critically ill patients can actually tolerate an ultrafiltration rate of 1000mL/h [conventional and short daily dialysis (SDD)]. The sustained low efficiency (SLED) IHD variant

TABLE 33.6. "Typical" Parameters for IHD Variants.

	Conventional	*SLED*	*Short daily*
Hemodialyzer	Hi-Efficiency/ Flux	Hi-Flux	Hi-Flux
Treatment duration (h)	3–4.5	6–8	2–2.5
Treatment frequency (per week)	3	6	5
Blood flow rate (Bf) (mL/min)	400–500	250–300	400
Dialysate flow rate (Df) (mL/min)	700	300	700
Bf/Df	0.6	1	0.6
Ultrafiltration rate (mL/h)	1000	150–400	1000
Anticoagulation	Heparin/ none	Heparin/ other	Heparin/ none
Total blood processed (L/week)	270	600	300

IHD, intermittent hemodialysis; SLED, sustained low efficiency dialysis.

model may achieve between 900 and 3000 mL of ultrafiltration per day at more tolerable hourly rates. Therefore, a second selection consideration is how much fluid a patient is receiving per day and how much needs to be removed. Although it may be possible to use an IHD variant, a continuous therapy may be a better choice for hemodynamically unstable patients. IHD is the superior choice when "clearance" is necessary in a relatively short period of time (i.e., the patient with hyperkalemia, other acute electrolyte abnormalities, or dialyzable drug intoxication).

Preparing a Patient for Intermittent Hemodialysis: Access Selection

There are a number of temporary access options for performing effective IHD.[52] Access placement is often unnecessary in chronic renal failure patients undergoing IHD. However, it is not uncommon for access (i.e., fistula or graft) to clot during a period of hypotension; temporary access creation then becomes necessary. Catheters are typically dual lumen; they have two distinct side-by-side channels for blood removal into the dialysis system (so-called arterial side) and blood return from the dialysis system to the patient (so-called venous side). Basically, two types of immediate-use catheters are available. Catheters may be tunneled and have a subcutaneous cuff for fixation and to prevent infection, or they may be uncuffed (Figure 33.4). The latter catheters are typically placed at the bedside in either the groin or neck [i.e., external jugular, internal jugular (right side is preferred), or femoral vein]. The subclavian vein is less desirable because of the associated stenosis and thrombosis risk, which may compromise chronic access placement.[53] Cuffed catheters, generally thought of for more chronic use, require placement with fluoroscopic guidance. Patients with abnormal clotting studies (e.g., prolonged prothrombin time) may require preadministration of several units of fresh-frozen plasma before catheter placement. Similarly, patients with platelet counts less than 50,000 mm^3 should receive a platelet transfusion before placement. Uncuffed catheters, especially in the femoral vein, need to be changed every 7 to 10 days. The blood flow through an uncuffed catheter may be "positional" (i.e., with a change in a patient's position), or the location of the catheter in the vein may change and limit achievable withdrawal blood flow rates (arterial side) or return blood flow rates to the patient (venous side). Cuffed catheters do not require changing and, if cared for properly, may be used for months. Between treatments, both types of catheters are filled with an anticoagulant (e.g., heparin or citrate)[54] to prevent clotting. A patient who develops sepsis, as is not uncommon in the ICU, requires removal of either type of catheter. On the other hand, an infected patient who requires dialysis should always initiate RRT with an uncuffed catheter, which may be removed after treatment completion and reinserted as necessary.

Either type of catheter may clot or become infected. Infection of the catheter mandates removal and then replacement, preferably at a different site, when the infection is controlled. Blood flow through catheters is typically less than 350 mL/min, although some newer configurations may allow higher blood flow rates. An additional catheter-related characteristic that may limit treatment efficacy is so-called reflow or recirculation (see Figure 33.4).[55] In most catheters, the ports of entry and egress to the arterial and from the venous channels are separated by approximately 1 cm and are on opposite sides of the catheter. Mechanical limitation to either blood withdrawal or return may increase turbulence and divert an excessive amount of "returning" (venous) dialyzed blood into the withdrawal (arterial) port, diluting "nondialyzed" blood from the patient that is just entering the dialysis circuit. Thus, treatment efficiency, the actual amount of "new" blood being cleaned during the treatment, is decreased. Reflow should be suspected if, several hours after a treatment, blood chemistries (e.g., urea nitrogen, creatinine, or potassium concentrations) remain elevated. Reflow can be quantified[56] and may be more common with femoral than internal jugular catheters.[56] Recirculation can be minimized in femoral catheters if they are at least 19 cm long.[57]

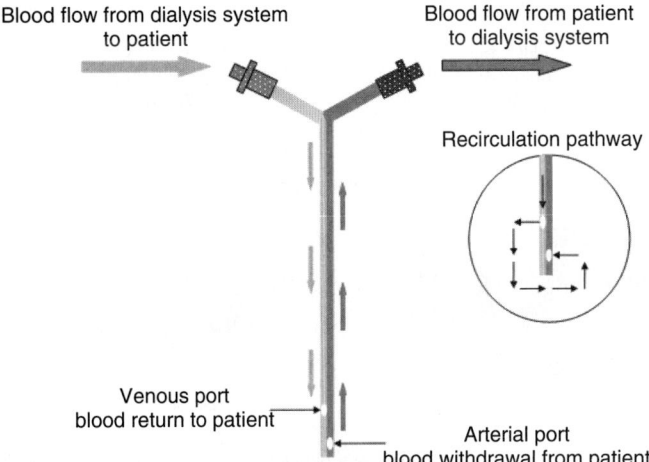

FIGURE 33.4. Schematic of typical acute, uncuffed dialysis catheter. *Inset* traces the recirculation pathway from the venous to the arterial port.

Selecting a Dialyzer

There are basically two types of dialyzers available for use in the circuit illustrated in Figure 33.3, the so-called high-flux and high-efficiency dialyzers. The difference is illustrated in Figure 33.5. The clearance of different size molecules is presented as a function of blood flow for representative examples of the two types of dialyzers. High-flux dialyzers, the dialyzers of choice, provide greater clearance for larger molecules (e.g., vitamin B_{12} compared to smaller molecules, such as urea) at a given blood flow rate. Both types of dialyzers can be used at the same high blood flow rates, but note that doubling the blood flow rate does not double clearance.

Most high-flux dialyzers that are used in the ICU are made from a polymer (e.g., polysulfone, polyacrilonitrile, or cellulose triacetate) and are quite biocompatible (i.e., passage of blood through these dialyzers does not provoke substantial production of inflammatory mediators). Inflammatory mediator production, during treatment, has resulted in pulmonary decompensation or may affect recovery from ARF.[58,59] This problem has become a moot point because noncompatible dialyzers (made from cellulose and some of its derivatives) are no longer being used for the most part. The tendency to clot during a treatment may also be an important selection consideration. In a number of intensive care settings (e.g., postoperative, active bleeding) IHD treatments can be performed without any intratreatment anticoagulation (e.g., heparin).[60] However, clotting during a treatment is not solely a function of biocompatibility and may be determined by other physical determinants of the dialyzer, including blood volume and surface area. Experience using different dialyzers becomes the guide to selection.

Additional Considerations When Writing an Intermittent Hemodialysis Prescription

Each prescription for an IHD session should be written with a specific goal in mind. What does the treatment need to accomplish (i.e., clearance, ultrafiltration, or both)? Most of the clearance achieved during an IHD session is through diffusion. In general, longer treatment sessions at higher blood flow rates will increase diffusive clearance. A sampling of available premixed dialysate solutions is illustrated in Table 33.7. Dialysate solutions contain no urea, creatinine, uric acid, or phosphorus to maximize the potential for their clearance. Potassium concentration is below "typical" serum concentrations, and can be zero if necessary or increased to 3 mEq/L to avoid excessive potassium lowering. Calcium-free dialysate may be selected to treat hypercalcemia. Virtually all treatments use a bicarbonate-based dialysate. Bicarbonate will diffuse into the blood compartment at the same time that organic and inorganic acids (i.e., lactate, phosphates) are cleared. The dialysate bicarbonate concentration can be varied (30–40 mEq/L) to help correct metabolic acidosis or alkalosis. If a patient has marginal blood pressure or is pressor dependent, hemodialysis treatments can be prescribed to perform only clearance with no ultrafiltration. IHD ultrafiltration rates for chronic stable patients can exceed 1000 mL/h. A hypotensive, fluid-overloaded patient in an ICU is not likely to tolerate fluid removal at this rate. However, there are times that even patients with marginal or hypotensive blood pressures need urgent ultrafiltration. Suggestions for techniques to support blood pressure during intermittent hemodialysis are listed in Table 33.8.[61–66] An important consideration for managing intradialytic hypotension is to anticipate that it may occur. The treatment prescription should be written from the start, including any of the suggested interventions. Using these interventions only after a patient has become hypotensive during a treatment will diminish the likelihood of an effective treatment.

Patients receiving HD treatments typically require anticoagulation to prevent system clotting. The most commonly used anticoagulant is heparin. A typical 80-kg patient, assuming a 20 IU/kg bolus of heparin at the start of a treatment and then an hourly infusion rate of 10 IU/kg, would receive approximately 4800 IU heparin by the end of a 4-h treatment. Although this is a relatively small amount of heparin when compared to what is used for therapeutic anticoagulation for venous thromboembolic disease, it is enough to cause bleeding in a patient at risk. Thus, dialysis treatments without anticoagulation are common in the ICU. Considerations for performing an anticoagulant-free treatment include selecting a dialyzer with a lower likelihood of spontaneous clotting and then flushing the dialyzer with saline at frequent intervals during the treatment (i.e., every 30 min). Treatments with no anticoagulation are prescribed commonly: during the first 72 h after surgery, when a patient is bleeding actively or there is concern for precipitating bleeding (e.g., thrombocytopenia, coagulopathy as in liver failure), and for a patient who devel-

TABLE 33.7. Sample Electrolyte and Glucose Concentrations in Available Premixed Hemodialysate.

	Standard	*Low K*	*High K*	*0 Ca*
Na (mEq/L)	137	137	137	137
K (mEq/L)	2.0	0	3.0	2.0
Cl (mEq/L)	105.8	103.2	106.8	102.8
HCO_3 (mEq/L)	33	33	33	33
Acetate (mEq/L)	4.0	4.0	4.0	4.0
Mg (mEq/L)	0.75	0.75	0.75	0.75
Ca (mEq/L)	3.0	2.5	3	0
Dextrose (mg/day)	200	200	200	200

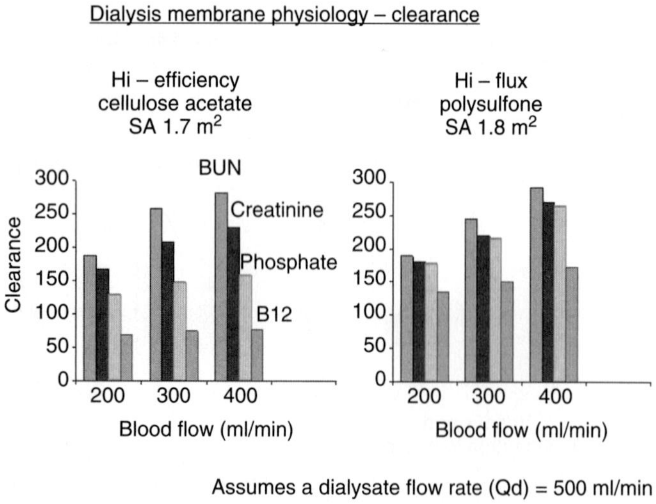

FIGURE 33.5. A comparison of clearance of different-sized molecules in representative high-efficiency and high-flux dialyzers. SA, surface area.

TABLE 33.8. Recommendations for Preventing Intradialytic Hypotension.

Suggestions	*Explanation*
Increase dialysate Na	Most IHD machines have programs to allow sodium modeling, i.e., starting a treatment at higher Na levels (≥145 mEq/L) and then lowering dialysate Na to physiological levels by the end of the treatment. The effect is to avoid fluid shifts that may occur by lower serum Na levels.
Vary ultrafiltration (UF) rates during the treatment	Prescribe 60%–70% of planned UF during the first 50% of the treatment when extravascular fluid mobilization is more likely to occur; this can be performed in conjunction with the sodium modeling mentioned above.
Decreasing treatment temperature	Decreasing treatment temperature to as low as 35°C promotes vasoconstriction to maintain blood pressure.
Intratreatment hyperosmotic or hyperoncotic infusions	Administration of 25% albumin or mannitol during a treatment promotes extravascular fluid transfer into the intravascular space.
Pharmacotherapy	Pretreatment alpha agonists, i.e., midodrine or intratreatment vasoconstrictors, e.g., norepinephrine and dopamine, will raise blood pressure.

See text for abbreviations.

ops a heparin-induced thrombocytopenia syndrome (HITS) during an illness. Although HITS patients may be dialyzed using alternative anticoagulants (i.e., argatroban[67] or citrate[68]), in our experience a treatment without anticoagulation is simpler, as effective, and preferred.

Quantifying Intermittent Hemodialysis in the Critical Care Setting

A number of parameters have been developed to quantify both individual IHD treatments and "adequate" therapy for chronic, dialysis-dependent patients. However, these parameters have not been applied critically to the acute care setting (for either ARF or ESRD). Limited evidence supports the use of daily treatments to improve both recovery from ARF and associated morbidity and mortality.[14] Metabolic abnormalities that persist in spite of initiation of IHD treatment including hyperkalemia, metabolic acidosis, and azotemia (i.e., urea nitrogen levels greater than 100 mg/dL) suggest inadequate therapy; this may be the result of either inefficient treatments, quantified by measuring a treatment urea reduction ratio (URR) [(predialysis BUN–postdialysis BUN)/predialysis BUN)],[69] where a URR of at least 65% reflects an adequate treatment, or the need for a more intensive therapeutic prescription to match a patient's protein catabolic rate.

Extracorporeal Continuous Renal Replacement Therapy

Extracorporeal CRRTs (i.e., non-PD CRRTs) developed because critically ill, renal failure patients with marginal hemodynamics still needed ultrafiltration in spite of requiring large fluid volumes to provide nutrition and fluid resuscitation. The high ultrafiltration rates necessary to maintain fluid balance using IHD treatments were associated with hypotension and inadequate treatment. As a result, a simple system was conceived that could accomplish these objectives over a longer period of time at a slower fluid removal rate.[70]

A diagram of the original arteriovenous system[70] is illustrated in Figure 33.6. Arterial and venous lines were inserted (typically in the femoral artery and vein) and a dialyzer was connected between them. Blood pressure was the driving force for the system. The rate of ultrafiltrate formation was based on the dialyzer permeability. Pressure provided by the clamp on the ultrafiltrate line could modify ultrafiltration (provide resistance) to achieve the desired hourly rate. There were no safety features, arterial access was considered a bleeding risk, and hypotension limited efficacy.

The follow-up, evolutionary design for a venovenous hemofiltration system included pumps to ensure blood flow, safety alarms, and matched replacement fluid and ultrafiltration. Dialysate was added to improve clearance further. Figure 33.6 depicts replacement fluid being added to the blood pathway before it enters the filter (prefilter setup). Administration of replacement fluid "postfilter" is also possible in many systems, as is a mixture of pre- and postfilter replacement.

The system illustrated in Figure 33.7 may be used to provide hemofiltration (convective dialyzer clearance to produce large amounts of an ultrafiltrate that is at least partially replaced using pre- or postfilter replacement fluid), which is referred to as continuous venovenous hemofiltration (CVVH). The system can also provide dialysis (use of a dialysate to provide diffuse clearance) in addition to the desired ultrafiltration, which is referred to as continuous venovenous hemodialysis (CVVHD). Also possible is the production of relatively small amounts of ultrafiltrate (using no replacement fluid or dialysate), or slow continuous ultrafiltration (SCUF). All these variations can be combined into one treatment, referred to as continuous venovenous hemodiafiltration (CVVHDF). With the exception of the replacement fluid, these provided variations are simply IHD over a prolonged treatment time. Selecting ultrafiltration rates between 50 and 250 mL/h will provide up to 6000 mL ultrafiltrate formation

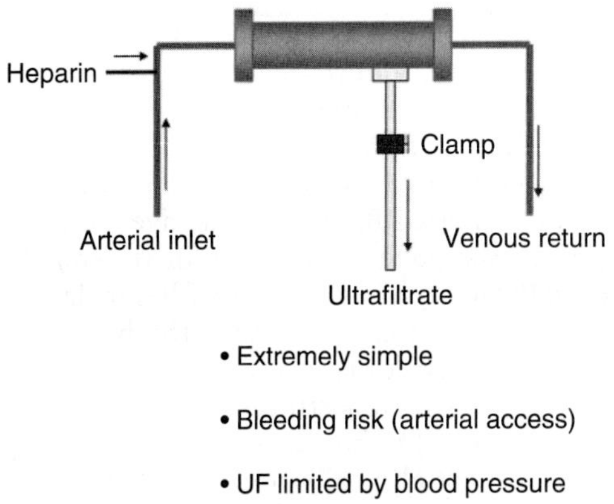

FIGURE 33.6. Continuous arteriovenous hemofiltration (CAVH). *UF*, ultrafiltration.

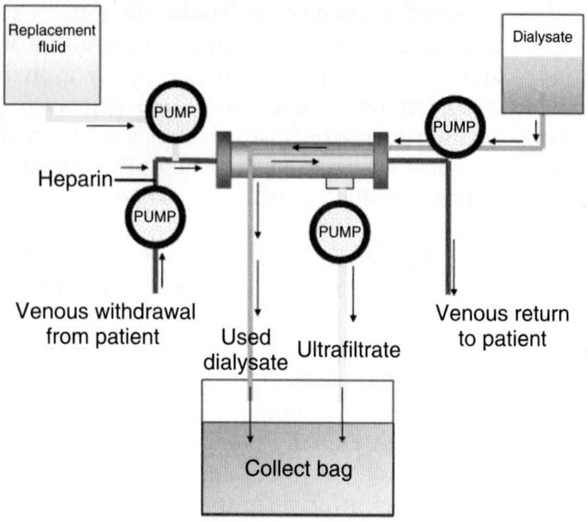

FIGURE 33.7. Schematic for a continuous venovenous hemodiafiltration (CAVH/HD) system including prefilter replacement fluid.

in 24h, which is equivalent to attempting to remove 1500mL fluid per hour during a 4-h IHD treatment.

A theoretical calculation of the urea clearance for a CVVH treatment with replacement fluid of 1000mL/h and no additional ultrafiltration is illustrated in Figure 33.8. In the CRRT system, clearance is determined by the total amount of fluid collected regardless of whether the clearance is diffusive (dialysate) or convective (replacement fluid). For a small molecule such as urea, the concentration in the ultrafiltrate is nearly equal to the blood concentration. In this example, the volume of blood "cleaned" by the replacement fluid per unit of time is equal to the volume of replacement fluid (see calculation in diagram). The calculation for dialysate related clearance is very similar for small molecules such as urea. In the absence of additional ultrafiltration, it is equivalent to the volume of dialysate used per unit of time. Clearances of larger or largely protein-bound molecules are less. Adding dialysate (or additional replacement fluid) at the rate of 1000mL/h to the current treatment essentially doubles urea clearance. Even considering an error of 10% to 20%, a reasonable estimate of urea clearance can be made.

Selecting an Extracorporeal Renal Replacement Therapy Variant

As per original intent, CRRT treatments are generally recommended to provide ultrafiltration and clearance for patients with marginal hemodynamics. The SCUF variant has been applied to diuretic-resistant patients with congestive heart failure.[25] In addition to its cost and complexity, questions remain about using CRRT to prevent dye-induced ARF.[10,71] CRRT may be the preferred method for treating ARF when compared to PD in some settings.[72] Prefilter replacement fluid administration during CVVH dilutes the blood pathway in the dialyzer and provides less efficient clearance when compared to treatments with postfilter replacement fluid administration. However, the difference in clearance between the two is generally not clinically important.[73] Prefilter replacement fluid administration may be preferred for patients with a tendency to clot or in whom anticoagulant-free treatments are attempted.[74] The prefilter setup has the advantage of flushing the dialyzer constantly with replacement fluid. Assuming a blood flow of 200mL/min, a prefilter replacement fluid flow rate of 2L/h is equivalent to 15% of the blood flow rate (similar consideration relative to clearance). Administration of replacement fluid into the blood pathway before it enters the dialyzer facilitates ultrafiltration. With postfilter replacement fluid administration, ultrafiltration rates are more limited because blood viscosity increases in the dialyzer as fluid is removed.

Patients with an adequate blood pressure and for whom there is a contraindication to anticoagulant use may be treated better with IHD. IHD anticoagulant-free treatments may require periodic dialyzer flushes with saline. Trying to accomplish this during CRRT treatment is too labor intensive in the context of the overall nursing care of a critically ill patient. Hypotensive patients who cannot be anticoagulated may be considered for PD (e.g., postoperative patients who require immediate treatment and who have not just undergone abdominal surgery).

Preparing a Patient for Extracorporeal Continuous Renal Replacement Therapy: Access Selection

The majority of CRRT patients are treated for ARF and its renal-related complications (i.e., fluid overload, electrolyte imbalance). Cuffless, dual-lumen catheters, designed for temporary use and described previously in the foregoing section, "Preparing a Patient for IHD: Access Selection," may be inserted at the bedside and used immediately. Coagulation studies should be checked, but no other specific patient preparation is necessary. On occasion, cuffless catheters may have to be placed in patients with sepsis. Portable ultrasound guidance may be available and useful for difficult patients.[75] As already described, catheters may be placed in the groin or neck area.

Use of chronic IHD access (e.g., fistulas, grafts) is generally not recommended, with the exception of the cuffed catheters described above, when chronic hemodialysis patients require CRRT treatments. Potential problems including infection, dislodged or infiltrated needles, and access clotting

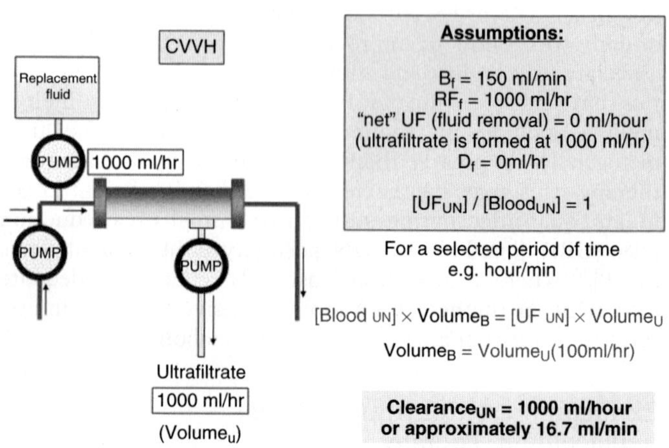

FIGURE 33.8. The assumptions and calculations to estimate clearance provided by a modeled continuous venovenous hemofiltration (CVVH) treatment. See text for abbreviations.

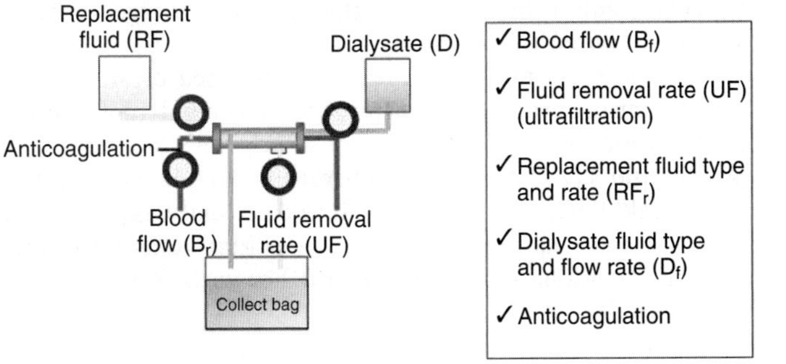

FIGURE 33.9. Parameters that need to be specified to provide effective continuous renal replacement therapy (CRRT).

can occur and compromise the chronic access. Temporary catheter placement is preferred.

Additional Considerations When Writing an Extracorporeal Renal Replacement Therapy Prescription

Selection of a specific dialyzer is generally not a consideration when initiating CRRT treatment. Most systems include a high-flux dialyzer and tubing cartridge. However, some of the newer systems are more flexible, and the tubing is compatible with commonly used IHD dialyzers. Practically, selecting a specific dialyzer is probably not necessary unless one is attempting a treatment with no anticoagulation and one dialyzer may be less likely to clot than others that are available.

Parameters that need to be specified for a CRRT treatment are presented in the checklist in Figure 33.9. Blood flow rate (B_f) selection may vary, typically up to about 200 mL/min although some systems will permit higher flow rates. Blood flow rates less than 150–200 mL/min make little sense. The blood pathway illustrated in Figure 33.10 (including the patient's intravascular volume and excluding replacement fluid) has a fixed volume, regardless of blood flow rate. Faster flow rates are not associated with hypotension during treatment. However, slower flow rates are associated with a greater likelihood of clotting of the system. Clearance and ultrafiltration rate (i.e., the two major CRRT treatment goals) are independent of blood flow rate at this speed. However, clearance is dependent on both replacement fluid rate and dialysate flow rate. During an IHD treatment, dialysate flow rate (D_f) is often 50% faster than B_f, and clearance improves at faster B_f. During CRRT treatments, the reverse occurs, and B_f is often a multiple of D_f or replacement fluid rates (RF_r). Thus, higher blood flow rates provide no additional advantage.

Replacement fluid is typically an isotonic crystalloid solution containing a physiological concentration of sodium bicarbonate (i.e., 30–40 mEq/L). Potassium, typically 0–4 mEq/L, calcium at 3 mEq/L, and magnesium at 1 mEq/L may be added as necessary.[76] In some institutions, commercially premixed, sterile dialysate is used. At this time, the U.S. Food and Drug Administration (FDA) has not approved the use of sterile dialysate solutions for use as replacement fluid. In severe metabolic acidosis, isotonic sodium bicarbonate (150 mEq/L) has been used as replacement fluid. Especially when used in a prefilter configuration, it is not clear that this is an efficient way to administer sodium bicarbonate and affect patient outcome. Because the replacement fluid rate contributes significantly to overall procedure clearance, it rarely makes sense to use less than 1000 mL/h of replacement fluid and rates varying up to approximately 3000 mL/h (38 mL/kg/h for an 80-kg patient[77] are common. In addition, higher prefilter replacement fluid flow rates provide greater volumes of fluid with which to flush the dialyzer and help prevent clotting.

Premixed dialysate solution is available that includes physiological levels of bicarbonate, calcium, and magnesium. Instead of bicarbonate, older formulations included large concentrations of other anions (i.e., acetate or lactate). Potassium can be added to the dialysate as necessary (typically 0–4 mEq/L). Dialysate is a source of bicarbonate administration during a treatment. Similar to the quantification of

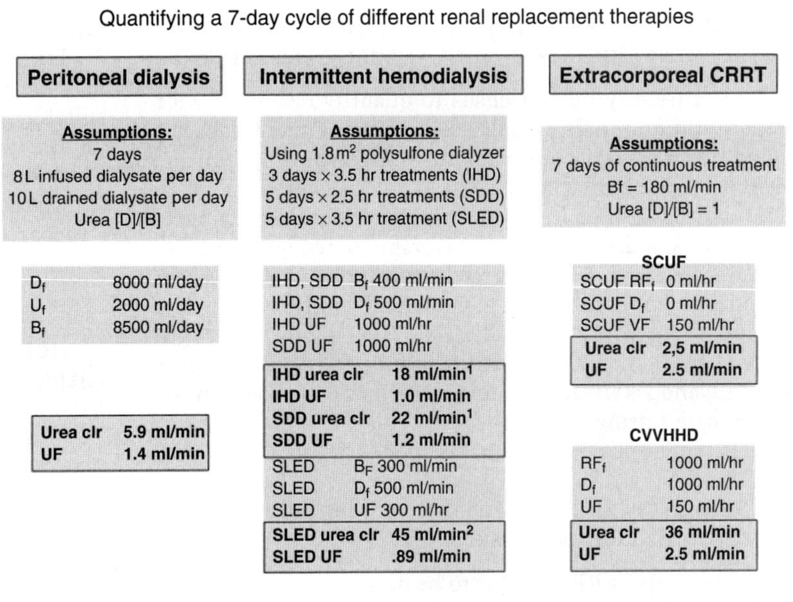
Quantifying a 7-day cycle of different renal replacement therapies
Peritoneal dialysis
Intermittent hemodialysis
Extracorporeal CRRT
Assumptions:
7 days
8 L infused dialysate per day
10 L drained dialysate per day
Urea [D]/[B]
Assumptions:
Using 1.8 m² polysulfone dialyzer
3 days × 3.5 hr treatments (IHD)
5 days × 2.5 hr treatments (SDD)
5 days × 3.5 hr treatment (SLED)
Assumptions:
7 days of continuous treatment
Bf = 180 ml/min
Urea [D]/[B] = 1
D_f 8000 ml/day
U_f 2000 ml/day
B_f 8500 ml/day
Urea clr 5.9 ml/min
UF 1.4 ml/min
IHD, SDD B_f 400 ml/min
IHD, SDD D_f 500 ml/min
IHD UF 1000 ml/hr
SDD UF 1000 ml/hr
IHD urea clr 18 ml/min¹
IHD UF 1.0 ml/min
SDD urea clr 22 ml/min¹
SDD UF 1.2 ml/min
SLED B_F 300 ml/min
SLED D_f 500 ml/min
SLED UF 300 ml/hr
SLED urea clr 45 ml/min²
SLED UF .89 ml/min
SCUF
SCUF RF_f 0 ml/hr
SCUF D_f 0 ml/hr
SCUF VF 150 ml/hr
Urea clr 2,5 ml/min
UF 2.5 ml/min
CVVHHD
RF_f 1000 ml/hr
D_f 1000 ml/hr
UF 150 ml/hr
Urea clr 36 ml/min
UF 2.5 ml/min
Assumptions for urea clearance: (1) IHD, SDD 290ml/min (2) SLED 250 ml/min

FIGURE 33.10. A comparison of the clearance and ultrafiltration provided by prescriptions for different renal replacement therapies. As in practice, not all therapies are administered every day. To compare their effectiveness, calculations are based on a 7-day period during which treatments have been given for part or all of that time. For intermittent therapies, these values may be significantly less than intra-treatment clearance and ultrafiltration. See text for abbreviations.

convective clearance provided by replacement fluid, dialysate may provide a substantial amount of diffusive clearance during a treatment. Dialysate flow rates are typically between 1000 and 2000 mL/h.

The CRRT prescription may be based on the volume of replacement fluid, dialysate, or a combination of the two.[77] The prescription may also be based on a modeled urea clearance determination. The latter may be a useful starting point for estimating systemic antibiotic administration (i.e., dosing according to the clearance provided with modification based on measured serum drug concentrations). Ultrafiltration is independent of either replacement fluid or dialysate flow rate.

Anticoagulation with heparin is the standard during most CRRT treatments. Typically a heparin bolus (20 IU/kg) is administered at the start of a treatment, followed by an hourly infusion (10 IU/kg). The dose is adjusted to maintain an activated partial thromboplastin time of approximately twice the upper limit of normal. Patients may develop heparin-induced thrombocytopenia (HIT) or other heparin allergies. Alternatives to heparin include argatroban[78] and citrate infusions[79]; the latter is particularly labor intensive and the former is expensive.

Treatments with no anticoagulation may be attempted for patients who are bleeding actively, thrombocytopenic, or otherwise coagulopathic.[80] In spite of abnormal clotting parameters, clotting of the system may still occur. Prefilter replacement fluid administration (approximately 2000 mL/h) at a blood-flow of at least 180–200 mL/min may help prevent clotting.

Laboratory studies need to be performed during therapy to evaluate the hemogram, including platelet count, anticoagulation status, and biochemical studies including electrolytes, calcium, magnesium, creatinine, and urea nitrogen concentrations. Anticoagulation and chemistries are checked every 6 h for the first 48 h and then less frequently if treatment parameters remain unchanged. A hemogram once per 24 h is sufficient. Chemistries from aliquots of used dialysate and ultrafiltrate (note collection bag in Figure 33.10) may be analyzed to measure clearances (i.e., urea, creatinine, phosphorus).

Quantifying Extracorporeal Continuous Renal Replacement Therapy in the Critical Care Setting

There is currently no consensus to quantify optimal CRRT therapy and few trials actually comparing different "doses." A single center study comparing 20 mL/kg/h, 35 mL/kg/h, and 45 mL/kg/h hemofiltration prescriptions resulted in 41%, 57%, and 58% patient survival, respectively, 15 days after treatment was discontinued.[77] Favorable outcomes have not been associated with higher treatment volumes in all studies[81]; variable patient entry criteria and overall survival make data difficult to interpret. Hemofiltration rates of 20–35 mL/kg/h for typical 60-kg (1200 mL and 2100 mL) and 80-kg patients (1600 mL and 2800 mL) are being prescribed commonly in the critical care setting.

A Comparison of the Continuous Therapies and Intermittent Hemodialysis

Different forms of RRT appear to be better choices for different clinical situations. However, despite what may appear to be better suitability, no best therapy has emerged to date when compared to the others.

Figure 33.10 provides models of the urea clearance and ultrafiltration provided by representative renal replacement prescriptions for some continuous therapies including PD, SCUF, and CVVHHD and intermittent therapies including "classical" IHD, so-called daily short daily dialysis (SDD), and SLED. These examples include representative assumptions. The prescriptions may be varied further with somewhat different results.

Peritoneal dialysis provides the least amount of clearance when compared to the other therapies but comparable ultrafiltration. It affects hemodynamics little and is suitable for hypotensive patients and for treatments when anticoagulation should be avoided. In addition, continuous PD is the least expensive and least technically demanding RRT and may be particularly effective for some cardiothoracic surgery patients immediately after surgery. Although it may not be entirely accurate to compare PD clearance to the clearance provided by other renal replacement therapies, it would seem less suited for severely catabolic patients or patients with markedly abnormal biochemistries, such as severe hyperkalemia or hypercalcemia. PD is typically premixed with lactate as the predominant anion and may not be the best choice for liver failure patients who have difficulty converting lactate to bicarbonate. PD also may not be suitable for patients with recent abdominal surgery or marginal pulmonary function.

IHD therapies provide high levels of intratreatment clearance (see Table 33.6) and may be particularly useful to treat certain electrolyte abnormalities (i.e., hyperkalemia). It is unlikely that many truly critically ill patients will tolerate an ultrafiltration rate of 1000 mL/h. With the exception of the SLED model, IHD treatments do not lend themselves to patients who require large amounts of fluid and concomitant ultrafiltration as well as some other RRTs; this is particularly the case for patients with marginal blood pressure. IHD treatments may be particularly useful for "stable" patients in an ICU, providing reasonable clearance and ultrafiltration. As with PD, IHD also can be done easily and effectively with no anticoagulation. The SLED IHD variant provides excellent overall clearance and more broadly applicable ultrafiltration rates for unstable, critically ill patients.

Extracorporeal CRRT treatment variants provide excellent clearance and ultrafiltration rates and are particularly suitable for patients with borderline blood pressure who require substantial amounts of fluid administration and ultrafiltration. However, they are quite labor intensive, especially if citrate is used as an anticoagulant or treatment with no anticoagulation is being attempted.

Conclusion and Recommendations: Integrating Renal Replacement Therapy into Critical Care Management

Critically ill patients typically require RRT for the management of fluid and electrolyte abnormalities. Before initiation, less invasive therapeutic interventions (e.g., diuretics, ion-exchange resins) should be considered. RRT is typically initiated and titrated to maintain a pretreatment blood urea nitrogen concentration less than 100 mg/dL and optimized

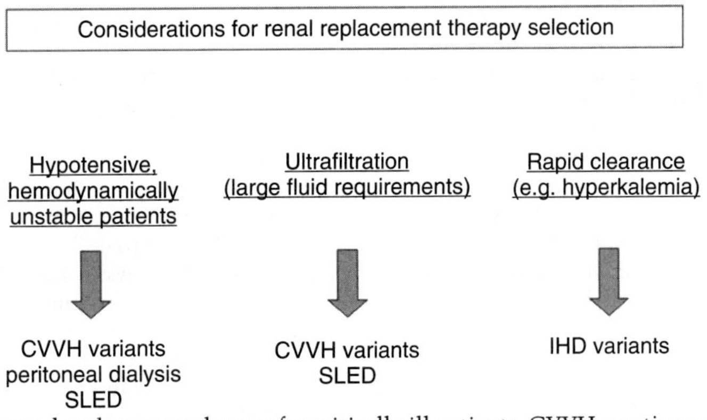

FIGURE 33.11. A guide for selecting renal replacement therapy for critically ill patients. CVVH, continuous venovenous hemofiltration; SLED, sustained low efficiency dialysis; IHD intermittent hemodialysis.

fluid and electrolyte balance. In the critical care setting, extrarenal, azotemia-related organ dysfunction (i.e., uremia including encephalopathy, bleeding) are less common considerations for initiating therapy. In fact, by accepting a urea nitrogen concentration of 100mg/dL as the trigger to start treatment, most of the clinical manifestations of uremia, as described in textbooks, are more of historical interest than likely clinical events. In many cases, because of comorbidities and case complexity, it is difficult to define a specific uremic causality for many of the symptoms (e.g., encephalopathy) for which therapy may be initiated. In such cases, it then is often difficult to judge response to therapy.

A summary guide to RRT selection is illustrated in Figure 33.11. Recent comparative trials may help inform the decision (Table 33.9).[14,77,82–84] These recommendations should be guided by availability and operator experience. Attention to therapy should be accompanied by attention to the potential recovery of renal function for those critically ill patients who develop ARF. Recovery may be months after RRT has been initiated. Attention to increasing urine output or decreasing creatinine and urea nitrogen concentrations may prompt reexamination of renal function including increasing the interval between treatments and periodic assessment of renal function.

TABLE 33.9.
Prospective Trials of Renal Replacement Therapy for Acute Renal Failure.

Author (reference number)	*Design*	*Main findings*	*Comment*
Schiffl[14]	RCT of 3× weekly vs. 6× weekly hemofiltration. Hemodynamically unstable patients excluded.	Mortality 46% for 3× weekly vs. 28% for 6× weekly ($P = 0.01$). Odds ratio for death 3.92 (1.68–9.18). Higher APACHE III score, oliguria, and sepsis as the cause of renal failure also predicted mortality.	Exclusion of unstable patients introduced bias; 3× weekly group may have been underdialyzed (time-averaged BUN concentration, 104mg/dL).
Ronco[77]	RCT of different doses of ultrafiltration during CVVH (20mL/kg/h vs. 35mL/kg/h vs. 45mL/kg/h). Endpoint: 15-day survival after CVVH stopped.	Higher ultrafiltration rates [adjusted hazard ratio for 35-mL group, 0.51 (0.36–0.72); for 45-mL group, 0.49 (0.35–0.69)].	Surgical patients 95% of groups, trauma patients 10% of groups. Short-duration follow-up at end of treatment.
Cho[82]	Multicenter, observational prospective trial. Treatment assignment at discretion of treating physicians. 398 patients enrolled; 206 received CRRT.	Adjusted relative risk of death for CRRT, 1.82 (1.26–2.62). Further adjustment by propensity score for receipt of CRRT did not alter the estimate [RR 1.92 (1.92–2.89)].	One center enrolled nonconsecutive patients to avoid single-center overpresentation. Assignment of treatment modality significantly different by center.
Vinsonneau[83]	RCT of IHD vs. CVVHDF for acute renal failure in multiple organ dysfunction syndrome. Endpoint: 60-day survival.	No survival difference [(mortality rate, 32% vs. 33%), 95% CI, −8.8, 11.1]. Survival improved over time in the IHD group, but not in the CVVHDF group, as the study progressed.	No comprehensive comparison of the delivered dose of dialysis with both methods.
Baldwin[84]	Pilot RCT of CVVH vs. extended IHD. Endpoints were solute clearance and control of acidosis.	Clearance of urea, creatinine, and electrolytes was similar. Acidosis was corrected better by CVVH.	Small study ($n = 16$). Utility of solute clearance data to relevant clinical outcomes is uncertain.

APACHE III, acute physiology and chronic health evaluation-III; CVVH, continuous venovenous hemofiltration; CRRT, continuous renal replacement therapy; CVVHDF, continuous venovenous hemodiafiltration; IHD, intermittent hemodialysis; RCT, randomized controlled trial.

References

1. Schetz M. Non-renal indications for continuous renal replacement therapy. Kidney Int Suppl 1999;72:S88–S94.
2. van Deuren M, van der Meer JW. Hemofiltration in septic patients is not able to alter the plasma concentration of cytokines therapeutically. Intensive Care Med 2000;26:1176–1178.
3. Brivet FG, Kleinknecht DJ, Loirat P, Landais PJ. Acute renal failure in intensive care units: causes, outcome, and prognostic factors of hospital mortality; a prospective, multicenter study. French Study Group on Acute renal failure. Crit Care Med 1996;24:192–198.
4. de Mendonca A, Vincent JL, Suter PM, et al. Acute renal failure in the ICU: risk factors and outcome evaluated by the SOFA score. Intensive Care Med 2000;26:915–921.
5. Clermont, G, Acker CG, Angus DC, et al. Renal failure in the ICU: comparison of the impact of acute renal failure and end-stage renal disease on ICU outcomes. Kidney Int 2002;62:986–996.
6. Liano F, Junco E, Pascual J, et al. The spectrum of acute renal failure in the intensive care unit compared with that seen in other settings. The Madrid Acute Renal Failure Study Group. Kidney Int Suppl 1998;66:S16–S24.
7. Kellum JA, Mehta RL, Angus DC, et al. The first international consensus conference on continuous renal replacement therapy. Kidney Int 2002;62:1855–1863.
8. Hoste EA, De Waele JJ. Physiologic consequences of acute renal failure on the critically ill. Crit Care Clin 2005;21: 251–260.
9. Marsh JD, Margolis TI, Kim D. Mechanism of diminished contractile response to catecholamines during acidosis. Am J Physiol 1988;254:H20–H27.
10. Marenzi G, Marana I, Lauri G, et al. The prevention of radiocontrast-agent-induced nephropathy by hemofiltration. N Engl J Med 2003;349:1333–1340.
11. Rabb H, Wang Z, Nemoto T, et al. Acute renal failure leads to dysregulation of lung salt and water channels. Kidney Int 2003;63:600–606.
12. Kelly KJ. Distant effects of experimental renal ischemia/reperfusion injury. J Am Soc Nephrol 2003;14:1549–1558.
13. Levy EM, Viscoli CM, Horwitz RI. The effect of acute renal failure on mortality. A cohort analysis. JAMA 1996;275:1489–1494.
14. Schiffl H, Lang SM, Fischer R. Daily hemodialysis and the outcome of acute renal failure. N Engl J Med 2002;346:305–310.
15. National Kidney Foundation. K/DOQI clinical practice guidelines for chronic kidney disease: evaluation, classification and stratification. Am J Kidney Dis 2003;29(suppl 1):S17–S31.
16. Winchester JF, Kitiyakara C. Use of dialysis and hemoperfusion in treatment of poisoning. In: Daugirdas J, Blake PG, Ing T, eds. Handbook of Dialysis. 3rd edition. Philadelphia, Lippincott Williams & Wilkins 2000;263–280.
17. Reuler JB, Parker RA. Peritoneal dialysis in the management of hypothermia. JAMA 1978;240:2289–2290.
18. Zavada E. Treatment of profound hypothemia with peritoneal dialysis. Dial Transplant 1980;9:255–258.
19. Ranson J, Spencer FC. The role of peritoneal lavage in severe acute pancreatitis. Ann Surg 1977;187:565–575.
20. Wall AJ. Peritoneal dialysis in the treatment of severe acute pancreatitis. Med J Aust 1965;2:281–283.
21. Gjessing J. Peritoneal dialysis in severe acute hemorrhagic pancreatitis. Acta Chir Scand 1967;133:645–647.
22. Mayer AD, McMahon MJ, Corfield AP, et al. Controlled clinical trial of peritoneal lavage for the treatment of severe acute pancreatitis. N Engl J Med 1985; 312:399–404.
23. Grootendorst AF, van Bommel EF, van der Hoven B. High volume hemofiltration improves right ventricular function in endotoxin-induced shock in the pig. Intensive Care Med 1992;18:235–240.
24. Hoffmann JN, Hartl WH, Deppisch R, et al. Effect of hemofiltration on hemodynamics and systemic concentrations of anaphylatoxins and cytokines in human sepsis. Intensive Care Med 1996;22:1360–1367.
25. Ronco C, Ricci Z, Brendolan A, et al. Ultrafiltration in patients with hypervolemia and congestive heart failure. Blood Purif 2004;22:150–163.
26. Cole L, Bellomo R, Hart G, et al. A phase II randomized, controlled trial of continuous hemofiltration in sepsis. Crit Care Med 2002;30:100–106.
27. Sharma A, Hermann DD, Mehta RL. Clinical benefit and approach of ultrafiltration in acute heart failure. Cardiology 2001;96:144–154.
28. Marenzi G, Agostoni P. Hemofiltration in heart failure. Int J Artif Organs 2004;27:1070–1076.
29. Vogt B, Ferrari P, Schönholzer C, et al. Prophylactic hemodialysis after radiocontrast media in patients with renal insufficiency is potentially harmful. Am J Med 2001;111:692–698.
30. Abdeen O, Mehta RL. Dialysis modalities in the intensive care unit. Crit Care Clin 2002;18:223–247.
31. Hyman A, Mendelssohn DC. Current Canadian approaches to dialysis for acute renal failure in the ICU. Am J Nephrol 2002;22:29–34.
32. Gokal R, Khanna R, Krediet RT, Nolph KD, eds. Textbook of Peritoneal Dialysis, 2nd ed. Dordrecht: Kluwer. Academic Publishers, 2000.
33. Leypoldt JK. Solute transport across the peritoneal membrane. J Am Soc Nephrol 2002;13(suppl 1):S84–S91.
34. Rippe B, Rosengren BI, Venturoli D. The peritoneal microcirculation in peritoneal dialysis. Microcirculation 2001;8:303–320.
35. Fischbach M, Dheu C, Helms P, et al. The influence of peritoneal surface area on dialysis adequacy. Perit Dial Int 2005;25(suppl 3):S137–S140.
36. Miyata T, van Ypersele de Strihou C, Imasawa T, et al. Toward better dialysis compatibility: advances in the biochemistry and pathophysiology of the peritoneal membranes. Kidney Int 2002;61:375–386.
37. Sobiecka D, Waniewski J, Weryński A, Lindholm B. Peritoneal fluid transport in CAPD patients with different transport rates of small solutes. Perit Dial Int 2004:24:240–251.
38. Flanigan M, Gokal R. Peritoneal catheters and exit-site practices toward optimum peritoneal access: a review of current developments. Perit Dial Int 2005;25:132–139.
39. Daugirdas JT, Blake PG, Ing TS. Handbook of dialysis, 3rd ed. New York: Lippincott Williams & Wilkins, 2001:333–343.
40. Smit W, Struijk DG, Ho-Dac-Pannekeet MM, Krediet RT. Quantification of free water transport in peritoneal dialysis. Kidney Int 2004;66:849–854.
41. Ronco C, Clark W. Factors affecting hemodialysis and peritoneal dialysis efficiency. Semin Dial 2001;14:257–262.
42. Piraino B, Bailie GR, Bernardini J, et al.; ISPD Ad Hoc Advisory Committee. Peritoneal dialysis-related infections recommendations: 2005 update. Perit Dial Int 2005;25:107–131.
43. Thodis E, Passadakis P, Ossareh S, et al. Peritoneal catheter exit-site infections: predisposing factors, prevention and treatment. Int J Artif Organs 2003;26:698–714.
44. Bernardini J, Bender F, Florio T, et al. Randomized, double-blind trial of antibiotic exit site cream for prevention of exit site infection in peritoneal dialysis patients. J Am Soc Nephrol 2005;16:539–545.
45. Sieberth HG, Kierdorf HP. Is cytokine removal by continuous hemofiltration feasible? Kidney Int Suppl 1999;72:S79–S83.
46. de Vries PM, Olthof CG, Solf A, et al. Fluid balance during haemodialysis and haemofiltration: the effect of dialysate sodium and a variable ultrafiltration rate. Nephrol Dial Transplant 1991;6:257–263.

47. Fauchald P. Effects of ultrafiltration on body fluid volumes and transcapillary colloid osmotic gradient in hemodialysis patients. Contrib Nephrol 1989;74:170–175.
48. Pierratos A. Daily hemodialysis: why the renewed interest? Am J Kidney Dis 1998;32(6 suppl 4):S76–S82.
49. Marshall MR, Ma T, Galler D, et al. Sustained low-efficiency daily diafiltration (SLEDD-f) for critically ill patients requiring renal replacement therapy: towards an adequate therapy. Nephrol Dial Transplant 2004;19:877–884.
50. Van Biesen W, Vanholder R, Lameire N. Dialysis strategies in critically ill acute renal failure patients. Curr Opin Crit Care 2003;9:491–495.
51. Marshall MR, Golper TA, Shaver MJ, et al. Sustained low-efficiency dialysis for critically ill patients requiring renal replacement therapy. Kidney Int 2001;60:777–785.
52. Weijmer MC, ter Wee PM. Temporary vascular access for hemodialysis treatment. Current guidelines and future directions. Contrib Nephrol 2004;142:94–111.
53. Schillinger F, Schillinger D, Montagnac R, Milcent T. Post catheterisation vein stenosis in haemodialysis: comparative angiographic study of 50 subclavian and 50 internal jugular accesses. Nephrol Dial Transplant 1991;6:722–724.
54. Ponikvar R. Hemodialysis catheters. Ther Apher Dial 2005; 9:218–222.
55. Warren SE, O'Connor DT, Steinberg SM. Recirculation: a uremic syndrome complicating the use of prosthetic arteriovenous fistulas for hemodialysis. J Dial 197;2:251–259.
56. Little MA, Conlon PJ, Walshe JJ. Access recirculation in temporary hemodialysis catheters as measured by the saline dilution technique. Am J Kidney Dis 2000;36:1135–1139.
57. NKF-K/DOQI Clinical Practice Guidelines for Vascular Access: update 2000. Am J Kidney Dis 2001;37(1 suppl 1):S137–S181.
58. Craddock PR, Fehr J, Brigham KL, et al. Complement and leukocyte-mediated pulmonary dysfunction in hemodialysis. N Engl J Med 1977;296:769–774.
59. Hakim RM, Wingard RL, Parker RA. Effect of the dialysis membrane in the treatment of patients with acute renal failure. N Engl J Med 1994;331:1338–1342.
60. Ludlow MK. Heparin-free dialysis. ANNA J 1989;16:295–298.
61. Raja RM, Po CL. Plasma refilling during hemodialysis with decreasing ultrafiltration. Influence of dialysate sodium. ASAIO J 1994;40:M423–M425.
62. Coli L, Ursino M, Donati G, et al. Clinical application of sodium profiling in the treatment of intradialytic hypotension. Int J Artif Organs 2003;26:715–722.
63. Sherman RA, Rubin MP, Cody RP, Eisinger RP. Amelioration of hemodialysis-associated hypotension by the use of cool dialysate. Am J Kidney Dis 1985;5:124–127.
64. Splendiani G, Costanzi S, Passalacqua S, et al. Sodium and fluid modulation in dialysis: new approach. Nephron 2001;89:377–380.
65. Van der Sande FM, Luik AJ, Kooman JP, et al. Effect of intravenous fluids on blood pressure course during hemodialysis in hypotensive-prone patients. J Am Soc Nephrol 2000;11:550–555.
66. Emili S, Black NA, Paul RV, et al. A protocol-based treatment for intradialytic hypotension in hospitalized hemodialysis patients. Am J Kidney Dis 1999;33:1107–1114.
67. Murray PT, Reddy BV, Grossman EJ, et al. A prospective comparison of three argatroban treatment regimens during hemodialysis in end-stage renal disease. Kidney Int 2004;66:2446–2453.
68. Apsner R, Buchmayer H, Gruber D, Sunder-Plassmann G. Citrate for long-term hemodialysis: prospective study of 1,009 consecutive high-flux treatments in 59 patients. Am J Kidney Dis 2005;45:557–564.
69. Kessler E, Ritchey NP, Castro F, et al. Urea reduction ratio and urea kinetic modeling: a mathematical analysis of changing dialysis parameters. Am J Nephrol 1998;18:471–477.
70. Kramer P, Schrader J, Bohnsack W, et al. Continuous arteriovenous haemofiltration. A new kidney replacement therapy. Proc Eur Dial Transplant Assoc 1981;18:743–749.
71. Gabutti L, Marone C, Monti M, et al. Does continuous venovenous hemodiafiltration concomitant with radiological procedures provide a significant and safe removal of the iodinated contrast ioversol? Blood Purif 2003;21:152–157.
72. Phu NH, Hien TT, Mai NT, et al. Hemofiltration and peritoneal dialysis in infection-associated acute renal failure in Vietnam. N Engl J Med 2002;347:895–902.
73. Uchino S, Fealy N, Baldwin I, et al. Pre-dilution vs. post-dilution during continuous veno-venous hemofiltration: impact on filter life and azotemic control. Nephron Clin Pract 2003;94:c94–c98.
74. Gilman CM, Coffel BE, Gunn SK. Continuous venovenous hemofiltration: a cost-effective therapy for the pediatric patient. ANNA J 1997;24:337–341.
75. Lin BS, Huang TP, Tang GJ, et al. Ultrasound-guided cannulation of the internal jugular vein for dialysis vascular access in uremic patients. Nephron 1998;78:423–428.
76. Locatelli F, Pontoriero G, Di Filippo S. Electrolyte disorders and substitution fluid in continuous renal replacement therapy. Kidney Int Suppl 1998;66:S151–S155.
77. Ronco C, Bellomo R, Homel P. Effects of different doses in continuous veno-venous haemofiltration on outcomes of acute renal failure: a prospective randomised trial. Lancet 2000;356:26–30.
78. Tang IY, Cox DS, Patel K, et al. Argatroban and renal replacement therapy in patients with heparin-induced thrombocytopenia. Ann Pharmacother 2005;39:231–236.
79. Schneider T, Heuer B, Delle A, Boesken WH. Continuous haemofiltration with r-hirudin (lepirudin) as anticoagulant in a patient with heparin induced thrombocytopenia (HIT II). Wien Klin Wochenschr 2000;112:552–555.
80. Tan HK, Baldwin I, Bellomo R. Continuous veno-venous hemofiltration without anticoagulation in high-risk patients. Intensive Care Med 2000;26:1652–1657.
81. Bouman CS, Oudemans-Van Straaten HM, Tijssen JG, et al. Effects of early high-volume continuous venovenous hemofiltration on survival and recovery of renal function in intensive care patients with acute renal failure: a prospective, randomized trial. Crit Care Med 2002;30:2205–2211.
82. Cho KC, Himmelfarb J, Pagainini E, et al. Survival by dialysis modality in critcally ill patients with acute kidney injury. J Am Soc Nephrol 2006;17:3132–3138.
83. Vinsonneau C, Camus C, Combes A, et al. Hemodiafe Study Group. Continuous venovenous hemodiafiltration versus intermittent haemodialysis for acute renal failure in patients with multiple-organ dysfunction syndrome: a multivariate randomized trial. Lancet 2006;368:379–385.
84. Baldwin I, Naka T, Koch B, et al. A pilot randomized controlled comparison of continuous veno-venous haemofiltration and extened daily dialysis with filtration: effect on small solutes and acid-base balance. Intensive Care Med 2007;33:830–835.

34

Open Abdomen

Claudia E. Goettler and Michael F. Rotondo

During the past century, a gradual understanding has developed of the abdomen as a compartment. Although compartment syndrome is common and anticipated in calf muscle compartments, any closed, nondistensible body space will develop increased intracompartmental pressure when there is an increase in the contents of that compartment. When the increase in pressure results in clinically meaningful physiological changes, the term *compartment syndrome* is used.

The abdomen is encased in a relatively rigid structure of muscles and fascia that does not allow for a rapid increase in volume. Although it is possible to increase the size of the abdominal compartment over time with small, gradual increases in pressure, rapid volume increases result in rapid pressure increases, with disastrous physiological consequences.

Intraabdominal Hypertension and the Abdominal Compartment Syndrome

History

Increased intraabdominal pressure (IAP) was first noted to be pathological in the 1860s by Marey and Burt, who found that increased intraabdominal pressure eventually leads to respiratory failure and death. As with many advances in medical science, these observations were largely ignored and only rediscovered in the past two decades.

In 1911, Emerson showed in animal models that intraabdominal hypertension (IAH) caused cardiovascular collapse. Thoringon showed in 1923 that treatment with decompression resulted in restoration of urinary output. In 1947, Bradley and Gross described the clinical triad of *abdominal compartment syndrome* (ACS) (increased airway pressure, hypotension, oliguria) during the treatment of gastroschisis, when it was recognized that forcibly returning the abdominal contents into a space too small to contain them could be disastrous.[1] These findings were again essentially ignored until redescribed in the 1980s by Kron and Richardson, who also first used the term abdominal compartment syndrome.[2] The phenomenon of ACS is still not commonly recognized and understood by many physicians today.[1]

Historically, data for this disorder have come from the pediatric surgical (gastroschisis), morbid obesity, and trauma literatures. An increasing body of experimental research is evolving from the now routine elective induction of IAH: laparoscopy. As patients undergoing laparoscopy are otherwise healthy patients, and confounding variables such as carbon dioxide absorption must be taken into account, the utility of extrapolating this research to the ill or injured patient with IAH remains unknown.

Although there has been a large increase in the amount of literature published about IAH and ACS, these are mostly small studies, with few data from prospective randomized trials. Hence, although the pathophysiology is beginning to be understood, the exact clinical consequences of the findings and optimal treatment options remain to be elucidated. As "damage control" surgery increases in the trauma and general surgery arena, and as critical care continues to improve, greater numbers of previously unsalvageable patients are surviving and developing the complications of increased intraabdominal pressure. The understanding of this complex entity represents one of the greatest advances and challenges in surgery and critical care in the past decade.

Abdominal Pressure

Under normal circumstances, pressure within the abdomen is low, typically less than 10 mmHg. Pressure increases acutely but transiently with any increase in muscle tension, such as with the Valsalva maneuver. In hospitalized patients, the mean intraabdominal pressure is 6.5 mmHg, with elevated pressures correlated to elevated body mass index (BMI).[3]

Gradual increases in abdominal pressures do not cause immediate clinical problems, largely because of compensation by gradual stretching of the abdominal wall fascia and musculature. In pregnancy, obesity, and ascites, pressures within the abdomen are typically 10 to 20 mmHg. These patients begin to have the early physiological findings of IAH, such as cephalad displacement of the diaphragm and decreased functional residual capacity.[4] In patients with cirrhotic ascites, increases in cardiac output and urine production after paracentesis are common. Studies also show that portal venous pressures and venous collateral flow increase with increased intraabdominal pressure.[5]

"Chronic abdominal compartment syndrome" is likely responsible for many of the comorbidities of obesity. Increased bladder intravesical pressure results in stress incontinence, increases in cardiac filling pressure and intrathoracic pressures cause obesity-hypoventilation syndrome, and high cerebrospinal fluid pressure results in pseudotumor cerebri. All these conditions resolve or improve with weight loss. Systemic hypertension, incisional hernia, gastroesophageal reflux, and lower extremity venous stasis have all been linked to obesity and are more common in patients with higher abdominal pressures.[6] Chronic abdominal compartment syndrome may also be a cause of preeclampsia in pregnancy, as it is more common in first pregnancies, twin pregnancies, and pregnancy in obesity, all related to higher intraabdominal pressures.[7] Canine studies of chronically increased intraabdominal pressure show increases in blood pressure, supporting these suppositions.[8] Additionally, all these findings can be worsened by pneumoperitoneum in the obese patient; hence, laparoscopy results in greater physiological changes than in lean patients.[9]

Pediatric surgeons recognized that the high mortality rate for closure of abdominal wall defects was the consequence of compression of viscera during attempts to return abdominal contents that had lost the "right of domain." Similar findings occur in adults with repairs of massive abdominal wall hernia.[10] Development of silo techniques for gradual abdominal stretching reduced mortality significantly. Additionally, recent studies recommend following intraabdominal pressure as a guide for closure in a single stage or the degree of silo reduction that can be accomplished safely at any one time. The care of these infants has improved, but it is difficult to extrapolate these findings to the intensive care unit (ICU) population, because the initial degree of physiological insult and the distensibility of the abdominal wall are frequently different.[11,12]

Intraabdominal Hypertension

Intraabdominal hypertension occurs when the abdominal contents increase in volume acutely in excess of the capacity of the abdominal cavity and beyond the normal capacity of the abdominal wall to stretch. Pressures greater than 10 mmHg are considered abnormal and are termed IAH. The causes of this phenomenon are myriad but can be assigned to several general groups (Table 34.1).

TABLE 34.1. Causes of Increased Intraabdominal Pressure.

Category	*Trauma or surgery*	*Medical*
Abdominal contents	Blood Resuscitation fluid (ascites, tissue edema) Packs (iatrogenic)	Resuscitation fluid (e.g., cardiac arrest) Tumor (carcinomatosis or malignant ascites) Ascites with rapid accumulation
Retroperitoneal contents	Blood (ruptured abdominal aortic aneurysm, pelvic fracture) Pancreatic edema	Blood (spontaneous retroperitoneal hematoma) Tumor Pancreatic edema
Intestinal distension	Intestinal edema Intestinal contents (obstruction)	Intestinal edema Intestinal contents (ileus)
External compression	Burn eschar Tight abdominal closure Compression garment (antishock trousers)	

Measuring Abdominal Pressure

Diagnosis of IAH is initially based on clinical suspicion. Clinical examination would be convenient for detecting IAH; however, physical examination correlates poorly with abdominal pressures. In a blinded, prospective trial of high-risk trauma patients, clinical assessment demonstrated a sensitivity of 56%, a specificity of 87%, and an accuracy of 84% for significantly increased IAP of 15 mmHg.[13] Abdominal circumference, studied in a similar patient population, also correlated poorly with IAP. Hence, patients may have meaningful elevations in IAP without clinically notable abdominal distension.

IAP is measured easily by noninvasive means. The most commonly used technique is to measure intravesicular pressure utilizing the urinary catheter. Fifty to 100 mL sterile saline is instilled into the urinary bladder and the catheter is clamped, providing a static column of fluid in equilibrium with the abdominal cavity.[2] The pressure is measured with a transduced catheter system through the urinary catheter sampling port, with the pressure transducer placed at the pubic symphysis; this provides a simple, reliable, reproducible measurement that correlates with directly measured IAP in both human and animal studies.[14,15] Care must be taken to keep a closed system to prevent bacterial contamination, the risk of which is increased by the use of stopcocks. Potential disadvantages of this method are inability to measure after bladder surgery or repair and interference with accurate measurement of urinary output. Indistensibility of the bladder, as seen in chronically aneuric patients, or overfilling with instilled saline, will artificially increase the pressure measured. Although there are no clear data to this effect, it can be expected that extrinsic compression of the bladder as a result of packing or pelvic hematoma may cause a false increase of measured bladder pressure.[16] Despite these concerns, urinary bladder pressure monitoring is the most commonly utilized technique for IAP measurement.

Gastric pressure monitoring is done via a nasogastric, orogastric, or gastrostomy tube. As the gastroesophageal junction does not form a tight seal, it is difficult to maintain a column of fluid.[17] Tonometers utilizing a small intragastric balloon and a dry (air) transducer have been described, but these are position–dependent and require frequent recalibration. Rectal and uterine pressure measurements have also been described but are not recommended.[16] Inferior vena caval pressure measurements require central venous access and have relatively poor correlation to abdominal pressure because of intravascular dynamics.[18] Computed tomographic diagnosis of a "round belly sign" (anteroposterior to transverse abdominal diameter ratio greater than 1:0.8), with associated vena caval compression, renal compression, and occasionally inguinal herniation, is both sensitive and specific for IAH, although this is not recommended as a primary diagnostic modality.[19–21]

Abdominal Compartment Syndrome

As described earlier, IAH is defined as IAP greater than 10mmHg. The importance of increased IAP is variable depending on the clinical situation. Standard laparoscopy CO_2 insufflation pressures exceed the IAH threshold, yet are only rarely associated with clinical problems. Abdominal hypertension and ACS lie along a continuum; there is no general consensus as to a defining pressure for each.

The diagnosis of ACS requires both increased IAP as well as clinical compromise. It is typically described by the triad of increased pulmonary ventilatory pressures, oliguria, and hypotension. The magnitude of abdominal pressure necessary to generate this clinical triad is variable; the clinical findings are more important than the absolute number. Burch et al. (Table 34.2) described a grading scale that allows development of treatment algorithms as well as comparisons among studies.[22]

Risk factors for Abdominal Compartment Syndrome

ACS is a complication associated with high mortality, and thus rapid diagnosis is paramount. The most common presentation of IAH is after trauma, but this complication occurs in only a subset of patients. ACS occurs in about one-third of "damage control" surgery patients, with no differentiating factors on the basis of demographics, injury severity, initial vital signs, or laboratory data. Various risk factors, including hemorrhagic shock, damage control, fascial closure after damage control, and a high abdominal trauma index score have been associated with development of ACS. Several physiological variables have been identified as predictors, including high peak airway pressure and low gastric mucosal pH; however, these findings more likely are results of the IAH and merely early indicators.[23] There is also evidence that excessive fluid resuscitation increases rates of IAH and ACS. The amount of volume required to place patients at high risk of ACS varies among studies, but volumes exceeding 10L crystalloid, 10 units red blood cell concentrates, 0.25L/kg crystalloid, or 6L crystalloid in 6h or 6 units of red blood cell concentrates in 6h have all been associated. Balogh et al. compared standardized, protocol-based resuscitation to normal or supranormal oxygen delivery parameters. More crystalloid volume and blood were required to achieve supranormal oxygen delivery, and this group had essentially double the incidence of IAH, ACS, multiple organ dysfunction syndrome, and death. Hence, although optimal resuscitation is necessary, too much may be deadly.[24] Clearly, patients requiring large volumes of fluid are at risk, but large resuscitation requirements are as much a symptom of the development of ACS as a cause.

TABLE 34.2. Grades of Intraabdominal Hypertension.

Grade	*Bladder pressure (mmHg)*
I	10–15
II	16–25
III	26–35
IV	>35

Incidence of Abdominal Compartment Syndrome

The rate of ACS ranges between 5% and 30%, depending on the population studied and the precise definition of ACS. In a review of 311 damage control trauma patients, the incidence was 5.5%, with 30% caused by visceral edema and 70% by bleeding. All patients with ACS had primary abdominal closure during the initial operation.[25] In a mixed group of trauma patients, a 2% incidence of IAH was found in 706 patients. Nearly one-half had resolution of their abdominal pressures, whereas the remainder progressed to ACS. Despite decompression, all the patients with ACS eventually died.[26] A 1-day prevalence study of medical and surgical ICU patients found 50% had IAH and 8% had ACS. The parameter most associated was elevated BMI, with massive fluid resuscitation and coagulopathy of lesser importance.[27] Thus, the trauma population may have the highest incidence of ACS as a consequence of its increased recognition. The most common cause of IAH in nontrauma surgical patients is the ruptured abdominal aortic aneurysm, but case reports have associated essentially all surgical and abdominal pathology with the development of ACS. Increasing attention to ACS has revealed it to be common (32%) and morbid (e.g., prolonged ventilation, increased mortality, and decreased graft function in liver transplantation patients).[28] Additionally, ACS has been described in multiple medical conditions. A study of 405 ICU patients revealed an overall incidence of IAH of 17.5%. Emergency surgical patients had an incidence of 39%, whereas medical patients had an incidence of 20% and elective surgical patients, 6%.[27]

Secondary ACS also has been described, being defined as the development of IAH without abdominal pathology[29]; this is an uncommon, and difficult to diagnose, group of patients. Secondary IAH tends to occur in patients requiring massive volume resuscitation after an ischemic event. As these are often not surgical patients and there is no abdominal injury, the diagnosis is not suspected early, and discovery and treatment are delayed. In a review of ICU trauma patients, secondary ACS was seen in 0.5% of patients, but it is likely more frequent and not recognized. Delayed decompression resulted in increased mortality with average time to decompression being 3h for survivors versus 25h for nonsurvivors.[30] All patients underwent massive resuscitation after shock. Despite decompression, the mortality of secondary ACS was 38% in trauma patients and 100% in nontrauma patients, although ACS clearly is coincident to an already high mortality disease process. Additionally, although decompression occurred rapidly after diagnosis, diagnosis was delayed by 11h after trauma and 16h in other patients because of lack of clinical suspicion without a history of abdominal pathology.[31]

After a number of case reports of fatal secondary ACS in burn patients, a small prospective evaluation was conducted of burns greater than 20% total body surface area (TBSA). In 7 of 10 patients, IAH developed; 2 patients progressed to ACS that required decompression.[32] In a retrospective review of burn patients with ACS, an overall 1% incidence was found. The patients developing ACS had an average 70% TBSA burn and survival of 40%.[33]

Physiological Effects of Increased Abdominal Pressure

Cardiovascular

The cardiovascular effects of IAP were first described by Cullen et al. in a small clinical series.[34] Hypotension is the most obvious finding and is recognized as part of the ACS clinical triad. It is, however, a late finding of the disease process. Other studies are listed in Table 34.3.[15,34–45] Because of compression of vascular beds, peripheral vascular resistance is increased. Venous return via the inferior vena cava is decreased by high abdominal and thoracic pressures. Cardiac compression, whether from intrathoracic pressure or abdominal compression, results additionally in decreased production of atrial natiuretic peptide and increased fluid sequestration, resulting in increasing lung water and potentially worsened visceral edema.

Despite ongoing volume resuscitation, cardiac index is typically not improved. This lack of response to volume loading may be the first sign of impending ACS. Additionally, futile attempts to improve cardiac performance with additional fluid result in increasing interstitial and visceral edema and worsening of IAP. Patients with ACS have artificially elevated high pulmonary artery occlusion pressures (PAOP) and high central venous pressures (CVP) from high intrathoracic pressures that correlate poorly with actual volume status. Several studies have demonstrated that right ventricular end-diastolic volume index is the best measure of volume status in patients with IAH.

All series demonstrate that release of abdominal compartment results in prompt restoration of blood pressure and may reveal a relative hypovolemia as PWP and CVP decrease precipitously. Hence, in ACS, patients have decreased intravascular volume, despite high CVP and severe edema. Third-space fluid losses are the result of cytokine release and decreased transmural atrial pressure, which induces fluid retention.

All the foregoing conditions result in a vicious cycle of hypotension, treated with volume resuscitation, resulting in fluid sequestration and worsening ACS. Additionally, there is extensive evidence to support ACS as part of a "second-hit" phenomenon, as all the physiological sequelae are worsened when ACS occurs in conjunction with hypovolemia, shock/reperfusion, or inhalational anesthesia.

Pulmonary

The second component of the ACS triad is high peak airway pressures. Clinically, this presents as difficulty with oxygenation and ventilation. Initially, this was believed to be caused by cephalad movement of the diaphragm from IAP, which alone results in a 40% to 50% decrease in pulmonary compliance. Although clearly part of the pathophysiology, several other factors are important (Table 34.4).[46–49] The decreased excursion of the diaphragm results in less negative pressure within the chest, particularly in the lower lung, with ventilation in these areas becoming mismatched with blood flow, leading to increased physiological dead space and shunt.

Patients with ACS have undergone aggressive fluid resuscitation for hypotension and are typically quite edematous. Resulting decreased chest wall compliance increases the work of breathing. Also, several studies have shown increased lung water, even in the face of normal PAOP and cardiac output, because of third-space losses, both from cytokine release and increased intrathoracic vascular pressures. Decreased lung compliance results, exacerbating the inspiratory pressures needed for lung expansion.

Positive end-expiratory pressure (PEEP) must be considered carefully in patients who are developing IAH. IAP and PEEP both result in increased intrathoracic pressures and decreased venous return. Hence, IAP and PEEP act in concert to decrease cardiac return and cause hypotension. Additionally, compression of the heart may contribute to decreased cardiac output and worsening of visceral blood flow. Hence, PEEP should be decreased as much as possible in patients with IAH, and a high PEEP requirement must be considered as a factor when deciding on the appropriate treatment of any specific level of IAP.

Last, cytokine release caused by either the initial injury or ACS places this patient population at high risk for the development of acute respiratory distress syndrome (ARDS), further complicating the pulmonary management.

Renal

The third component of the triad of ACS is impaired renal function, seen clinically as oliguria. In 1876, Wendt reported decreased urine flow in association with increased IAP.[50] More recent data are presented in Table 34.5.[17,51–58] Oliguria is typically seen at an IAP of 15 to 20 mmHg, and anuria occurs at 30 mmHg. The renal impairment is independent of volume expansion and the maintenance of normal cardiac output. Additionally, the incidence of renal insufficiency increases with increasing abdominal pressure. Neither is ureteral compression the cause of oliguria, as ureteral stenting fails to correct oliguria. Compression of the renal parenchyma has been studied in several ways with conflicting results. Compression of the renal veins clearly results in oliguria in ACS, presumptively the result of renal venous hypertension and consequent decreased renal blood flow. Endocrine changes such as increased production of vasopressin and aldosterone may contribute variably to oliguria and may also account for the hypertension and nephrotic syndrome seen in patients with chronically elevated abdominal pressure.

No study has been definitive, but it is likely that the oliguria of IAH is a result of decreased cardiac output and renal venous compression with renovascular hypertension. Renal parenchymal compression and vasoactive hormone secretion likely cause only minor effects in acute IAH.

Splanchnic Circulation

All factors of the triad of ACS become apparent clinically, but the changes that are not readily apparent may be even more

TABLE 34.3.
Intraabdominal Pressure (IAP) Effects on the Cardiovascular System.

Author, year	*Study population*	*Study characteristics (Grade of Evidence, for Clinical Studies)*	*Findings*
Cheatham 1999[35]	ICU patients with ACS before and after decompression	Concurrent observation (II)	PAOP and CVP do not correlate well with CO and are poor predictors of volume status. Right ventricular end-diastolic volume index is the best indicator of volume status.
Balogh 2003[36]	"High-risk" trauma patients	Retrospective review of therapy with a standardized protocol (III)	In patients who developed ACS, volume loading increased PAOP but not CO. Lack of response to volume loading can be used to predict likely onset of ACS. ACS group required more crystalloid and blood infusion.
Schachtrupp 2003[37]	Pigs with ACS, evaluated intravascular volumes	Controlled, compared to baseline	Despite fourfold increase in CVP, total circulating blood volume decreased by 67%, increased hematocrit, 27% decreased CO, increased extravascular lung water volume.
Simon 1997[38]	Pigs with ACS with or without prior hemorrhage and resuscitation	Controlled, compared to baseline	Prior hemorrhage resulted in more severe decline in cardiac and pulmonary function despite resuscitation—ACS acts as a "second hit."
Chang 1998[39]	ICU patients with ACS before and after decompression	Concurrent observation (II)	Abdominal decompression results in decreased IAP, increased filling pressures best monitored by RVEDVI. PAOP is a poor predictor of volume status in ACS due to decreased cardiac compliance. Decompression reduced pulmonary shunt fraction, improved dynamic compliance, urine output, and gastric mucosal pH.
Shelly 1987[40]	Orthotopic liver transplant patients	Case series (III)	Report of immediate hemodynamic changes at release of ACS: hypotension, decreased SVR and PAOP, increased CO.
Robotham 1985[42]	Dogs with external abdominal compression and open chest on right heart bypass	Controlled, compared to baseline	With the bypass removing changes from venous return, increased abdominal pressure resulted in increased aortic and left atrial pressures and decreased flow in the aorta.
Cullen 1989[34]	Patients with ACS	Case series (III)	Patients before decompression had small to normal left ventricular end-diastolic volume, normal ejection fraction, and high right and left atrial filling pressures, but clinically appeared hypovolemic. They required high ventilatory pressures and oxygen and were oliguric. With abdominal decompression, filling pressures, cardiac output, and stroke volume increased significantly with improved oxygenation, ventilation, and urine output.
Ivankovich 1975[41]	Dogs with induced IAP	Controlled, compared to baseline	Increased abdominal pressure resulted in increased mean arterial, right atrial, pleural and femoral vein pressures with 60% reduction in cardiac output and vena caval flow. Calculated transmural right atrial pressure decreased, resulting in volume retention.
Diamant 1978[43]	Dogs with induced IAP	Controlled, compared to baseline	IAP to 40 torr during normovolemia results in 35% reduction in cardiac output correlated with decreased inferior vena caval blood flow. Hypovolemia and or inhalational anesthesia resulted in a further 26%–43% decrease.
Kelman 1972[44]	Laparoscopy patients	Controlled, compared to baseline (II)	Femoral venous pressure and central venous pressure increased with IAP. A small increase in cardiac output and intrathoracic pressure was also seen. With higher IAP to 40 cm H_2O, CVP, cardiac output, and MAP decreased with increased heart rate.
Kashtan 1981[45]	Dogs with induced IAP	Controlled, compared to baseline	IAP to 40 mmHg resulted in 53% decreased cardiac output in hypovolemic dogs, 17% decrease in normovolemia and 50% increase in hypervolemia.
Ridings 1995[15]	Pigs with IAP to 25 mmHg	Controlled, compared to baseline	Bladder pressures correlated with IAP. CI decreased, and PAOP, PA, and pleural pressures increased. Worsened PaO_2 and $PaCO_2$. CI improved with volume resuscitation, despite elevated PAOP.

ICU, intensive care unit; ACS, abdominal compartment syndrome; PAOP, pulmonary artery occlusion pressure; CVP, central venous pressure; CI, cardiac index; CO, cardiac output; IAP, intraabdominal pressure; PA, pulmonary artery; MAP, mean arterial pressure; IAH, intraabdominal hypertension; SVR, systemic vascular resistance; torr, mmHg; RVEDVI, right ventricular end-diastolic volume index.

TABLE 34.4.
Intraabdominal Pressure Effects on the Pulmonary System.

Author, year	*Study population*	*Study characteristics*	*Findings*
Murtoh 1991[46]	Pigs with induced IAP	Controlled, compared to baseline	IAP results in elevation of the diaphragm with 40% reduction in functional residual capacity but also results in decreased tidal compliance, resulting in both decreased expansion and a shift to less negative pleural pressures in the lower lung fields, resulting in less uniformity of ventilation.
Kotzampassi 2000[47]	Pigs with IAH at various levels of PEEP	Controlled, compared to baseline	PEEP and IAH have additive effects with decreased flow in the SMA by 35%, mucosal microcirculation by 31%, mucosal pH to 7.1, hepatic artery flow reduced 33% and portal flow 24%.
Oda 2002[48]	Pigs with shock, ACS, and both	Control group, five pigs per group	Measurements of cytokines, myeloperoxidase, and lung white cells indicate that the combination of shock and ACS results in more severe lung injury, likely due to cytokines, than either alone.
Buchard 1985[49]	Dogs with induced IAP at various levels of PEEP	Controlled, compared to baseline	Combination of PEEP and IAP results in significant decrease in CO, increase in PAOP and CVP and lactate. ?Changed hepatic metabolism of lactate.

ACS, abdominal compartment syndrome; IAH, intraabdominal hypertension; IAP, intraabdominal pressure; PEEP, positive end-expiratory pressure; SMA, superior mesenteric artery; CO, cardiac output; CVP, central venous pressure; PAOP, pulmonary artery occlusion pressure.

important. As first described by Caldwell and Ricotta[59] in an early animal model, IAP results in visceral ischemia. Further studies (Table 34.6)[17,58–75] demonstrate that flow to all abdominal viscera, except the adrenal glands, is decreased by 50% or more. This decrease in flow is independent of cardiac output. Additional clinical evidence demonstrates decreased gastric and intestinal mucosal pH.

These decreases in flow and intestinal ischemia result in cytokine release, ischemia/reperfusion injury, and possibly bacterial translocation. Hence, ACS is likely a cause of multiple organ dysfunction syndrome. Additionally, intestinal anastomotic failure is associated with ACS, likely because of bowel ischemia.[60]

Intracranial Pressure

Several case reports, a small series,[76] and some animal data indicate that the increased intrathoracic venous pressure

TABLE 34.5.
Intraabdominal Pressure Effects on the Renal System.

Author, year	*Study population*	*Study characteristics*	*Findings*
Sugrue 1995, 1999[17,51]	ICU patients	Concurrent observation	40% of 263 patients developed IAH (>18 mmHg). Renal impairment was more common with IAH (32% vs. 14%). Factors related to development of renal dysfunction were hypotension, age greater than 60 years, sepsis, and IAH in order of clinical significance.
Doty 1999[52]	Pigs with renal vein constriction	Controlled, compared to baseline	Decreased renal artery blood flow and glomerular filtration independent of cardiac index. Increased aldosterone and renin.
Weibe 2004[53]	Renal transplant patient with IAH due to very large kidney	Case report	Reversal of diastolic arterial flow was an early sign of increased abdominal pressure on the kidney and resolved with release of pressure.
Doty 2000[54]	Pigs with direct renal parenchymal compression	Controlled, compared to baseline	No change in GFR, renal blood flow, renin, or aldosterone production.
Stone 1977[55]	Rhesus monkeys with aortic cross-clamp-induced renal ischemia	Controlled against the contralateral kidney	Removing the renal capsule decreased the loss of function as measured by creatinine clearance.
Harman 1982[56]	Dogs with induced IAP	Controlled, compared to baseline	Increased IAP results in decreased renal blood flow and glomerular filtration to 25% of baseline at 20 mmHg IAP and to aneuria at 40 mmHg IAP. Restoration of cardiac output does not prevent renal dysfunction.
Bradley 1947[57]	Human experimental subjects with external abdominal compression	Controlled, compared to baseline	Increased IAP to 20 mmHg results in increased renal venous pressure (decreased flow gradient across the parenchyma), decreased renal plasma flow, GFR, and filtration fraction, increased water reabsorption, and urinary concentration.
Biancofiore 2002[58]	Liver transplant patients	Concurrent observation	Patients with IAP greater than 25 mmHg had a significantly higher rate of renal failure.

ICU, intensive care unit; IAH, intraabdominal hypertension; IAP, intraabdominal pressure; GFR, glomerular filtration rate.

TABLE 34.6.
IAP Effects on the Splanchnic Circulation.

Author, year	*Study population*	*Study characteristics (Grade of Evidence if a Clinical Study)*	*Findings*
Caldwell 1987[59]	Dogs with induced IAP	Controlled, compared to baseline	HR, R atrial pressure, PAOP, MAP SVR, and hematocrit increased and CO decreased with IAP and returned to baseline with release. Organ flow by microspheres decreased to all intraabdominal organs by greater than 50% (omentum, esophagus, stomach, duodenum, jejunum, ileum, colon, pancreas, gallbladder, liver, spleen, renal cortex) except the adrenal gland, which had increased flow. Organ blood flow index calculation shows decline in flow independent of the decrease in CO.
Diebel 1992[61]	Pigs with induced IAP	Controlled, compared to baseline	Mesenteric blood flow decreased to 73%, intestinal blood flow decreased to 61% at 20 mmHg, 31% and 28%, respectively, at 40 mmHg with severe mucosal ischemia by intestinal mucosal pH.
Diebel 1992[62]	Pigs with induced IAP	Controlled, compared to baseline	Hepatic arterial blood flow decreased to 45%, portal blood flow to 65%, and hepatic microcirculatory flow decreased to 71% of normal at 20 mmHg. Further decreases to 30%, 48%, and 48%, respectively, were seen at 40 mmHg, despite maintained MAP and CO.
Eleftheriadis 1996[63]	Rats with IAP at 15 mmHg pneumoperitoneum	Randomized control group	No change in MAP, decreased jejunal microcirculation, and gut metabolic activity. Increased malondialdehyde concentrations in gut mucosa, liver, spleen, and lung indicating free radical formation. Bacterial translocation to mesenteric lymph nodes, liver, and spleen.
Diebel 1997[64]	Rats with induced IAP	Controlled, compared to baseline	Decreased mesenteric flow and presence of bacterial translocation with IAP of 20–25 mmHg.
Sugrue 1996[65]	Human abdominal surgery patients	Concurrent observation (II)	Half the patients had abnormally low gastric mucosal pH. Those patients were 11 times more likely to have elevated IAP. Both findings predicted increased risk for hypotension, intraabdominal sepsis, renal impairment, need for repeat laparotomy, and death.
Freidlander 1998[66]	Pigs with induced IAH with and without hemorrhage and resuscitation	Controlled, compared to baseline	SMA flow decreases with increasing levels of IAP. This decrease is greater with prior hemorrhage and greater than explained by the decrease in CO.
Nakatani 1998[67]	Rabbits with induced IAH	Controlled, compared to baseline	Hepatic flow decrease at 20 mmHg abdominal pressure did decrease sinusoidal blood flow but did not change energy expenditure. At 30 mmHg, reduced mitochondrial energy expenditure was seen, likely from cellular hypoxia, and was not ameliorated by increased oxygen administration.
Andrei 1998[68]	Laparoscopy patients	Retrospective (III)	Liver-associated enzymes increased statistically more after laparoscopic cholecystectomy than open cholecystecomy, although without clinical significance.
Andrei 1999[69]	Laparoscopy patients	Case reports (III)	Intestinal ischemic necrosis after laparoscopic surgery attributed to increased IAP.
Doty 2002[70]	Pigs with hypotension and IAH	Controlled, compared to baseline	No increase in bacterial translocation.
Ivatury 1998[71]	Trauma patients	Retrospective (III)	IAP resulted in decreased gastric mucosal pH. Closure of the abdomen results in decreased rate of IAH (22% vs. 52%). MODS and death were decreased with mesh closure.
Sugrue 1995[17]	Abdominal surgery patients	Concurrent observation (II)	Elevated IAP present in 33% of patients, renal failure developed in 33% of patients, and 69% of patients with elevated IAP developed renal failure and increased risk for death.
Hsu 2004[72]	Rats with induced IAP to 30 mmHg	Control group	After induction of IAH, isolated hepatocytes had depleted glutathione, indicating ischemia-reperfusion injury.
Rasmussen 1995[73]	Pigs with pneumoperitoneum	Control group	66% portal venous flow, and increased portal and hepatic vascular resistance (360% and 650% increase), with IAP 25 mmHg.
Bongard 1995[74]	Pigs with IAP from helium	Controlled, compared to baseline	Bowel tissue oxygen decreased by 25% at 15 mmHg and by 50% at 25 mmHg. Although there was also a change in cardiac output and mixed venous oxygen, there was no change in subcutaneous oxygen levels.
Pusajo 1994[75]	Surgical ICU patients	Concurrent observation (II)	Patients with IAP less than 10 mmHg had significantly higher gastric pH and urine output than those with IAP greater than 10 mmHg. Additionally, there was a higher rate of reoperation (30% vs. 0%), MODS (80% vs. 20%), sepsis (50% vs. 9%), and mortality (50% vs. 9%) in patients with elevated IAP.

ICU, intensive care unit; IAH, intraabdominal hypertension; IAP, intraabdominal pressure; HR, heart rate; PAOP, pulmonary artery occlusion pressure; MAP, mean arterial pressure; SVR, systemic vascular resistance; CO, cardiac output; SMA, superior mesenteric artery; MODS, multiple organ dysfunction syndrome.

TABLE 34.7.
Effect of IAP on Intracranial Pressure (ICP).

Author, year	*Study population*	*Study characteristics*	*Findings*
Citerio 2001[78]	Head injury patients with external abdominal compression	Concurrent observation	Increased IAP resulted in increases in CVP, jugular pressure, and ICP and MAP. There was no change in CPP.
Bloomfield 1995[79]; Ertel 2000[25]	ICU patients	Case reports	Intractable ICP responded to decompression of elevated IAP.
Bloomfield 1996, 1997[80,81]	Pigs with induced IAP	Controlled, compared to baseline	ICP increased with increasing IAP, sternotomy reduced ICP independent of IAP, indicating transmitted thoracic venous pressure.
Josephs 1994[82]	Pigs with induced elevated ICP and IAP	Controlled, compared to baseline	ICP increased with increased IAP caused by pneumoperitoneum. Laparoscopy in patients with head injury is potentially hazardous.

ICU, intensive care unit; IAH, intraabdominal hypertension; IAP, intraabdominal pressure; ICP, intracranial pressure; CVP, central venous pressure; MAP, mean arterial pressure; CPP, cerebral perfusion pressure.

induced by IAH is transmitted to the cranium, and resulting in elevated intracranial pressure (ICP) (Table 34.7).[25,78–82] Decompression of even low levels of IAP (mean, 27 mmHg) in head-injured patients resulted in prompt decreases in ICP. All patients with elevated ICP that persisted after decompression died, whereas the remaining patients survived to be discharged to a rehabilitation facility. Early decompression of the abdomen should thus be considered in patients with intractable elevations in ICP, possibly at levels lower than with isolated abdominal injury.

Indeed, there is speculation that the effect of IAP on ICP may result in a hormonal cascade that induces many of the physiological findings of ACS, rather than just a mechanical effect of the IAP.[77]

Abdominal Wall

The abdominal wall is very important in the development of IAH, as its capability for expansion is not linear. With greater distension, the degree of elasticity reduces rapidly, such that large increases in pressure will result in only slight increases in volume. Clinically, this means that when using intermittent measurement of IAP, more frequent measurements should be taken to avoid missing a rapid and dangerous pressure increase (Table 34.8).[84,85]

In addition to affecting IAP, the abdominal wall is affected as an organ by the pressure. Increasing IAP results in decreased epigastric blood flow, with resultant ischemia of the abdominal wall. Diebel et al.[83] found that rectus sheath blood flow in swine decreased by 42% at 10 mmHg IAP and by 80% at 40 mmHg; this results in the potential of necrosis or fascial dehiscence. Hence, attempts to close the abdomen under tension results in two insults to the abdominal wall, one from the tension at the sutures and another from the relative ischemia from increased IAP. The result may be necrosis and even more difficulty in closing the abdominal wall in the future.

Other

Specific effects of ACS on neuroendocrine function remain to be determined. There are some conflicting clinical and basic science data that reflect changes in hormone concentrations, specifically vasopressin, renin, and aldosterone.[77] It is likely that all endocrine systems are affected in some way. On a molecular level, changes in gene expression have also been studied, although the clinical consequences of these are unknown (Table 34.9).[88–90]

Another effect attributed to ACS, but not yet shown in clinical or laboratory studies, is deep venous thrombosis caused by vena cava compression and pooling of blood in the lower extremities. Release of ACS may place these patients at increased risk of pulmonary embolism as normal venous flow resumes.[86] Additionally, there is a case report attributing lower extremity arterial graft failure to ACS.[87]

TABLE 34.8.
IAP Effect on Abdominal Wall.

Author, year	*Study population*	*Study characteristics*	*Findings*
Barnes 1985[84]	Dogs with induced IAP	Controlled, compared to baseline	Abdominal compliance decreased to minimal at 40 mmHg pressure and is nonlinearly decreased. Cardiac output and stroke volume reduced 36% and flow to the celiac, superior mesenteric, renal, and femoral arteries decreased by 42%, 61%, 70%, and 65%, respectively. Oxygen consumption, pH, and PO_2 decreased.
Obied 1995[85]	Laparoscopic cholecystectomy patients	Controlled, compared to baseline	Abdominal insufflation resulted in 50% decreased compliance at 16 mmHg. Rectal and gastric pressures were found to be position-dependent and less reliable than bladder pressures.

TABLE 34.9.
IAP Effect on Endocrine and Cytokine Function.

Author, year	*Study population*	*Study characteristics*	*Findings*
Edil 2003[88]	Rats with induced IAH	Controlled, compared to baseline	Overall decreased gene expression, decrease in upregulated genes, and increase in downregulated genes.
Rezende-Neto 2002[89]	Rats with IAH and hypotension	Controlled, compared to baseline	Induction of proinflammatory cytokines, likely cause for MODS, although also had hypotension as potential cause.
Le Roith 1982[90]	Dogs with induced IAP	Controlled, compared to baseline	IAP to 80 mmHg resulted in double baseline production of vasopressin; this was prevented with infusion of dextran to normalize cardiac output.

IAH, intraabdominal hypertension; IAP, intraabdominal pressure; MODS, multiple organ dysfunction syndrome.

Clinical Outcomes of Increased Intraabdominal Pressure and Abdominal Compartment Syndrome

As ACS has become increasingly recognized, the natural history is no longer described because treatment occurs after recognition of the syndrome. However, past experience has shown clearly that multiple organ dysfunction syndrome and death are the inevitable result of delayed treatment.

Despite our increased understanding of ACS, it is not clear at exactly what level of abdominal pressure dangerous clinical changes occur. Indeed, the crucial number probably varies from patient to patient, depending on the clinical scenario and individual response. The hemodynamic effects and clinical organ dysfunction are worsened with increasing pressures, and at some point become critical. Utilizing the grading scale described earlier, Table 34.10 displays the degree of concurrent organ dysfunction.[91]

Given the mortality of organ failure in the ICU, it is hardly surprising that untreated ACS carries such high mortality. A large ICU study demonstrated dramatically increased mortality with IAH (65% vs. 8%), and that the mortality risk was increased for the ICU stay as well as the hospital stay. In multivariate analysis, IAH was also a risk factor for prolonged mechanical ventilation, renal failure, renal replacement therapy, and prolonged ICU and hospital stay. IAP as low as 12 mmHg was found to cause significant risk of mortality and organ dysfunction.[92]

Prevention of IAH and ACS

Prevention of IAH and ACS is by far the best method of preventing further injury to these precarious patients. In a retrospective study of 52 damage control patients, ACS occurred in 80% of those whose fascia was closed, with an associated 90% rate of ARDS or multiple organ dysfunction syndrome (MODS). In those patients in whom skin only was closed, the incidence of ACS was 24%, with ARDS or MODS in 36%. Closure with a temporary prosthesis or transitional dressing, in this case the "Bogota bag" (a sheet of polyvinyl chloride cut from an intravenous fluid bag), reduced the incidence of ACS to 18%, but with 47% ARDS/MODS. The development of ACS increased the incidence of ARDS/MODS to 42% versus 12% in the non-ACS group; the development of ARDS/MODS increased mortality from 12% to 42%.[93] Similar studies show low rates of IAH or ACS (0%–22%) and decreased rates of MODS and death by not closing the fascia in high-risk cases.[71,94]

It is not possible to predict with complete certainty which patients are going to progress to IAH or ACS, so leaving the abdomen open should be considered for all patients undergoing emergency laparotomy and all patients with shock or hemodynamic instability during laparotomy.[95,96] Any patients with extensive visceral or retroperitoneal edema and any in which approximation of the fascia is difficult should be considered for a temporary closure method. The risk of maintaining the abdomen open after the first operation is relatively low. The patient will require deep sedation, and hence ICU care and mechanical ventilation, and at least one further operative procedure. The risk of closure and development of IAH and/or ACS is potential organ failure and death. Thus, when in doubt, it is safer to maintain an open abdomen in unstable and critically ill laparotomy patients. The risk of peritonitis is low, and antibiotic prophylaxis is not required for the open abdomen regardless of whether a temporary prosthesis is placed. Additionally, temporary closure allows rapid termination of operative procedures and transfer to the ICU for further resuscitation if the patient is unstable or has developed the "lethal triad" of hypothermia, coagulopathy, and acidosis.

Speculation regarding the use of colloid resuscitation to prevent development of IAH or to prevent worsening of IAH to ACS is completely unsupported, not even by preliminary data; therefore, current resuscitation regimens that emphasize administration of crystalloid solutions should not be modified for possible or actual IAH.

TABLE 34.10. Organ Dysfunction Associated with ACS by Grade.

Grade of ACS	*Bladder pressure (mmHg)*	*Renal dysfunction*	*Pulmonary dysfunction*	*Cardiovascular dysfunction*
I	10–15	0%	0%	0%
II	15–25	0%	40%	20%
III	25–35	65%	78%	65%
IV	>35	100%	100%	100%

Treatment of IAH and ACS

Treatment is necessary for IAH, but the absolute level of pressure requiring therapy and the optimal therapy for each level of pressure remain a matter of debate. The patient's overall physiological status is more important than the numerical value of the pressure, although it must be remembered that even at low levels of IAH, ischemia is occurring that is not clinically apparent.

All patients with elevation of IAP must be observed closely. Serial urinary bladder pressures should be checked and optimal fluid balance maintained. It must be remembered that fluid balance is difficult to assess in this patient population because PAOP and CVP begin to increase despite inadequate intravascular volume. In addition, excessive volume resuscitation will result in worsened visceral edema, creating a difficult clinical balance. Hence, the endpoints of resuscitation must be monitored as well, such as clearance of acidosis, restoration of cardiac output, or normalized right ventricular end-diastolic index. Patients should be monitored for the development of clinical sequelae of ACS, particularly the triad of hypotension, oliguria, and elevated peak airway pressures.

Abdominal perfusion pressure has been studied as a determinant of survival in IAH, the hypothesis being that abdominal pressure alone is not sufficient to determine effects on the patient's physiology. Abdominal perfusion pressure is defined as mean arterial blood pressure minus the IAP. In a hypotensive patient, lower levels of IAH may therefore be threatening, mirroring the concept of cerebral perfusion pressure, which is widely measured in brain-injured patients. This is likely also the reason that patients with chronically elevated abdominal pressure do not suffer clinical consequences—mean arterial pressure increases to compensate. Maintenance of abdominal perfusion pressure resulted in an 85% prediction of survival in one series of patients with IAH.[97]

Neuromuscular blockade should be considered for all patients with elevated IAP, certainly grade II and above. Induced paralysis provides maximal abdominal wall compliance and also removes confounding variables such as asynchronous ventilation, which may lead to overestimation of the actual abdominal pressure. However, pharmacotherapy should not delay surgical decompression if the patient's IAP or clinical circumstances warrant.[98]

Medical management of IAH (not ACS) has been described utilizing vasopressor support and diuresis. Although successful in lowering bladder pressures and correcting hypotension, this intervention likely results in increased visceral ischemia consequent to vasoconstriction and hence is not recommended. Limited success of nonsurgical management of IAH in patients who are not considered to be candidates for open abdomen management, because of either a "frozen abdomen" or end-of-life decision making, have been reported. As such, there are no data outside of isolated anecdotal experience.

In patients with secondary ACS, hence without abdominal pathology, the use of peritoneal catheters or paracentesis to remove fluid has been sufficient to reduce IAH and prevent the development of ACS in selected patients. Particularly, this has been described in burned patients.[33] This therapy seems to be effective in about one-half of patients with IAH, preventing progression to ACS.[99] Escharotomy has also been shown to reduce IAP when the burn eschar is believed to contribute to decreased abdominal wall compliance and should be considered as a first-line treatment modality for selected patients.[32,100]

Several recent small studies have examined other less invasive methods to reduce IAP. External negative abdominal pressure shows some promise in animal studies; however, IAH was artificially created in an otherwise healthy animal. Use in ICU patients remains to be investigated.[101]

In patients with primary abdominal pathology, the development of IAH or ACS must be considered a harbinger of hemorrhage, missed injury, or worsening of the inciting disease process. Additionally, ACS in the surgical patient has been associated with the finding of necrotic bowel at decompression. This finding may result from ACS causing decreased visceral perfusion, or the converse may be true; high volume requirements induced by intestinal ischemia, leading to development of ACS.[102,103]

It is agreed by most intensive care physicians that treatment of ACS (i.e., IAH with clinical deterioration) and IAH with pressures greater than 35 mmHg regardless of symptomatology mandate abdominal decompression. Many centers have the capability to perform bedside surgery in the ICU when the patient is deemed too unstable to transport. However, if bleeding or bowel resection is likely, the operating room is a safer place to perform decompression. Despite isolated case reports of lateral releasing incisions, only a formal midline laparotomy can reliably provide decompression of the abdominal compartment.

Abdominal decompression is clearly the method of choice for relieving IAP, but it is not without risks. Immediately upon decompression, a "reperfusion syndrome" occurs with washout of by-products of anaerobic metabolism or unquenched reactive oxygen species (ROS) resulting from reintroduction of oxygen to ischemic tissue; this may result in worsening hemodynamic instability and even asystole that is refractory to resuscitation.[104] Even if hemodynamics remain stable, ischemia-reperfusion injury to viscera (e.g., liver, lung, stomach) caused by ROS may cause severe MODS. Predecompression resuscitation with volume and consideration for bicarbonate or mannitol loading should be undertaken, similar to unclamping during aortic surgery. The search has begun for the "magic bullet" to prevent the injury induced by reperfusion. In rats, utilizing induced IAH, octreotide and melatonin mitigated against oxidant injury, but survival was not measured and the data must be considered preliminary.[105,106]

IAH and ACS are more likely to develop in patients with closed abdominal fascia, but it is also possible to develop increased pressure with a temporary abdominal closure, especially if the abdomen is packed for hemostasis. Despite an initially loose temporary closure, ongoing monitoring for IAH is necessary as development of "recurrent" ACS has been described within a temporary abdominal containment dressing. In a retrospective analysis of these patients, the mortality was 60%, compared with a rate of 7% among patients who had an open abdomen but did not develop recurrent ACS.[107]

Based on ACS grades, one management schema is described in Table 34.11. It is crucial to provide aggressive resuscitation, but to temper it with reasonable targeted endpoints so as to reduce abdominal and retroperitoneal edema

TABLE 34.11. Management of ACS Based on Grade.

Grade	*Bladder pressure (mmHg)*	*Treatment recommendations*
I	10–15	Normovolemic resuscitation, consider neuromuscular blockade.
II	15–25	Hypervolemic resuscitation with neuromuscular blockade.
III	25–35	Release of abdominal fascia in intensive care unit.
IV	>35	Release of abdominal fascia in operating room.

Source: From Burch JM, Moore EE, Morre FA, Fancoise R. The abdominal compartment syndrome. Surg Clin North Am 1996;76: 833–842.[22]

formation. Additionally, frequent monitoring and prompt treatment of IAH are required to prevent the development of the ischemic sequelae of ACS. Opening the abdomen is not without risk, but development of full-blown ACS is essentially always fatal.

Managing the Open Abdomen

The foregoing discussion has concentrated on ACS, but there are other reasons for maintaining an open abdomen, which include severe peritonitis requiring serial abdominal washouts, ischemic viscera requiring a second-look laparotomy, removal of packs used for hemostasis, or serial debridements for pancreatic necrosis. Avoiding multiple closures of the fascia results in decreased fascial injury and loss and preserves the ability to close the abdomen with native tissue in the future.

With the decision to keep an abdomen open, several additional concerns develop, including how to keep the viscera within the abdomen and when and how to close the abdomen. As most of the data from the literature consist of case series with essentially no prospective trials, the following discussion consists mainly of the options available and the experience of individual surgeons and centers with these options.

Temporary Abdominal Containment

Temporary abdominal containment methods are used until the abdomen can be closed, either by delayed primary closure or by a transitional closure. Many methods have been described but, optimally, containment will keep the abdominal viscera inside, prevent further contamination of the peritoneal cavity, and be large enough to cover protruding viscera without increasing IAP (Fig. 34.1). Rapid application and reopening and inexpensive materials are best. A dressing that provides for egress of peritoneal fluid but prevents leakage allows for accurate measurement of fluid balance and facilitates skin care. Most important is that the material in contact with the intestines is nonadherent to prevent injury.

Skin closure only results in a watertight seal and may be used occasionally as a permanent closure with eventual repair of the ventral hernia. Closure is rapid and does not use prosthetic material, but provides little increase in abdominal volume, and hence is typically not used for a patient with or at risk for ACS.

Interposition methods of closure provide coverage for any amount of intestinal protuberance. By preventing development of, or treating ACS, they have been shown to decrease the incidence of MODS, ACS, abscess, necrotizing fasciitis, and fistula, and to improve outcome in retrospective reviews of a diverse group of patients.[93,108,109] A variety of materials can be used that may be attached to fascia or skin. Enough laxity must be provided to prevent later development of recurrent IAH.

The most common[110] and least expensive[111] option is the "Bogota bag." An opened sterilized intravenous solution bag, usually a 3-Liter irrigation bag, is sewn into the abdominal defect; this has the advantage of transparency, which allows the abdominal contents to be inspected, but it does not provide a watertight seal and requires time to sew it in place. At repeat laparotomy, as it can be opened down the middle and then reclosed with a continuous suture.

Mesh of all types has been described; however, none is watertight. Vicryl (polyglactic acid; Ethicon, Somerville, NJ) or Dexon (polyglycolic acid; Davis & Geck, Danbury, CT) meshes may tear unless multiple layers are placed, resulting in evisceration. Polypropylene mesh (Marlex; Bard, Billerica, MA; Prolene; Ethicon, Somerville, NJ; Surgipro; US Surgical, Norwalk, CT) is abrasive and will adhere to bowel, resulting in fistulae in 12% to 50% of patients.[112] GoreTex (polytetrafluoroethylene; Gore, Flagstaff, AZ) is quite expensive and may become infected if left uncovered.

Additional drawbacks to all types of interposition dressings are increased time for implantation and fascial injury. Added time needed in the operating room to sew the material in place may be life threatening to a critically ill, damage control patient. The material must be sewn to either skin or fascia, and these sutures may result in damage to already ischemic abdominal wall structures. Loss of fascia or skin makes later definitive closure more difficult.

Our preferred method for temporary abdominal containment is an adhesive vacuum dressing ("Vac-Pac"). This

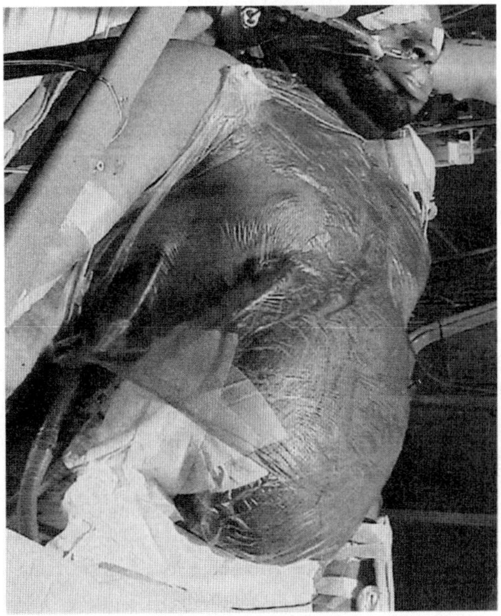

FIGURE 34.1. Protuberance of abdominal contents in early damage control abdomen.

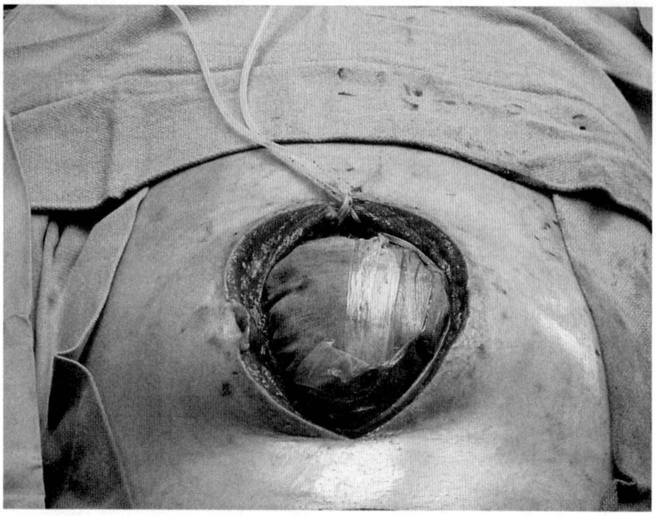

FIGURE 34.2. "Vac-Pac" application with insertion of plasticized towel and drains.

dressing consists of a nonadhesive, soft, clear plastic layer tucked under the abdominal wall against the bowels and covered by roll gauze containing closed-suction drains that allows fluid out of the abdomen and maintains negative pressure within the dressing and abdomen. A large adhesive drape is then placed over this and the anterior abdominal wall, with the drains placed to low continuous suction. The dressing can be applied rapidly, will cover abdominal contents of any size, costs about $40 (U.S.), is watertight, and can be reopened rapidly if IAH or the need for reexploration develop (Fig. 34.2, 34.3).

Resuscitation

With ongoing resuscitation in the ICU, patients often receive large volumes of fluid or blood products, which may result in edema of the intraabdominal contents. Thus, frequent measurement of bladder pressures should continue until the patient is physiologically stable.

The majority of patients will stabilize quickly and normalize their physiological and laboratory parameters. These patients can usually return to the operating room in 24 to 36h for unpacking, definitive operative repair, and primary closure if possible without tension. If there is evidence of ongoing visceral edema, or if a subsequent operation is planned, another temporary dressing is applied.

A small group of patients will not have normalization of their hemodynamics despite appropriate resuscitation. The potential reasons for this include bleeding, missed injury, and missed ACS. These patients will require early reexploration, either at the bedside or in the operating room with another temporary dressing thereafter.

Managing and Changing Temporary Closure

Temporary abdominal containment dressings cannot be left in place indefinitely. However, the optimal duration between changes has not been determined. Patients with packs for hemostasis, a need for serial debridement or washout, and patients requiring reestablishment of intestinal continuity should return to the operating room as soon as possible for these procedures. Serial washouts or maintenance dressings while waiting for visceral edema to subside can be done in a sterile manner in the ICU. The more frequently these dressings are changed, the greater the risk of bowel injury from manipulation, but not changing the dressings may result in increased risk of infection, particularly with packing in place. Generally, every other or every third day is adequate.

With each dressing change, a decision should be made as to timing of closure. Patients who have a rapid decrease in their edema may be considered for delayed primary closure, which is the optimal method of closure. The longer the abdomen is left open, however, the less likely this can be accomplished as there is progressive loss of abdominal domain, increasing the likelihood that a transitional closure will be necessary. In total, 50% to 70% of open abdomen patients will be able to undergo delayed primary closure, with the remainder requiring a transitional closure.[113]

Transitional Closure

Closure should be accomplished as soon as possible to decrease the metabolic demand of serial abdominal explorations and a large open wound. In patients who remain too edematous to close the abdomen without causing IAH, several methods of transitional closure exist. The placement of an absorbable interposition mesh to the skin or fascia is safe and simple. Closure should not be tight, or tearing of the mesh with evisceration or IAH may result. This method does little to maintain abdominal domain as the mesh has low distensibility. It is safe for use in the presence of infection, and the risk of fistulation is low (5%).[110,112,113] Wet dressings over the mesh encourage formation of granulation tissue that will accept a split-thickness skin graft (Fig. 34.4). Although the patient is left with a large ventral hernia that will eventually require complex closure, it is the most rapid and safest method to facilitate rehabilitation and restoration of positive nitrogen balance.

Although strong enough to maintain containment, polypropylene mesh is less likely to be incorporated in an infected field and has a high rate of intestinal fistula development.

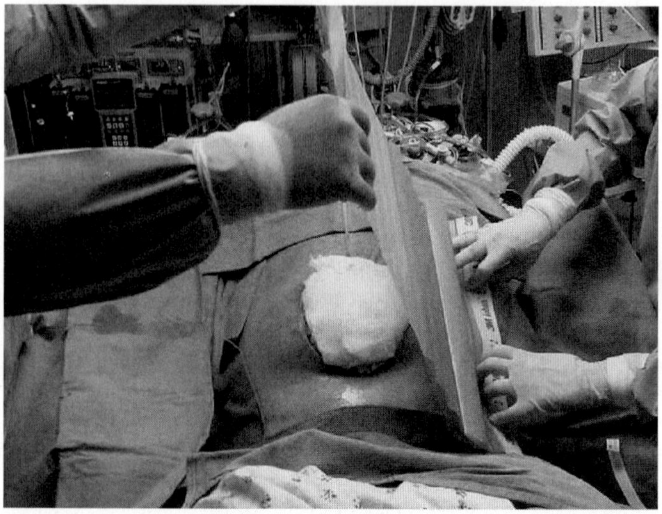

FIGURE 34.3. "Vac-Pac" cover dressing over fluffed gauze.

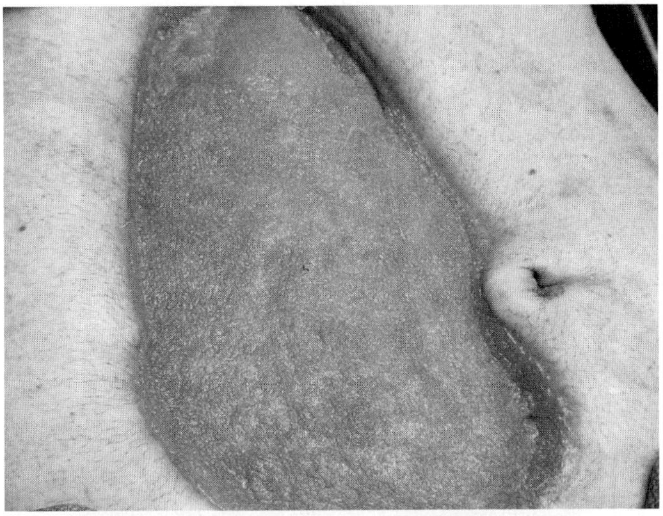

FIGURE 34.4. Mesh transitional closure polyglactin 910 after granulation.

Polytetrafluoroethylene mesh is strong and nonadherent, with a very low fistula rate; however, the risk of infection is high if not covered immediately with tissue.[94] Methods of closure with soft tissue advancement flaps (abdominal component separation) with or without mesh have been described but have a high failure rate in critically ill and malnourished patients because of the metabolic strain of such an extensive procedure; thus, the technique is best reserved for delayed definitive closure of recovered patients.

Attempts to draw the fascia together for delayed primary closure have been described, varying from silo creation, retention sutures, serial mesh tightening, and hook-and-loop fabrics.[114–116] Modest success has been described with all these series, although the advantage of avoiding a mandatory second procedure is outweighed by several substantial drawbacks. Any attempt to bring the fascia together under tension may result in abdominal wall complications, such as fascial ischemia, tearing, necrosis, or hernia formation, if indeed IAH/ACS is avoided. Any attempt to close fascia under tension in the critically ill patient population may result in increased IAP, and the physiological consequences may be dire or even lethal. The rate of successful primary closure in these diverse populations is about 52%,[117] not significantly different from regular delayed primary closure.

Tubes and Stomas

Development and resolution of visceral and abdominal wall edema results in ongoing changes in the topography of the abdomen, which causes particular difficulty as drains and feeding tubes may pull out and stomata may withdraw into the abdomen or become ischemic because of tension on the mesentery. For these reasons, avoidance of artificial openings in the abdominal wall is optimal. Despite the risk of anastomotic dehiscence, many surgeons choose to perform a primary bowel anastomosis rather than bring out a stoma.[96,104]

Nasoduodenal feeding is preferred to feeding tubes placed operatively. Nasogastric feeding may be just as safe and effective with the adjunctive use of promobility agents (e.g., erythromycin) and positioning of the patient in the head-up position. Drains should have slack tubing, and all transabdominal tubes and stomas should be brought out as lateral as possible to prevent scarring to the rectus muscle, which can make later definitive closure more difficult.

Fistulae

Enterocutaneous fistulae develop in 1% to 15% of patients with open abdomen management, depending on the initial pathology and the method of abdominal containment.[94] These fistulae are a major cause of morbidity. Because there is no intervening tissue, they usually form to the mesh and have been called *entero-atmospheric fistula*. Because there is usually no overlying tissue to collapse on the tract as drainage decreases, they have only about a 25% rate of closure without surgery,[117] and, as these occur in a granulating bed, fitting a collection appliance is difficult.

Prevention of fistulization is usually possible with gentle bowel handling and interposition of the omentum over the intestines whenever possible. Anastomoses should not be left exposed in the wound. Transitional or definitive closure as soon as possible reduces the number of dressing changes. Dressings over the mesh must be kept moist; petrolatum gauze can also be used to prevent adhesion to intestinal serosa. Skin grafting is also protective and should be placed as soon as sufficient tissue granulation has occurred.[93]

When a fistula develops, standard management is bowel rest and parenteral nutrition. Fistula output control may require placement of a suction drain at the site. Early skin grafting around the fistula is beneficial as, even though some loss of engrafted skin can be expected, a mature skin graft around the fistula will allow placement of an appliance to manage secretions.

Although small or initially low-output (300–500 mL/day) or even high-volume fistulae may close with nonoperative management, larger fistulae will usually not close without surgery, usually resection and anastomosis of the involved segment of intestine. The patient should be allowed to recover completely from the initial disease process, regain positive nitrogen balance, and be ready for definitive abdominal closure, at which time fistula resection, anastomosis, and abdominal wall closure can be completed in a single operation with an optimal chance for success.

Definitive Abdominal Wall Repair

Definitive abdominal wall reconstruction should be attempted when the patient has recovered from the initial disease process, is repleted nutritionally, and intraabdominal adhesions have softened; this usually requires 6 to 12 months from the last operation. An abdominal binder helps provide comfort and maintains abdominal domain in the interim. Additionally, physical therapy, cessation of substance abuse and smoking, and psychological counseling may be helpful.

When it is apparent that the underlying bowel has separated from the mesh and skin graft, based on physical ability to "pinch" the skin (Figure 34.5), and sufficient weight gain for subcutaneous flaps has developed, the patient is considered for closure. Patients with a stoma may be evaluated for restoration of intestine as a separate initial operation or at the same time as abdominal closure. The majority of patients are closed by rectus component separation with occasional mesh

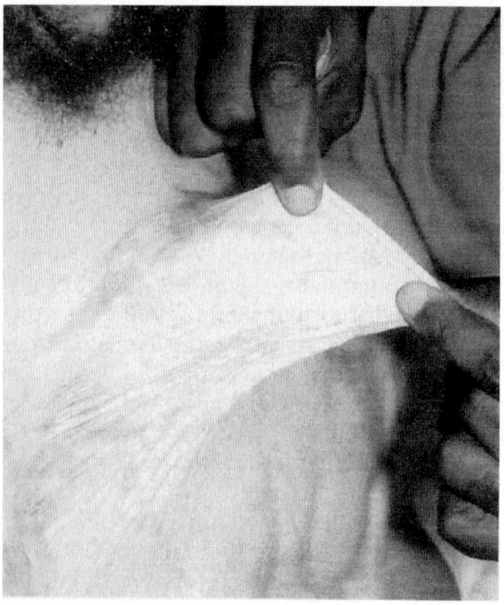

FIGURE 34.5. "Pinch" test for readiness for reconstruction.

reinforcement (Figures 34.6, 34.7). In patients with substantial loss of abdominal domain, seen most often in patients waiting for more than a year for reconstruction,[112] plastic surgical techniques such as tissue expanders may be needed (Figure 34.8).

Management with an open abdomen is lifesaving in a group of patients in extremis, although it leads to a prolonged hospital course and potential for many severe complications. Patients with a skin-grafted ventral hernia perceive a decreased level of physical, social, and emotional health; these perceptions return to the baseline of the healthy general population after definitive abdominal closure. Seventy-eight percent of previously employed patients return to work. The morbidity is substantial, but the majority of patients can eventually be expected to return to near-normal lifestyles after open abdomen management.[118]

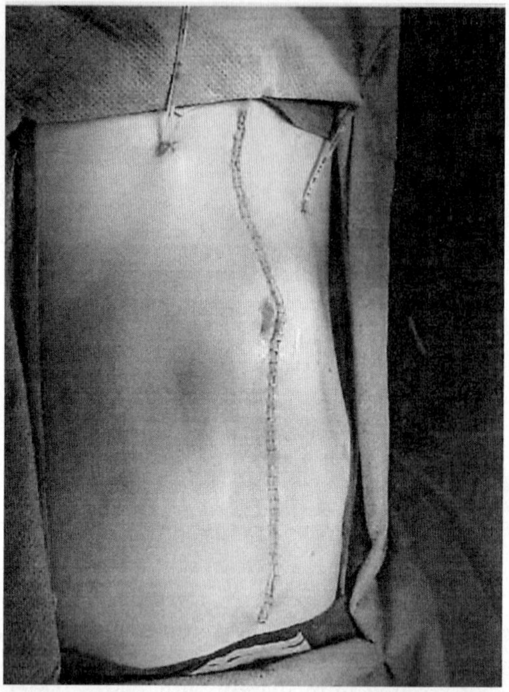

FIGURE 34.7. Case shown in Figures 34.5 and 34.6 after reconstruction with separation of components.

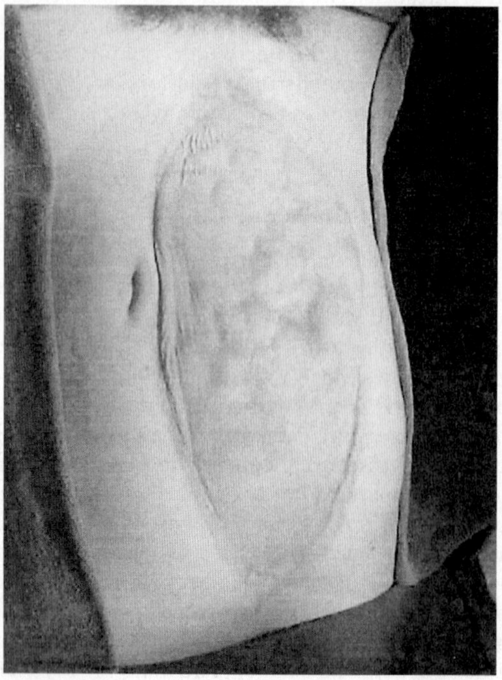

FIGURE 34.6. Case shown in Figure 34.5 before reconstruction.

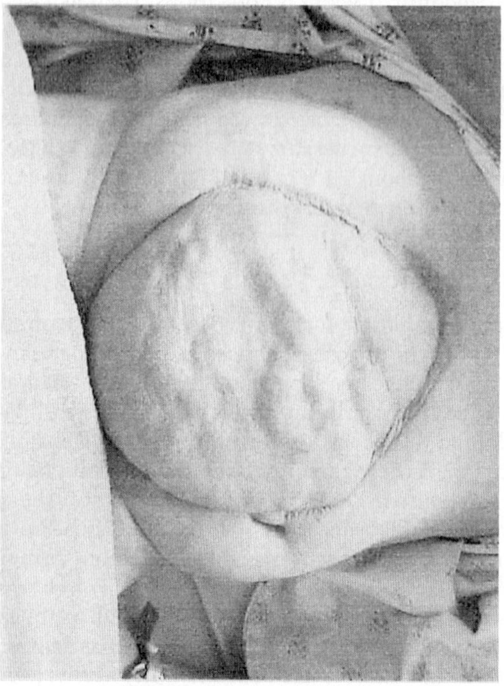

FIGURE 34.8. Loss of abdominal domain.

Conclusion

Intraabdominal hypertension may progress to ACS with the clinical triad of hypotension, oliguria, and high peak airway pressure. This syndrome causes a predictable and preventable cycle of ischemia and reperfusion injury. Risk factors remain poorly understood but include damage control surgery and large volumes of resuscitation fluid. Observed hemodynamics overestimate the quality of resuscitation, with the most accurate measure of volume status being right ventricular end-diastolic volume index. Definitive treatment is by surgical decompression of the abdomen. The exact level of abdominal pressure at which this is necessary is unclear, but pressures greater than 35 mmHg mandate decompression. Methods for earlier "subclinical" detection are needed as multiple effects of ischemia occur before the overt presentation of the clinical triad.

Managing the open abdomen is a challenge. Careful bowel handling, prevention of injury to the fascia, prevention of recurrent IAH, and early transitional closure are necessary to minimize complications. Time for physical and nutritional recovery is paramount for successful definitive closure.

References

1. Ivatury RR, Sugerman HJ. Abdominal compartment syndrome: a century later, isn't it time to pay attention? Crit Care Med 2000;28:2137–2138.
2. Kron IL, Harman PK, Nolan SP. The measurement of intra-abdominal pressure as a criterion for abdominal re-exploration. Ann Surg 1984;199:28–30.
3. Sanchez NC, Tenofsky PL, Dort JM, Shen LY, Helmer SD, Smith RS. What is normal intra-abdominal pressure? Am Surg 2001;67: 243–47.
4. Pelosi P, Croci M, Ravagnan I, et al. Respiratory system mechanics in sedated, paralyzed morbidly obese patients. Appl Physiol 1997;82:811–818.
5. Luca A, Cirera I, Garcia-Pagan CJ, et al. Hemodynamic effects of acute changes in intra-abdominal pressure in patients with cirrhosis. Gastroenterology 1994;104:222–227.
6. Sugerman HJ, DeMaria EJ, Felton III WL, Nakatsuka M, Sismanis A. Increased intra-abdominal pressure and cardiac filling pressures in obesity-associated pseudotumor cerebri. Neurology 1997;49:507–511.
7. Sugarman HJ. Effects of increased intra-abdominal pressure in severe obesity. Obesity surgery. Surg Clin N Am 2001;81:1063–1076.
8. Bloomfield GL, Sugerman HJ, Blocher CT, Gehr TWB, Sica DA. Chronically increased intra-abdominal pressure produces systemic hypertension in dogs. Int J Obes 2000;24:819–824.
9. Nguyen NT, Wolfe BM. The physiologic effects of pneumoperitoneum in the morbidly obese. Ann Surg 2005;241:219–226.
10. Pierri A, Munegato G, Carraro L, Zaccaria F, Tiso I, Zotti EF. Hemodynamic alterations during massive incisional hernioplasy. JACS 1995;181:299–302.
11. Wesley JR, Drongowski R, Coran, AG. Intragastric pressure measurement: a guide for reduction and closure of the silastic chimney in omphalocele and gastroschisis. J Pediatr Surg 1981;16:264–270.
12. Lacey SR, Carris LA, Beyer J III, Azizkhan RG. Bladder pressure monitoring significantly enhances care of infants with abdominal wall defects: a prospective clinical study. J Pediatr Surg 1993;28:1370–1375.
13. Kirkpatrick AW, Brenneman FD, McLean RF, Rapanos T, Boulanger BR. Is clinical examination an accurate indicator of raised intra-abdominal pressure in critically injured patients? Can J Surg 2000;43:207–211.
14. Engum SA, Kogon B, Jensen E, Isch J, Balanoff C, Grosfeld JL. Gastric tonometry and direct intraabdominal pressure monitoring in abdominal compartment syndrome. J Pediatr Surg 2002;37: 214–218.
15. Ridings PC, Bloomfield GL, Blocher CR, Sugerman HJ. Cardiopulmonary effects of raised intra-abdominal pressure before and after intravascular volume expansion. J Trauma 1995;39:1071–1074.
16. Malbrain MLNG. Different techniques to measure intra-abdominal pressure (IAP): time for a critical re-appraisal. Intensive Care Med 2004;30:357–371.
17. Sugrue M, Buist MD, Hourihan F, et al. Prospective study of intra-abdominal hypertension and renal function after laparotomy. Br J Surg 1995;82:235–238.
18. Richardson JD, Trinkle JK. Hemodynamic and respiratory alterations with increased intra-abdominal pressure. J Surg Res 1976; 20:401–404.
19. Pickhardt PJ, Shimony JS, Heiken JP, Buchman TG, Fischer AJ. The abdominal compartment syndrome: CT findings. AJR 1999; 173:575–579.
20. Epelman M, Soudack M, Engel M, Beck R. Abdominal compartment syndrome in children: CT findings. Pediatr Radiol 2002; 32:319–322.
21. Wachsberg RH, Sebastiano LLS, Levine CD. Narrowing of the upper abdominal inferior vena cava in patients with elevated intraabdominal pressure. Abdom Imaging 1998;23:99–102.
22. Burch JM, Moore EE, Morre FA, Fancoise R. The abdominal compartment syndrome. Surg Clin N Am 1996;76:833–842.
23. McNelis J, Marini CP, Jurkiewecz A, et al. Predictive factors associated with the development of abdominal compartment syndrome in the surgical intensive care unit. Arch Surg 2002; 137:133–136.
24. Balogh Z, McKinley BA, Cocanour CS, et al. Supranormal trauma resuscitation causes more cases of abdominal compartment syndrome. Arch Surg 2003;138:637–643.
25. Ertel W, Oberholzer A, Platz A, Stocker R, Trentz O. Incidence and clinical pattern of the abdominal compartment syndrome after "damage-control" laparotomy in 311 patients with severe abdominal and/or pelvic trauma. Crit Care Med 2000;28:1747–53.
26. Hong JJ, Cohn SM, Perez JM, Colich MO, Brown M, McKenney MG. Prospective study of the incidence and outcome of intra-abdominal hypertension and the abdominal compartment syndrome. Br J Surg 2002;89:591–596.
27. Malbrain MLNG, Chiumello D, Pelosi P, et al. Prevalence of intra-abdominal hypertension in critically ill patients: a multicentre epidemiological study. Intensive Care Med 2004;30:822–829.
28. Biancofiore G, Bindi ML, Romanelli AM, et al. Intra-abdominal pressure monitoring in liver transplant recipients: a prospective study. Intensive Care Med 2003;29:30–36.
29. Kopelman T, Harris C, Miller R, Arrillaga A. Abdominal compartment syndrome in patients with isolated extraperitoneal injuries. J Trauma 2000;49:744–749.
30. Maxwell RA, Fabian TC, Croce MA, Davis KA. Secondary abdominal compartment syndrome: an under-appreciated manifestation of severe hemorrhagic shock. J Trauma 1999;47:995–999.
31. Biffl WL, Moore EE, Burch JM, Offner PJ, Franciose RJ, Johnson JL. Secondary abdominal compartment syndrome is a highly lethal event. Am J Surg 2001;182:645–648.
32. Ivy ME, Atweh NA, Palmer J, Posseti PP, Pineau M, D'Aiuto M. Intra-abdominal hypertension and abdominal compartment syndrome in burn patients. J Trauma 2000;49:387–391.
33. Hobson KG, Young KM, Ciraulo A, Palmieri TL, Greenhalgh DG. Release of abdominal compartment syndrome improves

survival in patients with burn injury. J Trauma 2000;53:1129–1134.
34. Cullen DJ, Coyle JP, Teplick R, Long MC. Cardiovascular, pulmonary, and renal effects of massively increased intra-abdominal pressure in critically ill patients. Crit Care Med 1989;17:118–121.
35. Cheatham ML, Safesak K, Block EFJ, Nelson LD. Preload assessment in patients with an open abdomen. J Trauma 1999;46:16–22.
36. Balogh Z, McKinley BA, Cacanour CS, Kozar RA, Cox CS, Moore FA. Patients with impending abdominal compartment syndrome do not respond to early volume loading. Am J Surg 2003;186:602–608.
37. Schachtrupp A, Graf J, Tons C, Hoer J, Fackeldey V, Schumpelick V. Intravascular volume depletion in a 24-hour porcine model of intra-abdominal hypertension. J Trauma 2003;55:734–740.
38. Simon RJ, Friedlander MH, Ivatury RR, DiRaimo R, Machiedo GW. Hemorrhage lowers the threshold for intra-abdominal hypertension-induced pulmonary dysfunction. J Trauma 1997;42:398–405.
39. Chang MC, Miller PR, D'Agostino R, Meredith JW. Effects of abdominal decompression on cardiopulmonary function and visceral perfusion in patients with intra-abdominal hypertension. J Trauma 1998;44:440–445.
40. Shelly MP, Robinson AA, Hesford JW, Park GR. Haemodynamic effects following surgical release of increased intra-abdominal pressure. Br J Anaesth 1987;59:800–805.
41. Ivankovich AD, Miletich DJ, Albrecht RF, Heyman HJ, Bonnet RF. Cardiovascular effects of intraperitoneal insufflation with carbon dioxide and nitrous oxide in the dog. Anesthesiology 1975;42:281–287.
42. Robotham JL, Wise RA. Bromberger-Barnea B. Effects of changes in abdominal pressure on left ventricular performance and regional blood flow. Crit Care Med 1985;13:803–809.
43. Diamant M, Benumof JL, Saidman LJ. Hemodynamics of increased intra-abdominal pressure. Anesthesiology 1978;48:23–27.
44. Kelman GR, Swapp GH, Smith I, Benzie RJ, Gordon NLM. Cardiac output and arterial blood-gas tension during laparoscopy. Br J Anesth 1972;44:1155–1161.
45. Kashtan J, Green JF, Parsons EQ, Holcroft JW. Hemodynamic effects of increased abdominal pressure J Surg Res 1981;30:249–222.
46. Murtoh T, Lamm WJE, Embree LJ, Hilebrandt J, Albert RK. Abdominal distension alters regional pleural pressure and chest wall mechanics in pigs in vivo. J Appl Physiol 1991;70:2611–2618.
47. Kotzampassi K, Paramythiotis D, Eleftheriadis E. Deterioration of visceral perfusion caused by intra-abdominal hypertension in pigs ventilated with positive end-expiratory pressure. Surg Today 2000;30:987–992.
48. Oda J, Ivatury RR, Blocher CR, Malhotra AJ, Sugerman HJ. Amplified cytokine response and lung injury by sequential hemorrhagic shock and abdominal compartment syndrome in a laboratory model of ischemia-reperfusion. J Trauma 2002;52:625–632.
49. Buchard KW, Ciombor DM, McLeod MK, Slotman GJ, Gann DS. Positive end expiratory pressure with increased intra-abdominal pressure. Surg Gynecol Obstet 1985;161:313–318.
50. Wendt EC. Uber den Einflus des intra-abdominellen Druckes auf dies Absonderungsgeschwingigkeit des Hames. Arch Heilkd 1876;17:527.
51. Sugrue M, Jones F, Deane SA, Bishop G, Bauman A, Hillman K. Intra-abdominal hypertension is an independent cause of postoperative renal impairment. Arch Surg 1999;134:1082–1085.
52. Doty JM, Saggi BH, Sugerman HJ, et al. Effect of increased renal venous pressure on renal function. J Trauma 1999;47:1000–1003.
53. Wiebe S, Kellenberger CJ, Khoury A, Miller SF. Early Doppler changes in a renal transplant patient secondary to abdominal compartment syndrome. Pediatr Radiol 2004;34:432–434.
54. Doty JM, Saggi GH, Blocher CR, et al. Effects of increased renal parenchymal pressure on renal function. J Trauma 2000;48:874–877.
55. Stone HH, Fulenwider JT. Renal decapsulation (decaps) in the prevention of post-ischemic oliguria. Ann Surg 1977;186:343–355.
56. Harman PK, Kron IL, McLachlan HD, Freedlender AE, Nolan SP. Elevated intra-abdominal pressure and renal function. Ann Surg 1982;196:594–597.
57. Bradley SE, Bradley GP. The effect of increased intra-abdominal pressure on renal function in man. J Clin Invest 1947;26:1010-22.
58. Biancofiore G, Bindi L, Romanelli AM, et al. Renal failure and abdominal hypertension after liver transplantation: determination of critical intra-abdominal pressure. Liver Transplant 2002;8:1175–1178.
59. Caldwell CB, Ricotta JR. Changes in visceral blood flow with elevated intraabdominal pressure. J Surg Res 1987;43:14–20.
60. Behrman SW, Bertken KA, Stefanacci HA, Parks SN. Breakdown of intestinal repair after laparotomy for trauma: incidence, risk factors, and strategies for prevention. J Trauma 1998;45:227–233.
61. Diebel LN, Dulchavsky SA, Wilson RF. Effect of increased intra-abdominal pressure on mesenteric arterial and intestinal mucosal blood flow. J Trauma 1992;33:45–49.
62. Diebel LN, Wilson RF, Dulchavsky SA, Saxe J. Effect of increased intra-abdominal pressure on hepatic arterial, portal venous, and hepatic microcirculatory blood flow. J Trauma 1992;33:279–283.
63. Eleftheriadis E, Kotzampassi K, Papanotas K, Heliadis N, Sarris K. Gut ischemia, oxidative stress and bacterial translocation in elevated abdominal pressure in rats. World J Surg 1996;20:11–16.
64. Diebel LN, Culchavsky SA, Brown WJ. Splanchnic ischemia and bacterial translocation in the abdominal compartment syndrome. J Trauma 1997;43:852–855.
65. Sugrue M, Jones F, Lee A, et al. Intraabdominal pressure and gastric intramucosal pH: is there an association? World J Surg 1996;20:988–991.
66. Friedlander MH, Simon RJ, Ivatury R, DiRaimo R, Machiedo GW. Effect of hemorrhage on superior mesenteric artery flow during increased intra-abdominal pressures. J Trauma 1998;45;433–439.
67. Nakatani T, Sakamoto Y, Kaneko I, Ando H, Kobayashi K. Effects of intra-abdominal hypertension on hepatic energy metabolism in a rabbit model. J Trauma 1998;44:446–453.
68. Andrei VE, Shein M, Margolis M, Rucinski JC, Wise L. Liver enzymes are commonly elevated following laparoscopic cholecystectomy: is elevated intra-abdominal pressure the cause? Dig Surg 1998;15:256–259.
69. Andrei VE, Schein M, Wise L. Small bowel ischemia following laparoscopic cholecystectomy. Dig Surg 1999;16:522–524.
70. Doty JM, Oda J, Ivatury RR, Blocher CR, Christie GE, Yelon JA, Sugerman HJ. The effects of hemodynamic shock and increased intra-abdominal pressure on bacterial translocation. J Trauma 2002;52:13–17.
71. Ivatury RR, Porter JM, Simon RJ, Islam S, John R, Stahl WM. Intra-abdominal hypertension after life-threatening penetrating abdominal trauma: prophylaxis, incidence, and clinical relevance to gastric mucosal pH and abdominal compartment syndrome. J Trauma 1998;44:1016–1023.
72. Hsu YP, Chen RJ, Fang JF, et al. Increased susceptibility to oxidant injury in hepatocytes from rats with intra-abdominal hypertension. J Trauma 2004;57:569–575.

73. Rasmussen I, Berggren U, Aevidsson D, Ljungdahl M, Haglund U. Effects of pneumoperitoneum on splanchnic hemodynamics: an experimental study in pigs. Eur J Surg 1995;161:819–826.
74. Bongard F, Pianim N, Cubecz S, Klein SR. Adverse consequences of increased intra-abdominal pressure on bowel tissue oxygen. J Trauma 1995;39:519–525.
75. Pusajo JF, Bumaschny E, Agurrola A, et al. Postoperative intra-abdominal pressure: its relation to splanchnic perfusion, sepsis, multiple organ failure and surgical reintervention. Intensive Surg Crit Care Dig 1994;13:2–4.
76. Joseph DK, Dutton RP, Aarabi B, Scalea TM. Decompressive laparotomy to treat intractable intracranial hypertension after traumatic brain injury. J Trauma 2004;57:687–695.
77. Rosin D, Rosenthal RJ. Adverse hemodynamic effects of intra-agdominal pressure—is it all in the head? J Surg Invest 2000;2:335–345.
78. Citerio G, Vascotto E, Villa F, Celotti S, Pesenti A. Induced abdominal compartment syndrome increases intracranial pressure in neurotrauma patients: a prospective study. Crit Care Med 2001;29:1466–1471.
79. Bloomfield GL, Dalton JM, Sugerman HJ, et al. Treatment of increasing intracranial pressure secondary to the acute abdominal compartment syndrome in a patient with combined abdominal and head trauma. J Trauma 1995;39:1168–1170.
80. Bloomfield GL, Ridings PC, Blocher CR, Marmarou A, Sugerman HJ. Effects of increased intra-abdominal pressure upon intracranial and cerebral perfusion pressure before and after volume expansion. J Trauma 1996;40:936–943.
81. Bloomfield GL, Ridings PC, Blocher CL, et al. A proposed relationship between increased intra-abdominal, intrathoracic, and intracranial pressure. Crit Care Med 1997;25:496–503.
82. Josephs LG, Este-McDonald JR, Birkett DH, Hirsch EF. Diagnostic laparoscopy increases intracranial pressure. J Trauma 1994;36:815–819.
83. Diebel L, Saxe J, Dulchavsky S. Effect of intra-abdominal pressure on the abdominal wall blood flow. Am Surg 1992;58:573.
84. Barnes GE, Laine GA, Giam PY, Smith EE, Granger HJ. Cardiovascular responses to elevation of intra-abdominal hydrostatic pressure. Am J Physiol 1985;248:R208–R213.
85. Obeid F, Saba A, Fath J, et al. Increases in intra-abdominal pressure affect pulmonary compliance. Arch Surg 1995;130:544–548.
86. MacDonnell SPJ, Lalude OA, Davidson AC. Letter to the editor. JACS 1996;183:19–20.
87. Biffl WL, Moore EE, Burch J. Femoral arterial graft failure caused by the secondary abdominal compartment syndrome. J Trauma 2001;50:740–742.
88. Edil GH, Tuggle DW, Puffinbarger NK, Mantor PC, Palmer GW, Knutson ZA. The impact of intra-abdominal hypertension on gene expression in the kidney. J Trauma 2003;55:857–859.
89. Rezende-Neto JB, Moore EE, De Andrade MVM, et al. Systemic inflammatory response secondary to abdominal compartment syndrome: stage for multiple organ failure. J Trauma 2002;53:1121–1128.
90. Le Roith D, Bark H, Nyska M, Glick SM. The effect of abdominal pressure on plasma antidiuretic hormone levels in the dog. J Surg Res 1982;32:65–69.
91. Meldrum DR, Moore FA, Moore EE, Francoise RJ, Sauala A, Burch JM. Prospective characterization and selective management of the abdominal compartment syndrome. Am J Surg 1997;174:667–673.
92. Malbrain M. Abdominal pressure in the critically ill: measurement and clinical relevance. Intensive Care Med 1999;25:1453–1458.
93. Offner PJ, de Souza AL, Moore EE, et al. Avoidance of abdominal compartment syndrome in damage-control laparotomy after trauma. Arch Surg 2001;136:676–681.
94. Mayberry JC, Mullins RJ, Crass RA, Trunkey DD. Prevention of abdominal compartment syndrome by absorbable mesh prosthesis closure. Arch Surg 1997;132:957–962.
95. Rotondo MF, Schwab CW, McGonigal MD, et al. "Damage control": an approach for improved survival in exsanguinating penetrating abdominal injury. J Trauma 1993;35:375–383.
96. Johnson JW, Gracias VH, Schwab CW, et al. Evolution in damage control for exsanguinating penetrating abdominal injury. J Trauma 2001;51:261–269.
97. Cheatham ML, Whiet MW, Sagraves SG, Johnson JL, Block EFJ. Abdominal perfusion pressure: a superior parameter in the assessment of intra-abdominal hypertension. J Trauma 2000;49:621–627.
98. Macalino JU, Goldman RK, Mayberry JC. Medical management of abdominal compartment syndrome: case report and a caution. Asian J Surg 2002;25:244–246.
99. Latenser BA, Kowal-Vern A, Kimball K, Chakrin A, Dujovny N. A pilot study comparing percutaneous decompression with decompressive laparotomy for acute abdominal compartment syndrome in thermal injury. J Burn Care Rehabil 2002;23:190–195.
100. Tsoutsos D, Rodopoulou S, Kermidas E, Lagios M, Stamatopoulos K, Ioannovich J. Early escharotomy as a measure to reduce intraabdominal hypertension in full-thickness burns of the thoracic and abdominal area. World J Surg 2003;27:1323–1328.
101. Bloomfield G, Saggi B, Blocher C, Sugerman H. Physiologic effects of externally applied continuous negative abdominal pressure for intra-abdominal hypertension. J Trauma 1999;46:1009–1014.
102. McNelis J, Soffer S, Marini CP, et al. Abdominal compartment syndrome in the surgical intensive care unit. Am Surg 2002;68:18–23.
103. Williams M, Simms HH. Abdominal compartment syndrome: case reports and implication for management in critically ill patients. Am Surg 1997;63:555–558.
104. Morris JA Jr, Eddy VA, Blinnman TA, Rutherford EJ, Sharp KW. The staged celiotomy for trauma: issues in packing and reconstruction. Ann Surg 1993;217:576–586.
105. Sener G, Kacmaz A, User Y, Ozkan S, Tilki M, Yegen BC. Melatonin ameliorates oxidative organ damage induced by acute intra-abdominal compartment syndrome in rats. J Pineal Res 2003;35:163–168.
106. Kacmaz A, Polat A, User Y, Tilki M, Ozkan S, Sener G. Octreotide improves reperfusion-induced oxidative injury in acute abdominal hypertension in rats. J Gastrointest Surg 2004;8:113–119.
107. Gracias VH, Braslow B, Johnson J, et al. Abdominal compartment syndrome in the open abdomen. Arch Surg 2002;137:1198–1300.
108. Oelschlager BK, Boyle EM, Johansen K, Meissner MH. Delayed abdominal closure in the management of ruptured abdominal aortic aneurysms. Am J Surg 1997;173:411–415.
109. Rasmussen TE, Hallett JW, Noel AA, et al. Early abdominal closure with mesh reduces multiple organ failure after ruptured abdominal aortic aneurysm repair: guidelines from a 10-year case-control study. J Vasc Surg 2002;35:246–253.
110. Mayberry JC. Bedside open abdominal surgery. Critical Care Clin 2000;16:151–172.
111. Ghimenton F, Thomson SR, Muckart DJJ, Burrows R. Abdominal content containment: practicalities and outcome. Br J Surg 2000;87:106–109.
112. Jernigan TW, Fabian TC, Croce MA, et al. Staged management of giant abdominal wall defects. Ann Surg 2003;238:349–357.
113. Barker DE, Kaufman HJ, Smith LA, Ciraulo DL, Richart CL, Burns RP. Vacuum pack technique of temporary abdominal closure: a 7-year experience with 112 patients. J Trauma 2000;48:201–206.

114. Wittmann DH, Aprahamian C Bergstein JM. Etappenlavage. Advanced diffuse peritonitis managed by planned multiple laparotomies utilizing zippers, slide fastener, and Velcro analogue for temporary abdominal closure. World J Surg 1990;14:218–226.
115. Kafie FE, Tessier DJ, Williams RA, et al. Serial abdominal closure technique (the "SAC" procedure): a novel method for delayed closure of the abdominal wall. Am Surg 2003;69:102–105.
116. Koniaris LG, Hendrickson RJ, Drugas G, Abt P, Shoeniger LO. Dynamic retention. A technique for closure of the complex abdomen in critically ill patients. Arch Surg 2001;136:1359–1362.
117. Tremblay LN, Feliciano DV, Schmidt J, et al. Skin only or silo closure in the critically ill patient with an open abdomen. Am J Surg 2002;182:670–675.
118. Cheatham ML, Safcsak K, Llerena LE, Morrow CE Jr, Block EFJ. Long-term physical, mental and functional consequences of abdominal decompression. J Trauma 2003;56:237–242.

35

Principles of Surgical Rehabilitation

Michael W. O'Dell and Tammy Noren

Definition and Philosophy of Rehabilitation Medicine

Rehabilitation is the branch of medicine that addresses the maximization of human performance. Because rehabilitation interventions differ widely among various clinical settings, the definition of "performance" might be as sophisticated as the speed of an elite athlete following a musculoskeletal injury or as basic as bed mobility in a patient with catastrophic brain or spinal cord injury. However, interventions in both settings focus on improving performance at some level. Performance activities required to move more effectively in the environment or to care for one's self are termed "functional activities," or function. Maximization of function is the primary endpoint in nearly all rehabilitation in a surgical setting. Advances in surgical and medical care during the past decades have substantially decreased mortality from many types of illness and injury. These achievements magnify the importance of rehabilitation professionals in the initial mobilization of surgical patients in the hospital and management of residual functional deficits after discharge.

The 1980 World Health Organization (WHO) International Classification of Impairment, Disability, and Handicaps[1] serves as a helpful philosophical framework to discuss the relationships between (1) illness and performance and (2) rehabilitation medicine and surgery. Table 35.1 outlines the WHO terminology and interventions within the context of a person with a C7 traumatic spinal cord injury. Ultimately, all branches of medicine strive to improve quality of life by maximizing performance, that is, minimizing disability. Surgery improves performance by the direct treatment of disease, such as the removal, repair, replacement, or reconstruction of abnormal or injured tissues. Internal medicine does the same with the use of medications and various procedures. However, interventions in rehabilitation medicine often occur directly at the level of functional performance and may have no appreciable impact on the underlying disease process or injury (see Table 35.1 for examples of rehabilitation interventions for disability and handicap).

Treatment of functional performance uses several basic strategies,[2] including techniques to enhance recovery of affected or diseased systems,[3] to use compensatory techniques to utilize fully the nonaffected systems that remain intact,[4] to prevent further disability during treatment,[5] to use adaptive equipment to facilitate function of an extremity,[6] to modify or match the environment with a person's capabilities, and to understand the importance of patient motivation, cognitive deficits, depression, and anxiety in the rehabilitation process[7] (see Table 35.2; adapted from DeLisa et al.[2]). Implementing one or several of these strategies results in greater independence in mobility or self-care, even if the disease process itself is likely unaffected.

Rehabilitation Team Members

Rehabilitation professionals work as a team to maximize independence. Patient, family, and team should realize that, in some cases of severe disease or injury, "maximizing," rather than "normalizing," performance may be the only realistic endpoint of treatment.[2] Physical therapy (PT) focuses on locomotion in the form of bed mobility, transfers, ambulation with or without an assistive device, and manual or motorized wheelchair mobility. Occupational therapy (OT) is concerned with activities of daily living (ADL, such as bathing, dressing, feeding, and grooming) and instrumental-ADL (higher-level skills such as cooking, home maintenance, use of public transportation). OT professionals also have special training in functional cognition, visual rehabilitation, and swallowing evaluation. Some PT and OT have expertise in the evaluation

TABLE 35.1. World Health Organization Classification of Human Disablement (1980).[a]

Case description: Consider a 26-year-old construction worker with complete C7 spinal cord injury from a fall. He has a wife, was planning on having children, and lives in a three-story walk-up apartment.

Term	*Level of dysfunction*	*Example*	*Interventions*
Disease	Cellular	Spinal cord edema, petechial hemorrhages, secondary injury from calcium influx into parenchymal cells	**Surgery:** methylprednisolone, adequate oxygenation and supportive care **Rehabilitation:** none
Impairment	Organ system (i.e., signs and symptoms)	**Acute:** unstable cervical spine fracture, paraplegia, complete sensory loss **Chronic:** spastic hypertonia, flexion contractures of hips and knees, depression	**Surgery:** acute: surgical fixation of spine, traction; chronic: functional tendon transfers, surgical management of decubiti, placement of intrathecal baclofen pump **Rehabilitation:** acute: stretching, range of motion, positioning, cushions to prevent skin breakdown, splints, strengthen arms; chronic: home stretching and exercise program, functional splints, spasticity medications or injections, mood counseling or treatment
Disability	Person (i.e., performance)	Unable to move in bed, unable to stand or ambulate, unable to transfer into a wheelchair, unable to feed self or perform lower extremity bathing and dressing	**Rehabilitation:** wheelchair mobility, transfer training with sliding board, adaptive equipment for dressing and bathing, education in self bowel and bladder management, monitor skin status **Surgery:** routine follow-up for interventions outlined above
Handicap	Society, roles	Unable to support family as a construction worker, cannot return to non-elevator-accessible home, sexual dysfunction impacting family planning	**Rehabilitation:** social service support for housing and job retraining, electroejaculation for pregnancy, explore wheelchair-level activities to interact with children **Surgery:** none

[a]*Source:* World Health Organization. International Classification of Impairments, Disability, and Handicaps. Geneva: WHO, 1980.[1]

and treatment of vestibular disorders with dizziness. The speech-language pathologist assesses and treats communication (aphasia, dysarthria, and dysphonia), cognitive disorders, and in many cases, swallowing. Rehabilitation medicine physicians (physiatrists) are trained to assess the relationships between impairment and disability and how a patient's medical status will impact the treatment of those deficits by the rehabilitation team. In the inpatient rehabilitation setting, the physiatrist directs the team in a coordinated and goal-directed plan of care. Rehabilitation services are often pro-

TABLE 35.2. Categories of Rehabilitation Intervention for Disability.

Intervention category	*Example*	*Result*
Prevent further disability	Serial casting Early bladder training Nighttime hand splint	Improved ROM Fewer UTI Improved ROM, less pain
Enhance *affected* systems	Constraint-induced therapy Neuromuscular stimulation Discontinue detrimental drugs	Improved strength, movement Improved strength, movement Improved rate of recovery
Enhance *unaffected* systems	Strengthen arms Left-handed writing/dressing	Compensate for paraparesis Compensate for right hemiplegia
Adaptive equipment and prostheses	Below-knee prostheses Walker, cane Sliding board	Facilitate ambulation in BKA Improved safety and endurance Improved safety and independence of transfers
Environmental modification	Install grab bars in home bathroom Install ramp into home	Improved safety and independence Decreased burden of care, increase independence
Psychological techniques	Initiation of antidepressant Using written instructions	Improved participation in and benefit from therapy Facilitate carryover with poor auditory comprehension/memory

ROM, range of motion; UTI, urinary tract infections; BKA, below-knee amputation.

Source: Adapted from DeLisa JA, Currie DM, Martin GM. Rehabilitation medicine: past, present and future. In: DeLisa JA, ed. Physical Medicine and Rehabilitation: Principles and Practice, 3rd ed. Philadelphia: Lippincott, 1998:3–32.[2]

vided without the direct involvement of a rehabilitation medicine physician. However, in certain circumstances, direct consultation is particularly useful. For example, a patient with a moderate traumatic brain injury may have bilateral lower extremity spastic hypertonia, ankle contractures, pain from a concomitant fracture, and hemiparesis with resultant severe ambulation deficits. A physiatrist may be helpful in delineating the extent to which each impairment contributes to the ambulation deficit. Management suggestions can then be made to both the surgical team and therapy staff. It is common for the physiatrist to recommend discharge venues for further rehabilitation such as acute or subacute rehabilitation, outpatient therapy, or home care. Consultation may also be helpful in surgical planning, for example, how a patient's cardiovascular limitations might impact prosthetic training in an amputee or the functional choice of a tendon for transfer.

When providing orders for either inpatient or outpatient PT and OT, the surgeon or surgeon-in-training should clearly provide the diagnosis for treatment, the frequency and duration of treatment, and delineate any precautions or special monitoring required of the therapist (e.g., weight-bearing restrictions, range-of-motion limitations, parameters for vital signs with activity).

Progression of Mobility Following Surgery

The role of rehabilitation evolves dramatically following surgery (Table 35.3), serving both a preventive and therapeutic role. There may be little or no rehabilitation involvement for the critically ill patient who will not tolerate additional activity physiologically. Activities progress from passive prevention of complications to active bed mobility in the intensive care unit (ICU), through short-distance ambulation and home independence on the general hospital floor to community reentry in the outpatient setting. For a subset of substantially impaired patients, acute or subacute inpatient rehabilitation may be appropriate. In these settings, mobilization and self-care skills are the primary focus of hospitalization. Treatment interventions include manual techniques, therapeutic exercise, functional mobility activities, adaptive equipment, bracing, gait training, and patient/family education.

Consequences of Immobility

In the mid-20th century, bed rest and prolonged immobilization were prescribed commonly as treatment. Although warranted in certain conditions (e.g., fractures, back pain), immobilization is now understood to have detrimental consequences (Fig. 35.1).[8] Even after only 72h, the deleterious effects of bed rest have already commenced in several systems.[9] Muscle strength can decline by as much as 1.5% per day after strict bed rest, with the greatest loss after the first week (as much as 40%.)[10] Type I muscle fibers used for transfers and ambulation appear to be affected disproportionately.[11] Even when strength is decreased only mildly, poor endurance can still be a primary functional limitation. Both the central and peripheral cardiovascular systems are altered, with increased heart rate and decreased stroke volume and cardiac size. Close communication with the surgical team

TABLE 35.3. Evolution of Surgical Rehabilitation Interventions.

Time period	*Typical surgical activities*	*Typical rehabilitation activities*
ICU: medically unstable	Stabilization of vital signs and hemorrhage, mechanical ventilation, surgical stabilization of injury	None (if medically unstable), passive ROM by nursing staff
ICU: medically stable	Ventilation weaning, treatment of infections, further surgical interventions as needed, nutritional supplementation	Active ROM, positioning and splinting of limbs to prevent contracture, bed mobility to facilitate pressure relief, bedside sitting, standing, steps
Medical-surgical floor	Adjustment of oral medications, further nonemergent diagnostic or therapeutic testing, observation of surgical wounds for healing	Short-distance ambulation training, strengthening, endurance, education on precautions or restrictions, ADL training, assess safety for home discharge or need for further rehabilitation
Acute *inpatient* rehabilitation	Occasional follow-up on IRU to monitor wound healing, medication adjustment, late surgical complications	*Primary focus* (3h/day) on home-level mobilization, self-care training: household-level ambulation with assistive device, transfer training, wheelchair use, use of prosthetic device, bathing, dressing; expect 1- to 3-week length of stay and need for daily medical care
Subacute inpatient rehabilitation	Surgical F/U for late complications of surgery and medication adjustments, transport from skilled nursing facility to clinic	Substantial focus (1–2h/day) on household-level mobilization along with general convalescence, does not require daily medical care
Outpatient rehabilitation	Routine outpatient F/U as needed, may have been discharged from surgical care	Focus on community-level ambulation and home maintenance skills, high-level endurance, balance, and strengthening; transportation sometimes limited

ICU, intensive care unit; IRU, inpatient rehabilitation unit; ADL, activities of daily living; ROM, range of motion; F/U, follow-up.

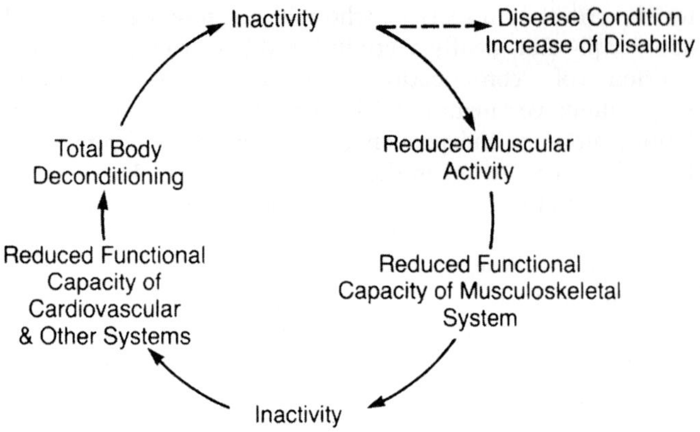

FIGURE 35.1. The cycle of immobility demonstrates diminished muscular and cardiovascular reserves, which make mobilization more difficult. (From DeLisa JA, Currie DM, Martin GM,[2] by permission of Lippincott.)

is required to determine the appropriate time to initiate mobilization.

Intensive Care Unit

Even the most basic mobilization will help counteract the effects of prolonged bed rest and maintain or improve strength, functional ability, and endurance. Depending on medical stability, the focus of rehabilitation in the ICU is the patient's ability to roll, shift weight, grab, sit, and stand. Ambulation may or may not be part of the treatment. Particularly with prolonged ICU stays, initial interventions are rather passive, including an evaluation of positioning and the need for splinting devices to maintain joint integrity and prevent skin breakdown. Active participation begins with exercises and positioning to enhance breathing, active and passive range of motion to prevent contracture, and therapeutic bed activities to build strength and endurance. If symptoms and vital signs are stable, functional mobility is initiated in a hierarchical fashion. For example, bed mobility progresses from rolling with to rolling without a side rail to sitting, as muscle strength and endurance improve. The transition from a supine to sitting position can be especially challenging. Incisional pain and truncal muscle weakness may result in increased time and effort to perform these tasks. Adequate pain control is mandatory to initiate mobilization. Relaxation techniques such as guided meditation, mental imagery, and deep breathing may help decrease pain. Self-administered splinting techniques using a pillow are helpful to decrease incisional pain during movement.

Once sitting, therapists will then have the patient perform therapeutic activities as a precursor to performing standing and out-of-bed activities. As the patient progresses and more complex activities are performed, other underlying weaknesses or pathologies may become apparent (i.e., peroneal neuropathy, inflammation or trauma at joints, cognitive or visual deficits). PT/OT may be the first disciplines to identify these impairments and report to the surgical team in case further evaluation is required.

In the event that the patient is unable to tolerate sitting on the edge of the bed, other methods may be used. Elevating the head of the bed for progressively longer periods of time can help with orthostasis and give a head start to assuming a sitting position. Hospital beds that flex upward at the head and downward at the foot, converting into a chair-like apparatus, allow the benefits of maintaining an upright posture even though weakness or fatigue prevent positioning. Benefits of sitting include increased activation of trunk musculature, increased weight-bearing through pelvis and legs, a heightened level of arousal, and the potential for interaction with the environment.

Rehabilitation interventions in the ICU can help address pulmonary issues as well.[12] Mechanical ventilation is not a contraindication to participate in rehabilitation, assuming the patient is oxygenated adequately. If the patient is already utilizing accessory muscles (trapezius or scalene muscles) or is tachypnic at more than 35 breaths/min, therapy may not be appropriate. For patients initiating some degree of spontaneous breathing, PT can assist the patient to develop a more efficient breathing pattern using manual techniques to improve lung aeration, rib cage expansion, diaphragm capacity, and decreased accessory muscle use. An abdominal binder increases intraabdominal pressure and may allow the diaphragm to work more effectively.

Constant monitoring is required with any patient who is medically tenuous or on mechanical ventilation. Participation will fluctuate session to session, with respiratory and heart rates and oxygen saturation levels indicating how well a patient is tolerating treatment. The impact of medications and pain on heart rate must also be considered.

Arousal level is also a frequent limitation. Elevating the head of the bed to stimulate the reticular activating system, repositioning, and stimulation with deep pressure, sounds, and smells are all used to enhance responsiveness. For patients with neurological disease, the use of a standardized assessment scale is recommended, for example, the Coma Recovery Scale.[13] For the agitated patient, relaxation techniques, reorientation, and decreasing environmental stimulation may be attempted before pharmacological treatment.

Medical-Surgical Floor

After medical stabilization and transfer to the floor, rehabilitation becomes a more integral part of the recovery and discharge process. The focus of therapy here is progression to medium-level functional skills such as standing, transfers, short-distance ambulation, stair climbing, and ADL, all of which are needed for home discharge. Accurate assessment of these skills are key factors in discharge planning. The identification of patients who are not likely to achieve independence, with or without supervision, should prompt a referral for acute or subacute rehabilitation. Medical and functional limitations such as poor endurance and balance, pain, and weakness should be distinguished from psychological barriers, such as fear, anxiety, malingering, or manipulation.

Gait training begins with dynamic standing activities, such as reaching or lateral weight shifts. Activities outside the base of support may reveal unrecognized, high-level balance deficits or weakness. For example, a patient may compensate for weak hip extensors by either assuming a forward flexed posture or increased lumbar lordosis to improved stability in standing. The functional sequelae of specific muscle weakness can be alleviated with braces, such as an ankle-foot orthosis for dorsiflexion weakness. Fear of falling is common, especially for elderly patients after a prolonged hospitalization, and can be ameliorated with an assistive device to increase stability and normalize gait patterns. The appropriate device should provide the greatest stability but be least restrictive for the patient. For example, although a standard walker provides more stability than a rolling walker, the latter provides a much greater degree of mobility. A cane can be used for minimal balance deficits to provide an additional point of contact and increase the base of support. With improved confidence comes greater activity to enhance endurance and stamina. A strong patient–therapist relationship greatly facilitates progress.[14] As in the ICU, constant monitoring of symptoms and vital signs dictates the rate of progression. Not surprising, therapists with more experience tend to be more aggressive in their treatment approach and advancing functional activities. Stair training is generally provided only if required for home discharge. Upon discharge, a patient may require referral for home services including PT and OT to allow the patient to participate in community activities and regain or maximize functional independence. Home therapy is an excellent opportunity to tailor treatment to a familiar and consistent environment.

Outpatient Setting

Referral to outpatient PT or OT is indicated when functional needs lie in the higher realm of community reintegration (rather than home activities) and is common for patients with neurological and more long-term impairment. Many hospitals have protocol-driven, specialized programs in cardiac and pulmonary rehabilitation. Outpatient interventions differ in intensity more than character. Programs may utilize weight training for strengthening and treadmills and stationary bicycles for aerobic conditioning. Gait training focuses not only on endurance and distance but also fine-tuning of abnormal gait patterns because of weakness, contracture, pain, or fear. OT shifts to a focus on higher-level home management (e.g., laundry, meal preparation, home maintenance, money management). Pain reduction techniques utilize therapeutic hot and cold, massage, and electrical stimulation. Pool therapy is used to help normalize movement patterns when weakness or joint pain are limitations. Scar management, especially in patients with burns and amputations, includes use of over-the-counter and custom-made pressure dressings and manual scar mobilization to decrease connective tissue adhesions.

Surgical Rehabilitation Principles: Specific Diagnoses

Burn Injuries

There may be no other area where surgeons, nurses, and rehabilitation professionals work so closely together over such long periods of time as after burn injuries. The primary interventions by rehabilitation professionals address range of motion, mobility, and scar management.[15] In the initial days after a severe burn, patients often assume an adducted and flexed posture to minimize pain; therefore, positioning and splinting tend to emphasize abduction and extension of the extremities.[16] In general, exposed tendons should be splinted in the slack position to minimize risk of rupture and exposed joints placed in a functional position (assuming they will eventually ankylose). Serial casting can improve range in joints and tissues already contracted, with the best clinical results commonly seen at the elbow.[17] Continuous passive motion devices are used to improve range in the hand[18] and other joints.[16]

Burns to the hand are functionally devastating. Chronic edema and inelastic eschar underlie the deformity known as "claw" hand. Exposed digital tendons and joints can lead to boutonniere and swan neck deformities, mallet finger, and anklyosed joints.[15] After substantial healing has occurred, warm paraffin baths are employed, providing both heat to facilitate active and passive ROM and lubrication to soften skin and scar tissue. Static, or immobile, splints are used for prolonged stretching of contracted tissue, or tissue at risk for contracture, and are often worn at night. Dynamic splints, made with movable parts, are used primarily at the hand to take advantage of residual ROM and strength, and are specifically constructed to facilitate functional movements, such as grasp or pinch (Fig. 35.2).

Mobilizing a burn patient from bed can be extremely difficult because of pain, fear of falling, recent skin grafting, cognitive deficits, or severe deconditioning and weakness. Although many burn units wait 5 days, a recent class I study demonstrated that ambulation as early as 3 days post-lower extremity skin grafting will facilitate mobility without risk to the grafts.[19] Using a modified tilt table may help a patient acclimate gradually to an upright position (avoiding orthostatic hypotension), increase cardiopulmonary endurance, improve overall strength, and regain self-confidence.[20] Peripheral and mononeuropathies[21] and heterotopic ossification[22] complicate both mobilization and ROM.

Scar management is the active modification and remodeling of tissue that occurs later in the hospital stay or in the outpatient setting. It should be distinguished from more acute wound care that focuses on prevention of infection and debridement of nonviable tissue. Therapists facilitate scar management using various techniques including manual soft tissue mobilization, application of pressure garments,

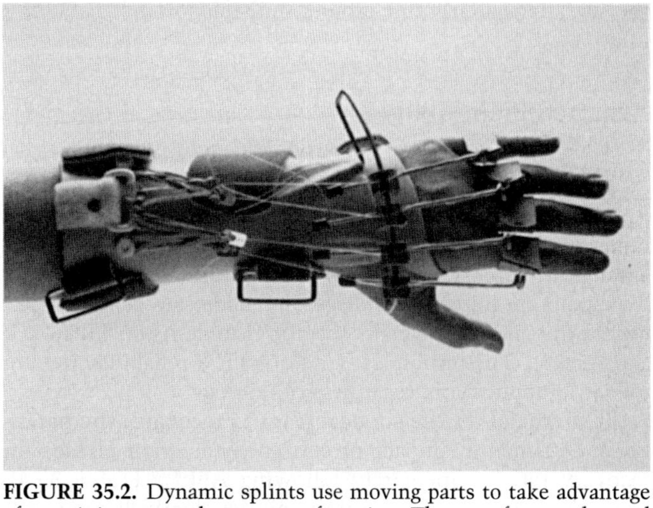

FIGURE 35.2. Dynamic splints use moving parts to take advantage of remaining strength or range of motion. They are frequently used in hand injuries and burns.

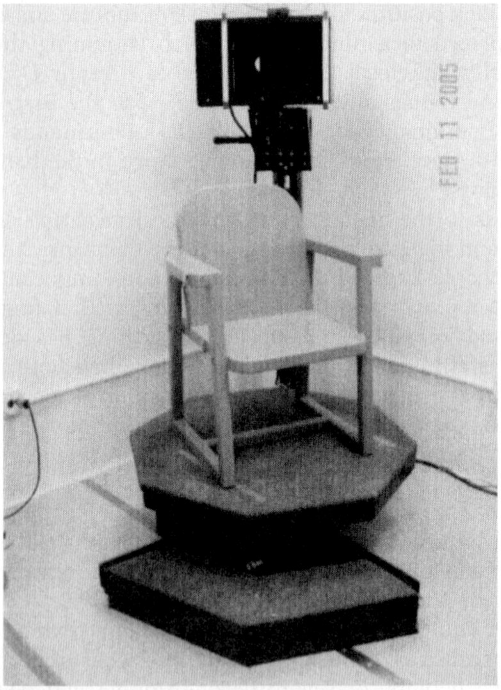

FIGURE 35.3. Apparatus for making facial masks in burns shows the Cyberware 3030 PS/RGB scanning system (Total Contact, Inc., Germantown, OH) machine that uses LASAR technology to generate extremely accurate, clear facial pressure masks to remodel scars following facial burns. The scanner above the chair makes a detailed, digital topographic depiction of the face from which a transparent mask can be fabricated.

massage, stretching, casting, and splinting. Pressure strategies for scar management at the face are particularly difficult because of its irregular contour and crucial cosmetic importance.[16] Transparent facial pressure masks can be created by either plaster molds or, more recently, using digital light technology (Fig. 35.3).[23] Patients must embrace the importance of long-term rehabilitation that includes antagonist muscle strengthening used to combat scar and contracture formation and ongoing stretching along the entire length of the scar, particularly if it crosses multiple joints.[15]

Acquired Brain Injury

General Issues in Neurological Rehabilitation

Acquired brain injury (ABI) refers to adult cerebral disease or injury including traumatic brain injury (TBI), aneurysmal subarachnoid hemorrhage (SAH), brain tumors, stroke, and hypoxic brain injury. This discussion addresses general treatment principles followed by specific comments on TBI, SAH, and tumors. The principles of neurological rehabilitation are robust in application, regardless of etiology.

It is crucial for the surgical team to recognize the potentially detrimental impact of certain medication classes on recovery rates immediately following ABI[24–26] (Table 35.4). Animals with experimental brain injuries clearly demonstrate slower recovery rates when given neuroleptics,[27] benzodiazepines,[28] centrally acting antihypertensives,[29] and the antiepileptics phenytoin[26] and phenobarbital.[30] Clinical studies have demonstrated delayed motor recovery after stroke with benzodiazepines (Class III data),[31] delayed cognitive recovery in TBI with phenytoin (Class I data),[25] and delayed intellectual development in children receiving phenobarbital (Class I data).[32] Seizure prophylaxis in TBI should be limited to 1 week only (Class I data).[33,34] Prophylaxis data in SAH are weak, at best,[35] and prophylaxis appears to be ineffective altogether in brain tumors.[36,37] Reasonable substitutions are available for these four medication classes, as outlined in Table 35.5. Alternatively, solid animal data[24,27,38] and initial human studies suggest that neurostimulants can enhance motor, functional, and language recovery following TBI,[39–41] stroke,[42,43] and brain tumors.[44] Allowing animals to practice a motor task in conjunction with neurostimulants (generally interpreted as a "rehabilitation" equivalent) consistently improves recovery.[24,27,45,46]

Rehabilitation interventions in ABI are focused on symptoms, rather than etiology. Speech pathologists provide interventions for aphasia (language deficits), dysarthria (articulation deficits), dysphonia (sound production deficits), and verbal apraxia (motor planning deficits). Although objective efficacy data are sparse,[47] aphasia treatment includes verbal and visual cues to prompt accurate verbal production ("stimulation-facilitation"), identification and application of compensatory strategies, and language initiation using right brain circuitry (melodic intonation therapy), among others.[4] Communication deficits following TBI and SAH are often "cognitive-linguistic," presenting with confabulation or sexually/socially inappropriate comments because of frontal lobe disinhibition (pragmatic deficits). PT and OT facilitation of motor recovery includes extremity weight-bearing to elicit sensory and proprioceptive feedback, guided movement of weak limbs to reinforce normal movement patterns, functional electrical stimulation, and aggressive stretching to improve both spastic hypertonia and contracture that may limit movements.[4,48] Stretching is vastly underutilized as a method to prevent contracture and decrease muscle tone (Fig. 35.4). Other methods of interest include use of robotics,[49] partial weight-bearing suspension devices (Fig. 35.5),[50] and "constraint-induced movement therapy," where an intact limb is restrained to force the patient to use the paretic side.[51] Hypertonia can limit ambulation and ADL, and is treated acutely with oral medications, and more chronically with phenol and botulinum toxin injections if focal, or placement of an intrathecal baclofen pump if severe and generalized.[52] Neglect, seen with right brain damage, is defined as the failure to attend to one side of space. Strategies to address neglect include verbal and tactile cueing to the affected side, and standing or presenting information on the right side to elicit visual scanning to the left, although the ultimate impact on disability is unclear.[53] Cognitive problems can be difficult to identify during periods of critical illness during mechanical ventilation, neuromuscular blockade, and sedation. As already mentioned, therapists are often the first team members to discover cognitive deficits during transfers, ambulation, or self-care activities that require attention, carryover, and multistep planning. Cognitive rehabilitation remains controversial[54] but uses strategies geared toward reducing complex cognitive processes into manageable subcomponents. Feedback and self-monitoring gradually improve

TABLE 35.4

Selected Evidence-Based Trials for Medications Management in Acquired Brain Injury.

Trial, year, reference	*Medication/population*	*Class*	*Randomized groups (n)*	*Follow-up*	*Major endpoint*	*Comments*
Potentially detrimental medications:						
Dikman 1991[25]	Phenytoin in TBI	I	208, treatment 196, placebo	2 years	Phenytoin impaired cognitive performance at 1 month, no difference at 1 year	Detrimental effect more prominent in early and severe TBI
Farwell 1990[32]	Phenobarbital in children with febrile seizures	I	108, treatment 109, placebo	2.5 years	Children receiving phenobarbital had mean intelligence quotients 8.4 points lower, still 5.2 points lower 6 months after drug stopped	Assumes aspects of developing brain in children may reflect healing brain in an adult after ABI
Temkin 1990[33]	Phenytoin for seizure prophylaxis in TBI	I	208, treatment 196, placebo	2 years	No benefit to phenytoin for seizure prevention in TBI after 7 days	Given detrimental impact on cognition as above, clear that drug should be stopped by day 8
Goldstein 1995[31]	Several drugs in stroke	II	NA: prospective study of 96 subjects, 37 in detrimental and 56 in neutral drug group	3 months	Lower functional scores (Barthel Index) and worse motor recovery in patients receiving detrimental medications	Not randomized, but post hoc analysis showed nearly identical baseline characteristics; data are best to support detrimental impact of benzodiazepines
Potentially advantageous medications:						
Walker-Batson 2001[43]	Dextroamphetamine for aphasia in stroke	I	12, treatment 9, placebo	6 months	Better performance on standardized aphasia measures after 10 doses/treatments, difference continued at 6 months but not statistically significant	Highly selected patients within 16–45h of stroke, 10-mg drug used with speech therapy sessions, no side effects occurred
Cristosomo 1988[42]	Amphetamine for motor recovery in acute stroke	I	4, treatment 4, placebo	3 days	Better motor scores after single dose of 10mg	Small *N*, highly selected patients more than 10 days from stroke, drug timed in conjunction with physical therapy, short follow-up
Plenger 1996[39]	Methylphenidate for recovery in TBI	I	10, treatment 13, placebo	3 months	At 30 days ($n = 12$) better functional and neuropsychological scores with drug, no difference at 90 days ($n = 9$)	Significant dropout, ? bias, patients on neurosurgical service, drugs may increase rate of but not ultimate recovery
Whyte 2004[41]	Methylphenidate for recovery and attention deficit in TBI	I	34, randomized, repeated crossover design (3 cycles)	6 weeks	Benefit from methylphenidate in a variety of attention tasks, effect sizes in small to medium range	Dose 0.6mg/kg/day, complicated assessment and analysis using chronic, TBI outpatients
Kaelin 1996[40]	Methylphenidate for recovery in TBI	III	NA: $n = 9$ (open, prospective crossover design)	3 weeks	Drug increased rate of functional and (basic) cognitive measures over natural recovery	Study in inpatient rehabilitation, suggests drug effect continues after discontinued
Meyer 1998[44]	Methylphenidate for mood, cognition and function in brain tumors	III	NA: case series of 26, testing pre- and post-drug treatment	Unclear, ? weeks	Improvements in a variety of standardized neuropsychological and mood tests, functional independence measure	Poor dose standardizations from 20 to 60mg/day, treatment duration unclear, ? better response at higher doses

TBI, traumatic brain injury; ABI, acquired brain injury; kg, kilogram; mg, milligram; NA, not applicable.

This evidence-based table represents selected clinical studies suggesting both detrimental and advantageous effects of medications following acquired brain injury.

TABLE 35.5. Substitutions for Potentially Detrimental Medications in Acquired Brain Injury.

Detrimental medication	*Possible substitution*	*Comments*
Phenobarbital, phenytoin	Levetiracetam, lamotrigene, topiramate, valproic acid, carbamazepine	Few clinical data on newer agents, valproic acid has no cognitive ill effect in TBI[25]
Benzodiazepines: sleep	Zolpidem, trazadone	Enteral only
Benzodiazepines: agitation	Propranolol, trazadone, buspirone, amantadine, valproic acid, carbamazepine, lithium	Other than propranolol, few data to support any one agent, all agents anecdotally reported helpful
Neuropeptics: agitation	Olanzapine, risperidone	Third-generation neuroleptics probably less detrimental, few data
Metoclopramide: gastrointestinal prokinetic effect	Erythromycin	Metoclopramide is chemically related to neuroleptic medications
Centrally acting antihypertensives (clonidine, etc.)	ACE-I, calcium channel and beta-blockers	Good animal data to support slowing of neurological recovery

TBI, traumatic brain injury; ACE-I, angiotensin-converting enzyme inhibitor.

This table outlines possible substitutions for potentially detrimental medications following acquired brain injury. Substitution may not be possible in certain clinical circumstances.

performance and generalize to broader, more functionally relevant tasks.

Traumatic Brain Injury

TBI is a heterogeneous diagnosis, ranging from mild injury with no loss of consciousness to patients with coma and vegetative state. Physiatry consultation may contribute to a shorter acute care length of stay.[55] The length of posttraumatic amnesia (time from injury to return of ongoing memory) is probably the best predictor of functional outcome.[56] Diffuse axonal injury is associated with attention deficits, a slower rate of recovery, and a longer duration of unconsciousness and posttraumatic amnesia.[4] Cerebral contusions commonly occur at the frontal and temporal poles, accounting for the typical symptoms of behavioral disinhibition and memory deficits, respectively.[4] Impulsiveness and disinhibition greatly complicate mobilization in concomitant pelvic and lower extremity fractures when weight-bearing restrictions are required. Agitation is associated with hypoxia, pain, impaired cognition (from either injury or sedating medications), sleep deprivation, and posttraumatic psychosis, among other manifestations. Impaired cognition may be a primary contributing

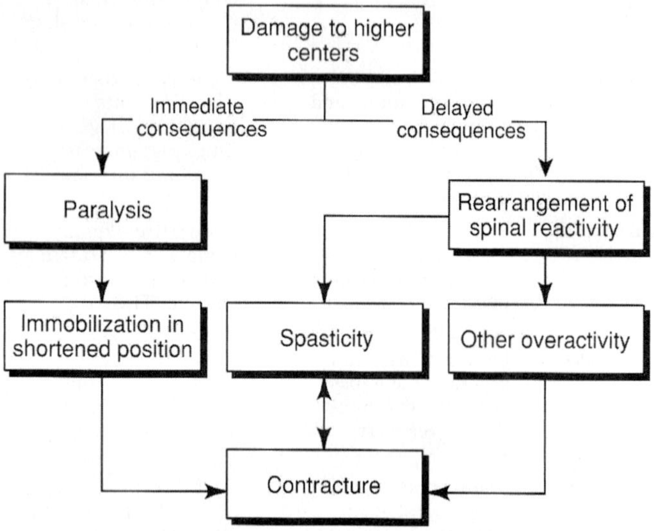

FIGURE 35.4. Relationships among tone, contracture, and stretching. Both weakness and spastic hypertonia contribute to contracture in central nervous system disease and injury. Stretching is greatly underestimated as a treatment for reducing hypertonia and should be an integral part of rehabilitation efforts. (From Gracies JM, Nance P, Elovic E, McGuire J, Simpson DM,[48] by permission of John Wiley & Sons, Inc.)

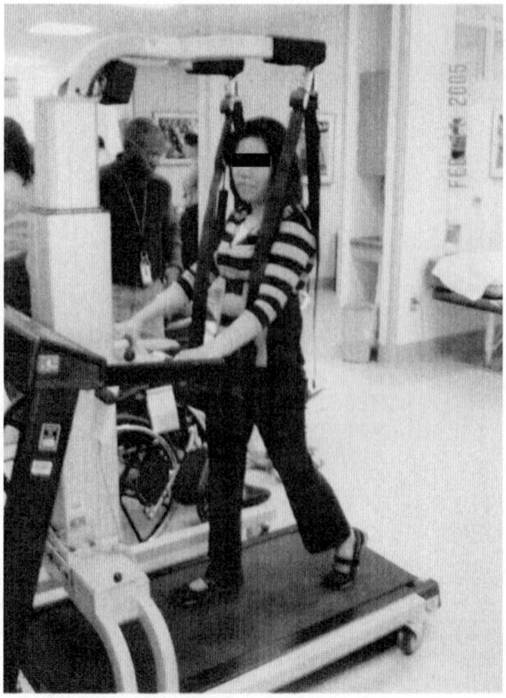

FIGURE 35.5. Device for partial weight-bearing suspension, such as the one pictured, suspend patients above a treadmill (or floor) to decrease weight-bearing in patients with cerebral or spinal cord injury. This apparatus may allow muscles too weak to support joint movement with full weight-bearing to do so now. The devices also take advantage of spinal cord reflexes used in walking.

factor to agitation and underscores the need to minimize sedating medications. First-generation neuroleptics should be used only as a last resort because of concerns, as discussed. Third-generation neuroleptic agents may be less detrimental.[57] The best data for the pharmacological treatment of agitation are for propranolol, although hypotension and bradycardia are frequent side effects.[58] Other alternatives are outlined in Table 35.5. Interventions for persons in coma or vegetative state are not well studied[59] but reasonably include physical management, aggressive medical and nursing care, medication trials (usually neurostimulants or dopamine agonists), and directed stimulation of the senses as an assessment method.[60] Following mild TBI, 10% to 20% of patients will develop "post-concussive disorder," characterized by continued symptoms such as headache, dizziness, and memory and attention deficits. Neuropathology, psychopathology, and secondary gain may all contribute to the clinical presentation.[61]

Subarachnoid Hemorrhage

Patients with SAH are distinguished by the potential for multiple neurological deficits: the initial parenchymal hemorrhage, infarctions from vasospasm, surgical morbidity, and hydrocephalus.[35] Poor Hunt and Hess scores do not appear to predict functional outcome following rehabilitation and should not discourage referral for rehabilitation in appropriate cases.[62] Anterior communicating artery aneurysm rupture sometimes presents with amnesia, confabulation, and personality changes—the so-called *A-Comm syndrome*—with generally intact motor function.[63] Patients following SAH show similar functional gains to groups with stroke and TBI in an inpatient rehabilitation setting.[62]

Brain Tumors

Brain tumor pathology substantially alters the rehabilitation approach because patients with less aggressive tumors (i.e., meningioma) may have long-term educational and vocational reintegration goals.[64] In aggressive disease (glioblastoma multiforme), functional mobility in the home setting and training for family members or caretakers may be the focus.[64] Patients with brain tumors also achieve comparable functional gain, as do TBI and stroke patients in inpatient rehabilitation, even while receiving radiation therapy.[65] Depression or anxiety can be intrinsic or secondary to steroids and should be treated if participation is impacted. Methylphenidate, up to 60mg/day, may be helpful for mood and function.[44]

Spinal Cord Injury

During the past 20 years, effective initial management and rehabilitation have resulted in a substantial decrease in mortality and morbidity among persons with spinal cord injuries (SCI).[4] SCI can be of traumatic or nontraumatic etiology (e.g., neoplasm, severe degenerative spine disease, vascular injury).[66] The initial surgical care of traumatic SCI involves management of vital functions (hypotension, hypothermia, respiratory compromise, bradycardia), closed spine reduction, or operative stabilization of the spine. The initial neurological assessment is crucial, relying on the standardized examination revised by the American Spinal Injury Association (ASIA) in 2002 (Figure 35.6).[67] Twenty-eight dermatomes and 10 muscle groups are assessed on each side of the body. After determining whether anal contraction is present, the injury can then be classified by neurological level, whether complete or incomplete (defined as the presence of motor or sensory function below the neurological level of injury), and whether a "zone of partial preservation" is present. The ASIA nomenclature designates a spinal level (e.g., C5) followed by the letter A if complete or B through E designating the type of incomplete injury.[67]

The initial muscle strength, and level and degree of injury, with or without neuroimaging and electrophysiological studies, are used for prognostication of neurological recovery and eventual functional outcome.[68] Compared with traumatic SCI, persons with nontraumatic etiologies tend to be older (>40 years), present with incomplete injuries, and as paraparesis rather than tetraparesis.[69]

Several interventions in the surgical ICU and on the floor can improve function and future rehabilitation efforts. Aggressive, early management of medical complications is associated with more successful inpatient rehabilitation and lower overall costs.[70] Aggressive range of motion to prevent contracture at the proximal limbs and ankles will decrease pain and facilitate functional performance should motor function return. Observation or report of a red, swollen joint with rapid loss of range below the neurological level of injury should prompt an investigation for heterotopic ossification.[71] Heterotopic ossification is most common at the hip, knee, or shoulder joints, but sensory loss may limit pain as a presenting symptom. Early splinting of the upper extremities may thwart the development of hand contractures. Splinting can also facilitate functional grip in C6 injuries with intact wrist extensors, as with the so-called tenodesis splint (Figure 35.7).[6] Depression is common and should be treated if it interferes with therapy participation.[70] Because of orthostasis and weakness, standing may need to be initiated on a tilt table with abdominal binders and lower extremity support stockings. Other rehabilitation methods include partial weight-bearing treadmill training (see Figure 35.4), use of functional electrical stimulation of affected muscles, and advances in wheelchair cushion and seating systems.[72]

Chronic problems include autonomic hyperreflexia with lesions above T6, usually manifesting beyond 1 month postinjury and presenting with headache and sweating above the level of injury, hypertension, and bradycardia. Immediate treatment is mandatory and includes loosening of tight clothing, bladder catheterization to relieve urinary retention, and use of topical nitrates or other pharmacological agents if the systolic blood pressure remains above 150mmHg.[66] Although spastic hypertonia can occasionally be beneficial, most times it contributes to contracture, pain, and poor wheelchair positioning, increasing the risk for decubitus ulceration.[66] In chronic SCI, surgeons may be involved in managing decubiti, tendon lengthening, and other functional orthopedic procedures, or in the placement of intrathecal baclofen pumps for management of refractory spastic hypertonia.[73]

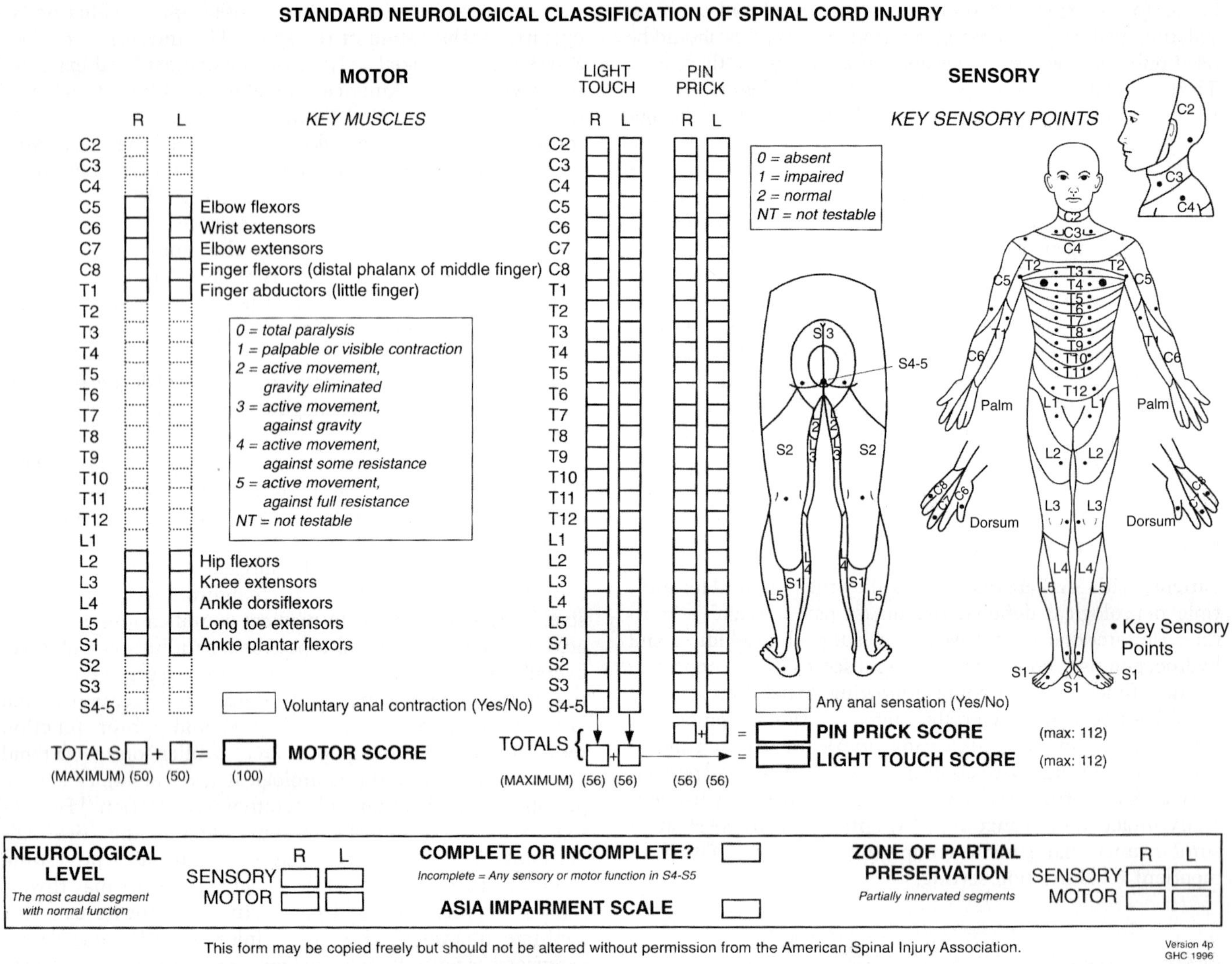

STANDARD NEUROLOGICAL CLASSIFICATION OF SPINAL CORD INJURY

MOTOR — KEY MUSCLES

	R	L	
C2			
C3			
C4			
C5			Elbow flexors
C6			Wrist extensors
C7			Elbow extensors
C8			Finger flexors (distal phalanx of middle finger)
T1			Finger abductors (little finger)
T2			
T3			
T4			
T5			
T6			
T7			
T8			
T9			
T10			
T11			
T12			
L1			
L2			Hip flexors
L3			Knee extensors
L4			Ankle dorsiflexors
L5			Long toe extensors
S1			Ankle plantar flexors
S2			
S3			
S4-5			

> 0 = total paralysis
> 1 = palpable or visible contraction
> 2 = active movement, gravity eliminated
> 3 = active movement, against gravity
> 4 = active movement, against some resistance
> 5 = active movement, against full resistance
> NT = not testable

☐ Voluntary anal contraction (Yes/No)

TOTALS ☐ + ☐ = ☐ **MOTOR SCORE**
(MAXIMUM) (50) (50) (100)

LIGHT TOUCH / PIN PRICK

	R	L		R	L
C2					
C3					
C4					
C5					
C6					
C7					
C8					
T1					
T2					
T3					
T4					
T5					
T6					
T7					
T8					
T9					
T10					
T11					
T12					
L1					
L2					
L3					
L4					
L5					
S1					
S2					
S3					
S4-5					

> 0 = absent
> 1 = impaired
> 2 = normal
> NT = not testable

☐ Any anal sensation (Yes/No)

TOTALS { ☐ ☐ } = ☐ **PIN PRICK SCORE** (max: 112)
☐ + ☐ = ☐ **LIGHT TOUCH SCORE** (max: 112)
(MAXIMUM) (56) (56) (56) (56)

SENSORY — KEY SENSORY POINTS

• Key Sensory Points

NEUROLOGICAL LEVEL		R	L	COMPLETE OR INCOMPLETE? ☐		ZONE OF PARTIAL PRESERVATION		R	L
The most caudal segment with normal function	SENSORY	☐	☐	Incomplete = Any sensory or motor function in S4-S5		Partially innervated segments	SENSORY	☐	☐
	MOTOR	☐	☐	**ASIA IMPAIRMENT SCALE** ☐			MOTOR	☐	☐

This form may be copied freely but should not be altered without permission from the American Spinal Injury Association.

Version 4p
GHC 1996

FIGURE 35.6. The American Spinal Injury Association Neurological Assessment should be completed on all patients with spinal cord injury (SCI). In traumatic SCI, scores can be used to assist with prognostication of functional outcomes.

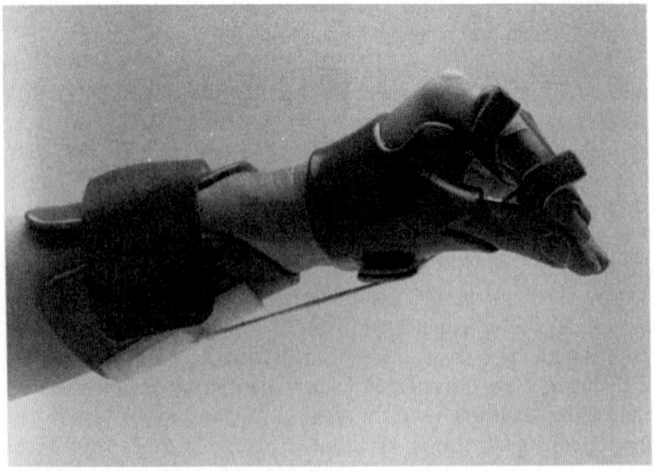

FIGURE 35.7. Tenodesis splints redirect forces from intact wrist extensors to the finger flexors, resulting in a grasping motion that can be used as functional grip in selected circumstances.

Multiple Orthopedic Trauma and Joint Replacements

The basic tenets of rehabilitation in brain injury, SCI, or amputation apply equally to those injuries in the presence of multiple orthopedic or visceral injuries. Surgical management facilitating the earliest possible mobilization appears advantageous in terms of both functional outcome[74] and possibly survival.[75] Beyond the initial life- and limb-saving management in the emergency department and ICU, as many as 75% of multiple trauma survivors experience a decrement in quality of life 1 year postinjury, with deficits in physical mobility quite common.[76] Musculoskeletal disability and pain are particularly common, especially in cases of simultaneous pelvic and appendicular fractures.[77] Because of the importance of these musculoskeletal injuries, rehabilitation professionals can provide an additional set of "eyes and hands" for the identification of secondary, non-life-threatening injuries (especially unrecognized fractures and peripheral nerve injuries).[78,79] Identification may occur during treatment when a therapist notes bruises, abrasions, or weakness during mobilization, more formally during a physiatry consultation, or later during the inpatient rehabilitation admission. The association of TBI and alcohol appears to increase the likelihood of unrecognized injuries.[78,80] The team should assume a peripheral nerve injury has occurred distal to any fracture until proven otherwise. Brachial plexus injuries are seen more commonly in motorcycle and snowmobile injuries compared with other motor vehicle collisions.[80] Grip strength is served primarily by the C8 and T1 nerve roots and cannot be used to rule out an injury to the upper trunk plexus, which innervates the shoulder musculature via C5 and C6. Nerve injuries occur in 10% to 15% of pelvic fractures, with the L5 and S1 roots involved frequently.[81]

With more than 340,000 cases annually in the United States (year 2000),[82] hip fracture is a major source of morbidity and mortality, especially in the geriatric population. Although earlier surgery may decrease hospital length of stay, pain, and complications, it does not appear to greatly impact functional outcome.[83] Mobilization should begin immediately, following medical stabilization, and is associated with better outcomes and shorter surgical lengths of stay without increased complications.[84,85] How quickly mobility is advanced will depend on comorbidities present and postoperative complications. Adequate pain control is crucial in the acute mobilization process, and careful monitoring of mental status and constipation will prevent either from delaying progress. Patients with limited social supports, challenging home environments (e.g., stairs rather than elevator access), or substantial comorbidities may benefit from an inpatient rehabilitation admission. Rehabilitation length of stay is increased by the presence of a premorbid neurological impairment,[86] decreased cognition, or depression (mediated by decreased participation).[87] The majority of patients will return to their baseline in basic mobility and ADL within 6 weeks,[88] but a hip fracture marks the beginning of a slow functional decline in selected patients. Extended outpatient physical therapy in the several months after fracture clearly improves outcomes[89] but is logistically difficult for many elders because of transportation and payment.[90]

Total knee (TKA) and hip arthoplasty (THA) are among the most common orthopedic procedures in the United States, with more than 250,000 hip replacements alone annually.[91] The postoperative mobilization of these patients has changed enormously over the past two decades, with strong trends for earlier initiation of activity, ambulation, and discharge from the surgical service.[91] Although appealing intuitively, data on physical conditioning and rehabilitation before joint replacement surgery are mixed.[92–94] Recent changes in federal regulations for inpatient rehabilitation facilities are restricting the number of patients with single joint replacements cared for in this setting.[95] Given that bilateral replacements are favored under the new rules, it is encouraging that outcomes are similar, costs are lower, and rehabilitation need is greater compared to two-stage procedures.[96,97] Although the relative merits of inpatient rehabilitation in an acute versus subacute setting for TKA/THA are not entirely clear, among those patients receiving inpatient rehabilitation, class I data have shown outcome to be superior for those transferred earlier after surgery (3 versus 7 days).[98]

For THA, the immediate postoperative rehabilitation focuses on mobilization, strengthening (especially hip abductors), flexibility, and education on adherence to weight-bearing limitations and hip precautions so as to prevent dislocation of the prostheses.[94] Rehabilitation outcome is similar between first-time and revised THA.[99] Adequate pain control, timed carefully to ensure maximal drug levels during activity in therapy, is ideal. Although PT oversees mobilization, OT plays an important role in the evaluation and provision of adaptive equipment for lower extremity dressing and hygiene and for the home, such as raised toilet seats and tub benches.[94]

Fewer precautions are inherent in the rehabilitation of TKA, but in many cases pain control is more difficult. Long-acting narcotics for TKR may provide better pain control and facilitate improved ROM.[100] Maintaining adequate ROM is essential to the long-term success of TKA and is a primary focus of rehabilitation intervention. Generally, 65° knee flexion is required for normal gait and 105° to rise from a low chair.[94] Continuous passive motion (CPM) machines are employed frequently in the acute and rehabilitation phases of TKR to lower the rate of surgical manipulation, increase active knee flexion earlier, and decrease length of stay in combination with PT. However, long-term outcome is probably not affected with CPM.[101]

Cardiac and Pulmonary Rehabilitation in Surgery

In addition to cardiothoracic surgeons, general and other surgeons will care for patients with substantial cardiopulmonary disease as either comorbidities or complications of treatment [e.g., perioperative myocardial infarction (MI), need for prolonged mechanical ventilation]. Cardiac rehabilitation (CR) and pulmonary rehabilitation (PR) extend far beyond exercises to include education in nutrition, risk factor modification, weight control, and psychosocial (stress) management.[102–104]

Cardiac rehabilitation is commonly initiated following MI, coronary artery bypass grafting (CABG), valve replacement, heart transplantation, and for patients with congestive heart failure (CHF). Rehabilitation starts in the hospital during the immediate postoperative or postinfarction period ("inpatient phase") and focuses on gentle, monitored mobilization [up to 2 metabolic equivalents (METs); 1 MET equals 3.5 mL/kg-min oxygen consumption], education on energy conservation techniques for ADL, maintaining muscle tone, endurance, and active ROM of joints. Isometric activities are avoided given the disproportional increases in blood pressure.[102] After discharge, during the "outpatient phase," CR includes a combination of exercises for flexibility, aerobic conditioning (i.e., stationary bike or treadmill), and resistance exercises (weight training.) A monitored CR program should be sought for patients with an ejection fraction >25%, major complications or comorbidities, symptoms or electrocardiogram changes with exercise, or those who are unable to monitor themselves.[105] Functional exercise testing is recommended for the development of a safe and effective outpatient exercise regimen.[102]

Rehabilitation following heart transplantation is a special circumstance. The response to exercise in a denervated, transplanted heart is characterized by a blunted increase in heart rate and blood pressure at the initiation of exercise. This response necessitates a gradual onset of activity to allow peripheral catecholamines to enhance the cardiac response.[106] Class I data (albeit in a small sample)[107] indicate that, when initiated early after transplantation, CR results in increased capacity for physical work at 1 year. Congestive heart failure often precedes cardiac transplantation; a substantial medical literature supports the benefit of exercise in persons with CHF.[103,108,109] Long-duration, low-intensity exercise designed to see fatigue, not dyspnea, as the limiting symptom is recommended.[102] Cardiac rehabilitation also has been suggested as a beneficial component of care following CABG.[110] Class II data with a 10-year follow-up point to significantly fewer cardiac events (18.4% vs. 34.7%), hospital readmissions (103 vs. 342), and hospital days (541 vs. 2556) among CABG patients provided access to CR.[111] A smaller study suggests that a once-weekly program did not provide the benefit seen in more intense, thrice-weekly programs.[112]

Pulmonary rehabilitation is also both a therapeutic and educational process utilized in patients with intrinsic pulmonary disease or chronic neuromuscular diseases, used in conjunction with inhalers, secretion management, and nutritional and oxygen supplementation.[104] Breathing exercises include diaphragmatic and "pursed-lip" breathing techniques that maximize use of the rib cage muscles to decrease dead space ventilation. Reconditioning exercises use aerobic activities and upper extremity activities to strengthen accessory respiratory muscles.[104] Inclusion of lower extremity training is required for improvements in either function or symptoms,[113] and positive results can be seen even in severe disease.[114,115]

Amputation

Successful rehabilitation of the patient with an amputation requires a combination of excellent surgical and rehabilitative care and applied biomechanics. In addition to PT and OT, the prosthetist is crucial in this process and is included in all aspects of prosthetic planning and fitting.[116] Trauma is the most common etiology for upper extremity limb loss and vascular disease, by far, the most frequent for lower extremity limb loss. Tumor accounts for a small percentage of both.[116]

The rehabilitation team, especially the physiatrist, may be helpful in several aspects of the presurgical planning, such as identifying problematic issues with prosthetic fitting for a given amputation level and estimating how comorbidities (e.g., cardiovascular disease, vascular disease in the remaining limb, cognitive deficits, visual loss) might impact the ultimate functional prognosis.[116] As a rule, functional household and community ambulation declines significantly with more proximal (i.e., above-knee) amputations.[117,118] There are many patients for whom functional ambulation is clearly not a realistic goal, but borderline cases are usually fit with a limb and training attempted.[116]

There are technical aspects of surgery that facilitate a smooth fitting and training process. The surgical team should keep in mind that distal tissues of the residual limb will now be the weight-bearing surface for gait. Amputation might best be viewed as a "reconstructive," rather than a salvage, procedure.[116] Careful attention to beveling of the distal, remaining bone, placement of the skin incision in a non-weight-bearing position, adequate retraction of nerve endings to prevent neuroma formation, and allocating the appropriate soft tissue padding are all crucial to success.[116]

Postoperatively, the rehabilitation team focuses on pain control, reduction of swelling and edema, residual limb reshaping, wound healing, and early cardiovascular and musculoskeletal conditioning to prepare eventual fitting and ambulation.[119] Although pain and swelling encourage a flexed posture of the leg after surgery, range at the knee and hip must be preserved so as to not alter the biomechanics of the eventual prosthesis. OT plays a vital role in adapting skills for household activities in lower extremity amputation and plays the central role in training and fitting in upper extremity loss. Regardless of the extremity, aggressive strengthening of the proximal musculature will aid in controlling and propelling the prosthetic device.

The team should understand the patient's desired activity level, recreational and vocational goals and interests, and motivation to learn before prosthetic fitting. Comorbidities are often a limitation, even if motivation is not. As a rule, the patient with adequate cardiovascular reserve to ambulate with a walker or, especially, crutches, without the prosthesis, likely has the reserve to be a functional ambulatory patient with the prosthesis. Permanent prosthetic fitting is often delayed for a few months after surgery while a temporary device is used. This time allows the residual limb to "mature" for weight-bearing and allows more time for improvement of overall strength and endurance. Finally, phantom pain should be distinguished from phantom sensation. The latter is nearly universal and is not perceived by the patient as discomfort, but rather a "presence" that dissipates over time. Mental imagery by "exercising the missing limb" can sometimes help. Phantom pain is much less common; treatment includes medications (e.g., tricyclic antidepressants, antiepileptic agents, mexilitine), relaxation techniques, transcutaneous electrical nerve stimulation, compressive wraps, and ensuring adequate residual limb healing and prosthetic fitting.[116]

References

1. World Health Organization. International Classification of Impairments, Disability, and Handicaps. Geneva: WHO, 1980.
2. DeLisa JA, Currie DM, Martin GM. Rehabilitation medicine: past, present and future. In: DeLisa JA, ed. Physical Medicine and Rehabilitation: Principles and Practice, 3rd ed. Philadelphia: Lippincott, 1998:3–32.
3. Bolton DA, Cauraugh JH, Hausenblas HA. Electromyogram-trigger neuromuscular stimulation and stroke motor recovery of arm/hand function: a meta-analysis. J Neurol Sci 2004;223:121–127.
4. Dobkin BH. The Clinical Science of Neurological Rehabilitation, 2nd ed. Oxford: Oxford University Press, 2003.
5. Mortenson PA, Eng JJ. The use of casts in the management of joint mobility and hypertonia following brain injury in adults: a systemic review. Phys Ther 2003;83:648–658.
6. Uustal H. Upper extremity orthotics. In: DeLisa JA, ed. Physical Medicine and Rehabilitation: Principles and Practice, 4th ed. Philadelphia: Lippincott, 2005:1368–1376.
7. Carter BS, Buckley DRN, Ferraro R, et al. Factors associated with reintegration to normal living after subarachnoid hemorrhage. Neurosurgery 2000;46:1326–1334.
8. Allen C, Glasziou P, Del Mar C. Bed rest: a potentially harmful treatment needing more careful evaluation. Lancet 1999;354: 1229–1233.

9. Convertino VA, Bloomfield SA, Greenleaf JE. An overview of the issues: physiologic effects of bedrest and restricted physical activity. Med Sci Sports Exerc 1997;29:187–190.
10. Bloomfield SA. Changes in musculoskeletal structure and function with prolonged bed rest. Med Sci Sports Exerc 1997;29:197–206.
11. Topp R, Ditmyer M, King K, Doherty K, Hornyak. The effect of bed rest and potential of prehabilitation on patients in the intensive care unit. AACN Clin Issues 2002;13:263–276.
12. Nava S, Ambrosino N. Rehabilitation in the ICU: the European phoenix. Intensive Care Med 2000;26:841–844.
13. O'Dell MW, Jasin P, Lyons N, Stivers M, Meszaros F. Standardized assessment instruments for minimally-responsive, brain-injured patients. Neurorehabilitation 1996;6:45–55.
14. George S, Fritz J, Bialosky J, Donald D. The effect of a fear-avoidance-based physical therapy intervention for patients with acute low back pain: results of a randomized clinical trial. Spine 2003;28:2551–2560.
15. Helm PA, Kowalske K, Head M. Burn rehabilitation. In: DeLisa JA, ed. Physical Medicine and Rehabilitation: Principles and Practice, 4th ed. Philadelphia: Lippincott, 2005:1867–1889.
16. Young A. Rehabilitation of burn injuries. Phys Med Rehabil Clin 2002;13:85–108.
17. Bennett GB, Helm P, Purdue GF, Hunt JL. Serial casting: a method for treating burn contracture. J Burn Care Rehabil 1989;10:543–545.
18. Covey MH, Dutcher K, Marvin JA, Heimbach DM. Efficacy of continuous passive motion devices with hand burns. J Burn Care Rehabil 1988;9:397–400.
19. Kowalske KJ, Purdue G, Hunt J, et al. Early ambulation following skin grafting of lower extremity burns: a randomized controlled trial. Proc Am Burn Assoc 1993;25:102.
20. Trees DW, Ketelsen CA, Hobbs JA. Use of a modified tilt table for pre-ambulation strength training as an adjunct to burn rehabilitation: a case series. J Burn Care Rehabil 2003;24: 97–103.
21. Kowalske K, Holavanahalli R, Helm P. Neuropathy after burn injury. J Burn Care Rehabil 2001;22:353–357.
22. Tsionos I, Leclercq C, Rochet JM. Heterotopic ossification of the elbow in patients with burns. Results after early excision. J Bone Joint Surg Br 2004;86:396–403.
23. Lin J, Nagler W. Use of surface scanning for creation of transparent facial orthoses: a report of two cases. Burns 2003;29:599–602.
24. Goldstein LB. Neuropharmacology of TBI-induced plasticity. Brain Inj 2003;17:685–694.
25. Dikman SS, Temkin NR, Miller B, Machamer J, Winn HR. Neurobehavioral effects of phenytoin prophylaxis of posttraumatic seizures. JAMA 1991;265:1271–1277.
26. Brailowsky S, Knight RT, Efron R. Phenytoin increases the severity of cortical hemiplegia in rats. Brain Res 1986;376:71–77.
27. Feeney DM, Gonzalez A, Law WA. Amphetamine, haloperidol, and experience interact to affect rate of recovery after motor cortex injury. Science 1982;217:855–857.
28. Shallert T, Hernandez TD, Barth TM. Recovery of function after brain damage: severe and chronic disruption by diazepam. Brain Res 1986;379:104–111.
29. Goldstein LB, Davis JN. Clonidine impairs recovery of beam-walking after a sensorimotor cortex lesion in the rat. Brain Res 1990;508:305–309.
30. Hernandez TD, Holling LC. Disruption of behavioral recovery by the anticonvulsant phenobarbitol. Brain Res 1994;635:300–306.
31. Goldstein LB. Sygen in acute stroke study investigation: common drugs may influence motor recovery after stroke. Neurology 1995;45:865–871.
32. Farwell JR, Young JL, Hirtz DG, et al. Phenobarbital for febrile seizures: effects on intelligence and on seizure occurrence. N Engl J Med 1990;322:364–369.
33. Temkin NR, Dikman SS, Wilensky AJ, et al. A randomized, double-blind study of phenytoin for the prevention of post-traumatic seizures. N Engl J Med 1990;323:497–502.
34. Temkin NR, Dikman SS, Anderson GD, et al. Valproate therapy for prevention of posttraumatic seizures: a randomized trial. J Neurosurg 1999;91:593–600.
35. Mayberg MR, Batjer HH, Dacey R, et al. Guidelines for the management of aneurismal subarachnoid hemorrhage. Circulation 1994;90:2592–2605.
36. Glanz MJ, Cole BF, Friedberg MH, et al. A randomized, blinded, placebo-controlled trial of divalproex sodium prophylaxis in adults with newly diagnosed brain tumors. Neurology 1996;46:985–991.
37. Glanz MJ, Cole BF, Forsyth PA, et al. Practice parameter: anticonvulsant prophylaxis in patients with newly diagnosed brain tumors. Neurology 2000;54:1886–1893.
38. Kline AE, Yan HQ, Bao J, Marian DW, Dixon CE. Chronic methylphenidate treatment enhances water maze performance following traumatic brain injury in rats. Neurosci Lett 2000;280:163–166.
39. Plenger PM, Dixon CE, Castillo RM. Subacute methylphenidate treatment for moderate to moderately severe traumatic brain injury: a preliminary double-blind, placebo-controlled study. Arch Phys Med Rehabil 1996;77:536–540.
40. Kaelin DL, Cifu DX, Matthies B. Methylphenidate effect on attention deficit in the acutely brain-injured adult. Arch Phys Med Rehabil 1996;77:6–9
41. Whyte J, Hart T, Vaccaro M, et al. Effects of methylphenidate on attention deficits after traumatic brain injury: a multidimensional, randomized controlled trial. Am J Phys Med Rehabil 2004;83:401–420.
42. Cristosomo EA, Duncan PW, Propst M, Dawson DV, David JN. Evidence that amphetamine with physical therapy promotes recovery of motor function in stroke patients. Ann Neurol 1988;23:94–97.
43. Walker-Batson D, Curtis S, Natarajan R, et al. A double-blind, placebo-controlled study of the use of amphetamine in the treatment of aphasia. Stroke 2001;32:2093–2098.
44. Meyers CA, Weitzner MA, Valentine AD, Levin VA. Methylphenidate therapy improves cognition, mood, and function of brain tumor patients. J Clin Oncol 1998;16:2522–2527.
45. Goldstein LB, Davis JN. Post-lesion practice and amphetamine-facilitated recovery of beam-walking in the rat. Restor Neurol Neurosci 1990;1:311–314.
46. Will B, Galani R, Kelche C, Rosenzweig MR. Recovery from brain injury in animals; relative effect of environmental enrichment, physical exercise, and formal training (1990–2002). Prog Neurobiol 2004;72:167–182.
47. Greener J, Enderby P, Whurr R. Speech and language therapy for aphasia following stroke. Cochrane Database Syst Rev 2000;2: CD0000425.
48. Gracies JM, Nance P, Elovic E, McGuire J, Simpson DM. Traditional pharmacological treatments for spasticity. Part 1. Local treatments. Muscle Nerve 1997;Suppl 6:S61–S91.
49. Hesse S, Schmidt H, Werner C, Bardeleben A. Upper and lower extremity robotic devices for rehabilitation and for studying motor control. Curr Opin Neurol 2003;16:705–710.
50. Barbeau H, Visintin M. Optimal outcomes obtained with body-weight support combined with treadmill training in stroke subjects. Arch Phys Med Rehabil 2003;84:1458–1465.
51. Wolf SL, Winstein CL, Miller JP, et al. Effect of constraint-induced movement therapy on upper extremity function 3–9 months after stroke. JAMA 2006;296:2095–2104.
52. Elovic E, Bogey R. Spasticity and movement disorder. In: DeLisa JA, ed. Physical Medicine and Rehabilitation: Principles

and Practice, 4th ed. Philadelphia: Lippincott, 2005:1427–1446.
53. Bowen A, Lincoln NB, Dewey M. Cognitive rehabilitation for spatial neglect following stroke. Cochrane Database Syst Rev 2002;2:CD03586.
54. Cicerone K, Dahlberg C, Kalmar K, et al. Evidence-based cognitive rehabilitation: recommendations for clinical practice. Arch Phys Med Rehabil 2000;81:1596–1615.
55. Wagner AK, Fabio T, Zafonte RD, et al. Physical medicine and rehabilitation consultation: relationships with acute functional outcome, length of stay, and discharge planning after traumatic brain injury. Am J Phys Med Rehabil 2003;82:526–536.
56. Greenwood R. Value of recording duration of post-traumatic amnesia. Lancet 1997;349:1041–1042.
57. Elovic EP, Lansang R, Li Y, Ricker JH. The use of atypical antipsychotics in traumatic brain injury. J Head Trauma Rehabil 2003;18:177–195.
58. Felminger S, Greenwood RJ, Oliver DL. Pharmacological management for agitation and aggression in people with acquired brain injury. Cochrane Database Syst Rev 2003;1:003299.
59. Lombardi F, Taricco M, DeTanti A, Telaro E, Liberati A. Sensory stimulation for brain injured individuals in coma or vegetative state. Cochrane Database Syst Rev 2002;2:001427.
60. O'Dell MW, Rigg RV. Management of the minimally responsive patient. In: Horn LJ, Zasler ND, eds. Medical Rehabilitation of Traumatic Brain Injury. St. Louis: Mosby, 1996:103–131.
61. Ruff R. Two decades of advances in understanding of mild traumatic brain injury. J Head Trauma Rehabil 2005;20:5–18.
62. O'Dell MW, Watanabe TK, DeRoos ST, Kager C. Functional outcome after inpatient rehabilitation in persons with subarachnoid hemorrhage. Arch Phys Med Rehabil 2002;83:678–682.
63. DeLuca J, Diamond BJ. Aneurysm of the anterior communicating artery: a review of neuroanatomical and neuropsychological sequelae. J Clin Exp Neuropsychol 1995;17:100–121.
64. Bell K, O'Dell MW, Barr K, Yablon S. Rehabilitation of the patient with brain tumor. Arch Phys Med Rehabil 1998;79:S37–S46.
65. O'Dell MW, Barr K, Spanier D, Warnick R. Functional outcome of inpatient rehabilitation in persons with brain tumors. Arch Phys Med Rehabil 1998;79:1530–1534.
66. Kirshblum S. Rehabilitation of spinal cord injury. In: DeLisa JA, ed. Physical Medicine and Rehabilitation: Principles and Practice, 4th ed. Philadelphia: Lippincott, 2005:1715–1751.
67. American Spinal Injury Association. International Standards for Neurological Classification of Spinal Cord Injury. Chicago: American Spinal Injury Association, 2002.
68. Kirshblum S, O'Connor KC. Predicting neurological recovery in traumatic spinal cord injury. Arch Phys Med Rehabil 1998;79:1456–1466.
69. McKinley WO, Seel RT, Hardman JT. Non-traumatic spinal cord injury: incidence, epidemiology, and functional outcome. Arch Phys Med Rehabil 1999;80:619–623.
70. Kirshblum S, Ho C, Drum E, et al. Rehabilitation after spinal cord injury. In: Kirshblum S, Campagnolo, DeLisa JE, eds. Spinal Cord Medicine. Philadelphia: Lippincott, 2002:275–298.
71. Van Kuiik AA, Geurts ACH, van Kuppevelt HJM. Neurogenic heterotopic ossification in spinal cord injury. Spinal Cord 2002;40:313–326.
72. Kirshblum S. New rehabilitation interventions in spinal cord injury. J Spinal Cord Med 2004;27:342–350.
73. Plassat R, Perrouin VB, Menei P, et al. Treatment of spasticity with intrathecal bacolfen administration: long-term follow-up, review of 40 patients. Spinal Cord 2004;42:686–693.
74. Plaisier BR, Meldon SW, Super DM, Malangoni MA. Improved outcome after fixation of acetabular fractures. Injury 2000;31:81–84.
75. Latenser BA, Gentilello LM, Tarver AA, Thalgott JS, Batdorf JW. Improved outcome with early fixation of skeletally unstable pelvic fractures. J Trauma Inj Infect Crit Care 1991;31:28–31.
76. Dimopoulou I, Anthi A, Mastora Z, et al. Health-related quality of life and disability in survivors of multiple trauma one year after intensive care unit discharge. Am J Phys Med Rehabil 2004;83:171–176.
77. Mkandawire NC, Boot DA, Braithwaite IJ, Patterson M. Musculoskeletal recovery 5 years after severe injury. Long-term problems are common. Injury 2002;33:11–115.
78. Ward WG, Nunley JA. Occult orthopedic trauma in the multiply injured patient. J Orthop Trauma 1991;5:308–312.
79. Noble J, Munro CA, Prasad V. Analysis of upper and lower extremity peripheral nerve injuries in a population of patients with multiple injuries. J Trauma Inj Infect Crit Care 1998;45:116–122.
80. Midha R. Epidemiology of brachial plexus injuries in a multitrauma population. Neurosurgery 1997;40:1182–1189.
81. Kellam JF, Mayo KL. Pelvic ring fractures. In: Browner BD, Jupiter JB, Levine AM, Trafton PG, eds. Skeletal Trauma: Basic Science, Management, and Reconstruction. Philadelphia: Saunders, 2003:1052–1108.
82. U.S. Department of Health and Human Services. Surveillance for selected public health indicators affecting older adults: United States. MMWR 1999;48:33–34.
83. Orosz GM, Magaziner J, Hannan EL, et al. Association of timing of surgery for hip fracture and patient outcomes. JAMA 2004;291:1738–1743.
84. Day GA, Swanson C, Yelland C, et al. Surgical outcomes of a randomized prospective trial involving patients with a proximal femoral fracture. Aust N Z J Surg 2001;71:11–14.
85. Huusko TM, Karppi P, Avikainen V, Kautiainen, Sulkava R. Intensive rehabilitation of hip fractures: a randomized controlled trial. Acta Orthop Scand 2002;73:425–431.
86. DiMonaco M, Vallero F, DiMonaco F, Cavanna A. Functional recovery and length of stay after hip fracture in patients with neurological impairment. Am J Phys Med Rehabil 2003;82:143–148.
87. Lenze EJ, Munin MC, Dew MA, et al. Adverse effects of depression and cognitive impairment on rehabilitation participation and recovery from hip fracture. Int J Geriatr Psychiatry 2004;19:472–278.
88. Cifu DX. Rehabilitation of hip fractures. PMR State Art Rev 1995;9:125–139.
89. Binder EF, Brown M, Sinacore DR, et al. Effects of extended outpatient rehabilitation after hip fractures: a randomized controlled trial. JAMA 2004;292:837–846.
90. Peterson MGE, Ganz SB, Allegrante JP, Cornell CN. High-intensity exercise following hip fracture. Top Geriatr Rehabil 2004;4:273–284.
91. Ganz SB. A historic look at functional outcome following total hip and knee arthroplasty. Top Geriatr Rehabil 2004;20:236–252.
92. McGregor AH, Rylands H, Owen A, Dore CJ, Hughes SP. Does preoperative hip rehabilitation improve recovery and patient satisfaction? J Arthroplasty 2004;19:464–468.
93. Beaupre LA, Lier D, Davies DM, Johnston DB. The effect of a preoperative exercise and educations program on functional recovery, health related quality of life, and health service utilization following primary total knee arthroplasty. J Rheum 2004;31:1166–1173.
94. Brander VA, Stulberg SD. Rehabilitation after lower limb joint reconstruction. In: DeLisa JA, ed. Physical Medicine and Rehabilitation: Principles and Practice, 4th ed. Philadelphia: Lippincott, 2005:855–872.
95. Center for Medicare and Medicaid Services (CMS). Medicare program: changes to the criteria for being classified as an inpatient rehabilitation facility. Final rule. Fed Reg 2004;69:25752–25776.

96. Maccaulay W, Salvati EA, Sculco TP, Pellicci PM. Single stage bilateral hip arthroplasty. J Am Acad Orthop Surg 2002;10:217–221.
97. Macario A, Schilling BA, Rubio R, Goodman S. Economics of one-stage versus two-staged bilateral total knee arthroplasties. Clin Orthop Relat Res 2003;414:149–156.
98. Munin MC, Rudy TE, Gyynn NW, Crossett LS, Rubash HE. Early inpatient rehabilitation after elective hip and knee arthroplasty. JAMA 1998;279:847–852.
99. Walker WC, Keyser-Marcus LA, Cifo DX, Chaudhri M. Inpatient interdisciplinary rehabilitation after total hip arthroplasty surgery: a comparison of revision and primary total hip arthroplasty. Arch Phys Med Rehabil 2001;82:129–133.
100. Chevelle A, Chen A, Oster G, McGarry L, Narcessian E. A randomized trial of controlled-release oxycodone during inpatient rehabilitation following unilateral total knee arthroplasty. J Bone Joint Surg 2001;83A:572–576.
101. Milne S, Brosseau L, Robinson V, et al. Continuous passive motion following total knee arthroplasty. Cochrane Database Syst Rev 2003:2:CD004260.
102. Shah SK. Cardiac rehabilitation. In: DeLisa JA, ed. Physical Medicine and Rehabilitation: Principles and Practice, 4th ed. Philadelphia: Lippincott, 2005:1811–1841.
103. Stewart KJ, Badenhop D, Brubaker PH, Keteyian SJ, King M. Cardiac rehabilitation following percutaneous revascularization, heart transplant, heart valve surgery, and chronic heart failure. Chest 2003;123:2104–2111.
104. Bach J. The Rehabilitation of the Patient with Respiratory Dysfunction. In: DeLisa JA, ed. Physical Medicine and Rehabilitation: Principles and Practice, 4th ed. Philadelphia: Lippincott, 2005:1843–1866.
105. Wenger NK, Friesen M, Smith LK, et al. Cardiac rehabilitation as secondary prevention. Clinical practice guideline. Quick look reference for clinicians #17. AHCPR publication 96–0673. Rockville, MD: Agency for Health Care Policy and Research, 1995:1–23.
106. Mettauer B, Zhao QM, Epailly E, et al. VO_2 kinetics reveals a central limitation at the onset of subthreshold exercise in heart transplantation recipients. J Appl Physiol 2000;88:1228–1238.
107. Kobashigawa JA, Leaf DA, Lee N, et al. A controlled trial of exercise rehabilitation after heart transplantation. N Engl J Med 1999;340:272–277.
108. Pina IL, Apstein CS, Balady GJ, et al. Exercise and heart failure. A statement from the American Heart Association Committee on Exercise, Rehabilitation, and Prevention. Circulation 2003;107:1210–1225.
109. Rees K, Taylor RS, Singh S, Coats AJ, Ebrahim S. Exercise based rehabilitation for heart failure. Cochrane Database Syst Rev 2004;3:CD003331.
110. Charlson ME, Isom OW. Care after coronary-artery bypass surgery. N Engl J Med 2003;348:1456–1463.
111. Hedback B, Perk J, Hornblad M, Ohlsson U. Cardiac rehabilitation after coronary artery bypass surgery: 10-year results on mortality, morbidity, and readmissions to hospital. J Cardiovasc Risk 2001;8:153–158.
112. Wright DJ, Riley R, Marshall P, Tan LB. Is early, low level, short term exercise cardiac rehabilitation following coronary artery bypass surgery beneficial. A randomized controlled trial. Heart 2002;88:83–84
113. Rochester CL. Exercise training in chronic obstructive pulmonary disease. J Rehabil Res Del 2003;40(5 suppl 2):59–80.
114. Palmer SM, Tapson VE. Pulmonary rehabilitation in the surgical patient. Lung transplantation and lung volume reduction surgery. Respir Care Clin N Am 1998;4:71–83.
115. Decramer M. Treatment of chronic respiratory failure: lung volume reduction surgery versus rehabilitation. Eur Respir J Suppl 2003;47:47s–67s.
116. Gitter A, Bosker G. Upper and lower extremity prosthetics. In: DeLisa JA, ed. Physical Medicine and Rehabilitation: Principles and Practice, 4th ed. Philadelphia: Lippincott, 2005:1325–1354.
117. Nehler MR, Coll JR, Hiatt WR, et al. Functional outcome in a contemporary series of major lower extremity amputations. J Vasc Surg 2003;38:7–14.
118. Davies B, Datta D. Mobility outcome following unilateral lower limb amputation. Prosthet Orthot Int 2003;27:186–190.
119. Esquenazi A, DiGiacomo R. Rehabilitation after amputation. J Am Podiatric Assoc 2001;91:13–22.

SECTION THREE

Care of Unique Populations

36

Pediatric Surgery

Russell K. Woo and Craig T. Albanese

The care of surgical diseases in children has long been recognized as a unique field of medicine. The first credited textbook of pediatric surgery was published in 1563 by the Swiss surgeon Felix Wurtz.[1] This was later followed in the 1860s by pediatric surgical texts published by Forster of England and Guersant of France[2,3] In the United States, the first textbook of pediatric surgery was published by Kelly in 1909.[4] Today, following the footsteps of these early developments, the field of pediatric surgery has grown significantly in both scientific understanding and clinical expertise. Advances in prenatal evaluation, neonatal care, diagnostic techniques, anesthesia, and clinical management have enhanced the care of the pediatric surgical patient.[5] Compared to adult patients, infants and children possess their own distinct physiological characteristics that must govern their care. In addition, the disease processes that afflict these patients are clearly distinct from the common disorders of adulthood. The purpose of this chapter is to provide an overview of pediatric surgery, focusing on the unique physiological characteristics of children that govern their preoperative and postoperative management, as well as reviewing the current issues in the diagnosis and management of the major pediatric surgical diseases.

Preoperative and Postoperative Management

The neonate, infant, child, and adolescent differ significantly from each other and from the adult. The most distinctive and rapidly changing physiological characteristics occur during the neonatal period because of the newborn infant's adaptation from complete placental support to the extrauterine environment, differences in the physiological maturity of individual neonates, the small size of these patients, and the demands of growth and development.[6] Recent advances in neonatal care have resulted in the survival of increasing numbers of extremely low birth weight infants. Extreme prematurity magnifies the already dynamic and relatively fragile physiology of the newborn period, predisposing these tiny infants to physiological derangements in temperature regulation, fluid and electrolyte homeostasis, glucose metabolism, hematological regulation, and immune function. In addition, physiological and anatomic organ system immaturity makes the preterm neonate vulnerable to specific problems such as intraventricular hemorrhage, hyaline membrane disease, and hyperbilirubinemia. From a surgical standpoint, these dynamic and fragile physiological parameters are often the primary components that dictate the preoperative and postoperative management of the neonatal surgical patient. This section focuses on the physiology of the neonate undergoing surgery, highlighting the practical considerations of preoperative and postoperative management as well as special considerations relevant to specific disease states.

Low Birth Weight Infants

Neonates may be classified according to their level of maturation (gestational age) and development (weight) (Tables 36.1, 36.2). This classification is important because the physiology of neonates may vary significantly depending on these parameters.

Under this classification system, a term, appropriate for gestational age, infant is born between 37 and 42 weeks gestation with a birth weight greater than 2500g. However, in the United States, approximately 7% of all babies do not meet these criteria as a consequence of prematurity or intrauterine

TABLE 36.1. Newborn Classification by Maturation (Age).

Classification	*Age at birth*
Preterm	Birth before 37 weeks gestation
Term	Birth between 37 and 42 weeks gestation
Post term	Birth after 42 weeks gestation

TABLE 36.2. Newborn Classification by Development (Weight).

Classification	*Birth weight*
Small for gestational age	Birth weight below 10th percentile
Appropriate for gestational age	Birth weight between 10th and 98th percentile
Large for gestational age	Birth weight greater than 98th percentile

growth retardation. From a clinical standpoint, neonates born weighing less than 2500g are broadly classified as *low birth weight* (LBW) infants. Further subclassification into moderately low birth weight, very low birth weight, and extremely low birth weight infants have been used for epidemiological and prognostic purposes (Table 36.3). Using this terminology, low birth weight infants may be preterm and appropriate for gestational age, term, but small for gestational age, or both. This distinction is important in that the overall prognosis and potential risks may be significantly different for the different populations.

Preterm Infant

By definition, *preterm infants* are born before 37 weeks gestation. They generally have body weights appropriate for their age, although they may also be small for their gestational age. If the gestational age is not accurately known, the prematurity of an infant can be confirmed by physical examination. The principal features of preterm infants are a head circumference below the 50th percentile; thin, semitransparent skin with an absence of plantar creases; soft and malleable ears with poorly developed cartilage; absence of breast tissue; undescended testes (testicular descent begins around the 32nd week of gestation); with a flat scrotum in boys and relatively enlarged labia minora and small labia majora in girls.

In addition to these physical characteristics, several physiological abnormalities exist in preterm infants. These abnormalities are often a result of unfinished fetal developmental tasks that normally enable an infant to successfully transition from intrauterine to extrauterine life. These tasks, which include renal, skin, pulmonary, and vascular maturation, are usually completed during the final weeks of gestation. The more premature the infant, the more fetal tasks are left unfinished and the more vulnerable the infant.

This physiological and anatomic vulnerability sets the preterm infant up for several specific and clinically significant problems:

1. Central nervous system (CNS) immaturity, leading to episodes of apnea and bradycardia, and a weak suck reflex.
2. Pulmonary immaturity, leading to surfactant deficiency that can result in hyaline membrane disease (HMD).
3. Cerebrovascular immaturity leading to fragile, unsupported cerebral vessels that lack the ability to autoregulate; this predisposes the preterm infant to intraventricular hemorrhage (IVH), the most common acute brain injury of the neonate.
4. Skin immaturity leading to an underdeveloped stratum corneum with significant transepithelial water loss (TEWL); this complicates the thermal regulation and fluid status management of the infant.
5. Gastrointestinal (GI) underdevelopment causing inadequate GI absorption and the risk of necrotizing enterocolitis.
6. Impaired bilirubin metabolism causing predominantly indirect hyperbilirubinemia.
7. Cardiovascular immaturity leading to a patent ductus arteriosus or patent foramen ovale. These retained elements of the fetal circulation can cause persistent left-to-right shunting and cardiac failure.

From a practical standpoint, the care of the preterm infant must therefore be directed at preventing and/or treating these specific problems. Episodes of apnea and bradycardia are common and may occur spontaneously or as nonspecific signs of problems such as sepsis or hypothermia. Prolonged apnea with significant hypoxemia leads to bradycardia and ultimately to cardiac arrest. All preterm infants should therefore undergo apnea monitoring and electrocardiographic pulse monitoring, with the alarm set at a minimum pulse rate of 90 beats/min. In the neonate with respiratory difficulties, chest radiography will help to detect hyaline membrane disease and cardiac failure. The lungs and retinas of preterm infants are very susceptible to high oxygen levels, and even relatively brief exposures may result in various degrees of pulmonary hyaline membrane disease and retinopathy of prematurity. Infants receiving oxygen therefore require continuous pulse oximetry monitoring, with the alarm set between 85% and 92%. The preterm infant may also be unable to tolerate oral feeding because they have a weak suck reflex, necessitating intragastric tube feeding or total parenteral nutrition. Finally, impaired bilirubin metabolism may necessitate serum bilirubin monitoring for rising levels of unconjugated bilirubin; this may require phototherapy or exchange transfusion.

Small for Gestational Age Infant

Infants whose birth weight is below the 10th percentile are considered to be small for gestational age (SGA). SGA new-

TABLE 36.3. Alternative Newborn Classification by Weight.

Classification	*Birth weight*	*Percent of premies*	*Mortality rate vs. term infants*
Low birth weight	Birth weight <2500g	—	—
• Moderately low birth weight	Birth weight between 2500g and 1501g	82%	40 times higher mortality
• Very low birth weight	Birth weight between 1500g and 1001g	12%	200 times higher mortality
• Extremely low birth weight	Birth weight <1000g	6%	600 times higher mortality

TABLE 36.4. Common Conditions Associated with Intrauterine Growth Retardation.

Age at delivery	*Condition*
Preterm	Placental insufficiency Discordant twin Chronic maternal hypertension Intrauterine infection, Toxemia
Term	Congenital anomaly, Microcephaly
Post term	Placental insufficiency

borns are thought to be a product of restricted intrauterine growth as a result of placental, maternal, and fetal abnormalities. Table 36.4 lists several conditions that may lead to intrauterine growth retardation. It should be noted that not all infants in this group are truly growth retarded and therefore at higher risk. Some infants are simply born small as a result of a variety of factors including race, ethnicity, sex, and geography. It is therefore important to differentiate these infants from those whose relatively low birth weight is a result of a genetic or intrauterine abnormality.

SGA infants can be divided into two broad categories: the symmetrical SGA infant and the asymmetrical SGA infant. This distinction is based primarily on when in the gestational period fetal growth was actually restricted. If fetal growth is restricted during the first half of pregnancy, when cellular hyperplasia and differentiation lead to tissue and organ formation, the neonate is generally a symmetrical SGA infant. Fetal factors such as genetic dwarfism, chromosomal abnormalities, congenital abnormalities, inborn errors of metabolism, and fetal infection, as well as maternal factors such as genetics, toxin ingestion, and substance abuse, are all causative etiologies. Although only 30% of SGA infants fall into this group, they have the highest morbidity and mortality rates.

In contrast, asymmetrical SGA infants are those who experience restriction in intrauterine growth during the last half of gestation, often during the third trimester; this is usually the result of an inadequate nutrient supply. An example of this is twin gestations. Although both infants may be full term at birth, they generally have a low birth weight because the placental mass/function is inadequate to meet the growth demands of both fetuses. Other causes of asymmetrical growth retardation include maternal conditions that reduce uteroplacental blood flow such as hypertension, toxemia, and cardiac and renovascular disorders.

In general, SGA infants have a body weight that is low for their gestational age, although their body length and head circumference are appropriate. The SGA infant is older and developmentally more mature than a preterm infant of equivalent weight. They therefore face significantly different physiological problems. Because of the longer gestational period and resultant well-developed organ systems, the metabolic rate of the SGA infant is much higher in proportion to body weight than a preterm infant of similar overall weight. Fluid and caloric requirements are therefore increased. Intrauterine malnutrition results in a relative lack of body fat and decreased glycogen stores. In fact, body fat levels in SGA infants are often below 1% of their total body weight. This, coupled with their relatively large surface area, greatly predisposes these infants to hypothermia and hypoglycemia. Close monitoring of blood sugar level is therefore essential. In addition, polycythemia is common in SGA infants because of increased red blood cell volumes. Occurring in 15% to 40% of asymmetrical SGA babies, polycythemia may lead to hyperviscosity syndrome characterized by respiratory distress, tachycardia, pleural effusions, and the risk of venous thrombosis, which requires frequent monitoring of the infant's hematocrit level and possibly plasma exchange transfusions. Last, fetal asphyxia and distress caused by inadequate placental support may lead to passage of meconium in utero, resulting in an increased risk of meconium aspiration syndrome in SGA infants if the material is aspirated during labor and delivery. The perioperative management of these conditions is detailed in the following sections. Although the SGA infant is at a significant risk for morbidity and mortality associated with these syndromes, their adequate length of gestation puts them at a relatively lower risk for many of the conditions that affect preterm infants such as retinopathy of prematurity, intraventricular hemorrhage, and hyaline membrane disease.

Physiological Considerations in the Perioperative Care of the Neonate

As stated previously, the dynamic physiological changes that occur during the neonatal period significantly influence the preoperative and postoperative care of the newborn surgical patient. In particular, physiological derangements in temperature regulation, glucose metabolism, hematological regulation, immune function, and fluid and electrolyte homeostasis often dictate perioperative management.

Thermoregulation

Neonates are susceptible to heat loss because of their large surface area, low body fat to body weight ratio, and limited heat sink capacity resulting from their small size. In addition, neonates have a relatively high thermoneutral temperature zone. The optimal thermal environment (thermoneutrality) is defined as a range of ambient temperatures in which an infant, at a minimal metabolic rate, can maintain a constant normal body temperature by vasomotor control. The environmental temperature must be maintained near the appropriate thermoneutral zone for each individual. In adults, this critical temperature range is 26° to 28°C whereas in the term infant it is 32° to 34°C. In the low birth weight infant, this critical range is even higher at 34° to 35°C.

Mechanisms of Heat Loss

In the neonate, heat loss may occur by evaporation, conduction, convection, and radiation. Evaporative heat loss occurs as a result of transepithelial water loss and depends on the gestational age of the infant, the relative humidity, and other environmental conditions. In addition, the presence of liquid in contact with an infant's skin also contributes to evaporative heat loss. Conductive heat loss occurs when an infant's skin is in contact with a solid object of lower temperature, causing heat to flow from the infant to the object at a rate dependent on the temperature difference between the two as well as the insulating properties of the baby and the object. Similarly, convective heat loss occurs when the ambient air temperature is less than the infant's skin temperature. Convective heat loss depends on the temperature gradient between the infant's skin and the air as well as the speed of the air

TABLE 36.5. Types of Heat Loss in the Neonate.

Type of heat loss	*Mechanism*	*Prevention*
Evaporation	• Transepithelial water loss • Skin in contact with wet surface	• Humidity • Plastic sheets
Conduction	• Direct skin contact with a cooler object	• Insulating padding
Convection	• Air currents in contact with the infant	• Warming incubator air
Radiation	• Radiation of heat to a cooler surface not in direct contact with the infant	• Double-walled incubators

current over the infant. Last, radiant heat loss occurs via the passage of infrared rays from the infant's skin to a cooler surface, such as the incubator or nursery wall. This type of heat loss is often the most difficult to control. Table 36.5 details the types of heat loss affecting the neonate.

Thermogenesis in the Neonate

Neonates generate heat by increasing metabolic activity, which can occur via shivering, as in adults, or via nonshivering thermogenesis using brown fat. This distinction has practical consequences because brown fat may be rendered inactive by pressors or anesthetic and neuromuscular blocking agents.[7] Brown fat stores may also be depleted by poor nutritional intake, such as in an SGA infant. When an infant is exposed to cold, metabolic work increases above basal levels and calories are consumed to maintain body temperature. If prolonged, this effort depletes the limited energy reserves of the neonate and predisposes to hypothermia and increased mortality.

Practical Considerations The environmental temperature of the neonate is best controlled in an incubator by monitoring the ambient temperature and maintaining it at thermoneutrality. Inside the incubator, clothing on the infant can increase insulation, reducing radiant and convective heat loss. In particular, covering the head with an insulated hat can reduce heat loss and total metabolic activity during cold stress by up to 15%. Similarly, conductive heat loss is minimized by the use of insulating padding. The incubators themselves are plastic-walled containers that warm the infant by convection. The air in the incubator is heated by a heating element and then circulated by a fan. A servosystem regulates incubator temperature according to the patient's skin temperature monitored by a skin probe. In this manner, the infant's skin temperature is maintained at a relatively constant value. Double-walled incubators minimize radiant heat loss by maintaining the inner wall of the incubator at the same temperature as the air temperature inside the incubator. Finally, humidity can be provided to the incubator environment, thereby reducing evaporative heat loss.

Optimal air temperatures for individual infants vary with the gestational age and condition of the infant as well as with specific environmental factors such as humidity and airflow. Standard nomograms are available that aid in determining the appropriate incubator temperature necessary to achieve thermoneutrality.[8] Term infants usually require the incubator air temperature to be 32° to 34°C. Low birth weight infants may require temperatures at or above 35°C.

In contrast to fully enclosed incubators, radiant warmers provide open access and visibility to the infants. Their use has become common for ill neonates who need frequent manipulation. Radiant warmers generate heat by means of an overhead panel that produces heat in the infrared range. However, these warmers do not prevent heat loss by convection and often lead to higher evaporative water and heat losses. This evaporative heat loss may be reduced by plastic sheets.

The feedback mechanisms of both incubators and radiant warmers are used to maintain an infant's skin temperature in the normal range. The normal skin temperature for a term infant is 36.2°C and that for a low birth weight infant is 36.5°C. Increased metabolic activity can be detected by comparing skin and rectal temperatures, which normally differ by 1.5°C. A decreasing skin temperature with a constant rectal temperature suggests that the metabolic rate has increased to maintain the core temperature.

In a cold environment, such as the operating room or radiology suite, heat loss may be reduced by wrapping the head, extremities, and as much of the trunk as possible in clothing, plastic sheets, or aluminum foil. A plastic sheet placed beneath the infant decreases the humidity of the microenvironment between it and the sheet. Any exposed intestine (e.g., gastroschisis) should be wrapped in plastic. An overhead infrared heating lamp should be focused on the infant during induction of anesthesia, preparation for operation, and at the termination of the operation. Solutions used for skin cleansing as well as intracorporeal irrigation should be warmed.

Glucose Homeostasis

The fetus receives glucose from its mother by facilitated placental diffusion; very little is derived from fetal gluconeogenesis. The limited liver glycogen stores accumulated during the later stages of gestation are rapidly depleted within 2 to 3h after birth. The blood glucose level of the infant then depends on the neonate's capacity for gluconeogenesis, the adequacy of substrate stores, and the energy requirements of the infant. Of note, the neonate's ability to synthesize glucose from fat or protein substrates is severely limited, necessitating the intake of exogenous carbohydrates to maintain adequate blood glucose levels.

Hypoglycemia

The risk of developing hypoglycemia is high in low birth weight infants (especially SGA infants), those born to toxemic or diabetic mothers, and those requiring surgery who are unable to take oral nutrition and who have the additional metabolic stresses of their disease and the surgical procedure. The clinical features of hypoglycemia are nonspecific and include a weak or high-pitched cry, cyanosis, apnea, jitteriness or trembling, apathy, and seizures. The differential diagnosis includes other metabolic disturbances or sepsis. More than 50% of infants with symptomatic hypoglycemia suffer significant neurological damage. Neonatal hypoglycemia is defined as a serum glucose level less than 1.66 mmol/L in the full-term infant and less than 1.11 mmol/L in the low birth weight infant. However, neurological abnormalities have been reported with higher blood glucose levels. Older children, particularly those with depleted stores and severe metabolic demands, are also at risk of hypoglycemia.

Practical Considerations All pediatric surgical patients, particularly neonates, are monitored for hypoglycemia. To avoid delay, blood glucose levels can be rapidly determined in the neonatal unit using blood glucose reagent strips activated by using blood from a heel stick. This method may be correlated at intervals with serum glucose determinations, the frequency depending on the stability of the patient. Any intravenous fluids administered should contain at least 10% dextrose. If non-dextrose-containing solutions such as blood or plasma are being administered, close monitoring of the blood glucose level is essential. Hypoglycemia should be treated urgently with intravenous 50% dextrose, 1–2 mL/kg, and maintenance intravenous dextrose, 10% to 15%, 80–100 mL/kg for each 24 h.

Hyperglycemia

Hyperglycemia is commonly a problem of very low birth weight infants on parenteral nutritional support because they have a lower insulin response to glucose. Hyperglycemia may lead to intraventricular hemorrhage and renal water and electrolyte loss from glycosuria. Prevention of hyperglycemia is by small and gradual incremental changes in the glucose concentration and infusion rate.

Hematological Regulation

Total blood, plasma, and red cell volumes are higher during the first few hours after birth than at any other time in an individual's life. The levels may be further increased if a significant placental transfusion takes place at delivery (delayed cord clamping). Several hours after birth, plasma shifts out of the circulation and total blood and plasma volumes decrease. The high red blood cell volume persists, decreasing slowly to reach adult levels by the third postnatal month. Age-related estimations of blood volume are summarized in Table 36.6.

Polycythemia

In addition to SGA infants, neonatal polycythemia occurs in infants of diabetic mothers and infants of mothers with toxemia of pregnancy. In the neonate, polycythemia is defined as a central venous hematocrit greater than 65% or a hemoglobin level greater than 22 g/dL. Values at or above this threshold may be associated with high blood viscosity, which is further increased by a fall in body temperature. Partial exchange transfusion may be indicated because hyperviscosity is associated with CNS and GI tract disorders.

TABLE 36.6. Estimation of Blood Volume.

Age	*Blood volume (mL/kg)*
Preterm infants	85–100
Term infants	85
1–3 months	75
3 months to adult	70

Adapted from Rowe P.[12] The Harriet Lane Handbook, 11th ed. Chicago: Year Book Medical Publishers, 1987.

Anemia

In the neonate, anemia is generally caused by hemolysis, blood loss, or decreased erythrocyte production. Hemolytic anemia in the newborn is most often caused by placental transfer of maternal antibodies that destroy the infant's erythrocytes. Significant hemolytic anemia is most commonly the result of Rh incompatibility producing jaundice, pallor, hepatosplenomegaly, and in severe cases, *hydrops fetalis*. In addition, congenital infections, inherited hemoglobinopathies, and thalassemias may all manifest as hemolytic anemia in the newborn period. In severe cases, these conditions may require exchange transfusions.

In addition to hemolysis, severe anemia in the neonate may be secondary to acute hemorrhage, which can occur as a result of placental abruption or in utero internal bleeding into the intraventricular, intraabdominal, subgaleal, or mediastinal space. Twin-twin transfusion syndrome may also result in severe anemia in the "donor" cotwin. Last, anemia of prematurity resulting from decreased red blood cell production is another cause of significant neonatal anemia; this occurs in preterm infants born before a gestational age of 30 to 34 weeks, before erythropoietin release by the kidneys has occurred.

Given an infant with a normal blood volume, mild blood loss, defined as less than 10% of blood volume, does not require transfusion. The following equation is used to determine allowable blood loss, that is, the amount of blood that can be lost before transfusion is required: estimated blood volume × (actual hematocrit − lowest allowable hematocrit), multiplied by 3 because there is an approximate 3:1 ratio of blood to red blood cells. For example, a 10-kg, 2-year-old child with an initial hematocrit of 45% would have an allowable blood loss of 120 mL: $[(80\,\text{mL/kg} \times 10\,\text{kg}) \times (0.45 - 0.30)] \times 3 = 120\,\text{mL}]$.[9] A transfusion of packed red blood cells at a volume of 10 mL/kg usually raises the hematocrit 3%–4%. Only warmed, fresh (<3 days old) whole blood or packed red cells should be transfused.

Hemoglobin

Infant erythopoiesis does not occur before approximately 2 to 3 months of age. Until that time, fetal hemoglobin represents most of the circulating hemoglobin in the neonate; this is significant in that the high proportion of fetal to adult hemoglobin in the neonate shifts their hemoglobin dissociation curve to the left. Because fetal hemoglobin has a higher affinity for retaining oxygen, lower peripheral oxygen levels are needed to release and deliver oxygen from fetal blood to the receiving tissues.

Coagulopathy

The routine administration of vitamin K to all neonates to prevent hypoprothrombinemia and hemorrhagic disease is established practice. However, this may be overlooked during the activities attendant on major congenital anomalies or conditions requiring urgent surgical evaluation. When in doubt, 1.0 mg vitamin K should be administered by intramuscular or intravenous injection.

Jaundice

Heme pigments, notably hemoglobin, are catabolized in the spleen and liver to produce bilirubin. The bilirubin is conjugated with glucoronic acid in the liver, forming a water-soluble substance that is excreted via the biliary system into the intestine. In the fetus, the lipid-soluble, unconjugated (indirect) bilirubin is cleared across the placenta. In the fetal intestine, beta-glucoronidase hydrolases conjugate bilirubin, which is then reabsorbed for transplacental clearance. Circulating unconjugated bilirubin is bound to albumin.

The neonate's capacity for conjugating bilirubin is not fully developed and may be exceeded by the bilirubin load, resulting in transient physiological jaundice that reaches a maximum at the age of 4 days but returns to normal levels by the sixth day. Usually the maximum bilirubin level does not exceed 170 μmol/L. Physiological jaundice is particularly likely to occur in SGA and preterm infants in whom a higher and more prolonged hyperbilirubinemia may be encountered.

High serum levels of unconjugated bilirubin may cross the immature blood–brain barrier in the neonate and can act as a neural poison leading to kernicterus. This condition, in its most severe form, is characterized by athetoid cerebral palsy and sensorineural hearing loss. Predisposing factors are hypoalbuminemia, acidosis, cold stress, hypoglycemia, caloric deprivation, hypoxemia, and competition for bilirubin-binding sites by drugs (e.g., furosemide, digoxin, and gentamicin) or free acids.

Practical Considerations Clinical jaundice is apparent at serum bilirubin levels of 120 to 135 μmol/L. A rapid rise early in the neonatal period suggests hemolysis, secondary to inherited enzyme defects or to maternal–neonatal blood group incompatibilities. Prolonged hyperbilirubinemia is often associated with an increase in conjugated bilirubin caused by biliary obstruction or hepatocellular dysfunction. Breast milk jaundice commonly appears between 1 and 8 weeks of age. Mild indirect hyperbilirubinemia occurs with pyloric stenosis and quickly disappears after pyloromyotomy. Intestinal obstruction can intensify jaundice by increasing the enterohepatic circulation of bilirubin. Finally, jaundice is an early and important sign of septicemia.

If hemolysis is suspected, serial hematocrit estimations, reticulocyte counts, peripheral blood smears, and a Coomb's test are appropriate. Evaluation of neonatal sepsis includes hematocrit, white blood cell count and differential platelet count, chest radiography, and cultures of blood, urine, and cerebrospinal fluid.

Phototherapy is widely used prophylactically in high-risk neonates. This therapy decreases the serum bilirubin levels by photodegradation of bilirubin in the skin into water-soluble products. It is continued until the total serum bilirubin level is less than 170 μmol/L and falling. The timing of phototherapy is based on the level of indirect bilirubin and the weight of the patient. Exchange transfusion is indicated if the indirect bilirubin level exceeds 340 μmol/L. The precise indications vary according to the individual patient, and in very low birth weight infants exchange transfusion is indicated at much lower serum bilirubin levels. Factors increasing the risk of kernicterus also influence the indications for exchange transfusion.

Immune Function

As a group, neonates are particularly vulnerable to bacterial infections during the first 4 weeks of life, which may be the consequence of maternal factors as well as intrinsic deficiencies in their host defense system. Maternal factors independently associated with a higher incidence of neonatal sepsis include premature onset of labor, prolonged rupture of membranes (more than 24 h), chorioamnionitis, colonization of the genital tract with pathogenic bacteria such as group B streptococci, and urinary tract infection.[10] In general, these factors increase the risk of neonatal infection by exposing the neonate to bacterial pathogens during gestation as well as during delivery. Neonatal factors, many of which are transient, include a diminished neutrophil storage pool, abnormal neutrophil and monocyte chemotaxis, decreased cytokine and complement production, and diminished levels of type-specific immunoglobulins including IgG, secretory IgA, and IgM.[10] Overall, these factors lead to a significantly impaired host defense mechanism in the neonate with compromised anatomic barriers. Furthermore, these deficiencies appear to be more severe in low birth weight infants.

Practical Considerations The impaired immune function and compromised anatomic barriers of neonates may contribute to postoperative infection rates in the newborn surgical patient. Specifically, wound infections, as well as infections precipitated by indwelling catheters, may complicate the perioperative course of the neonate. For this reason, many surgeons advocate the use of prophylactic, broad-spectrum antimicrobials in neonatal surgical patients. Although this practice may be common, it should be noted that the specific antibiotics used as well as the duration of antibiotic therapy are very site- and surgeon-specific parameters. At this time, there are no conclusive studies supporting the use of any particular regimen. Therefore, the prophylactic use of antibiotics in these patients must be determined on a case-by-case and surgeon-by-surgeon basis.

Fluid and Electrolyte Homeostasis

Fetal Total Body Water

In the fetus, total body water (TBW) constitutes 94% of the body weight during early gestation. As the fetus grows, this percentage progressively diminishes to a value of 78% at term. This then decreases further by approximately 3% to 5% during the first 5 days of life, eventually reaching adult levels by 9 months to 1 year of age. In addition to total body water, extracellular water (ECW) also declines until 1 to 3 years of age. In the term infant, ECW is often 40% of birth weight at 5 days. By 3 months of age, this value decreases to 33%, stabilizing at adult values of 20% to 25% by 1 to 3 years of age. Conversely, fetal intracellular water (ICW) slowly increases during gestation and the neonatal period. At 20 weeks gestation, ICW is around 25%; this increases to 33% at the time of birth, finally reaching adult levels around 44% by 3 months of age.

These fluid shifts are important because the neonate must complete these water redistribution tasks to go effectively from the intrauterine to the extrauterine environment. Under normal conditions, these changes in fetal body water progress in an orderly fashion in utero and after birth. If this process is interrupted by premature birth or intrauterine growth retardation, specific tasks my be left unfinished, predisposing the infant to increased risk for developing serious complications such as necrotizing enterocolitis, patent ductus arteriosus, and congestive heart failure.

Renal Function

Renal function is significantly impaired in the neonate. Compared to adults, the newborn infant has a relatively low renal blood flow and plasma flow and a high renovascular resistance. In fact, only 6% of the newborn's cardiac output is directed toward the kidneys, in contrast to the 25% of cardiac output in adults. Overall, these factors lead to a relatively decreased glomerular filtration rate (GFR) in neonates. In term infants, the GFR rises rapidly during the first 3 months of life, nearing adult levels by 12 to 24 months of age. In premature infants, this process is delayed, and GFR may lag behind the term infant.

In addition to GFR, the concentration capacity of the neonatal kidney is significantly lower than that of the adult kidney. Specifically, although the adult kidney can concentrate urine up to 1200 mOsm/kg, the neonatal kidney is only able to achieve 500–600 mOsm/kg. Furthermore, newborn renal tubules are particularly insensitive to the effects of antidiuretic hormone (ADH) compared to adults. Similarly, newborn tubules respond to a lesser degree to aldosterone than adult tubules. This blunted response is magnified in preterm infants. In addition, preterm infants are at a significant risk for salt wasting, which may lead to further growth retardation as sodium appears to be a permissive growth factor.

Practical Considerations for Fluid Management in the Neonate

Effective fluid and electrolyte management involves (1) calculating the fluid and electrolyte requirements for maintaining metabolic functions; (2) replacing fluid losses (third space, evaporative, insensible); and (3) considering preexisting fluid deficits or excesses. Taking these factors into consideration, a tentative program is devised for fluid and electrolytes administered for a finite period of time, usually 8h, although shorter intervals may be required in critically ill patients. The response of the patient is then closely monitored and the treatment program adjusted accordingly.[6,11]

Calculating Maintenance Needs

The neonate's basic maintenance requirement for water is the volume required for growth, renal excretion (renal water) and replacing losses from the skin, lungs, and stool. Stool water loss has been estimated at 5 to 10mL per 420 J expended, the lower figure applying to those patients not being fed. In the surgical patient with postoperative ileus, stool water loss is usually insignificant. Growth is inhibited during periods of severe stress and is also not a major factor under these conditions. The basal fluid maintenance requirement is therefore renal water plus insensible loss. Requirements during the first day of life are unique because of the greatly expanded extracellular fluid volume in the neonate, which decreases after 24h. In addition, neonates with intestinal obstruction are not hypovolemic as a result of intrauterine adjustments across the placenta. During these first 24h, basic maintenance fluid should not exceed 90mL/kg in preterm infants weighing less than 1000g or of less than 32 weeks gestation. In larger infants, maintenance fluid rates should not exceed 75mL/kg.

The basic electrolyte and energy requirements are provided by NaCl (2–5mEq/kg/day) in 5% or 10% dextrose with the addition of potassium (2–3mEq/kg/day) once urine production has been established. Calcium gluconate (1–2g/L fluid) may be added, especially in preterm infants.

Renal Water The volume of water required for excretion by the kidney depends on the renal solute load and the renal concentrating ability of the individual. The solute load that the kidneys must excrete is derived from the endogenous tissue catabolism and exogenous protein and electrolyte intake. The osmolar load is thus reduced by growth and increased by tissue necrosis, high osmolar feeds, and infusions. The volume of fluid administered should be sufficient to allow excretion of the solute load at an isotonic urine osmolality of 280 mOsm/dL.[6] It is important to understand that there is no "normal" urine output for neonates because the osmolar load is highly variable in newborns. The calculated ideal urine output, representing the renal water required to excrete an osmolar load, is also therefore variable.

Insensible Losses Invisible continuing loss of water occurs from the lungs (respiratory water loss) and through the skin (transepithelial water loss) and constitutes the insensible water loss (IWL). Respiratory water loss (RWL) accounts for approximately one-third of IWL in infants older than 32 weeks gestation and is approximately 5mL/kg body weight per 24h at a relative humidity of 50%. Transepithelial water loss (TEWL) for a full-term infant in a thermoneutral environment is approximately 7mL/kg body weight. The insensible water loss for a full-term infant in the thermoneutral environment at 50% humidity is therefore 12mL/kg per 24h.

The main factors that affect IWL are the gestational age of the infant and the relative humidity of the environment. For infants of 25 to 27 weeks gestation, TEWL has been estimated at 128mL/kg per 24h at 50% relative humidity. The relative humidity has a marked inverse effect on TEWL, which decreases to almost zero as the relative humidity approaches 100%. Plastic sheets may be used to increase the relative humidity around the infant and reduce TEWL by 50% to 70%. Conversely, radiant warmers and phototherapy increase IWL. This loss is magnified in the preterm infant.

Management Program The most commonly used method of calculating fluid requirements is based on body weight (Table 36.7). However, because of the many factors affecting maintenance requirements, there is no close or constant relationship between body weight and fluid and electrolyte needs. Thus, many surgeons advocate the use of a dynamic approach to fluid management. Such approaches generally begin with the administration of an initial fluid volume that

TABLE 36.7. Calculation of Maintenance Fluid Requirements.

Body weight (kg)	*Fluid volume per 24h*
1–10	100mL/kg
11–20	1000mL + 50mL for each 1kg over 10kg
>20	1500mL + 20mL for each 1kg over 20kg

is safe for the patient's status. This initial volume is essentially a "best guess" volume. The effects of this volume on the patient's physiology are then monitored and appropriate changes are made.

Calculation of Additional Losses

External losses from intestinal drainage, fistulas, and drainage tubes are directly measured and replaced volume for volume with an appropriate electrolyte solution. In neonates it is wise to measure the electrolytes in the fluid to more accurately guide replacement. Protein-rich losses (e.g., pleural fluid from chest tubes) are replaced with albumin solutions or fresh-frozen plasma. Internal losses into body cavities or tissues (third space losses) cannot be measured, and adequate replacement of these losses depends on careful monitoring of the patient's response to fluid therapy.

Considering Preexisting Fluid Deficits or Excesses

In addition to addressing maintenance requirements and additional losses, the fluid management of the neonate should include an assessment of any preexisting fluid deficits or excesses. Preexisting deficits may be caused by in utero or intrapartum hemorrhage as well as third space losses. Preexisting excesses may be secondary to prematurity leading to a high total body water content. In all these cases, the preexisting condition should be considered when determining a fluid management plan.

Monitoring the Fluid and Electrolyte Program

Once a fluid and electrolyte management program has been initiated, proper monitoring must occur to identify the newborn's response. In this manner, therapy may be adjusted dynamically to meet the specific needs of each neonate. The newborn's response to a fluid and electrolyte program may be monitored by clinical examination, body weight measurements, and urine volume and composition measurements.

Clinical Features Severe isotonic and hypovolemic dehydration results in poor capillary filling and collapse of peripheral veins. The skin is cool and mottled, with reduced turgor; the mucous membranes are dry, and the anterior fontanelle is sunken. These findings occur with 10% body fluid losses in an infant of more than 28 days of age and with 15% losses in a neonate. Hypertonic dehydration is more difficult to detect clinically because the decrease in circulating blood volume is considerably less than the total loss of body fluids. Signs of shock occur late, and CNS signs such as lethargy, stupor, and seizures predominate.

Body Weight Serial measurements of body weight are a useful guide to total body water in the neonate. Fluctuations over a 24-h period are primarily related to loss or gain of fluid; 1 g body weight being approximately equal to 1 mL water. Errors occur if changes in clothing, dressings, tubes, and standard intravenous arm/leg boards are not accounted for and if weighing scales are not regularly calibrated.

Urine Volume and Composition If the volume of fluid administered is inadequate, urine volume falls and its concentration increases. If excess fluid is administered, the opposite occurs. One should aim to achieve a urine output that will maintain a urine osmolality of approximately 280 mOsm/dL. In neonates, this usually results in a urine output of 2 mL/kg/h. For infants and older children, hydration is adequate if the urine output is 1–2 mL/kg/h with an osmolality of 280–300 mOsm/kg. Serial hematocrit determinations, in the absence of hemolysis or bleeding, also suggest a loss or gain of plasma water.

When the osmolar load is large, for example, with extensive tissue destruction or with infusion of high osmolar solutions, urine flow may have to be increased to provide adequate renal clearance. Accurate measurements of urine flow and concentration are fundamental to the management of critically ill infants and children. In this situation, the insertion of an indwelling urinary catheter is recommended.

The specific gravity of the urine is a reliable indicator of hypertonicity (>1.012 specific gravity) and hypotonicity (<1.008 specific gravity) but is unreliable if urine is in the isotonic range (1.009–1.011 specific gravity). When fluid monitoring is critical, urine osmolality estimations provide more precise information than specific gravity. An increase in osmolality suggests that too little water or too much electrolyte has been given. A fall in osmolality suggests that sodium replacement is inadequate or that too much water has been administered. An unexpected change in osmolality, particularly an increase, requires immediate determination of serum levels of electrolytes, blood urea nitrogen, and glucose values and a calculation of the osmolality. Serum osmolality can be measured directly or calculated by the formula:

$$\text{Osmalility} = \text{serum sodium} \times 1.86 + (\text{blood urea nitrogen}/2.8) + (\text{glucose}/18) + 5$$

From this equation, it is possible to determine whether the rise in osmolality is caused by an increase in serum sodium, the development of hyperglycemia, or high blood urea nitrogen. Occasionally the measured serum osmolality is higher than the calculated osmolality, suggesting that the increase in serum osmolality is caused by some unidentified osmolar active substance such as a metabolic byproduct resulting from sepsis, shock, or radiopaque contrast material.

A rising blood urea nitrogen level and falling urine output may be caused by acute renal failure or prerenal oliguria with azotemia resulting from hypovolemia. The distinction between these two states is important for appropriate treatment. Initially, the response to a fluid challenge of 20 mL/kg 5% dextrose and sodium chloride over 1 h is monitored. If oliguria persists, the sodium, creatinine, and osmolality levels in both blood and urine are determined. The fractional excretion of sodium (Fe_{Na}) is calculated using the formula:

$$Fe_{Na} = (\text{urine Na}/\text{serum Na}) / (\text{urine creatinine}/\text{xerum creatinine}) \times 100$$

A normal Fe_{Na} is 2% to 3%. A value below 2% implies prerenal azotemia and a value above 3% implies renal failure.

Calcium and Magnesium Homeostasis

In addition to fluid and sodium management, calcium and magnesium homeostasis are clinically significant challenges in the newborn surgical patient. The fetus receives calcium by active transport across the placenta, 75% of the total requirement being transferred after the 18th week of gestation. Hypocalcemia, defined as a serum level of ionized calcium below 1.0mg/100mL, is most likely to occur 24 to 48h after birth. Causes include decreased calcium stores, decreased renal phosphate excretion, and relative hypoparathyroidism secondary to suppression by high fetal calcium levels. Low birth weight infants are at a great risk (particularly if they are preterm), as are those born of a complicated pregnancy or delivery (e.g., diabetic mother) or those receiving bicarbonate infusions. Exchange transfusions or the rapid administration of citrated blood may also lead to hypocalcemia. The symptoms of hypocalcemia are nonspecific and include jitteriness, high-pitched crying, cyanosis, vomiting, twitching, and seizures. Diagnosis is confirmed by determining the serum calcium level. However, the ionized fraction of the serum calcium may be low, resulting in clinical hypocalcemia without a great reduction in total serum calcium. Therefore, evaluation of the serum ionized calcium level is often useful.

Practical Considerations Hypocalcemia is prevented by adding calcium gluconate to daily maintenance therapy, 1–2g/24h intravenously or 2g/24h by mouth.[12] Symptomatic hypocalcemia is treated by intravenous administration of 10% calcium gluconate in a dose of 1–2mL/kg over 10min; the rate should not exceed 1mL/min.

Infants at high risk for hypocalcemia are also at risk for hypomagnesemia. In fact, the two conditions may coexist. If there is no response to attempted correction of a documented calcium deficiency, hypomagnesemia should be suspected and serum magnesium levels measured. Hypomagnesemia is corrected by administering 50% magnesium sulfate, 0.2mEq/kg every 6h intravenously, followed by oral magnesium sulfate 30mEq/day.

Although most seizures that occur in the neonatal period have a cerebral cause and are not secondary to hypoglycemia or hypocalcemia, hypocalcemia should be suspected in high-risk infants, particularly after surgery. Immediate blood glucose determination and serum glucose and calcium measurements should therefore be performed in a "jittery" neonate. Treatment should be prompt, with intravenous glucose when hypoglycemia is suspected, followed by intravenous calcium if symptoms persist.

General Considerations in the Perioperative Care of the Neonate

Invasive Monitoring

Because of the dynamic physiology of the neonatal period, newborn surgical patients should be monitored continuously in the neonatal unit. As already described, transcutaneous pulse oximetry is useful for monitoring episodes of apnea and bradycardia, which can be common in the preterm infant. In addition, accurate monitoring of fluid status often requires an indwelling urinary catheter and frequent laboratory evaluations.

Invasive monitoring and access in the newborn can be achieved through the umbilical vessels as they are relatively accessible in this population. Specifically, umbilical venous catheters provide central venous access. A 3.5 Fr. catheter is required for infants less than 1500g; those 1500 to 3500g can accommodate a 5 Fr. catheter. Umbilical artery catheters may be indicated in infants with significant respiratory distress or any infant who may require frequent blood sampling. These catheters usually enter the aorta through the internal iliac arteries: 3.5 Fr. catheters are used in infants weighing less than 1200g and 5 Fr. catheters are used in infants weighing more than 1200g.

Nutrition

In the neonatal surgical patient, proper nutrition must be delivered to meet their relatively large energy requirements. Specifically, neonates require a large energy intake because of their high basal metabolic rate, requirements for growth and development, energy needs to maintain body heat, and their limited energy reserves. These requirements vary according to age and environmental factors and are significantly increased by cold stress, surgical procedures, infections, and injuries. Energy requirements are increased 10% to 25% by surgery, more than 50% by infections, and 150% by burns.[13] Energy reserves are limited in the neonate, whose liver glycogen stores are usually consumed in the first 3h of life. These limited reserves are even more restricted in the preterm and SGA infant.

The energy needs of individual newborns can be calculated according to the requirements for basal metabolism plus growth. Table 36.8 lists the energy requirements of children by age group. Consideration must also be given to the adequacy of energy reserves in the presence of stress factors such as cold, infection and trauma, and surgery. Protein should be administered at a rate of 2–3g/kg/24h to achieve a normal weigh gain of 10–15g/kg/24h; 30% to 40% of the total nonprotein calories should be provided as fat.

Enteral Nutrition

The best means of providing calories is via the GI tract either by mouth, or nasogastric or nasojejunal feeding tube, or through a surgically placed gastrostomy or jejunostomy tube. Gastric feeding is preferable because it allows for normal digestive processes and hormonal responses, a greater tolerance for larger osmotic loads, and a low incidence of dumping. Breast or bottle feeding is preferable for infants, usually more than 32 to 34 weeks gestation, who have a coordinated suck

TABLE 36.8. Energy Requirements of Various Age Groups.

Age at delivery	*Energy required per 24h (J)*
Basal metabolism: full-term infant:	
Birth	134
2 weeks	202
1 year	168
Teen	97
Growth calories:	
Birth	139
3 months	76
6 months	50
1 year	50
Teen	76
Total calories (maintenance and growth):	
Neonatal term (0–4 days)	462–504
Low birth weight infant	504–546
3–4 months	420–445
5–12 months	420
1–7 years	378–315
7–12 years	315–252
12–18 years	252–126

and swallow mechanism. Gavage feeding is indicated for infants with an impaired coordinated suck and swallow mechanism, or for supplementation for those infants with a high metabolic rate who cannot gain weight with oral feeding alone and is performed by passing a 5 Fr. silastic or polyethylene feeding tube into the stomach. The use of nasoduodenal or nasojejunal tubes is reserved for infants who cannot tolerate intragastric feeding (e.g., delayed gastric emptying, gastroesophageal reflux, depressed gag reflex). A silastic mercury-tipped feeding tube (length: tip of nose to knee) is passed through the nose into the stomach. Transpyloric tube placement can be accomplished by one of two methods: placement of a mercury-weighted tube into the stomach, positioning the patient right side down, and administering a prokinetic agent if gastric peristalsis does not propel the tube into the duodenum; or fluoroscopic placement. It is mandatory to confirm proper tube placement by aspirating and obtaining a chest radiograph.

A prolonged delay or inability to initiate oral feeding mandates placement of a gastrostomy or a jejunostomy tube placed during open surgery, or laparoscopic surgery, or by a percutaneous approach aided by either gastroscopy or fluoroscopy.

PARENTERAL NUTRITION

The indications for parenteral feeding include the following: extremely low birth weight infant, surgical GI tract abnormalities with prolonged postoperative ileus (gastroschisis, necrotizing enterocolitis), short gut syndrome following extensive bowel resection, chronic diarrhea (malabsorption syndrome), inflammatory bowel disease, severe acute alimentary disorders (pancreatitis, necrotizing enterocolitis), chylothorax, intestinal fistulae, and persistent vomiting associated with cancer chemotherapy.[14]

Short-term or supplemental, relatively low calorie, parenteral nutrition may be administered via a peripheral vein. However, concentrated glucose solutions greater than 15% will thrombose a peripheral vein, so peripheral parenteral nutrition is limited to 12.5% dextrose solution. In contrast, central venous administration allows the large blood flow to immediately dilute the solution. Central venous access can be obtained either percutaneously or via cutdown. The tip of the catheter should be at the superior vena cava/right atrial junction as judged by fluoroscopy. A postprocedure chest radiograph is mandatory to rule out pneumothorax. The daily component requirements for total parenteral nutrition (TPN) are detailed in Table 36.9.

Initiating TPN

CARBOHYDRATES. Begin neonates at 4–6 mg/kg/min dextrose, infants and children at 7–8 mg/kg/min. Increase by 2 mg/kg/min every day until the goal of 10–12 mg/kg/min is reached. Do not exceed 12.5% dextrose in peripheral veins. Central veins can tolerate up to 30% dextrose.

PROTEIN. Begin neonates and infants at 0.5 g/kg/day and advance by 0.5–1.0 g/kg/day until 3 g/kg/day. Do not exceed 10% to 12% of total daily caloric intake. Start children at 1 g/kg/day and advance 1 g/kg/day until 3 g/kg/day is reached. Protein intake should be restricted in patients who cannot tolerate a large nitrogen load (e.g., patients with renal insufficiency).

TABLE 36.9. Total Parenteral Nutrition Requirements.

Component	*Neonate*	*6 months–10 years*	*More than 10 years*
Calories (kcal/kg/day)	90–120	60–105	40–75
Fluid (mL/kg/day)	120–180	120–150	50–75
Dextrose (mg/kg/min)	4–6	7–8	7–8
Protein (g/kg/day)	2–3	1.5–2.5	0.8–2.0
Fat (g/kg/day)	0.5–3.0	1.0–4.0	1.0–4.0
Sodium (mEq/kg/day)	3–4	3–4	3–4
Potassium (mEq/kg/day)	2–3	2–3	1–2
Calcium (mg/kg/day)	80–120	40–80	40–60
Phosphate (mg/kg/day)	25–40	25–40	25–40
Magnesium (mEq/kg/day)	0.25–1.0	0.5	0.5
Zinc (μg/kg/day)	300	100	3 mg/day
Copper (μg/kg/day)	20	20	1.2 mg/day
Chromium (μg/kg/day)	0.2	0.2	12 mg/day
Manganese (μg/kg/day)	6	6	0.3 mg/day
Selenium (μg/kg/d)	2	2	10–20/day

FAT. Begin neonates at 0.5 g/kg/day, infants and children at 1.0 g/kg/day, and advance 0.5–1.0 g/kg/day as a continuous infusion until the goal of 3.0 g/kg/day. Contraindications to lipid infusion include allergy to egg yolk phospholipids and fat metabolism abnormalities (e.g., hyperlipidemia, lipoid nephrosis). Thrombocytopenia is a relative contraindication to lipids (intralipid may interfere with platelet function). Do not exceed 1 g/kg/day in premature infants with hyperbilirubinemia (free fatty acids can displace bilirubin from albumin). Intralipids must account for at least 2% of the caloric requirements to prevent essential fatty acid deficiency.

Pain Management

Postoperative pain management in the newborn surgical patient may be challenging. In particular, the use of opioid analgesics in the neonate must be monitored carefully. As a group, neonates have a narrower therapeutic window for postoperative morphine analgesia than older age groups. In addition, neonates treated with opioids exhibit variable pharmacokinetics and are at a high risk for respiratory depression.[15] Despite these challenges, postoperative opiate analgesia can be effectively used to control pain in neonates. However, this requires close monitoring and may necessitate consultation with a pain management service. In addition to opiate analgesics, acetaminophen and nonsteroidal antiinflammatory agents may be used to for pain control. In particular, acetaminophen has had a long safety record in newborn patients.

Gastrointestinal Decompression

The importance of gastric decompression in the neonate undergoing surgery cannot be overemphasized. The distended stomach carries the risk of aspiration and pneumonia, and may impair diaphragmatic excursions, resulting in respiratory distress. With congenital diaphragmatic hernia, ventilation is progressively impaired as the herniated intestine becomes distended with air and fluid. With gastroschisis, omphalocele, and diaphragmatic hernia, the ability to reduce the herniated intestine into the abdominal cavity is impaired by intestinal distension, which may be alleviated by adequate orogastric or nasogastric decompression. A double-lumen sump tube, such as a Replogle tube, is preferred, utilizing low continuous suction. If a single-lumen tube is used, intermittent aspiration is required. The correct position of the tube in the stomach is confirmed by carefully measuring the tube before insertion, by noting the nature of the aspirate, and by radiography. The tube should be carefully taped to avoid displacement. The use of gastrostomy tubes for postoperative gastric decompression is decreasing in popularity, but should be considered when prolonged postoperative gastric or intestinal stasis is anticipated.

Diagnostic Studies

Most laboratory tests pose an additional burden to the already stressed neonate. Therefore, diagnostic studies should be restricted to those essential for diagnosis and proper management. The volume of blood drawn for laboratory tests should be documented as these small volumes cumulatively represent significant loss in a small infant.

When the patient is transferred to other departments for investigational procedures, monitoring and resuscitation equipment should be available with a surgeon in attendance. All studies should be performed with minimal disturbance, taking steps to prevent heat loss. Before using hyperosmolar radiopaque contrast materials, intravenous fluids must be administered and fluid deficits corrected, regardless of the route of administration. To counteract the osmotic effect of the contrast medium, an intravenous infusion of sodium chloride 34 mEq/L at twice the maintenance rate should be given during the radiographic study and for 2 to 4 h afterward. During this period the patient should be carefully monitored as already described.

Antimicrobial Therapy

Deficiencies in the immune system of the newborn infant render it vulnerable to major bacterial insults. Prophylactic antimicrobial therapy is advised for infants undergoing major surgery, particularly of the GI tract or genitourinary (GU) system. Adequate coverage is provided by combining a penicillin (e.g., ampicillin) or first-generation cephalosporin (e.g., cefazolin) with an aminoglycoside (e.g., gentamicin). Clindamicin or metronidazole is added when anaerobic coverage is deemed necessary. Alternatively, single-drug therapy using a broad-spectrum cephalosporin (e.g., cefoxitin) may be appropriate. Antibiotics are commenced before the operation and may be discontinued postoperatively at the surgeon's discretion.

Preoperative NPO Guidelines

Patients Younger than 6 Months. No food or formula 4 h before the procedure. Children may continue to have breast milk and clear liquids (water, Pedialyte, glucose water, or apple juice) until 2 h before the procedure.

Patients from 6 Months to 18 Years. Nothing to eat or drink after midnight except clear liquids (water, apple juice, Pedialyte, plain Jell-o, popsicles, white grape juice), which can be continued until 2 h before the procedure.

Patients Older than 18 Years. Nothing to eat or drink after midnight except clear liquids (water, apple juice, plain Jell-o, popsicles) until 4 h before the procedure.

TABLE 36.10. Bowel Preparation Before Elective Pediatric Surgery.

Inpatient preparation	• Begin prep at noon or sooner, the day before surgery • Place a small nasogastric (NG) feeding tube if unable to take Golytely orally • Administer Reglan (unless contraindicated) • Dose: 0.1–0.2 mg/kg/dose (maximum of 0.8 mg/kg over 24 h); may give per NG q 4 h • Begin Golytely 25 mL/kg/h by NG tube for 4 h or until effluent is clear • Clears or Pedialyte by mouth ad lib until n.p.o.
Outpatient preparation	**Patients over 1 year of age:** • Clear liquids only the day before surgery. Examples: Pedialyte, glucose water, juice without pulp, clear broths, Gatorade, tea, boullion, water, popsicles, Jell-o **Alternative for children over 1 year of age with history of moderate to severe constipation:** • Magnesium citrate (1 oz./year of age, maximum 10 oz.) by mouth, once in the evening for 2 days before surgery • Start clear liquids 24 h before surgery **Patients 12–16 years of age add:** Dulcolax 5 mg PO daily × 2 days **Patients over 16 years of age add:** Dulcolax 10 mg PO daily × 2 days

Bowel Preparation Instructions

The bowel is mechanically cleansed for elective bowel resection. There is varied opinion as to whether a bowel preparation is needed for certain procedures, as well as what to use to accomplish it, and whether to do it at home or in the hospital. Examples of inpatient and outpatient regimens are detailed in Table 36.10.

Lateral Neck Masses

The differential diagnosis of a laterally presenting neck mass is extensive and includes branchial cleft remnants, lymphangioma, dermoid cyst, epidermoid cyst, hemangioma, lymphadenitis, leukemia, torticollis, neurofibroma, lipoma, metastatic tumor to the cervical lymph nodes, parotid tumor, and tumors of dentigerous origin. Of these, branchial cleft remnants, lymphangioma (cystic hygroma), lymphadenitis, and torticollis are discussed.

Branchial Cleft Cysts, Sinuses, and Remnants

The branchial arches develop and partially regress all during the first 6 weeks of life.[16] They are composed of endodermal pouches on the pharyngeal wall and are noted externally by the presence of ectodermal clefts. The dorsal portion of the first cleft becomes the external auditory canal; the other clefts are obliterated. The first, third, and fourth pharyngeal pouches persist as adult organs. The first pouch becomes the eustachian tube, the middle ear cavity, and the mastoid air cells. The second pouch incompletely regresses and becomes the palatine tonsil and the supratonsillar fossa. The third pouch forms the superior parathyroid; the fourth forms the inferior parathyroid and the thymus glands. Cysts developing from branchial structures usually appear later in childhood as opposed to sinuses, fistulae, and cartilaginous remnants. Incomplete sinus tracts are mere dimples in the skin, which are often associated with a small segment of ectopic cartilage. Approximately 15% are bilateral, and one frequently observes similar lesions in siblings.

Anomalies of the First Branchial Cleft

These anomalies are rare and often present in adulthood as a small cyst lying close to the parotid gland. During infancy, this anomaly is usually noted as a draining sinus located anterior to the ear. Excision should be undertaken cautiously because the tract extends to the external auditory canal, placing the branches of the facial nerve at risk for injury.

Anomalies of the Second Branchial Cleft

These are the most common lesions, arising in the mid- or lower neck, along the anterior border of the sternocleidomastoid muscle. A cyst, sinus, or fistula may be present. The fistula tract classically extends from the skin opening, deep to the platysma, superiorly beneath the stylohyoid and digastric muscles at the level of the hyoid bone, passes over the hypoglossal and glossopharyngeal nerves and between the bifurcation of the carotid artery, and passes medially to enter the lateral pharyngeal wall.

Anomalies of the Third Branchial Cleft

These are extremely rare and, similar to the second branchial cleft remnant, are located along the anterior border of the sternocleidomastoid muscle. However, these are usually lower on the neck and the fistula tract, when present, passes lateral to the carotid artery bifurcation rather than through it and enters the piriform sinus.

Treatment

Rarely are branchial cleft anomalies cosmetically unappealing. Rather, they should be excised early in life, shortly after diagnosis, because repeated infection is quite common, making resection more difficult. When infection occurs, antibiotic therapy and often incision and drainage are indicated. The definitive excision is staged, approximately 6 weeks later, giving the inflammation adequate time to resolve, thus assuring a complete resection. Every effort should be made to excise the entire cyst wall or fistula tract (including the skin punctum, if present) as recurrence and infection are common with incomplete removal.

Lymphangioma (Cystic Hygroma)

These hygromas are benign multilobular, multinodular cystic masses lined by endothelial cells. They result from maldevelopment of the lymphaticovenous sacs.[17] Eventually, sequestrations of lymphatic tissue develop that do not communicate with the normal lymphatic system. Fifty percent to 65% appear at birth, 90% by the second year of life. They are located most commonly in the posterior triangle of the neck (75%) (Fig. 36.1); axilla (20%); and mediastinum, retroperitoneum, pelvis, and groin (5%). Neck hygromas may communicate beneath the clavicle with an axillary hygroma, mediastinal hygroma, or rarely both. The majority are asymptomatic, although large lesions invading the floor of the mouth may cause symptoms referable to pharyngeal and/or upper airway obstruction. The skin is never involved; these lesions grow along fascial planes and around neurovascular structures.

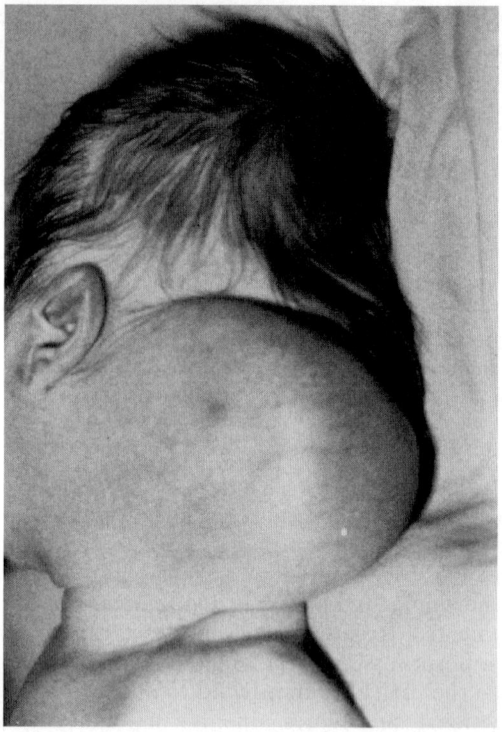

FIGURE 36.1. Typical neonatal lymphangioma arising from the posterior cervical triangle. (Reproduced with permission from Seminars in Pediatric Surgery 1994;(3):147–159.)

There are two modes of treatment that are chosen based on imaging [computed tomography (CT) or magnetic resonance imaging (MRI)] studies; sclerotherapy and excision. Intralesional injection of a sclerosing agent is most effective for unilocular cysts. Examples of agents that have been used are OK-432 (a lyophilized mixture of *Streptococcus pyogenes* and penicillin G potassium) and bleomycin.[18–20] Excision is carried out with bipolar cautery to ensure a hemostatic dissection and decrease the incidence of lymph leak and nerve injury. Intraoperative cyst rupture increases the difficulty of the dissection because the thin-walled empty cyst is difficult to identify and the margins are obscured. The recurrence rate is low (10%) if all microscopic disease is resected. When gross disease is left, recurrence occurs in up to 100%.

Cervical Lymphadenitis

Cervical adenitis is an inflammatory enlargement of one or more lymph nodes of the head and neck.[21] There is tenderness, erythema, fever, and leukocytosis. It is often secondary to an acute staphylococcal or streptococcal infection originating in the upper respiratory tract, scalp, ear, or neck. Treatment is with antibiotics, warm compresses, and surgical drainage when the lymph node(s) become fluctuant.

A more indolent form of cervical adenitis is caused by nontuberculous (atypical) mycobacteria and cat scratch disease. Nontuberculous adenitis is a local process without systemic involvement. There is unilateral nontender enlargement of submandibular/submaxillary lymph nodes, often with a draining sinus, that is refractory to antibiotic therapy. Excisional biopsy is indicated. Cat scratch disease is benign and self-limited. After 3 to 5 days, a characteristic papule appears at the site of inoculation. Adenopathy and mild constitutional symptoms evolve over 1 to 2 weeks. Suppuration is rare, and resolution occurs without treatment.

More obscure causes of cervical adenitis include tuberculous adenitis, *Actinomyces israelii*, toxoplasmosis, *Francisella tularensis*, Epstein–Barr virus, *Yersinia enterocolitica*, *Nocardia* sp., and fungi.

Torticollis

Torticollis occurs in newborns and results from fibrosis and shortening of the sternocleidomastoid muscle, producing a "tumor" in the muscle that causes the face to turn toward the contralateral side and the head to tilt toward the ipsilateral shoulder.[22] Increasing facial and cranial asymmetry results from this abnormal positioning. Facial hemihypoplasia and plagiocephaly (flattening of the ipsilateral posterior skull) occurs in untreated cases, usually within 6 months. The etiology is unclear and most likely results from birth trauma. Passive range-of-motion exercises, coupled with a change in the infant's feeding position, will cure most. Often the "tumor" disappears well before full range of motion is acquired. The only indication for operation (division of the muscle) is facial hemihypoplasia.

Midline Neck Masses

These masses usually present in children more than 6 months old and are often thyroglossal duct cysts/sinuses, dermoid/epidermoid inclusion cysts, or goiter. Less common differential diagnoses are ectopic midline thyroid, pyramidal lobe of the thyroid, thyroid adenoma of the isthmus, carcinoma of the thyroid with a pretracheal nodal metastasis, dermoid or seabaceous cyst, lipoma, and submental lymphadenitis. In contrast, cervical teratoma and lymphangioma are the most common midline neck masses in the newborn. They are often quite large and may threaten the airway.

Thyroglossal Duct Cysts and Sinuses

Thyroglossal duct remnants are three times more common than branchial cleft remnants. The majority are noted before the age of 5 years and 75% are cysts, 25% draining sinuses. These develop as the thyroid diverticulum descends from the foramen cecum of the tongue, often through the midline of the developing hyoid bone.[16] The thyroid diverticulum remains connected to the foramen cecum by the thyroglossal duct. Normally the duct disappears by the time the thyroid reaches its final position. When the thyroid descends fully but elements of the duct persist, a thyroglossal duct cyst may develop. Thyroid tissue (often dysgenetic) may be present in the cyst or the along the sinus tract. Because the mass is located within the strap muscles and may be attached to the base of the tongue, it moves with deglutition or when the tongue is protruded.

Complete excision is indicated because of the risk of acute or chronic infection and the possibility of papillary carcinoma arising from dysgenetic ectopic thyroid tissue later in adulthood. The procedure should include excision of the cyst and the entire tract upward to the base of the tongue. The central portion of the hyoid bone should be removed because the duct often passes through this structure. Recurrences occur when the hyoid is not removed or when the cyst was previously infected and/or drained. If thyroid tissue is noted in the resected specimen, thyroid scanning is indicated to identify those children in whom there is no other thyroid tissue remaining as they require lifelong thyroid hormone replacement therapy.

Inclusion Cysts

Inclusion cysts occur when ectodermal elements become trapped beneath the skin at sites of embryonic fusion lines.[23,24] These often contain sebum, hair follicles, connective tissue, and papillae. They are commonly noted in the supraorbital region or just above the sternal notch. Removal is justified to confirm the diagnosis and to avoid infection.

Congenital Anomalies of the Lung

Congenital Cystic Adenomatoid Malformation

Congenital cystic adenomatoid malformations (CCAM) are cystic, solid, or mixed intrapulmonary hamartomas that communicate with the normal tracheobronchial tree and do not have an anomalous blood supply.[25] Embryologically, they arise from excessive proliferation of cartilage and mucous gland-deficient bronchial structures without alveoli. They are most often lobar and are classified radiologically based on cyst size[26,27]; type I are large (>2 cm) cysts, type II are smaller cysts (<2 cm), and type III have cysts that are so small as to impart a solid appearance. Histologically, a CCAM may be found in conjunction with a pulmonary sequestration. The majority of these lesions are lobar and can be identified prenatally by ultrasound. The prenatal natural history can be quite variable.[28] Some may grow so large and produce such severe mediastinal shift that heart failure and hydrops results. If the mass is not resected (either via in utero surgery or after emergency cesarean delivery), death ensues in virtually 100%. Others may remain the same size or regress considerably. Those children in whom hydrops did not occur before birth may be born asymptomatic (small lesions) or have variable degrees of respiratory distress caused by compression of the ipsilateral normal lung. Asymptomatic children may be observed, but resection (pulmonary lobectomy) is recommended because these lesions often become infected and there are case reports of malignant transformation occurring in untreated, long-standing cysts.[29]

Pulmonary Sequestration

This cystic lung lesion is most commonly noted in the lower left hemithorax. It has an aberrant arterial supply, usually from the infradiaphragmatic aorta and venous drainage, that is either pulmonary or systemic.[30] There is an extralobar variant that has its own investing pleura but no communication with the tracheobronchial tree. In contrast to prenatally diagnosed CCAMs, sequestrations rarely grow large enough to produce hydrops and in utero demise. Children with extralobar sequestrations are usually asymptomatic at birth and have been diagnosed either prenatally or by chest radiograph demonstrating a radiopaque mass in the lower hemithorax. These are often associated with congenital diaphragmatic hernia and are noted incidentally during repair of the diaphragmatic defect. The intralobar variant is enveloped within the visceral pleura of the adjacent normal lung and has common alveolar communications, predisposing it to infection and lung abscess formation. Treatment is by excision of the sequestration; this may or may not require lower lobectomy, depending on the degree of inflammation.

Congenital Lobar Emphysema

Congenital lobar emphysema (CLE) consists of hyperinflation of a single lobe, usually the upper or middle lobes.[31] There are a variety of causes such as bronchial obstruction (deficient bronchial cartilage support, redundant mucosa, bronchial stenosis, bronchial compression by anomalous vessels or mediastinal mass, mucous plug), a polyalveolar lobe (large number of abnormal alveoli that are prone to expansion), or hypoplastic emphysema (reduced number of bronchi and alveoli with increased air space size).

Infants with CLE usually do not present with respiratory distress for several days or weeks. Many infants, however, present with mild tachypnea at birth. In only 5% of cases do symptoms develop after 6 months of life. Most of the babies require excision of the affected lobe because of progressive hyperinflation. At thoracotomy, the large, overdistended lobe characteristically "pops out" when the ribs are separated. Anesthesia should not be started until all surgical personnel are present and prepared for emergency thoracotomy because positive pressure ventilation may acutely enlarge the emphysematous lobe, thereby compressing the normal lung tissue and heart.

Mediastinal Masses

Mediastinal masses are relatively common in infants and children and can be classified according to the compartment of the mediastinum from which they arise.[32] The most common mediastinal mass is a posterior mediastinal neurogenic tumor.

Anterior Mediastinal Masses

1. Thymic cysts and thymomas are rare and account for 5% of cases.
2. Lymphoma accounts for approximately 10% and is either Hodgkin's or non-Hodgkin's variety. About 40% to 60% of children with Hodgkin's disease present with an anterior mediastinal mass.
3. Teratoma (15%) may be cystic, solid, and may also be found within the pericardium; approximately 20% are malignant.
4. Lymphangioma occur in 7% and most commonly extend caudally from the neck into the mediastinum; these rarely arise primarily in the mediastinum.

Middle Mediastinal Masses

1. Bronchogenic cysts (15%): these extrapulmonary cysts are located in either the paratracheal or juxtahilar regions. The intrapulmonary variant has airway connections and is thus prone to infection. They are three times more common on the right side than on the left.
2. Pericardial cysts are rare, are almost always asymptomatic, and are usually an incidental chest radiograph finding.

Posterior Mediastinal Masses

1. Neurogenic tumors (see Childhood Tumors section) account for 33% and include neuroblastoma, ganglioneuroblastoma, ganglioneuroma, neurofibroma, and neurofibrosarcoma. Common symptoms include respiratory distress (via tracheal or lung compression), Horner's syndrome, and pain.
2. Enterogenous cysts (28%) are esophageal duplica-tions that often contain ectopic gastric tissue (see GI duplications below). They are termed neurenteric cysts when there is an associated cervical or thoracic vertebral anomaly. They can end blindly (above or below the diaphragm) or may communicate with the jejunum. Ten percent to 15% are associated with a separate intraabdominal GI duplication.

Congenital Diaphragmatic Hernia

Congenital diaphragmatic hernia (CDH) is a highly lethal and morbid disease that affects 1 in 2000 live births.[33] Anatomically, CDH results from an embryological fusion defect, allowing herniation of intraabdominal contents into the chest. Failure of posterolateral fusion of the various components comprising the diaphragm leads to a persistent pleuroperitoneal canal, the foramen of Bochdalek. Diaphragmatic fusion occurs just before the return of the intestinal tract into the abdomen following its physiological herniation (10–12 weeks gestation). The hernia is most common on the left side (90%), with a rate of associated anomalies of 20% (chromosomal abnormalities, neural tube defects, and congenital heart disease). Pulmonary hypoplasia is believed to occur when the developing fetal lungs are compressed by the herniated abdominal viscera, limiting the number of bronchopulmonary generations.[34,35] An alternate theory based on experimental studies with nitrofen-induced CDH in rodents suggests that pulmonary hypoplasia may be a separate developmental defect not related to the mass effect of viscera on the developing lungs.[36] Herniation of gut through the diaphragmatic defect prevents normal intestinal rotation and fixation, accounting for the almost universal presence of intestinal rotational anomalies in infants with CDH. The size of the defect ranges from a small slit to complete diaphragmatic agenesis. Commonly, the posterolateral diaphragmatic rim is represented by a thin ridge of muscle under the peritoneum, or it may be completely absent. The anteromedial diaphragmatic rim is usually intact. A hernia sac can be found in up to 20% of patients and may be associated with an improved survival.

Physiologically, children born with CDH frequently develop respiratory distress from pulmonary hypoplasia and/or persistent fetal circulation with pulmonary hypertension. The development of symptoms in CDH correlates with the degree of pulmonary hypoplasia and pulmonary hypertension. The abdomen is classically scaphoid. Breath sounds may be absent on the ipsilateral side, and cardiac sounds may be distant. The babies are usually symptomatic in the delivery room with tachypnea, grunting respirations, retractions, and cyanosis and may require urgent intubation. The radiographic findings include air-filled loops of bowel in the hemithorax, a paucity of gas within the abdomen, radiopaque hemithorax if the bowel does not contain a significant amount of gas or if the liver occupies the majority of the hemithorax, contralateral mediastinal shift with compression of the contralateral lung, loss of normal ipsilateral diaphragmatic contour, and the nasogastric tube may coil in the hemithorax. The radiographic differential diagnosis includes congenital cystic lung diseases (e.g., cystic adenomatoid malformation), congenital lobar emphysema, pulmonary sequestration, diaphragmatic eventration, and unilateral pulmonary agenesis.

Prenatal diagnosis is occurring more and more frequently and allows the mother and fetus to be referred to an institution where sophisticated perinatal and pediatric surgical units are available. Treatment before birth has been studied in two randomized trials and was found to be no more efficacious than treatment after birth.[37,38] Treatment includes prompt orotracheal intubation after sedation and paralysis. Avoid bag-mask ventilation, even for brief periods, as the gut may distend with air. Administer 100% oxygen; peak inspiratory pressures >35 mmHg should be avoided, if possible. Insert a sump gastric tube and place it on low continuous suction. Monitor pre- and postductal oxygen saturations and treat right-to-left shunting (pulmonary hypertension) (Table 36.11). Persistent pulmonary hypertension may respond only to extracorporeal membrane oxygenation (ECMO) support.

Repair of the diaphragmatic defect is not a surgical emergency and should be performed once the infant has stabilized and has demonstrated minimal to no pulmonary hypertension (usually more than 48 h postnatally). Early reduction and repair has been shown to transiently worsen pulmonary function by decreasing the pulmonary compliance and increasing airway reactivity[39] A subcostal incision on the affected side should be performed, although some surgeons prefer a transthoracic approach, particularly for right-sided defects. The herniated abdominal contents should be carefully reduced from the chest. There may be a negative pressure "seal" that can be relieved by placement of a right-angled retractor below the anterior edge of the diaphragm, into the chest, and gently pulling upward. Reduction of the liver in right-sided defects can be very challenging and may require evisceration of all the abdominal contents as well as complete incision of the falciform and triangular ligaments. A hernia sac may be present and must be excised before closure to avoid a postoperative cystic collection that may enlarge, producing a mass effect. Primary diaphragmatic closure using interrupted nonabsorbable sutures can be performed if the defect is small. If the defect is too large for a primary closure, then a prosthetic patch (e.g., Gore-Tex) should be inserted and sutured around the ribs of the posterolateral body wall.

TABLE 36.11. Treatment of Pulmonary Hypertension.

Goal	*Treatment*
Oxygenate	Mechanical ventilation, F_IO_2 1.0
Correct acidosis	Hyperventilate Sodium bicarbonate (or THAM if retaining CO_2)
Correct malperfusion	Adequate volume replacement as needed Inotropic agents: dopamine, dobutamine
Sedation/paralysis	Fentanyl infusion, neuromuscular blockade (vecuronium)
Pulmonary vasodilation	Nitric oxide?
Correct hypocalcemia	Intravenous calcium supplements ($CaCl_2$, Ca gluconate)

THAM, tromethamine.

The majority of children with CDH who survive the neonatal period and are successfully extubated enjoy relatively normal lives. In the long term, there are a number of probably clinically insignificant physiological abnormalities such as a reduction in total lung volume, restrictive or obstructive lung disease, and abnormal lung compliance. A small subset of patients survive as "pulmonary cripples" and remain oxygen- or ventilator dependent, often requiring tracheostomies. Recurrent diaphragmatic hernia occurs in 10% to 20% of infants and should be considered in any child with a history of CDH who presents with new GI or pulmonary symptoms. Standard anteroposterior and lateral chest radiographs are diagnostic. Recurrence is most common when a prosthetic patch is used for the repair. As there may be deficient periesophageal muscular tissue or an abnormal orientation of the gastroesophageal junction, gastroesophageal reflux is common. It is most commonly treated nonoperatively, but refractory cases may require an antireflux procedure.

Foramen of Morgagni Hernia

The foramen of Morgagni (or space of Larrey) represents the junction of the septum transversum, the lateral portion of the diaphragm, and the anterior thoracic wall and allows the passage of the superior epigastric vessels. This anterior diaphragmatic defect accounts for only 2% of diaphragmatic hernias. They are most commonly right parasternal but may be left parasternal, retrosternal, or bilateral.[40] This defect, when noted in newborns, can be associated with the pentalogy of Cantrell[41]; this is a disorder with considerable morbidity and mortality that consists of the diaphragmatic defect, distal sternal cleft, epigastric omphalocele, apical pericardial defect, and congenital heart disease (usually a septal defect). Typically, however, children are asymptomatic and the defect is discovered later in life on a chest radiograph taken for reasons unrelated to the hernia. The lateral chest radiograph demonstrating an air-filled mass extending into the anterior mediastinum is pathognomonic. Repair is indicated in the asymptomatic patient for reasons of the risk of bowel incarceration or strangulation. The viscera are reduced and any associated hernia sac excised. The defect is closed by suturing the posterior rim of the diaphragm to the posterior rectus sheath (as there is no anterior diaphragm). Large defects require a prosthetic patch. There is no associated pulmonary hypoplasia or hypertension. Thus, excluding patients with the pentalogy of Cantrell, survival is 100%.

Eventration of the Diaphragm

Diaphragmatic eventration is an abnormally elevated portion of the diaphragm or, most commonly, hemidiaphragm. It may be congenital (usually idiopathic, but can be associated with congenital myopathies or intrauterine infections) or acquired (as a result of phrenic nerve injury during forceps delivery or thoracotomy).[42] There is a variable absence of diaphragmatic muscle, at which point its distinction from a CDH with a persistent hernia sac is obscure. The elevated hemidiaphragm produces abnormalities of chest wall mechanics with impaired pulmonary function. Respiratory distress and pneumonia are frequent presenting symptoms, although GI symptoms such as vomiting or gastric volvulus may occur.

The diagnosis is made by chest radiograph and confirmed by fluoroscopy or ultrasound, which demonstrates paradoxical movement of the diaphragm during spontaneous respiration. Incidentally discovered small, localized eventrations do not need to be repaired. Eventrations that are large or which are associated with respiratory symptoms should be repaired by plicating the diaphragm using interrupted nonabsorbable sutures. In cases of complete eventration, a prosthetic patch may be required.

Congenital Chest Wall Deformities

Congenital chest wall deformities are a heterogeneous group of disorders noted in infants and adults that commonly consist of bony and cartilaginous absence or deformity, often associated with musculoskeletal abnormalities.

Sternal Defects

Simple Cleft Sternum

Simple cleft sternum results from a failure of the embryonic sternal bars to unite and fuse, typically involving the manubrium and varying lengths of the body. Rarely is the entire sternum bifid. Patients are usually asymptomatic. Operative correction is performed in the neonatal period as the chest wall is so pliable and consists of simple suture approximation of the sternal halves.

Cleft Sternum with True Ectopia Cordis

Cleft sternum with true ectopia cordis consists of varying degrees of upper sternal cleft associated with ectopia cordis or a "bare" heart (no investing pericardium) that is located outside the chest wall, via the cleft. Intrinsic congenital heart disease (CHD) is common, as are extracardiac anomalies including cleft lip, cleft palate, hydrocephalus, and other CNS disorders. This defect is generally incompatible with life because of the severe congenital heart lesion(s).

Cleft Sternum with Thoracoabdominal Ectopia Cordis (Pentalogy of Cantrell)

There are five components to this disorder, cleft sternum with thoracoabdominal ectopia cordis; minimal distal sternal cleft, ventral diaphragmatic defect (central tendon defect), epigastric abdominal wall defect (omphalocele), CHD, and apical pericardial defect. Because the heart is not completely outside the mediastinum and retains most of its investing pericardium, this is not considered true ectopia cordis. The CHD is typically not severe (usually a septal defect). The mortality is appreciable and is related to the huge upper abdominal wall defect and the cardiorespiratory compromise that results from attempted closure.

Pectus Excavatum

Pectus excavatum is a depression deformity and is the most common congenital chest wall abnormality, occurring in 1 in 300 live births, with a 3:1 male predominance. It is associated with other musculoskeletal disorders (Marfan's syndrome, Poland's anomaly, scoliosis, clubfoot, syndactylism), and 2% have CHD. There is a familial form. It results from unbalanced posterior growth of costal cartilages that are often fused, bizarrely deformed, or rotated.[43] The body of the sternum secondarily exhibits a prominent posterior curvature, usually involving its lower half (Fig. 36.2). Asymmetrical deformities are common, particularly with sternal rotation to the right. It is identified during infancy in 90%. The depression progresses during childhood, becoming most pronounced during the growth spurt of puberty. The physio-

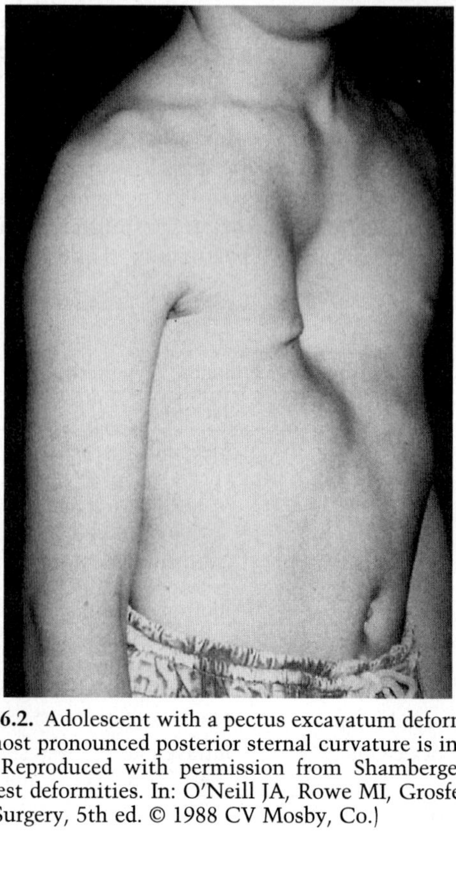

FIGURE 36.2. Adolescent with a pectus excavatum deformity. Note that the most pronounced posterior sternal curvature is in the lower one-half. (Reproduced with permission from Shamberger R. Congenital chest deformities. In: O'Neill JA, Rowe MI, Grosfeld JL, eds. Pediatric Surgery, 5th ed. © 1988 CV Mosby, Co.)

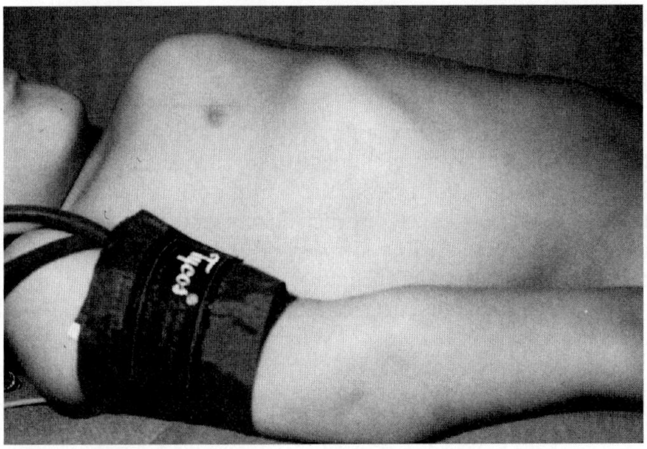

FIGURE 36.3. Severe pectus carinatum deformity.

logical data implicating adverse cardiopulmonary effects as a result of deformity are controversial and contradictory.[44] In general, there is no cardiopulmonary benefit after chest wall repair except in rare instances when the deformity is extensive. Otherwise, the repair is performed solely to improve appearance. However, the psychosocial benefits of repair of this often embarrassing deformity cannot be minimized.

There is no standard age for repair. Traditionally, an open repair is performed in which the abnormal cartilages are resected and the sternum is often fractured and fixed in a corrected position (often with a Kirschner wire or steel strut).[45] Recently, a minimal access technique has been proposed by Nuss et al.[46] in which a preformed sternal strut is passed, either blindly or with thoracoscopic assistance, under the chest wall muscles, into each hemithorax, and across the mediastinum under the sternum via two small incisions in the midaxillary line. The curve bar is passed upside down and "flipped" into position under the sternum, effectively lifting the sternum and chest wall into a corrected position. The bar is left in place for 2 years, and the children can resume activity in 3 months. The recurrence rate for the open procedure is less than 3%; there are not enough long-term follow-up data to assess the Nuss technique presently.

Pectus Carinatum

Pectus carinatum is a protrusion deformity, also referred to as pigeon or chicken breast[47] (Fig. 36.3). It is approximately 10 times less frequent than depression deformities. It results from overgrowth of costal cartilages, with forward buckling and secondary deformation of the sternum. Atypical and asymmetrical forms with rotation are common. There is a familial form. It is associated with Marfan's disease, neurofibromatosis, Poland's disease, and Morquio's disease. The defect does not affect cardiopulmonary function. In contrast to pectus excavatum, the deformity is typically mild or nearly imperceptible in early childhood and becomes increasingly prominent during the rapid growth in early puberty.

There is no cardiorespiratory compromise with this deformity, and repair is performed solely for an improved cosmetic appearance. The deformed cartilages are resected, leaving the costochondral membranes (perichondrium) intact.[48] Sternal fracture usually is not necessary. To ensure that the costal cartilages grow back on a straighter line, reefing sutures are placed in the costochondral membranes. The costal cartilages regenerate within 6 weeks. A thorough procedure will produce an excellent cosmetic result in nearly 100% of cases. Recurrences are rare.

Congenital Anomalies of the Esophagus

Anomalies of the esophagus, namely esophageal atresia, tracheoesophageal fistula, and their variants, are potentially life threatening in the newborn period.[49] Shortly after birth, the infant with esophageal atresia is noted to have excessive salivation and repeated episodes of coughing, choking, and cyanosis, and attempts at feeding are unsuccessful. Those with an associated tracheoesophageal fistula are prone to gastric reflux into the tracheobronchial tree with resulting chemical tracheobronchitis and pneumonia, especially if they are on mechanical ventilatory support. The diagnosis is confirmed by demonstrating that a small feeding tube coils in the upper esophageal pouch on a plain radiograph. A contrast study is almost never indicated. Bronchoscopy is the most sensitive means of identifying a tracheoesophageal fistula. The rare esophageal atresia variant, in which there is no tracheoesophageal fistula ("pure" atresia), can be confirmed by the absence of gas in the GI tract on plain radiograph. There is a 50% to 70% incidence of associated anomalies, namely, cardiac [patent ductus arteriosus (PDA), septal defects], GI (imperforate anus, duodenal atresia), GU, and skeletal. The VACTERL association (*v*ertebral, *a*norectal, *c*ardiac, *t*racheo-*e*sophageal, *r*enal, and *l*imb anomalies) is present in 25% of cases.

The classification is based on the presence or absence of an esophageal atresia and the presence and location of a fistula(e). These are listed below in descending order of their frequency (Fig. 36.4). Historically, they have been classified as types A through E:

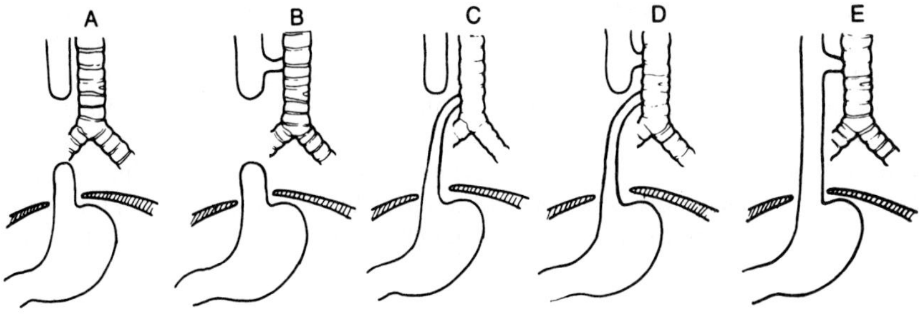

FIGURE 36.4. **A.** Pure (long gap) esophageal atresia. **B.** Esophageal atresia with proximal tracheoesophageal fistula. **C.** Esophageal atresia with distal tracheoesophageal fistula. **D.** Esophageal atresia with proximal and distal fistulae. **E.** Tracheoesophageal fistula without esophageal atresia. (From Grosfeld JL. Pediatric surgery. In: Sabiston DJ, ed. Textbook of Surgery, 1991, by permission of WB Saunders.)

1. Esophageal atresia with distal tracheoesophageal fistula (type C, 85% of cases). The distal tracheoesophageal fistula ends in the distal one-third of the trachea or in the carina.
2. Pure esophageal atresia (type A, 8%–10%). This is referred to as "long gap atresia" as the distal esophageal pouch is remote from the upper pouch, usually just above the diaphragm.
3. Tracheoesophageal fistula without esophageal atresia (type E, 4%–5%). The fistula, unlike the type C variant, is usually located in the cervical region. It is often termed an "H"-type fistula, although in reality the anatomic configuration resembles an "N," with the entrance into the esophagus as the most cephalad point.
4. Esophageal atresia with proximal and distal fistulae (type D, 2%). In contrast to the H-type fistula, the proximal fistula is usually from the distal portion of the upper esophagus.
5. Esophageal atresia with proximal tracheoesophageal fistula (type B, 1%). There may or may not be a long gap between the esophageal segments.

Treatment begins with stabilization of the child and assessment for associated anomalies. A Replogle sump suction catheter should be placed in the upper esophageal pouch and the head of the bed elevated. An echocardiogram is required to determine the position of the aortic arch because a right-sided arch makes the standard right thoracotomy repair difficult. The goal of operative therapy is to divide and ligate the fistula and repair the atresia in one stage. This procedure is usually performed using a right posterolateral thoracotomy with an extrapleural dissection, although the thoracoscopic approach is gaining favor.[50] Staged operations are reserved for extremely premature babies and those with severe anomalies or long gaps between the esophageal pouches. A staged procedure involves either division of the fistula alone, or creation of a cervical esophagostomy and insertion of a feeding gastrostomy tube for those with long gap atresia (type A). A feeding gastrostomy tube is no longer routinely inserted except when the esophageal repair is under extreme tension, when there is long gap atresia not amenable to single-stage repair, and when there are severe associated anomalies (e.g., congenital heart disease). A transanastomotic feeding tube is placed for postoperative feeding, pending the demonstration of a leak-free anastomosis by esophagram obtained 7 days after surgery.

There are several strategies for repairing long gap esophageal atresia without fistula: these include cervical esophagostomy and gastrostomy tube, followed several months later by esophageal replacement (colon or stomach interposition); gastrostomy tube alone with intermittent bougienage and stretching of the upper esophageal pouch, followed by primary esophageal anastomosis; and immediate interposition graft.[51]

Immediate postoperative complications include anastomotic leak, stricture, and recurrent fistula. Long-term complications include gastroesophageal reflux (GER), dysphagia caused by the intrinsically poor esophageal motility in these children, and tracheomalacia from in utero tracheal compression by the large proximal esophageal pouch and/or from the repair of the fistula.

Gastrointestinal Tract Abnormalities

Gastroesophageal Reflux

Gastroesophageal reflux is physiological at birth because the lower esophageal sphincter does not mature for approximately 2 months; this accounts for the commonly noted regurgitation (chalazia, or "wet" burps) during and after feeds in a normal newborn. Although most GER is idiopathic, GER is found in association with neurological disorders, esophageal atresia, CDH, delayed gastric emptying, and abdominal wall defects.

The symptoms of GER in infants and children are protean.[52,53] The most common is vomiting, which can cause failure to thrive, aspiration pneumonia, apnea, bronchospasm that is confused with asthma, and laryngospasm which may lead to sudden infant death. Reflux may produce esophagitis, which can lead to heartburn, dysphagia, and odynophagia. Long-standing GER can cause occult esophageal bleeding, esophageal stricture, and Barrett's metaplasia. The gold standard diagnostic test is lower esophageal 24-h pH monitoring.[53] An upper GI series is less sensitive but is used to rule out other disorders (e.g., intestinal malrotation) and to assess for esophageal stricture. Upper endoscopy is useful to diagnose and monitor the inflammatory changes in the distal esophagus. Gastric emptying may be assessed by technetium pertechnetate scan. There is little role for esophageal manometric studies in children, except for those in whom one suspects achalasia or diffuse esophageal spasm.

Nonoperative treatment is successful in most cases. For infants, thickening the feeds with rice cereal and upright positioning during and shortly after feeding is effective. Persistent symptoms mandate drug therapy with an antacid (e.g., H_2 blocker or proton pump inhibitor) with or without a prokinetic agent (e.g., Reglan). The indications for operation are failure of medical therapy, complications while on medical treatment (e.g., recurrent pneumonia), severe esophagitis, Barrett's esophagitis, esophageal stricture, or significant bleeding.[54] The gold standard antireflux surgical procedure is the Nissen fundoplication,[55] although some advocate the Thal partial fundoplication.[56] Controversy exists as to whether to assess for delayed gastric emptying. There are growing data that suggest that the "funneling" effect of the fundoplication promotes gastric emptying, even in the face of known delayed emptying. Gastric emptying is most often delayed in neurologically impaired children.

In recent years, the traditional open approach to antireflux operations has been gradually replaced by the more cosmetic and better visualized laparoscopic procedure.[57] At this time, most data from the pediatric population regarding laparoscopic antireflux procedures consist of retrospective case series. Evaluating the efficacy of the laparoscopic approach is not straightforward in children as parameters such as symptom control and satisfaction rates are difficult to obtain and may be confounded by a number of variables (patient age, neurological impairment, and other congenital abnormalities). Because of this, many studies have evaluated the effectiveness of laparoscopic antireflux procedures in relationship to the development of recurrent GER as well as wrap failure.

Based on review of the large (more than 100 patients) retrospective case series published to date, recurrent GER has been reported to occur in 2% to 6% of pediatric patients after laparoscopic antireflux operations.[58,59] Differences vary from series to series, with variables including the type of operation performed (e.g., Nissen versus Thal fundoplication). In contrast, failure rates reported for open Nissen fundoplication have been reported to range from 20% to 47%.[60–64] Wrap failure most commonly occurs as a result of crural breakdown and migration of the wrap into the chest through the resulting hiatal hernia. In the adult population, wrap migration has been reported to occur in 20% of patients whereas the pediatric literature displays failure rates from 2% to 5%.[65,66] Furthermore, wrap migration appears to occur more commonly in neurologically impaired children, presumably as a result of increased abdominal pressure from retching and concomitant seizure disorders. Symptomatic dysphagia, which is the most common postoperative complaint in the adult population, appears to be significantly less prevalent in children, likely because infants tend to consume a primarily liquid diet, transitioning to solid foods well after postoperative edema in the distal esophagus is no longer a concern.

Table 36.12 summarizes the published series to date reviewing large experiences (more than 100 patients) with laparoscopic antireflux procedures. At this time all reports consist of retrospective case series with relatively short-term follow-up. Multiple operations are utilized including Nissen, Nissen–Rosetti, Thal, and Toupet fundoplications. Overall, recurrence of GER, complication rates, and conversion rates appear favorable. In total (more than 1500 patients), only 4 deaths have been reported: 1 operative, 3 postoperative. Although these studies are retrospective and do not directly compare the laparoscopic to open approach, they indicate that the laparoscopic operations represent at least as safe and an equivalent alternative to the traditional open approach.

Pyloric Stenosis

Pyloric stenosis is the most common surgical disorder producing emesis in infancy. The symptoms are of gastric outlet obstruction and are caused by concentric hypertrophy of the pyloric muscle with progressive narrowing of the pyloric canal. The disease evolves postnatally because it is rare in preterm infants, and symptoms are usually absent in the first week of life. It is usually diagnosed in the first 3 to 6 weeks after birth. It is most common in Caucasians, least common in Asians, and there is a male-to-female ratio of 4:1. There is a familial predilection, particularly if the mother has been afflicted.

Clinically, there is progressive, forceful nonbilious emesis. The vomiting occurs immediately or within 30 to 45 min of the last feeding and consists of undigested formula with thick curds. Brownish or coffee-ground material may be present, suggesting gastritis. Affected infants are voraciously hungry after vomiting and will eagerly take to the bottle or nurse. The differential diagnosis is overfeeding (most common), formula intolerance, GER, pyloric duplication, antral web, CNS lesion with increased intracranial pressure, and salt-wasting andrenogenital syndrome. Infants are often dehydrated with sunken fontanelles, dry mucous membranes, and poor skin turgor. Jaundice (elevated indirect bilirubin) may be present as a result of decreased glucuronyl transferase activity. A firm, mobile hypertrophic pylorus, or "olive," is palpated by an experienced examiner in 90% of cases, provided the child is relaxed and the stomach is decompressed. Diagnostic imaging is required only if the olive cannot be palpated. Ultrasonography is the most sensitive test, although a negative study is nondiagnostic for other entities. An upper GI contrast study can provide anatomic and functional details. Plain abdominal radiographs are never indicated. Prolonged vomiting of gastric fluid can result in a hypochloremic, hypokalemic metabolic alkalosis. Hydrogen and chloride ion-rich

TABLE 36.12.
Large (More Than 100 patients) Published Series of Pediatric Laparoscopic Fundoplication for Gastroesophageal Reflux Disease (GERD).

Author/year	*Study design*	N	*Antireflux procedure*	*Recurrence of GER*	*Complication rates*	*Conversion rates*	*LOS*	*TTF*	*Operation time*
Georgeson 1998[57]	Retrospective case series	389	201 Toupet 188 Nissen	6.1% Toupet 3.5% Nissen	2 deaths (1 operative)	3.3%	~3 days	N/A	~60 min
Esposito 2000[137]	Retrospective case series	289	148 Nissen-Rossetti 141 Toupet	2.10%	Intraoperative, 5.1% Postoperative, 3.4%	1.3%	N/A	N/A	70 min
Montupet 2001[138]	Retrospective case series	284	Thal	2.10%	Intraoperative, 0% Postoperative, 1%	N/A	N/A	~3 days	~60 min
Rothenberg 1998[66]	Retrospective case series	220	Nissen	3.40%	Intraoperative, 2.6% Postoperative, 7.3%	1.0%	1.6 days	N/A	82 min
Allal 2001[139]	Retrospective case series	142	56 Toupet 83 Nissen	4.20%	Intraoperative, 0.5% Postoperative, 2%; 1 death	2.1%	3 days	N/A	105 min
Iglesias 2001[140]	Retrospective case series	104	Nissen	2.90%	Major, 12.7%; 1 death	1.0%	More than 10 days	~3 days	60 min
Ostlie 2003[141]	Retrospective case series	154	Nissen	2%	Intraoperative, 0% Postoperative, 2%	0%	2.8 days	~1 day	90 min

N/A, not available; LOS, length of stay; TTF, time to feed.

gastric fluid is lost by prolonged vomiting. The kidney attempts to maintain a normal serum pH by excreting alkaline urine. Hypokalemia results from K^+ loss in the urine as the cations are excreted with bicarbonate and cellular uptake of K^+ in exchange for hydrogen ions in the face of an alkaline serum. With continued vomiting, the kidney attempts to maintain volume by reabsorbing sodium in exchange for hydrogen ions, producing a paradoxical aciduria. The fluid and electrolyte abnormalities are corrected using D5 0.45% normal saline at 150–175 mL/kg/day. Potassium (20 mEq/L) is added after the child voids. The volume of resuscitation fluid is adjusted based on the child's urine output, urine specific gravity, and vital signs.

The timing of operation is dictated solely by the fluid and electrolyte status. Surgery may be undertaken when an adequate amount (1–2 mL/kg/h) of nonconcentrated (specific gravity ≤1.012) urine is established and the serum chloride and potassium are corrected. The surgical repair consists of an extramucosal myotomy beginning 1–2 mm proximal to the pyloroduodenal junction and extending onto the antrum. There are three approaches to the pylorus: a right upper quadrant transverse skin incision, a circumumbilical or intraumbilical skin incision, or a laparoscopic approach with the camera in the umbilicus and the two working instruments placed directly through the abdominal wall.[67,68] Regardless of technique, a complete myotomy will allow independent movement of the upper and lower muscular edges. If the mucosa is entered (usually on the duodenal side), it can be closed with fine nonabsorbable suture and an omental patch. Large perforations are managed by closing the pyloromyotomy, rotating the pylorus 90°, and repeating the myotomy.

Multiple postoperative feeding schedules have been described, ranging from immediate full feeds to delayed feeds with incremental advances in volume, stemming from the observation that nearly all patients with pyloric stenosis vomit after surgery, presumably as a consequence of gastric ileus, gastritis, GER, or all of these. An incomplete pyloromyotomy (usually on the antral side) is suspected when vomiting persists after 2 weeks postoperatively. Pyloric stenosis never recurs, and there is a uniformly excellent outcome.

Intestinal Obstruction in the Newborn

As fetuses continually swallow amniotic fluid into their GI tracts and excrete it via the urine, intestinal obstruction may be noted on prenatal ultrasound by the presence of polyhydramnios (increased amniotic fluid level). The presence of polyhydramnios correlates with the level of the obstruction; it is most common with proximal GI tract obstruction (e.g., esophageal and duodenal atresia), is rarely noted with ileal atresia, and is never noted in association with anorectal obstruction (e.g., rectal atresia).

After birth, vomiting is the principal symptom, and it is bile stained if the obstruction is distal to the ampulla of Vater. It is important to note that newborn bilious vomiting is pathological until proven otherwise. On physical examination, the presence and degree of abdominal distension depend on the level of the obstruction and should be noted. For example, there is no significant distention with duodenal obstruction versus massive distension with colonic obstruction (e.g., Hirschsprung's disease). A careful perineal examination should be performed to assess if an anus is present, patent, and in the normal location. Meconium, the first newborn stool, is passed in the first 24 h of life in 94% of normal full-term infants and by 48 h in 98%.[12] Failure to pass meconium may be indicative of lower GI tract obstruction.

Nonbilious emesis is caused by esophageal atresia, proximal duodenal obstruction (see below), antral web, pyloric atresia, or gastric duplication. Depending on the plain abdominal radiograph, an upper GI series may or may not be needed before operative intervention. Bilious emesis may be caused by distal duodenal obstruction, jejunal or ileal atresia, intestinal malrotation (with either obstructing peritoneal bands or volvulus), meconium plug syndrome, meconium ileus syndrome, small left colon syndrome, Hirschsprung's disease, rectal atresia, or imperforate anus. Because the plain abdominal radiograph in a newborn cannot differentiate small bowel from large bowel in an infant with multiple distended bowel loops, the most common test in the workup of bilious emesis is the contrast enema. It can be both diagnostic and therapeutic (e.g., wash out a meconium plug).

Duodenal Obstruction

Duodenal obstruction can be complete (e.g., atresia) or partial (e.g., stenosis).[69] The various causes are idiopathic atresia (failure of canalization), annular pancreas, preduodenal portal vein, or peritoneal bands (Ladd's bands) from malrotation. There may also be a mucosal web or diaphragm that can partially (perforated web) or completely obstruct the duodenum. Approximately one-third of babies with duodenal atresia or stenosis have trisomy 21 (Down's syndrome). Patients present with bilious emesis and the presence of a "double bubble" on plain abdominal radiographs (Fig. 36.5). Rarely are contrast studies needed preoperatively. Treatment is by duodenoduodenostomy with tapering of the proximal, hugely dilated duodenum (tapering duodenoplasty) because this overstretched bowel segment has impaired aboral progression of ingested feedings. In contrast, an obstructing duodenal web is simply excised. Obstruction from Ladd's bands requires division of the bands and correction of the malrotation (see fol-

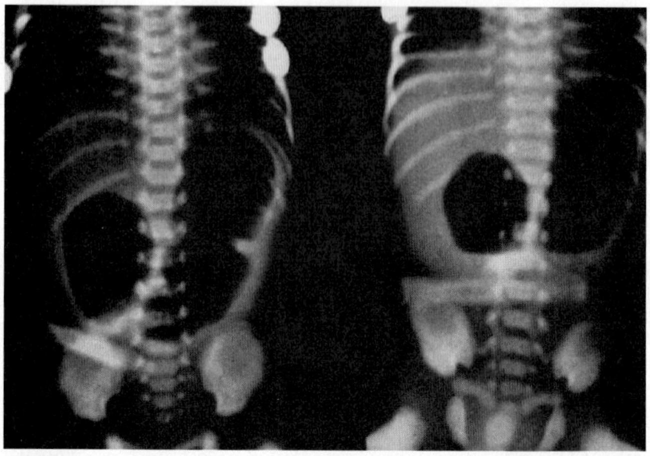

FIGURE 36.5. Plain abdominal radiographs demonstrating a gas-filled stomach and proximal duodenum ("double bubble"), indicative of proximal duodenal obstruction. The radiograph on the *left* was taken with the baby supine; in the one on the *right*, the child is upright.

lowing). The distal bowel must be irrigated and assessed for intrinsic obstruction (1%–3% incidence).

Disorders of Intestinal Rotation

Disorders of intestinal rotation are classified in four ways: incomplete rotation (the most common—also termed malrotation), nonrotation, reversed rotation (the least common), and anomalous mesenteric fixation.[70,71] To understand the four types of abnormal anatomy, one must acknowledge the series of fetal events that lead to normal intestinal rotation and fixation. The fetal intestine begins as a somewhat straight tube that grows faster than the abdominal cavity and thus herniates into the body stalk (future umbilicus) at about week 4 to 6 weeks gestation. At 10 to 12 weeks gestation, the bowel returns to the abdominal cavity where it will rotate and fixate. The duodenojejunal portion undergoes a counterclockwise 270° rotation posterior to the superior mesenteric artery (SMA) and fixes to the posterior body wall as the ligament of Treitz at the level of the 12th thoracic vertebra, to the left of the midline above the level of the pylorus. The cecocolic portion also rotates 270°, but anterior to the SMA, and becomes fixed in the right lower quadrant at the level of the 5th lumbar vertebra.

Incomplete rotation may affect the duodenojejunal portion, the cecocolic portion, or both. Because only partial rotation occurs, the bowel is fixed posteriorly by a relatively narrow mesenteric base that is prone to twisting (volvulus). Volvulus occurs around the SMA in a clockwise direction and can lead to gangrene of the entire midgut, heralded by abdominal distension, bloody stools, and often hematemesis. It presents either acutely in infancy or as a chronic intermittent obstruction (intermittent volvulus) in older children. The partial rotation of the cecum may result in duodenal obstruction by Ladd's bands, which are peritoneal folds that serve to fix the cecum to the posterior body wall; if rotation halts in the right upper quadrant, these bands will stretch out over and obstruct the third portion of the duodenum. Using an upper abdominal transverse incision, the volvulus should be untwisted in a counterclockwise direction. Incomplete intestinal rotation is managed by division of Ladd's bands, division of any intermesenteric adhesions, straightening the duodenum as much as possible, and placing the cecum on the left side of the abdomen. In essence, one is creating nonrotated intestinal anatomy, much as in early fetal life. Appendectomy is advocated based on the abnormal final position of the appendix.

With nonrotation of the intestine, the midgut is "suspended" from the superior mesenteric vessels; the majority of the small intestine lies on the right side of the abdomen, the large bowel on the left. It is often noted in patients with CDH, gastroschisis, and omphalocele. This anatomy is less prone to volvulus compared to the incomplete rotation variant. In reversed rotation, the duodenojejunal bowel rotates varying degrees in a clockwise direction about the SMA. The cecocolic portion may rotate clockwise or counterclockwise, anterior or posterior to the SMA. Anomalous mesenteric fixation accounts for internal mesenteric and paraduodenal hernias. The bowel may rotate normally but fixes to the abdominal wall abnormally. Excessive cephalad rotation of the duodenojejunal portion results in obstruction of the third portion of the duodenum in thin patients (SMA syndrome).

Atresia of the Jejunum, Ileum, and Colon

In contrast to duodenal atresia, more distal intestinal atresias are caused not by a failure of canalization but by a mesenteric vascular accident with resultant aseptic resorption of the bowel, usually later in gestation. The spectrum of anomalies (Fig. 36.6) ranges from a stenosis or mucosal web (type I), a fibrous cord between two bowel ends (type II), blind-ending proximal and distal bowel loops with a V-shaped mesenteric defect (type IIIa), and multiple atresias of any kind (type IV).[72] Type IIIb is the rarest and is associated with short bowel syndrome. It is termed the apple peel deformity or Christmas tree deformity, in which there is a blind-ending proximal jejunum, absence of a large portion of the midgut, and a terminal ileum that is coiled around its ileocolic blood supply. The most common site of atresia is the ileum, followed by the jejunum and the colon. Bilious emesis is uniform. Because the atresia is believed to be a late gestational event, these babies often pass a normal meconium stool after birth. Plain radiographs demonstrating only a few dilated bowel loops are indicative of a proximal obstruction, and a contrast study is not required. If many loops are dilated, a contrast enema will help differentiate a distal small bowel atresia from a potentially nonoperative cause of obstruction such as meconium plug syndrome (see below).

At operation, the distal portion of the proximal blind-ending bowel segment is disproportionately dilated and should be resected because it is functionally abnormal and

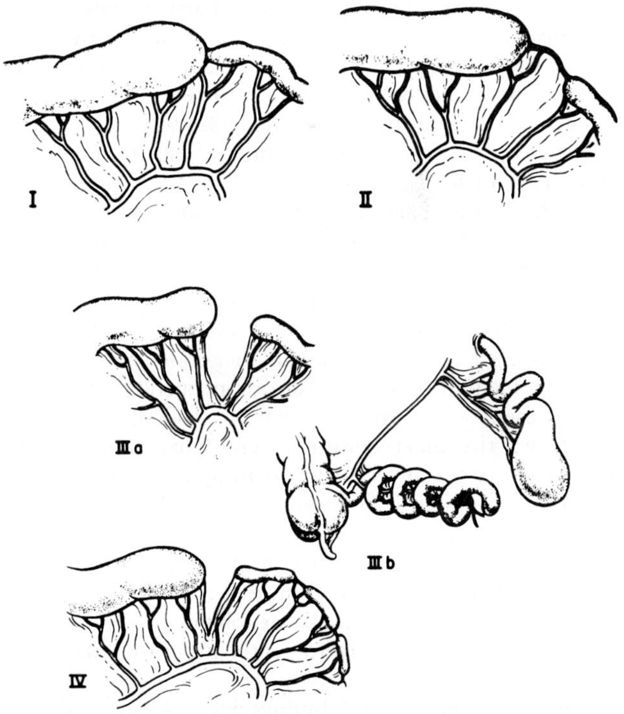

FIGURE 36.6. The anatomical spectrum of intestinal atresia. Type *I* is a stenosis or mucosal web; type *II*, a fibrous cord between two bowel ends; type *IIIa*, blind-ending proximal and distal bowel loops with a V-shaped mesenteric defect. Type *IIIb* (apple peel deformity or Christmas tree deformity) consists of a blind-ending proximal jejunum, absence of a large portion of the midgut, and a terminal ileum that is coiled around its ileocolic blood supply; type *IV*, multiple atresias of any kind. (From Grosfeld JL. Pediatric surgery. In: Sabiston DJ, ed. Textbook of Surgery, 1991, by permission of WB Saunders.)

atonic. If this is a long segment of proximal jejunum, the antimesenteric portion of the bowel should be tapered over a large tube using a stapler or a running suture. There is always a discrepancy in bowel diameter between the proximal and distal ends, so an end-to-side or end-to-oblique anastomosis is necessary.

Duplications of the Gastrointestinal Tract

Duplications are rare congenital cystic abnormalities of the GI tract that have been reported to occur anywhere from the mouth to the anus. They originate on the mesenteric side of the associated alimentary tract and shared a common blood supply with the native bowel.[73]

Based upon embryology, duplications have been categorized into foregut, midgut, and hindgut. Foregut duplications include the pharynx, respiratory tract, esophagus, stomach, and the first portion and proximal half of the second portion of the duodenum. Midgut duplications include the distal half of the second part of the duodenum, the jejunum, ileum, cecum, appendix, the ascending colon, and the proximal two-thirds of the transverse colon. The hindgut is composed of duplications of the distal third of the transverse colon, the descending and sigmoid colon, the rectum, anus, and components of the urological system. In one series, 39% of duplications involved the foregut while 61% represented duplications of both mid- and hindgut.[74]

Duplication cysts are spherical or tubular in shape and share a common seromuscular coat and similar mucosal lining as the normal adjacent GI tract. Further, they are typically located on the dorsal or mesenteric side of the native bowel.[75] Heterotopic gastric mucosa is seen in up to one-third of these lesions and may result in severe ulceration, bleeding, and eventual perforation. Communication with the lumen of the gut is more common with tubular duplications. Eighty-five percent of duplications are diagnosed before age 2 and 60% by 6 months of age. Vertebral anomalies are seen in 21% of patients, whereas other congenital anomalies are encountered in 48% of patients with alimentary tract duplications.

The signs and symptoms of alimentary tract duplications are not unique and therefore may be confused with other GI tract pathology. Although many duplications remain "silent" and are incidentally discovered during an operative procedure, others present with severe GI distress. Abdominal pain and melena are the most common symptoms, and a mobile abdominal mass may be palpated in approximately half of patients. Accumulation of secretions within the duplication can cause intense pain and potential obstruction from compression of the adjacent bowel lumen. Heterotopic gastric mucosa is present in up to one-third of duplications; as such, patients may develop occult or obvious blood loss or frank perforation secondary to peptic ulceration within the duplication.

Specific complaints and findings may also be attributable to the location of the duplication. Foregut duplications may present with vomiting, respiratory distress, failure to thrive, dysphagia, and hematemesis. Gastric and duodenal lesions typically present with a palpable abdominal mass and may cause vomiting, abdominal distension, melena, and peritonitis following perforation. Gastric outlet obstruction mimicking hypertrophic pyloric stenosis is also a common presentation of these duplications.

Midgut duplications are frequently associated with abdominal distension, vomiting, and melena. Other less common symptoms include pain, peritonitis, and diarrhea. These duplications are often difficult to identify preoperatively as they can easily mimic acute appendicitis. Additionally, they can cause an intussusception and thereby obscure the diagnosis. Duplications of the hindgut may present with vomiting, constipation, diarrhea, or abdominal distension.

The treatment for the majority of intraabdominal duplications is excision. Before operative intervention, plans for intraoperative radiography, which may include scintigraphy, ultrasonography, and cholangiography should be made. The location and association of the lesion to its native structures will help determine the appropriate surgical procedure. Extreme care must be taken to recognize the common blood supply between the duplication cyst and the adjacent native bowel. Additionally, the presence of heterotopic gastric mucosa will negate the ability to perform an internal drainage procedure because of the risk of secondary ulceration and possible hemorrhage.[74]

Meckel's Diverticulum

A Meckel's diverticulum is present in 1% to 3% of the population and is the most common remnant of the omphalomesenteric duct.[76] It is located 10 to 90 cm from the ileocecal valve and may contain ectopic gastric (most common) or ectopic pancreatic tissue. The lifelong risk of complications is 4%, and 40% of these cases occur in children under 10 years of age. Complications include bleeding (40%), intussusception (20%), diverticulitis or peptic perforation (15%), umbilical fistula (15%), intestinal obstruction (7%), and abscess (3%). Bleeding is the most serious complication and most often occurs in children younger than 5 years. It is often massive, seldom occult. Contrast studies rarely outline the diverticulum. The diagnosis is often made by a technetium-99m pertechnetate scan, which demonstrates uptake of the tracer by ectopic gastric parietal cells. The sensitivity of the scan is increased with pretreatment by either cimetidine or pentagastrin. Resection can be accomplished by laparotomy or laparoscopically. The diverticulum is easily excised using a surgical stapler or Endoloop if the base is narrow.

Anorectal Anomalies: Imperforate Anus

Anomalies of the rectum develop as a result of the faulty division of the cloaca into the urogenital sinus. The sphincters and levator muscle complex as well as the sacral nerves are affected to varying degrees. Therefore, a "perfect" surgical repair may not result in perfect continence.[77] There is a wide range of anomalies, many of which can be simply classified as either "low" or "high" based on physical examination and imaging studies (Figs. 36.7–36.10). Low defects are defined by an orifice that is visible at the perineum but is not in the normal location or is partially covered in the normal location. In males, the orifice is anywhere on the perineum, including the median raphe of the scrotum, or it may simply be a covered anus in which there is an incomplete epithelial membrane over the anus. In females, the orifice is either at the perineal body, fourchette, vestibule, or distal vagina. These babies often have well-developed perineal/gluteal musculature and rarely have sacral vertebral anomalies. High defects

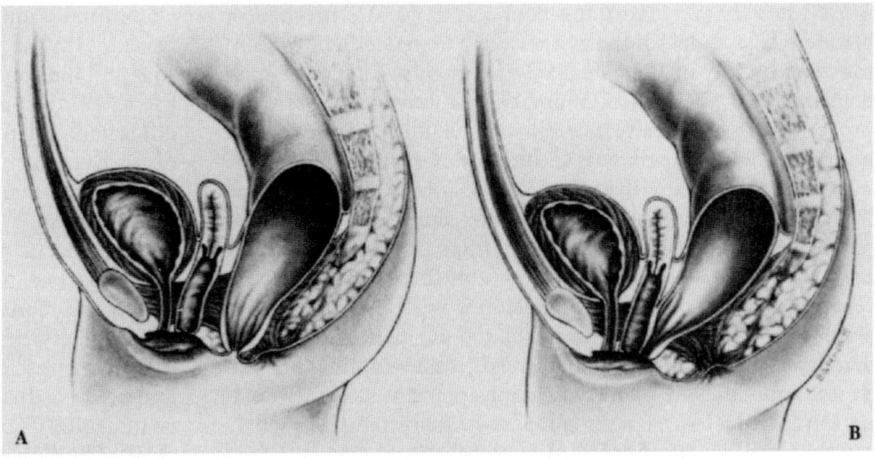

A B

FIGURE 36.7. A. Low female anomaly. Perineal fistula. **B.** Low female anomaly. Fourchette/vestibule fistula. (Reproduced with permission from Pena A. Surgical Management of Anorectal Malformations. New York: Springer-Verlag, 1992.)

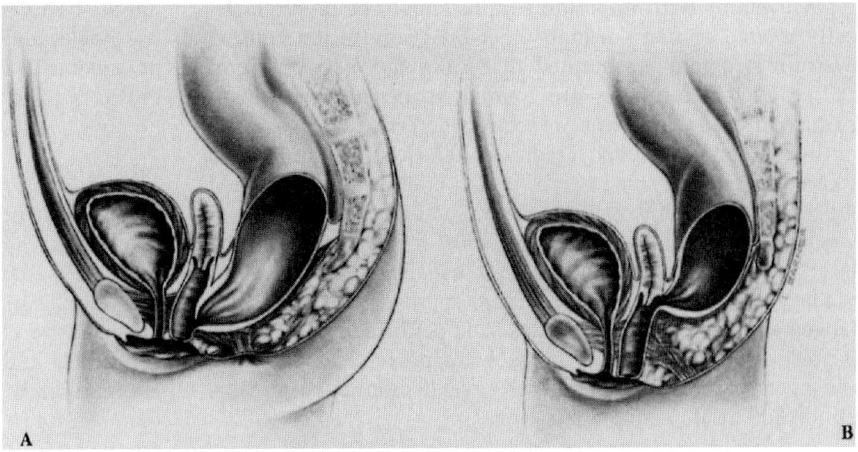

A B

FIGURE 36.8. A. High female anomaly. Low vaginal fistula. **B.** High female anomaly. High vaginal fistula. (Reproduced with permission from Pena A. Surgical Management of Anorectal Malformations. New York: Springer-Verlag, 1992.)

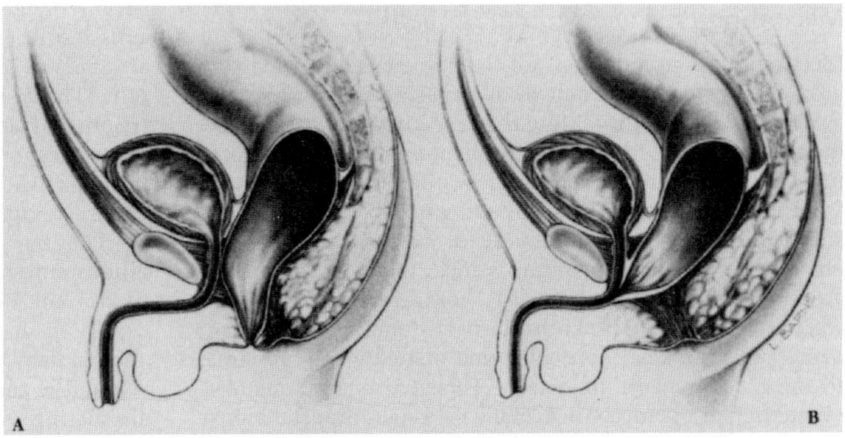

A B

FIGURE 36.9. A. Low male anomaly. Perineal fistula. **B.** Rectobulbar urethra fistula. (Reproduced with permission from Pena A. Surgical Management of Anorectal Malformations. New York: Springer-Verlag, 1992.)

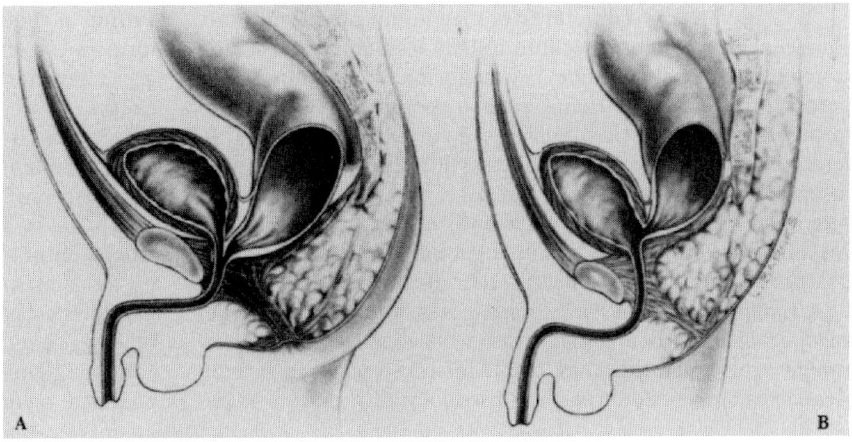

A B

FIGURE 36.10. A. High male anomaly. Rectoprostatic urethra fistula. **B.** High male anomaly. Rectobladder neck fistula. (Reproduced with permission from Pena A. Surgical Management of Anorectal Malformations. New York: Springer-Verlag, 1992.)

most often have a fistulous connection to the urethra or bladder neck (males) or the upper vagina (females). The rectum may end blindly in 10% of cases. The most severe of the high deformities is the cloacal anomaly, also termed a persistent urogenital sinus. There is only one visible orifice on the perineum; within it there is a common channel between the vagina and urethra with the rectum opening into the vagina. Patients with high imperforate anus often have deficient pelvic and gluteal musculature, a high incidence of sacral anomalies, and a poor prognosis for continence after surgical repair. Imperforate anus is associated with the VACTERL syndrome. The most common isolated association is genitourinary (e.g., unilateral renal agenesis, vesicoureteral reflux). Sacral anomalies by plain radiographs warrant a further evaluation by MRI to assess for spinal cord abnormalities such as a tethered filum terminale or lipomeningocele.

All infants with imperforate anus should be prophylactically treated against a urinary tract infection until a voiding cystourethrogram is obtained that rules out vesicoureteral reflux. Low deformities are treated by perineal anoplasty using a muscle stimulator to precisely determine the location of the sphincter complex. Traditionally, a high deformity was treated by a three-stage repair, which consisted of a divided loop colostomy, a posterior sagittal anorectoplasty 4 to 6 weeks later, and closure of the colostomy several months later.[53] Fistulae to the bladder neck usually require division via laparotomy. Recently, the staged approach has been challenged and a one-stage repair has been performed by both the posterior sagittal[78] and a laparoscopic approach.[79] In all cases, the neoanus must be dilated for several months to prevent circumferential cicatrix formation.

Meconium Plug and Meconium Ileus

Meconium plug syndrome, or neonatal small left colon syndrome, is believed to result from transient colonic immaturity-related dysmotility. More than 50% of these babies were born to diabetic mothers. In some, hypermagnesemia is noted in response to maternal magnesium sulfate administration to treat preeclampsia. Infants present with abdominal distension, bilious emesis, and failure to pass meconium. The obstructing plug of meconium is most often located in and around the splenic flexure. The contrast enema, using a water-soluble agent, is both diagnostic and therapeutic. It demonstrates a small left colon and dilated bowel proximal to the meconium filling defects. Persistent symptoms after evacuation of the meconium mandate a suction rectal biopsy to rule out Hirschsprung's disease.

It is important to differentiate meconium plug syndrome from meconium ileus. Meconium ileus results from obstruction of the terminal ileum by abnormal meconium. Ten percent to 33% of patients with meconium ileus have a family history of cystic fibrosis.[56] The presentation is no different from that of meconium plug syndrome, Hirschsprung's disease, or distal intestinal atresia. Characteristically, the proximal ileum is greatly dilated and contains thick, viscous meconium, while the terminal ileum is collapsed and obstructed by thickly packed round mucous pus that resembles rabbit stool pellets. In some cases, the weight of the meconium-filled ileum may cause a localized volvulus (not midgut volvulus); this may result in intestinal obstruction, ileal atresia, or perforation with pseudocyst formation. Plain abdominal radiographs show dilated bowel loops, and air mixed with the viscous meconium conveys a ground-glass or soap-bubble appearance. There are no air–fluid levels because the thick meconium fails to layer rapidly. There may be calcifications on the plain film if an antenatal perforation has occurred. A contrast enema is both diagnostic and potentially therapeutic. It shows a microcolon, and reflux into the ileum demonstrates a small-caliber terminal ileum with multiple filling defects. Further reflux demonstrates a large-caliber ileum packed with meconium. Initial treatment is with a hypertonic contrast enema mixed with a mucolytic agent (e.g., *N*-acetylcysteine). This treatment draws hypotonic fluid into the intestinal lumen, so the infant must be kept well hydrated. If this fails to relieve the obstruction, laparotomy is indicated. The ileum is opened and, if possible, flushed clear. The bowel can be reanatomosed or brought out as a double-barrel stoma. Alternatively, a T-tube may be placed in the bowel and brought out the anterior abdominal wall for postoperative irrigations. All patients should be evaluated for cystic fibrosis.

Hirschsprung's Disease

Congenital intestinal aganglionosis (Hirschsprung's disease) results from a failure of craniocaudal migration of neuroblasts that are destined to become the parasympathetic ganglion cells of the intestine. The absence of ganglion cells always begins just proximal to the dentate line, never skips intestinal segments, and extends proximally for varying lengths. In approximately 75% of cases, the disease is limited to the rectosigmoid colon. Five percent of cases involve the entire colon (total colonic aganglionosis), and 5% can involve varying lengths of small intestine. The absence of ganglion cells results in a functional obstruction because the affected area fails to relax as a consequence of unopposed sympathetic tone. The disease may run in families and is associated with trisomy 21 and congenital heart disease. Males are affected four times more frequently than females when the disease is limited to the rectosigmoid. Longer lengths of disease and the familial forms favor females.

The typical neonate with Hirschsprung's disease has bilious emesis, abdominal distension, and passes little or no meconium. Rectal examination of the infant may produce an expulsion of stool and air. Short segments of disease may allow a baby to escape diagnosis for weeks, months, or even years. The older patients present with chronic constipation alternating with diarrhea and failure to thrive. Children with constipation from Hirschsprung's disease do not exhibit soiling of their diapers or undergarments, distinguishing this form of constipation from idiopathic constipation (encopresis). The differential diagnosis includes all the aforementioned causes of neonatal mechanical obstruction along with a variety of functional causes such as hypermagnesemia, hypocalcemia, hypokalemia, and hypothyroidism. Untreated Hirschsprung's disease may lead to enterocolitis, characterized by fever, abdominal distension, and foul-smelling watery stools. Enterocolitis is the principal cause of neonatal mortality associated with Hirschsprung's disease.

Plain abdominal radiographs demonstrate dilated loops of bowel. A contrast enema is the imaging test of choice. Typically, it demonstrates a transition zone in which there is proximal colonic dilation and distal narrowing, most evident

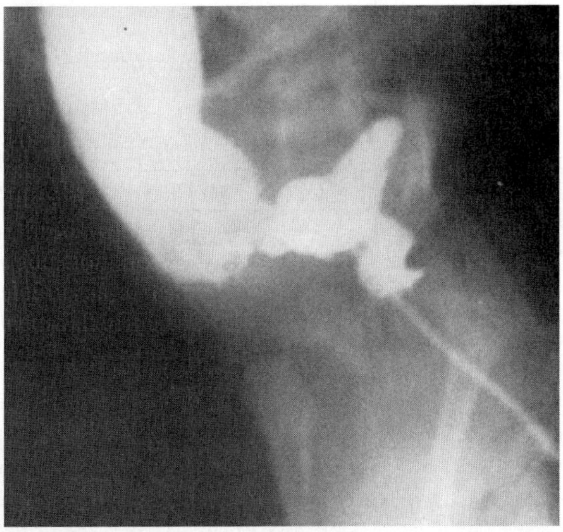

FIGURE 36.11. Lateral view of a contrast enema from a baby with Hirschsprung's disease shows distal rectosigmoid narrowing with proximal dilation of the colon.

in the lateral projection (Fig. 36.11), in contrast to a normal neonate's rectum, which is the widest portion of the colon. The transition zone may be difficult to identify in the first weeks of life because the newborn's normally liquid stool may pass through the aganglionic bowel. Contrast (e.g., barium) is usually retained for prolonged periods (>24 h) after the initial study.

The definitive diagnosis is made by rectal biopsy, a painless bedside procedure in which the mucosa and submucosa are sampled beginning 1 cm above the dentate line. Serial sections demonstrate an absence of ganglion cells, hypertrophied nerve trunks, and increased acetylcholinesterase staining. If sampling error occurs, it can be repeated or a full-thickness biopsy performed under general anesthesia in the operating room. Although not indicated in neonates, manometric studies will show a failure of relaxation of the internal sphincter following balloon distension of the rectum.

Traditionally, the surgical treatment was staged and consisted of a leveling colostomy followed several months later by resection of the aganglionic bowel and one of three pull-through procedures.[80] Recently, there has been a trend toward performing a single-stage procedure (no colostomy) in the newborn period.[81] This paradigm is as follows: bowel obstruction and mild enterocolitis (if present) may be relieved by placement of a large (30 Fr.) rectal tube and repeated warmed saline irrigations in 10 mL/kg aliquots preoperatively. Infants with moderate to severe enterocolitis should be treated with a diverting colostomy. At the time of surgery, frozen section analysis of the colonic muscle is required to establish the correct (ganglionic) level for the stoma. Those infants who are not ill may undergo any one of three effective operative procedures: Swenson operation, Duhamel operation, and Soave operation. The main operative principles for these procedures are removal of most or all of the aganglionic bowel while preserving the surrounding nerves to the pelvic organs, and anastomosing ganglionic bowel (confirmed by frozen section analysis) to the rectum 0.5 to 1.0 cm above the dentate line. In contrast to the Swenson and Soave procedures, the Duhamel operation leaves a cuff of aganglionic rectum along which the ganglionic bowel is stapled, creating a mini-reservoir. Historically, the operations have been performed via a low transverse abdominal incision. However, a laparoscopic-assisted operation is quickly becoming the method of choice.[82] A solely transanal mucosectomy has been used for those babies with short segment disease.[83]

Necrotizing Enterocolitis

Necrotizing enterocolitis (NEC) is the most serious and frequent GI disorder of predominantly premature infants, with a median onset of 10 days after birth. Although the true incidence of NEC is unknown, it appears to be increasing given the recent therapeutic advancements in neonatal intensive care that have allowed smaller and smaller babies to survive. In the United States, NEC accounts for 1% to 7% of all neonatal intensive care admissions or 1 to 3 cases per 1000 births.[84,85] Despite years of investigation, the pathogenesis of NEC remains unclear. Prematurity continues to be the most consistent and important risk factor.[86] Strong evidence exists that infection in a vulnerable host plays the key role in the pathogenesis of NEC.[87] In addition, the initiation of enteral feedings has been accepted as an important risk factor for the development of NEC as approximately 90% of infants develop the disease after being fed whereas only 10% develop the disease before feedings.[86,88] Overall, the development of NEC appears to be multifactorial, involving some aspects of mucosal compromise, pathogenic bacteria, and feedings combined in a susceptible host leading to bowel injury and an inflammatory cascade.

In children who develop NEC, the most common site of involvement is the terminal ileum, followed by the colon. Together, the large and small bowel are involved in 44% of cases. Pan-necrosis is the most fulminating form of the disease and is characterized by involvement of greater than 75% of the length of the intestine. Mucosal cellular injury causes necrosis and ulceration, followed by edema and hemorrhage of the submucosa, muscularis, and then serosa. Full-thickness necrosis often leads to perforation. Gas-producing bacteria in the intestinal wall may lead to pneumatosis, a finding that may be noted on gross examination as well as on plain abdominal radiographs.

Clinical findings include abdominal distension; feeding intolerance; palpable abdominal mass; and abdominal wall edema, erythema, and crepitus. Rectal bleeding is frequent but seldom massive.[89] A variety of nonspecific clinical findings suggest physiological instability, such as apnea, bradycardia, hypoglycemia, temperature instability, and lethargy. Plain abdominal radiographs (supine and either left lateral decubitus or cross-table lateral views) may demonstrate pneumatosis, portal vein air, or pneumoperitoneum. There is virtually no role for contrast studies to evaluate the acute disease.

Initial treatment consists of cessation of feeds, broad-spectrum antibiotics, gastric suction, and correction of hypovolemia, acidosis, and electrolyte abnormalities. The only absolute indication for operation is pneumoperitoneum. Relative indications are portal vein air, clinical deterioration, a fixed intestinal loop on serial radiographs, erythema of the abdominal wall, an abdominal mass, and a paracentesis demonstrating bacteria on Gram stain. At laparotomy, all necrotic bowel is resected and the proximal bowel is made into a stoma. Rarely is primary anastomosis safe. Late complications

TABLE 36.13.
Published Data Comparing Laparotomy (LAP) to Primary Peritoneal Drainage (PPD) for the Treatment of Perforated Necrotizing Enterocolitis (NEC).

	LAP				PPD			
Study	*No.*	*GA (weeks)**	*BW (g)**	*Survival rate (%)*	*No.*	*GA (weeks)**	*BW (g)**	*Survival rate (%)*
Cheu et al.[142]	41	32	1875	31 (76)	51	29	1158	18 (35)
Takamatsu et al.[143]	3	3	3	3	4	27	808	4 (100)
Morgan et al.[144]	20	32	1854	18 (90)	29	27	994	23 (79)
Azarow et al.[145]	42	31	1700	24 (57)	44	28	1100	27 (61)
Snyder et al.[146]	91	31	1628	52 (57)	12	29	1134	3 (25)
Lessin et al.[147]	3	3	3	3	9	25	615	6 (67)
Ahmed et al.[148]	22	35	2271	19 (86)	23	27	910	10 (43)
Rovin et al.[149]	10	29	1274	9 (90)	18	28	1118	16 (89)
Downard et al.[150]	9	30	1510	7 (78)	24	26	794	19 (79)
Dimmitt et al.[151]	9	26	807	5 (56)	17	25	677	7 (41)

No., number of patients; GA, gestational age; BW, birth weight.
*Mean (SEM).
Source: Moss R, Dimmit R, Henry C, Geraghty N, Efron B.[91] A meta-analysis of peritoneal drainage versus laparotomy for perforated necrotizing enterocolitis. Journal of Pediatric Surgery 2001;36(8):1210–1213.

of NEC include short bowel syndrome and stricture formation in the distal, defunctionalized bowel (usually the left colon). For this reason, a contrast enema is used to evaluate the defunctionalized distal bowel before closing the stoma.

Another strategy that is gaining acceptance for those with documented intestinal perforation is bedside peritoneal drainage using a penrose drain inserted under general anesthesia.[90] In a recent review, Moss et al. performed a meta-analysis of 10 published studies from 1978 to 1999 comparing laparotomy to primary peritoneal drainage for the treatment of perforated necrotizing enterocolitis.[91] The authors of the studies were contacted and all available raw patient data were obtained and included in the analysis. In all, the analysis included the results of 475 different patients, 244 undergoing laparotomy and 231 undergoing primary peritoneal drainage. However, the mean birth weight and gestational ages were far lower and younger in the patients undergoing laparotomy. The authors used logistic regression to control to determine the relative survival rate after laparotomy or primary peritoneal drainage, controlling for the effects of institution and gestational age. Overall, they found that the combined probability of survival did not show an advantage for either laparotomy or primary peritoneal drainage. No significant differences were found even after analysis of the obtained raw patient data as well as correction for birth weight. The authors concluded that, based on the available data, it was not possible to determine if laparotomy or primary peritoneal drainage led to better survival. In response to these questions, a randomized multicenter clinical trial is currently underway to determine the best treatment for these children. Table 36.13 details the 10 published studies comparing laparotomy versus primary peritoneal drainage for the treatment of infants with perforated NEC.

Intussusception

Intussusception (Fig. 36.12) is the most common cause of intestinal obstruction in children under 2 years of age. The peak incidence is 6 to 12 months, and there is a 3:1 male predominance. It is defined by the telescoping of a segment of proximal bowel (intussusceptum) into the adjacent distal bowel (intussuscipiens). It is typically idiopathic and involves the terminal ileum and right colon (ileocolic intussusception). In most cases, hypertrophied Peyer's patches are noted to be a leading point. Ileoileal, ileoileocolic, jejunojejunal, and colocolic intussusception have been described. Organic causes that act as lead points are most common in the older (>2 years) patients and include Meckel's diverticulum, hemangioma, polyp, intramural hematoma (Henoch–Schönlein purpura), lymphoma, inspissated stool (cystic fibrosis

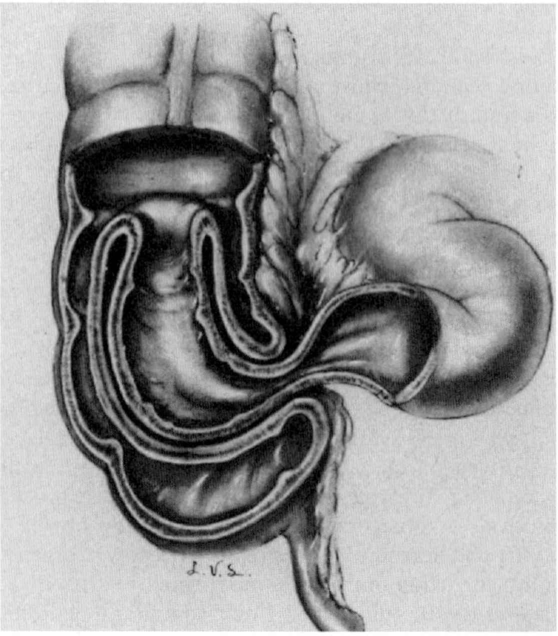

FIGURE 36.12. Ileocolic intussusception. (Reproduced with permission from de Lorimier AA. Pediatric surgery. In: Way LW, ed. Current Surgical Diagnosis and Treatment, 1994, Appleton & Lange.)

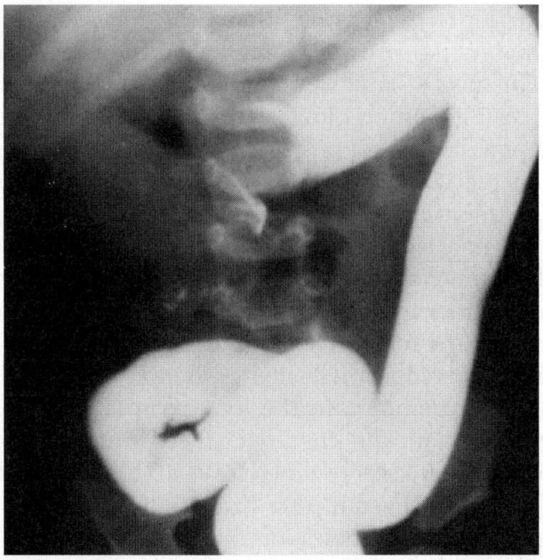

FIGURE 36.13. Contrast enema demonstrating obstruction to retrograde flow of barium by a filling defect (intussusceptum) in the mid-transverse colon.

patients), and enteric duplication. Rarely, intussusception may result from differential return of bowel function, typically after retroperitoneal surgery.

The characteristic clinical presentation is one of crying and drawing the legs upward, alternating with periods of apparent well-being or even lethargy. Reflex vomiting may occur, but vomiting from bowel obstruction is a late finding. Blood and mucus in the stool are noted in one-third of patients and have a characteristic "currant jelly" appearance. A mass may be palpable where the intussusceptum ends. For example, a typical ileocolic intussusception ends at the level of the hepatic flexure so there would be a right upper quadrant mass. Contrast enema is both diagnostic and therapeutic in more than 90% of cases (Fig. 36.13). The contrast agent may be either barium or air.[92] If barium is used, the column of contrast should not exceed 3.5 feet above the sedated patient to minimize the risk of perforation. When air is used as the contrast agent, it is pumped into the colon at a pressure of 60 to 80 mmHg (maximum, 120 mmHg). A successful study reduces the intussusceptum and demonstrates reflux of barium or air into the terminal ileum. Several attempts should be made before taking the child to surgery.

The indications for operation are peritonitis, bowel perforation, and inability to completely reduce the intussusceptum using contrast. The procedure may be performed either by laparotomy or laparoscopy. The intussusceptum is reduced manually and appendectomy performed. Occasionally, bowel resection with primary anastomosis is required for gangrene because of longstanding obstruction.

Biliary Tract Anomalies

Neonatal Jaundice

Neonatal jaundice is common and physiological for the first 7 to 10 days of life. It is principally caused by immaturity of the hepatic enzyme glucuronyl transferase and results in a predominantly indirect hyperbilirubinemia. Jaundice persisting after 2 weeks following birth is pathological, often associated with a rise in the direct bilirubin fraction, and mandates prompt evaluation. The most frequent causes of prolonged jaundice in infancy are biliary atresia, a variety of hepatitides, and choledochal cyst. The differential diagnosis of neonatal jaundice is summarized in Table 36.14.

The workup of neonatal jaundice consists of an analysis of liver function tests, complete blood count, metabolic and serological screening, and ultrasound. Depending on these results, hepatobiliary nuclear scanning and/or liver biopsy may be indicated. In those cases where a firm diagnosis has not been established using the aforementioned tests, intraoperative cholangiography is indicated.

Biliary Atresia

Biliary atresia is the absence of patent bile ducts draining the liver.[93] The atretic ducts consist of solid fibrous cords that may contain islands of biliary epithelium. The disease is progressive postnatally because infants are rarely born with remarkable jaundice. The extent of ductal involvement may vary greatly. There are three anatomic patterns of obstruction: (1) the proximal extrahepatic bile ducts are patent and the ducts distal to the cystic duct are obliterated; (2) the gallbladder, cystic duct, and common bile duct are patent and the proximal hepatic ducts are occluded; and (3) the entire ductal system is obstructed, noted in 83% of infants. Liver biopsy demonstrates proliferation of the bile canaliculi containing inspissated bile. Over time, the failure to excrete bile from the liver results in progressive periportal fibrosis and obstruction of the intrahepatic portal veins, resulting in biliary cirrhosis.

Neonates with biliary atresia are usually healthy appearing and active, in contrast to those with neonatal hepatitis. Jaundice is progressive and is a result of a predominantly direct hyperbilirubinemia. The urine is dark from bilirubin and the stools are light (acholic). Firm hepatomegaly appears by 4 weeks. Ascites and portal hypertension do not become manifest for several months. Ultrasonography may demon-

TABLE 36.14. Differential Diagnosis of Neonatal Jaundice.

ABO, Rh, and rare blood group incompatibilities:
Breast-feeding
Sepsis
Metabolic disorders
Alpha-1-antitrypsin deficiency
Gaucher's disease
Galactosemia
Tyrosinemia
Hypothyroidism
Cystic fibrosis
Criglar–Najjar syndrome
Gilbert's disease
Hepatitis
Biliary atresia
Choledochal cyst
Inspissated bile syndrome
Parenteral alimentation cholestasis
Alagille's syndrome
Byler's disease
Pyloric stenosis

strate absence or inability to visualize a contracted gallbladder. There is no intrahepatic biliary dilation with biliary atresia. A technetium 99m-labeled iminodiacetate compound scintiscan (e.g., HIDA, DISIDA) will demonstrate uptake but no intestinal excretion. Percutaneous liver biopsy may be necessary to distinguish biliary atresia from neonatal hepatitis, although there is considerable histological overlap in advanced cases. Unless the workup has conclusively diagnosed another entity, all children suspected of having biliary atresia should undergo operative cholangiography with the intention of proceeding to exploration of the porta hepatis.

Confirmed biliary atresia requires hepatic portoenterostomy (Kasai procedure.)[94] The scarred bile ducts and gallbladder are removed, and a Roux-en-Y limb of jejunum is sutured to an area of the hilum bounded laterally by the hepatic artery branches. It is important to dissect any scar off the portal ,nd its branches so the Roux limb can be sutured to as large a hilar surface as possible. A liver biopsy should also be performed. Other biliary conduits have been used such as the appendix and jejunal limbs with surgically created antireflux-ing valves. A good long-term outcome is related to a meticulously performed procedure, age at operation less than 2 months, absence of cirrhosis at the time of operation, the presence of microscopic ductules in the hepatoduodenal ligament, and whether adequate bile flow was established.[95] In general, 33% will have excellent bile flow and do not develop liver failure, 33% never have bile flow and require early liver transplantation, and 33% have initially good bile flow, but months to years later develop progressive biliary cirrhosis requiring liver transplantation. Patients in whom bile flow was established are at lifelong risk of cholangitis, which is a source of major morbidity and rehospitalization and is often treated prophylactically after operation with a once-daily oral antibiotic (e.g., trimethoprim-sulfamethoxazole).

Choledochal Cyst

Choledochal cysts are dilations or diverticuli of all or a portion of the common bile duct. The incidence is estimated from 1 in 13,000 to 1 in 2,000,000.[96] There is a female predominance (3:1) and they are more common in Asians, with a large majority of the reported cases originating from Japan.

Choledochal cysts are classified into one of five subtypes.[97] Type I is a fusiform dilation of the extrahepatic bile duct. Type II is a saccular outpouching of the common bile duct. Type III is referred to as a choledochocele and is a wide-mouth dilation of the common duct at its confluence with the duodenum. Type IV is a cystic dilation of both the intra- and extrahepatic bile ducts. Type V consists of lakes of multiple intrahepatic cysts with no extrahepatic component, and when type V is associated with hepatic fibrosis, it is termed Caroli's disease. Type I and type IV are the most common. Caroli's disease is associated with type V, appears to be a congenital syndrome, and often follows an autosomal recessive pattern of inheritance in association with various other anomalies, such as polycystic kidney disease and renal tubular ectasia.[98]

There are several theories to explain the development of the common forms of choledochal cysts The increased incidence in girls and in Asians suggests a genetic etiology causing a primary congenital ductal ectasia. Nevertheless, familial cases have not been described, and an alternative explanation for geographic increases in incidence indicates that an infectious agent may be involved.[96] Alternatively, cystic dilation may be a result of embryological obstruction of the bile duct.[99] Another popular theory postulates that an anomalous entry of the pancreatic duct into the common bile duct results in a long common channel and reflux of potentially injurious activated pancreatic enzymes into the bile duct.[100] The long common channel theory is attractive, but the abnormal long common channel anatomy has been demonstrated by cholangiography in only 65% to 80% of patients.

If left untreated, choledochal cysts may cause cholangitis and cholangiocarcinoma in the long term. The risk of cholangiocarcinoma in the first decade of life is only 0.7%; however, this increases to about 14% at 20 years and is postulated to increase even further throughout life.[101] It has been suggested that type III cysts, or choledochoceles, represent a form of duodenal duplication and therefore do not share the malignant potential of the other bile duct cysts.

The classic presentation of a choledochal cyst is the triad of abdominal pain, jaundice, and an abdominal mass. However, in children, the complete triad proves to be the exception rather than the rule. Ultrasonography is increasingly responsible for detecting choledochal cysts in the fetus. Neonates more commonly present with asymptomatic jaundice (predominantly direct hyperbilirubinemia) or an abdominal mass. As children grow older, the cyst may become painful or infected. In adults, an abdominal mass is rarely appreciated, and patients present more commonly with symptoms of cholangitis and/or pancreatitis. On rare occasions, children have been described with bile peritonitis secondary to perforation of a choledochal cyst. An ultrasound usually confirms the diagnosis, although radionuclide scanning, MRI, and endoscopic retrograde cholangiopancreatography (ERCP) have also been used.

Historically, choledochal cysts were treated with internal drainage by anastomosis of the cyst wall to the stomach, duodenum, or small bowel. Internal drainage procedures have an unacceptably high morbidity, including persistent biliary stasis with the development of sludge, stones, cholangitis, chronic inflammatory fibrosis, and anastomotic stricture. Furthermore, the unresected cyst is capable of malignant degeneration. Presently, the gold standard operation consists of complete cyst excision with Roux-en-Y hepaticojejunostomy. Distally, the common bile duct is transected just above the pancreatic duct, limiting the amount of residual biliary tissue at risk for malignancy.

The results of choledochal cyst excision with hepaticojejunostomy reconstruction are consistently excellent, but these children do require lifelong follow-up because of the risk of anastomotic stricture and intrahepatic stone formation.

Abdominal Wall Defects

Omphalocele

Omphalocele is a midline abdominal wall defect noted in 1 in 5000 live births. The abdominal viscera (commonly liver and bowel) are contained within a sac composed of peritoneum and amnion, from which the umbilical cord arises at

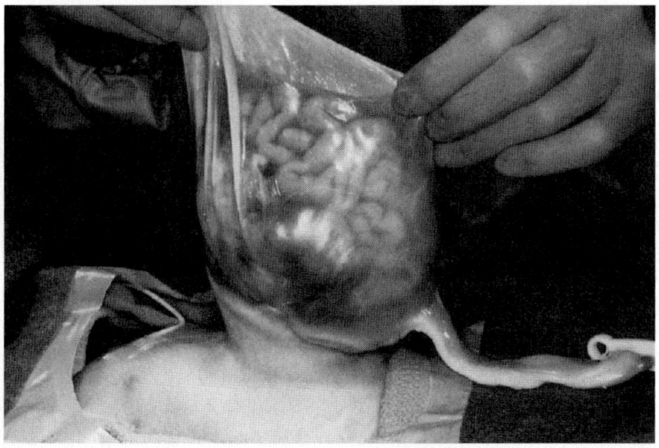

FIGURE 36.14. Neonate with an omphalocele. The liver and bowel herniated through a midline abdominal wall defect and are contained within a sac of amnion and chorion from which the umbilical cord emanates.

the apex and center[102] (Fig. 36.14). When the defect is less than 4 cm it is termed a hernia of the umbilical cord and when greater than 10 cm it is termed a giant omphalocele. Associated abnormalities occur in 30% to 70% and include, in descending order of frequency, chromosomal abnormalities (trisomy 13, 18, 21), congenital heart disease, Beckwith–Wiedemann syndrome (hyperinsulinism, gigantism, macroglossia), cloacal exstrophy (hypogastric omphalocele, open hemibladders separated by a vesicointestinal fissure, ambiguous genitalia), pentalogy of Cantrell (see chest wall deformities, above), and prune belly syndrome (absent abdominal wall muscles, genitourinary abnormalities, cryptorchidism).

After delivery, the omphalocele is covered by placing the baby's lower extremities and torso within a sterile bag (bowel bag) or placing Saran wrap around the defect to minimize heat and water loss. Intravenous fluids are administered and nasogastric suction commenced. Emergency operation is not necessary, so a thorough physical examination and workup for associated anomalies are performed. The primary goal of surgery is to return the viscera to the abdominal cavity and close the defect. The success of primary closure is predicated on the size of the defect and the size of the abdominal and thoracic cavities. It is wise to leave the sac in situ because primary closure may not be possible and thus one has maintained the best biological dressing for the viscera. If the viscera reduce but abdominal wall closure is not possible, there are two options: staged repair and prosthetic patch repair. A staged repair aims to create a protective extraabdominal extension of the peritoneal cavity (termed a silo), allowing gradual reduction of the viscera and gradual abdominal wall expansion using two parallel sheets of reinforced silastic sheeting sutured to the fascial edges or a preformed, spring-loaded silo. A prosthetic patch repair can be used to bridge a wide fascial gap and the skin is closed over the patch. In rare cases, nonoperative treatment is indicated because of the presence of a giant omphalocele or severe associated anomalies (e.g., pentalogy of Cantrell). The aim is to allow the sac to dry and form an eschar, allowing epithelialization to occur over the ensuing 16 to 20 weeks. The result is a ventral hernia that is repaired electively when the patient is stable. A silo repair is managed by daily manual reduction at the bedside. Complete reduction usually takes 5 to 7 days, and then the defect is primarily closed. The outcome is excellent when there are no serious associated anomalies.

Gastroschisis

Compared to an omphalocele, a gastroschisis is a much smaller, right paramedian defect without an investing sac[102] (Fig. 36.15). It is twice as common as omphalocele, and the hernia contains gut and pelvic organs but not the liver. Forty percent of affected infants are born prematurely or are small for gestational age. The bowel may be edematous, matted, foreshortened, and have extensive fibrin coating or "peel" because of amniotic peritonitis. In both omphalocele and gastroschisis, nonrotation of the gut is common. In contrast to omphalocele, associated anomalies are rare; the most common is intestinal atresia (10%–15%).

At delivery, the bowel should be assessed for ischemia from obstructed mesenteric vessels herniating out a small defect or for a volvulus. The infant should be placed on his or her side to prevent "kinking" of the mesentery as it drapes over the abdominal wall. The bowel is covered with a sterile bag, as already described, and the GI tract is decompressed with a gastric tube. In contrast to omphalocele, urgent repair is necessary. Primary closure is often possible except when the abdominal cavity is small or there is significant edema and thickening of the bowel and mesentery. It is important to irrigate the colon free of meconium before attempting reduction and repair. If an intestinal atresia is noted, there are three options: (1) no immediate treatment, reduce the bowel, and reoperate in 2 to 4 weeks and either repair or create a stoma; (2) immediate stoma (beware of possible contamination of the silo, if present); and (3) resection and primary anastomosis (least likely). A staged silo repair and/or prosthetic patch closure of the fascia may be necessary, as described above for an omphalocele.

In contrast to infants with omphalocele, those with repaired gastroschisis have a predictably prolonged ileus (2–6 weeks) and require central parenteral nutrition. If bowel function does not return in 4 to 6 weeks, obtain a contrast study to rule out an obstruction from inspissated meconium or an intestinal atresia not noted during the initial surgery because of the extensive inflammation and matting of the bowel loops.

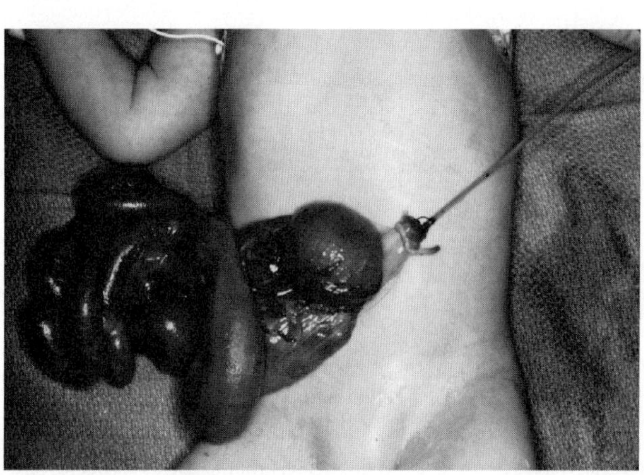

FIGURE 36.15. Neonate with a gastroschisis. The defect is to the *right* of the umbilical cord and the bowel has no investing sac. Note the edema of the bowel wall and the dilated stomach adjacent to the umbilical cord.

Umbilical Hernia

An umbilical fascial defect is very common in newborns. The highest incidence is in preterm infants and those of African-American descent. In most children (95%), a defect less than 1.5 cm will progressively diminish in size and eventually close[103]; this may take months or years. Unlike inguinal hernias, complications (incarceration, strangulation) from umbilical hernias are extremely rare. Repair of the defect is indicated when the defect is larger than 1.5 cm or the child is 4 years or older because defects in these children are not likely to close spontaneously.

Inguinal and Scrotal Disorders

Inguinal Hernia and Hydrocele

Inguinal hernia is a common condition in infancy and childhood.[104] Differing from hernias in adulthood, these hernias nearly exclusively result from a patent processus vaginalis (indirect hernia) and not a weakness in the floor of the inguinal canal (direct hernia). The processus vaginalis follows the descent of the testis into the inguinal canal. Failure of obliteration of the processus may lead to a variety of anomalies including scrotal hernia, inguinal hernia, communicating hydrocele, noncommunicating hydrocele, hydrocele of the spermatic cord, and hydrocele of the tunica vaginalis (Fig. 36.16).

The incidence of a clinically detectable inguinal hernia varies with gestational age: 9% to 11% in preterm infants and 3% to 5% for full-term infants. They occur on the right side 60% (because of later descent of the right testis), left 30%, and bilaterally 10%, and are more common in males. Conditions associated with an increased risk of inguinal hernia include prematurity, family history, abdominal wall defects, cryptorchidism, intersex anomalies, connective tissue disorders, and ascites from any cause (e.g., ventriculoperitoneal shunt, peritoneal dialysis, liver disease). The usual presentation is a nontender mass in the inguinal region (Fig. 36.17). The hernia is often appreciated only when the child strains or cries. One must always locate the position of the testis during an examination for a hernia because an inguinal bulge caused by an undescended or retractile testis may be mistaken for a hernia. Commonly, testicular hydroceles are mistaken for hernias. The hallmark of the hydrocele is that one can palpate the normal spermatic cord above the level of the hydrocele. Transillumination is not reliable in the newborn because intestine and fluid transilluminate equally well. It may be difficult to distinguish between a large inguinoscrotal hydrocele and an incarcerated hernia. In the first 2 months of life, one can palpate the area of the internal ring by digital rectal examination and potentially feel the bowel entering the internal ring. In general, hydroceles that do not communicate with the peritoneal cavity are physiological, and most resolve within 1 year. Those that persist after 1 year or those which demonstrate changes in size (communicating hydrocele) should be repaired.

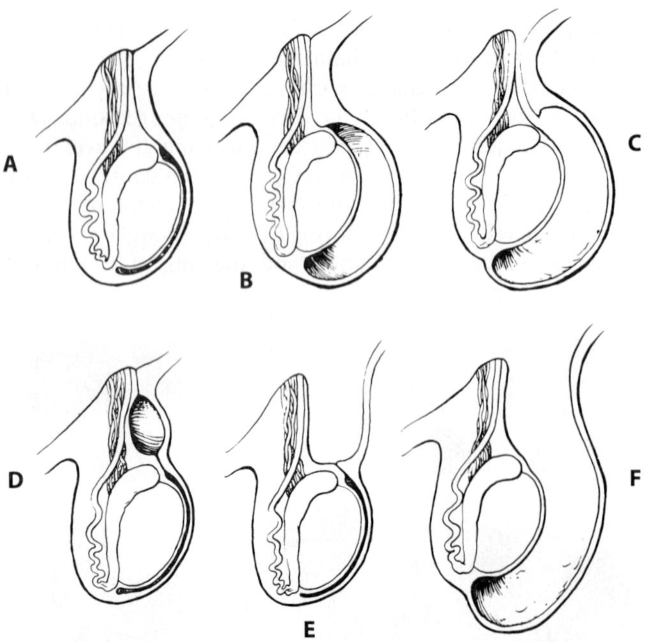

FIGURE 36.16. Spectrum of inguinoscrotal disorders. **A.** Normal anatomy. The processus vaginalis is obliterated and there is a small remnant, the tunica vaginalis, adjacent to the posterior surface of the testis. **B.** Scrotal hydrocele. **C.** Communicating hydrocele. Note the proximal patency of the processus vaginalis. **D.** Hydrocele of the spermatic cord. **E.** Inguinal hernia. B Inguinoscrotal hernia. (Reproduced with permission from Rowe MI. Inguinal and serotal disorder. In: Essentials of Pediatric Surgery, 1995, by permission of CV Mosby Co.)

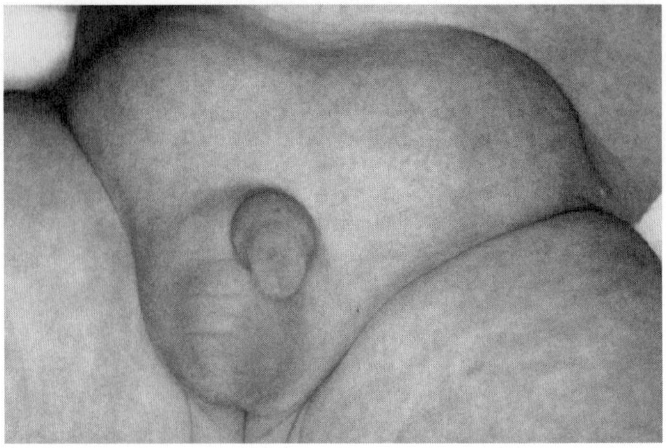
FIGURE 36.17. Bilateral inguinal hernias in a neonate. This baby also has an undescended testicle on the left as characterized by a flat left hemiscrotum without rugae.

All inguinal hernias in children should be repaired shortly after diagnosis to prevent incarceration (nonreducible viscera in the hernia sac), strangulation (vascular compromise to the incarcerated bowel), or injury to the ipsilateral testis from compression of the spermatic cord by the incarcerated bowel. An incarcerated hernia can usually be reduced before surgery. If the initial manual reduction is unsuccessful, the child should be sedated and reduction reattempted. After reduction, repair is delayed 48 to 72 h to allow the edema to subside.

At operation, a small inguinal crease incision is made, the external oblique opened, and the anteromedially positioned hernia sac is dissected free from the cord structures and ligated flush with the internal ring (high ligation). Distally, as much sac is removed as possible and any remnant is left open to drain. Historically, it was recommended that all boys under 2 years of age and all girls under 5 years undergo operative exploration of the contralateral inguinal canal in search of a clinically silent patent processus vaginalis.[105] This approach has been replaced, in large part, by laparoscopic exploration[106,107]; this is performed either through the ipsilateral hernia sac, through the umbilicus, or in line with the internal ring (at the lateral border of the hemirectus muscle) using a needlescope. If a patent processus vaginalis is demonstrated laparoscopically, then a second inguinal incision is made and the procedure repeated as described earlier. The incidence of complications from inguinal hernia repair (recurrence, wound infection, and damage to the spermatic cord) should be 2% or less.

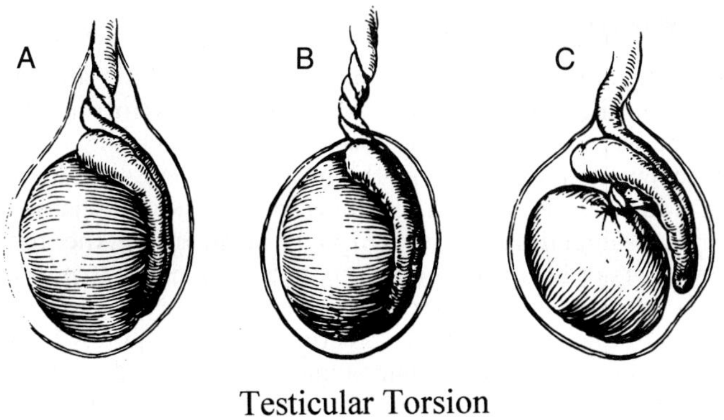

FIGURE 36.18. Three anatomical variants of testicular torsion. **A.** Intravaginal. **B.** Extravaginal. **C.** Torsion around a long epididymal mesentery.

Disorders of the Testes

Cryptorchidism

By the eighth month of gestation, testicular descent should be complete. The incidence of undescended or partially descended testis is 1% to 2% in full-term infants and up to 30% in premature babies. The cryptorchid testis may be located in the inguinal canal, in the peritoneal cavity, or anywhere on the lower abdomen, thigh, and perineum (ectopic testis). The cryptorchid testis may continue to descend into the scrotum up to 1 year after birth. Operation is indicated after 1 year because degenerative changes begin to take place in these testes that may impair spermatogenesis and lead to malignant transformation. Additionally, cryptorchid testes are more prone to trauma and torsion, often have an associated inguinal hernia, and may cause adverse psychosocial effects The incidence of testicular cancer in a cryptorchid testis (30 times higher than the normal population) is not lessened by repair, but a scrotal testicle can be more reliably examined for a testicular mass later in life.

The differential diagnosis includes retractile testis (a normal testis that has a hyperreactive cremasteric reflex and can be manually pulled into the mid-hemiscrotum), ectopic testis, and absent testis (usually because of in utero torsion). Between 6 and 12 months of age, orchiopexy using the dartos pouch technique is performed.[108] If the testis is not palpable when the child is anesthetized, laparoscopy should be performed before making an inguinal incision to allow for identification of an abdominal testis or the diagnosis of an absent testis. A two-stage repair (clip or laser the spermatic artery and vein, followed by positioning in the scrotum 6–8 weeks later) is indicated for a high intraabdominal testis. If spermatic cord structures are seen entering the inguinal ring, an inguinal incision is then made.

Testicular Torsion

Testicular torsion is most frequent in late childhood and early adolescence, although the range is from fetus to newborn.[109] Anatomically, there are two forms of testicular torsion: intravaginal torsion (bell-clapper deformity), the most common form, and extravaginal torsion, which occurs principally in neonates and in children with an undescended testis (Fig. 36.18). Rarely, the testis may twist on a long epididymal mesentery. In children, testicular torsion is either idiopathic or occurs after activity or trauma. There is acute scrotal or testicular pain that may radiate to the lower abdomen. Progressive swelling, edema, and erythema of the hemiscrotum occur. The testicle is exquisitely tender on palpation. The testicle may be foreshortened, the epididymis may lie anteriorly, and the cremasteric reflex may be absent, although these signs can be difficult to elicit. Fetal or neonatal torsion is probably responsible for the "absent" testis noted during the workup of cryptorchidism. Testicular salvage after neonatal torsion is rare.

Torsion of the testicular appendices[110] (vestigial Müllerian duct structures) and epididymitis may mimic testicular torsion. With epididymitis, there is often pyuria, voiding symptoms, and fever. Torsion of a testicular appendix often has a gradual onset, and careful palpation may reveal point, rather than diffuse, tenderness. There may be a visible necrotic lesion on scrotal transillumination (blue dot sign).

The diagnosis of testicular torsion is made principally on clinical grounds. Although one may utilize Doppler ultrasonography and radionuclide scanning to aid in the diagnosis, these tests are time consuming and, in the case of ultrasound, not very specific. If the diagnosis is strongly suspected, the best "test" is operative scrotal exploration. The testicular salvage rate if detorsion is performed within 6h of symptoms is up to 97% versus less than 10% if more than 24h have elapsed. At operation, the testicle is detorsed and, if viable, it is fixed to the hemiscrotum in three places. The contralateral testicle is at risk for torsion because the testicular anatomy tends to mirror itself, so a contralateral orchiopexy should be performed in all cases. Torsion of the testicular appendices tends to be self-limiting because necrosis and autoamputation usually occur. Treatment is with warm baths, limited activity, and an antiinflammatory agent. If significant pain persists after 2 to 3 days, the appendix has not autoamputated and excision is indicated.

Cutaneous Vascular Anomalies

Cutaneous vascular anomalies constitute a group of congenital and acquired vascular malformations of the skin. They are present in 2.6% of all newborns. These anomalies are broadly divided into two categories: hemangiomas and vascular malformations.[111] They are most precisely classified by the biological activity of the endothelium.

Hemangiomas

Hemangiomas demonstrate endothelial hyperplasia and are seen in children and adults but behave differently at different ages. Hemangiomas are much more common than vascular malformations. In the neonatal period, hemangiomas can be subclassified according to their growth phase. A rapid proliferating phase is usually seen during the first few years of life, followed by the involuting phase that may last several years. Their clinical appearance depends on depth of the lesion; superficial dermis lesions (capillary hemangiomas, strawberry hemangiomas) appear raised and profoundly erythematous with an irregular texture, whereas deep lesions (cavernous hemangiomas) appear smooth, slightly raised, with a bluish hue or a faint telangiectatic pattern on the overlying skin. Mixed lesions are often noted (capillary-cavernous hemangiomas). Twenty percent of patients have multiple lesions. Complications from hemangiomas consist of ulceration (during proliferative phase), bleeding, thrombocytopenia (Kasabach–Merritt syndrome), consumptive coagulopathy, high output heart failure, visual field encroachment, airway obstruction, and minor skeletal distortions.

Fifty percent will involute without treatment by age 5 years, 70% by 7 years. The remainder will slowly resolve by age 10 to 12 years. Steroid therapy hastens the rate of proliferation of hemangiomas by 30% to 90% and is indicated for complicated lesions (i.e., those causing severe physiological or anatomical abnormalities).

Cutaneous Vascular Malformations

Vascular malformations have normal endothelial cell turnover and tend to grow with the child. These lesions are structural anomalies that are considered errors in vascular morphogenesis. They are usually visible at birth but may take years or even decades to manifest. They are separated into low- and high-flow variants, and further classified according to the type of vascular channel abnormality: capillary, venous, arterial, and mixed malformations. Capillary and venous malformations are low-flow variants; arterial and mixed arterial/venous are high-flow variants.

Capillary malformations consist of port-wine stain (nevus flammeus), nevus flammeus neonatorum (angel's kiss), nevus flammeus nuchae (stork bite, salmon patch), angiokeratomas, telangiectasias [spider, hereditary hemorrhagic telangiectasia (Rendu–Osler–Weber syndrome)]. They are prone to infection and are treated aggressively with intravenous antibiotics. A compression garment should be used if anatomically feasible. Some lesions can be excised or injected with a sclerosing solution.

Venous malformations have a wide spectrum of appearances ranging from simple varicosities to complex deep lesions that may be located in deeper tissues (e.g., bone, muscle, salivary gland). Pain is often related to thrombosis within the lesion. Radiographic imaging delineates the nature and extent of the lesion (angiogram, CT, MRI). Photocoagulation or YAG laser may be effective for superficial lesions. Resection is the definitive treatment because it can reduce bulk, improve contour and function, and control pain. It is limited by anatomic boundaries, and multiple staged procedures may be required.

Arterial and arteriovenous malformations have multiple small fistulae surrounded by abnormal tissues and can cause high-output cardiac failure. They are most common in the head and neck region (especially intracerebral). There is pain and overlying cutaneous necrosis. Adjacent osseous structures are often destroyed. Selective embolization is used either as palliation or presurgically to limit hemorrhage. Excision, when possible, is the procedure of choice.

Combined vascular malformations and hypertrophy syndromes consist of Klippel–Trenaunay–Weber syndrome (combined capillary-lymphatic venous malformation associated with lower limb hypertrophy), Parkes–Weber syndrome (upper limb arteriovenous shunting), Marffucci's syndrome (low-flow vascular malformations and multiple extremity enchondromas with hypoplastic long bones), and Sturge–Weber syndrome (upper facial port-wine stain and vascular anomalies of the choroid plexus and leptomeninges).

Childhood Tumors

Neuroblastoma

Neuroblastoma is the most common tumor in infants less than 1 year of age and the second most common solid tumor of childhood (after brain tumors).[112] Approximately 60% of all cases occur in children less than 2 years of age and 97% before age 10. The most common site for primary disease is in the abdomen (adrenal), followed by the thorax, pelvis, and, occasionally, head and neck. They may reach massive size and violate tissue planes such that they envelop major blood vessels, their branches, and other important structures (e.g., ureter), making primary resection potentially hazardous. Large tumors may have calcifications because of hemorrhage and necrosis. They contain small blue round cell tumors and thus must be differentiated from peripheral neurectodermal tumors, Ewing's sarcoma, rhabdomyosarcoma, and lymphoma. They may show the full range of maturation from neuroblastoma to ganglioneuroblastoma to ganglioneuroma.

Several molecular and cellular characteristics of neuroblastic tumors are prognostically important. The most important is the high incidence of amplification of the protooncogene n-*myc*, seen in approximately 30% of tumors. Amplification of n-*myc* (more than 10 copies) adversely correlates with prognosis, independent of clinical stage. Other genetic abnormalities include a deletion of the short arm of chromosome 1 and the tendency for hyperdiploid tumors to have an improved prognosis over diploid tumors. Using the Shimada index, well-differentiated, stroma-rich tumors have a favorable prognosis. Eighty-five percent to 90% secrete high levels of the catecholamine metabolites vanillylmandelic acid (VMA) and homovanillic acid (HVA); an elevated ratio of VMA to HVA correlates with an improved outcome in patients with advanced disease. Other biochemical indicators of advanced disease include neuron-specific enolase, serum ferritin, serum ganglioside Gd2, and serum lactate dehydrogenase.

Symptoms are site specific. The most common is pain (from the primary or metastatic disease). Other symptoms include failure to thrive, malaise, fever, weight loss, and anorexia. Children frequently appear "ill" at the time of diagnosis. Constipation and urinary retention are signs of pelvic disease. Orbital metastases commonly present with periorbital ecchymoses and proptosis ("raccoon eyes"). Spinal canal involvement may present with acute paralysis because of compression. The opsomyoclonus syndrome is an acute cerebellar encephalopathy characterized by ataxia, opsoclonus ("dancing eyes"), myoclonus, and dementia. It occurs in association with approximately 3% of all neuroblastomas, and is usually associated with a good prognosis, although the neurological abnormalities tend to persist after successful treatment of the primary tumor. Infants with stage 4-S disease (Table 36.15) may display cutaneous metastases ("blueberry muffin" lesions) or respiratory embarrassment secondary to massive hepatomegaly from tumor infiltration.

Imaging includes a chest radiograph, skeletal survey, and bone scan. Neuroblastoma is the most common abdominal tumor to demonstrate calcifications (50%) before chemotherapy. The CT scan is instrumental in making the diagnosis and in determining resectability. CT myeleography is useful in assessing tumor within the spinal canal and spinal cord compression. MRI is as sensitive as CT scanning in terms of assessing tumor size and resectability, but has the added advantage of being superior to CT in assessing vessel encasement, vessel patency, and spinal cord compression. MRI can also demonstrate bone marrow involvement in selected cases. I-Meta-iodobenzylguanidine nuclear scanning is very sensitive in detecting tumors that concentrate catecholamines and has been useful in the diagnosis of primary, residual, and metastatic disease in patients with neuroblastoma. The staging systems are surgical and anatomically based, and all have prognostic value. The most recent is the International Neuroblastoma Staging System (see Table 36.15).

TABLE 36.15. International Neuroblastoma Staging System and Estimated Survival Rates.

Stage	*Characteristics*	*Survival*
Stage 1	Localized tumor confined to the area of origin; complete gross excision, with or without microscopic residual disease; identifiable ipsilateral and contralateral lymph nodes negative microscopically.	100%
Stage 2A	Unilateral tumor with incomplete gross excision; identifiable ipsilateral nonadherent lymph nodes negative microscopically.	80%
Stage 2B	Unilateral tumor with complete or incomplete gross excision; with positive ipsilateral nonadherent lymph nodes; identifiable contralateral lymph nodes negative microscopically.	70%
Stage 3	Tumor infiltrating across the midline (vertebral column) with or without regional lymph node involvement; or unilateral tumor with contralateral regional lymph node involvement; or midline tumor with bilateral regional lymph node involvement or extension by infiltration.	40%
Stage 4	Dissemination of tumor to distant lymph nodes, bone, bone marrow, liver, or other organs (except as defined in stage 4-S).	15%
Stage 4-S	Localized primary tumor as defined for stage 1 or 2 with dissemination limited to liver, skin, and/or bone marrow (<10% tumor) in infants younger than 1 year.	85%

The diagnosis rests upon the demonstration of immature neuroblastic tissue obtained by tissue or bone marrow aspirate and biopsy. Tissue is obtained by biopsy (either by laparotomy or laparoscopically), which allows accurate determination of resectability and assures that adequate tissue (1 g or 1 cm^2) is available for determination of tumor markers, cytological studies, and the special stains required for accurate diagnosis and staging. Needle biopsy is used when open biopsy is hazardous.

Primary excision is attempted whenever possible; sacrifice of major structures, such as intraabdominal organs or vessels, is not warranted at the first operation. Gross total excision is attempted, but negative microscopic tumor margins are not necessary. Tumors that are not safely resectable at diagnosis should be biopsied, along with any visible lymph nodes. Cyclic chemotherapy with or without radiation therapy frequently results in shrinkage and maturation of the tumor, allowing for later attempts at more aggressive resection. Removal of all residual disease is the goal, and a more radical approach is warranted. Abdominal midline tumors frequently encase the aorta, vena cava, and visceral vessels, making resection hazardous. The cavitron ultrasonic dissector (CUSA) has been useful in these cases. Basic tenets of tumor surgery need to be violated to remove tumors that encase major vessels: the tumor is often "split" to uncover and dissect major vessels and their branches. Lymph node sampling is a required component of most staging protocols; gross appearance alone is not adequate (false-negative and -positive rates up to 25%). The use of intraoperative radiation therapy is controversial. Liver biopsy is a part of the staging evaluation in all patients with an abdominal primary.

Bone marrow transplantation is used for patients with stage 3 and 4 disease who are at high risk by virtue of their age, stage, or biological characteristics of their tumor.[113] Patients receive sublethal doses of chemotherapeutic agents and total body irradiation, then are "rescued" with either allogeneic bone marrow or, more commonly, with purged autologous bone marrow.

Wilms Tumor

Wilms tumor is the most common childhood intraabdominal tumor.[114] Seventy-five percent of children are less than 5 years old, the peak incidence is 2 to 3 years of age. It is associated with aniridia, hemihypertrophy, and the Beckwith–Wiedemann syndrome. The constellation of Wilms tumor, aniridia, genitourinary anomalies, and mental retardation (WAGR syndrome) and the Denys–Drash syndrome (mental retardation, pseudohermaphroditism, renal disease, and Wilms tumor) are associated with a deletion of 11p13.[115]

Children are healthy appearing and present with an asymptomatic abdominal mass. It is not uncommonly detected during the workup of seemingly trivial trauma-induced hematuria. The physical findings are generally limited to a large, nontender mass. Ascites may be present in advanced cases.

There are no specific tumor markers. Imaging is required to determine the extent of the mass, to assess for bilateral disease, venous invasion, and metastases, and to confirm contralateral renal function; this is accomplished with an abdominal ultrasound and a CT scan of the chest and abdomen. The most important determinants of outcome for children are

TABLE 36.16. Wilms Tumor Staging System.

Stage	*Characteristics*
Stage I	Tumor limited to kidney and completely excised. The surface of the renal capsule is intact and the tumor was not ruptured before removal. There is no residual tumor.
Stage II	Tumor extends through the perirenal capsule but is completely excised. There may be local spillage of tumor confined to the flank or the tumor may have been biopsied. Extrarenal vessels may contain tumor thrombus or be infiltrated by tumor.
Stage III	Residual nonhematogenous tumor confined to the abdomen: lymph node involvement, diffuse peritoneal spillage, peritoneal implants, tumor beyond surgical margin either grossly or microscopically, or tumor not completely removed.
Stage IV	Hematogenous metastases to lung, liver, bone, brain, etc.
Stage V	Bilateral renal involvement at diagnosis; each kidney should be staged separately.

histopathology and tumor stage. Histopathologically, there are two prognostic groups: favorable and unfavorable. Unfavorable types display varying degrees of anaplasia. Staging is based on surgical and pathological aspects of the tumor (Table 36.16).

Surgical excision can often be accomplished without any preoperative treatment. The aim of surgery is to completely remove the tumor (nephrectomy) without spill and determine the stage by virtue of its size, extent, and lymph node involvement. Tumor rupture with gross spillage portends a sixfold increase in risk of local recurrence and requires the use of postoperative external-beam radiation. Palpation of the renal veins and inferior vena cava is performed to detect tumor thrombus. The contralateral kidney must be examined and palpated. Bilateral involvement (6%) is a contraindication to primary nephrectomy. Suspicious lesions in the opposite kidney are biopsied. Bilateral disease mandates "nephron-sparing" surgery (see following). If the tumor is too large for safe resection, it is biopsied, along with regional lymph nodes. Chemotherapy with or without radiation therapy usually results in a significant reduction in tumor size and allows subsequent resection. Preoperative chemotherapy is administered to patients with intracaval tumor thrombus; complete dissolution is the rule with one or two cycles.[114]

The treatment of bilateral disease is individualized, with the goal of eradicating tumor while preserving the maximal amount of functional renal mass. After bilateral biopsy, the child is treated according to the most advanced stage. Delayed reexploration determines the response to treatment, and renal-preserving resection is performed.

The overall survival is 85%, and most patients are cured. Survival correlates with stage. The 4-year survival with respect to age and histology is presented in Table 36.17.

Rhabdomyosarcoma

Rhabdomyosarcoma is a childhood malignancy that arises from embryonic mesenchyme with the potential to differentiate into skeletal muscle.[116] It is the most common pediatric soft tissue sarcoma and is the third most common solid malignancy. It accounts for 4% to 8% of all malignancies and 5% to 15% of all solid malignancies of childhood.

The age distribution is bimodal: the first peak is between 2 to 5 years and the secondary peak between 15 and 19 years. Fifty percent present before 5 years, and 6% in infancy. There is an increased incidence in patients with neurofibromatosis, the Beckwith–Wiedemann syndrome, and Li–Fraumani cancer-family syndrome.

Most studies divide rhabdomyosarcoma into distinct histological groups: favorable, intermediate, and unfavorable. Favorable types (5%) include the sarcoma botryoides and spindle-cell variants. Botryoid tumors typically present in young children from within visceral cavities (e.g., vagina), whereas spindle-cell types have a predilection for paratesticular sites. Intermediate prognosis tumors (50%) are of the embryonal type. Unfavorable prognosis tumors (20%) include alveolar and undifferentiated tumors. Alveolar tumors arise from the extremities, trunk, and perineum. Undifferentiated tumors arise from the extremity and head and neck sites. Thirteen percent cannot be adequately characterized and are labeled "small, round cell sarcoma, type indeterminant."

The clinical presentation varies with the site of origin of the primary tumor, age, and the presence or absence of metastatic disease. The majority of symptoms are secondary to the effects of tumor compression or by the presence of a mass. The most common site is the head and neck region (35%); these are subdivided into orbital (10%), parameningeal (15%), and nonparameningeal (10%) sites. They are usually embryonal and present as asymptomatic masses or functional deficits. Genitourinary rhabdomyosarcoma (26%) are divided into two groups: bladder/prostate (10%) and nonbladder/prostate, including paratesticular sites, perineum, vulva, vagina, and uterus (16%). The most common histological type is embryonal, although botryoid tumors and spindle-cell tumors are seen more frequently here than in any other site. These tumors may be so massive as to make determination of the primary tumor site impossible. There is a propensity for early lymphatic spread in GU primary tumors. Bladder/prostate tumors frequently present with urinary retention or hematuria, whereas vaginal and uterine tumors present with vaginal bleeding or discharge or with a mass exiting the vagina. Extremity rhabdomyosarcomas (1%) are more common in the lower than upper extremity. These tumors are usually of the alveolar variety, with a high incidence of regional nodal involvement and distal metastases. "Other" sites account for 20%; the most common are the thorax, diaphragm, abdominal and pelvic walls, and intraabdominal or intrapelvic organs.

Staging is determined by the histological variant and the primary site; the extent of disease is mandatory as each has

TABLE 36.17. Four-Year Survival for Wilms Tumor.

Stage	*Four-year survival*
Stage I/FH	98%
Stage I-III/UH	68%
Stage II/FH	90%–95%
Stage III/FH	85%–90%
Stage IV/FH	78%–86%
Stage IV/UH	52%–58%

FH, favorable histology; UH, unfavorable histology.

TABLE 36.18. Intergroup Rhabdomyosarcoma Study Clinical Group Staging System.

Group	*Characteristics*
Group I	Localized disease, completely removed a. Confined to muscle or organ of origin b. Infiltration outside organ or muscle of origin; regional nodes not involved
Group II	Total gross resection with evidence of regional spread a. Grossly resected tumor with microscopic residual b. Regional disease with nodes, completely involved resected with no microscopic residual c. Regional disease with involved nodes, grossly resected, but with evidence of microscopic residual and/or histological involvement of the most distal regional node in the dissection
Group III	Incomplete resection, or biopsy with presence of gross disease
Group IV	Distant metastases

an important influence on the choice of treatment and on prognosis. CT or MRI scanning is essential to evaluate the primary tumor and its relationship to surrounding structures. A clinical grouping system was designed by the Intergroup Rhabdomyosarcoma Study Group (IRS) to stratify different extents of disease to compare treatment and outcome results (Table 36.18). It is based on pretreatment and operative outcome and does not account for the biological differences or the natural history of tumors arising from different primary sites.

The surgical management is site specific and includes complete wide excision of the primary tumor and surrounding uninvolved tissue while preserving cosmesis and function. Incomplete excision (beyond biopsy) or tumor debulking is not beneficial, and severely mutilating or debilitating procedures should not be performed. Tumors not amenable to primary excision should be amply biopsied and then treated with neoadjuvant therapies; secondary excision is then performed and is associated with a better outcome than partial or incomplete excisions. Clinically suspicious lymph nodes should be excised or biopsied; excision of clinically uninvolved nodes is site specific. Primary reexcision has been shown to improve outcome in patients where microscopic margins are positive, where the initial procedure was not a formal "cancer" resection, or where malignancy was not suspected preoperatively.[117]

Liver Neoplasms

Tumors of the liver are uncommon in childhood (2% of all pediatric malignancies). More than 70% of pediatric liver masses are malignant. The majority of hepatic malignancies are of epithelial orgin; most benign lesions are vascular in nature.[118]

Hepatoblastoma

Hepatoblastomas account for almost 50% of all liver masses in children and approximately two-thirds of malignant tumors. The majority are seen in children less than 4 years of age, and two-thirds are noted before 2 years of age. The Beckwith–Wiedemann syndrome, hemihypertrophy, the fetal alcohol syndrome, and parenteral nutrition administration in infancy all increase the risk of hepatoblastoma.

The most common finding is an asymptomatic abdominal mass or diffuse abdominal swelling in a healthy-appearing child. There may be obstructive GI symptoms secondary to compression of the stomach or duodenum, or acute pain secondary to hemorrhage into the tumor. Physical examination reveals a nontender, firm mass in the right upper quadrant or midline that moves with respiration. Advanced tumors present with weight loss, ascites, and failure to thrive. Approximately 10% of males present with isosexual precocity secondary to tumor secretion of beta-human chorionic gonadotropin (β-hCG). Laboratory studies reveal nonspecifically elevated liver function tests and a mild anemia. Thrombocytosis of unknown etiology is occasionally seen. Alpha-fetoprotein (AFP) is significantly elevated in 90% to 95%. This marker is also associated with other malignant lesions such as germ cell tumors, but levels are lower. Serial serum AFP measurements are used to monitor patients for tumor recurrence. Levels fall to normal after curative resection. Abdominal ultrasound demonstrates a solid, usually unilobar (right lobe most common) lesion of the liver but lacks sufficient detail to determine resectability. An abdominal CT scan using intravenous contrast is currently the imaging procedure of choice, both for diagnosis and for planning therapy. The CT scan demonstrates the tumor's proximity to major vascular and hilar structures. The typical CT appearance is a solid, solitary mass with lower attenuation levels than the surrounding liver. MRI has proven to be very useful in defining the patency of vascular structures but is not used routinely. The definitive diagnosis requires a tissue biopsy. Although this can be performed percutaneously, there are reports of "seeding" of the biopsy tract. It is preferable to perform an open biopsy of the lesion with assessment of resectability. If the lesion is not primarily resectable, then vascular access is obtained during the same anesthesia for subsequent chemotherapy. A surgical staging system for childhood hepatic malignancies is noted in Table 36.19.

Complete surgical resection is the major objective of therapy and is the only chance for cure.[119] Approximately 60% of patients have primarily resectable lesions. A lobectomy or extended lobectomy (trisegmentectomy) is usual, but segmental (nonanatomic) resection of small, isolated tumors may be possible. Careful preoperative evaluation and planning has made liver resection in children a safe procedure, with a low mortality rate (<5%) in the hands of an experienced surgeon. Adequate exposure can be obtained via an extended subcostal or bilateral subcostal incision, although large, bulky lesions may require an extension into the right hemithorax to gain adequate vascular control during the dissection. Ascitic fluid is obtained for cytology. If the lesion is deemed unresectable, the tumor is biopsied. If the lesion is

TABLE 36.19. Hepatic Tumor Staging.

Stage	*Characteristics*
Stage I	Tumor localized and completely resected
Stage II	Tumor resected with microscopic residual disease
Stage III	Unresectable tumor or gross residual disease
Stage IV	Metastatic disease

made resectable following chemotherapy, a lobectomy or trisegmentectomy is performed. Intraoperative cholangiography is helpful to verify the integrity of the remaining biliary tree. Postoperative complications include bleeding, biliary fistula, subphrenic fluid collections or abscess, and inadvertent injury to the biliary tree. Hepatic regeneration occurs quickly, and hepatic insufficiency is rare if 25% or more of the liver parenchyma remains.

Hepatic transplantation is used for unresectable disease where chemotherapy has failed to allow complete resection but no demonstrable metastases exist.[120] Long-term follow-up is required before this becomes an accepted alternative treatment.

The overall survival for all children with hepatoblastoma is approximately 50%. The best survival (90%) is seen in patients with stage I tumors who receive adjunctive chemotherapy after complete excision. Survival decreases as the surgical stage increases, although long-term survival approaches 60% to 70% in patients with unresectable disease who receive chemotherapy.

Hepatocellular Carcinoma

Hepatocellular carcinoma is less common than hepatoblastoma and typically presents in older children and adolescents (median age, 10 years). It is associated with preexisting chronic hepatitis, cirrhosis because of hepatitis B virus, and other causes of childhood cirrhosis (tyrosinemia, biliary cirrhosis, alpha-1-antitrypsin deficiency, type 1 glycogen storage disease), and cirrhosis caused by long-term parenteral nutrition. Signs and symptoms consist of an abdominal mass or diffuse swelling, abdominal pain, weight loss, anorexia, and jaundice. The serum AFP level is elevated in 50%, although the absolute levels are lower than in patients with hepatoblastoma. The diagnostic studies, staging, and treatment are similar to hepatoblastoma.[119] Only 15% and 20% of hepatocellular carcinomas are resectable because of multicentricity, bilobar involvement, portal vein invasion, and lymphatic metastases. Fibrolamellar hepatocellular carcinoma is a variant in younger patients with a high rate of resectability and a better prognosis. The overall long-term survival is poor (15%), even for resectable disease. The role of liver transplantation remains unclear.

Hemangioma

Hemangioma is the most common benign pediatric hepatic lesion.[121] These are solitary (cavernous hemangioma) or multiple (infantile hemangioendothelioma), involving the bulk of the liver. Isolated cavernous hemangiomas are not often associated with cutaneous hemangiomas, whereas infantile hemangioendotheliomas commonly have hemangiomata in other parts of the body or integument. Patients with a solitary hemangioma frequently have no symptoms or present with a mass. Infrequently there is intratumor hemorrhage or rupture resulting in abdominal pain. Infants with hemangioendothelioma commonly present with massive hepatomegaly and high-output cardiac failure from arteriovenous shunting. Approximately 40% develop the Kasabach–Merritt syndrome.

The diagnosis is made by red blood cell-labeled radionuclide or dynamic abdominal CT scanning. The CT scan demonstrates increased filling and rapid venous phase from arteriovenous shunting. Angiography is unnecessary, and percutaneous biopsy is contraindicated.

Treatment is not necessary in an asymptomatic child. Patients with congestive heart failure and/or thrombocytopenia are treated with corticosteroids, digoxin, and diuretics. Refractory patients benefit from hepatic artery embolization. External-beam radiation reduces hepatic size and controls symptoms. Their large size and diffuse involvement may preclude resection. Disease limited to one lobe can be surgically removed. Hemangioendotheliomas may undergo malignant degeneration into angiosarcoma.

Hepatic Adenoma

Hepatic adenoma is a benign lesion that accounts for less than 5% of all pediatric liver tumors.[122] The incidence is higher in adolescent females (associated with estrogen-containing oral contraceptives) and younger children with glycogen storage diseases. It presents as an asymptomatic mass; occasionally acute abdominal pain results from tumor rupture and bleeding. Abdominal CT scan demonstrates a well-circumscribed mass, usually confined to the right lobe. AFP levels and liver function tests are normal. The major management problem is the inability to differentiate adenomas from hepatocellular carcinoma. Thus, excision is recommended.

Focal Nodular Hyperplasia

Focal nodular hyperplasia is a well-circumscribed, nonencapsulated nodular liver mass. Its etiology is obscure, but there is an association with oral contraceptive use.[122] It presents as an asymptomatic hepatic mass or abdominal pain (from rupture or bleeding). Ultrasonography and CT scan demonstrate a solid mass, but one cannot differentiate it from an adenoma or malignancy without a biopsy. If the diagnosis can be made by biopsy (percutaneous or open), no further treatment is needed.

Mesenchymal Hamartoma

Mesenchymal hamartoma is an uncommon benign lesion presenting in the first year of life as an asymptomatic large solitary mass usually confined to the right lobe of the liver.[123] The CT scan demonstrates a well-defined tumor margin and minimal to no contrast enhancement. The treatment is surgical wedge resection; lobectomy is rarely required.

Teratomas

Teratomas are embryonal neoplasms derived from totipotential cells containing tissue from at least two of three germ layers (ectoderm, endoderm, mesoderm). Approximately 80% are found in females. They are typically midline or para-axial tumors[124] and are distributed in the following regions: sacrococcygeal (57%), gonadal (29%), mediastinal (7%), cervical (3%), retroperitoneal (4%), and intracranial (3%). Other sites are rare. Nongonadal teratomas present in infancy and gonadal in adolescence. Twenty-one percent are malignant.

The serum AFP level is elevated in tumors containing malignant endodermal sinus (yolk sac) elements. Serial AFP levels are a marker for recurrence. β-hCG is produced from those containing malignant choriocarcinoma tissue. Rarely, enough β-hCG is produced to cause precocious puberty.

Elevated AFP and β-hCG levels in histologically benign tumors indicate an increased risk of recurrence and malignant transformation, particularly with "immature" benign teratomas.

Sacrococcygeal Teratomas

The majority of sacrococcygeal teratomas present in the newborn period and can be detected by prenatal ultrasound. Females predominate, and a history of twins is common. Pregnancy may be complicated by high-output cardiac failure via arteriovenous shunting within the tumor, polyhydramnios, and hydrops fetalis leading to fetal demise. Fetal surgery has been utilized successfully in those with second-trimester hydrops. The tumors are classified according to location: type I, predominantly external (46%); type II, external mass and presacral component (35%); type III, visible externally, but predominantly presacral (9%); and type IV, entirely presacral, not visible externally (10%).

Treatment is excision of the tumor and coccyx[125]; type I and II lesions are resected from the perineal approach, and type III and IV lesions require a combined intraabdominal and perineal resection. The majority (97%) of newborn sacrococcygeal teratomas are benign and do not require adjuvant therapy. Follow-up requires serial AFP levels and physical examination, which include a digital rectal examination. Recurrent tumors are excised. The greatest risk factor for malignancy is age at diagnosis. The malignancy rate is approximately 50% to 60% after 2 months of age. Malignant tumors are often treated with surgery and chemotherapy. The 5-year survival for malignant germ cell tumors arising from a sacrococcygeal teratoma is approximately 50%.

Mediastinal Teratomas

Mediastinal teratomas account for approximately 20% of all pediatric mediastinal tumors.[124] They usually arise in the anterior mediastinum, although intrapericardial and cardiac lesions have been reported. Symptoms include respiratory distress, chronic cough, chest pain, and wheezing. Males with β-hCG-producing tumors may display precocious puberty. Cardiac failure may develop from compression or pericardial effusion. The chest radiograph demonstrates a calcified (35%) anterior mediastinal mass. Ultrasonography delineates cystic and solid components. General anesthesia should not be induced until a CT scan evaluation of the airway has been obtained, because the supine position coupled with a loss of airway tone from the anesthetic agent(s) may allow the anterior mass to obstruct the distal trachea, making the rapid establishment of an airway nearly impossible. If significant airway compression is present, an awake needle biopsy under local anesthesia followed by radiation therapy and/or chemotherapy is indicated. The definitive treatment is complete resection.

Cervical Teratomas

Cervical teratomas are rare neonatal neck masses which, by virtue of their large size, frequently result in respiratory distress. Calcifications may be seen on a plain radiograph and a mixed cystic/solid appearance on ultrasound. The rapid establishment of an endotracheal airway may be necessary. Tracheostomy is hazardous because of the distortion of landmarks by the large mass. Treatment is complete excision.

Pediatric Trauma

Trauma is a significant cause of morbidity and mortality among children worldwide. In the United States, trauma was identified as the leading cause of mortality among children 30 years ago. Today, this statistic remains unchanged, with approximately 15,000 to 20,000 childhood deaths occurring each year because of trauma alone.[126–128] Furthermore, more than 1.5 million childhood injuries occur each year, leading to approximately 500,000 hospitalizations.[126,128] With respect to trauma in general, more than 25% of all major injuries occur in patients under the age of 18.[126–128] Pediatric trauma is a multidisciplinary field requiring the collaboration of emergency room physicians, pediatricians, and multiple pediatric surgical specialists. However, the primary responsibility for the evaluation and care of the pediatric trauma patient falls to the pediatric general surgeon.

Evaluation and Resuscitation of the Pediatric Trauma Patient

Compared to adults, children have distinct anatomic and physiological differences that impact their response to injury and influence their evaluation and treatment. Specifically, children have a smaller mass to body surface area ratio, a less-rigid skeleton, and more-elastic connective tissue.[129] Overall, this leads to relatively vulnerable abdominal and thoracic structures because energy transmitted during trauma delivers a greater force per unit volume to less-developed protective structures. This vulnerability often leads to multisystem injuries in the pediatric patient. Examples include hepatic, splenic, and pulmonary injuries as a result of blunt trauma to the chest—the pliable ribs of the child are less protective. In addition, the higher surface area to body mass ratio of children make them more susceptible to heat loss and insensible fluid loss; this has significant implications with regard to resuscitation and may compound the physiological alterations associated with the traumatic injuries themselves.

Taking these factors into consideration, the evaluation and resuscitation of the pediatric trauma patient follows well-established guidelines detailed in the Advanced Trauma Life Support (ATLS), The Pediatric Emergency Medicine Resource, and the Pediatric Advanced Life Support courses. These guidelines are part of the standard training of the pediatric surgeon and are beyond the scope of this chapter. However, several highlights are covered.

Analogous to the care of adult trauma patients, the early evaluation of pediatric trauma patients follows the standard "ABCDE" (airway, breathing, circulation, disability, exposure) format detailed in the ATLS guidelines. With respect to airway, several critical aspects distinguish the care of the injured child.[129] In very young children, there is a significant disproportion between the cranium and midface; this results in a tendency for the neck to flex when a child is in the supine position, often obstructing the posterior pharynx. In addition, the larynx of the young child is often more anterior compared to older children and adults. Similarly, the soft tissues of the head and neck of a child may be significantly different from those of the adult. In particular, the relatively large tongue of infants may contribute to decreased visibility during laryngoscopy and may lead to frank airway obstruction. The epiglottis of children is more prominent and rigid than adults. The trachea of the child is short, and the cricoid ring represents the narrowest portion of the airway in children up to approximately 8 years of age. Overall, all these anatomic characteristics influence the airway management of the pediatric trauma patient. Specifically, traditional teaching dictates the use of uncuffed endotracheal tubes in children less than 8 years of age as the cricoid ring is thought to be a natural sealing point around the endotracheal tube. However, the use of cuffed tubes to decrease the risk of aspiration has recently gained popularity. In addition, the small anatomy of children under 11 years of age means the creation of a surgical airway, namely, emergent cricothyroidotomy, is rarely indicated because of the small target size of the cricothyroid membrane and the risk to nearby structures. Instead, needle cricothyroidotomy with jet insufflation is recommended when bag-valve and orotracheal ventilation are unsuccessful.

With regard to breathing, the normal respiratory rate of children decreases with age, with infants breathing around 60 breaths per minute and older children down to 20 breaths per minute. Proper ventilation of the pediatric trauma patient is of utmost importance because hypoventilation can lead to profound respiratory acidosis and is the most common etiology of cardiac arrest in children. To achieve adequate ventilation, appropriate tidal volumes range from 7 to 10 mL/kg.[129] The treatment of pneumothoraces may require needle thoracostomy at the second intercostal space at the midclavicular line or standard tube thoracostomy at the fifth intercostal space at the anterior axillary line.

Assessment of circulation and shock in the pediatric trauma patient may be difficult. The accepted ranges for vital signs vary significantly with age and are readily available in any pediatric text. As a rule of thumb, ATLS guidelines state that the systolic blood pressure for a child should be approximately 8 mmHg plus twice the age in years.[129] Compared to adults, children have a larger physiological reserve and often manifest the physical signs of hypovolemic shock much later. In addition, the relatively large head size of children leads to a higher incidence of head trauma, often decreasing the value of mental status changes in the assessment of shock. Finally, the lower overall blood volume of children can lead to significant physiological derangements with relatively small actual blood losses. The treatment of hypovolemic shock in the pediatric patient follows standard principles, with warmed crystalloid used as a first-line agent. Typical boluses are administered in 20-ml/kg increments. If the signs of shock do not resolve and/or significant blood loss is recognized, type-specific or O-negative blood is administered. The patient's urine output is an indicator of volume status, with normal urine output being more than 2 mL/kg/h in children less than 1 year of age and 1 to 1.5 mL/kg/h in older children and adolescents.[129] Venous access is secured peripherally. If this is unsuccessful, and emergency access is necessary, intraosseus access in the proximal tibia below the tuberosity or in the distal femur can be used for children under 6 years of age. Saphenous vein cutdowns (ankle or groin) and central venous access are also options.

As already stated, head injuries are particularly common among pediatric trauma patients, with more than 95,000 cases of pediatric traumatic brain injury in the United States each year.[130] The appropriate assessment and treatment of neurological disability is of great importance in the injured child. Historically, children with head injuries were often treated with a volume restrictive approach based on concerns that aggressive resuscitation may lead to increased intracranial pressures and worsen neurological injury. Today, these approaches are generally considered to be incorrect, as hypotension has been shown to be profoundly detrimental to the head-injured child. Specifically, it has been shown that pediatric trauma patients with a presenting Glasgow Coma Score (GCS) of 6 to 8 have a significantly higher mortality rate if they are also hypotensive.[130] Therefore, aggressive resuscitation and treatment of hypotension are vital to the care of the head-injured child.

The assessment of neurological injury is based on physical examination. CT scan of the head is often useful in patients suspected of intracranial injury because elevated intracranial pressure (ICP) may occur in children without any significant signs or symptoms. Patients with changes in mental status or affect may be at high risk for intracranial injury. Intubation is indicated in patients with a GCS of 8 or less or a GCS motor score of 2 or less. Antiepileptics (phenobarbitol, phenytoin, diazepam) may be administered to the brain-injured patient. Efforts to decrease ICP using diuretics (lasix, mannitol) may be performed but should be used with caution as they may exacerbate hypotension.

Finally, exposure including a complete examination of the patient's front and back is important. This examination also includes the identification of any injurious environmental factors to which the child may have been exposed. Last, it is important to maintain an adequate thermal environment using heating devices or blankets throughout the trauma survey.

Pediatric Closed Head Injury

Head injury accounts for nearly 7000 childhood deaths in the United States each year.[130] Common injuries in children include concussions, diffuse axonal injury, contusions, epidural hematomas, subdural hematomas, and skull fractures.

Concussions

A concussion may be defined as the mild end of a group of injuries resulting from angular acceleration-deceleration forces that result in a transient loss of consciousness, followed by a return of normal mental function. In children, concussions may occur after falls, collisions, or impacts with moving objects, and may present with a variety of symptoms including headaches, blurry vision, irritability, and decreased attention. No absolute guidelines exist for the workup and treatment of children suspected to have a concussion. In general, CT scan of the head is indicated in children with persistent symptoms. If this does not reveal any other injury but the patient's symptoms persist, admission and observation may be warranted. Children whose symptoms resolve and return to a baseline level of mental function can often be discharged with instructions to the parents to seek medical attention if symptoms return.

Diffuse Axonal Injury

Diffuse axonal injury (DAI) occurs when shear strains applied to the brain cause axonal tears in a characteristic distribution. This injury commonly caused by severe angular or rotational acceleration-deceleration forces. CT scan or MRI may display characteristic small hemorrhages within the brain. Typically, DAI is characterized by an immediate loss of consciousness associated with decerebrate or decorticate posturing. Hypertension, hyperhydrosis, and hyperthermia may also be seen. Similar to other closed head injuries, DAI is often managed nonsurgically with supportive care and management of intracranial pressures.

Cerebral Contusion

Cerebral contusions are observed in up to 30% of patients with severe head injury.[130] They may be focal or diffuse and may occur with or without direct contact to the head. Contusions can occur underlying a point of external injury (coup contusions) such as under a skull fracture or may occur at a location remote from a point of contact (countercoup contusions) because of forces between the brain and the skull. Cerebral contusions may exhibit significant swelling of the injured tissue as well as adjacent tissues because of toxic metabolite release from the injured brain. This swelling typically peaks at 4 to 6 days postinjury. Medical management of cerebral contusions involves supportive care and management of intracranial pressure. Progressive mass effect may require surgical decompression.

Epidural Hematoma and Subdural Hematoma

Epidural hematomas (EDH) and subdural hematomas (SDH) in children under 3 years of age are caused by falls, motor vehicle accidents, bicycle accidents, and child abuse. As children reach adolescence, the incidence of head trauma from motor vehicle accidents and bicycle accidents increases while the incidence from falls decreases. In addition, assault becomes a more common cause of these injuries in the adolescent population.

Epidural hematomas are usually caused by a tear in the middle meningeal artery. Once considered neurosurgical emergencies, EDHs have recently been managed nonsurgically in neurologically intact patients. In children, EDHs may show spontaneous regression and resorption in 4 to 6 weeks. Craniotomy and evacuation of the hematoma is indicated in patients with focal neurological deficits, increasing lethargy, and signs of brainstem compression.

Similarly, small subdural hematomas in children with few to no neurological symptoms may be managed conservatively. Craniotomy and evacuation of the hematoma are indicated in patients with large SDHs who display neurological deficit. Compared to EDHs, SDHs are more commonly associated with underlying parenchymal injury to the brain.

Skull Fractures

Skull fractures are noted in 8% to 41% of head-injured children. Linear skull fractures account for 75%[130]; these are not often associated with underlying brain injury and commonly heal within 1 to 2 months. Depressed skull fractures occur in 7% to 10% and often require surgery; these are commonly caused by falls, motor vehicle and bicycle accidents, and birth injury. Operative intervention is indicated for grossly contaminated fractures, underlying symptomatic hematomas, intracerebral bone fragments, cerebrospinal fluid (CSF) leak, and associated neurological deficits.

Management of Severe Pediatric Traumatic Brain Injury

In a recent issue of seminars in pediatric surgery, guidelines for the management of severe traumatic brain injury in children were reviewed.[130] Highlights include the following:

- *Airway management and resuscitation*
  - Airway control should be obtained in children with a GCS of 8 or less.
  - Hypoxia and hypotension must be identified and treated immediately.
- *ICP monitoring and management*
  - ICP monitors recommended in infants and children with a GCS of 8 or less.
  - ICP monitoring may be indicated in children in whom sedation, neuromuscular blockade, or anesthesia do not allow for serial neurological examination.
  - Treatment should be considered for ICP above 20 to 25 mmHg.
  - Cerebral perfusion pressure (CPP) should be maintained above 40 mmHg.
  - Options for ICP management include drainage, neuromuscular blockade, sedation, administration of hypertonic saline, mannitol with serum osmolality maintained at less than 320 mOsm/L, and barbiturate-induced coma.
  - Chronic hyperventilation should be avoided because of hypocapnia-induced vasoconstriction and compromise of cerebral blood flow.
- *Anticonvulsant prophylaxis*
  - The use of prophylactic anticonvulsants to prevent posttraumatic seizures has not been well studied.
  - The use of prophylactic anticonvulsants to prevent early (within 7 days of injury) posttraumatic seizures may be considered.
  - The use of prophylactic anticonvulsants to prevent late (after 7 days of injury) posttraumatic seizures is not recommended.

Thoracic Injury in Children

Thoracic injuries represent a major source of morbidity and mortality among children, occurring in 4% to 6% of children hospitalized for trauma and accounting for 25% of pediatric trauma deaths.[131] Penetrating thoracic trauma in children and adolescents is often severe and is most commonly caused by gunshot wounds, although knife wounds and impalement injuries occur.[132] Chest radiographs and CT scans (in stable patients) are useful in determining the trajectory of injury and in identifying possible organ damage. Hemothorax and pneumothorax are the most common injury patterns seen. After airway management, needle decompression and/or tube thoracostomy is usually indicated. Thoracotomy is indicated in patients with immediate chest tube output of 20% of their estimated blood volume or 2 mL/kg/h or more of persistent output. The indications for ER thoracotomy (ERT) in children are unclear. ERT may be useful in children with suspected cardiac tamponade from penetrating trauma. Such tamponade should be treated with a vertical incision above and parallel to the phrenic nerve. Myocardial lacerations may be repaired primarily using polypropylene suture.

Blunt thoracic injury accounts for 80% to 85% of all pediatric thoracic injuries.[131] These injuries commonly occur as a result of motor vehicle accidents, pedestrian accidents, and falls. In children, pulmonary contusions, rib fractures, and pneumothoraces are the most common chest injuries. Injuries to the heart, great vessels, tracheobronchial tree, diaphragm, and esophagus are rare. Overall, less than 10% of pediatric blunt chest injuries require surgical intervention. However, the presence of thoracic injuries in children with multiple injuries is associated with a 20-fold increase in mortality compared to children without chest trauma.

Management of blunt thoracic trauma in children requires an understanding of the anatomic and physiological differences between children and adults.[131] Compared to an adult, a child's chest wall is extremely compliant because of incomplete ossification of the ribs and a greater overall collagen content. This compliance means that significant amounts of energy may be transferred to the chest wall and intrathoracic contents without a resultant fracture. In fact, rib fractures occur in only half of children with pulmonary contusions. Similarly, the mediastinum of young children is very mobile compared to that of adults. This can lead to significant mediastinal shift with injuries such as hemothorax, pneumothorax, or diaphragmatic rupture. Eventually, this may result in decreased venous return to the heart and impaired cardiac output because of displacement of the heart and great vessels. From a metabolic standpoint, children consume more oxygen per kilogram of body weight compared to adults. This factor, combined with a relatively decreased pulmonary functional residual capacity, makes children particularly sensitive to the development of hypoxemia with chest injury.

Evaluation of a child with a blunt chest injury follows standard ATLS principles. A high index of suspicion is critical for the early detection and management of blunt thoracic trauma as injuries are often not apparent on initial examination. Signs and symptoms associated with thoracic injuries include chest wall crepitus, subcutaneous emphysema, diminished breath sounds, and varying degrees of respiratory compromise evidenced by nasal flaring, retractions, tachypnea, dyspnea, and low oxygen saturation by transcutaneous pulse oximetry. Standard anteroposterior chest radiographs are a valuable tool in the evaluation of possible thoracic trauma and have been found to be abnormal in 60% to 90% of children with significant injuries.[131] If a widened or abnormal mediastinum is demonstrated on chest radiograph, helical CT scan of the chest is warranted to rule out aortic injury. In addition, the chest CT scan is useful in identifying injuries not appreciated on plain films such as pulmonary contusion or rib fractures. Recent data suggest that the chest CT scan may identify additional thoracic injuries in up to 15% of patients with a normal chest X-ray.[131]

The management of thoracic trauma varies depending on the pattern of injury and organs affected. A complete discussion of thoracic trauma is beyond the scope of this chapter. However, the common blunt thoracic injuries are highlighted.

Rib Fractures and Chest Wall Injuries

Because of the compliance of their chest walls, rib fractures are relatively rare (1%–2%) in children. When present, they are often an indicator of significant trauma and have been associated with a trauma mortality of 43% to 50%.[131] Moreover, first rib fractures are uncommon and may be associated with significant vascular injuries. In patients under 3 years old, rib fractures are often because of child abuse, with a positive predictive value of 95% to 100% in patients for whom motor vehicle collisions or predisposing medical conditions can be ruled out.[131] Management of rib fractures is nonsurgical, consisting of pulmonary toilet and pain management.

Pulmonary Contusions

Pulmonary contusions result in alveolar disruption, hemorrhage, and interstitial edema. The presentation of pulmonary contusions varies from radiographic abnormality alone to severe respiratory distress requiring mechanical ventilation. The process of inflammation and swelling associated with such injury often peaks at 24 to 48 h, with radiographic changes often becoming apparent 4 to 6 hours postinjury. Thus, significant pulmonary contusions cannot be ruled out by a normal chest radiograph, although such studies are abnormal in 67% to 90% of children with the injury.[131] Helical chest CT scan can be helpful in diagnosing and characterizing pulmonary contusions. Clinically, pulmonary contusions can lead to significant ventilation/perfusion mismatches, intrapulmonary shunting, atelectasis, and consolidation. Serious complications of these injuries include pneumonia (20%), acute respiratory distress syndrome (5%–20%), and death (15%–20%).[131] Management is usually supportive, consisting of pulmonary toilet, pain control, judicious fluid management to minimize alveolar edema, and sometimes assisted venitilation. Approximately 20% to 37% of children with pulmonary contusions require mechanical ventilation.[131] With appropriate treatment, most pulmonary contusions resolve within 7 to 10 days.

Pneumothorax and Hemothorax

As stated previously, the relatively mobile mediastinum of children makes them particularly sensitive to hemodynamic compromise as a result of pneumothorax. As in adults, pneumothoraces are most commonly treated with tube thoracostomy. Hemothorax is noted in 13% to 29% of children suffering from blunt chest trauma.[131] Bleeding is most commonly from a pulmonary parenchymal laceration or a lacerated intercostal vessel. Tube thoracostomy is indicated in these cases to provide prompt evacuation of the intrapleural blood. Retained blood in the pleural space may lead to empyema or fibrothorax and should be evacuated within 1 week of injury.

Tracheobronchial Injuries

Tracheobronchial injuries in children are rare (0.7%–2.8%).[131] The most common mechanisms for these injuries include motor vehicle accidents, pedestrian accidents, falls, and crush injuries. These injuries are generally severe, with an approximately 30% mortality, half of which occurs within the first hour after injury. Anatomically, tracheobronchial ruptures usually occur within 2.5 cm of the carina because of anterior–posterior compressive forces. Tracheobronchial injuries may present with pneumothorax, hemothorax, hemoptysis, or subcutaneous emphysema. Patients may initially display minimal symptoms or may be in acute respiratory distress. Chest radiograph and CT scan rarely demonstrate a clear disruption of the tracheobronchial tree, although pneumothorax or hemothorax may be easily visualized. A high index of suspicion is the key to prompt diagnosis, with suggestive clinical signs including failure of a pneumothorax to resolve with tube thoracostomy, persistent air leak, and persistent pneumomediastinum. Bronchoscopy is useful in diagnosing and determining the location of the injury so that an endotracheal tube may be passed beyond it for ventilation. Treatment of tracheobronchial injuries is based on the size of the injury and the respiratory stability of the patient. Injuries encompassing less than one-third the diameter of the bronchus in clinically stable patients may be managed nonsurgically. Larger injuries, or injuries in those clinically unstable (e.g., unable to adequately ventilate, increasing pneumothorax despite thoracostomy) may require operative intervention ranging from primary repair to pulmonary resection depending on the extent of the injury and potential concomitant injuries. Complications include pulmonary infections, bronchial stenosis, and bronchopleural fistulae.

Aortic Injury

Blunt aortic injury (BAI) is rare (1%) in children. Compared to adults, thoracic aortic injuries were found in only 2% to 5% of children dying of blunt trauma on autopsy versus 15% to 17%.[131] These injuries are most commonly a result of motor vehicle accidents (usually improper use of restraint belts), pedestrian accidents, and falls. The majority die at the scene of the accident or during transport. However, children who remain alive until diagnosis have a survival of 67% to 91%.[131] Injuries commonly occur at the aortic isthmus distal to the left subclavian artery (at the level of the ligamentum arteriosum). Chest radiograph findings that indicate the potential for BAI include a widened mediastinum, first rib fracture, and loss of the normal aortic contour. Aortic arch angiography is still the gold standard for the diagnosis of BAI, although helical CT scan with CT angiogram has become increasingly utilized. In addition, transthoracic echocardiography and intravascular ultrasound have been advocated as diagnostic adjuncts in patients in whom angiography is equivocal. At this time, operative repair of BAI remains the standard of care.

Tight preoperative blood pressure control is important for decreasing the risk of injury extension or aortic rupture. Postoperative paraplegia is a complication of thoracic aortic repair; it can occur in 5% to 17% of patients and is associated with aortic cross-clamp times greater than 30 min.[131] In children, primary repair is preferable to interposition graft, when possible, because of the possibility of aortic pseudocoarctation as a result of postoperative growth. If an interposition graft is necessary, the largest graft size possible should be used. In patients in whom concomitant injuries preclude operative aortic repair, delayed aortic repair or expectant management may be considered. In these cases, aggressive blood pressure control and serial imaging to monitor for changes in aortic hematoma are keys to successful management. Last, endovascular stent grafts to repair thoracic aortic injuries in adults and children have been used, although experience is extremely limited.

Cardiac Contusions

Blunt cardiac injury (BCI) in children ranges from 0.3% to 4.6%.[131] By far the most common blunt injuries to the heart are cardiac contusions, accounting for 95% of all BCIs. Cardiac rupture accounts for the other 5% of injuries, with an extremely low survival rate. The clinical presentation of cardiac contusion is variable, ranging from isolated electrocardiographic (ECG) changes to dysrhythmias and hypotension. The diagnosis can be difficult. ECG, cardiac enzymes, and echocardiography have been advocated as diagnostic methods. The management of cardiac contusion is supportive. Patients should be monitored (cardiac monitoring) until hemodynamic stability and cardiac rhythm abnormalities have been resolved. Dysrhythmias are treated pharmacologically. Most children do well with minimal long-term sequelae from the injury.

Commotio cordis is a rare condition most commonly seen in 12- to 13-year-old children in whom sudden death occurs after blunt impact to the chest wall without evidence of significant injury. The injury commonly occurs during sports and is thought to be caused by ventricular fibrillation triggered by blunt impact to the chest during cardiac repolarization. The overall mortality rate for commotio cordis is approximately 16%. The treatment is prompt cardiac defibrillation and supportive care.

Abdominal Injuries in Children

Penetrating abdominal injuries in children are most commonly the result of gunshot wounds and stab wounds, although impalement injuries do occur.[132] In general, these injuries require surgical intervention. The initial evaluation and treatment follow standard ATLS guidelines. Diagnostic tools include chest and abdominal radiographs to determine bullet trajectory and to identify retained foreign bodies. Concomitant chest injury should also be ruled in or out. CT scan and laparoscopy have been advocated in cases where it is unclear if the peritoneal cavity has been violated. The management of penetrating abdominal trauma depends on the particular organs injured. Solid organ injuries (e.g., liver, spleen) can typically be treated with packing and local hemostatic maneuvers, although resection may be required for severe injuries. In the pediatric population, the risk of postsplenectomy sepsis favors splenic salvage when possible. Similarly, the management of penetrating trauma to the GI tract is based on the location and extent of injury. Isolated injuries with minimal blast effect may be managed with debridement and primary repair, taking care to ensure normal bowel caliber. Larger injuries or multiple nearby injuries may require resection and reconstruction. Based on the adult literature, most colonic injuries are managed with primary repair or resection with primary reconstruction. A colostomy is created in unstable patients or in patients with complex injuries. However, data regarding these approaches are sparse in the pediatric population.

Blunt abdominal trauma often is most commonly caused by motor vehicle accidents and falls. Overall, approximately 8% of all children suffering from blunt trauma sustain trauma to the abdomen.[133] Most commonly, the solid organs (liver, spleen, kidney) are affected. Initial evaluation follows ATLS guidelines. The abdominal CT scan is the most commonly employed imaging study for the evaluation of pediatric blunt abdominal trauma. Such CT scans are performed with intravenous contrast. The use of oral contrast, although useful in diagnosing duodenal injuries, carries the risk of aspiration in the child with a head injury. Focused abdominal sonography (FAST) examination in the emergency department has gained wide acceptance for the evaluation of adult trauma patients. However, its use in children by pediatric trauma surgeons has been limited; this may be secondary to high rates of solid organ injury without hemoperitoneum (up to 40%). At this time, its role appears to be as a replacement for diagnostic peritoneal lavage in multiply injured patients too unstable to undergo CT scanning.

The management of blunt abdominal trauma in children is based on the clinical stability of the patient. Physiological signs of ongoing hemorrhage such as refractory hemodynamic instability or progressive transfusion requirements require prompt operative exploration. In the adult population, radiographic predictors for the need for surgery versus nonoperative management such as the presence of a "contrast blush," the radiographic "injury grade," or the location and quantity of free peritoneal fluid have been studied. However, the utility of these findings to guide operative versus nonoperative management in the hemodynamically stable pediatric trauma patient is unclear.

Splenic Injury

Over the past few decades, the nonoperative management of blunt solid organ injuries in children has gained widespread acceptance. Of the solid abdominal organs, the spleen is the most frequently injured. Although numerous variations exist for the specific management of these injuries, a nonoperative approach is successful in more than 90% of patients with grade I to grade IV injuries.[133] Up to 40% of children with grade V injuries can be managed nonoperatively. The nonoperative approach decrease, morbidity, transfusion requirements, and long-term infectious complications. The specifics of management such as length of hospital stay, length of outpatient convalescence, and frequency of follow-up imaging are variable. For patients with low-grade injuries, there is a recent trend toward decreased hospital days (often only 3 days) and the use of nonmonitored, general ward beds instead of an intensive care setting. For the minority of patients who fail nonoperative management, splenectomy is the primary surgical treatment, although an attempt is made to repair the spleen, if possible. In addition, the use of endovascular embolization to control bleeding has been reported. Patients who require splenectomy need vaccination against the encapsulated organisms *Streptococcus pneumonia*, *Haemophilus influenzae* type b, and *Nisseria meningitides*.

Liver Injury

Injuries to the liver are the most frequent cause of death in children sustaining blunt abdominal trauma. Similar to splenic injuries, the majority of blunt hepatic injuries are managed nonoperatively, and the decision to operate is predicated on the patient's hemodynamic status. Radiographic injury scoring systems do correlate with outcome in children. For patients who require operative intervention, packing and damage control/hemostatic techniques are employed. Complications of nonoperative management include persistent bile leak, biloma formation, and hemobilia.

Renal Injury

Children are particularly vulnerable to blunt renal trauma because of the relatively large size of the kidney and relatively less protective Gerota's fascia compared to adults. Nonoperative management of renal injuries has a high success rate in the pediatric population. In fact, renal salvage rates of nearly 90% have been reported in large series of children with blunt renal injuries treated nonoperatively.[133] Similar series in adults have reported operative rates of approximately 85% across all injury grades. Furthermore, favorable results with nonoperative management have been reported in children with severe injuries including injuries associated with collecting system disruption, renovascular injury, and urinary extravasation. Delayed complications such as impaired renal function, urinomas, and renovascular hypertension are rare. When persistent, these complications may require nephrectomy.

Pancreas Injury

Blunt pancreatic injury occurs in 3% to 12% of children sustaining blunt abdominal trauma and is the most common cause of pancreatitis in children.[133] Common mechanisms of injury include child abuse and bicycle handlebar injuries. The diagnosis of pancreatic injury is often difficult, as initial serum enzyme evaluation and abdominal CT scanning may underestimate the extent of injury. In addition, elevated pancreatic enzyme levels poorly correlate with injury severity. Pancreatic injury is often managed nonoperatively. Nonoperative management includes bowel rest (with or without nasogastric decompression) and parenteral nutrition. Healing of the injury is documented with an imaging study (ultrasound or CT scan). Pancreatic pseudocyst formation is a complication that occurs in up to 10% of patients treated nonoperatively. These pseudocysts may be treated by percutaneous drainage, distal pancreatectomy, or an enteric drainage procedure.

Hollow Viscus Injury

Intestinal injury has been reported to occur in 1% to 15% of children suffering from blunt trauma.[134] Approximately 14% of all intraabdominal injuries in children are hollow organ injuries. These injuries are associated with a mortality rate of 15%. This relatively high mortality rate is likely caused by the high frequency of associated nonintestinal injuries, namely, traumatic brain injuries.

The most common mechanism of blunt hollow viscus injury in children is motor vehicle accidents, followed by bicycle accidents and abuse. In a review of a 12-year experience at one pediatric trauma center, Canty et al.[135] reported 79 blunt injuries to the GI tract; 19% were from seatbelts, 13% from bicycle handlebars, and 19% from abuse. Intestinal injury rates are increasing as a consequence of mandatory use of vehicle restraints. When improperly positioned on a child, a lap belt transmits energy to the abdomen instead of the bony pelvis. During rapid deceleration, the lap belt compresses the intraabdominal organs against the spine, resulting in bowel and/or mesenteric injuries. Lumbar spine fractures (Chance fracture) are common during deceleration/flexion injuries. The most common site of blunt hollow viscus injury is the small intestine. It often occurs near fixation points, such as the ligament of Treitz or the ileocecal valve.[134] In their reviews of large series at pediatric trauma centers, Canty et al.[135] and Galifer et al.[136] found the jejunum or ileum to be the most common site of damage, followed by the duodenum, colon, and finally, stomach.

The diagnosis of hollow viscus injury caused by blunt trauma in children is often difficult. Delays in diagnosis are common, necessitating a high index of suspicion to facilitate early diagnosis and treatment. Overall, the diagnosis of these injuries is clinical, based on a conglomeration of factors (physical examination, imaging, observation). Physical examination may or may not demonstrate peritoneal signs even in the presence of an intestinal leak. In children with blunt intestinal perforation, fewer than 50% were noted to have peritoneal signs on examination.[134] In children involved in motor vehicle accidents, abdominal wall ecchymosis (seat belt sign) may be associated with a high incidence of significant injury to the intestine and/or lumbar spine.

In addition to physical examination, vital sign abnormalities (temperature, heart rate, urine output, etc.) and adjunctive laboratory studies (complete blood count) may also be useful in evaluating the child with potential blunt intestinal trauma, although normal values do not preclude significant injury. Similarly, imaging studies are used in the evaluation of potential blunt intestinal trauma. Abdominal CT scan imaging is the preferred study, permitting accurate evaluation of the solid abdominal organs as well as the GI tract. The utility of oral contrast is still debated. Current evidence suggests that oral contrast does not increase the diagnostic accuracy of CT imaging and may only serve to delay the time required to complete the scan. CT findings suggestive of intestinal injuries have been described and include bowel wall thickening and enhancement, mesenteric stranding, and free fluid without associated solid visceral injury. Although these findings may increase the suspicion of injury, their presence alone is not an indication for laparotomy.

Because of the limitations of noninvasive imaging, peritoneal lavage has been advocated as a means of early diagnosis. However, this procedure is invasive and is associated with a significant nontherapeutic laparotomy rate (20%–40%).[134] Laparoscopy has been used as a tool for the evaluation of potential blunt intestinal injuries in patients with an abnormal physical examination and CT findings. The absence of all the aforementioned findings does not preclude significant GI tract injury. Therefore, all children with suspected blunt intestinal injuries should be observed for the development of physical findings (e.g., peritonitis).

During the operation for blunt intestinal injury, hemorrhage is controlled as concomitant solid organ injury is common. The site of intestinal injury is repaired, debrided, or resected. Blunt injury to the small intestine in children requires inspection of the entire bowel and mesentery. The type of repair is dictated by the extent of injury. Injuries involving less than 50% of the bowel circumference are debrided and repaired primarily in a transverse fashion. Perforations involving greater than 50% of the bowel circumference require resection and primary anastomosis. Gastric wounds can often be debrided and repaired primarily.

A duodenal injury is most commonly a hematoma. In the absence of perforation, it is managed nonoperatively. Nonoperative management consists of supportive care, including nasogastric decompression and total parenteral nutrition, as the hematoma often causes partial or complete obstruction. Resolution of this obstruction often occurs within 10 days. Duodenal perforation requires repair and/or exclusion.

The management of colonic injuries has been extensively studied in the adult literature. In the adult population, primary repair appears to be preferable to colostomy and is associated with fewer complications. This approach is likely applicable in the pediatric population but has not been extensively studied.

Maternal-Fetal Surgery

Advanced fetal diagnostic techniques (e.g., chorionic villous sampling, amniocentesis) and serial imaging (e.g., ultrasound, magnetic resonance imaging) have led to an increased understanding of the natural history and outcome of many genetic and congenital anomalies. However, before the 1980s, obstetricians and perinatologists could only observe helplessly as these disease processes took their toll, counseling parents on potentially grim prognoses. When such a fetus survived to birth, pediatricians were then left to care for an infant with devastating medical problems that were untreatable or only partly treatable at this later stage of development. This dilemma fostered basic science and clinical research aimed at understanding and treating congenital diseases during the fetal period. From this research, the field of fetal therapy, and more specifically, maternal-fetal surgery emerged.

Although the majority of fetuses with anomalies amenable to surgery are best served by planned delivery and care after birth, there are highly select fetuses in whom an untreated anomaly will result in death in utero or shortly after birth. Prenatal intervention has, in large part, been predicated on those anomalies that result in either low- or high-output cardiac failure resulting in hydrops, defined as skin and/or nuchal edema or fluid accumulation in two of three body cavities (pleura, pericardium, peritoneum). As the understanding of fetal disease improves, an increasing number of fetal anomalies, including nonlethal anomalies, are being considered amenable to fetal intervention. Currently, anomalies such as cystic adenomatoid malformation, sacrococcygeal teratoma, twin–twin transfusion syndrome, and twin reversed arterial perfusion (TRAP) sequence, obstructive uropathy, select heart anomalies, and congenital diaphragmatic hernia may be treated during the prenatal period. Table 36.20 lists the congenital anomalies that have been treated prenatally.

Compared to other fields of surgery, maternal-fetal surgery is unique in that the risks and benefits of a potential intervention have to be considered for two patients, the mother and the fetus. The prerequisites for consideration of intervention include the absence of severe associated anomalies; a normal karyotype; and the presence of a correctable lesion that if uncorrected will lead to fetal death or irreversible organ dysfunction before birth. Although the risk–benefit ratio may be clear for the fetus, the situation is less clear for the mother. Without antenatal treatment, the risks to the mother are little more than that of the pregnancy alone. With fetal intervention, the risks of preoperative evaluation including

TABLE 36.20. Applications of Fetal Surgery.

Defect	*Effect on development*		*Open hysterotomy procedure*	*Fetoscopic procedure*
Lethal anomalies:				
Placental vascular anomalies				
Twin-twin transfusion syndrome (TTTS)	Vascular steal through placenta	→ Fetal hydrops/demise Surviving twin with severe morbidity	Fetectomy	Photocoagulation of chorangiopagus
Twin reversed arterial perfusion syndrome (TRAP)	Normal cotwin heart pumps for both twins	→ High output cardiac failure, hydrops	Fetectomy	Selective reduction via umbilical cord ligation or radiofrequency needle
Obstructive uropathy	Hydronephrosis Lung hypoplasia	→ Renal failure Pulmonary failure	Vesicostomy	Vesicoamniotic shunt Valve ablation
Congenital diaphragmatic hernia	Lung hypoplasia	→ Pulmonary failure	Complete repair Temporary tracheal occlusion	Temporary tracheal occlusion (PLUG)
Cystic adenomatoid malformation/ sequestration	Lung hypoplasia or hydrops	→ Respirator insufficiency Fetal hydrops/demise	Pulmonary lobectomy	Radiofrequency ablation
Sacrococcygeal teratoma	High-output heart failure	→ Fetal hydrops/demise	Debulk Complete resection	Laser vascular occlusion Radiofrequency ablation
Complete heart block	Low-output failure	→ Fetal hydrops/demise	Pacemaker	Pacemaker
Pulmonary/aortic stenosis	Ventricular hypertrophy	→ Heart failure Single ventricle physiology	Valvuloplasty	Catheter valvuloplasty
Pericardial teratoma	Heart failure	→ Fetal hydrops/demise	Resection	—
Ebstein's anomaly	Heart failure Pulmonary hypoplasia	→ Fetal hydrops/demise Pulmonary failure	Valve repair and atrial reduction	—
Congenital high airway obstruction syndrome	Overdistension by lung fluid	→ Fetal hydrops/demise	Tracheostomy EXIT strategy	Tracheostomy
Obstructive hydrocephalus	Hydrocephalus	→ Brain damage	Ventriculoamniotic shunt Ventriculoperitoneal shunt	Ventriculoamniotic shunt
Nonlethal abnormalities:				
Myleomeningocele	Chiari formation Exposed spinal cord Hydrocephalus	→ Paralysis Neurogenic bladder/ bowel Orthopedic anomalies	Repair	Repair
Tension hydrothorax	Lung hypoplasia	→ Respiratory failure	—	Serial thoracocenteses Thoracoamniotic shunt
Cleft lip/palate	Facial defect	→ Persistent deformity	Repair	Repair
Previable premature rupture of membranes	Preterm labor	→ Fetal demise Fetal/maternal infection	—	Amniopatch Amniograft
Gastroschisis	Bowel exteriorization	→ Bowel preivisceritis Prolonged ileus	—	Amnioexchange
Amniotic bands	Limb/digit/umbilical cord constriction	→ Limb/digit deformity or amputation Fetal demise (cord occlusion)	—	Laser separation of bands

amniocentesis, chorionic villous sampling, and percutaneous umbilical blood sampling, as well as the risks of an operation, must be considered. In addition, maternal comorbidities and psychosocial support structure must be taken into account. Although there have been no reported maternal deaths during or after fetal surgery, complications such as bleeding, wound infection, preterm labor, deep venous thrombosis, and pulmonary embolus have occurred.

At this time, several techniques have been utilized to perform fetal surgery. Overall, these techniques involve a method of accessing the fetus and represent an evolution of surgical technique toward a less invasive approach. The open hysterotomy technique involves a low transverse skin incision or vertical midline incision followed by a stapler-made hysterotomy. The ex utero intrapartum treatment (EXIT) procedure is another strategy that is used principally for late-

TABLE 36.21.
Prospective Randomized Clinical Trials in Fetal Surgery for Severe Congenital Diaphragmatic Hernia.

Trial	*Experimental group*	*Control group*	*Survival rates*
Harrison et al. 1997[37]	4: Fetal open hysterotomy repair	7: Postnatal supportive therapy and repair	Experimental: 75% Control: 86%
Harrison et al. 2003[38]	11: Fetoscopic balloon tracheal occlusion	13: Postnatal supportive therapy and repair	Experimental: 77% Control: 73%

gestation fetuses with potential airway obstruction from a neck mass such as a teratoma or lymphangioma. It is similar to a cesarean delivery, except myometrial bleeding is controlled and the umbilical cord is not cut until an airway is obtained, either by orotracheal intubation, tracheostomy, or mass resection followed by intubation or tracheostomy. Once a definitive airway is obtained, the umbilical cord is cut and the patient is from placental support to mechanical support. Fetoscopy and endoscopic instrumentation are used for select procedures (e.g., laser coagulation for twin–twin transfusion syndrome). During the procedure, the turbid amniotic fluid is replaced with lactated Ringer's solution to enable videoscopic visualization. Two or three trocars are used.

Although the clinical experience with fetal surgery is growing, it is still relatively limited because most anomalies amenable to fetal surgery are relatively rare, even at the busiest centers. Because of this, published clinical data regarding fetal surgery have primarily consisted of case series demonstrating the safety and feasibility of fetal surgical operations. To date, only two randomized prospective clinical trials have been completed investigating the efficacy of fetal surgical treatment of CDH. Published in 1997 by Harrison et al.,[37] the first trial compared fetal repair of a CDH via an open hysterotomy approach to standard postnatal care and surgery. The second trial, published in 2003,[38] compared fetoscopic balloon tracheal occlusion to induce lung growth for fetuses with severe CDH to postnatal care. In both trials, no statistically significant difference was found between the two treatment groups. Table 36.21 summarizes the results of these trials. In addition to these trials, ongoing prospective randomized trials exist for fetal surgical treatment of myelomeningocele and twin–twin transfusion syndrome. Overall, the clinical evidence regarding the efficacy of fetal surgery compared to conventional treatments is still sparse, and more data are needed. However, as scientific knowledge of fetal anomalies as well as clinical experience with fetal surgical techniques improves, the prenatal treatment of congenital diseases may become an increasingly utilized treatment option.

References

1. Grosfeld JL. Pediatric surgery. In: Sabiston DC, Lyerly HK, eds. Textbook of Surgery: The Biological Basis of Modern Surgical Practice, 15th ed. Philadelphia: Saunders, 1997:1234–1274.
2. Forster J. The Surgical Diseases of Children. London: John W. Parker & Son, 1860.
3. Guersant P. Notices sur la Chirurgie des Infants. Paris: Asselin: 1864.
4. Kelley S. Surgical Diseases of Children: A Modern Treatise on Pediatric Surgery. New York: E.B. Treat, 1909.
5. Grosfeld J. Pediatric Surgery. In: Sabiston DJ, ed. Textbook of Surgery: The Biological Basis of Modern Surgical Practice. Philadelphia: Saunders, 1997.
6. Rowe MI. The newborn as a surgical patient. In: O'Neill J, Rowe M, Grosfeld J, Fonkalsrud E, Coran A, eds. Pediatric Surgery, 5th ed. St. Louis: Mosby Year-Book, 1998:43–58.
7. Albanese CT, Nour BM, Rowe MI. Anesthesia blocks nonshivering thermogenesis in the neonatal rabbit. J Pediatr Surg 1994;29(8):983–986.
8. Sauer PJ, Dane HJ, Visser HK. New standards for neutral thermal environment of healthy very low birthweight infants in week one of life. Arch Dis Child 1984;59(1):18–22.
9. Lockhart C. Maintenance of general anesthesia. In: Gregory G, ed. Pediatric Anesthesia, 2nd ed. New York: Churchill Livingstone, 1989:575–576.
10. Ford H, Rowe M. Sepsis and related considerations. In: O'Neill J Jr, Rowe M, Grosfeld J, Fonkalsrud E, Coran A, eds. Pediatric Surgery, 5th ed. St. Louis: Mosby Year-Book, 1998:135–155.
11. Bell EF, Oh W. Fluid and electrolyte balance in very low birth weight infants. Clin Perinatol 1979;6(1):139–150.
12. Rowe P. The Harriet Lane Handbook, 11th ed. Chicago: Year Book Medical, 1987.
13. Chwals WJ, Letton RW, Jamie A, Charles B. Stratification of injury severity using energy expenditure response in surgical infants. J Pediatr Surg 1995;30(8):1161–1164.
14. Taylor L, O'Neill JA Jr. Total parenteral nutrition in the pediatric patient. Surg Clin N Am 1991;71(3):477–491.
15. Landsman I, Cook D. Pediatric anesthesia. In: O'Neill J Jr, Rowe MG, Grosfeld JL, Fonkalsrud E, Coran A, eds. Pediatric Surgery, 5th ed. St. Louis: Mosby Year-Book, 1998:197–228.
16. Gray S, Skandalakis J. The pharynx and its derivatives. In: Embryology for Surgeons: The Embryological Basis for the Treatment of Congenital Defects. Baltimore: Williams & Wilkins, 1994:17–64.
17. Tran Ngoc N, Tran Xuan N. Cystic hygroma in children: a report of 126 cases. J Pediatr Surg 1974;9(2):191–195.
18. Tanigawa N, Shimomatsuya T, Takahashi K, et al. Treatment of cystic hygroma and lymphangioma with the use of bleomycin fat emulsion. Cancer (Phila) 1987;60(4):741–749.
19. Ogita S, Tsuto T, Nakamura K, Deguchi E, Tokiwa K, Iwai N. OK-432 therapy for lymphangioma in children: why and how does it work? J Pediatr Surg 1996;31(4):477–480.
20. Ogita S, Tsuto T, Tokiwa K, Takahashi T. Intracystic injection of OK-432: a new sclerosing therapy for cystic hygroma in children. Br J Surg 1987;74(8):690–691.
21. Bodenstein L, Altman RP. Cervical lymphadenitis in infants and children. Semin Pediatr Surg 1994;3(3):134–141.
22. Armstrong D, Pickrell K, Fetter B, Pitts W. Torticollis: an analysis of 271 cases. Plast Reconstr Surg 1965;35:14–25.
23. May M. Neck masses in children: diagnosis and treatment. Pediatr Ann 1976;5(8):518–535.
24. McAvoy JM, Zuckerbraun L. Dermoid cysts of the head and neck in children. Arch Otolaryngol 1976;102(9):529–531.

25. Neilson IR, Russo P, Laberge JM, et al. Congenital adenomatoid malformation of the lung: current management and prognosis. J Pediatr Surg 1991;26(8):975–980; discussion 980–971.
26. Adzick NS, Harrison MR. Management of the fetus with a cystic adenomatoid malformation. World J Surg 1993;17(3):342–349.
27. Adzick NS, Harrison MR, Crombleholme TM, Flake AW, Howell LJ. Fetal lung lesions: management and outcome. Am J Obstet Gynecol 1998;179(4):884–889.
28. Stocker J, Madewell J, Drake R. Congenital cystic adenomatoid malformation of the lung. Hum Pathol 1977(8):155–171.
29. Benjamin DR, Cahill JL. Bronchioloalveolar carcinoma of the lung and congenital cystic adenomatoid malformation. Am J Clin Pathol 1991;95(6):889–892.
30. Lopoo JB, Goldstein RB, Lipshutz GS, Goldberg JD, Harrison MR, Albanese CT. Fetal pulmonary sequestration: a favorable congenital lung lesion. Obstet Gynecol 1999;94(4):567–571.
31. Stigers KB, Woodring JH, Kanga JF. The clinical and imaging spectrum of findings in patients with congenital lobar emphysema. Pediatr Pulmonol 1992;14(3):160–170.
32. Grosfeld JL, Skinner MA, Rescorla FJ, West KW, Scherer LR III. Mediastinal tumors in children: experience with 196 cases. Ann Surg Oncol 1994;1(2):121–127.
33. Puri P. Congenital diaphragmatic hernia. Curr Probl Surg 1994;31(10):787–846.
34. Adzick NS, Outwater KM, Harrison MR, et al. Correction of congenital diaphragmatic hernia in utero. IV. An early gestational fetal lamb model for pulmonary vascular morphometric analysis. J Pediatr Surg 1985;20(6):673–680.
35. Harrison MR, Adzick NS, Flake AW, et al. Correction of congenital diaphragmatic hernia in utero: VI. Hard-earned lessons. J Pediatr Surg 1993;28(10):1411–1417; discussion 1417–1418.
36. Allan DW, Greer JJ. Pathogenesis of nitrofen-induced congenital diaphragmatic hernia in fetal rats. J Appl Physiol 1997;83(2):338–347.
37. Harrison MR, Adzick NS, Bullard KM, et al. Correction of congenital diaphragmatic hernia in utero VII: a prospective trial. J Pediatr Surg 1997;32(11):1637–1642.
38. Harrison MR, Keller RL, Hawgood SB, et al. A randomized trial of fetal endoscopic tracheal occlusion for severe fetal congenital diaphragmatic hernia. N Engl J Med 2003;349(20):1916–1924.
39. Nakayama DK, Motoyama EK, Tagge EM. Effect of preoperative stabilization on respiratory system compliance and outcome in newborn infants with congenital diaphragmatic hernia. J Pediatr 1991;118(5):793–799.
40. Pokorny WJ, McGill CW, Harberg FJ. Morgagni hernias during infancy: presentation and associated anomalies. J Pediatr Surg 1984;19(4):394–397.
41. Cantrell J, Haller J, Ravitch M. A syndrome of congenital defect involving the abdominal wall, sternum, diaphragm, pericardium, and heart. Surg Gynecol Obstet 1958;107:602–614.
42. Smith CD, Sade RM, Crawford FA, Othersen HB. Diaphragmatic paralysis and eventration in infants. J Thorac Cardiovasc Surg 1986;91(4):490–497.
43. Ravitch M. Congenital Deformities of the Chest Wall and Their Operative Correction. Philadelphia: Saunders, 1977.
44. Shamberger RC, Welch KJ. Cardiopulmonary function in pectus excavatum. Surg Gynecol Obstet 1988;166(4):383–391.
45. Bentz ML, Rowe MI, Wiener ES. Improved sternal fixation in the correction of pediatric pectus excavatum. Ann Plast Surg 1994;32(6):638–641.
46. Nuss D, Kelly RE Jr, Croitoru DP, et al. A 10-year review of a minimally invasive technique for the correction of pectus excavatum. J Pediatr Surg 1998;33:545–552.
47. Ravitch M. Protrusion Deformities. Pediatric Surgery, 4th ed. St. Louis: Mosby Year-Book, 1986.
48. Shamberger RC, Welch KJ. Surgical correction of pectus carinatum. J Pediatr Surg 1987;22(1):48–53.
49. Harmon C, Coran A. Congenital anomalies of the esophagus. In: O'Neill J Jr, Rowe M, Grosfeld J, Fonkalsrud E, Coran A, eds. Pediatric Surgery, 5th ed. St. Louis: Mosby Year-Book, 1998:941–967.
50. Rothenberg SS. Thoracoscopic repair of esophageal atresia and tracheo-esophageal fistula. Semin Pediatr Surg 2005;14(1):2–7.
51. Lipshutz GS, Albanese CT, Jennings RW, Bratton BJ, Harrison MR. A strategy for primary reconstruction of long gap esophageal atresia using neonatal colon esophagoplasty: a case report. J Pediatr Surg 1999;34(1):75–77; discussion 77–78.
52. Boyle JT. Gastroesophageal reflux in the pediatric patient. Gastroenterol Clin N Am 1989;18(2):315–337.
53. Hassall E. Decisions in diagnosing and managing chronic gastroesophageal reflux disease in children. J Pediatr 2005;146(3 suppl):S3–S12.
54. Schier F. Indications for laparoscopic antireflux procedures in children. Semin Laparosc Surg 2002;9(3):139–145.
55. Kazerooni NL, VanCamp J, Hirschl RB, Drongowski RA, Coran AG. Fundoplication in 160 children under 2 years of age. J Pediatr Surg 1994;29(5):677–681.
56. Ashcraft KW, Holder TM, Amoury RA, Sharp RJ, Murphy JP. The Thal fundoplication for gastroesophageal reflux. J Pediatr Surg 1984;19(4):480–483.
57. Georgeson KE. Laparoscopic fundoplication and gastrostomy. Semin Laparosc Surg 1998;5(1):25–30.
58. Ashcraft KW, Holder TM, Amoury RA. Treatment of gastroesophageal reflux in children by Thal fundoplication. J Thorac Cardiovasc Surg 1981;82(5):706–712.
59. Hunter JG, Smith CD, Branum GD, et al. Laparoscopic fundoplication failures: patterns of failure and response to fundoplication revision. Ann Surg 1999;230(4):595–604; discussion 604–596.
60. Martinez DA, Ginn-Pease ME, Caniano DA. Sequelae of antireflux surgery in profoundly disabled children. J Pediatr Surg 1992;27(2):267–271; discussion 271–263.
61. Martinez DA, Ginn-Pease ME, Caniano DA. Recognition of recurrent gastroesophageal reflux following antireflux surgery in the neurologically disabled child: high index of suspicion and definitive evaluation. J Pediatr Surg 1992;27(8):983–988; discussion 988–990.
62. Pearl RH, Robie DK, Ein SH, et al. Complications of gastroesophageal antireflux surgery in neurologically impaired versus neurologically normal children. J Pediatr Surg 1990;25(11):1169–1173.
63. Smith CD, Othersen HB Jr, Gogan NJ, Walker JD. Nissen fundoplication in children with profound neurologic disability. High risks and unmet goals. Ann Surg 1992;215(6):654–658; discussion 658–659.
64. Taylor LA, Weiner T, Lacey SR, Azizkhan RG. Chronic lung disease is the leading risk factor correlating with the failure (wrap disruption) of antireflux procedures in children. J Pediatr Surg 1994;29(2):161–164; discussion 164–166.
65. Chung DH, Georgeson KE. Fundoplication and gastrostomy. Semin Pediatr Surg 1998;7(4):213–219.
66. Rothenberg SS. Experience with 220 consecutive laparoscopic Nissen fundoplications in infants and children. J Pediatr Surg 1998;33(2):274–278.
67. Leinwand MJ, Shaul DB, Anderson KD. The umbilical fold approach to pyloromyotomy: is it a safe alternative to the right upper-quadrant approach? J Am Coll Surg 1999;189(4):362–367.
68. Rothenberg S. Laparoscopic pyloromyotomy: the slice and pull technique. Pediatr Endosurg Innov Tech 1997;1:39–41.
69. Grosfeld JL, Rescorla FJ. Duodenal atresia and stenosis: reassessment of treatment and outcome based on antenatal diagnosis, pathologic variance, and long-term follow-up. World J Surg 1993;17(3):301–309.
70. Touloukian R, Smith E. Disorders of rotation and fixation. In: O'Neill J Jr, Rowe M, Grosfeld J, Fonkalsrud E, Coran A Jr, eds.

Pediatric Surgery, vol 2. St. Louis: Mosby-Year Book, 1998:1199–1222.
71. Rescorla FJ, Shedd FJ, Grosfeld JL, Vane DW, West KW. Anomalies of intestinal rotation in childhood: analysis of 447 cases. Surgery (St. Louis) 1990;108(4):710–715; discussion 715–716.
72. Grosfeld JL, Ballantine TV, Shoemaker R. Operative mangement of intestinal atresia and stenosis based on pathologic findings. J Pediatr Surg 1979;14(3):368–375.
73. Ladd W. Duplications of the alimentary tract. South Med J 1937;30:363–371.
74. Ildstad ST, Tollerud DJ, Weiss RG, Ryan DP, McGowan MA, Martin LW. Duplications of the alimentary tract. Clinical characteristics, preferred treatment, and associated malformations. Ann Surg 1988;208(2):184–189.
75. Wrenn E. Tubular duplication of the intestine. Surgery (St. Louis) 1962;52:494–498.
76. St-Vil D, Brandt ML, Panic S, Bensoussan AL, Blanchard H. Meckel's diverticulum in children: a 20-year review. J Pediatr Surg 1991;26(11):1289–1292.
77. Pena A, Hong A. Advances in the management of anorectal malformations. Am J Surg 2000;180(5):370–376.
78. Pena A, Devries PA. Posterior sagittal anorectoplasty: important technical considerations and new applications. J Pediatr Surg 1982;17(6):796–811.
79. Georgeson KE, Inge TH, Albanese CT. Laparoscopically assisted anorectal pull-through for high imperforate anus—a new technique. J Pediatr Surg 2000;35(6):927–930; discussion 930–921.
80. Rescorla FJ, Morrison AM, Engles D, West KW, Grosfeld JL. Hirschsprung's disease. Evaluation of mortality and long-term function in 260 cases. Arch Surg 1992;127(8):934–941; discussion 941–932.
81. Langer JC, Fitzgerald PG, Winthrop AL, et al. One-stage versus two-stage Soave pull-through for Hirschsprung's disease in the first year of life. J Pediatr Surg 1996;31(1):33–36; discussion 36–37.
82. Georgeson KE, Cohen RD, Hebra A, et al. Primary laparoscopic-assisted endorectal colon pull-through for Hirschsprung's disease: a new gold standard. Ann Surg 1999;229(5):678–682; discussion 682–673.
83. Albanese CT, Jennings RW, Smith B, Bratton B, Harrison MR. Perineal one-stage pull-through for Hirschsprung's disease. J Pediatr Surg 1999;34(3):377–380.
84. Guthrie S, Gordon P, Thomas V. Necrotizing enterocolitis among neonates in the United States. J Perinatol 2003;23:278.
85. Hallstrom M, Koivisto A, Janas M. Frequency of and risk factors for necrotizing enterocolitis in infants born before 33 weeks of gestation. Acta Paediatr 2003;92:111.
86. Kliegman R, Fanaroff A. Neonatal necrotizing enterocolitis. N Engl J Med 1984;310:1093.
87. Albanese C, Rowe R. Necrotizing enterocolitis. In: O'Neill J Jr, Rowe M, Grosfeld J, Fonkalsrud E, Coran A Jr, eds. Pediatric Surgery, vol 2. St. Louis: Mosby-Year Book, 1998:1297–1320.
88. Marchildon M, Buck B, Abdenour G. Necrotizing enterocolitis in the unfed patient. J Pediatr Surg 1982;17:620.
89. Grosfeld JL, Cheu H, Schlatter M, West KW, Rescorla FJ. Changing trends in necrotizing enterocolitis. Experience with 302 cases in two decades. Ann Surg 1991;214(3):300–306; discussion 306–307.
90. Ein SH, Shandling B, Wesson D, Filler RM. A 13-year experience with peritoneal drainage under local anesthesia for necrotizing enterocolitis perforation. J Pediatr Surg 1990;25(10):1034–1036; discussion 1036–1037.
91. Moss R, Dimmit R, Henry C, Geraghty N, Efron B. A meta-analysis of peritoneal drainage versus laparotomy for perforated necrotizing enterocolitis. J Pediatr Surg 2001;36(8):1210–1213.
92. Meyer JS, Dangman BC, Buonomo C, Berlin JA. Air and liquid contrast agents in the management of intussusception: a controlled, randomized trial. Radiology 1993;188(2):507–511.
93. Hays D. Biliary Atresia. Cambridge: Harvard University Press, 1980.
94. Lilly JR, Karrer FM, Hall RJ, et al. The surgery of biliary atresia. Ann Surg 1989;210(3):289–294; discussion 294–286.
95. Kasai M, Watanabe I, Ohi R. Follow-up studies of long-term survivors after hepatic portoenterostomy for "noncorrectible" biliary atresia. J Pediatr Surg 1975;10(2):173–182.
96. O'Neill JA Jr. Choledochal cyst. Curr Probl Surg 1992;29(6):361–410.
97. Todani T, Watanabe Y, Narusue M, Tabuchi K, Okajima K. Congenital bile duct cysts: classification, operative procedures, and review of thirty-seven cases including cancer arising from choledochal cyst. Am J Surg 1977;134(2):263–269.
98. Pinto RB, Lima JP, da Silveira TR, Scholl JG, de Mello ED, Silva G. Caroli's disease: report of 10 cases in children and adolescents in southern Brazil. J Pediatr Surg 1998;33(10):1531–1535.
99. Ando H, Kaneko K, Ito F, et al. Surgical removal of protein plugs complicating choledochal cysts: primary repair after adequate opening of the pancreatic duct. J Pediatr Surg 1998;33(8):1265–1267.
100. Han SJ, Hwang EH, Chung KS, Kim MJ, Kim H. Acquired choledochal cyst from anomalous pancreatobiliary duct union. J Pediatr Surg 1997;32(12):1735–1738.
101. Shian WJ, Wang YJ, Chi CS. Choledochal cysts: a nine-year review. Acta Paediatr 1993;82(4):383–386.
102. Meller JL, Reyes HM, Loeff DS. Gastroschisis and omphalocele. Clin Perinatol 1989;16(1):113–122.
103. Lassaletta L, Fonkalsrud EW, Tovar JA, Dudgeon D, Asch MJ. The management of umbilical hernias in infancy and childhood. J Pediatr Surg 1975;10(3):405–409.
104. Grosfeld JL. Current concepts in inguinal hernia in infants and children. World J Surg 1989;13(5):506–515.
105. Weber T, Tracy TJ. Groin hernias and hydrocele. In: Ashcraft K, Holder T, eds. Pediatric Surgery, 2nd ed. Philadelphia: Saunders, 1993:562–570.
106. Fuenfer MM, Pitts RM, Georgeson KE. Laparoscopic exploration of the contralateral groin in children: an improved technique. J Laparoendosc Surg 1996;6(suppl 1):S1–S4.
107. Yerkes EB, Brock JW III, Holcomb GW III, Morgan WM III. Laparoscopic evaluation for a contralateral patent processus vaginalis: part III. Urology 1998;51(3):480–483.
108. Elder JS. The undescended testis. Hormonal and surgical management. Surg Clin N Am 1988;68(5):983–1005.
109. Williamson RC. Torsion of the testis and allied conditions. Br J Surg 1976;63(6):465–476.
110. Skoglund RW, McRoberts JW, Ragde H. Torsion of testicular appendages: presentation of 43 new cases and a collective review. J Urol 1970;104(4):598–600.
111. Low DW. Hemangiomas and vascular malformations. Semin Pediatr Surg 1994;3(2):40–61.
112. Matthay KK. Neuroblastoma: a clinical challenge and biologic puzzle. CA Cancer J Clin 1995;45(3):179–192.
113. Chamberlain RS, Quinones R, Dinndorf P, Movassaghi N, Goodstein M, Newman K. Complete surgical resection combined with aggressive adjuvant chemotherapy and bone marrow transplantation prolongs survival in children with advanced neuroblastoma. Ann Surg Oncol 1995;2(2):93–100.
114. Ritchey ML, Kelalis PP, Haase GM, Shochat SJ, Green DM, D'Angio G. Preoperative therapy for intracaval and atrial extension of Wilms tumor. Cancer (Phila) 1993;71(12):4104–4110.
115. Green DM, D'Angio GJ, Beckwith JB, et al. Wilms tumor. CA Cancer J Clin 1996;46(1):46–63.
116. Wiener ES. Rhabdomyosarcoma: new dimensions in management. Semin Pediatr Surg 1993;2(1):47–58.
117. Hays DM, Lawrence W Jr, Wharam M, et al. Primary reexcision for patients with "microscopic residual" tumor following initial excision of sarcomas of trunk and extremity sites. J Pediatr Surg 1989;24(1):5–10.

118. Weinberg AG, Finegold MJ. Primary hepatic tumors of childhood. Hum Pathol 1983;14(6):512–537.
119. Wheatley JM, LaQuaglia MP. Management of hepatic epithelial malignancy in childhood and adolescence. Semin Surg Oncol 1993;9(6):532–540.
120. Tagge EP, Tagge DU, Reyes J, et al. Resection, including transplantation, for hepatoblastoma and hepatocellular carcinoma: impact on survival. J Pediatr Surg 1992;27(3):292–296; discussion 297.
121. Selby DM, Stocker JT, Waclawiw MA, Hitchcock CL, Ishak KG. Infantile hemangioendothelioma of the liver. Hepatology 1994;20(1 pt 1):39–45.
122. Cherqui D, Rahmouni A, Charlotte F, et al. Management of focal nodular hyperplasia and hepatocellular adenoma in young women: a series of 41 patients with clinical, radiological, and pathological correlations. Hepatology 1995;22(6):1674–1681.
123. Chandra RS, Kapur SP, Kelleher J Jr, Luban N, Patterson K. Benign hepatocellular tumors in the young. A clinicopathologic spectrum. Arch Pathol Lab Med 1984;108(2):168–171.
124. Rescorla FJ, Breitfeld PP. Pediatric germ cell tumors. Curr Probl Cancer 1999;23(6):257–303.
125. Schropp KP, Lobe TE, Rao B, et al. Sacrococcygeal teratoma: the experience of four decades. J Pediatr Surg 1992;27(8):1075–1078; discussion 1078–1079.
126. Potoka D, Schall L, Gardner M, Stafford P, Peitzman A, Ford H. Impact of pediatric trauma centers on mortality in a statewide system. J Trauma Injury Infect Crit Care 2000;49(2):237–245.
127. Rivera F. Pediatric injury control in 1999: where do we go from here? Pediatrics 1999;103:883–888.
128. Schafermeyer R. Pediatric trauma. Emerg Med Clin N Am 1993;11:187–205.
129. DeRoss AL, Vane DW. Early evaluation and resuscitation of the pediatric trauma patient. Semin Pediatr Surg 2004;13(2):74–79.
130. Khoshyomn S, Tranmer BI. Diagnosis and management of pediatric closed head injury. Semin Pediatr Surg 2004;13(2):80–86.
131. Sartorelli KH, Vane DW. The diagnosis and management of children with blunt injury of the chest. Semin Pediatr Surg 2004;13(2):98–105.
132. Cotton BA, Nance ML. Penetrating trauma in children. Semin Pediatr Surg 2004;13(2):87–97.
133. Keller MS. Blunt injury to solid abdominal organs. Semin Pediatr Surg 2004;13(2):106–111.
134. Bruny JL, Bensard DD. Hollow viscous injury in the pediatric patient. Semin Pediatr Surg 2004;13(2):112–118.
135. Canty TG Sr, Canty TG Jr, Brown C. Injuries of the gastrointestinal tract from blunt trauma in children: a 12-year experience at a designated pediatric trauma center. J Trauma 1999;46(2):234–240.
136. Galifer RB, Forgues D, Mourregot A, et al. Blunt traumatic injuries of the gastrointestinal and biliary tract in childhood. Analysis of 16 cases. Eur J Pediatr Surg 2001;11(4):230–234.
137. Esposito C, Montupet P, Amici G, Desruelle P. Complications of laparoscopic antireflux surgery in childhood. Surg Endosc 2000;14(7):622–624.
138. Montupet P, Mendoza-Sagan M, DeDreuzy O. Laparoscopic Toupet fundoplication in children. Pediatr Endosurg Innov Tech 2001;5:305–308.
139. Allal H, Captier G, Lopez M, Forgues D, Galifer RB. Evaluation of 142 consecutive laparoscopic fundoplications in children: effects of the learning curve and technical choice. J Pediatr Surg 2001;36(6):921–926.
140. Iglesias J, Kogut K, Owings E. Safety and efficacy of laparoscopic Nissen fundoplication in early infancy. Pediatr Endosurg Innov Tech 2001;5:379–384.
141. Ostlie DJ, Miller KA, Woods RK, Holcomb GW III. Single cannula technique and robotic telescopic assistance in infants and children who require laparoscopic Nissen fundoplication. J Pediatr Surg 2003;38(1):111–115; discussion 115–116.
142. Cheu HW, Sukarochana K, Lloyd DA. Peritoneal drainage for necrotizing enterocolitis. J Pediatr Surg 1988;23(6):557–561.
143. Takamatsu H, Akiyama H, Ibara S, Seki S, Kuraya K, Ikenoue T. Treatment for necrotizing enterocolitis perforation in the extremely premature infant (weighing less than 1,000 g). J Pediatr Surg 1992;27(6):741–743.
144. Morgan LJ, Shochat SJ, Hartman GE. Peritoneal drainage as primary management of perforated NEC in the very low birth weight infant. J Pediatr Surg 1994;29(2):310–314; discussion 314–315.
145. Azarow KS, Ein SH, Shandling B, Wesson D, Superina R, Filler RM. Laparotomy or drain for perforated necrotizing enterocolitis: who gets what and why? Pediatr Surg Int 21 1997;12(2/3):137–139.
146. Snyder CL, Gittes GK, Murphy JP, Sharp RJ, Ashcraft KW, Amoury RA. Survival after necrotizing enterocolitis in infants weighing less than 1,000 g: 25 years' experience at a single institution. J Pediatr Surg 1997;32(3):434–437.
147. Lessin MS, Luks FI, Wesselhoeft CW Jr, Gilchrist BF, Iannitti D, DeLuca FG. Peritoneal drainage as definitive treatment for intestinal perforation in infants with extremely low birth weight (<750 g). J Pediatr Surg 1998;33(2):370–372.
148. Ahmed T, Ein S, Moore A. The role of peritoneal drains in treatment of perforated necrotizing enterocolitis: recommendations from recent experience. J Pediatr Surg 1998;33(10):1468–1470.
149. Rovin JD, Rodgers BM, Burns RC, McGahren ED. The role of peritoneal drainage for intestinal perforation in infants with and without necrotizing enterocolitis. J Pediatr Surg 1999;34(1):143–147.
150. Downard C, Curran T, Campbell T. Peritoneal drainage for neonatal intestinal perforation. Presented at 33rd Annual Meeting of the Pacific Association of Pediatric Surgeons, Las Vegas, NV, 2000.
151. Dimmitt RA, Meier AH, Skarsgard ED, Halamek LP, Smith BM, Moss RL. Salvage laparotomy for failure of peritoneal drainage in necrotizing enterocolitis in infants with extremely low birth weight. J Pediatr Surg 2000;35(6):856–859.

37

Surgery in the Immunocompromised Patient

John Mihran Davis and Kathleen King Casey

It is currently estimated that more than 40 million people worldwide are infected with the human immunodeficiency virus (HIV). Although there is no end in sight to the epidemic, current therapeutics have significantly altered the course of the illness. HIV-infected people are much more likely to live longer, less likely to die of opportunistic infections, and more likely to present to the surgical community with relatively well-preserved immune function. Physicians must be not only armed with knowledge on how to protect themselves from inadvertent infection but possess a basic understanding of the disease process and treatment. Patients present with malignancies, end-organ failures, and treatment-related toxicities as well as those illnesses expected in any adult population regardless of immune function. Surgical intervention is routine, and outcome will be influenced by how well we define preoperative risk and understand optimum perioperative management.

The concept of evidence-based medicine is predicated on the availability of clinical evidence gleaned from systematic research coupled with individual clinical experience. More than two decades into the HIV/acquired immunodeficiency syndrome (AIDS) epidemic, there is still a paucity of systematic research and very few centers that have extensive clinical experience with performing surgery on HIV-infected individuals. A thorough review of the literature reveals that the bulk of the articles dealing with surgery and HIV concentrate on issues of risk of transmission in the workplace and not patient care.

Even within the realm of antiretroviral management, evidence-based medicine has been slow to evolve. The urgency to develop antiretroviral agents resulted in an entirely new approach at the Food and Drug Administration (FDA) toward accelerating the approval process for therapeutic agents and allowing clinical use earlier in the approval process. The current standard of care involving a three-drug antiretroviral regimen only came into use in 1996. Until recently, a 48-week protocol was perceived as a "long-term" study. It is only in the past 2 years that clinical trial data have provided conclusions that predict inferiority or toxicity with particular regimens. We now know that the use of stavudine and (d4T) didanosine (ddl), simultaneously, increases the likelihood of lactic acidosis. Studies have also been able to document the clinical inferiority of triple nucleoside regimens in patients with high viral loads.

Drug Therapy Toxicities and Postexposure Prophylaxis

All healthcare professionals who have occupational exposure to blood are at risk of acquiring HIV infection. Over the past two decades myriad innovations in safer needle devices, barrier protections, and safer practices have been introduced to minimize exposure to blood. Percutaneous injury is the most common mechanism of transmission. The pooled data from 21 prospective studies estimate the risk of percutaneous acquisition associated with needles and other contaminated devices to be 0.2%.[1] Variable influences thought to favor the transmissibility of infection are hollow-bore needles and a high HIV viral load in the source patient, but undoubtedly there are other host variables, such as cytoxic T-lymphocyte response, and perhaps T-cell C3a/C5a receptors that may also influence the outcome. It is important to counsel the exposed healthcare worker as to his/her individual risk at the time of the incident.

Mucocutaneous exposures accounted for about 12% of the HIV infections reported to the Centers for Disease Control (CDC) as occupationally related by 1992.[2] The risk associated with such exposures is very difficult to quantify as many go unreported and those reported may differ substantially in characteristics of exposure. The estimated risk of mucocutaneous exposure is believed now to be approximately 0.09%.

Proper management of occupational blood exposure focuses on a thorough assessment of the type of exposure, the source patient, and prompt counseling of the exposed healthcare worker. Is the source HIV infected? What type of exposure occurred? Is antiretroviral therapy appropriate in the exposed healthcare worker (HCW)? It is thought that to be efficacious such therapy should be administered within a 4-h window after exposure; consequently, time is of the essence.

Establishing the source's HIV status should be done whenever possible. Fortunately rapid HIV testing is commercially available and should be employed if the source's status is unknown. The SUDS (Single Use Diagnostic System) HIV-1 test manufactured by Abbot-Murex Diagnostics is a rapid test requiring about 15 min to perform. It is highly sensitive such that a negative test is reliable evidence against the presence of HIV infection. With the new enzyme-linked immunosorbent assay (ELISA) tests, the window between infection and a positive test is thought to be only a few days. Therefore, unless there was a clinical suspicion of acute retroviral syndrome in the source, a negative SUDS result should be taken to mean the HCW was not exposed and HIV postexposure prophylaxis (PEP) is unnecessary.

If the source cannot be promptly tested, or the source is confirmed to be positive, further assessment of the injury is required. The likelihood of transmission is thought to be increased when a hollow-bore device caused a deep injury from a patient whose viral load is high. In the case control study done by the CDC,[3] it was noted that death of the HIV-positive source within 2 months of exposure was associated with an increased likelihood of infection. We now presume this is a surrogate marker for a high viral load, but these data were collected before viral loads or highly active antiretroviral therapy (HAART) were part of the standard of care for HIV-infected patients. In accidents involving other devices such as suture needles and mucous membrane exposure, the risk of transmission is very low, but not zero. It is important to mention that transmission has been reported even when viral loads were nondetectable (Table 37.1).

Each case warrants unique risk analysis as antiretroviral drugs used for prophylaxis are not without side effects; these can be merely nausea, diarrhea, or headache, but serious side effects such as rashes, nephrolithiasis, hepatitis, hyperglycemia, and pancytopenia have been reported (Table 37.2). When nevirapine was included as a prophylactic agent serious hepatotoxicity occurred and necessitated a liver transplant in one person. We now know that nevirapine poses a serious hepatic risk to anyone with immune competence, but when it is used therapeutically it can quickly drop the viral load in infected individuals. In fact, it is still a mainstay of perinatal vertical transmission intervention when no prenatal care has been available, for that very reason.

In 1995, Julie Gerberding published a review article in the *New England Journal of Medicine* discussing management of occupation exposures to blood-borne viruses.[4] This article stressed that there was a paucity of data regarding the utility of PEP with zidovudine. The argument to take zidovudine was mainly the biological plausibility that it might interfere with transmission by keeping the viral replication in check to allow the cellular immune system to respond to a relatively small inoculum and thereby avoid established infection. There were no controlled data, and Dr. Gerberding stated it should not be regarded as the standard of care given the uncertainties about the efficacy and safety of zidovudine in this setting. Despite this, its use became widespread, and by the time she wrote another review on the subject in 2003, antiretroviral therapy had become the standard of care.[5]

The 2001 U.S. Public Health guidelines recommend a 4-week regimen of two drugs be started as soon as possible after HIV exposure by mucosal routes. If the injury includes damage by a hollow-bore needle, associated with a deep injury, or caused by a device that had directly entered an artery or vein,

TABLE 37.1. Possible Antiretroviral Regimens for Occupational Exposure to Human Immunodeficiency Virus (HIV).

Preferred regimens	
NNRTI based	Efavirenz[a] plus (lamivudine or emtricitabine) plus (zidovudine or tenofovir)
Protease inhibitor (PI) based	Lopinavir/ritonavir (coformulated as Kaletra) plus (lamivudine or emtricitabine) plus zidovudine
Alternative regimens	
NNRTI based	Efavirenz plus (lamivudine or emtricitabine) plus abacavir or didanosine or stavudine[b]
PI based	Atazanavir plus (lamivudine or emtricitabine) plus (zidovudine or stavudine or abacavir or didanosine) or (tenofovir plus ritonavir, 100 mg/day)
	Fosamprenavir plus (lamivudine or emtricitabine) or (abacavir or tenofovir or didanosine)
	Fosamprenavir/ritonavir[c] plus (lamivudine or emtricitabine) plus zidovudine or stavudine or abacavir or tenofovir or didanosine)
	Indinavir/ritonavir[c,d] plus (lamivudine or emtricitabine) plus (zidovudine or stavudine or abacavir or tenofovir or didanosine)
	Lopinavir/ritonavir (coformulated at Kaletra) plus (lamivudine or emtricitabine) plus (stavudine or abacavir or tenofovir or didanosine)
	Nelfinavir plus (lamivudine or emtricitabine) plus (zidovudine or stavudine or abacavir or tenofovir or didanosine)
	Saquinavir (hgc or sgc)/ritonavir[a] plus (lamivudine or emtricitabine) plus (zidovudine or stavudine or abacavir or tenofovir or didanosine)
Triple NRTI	Abacavir plus lamivudine plus zidovudine (only when an NNRTI- or PI-based regimen cannot or should not be used)

NNRTI, nonnucleoside reverse transcriptase inhibitor; NRTI, nucleoside reverse transcriptase inhibitor; sgc, soft-gel saquinavir capsule (Fortovase); hgc, hard-gel saquinavir capsule (Invirase).

[a]Efavirenz should be avoided in pregnant women and women of childbearing potential.

[b]Higher incidence of lipoatrophy, hyperlipidemia, and mitochondrial toxicities associated with stavudine than with other NRTIs.

[c]Low-dose (100–400 mg) ritonavir.

[d]Use of ritonavir with indinavir might increase risk for renal adverse events.

Source: U.S. Department of Health and Human Services. Guidelines for the Use of Antiretroviral Agents in HIV-Infected Adults and Adolescents, October 29, 2004 revision. Available at http://www.aidsinfo.nih.gov/guidelines/default_db2.asp?id=50. This document is updated periodically; refer to Web site for updated versions.

TABLE 37.2. Adverse Effects of Antiretroviral Therapies.

Reaction	*Drug*
Cutaneous:	
Hypersensitivity reaction	ABC
Skin rash	NVP, EFV, DLV
	ABC, APV, f-APV, ATV
	TPV/RTV
Stevens–Johnson syndrome	NVP, EFV, DLV
Toxic epidermal necrosis	APV, f-APV, ABC
	ZDV, ddI, IDV, LPV/r
	ATV
Hematological:	
Bone marrow suppression	ZDV
Increased bleeding episodes in hemophilia	All PIs
Gastrointestinal:	
GI intolerance	All PI's, ZDV, ddI
Hepatic necrosis	NVP
Hepatitis	All NRTIs, NNRTIs, and PIs
Hyperbilirubinemia	IDV, ATV
Pancreatitis	ddI, ddI + d4T
Metabolic:	
Fat maldistribution	PIs, d4T
Hyperlipidemia	All PIs except ATV, d4T, ±EFV
Mitochondrial toxicity (with lactic acidosis/steatosis)	d4T most frequently implicated
	All NRTIs especially d4T, ddI, ZDV
Osteonecrosis	All PIs
Musculoskeletal:	
Myopathy	ZDV
Nephrotoxicity:	
Interstitial nephritis	TDF
Renal stones	IDV
Neurotoxicity:	
CNS effects	EFV
Lactic acidosis with ascending neuromuscular weakness	d4T
Peripheral neuropathy	ddI, d4T, ddc

For definitions of drug acronyms, see Table 37.3.

the addition of a third drug to the regimen was recommended. This change has come about primarily because of the success of perinatal intervention to prevent vertical transmission of HIV. Through the use of antepartum and postpartum antiretrovirals, the vertical transmission rate has been reduced by 90%. The true relevance of these data to occupational exposure is not known. It is clear, however, that with the relatively low risk of transmission from occupational injury it is unlikely that the numbers would ever be sufficient to power a placebo-controlled trial to prove or disprove efficacy. As it has now become the standard of care, it is unlikely that any controlled study will ever be performed. It remains now to refine treatment as to which drugs, for how long, and how many should be used.

In 2004 a paper was published by Bassett et al. regarding the statistical benefit of two-drug versus three-drug regimens.[5] As the number of side effects in a three- versus two-drug regimen is greater, fewer people are likely to complete prophylaxis, perhaps negating any beneficial effect of the third drug. There is no evidence that a three-drug regimen is more efficacious in preventing transmission. Its recommendation is based upon the assumption that maximal viral suppression would be most likely to prevent infection. Furthermore, with antiretroviral resistance increasing, perhaps a more specific

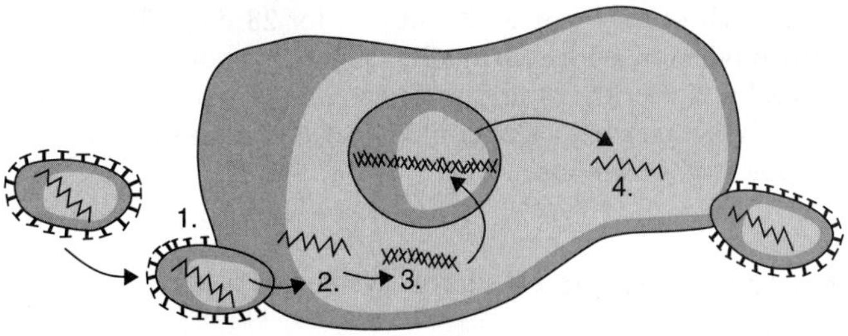

FIGURE 37.1. A diagram showing the invasion and reproduction of human immunodeficiency virus (HIV) in a lymphocyte. *1*, HIV enters the CD4 lymphocyte; *2*, the virus reverse transcriptase converts its RNA to DNA; *3*, HIV enters the nucleus and inserts its DNA into the host DNA; *4*, new HIV leaves the cell. Sites of action of antiretroviral drugs are identified by the numbers: *1* is the site of the entry where fusion inhibitors work, *2* is the site where nonnucleoside reverse transcriptase and nucleoside reverse transcriptase drugs work; *4* is the site of action of protease inhibitors.

selection of agents is warranted based on the knowledge of the source's antiretroviral history (shown schematically in Fig. 37.1 and in Table 37.3). If available, consultation should be sought with the source's medical provider.

As antiretroviral agents are not without harmful side effects, underlying conditions in the healthcare worker must be taken into consideration as well. Anemia, hepatitis, hyperglycemia, and nephrolithiasis are a few of the potential side effects. The only agent identified as not a candidate for use in a PEP regimen is Nevirapine.

The 1998 CDC Guidelines had suggested zidovudine and 3TC for a two-agent therapy, now available as Combivir. They added indinavir or nelfinavir as the third drug. In 2001, the guidelines left the choice more open to expertise. Truvada (tenofovir/FTC) once a day with or without efavirenz is an attractive choice currently. However, the increasing prevalence of the 184 mutation among antiretroviral-experienced patients may make both FTC and 3TC ineffective. Local expertise should be sought. Ideally, prophylaxis should begin

TABLE 37.3. Antiretroviral Therapies.

Nucleoside reverse transcriptase inhibitors (NRTI):	
Abacavir	ABC
Didanosine	ddI
Emtricitabine	FTC
Lamivudine	3TC
Stavudine	d4T
Zalcitabine	Ddc
Zidovudine	ZDV
Tenofovir	TDF
Entry inhibitors:	
Enfuvirtide	T-20
Nonnucleoside reverse transcriptase inhibitors (NNRTI):	
Delavirdine	DLV
Efavirenz	EFV
Nevirapine	NVP
Protease inhibitors (PI):	
Amprenavir	APV
Atazanavir	ATZ
Fos-amprenavir	f-APV
Indinavir	IDV
Lopinavir/Rit	LPV/r
Nelfinavir	NLF
Saquinavir	SQV
Tripanzvir/rit	TRP/rit
Darunavir/rit	DRN/rit

within 4h of exposure and continue for 28 days. Testing for seroconversion with routine ELISA assays should be done at 6 weeks, 3 months, and 6 months. There is no defined role for polymerase chain reaction (PCR)-RNA assays in monitoring for seroconversion.

Protection from Disease Transmission

An ongoing concern on the part of healthcare workers, in general, and surgeons in particular, is that of disease transmission. However, it is evident that the microorganisms infecting AIDS patients are not particularly contagious, providing proper precautions are taken (Table 37.4). One major concern for surgeons, operating room committees, infection control committees, and clinicians involved with endoscopy is how to effectively clean instruments, equipment, or other inanimate objects to be used with AIDS patients. Agents that are effective against mycobacteria, the most resistant group of organisms, are also the agents considered most effective against other bacterial and viral pathogens.[6,7] (A complete list of agents and their efficacies can be obtained from the Disinfectants Branch, Office of Pesticides, United States Environmental Protection Agency, 401 M Street, S.W., Washington, DC 20460.)

Agents are classified according to whether they are to be used for sterilization, disinfection, or antisepsis.[8] Agents that sterilize inanimate objects kill all microbial organisms as well as bacterial endospores. Disinfectants are not quite as effective in that they are not capable of killing bacterial spores. In many cases, an agent may serve as a disinfectant when placed in contact for a short time with the object requiring cleansing. The same agent may be capable of sterilizing surgical instruments when exposed to them for longer periods. Disinfectants are subclassified as having high-level, intermediate-level, and low-level germicidal activity. High-level agents are effective against bacterial spores. Intermediate-level disinfectants are less effective against spores but are mycobactericidal. Low-level disinfectants do not kill mycobacteria and some fungi. Antiseptic agents are used on tissue and therefore must be less toxic than sterilants or disinfectants.

According to the current recommendations from the CDC, agents classified by the U.S. Environmental Protection Agency as sterilants can be used for sterilization or high-level disinfection, depending on contact time. All instruments entering the bloodstream or other sterile tissues should be sterilized before use. Instruments that contact mucosal surfaces, such as endoscopes, should receive high-level disinfection, which can be achieved with solutions of glutaraldehyde (2%), hydrogen peroxide (3%–6%), or formaldehyde (1%–8%).

TABLE 37.4. Precautions Healthcare Workers Should Take When Handling Infectious Materials.

1. Wear gloves when handling body fluids.
2. Wear a gown to prevent contamination of clothing.
3. Wash hands after contact with body fluids.
4. Place fluid from a potentially contaminated host in two impervious containers.
5. Clean spills with either a 1:10 dilution of 5.25% sodium hypochlorite in water or with some other type of sterilant.
6. Wear masks and protective eyeglasses when there is a possibility of aerosolization of material.

Transfusions

Additional screening policies at the time of blood donation has reduced the risk of receiving a contaminated unit of blood. It is currently estimated that the risk of receiving a unit of blood that is contaminated with HIV is 1 in 1 million.[9]

Transplantation

Because it is known that HIV is present in semen, blood, urine, tears, breast milk, cerebrospinal fluid, and saliva, and because it is suspected that HIV can be present in all secretions and excretions as well as all body tissues,[10] potential donors of tissue for transplantation must be tested for HIV to prevent inadvertent transfer of the virus. (The risk of transmitting the virus by artificial insemination has also been documented and should be considered whenever artificial insemination is planned.[11])

Healthcare Workers

In 1989, the CDC recommended that universal precautions be adopted as a strategy for interacting with all patients to prevent accidental HIV transmission in the healthcare setting.[12–15] Hospital personnel who come in contact with patients' tissues, blood, body fluids, or excreta must use barrier precautions. Even healthcare workers who do not have exfoliative dermatitis or an open wound should wear gloves during patient care. Evidence suggests that the affinity of HIV for Langerhans' cells may permit the virus to invade a host through apparently intact skin or mucous membranes.[16] As part of any operative procedure on HIV-infected patients, all operating room, nursing, and anesthesia personnel, as well as employees of surgical pathology laboratories and any other laboratories, should use universal precautions for handling equipment and specimens. Employees in ancillary areas, such as housekeeping and dietary services, and the venipuncture team need to be trained in the use of universal precautions (see Table 37.4).

Exposures to the virus in the workplace are preventable provided appropriate precautions are in place.[17] Most injuries result from carelessness in handling sharp objects, such as needles and scalpels. Self-inflicted puncture incurred in the course of recapping used needles is the most common cause of inadvertent exposure to HIV and is the most dangerous because of the potential volume of blood in the needle and attached syringe that can serve as an inoculum. Newly designed syringes and needles with automatic self-capping tips have become recently available, as well as scalpels with blade covers. These newer technologies should reduce the accidental injuries. As of 2002 the Occupational Safety and Health Administration (OSHA) has mandated that each institution must maintain records of where and how injuries occur to prevent them in the future.

The use of double gloves by the surgeon has been extensively studied in several prospective randomized trials. These studies have shown a surgeon who uses double gloves significantly reduces the chance of contact with patient blood.[18–20] However, none of the studies showed that the double gloves either reduced disease transmission from the patient to the surgeon or reduced the subsequent infection rate of the patient.

Transmission from Surgical Personnel

The HIV-infected surgeon poses an immeasurable risk that he or she will transmit the virus to their patient. Although this concern has been well publicized,[21] there is only one documented report of transmission from a surgeon to patient.[22] Furthermore, the Centers for Disease Control and Prevention has not recommended restricting HIV-positive surgeons from operating.[23] Suspected hepatitis C virus (HCV) transmission has occurred from a surgeon to a patient in which the transmission similarly occurred after the diagnosis in the surgeon. Because these transmissions occurred before the diagnosis of the involved individual, editorial review suggested, rather than promoting the restriction of the surgeon's practice, promoting better barriers to minimize exposure between the surgeon and the patient.

In contrast to HIV surgeon-to-patient transmission, hepatitis B virus (HBV) transmission from surgeon to patient is a more significant concern. In a well-documented report involving a nonimmunized cardiac surgeon who acquired HBV infection in the workplace, transmission of the virus occurred in 19 (13%) of 122 patients on whom the surgeon operated over a 12-month period.[24] The surgeon was positive for hepatitis B_e antigen (HB_eAg), and sweat from inside his glove was found to contain HBV antigen as well as HBV DNA. No deficiencies were found in the surgeon's infection control practice by the CDC, which suggested that the virus might have spread through microperforations in his gloves. This case did not receive the same publicity that cases of HIV transmission have received in the lay press. However, its significance is clear: contact between healthcare workers who are HBV (HB_eAg) positive and patients should be restricted. The risk of transmission of HCV from the surgeon to the patient in the operating room is very small. A single well-documented case report is the best evidence that it can occur and supports the concept of improved intraoperative techniques to prevent intraoperative exposure of surgeon and patient blood.

Risks to Surgeons

Since 1985 when HIV testing became available, 23,212 healthcare workers acquired HIV in the workplace. Fifty-seven healthcare workers had a negative HIV test at the time of the injury, followed by a documented conversion to HIV or AIDS without having another risk factor. These healthcare workers are listed as "possible" occupationally acquired HIV. No surgeon has had a documented conversion following a needlestick injury in the operating room. Six surgeons have suspected HIV transmission, having no other high-risk behavior than their surgical profession.

The risk to a surgeon of acquiring an HIV infection while treating a patient who has undetected AIDS is quite low.[17,23] The CDC initially evaluated nearly 1500 healthcare workers who cared for AIDS victims. Serum samples were taken from these workers when they first began to work with immunocompromised patients and were stored in anticipation of a test for HIV. Of these workers, 666 were exposed to HIV through needle sticks or through cuts from sharp instruments. When tests were performed on these exposed individuals, none were found to have seroconverted after their exposure to HIV. However, two healthcare workers who had had no baseline blood sample drawn did show a positive antibody test after an injury. Because they did not belong to a known risk group for AIDS, they were believed to have generated antibody to HIV as a result of exposure in the workplace. On the basis of this study, the risk to a healthcare worker of acquiring HIV infection after an accidental needle-stick exposure was concluded to be 2 divided by 666, or 0.3%. A follow-up study found the rate of infection to be 0.5%.[25] Subsequent surveillance of healthcare workers identified 151 individuals who acquired HIV infection in the workplace[17] had proven seroconversion and 102 were HIV positive, with no HIV-negative baseline serum sample.

A serosurvey of 770 surgeons practicing in two inner-city areas where more than 3000 cases of AIDS have been reported was recently conducted by the CDC.[26] Accompanying the assay for HIV, HBV, and HCV was a questionnaire designed to elucidate the various practice patterns of the surgeons tested. One (0.13%) of the 770 surgeons was HIV positive; he had practiced for more than 25 years and performed more than 300 operations in the past year. The study did not specify how the surgeon acquired HIV, except to note that he did not participate in high-risk behavior. To date, there has been no documented seroconversion in OR personnel after a solid-bore needle injury in the operating room (http//www.cdc.gov/ncidod/hip/BLOOD/hivpersonell.htm).

Transmission via skin contact with body fluids was documented in the case of a woman whose infant had received multiple transfusions, one of which was from an HIV-infected donor. The baby had received the contaminated transfusion at 3 months of age. The presence of HIV antibody in the mother was not determined until 1 year later, at which time an ELISA result was positive. The mother was closely involved with the baby's care and took no precautions against contact with the child's blood and body fluids. Seventeen months after the child received the infected blood transfusion, the mother seroconverted. No other risk factors accounted for the change in the mother's HIV antibody titer.[27]

Centers for Disease Control Reclassification of HIV Infection

In 1993 the Centers for Disease Control and Prevention (CDC) revised the classification of the HIV-infected adult and adolescent. At that time a CD4 (T-helper lymphocyte) count of less than 200 cells/μl was recognized as an indicator of AIDS regardless of the symptoms. Once a patient has been classified into a given group, they will not be reclassified to a more favorable category, even if their symptoms resolve or the CD4 count rises. However, if the disease progresses or the CD4 count deteriorates, they will be reclassified into the next less favorable group. This system allows for uniformity in patient classification for research trials, scientific communication, and, most of all, facilitates formulation of healthcare policy and strategy. Unfortunately, the system does not take into account the immune reconstitution that occurs with highly active antiretroviral therapy (HAART). A number of studies have been done now to show that secondary prophylaxis for *Pneumocystis* pneumonia, cytomegalovirus (CMV) retinitis, toxoplasmosis encephalitis, and cryptococcal meningitis may be safely discontinued in patients whose CD4 counts have risen and remained above 200 cells/μl due to HAART. Therefore, patients originally classified as AIDS based on their CD4 count or level of immunocompromise may no longer be expected to behave, after successful treatment with antiretrovirals, as they would have based on their original CDC classification.

Even more recent studies evaluating surgical infection rates in gynecological procedures have only been able to correlate increased infection rates with the current CD4 count showing that a CD4 level below 200 cells/μl at the time of the procedure is an independent risk factor for surgical complications. The previous nadir has not been shown to influence the outcome.

Diagnosis

The enzyme-linked immunosorbent assay (ELISA) and the Western blot assay are designed to detect the presence of HIV antibody in serum. The ELISA test is considered very sensitive (i.e., its false-negative rate is low, 93%–100%). The specificity of a repeatedly reactive ELISA approaches 99%. The weakness of the ELISA test is that some individuals have antibodies that react with HIV antigens but are not specific for HIV. The Western blot assay is a more specific test but is cumbersome and a less sensitive assay. It is therefore used most effectively in confirming ELISA results, but it is not a good screening test. Most blood banks will not use blood that has demonstrated a positive ELISA reaction even if HIV antibody was not detected by Western blotting.[28]

On August 8, 1995, the Food and Drug Administration recommended that all blood donated for transfusion be screened for the p24 antigen (the core structural protein of HIV).[29] With the current test for HIV, there is a so-called window period of 25 days between infection and seroconversion. It has been estimated that since 1985, when all banked blood was tested for HIV, 35 patients have contracted HIV infection because the donor blood was collected from an HIV-infected individual during this window period.[30,31] Additional laboratory tests that may help in the diagnosis of patients who are believed to have HIV infection but in whom HIV antibody screening yields negative results include DNA PCR, antigen testing after immune complex disruption, and RNA reverse transcriptase PCR.[31] The SUDS (single use diagnostic system by Murex Diagnostics) provides a rapid ELISA technology that can yield a reliable result in 15 min. A positive SUDS must still be confirmed by Western blot. This assay is especially useful in occupational injury investigation.

Care of HIV-Infected Patients: Surgical Issues

General

The HIV-infected patient usually presents the surgeon with three clinical problems that relate to the general immunodeficiency of the individual. The surgeon first needs to be aware of the patient's level of immunosuppression because this has the greatest bearing on the patient's outcome. For example, the risk of a complication after treating a patient with HIV and normal CD4 counts who has a perforated appendix is comparable to patients without an HIV infection. The infectious risks in a patient with AIDS (<200 cells/mm^3) are more related to an opportunistic organism associated with severe immunosuppression and not the common pathogens.[32–36] Renal failure and cardiac dysfunction are also problems that arise as a complication of HIV infection. There is a specific HIV-related nephropathy that occurs in up to 10% of HIV-infected patients. The renal disease may also exist as a consequence of other underlying causes such as drug toxicity (pentamidine, foscarnet, and aminoglycosides cause acute tubular necrosis; acyclovir, indinavir, and sulfadiazine cause intratubular obstruction). Until recently the risk of cardiac disease in HIV-infected patients has not been as well documented as renal failure. As HIV-infected patients are living longer, the problems of acquired heart disease have been increasingly appreciated.

The incidence of malignancy has also been increasingly recognized during the past two decades. Initially, AIDS-defining tumors, B-cell lymphoma and Kaposi's sarcoma, were associated with HIV and thought to relate to the immunosuppression of the host. Increasingly large numbers of tumors have been associated with HIV infection, including squamous cancer of the cervix, squamous cell cancer of the anus, and lung cancer. It is believed that at some point after HIV infestation, activation of oncogenes and loss of tumor suppressor genes give rise to microsatellite alterations, which are highly pleomorphic segments of DNA associated with tumor growth. The treatment options for these patients require the input of oncology and infectious disease, as well as surgery. Three principal concerns must be considered when evaluating patients who have both HIV and cancer: first, the HIV infection must be managed; second, the malignant disorder must be treated; and finally the underlying immunodeficiency must be considered in relation to the cancer and the HIV infection. The role of the surgeon in the management of these chronically, and sometimes critically, ill patients includes performing diagnostic biopsies, giving supportive care, and managing complications of malignant or infectious processes. These complications include a number of nonsurgical gastrointestinal problems, such as gonococcal proctitis and a fulminant watery diarrhea caused by *Cryptosporidium*.[32,37]

Pathogenesis of HIV Infection

Identified in 1985, HIV is an RNA virus, belonging to the retrovirus family, with the potential of causing neoplasia. This group of viruses was first identified in 1911 by the American pathologist Rous, who described their association with malignancies in animals.[38] Human T-cell lymphotropic virus type I (HTLV-I), a retrovirus related to HIV, has been identified as causing leukemia in humans.[39]

The unique characteristic of retroviruses, such as HIV and HTLV, is the enzyme reverse transcriptase, which allows the virus to transcribe viral RNA to the host's DNA. The virus can synthesize double-stranded DNA from single-stranded DNA that has been liberated from the RNA–DNA hybrid. This double-stranded DNA inserts itself into the host's nucleus and serves as a template for viral replication. Thus, whenever the infected host cell synthesizes proteins, new HIV particles are reproduced and disseminated in the host. During this process, the virus also kills the cell in which it resides. Because the CD4, or T-helper, cell is targeted by the HIV, loss of this important cell mediator results in the profound immune dysfunction.

Specific Cancer Issues

The association of cancer with AIDS was established with the initial case descriptions in 1981 of immunodeficiency in gay men with Kaposi's sarcoma. Subsequently, intermediate- or high-grade B cell non-Hodgkin's lymphoma was seen with increasing frequency, as was cancer of the cervix uteri. These cancers have subsequently been referred to as AIDS-defining cancers (ADC). Although failing immune function and the development of malignancy appear to be directly related for the ADC, the actual relationship is not that simple.[40–53] For example, cervical cancer has been shown to occur in immunocompetent individuals who are HIV infected (Table 37.5). Other cancers have been seen with increasing frequency in HIV-infected patients, and the specific relationships with immune suppression in still being defined. As yet the data for individual cancers that are not AIDS-defining cancers (NADC) have been evaluated on a limited basis. It is clear that there is an increased risk in HIV patients to develop some form of cancer; however, this risk varies significantly depending on the part of the world where the study was done (see Table 37.6). One interesting trend is that breast cancer is decreased in incidence in HIV-infected patients.

Kaposi's Sarcoma

The incidence of Kaposi's sarcoma has declined since the early 1980s and most dramatically after the introduction of highly active antiretroviral therapy (HAART). The pathogenesis of Kaposi's sarcoma (KS) in immunosuppressed patients became clearly defined in the early 1990s with the discovery of human herpesvirus (HHV-8), which is also known as KS-associated herpesvirus (KSHV). For more than two-thirds of the patients, HAART is sufficient for the treatment of KS. In those patients who do not respond, the clinical management of localized KS is radiation therapy. For the small number of patients (about 5%) with generalized KS who do not respond to HAART therapy with rapidly progressing, life-threatening KS, systemic chemotherapy is used. The combination of the chemotherapy agents bleomycin and vincristine, with or without doxorubicin, is the standard therapy. These patients need to be followed carefully for immunosuppression and maybe also treated with recombinant hematopoietic growth factors to prevent bacterial infections.

TABLE 37.5. AIDS Defining Cancers.

Cancer	*Immune related*
Lymphomas	
NHL	Yes
High grade	Yes
Immunoblastic	Yes
Burkitt	No
Other high grade	No
Intermediate grade	Yes
Low grade	No
Other unspec	Yes
CNS	Yes
Other cancers	
Cervical	No
Kaposi's	Yes

NHL, non-Hodgkin's lymphoma; CNS, central nervous system.

TABLE 37.6. Incidence of Non-AIDS Defining Cancer.

Cancer	*Grulich SIR*[a]	*Herida SIR*[a]	*Frisch SIR*[a]
Study country	Australia	France	United States
Lung	1.4	2	4.5
Hodgkin's	8	31	11.5
Oral pharynx	2.5	1	ND
Lip	ND	ND	3.1
Anus	37	1.1	33
Prostate	1	0.5	.7
Melanoma	1.3	1	1.3
Testis	1.7	ND	2
Breast	1.3	ND	1.1
CNS tumors	1.8	ND	3.5

CNS, central nervous system; ND, not documented.

[a]SIR, Standard Incidence Rates: calculated number of cases in HIV-positive patients compared to the incidence of the general population.

Non-Hodgkin's Lymphoma

In contrast to KS, which has decreased in incidence, especially since the advent of HAART, non-Hodgkin's lymphoma (NHL) has increased. In 1986 the CDC recognized NHL as an AIDS-defining cancer (ADC). These tumors appear most commonly at the end stages of AIDS when patients are most immunosuppressed. NHL is clearly a more difficult entity to manage. Surgeons are involved for lymph node biopsy to obtain adequate tissue sampling for flow cytometry of the lymph node. While the relative risk for acquiring Kaposi's is increased up to 10-fold, the increase of NHL in the HIV population compared to age-matched controls is increased as much as 400-fold for intermediate- and high-grade NHL. It is suspected that the incidence of NHL is tremendously underestimated because a number of central nervous system (CNS) lymphomas are diagnosed only at the time of autopsy and a large number of patients who develop NHL do so at the end stage of their HIV infection and therefore are undocumented. It is suspected that the introduction of HAART, while having reduced the incidence of KS, has not significantly affected the development of NHL. In addition, the treatment for NHL has challenged oncologists because standard chemotherapy more adversely affects patients who are at the end stage of their immunosuppression.

Cancer of the Cervix Uteri

The third type of AIDS-defining malignancy is cervical cancer, associated with chronic human papilloma virus (HPV) infection. Risk factors include multiple sex partners, cigarette smoking, and other sexually transmitted diseases. The highest rates of cervical cancer are found in women who are professional sex workers rather than patients who acquired their HIV infection heterosexually. Clinical management requires heightened surveillance practices and, should a cancer occur, standard therapeutic recommendations for non-HIV-infected patients apply to patients with HIV-associated cervical cancer.

Non-AIDS-Defining Cancers in Patients with HIV Infections

Many data have accrued during the past 8 to 10 years identifying HIV-positive patients to be at greater risk for developing cancers other than the three cancers identified as AIDS-defining malignancies. The data are based on a number called the Standardized Incidence Ratio (SIR), which is the calculated number of cases identified in HIV-positive patients compared to the incidence of the cancer in question based on age- and sex-specific data from the general population. The overall risk of developing a number of different cancers in the presence of HIV is approximately double that of the population at large. The cancers that have been most extensively studied include lung, prostate, Hodgkin's oropharyngeal, anal, melanoma, testis, and CNS cancer.

In some cases the increased rate of cancer is not related to the declining immunity. For example, it is generally believed that the increase in the rate of lung cancer is associated with the 90% use of tobacco in HIV-affected patients. Nearly all lung cancers in the HIV population are adenocarcinoma. However, in the general population lung cancers are evenly divided between oat cell adenocarcinoma and squamous cell carcinoma. The data suggest that HIV disease alone is not the major factor causing the increase in this cancer. Another cancer with a very high incidence in HIV-infected males is anal cancer, which is caused by HPV, which is also associated with genital warts. Studies are now under way to evaluate the efficacy of anal Papanicolaou smears for early detection.

The rates of ADC and NADC have been studied as a function of the patients' CD4 counts. The study was conducted by reviewing registries in the United States. As the CD4 counts fell from progression of HIV disease, the rates of eight cancers were analyzed (see Table 37.5). Falling immune function affected only oropharyngeal cancer rates. Anal cancer was not affected by lowered immune function, and similarly cancer of the cervix uteri was not affected. The relation-ship between failing immune system and development of Hodgkin's disease, however, has been directly documented. Specifically, when T-cell counts fall to less than 300, this is associated with a higher rate of development of Hodgkin's lymphoma.

A prospective analysis of deaths from HIV disease in 2000 in France showed that 28% of all the 964 HIV deaths were related to cancer. NHL was the most common cancer in the patients who died of ADC. A little more than half of the deaths (55%) were caused by ADC, but a surprising 45% were caused by NADC. The most common cause was respiratory cancer, 19% overall, followed by hepatocellular cancer (HCC), 7% overall. The relationship between HCC and HIV disease is understudied: for example, the National Cancer Institute (NCI) study did not even list HCC in its analysis. Because many of the HIV-infected patients are coinfected with HBV and HCV, the risk of HCC in HIV-infected patients will probably be a developing issue to follow.

Miscellaneous Surgical Interventions

Enlarged Spleen

The role of splenectomy in patients with marked splenomegaly or with thrombocytopenia must be individualized. Some believe that coinfections such as HCV play a role in the development of HIV-related immune thrombocytopenia purpura (ITP). Thrombocytopenia occurs in AIDS patients as a result of the circulating immune complex deposition on platelets rather than as a result of a specific antiplatelet antibody.[41,42] Splenectomy has been extremely successful in managing these patients, with a success rate greater than 90%. Occasionally, patients with debilitating fevers associated with significantly enlarged spleens experience dramatic palliation after splenectomy. Some data indicate that splenectomy favors a slower progression of the HIV dissemination and progression to AIDS.[43] In patients with massive splenomegaly and fever, simple splenomegaly is sometimes difficult to distinguish from abscess or parenchymal necrosis. In addition, splenectomy may be indicated in instances in which there is merely a likelihood of injury and in those in which a large spleen compresses the stomach, thereby contributing to the patient's malnutrition.

Implantable Venous Access Devices

A request frequently directed to the general surgeon from the primary care physician, the infectious disease consultant, or the hematologist caring for an AIDS patient is for placement of an indwelling central catheter. Long-term venous access for treating fungal infections or, occasionally, for nutritional support in patients with debilitating diarrhea syndromes can significantly enhance the delivery of care to these patients. However, line placement often occurs when the patient is febrile, as a result of either the underlying infectious problem or treatment with amphotericin B. Therefore, the surgeon should keep a close watch postoperatively to ensure that fevers are not related to an infected catheter. Although the presence of a catheter-related infection is as high as 30%, mortality is not affected.[44] The high rate of infection relates in part to the high incidence of staphylococcus colonization in these patients.

Lymphadenopathy

Another group of HIV-infected patients defined by the CDC includes those with persistent generalized lymphadenopathy, that is, palpable lymphadenopathy measuring more than 1 cm in diameter in at least two extrainguinal sites and persisting for longer than 3 months. Before the availability of HIV antibody testing, the relation of this lymphadenopathy to systemic manifestations of immunosuppression (systemic symptoms, neurological symptoms, secondary infections, or cancers) was not known. It is now clear that lymphadenopathy is part of the general clinical spectrum associated with HIV infection, and that opportunistic infection, Kaposi's sarcoma, or large cell lymphoma will develop in some, if not all, lymphadenopathy patients. The precise reason why lymphadenopathy occurs in some but not all patients who acquire HIV infection is not known.

The role of lymph node biopsy in these patients is currently of academic interest only since the development of serological tests to diagnose HIV infection.[54] The histological appearance of a clinically enlarged lymph node has prognostic value (see following); however, when the decision whether to perform a lymph node biopsy is being made, the value of the biopsy findings must be weighed against the value of the information that can be obtained by means of clinical staging with lymphocyte helper:suppressor T-cell ratios and total lymphocyte counts. The total number of helper T cells in the circulation has been correlated with the risk of AIDS in patients with generalized lymphadenopathy[55–58]; the Walter Reed classification provides the most detailed clinical staging system.[57,58] Should the clinical condition warrant, a lymph node biopsy may help in the diagnosis of an opportunistic infection. Performing a gallium scan to locate the most suspicious node[54,59] can enhance the yield of the biopsy.

Once a lymph node is removed from an HIV-infected patient and before the tissue is removed from the operative field, the surgeon should place representative specimens in sterile containers for routine bacterial culture, culture, and smear for tuberculosis, fungal culture, and viral culture. Tissue from the same lymph node should then be delivered to the pathologist as quickly as possible. It is important that culture material from the same lymph node be examined microscopically because granulomas or actual organisms may be detected before the culture results are available. Data from the pathologist may aid the microbiology laboratory staff in its handling of the cultures.

The pathologist needs to receive the fresh, gently handled specimen, in saline, as soon after the biopsy as possible for two important reasons. First, because the tissue is not in formalin, it will rapidly autolyze if not processed immediately. Second, the pathologist must have the tissue when it is fresh to perform lymphocyte marker studies if the diagnosis is lymphoma. Because different lymphomas respond to different chemotherapeutic regimens, the cell type of the lymphoma is critical. Most surgical pathology laboratories are equipped to perform membrane marker studies on lymph node tissue.

Gastrointestinal Diseases

Cryptosporidiosis and cytomegalovirus infection of the biliary tree have been reported to cause both acute cholecystitis and acute cholangitis, necessitating emergency surgical interventions. It is suggested that choledochoenteric bypass provides the best palliation in these patients. It is not known, however, whether the biliary tree is ever cleared of the infectious pathogens. *Candida* infection and Kaposi's sarcoma have also caused cholangitis, necessitating bypass surgery.[34] Because the gallbladder can be infected with a variety of unusual pathogens in more than 50% of HIV-infected patients, the gallbladder wall should be sent for culture and the pathologist should be alerted to process the tissue with special stains.[60,61]

Acute perforations of the gastrointestinal tract from cytomegalovirus infection, cryptosporidiosis, and candidiasis, as well as from necrotic lymphoma, have been reported.[35,46,47] Obstruction of the gastrointestinal tract caused by Kaposi's sarcoma or lymphoma may also be an indication for resection, bypass, or colostomy. One study of AIDS patients requiring a laparotomy identified four distinct clinical syndromes that called for surgical intervention: (1) peritonitis secondary to cytomegalovirus enterocolitis and perforation, (2) non-Hodgkin's lymphoma of the gastrointestinal tract (usually the terminal ileum), presenting as obstruction or bleeding, (3) Kaposi's sarcoma of the gastrointestinal tract, and (4) mycobacterial infection of the retroperitoneum or the spleen.[62]

Another gastrointestinal lesion that has been increasingly associated with homosexual men who are HIV infected is squamous cell carcinoma of the anus (SCCA). It is estimated that the risk of developing SCCA is nearly 25 times greater in the HIV-infected homosexual male than in the population in general. The underlying relationship is not well understood because the development is not related to the time of the HIV infection. Some believe that human papilloma virus 16 and human papilloma 18 are important cofactors in the evolution of SCCA.[63,64]

References

1. Ippolito G, Puro V, DeCarli G. The risk of occupational human immunodeficiency virus infection in healthcare workers. Italian Multicenter Study. The Italian Study Group on Occupational Risk of Human Immunodeficiency Virus. Arch Intern Med 1993;153:1451–1458.
2. Gerberding J. Management of occupational exposure to blood-borne virus. N Engl J Med 1995;332:444–451.
3. Update: acquired immunodeficiency syndrome United States, 1981–1988. MMWR 1989;38:229.
4. Gerberding JL. Clinical practice. Occupational exposure to human immunodeficiency virus in healthcare settings. N Engl J Med 2003;348:826–833.
5. Bassett IV, Freedberg SA, Walensky DP. Two drugs or three? Balancing efficacy, toxicity, and resistance in post-exposure prophylaxis or occupational exposure to HIV. Clin Infect Dis 2004;39:395–401.
6. Sterilization, disinfection, and antisepsis in the hospital. In: Lenette EH, Balows A, Hausler W, et al, eds. Manual of Clinical Microbiology, 4th ed. Washington, DC: American Society for Microbiology, 1985:129.
7. http//www.gov/oppad001/pdf_files/workplan.2005.pdf.
8. Jawetz EMJ, Adelberg EA. Antimicrobial chemotherapy. In: Review of Medical Microbiology, 15th ed. Los Altos: Lange Medical, 1982:117.
9. Dodd RY, Notari EP, Stammer SL. Current prevalence and incidence of infectious disease markers and estimated window period risk in the American Red Cross blood donor population. Transfusion 2002;42:975.
10. Ho DD, Byington RE, Schooley RT, et al. Frequency of isolation of HTLV-III virus from saliva in AIDS. N Engl J Med 1985; 313:1606.
11. Morgan J, Nolan J. Risks of AIDS with artificial insemination. N Engl J Med 1986;314:386.
12. Recommendations for prevention of HIV transmission in health-care settings. MMWR 1987;36(suppl 2S):1.
13. Guidelines for prevention of transmission of human immunodeficiency virus and hepatitis B virus to health-care and public-safety workers. MMWR 1989;38(suppl S-6):1.
14. Update: acquired immunodeficiency syndrome and human immunodeficiency virus infection among health-care workers. MMWR 1988;37:229.

15. Recommendations for preventing transmission of FHV and HBV to patients during exposure-prone invasive procedures. MMWR 1991;40(suppl RR-8):1.
16. Braathen LR, Ramirez G, Kunze RO, et al. Langerhans cells as primary target cells for HIV infection (letter). Lancet 1987;2:1094.
17. McCray E. Occupational risk of the acquired immunodeficiency syndrome among health care workers. N Engl J Med 1986;314:1127.
18. Gerberding JL, Littell C, Tarkington A, et al. Risk of exposure of surgical personnel to patients' blood during surgery at San Francisco General Hospital. N Engl J Med 1990;322:1788.
19. Quebbeman EJ, Telford GL, Wadsworth K, et al. Double gloving: protecting surgeons from blood contamination in the operating room. Arch Surg 1992;127:213.
20. Tanner J, Parker H. Double-gloving to reduce surgical cross-infection. Cochrane Database Syst Rev 2005;I.
21. Gerbert B, Maguire BT, Hulley SB, Coates TJ. Physicians and acquired immunodeficiency syndrome: what patients think about human immunodeficiency virus in medical practice. JAMA 1989;262:1969.
22. Gerberding JL. Clinical practice. Occupational exposure to HIV in health care setting. N Engl J Med 2003;348:826–833.
23. Summary: recommendations for preventing transmission of infection with human T-lymphotropic virus type III/lymphadenopathy-associated virus in the workplace. MMWR 1985; 34:681.
24. Harpaz R, Seidlein L von, Averhoff FM, et al. Transmission of hepatitis B virus to multiple patients from a surgeon without evidence of inadequate infection control. N Engl J Med 1996;334:549–554.
25. The CDC Cooperative Needlestick Surveillance Group. Surveillance of health care workers exposed to blood from patients infected with the human immunodeficiency virus. N Engl J Med 1988;319:1118.
26. Panlilio AL, Shapiro CN, Schable CA, et al. Serosurvey of HIV, HBV, HCV infection among hospital-based surgeons. J Am Coll Surg 1995;180:16.
27. Apparent transmission of human T-lymphotropic virus type III/lymphadenopathy-associated virus from a child to a mother providing health care. MMWR 1996;35:76–79.
28. Edlin BR, Irwin KL, Faruque S, et al. Intersecting epidemics: crack cocaine use and HIV infection among inner-city young adults. N Engl J Med 1994;331:1422–1427.
29. Public Health Service. Recommendations for Donor Screening with a Licensed Test for HIV-I Antigen. U.S. Department of Health and Human Services. Rockville, MD: Food and Drug Administration, 1995.
30. U.S. Public Health Service guidelines for testing and counseling blood and plasma donors for human immunodeficiency virus type I antigen. MMWR 1996;45(R-22):1.
31. Persistent lack of detectable HIV-I antibody in a person with HIV infections, Utah, 1995. MMWR 1996;45:182.
32. Sexually transmitted diseases. In: Rubenstein FD, ed. Scientific American Medicine, section 7, subsection XXII. New York: Scientific American, 1990.
33. Margulis SJ, Honig CL, Soave R, et al. Biliary tract obstruction in the acquired immunodeficiency syndrome. Ann Intern Med 1986;105:207.
34. Robinson G, Wilson SE, Williams RA. Surgery in patients with acquired immunodeficiency syndrome. Arch Surg 1987; 122:170.
35. Barone JE, Gingold BS, Nealon TF, Arvnatis ML. Abdominal pain in patients with acquired immune deficiency syndrome. Ann Surg 1986;204:619–623.
36. Davis JM, Mouradian J, Fernandez RJ, et al. Acquired immune deficiency syndromes surgical perspective. Arch Surg 1984;119:90.
37. Rubin R. Acquired immunodeficiency syndrome. In: Rubenstein FD, ed. Scientific American Medicine, section 7, subsection XXII. New York: Scientific American, 1990.
38. Rous P. Transmission of a malignant growth by means of cell-free filtrate. JAMA 1911;56:198.
39. Robert-Guroff M, Nakao Y, Notake K, et al. Natural antibodies to human retrovirus HTLV in a cluster of Japanese patients with adult T-cell leukemia. Science 1982;215:975.
40. Martin F, Grulich E, Johanseman AC. Cancer in the population-based cohort of men and women registered homosexual partners. Am J Epidemiol 2003;157:966–972.
41. Chiao E, Krown S. Update on non-acquired immunodeficiency syndrome defining malignancies. Curr Opin Oncol 2003;15:389–397.
42. Berretta M, Cinelli R, Martoletto F, Sbina M, Baccatr E, Tirelli U. Therapeutic approaches to AIDS-related malignancy. Oncogene 2003;22:6646–6659.
43. Tsoukas CM, Bernard NF, Abrahamowicz M. Effect of splenectomy on slowing human immunodeficiency virus disease progression. Arch Surg 1998;133:25–31.
44. Dega H, Eliaszewicz M, Gisselbrecht M, et al. Infections associated with totally implantable venous access devices (TIVAD) in human immunodeficiency virus-infected patients. J AIDS Hum Retrovirol 1996;13:146–154.
45. Frisch M, Biggar R, Engles E, Goedert J. Association of cancer with AIDS-related immunosupression in adults, JAMA 2002;285:1736–1745.
46. Grulich AE, Li Y, McDonald A, Correll PKL, Law M, Kalgor JM. Rates of non-AIDS-defining cancers in people with HIV infection before and after AIDS diagnosis. AIDS 2002;16:1155–1161.
47. Hoffman C, Wolf E, Fatkenheuer G, et al. Response to highly active retroviral therapy strongly predicts outcome in patients with AIDS-related lymphoma. AIDS 2003;17:1521–1529.
48. Mbulaiteye S, Biggar R, Goedert J, Engel E. Immune deficiency and risk of malignancy among persons with AIDS. J AIDS 2003;32:527–533.
49. Herida M, Mary-Kraus M, Kaphan R, et al. Incidence of non-AIDS defining cancers before and during the highly active retroviral therapy era in a cohort of human immunodeficiency virus-infected patients. J Clin Oncol 2003;21:3447–3453.
50. Sriplung H, Parkin D. Trends in the incidence of immunodeficiency syndrome-related malignancies in Thailand. Cancer (Phila) 2004;101:2660–2666.
51. Shahul E, Abdullah A, McKenna M, Hamers F. AIDS-defining cancers in Western Europe, 1994–2001. AIDS Patient Care 2004;18:501–508.
52. Bonnet F, Lewden C, May T, et al. Malignancy-related causes of death in human immunodeficiency virus-infected patients in the era of highly active retroviral therapy. Cancer (Phila) 2004;101:317–324.
53. Morton F, Biggar R, Engels E, Goedert J. Association of cancer with AIDS-related immunosuppression in adults. JAMA 2001;35:1736–1745.
54. Nugent P, O'Connell TX. The surgeon's role in treating acquired immunodeficiency syndrome. Arch Surg 1986;121:1117–1120.
55. Kaplan JE, Spira TJ, Fishbein DB, Pinsky PF, Schonberger LB. Lymphadenopathy syndrome in homosexual men: evidence for continuing risk of developing the acquired immunodeficiency syndrome. JAMA 1987;257:335.
56. Goedert JJ, Biggar RJ, Melbye M, et al. Effect of T4 count and cofactors on the incidence of AIDS in homosexual men infected with human immunodeficiency virus. JAMA 1987;257:331.
57. Redfield RR, Burke DS. HIV infection: the clinical picture. Sci Am 1988;259:70–78.
58. Redfield RR, Wright DC, Tramont EC. The Walter Reed staging classification for HTLV-IIII/LAV infection. N Engl J Med 1986;314: 131–132.

59. Fernandez R, Mouradian J. Metroka C, et al. The prognostic value of histopathology in persistent generalized lymphadenopathy in homosexual men. N Engl J Med 1983;309:185.
60. French AL, Beaudet LM, Benator DA, et al. Cholecystectomy in patients with AIDS: clinicopathologic correlations in 107 cases. Clin Infect Dis 1995;21:852–858.
61. Kavin H, Jonas RB, Chowdhury L, et al. Acalculous cholecystitis and cytomegalovirus infection in the acquired immunodeficiency syndrome. Ann Intern Med 1986;104:53–54.
62. Wilson SE, Robinson G, Williams RA, et al. Acquired immune deficiency syndrome (AIDS): indications for abdominal surgery, pathology, and outcome. Ann Surg 1989;210:428.
63. Benator DA, French AL, Beaudet LM, et al. Isospora belli infection associated with acalculous cholecystitis in a patient with AIDS. Ann Intern Med 1994;121:663–664.
64. Lorenz HP, Wilson W, Leigh B, et al. Squamous cell carcinoma of the anus and HIV infection. Dis Colon Rectum 1991;34:336–338.

38

Evidence-Based Bariatric Surgery

John Morton

Obesity as a Global Epidemic

An obesity epidemic exists throughout the developed and much of the developing world.[1–4] Obesity, typically measured as body mass index (BMI) of 30 kg/m^2 or higher, has three subclasses: obesity 1 (30–34.9); obesity 2 (35–39.9); and extreme obesity (>40). Extreme or morbid obesity is increasing particularly rapidly in the United States and may have the potential of decreasing life expectancy.[5–7] From 1986 to 2000, the prevalence of BMI of 30 or more doubled, whereas that of BMI of 40 or more quadrupled, and even extreme obesity, BMI of 50 or more, increased fivefold.[2] Of particular concern is the alarming increasing prevalence of obesity among children, suggesting that the epidemic will worsen before it improves.[1]

In the United States, 32% of adults and 17% of children and adolescents are classified as obese.[1,8] When tracked over time, there has been a slow but steady rise in the percent of Americans classified as obese over the past several decades. Between 1980 and 2002, obesity prevalence doubled in adults aged 20 years or older, and obesity prevalence tripled in children and adolescents aged 6 to 19 years. However, over time there has also been a distinctively greater increase in the growth rates for the higher weight (BMI) categories. For instance, between the mid-1980s and 2000, the prevalence of BMI of 40 or greater quadrupled from about 1 in 200 adult Americans to 1 in 50. At the same time, those individuals with BMI of 50 or greater were five times more common in America, from about 1 in 2000 in the year 1985 to 1 in 400 in the year 2000.

Other countries have also witnessed rising rates of obesity, including Canada. In the adult Canadian population, the prevalence of obesity was 6% in 1985, increasing to 15% by 1998.[9] Indeed, worldwide, there are some 300 million obese people, a problem seen not only in industrialized countries but in developing nations also.[4]

Importantly, the prevalence of morbid obesity (BMI of 40 or more) in 2003–2004 was estimated to be 2.8% in men and 6.9% in women, based on nationally representative sampling.[1] Based on the 2004 U.S. adult population of 103 million men and 109 million women (http://www.census.gov/popest/national/asrh/NC-EST2004-sa.html; accessed December 2006), there were approximately 2.9 million men and 7.5 million women (totaling 10.4 million people) with morbid obesity in America in 2004. Other estimates indicate that more than 1 million adolescents and young adults may be affected with extreme obesity.[10] Because comorbidities and resulting healthcare expenditures are much higher among morbidly obese individuals, these trends warrant special attention and serious consideration of effective interventions, such as bariatric surgery.[11,12]

Obesity: Comorbidities and Mortality

Epidemiological studies have demonstrated that increasing BMI is a causative factor in many life-threatening comorbidities, including type 2 diabetes, cardiovascular disease, and cancer. Body mass index has been established as an independent risk factor for premature mortality (Fig. 38.1).[6,13] Obesity

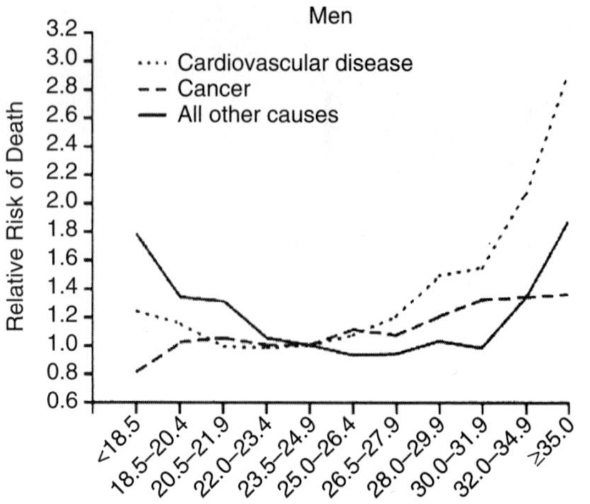

FIGURE 38.1. Body mass index has been established as an independent risk factor for premature mortality. (From Calle EE, Thun MJ, Petrelli JM,[5] by permission of New England Journal of Medicine.)

is a major independent risk factor for the development of type 2 diabetes and has caused the rapid increase in the prevalence of type 2 diabetes.[2] In the United States, the majority diagnosed with type 2 diabetes are overweight, with 50% obese (i.e., BMI >30 kg/m^2) and 9% morbidly obese (BMI >40 kg/m^2).[5] This twin epidemic of obesity and diabetes carries severe consequence for premature mortality.[14,15]

With the increase in the prevalence of obesity comes an accompanied increase in the comorbid diseases and conditions attributable to obesity. Obesity adversely impacts every organ system in the human body, contributing to organ dysfunction, disability, and excess mortality.

Obesity is an independent risk factor for cardiovascular disease[16–18] as well as contributing to increased risk through its effect on other known risk factors such as hypertension, diabetes, hyperlipidemia, inflammatory markers, and a prothrombotic state. Hypertension is about six times more frequent in the obese compared to lean men and women,[18] and in the Framingham study, excess weight accounted for 40% to 70% of the occurrence of hypertension.[18] A 10-kg increase in weight is associated with a 3.0 mmHg increase in systolic blood pressure and a 2.3 mmHg increase in diastolic blood pressure, which translates into a 12% increased risk for coronary heart disease (CHD) and a 24% increased rate for stroke.[18] Diabetes is an established risk factor for CHD, and excess weight accounts for an estimated 70% of the diabetes risk in the United States. Modest weight loss results in an improvement in diabetes and insulin resistance. A study of diabetics by Lean et al. suggested that each kilogram of weight loss was associated with 3 to 4 months of extra survival.[12] Dyslipidemia, another major risk factor for CHD, is also increased in obesity. The prevalence of elevated cholesterol is 22% in obese men and 27% in obese women, compared to 13% in adults who are not overweight.[8] The lipid profile observed in the obese is particularly harmful, with elevated fasting triglycerides, low high density lipoprotein (HDL) cholesterol, and increased atherogenic small, dense, low density lipoprotein (LDL) cholesterol.[19]

Numerous respiratory conditions are associated with obesity, including asthma, obstructive sleep apnea, pulmonary hypertension, and the obesity-hypoventilation syndrome. The prevalence of sleep-disordered breathing rises dramatically in obese subjects.[20] Left ventricular hypertrophy, pulmonary hypertension, and CHD risk factors all contribute to an increased risk of congestive heart failure in the morbidly obese, as well as increased risk of fatal arrhythmias.[16]

Higher BMI is associated with increased mortality from cancers of the esophagus, colon, liver, gallbladder, pancreas, and kidney, as well as cancers of the stomach and prostate in men and cancers of the breast, uterus, cervix, and ovaries in women.[5] Men with a BMI of 40 or more had a 52% higher death rate from cancer and women a 62% higher death rate compared to individuals of normal weight.

Obesity increases the risk of death 50% to 100% from all causes compared to normal weight individuals, as well as increasing the mortality risk from cardiovascular disease.[5] Young white men with a BMI of 45 or more have a 13-year reduction in life expectancy, with a 20-year reduction in young black males.[10]

Numerous other diseases and conditions are increased in obese individuals that may adversely impact quality of life and activities of daily living, including gastroesophageal reflux, venous insufficiency, urinary incontinence, osteoarthritis and back pain, pseudotumor cerebri, menstrual irregularities and infertility, and nonalcoholic liver disease.[21–24]

Nonmedical Consequences of Obesity

Obesity has a major impact on individuals as well as society as a whole, beyond the direct effects of obesity related comorbid disease. The Nurses Health Study demonstrated that weight gain over a 4-year period was associated with decreased physical function in middle-aged and older women, as well as reduced vitality and increased bodily pain.[25] Obesity results in limitations in activities of daily living compared to normal weight individuals.[22] Psychosocial consequences of obesity include fewer years of education, lower family income, and higher poverty rates. Obese patients are subjected to social rejection, negative stereotyping, and discrimination. Numerous studies have demonstrated lower self-esteem and a more negative body image in obese children and adolescents. Adults seeking treatment for obesity demonstrate a fourfold increase in prevalence of childhood sexual abuse and a twofold increase in nonsexual abuse.[26]

Costs to society attributable to obesity include healthcare expenses and loss of productivity. In 1995, the societal cost of obesity was estimated to be $99.2 billion in the United States.[11] Because of the increased prevalence of obesity and inflation since 1995, current estimates approach $200 billion, surpassing the economic costs of cigarette smoking.

Medical Treatment of Obesity

Tremendous resources are expended on diets and weight reduction plans, with $30 billion annually spent on commercial weight loss programs alone.[11] Unfortunately, there is no evidence demonstrating long-term success with medical, pharmacological, diet, exercise, and behavioral therapies. The majority of reported trials consist of short-term studies ranging from 10 weeks to 1 year, with an average weight loss of less than 15 kg.[27] Combined diet and behavior modification programs appear to provide the greatest benefit, although results in the severely obese remain poor. Sustained weight reduction requires lifelong behavior modification, and weight regain after completion of a dietary/behavior modification program occurs in the majority of severely obese individuals. Weight regain in the morbidly obese after dieting is not a lack of willpower or moral failure. Postdieting weight regain in the morbidly obese may be attributed to physiological drives such as an increase in ghrelin, the appetite hormone.[28]

A regular exercise program has been demonstrated to be essential for maintaining weight loss. NIH/NHLBI guidelines state that weight loss and weight maintenance therapy should employ the combination of low-calorie diets, increased physical activity, and behavior therapy. Weight loss drugs may be used as part of a comprehensive weight loss program for patients with a BMI of 30 or more and for patients with a BMI of 27 or more with concomitant obesity-related risk factors or diseases.[29] Dietary and behavior therapy, along with physical activity, must be continued indefinitely for maintenance of weight loss.[30,31]

Medications currently available for the treatment of obesity include phentermine, orlistat, sibutramine, and, the most recent, rimonabant.[32] Although these agents appear to improve the results of dietary and behavioral therapy, the degree of weight reduction is inadequate in severely obese patients, and weight regain is typical following the cessation of pharmacotherapy.[30] In addition, all weight reduction therapies require lifelong use given that obesity is a chronic disease. Even short-term use of any medication may carry risk, as evidenced by the cautionary tale of Fen-Phen.[33] Despite the poor long-term results of nonsurgical weight loss programs, attempts at weight reduction should be encouraged in all overweight or obese patients. Even a modest weight reduction (5%–10%) produces significant health benefits with regard to blood glucose, blood pressure, and lipid profiles.[12]

Surgical Patient Selection

The indications for gastrointestinal surgery for severe obesity were outlined in the 1991 NIH Consensus Development Statement.[34] Candidates for operative intervention should have a BMI greater than 40 kg/m^2 or a BMI greater than 35 kg/m^2 when associated with comorbid conditions. Sleep apnea, diabetes mellitus, hypertension, and functional impairments limiting employment or activities of daily living are the more common indications in patients with a BMI between 35 and 40 kg/m^2. The two operations recommended by the 1991 NIH Consensus Conference on Surgery for Morbid Obesity are gastric bypass and vertical banded gastroplasty. In addition, the consensus panel recommended that a surgeon with substantial experience with the appropriate procedure should perform the surgery, working in a clinical setting capable of supporting all aspects of management and assessment. Lifelong medical surveillance after the surgical procedure is necessary.[34] There have been calls to update the 1991 NIH Consensus Conference given the newer procedures, increased clinical evidence, and the long-term efficacy and complications associated with vertical banded gastroplasty. Evaluations of the benefits of surgically induced weight loss must be balanced by the potential risk of surgery.

The NIH panel did not give recommendations regarding bariatric surgery in adolescents because of the insufficient study in this population. The increasing epidemic of childhood obesity as well as mounting evidence of the effectiveness of bariatric surgery in the pediatric population has led to a reappraisal of this topic.[35] Current guidelines suggest that bariatric surgery may be considered in adolescents with a BMI of 50 kg/m^2 or more or a BMI of 40 or more with associated comorbidities. In addition, patients should have attained or nearly attained physical maturity, demonstrate decisional capacity, be willing and capable of adhering to nutritional guidelines, and have a supportive family environment.[35]

Medical Versus Surgical Treatment of Morbid Obesity

Weight loss surgery has existed since 1954, highlighting the chronic need for effective therapy for the morbidly obese. All weight loss surgeries can be generally grouped into three categories: restrictive, malabsorptive, or a combination of the two.

Restrictive weight loss surgery relies on the premise that limiting volume of food intake will lead to lesser caloric intake. Restrictive weight loss procedures consist of vertical banded gastroplasty, adjustable gastric banding, and sleeve gastrectomy. Malabsorptive procedures include jejenual-ileal bypass, biliopancreatic diversion, and duodenal switch operations. Malabsorptive operations engender weight loss through less absorption of calories as a result of a shorter common channel of both digestive enzymes and food flow. A combined restrictive and malabsorptive operation includes Roux-en-Y gastric bypass (RNYGB). There are data from a few randomized trials to support indications for which type of surgery is most appropriate (Tables 38.1, 38.2). In addition, there are varying degrees of medical evidence and long-term outcomes for each procedure.[36–38] However, there is a clear preponderance of evidence for all weight loss surgeries to be greatly superior to traditional weight loss therapies in promoting weight reduction and resolution of comorbidities such as diabetes (Table 38.3).[36–41] These sterling results and the lack of an alternative have no doubt contributed to the tremendous growth seen in bariatric surgery (Figs. 38.2, 38.3). In the United States, the leading operation performed for weight loss is gastric bypass, whereas in the rest of the world, adjustable gastric banding is most frequently performed[42,43] (Table 38.4). Given the effectiveness of bariatric surgery, surgical management of morbid obesity has grown tremendously. In the year 2002–2003, worldwide 146,301 bariatric surgery operations were performed by 2,839 bariatric surgeons, and 103,000 of these operations were performed in the United States and Canada by 850 surgeons.[3]

The comparative trials that have been performed for medical versus surgical management for morbid obesity are few but telling. The Program on the Surgical Control of the Hyperlipidemias (POSCH) trial randomized patients to either medical management or the jejenual-ileal bypass (JIB) with modification of serum lipids as the primary endpoint.[40] Although the JI bypass is no longer performed because of concerns about liver deterioration, the results from the trial are striking, with significant reductions in both lipid profiles and mortality.[40] Christou et al. also found a decided advantage

TABLE 38.1.
Comparative Surgical Trials, 1977–1989.

Level of evidence	*Trial*	*Outcome*
I	Griffen (1977)[44] RNYGB (R) vs. JIB (J)	Complications 62.5 (R) vs. 48 (J)% 75% progression of liver disease with JIB
I	Laws (1980)[45] RNYGB (R) vs. horizontal gastroplasty (H)	35% (R) vs. 16% (H) reduction in original body weight
I	Pories (1982)[46] RNYGB (R) vs. (H)	40% (R) vs. 20% (H) reduction in original body weight
I	Naslund (1986)[48] RNYGB (R) vs. gastroplasty (G)	RNYGB with increased weight loss and complications
I	Sugerman (1986)[49] RNYGB (R) vs. VBG (V)	% EWL, 68% (R) vs. 43% (V)
I	Andersen (1989)[47] VBG (V) vs. H	Weight loss: VBG > H

RNYGB, Roux-en-Y gastrointestinal bypass; JIB, jejeunal-ileal bypass; VBG, vertical banded gastroplasty; HG, horizontal gastroplasty; EWL, excess weight loss.

for surgery in the management of morbid obesity.[41] In this study, morbidly obese patients in the province of Quebec were followed through all levels of care including clinic visits. Surgically treated morbidly obese patients were matched by age, gender, and comorbidity to medically managed patients. At 5 years, huge reductions in healthcare utilization, costs, and mortality were found. In this Quebec study, an 89% mortality risk reduction was demonstrated.

A well-designed randomized clinical trial between laparoscopic adjustable gastric banding and traditional medical management for morbid obesity also found a similar decided advantage for bariatric surgery over medical management.[39] In this study, 80 adults with mild to moderate obesity (BMI, 30–35 kg/m^2) were randomized to nonsurgical intervention (VLCD [very low carbohydrate diet], orlistat, and lifestyle change) or to surgical intervention (gastric banding); surgical treatment was statistically significantly more effective than nonsurgical therapy in reducing weight, resolving the metabolic syndrome, and improving quality of life during a 24-month treatment program. At 2-year follow-up, laparoscopic adjustable gastric banding achieved a remarkable 87% excess weight loss in contrast to a 22% excess weight loss for traditional medical management.

The Swedish Obese Subjects (SOS) study also found very favorable results for bariatric surgery.[36] With 12-year follow-up, percent weight change for surgically treated patients was a 23% decrease in contrast to 1.6% weight increase for medically managed patients. Differences in surgical techniques, as detailed later, also resulted in differences in outcomes.

TABLE 38.2.
Comparative Surgical Trials, 1989–2006.

Level of evidence	*Trial*	*Outcome*
I	Hall (1990)[50] Adelaide study HG vs. VG vs. RNYGB	3 years, % EWL > 50 HG, 17% VG, 48% RNYGB, 67%
II	Weber (2004)[51] LRNYGB vs. LAP-BAND	2 years, % EWL 54 (R) vs. 42 (LB)
II	Sjostrom (2004)[36] RNYGB vs. VBG vs. LB	10 years, % weight change 25.1%, RNYGB 16.5%, VBG 13.2%, LB
I	Olbers (2006)[55] LRNYGB vs. LAP VBG	1 year, % EWL 78% (R) vs. 63% (V)
I	Nilsell (2001)[53] Lap-Band (LB) vs. LAP VBG (V)	Weight loss, kg 43 (LB) vs. 35 (V)
I	Morino (2003)[54] Lap-Band (LB) vs. LAP VBG (V)	3 years, % EWL 39% (LB) vs. 59% (V) Late complications 33% (LB) vs. 14% (V)
II	Skroubis (2006)[52] RNYGB vs. BPD	2 years, % EWL 72% (R) vs. 83% (BPD)

LAP, laparoscopy; BPD, biliopancreatic diversion.

TABLE 38.3.
Medical Versus Surgical Treatment of Obesity.

Level of evidence	*Trial*	*Outcome*
I	O'Brien (2006)[39] Medical treatment (MT) vs. laposcopic adjustable gastric banding (LB)	% EWL, 2 years 21.8% (MT) vs. 87.2% (LB)
I	Buchwald (2004)[37] POSCH (diet vs. JIB)	18-year follow-up 20% mortality reduction with surgery
II	Christou (2004)[41] Quebec study RNYGB vs. control	5-year follow-up 89% mortality reduction with surgery
II	Sjostrom (2004)[36] Medical (MT) vs. surgical treatment (ST)	% EWL, 12 years 0.15% increase (MT) vs. 23.4% decrease (ST)

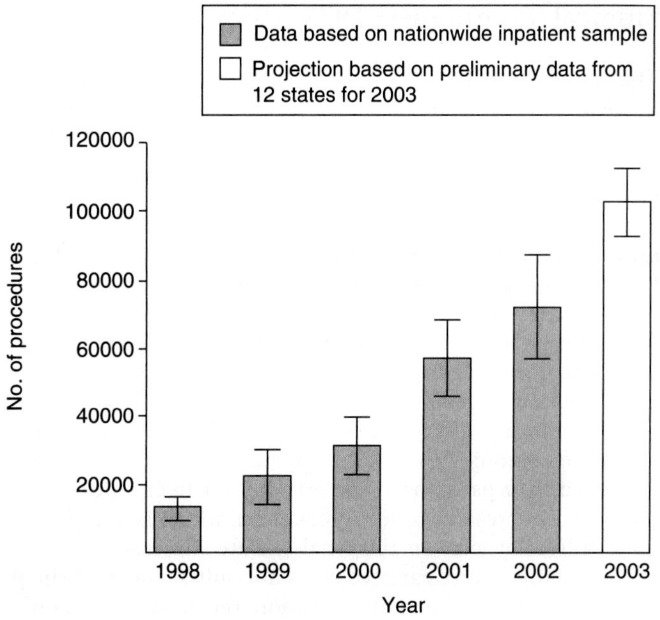

FIGURE 38.2. National trends in annual numbers of bariatric procedures from 1998 to 2003. (From Santry HP, Gillen DL, Lauderdale DS,[42] by permission of Journal of the American Medical Association.)

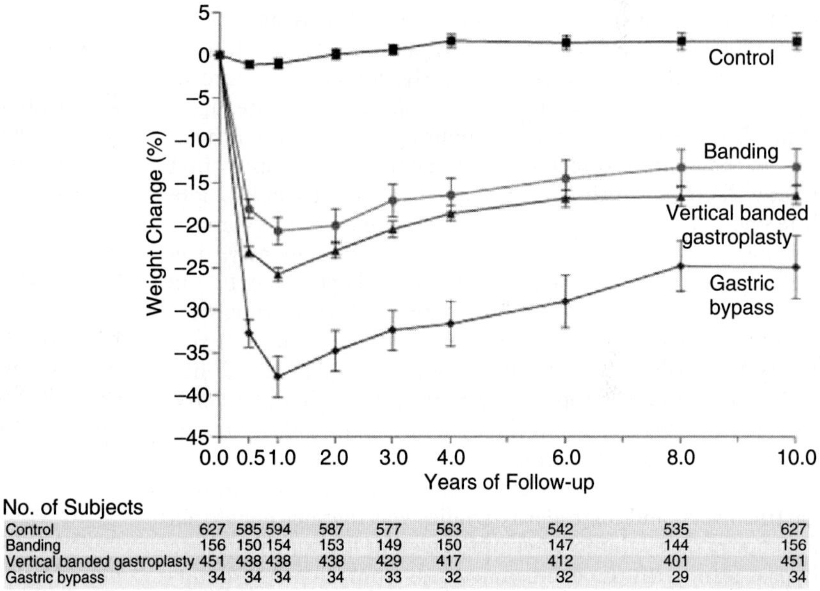

FIGURE 38.3. Percent of weight change by procedure. (From Sjostrom L, Lindroos AK, Peltonen M, et al.,[36] by permission of New England Journal of Medicine.)

TABLE 38.4. Types of Bariatric Surgical Procedures Performed in the United States from 1998 to 2002 Based on Data from the Nationwide Inpatient Sample.

	No. (%) of procedures					
Procedure type	*1998*	*1999*	*2000*	*2001*	*2002*	*P value for trend*[a]
Gastric bypass	10,675 (79.9)	20,421 (89.5)	27,497 (88.5)	48,507 (85.4)	63,538 (88.0)	0.27
Gastroplasty[b]	3,296 (24.7)	2,097 (9.2)	4,357 (14.0)	6,247 (11.0)	5,369 (7.4)	0.01
Malabsorptive[c]	990 (7.4)	1,277 (5.6)	3,684 (11.9)	4,732 (8.3)	7,495 (10.4)	0.64
Gastrectomy[d]	258 (1.9)	721 (3.2)	495 (1.6)	2,186 (3.8)	3,082 (4.3)	0.30
Other^	43 (0.3)	31 (0.1)	70 (0.2)	303 (0.5)	1,446 (1.9)	0.13
Total no. of procedures	13,365	22,809	31,082	56,781	72,177	<0.001

The numbers in the columns do not add up becasue they are survey-weighted estimates.

[a]In the proportion of total procedures.

[b]Includes vertical banded gastroplasty and adjustable gastric banding.

[c]Includes duodenal switch, pancreatic diversion, and isolated intestinal bypass.

[d]Includes sleeve gastrectomy and any isolated partial gastrectomy.

[e]Includes gastric bubble insertion and nonspecified stomach procedures.

Source: From Santry HP, Gillen DL, Lauderdale DS,[42] by permission of JAMA.

Surgical Techniques: 1977–1989

The gains seen in bariatric surgery have resulted from lessons learned via previous experience. Bariatric surgery has been a fertile area for investigation regarding its efficacy and indication. Early comparative trials (1977–1989) had several long-lasting implications (see Table 38.2).[44–50] A landmark study comparing jejenual-ileal (JI) and gastric bypass found a significant increase in liver complications with the JI bypass.[44] Liver pathology worsened in many JI bypass patients to the stage of cirrhosis. A lingering misconception regarding the deterioration of hepatic function after a JI bypass is that the cause for the derangement was rapid weight loss. Griffen et al.[44] demonstrated that weight loss per se was not the cause of liver failure given that gastric bypass did not cause worsened liver pathology in this comparative trial but actually improved liver pathology. The etiology for liver failure after JI bypass is increased oxalate production, which is manifested in both liver deposition and renal oxalate stones.

These initial comparative trials not only repudiated the JI bypass but also called into question the other commonly performed weight loss procedure in the 1970s and 1980s, the horizontal and vertical gastroplasty. Several randomized controlled trials asserted the primacy of the Roux-en-Y gastric bypass over gastroplasty.[45–49] Better weight loss and fewer revisions were noted with gastric bypass in comparison with gastroplasty. A key component for the long-term failure of gastroplasty is the dubious reliance of the procedure upon staple lines remaining intact without transaction. It has been shown that a nontransected staple line in the gastrointestinal tract will open over time.[50] This fact of a nontransected staple line opening over time is actually an implicit component of a pyloric exclusion for duodenal trauma. Consequently, it is not surprising that the gastroplasty may fail over time. In one comparative trial between horizontal and vertical gastroplasty, better weight loss was seen with the vertical gastroplasty.[47] This difference in weight loss is caused by the ability of the horizontal gastroplasty to distend more than the vertical gastroplasty, given that the horizontal gastroplasty incorporated the fundus, which is the most distensible part of the stomach. Another interesting finding from the comparative gastric bypass and gastroplasty studies was that neither stoma size nor pouch volume determined weight loss in the gastric bypass arm, with the exclusion of the stomach as the determining factor for the supremacy of the gastric bypass.[45–49] These initial comparative trials secured gastric bypass superiority among bariatric surgeries. Further comparative trials performed from 1989 to 2006 also reinforced the role of gastric bypass as a gold standard for bariatric surgery (see Table 38.2).

Surgical Techniques: 1989–2006

The Adelaide study of 1989 randomized patients to either horizontal gastroplasty, vertical gastroplasty, or Roux-en-Y gastric bypass.[50] This well-designed study found superior weight loss at 3 years for gastric bypass. At 3 years, the percent of patients who had lost more than 50% of their excess weight was greatest for gastric bypass (67%), followed by both vertical (48%) and horizontal gastroplasty.

The best comparative study between different surgical techniques remains the Swedish Obese Subjects Study.[36] This was a prospective study that, even though it was not randomized, had well-matched controls, large numbers, and a long follow-up. In the SOS, the mean changes in weight and risk factors were more favorable among the subjects treated by gastric bypass than among those treated by adjustable gastric banding or vertical banded gastroplasty. The maintained weight change over 10 years was 25% in the gastric bypass subgroup. Another study by Weber et al. also found an advantage for gastric bypass in comparison to gastric banding.[51] When comparing gastric bypass to biliopancreatic diversion (BPD)/duodenal switch, it is apparent that the duodenal switch has slightly better weight loss than the gastric bypass, particularly in larger patients.[37,52] However, this modest increment in weight loss must be balanced with the potential for more complications in this higher-risk operation.[38]

Other comparative surgical trials have included comparison of laparoscopic adjustable gastric banding versus laparoscopic vertical gastroplasty.[53–56] The evidence here is mixed, with few long-term data and lingering concerns about the need for either remedial band operations and potential for staple disruption for the vertical gastroplasty.

Benefits of Weight Loss Surgery: Weight Loss

The degree of weight loss associated with bariatric surgery is dependent upon which operation is employed. Recently, several studies have provided considerable information regarding weight loss after surgery. In the Swedish Obese Subjects (SOS) Study, which compared medically and surgically treated obese patients, there were striking differences between the two groups regarding weight loss.[36] At 10 years the conventionally treated group had a 1.6% increase in total weight while the surgically treated group saw a 24% decrease in total weight. Among the different surgical procedures performed in the SOS Study, the highest amount of total weight loss was for gastric bypass (25%), followed by vertical banded gastroplasty (17%) and adjustable gastric banding (13%) (see Table 38.4).

Two important studies have reviewed the entire published medical literature regarding bariatric surgery. These two meta-analyses provide strong validation for the efficacy of weight loss surgery. The outcomes after surgically induced weight loss published in the last years are impressive.[37,38] The meta-analysis by Buchwald et al. found that the degree of weight loss is lowest for restrictive procedures and highest for malabsorptive procedures.[37] In this meta-analysis of 22,094 patients (mean age, 47 years; mean BMI, 46.9; 72.6% women), the mean percentage of excess weight loss was 61.2% for all patients (Table 38.5). Excessive weight loss was higher for patients who underwent gastric bypass (61.6%) or gastroplasty (68.2%) compared with those who received gastric banding (47.5%). Similar results for weight loss were reported by Maggard et al. in the *Annals of Internal Medicine*.[38] In this study, weight loss in kilograms for at least 3 years postoperatively was as follows: gastric banding (35 kg), gastroplasty (32 kg), biliopancreatic diversion/duodenal switch (53 kg), and gastric bypass (42 kg).

It is clearly evident that weight loss surgery leads to profound weight loss that varies depending on the type of surgery.

TABLE 38.5. Efficacy Outcomes for Weight Reduction.[a]

Outcome measure	*No. of patients evaluatated*	*No. of treatment groups*	*Mean change (95% confidence interval)*[b]	*Weighted mean change (range of mean change)*
Total population[c]				
Absolute weight loss (kg)	7,588	83	−39.71 (−42.23 to −37.19)	−40.53 (−70.0 to 9.0)
BMI decrease	8,232	96	−14.20 (−15.13 to −13.27)	−14.01 (−27.0 to −4.10)
Initial weight loss	1,386	9	−32.64% (−36.39% to −28.89%)	−35.58% (−39.0% to −20.90%)
Excess weight loss	10,172	67	−61.23% (−64.40% to −68.06%)	−64.67% (−93.0% to −32.0%)
Gastric banding				
Absolute weight loss (kg)	482	13	−28.64 (−32.77 to −24.51)	−32.36 (−45.40 to −13.10)
BMI decrease	1,959	25	−10.43 (−11.52 to −9.33)	−10.83 (−16.40 to −4.70)
Excess weight loss	1,848	12	−47.45% (−54.23% to −40.68%)	−49.50% (70.0% to −32.0%)
Gastric bypass				
Absolute weight loss (kg)	2,742	20	−43.48 (−48.14 to −36.82)	−47.06 (−62.70 to −21.0)
BMI decrease	2,705	22	−16.70 (−18.43 to −14.98)	−17.10 (−25.0 to −8.0)
Initial weight loss	969	4	−34.93% (−35.61% to −34.26%)	−34.97% (−36.20% to −31.40%)
Excess weight loss	4,204	22	−61.56% (−66.45% to −56.68%)	−68.11% (−77.0% to −33.0%)
Gastroplasty				
Absolute weight loss (kg)	936	28	−39.82 (−44.74 to −34.90)	−39.45 (−70.0 to −9.0)
BMI decrease	942	27	−14.20 (−16.14 to −12.27)	−14.50 (−22.60 to −4.10)
Initial weight loss	27	2	−24.35% (−31.31% to −17.40%)	−25.90% (−28.0% to −20.90%)
Excess weight loss	506	15	−68.17% (−74.81% to −61.53%)	−69.15% (−93.0% to −48.0%)
Biliopancreatic diversion or duodenal switch				
Absolute weight loss (kg)	1,282	10	−46.39 (−51.58 to −41.20)	−45.96 (−64.20 to −33.0)
BMI decrease	984	12	17.99 (−19.40 to −16.59)	−16.75 (−27.0 to −13.10)
Initial weight loss	311	2	−38.98% (−40.01% to −37.94%)	−36.97% (−39.0% to −38.20%)
Excess weight loss	2,480	7	−70.12% (−73.91 to −66.34%)	−72.09% (−75.0% to −62.0%)

Includes standard and long-limb procedures with additional components (e.g., gastroplasty, band).

[a]Body mass index (BMI) is calculated as weight in kilograms divided by the square of height in meters.

[b]Comparison across studies significant ($P < 0.01$) for heterogeneity except for inital weight loss for gastric bypass and biliopancreatic diversion or duodenal switch.

[c]Includes gastric banding, gastric bypass, gastroplasty, biliopancreatic diversion or duodenal switch, as well as mixed groups and other less common procedures (biliary intestinal bypass, ileogastrostomy, jejunoileal bypass, and unspecified bariatric surgery).

Source: From Buchwald H, Avidor Y, Braunwald E, et al.,[40] by permission of JAMA.

The weight loss engendered by bariatric surgery also leads to numerous downstream benefits such as comorbidity resolution, quality of life improvement, and increased lifespan.

Benefits of Weight Loss Surgery

Comorbidity Resolution

Weight loss surgery is a singular medical intervention that has the unique ability to reverse or improve the numerous medical conditions associated with obesity.

The leading cause of death in the United States remains stroke and heart disease, with 300,000 patients dying annually. The primary medical conditions contributing to this devastating human toll are diabetes, hypertension, and hyperlipidemia. These three comorbidities, along with visceral obesity, constitute the metabolic syndrome that is a strong risk factor for cardiovascular mortality.[13] All three of these cardiovascular risk factors improved, as described in an important *Annals of Surgery* publication by Schauer et al.[23] regarding laparoscopic gastric bypass with the following resolution rates: diabetes (82%), hypertension (70%), and hyperlipidemia (63%) (Table 38.6).

The Swedish Obese Subjects (SOS) Study provided further demonstration of the ameliorative effect of bariatric surgery. At 10 years in the SOS study, surgically treated obese patients had substantial improvements in their cardiac risk factors in comparison to nonsurgically treated obese patients.[36] Surgically treated obese patients had 25% reduction in hypertension, 43% improvement in HDL, and 75% reduction in diabetes in comparison to the medically treated group.

As noted in the two previous studies, bariatric surgery reverses, ameliorates, or eliminates major cardiovascular risk factors, including diabetes, hypertension, and lipid abnormalities.[23,37] Moreover, large epidemiological follow-up studies have shown that obesity per se increases cardiovascular risk, independent of other associated traditional cardiovascular risk factors.[15–17] Obesity clearly carries a mechanism for metabolic cardiac risk. This mechanism follows adipose tissue as the predominant site of fat stores. Increasing obesity results in an overload of lipids within the body's natural storage sink (i.e., the adipocyte), followed by the necessary deposition of fat within ectopic sites such as muscle, liver, and pancreas. The resulting metabolic derangements are associated with insulin resistance, central obesity, and chronic inflammation as adipose tissue acts as an endocrine organ, producing and secreting a host of biological mediators.

There is now increasing evidence that these less well characterized atherogenic biomarkers or mediators have an important role in obesity-related cardiovascular risk, such as chronic inflammation, endothelial dysfunction, and hypercoagulation.[57–67] These recent studies have shown that weight loss induced by surgery results in an impressive reduction of

TABLE 38.6. Change in Obesity-Related Comorbidity.

Comorbidity	*Total*	*Percent aggravated*	*Percent unchanged*	*Percent improved*	*Percent resolved*
OA/DJD	64	2	10	47	41
Hypercholesterolemia	62	0	4	33	63
GERD	58	0	4	24	72
HTN	57	0	12	18	70
Sleep apnea	44	2	5	19	74
Hypertriglyceridemia	43	0	14	29	57
Depression	36	8	37	47	8
Peripheral edema	31	0	4	55	41
Urinary incontinence	18	0	11	39	44
Asthma	18	6	12	69	13
Diabetes	18	0	0	18	82
Migraine headaches	7	0	14	29	57
Anxiety	7	0	50	17	33
Venous insufficiency	7	0	71	29	0
Gout	7	0	14	14	72
CAD	5	0	0	75	25
COPD	3	0	33	67	0
CHF	3	0	33	67	0
OHS	2	0	0	50	50

CAD, coronary heart disease; CHF, congestive heart failure; COPD, chronic obstructive pulmonary disease; GERD, gastroesophageal reflux disease; HTN, hypertension; OA/DJD, osteoarthritis/degenerative joint disease; OHS, obesity hypoventilation syndrome.

Source: From Schauer PR, Ikramuddin S, Gourash WC, et al.,[23] by permission of Annals of Surgery.

insulin resistance, reduces relevant markers [C-reactive protein (CRP), interleukin 6, interleukin 18, sCD40L] of chronic vascular inflammation, and decreases well-established cardiac risk factors that have been shown to be important predictors of cardiovascular morbidity and mortality. In addition, surgery improves endothelial dysfunction and reduces key factors responsible for the increased atherothrombotic risk of the morbidly obese patients, such as tissue factor, Factor VII, and PAI-1. One study found clear, consistent, and convincing resolution of every conventional risk factor at 1 year after gastric bypass surgery.[68]

Enternal nutrition diet gastric bypass has assembled the most evidence for resolution of comorbidities. However, all weight loss surgeries promote resolution of these important medical problems. Each procedure has a different degree of improvement for different comorbidities, as demonstrated by the *JAMA* article by Buchwald et al.[37] For diabetes, each procedure has the following resolution rate: banding (48%), gastroplasty (68%), gastric bypass (84%), and biliopancreatic diversion/duodenal switch (98%). Hyperlipidemia is another cardiac risk factor that is improved by each weight loss surgery by different amounts: banding (71%), gastroplasty (81%), gastric bypass (94%), and biliopancreatic diversion/duodenal switch (99%). Finally, hypertension is also resolved by the following procedures at the accompanying rates: banding (38%), gastroplasty (73%), gastric bypass (75%), and biliopancreatic diversion/duodenal switch (81%).

Beyond the tremendous improvement in cardiac risk factors, weight loss surgery also provides enormous enhancement of the myriad medical problems that obesity engenders. An important health concern associated with obesity is sleep apnea, which carries significant health risk, including premature death. Fortunately, weight loss surgery also improves sleep apnea, as demonstrated here:[20] banding (95%), gastroplasty (77%), gastric bypass (87%), and biliopancreatic diversion/duodenal switch (95%). Joint disease is a leading health concern that severely decreases both personal satisfaction and work productivity. Schauer et al. demonstrated 88% resolution or improvement of joint disease for morbidly obese patients undergoing laparoscopic gastric bypass.[23]

In addition, the leading digestive health complaint, gastroesophageal reflux disease, is cured or improved at a 96% rate.[23] The most prevalent liver disease, nonalcoholic fatty liver disease, is very commonly associated with morbid obesity and is also very often improved by weight loss surgery.[24]

Furthermore, weight loss surgery has been demonstrated to either eliminate or improve the following health conditions: venous stasis disease, gout, asthma, pseudotumor cerebri, urinary incontinence, and infertility.[23]

Survival

Given the tremendous improvement in health that weight loss surgery provides, it is apparent that weight loss surgery will have an impact on survival. Weight loss and comorbidity resolution each contribute to increased survival for the surgically treated morbidly obese patient. Three studies have demonstrated improved survival after gastric bypass surgery. Flum et al. noted a 33% reduction in mortality for morbidly obese patients who underwent surgery versus morbidly obese patients who were treated medically.[68] MacDonald et al. also provided clear evidence for a survival benefit in the surgically treated morbidly obese patient.[69] This retrospective analysis of 232 type 2 diabetic patients with morbid obesity (mean BMI, 50), who underwent either gastric bypass operation (n = 154) or did not undergo surgery (n = 78) demonstrated a mortality rate of only 9% in the surgical group during the 9-year follow-up compared with 28% in the nonsurgical control group.[12] Patients in the control group had 4.5 times the incidence of death of patients in the surgical group. Notably, the improvement in the mortality rate in the surgical group was primarily the result of a decrease in the number of cardiovascular deaths. A decisive conclusion regarding the survival benefit conferred by gastric bypass surgery is provided by a population-based study from Quebec, Canada (Table 38.7).[41] Christou and colleagues were able to follow morbidly obese patients who were either medically or surgically treated through all aspects of medical care. This observational two-cohort study compared the outcome of 1035 severely obese patients who underwent bariatric surgery with a control group of 5746 age- and gender-matched severely obese patients who had not undergone weight reduction surgery.[41] The mortality rate in the bariatric surgery cohort was 0.68% compared with 6.17% in controls, which translated to a tremendous 89% reduction in the relative risk of death.

Long-term outcome data of a controlled surgical intervention study of obesity (the SOS study) were recently reported by Lars Sjöström at the International Federation of Surgery for Obesity Congress in Sydney as well as at the European Diabetes (EASD) Congress in Copenhagen.[70] In the SOS trial, a surgical group of 2010 patients (matched by age, gender, BMI, and comorbidities) was compared with a nonsurgical control group consisting of 2037 patients, and both groups were followed for 15 years. Surgically induced weight loss frequently resolved or markedly improved diabetes, reduced myocardial infarction by 43%, and provided a 31% reduction in overall mortality. In this single trial, weight loss induced by bariatric surgery had no effect on incidence of stroke. Interestingly, the benefit in the reduction of myocardial infarction and overall mortality was almost exclusively seen in diabetic patients. The less impressive effects observed in the nondiabetic patients of the SOS study might be explained by the fact that the cardiovascular risk factor profile is frequently quite favorable in morbidly obese subjects despite the accumulation of more than 40 kg excess fat.[71] Another possible explanation for the comparatively lower benefit achieved by nondiabetic patients may be the multiple procedures being offered in the surgical arms (gastric bypass, vertical banded gastroplasty, adjustable gastric banding). The postoperative mortality for all procedures was low and was kept at approximately 0.25%.

Quality of Life

Quality of life in the morbidly obese patient is clearly diminished for reasons of self-image, economic discrimination, lack of medical access, and societal lack of acceptance. Of note, weight loss surgery is also equally powerful in reversing poor quality of life as it is in resolving medical problems. There is ample evidence to demonstrate improvement in quality of life after weight loss surgery. The most accepted survey in medicine for quality of life is the SF36, which has been demonstrated to improve sharply after bariatric surgery.[72] Also, disease-specific quality of life instruments have also shown improvement after surgery.[73] Finally, depression is a disease that can severely impair quality of life. A measure of depression, the Beck Depression Index, has been demonstrated to decline by half following weight loss surgery.[74]

Cost-Effectiveness

Given the dramatic effects upon comorbidities that bariatric surgery renders, it is apparent that bariatric surgery can also provide reduction in healthcare costs (Table 38.8). This reduction in healthcare costs has been demonstrated in the province of Quebec where surgically treated patients incurred $6000 CN less in healthcare costs versus morbidly obese patients treated nonsurgically.[75] Two studies demonstrated that in the first year after gastric bypass healthcare costs increased.[76,77] This increase in costs decreased over time, and the initial increase may be caused by a "pent-up" demand for medical services that were not provided to patients while they were morbidly obese.[78] Two cost-effectiveness analyses demonstrated that bariatric surgery is a dominant strategy with a range of $5,000 to $35,600 per Quality Adjusted Life

TABLE 38.7. Five-Year Morbidity and Mortality.

	Cohort							
	Bariatric surgery		*Controls*		*Relative risk reduction*			
Condition/disease	*Number*	*%*	*Number*	*%*	*Estimate*	*95%*	*CI*	*P value*
Blood and blood-forming organs	4	0.39	41	0.72	0.54	0.19	1.50	0.230
Cancer	21	2.03	487	8.49	0.24	0.17	0.39	0.001
Cardiovascular and circulatory	49	4.73	1530	26.69	0.18	0.12	0.22	0.001
Digestive	377	36.43	1414	24.66	1.48	1.42	1.78	0.001
Endocrinological	98	9.47	1566	27.25	0.35	0.32	0.38	0.001
Genitourinary	77	7.44	551	9.61	0.77	0.63	0.97	0.027
Infectious diseases	90	8.70	2140	37.33	0.23	0.17	0.25	0.001
Musculoskeletal	50	4.83	682	11.90	0.41	0.32	0.55	0.001
Nervous system	25	2.42	228	3.98	0.61	0.44	0.93	0.010
Psychiatric and mental	45	4.35	470	8.20	0.53	0.41	0.73	0.001
Respiratory	28	2.71	651	11.36	0.24	0.17	0.36	0.001
Skin	38	3.67	305	5.32	0.69	0.48	0.96	0.027
Mortality	7	0.68	354	6.17	0.11	0.04	0.27	0.001

Source: From Christou NV, Sampalis JS, Liberman M, et al.,[41] by permission of Annals of Surgery.

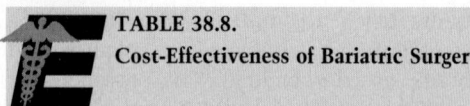

TABLE 38.8.
Cost-Effectiveness of Bariatric Surgery.

Level of evidence	*Trial*	*Outcome*
I	Clegg (2003)[79]	22,000/QALY
II	Craig (2002)[80]	5–16, 100/QALY women 10–35, 600/QALY men
III	Sampalis (2004)[75]	$6000 (CN) decrease in healthcare costs/patient

QALY, quality adjusted life year.

Year (QALY).[79,80] Both studies show that bariatric surgery provides a QALY at lower rate than $50,000, the common marker of cost-effectiveness. A short-term time perspective such as 1 year underestimates the entire economic benefit of bariatric surgery. If payers take a short-term view, they may be tempted to avoid providing coverage for bariatric surgery. The ruling by the Centers of Medicare and Medicaid Services to provide coverage for bariatric surgery and state-mandated coverage for bariatric procedures serve as legislative rebuffs to a short-sighted view of bariatric surgery.[81] True cost-effectiveness must utilize a societal perspective that fully takes into account the salutary effect of bariatric surgery on long-term health and economic productivity.

Risks of Weight Loss Surgery

There is clear and convincing evidence that bariatric surgery is a powerful therapy in treating morbid obesity and its health consequences. The ideal target population for bariatric surgery are morbidly obese patients with diabetes and metabolic syndrome because of the enormous benefit derived by surgical treatment and the large risk of premature mortality engendered by diabetes and metabolic syndrome.[13] Given the paucity of alternative treatments for weight loss in this challenging population, early and prompt surgical referral of the morbidly obese patient with diabetes and metabolic syndrome is needed. Despite the high prevalence of comorbidity in this population, bariatric surgery can provide tertiary prevention of the complications of obesity.

Patient education and selection are important components in long-term success of bariatric surgery. Although surgery provides important physiological reinforcement of a healthier lifestyle, patients must still make critical changes in their dietary, exercise, and sleep habits. Preoperative education ensures that patients are prepared to make these substantial changes in lifestyle.[82] Surgery remains a tool, not a cure, for the morbidly obese patient in their change in lifestyle. These habits are critical given that morbid obesity is a chronic disease and requires lifelong maintenance. Identification of preoperative characteristics of success after surgery remains elusive, and the best determinant of postoperative success is both patient and programmatic commitment.[82–85]

The risk of complications may temper some enthusiasm for bariatric surgery. There are demonstrated differences between surgical techniques and outcomes (Table 38.9).[35] The most concerning risk after weight loss surgery is mortality. Based on meta-analysis by Maggard et al., mortality ranges depend upon the procedure performed.[38] The average mortality with ranges is presented for the different procedures as follows: banding (0.4%, 0.01%–2.1%), gastroplasty (0.2%, 0%–16.8%), gastric bypass (1%, 0.2%–2.5%), and biliopancreatic diversion/duodenal switch (0.9%, 0.01%–1.3%).

In addition to mortality, there may also be complications from weight loss surgery such as anastomotic leak or stenosis, pulmonary embolus, bleeding, nutritional deficiencies, wound complications, bowel obstructions, ulcers, hernias, and respiratory, cardiac, and implant device-related complications. The degree of complications again varies depending on the type of procedure, as follows: banding (7%), gastroplasty (18%), gastric bypass (17%), and biliopancreatic diversion/duodenal switch (38%).[35]

Many of the reported studies regarding morbidity and mortality had been previously completed before many improvements in the current surgical technique.[72] In addition, surgeon and hospital experience can also mitigate the risk associated with weight loss surgery.[86–92] Among the different surgical procedures, the rate of complications is inversely proportional to the amount of weight loss produced

TABLE 38.9. Mortality Analysis for Surgical Procedures.

	Early or time-unspecified deaths[a]				*Late deaths*[b]			
	Controlled trials		*Case series*		*Controlled trials*		*Case series*	
Procedure	*Mortality rate (%)*	*Studies/ patients (no.)*	*Mortality rate (%)*	*Studies/ patients (no.)*	*Mortality rate (%)*	*Studies/ patients (no.)*	*Mortality rate (%)*	*Studies/ patients (no.)*
RYGB	1.0 (0.5–1.9)	15/907	0.3 (0.2–0.4)	50/11,290	1.1 (0.4–2.5)	9/524	0.6 (0.4–0.8)	24/5,411
VBG	0.2 (0–1.4)[c]	11/401	0.3 (0.1–0.5)	33/4,091	0.0 (0–16.8)[c]	1/20	0.6 (0.4–1.0)	20/2,638
Adjustable gastric banding	0.4 (0.01–2.1)	6/268	0.02 (0–0.78)[c]	35/9,222	NR	0/0	0.1 (0.02–0.2)	11/3,975
BPD	NR	0/0	0.9 (0.5–1.3)	7/2,808	NR	0/0	0.3 (0.01–0.6)	4/2,362

Values in parentheses are 95% CI unless otherwise indicated.

BPD, biliopancreatic diversion; NR, not reported; RYGB, Roux-en-Y gastric bypass; VBG, vertical banded gastroplasty.

[a]Early, less than 30 days from procedure or designated "early" in the original report.

[b]Late, more than 30 days from procedure or designated "late" in the original report.

[c]One-sided 97.5% CI.

Source: From Maggard M, Lisa R, Sugarman L, et al.,[38] by permission of Annals of Internal Medicine.

by each surgery.[38] Beyond the type of procedure, there are identified risk factors for complications after bariatric surgery including age, gender, BMI, comorbidities, and insurance status.[67,93–101] It should be noted that the best demonstrated and most protective effect against complications is an experienced surgeon and hospital.[86–92] In addition, complications may not affect long-term weight loss, which is the outcome that best predicts long-term mortality risk.[102]

Age has been repeatedly demonstrated to be a factor influencing outcome after bariatric surgery. However, in a study examining bariatric surgery outcomes for Medicare patients, the rate of complications for those less than 65 and more than 65 years of age equalized when patients were treated by experienced surgeons.[103] Male gender has also been identified as a risk factor for complications after bariatric surgery. Male gender may lead to more complications because of increased technical difficulty caused by a higher BMI, more visceral fat, and potentially more advanced comorbidities.[91,93,94] In the United States, 82% of bariatric surgery patients are women.[42] The proportion of men undergoing bariatric surgery does not reflect the gender distribution of morbid obesity. Clearly, male morbidly obese patients are seeking surgical care less often, which may be the result of general decreased access to care by men as well as a greater social acceptance of the morbidly obese male. Increased BMI is also recognized as a risk factor for complications, primarily because of technical ability to complete the operation and the potential for worsened comorbidity in these patients.[93–95] Finally, certain comorbidities have been demonstrated to increase complication rates including diabetes, chronic obstructive pulmonary disease (COPD), sleep apnea, and hypertension.[93–95,103] Studies have substantiated the risk of Medicare insurance status upon bariatric surgery outcomes.[68,93–95] Most likely, Medicare insurance status is a proxy for age, socioeconomic status, and disability. Although patients with the most risk factors carry the most risk for surgery, those high-risk patients may also derive the most benefit from bariatric surgery given the disease burden they carry.[78]

Volume and Outcomes of Bariatric Surgery

The volume–outcome relationship in weight loss surgery has been amply shown in different practice settings (Fig. 38.4).[86–92] Clearly, there is a benefit in having this complex and demanding surgery performed by experienced and committed surgeons operating in a dedicated healthcare facility.

All the previously mentioned perioperative risk factors are not modifiable, with the exception of either surgeon or hospital volume status. As mentioned earlier, the single, consistent protective factor for complications is both surgeon and hospital volume. For gastric bypass surgery, it has been demonstrated that a high-volume surgeon and high-volume hospital lead to decreased morbidity and mortality.[86–92] In the United States, this volume outcome effect has been recognized by the Centers for Medicare and Medicaid Services, which now requires that Medicare patients undergo surgery only at Bariatric Surgery Centers of Excellence.[103] Numerous criteria constitute a Bariatric Surgery Center of Excellence, but the primary criteria are surgeon volume greater than 50 cases and hospital volume greater than 125 cases annually. Although a referral to a Bariatric Surgery Center of Excellence

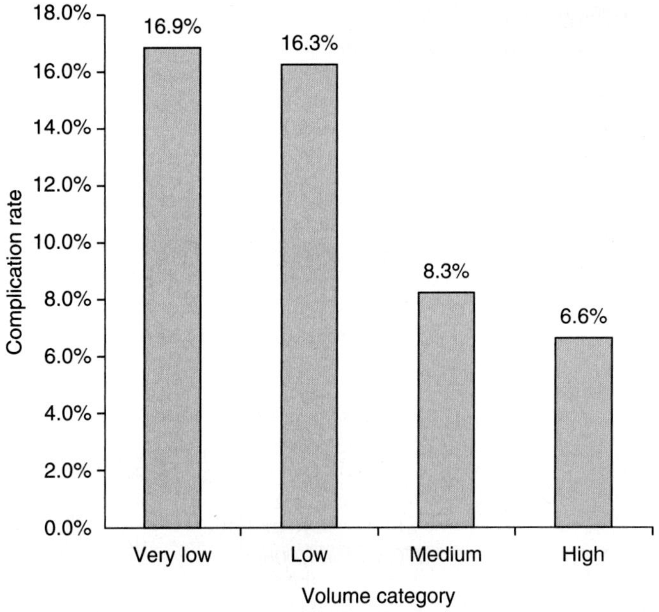

FIGURE 38.4. Complication rates (crude) by volume category (very low, <50 cases per year; low, 50–99 cases per year; medium, 100–199 cases per year; high, >200 cases per year. (From Liu JH, Zingmond D, Etzioni DA, et al.,[86] by permission of American Surgeon 2003;69:823–828.)

may lead to decreased morbidity and mortality, this referral pattern must be balanced with appropriate and sufficient access to care for a vulnerable population without other therapeutic options.

Surgical volume is a surrogate measure for a wide expanse of practice patterns that determine best outcomes. More research is required to determine which practice patterns most affect outcomes, including preoperative weight loss, advanced surgical training, and surgical assistant status.[99–101] Given this need for further research, clinically derived, prospectively maintained databases regarding bariatric surgery are required.[103,104]

Technique and Practice Patterns: Gastric Bypass

In addition to volume status, different surgical techniques and practice patterns can influence outcomes in bariatric surgery. In the practice of gastric bypass surgery, certain refinements in technique have demonstrated clear improvement over previous iterations of bariatric surgery. The most revolutionary change in bariatric surgery has been the advent of the laparoscopic approach. It is apparent that the seminal laparoscopic approach fueled the explosive growth of bariatric surgery.[37,38]

Several randomized trials have compared the laparoscopic and open approach to gastric bypass (Table 38.10).[105–108] In each circumstance, the laparoscopic approach has decidedly demonstrated an advantage over the traditional open approach on the basis of postoperative pain, length of stay, return to work, and decreased pulmonary-related, diagnostic ability-related,[109] and wound-related complications. Similar to other laparoscopic experience, the increased operative costs with laparoscopic bariatric surgery are offset by a decreased length

TABLE 38.10.
Gastric Bypass Techniques.

Level of evidence	*Trial*	*Outcome*
I	Westling (2001)[107] Laparoscopic vs. open gastric bypass	Laparoscopic approach with decreased LOS/pain and increased reoperation
I	Lujan (2004)[106] Laparoscopic vs. open gastric bypass	Equivalent % EWL Laparoscopic approach with decreased LOS and wound complications
I	Nguyen (2001)[72] Laparoscopic vs. open gastric bypass	Equivalent % EWL Laparoscopic approach decreases LOS and wound-related and pulmonary complications
I	Inabet (2005)[112] Long vs. short Roux limb (BMI < 50)	Equivalent % EWL Longer limb with increased internal hernia rate
I	Brolin (1991)[110] Long (LL) vs. short (SL) Roux limb (superobese)	EWL > 50% (83% LL vs. 50% SL)
I	Choban (2002)[111] LL vs. SL Roux limb	Equivalent % EWL, BMI < 50% EWL, LL > SL, BMI > 50
II	Christou (2006)[113] Long vs. short Roux limb	10 years follow-up % EWL equivalent
II	Fobi (2001)[114] Stapled (S) vs. complete transection (T) gastric pouch and remnant	Gastric–gastric fistula rate 32% (S) vs. 4% (T)

LOS, length of stay.

of stay. Although the laparoscopic approach has decided advantages over the open technique, there is also an accompanying learning curve that must be surmounted before these benefits are accrued.[106,107]

Other Level I evidence regarding gastric bypass techniques includes trials examining appropriate Roux limb length and complete transection versus stapled partition of the gastric remnant and pouch (see Table 38.10). Initial enthusiasm was present for a longer (150-cm) Roux limb length for the obese patient in the hope that a longer Roux limb might engender more malabsorption and potential weight loss.[110,111] No convincing evidence exists that a longer Roux limb in bariatric patients with a BMI less than 50 creates more weight loss, and this choice might have a propensity for more internal hernias.[112] For bariatric patients with a BMI greater than 50, two randomized controlled trials support the premise that a longer Roux limb leads to increased weight loss in the first year after surgery.[110,111] However, longer follow-up comparing standard and long Roux limb gastric bypass cases does not show a persistent difference in weight loss.[113]

Another advance in gastric bypass surgical technique has been the advocacy of complete transection of the gastric pouch from the gastric remnant. One comparative trial showed that complete transection versus stapled partitioning of the gastric pouch and remnant dramatically reduced the formation of gastric–gastric fistulas, a potential cause of pouch gastric ulcers and late weight regain.[114]

Another area of improvement in the provision of gastric bypass surgery includes appropriate practice patterns (Table 38.11). A feared complication of bariatric surgery is

TABLE 38.11.
Gastric Bypass Practice Patterns.

Level of evidence	*Trial*	*Outcome*
I	Kalfarentzos (2001)[116] 5,000 vs. 10,000U heparin	Equivalent venous thrombotic events and bleeding complications Weight loss equivalent
I	Alami (2007)[102] Preoperative weight loss (10% vs. standard)	Equivalent complications and postoperative weight loss
I	Morton (2007)[96] Local anesthesia pump, marcaine vs. saline, laparoscopic RNYGB	Equivalent pain scores, use of narcotic
I	Brolin (1998)[120] Fe supplementation vs. placebo	Fe deficiency less with supplementation Anemia rates equivalent
I	Miller (2003)[118] Prophylactic Actigall (A) vs. placebo (P)	1-year gallstone rate, 22% (P) vs. 3% (A)
I	Sugerman (1995)[119] Actigall vs. placebo	1-year gallstone rate, 32% (P) vs. 2% (A)

TABLE 38.12.
Adjustable Gastric Banding Technique Trials.

Level of evidence	*Trial*	*Outcome*
I	Weiss (2002)[122] Placement of band Gastric vs. esophagogastric (EG)	Less functional impairment with EG placement
I	Kirchmayr (2004)[126] Bolus vs. stepwise adjustment	Equivalent % EWL Bolus technique with less resource utilization
I	O'Brien (2005)[125] Perigastric (PG) vs. pars flaccida (PF) placement	Equivalent % EWL PF with less prolapse
I	Blanco-Engert (2003)[127] Lap-Band (LB) vs. heliogast (HG)	1-year % EWL 41.7% (LB) vs. 28.3% (HG)
I	Suter (2005)[129] Lap-Band (LB) vs. SAGB	Equivalent % EWL Morbidity 0% (LB) vs. 8.8% (SAGB)
I	Ponson (2002)[128] Lap-Band vs. SAGB	Equivalent % EWL
I	de Wit (1999)[121] Laparoscopic vs. open placement of adjustable gastric band	Equivalent % EWL Open technique with increased LOS, readmissions

SAGB, standard anatomic gastric bypass.

pulmonary embolus,[115] with one study demonstrating appropriate heparin dosing.[116] Postoperative pain in the laparoscopic approach is certainly reduced in comparison with the open technique but not eliminated. A randomized study utilizing a local anesthesia infusion pump did not demonstrate an advantage in laparoscopic gastric bypass surgery.[117] A consistent complication of surgically induced rapid weight loss is the formation of gallstones and gallstone-related complications. Two multicenter randomized controlled trials (RCTs) proved that Actigall prophylaxis is highly effective in reducing the onset of gallstone formation after gastric bypass surgery.[118,119] When patients are fully compliant, postoperative Actigall reduces gallstone formation from 32% to 2%.[119]

Micronutrient supplementation after any malabsorptive surgery is critical. For gastric bypass surgery, multivitamin and B_{12} replacement are critical and lifelong. Calcium and iron supplementation, particularly in female bariatric surgery patients, is also important in preventing osteoporosis and anemia. One randomized trial found that iron supplementation intuitively avoided iron deficiencies but did not decrease postoperative anemias.[120] More malabsorptive procedures such as the duodenal switch might additionally require fat-soluble vitamin supplementation and even inpatient protein supplementation.[38]

Preoperative weight loss is another practice pattern of interest. One randomized trial did not support the contention that preoperative weight loss leads to fewer postoperative complications and more weight loss.[121] Drawbacks to the mandate of preoperative weight loss are the inability of superobese or insulin-dependent diabetics to lose weight and an unfortunate willingness by insurers to use this mandate to bar worthy surgical candidates from a needed therapy. Clearly, weight loss of any amount and by any safe means is advantageous and merits support. However, inability to lose weight before bariatric surgery should be seen as an opportunity for education and not as an impediment to lifesaving surgery.

Technique and Practice Patterns: Adjustable Gastric Banding

In addition to gastric bypass, the practice of adjustable gastric banding has also seen numerous clinical trials that have aided its outcomes (Table 38.12). As has been repeatedly demonstrated in other comparative trials, the laparoscopic approach has clear and decided advantages over the open technique for adjustable gastric banding.[122] The appropriate level of placement of the band has been confirmed to be gastric rather than esophagogastric given the propensity of the latter approach to cause lower esophageal dysfunction.[123,124] The long-term effect of adjustable gastric banding on esophageal dysfunction is a potential concern that has not been borne out by one large case series.[123,124] Periodic surveillance by upper gastrointestinal radiography after adjustable gastric banding appears prudent.

Band slippage and prolapse is certainly lessened when a pars flaccida technique is employed rather than the initial perigastric technique.[125] The appropriate method of postoperative band adjustment is far from settled, requiring multiple variables including patient compliance, weight loss, and physiology. One RCT demonstrated that a simple one-time bolus adjustment in contradistinction to the stepwise approach resulted in equivalent weight loss and less resource utilization.[126] In addition, there are Level I data supporting the Lap-Band versus other adjustable gastric bands.[127–129]

Sleeve Gastrectomy

A relatively new approach to surgically induced weight loss is the vertical sleeve gastrectomy. As often occurs in medicine, a new approach is implemented by chance. Initially, the sleeve gastrectomy was designed as the first stage of a duodenal switch in supermorbidly obese patients who were considered too high risk for a single-stage duodenal switch.

TABLE 38.13.
Sleeve Gastrectomy Trials.

Level of evidence	*Trial*	*Outcome*
I	Himpens (2006)[132] Laparoscopic gastric sleeve resection (SG) vs. Laparoscopic adjustable gastric band (LB)	% EWL, 66 (SG) vs. 48% (LB)
II	Gagner (2005) Sleeve gastrectomy (SG) vs. intragastric balloon (IGB)	% EWL, 6 months 35% (SG) vs. 24% (IGB)

Follow-up of these patients who underwent an initial sleeve gastrectomy indicated they had sufficient weight loss to the point that many patients did not pursue further intervention.[130] The amount of weight loss after a sleeve gastrectomy is very dependent upon the size of the sleeve created. As a result, there has been a great deal of variation in weight loss after a sleeve gastrectomy.[130,131] In addition, longer-term data are required of the sleeve gastrectomy particularly in regard to complications, weight loss, and micronutrient supplementation. However, the vertical sleeve gastrectomy has the allure of surgical weight loss without an anastomosis and need for postoperative adjustment. Two controlled trials with the sleeve gastrectomy indicated that it was superior to both the adjustable gastric band and intragastric balloon (Table 38.13).[132,133]

Intragastric Balloon

Many efforts have been made to provide a nonsurgical solution to morbid obesity. Given the ready access to the stomach provided by the endoscope, it has been an obvious choice to provide an obesity solution endoscopically. The first attempt at endoscopic obesity intervention is the intragastric balloon (IGB), the first iteration being the Garren–Edwards balloon. Initial trials for the intragastric balloon found very high device failure rates and minimal weight loss (Table 38.14).[134–138] These poor early results led to the balloon being withdrawn from the U.S. market. This lack of efficacy for the intragastric balloon caused a skepticism that remains, with no intragastric balloon currently being approved by the U.S. Food and Drug Administration (FDA).

Since the initial inception of the balloon, several device improvements have been made and much better weight loss has been seen.[139] Concerns regarding intragastric balloon (IGB) efficacy and safety remain. The IGB has been implanted extensively in Europe but is indicated only for 6 months. Given the chronicity of obesity as a disease, this short-term indication certainly mutes enthusiasm for the IGB. In addition, complications such as gastric ulcers, device migration, and aspiration remain a concern. Clearly, the appeal of the IGB is its ease of placement and generally low complication rate. These advantages must be tempered by its short-term use, and further study is needed to demonstrate its appropriate role in the management of morbid obesity.

TABLE 38.14.
Intragastric Balloon Trials.

Level of evidence	*Trial*	*Outcome*
I	Genco (2006)[139] Balloon vs. sham, crossover	% EWL, 3 months 34% vs. 2.1%
I	Galiebeter (1990) Garren–Edwards balloon, deflation vs. inflation	1 month, NS
I	Mathus–Vliegen (2005)[138] Balloon vs. sham	2 years, BMI loss 12% vs. 5%
I	Ramhamadany (1989) Balloon vs. sham	3 months, kilogram loss 7.33 vs. 3.33
I	Lindor (1987)[135] Sham vs. balloon	90% device failure 6 kg vs. 2.8 kg at 3 months
II	Marshall (1990)[136] Taylor balloon	11.6-kg loss at 4 months 100% device failure

Gastric Pacing

A new approach to morbid obesity is gastric pacing. Dr. Valerio Cigaina recognized that by mimicking the disease state of a gastric ectopic pacemaker, weight loss without permanent gastrointestinal alteration could be attained. He performed animal pacing studies demonstrating that peristalsis could be altered and cause reduced feed intake and weight loss. Dr. Cigaina followed his animal work with the first human gastric stimulator implant in December 1995 in a patient who had more than 50% excess weight loss.[140]

Since these initial results, gastric pacing has continued to progress with three controlled trials (Table 38.15).[141,142] The weight loss engendered by gastric pacing in these trials was modest, at 20% to 23% excess weight loss in comparison to other established surgical treatments for morbid obesity. An interesting concept arose from one of the trials that was a predictive model for weight loss. This predictive model, BaroScreen, when implemented raised the percent excess weight loss to 40%. This interesting finding had not been previously demonstrated in bariatric surgery, which has long sought to find predictors of success after bariatric surgery.[83]

TABLE 38.15.
Pacing Trials.

Level of evidence	*Trial*	*Outcome*
II	Loss (2004)	EWL, 15 months, 21%
II	Digest (2002)	EWL, 16 months, 23% 40% screening
I	0–01 (2001)	EWL, 29 months, 20% 40% screening
II	Cigaina (2002)	% EWL, 24%, 24 months

Special Populations

The Elderly

The twin demographic trends of obesity and aging ensure that bariatric surgery in the elderly must be considered. However, operative risk of bariatric surgery can be expected to increase with increasing age while the potential benefits of surgery on life expectancy decrease. Surgically induced weight loss can improve or cure comorbid illness while improving quality of life in the elderly, justifying bariatric surgery in older populations. Flum, in a retrospective cohort study of the Medicare National Claims database, demonstrated increased mortality in patients 65 or more years of age compared to younger patients undergoing bariatric surgery, with a fivefold increase in mortality in patients 75 years of age or older compared to patients aged 65 to 74 years.[97] Importantly, this study demonstrated that mortality was not increased in older patients when the procedures were performed by more experienced surgeons. Single-institution series confirm the fact that bariatric surgical procedures can be performed safely, with low perioperative mortality, in the elderly while reducing obesity-related comorbidity.[143]

Superobese

Superobesity is defined as a BMI of 50 kg/m^2 or more. Increasing BMI has been demonstrated to be an independent risk factor for perioperative morbidity and mortality following bariatric surgery. Patients with massive superobesity have higher perioperative risk but also see the greatest benefit in quality of life with bariatric surgery, whereas nonsurgical attempts at weight reduction are particularly unsuccessful in this population. Laparoscopic procedures become technically more difficult with increasing BMI in the superobese, so controversy exists as to the optimal procedure in these patients. Gastric bypass, biliopancreatic diversion, and laparoscopic adjustable gastric banding have been advocated in the superobese, with good results with laparoscopic approaches.[144–147] Simplified or staged procedures utilizing laparoscopic sleeve gastrectomy have been advocated in the superobese to reduce operative risk, but long-term data regarding the efficacy of this approach are lacking.

Adolescents

Obesity has a number of serious consequences for adolescents. Follow-up of more than 200,000 children over a 30-year period showed that teenagers with the highest BMI values were twice as likely to die during the following 30 years.[148]

Childhood obesity also confers a significantly increased risk of hypertension, hypercholesterolemia, hypertriglyceridemia, hyperinsulinemia, and atherosclerosis compared to normal weight children.[149] Additionally, type 2 diabetes mellitus has also been increasingly diagnosed in adolescents, particularly among the obese, with a 10-fold increase in incidence over recent decades.[150] Obstructive sleep apnea syndrome also occurs more frequently in obese children and has serious adverse effects on daytime learning and quality of life.[151]

The psychosocial consequences of severe pediatric obesity are equally profound.[150,151] Obese adolescents are more stigmatized and victimized by peers and have fewer friendships than do lean adolescents. Studies of obese adult women have found that obesity in the emerging adult years is associated with completing fewer years of advanced education, lower family income, lower rates of marriage, and lower life satisfaction with work and close interpersonal relationships. Finally, as compared to adolescents within a normal weight range, obese adolescents have a health-related quality of life that is quite poor, indistinguishable from that of children with cancer.[150]

It is clear that once an adolescent has become extremely obese and has failed traditional and available weight loss options, there is little chance that a healthy weight will be achieved and maintained in the absence of drastic intervention, regardless of whether surgical consideration is delayed until adulthood. Consequently, bariatric surgery guidelines for adolescents were published in 2004.[152] From the limited studies available, it is likely that young adults will reap similar health benefits of surgically induced weight loss.[153]

Pregnancy

Pregnancy outcomes for obese women in general are poorer than those of women of normal BMI. There is an increased chance of certain complications such as gestational diabetes mellitus, high blood pressure, preeclampsia, fetal macrosomia, cesarean deliveries, and anesthesia-related complications. Many obese women of childbearing age are seeking bariatric surgery. Consequently, there may be concerns regarding the effect of bariatric surgery on birth-related events. However, review of the literature is generally reassuring. One large study of pregnancy outcomes in nearly 300 bariatric patients showed that previous bariatric surgery was not associated with adverse outcome around the time of delivery.[154] The study showed that rates of perinatal death, congenital malformations, and health at the time of birth were similar in patients with and without a maternal history of previous bariatric surgery. Similar positive fetal-maternal outcomes were noted after gastric banding.[155]

Regardless of pregnancy, all bariatric surgery patients must maintain lifelong nutritional maintenance including sufficient protein and micronutrient supplementation. A few reports have described nutritional complications for bariatric patients who have become pregnant. The most severe of such complications included inadequate fetal growth and fetal malformations.[156]

In particular, bariatric patients who become pregnant are at increased risk for anemia and their fetuses at risk of poor brain and spinal cord development because of insufficient dietary intake iron, folate, and vitamin B_{12}. With proper supplementation and surveillance, these nutritional deficiencies can be prevented.

Conclusion

Obesity is a worldwide epidemic with serious medical and economic consequences. The only effective and enduring therapy for morbid obesity is weight loss surgery. Weight loss surgery is most effective with proper patient selection and an appropriately trained surgical team. Weight loss surgery has the unique ability to solve many different health concerns through a single intervention. Strong evidence supports the well-known benefits of weight loss surgery including weight loss, comorbidity resolution, quality of life improvement, and increased lifespan. Certain risks exist for weight loss surgery that can be mitigated by surgical experience and patient selection, education, and lifelong surveillance. Special populations of the morbidly obese require particular consideration when performing weight loss surgery. Weight loss surgery is a life-saving intervention for the right patients and in the right hands.

References

1. Ogden CL, Carroll MD, Curtin LR, McDowell MA, Tabak CJ, Flegal KM. Prevalence of overweight and obesity in the United States, 1999–2004. JAMA 2006;295:1549–1555.
2. Leibson CL, Williamson DF, Melton LJ III, et al. Temporal trends in BMI among adults with diabetes. Diabetes Care 2001; 24:1584–1589.
3. Buchwald H, Williams SE. Bariatric surgery worldwide 2003. Obes Surg 2004;14:1157–1164.
4. Yoon K, Lee J-H, Kim J-W, et al. Epidemic obesity and type 2 diabetes in Asia. Lancet 2006:368:1681–1686.
5. Calle EE, Thun MJ, Petrelli JM. Body-mass index and mortality in a prospective cohort of US adults. N Engl J Med 1999;341:1097–1105.
6. Olshansky SJ, Passaro DJ, Hershow RC, et al. A potential decline in life expectancy in the United States in the 21st century. N Engl J Med 2005;352:1138–1145.
7. Pinhas-Hamiel O, Dolan LM, Daniels SR, Standford D, Khoury PR, Zeitler P. Increased incidence of non-insulin diabetes among adolescents. J Pediatr 1996;128(5):608–615.
8. Brown CD, Higgins M, Donato KA, et al. Body mass index and prevalence of hypertension and dyslipidemia. Obes Res 2000;348: 1625–1638
9. Engeland A, Bjørge T, Søgaard AJ, Tverdal A. Body mass index in adolescence in relation to total mortality. Am J Epidemiol 2003;157(6):517–523.
10. Fontaine KR, Redden DT, Wang C, et al. Years of life lost due to obesity. JAMA 2003;289:187–193.
11. Wolf AM, Colditz GA. Current estimates of the economic cost of obesity in the United States. Obes Res 1998;6:97–106.
12. Lean MEJ, Powrie JK, Anderson AS, et al. Obesity, weight loss, and prognosis in type 2 diabetes. Diabet Med 1990;7:228–233.
13. Malik S, Wong ND, Franklin SS, et al. Impact of the metabolic syndrome on mortality from coronary heart disease, cardiovascular disease, and all causes in United States adults. Circulation 2004;110:1245–1250.
14. Poirier P, Giles TD, Bray GA, et al. Obesity and cardiovascular disease: pathophysiology, evaluation, and effect of weight loss. Circulation 2006;113:898–918.
15. Kim KS, Owen WL, Williams D, Adams-Campbell LL. A comparison between BMI and conicity index on predicting coronary heart disease: the Framingham Heart Study. Ann Epidemiol 2000;10:424–431.
16. Jonsson S, Hedblad B, Engstrom G, Nilsson P, Berglund G, Janzon L. Influence of obesity on cardiovascular risk. Twenty-three-year follow-up of 22,025 men from an urban Swedish population. Int J Obes 2002;26:1046–1053.
17. Stamler R, Stamler J, Riedlinger WF, et al. Weight and blood pressure: findings in hypertension screening of 1 million Americans. JAMA 1978;240:1607–1610.
18. Garrison RJ, Kannel WB, Stokes J III, Castelli WP. Incidence and precursors of hypertension in young adults: the Framingham Study. Prev Med 1987;16:235–251.
19. Dixon JB, O'Brien P. A disparity between conventional lipid and insulin resistance markers at body mass index levels greater than 34 kg/m^2. Int J Obes Relat Metab Disord 2001;25:793–797.
20. Vgontzas AN, Tan TL, Bixler EO, et al. Sleep apnea and sleep disruption in obese patients. Arch Intern Med 1994;154:1705–1711.
21. Clinical guidelines on the identification, evaluation, and treatment of overweight and obesity in adults: the evidence report. National Institutes of Health. Obes Res 1998;(suppl 2):51S–S209.
22. Houston DK, Stevens J, Cai J, et al. Role of weight history on functional limitations and disability in late adulthood: the ARIC study. Obes Res 2005;13:1793–1802.
23. Schauer PR, Ikramuddin S, Gourash WC, Ramanathan R, Luketich J. Outcomes after laparoscopic Roux-en-Y gastric bypass for morbid obesity. Ann Surg 2000;232:515–529.
24. Klein S, Mittendorfer B, Eagon JC, et al. Gastric bypass improves metabolic and hepatic abnormalities associated with non-alcoholic liver disease. Gastroenterology 2006;130(6):1564–1572.
25. Fine JT, Colditz GA, Coakley EH, et al. A prospective study of weight change and health-related quality of life in women. JAMA 1999;282:2136–2142.
26. Fellitti VJ. Childhood sexual abuse, depression, and family dysfunction in adult obese patients. South Med J 1993;86:732–736.
27. Miller WC, Koceja DM, Hamilton EJ. A meta-analysis of the past 25 years of weight loss research using diet, exercise or diet plus exercise intervention. Int J Obes Relat Metab Disord 1997;21(10):941–947.
28. Cummings DE, Weigle DS, Frayo RS, et al. Plasma ghrelin levels after diet-induced weight loss or gastric bypass surgery. N Engl J Med 2002;346(21):1623–1630.
29. Li Z, Maglione M, Tu W, et al. Meta-analysis: pharmacologic treatment of obesity. Ann Intern Med 2005;142(7):532–546.
30. Anderson JW, Grant L, Gotthelf L, Stifler LT. Weight loss and long-term follow-up of severely obese individuals treated with an intense behavioral program. Int J Obes 2006;443–450.
31. Nordmann AJ, Nordmann A, Briel M, et al. Effects of low-carbohydrate vs. low-fat diets on weight loss and cardiovascular risk factors: a meta-analysis of randomized controlled trials. Arch Intern Med 2006;166(3):285–293.
32. Despres JP, Golay A, Sjostrom L. Effects of rimonabant on metabolic risk factors in overweight patients with dyslipidemia. N Engl J Med 2005;353(20):2121–2134.
33. Volmar KE, Hutchins GM. Aortic and mitral fenfluramine-phentermine valvulopathy in 64 patients treated with anorectic agents. Arch Pathol Lab Med 2001;125(12):1555–1561.
34. Consensus Development Conference Panel. Gastrointestinal surgery for severe obesity. Ann Intern Med 1991;115(12):956–961.
35. Inge TH, Krebs NF, Garcia VF, et al. Bariatric surgery for severely overweight adolescents: concerns and recommendations. Pediatrics 2004;114:217–223.
36. Sjostrom L, Lindroos AK, Peltonen M, et al. Lifestyle, diabetes, and cardiovascular risk factors 10 years after bariatric surgery. N Engl J Med 2004;351:2683–2693.
37. Buchwald H, Avidor Y, Braunwald E, et al. Bariatric surgery: a systematic review and meta-analysis. JAMA 2004;292:1724–1737.
38. Maggard MA, Shugarman LR, Suttorp M, et al. Meta-analysis: surgical treatment of obesity. Ann Intern Med 2005;142:547–559.
39. O'Brien PE, Dixon JB, Laurie C, et al. Treatment of mild to moderate obesity with laparoscopic adjustable gastric banding or an intensive medical program: a randomized trial. Ann Intern Med 2006;144:625–633.
40. Buchwald H, Varco RL, Boen JR, et al. Effective lipid modification by partial ileal bypass reduced long-term coronary heart disease mortality and morbidity: five-year posttrial follow-up

report from the POSCH. Arch Intern Med 1998;158(11):1253–1261.
41. Christou NV, Sampalis JS, Liberman M, et al. Surgery decreases long-term mortality, morbidity, and health care use in morbidly obese patients. Ann Surg 2004;240:416–423; discussion 423–424.
42. Santry HP, Gillen DL, Lauderdale DS. Trends in bariatric surgical procedures. JAMA 2005;294:1909–1917.
43. Trus TL, Pope GD, Finlayson SRG. National trends in utilization and outcomes of bariatric surgery. Surg Endosc 2005; 19(5):616–620.
44. Griffen WO Jr, Young VL, Stevenson CC. A prospective comparison of gastric and jejunoileal bypass procedures for morbid obesity. Ann Surg 1977;186(4):500–509.
45. Laws HL, Piantadosi S. Superior gastric reduction procedure for morbid obesity: a prospective, randomized trial. Ann Surg 1981;193(3):334–340.
46. Pories WJ, Flickinger EG, Meelheim D, et al. The effectiveness of gastric bypass over gastric partition in morbid obesity: consequence of distal gastric and duodenal exclusion. Ann Surg 1982;196(4):389–399.
47. Andersen T, Pedersen BH, Dissing I, et al. A randomized comparison of horizontal and vertical banded gastroplasty: what determines weight loss? Scand J Gastroenterol 1989;24(2):186–192.
48. Naslund I, Wickbom G, Christoffersson E, et al. A prospective randomized comparison of gastric bypass and gastroplasty. Complications and early results. Acta Chir Scand 1986;152:681–689.
49. Sugerman HJ, Starkey JV, Birkenhauer R. A randomized prospective trial of gastric bypass versus vertical banded gastroplasty for morbid obesity and their effects on sweets versus non-sweets eaters. Ann Surg 1987;205(6):613–624.
50. Hall JC, Watts JM, O'Brien PE, et al. Gastric surgery for morbid obesity. The Adelaide Study. Ann Surg 1990;211(4):419–427.
51. Weber M, Muller MK, Bucher T, et al. Laparoscopic gastric bypass is superior to laparoscopic gastric banding for treatment of morbid obesity. Ann Surg 2004;240(6):975–982; discussion 982–983.
52. Skroubis G, Anesidis S, Kehagias I, et al. Roux-en-Y gastric bypass versus a variant of biliopancreatic diversion in a nonsuperobese population: prospective comparison of the efficacy and the incidence of metabolic deficiencies. Obes Surg 2006;16(4):488–495.
53. Nilsell K, Thorne A, Sjostedt S, et al. Prospective randomised comparison of adjustable gastric banding and vertical banded gastroplasty for morbid obesity. Eur J Surg 2001;167(7):504–509.
54. Morino M, Toppino M, Bonnet G, et al. Laparoscopic adjustable silicone gastric banding versus vertical banded gastroplasty in morbidly obese patients: a prospective randomized controlled clinical trial. Ann Surg 2003;238(6):835–842; discussion 841–842.
55. Olbers T, Bjorkman S, Lindroos A, et al. Body composition, dietary intake, and energy expenditure after laparoscopic Roux-en-Y gastric bypass and laparoscopic vertical banded gastroplasty: a randomized clinical trial. Ann Surg 2006; 244(5):715–722.
56. Olbers T, Fagevik-Olsen M, Maleckas A, et al. Randomized clinical trial of laparoscopic Roux-en-Y gastric bypass versus laparoscopic vertical banded gastroplasty for obesity. Br J Surg 2005;92(5):557–562.
57. Primrose JN, Davies JA, Prentice CR, Hughes R, Johnston D. Reduction in factor VII, fibrinogen and plasminogen activator inhibitor-1 activity after surgical treatment of morbid obesity. Thromb Haemost 1992;68:396–399.
58. Kopp CW, Kopp HP, Steiner S, et al. Weight loss reduces tissue factor in morbidly obese patients. Obes Res 2003;11:950–960.
59. Hanusch-Enserer U, Cauza E, Spak M, et al. Improvement of insulin resistance and early atherosclerosis in patients after gastric banding. Obes Res 2004;12:284–291.
60. Schernthaner GH, Kopp HP, Kriwanek S, et al. Effect of massive weight loss induced by bariatric surgery on serum levels of interleukin-18 and monocyte-chemoattractant-protein-1 in morbid obesity. Obes Surg 2006;16:709–715.
61. Schernthaner GH, Kopp HP, Krzyzanowska K, et al. Soluble CD40L in patients with morbid obesity: significant reduction after bariatric surgery. Eur J Clin Invest 2006;36:395–401.
62. Krzyzanowska KA, Mittermayer F, Kopp HP, Wolzt M, Schernthaner G. Weight loss reduces circulating asymmetrical dimethylarginine concentrations in morbidly obese women. J Clin Endocr Metab 2004;89:6277–6281.
63. Kopp HP, Spranger J, Möhlig M, Krzyzanowska K, Pfeiffer AFH, Schernthaner G. Effect of weight loss on plasma levels of adiponectin in association with markers of chronic subclinical inflammation and the insulin resistance syndrome in obese subjects. Int J Obes 2005;29:766–771.
64. Blankenberg S, Tiret L, Bickel C, et al. Interleukin-18 is a strong predictor of cardiovascular death in stable and unstable angina. Circulation 2002;106:24–30.
65. de Lemos JA, Morrow DA, Sabatine MS, et al. Association between plasma levels of monocyte chemoattractant protein-1 and long-term clinical outcomes in patients with acute coronary syndromes. Circulation 2003;107:690–695.
66. Heeschen C, Dimmeler S, Hamm CW, et al. Soluble CD40 ligand in acute coronary syndromes. N Engl J Med 2003;348:1104–1111.
67. Williams B, Hagedorn J, Lawson E, et al. Gastric bypass reduces biochemical cardiac risk factors. Surg Obes Relat Dis 2007;3(1):8–13.
68. Flum DR, Dellinger EP. Assessing the impact of bariatric surgery on survival. J Am Coll Surg 2004;199:543–551.
69. MacDonald KG Jr, Long SD, Swanson MS, et al. The gastric bypass operation reduces the progression and mortality of non-insulin-dependent diabetes mellitus. J Gastrointest Surg 1997;1:213–220.
70. Sjöström L. Bariatric surgery in diabetic patients—what is the evidence? Presented at 42nd EASD Meeting, Copenhagen, 2006.
71. Barakat HA, Mooney N, O'Brien K, et al. Coronary heart disease risk factors in morbidly obese women with normal glucose tolerance. Diabetes Care 1993;16:144–149.
72. Nguyen NT, Goldman C, Rosenquist CJ, et al. Laparoscopic versus open gastric bypass: a randomized study of outcomes, quality of life, and costs. Ann Surg 2001;234(3):279–289.
73. Dymek M, le Grange D, Neven K, Alverdy J. Quality of life after gastric bypass surgery: a cross-sectional study. Obes Res 2002; 10:1135–1142.
74. Dixon J, Dixon M, O'Brien P. Depression in association with severe obesity changes with weight loss. Arch Intern Med 2003;163:2058–2065.
75. Sampalis JS, Liberman M, Auger S, et al. The impact of weight reduction surgery on health-care costs in morbidly obese patients. Obes Surg 2004;14(7):939–947.
76. Zingmond DS, McGory ML, Ko CY. Hospitalization before and after gastric bypass surgery. JAMA 2005;294:1918–1924.
77. Encinosa WE, Bernard DM, Chen CC, et al. Healthcare utilization and outcomes after bariatric surgery. Med Care 2006; 44(8):706–712.
78. Wolfe B, Morton J. Weighing in on bariatric surgery: procedure use, readmission rates, and mortality. JAMA 2005;294(15):1960–1963.
79. Clegg A, Colquitt J, Sidhu M, et al. Clinical and cost effectiveness of surgery for morbid obesity: a systematic review and economic evaluation. Int J Obes Relat Metab Disord 2003; 27(10):1167–1177.

80. Craig BM, Tseng DS. Cost-effectiveness of gastric bypass for severe obesity. Am J Med 2002;113(6):491–498.
81. Vanek VW. State laws on insurance coverage for bariatric surgery: help or a hindrance? Surg Obes Relat Disord 2005; 1(4):424–429.
82. Giusti V, De Lucia A, Di Vetta V, et al. Impact of preoperative teaching on surgical option of patients qualifying for bariatric surgery. Obes Surg 2004;14:1241–1246.
83. Van Hout GC, Verschure SK, van Heck GL. Psychosocial predictors of success following bariatric surgery. Obes Surg 2005;15:552–560.
84. Delin CR, Watts JM, Bassett DL. An exploration of the outcomes of gastric bypass surgery for morbid obesity: patient characteristics and indices of success. Obes Surg 1995;5(2):159–170.
85. Dixon JB, Dixon ME, O'Brien PE. Pre-operative predictors of weight loss at 1-year after Lap-Band surgery. Obes Surg 2001;11(2):200–207.
86. . Liu JH, Zingmond D, Etzioni DA, et al. Characterizing the performance and outcomes of obesity surgery in California. Am Surg 2003;69:823–828.
87. Nguyen NT, Paya M, Stevens CM, Mavandadi S, Zainabadi K, Wilson SE. The relationship between hospital volume and outcome in bariatric surgery at academic medical centers. Ann Surg 2004;240:586–593.
88. Courcoulas A, Schuchert M, Gatti G, Luketich J. The relationship of surgeon and hospital volume to outcome after gastric bypass surgery in Pennsylvania: a 3-year summary. Surgery (St. Louis) 2003;134:613–621.
89. Fernandez AZ Jr, Demaria EJ, Tichansky DS, et al. Multivariate analysis of risk factors for death following gastric bypass for treatment of morbid obesity. Ann Surg 2004;239:698–703.
90. Poulose BK, Griffin MR, Zhu Y, et al. National analysis of adverse patient safety events in bariatric surgery. Am Surg 2005;71:406–413.
91. Livingston EH, Ko CY. Assessing the relative contribution of individual risk factors on surgical outcome for gastric bypass surgery: a baseline probability analysis. J Surg Res 2002;105:48–52.
92. Ballantyne GH, Svahn J, Capella RF, et al. Predictors of prolonged hospital stay following open and laparoscopic gastric bypass for morbid obesity: body mass index, length of surgery, sleep apnea, asthma, and the metabolic syndrome. Obes Surg 2004;14(8):1042–1050.
93. Benotti PN, Wood GC, Rodriguez H, et al. Perioperative outcomes and risk factors in gastric surgery for morbid obesity: a 9-year experience. Surgery (St. Louis) 2006;139(3):340–346.
94. Livingston EH, Huerta S, Arthur D, et al. Male gender is a predictor of morbidity and age a predictor of mortality for patients undergoing gastric bypass surgery. Ann Surg 2002;236(5):576–582.
95. Livingston EH, Langert J. The impact of age and Medicare status on bariatric surgical outcomes. Arch Surg 2006;141(11):1115–1120; discussion 1121.
96. Morton JM, Hagedorn J, Encarnacion B, et al. Post-operative gastric bypass complications do not affect weight loss. Presented at 11th Annual IFSO Meeting, Sydney, Australia, August 2006.
97. Flum DR, Salem L, Elrod JAB, et al. Early mortality among Medicare beneficiaries undergoing bariatric surgery. JAMA 2005;294:1903–1908.
98. http://www.cms.hhs.gov/mcd/viewdecisionmemo.asp?id=160 (accessed Dec. 2006).
99. Hsu GP, Morton JM, Jin L, Safadi BY, Satterwhite TS, Curet MJ. Laparoscopic Roux-en-Y gastric bypass: differences in outcome between attendings and assistants of different training backgrounds. Obes Surg 2005;15:1104–1110.
100. Schauer P, Ikramuddin S, Hamad G, Gourash W. The learning curve for laparoscopic Roux-en-Y gastric bypass is 100 cases. Surg Endosc 2003;17:212–215.
101. Ballantyne GH, Ewing D, Capella RF, et al. The learning curve measured by operating times for laparoscopic and open gastric bypass: roles of surgeon's experience, institutional experience, body mass index and fellowship training. Obes Surg 2005; 15(2):172–182.
102. Alami RS, Morton JM, Schuster R, Lie J, Sanchez BR, Curet MJ. Is there a benefit to pre-operative weight loss in gastric bypass patients? A prospective randomized trial. Surg Obes Relat Disord 2007;3(2):141–145; discussion 145–146.
103. Nguyen NT, Morton JM, Wolfe BM, Schirmer B, Ali M, Traverso LW. The SAGES Bariatric Surgery Outcome Initiative. Surg Endosc 19:1429–1438, 2005
104. Hutter M, Crane M, Keenan M. Data collection systems for weight loss surgery: an evidence-based assessment. Obes Res 2005;13(2):301–305.
105. Puzziferri N, Austrheim-Smith IT, Wolfe BM, Wilson SE, Nguyen NT. Three-year follow-up of a prospective randomized trial comparing laparoscopic versus open gastric bypass. Ann Surg 2006;243:181–188.
106. Lujan JA, Frutos MD, Hernandez Q, et al. Laparoscopic versus open gastric bypass in the treatment of morbid obesity: a randomized prospective study. Ann Surg 2004;239(4):433–437.
107. Westling A, Gustavs.son S. Laparoscopic vs. open Roux-en-Y gastric bypass: a prospective, randomized trial. Obes Surg 2001;11(3):284–292.
108. Brolin RE. Laparoscopic versus open gastric bypass to treat morbid obesity. Ann Surg 2004;239(4):438–440.
109. Sanchez BR, Morton J, Curet MJ, Alami RS, Safadi BY. Incidental finding of gastrointestinal stromal tumors (GISTs) during laparoscopic gastric bypass. Obes Surg 2005;10(15):1384–1388.
110. Brolin RE, Kenler HA, Gorman JH, et al. Long-limb gastric bypass in the superobese. A prospective randomized study. Ann Surg 1992;215(4):387–395.
111. Choban PS, Flancbaum L. The effect of Roux limb lengths on outcome after Roux-en-Y gastric bypass: a prospective, randomized clinical trial. Obes Surg 2002;12(4):540–545.
112. Inabnet WB, Quinn T, Gagner M, et al. Laparoscopic Roux-en-Y gastric bypass in patients with BMI <50: a prospective randomized trial comparing short and long limb lengths. Obes Surg 2005;15(1):51–57.
113. Christou NV, Look D, Maclean LD. Weight gain after short- and long-limb gastric bypass in patients followed for longer than 10 years. Ann Surg 2006;244(5):734–740.
114. Fobi MA, Lee H, Igwe D Jr, et al. Prospective comparative evaluation of stapled versus transected silastic ring gastric bypass: 6-year follow-up. Obes Surg 2001;11(1):18–24.
115. Sapala JA, Wood MH, Schuhknecht MP, et al. Fatal pulmonary embolism after bariatric operations for morbid obesity. Obes Surg 2003;13:819–825.
116. Kalfarentzos F, Stavropoulou F, Yarmenitis S, et al. Prophylaxis of venous thromboembolism using two different doses of low-molecular-weight heparin (nadroparin) in bariatric surgery: a prospective randomized trial. Obes Surg 2001;11(6):670–676.
117. LaMasters T, Lau J, Lemmens H, Morton JM. Use of local anesthetic infusion pump in laparoscopic Roux-en-Y gastric bypass: a prospective double-blinded randomized placebo controlled trial. Surg Endosc 2007, in press.
118. Miller K, Hell E, Lang B, et al. Gallstone formation prophylaxis after gastric restrictive procedures for weight loss: a randomized double-blind placebo-controlled trial. Ann Surg 2003;238(5):697–702.
119. Sugerman Hj, Brewer WH, Shiffman ML, et al. A multicenter, placebo-controlled, randomized, double-blind, prospective trial of prophylactic ursodiol for the prevention of gallstone formation following gastric-bypass-induced rapid weight loss. Am J Surg 1995;169(1):91–96; discussion 96–97.
120. Brolin RE, Gorman JH, Gorman RC, et al. Prophylactic iron supplementation after Roux-en-Y gastric bypass: a prospective,

double-blind, randomized study. Arch Surg 1998;133(7):740–744.
121. de Wit LT, Mathus-Vliegen L, Hey C, et al. Open versus laparoscopic adjustable silicone gastric banding: a prospective randomized trial for treatment of morbid obesity. Ann Surg 1999; 230(6):800–805; discussion 805–807.
122. Weiss HG, Nehoda H, Labeck B, et al. Adjustable gastric and esophagogastric banding: a randomized clinical trial. Obes Surg 2002;12(4):573–578.
123. Ren CJ, Weiner, Allen JW. Favorable early results of gastric banding for morbid obesity: the American experience. Surg Endosc 2004;18(3):543–546.
124. DeMaria EJ, Sugerman HJ, Meador JG, et al. High failure rate after laparoscopic adjustable silicone gastric banding for treatment of morbid obesity. Ann Surg 2001;233(6):809–818.
125. O'Brien PE, Dixon JB, Laurie C, et al. A prospective randomized trial of placement of the laparoscopic adjustable gastric band: comparison of the perigastric and pars flaccida pathways. Obes Surg 2005;15(6):820–826.
126. Kirchmayr W, Klaus A, Muhlmann G, et al. Adjustable gastric banding: assessment of safety and efficacy of bolus-filling during follow-up. Obes Surg 2004;14(3):387–391.
127. Blanco-Engert R, Weiner S, Pomhoff I, et al. Outcome after laparoscopic adjustable gastric banding, using the Lap-Band and the Heliogast band: a prospective randomized study. Obes Surg 2003;13(5):776–779.
128. Ponson AE, Janssen IM, Klinkenbijl JH. Laparoscopic adjustable gastric banding: a prospective comparison of two commonly used bands. Obes Surg 2002;12(4):579–582.
129. Suter M, Giusti V, Worreth M, et al. Laparoscopic gastric banding: a prospective, randomized study comparing the Lapband and the SAGB: early results. Ann Surg 2005;241(1):55–62.
130. Cottam D, Qureshi FG, Mattar SG, et al. Laparoscopic sleeve gastrectomy as an initial weight-loss procedure for high-risk patients with morbid obesity. Surg Endosc 2006;20(6):859–863.
131. Roa PE, Kaidar-Person O, Pinto D, et al. Laparoscopic sleeve gastrectomy as treatment for morbid obesity: technique and short-term outcome. Obes Surg 2006;16(10):1323–1326.
132. Himpens J, Dapri G, Cadiere GB. A prospective randomized study between laparoscopic gastric banding and laparoscopic isolated sleeve gastrectomy: results after 1 and 3 years. Obes Surg 2006;16(11):1450–1456.
133. Milone L, Strong V, Gagner M. Laparoscopic sleeve gastrectomy is superior to endoscopic intragastric balloon as a first stage procedure for super-obese patients (BMI > or = 50). Obes Surg 2005;15(5):612–617.
134. Kirby DF, Wade JB, Mills PR, et al. A prospective assessment of the Garren–Edwards gastric bubble and bariatric surgery in the treatment of morbid obesity. Am Surg 1990;56(10):575–580.
135. Lindor KD, Hughes RW Jr, Ilstrup DM, et al. Intragastric balloons in comparison with standard therapy for obesity—a randomized, double-blind trial. Mayo Clin Proc 1987;62(11):992–996.
136. Marshall JB, Schreiber H, Kolozsi W, et al. A prospective, multicenter clinical trial of the Taylor intragastric balloon for the treatment of morbid obesity. Am J Gastroenterol 1990;85(7):833–837.
137. Mathus-Vliegen EM, Tytgat GN, Veldhuyzen-Offermans EA. Intragastric balloon in the treatment of super-morbid obesity. Double-blind, sham-controlled, crossover evaluation of 500-milliliter balloon. Gastroenterology 1990;99(2):362–369.
138. Mathus-Vliegen EM, Tytgat GN. Intragastric balloon for treatment-resistant obesity: safety, tolerance, and efficacy of 1-year balloon treatment followed by a 1-year balloon-free follow-up. Gastrointest Endosc 2005;61(1):19–27.
139. Genco A, Cipriano M, Bacci V, et al. BioEnterics intragastric balloon (BIB): a short-term, double-blind, randomised, controlled, crossover study on weight reduction in morbidly obese patients. Int J Obes (Lond) 2006;30(1):129–133.
140. Cigaina VV, Pinato G, Rigo V, et al. Gastric peristalsis control by mono situ electrical stimulation: a preliminary study. Obes Surg 1996;6(3):247–249.
141. De Luca M, Segato G, Busetto L, et al. Progress in implantable gastric stimulation: summary of results of the European multicenter study. Obes Surg 2004;14(suppl 1):S33–S39.
142. Shikora SA. "What are the Yanks doing?" the U.S. experience with implantable gastric stimulation (IGS) for the treatment of obesity: update on the ongoing clinical trials. Obes Surg 2004;14(suppl 1):S40–S48.
143. Sugerman HJ, DeMaria EJ, Kellum JM, et al. Effects of bariatric surgery in older patients. Ann Surg 2004;240:243–247.
144. Fielding GA. Laparoscopic adjustable gastric banding for massive superobesity (>60 body mass index kg/m^2). Surg Endosc 2003;17:1541–1545.
145. Dolan K, Hatzifotis M, Newbury L. A comparison of laparoscopic adjustable gastric banding and biliopancreatic diversion in superobesity. Obes Surg 2004;14:165–169.
146. Mongol P, Chosidow D, Marmuse JP. Laparoscopic gastric bypass versus laparoscopic adjustable gastric banding in the superobese: a comparative study of 290 patients. Obes Surg 2005;15:76–81.
147. Regan JP, Inabnet WB, Gagner M, et al. Early experience with 2-stage laparoscopic Roux-en-Y gastric bypass as an alternative in the super-super obese patient. Obes Surg 2003;13:861–864.
148. Must A, Jacques PF, Dallal GE, Bajema CJ, Dietz WH. Long-term morbidity and mortality of overweight adolescents. A follow-up of the Harvard Growth Study of 1922 to 1935. N Engl J Med 1992;327(19):1350–1355.
149. Freedman DS, Dietz WH, Srinivasan SR, Berenson GS. The relationship of overweight to cardiovascular risk factors among children and adolescents: the Bogalusa Heart Study. Pediatrics 1999;103(6):1175–1182.
150. Schwimmer JB, Burwinkle TM, Varni JW. Health-related quality of life of severely obese children and adolescents. JAMA 2003;289(14):1813–1819.
151. Gortmaker SL. Social and economic consequences of overweight in adolescence and young adulthood. N Engl J Med 1993; 329(14):1008–1012.
152. Inge TH, Krebs NF, Garcia VF, et al. Bariatric surgery for severely overweight adolescents: concerns and recommendations. Pediatrics 2004;114(1):217–223.
153. Lawson ML. One year outcomes of Roux-en-Y gastric bypass for morbidly obese adolescents. J Pediatr Surg 2006;41(1):137–143.
154. Sheiner E, Levy A, Silverberg D, et al. Pregnancy after bariatric surgery is not associated with adverse perinatal outcome. Am J Obstet Gynecol 2004;190(5):1335–1340.
155. Martin LF, Finigan KM, Nolan TE. Pregnancy after adjustable gastric banding. Obstet Gynecol 2000;95(6):927–930.
156. Martin L. Gastric bypass as a maternal risk factor for neural tube defects. Lancet 1988;1(8586):640–641.

39

Surgical Care of the Pregnant Patient

Erika J. Lu and Myriam J. Curet

One of the greatest challenges that confront the surgeon is the care of the pregnant patient. Outcomes of disease management affect two patients, both the mother and the fetus. In addition, physiological changes during pregnancy alter classic complaints, presentations, and treatments. Abdominal emergencies in the gravid woman are frequently difficult to diagnose, and management of cases that are straightforward in the nonpregnant patient become complicated in the pregnant state.

This chapter reviews the physiological changes that affect the diagnosis and management of the acute abdomen in pregnancy. Common surgical conditions are reviewed. Particular discussion is dedicated to the use of minimally invasive surgery in pregnancy, as operative laparoscopy has become increasingly common in pregnant women during the past decade.

Physiological Changes in Pregnancy

Physiological changes unique to pregnancy alter the patterns of evaluation for the gravid surgery patient. Changes in cardiac, respiratory, renal, and gastrointestinal physiology are important concepts to keep in mind when evaluating the pregnant patient (Table 39.1).

Cardiac Changes

Increased Maternal Blood Volume

During pregnancy, there is a 30% to 50% increase in plasma volume with a lesser expansion in red blood cell mass; this results in dilutional anemia, or a physiological anemia of pregnancy. By the second trimester, a hematocrit of 30% to 35% is normal. This increase in maternal blood volume allows the pregnant woman to tolerate blood loss better, but mild to moderate blood loss may occur before physical manifestations appear. As much as 2 L, or 30% of the total blood volume, may be lost before hemodynamic alterations such as tachycardia or hypotension appear.[1] This loss is clinically significant because a pregnant patient demonstrating signs of hypovolemia may already be significantly volume depleted.

Vascular Alterations

Cardiac output increases by 30% to 50% in pregnancy, peaking late in the second trimester.[2] Concurrently, there is a drop in systemic vascular resistance, causing a 5 to 10 mmHg decrease in systolic blood pressure and a 10 to 20 mmHg decrease in diastolic blood pressure. The combination of increased cardiac output and decreased systemic vascular resistance (SVR) results in an increase in resting pulse of 10 to 15 beats/min over baseline.

During surgical evaluation of the gravid patient, it is important to understand the effects of the gravid uterus on cardiac output. After 20 weeks gestation, the uterus is at the level of the bifurcation of the great vessels (at the level of the umbilicus). In the supine position, the gravid uterus compresses the inferior vena cava, reducing venous return and thereby reducing preload and cardiac output by as much as 25% to 30%. Even without the presence of pathology, 10% of pregnant women near term can develop a "physiological" hypotensive syndrome, with dizziness and syncope, secondary to pressure on the vena cava. Therefore, when evaluating the pregnant surgical patient, it is useful to displace the uterus via left lateral tilt or manual displacement to avoid this hypotensive state.

Hemostatic Alterations

The presence of higher levels of serum estrogen during pregnancy causes an increase in liver production of Factors II, VII, VIII, IX, X, and fibrinogen; this results in a hypercoagulable state in which there is a four- to sixfold increase in the risk of thromboembolism. In addition, positioning of the patient in reverse Trendelenburg during laparoscopic surgery decreases venous return, thereby increasing the risk of deep venous thrombosis (DVT). Therefore, DVT prophylaxis is an important part of perioperative care in the pregnant patient.[3]

Platelet counts are mildly decreased during pregnancy but usually fall in within the normal range. White blood cell

TABLE 39.1. Physiological Changes During Pregnancy.

Blood volume	↑	Decrease by 30%–50%
Hematocrit	↓	30%–35% normal
SVR	↓	↓ in SBP by 5–10 mmHg, ↓ in DBP by 10–20 mmHg
Heart rate	↑	Increase by 10–15 bpm
Clotting factors	↑	Increase in Factors II, VII, VIII, IX, X, fibrinogen
WBC	↑	10,000–14,000 normal
Platelets	↓	Low to normal
FRC	↓	
Minute ventilation	↑	

SVR, systemic vascular resistance; WBC, white blood cells; FRC, functional residual capacity.

counts of 10,000 to 14,000 are normal in the pregnant patient and increase to 15,000 to 18,000 in the third trimester, making evaluation of infectious abdominal processes difficult during late pregnancy.

Respiratory Changes

During pregnancy, the mother is essentially breathing for two individuals and her respiratory requirements increase, which is reflected in a higher minute ventilation and tidal volume. Each of these parameters may increase by 30% to 40%.[2] With this physiological hyperventilation, there is a partially compensated respiratory alkalosis, with decreased pCO_2 to approximately 30 mmHg and decreased HCO_3. Consequently the mother has less buffering capacity for metabolic acidosis. In addition, it has been shown that the fetus is typically slightly more acidotic than the mother.[4]

Decreased functional residual capacity occurs as a result of compression by the gravid uterus. As a result, the mother has a lower threshold for hypoxemia and atelectasis becomes more common.

Gastrointestinal Changes

Hormonal changes during pregnancy cause digestive changes secondary to progesterone-mediated smooth muscle relaxation. Gastroesophageal reflux is common as the tone of the lower esophageal sphincter decreases. Up to 30% to 70% of pregnant women complain of reflux symptoms, especially during the third trimester. These changes increase the risk of aspiration with general anesthesia.[3] Bowel peristalsis decreases, prolonging the period of postoperative ileus following laparotomy, an important consideration in managing the advancement of postoperative diet. Decrease in gastrointestinal motility also leads to increased frequency of nausea and vomiting. Progesterone-induced smooth muscle relaxation also affects the gallbladder, making stasis more common and increasing the risk of cholecystitis.

Anatomic changes occur that are related to the cephalad displacement of abdominal contents by the gravid uterus. The appendix is displaced progressively upward, making the diagnosis of appendicitis by physical examination more difficult. Additionally, laxity of the abdominal muscles during late pregnancy makes it difficult to appreciate the physical findings of peritoneal irritation such as guarding and rebound tenderness.[3]

Renal Changes

The renal collecting system progressively dilates as a result of progesterone-mediated smooth muscle relaxation. Hydroureter and urinary stasis are common. Thus, when evaluating the acute abdomen, it is important to rule out the presence of a urinary tract infection or pyelonephritis.

Diagnostic Imaging

The selection of diagnostic imaging studies in the pregnant patient is frequently a source of anxiety for the patient and surgeon. The use of diagnostic radiology is often curtailed because of the fear of fetal injury and the availability of safer alternatives such as magnetic resonance imaging (MRI) and ultrasound. Fortunately, most radiologic studies are quite benign and expose the fetus to relatively low doses of radiation, typically less than 1 rad. In certain situations, diagnostic radiology is an unavoidable part of evaluation of the pregnant surgical patient, and the benefits of such procedures should be weighed against an accurate assessment of the risk.

Diagnostic imaging that exposes the fetus to less than 5 rad is not believed to cause birth defects, intrauterine growth retardation, or spontaneous abortion, even during the first trimester. Although there is concern about teratogenicity of exposure between 5 and 10 rad, serious risk to the fetus is only known to occur above 10 rad.[5] Direct fetal irradiation of greater than 10 rad is associated with microcephaly, intrauterine growth retardation, developmental delay, and even fetal death. Lead shielding of the abdomen should be used whenever possible to reduce the dose of radiation to the fetus.

Conventional X-ray examinations expose the fetus to less than 0.2 rad. Computed tomography exposes the fetus to higher doses of radiation, as outlined in Table 39.2.[6]

The American College of Obstetricians and Gynecologists has outlined the following guidelines for radiographic examination or exposure during pregnancy.[7]

- Pregnant patients should be counseled that exposure from a single radiographic procedure does not result in harmful effects to the fetus. Specifically, exposure of less than 5 rad is not associated with an increased risk of fetal anomalies or spontaneous abortion.
- Concern about potential adverse effects of high-dose ionizing radiation should not prevent medically indicated diagnostic imaging.
- During pregnancy, nonionizing imaging procedures such as ultrasound and MRI should be considered whenever possible.

TABLE 39.2. Approximate Fetal Doses from Common Diagnostic Procedures.

Procedure	*Fetal exposure (rad)*
Chest radiograph (two views)	0.00002–0.00007
Abdominal radiograph (one view)	0.1–0.4
Computed tomography (CT) of the chest	0.6–0.96
Computed tomography (CT) of the abdomen	0.8–4.9
Computed tomography (CT) of the pelvis	2.5–7.9

Common General Surgery Problems in Pregnancy

Appendicitis

Appendicitis is the most common nongynecological cause of the acute abdomen during pregnancy, appearing in 1 in 1500 pregnancies.[8] Unfortunately, it is also the most commonly delayed surgical intervention secondary to its difficult diagnosis and a general reluctance to operate unnecessarily on a gravid patient. The reported incidence of complications varies widely, but delay in diagnosis and subsequent appendiceal perforation is the cause of preterm labor and fetal loss in as many as 36% of cases.[8–10] Early diagnosis and surgical intervention prevent fetal loss, with only a 1% to 5% fetal loss rate in unperforated cases.[11] Some authors suggest that delay of more than 24h in surgical intervention results in perforation in two-thirds of the patients[12]; this is of particular concern during the third trimester, when the incidence of perforative appendicitis is highest and fetal viability is the most likely. Appendiceal rupture is twice as common during the third trimester as in the first and second trimesters (69% versus 31%).[13]

Maternal mortality from appendicitis is now a rarity and usually associated with significant surgical delay. The incidence of mortality has dropped sharply over the past 30 years to nearly zero, likely secondary to prompt surgical intervention and improved antibiotic coverage.[10]

When appendicitis is suspected, the decision to operate should be based on clinical grounds, just as in the nonpregnant patient. Larger series quote a negative laparotomy rate of 20% to 35%, with greater accuracy of diagnosis in the first trimester.[10]

Clinical Presentation

The diagnosis of appendicitis during pregnancy is challenging because the hallmarks of appendicitis such as anorexia, nausea, vomiting, and leukocytosis are present in the normal obstetric population. The most reliable symptom in pregnant patients with appendicitis is right lower quadrant pain.[14] Classic teaching suggests that this pain moves from the right lower quadrant in first-trimester presentations toward the right upper quadrant in third-trimester presentations. This migration was described in 1932 by Baer et al., who used barium radiographs to demonstrate cephalad displacement of the appendix by the expanding uterus.[15] However, clinical series have not confirmed this assertion, and the most frequent location of pain remains in the right lower quadrant, regardless of trimester.[14] Rebound tenderness and guarding are not particularly specific to the diagnosis of appendicitis in the gravid patient secondary to the laxity of abdominal musculature in the latter half of pregnancy.[3] Fever is not present in the majority of pregnant patients with appendicitis; up to 70% of patients have temperatures below 99.6°F.[16]

Interpretation of laboratory data in the pregnant patient is associated with several pitfalls. Assessment of the white blood cell may not be helpful as a consequence of the physiological leukocytosis present in normal pregnancy, especially during the third trimester. Elevated neutrophil counts traditionally suggest infectious etiologies, but one study found that only 59% of patients with proven appendicitis had leftward shift.[16] The same authors suggest that urinalysis can also be misleading, with approximately 20% of women with appendicitis having abnormal results, leading to the incorrect diagnosis of urinary tract infection.[16] Recent series have questioned the utility of using laboratory tests to confirm or reject the diagnosis of appendicitis at all.[14]

Imaging

Ultrasound is the initial imaging modality of choice in the pregnant patient. It has a sensitivity of 86% in the nonpregnant patient, with similar accuracy in the first and second trimesters of pregnancy.[3] During the third trimester, ultrasound examination is technically difficult and may be nondiagnostic. In these cases, helical CT should be considered. It can be performed in 15min and exposes the fetus to only 0.3rad.[10] In a recent study of seven patients with suspected appendicitis, helical CT identified the two cases of pathologically proven appendicitis and allowed surgery to be avoided in the remaining five cases.[17] Larger studies are needed to validate the initial favorable result of helical CT in diagnosing appendicitis in pregnancy.

Management

When a pregnant patient is to undergo surgery, timely consultation among appropriate services such as surgery, obstetrics, and neonatology should take place. Positioning of the patient involves left lateral tilt with a hip roll to minimize aortocaval compression and to optimize blood flow to the fetus.

Various incisions have been described for open appendectomy in the pregnant patient. The most popular is a muscle-splitting incision over the point of maximal tenderness, which is of particular significance in the second and third trimesters. Paramedian and midline vertical incisions should be used if there is significant doubt as to the diagnosis to gain easier access to the left adnexa. Uterine manipulation should be avoided to decrease the risk of uterine irritability and preterm labor.

Laparoscopic appendectomy is an option for women up to 28 weeks gestation, before the size of the gravid uterus prevents visualization of the operative field. The patient should be positioned in the left lateral decubitus position as with open surgery. Also, minimizing the degree of reverse Trendelenburg positioning will further reduce uterine compression. In patients in their first trimester of pregnancy, trocar placement is similar to that in the nonpregnant patient. As pregnancy progresses, increasing uterine size may require changes in port site placement. When the fundal height reaches that of the umbilicus or higher, initial placement of the camera port is recommended at the subxiphoid space. After visual exploration of the abdomen, additional trocar ports may be placed under direct visualization, typically in the right upper and lower quadrants.[18] Special precautions unique to laparoscopic surgery are detailed in subsequent sections.

External fetal monitoring should be considered intraoperatively if the gestational age is in the range of fetal viability (more than 24 weeks gestation). In open laparotomy, a sterile plastic bag may be wrapped around the fetal heart rate monitor and displaced from the skin incision. In laparoscopic surgery, intraoperative fetal monitoring should always be performed regardless of gestational age so that if fetal tachycardia develops, pneumoperitoneum can be desufflated in an attempt to correct the problem. With laparoscopy, transvaginal ultrasound should be used, because with transabdominal ultrasound monitoring, the signal is lost during abdominal insufflation.[19]

In cases where perforation has occurred, a critical part of therapy is the use of copious irrigation and broad-spectrum antibiotics with anaerobic coverage. The use of intraperitoneal drains is advocated in these cases.[10]

Preterm contractions are common after appendectomy, occurring in approximately 80% of patients. However, preterm labor with cervical changes and subsequent preterm delivery is relatively uncommon, occurring in 5% to 14% of patients.[14] Although tocolytic agents have not been shown to be helpful in preventing preterm delivery, they are frequently used.

Symptomatic Cholelithiasis

Cholecystitis is the second most common nongynecological condition requiring surgery during pregnancy, occurring in 1 of 1600 pregnancies.[13] The overall incidence of biliary tract disease during pregnancy ranges from 0.05% to 0.3%.[20,21] Numerous studies have demonstrated that multiparity and abnormal gallbladder motility during pregnancy increase the risk of developing gallstones.[22,23]

When facing the gravid patient with biliary tract disease, the outcomes of medical and surgical management must be considered. There is consensus that surgical intervention is needed in cases of obstructive jaundice, acute cholecystitis failing medical management, gallstone pancreatitis, or suspected peritonitis.[20,22,24] In contrast to chronic cholecystitis, gallstone pancreatitis is associated with a significant maternal mortality rate, 15% to 60%, and a fetal mortality rate near 60%,[21] and timely surgical intervention is warranted. However, the management of symptomatic cholelithiasis remains controversial with regard to medical versus surgical management.

Clinical Presentation

Pregnant patients with symptomatic cholelithiasis present with the same symptoms as nonpregnant patients, such as nausea, vomiting, and the acute onset of stabbing right upper quadrant or midabdominal pain. Murphy's sign, with tenderness on deep inspiration under the right costal margin, is less common in the pregnant patient.

Laboratory studies of serum transaminases and direct bilirubin can be elevated in biliary tract disease. Alkaline phosphatase is elevated during normal pregnancy secondary to high serum estrogen levels and is therefore less helpful in diagnosis. Leukocytosis is also a part of normal pregnancy and is not helpful in differentiating between biliary colic and acute cholecystitis.

Imaging

Ultrasound is the diagnostic modality of choice in pregnancy because of its noninvasiveness, speed, and accuracy. It has a sensitivity of 95% for detecting gallstones and usually yields good views of the gallbladder even without fasting.[25]

Medical Management

Traditionally, treatment of symptomatic cholelithiasis and acute cholecystitis during pregnancy has been medical, particularly during the third trimester. Conservative treatment involves the use of supportive intravenous hydration, bowel rest with nasogastric suction and NPO status, and narcotics. Antibiotics are indicated for signs of cholecystitis or infection. Surgery was usually reserved for refractory cases failing medical management after several days, or for patients with recurrent bouts of biliary colic. Recent studies have challenged this approach in favor of more aggressive early surgical intervention.

Surgical Management

Since the late 1980s, several authors have argued that early surgical management of biliary colic resulted in better pregnancy outcomes than in medically managed patients.[26–28] A recent study suggests that pregnant patients with symptomatic cholelithiasis have a high rate of symptomatic relapse during pregnancy, with more severe disease during relapse, including choledocholithiasis and gallstone pancreatitis.[28]

The safest time to operate on the pregnant patient is during the second trimester, when the risks of teratogenesis, miscarriage, and preterm delivery are lowest. During the second trimester, the miscarriage rate is only 5.6%, compared to 12% in the first trimester.[18] In addition, the rates of preterm labor and premature delivery are 0% during the second trimester, compared to 40% in the third trimester.[18] Finally, the risk of teratogenesis seen in the first trimester is no longer present by the second trimester, and the gravid uterus does not obscure the operative field during the second trimester as it does during the third.[18] Patients presenting in the first or third trimesters should be managed medically and offered elective cholecystectomy in the second trimester or immediately postpartum. Any patient whose clinical condition deteriorates despite medical therapy should undergo cholecystectomy or cholecystostomy regardless of the trimester.[29]

Uncomplicated open cholecystectomy is associated with 0% maternal mortality, 5% fetal death, and 7% preterm labor.[30] Percutaneous cholecystostomy can be an effective management option that avoids the use of general anesthesia but is infrequently performed.

Laparoscopic biliary tract surgery has emerged as a safe option for cholecystectomy during pregnancy. Since it was first performed in a pregnant patient in 1991, numerous authors have suggested that it reduces postoperative pain and recovery time, results in less fetal exposure to narcotics, and decreases the risk of incisional hernias compared to open cholecystectomy.[18,19] It is more likely to be technically feasible later in pregnancy than laparoscopic appendectomy because the uterus does not obscure the operative field, even during the third trimester. In general, 28 weeks gestation appears to be the limit for successful completion of laparoscopic surgery. The camera port should be placed using an open Hasson technique cephalad to the uterine fundus or in the subxiphoid position. Use of the Veress needle is contraindicated in pregnancy. Three other ports should be placed under direct visualization: a 10-mm trocar in the subxiphoid space and 5-mm trocars in the right upper and lower quadrants. Cholangiography should be performed selectively with a single film and use of lead shielding to protect the fetus from radiation exposure.[31] Conversion to open cholecystectomy should always be performed if intraoperative conditions make continued laparoscopic surgery unsafe.[32]

Laparoscopy in Pregnancy

Laparoscopic surgery has revolutionized the field of general surgery over the past 15 years. Numerous studies have shown that the advantages of minimally invasive surgery, including decreased pain, shorter hospitalization, and quicker return to normal activity, apply to the pregnant population.[18,30,33] Historically, most surgeons considered pregnancy to be a contraindication to laparoscopy. However, recent literature has demonstrated that minimally invasive surgery can be performed safely during pregnancy with acceptable maternal and fetal morbidity.[18–22,24,28,31,34,35–38] As with open surgery, the safest time to perform laparoscopic surgery in the pregnant patient is during the second trimester when the risks of teratogenesis, spontaneous abortion, and premature delivery are lowest. There are more than 50 reports in the English-language literature documenting the use of laparoscopic cholecystectomy during pregnancy. The largest series are documented in Table 39.3, which summarizes 171 cases with only 1 fetal loss. To date, more than 320 laparoscopic cholecystectomies in pregnant patients have been reported in the English literature. The large majority have been performed in the second trimester. Average operative time was slightly less than 70min (range, 30–106min), and average length of stay was slightly less than 2 days (range, 1–7 days). Of 268 babies delivered at time of publication, 10 were premature and 1 was born with hyaline membrane disease at 37 weeks gestation. The remaining 257 were full term and healthy. Seven of these experienced preterm labor, which was controlled with tocolytics. There was 1 case that resulted in both maternal and fetal death. In addition, 5 fetal deaths have been reported (fetal mortality rate, 1.9%), 1 of which occurred after conversion. This rate compares favorably with a 5% rate of fetal loss in open cholecystectomy for uncomplicated biliary tract disease.[20,21,26] The study with the highest fetal mortality rate was reported by Amos et al.,[36] who noted 3 fetal losses among 4 patients who underwent laparoscopic cholecystectomy. Although this series addresses the risks of laparoscopy, it should be noted that the pregnancies that resulted in fetal death involved long operative times and complicated biliary tract disease such as gallstone pancreatitis, which is inherently associated with a fetal loss rate up to 60%.[21,28]

To date, there have been 20 published reports of pregnant patients undergoing laparoscopic appendectomies. Those reports including at least 3 patients are described in Table 39.4.[48–58] Among the 123 patients described, the majority of cases were performed in the second trimester; average operative time has been nearly 1h (range, 25–90min), with a mean length of stay of nearly 4 days (range, 1–11 days). Seven fetal deaths have been reported, 3 secondary to uterine infection, 2 of which were misdiagnosed preoperatively as appendicitis and 1 caused by pneumoamnion after uterine puncture with a Veress needle. Eight patients delivered prematurely while at least 110 patients delivered healthy term infants. Four of these patients experienced preterm labor, which was controlled with tocolytics.

Additional data on pregnant patients undergoing laparoscopic surgery are reported by Reedy et al.,[48] who presented the results of a survey sent to members of the Society of Laparoendoscopic Surgeons regarding their experiences with laparoscopic procedures in pregnant patients. Two spontaneous abortions occurred among 199 patients undergoing lapa-

TABLE 39.3.
Reported Cases of Laparoscopic Biliary Tract Surgeries During Pregnancy Trimester.

Source	Number of patients	First: no. of patients	Second: no. of patients	Third: no. of patients	Preterm delivery (PTD) (%)	Mean gestational age of PTD	Number of fetal deaths	Level of evidence[a]
Rollins et al.[39]	31	3	19	9	6 (20%)	33.8 weeks	1	II
Affleck et al.[40]	42	3	28	11	5 (11.9%)	35.5 weeks	0	II
Muench et al.[41]	16	9	6	1	0	—	0	III
Sungler et al.[42]	9	0	8	1	0	—	0	III
Cosenza et al.[35]	12	—	—	—	0	—	0	II
Daradkeh et al.[43]	16	2	10	4	0	—	0	III
Graham et al.[44]	6	2	4	0	0	—	0	III
Glasgow et al.[45]	14	3	11	0	1	35 weeks	0	III
Gouldman et al.[24]	8	1	7	0	0	—	0	III
Lu et al.[28]	6	0	6	0	0	—	0	III
Comitalo et al.[46]	4	0	4	0	1	37 weeks	0	III
Soper et al.[34]	5	0	5	0	0	—	0	III
Morrell et al.[47]	5	0	5	0	2	33 weeks	0	III
Lanzafame[22]	5	0	3	2	0	—	0	III

[a]Clinical studies are classified according to the design of study and the quality of the resulting data: Class I, prospective, randomized studies; Class II, prospective, nonrandomized or case-controlled retrospective studies; Class III, retrospective analyses without case controls.

TABLE 39.4.
Reported Cases of Laparoscopic Appendectomy During Pregnancy Trimesters.

Source	Number of patients	1st: no. of patients	2nd: no. of patients	3rd: no. of patients	Preterm delivery (PTD) (%)	Mean gestational age of PTD (weeks)	No. of fetal deaths	Level of evidence[a]
Schreiber[50]	6	2	4	0	NI	—	0	III
Andreoli et al.[51]	5	0	5	0	1	35	0	II
Amos et al.[36]	3	0	3	0	NI	—	1	III
Curet et al.[18]	4	(4)	(4)	0	0	—	0	II
Gurbuz and Peetz[52]	5	2	0	3	0	—	0	II
Lemaire and van Erp[53]	4	1	3	0	0	—	0	III
Affleck et al.[40]	19	6	9	4	3	35.7	0	II
de Perrot et al.[54]	6	2	3	1	1	36	2	III
Rizzo[55]	4	0	4	0	0	—	0	III
Rollins et al.[39]	28	6	13	9	2	33.5	0	II
Carver et al.[56]	17	5	12	0	0	—	2	II
Wu et al.[57]	11	4	6	1	0	—	1	III
Halkic et al.[58]	11	NI	NI	NI	0	—	0	III

NI, not indicated.

[a]Clinical studies are classified according to the design of study and the quality of the resulting data: Class I, prospective, randomized studies; Class II, prospective, nonrandomized or case-controlled retrospective studies; Class III, retrospective analyses without case controls.

roscopic cholecystectomy; 1 patient among 567 undergoing laparoscopic appendectomy experienced a spontaneous abortion. All spontaneous abortions occurred in patients who had surgery in the first trimester. These data too support a favorable comparison of laparoscopic surgery to open surgery in pregnant patients. Graham et al. reviewed the literature on laparoscopic cholecystectomy during pregnancy to correlate adverse outcomes with gestational age at surgery.[49] They found that, in all three trimesters, the rates of fetal loss were equal to or less than those seen with open cholecystectomy for the same trimester. These data suggest that laparoscopic surgery is safe in all three trimesters of pregnancy, with no increase in fetal morbidity or mortality rates.

In addition to the safety of laparoscopy in pregnancy, there are the added benefits of decreased preterm delivery secondary to decreased uterine manipulation and decreased fetal depression secondary to decreased narcotic use.[19,33] This factor has popularized operative laparoscopy for various indications during pregnancy, including appendicitis and cholecystitis.

The proven benefits of laparoscopic surgery during pregnancy must be weighed against the risks. In addition to its technical difficulty as a result of the gravid uterus, the surgeon must consider the unknown risks of fetal acidosis caused by carbon dioxide absorption, decreased uterine blood flow caused by increased intraabdominal pressure, and fetal hypotension from decreased maternal cardiac output.

The concern for fetal hypotension with pneumoperitoneum is theoretical, but it is not believed to be of clinical significance given the presence of increased intraabdominal pressure with maternal Valsalva, coughing, and straining.[34] Although there are no reports of deleterious effects of pneumoperitoneum gas on the human fetus, animal studies have raised concern for fetal acidosis. Pregnant baboons and ewes showed maternal respiratory acidosis leading to fetal respiratory acidosis with the use of carbon dioxide pneumoperitoneum.[4,37] These disturbances persisted despite attempts to correct the problem by adjusting the maternal respiratory rate. In pregnant ewes, fetal tachycardia, fetal hypertension, an increase in intrauterine pressure, and a decrease in uterine blood flow were seen. Despite this, the animals delivered full-term, healthy lambs after 1 h of carbon dioxide intraabdominal insufflation at 15 mmHg. Interestingly, the physiological changes demonstrated by the pregnant ewes with CO_2 pneumoperitoneum are not present with nitrous oxide insufflation. Use of nitrous oxide as an insufflating gas in pregnant humans has not yet been evaluated but may prove to be a safer alternative to carbon dioxide.

The following practice guidelines are based on the SAGES Guidelines of Laparoscopic Surgery During Pregnancy.[38] They should be followed when performing minimally invasive surgery in the pregnant patient to mimimize adverse effects on the mother or fetus.

1. Obstetric consultation should be obtained to aid in perioperative management.
2. When possible, surgery should be deferred until the second trimester, when the risk to the fetus is lowest.
3. Aspiration precautions should be taken, because the pregnant woman has a decreased lower esophageal sphincter pressure and delayed gastric emptying.
4. The patient should be placed in left lateral decubitus position with minimal reverse Trendelenburg to decrease uterine compression of the inferior vena cava.
5. Antiembolic stockings should be used to prevent deep venous thrombosis, especially given the increased levels of clotting factors and fibrinogen creating a procoagulable state during pregnancy.
6. Utilize an open Hasson technique for entering the abdominal cavity. Although several authors have successfully used the Veress needle, puncture of the uterus has been

reported. There is a higher risk of abdominal visceral injury with increasing gestational age, making the Veress needle contraindicated.

7. Maintain carbon dioxide pneumoperitoneum at 12–15 mmHg, keeping intraabdominal pressure at the minimum level to achieve adequate visualization.

8. Maternal end-tidal CO_2 should be continuously monitored and maintained at 25–30 mmHg to minimize maternal and thereby fetal acidosis. Prompt adjustments to the minute ventilation are critical.

9. If the fetus is of viable gestational age, continuous fetal monitoring should be employed. Transvaginal ultrasound is often needed because transabdominal ultrasound is made difficult by the presence of pneumoperitoneum. If there is evidence of fetal distress, pneumoperitoneum should be released immediately. If the fetus is not of viable gestational age, then preoperative and postoperative fetal heart tones should be documented.

10. Lead shielding of the fetus should be utilized whenever cholangiography is used. Fluoroscopy should be limited.

11. Minimize operative time. Several studies have shown an increase in $PaCO_2$ with increased operative time.

Conclusion

Surgical diseases occurring during pregnancy are difficult cases that all general surgeons face. When evaluating the gravid surgical patient, it is important to keep in mind the unique physiological changes during pregnancy that affect management. With symptoms such as nausea and vomiting common during pregnancy, and with limitations on the use of radiography, acute illnesses such as appendicitis may be difficult to diagnose. When caring for a pregnant patient, it is always preferable to operate in the second trimester if the case may be delayed, as with uncomplicated biliary tract disease. When considering surgical approaches, laparoscopy offers significant advantages, with good maternal and fetal outcomes when guidelines for safety are followed.

References

1. Van Hook JW. Trauma in pregnancy. Clin Obstet Gynecol 2002;45(2):414–424.
2. Stone K. Acute abdominal emergencies associated with pregnancy. Clin Obstet Gynecol 2002;45:553–561.
3. Martin C, Varner MW. Physiologic changes in pregnancy: surgical implications. Clin Obstet Gynecol 1994;37:241–255.
4. Hunter JG, Swanstrom L, Thornburg K. Carbon dioxide pneumoperitoneum induces fetal acidosis in a pregnant ewe model. Surg Endosc 1994;4:268–271.
5. Schwartz HM, Reichling BA. Hazards of radiation exposure for pregnant women. JAMA 1978;239:1907–1909.
6. Lowe SA. Diagnostic radiography in pregnancy: risks and reality. Aust N Z J Obstet Gynecol 2004;44:191–196.
7. Guidelines for diagnostic imaging during pregnancy. In: Committee Opinion. Washington, DC: American College of Obstetricians and Gynecologists, 1995.
8. Babaknia A, Parsa H. Appendicitis during pregnancy. Obstet Gynecol 1977;50:40–44.
9. Horowitz MD, Gomez GA, Santiesteban R. Acute appendicitis in pregnancy. Arch Surg 1995;120:1362–1367.
10. Sharp HT. The acute abdomen during pregnancy. Clin Obstet Gynecol 2002;43:405–413.
11. Firstenberg MS, Malangoni MA. Gastrointestinal surgery during pregnancy. Gastroenterol Clin N Am 1998;27:73–88.
12. Tamir IL, Bongard FS, Klein SR. Acute appendicitis in the pregnant patient. Am J Surg 1990;160:571–576.
13. Weingold AB. Appendicitis in pregnancy. Clin Obstet Gynecol 1983;26:801–809.
14. Mourad J, Elliot JP, Erickson L. Appendicitis in pregnancy: new information that contradicts long-held clinical beliefs. Am J Obstet Gynecol 2000;182:1027–1029.
15. Baer JL, Reirs RA, Arens RA. Appendicitis in pregnancy with changes in position and axis of the normal appendix in pregnancy. JAMA 1932;52:1359–1364.
16. Masters K, Levine BA, Gaskill HV. Diagnosing appendicitis during pregnancy. Am J Surg 1984;148:768.
17. Castro MA, Shipp TD, Castro EE. The use of helical computed tomography in pregnancy for the diagnosis of acute appendicitis. Am J Obstet Gynecol 2001;184:184–185.
18. Curet MJ, Allen D, Josloff RK, et al. Laparoscopy during pregnancy. Arch Surg 1996;131:546–551.
19. Hart RO, Tamadon A, Fitzgibbons RJ, Fleming A. Open laparoscopic cholecystectomy in pregnancy. Surg Laparosc Endosc 1993;3:13–16.
20. McKellar DP, Anderson CT, Boynton CJ, Peoples JB. Cholecystectomy during pregnancy without fetal loss. Surg Gynecol Obstet 1992;174:465–468.
21. Printen KJ, Ott RA. Cholecystectomy during pregnancy. Am J Surg 1978;44:432–434.
22. Lanzafame RJ. Laparoscopic cholecystectomy. Surgery (St. Louis) 1995;118:627–631.
23. Scott LD. Gallstone disease and pancreatitis in pregnancy. Gastroenterol Clin N Am 1992;21:803–815.
24. Gouldman JW, Sticca RP, Rippon MB, McAlhany JC. Laparoscopic cholecystectomy in pregnancy. Am Surg 1998;64:93–98.
25. Stauffer RA, Adams A, Wygal J. Gallbladder disease in pregnancy. Am J Obstet Gynecol 1982;6:661–664.
26. Dixon NP, Faddis DM, Silberman H. Aggressive surgical management of cholecystitis during pregnancy. Am J Surg 1987;154:292–294.
27. Lee S, Bradley JP, Mele MM. Cholelithiasis in pregnancy: surgical versus medical management. Obstet Gynecol 2000;95:S70–S71.
28. Lu EJ, Curet MJ, El-Sayed YY, Kirkwood KS. Medical versus surgical management of biliary tract disease in pregnancy. Am J Surg 2004;188:755–759.
29. Weber RA, Smith RW, Wright RC. Percutaneous cholecystostomy during pregnancy: a new treatment for acute cholecystitis in pregnancy? Contemp Surg Resident 1993;1:21–23.
30. Curet MJ. Laparoscopy during pregnancy. In: Scott-Conner CEH, ed. The Sages Manual. New York: Springer, 1999:98–103.
31. Chandra M, Shipro SJ, Gordon LA. Laparoscopic cholecystectomy in the first trimester of pregnancy. Surg Laparosc Endosc 1994;4:68–69.
32. Barone JE BS, Chen S, Tsai J. Outcome study of cholecystectomy during pregnancy. Am J Surg 1999;177:232–236.
33. Bisharah M, Tulandi T. Laparoscopic surgery in pregnancy. Clin Obstet Gynecol 2003;46:92–97.
34. Soper NJ, Hunter J, Petrie RH. Laparoscopic cholecystectomy during pregnancy. Surg Endosc 1992;6:115–117.
35. Cosenza CA, Saffari B, Jabbour N, et al. Surgical management of biliary gallstone disease during pregnancy. Am J Surg 1999;178:545–548.
36. Amos JD, Schorr SJ, Norman PF, et al. Laparoscopic surgery during pregnancy. Am J Surg 1996;171:435–437.
37. Reedy MB, Galan HL, Bea JD, Carnes A, Knight AB, Kuehl TJ. Laparoscopic insufflation in the gravid baboon: maternal and fetal effects. J Am Assoc Gynecol Laprosc 1995;2:399–406.

38. Guidelines for laparoscopic surgery during pregnancy. Society of American Gastrointestinal Endoscopic Surgeons (SAGES). Surg Endosc 1998;12:189–190.
39. Rollins MD, Chan KJ, Price RR. Laparoscopy for appendicitis and cholelithiasis during pregnancy. Surg Endosc 2004;18:237–241.
40. Affleck DG, Handrahan DL, Egger MJ, Price RR. The laparoscopic management of appendicitis and cholelithiasis during pregnancy. Am J Surg 1999;178:523–529.
41. Muench J, Albrink M, Seragini F, Rosemurgy A, Carey L, Murr MM. Delay in treatment of biliary disease during pregnancy increases morbidity and can be avoided with safe laparoscopic cholecystectomy. Am Surg 2001;67:539–542.
42. Sungler P, Heinerman PM, Steiner H, et al. Laparoscopic cholecystectomy and interventional endoscopy for gallstone complications during pregnancy. Surg Endosc 2000;14:267–271.
43. Daradkeh S, Sumrein I, Daoud F, Zaiden K, Abu-Khalaf M. Management of gallbladder stones during pregnancy: conservative treatment or laparoscopic cholecystectomy? Hepatogastroenterology 1999;46:3074–3076.
44. Graham G, Baxi L, Tharakan T. Laparoscopic cholecystectomy during pregnancy: a case series and review of the literature. Obstet Gynecol Surv 1998;53:566–574.
45. Glasgow RE, Visser BL, Harris HW, Patti MG, Kilpatrick SJ, Mulvihill SJ. Changing management of gallstone disease during pregnancy. Surg Endosc 1998;12:241–246.
46. Comitalo JB, Lynch D. Laparoscopic cholecystectomy in the pregnant patient. Surg Laparosc Endosc 1994;4:268–271.
47. Morrell DG, Mullins JR, Harrison PB. Laparoscopic cholecystectomy during pregnancy in symptomatic patients. Surgery (St. Louis) 1992;112:856–859.
48. Reedy MB, Galan HL, Richards WE, et al. Laparoscopy during pregnancy: A survey of laparoendoscopic surgeons. J Reprod Med 1997;42:33–38.
49. Graham G, Baxi L, Tharakan T. Laparoscopic cholecystectomy during pregnancy: a case series and review of the literature. Obstet Gynecol Surg 1998;53:566–574.
50. Schreiber JH. Laparoscopic appendectomy in pregnancy. Surg Endosc 1990;4:100–102.
51. Andreoli M, Servakov M, Meyers P, Mann WJ Jr. Laparoscopic surgery during pregnancy. J Am Assoc Gynecol Laparosc 1999;6:229–233.
52. Gurbuz AT, Peetz ME. The acute abdomen in the pregnant patient: is there a role for laparoscopy? Surg Endosc 1997;11:98–102.
53. Lemaire BM, van Erp WF. Laparoscopic surgery during pregnancy. Surg Endosc 1997;11:1216–1217.
54. de Perrot M, Jenny A, Morales M, Kohlit M, Morel P. Laparoscopic appendectomy during pregnancy. Surg Laparosc Endosc Percutan Tech 2000;10:368–371.
55. Rizzo AG. Laparoscopic surgery in pregnancy. J Laparoendosc Adv Surg Tech A 2003;13:11–15.
56. Carver TW, Antevil J, Egan JC, Brown CV. Appendectomy during early pregnancy: what is the preferred surgical approach? Am Surg 2005;71:809–812.
57. Wu JM, Chen KH, Lin HF, Tseng LM, Tseng SH, Huang SH. Laparoscopic appendectomy in pregnancy. J Laparoendosc Adv Surg Tech A 2005;15:447–450.
58. Halkic N, Tempia-Caliera AA, Ksontini R, Suter M, Delaloye JF, Vuilleumier H. Laparoscopic management of appendicitis and symptomatic cholelithiasis during pregnancy. Langenbecks Arch Surg 2006;391:467–471.

40

Palliative and End-of-Life Care

Sharon M. Weinstein and Olivia Walton

The World Health Organization defines palliative care as "an approach to care that improves quality of life of patients facing life-threatening illness and their families, through the prevention and relief of suffering by means of early identification and impeccable assessment and treatment of pain and other problems, physical, psychosocial, and spiritual."[1] In contemporary discussions of healthcare, the topics of "palliative care" and "end-of-life care" are prominent. Although palliative medicine specialists have become more widely available for consultation, the care of seriously ill and dying patients is central to the entire practice of medicine, including surgery. However, fear of treating patients at end of life is experienced by many healthcare providers. Providers are generally not formally prepared to manage dying as a normal process. Caring for this population entails complex decisions that may seem to contradict the intent to cure. However, it is recognized that the essential goal of medicine is to relieve suffering, and that caring well for these patients and their families can be a hopeful and healing process.

Given the extensive needs of patients with life-threatening illness, the central assumption of palliative care, and, ultimately, managing death, is that the treatment of patients be carried out in a comprehensive, intensive, and compassionate manner. Three elements define clinical palliative care: (1) medical symptom management, (2) psychosocial and spiritual support of the patient and family, and (3) advanced care planning.[2] An integrated palliative care model requires treatment of patients starting at the time of diagnosis and continuing throughout the course of illness: during treatment to cure, in disease relapse, or through disease progression to death.

Regardless of prognosis, soon after receiving a diagnosis of a life-threatening condition most patients require interventions that are directed against the disease, medical supportive care, and palliative care aimed at relief of symptoms (the integrated model). However, as disease progresses toward death, the goals of care for the terminally ill patient shift away from cure-oriented medical treatment to those aimed at providing comfort and dignity at end of life. The goals of care attempt to optimize supportive care and relief of symptoms. Specifically, goals shift to relief of pain and other distressing symptoms, maintenance of function, support of family and personal relationships, avoidance of impoverishment, and attentiveness to meaningful activities and spiritual issues.[3] This focus allows patients to voice concerns about the burden of life-prolonging interventions and fears about the dying process; it also emphasizes provider–patient communication and enhancing quality of life.

Very dynamic physiological changes occur as a terminally ill patient approaches death, and progressing symptoms require intensification of care. In the Study to Understand Prognosis and Preferences for Outcomes and Risks of Treatment, at least 50% of patients were reported by their families to have had severe pain in the last 4 weeks of life.[4] A review of the current literature indicates that the prevalence rates of pain and other distressing symptoms during the last weeks of life range from 20% to 87%, and that most patients have more than 10 symptoms that require medical management.[5–7] Palliative care and end-of-life care therefore require frequent comprehensive assessment and demand that medical decisions be considered thoughtfully. Last, although the goals of palliative care and end-of-life care are patient focused, they should also address family concerns and the family's interpretation of the patient's symptoms. As families watch loved ones suffer, it is important that healthcare providers understand what a family is observing and provide education and support as needed.

Surgeons play varied clinical roles. They may act as the primary treating physician for patients with conditions that are curable by surgical intervention. They provide intensive care of critically ill surgical patients, in some of whom death is anticipated. Surgeons may also act as partners in the management of patients with many different life-limiting illnesses, such as cancer. They may be called upon to evaluate patients with advanced illness for palliative surgical intervention. The fundamental principles of palliative care should be understood by surgeons and applied in the different settings in which they practice, whether they are acting in a primary or a partnering role.

TABLE 40.1. Palliative Care Core Competencies for Surgeons.

Patient care
Medical knowledge
Communication
Professionalism
Systems-based practice

Source: Robert Wood Johnson Foundation, Office of Promoting Excellence in End-of-Life Care. Executive Summary of the Report from the Field. Surgeons Palliative Care Workgroup. J Am Coll Surg 2003;196(5):807–813.

During the past decade, numerous policy statements and guidelines have been developed for palliative care in the United States[8,9] (Table 40.1). The principles of hospice have been adopted in a wider setting, and there is growing appreciation for the need for palliative medicine specialists. At the same time, palliative medicine specialists have worked to bring fundamental knowledge and skills to all physicians.

Despite the fact that palliative care and end-of-life care are central to the practice of medicine, historically these topics have not been included in surgical textbooks. Surgical textbooks serve as an important education and reference resource, and often address disease epidemiology, prognosis, progression, and medical interventions. However, symptom management at end of life, medical decision making at end of life, advance care planning, and the effects of death and dying on both family and surgeon are often not included.[10] Because dying patients and death are encountered frequently in surgical practice, this textbook endeavors to address the topic and better prepare the surgeon to participate in the care of seriously ill and dying patients.

The Role of the Surgeon in Palliative and End-of-Life Care

Multispecialty, interdisciplinary care of seriously ill and dying patients is now standard practice. This care requires teamwork in both the inpatient and outpatient settings. Surgeons need to relate to other physicians, nurses, mental health professionals, spiritual advisors, and clinical support staff of various disciplines. Extensive discussions with patients, families, and other healthcare professionals in this setting require time and patience.[11,12]

It is important for surgeons to characterize planned operations as either curative or palliative. In one study of patients with advanced cancer, surgeons identified planned operations before surgery as either curative or palliative and estimated patient survival time. These surgeons identified 22 operations (37%) as palliative and 37 (63%) as curative. The median overall survival time was 14.9 months, and it did not differ between curative and palliative operations. Surgical morbidity was high and also did not differ between the two groups: 56% of patients were symptomatic before surgery and major symptom resolution was achieved after surgery in 79%.[13]

When presenting with advanced disease that requires palliative interventions, the patient must be assessed with the intent of resolving chief complaints; controlling pain or morbidity of disease and therapy; and improving quality of life. The surgeon is in a unique position to care for terminally ill patients through the appropriate use of palliative procedures. Both operative and nonoperative procedures can be used with noncurative intent for the purpose of relieving specific symptoms. After assessing the patient, the surgeon recommends the intervention that will best maximize symptom relief and minimize complications. When a procedure is then selected and performed with palliative intent, treatment goals must be clearly defined and communicated between patient and family. Because palliative care requires a patient approach defined in terms of the patient's individual needs, identical procedures may achieve dramatically different results in different patients. Because treatment choices can greatly affect a patient's final days, effective palliation of terminally ill patients demands the highest level of surgical judgment.[14] It has been suggested that, during initial consultation, each patient should be asked to state the problem that he or she wants palliated by the procedure. The terminally ill patient's family members should also be included in this conversation, and additional expectations, opinions, or concerns should be elicited from them. Patients may acknowledge the palliative intent of the proposed procedure and also express a hope that the procedure is curative or that there will be no evidence of disease found at the time of surgery. In one study, 38% of patients undergoing palliative procedures stated that they also sought a prolongation of life, and 27% of patients reported that they did not expect to survive the proposed procedure. The preoperative assessment is important because the goals of the patient, family, and surgeon should match.[15] Factors contributing to variability of patients' expectations have yet to be elaborated.

Recent reports of specific palliative surgical approaches are evidence of the evolving appreciation for the important role surgeons can play in the care of patients with very advanced disease, for example, stereotactic radiosurgery for melanoma metastatic to brain[16] and complications of advanced colon cancer. In colorectal cancer, resection or other operative procedures of the colon or rectum may be performed for the following indications: bowel obstruction, active hemorrhage, severe anemia from gastrointestinal bleeding, intractable pain, and perforation of colon. In one study of 74 patients with colorectal cancer, 49/74 (66%) underwent an operation and 25 were managed nonoperatively. The average survival was 11.2 months for operative patients versus 6.5 months for nonoperative patients ($P > 0.05$). The authors concluded that many patients who present with metastatic disease will benefit from palliative operations with relatively short hospitalizations and reasonable survival[17] (Table 40.2).

It is important to recognize that some patients may have surgically correctable problems unrelated to their terminal illness, but that decision analyses pertaining to surgical choices for these conditions must incorporate considerations related to the terminal condition.

Last, although other experts may have the primary responsibility for providing medical care of the seriously ill patient, surgeons should have a minimum of expertise in perioperative symptom control, particularly the control of pain and nausea. Advances in symptom management continue, and it behooves the practicing surgeon to stay up to date with general knowledge, for example, in the clinical pharmacology of opioids.

TABLE 40.2. Palliative Surgical Interventions.

General Goals:
Reconstruction
Restoration of function
Relief of hollow organ obstruction
Stenting
Repair of fistula
Symptom control
Disease control
Debulking resection
Amputation
Endoscopic ablation
Percutaneous ablation
Chemoembolization
Control of hemorrhage, discharge, odor
Wound management
Specific Procedures:
Brain
Cerebrospinal fluid shunt
Stereotactic radiosurgery
Craniotomy
Respiratory
Tracheotomy
Pulmonary drain
Thoracentesis
Mediastinal mass resection
Cardiac
Cardiocentesis
Removal of pericardium
Gastrointestinal
Relief of gastrointestinal obstructions
Fistula repair
Paracentesis
Placement of feeding tube
Genitourinary
Fistula repair
Renal stents
Urinary diversion
Spine
Laminectomy
Decompression of spinal cord or cauda equina
Stabilization
Vertebroplasty
Kyphoplasty
Bone
Fracture stabilization

Source: Data from Berger AM, Portenoy RK, Weissman DE, eds. Principles and Practice of Palliative Care and Supportive Oncology, 2nd ed. Philadelphia: Lippincott Williams & Wilkins, 2002.

Ethical Considerations

Ethical considerations arise in relationship to declining to intervene and withdrawing specific medical interventions. Advance care planning is essential to preventing unwanted interventions, but, perhaps more importantly, to supporting families when they act as surrogate decision makers and choose to decline or stop specific interventions. Clinicians should elicit values and preferences for end-of-life care, provide education about the dying process, and guide discussions leading to the signing of relevant legal documents, that is, Advance Directives.

High-quality palliative care and end-of-life care are delivered in the context of excellent therapeutic relationships. Therefore, the success of care being delivered is dependent on the nature of that relationship. The intrinsic aim of such care is the relief of suffering ("quarternary prevention"), and the extrinsic aims are relief of physical, psychological, social, and spiritual distress. Healthcare professionals have an obligation to provide treatments that carry a favorable balance of benefits to burdens or risks. If the balance is very favorable, then it is obligatory to offer those treatments with the appropriate advice. In many circumstances, the balance of benefits to burdens or risks is not marked in either direction and treatments are regarded as optional; these decisions may be harder for patients and families to make. Finally, treatments that have only a minimal chance of benefit but which in the particular case entail overwhelming burdens or risks should not be provided at all. It could be said that we have an obligation not to provide such treatments.

The moral problems that arise in palliative care and end-of-life care regarding treatments intended primarily to prolong or sustain life relate to the balance between the benefit and the burdens of treatment. Great value is placed on prolonging life in our society. The lives of patients are entrusted to their healthcare professionals, but we do not have a duty to attempt to extend life at all costs. In certain circumstance, it is ethical for providers not to offer life-prolonging treatment: if the treatment is considered futile; when burdens and risks greatly outweigh benefits of the treatment; when treatment will not further the patient's total good; and when treatments are not available for reasons of resource constraints. This last aspect may pose the most difficult dilemmas for physicians. However, a more extensive discussion of these ethical issues is beyond the scope of this chapter.

Healthcare professionals practicing palliative and end-of-life care will encounter troubling cases. It is important for the individual professional to seek opportunities to read, reflect, and discuss these as they arise. In this way we not only protect ourselves from professional "burnout," we also advance the practices of palliative and end-of-life care.

Surgeons are strongly encouraged to be familiar with principles of medical ethics and to participate in family conferences, interdisciplinary treatment planning meetings, and ethics committees.

Conclusion

Surgeons have a vital role to play in the multidisciplinary, interspecialty care of the seriously ill patient and the family. In doing so, they face many challenges. "But as the challenges are great, when done well, so are the rewards."[18] These rewards derive from knowing that we have contributed to enhancing the quality of life of patients and families, and that, along with our colleagues, we have served humanity in the best way possible.

References

1. WHO Expert Committee: Cancer Pain Relief and Palliative Care Report of the World Health Organization. Geneva: WHO, 1998.
2. Weinstein SM. Integrating palliative care in oncology. Cancer Control 2001;8(1):32–35.
3. Schwenzer KJ. How to offer comfort and symptom relief to dying patient. J Crit Illness 1998;13:381–392.
4. Covinsky KE, Fuller JD, Yaffe K, et al. Communication and decision-making in seriously ill patients: findings of the SUPPORT project. The Study to Understand Prognoses and

Preferences for Outcomes and Risks of Treatments. J Am Geriatr Soc 2000;48:S187–S193.
5. Donnely S, Walsh D. The symptoms of advanced cancer. Semin Oncol 1995;22(suppl 3):67–72.
6. Kaiser HE, Brock DB. Comparative aspects of the quality of life in cancer patients. In Vivo 1992;5(2):83–92.
7. Coyle N, Adelhardt J, Foley KM, Portenoy RK. Character of terminal illness in the advanced cancer patient: pain and other symptoms during the last four weeks of life. J Pain Symptom Manag 1990;46:870–872.
8. Field MJ, Cassel CK, eds. Approaching Death: Improving Care at the End of Life. Washington, DC: Institute of Medicine, National Academy Press, 1997.
9. Foley KM, Gelbrand H. Improving Palliative Care for Cancer. Washington, DC: National Academy Press, 2001.
10. Easson AM, Crosby JA, Librach SL. Discussion of death and dying in surgical textbooks. Am J Surg 2001;182(1):34–39.
11. Lee K, Purcell G, Hinsaw D, Krouse R, Ballus M. Clinical palliative care for surgeons. Part I. J Am Coll Surg 2004;198(2):303–319.
12. Lee K, Purcell G, Hinsaw D, Krouse R, Ballus M. Clinical palliative care for surgeons. Part II. J Am Coll Surg 2004;198(3):477–491.
13. McCahill LE, Smith DD, Borneman T, et al. A prospective evaluation of palliative outcomes for surgery of advanced malignancies. Ann Surg Oncol 2003;10(6):654–663.
14. Cullinane CA, Borneman T, Smith DD, Chu DZJ, Farrell BR, Wagman LD. The surgical treatment of cancer: a comparison of resource utilization following procedures performed with curative and palliative intent. Cancer (Phila) 2003;98(10):2266–2273.
15. Miner TJ, Jaques DP, Shriver CD. A prospective evaluation of patients undergoing surgery for the palliation of advanced malignancy. Ann Surg Oncol 2002;9:696–703.
16. Wong SL, Coit DG. Role of surgery in patients with stage IV melanoma. Curr Opin Oncol 2004;16(2):155–160.
17. Cummins ER, Vick DK, Poole GV. Incurable colorectal carcinoma: the role of surgical palliation. Am J Surg 2004;70(5):433–437.
18. Whooley BP, Milch RA, Gibbs JF. Palliative surgery. In: Berger AM, Portenoy RK, Weissman DE, eds. Principles and Practice of Palliative Care and Supportive Oncology, 2nd ed. Philadelphia: Lippincott Williams & Wilkins, 2002:719.

SECTION FOUR

Gastrointestinal and Abdominal Surgery

41 History of Surgery of the Gastrointestinal Tract

Sean J. Mulvihill and Haile T. Debas

Four salient points can be made in any discussion of the history of gastrointestinal surgery. First, major contributions in surgical technique have been made by individual surgeons who were giants in their times. These individuals had the insight to translate scientific observations and knowledge of pathophysiology into advances in patient care. Second and equally important, the evolution of the field has been furthered by advances in allied fields, including anesthesia and critical care, radiology, gastroenterology, and bioengineering. Indeed, complex care in gastrointestinal surgery is increasingly delivered by teams of experts from all these fields. Third, the field of gastrointestinal surgery has evolved without the benefit of organized, structured training programs. The need for specialized training in complex gastrointestinal surgery is becoming increasingly appreciated, and such training is likely to be demanded by better-informed consumers if we fail to provide it. Fourth, advances in pharmacology and microbiology have had a profound effect on both the incidence and safety of surgical procedures. A poignant example is the virtual disappearance of elective surgery for peptic ulcer because of the discovery of powerful acid-suppressing pharmaceutical agents as well as recognition of the etiological significance of *Helicobacter pylori* eradication. Similarly, antimicrobial therapy has increased the safety of colon resection and other major operations.

Gastrointestinal Surgery Has Benefited from Technological Advances

The evolution of gastrointestinal surgery has been profoundly affected by technological advances in surgical and imaging techniques (Table 41.1), three of which have had an especially important role: fiber-optic endoscopy, diagnostic and interventional radiology, and videoendoscopic surgery. Endoscopic control of bleeding peptic ulcer has greatly reduced the need for emergency surgery. Similarly, endoscopic papillotomy and extraction of common bile duct stones have changed the indications for choledocholithotomy. In the colon, colonoscopic polypectomy has made open polypectomy a rare operation.

Advances in diagnostic radiology have provided the surgeon with more accurate information, permitting more precise diagnosis as well as careful selection and planning of surgical procedures. Not so long ago, gastrointestinal surgeons depended largely on plain abdominal films and barium studies for this purpose. The situation was significantly improved with the development of fluoroscopy in 1896, but it was the more recent advent of ultrasonography, computed tomography (CT), and magnetic resonance imaging (MRI) that has brought about the great revolution in diagnostic radiology. Similarly, the introduction of digital angiography and the combination of selective angiography with CT scan have greatly enhanced imaging of tumors and their blood supply. The rapidly developing field of three-dimensional CT scanning will complement or even replace diagnostic colonoscopy. Similarly, magnetic resonance cholangiopancreatography (MRCP) has the potential to replace diagnostic endoscopic retrograde cholangiopancreatography (ERCP).

Interventional radiology has contributed immensely to the surgical care of patients with gastrointestinal disease. Most intraabdominal abscesses and fluid collections can now be treated percutaneously without resorting to laparotomy. In recent years, the mortality rate following major abdominal operations, such as pancreaticoduodenectomy, has dropped dramatically, in part because postoperative complications can be managed with these techniques. The ability of the radiologist to thread catheters into abdominal vessels and across vascular beds has also had significant impact. The best example is the advent of transjugular intrahepatic portasystemic shunts (TIPS) in 1989. This technique has had a significant influence on surgical portasystemic shunting, particularly as a bridge to reduce portal pressure and stop variceal bleeding before liver transplantation.

Perhaps the most revolutionary development has been the advent of minimally invasive surgery. In two areas in

TABLE 41.1. Impact of Technological Advances on Gastrointestinal Surgery.

Fiber-optic endoscopy	
	Improved diagnosis and biopsy of tumors
Interventional endoscopy	
	Sclerotherapy of bleeding esophageal varices
	Injection and cautery control of bleeding peptic ulcer
	Gastrostomy
	Endoscopic retrograde cholangiography
	Endoscopic papillotomy
	Polypectomy
Imaging technology	
	Ultrasonography
	Computed tomography
	Magnetic resonance imaging
	Three-dimensional computed tomography
	Subselective angiography
	Digital angiography
Interventional radiology	
	Percutaneous biopsy
	Percutaneous drainage (abscess, fluid collection)
	Percutaneous embolization for hemorrhage
	Feeding jejunostomy
	Bowel decompression
	TIPS (transjugular intrahepatic portasystemic shunt)
Minimally invasive surgery	
	Laparoscopic cholecystectomy and common bile duct exploration
	Laparoscopic fundoplication and hiatal hernia repair
	Laparoscopic and thoracoscopic Heller myotomy
	Laparoscopic excision of hepatic cysts
	Laparoscopic transgastric cystgastrostomy
	Laparoscopic appendectomy and colectomy
	Laparoscopic splenectomy and adrenalectomy
	Laparoscopic inguinal hernia repair
Future	
	Robotic surgery
	Virtual reality
	Miniaturization

particular—cholecystectomy and surgery for gastroesophageal reflux—the laparoscopic approach has replaced open surgery as the routine procedure. Future advances in instrumentation, miniaturization, robotics, and virtual reality are likely to have even greater ramifications in coming years.

In subsequent paragraphs, the history of gastrointestinal surgery is recounted, organized around specific organs. Vignettes of interesting historical milestones are recounted in sidebars. A theme of milestone contributions by surgical scientists who bridged the gap between laboratory and bedside is developed using specific examples.

History of Esophageal Surgery

Reflux Esophagitis and Hiatal Hernia

With the advent of barium examination of the upper gastrointestinal tract, the frequent association of sliding hiatal hernia with gastroesophageal reflux disease (GERD) was recognized. This anatomical abnormality became the focus of treatment. As a result, surgery for hiatal hernia was directed at repairing the anatomical defect with reduction of the hernia, narrowing the hiatus by approximating the crura, and performing some type of gastropexy to anchor the stomach below the diaphragm. Several approaches evolved to accomplish this repair (Table 41.2). The best known of the anatomical defect-correcting operations was the Allison repair.[1] It is of interest that Allison was the first to coin the term *reflux esophagitis*, demonstrating his understanding of gastroesophageal reflux as the cause of esophageal inflammation. The recognition of an incompetent or hypotensive lower esophageal sphincter (LES) as the underlying cause of reflux had to await the development of esophageal manometry. Charles Code from the Mayo Clinic[2] was a pioneer in the development of esophageal motility studies and in defining the LES, the normal contractile pattern of the body of the esophagus, and the upper esophageal sphincter (UES).

These advances in our understanding of esophageal physiology heralded the era of operations designed to restore continence by increasing the LES pressure (LESP). Of these operations, the best known are the Nissen fundoplication, the Hill posterior gastropexy, and the Belsey Mark IV, introduced by Skinner and Belsey. The Nissen and Belsey repairs increase LESP by wrapping the gastric fundus around the lower esophagus totally or partially, respectively. Nissen (Fig. 41.1) began his experience with a transabdominal approach to fundoplication in 1955, using a 360° wrap of fundus around the lower esophagus.[3] The Belsey operation is performed through a left posterolateral thoracotomy and involves a 240° fundoplication.[4] The Hill repair differs in that the emphasis is on restoration of the posterior fixation of the gastroesophageal junction within the abdomen.[5] This technique restores a length of subdiaphragmatic esophagus to be subjected to positive intra-abdominal pressure, thereby improving LESP.

Of equal importance to manometry in understanding the pathophysiology of reflux was the development of techniques to assess the role of acid in the esophagus. It had been difficult to differentiate symptoms related to reflux from those of other foregut disorders before the Bernstein acid perfusion test was employed to verify the etiology.[6] The development by Tuttle and Grossman[7] of an intraesophageal pH probe significantly improved diagnosis and led to the introduction by Skinner and Booth[8] of the standard acid reflux test (SART).

TABLE 41.2. Milestones in Hiatal Hernia Surgery.

What	*Who*	*When*
Surgical repair		
Allison repair	Allison	1951
Total fundoplication	Nissen	1961
Posterior gastropexy	Hill	1960s
Belsey Mark IV	Skinner and Belsey	1967
Gastroplasty and fundoplication	Pearson et al.	1987
Physiological studies		
Manometry	Texter et al.	1957
Acid perfusion test	Bernstein and Baker	1958
Intraesophageal pH electrode	Tuttle and Grossman	1958
Esophageal manometry	Code	1967
Standard acid reflux test (SART)	Skinner and Booth	1970
24-hour pH monitoring	Johnson and DeMeester	1974
Technetium-99m radionuclide scanning	Fisher et al.	1976

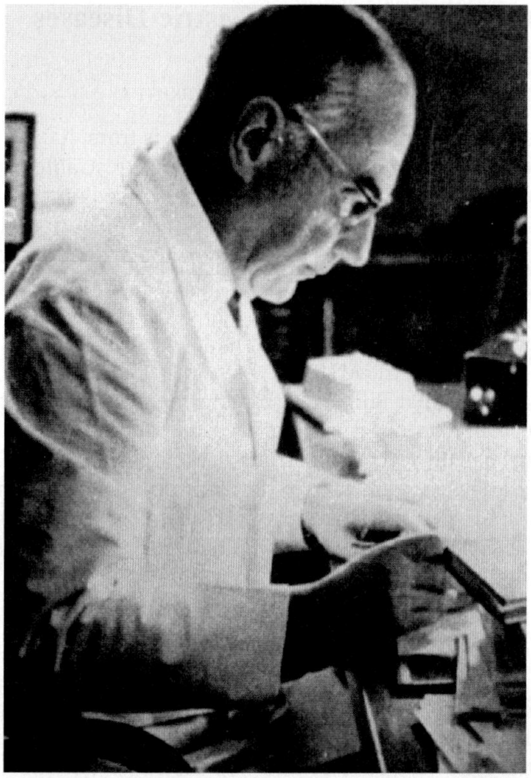

FIGURE 41.1. Rudolph Nissen (b. 1896) developed a transabdominal approach to fundoplication in 1955 using a 360° wrap of the gastric fundus around the lower esophagus. Referred to as the Nissen fundoplication, it is one of the better-known procedures for restoring sphincter continence by increasing the lower esophageal sphincter pressure (LESP). (Figure provided courtesy of the National Library of Medicine.)

Further evolution led to the best assessment of symptomatic acid reflux, now accomplished in a standard way by the use of ambulatory 24-h pH monitoring, perfected by Johnson and DeMeester.[9]

The combined use of esophageal manometry and pH studies became important both in selecting an antireflux operation and in evaluating postoperative results. The demonstration of an aperistaltic or hypomotile esophagus, for example, may contraindicate the use of a total wrap, as performed in the Nissen procedure. Chronic esophagitis can occasionally result in the development of a shortened esophagus. Pearson and colleagues at the University of Toronto popularized the Collis gastroplasty as an esophagus-lengthening procedure for this situation.[10] Fundoplication could then be performed around the neoesophagus to restore sphincter competence. The most recent advance in surgery for reflux esophagitis is the minimally invasive approach. Indeed, the laparoscopic approach is increasingly preferred for performing antireflux procedures and hiatal hernia repair.

Disorders of Esophageal Motility

Esophageal Diverticula

Esophageal diverticula are associated with underlying motility disorders. Until the advent of esophageal manometry, however, surgical correction of esophageal diverticula, like operations for hiatal hernia, was directed solely at the anatomical abnormality. It is now generally accepted that a Zenker's diverticulum is associated with failure of relaxation of the UES with deglutition, and epiphrenic diverticula are associated with underlying esophageal spasm, achalasia, or other functional disorders. Failure to recognize and treat the underlying motility disorder leads to persistent symptoms and recurrent diverticula. Allen and Clagget in 1965 and Belsey in 1966 recognized this and advocated the performance of cricopharyngeal myotomy to treat Zenker's diverticulum.[11] Similarly, by 1980, a Mayo Clinic study recommended correction of the underlying motility disorder with excision of epiphrenic diverticula. Failure to do this resulted in increased dehiscence at the diverticulectomy site.[12]

Achalasia

First coined by Sir Cooper Perry in 1915, *achalasia* is a Greek term meaning failure or lack of relaxation. Treatment of achalasia has evolved from simple bougienage, used by Thomas Willis in the 17th century, to forceful dilation and disruption of the LES by pneumatic or hydrostatic dilators. In 1914, Ernst Heller (1877–1964), of Leipzig, described a procedure for achalasia involving myotomy on both sides of the distal esophagus.[13] By 1920, at the German Surgical Congress, he had reported 20 patients operated on without mortality. In 1923, Zaaijer reported a modification that included a single myotomy.[14] Despite its simplicity and evident superiority to other treatment options, Heller's myotomy was slow to be accepted. It was not until 1949, when Norman Barrett and R.H. Franklin recounted the failure of cardioplasty or esophagogastrostomy and their own good results with myotomy that the operation became the standard.[15] Ellis and associates contributed significantly to the treatment of this disease, advocating a limited extension of the myotomy onto the stomach to prevent postoperative reflux.[16]

Most recently, myotomy is performed either thoracoscopically or laparoscopically, and the minimally invasive approach is emerging as the operation of choice.[17] The use of esophageal motility studies has enabled us to define various other motility disorders, including diffuse esophageal spasm, the nutcracker esophagus, the hypertensive LES, and a number of nonspecific disorders, including scleroderma.

Esophageal Resection

Early attempts at esophageal surgery were significantly limited by difficulties related to maintenance of ventilation under anesthesia. Rudolf Matas is credited with introducing tracheal insufflation, a technique perfected by Meltzer and Auer in 1909.[18,19] Theodore Billroth (Fig. 41.2) probably performed the first successful resection of the cervical esophagus in dogs in 1871, and by 1877, Czerny is thought to have performed a similar operation in a patient. By 1908, Voeckler had performed an esophagogastrectomy with anastomosis, using an abdominal approach for a tumor at the cardia. Successful resection of the thoracic esophagus was first accomplished in 1913 by Torek.[20] His reconstruction involved a cervical esophagostomy and gastrostomy without anastomosis and no restoration of gastrointestinal continuity.

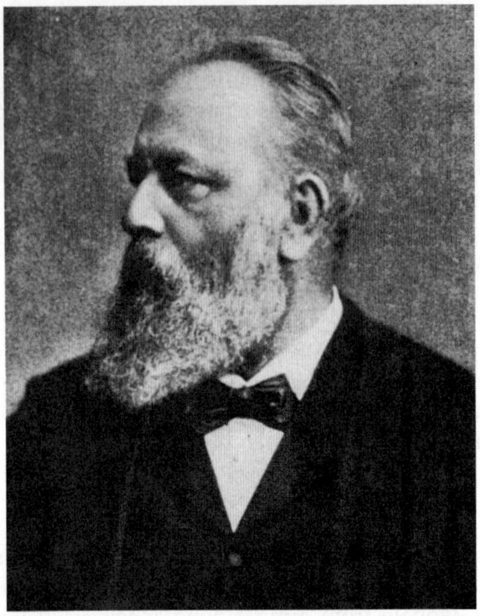

FIGURE 41.2. German surgeon Theodor Billroth (1829–1894) performed the first successful gastroenterostomy (with his assistant Anton Wölfer) and the first successful gastrectomy, both in 1881. A composer of music and friend of Johannes Brahms, Billroth is known for his teaching of many great students, his humility, and his publication of his surgical failures as well as successes. (Figure provided courtesy of the National Library of Medicine.)

It was not until 1933 that resection with anastomosis was successfully performed for carcinomas of the distal third of the esophagus by Ohsawa and, later, Adams and Phemister.[21,22] Resection of midthird cancers proved more difficult because left thoracotomy did not provide adequate exposure. In 1946, Lewis described a new operation that used both an abdominal and right thoracic approach to resect midthird lesions, with esophagogastrostomy near the level of the azygous vein in the right chest.[23]

A major limitation of intrathoracic anastomosis was leakage, leading to mediastinitis and death. This problem led to a safer approach with cervical anastomosis.[24] A major contribution was the recognition of the possibility of esophageal dissection via the abdomen, blunt or transhiatal esophagectomy, popularized by Kirk in 1974 and Orringer in 1978. The group at the University of Michigan has published material on the largest and best experience with this operation.[25] A summary of milestones in esophageal surgery is given in Table 41.3.

TABLE 41.3. Milestones in Esophageal Surgery.

What	Who	When
Esophageal motility		
Heller myotomy for achalasia	Heller	1913
Modified Heller	Zaaijer	1923
Cricopharyngeal myotomy for Zenker's diverticulum	Belsey	1966
Esophageal resection		
Cervical esophagectomy	Billroth	1871
Thoracic esophagectomy	Torek	1915
Esophagogastrectomy	Ohsawa	1933
Ivor Lewis esophagectomy	Lewis	1946
Transhiatal esophagectomy	Orringer	1993

Peptic Ulcer and Other Gastric Diseases

Gastroenterostomy and Gastrectomy

The earliest reference to gastric surgery is from 400 BC, when Aesculapius cut out a stomach ulcer in a restrained patient and sewed him up again. The case is inscribed on the second pillar in the Temple of Aesculapius at Epidaurus, Greece. Péan (1879) and Rydigier (1880) performed pylorectomies, but their patients died. Modern surgical techniques began to appear in the late 19th century (Table 41.4). In 1881, Theodor Billroth (1829–1894) and his assistant, Anton Wölfler (1850–1917), performed the first successful gastroenterostomy,[26] and in that same year Billroth also performed the first successful gastrectomy on a patient with gastric cancer.[27] In his first operations, Billroth reconstructed the gastrointestinal tract with a gastroduodenostomy (Billroth I), but by 1885 he had performed gastrojejunostomy after distal gastrectomy (Billroth II). Others credited with popularizing gastroenterostomy include Doyen (1892) and Rydigier (1884).[28]

Total Gastrectomy

Carl Schlatter (1864–1934) was the first to successfully perform total gastrectomy in a 56-year-old woman with gastric cancer in Zurich in 1897. This patient lived some 14 months following surgery and was the subject of subsequent investigation of digestion and metabolism at the University of Zurich. By 1929, only 67 cases of total gastrectomy had been reported, with an operative mortality rate of 54%.[29]

The Roux-Y Modification

Shortly after the initial descriptions of gastroenterostomy for peptic ulcer or gastric cancer, the problem of postoperative bilious vomiting was recognized. This was thought to be related to the reentry of bile and food into the stomach via the afferent limb (circulus vitiosus or vicious circle). By 1897, Cesar Roux, professor of surgery in Lausanne, Switzerland, described his famous "Roux ansa en Y" as an alternative to loop gastroenterostomy.[30,31] Roux's operation prevented

TABLE 41.4. Milestones in Peptic Ulcer Therapy.

What	Who	When
Gastroenterostomy	Billroth, Wölfler	1881
Gastrectomy	Billroth	1881
Truncal vagotomy (first successfully performed)	Latarjet	1921
Truncal vagotomy (popularized procedure)	Dragstedt	1943
Selective gastric vagotomy (first successfully performed)	Franksson	1948
Selective gastric vagotomy (popularized procedure)	Kennedy	1969
Highly selective vagotomy (first successfully performed)	Holle	1969
Highly selective vagotomy (popularized procedure)	Johnston	1970
H_2-receptor antagonists	Black	1972
Discovered *Helicobacter pylori*	Marshall, Warren	1983

bilious vomiting but was complicated by stomal ulceration in patients with peptic ulcer disease. Renewed interest in the procedure occurred in the middle of this century when the concept was applied to biliary, pancreatic, and esophageal reconstruction.

Vagotomy

In the first half of this century, gastroenterostomy and gastrectomy were commonly used to treat benign ulcer disease. The recurrence rate and undesirable sequelae of these procedures became widely recognized. Based on the understanding that the vagus nerves control acid secretion, in 1921 the French surgeon Latergết performed the first reported case of vagotomy.[32] This operation did not come into favor, however, until 1943 when Lester Dragstedt from the University of Chicago popularized it for the treatment of peptic ulcer.[33] Initially, he did not perform a drainage procedure, and up to a third of his patients developed problems of delayed gastric emptying and stasis gastric ulcer. This observation led him to advocate the addition of a drainage procedure (pyloroplasty or gastrojejunostomy) to truncal vagotomy. The next 30 years saw progressive refinement of vagotomy to make it more selective. Selective gastric vagotomy was first reported in 1948 by Franksson.[34] Because the entire stomach was denervated in this operation, a drainage procedure was still required. In 1969, however, highly selective vagotomy for peptic ulcer (also known as parietal cell or proximal gastric vagotomy) was popularized by Kennedy, Johnston, and others.[35,36] Only the parietal cell portion of the stomach was denervated in highly selective vagotomy, so antropyloric motility was unaffected, and drainage procedures were unnecessary.

Medical Therapy for Ulcer

In a quirk of history, the introduction of the most "physiological" operation for peptic ulcer, highly selective vagotomy, was followed closely by the discovery of potent acid-suppressing drugs. First came the discovery of the histamine H_2-receptor antagonists, for which Sir James Black won a Nobel Prize, then that of the even more potent proton pump inhibitors. With the advent of these two powerful agents, elective surgery for peptic ulcer disease has all but disappeared. Medical therapy, however, appears to have had little effect on the prevalence of the complications of perforation and bleeding and the need for emergent surgery to treat peptic ulcer disease.

Important as the acid-inhibitory drugs have been in peptic ulcer therapy, the real revolution occurred with the discovery by Marshall and Warren in 1983 of *Helicobacter pylori* (HP) and its etiological significance in peptic ulceration.[37] For the first time, it became possible to cure patients using antimicrobial agents to eradicate HP, which is now believed to have etiological significance in 90% of patients with duodenal ulcer and 80% with gastric ulcer. The long-term effect of HP eradication on complications of peptic ulcer and prevalence of emergency ulcer surgery has yet to be established. Not all peptic ulcers are caused by HP. Increasingly, the etiological importance of nonsteroidal antiinflammatory drugs (NSAIDs) has become evident, particularly in cases of bleeding and perforation.

History of Biliary Tract Surgery

Early History

Gallstones, the most common disorder of the biliary tract, have been found in the remains of a Mycenaean male skeleton, circa 1600–1500 BC. Similarly, a preserved Egyptian mummy, circa 1500 BC, was found to have a gallbladder containing some 30 radiopaque gallstones.[38] This mummy was housed in the Museum of the Royal College of Surgeons in London but was unfortunately destroyed in Nazi bombing during World War II.

The first publication describing pathology recognizable as gallstones was written by Alexander Trallianus (525–605), a Greek physician, who described concretions within the bile ducts. With the revival of anatomical dissection in Italy, Beniveni (ca. 1440–1502) and Vesalius (1514–1564) identified gallstones and their clinical sequelae. Expulsion of stones in the gastrointestinal tract through vomitus or stool was recognized in 1586 by Marcellus Donatus, who published an important treatise on biliary tract pathology. Despite this history, gallbladder symptoms in women were attributed to hysteria by Thomas Syndenham (1624–1689), the famous English physician. Gallstone disease has affected the leaders of civilization, ranging from Alexander the Great, who succumbed to an illness suggestive of acute cholecystitis in 323 BC,[39] to Lyndon Baines Johnson, who underwent cholecystectomy while president of the United States.

Early Attempts at Treatment

Treatment of gallstones was initially limited to cholecystostomy, usually attributed to Fabricius Hildanus (1560–1624) of Bern in 1618. By 1667, Teckoy, in Leyden, had performed experiments in dogs and concluded that the gallbladder was not necessary for life. Drainage of the gallbladder by trocar was performed in 1743 by Jean Louis Petit (1674–1760).[40] Few subsequent advances in the treatment of gallbladder disease occurred until 1867, when John Bobbs of Indiana successfully performed cholecystostomy and stone removal in a young woman under chloroform anesthesia. She was reported to live for some 45 years postoperatively and attended a meeting of the American Medical Association as a testament to the success of this treatment. Nearly simultaneous reports of cholecystostomy were also given by James Marion Sims of South Carolina and Lawson Tait of England in 1878.

The first cholecystectomy was probably performed by Carl Langenbuch at Lazarus Hospital in Berlin on July 15, 1882. Langenbuch had studied the gallbladder in the autopsy room, found it absent in horses and elephants, and concluded it was not necessary for survival. His first patient was a 43-year-old man who suffered intermittent attacks of vomiting and pain once or twice per year. He had intermittent jaundice, a palpable gallbladder, and gallstones had been found in his stool. At the time of surgery, his symptoms had progressed to daily pain, vomiting, and "stubborn" constipation. At operation, a thickened gallbladder wall and two small cholesterol stones were discovered. After the gallbladder was removed, the patient had relatively rapid convalescence and relief of pain.[41] Langenbuch is attributed with the quotation, still relevant today, that the gallbladder should be removed

HISTORICAL VIGNETTE 41.1. Incisions in Abdominal Surgery.

Incision	*Description*
Kocher incision	Right upper quadrant subcostal incision for biliary tract surgery
Kehr incision	Subcostal incision with midline cephalad extension for biliary tract or splenic operations
Rockey-Davis incision	Muscle-splitting right lower quadrant incision for appendicitis
Pfannenstiehl incision	Lower transverse skin incision with midline fascial opening classically used for cesarean section
Midline incision	Division of the linear alba in the midline, allowing rapid access to the abdominal cavity
Bilateral subcostal incision	Useful for hepatic, pancreatic, and complex biliary surgery
Thoracoabdominal incision	Extension of laparotomy incision into left or right chest
Coller incision	Oblique left upper quadrant to right lower quadrant (saber-slash) incision popularized at the University of Michigan

"not because it contains stones, but because it forms them."

Hans Kehr, a German surgeon in Halberstadt, contributed to the development of biliary tract surgery through his large experience, his careful record keeping of operations, and the publication of his results. A common biliary tract incision is named for him (Historical Vignette 41.1). In 1910, he moved to Berlin and prepared the second of his two books on biliary tract surgery, *The Practice of Biliary Tract Surgery in Words and Pictures*. He succumbed to sepsis related to a finger infection arising from an intraoperative injury in 1916. Kehr is credited with development of the T tube, which is still known in Europe as the Kehr tube.[42]

Development of Radiographic Techniques

Identification of biliary tract pathology was limited to clinical symptoms and intraoperative findings until the development of x-rays by Wilhelm Roentgen (1845–1923) in 1895. He was a professor of physics at the University of Wurzburg at the time of his discovery. Shortly thereafter, the first identification of radiopaque gallstones was made by Buxbaum of Austria. Imaging of the biliary tree began in 1924 with cholecystography by Evarts Graham and Warren Cole.[43,44] Cole, a young resident, and Graham, his professor, collaborated with Mallinckrodt Chemical Works in St. Louis to develop a compound excreted and concentrated in bile. Subsequent efforts at intraoperative cholangiography by Mirizzi and Losada of Argentina in 1932 via direct puncture of the gallbladder and transhepatic cholangiography in 1952 by Carter and Saypol[45] evolved into the familiar techniques of today.

Common Bile Duct Pathology

One of the first descriptions of common bile duct pathology was the report of cholangitis by Jean Martin Charcot (1825–1893). Charcot, a French physician, was a student of Claude Bernard and practiced at Salpetriere, a 4000-bed women's hospital. In 1877, he published the clinical symptoms associated with passage of common duct stones that we now know as Charcot's triad—right upper quadrant pain, fever with chills, and jaundice. These clinical findings were extended by Telfer Reynolds, a hepatologist in Los Angeles, who recognized the presence of hypotension and altered mental status related to sepsis in cholangitis. Charcot also described the neuropathic arthritis in syphilis that bears his name (Charcot's joint) and Charcot-Leyden crystals (eosinophilic debris in the sputum of asthmatics).[46]

Ludwig Courvoisier (1843–1918) of Basel recognized the reservoir effect of the gallbladder, leading to massive distention in the setting of distal malignant obstruction, as in pancreatic cancer. We know this clinical feature of a palpable gallbladder in malignant biliary obstruction as the Courvoisier sign. He was also one of the first to describe common bile duct exploration via choledochotomy in 1890. The American surgeon William Halsted died in 1922 following complications from his own two bile duct operations (Historical Vignettes 41.2 and 41.3).

Laparoscopic Era

Laparoscopic cholecystectomy grew out of initial experience with diagnostic laparoscopy and pelviscopy by gynecologists, including Kurt Semm of Germany. The first laparoscopic gallbladder operation was performed in 1987 by Mouret of Lyon. This unpublished experience was followed shortly by reports from other European surgeons.[47,48] The initial US experience was reported by Reddick and Olsen[49] shortly thereafter. Although this development was initially met with great skepticism, the advantages, including decreased incisional pain, shortened hospital stay, and rapid return to full physical activities, led to rapid acceptance by the lay public and the medical community.[50] By the early to mid-1990s, the laparoscopic approach had become the preferred method of chole-

HISTORICAL VIGNETTE 41.2. Halsted and the Common Bile Duct.

An ironic historical vignette involves one of America's most prominent surgeons, William Stewart Halsted, and his travails with the common bile duct.[40,99] Halsted operated on his first patient with gallstones in 1882; the patient was his own mother. She was quite ill, and her physicians were undecided regarding the best course of action. Halsted found her jaundiced with a very tender right upper abdominal quadrant. He proceeded with an operation, finding an empyema of the gallbladder. He performed a cholecystostomy with removal of seven stones. She subsequently continued to suffer jaundice and at the time of her death 2 years later, she was found to have a markedly dilated bile duct. Another of Halsted's patients, a middle-aged man with hemorrhagic pancreatitis, was studied at autopsy by Opie, who found a small gallstone impacted at the ampulla of Vater, leading to the formulation of his obstructing gallstone theory of the pathogenesis of pancreatitis.[72] Halsted himself developed abdominal pain and jaundice at age 68 and underwent operation by Dr. Richard Follis at Johns Hopkins in 1917. At operation, numerous common bile duct calculi were found, including one impacted at the ampulla. A cholecystectomy and common bile duct exploration were performed, complicated by a postoperative bile leak. In 1922, Halsted suffered another attack of cholangitis and underwent reoperation by George Heuer and Mont Reid. Another common duct stone was removed, but postoperatively he developed pneumonia, erosive gastritis, and Vincent's angina, leading to his death on September 22, 1922.

HISTORICAL VIGNETTE 41.3. The Development of Rubber Gloves.

In 1913, William Stewart Halsted published an account of the development of rubber gloves in the United States.[100] At that time, operations were performed barehanded, with disinfectants such as carbolic acid used to sterilize the operating team's skin. He described the problem of dermatitis that his operating room nurse, Miss Carolyn Hampton, experienced from the solution of mercuric chloride used as a disinfectant in his operating room. In his words, "As she was an unusually efficient woman, I gave the matter my consideration . . ." He prevailed on the Goodyear Rubber Company to manufacture two pair of thin rubber gloves with gauntlets as a trial, and "these proved to be so satisfactory that additional gloves were ordered." This occurred in 1889 or 1890. Miss Hampton later became Halsted's wife. Others, including J. Mikulicz and, separately, von Zoege-Manteuffel, both of Germany, are credited with reports describing the use of gloves around 1897.[101] This background, however, indicates that the motivation for introducing gloves was to protect the operator's skin from the harsh nature of disinfectants. It is remarkable to consider how relatively recently the policy of universal precautions, including the use of gloves to protect the health professional from patients' blood-borne disease, has come to pass.

cystectomy for most patients. This change, however, did not come without a cost, as the rate of certain complications, especially bile duct injury, was higher with the laparoscopic approach.[51] Laparoscopic cholecystectomy supplanted other developing approaches to treat gallstone disease, including lithotripsy and dissolution agents.[52]

As laparoscopic cholecystectomy emerged as a valid treatment for cholelithiasis, general surgeons felt that their role was threatened by gynecologists and gastroenterologists with previous laparoscopic experience. This concern challenged hospitals to develop credentialing standards for privileges in laparoscopic surgery. Professional societies, such as the Society of American Gastrointestinal Endoscopic Surgeons (SAGES), led the way in developing standards in this area, and laparoscopic cholecystectomy remained firmly in the province of the general surgeon.

History of Liver Surgery

Early History

The origins of liver surgery can be traced to early beliefs regarding the spiritual importance of this unique organ. In Babylonia (ca. 2000 BC), the livers of sacrificed sheep were used to divine the future. Clay models of these livers were made, one of which survives on display in the British Museum.[38] Roman philosophers such as Cicero similarly used markings on the livers of sacrificed sheep and goats to divine the wisdom of government policies. In ancient Mesopotamia, the liver was thought to be the seat of the soul, full as it is with blood, the symbol of life itself. In Egypt, pharaohs were embalmed with special attention to certain organs, including the liver, to ensure their place in the afterlife.

An understanding of the function of the liver was slow in developing. By 300 BC, in the reign of Ptolemy I of Egypt, Celsus of Alexandria had studied liver anatomy through dissections and concluded that it played a necessary role in maintaining life. The first written description of jaundice is attributed to the Roman physician Soranus of Ephesus (ca. 100 AD), but at that time the major function of the liver was thought to relate to the manufacture of blood. Galen, physician to the Roman emperors (131–201 AD), advanced early theories of the role of the liver in digestion. He understood bile to be one of the four humors but mistakenly thought it formed in the gallbladder.

It was not until the 17th century that Bartholin (1616–1680) described the function of the liver as related to excretion of bile. In 1900, Nicholas Augustin Gilbert (1858–1927), professor of medicine at the Hôpital de l'Hôtel-Dieu in Paris, described benign familial icterus.[53] We know this condition to be unconjugated hyperbilirubinemia without underlying liver disease.

Early Attempts at Treatment

Intervention for liver disorders was largely limited to debridement of protruding liver in spear and sword wounds in ancient cultures. In ancient Greece, incision and drainage of liver abscess was described by Hippocrates (ca. 480 BC). Lawson Tait in 1880 described drainage of echinococcal cysts of the liver.[54] In 1887, Carl von Langenbuch performed the first documented successful liver resection, removal of a pedicled tumor from the left lobe of a 30-year-old woman.[55] Although she suffered postoperative hemorrhage and required reoperation, she eventually recovered. As Ambrose Paré (1510–1590) the great French barber-surgeon described in his classic treatise, "When the liver is wounded, much blood commeth out."[56] At the turn of the century, hemorrhage and death remained major problems with any intervention for liver disease. Tilton, for example, in 1905 described a mortality rate of 44% for operations for liver trauma.[57] An early experience with liver resection was tabulated by William Keen, chair of the department of surgery at Jefferson Medical College in Philadelphia.[58] At that time, cautery, large mattress sutures, and constricting loops around pedicled tumors were the main hemostatic techniques. Mortality rates were high, even into the 1960s, when Brunschwig described mortality rates for right and left lobectomy of 50% and 18%, respectively.[59]

Liver Resection

The modern era of liver resection was predicated on careful study of the anatomy of the liver and application of that knowledge in the operating room. Although Glisson, in 1654, first described the vascular anatomy of the liver through corrosion casting techniques, this knowledge was largely ignored by early liver surgeons. Pringle, in 1908, emphasized the unique feature of liver anatomy allowing control of vascular inflow by occlusion at the hepatoduodenal ligament, the maneuver that now bears his eponym.[60] Nonanatomical resections were common until 1954, when Couinard, from France, classified segmental liver anatomy.[61] At about that time, his countrymen Lortat-Jacob and Robert reported their experience with "anatomic" liver resection, and they are often credited with being the first with this approach.[55]

In the subsequent 40 years, new tools, including intraoperative ultrasonography and the ultrasonic dissector, have improved the technical aspects of liver surgery. Modern blood-banking techniques have made transfusion safer and correction of coagulopathy with specific blood products possible. Postoperative care of these patients has been improved by better understanding of the metabolic derangements related to major liver resection and by the development of intensive care units. These developments have made liver resection dramatically safer. Today, population studies show that the operative mortality rate for liver resection in the absence of cirrhosis has improved to about 3%, but this increases to 15% for tumors such as hepatocellular carcinoma.[62]

Portal Hypertension

Surgery for portal hypertension began with Nicolai Vladirmirovich Eck, who performed the first portacaval anastomosis in 1877. Little clinical success with this operation was reported until the middle of the 20th century, with reports from Blakemore, Whipple, and others.[63–65] The mortality rate for shunt operations at this time ranged from 25% to 40%. In survivors, hepatic encephalopathy was increasingly recognized as a clinical problem.

In the 1960s, Warren and colleagues studied this problem and concluded that total diversion of blood flow from the liver was key to the pathophysiology of hepatic encephalopathy. They designed a shunt that preserved hepatic blood flow but decompressed esophageal varices and prevented variceal hemorrhage. This became known as the distal splenorenal, or Warren, shunt.[66] Encephalopathy in patients undergoing the Warren shunt was much reduced compared to the portacaval shunt. The technical demands of the Warren shunt precluded its use in the emergency setting, and because portal hypertension in the bowel mesentery is not relieved, ascites remains a contraindication. Orloff is credited with developing systems to improve outcome of shunt operations in the emergency setting.[67] These operations, however, have largely been supplanted by radiological techniques for intrahepatic creation of an anastomosis between portal and hepatic vein branches via a percutaneous approach (TIPS).[68]

Liver Transplantation

The era of liver transplantation is unique, as the founders of the field are still active clinicians and scientists. On March 1, 1963, Tom Starzl and his colleagues in Denver performed the first liver transplantation in a human, a 3-year-old child with biliary atresia. Although this patient died, the field rapidly developed, with groups headed by Roy Calne in Cambridge, F.D. Moore in Boston, and others. In addition to the formidable technical challenges posed by liver transplantation, advancement in the field was stymied by the difficulties related to organ rejection. By 1971, 102 liver transplants had been performed, and only 12 patients had survived. This picture changed with the introduction in 1980 of cyclosporine as an immunosuppressive.[69]

Now, liver transplantation is performed in 3700 patients per year in the United States alone, with 123 active centers. A major limitation is availability of donor organs, with some 6000 suitable liver transplant candidates now on waiting lists. Major advances continue, with the development of split liver transplantation and the use of organs from living related donors. On the horizon is xenotransplantation, which offers the potential for an unlimited organ supply. With these technical developments, however, new ethical dilemmas have emerged, requiring thoughtful analysis and collaboration among clinicians, scientists, patients, payors, and government.

History of Pancreatic Surgery

Recognition of Pancreatic Function and Disorders

The pancreas was a mysterious organ, and physicians had a poor understanding of its functions well into the 19th century. Johann Georg Wirsung (1589–1643)[70] made one of the first descriptive studies of the pancreas in 1642 with a copperplate engraving showing the anatomy of the pancreatic duct. Despite the Papal Bull of 1300 forbidding human dissection, such activity was common in Padua, Italy, thanks to the leadership of Andreas Vesalius (1514–1564). Wirsung was a student of anatomy and held the position of Prosector in Padua, with responsibility for preparing cadavers for dissection and public demonstration. It was in the course of this work that he discovered the duct, but he had no idea of its function or significance. His copperplate engraving is on display at the University of Padua today. Wirsung met an untimely end at the hands of a rival, Giacomo Cambier, shortly after his discovery of the duct that now bears his name.[71]

Little was known of the function of the pancreas until Claude Bernard (1813–1878) established pancreatic fistulas to study secretion. He demonstrated the effect of pancreatic juice on emulsification of fatty foods, conversion of starch to sugar, and digestion of protein. Although P. Langerhans had described the histological appearance of islet cells in the pancreas in 1869, it was not until the studies of Banting and Best in 1922 that the role of the pancreas in insulin secretion and glucose metabolism was understood (Historical Vignette 41.4).

Acute Pancreatitis

Acute pancreatitis in humans was first described by Edward Klebs in 1870. By 1889, Reginald Fitz had called attention to the hemorrhagic complications of necrotizing pancreatitis with a report of 15 patients. Grey-Turner and

HISTORICAL VIGNETTE 41.4. The Discovery of Insulin.

In the summer of 1921, F.G. Banting, a general surgeon just out of military service, approached Macleod, professor of physiology at the University of Toronto, with a new idea. His plan was to isolate the islets of Langerhans by ligating the pancreatic duct in vivo and preferentially destroying acinar cells. Macleod accepted Banting to work on the project but then left for Scotland on a 1-year sabbatical absence. Banting recruited a bright medical student, C.H. Best, to work with him. Together, over the course of several months, Banting and Best isolated the islets, prepared an extract, and demonstrated that intravenous administration of the extract to a previously pancreatectomized dog resulted in immediate reversal of diabetes.

Macleod returned from Scotland just in time for the public announcement of this momentous discovery and to take credit for the work. By 1922, the first human patient with diabetes was successfully treated with insulin and, in 1923, the Nobel Prize for Medicine was awarded. The award was made to Banting and Macleod, and Best was left out. Despite Banting's outrage, the Nobel Committee would not reverse its decision. Instead, Banting graciously shared his award with the medical student. Now, when historians refer to the discoverers of insulin, they talk about Banting and Best.

Cullen expanded on these clinical descriptions of pancreatitis by noting the ecchymoses in the flank and periumbilical areas, respectively, from retroperitoneal hemorrhage. These clinical descriptions were paralleled by early attempts to define the pathophysiology of pancreatitis. Claude Bernard, for example, studied retrograde injection of bile into the pancreatic duct as a model of pancreatitis. This concept was refined by E.L. Opie, the Johns Hopkins pathologist, who in 1901 identified stone impaction at the ampulla of Vater obstructing the common channel as a cause of hemorrhagic pancreatitis.[72] Along this same line of thinking, in 1948 Lium and Maddock developed a model of pancreatitis induced by pancreatic duct ligation with stimulated secretion.[73]

By this time it began to become clear, however, that in only a few cases of pancreatitis could a stone be found at the ampulla at the time of the attack. In a landmark study, Acosta and Ledesma of Argentina found that 90% of patients with acute biliary pancreatitis excreted gallstones in the stool within a week or so following the attack, compared to only 10% to 15% of patients with biliary colic.[74] This study was soon followed by one from the United States by Kelly, replicating the findings.[75] These studies emphasized the transient nature of the ampullary obstruction related to gallstone passage and guided therapy directed at the common bile duct in subsequent years.

John H.C. Ranson (1938–1995), professor and chief of general surgery at New York University, contributed greatly to our understanding of pancreatitis by identifying the 11 signs of severity that now bear his acronym.[76] This tool, still useful today, allows prediction of outcome, comparisons of results between hospitals, and assessment of new therapies. Along with efforts by Ranson, Imrie, and others to quantify the severity of pancreatitis came renewed efforts at improving outcome, especially with such measures as better fluid resuscitation, trials of antibiotics, improved intensive care and ventilatory management, and peritoneal lavage. With these efforts, a change in the nature of pancreatitis has occurred, with fewer early deaths and a virtual disappearance of hemorrhage as an acute complication, but conversely greater recognition of the problem of late infection as a cause of mortality.

Chronic Pancreatitis

Surgery for chronic pancreatitis has been a relatively recent undertaking. In the mid-1960s, Doubilet and Mulholland described transduodenal sphincterotomy for chronic pancreatitis, with the idea that, at least in some patients, stenosis or stricture at the sphincter of Oddi played an important role. The high failure rate with this operation, however, led to its abandonment as a routine procedure, a lesson endoscopists of today should remember. In 1965, P. Mallet-Guy of Lyon recommended ganglionectomy, the precursor of our percutaneous celiac plexus block of today. An important advance for managing ductal obstruction and dilation in chronic pancreatitis was described by Charles Puestow of Chicago. His longitudinal pancreaticojejunostomy, although modified over the years, remains a safe and reasonably effective surgical treatment for this vexing disease. Duodenal-sparing resective techniques, such as those described by Beger and Frey, as well as standard operations such as pancreaticoduodenectomy, have reasonable track records in terms of pain control but pose greater operative risk and more long-term problems such as diabetes than do drainage procedures.

Pancreaticoduodenectomy

Allen Oldfather Whipple (1881–1963)[77] is well known for his contributions to pancreatic surgery, including pancreaticoduodenectomy. Whipple was born in Iran to Puritan missionary parents. He served as chair of surgery at Presbyterian Hospital in New York from 1921 to 1946. At the time of his landmark report of pancreatic head resection for carcinoma of the ampulla of Vater in 1935, such operations were unsuccessful because of the complications related to preoperative jaundice, technical problems such as hemorrhage, and postoperative anastomotic leakage and infection. Whipple described a two-stage procedure, beginning with biliary and gastric bypass to relieve jaundice and restore nutrition, followed 2 to 3 weeks later by resection and pancreatic anastomosis (Fig. 41.3).[78] Others, including Brunschwig, published similar descriptions. By 1940, Whipple, along with others such as Trimble, had modified his procedure to one stage.[79] Traverso and Longmire in 1978 published their description

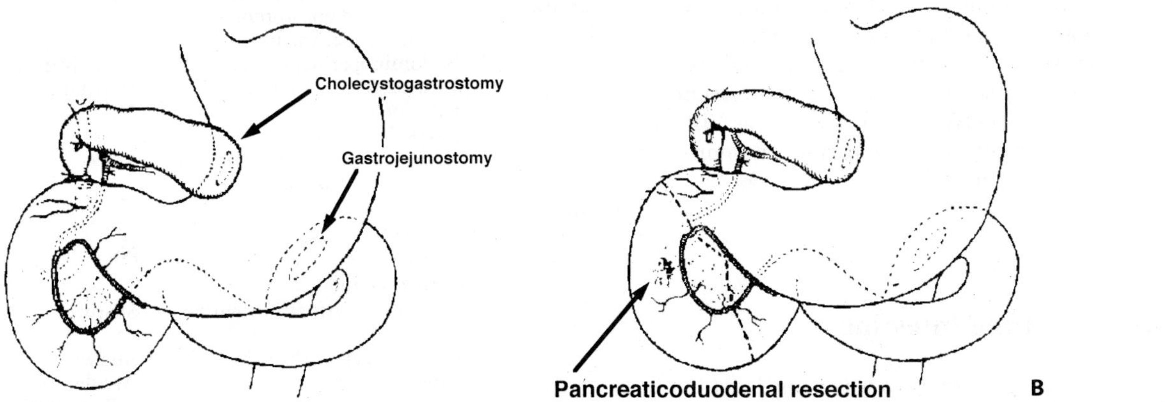

FIGURE 41.3. A technique for two-stage pancreaticoduodenectomy was described by Allen Oldfather Whipple in 1935. At the time, such operations were unsuccessful because of the complications related to preoperative jaundice, technical problems such as hemorrhage, and postoperative anastomotic leakage and infection. Whipple described a two-stage procedure, beginning with biliary and gastric bypass to relieve jaundice and restore nutrition (**A**), followed 2 to 3 weeks later by resection and pancreatic anastomosis (**B**). (Reprinted with permission from Whipple AO, Parsons WB, Mullins CR. Treatment of carcinoma at ampulla of Vater. *Annals of Surgery* 1935;102:763–779.[78])

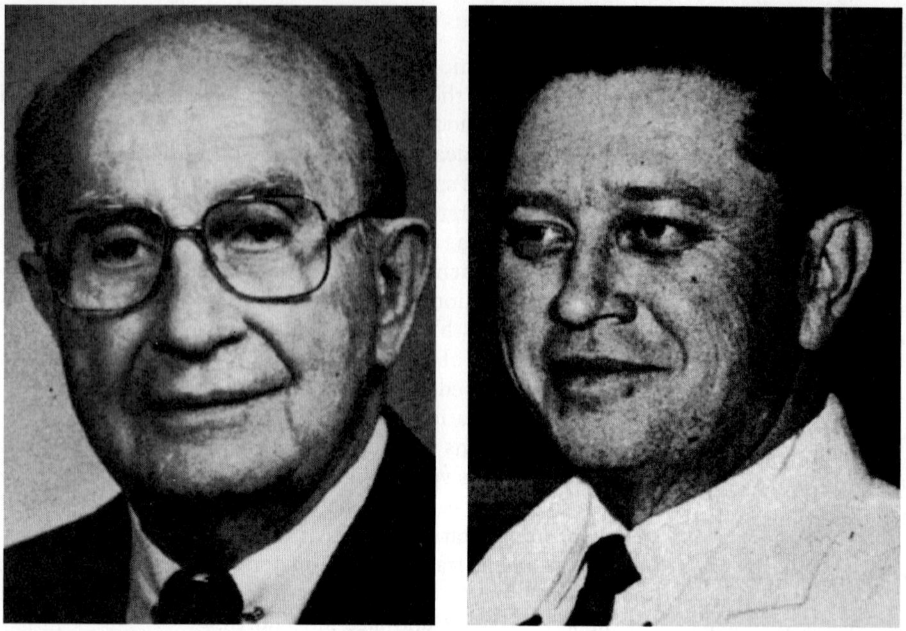

FIGURE 41.4. Robert Zollinger (*left*) and Edwin Ellison (*right*) in 1955 described the peculiar association of virulent peptic ulcer disease with a pancreatic islet cell adenoma, known today as Zollinger-Ellison syndrome. (Reprinted with permission from *Surgery* 1991;109:377–398.)

of a modification of the Whipple resection with pyloric preservation.[80]

Islet Cell Tumors

The history of islet cell tumors of the pancreas is a fascinating study of linkage of clinical observations, physiological experiments, and biochemical isolation of gut peptides to arrive at an understanding of the nature of these tumors. The term *islet cell adenoma* was coined by A.G. Nichols in 1902, but the first successful resection of such a tumor is credited to Roscoe Graham, who excised an insulinoma in 1929. Allen O. Whipple, of pancreaticoduodenectomy fame, described the clinical symptoms of insulinoma in 1938, noting that "'Attacks' come on in the fasting period . . . the blood sugar levels are always below 50 milligrams percent . . . victims . . . brought back to a normal state . . . on administration of sugar."[81] Robert Zollinger and Edwin Ellison from Ohio State (Fig. 41.4) described the peculiar association of virulent peptic ulcer disease with a pancreatic islet cell adenoma in 1955, but it was not until 1965 that a radioimmunoassay for gastrin was developed by James McGuigan. Verner and Morrison published their experience with massive secretory diarrhea, hypokalemia, and acidosis in association with an islet cell tumor in 1958. We now know this as VIPoma. The clinical era of gastrointestinal endocrinology spurred scientists to study the gut peptides causing these disorders and, along the way, unravel many mysteries surrounding the regulation of gut function.

Diseases of the Intestine

Repair of intestinal injuries was considered invariably hopeless from the times of Hippocrates (460–370 BC) to those of Ruggero da Frugardo. "If a part of the tender intestine is wounded," the latter wrote, "it is better to leave the treatment to God than to man, since death will follow it too soon."[82] This pessimism gradually disappeared as safe techniques evolved for intestinal suturing and anastomosis, which enabled surgeons to operate with confidence to close perforations, relieve obstruction, and resect tumors or diseased intestinal segments (Table 41.5).

Pharmacological, Nutritional, and Technical Advances in Bowel Surgery

A number of ancillary developments must be mentioned because of their contribution to the development of safe and

TABLE 41.5. Milestones in Intestinal Surgery and Suturing Techniques.

What	*Who*	*When*
Surgery		
First successful colostomy to treat transverse colon injury	Saccher	1720
Resection of strangulated bowel and anastomosis over animal trachea	Duverger	1757
Abdominoperineal resection	W. E. Miles	1908
Two-stage colon resection	Hartmann	1921
Exteriorized resection	Mikulicz	1952
Brooke's ileostomy	Brooke	1956
Kock's continent ileostomy	Kock	1969
Ileoanal continent pouches:		
J-pouch	Utsunomiya	1980
S-pouch	Parks	1980
W-pouch	Nicholls	1985
Suturing techniques		
Closure of perforation with ants	Susrutra	6th century BC
Use of sheep gut suture	Rhazes	10th century
Closure of intestinal perforation with silk suture	Arculanus, Bertapaglia	1400
Lembert suture technique	Lembert	1826
Two-layer anastomosis	Czerny	1830s
Murphy button	Murphy	1892
Stapling technique	Ravitch	1958

TABLE 41.6. Key Ancillary Contributions to Intestinal Surgery.

Microbiology and antibiotics
Importance of anaerobic bacteria in peritoneal sepsis
Bacteriological bowel preparation
Perioperative use of antibiotics
Technology
Stapling devices
Stapled anastomosis
Percutaneous jejunostomy/gastrostomy
Fiberscopic endoscopy
Nutrition
Total parenteral nutrition
Elemental diet

effective techniques in gastrointestinal surgery (Table 41.6). The use of antibiotics, both parenteral and enteral, has played an important role in facilitating increasingly major operations on the intestines. Antimicrobial therapy has perhaps contributed most to surgery of the large intestine. The recognition of anaerobic bacteria as a significant factor in the pathogenesis of peritonitis and intraperitoneal abscess has led to the use of appropriate antibiotics. Also significant has been the realization that large-bowel surgery requires bacteriological as well as mechanical preparation. In this respect, the Condon-Nichols bowel preparation regimen must be mentioned.[83]

Stapling devices have significantly shortened the duration of surgical procedures, particularly those involving an intestinal anastomosis. Surgery is grateful to the pioneering work of Mark Ravitch in the development of stapling devices and the stapled intestinal anastomosis.[84] Similarly, we have benefited significantly from our ability to perform gastrostomy and jejunostomy percutaneously. As mentioned in the introduction, fiber-optic endoscopy has played an important role in the diagnosis and preoperative evaluation of intestinal diseases such as cancer, polyps, and inflammatory bowel disease (IBD).

It is with great pride that, as surgeons, we recognize the development of total parenteral nutrition (TPN), a pioneering contribution of Jonathan Rhoads and Stanley Dudrick.[85] A resident in Rhoads's laboratory at the University of Pennsylvania, Dudrick worked to solve the problem of providing intravenous nutrition in a canine model. They showed, for the first time, that normal growth and development of beagle puppies was possible with no oral intake and complete nutritional sustenance by vein. Milestones in the development of TPN included identification and provision of essential amino and fatty acids, calculation of vitamin and trace mineral requirements, and the practical problem of achieving durable venous access for these hypertonic solutions. Today, TPN has facilitated maintaining nutrition in surgical patients who are unable to use the enteral route for short or long periods of time, preoperatively or postoperatively.

Intestinal Obstruction

The evolution of safe therapy for intestinal obstruction is of great historical importance. The key to successful surgical treatment was an understanding of the basic pathophysiology (Historical Vignette 41.5). Critical concepts included the importance of distension and swallowed air; the loss of fluid not only through vomiting but also within the bowel lumen, bowel wall, and peritoneum; the importance of distension and volvulus in vascular compromise; and invasion of the ischemic bowel wall by bacteria and their transmigration to the peritoneum and into the bloodstream.

HISTORICAL VIGNETTE 41.5. William Beaumont and Early Studies of Gastric Physiology.

A milestone in our understanding of gastric physiology occurred on June 6, 1822, when William Beaumont (1785–1853), an army surgeon stationed at Fort Mackinac, Michigan, was called to see a patient who had suffered an accidental gunshot wound to the abdomen. The patient, 19-year-old Alexis St. Martin, had a large wound in the left upper abdomen, including a gastric laceration "pouring out the food he had taken for breakfast." It took 2 years for him to recover, but he was left with a 2.5-inch gastrocutaneous fistula, from which "food and drink constantly exuded, unless prevented by a tent, compress and bandage."[102] Beaumont began a series of studies of gastric physiology via this fistula, culminating in his book, *Experiments and Observations on the Gastric Juice and the Physiology of Digestion*, published in 1833. This book is regarded as the greatest surgical text from that era. Curiously, Beaumont entered into a series of formal contracts with St. Martin for these studies, an example of which is on display at the Washington University School of Medicine in St. Louis. This was the first documented instance of formal, written, informed consent so familiar to us today.

Although many surgeons have made contributions in this area, we credit Owen Wangensteen (Fig. 41.5) perhaps more than anyone else with establishing the modern treatment for intestinal obstruction. Wangensteen (1898–1981) was chair of the department of surgery at the University of Minnesota

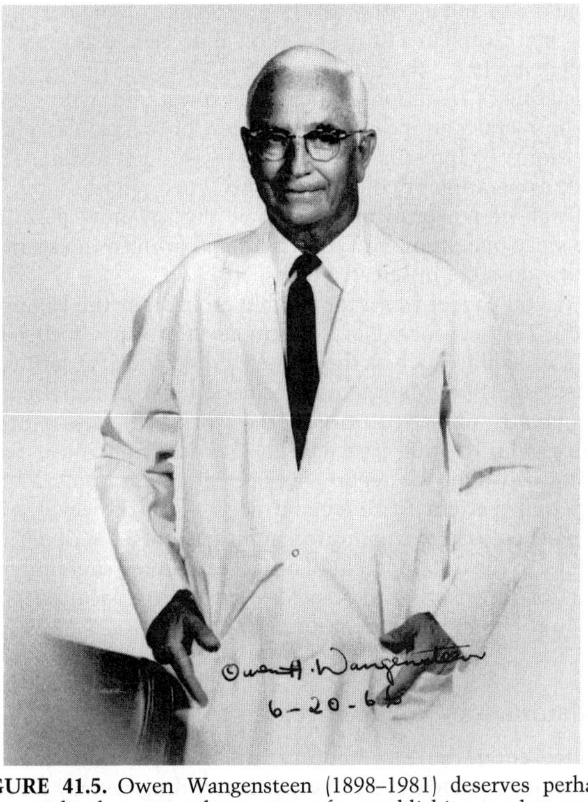

FIGURE 41.5. Owen Wangensteen (1898–1981) deserves perhaps more credit than any other surgeon for establishing modern treatment for intestinal obstruction. Chair of the University of Minnesota department of surgery from 1930 to 1967, Wangensteen developed many surgical techniques that helped reduce the death rate from intestinal obstruction. (Figure provided courtesy of Mary W. Brink.)

from 1930 to 1967. In the 1920s, death from intestinal obstruction was frequent, and Wangensteen took on this problem as one of his first research projects. His seminal contributions include the use of nasogastric suction, the importance of fluid resuscitation, the role of electrolyte and acid–base disturbance in high small-bowel obstruction, and the need for emergent operation in cases of complete small-bowel obstruction.[86] These and other achievements led to a decline in mortality, from 40% to 50% in the early 1930s to about 10% in the 1950s. In 1963, Zollinger and associates observed that a delay in surgery of more than 24h doubled the mortality in acute small-bowel obstruction.[87] These principles, so familiar to us today, came into being because of the translation of laboratory investigation by surgeon-scientists such as Wangensteen to the bedside of their patients.

Diverticulitis and Carcinoma

The leading causes of large-bowel obstruction are diverticulitis and carcinoma. Here, also, surgical therapy has undergone a remarkable evolution. By 1880, only 10 colectomies had been reported. The high mortality following colectomy was the result of sepsis associated with anastomotic dehiscence. The emergency treatment for complications of diverticulitis provides a good illustration of how colon surgery has evolved.

During the 1950s and 1960s, the treatment of choice for obstruction or localized perforation caused by diverticulitis was a three-stage procedure. First, a diverting transverse loop colostomy was performed, followed by resection of the diseased colon and anastomosis in 6 to 8 weeks. The colostomy was then closed in a third operation after the anastomosis had healed. In 1921, Hartmann proposed a two-stage operation consisting of resection of the diseased sigmoid, with closure of the rectal stump and construction of an end-descending colostomy.[88] Intestinal continuity was then restored in a second operation by coloproctostomy 2 to 6 months later. The addition of powerful antimicrobial therapy now permits a one-stage operation with resection, and primary anastomosis is now possible in selected cases.

Rectal cancer was a formidable problem at the beginning of the 20th century. Early treatment efforts had focused on local excisions, such as the transsacral approach described by Kraske in 1885. Management of patients with rectal cancer was greatly improved through the work of Professor Ernest Miles, who in 1908 first described abdominoperineal resection. Soon after his report, his operation was applied to all resectable patients with rectal cancer. Today, however, a permanent colostomy is required in only about 15% of patients thanks to the development of other techniques, including low anterior resection with stapled anastomosis, local excision, fulguration, and laser ablation.

Inflammatory Bowel Disease

As we enter the 21st century, we neither understand the cause of nor have a completely effective drug therapy for IBD. Surgery continues to play a major role in the management of these patients, both to handle local complications related to the inflammatory process such as perforation and stricture and to prevent late complications such as carcinoma.

Crohn's Disease

Crohn's disease was probably first described in a patient by Morgagni in 1761. The classic description, however, was provided in 1932 by Crohn, Ginzburg, and Oppenheimer from Mount Sinai Hospital in New York.[89] The disease requires surgical attention either as an acute disease, when it affects the terminal ileum and presents as acute abdomen, or as a chronic disease that has reached the point of complication or intractability. Several historical controversies in the surgical treatment of Crohn's disease have been resolved with time. It is now generally accepted that, when the disease first presents as an acute abdomen, appendectomy is performed so long as the cecum is not involved, but resection is not performed. The controversy was more heated on the subject of chronic Crohn's disease, especially on the issues of whether to resect or bypass and how much bowel to resect. Francis Moore advocated resection of the diseased terminal ileum with ileotransverse colostomy. Crohn and associates, however, advised bypass without resection but with end-to-side ileotransverse colostomy. With time, it became clear that the bypass procedure lessens neither the progression of the disease nor its complications. With respect to the extent of bowel to resect, the earlier dogma that resection margins should be microscopically disease free has been abandoned in the interest of preserving bowel. Indeed, the 1980s saw the introduction with good results of stricturoplasty to minimize bowel resection.

Chronic Ulcerative Colitis

Even though chronic ulcerative colitis (CUC) was first recognized by Samuel Wilks at Guy's Hospital in 1859, the first complete description of the disease was given by Sir Arthur Hurst in 1909. Alfred Strauss of Chicago described one of the earliest treatments for ulcerative colitis, ileostomy for fecal diversion. Surgical treatment has evolved from the "double-barreled ileostomy" advocated by Truelove et al. in 1965 to total colectomy with permanent ileostomy of the Brooke's variety or the continent Kock's pouch[90] and now to total colectomy with mucosal proctectomy and ileoanal anastomosis using an ileal reservoir.[91–93] The last procedure, although associated with such complications as impotence and "pouchitis," has emerged as the treatment of choice. As in peptic ulcer disease, revolutionary developments in therapy for both Crohn's disease and ulcerative colitis await the understanding of the cause of these diseases and the development of drugs targeted at prevention and cure.

Peritonitis and Intraabdominal Abscess

Primitive medicine was not rational by our standards. No better example can be given than the attempts at bloodletting for serious illness such as infection in an attempt to let the evil humors escape. One hopes that future historians do not look on our own meager therapeutic efforts with a similar cynicism. Hippocrates offered one of the first clinical descriptions of a patient with peritonitis, including the associated volume depletion, tachycardia, shallow breathing, abdominal muscular guarding, and tenderness.[94] Pasteur in 1863 described his germ theory of disease, followed by Robert Koch, who in 1882 identified his postulates requiring fulfillment to be certain of a microorganism's role in disease.

Semmelweis and Lister are credited with the first clinical applications of infection control practices so familiar to us today. Weinberg in France and Altemeir in the United States were among the first to recognize the polymicrobial nature of intraabdominal infection and the role of anaerobic organisms.[95,96]

Martin Kirschner (1897–1942), professor of surgery in Königsberg, Germany, contributed greatly to treatment of patients with peritonitis by defining several management principles; these include early operation with gentle technique, orientation of the incision over the focus of infection, identification and control of the infection source, saline irrigation to remove infected debris, avoidance of mechanical emptying of the bowel or stoma formation, and the inefficacy of drainage of the entire peritoneal cavity.[94] Following these principles reduced mortality from peritonitis from 80%–100% to 20%–30%.

By the 1970s, the development of antibiotics was accelerating. The sepsis syndrome and multiple organ failure in the absence of continued active bacterial infection was increasingly recognized as a cause of death.[97,98] These developments heralded the modern era of surgical infectious disease as improved understanding of the host cytokine response has led to novel treatment strategies including tumor necrosis factor (TNF) and interleukin-6 (IL-6) antibodies.

References

1. Allison PR. Reflux esophagitis, sliding hiatal hernia and the anatomy of repair. Surg Gynecol Obstet 1951;92:419.
2. Code CF. Alimentary canal. In: Society AP, ed. Handbook of Physiology. Section 6. Baltimore: Williams & Wilkins, 1967–1968.
3. Nissen R. Gastropexy and fundoplication in surgical treatment of hiatal hernia. Am J Dig Dis 1961;6:954.
4. Skinner DB, Belsey RHR. Surgical management of esophageal reflux and hiatus hernia: long-term results with 1030 cases. J Thorac Cardiovasc Surg 1967;53:33–54.
5. Hill LD, Velasco M, Russell COH, et al. Results of Hill antireflux operation before and after intraoperative manometry. Gastroenterology 1981;80:1176.
6. Bernstein LM, Baker LA. A clinical test for esophagitis. Gastroenterology 1958;34:760.
7. Tuttle SG, Grossman MI. Detection of gastroesophageal reflux by simultaneous measurement of intraluminal pressure and pH. Proc Soc Biol Med 1958;98:225.
8. Skinner DB, Booth D. Assessment of distal esophageal function in patients with hiatus hernia and/or gastroesophageal reflux. Ann Surg 1970;172:627–637.
9. Johnson LF, Demeester TR. Twenty-four hour pH monitoring of the distal esophagus. Am J Gastroenterol 1974;62: 325–332.
10. Pearson FG, Cooper JD, Patterson GA, et al. Gastroplasty and fundoplication for complex reflux problems. Ann Surg 1987;206:473–481.
11. Belsey R. Functional diseases of the esophagus. J Thorac Cardiovasc Surg 1966;52:164–188.
12. Debas HT, Payne WS, Cameron AJ, Carlson HC. Physiopathology of lower esophageal diverticulum and its implications for treatment. Surg Gynecol Obstet 1980;151:593–600.
13. Heller E. Extramokose kardioplastik beim chronischen kardiospasmus mit dilatation des oesophagus. Mitt Grenzgeb Med Chir 1914;27:141–149.
14. Zaaijer JH. Cardiospasm in the aged. Ann Surg 1923;77:615.
15. Barrett NR, Franklin RH. Concerning the unfavourable late results of certain operations performed in the treatment of cardiospasm. Br J Surg 1949;37:194–202.
16. Ellis FH, Crozier RE, Watkins E. Operations for esophageal achalasia: results of esophagomyotomy without an antireflux operation. J Thorac Cardiovasc Surg 1984;88:344–351.
17. Pellegrini CA, Leichter R, Patti M, et al. Thoracoscopic esophageal myotomy in the treatment of achalasia. Ann Thorac Surg 1993;56:680–682.
18. Meltzer SJ, Auer J. Continuous respiration without respiratory movements. J Exp Med 1909;11:622–625.
19. Matas R. Intralaryngeal insufflation for the relief of acute surgical pneumothorax: its history and methods with a description of the latest devices for this purpose. JAMA 1900;34: 1468–1473.
20. Torek F. The first successful case of resection of the thoracic portion of the esophagus for carcinoma. Surg Gynecol Obstet 1913;16:614.
21. Franklin RH. Milestones in oesophageal surgery. Proc R Soc Med 1971;64:257–260.
22. Ohsawa T. The surgery of the esophagus. Arch Jpn Chir 1933;10:605.
23. Lewis I. The surgical treatment of carcinoma of the oesophagus with special reference to a new operation for growths of the middle third. Br J Surg 1946;34:18.
24. McKeown KC. Trends in oesophageal resection for carcinoma with special reference to total oesophagectomy. Ann R Coll Surg Engl 1972;51:213–239.
25. Orringer MB, Stirling MC. Transhiatal esophagectomy for benign and malignant disease. J Thorac Cardiovasc Surg 1993;105: 265–276.
26. Wölfler A. Gastro-enterostomie. Zentralb Chir 1881;8: 705–708.
27. Billroth T. Wien Med Wochenschr Gastrectomie 1881;31:162.
28. Ravitch MM. The reception of new operations. Ann Surg 1984;200:231–246.
29. Finney JMT, Rienhoff WF Jr. Gastrectomy. Arch Surg 1929;18:140–162.
30. Ikard RW. The Y anastomosis of Cesar Roux. Surg Gynecol Obstet 1989;169:559–567.
31. Roux C. De la gastroenterostomie. Rev Gynecol Chir Abdomen 1897;1:67–122.
32. Latarjet A, Wertheimer P. Quelques results de l'inervation gastrique. Presse Med 1923;2:993.
33. Dragstedt LR, Owens FMJ. Supradiaphragmatic section of the vagus nerves in treatment of duodenal ulcer. Proc Soc Exp Biol Med 1943;53:125.
34. Franksson C. Selective abdominal vagotomy. Acta Chir Scand 1948;96:409.
35. Johnston D, Wilkinson AR. Highly selective vagotomy without a drainage procedure in the treatment of duodenal ulcer. Br J Surg 1970;57:289–296.
36. Kennedy T, Johnston GW, Macrae KD, et al. Proximal gastric vagotomy: interim results of a randomized controlled trial. Br Med J 1975;2(5966):301–303.
37. Marshall BJ, Warren JR. Unidentified curved bacilli in the stomach of patients with gastritis and peptic ulceration. Lancet 1984;1(8390):1311–1315.
38. Rubio PA. The history of gallbladder surgery. Contemp Surg 1996;48:230–236.
39. Gordon-Taylor G. On gallstones and their sufferers. Br J Surg 1937;25:241–251.
40. Beal JM. Historical perspective of gallstone disease. Surg Gynecol Obstet 1984;158:181–189.
41. Ellis H. Cases from out of the past: Carl Langenbuch. Contemp Surg 1991;38:39–42.
42. Morgenstern L. Hans Kehr: not first, but foremost. Surg Endosc 1993;7:152–154.

43. Cole WH. The development of cholecystography: the first 50 years. Am J Surg 1978;136:541–560.
44. Graham E, Cole WH. Roentgenologic examination of the gallbladder: preliminary report of a new method utilizing the intravenous injection of tetrabromophenolphthalein. JAMA 1924;82: 613–614.
45. Carter RF, Saypol GM. Transabdominal cholangiography. JAMA 1952;148:253–255.
46. Haubrich WS. Charcot of Charcot's triad. Gastroenterology 1998;115:541.
47. Perissat J, Collet DR, Belliard R. Gallstones: laparoscopic treatment, intracorporeal lithotripsy followed by cholecystostomy or cholecystectomy—a personal technique. Endoscopy 1989; 21(suppl):373–374.
48. Dubois F, Icard P, Berthelot G, et al. Coelioscopic cholecystectomy. Preliminary report of 36 cases. Ann Surg 1990;211: 60–62.
49. Reddick EJ, Olsen DO. Laparoscopic laser cholecystectomy. A comparison with mini-lap cholecystectomy. Surg Endosc 1989;3:131–133.
50. NIH Consensus Conference. Gallstones and laparoscopic cholecystectomy [review]. JAMA 1993;269:1018–1024.
51. Way LW. Bile duct injury during laparoscopic cholecystectomy [editorial; comment]. Ann Surg 1992;215(3):195.
52. McSherry CK. The results of the EDAP multicenter trial of biliary lithotripsy in the United States. The EDAP Investigators Group. Surg Gynecol Obstet 1991;173:461–464.
53. Haubrich WS. Gilbert of Gilbert's syndrome. Gastroenterology 1998;115:821.
54. Tait L. Case of hydatids of the liver, treated by abdominal section and drainage. Br Med J 1880;2:975.
55. Foster JH. History of liver surgery. Arch Surg 1991;126: 381–387.
56. Paré A. The Apologie and Treatise of Ambrose Paré. New York: Dover, 1968.
57. Tilton BT. Some considerations regarding wounds of the liver. Ann Surg 1905;41:20.
58. Keen WW. Report of a case of resection of the liver for removal of a neoplasm with a table of 76 cases of resection of the liver for hepatic tumors. Ann Surg 1899;30:267.
59. Brunschwig A. Hepatic lobectomy for metastatic cancer. Cancer (Phila) 1963;16:277–282.
60. Pringle JH. Notes on the arrest of hepatic hemorrhage due to trauma. Ann Surg 1908;48:541.
61. Couinard C. Lobes de segments hepatiques: notes sur architecture anatomique et chirurgicale du foie. Presse Med 1954; 62:709.
62. Glasgow R. Surg Forum 1998.
63. Illis DSE, Linton RR, Jones CM. Effect of venous shunt surgery on liver function in patients with portal hypertension. A follow-up study of 125 patients operated upon in the last 10 years. N Engl J Med 1956;254:931–936.
64. Blakemore AH. Portacaval shunt for portal hypertension: follow-up results in cases of cirrhosis of the liver. JAMA 1951; 145:1335–1339.
65. Whipple AO. The problem of portal hypertension in relation to the hepatosplenopathies. Ann Surg 1945;122: 449–475.
66. Warren WD, Zeppa R, Fomon JJ. Selective trans-splenic decompression of gastroesophageal varices by distal splenorenal shunt. Ann Surg 1967;166:437–455.
67. Orloff MJ, Orloff MS, Rambotti M, et al. Is portal-systemic shunt worthwhile in Child's class C cirrhosis? Long-term results of emergency shunt in 94 patients with bleeding varices. Ann Surg 1992;216:256–266; discussion 266–268.
68. Rosch J, Hanafee WN, Snow H. Transjugular portal venography and radiologic portacaval shunt: an experimental study. Radiology 1969;92:1112–1114.
69. Jamieson NV, Tan L, Jamieson I, et al. Neoral in liver transplantation. Transplant Proc 1996;28:2229–2231.
70. Howard JM, Hess W, Traverso W. Johann Georg Wirsüng (1589–1643) and the pancreatic duct: the prosector of Padua, Italy. J Am Coll Surg 1998;187:201–211.
71. Carter R. Assassination of Johann Georg Wirsung (1589–1643): mysterious medical murder in Renaissance Padua. World J Surg 1998;22:324–326.
72. Opie EL. The etiology of acute hemorrhagic pancreatitis. Bull Johns Hopkins Hosp 1901;12:182–188.
73. Lium R, Maddock S. Etiology of pancreatitis: experimental study. Surgery (St. Louis) 1948;24:593–604.
74. Acosta JM, Ledesma CL. Gallstone migration as a cause of acute pancreatitis. N Engl J Med 1974;290(9):484–487.
75. Kelly TR. Gallstone pancreatitis: pathophysiology. Surgery (St. Louis) 1976;80:488–492.
76. Ranson JH, Rifkind KM, Turner JW. Prognostic signs and non-operative peritoneal lavage in acute pancreatitis. Surg Gynecol Obstet 1976;143:209–219.
77. Chen TSN, Chen PSY. The Whipples and their legacies in medicine. Surg Gynecol Obstet 1993;176:501–506.
78. Whipple AO, Parsons WB, Mullins CR. Treatment of carcinoma of ampulla of Vater. Ann Surg 1935;102:763–779.
79. Trimble IR, Parsons JW, Sherman CP. A one-stage operation for the cure of the carcinoma of Vater and of the head of the pancreas. Surg Gynecol Obstet 1941;73:711–722.
80. Traverso LW, Longmire WP Jr. Preservation of the pylorus in pancreaticoduodenectomy. Surg Gynecol Obstet 1978;146: 959–962.
81. Whipple AO. Hyperinsulinism in relation to pancreatic tumors. Surgery (St. Louis) 1944;16:289–305.
82. Zimmerman LM, Veith I. Great Ideas in the History of Surgery. Baltimore: Williams & Wilkins, 1961.
83. Clarke JS, Condon RE, Bartlett JG, et al. Preoperative oral antibiotics reduce septic complications of colon operations: results of prospective, randomized, double-blind clinical study. Ann Surg 1977;186:251–259.
84. Ravitch MM, Steichen FM. Contemporary stapling instruments and basic mechanical suturing techniques. Surg Clin North Am 1984;64:425–440.
85. Dudrick SJ, Wilmore DW, Vars HMR, et al. Long-term total parenteral nutrition with growth, development and positive nitrogen balance. Surgery (St. Louis) 1968;64:134–142.
86. Wangensteen OH. Acute bowel obstruction: its recognition and management. N Engl J Med 1938;219:340–348.
87. Zollinger R, Kinsey D, Grant G. Intestinal obstruction. Postgrad Med 1963;33:165–171.
88. Hartmann H, Quenu E. Chirurgie du rectum. Paris: Steinheil, 1931.
89. Crohn B, Ginzburg L, Oppenheimer G. Regional enteritis: a pathological and clinical entity. JAMA 1932;99:1323.
90. Kock NG. Intra-abdominal "reservoir" in patients with permanent ileostomy. Preliminary observations on a procedure resulting in fecal "continence" in five ileostomy patients. Arch Surg 1969;99:223–231.
91. Nicholls RJ, Pezim ME. Restorative proctocolectomy with ileal reservoir for ulcerative colitis and familial edematous polyposus: a comparison of three reservoir designs. Br J Surg 1985;72: 470–474.
92. Martin LW, LeCoultre C, Schubert WK. Total colectomy and mucosal protectomy with preservation of continence in ulcerative colitis. Ann Surg 1977;186:477–480.
93. Utsunomiya J, Iwama T, Imago M. Total colectomy, mucosal proctectomy and ileoanal pull-through. Dis Colon Rectum 1980;23:459–466.
94. Hau T. Biology and treatment of peritonitis: the historic development of current concepts. J Am Coll Surg 1998;186: 475–484.

95. Weinberg M, Prevot AR, Davesne J, et al. Recherches sur la bacteriologie et la serotherapie des appendicites aigues. Ann Int Pasteur 1928;42:1167–1241.
96. Altemeier WA. The bacterial flora of acutely perforated appendicitis with peritonitis: a bacteriologic study based on one hundred cases. Ann Surg 1938;107:517–528.
97. Baue AE. Multiple, progressive, or sequential organ failure: a syndrome for the 1970s. Arch Surg 1975;110:779–781.
98. Eiseman B, Beart R, Norton L. Multiple organ failure. Surg Gynecol Obstet 1977;144:323–326.
99. Morgenstern L. Halsted's nemesis: the common bile duct. Surg Endosc 1994;8:1165–1167.
100. Halsted WS. Ligature and suture material: introduction of gloves. JAMA 1913;60:1123.
101. Day SB. Postscript to the surgical legend of William Stewart Halsted and the introduction of rubber gloves to surgery. Surg Gynecol Obstet 1963;117:121–122.
102. Rutkow IM. Beaumont and St. Martin: a blast from the past. Arch Surg 1998;133:1259.

42

Assessment of Acute Abdominal Symptoms

William P. Schecter

Acute Abdomen

The diagnostic evaluation of the patient with acute abdominal pain is one of the most interesting and challenging problems in clinical medicine. Changes in technology in the past 25 years (ultrasonography, computed tomographic [CT] scanning, magnetic resonance imaging [MRI], diagnostic peritoneal lavage, and laparoscopy) have improved our ability to "see" into the abdomen. Nevertheless, the abdomen remains very much a "black box" for the clinician on the front line. Surgery is still awaiting the development of an imaging test of sufficient accuracy to revolutionize the evaluation of the acute abdomen much as the head CT scan changed forever the fields of neurology and neurosurgery. A careful history and physical examination by an experienced surgeon, together with judicious use of laboratory and currently available imaging studies, remain the best method of evaluation at present.

The surgeon evaluating a patient with an acute abdomen is asking two specific questions: (1) what is the diagnosis? and (2) does the patient require an emergency laparotomy? The goal of the following discussion is to describe the process by which the surgeon attempts to answer these two questions.

History

A careful, complete history is essential to avoid serious mistakes. Approach the patient with an open mind and do not jump to early, unwarranted conclusions. The time course, nature, location, and radiation of pain are important clues. The sudden onset of severe pain (the patient can often state the precise time of onset) is associated with hollow viscus perforation. The gradual progression of intermittent spasmodic pain is characteristically associated with hollow viscus obstruction. Epigastric pain radiating to the back is a common complaint in patients with pancreatitis. Colicky flank pain radiating to the groin is typical in patients with renal colic. Ask the patient specifically about a change in the location of the pain (shifting pain). Generalized abdominal pain shifting to a specific location is an important finding. The usual mechanism is the initial development of poorly localized visceral pain caused by distention and ischemia of the abdominal viscera with subsequent irritation of the somatically innervated parietal peritoneum as the inflammatory process progresses, thereby causing localization of the pain.

Ask about nausea, vomiting, and hematemesis. What color is the vomitus? Clear vomitus may indicate gastric outlet obstruction. Feculent emesis, on the other hand, often indicates a distal bowel obstruction. What is the relationship of the vomiting to the other symptoms and signs? Early extensive vomiting associated with a scaphoid abdomen indicates high small-bowel obstruction. Late or absent vomiting associated with abdominal distension indicates distal small-bowel or colonic obstruction.

Are the bowel movements regular? What is their color and consistency? Inquire about symptoms of dysuria, frequency, or hematuria. Has the urine changed color (possibly indicating excretion of metabolites of bilirubin)? In women, a careful menstrual and obstetric history is essential. What is the relationship of the pain to the menstrual cycle? Could the patient be pregnant? Inquire about alcohol and drug use and recent injuries or accidents. I usually ask patients if they have ever heard the word *pancreatitis*. Most patients who have had previous pancreatitis are familiar with this term. Finally, a careful cardiac and respiratory history can help to identify nonsurgical causes of abdominal pain.

Physical Examination

The patient with acute abdominal pain requires a complete physical examination. I usually begin my exam of the patient during the history. I hold the patient's hand during the interview and assess the rate and quality of the pulse while looking at the patient's eyes and the manner of response to my questions. A rapid, thready pulse and a "worried look" or glazed disinterested response to questions should raise the suspicion of serious illness.

Deep palpation has little or no role in the initial assessment of the patient with peritonitis. The goal of the examination is to move the peritoneum with minimum force to see if the patient experiences pain. First, inspect the abdomen and note whether it is scaphoid or distended. Ask the patient to cough before touching the abdomen. Cough tenderness, particularly cough tenderness that localizes to a specific abdominal location, is an important sign of peritoneal irritation.

If the patient has an umbilical hernia, the peritoneum lies adjacent to the skin of the umbilicus. Gently tap over the umbilical hernia to see if pain is elicited. Gently scratch the skin of the four abdominal quadrants. Rarely, hyperesthesia of the skin is present over the area of peritoneal irritation. Next, apply graded stimuli to the four abdominal quadrants. "Guarding" or rigidity of the abdomen wall musculature may result from peritonitis. Start by "jiggling" the skin with your fingers, gently palpate, and then percuss to apply a firmer controlled stimulus. Finally, deep palpation should be done followed by quick release to assess direct and referred rebound tenderness, two important signs of peritoneal irritation akin to cough tenderness.

Examine the patient for flank and costovertebral angle tenderness indicative of renal colic or pyelonephritis. Search for abdominal wall hernias and examine the scrotum and testicles in men. Sometimes torsion of the testicle or epididymitis can present as lower abdominal pain in embarrassed and frightened young men.

Auscultation can be useful in patients with suspected bowel obstruction. The characteristic high-pitched "auscultatory rush" of a peristaltic wave vainly attempting to propel intestinal chyme beyond a point of obstruction supports the diagnosis of mechanical obstruction. Although bowel sounds are said to be absent in diffuse peritonitis, I do not find abdominal auscultation helpful in assessing most cases because a "quiet" abdomen can be normal, and a patient with "active bowel sounds" can have abdominal pathology requiring emergency surgery. The digital rectal exam usually identifies rectal and pelvic masses. The presence of blood or edema and air in the rectal ampulla are also important diagnostic clues.

In women, a vaginal speculum and bimanual and pelvic examination are important to evaluate the possibility of pregnancy, tubal pregnancy, endometriosis, and pelvic inflammatory disease. The diagnosis of pelvic inflammatory disease may be subtle. Not all patients have exquisite cervical motion tenderness when examined. Adnexal masses can be difficult to palpate in patients who are guarding or who are obese. Pelvic ultrasonography, an abdominal CT scan, or diagnostic laparoscopy may be necessary to make the diagnosis in patients with subtle signs of gynecological disease causing acute abdominal pain.

Laboratory Evaluation

Routine laboratory evaluation for the patient with an acute abdomen should include a complete blood count, a urinalysis, and an assessment of renal function (measurement of the serum urea nitrogen [BUN] and serum creatinine). The serum electrolytes are usually measured along with the BUN and creatinine. Measurement of the electrolytes is mandatory if there has been a prolonged period of vomiting. The serum lipase should be measured if there is any question of pancreatitis. Measure serum alkaline phosphatase, bilirubin, and serum transaminase levels if liver or biliary tract disease is a possibility. Women in their reproductive years should have a pregnancy test.

Radiology of the Acute Abdomen

The approach to the radiologic assessment of the patient with acute abdomen pain is in transition as the result of changes in technology permitting accurate imaging of most intraabdominal organs. Although accurate diagnosis remains very much a clinical art at present,[1] further improvements in imaging technology hold the promise of precision in preoperative diagnosis for most conditions, including hollow viscus perforation and ischemia.

The traditional radiologic evaluation begins with an upright chest film and flat plate and upright abdominal films. The chest film can rule out pneumonia and pleural effusion as a cause of upper abdominal pain. Occasionally, a dehydrated patient with pneumonia and upper abdominal pain will have a clear chest x-ray. The pulmonary infiltrate becomes apparent only after rehydration with intravenous fluids. The upright chest film is also an excellent test for demonstrating free intraperitoneal air (Fig. 42.1). Search the x-ray carefully below the diaphragm for the characteristic radiolucent line indicating extraluminal air, easiest to see between the liver and the right hemidiaphragm. If an upright chest film is impossible to obtain because of the severity of the patient's illness, then free air may be demonstrated by turning the patient to the left lateral decubitus position and waiting a few minutes. The extraluminal air will rise and be evident as a radiolucent line between the abdominal wall and the right lobe of the liver after shooting a cross-table lateral x-ray.[2] A word of caution: Although most cases of pneumoperitoneum are caused by gastrointestinal perforation, rupture of bronchi and alveolar membranes causing air to dissect from the chest into the peritoneal cavity, pneumatosis cystoides intestinalis, and intraabdominal infection caused by gas-forming organisms can also occasionally cause pneumoperitoneum.[3] Although abdominal films are useful in demonstrating bowel distention and foreign bodies, they are overall not sensitive in the evaluation of the patient with an acute abdomen.[4]

Pelvic ultrasonography is an important imaging test in the evaluation of women with lower abdominal pain. Using the distended urinary bladder as an acoustic window, the uterus and adnexae can usually be accurately examined, permitting diagnosis of intrauterine pregnancy, tubal pregnancy, tuboovarian abscess, and pelvic inflammatory disease. In my experience, the pelvic ultrasound is most useful in distinguishing appendicitis from gynecological diseases causing right lower quadrant pain in women.[5]

Appendicitis itself can be diagnosed by abdominal ultrasonography. The technique requires a committed, experienced sonographer. In most normal patients, the appendix cannot be visualized sonographically. Visualization of the appendix suggests the diagnosis of appendicitis.[6] The use of appendiceal ultrasonography as an adjunct to clinical

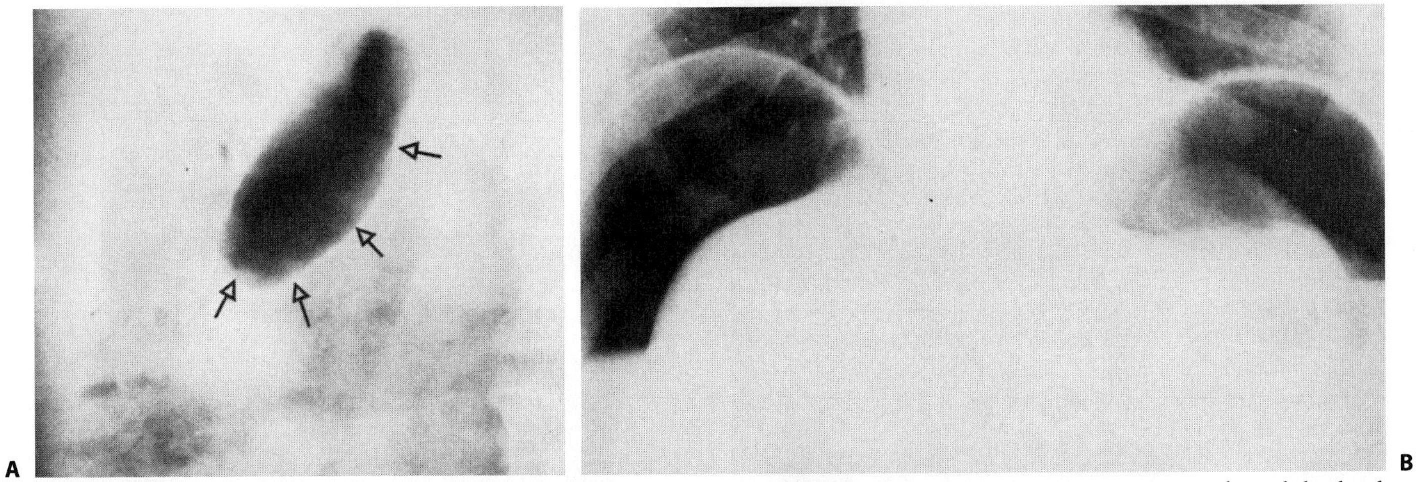

FIGURE 42.1. Free intraperitoneal air. (**A**) Supine. Although no increased lucency is directly apparent, it is revealed by the visualized density of the wall of a small-bowel loop. This presents as a subtle white line around the gas-containing lumen (arrows). (**B**) Erect film documents considerable free air. At surgery, a perforated duodenal ulcer was found. (Reproduced with permission from Meyers and Oliphant,[32] © 1974 Year Book Medical Publishers.)

evaluation improves diagnostic accuracy; however, ultrasonography cannot completely exclude the diagnosis if the surgeon has a high index of suspicion.[7]

Ultrasonography is the initial imaging test of choice in the evaluation of right upper quadrant pain.[8] The exam usually provides accurate information about the gallbladder and the common bile duct. The kidney can be visualized to look for nephrolithiasis or hydronephrosis in patients with flank pain.

Ultrasonography by surgeons in the trauma resuscitation room is rapidly becoming a standard test to diagnose the presence of intraabdominal hemorrhage and hemopericardium after blunt and penetrating torso trauma.[9] There are several problems with ultrasonography, however. It is not useful in the evaluation of patients with a distended abdomen because air does not conduct sound waves well. The quality of the information obtained from ultrasonography is highly dependent on the skill of the sonographer performing and interpreting the examination.

The CT scan provides the best anatomical information about the acute abdomen. The peritoneum is composed of a layer of polyhedral-shape squamous cells approximately 3 mm thick and may be viewed anatomically as a closed sac that allows for the free movement of abdominal viscera. Adherent to the anterior and lateral abdominal walls, the peritoneum invests the intraabdominal viscera in such a way as to form the mesentery for the small and large bowel, a peritoneal diverticulum posterior to the stomach (the lesser sac) and a number of spaces or recesses in which blood, fluid, or pus can localize in response to various disease processes (Fig. 42.2).

Fluid can therefore collect in (1) the right and left subphrenic spaces (left more commonly than right) (Fig. 42.3); (2) the subhepatic space (posterior to the left lobe of the liver) (Fig. 42.4); (3) Morrison's pouch (adjacent to the gallbladder) (Fig. 42.5); (4) the lesser sac (usually in response to pancreatitis or pancreatic injury) (Fig. 42.6); (5) the left and right gutters (lateral to the left and right colon, respectively) (Fig. 42.7); (6) the pelvis (Fig. 42.8); and (7) the interloop spaces (between the loops of intestine) (Fig. 42.9). Search these areas when studying an abdominal CT much as a surgeon would inspect them during the course of a complete exploratory laparotomy.

The introduction of the helical (spiral) abdominal CT scan has reduced the time of the scan to less than 5 min and vastly improved the quality of the images by reducing respiratory misregistration.[3] The role of the CT scan in the overall eval-

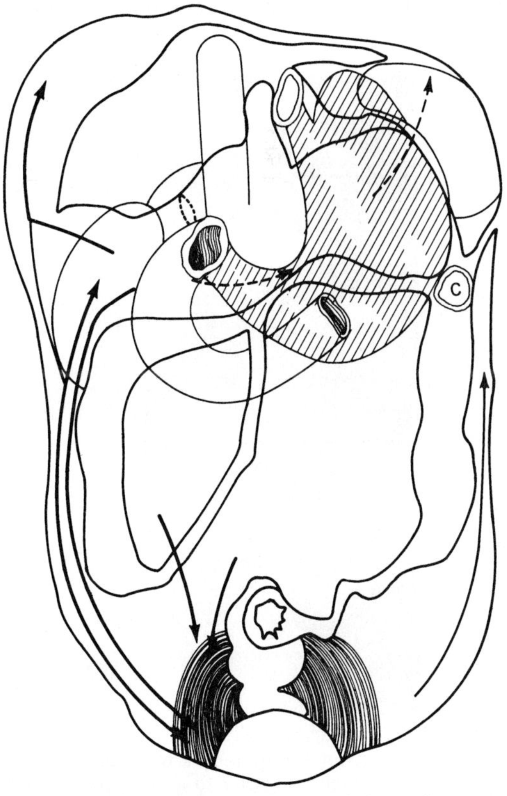

FIGURE 42.2. Diagram of the pathways of flow of intraperitoneal exudates. Broken arrows indicate spread anterior to the stomach to the left subphrenic area. C, splenic flexure of colon. (Modified from Meyers and Oliphant,[32] © 1974 Year Book Medical Publishers.)

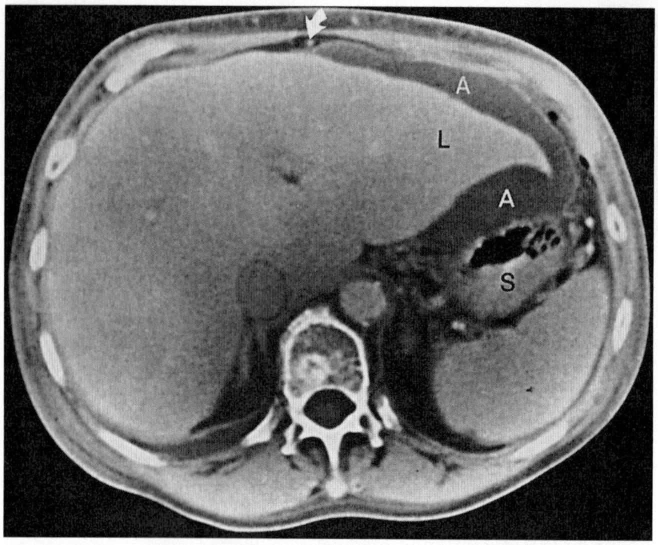

FIGURE 42.3. Left subphrenic abscess secondary to anterior perforation of a gastric ulcer. The abscess (A) is bordered by the falciform ligament (arrow), the anterior peritoneal reflection of the stomach (S), and the liver (L). Gas is present around the pars transversus of the left portal vein. (Courtesy of Richard Gore, MD, Evanston Hospital, Evanston, IL.)

uation of the patient with the acute abdomen is evolving. The CT scan provides highly accurate anatomical information about the liver, spleen, kidney, ureter, and bladder (if a retrograde cystogram is performed during the CT scan). It is an excellent test for the identification of intraabdominal abscesses.[10] It is a useful test in diagnosing pancreatitis and pancreatic injury after trauma. Previous generations of CT scanners did not provide accurate information about hollow viscus perforation or injury. I have seen several patients die due to a delay in laparotomy because their surgeons believed the negative CT findings in spite of deterioration in the abdominal physical findings and hemodynamic stability. The

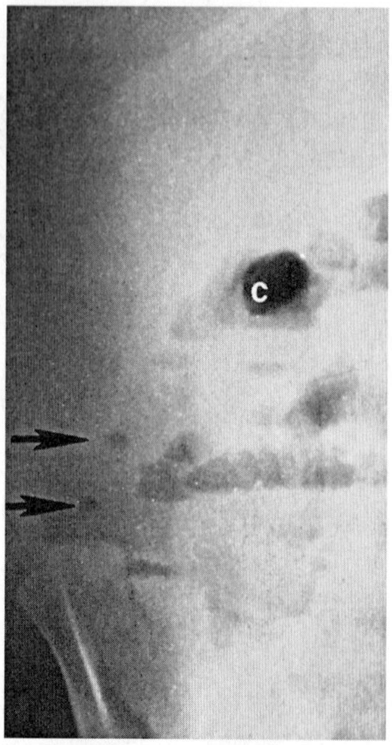

FIGURE 42.4. Right paracolic and anterior subhepatic abscesses, postappendectomy. Exudate containing a few gas bubbles (arrows), extends up the right paracolic gutter to a subhepatic abscess. This depresses the proximal transverse colon (C) and, by lifting the edge of the liver from its bed of extraperitoneal fat, results in loss of visualization of the hepatic angle. (Modified from Meyers and Oliphant,[32] © 1974 Year Book Medical Publishers.)

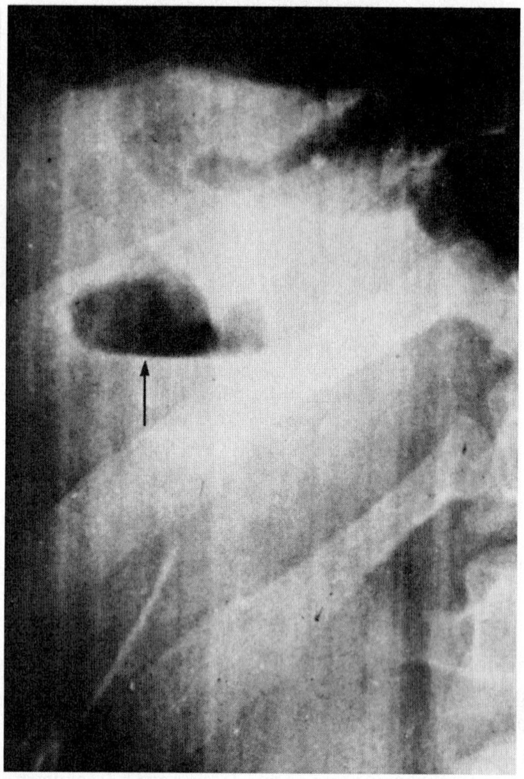

FIGURE 42.5. Abscess of Morison's pouch. Erect view identifies a conspicuous air–fluid level (arrow) characteristically in relation to the upper pole of the right kidney at the level of the 11th rib. (Reprinted with permission from Meyers,[33] © 1994 Springer-Verlag, New York.)

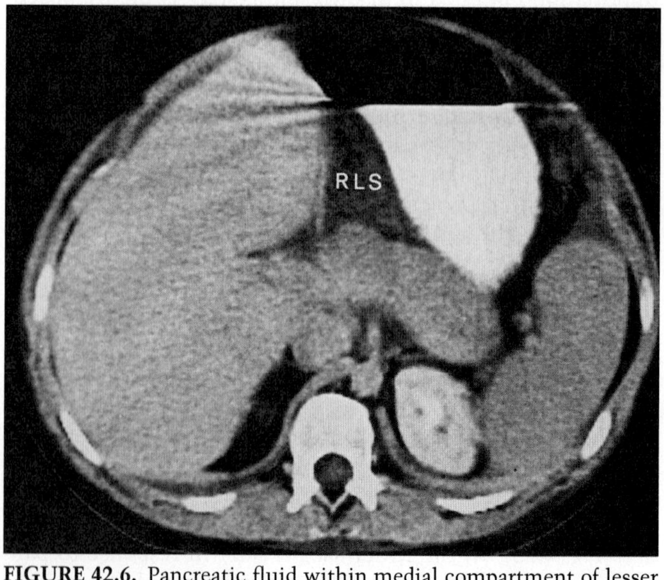

FIGURE 42.6. Pancreatic fluid within medial compartment of lesser sac. In this patient with acute pancreatitis, there is fluid loculation within the right (medial) compartment of the lesser sac (RLS). (Reprinted with permission from Meyers,[33] © 1994 Springer-Verlag, New York.)

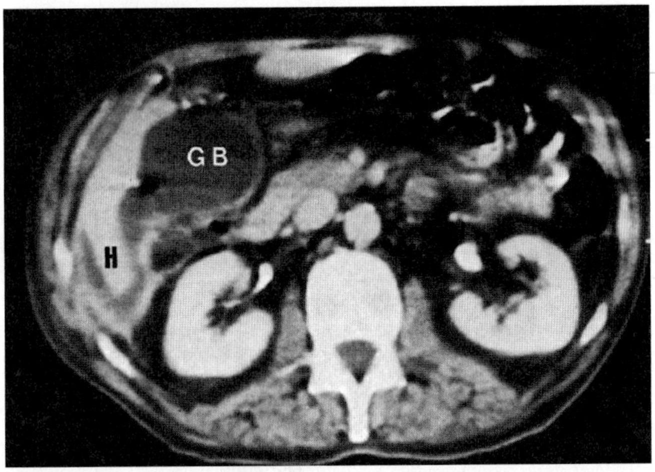

FIGURE 42.7. Infected fluid in Morison's pouch and right paracolic gutter. Secondary to perforation of the gallbladder (GB) from emphysematous cholecystitis, CT demonstrates fluid pooling in posterior subhepatic space and right paracolic gutter. The collection surrounds the hepatic angle (H), explaining the loss of visualization by conventional radiologic techniques in these circumstances. (Reprinted with permission from Meyers,[33] © 1994 Springer-Verlag, New York.)

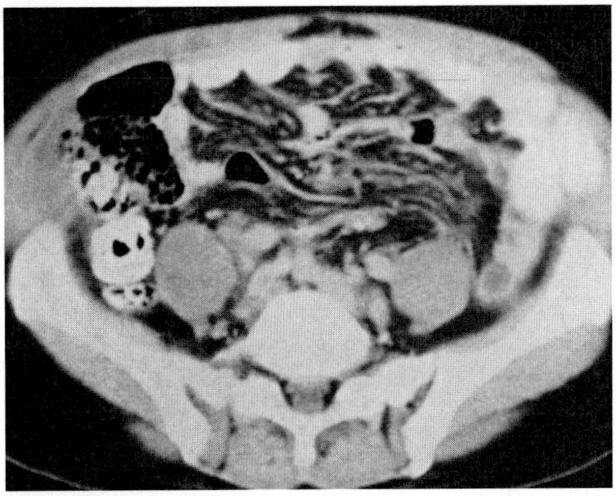

FIGURE 42.9. Intestinal borders. This example of tuberculous peritonitis illustrates the radiation of thickened vessels coursing through the mesentery to the mesenteric borders of multiple small-bowel loops. (Courtesy of Emil Balthazar, MD, Bellevue Hospital, New York, NY; reprinted with permission from Meyers,[33] © 1994 Springer-Verlag, New York.)

spiral abdominal CT, however, can detect small amounts of intraperitoneal fluid associated with a hollow viscus injury[11] and has improved the accuracy of this preoperative diagnosis.

Because of the ease and speed of the test, many patients with acute abdominal pain have already undergone a spiral abdominal CT scan ordered by the emergency physician before the surgeon is consulted. Some of these patients have obvious indications for surgery and are unnecessarily exposed to radiation. However, studies in both the adult and elderly adult populations suggest that the liberal use of abdominal CT scan in patients with an acute abdomen alters both the diagnosis and therapy in one-third to one-half of the patients. The major effect is avoidance of a nontherapeutic laparotomy.[12,13]

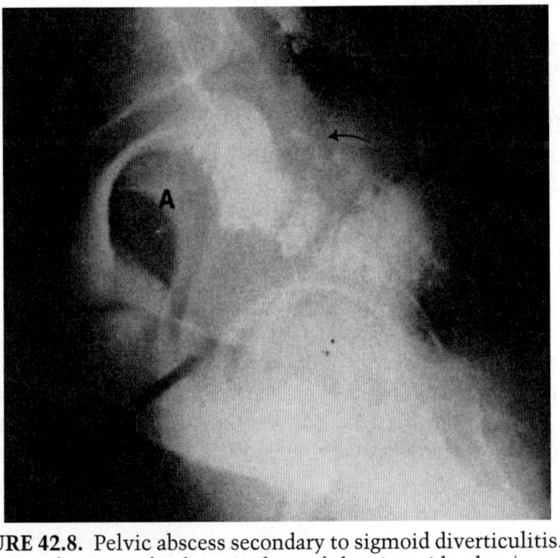

FIGURE 42.8. Pelvic abscess secondary to sigmoid diverticulitis. Following perforation of a diverticulum of the sigmoid colon (arrow) in the left lower quadrant, drainage into the pelvis results in an abscess (A) in the pouch of Douglas, shown by its characteristic compression on the rectosigmoid junction. (Reprinted with permission from Meyers,[33] © 1994 Springer-Verlag, New York.)

Differential Diagnosis of the Acute Abdomen

After reviewing the history, physical exam, and appropriate laboratory and radiologic data, the surgeon must develop a differential diagnosis and decide whether the patient requires surgery. Serial abdominal examinations searching for evolving peritoneal signs and repeat measurements of the white blood cell count are critical if the diagnosis is uncertain. Several variables determine the speed of the diagnostic evaluation, the diagnoses to be considered, and the necessity for exploratory laparotomy in the absence of a definitive diagnosis. These variables are (1) the hemodynamic stability of the patient, (2) the presence or absence of a rigid abdomen on physical examination, (3) the character and anatomical location of the abdominal pain, and (4) the deterioration or improvement in symptoms, signs, and laboratory data during the period of observation.[1]*

The hemodynamically unstable patient with acute abdominal pain presents a surgical emergency and requires rapid evaluation and treatment (Fig. 42.10). The first priority is to consider the diagnosis of a leaking abdominal aortic aneurysm (AAA). These patients have diffuse pain radiating to the back. A pulsatile, expansile, abdominal mass may be palpable. However, the aneurysm is often not palpable in the obese patient or the patient who is guarding because of pain. An abdominal ultrasound or CT scan can confirm the diagnosis. The patient should be transported to the operating room as soon as the diagnosis is made. Attempts to fluid

*I owe the discussion of the protocol for evaluation of patients based on hemodynamic stability and abdominal rigidity to algorithms published by Ronald F. Martin and Ricardo L. Rossi cited in reference 1.

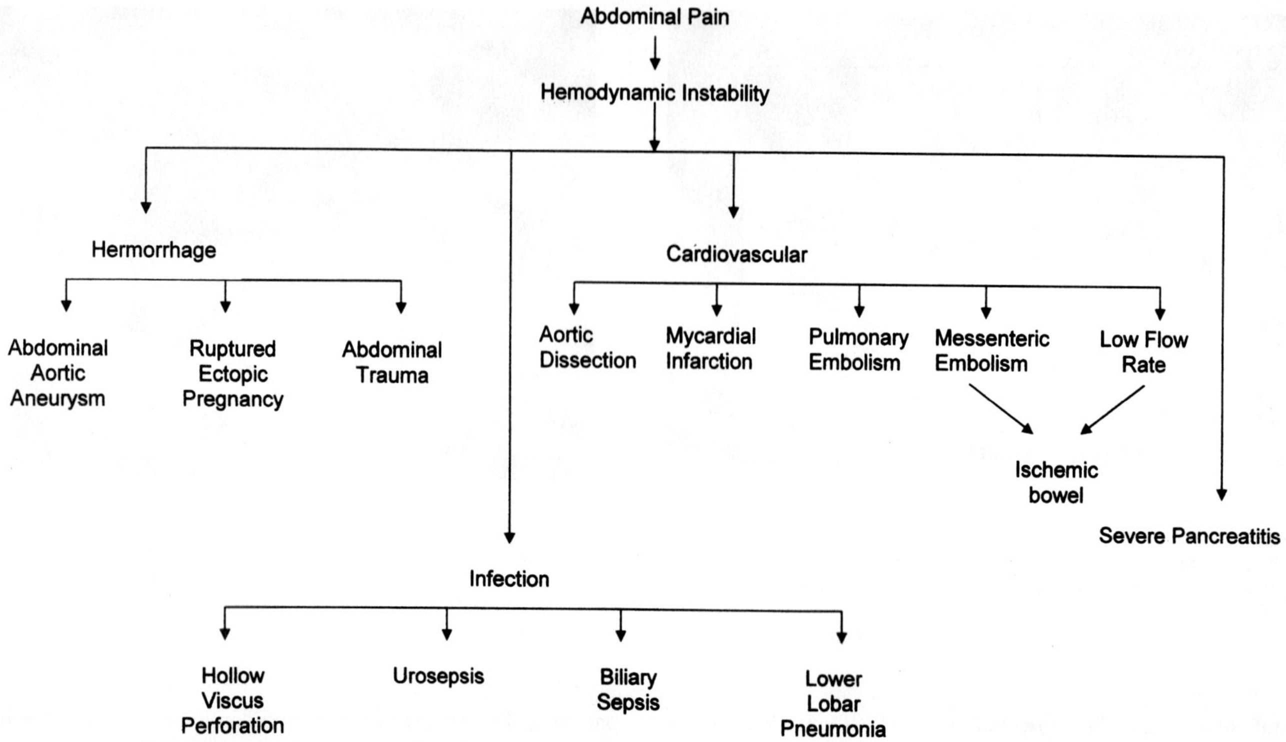

FIGURE 42.10. Diagnostic algorithm for acute abdominal pain in the hemodynamically unstable patient.

resuscitate patients with a leaking AAA in the emergency department are counterproductive because they both delay definitive treatment and may lead to free intraperitoneal rupture and death by raising the blood pressure.[14] If the patient does not have an AAA, then fluid resuscitation should begin immediately. In these cases, both the treatment and the diagnostic evaluation proceed in parallel. Patients with intraperitoneal or retroperitoneal hemorrhage require resuscitation and control of hemorrhage in the operating room, in the interventional radiology suite, or in the intensive care unit (ICU) depending on the source of the bleeding and the response to fluid resuscitation. Discussion of the resuscitation of the patient with abdominal sepsis is beyond the scope of this chapter. However, I would emphasize that the emergency department is not the appropriate place for a prolonged evaluation of the unstable patient. These patients should be transported to the operating room or the ICU as soon as feasible for assessment and treatment.

In general, hemodynamic instability caused by peritonitis is a late development occurring in patients with hollow viscus perforation, prolonged obstruction, or intestinal ischemia. Urosepsis should always be considered as it is a common cause of hemodynamic instability, particularly in the elderly patient, and does not require laparotomy. Patients with pyelonephritis usually have costovertebral angle tenderness or flank pain. Elderly septic men with lower abdominal pain may have massive distension of the bladder from prostatic hypertrophy, which can be diagnosed by dullness to percussion of the lower abdomen. A Foley catheter, antibiotics, and fluids will usually solve the acute problem.

Another relatively common cause of hemodynamic instability in the septic elderly patient is cholangitis. Occasionally, these patients are obtunded and do not exhibit the usual findings of the right upper quadrant pain, chills, and fever. Patients with severe sepsis can present with hypothermia. Most of these patients have jaundice, hyperbilirubinemia, and ultrasonographic evidence of extrahepatic biliary obstruction. The first line of treatment is antibiotics and biliary drainage. Nasobiliary drainage established by endoscopic cholangiopancreatography is the preferred method of drainage. The patient should be resuscitated and undergo elective biliary surgery when completely stable. The hemodynamically stable patient with a rigid abdomen and peritoneal signs should be studied with an upright chest x-ray and plain and upright abdominal x-rays. Most of these patients are candidates for an abdominal CT scan. The plain and upright abdominal x-rays can be eliminated if the patient proceeds directly to abdominal CT. Patients with evidence of hollow viscus perforation or obstruction should undergo immediate abdominal exploration.

If the abdomen is soft without generalized peritoneal signs, then a reasonable differential diagnosis can be developed based on the nature and the location of the abdominal pain (Table 42.1). Poorly localized abdominal pain, particularly severe abdominal pain out of proportion to the findings on physical examination, suggests the diagnosis of bowel ischemia. Pain caused by obstructive processes (bowel obstruction and appendicitis), visceral inflammation (inflammatory bowel disease, enteritis, or colitis), and retroperitoneal disease (pancreatitis) may initially present as poorly localized abdominal pain transmitted by the visceral C fibers. Localization occurs when the somatically innervated parietal peritoneum becomes inflamed.

Abdominal pain can localize to the (1) epigastrium, (2) right upper quadrant, (3) left upper quadrant, (4) right lower quadrant, (5) left lower quadrant, and (6) the right and left flanks. The location of the pain is an important clue to the diagnosis. However, the surgeon who undertakes a true exploratory laparotomy must be prepared to handle the entire

TABLE 42.1. Common Locations and Corresponding Diagnosis in Abdominal Pain.

Epigastrium	Right upper quadrant and flank
Abdominal aortic aneurysm	Cholecystitis
Colon carcinoma	Choledocholithiasis
Duodenal ulcer	Gastric ulcer
Early appendicitis	Intestinal obstruction
Gastritis	Pancreatitis
Mesenteric ischemia	Penetrating ulcer
Pancreatitis	Pyelonephritis
Penetrating ulcer	Renal colic
Retrocecal appendicitis	
Left upper quadrant and flank	Right lower quadrant
Bowel obstruction	Appendicitis
Diverticulitis	Bowel obstruction
Pyelonephritis	Cholecystitis
Renal colic	Diverticulitis
Splenic enlargement	Hernia
Leaking aneurysm	
Psoas abscess	
Pyelonephritis	
Left lower quadrant	
Abdominal wall hematoma	
Bowel obstruction	
Diverticulitis	
Hernia	
Leaking aneurysm	
Pyelonephritis	
Geriatric abdominal pain	
Mesenteric ischemia	

Source: Modified with permission from Caesar, Emerg Med Rep 1994;3(20): 191–202.

spectrum of intraabdominal pathology because of the imprecision of current diagnostic techniques.

Upper abdominal pain localizing to either the epigastrium or the right or the left upper quadrant may be caused by diseases of the myocardium (infarction, pericarditis); lungs (pneumonia, pleuritis, pleural effusion, empyema, pulmonary infarction); peptic ulcer disease; and pancreatitis. Subphrenic abscesses may also cause left or right upper abdominal pain and are frequently associated with sympathetic pleural effusions and occasionally associated with hiccups. Pain localizing to the right upper quadrant is classically associated with hepatobiliary disease (cholangitis, biliary colic, cholangitis, hepatitis). Appendicitis, particularly a long retrocecal inflamed appendix, can present with right upper quadrant pain. Right-sided pyelonephritis or nephrolithiasis can also cause right upper quadrant pain. A careful physical examination, however, will usually elicit more tenderness in the right flank than the right upper quadrant in these cases.

Splenomegaly, ruptured spleen, pancreatitis, and pancreatic pseudocysts are diagnoses that should be considered in patients with left upper quadrant pain. Patients with irritation of the left hemidiaphragm may also have referred pain to the left shoulder.

Lower abdominal pain can be caused by musculoskeletal injury, rectus sheath hematoma (particularly in patients receiving anticoagulation medication), ileopsoas muscle abscess (the ipsilateral hip is usually held in flexion[15]), and ureterolithiasis. Appendicitis commonly presents with a history of generalized abdominal pain subsequently localizing to the right lower quadrant. Meckel's diverticulitis, diverticulitis of the right colon, mesenteric adenitis, and regional enteritis (Crohn's disease) must be considered in the differential diagnosis. A history of diarrhea with mucus or blood in the stool is usually present with active Crohn's disease causing right lower quadrant pain. Occasionally, the surgeon can be fooled by a patient with a perforated duodenal ulcer who presents with right lower quadrant pain. In such cases, the duodenal contents pool in the right gutter adjacent to the cecum, causing irritation of the parietal peritoneum. At laparotomy, bile-stained fluid is found without evidence of appendicitis or Meckel's diverticulitis.

Acute cholecystitis can sometimes present with right lower quadrant pain. A careful history and physical examination, together with an ultrasound examination, should lead to the correct preoperative diagnosis in most cases. The distinction between appendicitis and right lower quadrant pain caused by gynecological disease in women, however, is often difficult. Pelvic inflammatory disease, tuboovarian abscesses, ectopic pregnancy, endometriosis, and even mittelschmerz should be considered on the differential diagnosis. The pelvic ultrasound examination is currently the most important test for diagnosing gynecological disease in patients with acute abdominal pain. However, the role of the helical CT scan is becoming increasingly important in the evaluation of patients with right lower quadrant pain. The differential diagnosis of left lower quadrant pain is similar to that for right lower quadrant pain except that diverticulitis replaces appendicitis as the most common diagnosis in the differential. Neoplasm and bowel obstruction should also be considered.

Abdominal distension and obstipation suggest the diagnosis of bowel obstruction. The obstruction may be located in the small or large intestine. Patients with large-bowel obstruction have a dilated colon usually visible on the plain film of the abdomen. The goals of the evaluation are determination of the precise location of the obstruction, assessment of whether the obstruction is partial or complete, determination of whether emergency surgery or conservative management is required, and ultimately diagnosis of the precise cause of the obstruction.

The history elicits the duration of symptoms, the presence of nausea or vomiting, and whether the patient has recently passed flatus. A careful review of previous operations, weight loss, or previous diagnoses of malignancy or endometriosis may reveal important clues. The physical examination should include a careful search for incarcerated hernias, peritoneal signs, or localized abdominal pain and fever. The absence of air in the rectal ampulla is an important sign of complete obstruction. Leukocytosis may indicate ischemia resulting from closed-loop obstruction.

Examine the abdominal plain films carefully for signs of air in the colon or colonic distention. A large air-filled loop of colon located between the left lower and right upper quadrants suggests the diagnosis of sigmoid volvulus. Conversely, a dilated loop of colon between the right lower and left upper quadrants suggests cecal volvulus. Search the abdominal film for air in the wall of the colon (pneumatosis cystoides intestinalis), a sign of ischemic bowel due to mesenteric vessel obstruction caused by the volvulus. Volvulus can often be treated by sigmoidoscopic or colonoscopic decompression. However, extreme caution must be exercised to avoid colon perforation. It is far better to achieve safe surgical decompression than to unwisely persist with a prolonged difficult endoscopy that may result in massive fecal contamination of the peritoneal cavity due to perforation. A gentle water-soluble contrast enema can be used to identify the point of obstruction. Barium should *never* be used in this clinical situation because of the risk of perforation.

Small-bowel obstruction is suggested by a plain film with multiple air–fluid levels and the absence of air in the colon. Peritoneal signs, localized abdominal pain, fever, and leukocytosis are absolute indications for exploration. A patient with a distended abdomen who has recently passed flatus may be only partially obstructed. If the patient appears to be partially obstructed, then nasogastric decompression, fluid resuscitation, and serial abdominal examinations are appropriate initial therapy.

Pitfalls in the Assessment of the Acute Abdomen

The physician evaluating a patient with acute abdominal pain has an important responsibility. The art of history and physical examination is of paramount importance; the precision of the diagnostic radiologic and laboratory tests are not yet up to the task; and the consequences of error can be disastrous. Complaints of abdominal pain must be taken seriously. Any patient with acute abdominal pain of 6h duration should be admitted for serial abdominal examinations and observation. Remember, peritonitis is a process in evolution. A one-time "snapshot" abdominal examination can be misleading. The progression or resolution of physical findings and laboratory parameters under observation is extremely important. If you are concerned, then admit the patient. If you decide to send the patient home, then call them (by telephone) 4 to 8h later to inquire about their symptoms. Initial underestimation of the severity of an intraabdominal process is understandable and acceptable as long as you assume the personal responsibility for patient follow-up and intervene promptly if the patient's condition deteriorates.

Unusual Nonoperative Causes of Abdominal Pain

A number of diseases can cause abdominal pain and simulate an acute surgical abdomen but do not require surgery.[16]

Neurological Causes of Abdominal Pain

Varicella zoster viral infections can cause radiating pain and hyperesthesia along the dermatome of an intercostal nerve followed by a typical vesicular rash 5 to 7 days after the onset of symptoms. "Shingles" is usually a self-limited disease treated by analgesics. Treatment with acyclovir is indicated in severe cases. Occasionally, a herniating disk producing compression radiculopathy causes confusing symptoms of abdominal wall pain. A CT scan or MRI will make the definitive diagnosis.

Pain Caused by Toxic Substance Ingestion

Ingestion of toxic substances such as iron, lead, poisonous mushrooms, and alcohol (ethanol, isopropanol, and methanol) all cause crampy abdominal pain often associated with diarrhea. Patients withdrawing from opiates (heroin) have abdominal pain as a characteristic part of the withdrawal symptoms.

Endocrine Causes of Abdominal Pain

Endocrine and metabolic diseases can cause abdominal pain. Glucocorticoid deficiency (Addison's disease) presents with hypotension, tachycardia, weakness, fatigue, and crampy abdominal pain (50% of cases). The etiology may be diseases of the hypothalamus causing reduction in corticotropin (ACTH) secretion (infarction, tumor, infiltrative disease); diseases of the adrenal gland (tumor, infection, hemorrhagic infarction, infiltration disorders); and withdrawal of steroids in patients receiving chronic steroid therapy. Glucocorticoid therapy results in resolution of the abdominal pain.

Hypercalcemia can cause diffuse symptoms, including crampy abdominal pain. Hypercalcemia is also associated with other causes of abdominal pain, including peptic ulcer disease, pancreatitis, and nephrolithiasis. Severe hypercalcemia is associated with hypovolemia, altered mental states, muscle cramps, and cardiac arrhythmias. Emergency treatment with normal saline, furosemide, and a bisphosphonate (pamidronate or zoledronic acid) is required for rapid control of hypercalcemia.

Diabetic ketoacidosis sometimes presents with acute abdominal pain. The mechanism is poorly understood. More often, the patient develops ketoacidosis as a consequence of pulmonary, intraabdominal (urinary tract, biliary tract), or soft tissue infection. Treatment consists of restoration of intravascular volume, correction of hyperglycemia and the electrolyte imbalance, and identification and treatment of the source of infection.

Genetic Disorders Causing Abdominal Pain

Familial Mediterranean fever is an autosomal recessive genetic disease characterized by recurrent episodes of abdominal pain, peritoneal inflammation, and fever. Other serosal membranes such as the pleura, pericardium, and meninges also become intermittently inflamed. A family history and history of recurrent attacks are important in establishing the diagnosis. Laparoscopic appendectomy has been advocated as a way to reduce diagnostic uncertainty in these patients.[17]

Porphyria is a term referring to a group of autosomal dominant disorders caused by defective heme synthesis. Neurotoxic intermediates of heme metabolism (porphyrins) accumulate that cause abdominal pain, ileus, changes in mental status, psychiatric disturbance, muscle weakness, and skin photosensitivity. The diagnosis is made by a false-positive test for urobilinogen on the urinary dipstick test (porphobilinogen cross-reacts with urobilinogen). If the patient has a normal serum bilirubin and a positive dipstick test for urobilinogen, then porphyria should be suspected.[18]

Sickle cell anemia is an autosomal recessive disease of the hemoglobin molecule resulting in red cell deformation and clotting in the microcirculation under hypoxic conditions. Patients have multiple sickle cell crises throughout their lives. The symptoms of sickle cell crisis may vary but often are characteristic for each patient. Abdominal pain is a frequent symptom. The diagnostic challenge is the distinction between abdominal pain caused by reversible ischemia and bowel infarction. Ask the patient whether current symptoms are typical of the crises experienced in the past. Treatment includes volume expansion, oxygenation, and analgesics followed by serial abdominal examinations. Pain that fails to resolve should raise the suspicion of bowel infarction. Sickle cell anemia is also associated with cholecystitis caused by bilirubin stones, splenomegaly caused by sequestration of damaged red cells, and splenic infarction. These entities also cause abdominal pain but are usually not associated with sickle cell crises.

Mesenteric vasculitis caused by a number of immune-mediated diseases can cause acute abdominal pain. The disease that classically causes diagnostic confusion is Henoch-Schonlein purpura (HSP), an autoimmune disseminated vasculitis, primarily occurring in young children, characterized by complaints of abdominal pain, joint pain, and a characteristic purpuric rash. The symptoms often begin several weeks after a streptococcal upper respiratory infection or infectious diarrhea. Most children also have associated renal vasculitis manifested by hematuria and proteinuria on urinalysis.

Special Situations

The Acute Abdomen in the Elderly

Some geriatric patients are poor historians because of either confusion accompanying serious illness or senile dementia. Close family members and caretakers are extremely important when present, but unfortunately many senior citizens in our society are increasingly left to fend for themselves, leading to late presentation. The abdominal examination can also be misleading. The signs of peritoneal irritation that are so important in the evaluation of the younger patient are often absent in geriatric patients. A "surgical abdomen" should be suspected in all elderly patients who present with abdominal pain and distension or obtundation and sepsis regardless of the absence of peritoneal signs. Bowel ischemia, biliary and urosepsis, bowel obstruction, and occult appendicitis are all common diagnoses that should be considered (Table 42.1).

The Acute Abdomen in the Intensive Care Unit

The evaluation of the sedated, intubated ICU patient is challenging. There are four situations in which an acute abdomen presents in the ICU patient.

1. Patient "found down": Many patients are admitted to the medical ICU after they are found unconscious at home for variable periods of time. These patients are usually septic, acidotic, and often hypothermic. Bowel ischemia, either as a cause of the problem or a consequence of the low-flow state, should be considered. Abdominal CT scan and diagnostic laparoscopy are assuming an increasingly important role in the workup of this clinical situation.

2. Missed injury: Multiple-trauma patients (often with head, chest, and extremity injuries) are usually screened with an abdominal CT scan. In the absence of definitive indications for laparotomy, most of these patients are observed—usually in the ICU. If the patient is behaving in a manner unanticipated by the extent of the known injuries (e.g., hemodynamic instability, large intravenous volume requirement, progressive hypoxemia, unexplained blood requirement), then the possibility of a missed injury should be considered. Prolonged delay in laparotomy in these cases will lead to a significant increase in morbidity and mortality.

3. Postoperative surgical complications: Postoperative hemorrhage, obstruction, anastomotic leak, and intraabdominal abscess formation are all potential complications of abdominal surgery. Hemorrhage is usually an early complication, whereas obstruction, anastomotic leak, and intraabdominal abscess present days to weeks after surgery. The physical examination is confusing because pain and distension caused by incisions and surgical manipulation are difficult to distinguish from peritonitis and intra-abdominal abscess. Fever, leukocytosis, tachycardia, and an inability to tolerate enteral tube feedings may be the only signs of an occult abscess. The abdominal CT scan is a critical tool in this situation as it permits accurate identification and often drainage of localized collections of intraabdominal pus without resorting to repeat laparotomy.

4. Abdominal complications of intensive care: Acalculous cholecystitis and perforation or hemorrhage due to stress ulceration of the stomach or duodenum are the most common causes of the acute abdomen as a consequence of the ICU experience. Early enteral feedings and ulcer prophylaxis with H_2 blockers or sucralfate significantly reduce the incidence of stress ulceration.[19] A complete daily physical examination is essential for the early identification of subtle changes in the abdominal findings.

Planned Abdominal Reexploration

Planned abdominal reexploration is assuming an increasingly important role in the management of selected patients. There are four situations for which planned reexploration is helpful: (1) "second-look" laparotomy following resection for intestinal infarction; (2) planned repeat laparotomy to ensure peritoneal toilet in a patient with severe (usually fecal) peritonitis; (3) reexploration after "damage control" laparotomy; and (4) reexploration and closure of a patient with abdominal compartment syndrome.

1. Second-look laparotomy for bowel ischemia: Intestinal ischemia is a disease process in evolution. Despite a careful inspection and Wood's lamp ultraviolet examination of the bowel after intravenous fluorescein to assess intestinal viability, the surgeon often cannot be completely sure of the viability of the remaining intestine after resection for ischemia. In this situation, a second-look laparotomy 24 to 48h after the first operation is prudent.[20]

2. Peritoneal toilet: Patients with severe fecal peritonitis of long-standing duration may benefit from repeated trips to the OR every 24 to 48h for peritoneal irrigation until the effluent becomes clear.[21] Usually, a relatively clean peritoneal cavity can be achieved after two or three trips to the OR. The indications for this method of treatment are not clear, and the efficacy is not definitely proven. Patients who remain unstable hemodynamically with extensive free fecal peritonitis are potential candidates for repeat peritoneal toilet. The surgeon may elect to delay fascial closure to facilitate access to the peritoneal cavity and avoid closing the fascia under tension. When possible, the skin can be closed temporarily over the bowel or a temporary soft, nonadherent prosthetic material can be used.[22] Use of a Marlex mesh placed directly

on distended bowel in this clinical situation increases the risk of fistula formation.

3. Reexploration after damage control laparotomy: Hemodynamically unstable, acidotic, hypothermic, coagulopathic patients with major intraabdominal injuries require rapid control of hemorrhage (often with intraabdominal packing) and closure or resection of hollow viscus injuries. Temporary abdominal closure before intestinal reconstruction allows time for continued resuscitation, patient rewarming, and correction of the coagulopathy in the ICU. The patient can then be returned to the operating room in 12 to 24h for reexploration and appropriate intestinal reconstruction under stable conditions. Damage control laparotomy with planned reexploration plays an important role in the salvage of selected unstable patients.[23]

4. Abdominal compartment syndrome: The abdominal compartment syndrome occurs when intraabdominal pressure increases to a level resulting in oliguria, hypoperfusion of the intraabdominal viscera, inadequate mechanical ventilation despite high peak inspiratory pressures, and collapse of the vena cava and renal veins (as seen on abdominal CT scan). Clinically, the abdomen is rigid. The urinary bladder pressure measured by transducing the pressure in the Foley catheter approximates the intraabdominal pressure. An elevated urinary bladder pressure (30mmHg) is an objective sign of abdominal compartment syndrome. The syndrome usually occurs after massive abdominal injuries and prolonged resuscitation. Loose abdominal closure with a temporary nonadherent prosthetic material decompresses the high intraabdominal pressure. The abdominal compartment syndrome can also occur after severe peritonitis or occasionally after massive fluid resuscitation for extra-abdominal sepsis (e.g., toxic shock syndrome). Planned reoperation to close the abdomen after reduction of the distension and edema is required. Often, the abdomen cannot be closed, and temporary split-thickness skin graft coverage of the abdominal viscera for a period of 6 months to 1 year is necessary before elective ventral herniorrhaphy.[24]

The Acute Abdomen in the Tropics

A variety of bacterial and parasitic diseases endemic to tropical regions are potential causes of an acute surgical abdomen. Surgeons practicing in the United States and western Europe may have occasion to treat these diseases.

Typhoid fever: *Salmonella typhi* causes a severe enteritis with enlargement of Peyer's patches. Perforation of the terminal ileum due to typhoid fever is a common problem in endemic areas of the developing world. The patient has a history of crampy abdominal pain and fever progressing to frank peritonitis. Classically, the pulse is disproportionately low in comparison to the high fever. Rose spots (a subtle pink rash, usually on the abdomen) sometimes accompany the other symptoms. Laparotomy, closure of the perforation, peritoneal toilet, and antibiotics constitute the treatment of choice. Unfortunately, peritonitis associated with typhoid fever has a high mortality.

Amebiasis: The most common presentations of amebiasis are amebic colitis (characterized by diarrhea, crampy abdominal pain, and colonic mucosal ulcers) and amebic liver abscess. Extensive amebic colitis can lead to colon infarction and perforation, causing acute peritonitis. Rupture of an amebic liver abscess can also cause acute peritonitis.

Ascariasis: Infestation with *Ascaris lumbricoides* (roundworms) can result in common bile duct obstruction due to worms entering the duct via the ampulla of Vater. However, *Ascaris* more commonly causes small-bowel obstruction in children. Treatment consists of enterotomy, removal of the "ball of worms" causing the obstruction, and mebendazole.

The Acute Abdomen in the Patient Infected with Human Immunodeficiency Virus

An increasing number of patients presenting with acute abdominal pain have concomitant human immunodeficiency virus (HIV) infection because of the increasing prevalence of HIV. Many cases of abdominal pain are due to nonoperative causes, such as splenomegaly, hepatomegaly, pancreatitis, and enterocolitis caused by opportunistic infections. However, HIV-infected patients also develop acute surgical abdomens caused by disease processes both related and unrelated to the underlying HIV infection. In the absence of obvious peritoneal signs, a CT scan is advisable in most HIV-infected patients before surgery to rule out a nonoperative cause of the pain. In a review of our cases published in 1994, we found that approximately 40% of HIV-infected patients with acute surgical abdomens have diagnoses directly related to their immunocompromised state (e.g., perforated colon from cytomegalovirus [CMV] colitis, CMV cholecystitis, bowel obstruction from lymphoma, etc.).[25] The remaining diagnoses result from common causes of the acute abdomen.

The outcome after emergency laparotomy in HIV-infected patients is a function of the preoperative physiological condition of the patient (muscle mass, exercise tolerance, and immune status) and the nature and extent of the disease causing the acute abdomen. The overall mortality rate for 57 AIDS patients undergoing 63 emergency laparotomies was 12% in a series from the San Francisco General Hospital.[25] Since the introduction of highly active antiretroviral therapy in 1996, we have seen few patients in San Francisco requiring surgery for acute abdominal pain caused by HIV-related intraabdominal disease. No patient should be denied surgical therapy solely on the basis of the diagnosis of HIV infection.[26]

The Acute Abdomen in Pregnancy

Pregnancy complicates the evaluation and management of the acute abdomen for several reasons. First and foremost, there is a natural reluctance to explore the abdomen of a pregnant woman in the face of diagnostic uncertainty. However, allowing the patient to progress to advanced peritonitis will almost certainly result in loss of the fetus and possibly the mother as well.

The enlarging uterus alters the intraabdominal location of adjacent organs. The cecum is pushed into the right upper quadrant, making assessment of the physical findings more difficult. If appendicitis is suspected, then the incision should be centered over the point of maximum tenderness rather than over McBurney's point to optimize exposure.

The surgeon has two patients, the mother and the fetus. If laparotomy is indicated, then the surgeon should work in concert with the obstetrician and the anesthesiologist to monitor the fetus and provide tocolytic therapy to prevent premature labor and delivery.[27]

Laparotomy or Laparoscopy

The recent expansion of both diagnostic and therapeutic laparoscopy has added a new tool to the surgical armamentarium. Laparoscopy usually allows a good view of the uterus and adenexae, the appendix and cecum, the gallbladder, the stomach, the pylorus, and the first portion of the duodenum. Laparoscopic appendectomy[28,29] and closure of perforated duodenal ulcers[30] have become common procedures, and laparoscopic cholecystectomy is now the standard of care. Laparoscopy can be used to assess intestinal viability if bowel ischemia is suspected, although interpretation of the findings is difficult in the absence of clear-cut gangrenous bowel. Unfortunately, laparoscopic technology has not yet developed to the point at which the average surgeon can adequately examine the entire bowel. Furthermore, in cases of intestinal obstruction, there is a significant risk of bowel injury during trocar insertion and bowel perforation during intestinal manipulation with the instruments currently available.

Laparoscopy certainly has a role in the management of the acute abdomen, and that role will increase as technology improves and experience increases. At the present time, the choice of diagnostic laparoscopy versus exploratory laparotomy when the diagnosis is unknown depends on the experience and judgment of the individual surgeon.[31]

The evaluation and management of the patient with an acute abdomen remain one of the most challenging problems in clinical medicine. Cultivation of the clinical skills of history and physical examination, maintenance of a high index of suspicion, and the assumption of personal responsibility for patient follow-up are essential for achieving the best results.

References

1. Martin RF, Rossi RL. The acute abdomen: an overview and algorithm. Surg Clin North Am 1997;77:1227.
2. Gypta H, Dupuy DE. Advances in imaging the acute abdomen. Surg Clin North Am 1997;77:1245–1283.
3. Omori H, Asahi H, Inoue Y, et al. Pneumoperitoneum without perforation of the gastrointestinal tract. Dig Surg 2003;20:334–338.
4. Ahn SH, Mayo-Smith WW, Murphy BL, et al. Acute non-traumatic abdominal pain in adult patients: abdominal radiography compared with CT evaluation. Radiology 2002;225:159–164.
5. Fa EM, Cronan EJ. Compression ultrasonography as an aid in the differential diagnosis of appendicitis. Surg Gynecol Obstret 1989;169:290–298.
6. Chen SC, Chen KM, Wang SM, Chang KJ. Abdominal ultrasound screen of clinically diagnosed or suspected appendicitis before surgery. World J Surg 1998;22:449–452.
7. Wade DS, Marrow SE, Balsaraza ZN, et al. Accuracy of ultrasound in the diagnosis of acute appendicitis compared with the surgeon's clinical impression. Arch Surg 1993;128:1039–1044.
8. Carroll BA. Preferred imaging techniques for the diagnosis of cholecystitis and cholelithiasis. Ann Surg 1989;210:1–12.
9. Healey MA, Simons RK, Winchell RJ, et al. A prospective evaluation of abdominal ultrasound in blunt trauma: is it useful? J Trauma 1996;40:875–883.
10. Goletti O, Lippolis PV, Chiarugi M, et al. Percutaneous ultrasound guided drainage of intra-abdominal abscesses. Br J Surg 1993;80:336–339.
11. Livingston DH, Lavery RF, Passannante MR, et al. Admission or observation is not necessary after a negative abdominal computed tomography scan in patients with blunt abdominal trauma: results of a prospective multi-institutional trial. J Trauma 1998;44:273–280.
12. Chambers A, Halligan S, Goh V, et al. Therapeutic impact of abdomino-pelvic computed tomography in patients with acute abdominal symptoms. Acta Radiol 2004;45:248–253.
13. Esses D, Birnbaum A, Bijur P, et al. Ability of CT to alter decision making in elderly patients with acute abdominal pain. Am J Emerg Med 2004;22:270–272.
14. Adam DJ, Bradbury AW, Stuart WP, et al. The value of computed tomography in the assessment of suspected ruptured abdominal aortic aneurysm. J Vasc Surg 1998;27:431–437.
15. Schecter W, Rintel T, Slutkin G, et al. Tropical pyomyositis of the iliacus muscle. Am J Trop Med Hyg 1983;34:809–811.
16. Roy S, Weimersheimer P. Non-operative causes of abdominal pain. Surg Clin North Am 1997;77:1433–1454.
17. Reissman P, Durst AL, Rivkind A, et al. Elective laparoscopic appendectomy in patients with familial Mediterranean fever. World J Surg 1994;18:139–141.
18. Lim H. The porphyrias. Clin Dermatol 1996;14:375–387.
19. Cook D, Guyatt G, Marshall J, et al. A comparison of sucralfate and ranitidine for the prevention of upper gastrointestinal bleeding in patient requiring mechanical ventilation. Canadian Critical Care Trials Group. N Engl J Med 1998;338:791–797.
20. Montgomery RA, Venbrux AC, Bulkley GB. Mesenteric vascular insufficiency. Curr Probl Surg 1997;34:941–1028.
21. Butler JA, Huang J, Wilson SE. Repeated laparotomy for postoperative intra-abdominal sepsis: an analysis of outcome predictors. Arch Surg 1987;122:702–706.
22. Sleeman D, Sosa JL, Gonzalez A, et al. Reclosure of the open abdomen. J Am Coll Surg 1995;180:200–204.
23. Hirschberg A, Wall MJ Jr, Mattox KL. Planned reoperation for trauma: a 2-year experience with 24 consecutive patients. J Trauma 1994;37:365–369.
24. Mayberry JC, Mullins RJ, Crass RA, Trunkey DD. Prevention of abdominal compartment syndrome by absorbable mesh prosthesis closure. Arch Surg 1997;132:957–961.
25. Whitney TM, Brunell W, Russell TR, et al. Emergent abdominal surgery in AIDS: experience in San Francisco. Am J Surg 1994;168:239–243.
26. Schecter WP. Surgical care of the HIV-infected patient: a moral imperative. Camb Q Healthcare Ethics 1992;1:223–228.
27. Fallon WF, Newman JS, Fallon GL, Malangoni MA. The surgical management of intraabdominal inflammatory conditions during pregnancy. Surg Clin North Am 1995;75:15–31.
28. Pier A, Gotz F, Bacher C, et al. Laparoscopic appendectomy. World J Surg 1993;17:29–33.
29. Ortega AE, Hunter JG, Peters JH, et al. A prospective randomized comparison of laparoscopic appendectomy with open appendectomy. Laparoscopic appendectomy study group. Am J Surg 1995;169:208–212.
30. Lau WY, Leung KL, Kwong KH, et al. A randomized study comparing laparoscopic versus open repair of perforated peptic ulcer using suture or sutureless technique. Am Surg 1996;224:131–138.
31. Memon MA, Fitzgibbons RJ. The role of minimal access surgery in the acute abdomen. Surg Clin North Am 1997;77:1333–1353.
32. Meyers MA, Oliphant M. Pitfalls and pickups in plain-film diagnosis of the abdomen. 1974;4(2):1–37.
33. Meyers MA. Dynamic Radiology of the Abdomen. 4th ed. New York: Springer-Verlag 1994.

43

Principles of Minimally Invasive Surgery

Theodore N. Pappas and Alison M. Fecher

The historical development of laparoscopy can be traced to early in the 19th century when Bozzini, an Italian physician living in Germany, first examined the abdominal cavity using reflected candlelight.[1] In 1901, George Kelling, a German, described the establishment of a pneumoperitoneum (PNP) and trocar placement through which a cystoscope was placed. In the early 1930s throughout Europe, modern laparoscopy was popularized by Kalk, who used room air to create a PNP.[2,3] Laparoscopy was initially applied in gynecological procedures, and it was not until 1991 that general surgeons began to take notice when Muhe introduced the first laparoscopic cholecystectomy (LC) in Germany.[4]

The excellent preliminary results achieved by the pioneers of laparoscopic cholecystectomy, coupled with a groundswell of support in the lay press, led to the convening of a National Institutes of Health Consensus Conference in 1992 to consider the position of laparoscopic cholecystectomy. This panel concluded that LC was a bona fide alternative to open cholecystectomy (OC).[5] Additional laparoscopic applications for a variety of surgical procedures have subsequently been described. Semm performed the first laparoscopic appendectomy in 1983, and laparoscopic fundoplication was introduced by Geagea in 1991.[6]

The purpose of this chapter is to provide an overview of the field of laparoscopic surgery and to provide reference to relevant clinical and experimental literature. Considerable research efforts have been published by a variety of research groups to describe the physiological response to PNP and document measurable outcomes for evaluating the position of current and future laparoscopic procedures. Although the tremendous efforts made toward describing the physiological response to PNP have already answered several questions, this research, as is often the case, has raised several additional provocative questions. For instance, is laparoscopy safe under certain circumstances, such as sepsis or pregnancy? Also, what is the relationship between PNP and cancer? Who should perform these procedures? Where, when, and how should the training take place? The following discussion reviews the available literature that describes the physiological response to PNP and the current position of laparoscopic surgery within the field of surgery.

Equipment

Laparoscopic surgery is defined by its instrumentation, and advancements in equipment have been largely driven by industry. The equipment required for basic laparoscopy can be grouped into three categories: image production, peritoneal access devices, and instrumentation. With the rising cost of health care, many debates have centered on the issue of disposable versus reusable access devices and instrumentation. Because functional equipment is available in both disposable and reusable forms, most decisions regarding these issues have been based on a cost analysis.

Cost

An instrument's or procedure's true value is defined as quality divided by cost. Traverso explained that surgeons should be primarily interested in the quality of a new procedure, followed by its value.[7] *Quality* is defined as a procedure's clinical effectiveness; for example, does the stapler staple effectively? Therefore, when trying to discern the true value of a certain device, it must first be determined that the clinical effectiveness of the device is similar to that of the accepted standard. If so, then the true value of the instrument will reside in its cost.[7] As surgeons, especially laparoscopists, have become increasingly responsible for cost control, accurate definitions are necessary[8] (Table 43.1). Certainly, the convenience of disposable instrumentation is readily apparent; however, with costs factored into the equation for true value, the position of reusables will be increasingly defined.[9] Laparoscopic surgeons must work closely with industry to continue to develop appropriate cost-effective advancements in laparoscopic equipment and instrumentation.

TABLE 43.1. Categories of Costs and Examples.

Direct costs (patient related)	*Indirect costs (overhead)*
Fixed costs: Nurse managers Do not change with procedure volume	Mortgage Amoritzed OR equipment
Variable costs: OR nurse salaries Increase with procedure volume	Employee benefits Disposable equipment Administrative salaries Marketing expenses

Direct costs are *controllable* because the hospital can choose how much to spend on each patient's procedure through efficient application of nurses and equipment. Indirect costs are *uncontrollable* because they remain the same day after day and are not influenced to any appreciable extent by patient volumes.

Source: From Traverso,[8] by permission.

Access Devices

Access to the peritoneal cavity is gained using the closed, Veress needle technique or the open, Hasson technique. The closed technique first calls for the Veress needle (fashioned with a safety shield) to be placed through a small cutaneous incision. Next, the abdominal wall is grasped and lifted as the needle is placed through the abdominal fascia and into the peritoneal cavity. Proponents of this technique claim that it is safer, easier, and quicker than alternatives. The open technique, similar to that used for open diagnostic peritoneal lavage, provides peritoneal access under direct visualization. Although the open technique is often claimed to be safer,[10] both techniques have been associated with complications and serious injuries. The experience and training of the surgeon as well as the specific clinical setting should guide the choice of devices. However, most would agree that the open technique is superior in patients who have undergone previous abdominal surgery or in other special circumstances, such as in pregnancy.

With the recent increased interest in hand-assisted laparoscopic surgery, handports should also be included in the access devices. Hand-assisted laparoscopic surgery involves a small (6- to 8-cm) incision, which after the application of the handport and establishment of PNP allows insertion of the surgeon's hand into the peritoneal cavity.[11] The access incision can also be used for specimen retrieval, performance of intestinal anastomoses, and so on. Hand-assisted techniques are used in complex procedures and frequently in the early stages of the learning curve for a procedure. Their use in colorectal surgery has been shown to decrease operative times compared to conventional laparoscopic procedures, maintaining most of the advantages of minimally invasive surgery.[12]

Gases

Once access has been gained to the peritoneal cavity, a working space is created through insufflation or by mechanical lifting. In most centers, CO_2 is the insufflation gas of choice. Advantages of CO_2 include its noncombustible nature (allowing for the use of electrocautery) and its high solubility (allowing for easy expiration via the lungs). However, because the absorbed CO_2 is converted to H_2CO_3 in the bloodstream, the extra hydrogen ion is responsible for lowering the plasma pH, which can lead to several physiological consequences, as described later. Consequently, other gases with varying properties have been used (Table 43.2). Nitrous oxide has the advantage of causing less peritoneal irritation; however, its propensity for combustion makes it inappropriate for use in conjunction with electrocautery.[13] Like nitrous oxide, helium is inert; however, it is noncombustible. The main drawback for helium lies in its insoluble nature and potential for air embolism. The use of wall lifters may be necessary in certain procedures, such as laparoscopic liver surgery, for which the risk of gas embolism is higher. The routine use of wall lifters is less practical and of questionable clinical benefit.

Trocars

Following insufflation, additional trocars are placed under direct visualization. In general, the trocars should be arranged in a triangle so that the instruments are moving toward the operative field in the same direction as the laparoscope. The trocars should be placed far enough apart (8–10cm) to allow for easy external access and to avoid unnecessary internal interactions or "swordfighting." In general, three to five trocars are adequate to accomplish most laparoscopic procedures, with the exact number dictated by the individual procedure. Within the trocar, there is a sheath-valve mechanism that maintains PNP when cannulated with an instrument and during instrument exchanges. The trocar also incorporates a mechanism to secure its place within the abdominal wall. The use of radially expanding (i.e., noncutting) trocars has also been described, reportedly resulting in smaller fascial defects and potentially a lower incidence of trocar site hernias.[14]

Image Production

Laparoscopic surgery is dependent on adequate visualization of the operative field. The standard 0° Hopkins rod-lens laparoscope ranges in size between 5 and 10mm in outer diameter with oblique viewing scopes (30° and 45°) also available. The light originates from a high-intensity external source and is transmitted in a zigzag pattern along a fiber-optic cable to an attachment on the laparoscope with subsequent transmission through the laparoscope to the operative field. The illuminated image is then interpreted by a camera that is mounted on the extracorporeal end on the laparoscope. Presently, most institutions employ three chip or CCD (charge-coupled

TABLE 43.2. Characteristics of Different Pneumoperitoneum Gases.

	Carbon dioxide	*Nitrous oxide*	*Air*	*Argon*	*Helium*	*Oxygen*
Inert	—	Yes	Yes	Yes	Yes	No
Combustible	No	Yes	Yes	No	No	Yes
Water soluble	Yes	No	No	No	No	No
Peritoneal irritation (abdominal pain)	Yes	No	Yes	No	No	Yes

Source: From Lacy et al.,[160] by permission.

device) video cameras, with one chip used for each of three colors (R, red; G, green; B, blue). The image from each of these chips is regenerated on a high-resolution RGB monitor to allow the entire operating team to visualize the operative field.[15] The video image can be recorded using a standard videotape or DVD equipment for later viewing or for teaching purposes. The inherent disadvantage of such a system is the creation of a two-dimensional image and subsequent loss of depth perception. Systems for three-dimensional imaging are available but remain under development.[16]

Instrumentation

A basic laparoscopic instrument set should include graspers, dissectors, scissors, and a needle holder. In addition, most procedures also require a clip applier, stapling or suturing device, and the suction/irrigator. Advanced procedures employ more specialized instrumentation that may include a specimen retrieval bag or specialized graspers and retractors. A wide variety of instruments is available from several manufacturers; a detailed discussion of the advantages or disadvantages of the various instruments is beyond the scope of this chapter.

The major advances in laparoscopic instrumentation in recent years have been in the development of intracorporeal suturing devices (Fig. 43.1) and ultrasonic coagulating instruments. Commercially available stitching devices require specialized suture delivery systems and, with appropriate practice, are easy to use.[17] The ultrasonic scalpel works by tamponading the blood vessel between the jaws of the instrument and sealing the vessel via denaturing the hydrogen bonds in the tissue and vessels forming a coagulum. The advantage of these instruments lies in their ability to achieve precise cutting with minimal lateral thermal tissue damage.[18] An alternative system for transection of tissue and vessels is the electrothermal bipolar vessel sealer (EBVS), which causes the collagen and elastin to denature and the pressure of the wall being opposed allows the protein in the vessel walls to seal together. Vessel burst pressure has been tested and is shown to be safe up to 7mm with the EBVS system and up to 3mm with the ultrasonic system.[19,20]

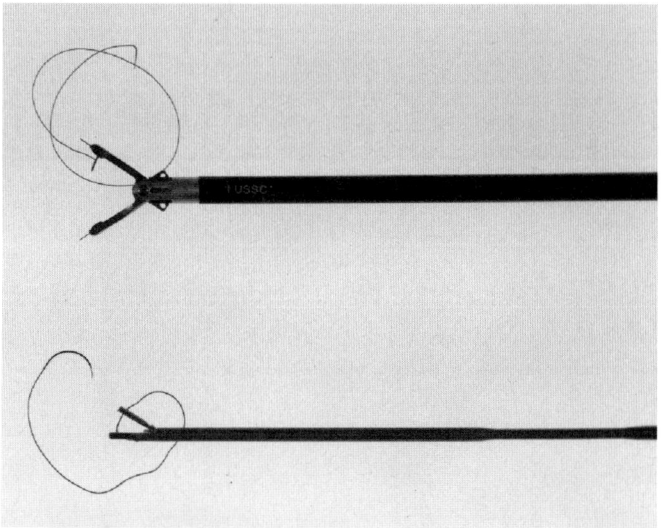

FIGURE 43.1. Intracorporeal suturing devices. Endostitch (US Surgical Corp., Norwalk, CT) and Suture Assist (Ethicon Endo-Surgery; Somerville, NJ).

Physiology of Pneumoperitoneum

The term *pneumoperitoneum* (*pneuma*: air; *peri*: around; *teinein*: to stretch) comes from Greek origins and is defined as the presence of gas within the peritoneal cavity. In some reports, the physiology of PNP has been considered synonymously with the physiology of laparoscopy. Similarly, as the clinical indications for procedures performed within the extraperitoneal space become better defined, a distinction must be made between extraperitoneal and intraperitoneal insufflation. Within this section, the term *pneumoperitoneum* (PNP) refers to the physiological changes associated with intraperitoneal carbon dioxide insufflation unless otherwise specified.

A wide variety of systemic manifestations are associated with the creation of PNP. Systemic effects on the cardiovascular, pulmonary, gastrointestinal, neurological, and immune systems have been described in both clinical and experimental studies. As with any patient experiencing either surgery or trauma, there are normal physiological and metabolic changes that are directly proportional to the degree of physical insult. These systemic changes, collectively referred to as the *acute-phase response*, have been well documented following traditional open surgical procedures. The laparoscopic approach to surgery involves limited abdominal access, less systemic stress, and subsequently a blunted acute-phase response. In recent years, this response has become increasingly qualified and quantified through a significant amount of research. It is only through the description of this physiological response during and following laparoscopy that the role of laparoscopic interventions (i.e., mechanical lifting, various intraabdominal pressures [IAPs]) in special, clinical situations (i.e., COPD [chronic obstructive pulmonary disease], pregnancy, and cancer) will become more appropriately defined.

Circulatory Effects

Cardiovascular

Pneumoperitoneum significantly and reproducibly affects the venous and arterial systems, and these effects have been described both clinically and in the laboratory (Tables 43.3, 43.4, and 43.5). These hemodynamic alterations result from increased IAP and volume and, to a lesser extent, systemic hypercarbia. In the supine patient, the main pressure–volume effect of intraperitoneal insufflation to approximately 10 to 20mmHg is to simultaneously decrease preload and increase afterload. In turn, several authors have reported a subsequent decrease in cardiac output (CO). The extent, cause, and clinical significance of this reduction of CO have each been well studied.

Preload

Several studies have measured the physiological effects of PNP on the venous system, with specific attention to its effects on cardiac filling pressures and pulmonary vasculature. These studies have shown that there is an increase in

TABLE 43.3.
Prospective Clinical Studies (Level II Evidence) of Hemodynamic Responses to Carbon Dioxide Pneumoperitoneum in Healthy Adults Compared to a Control Group Postinduction.

Author	*Year*	*n*	*Mean age of study group*	*Procedure*	*IAP (mmHg)*	*Time after PNP (min)*	*CVP*	*MAP*	*SVR*	*CI*	*HR*	*SV*	*PCWP*	*Author's conclusions*
Odeberg et al.[24]	1994	11	41	LC	15	30	NC	↑	↑	NC	NC		NC	PNP causes signs of elevated preload and afterload
Dorsay et al.[25]	1995	14	18–58[a]	LC	15	—		↑		↓	↑	↓		Combination of CO_2 PNP, head-up position adversely affects CI
Girardis et al.[34]	1996	12	48	LC	10–15	20		NC	NC	NC	NC	NC		CO_2 PNP does not induce significant changes in cardiopulmonary function
Köksoy et al.[166]	1995	21	51	LC	12–15	20		NC	↑	↓	NC	↓		No significant changes in routine hemodynamic parameters
Kubota et al.[167]	1993	48	53	LC	10	30				NC			NC	10 mmHg PNP; no crucial problems in cardiac function
Liu et al.[168]	1991	16	40	LC	15	—		↑		NC				Significant cardiovascular changes with laparoscopy
Myre et al.[23]	1997	7	28–72[a]	LC/flat	15	10	q	↑	↑	NC	NC		↓	LV filling pressure, estimated by PCWP, cannot be used as an indicator of LV dilation
Gannedahl et al.[27]	1996	8	37	LC	11–13	—	NC	↑	↑	NC	NC		NC	LV volume is increased during PNP; PCWP does not correlate linearly with changes in volume indices of LV filling
Mclaughlin et al.[28]	1995	18	46	LC	15	30	↑	↑	↑	↓	NC			Significant and reversible decreases in cardiac performance
Hashimoto et al.[26]	1993	8	52	LC	12	20	↑	↑	↑					Cardiopulmonary changes at an IAP of 12 mmHg
Hirvonen et al.[169]	1995	20	44	GL[b]	13–16	20	↑	NC		↓	NC		↑	Head-down position increased CVP, PCWP, PA; decreased CO; PNP increased these pressures mostly in the beginning of the laparoscopy, and CO decreased toward the end
Marshall et al.[33]	1972	7	21–38[a]	GL	15–20	<20	↑	↑		NC	↑			Vagal activity is a major factor in the rise of CVP during laparoscopy
Motew et al.[170]	1973	12	24–43[a]	GL	20	<20	↑	↑	↑	NC	NC			IAP.20 mmHg potentially dangerous

CI, cardiac index/cardiac output; CO, cardiac output; CVP, central venous pressure; GL, gynecological laparoscopy/Trendelenberg; HR, heart rate; IAP, intraabdominal pressure; LC, laparoscopic cholecystectomy/reverse Trendelenberg; LV, left ventricle; MAP, mean arterial pressure; NC, no change; PCWP, pulmonary capillary wedge pressure; PNP, pneumoperitoneum; SV, stroke volume; SVR, systemic vascular resistance.

[a]Range.

[b]Control group measured preinduction.

TABLE 43.4.
Prospective Clinical Studies (Level II Evidence) of Hemodynamic Responses to Carbon Dioxide Pneumoperitoneum in Adults with Cardiopulmonary Disease.

Author	*Year*	*n*	*Mean age of study group (yr)*	*Procedure*	*IAP (mmHg)*	*Time after PNP (min)*	*Control group (–induction)*	*Design*	*CVP*	*MAP*	*SVR*	*CI*	*HR*	*SV*	*PCWP*	*Author's conclusions*
Iwase et al.[171]	1992	19	61	LC	12	30	—	5 patients heart disease vs. 14 patients control	NC	NC		↓			NC	LC is feasible in patients with heart disease
Zollinger et al.[40]	1997	22	72	LC	14	—	Post	10 patients ASA III vs. 12 patients control	↑	↑	↑	NC	NC	NC	↑	CO_2 PNP is associated with significant but relatively benign hemodynamic changes; anesthesia for LC may be performed safely in elderly ASA class III patients
Dhoste et al.[36]	1996	16	81	LC	12	30	Pre	ASA III		↑	↑	↓	NC	↓		PNP to 12 mmHg with 10° RT can be accomplished with cardiovascular stability
Harris et al.[39]	1996	12	66	LCL	14–16	20	Post	Cardiac and pulmonary disease	↑	↑	NC	NC	NC	NC	↑	In an elderly population with significant coexisting cardiopulmonary disease, intraoperative maneuvers required for LCL resulted in alterations of cardiovascular performance
Hein et al.[37]	1997	17	58	LC	15	25	Pre	ASA III, IV	↑	NC	NC	↓	NC		NC	LC in patients with severe cardiac dysfunction results in significant hemodynamic changes
Safran et al.[32]	1993	15	74	LC	15	Immediate	Pre	ASA III, IV	↑	↑	↑	↓	NC		NC	Laparoscopy presents serious hemodynamic stress but it can be performed safely in high-risk patients, using aggressive intraoperative monitoring

CI, cardiac index; CVP, central venous pressure; HR, heart rate; LCL, laparoscopic colectomy; MAP, mean systemic arterial pressure; NC, no significant change; PCWP, pulmonary capillary wedge pressure; SV, stroke volume; SVR, systemic vascular resistance; ASA III, severe systemic disease that is not incapacitating; ASA IV, severe systemic disease that is a constant threat to life; 10 RT, 10 degrees reverse-trendelenberg..

TABLE 43.5.
Randomized Controlled Animal Studies (Level I Evidence) of Hemodynamic Responses to Laparoscopy Compared to Postinduction Control.

Author	*Year*	*n*	*Animal/procedure*	*Gas*	*Length of PNP (min)*	*IAP (mmHg)*	*Study groups*	*CVP*	*MAP*	*SVR*	*CO*	*HR*	*SV*	*PCWP*	*Author's conclusions*
Baseline															
Windenberger et al.[29]	1995	9	Pigs	CO_2	5	10–14		↑	↑		↑	↓	↑		Abdominal PNP was associated with increased CO, cardiac contractility, and MAP The sharp initial rise of MAP could be the effect of a mechanical action, whereas sustained hemodynamic alterations would involve complex regulatory mechanisms like an increase of sympathetic activity, baroreceptor control, or a response to acidosis
Ortega et al.[35]	1996	12	Pigs	CO_2	60	15		NC	NC	↓	↑	NC	↑	NC	Complex interactions between the mechanical and systemic effects of the CO_2 PNP on venous return
Talamini et al.[172]	1997	7	Pigs	CO_2	60	15		↑	NC	NC	NC			↑	A significant reduction in CO occurs after surgical disruption of the esophageal hiatus during LNF
Ho et al.[30]	1995	8	Pigs	CO_2	60	15		NC	↑		NC	NC	↓		Accumulation of CO_2 is associated with an increase in MAP
Access															
Horvath et al.[173]	1998	24	Pigs/colectomy		30	15	Open	NC	NC		NC	NC	NC	NC	The effects of laparoscopic surgery and open surgery on hemodynamic responses are minimal, and no one method is superior to another
							CO_2 PNP	↑	NC		↑	NC	NC	NC	
							He PNP	↑	NC		NC	NC	NC	↑	
							Gasless litter	↑	NC		↑	NC	NC	↑	
Rademaker et al.[174]	1995	8	Pigs		30	15	CO_2 PNP	↑	↑		NC	NC		↑	In contrast with CO_2 PNP, laparoscopy using abdominal wall retraction was not associated with adverse effects on hemodynamics or gas exchange
							Gasless litter	NC	NC		NC	NC		↑	
Davidson et al.[175]	1996	16	Pigs		40	12	CO_2 PNP				NC			NC	Neither He PNP or the litter have significant deleterious pulmonary or hemodynamic effects
							He PNP				NC			NC	
							Gasless litter				NC			NC	

Pressures														
Ishizakl et al.[21]	1993	21	Dogs	CO_2	60		8 mmHg	NC	NC	NC	NC	NC			IAP from 8 to 12 mmHg is recommended for laparoscopic surgery to avoid complications caused by hemodynamic derangements
							12 mmHg	NC	NC	NC	NC	NC			
							16 mmHg	NC	NC	↑	↓	NC			
Liem et al.[41]	1994	4	Piglets	CO_2	60		10 mmHg	↑	NC			NC			CVP increased in proportion of increase in IAP
							15 mmHg	↑	NC			NC			
Marathe et al.[22]	1996	10	Dogs	CO_2	20		5 mmHg	↑	NC		NC	NC			In the dog, any hemodynamic alterations induced by CO_2 PNP are secondary to altered LV preload
							15 mmHg	↑	NC		NC	NC			
							25 mmHg	↑	NC		↓	NC			
Special conditions															
Bannenberg et al.[42]	1997	16	Pigs	CO_2	10	15	Intraperitoneal PNP	↑	↑		↑	NC		↑	CVP, PCWP increased faster in intraperitoneal group; extraperitoneal PNP might result in less cardiovascular impairment than intraperitoneal PNP
							Extraperitoneal PNP	NC	NC		NC	NC		NC	
Ho et al.[43]	1993	32	Pigs/subjected to hemorrhage	CO_2	60	15	No hemorrhage		↑		NC				Fluid resuscitation to baseline MAP did not maintain hemodynamics once CO_2 pneumo was begun; CO_2 PNP for diagnostic laparoscopy may be hazardous in acutely hypovolemic subjects
							10 cc/kg continuous bleeding for 1 h		↓		↓		↓		
							20 cc/kg continuous bleeding for 1 h		↓		↓		↓		
							20 cc/kg continuous bleeding for 1 h and fluid resuscitation		↓		↓		↓		
Moffa et al.[176]	1993	5	Pigs/subjected to PEEP	CO_2	10	15	5 cmH_2O PEEP	↑	↑	NC	↓	NC	↓	NC	CO_2 PNP increases afterload and exacerbates the adverse effects of PEEP
							10 cmH_2O PEEP	↑	↑	NC	↓	NC	↓	NC	
							20 cm H_2O PEEP	↑	↑	NC	↓	NC	↓	NC	
Luz et al.[177]	1994	10	Dogs/Laparoscopic pelvic lymphadenectomy	CO_2	—		10 mmHg		NC		NC			NC	An increase in IAP up to 15 mmHg had no effect on the cardiovascular system; however, the combination of an increased IAP with PEEP markedly depressed hemodynamic variables
							10 mmHg, 8 PEEP		↓		NC			↑	
							15 mmHg		NC		NC			NC	
							15 mmHg, 8 PEEP		↓		NC			↑	

CO, cardiac output, CO_2, carbon dioxide; CVP, central venous pressure; He, helium; HR, heart rate; IAP, intraabdominal pressure; MAP, mean arterial pressure; NC, no change; NO_2, nitrous oxide; PCWP, pulmonary capillary wedge pressure; PEEP, positive end expiratory pressure; PNP, pneumoperitoneum; SV, stroke volume; SVR, systemic vascular resistance.

central venous pressure (CVP) and pulmonary capillary wedge pressure (PCWP) but a concurrent decrease in stroke volume (SV). The rise in measured CVP is the result of an increase in IAP that directly compresses the low-pressure vasculature, such as the abdominal vena cava.[21]

The effects of PNP on cardiac parameters have been investigated via transesophageal echocardiography (TEE) and pulmonary artery thermodilution catheters. In dogs, Marathe et al. used TEE and direct cannulation of the external jugular vein, left ventricle, and pericardial space to show that an IAP of 15 mmHg or greater resulted in a significant decrease in left ventricular end-diastolic volume (preload) without a concomitant effect on left ventricular contractility.[22] In patients similarly insufflated and undergoing LC, Myre et al., using TEE with multiplane images, showed an increase in PCWP (10–17 mmHg, median 70%) with no change in the left ventricular diastolic area index.[23] Therefore, perhaps paradoxically, the increase in CVP and PCWP actually results in decreased cardiac filling pressures or preload.

Afterload

Most of the reported studies have shown an increase in both mean arterial pressure (MAP) and systemic vascular resistance (SVR) with moderate degrees of PNP. This increase in afterload, as reflected by an elevated MAP and a calculated increase in SVR, has been demonstrated in several human[24–28] and animal studies.[29,30] Most authors believe that the increase in afterload in conjunction with PNP is the result of two factors: the release of humoral factors (catecholamines and vasopressin) soon after commencing insufflation and direct aortic compression due to increased IAP.[31,32] There can also be a marginal[33] increase in heart rate (HR) associated with PNP that is typically short-lived and most likely the result of early catecholamine release following induction.

Finally, PNP has effects on CO. *Cardiac output* is defined as the product of HR and SV. Several authors have reported a decrease in CO with PNP.[25,28] In these reports, patients undergoing LC at an insufflation pressure of 15 mmHg had a reduction in cardiac index between 3% and 29%. However, in similar studies others reported no change in CO with moderate PNP.[24,27,34] In experimental animals similarly insufflated, several studies have shown not a decrease but actually an increase in CO.[29,35]

The difference in CO response to PNP among these various studies is most likely secondary to a difference in blood vessel distensibility among individuals and between species (i.e., atherosclerotic arteries are less-distensible vessels that result in an increase in afterload and a decrease in CO). Studies such as these have raised concern for the safety of PNP in patients with a known compromised cardiopulmonary system. However, the hemodynamic alterations seen in patients with known cardiopulmonary disease were similar to those reported in healthy adults. Therefore, although there was a mild[36–38] or minimal[39,40] decrease in CO, most agree that the effects of PNP on CO are clinically insignificant. It must be emphasized, however, that it is only with adequate hemodynamic monitoring and conscientious anesthetic management that untoward clinical outcomes can be reproducibly avoided in patients with cardiopulmonary disease.

Patient positioning and duration of insufflation are additional factors influencing various hemodynamic parameters measured during PNP. Gannedahl et al. studied hemodynamic variables in eight healthy patients undergoing PNP in various patient positions. Throughout the various position changes, minimal changes were seen in either MAP or CO. However, parameters directly reflecting changes in preload were significantly altered with patient repositioning. Reverse-Trendelenberg (head-up) positioning combined with PNP, as in LC, counteracts the effects of PNP by causing a decrease in CVP and PCWP in comparison to the supine patient. Likewise, Trendelenberg (head-down) positioning combined with PNP, as in gynecological procedures, causes an increase in measured CVP and PCWP when compared to supine positioning.[27] Although some warn that head-up positioning may compromise CO by decreasing preload,[24] the incidence of documented clinically significant sequelae in such patients is low (see Table 43.5). Again, appropriate anesthetic management must be emphasized.

In animal studies targeting various insufflation pressures, there appears to be a proportional increase in CVP with insufflation pressure.[22,41] Similarly, intraperitoneal insufflation seems to have a more dramatic physiological effect on CVP and PCWP than does extraperitoneal insufflation.[42] Various special clinical circumstances have also been investigated by using laboratory animals. For example, there has been debate regarding whether it is safe to subject hypovolemic trauma patients to PNP. Ho et al. studied this issue in pigs subjected to controlled, varying levels of hemorrhagic shock and found that diagnostic laparoscopy may be hazardous in hypovolemic animals. During PNP, both SV and CO decreased with mild (10 mL/kg) and moderate (20 mL/kg) hemorrhage, and although these parameters initially responded to fluid resuscitation, they quickly fell to levels similar to unresuscitated animals.[43]

Splanchnic/Hepatic/Renal

Just as PNP has been shown to decrease cardiac venous return, studies have also illustrated that an increase in IAP similarly affects the perfusion of many abdominal organs. These effects may occur locally before the recognition of the aforementioned systemic hemodynamic effects. The effects of PNP on specific mesenteric beds have been specifically illustrated through direct cannulation of these vessels in experimental animals. For instance, in pigs outfitted with gastric tonometry, Knolmayer et al.[44] showed that a PNP in excess of 15 mmHg significantly decreased gastric blood flow and subsequently lowered intramucosal gastric pH without affecting CO or arterial lactate levels.[44] In dogs, Caldwell and Ricotta showed that during PNP there is a trend toward a decrease in absolute blood flow to all intraabdominal and extra-abdominal organs except the retroperitoneally located adrenal gland, and that this decrease was significant for the omentum, esophagus, stomach (and gastric mucosa), duodenum, and jejunum.[45]

Both hepatic and renal perfusion are decreased with increasing IAP (Fig. 43.2). Using an ultrasonic blood flowmeter in dogs, Ishizaki et al. reported an increase in portal venous pressure and a decrease in portal venous and hepatic artery flow in parallel with an increase in IAP. Total hepatic blood flow was significantly decreased after 30 min of insufflation.[21] Other experimental models have confirmed these results.[46] Similarly, laser Doppler flowmetry of the renal arteries of pigs showed there is a significant decrease in renal perfusion with an IAP of 15 mmHg.[47] This was confirmed when renal hemo-

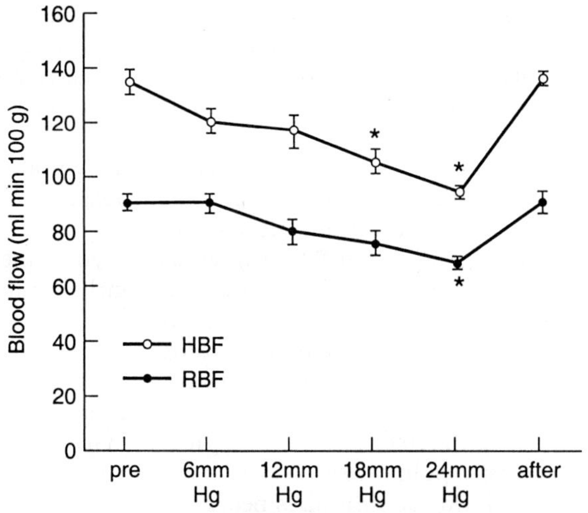

FIGURE 43.2. Changes in hepatic blood flow (HBF) and renal blood flow (RBF) with increasing intraperitoneal pressure. Hepatic blood flow was significantly reduced at pressures of 18 and 24 mmHg, and renal blood flow was significantly decreased at a pressure of 24 mmHg. Values are expressed as mean ± SE. *pre*, preinsufflation; *after*, after CO_2 evacuation; *, $P < .05$ versus each control value. (From Hashikura et al.,[46] by permission.)

dynamics during intraperitoneal insufflation, extraperitoneal insufflation, and use of a lifting mechanism were directly compared. Significant renal hemodynamic changes were elicited in both the gaseous groups but not in the gasless laparoscopy group.[48] However, the clinical implications of decreased renal perfusion are less apparent. Miki et al. compared the intraoperative renal function of patients undergoing LC (IAP, 12 mmHg) to LC patients for whom the retraction method (IAP, 4 mmHg) was used. Urine output, effective renal plasma flow (ERPF), and glomerular filtration rate (GFR) were each decreased in the former group as compared to the latter, suggesting that a retraction method may prevent transient renal dysfunction.[49] In another study, when patients undergoing LC (IAP, 12 mmHg) were compared to a minilaparotomy group, urine output, ERPF, and GFR were similarly decreased in the laparoscopy group.[50] However, this transient decrease in intraoperative blood flow does not produce significant renal dysfunction postoperatively. Preoperative and postoperative serum urea nitrogen and creatinine concentrations were not different in a group of patients undergoing LC or pelvic lymph node dissection.[51] Prospective studies involving patients with documented preoperative compromised renal function undergoing PNP are currently unavailable.

Coagulation Effects

Virchow's triad of hypercoagulability, venous stasis, and trauma are the three main factors responsible for venous thromboembolism. Laparoscopic surgery entails the same risks of thromboembolism as the traditional approach; however, some have postulated that certain risk factors, namely venous stasis caused by PNP and hypercoagulability, pose a greater threat to the patient undergoing a laparoscopic procedure.

The increase in IAP causes compression on the abdominal inferior vena cava, a subsequent rise in CVP, and a decrease in lower extremity venous return. As a result, venous stasis, a known risk factor for deep vein thrombosis (DVT), occurs in the lower extremities. Venous stasis was confirmed by Jorgensen et al. by using an ultrasound flow probe in pigs to measure femoral venous flow. These authors found that venous outflow was markedly and significantly depressed as IAP was increased from 10 to 20 mmHg.[52] Clinically, during LC and laparoscopic antireflux procedures, reverse-Trendelenberg (head-up) positioning further predisposes the patient to venous stasis and the subsequent development of DVT. Millard et al. studied the femoral veins of 20 consecutive patients undergoing LC and found a significant reduction in common femoral venous flow.[53] In general, surgical intervention induces a postoperative hypercoagulable state, and similar results of hypercoagulability have been noted following both LC and OC.[54] As a result, this hypercoagulable state following laparoscopy may be due in part to the body's response to general anesthesia and indirectly to venous stasis.[55]

Although there is an increased theoretical risk of DVT following laparoscopic procedures, clinically this complication is infrequently realized. The incidence of DVT following OC is between 5% and 10% depending on how it was detected and whether the patient received prophylaxis.[55,56] In turn, of 1200 open cholecystectomies, there were 4 cases of pulmonary embolism (PE).[57] The true incidence of DVT and subsequent PE following LC has yet to be established.[55] However, in one series of 77,604 patients undergoing LC, there were only 3 deaths attributable to PE.[58] The incidence of DVT and PE seem to be lower than for comparable conventional procedures, but randomized data are not yet available.

Regardless of the low reported risk of death from PE following LC, the provocative theoretical increased risk for DVT/PE have prompted the drafting of policies for DVT prophylaxis during laparoscopic procedures. In 1993, of 3500 fellows of the American College of Surgeons, 1018 responded to a survey querying their approach to DVT prophylaxis during LC. This survey showed that among those responding to the survey a similar approach (graduated compression stockings, sequential compression stockings [sequential compression devices, SCDs], or low molecular weight heparin) was employed for OC and LC patients.[59] Shwenk et al., in a prospective, randomized trial involving 50 patients (25 patients with SCDs [+SCD] and 25 without [–SCDs]), studied the effectiveness of pneumatic SCDs in preventing venous stasis during LC. These authors found that peak flow velocity in the femoral vein decreased less from the baseline value in the +SCD group as compared to the –SCD group, supporting the routine use of SCDs.[60] Finally, in a study of eight consecutive patients undergoing laparoscopic herniorrhaphy, flow in the common femoral vein was reduced with intraperitoneal insufflation but not with preperitoneal insufflation.[60] With the dramatic increase of laparoscopic bariatric procedures, the issue of DVT prophylaxis was reexamined[61] as these patients are at increased risk for thromboembolic complications. Most authors agree that pharmacologic prophylaxis is indicated,[62] frequently in increased doses, after appropriate adjustment for the patient's weight.[63]

The theoretical risk of thromboembolism during laparoscopy, coupled with the measured decreased femoral venous flow without SCDs, make it prudent to recommend DVT prophylaxis for all patients who are approached laparoscopically. The low rate of documented DVT/PE in these patients is most likely the result of conscientious DVT prophylaxis. In patients at high risk for thrombosis, the benefits of laparoscopy must be weighed against the risks of thromboembolism.

Pulmonary Effects

The pulmonary system is influenced by PNP both mechanically and chemically. In general, the intraoperative and postoperative respiratory embarrassment experienced by the patient undergoing a laparoscopic procedure is markedly less than for those undergoing the more traditional open approach. These pulmonary effects have been delineated using spirometry/pulmonary function tests and blood gas analysis.

From a mechanical standpoint, as IAP is increased intraoperatively the diaphragm is shifted in the cephalad direction, which increases intrathoracic pressure. This reduced, paradoxical diaphragmatic movement in the face of increased intrathoracic pressure leads to an increase in peak airway pressure[64] and the collapse of alveoli. As a result, forced residual capacity (FRC) is decreased.[65] Concurrently, there is also a decrease in tidal volume[66] as well as a decrease in compliance of both the lung and chest wall,[64,67] leading to an overall increase in the work of breathing to maintain constant minute ventilation volume.[68] The addition of positive end-expiratory pressure (PEEP) is a helpful ventilatory adjunct during conventional surgery to help recruit alveoli and to prevent further alveolar collapse. However, the hemodynamic implications of additional PEEP during PNP are complex. Increasing levels of PEEP coupled with abdominal insufflation have been shown to cause an increase in the MAP of pigs[69] and a decrease in dogs.[70] Although the direct implications of additional PEEP during PNP are controversial, there is clearly more hemodynamic instability with increasing levels of PEEP.

Hypercapnia is another pulmonary concern requiring the attention of anesthesiologists during laparoscopic cases. Hypercapnia is defined as an increase in the plasma CO_2 concentration and may occur intraoperatively because CO_2 can easily diffuse across the peritoneal lining.[71] In healthy patients, as CO_2 is absorbed (i.e., $Paco_2$ increases), the respiratory rate increases and CO_2 is expired through the lungs (i.e., $Paco_2$ increases). Wahba et al. showed that minute ventilation had to be increased by 12% to 16% to maintain eucapnia.[72] In unhealthy patients, or in patients unable to spontaneously increase their respiratory rate (i.e., anesthetized, intubated patients), the dissolved CO_2 in the blood is not effectively eliminated, and this can lead to systemic acidosis. Mild hypercapnia has few significant hemodynamic effects. However, severe hypercapnia (50–70mmHg) can result in systemic hypotension by decreasing CO and SV, given that hypercarbia is both a myocardial depressant and a vasodilator.[73] Because end-tidal CO_2 underestimates $Paco_2$ during PNP and is increasingly unreliable as $Paco_2$ increases,[72] invasive blood gas analysis is imperative in patients in whom minimal hypercarbia could be detrimental.

There are several well-done studies of patients undergoing cholecystectomy that illustrate that LC causes less postoperative pulmonary embarrassment than OC. Pulmonary function tests administered to patients 1 to 2 days postoperatively show a smaller reduction in forced vital capacity (FVC), forced expiratory volume in 1 s (FEV_1), and peak expiratory flow rate (PEFR) following LC as compared to OC. McMahon et al. reported a smaller reduction of mean PEFR in LC compared to open (64% vs. 49%; $P < .001$).[74] In addition, spirometry values returned to preoperative values 4 to 10 days sooner in patients undergoing LC.[75] Postoperative atelectasis and hypoxia are reduced after LC as compared to OC,[75] although postoperative atelectasis or effusion can be shown on chest x-ray in 7 of 20 patients following LC.[76] A decrease in oxygen saturation was one-third less after LC compared to OC on postoperative day 1,[75] and P_aO_2 values, expressed as median change reduction from baseline, were significantly less for LC (−2) versus OC (−20) on postoperative day 2.[77] The majority of studies showed no difference in postoperative CO_2 retention for LC compared to OC. Clearly, the laparoscopic approach to cholecystectomy causes less pulmonary embarrassment than the traditional open approach. In patients with known chronic pulmonary disease, however, conscientious monitoring during anesthesia is necessary.

Effects on Intestinal Function

Many studies have documented an earlier return of bowel function after laparoscopic procedures compared to open procedures.[78,79] Garcia-Caballero et al. found that flatus and bowel movement occurred significantly sooner after LC as compared to OC (10 and 36h vs. 60 and 96h, respectively).[79] However, there are conflicting animal studies reporting on the return of intestinal myoelectric activity following LC. Some evidence supports a faster return of intestinal myoelectric activity,[80] while other does not.[81] With the development of laparoscopic colon procedures, interest has surfaced regarding whether laparoscopic colon resection results in a faster return of bowel function compared to an open procedure. Although laparoscopic colon resection may afford the patient less postoperative pain[82] and shorter hospitalization,[83] there seems to be no improvement in myoelectric activity.[79] In canine models for colon resection, transit studies favor laparoscopy,[84] but measurements of intestinal myoelectric activity showed no difference.[85]

Effects on Neurological Function

Cerebral blood flow depends on cerebral perfusion pressure, which is calculated as MAP minus intracranial pressure (ICP). Mortality is increased with elevated, uncontrolled levels of ICP, and cerebral blood vessels constrict in response to hypocapnia.[86] Animal studies directly measuring ICP showed a linear increase in ICP with rising levels of IAP. This trend also became worse following Trendelenberg (head-down) positioning.[87,88] These physiological changes are the result of mechanical pressure forces as well as the transperitoneal diffusion of CO_2. Abdominal insufflation results in decreased lumbar venous plexus drainage and increased MAP, both of which may contribute to the rise in ICP. In pigs outfitted for direct lumbar spinal pressure transducers, Halverson et al. showed an increase in lumbar spinal pressure with PNP.[88] Chemically, as $Paco_2$ levels rise during PNP, concomitant reflex cerebral vasodilation occurs that allows for an increase in cerebral blood flow and ICP. Fujii et al. studied 10 patients undergoing LC and showed an increase in cerebral blood flow velocity with increasing levels of P_aCO_2.[89] There are limited reports of neurological deterioration with PNP[90]; however, laparoscopic intervention should be discouraged in patients

TABLE 43.6.
Level II Human Studies on the Metabolic and Immune Responses to Laparoscopic Versus Open Cholecystectomy.

Factor	*LC*	*OC*
Catecholamines[92]	↑	↑↑
Cortisol[161]	↑	↑↑
Glucose[92]	↑	↑↑
IL-6[95,162,163]	↑	↑↑
WBC[164]	↑	↑↑
CRP[161–163]	↑	↑↑
TNF[164]	↑	↑↑
DTH[165]	↓	↓↓

CRP, C-reactive protein; DTH, delayed-type hypersensitivity; LC, laparoscopic cholecystectomy; IL-6, interleukin-6; OC, open cholecystectomy; WBC, white blood cell count.

in whom a marginal increase in ICP could be devastating (i.e., patients with head trauma).

Metabolic and Immune Effects

Postoperative and posttraumatic immunosuppression have been extensively studied.[91] It is well known that the extent of surgical intervention or trauma leads to a proportional acute-phase inflammatory response and postoperative immunosuppression. The acute-phase response is a biochemical defense that includes mobilized cytokines and cells of inflammation (i.e., white blood cells, macrophages). This reaction may be accompanied by an elevated blood glucose, an increase in free fatty acids, and a liberation of catecholamines.

In general, laparoscopy causes a blunted acute-phase and catabolic response compared to open surgery. In studies comparing LC to OC, LC caused a more modest increase in catecholamines (norepinephrine, epinephrine, dopamine), cortisol, and glucose (Table 43.6). Not only were levels of these stress indicators significantly less throughout the operative procedure, but also they returned to baseline faster following LC as compared to OC[92] (Fig. 43.3). Similarly, other markers of inflammation, including erythrocyte sedimentation rate, C-reactive protein,[93] interleukin-6 (IL-6), white blood cell count, and tumor necrosis factor,[94,95] were each increased less following LC as compared to OC.[96] There is also less catabolism following laparoscopy as compared to open surgery. Bouvy et al. studied the level of catabolism in rats following open or laparoscopic bowel surgery by measuring serum insulin-like growth factor-1 (IGF-1) levels and found a significantly lower IGF-1, less catabolism, in the laparoscopic group.[97]

Both systemic and local immune responses have been studied during PNP. Systemically, delayed-type hypersensitivity (DTH), a marker for cell-mediated immunity, is less depressed following laparoscopic procedures.[98] In a pig model, Bressler et al. reported T-cell-related immune function as measured by DTH to be better preserved following laparoscopic as compared to open colon resection.[94] Similarly, Brune et al. compared LC and OC in a prospective study and showed that, although the antigen-presenting capacity of monocytes remained normal in both groups, T-cell stimulation was observed after OC but not after LC.[99] Others have reported similar results.[100,101]

Trocar site tumor recurrences following laparoscopy have prompted research into the local effects of PNP on the peritoneal environment. Because CO_2 forms carbonic acid in an aqueous environment, the pH of the peritoneal milieu drops after the induction of CO_2 PNP. It has been speculated that this change in pH may affect the biochemical and cellular immune function inherent to the peritoneal cavity. In vitro functional assays have shown CO_2 to decrease the function of peritoneal macrophages of experimental animals as well as to decrease the spontaneous release of cytokines from human macrophages.[102,103] Tung et al., using open versus laparoscopic gut manipulation in mice, also showed less local inflammatory response with laparoscopy by demonstrating that there was increased serum and gut mucosal IL-6 in the open group compared to laparoscopy.[104] Further experimental and clinical efforts are necessary to better understand the effects of PNP on intraperitoneal immunity and to help clarify a relevent clinical endpoint.

Special Circumstances Concerning Pneumoperitoneum

Under certain physiological conditions, laparoscopy may be contraindicated. Initially, many believed that patient characteristics such as previous abdominal surgery, obesity, acute inflammation, and existing cardiopulmonary disease were absolute contraindications for a laparoscopic procedure. However, as experience has been gained and more advanced instrumentation has become available, several of these

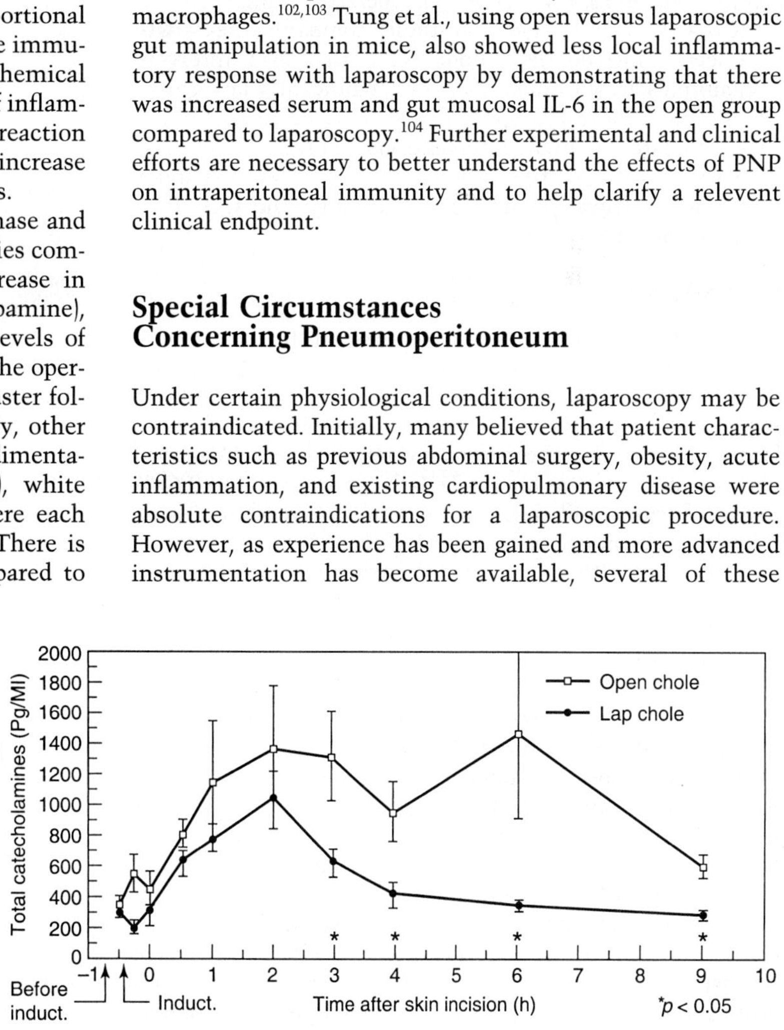

FIGURE 43.3. Changes in total plasma catecholamine concentration (mean ± SEM) after open and laparoscopic cholecystectomy. (From Schauer and Sirnek,[159] by permission.)

contraindications have been challenged. For example, mostly as a result of increased operator experience with the laparoscopic view, laparoscopic interventions for acute cholecystitis have become increasingly successful. However, laparoscopic interventions performed in septic laboratory animals have produced cloudy results and require further study.[105] Other special circumstances, which have been even more extensively studied in conjunction with laparoscopy, include cancer and pregnancy.

Pneumoperitoneum and Cancer

Host immunity and cancer should be considered simultaneously. The systemic immune system seems to be better preserved following laparoscopy; however, some studies demonstrate that CO_2 PNP actually encourages tumor growth intraperitoneally. The initial reports documenting an increased risk of trocar site tumor recurrence following laparoscopic cancer procedures led some investigators to question the safety of CO_2 PNP in oncological patients. A discussion of PNP and cancer can be divided into systemic and local oncological effects of PNP.

Systemic Oncological Effects

Both laparotomy and laparoscopy encourage tumor growth. However, in several animal studies, it appears that full laparotomy encourages systemic postoperative tumor growth more than CO_2 PNP. In animal studies comparing the growth of injected intradermal tumor cells, the open intervention animals grew tumors that were significantly larger than CO_2 PNP and control groups.[106] Likewise, several other studies that compared similar interventions showed a stepwise increase in postoperative tumor size or proliferation index from the anesthesia/control group through the CO_2 PNP group to the laparotomy group.[107,108]

Port Site Metastasis

Several early reports claimed an increase in the incidence of port site tumor recurrences following laparoscopic tumor resection as compared to incisional tumor recurrences following traditional surgery.[109–112] In fact, these initial efforts of laparoscopic colon cancer resection reported an incidence of port site metastases as high as 21%,[113] as compared to a 0.69% to 3.3% incidence of abdominal wound recurrence following traditional resection for colorectal cancer.[114]

However, with an increase in experience with laparoscopic colon resection, more recent reports claim that these rates of trocar site recurrences were largely overestimated. Several large series have documented trocar site tumor recurrence as low as 2%.[82,115–117] In one study of 208 cases of laparoscopic colon resections, there were 3 cases of port site recurrence after a minimum follow-up of 1 year.[117] Similarly, in another prospective, randomized trial that included 109 patients and compared laparoscopic and conventional techniques of bowel resection for colorectal cancers or polyps, there were no instances of port site metastases in the laparoscopic group after a median follow-up of 1.5 years.[118] Another prospective, comparative study of open versus laparoscopic colon resection (n = 224 vs. 191, respectively) also reported no cases of trocar implants in the laparoscopic group after 5 years of follow-up.[119] It appears that the true incidence of port site recurrences is close to that of incisional recurrences after open surgery.[120]

As the true incidence of port site tumor recurrence becomes increasingly defined, experimental studies have provided insight into the pathophysiology behind this phenomenon. In general, port site recurrences seem to be more of an issue in animal models than in most human studies. In animal studies comparing laparoscopy to open resection, the incidence of trocar site tumor recurrence is considerably higher following CO_2 PNP. In a hamster model of intraperitoneally injected human colon cancer cells, trocar site implantation tripled following laparotomy with the addition of CO_2 PNP as compared to laparotomy alone (26% vs. 75%).[112] Reports such as these have continued to raise skepticism regarding the safety of laparoscopy for oncological procedures, and several hypotheses have been developed to explain this increased occurrence. Most researchers agree that because systemic immunological and antioncological effects appear to be well preserved with laparoscopy, the increased port site tumor implantation demonstrated in these studies is most likely caused by a direct effect of PNP on the peritoneum, an effect that allows for the implantation of tumor. At the Second International Laparoscopic Physiology Conference, held in Frankfurt, Germany, efforts from several laparoscopic animal research laboratories were presented to address the possible origins of port site tumor recurrences[106] (Fig. 43.4).

The first two hypotheses highlight the biochemical effects of CO_2 PNP. As mentioned, there is well-designed experimental evidence demonstrating that the acidic environment created with CO_2 PNP is harmful to the peritoneal macrophage, and as a result there is ineffective tumor cell clearance.[102] Others believe that CO_2 actually has a stimulatory effect on tumor growth.[121] For instance, intradermally injected tumor cells were more easily established and grew more aggressively following laparotomy than after CO_2 insufflation.[122]

Clearly, tumor recurrence requires the presence of tumor cells at the trocar site, and direct contact between the solid tumor and the port site enhances port site tumor growth[123]; this contact could occur by removing the pathological speci-

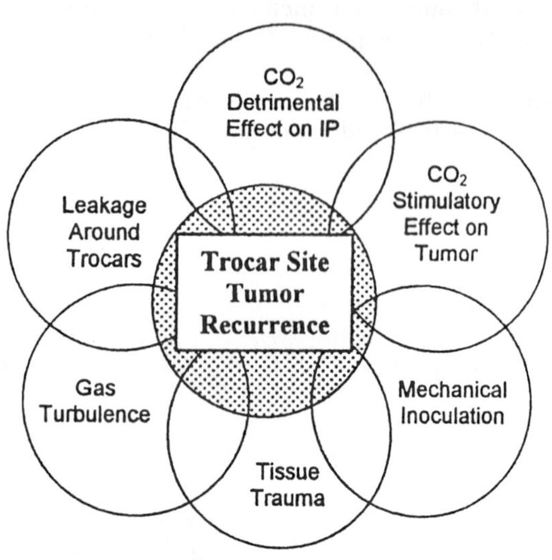

FIGURE 43.4. Factors influencing trocar site tumor recurrence. IP, intraperitoneal immunity.

men through an unprotected trocar site. Investigators who have treated trocar sites with various materials that deter cell adherence and prevent tumor implantation (i.e., heparin, taurolidin) have reported varying results.[124] Evidence also exists showing that more trauma to the trocar site encourages tumor growth. In animals with trocar sites that were crushed with a surgical clamp before trocar insertion, there were greater numbers of port site metastases in the crushed sites as compared to other, noncrushed sites.[125] Further support for a mechanical cause as responsible for port site tumors was demonstrated in a human study in which CO_2 insufflation was found to contain very low levels of free-floating tumor cells even in the presence of massive contamination.[126] Although some studies supported the chimney effect (gas leakage around trocars),[125] the small clumps of cells found in the smoke during laparoscopy were not malignant,[127] and aerosols of tumor cells are not likely to form.[128,129] Further reports specifically implicating gas turbulence include studies in which gasless laparoscopy caused less abdominal wall metastasis than CO_2 PNP.[123,130] A specimen containing or potentially containing cancer should be carefully manipulated and removed through a protected wound.

TABLE 43.7.
Vascular and Bowel Injuries During 77,604 Laparoscopic Cholecystectomies (Level III Evidence).

Injury site	*No. of patients (%)*	*No. of patients requiring laparotomy*
Vascular		
Retroperitoneal vessels		
Aorta	13	12
Inferior vena cava	5	3
Iliac artery	11	10
Iliac vein	7	6
Total	36 (0.05)	31
Portal vessels		
Hepatic artery	44	36
Cystic artery	73	63
Portal vein	5	4
Total	122 (0.16)	103
Other intraabdominal vessels	35 (0.05)	24
Total vascular	193 (0.25)	158
Bowel		
Small intestine	57	42
Colon	35	26
Duodenum	12	12
Stomach	5	5
Total	109 (0.14)	85

Source: From Deziel et al.,[58] by permission.

Pneumoperitoneum and Pregnancy

If surgery during pregnancy is unavoidable, then the optimal time period for such intervention is during the second trimester. Second-trimester operative intervention avoids the potential disruption of organogenesis during the first trimester and possible labor induction during the third. For the safety of both mother and fetus, operative time should be kept to a minimum, and the fetus should be monitored intraoperatively. The typical indications for laparoscopic surgical intervention during pregnancy include acute appendicitis, acute cholecystitis, ectopic pregnancy, and ovarian torsion. When operating on the pregnant patient, three unique physiological factors must be considered: maternal physiological alterations with pregnancy, uteroplacental blood flow, and the overall well-being of the fetus[131] (Fig. 43.5).

There are few studies presently available to delineate the effects of PNP on the developing fetus or the pregnant mother. The limited evidence that is available supports the safety of laparoscopy during pregnancy. In a retrospective study, Reedy et al. reviewed a 20-year period of 2,015,000 delivery records in Sweden and found 2,181 laparoscopic interventions and 1,522 laparotomies during pregnancy. When these two groups were compared, these authors found no difference in fetal outcome in singleton pregnancies between 4 and 20 weeks of gestation.[132] In one 6-year case-controlled study comparing 16 pregnant patients during the first or second trimester undergoing laparoscopic surgery (4 appendectomies and 12 cholecystectomies) to 18 similar patients undergoing laparotomy (7 appendectomy and 11 cholecystectomy), the authors found no difference in morbidity or mortality.[133] Prospective data documenting the safety of laparoscopic general surgical interventions during pregnancy are presently not available. Experimental animal evidence supporting laparoscopy during pregnancy is also limited.

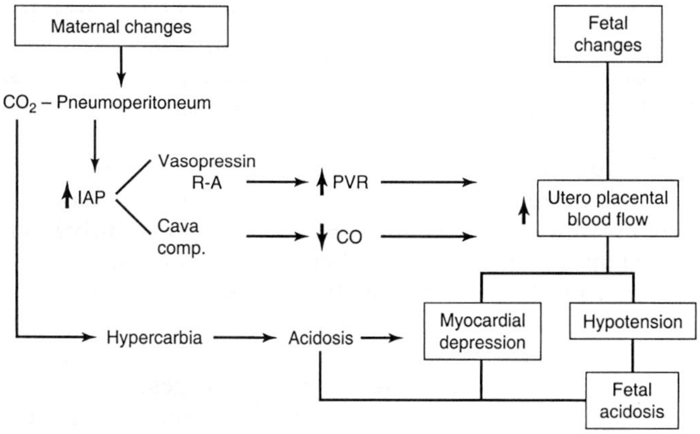

FIGURE 43.5. Maternal and fetal changes in pneumoperitoneum during pregnancy. (From Silva and Platt,[131] by permission.)

Complications of Laparoscopy

Fortunately, major complications occur in well under 1% of laparoscopic procedures, with an overall mortality of 4 to 8 deaths per 100,000 procedures.[134] However, the minimally invasive nature of laparoscopy does not eliminate the potential for serious surgical complications. Several categories of complications unique to laparoscopy include complications related to needle and trocar site insertion,[134] those specific to insufflation, and the establishment of PNP and those related to the use or misuse of specialized laparoscopic equipment. Most of the data illustrating the complications during laparoscopy have been accumulated during LC (Table 43.7). The overall morbidity rate for needle and trocar complications is between 0.2% and 0.5%, with mortality rates of 0.0033% to 0.1%.[135–137]

The placement of the first trocar or Veress needle accounts for the majority of these injuries.[138] Because the Veress needle is placed blindly through a small skin incision, it can inadvertently puncture blood vessels or abdominal viscera. As a result, many operators opt for the open approach as originally described by H.M. Hasson.[139] Using this technique, the fascia is directly visualized and incised. However, despite using the utmost care, the overall incidence of visceral injuries with the open approach is approximately 0.1%.[58] The organ most likely injured is the small bowel (52%), followed by colon, duodenum, and stomach (32%, 11%, and 4.5%, respectively).[58] Bladder perforation can occur any time; however, this complication occurs most frequently during laparoscopic procedures in patients who have had previous surgery. Bladder perforation can be recognized by bubbling within the urine collection bag.

Vascular injuries are reported less frequently[140] but if unrecognized can be devastating. The placement of additional trocars can lead to bleeding from abdominal wall vessels, especially the epigastric vessels. The reported incidence of hemorrhage caused by injury of the epigastric vessels during trocar insertion ranges between 0.25% and 6.0%.[141] These injuries can be controlled with electrocautery, by tamponade using a balloon-tipped catheter that is pulled against the abdominal wall, or by enlargement of the incision for suture ligation.

Port site infection occurs in fewer than 1% of patients. The risk factors for port site infection are the same as for any incision, including poor nutrition, obesity, and diabetes mellitus. Port site infection can lead to hernia development. The overall incidence of port site herniation is relatively low, with larger trocar sites posing the highest risk. The umbilical trocar is the most common site of herniation, occurring in 0.1% of patients undergoing LC.[135] Inappropriate closure of a trocar site can lead to the development of a trocar site hernia. All trocar sites measuring 10mm or greater should be sutured closed, unless created with a dilating, noncutting trocar.

Abdominal gas insufflation has been implicated as the cause of unusual laparoscopic complications. The diffusion of CO_2 into the bloodstream or its direct introduction into the vascular system can lead to cardiac dysrythmias or embolization.[142–145] Large volumes of intravascular CO_2 can lead to sudden cardiac collapse by forming a gas lock in the right ventricular outflow tract. The signs of CO_2 embolization include hypotension, cyanosis, arrhythmia, and "millwheel" murmur that can be heard through an esophageal stethoscope. Fortunately, CO_2 embolization during laparoscopy is rare, with an incidence of 0.002% to 0.016%.[143] When it occurs, treatment entails release of the PNP and repositioning the patient in the left lateral decubitus position, head down, to float the gas bubble into the right atrium, thus avoiding obstruction of the pulmonary outflow tract.

Inappropriate patient positioning and misuse of the specialized laparoscopic equipment can also lead to complications. The lithotomy position, often used during antireflux procedures or colon resections, can cause nerve stretching and ischemia that can lead to femoral neuropathy.[146] As discussed, head-up and head-down positioning can each have cardiovascular implications. Proper functioning of all laparoscopic equipment should be ensured before beginning the operation. Unless on standby, the laparoscopic light source should be immediately attached to the laparoscope. If left unattached, then surgical drape combustion is possible. Instrumentation should be periodically inspected for proper functioning and intact insulation.

TABLE 43.8. Avoiding Complications During Laparoscopy.

Training
Patient selection
Room setup
Port placement (site/technique)
Visualization (equipment/blood or debris)
Familiarity with anatomical landmarks
Early consultation

All operating personnel should be acquainted with the proper applications for the basic instrumentation. For instance, the laparoscopic grasper has many applications. As a result, the jaws are designed for secure fastening (with teeth) or for visceral manipulation (smooth). To avoid intestinal perforation, only smooth graspers should be used for intestinal manipulation. Bowel injuries have also been reported by careless application of the suction[147] and irrigation stream. Because these devices are deployed with considerable force, the suction or irrigator should not be directed toward recently applied clips (i.e., cystic duct).

Finally, thermal injuries from electrocautery can result from careless application, defective insulation, or improper grounding. The extent of such injury is directly related to the magnitude of current and the length of time that such current is applied. In 1993, a survey of 500 physician respondents at the American College of Surgeons meeting was conducted, and 18% of these physicians reported laparoscopic complications that they attributed to electrosurgery. It is safest to use properly insulated electrocautery instruments and short bursts of current to avoid thermal injuries. Attention to detail in laparoscopy, just as in all surgical procedures, avoids most complications (Table 43.8).

Training and Credentialing in Laparoscopic Surgery

Surgical training is evolving. As laparoscopic techniques become more refined, they are increasingly important in general surgeons' practices. Indeed, general surgery is becoming more and more synonymous with laparoscopic surgery. Mostly because of the widespread acceptance of both LC and fundoplication, both basic and advanced laparoscopic techniques have been increasingly integrated into surgical residency programs. At the same time, private industry has propagated an explosion in the production of advanced laparoscopic instrumentation. These two developments, coupled with public pressure for minimally invasive techniques, spearheaded an evolution in surgical education. The hands, and in turn the working end of the instrument, of the trainer and trainee are now separated from each other by the patient's abdominal wall, and the surgical action is concurrently interpreted on the inanimate two-dimensional monitor.

As a result, influence of the trainer over the trainee is more reliant on the verbal commands of the instructor than ever before. The trainer is less able to physically guide the trainee's hands through the preliminary stages of an operation, and as a result, there is increasing pressure to move the education of basic laparoscopic skills outside the clinical operating room. The student laparoscopist must now become acquainted with the change in depth perception, the point of view of the laparoscope, as well as basic technical skills (laparoscopic suturing and knot tying) outside the clinical operating room. The paradigm for laparoscopic surgical education is evolving from the traditional surgical learning cliché of "see one, do one, teach one" to "see one, practice one, do one."

The "practice one" step in laparoscopic skills education has been addressed through a variety of methods. Considerable effort has been expended to define the essential laparoscopic skills as well as the best method for educating students in these techniques. Since it was founded, the Society of American Gastrointestinal Endoscopic Surgeons (SAGES) has actively developed guidelines for the organized integration of laparoscopy into surgical residency programs. This group has divided laparoscopic procedures into two categories: basic (diagnostic laparoscopy, cholecystectomy, and appendectomy) and advanced (everything else).[148] Presently, the majority of general surgery residents in the United States are being exposed to basic laparoscopic techniques by faculty with adequate and often exceptional experience. The importance of basic laparoscopy in undergraduate surgical education is emphasized by the American Board of Surgery (ABS), which now requires experience with LC during a surgical residency to qualify for certification. The plan to maintain laparoscopic training within the 5-year general surgery residency program has been emphasized by the ABS and echoed by SAGES.[149]

With regard to advanced laparoscopic techniques, training of both educators and residents remains a challenge. Advanced techniques such as antireflux procedures, solid organ surgery, and colon procedures require proficiency in both basic and advanced laparoscopic skills. In addition, the risk for significant operative complication is also increased. The faculty presently teaching advanced laparoscopic procedures have gained this experience in a variety of ways, including independent experience, weekend courses, visiting surgeon proctoring, and telementoring. These methods of education have had varying success.[150,151] To provide standards for these training methods as well as documentation for proficiency, SAGES has developed guidelines for granting privileges in laparoscopic surgery. According to SAGES, to sponsor an advanced laparoscopic training program, the educating surgeon "should demonstrate proficiency in laparoscopic procedures and clinical judgment equivalent to that obtained in a surgical residency program."[152] It is only after educators well versed in advanced laparoscopic techniques become more available that advanced laparoscopic experience will become commonplace in surgical residency programs across the country.

With a residency program, in-house skills labs and inanimate trainers are now staples in the education of basic laparoscopic skills,[153,154] the result of educational research that has documented the benefit of these media for laparoscopic skill acquisition. Rosser et al. described a method of training that includes specific drills (rope pass, cup drop, and triangle transfer), which translates to improved performance in more complex laparoscopic skills such as suturing.[155,156] In most institutions, these skill stations are located in-house with continuous availability. However, in conjunction with the development of more efficient microprocessors, these simulators are becoming increasingly compact and portable. In addition, more advanced learning materials such as CD-ROMs, the Internet, and virtual reality have also been shown to be effective in laparoscopic surgical education.[151,157] Operating room experience in laparoscopy can also be targeted within a residency program toward residents with a particular interest in pursuing a career in general surgery. As advanced laparoscopic procedures become more commonplace, individual program directors should have the flexibility to direct these residents toward advanced laparoscopic cases.[149] In the interim, training in advanced laparoscopy is offered in postresidency educational venues such as fellowship programs.

Postresidency training experiences programs can be divided into two categories: private apprenticeships for those seeking practical experience and academic fellowships designed for physicians seeking more experience in advanced laparoscopic techniques combined with academic or research experience. Guidelines for laparoscopic fellowships have been delineated by SAGES,[158] and just as in other fellowships, the training of advanced laparoscopists should not detract from the training of residents of that particular residency program. To prepare future educators, academic fellowships should not only include an emphasis on achieving appropriate clinical skills but also place particular emphasis on laparoscopic research (both basic science and clinical) and advanced education in information technology.

Future

In the near future, advancement in minimally invasive surgery will occur in three areas: instrumentation, education, and basic science/outcomes research. As instruments and optics become smaller and more reliable, the place for this instrumentation will become better defined. Advancements in instrumentation will also lead to more sophisticated robotics that will not only assist surgery but also allow operators to perform surgery from remote locations or advance the ability to teleproctoring learning surgeons. Advancement in robotics coupled with information technology will further enhance surgical education. This arrangement allows expert technical consultation to be available both in and outside the operating room. Advancement in virtual reality has great potential to change the way we presently think of surgical education. More advanced simulators will allow surgeons the opportunity to practice a laparoscopic surgical case before attempting it in a patient. Finally, the creation of more sophisticated databases coupled with surgeons more acquainted with information technology will lead to a greater ease in collaboration and quicker, more effective clinical trials.

Acknowledgment. We would like to thank the previous edition's authors, Dr. Chekan and Dr. Pappas. We also thank Thomas J. Birdas, MD; Amjad Ali, MD; Erik Clary, DVM; Gray Hughes, MD; and Maureen Fina for their editing and clerical efforts. We also thank Robert Anderson, MD, for his ongoing support.

References

1. Bozzini P. Lichtleiter, eine Erfindung zur Anschauung innerer Teile und Krankheiten. J Prak Heilkd 1806;24:107.

2. Berci G. History of pneumoperitomeum. In: Rosenthal R, Friedman R, Phillips E, eds. The Physiology of Pneumoperitoneum. New York: Springer, 1998:1–6.
3. Kalk H. Erfahrungen mit der Laparoskopie. Stuttgart: Thieme; 1929.
4. Muhe E. [Laparoscopic cholecystectomy—late results]. Langenbecks Arch Chir Suppl Kongressbd 1991:416–423.
5. Gollan J, Kalser S, Pitt H, Strasberg S. NIH Consensus Development Conference statement on gallstones and laparoscopic cholecystectomy. Am J Surg 1993;165:390–396.
6. Geagea T. Laparoscopic Nissen's fundal plication is feasible. Can J Surg 1991;34:313.
7. Traverso LW. Technology and surgery. Dilemma of the gimmick, true advances, and cost effectiveness. Surg Clin North Am 1996;76:129–138.
8. Traverso LW. The laparoscopic surgical value package and how surgeons can influence costs. Surg Clin North Am 1996;76:631–639.
9. DesCoteaux JG, Tye L, Poulin EC. Reuse of disposable laparoscopic instruments: cost analysis. Can J Surg 1996;39:133–139.
10. McKernan JB, Champion JK. Access techniques: Veress needle—initial blind trocar insertion versus open laparoscopy with the Hasson trocar. Endosc Surg Allied Technol 1995;3:35–38.
11. Nakajima K, Lee SW, Cocilovo C, et al. Hand-assisted laparoscopic colorectal surgery using GelPort. Surg Endosc 2004;18:102–105.
12. Kang JC, Chung MH, Chao PC, et al. Hand-assisted laparoscopic colectomy versus open colectomy: a prospective randomized study. Surg Endosc 2004;18:577–581.
13. El-Kady AA, Abd-El-Razek M. Intraperitoneal explosion during female sterilization by laparoscopic electrocoagulation. A case report. Int J Gynaecol Obstet 1976;14:487–488.
14. Bhoyrul S, Payne J, Steffes B, Swanstrom L, Way LW. A randomized prospective study of radially expanding trocars in laparoscopic surgery. J Gastrointest Surg 2000;4:392–397.
15. Bordelon B, Hunter J. Endoscopic technology. In: Greene F, Ponsky J, eds. Endoscopic Surgery. Philadelphia: Saunders; 1994:6–18.
16. Dion YM, Gaillard F. Visual integration of data and basic motor skills under laparoscopy. Influence of 2-D and 3-D video-camera systems. Surg Endosc 1997;11:995–1000.
17. Madan AK, Frantzides CT, Tebbit CL, Park WC, Kumari NV, Shervin N. Evaluation of specialized laparoscopic suturing and tying devices. J Soc Laparoendosc Surg 2004;8:191–193.
18. McCarus SD. Physiologic mechanism of the ultrasonically activated scalpel. J Am Assoc Gynecol Laparosc 1996;3:601–608.
19. Harold KL, Pollinger H, Matthews BD, Kercher KW, Sing RF, Heniford BT. Comparison of ultrasonic energy, bipolar thermal energy, and vascular clips for the hemostasis of small-, medium, and large-sized arteries. Surg Endosc 2003;17:1228–1230.
20. Takada M, Ichihara T, Kuroda Y. Comparative study of electrothermal bipolar vessel sealer and ultrasonic coagulating shears in laparoscopic colectomy. Surg Endosc 2004;19:226–228.
21. Ishizaki Y, Bandai Y, Shimomura K, Abe H, Ohtomo Y, Idezuki Y. Changes in splanchnic blood flow and cardiovascular effects following peritoneal insufflation of carbon dioxide. Surg Endosc 1993;7:420–423.
22. Marathe US, Lilly RE, Silvestry SC, et al. Alterations in hemodynamics and left ventricular contractility during carbon dioxide pneumoperitoneum. Surg Endosc 1996;10:974–978.
23. Myre K, Buanes T, Smith G, Stokland O. Simultaneous hemodynamic and echocardiographic changes during abdominal gas insufflation. Surg Laparosc Endosc 1997;7:415–419.
24. Odeberg S, Ljungqvist O, Svenberg T, et al. Haemodynamic effects of pneumoperitoneum and the influence of posture during anaesthesia for laparoscopic surgery. Acta Anaesthesiol Scand 1994;38:276–283.
25. Dorsay DA, Greene FL, Baysinger CL. Hemodynamic changes during laparoscopic cholecystectomy monitored with transesophageal echocardiography. Surg Endosc 1995;9:128–133; discussion 133–134.
26. Hashimoto S, Hashikura Y, Munakata Y, et al. Changes in the cardiovascular and respiratory systems during laparoscopic cholecystectomy. J Laparoendosc Surg 1993;3:535–539.
27. Gannedahl P, Odeberg S, Brodin LA, Sollevi A. Effects of posture and pneumoperitoneum during anaesthesia on the indices of left ventricular filling. Acta Anaesthesiol Scand 1996;40:160–166.
28. McLaughlin JG, Scheeres DE, Dean RJ, Bonnell BW. The adverse hemodynamic effects of laparoscopic cholecystectomy. Surg Endosc 1995;9:121–124.
29. Windberger U, Siegl H, Ferguson JG, et al. Hemodynamic effects of prolonged abdominal insufflation for laparoscopic procedures. Gastrointest Endosc 1995;41:121–129.
30. Ho HS, Saunders CJ, Gunther RA, Wolfe BM. Effector of hemodynamics during laparoscopy: CO_2 absorption or intra-abdominal pressure? J Surg Res 1995;59:497–503.
31. Joris JL, Noirot DP, Legrand MJ, Jacquet NJ, Lamy ML. Hemodynamic changes during laparoscopic cholecystectomy. Anesth Analg 1993;76:1067–1071.
32. Safran DB, Orlando R 3rd. Physiologic effects of pneumoperitoneum. Am J Surg 1994;167:281–286.
33. Marshall RL, Jebson PJ, Davie IT, Scott DB. Circulatory effects of carbon dioxide insufflation of the peritoneal cavity for laparoscopy. Br J Anaesth 1972;44:680–684.
34. Girardis M, Broi UD, Antonutto G, Pasetto A. The effect of laparoscopic cholecystectomy on cardiovascular function and pulmonary gas exchange. Anesth Analg 1996;83:134–140.
35. Ortega AE, Richman MF, Hernandez M, et al. Inferior vena caval blood flow and cardiac hemodynamics during carbon dioxide pneumoperitoneum. Surg Endosc 1996;10:920–924.
36. Dhoste K, Lacoste L, Karayan J, Lehuede MS, Thomas D, Fusciardi J. Haemodynamic and ventilatory changes during laparoscopic cholecystectomy in elderly ASA III patients. Can J Anaesth 1996;43:783–788.
37. Hein HA, Joshi GP, Ramsay MA, et al. Hemodynamic changes during laparoscopic cholecystectomy in patients with severe cardiac disease. J Clin Anesth 1997;9:261–265.
38. Safran D, Sgambati S, Orlando R 3rd. Laparoscopy in high-risk cardiac patients. Surg Gynecol Obstet 1993;176:548–554.
39. Harris SN, Ballantyne GH, Luther MA, Perrino AC Jr. Alterations of cardiovascular performance during laparoscopic colectomy: a combined hemodynamic and echocardiographic analysis. Anesth Analg 1996;83:482–487.
40. Zollinger A, Krayer S, Singer T, et al. Haemodynamic effects of pneumoperitoneum in elderly patients with an increased cardiac risk. Eur J Anaesthesiol 1997;14:266–275.
41. Liem T, Applebaum H, Herzberger B. Hemodynamic and ventilatory effects of abdominal CO_2 insufflation at various pressures in the young swine. J Pediatr Surg 1994;29:966–969.
42. Bannenberg JJ, Rademaker BM, Froeling FM, Meijer DW. Hemodynamics during laparoscopic extra- and intraperitoneal insufflation. An experimental study. Surg Endosc 1997;11:911–914.
43. Ho HS, Saunders CJ, Corso FA, Wolfe BM. The effects of CO_2 pneumoperitoneum on hemodynamics in hemorrhaged animals. Surgery 1993;114:381–387; discussion 387–388.
44. Knolmayer TJ, Bowyer MW, Egan JC, Asbun HJ. The effects of pneumoperitoneum on gastric blood flow and traditional hemodynamic measurements. Surg Endosc 1998;12:115–118.
45. Caldwell CB, Ricotta JJ. Changes in visceral blood flow with elevated intraabdominal pressure. J Surg Res 1987;43:14–20.
46. Hashikura Y, Kawasaki S, Munakata Y, Hashimoto S, Hayashi K, Makuuchi M. Effects of peritoneal insufflation on hepatic and renal blood flow. Surg Endosc 1994;8:759–761.

47. Chiu AW, Chang LS, Birkett DH, Babayan RK. A porcine model for renal hemodynamic study during laparoscopy. J Surg Res 1996;60:61–68.
48. Chiu AW, Chang LS, Birkett DH, Babayan RK. The impact of pneumoperitoneum, pneumoretroperitoneum, and gasless laparoscopy on the systemic and renal hemodynamics. J Am Coll Surg 1995;181:397–406.
49. Miki Y, Iwase K, Kamiike W, et al. Laparoscopic cholecystectomy and time-course changes in renal function. The effect of the retraction method on renal function. Surg Endosc 1997; 11:838–841.
50. Iwase K, Takenaka H, Ishizaka T, Ohata T, Oshima S, Sakaguchi K. Serial changes in renal function during laparoscopic cholecystectomy. Eur Surg Res 1993;25:203–212.
51. Chang DT, Kirsch AJ, Sawczuk IS. Oliguria during laparoscopic surgery. J Endourol 1994;8:349–352.
52. Jorgensen JO, Gillies RB, Lalak NJ, Hunt DR. Lower limb venous hemodynamics during laparoscopy: an animal study. Surg Laparosc Endosc 1994;4:32–35.
53. Millard JA, Hill BB, Cook PS, Fenoglio ME, Stahlgren LH. Intermittent sequential pneumatic compression in prevention of venous stasis associated with pneumoperitoneum during laparoscopic cholecystectomy. Arch Surg 1993;128:914–918; discussion 918–919.
54. Vander Velpen G, Penninckx F, Kerremans R, Van Damme J, Arnout J. Interleukin-6 and coagulation-fibrinolysis fluctuations after laparoscopic and conventional cholecystectomy. Surg Endosc 1994;8:1216–1220.
55. Caprini JA, Arcelus JI. Prevention of postoperative venous thromboembolism following laparoscopic cholecystectomy. Surg Endosc 1994;8:741–747.
56. Bergqvist D, Matzsch T, Jendteg S, Lindgren B, Persson U. The cost-effectiveness of prevention of post-operative thromboembolism. Acta Chir Scand Suppl 1990;556:36–41.
57. Morgenstern L, Wong L, Berci G. Twelve hundred open cholecystectomies before the laparoscopic era. A standard for comparison. Arch Surg 1992;127:400–403.
58. Deziel DJ, Millikan KW, Economou SG, Doolas A, Ko ST, Airan MC. Complications of laparoscopic cholecystectomy: a national survey of 4,292 hospitals and an analysis of 77,604 cases. Am J Surg 1993;165:9–14.
59. Caprini JA, Arcelus JI, Hoffman K, et al. Prevention of venous thromboembolism in North America: results of a survey among general surgeons. J Vasc Surg 1994;20:751–758.
60. Schwenk W, Bohm B, Fugener A, Muller JM. Intermittent pneumatic sequential compression (ISC) of the lower extremities prevents venous stasis during laparoscopic cholecystectomy. A prospective randomized study. Surg Endosc 1998;12:7–11.
61. Wu EC, Barba CA. Current practices in the prophylaxis of venous thromboembolism in bariatric surgery. Obes Surg 2000;10:7–13; discussion 14.
62. Nguyen NT, Owings JT, Gosselin R, et al. Systemic coagulation and fibrinolysis after laparoscopic and open gastric bypass. Arch Surg 2001;136:909–916.
63. Miller MT, Rovito PF. An approach to venous thromboembolism prophylaxis in laparoscopic Roux-en-Y gastric bypass surgery. Obes Surg 2004;14:731–737.
64. Volpino P, Cangemi V, D'Andrea N, Cangemi B, Piat G. Hemodynamic and pulmonary changes during and after laparoscopic cholecystectomy. A comparison with traditional surgery. Surg Endosc 1998;12:119–123.
65. Drummond GB, Martin LV. Pressure–volume relationships in the lung during laparoscopy. Br J Anaesth 1978;50:261–270.
66. Simonneau G, Vivien A, Sartene R, et al. Diaphragm dysfunction induced by upper abdominal surgery. Role of postoperative pain. Am Rev Respir Dis 1983;128:899–903.
67. Fahy BG, Barnas GM, Flowers JL, Nagle SE, Njoku MJ. The effects of increased abdominal pressure on lung and chest wall mechanics during laparoscopic surgery. Anesth Analg 1995;81:744–750.
68. Sharma KC, Brandstetter RD, Brensilver JM, Jung LD. Cardiopulmonary physiology and pathophysiology as a consequence of laparoscopic surgery. Chest 1996;110:810–815.
69. Moffa SM, Quinn JV, Slotman GJ. Hemodynamic effects of carbon dioxide pneumoperitoneum during mechanical ventilation and positive end-expiratory pressure. J Trauma 1993;35:613–617; discussion 617–618.
70. Luz CM, Polarz H, Bohrer H, Hundt G, Dorsam J, Martin E. Hemodynamic and respiratory effects of pneumoperitoneum and PEEP during laparoscopic pelvic lymphadenectomy in dogs. Surg Endosc 1994;8:25–27.
71. Fitzgerald SD, Andrus CH, Baudendistel LJ, Dahms TE, Kaminski DL. Hypercarbia during carbon dioxide pneumoperitoneum. Am J Surg 1992;163:186–190.
72. Wahba RW, Mamazza J. Ventilatory requirements during laparoscopic cholecystectomy. Can J Anaesth 1993;40:206–210.
73. Smith I, Benzie RJ, Gordon NL, Kelman GR, Swapp GH. Cardiovascular effects of peritoneal insufflation of carbon dioxide for laparoscopy. Br Med J 1971;3:410–411.
74. McMahon AJ, Russell IT, Ramsay G, et al. Laparoscopic and minilaparotomy cholecystectomy: a randomized trial comparing postoperative pain and pulmonary function. Surgery 1994; 115:533–539.
75. Schauer PR, Luna J, Ghiatas AA, Glen ME, Warren JM, Sirinek KR. Pulmonary function after laparoscopic cholecystectomy. Surgery 1993;114:389–397; discussion 397–399.
76. Torrington KG, Bilello JF, Hopkins TK, Hall EA Jr. Postoperative pulmonary changes after laparoscopic cholecystectomy. South Med J 1996;89:675–678.
77. Eden CG, Haigh AC, Carter PG, Coptcoat MJ. Laparoscopic nephrectomy results in better postoperative pulmonary function. J Endourol 1994;8:419–422; discussion 422–423.
78. Litwin DE, Girotti MJ, Poulin EC, Mamazza J, Nagy AG. Laparoscopic cholecystectomy: trans-Canada experience with 2201 cases. Can J Surg 1992;35:291–296.
79. Garcia-Caballero M, Vara-Thorbeck C. The evolution of postoperative ileus after laparoscopic cholecystectomy. A comparative study with conventional cholecystectomy and sympathetic blockade treatment. Surg Endosc 1993;7:416–419.
80. Schippers E, Ottinger AP, Anurov M, Polivoda M, Schumpelick V. Laparoscopic cholecystectomy: a minor abdominal trauma? World J Surg 1993;17:539–542; discussion 543.
81. Ludwig KA, Frantzides CT, Carlson MA, Grade KL. Myoelectric motility patterns following open versus laparoscopic cholecystectomy. J Laparoendosc Surg 1993;3:461–466.
82. Ballantyne GH. Laparoscopic-assisted colorectal surgery: review of results in 752 patients. Gastroenterologist 1995;3: 75–89.
83. Liberman MA, Phillips EH, Carroll BJ, Fallas M, Rosenthal R. Laparoscopic colectomy versus traditional colectomy for diverticulitis. Outcome and costs. Surg Endosc 1996;10:15–18.
84. Davies W, Kollmorgen CF, Tu QM, et al. Laparoscopic colectomy shortens postoperative ileus in a canine model. Surgery 1997;121:550–555.
85. Carlson MA, Frantzides CT. Canine intestinal myoelectric activity after open versus laparoscopically assisted right hemicolectomy. Am J Surg 1997;174:79–82.
86. Pitts LH, Martin N. Head injuries. Surg Clin North Am 1982;62:47–60.
87. Rosenthal RJ, Hiatt JR, Phillips EH, Hewitt W, Demetriou AA, Grode M. Intracranial pressure. Effects of pneumoperitoneum in a large-animal model. Surg Endosc 1997;11:376–380.
88. Halverson A, Buchanan R, Jacobs L, et al. Evaluation of mechanism of increased intracranial pressure with insufflation. Surg Endosc 1998;12:266–269.

89. Fujii Y, Tanaka H, Tsuruoka S, Toyooka H, Amaha K. Middle cerebral arterial blood flow velocity increases during laparoscopic cholecystectomy. Anesth Analg 1994;78:80–83.
90. Paulson GW, DeVoe K Jr. Neurological complications of laparoscopy. Am J Obstet Gynecol 1981;140:468–469.
91. Lennard TW, Shenton BK, Borzotta A, et al. The influence of surgical operations on components of the human immune system. Br J Surg 1985;72:771–776.
92. Schauer PR, Sirinek KR. The laparoscopic approach reduces the endocrine response to elective cholecystectomy. Am Surg 1995;61:106–111.
93. McMahon AJ, O'Dwyer PJ, Cruikshank AM, et al. Comparison of metabolic responses to laparoscopic and minilaparotomy cholecystectomy. Br J Surg 1993;80:1255–1258.
94. Bressler M, Whelan RL, Halverson A, Treat MR, Nowygrod R. Is immune function better preserved after laparoscopic versus open colon resection? Surg Endosc 1994;8:881–883.
95. Kloosterman T, von Blomberg BM, Borgstein P, Cuesta MA, Scheper RJ, Meijer S. Unimpaired immune functions after laparoscopic cholecystectomy. Surgery 1994;115:424–428.
96. Mealy K, Gallagher H, Barry M, Lennon F, Traynor O, Hyland J. Physiological and metabolic responses to open and laparoscopic cholecystectomy. Br J Surg 1992;79:1061–1064.
97. Bouvy ND, Marquet RL, Tseng LN, et al. Laparoscopic versus conventional bowel resection in the rat. Earlier restoration of serum insulin-like growth factor 1 levels. Surg Endosc 1998;12:412–415.
98. Buunen M, Gholghesaei M, Veldkamp R, Meijer DW, Bonjer HJ, Bouvy ND. Stress response to laparoscopic surgery: a review. Surg Endosc 2004;18:1022–1028.
99. Brune IB, Wilke W, Hensler T, Feussner H, Holzmann B, Siewert JR. Normal T lymphocyte and monocyte function after minimally invasive surgery. Surg Endosc 1998;12:1020–1024.
100. Gutt CN, Kuntz C, Schmandra T, et al. Metabolism and immunology in laparoscopy. First Workshop on Experimental Laparoscopic Surgery, Frankfurt, 1997. Surg Endosc 1998;12:1096–1098.
101. Berguer R, Dalton M, Ferrick D. Adrenocortical response and regional T-lymphocyte activation patterns following minimally invasive surgery in a rat model. Surg Endosc 1998;12:236–240.
102. West MA, Hackam DJ, Baker J, Rodriguez JL, Bellingham J, Rotstein OD. Mechanism of decreased in vitro murine macrophage cytokine release after exposure to carbon dioxide: relevance to laparoscopic surgery. Ann Surg 1997;226:179–190.
103. Carozzi S, Caviglia PM, Nasini MG, Schelotto C, Santoni O, Pietrucci A. Peritoneal dialysis solution pH and Ca^{2+} concentration regulate peritoneal macrophage and mesothelial cell activation. Asaio J 1994;40:20–23.
104. Tung PH, Wang Q, Ogle CK, Smith CD. Minimal increase in gut-mucosal interleukin-6 during laparoscopy. Surg Endosc 1998;12:409–411.
105. Jacobi CA, Krahenbuhl L, Blochle C, Bonjer HJ, Gutt CN. Peritonitis and adhesions in laparoscopic surgery. First Workshop on Experimental Laparoscopic Surgery, Frankfurt 1997. Surg Endosc 1998;12:1099–1101.
106. Whelan RL, Allendorf JD, Gutt CN, et al. General oncologic effects of the laparoscopic surgical approach. 1997 Frankfurt International Meeting of Animal Laparoscopic Researchers. Surg Endosc 1998;12:1092–1095.
107. Allendorf JD, Bessler M, Whelan RL, et al. Better preservation of immune function after laparoscopic-assisted versus open bowel resection in a murine model. Dis Colon Rectum 1996;39: S67–S72.
108. Bouvy ND, Marquet RL, Jeekel J, Bonjer HJ. Laparoscopic surgery is associated with less tumour growth stimulation than conventional surgery: an experimental study. Br J Surg 1997;84:358–361.
109. Cirocco WC, Schwartzman A, Golub RW. Abdominal wall recurrence after laparoscopic colectomy for colon cancer. Surgery 1994;116:842–846.
110. Fodera M, Pello MJ, Atabek U, Spence RK, Alexander JB, Camishion RC. Trocar site tumor recurrence after laparoscopic-assisted colectomy. J Laparoendosc Surg 1995;5:259–262.
111. Jacquet P, Averbach AM, Jacquet N. Abdominal wall metastasis and peritoneal carcinomatosis after laparoscopic-assisted colectomy for colon cancer. Eur J Surg Oncol 1995;21:568–570.
112. Jones DB, Guo LW, Reinhard MK, et al. Impact of pneumoperitoneum on trocar site implantation of colon cancer in hamster model. Dis Colon Rectum 1995;38:1182–1188.
113. Wexner SD, Cohen SM. Port site metastases after laparoscopic colorectal surgery for cure of malignancy. Br J Surg 1995;82:295–298.
114. Hughes ES, McDermott FT, Polglase AL, Johnson WR. Tumor recurrence in the abdominal wall scar tissue after large-bowel cancer surgery. Dis Colon Rectum 1983;26:571–572.
115. Lord SA, Larach SW, Ferrara A, Williamson PR, Lago CP, Lube MW. Laparoscopic resections for colorectal carcinoma. A 3-year experience. Dis Colon Rectum 1996;39:148–154.
116. Lacy AM, Delgado S, Garcia-Valdecasas JC, et al. Port site metastases and recurrence after laparoscopic colectomy. A randomized trial. Surg Endosc 1998;12:1039–1042.
117. Ramos JM, Gupta S, Anthone GJ, Ortega AE, Simons AJ, Beart RW Jr. Laparoscopy and colon cancer. Is the port site at risk? A preliminary report. Arch Surg 1994;129:897–899; discussion 900.
118. Milsom JW, Bohm B, Hammerhofer KA, Fazio V, Steiger E, Elson P. A prospective, randomized trial comparing laparoscopic versus conventional techniques in colorectal cancer surgery: a preliminary report. J Am Coll Surg 1998;187:46–54; discussion 54–55.
119. Franklin ME Jr., Rosenthal D, Abrego-Medina D, et al. Prospective comparison of open vs. laparoscopic colon surgery for carcinoma. Five-year results. Dis Colon Rectum 1996;39:S35–S46.
120. Curet MJ. Port site metastases. Am J Surg 2004;187:705–712.
121. Jacobi CA, Sabat R, Bohm B, Zieren HU, Volk HD, Muller JM. Pneumoperitoneum with carbon dioxide stimulates growth of malignant colonic cells. Surgery 1997;121:72–78.
122. Allendorf JD, Bessler M, Kayton ML, et al. Increased tumor establishment and growth after laparotomy versus laparoscopy in a murine model. Arch Surg 1995;130:649–653.
123. Bouvy ND, Marquet RL, Jeekel H, Bonjer HJ. Impact of gas(less) laparoscopy and laparotomy on peritoneal tumor growth and abdominal wall metastases. Ann Surg 1996;224:694–700; discussion 700–701.
124. Goldstein DS, Lu ML, Hattori T, Ratliff TL, Loughlin KR, Kavoussi LR. Inhibition of peritoneal tumor-cell implantation: model for laparoscopic cancer surgery. J Endourol 1993;7:237–241.
125. Kazemier G, Bonjer HJ, Berends FJ, Lange JF. Port site metastases after laparoscopic colorectal surgery for cure of malignancy. Br J Surg 1995;82:1141–1142.
126. Reymond MA, Wittekind C, Jung A, Hohenberger W, Kirchner T, Kockerling F. The incidence of port-site metastases might be reduced. Surg Endosc 1997;11:902–906.
127. Champault G, Taffinder N, Ziol M, Riskalla H, Catheline JM. Cells are present in the smoke created during laparoscopic surgery. Br J Surg 1997;84:993–995.
128. Whelan RL, Sellers GJ, Allendorf JD, et al. Trocar site recurrence is unlikely to result from aerosolization of tumor cells. Dis Colon Rectum 1996;39:S7–S13.
129. Allardyce RA, Morreau P, Bagshaw PF. Operative factors affecting tumor cell distribution following laparoscopic colectomy in a porcine model. Dis Colon Rectum 1997;40:939–945.
130. Watson DI, Mathew G, Ellis T, Baigrie CF, Rofe AM, Jamieson GG. Gasless laparoscopy may reduce the risk of port-site metas-

tases following laparascopic tumor surgery. Arch Surg 1997; 132:166–168; discussion 169.
131. Silva J, Platt L. Laparoscopic surgery during pregnancy. In: Rosenthal R, Friedman R, Phillips E, eds. The Pathophysiology of Pneumoperitoneum. New York: Springer; 1998.
132. Reedy MB, Kallen B, Kuehl TJ. Laparoscopy during pregnancy: a study of five fetal outcome parameters with use of the Swedish Health Registry. Am J Obstet Gynecol 1997;177:673–679.
133. Curet MJ, Allen D, Josloff RK, et al. Laparoscopy during pregnancy. Arch Surg 1996;131:546–550; discussion 550–551.
134. Phillips JM, Hulka JF, Hulka B, Corson SL. 1979 AAGL membership survey. J Reprod Med 1981;26:529–533.
135. Larson GM, Vitale GC, Casey J, et al. Multipractice analysis of laparoscopic cholecystectomy in 1983 patients. Am J Surg 1992;163:221–226.
136. Frenkel Y, Oelsner G, Ben-Baruch G, Menczer J. Major surgical complications of laparoscopy. Eur J Obstet Gynecol Reprod Biol 1981;12:107–111.
137. Yuzpe AA. Pneumoperitoneum needle and trocar injuries in laparoscopy. A survey on possible contributing factors and prevention. J Reprod Med 1990;35:485–490.
138. Oshinsky GS, Smith AD. Laparoscopic needles and trocars: an overview of designs and complications. J Laparoendosc Surg 1992;2:117–125.
139. Hasson HM. A modified instrument and method for laparoscopy. Am J Obstet Gynecol 1971;110:886–887.
140. Nordestgaard AG, Bodily KC, Osborne RW Jr, Buttorff JD. Major vascular injuries during laparoscopic procedures. Am J Surg 1995;169:543–545.
141. Loffer FD, Pent D. Indications, contraindications and complications of laparoscopy. Obstet Gynecol Surv 1975;30:407–427.
142. Cottin V, Delafosse B, Viale JP. Gas embolism during laparoscopy: a report of seven cases in patients with previous abdominal surgical history. Surg Endosc 1996;10:166–169.
143. Gomar C, Fernandez C, Villalonga A, Nalda MA. Carbon dioxide embolism during laparoscopy and hysteroscopy. Ann Fr Anesth Reanim 1985;4:380–382.
144. Yacoub OF, Cardona I Jr, Coveler LA, Dodson MG. Carbon dioxide embolism during laparoscopy. Anesthesiology 1982;57: 533–535.
145. Ostman PL, Pantle-Fisher FH, Faure EA, Glosten B. Circulatory collapse during laparoscopy. J Clin Anesth 1990;2:129–132.
146. Hershlag A, Loy RA, Lavy G, DeCherney AH. Femoral neuropathy after laparoscopy. A case report. J Reprod Med 1990;35:575–576.
147. Riedel HH, Lehmann-Willenbrock E, Mecke H, Semm K. The frequency distribution of various pelviscopic (laparoscopic) operations, including complications rates—statistics of the Federal Republic of Germany in the years 1983–1985. Zentralbl Gynakol 1989;111:78–91.
148. Integrating advanced laparoscopy into surgical residency training. Surg Endosc 1998;12:374–376.
149. SAGES position statement on advanced laparoscopic training. Surg Endosc 1998;12:377.
150. Satava RM. Proctors, preceptors, and laparoscopic surgery. The role of "proctor" in the surgical credentialing process. Surg Endosc 1993;7:283–284.
151. Schulam PG, Docimo SG, Saleh W, Breitenbach C, Moore RG, Kavoussi L. Telesurgical mentoring. Initial clinical experience. Surg Endosc 1997;11:1001–1005.
152. Granting of privileges for gastrointestinal endoscopy by surgeons. Society of American Gastrointestinal Endoscopic Surgeons (SAGES). Surg Endosc 1998;12:381–382.
153. Derossis AM, Bothwell J, Sigman HH, Fried GM. The effect of practice on performance in a laparoscopic simulator. Surg Endosc 1998;12:1117–1120.
154. Mori T, Hatano N, Maruyama S, Atomi Y. Significance of "hands-on training" in laparoscopic surgery. Surg Endosc 1998; 12:256–260.
155. Rosser JC, Rosser LE, Savalgi RS. Skill acquisition and assessment for laparoscopic surgery. Arch Surg 1997;132:200–204.
156. Rosser JC Jr, Rosser LE, Savalgi RS. Objective evaluation of a laparoscopic surgical skill program for residents and senior surgeons. Arch Surg 1998;133:657–661.
157. Gandsas A, Altrudi R, Pleatman M, Silva Y. Live interactive broadcast of laparoscopic surgery via the Internet. Surg Endosc 1998;12:252–255.
158. Framework for post-residency surgical education and training—a SAGES guideline. Available at: http://www.sages.org/sagespublication.php?doc=17. Accessed January 22, 2005.
159. Schauer PR, Sirnek KR. The laparoscopic approach reduces the endocrine response to elective cholecystectomy. Am Surg 1995;61:106.
160. Lacy A, Sala Blanch X, Visa J. Alternative gases in laparoscopic surgery. In: Rosenthal RJ, Friedman RL, Phillips EH, eds. The Physiology of Pneumoperitoneum. New York: Springer-Verlag; 1998.
161. Dominioni L, Cuffari S, Giudce G, Carcano G, Nicora L, Dionigi R. The acute phase response after laparoscopic cholecystectomy and after open cholecystectomy. Hepatico-Pancreatico-Biliary Surg 1993;6:65.
162. Cho JM, LaPorta AJ, Clark JR, Schofield MJ, Hammond SL, Mallory PL. Response of serum cytokines in patients undergoing laparoscopic cholecystectomy. Surg Endosc 1994;8:1380.
163. Ueo H, Honda M, Adachi M, et al. Minimal increase in serum interleukin-6 levels during laparoscopic. Am J Surg 1994;168:358–360.
164. Redmond HP, Watson RWG, Houghton T, Condron C, Watson RGK, Bouchier-Hayes D. Immune function in patients undergoing open versus laparoscopic cholecystectomy. Arch Surg 1994;129:1240.
165. Trokel MJ, Bessler M, Treat MR, Whelan RL, Nowygrod R. Preservation of immune response after laparoscopy. Surg Endosc 1994;8:1385–1387; discussion 1387–1388.
166. Köksoy C, Kuzu MA, Kurt I, et al. Haemodynamic effects of pneumoperitoneum during laparoscopic cholecystectomy: a prospective comparative study using bioimpedance cardiography. Br J Surg 1995;82:972–974.
167. Kubota K, Kajiura N, Teruya M, et al. Alterations in respiratory function and hemodynamics during laparoscopic cholecystectomy under pneumoperitoneum. Surg Endosc 1993;7:500–504.
168. Liu SY, Leighton T, Davis I, Klein S, Lippmann M, Bongard F. Prospective analysis of cardiopulmonary responses to laparoscopic cholecystectomy. J Laparoendosc Surg 1991;1:241–246.
169. Hirvonen EA, Nuutinen LS, Kauko M. Hemodynamic changes due to Trendelenburg positioning and pneumoperitoneum during laparoscopic hysterectomy. Acta Anaesthesiol Scand 1995;39:949–955.
170. Motew M, Ivankovich AD, Bieniarz J, Albrecht RF, Zahed B, Scommegna A. Cardiovascular effects and acid-base and blood gas changes during laparoscopy. Am J Obstet Gynecol. 1973;115:1002–1012.
171. Iwase K, Takenaka H, Yagura A, et al. Hemodynamic changes during laparoscopic cholecystectomy in patients with heart disease. Endoscopy 1992;24:771–773.
172. Talamini MA, Mendoza-Sagaon M, Gitzelmann CA, et al. Increased mediastinal pressure and decreased cardiac output during laparoscopic Nissen fundoplication. Surgery 1997;122: 345–353.
173. Horvath KD, Whelan RL, Lier B, et al. The effects of elevated intraabdominal pressure, hypercarbia, and positioning on the hemodynamic responses to laparoscopic colectomy in pigs. Surg Endosc 1998;12:107–114.

174. Rademaker BM, Meyer DW, Bannenberg JJ, Klopper PJ, Kalkman CJ. Laparoscopy without pneumoperitoneum. Effects of abdominal wall retraction versus carbon dioxide insufflation on hemodynamics and gas exchange in pigs. Surg Endosc 1995;9:797–801.
175. Davidson BS, Cromeens DM, Feig BW. Alternative methods of exposure minimize cardiopulmonary risk in experimental animals during minimally invasive surgery. Surg Endosc 1996;10:301–304.
176. Moffa SM, Quinn JV, Slotman GJ. Hemodynamic effects of carbon dioxide pneumoperitoneum during mechanical ventilation and positive end-expiratory pressure. J Trauma 1993;35:613–618.
177. Luz CM, Polarz H, Böhrer H, Hundt G, Dörsam J, Martin E. Hemodynamic and respiratory effects of pneumoperitoneum and PEEP during laparoscopic pelvic lymphadenectomy in dogs. Surg Endosc 1994;8:25–27.

44A

Esophagus
Benign Diseases of the Esophagus

C. Daniel Smith and David A. McClusky III

Anatomy

General

The esophagus is a muscular tube lined with nonkeratinizing squamous epithelium that starts as a continuation of the pharynx and ends as the cardia of the stomach. The esophagus is fixed only at its upper and lower ends, the upper end being firmly attached to the cricoid cartilage and the lower end to the diaphragm. This lack of fixation throughout its length allows the esophagus both transverse and longitudinal mobility. This mobility is important in normal esophageal function as well as pathological states, which can easily displace the esophagus or require extensive surgical mobilization for correction.

Course

Although the esophagus lies in the midline, it does not follow a straight vertical course from pharynx to stomach but rather deviates to the left of midline as it courses through the neck and upper thorax and slightly to the right of midline in the midportion of the thorax near the tracheal bifurcation. It is this deflection to the right of midline that dictates a right thoracotomy when transthoracic esophagointestinal anastomosis is necessary. In the lower portion of the thorax, the esophagus again deviates to the left of midline as it passes behind the heart and through the diaphragmatic hiatus. Overall, the esophageal axis through the chest is vertical. Any distortion of this vertical axis strongly suggests malignancy with mediastinal invasion and retraction. In addition, the esophagus has anteroposterior deflections that correspond to the curvatures of the cervical and thoracic spine. At its distal end, the esophagus leaves the normal curvature of the spine and deviates anteriorly to pass through the diaphragmatic hiatus.

In its course from the pharynx to the stomach, the esophagus passes through three compartments: the neck, thorax, and abdomen. The cervical portion of the esophagus is approximately 5 cm in length and courses between the trachea and the vertebral column, passing into the chest at the level of the sternal notch. The thoracic esophagus is approximately 20 cm long and courses behind the tracheal bifurcation and heart before entering the abdominal cavity at about the level of the xiphoid process of the sternum. The abdominal portion of the esophagus is approximately 2 cm in length and is surrounded by the phrenoesophageal ligament. This phrenoesophageal membrane provides an airtight seal between the thoracic and abdominal cavities and must be strong enough to resist abdominal pressure, yet flexible enough to move with the pressure changes and movements incidental to breathing and swallowing. The phrenoesophageal ligament is comprised of pleura, subpleural (endothoracic) fascia, phrenoesophageal fascia, transversalis fascia, and peritoneum (Fig. 44A.1).

Length

The length of the esophagus is defined anatomically as the distance from the cricoid cartilage to the gastric orifice. In the adult male, this length is from 22 to 28 cm and averages 2 cm shorter in the female; esophageal length varies more with individual height than sex. Because the precise location of the cricoid cartilage is difficult to determine, the length of the esophagus is more commonly measured as the distance from the incisors to the gastric inlet. This distance is easily determined during esophagoscopy and averages 40 cm. Finally, the length of the esophagus as measured manometrically is the

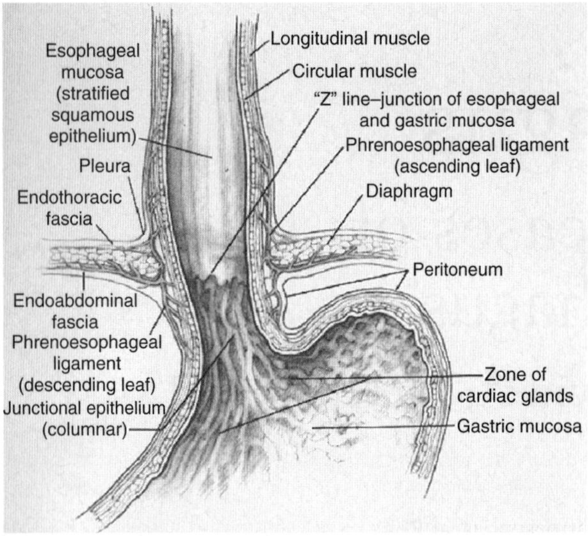

FIGURE 44A.1. Anatomical relationships of the distal esophagus and phrenoesophageal ligament. (From Gray,[272] with permission.)

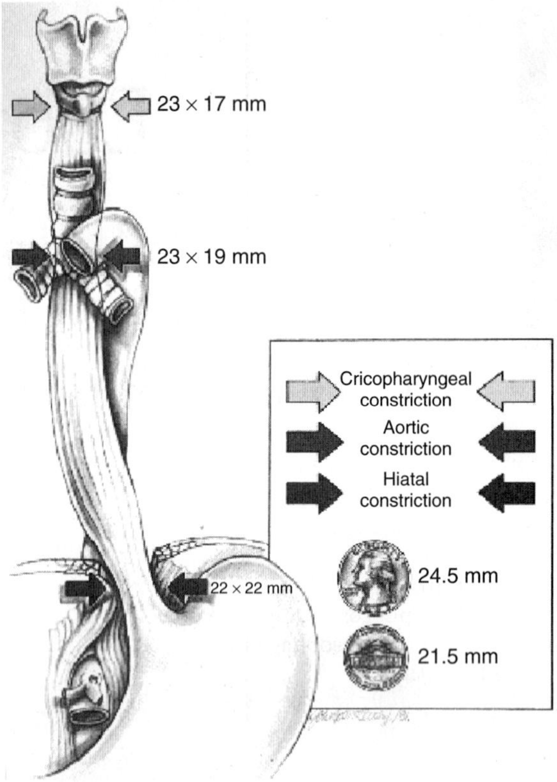

FIGURE 44A.2. Normal constrictions of the esophagus. (From Gray et al.,[272] with permission.)

distance from the cricopharyngeus to the lower esophageal sphincter (LES).

Normal Constrictions

At rest, the esophagus is collapsed and in its proximal two-thirds is flat with a diameter of 2.3 × 1.9 cm. At its lower end, the esophagus is rounded with a diameter of 2.2 × 2.2 cm. Compression by adjacent structures or muscles causes normal constrictions (Fig. 44A.2) that are evident on a barium esophagogram or during esophagoscopy. The most proximal constriction represents the narrowest portion of the entire gastrointestinal (GI) tract and occurs at the beginning of the esophagus where the cricopharyngeal musculature is located. The next constriction is located 20 cm from the incisors and is the result of indention of the esophagus by the aortic arch and the left mainstem bronchus. The lowermost narrowing, which is not constant, is located at about 44 cm from the incisors and is caused by the gastroesophageal sphincter mechanism. Ingested foreign bodies tend to lodge at these points of normal constriction; also, the transit of swallowed corrosives slows at these narrowings, leading to prominent mucosal injury at these sites.

Structure

The esophagus consists primarily of three layers (Fig. 44A.3). The outer layer, the muscularis externa, comprises the chief muscles of the esophagus and is made up of an internal circular muscle layer and an external longitudinal muscle layer. In the upper third of the esophagus, both layers are primarily striated (voluntary) muscle fibers. In the middle third of the esophagus, striated and smooth (involuntary) muscle fibers are intermingled, and in the lower third, smooth muscle fibers predominate. Most of the clinically significant esophageal motility disorders involve only the smooth muscle portion of the esophagus; thus, esophageal myotomy for the management of most esophageal motor disorders needs only to extend along the lower esophagus. Two bundles of longitudinal muscle fibers diverge and meet in the midline of the posterior esophageal wall 3 cm below the cricoid cartilage. This V-shaped area along the posterior wall of the proximal esophagus covered only with circular muscle fibers represents a potential weak area for subsequent diverticula formation (see the section Esophageal Diverticula). The esophagus is lined internally with a thick layer of nonkeratinizing, stratified squamous epithelium continuous with the lining of the oral pharynx. The squamous epithelium of the esophagus meets the junctional columnar epithelium of the gastric cardia in a sharp transition called the Z-line, typically located

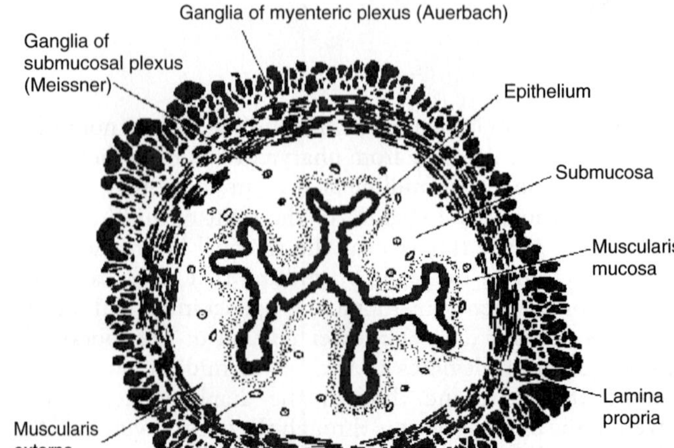

FIGURE 44A.3. Cross section of the esophagus showing the layers of the wall. (From Jamieson,[273] with permission.)

at or near the physiological LES. The submucosa contains elastic and fibrous tissue and is the strongest part of the esophageal wall. It is this layer that contains the lamina propria, which the surgeon relies on for a sound esophageal anastomosis. Meissner's plexus of nerves also resides within the submucosal layer.

Vessels

Arterial

The arterial blood supply to the esophagus is segmental with three main sources supplying the upper, middle, and lower sections of the esophagus (Fig. 44A.4). The cervical esophagus receives blood from the superior thyroidal artery as well as the inferior thyroidal artery of the thyrocervical trunk, and both sides communicate through a rich collateral network. The thoracic portion of the esophagus is supplied proximally by two to three bronchial arteries and distally from esophageal arteries arising directly from the aorta. The abdominal esophagus receives blood from branches of the left gastric and inferior phrenic arteries. At some distance from the esophagus, these main arteries divide into minute branches, and after entering the wall of the esophagus, arterial branches assume right angles to their entry point, thereby establishing a longitudinal anastomosing network of vessels. This early branching and extensive collateralization between the cervical, thoracic, and gastric segments desegmentalizes the esophageal blood supply, thereby enabling mobilization of the esophagus from the stomach to the aortic arch with little ischemic effect. This rich blood supply is more than adequate for intramural anastomosis, and poor technique rather than poor blood supply is usually responsible for anastomotic failures.

Venous

The venous drainage of the esophagus follows the arterial capillary network. Longitudinally oriented periesophageal

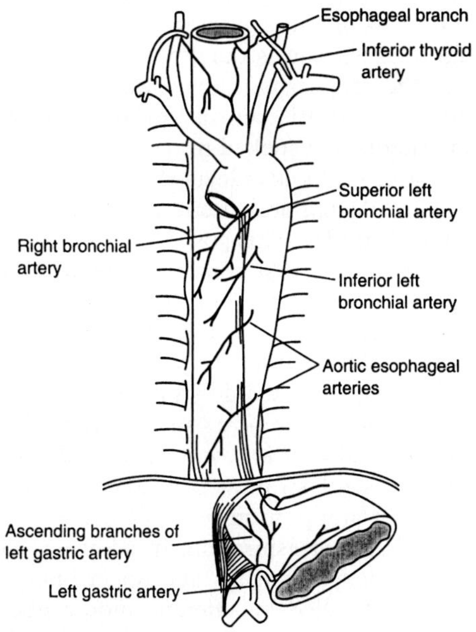

FIGURE 44A.4. Arterial blood supply of the esophagus. (From Shields,[274] with permission.)

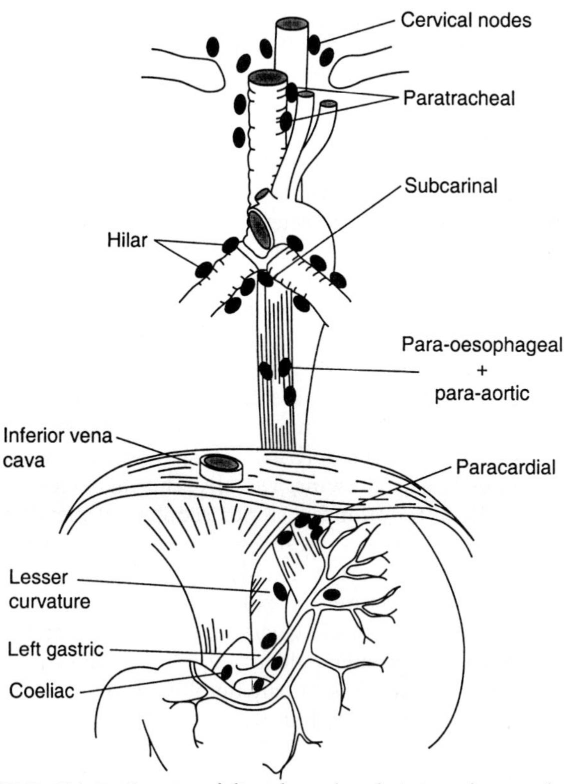

FIGURE 44A.5. Groups of lymph nodes draining the esophagus. (From Jamieson,[273] with permission.)

venous plexi return blood in the cervical esophagus to the inferior thyroid vein; in the thoracic esophagus to the bronchial, azygous, and hemiazygous veins; and in the abdominal esophagus to the coronary vein. Because the submucosal venous networks of the esophagus and stomach are in continuity with each other, portal venous obstruction may lead to collateralization through the esophageal venous plexus and subsequent esophageal varices.

Lymphatic

The lymphatic drainage of the esophagus is abundant and forms a dense submucosal plexus. Flow of lymph runs longitudinally, coursing cephalad in the upper two-thirds of the esophagus and caudad in the lower third. Because this lymphatic system is not segmental, lymph can travel a long distance in this plexus before traversing the muscle layer and entering the regional lymph nodes. As a consequence, free tumor cells of the upper esophagus can metastasize to superior gastric nodes, or conversely, a cancer of the lower esophagus can metastasize to superior mediastinal nodes. More commonly, the lymphatic drainage from the upper esophagus courses primarily into the cervical and peritracheal lymph nodes, while that from the lower thoracic and abdominal esophagus drains into the retrocardiac and celiac nodes (Fig. 44A.5).

Innervation

The esophageal neural branches are secretomotor to glands and motor to muscular layers. The esophagus has both sympathetic and parasympathetic innervation. The sympathetic nerve supply is through the cervical and thoracic sympathetic chain running downward just lateral to the spine, and the cardiobronchial and periesophageal splanchnic nerves are derived from the celiac plexus and ganglia. The parasympathetic innervation of the pharynx and esophagus is primarily through the vagus nerve. Although it carries both afferent and efferent fibers, the proportion of efferent fibers in the vagus is small in relation to the sensory component. In the neck, the superior laryngeal nerves arise from the vagus nerve and divide into the external and internal laryngeal branches. The external laryngeal nerve innervates the cricothyroid muscle and in part the inferior pharyngeal constrictor, while the internal laryngeal nerve provides sensation to the pharyngeal surface of the larynx and base of the tongue. Injury to the recurrent laryngeal nerve may cause both hoarseness and upper esophageal sphincter (UES) dysfunction with secondary aspiration during swallowing. Distally, the vagal trunks contribute to the anterior and posterior esophageal plexi, and at the diaphragmatic hiatus, these plexi fuse to form the anterior and posterior vagus nerves. Finally, a rich intrinsic nervous supply called the myenteric plexus exists between the longitudinal and circular muscle layers (Auerbach's plexus) and in the submucosa (Meissner's plexus). It appears that this intraesophageal innervation is in part involved in the fine motor control of the esophagus, but exact mechanisms of control remain unknown.

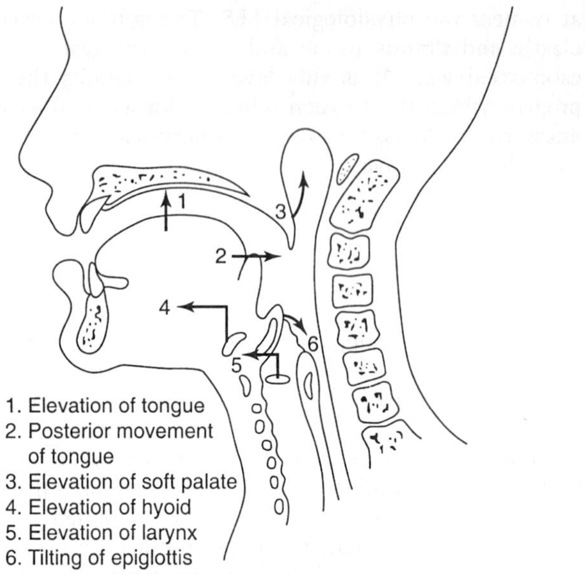

FIGURE 44A.6. Sequence of events during the pharyngeal phase of swallowing. (From Zuidema and Orringer,[275] with permission.)

Physiology

The esophagus is the first segment of the alimentary tract and the conduit between the mouth and stomach. Passage of food and drink from mouth to stomach requires a well-orchestrated series of neuromotor events. The first one-third of the distance between lips and stomach is made up of the mouth and hypopharynx; the remaining two-thirds consists of the esophagus. As nicely detailed by DeMeester et al.,[1] the mechanism of swallowing is mechanically analogous to a piston pump and cylinder with three valves that propels a bolus into a worm drive with a single valve (Table 44A.1). Failure of the pump, valves, or worm drive leads to mechanical abnormalities in swallowing such as difficulty in propelling food from mouth to stomach or regurgitation of food into the oral pharynx, nasopharynx, or esophagus.

Once initiated, swallowing is entirely a reflex. The tongue acts like a piston propelling the bolus into the posterior oral pharynx and forcing it into the cylinder of the hypopharynx. With this piston-like movement of the tongue posteriorly, the soft palate is elevated, sealing the passage between the oral pharynx and the nasopharynx. The closing of the valve of the soft palate prevents dissipation of the pressure generated within the pharyngeal cylinder through the nasopharynx and nose. Nearly concomitant with this, the hyoid bone and larynx move upward and anteriorly, bringing the epiglottis under the tongue and sealing the opening of the larynx to prevent aspiration (Fig. 44A.6). This sequence, the pharyngeal phase of swallowing, occurs within 1.5 s of initiation of a swallow. Dysfunction or paralysis of any of these interrelated actions, such as following a cerebrovascular accident, leads to discoordinated movements and regurgitation of food into the nasopharynx or aspiration.

TABLE 44A.1. Mechanical Analogies in Swallowing.

Mechanical mechanism	*Functional equivalent*
Piston pump	Tongue
Cylinder	Pharynx
Three valves	Soft palate Epiglottis Cricopharyngeus
Worm drive	Esophagus
Single valve	Lower esophageal sphincter

During the *pharyngeal phase* of swallowing, the pressure in the hypopharynx quickly rises to at least 60 mmHg, creating a sizable pressure difference between the hypopharyngeal and the less-than-atmospheric midesophageal or intrathoracic pressure. With this pressure gradient, when the cricopharyngeus or UES relaxes, food is quickly moved from the hypopharynx into the esophagus. In this way, the bolus is both pushed through peristaltic contraction of the posterior pharyngeal constrictors and sucked into the thoracic esophagus. Immediately after the bolus clears the UES, the UES closes to an immediate closing pressure of approximately twice its resting level of 30 mmHg. This post-UES contraction initiates a migrating contraction that continues down the esophagus as a primary peristaltic wave (Fig. 44A.7). The high closing pressure and progression of the peristaltic wave prevents reflux of the bolus back into the pharynx. Shortly after the peristaltic wave has migrated down the esophagus, the pressure of the UES quickly returns to its resting level. These neuromotor events always follow a rigidly ordered pattern of outflow for successful swallowing. Cerebral vascular accidents may disrupt any portion of this complex mechanism, leading to dysphagia or aspiration. In addition, the striated muscles of the cricopharyngeus and upper one-third of the esophagus are controlled by efferent motor fibers via the vagus nerve and its recurrent laryngeal branches. Damage to this neural pathway by disease (malignancy) or operative trauma may also lead to discoordinated pharyngeal swallowing and aspiration.

Once the bolus of food is propelled into the proximal esophagus, the "worm drive" of the esophagus functions to propel the food distally and into the stomach. This *esophageal phase* of swallowing requires well-coordinated motor activity to propel the food from the negative-pressure (26-mmHg) environment of the chest to the positive-pressure (16-mmHg) environment of the stomach. Peaks of a *primary* peristaltic contraction result in an occlusive pressure wave varying from 30 to 100 mmHg, with this primary peristaltic contraction moving down the esophagus at 2 to 4 cm per second (see Fig. 44A.7). The transit time from initiation of a swallow to the bolus reaching the distal esophagus is about 9 s.

A second type of peristaltic wave (*secondary* peristalsis) is not triggered by voluntary swallowing but rather refers to peristaltic waves that usually appear after esophageal dilation either from a retained bolus or from active distention of the esophagus. These secondary contractions occur without any movements of the mouth or pharynx and can occur as independent local reflexes to clear the esophagus of ingested material left behind after the passage of the primary wave. A third pattern of contractile activity, *tertiary* contractions, occurs after voluntary swallows or spontaneously between swallows. Tertiary contractions are nonpropulsive, generate peak pressures in the range of 10 to 13 mmHg, and follow 3% to 4% of all swallows.

The LES acts as the valve at the end of the worm drive of the esophageal body and provides a pressure barrier between the esophagus and stomach. Although an anatomical LES does not exist, the architecture of the muscle fiber at the junction of the esophagus and the stomach helps explain some of the sphincter-like activity of the LES. The resting tone of the LES is approximately 20 mmHg and resists reflux of gastric content into the lower esophagus. With initiation of a pharyngeal swallow, the LES pressure decreases to allow the primary peristaltic wave to propel the bolus into the stomach. A pharyngeal swallow that does not initiate a peristaltic contraction leads to relaxation of the LES, allowing reflux of gastric juice into the distal esophagus. This effect may be one explanation for the observation of spontaneous lower esophageal relaxation thought by some to be causative in gastroesophageal reflux (GER) disease. The coordinated activity of the pharyngeal swallow and LES relaxation appears to be in part vagally mediated.

The LES's intrinsic myogenic tone can be affected by both neural and hormonal mechanisms. In addition, diet and medications can alter LES function (Table 44A.2).

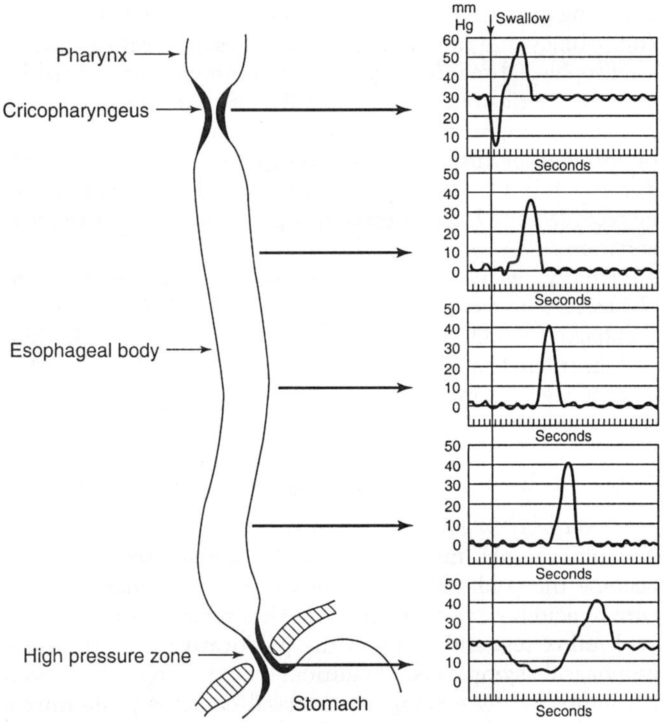

FIGURE 44A.7. Intraluminal esophageal pressures in response to swallowing. (From Waters and DeMeester,[276] with permission.)

TABLE 44A.2. Neural, Hormonal, and Dietary Factors Thought to Affect Lower Esophageal Sphincter (LES).

Increase LES pressure
Cholinergics
Prokinetics
α-agonists
β-blockers
Gastrin
Motilin
Bombesin
Substance p
Decrease LES Pressure
α-blockers
β-blockers
Calcium channel blockers
Cholecystokinin
Estrogen
Progesterone
Somatostatin
Secretin
Caffeine (chocolate, coffee)
Fats

Assessment of Esophageal Function

Although the esophagus is a hollow tube functioning primarily as a conduit between the mouth and stomach, its anatomical course through three body compartments, its complex neuromotor mechanisms for propelling a bolus from mouth to stomach, and its juxtaposition to the stomach's harsh intraluminal environment lead to a wide variety of esophageal disorders. Several diagnostic tests are available to evaluate patients with esophageal disease. Remembering the anatomical and physiological features of the esophagus, these tests can be divided into (1) tests to detect structural abnormalities, (2) tests to detect functional abnormalities, (3) tests to assess esophageal exposure to gastric content, and (4) tests to provoke esophageal symptoms (Table 44A.3).

Assessment of Structural Abnormalities

Radiologic Studies

Contrast Esophagogram

The simplest and often first diagnostic test for esophageal disease is a contrast esophagogram, most commonly a barium

TABLE 44A.3. Assessment of Esophageal Function.

Condition	*Diagnostic test*
Structural abnormalities	Barium swallow
Endoscopy	
Chest x-ray	
CT scan	
Cine fluoroscopy	
Endoscopic ultrasound	
Functional abnormalities	Manometry (stationary and 24h) Transit studies Multichannel intraluminal impedance (MII)
Esophageal exposure to gastric content	24-h pH monitoring Bravo wireless pH probe
Combined	MII-Manometry MII-pH
Provoke esophageal symptoms	Acid perfusion (Berstein) Edrophonium (Tensilon) Balloon distension
Others	Gastric analysis Gastric-emptying study Gallbladder ultrasound

swallow. Structural abnormalities including diverticula, narrowing or stricture, ulcers, and hiatal or paraesophageal hernias can all be nicely demonstrated with an esophagogram. Use of fluoroscopy with videotaped recordings during both a liquid and a solid contrast swallow increases the accuracy in identifying subtle abnormalities. Abnormalities of esophageal motility or GER can be seen during a barium swallow, but these disorders are more appropriately diagnosed using other tests.

Other Radiologic Studies

Plain chest x-ray films may reveal changes in cardiac silhouette or tracheobronchial location suggesting esophageal disorders. Computed tomographic (CT) scan of the chest or magnetic resonance imaging (MRI) may also be useful in assessing lesions thought to be malignancies identified with barium swallow or endoscopy. Finally, a modified barium study in the lateral projection under cine fluoroscopy may be especially useful in identifying mechanical disorders of the pharyngeal swallowing mechanism.

Endoscopy

Most patients with esophageal symptomatology should undergo esophagoscopy. All patients with dysphagia should undergo esophagoscopy, even in the presence of a normal barium swallow. A barium swallow performed before esophagoscopy helps the endoscopist to focus on any subtle radiographic findings and helps to prevent endoscopic misadventures with anatomic abnormalities such as esophageal diverticula.

For the initial assessment, the flexible esophagoscope allows a safe, thorough assessment, which can be performed quickly in an outpatient setting with high patient tolerance and acceptance. The mucosa of the entire esophagus, stomach, and duodenum should be carefully inspected. Any areas of mucosal irregularity or abnormality should be photodocumented and biopsied. Retroflex views within the stomach of the gastroesophageal junction (GEJ) should note the presence of hiatal hernia. The location of the transition from squamous mucosa to columnar gastric mucosa (Z-line) should be noted as the distance from the incisors to this point of transition. Known esophageal diverticula can be investigated endoscopically; however, great care should be taken because diverticula can easily be perforated.

Rigid esophagoscopy is rarely indicated and remains a tool used primarily in the operating room when cricopharyngeal or cervical esophageal lesions prevent passage of a flexible scope or when biopsies deeper than those obtainable with flexible endoscopy are needed to stage disease and plan resective therapy for malignancy.

More recently, endoscopic ultrasound (EUS) allows characterization and staging of esophageal lesions by imaging the layers of the esophageal wall and surrounding structures to identify depth of tumor invasion, periesophageal lymphadenopathy, and EUS-guided fine-needle aspiration of lymph nodes.

Assessing Functional Abnormalities

Esophageal Manometry

In recent years, esophageal manometry has become widely available and used to examine the motor function of the esophagus and the LES. Manometry is indicated when a motor abnormality is suspected on the basis of symptoms of dysphagia or odynophagia and the barium swallow and esophagoscopy do not show an obvious structural abnormality. Manometry is essential to confirm the diagnosis of primary esophageal motility disorders of achalasia, diffuse esophageal spasm, nutcracker esophagus, and hypertensive LES. It may be useful in identifying nonspecific esophageal motility disorders and motility abnormalities secondary to systemic diseases of scleroderma, dermatomyositis, polymyositis, or mixed connective tissue disease. Finally, in patients with symptomatic GER, manometry is particularly useful in assessing preoperative esophageal clearance mechanisms and competency and function of the distal esophageal sphincter.

Esophageal manometry is most commonly performed by passing a series of catheters nasally into the stomach while measuring pressure through a pressure-sensitive transducer or with autoperfused open-tipped catheters attached to transducers. Over 1 to 2h, esophageal body and LES function can be recorded and later assessed using computer-based analysis software.

Finally, esophageal transient scintigraphy proposes to objectively assess transit of a swallowed bolus through the esophagus, which would most accurately objectify normal and disordered esophageal function. The clinical use of such an esophageal "emptying study" remains unclear, and transit scintigraphy presently remains a research tool.

Assessing Esophageal Exposure to Gastric Content

Ambulatory pH Monitoring

Ambulatory pH monitoring in the distal esophagus has become the gold standard for quantitating esophageal exposure to acidic gastric content. This has replaced the standard acid reflux test and many of the provocative tests to assess esophageal symptoms. Traditionally, this test has been accomplished by placing a transnasal catheter containing a pH probe 5cm proximal to the manometrically identified distal esophageal sphincter. The esophageal pH at this loca-

TABLE 44A.4. Normal Values for Esophageal Exposure to pH <4.0 (n = 550).

Component	*Mean*	*SD*	*95%*
Total time (min)	1.51	1.36	4.45
Upright time (min)	2.34	2.34	8.42
Supine time (min)	0.63	1.00	3.45
Number of episodes	19.00	12.76	46.90
Number of episodes > 5 min	0.84	1.18	3.45
Longest episode	6.74	7.85	19.80

Source: From DeMeester and Stein.[280]

tion is then recorded continuously throughout a 24-h cycle while the patient continues his or her normal routine, including eating and usual activities. A catheter-free wireless pH monitoring system (Bravo) has now been developed that allows for 24- to 48-h ambulatory monitoring via a endoscopically placed probe that is secured to the esophageal mucosa.[2] After 48h, the catheter naturally detaches from the mucosa and is passed through the GI tract. In both studies, during the test the patient maintains a diary and records body positions, meals, and symptoms so that esophageal exposure to acid can be correlated with symptoms. At the completion of the test, the results are tallied and compared to normal values for esophageal exposure to acid (Table 44A.4). An episode of acid reflux is defined as pH less than 4.0 in the distal esophagus.

Ambulatory pH monitoring is indicated for patients who have typical symptoms of GER for whom other diagnostic tests are equivocal; atypical symptoms of GER such as noncardiac chest pain; persistent cough, wheezing, or unexplained laryngitis; or previously failed esophageal or gastric surgery with recurrent symptoms.

Provocation of Esophageal Symptoms

The acid perfusion test (Bernstein test), edrophonium (Tensilon) test, and balloon distension test to identify a relationship between symptoms and esophageal exposure to acid or motor abnormalities have been virtually replaced by 24-h ambulatory pH monitoring and esophageal manometry. The acid perfusion test is done by instilling 0.1 N HCl into the distal esophagus while the patient reports any symptoms developing during infusion. A placebo is similarly infused to differentiate symptom occurrence. In the edrophonium test, edrophonium hydrochloride is injected intravenously at a dose of 80 μg/kg. The acetylcholinase inhibitor edrophonium induces esophageal contractions, and a positive test is defined as replication of the patient's chest pain within 5 min of injection. The test is placebo controlled, and placebo should not reproduce the patient's typical chest pain. Finally, in the balloon distension test an inflatable balloon is positioned 10 cm below the UES. This balloon is gradually inflated with air and esophageal motility is simultaneously monitored. This test is considered positive when typical symptoms are reproduced with gradual distension of the balloon. Again, 24-h ambulatory pH testing and esophageal manometry have made these tests primarily of historical and academic interest only.

In evaluating a patient with esophageal symptoms, it is also important to consider the impact gastroduodenal dysfunction may have on normal lower esophageal function and other common GI problems that can mimic lower esophageal disease. A gastric-emptying study, right upper quadrant ultrasound, and cholescintigraphy may all be indicated in patients with symptomatology suggestive of esophageal disorders to rule out gastroparesis or gallbladder disease.

Combined Assessment of Structural and Functional Abnormalities and Exposure to Gastrointestinal Content

The increased availability of multichannel intraluminal impedance (MII) catheter studies has provided clinicians with a new means of evaluating esophageal bolus transit without the use of cine fluoroscopy.[3–5] An MII catheter consists of an alternating current source connected to a series of metal rings located along segments of the esophageal lumen. The impedance within a given segment is then determined by measuring the electrical resistance as a substance passes through the current established by the rings. Impedance and resistance have an inverse relationship such that a substance with minimal resistance, like air, will register a high impedance. Conversely, as fluid passes through this current, the impedance will drop. Thus, a fluid bolus can be detected as it progressively traverses segments of rings during the course of a swallow. The retrograde progression of a reflux episode can also be monitored in this fashion.

With the additional information it can provide, MII has also been combined with catheters measuring esophageal manometry (MII-EM) and pH (MII-pH), allowing for a more complete evaluation of patients with esophageal motility disorders and GER.[6,7] Combined MII-EM catheters were approved for clinical use by the Food and Drug Administration (FDA) in 2002 and have helped identify subsets of patients who have been difficult to evaluate using traditional methods. Examples include patients with ineffective esophageal motility and normal bolus transit, patients with dysphagia after fundoplication, and those with abnormal bolus transit of solids but not liquids.[8] Likewise, combined MII-pH catheters have helped further characterize patients with symptomatic nonacid GER, symptomatic gas or gas/liquid reflux, and persistent symptoms on proton pump inhibitor (PPI) therapy.[9,10] Although the utility and therapeutic implications of these new findings are still under review, combined MII-EM and MII-pH studies continue to help physicians refine their knowledge of the various manifestations of esophageal disease.

Assessment of Esophageal Symptoms

Appropriate identification and evaluation of esophageal abnormalities relies on a thorough understanding of the patient's symptoms and how these symptoms relate to various disorders. Table 44A.5 lists patient symptoms that may be attributable to esophageal disorders. The occasional occurrence of any of these symptoms is common in everyone and usually does not indicate disease. However, frequent and persistent symptoms, especially those of heartburn, dysphagia, or odynophagia, should immediately suggest an esophageal cause that requires further investigation and treatment.

TABLE 44A.5. Patient Symptoms and Likely Etiologies.

Symptom	*Definition*	*Likely etiology*
Heartburn	Burning discomfort behind breast bone Bitter acidic fluid in mouth Sudden filling of mouth with clear/salty fluid	Gastroesophageal reflux (GER)
Dysphagia Inflammatory process Diverticula Tumors	Sensation of food being hindered in passage from mouth to stomach	Motor disorders
Odynophagia	Pain with swallowing	Severe inflammatory process
Globus sensation	Lump in throat unrelated to swallowing	
Chest pain Motor disorders Tumors	Mimics angina pectoris	GER
Respiratory symptoms Diverticula Tumors	Asthma/wheezing, bronchitis, hemoptysis, stridor	GER
Ear/nose/throat symptoms Diverticula	Chronic sore throat, laryngitis, halitosis, chronic cough	GER
Rumination Inflammatory process Diverticula Tumors	Regurgitation of recently ingested food	Achalasia into mouth

Motor Disorders of the Esophagus

Disordered motor function of either the pharyngeal or esophageal phase of swallowing leads to a variety of swallowing disorders, with the primary clinical manifestation being dysphagia. The development and widespread use of esophageal manometry has allowed the characterization of both normal and abnormal motor function of the esophagus.

Disordered Pharyngeal Swallowing

Diseases affecting pharyngoesophageal function produce a characteristic type of dysphagia. Patients experience the more universally understood symptom of "difficulty in swallowing," with difficulty propelling food out of the mouth and through the hypopharyngeal region into the esophageal body. Aspiration or nasopharyngeal regurgitation are frequent outcomes.

Disorders of the pharyngoesophageal phase of swallowing are rare and are usually a consequence of (1) inadequate oral pharyngeal bolus transit, (2) inability to pressurize the pharynx, (3) inability to elevate the larynx, or (4) discoordination of the cricopharyngeus. Table 44A.6 lists conditions that can disrupt the carefully coordinated steps in the pharyngeal phase of swallowing.

TABLE 44A.6. Classification of Disordered Pharyngeal Phase of Swallowing.

Muscular diseases (dermatomyositis, polymyositis, etc.)
Central nervous system disease (cerebrovascular accident, multiple sclerosis, amyotrophic lateral sclerosis (AMLS), brainstem tumor, etc.)
Miscellaneous Structural lesions Cricopharyngeus dysfunction

Diagnosis

The diagnosis of disordered pharyngoesophageal swallowing relies on a strong suspicion of disordered swallowing based on a carefully taken history. Dysphagia immediately following initiation of a swallow, associated with coughing or nasopharyngeal regurgitation, will predominate. This should be distinguished from globus sensation, in which the patient has the feeling of fullness in the throat that is not associated with swallowing.

The short duration of the oropharyngeal phase of swallowing makes the evaluation of abnormalities in this region difficult using conventional radiographic or manometric techniques. The single most objective measure in assessing oropharyngeal dysfunction is the modified barium swallow in which the barium is thickened, and during swallowing a fluoroscopic recording in the lateral projection is made to document bolus passage from the mouth, through the oral pharynx, and into the esophageal body. Careful slow-motion review of this study allows identification of abnormalities in any of the previously listed steps of oropharyngeal swallowing. In addition, all patients should undergo an endoscopic evaluation to rule out structural abnormalities or malignancy.

Treatment

Once identified, most disorders of pharyngoesophageal swallowing are managed with diet modification and swallowing retraining. Cricopharyngeus dysfunction may lead to conditions amenable to operative therapy (see section on esophageal diverticula).

Disordered Esophageal Body and Lower Esophageal Sphincter

Motor disorders of the esophageal body or LES lead to a variety of functional abnormalities of the esophagus.

TABLE 44A.7. Motor Disorders of the Esophagus.

Primary
Achalasia
Spastic disorders
Diffuse and segmental spasm
Nutcracker esophagus
Hypertensive LES
Secondary
Collagen vascular diseases
Scleroderma, polymyositis, dermatomyositis, systemic lupus erythematosus, mixed connective tissue disease
Idiopathic intestinal dysmotility/pseudoobstruction
Neuromuscular diseases
Multiple sclerosis, Huntington's chorea, amyotrophic lateral sclerosis, myotonic dystrophy, cerebrovascular accident
Endocrine and metabolic
Diabetes, hypothyroidism, myasthenia gravis
Other
Trauma or operative nerve injury, radical neck surgery/radiation

These disorders can be either primary or secondary (Table 44A.7).

Achalasia

Achalasia is characterized by an absence of esophageal peristalsis and failure of the LES to completely relax on swallowing. Primary achalasia is the result of one or more neural defects, with the most common neuroanatomical change being the decrease or loss of myenteric ganglion cells or function.[2,11,12] Investigations of patients with vigorous achalasia, considered by most to be an early stage in the disease process, have revealed only mild inflammation and preservation of myenteric ganglion cells,[13] suggesting that achalasia develops as a primary inflammatory process that progresses from neuritis and ganglionitis to fibrosis with secondary ganglion cell and nerve damage. This may be triggered by an autoimmune process as associations with class II major histocompatibility complex antigens such as HLA-DQw1, HLA-DQB1 and HLA-DRB1 have been noted.[14,15]

Histological analysis has revealed selective inhibitory denervation of vasoactive peptide and nitric-oxide-producing neurons of Auerbach's plexus as well as Wallerian degeneration within the vagus nerve.[16,17] These findings support the hypothesis that the pathophysiology of achalasia is based on a decrease in inhibitory innervation in the esophageal body and LES, leading to an imbalance between the inhibitory and excitatory cholinergic tone of the LES. Such an imbalance may be responsible for the absence of LES relaxation characteristic of achalasia as well as the aperistalsis observed within the smooth muscle portion of the esophagus.[18–21] However, a full understanding of the morphological changes in achalasia is limited by the fact that most studies rely on tissue specimens from esophageal resections most commonly performed for end-stage disease. As newer animal and cellular models are developed, the underlying pathophysiology of achalasia remains under active investigation.

Achalasia has an incidence of 0.4 to 1.1 per 100,000 and a prevalence of 8 per 100,000. Given the limited access to manometry in community settings worldwide, these figures are based on primarily retrospective reviews of hospital records. Overall, this is likely to underestimate the true incidence worldwide.[22] It has been described in those from infants to the elderly, with the majority of patients presenting between the ages of 20 and 40 years. There is no sex predilection. Familial cases have been identified,[23,24] primarily in the pediatric population, with the role of genetic factors remaining unclear. The autosomal recessive disorder known as Allgrove syndrome (consisting of achalasia, alacrima, and Addison deficiency) has been linked to mutations of the AAAS gene located on chromosome 12q13. Although reports of disease presentation within the second and third decades of life have been noted,[25–27] the relationship between the AAAS gene and primary achalasia have not been established.

Achalasia is considered a risk factor for esophageal malignancy.[28,29] It is estimated that squamous cell carcinoma develops on average 20 years after initial diagnosis in approximately 5% of patients with achalasia. Esophageal carcinoma presents in achalasia approximately 10 years earlier than in the general population, and the prognosis of esophageal carcinoma in achalasia patients is worse than that in the general population, possibly because early symptoms of malignancy mimic achalasia and delay diagnosis.

Diagnosis

Patients typically present with solid food dysphagia and varying degrees of liquid dysphagia. Often, exacerbation of their dysphagia is brought on with ingestion of cold liquids or emotional stress. Symptom onset is gradual, with the average duration of dysphagia before presentation 2 years; 60% to 90% of patients report experiencing regurgitation, and nearly half complain of chest pain. Long-standing disease may be accompanied by heartburn as a result of bacterial fermentation of food retained in the dilated esophagus.[30] A diverticulum of the distal esophagus may develop secondary to the chronic functional obstruction at the LES.

Despite its rarity, the diagnosis of achalasia is seldom difficult.[31,32] The typical symptoms of dysphagia and regurgitation prompt the performance of a barium swallow, revealing the typical bird's beak deformity in the distal esophagus with more proximal esophageal dilation (Fig. 44A.8); 90% of

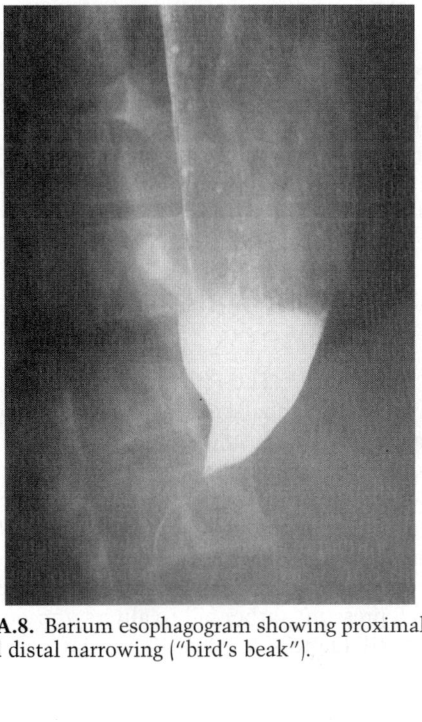

FIGURE 44A.8. Barium esophagogram showing proximal esophageal dilation and distal narrowing ("bird's beak").

patients with achalasia have this typical radiographic finding.[33] This typical esophagogram may also be found with *pseudo-achalasia*, a condition in which compression by intrinsic or extrinsic masses may mimic the classic radiographic findings of achalasia.[34] Pseudoachalasia is typically seen with gastroesophageal malignancies or as part of a paraneoplastic syndrome.[35,36] Finally, vigorous achalasia, an early stage of achalasia, may present with strong tertiary esophageal contractions resulting in a radiographic appearance similar to diffuse esophageal spasm.[37]

Even with the typical patient presentation and radiographic findings, upper GI endoscopy is vital to rule out causes of pseudoachalasia and to investigate the esophageal mucosa and integrity of the GEJ before initiating any therapy (e.g., the finding of candidiasis would dictate antifungal therapy before further treatment of achalasia). The classic endoscopic picture is that of a dilated, patulous esophageal body tapering down to a puckered LES that fails to open with air insufflation. However, the endoscope usually passes the LES easily with minimal force or pressure.

Esophageal manometry remains the gold standard for diagnosing achalasia, characterized by absent peristalsis in the distal smooth muscle segment of the esophagus with incomplete LES relaxation.[38] While an elevated LES pressure (greater than 35 mmHg) may be seen, it is the incomplete sphincter relaxation that is characteristic, occurring in more than 80% of patients with achalasia. The manometric finding of normal esophageal motility should prompt an aggressive search for a tumor that may be causing pseudoachalasia. Generally, a CT scan of the chest or endoscopic ultrasonography of the distal esophagus will identify the cause of pseudoachalasia.

Additional studies may be helpful in confirming the diagnosis of achalasia. Radionuclide studies using a labeled semisolid meal have been used to demonstrate impaired esophageal transit.[39] This study lacks the specificity of manometry[26] but has been used by some when manometry was not available or to objectively assess the response to therapy.

Treatment

The primary therapies for achalasia, aimed at decreasing LES resistance to the passage of a swallowed bolus, include (1) pharmacological therapy, (2) botulinum toxin (Botox) injection into the LES, (3) balloon dilation of the LES, or (4) operative myotomy. Predictors of long-term response to therapy include an LES pressure less than 10 mmHg or 50% to 90% esophageal emptying at 2 min after upright swallowing of a radiolabeled liquid meal.[40] Although these measures have investigational use, to date the most clinically useful measure of successful treatment of achalasia is the elimination of dysphagia.

Pharmacotherapy. The agents traditionally used to treat patients with achalasia have been smooth muscle relaxants aimed at decreasing LES tone, including calcium channel blockers (nifedipine, verapamil); opioids (loperamide); nitrates (isorsorbide dinitrate); and anticholinergics (cimetropium bromide). In prospective randomized trials, each of these medications has been shown to reduce LES tone in patients with achalasia.[41–49] These drugs, while effective in reducing LES pressure, either fail to alter symptoms[49] and are poorly tolerated due to side effects[43,48] or have no sustainable effects.[44,47] Given these results and the excellent results obtained with other modes of therapy, pharmacotherapy is best reserved as an adjunct to the other therapies or for those patients not candidates for other, more effective treatments.

Botulinum Toxin. Botulinum toxin (Botox) is a potent inhibitor of acetylcholine release from presynaptic nerve terminals and has been used in the management of skeletal disorders such as blepharospasm and dystonias with minimal side effects. Recently, Botox (between 50–200 IU) endoscopically injected into the LES has been used in the management of achalasia to decrease resting LES tone (Table 44A.8).

Botox appears to be a fairly effective form of therapy, at least in the short term. Advantages include its safety, ease of administration, and minimal side effects. Disadvantages include the lack of response in approximately one-third of patients, the need for multiple injections to possibly effect a long-term response, and decreasing response after multiple injections. Of particular concern to surgeons is the impact Botox injection may have on future operative myotomy. Obliteration of the dissection plane between the submucosa and muscular layer may increase the likelihood of esophageal perforation during operative myotomy (Table 44A.9).[50,51]

The exact role of Botox injection in the overall management of achalasia remains to be defined. It may be particularly useful in patients who are not candidates for other therapies with proven long-term results. Specifically, several prospective studies have evaluated the utility of Botox injection in the elderly. Bassotti and colleagues reviewed their experience in 33 patients (aged 81–94) noting that 78% of patients had alleviation of symptoms after 1 year.[52] Notably, 54% of patients continued to be symptom free after 2 years. This finding is consistent with those of Zarate et al., who noted that the mean duration of symptom relief in patients over 65 was approximately 14 months.[53]

Esophageal Dilation. Pneumatic dilation is considered the standard nonoperative therapy for achalasia. In many

TABLE 44A.8.

Selective Review of Cited Experiences Using >80 U Botulinum Toxin (Botox) for Treatment of Adults with Achalasia (Studies with 20 or More Subjects).

Author	*Year*	*No. patients*	*Response 1 mo (%)*	*Response 6 mo (%)*
Pasricha[177]	1995	31	90	66
Fishman[178]	1996	60	70	—
Cuilliére[179]	1997	55	75	60
Wehrmann[180]	1999	20	80	70
Kolbasnik[181]	1999	30	77 (3 mo)	57
Prakash[182]	1999	42	80	81
Annese (100 U[a])[183]	1999	38	84	57
Annese (200 U)[183]	1999	40	88	36
Allescher[184]	2000	23	83	30 (24 mo)
Storr[185]	2002	40	7 (3 mo)	7
D'Onofrio[186]	2002	37	84	65
Martinek[187]	2003	49	83	41 (22 mo)

p, prospective clinical series; pr, prospective randomized trial.
[a]Study with different groups based on treatment dose.

TABLE 44A.9.
Review of Cited Experience with Operative Myotomy After Prior Endoscopic Therapy.

Author	*No. patients*	*Type of treatment*	*Results*
Ferguson[188] 1996	49	PD	No perforations; no difficulties in dissection
Morino[189] 1997	7	PD	28% esophageal perforation rate
Horgan[190] 1999	34	PD/Botox	13% esophageal perforation rate in Botox group; 2.4% perforation rate in non-Botox with previous PD; 53% difficult dissection in Botox group
Patti[191] 1999	28	PD/Botox	5% esophageal perforation rate in pneumatic dilation group; 0% perforation in nonresponding Botox group; 50% esophageal perforation rate in responding Botox group
Ponce[192] 1999	31	PD	6% esophageal "small mucosal breach"
Gockel[193] 2004	19	PD	No intraoperative or postoperative complications
Rosemurgy[194] 2005	207	PD/Botox	5% esophageal perforation rate
Portale[195] 2005	45	PD/Botox	Perforation rate: 5.3% pneumatic dilation, 3.8% Botox ± PD, 3.9% primary surgery
Smith[196] 2006	154	PD/Botox	9.7% gastric and esophageal perforations; 19.5% failure of myotomy

Botox, botulinum toxin; PD, pneumatic dilation.

institutions, it is considered the overall treatment of choice. The objective of forced dilation of the esophagus is to break the muscle fibers of the LES and thereby decrease LES tone. Response to pneumatic dilatation is variable, with most studies documenting response rates between 60% and 80%.[54–58] However, a decrease in LES pressure does not always correspond to improvement in clinical symptoms,[59] and up to 50% of patients with initial good response to dilation have recurrence of their symptoms within 5 years of treatment.[60] Fortunately, patients who respond to dilation appear to respond equally well to a second session. Although pneumatic balloon dilation is considered by many to be the most effective nonoperative therapy for achalasia, dilation carries a risk of esophageal perforation with devastating effects, and the long-term effectiveness of dilation falls short of the long-term results following operative myotomy (Table 44A.10). Given these findings, dilation may be appropriate in select patients who require only a short-term response (limited life expectancy).

TABLE 44A.10.
Review of Cited Experience Using Balloon Dilation Versus Operative Myotomy for Treatment of Achalasia.

Author	*No. patients*	*Results*
Felix[197] 1998 (pr)	40	Myotomy, lower LESP, less GER; otherwise, no difference
Csendes[198] 1989 (pr)	81	Myotomy, 95% improved at 65 mo Dilation, 65% improved at 58 mo
Moreno-Gonzalez[199] 1988 (ret, multi)	1416 320	Myotomy, 82% improved Dilation, 65% improved
Okike[200] 1979 (ret)	468 431	Myotomy, 85% improved Dilation, 65% improved

GER, gastroesophageal reflux; LESP, lower esophageal sphincter pressure; multi, multi-institutional; Pr, prospective randomized; ret, retrospective.

As with Botox, prior pneumatic dilation may make subsequent operative myotomy technically more difficult as the result of esophageal scarring. The impact of morphologic changes associated with both pneumatic dilation and Botox injection on the course of operative myotomy has been addressed in several prospective series. In the larger series, the GI perforation rate was significantly higher than with operative myotomy alone (5%–10% vs. 3%–4%), with eventual myotomy failure rates reaching 20%.[51,61] Given these findings, operative myotomy is more frequently advocated as the procedure of choice.[62]

Operative Myotomy. Operative myotomy involves dividing the muscle layers of the LES while preserving the integrity of the esophageal mucosa (Fig. 44A.9). A dissection

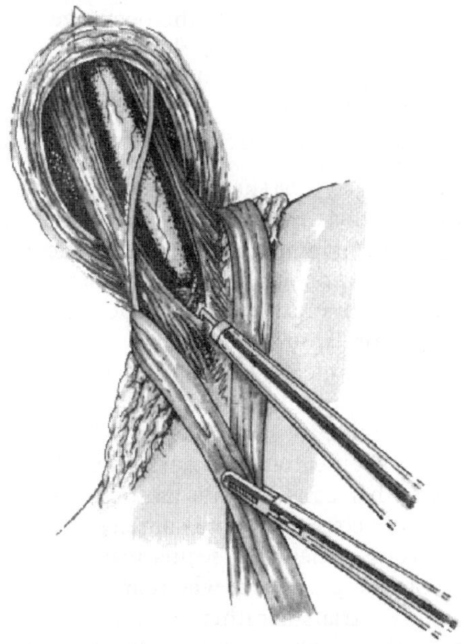

FIGURE 44A.9. Esophageal myotomy for the treatment of achalasia (Heller myotomy). (From Hunter and Richardson,[277] with permission.)

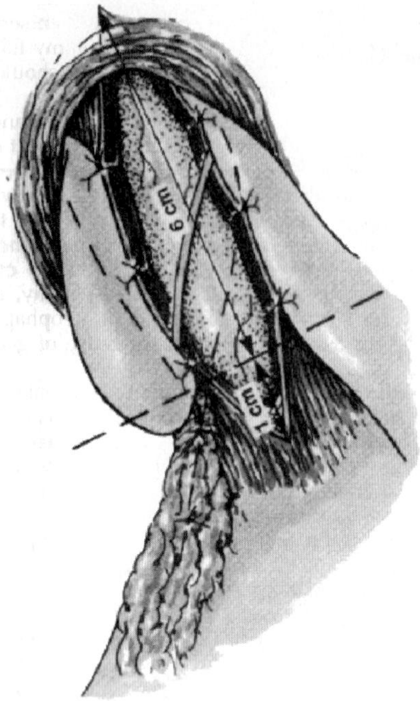

FIGURE 44A.10. One hundred eighty degree fundoplication performed in association with esophageal myotomy. (From Hunter and Richardson,[277] with permission.)

plane is usually easily developed in the submucosa where the overlying muscle fibers can be transected. An antireflux procedure often accompanies the esophageal myotomy (Fig. 44A.10). The length of the myotomy should extend 6 to 7 cm above the GEJ with distal extension 1 to 3 cm onto the stomach. A more aggressive distal extension (up to 3 cm) has been associated with less postoperative dysphagia and a more marked decrease in LES pressure.[63] Esophageal myotomy has been performed either through the chest or abdomen, using both open and minimally invasive techniques.

Although the results of operative myotomy by nearly all reports are superior to other modes of therapy, there remain several unanswered questions in the operative management of achalasia. A careful review of the data just summarized raises several issues: (1) Who should be offered operative myotomy? (2) Which operative approach should be used? (3) Should an antireflux procedure accompany a myotomy?

Who Should Be Offered Operative Myotomy? A careful review of the data does not answer the question of who should be offered operative myotomy. Generally, there are four groups for whom one should consider myotomy. The first is young patients for whom a single intervention with the best long-term result is the most effective overall. Pneumatic dilation is clearly less effective in younger patients, and because of the short duration of its effect, treatment with Botox is less desirable for young patients. The second group is those who have failed either Botox or pneumatic dilation. It is not clear what constitutes a failure of these therapies because they can be repeated with some increase in response with successive treatments. It seems reasonable to offer an operative myotomy to a patient who is an operative candidate and has failed two trials of either nonoperative therapy. The third group is patients who are at excessive risk for esophageal perforation with pneumatic dilation, including patients with a tortuous esophagus, esophageal diverticula, or previous GEJ surgery. These same conditions will also limit endoscopic access for Botox injection. Finally, there is an increasing number of patients who are looking for more lasting therapy and wish to avoid multiple interventions. The success of laparoscopic approaches to GER and hiatal hernia is now prompting patients to seek out "minimally invasive" therapies that have a low complication rate and lasting results for achalasia.

Which Technique of Operative Myotomy Should Be Used? Excellent results have been obtained with both the open transthoracic and the transabdominal approaches. Recent success with laparoscopic myotomy has shown the laparoscopic approach to be comparable to open myotomy, with enhanced postoperative recovery and shorter hospital stay.[64] The laparoscopic approach has nearly replaced the open transabdominal approaches. Similarly, the excellent results with open transthoracic myotomy have been reproduced with a thoracoscopic approach, thereby minimizing the postoperative consequences of a thoracotomy. Failures following a thoracic approach have largely been related to the development of GER because most transthoracic techniques are not accompanied by an antireflux procedure.

Which approach is used depends on the individual surgeon's comfort and experience in performing any of these techniques. The data do not clearly support any technique over another, although the laparoscopic technique of operative myotomy currently appears to be the most widely applied and reproducible. This trend will continue as surgeons become more familiar with minimally invasive techniques, newer instumentation is developed, and new modes of therapy are realized (e.g., robotic and computer-enhanced techniques).[65,66] Performance of safe and effective cardiomyotomy continues to be a source of active investigation.

Should an Antireflux Procedure Accompany Myotomy? The two most common reasons for a poor outcome following operative myotomy are persistent dysphagia or GER. The occurrence of each of these may reflect differences in operative approach or technique. Typically, a transabdominal myotomy is likely to be carried not only across the LES but also down onto the cardia of the stomach for a distance of 3 cm. In those series in which a transabdominal myotomy without an antireflux procedure is performed, rates of postoperative dysphagia are low and of GER are high. When an antireflux procedure is added, GER rates decrease. Conversely, a transthoracic myotomy is likely to go across the LES and for a shorter distance along the gastric cardia (typically 1 cm). When a shorter distal myotomy is performed, GER rates are lower, and dysphagia rates are increased. The use of a fundoplication adds operative time, and its use has primarily been based on surgeon preference. Further, the evidence suggested by a number of retrospective and prospective reviews has done little to settle the controversy (Table 44A.11).

However, two recent randomized prospective controlled trials have revealed that a significant number of patients undergoing cardiomyotomy with a distal extension of greater than 1 cm experience a significantly higher number of reflux episodes if a fundoplication is not included. Results based on both objective (pH probe, esophagogastroduodenoscopy [EGD]) and subjective (symptom scores of GER and dysphagia) measures have now led many to advocate for the addition of a

TABLE 44A.11.
Review of Studies Evaluating Antireflux Procedure After Heller Myotomy (>20 patients, >12 month follow-up).

Author	*Year*	*No. patients*	*Type of fundoplication*	*Length of distal myotomy*	*% with GER pH*	*% GER symptoms*
Peracchia[201]	1995	40	Anterior	2 cm	7.5 (3/40)	0 (0/40)
Raiser[202]	1996	35	6 anterior/29 posterior	2–3 cm	0 (0/18)	78 (14/18)
Hunger[203]	1997	39	7 anterior/32 posterior	1 cm	—	(1/37)
Morino[189]	1997	21	Anterior	2 cm	6 (1/17)	0 (0/17)
Kumar[204]	1998	19	None	1 cm	7 (1/15)	7 (1/15)
Patti[205]	1999	133	25 anterior/8 posterior	1–1.5 cm	17 (6/35)	—
Richards[206]	1999	30	None	1 cm	7 (1/14)	13 (2/16)
Stewart[207]	1999	55	3 anterior/2 posterior	2 cm	14 (1/7)	10 (5/49)
Zaninotto[208]	2000	100	Anterior	1–1.5 cm	7 (5/76)	3 (3/100)
Yamamura[209]	2000	24	Anterior	1–1.5 cm	14 (1/7)	0
Oelschlager[210]*	2003	52	Anterior	1.5 cm	32 (6/19)	44 (14/32)
Oelschlager[210]	2003	58	Posterior	3 cm	54 (13/24)	22 (11/50)
Falkenbach[211]* (RCT)	2003	10	None	2–3 cm	100 (9/9)	70 (7/10) (requiring medications)
Falkenback[211] (RCT)	2003	10	360°	–3 cm	25 (2/8)	11 (1/9) (requiring medications)
Richards[212]* (RCT)	2004	21	1–2 cm	None	48 (10/21)	—
Richards[212] (RCT)	2004	22	1–2 cm	Anterior	9 (2/22)	—
Diamantis[213]	2006	33	None	5 mm	0	0

*, separate group from trial; RCT, randomized controlled trial.

fundoplication after every cardiomyotomy.[67–69] Given that technique continues to vary worldwide, the optimal type of fundoplication after cardiomyotomy remains to be determined. Currently, most centers add either an anterior (Dor) or posterior (Toupet) fundoplication to the procedure.

Spastic Disorders of the Esophagus

Spastic disorders of the esophagus are primarily disorders defined by manometric abnormalities in the smooth muscle segment of the esophagus. These smooth muscle "spasms" typically consist of tertiary contractions that are simultaneous, repetitive, nonperistaltic, and often of prolonged duration and increased power. Spastic disorders of the esophagus are classically discussed as four distinct entities (diffuse esophageal spasm, nutcracker esophagus, hypertensive LES, and nonspecific esophageal motility dysfunction), but reports of evolution of one motility pattern into another suggest that these separate disorders may be within a single spectrum of motor dysfunction.

Diagnosis

Dysphagia and chest pain are the dominant presenting symptoms, with chest pain occurring in 80% to 90% of patients and dysphagia in 30% to 60%. Symptoms are often brought on by psychological or emotional stress, and before the widespread availability of esophageal motility testing many patients carried psychiatric diagnoses before their esophageal condition was identified. Often, the diagnosis of a spastic esophageal disorder becomes one of exclusion as cardiac causes on the potential role of acid reflux as an explanation for the symptom complex are ruled out. Esophageal manometry remains the gold standard for diagnosing spastic esophageal disorders (Table 44A.12).

Despite this manometric classification, the causal relationship between abnormalities in manometric parameters and symptoms remains weak. Some investigators have suggested that abnormalities on esophageal motility testing may, at best, suggest a possible cause of a patient's symptoms, with a diagnostic yield as low as 28%. Despite these controversies, it is helpful to separate these entities when considering treatment options.

Treatment

Approaches to the treatment of esophageal spastic disorders are aimed at ameliorating symptoms. Strategies have included those same therapies applied to achalasia and include phar-

TABLE 44A.12. Manometric Criteria for Spastic Motor Disorders of the Esophagus.

Diffuse esophageal spasm Intermittent normal peristalsis	Simultaneous contractions (>10% of wet swallows)
Nutcracker esophagus Normal peristalsis	High-amplitude contractions (>180 mmHg)
Hypertensive LES Normal LES relaxation Normal peristalsis	High resting LES pressure (>45 mmHg)
Nonspecific motor dysfunction Low-amplitude contractions (<30 mmHg) Abnormal waveforms Body aperistalsis with normal LES	Frequent nonpropagated or retrograde contractions

LES, lower esophageal sphincter.

macotherapy, Botox injection into the LES, balloon dilation, or operative myotomy. Due to the rarity of these conditions and the difficulty in their diagnosis, no data exist on which to base definitive statements regarding treatment. After a thorough workup and exclusion of other conditions, a trial of pharmacotherapy with smooth muscle relaxants (calcium channel blockers, nitrates, and anticholinergics) is reasonable. Because there is often a psychoemotional aspect to symptomatic episodes, reassurance and support are vital components in the care of these patients. Select patients may benefit from nonpharmacotherapy. Favorable responses to dilation and Botox have been reported in patients with diffuse esophageal spasm and hypertensive LES. Operative myotomy may be particularly effective in those with hypertensive LES and less so in patients with segmental spasm and nutcracker esophagus. Most of these patients are best treated by GI specialists (both medical and surgical) with extensive experience in managing these challenging problems.

Esophageal Diverticula

An esophageal diverticulum is an epithelial-lined mucosal pouch that protrudes from the esophageal lumen. Most esophageal diverticula are acquired and occur in adults. Esophageal diverticula are classified according to their location (pharyngoesophageal, midesophageal, or epiphrenic); the layers of the esophagus that accompany them (true diverticulum, which contain all layers, or false diverticulum, containing only mucosa and submucosa); or mechanism of formation (pulsion or traction) (Table 44A.13). Most esophageal diverticula are pulsion diverticula and are the consequence of elevated intraluminal pressure forcing the mucosa and submucosa to herniate through the esophageal musculature. Less commonly, traction diverticula develop that result from periesophageal inflammatory process adhering to the esophagus and subsequently pulling the esophageal wall as the inflammation heals and retracts. Pharyngoesophageal and epiphrenic diverticula are pulsion diverticula that are generally associated with abnormal esophageal motility, whereas midesophageal diverticula are usually traction diverticula resulting from inflammatory changes in mediastinal lymph nodes.

Pharyngoesophageal Diverticulum (Zenker's)

In 1878, Zenker reported on 27 cases of pharyngoesophageal diverticulum, and thus his name became associated with this entity. This is the most common of the esophageal diverticula, with a prevalence between 0.01% and 0.11%. It is a condition of the elderly, with 50% of cases occurring during the seventh and eighth decades of life. Pharyngoesophageal diverticula consistently arise within the inferior pharyngeal constrictor, between the oblique fibers of the thyropharyngeus muscle and through or above the more horizontal fibers of the cricopharyngeus muscle (the UES) (Fig. 44A.11). The point of transition in the direction of these muscle fibers represents an area of potential weakness in the posterior pharynx (Killian's triangle). Pharyngoesophageal diverticula appear to be acquired, as evidenced by the predominance in the elderly. Despite the acceptance of this acquired etiology, there remains considerable debate regarding the exact pathophysiology of pharyngoesophageal diverticulum formation. What most do agree on is that some degree of incoordination in the swallowing mechanism is the basis for the formation of these diverticula, with an abnormally high intrapharyngeal pressure leading to protrusion of esophageal mucosa and submucosa through Killian's triangle with subsequent diverticulum formation.

TABLE 44A.13. Classification of Esophageal Diverticula.

Diverticulum	*Location*	*Mechanism*	*Type*
Pharyngoesophageal	UES	Pulsion	False
Midesophageal	Tracheal bifurcation	Traction	True
Epiphrenic	Distal esophagus	Pulsion	False

UES, upper esophageal sphincter.

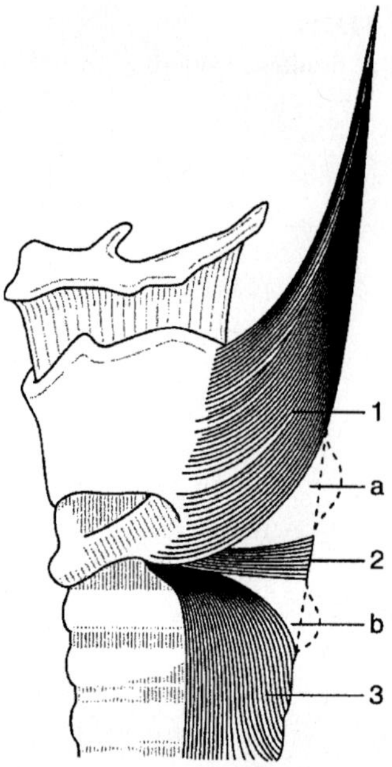

FIGURE 44A.11. The lateral aspect of the pharyngoesophageal junction: (a) site of origin of pharyngoesophageal diverticula; (b) lower weak area; (1) oblique fibers of the inferior pharyngeal constrictor; (2) cricopharyngeal muscle; (3) muscularis of the esophagus. (From Terracol and Sweet,[278] with permission.)

Inadequacies in modern esophageal manometric testing and the rapidity of the pharyngeal phase of swallowing have prevented definitive characterization of the underlying cause of these diverticula. The variety of approaches to the treatment of pharyngoesophageal diverticula reflects the uncertainty of its cause.

Diagnosis

The presenting symptoms of pharyngoesophageal diverticulum are usually characteristic and consist of cervical esophageal dysphagia, regurgitation of bland undigested food, frequent aspiration, noisy deglutition (gurgling), halitosis, and voice changes. Dysphagia is present in 98% of patients, and pulmonary aspiration is a serious consequence, occurring in up to one-third of patients. Cancer has been reported in a pharyngoesophageal diverticulum, but the frequency of this occurrence is no higher than that in the general population.

The diagnosis of pharyngoesophageal diverticulum is easily made with a barium esophagogram (Fig. 44A.12). Endos-

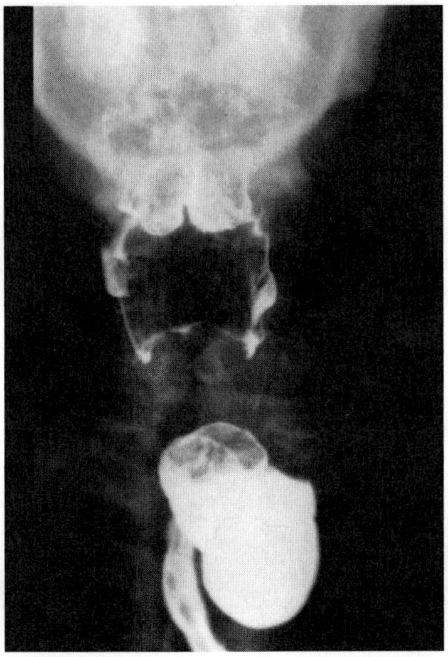

FIGURE 44A.12. Barium esophagogram showing pharyngoesophageal diverticulum.

copy, 24-h pH monitoring, and esophageal manometry are not indicated unless some feature of the symptoms or the esophagogram raise suspicion of other conditions (malignancy or GER). Although these diverticula can reach impressive sizes, it is the degree of UES dysfunction that determines the severity of symptoms, not the absolute size of the diverticulum. In most symptomatic cases, treatment is indicated regardless of the size of the diverticulum.

Treatment

As is the case with all pulsion diverticula, the proper treatment must be directed at relieving the underlying neuromotor abnormality responsible for the increased intraluminal pressure and then managing the diverticulum. Most techniques described have employed division of the cricopharyngeus muscle followed by resection, imbrication, obliteration, or fenestration of the diverticulum (Table 44A.14).

TABLE 44A.14. Treatment Options for Pharyngoesophageal Diverticula.

Treatment	*Description*
Endoscopic diverticulotomy	Endoscopic division of cricopharyngeus and common wall between diverticulum and esophagus (electrocautery, stapler, laser, etc.)
Operative myotomy and diverticulectomy	Cricopharyngeal myotomy and excision of diverticulum
Operative myotomy and diverticulopexy	Cricopharyngeal myotomy and mobilization of sac with suture fixation of the sac above neck of diverticulum
Operative myotomy alone	Cricopharyngeal myotomy only

There are no prospective randomized studies assessing the various treatments available for pharyngoesophageal diverticula. Of the retrospective studies comparing open versus endoscopic therapy, greater than 75% of patients have good results regardless of method. However, there is a trend toward a significantly higher success rate using the open approach.[70–72] Given their retrospective nature and relatively short follow-up, it remains difficult to draw final conclusions.[73] A summary of the available treatments and results available from retrospective reviews is presented in Table 44A.15. Most approaches to management agree that relief of the relative obstruction distal to the pouch through cricopharyngeal myotomy is the most important aspect of treatment. Early surgical strategies using diverticulectomy only, without myotomy, had high failure rates because of esophageal leaks from the suture line or from recurrence.[74]

TABLE 44A.15.
Summary of Results in Managing Pharyngoesophageal Diverticula.

Author	*No. patients*	*Results*	*Comments*
Endoscopic diverticulotomy			
Mattinger[214] 2002	52	85% improved	CO_2 laser
Mulder[215] 1999	167	100% improved	APC laser
Narne[216] 1999	102	96% success	Stapled
Peracchia[217] 1998	95	97% success	Stapled
Scher[218] 1998	34	94% improved	Two failures re-treated successfully endoscopically
Von Doersten[219] 1997	40	92.5% improved	
Lippert[220] 1997	37	97% improved	Laser endoscopic
Ishioka[221] 1995	42	100% improved	One to five "sessions" necessary
Wouters[222] 1992	508	92.1% improved	
Myotomy and diverticulectomy			
Gutschow[223] 2002	47	98% success	Open (most myotomy + diverticulectomy)
Bonafede[224] 1997	56	89% improved	
Witterick[225] 1995	18	83% improved	Four redos
Laing[226] 1995	65	93% improved	
Myotomy and diverticulopexy			
Lerut[227] 1992	94	92% improved	
Myotomy alone			
Schmit[228] 1992	48	87% improved	Local anesthesia
Payne[229] 1992	25	96% success	Small pouch (<4cm)

There is at present no long-term follow-up study showing the superiority of one treatment over another. Endoscopic diverticulectomy appears to be a reasonable initial therapy for most patients. Those with a small (<2 cm) symptomatic diverticulum that is difficult to approach endoscopically or a large (>10 cm) pouch extending into the mediastinum may best be served with an operative myotomy alone.[75]

Midesophageal Diverticulum

Midesophageal diverticula are rare and most commonly associated with mediastinal granulomatous disease (histoplasmosis or tuberculosis). They are thought to arise because of adhesions between inflamed mediastinal lymph nodes and the esophagus. By contraction, the adhesions exert "traction" on the esophagus with eventual localized diverticulum development. These are true diverticula, with all layers of the esophagus present in the diverticulum. Some midesophageal diverticula are related to motility disorders and represent more classic pulsion features (typically larger, false diverticulum).

Diagnosis/Treatment

A midesophageal diverticulum is typically asymptomatic and diagnosed incidentally on a barium esophagogram for other reasons. When such an asymptomatic diverticulum is found, no treatment is necessary. In patients with symptoms, esophageal manometry is indicated to search for an esophageal motor disorder. Symptomatic diverticula require treatment. When associated with an esophageal motility disorder, a small diverticulum may be treated with esophageal myotomy only. Larger diverticula usually require an accompanying resection or diverticulopexy. In the absence of a motor abnormality, diverticulectomy alone is indicated. Diverticulectomy with or without myotomy usually requires a transthoracic approach, either open or thoracoscopic.

Epiphrenic (Pulsion) Diverticulum

A fairly rare condition, an epiphrenic diverticulum typically occurs within the distal 10 cm of the esophagus and is a pulsion type. It is most commonly associated with esophageal motor abnormalities (achalasia, hypertensive LES, diffuse esophageal spasm, nonspecific motor disorders) but may be the result of other causes of increased esophageal pressure.

Diagnosis/Treatment

Most epiphrenic diverticula are symptomatic because of the underlying esophageal motor disorder. Diagnosis of the diverticulum is made during barium esophagogram (Fig. 44A.13). Manometry, esophagoscopy, and 24-h pH testing may be necessary to diagnose associated conditions and direct specific treatments. Most epiphrenic diverticula require esophageal myotomy extending from the neck of the diverticulum onto the gastric cardia for a distance of 1.5 to 3.0 cm (see section on myotomy for achalasia). Diverticulectomy, fundoplication, or repair of hiatal hernia may also be necessary depending on the size of the diverticulum or associated conditions. No prospective data or large clinical experiences are available on which to base specific treatment recommendations.

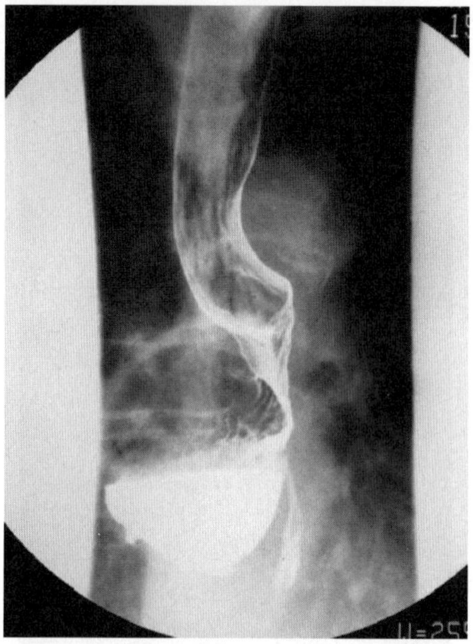

FIGURE 44A.13. Barium esophagogram showing epiphrenic diverticulum.

Gastroesophageal Reflux

Definition

Gastroesophageal reflux (GER) is defined as the failure of the antireflux barrier, allowing abnormal reflux of gastric contents into the esophagus.[76,77] It is a mechanical disorder that is caused by a defective LES, a gastric-emptying disorder, or failed esophageal peristalsis. These abnormalities result in a spectrum of disease ranging from the symptom of "heartburn" to esophageal tissue damage with subsequent complications. As diagnostic tools have become more widely available and applied, a host of extraesophageal manifestations of GER are also increasingly identified (e.g., asthma, laryngitis, dental breakdown).

Gastroesophageal reflux is an extremely common condition, accounting for nearly 75% of all esophageal pathology. Nearly 44% of Americans experience monthly heartburn, and 18% of these individuals use nonprescription medication directed against GER.[78] With a prevalence of nearly 19 million cases per year with an associated total cost of care of $9.8 billion in the United States, GER is clearly a significant public health concern.[79]

Pathophysiology: Antireflux Mechanism

Although the exact nature of the antireflux barrier is incompletely understood, the current view is that the LES, the diaphragmatic crura, and the phrenoesophageal ligament are key components.[80,81] Dysfunction of the LES is the most common cause of GER. A popular model proposed by DeMeester details three factors that determine the competence of the LES: (1) resting LES pressure, (2) resting LES length, and (3) abdominal length of the LES (Table 44A.16).

Dysfunction of the LES may be either physiological and transient or pathological and permanent. Nearly everyone experiences physiological reflux, most commonly following

TABLE 44A.16. Features of an Incompetent Lower Esophageal Sphincter.

LES characteristics	*Incompetent if:*
Resting LES pressure	<6 mmHg
Resting LES length	<2 cm
Length intraabdominal LES	<1 cm

LES, lower esophageal sphincter.

a meal, which is related to gastric distension. Postprandial gastric distension results in pressure against the LES, stretching and pulling the sphincter open while shortening the LES length. The resulting incompetence of the LES leads to transient periods of reflux. These transient episodes of reflux are relieved with gastric venting (belching) or when the stomach empties normally. Overeating exacerbates these episodes, and the high-fat Western diet may delay gastric emptying, thereby extending the duration of these transient episodes. There is accumulating evidence to suggest that this phenomenon of gastric-related transient physiological reflux leads to enough esophageal injury and subsequent LES dysfunction to progress to more permanent and pathological reflux.

Permanent failure of the LES occurs when there is structural damage to the components of the LES (resting pressure, overall length, and intraabdominal length). Any or all of these components of LES function interrelate to provide a structural barrier against reflux. Several mechanisms may account for permanent structural failure. The most popular theory proposes that, over time, physiological reflux leads to enough persistent esophageal inflammation to result in a structurally defective LES and resulting LES hypotension. However, a specific histopathological mechanism to support this proposal is lacking. As detailed above, the second component of the LES, overall sphincter length, is shortened during gastric distension, thereby further impacting LES structural function. Finally, weakening of the phrenoesophageal ligament and the development of a hiatal hernia displaces the LES into the chest, thereby altering the intraabdominal location and length of the LES. The underlying cause of hiatal hernia may relate to gastric factors (overeating) or intraabdominal factors (increased intraabdominal pressure). If one component is abnormal, then the probability of GER is 73%. If two components are abnormal, then this increases to 74%, and if all three are abnormal, 92%. Because the probability of GER does not reach 100% with complete LES dysfunction, there are clearly other components of the antireflux barrier.

Other factors affecting the pathological nature of GER include the esophageal clearance mechanism (peristalsis), the nature of the gastric refluxate, underlying gastric motor abnormalities, and mucosal protective mechanisms.[82] Poor esophageal motility and clearance prolong exposure of the esophageal mucosa to the refluxate. Hyperacidic refluxate may induce more injury, although there is mounting evidence that alkaline reflux may induce a more severe, asymptomatic esophageal injury. Gastric-emptying disorders lead to gastric distension and induce reflux through mechanical effects on the LES. Abnormalities in the esophageal mucosal protective mechanisms such as submucosal gland secretions or the quality and quantity of swallowed saliva for acid neutralization may also have an impact on esophageal acid exposure.

Finally, the diaphragmatic crura appear to play a role in the antireflux barrier. Some investigators have demonstrated a direct correlation between crural pressure and electromyographic activity of the LES, and that LES pressure can increase even when the smooth muscle of the LES is relaxed chemically.[83,84] Despite all these proposed mechanisms for GER, our understanding of the antireflux barrier and LES function, the genesis of GER, and the resulting injury is at best incomplete.

Consequences of Reflux

Gastroesophageal reflux may lead to symptoms related to the reflux of gastric content into the esophagus, lungs, or oropharynx or to damage to the esophageal mucosa and respiratory epithelium with subsequent changes related to repair, fibrosis, and reinjury. Manifestations of GER are typically classified as esophageal and extraesophageal. Esophageal manifestations of GER include heartburn, chest pain, water brash, or dysphagia (see Table 44A.5). Dysphagia often suggests a complication of GER such as esophagitis and ulceration, stricture, or Barrett's metaplastic changes. Extraesophageal manifestations are generally pulmonary, resulting from pulmonary aspiration of refluxate, or a vagally mediated reflex that induces bronchospasm when refluxate stimulates the distal esophagus. Other extraesophageal manifestations include chronic cough, laryngitis, dental damage, and chronic sinusitis.

With a better understanding of GER and new therapies for eliminating symptoms, fewer patients are presenting with complications of GER. However, those with complicated GER (grade IV esophagitis, stricture, or Barrett's mucosa) have more severe reflux, suggesting a mechanically defective LES as a major etiological factor. This problem has been the basis of offering operative therapy for complicated GER.

Diagnosis

The clinical diagnosis of GER is fairly straightforward if the patient reports the classic symptom of heartburn that is readily relieved after ingesting antacids. Many patients with this classic presentation will have been treated by their primary care physician with an empiric trial of H_2 blockers or, more commonly, PPIs. Other typical symptoms of GER include regurgitation or dysphagia. Recently, it has been appreciated that chest pain, asthma, laryngitis, recurrent pulmonary infections, chronic cough, and hoarseness may be associated with reflux, and this association is leading to increasing numbers of patients with these *atypical* GER symptoms to be evaluated for reflux. As many as 80% of patients with asthma have endoscopic evidence of GER,[85] and 50% of patients in whom a cardiac cause of chest pain has been excluded have acid reflux as a cause of their pain. Otolaryngologists are beginning to make primary referrals for the treatment of GER based on chronic laryngitis and evidence of acid-induced vocal cord damage, and dentists are identifying dental damage from chronic acid reflux.

A careful history should confirm both typical and atypical symptoms of GER and any response to medical therapy. Atypical symptoms, no response to high doses of PPIs, or patients with dysphagia, odynophagia, GI bleeding, or weight loss suggest complications of GER, or another disease process entirely, and should prompt a more thorough symptom-directed workup to look for another explanation for symptoms.

In a patient with typical symptoms, endoscopic findings of esophageal erosions, ulcers, or columnar-lined esophagus are fairly specific for GER. During EGD, esophageal mucosal biopsy should be obtained to confirm esophagitis, and esophageal length and the presence of a hiatal hernia or stricture can be assessed and may eliminate the need for a confirmatory barium swallow. With these findings, no other tests beyond EGD are necessary to diagnose GER. However, in many patients the EGD will be normal due to empiric treatment of symptoms by primary care physicians. In this setting, 24-h pH testing is necessary to objectively establish the diagnosis of GER.

Ambulatory 24-h pH monitoring has been regarded as the gold standard in diagnosing GER and is of unquestionable benefit in patients for whom the diagnosis is unclear or in those with nonerosive esophagitis. However, this test is lengthy, cumbersome, and uncomfortable, particularly for patients with severe GER, who must stop antisecretory medication for 5 to 10 days before the test. Ambulatory pH monitoring is not mandatory in patients with typical reflux symptoms and erosive esophagitis on EGD. It should be performed, however, when an objective diagnosis of GER is lacking. Barium swallow is the test of choice in evaluating the patient with dysphagia, suspected stricture, paraesophageal hernia, or shortened esophagus. Other studies may be helpful in difficult cases, such as gastric testing including gastric emptying or secretion studies in patients with significant bloating, nausea, or vomiting.

Treatment

There is considerable debate regarding optimal treatment of GER. With as many as 10% of Americans experiencing daily heartburn and the recently recognized impact this condition has on an individual's quality of life, it is no surprise that there is a tremendous amount of interest and effort going into understanding this condition and establishing treatment algorithms that are effective and cost-efficient. Since 1997, more than 2500 citations in the medical literature have concerned GER, an indication of the amount of effort and research directed toward GER.

Medical

The principles of nonoperative management of GER include lifestyle modifications, medical therapy to control symptoms, and identification of those patients who would be best served with an antireflux operation. Although lifestyle modifications have always been the initial step in therapy, only those patients with mild and intermittent symptoms seem to benefit from lifestyle changes alone. Most patients who seek medical advice will be best treated either medically or surgically.

Selection of a particular medical regimen depends on the severity of GER, effectiveness of the proposed therapy, cost, and convenience of the regimen. Numerous trials have shown that short-term treatment of GER with acid suppression regimens can effectively relieve symptomatic GER and heal reflux esophagitis; however, levels of success depend on the type, duration, and dosage of antisecretory therapy. Recurrence of esophagitis and symptoms is frequently observed; thus, treatment strategies based on effectiveness and outcome must be based on benefits achieved in long-term follow-up. Unfortunately, data on long-term outcomes for patients with GER are sparse. It appears, however, that reflux symptoms disappear only in a minority of patients with GER,[86] and patients who present with erosive esophagitis predictably follow a course of multiple relapses of the disorder. Proton pump inhibitors have profoundly changed the medical treatment of GER. Rates of healing of esophagitis have dramatically improved with PPIs when compared to H_2 receptor antagonists (H_2RAs) (Table 44A.17). However, the cost of PPIs has led many to recommend their use in only complicated or refractory GER.

TABLE 44A.17.
Healing Rates of Esophagitis: PPI Versus H_2RA.

Author	*Regimen*	*Healing rates (%)*
Klinkenberg-Knol[230] 1987	Omeprazole, 60 mg QD	88[a]
	Ranitidine, 150 mg BID	38
Havelund[231] 1988	Omeprazole, 40 mg QD	95
	Ranitidine, 150 mg BID	70
Sandmark[232] 1988	Omeprazole, 20 mg QD	85
	Ranitidine, 150 mg BID	50
Vantrappen[233] 1988	Omeprazole, 40 mg QD	96
	Ranitidine, 150 mg BID	52
Lundell[234] 1990	Omeprazole, 40 mg QD	90
	Ranitidine, 150 mg BID	47

H_2RA, H_2 receptor antagonist; PPI, proton pump inhibitor.
[a]$P < .05$.

Historical treatment algorithms have used a stepwise approach using the least-effective regimen first and intensifying therapy only if necessary. With the availability of strong antacids over the counter and public awareness of GER and its treatment, many patients self-medicate for long periods of time before seeking medical attention. Thus, presently it may be appropriate to immediately escalate therapy to the most effective medical regimen or surgery. The associated costs of these more effective regimens cannot be overlooked when initiating treatment. There are no contemporary prospective studies from which to make definitive recommendations regarding medical management of GER or medical versus surgical management. Treatment algorithms based on endoscopic findings are shown in Figures 44A.14 and 44A.15.

Surgical

Medical therapy is the first line of management for GER. Esophagitis heals in approximately 90% of cases with intensive medical therapy. However, medical management does not address the condition's mechanical etiology; thus, symptoms recur in more than 80% of cases within 1 year of drug withdrawal.[78] In addition, although medical therapy may effectively treat the acid-induced symptoms of GER, esophageal mucosal injury may continue because of ongoing alkaline reflux.[87] Because GER is a chronic condition, medical therapy involving acid suppression or promotility agents may be

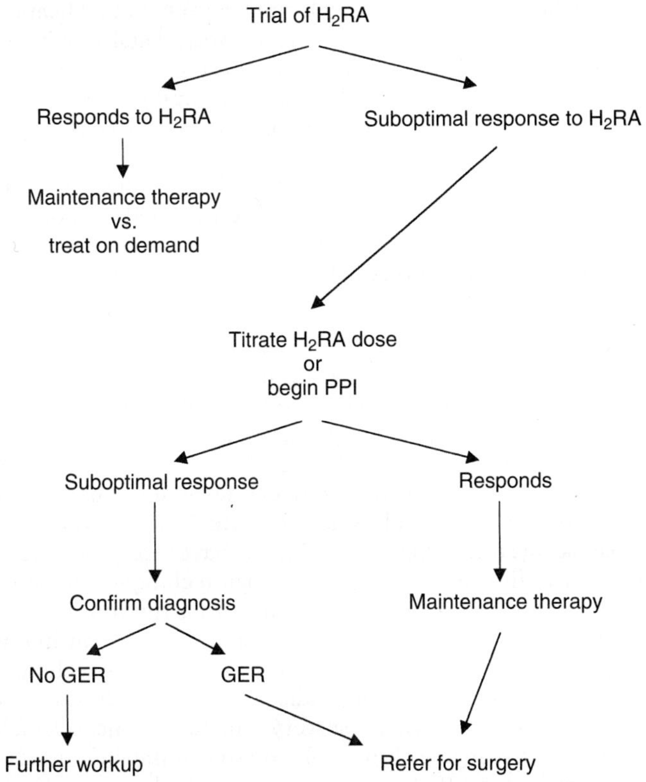

FIGURE 44A.14. Management algorithm for treatment of uncomplicated gastroesophageal reflux (based on endoscopic findings). GER, gastroesophageal reflux; H_2RA, H_2 receptor antagonist; PPI, proton pump inhibitor. (After Fennerty et al.[279])

required for the rest of a patient's life. The expense and psychological burden of a lifetime of medication dependence, undesirable lifestyle changes, uncertainty regarding the long-term effects of some newer medications, and the potential for persistent mucosal changes despite symptomatic control, all make surgical treatment of GER an attractive option. Surgical therapy, which addresses the mechanical nature of this condition, is curative and durable in 85% to 93% of patients.[88–93] Chronic medical management may be most appropriate for patients with limited life expectancy or comorbid conditions that would prohibit safe surgical intervention.

Historically, antireflux surgery was recommended only for patients with refractory or complicated GER.[94,95] Through the early 1990s, several major developments have changed our thinking regarding the long-term management of patients with GER. First, the introduction of PPIs provided a truly effective medical therapy for GER. Therefore, few patients have "refractory" GER. Second, laparoscopic surgery became available. The rapid postoperative recovery seen with laparoscopic cholecystectomy is now feasible following antireflux procedures. Third, the widespread availability and use of ambulatory pH monitoring has dramatically improved our ability to recognize true GER and select patients for long-term therapy. Finally, we have realized that patients with GER have a greatly impaired quality of life, which normalizes with successful treatment.[96]

With this, the management goals of GER have changed. Rather than focusing therapy only on *controlling* symptoms, modern treatment of GER aims to *eliminate* symptoms, improve a patient's quality of life, and institute a lifelong plan for management. In the 1990s, controlled trials that compared medical and surgical therapy of GER favored surgical therapy.[94,97] Within these prospective randomized comparisons, surgical treatment was significantly more effective than medical therapy in improving symptoms and endoscopic signs of esophagitis for as long as 2 years. Other longitudinal studies reported good-to-excellent long-term results in 80% to 93% of surgically treated patients.[98–107]

Although the goal of eliminating symptoms remains the primary concern, long-term follow-up of the controlled trials of the 1990s has raised questions regarding the durability of symptom control after antireflux surgery. In a follow-up to their original publication in 1992, Spechler and colleagues noted that 62% of those patients in the surgical treatment group participating in follow-up analysis took antireflux medications regularly. In addition, they found no significant difference between the medical and surgical groups in the rate of esophagitis, esophageal strictures, esophageal cancer, or overall satisfaction.[108] Others have noted a similar number of patients requiring antisecretory medications more than 10 years following surgery.[109,110] Given a small, but not insignificant, mortality rate of 0.3% and the known associations with medium- to long-term postprandial bloating and diarrhea in up to 30%–45% of patients, this has led to a reappraisal of the role of antireflux surgery.[111,112] Ultimately, these data have helped patients become more informed about their choices in instituting a lifelong management plan.

Considering the treatment goals just listed, it is appropriate to ask: (1) Who should be considered for antireflux surgery? (2) Which preoperative tests are necessary? (3) Which operation should be performed?

WHO SHOULD BE CONSIDERED FOR ANTIREFLUX SURGERY? Although it appears that the indications for antireflux surgery

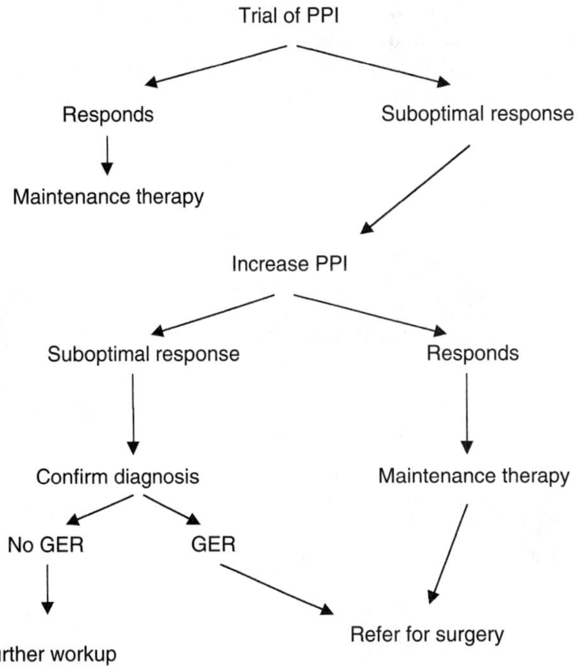

FIGURE 44A.15. Management algorithm for treatment of complicated gastroesophageal reflux (based on endoscopic findings). GER, gastroesophageal reflux; PPI, proton pump inhibitor. (After Fennerty et al.[279])

have changed, this should not be true. There remain two clear indications. First, antireflux surgery should be considered in patients who have failed intensive medical therapy; with the advent of PPIs, true medical failures are unusual. Second, and more commonly, antireflux surgery should be offered to patients whose symptoms recur immediately after stopping medications and thus require long-term daily medication. Many patients want to avoid the cost, inconvenience, and side effects of long-term daily medication and are eager to find alternatives that will effectively control symptoms and preserve their quality of life. Antireflux surgery effectively relieves symptoms in 93% of patients, returning an individual's quality of life to normal.[93,113]

Occasionally, GER presents atypically with chest pain, asthma, chronic cough, or hoarseness. Patients with these atypical symptoms usually improve with antireflux surgery; however, appropriate patient selection can be difficult.[114] Ambulatory pH monitoring has been thought to provide the most objective way to select these patients for surgery, but an abnormal pH study does not correlate well with symptom relief following antireflux surgery. Therefore, a trial of medical therapy with resolution of symptoms remains the best way to prove an association between GER and an individual's atypical symptoms. When such an association exists, antireflux surgery is indicated.

Finally, complications of GER such as Barrett's esophagus and esophageal stricture should not alter the approach to long-term management of these patients. However, patients with these complications usually have more severe disease and consequently require more intensive medical therapy, which may necessitate early surgical referral.

WHICH PREOPERATIVE TESTS ARE NECESSARY? The preoperative evaluation should both justify the need for surgery and direct the operative technique to optimize outcome. At a minimum, all patients considered for surgery should undergo a thorough history and physical exam, EGD, and esophageal manometry.[115]

Esophageal manometry allows evaluation of the LES and is diagnostic in differentiating GER from achalasia. Equally important is its use in assessing esophageal body pressures and identifying individuals with impaired esophageal clearance who may not do as well with a 360° fundoplication. Reliable esophageal clearance occurs with distal esophageal contractions of 30 to 40 mmHg. In those patients who have impaired peristalsis, as evidenced by mean distal esophageal pressures of 30 mmHg or less or esophageal peristalsis in 60% or fewer of wet swallows, many advocate modifying the surgical approach by performing a partial fundoplication (270° wrap). Finally, an entirely normal esophageal manometry may occur in patients with GER, but one should consider further testing when this is found.

WHICH ANTIREFLUX PROCEDURE SHOULD BE PERFORMED? The goal of antireflux surgery is to establish effective LES pressure. To realize this goal, most surgeons believe it necessary to position the LES within the abdomen where the sphincter is under positive (intraabdominal) pressure and to close any associated hiatal defect.[116] To accomplish this, various safe and effective surgical techniques have been developed (Fig. 44A.16). Since the late 1980s, advances in laparoscopic technology and technique have nearly eliminated open antireflux surgery. The laparoscopic techniques reproduce their open counterparts while eliminating the morbidity of an upper midline laparotomy incision.[117] Open antireflux operations remain indicated when the laparoscopic technique is not available or is contraindicated. Contraindications to laparoscopic antireflux surgery include uncorrectable coagulopathy, severe chronic obstructive pulmonary disease, and pregnancy. Previous upper abdominal operation, in particular prior open antireflux surgery, is a relative contraindication to a laparoscopic approach and should only be undertaken by experienced laparoscopic surgeons.

The laparoscopic Nissen fundoplication has emerged as the most widely accepted and applied antireflux operation.[113,118–123] In many centers, it is the antireflux procedure of choice in patients with normal esophageal body peristalsis. Key elements of the procedure include the complete dissection of the esophageal hiatus and both crura, mobilization of the gastric fundus by dividing the short gastric vessels, closure of the associated hiatal defect, creation of a tensionless 360° gastric wrap at the distal esophagus around a 50- to 60-French intraesophageal dilator, limiting the length of the wrap to 1.5 to 2.0 cm, and stabilizing the wrap to the esophagus by partial-

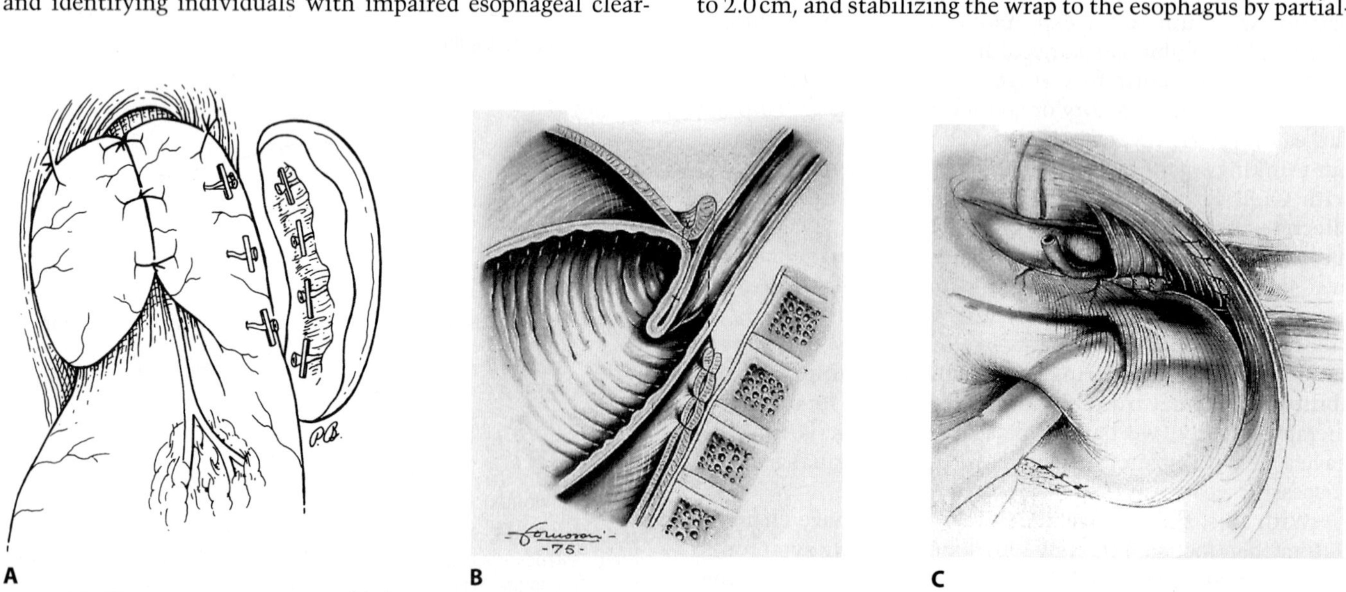

A B C

FIGURE 44A.16. Depiction of (**A**) Nissen 360° fundoplication; (**B**) Belsey 270° fundoplication; and (**C**) Hill posterior gastropexy.

thickness bites of the esophagus during creation of the wrap. Although widely accepted, these key elements have not been tested in prospective randomized trials.

Early complications have mostly been minor and infrequent. Transient dysphagia occurs in nearly 50% and resolves within 3 weeks of surgery. An infrequent early problem, but one of greater concern, has been postoperative nausea and retching. During episodes of retching, breakdown of the fundoplication can occur. Therefore, postoperative nausea should be treated aggressively. Late complications of wrap migration and paraesophageal herniation may also be related to postoperative retching but more likely result from failure to close the esophageal hiatus or a shortened esophagus. Long-term dysphagia is emerging in 10% to 15% of patients but is well accepted by patients in the context of GER symptom control. When a shortened esophagus is encountered, an esophageal lengthening procedure (Collis gastroplasty) should be used. Esophageal lengthening is rarely indicated, and its use should be balanced with the findings that 80% of patients develop uncontrollable esophagitis or pathologic esophageal acid exposure.[124]

The Toupet fundoplication (Fig. 44A.17) is identical to the Nissen except that the fundoplication is a 270° wrap rather than a 360° wrap. The gastric fundus is brought posterior to the esophagus and sutured to either side of the esophagus, leaving the anterior surface bare. This 270° fundoplication has the theoretical advantage of limiting postoperative bloating and dysphagia, especially in those with impaired esophageal body peristalsis. Many centers use the Toupet procedure exclusively in patients with abnormal esophageal peristalsis identified during preoperative esophageal manometry. Some have advocated the routine use of the Toupet fundoplication on all GER patients, which could eliminate the need for preoperative esophageal manometry in many patients. However, it appears that a partial fundoplication is not as durable as a total fundoplication, and its use in the most severe cases (grade IV esophagitis, Barrett's esophagus, stricture) is in question.[125]

Regardless of the technique used, the eightfold increase in the use of antireflux surgery since 1990 has also exposed a larger cohort of patients in whom the procedure has failed. Failure rates range from 2% to 30% depending on the definition of failure. In select cases (e.g., patients with symptomatic recurrent reflux), revisional fundoplication is offered, with most centers reporting a 3%–5% reoperation rate and a 65%–90% success rate. Wrap herniation is the leading cause of failure requiring reoperation, while wrap disruption, wrap slippage, too tight a fundoplication, and an undiagnosed motility disorder prior to the initial fundoplication are also frequently observed (Table 44A.18).[126]

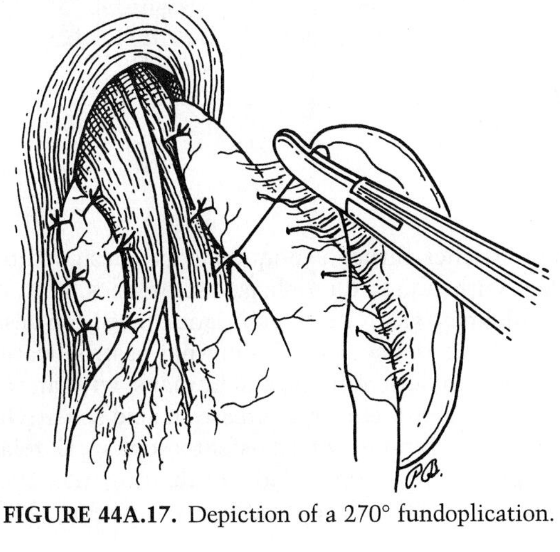

FIGURE 44A.17. Depiction of a 270° fundoplication.

To summarize, antireflux surgery is indicated in any patient with GER refractory to medical management or who has symptom recurrence when medicine is withdrawn. In many patients with classic symptoms, an EGD and esophageal manometry are all the preoperative testing necessary. Additional tests are confirmatory in difficult cases. The laparoscopic Nissen fundoplication is both safe and effective in the long-term management of nearly all patients with chronic GER. The Toupet fundoplication may be best used in patients with impaired esophageal body peristalsis.

Endoscopic Endoluminal Therapy

Despite the advances made with the advent of laparoscopy, an ideal treatment for GER that permanently alleviates symptoms, protects against esophageal erosion, and prevents malignant progression while minimizing the risk or therapy after one application remains elusive. The search for this ideal therapy has led to the development of less-invasive alternatives to medical and surgical therapy utilizing endoscopy-based endoluminal approaches. Now, those patients searching for a nonpharmacologic solution who wish to avoid surgery can opt for procedures that require no skin incisions and are often performed on an outpatient basis. The inherent allure of this approach has led several groups within industry to develop therapies designed to alter the anatomy or physiology of the GEJ via the delivery of radio-frequency energy to the GEJ, injection or implantation of devices into the cardia and LES, or suture plication of the proximal stomach.[127]

The clinical uses of radio-frequency energy have been well known for decades, ranging from the treatment of benign prostatic hyperplasia to hepatic tumor ablation. The delivery of radio-frequency energy to the esophagus and gastric cardia at a temperature of 65°C has been shown to cause collagen contraction and eventual tissue shrinkage, leading to scarring at the GEJ and neurolysis in the same region. Although a clear understanding of the mechanism of action remains to be determined, it is thought that these anatomic changes induced by radio-frequency energy delivery decrease the frequency of transient LES relaxation episodes either via interference of afferent nerve signals to the brain or by decreasing the stimulation of gastric cardia mechanoreceptors through fibrosis or direct ablation.[128–130]

In 1984, O'Conner injected Teflon paste into the EGJ of five dogs with a surgically incompetent LES in an attempt to reverse GER from within the distal esophagus. He noted that all reversed the preinjection levels of esophagitis with an improvement in reflux volume.[130a] Since that time, the concept of reversing GER using an injectable substance at the LES has been actively investigated. Like radio-frequency ablation, no clear mechanism of action has been established. However, studies using an ethylene vinyl alcohol copolymer with tantalum dissolved in dimethyl sulfide (Enteryx, Boston Scientific Corp., Natick, MA) injected into a porcine model led to an initial inflammatory reaction with eventual circum-

TABLE 44A.18.
Review of Cited Reports of Surgical Revision After Failed Fundoplication.

		Etiology of failure					
Author	*No.*	*Herniation*	*Disrupted wrap*	*Displaced/ slipped wrap*	*Esophageal motor disorder*	*Other*	*Results*
Stein[235] 1996	105/71[a]	6	48	24	10	Tight fundoplication (11); Gastric denervation (6)	86% good-to-excellent results
Floch[236] 1999	46	31	20	5	2	Other (2)	Decrease in well-being score from 8.6 to 2.9; 89% patient satisfaction
Soper[237] 1999	20/8[a]	13	1	1	—	—	—
Pointner[238] 1999	30	—	—	—	—	—	Increase in LES from 2.7 to 12.29 after 1 year; decreased DeMeester score from 57.3 to 12.2 after 1 year; QOL increase from 86.7 to 123.1 after 1 year
Awad[239] 2001	37	6	8	—	2	Tight fundoplication (7); total anatomical disruption (5); hiatal stenosis (2); other (3)	68% good-to-excellent results
Heniford[240] 2002	55	29	19	—		Too tight (3); anatomically normal (4)	92.5% good-to-excellent results with regard to dysphagia/ reflux symptoms
Granderath[241] 2003	27	—	—	—	—	—	93% very good satisfaction, 92.6% heartburn free, 93% without medications, improved QOL
Rosemurgy[242] 2004	64	52	32	13	—	Too tight (1)	79% good-to-excellent outcomes with patients with pre-operative heartburn, 73% satisfied
Byrne[243] 2005	118	26	35	6	—	Loose (2)	84% DeMeester score 0–1, 25/32 patients with dysphagia improved, 87% regurgitation score 0–1
Smith[244] 2005	300	121	16	28	—	Crural stenosis (4); twisted wrap (10); misplaced wrap (1); other (1); unknown (41)	73%–89% absent or mild heartburn/dysphagia/chest pain score; 16% unsatisfied; 17% using antisecretory medications on follow-up
Iqbal[245] 2006	104	52	43	18	1	Stenosis (5); hypertensive fundoplication (24); inadequate esophageal length (16)	Symptom resolution: 74% (dysphagia), 75% (heartburn), 85% (regurgitation), 94% (chest pain)

QOL, quality of life.
[a]Patients with recurrent reflux/patients undergoing reoperation.

ferential granulation and fibrous capsule formation (around the implant). It is hypothesized that this decreased the distensibility of the esophagus and gastric cardia, preventing shortening of the LES and possibly decreasing the number of transient lower esophageal relaxation episodes.[131–133]

The creation of intraluminal gastric pleats at the GEJ is intended to mimic the effects of a gastric fundoplication by revising the anatomic alterations affecting the gastric cardia caused by chronic GER. This is done via the deployment of staples or stitches through unique devices designed to work in tandem with standard esophagogastroscopes. Both partial- and full-thickness gastropexy techniques have been described. The physiologic impact of intraluminal gastroplication has been observed in both animals and humans, with an immediate increase in LES pressure, decrease in acid sensitivity, and decrease in the number of transient esophageal relaxation episodes detected. In one study evaluating the effects of partial-thickness suture application in humans, 24-h acid

TABLE 44A.19.
Cited Cohort Studies Evaluating Endoscopic Endoluminal Therapies.

Author	No. patients	Months follow-up	Significant improvements	No significant change
Radio-frequency ablation				
Richards[246] 2001	25	3	QOL	
Triadafilopoulos[247] 2002	118	12	Symptom, QOL, PPI usage, pH, manometry, esophagitis grade	
Houston[248] 2003	41	6	QOL, pH	LESP
Go[249] 2004	50	10		QOL
Injection therapy				
Johnson[250] 2003 (Enteryx)[a]	85	6	QOL	LESP
Cohen[251] 2005 (Enteryx)	64	24	PPI usage	
Schumacher[252] 2005 (Enteryx)	93	12	PPI usage, QOL	pH, LESP
Fockens[253] 2004 (Gatekeeper)[b]	68	6	QOL, pH, LESP	
Gastroplication				
Pleskow[254] 2004 (full thickness)	64	6	QOL, pH	LESP
Arts[255] 2005 (EndoCinch)	20	12	QOL, pH	
Chen[256] 2005 (EndoCinch)	85	24	Symptoms, pH	LESP

LESP, lower esophageal sphincter pressure; QOL, quality of life.
[a]Enteryx is no longer available.
[b]Gatekeeper was never commercially released.

exposure time decreased significantly at both 6 and 12 months, despite findings that only one plication was visible in 6 of 15 patients. This may be explained by the eccentric thickening of smooth muscle adjacent to suture sites noted after placement.[134,135]

Evidence regarding the effectiveness and safety of these procedures is still accumulating, primarily in the setting of proof-of-concept, small case-study, cohort, or sham-comparison studies. Early results from cohort studies are promising, with therapies demonstrating improvements in quality of life (between 50% and 75% improvement), postprocedure symptom scores, PPI use (up to 40%–75%), 24-h pH (16%–33% time pH < 4.0 improvement), and LES pressure (Table 44A.19). Randomized data reveals a trend in improvement of quality-of-life scores and medication use, with two studies noting improvements on objective evaluation (pH, EGD/esophagitis score/manometry) (Table 44A.20).

These findings suggest that endoluminal therapy may primarily play a future role in reducing symptoms and medication usage, with further evaluation required to fully understand the effects on the histopathological changes associated with GER. Follow-up has been limited to 2 years, limiting conclusions regarding the durability of the therapeutic effect. To date, one case-control comparison of endoscopic suturing with laparoscopic Nissen fundoplication has been published. In this study, 27 endoscopic plication patients were followed for 6 weeks, with results compared to 27 case-matched patients who underwent a previous laparoscopic 360° fundoplication. Although median symptom score (gastroesophageal reflux disease [GERD]-Health related quality of life) improved in both groups with no statistical differences noted, there were more patients satisfied after operative intervention (78% vs. 96%).[136]

As with any new therapy, questions of safety remain unanswered. Data from FDA phases III and IV only recently have come under evaluation. Market forces are also having an impact on the availability of these therapies outside clinical trials as several injectable devices have been pulled from

TABLE 44A.20.
Cited Randomized Controlled Sham Trials Regarding Endoscopic Endoluminal Therapy for Gastroesophageal Reflux.

Author	Procedure	No. patients	Months follow-up	Significant improvement	No difference
Corley[257] 2003	RFA	64	6	QOL, PPI use	pH, esophagitis grade
Deviere[258] 2005	Injection (Enteryx)[a]	64	3	QOL, PPI use	pH, SF-36 score
Cohen[251] 2005	Injection (Enteryx)	62	3	QOL, pH	—
Park[259] 2005	Gastropexy (EndoCinch)	47	12	—	QOL, pH, PPI use
Schwartz[260] 2005	Gastropexy (EndoCinch)	45	3	Heartburn score, PPI use	QOL, pH, manometry
Schwartz[261] 2007	Gastropexy (EndoCinch)	60	3, 6, 12	Symptom, medication use, QOL	pH, manometry

PPI, proton pump inhibitor; QOL, quality of life; RFA, radio-frequency ablation.
[a]Enteryx is no longer available.

clinical use, and the company producing GEJ radio-frequency delivery devices has stopped production. Until more data are accumulated, recommendations regarding the widespread use of endoluminal therapies for GER disease outside clinical trials cannot be made, particularly in patients with hiatal herniation, Barrett's esophagus, or multiple comorbidities.[127] There is still promise that endoluminal therapies may serve as a means of symptom control as a bridge to definitive therapy, as an alternative in mild-to-moderately symptomatic patients who do not desire surgery, as a more permanent therapeutic option for those who cannot tolerate surgical intervention, or as a less-involved method of helping patients with recurrent reflux after antireflux surgery.

TABLE 44A.21. Features Suggesting Intestinal Metaplasia of the Esophagus.

Clinical features	*Long-standing or severe gastroesophageal reflux symptoms*
Endoscopic features A jagged, irregular squamocolumnar junction A prominent squamocolumnar junction Discrete patches of columnar epithelium in distal esophagus	Long segments of columnar epithelial lining (>3 cm)
Histological features	Intestinal metaplasia (not gastric or junctional)

Barrett's Esophagus

Special mention is necessary for Barrett's esophagus. In 1950, Norman Barrett described the condition in which the tubular esophagus becomes lined with metaplastic columnar epithelium that is at risk for adenocarcinoma, rather than the normal squamous epithelium. Most recently, it has been recognized that the specialized intestinal metaplasia (not gastric-type columnar changes) constitutes true Barrett's esophagus, with a risk of progression to dysplasia and adenocarcinoma.

This abnormality occurs in 7% to 10% of people with GER and may represent the end stage of the natural history of GER. Clearly, Barrett's esophagus is associated with a more profound mechanical deficiency of the LES, severe impairment of esophageal body function, and marked esophageal acid exposure.[137] In contrast, some patients are asymptomatic and have only short segments of columnar-lined epithelium in the distal esophagus (<3 cm), which does not have this same strong association with GER. In addition, there seems to be a lower incidence of metaplastic epithelium in these "short segments" of Barrett's and therefore a lower malignancy potential.

There remains considerable debate regarding the significance of short-segment Barrett's esophagus, and identifying those patients with so-called short-segment Barrett's remains problematical because endoscopically localizing the precise anatomical esophagogastric junction is difficult, and metaplastic epithelium (and therefore malignant potential) can exist even in these short segments. Recommendations for identifying Barrett's esophagus are detailed in Table 44A.21. The endoscopic feature most strongly associated with intestinal metaplasia is the finding of long segments of esophageal columnar lining, with more than 90% of patients with greater than 3 cm of esophageal columnar lining having intestinal metaplasia.

Endoscopically, obvious Barrett's esophagus with intestinal metaplasia is a major risk factor for adenocarcinoma of the esophagus, with the annual incidence of adenocarcinoma in this condition estimated at approximately 0.8%, 40 times higher than in the general population. Once high-grade dysplasia is identified in more than one biopsy from columnar-lined esophagus, nearly 50% of patients already harbor a foci of invasive cancer. This frequency is the basis for recommending careful endoscopic surveillance in patients with Barrett's esophagus with intestinal metaplasia and esophagectomy when high-grade dysplasia is identified.[138,139]

Treatment goals for patients with Barrett's esophagus are similar to those for patients with GER, that is, relief of symptoms and arrest of ongoing reflux-mediated epithelial damage. In addition, those with Barrett's esophagus, regardless of type of treatment (surgical or medical), require long-term endoscopic surveillance with biopsy of columnar segments to identify progressive metaplastic changes or progression to dysplasia.[140,141]

Several studies have compared medical and surgical therapy in patients with Barrett's esophagus (Table 44A.22). These data support the notion that Barrett's esophagus is associated with more severe and refractory GER, and antireflux surgery is effective at alleviating these symptoms in 75% to 92% of patients.[142,143] However, many patients are asymptomatic (perhaps explaining why they have such advanced sequelae of GER), and there is mounting evidence to suggest that an alkaline refluxate may be as damaging as acid reflux.[144] For these reasons, correction of the mechanically defective

TABLE 44A.22.
Medical Versus Surgical Treatment of Barrett's Esophagus.

	No. patients		*Symptom control*		*Stricture/esophagitis*	
Author	*Medical*	*Surgical*	*Medical*	*Surgical*	*Medical*	*Surgical*
Attwood[262] 1992 (p)[a]	26	19	22%	81%	38%	21%
Oritz[263] 1996 (pr)	27	32	85%	89%	53%/45%	5%/15%
Sampliner[264] 1994 (p)	27	—	70%	—	50%	—
Csendes[265] 1998 (pr)	—	152	—	46%	—	64%

p, prospective; pr, prospective randomized; ret, retrospective.
[a]Before availability of proton pump inhibitors.

TABLE 44A.23.
Antireflux Surgery and Regression of Barrett's Esophagus.

Author	*No. patients*	*Years of follow-up*	*Q length Barrett's*	*No Barrett's*	*Cancer*
Skinner[266] 1983	10	4	1	1	0
Williamson[267] 1990	37	4.2	4	0	
Martinez[268] 1992	16	6.6	0	0	3
Sagar[269] 1995	56	5.5	24	5	0
Oritz[263] 1996	32	5	8	0	1
Total	151		37	6	4

antireflux barrier may be especially important in these patients.

Although symptom control in these patients suggests control of ongoing damage, the ultimate goal in therapy is to change the natural history in Barrett's of progression to adenocarcinoma. With this goal, several questions arise: (1) Does antireflux surgery result in regression of Barrett's epithelium? (2) Does antireflux surgery prevent progression of metaplastic changes? (3) Is there a role for antireflux surgery accompanied by other therapies for metaplastic or dysplastic epithelium?

Does Antireflux Surgery Result in Regression of Barrett's Epithelium? Operative therapy corrects the mechanically defective antireflux barrier and therefore might be expected to have a higher likelihood than medical therapy alone of inducing regression of Barrett's epithelium. The results in five operative series following a total of 151 patients over 4 to 6 years are detailed in Table 44A.23. Complete regression occurred in only 6 patients, with all but 1 coming from one series. Thirty-one patients showed some decrease in the length of Barrett's, but only 6 had a decrease in length of more than 1 cm. Furthermore, 6 patients went on to develop adenocarcinoma of the esophagus. Clearly, current evidence suggests that neither medical nor surgical therapy result in regression of Barrett's epithelium.[145]

Does Antireflux Surgery Prevent Progression of Metaplastic Changes? There is growing evidence suggesting that antireflux surgery may prevent progression of Barrett's changes and thereby protect against dysplasia and malignancy. Three recent studies are summarized in Table 44A.24. In the series reported by McDonald from the Mayo Clinic, three cancers occurred over an 18.5-year follow-up period, all within the first 3 years after operation. The clustering of these three cases within the first 3 years of follow-up suggests that these patients may have already progressed to dysplasia at the time of operation. These are strong data in support of the favorable impact of operative therapy on the natural history of Barrett's esophagus.

TABLE 44A.24.
Antireflux Surgery and Progression of Barrett's to Dysplasia or Adenocarcinoma.

	No. patients		*Development of dysplasia*	
Author	*Medical*	*Surgical*	*Medical*	*Surgical*
Polepalle[270] 1990	152	29	19%	3.4%
Oritz[263] 1996	27	32	22%	3.1%
McDonald[271] 1996	—	118	—	2.5%

Is There a Role for Antireflux Surgery Accompanied by Other Therapies for Metaplastic or Dysplastic Epithelium? Combination therapy, that is, pharmacological or operative control of acid reflux plus endoscopic ablation of Barrett's mucosa, is having encouraging preliminary results.[146,147] These early experiences suggest that the ablated areas reepithelialize with more normal squamous mucosa. Ablative therapies have included laser ablation, photodynamic therapy, and cryotherapy. This exciting early work needs further study before becoming a clinical standard.

Diaphragmatic Hernia

To complete its course from mouth to stomach, the esophagus must traverse the diaphragm. The site of transit of the esophagus from chest into the abdomen, the esophageal hiatus, is the site of a variety of defects (Fig. 44A.18).

A type I hiatal hernia, also known as a sliding hiatal hernia, consists of a simple herniation of the GEJ into the chest. The phrenoesophageal ligament is attenuated, and there is no true hernia sac. This, the most common of the hiatal hernias, is more common in women and in the fifth

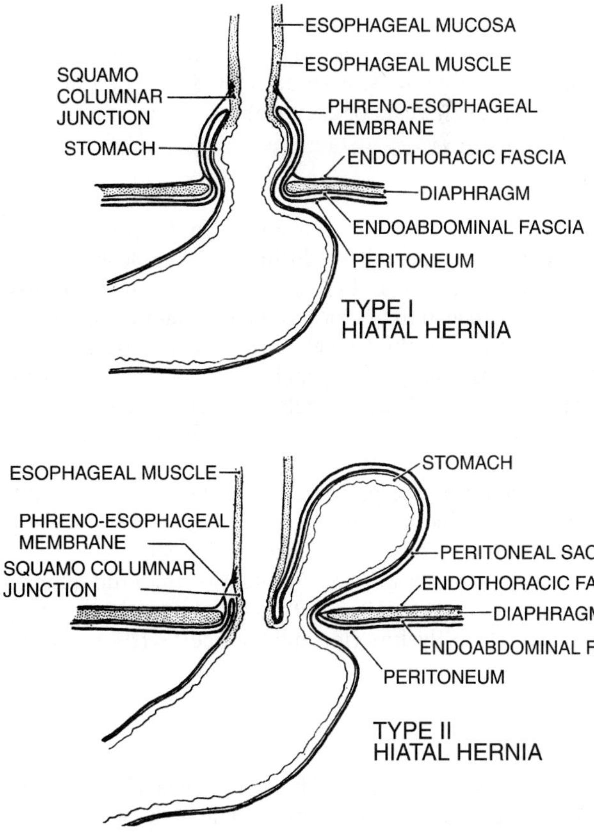

FIGURE 44A.18. Classification of hiatal hernia.

and sixth decades of life. With a type II hiatal hernia, commonly referred to as a *paraesophageal hernia*, the GEJ remains at the esophageal hiatus, while the gastric fundus herniates alongside the esophagus into the chest. The type III hiatal hernia is a combination of type I and type II hernias, with the esophagogastric junction displaced into the chest along with the gastric fundus and body. Paraesophageal hernias (types II and III) have a true hernia sac accompanying the herniated stomach. Finally, some have characterized a type IV hernia as an advanced stage of paraesophageal hernia in which the entire stomach and other intraabdominal content (e.g., colon, spleen) are herniated into the chest, although use of this fourth classification is not widely accepted.

Although the exact prevalence of hiatal hernia remains unknown, it is clear that it is a relatively common abnormality and is the most common finding reported on barium studies of the upper GI tract. The difficulty in establishing the incidence of hiatal hernia lies in the fact that a large number of patients with hiatal hernia are asymptomatic, and the diagnosis is often made incidentally during investigation of other GI problems.

The underlying etiology of esophageal hiatal hernias remains unclear. Some investigators try to characterize hiatal hernias as acquired or congenital based on the age of patient presentation, with acquired hernias presenting at later ages and congenital earlier, but the age at presentation is more likely a function of symptoms than hernia presence. Clearly, confounding data are available from which to guess about etiology. What is clear is that attenuation of the phrenoesophageal membrane allows the esophagogastric junction to migrate through a patulous hiatus into the chest, whereas type II hernias occur through a defect in the esophageal hiatus anterior to the esophagus while the esophagogastric junction remains fixed. The nature of these defects remains unknown. Both sliding and paraesophageal hernias are found predominantly in older individuals, with up to 50% of type I hernias found in patients 50 years of age or older.

Diagnosis

Most type I and III hiatal hernias are diagnosed incidentally during a contrast upper GI or during upper endoscopy performed for other reasons. Type II hernias can be similarly diagnosed but are also frequently found on a radiograph of the chest showing an air–fluid level in the mediastinum or the left chest. Occasionally, the inability to pass a nasogastric tube or a contrast study of the colon reveals a twisted intrathoracic stomach or colon, leading to the diagnosis of a type III hernia.

When symptoms are present, sliding hernias have a different presentation compared to paraesophageal hernias. Paraesophageal hernias tend to produce more dysphagia, chest pain, bloating, and respiratory problems than do sliding hernias. Symptoms associated with a sliding hernia are more often related to LES dysfunction and include heartburn, regurgitation, and dysphagia.

Treatment

Because hiatal hernia is a purely mechanical abnormality, there is no nonoperative treatment. The risk of bleeding, incarceration, strangulation, perforation, and death with paraesophageal hernias is such that when a type II or type III hernia is identified, operative repair should be performed.[148] In contrast, a significant number of patients with type I hiatal hernias are asymptomatic and remain so throughout the remainder of their life. Therefore, the presence of a sliding hiatal hernia alone does not mandate intervention. However, those patients with a type I hernia and GER, chest pain, dysphagia, regurgitation, or other symptoms referable to their hernia should undergo symptom-specific workup and may be best served with an operative repair. An often-overlooked complication of hiatal hernia is occult GI bleeding, thought to result from the mechanical trauma of the stomach herniating back and forth, into and out of the chest, causing subtle linear erosions in the proximal stomach that slowly bleed and lead to anemia.[149,150]

Operative correction of esophageal hiatal hernia should (1) return the herniated content to its anatomically correct position below the diaphragm, (2) repair the hernia defect, and (3) prevent recurrence while minimizing associated morbidity. There are a number of proven operations that can be performed through the chest or abdomen to accomplish these goals. Questions remain regarding the need for an accompanying antireflux procedure and the method of abdominal or thoracic access.

Are Hiatal Hernia and Gastroesophageal Reflux Associated? Many surgeons believe that, by allowing the LES to reside within the negative-pressure environment of the chest, a hiatal hernia plays an important role in the pathogenesis of GER. In support of this feeling is the finding that 50% of patients with GER have an associated sliding hiatal hernia.[151] On the other hand, approximately one-third of patients with a hiatal hernia do not have evidence of GER, and this number may far exceed one-third because the number of patients with asymptomatic hernias who did not seek medical care may be vastly underestimated. It appears that the presence of an endoscopically reducible sliding hiatal hernia does not change LES function enough to result in abnormal GER, whereas an unreducible LES will.[152–156] On the other hand, abnormal GER in the presence of a sliding hiatal hernia results in more severe GER and impaired esophageal clearance.[157] Sliding hiatal hernia alone presently appears not causative of GER, but the presence of a hiatal hernia in patients with GER magnifies this condition and its sequelae.

Should an Antireflux Procedure Accompany All Hiatal Hernia Repairs? Whether to include an antireflux procedure with all hiatal hernia repairs remains controversial, especially when dealing with a type II paraesophageal hernia. Because most sliding-type hernias are repaired on the basis of symptoms, adding an antireflux procedure seems more straightforward because of the prevalence of reflux symptoms in type I and III hernias. In contrast, most patients who have type II hernias do not have reflux symptoms, and an antireflux operation for these patients may add little benefit to the outcome. However, with careful questioning, many patients with type II hernias give a history of GER symptoms that spontaneously abated, suggesting an anatomical change (perhaps hernia development) leading to this resolution of symptoms. Recent data from small series are suggesting that

GER may be more prevalent in type II hernia than was earlier recognized.[158–160]

The role of fundoplication in patients with type II paraesophageal hernia remains controversial. Conventional thinking suggests that because the LES is located within the abdomen, it is competent, and fundoplication is unnecessary. On the other hand, a key principle in repairing a hiatal hernia is to anchor the stomach within the abdomen to help prevent recurrence, and some surgeons are now using a fundoplication to serve as this anchor (the wrap buttresses against the hernia repair and holds the distal esophagus and stomach intra-abdominally). In up to one-third of patients, adding fundoplication may avert the unmasking of GER following repair. This rationale is leading many surgeons to use fundoplication routinely for all hiatal hernia repairs. Early data suggest that this is a safe and effective means of managing paraesophageal hernias. However, few studies have objectively evaluated addition of an antireflux procedure to hiatal hernia repair, and there are limited data available to definitively answer this question.

Should Hiatal Hernias Be Repaired Laparoscopically? The role of laparoscopy in repairing hiatal hernias has recently been challenged. Anecdotal data suggest that hernia recurrence is higher following laparoscopic repair than after traditional open hiatal hernia repair. The proposed basis for this is the relative absence of intraabdominal adhesions that accompanies laparoscopic hernia repair as compared to open operations. The absence of these adhesions to anchor the stomach and distal esophagus allows the stomach to more readily "slip" back through the esophageal hiatus and into the chest than would be the case with the adhesions associated with open repairs. These anecdotal experiences need further investigation before any conclusions regarding route of abdominal access for repair of hiatal hernia can be made.

Esophageal Perforation/Injury

The most common cause of esophageal injury or perforation is instrumentation of the esophagus during diagnostic or therapeutic procedures. Esophageal injury may also result from ingestion of a caustic substance (either accidental or intentional), ingestion of a foreign body, profound retching, progression of disease (malignancy), or external trauma.

Perforation

The expansion of uses for esophagogastroscopy has elevated instrumentation of the esophagus to the most common cause of esophageal perforation. From simple passage of a flexible scope through the cervical esophagus and into the stomach, to interventions such as endoscopic dilation of benign and malignant strictures, injection of esophageal varices, laser or photodynamic ablation of Barrett's mucosa, or chemical injection of the LES for achalasia, all have led to esophageal perforation of varying clinical significance. Other less-common causes include barotrauma from violent retching (Boerhaave syndrome) or blunt trauma, penetrating injuries to the neck or chest, swallowed foreign body, advanced malignancy, or operative injury.

Diagnosis

Regardless of the cause, esophageal perforation is a true emergency requiring immediate recognition and treatment. A high index of suspicion, especially when an iatrogenic cause is suspected, allows early diagnosis of esophageal perforation. Early diagnosis is the key to obtaining the most favorable outcome of treatment. Difficulties during diagnostic or therapeutic endoscopy should raise one's suspicion of an injury, and immediate postprocedure pain or subcutaneous emphysema should prompt an immediate and thorough investigation for perforation.

Abnormalities on chest radiography are variable and should not be relied on to diagnose esophageal perforation. Air within the soft tissues of the mediastinum or neck indicates perforation but fails to localize the site and magnitude of perforation. The diagnosis is best made with a contrast esophagogram. Water-soluble contrast is initially administered, followed by dilute barium if the initial swallow fails to reveal a perforation.[161] Barium provides much better mucosal detail than water-soluble contrast, and the risk of missing a perforation far outweighs the risks of barium extravasation in the neck or mediastinum. If a perforation is demonstrated with water-soluble contrast, then barium is unnecessary and should be avoided.

When there is a high suspicion of perforation but the esophagogram fails to identify it, a chest CT may be helpful by demonstrating air in the soft tissues of the neck or mediastinum or a hydrothorax or pneumothorax.[162] Again, an esophagogram has the highest certainty of demonstrating both the site and magnitude of perforation and may need to be repeated to plan subsequent management. The risks of further injury or increased spillage and soiling mean there is virtually no role for esophagoscopy in diagnosing esophageal perforation.

Treatment

The key to optimum management of esophageal perforation (Fig. 44A.19) is early recognition and treatment. When esophageal perforation occurs intraoperatively, immediate primary closure should be performed, with drainage of the operative field over closed-suction drains. In this setting, outcomes are excellent, with 98% survival and success.[163–167] Otherwise, immediate treatment is first aimed at minimizing bacterial and chemical contamination of the neck or mediastinum and restoring intravascular volume. Oral intake is withheld, and broad-spectrum intravenous antibiotics are given.

The best outcome is obtained when the perforation has occurred less than 24 h previously and can be closed primarily (80% to 90% survival). Critical to this success is the viability of the tissue for closure, debridement of any necrotic or stained tissue, and drainage of the field. Occasionally, cervical esophageal perforations can be managed with drainage alone, especially when the perforation is small, making intraoperative localization difficult or hazardous. When the perforation has been present more than 24 h, survival decreases to less than 50%, regardless of whether the perforation is managed by closure and drainage or by drainage alone. In this setting, the decision whether to close the perforation, resect the involved segment of esophagus, or merely drain the area and divert enteric flow proximally and distally (esophagostomy,

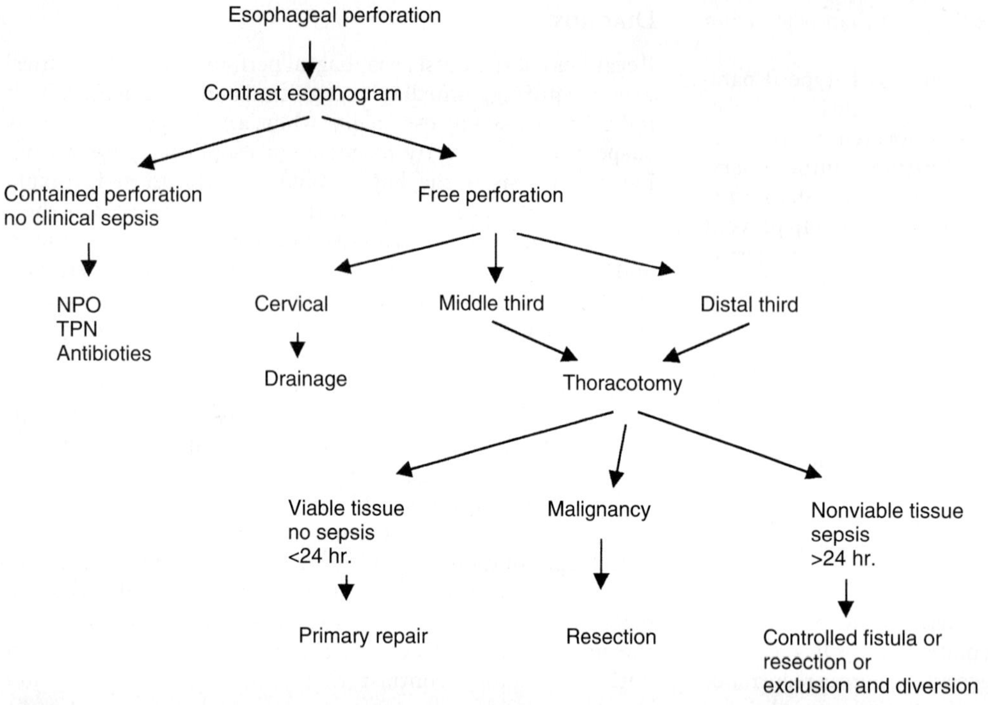

FIGURE 44A.19. Treatment algorithm for esophageal perforation.

tube gastrostomy, and feeding jejunostomy) is individualized on the basis of the size of the perforation, extent of tissue devitalization, and associated sepsis. In many of these extreme cases, rapid control of ongoing soilage and sepsis is the only hope for survival.

In select circumstances, nonoperative management is appropriate: (1) contrast esophagogram demonstrates a perforation that is contained within the mediastinum and drains well back into the esophagus, (2) associated symptoms are mild, and (3) there is no clinical evidence of sepsis.[168] In this setting, oral intake is withheld for 7 to 14 days, hyperalimentation is given, and gastric antisecretory medication is administered. Any decline in clinical course mandates immediate operative management. Free perforation into the pleural cavity contraindicates nonoperative management.

Because esophageal perforation is infrequent, there are no prospective studies comparing various treatments. Several retrospective reviews applying each of the foregoing strategies has led to the formulation and application of the management algorithm detailed in Figure 44A.19.

Injury

Each of the causes of esophageal perforation detailed here can lead to esophageal injury without perforation. Caustic ingestion and violent retching, resulting in upper GI bleeding (Mallory-Weiss tear), present unique features and management.

Caustic Ingestion

Typically, caustic ingestion takes on two separate patterns of injury depending on the underlying nature of the ingestion. Accidental ingestion usually occurs in children or the mentally impaired, and consequently smaller quantities of caustic are ingested, with resulting injuries of less magnitude. In contrast, in adults and teenagers ingestion is more commonly deliberate, with larger quantities of caustic ingested and more pronounced and devastating injuries. Although acid is occasionally ingested, the immediate mucosal burn with acids minimizes its ingestion. In contrast, alkalies result in a slower and delayed mucosal burn, allowing ingestion of larger amounts of substance before pain prevents swallowing.[169]

Diagnosis

Because a history of caustic ingestion is usually known at initial presentation, diagnostic maneuvers center on assessing the extent and magnitude of injury. Pain in the mouth and sternal region, hypersalivation, odynophagia, and dysphagia suggest ingestion rather than attempted ingestion. Contrast esophagogram is not a reliable way to assess acute esophageal injury but is necessary in later follow-up to identify strictures. Esophagogastroscopy is the single-best maneuver when performed early after presentation, allowing confirmation of significant caustic ingestion and grading of the severity of the injury[170] (Table 44A.25).

Treatment

Treatment must address both the immediate and long-term consequences of caustic ingestion. The immediate

TABLE 44A.25. Endoscopic Grading of Caustic Esophagogastric Injury.

First-degree burn	Mucosal hyperemia and edema
Second-degree burn	Mucosal ulceration; exudates and pseudomembrane formation
Third-degree burn	Mucosal sloughing; deep ulceration; massive hemorrhage; perforation; obstruction by edema

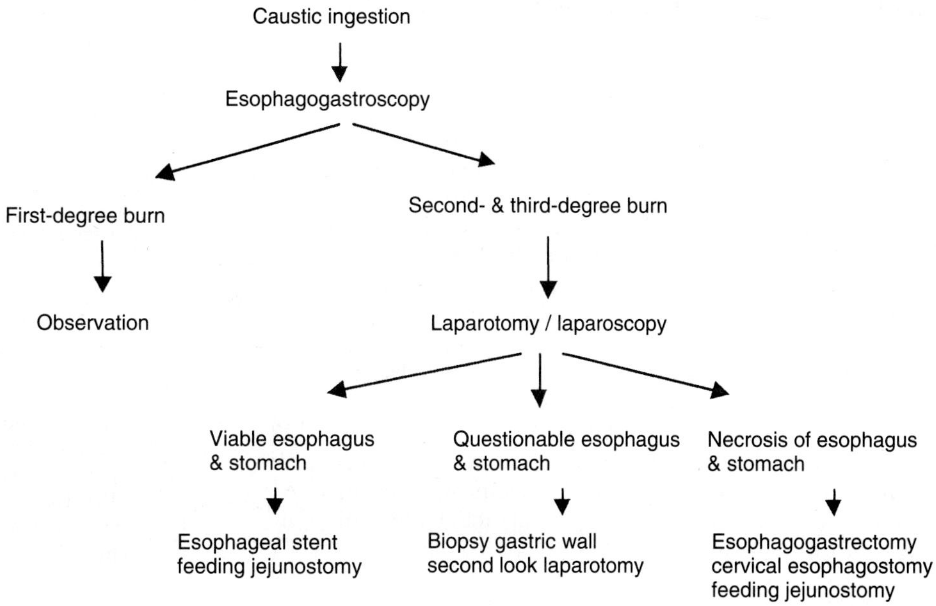

FIGURE 44A.20. Treatment algorithm for caustic ingestion.

treatment focuses on fluid resuscitation and initiation of broad-spectrum antibiotics.[171] Early intubation may be necessary because loss of the airway can rapidly develop after significant laryngeal or epiglottic injury. Neutralization of the corrosive risks exothermic reactions and exacerbation of the mucosal injury and should be avoided. Emetics reexpose the esophagus to the corrosive agent and are contraindicated, and nasogastric intubation is not recommended because of the risk of perforating the friable esophagus. During this acute phase, operative treatment is based on endoscopic grading of injury and intraoperative assessment of extent of injury and tissue viability (Fig. 44A.20). Laparoscopy and thoracoscopy are allowing minimally invasive means of making this assessment.

Once the acute phase has passed, management focuses on prevention and treatment of strictures. Although antibiotics and corticosteroids used in the acute phase decrease the occurrence of esophageal stricture in animals, a controlled trial in humans failed to show any benefit of corticosteroids.[172] This lack of proven benefit and the potential side effects of steroids argue against their routine use. In addition, prospective studies using prophylactic dilation or early stent placement have not proven any benefit in preventing stricture formation. In contrast, retrospective experiences with early dilation started during the acute phase of management gave excellent results in up to 78% of patients, while only 21% of those who had strictures dilated only when they became symptomatic had excellent results. However, 5% of those undergoing early dilation died during treatment, while only 0.9% died during symptomatic treatment. Therefore, routine use of early dilation cannot be recommended.

Occasionally, optimal management of strictures requires operative resection or esophagoplasty. Operative intervention is indicated when (1) there is complete stenosis in which all attempts have failed to establish a lumen, (2) there is marked irregularity and pocketing on esophagogram, (3) severe periesophageal reaction or mediastinitis develops with dilation, (4) a fistula forms, (5) a lumen cannot be maintained with repeated dilation, or (6) the patient is unable to undergo repeated dilation for a prolonged period of time.[173,174] Esophageal reconstruction needs to be individualized, including decisions regarding conduit for replacement and location of replacement. In most cases, the damaged esophagus should be resected because the retained esophagus can develop into a mucocele, and there is a risk of esophageal carcinoma developing in the native damaged esophagus. However, when the native esophagus is severely damaged and inflamed, an extraanatomical route may be beneficial to keep the neoesophagus out of the inflamed field. The ideal conduit for esophageal replacement, in order of preference, is (1) colon, (2) stomach, and (3) jejunum.

Mallory-Weiss Tear

During vomiting, significant intragastric pressures are generated. Fortunately, the extragastric pressure usually equals intragastric pressure, thereby minimizing the stretching of the gastric wall. When there is a paraesophageal hernia and the LES is fixed within the abdomen, these intragastric pressures are transmitted to the supradiaphragmatic portion of the gastric wall, resulting in a mucosal tear with subsequent bleeding. Bleeding can be profuse and mimic a bleeding duodenal ulcer or varices. A history of retching immediately before an upper GI bleed should raise the suspicion of a Mallory-Weiss tear.[175]

Immediate esophagogastroscopy is usually diagnostic, showing a proximal source of bleeding and no esophageal varices.[176] Treatment is supportive, with gastric lavage and decompression, maintenance of intravascular volume, and transfusion to replace blood loss. Bleeding is usually self-limited. Rarely, laparotomy is indicated for ongoing blood loss and hemodynamic instability. At laparotomy, a gastrotomy and oversewing of mucosal tears arrests bleeding.

Miscellaneous

Schatzki's Ring

Schatzki's ring is a thin submucosal circumferential ring in the lower esophagus at the squamocolumnar junction. It is often associated with a hiatal hernia. The etiology of a Schatzki's ring remains unclear, but there appears to be an association with ingestion of pills known to be injurious to the esophageal mucosa and with GER, suggesting that this is an acquired lesion related to esophageal mucosal damage.

Clinical symptoms associated with Schatzki's ring are self-limited episodes of dysphagia during hurried ingestion of dry and solid foods. The best treatment of Schatzki's ring in patients who do not have GER is dilation. Often, a single dilation is sufficient for long-term symptom relief. In patients with a ring related to GER, dilation accompanied by an antireflux procedure is necessary to provide relief and avoid the need for future dilations.

Scleroderma

Scleroderma is a systemic collagen-vascular disease, with 80% of patients having some degree of esophageal involvement. In the GI tract, the predominant feature is smooth muscle atrophy with resulting sphincter and motor dysfunction. Most commonly, the LES mechanism is weakened, and esophageal peristalsis in the smooth muscle-lined distal esophagus is impaired. The result is reflux esophagitis with subsequent stricture formation and esophageal shortening.

Heartburn and dysphagia are frequent presenting complaints, and the barium esophagogram often reveals stricture with proximal esophageal dilation. Endoscopy confirms esophagitis, and esophageal manometry typically shows preservation of the motor activity of the striated muscle-lined proximal esophagus, absence of motor activity in the distal esophagus, and a hypotensive LES. When planning management, a gastric-emptying study should be performed to assess the magnitude of gastric dysfunction.

Medical treatment with antacids and prokinetics frequently fails. An antireflux procedure may be the best method to arrest reflux but may eventually lead to worsening dysphagia as the disease progresses. Esophageal shortening requires a Collis esophageal lengthening accompanied by an antireflux procedure. If the esophagitis is severe and accompanied by a significantly delayed gastric emptying or there has been a previous failed antireflux operation, then total gastrectomy with Roux-en-Y esophagojejunostomy affords the best results.

Plummer-Vinson Syndrome

The Plummer-Vinson clinical syndrome is uncommon and is characterized by dysphagia associated with atrophic oral mucosa, spoon-shaped fingers with brittle nails, and chronic iron deficiency anemia. It characteristically occurs in middle-aged edentulous women and is more common in Scandinavian countries. Radiographic and endoscopic studies reveal a fibrous web just below the cricopharyngeus muscle as the cause of the dysphagia. It is now thought that this web is a medication-induced acquired lesion, likely related to the iron replacement many of these patients are receiving.

Treatment of the dysphagia is dilation of the web. Careful long-term follow-up is necessary because 100% of these patients will eventually develop malignant lesions of the oral mucosa, hypopharynx, and esophagus.

References

1. DeMeester T, Stein H, Fuchs K. Physiologic diagnostic studies. In: Zuidema G, Orringer M, eds. Shackelford's Surgery of the Alimentary Tract. Vol. 1. Philadelphia: Saunders; 1991:94–126.
2. Ward E, Devault K, Bouras E, et al. Successful oesophageal pH monitoring with a catheter-free system. Aliment Pharmacol Ther 2004;15:449–454.
3. Blom D, Mason R, Balaji N, et al. Esophageal bolus transport identified by simultaneous multichannel intraluminal impedance and monofluoroscopy. Gastroenterology 2001;120:P103.
4. Sliny J. Intraluminal multiple electric impedance procedure for measurement of gastrointestinal motility. J Gastrointest Motil 1991;3:151–162.
5. Imam H, Baker M, Shay S. Concurrent video-esophagogram, impedance monitoring and manometry in the assessment of bolus transit in normal subjects [abstract]. Gastroenterology 2004;126(suppl 2):A638.
6. Tutuian R, Vela M, Balaji N, et al. Esophageal function testing using combined multichannel intraluminal impedance and manometry. Multicenter study of healthy volunteers. Clin Gastroenterol Hepatol 2003;(1):174–182.
7. Shay S, Tutuian R, Sifrim D, et al. Twenty-four hour ambulatory simultaneous impedance and pH monitoring: a multicenter report of normal values in 60 healthy volunteers. Am J Gastroenterol 2004;99:1037–1043.
8. Tutuian R, Castell D. Clarification of the esophageal function defect in patients with manometric ineffective esophageal motility: studies using combined impedance-manometry. Clin Gastroenterol Hepatol 2004;2:230–236.
9. Tamhankar A, Peters J, Portale G, et al. Omeprazole does not reduce gastroesophageal reflux: new insights using multichannel intraluminal impedance technology. J Gastrointest Surg 2004;8:888–896.
10. Mainie I, Tutuian R, Agrawal A, et al. Symptoms on PPI therapy associated with non-acid reflux GERD. Am J Gastroenterol 2004;99(suppl):S14.
11. Goldblum J, Whyte R, Orringer M, et al. Achalasia. A morphologic study of 42 resected specimens. Am J Surg Pathol 1994;18:327–337.
12. Csendes A, Smok G, Braghetto I, et al. Gastroesophageal sphincter pressure and histological changes in distal esophagus in patients with achalasia of the esophagus. Dig Dis Sci 1985;30:941–945.
13. Goldblum J, Rice T, Richter J. Histopathologic features in esophagomyotomy specimens from patients with achalasia. Gastroenterology 1996;111:648–654.
14. Verne G, Hahn A, Peneau B, et al. Association of HLA-DR and DQ alleles with idiopathic achalasia. Gastroenterology 1999;117:26–31.
15. Wong R, Maydonovitch C, Metz S, Baker J. Significant DQw1 association in achalasia. Dig Dis Sci 2004;34:349–352.
16. Cassella R, Ellis F, Brown A. Fine-structure changes in achalasia of the esophagus. I. Vagus nerves. Am J Pathol 1965;46:279.
17. Singaram C, Koch J, Gaumnitz E, et al. Nature of neuronal loss in human achalasia. Gastroenterology 1996;110:A259.
18. Aggestrup S, Uddman R, Sundle F, et al. Lack of vasoactive intestinal polypeptide nerves in esophageal achalasia. Gastroenterology 1983;84:924–927.
19. Behar J BP. Effect of cholecystokinin-octapeptide on lower esophageal sphincter. Gastroenterology 1977;73:57–61.
20. Dodds W, Dent J, Hogan W, et al. Effect of atropine on esophageal motor function in humans. Am J Physiol 1981;240:G290-G296.

21. Guelrud M, Rossiter A, Souney P, et al. The effect of vasoactive intestinal polypeptide on the lower esophageal sphincter in achalasia. Gastroenterology 1992;103:377–382.
22. Podas T, Eaden J, Mayberry M, Mayberry J. Achalasia: a critical review of epidemiological studies. Am J Gastroenterol 1998;93:2345–2347.
23. Chawla K CS, Alexander LL. Familial achalasia of the esophagus in mother and son: a possible pathogenetic relationship. J Am Geriatr Soc 1979;11:519–521.
24. Nihoul-Fekete C, Bawab F, Lortat-Jacob S, et al. Achalasia of the esophagus in childhood. Surgical treatment in 35 cases, with special reference to familial cases and glucocorticoid deficiency association. Hepatogastroenterology 1991;38:510–513.
25. Ehrich E, Aranoff G, Johnson W. Familial achalasia associated with adrenocortical insufficiency, alacrima, and neurological abnormalities. Am J Med Genet 1987;6:637–644.
26. Pedreira C, Zacharin M. Allgrove syndrome: when a recognizable paediatric disorder occurs in adulthood. Med J Aust 2004;180:74–75.
27. Weber A, Wienker T, Jung M, et al. Linkage of the gene for triple A syndrome to chromosome 12q13 near the type II keratin gene cluster. Hum Mol Genet 1996;5:2061–2066.
28. Meijssen M, Tilanus H, Blankenstein MV, et al. Achalasia complicated by oesophageal squamous cell carcinoma: a prospective study in 195 patients. Gut 1992;33:155–158.
29. Streitz JJ, Ellis F, Gibb S, et al. Achalasia and squamous cell carcinoma of the esophagus: analysis of 241 patients. Ann Thorac Surg 1995;59:1604–1609.
30. Crookes PF, Corkill S, DeMeester TR. Gastroesophageal reflux in achalasia. When is reflux really reflux? Dig Dis Sci 1997;42:1354–1361.
31. Birgisson S, Richter JE. Achalasia: what's new in diagnosis and treatment? Dig Dis Sci 1997;15:1–27.
32. Ferguson MK. Achalasia: current evaluation and therapy. Ann Thorac Surg 1991;52:336–342.
33. Schima W, Stacher G, Pokieser P, et al. Esophageal motor disorders: videofluoroscopic and manometric evaluation-prospective study in 88 symptomatic patients. Radiology 1992;185:487–491.
34. Tracey JP, Traube M. Difficulties in the diagnosis of pseudoachalasia. Am J Gastroenterol 1994;89:2014–2018.
35. Rozman RW Jr, Achkar E. Features distinguishing secondary achalasia from primary achalasia. Am J Gastroenterol 1990; 85:1327–1330.
36. Campos CT, Ellis FH Jr, LoCicero J III. Pseudoachalasia: a report of two cases with comments on possible causes and diagnosis. Dis Esophagus 1997;10:220–224.
37. Goldenberg SP, Burrell M, Fette GG, et al. Classic and vigorous achalasia: a comparison of manometric, radiographic, and clinical findings. Gastroenterology 1991;101:743–748.
38. Couturier D, Samama J. Clinical aspects and manometric criteria in achalasia. Hepatogastroenterology 1991;38:481–487.
39. Marshall JB, Bodnarchuk G, Singh A. Supine and upright radionuclide esophageal transit before and after treatment for achalasia. Clin Nuclear Med 1994;19:683–686.
40. Stacher G, Schima W, Bergmann H, et al. Sensitivity of radionuclide bolus transport and videofluoroscopic studies compared with manometry in the detection of achalasia. Am J Gastroenterol 1994;89:1484–1488.
41. Bortolotti M, Labo G. Clinical and manometric effects of nifedipine in patients with esophageal achalasia. Gastroenterology 1981;30:39–44.
42. Bortolotti M, Coccia G, Brunelli F, et al. Isosorbide dinitrate or nifedipine: which is preferable in the medical therapy of achalasia? Ital J Gastroenterol 1994;26:379–382.
43. Ferreira-Filho LP, Patto RJ, Troncon LE, et al. Use of isosorbide dinitrate for the symptomatic treatment of patients with Chagas' disease achalasia. A double-blind, crossover trial. Braz J Med Biol Res 1991;24:1093–1098.
44. Marzio L, Grossi L, DeLaurentis MF, et al. Effect of cimetropium bromide on esophageal motility and transit in patients affected by primary achalasia. Dig Dis Sci 1994;39:1389–1394.
45. Nasrallah SM, Tommaso CL, Singleton RT, et al. Primary esophageal motor disorders: clinical response to nifedipine. South Med J 1985;78:312–315.
46. Penagini R, Bartesaghi B, Zannini P, et al. Lower oesophageal sphincter hypersensitivity to opioid receptor stimulation in patients with idiopathic achalasia. Gut 1993;34:16–20.
47. Penagini R, Bartesaghi B, Negri G, et al. Effect of loperamide on lower oesophageal sphincter pressure in idiopathic achalasia. Scand J Gastroenterol 1994;29:1057–1060.
48. Traube M, Dubovik S, Lange RC, et al. The role of nifedipine therapy in achalasia: results of a randomized, double-blind, placebo-controlled study. Am J Gastroenterol 1989;84:1259–1262.
49. Triadafilopoulos G, Aaronson M, Sackel S, et al. Medical treatment of esophageal achalasia. Double-blind crossover study with oral nifedipine, verapamil, and placebo. Dig Dis Sci 1991;36:260–267.
50. Eaker EY, Gordon JM, Vogel SB. Untoward effects of esophageal botulinum toxin injection in the treatment of achalasia. Dig Dis Sci 1997;42:724–727.
51. Smith C, Stival A, Howell L, Swafford V. Endoscopic therapy for achalasia before Heller myotomy results in worse outcomes than Heller myotomy alone. Ann Surg 2006;243:579–586.
52. Bassotti G, D'Onofrio V, Battaglia E, et al. Treatment with botulinum toxin of octo-nonagenerians with oesophageal achalasia: a 2-year follow-up study. Aliment Pharmacol Ther 2006;23:1615–1619.
53. Zarate N, Mearin F, Baldovino F, et al. Achalasia treatment in the elderly: is botulinum toxin injection the best option? Eur J Gastroenterol Hepatol 2002;14:285–290.
54. Nair LA, Reynolds JC, Parkman HP, et al. Complications during pneumatic dilation for achalasia or diffuse esophageal spasm. Analysis of risk factors, early clinical characteristics, and outcome. Dig Dis Sci 1993;38:1893–1904.
55. Parkman HP, Reynolds JC, Ouyang A, et al. Pneumatic dilatation or esophagomyotomy treatment for idiopathic achalasia: clinical outcomes and cost analysis. Dig Dis Sci 1993;38:75–85.
56. Kadakia SC, Wong RK. Graded pneumatic dilation using Rigiflex achalasia dilators in patients with primary esophageal achalasia. Am J Gastroenterol 1993;88:34–38.
57. Barnett JL, Eisenman R, Nostrant TT, et al. Witzel pneumatic dilation for achalasia: safety- and long-term efficacy. Gastrointest Endosc 1990;36:482–485.
58. Okike N, Payne WS, Neufeld DM, et al. Esophagomyotomy versus forceful dilation for achalasia of the esophagus: results in 899 patients. Ann Thorac Surg 1979;28:119–125.
59. Kim CH, Cameron AJ, Hsu JJ, et al. Achalasia: prospective evaluation of relationship between lower esophageal sphincter pressure, esophageal transit, and esophageal diameter and symptoms in response to pneumatic dilation. Mayo Clin Proc 1993;68:1067–1073.
60. Eckardt VF, Aignherr C, Bernhard G. Predictors of outcome in patients with achalasia treated by pneumatic dilation. Gastroenterology 1992;103:1732–1738.
61. Rosemurgy A, Villadolid D, Thometz D, et al. Laparoscopic Heller myotomy provides durable relief from achalasia and salvages failures after Botox or dilation. Ann Surg 2005;241:725–733; discussion 733–735.
62. Spiess A, Kahrilas P. Treating achalasia: from whalebone to laparoscope. JAMA 1998;280:638–642.
63. Oelschlager B, Chang L, Pellegrini C. Improved outcome after extended gastric myotomy for achalasia. Arch Surg 2003;138:490–497.
64. Ancona E, Anselmino M, Zaninotto G, et al. Esophageal achalasia: laparoscopic versus conventional open Heller-Dor operation. Am J Surg 1995;170:265–270.

65. Melvin WS, Dundon JM, Talamini M, Horgan S. Computer-enhanced robotic telesurgery minimizes esophageal perforation during Heller myotomy. Surgery 2005;138:553–558; discussion 558–559.
66. Melvin WS, Needleman BJ, Krause KR, et al. Computer-assisted robotic Heller myotomy: initial case report. J Laparoendosc Adv Surg Tech A 2001;11:251–253.
67. Diamantis T, Pikoulis E, Felekouras E, et al. Laparoscopic esophagomyotomy for achalasia without a complementary antireflux procedure. J Laparoendosc Adv Surg Tech A 2006;16:345–349.
68. Falkenback D, Johnson J, Oberg S, et al. Heller's esophagomyotomy with or without a 360 degrees floppy Nissen fundoplication for achalasia. Long-term results from a prospective randomized study. Dis Esophagus 2003;16:284–290.
69. Richards WO, Torquati A, Holzman MD, et al. Heller myotomy versus Heller myotomy with Dor fundoplication for achalasia: a prospective randomized double-blind clinical trial [see comment]. Ann Surg 2004;240:405–412; discussion 412–415.
70. Zaninotto G, Narne S, Costantini M, et al. Tailored approach to Zenker's diverticula. Surg Endosc 2003;17:129–133.
71. Gutschow C, Hamoir M, Rombaux P, et al. Management of pharyngoesophageal (Zenker's) diverticulum: which technique? Ann Thorac Surg 2002;74:1677–1683.
72. Smith S, Genden E, Urken M. Endoscopic stapling technique for the treatment of Zenker diverticulum versus standard open-neck technique. Arch Otolaryngol Head Neck Surg 2002;128:141–144.
73. Costantini M, Zaninotto G, Rizzetto C, et al. Oesophageal diverticula. Best Practice and Research Clinical Gastroenterology 2004;18:3–17.
74. Siewert JR, Blum AL. The oesophagus. Part I: surgery at the upper oesophageal sphincter, tubular oesophagus and lower oesophageal sphincter. Clin Gastroenterol 1979;8:271–291.
75. Aly A, Devitt P, Jamieson G. Evolution of surgical treatment for pharyngeal pouch. Br J Surg 2004;91:657–664.
76. Patti MG, Bresadola V. Gastroesophageal reflux disease: basic considerations. Probl Gen Surg 1996;13:1–8.
77. Wetscher GJ, Redmond EJ, Vititi LMH. Pathophysiology of gastroesophageal reflux disease. In: Hinder RA, ed. Gastroesophageal Reflux Disease. R.G. Landes: Austin, TX, 1993.
78. Klingman RR, Stein HJ, DeMeester TR. The current management of gastroesophageal reflux. Adv Surg 1991;24:259–291.
79. Sandler R, Everhart J, Donowitz M, et al. The burden of selected digestive diseases in the United States. Gastroenterology 2002;122:1500–1511.
80. Ireland AC, Holloway RH, Toouli J, et al. Mechanisms underlying the antireflux action of fundoplication. Gut 1993;34:303–308.
81. Little AG. Mechanisms of action of antireflux surgery: theory and fact. World J Surg 1992;16:320–325.
82. Orlando RC. The pathogenesis of gastroesophageal reflux disease: the relationship between epithelial defense, dysmotility, and acid exposure. Am J Gastroenterol 1997;92:14–18.
83. Mittal RK, Rochester DF, McCallum RW. Sphincteric action of the diaphragm during a relaxed esophageal sphincter. Am J Physiol 1989;256:G139–G144.
84. Mittal RK, Rochester DF, McCallum RW. Electrical and mechanical activity in the human lower esophageal sphincter during diaphragmatic cotraction. J Clin Invest 1988;81:1182–1189.
85. Sontag SJ. Gastroesophageal reflux and asthma. Am J Med 1997;103:84S–90S.
86. Shindlebeck NE, Klauser AG, Berghammer G, et al. Three-year follow-up with patients with gastroesophageal reflux disease. Gut 1992;33:1016–1019.
87. Vaezi MF, Richter JE. Synergism of acid and duodenogastroesophageal reflux in complicated Barrett's esophagus. Surgery (St Louis) 1995;117:699–704.
88. Hill LD. An effective operation for hiatal hernia: an eight year appraisal. Ann Surg 1967;166:681.
89. Luostarinen M. Nissen fundoplication for reflux esophagitis. Long-term clinical and endoscopic results in 109 of 127 consecutive patients. Ann Surg 1993;217:329–337.
90. Shirazi SS, Schulze K, Soper RT. Long-term follow-up for treatment of complicated chronic reflux esophagitis. Arch Surg 1987;122:548–552.
91. Anvari M, Allen C. Five-year comprehensive outcomes evaluation in 181 patients after laparoscopic Nissen fundoplication. J Am Coll Surg 2003;196:51–59.
92. Bammer T, Hinder R, Kluas A, et al. Five- to eight-year outcome of the first laparoscopic fundoplications J Gastrointest Surg 2001;5:42–48.
93. Terry M, Smith CD, Branum GD, et al. Outcomes of laparoscopic fundoplication for gastroesophageal reflux disease and paraesophageal hernia. Surg Endosc 2001;15:691–699.
94. Spechler SJ. Comparison of medical and surgical therapy for complicated gastroesophageal reflux disease in veterans. N Engl J Med 1992;326:786–792.
95. Richter JE, Castell DO. Gastroesophageal reflux: pathogenesis, diagnosis and therapy. Ann Intern Med 1989;97:93–103.
96. Laycock W, Mauren S, Waring JP. Improvement in quality of life measures following laparoscopic antireflux surgery. Gastroenterology 1995;108:A244.
97. DeMeester TR, Bonavina L, Albertucci M. Evaluation of primary repair in 100 consecutive patients. Ann Surg 1986;204:9–20.
98. Donohue PE, Samelson S, Nyhus LM, et al. The Nissen fundoplication. Effective long-term control of pathologic reflux. Arch Surg 1985;120:663–667.
99. Ellis FH. The Nissen fundoplication. Ann Thorac Surg 1992;54:1231–1235.
100. Grande L, Toledo-Pimentel V, Manterola C, et al. Value of Nissen fundoplication in patients with gastro-oesophageal reflux judged by long-term symptom control. Br J Surg 1994;81:548–550.
101. Johansson J, Johnsson F, Joelsson B, et al. Outcome 5 years after 360 degree fundoplication for gastro-oesophageal reflux disease. Br J Surg 1993;80:46–49.
102. Luostarinen M, Isolauri J, Laitinen J, et al. Fate of Nissen fundoplication after 20 years. A clinical, endoscopical, and functional analysis. Gut 1993;34:1015–1020.
103. Macintyre IM, Goulbourne IA. Long-term results after Nissen fundoplication: a 5–15-year review. J R Coll Surg Edinb 1990;35:159–162.
104. Martin CJ, Cox MR, Cade RJ. Collis-Nissen gastroplasty fundoplication for complicated gastrooesophageal reflux disease. Aus N Z J Surg 1992;62:126–129.
105. Mira-Navarro J, Bayle-Bastos F, Frieyro-Segui M, et al. Long-term follow-up of Nissen fundoplication. Eur J Pediatr Surg 1994;4:7–10.
106. Pope C. The quality of life following antireflux surgery. World J Surg 1992;16:355–358.
107. Thor KBA, Silander T. A long-term randomized prospective trial of the Nissen—procedure versus a modified Toupet technique. Ann Surg 1989;210:719–724.
108. Spechler S, Lee E, Ahnen D, et al. Long-term outcome of medical and surgical therapies for gastroesophageal reflux disease: follow-up of a randomized controlled trial. JAMA 2001;9:2331–2338.
109. Fernando H, Luketich N, Christie, et al. Outcome of laparoscopic Toupet compared to laparoscopic Nissen fundoplication. Surg Endosc 2002;16:902–905.
110. Liu J, Woloshin W, Laycock W, Schwartz L. Late outcome after laparoscopic surgery for gastroesophageal reflux. Arch Surg 2002;137:397–401.
111. Richter J. Let the patient beware: the evolving truth about laparoscopic antireflux surgery. Am J Med 2003;114:71–73.

112. Rantanen TK, Salo JA, Sipponen JT. Fatal and life-threatening complications in antireflux surgery: analysis of 5,502 operations [see comment]. Br J Surg 1999;86:1573–1577.
113. Hunter JG, Trus TL, Branum DG, et al. A physiologic approach to laparoscopic fundoplication for gastroesophageal reflux disease. Ann Surg 1996;223:673–687.
114. Waring JP, Lacayo L, Hunter J, et al. Chronic cough and hoarseness in patients with severe gastroesophageal reflux disease. Diagnosis and response to therapy. Dig Dis Sci 1995;40:1093–1097.
115. Waring JP, Hunter JG, Oddsdottir M, et al. The preoperative evaluation of patients considered for laparoscopic antireflux surgery. Am J Gastroenterol 1995;90:35–38.
116. Smith CD, Fink AS, Applegren K. Guidelines for surgical treatment of gastroesophageal reflux disease (GERD). Society of American Gastrointestinal Endoscopic Surgeons (SAGES). Surg Endosc 1998;12:186–188.
117. Eshraghi N, Farahmand M, Soot SJ, et al. Comparison of outcomes of open versus laparoscopic Nissen fundoplication performed in a single practice. Am J Surg 1998;175:371–374.
118. Anvari M, Allen C, Borm A. Laparoscopic Nissen fundoplication is a satisfactory alternative to long-term omeprazole therapy. Br J Surg 1995;82:938–942.
119. Champault G. Gastroesophageal reflux. Treatment by laparoscopy: 940 cases—French experience. Ann Chir 1994;48:159–164.
120. Hinder RA, Filipi CJ, Wetscher G, et al. Laparoscopic Nissen fundoplication is an effective treatment for gastroesophageal reflux disease. Ann Surg 1994;220:472–481; discussion 481–483.
121. Anvari M, Allen C. Laparoscopic Nissen fundoplication: 2-year comprehensive follow-up of a technique of minimal paraesophageal dissection. Ann Surg 1998;227:25–32.
122. Bloomston M, Zervos E, Gonzalez R, et al. Quality of life and antireflux medication use following laparoscopic Nissen fundoplication. Am Surg 1998;64:509–513; discussion 513–514.
123. McKernan JB, Champion JK. Minimally invasive antireflux surgery. Am J Surg 1998;175:271–276.
124. Lin E, Swafford V, Chadalavada R, et al. Disparity between symptomatic and physiologic outcomes following esophageal lenghtening procedures for antireflux surgery. J Gastrointest Surg 2004;8:31–39.
125. Farrell TM, Smith CD, Archer SB, et al. Heartburn is more likely to recur after Toupet fundoplication than Nissen fundoplication. Am J Surg 2000;66:1–9.
126. Smith CD, McClusky DA, Murad AR, et al. When fundoplication fails: redo? Ann Surg 2005;241:861–869.
127. Falk GW, Fennerty MB, Rothstein RI. AGA Institute technical review on the use of endoscopic therapy for gastroesophageal reflux disease. Gastroenterology 2006;131:1315–1336.
128. Kahrilas P. Radiofrequency therapy of the lower esophageal sphincter for treatment of GERD. Gastrointest Endosc 2003;57:723.
129. Kim M, Holloway R, Dent J, Utley D. Radiofrequency energy delivery to the gastric cardia inhibits triggering of transient lower esophageal sphincter relaxation and gastroesophageal reflux in dogs. Gastrointest Endosc 2003;57:17.
130. Utley D, Kim M, Vierra M, Triadfilopoulos G. Augmentation of lower esophageal sphincter pressure and gastric yield pressure after radiofrequency energy delivery to the gastroesophageal junction: a porcine model. Gastrointest Endosc 2001;52:81.
131. Fockens P, Bruno M, Gabbrielli A, et al. Endoscopic augmentation of the lower esophageal sphincter for the treatment of gastroesophageal reflux disease: a multicenter study of the Gatekeeper reflux repair system. Endoscopy 2004;36:682.
132. Mason RJ, Hughes M, Lehman GA, et al. Endoscopic augmentation of the cardia with a biocompatible injectable polymer (Enteryx) in a porcine model. Surg Endosc 2002;16:386–391.
133. Peters JH, Silverman DE, Stein A. Lower esophageal sphincter injection of a biocompatible polymer: accuracy of implantation assessed by esophagectomy. Surg Endosc 2003;17:547–550.
134. Martinez-Serna T, Davis RE, Mason R, et al. Endoscopic valvuloplasty for GERD. Gastrointest Endosc 2000;52:663–670.
135. Tam WC, Holloway RH, Dent J, et al. Impact of endoscopic suturing of the gastroesophageal junction on lower esophageal sphincter function and gastroesophageal reflux in patients with reflux disease. Am J Gastroenterol 2004;99:195–202.
136. Velanovich V, Ben-Menachem T, Goel S. Case-control comparison of endoscopic gastroplication with laparoscopic fundoplication in the management of gastroesophageal reflux disease: early symptomatic outcomes. Surg Laprosc Endosc Percutan Tech 2002;12:219–223.
137. Peters JH. The surgical management of Barrett's esophagus. Gastroenterol Clin North Am 1997;26:647–668.
138. Edwards MJ, Gable DR, Lentsch AB, et al. The rationale for esophagectomy as the optimal therapy for Barrett's esophagus with high-grade dysplasia. Ann Surg 1996;223:585–589; discussion 589–591.
139. Heitmiller RF, Redmond M, Hamilton SR. Barrett's esophagus with high-grade dysplasia. An indication for prophylactic esophagectomy. Ann Surg 1996;224:66–71.
140. Sampliner RE. Practice guidelines on the diagnosis, surveillance, and therapy of Barrett's esophagus. The Practice Parameters Committee of the American College of Gastroenterology. Am J Gastroenterol 1998;93:1028–1032.
141. Spechler SJ. Esophageal columnar metaplasia (Barrett's esophagus). Gastrointest Endosc Clin North Am 1997;7:1–18.
142. McDonald ML, Trastek VF, Allen MS, et al. Barretts's esophagus: does an antireflux procedure reduce the need for endoscopic surveillance? J Thorac Cardiovasc Surg 1996;111:1135–1138; discussion 1139–1140.
143. DeMeester TR, Attwood SE, Smyrk TC, et al. Surgical therapy in Barrett's esophagus. Ann Surg 1990;212:528–540; discussion 540–542.
144. Csendes A, Braghetto I, Burdiles P, et al. A new physiologic approach for the surgical treatment of patients with Barrett's esophagus: technical considerations and results in 65 patients. Ann Surg 1997;226:123–133.
145. Wetscher GJ, Profanter C, Gadenstatter M, et al. Medical treatment of gastroesophageal reflux disease does not prevent the development of Barrett's metaplasia and poor esophageal body motility. Langenbecks Arch Chir 1997;382:95–99.
146. Sampliner RE. Ablation of Barrett's mucosa. Gastroenterologist 1997;5:185–188.
147. Sampliner RE. New treatments for Barrett's esophagus. Semin Gastrointest Dis 1997;8:68–74.
148. Skinner DB, Belsey RHR. Surgical management of esophageal reflux and hiatus hernia: long-term results—with 1030 patients. J Thorac Cardiovasc Surg 1967;53:33.
149. Moskovitz M, Fadden R, Min T, et al. Large hiatal hernias, anemia, and linear gastric erosion: studies of etiology and medical therapy. Am J Gastroenterol 1992;87:622–626.
150. Landreneau RJ, Johnson JA, Marshall JB, et al. Clinical spectrum of paraesophageal herniation. Dig Dis Sci 1992;37:537–544.
151. Berstad A, Weberg R, Froyshov Larsen I, et al. Relationship of hiatus hernia to reflux oesophagitis. A prospective study of coincidence, using endoscopy. Scand J Gastroenterol 1986;21:55–58.
152. Sloan S, Rademaker AW, Kahrilas PJ. Determinants of gastro-esophageal junction incompetence: hiatal hernia, lower esophageal sphincter, or both? Ann Intern Med 1992;117:977–982.
153. Mattioli S, D'Ovidio F, Di Simone MP, et al. Clinical and surgical relevance of the progressive phases of intrathoracic migration of the gastroesophageal junction in gastroesophageal reflux disease. J Thorac Cardiovasc Surg 1998;116:267–275.

154. Kasapidis P, Vassilakis JS, Tzovaras G, et al. Effect of hiatal hernia on esophageal manometry and pH-metry in gastroesophageal reflux disease. Dig Dis Sci 1995;40:2724–2730.
155. Petterson GB, Bombeck CT, Nyhus LM. The influence of hiatal hernia on lower esophageal sphincter function: an experimental study. Ann Pediatr Surg 1981;193:214–220.
156. DeMeester TR, Lafontaine E, Joelsson BE, et al. Relationship of a hiatal hernia to the function of the body of the esophagus and the gastroesophageal junction. J Thorac Cardiovasc Surg 1981;82:547–558.
157. Sloan S, Kahrilas PJ. Impairment of esophageal emptying with hiatal hernia. Gastroenterology 1991;100:596–605.
158. Mittal RK. Hiatal hernia and gastroesophageal reflux: another attempt to resolve the controversy. Gastroenterology 1993; 105:941–943.
159. Casabella F, Sinanan M, Horgan S, et al. Systematic use of gastric fundoplication in laparoscopic repair of paraesophageal hernias. Am J Surg 1996;171:485–489.
160. Fuller CB, Hagen JA, DeMeester TR, et al. The role of fundoplication in the treatment of type II paraesophageal hernia. J Thorac Cardiovasc Surg 1996;111:655–661.
161. Buecker A, Wein BB, Neuerburg JM, et al. Esophageal perforation: comparison of use of aqueous and barium-containing contrast media. Radiology 1997;202:683–686.
162. Lee S, Mergo PJ, Ros PR. The leaking esophagus: CT patterns of esophageal rupture, perforation, and fistulization. Crit Rev Diagn Imaging 1996;37:461–490.
163. Enns R, Branch MS. Management of esophageal perforation after therapeutic upper gastrointestinal endoscopy. Gastrointest Endosc 1998;47:318–320.
164. Wetstein L, Duerr A, Wagner RB. Esophageal perforation. Ann Thorac Surg 1998;65:875–876.
165. Bufkin BL, Miller JI Jr, Mansour KA. Esophageal perforation: emphasis on management. Ann Thorac Surg 1996;61:1447–1451; discussion 1451–1452.
166. Reeder LB, DeFilippi VJ, Ferguson MK. Current results of therapy for esophageal perforation. Am J Surg 1995;169:615–617.
167. Whyte RI, Iannettoni MD, Orringer MB. Intrathoracic esophageal perforation. The merit of primary repair. J Thorac Cardiovasc Surg 1995;109:140–144; discussion 144–146.
168. Altorjay A, Kiss J, Voros A, et al. Nonoperative management of esophageal perforations. Is it justified? Ann Surg 1997;225:415–421.
169. Zargar SA, Kochhar R, Nagi B, et al. Ingestion of strong corrosive alkalis: spectrum of injury to upper gastrointestinal tract and natural history. Am J Gastroenterol 1992;87:337–341.
170. Zargar SA, Kochhar R, Mehta S, et al. The role of fiberoptic endoscopy in the management of corrosive ingestion and modified endoscopic classification of burns. Gastrointest Endosc 1991;37:165–169.
171. Andreoni B, Farina ML, Biffi R, et al. Esophageal perforation and caustic injury: emergency management of caustic ingestion. Dis Esophagus 1997;10:95–100.
172. Anderson KD, Rouse TM, Randolph JG. A controlled trial of corticosteroids in children with corrosive injury of the esophagus. N Engl J Surg 1990;323:637–640.
173. Altorjay A, Kiss J, Voros A, et al. The role of esophagectomy in the management of esophageal perforations. Ann Thorac Surg 1998;65:1433–1436.
174. Berthet B, Castellani P, Brioche MI, et al. Early operation for severe corrosive injury of the upper gastrointestinal tract. Eur J Surg 1996;162:951–955.
175. Pate JW, Walker WA, Cole FH Jr, et al. Spontaneous rupture of the esophagus: a 30-year experience. Ann Thorac Surg 1989; 47:689–692.
176. Bharucha AE, Gostout CJ, Balm RK. Clinical and endoscopic risk factors in the Mallory-Weiss syndrome. Am J Gastroenterol 1997;92:805–808.
177. Pasricha P, Ravich W, Hendrix T, et al. Intrasphincteric botulinum toxin for the treatment of achalasia. N Engl J Med 1995;332:774–778.
178. Fishman V, Parkman H, Schiano T, et al. Symptomatic improvement in achalasia after botulinum toxin injection of the lower esophageal sphincter. Am J Gastroenterol 1996;91:1724–1730.
179. Cuillière C, Ducrottè P, Zerbib F, et al. Achalasia: outcome of patients treated with intrasphincteric injection of botulinum toxin. Gut 1997;41:87–92.
180. Wehrmann T, Kokabpick H, Jacobi V, et al. Long-term results of endoscopic injection of botulinum toxin in elderly achalasic patients with tortuous megaesophagus or epiphrenic diverticulum. Endsocopy 1999;31:352–358.
181. Kolbasnik J, Waterfall W, Fachnie B, et al. Long-term efficacy of botulinum toxin in classical achalasia: a prospective study. Am J Gastroenterol 1999;94:3434–3439.
182. Prakash C, Feedland K, Chan M, Clouse R. Botulinum toxin injections for achalasia symptoms can approximate the short term efficacy of a single pneumatic dilation: a survival analysis approach. Am J Gastroenterol 1999;94:328–333.
183. Annese V, Bassotti G, Coccia G, et al. Comparison of two different formulations of botulinum toxin A for the treatment of oesophageal achalasia. The Gismad Achalasia Study Group. Aliment Pharmacol Ther 1999;13:1347–1350.
184. Allescher H, Storr M, Seige M, et al. Treatment of achalasia: botulinum injection versus pneumatic balloon dilation. A prospective study with long-term follow-up. Endoscopy 2001; 33:1007–1117.
185. Storr M, Born P, Frimberger E, et al. Treatment of achalasia: the short-term response to botulinum toxin injection seems to be independent of any kind of pretreatment. BMC Gastroenterol 2002;2:19.
186. D'Onofrio V, Miletto P, Leandro G, Iaquinto G. Long-term follow-up of achalasia patients treated with botulinum toxin. Dig Liver Dis 2002;34:105–110.
187. Martinek J, Siroky M, Plottova Z, et al. Treatment of patients with achalasia with botulinum toxin: a multicenter prospective cohort study. Dis Esophagus 2003;16:204–209.
188. Ferguson M, Reeder L, Olak J. Results of myotomy and partial fundoplication after pneumatic dilation for achalasia. Ann Thorac Surg 1996;62:327–330.
189. Morino M, Rebecchi F, Festa V, Garrone C. Preoperative pneumatic dilation represents a risk factor for laparoscopic Heller myotomy. Surg 1997;11:359–361.
190. Horgan S, Hudda K, Eubanks T, et al. Does botulinum toxin injection make esophagomyotomy a more difficult operation? Surg Endosc 1999;13:576–579.
191. Patti M, Feo C, Arcerito M, et al. Effects of previous treatment on results of laparoscopic Heller myotomy for achalasia. Dig Dis Sci 1999;44:2270–2276.
192. Ponce J, Juan M, Garrigues V, et al. Efficacy and safety of cardiomyopathy in patients with achalasia after failure of pneumatic dilation. Dig Dis Sci 1999;44:2277–2282.
193. Gockel I, Junginger T, Bernhard G, Eckardt V. Heller myotomy for failed pneumatic dilation in achalasia. Ann Surg 2004;293: 371–377.
194. Rosemurgy A, Villadolid D, Thometz D, et al. Laparoscopic Heller myotomy provides durable relief from achalasia and salvages failures after Botox or dilation. Ann Surg 2005;241:725–735.
195. Portale G, Costantini M, Rizzetto C, et al. Long-term outcome of laparoscopic Heller-Dor surgery for achalasia: Possible detrimental role of previous endoscopic treatment. J Gastrointest Surg 2005;9:1332–1339.
196. Smith C, Stival A, Howell L, Swafford V. Endoscopic therapy for achalasia before Heller myotomy results in worse outcomes than Heller myotomy alone. Ann Surg 2006;243:579–586.
197. Felix VN, Cecconello I, Zilberstein B, et al. Achalasia: a prospective study comparing the results of dilatation and myotomy. Hepatogastroenterology 1998;45:97–108.

198. Csendes A, Braghetto I, Henriquez A, et al. Late results of a prospective randomised study comparing forceful dilatation and oesophagomyotomy in patients with achalasia. Gut 1989;30:299–304.
199. Moreno-Gonzalez E, Garcia Alvarez A, Landa Garcia I, et al. Results of surgical treatment of esophageal achalasia. Multicenter retrospective study of 1856 cases. GEEMO (Groupe Europeen Etude Maladies Oesophageennes) Multicentric Retrospective Study. Int Surg 1988;73:69–77.
200. Okike N, Payne WS, Neufeld DM, et al. Esophagomyotomy versus forceful dilation for achalasia of the esophagus: results in 899 patients. Ann Thorac Surg 1979;28:119–125.
201. Peracchia A, Rosati R, Bona S, et al. Laparoscopic treatment of functional diseases of the esophagus. Int Surg 1995;80:336–340.
202. Raiser F, Perdikis G, Hinder R, et al. Heller myotomy via minimal-access surgery. An evaluation of antireflux procedures. Arch Surg 1996;131:593–597.
203. Hunger J, Trus T, Branum G, Waring J. Laparoscopic Heller myotomy and fundoplication for achalasia. Ann Surg 1997;225:655–664.
204. Kumar V, Shimi S, Cuschieri A. Does laparoscopic cardiomyotomy require an antireflux procedure? Endsocopy 1998;30:8–11.
205. Patti M, Pellegrini C, Horgan S, et al. Minimally invasive surgery for achalasia: an 8-year experience with 168 patients. Ann Surg 1999;230:587–593.
206. Richards W, Clements R, Wang P, et al. Prevalence of gastroesophageal reflux after laparoscopic Heller myotomy. Surg Endosc 1999;13:1010–1014.
207. Stewart K, Finley R, Clifton J, et al. Thoracoscopic versus laparoscopic modified Heller myotomy for achalasia: efficacy and safety in 87 patients. J Am Coll Surg 1999;189:164–169.
208. Zaninotto G, Costantini M, Molena D, et al. Treatment of esophageal achalasia with laparoscopic Heller myotomy and Dor partial anterior fundoplication: prospective evaluation of 100 consecutive patients. J Gastrointest Surg 2000;4:282–289.
209. Yamamura M, Gilster J, Myers B, et al. Laparoscopic Heller myotomy and anterior fundoplication for achalasia results in a high degree of patient satisfaction. Arch Surg 2000;135:902–906.
210. Oelschlager B, Chang L, Pellegrini C. Improved outcome after extended gastric myotomy for achalasia. Arch Surg 2003;138:490–497.
211. Falkenback D, Johansson J, Oberg S, et al. Heller's esophagomyotomy with or without a 360 degrees floppy Nissen fundoplication for achalasia. Long-term results from a prospective randomized study. Dis Esophagus 2003;16:284–290.
212. Richards WO, Torquati A, Holzman MD, et al. Heller myotomy versus Heller myotomy with Dor fundoplication for achalasia: a prospective randomized double-blind clinical trial [see comment]. Ann Surg 2004;240:405–412; discussion 412–415.
213. Diamantis T, Pikoulis E, Felekouras E, et al. Laparoscopic esophagomyotomy for achalasia without a complementary antireflux procedure. J Laparoendosc Adv Surg Tech A 2006;16:345–349.
214. Mattinger C, Hormann K. Endoscopic diverticulostomy of Zenker's diverticulum: management and complications. Dysphagia 2002;17:34–39.
215. Mulder C, Costamagna G, Sakai P. Zapping Zenker's diverticulum: gastroscopic treatment. Can J Gastroenterol 1999;13:405–407.
216. Narne S, Cutrone C, Bonavina L, et al. Endoscopic diverticulotomy for the treatment of Zenker's diverticulum: results in 102 patients with staple assisted endoscopy. Ann Otol Rhinol Laryngol 1999;108:810–815.
217. Peracchia A, Bonavina L, Narne S, et al. Minimally invasive surgery for Zenker diverticulum: analysis and results in 95 consecutive patients. Arch Surg 1998;133:695–700.
218. Scher RL, Richtsmeier WJ. Long-term experience with endoscopic staple-assisted esophagodiverticulostomy for Zenker's diverticulum. Laryngoscope 1998;108:200–205.
219. Von Doersten PG, Byl FM. Endoscopic Zenker's diverticulotomy (Dohlman procedure): 40 cases reviewed. Otolaryngol Head Neck Surg 1997;116:209–212.
220. Lippert BM, Folz BJ, Gottschlich S, et al. Microendoscopic treatment of the hypopharyngeal diverticulum with the CO_2 laser. Lasers Surg Med 1997;20:394–401.
221. Ishioka S, Sakai P, Maluf Filho F, et al. Endoscopic incision of Zenker's diverticula. Endoscopy 1995;27:433–437.
222. Wouters B, van Overbeek JJ. Endoscopic treatment of the hypopharyngeal (Zenker's) diverticulum. Hepatogastroenterology 1992;39:105–108.
223. Gutschow C, Hamoir M, Rombaux P, et al. Management of pharyngoesophageal (Zenker's) diverticulum: which technique? Ann Thorac Surg 2002;74:1677–1683.
224. Bonafede JP, Lavertu P, Wood BG, et al. Surgical outcome in 87 patients with Zenker's diverticulum. Laryngoscope 1997;107:720–725.
225. Witterick IJ, Gullane PJ, Yeung E. Outcome analysis of Zenker's diverticulectomy and cricopharyngeal myotomy. Head Neck 1995;17:382–388.
226. Laing MR, Murthy P, Ah-See KW, et al. Surgery for pharyngeal pouch: audit of management with short- and long-term follow-up. J R Coll Surg Edinb 1995;40:315–318.
227. Lerut T, van Raemdonck D, Guelinckx P, et al. Zenker's diverticulum: is a myotomy of the cricopharyngeus useful? How long should it be? Hepatogastroenterology 1992;39:127–131.
228. Schmit PJ, Zuckerbraun L. Treatment of Zenker's diverticula by cricopharyngeus myotomy under local anesthesia. Am Surg 1992;58:710–716.
229. Payne WS. The treatment of pharyngoesophageal diverticulum: the simple and complex. Hepatogastroenterology 1992;39:109–114.
230. Klinkenberg-Knol EC, Jansen JM, Festen HP, et al. Double-blind multicentre comparison of omeprazole and ranitidine in the treatment of reflux oesophagitis. Lancet 1987;1:349–351.
230a. O'Connor KW, Madison ST, Smith DJ, et al. An expeimental endoscopic technique for reversing gastroesophageal reflux in dogs by injecting inert material in the distal esophagus. Gastrointest Endosc 1984;30:275–280.
231. Havelund T, Laursen LS, Skoubo-Kristensen E, et al. Omeprazole and ranitidine in treatment of reflux oesophagitis: double blind comparative trial. Br Med J Clin Res Ed 1988;296:89–92.
232. Sandmark S, Carlsson R, Fausa O, et al. Omeprazole or ranitidine in the treatment of reflux esophagitis. Results of a double-blind, randomized, Scandinavian multicenter study. Scand J Gastroenterol 1988;23:625–632.
233. Vantrappen G, Rutgeerts L, Schurmans P, et al. Omeprazole (40 mg) is superior to ranitidine in short-term treatment of ulcerative reflux esophagitis. Dig Dis Sci 1988;33:523–529.
234. Lundell L, Backman L, Ekstrom P, et al. Omeprazole or high-dose ranitidine in the treatment of patients with reflux oesophagitis not responding to "standard doses" of H_2-receptor antagonists. Aliment Pharmacol Ther 1990;4:145–155.
235. Stein HJ, Feussner H, Siewert JR. Failure of antireflux surgery: causes and management strategies. Am J Surg 1996;171:36–39; discussion 39–40.
236. Floch NR, Hinder RA, Klingler PJ, et al. Is laparoscopic reoperation for failed antireflux surgery feasible? Arch Surg 1999;134(7):733–737.
237. Soper N, Dunnegan D. Anatomic fundoplication failure after laparoscopic antireflux surgery. Ann Surg 1999;229:669–676.
238. Pointner R, Bammer T, Then P, Kamolz T. Laparoscopic refundoplications after failed antireflux surgery. Am J Surg 1999;178(6):541–544.
239. Awad Z, Anderson P, Sato K, et al. Laparoscopic reoperative antireflux surgery. Surg Endosc 2001;15:1401–1407.

240. Heniford BT, Matthews BD, Kercher KW, et al. Surgical experience in 55 consecutive reoperative fundoplications. Am Surg 2002;68:949–954; discussion 954.
241. Granderath FA, Kamolz T, Schweiger UM, Pointner R. Failed antireflux surgery: quality of life and surgical outcome after laparoscopic refundoplication. Int J Colorectal Dis 2003;18:248–253.
242. Rosemurgy AS, Arnaoutakis DJ, Thometz DP, et al. Reoperative fundoplications are effective treatment for dysphagia and recurrent gastroesophageal reflux. Am Surg 2004;70:1061–1067.
243. Byrne JP, Smithers BM, Nathanson LK, et al. Symptomatic and functional outcome after laparoscopic reoperation for failed antireflux surgery. Br J Surg 2005;92:996–1001.
244. Smith CD, McClusky DA, Murad AR, et al. When fundoplication fails: redo? Ann Surg 2005;241:861–869.
245. Iqbal A, Awad Z, Simkins J, et al. Repair of 104 failed anti-reflux operations. Ann Surg 2006;244:42–51.
246. Richards W, Scholz S, Khaitan L, et al. Initial experience with the Stretta procedure for the treatment of gastroesophageal reflux disease. J Laparoendosc Adv Surg Tech 2001;11:267.
247. Triadafilopoulos G, DiBaise JK, Nostrant TT, et al. The Stretta procedure for the treatment of GERD: 6 and 12 month follow-up of the US open label trial. Gastrointest Endosc 2002;55:149–156.
248. Houston H, Khaitan L, Holzman M, Richards WO. First year experience of patients undergoing the Stretta procedure. Surg Endosc 2003;17:401–404.
249. Go MR, Dundon JM, Karlowicz DJ, et al. Delivery of radiofrequency energy to the lower esophageal sphincter improves symptoms of gastroesophageal reflux. Surgery 2004;136:786–794.
250. Johnson DA, Ganz R, Aisenberg J, et al. Endoscopic implantation of enteryx for treatment of GERD: 12-month results of a prospective, multicenter trial. Am J Gastroenterol 2003;98:1921–1930.
251. Cohen LB, Johnson DA, Ganz RA, et al. Enteryx implantation for GERD: expanded multicenter trial results and interim post-approval follow-up to 24 months. Gastrointest Endosc 2005;61:650–658.
252. Schumacher B, Neuhaus H, Ortner M, et al. Reduced medication dependency and improved symptoms and quality of life 12 months after Enteryx implantation for gastroesophageal reflux. J Clin Gastroenterol 2005;39:212–219.
253. Fockens P, Bruno M, Gabbrielli A, et al. Endoscopic augmentation of the lower esophageal sphincter for the treatment of gastroesophageal reflux disease: a multicenter study of the Gatekeeper reflux repair system. Endoscopy 2004;36:682.
254. Pleskow D, Rothstein R, Lo S, et al. Endoscopic full-thickness plication for the treatment of GERD: 12-month follow-up for the North American open-label trial. Gastrointest Endosc 2005;61:643–649.
255. Arts J, Lerut T, Rutgeerts P, et al. A 1-year follow-up study of endoluminal gastroplication (Endocinch) in GERD patients refractory to proton pump inhibitor therapy. Dig Dis Sci 2005;50:351–356.
256. Chen YK, Raijman I, Ben-Menachem T, et al. Long-term outcomes of endoluminal gastroplication: a US multicenter trial. Gastrointest Endosc 2005;61:659–667.
257. Corley DA, Katz P, Wo JM, et al. Improvement of gastroesophageal reflux symptoms after radiofrequency energy: a randomized, sham-controlled trial. Gastroenterology 2003;125:668–676.
258. Deviere J, Costamagna G, Neuhaus H, et al. Nonresorbable copolymer implantation for gastroesophageal reflux disease: a randomized sham-controlled multicenter trial. Gastroenterology 2005;128:532–540.
259. Park P, Hall-Angeras M, Ohlin B, et al. A prospective, multicenter, randomized, single-blind, parallel group study on the comparison between endoscopic cardia suturing and sham operation as a treatment of patients with gastroesophageal reflux symptoms. Gastroenterology 2005;128 (suppl 2): A-95.
260. Schwartz M, Wellink H, Gooszen H, et al. A blinded, randomized, sham-controlled trial of endoscopic gastroplication for the treatment of gastro-esophageal reflux disease (GERD): preliminary results. Gastrointest Endosc 2005;61:AB95.
261. Schwartz M, Wellink H, Gooszen H, et al. Endoscopic gastroplication for the treatment of gastro-oesophageal reflux disease: a randomized, sham-controlled trial. Gut 2007;56:20–28.
262. Attwood SE, Barlow AP, Norris TL, et al. Barrett's oesophagus: effect of antireflux surgery on symptom control and development of complications. Br J Surg 1992;79:1050–1053.
263. Ortiz A, Martinez de Haro LF, Parrilla P, et al. Conservative treatment versus antireflux surgery in Barrett's oesophagus: long-term results of a prospective study. Br J Surg 1996;83:274–278.
264. Sampliner RE. Effect of up to 3 years of high-dose lansoprazole on Barrett's esophagus. Am J Gastroenterol 1994;89:1844–1848.
265. Csendes A, Braghetto I, Burdiles P, et al. Long-term results of classic antireflux surgery in 152 patients with Barrett's esophagus: clinical, radiologic, endoscopic, manometric, and acid reflux test analysis before and late after operation. Surgery (St Louis) 1998;126:645–657.
266. Skinner DB, Walther BC, Riddell RH, et al. Barrett's esophagus. Comparison of benign and malignant cases. Ann Surg 1983;198:554–565.
267. Williamson WA, Ellis FH Jr, Gibb SP, et al. Effect of antireflux operation on Barrett's mucosa. Ann Thorac Surg 1990;49:537–541; discussion 541–542.
268. Martinez de Haro LF, Ortiz A, Parrilla P, et al. Long-term results of Nissen fundoplication in reflux esophagitis without strictures. Clinical, endoscopic, and pH-metric evaluation. Dig Dis Sci 1992;37:523–527.
269. Sagar PM, Ackroyd R, Hosie KB, et al. Regression and progression of Barrett's oesophagus after antireflux surgery. Br J Surg 1995;82:806–810.
270. Polepalle SC, McCallum RW. Barrett's esophagus. Current assessment and future perspectives. Gastroenterol Clin North Am 1990;19:733–744.
271. McDonald ML, Trastek VF, Allen MS, et al. Barretts's esophagus: does an antireflux procedure reduce the need for endoscopic surveillance? J Thorac Cardiovasc Surg 1996;111:1135–1138; discussion 1139–1140.
272. Gray SW, Skandalakis JE, McClusky DA. Atlas of Surgical Anatomy for General Surgeons. Baltimore: Williams & Wilkins; 1985.
273. Jamieson GG, ed. Surgery of the Esophagus. Edinburgh: Churchill Livingstone; 1988:19–35.
274. Shields TW, ed. General Thoracic Surgery. 3rd ed. Philadelphia: Lea & Febiger; 1989:84.
275. Zuidema GD, Orringer MD, eds. Shackelford's Surgery of the Alimentary Tract. Vol. 1, 3rd ed. Philadelphia: Saunders; 1991:95.
276. Waters PF, DeMeester TR. Foregut motor disorders and their surgical management. Med Clin North Am 1981;65:1238.
277. Hunter JF, Richardson WS. Surgical management of achalasia. Surg Clin North Am 1997;77:993–1015.
278. Teracol J, Sweet RH. Diseases of the Esophagus. Philadelphia: Saunders; 1958.
279. Fennerty MB, Castell D, Fendrick AM, et al. The diagnosis and treatment of gastroesophageal reflux disease in a managed care environment. Suggested disease management guidelines. Arch Intern Med 1996;156:477–484.
280. DeMeester TR, Stein HJ. Gastroesophageal reflux disease. In: Moody FG, ed. Surgical Treatment of Digestive Disease. 2nd ed. Chicago: Mosby Year Book; 1989:68.

44B

Malignant Tumors of the Esophagus

Gail Darling

Carcinoma of the esophagus is the 10th leading cause of cancer deaths in North America. The incidence varies considerably from 5 per 100,000 in most Western countries to as high as 100 per 100,000 in some countries such as Iran, Japan, China, and other countries in the "esophageal cancer belt." The estimated 5-year survival for cancer of the esophagus is 10%. Adenocarcinoma, previously rare, is increasing in incidence in Western countries by approximately 5%–10% per year[1,2] and is now the dominant cell type in patients in North America and Europe, although squamous cell carcinoma still dominates globally. In a recent series of patients with esophageal cancer from the Mayo Clinic,[3] adenocarcinoma was present in 85.5%. Adenocarcinoma and squamous cell cancer account for almost all cases. Leiomyosarcoma, lymphoma, small-cell carcinoma, and melanoma occur rarely.

Etiology

The etiologic factors associated with squamous cell cancer of the esophagus include smoking; alcohol abuse; poor nutrition; dietary carcinogens (nitrates, nitrites); vitamin deficiencies (C, E, B); mineral deficiencies (selenium, zinc, molybdenum); caustic injury; achalasia; Plummer-Vinson syndrome; celiac disease; previous radiation; history of head and neck cancer; tylosis; and p53 mutations or overexpression.

The factors associated with adenocarcinoma include Barrett's esophagus, severe gastroesophageal reflux disease (GERD) and obesity.[4]

Presentation

The most common presenting symptom is dysphagia. This usually is indicative of locally advanced disease since the esophageal lumen must be significantly compromised (>50%) before dysphagia occurs. Other symptoms may include anorexia, weight loss, odynophagia, chest or back pain, melena or hematemesis, and occasionally hoarseness. Unfortunately, almost half of patients will have metastatic disease at the time of initial presentation and have an estimated survival of 4–8 months. A small fraction of patients will be identified with early-stage cancer either through Barrett's surveillance programs or when endoscoped for other reasons.

The evaluation of a patient with dysphagia requires barium swallow or esophagogastroduodenscopy. Although a barium swallow is useful, endoscopy is essential to confirm the diagnosis and obtain tissue for histology. Bronchoscopy should be performed for tumors at or above the level of the tracheal carina to rule out airway invasion.

Adenocarcinoma usually occurs in the lower esophagus, with 79% in the lower third, 18% in the middle third, and 3% in the upper third,[5] whereas squamous cancer is more common in the middle and upper thirds.

Staging

CT scanning is used to evaluate the extent of the primary tumor and to determine the presence of nodal or distant metastatic disease. Loss of the fat plane between the esophagus and adjacent structures is suggestive of invasion, as is the finding of greater than 90° of contact. However, even these radiologic signs are not foolproof.

Stage-specific therapies previously have not been used for esophageal cancer, so precise staging has been less important for this tumor than many others. However, Rice et al. advocated for treatment strategies based on the stage of disease, offering immediate surgery to those with early disease, postoperative therapy if positive nodes are found, and preoperative chemoradiotherapy to those with more advanced disease at time of presentation. Hence, more accurate staging tests are required.[6]

Endoscopic ultrasound (EUS) has been found to be useful in evaluating the depth of penetration of the primary tumor

TABLE 44B.1. Staging of Lymph Nodes by Endoscopic Ultrasound (EUS) Versus EUS-FNA.

	EUS	*EUS-FNA*	*P value*
Sensitivity	63%	93%	.01
Specificity	81%	100%	NS
Accuracy	70%	93%	0.02

EUS-FNA, endoscopic ultrasound-fine needle aspiration; NS, not significant.

Source: From Vasquez-Sequeiros et al.,[10] by permission of *Gastrointestinal Endoscopy*.

and thus establishing the T stage prior to treatment. The overall accuracy for EUS staging of the primary tumor ranges from 50.0% to 81.3%. Accuracy is improved if endoscopic information is available unless the tumor completely obstructs the esophageal lumen.[7] Endoscopic ultrasound can reliably distinguish T1/T2 from T3/T4 but is most accurate for the latter.[7,8] Celiac and mediastinal nodes can be assessed by EUS, but accuracy is higher for celiac nodes. The sensitivity of EUS for nodal disease is 89%, with 75% specificity and overall accuracy of 80%.[9] Accuracy may be increased by EUS-guided needle biopsy (EUS-FNA)[10] (Table 44B.1).

Positron emission tomography (PET) has demonstrated promise in staging of esophageal cancer. It is most useful in detecting distant metastatic disease, for which it has been found to detect metastatic sites not identified by conventional staging in 15% of patients.[11] However, the regional nodes close to the tumor are not easy to assess because of the intense uptake by the primary tumor itself, which obscures adjacent lymph nodes. Similarly, it is not as useful as EUS in determining T stage.[12] Integrated PET/computed tomography (CT) has improved diagnostic accuracy over PET alone.[13] Discordance between PET and CT findings are clinically relevant about half of the time.[14] Comparison of PET, CT, and EUS suggests that these are complimentary staging techniques[12,15] (Table 44B.2).[15]

Laparoscopic and thoracoscopic staging has been advocated by Krasna and others[16] but has not been universally accepted. Surgical staging can clearly identify nodal disease, with sensitivity of 63%–85%, specificity of 100%, and overall accuracy of 93%–94%. Also, it allows evaluation of the extent of the primary tumor.[17] It is most useful in the setting of neoadjuvant therapies. However, the combination of PET, EUS-FNA (fine needle aspiration), and CT appear to provide similar data.

Using decision analysis, Wallace and colleagues determined that EUS with FNA and PET was the most effective staging strategy in terms of quality-adjusted life years. The use of EUS-FNA with CT was almost as effective but was more cost-effective.[18]

TABLE 44B.2. Comparison of Positron Emission Tomography (PET), Computed Tomography (CT), and Endoscopic Ultrasound (EUS).

	PET	*CT*	*EUS*
T detection sensitivity (%)	83	67	100
T stage accuracy (%)		63	
N stage			
Sensitivity (%)	37	47	89
Specificity (%)	100	92	54
Accuracy (%)	63	66	75
M stage			
Sensitivity (%)	47	33	
Specificity (%)	89	96	
Accuracy (%)	74	74	

Source: From Rasanen JV, Sihvo EI, Knuuti MJ, Minn HR, et al.[15]

Staging of Esophageal Carcinoma

The staging system for esophageal cancer is shown in Table 44B.3. There is a proposal to revise the staging system, but this has not been adopted yet.

TABLE 44B-3. Definition of TMN, Stage Grouping, Histopathologic Type, and Histologic Grade for Esophageal Carcinoma.

Definition of TMN			
Primary Tumor (T)			
TX	Primary tumor cannot be assessed		
T0	No evidence of primary tumor		
Tis	Carcinoma *in situ*		
T1	Tumor invades lamina propria or submucosa		
T2	Tumor invades muscularis propria		
T3	Tumor invades adventitia		
T4	Tumor invades adjacent structures		
Regional Lymph Nodes (N)			
NX	Regional lymph nodes cannot be assessed		
N0	No regional lymph node metastasis		
N1	Regional lymph node metastasis		
Distant Metastasis (M)			
MX	Distant metastasis cannot be assessed		
M0	No distant metastasis		
M1	Distant metastasis		
Tumors of the lower thoracic esophagus:			
M1a	Metastasis in celiac lymph nodes		
M1b	Other distant metastasis		
Tumors of midthoracic esophagus:			
M1a	Not applicable		
M1b	Nonregional lymph node and/or other distant metastasis		
Tumors of upper thoracic esophagus:			
M1a	Metastasis in cervical lymph nodes		
M1b	Other distant metastasis		
Stage Grouping			
Stage 0	Tis	N0	M0
Stage I	T1	N0	M0
Stage IIA	T2	N0	M0
	T3	N0	M0
Stage IIB	T1	N1	M0
	T2	N1	M0
Stage III	T3	N1	M0
	T4	Any N	M0
Stage IV	Any T	Any N	M1
Stage IVA	Any T	Any N	M1a
Stage IVB	Any T	Any N	M1b

Source: Used with the permission of the American Joint Committee on Cancer (AJCC), Chicago, Illinois. The original source for this material is the *AJCC Cancer Staging Manual, Sixth Edition* (2002) published by Springer Science and Business Media LLC, www.springerlink.com.

TABLE 44B.4.
Operative Mortality, Morbidity, and Survival for Esophagectomy for Cancer.

Author	*Year*	*N*	*Operation*	*Mortality (%)*	*Survival (%)*			*Median survival (mo)*
					3 yr	*4 yr*	*5 yr*	
Guili[69]	1980	2,400	TTE	30				
Earlan[70]	1980	87,783	TTE	33				
Posthlethwait[71]	1983	164	TTE	12.8				
Ellis[72]	1983	167	TTE	1.3			21.7	17.3
Orringer[20]	1984	100	THE	6	22	17		
Katariya[73]	1994	1,353	THE	7.1				
Orringer[74]	1999	800	THE	4.2		23		
Ellis[25]	1999	455	TTE	3.3		24.7		
Altorki[26]	1999	103	En bloc	4.8		46		
Visbal[3]	2001	220	I-L			25.2	22.8	
Altorki[77]	2002	80	3 field	3		51		
Casson[35]	2002	91		4.4				
Hulscher[24]	2002	111	TTE	4		39	24	
Hulscher[24]	2002	94	THE	2		29	21.6	
Bailey[78]	2003	1,777		9.8				

THE, transhiatal esophagectomy; TTE, transthoracic esophagectomy.

Treatment of Esophageal Cancer

Surgery

Surgery is the primary treatment for esophageal cancer. Surgery provides excellent palliation of dysphagia, provides local control, and allows patients to eat comfortably until death. In those fit for surgery, 13.5%–51% will be cured of their cancer. Most surgical series report 5-year survival of approximately 25%, but higher rates have been reported with more extensive surgery (Table 44B.4). The mortality of esophagectomy performed by experienced high-volume surgeons in high-volume centers is less than 5%, although in a recent study of patterns of care, the mortality across the United States averaged 10.5%.[19] This represents a significant improvement over the years since the 1960s, when the mortality of esophagectomy was approximately 30% (Table 44.B4). Nevertheless, the mortality varies considerably depending on the practice volume of both surgeon and hospital. Even though mortality is lower, the morbidity of esophagectomy is still considerable, with 40%–50% of patients experiencing one or more postoperative complications (Table 44B.5).

Surgery is the treatment of choice for tumors of the mid- and distal esophagus, including the gastroesophageal junction, in patients who are medically fit for esophagectomy. Radiation may be used for those who are deemed medically inoperable or who chose not to have surgery and is generally the treatment of choice for tumors of the upper third of the esophagus. For upper-third tumors, outcomes are similar with either radiation or surgery; however, radiation allows preser-

TABLE 44B.5.
Morbidity of Esophagectomy for Cancer.

Author	*Year*	*N*	*Leaks (%)*	*RLN (%)*	*Resp (%)*	*Afib/MI (%)*	*Chylothorax (%)*	*Total (%)*
Orringer[20]	1984	100	5	4	3			
Visbal[3]	2001	220	4.5	0.9		17.3/2.2	1.8	37.7
Bailey[78]	2003	1,777			21.4	/1.2		49.5
Orringer[74]	1999	800	13	7			<1	
Posthlethwait[71]	1983	162	3		10.5	/1.2		
Ellis[72]	1983	167	3.5					21.5
Altorki[76]	1999	103						40
Altorki[77]	2002	80	11.2	8.8	26.2		1.2	51
Casson[35]	2002	91	16.5					36.3

Afib, atrial fibrillation; MI, myocardial infarction; Resp, respiratory complications; RLN, recurrent laryngeal nerve injury.

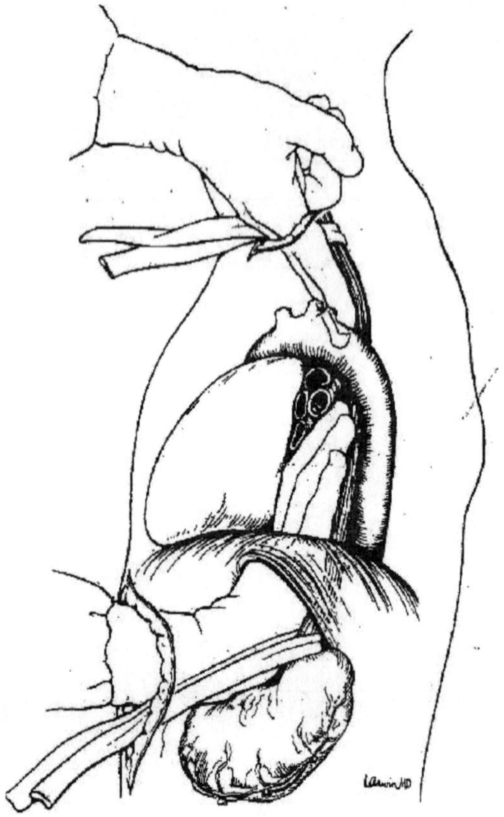

FIGURE 44B.1. Transhiatal dissection of the plane anterior to the esophagus. (From Orringer.[78])

vation of the larynx. Surgery may be used as salvage in those who fail radiotherapy.

Controversies in Esophageal Surgery

Controversies in esophageal surgery include the choice of operative approach; the choice of conduit (stomach or colon); the route of the conduit (retrosternal or posterior mediastinum); whether to tubularize the stomach; the location of the anastomosis (chest or neck); whether to perform a pyloric drainage procedure; the choice of hand-sewn or stapled anastomosis; the extent of lymphadenectomy; and whether to combine surgery with chemotherapy or radiation or both.

Operative Approaches

The operative approaches to esophagectomy include the Ivor-Lewis (also known as Lewis-Tanner), the McKeown, transhiatal, radical en bloc, minimally invasive surgery (MIS), and left thoracoabdominal with either an intrathoracic or left neck anastomosis.

The Ivor-Lewis procedure consists of a laparotomy and right thoracotomy with an intrathoracic anastomosis at or just above the level of the azygous vein. The McKeown approach uses a right thoracotomy for resection of the entire thoracic esophagus, a laparotomy to prepare the gastric conduit, and a neck incision to perform the anastomosis.

A transhiatal esophagectomy (THE) avoids a thoracotomy by dissecting the thoracic esophagus through the esophageal hiatus via a laparotomy incision from below and via a neck incision from above, with the anastomosis in the neck[20] (see Fig. 44B.1).

Another approach is to use a left thoracoabdominal incision to dissect the esophagus and prepare the gastric conduit, which may then be anastomosed to the esophageal remnant in the chest or in the neck via a separate neck incision. A higher anastomosis is preferred to obtain adequate margins and to provide better functional results with less reflux. The en bloc resection proposed by Skinner includes resection of adjacent pleura, pericardium, thoracic duct, and a cuff of diaphragm with extensive lymph node dissection, including the azygous vein and adjacent intercostal vessels.[21]

More recently, minimally invasive approaches using laparoscopy alone or combined laparoscopy and thoracoscopy with a cervical incision for completion of the anastomosis have been developed in selected centers.[22]

The THE, by avoiding a thoracotomy, is associated with fewer respiratory complications, whereas the transthoracic approach in all its various modifications allows wider dissection, removal of adjacent tissues, and more complete lymphadenectomy. A meta-analysis of 50 publications, including 3942 patients, compared the two approaches. However, there were only six prospective trials, of which three were randomized trials. This analysis showed no significant overall difference in survival between the two approaches, with a 5-year survival of 21.7%–23%. However, in the studies that directly compared the two approaches,[23] there was a statistically significant improvement in 5-year survival in the transthoracic group (transthoracic esophagectomy, TTE) versus the transhiatal group (THE): 35.2% versus 24.9%, relative risk (RR) 1.41, 95% CI 1.68–1.89 (see Table 44B.6). In the largest prospective randomized trial, including 220 patients, comparing TTE versus THE, 5-year overall survival was 39% in the transthoracic resection group versus 29% in the transhiatal group (95% CI –3 to 23, $P = .12$), although the morbidity of the transhiatal approach was less[24] (see Fig. 44B.2). Although the survival difference did not reach statistical significance, there was a clear trend in favor of the more extensive approach (see Table 44B.7).

Proponents of the transhiatal approach argue that once esophageal cancer has spread to lymph nodes, it is not curable by surgery; therefore, the increased morbidity of the transthoracic approach is not justified. However, the improved survival in series using more extensive lymph node dissection that include periesophageal tissues suggests that more radical surgery may be beneficial. In addition, in Hulscher et al.'s randomized trial, the increased early pulmonary complications did not translate into significant adverse events or pro-

TABLE 44B.6. Meta-analysis of Transthoracic Esophagectomy (TTE) Versus Transhiatal Esophagectomy (THE).[23]

	TTE	*THE*	*RR*	*95% CI*
In-hospital mortality (%)	9.2	5.7	1.60	1.42–1.89
Complications:				
Anastomotic leak (%)	7.2	13.6	0.53	0.45–0.63
Vocal cord paralysis (%)	3.5	9.5	0.36	0.27–0.47
Chyle leak (%)	2.4	1.4	1.70	2.72–10.5
Respiratory (%)	18.7	12.7	1.47	1.29–1.68
Cardiac (%)	6.6	19.5	0.34	0.27–0.41
Survival (%)				
3 year	26.7	25.6	1.83	0.70–4.78
5 year	23.0	21.7	1.06	0.96–1.18

Source: From Hulscher,[23] by permission of *Annals of Thoracic Surgery.*

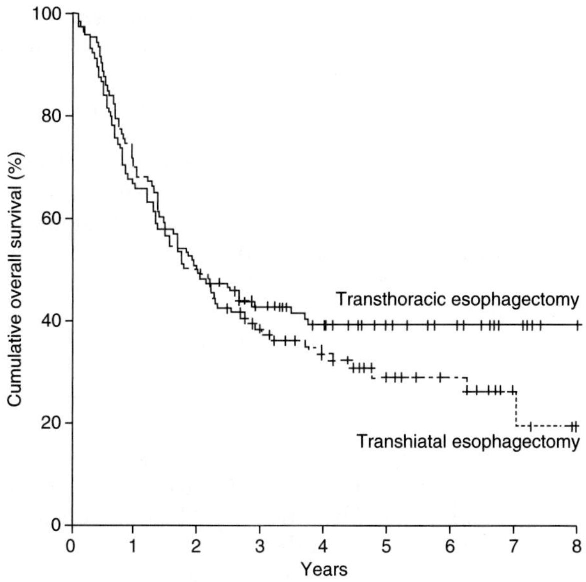

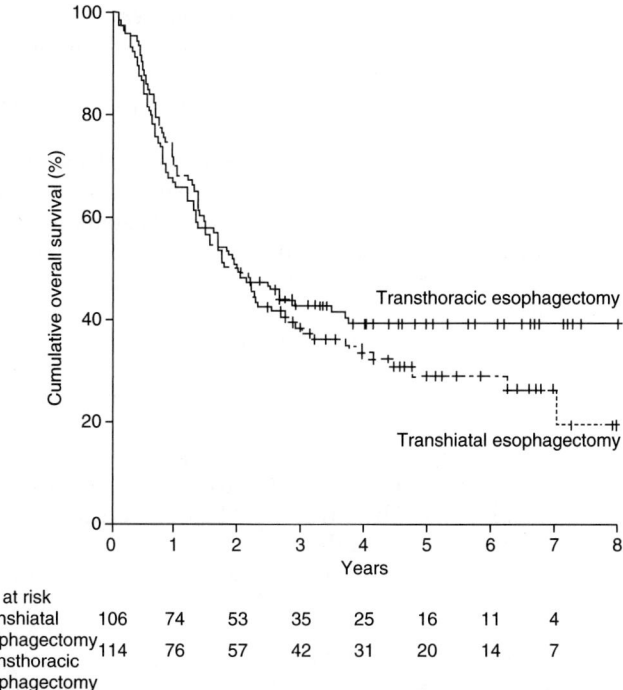

No. at risk								
Transhiatal esophagectomy	106	74	53	35	25	16	11	4
Transthoracic esophagectomy	114	76	57	42	31	20	14	7

FIGURE 44B.2. Kaplan-Meier curves showing overall survival among patients randomly assigned to transhiatal esophagectomy or transthoracic esophagectomy with extended en bloc lymphadenectomy. (From Hulscher,[24] by permission from The New England Journal of Medicine.)

longed length of stay.[25] Furthermore, the hospital mortality for a radical en bloc resection has decreased from 11%[21] to approximately 5%.[24–27]

For tumors at the gastroesophageal junction or in the lower third of the esophagus, several operative approaches may be appropriate depending on surgeon preference, including transhiatal, Ivor-Lewis, minimally invasive techniques (MIS), left thoracoabdominal, or radical en bloc. For tumors of the midesophagus, the McKeown, Ivor-Lewis, or radical en bloc approach may be used. The MIS techniques may also be used. The transhiatal approach has been used for midesophageal tumors by some but is not widely recommended.

Technical Considerations in Esophagectomy

Route of Reconstruction. The gastric conduit may be placed either in the bed of the resected esophagus or substernally. Although a meta-analysis of six randomized trials concluded that there was no significant difference between the two, consideration should be given to the retrosternal route if an R0 resection cannot be accomplished as local recurrence is unlikely to affect the function of the conduit if it is retrosternal.[28] There was a suggestion of increased mortality (RR 0.56, 95% CI 0.17–1.82) and increased morbidity (cardiac RR 0.43, 95% CI 0.17–1.12; pulmonary RR 0.67, 95% CI 0.34–1.33) with the retrosternal route. When the retrosternal route is chosen, most surgeons will resect the sternoclavicular joint or portion of sternum to reduce the risk of compression of the conduit by the thoracic inlet, which may compromise arterial blood supply or venous drainage. From a functional perspective, the posterior mediastinal route is the shortest and straightest. This lack of angulation allows more comfortable swallowing.

Choice of Reconstruction. The stomach is the preferred conduit for reconstruction based on its reliable blood supply, adequate length, and simplicity of reconstruction with only one anastomosis. There is some controversy whether the whole stomach should be used or a gastric tube created and whether the width of the tube affects function. Proponents of a narrow tube believe it empties better and is less likely to become overdistended and tortuous. However, in a nonrandomized study, Collard et al. reported increased anastomotic fistula (7.9% vs. 1%, $P = .0209$), strictures (22.3% vs. 6%, $P = .0008$), as well as significantly increased problems with eating associated with tubularized stomach versus whole stomach.[29] With either choice, it is important to resect the lymph nodes along the lesser curvature extending to the left gastric artery.

Alternatives to stomach include the colon (right or left) or jejunum. The colon has adequate length to replace the entire esophagus.[30] The jejunum is more useful for short segments and may be used either as a pedicled or free graft with microvascular reconstruction.[31–33]

Anastomotic Techniques. The anastomotic leak rate after esophagogastric anastomoses remains a significant problem in most centers. There are three techniques currently used: hand sewn and stapled using either a circular stapler or a linear stapler. The use of linear staplers in a side-to-side technique was popularized by Orringer et al.[34] Using this technique, they reported a significant decrease in anastomotic leaks from 13% to 2.7%. Casson et al. also reported a decrease in anastomotic leak rate from 22.6% to 7.9% after adopting the side-to-side stapled technique. With a decrease in anastomotic leaks, there was an accompanying decrease in strictures from 17.0% with hand-sewn anastomoses to 7.9% in patients with stapled anastomoses.[35] A further modification of the side-to-side stapled anastomosis has been popularized by Rice and coworkers and is also associated with reduced leaks.[36]

A meta-analysis of randomized trials comparing hand-sewn versus stapled anastomoses found no significant difference in terms of leaks (RR 0.79, 95% CI 0.44–1.42, $P = .43$) or strictures (RR 0.99, 95% CI 0.55–1.77, $P = .97$), although there is a suggestion of increased strictures with circular staplers.[37,38]

The site of the anastomosis in the neck versus chest is a confounding factor in comparing leak rate. A randomized prospective trial comparing cervical to intrathoracic anastomoses reported a leak rate of 26% versus 4% ($P < .002$). The

TABLE 44B.7. Transthoracic Versus Transhiatal Esophagectomy.

	Transthoracic	*Transhiatal*
5-year survival (%)	39	29
5-year disease-free survival (%)	39	27
Local recurrence	12	14
Operative mortality (%)	4	2
Blood loss (mL)	1402	847
Hospital length of stay (days)	19	15
Respiratory complications (%)	57	27
Cardiac complications (%)	26	16
Anastomotic leaks (%)	15	14

Source: From Hulscher,[24] with permission from *Annals of Thoracic Surgery.*

cervical anastomosis was also associated with a higher stricture rate of 23% versus 14%.[39] Indeed, anastomotic leak is clearly identified as an independent risk factor for the development of stricture, as is the use of circular stapling techniques.[40] The cervical anastomosis has been used by many surgeons because a leak in the neck is rarely life threatening, whereas an intrathoracic leak is associated with significant morbidity and mortality. However, the cervical anastomotic leak can have catastrophic consequences, such as fistula into the airway or osteomyelitis, as reported by Iannettoni et al.[41]

Resection Margins

The ideal length of the proximal resection margin is 10 cm based on data from Wong, which demonstrated no anastomotic recurrences with a resection margin of 10 cm.[42] The distal margin should be 5 cm based on anatomic studies demonstrating microscopic spread distally of 4 cm or less.[43]

Role of Pyloric Drainage Procedures

The use of a drainage procedure is favored by many surgeons after esophagectomy, but others argue against it based on the finding that only one-third of patients will have problems with delayed emptying if a drainage procedure is not performed. However, a meta-analysis of three randomized trials reported a significant benefit in favor of pyloric drainage versus no drainage in terms of early gastric outlet obstruction (RR = 0.18, 95% CI 0.03–0.97, $P = .046$), although there was no difference in any other outcomes.[44] In the largest randomized study of 200 patients comparing pyloroplasty to no drainage, there were increased complications in the no-drainage group; these complications consisted of early (13 patients) and late (5 patients) gastric outlet obstruction and pulmonary complications (4 patients), including 2 cases of fatal aspiration pneumonia. In addition, patients who did not have a drainage procedure had significantly ($P < .01$) more frequent and severe problems eating. The authors concluded that a drainage procedure should be performed.[45] A subsequent randomized trial by the same group found no difference between pyloroplasty and pyloromyotomy.[46]

Combined Modality Therapy

In an effort to improve outcomes, and encouraged by results in other solid tumors, many investigators are using combined modality therapy.

Chemotherapy

Preoperative Chemotherapy and Surgery

The evidence regarding the role of preoperative chemotherapy is conflicting (Table 44B.8). The two largest randomized trials of neoadjuvant chemotherapy have reported opposite results. The Medical Research Council (MRC) Oesophageal Cancer Working Group administered two cycles of cisplatin and infusional 5-fluorouracil (5FU) prior to surgery versus surgery alone in patients with resectable esophageal cancer. Overall survival was better in the chemotherapy plus surgery group (hazard ratio [HR] 0.79, 95% CI 0.67–0.93, $P = .004$) without any increase in perioperative complications. Median survival also favored the neoadjuvant chemotherapy arm at 16.8 months versus 13.3 months (95% CI 30–196), respectively.[47] The trial reported by Kelsen et al. using three cycles of cisplatin and 5FU preoperatively versus surgery alone found no significant difference in survival between the two arms of the study. The median survival was 14.9 months for the chemosurgery arm and 16.1 months for the surgery-alone arm ($P = .53$).[48]

However, in a systematic review of 11 randomized controlled trials including 2051 patients treated with preoperative chemotherapy plus surgery versus surgery alone, improved survival after 3 years was demonstrated in patients receiving preoperative chemotherapy, which reached statistical significance at 5 years with a 44% increase in survival (RR 1.44, 95% CI 1.05–1.97, $P = .02$).[49] This most recent review is at odds with previous meta-analyses and systematic reviews, which all failed to demonstrate an improvement in survival with induction chemotherapy.[50–52] Both the review by Urschel et al.[51] and the previous review by Malthaner and Fenlon[50] did not include the results of the MRC trial or updated results of other small trials. The MRC trial had sufficient power to change the conclusion of the most recent review.[49] However, this was not the only factor, as pointed out in this review. When only the most recent trials (>1990) were included in the review, there was a survival advantage but only at 5 years (RR 1.44, 95% CI 1.05–1.97). If the trials that included postoperative chemotherapy as well as preoperative chemotherapy were excluded from the analysis, then the survival advantage at 5 years was even greater (71%), whereas there was still no benefit at 1, 2, and 3 years. Based on these data, it appears that preoperative chemotherapy is of benefit in terms of long-term survival.

Whereas the previous trials all used a combination of cisplatin and 5FU, a more recent trial used a strategy of three cycles of preoperative and three cycles of postoperative chemotherapy with epirubicin, cisplatin, and 5FU. This randomized trial reported a significant survival advantage for the group receiving chemotherapy, with a HR for death of 0.75 (CI 0.60–0.93, $P = .009$) for the chemotherapy arm. The 5-year survival was 36% for the chemotherapy group versus 23% for the surgery-alone group. Patients eligible for the trial were those with resectable gastric cancer, but 30% of those included in the trial had tumors of the lower esophagus or gastroesophageal junction. Only 42% of patients completed all six cycles, whereas 91% completed the preoperative chemotherapy. This trial has influenced practice, and although the treatment plan included both pre- and postoperative chemotherapy, it appears that patients benefit even if they do not complete the postoperative portion.[53] Whether the postoperative chemotherapy is detrimental is unclear. The previous meta-analyses suggested that it was not beneficial, but did not include the long-term results of the most recent trials.

Postoperative Chemotherapy

Of three randomized trials of postoperative chemotherapy reported,[54–56] only one demonstrated any survival benefit, with improved 5-year disease-free survival (45% vs. 55%, $P = .037$) but not overall survival (52% vs. 61%, $P = .13$).[56] A meta-analysis of the three trials showed no benefit (RR 0.94, 95% CI 0.74–1.18, $P = .60$) but did not include the long-term results of the most recent Ando trial or the results of the MAGIC trial.[57]

Postoperative Chemoradiotherapy

There are few studies of postoperative chemoradiotherapy following esophagectomy. However, in a study using the

TABLE 44B.8.
Randomized Trials of Preoperative Chemotherapy Versus Surgery Alone.

Author	*Trial design*	*Level of evidence*	*N*	*Chemotherapy*	*Median survival (mo)*		*2-year survival (%)*		*Mortality*	*Comments*
					CS	S	CS	S		
Kelsen[48]	RCT	I	440	CDDP, 5FU	14.9	16.1	35	37	6	71% completed all 3 cycles of chemo, 83% received 2 cycles; R0 resection rate only 62% in CS, 59% in S; RR (death) = 1.07 for CS, 95% CI 0.87–1.32, $P = .49$
MRC[47]	RCT	I	802	CDDP, 5FU	16.8	13.3	43	34	10	96% received chemo, 81% received both cycles; preop RT 9% both groups; R0 resection rate 60% for CS, 53% for S; overall survival favored CS: HR 0.79, 95% CI 0.67–0.93, $P = .004$
Law[80]	RCT	I	147	CDDP, 5FU	16.8	13.0	41	31	8.3–8.7	Only squamous cell cancer; 85% received both cycles of chemo; no statistically significant difference in survival except in responders, although curves do separate; recurrence rate 72% for S vs. 48% for CS at 17 months of follow-up ($P = .005$)
Ancona[81]	RCT	II	96	CDDP, 5FU	25.0	24.0	50	50	4.2	Only squamous cell cancer; 68% received all 3 cycles of chemotherapy, 28% received 2 cycles; R0 resection 79% for CS vs. 75% for S; no difference in survival between the two groups ($P = .45$)
Schlag[83]	RCT	II	46	CDDP, 5FU	10.0	10.0			19 (CS) vs. 10	Squamous cell cancer only; increased operative mortality for CS; not truly randomized as patients could refuse their treatment allocation; increased operative mortality in CS led to premature closure of the trial; no difference in survival
Maipang[83]	RCT	II	24	CDDP, VB, Bleo	17.0	17.0	36	40		Squamous cell cancer only; 66% completed chemotherapy, 17% chemotherapy related deaths related to erosion of tumor into airway or aorta; operative mortality not stated; overall survival no difference
Cunningham[53a]	RCT	I	503	CDDP, 5FU, E	24	20	50	42	5.6–5.9	Included gastric cancers, lower esophageal cancers, and gastroesophageal junction cancers; 91% received all 3 preop cycles of chemotherapy; 41.6% completed all 6 cycles (3 preop and 3 postop); R0 resection 69% for CS vs. 66% for S-alone group; no increase in operative mortality or morbidity for CS; significant improvement in survival in CS vs. S: HR (death) 0.75, 95% CI 0.60–0.93, $P = .009$; 5-year survival 36% vs. 23%; HR (progression) 0.66, 95% CI 0.53–0.81, $P < .001$

CDDP, Cisplatinum; CS, chemosurgery; E, Epirubicin; 5FU, 5-fluorouracil; HR, hazard ratio; RCT, randomized controlled trial; RT, radiation therapy; S, Surgery alone.

[a]Data not stated, interpolated from published survival curves.

Source: From Malthaner et al.[49,53,57]

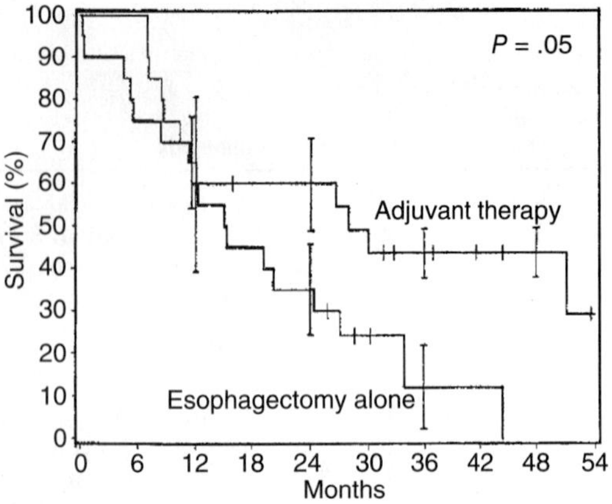

FIGURE 44B.3. Propensity-matched survival among patients receiving adjuvant chemoradiation compared with surgery alone. (From Rice.[58])

technique of propensity matching, Rice et al. reported a significant improvement in survival in patients treated with postoperative radiation (50.4–59.4 Gy) and concurrent chemotherapy with cisplatin and infusional 5FU.[58] Patients treated with postoperative chemoradiotherapy versus surgery alone had a median survival of 28 versus 15 months ($P = .05$), 4-year survival of 65% versus 44% ($P = .05$), and recurrence-free survival of 22 versus 10 months ($P = .02$) (see Fig. 44B.3).

A trial of postoperative chemoradiation with 5FU and leucovorin with concurrent radiation therapy (RT) of 45 Gy for gastric cancer demonstrated significant survival advantage for the combined-modality arm. Median survival was 27 months for surgery alone versus 36 months for combined-modality therapy (HR 1.35, 95% CI 1.23–1.86, $P < .001$). Although this was primarily a trial of gastric cancer, 7% of those included had cancers of the gastric cardia, which by definition are tumors of the gastroesophageal junction.[59]

Radiation and Surgery

Preoperative Radiation

Radiation has been used prior to surgery in an effort to improve both local control and long-term survival. A meta-analysis of five randomized trials of surgery plus preoperative radiation versus surgery alone, including 1147 patients with predominantly squamous cancers, reported an 11% reduction in risk of death using preoperative radiation, with an absolute survival benefit of 4% at 5 years, but this did not reach statistical significance ($P = .062$)[60] (see Fig. 44B.4).

Postoperative Radiation

A meta-analysis including data from four small randomized trials of surgery plus postoperative radiotherapy versus surgery alone found no significant reduction in the risk of death at 1 year with postoperative radiation (RR 1.32, 5% CI 0.99–1.77, $P = .06$).[57] A more recent randomized trial of 495 patients with squamous cell cancer treated postoperatively with 50–60 Gy reported 5-year overall survival of 31.7% (surgery alone) versus 41.3% (surgery plus RT), which was not statistically significant. However, there was a survival advantage for stage III patients.[61]

Radiation Alone

Radiotherapy is effective in the treatment of esophageal cancer. However, in two randomized trials comparing surgery to radiation alone, survival was better with surgery.[62,63] Survival at 5 years with radiation alone is 0%–6%[64] but may be higher for upper-third cancers.

Radiation Plus Chemotherapy

The addition of chemotherapy to radiation was clearly proven to be superior to radiation alone based on the Radiation Therapy Oncology Group (RTOG) 85-01 trial comparing radiation alone to radiation plus concomitant cisplatin and 5FU.[63] The 5-year survival with RT alone was 0% versus 26% for RT plus chemotherapy. Local recurrence was also reduced with combined therapy, from 37% with RT alone to 26% with chemotherapy/RT. For upper-third cancers, 5-year survival with chemoradiation may reach 49%.[65]

In an attempt to determine whether increasing the dose of radiation would improve survival or local control, RTOG 94-05 randomized patients with adenocarcinoma or squamous cancer of the esophagus to concurrent chemotherapy with cisplatin and infusional 5FU with either 64.8 or 50.4 Gy of radiotherapy, but there were no significant differences between the two arms with respect to median survival, locoregional failure, or persistence of disease.[66]

A meta-analysis of eight trials of concomitant chemotherapy/RT versus RT alone and five trials of sequential

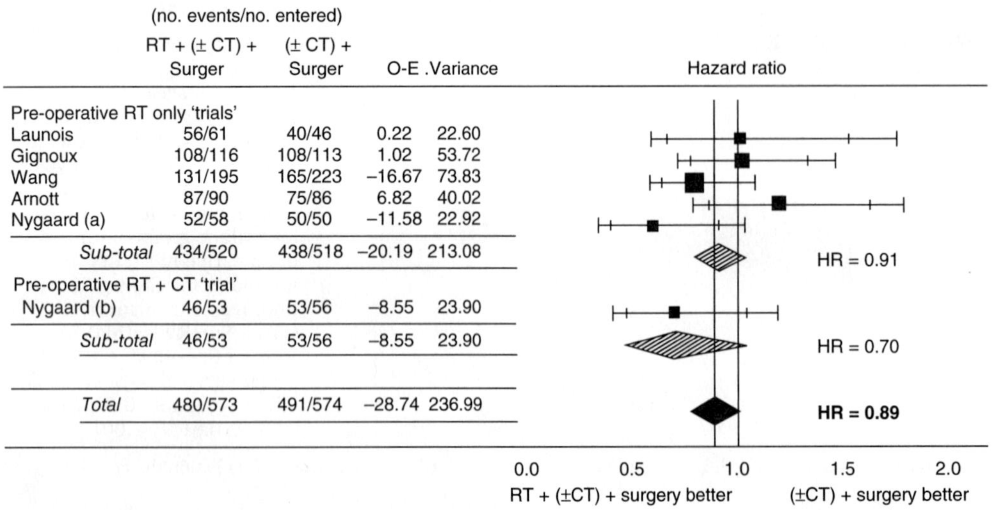
(no. events/no. entered)
RT + (± CT) + Surger
(± CT) + Surger
O-E .Variance
Hazard ratio
Pre-operative RT only 'trials'
Launois 56/61 40/46 0.22 22.60
Gignoux 108/116 108/113 1.02 53.72
Wang 131/195 165/223 −16.67 73.83
Arnott 87/90 75/86 6.82 40.02
Nygaard (a) 52/58 50/50 −11.58 22.92
Sub-total 434/520 438/518 −20.19 213.08
HR = 0.91
Pre-operative RT + CT 'trial'
Nygaard (b) 46/53 53/56 −8.55 23.90
Sub-total 46/53 53/56 −8.55 23.90
HR = 0.70
Total 480/573 491/574 −28.74 236.99
HR = 0.89
0.0 0.5 1.0 1.5 2.0
RT + (±CT) + surgery better
(±CT) + surgery better

FIGURE 44B.4. Meta-analysis of preoperative radiotherapy with or without chemotherapy versus surgery with or without chemotherapy. The overall hazard ratio (HR) estimate of the effect of preoperative radiotherapy was 0.89. (From Arnott,[60] by permission of Int J Radiat Oncol Biol Phys.)

chemotherapy/RT versus RT alone demonstrated improved survival (1-year mortality OR 0.61, 95% CI 0.44–0.84, $p < .00001$) and local control (OR 0.52, 95% CI 0.31–0.89, $P = .004$) with combined therapy. Concomitant therapy was superior to sequential and has been accepted as the standard of care.[67]

Surgery and Preoperative Chemoradiation

The approach of surgery and preoperative chemoradiation has been successful in other tumor sites and offers several potential advantages. Preoperative therapy has the potential to reduce tumor size, potentially reduce tumor seeding at the time of resection, and decrease the RT dose since the tumor vascularity is undisturbed and therefore is less likely to be hypoxic; the use of radiosensitizing chemotherapeutic agents may increase the therapeutic ratio for a given dose of RT. A multitude of phase II trials have reported improved survival with this approach. Unfortunately, of the six fully published randomized controlled trials utilizing this approach only one demonstrated a clear survival benefit in favor of the combined modality approach (see Table 44B.9). When the data from

TABLE 44B.9.
Randomized Trials of Neoadjuvant Chemoradiation and Surgery Versus Surgery Alone.

Trial	*Year*	*Level of evidence*	*N*	*Chemotherapy*	*Radiation (GY)*	*Median survival (mo)*		*3-yr survival (%)*		*Percentage mortality*	*Comments*
						CRTS	S	CRTS	S		
Nygaard[84]	1992	II	103	CDDP, Bleo	35	7	7	17	9	5	Sequential RT; no difference in survival, $P = .30$
Apinop[85]	1994	II	69	CDDP, 5FU	40	9.7	7.4	26	20		Concurrent RT; no difference in survival, $P = .40$
Le Prise[86]	1994	II	86	CDDP, 5FU	20	11	11	19	14	8.5 vs. 7	Concurrent RT; no difference in survival, $P = .56$
Walsh[87]	1996	II	113	CDDP, 5FU	40	11	32			6	Concurrent RT; survival improved with preop chemo/RT, $P = .01$, but survival in surgery-alone arm inferior compared with other studies (6% at 3 years); trial stopped early because of improved results in CRTS
Bosset[88]	1997	I	282	CDDP	37	18.6	18.6	39	37	12 vs. 4	Concurrent RT split course; no survival difference, $P = .78$, but longer disease-free interval, lower cancer-related deaths, more R0 resections with CRTS; trial stopped early because of increased mortality in CRTS arm
Urba[89]	2001	II	100	CDDP, VB, 5FU	45	17.6	16.9	30	16	2 vs. 4	Concurrent RT; no survival difference, $P = .15$, HR 0.73 (95% CI 0.48–1.12); decreased local failure with CRTS 19% vs. 42%, $P = .02$
Burmeister[90]	2002	I	256	CDDP, 5FU	35	21.7	18.5				Concurrent RT

Bleo, bleomycin; CDDP, cisplatinum; CRTS, chemoradiation surgery; 5FU, 5-fluorouracil; HR, hazard ratio; RT, radiation therapy; S, surgery; VB, vinblastine.

Source: From Malthaner et al.[57]

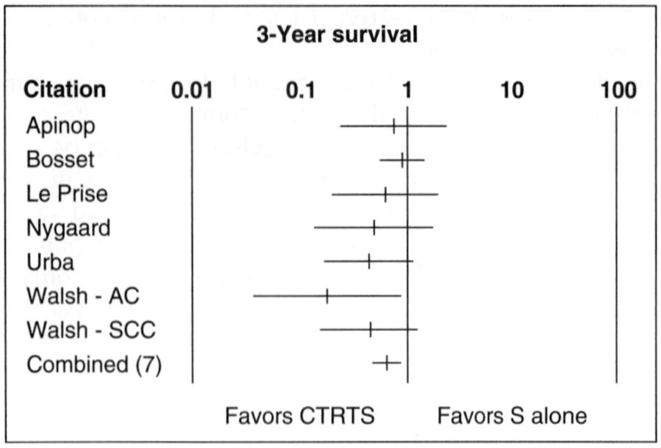

FIGURE 44B.5. Meta-analysis of trials comparing chemoradiation surgery to surgery alone. Three-year survival (OR 0.66, 95% CI 0.47–0.92, $P = .016$). AC, adenocarcinoma; CTRTS, chemotherapy, radiation therapy, surgery; S, surgery; SCC, squamous cell carcinoma. (From Urschel.[68])

these trials plus three others published in abstract form only were combined in a meta-analysis, a survival benefit was demonstrated but only after 3 years[68] (see Fig. 44B.5). The odds ratio for survival at 3 years was 0.66 (95% CI 0.47–0.92, $P = .016$) in favor of combined treatment. The odds ratio was even stronger if only trials using concomitant chemotherapy/RT were considered (OR 0.45, 95% CI 0.26–0.79, $P = .005$), whereas trials using sequential therapy did not show any benefit. It is notable that all these trials were small and underpowered; however, an attempt to mount an adequately powered multicenter trial failed to accrue because neoadjuvant chemoradiation has been adopted in many centers as the standard of care for locally advanced tumors despite the relatively weak evidence.

Approach to the Patient with Esophageal Cancer

In the past, there was only one treatment option for patients with esophageal cancer: surgery. If the patient was not fit for surgery or had metastatic disease, then radiation was used. Even though precise stage-specific treatment algorithms are still lacking in this disease, there are some generalized algorithms that may be applied (see Table 44B.10).

Patients with clinical T1N0M0 disease are frequently cured by surgery alone. For such patients, delaying surgery to give induction therapy cannot be justified. A similar approach could be used for clinical T2N0M0. If after resection a higher stage is found on pathological examination, then consideration could be given to adjuvant chemoradiotherapy based on the work of Rice et al.[58]; however, this cannot yet be accepted as the standard of care. Nonetheless, there is support for such an approach based on the experience in gastric cancer.[59]

In the patient with clinical T3N0M0, T1N1M0, or T2N1M0 disease, the best evidence suggests that induction therapy with chemoradiation followed by surgery is appropriate. Although cisplatin and 5FU have been the most extensively studied combination, other drugs show promise. Whether induction chemoradiotherapy is superior to induction chemotherapy alone is unknown. Induction chemotherapy will become more widely used based on two positive large randomized trials and meta-analysis.

In patients with more advanced but technically resectable disease (T4N0-1M0, TNM1A), the appropriate treatment is more controversial. The likelihood of cure with this stage of disease is low. Such patients may be treated with surgery alone as the best palliation, with induction chemoradiotherapy followed by surgery, or with chemoradiation alone. Surgery offers the best chance of local control and hence long-term palliation if an R0 resection can be achieved.

In patients with distant metastatic disease, resection is not indicated. Alternative techniques for palliating dysphagia are more appropriate, including esophageal stents, laser, photodynamic therapy, or radiation. Chemotherapy may be beneficial in short-term control of disease progression.

Conclusion

Esophageal cancer remains highly lethal. Esophagectomy provides the best chance of long-term survival for appropriate patients. Improvements in operative technique and postoperative care as well as better patient selection have reduced the operative mortality for esophagectomy. However, the operative mortality remains relatively high compared to other

TABLE 44B.10.
Comparison of Treatment Alternatives by Meta-analyses.

Reference	*Treatments*	*OR*	*95% CI*	*P*	*Comments*
Urschel[51]	Preop chemo/RT vs. surgery	HR (death) 0.45	0.26–0.76	.005	Weak evidence, small trials, all tend to benefit but only one positive, but standard of care in many centers
Malthaner[49]	Preop chemo vs. surgery	RR (survival) 1.44	1.05–1.97	.02	Strong evidence from 2 large RCTs
Malthaner[57]	Postop chemo vs. surgery	RR (death) 0.94	0.74–1.18	.60	Small trials, weak evidence
Arnott[60]	Preop RT vs. surgery	RR (death) 0.89	0.78–1.01	.062	Strong evidence but weak benefit
Malthaner[57]	Postop RT vs. surgery	RR (death) 1.32	0.91–1.77	.06	No benefit
Wong[67]	Chemo/RT vs. RT	RR (death) 0.61	0.44–0.84	$P < .00001$	Chemo/RT is standard of care for nonoperative treatment

HR, hazard ratio; RR, relative risk; RT, radiation therapy.

complex operative procedures except in centers of excellence. Even in such centers with experienced surgeons performing the highest volumes, morbidity remains significant. Long-term survival after esophagectomy may be improved by including regional lymphadenectomy and periesophageal tissues in the resection, but significant improvements in survival require combined-modality therapy. The optimum combination of therapy has yet to be determined, and much research remains to be done. Improved staging with EUS and PET should allow the development of stage-specific treatment strategies such as exist for other tumor types.

References

1. Blot WJ, Devesa SS, Kneller RW, et al. Rising incidence of adenocarcinoma of the esophagus and gastric cardia. JAMA 1991; 265:1287–1289.
2. Blot WJ, Devesa SS, Fraumenii JF. Continued climbs in rates of esophageal adenocarcinoma: an update. JAMA 1993;270: 1320.
3. Visbal AL, Allen MS, Miller DL, Trastek VF, Pairolero PC. Ivor Lewis esophagogastrectomy for esophageal cancer. Ann Thorac Surg 2001;71:1803–1808.
4. Lagergren J, Bergstrom R, Lindgren A, Nyren O. Symptomatic gastroesophageal reflux as a risk factor for esophageal adenocarcinoma. N Engl J Med 1999;340:825–831.
5. Yang PC, Davis S. Incidence of cancer of the esophagus in the United States by histologic type. Cancer 1988;61:612.
6. Rice TW, Blackstone EH, Adelstein DJ, et al. Role of clinically determined depth of tumor invasion in the treatment of esophageal carcinoma. J Thorac Cardiovasc Surg 2003;125:1091–1102.
7. Meining A, Dittler HJ, Wolf A, et al. You get what you expect? A critical appraisal of imaging methodology in endosonographic cancer staging. Gut 2002;50:599–603.
8. Kelly S, Harris KM, Berry E, et al. A systematic review of the staging performance of endoscopic ultrasound in gastro-oesophageal carcinoma. Gut 2001;49:534–539.
9. Catalano MF, Sivak MV Jr, Rice T, et al. Endosonographic features predictive of lymph node metastases. Gastrointest Endosc 1994;40:442.
10. Vasquez-Sequeiros E, Norton ID, Clain JE, et al. Impact of EUS guided fine needle aspiration in lymph node staging inpatients with esophageal carcinoma. Gastrointest Endosc 2001;53:751–757.
11. Downey RJ, Akhurst T, Ilson D, et al. Whole body 18FDG-PET and the response of esophageal cancer to induction therapy: the results of a prospective trial. J Clin Oncol 2003;21:428–432.
12. Lowe VJ, Booya F, Fletcher JG, et al. Comparison of positron emission tomography, computed tomography, and endoscopic ultrasound in the initial staging of patients with esophageal cancer. Mol Imaging Biol 2005;7:422–430.
13. Yuan S, Yu Y, Chao KS, et al. Additional value of PET/CT over PET in assessment of locoregional lymph nodes in thoracic esophageal squamous cell cancer. J Nucl Med 2006;47:1255–1259.
14. Stahl A, Stollfuss J, Ott K, et al. FDG PET and CT in locally advanced adenocarcinomas of the distal oesophagus. Clinical relevance of a discordant PET finding. Nucl Med 2005;44:249–255.
15. Rasanen JV, Sihvo EI, Knuuti MJ, et al. Prospective analysis of accuracy of positron emission tomography, computed tomography and endoscopic ultrasonography in staging of adenocarcinoma of the esophagus and esophagogastric junction. Ann Surgical Oncol 2003;10:954–960.
16. Krasna MJ, Reed CE, Jaklitsch MT, et al. Thoracoscopic staging of esophageal cancer: a prospective, multiinstitutional trial. Cancer and Leukemia Group B Thoracic Surgeons. Ann Thorac Surg 1995;60:1337–1340.
17. Krasna MJ, et al. The role of thoracoscopic staging of esophageal cancer patients. Eur J Cardiovasc Surg 1999;16(suppl 1):S31.
18. Wallace MB, Nietert PJ, Earle C, et al. An analysis of multiple staging management strategies for carcinoma of the esophagus: computed tomography, endoscopic ultrasound, positron emission tomography, and thoracoscopy/laparoscopy. Ann Thorac Surg 2002;74:1026–1032.
19. Dimick JB, Wainess RM, Upchurch GR Jr, Iannettoni MD, Orringer MB. National trends in outcomes for esophageal resection. Ann Thorac Surg 2005;79:212–218.
20. Orringer MB. Transhiatal esophagectomy without thoracotomy for carcinoma of the thoracic esophagus. Ann Surg 1984;200:282–288.
21. Skinner DB. En bloc resection for neoplasms of the esophagus and cardia. J Thorac Cardiovasc Surg 1983;85:59–71.
22. Luketich JD, et al. Minimally invasive esophagectomy: outcomes in 2222 patients. Ann Surg 2003;238:486.
23. Hulscher JB, Tijssen JG, Obertop H, et al. Transthoracic versus transhiatal resection for carcinoma of the esophagus: a meta-analysis. Ann Thorac Surg 2001;72:306–313.
24. Hulscher JB, van Sandick JW, de Boer AG, et al. Extended transthoracic resection compared to limited transhiatal resection for adenocarcinoma of the esophagus. N Engl J Med 2002;347:1662–1669.
25. Altorki N, Girardi L, Skinner DB. En bloc esophagectomy improves survival for stage III esophageal cancer. J Thorac Cardiovasc Surg 1997;114:948–956.
26. Hagan JA, DeMeester SR, Peters JH, et al. Curative resection for esophageal adenocarcinoma: analysis of 100 enbloc esophagectomies. Ann Surg 2001;234:520–531.
27. Siewert JR, Stein HJ, Feith M, et al. Histologic tumor type is an independent prognostic parameter in esophageal cancer: lessons from more than 1000 consecutive resection at a single center in the Western world. Ann Surg 2001;234:360–369.
28. Urschel JD, Urschel DM, Miller JD, et al. A meta-analysis of randomized controlled trials of route of reconstruction after esophagectomy for cancer. Am J Surg 2002;182:470–475.
29. Collard J-M, Tinton N, Malaise J, Romagnoli R, Otter J-B, Kestens PJ. Esophageal replacement: gastric tube or whole stomach? Ann Thorac Surg 1995;60:261–267.
30. Posthlethwaite RW. Colonic interposition for esophageal substitution: collective review. Surg Gynecol Obstet 1983; 156:377.
31. Gaissert HA, et al. Short-segment intestinal interposition of the distal esophagus. J Thorac Cardiovasc Surg 1993;106:860.
32. Heitmiller RF, et al. Long segment substernal jejunal esophageal replacement with internal mammary vascular augmentation. Dis Esophagus 2000;13:240.
33. Chen HC, Tang YB. Microsurgical reconstruction of the esophagus. Semin Surg Oncol 2000;19:235.
34. Orringer MB, Marshall B, Iannettoni MD. Eliminating the cervical esophagogastric anastomotic leak with a side-to-side stapled anastomosis. J Thorac Cardiovasc Surg 2000;119:277–288.
35. Casson AG, Porter GA, Veugelers PJ. Evolution and critical appraisal of anastomotic technique following resection of esophageal adenocarcinoma. Dis Esophagus 2002;15:296–302.
36. Ercan S, Rice TW, Murthy SC, Rybicki LA, Blackstone EH. Does esophagogastric anastomotic technique influence the outcome of patients with esophageal cancer? J Thorac Cardiovasc Surg 2005;129:623–631.
37. Urschel JD, Blewett CJ, Bennett WF, et al. Handsewn or stapled esophagogastric anastomoses after esophagectomy for cancer: meta-analysis of randomized controlled trials. Dis Esophagus 2001;14:212–217.
38. Beitler AL, Urschel JD. Comparison of stapled and hand-sewn esophagogastric anastomoses. Am J Surg 1998;175:337–340.

39. Chasseray VM, Kiroff GK, Buard JL, Launois B. Cervical or thoracic anastomosis for esophagectomy for carcinoma. Surg Gyn Obstet 1989;169:55–62.
40. Honkoop P, Siersema PD, Tilanus HW, Stassen LPS, Hop WCJ, van Blankenstein M. Benign anastomotic strictures after transhiatal esophagectomy and cervical esophagogastrostomy: risk factors and management. J Thorac Cardiovasc Surg 1996;111:1141–1148.
41. Iannettoni MD, Whyte RI, Orringer MB. Catastrophic complications of the cervical esophagogastric anastomosis. J Thorac Cardiovasc Surg 1995;110:1493–1501.
42. Wong J. Esophageal resection for cancer: the rationale of current practice. Am J Surg 1997;153:18.
43. Burgess HM, et al. Carcinoma of the esophagus: clinicopathologic study. Surg Clin North Am 1991;31:965.
44. Urschel JD, Blewett CJ, Young JE, et al. Pyloric drainage (pyloroplasty) or no drainage in gastric reconstruction after esophagectomy: a meta-analysis of randomized controlled trials. Dig Surg 2002;19:160–164.
45. Fok M, Cheng SW, Wong J. Pylorplasty versus no drainage in gastric replacement of the esophagus. Am J Surg 1991;162:447–452.
46. Law S, Cheung MC, Fok M, Chu KM, Wong J. Pyloroplasty and pylormyotomy in gastric replacement of the esophagus after esophagectomy: a randomized trial. J Am Coll Surg 1997;184:630–636.
47. Medical Research Council Oesophageal Working Group. Surgical resection with or without preoperative chemotherapy in oesophageal cancer: a randomized trial. Lancet 2002;359:1727–1733.
48. Kelsen DP, Ginsberg RJ, Pajak TF, et al. Chemotherapy followed by surgery compared with surgery alone for localized esophageal cancer. N Engl J Med 1998;339:1979–1984.
49. Malthaner R, Fenlon D. Preoperative chemotherapy for resectable thoracic esophageal cancer. (Cochrane Review) In: The Cochrane Library Issue 1. Chichester, UK: John Wiley and Sons Ltd., 2004.
50. Malthaner R, Fenlon D. Preoperative chemotherapy for resectable thoracic esophageal cancer. Cochrane Database Syst Rev 2001;1(1):1699.
51. Urschel JD, Vasan H, Blewett CJ. A meta-analysis of randomized controlled trials that compared neoadjuvant chemotherapy and surgery to surgery alone for resectable esophageal cancer. Am J Surg 2002;183:274–279.
52. Bhansali MS, Vaidya JS, Bhatt RG, Patil PK, Badwe RA, Desai PB. Chemotherapy for carcinoma of the esophagus: a comparison of evidence from meta-analyses of randomized trials and of historical control studies. Ann Oncol 1996;7:355–359.
53. Cunningham D, Allum WH, Stenning SP, et al. and the MAGIC trial participants. Perioperative chemotherapy versus surgery alone for resectable gastroesophageal cancer. N Engl J Med 2006;355:11–20.
54. Pouliquen X, Levard H, Hay JM, et al. 5-Fluorouracil and cisplatin therapy after palliative surgical resection of squamous cell carcinoma of the esophagus. A multicenter randomized trial. French Association for Surgical Research. Ann Surg 1996;223:127–133.
55. Ando N, Iizuka T, Kakegawa T, et al. A randomized trial of surgery with and without chemotherapy for localized squamous carcinoma of the thoracic esophagus: the Japan Clinical Oncology Group Study. J Thorac Cardiovasc Surg 1997;114:205–209.
56. Ando N, Iizuka T, Ide H, et al. Surgery plus chemotherapy compared to surgery alone for localized squamous cell carcinoma of the thoracic esophagus: a Japan Clinical Oncology Group Study JCOG 9204. J Clin Oncol 2003;21:4592–4596.
57. Malthaner R, Wong RKS, Rumble RB, Zuraw L. Neoadjuvant or adjuvant therapy for resectable esophageal cancer. Practice Guideline Report 2-11. Program in Evidence Based Care, Cancer Care Ontario, 2002. Available at: http://www.cancercare.on.ca/access_PEBC.htm.
58. Rice TW, Adelstein DJ, Chidel MA, et al. Benefit of postoperative adjuvant chemoradiotherapy in locoregionally advanced esophageal carcinoma. J Thorac Cardiovasc Surg 2003;126:1590–1596.
59. MacDonald J, Smalley S, Benedetti J, et al. Chemoradiotherapy after surgery compared with surgery alone for adenocarcinoma of the stomach or gastroesophageal junction. N Engl J Med 2001;345:725.
60. Arnott SJ, Duncan W, Gignoux M, et al. Preoperative radiotherapy for esophageal carcinoma. Cochrane Database Syst Rev 2000;4:CD001799.
61. Xiao ZF, Yang ZY, Liang J, et al. Value of radiotherapy after radical surgery for esophageal carcinoma: a report of 495 patients. Ann Thorac Surg 2003;75:331–336.
62. Fok M, McShane J, Law SYK, Wong J. Prospective randomized study in the treatment of oesophageal carcinoma. Asian J Surg 1994;17:223–229.
63. Badwe RA, Sharma V, Bhansall MS, et al. The quality of swallowing for patients with operable esophageal carcinoma. Cancer 1999;85:763–768.
64. Cooper JS, Guo MD, Herskoviv A, et al. Chemoradiotherapy of locally advanced esophageal cancer: long-term follow-up of a prospective randomized trial (RTOG 85-01). Radiation Therapy Oncology Group. JAMA 1999;281:1623–1627.
65. Denham JW, Steigler A, Kilmurray J, et al. Relapse patterns after chemo-radiation for carcinoma of the oesophagus. Clin Oncol (R Coll Radiol) 2003;15:98–108.
66. Minsky BD, Pajak TF, Ginsberg RJ, et al. INT 0123 (Radiation Therapy Oncology Group 94-05) phase III trial of combined modality therapy for esophageal cancer: high dose versus standard-dose radiation therapy. JCO 2002;20:1167–1174.
67. Wong RKS, Malthaner RA, Zuraw L, et al. Cancer Care Ontario Practice Guidelines Initiative Gastrointestinal Cancer Disease Site Group. Combined modality radiotherapy and chemotherapy in the non-surgical management of localized carcinoma of the esophagus. Int J Radiat Oncol Biol Phys 2003;55(4):930–942.
68. Urschel JD, Vasan H. A meta-analysis of randomized controlled trials that compared neoadjuvant chemoradiation and surgery to surgery alone for resectable esophageal cancer. Am J Surg 2003;185:538–543.
69. Guili R, Gignoux M. Treatment of carcinoma of the esophagus. Ann Surg 1980;192;44–52.
70. Earlam R, Cunha-Melo JR. Oesophageal squamous cell carcinoma. A critical review of surgery. Br J Surg 1980;67:381–390.
71. Posthlethwait RW. Complications and deaths after operations for esophageal carcinoma. J Thorac Cardiovasc Surg 1983;85:827–831.
72. Ellis FH Jr. Carcinoma of the Esophagus. CA Cancer J Clin 1983;33:264.
73. Katariya K, et al. Complications of transhiatal esophagectomy. J Surg Oncol 1994;57:157.
74. Orringer MB, Marshall B, Iannettoni MD. Transhiatal esophagectomy: clinical experience and refinements. Ann Surg 1999;230:392.
75. Ellis FH Jr. Standard resection for cancer of the esophagus and cardia. Surg Oncol Clin Am 1999;8:279–294.
76. Altorki NK. The rationale for radical resection. Surg Oncol Clin N Am 1999;8:295–305.
77. Altorki NK, Kent M, Ferrara C, Port J. Three field lymph node dissection for squamous and adenocarcinoma of the esophagus. Ann Surg 2002;236:177–183.
78. Bailey SH, Bull DA, Harpole DH, et al. Outcomes after esophagectomy: a ten year prospective cohort. Ann Thorac Surg 2003;75:217–222.

79. Orringer MB. In Glenn's Thoracic and Cardiovascular Surgery (5th ed.) Norwalk, Connecticut: Appletion & Lange, 1991;53:801.
80. Law S, Fok M, Chow S, Chu KM, Wong J. Preoperative chemotherapy versus surgical therapy alone for squamous cell carcinoma of the esophagus: a prospective randomized trial. J Thorac Cardiovasc Surg 1997;114:210–217.
81. Ancona E, Ruol A, Santi S, et al. Only pathologic complete response to neoadjuvant chemotherapy improves significantly the long term survival of patients with resectable esophageal squamous cell carcinoma: final report of a randomized, controlled trial of preoperative chemotherapy versus surgery alone. Cancer 2001;91:2165–2174.
82. Schlag PM. Randomized trial of preoperative chemotherapy for squamous cell cancer of the esophagus. The Chirurgische Arbeitsgemeinschaft Fuer Onkologie der Deutschen Gesellschaft Fuer Chirurgie Study Group. Arch Surg 1992;127:1446–1450.
83. Maipang T, Vasinanukorn P, Petpichetchian C, et al. Induction chemotherapy in the treatment of patients with carcinoma of the esophagus. J Surg Oncol 1994;56:191–197.
84. Nygaard K, Hagen S, Hansen HS, et al. Pre-operative radiotherapy prolongs survival in operable esophageal carcinoma: a randomized, multicenter study of pre-operative radiotherapy and chemotherapy. The second Scandinavian trial in esophageal cancer. World J Surg 1992;16:1104–1110.
85. Apinop C, Puttisak P, Preecha N. A prospective study of combined therapy in esophageal cancer. Hepatogastroenterology 1994;41:391–393.
86. Le Prise E, Etienne PL, Meunier B, et al. A randomized study of chemotherapy, radiation therapy and surgery versus surgery for localized squamous cell carcinoma of the esophagus. Cancer 1994;73:1779–1784.
87. Walsh TN, Noonan N, Hollywood D, Kelly A, Keeling N, Hennessy TP. A comparison of multimodal therapy and surgery for esophageal adenocarcinoma. N Engl J Med 1996;335:462–467.
88. Bosset JF, Gignoux M, Triboulet JP, et al. Chemoradiotherapy followed by surgery compared with surgery alone in squamous cell cancer of the esophagus. N Engl J Med 1997;337:161–167.
89. Urba SG, Orringer MB, Turrissi A, Iannettoni M, Forastiere A, Strawderman M. Randomized trial of preoperative chemoradiation versus surgery alone in patients with locoregional esophageal carcinoma, J Clin Oncol 2001;9:305–313.
90. Burmeister BH, Smithers BM, Gebski V, et al. Surgery alone versus chemoradiotherapy followed by surgery for resectable cancer of the oesophagus: a randomized controlled phase III trial. Lancet Oncol 2005;6:659–668.

45

Stomach and Duodenum

Robert E. Glasgow and Michael D. Rollins

Anatomy

Gross Anatomy

The stomach is a J-shaped dilation of the alimentary tract derived from the embryonic foregut. It lies in the left upper quadrant of the abdomen where the gastroesophageal junction is located to the left of the 10th thoracic vertebrae and crosses the midline at the pylorus, which is to the right of the L1 vertebral body. It is contiguous proximally with the esophagus and distally with the duodenum (Fig. 45.1). The stomach is fixed in two locations, the gastroesophageal junction and the retroperitoneal attachments at the duodenum. It can be divided into four anatomic regions (Fig. 45.2). The cardia is the most proximal region and is located just distal and to the left of the gastroesophageal junction. The fundus projects upward and is in contact with the left hemidiaphragm to the right of the spleen. The corpus, or body, is the largest portion of the stomach and is located below the fundus. The most distal portion of the stomach is the antrum. Its proximal boundary is an arbitrary line connecting the incisura angularis, which is located approximately two-thirds of the distance down the lesser curvature, to the greater curvature where the gastroepiploic arteries enter the stomach.

Vascular Supply

The stomach has a rich vascular supply with an extensive collateral network (Fig. 45.3). It is because of this collateral network that gastric tissue can remain viable after all but one of the major arteries that supply the stomach has been ligated. The majority of the stomach receives blood from branches of the celiac trunk, namely, the left gastric, common hepatic, and splenic arteries. The lesser curvature of the stomach is supplied by the left gastric artery from above and the right gastric artery (a branch of the common hepatic artery) from below. The greater curvature is supplied from above by the left gastroepiploic artery (a branch of the splenic artery) and from below by the right gastroepiploic artery (a branch of the gastroduodenal artery). In addition, the fundus and upper aspect of the greater curvature are supplied by the short gastric branches of the splenic artery. The superior aspect of the duodenum receives its blood supply from the anterior superior and posterior superior pancreaticoduodenal arteries, which originate from the gastroduodenal artery (a branch of the common hepatic artery). The inferior aspect of the duodenum is supplied by the anterior inferior and posterior inferior pancreaticoduodenal arteries, which are branches of the superior mesenteric artery. The arteries supplying the stomach terminate into capillaries, which form a rich submucosal vascular plexus. It is therefore possible to preserve gastric tissue from only one of the four major arterial branches, as is sometimes necessary with gastric procedures.

The venous and lymphatic drainage of the stomach corresponds to the arterial supply. The veins empty either directly into the portal vein or into one of its tributaries, the splenic or superior mesenteric veins. The left gastric vein (also known as the coronary vein) and the right gastric vein drain the lesser curvature of the stomach into the portal vein. The superior pancreaticoduodenal veins also empty into the portal vein. The left gastroepiploic vein drains into the splenic vein along with short gastric veins. The right gastroepiploic vein and the inferior pancreaticoduodenal veins drain into the superior mesenteric vein. Lymph drains into local nodal basins, eventually reaching the celiac artery and superior mesenteric artery major nodal collections. The lymphatics of the stomach form anastomoses within the gastric wall, which often results in the distant spread of disease processes involving the gastric lymphatics.

Innervation

The stomach receives both parasympathetic and sympathetic autonomic innervation. The left and right vagus nerves provide parasympathetic innervation to the stomach. During embryogenesis, the stomach rotates 90° such that the left and right vagus nerves become the anterior and posterior vagus

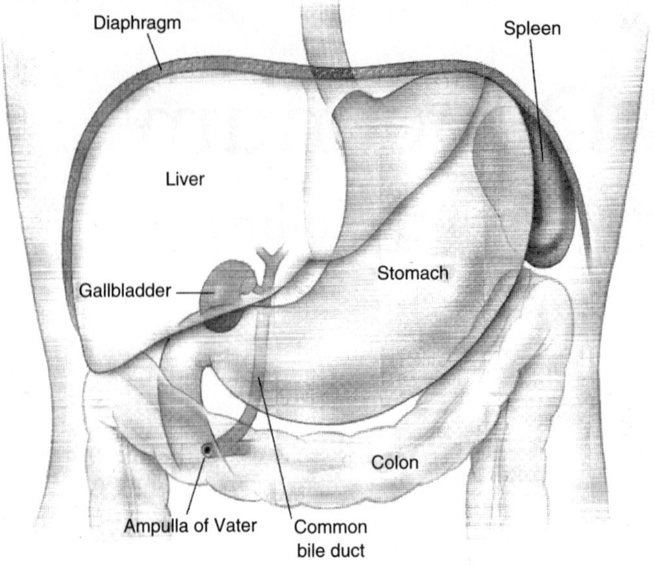

FIGURE 45.1. Anatomic relationships of the stomach. The esophagus emerges through the hiatus, where the abdominal esophagus and cardia are covered anteriorly by the left lobe of the liver. The spleen is intimately related to the gastric fundus through the short gastric vessels. The transverse colon is draped just inferior to the stomach and is connected to the stomach by the gastrocolic ligament, division of which provides access to the lesser sac. Distally, near the junction of the stomach and duodenum, important relationships exist with the gall bladder and common bile duct. Posterior to the stomach lies the lesser sac, containing the pancreas and splenic vessels. (From Debas.[252])

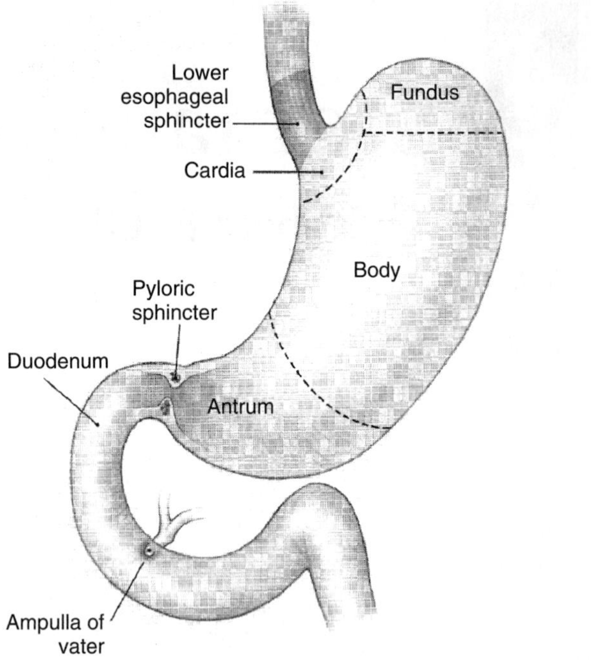

FIGURE 45.2. Anatomic regions of the stomach. The fundus and body of the stomach contain the parietal cell mass. The mucosa of the cardia is composed primarily of mucous and chief cells. The antral mucosa is the site of gastrin-secreting cells and contains no parietal cells. A transitional zone exists between the body and antrum, where gastric ulcers occur. (From Debas.[252])

nerves, respectively. Functionally, the anterior and posterior vagus nerves contain preganglionic nerve fibers from both the left and right vagus nerves as a result of the intrathoracic esophageal nerve plexus.

The anterior vagus nerve gives rise to a hepatic branch, which innervates the liver and gallbladder before becoming the anterior nerve of Latarget. The posterior vagus nerve gives rise to a celiac branch, which innervates the small bowel and colon before becoming the posterior nerve of Latarget. Both the anterior and posterior nerves of Latarget give off multiple fundic branches along the lesser curvature. These two main nerve trunks branch into multiple nerves at the incisura, forming the crow's foot, which terminates at the antrum. The crow's foot innervates the antrum and must be preserved during a highly selective vagotomy (HSV). The nerve of Grassi is an important nervous structure branching high on the posterior vagus nerve. It innervates the fundus and failure to divide this branch may result in ulcer recurrence following vagotomy. These preganglionic fibers synapse with the ganglia in the submucosal (Meissner's) and myenteric (Auerbach's) plexuses and subsequently become postganglionic nerve fibers, which innervate both secretory and motor components of the stomach (Fig. 45.4).

Sympathetic innervation of the stomach originates at the T6 to T8 spinal nerves. These preganglionic fibers synapse with the celiac ganglion and give rise to the postganglionic fibers, which follow the arterial supply of the stomach. Although these sympathetic fibers contain afferent pain fibers as well as motor fibers, they are of little importance in gastric surgery.

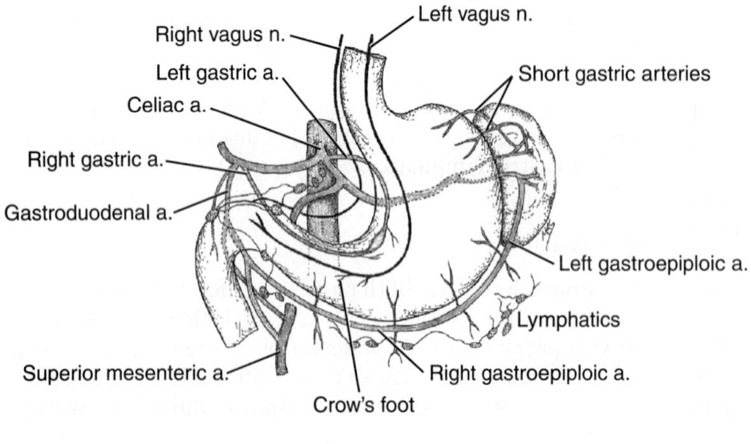

FIGURE 45.3. Neurovascular supply of the stomach. The stomach is richly vascularized by a highly redundant blood supply. Based on the celiac axis, the left and right gastric arteries supply the lesser curvature. The gastroepiploics supply the greater curvature. The gastroduodenal artery passes immediately behind the duodenum and may result in formidable bleeding should a duodenal ulcer perforate it. The lymphatics follow the arterial blood supply. The left (anterior) and right (posterior) vagi are depicted.

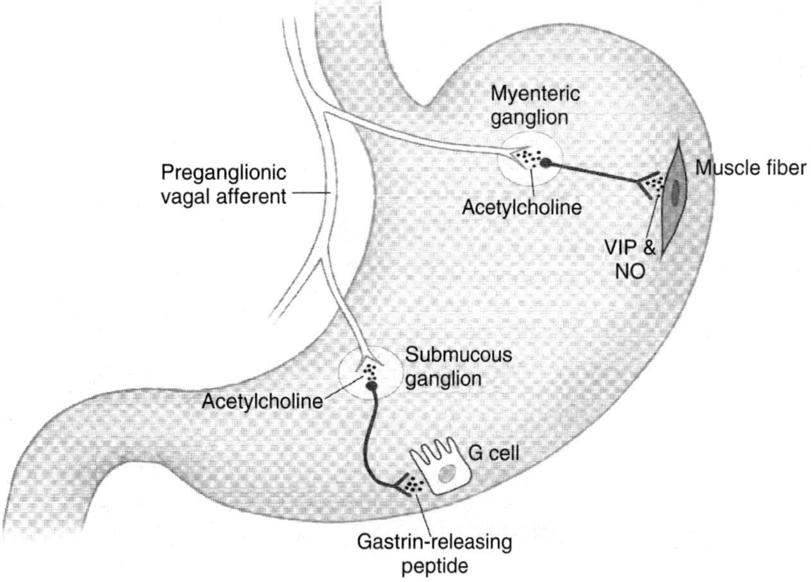

FIGURE 45.4. Vagal regulation of gastric function. Preganglionic vagal fibers terminate in the submucosal and myenteric ganglia of the stomach, where they are closely related to the postganglionic fibers, which supply the target cells (smooth muscle and epithelial). The neurotransmitter in the ganglia is acetylcholine. Relaxation of gastric smooth muscle fibers is caused by the release of vasoactive intestinal polypeptide (VIP) and nitric oxide (NO) at the neuromuscular junction. Postganglionic vagal regulation of gastrin release is accomplished through postganglionic peptidergic fibers that release gastrin-releasing peptide at the basal lateral surface of the G-cell. (From Debas.[252])

Microscopic Anatomy

The gastric wall is composed of four layers: mucosa, submucosa, muscularis propria, and serosa. The mucosa is the innermost layer, which consists of a columnar-lined epithelium, lamina propria, and muscularis mucosa. The surface epithelial lining is invaginated by gastric pits, which provide the gastric glands access to the lumen. The submucosa is rich in vascular, lymphatic, nervous, and connective tissue. The third layer is the thick muscularis propria, which contains fibers oriented in three directions: inner oblique, middle circular, and outer longitudinal. The final layer of the gastric wall is the serosa, which is the outer peritoneal covering.

Different types of specialized epithelial cells line the gastric glands in different anatomic regions of the stomach. The cardia contains cardiac glands that are populated by mucous, endocrine, and undifferentiated cells. Gastric (oxyntic) glands are the functional secretory unit of the gastric mucosa and are located in the fundus and body. These glands are populated by parietal, chief (peptic), endocrine, and mucous cells. The parietal cells are located predominantly in the neck of the gastric gland, whereas the chief cells are found in the base. Endocrine and mucous cells may be found throughout the gland. The antrum and pylorus make up the final region and are composed of pyloric glands, which contain endocrine, mucous, and gastrin-producing G cells.

Physiology

Acid Secretion

Gastric acid secretion is a complex event involving stimulatory and inhibitory signals from endocrine, paracrine, autocrine, and neural mechanisms. There are three phases of gastric acid secretion: cephalic, gastric, and intestinal. Vagal stimulation is a key initiator of gastric acid secretion during the cephalic phase. This is achieved directly by cholinergic innervation of the parietal cell and indirectly by the release of the hormone gastrin. The vagus enters the gastric wall along with arterial perforators and terminates at the myenteric plexus. Vagal stimulation of myenteric plexus interneurons results in the release of acetylcholine in close proximity to the parietal cells. Cholinergic stimulation of muscarinic receptors on the parietal cell (Fig. 45.5) causes an increase in intracellular calcium, which leads to hydrogen ion secretion via the H^+/K^+-ATPase (adenosine triphosphatase) pump (proton pump). The H^+/K^+-ATPase pump is located on the apical cell surface membrane and is capable of achieving a significant gradient of H^+ between the gastric lumen (pH 1.0) and the blood (pH 7.0).

Vagal fibers also act through interneurons to stimulate the release of gastrin from antral and pyloric G cells. Gastrin is one of the most important mediators of acid secretion during the gastric phase, which begins when food enters the stomach. The neurotransmitter thought to be responsible for the release of gastrin from the G cells is gastrin-releasing peptide (GRP or bombesin). However, a study involving a specific GRP receptor inhibitor in humans did not support this action.[1] Gastrin is released into the bloodstream and binds to gastrin receptors on the parietal cell, causing acid release. Furthermore, gastrin acts on enterochromaffin-like (ECL) cells, which are located close to the parietal cells in the oxyntic gland, thereby stimulating the release of histamine. Both vagal stimulation and gastrin act on mast cells to cause the release of histamine adjacent to parietal cells. Histamine then acts on histamine H_2 receptors of the parietal cell, causing increased H^+ release. Gastrin is also released when the pH in the gastric lumen rises above 3.0. This is a critical concept to understand when performing a vagotomy and antrectomy for peptic ulcer disease. Although vagotomy effectively reduces acid secretion from the parietal cell, if the antral G cell mass is incompletely resected, a stimulus for acid secretion remains.

The proton pump responsible for acid secretion is driven by two different mechanisms. Stimulation of acetylcholine and gastrin receptors on the parietal cell causes a rise in intracellular calcium, thereby activating phosphorylase kinase, which leads to the production of ATP. In contrast, stimulation of the histamine receptor results in increased adenylate cyclase activity. The increase in cyclic adenosine

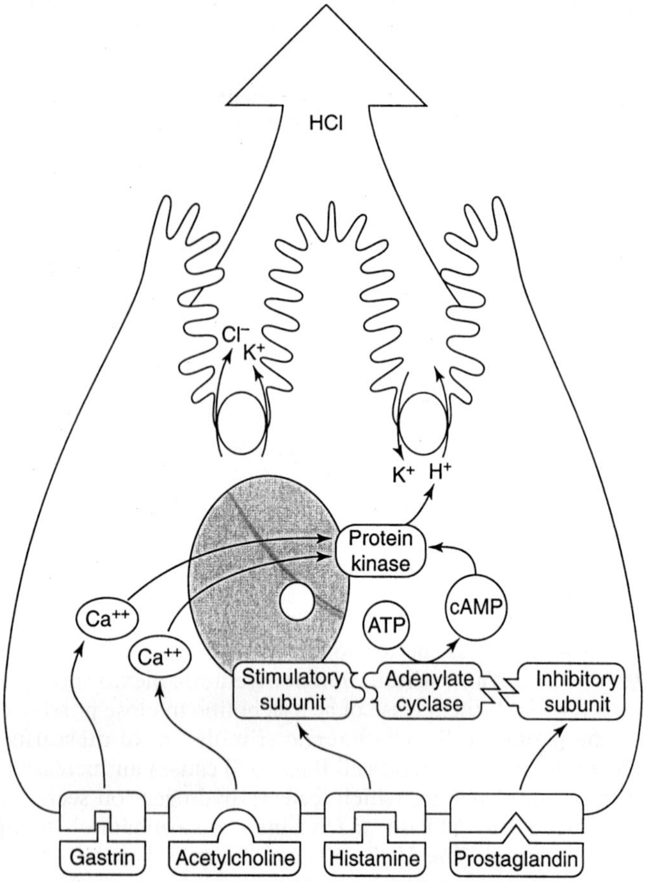

FIGURE 45.5. Parietal cell molecular signals regulating acid secretion. Both acetylcholine and gastrin bind to receptors on the basal surface of the parietal cell, raising intracellular calcium levels. The higher calcium stimulates protein kinase, which in turn activates the proton pump. Histamine binds its receptor, resulting in increased adenylate cyclase activity. The higher cAMP levels stimulate protein kinase, which causes increased proton pump activity. Prostaglandins act to inhibit acid secretion by adenylate cyclase inhibition.

monophosphate (cAMP) stimulates protein kinase, causing increased H^+/K^+-ATPase activity. Thus, the proton pump is the final common pathway for acid secretion, which explains the effectiveness of proton pump inhibitors (PPIs) in reducing acid production.

As mentioned, gastric acid secretion is controlled by a number of inhibitors. Somatostatin is produced in response to vagal stimulation by somatostatin-secreting D cells located in the fundus, antrum, and pylorus. Somatostatin acts in a paracrine fashion to reduce acid and gastrin production. In addition, somatostatin levels are increased in response to decreased pH in the antral lumen. When luminal pH falls below 3.0, somatostatin release is increased. This may be due to D-cell stimulation by calcitonin gene-related peptide. In contrast, when the pH of the lumen rises above 3.0, somatostatin release is inhibited, and gastrin is released, causing an increase in acid secretion. Prostaglandins may also act to inhibit gastric acid secretion via inhibition of adenylate cyclase within the parietal cell.

The duodenum plays an inhibitory role in gastric acid secretion during the intestinal phase of gastric acid secretion. When acidification of the duodenal lumen occurs, cholecystokinin (CCK) is released from duodenal endocrine cells, and secretin is released from duodenal S cells. Cholecystokinin inhibits gastric acid secretion by binding to CCK_A receptors on D cells, causing the release of somatostatin, which inhibits acid secretion by reducing histamine release from the ECL cells and inhibiting gastrin release from pyloric G cells. Furthermore, the presence of fat within the duodenal lumen reduces gastric acid secretion. Several other gastrointestinal (GI) peptides have been shown to inhibit gastric acid secretion, including peptide YY, gastric inhibitory peptide, neurotensin, pituitary adenylate cyclase-activating polypeptide, and vasoactive intestinal peptide.

Pepsin is secreted by the chief cells in the gastric gland as an inactive precursor, pepsinogen. Its release is stimulated by acetylcholine, histamine, gastrin, and secretin. Pepsinogen is converted to its active form pepsin by hydrochloric acid. The major physiologic function of pepsin is protein digestion. It becomes active at pH 2.0 to 4.0 but is irreversibly denatured at a neutral pH.

Bicarbonate, Mucous, and Intrinsic Factor Secretion

The gastric lumen is a purely acidic environment. The ability of the stomach to protect the gastric epithelium is the result of several mechanisms. The first is the highly impermeable membrane of the gastric surface, which prevents luminal acid from penetrating the gastric epithelium. In addition, tight intercellular junctions exist in the gastric epithelium to provide protection. Furthermore, the rich blood supply to the gastric mucosa aids in defense against the acidic environment. Finally, gastric surface cells secrete both bicarbonate and mucin. Bicarbonate secretion is stimulated by the vagus nerve and prostaglandin E_2 analogs. Secretion of these molecules creates a viscous mucous gel layer 0.2 to 0.6mm thick that covers the gastric epithelium. Thus, the microenvironment of the cell is maintained at a neutral pH of 7.0. Gastric acid secretion occurs through gastric pits that transiently penetrate the mucous gel layer. This facilitates the movement of acid into the lumen without disturbing the alkaline surface of the gastric epithelium. The loss of these gastric epithelial protective mechanisms contributes to the development of gastric ulceration.

The gastric mucosa is also responsible for the production of intrinsic factor. Intrinsic factor is a glycoprotein secreted by the parietal cells and is necessary for the absorption of vitamin B_{12} in the terminal ileum. Inhibitors of gastric acid secretion may reduce the production of intrinsic factor, although not to a degree that results in vitamin B_{12} deficiency. In contrast, chronic atrophic gastritis or total gastrectomy results in the absence of intrinsic factor, which leads to vitamin B_{12} deficiency and the development of pernicious anemia.

Motility

The functional anatomy of gastric emptying is divided into three regions: proximal stomach (cardia, fundus, proximal body); distal stomach (distal body and antrum); and pylorus. The proximal stomach functions as a storage area for ingested food and regulates the emptying of liquids, while the distal stomach functions to grind solid particles and regulates solid emptying.

The gastric pacemaker is located along the upper third of the greater curve of the stomach. Cyclic changes in potential are generated here at a frequency of three cycles per minute and propagate distally to the antrum. The gastric pacemaker is associated with the interdigestive motor cycles, which occur in the fasting state. These cycles are termed migrating motor complexes (MMCs). The MMCs are coordinated muscular contractions that clear the gastric lumen of residual particles during fasting. The gastric pacemaker is not responsible for the contractions during the fed state. In the fed state, contractions occur more frequently but are less powerful, with prolonged periods of contractile activity.

The rate of gastric emptying is dependent on the pressure gradient between the proximal stomach and duodenum. As swallowed food enters the stomach, the gastric fundus undergoes receptive relaxation. This occurs so that the gastric volume may increase without an increase in gastric pressure. The accommodation response is mediated by a vagovagal reflex. The fundus receives both excitatory cholinergic and inhibitory nitrergic input. During fasting, input is predominantly cholinergic, and the stomach is collapsed. Fundic distension stimulates mechanoreceptors, which send afferent signals to the brain. Efferent signals are then relayed to the fundus. The primary inhibitory neurotransmitter is nitric oxide, although vasoactive inhibitory peptide may be involved. In addition, serotoninergic receptors on nitrergic neurons of the enteric nervous system are involved in the inhibitory pathway. Vagotomy disrupts the vagal-mediated receptive relaxation, contributing to the dumping syndrome. With dumping, the accommodation response is lost, leading to rapid transit of food into the small bowel. Sympathetic nervous responses are generated by the presence of hyperosmolar substances within the lumen, causing abdominal cramping, diarrhea, heart palpitations, and dizziness, which are characteristic of dumping syndrome.

Antral contractions are the result of vagal stimulation. These contractions create an increase in intraluminal pressure, causing solids to be emptied into the duodenum. The antropyloric region ("antral mill") has the ability to discriminate solid particles according to size. Particles larger than 1 mm are reflected back into the antrum to be broken down into a smaller size. Vagotomy severely reduces antral contractions. It is for this reason that truncal vagotomy must be accompanied by a pyloroplasty to prevent a functional gastric outlet obstruction.

Gastric emptying of liquids differs from that of solids. Liquid emptying begins almost immediately following ingestion, although several factors may alter the rate. A larger volume of ingested liquid increases the rate of gastric emptying, whereas liquids with a higher osmolality or liquids containing protein, fats, and acid will slow emptying. In contrast, gastric emptying of solids is characterized by an initial lag phase followed by linear emptying. The lag phase is largely due to the trituration of solid particles occurring at the antral mill. This generally lasts for up to 1 h. Several factors alter the rate of solid emptying. Large particle size, high caloric content, and the presence of fats, triglycerides, or carbohydrates all prolong the lag phase, thus delaying gastric emptying. In addition, the presence of fat breakdown products within the duodenum is a potent inhibitor of gastric emptying. Moreover, the emptying of indigestible solids occurs by a different mechanism. Emptying of these substances takes place during the MMC through a relaxed pylorus rather than during the postprandial period.

Gastric emptying is regulated by both neural and hormonal mechanisms. The myenteric ganglia of the stomach receive direct vagal input (see Fig. 45.4). The vagus contains both excitatory and inhibitory fibers, which increase and decrease gastric tone, respectively, via specific neurotransmitters. Excitatory neurotransmitters causing contraction include acetylcholine and substance P, whereas vasoactive intestinal peptide and nitric oxide are inhibitory and cause muscle relaxation.[2] In addition, gastric emptying is influenced by a duodenal feedback mechanism. One of the central regulators of this is CCK. Cholecystokinin release is increased when the duodenum is exposed to acid, fats, and proteins as well as with duodenal distension, leading to a decrease in gastric emptying. Finally, the distal gut is thought to influence gastric emptying by the production of a hypothetical agent, enterogastrone. It is possible that this agent is peptide YY, which has been shown to decrease gastric emptying in a hormonal fashion.[3]

Peptic Ulcer Disease

Peptic ulcers are defects in the GI mucosa that extend through the muscularis mucosa. Peptic ulcer disease commonly refers to ulcers of the stomach, duodenum, or both. Historically, the pathogenesis of peptic ulcers was thought to be related to stress and diet. However, over the past two decades, research has demonstrated that the majority of peptic ulcers are associated with either the bacterium *Helicobacter pylori* or the use of nonsteroidal antiinflammatory drugs (NSAIDs).

Epidemiology

The incidence of peptic ulcer disease peaked in the first half of the 20th century and has been steadily declining since the late 1960s.[4] Although the frequency of uncomplicated peptic ulcer disease has declined, the rate of ulcer complications has not declined significantly and appears to be increasing in the elderly.[5] The ulcer incidence in *H. pylori*-infected individuals is 6- to 10-fold higher than for uninfected individuals, occurring at a rate of approximately 1% per year, with a lifetime ulcer prevalence of 10% to 20% in *H. pylori*-infected individuals.[6] The epidemiology of peptic ulcer disease closely reflects the incidence of *H. pylori* infection. In developing countries, most children become infected with the bacteria by the age of 10 years old, with prevalence rates greater than 80% by the age of 50. However, in developed countries such as the United States,[7] 10% of individuals between the ages of 18 and 30 years are infected, with the prevalence increasing to 50% in those over the age of 60.

Pathophysiology

Mucous Gel Layer

Gastric and duodenal epithelial cells are normally protected from acid and pepsin by a mucous layer as well as an unstirred water layer containing large amounts of bicarbonate. Gastric epithelial cells along with duodenal Brunner's glands secrete mucus and bicarbonate into the GI lumen. Furthermore, bicarbonate enters the unstirred water layer by diffusion from the blood. The blood flow provides energy and substrates necessary for mucosal defense mechanisms as well as the removal of acid that diffuses through uninjured mucosa. Additional acid protection is provided to the epithelial cells by a hydrophobic phospholipid layer within the mucus.

The gastric surface is highly impermeable due to the tight intercellular junctions of the gastric epithelium. These defense mechanisms result in the maintenance of a neutral pH on the gastroduodenal epithelial cell surface despite the highly acidic environment of the GI lumen.

When the defense mechanisms of the epithelium are overwhelmed, acid-peptic injury occurs. Superficial mucosal defects may be repaired by the migration of healthy cells within the mucous neck region in a process called rapid restitution,[8] whereas larger defects require regeneration of cells by cellular division.[9] Bicarbonate secretion in the proximal duodenum is impaired in patients with duodenal ulcers in response to acidification of the duodenum.[10] Eradication of *H. pylori* will return duodenal bicarbonate secretion to normal in patients with duodenal ulcers.[11] The mechanism by which *H. pylori* inhibits duodenal bicarbonate secretion is unclear but may be related to nitric oxide synthase activity.[12]

Helicobacter pylori

Helicobacter pylori is a gram-negative spiral, flagellated bacterium. Marshall and Warren first observed that gastritis was associated with an infection of spiral bacteria that has since become known as *H. pylori*.[13] *Helicobacter pylori* is able to survive the hostile environment of the stomach by producing large amounts of the enzyme urease. This enzyme catalyzes the breakdown of urea to alkaline ammonia and carbon dioxide, thus allowing the bacterium to protect itself from acid injury by surrounding itself with alkaline material. *Helicobacter pylori* appears to be transmitted by a fecal–oral route. Most adolescents and adults in developing countries are infected with *H. pylori*,[7] whereas in more developed nations as many as 50% of patients may be infected[14] by the age of 60.

Infection with *H. pylori* is a significant cause of gastroduodenal ulcers, with approximately 90%–95% of duodenal ulcers and 70%–75% of gastric ulcers attributable to the infection.[15] *Helicobacter pylori*-infected individuals may experience a 10% lifetime risk of developing peptic ulcer disease.[16] Although *H. pylori* infection is a significant cause of gastroduodenal ulcers, the exact mechanism by which the bacteria cause disease is incompletely understood. Two proposed mechanisms by which *H. pylori* leads to ulcer disease are (1) the host response to infection by this organism causes sufficient epithelial damage that luminal acid can access the tissue and create an ulcer and (2) infection impairs healing, and by eradicating the infection effective healing can proceed.[17] Moss and colleagues found that there were increased numbers of apoptotic cells in gastric tissue samples infected with *H. pylori*, and that eradication of the organism resulted in a decrease in the number of apoptotic cells.[18] The presence of apoptotic epithelial cells suggests a compromise in the epithelial barrier that could contribute to a breakdown in the cytoprotective mechanisms, leading to damage by luminal

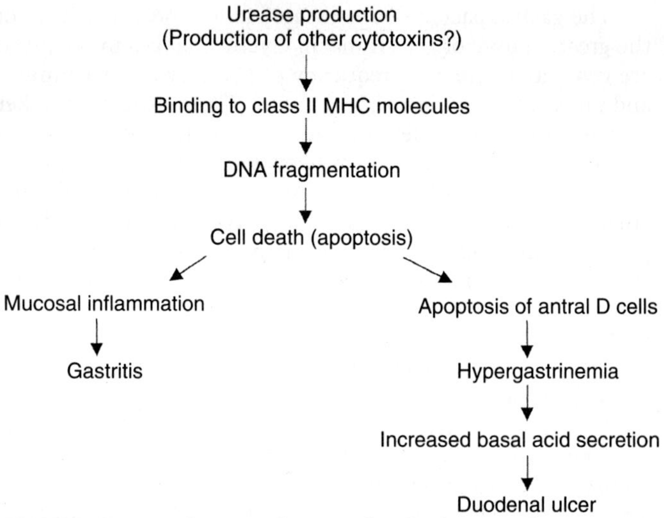

FIGURE 45.6. Mechanism of action of *Helicobacter pylori* as a cause of gastritis and duodenal ulcer. MHC, major histocompatibility complex. (From Debas.[252])

acid and pepsin,[17] metaplasia of gastric cells, and gastric atrophy and hypochlorhydria.[19] The pathophysiology of *H. pylori*-induced ulcer disease is illustrated in Figure 45.6.

Infection with *H. pylori* is almost always accompanied with superficial gastritis. In most persons, *H. pylori* infection is largely restricted to the gastric antrum. Antral gastritis leads to high levels of serum gastrin, increased acid output, and a propensity for duodenal ulcers. Others may develop a more widespread infection that involves the body of the stomach as well as the antrum. Persons who develop gastritis of the body of the stomach or a pangastritis are more likely to develop chronically decreased gastric acid output, gastric ulcers, and gastric cancer.

Inflammation is thought to be mediated by several mechanisms, including the induction of interleukin-8 (IL-8) production by direct contact between *H. pylori* and the gastric epithelium[20] and by *H. pylori* products such as urease, ammonia,[21] and the VacA protein.[22] A supposed virulence factor of *H. pylori* that increases the risk of developing gastroduodenal disease is the cagA gene, which encodes the CagA protein.[23] Persons infected with $cagA^+$ strains have a more intense inflammation in the stomach,[24] have higher amounts of mucosal IL-8,[25] and are more likely to have gastroduodenal ulceration than those who are $CagA^-$.[23,26]

Smoking

The general population risk of peptic ulcer disease attributable to cigarette smoking is approximately 23%.[27] Smoking has adverse effects on mucosal protective factors, and in rats, cigarette smoke has been shown to decrease gastric blood flow and angiogenesis at the ulcer margin as well as reduce gastric mucus synthesis.[28,29] Smoking and older age are associated with significantly reduced gastric and duodenal prostaglandin concentrations.[30] Cigarette smoking not only is a risk factor for peptic ulcer disease and its complications but also may inhibit the healing of peptic ulcers.

The excess of peptic ulcer disease in cigarette smokers may be explained by their increased susceptibility to *H. pylori* infection. One study demonstrated that the *H. pylori* prevalence was significantly higher in smokers (76%) than in nonsmokers (67%), with smokers experiencing a significantly higher ulcer risk than nonsmokers.[31] However, studies suggest that cigarette smoking does not increase the risk of peptic ulcer disease following successful eradication of *H. pylori*.[32,33]

Nonsteroidal Antiinflammatory Drugs

Nonsteroidal antiinflammatory drugs can injure the gastroduodenal mucosa through both topical and systemic effects and cause considerable morbidity and mortality related to gastric and duodenal ulcer disease. The NSAIDs primarily inhibit cyclooxygenase, thereby impairing the conversion of arachidonic acid to prostaglandins, prostacyclin, and thromboxanes. Gastric epithelium contains cyclooxygenase-1 (COX-1), an enzyme essential for prostaglandin synthesis and therefore gastric and duodenal cytoprotection.[34] Prostaglandins protect gastric and duodenal epithelium by preserving gastric mucosal blood flow and increasing mucus production and increasing bicarbonate secretion. The NSAIDs cause reduced prostaglandin synthesis, which can result in decreased epithelial secretion of mucus and bicarbonate, diminished mucosal blood flow, reduced mucosal proliferation, and subsequent peptic injury. A second isoform of the cyclooxygenase enzyme, COX-2, has been identified and is primarily involved in inflammation. Agents that block the COX-2 isoform appear to reduce tissue inflammation with less GI toxicity.[34–38]

Gastrinoma

In 1955, Zollinger and Ellison first described a syndrome of recurrent and often fatal GI hemorrhage that they proposed was the result of a pancreatic endocrine tumor. Zollinger-Ellison syndrome (ZES) consists of a triad of symptoms: severe peptic ulcer disease, gastric acid hypersecretion, and a non-β-cell gastrin-producing tumor of the pancreas. Gastrinomas are included in a larger group of tumors referred to as neuroendocrine tumors and may be part of the multiple endocrine neoplasia I (MEN I) syndrome in approximately one-third of patients. A fasting serum gastrin above 1000 pg/mL is virtually diagnostic of ZES, but in patients with only moderate elevations of fasting serum gastrin, a secretin stimulation test may be necessary to make the diagnosis. Certain conditions should increase suspicion of gastrinoma-associated ulcers. These include multiple ulcers, ulcers occurring distal to the duodenal bulb, a strong family history, peptic ulcers occurring in the absence of *H. pylori* or NSAID use, peptic ulcers in association with hypercalcemia or renal stones, ulcers refractory to medical therapy, ulcers that recur after surgery, and peptic ulcers in association with diarrhea, steatorrhea, or weight loss.

Classification

Gastric Ulcer

The term *peptic ulcer* includes both gastric and duodenal ulcerations. However, fundamental differences exist between these two entities that affect surgical therapy. Malignant gastric ulcers are indistinguishable from benign ulcers and therefore must be excised or biopsied. Furthermore, gastric ulcers tend to affect older individuals, which may increase perioperative morbidity and mortality.

TABLE 45.1. Classification of Gastric Ulcers According to Location, Symptoms, and Acid Secretion.

Type	*Location*	*Symptom*	*Acid secretion*
I	Gastric body on lesser curvature	Penetration	Normal or low
II	Gastric body and duodenal ulcer Obstruction Perforation	Hemorrhage	Elevated
III	Prepyloric Perforation	Hemorrhage	Elevated
IV	High on lesser curvature	Hemorrhage	Low
V	Anywhere on stomach		NSAID use

Gastric ulcers are classified into five categories. These are summarized in Table 45.1. Type I gastric ulcers are the most common and occur along the lesser curvature at the junction of the fundic and antral mucosa. This type of ulceration is generally associated with acid hyposecretion and can be treated with distal gastrectomy and Billroth I or II reconstruction. While Type I gastric ulcers are considered to be the consequence of inadequate mucosal defense rather than acid hypersecretion, many advocate the addition of vagotomy to the gastric resection. The Cleveland Clinic reviewed their experience with 349 patients operated on between 1950 and 1979 with a mean follow-up of 11.8 years. Of the patients, 55% had a gastric resection without vagotomy; 19.8% had gastric resection with vagotomy; and 20.3% had vagotomy, pyloroplasty, and wedge excision or biopsy of the ulcer. Operations were selected based on the type of ulcer (types I–IV), whether the surgeon suspected cancer preoperatively, whether the operation was elective or an emergency, and the age and general health of the patient (presence of significant comorbid disease). Long-term results were equivalent, with an ulcer recurrence rate of 4%.[39]

Type II gastric ulcers are found in the body of the stomach in conjunction with a duodenal ulcer, while type III gastric ulcers occur in the prepyloric region. Types II and III gastric ulcers are associated with increased acid secretion and should be managed with vagotomy and antrectomy, similar to duodenal ulcer patients. Type IV gastric ulcers are similar to type I gastric ulcers in that they tend to occur in the setting of acid hyposecretion. Type IV ulcers are located high on the lesser curve in close proximity to the gastroesophageal junction. Subtotal gastric resection for type IV ulcers is considered optimal, and reconstruction with a Roux-en-Y esophagogastrojejunostomy may be recommended.[40]

Duodenal Ulcer

Although *H. pylori* infection is a significant cause of duodenal ulceration, the exact mechanism by which *H. pylori* causes ulceration remains unclear. Duodenal ulceration is largely related to acid hypersecretion, but this is thought to be only part of the pathogenesis. It is likely the imbalance between duodenal acid load, mucosal defenses, and the buffering capacity of the duodenum in susceptible patients that leads to duodenal ulcer formation.[26] Further discussion regarding the pathogenesis of duodenal ulcer as it relates to specific factors, like *H. pylori* and NSAIDs, is presented above.

Stress Ulcer

Stress-related mucosal disease of the GI tract is a common problem as a result of severe physiologic stress among critically ill patients. Of critically ill patients, 75% to 100% demonstrate evidence of mucosal damage within 24h of admission to the intensive care unit (ICU).[41] A decrease in gastric blood flow as a result of a low intraluminal pH, hypoperfusion, and acidosis may be a major factor in stress-related mucosal lesions.[41] In the critically ill population, two types of stress-related mucosal disease commonly occur. The first consists of superficial erosions that are diffuse and have a low risk of clinically important bleeding. The second consists of deeper lesions that tend to be more focal and carry a greater risk of significant bleeding. *Clinically important bleeding* is defined as overt bleeding (hematemesis, hematochezia, melena) complicated by hemodynamic changes or the need for transfusions. This type of bleeding occurs in approximately 1% to 4% of critically ill patients.[42,43]

Risk factors for the development of stress-related mucosal disease have been identified as mechanical ventilation for longer than 48h and patients with a coagulopathy. Patients suffering from shock may also be at increased risk. In one large series, 3.7% of patients with risk factors experienced clinically significant bleeding, while only 0.1% of critically ill patients without these risk factors had clinically important bleeding.[44] This same study demonstrated that patients who suffered a clinically significant bleed had a higher mortality rate than those who did not (48.5% vs. 9.1%, respectively).[43]

Diagnostic Tests for Helicobacter pylori and Peptic Ulcers

Noninvasive Tests for Helicobacter pylori

Helicobacter pylori produces many enzymes that facilitate colonization. Urease is one such enzyme that allows the organism to metabolize urea into ammonia and carbamate to help neutralize luminal acid.[17,45] This reaction has been used for diagnosis of *H. pylori* infection and for follow-up after eradication therapy. The urea breath test is performed by having the patient ingest carbon-13 or -14-labled urea followed by breath collection 30 to 60min later. This method has proven clinically useful, with sensitivities and specificities for the diagnosis and assessment of patients after antimicrobial therapy higher than 95%. Urea breath test may confirm eradication of *H. pylori* within 6 weeks after therapy.[46] To reliably confirm eradication, PPIs must be discontinued at least 2 weeks prior to testing.

Direct fecal antigen detection is a relatively new and noninvasive means of diagnosis and follow-up testing for *H. pylori*. The sensitivity and specificity of enzyme immunoassay using polyclonal antibodies have been reported as approximately 89% and 94% to 95%, respectively.[47] Monoclonal stool antigen tests have also been developed and have demonstrated similar sensitivity and specificity to the polyclonal tests; diagnostic accuracy was 96%.[48] When using stool antigen tests for follow-up, it is necessary to wait up to 12 weeks to reliably confirm eradication of *H. pylori*.

Serologic tests are useful for the initial diagnosis of *H. pylori* infection but are less useful for diagnosing cure following therapy. Most patients infected with *H. pylori* produce an immune response composed primarily of immunoglobulin G (IgG). Overall sensitivity and specificity for enzyme-linked immunosorbent assay (ELISA) detection of serum IgG antibodies have been reported as 92% and 83%, respectively.[49] Whole-blood serologic IgG assays have been developed but have slightly decreased sensitivity and specificity compared to serum assays.[50] The accuracy of diagnostic methods for detecting *H. pylori* infection are presented in Table 45.2.[48,51]

TABLE 45.2. Accuracy of Diagnostic Tests for *Helicobacter pylori*.

Test	*Sensitivity (%)*	*Specificity (%)*	*PPV*	*NPV*
Invasive tests (endoscopy)				
Chronic inflammation	100	66	84	100
Acute inflammation	87	94	96	80
Warthin-Starry silver stain	93	99	99	89
Rapid urease test	90	100	100	84
Noninvasive tests				
Serum IgG antibody	91	97	95	85
Urea breath test	90	96	98	84
Fecal antigen detection	97	94	97	95

PPV, positive predictive valve; NPV, negative predictive valve.

Invasive Testing

Historically, barium contrast studies of the upper GI tract were the standard test for the diagnosis of peptic ulcer disease. Radiography has become less useful since the introduction of flexible endoscopy due to the higher sensitivity of endoscopy and the ability to obtain biopsy specimens. However, radiologic evaluation remains useful in select patients with complicated ulcer disease and may provide useful information about gastroduodenal anatomy. Double-contrast barium studies accurately identify peptic ulcers 80% to 90% of the time when compared with endoscopy.[52]

Peptic ulcers may display either benign or malignant radiographic features. Radiographic features of benign gastric ulcers include ulcer projection outside the lumen of the stomach; thickened, smooth, symmetrical folds that radiate to the ulcer crater; indentation on the wall of the stomach opposite the ulcer crater; smooth radiolucent band at the neck of the ulcer; and a thin, radiolucent line (Hampton line) at the rim of the ulcer crater where the mucosa has been undermined by the inflammatory process. In contrast, malignant ulcerations may demonstrate irregular collections of barium within an intraluminal mass as well as irregular and nonsymmetrical gastric folds.[53] Malignant gastric ulcers may appear radiographically benign approximately 3% to 5% of the time.[54]

Helicobacter pylori infection can usually be established during endoscopy by biopsy urease test, histology, or bacterial culture. However, endoscopy is not generally recommended solely for the purpose of establishing *H. pylori* infection. The American College of Gastroenterology has recommended that a urease test on an antral biopsy be performed as the first test in patients undergoing diagnostic endoscopy. The sensitivity and specificity of biopsy urease tests are 90% to 95% and 95% to 100%, respectively (Table 45.2).[55] Urease activity can be determined by using commercially available kits such as the Clotest. In patients taking PPIs, H_2 antagonists, antibiotics, or bismuth-containing compounds or in patients with recent GI bleeding, biopsy urease tests may have decreased sensitivity. In these patients, biopsies of both the antrum and fundus may increase the sensitivity of the test. Histology or serum antibodies may be used for the diagnosis of *H. pylori* if the urease test is negative and clinical suspicion of infection is high.[55] *Helicobacter pylori* culture and sensitivity testing may be indicated in patients with refractory disease given the increasing resistance of the organism to metronidazole and clarithromycin.[56]

Treatment of Peptic Ulcer

Medical Management

The PPIs are the most potent inhibitors of gastric acid secretion. Proton pump inhibitors are targeted at inhibiting the enzyme H± K± ATPase, which is the final step of acid secretion. They accumulate specifically and selectively in the secretory canaliculus of the parietal cell. The PPIs should be administered before the first meal of the day because the amount of H-K-ATPase present in the parietal cell is greatest after a prolonged fast.[57] Proton pump inhibitors should not be given together with H_2 receptor antagonists (H_2RAs), prostaglandins, or other antisecretory agents because of a reduction in their acid inhibitory effects when administered simultaneously.

The PPIs heal gastroduodenal ulcers more rapidly than H_2RAs, as demonstrated by two meta-analyses where pooled healing rates were 60% and 85% at 2 and 4 weeks, respectively, versus 40% and 75% for H_2RAs.[58,59] Studies have demonstrated the superior healing rates of PPIs compared to H_2RAs for gastroduodenal ulcers associated with NSAIDs when NSAIDs cannot be discontinued.[60,61]

Gastric Ulcers

There are differences between gastric and duodenal ulcers, such as a lower prevalence of *H. pylori* infection in gastric ulcer patients of 70% versus 90% with duodenal ulcer patients[62] and reduced gastric acid secretion in gastric ulcer patients compared to normal or increased acid secretion in duodenal ulcer patients.[63] A randomized controlled trial that studied the effects of *H. pylori* eradication on gastric ulcer healing randomly assigned patients to receive either a 1-week course of eradication therapy (120 mg bismuth subcitrate, 500 mg tetracycline, and 400 mg metronidazole, each given orally four times a day) or a 4-week course of omeprazole (20 mg orally per day). The mean size of gastric ulcers was 0.82 cm. At 5 weeks, *H. pylori* had been eradicated in 91% of the antibacterial treatment group and in 12.5% of the omeprazole group. The gastric ulcers were healed in 84.4% of the patients treated with antibacterial drugs and in 72.5% of those treated with omeprazole at 5 weeks. At 9 weeks, ulcers were healed in 96% of the antibacterial group and 92% of the PPI group. One year after treatment, recurrent gastric ulcers were detected in 4.5% of the antibacterial treatment group and in 52.2% of the omeprazole group. The authors concluded that in patients with *H. pylori* infection and gastric ulcers unrelated to the use of NSAIDs, 1 week of antibacterial therapy without acid suppression heals the ulcers as well as omeprazole and reduces the rate of their recurrence.[64]

Another randomized controlled trial compared 1-week triple therapy using PPI plus amoxicillin and clarithromycin to 8 weeks of therapy with a PPI alone for effect on large gastric ulcer healing. Healing rates in *H. pylori*-infected patients receiving triple therapy were 89% compared to 100% in the PPI-alone group for ulcers less than 1 cm. Healing occurred in 54% and 77% of patients with ulcers 1 to 1.5 cm (triple therapy vs. PPI, respectively) and 5% and 77% of patients with ulcers larger than 1.5 cm (triple therapy vs. PPI). *Helicobacter pylori* was eradicated in 84% of patients receiving triple therapy. The authors concluded that 1-week PPI-based triple therapy alone healed gastric ulcers smaller than 1 cm; however, this treatment was inadequate for larger ulcers. The authors recommended the use of additional acid suppressive therapy following triple therapy for larger gastric ulcers.[65]

The efficacy of three pantoprazole-based triple-therapy regimens for the eradication of *H. pylori* infection and gastric ulcer healing were tested in a multicenter, randomized study. *Helicobacter pylori*-positive patients with active gastric ulcers were randomized to receive pantoprazole (40 mg) (P) and two of three antibiotics: clarithromycin (500 mg) (C), metronidazole (500 mg) (M), or amoxicillin (1000 mg) (A). Triple therapy (PAC, PCM, PAM) was administered twice daily for 7 days, followed by pantoprazole until the ulcer had healed. The *H. pylori* eradication rates were 89% for PAC, 83% for PCM, and 76% for PAM. Healing rates after 4 weeks were 91% for PAM, 90% for PCM, and 88% for PAC, with healing rates increased to over 97% in all groups after 8 weeks. Successful eradication and the ulcer size (<15 mm) were significant predictors for healing after 4 weeks. Furthermore, 25 patients were found to have gastric neoplasms at the inclusion visit, with an additional 4 cases of gastric cancer diagnosed during the study. This finding emphasizes the need to perform additional endoscopy and histological evaluation in patients with gastric ulcers.[62]

The impact of pretreatment of *H. pylori* infection on gastric ulcer healing rates in patients receiving NSAIDs and antisecretory medications was evaluated in a prospective analysis of two identical double-blind, multicenter, parallel group studies. Patients were enrolled from 90 North American sites in primary care and referral centers. Patients were randomized to receive ranitidine (150 mg BID) or lansoprazole (15 mg or 30 mg once daily) for 8 weeks. In all three treatment groups, gastric ulcers were more likely to heal and heal faster if the individual was infected with *H. pylori*. Healing rates (regardless of *H. pylori* status) were significantly better in both lansoprazole groups than in the ranitidine group after 4 weeks and 8 weeks[66] but lower than healing rates reported following *H. pylori* eradication.

Duodenal Ulcers

The prevalence of *H. pylori* infection in patients with complicated duodenal ulcer disease appears to be lower than in patients with uncomplicated disease. Antisecretory therapy with H_2RAs is warranted in patients with duodenal ulcers who are not infected with *H. pylori*. The H_2RAs induce healing rates of 70% to 80% for duodenal ulcers after 4 weeks and 87% to 94% after 8 weeks of therapy.[67] The PPIs are also effective in inducing ulcer healing and may have the advantage of shorter healing times.[68] Maintenance acid suppression is recommended following *H. pylori* eradication in patients with complicated duodenal ulcers. Maintenance therapy can be stopped after 2 to 3 months if ulcer healing has occurred and *H. pylori* is eradicated.

Preexisting *H. pylori* infection is a risk factor for the development of duodenal ulcers. In the United States, the prevalence of *H. pylori* infection in duodenal ulcer patients appears to be less than in other areas, with one large study documenting infection in only 73% of patients.[69] All patients with duodenal ulcers associated with *H. pylori* infection should undergo eradication therapy, which reduces ulcer recurrence and complications.[70–73] Endoscopic recurrence of duodenal ulcers following eradication of *H. pylori* was 10% to 20% in two meta-analyses.[70,71]

In the United States, *H. pylori* resistance to clarithromycin, metronidazole, and amoxicillin is approximately 10%, 37%, and 1.4%, respectively.[74] Eradication rates with quadruple therapy are 3% to 6% higher than PPI triple therapy, largely due to the issue of antibiotic resistance. This has led some authors to conclude that quadruple therapy can be considered a first-line therapy for *H. pylori*.[75] A multicenter, randomized, controlled North American trial assessed efficacy of bismuth-based quadruple therapy with omeprazole, bismuth biscalcitrate, metronidazole, and tetracycline (OBMT) compared with triple therapy with omeprazole, amoxicillin, and clarithromycin (OAC) in treatment of patients with *H. pylori* infection and duodenal ulcers. Patients were randomly assigned to a 10-day course of OBMT or a 10-day course of OAC. Eradication was confirmed by two negative urea breath tests after more than 1 month and more than 2 months after therapy. Modified intent-to-treat eradication rates were 87.7% for OBMT and 83.2% for OAC. The authors discovered that OBMT therapy largely overcame *H. pylori* metronidazole resistance, which was present in 40% of patients in this study.[75] Similar *H. pylori* eradication rates were found when quadruple therapy was used as second-line therapy following a failed course of standard triple therapy including a PPI, clarithromycin, and amoxicillin.[76] Treatment regimens are discussed in Table 45.3.

There is clear evidence that eradication of *H. pylori* changes the natural history of peptic ulcer disease. In one meta-analysis, peptic ulcer recurrence was significantly less following treatment of *H. pylori*.[70] When *H. pylori* was eradicated, recurrent ulcer rates were 6% for duodenal ulcers and 4% for gastric ulcers compared to recurrence rates of 67% and 59%, respectively, when the organism was not eradicated.

Another meta-analysis that included 52 trials evaluated the clinical and economical benefits of *H. pylori* eradication in patients with gastric and duodenal ulcers who had a documented infection. After rigorous analysis, the authors concluded that *H. pylori* eradication therapy reduced the recurrence of peptic ulcer disease and was the most cost-effective therapy.[77]

TABLE 45.3. Recommended Treatment Regimens for *Helicobacter pylori* Infection (2 weeks).

Bismuth triple therapy	Bismuth 2 tablets QID Tetracycline 500 mg QID Metronidazole 500 mg TID
PPI triple therapy	Omeprazole 20 mg BID Amoxicillin 1000 mg BID Clarithromycin 500 mg BID
Quadruple therapy	Omeprazole 20 mg BID Bismuth 2 tablets QID Tetracycline 500 mg QID Metronidazole 500 mg QID

Idiopathic Peptic Ulcers

Once all known etiological factors have been excluded, there remains a group of patients with "idiopathic ulcers." The management of idiopathic peptic ulcers is not well defined; however, antisecretory drugs remain the mainstay of treatment to promote ulcer healing.[78]

Surgical Management

Operative therapy for peptic ulcer disease is classically indicated for bleeding, perforation, obstruction, and intractability. Some authors believe that the only indication for elective definitive surgical treatment of peptic ulcer disease is the patient with intractable recurrent symptoms of duodenal ulcer despite adequate medical treatment in the absence of *H. pylori* infection.[79] *Intractability* is generally defined as the failure of an ulcer to heal after 8–12 weeks of therapy or if patients relapse following discontinuation of therapy. In this setting, parietal cell vagotomy may be the procedure of choice. Additional indications for elective surgery may include suspicion of malignancy, intolerance or noncompliance with medical therapy, patients at high risk for ulcer complications (transplant recipients, steroid or NSAID dependency, giant ulcers), a strong ulcer diathesis, patient preference, and failure of nonoperative management of an ulcer complication. Finally, the cost of long-term antisecretory therapy is significant and may also be considered an indication for antiulcer surgery. Regardless of the indication for surgery, the fundamental goals of surgical therapy are to permit ulcer healing, prevent or treat ulcer complications, address the underlying ulcer diathesis, and minimize postoperative digestive sequelae.

Truncal vagotomy with antrectomy eliminates both the cephalic and gastric phases of acid secretion and results in a greater decrease in acid production compared to vagotomy with a drainage procedure. Vagotomy plus antrectomy and Billroth I or Billroth II reconstruction are shown in Figure 45.7. Vagotomy plus antrectomy decreases peak acid output by approximately 85% by removing the gastrin-secreting portion of the stomach. Several prospective trials have demonstrated that vagotomy with antrectomy is superior to vagotomy and drainage, with ulcer recurrence rates of 1%–2% following the former versus 10% with the latter.[80–84] Vagotomy with pyloroplasty is shown in Figure 45.8. Because truncal vagotomy sacrifices vagal innervation to the pancreas, small intestine, proximal colon, and hepatobiliary tree in addition to the stomach, a selective vagotomy was developed. Selective vagotomy spares the hepatic and celiac branches. However, compared to truncal vagotomy and drainage, selective vagotomy is inferior with regard to recurrence, dumping symptoms, diarrhea, pain, and dyspepsia and has fallen out of favor.

Highly selective vagotomy, also known as parietal cell vagotomy or proximal selective vagotomy, selectively eliminates the vagal innervation to acid-producing parietal cells and pepsin-producing chief cells of the fundus and body of the stomach while preserving innervation to the antrum and pylorus as well as the liver and small intestine. This is shown

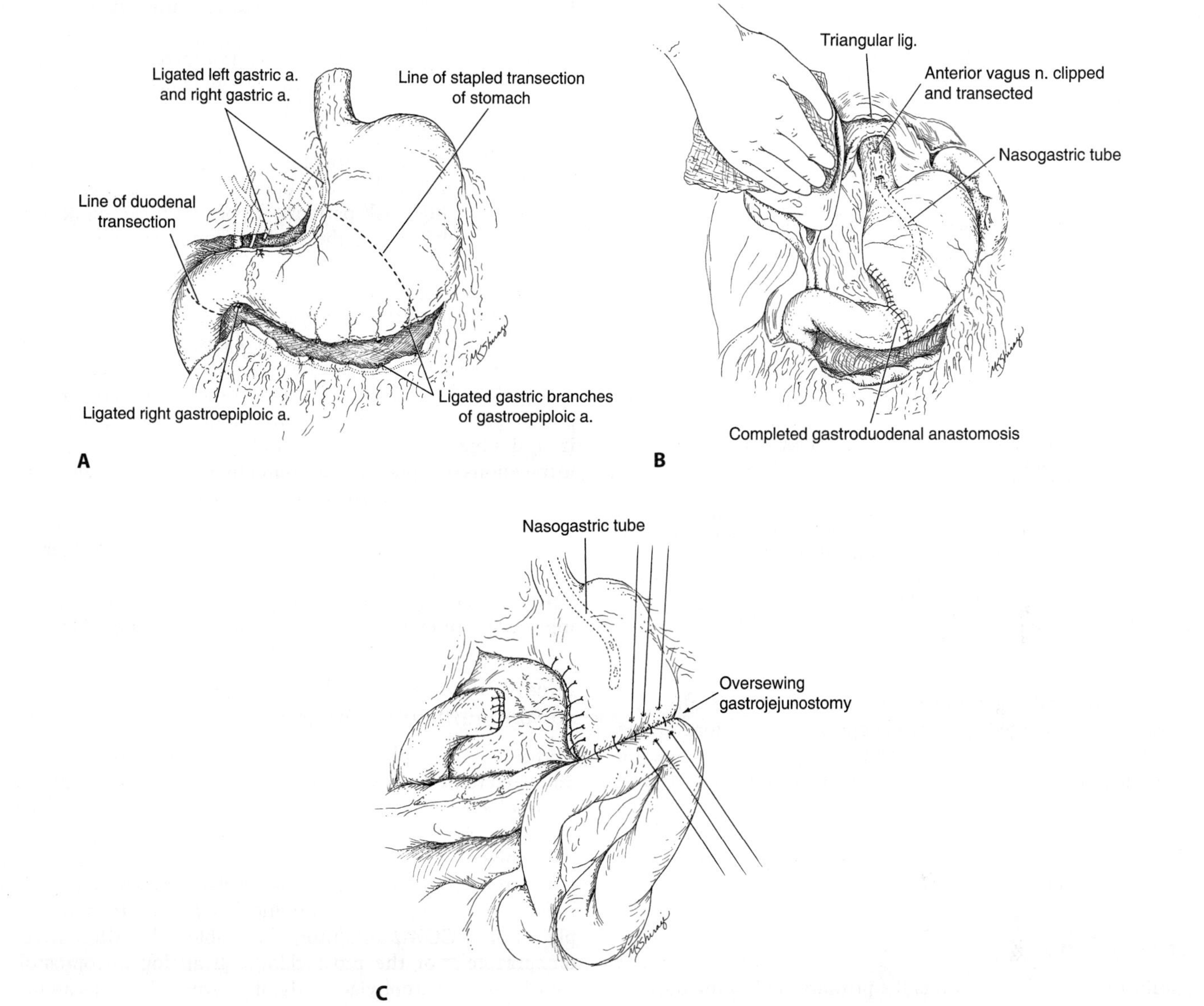

FIGURE 45.7. Vagotomy and antrectomy. **A.** The vagal trunks are identified and divided. The stomach is resected along a line from just above the incisura to the point along the greater curvature where the gastroepiploic vessels disappear or are at their closest approximation to the gastric wall. The duodenum is divided approximately 2 cm distal to the pylorus. **B.** The Billroth I reconstruction entails creation of a gastroduodenostomy. **C.** The Billroth II reconstruction is accomplished by closing the duodenal stump and the gastric remnant. The stomach is anastomosed to a loop of jejunum.

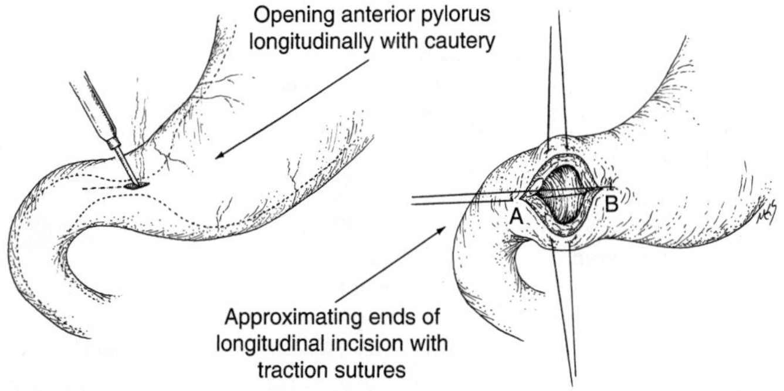

FIGURE 45.8. Vagotomy and pyloroplasty. Truncal vagotomy is followed by opening of the pylorus longitudinally. The ends of the longitudinal incision are closed transversely, creating a large opening at the pylorus.

in Figure 45.9. Therefore, a drainage procedure is unnecessary because the integrity of the antral mill and pyloric sphincter mechanism is preserved. Prospective randomized trials have demonstrated lower postoperative morbidity regarding post-vagotomy symptoms when HSV was compared to both truncal and selective vagotomy.[85,86] Although postoperative morbidity rates are lower following HSV, ulcer recurrence rates are higher. Studies have reported ulcer recurrence rates that range from 13% at 5 years[87] to 22% at 12 years.[88]

The differences between the various ulcer operations with regard to recurrence and morbidity are summarized in Table 45.4.[89] Anterior seromyotomy with posterior truncal vagotomy is an alternative to HSV that produces a similar reduction in acid secretion as HSV.[90] Furthermore, ulcer recurrence rates at 2 and 4 years following anterior seromyotomy with

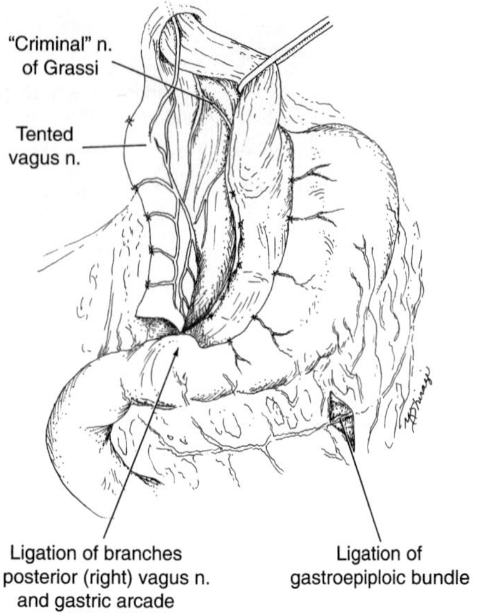

FIGURE 45.9. Parietal cell vagotomy. When performing a parietal cell vagotomy, the anterior and posterior vagal trunks are mobilized. The "criminal nerve of Grassi" is identified as it branches from the posterior vagus and is divided. The lesser curve is devascularized, the distal 5 cm of esophagus cleared of investing tissues, and the crow's foot preserved. Some advocate division of the gastroepiploic bundle, but the efficacy of this step is controversial.

posterior truncal vagotomy are similar to HSV.[91] Finally, laparoscopy has emerged as a surgical option not only for elective ulcer surgery but also for emergent complications of peptic ulcer disease. All of these surgical procedures, including parietal cell vagotomy and anterior seromyotomy with posterior truncal vagotomy, have been performed laparoscopically in the elective setting, with patients experiencing low recurrence rates and shorter hospital stays.

Stress Ulcer

Inhibition of acid secretion is the primary goal in the prevention and treatment of stress-related mucosal disease. Clinical trials demonstrated that mucosal injury may be prevented by maintaining intragastric pH above 3.5 to 5.0.[41,44,92] A meta-analysis performed by Cook et al. of 57 randomized controlled trials compared the ability of H_2RAs, antacids, and placebo to reduce the prevalence of clinically important bleeding in critically-ill patients.[44] The findings of this analysis suggested that H_2RAs reduced the likelihood of clinically significant bleeding by 50%.

A prospective randomized trial compared the efficacy of intravenous ranitidine to enteral omeprazole in mechanically ventilated patients and found that 31% of the patients in the ranitidine group experienced clinically significant bleeding compared to 6% in the omeprazole group.[93] Similarly, omeprazole has been found to be superior to both ranitidine and sucralfate in high-risk patients. Upper GI bleeding occurred in 10.5% and 9.3% of the ranitidine and sucralfate group, respectively, while no patients in the omeprazole group experienced bleeding.[94]

In patients with acute GI bleeding or those at risk for rebleeding after successful hemostasis, an intragastric pH above 6.0 should be maintained to prevent the dissolution of blood clots.[95] After successful endoscopic therapy, 15% to 20% of patients suffer from recurrent bleeding.[96] In a randomized, double-blind, crossover trial of 34 healthy volunteers, intravenous omeprazole was found to be superior to ranitidine in maintaining intragastric pH above 6.0, with a tolerance to ranitidine demonstrated on the second and third day of use.[97] Studies evaluating the efficacy of H_2RAs versus placebo[98,99] and PPIs versus placebo[96,100] suggest that PPIs are superior to H_2RAs as adjuvant therapy for preventing rebleeding following successful endoscopic treatment of acute ulcer bleeding.

Ulcers Associated with Nonsteroidal Antiinflammatory Drugs

Multiple factors place patients at increased risk for gastroduodenal toxicity from NSAIDs. The five most important risk factors have been identified as a prior history of an adverse GI event (ulcer, hemorrhage); age older than 60; high NSAID dose (twice normal); concurrent use of glucocorticoids; and concurrent use of anticoagulants.[101] Patients who are at high risk of developing NSAID-induced GI toxicity should be placed on a COX-2 inhibitor, if possible.[102,103] Alternatively, omeprazole[104] or the prostaglandin E analog misoprostol[105] may be started prophylactically. If a patient develops an ulcer while taking NSAIDs, then the agent should be stopped and therapy started with an H_2 receptor blocker or PPI.[104] Also, the patient should be tested for *H. pylori* and if positive started on eradication therapy. If a patient must remain on a nonselective NSAID such as aspirin for cardioprotective reasons after developing an ulcer, then a PPI should be started.[106]

TABLE 45.4. Results of Duodenal Ulcer Surgery.

	Highly selective vagotomy	*Truncal vagotomy with pyloroplasty*	*Truncal vagotomy with antrectomy*
Mortality rate (%)	0	0.5–1	2
Ulcer recurrence (%)	10	12	1–2
Gastric emptying			
Liquids	Accelerated	Accelerated	Accelerated
Solids	No change	Accelerated	Slowed
Dumping (%)			
Mild	<5	10	10–15
Severe	0	1	1–2
Diarrhea (%)			
Mild	<5	25	20
Severe	0	2	1–2

Complications of Peptic Ulcers

Perforation

The clinical presentation of a perforated duodenal ulcer may vary according to the location of the ulcer. Patients with ulcers that penetrate through the posterior duodenal wall generally present with bleeding, while anterior duodenal perforations cause the acute onset of severe, diffuse abdominal pain. When an anterior perforation occurs, free air within the abdominal cavity may be detected by plain or upright radiographs of the abdomen and chest in approximately 70% of cases.[107] Most patients who experience a perforation will have a history of peptic ulcer disease, and a detailed history will reveal ulcer symptoms in the majority of patients without known ulcer disease. However, chronically ill, elderly patients may be an exception to this presentation, with vague, poorly localized abdominal pain that has developed over days to weeks.

Most cases of duodenal ulcer perforation involve the anterior wall of the duodenal bulb, while the lesser curvature is commonly the sight of gastric ulcer perforation.[53] *Helicobacter pylori* and NSAIDs are the two major causes of perforated duodenal ulcers. Perforated ulcers are associated with NSAID use in one-third to one-half of patients[108,109] and more commonly occur in elderly patients. Smoking has also been associated with peptic ulcer perforation, and in patients younger than 75 years old it is a stronger risk factor than the use of NSAIDs.[110]

Perforated duodenal ulcers are commonly treated with an omental patch (Graham patch) or truncal vagotomy with pyloroplasty that incorporates the perforation. Simple patch closure (Fig. 45.10) may be appropriate in patients who have not been previously treated for peptic ulcer disease and who can take PPIs and antibiotics for *H. pylori*.[111,112] Perforations related to NSAID use may also be treated with patch closure if the drug can be discontinued. Simple closure of perforated peptic ulcer has been compared with definitive surgery in randomized clinical trials.[113–115] Ulcer recurrence rates were 61% following simple closure compared to 6% with a definitive operation.[79]

Recurrent ulcer disease after peptic ulcer perforation occurs mainly in patients infected with *H. pylori*.[116] This is

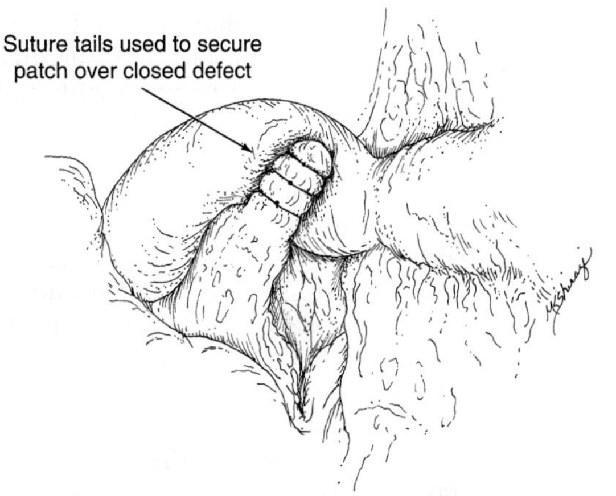

FIGURE 45.10. Graham patch for perforated duodenal ulcer. A row of sutures is used to close the duodenal defect. After the knots are tied, the tails are used to secure a tongue of omentum over the defect to reduce the chance for fistula should the closure fail.

supported by several studies that demonstrated low recurrence rates following simple closure of the ulcer with *H. pylori* eradication.[112,117–119] Therefore, patients presenting with perforated duodenal ulcers should be tested for *H. pylori* and if found to be positive treated with eradication therapy. In a study by Ng et al.[112] of patients presenting with perforation, 81% were shown to be infected by *H. pylori*. Patients were randomized to receive either a course of quadruple anti-*Helicobacter* therapy or a 4-week course of omeprazole alone. Follow-up endoscopy was performed 8 weeks, 16 weeks (if the ulcer did not heal at 8 weeks), and 1 year after hospital discharge for surveillance of ulcer healing and determination of *H. pylori* status. Initial ulcer healing rates were similar in the two groups (82% anti-*Helicobacter* vs. 87% omeprazole). However, after 1 year, ulcer relapse was significantly less common in patients treated with anti-*Helicobacter* therapy than in those who received omeprazole alone (4.8% vs. 38.1%, respectively).

Definitive ulcer surgery with an acid-reducing procedure should be considered in patients who will require continued use of nonselective NSAIDs or in whom compliance with *H. pylori* therapy is in doubt. One study that followed patients more than 10 years after truncal vagotomy and pyloroplasty for perforated duodenal ulcer reported a mortality rate of 5.5% with a recurrence rate of 8.8%. Operative mortality rates from perforated duodenal ulcers range from 5%[113] to more than 30% in the elderly.[120,121] Risk factors that increase mortality include a severe comorbidity, the presence of shock on admission, and a presentation delay of more than 24h.[113,121]

Patients who experience a gastric ulcer perforation tend to be elderly with significant comorbidities, which result in an increased mortality rate. Mortality rates following gastric perforation range from 10% to 40%.[122–125] The preferred surgical treatment is partial gastrectomy due to the risk of malignancy unless the patient is at high risk or becomes[126] unstable intraoperatively. If a distal gastrectomy cannot be performed, then the ulcer should be excised or biopsied and oversewn to rule out malignancy.

Laparoscopic repair of perforated peptic ulcers with an omental patch has been compared to open repair in randomized clinical trials.[122,127] While the earlier study failed to demonstrate any advantage to the laparoscopic approach other than decreased analgesic requirements, no significant differences in morbidity, reoperation rates, or mortality were demonstrated. Patients in the more recent study required fewer postoperative analgesics, experienced shorter hospital stays, and returned to normal activity earlier than patients undergoing the open procedure. The laparoscopic repair was also associated with shorter operative times. In addition, laparoscopy has been advocated as a diagnostic technique.

Hemorrhage

Upper GI hemorrhage commonly presents with hematemesis or melena. If the bleeding is massive, then the patient may present with hematochezia. The initial step in management of patients with acute upper GI hemorrhage is adequate initial and ongoing fluid resuscitation. Once the patient has been adequately resuscitated, endoscopy is performed to assess the cause and severity of the bleed. Peptic ulcers are the source of acute upper GI hemorrhage in 45%–50% of cases.[128,129]

Ulcers located along the lesser curve of the stomach and posterior duodenal bulb are at greater risk for severe bleeding and rebleeding due to the proximity of the left gastric artery and gastroduodenal artery, respectively. The mortality rate for bleeding peptic ulcers is approximately 6%–7%.[130]

Hemorrhage from a peptic ulcer will stop spontaneously in approximately 80% of cases.[131] Several stigmata of peptic ulcer bleeding may be identified endoscopically. These stigmata include an actively bleeding ulcer, a nonbleeding visible vessel, and an adherent clot at the base of the ulcer. The rebleeding rate for each of these findings is 90% to 100%, 40% to 50%, and 20% to 30% respectively.[132] Endoscopic therapy achieves hemostasis in more than 90% of cases.[133] Thermal coagulation, injection therapy, hemostatic clips, fibrin sealant, argon plasma coagulation, and combination therapy have all been described for the endoscopic treatment of bleeding peptic ulcers. The most commonly used endoscopic therapy is a combined modality with injection of an epinephrine-containing solution followed by thermocoagulation.[134] Compared with thermal coagulation alone, combination therapy with epinephrine injection followed by thermal coagulation achieves higher rates of initial hemostasis for actively bleeding ulcers.[135] The rebleeding rates may be as high as 18% if epinephrine injections alone are performed.[136] Patients with no clinical evidence of severe upper GI hemorrhage and a clean ulcer base are at low risk for experiencing a recurrent bleed and may be safely fed and discharged from the hospital following endoscopy.

Patients should receive antisecretory therapy following successful endoscopic hemostasis. In patients with a nonbleeding visible vessel or adherent clot, combination therapy with intravenous omeprazole plus endoscopic hemostasis is more effective in preventing recurrent bleeding than omeprazole alone.[137] One of the largest randomized controlled trials comparing intravenous omeprazole to placebo following endoscopic hemostasis found that recurrent bleeding was significantly lower in the omeprazole group (6.7% vs. 22.5%).[96] Patients with bleeding peptic ulcers should also be tested for *H. pylori*. A meta-analysis reported that recurrent bleeding from peptic ulcers occurred in only 1% of patients following successful *H. pylori* eradication compared with 5.6% in patients treated with maintenance antisecretory therapy alone.[138]

Generally accepted indications for surgery for peptic ulcer bleeding include hemodynamic instability despite aggressive resuscitation (>3-unit transfusion), failed endoscopic therapy, recurrent hemorrhage after initial endoscopic hemostasis, and continued slow bleeding requiring greater than 3 units per day of transfusion. In patients who rebleed after endoscopic therapy, the decision becomes one of repeat endoscopy or surgery. In one controlled trial, patients were randomized to repeat endoscopic therapy or surgery. Repeat endoscopy achieved long-term hemostasis in 73% of patients with similar mortality rates and lower morbidity rates compared to surgical intervention.[139] However, many patients who underwent repeat endoscopy required subsequent operations.

Acute bleeding from a posterior duodenal ulcer not controlled by endoscopy requires surgical intervention. The anterior surface of the postpyloric duodenum is opened longitudinally several centimeters. Direct pressure may be placed on the bleeding ulcer to allow resuscitation of the patient. The ulcer should then be oversewn at three separate sites: cephalad and caudad to the ulcer to ligate the gastroduodenal artery and a U-stitch placed through the base of the ulcer to ligate the transverse pancreatic artery. Once the bleeding is controlled by oversewing the ulcer, a truncal vagotomy and pyloroplasty using the Heineke-Mikulicz technique should be performed.[140] This technique, while commonly used, is not universally supported, however. A randomized controlled trial by Millat et al. concluded that patients undergoing emergency surgery for massive, persistent bleeding or recurrent bleeding from a duodenal ulcer should undergo distal gastric resection because of a lower postoperative recurrent bleeding rate compared to oversewing the ulcer and vagotomy.[141]

The unstable patient with a bleeding gastric ulcer requires ulcer excision or oversewing of the ulcer with biopsy. Excision of the ulcer is performed from within the gastric lumen through an anterior gastrotomy. Hemodynamically stable patients with a controlled bleed who will have a continued need for ulcerogenic medication postoperatively should undergo a definitive ulcer operation. A distal gastrectomy should be performed incorporating the ulcer along with bilateral truncal vagotomy. In patients with a type IV bleeding gastric ulcer, the left gastric artery may be ligated and the ulcer biopsied and oversewn through a high anterior gastrotomy.[142]

Gastric Outlet Obstruction

Patients with gastric outlet obstruction due to peptic ulcer disease typically present with nausea, vomiting, early satiety, bloating, indigestion, epigastric pain, and weight loss. Often, patients will have a hypochloremic, hypokalemic metabolic alkalosis as a result of chronic vomiting. Initial management of these patients includes nasogastric tube decompression, fluid resuscitation, and correction of electrolyte abnormalities. Approximately one-half of patients may initially respond to this regimen.[143]

Two underlying mechanisms have been proposed for gastric outlet obstruction. The first is related to the inflammation, edema, or muscular spasm that may accompany an acute ulceration. The second mechanism of obstruction is the scarring and fibrosis of chronic ulceration.[144,145] Upper GI radiography can provide useful information, although endoscopic inspection is warranted both for diagnosis and to rule out malignancy. Malignant obstruction has been reported in as many as 66% of patients. Patients presenting with malignant obstruction tend to be older and do not have a history of peptic ulcers or NSAID use.[146]

Patients that present with a gastric outlet obstruction secondary to peptic ulcer disease are commonly infected with *H. pylori*. The reported prevalence of *H. pylori* ranges from 33% to 69%[147,148] in some studies, with two studies demonstrating infection rates of 90% and 91%.[149,150] Reversal of gastric outlet obstruction has been reported following the eradication of *H. pylori* infection[151,152]; however, the time span from eradication of *H. pylori* to resolution of gastric outlet obstruction ranges from weeks to months.[150]

In patients who fail to respond to initial medical therapy and for whom malignancy has been ruled out, endoscopic balloon dilation may be useful.[147,153] Patients may require multiple endoscopic sessions,[154] but when *H. pylori* can be eradicated and NSAID use discontinued, a good long-term result may be achieved.

Surgery is generally indicated if obstruction fails to resolve after 72h of nonoperative management.[155] These patients usually require vagotomy and antrectomy to relieve the obstruction and to rule out malignancy. A randomized controlled trial was performed to examine the outcomes of 90 consecutive patients with gastric outlet obstruction secondary to a duodenal ulcer.[156] The three operations were the selective vagotomy with antrectomy, the HSV with gastrojejunostomy, and the HSV with Jaboulay (gastroduodenostomy) anastomosis. Postoperative gastric acid secretion was similar among the groups. Overall results were best with the HSV and gastrojejunostomy, while Jaboulay patients did the worst. Placement of a feeding jejunostomy tube at the time of surgery is due to postoperative gastric dysfunction, which occurs in 10% to 50% of patients.[157,158]

The laparoscopic management of gastric outlet obstruction secondary to duodenal ulceration has also been described. In one small series of 12 patients, truncal vagotomy with gastroenterostomy was performed, with patients experiencing good results, with a median follow-up of 6 months.[159]

Postgastrectomy Syndromes

Dumping Syndrome

The dumping syndrome is one of the most common causes of morbidity following gastric surgery. Between 25% and 50% of all patients who undergo gastric surgery have some symptoms of dumping, but these are disabling in only 1%–5%. The incidence of dumping symptoms varies according to the procedure performed. Significant dumping occurs in 5%–15% of patients following truncal vagotomy and drainage, 15%–20% of patients following partial gastrectomy, but fewer than 2% following proximal gastric vagotomy (PGV).[160]

The dumping syndrome has two forms, early and late, based on the onset of symptoms. The early form occurs within 10–30min of a meal and is characterized by both GI and vasomotor symptoms. Gastrointestinal symptoms include postprandial fullness, crampy abdominal pain, nausea, and explosive diarrhea. Vasomotor symptoms include diaphoresis, weakness, dizziness, flushing, palpitations, and an intense desire to lie down. Expression of these symptoms is variable among patients. Most, however, exhibit both GI and vasomotor manifestations. In the late form of dumping, symptoms arise 2–3h following a meal and are typical of hypoglycemia. These differences are summarized in Table 45.5. Approximately 75% of patients with dumping syndrome have symptoms of early dumping, while about 25% of patients have late symptoms. A few patients have both early and late dumping symptoms.

TABLE 45.5. Forms of Dumping Syndrome.

	Early dumping	*Late dumping*
Postprandial onset	10–30min	2–3h
Typical symptoms	Postprandial fullness Crampy abdominal pain Nausea Explosive diarrhea Diaphoresis Weakness Palpitations Flushing Dizziness	Diaphoresis Weakness Palpitations Flushing Dizziness

Pathophysiology

Dumping symptoms may occur following any gastric operation. The central factor responsible for the development of dumping appears to be the disruption of the normal regulation of gastric emptying. The emptying of a solid meal is regulated by the coordination of antral grinding and pyloric relaxation, whereas liquid emptying is largely controlled by the pressure differential between the fundus of the stomach and the duodenum. Gastric resection reduces fundic volume, with a secondary increase in basal fundic tone. Vagotomy increases gastric fundic tone and limits accommodation to a meal. These operations result in more rapid emptying of liquids. Similarly, operations in which the pylorus is removed, bypassed, or destroyed increase the rate of gastric emptying of solids, through both loss of coordinated antropyloric motility and loss of duodenal feedback inhibition of gastric emptying.

Early Dumping. Early dumping is thought to result from rapid emptying of hyperosmolar chyme into the small bowel. This leads to fluid shifts from the intravascular space into the intestinal lumen, resulting in small-bowel distention and an increase in both the amplitude and frequency of bowel contractions. This results in bloating, crampy abdominal pain, and diarrhea. Sequestration of fluid into the bowel depletes circulating blood volume, causing hypovolemia with tachycardia and lightheadedness.

Several gut hormones have been implicated in the pathogenesis of early dumping. The postprandial concentrations of enteroglucagon, glucose-dependent insulinotropic peptide (GIP), pancreatic polypeptide, vasoactive intestinal polypeptide, GRP, serotonin, bradykinin, motilin, and neurotensin are all increased in dumping patients as compared to asymptomatic patients following gastric surgery. Of these, neurotensin is the most likely agent involved in the pathogenesis of dumping. It has been shown to have both vasomotor and GI actions that mimic those seen in early dumping. However, proof that neurotensin or other peptides cause dumping symptoms is lacking.

Late Dumping. Late dumping most likely results from rapid gastric emptying, leading to delivery of unusually high carbohydrate concentrations to the proximal small bowel. The carbohydrates are rapidly absorbed, resulting in hyperglycemia and excessive insulin release. The cause of this increased insulin release is unclear but is thought to be related to the rapid absorption of luminal carbohydrates or to an enhanced incretin effect. Several peptides may play a role in mediating this incretin effect. These include CCK, enteroglucagon, GIP, and glucagon-like peptide (GLP). The increased insulin release causes a postprandial hypoglycemia approximately 2–3h following the meal. This reactive hypoglycemia leads to vasomotor symptoms characteristic of an insulin reaction.

Diagnosis

The diagnosis of dumping is based mainly on clinical history. A scoring system has been developed to assist in the differ-

TABLE 45.6. Sigstad Clinical Dumping Score.

Symptom	*Score*
Preshock, shock	+5
"Almost fainting," syncope, unconsciousness	+4
Desire to lie or sit down	+4
Breathlessness, dyspnea	+3
Weakness, exhaustion	+3
Sleepiness, drowsiness, yawning, apathy, falling asleep	+3
Palpitation	+3
Restlessness	+2
Dizziness	+2
Headache	+1
Feeling of warmth, sweating, pallor, clammy skin	+1
Nausea	+1
Fullness in the abdomen, meteorismus	+1
Borborygmi	+1
Eructation	−1
Vomiting	−4

A score of +7 or above suggests dumping; indices of +4 or less suggest other diagnoses.

entiation of dumping from other postgastrectomy syndromes (Table 45.6). Any patient with a history of gastric surgery who develops symptoms consistent with dumping warrants further evaluation. Despite the characteristic symptomatology, other postgastrectomy complications may mimic the presentation of dumping. To exclude these, patients should undergo an upper GI contrast study to exclude stomal obstruction or afferent loop syndrome. Upper endoscopy should also be done to exclude recurrent ulcer, reflux alkaline gastritis, or gastric remnant carcinoma. A radionuclide-labeled gastric-emptying study should be performed to document rapid gastric emptying and exclude gastric stasis. Falsely normal gastric emptying as measured by radionuclide scanning may be observed if the test meal is of insufficient volume to reproduce the patient's symptoms.

Treatment

Prevention. As with other postgastrectomy syndromes, prevention is the best form of treatment. In the surgical treatment of patients with peptic ulcer disease, PGV has the lowest risk of postoperative dumping syndrome and is the procedure of choice in our practice. Although the long-term ulcer recurrence rate after PGV is higher than after truncal vagotomy and antrectomy, management of recurrent ulcer is less problematic than management of dumping. If resection is required, then some surgeons have advocated the use of Roux-en-Y gastrojejunostomy as the drainage procedure of choice to minimize the risk of dumping symptoms. Roux-en-Y gastrojejunostomy clearly decreases the rate of gastric emptying when compared to pyloroplasty or loop gastrojejunostomy. Although this may be so, Roux-en-Y reconstruction has its own set of problems, including Roux stasis syndrome and obstruction. When feasible, Billroth I gastroduodenostomy is the preferred reconstruction after antrectomy as it most closely restores normal anatomy.

Medical Therapy. The majority of patients with the dumping syndrome have relatively mild symptoms that improve with time. Dietary modification is the mainstay of therapy, and most patients intuitively modify their diet appropriately to minimize their dumping symptoms. The best diet avoids simple carbohydrates and favors complex carbohydrates and dietary fiber. The patient should eat frequent, small meals and avoid liquids during a meal. Liquids may be taken an hour or later following the "dry" meal. For severe vasomotor symptoms, lying supine for 30 min postprandially may slow gastric emptying and increase venous return, thereby minimizing the likelihood of syncope.

Octreotide acetate, a long-acting somatostatin analog, is the most effective agent in the treatment of severe dumping symptoms. Octreotide ameliorates dumping by slowing gastric emptying, inhibiting insulin release, and decreasing enteric peptide secretion. Several anecdotal reports and randomized trials have documented the short-term efficacy of octreotide treatment in patients with severe dumping symptoms. These are summarized in Table 45.7.

In general, octreotide improves the symptoms in over 90% of patients with severe dumping unresponsive to other medical therapy. In all studies, acute octreotide therapy significantly decreased the symptom score, pulse rate, and plasma insulin when compared to placebo. It is unclear whether long-term octreotide will prove as beneficial as acute therapy. Steatorrhea is common with octreotide therapy due to inhibition of pancreatic exocrine secretion. This responds to oral pancreatic enzyme replacement. Other complications of octreotide treatment include hyper- or hypoglycemia, injection site pain, and cholelithiasis.

Surgical Therapy. For patients with debilitating dumping unresponsive to medical therapy or in patients unwilling to continue medical therapy, remedial surgery may be considered. A conservative approach is warranted, however, because most patients with dumping improve with time, and remedial surgery does not cure all patients. Many remedial operations for dumping syndrome have been described, including pyloric reconstruction, jejunal interpositions, conversion of Billroth II anastomosis to Billroth I gastroduodenostomy, and conversion to Roux-en-Y gastrojejunostomy. No controlled trials comparing the relative efficacy of these operations exist. Analysis of their efficacy is difficult as many of the procedures have good early results but are long-term failures.

For patients with dumping following pyloroplasty, pyloric reconstruction is the optimal remedial approach. In this operation, the pyloroplasty scar is identified and opened along its length. The sphincter muscle is identified and reapproximated. The incision is then closed longitudinally. This procedure has the advantages of simplicity and low risk. Interestingly, gastric stasis is unusual following pyloric reconstruction.[161]

Several types of small bowel segment interpositions for dumping syndrome have been described. These include an isoperistaltic jejunal segment interposed between the stomach and duodenum, creation of a 10-cm reversed jejunal segment interposed between the stomach and duodenum, and insertion of an antiperistaltic jejunal segment in the efferent limb of a Billroth II gastrojejunostomy or in a Roux-en-Y limb. Mixed results have been reported with these remedial operations, with good correction of dumping symptoms but a high rate of gastric outlet obstruction symptoms. It is clear that

TABLE 45.7.
Randomized, Double-Blinded, Placebo-Controlled, Crossover Trials of Octreotide Treatment for Severe Dumping Syndrome.

Author (year)	*n*	*Treatment*	*Symptom score*[a,b]	*Pulse rate (beats per min)*[a]	*Hematocrit (%)*[a]	*Plasma insulin*[a]
Hopman (1988)[245]	12	Control	11.7 ± 2.1	85 ± 7	41 ± 2	173 ± 16 (mU/L)
		Octreotide	4.6 ± 1.6[c]	67 ± 7[c]	41 ± 2	35 ± 9[c]
Tulassay (1989)[246]	8	Control	Severe in all patients	102 ± 3.5	43 ± 3.5	40 ± 3.2 (μE/mL)
		Octreotide	Alleviated in all patients	70 ± 2[c]	38 ± 1	11 ± 1[c]
Primrose (1990)[247]	10	Control	Severe in 10 of 10 patients	25 beats per min rise	4.5% rise	185 (mU/L)
		Octreotide	Improved in 9 of 10 patients	8 beats per min rise[c]	2.1% rise[c]	30 (mU/L)[c]
Geer (1990)[248]	10	Control	8.5 ± 0.5	87 ± 5		180 ± 50 (mU/L)
		Octreotide	1.7 ± 0.5[c]	66 ± 4[c]		20 ± 5[c]
Gray (1991)[249]	9	Control	15.7 ± 1.6	105 ± 6	41 ± 2	1162 ± 230 (pmol/L)
		Octreotide	4.6 ± 1.7[c]	80 ± 3[c]	39 ± 1	158 ± 29[c]
Hasler (1996)[250]	8	Control	Diarrhea: 3.5 ± 0.4 Pain: 2.0 ± 0.4 Lightheadedness: 3.8 ± 0.2 Palpitations: 3.2 ± 0.3	36 ± 6 beats per min rise	36.7 ± 0.6	87 ± 15 (U/mL)
		Octreotide	Diarrhea: 0[c] Pain: 1.3 ± 0.3 Lightheadedness: 1.0 ± 0.3[c] Palpitations: 0.8 ± 0.2[c]	17 ± 5 beats per min rise[c]	36.5 ± 0.4	26 ± 9 ((U/mL)[c]

[a]Mean ± standard error of the mean except where indicated.
[b]In the Hopman and Gray studies, a Sigstad dumping score was used; in the Geer study, a severity score of 0–10 was used; in the Hasler study, a severity score of 0–4 was used; in the Tulassay and Primrose studies, symptom relief was not quantified.
[c]Statistically significant ($p < 0.05$).

the reversed segment must be tailored to an appropriate length. Segments that are too short do not resolve the dumping symptoms, but segments constructed too long result in gastric retention. A 10-cm length appears ideal. Care must be taken to rotate the interposed segment only 180° and to avoid undue torsion of the mesentery. Mesenteric defects should be securely closed to avoid internal herniation.

Conversion of a Billroth II anastomosis to a Billroth I gastroduodenostomy improves dumping symptoms in about 75% of patients. The main advantage of this procedure is the restoration of the normal physiologic delivery of a meal into the duodenum. This operation, however, is occasionally technically difficult and fails to alleviate symptoms in a substantial minority of patients. Overall, conversion of a Billroth II to a Billroth I has been eclipsed by the relative simplicity of Roux-en-Y conversion.

There is support in the literature for conversion of a Billroth I or a Billroth II to a Roux-en-Y gastrojejunostomy as a remedial operation for dumping syndrome. In patients with previous Billroth I or Billroth II gastrectomy and medically resistant dumping, 85%–90% have favorable outcomes with Roux-en-Y conversion. In one of the larger series, Vogel et al. reported that 19 of 22 patients treated with Roux-en-Y conversion had a good result.[162] Of the three failures, only one was due to persistent dumping symptoms; the other two were due to the development of Roux stasis syndrome. This procedure has the advantage of simplicity when compared to jejunal interpositions, and it appears to have fewer undesirable long-term complications.

To summarize, remedial surgery for dumping syndrome should be considered for patients with medically unresponsive, severe symptoms. For patients with prior pyloroplasty, pyloric reconstruction is preferred. For patients with prior Billroth I or Billroth II gastrectomy, Roux-en-Y conversion is a simple and effective corrective operation. For patients who have previously undergone Roux-en-Y gastrojejunostomy, the best approach is construction of a 10-cm antiperistaltic jejunal segment within the Roux limb.

Postvagotomy Diarrhea

Up to 20% of patients undergoing truncal vagotomy complain of postoperative diarrhea, and it is debilitating in 1%–2%.[160] Its severe form is characterized by frequent, watery stools that are occasionally explosive. The diarrhea may be postcibal or continuous. In some patients, nocturnal diarrhea is problematic. Diarrhea following gastric surgery most commonly results from causes other than vagotomy. Thus, patients with early postoperative diarrhea should be initially investigated for causes such as bacterial overgrowth, pseudomembranous colitis, obstruction, inflammatory bowel disease, intestinal parasites, and malabsorption. The appropriate initial diagnostic tests should include fecal white blood cell count, stool culture, fecal *Clostridium difficile* titer, and occasionally sigmoidoscopy.

For patients with persistent diarrhea, further studies should be performed to exclude steatorrhea, partial intestinal obstruction, and inflammatory bowel disease. Appropriate diagnostic studies include 3-day fecal fat quantification, colonoscopy, upper GI barium contrast series with small-bowel follow through, and barium enema. Consideration should also be given to the possibility of laxative abuse. If this is suspected, then measurement of stool pH and magnesium concentration may be useful. If the workup is unrevealing, then the diarrhea may be due to dumping syndrome or vagotomy. These last conditions are diagnoses of exclusion. No specific tests are available to confirm that the diarrhea is, indeed, due to the gastric surgery.

The pathophysiology of postvagotomy diarrhea is unclear. Although to date there is no direct evidence, the most likely explanation is that truncal vagotomy interferes with central nervous system modulation of enteric nervous system control of gut motility and secretion. Rapid gastric emptying is often associated with the diarrhea, but normalization of gastric emptying by remedial surgery does not always correct the problem. Impaired gallbladder emptying and increased excretion of bile salts may be involved. Supportive evidence includes the finding of higher levels of fecal bile salts in patients with postvagotomy diarrhea compared to controls and the beneficial effect of cholestyramine, a bile acid-binding agent, in many patients.

Treatment

Medical Therapy. The medical treatment of postvagotomy diarrhea is similar to that recommended for patients with the dumping syndrome. Simple dietary changes, including small, frequent, dry meals and increased dietary fiber, may slow intestinal transit and therefore improve diarrhea. Opiates are beneficial through their inhibitory effect on intestinal transit. Cholestyramine improves diarrhea in the majority of patients. For patients unresponsive to these measures, octreotide, a long-acting somatostatin analog, may be tried. Octreotide, however, has had limited success in controlling severe postvagotomy diarrhea as it may exacerbate the diarrhea by inducing steatorrhea.

Surgical Therapy. For severe postvagotomy diarrhea unresponsive to medical therapy, remedial surgery may be considered. Although rapid gastric emptying is associated with the diarrhea, operations that slow gastric emptying are not usually curative. The most effective surgical strategies have focused on slowing small bowel transit. Construction of a 10-cm antiperistaltic jejunal segment located 100cm from the ligament of Treitz is effective in about two-thirds of patients. Sawyers et al., for example, reported on a series of 16 patients undergoing this procedure, with 14 having successful outcomes.[163] On the other hand, Cuschieri has reported that 12 of 13 patients in whom he performed this procedure had relief of diarrhea, but 10 required reoperation for pain and obstruction.[164]

The most important lesson learned regarding the treatment of postvagotomy diarrhea is that, like dumping, prevention is much simpler than treatment. Truncal vagotomy should be avoided if possible. The operation of choice in the elective management of patients with intractable duodenal ulcer is PGV.

Reflux Alkaline Gastritis

Alkaline reflux gastritis can occur in patients who have undergone removal, bypass, or destruction of the pyloric sphincter mechanism. Loss of pyloric function causes reflux of duodenal contents into the stomach, which may result in gastritis. Although some degree of reflux is seen in all patients following gastric surgery without significant sequelae, approximately 3% develop severe reflux alkaline gastritis. The majority of patients have a prior history of Billroth II reconstruction. However, Billroth I gastroduodenostomy and pyloroplasty are also associated with this syndrome.

Patients typically complain of persistent, burning, epigastric abdominal pain and nausea that are exacerbated by meal ingestion. Bilious emesis, often mixed with incompletely digested food, does not relieve the symptoms of pain and nausea. This feature distinguishes this condition from afferent loop syndrome, in which bilious emesis, void of foodstuff, relieves the patient's discomfort. Patients develop an avoidance to food, resulting in significant weight loss. In addition, chronic low-grade gastritis results in anemia, a common finding in these patients. Reflux alkaline gastritis is the most common postgastrectomy syndrome for which remedial surgery is performed.

Pathophysiology

Patients with reflux alkaline gastritis have extensive gastritis involving the entire gastric remnant on gross examination. The gastric mucosa has an erythematous, friable, inflamed, ulcerated appearance on endoscopic examination, usually with visible pooling of bile and duodenogastric reflux. Histologically, the mucosa is void of parietal cells, hemorrhagic, and superficially ulcerated. The first observation is responsible for the achlorhydria or hypochlorhydria seen in patients with alkaline gastritis. Intestinalization of gastric glands, an increase in mucin cells, and a chronic inflammatory infiltrate are commonly observed.

Although the association between duodenogastric reflux and the symptoms of alkaline reflux gastritis is clearly established, the exact pathogenesis of the gastritis is not clear. Some degree of reflux is seen in all patients following gastric surgery; however, only a small minority develop gastritis. Several reports have suggested that patients with alkaline gastritis have increased concentrations of bile acids in the refluxed duodenal juice, increased volume and frequency of reflux, increased concentration of specific bile acids like deoxycholic acid, or altered composition of bile acids and pancreatic enzymes. Others have suggested prolonged mucosal exposure to bile acids resulting from gastric dysmotility may play a role in the pathogenesis. Likewise, prolonged gastritis may exacerbate gastric hypomotility. Nevertheless, it appears that the mucosal injury is most likely caused by bile acids. Contact of bile acids with gastric mucosa results in breakdown of gastric mucosal barrier function, resulting in back diffusion of hydrogen ions. This causes mast cell disruption with release of serotonin, histamine, and other vasoactive amines that trigger the inflammatory changes characteristic of this condition.

Diagnosis

The diagnosis of reflux alkaline gastritis is based on a careful clinical history and endoscopic evidence of gastritis by gross and histologic appearance. Radiographic studies should be performed to exclude mechanical causes of epigastric pain, nausea, and vomiting, including recurrent ulcer, afferent loop syndrome, and so on. An analysis of gastric fluid to document the presence of hypo- or achlorhydria should be performed. If hyperchlorhydria is encountered, then hypergastrinemia from an undiagnosed ZES, retained antrum, or incomplete vagotomy should be excluded. Bile acid composition and concentration should be determined. Technetium scintigraphy with and without CCK stimulation can be used to quantify duodenogastric reflux. Provocative testing with alkaline solutions and bile acids may reproduce symptoms in afflicted patients and serve to identify patients who may benefit from remedial surgery. In patients considered for surgery, a solid-phase gastric-emptying study should be performed to exclude significant concomitant gastric dysmotility.

Treatment

Medical. The mainstays of medical therapy for alkaline reflux gastritis are prokinetic agents to improve gastric emptying and coating agents such as sucralfate to enhance gastric mucosal defense. No specific dietary or behavioral therapy is reliably successful. Attempts at binding bile acids with cholestyramine or aluminum-containing antacids have been unsuccessful.

Surgical. The goal of remedial surgery in patients with alkaline reflux gastritis is to prevent pancreaticobiliary secretions from refluxing into the gastric remnant. For patients with a prior history of Billroth I or Billroth II anastomosis, the best remedial choice is the conversion to a Roux-en-Y gastrojejunostomy with a Roux limb of sufficient length to prevent retrograde reflux, usually 45 to 60 cm. This procedure is 75% to 85% effective in treating reflux symptoms.[165] However, Roux-en-Y gastrojejunostomy has two major potential complications. First, Roux-en-Y gastrojejunostomy is ulcerogenic; therefore, a vagotomy must be performed if not done so in the initial operation. Second, approximately one-quarter of patients with reflux alkaline gastritis who undergo Roux conversion will develop the Roux stasis syndrome. This underscores the importance of adequate preoperative assessment of gastric emptying in patients with alkaline reflux gastritis. If significant preoperative gastroparesis is encountered, then a 90%–95% near-total gastrectomy should be performed with the Roux-en-Y gastrojejunostomy.

Others have advocated a Braun enteroenterostomy in patients at risk for Roux failure. In this procedure, the afferent and efferent limbs are anastomosed 30 to 60 cm away from gastroenterostomy in patients with a Billroth II anastomosis. Although the results with this procedure appear promising, it requires the presence of a long afferent limb.

For patients with reflux gastritis following truncal vagotomy and drainage, antrectomy with Roux-en-Y gastrojejunostomy should be performed. Antrectomy is necessary to minimize the risk of ulcer formation. For patients with a prior history of Billroth I gastroduodenostomy, a Roux-en-Y conversion should also be considered. Another option in this case is the Henley procedure, by which an isoperistaltic segment of jejunum is interposed between the gastric remnant and the duodenum. However, the results with this procedure have not been favorable.

The duodenal switch operation described by DeMeester has also been proposed in the treatment of patients with alkaline reflux gastritis. In this operation, the duodenum is divided 5 to 7 cm beyond the pylorus. The distal end is oversewn and the proximal end anastomosed end to end to a Roux-en-Y limb. Long-term results with this procedure are not available, but short-term results appear promising.

Stasis Syndromes

Stasis syndromes, including gastroparesis and the Roux syndrome, are well-recognized complications of gastric surgery. Postsurgical gastroparesis can occur following vagotomy or gastric resection. Two forms of postoperative delayed gastric emptying have been identified: an early form occurring in the immediate postoperative period and a late form occurring from weeks to years following surgery. The incidence of gastric atony varies with the indication for surgery and type of procedure initially performed. In patients operated on for gastric outlet obstruction, for example, the incidence of postsurgical gastroparesis is as high as 27% to 50%. Gastroparesis is seen in 1.4% of patients following vagotomy and drainage, in 2.4% to 9% of patients after vagotomy and antrectomy, and in 3% of patients following subtotal gastrectomy without vagotomy. Overall, the incidence of postsurgical gastroparesis is 2% to 3%.[160]

In patients who have previously undergone Roux-en-Y reconstruction, gastroparesis or stasis in the Roux limb are termed the *Roux syndrome*. The incidence of this syndrome has been reported to be as high as 25% to 30%. The incidence in patients who undergo Roux-en-Y diversion as a means of treating alkaline reflux gastritis is 10% to 50%.

Patients with postsurgical stasis syndromes present with postprandial epigastric fullness or bloating, early satiety, epigastric pain, nausea, and vomiting of incompletely digested food. Some patients develop bezoars. Patients may attempt to compensate for their condition by consuming only soft, semisolid foods or liquids. Weight loss and nutritional deficiencies often result.

The diagnosis of postsurgical stasis syndromes is one of exclusion as symptoms mirror those of other postgastrectomy syndromes. These include mechanical problems such as stomal obstruction from edema, kinking, or stricture; recurrent ulcer; and gastric stump carcinoma. In addition, symptoms may be confused with those of afferent or efferent limb syndrome or postoperative small-bowel obstruction. Functional problems, such as gastroparesis related to diabetes mellitus, may be confused with a postoperative complication. These conditions must be excluded prior to instituting therapy for presumed postsurgical stasis.

Afferent Limb Syndrome

The afferent limb syndrome occurs in rare patients following Billroth II gastrojejunostomy. In this condition, the limb of duodenum and jejunum responsible for proximal intestinal, biliary, and pancreatic drainage becomes partially or completely obstructed. The cause of this obstruction is mechanical and is usually related to excessive length. When the limb is too long, internal small-bowel herniation, kinking from redundancy or adhesions, loop volvulus, and intussusception can occur. In addition, obstruction at the gastrojejunostomy from recurrent ulceration, stricture formation, and carcinoma may cause the afferent limb syndrome.

Two forms of afferent limb syndrome have been described, acute and chronic. Acute afferent limb syndrome occurs in the early postoperative period, usually within the first week. Obstruction of the afferent limb leads to accumulation of intestinal, pancreatic, and biliary secretions within the proximal jejunal lumen. As luminal pressure increases, venous pressures are quickly exceeded, resulting in ischemia and pressure necrosis of the intestinal mucosa. Obstruction of pancreatic and biliary outflow may arise if luminal pressures are sufficiently elevated. Disruption of the duodenal stump may result.

The symptoms of acute afferent limb syndrome are abrupt in onset. Severe epigastric pain, nausea, nonbilious vomiting, tachycardia, and fever are uniformly present. Abdominal tenderness and fullness are usually present. If uncorrected, shock may ensue. Elevated serum amylase and liver function tests often confuse the clinician into believing postoperative pancreatitis or biliary pathology are the cause of the patient's deterioration. This leads to delay in appropriate surgical management. The diagnosis is confirmed by ultrasound or computed tomographic (CT) scan that reveals a fluid filled mass in the epigastrium. Acute afferent limb syndrome is a form of closed-loop obstruction and, as such, is a surgical emergency. Mortality rates associated with acute afferent limb syndrome approach 50%.[160]

Chronic afferent limb syndrome may occur at any point in time after the initial surgery. It results from intermittent, partial mechanical obstruction of the afferent limb. Patients typically present with postcibal epigastric discomfort, pain, and fullness. This results from the rapid accumulation of pancreatic, biliary, and duodenojejunal secretions within the limb in response to a meal. As intraluminal pressure exceeds the resistance to outflow caused by the obstruction, the patient experiences explosive bilious vomiting, usually void of foodstuff. This emesis relieves the patient of symptoms. These last two features distinguish chronic afferent limb syndrome from reflux alkaline gastritis, in which emesis usually contains undigested food and does not relieve the discomfort. A minority of patients develop bacterial overgrowth in the partially obstructed afferent limb, resulting in a blind-loop syndrome. Plain abdominal radiographs are usually nondiagnostic. Ultrasound or CT are the tests of choice. Endoscopy should be performed to exclude the presence of alkaline gastritis, recurrent ulcer, anastomotic stricture, and anastomotic carcinoma.

Patients with afferent limb syndrome require remedial surgery. In the average patient, this is best accomplished via conversion to a Roux-en-Y gastrojejunostomy. Alternatively, a Braun enteroenterostomy between the afferent and efferent limbs is effective in decompressing the obstructed afferent limb. In severely ill patients with acute obstruction, the afferent limb and duodenal stump must be examined for viability. In the rare patient with necrosis of the afferent limb, resection of the devitalized tissue, reconstruction of the afferent limb, bypass of the obstruction, and drainage of the duodenal stump are indicated. If extensive necrosis exists, then pancreaticoduodenectomy may be necessary. Afferent limb syndrome can be prevented by creation of a retrocolic gastrojejunostomy with a short (5- to 15-cm) afferent limb. All defects in the mesocolon or small bowel mesentery should be closed. The gastrojejunostomy should lie in a horizontal plane without kinks.

Malignant Gastric Tumors

Adenocarcinoma

Historically, gastric cancer has been one of the leading causes of cancer death worldwide. Worldwide, there is great geographic variation in the incidence of gastric cancer, with the highest rates seen in the Far East, especially Japan and Korea; Central America; and Eastern Europe and the lowest incidence in North America, North and South Africa, and Australia.[166] Fortunately, the incidence of gastric carcinoma is declining, especially in developed countries. In the United States, for example, the incidence of gastric cancer has decreased fourfold since 1930 to approximately 9 cases per 100,000 people.[167] Most patients present in the sixth to seventh decade in low-risk regions, while patients in high-risk regions present a decade earlier. In the United States, 39% of gastric cancers arise in the proximal stomach, 17% in the middle third, 32% in the distal third, and 12% involve the entire stomach.[168] The decline in the incidence of gastric cancer is attributed to a decline in the incidence of distal lesions. The incidence of cardial and gastroesophageal junction lesions has remained stable or increased.[169]

There are two major histological types of gastric cancer. The intestinal histology consists of cell groupings organized into glands, resembling intestinal mucosa. Intestinal-type tumors occur most frequently in the distal stomach and are seen more commonly in regions with a high incidence of gastric cancer. Cancer cells that have no specific organization characterize the diffuse histology. They tend to infiltrate the gastric wall, forming a thickened gastric wall but not a discrete mass. These lesions occur anywhere in the stomach but predominantly occur at the cardia. The incidence for diffuse tumors has been relatively constant over the years. Diffuse lesions occur in younger patients and are more clinically aggressive than intestinal-type lesions.

Like other GI malignancies, the pathogenesis of gastric cancer is thought to be a multistep process. Unlike colon cancer, however, the progression from normal mucosa to cancer is not well defined and likely represents an interaction between environmental factors and host predisposition to development of gastric cancer, including genetic and acquired factors. The pathogenesis is best characterized for intestinal-type cancers. Chronic inflammation is central in this process. Correa has postulated that, in response to environmental factors, normal mucosa becomes chronically inflamed, chronic active gastritis. This is followed by progression to atropic gastritis, intestinal metaplasia, dysplasia, and cancer.[170] Environmental factors, including chronic *H. pylori* infection, dietary factors such as high-salt or preserved food diets, chronic bile salt exposure, and cigarette smoking have been implicated in the pathogenesis of gastric cancer. Chronic *H. pylori* infection in the susceptible host is central in this process, with the World Health Organization declaring *H. pylori* a class 1 carcinogen. Host factors that likely play a role in making a patient prone to cancer include p53 mutations, microsatellite instability, polymorphisms in the interleukin-1β (IL-1β), IL-10, and tumor necrosis factor-α (TNF-α) genes, and alterations in the adenomatous polyposis pathways.[171]

The stomach's primary function is food storage. Consequently, it has the ability to significantly enlarge without necessarily being noticed by a patient. Because the sensation of a growing cancer is indistinguishable from that of food in the stomach, these tumors become very large before symptoms develop. Frequently, patients will present with anorexia, early satiety, weight loss, or other vague symptoms. Not uncommonly, patients with the most minimal symptoms will present with very large, metastatic tumors. A review of 18,365 gastric cancer patients by the American College of

TABLE 45.8. Presenting Symptoms for 18,365 Patients with Gastric Cancer Surveyed by the American College of Surgeons.

Symptom	*Frequency (%)*
Weight loss	61.6
Abdominal pain	51.6
Nausea	34.3
Anorexia	32.0
Dysphagia	26.1
Melena	20.1
Early satiety	17.5
Ulcer-type pain	17.1
Lower-extremity edema	5.9

Source: From Wanebo et al.[168]

Surgeons revealed that weight loss and abdominal pain were the most frequent presenting symptoms (Table 45.8).[168] The tumors can grow to considerable size before any symptoms develop. For this reason, patients often present with advanced-stage disease.

Overall survival for this disease is better in Japan, where it is common. Because of the high incidence, the Japanese have aggressive screening programs. The screening identifies small lesions that have a favorable prognosis following resection. Survival for various disease stages are roughly comparable between Japan and the West, such that the higher mortality in the West is accounted for by a higher proportion of advanced carcinomas.

Gastric cancers often bleed or obstruct. For this reason, patients with a limited extent of metastatic disease are good operative candidates, and if the primary tumor can be resected with acceptable risk, palliative resection should be considered.

Approximately one-half of gastric carcinomas present as an ulcerating lesion. The radiographic or gross appearance at endoscopy or laparotomy is indistinguishable from a benign gastric ulcer. For this reason, it is essential to biopsy all gastric ulcers to ensure that a malignancy is not missed. Another 25% of lesions present as large polyps. Superficial spreading carcinoma is an early lesion that is manifested by tumor confinement to the gastric mucosa and submucosa. These lesions have a favorable prognosis, but only 15% of the tumors present this way. Linitis plastica is a condition in which the entire stomach is indurated secondary to a desmoplastic reaction to the cancer. Linitis has a poor prognosis and fortunately only occurs in about 10% of gastric carcinoma cases. The main tools for diagnosis and staging of gastric cancer are endoscopy for diagnosis and CT to access metastatic disease.

Gastric remnant carcinoma is a clinical entity in which cancer develops in the remaining stomach following gastric resection. The risk appears greatest in patients more than 20 years following their initial gastric resection. In these patients, a threefold increase in the risk for gastric carcinoma was seen. The risk of gastric remnant carcinoma is fourfold higher following a Billroth II compared to a Billroth I reconstruction.[172] The cancers tend to occur at or just proximal the gastric anastomosis and tend to present as advanced lesions, with 2-year survivals of less than 10%.[173] Chronic bacterial overgrowth from hypochlorhydria with increased nitrite production, chronic reflux of bile and pancreatic juice, and atrophy secondary to loss of the gastric mucosal mitogen gastrin are thought to play a permissive role in the development of gastric remnant carcinoma.[171]

Surgical Resection

Surgical resection is the only curative treatment for gastric adenocarcinoma. The main points of discussion regarding gastrectomy for cancer include issues pertaining to the extent of gastric resection, extent of regional lymphadenectomy, and implications of adjacent organ involvement and resection. Prior to operation, a thorough staging of the patient is indicated to identify patients who may benefit from surgery, whether curative or palliative in nature. According to the National Comprehensive Cancer Network (NCNN) guidelines, preoperative staging should consist of a physical exam, routine laboratory evaluation, abdominal and pelvic CT scan, chest x-ray, and endoscopy with biopsy (http://nccn.org).

Gastric carcinoma invades adjacent organs, spreads via lymphatics, and can metastasize by hematogenous spread. Physical examination should consist of a search for signs of metastatic disease. Patients should be examined for Virchow's node in the left supraclavicular fossa, representing spread of the cancer via the thoracic duct, Sister Mary Joseph's node (periumbilical nodule suggestive of tumor of the peritoneal surface), and a Blumer's shelf (tumor mass in the cul-de-sac). Hematogenous spread of the cancer to the liver occurs in 30% of patients. Gastric cancer may also metastasize to the ovary, resulting in a Krukenberg tumor. These lesions are easily identified at surgery or by CT. Less frequently, metastases are found in the lungs or brain, causing associated pulmonary or neurologic symptoms.

A systematic approach to metastatic disease should be performed. Identification of metastatic lesions preoperatively is important because a planned curative resection will be downgraded to a palliative one, only used in carefully selected patients who have limited metastatic disease, with a tumor that can be removed with partial gastrectomy, and who are good operative candidates.

To facilitate staging prior to resection, diagnostic laparoscopy has been advocated by some authors and is included in the NCCN guidelines for staging prior to surgical resection.[174,175] Where metastatic disease is obvious based on preoperative staging or if the cancer is a very early stage lesion, laparoscopy is seldom beneficial.[174,175] During surgery, the tumor should be assessed for resectability by ensuring that the cancer has not spread into the adjacent pancreas, colon, or liver. Peritoneal metastases and ascites are obvious and preclude any type of surgery. Positive cytology of peritoneal washings is associated with advanced T stage and poorer prognosis.[176]

The extent of gastric resection is a function of the location and extent of stomach involvement with tumor. For curative intent, all gross and microscopic disease needs to be removed. Microscopic involvement of the resection margin is associated with anastomotic recurrence and poor survival.[177] As discussed in the section on reconstruction techniques, patients with distal lesions should undergo distal or subtotal gastrectomy. For midbody or proximal lesions and distal lesions for which less than 5 cm of proximal margin can be obtained and for lesions diffusely distributed in the stomach, total gastrectomy is indicated. For lesions that involve the

TABLE 45.9. Location for the Major Nodal Groups Relevant to Gastric Resection for Cancer.

Nodal group	*Location*
N1	Perigastric along the greater and lesser curves
N2	Adjacent to the celiac axis and its major branches: the common hepatic, splenic and left gastric arteries
N3	Hepatoduodenal ligament; retropancreatic region; celiac plexus; superior mesenteric artery
N4	Paraaortic area

caria of the stomach or encroach on the esophagogastric junction, an esophagogastrectomy may be needed.

In the past, the extent of resection depended on the extent of the resection of the nodal groups relevant to gastric resection for cancer (Table 45.9). Gastric R1 resections included gastrectomy and resection of the N1 nodal basin and omentum. Gastric R2 resections included gastrectomy plus the N2 nodal basin, and R3 the N3 nodes, and so on. This designation is confusing. It is preferable to reserve the R0 resection to mean all gross and microscopic disease removed, R1 all gross disease removed but residual microscopic disease, and R2 to indicate gross disease remaining. The term D1 implies resection of nodal tissue in the N1 distribution, D2 the N2 distribution, and so on. Similarly, the current staging system as adopted by the American Joint Commission reserves the N description to indicate the number of nodes present in the specimen rather than distinguishing nodes based on their anatomic location.

The current TNM staging is seen in Table 45.10. Previously, it was thought that splenectomy was necessary to ensure adequate tumor clearance. Splenectomy results in substantially increased perioperative morbidity without any clear survival benefit and is not recommended.[178,179]

Considerable controversy exists regarding the extent of lymph node dissection for gastric carcinoma. No consensus panels have been published; however, several well-designed and executed randomized controlled trials have been conducted. The Dutch Gastric Cancer Group in the Netherlands performed a randomized controlled trial of D1 versus D2 lymph node dissection in 996 patients at 80 cancer centers. Because results for D2 resection are dependent on the surgeon's experience, the study was done in collaboration with Japanese surgeons familiar with the operation who supervised the conduct of operations early in the study. A limited number of trained Dutch surgeons traveled to the various centers to ensure that the D2 dissections were performed appropriately. Morbidity in the D2 group was substantially higher than for the D1 patients; the operative complication rate for D2 patients was 43% compared to 25% for D1 dissections. Operative mortality was 10% for D2 and 4% for D1 patients. One flaw in the study was that D2 patients routinely underwent splenectomy, an aspect of the operation that is now known to be unnecessary. Higher morbidity for D2 dissections had been reported from most Western centers. Western patients have more frequent comorbid conditions and larger amounts of intraabdominal fat than Japanese patients, which might account for the higher complication rate. Seven-year survival in the Dutch study failed to demonstrate improved survival in D2 patients.[180] Even when corrected for the higher perioperative mortality for D2 patients, long-term survival was not impacted by D2 resection.[181]

During the course of this study there was an unanticipated improvement in stage-specific survival. When the study was begun, the investigators predicted 5-year survival to be 20% for D1 and 32% for D2 patients. The observed survival was substantially higher, 45% and 47%, respectively. This improvement results in part from improved staging but also from an unexpectedly high incidence of T1 (26%) and T2 (47%) cancers. The investigators also rejected a higher proportion of patients than previously because of distant metastases.

TABLE 45.10. Definition of TMN, Stage Grouping, Histopathologic Type, and Histologic Grade for Gastric Carcinoma.

Definition of TMN

Primary Tumor (T)	
TX	Primary tumor cannot be assessed
T0	No evidence of primary tumor
Tis	Carcinoma *in situ*: intraepithelial tumor without invasion of the lamina propria
T1	Invasion of lamina propria or submucosa
T2	Tumor invades muscularis propria or subserosa*
T2a	Tumor invades muscularis propria
T2b	Tumor invades subserosa
T3	Tumor penetrates serosa (visceral peritoneum) without invasion of adjacent structures**,***
T4	Tumor invades adjacent structures**,***

**Note:* A tumor may penetrate the muscularis propria with extension into the gastrocolic or gastrohepatic ligaments, or into the greater or lesser omentum, without perforation of the visceral peritoneum covering these structures. In this case, the tumor is classified T2. If there is perforation of the visceral peritoneum covering the gastric ligaments or the omentum, the tumor should be classified T3.

***Note:* The adjacent structures of the stomach include the spleen, transverse colon, liver, diaphragm, pancreas, abdominal wall, adrenal gland, kidney, small intestine, and retroperitoneum.

****Note:* Intramural extension to the duodenum or esophagus is classified by the depth of the greatest invasion in any of these sites, including the stomach.

Regional Lymph Nodes (N)	
NX	Regional lymph node(s) cannot be assessed
N0	No regional lymph node metastasis*
N1	Metastasis in 1 to 6 regional lymph nodes
N2	Metastases in 7 to 15 regional lymph nodes
N3	Metastases in more than 15 regional lymph nodes

**Note:* A designation of pN0 should be used if all examined lymph nodes are negative, regardless of the total number removed and examined.

Distant Metastasis (M)			
MX	Distant metastasis cannot be assessed		
M0	No distant metastasis		
M1	Distant metastasis		
Stage Grouping			
Stage 0	Tis	N0	M0
Stage IA	T1	N0	M0
Stage IB	T1	N1	M0
	T2a/b	N0	M0
Stage II	T1	N2	M0
	T2a/b	N1	M0
	T3	N0	M0
Stage IIIA	T2a/b	N2	M0
	T3	N1	M0
	T4	N0	M0
Stage IIIB	T3	N2	M0
Stage IV	T4	N1–3	M0
	T1–3	N3	M0
	Any T	Any N	M1

Source: TNM classification used with the permission of the American Joint Committee on Cancer (AJCC), Chicago, Illinois. The original source for this material is the *AJCC Cancer Staging Manual, Sixth Edition* (2002) published by Springer Science and Business Media LLC, www.springerlink.com.

TABLE 45.11.
Comparison of 5-Year Survival from the Dutch Study to American and Japanese Results.

	Dutch D1		*Dutch D2*		*United States*		*Japan*	
Stage	*No. cases*	*Survival*	*No. cases*	*Survival*	*No. cases*	*Survival*	*No. cases*	*Survival*
I	173 (46)	70	133 (40)	71	2,004 (17)	50	1453 (46)	91
II	105 (28)	38	66 (20)	42	1,796 (17)	29	377 (12)	72
III	86 (23)	12	111 (34)	23	3,945 (36)	13	693 (22)	44
IV	12 (3)	0	18 (5)	28	3,342 (31)	3	653 (21)	9
Total	380	45	331	47	11,087	19	3176	62

Note: This table compares the incidence and stage-specific survival from the randomized-prospective Dutch trial[180] (level I evidence). The Dutch trial had two arms: D1 and D2 dissection. A retrospective review of American Cancer centers derived from Wanebo et al.[168] provides the US experience for gastric cancer. The Japanese experience is from the retrospective review by Maruyama et al.[185] Data are presented as the number of patients; the percentages are in parentheses.

Table 45.11 compares the results from the Dutch study to reviews of large series of patients from the United States and Japan. Because gastric carcinoma is the most frequent cancer in Japan, aggressive screening programs are in place, which accounts for a larger proportion of early-stage disease. Also, there is a higher incidence of intestinal than diffuse histology cancers in Japan, with intestinal-type lesions having an inherently better prognosis. The Dutch study found significant stage migration for patients undergoing D2 resection; 30% of D2 resections were found to have nodal tissue previously unsuspected, resulting in reclassification to higher stages.[182] This shift accounts for the fewer stage II patients in the D2 group compared to the D1 group, whereas there were more stage III tumors in the D2 group. Thus, the American data include patients in lower TNM stage groups who would otherwise be included in a higher group had a D2 dissection been carried out. This difference accounts, in part, for the lower survival rate in the United States.

The Medical Research Council in Britain performed a multicenter randomized controlled trial comparing D1 and D2 resections. The extra morbidity was almost identical to that observed in the Dutch study, with a 46% complication rate for patients having a D2 resection compared to 28% for D1 resections. As with the Dutch trial, pancreas resection or splenectomy accounted for the excess morbidity.[183] There was no survival benefit from D2 resection: 5-year survival for D1 patients was 35%, and it was 33% for D2 patients. There was also no difference for disease-free survival.[184]

These studies were well designed and provide the strongest evidence thus far regarding the utility for D2 dissections. For Western patients, surgeons specifically trained to perform D2 dissections could not impact survival, in contrast to reports from Japan. However, there have not been any randomized controlled trials from Japan, and reports have been retrospective, observational studies.[185,186] In addition, the biology of Japanese gastric cancer appears to differ from that of the Western disease. Thus, for Western patients D2 resections are not necessary and would help only for improving disease staging. When performed, splenectomy or pancreatic resection should not accompany D2 dissection.

Reconstruction Techniques

Several reconstructive options are available that attempt to minimize functional problems associated with gastric resection. Following gastric resection, early satiety and anorexia result in less caloric intake with subsequent weight loss. Malabsorption following gastric resection occurs in part because of rapid food transit time through the small bowel and less contact with digestive enzymes. Dyspepsia, reflux, and bloating might also contribute to diminished food ingestion. Many of these symptoms result from the loss of gastric reservoir function. The standard operation for gastric cancer has been total gastrectomy with Roux-en-Y esophagojejunostomy for diffuse, cardia, fundus, and body lesions and subtotal gastrectomy with Billroth I or II reconstruction for antral lesions. Newer reconstructive techniques attempt to re-create the gastric reservoir function. Studies have been performed to determine if better functional results are obtained with subtotal gastrectomy without compromising survival.

Numerous reconstructive operations have been described in the literature. Most reports provide technical details of the operations with simple outcomes such as short-term complication and mortality rates. At best, these describe the feasibility of performing a technique, providing little insight into the real benefit of the new operation. Because these operations have been designed to improve functional outcomes following gastric resection, their assessment requires quality-of-life analysis or other measurements of functional status. Only a few of the newer operations have been studied in this manner. Few studies compared the different reconstructions in a randomized controlled fashion. Of those trials, each examined different types of operations or quantitated outcomes with unique measurement tools, precluding formal meta-analysis of these trials.

Subtotal gastrectomy has the theoretical disadvantage of less tumor clearance with potentially greater recurrence rate. For proximal and gastric midbody lesions, subtotal gastrectomy is impractical because the tumor cannot be adequately cleared, and the remaining gastric remnant would be too small to be of any functional value. For distal gastric lesions, subtotal gastrectomy is preferred. Cure rates are equivalent to total gastrectomy, with better functional results.[187,188]

Table 45.12 summarizes results of randomized trials comparing various reconstructions following distal gastrectomy. Billroth II reconstruction has been thought to be associated with better function results than Billroth I. A randomized trial comparing these two reconstructions following distal gastric resection for cancer found that the morbidity, perioperative mortality, and 5-year survival were equivalent. Most

TABLE 45.12.
Reconstructive Options Following Distal Gastrectomy (Level I Evidence).

Reconstruction type	*Outcome measurement*	*Results*	*Reference*
BI (n = 30) vs. BII (n = 32)	M&M, 5-year survival, digestive comfort	Same	Chareton[189]
RY to gastric remnant (n = 13) vs. total gastrectomy with RYEJ[a]	M&M, QOL	Mostly the same, except slightly less diarrhea following subtotal gastrectomy	Svedlund[188]
RY (n = 24) vs. BI (n = 26)	M&M, QOL	Longer hospital stay for RY secondary to Roux stasis, less inflammation in the gastric pouch in the RY patients	Ishikawa[251]

BI, BII, Billroth I, II, respectively; Ry, Roux-en-Y; RYEJ, Roux-en-Y esophagojejunostomy, M&M, morbidity and mortality.

[a]Not explicitly stated.

Note: This study had three arms. Thirteen patients underwent subtotal gastrectomy with Roux-en-Y esophagojejunostomy for distal lesions, and 20 underwent jejunal pouch interposition following total gastrectomy for proximal gastric lesions. Thirty-one had a Roux-en-Y reconstruction following total gastrectomy, some for proximal and others for distal lesions; the exact number of each was not specified.

notably, the functional results for these two reconstructions were the same, dispelling the notion that the Billroth II is superior.[189] Distal gastrectomy with Roux-en-Y gastrojejunostomy reconstruction has been compared to total gastrectomy with Roux-en-Y reconstruction. Theoretically, leaving a gastric remnant improves eating because of retention of some degree of gastric storage capacity. When these operations, which differed only by preservation of a gastric remnant, were compared, there was little functional difference.[188]

Patients who have undergone total gastrectomy frequently have difficulty maintaining their weight. As was discussed with reconstruction following distal gastrectomy, the loss of the gastric storage capacity is thought to reduce food ingestion. Several randomized trials have been performed investigating the relative merits of various reconstructive options following total gastrectomy (Table 45.13).

Jejunal interposition has been proposed, in theory, to reduce transit time for food down the jejunum. This change should reduce dumping and other functional problems associated with Roux-en-Y esophagojejunostomy reconstruction. When compared with quality-of-life and other functional assessment measurement tools, no differences between these two reconstructions could be found.[190] Creation of a jejunal pouch also did not improve outcomes compared to standard Roux-en-Y reconstruction.[188] Two relatively small studies have found modest benefits with an interposed pouch compared to a standard jejunal pouch or a Roux-en-Y esophagojejunostomy.[191,192] Taken together, these studies suggest that standard Roux-en-Y esophagojejunostomy provides equivalent results to any other reservoir-forming pouch. Thus, the pouches are an unnecessary addition to the reconstruction following total gastrectomy.[193]

Chemoradiotherapy

Historically, 75% of patients who present with gastric cancer have regional nodal involvement or metastatic disease at the time of diagnosis.[171] Furthermore, following resection, recurrence rates are high, with 49% developing local recurrence, 17% developing peritoneal recurrence, 21% developing locoregional disease, and 17% showing hematogenous spread.[194] While chemotherapy, radiotherapy, or chemoradiotherapy alone are not effective in the treatment of gastric cancer, the use of these modalities in combination with surgery shows promise. Combined adjuvant chemoradiotherapy has been shown to decrease local recurrence, distant relapse, and peritoneal carcinomatosis.

In one multicenter, double-armed, prospective randomized trial of adjuvant postoperative chemoradiotherapy comparing surgery alone versus surgery plus combined 5-fluorouracil (5FU)-based chemotherapy and 4500 cGy of radiotherapy, median survival in the treatment group was 36 months compared to 27 months in the surgery-alone group. The 3-year relapse-free survival was superior in the treatment group as well, 48% versus 31%.[195] More recently, periopera-

TABLE 45.13.
Reconstructive Options Following Total Gastrectomy (Level I Evidence).

Reconstruction type	*Outcome measurement*	*Results*	*Reference*
Jejunal interposition (n = 53) vs. RYEJ (n = 53)	M&M, 3-year survival	No differences	Fuchs[190]
Jejunal pouch with interposition (n = 10) vs. jejunal pouch (n = 10) vs. RYEJ (n = 10)	Nutritional measurements, food intake, gastric emptying	Higher weights and intake with pouch/interposition	Nakane[192]
Jejunal pouch (n = 20) vs. RYEJ (n = ?)[a]	M&M, QOL	No differences	Svedlund[188]

M&M, morbidity and mortality.

[a]Not explicitly stated. This study had three arms. Thirteen patients underwent subtotal gastrectomy with Roux-en-Y esophagojejunostomy, and 20 underwent jejunal pouch interposition following total gastrectomy for proximal gastric lesions. Thirty-one had a Roux-en-Y reconstruction, some following total gastrectomy for proximal lesions and others following subtotal gastrectomy; the exact number of each was not specified.

tive chemotherapy consisting of a regimen of epirubicin, cisplatin, and infused fluorouracil both preoperatively and following surgery decreased tumor size and stage and significantly improved progression-free and overall survival.[196] This has led to interest in applying current chemotherapy or chemoradiotherapy to the neoadjuvant setting, as seen in the current NCCN treatment guidelines for gastric cancer (http://nccn.org/professionals/physician_gls/PDF/gastric.pdf) Randomized data in support of this recommendation are lacking.

Hereditary Basis for Gastric Cancer

Gastric cancer has a hereditary basis in approximately 10% of patients, with a two- to threefold increased risk of cancer in first-degree relatives of patients with gastric cancer even after controlling for *H. pylori* status.[197–199] Gastric cancers are also seen in familial cancer syndromes. In familial adenomatous polyposis (FAP) and Gardner's syndrome, gastric polyps are found in 30% to 100% of patients[200] and are most commonly nonneoplastic fundic gland polyps.[201] Gastric adenomas occur in 5% of patients with FAP, usually developing in the distal stomach.[202] Fundic gland polyps are more common in the upper stomach. While patients with FAP have a lifetime risk of colon cancer approaching 100%, the risk of developing gastric cancer is rare, approximately 0.5%.[203] Patients with numerous gastric polyps should have representative biopsies performed. All adenomatous polyps should be excised endoscopically, which may require multiple sessions. In patients with FAP, upper GI endoscopy is recommended every 1–3 years beginning at age 20 or at the time of colectomy. Patients with hereditary nonpolyposis colorectal cancer (HNPCC) syndrome have an 11% chance of developing gastric cancer, usually the intestinal type. A possible link between Peutz-Jeghers syndrome and gastric cancer has been reported.[204] The majority of familial clusters of gastric cancer are more often related to clustering of *H. pylori* infection in susceptible kindreds.[205]

Gastrointestinal Stromal Tumors

Gastrointestinal stromal tumors (GIST) are mesenchymal tumors arising from the pacemaker cells of the GI tract known as the interstitial cells of Cajal. Of the GISTs, 70% arise in the stomach and demonstrate a wide spectrum of clinical aggressiveness, from benign to highly aggressive. The central histologic factor that distinguishes these lesions from other stromal tumors of the stomach is the presence of the KIT receptor tyrosine kinase.[206] More than 95% of GISTs express KIT, as manifest by positive immunohistochemical staining for the CD117 antigen. Of GISTs, 5% are CD117 negative but occur by a mutational activation of the related kinase, platelet-derived growth factor receptor-α.[207]

The mainstay of treatment for gastric GISTs is surgical resection. As these lesions typically do not spread to regional lymphatics, aggressive lymphadenectomy is not necessary. Either local resection for small lesions or formal resection for larger lesions or lesions abutting important anatomic landmarks in the stomach to achieve a R0 resection is needed. For unresectable lesions or to improve the potential for resection with less morbidity, neoadjuvant treatment with the tyrosine kinase inhibitor imatinib mesylate may be helpful. Neoadjuvant imatinib mesylate improves the chance for surgical resection in lesions felt to be unresectable secondary to the remarkable 70%–80% partial response GISTs show to this agent.[208] The role of imatinib mesylate in neoadjuvant and adjuvant treatment following surgical resection is under investigation.

Gastric Carcinoids

Gastric carcinoids arise from the neuroendocrine cells of the stomach. They account for fewer than 1% of gastric tumors and 2% of GI carcinoids.[209] Most of these lesions are well differentiated and maintain an appearance histologically similar to enterochromaffin cells, while others are poorly differentiated.

Three types of gastric carcinoid tumors have been described.[210] Type I occurs in patients with chronic atrophic gastritis with achlorhydria-induced hypergastrinemia. Type II is associated with ZES. Type III is sporadic. Types I and II result from the mitogenic effects of elevated serum gastrin on the enterochromaffin cell population of the stomach. The lesions generally appear as small lesions, occasionally multiple, in the fundus and body of the stomach with antral sparing. They are generally benign and can be managed endoscopically if the lesions are less than 1 to 2 cm in size or with observation. In the case of gastrinoma, resection of the primary tumor will result in involution of the gastric disease. In chronic atrophic gastritis with achlorhydria, some have advocated resection of the gastric antrum to eliminate the source of elevated gastrin with good results. Dominant lesions occasionally require localized surgical resection. Sporadic tumors tend to be solitary, are more likely to be truly invasive, and metastasize. Formal resection with lymph node dissection is indicated. The 5-year survival is less than 50%.[211]

Gastric Lymphoma

The stomach is the most common site of GI lymphoma. The most common types of gastric lymphoma are marginal zone B cell lymphoma of the mucosa-associated lymphoid tissue (MALT) type and diffuse large B-cell lymphoma, accounting for 40% and 45%–50% of gastric lymphomas, respectively. The MALT lymphomas are thought to arise from chronic *H. pylori* infection; these lymphomas regress in response to *H. pylori* treatment.

For disease limited to the mucosa and submucosa, as is the case in 90% of patients, antibiotics alone are sufficient.[212] In the rare case of more advanced disease with extension into the muscularis or serosa, nodal or adjacent organ involvement, disease refractory to antibiotics, or systemic disease, chemotherapy with or without radiotherapy should be considered in addition to *H. pylori* eradication. Surgery is seldom necessary, usually requiring a total gastrectomy, but is successful about 80% of the time. Historically, diffuse large B-cell lymphomas have been treated with surgery out of concern for perforation or bleeding during chemoradiotherapy.

As the risk of these untoward events happening is now thought to be insignificant, chemotherapy with cyclophosphamide, doxorubicin, vincristine, and prednisone (CHOP) with rituximab and 40–50 Gy of radiotherapy is thought to be standard management. Surgery is no longer the mainstay of the treatment of gastric lymphomas.[213]

Benign Gastric Neoplasms

Gastric Polyps

Although gastric polypoid lesions are uncommon, they are detected more often due to the increasing use of endoscopy for the evaluation of abdominal symptoms. Most polyps are asymptomatic. However, polyps may cause bleeding or obstruction if the polyp is ulcerated or large. Gastric polyps are identified in 2%–3% of all gastroscopic studies.[214] Once identified, it is necessary to biopsy or completely excise polyps by snare polypectomy for histologic assessment as well as perform careful examination of the entire gastric mucosa in search of a synchronous gastric carcinoma.

Hyperplastic polyps are among the most commonly observed gastric polyps, accounting for up to 75% of all gastric polyps. Histologically, they are characterized by elongation, branching, or cystic dilation of the gland. They are usually solitary, sessile lesions less than 1.5 cm in size. Hyperplastic polyps are believed to represent a regenerative response of normal mucosa to injury. The risk of developing dysplasia within a polyp is between 1.9% and 19%,[215] while the risk of developing adenocarcinoma within a polyp has been reported as 0% to 8%, with an average of 2.1%.[214] A solitary hyperplastic gastric polyp has also been associated with synchronous or metachronous gastric carcinoma in 1.2% to 28% of cases, while the risk of developing gastric carcinoma with multiple polyps is 3.6%.[216]

A high incidence of background mucosal disease has been demonstrated in patients with hyperplastic polyps.[215] They are commonly associated with atrophic gastritis, with *H. pylori* gastritis occurring in 50% to 90% of cases.[217] The disappearance of hyperplastic polyps has been demonstrated following eradication of *H. pylori*, suggesting a possible treatment strategy of *H. pylori* eradication followed by resection of persistent polyps.

Fundic gland polyps are nonneoplastic lesions and may account for up to 47% of all gastric polyps. They may occur sporadically or in polyposis syndromes. Histologically, they are characterized by dilated fundic glands forming small cysts. Endoscopically, they present as multiple, small, sessile lesions in the fundus and body surrounded by healthy gastric mucosa. While the cause of these lesions is unknown, they have been found in patients receiving long-term treatment with PPIs. Neither resection nor surveillance is required once the histologic diagnosis is confirmed.[218] Finally, it has been suggested that while fundic gland polyps themselves carry no malignant potential, they signal an increased risk of a patient having a colorectal adenoma or carcinoma.[214]

Inflammatory polyps account for 3% of gastric polyps and are most commonly located in the distal stomach. They have a characteristic whorl-like pattern of fibroblasts around vessels with infiltration of eosinophilic granulocytes. They do not undergo malignant change.

Adenomatous polyps are precancerous lesions that account for approximately 10% of gastric polyps.[219] These lesions are most commonly solitary, sessile, and located in the antrum. Adenomas usually appear in tubular or tubulovillous forms. Villous adenomas occur rarely in the stomach. The malignant potential of adenomatous polyps increases with larger polyps. Adenocarcinoma is detected in 24% to 60% of lesions greater than 2 cm, while in lesions less than 2 cm the risk is 4% to 23%.[218] The risk of developing adenocarcinoma in a polyp is also related to the polyp type. There is an increased risk of discovering adenocarcinoma in tubulovillous and villous adenomas compared to tubular adenomas in the stomach.[220] Coincident gastric carcinoma may occur in up to 25% of cases.[218]

Once discovered, adenomatous polyps should be excised. This can usually be performed with endoscopic snare polypectomy. However, if the lesion is not amenable to endoscopic excision, then numerous biopsies should be performed. If malignancy is detected, then the lesion should be excised with operative gastric wedge resection. Endoscopic surveillance should be performed 1 year after polypectomy and every 3 years after a negative endoscopic evaluation.[218]

Leiomyoma

Leiomyomas are the most common benign tumor of the stomach. They are generally a solitary, well-circumscribed lesion arising from the muscularis propria. While endoscopic biopsy is not always diagnostic due to the submucosal location of these lesions, endoscopic ultrasound is useful for characterization.[218] Leiomyomas are usually asymptomatic; however, when symptoms are present, bleeding is most common. Leiomyosarcomas may rarely develop in lesions greater than 2 to 3 cm in diameter. The diagnosis is made when 10 mitotic figures are seen per high-power field. Because of the rare occurrence of malignancy, the treatment for leiomyomas involves local excision with a 2–3 cm margin of gastric wall accompanied by frozen section.

Lipoma

Gastric lipomas are rare and usually asymptomatic. These submucosal lesions are most often solitary, with a yellowish color and located in the antrum.[218] Gastric lipomas require no specific treatment.

Other Gastric Conditions

Mallory-Weiss Syndrome

Mallory-Weiss tears are linear mucosal lacerations occurring most commonly along the lesser curvature of the stomach at the gastroesophageal junction. However, a smaller percentage of these lacerations may be located on the greater curve near the gastroesophageal junction or extend into the esophageal mucosa. The classic triad of the syndrome is retching, vomiting, and hematemesis, although a history of retching is obtained in only 29% of patients.[221] Mallory-Weiss syndrome is classically associated with alcoholics; however, more recently it has been described following coughing, childbirth, endoscopy, blunt abdominal trauma, and cardiopulmonary resuscitation.

Bleeding from Mallory-Weiss tears accounts for 5%–10% of all cases of upper GI bleeding.[222,223] Bleeding stops spontaneously in 80%–90% of patients, with less than a 5% incidence of rebleeding.[224] Initial management should be directed toward airway stabilization and fluid resuscitation. Endoscopy is essential for the diagnosis of Mallory-Weiss tears and has become the mainstay of treatment. Endoscopic therapy with coagulation techniques, injection, and banding has been shown to effectively stop bleeding. If endoscopy is unavailable, then angiographic intervention with the intra-arterial infusion of vasopressin or embolization may be performed successfully, although they carry additional risks. Surgical intervention is rarely required but should be performed in patients with ongoing bleeding following initial nonsurgical management.

Ménétrier's Disease

Ménétrier's disease, or hypoproteinemic hypertrophic gastropathy, is a rare premalignant condition of the stomach. It is characterized by thickened gastric folds, protein loss from the stomach, and hypochlorhydria. The gastric body and fundus along the greater curvature are commonly involved.[225] A number of other conditions may cause enlarged gastric folds, such as gastric lymphoma, gastric carcinoma, cytomegalovirus (CMV) and *H. pylori* gastritis, and granulomatous disease.

Ménétrier's disease appears to be an acquired disease of unknown etiology. Although the exact cause is unknown, infection with CMV and *H. pylori* has been implicated. In addition, recent evidence suggests a role of transforming growth factor-α and the epidermal growth factor (EGF) receptor in the pathogenesis of the disease.[226]

The predominant histologic findings include foveolar hyperplasia and cystic dilation, along with a decreased parietal cell mass and varying degrees of inflammation.[227] The varying degrees of lymphocytic infiltration reported throughout the literature is thought to be the result of confusion related to the diagnosis of Ménétrier's disease versus hypertrophic lymphocytic gastritis.

Symptoms include upper abdominal pain, weight loss, anorexia, nausea, vomiting, and diarrhea. Physical examination is usually unremarkable, with the exception of mild epigastric tenderness or signs of recent weight loss. Also, edema may be present if hypoproteinemia is severe. In addition to decreased serum albumin, there is a reduction in gastric acid secretion, which is thought to result from the decrease in parietal cell mass. Males are more frequently affected (3:1) and usually are diagnosed between 30 and 50 years of age. Diagnosis is made by barium swallow, which demonstrates enlarged gastric folds, and is confirmed by a full-thickness biopsy of the gastric wall. Ménétrier's disease may be self-limited in children. In adults with Ménétrier's disease, a primary concern is the development of cancer. A review of the literature demonstrated that 15% of the reported cases have been associated with carcinoma.[228]

The treatment of patients with Ménétrier's disease has been largely anecdotal. Medical therapies have included antacids, anticholinergics, antifibrinolytics, corticosteroids, octreotide, monoclonal antibodies against EGF receptor, and *H. pylori* eradication. The entire syndrome has been reported to regress with eradication of *H. pylori*; therefore, if *H. pylori* is present, it should be treated.

Surgery is reserved for intractable pain, symptoms related to hypoproteinemia, bleeding, obstruction, and cancer development. Relief of symptoms and normalization of serum protein almost always results from surgical treatment.[229] Although subtotal gastrectomy removing only the affected tissue has been recommended for the treatment of hypoproteinemia, complications such as marginal ulcer, persistent symptoms, and death from anastomotic dehiscence have been reported. Thus, total gastrectomy is the procedure of choice in patients who are able to tolerate the procedure. If the patient is unable to undergo surgical intervention, then close endoscopic surveillance must be performed.

Dieulafoy's Lesion

Dieulafoys's lesion is a "caliber-persistent artery" in the submucosa with a small overlying mucosal defect typically located in the proximal stomach, usually in the distribution of the left gastric artery.[230] Although most of these lesions are located in the stomach, they may also occur in the small intestine, colon, and rarely the esophagus.[231] Dieulafoys's lesion accounts for 0.3% to 6.7% of major upper GI bleeding, typically in the sixth to eighth decade of life.[231] Patients commonly present with intermittent GI bleeding, making endoscopic diagnosis challenging. When emergent endoscopy is required, Dieulafoy's lesion may be accurately diagnosed in only 49%–63% of cases.[232] An association between Dieulafoys's lesion and NSAID use, alcohol abuse, and peptic ulcer disease has been noted.[233] The pathogenesis is thought to be the result of hydrostatic forces of the large vessel along with a focal gastritis, which causes a mucosal defect and subsequent rupture of the artery into the lumen.

Historically, Dieulafoys's lesion was treated with gastric wedge resection. However, the consensus now seems to be that endoscopic management is the first-line therapy, with reported success rates ranging from 90% to 100%.[234–236] Multiple endoscopic therapeutic interventions have been described, including injection sclerotherapy, thermocoagulation, laser therapy, endoscopic band ligation, and hemoclip application.[233] Recurrent bleeding after endoscopic treatment occurs in 5.7%[235] to 33%[226] of patients. The lowest rates of rebleeding have been demonstrated when mechanical obliteration of the bleeding vessel using endoscopic banding and hemoclip application has been employed. Mortality rates following treatment of Dieulafoys's lesion have been reported as high as 26%, largely due to comorbid conditions.[233] If patients fail endoscopic management, then selective arterial embolization may be the treatment of choice, especially if the patients are poor surgical candidates. Surgical intervention is generally reserved for patients who have failed both endoscopic and angiographic therapy.

Bezoars

Bezoars are retained concretions of indigestible material that accumulate in the GI tract. They most commonly occur in the stomach but may also be found in the small bowel. Bezoars may be classified as phytobezoars, composed of food material that is nondigestable by humans; trichobezoars, composed of hair; medication bezoars (pharmacobezoars), composed of medications or medication vehicles; and lactobezoars, composed of congealed milk products of infant's formula. Phytobezoars are the most common type of bezoar.

Patients at greatest risk for bezoar formation are those with altered gastric anatomy and physiology as a result of surgery. A history of previous gastric surgery is present in 70%–90% of patients with bezoars.[237] Bezoar formation is more common following vagotomy and antrectomy, although any gastric surgery may predispose patients to their development. Phytobezoars have been reported in up to 20% of patients following antrectomy. The development of bezoars following gastric surgery is thought to be secondary to a reduction in gastric acidity, decreased gastric motility, and delayed gastric emptying.[238,239] Although gastroparesis is common in patients with bezoars who have no history of prior gastric surgery, others may demonstrate normal gastric emptying. Those with comorbid illnesses such as diabetes and end-stage renal disease requiring dialysis and mechanically ventilated patients are also at risk for bezoar formation.

Patients present with vague epigastric distress 80% of the time, with as many as 30% experiencing weight loss. Additional complaints include bloating, nausea, vomiting, dysphagia, and early satiety. Patients may also present with complications of bezoars, such as intestinal obstruction, gastric ulcer, upper GI hemorrhage, gastric perforation, or gastritis.[240] One study found gastric ulcers to be associated with large bezoars in 26% of patients.[241] Moreover, patients found to have an intestinal bezoar as the cause of obstruction will have a concurrent gastric bezoar 20% of the time.[242] Upper endoscopy is the diagnostic choice for identifying bezoars.[240] An upper GI contrast study may reveal the classic finding of a filling defect with a "bubbly" appearance; however, these studies may be falsely negative up to 76% of the time.[241]

Treatment of bezoars partially depends on the type of bezoar, with the ultimate goal removal and prevention of recurrence. If treatment is not administered, then mortality rates may be as high as 30% secondary to GI hemorrhage and perforation.[243] Current treatment strategies include observation, medical treatment with enzymes and prokinetic agents, endoscopic dissolution and mechanical disruption, and surgical removal. Small gastric bezoars may be amenable to conservative treatment; however, spontaneous resolution is rare and may take up to 10 months. Mechanical disruption and removal by endoscopy is successful 85%–90% of the time.[240] A number of chemicals have been used to dissolve bezoars with varying success. Other than gastric lavage with saline, 0.1 NHCl, and $NaHCO_3$, other agents include papain, *N*-acetylcysteine, cellulase, and Adolph's meat tenderizer. The most efficacious of these has been cellulase, with successful dissolution achieved in 83%–100% of the cases.[240]

Surgery is indicated when endoscopic management fails and for bezoar associated complications. Typically, operative intervention for bezoar extraction when endoscopic therapy has failed involves laparotomy with gastrostomy. However, there have been case reports using various laparoscopic techniques for removal of gastric bezoars.[244]

After successful dissolution or removal of a bezoar, prevention becomes an important issue because recurrence occurs in approximately 13% of cases.[241] Preventing recurrence must be directed toward the underlying pathology. Recommendations for preventing phytobezoars are to avoid raw citrus fruits, persimmons, and high-fiber foods. In addition, enzymatic dissolution agents may be taken with each meal. If gastric stasis is a component of bezoar formation, then prokinetic agents may be effective. Patients who develop trichobezoar and who have underlying psychiatric disorders may require specific therapy to prevent recurrence.

References

1. Hildebrand P, Lehmann FS, Ketterer S, et al. Regulation of gastric function by endogenous gastrin releasing peptide in humans: studies with a specific gastrin releasing peptide receptor antagonist. Gut 2001;49:23–28.
2. Debas HT, Mulvihill SJ. Neuroendocrine design of the gut. Am J Surg 1991;161:243–249.
3. Pappas TN, Debas HT, Taylor IL. Enterogastrone-like effect of peptide YY is vagally mediated in the dog. J Clin Invest 1986;77:49–53.
4. Sonnenberg A. The US temporal and geographic variations of diseases related to *Helicobacter pylori*. Am J Public Health 1993;83:1006–1010.
5. Fowler SF, Khoubian JF, Mathiasen RA, Margulies DR. Peptic ulcers in the elderly is a surgical disease. Am J Surg 2001;182:733–737.
6. Kuipers EJ, Thijs JC, Festen HP. The prevalence of *Helicobacter pylori* in peptic ulcer disease. Aliment Pharmacol Ther 1995;9(suppl 2):59–69.
7. Pounder RE, Ng D. The prevalence of *Helicobacter pylori* infection in different countries. Aliment Pharmacol Ther 1995;9(suppl 2):33–39.
8. Feil W, Klimesch S, Karner P, et al. Importance of an alkaline microenvironment for rapid restitution of the rabbit duodenal mucosa in vitro. Gastroenterology 1989;97:112–122.
9. Barnard JA, Beauchamp RD, Russell WE, et al. Epidermal growth factor-related peptides and their relevance to gastrointestinal pathophysiology. Gastroenterology 1995;108:564–580.
10. Isenberg JI, Selling JA, Hogan DL, Koss MA. Impaired proximal duodenal mucosal bicarbonate secretion in patients with duodenal ulcer. N Engl J Med 1987;316:374–379.
11. Hogan DL, Rapier RC, Dreilinger A, et al. Duodenal bicarbonate secretion: eradication of *Helicobacter pylori* and duodenal structure and function in humans. Gastroenterology 1996;110:705–716.
12. Fandriks L, von Bothmer C, Johansson B, et al. Water extract of *Helicobacter pylori* inhibits duodenal mucosal alkaline secretion in anesthetized rats. Gastroenterology 1997;113:1570–1575.
13. Marshall BJ, Warren JR. Unidentified curved bacilli in the stomach of patients with gastritis and peptic ulceration. Lancet 1984;1:1311–1315.
14. Parsonnet J. *Helicobacter pylori*: the size of the problem. Gut 1998;43(suppl 1):S6–S9.
15. Covacci A, Telford JL, Del Giudice G, et al. *Helicobacter pylori* virulence and genetic geography. Science 1999;284:1328–1333.
16. Parsonnet J. The incidence of *Helicobacter pylori* infection. Aliment Pharmacol Ther 1995;9(suppl 2):45–51.
17. Ernst PB, Gold BD. The disease spectrum of *Helicobacter pylori*: the immunopathogenesis of gastroduodenal ulcer and gastric cancer. Annu Rev Microbiol 2000;54:615–640.
18. Moss SF, Calam J, Agarwal B, et al. Induction of gastric epithelial apoptosis by *Helicobacter pylori*. Gut 1996;38:498–501.
19. Passaro DJ, Chosy EJ, Parsonnet J. *Helicobacter pylori*: consensus and controversy. Clin Infect Dis 2002;35:298–304.
20. Israel DA, Peek RM. Pathogenesis of *Helicobacter pylori*-induced gastric inflammation. Aliment Pharmacol Ther 2001;15:1271–1290.
21. Suzuki M, Miura S, Suematsu M, et al. *Helicobacter pylori*-associated ammonia production enhances neutrophil-dependent gastric mucosal cell injury. Am J Physiol 1992;263(5 pt 1):G719–G725.
22. Cover TL, Blaser MJ. Purification and characterization of the vacuolating toxin from *Helicobacter pylori*. J Biol Chem 1992;267:10570–10575.
23. Covacci A, Censini S, Bugnoli M, et al. Molecular characterization of the 128-kDa immunodominant antigen of *Helicobacter*

pylori associated with cytotoxicity and duodenal ulcer. Proc Natl Acad Sci U S A 1993;90:5791–5795.

24. Censini S, Lange C, Xiang Z, et al. Cag, a pathogenicity island of *Helicobacter pylori*, encodes type I-specific and disease-associated virulence factors. Proc Natl Acad Sci U S A 1996;93:14648–14653.
25. Yamaoka Y, Kita M, Kodama T, et al. *Helicobacter pylori* cagA gene and expression of cytokine messenger RNA in gastric mucosa. Gastroenterology 1996;110:1744–1752.
26. Chan FK, Leung WK. Peptic-ulcer disease. Lancet 2002;360:933–941.
27. Kurata JH, Nogawa AN. Meta-analysis of risk factors for peptic ulcer. Nonsteroidal antiinflammatory drugs, *Helicobacter pylori*, and smoking. J Clin Gastroenterol 1997;24:2–17.
28. Ma L, Chow JY, Cho CH. Cigarette smoking delays ulcer healing: role of constitutive nitric oxide synthase in rat stomach. Am J Physiol 1999;276(1 pt 1):G238–G248.
29. Ma L, Wang WP, Chow JY, et al. The role of polyamines in gastric mucus synthesis inhibited by cigarette smoke or its extract. Gut 2000;47:170–177.
30. Cryer B, Faust TW, Goldschmiedt M, et al. Gastric and duodenal mucosal prostaglandin concentrations in gastric or duodenal ulcer disease: relationships with demographics, environmental, and histological factors, including *Helicobacter pylori*. Am J Gastroenterol 1992;87:1747–1754.
31. Konturek SJ, Bielanski W, Plonka M, et al. *Helicobacter pylori*, non-steroidal anti-inflammatory drugs and smoking in risk pattern of gastroduodenal ulcers. Scand J Gastroenterol 2003;38:923–930.
32. Bardhan KD, Graham DY, Hunt RH, O'Morain CA. Effects of smoking on cure of *Helicobacter pylori* infection and duodenal ulcer recurrence in patients treated with clarithromycin and omeprazole. Helicobacter 1997;2:27–31.
33. Chan FK, Sung JJ, Lee YT, et al. Does smoking predispose to peptic ulcer relapse after eradication of *Helicobacter pylori*? Am J Gastroenterol 1997;92:442–445.
34. Feldman M, McMahon AT. Do cyclooxygenase-2 inhibitors provide benefits similar to those of traditional nonsteroidal anti-inflammatory drugs, with less gastrointestinal toxicity? Ann Intern Med 2000;132:134–143.
35. Bombardier C, Laine L, Reicin A, et al. Comparison of upper gastrointestinal toxicity of rofecoxib and naproxen in patients with rheumatoid arthritis. VIGOR Study Group. N Engl J Med 2000;343:1520–1528.
36. Goldstein JL, Silverstein FE, Agrawal NM, et al. Reduced risk of upper gastrointestinal ulcer complications with celecoxib, a novel COX-2 inhibitor. Am J Gastroenterol 2000;95:1681–1690.
37. Hawkey CJ, Tulassay Z, Szczepanski L, et al. Randomised controlled trial of *Helicobacter pylori* eradication in patients on non-steroidal anti-inflammatory drugs: HELP NSAIDs study. *Helicobacter* Eradication for Lesion Prevention. Lancet 1998;352:1016–1021.
38. Silverstein FE, Faich G, Goldstein JL, et al. Gastrointestinal toxicity with celecoxib versus nonsteroidal anti-inflammatory drugs for osteoarthritis and rheumatoid arthritis: the CLASS study: a randomized controlled trial. Celecoxib Long-term Arthritis Safety Study. JAMA 2000;284:1247–1255.
39. McDonald MP, Broughan TA, Hermann RE, et al. Operations for gastric ulcer: a long-term study. Am Surg 1996;62:673–677.
40. Csendes A, Braghetto I, Smok G. Type IV gastric ulcer: a new hypothesis. Surgery 1987;101:361–366.
41. Fennerty MB. Pathophysiology of the upper gastrointestinal tract in the critically ill patient: rationale for the therapeutic benefits of acid suppression. Crit Care Med 2002;30(6 suppl):S351–S355.
42. Cook D, Heyland D, Griffith L, et al. Risk factors for clinically important upper gastrointestinal bleeding in patients requiring mechanical ventilation. Canadian Critical Care Trials Group. Crit Care Med 1999;27:2812–2817.
43. Cook DJ, Fuller HD, Guyatt GH, et al. Risk factors for gastrointestinal bleeding in critically ill patients. Canadian Critical Care Trials Group. N Engl J Med 1994;330:377–381.
44. Cook DJ, Reeve BK, Guyatt GH, et al. Stress ulcer prophylaxis in critically ill patients. Resolving discordant meta-analyses. JAMA 1996;275:308–314.
45. Weeks DL, Eskandari S, Scott DR, Sachs G. A H^+-gated urea channel: the link between *Helicobacter pylori* urease and gastric colonization. Science 2000;287:482–485.
46. Versalovic J. *Helicobacter pylori*. Pathology and diagnostic strategies. Am J Clin Pathol 2003;119:403–412.
47. Monteiro L, de Mascarel A, Sarrasqueta AM, et al. Diagnosis of *Helicobacter pylori* infection: noninvasive methods compared to invasive methods and evaluation of two new tests. Am J Gastroenterol 2001;96:353–358.
48. Dore MP, Negrini R, Tadeu V, et al. Novel monoclonal antibody-based *Helicobacter pylori* stool antigen test. Helicobacter 2004;9:228–232.
49. Laheij RJ, Straatman H, Jansen JB, Verbeek AL. Evaluation of commercially available *Helicobacter pylori* serology kits: a review. J Clin Microbiol 1998;36:2803–2809.
50. Faigel DO, Magaret N, Corless C, et al. Evaluation of rapid antibody tests for the diagnosis of *Helicobacter pylori* infection. Am J Gastroenterol 2000;95:72–77.
51. Cutler AF, Havstad S, Ma CK, et al. Accuracy of invasive and noninvasive tests to diagnose *Helicobacter pylori* infection. Gastroenterology 1995;109:136–141.
52. Levine MS, Rubesin SE. The *Helicobacter pylori* revolution: radiologic perspective. Radiology 1995;195:593–596.
53. Spechler SJ. Peptic ulcer disease and its complications. In: Feldman M, Friedman LS, Sleisenger MH, eds. Sleisenger and Fordtran's Gastrointestinal and Liver Disease. Vol. 1. Philadelphia: Saunders; 2002:747–781.
54. Grossman MI. The Veterans Administration Cooperative Study on Gastric Ulcer. 10. Resume and comment. Gastroenterology 1971;61(suppl 2):635–638.
55. Howden CW, Hunt RH. Guidelines for the management of *Helicobacter pylori* infection. Ad Hoc Committee on Practice Parameters of the American College of Gastroenterology. Am J Gastroenterol 1998;93:2330–2338.
56. Osato MS, Reddy R, Reddy SG, et al. Pattern of primary resistance of *Helicobacter pylori* to metronidazole or clarithromycin in the United States. Arch Intern Med 2001;161:1217–1220.
57. Wolfe MM, Sachs G. Acid suppression: optimizing therapy for gastroduodenal ulcer healing, gastroesophageal reflux disease, and stress-related erosive syndrome. Gastroenterology 2000;118(2 suppl 1):S9–S31.
58. Holt S, Howden CW. Omeprazole. Overview and opinion. Dig Dis Sci 1991;36:385–393.
59. Poynard T, Lemaire M, Agostini H. Meta-analysis of randomized clinical trials comparing lansoprazole with ranitidine or famotidine in the treatment of acute duodenal ulcer. Eur J Gastroenterol Hepatol 1995;7:661–665.
60. Agrawal NM, Campbell DR, Safdi MA, et al. Superiority of lansoprazole versus ranitidine in healing nonsteroidal anti-inflammatory drug-associated gastric ulcers: results of a double-blind, randomized, multicenter study. NSAID-Associated Gastric Ulcer Study Group. Arch Intern Med 2000;160:1455–1461.
61. Yeomans ND, Tulassay Z, Juhasz L, et al. A comparison of omeprazole with ranitidine for ulcers associated with nonsteroidal antiinflammatory drugs. Acid Suppression Trial: Ranitidine versus Omeprazole for NSAID-associated Ulcer Treatment (ASTRONAUT) Study Group. N Engl J Med 1998;338:719–726.
62. Malfertheiner P, Kirchner T, Kist M, et al. *Helicobacter pylori* eradication and gastric ulcer healing—comparison of three pan-

toprazole-based triple therapies. Aliment Pharmacol Ther 2003;17:1125–1135.
63. Ruiz B, Correa P, Fontham ET, Ramakrishnan T. Antral atrophy, *Helicobacter pylori* colonization, and gastric pH. Am J Clin Pathol 1996;105:96–101.
64. Sung JJ, Chung SC, Ling TK, et al. Antibacterial treatment of gastric ulcers associated with *Helicobacter pylori*. N Engl J Med 1995;332:139–142.
65. Higuchi K, Fujiwara Y, Tominaga K, et al. Is eradication sufficient to heal gastric ulcers in patients infected with *Helicobacter pylori*? A randomized, controlled, prospective study. Aliment Pharmacol Ther 2003;17:111–117.
66. Campbell DR, Haber MM, Sheldon E, et al. Effect of *H. pylori* status on gastric ulcer healing in patients continuing nonsteroidal anti-inflammatory therapy and receiving treatment with lansoprazole or ranitidine. Am J Gastroenterol 2002;97:2208–2214.
67. Burget DW, Chiverton SG, Hunt RH. Is there an optimal degree of acid suppression for healing of duodenal ulcers? A model of the relationship between ulcer healing and acid suppression. Gastroenterology 1990;99:345–351.
68. Maton PN. Omeprazole. N Engl J Med 1991;324:965–975.
69. Ciociola AA, McSorley DJ, Turner K, et al. *Helicobacter pylori* infection rates in duodenal ulcer patients in the United States may be lower than previously estimated. Am J Gastroenterol 1999;94:1834–1840.
70. Hopkins RJ, Girardi LS, Turney EA. Relationship between *Helicobacter pylori* eradication and reduced duodenal and gastric ulcer recurrence: a review. Gastroenterology 1996;110:1244–1252.
71. Laine L, Hopkins RJ, Girardi LS. Has the impact of *Helicobacter pylori* therapy on ulcer recurrence in the United States been overstated? A meta-analysis of rigorously designed trials. Am J Gastroenterol 1998;93:1409–1415.
72. Marshall BJ, Goodwin CS, Warren JR, et al. Prospective double-blind trial of duodenal ulcer relapse after eradication of *Campylobacter pylori*. Lancet 1988;2:1437–1442.
73. Sonnenberg A, Olson CA, Zhang J. The effect of antibiotic therapy on bleeding from duodenal ulcer. Am J Gastroenterol 1999;94:950–954.
74. Meyer JM, Silliman NP, Wang W, et al. Risk factors for *Helicobacter pylori* resistance in the United States: the surveillance of *H. pylori* antimicrobial resistance partnership (SHARP) study, 1993–1999. Ann Intern Med 2002;136:13–24.
75. Laine L. Is it time for quadruple therapy to be first line? Can J Gastroenterol 2003;17(suppl B):33B–35B.
76. Perri F, Festa V, Merla A, et al. Randomized study of different "second-line" therapies for *Helicobacter pylori* infection after failure of the standard "Maastricht triple therapy." Aliment Pharmacol Ther 2003;18:815–820.
77. Ford AC, Delaney BC, Forman D, Moayyedi P. Eradication therapy in *Helicobacter pylori* positive peptic ulcer disease: systematic review and economic analysis. Am J Gastroenterol 2004;99:1833–1855.
78. Quan C, Talley NJ. Management of peptic ulcer disease not related to *Helicobacter pylori* or NSAIDs. Am J Gastroenterol 2002;97:2950–2961.
79. Millat B, Fingerhut A, Borie F. Surgical treatment of complicated duodenal ulcers: controlled trials. World J Surg 2000;24:299–306.
80. Goligher JC, Pulvertaft CN, De Dombal FT, et al. Clinical comparison of vagotomy and pyloroplasty with other forms of elective surgery for duodenal ulcer. Br Med J 1968;2:787–789.
81. Goligher JC, Pulvertaft CN, De Dombal FT, et al. Five to eight-year results of Leeds-York controlled trial of elective surgery for duodenal ulcer. Br Med J 1968;2:781–787.
82. Goligher JC, Pulvertaft CN, Irvin TT, et al. Five- to eight-year results of truncal vagotomy and pyloroplasty for duodenal ulcer. Br Med J 1972;1:7–13.
83. Jordan PH Jr, Condon RE. A prospective evaluation of vagotomy-pyloroplasty and vagotomy-antrectomy for treatment of duodenal ulcer. Ann Surg 1970;172:547–563.
84. Price WE, Grizzle JE, Postlethwait RW, et al. Results of operation for duodenal ulcer. Surg Gynecol Obstet 1970;131:233–244.
85. Hoffmann J, Jensen HE, Christiansen J, et al. Prospective controlled vagotomy trial for duodenal ulcer. Results after 11–15 years. Ann Surg 1989;209:40–45.
86. Jordan PH Jr, Thornby J. Twenty years after parietal cell vagotomy or selective vagotomy antrectomy for treatment of duodenal ulcer. Final report. Ann Surg 1994;220:283–293; discussion 293–296.
87. Macintyre IM, Millar A, Smith AN, Small WP. Highly selective vagotomy 5–15 years on. Br J Surg 1990;77:65–69.
88. Meisner S, Hoffmann J, Jensen HE. Parietal cell vagotomy. A 23-year study. Ann Surg 1994;220:164–167.
89. Mulholland MW, Debas HT. Chronic duodenal and gastric ulcer. Surg Clin North Am 1987;67:489–507.
90. Taylor TV, Lythgoe JP, McFarland JB, et al. Anterior lesser curve seromyotomy and posterior truncal vagotomy versus truncal vagotomy and pyloroplasty in the treatment of chronic duodenal ulcer. Br J Surg 1990;77:1007–1009.
91. Walia HS, Abd el-Karim HA. Anterior lesser curve seromyotomy with posterior truncal vagotomy versus proximal gastric vagotomy: results of a prospective randomized trial 3–8 years after surgery. World J Surg 1994;18:758–763.
92. Cook D, Guyatt G, Marshall J, et al. A comparison of sucralfate and ranitidine for the prevention of upper gastrointestinal bleeding in patients requiring mechanical ventilation. Canadian Critical Care Trials Group. N Engl J Med 1998;338:791–797.
93. Levy MJ, Seelig CB, Robinson NJ, Ranney JE. Comparison of omeprazole and ranitidine for stress ulcer prophylaxis. Dig Dis Sci 1997;42:1255–1259.
94. Spirt MJ. Acid suppression in critically ill patients: what does the evidence support? Pharmacotherapy 2003;23(10 pt 2):87S–93S.
95. Labenz J, Peitz U, Leusing C, et al. Efficacy of primed infusions with high dose ranitidine and omeprazole to maintain high intragastric pH in patients with peptic ulcer bleeding: a prospective randomised controlled study. Gut 1997;40:36–41.
96. Lau JY, Sung JJ, Lee KK, et al. Effect of intravenous omeprazole on recurrent bleeding after endoscopic treatment of bleeding peptic ulcers. N Engl J Med 2000;343:310–316.
97. Netzer P, Gaia C, Sandoz M, et al. Effect of repeated injection and continuous infusion of omeprazole and ranitidine on intragastric pH over 72h. Am J Gastroenterol 1999;94:351–357.
98. Walt RP, Cottrell J, Mann SG, et al. Continuous intravenous famotidine for haemorrhage from peptic ulcer. Lancet 1992;340:1058–1062.
99. Zuckerman G, Welch R, Douglas A, et al. Controlled trial of medical therapy for active upper gastrointestinal bleeding and prevention of rebleeding. Am J Med 1984;76:361–366.
100. Javid G, Masoodi I, Zargar SA, et al. Omeprazole as adjuvant therapy to endoscopic combination injection sclerotherapy for treating bleeding peptic ulcer. Am J Med 2001;111:280–284.
101. Lanza FL. A guideline for the treatment and prevention of NSAID-induced ulcers. Members of the Ad Hoc Committee on Practice Parameters of the American College of Gastroenterology. Am J Gastroenterol 1998;93:2037–2046.
102. Hooper L, Brown TJ, Elliott R, et al. The effectiveness of five strategies for the prevention of gastrointestinal toxicity induced by non-steroidal anti-inflammatory drugs: systematic review. BMJ 2004;329:948.

103. Jacobsen RB, Phillips BB. Reducing clinically significant gastrointestinal toxicity associated with nonsteroidal antiinflammatory drugs. Ann Pharmacother 2004;38:1469–1481.
104. Ekstrom P, Carling L, Wetterhus S, et al. Prevention of peptic ulcer and dyspeptic symptoms with omeprazole in patients receiving continuous non-steroidal anti-inflammatory drug therapy. A Nordic multicentre study. Scand J Gastroenterol 1996;31:753–758.
105. Silverstein FE, Graham DY, Senior JR, et al. Misoprostol reduces serious gastrointestinal complications in patients with rheumatoid arthritis receiving nonsteroidal anti-inflammatory drugs. A randomized, double-blind, placebo-controlled trial. Ann Intern Med 1995;123:241–249.
106. Cullen D, Bardhan KD, Eisner M, et al. Primary gastroduodenal prophylaxis with omeprazole for non-steroidal anti-inflammatory drug users. Aliment Pharmacol Ther 1998;12:135–140.
107. Shaffer HA Jr. Perforation and obstruction of the gastrointestinal tract. Assessment by conventional radiology. Radiol Clin North Am 1992;30:405–426.
108. Gunshefski L, Flancbaum L, Brolin RE, Frankel A. Changing patterns in perforated peptic ulcer disease. Am Surg 1990;56:270–274.
109. Lanas A, Serrano P, Bajador E, et al. Evidence of aspirin use in both upper and lower gastrointestinal perforation. Gastroenterology 1997;112:683–689.
110. Svanes C. Trends in perforated peptic ulcer: incidence, etiology, treatment, and prognosis. World J Surg 2000;24:277–283.
111. Datsis AC, Rogdakis A, Kekelos S, et al. Simple closure of chronic duodenal ulcer perforation in the era of *Helicobacter pylori*: an old procedure, today's solution. Hepatogastroenterology 2003;50:1396–1398.
112. Ng EK, Lam YH, Sung JJ, et al. Eradication of *Helicobacter pylori* prevents recurrence of ulcer after simple closure of duodenal ulcer perforation: randomized controlled trial. Ann Surg 2000;231:153–158.
113. Boey J, Choi SK, Poon A, Alagaratnam TT. Risk stratification in perforated duodenal ulcers. A prospective validation of predictive factors. Ann Surg 1987;205:22–26.
114. Hay JM, Lacaine F, Kohlmann G, Fingerhut A. Immediate definitive surgery for perforated duodenal ulcer does not increase operative mortality: a prospective controlled trial. World J Surg 1988;12:705–709.
115. Tanphiphat C, Tanprayoon T, Na Thalang A. Surgical treatment of perforated duodenal ulcer: a prospective trial between simple closure and definitive surgery. Br J Surg 1985;72:370–372.
116. Gisbert JP, Pajares JM. *Helicobacter pylori* infection and perforated peptic ulcer prevalence of the infection and role of antimicrobial treatment. Helicobacter 2003;8:159–167.
117. Alamowitch B, Aouad K, Sellam P, et al. [Laparoscopic treatment of perforated duodenal ulcer]. Gastroenterol Clin Biol 2000;24:1012–1017.
118. Metzger J, Styger S, Sieber C, et al. Prevalence of *Helicobacter pylori* infection in peptic ulcer perforations. Swiss Med Wkly 2001;131:99–103.
119. Tran TT, Quandalle P. [Treatment of perforated gastroduodenal ulcer by simple suture followed by *Helicobacter pylori* eradication]. Ann Chir 2002;127:32–34.
120. Blomgren LG. Perforated peptic ulcer: long-term results after simple closure in the elderly. World J Surg 1997;21:412–414; discussion 414–415.
121. Irvin TT. Mortality and perforated peptic ulcer: a case for risk stratification in elderly patients. Br J Surg 1989;76:215–218.
122. Lau WY, Leung KL, Zhu XL, et al. Laparoscopic repair of perforated peptic ulcer. Br J Surg 1995;82:814–816.
123. Hodnett RM, Gonzalez F, Lee WC, et al. The need for definitive therapy in the management of perforated gastric ulcers. Review of 202 cases. Ann Surg 1989;209:36–39.
124. Jordan PH Jr. Surgery for peptic ulcer disease. Curr Probl Surg 1991;28:265–330.
125. Herrington JL Jr, Sawyers JL. Gastric ulcer. Curr Probl Surg 1987;24:759–865.
126. Robles R, Parrilla P, Lujan JA, et al. Long-term follow-up of bilateral truncal vagotomy and pyloroplasty for perforated duodenal ulcer. Br J Surg 1995;82:665.
127. Siu WT, Leong HT, Law BK, et al. Laparoscopic repair for perforated peptic ulcer: a randomized controlled trial. Ann Surg 2002;235:313–319.
128. Mondardini A, Barletti C, Rocca G, et al. Non-variceal upper gastrointestinal bleeding and Forrest's classification: diagnostic agreement between endoscopists from the same area. Endoscopy 1998;30:508–512.
129. Silverstein FE, Gilbert DA, Tedesco FJ, et al. The national ASGE survey on upper gastrointestinal bleeding. II. Clinical prognostic factors. Gastrointest Endosc 1981;27:80–93.
130. Allan R, Dykes P. A study of the factors influencing mortality rates from gastrointestinal haemorrhage. Q J Med 1976;45:533–550.
131. Clason AE, Macleod DA, Elton RA. Clinical factors in the prediction of further haemorrhage or mortality in acute upper gastrointestinal haemorrhage. Br J Surg 1986;73:985–987.
132. Kankaria AG, Fleischer DE. The critical care management of nonvariceal upper gastrointestinal bleeding. Crit Care Clin 1995;11:347–368.
133. Van Dam J, Brugge WR. Endoscopy of the upper gastrointestinal tract. N Engl J Med 1999;341:1738–1748.
134. Savides TJ, Jensen DM. Therapeutic endoscopy for nonvariceal gastrointestinal bleeding. Gastroenterol Clin North Am 2000;29:465–487, vii.
135. Machicado GA, Jensen DM. Thermal probes alone or with epinephrine for the endoscopic haemostasis of ulcer haemorrhage. Baillieres Best Pract Res Clin Gastroenterol 2000;14:443–458.
136. Calvet X, Vergara M, Brullet E, et al. Addition of a second endoscopic treatment following epinephrine injection improves outcome in high-risk bleeding ulcers. Gastroenterology 2004;126:441–450.
137. Sung JJ, Chan FK, Lau JY, et al. The effect of endoscopic therapy in patients receiving omeprazole for bleeding ulcers with nonbleeding visible vessels or adherent clots: a randomized comparison. Ann Intern Med 2003;139:237–243.
138. Gisbert JP, Khorrami S, Carballo F, et al. Meta-analysis: *Helicobacter pylori* eradication therapy versus antisecretory non-eradication therapy for the prevention of recurrent bleeding from peptic ulcer. Aliment Pharmacol Ther 2004;19:617–629.
139. Lau JY, Sung JJ, Lam YH, et al. Endoscopic retreatment compared with surgery in patients with recurrent bleeding after initial endoscopic control of bleeding ulcers. N Engl J Med 1999;340:751–756.
140. Shope TR, Kauffman GL Jr. Duodenal ulcer. In: Cameron JL, ed. Current Surgical Therapy. Philadelphia: Elsevier Mosby; 2004:71–76.
141. Millat B, Hay JM, Valleur P, et al. Emergency surgical treatment for bleeding duodenal ulcer: oversewing plus vagotomy versus gastric resection, a controlled randomized trial. French Associations for Surgical Research. World J Surg 1993;17:568–573; discussion 574.
142. Sirinek KR, Bingener J, Richards ML. Benign gastric ulcer and stress gastritis. In: Cameron JL, ed. Current Surgical Therapy. Philadelphia: Elsevier Mosby; 2004:67–70.
143. Weiland D, Dunn DH, Humphrey EW, Schwartz ML. Gastric outlet obstruction in peptic ulcer disease: an indication for surgery. Am J Surg 1982;143:90–93.
144. Choudhary AM, Roberts I, Nagar A, et al. *Helicobacter pylori*-related gastric outlet obstruction: is there a role for medical treatment? J Clin Gastroenterol 2001;32:272–273.

145. Gisbert JP, Pajares JM. Review article: *Helicobacter pylori* infection and gastric outlet obstruction—prevalence of the infection and role of antimicrobial treatment. Aliment Pharmacol Ther 2002;16:1203–1208.
146. Shone DN, Nikoomanesh P, Smith-Meek MM, Bender JS. Malignancy is the most common cause of gastric outlet obstruction in the era of H_2 blockers. Am J Gastroenterol 1995;90:1769–1770.
147. Boylan JJ, Gradzka MI. Long-term results of endoscopic balloon dilatation for gastric outlet obstruction. Dig Dis Sci 1999;44:1883–1886.
148. Gibson JB, Behrman SW, Fabian TC, Britt LG. Gastric outlet obstruction resulting from peptic ulcer disease requiring surgical intervention is infrequently associated with *Helicobacter pylori* infection. J Am Coll Surg 2000;191:32–37.
149. Kate V, Ananthakrishnan N, Badrinath S, et al. *Helicobacter pylori* infection in duodenal ulcer with gastric outlet obstruction. Trop Gastroenterol 1998;19:75–77.
150. Taskin V, Gurer I, Ozyilkan E, et al. Effect of *Helicobacter pylori* eradication on peptic ulcer disease complicated with outlet obstruction. Helicobacter 2000;5:38–40.
151. de Boer WA, Driessen WM. Resolution of gastric outlet obstruction after eradication of *Helicobacter pylori*. J Clin Gastroenterol 1995;21:329–330.
152. Malik GM, Romshoo GHJ, Basu JA. *Helicobacter pylori* and gastric outlet obstruction. Am J Gastroenterol 1998;93: 2004.
153. Solt J, Bajor J, Szabo M, Horvath OP. Long-term results of balloon catheter dilation for benign gastric outlet stenosis. Endoscopy 2003;35:490–495.
154. DiSario JA, Fennerty MB, Tietze CC, et al. Endoscopic balloon dilation for ulcer-induced gastric outlet obstruction. Am J Gastroenterol 1994;89:868–871.
155. Zittel TT, Jehle EC, Becker HD. Surgical management of peptic ulcer disease today—indication, technique and outcome. Langenbecks Arch Surg 2000;385:84–96.
156. Csendes A, Maluenda F, Braghetto I, et al. Prospective randomized study comparing three surgical techniques for the treatment of gastric outlet obstruction secondary to duodenal ulcer. Am J Surg 1993;166:45–49.
157. Hom S, Sarr MG, Kelly KA, Hench V. Postoperative gastric atony after vagotomy for obstructing peptic ulcer. Am J Surg 1989;157:282–286.
158. McCallum RW, Polepalle SC, Schirmer B. Completion gastrectomy for refractory gastroparesis following surgery for peptic ulcer disease. Long-term follow-up with subjective and objective parameters. Dig Dis Sci 1991;36:1556–1561.
159. Wyman A, Stuart RC, Ng EK, et al. Laparoscopic truncal vagotomy and gastroenterostomy for pyloric stenosis. Am J Surg 1996;171:600–603.
160. Glasgow RE, Mulvihill SJ. Postgastrectomy syndromes. Probl Gen Surg 1997;14:132–152.
161. Cheadle WG, Baker PR, Cuschieri A. Pyloric reconstruction for severe vasomotor dumping after vagotomy and pyloroplasty. Ann Surg 1985;202:568–572.
162. Vogel SB, Hocking MP, Woodward ER. Clinical and radionuclide evaluation of Roux-en-Y diversion for postgastrectomy dumping. Am J Surg 1988;155:57–62.
163. Sawyers JL, Herrington JL Jr, Buckspan GS. Remedial operation for alkaline reflux gastritis and associated postgastrectomy syndromes. Arch Surg 1980;115:519–524.
164. Cuschieri A. Surgical management of severe intractable postvagotomy diarrhoea. Br J Surg 1986;73:981–984.
165. Zobolas B, Sakorafas GH, Kouroukli I, et al. Alkaline reflux gastritis: early and late results of surgery. World J Surg 2006;30:1043–1049.
166. Parkin DM. Epidemiology of cancer: global patterns and trends. Toxicol Lett 1998;102–103:227–234.
167. SEER Cancer Statistics Review 1975–2001. National Cancer Institute; 2004. Available at: http://seer.cancer.gov.
168. Wanebo HJ, Kennedy BJ, Chmiel J, et al. Cancer of the stomach. A patient care study by the American College of Surgeons. Ann Surg 1993;218:583–592.
169. Locke GR 3rd, Talley NJ, Carpenter HA, et al. Changes in the site- and histology-specific incidence of gastric cancer during a 50-year period. Gastroenterology 1995;109:1750–1756.
170. Correa P. Human gastric carcinogenesis: a multistep and multifactorial process—First American Cancer Society Award Lecture on Cancer Epidemiology and Prevention. Cancer Res 1992;52:6735–6740.
171. Houghton J, Wang TC. Tumors of the stomach. In: Feldman M, Friedman LS, Brandt LJ, eds. Sleisenger and Fordtran's Gastrointestinal and Liver Disease. Vol. 1. Philadelphia: Saunders; 2006:1139–1170.
172. Toftgaard C. Gastric cancer after peptic ulcer surgery. A historic prospective cohort investigation. Ann Surg 1989;210:159–164.
173. Schuman BM, Waldbaum JR, Hiltz SW. Carcinoma of the gastric remnant in a US population. Gastrointest Endosc 1984;30:71–73.
174. Sarela AI, Lefkowitz R, Brennan MF, Karpeh MS. Selection of patients with gastric adenocarcinoma for laparoscopic staging. Am J Surg 2006;191:134–138.
175. Yano M, Tsujinaka T, Shiozaki H, et al. Appraisal of treatment strategy by staging laparoscopy for locally advanced gastric cancer. World J Surg 2000;24:1130–1135; discussion 1135–1136.
176. Bentrem D, Wilton A, Mazumdar M, et al. The value of peritoneal cytology as a preoperative predictor in patients with gastric carcinoma undergoing a curative resection. Ann Surg Oncol 2005;12:347–353.
177. Shiu MH, Moore E, Sanders M, et al. Influence of the extent of resection on survival after curative treatment of gastric carcinoma. A retrospective multivariate analysis. Arch Surg 1987;122:1347–1351.
178. Wanebo HJ, Kennedy BJ, Winchester DP, et al. Role of splenectomy in gastric cancer surgery: adverse effect of elective splenectomy on longterm survival. J Am Coll Surg 1997; 185:177–184.
179. Yu W, Choi GS, Chung HY. Randomized clinical trial of splenectomy versus splenic preservation in patients with proximal gastric cancer. Br J Surg 2006;93:559–563.
180. Bonenkamp JJ, Hermans J, Sasako M, et al. Extended lymph-node dissection for gastric cancer. N Engl J Med 1999;340:908–914.
181. Pacelli F, Sgadari A, Doglietto GB. Surgery for gastric cancer. N Engl J Med 1999;341:538–539.
182. Bunt AM, Hermans J, Smit VT, et al. Surgical/pathologic-stage migration confounds comparisons of gastric cancer survival rates between Japan and Western countries. J Clin Oncol 1995;13:19–25.
183. Cuschieri A, Fayers P, Fielding J, et al. Postoperative morbidity and mortality after D1 and D2 resections for gastric cancer: preliminary results of the MRC randomised controlled surgical trial. The Surgical Cooperative Group. Lancet 1996;347:995–999.
184. Cuschieri A, Weeden S, Fielding J, et al. Patient survival after D1 and D2 resections for gastric cancer: long-term results of the MRC randomized surgical trial. Surgical Co-operative Group. Br J Cancer 1999;79:1522–1530.
185. Maruyama K, Okabayashi K, Kinoshita T. Progress in gastric cancer surgery in Japan and its limits of radicality. World J Surg 1987;11:418–425.
186. Noguchi Y, Imada T, Matsumoto A, et al. Radical surgery for gastric cancer. A review of the Japanese experience. Cancer 1989;64:2053–2062.

187. Gouzi JL, Huguier M, Fagniez PL, et al. Total versus subtotal gastrectomy for adenocarcinoma of the gastric antrum. A French prospective controlled study. Ann Surg 1989;209:162–166.
188. Svedlund J, Sullivan M, Liedman B, et al. Quality of life after gastrectomy for gastric carcinoma: controlled study of reconstructive procedures. World J Surg 1997;21:422–433.
189. Chareton B, Landen S, Manganas D, et al. Prospective randomized trial comparing Billroth I and Billroth II procedures for carcinoma of the gastric antrum. J Am Coll Surg 1996;183:190–194.
190. Fuchs KH, Thiede A, Engemann R, et al. Reconstruction of the food passage after total gastrectomy: randomized trial. World J Surg 1995;19:698–705; discussion 705–706.
191. Iivonen MK, Mattila JJ, Nordback IH, Matikainen MJ. Long-term follow-up of patients with jejunal pouch reconstruction after total gastrectomy. A randomized prospective study. Scand J Gastroenterol 2000;35:679–685.
192. Nakane Y, Okumura S, Akehira K, et al. Jejunal pouch reconstruction after total gastrectomy for cancer. A randomized controlled trial. Ann Surg 1995;222:27–35.
193. Espat NJ, Karpeh M. Reconstruction following total gastrectomy: a review and summary of the randomized prospective clinical trials. Surg Oncol 1998;7:65–69.
194. Roviello F, Marrelli D, de Manzoni G, et al. Prospective study of peritoneal recurrence after curative surgery for gastric cancer. Br J Surg 2003;90:1113–1119.
195. Macdonald JS, Smalley SR, Benedetti J, et al. Chemoradiotherapy after surgery compared with surgery alone for adenocarcinoma of the stomach or gastroesophageal junction. N Engl J Med 2001;345:725–730.
196. Cunningham D, Allum WH, Stenning SP, et al. Perioperative chemotherapy versus surgery alone for resectable gastroesophageal cancer. N Engl J Med 2006;355:11–20.
197. Brenner H, Arndt V, Sturmer T, et al. Individual and joint contribution of family history and *Helicobacter pylori* infection to the risk of gastric carcinoma. Cancer 2000;88:274–279.
198. La Vecchia C, Negri E, Franceschi S, Gentile A. Family history and the risk of stomach and colorectal cancer. Cancer 1992;70:50–55.
199. Palli D, Galli M, Caporaso NE, et al. Family history and risk of stomach cancer in Italy. Cancer Epidemiol Biomarkers Prev 1994;3:15–18.
200. Itzkowitz SH. Cancer prevention in patients with inflammatory bowel disease. Gastroenterol Clin North Am 2002;31:1133–1144.
201. Oberhuber G, Stangl PC, Vogelsang H, et al. Significant association of strictures and internal fistula formation in Crohn's disease. Virchows Arch 2000;437:293–297.
202. Offerhaus GJ, Giardiello FM, Krush AJ, et al. The risk of upper gastrointestinal cancer in familial adenomatous polyposis. Gastroenterology 1992;102:1980–1982.
203. Burt RW. Gastric fundic gland polyps. Gastroenterology 2003;125:1462–1469.
204. Howe JR, Mitros FA, Summers RW. The risk of gastrointestinal carcinoma in familial juvenile polyposis. Ann Surg Oncol 1998;5:751–756.
205. El-Omar EM, Oien K, Murray LS, et al. Increased prevalence of precancerous changes in relatives of gastric cancer patients: critical role of *H. pylori*. Gastroenterology 2000;118:22–30.
206. Hirota S, Isozaki K, Moriyama Y, et al. Gain-of-function mutations of c-kit in human gastrointestinal stromal tumors. Science 1998;279:577–580.
207. Heinrich MC, Corless CL, Duensing A, et al. PDGFRA activating mutations in gastrointestinal stromal tumors. Science 2003;299:708–710.
208. Scaife CL, Hunt KK, Patel SR, et al. Is there a role for surgery in patients with "unresectable" cKIT+ gastrointestinal stromal tumors treated with imatinib mesylate? Am J Surg 2003;186:665–669.
209. Gilligan CJ, Lawton GP, Tang LH, et al. Gastric carcinoid tumors: the biology and therapy of an enigmatic and controversial lesion. Am J Gastroenterol 1995;90:338–352.
210. Rindi G, Bordi C, Rappel S, et al. Gastric carcinoids and neuroendocrine carcinomas: pathogenesis, pathology, and behavior. World J Surg 1996;20:168–172.
211. Hou W, Schubert ML. Treatment of gastric carcinoids. Curr Treat Options Gastroenterol 2007;10:123–133.
212. Fischbach W, Goebeler-Kolve ME, Dragosics B, et al. Long term outcome of patients with gastric marginal zone B cell lymphoma of mucosa associated lymphoid tissue (MALT) following exclusive *Helicobacter pylori* eradication therapy: experience from a large prospective series. Gut 2004;53:34–37.
213. Collins RH. Gastrointestinal lymphomas. In: Feldman M, Friedman LS, Brandt LJ, eds. Sleisenger and Fordtran's Gastrointestinal and Liver Disease. Vol. 1. Philadelphia: Saunders; 2006: 565–587.
214. Oberhuber G, Stolte M. Gastric polyps: an update of their pathology and biological significance. Virchows Arch 2000;437:581–590.
215. Abraham SC, Singh VK, Yardley JH, Wu TT. Hyperplastic polyps of the stomach: associations with histologic patterns of gastritis and gastric atrophy. Am J Surg Pathol 2001;25:500–507.
216. Stolte M. Clinical consequences of the endoscopic diagnosis of gastric polyps. Endoscopy 1995;27:32–37; discussion 59–60.
217. Debongnie JC. Gastric polyps. Acta Gastroenterol Belg 1999; 62:187–189.
218. Burke CA, van Stolk RU. Diagnosis and management of gastroduodenal polyps. Surg Oncol Clin N Am 1996;5:589–607.
219. Stolte M, Sticht T, Eidt S, et al. Frequency, location, and age and sex distribution of various types of gastric polyp. Endoscopy 1994;26:659–665.
220. Nakamura T, Nakano G. Histopathological classification and malignant change in gastric polyps. J Clin Pathol 1985;38:754–764.
221. Graham DY, Schwartz JT. The spectrum of the Mallory-Weiss tear. Medicine (Baltimore) 1978;57:307–318.
222. Peura DA, Lanza FL, Gostout CJ, Foutch PG. The American College of Gastroenterology Bleeding Registry: preliminary findings. Am J Gastroenterol 1997;92:924–928.
223. Wilcox CM, Clark WS. Causes and outcome of upper and lower gastrointestinal bleeding: the Grady Hospital experience. South Med J 1999;92:44–50.
224. Hixson SD, Burns RP, Britt LG. Mallory-Weiss syndrome: retrospective review of eight years' experience. South Med J 1979;72:1249–1251.
225. Scharschmidt BF. The natural history of hypertrophic gastrophy (Menetrier's disease). Report of a case with 16 year follow-up and review of 120 cases from the literature. Am J Med 1977;63:644–652.
226. Burdick JS, Chung E, Tanner G, et al. Treatment of Menetrier's disease with a monoclonal antibody against the epidermal growth factor receptor. N Engl J Med 2000;343:1697–1701.
227. Komorowski RA, Caya JG. Hyperplastic gastropathy. Clinicopathologic correlation. Am J Surg Pathol 1991;15:577–585.
228. Wolfsen HC, Carpenter HA, Talley NJ. Menetrier's disease: a form of hypertrophic gastropathy or gastritis? Gastroenterology 1993;104:1310–1319.
229. Mulvihill SJ. Neoplasms of the stomach. In: Bell RH, Rikkers LF, Mulholland MW, eds. Digestive Tract Surgery: A Text and Atlas. Philadelphia: Lippincott-Raven; 1996:255–279.
230. Miko TL, Thomazy VA. The caliber persistent artery of the stomach: a unifying approach to gastric aneurysm, Dieulafoy's lesion, and submucosal arterial malformation. Hum Pathol 1988;19:914–921.

231. Norton ID, Petersen BT, Sorbi D, et al. Management and long-term prognosis of Dieulafoy lesion. Gastrointest Endosc 1999;50:762–767.
232. McGrath K, Mergener K, Branch S. Endoscopic band ligation of Dieulafoy's lesion: report of two cases and review of the literature. Am J Gastroenterol 1999;94:1087–1090.
233. Chandrashekar L, Brown RD, Venu RP. Management of Dieulafoy's lesion in the endoscopic era. J Clin Gastroenterol 2003;36:294–296.
234. Kasapidis P, Georgopoulos P, Delis V, et al. Endoscopic management and long-term follow-up of Dieulafoy's lesions in the upper GI tract. Gastrointest Endosc 2002;55:527–531.
235. Mumtaz R, Shaukat M, Ramirez FC. Outcomes of endoscopic treatment of gastroduodenal Dieulafoy's lesion with rubber band ligation and thermal/injection therapy. J Clin Gastroenterol 2003;36:310–314.
236. Yamaguchi Y, Yamato T, Katsumi N, et al. Short-term and long-term benefits of endoscopic hemoclip application for Dieulafoy's lesion in the upper GI tract. Gastrointest Endosc 2003;57:653–656.
237. Pfau PR, Ginsberg G.G. Foreign Bodies and Bezoars. Vol. 1, 7th ed. Philadelphia: Saunders; 2002.
238. Escamilla C, Robles-Campos R, Parrilla-Paricio P, et al. Intestinal obstruction and bezoars. J Am Coll Surg 1994;179:285–288.
239. Sanderson I, Ibberson O, Fish EB. Gastric phytobezoar following gastrectomy. Can Med Assoc J 1971;104:1115 passim.
240. Andrus CH, Ponsky JL. Bezoars: classification, pathophysiology, and treatment. Am J Gastroenterol 1988;83:476–478.
241. Diettrich NA, Gau FC. Postgastrectomy phytobezoars—endoscopic diagnosis and treatment. Arch Surg 1985;120:432–435.
242. Phillips MR, Zaheer S, Drugas GT. Gastric trichobezoar: case report and literature review. Mayo Clin Proc 1998;73:653–656.
243. Williams RS. The fascinating history of bezoars. Med J Aust 1986;145:613–614.
244. Yao CC, Wong HH, Chen CC, et al. Laparoscopic removal of large gastric phytobezoars. Surg Laparosc Endosc Percutan Tech 2000;10:243–245.
245. Hopman WP, Wolberink RG, Lamers CB, Van Tongeren JH. Treatment of the dumping syndrome with the somatostatin analogue SMS 201-995. Ann Surg 1988;207:155–159.
246. Tulassay Z, Tulassay T, Gupta R, Cierny G. Long-acting analogue of somatostatin—SMS 201-995—is highly effective in the prevention of clinical symptoms related to the dumping syndrome. Ann Surg 1989;210:250–252.
247. Primrose JN. Octreotide in the treatment of the dumping syndrome. Digestion 1990;45(suppl 1):49–58; discussion 58–59.
248. Geer RJ, Richards WO, O'Dorisio TM, et al. Efficacy of octreotide acetate in treatment of severe postgastrectomy dumping syndrome. Ann Surg 1990;212:678–687.
249. Gray JL, Debas HT, Mulvihill SJ. Control of dumping symptoms by somatostatin analogue in patients after gastric surgery. Arch Surg 1991;126:1231–1235; discussion 1235–1236.
250. Hasler WL, Soudah HC, Owyang C. Mechanisms by which octreotide ameliorates symptoms in the dumping syndrome. J Pharmacol Exp Ther 1996;277:1359–1365.
251. Ishikawa M, Kitayama J, Kaizaki S, et al. Prospective randomized trial comparing Billroth I and Roux-en-Y procedures after distal gastrectomy for gastric carcinoma. World J Surg 2005;29:1415–1420; discussion 1421.
252. Debas HT. Stomach and duodenum. In: Gastrointestinal Surgery. New York: Springer; 2004.

46

Pancreas

Robert E. Glasgow and Sean J. Mulvihill

Anatomy of the Pancreas

Embryology

The pancreas is derived as an outpouching of the primitive foregut endoderm in the region of the duodenum. It has two main embryologic components: (1) a dorsal bud, first identifiable at 4 weeks gestation, that goes on to become the body and tail of the gland and (2) a ventral bud that produces the head of the gland and the extrahepatic biliary system (Fig. 46.1). As these outpouchings grow, the ventral aspect rotates to fuse with the dorsal aspect by about the seventh week of gestation. The ductal system of the pancreas is derived from these two anlages. The embryonic ventral duct arises from the bile duct, drains with it into the duodenum at the major papilla, and fuses with the dorsal duct to drain the body of the gland as the main pancreatic duct of Wirsung. The embryonic dorsal duct persists as a separate structure in its proximal portion (duct of Santorini), draining into the duodenum at the minor papilla on the medial duodenal wall about 1–2 cm cephalad to the major papilla. In 5%–10% of people, the ventral and dorsal ducts fail to fuse, resulting in a condition known as *pancreas divisum*.[1] In this anatomical arrangement, the majority of pancreatic secretions are carried to the duodenum through the duct of Santorini and the minor papilla (Fig. 46.2).

The cells of the endocrine pancreas were thought, for many years, to derive from the neural crest. Pearse developed his theory of the origins of the islets, and other endocrine tissues, based on the observation that they shared the capacity to take up precursor amines, process them by decarboxylation, and manufacture peptide hormones.[2,3] This APUD (amine precursor uptake decarboxylation) theory was challenged and then refuted with microdissection techniques and molecular evidence that the islets arise from the primitive gut endoderm, not the neural crest. The expression of messenger RNA of islet hormones, including insulin, glucagon, and somatostatin, can be identified as early as 8–9 days after conception in the mouse, whereas exocrine enzymes such as carboxypeptidase and amylase are first found later.[4] Development of the exocrine pancreas requires the presence of endodermal and mesenchymal tissue, whereas islet development requires only endoderm.[5] This mesenchymal–epithelial interaction in the developing exocrine pancreas presumably leads to formation of intrapancreatic ductular structures and blood vessels.

The neurons innervating the pancreas are part of the enteric nervous system (ENS), best thought of as the third component of the autonomic nervous system. The ENS plays an important role in the regulation of secretion, motility, blood flow, and immune function in the gut. These neurons are derived, embryologically, from the neural crest. Neuroblasts from the vagal segment of the neural crest migrate in a craniocaudal direction down the gut during development, forming enteric ganglia in the pancreas and other organs. Migration of these neuroblasts is dependent on tyrosine kinase activity.

Developmental abnormalities of the pancreas are rare but can occasionally come to attention clinically. The risk of development of acute pancreatitis was shown to be increased in patients with pancreas divisum in some studies but not others.[1,6–9] The cause is thought to be the drainage of a large volume of pancreatic juice through a small duct of Santorini, perhaps in association with a stenotic minor papilla. Congenital pancreatic cysts are uncommon and usually solitary. Multiple congenital cysts can occur in the setting of polycystic kidney disease, von Hippel-Lindau syndrome, or cystic fibrosis. Heterotopic pancreatic tissue, termed *pancreatic rests*, are usually found in the proximal gastrointestinal tract, where they can contribute to ulceration or abdominal pain. Annular pancreas occurs when the ventral pancreas encircles

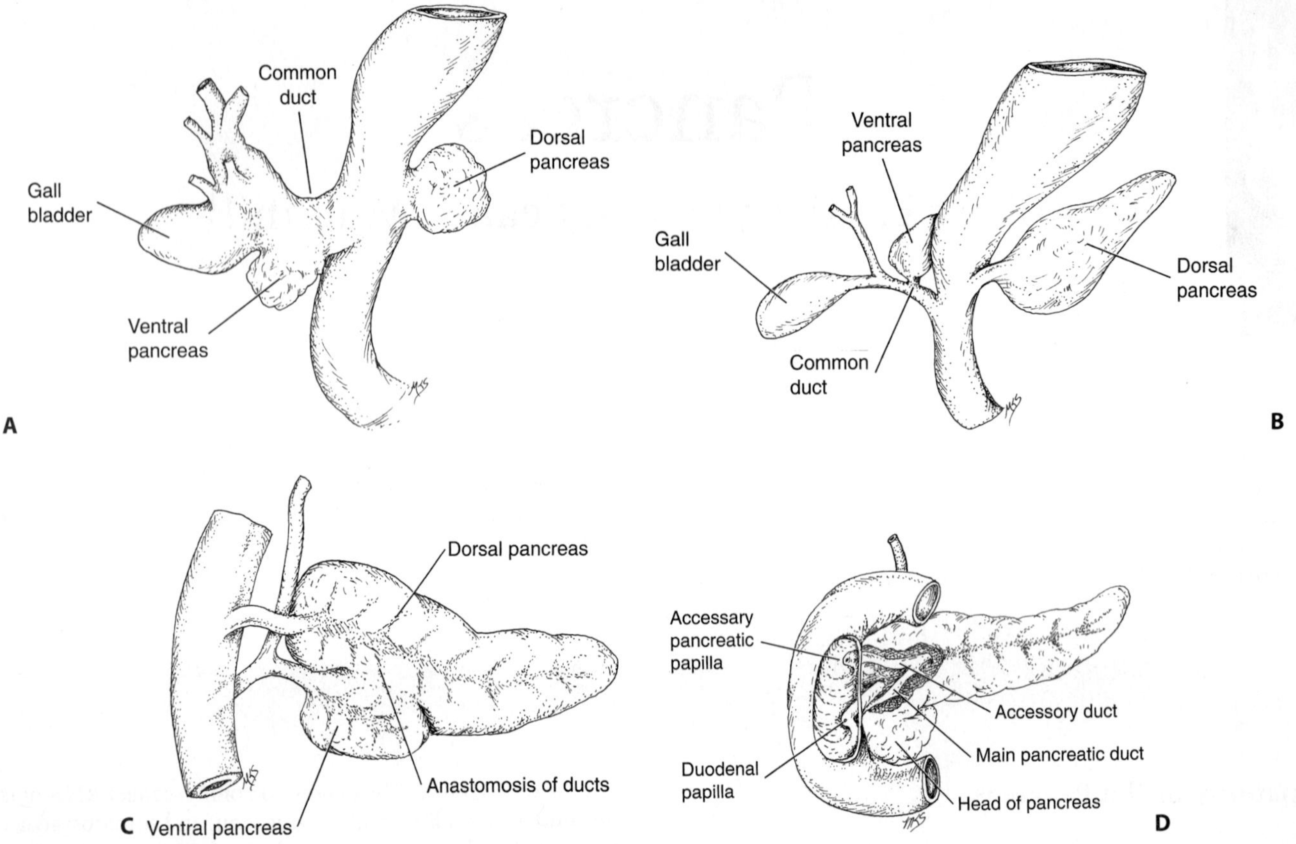

FIGURE 46.1. Embryologic development of the pancreas. The initial budding from the dorsal and ventral aspects of the foregut (**A**) is followed by clockwise rotation, beginning the C-loop of the duodenum and leading the dorsal bud to extend to the left and the ventral bud to extend to the right (**B**). By the seventh week of gestation, the ventral bud has continued to rotate around the foregut to fuse with the dorsal bud (**C**). The ductal system is beginning to develop at this time. (**D**) At term, there is fusion of the parenchyma, with the ventral bud forming the head and uncinate process of the pancreas and the dorsal bud forming the body, tail, and a portion of the head of the gland. The ductal system similarly fuses. The main pancreatic duct has a short common channel with the bile duct because of their common origin.

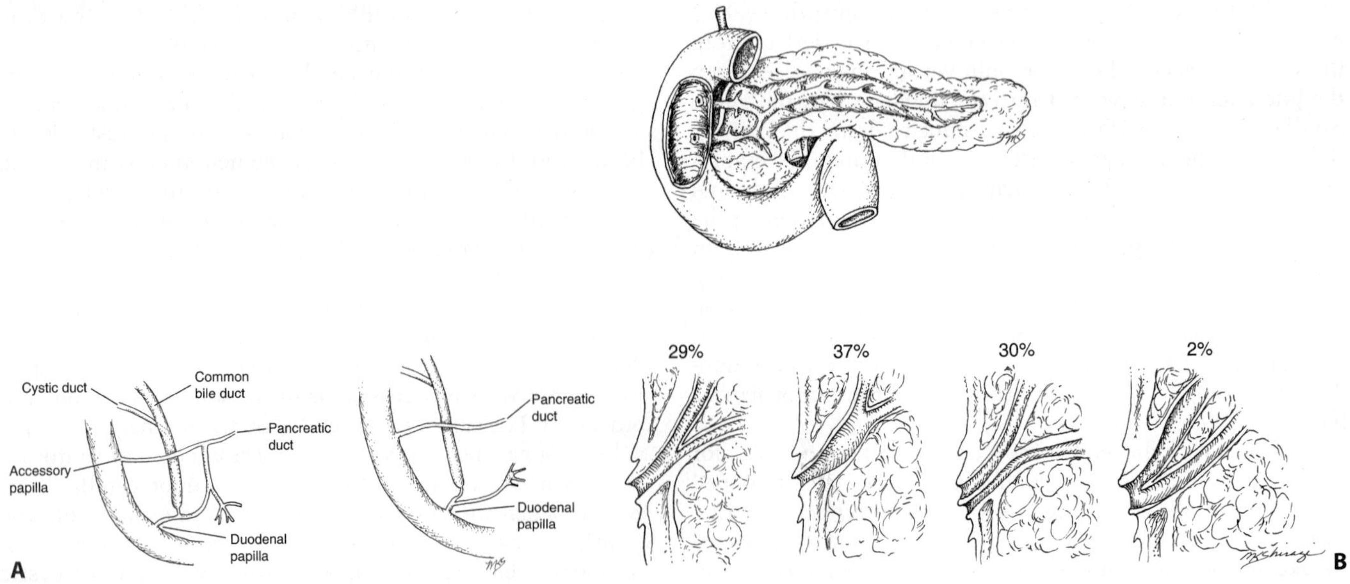

FIGURE 46.2. Pancreatic ductal anatomy. The pancreatic ductal anatomy is complex as a result of the embryologic origins from the ventral and dorsal buds. In most patients, the duct of Wirsung (the main pancreatic duct), drains the uncinate process, most of the head of the gland, and the body and tail (**A**). In a small fraction of patients, the ducts of the ventral and dorsal buds fail to fuse, leading to pancreas divisum (**B**). In this arrangement, the Wirsung's duct drains only the uncinate process and a portion of the head of the gland.

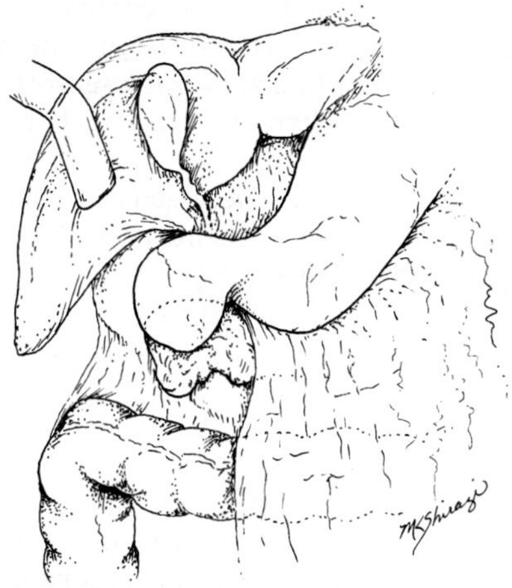

FIGURE 46.3. Annular pancreas. Annular pancreas is a congenital anomaly characterized by circumferential pancreatic tissue around the duodenum, occasionally leading to obstruction. It is best treated with duodenojejunostomy.

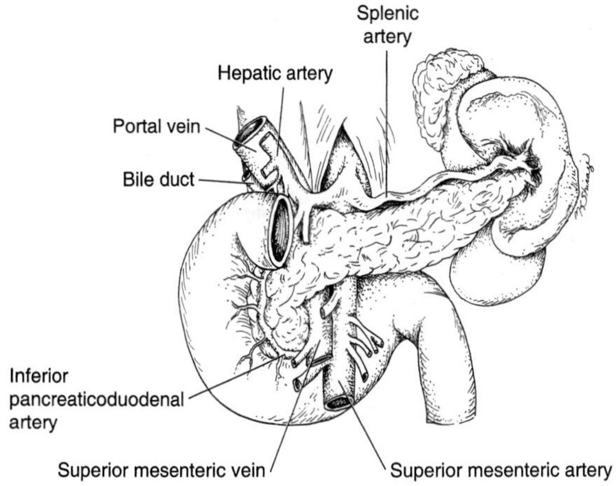

FIGURE 46.4. Anatomy of the pancreas. An anterior view of the pancreas, showing the major relationships with the duodenum, spleen, splenic artery, superior mesenteric artery, and superior mesenteric vein.

the duodenum, usually just proximal to the ampulla of Vater (Fig. 46.3). Annular pancreas may be an incidental finding or it may cause obstruction. An anomalous junction of the bile and pancreatic ducts near the ampulla of Vater has been associated with the presence of choledochal cysts and the development of acute pancreatitis.

Anatomic Relationships

The normal pancreas is about 15 cm in length, weighs approximately 120 g, and is located in the retroperitoneum, covered by a thin peritoneum (Fig. 46.4). The head of the gland lies nestled in the C-loop of the second part of the duodenum, and the tail of the gland extends obliquely into the hilum of the spleen. The superior mesenteric vein passes from the small-bowel mesentery toward the liver behind the neck of the pancreas, where it joins the splenic vein to become the portal vein. The inferior mesenteric vein similarly runs in a cephalad direction from the left colon mesentery behind the body of the pancreas near the ligament of Treitz to join the superior mesenteric and portal vein confluence. The splenic vein courses posterior to the body of the pancreas, and the splenic artery runs from its celiac origin to the spleen along the cephalad aspect of the pancreatic body. The body of the pancreas lies anterior to the left kidney and adrenal gland. The head of the pancreas lies anterior to the inferior vena cava, which can be exposed with the Kocher maneuver. The neck of the pancreas overlies the spine, where it is susceptible to injury in blunt abdominal trauma.

Blood Supply, Lymphatic Drainage, and Innervation

The pancreas has a redundant arterial blood supply, as shown in Figure 46.5. The head of the gland is supplied by paired (anterior and posterior) pancreaticoduodenal arteries, which course along the interface between the duodenum and the head of the pancreas. The celiac artery branches supply the right cephalic portion of the pancreatic head (dorsal anlag), the region around the intrapancreatic portion of the bile duct, and the first and second portions of the duodenum. The superior mesenteric artery branches supply the left caudal portion of the pancreatic head (ventral anlag) and the third and fourth

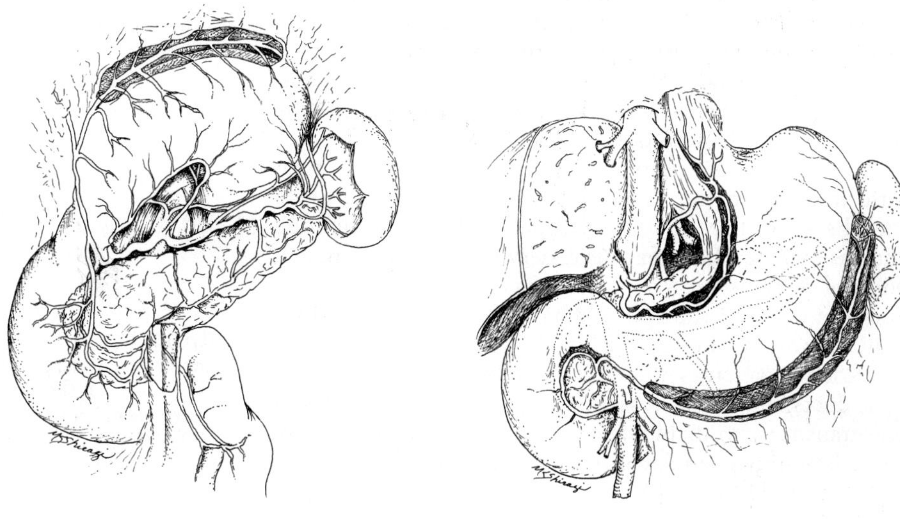

FIGURE 46.5. Blood supply to the pancreas. The pancreas has a rich blood supply from anterior and posterior pancreaticoduodenal arteries in the head of the gland and multiple small branches from the splenic artery in the body and tail.

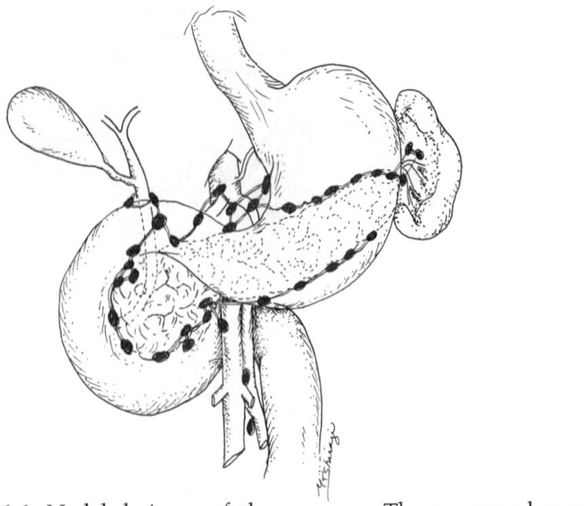

FIGURE 46.6. Nodal drainage of the pancreas. The pancreas has a rich lymphatic system, draining to pancreaticoduodenal, splenic, and hepatic nodes.

portions of the duodenum. The body of the gland is supplied by small branches from the splenic artery. The venous drainage of the pancreas is entirely into the portal vein. In the head and uncinate process of the pancreas, venous drainage is via small branches of the superior mesenteric and portal veins. Most of these branches enter the superior mesenteric and portal veins on their right lateral and posterior aspects. Usually, no veins drain from the neck of the gland to the anterior surface of the portal vein, making this plane of dissection safe during pancreaticoduodenectomy. The venous drainage from the body of the gland is into the splenic vein via small, unnamed branches.

The pancreas is drained by an extensive network of lymphatic channels, which coalesce into lymph nodes. These nodal drainage basins have importance in the treatment of patients with pancreatic cancer, for which nodal metastasis is common. Major draining nodal basins from the pancreas are shown in Figure 46.6. In the head of the gland, the initial drainage is to pancreaticoduodenal nodes, located near the groove between the pancreas and duodenum. Additional drainage is to nodes along the hepatoduodenal ligament, including those along the right lateral aspect of the portal vein and along the hepatic artery. Secondary drainage is seen to celiac and periaortic lymph nodes from the hepatic and gastroduodenal regions. From the uncinate process, drainage is toward the superior mesenteric arterial nodes and from there to the periaortic chain. From the body of the pancreas, drainage is mainly to nodes along the splenic artery and splenic hilum and from there to the celiac and periaortic nodes.

The pancreas is innervated extrinsically by parasympathetic fibers from the vagus nerve and sympathetic fibers from the splanchnic nerves. Ganglia are found within the pancreas, where these extrinsic nerves terminate on cell bodies of neurons intrinsic to the pancreas. These intrinsic neurons are part of the ENS and have abundant connections to the central nervous system via the vagal and splanchnic nerves. In the pancreas, these enteric neurons innervate acini, islets, ducts, and blood vessels. They largely use peptides as neurotransmitters, including vasoactive intestinal polypeptide, calcitonin gene-related peptide, neuropeptide Y, somatostatin, and others. In addition to efferent signals to the pancreas from the central nervous system, the pancreas has a rich network of afferent fibers, carrying sensory information centrally. These visceral afferent fibers largely pass via spinal nerves to the dorsal root ganglia, although the vagus nerves also contain afferent fibers. These sensory fibers are likely involved in pain perception in disorders such as chronic pancreatitis and pancreatic cancer.

Microscopic Anatomy

The pancreas is a finely nodular gland comprised of exocrine tissue (80% of the total mass), ducts, vessels, nerves, and connective tissue (18% of the total mass) and endocrine tissue, the islets of Langerhans (2% of the total mass). The exocrine portion of the gland is made up of pancreatic acinar cells, arranged in spherical masses termed *acini*, which in turn are grouped together as lobules. Pancreatic exocrine secretions are drained via small ductules originating in the acini, becoming progressively larger in the lobules and eventually emptying into the main pancreatic duct. The small ductules in the acini are lined by small, pale-staining centroacinar cells. The larger ducts are lined by columnar epithelium, with occasional goblet cells and argentaffin cells. The goblet cells secrete mucus. The argentaffin cells contain peptides important in the regulation of pancreatic secretion. The centroacinar and ductal epithelial cells contain the enzyme carbonic anhydrase and are responsible for the secretion of water and bicarbonate in pancreatic juice.

Pancreatic acinar cells are large and pyramidal shaped. Their basolateral aspect is in contact with nerves, blood vessels, and a connective tissue stroma, and their apical aspect converges on the central lumen of the acinus (Fig. 46.7) The apical aspect of acinar cells is packed with eosinophilic zymogen granules. These granules contain the enzymes manufactured by the extensive rough endoplasmic reticulum, found in the basolateral area of the cell, and packaged by the

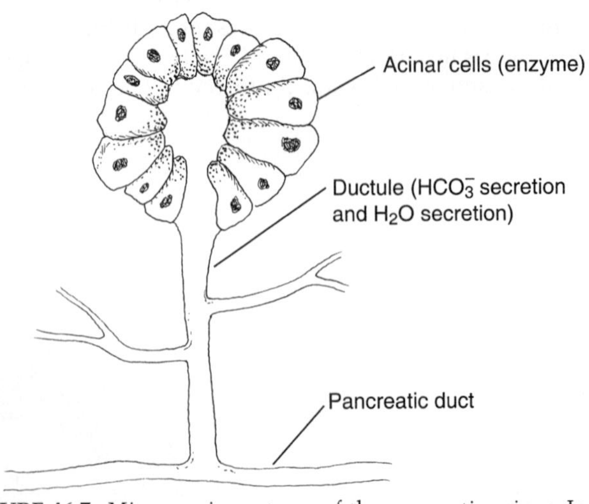

FIGURE 46.7. Microscopic anatomy of the pancreatic acinus. In the pancreatic acinus, the cells are arranged around a central ductule. The apical region of the acinar cells contains the machinery necessary for exocytosis of secretory granules. The basolateral surface of the acinar cell is exposed to a rich capillary bed. This region of the cell contains specific receptors for secretagogues such as cholecystokinin.

Golgi complex, a clear area located between the cell nucleus and the cell apex. The microscopic anatomy of the acinar cell changes cyclically in response to feeding or cholecystokinin (CCK) stimulation. With stimulation, the zymogen granules in the apex of the cell are depleted as they empty enzymes into the ductule lumen. Numerous mitochondria are found in the cell cytoplasm, providing the energy required for enzyme manufacture and release. George Palade and his colleagues were awarded the Nobel Prize in 1984 for their work describing the intracellular pathway of manufacture and secretion of proteins in the pancreatic acinar cell (Fig. 46.8).[10]

The islets of Langerhans are small islands of endocrine cells within a sea of exocrine tissue (Fig. 46.9). The pancreas contains approximately 1 million islets, distributed throughout the gland. The islets contain four endocrine cell types: (1) *B cells* account for 50%–80% of the total islet volume and contain insulin; (2) *PP cells* account for 10%–35% of the islet volume and contain pancreatic polypeptide; (3) *A cells* account for 5%–20% of the islet volume and contain glucagon; and (4) *D cells* account for less than 5% of the islet volume and contain somatostatin. Each cell produces only one peptide. Islets derived from the ventral embryonic bud tend to be rich in pancreatic polypeptide, whereas those from the dorsal bud tend to be rich in glucagon, for unknown reasons. During embryologic development, gastrin has been identified in the islets by immunochemical staining, but this expression is absent by term.

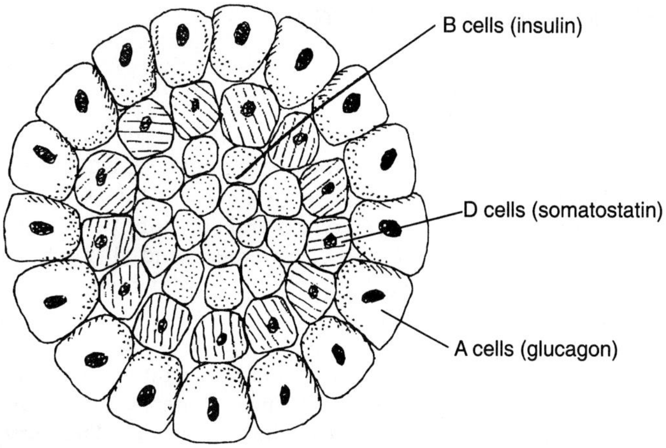

FIGURE 46.9. Microscopic appearance of the islets of Langerhans. The islets of Langerhans contain hormones, including insulin, glucagon, and somatostatin, involved in regulation of blood glucose levels. The islets are scattered throughout the pancreas within a sea of exocrine tissue. The islets can be well seen through the use of special immunoreactive stains, such as this one to chromogranin.

The islets have an important anatomical relationship to the acini, reflecting their role in regulation of exocrine as well as endocrine secretion. The islets are separated from the acini by a fine reticular layer. Acini surrounding the islets are distinguished from acini located away from islets by their larger cell and zymogen granule size. In addition, the islet blood supply is via a rich network of arterioles and capillaries in parallel with the acinar blood supply. The venous drainage from the islet, however, is arranged as a capillary portal system passing through nearby acini, presumably allowing a local influence of islet hormones such as insulin on acinar secretion (Fig. 46.10).

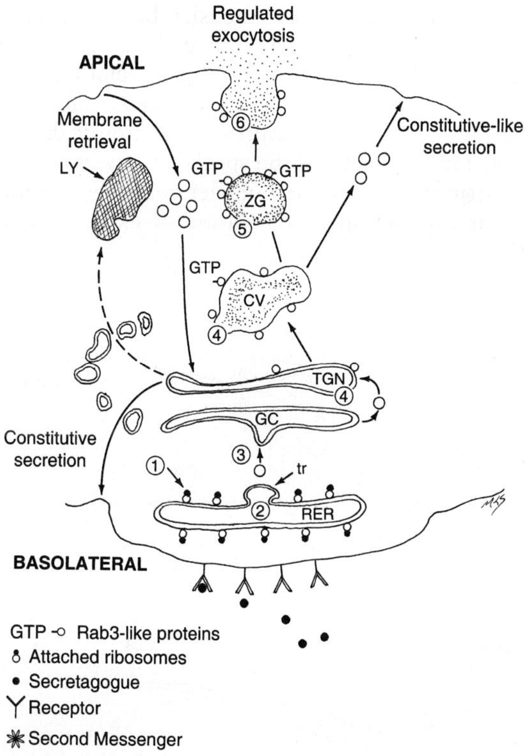

FIGURE 46.8. Pathway for the manufacture and secretion of enzymes in the pancreatic acinar cell. Palade and coworkers used the acinar cell as a model to identify the pathways of manufacture and secretion of enzymes. Pulse-chase techniques led them to identify the rough endoplasmic reticulum as the site of manufacture of proteins and the Golgi apparatus as the site of packaging into condensing granules.[10,201]

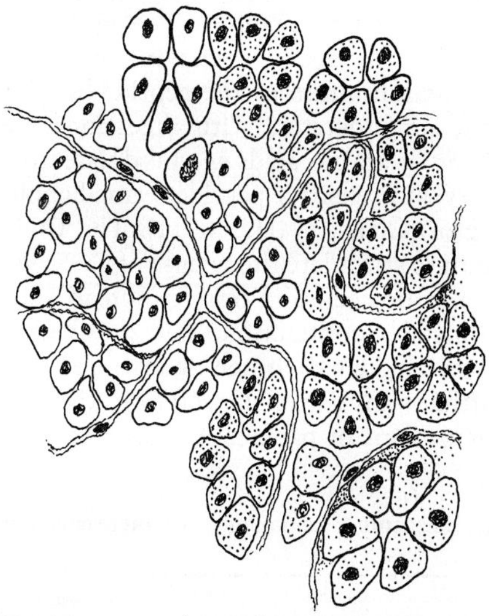

FIGURE 46.10. Anatomic relationships in the islet. The islets have a close relationship anatomically to the exocrine gland. Blood from the islet drains via a capillary bed to nearby exocrine lobules, influencing exocrine secretion. This anatomic arrangement is one clue to the presence of an islet-acinar axis regulating endocrine and exocrine secretion from the pancreas.

Physiology of the Pancreas

Exocrine Function

The pancreas has a major exocrine function in the production of digestive enzymes. These include (1) amylase, which functions in the breakdown of starches; (2) lipase, which functions to hydrolyze fatty acids; (3) trypsin and chymotrypsin, which function to degrade proteins in the meal; and (4) nucleases such as deoxyribonuclease and ribonuclease, which function to break down DNA and RNA, respectively. These enzymes are largely made and stored in the pancreas in an inactive form and are activated after secretion by the duodenal epithelial brush border enzyme enterokinase. Enterokinase hydrolyses trypsinogen to its active form, trypsin. The latter molecule in turn activates other proenzymes. To prevent damage from inadvertent intrapancreatic activation of digestive enzymes, a trypsin inhibitor is also secreted by the pancreas. The components of pancreatic juice and their normal concentrations are summarized in Tables 46.1 and 46.2.

Pancreatic juice is clear, colorless, and alkaline. In addition to its organic constituents, pancreatic juice contains a number of inorganic salts, including Na^+, K^+, Cl^-, and HCO_3^-. The concentrations of Cl^- and HCO_3^- are reciprocally linked according to the volume of secretion. The daily total volume of secretion of pancreatic juice is approximately 2.5 L. The hormone secretin, found in duodenal epithelium, is released in response to duodenal acidification and stimulates pancreatic water and bicarbonate secretion from pancreatic ductal and centroacinar cells, increasing pancreatic ductal flow from a basal rate of 0.2 mL/min to a maximal rate of 4 mL/min.

Secretin was the first hormone identified, through the 1902 efforts of Bayliss and Starling.[11] They found that duodenal acidification stimulated pancreatic exocrine secretion, and that this effect could be reproduced by intravenous injection of a crude extract of duodenal epithelium. This was the first documentation of the concept of an endocrine factor produced in one location and circulating through the bloodstream to affect another organ.

In the basal state, pancreatic enzyme secretion is minimal due to the tonic inhibition by the peptide hormone and neurocrine agent somatostatin. With ingestion of a meal, the presence of fat or amino acids in the duodenum stimulates release of a trypsin-sensitive peptide termed cholecystokinin-releasing factor (CCK-RF) (Fig. 46.11). The CCK-RF acts in the duodenum to stimulate the release of CCK, which in term stimulates enzyme secretion from pancreatic acinar cells as well as gallbladder contraction. The presence of activated trypsin in the duodenal lumen inactivates CCK-RF, thus reducing further stimulation of secretion. Cholecystokinin is the major stimulant of pancreatic exocrine secretion, but a number of other neurocrine agents are also involved, including acetylcholine, vasoactive intestinal polypeptide, gastrin-releasing peptide, and substance P. The main inhibitor of pancreatic exocrine secretion is somatostatin.

TABLE 46.1. Inorganic Components of Pancreatic Juice During Secretion.

Component	*Amount or concentration*
Water	1500–3000 mL per day
Sodium	140 mmol/L
Potassium	10 mmol/L
Chloride	20 mmol/L
Bicarbonate	110 mmol/L

TABLE 46.2. Pancreatic Digestive Enzymes.

Proteases
Trypsin
Chymotrypsin
Carboxypeptidases
Amylolytics
Amylase
Lipases
Lipase
Phospholipase A_2
Nucleases
Deoxyribonuclease (DNAse)
Ribonuclease (RNAse)

Endocrine Function

Besides secretion of digestive enzymes, a second major function of the pancreas is in regulation of blood glucose levels. The islets of Langerhans, which contain the endocrine cells of the pancreas, are distributed widely throughout the gland. Three main cell types make up the islets: alpha cells, which produce glucagon; beta cells, which produce insulin; and delta cells, which produce somatostatin. The organization of these cells within the islet follows a specific pattern, with the alpha cells rimming the outer part of the islet, beta cells making up the core, and delta cells distributed at the interface between the alpha and delta cells. The islet has a special venous drainage that bathes the acinar (exocrine) glands before entering the portal vein. These two features, the anatomic distribution of cells within the islet and the special islet venous drainage, likely contribute to regulation of islet hormone secretion and islet–acinar interaction in regulation of exocrine enzymes, respectively.

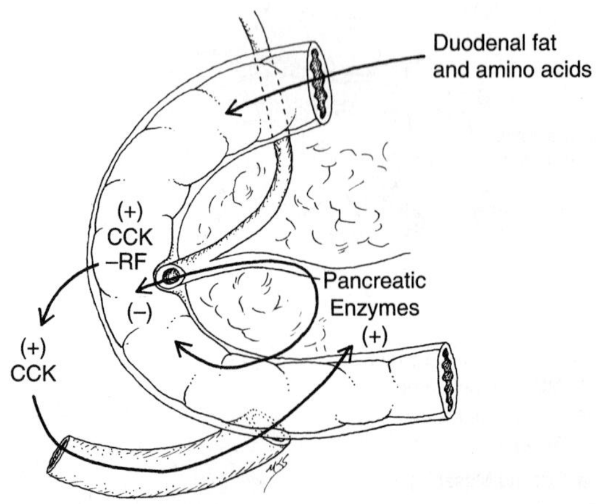

FIGURE 46.11. Mechanism of meal-stimulated pancreatic exocrine secretion. The presence of fat and protein in a meal stimulates the release of the trypsin-sensitive CCK-releasing factor from the duodenal epithelium, which in turn stimulates the release of CCK. The CCK acts hormonally to stimulate gallbladder contraction and enzyme secretion from the pancreatic acinar cells. When trypsinogen is activated in the duodenal lumen, it destroys CCK-releasing factor, reducing the degree of stimulation.

Acute Pancreatitis

Background

Acute pancreatitis is an inflammatory disorder of the pancreas with local and systemic manifestations. About 5000 new cases per year are seen in the United States, with an overall mortality rate of 10%, making pancreatitis a significant health problem.[12] Pancreatitis can be categorized as acute or chronic. The two forms can be differentiated by their differing clinical presentation and radiographic findings. An international symposium on pancreatitis held in Atlanta in 1992 reached consensus on terminology to describe various conditions related to pancreatitis (Table 46.3).[13]

Acute pancreatitis is best defined as an acute inflammatory disease of the pancreas with variable involvement of distant organs such as the lung, kidney, and heart. Two main pathologic forms of acute pancreatitis are recognizable: (1) a mild, interstitial or edematous pancreatitis characterized by interstitial edema and infiltration of polymorphonuclear cells and (2) a more severe necrotizing pancreatitis characterized by focal or diffuse necrosis of both the pancreatic parenchyma and adjacent soft tissue. The former is usually a self-limited process, whereas the latter commonly results in infection; systemic manifestations such as pulmonary, renal, or cardiac failure; and death.

The surgeon plays a key role in the management of patients with pancreatitis. This includes the management of the critically ill patient with severe pancreatitis in the intensive care unit setting; control of acute complications of the illness, such as infection and bleeding; and management of underlying causes of pancreatitis, particularly gallstones. To carry out this role, the surgeon needs broad knowledge of the pathophysiology, natural history, and treatment options of this complex illness.

TABLE 46.3. Definitions of Terminology in Pancreatitis.

Acute interstitial pancreatitis: A mild, self-limited form of pancreatitis characterized by interstitial edema and an acute inflammatory response without necrosis, local complications, or systemic manifestations such as organ failure.

Necrotizing pancreatitis: A severe form of acute pancreatitis characterized by locoregional tissue necrosis and systemic manifestations such as pulmonary, renal, or cardiac failure.

Sterile necrosis: Acute pancreatitis leading to tissue necrosis without supervening infection.

Infected necrosis: Acute pancreatitis with locoregional tissue necrosis complicated by bacterial or fungal infection.

Acute fluid collections: A fluid collection occurring early in the course of acute pancreatitis, located in or near the pancreas, and lacking an epithelial lining or a defined wall of granulation or fibrous tissue.

Pancreatic pseudocyst: A pancreatic or peripancreatic fluid collection with a well-defined wall of granulation tissue and fibrosis and absence of an epithelial lining. Pancreatic pseudocysts can arise in the setting of chronic pancreatitis, as a sequelae of an episode of necrotizing pancreatitis. One of the common complications of pseudocyst is the development of infection.

Pancreatic cysts: A fluid-filled pancreatic mass with an epithelial lining. These may be neoplastic lesions, such as serous cystadenomas or mucinous cystic tumors, or congenital cysts.

Pancreatic abscess: A circumscribed intraabdominal collection of pus, usually in proximity to the pancreas, containing little or no pancreatic necrosis, and arising as a consequence of necrotizing pancreatitis or pancreatic trauma.

Suppurative cholangitis: Bacterial infection within the biliary tree, associated with ductal obstruction, usually from a stone or stricture.

Adapted from the Atlanta Classification.

Source: From Bradley,[13] by permission of *Archives of Surgery*.

TABLE 46.4. Causes of Acute Pancreatitis.

Cause	*Relative frequency in the United States*
Gallstones	40%
Alcohol	30%
Idiopathic	15%
Metabolic:	5%
Hyperlipidemia	
Hypercalcemia	
Cystic fibrosis	
Anatomic and functional lesions:	<5%
Pancreas divisum	
Pancreatic duct strictures or tumors	
Ampullary stenosis or obstruction	
Sphincter of Oddi dysfunction	
Mechanical insults:	<5%
Blunt abdominal trauma	
Intraoperative injury	
Endoscopic retrograde cholangiopancreatography (ERCP)	
Drugs:	<5%
Azathioprine, thiazide diuretics, pentamidine, dideoxyinosine (ddI), sulfonamides, corticosteroids, furosemide	
Infections and toxins:	<5%
Mumps, viral hepatitis, cytomegalovirus, ascariasis, scorpion venom, anticholinesterase insecticides	
Ischemia:	Rare
Cardiac surgery	
Vasculitis	
Hereditary	Rare
Miscellaneous	Case reports
Burn injury	
Long-distance running	

Pathophysiology

Acute pancreatitis has many and varied underlying causes. Common causes of acute pancreatitis are listed in Table 46.4. A major challenge is to understand the cell biology underlying these varied inciting factors and linking this insult to the known local and systemic sequelae of the disease.

In gallstone pancreatitis, the Opie hypothesis, described by a pathologist at Johns Hopkins Hospital in the Halstead era, attributed the process to impaction of a stone at the papilla with subsequent reflux of bile into the pancreatic duct via the common channel. It was subsequently recognized that stone impaction rarely occurred, but that transient obstruction due to stone passage into the duodenal lumen was common. Gallstones can be recovered in the stool within a week of the onset of illness in about 90% of patients with gallstone pancreatitis, whereas patients with biliary colic seldom pass gallstones.[14,15] Thus, our current thinking attributes gallstone pancreatitis to transient obstruction of the common channel of the bile duct and pancreatic duct during passage of a stone. This transient obstruction may need to be accompanied by stimulated secretion, as with a fatty meal, or other unknown factors, to result in acute pancreatitis.

The mechanism of alcohol-related pancreatitis is unclear but may relate to a direct toxic effect of alcohol on the acinar cell, an effect by alcohol causing proteinaceous plugging of small pancreatic ductules, or an indirect effect of alcohol causing duodenitis, ampullary spasm, and reflux of bile into the pancreatic duct.[16] In hyperlipidemia, the mechanism of induction of pancreatitis is unclear, but generally very high triglyceride levels, above 1000 mg/dL, are thought to damage acinar or capillary membranes. In hypercalcemia, trypsin activation may occur in the acinar cell, initiating cell damage and tissue necrosis.

A number of lesions causing obstruction of the pancreatic duct are known to cause pancreatitis, including papillary stenosis, sphincter of Oddi dysfunction, and tumors. Although unproven, these obstructive lesions are hypothesized to cause ductal hypertension during periods of stimulated secretion, leading to acinar damage and inflammation. Endoscopic retrograde cholangiopancreatography (ERCP)-induced pancreatitis may relate to dye toxicity, but most cases are associated with overfilling of the ductal system (acinarization) or procedures such as sphincterotomy.[17–19]

At the cellular level, animal models of pancreatitis revealed several uniform findings (Fig. 46.12).[20] First, the normal process of exocytosis of secretory granules at the apical region of the acinar cell is blocked. Second, colocalization of zymogen granules and lysosomes occurs in the cytoplasm. Third, these fusion vacuoles migrate to the basolateral cell surface, where they may discharge their contents into the interstitium. The blockade of exocytosis in these models may explain the relative inefficacy of inhibitors of pancreatic exocrine secretion, such as glucagon, somatostatin, and octreotide, in the treatment of acute pancreatitis. Colocalization of zymogens with lysosomal enzymes may be important in inducing intracellular activation of trypsinogen, thought to be a key step in pathogenesis. Discharge of these activated enzymes into the interstitial space may hasten the development of an inflammatory response, edema, and necrosis. The contribution of the immune response to the pathophysiology of pancreatitis is under intensive study. It appears that immunocyte cytokine release likely plays a role in the systemic manifestations of severe pancreatitis, including respiratory failure, increased capillary permeability, and shock.

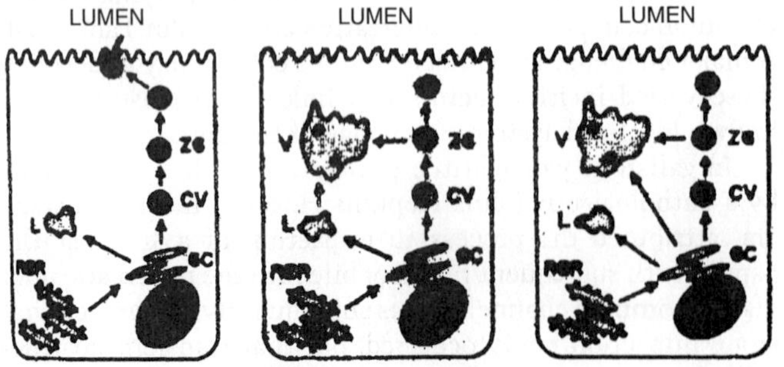

FIGURE 46.12. Cell biology of acute pancreatitis in animal models. The cell biology of pancreatitis has been difficult to study in the human, but several animal models have been developed. A common thread in early pancreatitis is inhibition of exocytosis, colocalization of secretory granules with lysosomes, and migration of these abnormal vesicles to the basolateral cell surface. (Adapted from Steer and Meldolesi.[20])

Clinical Presentation

The most prominent symptom in patients with acute pancreatitis is abdominal pain. Typically, the pain is located diffusely across the upper abdomen and radiates through to the back. In most patients, the onset of pain is relatively sudden, and may mimic other intraabdominal catastrophes such as perforated ulcer. The pain is usually severe and steady in nature, without the cramping characteristic of bowel obstruction or the waxing and waning course of renal colic. Nausea and vomiting frequently accompany the pain. Vomiting does not alleviate the pain.

On physical examination, the patient is usually found lying still in bed as movement exacerbates the discomfort. Low-grade fever is typically present at the outset of the illness, and high fevers to 39°C may be present within 2 or 3 days in severely afflicted patients. Tachycardia is commonly present, along with other signs of intravascular volume depletion. The abdomen is mildly distended, with tenderness and guarding in the upper quadrants. A picture of diffuse peritonitis can be seen in severe cases, usually without the board-like quality of perforated duodenal ulcer. Although not commonly seen today, occasional patients presenting with retroperitoneal hemorrhage have ecchymoses in the flanks (Grey Turner sign) or the periumbilical area (Cullen sign). Associated physical signs include diminished breath sounds with dullness at the lung bases from consolidation or effusion. In patients with gallstone pancreatitis, jaundice may be present, reflecting biliary obstruction from a gallstone. Pancreatitis related to alcohol ingestion may be accompanied by stigmata of chronic liver disease.

Diagnostic Evaluation

The most useful single test in the diagnosis of pancreatitis is the serum amylase level. Hyperamylasemia occurs early in the course of acute pancreatitis, and its return to normal levels generally follows the improving clinical course of uncomplicated patients. Hyperamylasemia is not specific for pancreatitis, however, as it has been described in a number of unrelated conditions (Table 46.5). The level of amylase elevation does not correlate with the severity of the illness. In the presence of hypertriglyceridemia, serum amylase levels may be falsely low.

Other blood tests useful in the diagnosis of pancreatitis include the white blood cell count, which is usually moderately elevated. In the presence of pancreatic necrosis, the white blood cell count may rise markedly. Hyperglycemia is common in acute pancreatitis, but nonspecific. Liver function tests are commonly transiently elevated in pancreatitis. A meta-analysis has shown that an alanine transaminase elevation greater than 150 IU/L has a 96% specificity for gallstone pancreatitis as opposed to other causes.[21] Serum lipase measurements are roughly as sensitive as amylase measurements in the diagnosis of acute pancreatitis. Lipase remains elevated somewhat longer in the course of illness than amylase, and it is somewhat more specific as lipase is not found in organs such as the salivary glands and ovaries. Other tests, including

TABLE 46.5. Causes of Hyperamylasemia.

Causes associated with acute abdominal pain	*Miscellaneous causes*
Acute pancreatitis	Mumps
Pancreatic ascites	Acute parotitis
Perforated viscus	Scorpion bites
Pancreatic pseudocyst	Ovarian cysts and tumors
Acute cholecystitis	Lung cancer
Small-bowel obstruction	Renal failure
Acute appendicitis	Macroamylasemia
Ruptured ectopic pregnancy	Endoscopic retrograde cholangiopancreatography
Acute salpingitis	Diabetic ketoacidosis
	Intracranial hemorrhage
	HIV infection

serum immunoreactive trypsin, phopholipase A_2, pancreatitis-associated protein, C-reactive protein, and pancreatic-specific protein have been described as markers for acute pancreatitis, but they are not in common clinical use. Serum calcium levels often fall in the course of pancreatitis. This is mainly due to a concomitant fall in serum albumin as serum ionized calcium levels remain normal in most patients.

Radiographic assessment of patients with pancreatitis should include right upper quadrant ultrasonography in those suspected of gallstones as the cause. In severely ill patients, computed tomography (CT) should be performed to assess the degree of necrosis present and identify fluid collections. Endoscopic ultrasound, magnetic resonance cholangiopancreatography, and ERCP play a diagnostic role in identifying certain causes of pancreatitis, such as gallstones, pancreas divisum, ductal strictures, and tumors, and ERCP plays a therapeutic role in selected patients with complicated gallstone pancreatitis.[22,23]

Measures of Severity of Pancreatitis

The severity of pancreatitis can be estimated with both clinical and radiographic criteria. The Ranson criteria for estimating severity are the most commonly used clinical system (Table 46.6). These 11 criteria were found, in multivariate analysis, to predict survival in patients with acute pancreatitis.[24,25] These criteria include five measured at the time of presentation and six others measured during the initial 48h of treatment. Patients with fewer than three of these criteria present were found to have uniformly good outcomes, whereas

TABLE 46.6. Ranson Criteria for Assessing Severity of Acute Pancreatitis.

Criteria at admission	*Criteria within the first 48h*
Age > 55 years	Drop in hematocrit >10%
White blood cell count >16,000/mm³	Fluid deficit >6000Ml
Serum glucose >200mg/dL	Serum calcium <8.0mg/dL
Serum LDH (lactate dehydrogenase) >350IU/L	Hypoxemia (Po_2 < 60mmHg)
Serum AST (aspartate aminotransferase) >250U/dL	Rise in BUN (serum urea nitrogen) >5mg/dL
	Base deficit >4mEq/L

From Ranson et al.,[24] by permission of *Surgical Gynecology and Obstetrics.*

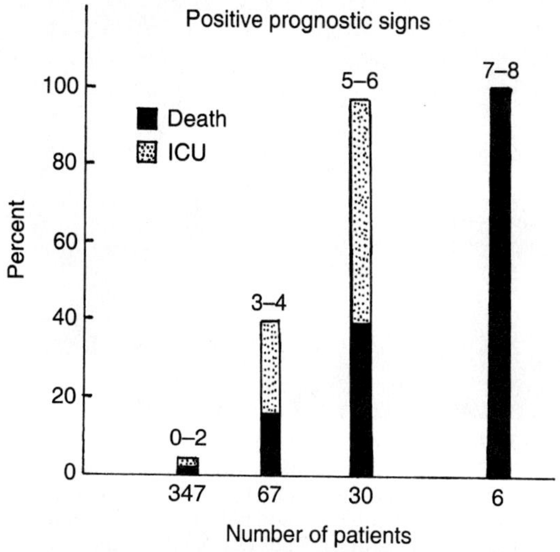

FIGURE 46.13. Mortality rate in acute pancreatitis related to Ranson's criteria. Ranson's criteria to estimate the severity of pancreatitis are useful clinically as they relate directly to the risk of patient death. (Data redrawn from Ranson et al.[24,25])

the mortality rate increased substantially in the presence of greater numbers of criteria (Fig. 46.13).

The Acute Physiology and Chronic Health Evaluation II (APACHE-II) Severity of Disease Classification System has also been used to predict outcome in acute pancreatitis.[26–30] This system has the advantage of repeated measurements over time. Scores less than 9 predict mild pancreatitis and high survival rates, whereas scores over 13 have a higher likelihood of mortality. The APACHE-II system is far more complex than Ranson's criteria, however, making it less commonly used.

The recognition of the importance of necrosis in determining outcome was recognized with the development of CT staging systems to estimate severity of pancreatitis.[27,31,32] Today, helical, or spiral, CT using rapid bolus intravenous contrast, 5-mm slice reconstruction, and a breath-hold technique gives the best pancreatic resolution. Necrosis in more than 50% of the gland, the presence of extensive peripancreatic fluid collections, and the presence of gas within the pancreas or adjacent soft tissue are all markers predicting poor outcome.[31] A typical scan depicting severe pancreatitis is shown in Figure 46.14.

Treatment of Pancreatitis

Mild-to-Moderate Acute Pancreatitis

Most patients with pancreatitis have a relatively mild, self-limited disease. The average patient with pancreatitis of mild-to-moderate severity should be initially supported with intravenous hydration and pain medications. Specific adjunctive treatments, such as inhibition of pancreatic secretion and antiproteases, do not improve the clinical course of the average patient.[33–35] Nasogastric tube suction, when used routinely, appears to have no benefit[36] but should be considered for patients with significant vomiting. In patients with gallstone pancreatitis, a laparoscopic cholecystectomy should be performed at a convenient time before discharge.[37] An intraoperative cholangiogram should be obtained during cholecys-

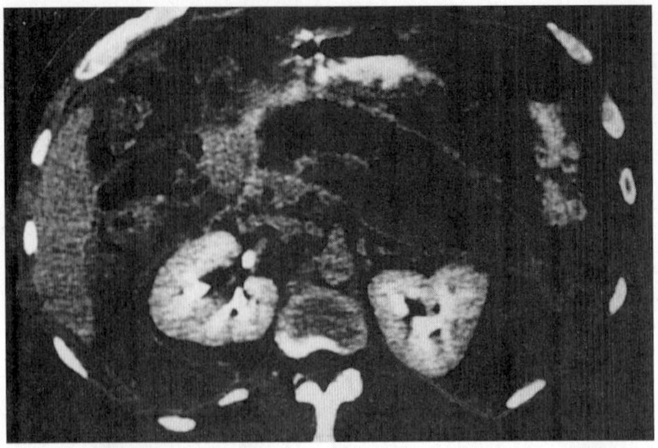

FIGURE 46.14. Computed tomography in necrotizing pancreatitis. Spiral CT with bolus intravenous contrast and thin-cut reconstruction through the pancreas is an important clinical tool in estimating the severity of acute pancreatitis and identifying complications, such as pseudocyst, abscess, and infected necrosis. In this scan, extensive necrosis is present in the body of the gland.

tectomy, and if common bile duct stones are found, a laparoscopic common bile duct exploration or postoperative endoscopic sphincterotomy with stone extraction should be performed. The outcome with this strategy is excellent, with common bile duct stones found in 7%–20% of patients.[38–42]

For patients with mild, interstitial pancreatitis, early cholecystectomy has been shown to reduce recurrent episodes of pancreatitis and overall patient morbidity. Conversion rates for laparoscopic cholecystectomy performed during the initial hospitalization for mild acute pancreatitis are 0%–15%, with morbidity and mortality rates similar to laparoscopic cholecystectomy for uncomplicated biliary colic.[38,40–43] Following an initial attack of mild gallstone pancreatitis, 25%–44% of patients managed nonoperatively can expect to have recurrent pancreatitis or other gallstone-related complications within 6 months.[44–46] Recurrent episodes of pancreatitis are likely to be more severe than the initial episode and associated with a higher rate of pancreatitis-associated morbidity and mortality.[47]

Severe Acute Pancreatitis

The patient with severe acute pancreatitis due to any cause is at risk for the development of complications for which surgical decision making plays a central role. Several recent advances have improved outcome in patients with severe pancreatitis, including (1) improved intensive care unit management of pulmonary, renal, and cardiac failure; (2) use of contrast-enhanced CT to improve staging and detect complications such as pancreatic infection; (3) improved nutritional support begun early in the course of the disease; (4) development of interventional radiologic techniques to manage certain complications; and (5) the availability of endoscopic sphincterotomy to treat impacted stones and cholangitis.

A small group of patients with severe acute pancreatitis may benefit from an early approach to clearing the common bile duct. This group is critically ill at presentation and fails to improve in the first 12–24h of treatment. If gallstones are confirmed radiographically by transabdominal or endoscopic ultrasound or magnetic resonance cholangiopancreatography (MRCP), an ERCP with sphincterotomy and stone extraction within the first 48h decreases mortality[48] (Table 46.7). Laparoscopic cholecystectomy is delayed until recovery from the pancreatitis. While preferably done during the same hospitalization, timing of surgery will depend on the patient's recovery and sufficient resolution of the retroperitoneal inflammation to allow for adequate exposure and safe dissection of gallbladder.

Sterile Necrosis

Necrotizing pancreatitis can produce necrotic areas of pancreas and retroperitoneal tissue without becoming infected. The clinical course of some of these patients is relatively benign, but in others the clinical course mimics that of patients with necrosis complicated by infection. If the patient is improving clinically, then conservative therapy is appropriate. If fever, leukocytosis, abdominal pain, ileus, or organ dysfunction are present, then CT-guided percutaneous aspiration of necrotic areas should be performed to rule out infection. If the Gram stain and culture of this material are sterile, bowel rest, total parenteral nutrition, analgesics, and intravenous antibiotics are appropriate treatment.[49,50]

Using this approach, Bradley and Allen,[51] for example, found that of 38 patients with necrosis, infection supervened in 27, and 11 were sterile. These 11 patients with sterile necrosis were managed nonoperatively and recovered without mortality, even in the face of pulmonary failure requiring mechanical ventilation. Similarly, in a retrospective study from Uhl, of 172 patients with sterile necrosis, about one-third were managed nonoperatively with admirably low

TABLE 46.7.
Randomized, Controlled Clinical Trials of Early Endoscopic Sphincterotomy in Gallstone Pancreatitis.

First author, reference, institution, year	*Patient groups*	*Mortality rate*	*Biliary sepsis rate*	*Comments*
Neoptolemos,[202] England, 1988	Early ERCP/ES (n = 59) Selective ERCP (n = 62)	1.7% ($P < .05$) 8.0%	6 of 25 severe pancreatitis patients ($P < .05$) 17 of 28 severe pancreatitis patients	Benefit confined to patients with severe pancreatitis; LOS also shortened by routine ERCP/ES
Fan,[203] Hong Kong, 1993	Early ERCP/ES (n = 97) Selective ERCP (n = 98)	5% (P = .4, NS) 9%	0% (P = .001) 12%	Benefit limited to patients with severe pancreatitis
Folsch,[204] European multicenter trial, 1995	Early ERCP/ES (n = 48) Selective ERCP (n = 52)	1% (NS) 2%	Cholangitis (odds ratio 3.3) and sepsis (odds ratio 3.5) slightly more frequent in selective group (NS)	No benefit observed with early, routine, endoscopic sphincterotomy

mortality (6.2%), whereas the two-thirds of patients managed operatively had a mortality of 13.1%.[52]

No randomized, controlled data exist to guide the clinician in this decision. In general, a worsening clinical course or failure to improve within 3 to 4 weeks are reasonable indications for debridement in the absence of infection. Persistent fever or stable organ system failure are not absolute indications for surgery, although a search for infection with fine-needle aspiration biopsy is warranted.

Necrotizing Pancreatitis with Infection

Infection can complicate severe acute pancreatitis as (1) infected pancreatic necrosis, (2) pancreatic abscess, (3) infected pseudocyst, and (4) acute suppurative cholangitis. These terms are defined in Table 46.3. Infected pancreatic necrosis is a fulminant infection occurring within the first 2 weeks of the onset of necrotizing pancreatitis. The reported incidence is 35%–40% in large series of patients with acute pancreatitis.[49,53] The usual pathogens are gram-negative rods from the gut, and in three-quarters of cases the infection is monomicrobial. The typical pathogens are shown in Table 46.8.

TABLE 46.8. Microbiology of Infected Pancreatic Necrosis.

Organism	*Frequency*
Escherichia coli	40%
Klebsiella	18%
Enterobacter	18%
Streptococcus	14%
Staphylococcus aureus	10%
Proteus	9%
Pseudomonas	8%
Bacteroides	8%
Enterococcus	8%
Candida	7%

Note: Numbers do not total 100% because of polymicrobial flora.
Source: Data from references 49, 58, and 205.

Randomized, controlled clinical data suggest that early, empiric antibiotic treatment in patients with severe acute pancreatitis decreases infectious complications and mortality (Table 46.9).[54] Mortality rates in infected necrosis as high as 25% have been reported in recent series.[49,55]

TABLE 46.9.
Randomized, Controlled Clinical Trials of Prophylactic Antibiotic Therapy in Necrotizing Pancreatitis.

First author, reference, year, center	*Patient groups*	*Infectious complications*	*Mortality rate*	*Comment*
Trials of intravenous antibiotics				
Pederzoli,[206] 1993, Italian multicenter trial	Imepenem (n = 41) Control (n = 33)	Pancreatic sepsis in 12.2% ($P < .01$) Nonpancreatic sepsis in 14.6% ($P < .01$) Pancreatic sepsis in 30.3% Nonpancreatic sepsis in 48.5%	7.3% (NS) 12.1%	Necrotizing pancreatitis only; imepenem has good penetration into pancreatic tissue; randomized, but not placebo controlled; significant improvement in pancreatic and other infection rates
Sainio,[207] 1995, Helsinki University	Cefuroxime (n = 30) Control (n = 30)	1.0 infections per patient ($P < .01$) 30% with pancreatic infection (NS) 1.8 infections per patient 40% with pancreatic infection	3.3% ($P = .03$) 23.3%	Enrollment of patients with necrotizing pancreatitis only; penetration data of cefuroxime unclear; good activity against expected pathogens; randomized, but not double blind or placebo controlled; only study to show improved mortality with intravenous antibiotics, but no improvement in pancreatic infection rate
Schwarz,[208] 1997, Chirurgische Clinik I	Ofloxacin and metronidazole (n = 13) Control (n = 13)	APACHE II scores (days 1, 5, 10) 15.0, 13.0, 9.5 11.5, 15.0, 16.0	0% 15%	Patients with acute necrotizing pancreatitis only; no difference in bacterial infection rates; significant improvements in mortality and overall clinical course
Nordback,[209] 2001, Johns Hopkins University	Imipenem (n = 25) Control (n = 33)	8% needed surgery 28% with complications 36% needed surgery 76% with complications	8% 15%	Reduction in infectious complications requiring surgery, major organ complications, and mortality
Isenmann,[210] 2004, German multicenter trial	Ciprofloxacin and metronidazole (n = 58) Control (n = 56)	12% 9%	5% 7%	No difference in the rate of systemic complications, infected necrosis, or mortality
Trials of selective gut decontamination				
Luiten,[211] 1995, Netherlands multicenter trial	Selective decontamination (n = 50) Control (n = 52)	Pancreatic infection in 18% ($P = .03$) Pancreatic infection in 38%	11 of 50, 22% ($P = .048$) 18 of 52, 35%	Enrollment criteria: Imrie score >3, Balthazar grade D or E Randomized, but not placebo controlled

In contrast, pancreatic abscess is less common, with an incidence of 2%, and generally does not develop until an average of 5 weeks following onset of pancreatitis.[13,56,57] Although the spectrum of responsible organisms is similar to that seen in infected pancreatic necrosis, multimicrobial involvement is far more common. Pancreatic abscess has a somewhat less-fulminant course and lesser mortality rate than infected necrosis.

Infection developing in preexisting pancreatic pseudocysts is a different problem and should be distinguished from infected necrosis or pancreatic abscess. These patients may develop a septic picture late in the course of pancreatitis. Infected pseudocysts generally are more indolent than infected necrosis or pancreatic abscess and commonly respond to external tube drainage and intravenous antibiotics.

Finally, cholangitis may complicate the course of acute pancreatitis if common bile duct obstruction occurs. This usually occurs in the setting of gallstone pancreatitis and may be fulminant. Relief of biliary obstruction by endoscopic papillotomy and stone extraction is the preferred management.

Patients with severe pancreatitis should undergo contrast-enhanced CT (CE-CT) examination. If hypoperfused areas suggestive of necrosis are identified and the patient's clinical condition is suggestive of infection, then CT-guided fine-needle aspiration is performed for Gram stain and culture to detect infection. In a series of 92 aspirations on 60 patients, Gerzof et al. found CT-guided aspiration to be free of complications with no false-positive examinations and a 2.4% rate of false-negative examinations.[58]

If infected pancreatic necrosis is identified, then the appropriate management is broad-spectrum intravenous antibiotics and immediate operative debridement. Techniques for subsequent management include closed passive (Penrose) drainage, closed-suction drainage, open packing (marsupialization), and peritoneal lavage. Multiple operative procedures are often required to debride the ongoing necrosis. Nonoperative drainage techniques are generally insufficient to adequately evacuate this necrotic tissue. No randomized data exist comparing these various treatment strategies, but good results have been reported in retrospective reviews with each technique.[55,59,60]

Peritoneal lavage is popular in some centers as an adjunctive therapy in patients with severe acute pancreatitis. The rationale for this treatment is the elimination of toxic substances that may collect within the peritoneal cavity during pancreatitis. It has been shown, for example, that proteolytic enzymes, complement, and various kinins are present in some patients.[61] Although early small, uncontrolled trials demonstrated some reduction in morbidity in patients treated with peritoneal lavage,[24,62] a larger, multicenter, randomized, controlled trial failed to show any benefit.[63]

Despite the serious nature of necrotizing pancreatitis with infection, the long-term results can be good. In a series of 40 patients requiring operative debridement at Duke University, the operative mortality rate was 18%. In follow-up, quality-of-life assessment with the Short Form-36 tool revealed comparable outcome of surviving patients to age-matched controls, patients with chronic pancreatitis treated medically, and patients with chronic pancreatitis managed surgically.[64]

Pancreatitis Complicated by Bleeding

Bleeding associated with acute necrotizing pancreatitis is a serious problem, with mortality rates in excess of 50%.[65] Bleeding may arise from extension of the necrotizing process into nearby major vessels, such as the gastroduodenal or splenic arteries, or from the gastrointestinal tract. The latter is usually secondary to severe stress gastritis or varices related to splenic vein thrombosis. Initial management of bleeding in this setting is by angiographic identification and embolization of the involved artery. Surgery is required if angiography is unsuccessful; however, these operations can be exceedingly difficult.[66] Fortunately, the incidence of hemorrhagic complications in severe acute pancreatitis is decreasing. This is thought to be due to improved early recognition and volume resuscitation of severely afflicted patients.

Management of Pancreatitis Associated with Pancreas Divisum

The incidence of pancreas divisum is about three- to fourfold higher in patients with recurring bouts of idiopathic pancreatitis than in unaffected controls. This has led to the suspicion that pancreatitis in these patients is due to a functional obstruction to pancreatic duct outflow at the minor papilla. Several small series of patients have suggested benefit from endoscopic minor papillotomy or pancreatic duct stent placement to reduce the incidence of recurrent pancreatitis. Patients who fail endoscopic therapy should be considered for surgical sphincteroplasty.

In a large series of patients with pancreas divisum and acute pancreatitis or "pancreatic pain" syndromes, 88 underwent minor duct sphincteroplasty. At a mean follow-up of 53 months, 70% of patients were improved, with the best results achieved in patients with stenotic accessory papillae and episodic attacks of acute pancreatitis.[67] This operation should probably be limited to patients with recurring bouts of abdominal pain associated with hyperamylasemia, ERCP evidence of pancreas divisum, and absence of evidence of gallstones or chronic pancreatitis.[68] Cholecystectomy is generally performed incidental to the sphincteroplasty.

Management of Patients with Pancreatitis and No Clear Cause

Occasional patients present with acute pancreatitis and no clear underlying cause (see Table 46.4). This has been called *idiopathic* pancreatitis, but this term should be reserved for those patients in whom the cause remains obscure after a thorough evaluation. Typically, the patient will have no history of significant alcohol ingestion, and an ultrasound examination shows no gallstones. In this setting, the clinician should review the patient's medication history to ensure that no offending agents have been administered. Serum calcium and lipid levels should be measured. A history of immunosuppression posing risk for infections such as cytomegalovirus should be sought. An ERCP should be considered to exclude the possibility of an occult pancreatic duct stricture or early neoplasm. Bile can be aspirated to identify microlithiasis. The pancreatogram may reveal pancreas divisum.

If these efforts are unrevealing, empiric laparoscopic cholecystectomy should be considered, especially if (1) the clinical course has been consistent with gallstone pancreatitis,

(2) there is a family history of gallstones, or (3) the patient's liver function tests were transiently abnormal. Under these circumstances, it is likely that occult cholelithiasis is the cause of the patient's symptoms. A common mistake is to assume that a negative ultrasound examination excludes gallstones, when in fact the false-negative rate is around 1.5%.[69]

Laparoscopic cholecystectomy is empirically a more attractive initial therapeutic step in this group of patients, compared to the alternatives, such as biliary manometry and endoscopic sphincterotomy for possible biliary dyskinesia.

Chronic Pancreatitis

Background

Chronic pancreatitis affects about 8 new patients per 100,000 population per year in the United States, with a prevalence of 26.4 cases per 100,000 population.[70] Autopsy series, however, suggest a higher prevalence of 0.04% to 5%. Chronic pancreatitis is characterized pathologically by parenchymal fibrosis, ductal strictures, and atrophy of acinar and islet tissue. Three subgroups of chronic pancreatitis have been described: (1) chronic calcific pancreatitis, (2) chronic obstructive pancreatitis, and (3) chronic inflammatory pancreatitis. The most common pattern is chronic calcific pancreatitis, usually related to alcohol ingestion and characterized by fibrosis, calcification in small ducts, and intraductal protein plugging. Chronic obstructive pancreatitis is commonly observed in the setting of pancreatic cancer, for which ductal obstruction by the tumor leads to dilation, acinar atrophy, and fibrosis. The least-common type is chronic inflammatory pancreatitis, usually associated with autoimmune diseases such as Sjögren's syndrome and sclerosing cholangitis.

Etiology

Most cases of chronic pancreatitis are due to excessive alcohol ingestion, in the range of 150g/day over many years.[70] Only about 10% of heavy drinkers develop chronic pancreatitis, however, so it is likely that other cofactors are required, such as a diet rich in fat and protein. The underlying pathophysiology of alcohol-related chronic pancreatitis remains unclear but probably involves ductal plugging and calcification related to abnormalities in pancreatic juice, including diminished lithosthatine (pancreatic stone protein) or GP2 concentrations.[71,72]

In tropical countries, chronic pancreatitis occurs in young individuals in the absence of alcohol ingestion, perhaps from dietary factors or micronutrient deficiency. These patients typically have marked ductal dilation and stone formation, with relative sparing of the parenchyma.

Several genes have been implicated in the pathogenesis of chronic pancreatitis.[73] These patients tend to present early in adult life. Gallstone disease does not result in chronic pancreatitis.

A better understanding of the causes of pain in chronic pancreatitis has been gained. In the past, increased intrapancreatic pressure was believed to be the main factor as ascertained from data obtained intraoperatively in patients undergoing ductal decompressive procedures.[74] Increased size and number of pancreatic neurons now is thought to be important, as are alterations in the type and amount of nociceptive neurotransmitters.[75,76] Increased nerve growth factor (NGF), its high-affinity receptor (TrkA), and immune cell infiltration appear to correlate with the degree of pancreatic fibrosis and intensity of pain in chronic pancreatitis.[75]

Clinical Presentation

There is no simple, accurate way to confirm the diagnosis of chronic pancreatitis. Clinical criteria for diagnosis include unrelenting epigastric abdominal pain that radiates through to the back, accompanied by nausea, poor appetite, and weight loss. The pain in chronic pancreatitis does not correlate well with the degree of anatomic abnormalities found radiographically. Occasional patients have a waxing-and-waning course. Typically, however, patients considered for surgical treatment have profound pain leading to narcotic dependence. Pancreatic exocrine insufficiency, resulting in steatorrhea, does not occur until about 90% of function is lost. Endocrine insufficiency, resulting in diabetes, does not occur until greater than 80% of the gland is destroyed. Because both insulin and glucagon secretion are lost with islet atrophy, the diabetes in chronic pancreatitis tends to be brittle and difficult to control.

The physical examination in patients with chronic pancreatitis is often unrevealing. Weight loss and malnutrition may be evident. Occasional patients may have concomitant chronic liver disease evident on examination. Epigastric tenderness is common. In the presence of a pseudocyst, a palpable mass may be found. Chronic pancreatitis complicated by biliary obstruction may result in jaundice. Splenomegaly suggests the possibility of splenic vein thrombosis. Malnutrition, in advanced cases, may be evident by temporal muscle wasting; dry, flaky skin; and brittle hair.

Diagnostic Evaluation

Routine laboratory investigation is not generally revealing in chronic pancreatitis. Serum amylase and lipase levels may be mildly elevated but are usually normal. Liver function tests are normal unless there is underlying liver disease or bile duct obstruction. Malnutrition may be revealed by decreased serum albumin levels. In patients with steatorrhea, fat malabsorption can be confirmed by Sudan staining of the stool or 72-h stool collection while the patient consumes a diet containing 100g of fat per day. Stool fat excretion of more than 7g/day is abnormal.

Imaging studies are performed to provide an assessment of the extent of disease. A plain film of the abdomen may detect calcification in the gland. An abdominal CT scan is useful to identify pancreatic calcification, masses suspicious for carcinoma, dilated ducts, and pseudocysts. Reported sensitivity of CT in the diagnosis of chronic pancreatitis ranges from 75% to 90%, with a specificity of 85% 100%.[77] Pancreatic calcification is a hallmark of the diagnosis of chronic pancreatitis, but the degree of calcification does not correlate well with the degree of exocrine insufficiency.

Magnetic resonance cholangiopancreatography or ERCP is necessary to determine the size and anatomy of the pancreatic duct, as well as unsuspected pathology such as biliary stricture and cancer. These studies allow patients to be categorized into those with "small-duct" disease and those with "large ducts." This is important in that those with large ducts are far more amenable to surgical correction.

Treatment

Surgery for chronic pancreatitis is indicated for disabling pain and obstruction of adjacent hollow viscera, commonly the bile duct or duodenum. For surgery to be effective, an identifiable anatomic lesion amenable to correction must be present. Options in surgical management broadly include drainage procedures, resective procedures, and nerve blocks. Successful treatment in terms of pain relief is improved in patients who cease alcohol and nicotine consumption.[78]

Disabling Pain

Pain is the usual reason for a patient with chronic pancreatitis to seek medical attention, and most treatment strategies are oriented around its relief. The severity of pain is a major factor in determining the advisability of surgery. In general, surgery is indicated if the pain interferes with the patient's ability to work, is refractory to pancreatic enzyme therapy, requires high doses of oral narcotics for control, and other possible causes for pain have been excluded. A number of factors must be considered in tailoring an operation to a specific patient, including, most importantly, the size and anatomy of the pancreatic duct, the distribution of pancreatitis in the gland, the presence of associated pseudocyst or biliary stricture, and the general condition of the patient.

If the preoperative assessment has demonstrated a dilated pancreatic duct (>6mm diameter) with or without associated strictures, then a drainage procedure of the duct is indicated. Conversely, if the duct is small (<6mm diameter), resectional surgery should be considered. Because of the relatively poor results in this latter group of patients and the morbidity of pancreatic resection, it should be considered only as a last resort.

Pancreatic Ductal Drainage

In patients with disabling pain and ERCP evidence of a dilated pancreatic duct, pancreatic ductal drainage is the procedure of choice. The best operation is longitudinal pancreaticojejunostomy, also known as the modified Puestow procedure (Fig. 46.15). In this operation, the anterior surface of the pancreas is exposed, and the location of the duct is identified. When necessary, this is aided by intraoperative ultrasonography.

The duct is opened longitudinally for most of its length. Stones and debris are removed as possible. An anastomosis is constructed between a Roux-Y limb of proximal jejunum and the pancreatic duct, usually in two layers. This operation has better results than the Duval procedure, or caudal pancreaticojejunostomy, in that the entire duct can be drained. Operative mortality rates for this operation are low, ranging from 0% to 4%. Relief of pain occurs in 80%–90% of patients when assessed within the first year, and in most series this is maintained at 5-year follow-up. Patients who cease consuming alcohol clearly do better than those who persist. Ductal drainage may prevent or delay further loss of exocrine or endocrine function.[79] Results from recent published series with long-term (>5-year) follow-up are shown in Table 46.10.

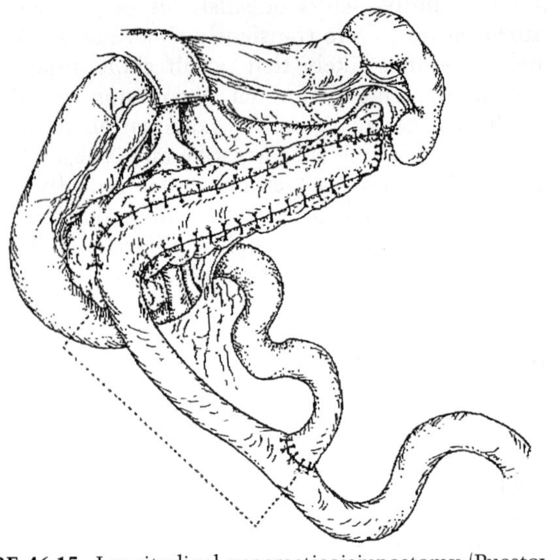

FIGURE 46.15. Longitudinal pancreaticojejunostomy (Puestow procedure). A 45-cm long Roux-Y limb of jejunum is brought through the mesocolon for a side-to-side anastomosis with the dilated pancreatic duct. This technique is useful in patients with chronic pancreatitis, pain, and a dilated ductal system. Results are poorer in nondilated (<6 mm) ducts.

Recent enthusiasm has been expressed for endoscopic pancreatic ductal stent placement to relieve pain in chronic pancreatitis. Approximately 50% of patients have clinical improvement in pain with intermediate follow-up.[80,81] Endoscopic stent placement has also been used in concert with shock wave lithotripsy for stone extraction. Stent dysfunction, such as occlusion or migration, is common. Unfortunately, pain relief wanes over time, and other studies have suggested that pancreatic stent placement induces changes consistent with chronic pancreatitis.[82,83] To date, no randomized data exist to document a benefit of endoscopic stenting over standard therapy.

Resectional Surgery for Chronic Pancreatitis

In a subset of patients with disabling pain and chronic pancreatitis, resection is appropriate. In general, resection is favored only in those patients with small ducts in whom all nonoperative measures have failed. Enthusiasm for resectional surgery is tempered by the significant complication rates and relatively poor long-term results. Options in resectional surgery include total pancreatectomy, distal (60%) resection, near-total (85%) distal resection, pancreaticoduodenectomy (Whipple resection), and duodenum-preserving pancreatic head resections (Beger and Frey procedures).

Total pancreatectomy is rarely justified as the long-term mortality rates are high. Instead, partial pancreatectomy of the most severely affected portion of the gland is favored. Most commonly, this requires near-total distal pancreatectomy, pancreaticoduodenectomy, or duodenum-preserving pancreatic head resections. The last operations are gaining increased acceptance because of the high late failure rate of distal resection and the emerging view that the diseased head of the gland acts as a "pacemaker" of symptoms.

TABLE 46.10.
Results of Longitudinal Pancreaticojejunostomy for Chronic Pancreatitis.

First author, reference center, year	*Number of patients*	*Operative mortality rate*	*Pain relief*	*Comment*
Class III data				
Partington,[212] Cleveland, 1960	7	0	Excellent in 4 of 7 patients	Partington and Rochelle modified the Puestow procedure by creating a longitudinal anastomosis between the pancreas and jejunum
Warshaw,[213] Massachusetts General Hospital, 1980	10	0	8 of 10 with substantial relief	Diabetes in 3 of 10 preoperatively and 5 of 10 postoperatively
Prinz,[214] Chicago, 1981	100	4%	80%	Diabetes present preoperatively in 30% and developed postoperatively in another 14%
Holmberg,[215] Sweden, 1985	51	0	Good to excellent in 65% of drinkers and 88% of abstinent patients	Mean 8-year follow-up
Munn,[216] Chicago, 1987	61	2%	84% of patients obtained pain relief	39% of patients had pseudocysts
Bradley,[217] Emory, 1987	46	0	Good 28% Fair 38% Poor 34%	8 late deaths at mean follow-up of 69 months
Nealon,[218] Galveston, 1988	41	0	Pain relief in 93%	87% of patients had postoperative weight gain 16% had progression of pancreatitis
Greenlee,[219] Chicago, 1990	50	2%	Complete in 42% Substantial in 40%	Follow-up 7.9 years
Adams,[220] South Carolina, 1994	85	0	"Good" in 24% "Fair" in 31% "Poor" in 45% Narcotic dependence in 35%	Diabetes requiring insulin in 23% of patients 42% continued to drink
Rios,[221] Charleston, 1998	17	0	Poor 76%	All with small-duct disease
Lucas,[222] Detroit, 1999	124	2/124	Substantial in 39% Complete in 61%	Diabetes in 13/124 preoperatively and 16/124 postoperatively
Sohn,[139] Baltimore, 2000	52	1.9%		
Nealon,[223] Galveston, 2001	124	0	86% off narcotics 91% without acute exacerbations	Follow-up 81 months; no patients without surgery had resolution; 4% complication rate

Relief of pain occurs in about 60% of patients at 5-year follow-up after pancreatic resection. Diabetes and steatorrhea are common long-term complications of all of these operations. Results of resectional surgery for chronic pancreatitis are summarized in Table 46.11.

Splanchnicectomy, Celiac Ganglionectomy, and Percutaneous Celiac Plexus Block

Nerve block or ablation procedures have had limited success in the management of patients with chronic pancreatitis. Recent results in chronic pancreatitis appear poorer than in pancreatic cancer, with fewer than half of patients achieving a durable reduction in pain.[84,85] Percutaneous celiac nerve block with phenol or alcohol and endoscopic ultrasound-guided techniques may have a role in the setting of a comprehensive pain management clinic.

More recently, thoracoscopic splanchnicectomy has been reported to give reasonable pain relief with minimal operative morbidity.[86–88] In this procedure, after placement of thoracoscopic ports, the greater and lesser splanchnic nerves are sectioned as they course from the spine to the abdomen. The nerves in the right and left chest can be dealt with sequentially with the patient in a prone position. As yet, no randomized data or long-term follow-up data are available to judge the relative merits of this procedure.

Obstruction of Adjacent Hollow Viscera

The most common adjacent hollow viscus affected by chronic pancreatitis is the intrapancreatic portion of the common bile duct, which occurs in 5%–10% of patients. The usual cause is fibrosis of the pancreatic parenchyma in the head of the gland, although on occasion the obstruction is due to pseudocyst. Patients may have obstructive jaundice or more subtle abnormalities of liver function tests, such as elevated alkaline phosphatase. Examinations by ERCP or MRCP reveal the

TABLE 46.11.
Results of Pancreatic Resection for Chronic Pancreatitis.

First author, reference, center, year	*Patient groups*	*Operative mortality rate*	*Pain relief*	*Diabetes*	*Comment*
Class I data					
Buchler,[224] Bern and Ulm, 1995	Beger procedure (n = 20) PPPD (n = 20)	0% 0%	75% pain free 40% pain free	Mean blood glucose 130 mg/dL 88 mg/dL	Weight gain 4.1 ± 0.9 kg 1.9 ± 1.2 kg
Izbicki,[225] Hamburg, 1995	Beger procedure (n = 20) Frey procedure (n = 22)	0% 0%	95% improvement 94% improvement	Impaired GTT in 90% Impaired in 86%	Quality of life improved significantly in both groups
Izbicki,[226] Hamburg, 1998	Beger procedure (n = 31) PPPD (n = 30)	3.2% 0%	94% improvement in pain score; global quality of life improved by 71% 95% improvement in pain score; global quality of life improved by 43%	—	Median follow-up 24 months
Strate,[227] Hamburg, 2005	Beger procedure (n = 38) Frey procedure (n = 36)	Late mortality 31% 32%	Pain score 11.25 11.25	Endocrine/exocrine insufficiency 56%/88% 60%/78%	9-year follow-up; no differences in late mortality, global quality of life, pain, endocrine or exocrine insufficiency
Class III data					
Braasch,[228] Lahey Clinic, 1978	Total pancreatectomy (n = 26)	0%	Improvement in 12 survivors	Diabetes in 100%	12 late deaths
Rossi,[229] Lahey Clinic, 1987	Whipple procedure (n = 73)	2.7%	Improved pain in 86% at 6 months	Diabetes in 37% at 6 months	17 late deaths, 4 related to diabetes
Beger,[230] Ulm, 1989	Beger procedure (n = 128)	0.8%	Complete pain relief in 71%	Worsening diabetes in 13.7%	Median follow-up 3.6 years Late mortality 4.7% Weight gain in 80% of patients
Easter,[231] Dundee, 1991	Pylorus-preserving total pancreatectomy (n = 8)	0%	Good pain relief in 6 of 8	Diabetes in 5/8 preoperatively and 8/8 postoperatively	One late death
Frey,[232] UC-Davis, 1994	Frey procedure (n = 50)	0%	Excellent in 74% Improved in 13% Unimproved in 13%	Progression of diabetes in 11%	5 late deaths Weight gain in 64%
Sawyer,[233] UC-Davis, 1994	Distal pancreatectomy, disease limited to body (n = 10) Distal pancreatectomy, disease present in head (n = 7)	0%	90% with excellent pain relief Unsatisfactory results in 6 of 7 patients	—	Best results in patients with small ducts (<5 mm) and disease limited to body and tail of gland
Martin,[234] Lahey Clinic, 1996	Pylorus-preserving Whipple procedure (n = 45)	2.2%	Mean preoperative pain score = 9.2/10 Mean pain score at 5-year follow-up = 1.1/10	21 of 45 (46%) at 5 years	92% of patients had improvement in pain at 5-year follow-up

TABLE 46.11. (continued)

First author, reference, center, year	*Patient groups*	*Operative mortality rate*	*Pain relief*	*Diabetes*	*Comment*
Rattner,[235] Massachusetts General Hospital, 1996	Distal pancreatectomy (n = 20)	5%	55% pain free 15% using narcotics intermittently 30% using narcotics continuously	—	Median follow-up "about 2 years"
Traverso,[236] Virginia Mason Clinic, 1997	Whipple procedure (n = 47) Total (n = 10)	0% 0%	Improved pain in 100%, 76% pain free	Diabetes in 32%	93% 5-year survival
Eddes,[237] Leiden, 1997	Beger procedure (n = 19)	0%	Pain relief in 86%	Insulin-dependent diabetes in 6 of 19	Oral glucose tolerance test unchanged pre- and postoperatively
Beger,[238] Ulm, 1999	Beger procedure (n = 504)	0.8%	Complete pain relief in 79%	New diabetes in 21%	9% readmission rate for pancreatitis
Sohn,[139] Baltimore, 2000	263 operations (Whipple, distal, Puestow, other)	1.9% early 11% late	20% reduction in narcotic use	19% increase in diabetes, 21% increase in exocrine insufficiency	Improvements in all aspects of quality of life

abnormality (Fig. 46.16). Use of CT or magnetic resonance imaging (MRI) is helpful to exclude an underlying carcinoma.

Endoscopic papillotomy or stenting is seldom curative. Jaundiced patients should be treated with choledochoduodenostomy. Thought should be given to the possibility of carcinoma, and brushings and biopsies are obtained as warranted. Occasionally, carcinoma is difficult to exclude, even at operation. In the presence of a mass, pancreaticoduodenectomy is usually the best course, even if biopsies do not confirm cancer. Rarely, patients with chronic pancreatitis can develop duodenal or transverse colonic obstruction. Occasionally, resection of the involved structure with the pancreas will be indicated, but these problems are more easily treated with bypass.

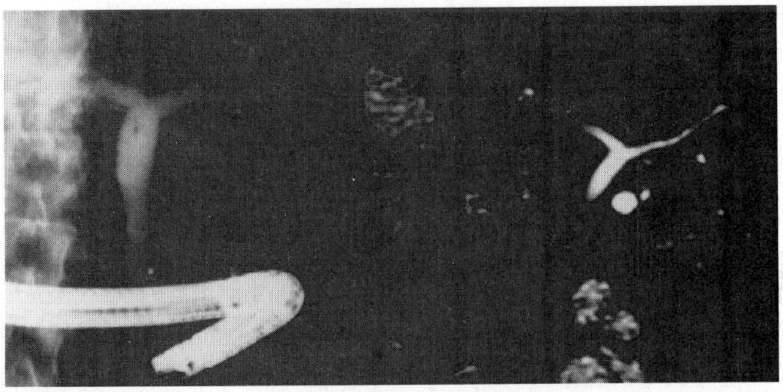

FIGURE 46.16. Endoscopic retrograde cholangiopancreatography (ERCP) and magnetic resonance cholangiopancreatogram (MRCP) in benign bile duct stricture from chronic pancreatitis. **A.** Magnetic resonance cholangiopancreatogram with coronal reconstruction showing a stricture of the intrapancreatic portion of the common bile duct without evidence of tumor in a patient with chronic pancreatitis. **B.** The ERCP from the same patient showing the smooth, tapered obstruction, suggesting a benign stricture.

Pancreatic Pseudocysts

Pseudocysts are among the most common complications of acute and chronic pancreatitis, occurring in 2%–10% of patients. In the United States, pancreatitis due to alcohol ingestion is the most common cause. Other etiologic factors include biliary, posttraumatic, and ERCP-induced pancreatitis. Severe acute pancreatitis of any cause, however, can occasionally result in development of a pseudocyst. In children, for example, abdominal trauma is the most common etiology. The management of patients with pseudocysts is challenging, in terms of both surgical decision making and the technical aspects of the operations. The natural history of pseudocysts has become better defined in recent years, and dramatic progress has been made in the development of therapeutic methods, including percutaneous, endoscopic, and laparoscopic approaches.

Terminology

Pancreatic pseudocysts are abnormal collections of fluid arising in the setting of acute or chronic pancreatitis or trauma. They can be located within the substance of the pancreas, adjacent to the gland, or even some distance away. An occasional pseudocyst will be found extending through the pelvis into the groin or cephalad into the mediastinum. The pseudocysts contain fluid rich in pancreatic secretions from a duct system disrupted by inflammation or trauma or obstructed by a stricture or stone. Pseudocysts differ from true cysts in that they lack an epithelial lining and have walls comprised of adjacent organs, fibrosis, and inflammatory granulation tissue.

In the past, the spectrum of disease following pancreatitis has been difficult to understand because of unclear terminology; words like *phlegmon*, *fluid collection*, and *acute* or *chronic pseudocysts* have been used incorrectly or inappropriately. The Atlanta International Symposium in 1992 reached agreement on terminology, based on clinical patient management, and provided working definitions for an acute pancreatic fluid collection, acute pseudocyst, chronic pseudocyst, and pancreatic abscess.[13] These definitions are summarized in Table 46.3.

Clinical Presentation

The most common symptom associated with pseudocysts is abdominal pain, which is present in 80%–90% of patients. The pain can be associated with chronic pancreatitis or can persist or recur after a bout of acute pancreatitis. Nausea, vomiting, early satiety, and weight loss are also common. Physical examination may reveal abdominal tenderness, a palpable epigastric mass (found in about 50% of patients), fever, jaundice, and ascites. The presenting signs and symptoms can be related to the mass effect of the pseudocyst itself or be from a complication of the pseudocyst. Complications arising from pseudocysts include hemorrhage, rupture, infection, or obstruction. Decisions regarding the advisability of treating a pseudocyst must balance the possibility of spontaneous resolution with observation against the risk of development of one of these potentially life-threatening complications.

Natural History of Pseudocysts

Until the 1950s, it was believed that pseudocysts seldom, if ever, resolved spontaneously, and that surgical intervention was warranted in all patients. Marsupialization and external drainage were the most common treatment methods, but the advantages of internal drainage were being recognized. By 1979, Bradley et al.[89] had studied the natural history of 93 patients with symptomatic pseudocysts prospectively with serial ultrasound examinations. In patients with a presumed duration of pseudocyst of less than 6 weeks, the rates of spontaneous resolution and complications were 40% and 20%, respectively. In contrast, in patients with a presumed pseudocyst duration of 7 to 12 weeks, the resolution rate was less than 10%, and the complication rate rose to 46%. In patients with pseudocysts observed from 13 to 18 weeks, spontaneous resolution was not observed, and the complication rate rose to 75%. These data influenced surgical thinking, with the conclusion that operative management of pseudocyst should not be delayed past the 6-week mark.

A weakness in the thinking regarding pseudocysts at this time was the failure to distinguish between those arising in the setting of acute versus chronic pancreatitis. In 1981, Crass and Way[90] retrospectively analyzed 68 patients with pseudocysts and concluded that symptomatic patients could be separated into two groups, those with symptoms arising in the setting of acute or chronic pancreatitis. They showed that acute pseudocysts have a high rate of spontaneous resolution, warranting delay in treatment, while chronic pseudocysts have a mature wall at presentation, and delay in operation only increased the risk of complication since the rate of resolution in this group was thought to be negligible. They recommended that acute pseudocysts should be treated with elective internal drainage after 6 weeks of observation, while chronic pseudocysts should be treated at the time of diagnosis. Their conclusions were supported by others.[91] Factors predicting failure of spontaneous resolution included (1) persistence for longer than 6 weeks, (2) evidence of chronic pancreatitis, (3) pancreatic duct abnormalities, and (4) a thick cyst wall on ultrasound examination.

More recently, two studies have suggested a greater frequency of spontaneous resolution of pseudocysts than previously suspected. Yeo et al.[92] followed 75 patients with CT evidence of pseudocysts. They managed 48% of the patients nonoperatively, while 52% required operative treatment because of persistent abdominal pain, enlargement, or complications. In contrast to earlier studies, only 1 of 36 patients managed expectantly developed a complication directly related to the pseudocyst, and 60% resolved without surgery. There were no deaths. Similarly, Vitas and Sarr[93] reported that, of 68 patients treated expectantly, 57% had spontaneous resolution, and only 9% suffered complications.

Because of the low incidence of complications and high rates of resolution with expectant management, these studies suggest that asymptomatic patients with pancreatic pseudocysts can be safely managed nonoperatively and followed by outpatient serial CT examinations. Intervention can be reserved for symptomatic patients, those with enlarging pseudocysts, and those who develop complications.

Treatment of Pseudocysts

Today, intervention for pseudocysts includes four main treatment options: percutaneous drainage, endoscopic drainage, laparotomy with internal drainage, or laparoscopic internal drainage. Occasionally, external drainage may be required via laparotomy. Resection is rarely indicated. These treatment options are discussed in turn.

Percutaneous Drainage

The advent of ultrasound and CT-guided catheterization via the Seldinger technique improved the safety and efficacy of percutaneous drainage. Now, percutaneous drainage is the preferred method of pseudocyst treatment in three specific circumstances: (1) treatment of critically ill patients who are not suitable candidates for surgery; (2) drainage of rapidly enlarging, immature peripancreatic fluid collections; and (3) drainage of infected pseudocysts. Percutaneous needle aspiration alone has an unacceptable failure rate of 70%–90%. Because of this, aspiration should be reserved for diagnostic purposes only. When the intent is therapeutic, a percutaneous 7- to 10-French pigtail catheter should be placed.

Percutaneous catheter drainage is much more effective than aspiration alone, with some reports of successful treatment in 60%–90% of patients.[94–97] Not all groups, however, have had good results with percutaneous drainage. Criado et al.,[98] for example, described only a 21% success rate at a mean 10-month follow-up, with 60% of patients eventually requiring a surgical procedure. Other studies have demonstrated higher mortality and morbidity rates in patients treated percutaneously compared to those undergoing operation.[99,100] In addition, those who fail percutaneous treatment tend to have complicated clinical courses, often requiring urgent surgical intervention with significant morbidity and mortality.[97,101]

Long-term results are best in patients treated for acute fluid collections or acute pseudocysts rather than chronic pseudocysts.[102] Similarly, patients in whom a ductal communication with the pseudocyst or ductal stenosis is identified have poorer outcome. Marked clinical improvement is usually promptly evident following percutaneous drainage of infected pseudocysts. No randomized data yet exist comparing percutaneous versus surgical treatment.

Endoscopic Drainage

Endoscopic drainage procedures for pseudocysts include transpapillary and transenteric techniques. Endoscopic retrograde cholangiopancreatography allows delineation of the pancreatic ductal anatomy and identification of communication between the ductal system and the pseudocyst. When a communication is identified, transpapillary stenting can be used to drain the pseudocyst into the duodenum. The combined published experience with 117 patients undergoing transpapillary drainage revealed technical success in 84% with a 9% recurrence rate.[103] Complications include bleeding, pancreatitis, and infection as well as stent-induced duct stricture.

In addition to transpapillary drainage, endoscopic transmural pseudocyst drainage techniques, including cystgastrostomy and cystduodenostomy, are feasible. Prerequisites for transmural drainage techniques include (1) cyst location in the pancreatic head or body; (2) a distance between the pseudocyst and the gastric or duodenal lumens of less than 1 cm; (3) a clear, bulging impression of the pseudocyst seen endoscopically from the gastric or duodenal lumen; and (4) firm adherence between the pseudocyst and enteric walls. Such criteria are met in about half of pseudocysts in the setting of chronic pancreatitis and in one-fourth of those with acute pancreatitis.[103,104]

Data describing results of these techniques are limited. Success rates range from 71% to 82% in large series.[103–105] Complications occur in one-third of patients, with a 10% incidence of major complications, including hemorrhage, perforation, and infection requiring additional surgical intervention. As in percutaneous treatment, patients who fail endoscopic treatment have a high likelihood of requiring urgent surgical invervention.[101]

The main difficulty with these techniques is that the catheter diameter may be insufficient to completely drain the pseudocyst cavity, especially if the material is thick or contains necrotic debris. Once the cavity has been contaminated by a communication to the gastrointestinal tract, incomplete drainage can result in a difficult problem of infected, necrotic debris. For this reason, the endoscopic approach is best in patients with chronic pseudocysts, and it has poorer outcomes in patients with acute pseudocysts and in those with necrosis.[104]

Internal Drainage via Laparotomy

Internal surgical drainage via laparotomy is the established benchmark by which all other techniques must be compared. Experience with operative drainage has defined a number of principles that must be followed to maximize success, including (1) cyst wall biopsy should be performed to rule out cystic neoplasm in patients with atypical presentations; (2) all necrotic material should be debrided from the cyst cavity; (3) the operative strategy must drain the entire pseudocyst cavity; and (4) any underlying ductal abnormalities must simultaneously be addressed. As new treatment options develop, the wise clinician will keep these principles in mind to avoid reproducing past errors.

Several options for surgical treatment of pseudocyst are available, including external drainage, internal drainage, and resection. The decision regarding which option is best must be individualized based on the patient's condition, the chronicity of the pseudocyst, anatomy of the pseudocyst, and associated lesions such as ductal strictures or pseudoaneurysms. The use of ERCP, CT, and angiography is helpful for preoperative planning, but ultimately the decision is made intraoperatively.

Internal drainage, including cystgastrostomy, Roux-en-Y cystjejunostomy, and cystduodenostomy, is the preferred surgical option, with recurrence and mortality rates less than 10%.[97,106–108] Of the internal drainage options, cystgastrostomy is preferable if the pseudocyst is in the lesser sac, is firmly adherent to the posterior stomach, and is small enough to allow for adequate dependent drainage. The cyst is approached from the lumen of the stomach, and the anastomosis between the cyst wall and stomach is sutured to provide hemostasis and prevent leakage.

The Roux-en-Y cystjejunostomy is the most versatile internal drainage technique. A Roux limb can be anastomosed side to side to the most dependent part of a pseudocyst arising in nearly any location. It can also be used to drain multiple cysts and to create a lateral pancreaticojejunostomy to the duct, if indicated.

Cystduodenostomy should be rarely used as an internal drainage method and only when no other technique is feasible. Care must be taken to avoid injury to the ampulla of Vater, bile and pancreatic ducts, and the gastroduodenal artery. Duodenal stenosis is sometimes problematic. A transduodenal approach is superior to laterolateral cystduodenostomy.

External drainage is indicated for immature cysts with walls that will not hold sutures, grossly infected cysts, and emergency situations, including hemorrhage and rupture. This procedure has high mortality and recurrence rates, most likely reflecting the high severity of illness in these patients.

Resection should be considered only in the rare situation of a small, chronic pseudocyst in the tail of the gland. Resection can be technically difficult due to the associated inflammatory reaction around the pseudocyst. The mortality and morbidity rates for resection are higher than for internal drainage.[109]

Laparoscopic Internal Drainage

The development of minimally invasive techniques in surgery has been extended to the treatment of pancreatic disorders, including enucleation and formal resection of tumors, debridement of necrotic tissue in acute pancreatitis, and internal drainage of pseudocysts. The available data exist only as case reports and small case series.[110,111] These limited data do not yet allow comparison of the minimally invasive approaches to percutaneous, endoscopic, or open surgical techniques.

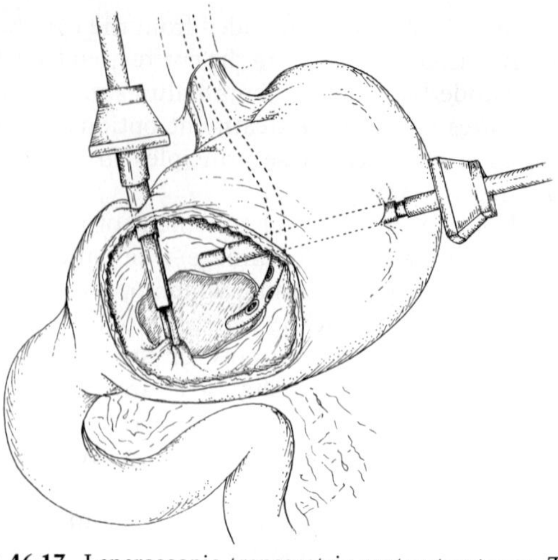

FIGURE 46.17. Laparoscopic transgastric cystgastrostomy. The preferred method of internal drainage of large pseudocysts occupying the lesser sac is laparoscopic transgastric cystgastrostomy. In this technique, a pneumoperitoneum is created to assess the relationship of the pseudocyst to the stomach. The stomach is then insufflated, and two or three trocars are passed through the abdominal wall into the gastric lumen. The pneumoperitoneum is then released. An incision is made through the posterior wall of the stomach into the pseudocyst cavity over a length of 5–6cm. The pseudocyst cavity is evacuated and debrided. To conclude the procedure, the pneumoperitoneum is reestablished, and the trocar sites on the gastric wall are sutured closed.

The most appealing of the minimally invasive approaches to pseudocysts is laparoscopic cystgastrostomy (Fig. 46.17). This can be done via an anterior gastrotomy, similar to its open counterpart; however, an intraluminal approach using the gastric lumen as the field of view has several advantages. In this procedure, a preliminary laparoscopy is performed, followed by transgastric intraluminal endoscopy. A direct incision is then made into the pseudocyst cavity, from the gastric lumen. After debridement of the pseudocyst cavity, the ports are backed out of the gastric lumen, a pneumoperitoneum is reestablished, and the gastric port sites are closed.

Roux-Y cystjejunostomy is also amenable to a laparoscopic approach using a stapled anastomosis between the jejunal limb and the pseudocyst cavity. Intraoperative ultrasonography is helpful to define the extent of the pseudocyst and plan the orientation of the anastomosis. A jejunojejunostomy is performed 45cm downstream of the cystjejunostomy, either at skin level in a laparoscopic-assisted approach or completely laparoscopically via a double-stapled technique.

Pancreatic Cancer

Background

In 2002, the incidence of carcinoma of the pancreas was 12.7/100,000 men and 9.9/100,000 women, making pancreatic cancer the 11th and 8th most common causes of cancer, respectively.[112] Each year in the United States 30,000 people will die from pancreas cancer, and 40,000 will die in Europe.[113,114] However, pancreatic cancer is the fourth leading cause of cancer death in men and women in the United States, behind lung, breast, prostate, and colorectal cancer. Surgery remains the only curative treatment. Although significant advances have been made in improving the safety of pancreatic cancer extirpation, only modest improvements have occurred in the overall 5-year survival rates. A number of pathologic and clinical factors have been identified that predict the prognosis of patients with this illness. These factors are reviewed in the following sections.

The cause of pancreatic cancer is unknown. Only a handful of epidemiologic factors have been associated with pancreatic cancer, and they play a role in the minority of patients. Cigarette smoking, for example, is associated with a statistically significant increase in risk of pancreatic cancer, with about a 3.3-fold increase in heavy users above nonsmokers.[115] Chronic pancreatitis similarly is associated with an increased risk.[116,117] The relationship of diabetes to pancreas cancer is complex as it may either be a primary risk factor or arise as a result of the cancer. Case-control series show that preexisting diabetes is associated with a twofold increased risk of pancreatic cancer.[118] On the other hand, some patients have new-onset diabetes as the first sign of pancreatic cancer.[119] This may be due to either pancreatic duct obstruction with the development of chronic pancreatitis or release and action of tumoral islet amyloid polypeptide, which has a diabetogenic effect. Prior gastrectomy is a minor risk factor for pancreatic cancer,[120] while other surgeries, such as cholecystectomy, are not.[121]

Progress in our understanding of the molecular basis of cancer has helped define genetic abnormalities underlying these tumors in some patients.[122] Mutations in K-ras oncogene have been described in up to 75% of patients.[123,124] Other oncogenes, such as C-*erb* B-12, HER2/neu, and Bcl-2, are also overexpressed in patients with pancreatic cancer.[125,126] Loss of p53 tumor suppressor function may be present in one-half of cases.[124,125] Similarly, mutations of the p16[127,128] and DPC4[129] tumor suppressor genes have been described. It is possible that the improved understanding of the molecular basis of pancreatic cancer will lead to novel prevention and treatment strategies.

Clinical Presentation

Pancreatic cancer, unfortunately, develops insidiously, and the majority of patients have advanced disease at the time of diagnosis. About 70% of tumors develop in the head of the gland, a location that often leads to stricture of the intrapancreatic portion of the common bile duct and the development of jaundice. The typical yellow discoloration of the sclera and skin is accompanied by dark, cola-colored urine and pale, clay-colored stools. Pruritis is a common and troubling symptom. In small, early tumors, the jaundice is painless, but larger, advanced lesions invade retroperitoneal nerves and cause abdominal and back pain. Weight loss is common, particularly in advanced lesions. Diabetes occurs in association with pancreatic cancer in about 20% of cases. In about 15% of cases, the tumor produces distortion of the duodenum, causing symptoms suggestive of gastric outlet obstruction. Rarely, acute pancreatitis due to pancreatic duct obstruction is the first sign of the presence of the tumor. Thus, in patients with acute pancreatitis and no clear underlying inciting event such as gallstones, alcohol ingestion, and the like, ERCP is useful to exclude an anatomic lesion.[130] Tumors of the body and tail do not typically involve the bile

TABLE 46.12. Evaluation of Liver Function Tests in Jaundice.

Test	*Source*	*Pattern in gallstone obstruction of the biliary tree*	*Pattern in malignant obstruction of the biliary tree*	*Pattern in acute hepatitis*
Total bilirubin	Red blood cell destruction, hepatocyte processing	Elevated, but typically less than 10 mg/Dl	Elevated, commonly more than 10 mg/dL	Elevated
Direct bilirubin	Conjugation by hepatocytes	Elevated	Markedly elevated	Mildly elevated
Indirect bilirubin	Red blood cell turnover, hepatocyte processing	Minimally elevated	Elevated	Elevated
Alkaline phosphatase	Biliary epithelial cells and bone	Elevated	Markedly elevated	Minimally elevated
Transaminases	Hepatocytes	Minimally elevated	Minimally elevated	Markedly elevated
Gamma glutamyl transferase	Biliary epithelial cells	Elevated	Markedly elevated	Minimally elevated

duct and seldom present with jaundice. These tumors grow until they involve splanchnic nerves, at which time the patient experiences a dull, visceral pain in the epigastrium radiating into the back.

Physical examination of the patient with pancreatic cancer typically reveals jaundice. As the jaundice progresses, the gallbladder distends and becomes palpable in the right midclavicular line at the costal margin (Courvoisier's sign). The tumor itself is rarely palpable. Weight loss is often evident on examination. In body and tail lesions, splenic vein thrombosis is common, and splenomegaly may be detected on examination. Advanced lesions may present with lymphadenopathy palpable in the left supraclavicular fossa (Virchow's node) or periumbilical area (Sister Mary Joseph's node). Carcinomatosis may reveal itself by the presence of ascites, palpable tumor in the omentum, or pelvic tumor palpable on rectal examination (Blumer's shelf). Extraabdominal signs of pancreatic cancer include deep venous thrombosis and migratory thrombophlebitis.

Diagnostic Evaluation

In the typical patient with painless jaundice, the initial goal is to differentiate obstructive jaundice from disorders of hepatocyte function, such as hepatitis. Evaluation of liver function tests is helpful (Table 46.12). When the clinical picture and pattern of blood test abnormality suggest obstructive jaundice, an imaging study of the biliary tree should be obtained. The two most commonly used screening studies today are ultrasound and CT.

Ultrasound has the advantages of being easily obtainable, inexpensive, and highly accurate for the diagnosis of gallstones. If the clinical suspicion is of obstructive jaundice related to gallstone passage, then a right upper quadrant ultrasound is the best approach. On the other hand, if the clinical picture is more suggestive of malignancy, such as the elderly patient with prolonged symptoms, associated weight loss, and markedly elevated bilirubin, CT has advantages over ultrasound. Despite being more expensive, CT allows identification and staging of a tumor causing biliary obstruction. For examination of the pancreas, a special pancreas CT protocol should be followed, including intravenous and oral administration of contrast, rapid spiral scanning, and reconstruction with 5- to 7-mm cuts through the pancreas.

Depending on the individual patient's situation, additional imaging information may be helpful. If the CT does not clearly identify the obstructing lesion, then ERCP usually identifies its location and extent in the bile duct.[18] Classically, pancreatic cancer is recognized at ERCP by the "double-duct sign" (Fig. 46.18), by which the tumor, arising in the pancreatic duct, eventually grows also to obstruct the bile duct in its intrapancreatic portion.

The sensitivity of ERCP in the diagnosis of pancreatic cancer is over 90%, but it should be recognized that small tumors and lesions in the uncinate process may be difficult to identify. Differentiation of ductal strictures due to pancreatic cancer or chronic pancreatitis can be difficult with ERCP. In general, the lesions of chronic pancreatitis tend to be more diffuse, whereas in pancreatic cancer the lesion is more focal. Brushings for cytologic evaluation of biliary strictures can be obtained, and for ampullary lesions, direct biopsy for histologic evaluation is possible. Other situations for which diagnostic ERCP is helpful include patients with peculiar pain syndromes or unexplained acute pancreatitis, for which an occult pancreatic duct stricture or tumor may be revealed.

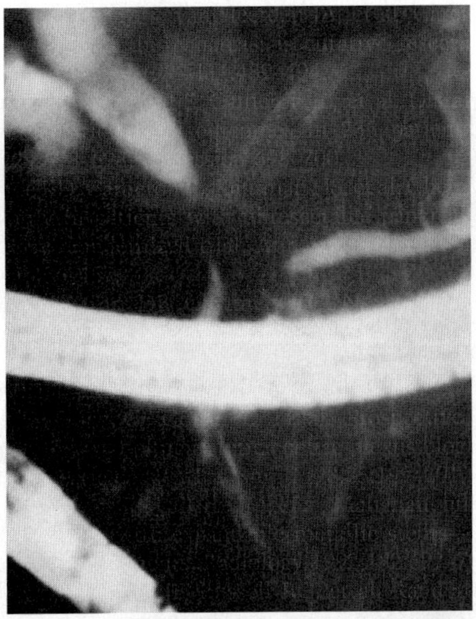

FIGURE 46.18. Double-duct sign in pancreatic cancer. Pancreatic cancer generally arises in the pancreatic duct, causing obstruction. As the tumor grows, it also obstructs the intrapancreatic portion of the common bile duct.

Today, MRCP is finding a role in hepatopancreaticobiliary imaging.[131,132] In this technique, a magnetic resonance scan is obtained, and the computer software is used to reconstruct the images in the desired planes. No special contrast material is required as the pancreatic and bile ducts are seen as bright white structures due to the presence of static fluid within them (Fig. 46.19) As the quality of the reconstructed images improves, MRCP has the potential to replace diagnostic ERCP as it is cheaper, safer, and less invasive.

Endoscopic ultrasonography has high reported sensitivity in the diagnosis of pancreatic cancer and can also help in staging, particularly in the assessment of the relationship of the tumor to the superior mesenteric and portal veins. Directed biopsies of the pancreatic head lesions for cytologic analysis can be obtained with an endoscopic needle using endoscopic ultrasonography for guidance.[133,134]

Additional staging studies may be warranted before treatment is begun. All patients should have a chest x-ray to exclude pulmonary metastases and occult cardiopulmonary disease that may affect the risk of operation. Nuclear medicine bone scans are appropriate for patients with new onset of bone pain. The frequency of bony metastases in the absence of advanced intraabdominal disease is low, however, making bone scans unnecessary as a routine preoperative measure. Similarly, head CT examinations to exclude brain metastases are indicated in patients with new onset of neurological symptoms but are unnecessary as a routine screening test.

Positron emission tomography (PET scanning) using labeled ^{18}fluorodeoxyglucose (^{18}FDG) has a potential role in identifying occult metastatic disease prior to treatment in patients with pancreatic cancer. This technology capitalizes on the increased uptake and retention of ^{18}FDG in malignant cells compared to normal tissue. This increased uptake depends in part on overexpression of glucose transport molecules in pancreatic cancer. Current technology allows for fusion of PET images with CT scans, allowing for more precise localization of ^{18}FDG avid tissues. Experience with this technology in staging pancreatic cancer suggests a sensitivity of 92% and specificity of 85%.[135,136] Use of ^{18}FDG-PET may be helpful in discriminating malignant pancreatic masses from those related to chronic pancreatitis—a distinction sometimes difficult radiographically or even by fine-needle aspiration cytology. Also, PET may be useful in surveillance for tumor recurrence.[137]

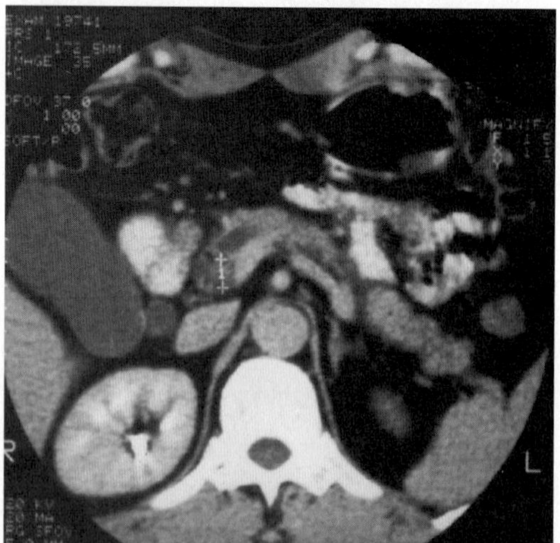

FIGURE 46.19. Magnetic resonance cholangiopancreatogram (MRCP) in pancreatic cancer. The MRCP in a patient with pancreatic cancer shows obstruction of the common bile duct and pancreatic duct in the setting of a mass lesion within the head of the pancreas.

Treatment of Patients with Pancreatic Cancer

Preoperative Biliary Drainage

Profound jaundice can be associated with coagulopathy, malabsorption, malnutrition, and immune dysfunction. These factors may adversely affect outcome of major surgery, such as pancreaticoduodenectomy. The development of transhepatic and endoscopic techniques for biliary drainage in the 1980s led to the hypothesis that preoperative drainage would improve outcome of major biliary surgery. However, results of a recent meta-analysis and large case series show no reduction in operative morbidity or mortality was achieved with preoperative drainage.[138–142] These data suggest that, as a routine, preoperative drainage is not advisable and may increase the risk of surgical site infections.[140,141] Correction of coagulopathy, the major surgical risk, can usually be achieved with vitamin K and, if necessary, fresh frozen plasma infusion.

Resection with Curative Intent

Surgical resection is the only potentially curative treatment for pancreatic cancer. For lesions arising in the head of the gland, the four main surgical options are the standard Whipple pancreaticoduodenectomy, pylorus-preserving pancreaticoduodenectomy, total pancreatectomy, and regional pancreatectomy. No convincing evidence demonstrates a survival advantage of one over another of these options. No randomized trials, however, have been undertaken. For lesions in the body and tail of the gland, distal pancreatectomy is the preferred approach.

The standard operation for periampullary malignancy, popularly known as the Whipple procedure, was conceived and first performed by Whipple in the United States in 1935 and by Kausch in Germany in 1912. In this operation, the head of the pancreas to the neck overlying the portal vein, the duodenum, gallbladder, intrapancreatic portion of bile duct, and antrum are resected en bloc with their associated lymph nodes. Reconstruction is via pancreaticojejunostomy, choledochojejunostomy, and gastrojejunostomy (Fig. 46.20). Traverso and Longmire in 1978 proposed preservation of the pylorus in the course of Whipple resection for benign or malignant disease with the goals of preservation of gastric function and reduction in the incidence of postoperative anastomotic ulceration.[143,144] Three randomized studies have shown no significant difference in perioperative outcomes and, more importantly, long-term or disease-free survival (Table 46.13).

The rationale for total pancreatectomy for carcinoma of the head of the pancreas is to eliminate multifocal disease, achieve wider lymphadenectomy, avoid spillage of tumor cells during transection of the pancreas, and avoid postoperative leakage from the pancreatic anastomosis. These theoretic advantages have not translated into improved operative mortality or long-term survival. Total pancreatectomy has a higher operative mortality rate in most series compared to

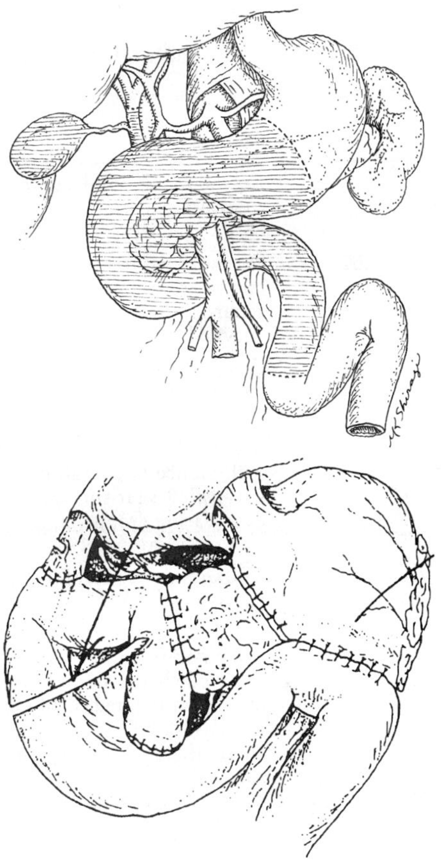

A

B

FIGURE 46.20. Pancreaticoduodenectomy. **A.** Localized tumors of the head of the pancreas, proximal duodenum, and distal bile duct are treated with pancreaticoduodenectomy. The classic operation includes an en bloc distal gastrectomy, duodenectomy, cholecystectomy, bile duct excision, and pancreatic head resection. Smaller tumors not involving the region of the first part of the duodenum can be treated with a pylorus-preserving resection, in which the antrum and pylorus are spared. **B.** Reconstruction following resection typically includes pancreaticojejunostomy, choledochojejunostomy, and duodenojejunostomy.

Whipple resection, and late deaths related to complications of brittle diabetes are problematic. In one recent representative review of over 1900 patients from the state of California, total pancreatectomy had a significantly higher operative mortality of 16% compared with 9% for Whipple resection.[145] In the Hopkins series, median survival in 201 patients was 16 months following Whipple resection, but only 10 months following total pancreatectomy.[146]

Fortner[147] advocated regional pancreatectomy for carcinoma of the pancreas, including en bloc total or subtotal pancreatectomy with radical lymph node dissection and portal vein resection. Operative mortality in these patients averaged 8%, with a median survival of 40 months. A recent single-institution randomized, controlled trial from Johns Hopkins comparing standard versus radical pancreaticoduodenectomy with extended lymph node dissection showed increased early morbidity with extended lymphadenectomy but no differences in long-term quality of life or survival.[148,149] Major vascular resection as a part of pancreaticoduodenctomy has been accomplished at the M.D. Anderson Cancer Center in Houston, with an acceptable operative mortality rate of 1.6% and survival rates similar to standard resection.[150,151]

Adjuvant Radiation and Chemotherapy

Approximately one-half of patients who undergo resection for pancreatic cancer will have regional recurrences without distant metastases, with the remainder developing metastatic disease with or without regional recurrence. Adjuvant therapy, therefore, must address the potential for both locoregional recurrence and metastatic disease. The effect of adjuvant therapy on cure rates in pancreatic cancer is controversial.[152–154] Data addressing its role are summarized in Table 46.14.

A recent meta-analysis of these studies demonstrated an overall improvement in 2- and 5-year survival for resected pancreatic cancer patients who received chemotherapy compared to resected patients who did not (38% and 19% for

TABLE 46.13.

Randomized, Controlled Clinical Trials Comparing Pylorus-Preserving Pancreaticoduodenectomy (PPPD) Versus Standard Whipple Procedure for Pancreatic Cancer.

First author,[239] center, year	*Patient groups*	*Operative mortality rate*	*Delayed gastric emptying*	*Survival*	*Comment*
Lin,[239] Taiwan, 1999	PPPD (n = 16) Whipple (n = 15)	1/16 (6%) 0/15 (0%)[a]	6/16 (38%) 1/15 (7%)	Not recorded	No differences in operative mortality, morbidity, OR time, blood loss; PPPD had higher delayed gastric emptying
Tran,[240] The Netherlands, 2004	PPPD (n = 87) Whipple (n = 83)	3/87 (3.4%) 6/83 (7.2%)[a]	22% 23%	Disease free/overall 6/12 months 7/11 months	No difference in operative morbidity, mortality, LOS, body weight; no difference in margin status, nodal harvest, disease-free and overall survival for periampullary cancer; no differences in the pancreatic cancer subset
Seiler,[241] Berne, 2005	PPPD (n = 64) Whipple (n = 66)	2% 3%	31% 45%[a]	19.2 months 18.2 months	No differences in perioperative morbidity and mortality; earlier return to normal work capacity in the PPPD, but no long-term differences in quality of life or survival

[a]Not significant.

TABLE 46.14.

Randomized, Controlled Trials of Adjuvant Therapy Following Potentially Curative Pancreaticoduodenectomy for Pancreatic Adenocarcinoma.

First author, reference, year, center	*Patient groups*	*Median survival*	*Comments*
Kalser,[242] Multicenter, 1985	Surgery + XRT + chemotherapy (5FU) (n = 21) Surgery alone (n = 22)	21 months 10.9 months	Prospective, randomized, multi-institutional trial
Bakkevold,[243] Scandinavian, 1993	Surgery + chemotherapy (doxorubicin, mitomycin, 5FU) (n = 30) Surgery alone (n = 31)	23 months (P = .02) 11 months	5-year survival did not differ (4% v 8%), suggesting chemotherapy delayed recurrence but did not improve survival
Lygidakis,[244] Athens, 1996	Surgery + intra-arterial immunochemotherapy (n = 40) Surgery alone (n = 40)	30 months 16.8 months	Marked improvement in survival in patients with nodal disease
Klinkenbijil,[245] The Netherlands, 1999	Surgery + XRT + chemotherapy (5FU) (n = 60) Surgery alone (n = 54)	17 months 13 months	No difference in overall median survival; 2-year survival 26% in the observation group versus 34% in the treatment group (NS)
Takada,[246] Tokyo, 2002	Surgery + chemotherapy (mitomycin, 5FU) (n = 81) Surgery alone (n = 77)	5-yr survival 11.5% 18%	No difference in overall or disease-free survival
Neoptolemos,[247,248] Liverpool, 2001, 2004	Surgery + chemotherapy (5FU) Surgery alone Surgery + XRT + chemotherapy (5FU) Surgery alone	5-year survival 21% 8% 10% 20%	Median survival in patients who received chemotherapy was 19.7 months compared to 14 months; the addition of radiotherapy to chemotherapy did not improve survival

treated patients vs. 28% and 12% for controls, respectively).[153] Median survival was also superior (19.0 vs. 13.5 months) compared to control patients. Resected patients who received adjuvant chemoradiotherapy had 2- and 5- year and median survivals of 30%, 12%, and 15.8 months, respectively, which were not significantly different from resected patients who did not receive treatment (34%, 17%, and 15.2 months, respectively). The addition of radiotherapy seemed to provide a modest benefit to patients with positive resection margins.

Intraoperative radiation therapy has been examined as an adjunct to resection and postoperative external beam radiation. Although most recent series demonstrated improved local control, intraoperative radiotherapy does not improve overall survival and therefore has not gained wide acceptance.[154,155]

Although no randomized data have been published, preliminary studies have demonstrated the safety and efficacy of preoperative (neoadjuvant) radiation and chemotherapy in patients with potentially resectable carcinoma of the pancreas.[156,157] Only one-third to one-half of patients enrolled in neoadjuvant trials eventually undergo resection. Recent data suggest that locoregional control of tumor is enhanced by preoperative chemoradiation, but that the majority of patients still succumb to systemic disease.[152] Pending results from randomized clinical trials, neoadjuvant chemoradiation should be considered investigational.

Cancer of the Pancreatic Body and Tail

Typically, patients with adenocarcinoma of the body and tail of the gland present with advanced disease, often unresectable, and have poor prognosis. By 1989, it was reported that only a handful of patients had survived more than 5 years following diagnosis and treatment.[158] Since then, a few groups have reported improved outcomes.[159–162] The resectability rate averages 10%. Operative mortality for distal pancreatectomy for cancer is less than that for pancreaticoduodenectomy, averaging 1% in all California hospitals.[145] In general, patients with body and tail lesions should be approached in the same manner as those with the more common lesion of the head of the gland. Those without evidence of metastatic disease or vascular invasion should be considered candidates for resection. Preliminary laparoscopy may be useful in identifying occult liver or peritoneal metastases and avoiding unnecessary laparotomy.

Palliative Treatment

The majority of patients with pancreatic cancer present with either locally advanced disease or metastases, making cure impossible at the present time. In this group of patients, the treatment goal is palliative. Palliative treatment has two main goals: to improve the quality of the patient's life and to increase life span. Quality of life is markedly affected by cancer pain as well as by complications of the tumor, such as biliary or gastric obstruction. The clinician should consider each of these issues in arriving at a treatment plan for an unresectable patient. Asymptomatic patients cannot be made to feel better by aggressive, ill-advised therapy.

Pain Relief

Careful attention should be paid to pain relief as evidence suggests that survival is prolonged when pain is well controlled.[163] Nonsteroidal antiinflammatory agents, oral and transdermal narcotics, and celiac plexus blocks are the main strategies. Unlike the situation in chronic pancreatitis, significant benefit can sometimes be gained by celiac block in patients with pancreatic cancer. In a meta-analysis summarizing 59 articles and 1145 patients, Eisenberg et al. found significant improvement in cancer pain in 89% of patients.[164] For most, the effect was durable. Side effects are uncommon. In a small, randomized, controlled trial, celiac plexus block was found to be more effective than standard pharmacologic therapy for pancreas cancer pain.[165]

Relief of Biliary Obstruction

Biliary obstruction is a common presentation of pancreatic malignancy. Options in palliation include surgical bypass, endoscopic stenting, and transhepatic stenting. Plastic stents in the range of 7-French to 10-French size have a median patency of 4 months. Expandable metallic stents are more expensive but have a median patency that exceeds median survival in this group of patients.[166] Randomized, controlled data are available comparing endoscopic or percutaneous stent placement versus surgical bypass for malignant biliary obstruction.[167] These data suggest that surgery carries a higher early morbidity and mortality rate compared to stenting, but stents have a high longer-term failure rate. There does not appear to be any significant difference in long-term survival between the two treatment options. Patients expected to live longer than 6 months or those requiring gastrojejunostomy for duodenal obstruction are probably best treated operatively. Those with widespread metastatic disease, and especially those with ascites and carcinomatosis, are best treated with stents.

Relief or Prevention of Duodenal Obstruction

Duodenal obstruction occurs in 10% to 20% of patients with pancreatic cancer.[168] The main palliative method is gastrojejunostomy. This can be accomplished laparoscopically or via open laparotomy. In one recent randomized, controlled trial of 87 highly selected patients with unresectable periampullary malignancy thought to be at low risk for gastric outlet obstruction, no difference in survival was observed in those with or without gastrojejunostomy (mean survival = 8.3 months in each group).[169] In 8 of the 43 patients (18%) without gastrojejunostomy, however, gastric outlet obstruction requiring treatment developed. Gastric outlet obstruction symptoms did not develop in those undergoing gastrojejunostomy. These data suggest that prophylactic gastrojejunostomy is indicated in patients with unresectable periampullary malignancy undergoing laparotomy. For patients with known unresectable tumors complicated by gastric outlet obstruction, laparoscopic gastrojejunostomy is a reasonable option. No randomized, controlled data comparing open to laparoscopic bypass are available. Endoscopic duodenal stenting can be considered for patients at high risk for surgery.[170]

Prolongation of Survival

Palliative radiation and chemotherapy have a limited role in patients with unresectable pancreatic cancer. A number of chemotherapy regimens for patients with advanced pancreatic cancer have been studied, but objective response rates are low. 5-Fluorouracil (5FU), mitomycin, and, more recently, gemcitabine-based protocols have shown some survival benefit, although improvements tend to be measured as a few months.[152] In a recent trial, patients with advanced pancreatic cancer treated with gemcitabine had a median survival of 5.7 months versus 4.4 months for patients treated with 5FU.[171] Improvements in quality of life, including pain control and dietary intake, were also observed. These data suggest that, at least in selected patients, cytotoxic chemotherapy may offer benefit. However, combining agents has not shown added promise.[172]

The role of radiation therapy in patients with unresectable pancreatic cancer is controversial. A combination of radiation (4000 or 6000cGy) and chemotherapy (5FU) is superior to radiation alone, with an approximate doubling of median survival rate to 40 weeks.[173] With continued accrual of patients, this trial showed a 40% survival at 1 year with combined modality therapy compared to 10% with radiation alone.[174] In a follow-up study, unresectable patients were randomized to combination chemotherapy using streptozocin, mitomycin, and 5FU versus radiation plus chemotherapy.[175] Median survival in the combined-modality group was significantly longer (42 weeks) than following chemotherapy alone (32 weeks). These studies suggest that a combination of chemotherapy and radiation is more effective than either therapy alone in patients with pancreatic cancer.

Prognosis

It is important to recognize that, although the outlook for patients with pancreatic cancer is poor, some patients achieve a substantial life span with optimal treatment. A number of clinical and pathologic factors have been shown to significantly predict prognosis. Recent series suggest 5-year survival is possible in about 20% of resected patients (Table 46.15).

Clinical Factors

Symptoms

Pancreatic cancer tends to grow insidiously, making late presentation common. Features on presentation such as back pain, abdominal pain, and weight loss suggest an advanced lesion, making resection less likely. Deep jaundice is known to increase the operative risk but does not appear to affect long-term survival if the cancer is resectable.[176,177] Other features, such as abdominal pain, steatorrhea, and thrombophlebitis, have not been shown to influence long-term survival.[178] Weight loss, long duration of symptoms, and the presence of anemia, while implying long-standing disease, were not predictors of long-term survival by univariate analysis if the patient could undergo resection.[176]

Blood Transfusion

A significant association between the use of perioperative blood transfusion and poorer survival has been identified for a number of malignancies, including colon cancer, breast cancer, and colorectal cancer metastatic to the liver. A similar relationship has been identified following surgery for pancreatic cancer. Cameron et al. found a median survival of 24.7 months in 41 patients undergoing pancreaticoduodenectomy for pancreatic cancer with two or fewer units of blood transfusion, while the survival of 40 patients receiving more than two units was 10.2 months.[179] This difference was highly significant and remained significant even after adjustment for tumor size. The reason for this relationship is not certain, but

TABLE 46.15.
Survival Following Pancreaticoduodenectomy for Pancreatic Adenocarcinoma: Recent Trials.

First author, reference, center, year	*Number of patients*	*Operative mortality*	*Median survival*	*5-year survival*	*Comments*
Trede,[249] 1990, Mannheim	N = 118	0	Not reported	36% in 76 patients with R0(–) resections, actual survival = 25%	One of the best reports of survival for pancreatic adenocarcinoma
Nitecki,[177] Mayo Clinic, 1995	N = 186	3%	17.5 months	6.8% (23% in subgroup with negative nodes)	12 patients initially classified as ductal adenocarcinoma found to have other diagnoses on rereview; mean follow-up 22 months
Nagakawa,[250] Japan, 1996	N = 53	9.4%	13 months	27.4%	Survival for GI cancers tends to be better in Japan than in Western series
Conlon,[251] Memorial Sloan-Kettering, 1996	N = 118	3.4%	14.3 months	10.2%	Resection for cure possible in 17% of all patients
Sohn,[252] Johns Hopkins, 2000	N = 526	2.3%	17 months	17%	Apparent improvement in survival with adjuvant chemoradiation, 30% positive resection margin

it has been proposed that blood transfusion induces immunosuppression that increases the risk of tumor recurrence.

Demographics

Patient demographic factors do not play strong roles in predicting prognosis following treatment of pancreatic cancer. In univariate analysis, factors such as gender, age, and race have not been found to be statistically significant predictors of survival. Similarly, factors such as alcohol intake history, smoking history, occupation, place of dwelling, and family history have not been shown to predict long-term survival.

Effect of Residual Disease

In large series of patients with pancreatic cancer, one of the strongest factors predicting survival is complete resection.[139,180,181] Population studies show that resection offers survival rates approximately twofold greater than palliative bypass procedures.[182] Similar data are available from single-institution studies, such as the Memorial Sloan-Kettering experience. In that study of 799 patients, the 5-year survival rate following resection was 24%, whereas no patient survived without resection.[183]

Residual disease present following resection is also a strong predictor of long-term mortality in patients with pancreatic cancer. In the Hopkins series, of 143 patients with negative resection margins, actuarial 5-year survival was 26%, but only 8% in 58 patients with positive margins.[146] This issue is important as, in a national survey of care of patients with pancreatic cancer undergoing resection, negative margins were achieved in only 8% of cases.[184] It is suspected, but not proven, that the quality of surgical resection could be improved by regionalization of patients to experienced centers.[185]

Pathologic Factors

Histologic Type

Ductal adenocarcinoma is the most common type of pancreatic cancer, accounting for 90%–95% of cases. Strictly speaking, this category excludes adenocarcinoma of the ampulla of Vater, which has a separate staging system, a different classification of histologic types, different biological and clinical associations, and a better overall prognosis. Pancreatic ductal adenocarcinoma is thought to arise directly from ductal epithelium, progressing through dysplasia and carcinoma in situ to invasive carcinoma, and its growth pattern typically includes the formation of ductal structures. A number of subtypes of ductal adenocarcinoma have been described, including mucinous noncystic carcinoma, signet ring cell carcinoma, adenosquamous carcinoma, mixed ductal-endocrine carcinoma, and anaplastic carcinoma. No significant differences in biological behavior or prognosis among different subtypes of ductal carcinoma have been identified.[186]

Certain other histologic types of epithelial tumors of the pancreas are regarded as both morphologically and biologically distinct from ductal adenocarcinoma. Included in this group are carcinomas with acinar cell differentiation (i.e., acinar cell carcinoma, acinar cell cystadenocarcinoma, and mixed acinar-endocrine carcinoma) and tumors with neuroendocrine differentiation (i.e., tumors formerly known as islet cell tumors and now more commonly termed pancreatic endocrine tumors). Acinar cell carcinomas are typically associated with aggressive biological behavior and poor prognosis. Pancreatic endocrine tumors vary widely in their biological behavior, from benign to highly virulent, but lack reliable histologic indicators of malignancy. Also included in this group of unique epithelial malignancies are intraductal mucinous papillary carcinoma and mucinous cystadenocarcinoma, both of which are associated with a better overall prognosis compared to ductal adenocarcinoma.

Intraductal papillary-mucinous carcinoma (known clinically as mucinous ductal ectasia) is a pancreatic ductal neoplasm that displays indolent behavior compared to typical ductal adenocarcinoma. It arises in a background of papillary adenomatous dysplasia within the pancreatic ductal system that is often multifocal or widespread and may represent true adenoma formation but is slow to undergo malignant transformation and slow to invade the duct wall once malignancy has developed. As its name implies, this tumor typically causes massive ductal dilation and obstruction symptoms long before invasive malignancy has developed; therefore, resection is usually curative. With the presence of invasive malignancy or lymph node metastases, however, the prognosis is apparently poor, and death from disease within a year of resection in such cases has been reported.

Mucinous cystadenocarcinomas also appear to arise in most cases from benign precursor lesions called mucinous cystic neoplasms (mucinous cystadenomas). Arguably, the overall favorable prognosis of mucinous cystadenocarcinomas compared to ductal adenocarcinoma may be related to earlier clinical presentation secondary to symptoms created largely by the precursor lesion.

Histologic Grade

Grading of ductal adenocarcinomas is somewhat subjective, and reports on the prognostic significance of histologic grade in pancreatic cancer often conflict. In most studies, a three- or four-tier grading system is usually employed as follows: grade 1 = well differentiated; grade 2 = moderately differentiated; grade 3 = poorly differentiated; and grade 4 = undifferentiated. Histologic grade is an expression of the relative degree of structural and functional differentiation of the tumor and is typically based on the amount of gland (duct) formation and mucin production. Nuclear atypia and mitotic activity may be included in the assessment. Generally, well-differentiated tumors display a high degree of gland formation, poorly differentiated tumors display little gland formation, and moderately differentiated tumors are intermediate between the two. Despite this degree of analytic subjectivity, histologic grade does correlate with survival by univariate and multivariate analysis.[178] In one multivariate analysis in which histologic grade was found to have independent prognostic significance, the 5-year survival was 50% for well-differentiated carcinomas and 10% for poorly differentiated carcinomas.[183]

Pathologic Tumor Stage

The stage of disease is currently the most powerful predictor of outcome among all defined prognostic factors in pancreatic cancer. The recognition of the direct strong relationship between stage of disease and outcome led to the development of the TNM staging system (Table 46.16). The TNM staging system has gained widespread acceptance, and the standardization of staging in pancreatic cancer has made it possible to compare variables in treatment such as methods of surgical resection and adjuvant radiation or chemotherapy. In the TNM system, a stage grouping is made up of three elements, one subcategory from each of the T, N, and M parameters. Because the subcategories of the T, N, and M parameters are precisely defined, the system is highly reproducible. Each of the T, N, and M categories and subcategories is based on features demonstrated to have independent prognostic significance. Nevertheless, the prognostic power of the TNM system is related to the combined data represented by the stage groupings rather than to the individual parameters alone. Currently, the observed postoperative 5-year survival following resection is about 38%, 15%, 10%, and 4% for stages I, II, III, and IV, respectively.[187]

Other Pathologic Factors

Several other pathologic features have been reported to have prognostic significance in pancreatic cancer. Among these,

TABLE 46.16. Definition of TNM, Stage Grouping, Histopathologic Type, and Histologic Grade of Exocrine Pancreas Carcinoma.

Definition of TMN

Primary Tumor (T)	
TX	Primary tumor cannot be assessed
T0	No evidence of primary tumor
Tis	Carcinoma *in situ**
T1	Tumor limited to the pancreas, 2 cm or less in greatest dimension
T2	Tumor limited to the pancreas, more than 2 cm in greatest diameter
T3	Tumor extends beyond the pancreas but without involvement of the celiac axis or the superior mesenteric artery
T4	Tumor involves the celiac axis or the superior mesenteric artery (unresectable primary tumor)
Regional Lymph Nodes (N)	
NX	Regional lymph nodes cannot be assessed
N0	No regional lymph node metastasis
N1	Regional lymph node metastasis
Distant Metastasis (M)	
MX	Distant metastases cannot be assessed
M0	No distant metastasis
M1	Distant metastasis

*This also includes the "PanInIII" classification

Stage Grouping

Stage 0	Tis	N0	M0
Stage IA	T1	N0	M0
Stage IB	T2	N0	M0
Stage IIA	T3	N0	M0
Stage IIB	T1	N1	M0
	T2	N1	M0
	T3	N1	M0
Stage III	T4	Any N	M0
Stage IV	Any T	Any N	M1

Source: Used with the permission of the American Joint Committee on Cancer (AJCC), Chicago, Illinois. The original source for this material is the *AJCC Cancer Staging Manual, Sixth Edition* (2002) published by Springer Science and Business Media LLC, www.springerlink.com.

histologic features such as small venous or lymphatic vessel invasion by tumor, perineural tumor invasion, round cell infiltration at the tumor periphery, and epithelial atypia in the surrounding uninvolved pancreatic ducts are reported to be associated with decreased survival. Diploid tumor cell DNA is correlated with increased tumor resectability and postoperative survival. Conversely, aneuploidy has shown a significant association with decreased survival. By univariate analyses, a significant association between low S-phase fraction (SPF) and increased survival was found in some studies[146,188] but not others.[189] Immunohistochemical studies of the oncogenes and oncogene products nucleoside diphosphate kinase/nm 23[190] and HER2/neu[126] and epidermal growth factor (EGF), its analog transforming growth factor-α (TGF-α), and EGF-receptor[191] in pancreatic ductal carcinoma have suggested that expression of these biomarkers may correlate with tumor aggressiveness. Thus far, however, the data are based on small numbers of cases and lack multivariate analysis.

Cystic Tumors of the Pancreas

Background

Cystic tumors of the pancreas are relatively uncommon but are important both because they generally have a better prognosis than solid pancreatic tumors and because they can be confused with pancreatic pseudocysts. Overall, about 80% of pancreatic cystic lesions are pseudocysts, and the minority, about 20%, are the lesions discussed in this section. Pseudocysts can generally be distinguished from other cystic lesions by the clinical situation in which they arise and by their radiographic appearance. Because most pseudocysts are best treated by internal drainage and other cystic lesions are best treated with resection, it is important to make this differentiation accurately. When the clinician is uncertain regarding the nature of the lesion, biopsy of the cyst wall with examination of its lining for epithelial elements is useful as these will be absent in pseudocysts but present in other cystic lesions. Cyst fluid analysis has limited usefulness in distinguishing among the diagnostic possibilities.

Simple (Congenital) Cysts

Simple cysts are thought to be congenital and are usually found in children. They tend to be solitary, unilocular, and lined by a simple cuboidal epithelium and probably arise as an abnormality of ductal development. They have no malignant potential. In adults, they cannot reliably be differentiated from mucinous cystadenomas radiographically; thus, when identified, they are best treated with excision. Formal pancreatectomy is not required.

Retention Cysts

Cysts can occur from obstruction of the pancreatic duct, as in pancreatitis, with progressive dilation of the obstructed segment of duct. Generally, the low cuboidal ductal epithelium is retained, but in most ways these lesions mimic pseudocysts. Most arise in the setting of chronic pancreatitis with ductal stricture or, less commonly, from an obstructing pancreatic cancer. Communication with the ductal system may be evident on ERCP.

Polycystic Disease of the Pancreas

Multiple pancreatic cysts can be present in association with polycystic kidney and liver disease, cystic fibrosis, and von Hippel-Lindau disease. About 10% of patients with polycystic kidney disease have pancreatic cysts. They generally are small and asymptomatic and do not require specific treatment. In cystic fibrosis, ductal plugging from thick secretions can lead to a form of retention cyst with ductal dilation proximal to the obstruction and parenchymal atrophy. Generally, these patients are not symptomatic from the pancreatic cysts, and no specific treatment is required. Von Hippel-Lindau disease is an autosomal dominant disorder associated with cerebellar tumors and retinal angiomas. Many of these patients have pancreatic cysts, which are lined by a cuboidal epithelium. Similar cysts can be found in the kidney, liver, and spleen.

Serous Cystadenoma

Serous cystadenomas are benign cystic tumors seen most often in middle-aged women. They average about 6 cm in size at the time of presentation. Symptoms commonly include vague abdominal pain. Many, however, are silent, and the lesion is discovered incidentally during a search for other pathology, such as gallstones. Jaundice and weight loss are rare. Radiographic assessment is key to their diagnosis. By ultrasonography, they generally appear as a complex low-density mass comprised of multiple small cysts separated by fine septae. Computed tomography shows a similar appearance and may identify a central stellate calcification in a "sunburst" pattern.

Treatment is excision. Formal pancreatectomy is generally not required. Pathologically, these lesions are found to contain thin, serous, fluid. The cysts are lined with flat cuboidal cells that stain richly for glycogen, but not mucin. Anaplastic features and tissue invasion are absent. Cure is achieved in nearly all patients with excision alone. Rare reported cases have had malignant transformation.

Mucinous Cystic Neoplasms

Mucinous cystic neoplasms are important to differentiate from serous cystadenomas because of the potential for malignancy in the former. The clinical presentation is similar to serous cystadenomas, with an apparent female preponderance. Most patients present with nonspecific abdominal pain, bloating, or an incidentally discovered mass. Jaundice is uncommon. Ultrasonography or CT show a large cystic mass similar in appearance to a pseudocyst. Unlike pseudocysts, however, patients with mucinous cystic neoplasms do not generally have a history of acute or chronic pancreatitis.[192] The lesions may include septae or have an irregular lumen. Occasionally, calcification will be seen in the cyst wall.

Treatment of mucinous cystic neoplasms is resection, including a margin of normal pancreas. For lesions in the body of the gland, this usually requires distal pancreatectomy. A splenic-preserving operation may be performed if there is no involvement of the splenic vessels or evidence of lymphadenopathy. If a suspicion of malignancy exists, then distal pancreatectomy and regional lymphadenectomy are indicated. For lesions in the head of the gland, pancreaticoduodenectomy may be required.

The prognosis of mucinous cystic neoplasms is generally good. In about 25% of cases, areas of malignancy will be identified in the cyst wall. Overall survival appears to be about 70% at 5 years. Most survivors, however, appear to be those without identified malignant elements.

Cystadenocarcinoma

Cystadenocarcinoma is the end stage of mucinous cystic neoplasm. These lesions tend to present as bulky cystic masses with irregular walls in the head or body of the pancreas. When found in the head of the gland, jaundice may be present. Those arising in the body of the gland tend to present with nonspecific symptoms, including abdominal and back pain, bloating, and weight loss. These lesions do not tend to be as invasive as typical ductal adenocarcinoma, and even bulky lesions may not invade the portal vein or hepatic artery. Treatment is resection. In the recent French multiinstitutional review of cystic neoplasms, the 5-year survival rate for patients with cystadenocarcinoma of the pancreas was 63%.[193]

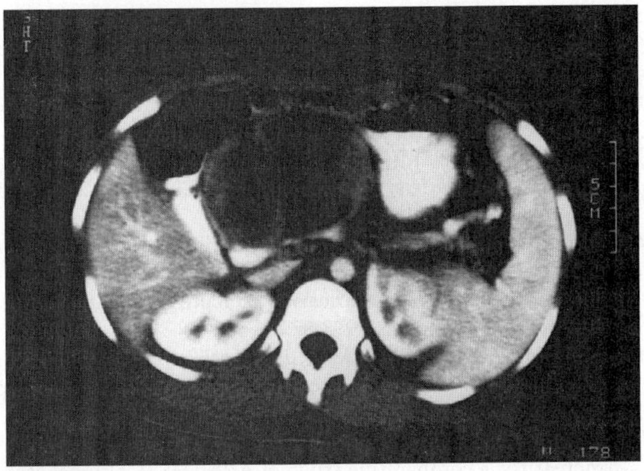

FIGURE 46.21. Computed tomography in a patient with a solid and cystic papillary neoplasm of the pancreas. This unusual lesion tends to arise in relatively young women and may attain a large size before detection. The lesion typically is well circumscribed and has both solid and cystic components. Resection is usually curative.

Solid and Cystic Papillary Neoplasm of the Pancreas

The solid and cystic papillary neoplasm is a rare lesion, typically arising in young women. The lesion tends to be large, averaging 10 cm in diameter. Most patients present with abdominal pain, and in many cases the lesions are confused with pseudocysts. Jaundice is rare. Computed tomography shows a large mass with heterogeneous solid and cystic components (Fig. 46.21). Treatment is resection. Although most patients are cured, rare reported cases have developed metastases, so this lesion should be considered a low-grade malignancy and be removed completely. Adjuvant chemotherapy and radiotherapy are not warranted.[194]

Intraductal Papillary Mucinous Tumors

Intraductal papillary mucinous tumor is a rare lesion, but increasingly recognized today. Many terms have been used to describe this lesion in the past, including mucinous ductal ectasia, ductectatic cystadenoma, mucin-producing ductal tumor, and the like. First reported in Japan, it is characterized by marked distension of the pancreatic duct with mucin with ductal epithelial mucinous hyperplasia, intraductal papillomas, and dysplasia. Cases have been described with progression to cancer.[195] Most patients present with features of pancreatitis, probably from ductal obstruction. Computed tomography demonstrates a cystic pancreatic mass, which may represent either ductal distension or an associated mucinous cystic neoplasm. Endoscopic retrograde cholangiopancreatography is key to the diagnosis and reveals extrusion of mucous through the papilla, a dilated and irregular ductal system, and filling defects within the duct.

Treatment of intraductal papillary mucinous tumor is with surgical resection. Although some cases have successfully been treated with local excision, because of its malignant potential, formal pancreatectomy is the preferred option. The prognosis is good, with better long-term survival than typical ductal adenocarcinoma.[196,197]

Other Tumors

Pancreatic Lymphoma

Pancreatic lymphomas are rare, especially as an isolated lesion.[198,199] More commonly, the pancreas is involved in non-Hodgkin's lymphoma as an incidental part of advanced intraabdominal and extraabdominal disease. Pancreatic lymphomas tend to present as bulky lesions with nonspecific symptoms, such as abdominal pain, that cannot be distinguished from those of pancreatic adenocarcinoma. A palpable abdominal mass is present in about one-half of patients. Despite their large size, jaundice is uncommon.

These tumors respond favorably to radiation and chemotherapy. Thus, suspicion of such a lesion warrants percutaneous fine-needle aspiration biopsy as a diagnosis of lymphoma makes surgical resection unnecessary. In general, palliative procedures such as biliary or gastric bypass are also unnecessary. Jaundice, if present, can be treated with an endoscopic stent prior to initiating radiation or chemotherapy. Gastric outlet obstruction is probably best treated with bowel rest and total parenteral nutrition as the obstruction is likely to rapidly regress as radiation and chemotherapy are begun.

Adenosquamous Carcinoma

Adenosquamous carcinoma tumors are rare, accounting for about 1% of pancreatic tumors. They are also known as squamous carcinoma of the pancreas, adenoacanthomas, or mucoepidermoid cancers. Normally, the pancreas does not contain any squamous or keratizing elements. Histologically, these tumors tend to have a mixture of squamous and columnar malignant cells. Tumors with purely squamous cell components may be metastatic to the pancreas. Patients tend to be elderly and present with advanced disease with jaundice or abdominal pain. Generally, these lesions cannot be distinguished from the more common ductal adenocarcinoma on the basis of clinical or radiographic criteria. Treatment is resection, but the prognosis is poor. In a recent review of the reported literature, summarizing 134 patients, the average survival was only 5.7 months.[200] Radiation and chemotherapy appear relatively ineffective.

Pancreatic Sarcomas

Pancreatic sarcomas are rare lesions, usually presenting as a bulky solid lesion in the body of the gland. Metastatic disease is commonly present at the time of diagnosis. Particular attention must be paid to excluding pulmonary metastases before considering surgical resection. If identified when localized, then radical distal pancreatectomy and splenectomy are warranted for lesions in the body and tail of the gland. Pancreaticoduodenectomy is indicated for lesions of the head of the gland.

References

1. Cotton PB. Pancreas divisum—curiosity or culprit? Gastroenterology 1985;89:1431–1435.
2. Pearse AG, Polak JM, Bloom SR. The newer gut hormones. Cellular sources, physiology, pathology, and clinical aspects. Gastroenterology 1977;72(4 pt 1):746–761.

3. Pearse AG. The cytochemistry and ultrastructure of polypeptide hormone-producing cells of the APUD series and the embryologic, physiologic and pathologic implications of the concept. J Histochem Cytochem 1969;17:303–313.
4. Gittes GK, Rutter WJ. Onset of cell-specific gene expression in the developing mouse pancreas. Proc Natl Acad Sci U S A 1992;89:1128–1132.
5. Gittes GK, Galante PE, Hanahan D, et al. Lineage-specific morphogenesis in the developing pancreas: role of mesenchymal factors. Development (Camb) 1996;122:439–447.
6. Kozarek RA, Ball TJ, Patterson DJ, et al. Endoscopic approach to pancreas divisum. Dig Dis Sci 1995;40:1974–1981.
7. Bernard JP, Sahel J, Giovannini M, et al. Pancreas divisum is a probable cause of acute pancreatitis: a report of 137 cases [see comments]. Pancreas 1990;5:248–254.
8. Delhaye M, Engelholm L, Cremer M. Pancreas divisum: congenital anatomic variant or anomaly? Contribution of endoscopic retrograde dorsal pancreatography. Gastroenterology 1985;89:951–958.
9. Richter JM, Schapiro RH, Mulley AG, et al. Association of pancreas divisum and pancreatitis, and its treatment by sphincteroplasty of the accessory ampulla. Gastroenterology 1981;81: 1104–1110.
10. Palade G. Intracellular aspects of the process of protein synthesis. Science 1975;189:347–358.
11. Bayliss WM, Starling EH. The mechanism of pancreatic secretion. J Physiol (Camb) 1902;28:325.
12. Mayerle J, Hlouschek V, Lerch MM. Current management of acute pancreatitis. Nat Clin Pract Gastroenterol Hepatol 2005;2:473–483.
13. Bradley ELD. A clinically based classification system for acute pancreatitis. Summary of the International Symposium on Acute Pancreatitis, Atlanta, GA, September 11–13, 1992. Arch Surg 1993;128:584–590.
14. Acosta JM, Ledesma CL. Gallstone migration as a cause of acute pancreatitis. N Engl J Med 1974;290:484–487.
15. Kelly TR. Gallstone pancreatitis: pathophysiology. Surgery (St. Louis) 1976;80:488–492.
16. Hanck C, Whitcomb DC. Alcoholic pancreatitis. Gastroenterol Clin North Am 2004;33:751–765.
17. Poon RT, Yeung C, Liu CL, et al. Intravenous bolus somatostatin after diagnostic cholangiopancreatography reduces the incidence of pancreatitis associated with therapeutic endoscopic retrograde cholangiopancreatography procedures: a randomised controlled trial. Gut 2003;52:1768–1773.
18. Shimizu S, Kutsumi H, Fujimoto S, et al. Diagnostic endoscopic retrograde cholangio-pancreatography. Endoscopy 1999;31:74–79.
19. Neuhaus H. Therapeutic pancreatic endoscopy. Endoscopy 2004;36:8–16.
20. Steer ML, Meldolesi J. The cell biology of experimental pancreatitis. N Engl J Med 1987;316:144–150.
21. Tenner S, Dubner H, Steinberg W. Predicting gallstone pancreatitis with laboratory parameters: a meta-analysis. Am J Gastroenterol 1994;89:1863–1866.
22. Scheiman JM, Carlos RC, Barnett JL, et al. Can endoscopic ultrasound or magnetic resonance cholangiopancreatography replace ERCP in patients with suspected biliary disease? A prospective trial and cost analysis. Am J Gastroenterol 2001;96:2900–2904.
23. Liu CL, Fan ST, Lo CM, et al. Comparison of early endoscopic ultrasonography and endoscopic retrograde cholangiopancreatography in the management of acute biliary pancreatitis: a prospective randomized study. Clin Gastroenterol Hepatol 2005;3:1238–1244.
24. Ranson JH, Rifkind KM, Turner JW. Prognostic signs and nonoperative peritoneal lavage in acute pancreatitis. Surg Gynecol Obstet 1976;143:209–219.
25. Ranson JH, Rifkind KM, Roses DF, et al. Prognostic signs and the role of operative management in acute pancreatitis. Surg Gynecol Obstet 1974;139:69–81.
26. McKay CJ, Imrie CW. Staging of acute pancreatitis. Is it important? Surg Clin North Am 1999;79:733–743.
27. De Sanctis JT, Lee MJ, Gazelle GS, et al. Prognostic indicators in acute pancreatitis: CT versus APACHE II. Clin Radiol 1997;52:842–848.
28. Dominquez-Munoz JE, Carballo F, Garcia MJ, et al. Evaluation of the clinical usefulness of APACHE II and SAPS systems in the initial prognostic classification of acute pancreatitis: a multicenter study. Pancreas 1993;8:682–686.
29. Larvin M, McMahon MJ. APACHE-II score for assessment and monitoring of acute pancreatitis [see comments]. Lancet 1989;2:201–205.
30. Wilson C, Heath DI, Imrie CW. Prediction of outcome in acute pancreatitis: a comparative study of APACHE II, clinical assessment and multiple factor scoring systems. Br J Surg 1990;77:1260–1264.
31. Balthazar EJ, Freeny PC, vanSonnenberg E. Imaging and intervention in acute pancreatitis. Radiology 1994;193:297–306.
32. Balthazar EJ, Robinson DL, Megibow AJ, et al. Acute pancreatitis: value of CT in establishing prognosis. Radiology 1990; 174:331–336.
33. Andriulli A, Leandro G, Clemente R, et al. Meta-analysis of somatostatin, octreotide and gabexate mesilate in the therapy of acute pancreatitis. Aliment Pharmacol Ther 1998;12:237–245.
34. Andriulli A, Caruso N, Quitadamo M, et al. Antisecretory versus antiproteasic drugs in the prevention of post-ERCP pancreatitis: the evidence-based medicine derived from a meta-analysis study. JOP 2003;4:41–48.
35. Seta T, Noguchi Y, Shimada T, Shikata S, Fukui T. Treatment of acute pancreatitis with protease inhibitors: a meta-analysis. Eur J Gastroenterol Hepatol 2004;16:1287–1293.
36. Sarr MG, Sanfey H, Cameron JL. Prospective, randomized trial of nasogastric suction in patients with acute pancreatitis. Surgery (St. Louis) 1986;100:500–504.
37. Z'graggen K, Uhl W, Friess H, Buchler MW. How to do a safe pancreatic anastomosis. J Hepatobiliary Pancreat Surg 2002; 9:733–737.
38. Griniatsos J, Karvounis E, Isla A. Early versus delayed single-stage laparoscopic eradication for both gallstones and common bile duct stones in mild acute biliary pancreatitis. Am Surg 2005;71:682–686.
39. Chang EG. Repair of common bile duct injury with the round and falciform ligament after clip necrosis: case report. JSLS 2000;4:163–165.
40. Tang E, Stain SC, Tang G, et al. Timing of laparoscopic surgery in gallstone pancreatitis. Arch Surg 1995;130:496–499.
41. Schwesinger WH, Page CP, Gross GW, et al. Biliary pancreatitis: the era of laparoscopic cholecystectomy. Arch Surg 1998;133: 1103–1106.
42. Bulkin AJ, Tebyani N, Dorazio RA. Gallstone pancreatitis in the era of laparoscopic cholecystectomy. Am Surg 1997;63:900–903.
43. Uhl W, Gloor B, Buchler MW. Pancreatic surgery. Curr Opin Gastroenterol 1999;15:410.
44. Ong AM, Bhayani SB, Hsu TH, et al. Bipolar needle electrocautery for laparoscopic partial nephrectomy without renal vascular occlusion in a porcine model. Urology 2003;62:1144–1148.
45. Burch JM, Feliciano DV, Mattox KL, et al. Gallstone pancreatitis. The question of time. Arch Surg 1990;125:853–859.
46. Cameron DR, Goodman AJ. Delayed cholecystectomy for gallstone pancreatitis: re-admissions and outcomes. Ann R Coll Surg Engl 2004;86:358–362.
47. Alimoglu O, Ozkan OV, Sahin M, Akcakaya A, Eryilmaz R, Bas G. Timing of cholecystectomy for acute biliary pancreatitis:

outcomes of cholecystectomy on first admission and after recurrent biliary pancreatitis. World J Surg 2003;27:256–259.
48. Ayub K, Imada R, Slavin J. Endoscopic retrograde cholangiopancreatography in gallstone-associated acute pancreatitis. Cochrane Database Syst Rev 2004 Oct 18;(4):CD003630.
49. Buchler MW, Gloor B, Muller CA, Friess H, Seiler CA, Uhl W. Acute necrotizing pancreatitis: treatment strategy according to the status of infection. Ann Surg 2000;232:619–626.
50. Uomo G, Visconti M, Manes G, et al. Nonsurgical treatment of acute necrotizing pancreatitis. Pancreas 1996;12:142–148.
51. Bradley ELD, Allen K. A prospective longitudinal study of observation versus surgical intervention in the management of necrotizing pancreatitis. Am J Surg 1991;161:19–24; discussion 24–25.
52. Rau B, Pralle U, Uhl W, et al. Management of sterile necrosis in instances of severe acute pancreatitis. J Am Coll Surg 1995; 181:279.
53. Beger HG, Krautzberger W, Bittner R, et al. Results of surgical treatment of necrotizing pancreatitis. World J Surg 1985;9:972–979.
54. Bassi C, Butturini G, Molinari E, et al. Pancreatic fistula rate after pancreatic resection. The importance of definitions. Dig Surg 2004;21:54–59.
55. Rau BM, Kruger CM, Schilling MK. Anti-cytokine strategies in acute pancreatitis: pathophysiological insights and clinical implications. Rocz Akad Med Bialymst 2005;50:106–115.
56. Beger HG, Büchler M, Bittner R, et al. Necrosectomy and postoperative local lavage in necrotizing pancreatitis. Br J Surg 1988;75:207–212.
57. vanSonnenberg E, Wittich GR, Chon KS, et al. Percutaneous radiologic drainage of pancreatic abscesses. AJR Am J Roentgenol 1997;168:979–984.
58. Gerzof SG, Banks PA, Robbins AH, et al. Early diagnosis of pancreatic infection by computed tomography-guided aspiration. Gastroenterology 1987;93:1315–1320.
59. Tsiotos GG, Luque-de Leon E, Seoreide JA, et al. Management of necrotizing pancreatitis by repeated operative necrosectomy using a zipper technique. Am J Surg 1998;175:91–98.
60. Fernandez-del Castillo C, Rattner DW, Makary MA, et al. Debridement and closed packing for the treatment of necrotizing pancreatitis. Ann Surg 1998;228:676–684.
61. Hartwig W, Werner J, Muller CA, Uhl W, Buchler MW. Surgical management of severe pancreatitis including sterile necrosis. J Hepatobiliary Pancreat Surg 2002;9:429–435.
62. Schroder T, Sainio V, Kivisaari L, et al. Pancreatic resection versus peritoneal lavage in acute necrotizing pancreatitis. A prospective randomized trial [see comments]. Ann Surg 1991;214:663–666.
63. Mayer AD, McMahon MJ, Corfield AP, et al. Controlled clinical trial of peritoneal lavage for the treatment of severe acute pancreatitis. N Engl J Med 1985;312:399–404.
64. Broome AH, Eisen GM, Harland RC, et al. Quality of life after treatment for pancreatitis [see comments]. Ann Surg 1996;223:665–670; discussion 670–672.
65. Stroud WH, Cullom JW, Anderson MC. Hemorrhagic complications of severe pancreatitis. Surgery (St. Louis) 1981;90:657–665.
66. Bergert H, Hinterseher I, Kersting S, Leonhardt J, Bloomenthal A, Saeger HD. Management and outcome of hemorrhage due to arterial pseudoaneurysms in pancreatitis. Surgery 2005;137:323–328.
67. Warshaw AL, Simeone JF, Schapiro RH, et al. Evaluation and treatment of the dominant dorsal duct syndrome (pancreas divisum redefined). Am J Surg 1990;159:59–64; discussion 64–66.
68. Bradley EL, Stephan RN. Accessory duct sphincteroplasty is preferred for long-term prevention of recurrent acute pancreatitis in patients with pancreas divisum. J Am Coll Surg 1996 Jul;183:65–70.
69. Chintapalli KN, Ghiatas AA, Chopra S, Escobar B, Esola CC, Dodd GD 3rd. Sonographic findings in cases of missed gallstones. J Clin Ultrasound 1999;27:117–121.
70. Steer ML, Waxman I, Freedman S. Chronic pancreatitis. N Engl J Med 1995;332:1482–1490.
71. Freedman SD, Sakamoto K, Venu RP. GP2, the homologue to the renal cast protein uromodulin, is a major component of intraductal plugs in chronic pancreatitis. J Clin Invest 1993;92:83–90.
72. Schmiegel W, Burchert M, Kalthoff H, et al. Immunochemical characterization and quantitative distribution of pancreatic stone protein in sera and pancreatic secretions in pancreatic disorders [see comments]. Gastroenterology 1990;99:1421–1430.
73. Teich N, Mossner J. Genetic aspects of chronic pancreatitis. Med Sci Monit 2004;10:RA325–RA328.
74. Bradley EL. Pancreatic duct pressure in chronic pancreatitis. Am J Surg 1982;144:313–316.
75. Di Sebastiano P, di Mola FF, Buchler MW, Friess H. Pathogenesis of pain in chronic pancreatitis. Dig Dis 2004;22:267–272.
76. Bockman DE, Buchler M, Malfertheiner P, et al. Analysis of nerves in chronic pancreatitis. Gastroenterology 1988;94:1459–1469.
77. Luetmer PH, Stephens DH, Ward EM. Chronic pancreatitis: reassessment with current CT. Radiology 1989;171:353–357.
78. Talamini G, Bassi C, Falconi M, et al. Pain relapses in the first 10 years of chronic pancreatitis. Am J Surg 1996;171:565–659.
79. Nealon WH, Thompson JC. Progressive loss of pancreatic function in chronic pancreatitis is delayed by main pancreatic duct decompression. A longitudinal prospective analysis of the modified Puestow procedure. Ann Surg 1993;217:458–466; discussion 466–468.
80. Brand B, Kahl M, Sidhu S, Nam VC, Sriram PV, Jaeckle S, Thonke F, Soehendra N. Prospective evaluation of morphology, function, and quality of life after extracorporeal shockwave lithotripsy and endoscopic treatment of chronic calcific pancreatitis. Am J Gastroenterol 2000;95:3428–3438.
81. Topazian M, Aslanian H, Andersen D. Outcome following endoscopic stenting of pancreatic duct strictures in chronic pancreatitis. J Clin Gastroenterol 2005;39:908–911.
82. Mallet-Guy PA. Late and very late results of resections of the nervous system in the treatment of chronic relapsing pancreatitis. Am J Surg 1983;145:234–238.
83. Kozarek RA. Pancreatic stents can induce ductal changes consistent with chronic pancreatitis. Gastrointest Endosc 1990;36:93–95.
84. Conwell DL, Vargo JJ, Zuccaro G, et al. Role of differential neuroaxial blockade in the evaluation and management of pain in chronic pancreatitis. Am J Gastroenterol 2001;96:431–436.
85. Gress FG, Hawes RH, Savides TJ, et al. Role of EUS in the preoperative staging of pancreatic cancer: a large single-center experience. Gastrointest Endosc 1999;50:786–791.
86. Buscher HC, Jansen JB, van Dongen R, Bleichrodt RP, van Goor H. Long-term results of bilateral thoracoscopic splanchnicectomy in patients with chronic pancreatitis. Br J Surg 2002;89:158–162.
87. Howard TJ, Swofford JB, Wagner DL, Sherman S, Lehman GA. Quality of life after bilateral thoracoscopic splanchnicectomy: long-term evaluation in patients with chronic pancreatitis. J Gastrointest Surg 2002;6:845–852.
88. Bradley EL 3rd, Bem J. Nerve blocks and neuroablative surgery for chronic pancreatitis. World J Surg 2003;27:1241–1248.
89. Bradley EL, Clements JL Jr, Gonzalez AC. The natural history of pancreatic pseudocysts: a unified concept of management. Am J Surg 1979;137:135–141.

90. Crass RA, Way LW. Acute and chronic pancreatic pseudocysts are different. Am J Surg 1981;142:660–663.
91. Warshaw AL, Rattner DW. Timing of surgical drainage for pancreatic pseudocyst. Clinical and chemical criteria. Ann Surg 1985;202:720–724.
92. Yeo CJ, Bastidas JA, Lynch-Nyhan A, et al. The natural history of pancreatic pseudocysts documented by computed tomography. Surg Gynecol Obstet 1990;170:411–417.
93. Vitas GJ, Sarr MG. Selected management of pancreatic pseudocysts: operative versus expectant management. Surgery (St. Louis) 1992;111:123–130.
94. D'Agostino HB, van Sonnenberg E, Sanchez RB, et al. Treatment of pancreatic pseudocysts with percutaneous drainage and octreotide. Work in progress. Radiology 1993;187:685–688.
95. D'Egidio A, Schein M. Percutaneous drainage of pancreatic pseudocyst: a prospective study. World J Surg 1991;16:141–146.
96. van Sonnenberg E, Wittich GR, Casola G, et al. Percutaneous drainage of infected and noninfected pancreatic pseudocysts: experience in 101 cases. Radiology 1989;170(3 pt 1):757–761.
97. Spivak H, Galloway JR, Amerson JR, et al. Management of pancreatic pseudocysts. J Am Coll Surg 1998;186:507–511.
98. Criado E, Destefano AA, Weiner TM, et al. Long term results of percutaneous catheter drainage of pancreatic pseudocysts. Surg Gynecol Obstet 1992;175:293–298.
99. Morton JM, Brown A, Galanko JA, et al. A national comparison of surgical versus percutaneous drainage of pancreatic pseudocysts: 1997–2001. J Gastrointest Surg 2005;9:15–20; discussion 20.
100. Heider R, Meyer AA, Galanko JA, et al. Percutaneous drainage of pancreatic pseudocysts is associated with a higher failure rate than surgical treatment in unselected patients. Ann Surg 1999;229:781–787.
101. Nealon WH, Walser E. Surgical management of complications associated with percutaneous and/or endoscopic management of pseudocyst of the pancreas. Ann Surg 2005;241:948–957.
102. Nealon WH, Walser E. Main pancreatic ductal anatomy can direct choice of modality for treating pancreatic pseudocysts (surgery vs. percutaneous drainage). Ann Surg 2002;235:751–758.
103. Beckingham IJ, Krige JE, Bornman PC, et al. Endoscopic management of pancreatic pseudocysts. Br J Surg 1997;84:1638–1645.
104. Baron TH, Harwood GC, Morgan ED, et al. Outcome differences after endoscopic drainage of pancreatic necrosis, acute pancreatic pseudocysts, and chronic pancreatic pseudocysts. Gastrointest Endosc 2002;56:7–17.
105. Edino ST, Yakubu AA. Experience with surgical internal drainage of pancreatic pseudocyst. J Natl Med Assoc 2006;98:1945–1948.
106. Becker WF, Pratt HS, Ganji H. Pseudocysts of the pancreas. Surg Gynecol Obstet 1968;127:744–747.
107. Grace PA, Williamson RC. Modern management of pancreatic pseudocysts. Br J Surg 1993;80:573–578.
108. Newell KA, Liu T, Aranha GV, et al. Are cystgastrostomy and cystjejunostomy equivalent operations for pancreatic pseudocysts? Surgery (St. Louis) 1990;108:635–639; discussion 639–640.
109. Howard TJ, et al. The role of pancreatic resection in the treatment of pancreatic pseudocysts. J Gastrointest Surg 1997;1:205–212.
110. Hauters P, Weerts J, Navez B, et al. Laparoscopic treatment of pancreatic pseudocysts. Surg Endosc 2004;18:1645–1648.
111. Obermeyer RJ, Fisher WE, Salameh JR, Jeyapalan M, Sweeney JF, Brunicardi FC. Laparoscopic pancreatic cystogastrostomy. Surg Laparosc Endosc Percutan Tech 2003;13:250–253.
112. Konner J, O'Reilly E. Pancreatic cancer: epidemiology, genetics, and approaches to screening. Oncology (Williston Park) 2002; 16:1615–1622, 1631–1632.
113. Parkin DM. Global cancer statistics in the year 2000. Lancet Oncol 2001;2:533–543.
114. Jemal A, Kulldorff M, Devesa SS, Hayes RB, Fraumeni JF Jr. A geographic analysis of prostate cancer mortality in the United States, 1970–89. Int J Cancer 2002;101:168–174.
115. Qiu D, Kurosawa M, Lin Y, et al. for the JACC Study Group. Overview of the epidemiology of pancreatic cancer focusing on the JACC Study. J Epidemiol 2005;15(suppl 2):S157–S167.
116. Haddock G, Carter DC. Aetiology of pancreatic cancer [see comments]. Br J Surg 1990;77:1159–1166.
117. Bansal P, Sonnenberg A. Pancreatitis is a risk factor for pancreatic cancer [see comments]. Gastroenterology 1995;109:247–251.
118. Everhart J, Wright D. Diabetes mellitus as a risk factor for pancreatic cancer. A meta-analysis. JAMA 1995;273:1605–1609.
119. Gullo L, Pezzilli R, Morselli-Labate AM. Diabetes and the risk of pancreatic cancer. Italian Pancreatic Cancer Study Group. N Engl J Med 1994;331:81–84.
120. Tascilar M, van Rees BP, Sturm PD, et al. Pancreatic cancer after remote peptic ulcer surgery. J Clin Pathol 2002;55:340–345.
121. Michaud DS. Epidemiology of pancreatic cancer. Minerva Chir 2004;59:99–111.
122. Hilgers W, Kern SE. Molecular genetic basis of pancreatic adenocarcinoma. Genes Chromosomes Cancer 1999;26:1–12.
123. Berthelemy P, Bouisson M, Escourrou J, et al. Identification of K-*ras* mutations in pancreatic juice in the early diagnosis of pancreatic cancer [see comments]. Ann Intern Med 1995;123:188–191.
124. Rall CJ, Yan YX, Graeme-Cook F, et al. Ki-*ras* and p53 mutations in pancreatic ductal adenocarcinoma. Pancreas 1996;12:10–17.
125. Bold RJ, et al. Prognostic factors in resectable pancreatic cancer: p53 and Bcl-2. J Gastrointest Surg 1999;3:263–277.
126. Lei S, Appert HE, Nakata B, et al. Overexpression of HER2-neu oncogene in pancreatic cancer correlates with shortened survival. Int J Pancreatol 1995;17:15–21.
127. Schutte M, Hruban RH, Geradts J, et al. Abrogation of the Rb/p16 tumor-suppressive pathway in virtually all pancreatic carcinomas. Cancer Res 1997;57:3126–3130.
128. Goldstein AM, Fraser MC, Struewing JP, et al. Increased risk of pancreatic cancer in melanoma-prone kindreds with p16INK4 mutations [see comments]. N Engl J Med 1995;333:970–974.
129. Hahn SA, Schutte M, Hoque AT, et al. DPC4, a candidate tumor suppressor gene at human chromosome 18q21.1. Science 1996;271:350–353.
130. Coyle WJ, Pineau BC, Tarnasky PR, et al. Evaluation of unexplained acute and acute recurrent pancreatitis using endoscopic retrograde cholangiopancreatography, sphincter of Oddi manometry and endoscopic ultrasound. Endoscopy 2002;34:617–623.
131. Schima W, Fugger R. Evaluation of focal pancreatic masses: comparison of mangafodipir-enhanced MR imaging and contrast-enhanced helical CT. Eur Radiol 2002;12:2998–3008.
132. Lopez Hanninen E, Amthauer H, Hosten N, et al. Prospective evaluation of pancreatic tumors: accuracy of MR imaging with MR cholangiopancreatography and MR angiography. Radiology 2002;224:34–41.
133. Jhala NC, Jhala DN, Chhieng DC, Eloubeidi MA, Eltoum IA. Endoscopic ultrasound-guided fine-needle aspiration. A cytopathologist's perspective. Am J Clin Pathol 2003;120:351–367.
134. Mertz HR, Sechopoulos P, Delbeke D, Leach SD. EUS, PET, and CT scanning for evaluation of pancreatic adenocarcinoma. Gastrointest Endosc 2000;52:367–371.
135. Heinrich S, Goerres GW, Schafer M, et al. Positron emission tomography/computed tomography influences on the management of resectable pancreatic cancer and its cost-effectiveness. Ann Surg 2005;242:235–243.
136. Rose DM, Delbeke D, Beauchamp RD, et al. ^{18}Fluorodeoxyglucose-positron emission tomography in the management of

patients with suspected pancreatic cancer. Ann Surg 1999;229:729–737; discussion 737–738.
137. Ruf J, Lopez Hanninen E, Oettle H, et al. Detection of recurrent pancreatic cancer: comparison of FDG-PET with CT/MRI. Pancreatology 2005;5:266–272.
138. Saleh MM, Norregaard P, Jorgensen HL, Andersen PK, Matzen P. Preoperative endoscopic stent placement before pancreaticoduodenectomy: a meta-analysis of the effect on morbidity and mortality. Gastrointest Endosc 2002;56:529–534.
139. Sohn TA, Yeo CJ. The molecular genetics of pancreatic ductal carcinoma: a review. Surg Oncol 2000;9:95–101.
140. Pisters PW, Hudec WA, Hess KR, et al. Effect of preoperative biliary decompression on pancreaticoduodenectomy-associated morbidity in 300 consecutive patients. Ann Surg 2001;234:47–55.
141. Povoski SP, Karpeh MS Jr, Conlon KC, et al. Association of preoperative biliary drainage with postoperative outcome following pancreaticoduodenectomy [see comments]. Ann Surg 1999;230:131–142.
142. Sewnath ME, Birjmohun RS, Rauws EA, Huibregtse K, Obertop H, Gouma DJ. The effect of preoperative biliary drainage on postoperative complications after pancreaticoduodenectomy. J Am Coll Surg 2001;192:726–734.
143. Traverso LW, Longmire WP Jr. Preservation of the pylorus in pancreaticoduodenectomy. Surg Gynecol Obstet 1978;146:959–962.
144. Traverso LW, Longmire WP Jr. Preservation of the pylorus in pancreaticoduodenectomy a follow-up evaluation. Ann Surg 1980;192:306–310.
145. Glasgow RE, Mulvihill SJ. Hospital volume influences outcome in patients undergoing pancreatic resection for cancer. West J Med 1996;165:294–300.
146. Yeo CJ, Cameron JL, Lillemoe KD, et al. Pancreaticoduodenectomy for cancer of the head of the pancreas. 201 patients. Ann Surgery 1995;221:721–731; discussion 731–733.
147. Fortner JG. Regional pancreatectomy for cancer of the pancreas, ampulla, and other related sites. Tumor staging and results. Ann Surg 1984;199:418–425.
148. Nguyen TC, Sohn TA, Cameron JL, et al. Standard versus radical pancreaticoduodenectomy for periampullary adenocarcinoma: a prospective, randomized trial evaluating quality of life in pancreaticoduodenectomy survivors. J Gastrointest Surg 2003;7:1–9; discussion 9–11.
149. Yeo CJ, Cameron JL, Lillemoe KD, et al. Pancreaticoduodenectomy with or without distal gastrectomy and extended retroperitoneal lymphadenectomy for periampullary adenocarcinoma, part 2: randomized controlled trial evaluating survival, morbidity, and mortality. Ann Surg 2002;236:355–366.
150. Bold RJ, et al. Major vascular resection as part of pancreaticoduodenectomy for cancer: radiologic, intraoperative, and pathologic analysis. J Gastrointest Surg 1999;3:233–243.
151. Tseng JF, Raut CP, Lee JE, et al. Pancreaticoduodenectomy with vascular resection: margin status and survival duration. J Gastrointest Surg 2004;8:935–949.
152. Neoptolemos JP, Cunningham D, Friess H, et al. Adjuvant therapy in pancreatic cancer: historical and current perspectives. Ann Oncol 2003;14:675–692.
153. Stocken DD, Buchler MW, Dervenis C, et al. Meta-analysis of randomised adjuvant therapy trials for pancreatic cancer. Br J Cancer 2005;92:1372–1381.
154. Crane CH, Beddar AS, Evans DB. The role of intraoperative radiotherapy in pancreatic cancer. Surg Oncol Clin N Am 2003;12:965–977.
155. Schwarz RE, Smith DD, Keny H, et al. Impact of intraoperative radiation on postoperative and disease-specific outcome after pancreatoduodenectomy for adenocarcinoma: a propensity score analysis. Am J Clin Oncol 2003;26:16–21.
156. Evans DB, Pisters PW, Lee JE, et al. Preoperative chemoradiation strategies for localized adenocarcinoma of the pancreas. Journal of Hepato-Biliary-Pancreatic Surg 1998;5:242–250.
157. Sasson AR, Wetherington RW, Hoffman JP, et al. Neoadjuvant chemoradiotherapy for adenocarcinoma of the pancreas: analysis of histopathology and outcome. Int J Gastrointest Cancer 2003;34:121–128.
158. Jordan GL Jr. Pancreatic resection for pancreatic cancer. Surg Clin North Am 1989;69:569–597.
159. Christein JD, Kendrick ML, Iqbal CW, Nagorney DM, Farnell MB. Distal pancreatectomy for resectable adenocarcinoma of the body and tail of the pancreas. J Gastrointest Surg 2005;9:922–927.
160. Brennan MF, Moccia RD, Klimstra D. Management of adenocarcinoma of the body and tail of the pancreas. Ann Surg 1996;223:506–511.
161. Dalton RR, Sarr MG, van Heerden JA, et al. Carcinoma of the body and tail of the pancreas: is curative resection justified? Surgery (St. Louis) 1992;111:489–494.
162. Lillemoe KD, Kaushal S, Cameron JL, et al. Distal pancreatectomy: indications and outcomes in 235 patients. Ann Surg 1999;229:693–698; discussion 698–700.
163. Lillemoe KD, Cameron JL, Kaufman HS, et al. Chemical splanchnicectomy in patients with unresectable pancreatic cancer. A prospective randomized trial. Ann Surg 1993;217:447–455; discussion 456–457.
164. Eisenberg E, Carr DB, Chalmers TC. Neurolytic celiac plexus block for treatment of cancer pain: a meta-analysis [published erratum appears in Anesth Analg 1995;811:213]. Anesth Analg 1995;80:290–295.
165. Polati E, Finco G, Gottin L, et al. Prospective randomized double-blind trial of neurolytic coeliac plexus block in patients with pancreatic cancer. Br J Surg 1998;85:199–201.
166. Gordon RL, Ring EJ, LaBerge JM, et al. Malignant biliary obstruction: treatment with expandable metallic stents—follow-up of 50 consecutive patients. Radiology 1992;182:697–701.
167. Smith AC, Dowsett JF, Russell RC, et al. Randomised trial of endoscopic stenting versus surgical bypass in malignant low bile duct obstruction. Lancet 1994;344:1655–1660.
168. Sarr MG, Cameron JL. Surgical management of unresectable carcinoma of the pancreas. Surgery (St. Louis) 1982;91:123–133.
169. Lillemoe KD, Cameron JL, Hardacre JM, et al. Is prophylactic gastrojejunostomy indicated for unresectable periampullary cancer? A prospective, randomized trial. Ann Surg 1999;230:322–330.
170. Lindsay JO, Andreyev HJ, Vlavianos P, Westaby D. Self-expanding metal stents for the palliation of malignant gastroduodenal obstruction in patients unsuitable for surgical bypass. Aliment Pharmacol Ther 2004;19:901–905.
171. Burris HA III, Moore MJ, Andersen J, et al. Improvements in survival and clinical benefit with gemcitabine as first-line therapy for patients with advanced pancreas cancer: a randomized trial [see comments]. J Clin Oncol 1997;15:2403–2413.
172. Adjei AA. Preclinical and clinical studies with combinations of pemetrexed and gemcitabine. Semin Oncol 2002;29(6 suppl 18):30–34.
173. Gastrointestinal Tumor Study Group. A multi-institutional comparative trial of radiation therapy alone and in combination with 5-fluorouracil for locally unresectable pancreatic carcinoma. Ann Surg 1979;189:205–208.
174. Gastrointestinal Tumor Study Group. Therapy of locally unresectable pancreatic carcinoma: a randomized comparison of high dose (6000 rad) radiation alone, moderated dose radiation (4000 rad 15-fluorouracil), and high dose radiation 15-fluorouracil. Cancer (Phila) 1981;48:1705–1710.
175. Gastrointestinal Tumor Study Group. Treatment of locally unresectable carcinoma of the pancreas: comparison of com-

bined-modality therapy (chemotherapy plus radiotherapy) to chemotherapy alone. J Natl Cancer Inst 1988;80:751–755.
176. Allema JH, Reinders ME, van Gulik TM, et al. Prognostic factors for survival after pancreaticoduodenectomy for patients with carcinoma of the pancreatic head region. Cancer (Phila) 1995;75:2069–2076.
177. Nitecki SS, Sarr MG, Colby TV, et al. Long-term survival after resection for ductal adenocarcinoma of the pancreas. Is it really improving? Ann Surg 1995;221:59–66.
178. Mannell A, van Heerden JA, Weiland LH, et al. Factors influencing survival after resection for ductal adenocarcinoma of the pancreas. Ann Surg 1986;203:403–407.
179. Cameron JL, Crist DW, Sitzmann JV, et al. Factors influencing survival after pancreaticoduodenectomy for pancreatic cancer. Am J Surg 1991;161:120–124.
180. Murr MM, Sarr MG, Oishi AJ, et al. Pancreatic cancer. CA Cancer J Clin 1994;44:304–318.
181. Lillemoe KD. Current management of pancreatic carcinoma. Ann Surg 1995;221:133–148.
182. Bramhall SR, Allum WH, Jones AG, et al. Treatment and survival in 13,560 patients with pancreatic cancer, and incidence of the disease, in the West Midlands: an epidemiological study [see comments]. Br J Surg 1995;82:111–115.
183. Geer RJ, Brennan MF. Prognostic indicators for survival after resection of pancreatic adenocarcinoma. Am J Surg 1993;165:68–72.
184. Janes RH Jr, Niederhuber JE, Chmiel JS, et al. National patterns of care for pancreatic cancer. Results of a survey of the Commission on Cancer. Ann Surg 1996;223:261–272.
185. Fong Y, Gonen M, Rubin D, Radzyner M, Brennan MF. Long-term survival is superior after resection for cancer in high-volume centers. Ann Surg 2005;242:540.
186. Eskelinen M, Lipponen P. A review of prognostic factors in human pancreatic adenocarcinoma. Cancer Detect Prevent 1992;16:287–295.
187. Yamamoto M, Saitoh Y, Hermanek P. Exocrine pancreatic carcinoma. In: Hermanek P, et al. eds. Prognostic Factors in Cancer. Berlin: Springer-Verlag; 1995:105–117.
188. Eskelinen M, Lipponen P, Marin S, et al. DNA ploidy, S-phase fraction, and G2 fraction as prognostic determinants in human pancreatic cancer. Scand J Gastroenterol 1992;27:39–43.
189. Alanen KA, Joensuu H, Klemi PJ, et al. Clinical significance of nuclear DNA content in pancreatic carcinoma. J Pathol 1990;160:313–320.
190. Nakamori S, Ishikawa O, Ohhigashi H, et al. Expression of nucleoside diphosphate kinase/nm23 gene product in human pancreatic cancer: an association with lymph node metastasis and tumor invasion. Clin Exp Metastasis 1993;11:151–158.
191. Yamanaka Y, Friess H, Kobrin MS, et al. Coexpression of epidermal growth factor receptors and ligands in human pancreatic cancer is associated with enhanced tumor aggressiveness. Anticancer Res 1993;13:565–570.
192. Martin I, Hammond P, Scott J, et al. Cystic tumours of the pancreas. Br J Surg 1998;85:1484–1486.
193. Le Borgne J, de Calan L, Partensky C. Cystadenomas and cystadenocarcinomas of the pancreas: a multiinstitutional retrospective study of 398 cases. French Surgical Association. Ann Surg 1999;230:152–161.
194. Mao C, Guvendi M, Domenico DR, et al. Papillary cystic and solid tumors of the pancreas: a pancreatic embryonic tumor? Studies of three cases and cumulative review of the world's literature. Surgery (St. Louis) 1995;118:821–828.
195. Brat DJ, Lillemoe KD, Yeo CJ, et al. Progression of pancreatic intraductal neoplasias to infiltrating adenocarcinoma of the pancreas. Am J Surg Pathol 1998;22:163–169.
196. Sugiyama M, Atomi Y. Intraductal papillary mucinous tumors of the pancreas: imaging studies and treatment strategies. Ann Surg 1998;228:685–691.
197. Rivera JA, Fernandez-del Castillo C, Pins M, et al. Pancreatic mucinous ductal ectasia and intraductal papillary neoplasms. A single malignant clinicopathologic entity. Ann Surg 1997; 225:637–644; discussion 644–646.
198. Bouvet M, Staerkel GA, Spitz FR, et al. Primary pancreatic lymphoma. Surgery (St. Louis) 1998;123:382–390.
199. Behrns KE, Sarr MG, Strickler JG. Pancreatic lymphoma: is it a surgical disease? Pancreas 1994;9:662–667.
200. Madura JA, Jarman BT, Doherty MG, et al. Adenosquamous carcinoma of the pancreas. Arch Surg 1999;134:599–603.
201. Palade GE. Structure and function at the cellular level. JAMA 1966;198:815–825.
202. Neoptolemos JP, Carr-Locke DL, London NJ, et al. Controlled trial of urgent endoscopic retrograde cholangiopancreatography and endoscopic sphincterotomy versus conservative treatment for acute pancreatitis due to gallstones. Lancet 1988;2:979–983.
203. Fan ST, Lai EC, Mok FP, et al. Early treatment of acute biliary pancreatitis by endoscopic papillotomy [see comments]. N Engl J Med 1993;328:228–232.
204. Folsch UR, Nitsche R, Ludtke R, Hilgers RA, Creutzfeldt W. Early ERCP and papillotomy compared with conservative treatment for acute biliary pancreatitis. The German Study Group on Acute Biliary Pancreatitis. N Engl J Med 1997;336:237–242.
205. Beger HG, Bittner R, Block S, et al. Bacterial contamination of pancreatic necrosis. A prospective clinical study. Gastroenterology 1986;91:433–438.
206. Pederzoli P, Bassi C, Vesentini S, et al. A randomized multicenter clinical trial of antibiotic prophylaxis of septic complications in acute necrotizing pancreatitis with imipenem. Surg Gynecol Obstet 1993;176:480–483.
207. Sainio V, Kemppainen E, Puolakkainen P, et al. Early antibiotic treatment in acute necrotising pancreatitis [see comments]. Lancet 1995;346:663–667.
208. Schwarz M, Isenmann R, Meyer H, et al. Antibiotic use in necrotizing pancreatitis. Results of a controlled study [in German]. Dtsch Med Wochenschr 1997;122:356–361.
209. Nordback I, Sand J, Saaristo R, et al. Early treatment with antibiotics reduces the need for surgery in acute necrotizing pancreatitis—a single-center randomized study. J Gastrointest Surg 2001;5:113–118; discussion 118–120.
210. Isenmann R, Runzi M, Kron M, et al. for the German Antibiotics in Severe Acute Pancreatitis Study Group. Prophylactic antibiotic treatment in patients with predicted severe acute pancreatitis: a placebo-controlled, double-blind trial. Gastroenterology 2004;126:997–1004.
211. Luiten EJ, Hop WC, Lange JF, et al. Controlled clinical trial of selective decontamination for the treatment of severe acute pancreatitis. Ann Surg 1995;222:57–65.
212. Partington PF, Rochelle REL. Modified Puestow procedure for retrograde drainage of the pancreatic duct. Ann Surg 1960;152:1037–1043.
213. Warshaw AL, Popp JW Jr, Schapiro RH. Long-term patency, pancreatic function, and pain relief after lateral pancreaticoduodenectomy for chronic pancreatitis. Gastroenterology 1980;79:289–293.
214. Prinz RA, Greenlee HB. Pancreatic duct drainage in 100 patients with chronic pancreatitis. Ann Surg 1981;194:313–320.
215. Holmberg JT. Chronic pancreatitis. Ann Surg 1985;160:3.
216. Munn JS, Aranha GV, Greenlee HB, et al. Simultaneous treatment of chronic pancreatitis and pancreatic pseudocyst. Arch Surg 1987;122:662–667.
217. Bradley ELD. Long-term results of pancreatojejunostomy in patients with chronic pancreatitis. Am J Surg 1987;153:207–213.
218. Nealon WH, Townsend CM Jr, Thompson JC. Operative drainage of the pancreatic duct delays functional impairment in

patients with chronic pancreatitis. A prospective analysis. Ann Surg 1988;208:321–329.
219. Greenlee HB, Prinz RA, Aranha GV. Long-term results of side-to-side pancreaticojejunostomy. World J Surg 1990;14: 70–76.
220. Adams DB, Ford MC, Anderson MC. Outcome after lateral pancreaticojejunostomy for chronic pancreatitis. Ann Surg 1994;219:481–487; discussion 487–489.
221. Rios GA, Adams DB, Yeoh KG, et al. Outcome of lateral pancreaticojejunostomy in the management of chronic pancreatitis with nondilated pancreatic ducts. J Gastrointest Surg 1998;2:223–229.
222. Lucas CE, McIntosh B, Paley D, et al. Chronic pancreatitis. Surgery (St. Louis) 1999;126:790.
223. Nealon WH, Matin S. Analysis of surgical success in preventing recurrent acute exacerbations in chronic pancreatitis. Ann Surg 2001;233:793–800.
224. Buchler MW, Friess H, Müller MW, et al. Randomized trial of duodenum-preserving pancreatic head resection versus pylorus-preserving Whipple in chronic pancreatitis. Am J Surg 1995;169:65–69; discussion 69–70.
225. Izbicki JR, Bloechle C, Knoefel WT, et al. Duodenum-preserving resection of the head of the pancreas in chronic pancreatitis. A prospective, randomized trial. Ann Surg 1995;221:350–358.
226. Izbicki JR, Bloeunle C, Broering DC, et al. Extended drainage versus resection in surgery for chronic pancreatitis: a prospective randomized trial comparing the longitudinal pancreaticojejunostomy combined with local pancreatic head excision with the pylorus-preserving pancreatoduodenectomy. Ann Surg 1998; 228:771–779.
227. Strate T, Taherpour Z, Bloechle C, et al. Long-term follow-up of a randomized trial comparing the Beger and Frey procedures for patients suffering from chronic pancreatitis. Ann Surg 2005;241:591–598.
228. Braasch JW, Vito L, Nugent FW. Total pancreatectomy of end-stage chronic pancreatitis. Ann Surg 1978;188:317–322.
229. Rossi RL, Rothschild J, Braasch JW, et al. Pancreatoduodenectomy in the management of chronic pancreatitis. Arch Surg 1987;122:416–420.
230. Beger HG, Büchler M, Bittner RR, et al. Duodenum-preserving resection of the head of the pancreas in severe chronic pancreatitis. Early and late results. Ann Surg 1989;209:273–278.
231. Easter DW, Cuschieri A. Total pancreatectomy with preservation of the duodenum and pylorus for chronic pancreatitis. Ann Surg 1991;214:575–580.
232. Frey CF, Amikura K. Local resection of the head of the pancreas combined with longitudinal pancreaticojejunostomy in the management of patients with chronic pancreatitis. Ann Surg 1994;220:492–504; discussion 504–507.
233. Sawyer R, Frey CF. Is there still a role for distal pancreatectomy in surgery for chronic pancreatitis? Am J Surg 1994;168: 6–9.
234. Martin RF, Rossi RL, Leslie KA. Long-term results of pylorus-preserving pancreatoduodenectomy for chronic pancreatitis. Arch Surg 1996;131:247–252.
235. Rattner DW, Fernandez-del Castillo C, Warshaw AL. Pitfalls of distal pancreatectomy for relief of pain in chronic pancreatitis. Am J Surg 1996;171:142–145; discussion 145–146.
236. Traverso LW, Kozarek RA. Pancreatoduodenectomy for chronic pancreatitis: anatomic selection criteria and subsequent long-term outcome analysis. Ann Surg 1997;226:429–434.
237. Eddes EH, Masclee AM, Gooszen HG, et al. Effect of duodenum-preserving resection of the head of the pancreas on endocrine and exocrine pancreatic function in patients with chronic pancreatitis. Am J Surg 1997;174:387–392.
238. Beger H. Chronic pancreatitis. Ann Surg 1999;230:512.
239. Lin PW, Lin YJ. Prospective randomized comparison between pylorus-preserving and standard pancreaticoduodenectomy. Br J Surg 1999;86:603–607.
240. Tran KT, Smeenk HG, van Eijck CH, et al. Pylorus preserving pancreaticoduodenectomy versus standard Whipple procedure: a prospective, randomized, multicenter analysis of 170 patients with pancreatic and periampullary tumors. Ann Surg 2004;240:738–745.
241. Seiler CA, Wagner M, Bachmann T, et al. Randomized clinical trial of pylorus-preserving duodenopancreatectomy versus classical Whipple resection-long term results. Br J Surg 2005;92:547–556.
242. Kalser MH, Ellenberg SS. Pancreatic cancer. Adjuvant combined radiation and chemotherapy following curative resection. Arch Surg 1985;120:899–903.
243. Bakkevold KE, Kambestad B. Morbidity and mortality after radical and palliative pancreatic cancer surgery. Risk factors influencing the short-term results. Ann Surg 1993;217:356–368.
244. Lygidakis NJ, Stringaris K. Adjuvant therapy following pancreatic resection for pancreatic duct carcinoma: a prospective randomized study. Hepato-Gastroenterology 1996;43:671–680.
245. Klinkenbijl JH, Jeekel J, Sahmoud T, et al. Adjuvant radiotherapy and 5-fluorouracil after curative resection of cancer of the pancreas and periampullary region: phase III trial of the EORTC gastrointestinal tract cancer cooperative group. Ann Surg 1999;230:776–782.
246. Takada T, Amano H, Yasuda H, et al. Is postoperative adjuvant chemotherapy useful for gallbladder carcinoma? A phase III multicenter prospective randomized controlled trial in patients with resected pancreaticobiliary carcinoma. Cancer 2002;95:1685–1695.
247. Neoptolemos JP, Stocken DD, Dunn JA, et al. Influence of resection margins on survival for patients with pancreatic cancer treated by adjuvant chemoradiation and/or chemotherapy in the ESPAC-1 randomized controlled trial. Ann Surg 2001;234:758–768.
248. Neoptolemos JP, Stocken DD, Friess H, et al. A randomized trial of chemoradiotherapy and chemotherapy after resection of pancreatic cancer [erratum in N Engl J Med 2004;351:726]. N Engl J Med 2004;350:1200–1210.
249. Trede M, Schwall G, Saeger HD. Survival after pancreatoduodenectomy. 118 consecutive resections without an operative mortality. Ann Surg 1990;211:447–458.
250. Nagakawa T, Nagamori M, Futakami F, et al. Results of extensive surgery for pancreatic carcinoma. Cancer (Phila) 1996;77:640–645.
251. Conlon KC, Klimstra DS, Brennan MF. Long-term survival after curative resection for pancreatic ductal adenocarcinoma. Clinicopathologic analysis of 5-year survivors. Ann Surg 1996;223:273–279.
252. Sohn TA, Yeo CJ, Cameron JL, et al. Resected adenocarcinoma of the pancreas-616 patients: results, outcomes, and prognostic indicators. J Gastrointest Surg 2000;4(6):567–569.

47

Biliary System

Hobart W. Harris

History

The history of biliary tract disease extends over 3500 years, but the birth of modern-day surgical intervention occurred little more than a century ago. Early Egyptians were aware of the liver and biliary system and assigned these organs significance for divining future events. The oldest recorded case of gallstones was in the mummified remains of the Princess of Amenen from Thebes, circa 1500 BC. At the time of her death, her well-preserved gallbladder contained at least 30 gallstones.

For more than a millennium after her demise, little changed regarding the largely mystical interpretation of the liver and biliary system. But, beginning with Hippocrates (400 BC) and extending through the time of Galen (AD 200), there gradually developed an appreciation for organ dysfunction and how this might result in disease.

In 1506, the detailed description of right upper quadrant abdominal pain associated with the presence of gallstones made by Antonio Benivieni (1440–1502) was published, representing the first correlation of biliary colic with autopsy findings. During the ensuing 250 years, a growing appreciation for human anatomy, combined with the hypothesis that biliary calculi could result from stasis within the gallbladder, culminated in the first reported cholecystectomy. In 1867, through a surgical misadventure, John Stough Bobbs of Indiana opened what he initially mistook for an ovarian cyst in a woman complaining of abdominal pain. No doubt to his surprise, the incision yielded several gallstones as the cystic structure was instead the gallbladder. After removing the stones, Bobbs closed the cholecystotomy incision, and the patient recovered.

During the 130 plus years since Bobbs's "cholecystectomy," advances in understanding biliary anatomy and the development of relevant surgical therapeutics have transpired at an amazing pace. Not only have most of the anatomical landmarks pertinent to biliary anatomy been described during the last two centuries, but also the operative procedures. And, innovation continues to revolutionize surgery of the biliary system, as shown by the recent advent of laparoscopic cholecystectomy.

Anatomy

In the extrahepatic biliary tree, the gallbladder (vesica fellea) is a hollow, piriform (L., pear-shaped) organ 7 to 10 cm in length, approximately 4 cm in diameter, and with a capacity of 30 to 60 mL (Fig. 47.1). At 4 weeks gestation, the human embryo develops a hepatic diverticulum within the foregut, subsequently forming the gallbladder and extrahepatic biliary ducts (Fig. 47.2). For descriptive purposes, the gallbladder is divided into a fundus, body, infundibulum, and neck. Attached to the liver by loose areolar connective tissue, the portion of the gallbladder not embedded within the liver substance is covered by visceral peritoneum. Small veins and lymphatics course between the gallbladder fossa and the gallbladder wall, connecting the lymphatic and venous drainage of the two organs. The shared lymphovascular drainage explains the spread of gallbladder inflammation and carcinoma to the liver. In addition, a small accessory bile duct may drain directly into the gallbladder (cholecystohepatic duct of Luschka) in a similar manner. During a cholecystectomy, these accessory ducts should be identified and ligated, if present, to prevent postoperative bile leaks. The gallbladder fossa anteriorly and the inferior vena cava posteriorly define the anatomical division between the right and left lobes of the liver.

The body of the gallbladder narrows toward the neck of the organ known as the infundibulum. Major portions of the body and infundibulum of the gallbladder are in juxtaposition to the first portion of the duodenum and the transverse colon. Inflammation of the gallbladder wall can result in the formation of adhesions between the gallbladder and the adjacent intestines, setting the stage for the creation of cholecystoenteric fistulas (e.g., a cholecystoduodenal fistula). The infundibulum of the gallbladder is attached to the first part of the duodenum by an avascular peritoneal reflection termed the

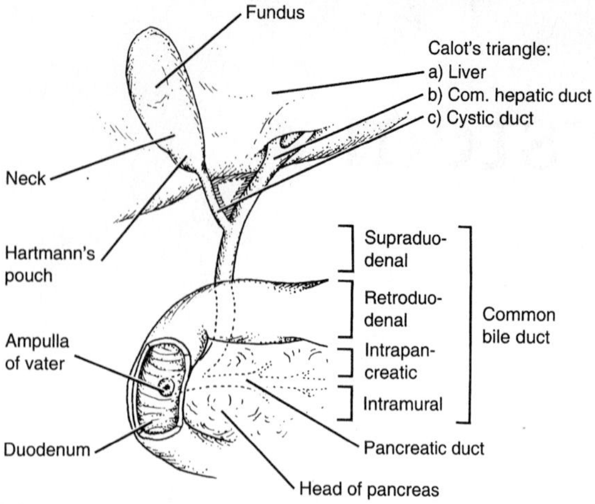

FIGURE 47.1. Anatomy of the gallbladder and bile ducts. (Redrawn with permission from Braasch and Tompkins.[140])

cholecystoduodenal ligament. This ligament is an inferior extension of the hepatoduodenal ligament and can be used during surgery as a landmark for the major vascular structures of the hepatic hilum. The infundibulum joins the cystic duct through the neck of the gallbladder, which is a short S-shaped structure, frequently curved on itself. Protruding from the lateral wall of the neck of the gallbladder, there may be a dilation termed Hartmann's pouch. Projecting in an infero-posterior direction toward the duodenum, gallstones frequently become lodged in this outpouching in such a way that if this area becomes inflamed it may adhere to and obstruct the cystic duct.

The cystic duct is a tubular structure attaching the gallbladder neck to the common hepatic duct. Its length varies from 1 to 5 cm and its diameter from 3 to 7 mm. The mucosa that lines the cystic duct is thrown into 4 to 10 spiral folds, the spiral valves of Heister. These valves prevent the ready passage of gallstones and excessive distension or collapse of the cystic duct despite wide variations in ductal pressure. It is important to keep the cystic duct patent at all times so that bile easily enters the gallbladder when the choledochal sphincter is closed and so that bile flows in the opposite direction down into the duodenum when the gallbladder contracts. The cystic duct may join the extrahepatic biliary tree in a variety of ways, including an angular, parallel, or spiral configuration (Fig. 47.3). In approximately 70% of people, the junction between the cystic and common hepatic ducts is angular,[1] occurring along the right lateral wall of the hepatic duct. However, the cystic duct can run parallel to the hepatic duct for as long as 6 cm before they merge. In such cases, the two ducts are often densely adherent and difficult to separate. When the ducts join in a spiral fashion, the cystic duct may circle either anterior or posterior to the hepatic duct, entering along the left lateral wall of the hepatic duct. This anatomical variant increases the risk of common bile duct injury when the cystic duct is dissected all the way to its junction with the hepatic duct.

The anatomical relationships of the extrahepatic biliary tree and its frequent variations are of importance to surgeons operating in this region. The variability applies to the gallbladder, the biliary ductal system, and their vascular supply. Although abnormalities of the gallbladder itself are uncommon, found in less than 3% of cases,[1] the range is broad. Gallbladder anomalies entail duplications, abnormalities of the gallbladder's shape, or variations in its attachment to the liver.[2,3] In rare instances, the gallbladder is completely embedded in the liver. Such intrahepatic gallbladders are usually located within the right lobe of the liver, close to the visceral surface. Congenital absence of the gallbladder, also rare, is frequently associated with atresia of additional segments of the extrahepatic biliary tree. As this is infrequently identified before operation, one must exclude the presence of an intrahepatic gallbladder before confirming this diagnosis.

A single cystic artery usually accomplishes the arterial supply to the gallbladder, but in 12% of cases double cystic

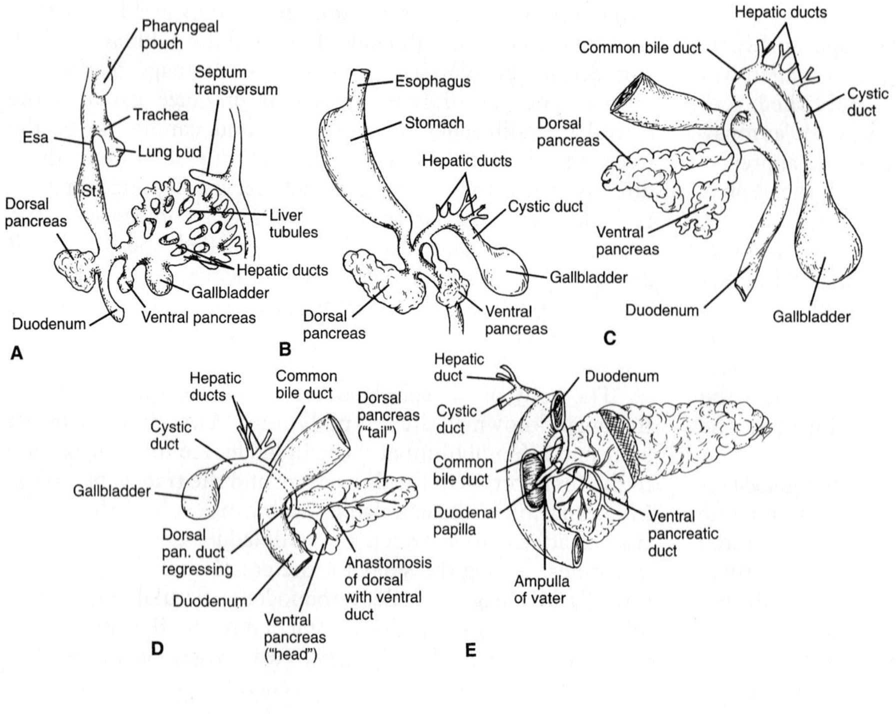

FIGURE 47.2. Development of the human biliary primordia. (**A**) Fifth week of development in a human embryo. (**B**) Sixth week of development. (**C**) Seventh week of development. (**D**) Maturation of the biliary system and pancreas. (**E**) Relationship of the biliary and pancreatic ductal systems. (Redrawn with permission from Patten,[141] © 1953 McGraw-Hill.)

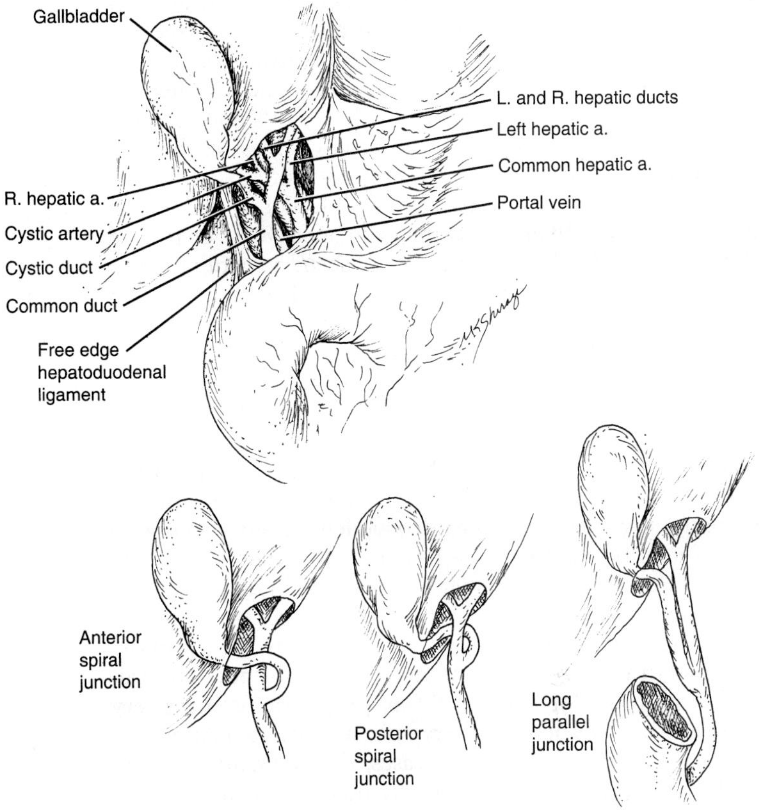

FIGURE 47.3. Variations in the anatomy of the cystic duct. (Adapted with permission from Lindner.[1])

arteries exist.[1,4] The origin and course of the cystic artery are highly variable; indeed, the course of this artery is one of the most variable in the body. In the majority (75%) of cases, the cystic artery originates from the proximal right hepatic artery and immediately divides into two branches: the superficial branch, which runs along the peritoneal surface of the gallbladder, and the deep branch, which runs along the gallbladder fossa between the gallbladder and liver (Fig. 47.4). The cystic artery usually lies superior to the cystic duct and passes posterior to the common hepatic duct. With this anatomical

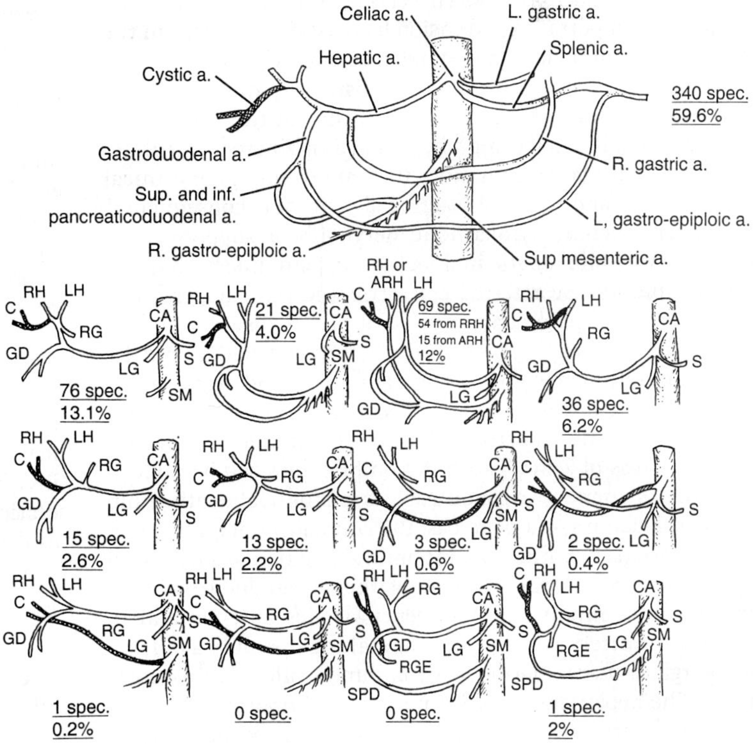

FIGURE 47.4. Variations in the anatomy of the cystic artery. The cystic artery is shaded in each drawing to highlight its variable origins. (Redrawn with permission from Braasch and Tompkins,[140] Mosby-Yearbook Co., © 1994.)

arrangement, the common hepatic duct, the liver, and the cystic duct define the boundaries of Calot's triangle (see Fig. 47.1). Located within this triangle are some structures of great importance to the surgeon: the cystic artery, the right hepatic artery, and the cystic duct lymph node. Calot's node is often involved with inflammatory or neoplastic disease of the gallbladder because this is one of the primary routes of lymphatic drainage. Lymph fluid from the gallbladder drains either directly into the liver across the gallbladder fossa or toward the common bile duct, where it can ascend toward nodes in the hilum of the liver or descend toward celiac axis nodes. In 25% of cases, the relationship between the arteries and bile ducts in the hilum of the liver varies widely (Fig. 47.4).

The cystic artery can originate from the following sites: an accessory or replaced right hepatic artery (12%), the left hepatic artery (6.2%), the gastroduodenal artery (2.6%), the common hepatic artery (2.2%), the proper hepatic artery (0.6%), the celiac axis (0.4%), or in rare cases, the superior mesenteric or superior pancreaticoduodenal artery.[2,4,5] Despite the variability, basic patterns do exist. More than 90% of the time, the cystic artery originates from the right hepatic artery, even though the latter vessel may have an anomalous origin. In addition, when the cystic artery originates to the left of the bile duct, it usually passes anteriorly to the bile duct. Regardless of its origin, in 7% to 10% of people the cystic artery parallels the right hepatic artery until just before it enters the right lobe of the liver. In these cases, the cystic artery is but a few millimeters long, and it may be easily confused with the right hepatic artery. Although ligation of a lobar hepatic artery is to be avoided, the usual concerns regarding consequent lobar degeneration or infarction are unwarranted. Unlike the arterial system, there are no named veins draining the gallbladder. As mentioned, some of the organ's venous return passes directly into the liver across the gallbladder fossa. The remaining venous drainage parallels the cystic duct lymphatics, forming venous networks along the common bile duct before joining the portal venous system. Occasionally, patients with portal hypertension have obvious varices in the area of the gallbladder and extrahepatic biliary tree.

Fibers from the sympathetic and parasympathetic nervous systems innervate the gallbladder. Although the nerves supplying the gallbladder and choledochal sphincter contribute to overall gallbladder function, they are of no major clinical significance and can be sacrificed without consequence. However, afferent sympathetic nerve fibers supplying the extrahepatic bile ducts include some pain fibers that are responsible for the referred epigastric and right upper quadrant abdominal pain characteristic of biliary disease.

As depicted in Figure 47.1, the common bile duct results from the confluence of the common hepatic and cystic ducts, varies in length from 5 to 17 cm, and is normally 3 to 8 mm in diameter, unless obstructed, when it can dilate to a diameter in excess of 2 cm. The common bile duct can be divided into four segments as a function of its anatomical relationship to the duodenum and pancreas: the supraduodenal, retroduodenal, intrapancreatic, and intramural segments. Enveloped within the peritoneal covering of the hepatoduodenal ligament, the common bile duct generally lies anterolateral to the hepatic artery and portal vein, making it readily available for surgical manipulation (e.g., common bile duct exploration). The hepatoduodenal ligament is an important anatomical landmark as it represents the right border of the

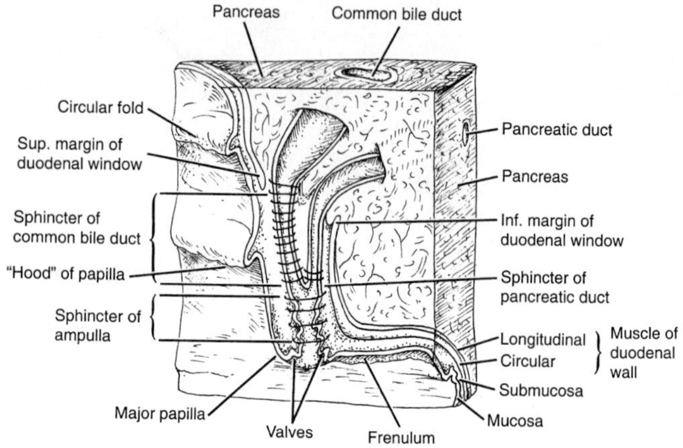

FIGURE 47.5. Sphincteric mechanism at the terminal end of the common bile duct. (Redrawn with permission from Way and Pelligrini,[142] W. B. Saunders Co., © 1987.)

hepatogastric ligament (lesser omentum) and defines the anterior border of the epiploic foramen of Winslow connecting the greater and lesser peritoneal cavities. In addition to yielding entry to the lesser sac, the foramen of Winslow enables the structures of the portal triad to be easily encircled and compressed (Pringle maneuver).

After the common duct descends posterior to the first part of the duodenum, it travels through the head of the pancreas, then for 1 to 2 cm obliquely within the medial wall of the second portion of the duodenum before forming a common channel with the main pancreatic duct (ampulla of Vater), which empties into the duodenal lumen through a mucosal papilla. The terminal portion of the common bile duct is encircled by a combination of circular and longitudinal smooth muscles, which serve to control the entry of biliopancreatic secretions into the proximal intestinal tract (Fig. 47.5). This muscular structure, termed the choledochalduodenal sphincter of Oddi, has a phasic resting tone ranging from a baseline of approximately 13 mmHg to as high as 200 mmHg. The contractile activity of the sphincter of Oddi demonstrates a cyclical pattern that varies in relationship to the intermittent myoelectric migratory complex (IMMC) of the intestinal tract, with the majority (85%) of peristaltic waves migrating in a caudal direction.

The common bile duct derives its blood supply not from any named blood vessels but rather from a complex network of interwoven small vessels derived predominantly from the cystic and the posterior pancreaticoduodenal arteries. Because there is no specific vessel to identify and preserve during dissections of the common bile duct, this tubular structure is vulnerable to ischemic injury. To avoid disrupting the fragile inconstant blood supply to the duct and thus increase the risk of postoperative bile leakage or stricture formation, it is critically important not to strip the common bile duct of the investing loose areolar tissue during its isolation and manipulation. The nerve supply to the common duct is the same as described for the gallbladder.

Physiology

The biliary tree is designed for the transport and storage of bile produced in the liver by hepatocytes and destined for the duodenal lumen to participate in the digestion of foodstuffs.

TABLE 47.1. Biliary Lipid Compositions of Gallbladder Bile.

Lipid component	*Controls*	*Cholesterol stones*	*Change (%)*
Biliary lipid (mol%)			
Bile salts	72.0	70.2	22.5
Phospholipids	21.1	20.6	22.4
Cholesterol	6.9	9.0	130
Cholesterol saturation index	1.00	1.32	132
Cholesterol : phospholipid ratio	0.34	0.46	135
Cholesterol : bile salt ratio	0.10	0.13	130

Source: Data from Thistle et al.[135] and Lamont and Carey.[136]

The pattern of bile flow throughout the biliary tree differs when a person is in the fasted versus the postprandial state. Under fasting conditions, biliary tree motility and thus bile flow are regulated by the IMMC and approximated by the cyclical activity of the duodenum.

Observations of the fasting gallbladder over time have shown a predictable pattern of filling, followed by gallbladder contraction and partial (15%–20%) emptying associated with increased plasma levels of motilin. In fact, during phase II of the IMMC (a period of increased duodenal and pancreatic activity), the gallbladder contracts along with the coordinated relaxation of the sphincter of Oddi. The specific function of the gallbladder's phasic activity during fasting is unclear but may represent a mechanism by which stasis of saturated bile and the attendant increased risk of gallstone formation is avoided. The enterohepatic circulation of bile acids predominantly regulates the overall production rate of bile by the liver. Thus, the rate of hepatic bile synthesis is inversely proportional to the amount of bile acid reclaimed from the terminal ileum and recycled to the liver.

Actual filling of the gallbladder results from the continuous production of bile by the liver in the face of a contracted sphincter of Oddi. As the pressure within the common bile duct exceeds that within the gallbladder lumen, hepatic bile enters the gallbladder via retrograde flow through the cystic duct, wherein it is rapidly concentrated. Within a few hours, the gallbladder mucosa, apparently by means of an active sodium-coupled transport mechanism, removes more than 90% of its water content, creating the more highly concentrated gallbladder bile. Consequently, the amount of electrolytes, lipids, bile salts, and pigments in gallbladder bile is significantly more concentrated than that found in hepatic bile (Table 47.1). As discussed elsewhere in this chapter, it is the relative concentrations of cholesterol, phospholipid, and bile salts that effectively determine the lithogenicity of bile.

Following a meal, the gallbladder contracts in response to both a vagally mediated cephalic phase of activity and the release of cholecystokinin (CCK), the major regulator of gallbladder function. During the following 60 to 120 min, approximately 80% to 90% of gallbladder bile is steadily emptied into the intestinal tract. The CCK, which was first identified in 1928, is localized to the proximal small intestine, especially the duodenal epithelial cells, where its release is stimulated by intraluminal fat, amino acids, and gastric acid and inhibited by bile. With a plasma half-life of less than 3 min, at least four different forms of CCK have been identified in plasma. Ranging in length from 8 to 58 amino acids, each form of CCK derives its physiological activity from the same C-terminal octapeptide. Cholecystokinin acts directly via smooth muscle receptors in the gallbladder wall, stimulating muscle contraction in direct proportion to its concentration and in a calcium-dependent as well as vagally mediated manner. In addition to stimulating gallbladder contractions, CCK acts to functionally inhibit the normal phasic motor activity of the sphincter of Oddi. By reducing the frequency and amplitude of the basal contractions, the sphincteric mechanism relaxes in coordination with gallbladder contraction, thus facilitating the delivery of bile into the proximal small intestine.

Gallbladder function is also influenced by other hormones, including vasoactive intestinal polypeptide (VIP), somatostatin, substance P, and norepinepherine. Both VIP and somatostatin inhibit contraction of the gallbladder, consistent with their inhibitory effects on gastrointestinal motility. The role of substance P, norepinepherine, and other neuropeptides in the regulation of gallbladder function remains to be elucidated.

Interestingly, the common bile duct contains very little if any smooth muscle, in only 20% of people. Therefore, the extrahepatic ducts do not actively contribute to bile flow. But, in addition to contraction of the gallbladder, the biliary canaliculi are thought to help pump bile out of the liver and into the intestine.

Diagnosis

Clinically significant symptoms originating from biliary tract pathology are common and generally are the result of obstruction, infection, or both. A thorough knowledge of how biliary tract diseases present is necessary for the clinician to accurately diagnose and manage these disorders. An appreciation for several fundamental tenets of pathophysiology proves invaluable to the evaluation of this patient population as many of the symptoms of biliary tract disease are nonspecific and can mimic other intraabdominal disorders. Specifically, as is true with any hollow tubular structure, the source of bile duct obstruction can be either extramural (pancreatic cancer), intramural (cholangiocarcinoma), or intraluminal (choledocholithiasis; Fig. 47.6). Similarly, as with infections elsewhere in the body, for an infection to develop within the biliary tree requires the following three components: a susceptible host, a sufficient inoculum, and stasis. Given these basic principles, the most common symptoms related to biliary tract disease are abdominal pain, jaundice, fever, and

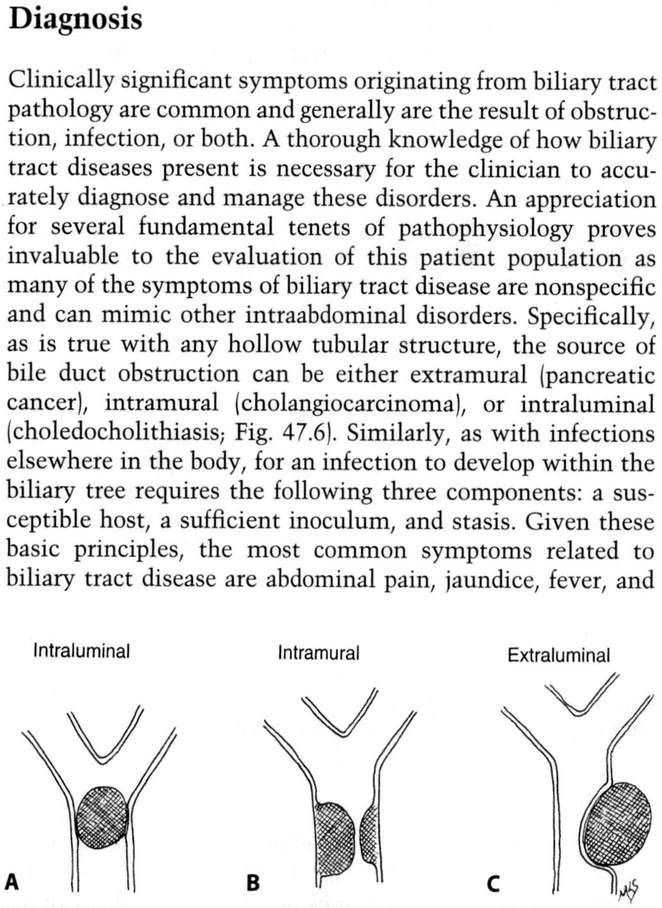

FIGURE 47.6. Mechanisms of bile duct obstruction. (**A**) Intraluminal obstruction (e.g., gallstones). (**B**) Intramural obstruction (e.g., cholangiocarcinoma). (**C**) Extraluminal obstruction (e.g., pancreatic neoplasm).

a constellation of constitutional complaints, including nausea, anorexia, weight loss, and vomiting.

Abdominal Pain

Gallstones and inflammation of the gallbladder are the most frequent causes of abdominal pain resulting from biliary tract disease. Acute obstruction of the gallbladder by calculi results in *biliary colic*, a misnomer in that the pain is not colicky but rather a constant abdominal pain typically localized to the epigastrium or right upper quadrant. Although the pain is often precipitated by eating fatty foods, it can also be triggered by eating other types of food or even begin spontaneously. Unlike intestinal colic, which presents in episodic waves lasting several minutes each, biliary colic is a more constant pain that gradually builds in intensity and can radiate to the back, interscapular region, or right shoulder. Many patients describe the pain as a band- or beltlike constriction of the upper abdomen that may be associated with nausea or vomiting. This recognizable type of abdominal pain results from a normal gallbladder contracting against a luminal obstruction, such as a gallstone impacted in the neck of the organ, the cystic duct, or common bile duct. Under the postprandial influence of CCK and the cholinergic cephalic phase of foregut motility, the essentially isometric contraction of gallbladder smooth muscle yields this characteristic pain. The episode of pain or "attack" resolves as either the diet-induced stimulus for increased gallbladder activity dissipates; the stone becomes dislodged, thereby alleviating the obstruction; or the spontaneous gallbladder wall spasm relaxes. Of note, this pain is visceral in nature, and often patients report a crescendo pattern of increasingly frequent and severe bouts of discomfort.

The pain of biliary colic is distinct from that associated with acute cholecystitis. Although biliary colic can also be localized to the right upper quadrant, the pain of acute cholecystitis is exacerbated by touch, somatic in nature, and often associated with the systemic findings of fever and leukocytosis. The transmural inflammation of the gallbladder provokes irritation of the adjacent visceral and parietal peritoneal surfaces. Therefore, any increases in wall tension or tactile pressure can stimulate nerve endings within the inflamed tissue, as evidenced by a positive *Murphy's sign*. This physical finding, of a patient abruptly stopping the inspiratory effort because of pain as the examiner palpates under the right costal margin, is indicative of acute cholecystitis. The clinical implication of acute cholecystitis is quite different from that of biliary colic. Although biliary colic is an episodic, even unpredictable, functional disorder of the gallbladder that many patients can live with for months to years, acute cholecystitis involves irreversible organ injury and activation of a locoregional inflammatory response, and it invariably requires a definitive therapeutic intervention.

Jaundice

When the serum concentration of bilirubin exceeds approximately 2.5 mg/dL, a yellowish discoloration of the sclera becomes evident (*scleral icterus*). A similar discoloration of the skin (*jaundice*) develops with serum bilirubin levels in excess of 5 mg/dL. Under both circumstances, the visible changes in color represent the deposition of bile pigments in the affected tissues. Jaundice resulting from biliary tract obstruction is presumably caused by the reflux of conjugated bilirubin directly across either the basement membrane of the hepatic sinusoids or damaged canaliculi. The rise in conjugated bilirubin (direct reacting) is in contrast to the increased levels of unconjugated bilirubin (indirect reacting) observed with hepatocellular injury. Interestingly, significant elevations of the total serum bilirubin level are indicative of common bile duct obstruction. In the absence of underlying hepatic dysfunction, the entire liver must be obstructed for a sufficient quantity of regurgitated bile to accumulate in the circulation, sclera, or skin because only a few functioning segments of liver are necessary to maintain normal serum bilirubin levels. As discussed later in this chapter, marked jaundice is considered an operative risk factor, and therefore its management should be carefully evaluated as various therapeutic options are considered.

Fever

Significant elevations in body temperature (≥38.0°C) due to biliary tract disease represent a systemic manifestation of an initially localized inflammatory process. Bacterial contamination of the biliary system is a common feature of acute cholecystitis or choledocholithiasis with obstruction and is to be expected following percutaneous or endoscopic cholangiography. Whether as components of ductal calculi or contaminants introduced during biliary tract instrumentation, fever results from the presence of bacteria within an obstructed biliary tree. Not only do these microorganisms proliferate in this static system, but also bacteria and endotoxin are refluxed into the systemic circulation, causing symptoms that can range from spiking fevers to septic shock. The combination of right upper quadrant abdominal pain, jaundice, and fever, known as *Charcot's triad*, signifies an active infection of the biliary system termed *acute cholangitis*. Patients suffering from acute cholangitis may not present with all these findings, but approximately two-thirds will. Virtually all patients have experienced all three symptoms at some point during their illness. Severely afflicted patients may also display an altered mental status and hypotension (*pentad of Reynolds*). Fever should be viewed as a signal that an otherwise localized disease process has progressed to a systemic illness.

Diagnostic Studies

Abdominal pain, jaundice, and fever are characteristic of biliary tract disease, but these signs and symptoms are also associated with other intraabdominal conditions, including peptic ulcers, acute pancreatitis, hepatitis, and diverticulitis. Thus, additional studies are necessary to confirm the biliary system as the source of the patient's problem, including specific laboratory tests and radiographic examinations.

Laboratory Tests

Simple biliary colic, in the absence of gallbladder wall pathology or common bile duct obstruction, does not produce abnormal laboratory test values. This condition is in many respects a functional disorder of the gallbladder caused by cystic duct obstruction and is not associated with organ injury. On the other hand, obstructive choledocholithiasis is commonly associated with an element of both liver dysfunction and acute cellular injury with resultant elevations in liver function tests.

In addition to hyperbilirubinemia (see Jaundice, earlier), the magnitude of which directly correlates with the severity and duration of the biliary system blockade, an increased serum alkaline phosphatase level is virtually pathognomonic of bile duct obstruction. Alkaline phosphatase is a membrane protein produced by bile canalicular cells in response to elevated ductal pressure, and it represents a sensitive and early cellular response to biliary tract obstruction. Serum transaminase (aspartate and alanine) levels can also be mildly elevated in biliary system disease, either because of direct injury of the liver adjacent to an inflamed gallbladder or from the effect of biliary sepsis on hepatocellular membrane integrity. Increased transaminase levels can be detected in serum when hepatocytes are injured as these cytoplasmic proteins subsequently leak across damaged plasma membranes. Leukocytosis with a predominance of neutrophils is often present with acute cholecystitis or cholangitis but is a nonspecific finding that does not distinguish these conditions from other infectious or inflammatory processes within the abdomen.

Radiographic Studies

Abdominal Radiographs

Although frequently obtained during the initial evaluation of abdominal pain, plain radiographs of the abdomen are seldom of significant diagnostic value. Only about 15% of gallstones contain enough calcium to render them radiopaque and thus visible on plain films of the abdomen. Calcium elsewhere within the peritoneal cavity, such as the wall of the gallbladder or the head of the pancreas, is noteworthy but is an uncommon explanation for acute abdominal pain. Rarely, one may identify pneumobilia (air within the biliary tree), which can indicate the presence of a severe bacterial infection. The most important value of plain abdominal films is the exclusion of other potential diagnoses, such as a perforated ulcer with free intraabdominal air or an intestinal obstruction with dilated loops of bowel and multiple air–fluid levels.

Ultrasonography

Surface ultrasound of the abdomen is an extremely useful and accurate method for identifying gallstones and pathological changes in the gallbladder consistent with acute cholecystitis. Abdominal ultrasound should be part of the routine evaluation of patients suspected of having gallstone disease, given the high specificity (>98%) and sensitivity (>95%) of this test for the diagnosis of cholelithiasis (Fig. 47.7). In addition to confirming the presence of gallstones within the gallbladder, ultrasound can also detail various signs of acute cholecystitis (thickening of the gallbladder wall, pericholecystic fluid) as well as gallbladder neoplasms. Due to overlying or adjacent bowel gas, accurate imaging of the extrahepatic bile ducts for signs of obstruction or the presence of stones can be difficult. Therefore, the absence of these findings on ultrasound is insufficient to exclude a diagnosis of choledocholithiasis (common bile duct stones). However, because intrahepatic ductal dilation is readily seen with ultrasound, this finding

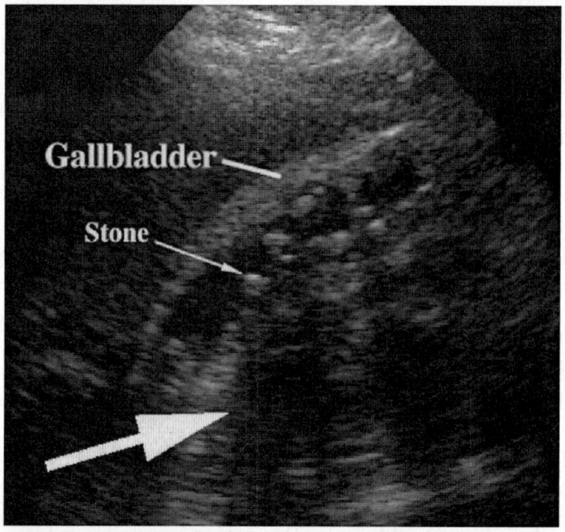

FIGURE 47.7. Ultrasonography of the gallbladder. The sonographic signs of gallstones include visible stones that produce acoustic shadowing (white arrow) and that move with the patient. (Courtesy of the Department of Radiology, UCSF.)

can serve to support the diagnosis of common duct stones with obstruction.

It is important to remember that while ultrasound is an excellent, noninvasive tool for the diagnosis of gallstone disease, it is not perfect. Gallstones can be present, yet difficult to document sonographically. A sensitivity of 95% means that in up to 5% of patients gallstones will be present but go undetected by this diagnostic modality. As cholelithiasis is a common condition, clinicians are likely to find themselves from time to time confronted by patients with clinical signs and symptoms characteristic of stone disease yet appearing normal on ultrasound examinations. Under such circumstances, it should be remembered that biliary sludge and microcalcifications are likely causes of biliary colic, acute cholecystitis, and acute pancreatitis that can escape ultrasound detection.[6]

Computed Tomography

Although abdominal computed tomographic (CT) scanning is probably the most informative single radiographic tool for examining intraabdominal pathology, its overall value for the diagnosis of biliary tract disease pales in comparison to ultrasonography. This disadvantage is largely because gallstones and bile appear nearly isodense on CT; that is, it is difficult to distinguish gallstones from bile unless the stones are heavily calcified. Therefore, CT documents the presence of gallstones within the biliary tree and gallbladder with a sensitivity of approximately 55% to 65%. However, abdominal CT is a powerful tool for evaluating biliary tract diseases when the differential diagnosis includes a question of hepatobiliary or pancreatic neoplasm, liver abscess, or hepatic parenchymal disease (e.g., biliary cirrhosis, organ atrophy).

Cholangiography

Defined as the mapping of bile ducts, *cholangiography* functionally involves the installation of contrast directly into the biliary tree and is the most accurate and sensitive method available to anatomically delineate the intra- and extrahepatic biliary tree. A cholangiogram is indicated when the diagnosis or therapy depends on a precise knowledge of biliary anatomy. Generally obtained to determine the location and extent of an intraluminal obstruction, diagnostic cholangiograms can be performed percutaneously, endoscopically, transabdominally (e.g., intraoperative cholangiogram), or through the use of intravenous or oral contrast material taken up and excreted by the liver into bile. The level and nature of the lesion, along with the patient's overall medical condition, are the primary guidelines that dictate which approach is preferred.

Percutaneous transhepatic cholangiography (PTC) requires a dilated intrahepatic ductal system and is invaluable for defining the upper extent of obstructing lesions. Endoscopic retrograde cholangiopancreatography (ERCP) is better suited for defining the lower limit of obstructing lesions, yet it also allows for the biopsy of any masses encountered for diagnostic purposes. Both approaches can be used to decompress the biliary tree and remove calculi.

Regardless of the approach, injection of contrast into an obstructed biliary system is commonly associated with transient bacteremias and occasionally precipitates an episode of frank sepsis. These risks are reduced through the use of broad-spectrum antibiotic prophylaxis, avoidance of high injection pressures, and by minimizing the total number of injections performed during the examination. Intravenous cholangiography is more popular in Europe than the United States and has the significant disadvantage of requiring normal liver function.

Magnetic resonance cholangiopancreatography (MRCP) is a recently developed, totally noninvasive imaging technique that can provide detailed anatomical information without the direct injection of contrast into the biliary system.[7] It obviates the need for physically manipulating the patient and thus promises to combine the convenience of CT with the data quality of traditional cholangiograms (Fig. 47.8). As this imaging method is new and incompletely proven, its overall role in the diagnosis of biliary system disease awaits further experience.

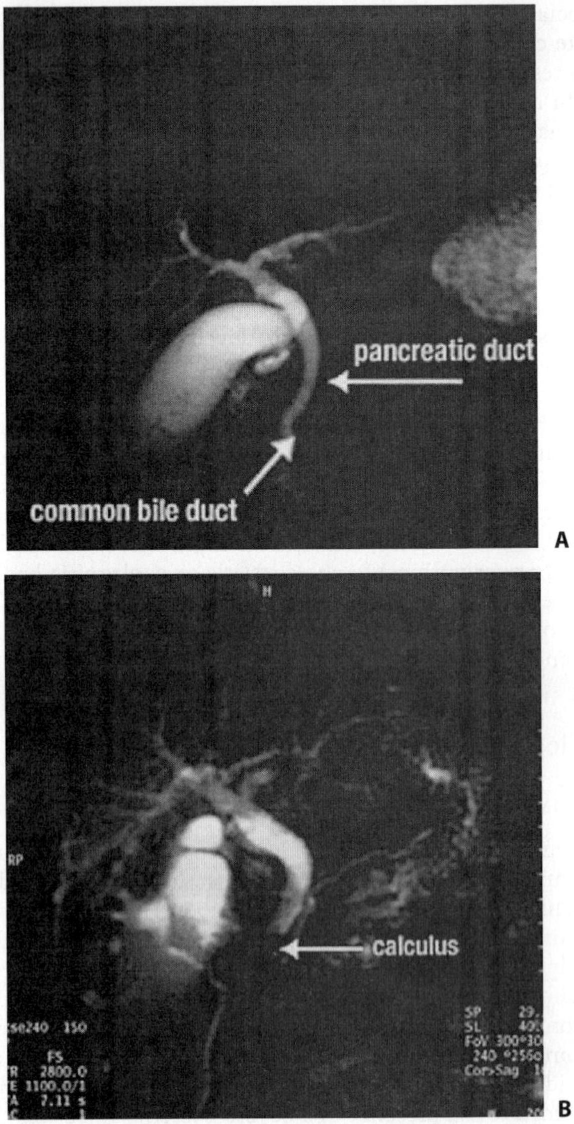

FIGURE 47.8. Normal (**A**) magnetic resonance cholangiopancreatogram and a gallstone obstructing the common bile duct (**B**). (Reprinted with permission from John V. Phillips, MD, Medical Director, Parkside MR Center, Lutheran General Hospital, Park Ridge, IL.)

Scintigraphy

Biliary scintigraphy is useful to visualize the biliary tree, assess liver and gallbladder function, and diagnose several common disorders with a sensitivity and specificity of 90% to 97%, respectively.[8] Although an excellent test to decide whether the common bile and cystic ducts are patent, biliary scintigraphy does not identify gallstones or yield detailed anatomical information. Commonly employed agents for this type of test are ^{99m}Tc-labeled iminodiacetic acid derivatives because these compounds are rapidly taken up by the liver and excreted into the bile.

To perform biliary scintigraphy, an appropriate agent is administered intravenously to a fasting patient, and the process of hepatic uptake and biliary excretion is monitored over time through the use of a gamma camera. This process generates a series of motion picture-like images that allow one to determine whether the extrahepatic bile ducts, including the cystic duct, are patent. Normally, the radioisotope is seen to concentrate within the liver, outline the extrahepatic biliary tree and gallbladder, and flow into the small intestine within approximately 30 to 45 min (Fig. 47.9A). Failure of the radiolabeled compound to fill the gallbladder, despite liver uptake and excretion into the small bowel, is considered diagnostic of acute cholecystitis; presumably, the gallbladder failed to fill because of an obstructed cystic duct (Fig. 47.9B).

False-negative studies can occur in patients with abdominal pain due to acalculous cholecystitis as the pathogenesis of this disease entity does not require cystic duct obstruction. Regardless, scintigraphy remains of diagnostic value in these patients because gallbladder imaging is usually abnormal secondary to edema and inflammation of the cystic duct. False positives can result from gallbladder stasis and poor filling, as seen with chronic cholecystitis, alcoholism, or extended administration of total parenteral nutrition (TPN).

Oral Cholecystography

The oral cholecystographic method of imaging the biliary system works via principles similar to scintigraphy but has

A

B

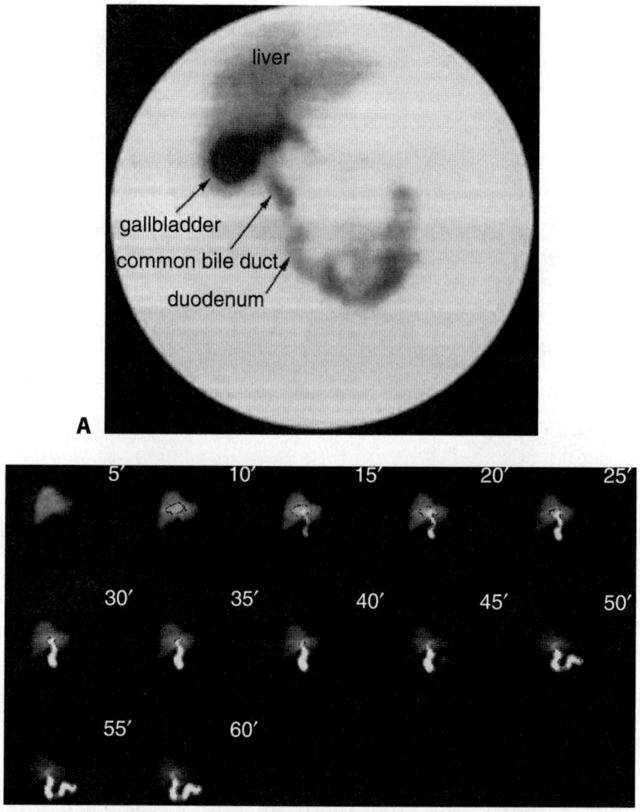

FIGURE 47.9. Hepatobiliary scintigraphy. (**A**) Normal (negative) study. (**B**) Positive study showing failure of the gallbladder to fill supporting a diagnosis acute cholecystitis. (Figures courtesy of UCSF Department of Nuclear Medicine.)

been largely supplanted by other more convenient or informative radiographic modalities. Instead of using a radiolabeled pharmaceutical, patients are given oral contrast pills 12 to 16h before the exam, during which time the peroral contrast material is absorbed by the small intestine, cleared by the liver, excreted into bile, and concentrated within the gallbladder. Subsequently, the gallbladder and common bile duct are visualized using traditional abdominal radiographs. Oral cholecystography generates images with much greater clarity and resolution than scintigraphy but requires more planning to perform and yields less-dynamic information. Disorders of the foregut (gastroparesis, small-bowel obstruction, and pancreatitis) or impaired liver function (hyperbilirubinemia) can all interfere with contrast absorption and thus generate a falsely negative exam.

Calculous Disease

Calculous disease of the biliary system is a common and significant medical problem throughout the world. While the frequency, type, and distribution of gallstones within the biliary tree vary among different populations of people, the presence of intraluminal calculi places all patients at risk for a range of clinically symptomatic conditions. Interestingly, the exact pathogenesis of gallstone disease is incompletely understood and remains the subject of intense study. Nonetheless, removal of the gallbladder has been the mainstay of therapy for symptomatic gallstones and has proven quite effective in most cases. Recent advances in our understanding of how calculi form and in surgical technology, however, have virtually revolutionized the approach to this widespread disease, dramatically expanding the therapeutic armamentarium available to physicians.

Pathogenesis

Classification of Gallstones

There are three types of gallstones: cholesterol, pigment, and mixed cholesterol and pigment stones. The distribution and location of biliary calculi varies throughout the world, undoubtedly reflecting different risk factors for their formation. In patients in the United States and most westernized countries, approximately 75% of gallstones are of the mixed type, 15% are pigment stones, and the remaining 10% pure cholesterol (Fig. 47.10). The stones are most commonly located within the gallbladder but can on occasion be found within the common bile duct or the liver or to have migrated into the intestinal tract. These findings are in stark contrast to those in other regions of the world, such as Southeast Asia, where the majority of biliary calculi are of the pigment variety and are most commonly located within the liver itself and not the gallbladder.

Such variation also applies to the overall incidence of gallstone disease. In the United States, about 12% of the population has cholelithiasis, with more than 950,000 new cases diagnosed each year, while in East Africa and other selected Third World countries the incidence is as low as 2% to 3%. The risk of developing biliary calculi throughout America and western Europe is directly proportional to a person's age and sex. While children and adolescents rarely have gallstones, by the seventh decade of life 10% of men and 25% of women have documented cholelithiasis.

Cholesterol-Enriched Gallstone Formation

The exact mechanism by which gallstones are formed is not fully understood, but calculi are likely the result of a complex, multifaceted alteration in hepatobiliary function (Table 47.2). Calculous disease has and continues to be the subject of intensive research. Yet, definitively detailing how stones develop has been significantly hampered by the absence of an appropriate animal model and the difficulties inherent in comprehensive longitudinal studies on humans, many of whom must be "normal" and thus either asymptomatic or without stones altogether. Regardless, the prevailing theory regarding the pathogenesis of cholesterol-enriched gallstones entails a multistep process that can be promoted by a variety of physiological, metabolic, or genetic variables.

Cholesterol-Supersaturated Bile

An early event in the process of gallstone formation is a change in the composition of bile, specifically a relative increase in the cholesterol content. Normally, bile is an isotonic combination of water, electrolytes, and organic macromolecules that is actively secreted by the liver. Designed to aid in the solubilization (emulsification) and subsequent absorption of dietary fats, the solute composition of bile includes bile salts, cholesterol, and phospholipids, predominantly phosphatidylcholine (lecithin). Bile salts are amphipa-

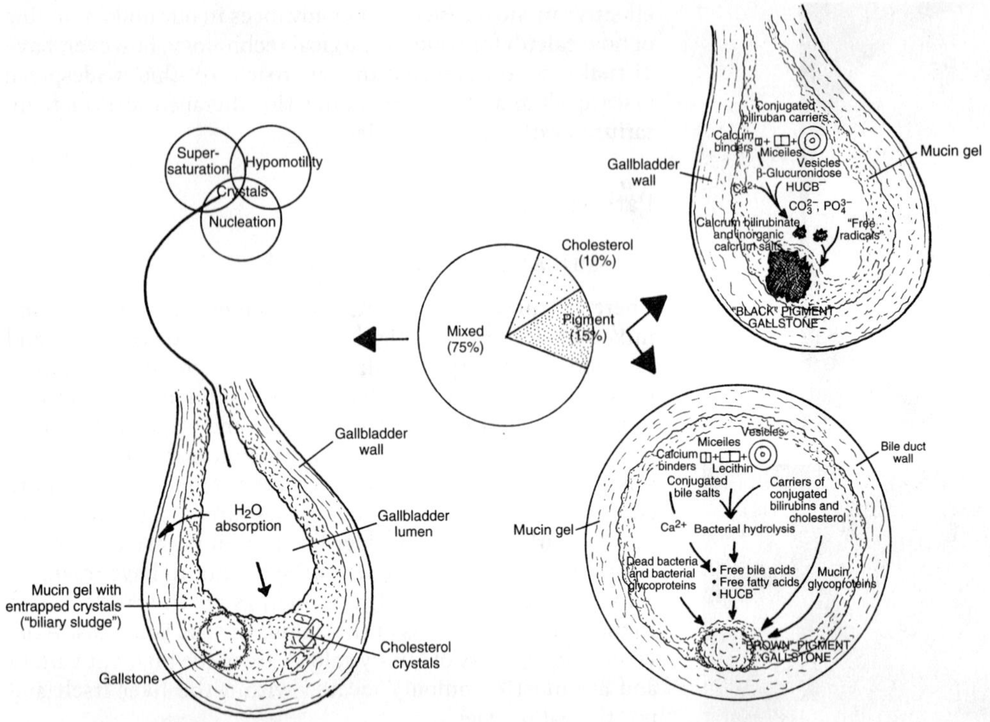

FIGURE 47.10. Pathogenesis of gallstones.

thic molecules (containing both hydrophobic and hydrophilic domains) that in concert with neutral lipids act as detergents, serving to break down dietary fats into smaller, more soluble micelles (Fig. 47.11).

The size and character of micelles formed, along with the efficiency with which this process takes place, are largely dependent on the ratio of cholesterol to bile salts to phospholipid present in the bile. Approximately 30 years ago Admirand and Small proposed the concept that when the relative concentration of cholesterol in bile exceeded its solubility constant, the excess lipid would precipitate and thus initiate gallstone formation.[9] The formation of cholesterol-

TABLE 47.2. Clinical Risk Factors Associated with Cholesterol Gallstones.

Risk factor	*Pathogenesis*
Age	Gallstone formation is a time-dependent process; 40 is the typical age at clinical diagnosis; possible age-related decrease in the conversion of cholesterol to bile salts
Gender	Female: male ratio 53:1; estrogens increase the uptake of plasma cholesterol by the liver with subsequent increased bile cholesterol saturation
Race and ethnicity	High risk: Pima Indians, other Native Americans, Hispanics, whites
	Low risk: Black Africans and African Americans
Genetics	Increased relative risks if parents, siblings, or first-degree relatives have gallstones
Obesity	Increased activity of hydroxy-methyl-glutaryl-CoA (HMG) reductase leads to increased cholesterol synthesis and bile cholesterol saturation
Crohn's disease	Decreased ileal resorption of bile salts
Total parenteral nutrition	Gallbladder stasis and distension; risk exacerbated in patients with Crohn's disease
Rapid weight loss	Intestinal bypass surgery and low-calorie, high-protein diets associated with high incidence of gallstones because of decreased bile salt secretion and gallbladder stasis

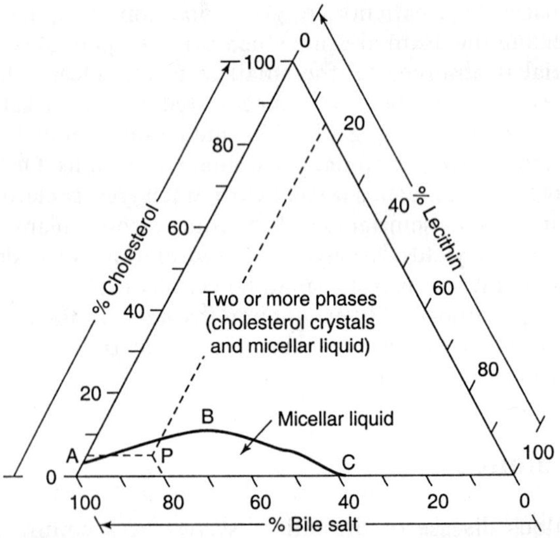

FIGURE 47.11. Solubility of the three major components of bile (bile salts, lecithin, and cholesterol) plotted on triangular coordinates. Point P represents bile composed of 80% bile salts, 5% cholesterol, and 15% lecithin. Line ABC represents the maximal solubility of cholesterol as a function of various bile salt and lecithin concentrations. When the combination of bile salts, cholesterol, and lecithin falls below the ABC line, the bile exists as a single-phase micellar liquid. When the constituents of bile are plotted above this line, however, there is supersaturation of cholesterol and the formation of cholesterol crystals. (Adapted with permission from Admirand and Small.[9])

supersaturated bile could, theoretically, result from either increased cholesterol synthesis or decreased bile salt or phospholipid secretion by the liver. This tripartite interrelationship among the concentrations of cholesterol, bile salts, and phospholipid in bile is commonly displayed graphically using triangular coordinates (see Fig. 47.11). As the molar ratio of cholesterol relative to either bile salts or phospholipid deviates from a relatively narrow range, the cholesterol solubilization capacity of bile is exceeded, resulting in rapid cholesterol crystal formation (see Table 47.1).

Bile cholesterol is commonly thought to exist as part of mixed micelles, with this nonpolar lipid concentrated within the hydrophobic core of these particles. There is, however, also evidence that as much as 70% to 80% of the cholesterol in bile actually exists in a vesicular form, distributed throughout the bilipid membrane of an unilamellar liposome. Although the macromolecular distribution of cholesterol between the micellar and vesicular forms varies according to bile concentration, it is interesting to speculate whether the different forms of cholesterol affect the overall lithogenicity of bile.

Gallstone Nucleation

Once bile has become supersaturated with cholesterol, the formation of a cholesterol-enriched gallstone presumably begins with a nucleation event. The precipitation of crystalline cholesterol is thought to occur via either the fusion or implosion of cholesterol-rich vesicles.[10,11] A variety of different crystal shapes has been recently identified in bile samples from numerous patients with gallstones.[12] These distinct cholesterol structures, including arcs/needles, spirals, tubes, and plates, may represent different stages in the nucleation process as well as the existence of different cholesterol crystallization pathways.

The possible contribution of gallbladder mucus to the formation of gallstones represents a fascinating example of how the different variables involved in the process of stone formation can be intricately interrelated. The concentration of deoxycholate is increased in cholesterol-supersaturated bile. This hydrophobic bile salt subsequently stimulates the hypersecretion of mucus glycoproteins by the gallbladder epithelium. The resultant increase in gallbladder mucus in turn may promote stone formation by the trapping of cholesterol microcrystals. While the cause-and-effect nature of this sequence of events is in part speculative, there are both animal and human data that correlate increased gallbladder mucus production with the formation of biliary calculi.

Other gallbladder-derived proteins are also thought to play a role in the pathogenesis of biliary calculi as both promoters and inhibitors of the process. A few of the nonmucin glycoproteins that can promote cholesterol nucleation include phospholipase C, α_1-acid glycoprotein, fibronectin, and immunoglobulin (Ig) M, IgA, and IgG. Inhibitors of stone formation secreted by the liver into bile include apolipoproteins A-1 and A-2 and a poorly characterized 120-kDa glycoprotein. Because the activities of these various proteins have been studied exclusively in vitro, their significance to in vivo disease has yet to be determined.

Gallbladder and Foregut Motility

Gallbladder stasis has long been associated with the formation of gallstones. Beyond the intuitive sense that a stagnant pool of supersaturated bile must promote nucleation and stone growth, there is a growing body of data to support the concept. Initially, clinicians associated gallbladder stasis with numerous clinical settings in which there was an increased risk of cholelithiasis, such as pregnancy, truncal vagotomy, and the extended use of TPN. Recently, using a combination of biliary ultrasound and scintigraphy, impairments in both postprandial and interdigestive gallbladder emptying have been carefully documented in many patients with symptomatic gallstones. Specifically, investigators have demonstrated that the volume of bile flow through the gallbladder during the postprandial period is dramatically reduced and leads to a large, flaccid gallbladder.[13,14] Many cholesterol stone patients also have increased fasting gallbladder volumes.

This last observation may represent the contribution of a more widespread motility disorder of the foregut to stone formation in selected patients. For example, women with gallstones were found to have significantly longer whole-gut transport times with only half the stool output as compared to stone-free patients. In addition, many gallstone patients were found to have longer cycles of the intestinal migrating motor complex (MMC) with disruption of motilin release. Although none of these alterations in motility are universal findings, they nonetheless underscore the importance of normal foregut physiology and contribute to our understanding of this common, yet complex, disease.

Gender and Genes

Gallstone disease is more common in women than in men at virtually all stages of life. Because this gallstone gender gap narrows by the eighth and ninth decades of life, it is likely the result of estrogen-induced changes in biliary lipid metabolism and gallbladder function. Evidence in support of a role for hormones in gallstone formation includes the observation that exogenously administered estrogen increases the incidence of cholesterol stones in both men and women. Also, estrogen may promote the supersaturation of bile by inhibiting the conversion of cholesterol to bile salts, thereby increasing the hepatic secretion of cholesterol into bile while simultaneously decreasing the secretion of bile salts. Last, pregnancy is associated with impaired gallbladder emptying and an overall increase in bile stasis. In the United States, the typical patient with symptomatic gallstones is "female, forty, fat, and fair."

The role of heredity in biliary calculous disease is not well understood. Although there are specific ethnic populations with widely divergent rates of cholelithiasis, exactly what accounts for these differences is not known. A most dramatic example of an ethnic risk factor for gallstone disease can be found among the Pima Indians of the American Southwest. By the third decade of life, approximately 80% of Pima women have documented gallstones. Analysis of bile from these women reveals extreme cholesterol supersaturation with concurrent alterations in hepatic cholesterol and bile salt secretion. There is also a high incidence of diabetes mellitus and obesity, two additional risk factors for cholelithiasis. The importance of genetics as a risk factor for gallstones is evident in studies of family history. A history of cholelithiasis in a first-degree relative doubles a person's risk of developing gallstones, and this genetic risk factor is greatest with a parental history of biliary calculi.[15]

Bile Calcium

Calcium has been recognized as a component of gallstones, especially pigment stones, for hundreds of years. In fact, approximately 15% of biliary calculi contain enough calcium as to be visible on plain radiographs of the abdomen. However, the role of calcium in the pathogenesis of gallstones is another uncertainty. Calcium was not originally thought to contribute to the formation of cholesterol stones, but recent studies have identified calcium carbonate within the core of these stones. Also, there are data showing that increased biliary calcium can promote cholesterol crystallization and gallstone nucleation via an unknown mechanism.

Obesity

Excess body fat is another independent risk factor for gallbladder disease. Studies using oral cholecystography or ultrasonography have documented a direct relationship between obesity and gallstones.[16–18] While the pathogenic mechanism linking obesity to cholelithiasis is unclear, it may involve alterations in lipid biogenesis with increased cholesterol synthesis. Regardless of mechanism, the relative risk of gallstones increases dramatically with morbid obesity.

Unifying Hypothesis

Even though the formation of cholesterol-enriched gallstones is a complex, multistep process, a unifying hypothesis has emerged in an attempt to further our understanding of this clinically important disease.[19] The hypothesis states that cholesterol hypersecretion, with its consequent biliary cholesterol supersaturation, places patients with either a genetic or metabolic susceptibility to form cholesterol stones at high risk (see Fig. 47.10). Theoretically, the chronic hypercholesterobilia has a pathological effect on the gallbladder wall muscle by incorporating excess cholesterol into the sarcolemma and thus leads to gallbladder and small intestinal hypomotility. At this point, a series of events may occur, any one of which can serve to promote cholesterol crystallization, including changes in gallbladder mucin production, further changes in bile composition, and the secretion of stone-promoting proteins by the liver. Once the nucleation event takes place, gallbladder hypomotility and stasis propagate further cholesterol deposition and stone growth. The testing of thermonuclear devices during the late 1950s and early 1960s enabled investigators to carbon date (measurement of ^{14}C) gallstones and determine that biliary calculi grow at a rate of 2 to 3 mm/year.[20] The study further revealed that gallbladder stones grow for an average of 8 years after the nucleation event before becoming symptomatic.

Pigment Stones

While only about 15% of gallstones in the United States are pigment stones, this type of biliary calculus is the predominant variety throughout the world. The sine qua non of pigment stones is their high concentration of bilirubin combined with low cholesterol content. These stones are usually mixed with a substantial amount of calcium bilirubinate and can be further categorized as either black or brown as a function of their gross appearance. Considerably less is known regarding the pathogenesis of pigment versus cholesterol-enriched gallstones, but some clinical and in vitro studies suggest that biliary infection and stasis play critical roles in their development.

TABLE 47.3. Pigmented Gallstones.

Characteristics	*Black*	*Brown*
Color	Black	Brownish-orange
Size	2–6 mm	5–30 mm
Consistency	Solid, rock-hard	Soft, sandy, sludge
Anatomical location	Gallbladder	Intra- and extrahepatic bile ducts
Geographic location	West and Asia	Predominantly Asia
Associated conditions	Hemolytic anemia, cirrhosis, alcoholism, extended TPN use, following ileal resection	Liver parasites, ductal strictures, biliary tract infections
Radiographic appearance	Radiopaque (70%)	Radiolucent
Etiology	Increased excretion unconjugated/deconjugation of bilirubin	Bacterial hydrolysis of conjugated bilirubin, possibly nucleated by ductal parasites or debris

Certainly, there appear to be different risk factors for developing black versus brown pigment gallstones. Black pigment stones are very dark in color, rock-hard in consistency, and commonly found in the gallbladders of patients with hemolytic disorders or chronic liver disease, after extended TPN use, or following ileal resection (Table 47.3). Under these circumstances, it is thought that an excessive load of bilirubin is delivered to or synthesized within the liver that far exceeds organ capacity to conjugate (and thus render water soluble) this macromolecule. Presumably, the unconjugated, relatively hydrophobic pigment is then directly secreted into bile, where it can precipitate with calcium carbonate.

As the name suggests, brown pigment gallstones are lighter in color and softer in consistency than black pigment stones and are commonly found within the liver or extrahepatic bile ducts of patients with biliary strictures or those born in Southeast Asia. Biliary infection and stasis caused by ductal obstruction are considered the critical etiological factors in brown pigment stone formation. In this case, the bacterial deconjugation of bile salts may create a lithogenic environment that is unique in composition but functionally not unlike that described for patients with hemolytic disorders.

Gallbladder Sludge and Microcalculi

The formation and clinical significance of gallbladder sludge is unclear, but it is observed with sufficient regularity to warrant mention.[21] Generally identified via abdominal sonography, sludge appears as echogenic material within the gallbladder, and it layers in the dependent area of the gallbladder yet does not generate the postacoustic shadows characteristic of gallstones. Commonly seen following prolonged fasting, sludge is thought to represent bile that has become concentrated within a relatively static gallbladder. In a study of patients on long-term TPN, the incidence of gallbladder sludge increased as a direct function of time. Within 3 weeks of starting TPN, 5% of patients developed sludge; by 4 to 6 weeks, the incidence had increased to 50%; and after 6 weeks, it was a universal finding.[22]

Although the natural history of gallbladder sludge is not known, it is not considered a pathological finding as it generally resolves with resumption of an oral diet. Yet, not infrequently gallbladder sludge is associated with the presence of microcalculi and contributes to the development of cholelithiasis and acute cholecystitis.[21,23] Cholesterol crystals can be identified microscopically in gallbladder or bile duct bile.

Clinical Syndromes

Gallstone disease continues to be a major health care problem in the United States and throughout selected parts of the world. There are more than 26 million Americans with gallstones, and although most of these people are asymptomatic, more than 700,000 cholecystectomies are performed each year. The total annual cost of medical care for patients suffering from biliary calculous disease is estimated at more than $7 billion. Still, not all gallstones require treatment. In fact, in the majority of patients (60%–80%) gallstones are completely asymptomatic. However, once symptoms develop patients are at risk for a wide range of problems, ranging from simple biliary colic to ascending cholangitis and septic shock.

Asymptomatic Gallstones

Once "silent" gallstones are discovered, the clinician is confronted with the question of what, if anything, to do about them. To logically address this question requires information regarding the natural history of asymptomatic gallstones. Data from several longitudinal studies reveal that approximately 10% to 20% of patients with silent gallstones go on to develop symptoms, most commonly biliary colic.[24–27] Serious symptoms or complications such as acute cholecystitis develop in these patients at a rate of 1% to 3% per year. These observations, combined with the fact that only 0.5% to 1.0% of patients die of complications from their silent gallstones, strongly suggest that asymptomatic gallstones generally follow a benign course.

A formal decision analysis performed to compare the consequences of prophylactic cholecystectomy versus expectant management for asymptomatic gallstones concluded that prophylactic surgery slightly decreased expected survival.[28] Using probability data on the natural history of silent gallstones, published mortality rates for cholecystectomy, and actuarial life tables, the analysis revealed that prophylactic surgery decreases average survival time. A 50-year-old man electing prophylactic cholecystectomy would lose 18 days of life, while a 30-year-old man would lose 4 days; the predictions are similar for women. Therefore, there is little role for the prophylactic medical or surgical treatment of asymptomatic gallstones. These interventions should be reserved for those patients who have experienced significant clinical symptoms, a calcified (porcelain) gallbladder, or gallbladder polyps.

Expectant management of asymptomatic gallstones in diabetic patients is somewhat controversial, with some clinicians proposing prophylactic surgery because of the morbidity and mortality associated with emergency surgery in this specific patient population. However, a recent prospective study assessed the natural history of gallstones in patients with non-insulin-dependent diabetes and concluded that, as with nondiabetic patients, prophylactic surgery is not advisable.[29] Asymptomatic diabetic patients developed symptomatic cholelithiasis (predominantly biliary colic) at a rate of approximately 3% per year. Because the risk of becoming symptomatic in diabetics is similar to that reported for the general population, prophylactic surgery is difficult to justify.

Acute Cholecystitis

One of the most common complications of symptomatic gallstones that requires surgical intervention is acute cholecystitis. This condition is thought to result from impaction of a gallstone in the cystic duct or neck of the gallbladder, thereby completely obstructing the organ. Consequently, the gallbladder becomes distended and somehow initiates a localized acute inflammatory reaction. The exact pathogenesis of acute cholecystitis is not well delineated, but the clinical syndrome begins with biliary colic-type pain. Biliary colic typically resolves over several hours, but the pain of acute cholecystitis persists and intensifies over days. Initially, the pain is vague and visceral in nature, but as the acute inflammation of the gallbladder becomes transmural, the visceral and adjacent parietal peritoneal coverings become irritated. At this point, the patient's discomfort is no longer vague and diffuse, but localizes to the right upper quadrant and is associated with guarding and rebound tenderness. As described earlier, the classical physical finding of acute cholecystitis is a positive Murphy's sign (inspiratory arrest on palpation of the right upper quadrant). Patients may also complain of nausea and vomiting, anorexia, and a low-grade fever. In many cases, the physical exam reveals a mass in the right upper quadrant. This mass or "phlegmon" represents the body's effort to wall off and compartmentalize the inflamed gallbladder using adjacent organs, including the greater omentum, first portion of the duodenum, and right colon.

Laboratory abnormalities are nonspecific but may reveal a mild leukocytosis and minor elevations in the liver function tests. The diagnosis is confirmed via abdominal ultrasound, with the findings of gallbladder wall thickening and pericholecystic fluid virtually pathognomonic. For further confirmation, the ultrasonographer can demonstrate a "sonographic Murphy's sign." With the ultrasound transducer placed directly over the distended gallbladder, the sonographer presses down in an effort to re-create the patient's discomfort. The source of pain from the gallbladder can thus be distinguished from other conditions, such as liver tenderness or hepatitis. Severe forms of acute cholecystitis can result in *gallbladder empyema*, in which the organ is filled with purulent bile and debris, and *emphysematous cholecystitis*, which is characterized by necrosis and gas within the wall of the gallbladder. The latter condition typically occurs in diabetic patients and demands aggressive decompression of the gall-

TABLE 47.4.
Clinical Trials Comparing Early Versus Delayed Surgery for Acute Cholecystitis.

Reference	*n*	*Study design*	*Level of evidence*	*Complications*	*Mortality*	*Findings/comments*
Linden and Sunzel 1970,[30] Sweden	140	Randomized, controlled trial	I	Early: 14.3% Delayed: 3.4%	Early: 0% Delayed: 0%	More than two-thirds of patients randomized to early surgery underwent operation within 10 days of diagnosis Low mortality in part the result of excluding 3 high-risk, elderly patients Noted that 17% of patients randomized to delayed surgery ultimately refused operation once acute symptoms resolved No difference in technical difficulty between early and delayed operations when the surgeon was experienced Early surgery (paradoxically) resulted in a 2-day-longer average length of stay, but fewer extended hospitalizations Concluded that early surgery avoids the hazards of diagnostic error, symptom recurrence during the waiting period, and shortened the convalescence period after early surgery
McArthur et al. 1975,[31] England	35	Randomized, controlled trial	I	Early: 40.0% Delayed: 29.4%	Early: 0% Delayed: 0%	Early surgery defined as immediately following confirmation of the diagnosis Reported no overall difference in the technical difficulty of early versus delayed cholecystectomy, but recommended that early surgery take place within 5 days of diagnosis Most complications were minor infections; Concluded that the major benefits of early surgery are the shortened hospitalization and the avoidance of the serious complications of conservative management, including gallbladder perforation and empyema.
Lahtinen et al. 1978,[32] Finland	100	Randomized, controlled trial	I	Early: 29.7% Delayed: 47.7%	Early: 0% Delayed: 9%	Noted a technically easier operation, shorter OR time (70 vs. 79 min), reduced wound infection rate (6% vs. 18%), and shorter postoperative hospital LOS (12 vs. 15 days) for early vs. delayed surgery High complication rates in both groups predominantly related to localized or systemic infection Authors recommend early surgery
Norrby et al. 1983,[34] Sweden	192	Randomized, controlled, multicenter, trial	I	Early: 14.9% Delayed: 15.4%	Early: 0% Delayed: 1.1%	Early surgery defined as operation within 7 days of symptoms Studied patients ≤75 years old, randomized by odd vs. even birthdays Complications were similar between the two groups, but early surgery reduced hospital length of stay by >6 days.
Sianesi et al. 1984,[35] Italy	471	Retrospective (1970–77) and prospective (1977–82) data	III	Early: 18.5% Delayed: 15%	Early: 0% Delayed: 1.6%	Study combined retrospective and prospective data, collected over 12 years, during which time patient management evolved Reported low incidence of biliary infection, low morbidity and mortality, and shorter hospitalization period Authors recommend early surgery, within 48–72 h of diagnosis
Ajao et al. 1991, Nigeria	81	Retrospective	III	Early: 41% Delayed: 12.5%	Early: 2.6% Delayed: 0%	Retrospective review over 12 months, compared early (≤48 h) versus delayed (7–14 days) surgery Prohibitive rate of complications reported early surgery including 7 (18%) common bile duct injuries; only complications reported were wound infections (23%) and duct injuries Authors recommend delayed surgery, recommendations seemingly specific to the practice environment and level of surgical experience
Summary/ totals	1019	—	—	Early: 21.0% Delayed: 16.5%	Early: 0.2% Delayed: 1.8%	Early surgery was technically more challenging with a higher complication rate, but shorter hospital stay and convalescence, more rapid return to work, and lower overall mortality than delayed surgery for acute cholecystitis

bladder to avoid gallbladder perforation, intraabdominal abscess formation, and progressive sepsis.

Once the diagnosis is confirmed, the patient is rehydrated, any metabolic abnormalities are corrected, and pain is controlled with analgesics. There is a commonly cited concern regarding the use of morphine and other opiates in the setting of biliary tract disease. These drugs can have a hypertensive effect on the sphincter of Oddi and thus potentially exacerbate a patient's condition. Despite the data in support of this contention, clinical practice suggests that completely avoiding the use of opiates in patients with biliary system disease is generally unnecessary.

Definitive treatment involves removal of the inflamed and irreversibly damaged gallbladder and its contents. Historically, surgeons recommended that the patient's gallbladder be allowed to "cool down" before performing a cholecystectomy, theoretically allowing the acute inflammation to resolve and thus render the procedure less technically demanding.

The results of several randomized, controlled trials comparing early versus delayed surgery for acute cholecystitis in more than 1000 patients are presented in Table 47.4. As a result of these data, it is now generally accepted that early cholecystectomy (within 24–48 h of making the diagnosis) is not only technically feasible but also the preferred method of treatment as it effectively short-circuits the illness. Although there is an increase in the morbidity rate for early as compared to delayed surgery (21.0% vs. 16.5%, respectively), the complications are generally minor, and the overall mortality rated is reduced. Furthermore, patients return to normal activities more quickly, they avoid the risk of recurrent gallbladder symptoms while awaiting surgery, and the total cost of the illness is reduced.[30–35] As with open cholecystectomy, several prospective randomized, controlled trials have also confirmed the advantage of early versus delayed laparoscopic surgery for acute cholecystitis provided the surgeon is experienced.[36,37]

Choledocholithiasis

When gallstones are confined to the gallbladder, they can cause pain and the localized inflammatory changes of acute cholecystitis but rarely result in any potentially life-threatening illnesses. Stones within the common bile duct, however, may produce a variety of symptoms, including jaundice, cholangitis, acute pancreatitis, or even systemic sepsis. Choledocholithiasis represents gallbladder stones that have migrated into the common bile duct via the cystic duct, stones that were left in the common duct following biliary tract surgery (retained stones), or stones that originated within the intra- or extrahepatic bile ducts primarily (Fig. 47.12). The overall incidence of choledocholithiasis is difficult to know, but up to 15% of patients who undergo gallbladder surgery are found to have common duct stones. Ductal stones are also a frequent component of other biliary system diseases, including benign biliary strictures, sclerosing cholangitis, and recurrent pyogenic cholangitis.

Numerous indicators have been examined for their ability to predict the presence of choledocholithiasis in patients with symptomatic gallstones.[38,39] Several indicators are highly specific, but only elevated bilirubin and alkaline phosphatase yield sensitivities greater than 50% (Table 47.5). In the final analysis, no perfect preoperative predictor of choledocholithiasis has been identified, but the presence of cholangitis, common bile duct stones on ultrasound, or preoperative jaundice are the indicators associated with the greatest discriminatory power (likelihood ratios).

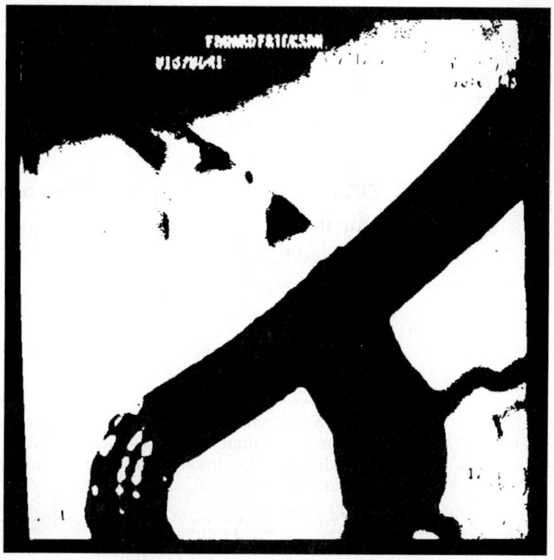

FIGURE 47.12. Endoscopic cholangiopancreatography in a patient with choledocholithiasis, as evidenced by multiple filling defects within the common bile duct. (Courtesy of J.P. Cello, MD, Department of Medicine, UCSF.)

Specific clinical syndromes and biochemical tests can suggest the presence of common duct stones, but they are definitively identified by radiographic evaluation of the biliary tree, including cholangiography. Considering the frequency with which calculi are found during cholecystectomy surgery, to avoid exposing every patient to the risks and costs of an intraoperative cholangiogram, a series of relative indications for performing this test have been developed. In addition to identifying patients at high risk for choledocholithiasis, these guidelines underscore the pathogenesis of common duct stone-related complications. Indications for cholangiography include palpable choledocholithiasis, a dilated common bile duct, elevated liver function tests, or a recent history of jaundice, cholangitis, or pancreatitis.

Cholangitis

In 1877, Charcot described the triad of abdominal pain, fever, and jaundice in patients suffering from cholangitis. This constellation of findings is most commonly caused by an obstructing stone lodged in the distal common bile duct. The abdominal pain results from elevated ductal pressures and distension of the gallbladder, and jaundice implies bilobar hepatic obstruction. If only a part of the liver is unobstructed, then these unaffected segments continue to conjugate and secrete bile and thus successfully compensate for the obstructed and dysfunctional portion of the organ. Fever represents a systemic response to a biliary tract infection. As the incidence of bactobilia ranges from 50% to 70% in patients with symptomatic gallstone disease (Table 47.6), the combination of an infectious inoculum in a closed (obstructed) space creates the environment necessary for clinical infection.

TABLE 47.5. Indicators of Choledocholithiasis.

Indicator	*Sensitivity*	*Specificity*	*Likelihood ratio*
Cholangitis	0.11	0.99	18.3
Choledocholithiasis on ultrasound	0.38	1.00	13.6
Preoperative jaundice	0.36	0.97	10.1
Dilated common bile duct on ultrasound	0.42	0.96	6.9
Jaundice	0.39	0.92	3.9
Elevated bilirubin	0.69	0.88	4.8
Elevated alkaline phosphatase	0.57	0.86	2.6
Pancreatitis	0.10	0.95	2.1
Acute cholecystitis	0.50	0.76	1.6
Elevated amylase	0.11	0.95	1.5

Note: Sensitivity describes the probability that a patient with common bile duct stones will exhibit an indicator; specificity describes the probability that a patient without common bile duct stones will not exhibit an indicator; likelihood ratios describe how much the odds of common bile duct stones will change when an indicator is present.

Source: From Abboud et al.[38]

Of note, cholangitis is a potentially life-threatening infection that can rapidly progress from mild fever and malaise to full-blown septic shock and multisystem organ failure over a matter of hours. The clinical volatility of this condition results from the relative ease with which bacteria and endotoxin under pressure can reflux from the bile duct lumen, cross the canalicular membrane, and enter the systemic circulation.

Beyond supportive measures and antibiotics, the treatment for cholangitis must include decompression of the obstructed biliary system. Recent prospective, randomized trials have shown that endoscopic decompression is associated with lower morbidity and mortality rates than open surgical procedures.[40–43] Another potentially serious clinical consequence of choledocholithiasis is acute (gallstone) pancreatitis. Discussed in greater detail elsewhere in this book, common duct stones can initiate a dysregulated inflammatory reaction in the pancreas by an incompletely understood mechanism.

The appropriate treatment for choledocholithiasis is entirely dependent on the clinical circumstances but generally entails removal of the common duct calculi and the gallbladder. Of note, small common duct stones (<5–6 mm in diameter) will likely spontaneously pass into the intestinal tract and therefore do not require treatment.[44,45] Stones discovered at the time of gallbladder surgery should be removed and a choledochostomy tube (T-tube) placed for 2 to 6 weeks. If common duct stones are identified in the perioperative period (i.e., before or after the cholecystectomy), then they can frequently be removed either endoscopically or percutaneously (Fig. 47.13). In special cases of choledocholithiasis, as in conjunction with benign strictures or recurrent pyogenic cholangitis, stone extraction is only part of an overall therapeutic strategy that must also address the associated ductal injury and fibrosis.

TABLE 47.6. Bacterial Organisms Found in the Bile of Patients with Symptomatic Gallstone Disease.

Organisms	*Percentage*
AEROBIC	**87**
Gram-positive	**21**
Streptococcus faecalis	15
Beta-hemolytic streptococci	2
Staphylococcus aureus	2
Staphylococcus albus	2
Gram-negative	**66**
Escherichia coli	39
Klebsiella aerogenes	11
Proteus spp.	7
Pseudomonas aeruginosa	2
Actinobacter spp.	2
ANAEROBIC	**13**
Gram-positive	**12**
Clostridium welchii	8
Anaerobic streptococci	4
Gram-negative	**1**
Bacterodies spp.	1

Source: From Alexander-Williams.[137]

Gallstone Ileus

Biliary calculi can produce many different symptoms, including changes in bowel function and motility. In addition to the nonspecific nausea and vomiting occasionally observed with simple biliary colic and frequently associated with acute cholecystitis, a gallstone ileus represents a unique type of small-bowel obstruction. As previously mentioned, during acute cholecystitis the body attempts to compartmentalize the inflammatory process by surrounding it with adjacent soft tissues. The resultant phlegmon is composed of omentum and nearby bowel, including the duodenum. If the inflammatory process is of sufficient intensity and duration, then the diseased gallbladder can form a fistulous communication with adjacent hollow organs. This process most commonly results in a cholecystoduodenal fistula but can also involve the colon, stomach, or more distal segments of the small intestine.

The gallstones responsible for a gallstone ileus are large, generally greater than 2 to 3 cm in diameter. When a stone of this size enters the intestinal tract through a cholecystoen-

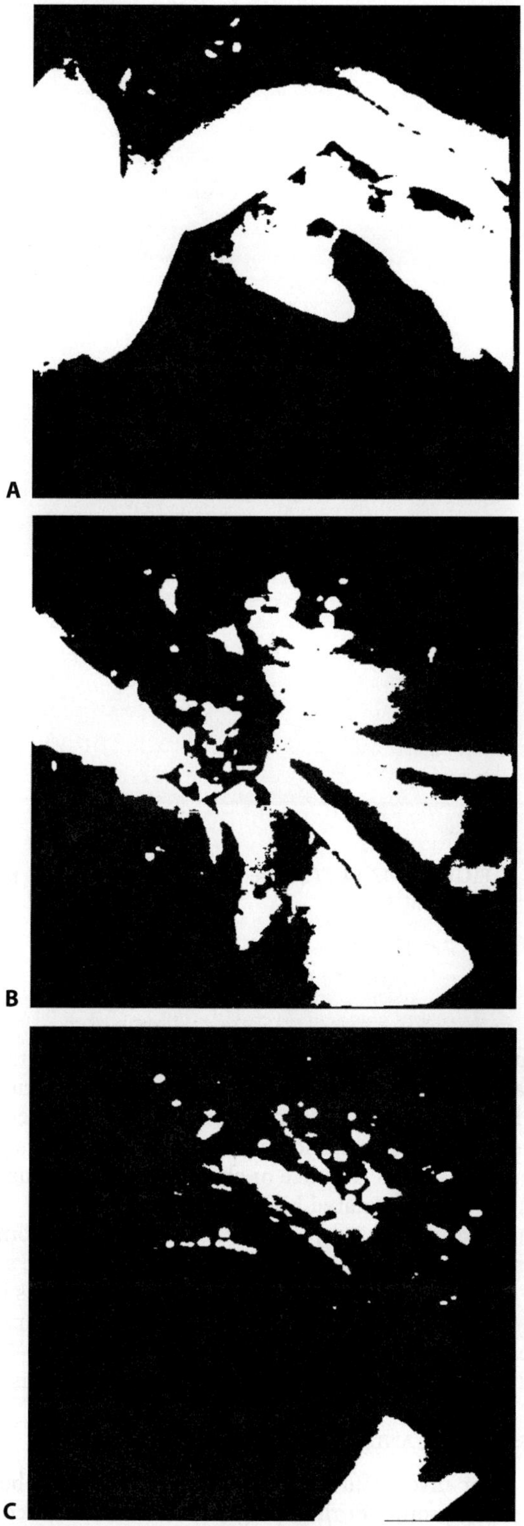

FIGURE 47.13. Endoscopic stone extraction. Cholangiocatheter entering the duodenal papilla (A). Extraction of a gallstone from the common bile duct (B). View of the intestinal lumen after the stone extraction. Note the duodenal papilla following performance of an endoscopic sphincterotomy (C). (Courtesy of J.P. Cello, MD, Department of Medicine, UCSF.)

teric fistula, it migrates distally until either it exits the rectum or becomes lodged in the narrowest segment of the bowel, the terminal ileum. The typical patient is an elderly woman with previous biliary colic who now presents with a "tumbling" bowel obstruction. The diagnosis of gallstone ileus should be suspected in patients presenting with bowel obstruction in the absence of an incarcerated hernia or a history of prior abdominal surgery.

Treatment entails an exploratory laparotomy not only to remove the stone causing the obstruction, but also to carefully inspect the remainder of the small intestine for additional calculi. Simultaneous removal of the gallbladder is ill advised. The gallbladder rarely (<4% of patients) causes future symptoms, and the morbidity and mortality of a frequently difficult prophylactic operation in an elderly patient are greater than that of leaving the organ in place.

Acalculous Cholecystitis

Acalculous cholecystitis is a rare but potentially lethal condition that involves acute transmural inflammation of the gallbladder in the absence of identifiable gallstones. In contrast to classical acute cholecystitis, its pathogenesis is likely the result of gallbladder ischemia rather than cystic duct obstruction. The typical patient is critically ill or septic, fasting, and found in the intensive care unit. Under these circumstances, bile stasis, activation of factor XII, endotoxins, and distension of the gallbladder can each contribute to the organ's diminished perfusion and predispose to irreversible injury.[46] Gangrene, empyema, and perforation more commonly complicate the course of acalculous cholecystitis than of acute cholecystitis resulting from gallstones, with an incidence approaching 75% and a mortality of approximately 40% in some series.[47]

Diagnosis of acalculous cholecystitis can be challenging as many of the patients are sedated and unable to actively participate in the history and physical examination. Cholecystectomy is the mainstay of therapy for acalculous cholecystitis. Prompt removal of the gallbladder is especially important when gangrene or empyema is suspected and there is impending perforation. Because the findings of biliary sonography and scintigraphy can be equivocal, percutaneous cholecystostomy is an appropriate method of diagnosis and treatment in lieu of cholecystectomy.

Recurrent Pyogenic Cholangitis

The complex biliary system disease recurrent pyogenic cholangitis, also known as oriental cholangiohepatitis, is endemic to Southeast Asia and seen with increasing frequency in the United States.[48] Characterized by the presence of intrahepatic (i.e., hepatolithiasis) and extrahepatic pigment stones in the absence of disease within the gallbladder, recurrent pyogenic cholangitis has been reported as the number one cause of acute abdominal pain in Hong Kong emergency rooms. As a result of the recent widespread immigration of Southeast Asians to the United States, the diagnosis of recurrent pyogenic cholangitis must be entertained when evaluating patients with biliary tract disease who were born in a country rimming the South China Sea (Fig. 47.14).

First described in 1930, the precise pathogenesis of recurrent pyogenic cholangitis is unknown. Although a variety of

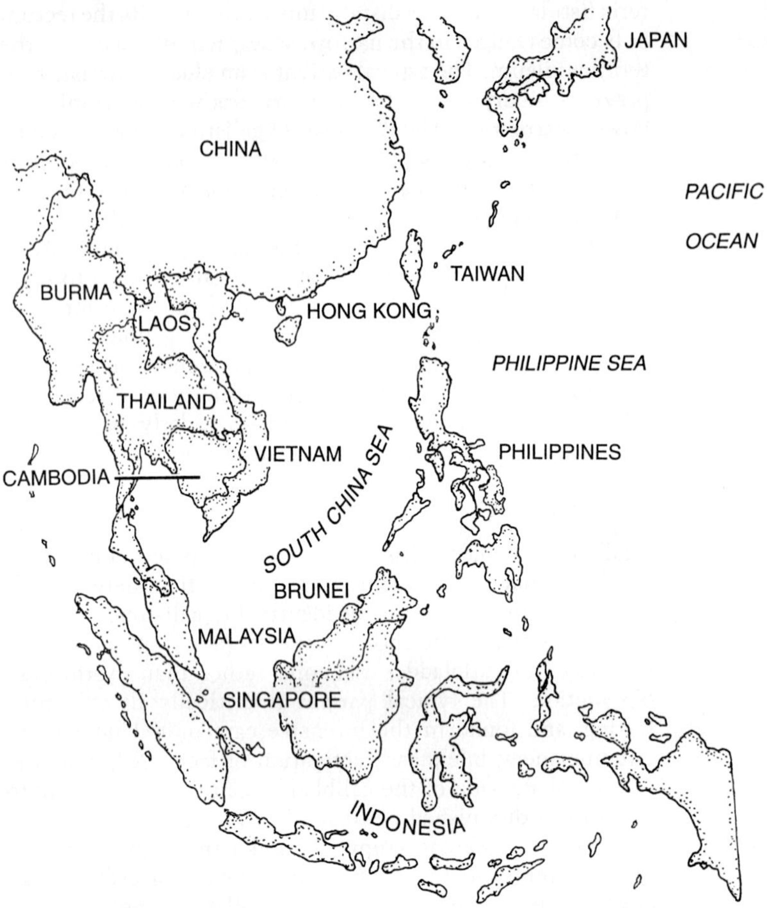

FIGURE 47.14. The geography of recurrent pyogenic cholangitis.

potential etiological factors have been evoked, including parasitic infections (*Clonorchis sinensis, Ascaris lumbricoides*), indolent bacterial infections, and protein malnutrition, the exact cause of the ductal ectasia and strictures and the intrahepatic stone formation characteristic of this disease remains a mystery.

Patients present with complaints of abdominal pain and fever. As there is usually segmental rather than complete bile duct obstruction, frank jaundice is uncommon. Even though these episodes may have been occurring over a period of several years to decades, the patient may only seek medical attention when the frequency and severity of the attacks become incapacitating. Treatment is aimed at decompression of the obstructed bile ducts and removal of as many stones and as much intraluminal debris as possible.

Mirizzi's Syndrome

First reported in 1948, Mirizzi's syndrome entails obstruction of the common bile duct by a stone impacted in the adjacent cystic duct or Hartmann's pouch. Although this condition is more prevalent in the elderly, it can occur in any patient with cholelithiasis. Two types have been described.[49] In type I, the hepatic duct is compressed by a large stone that has become impacted in the cystic duct or Hartmann's pouch. Associated inflammation may contribute to the stricture. In other patients (type II), the calculus has eroded into the hepatic duct, producing a cholecystocholedochal fistula. Certain anatomical variations seem to predispose to this condition, specifically a long cystic duct that runs parallel to the common duct or a low cystic–common duct junction.[50] Patients present with either painless jaundice or cholangitis, depending on the presence of contaminated bile.

The treatment for type I lesions is cholecystectomy, but awareness of this syndrome is important because the surgical removal of the gallbladder under these circumstances is associated with an increased incidence of bile duct injury. Management of type II strictures is best accomplished through partial cholecystectomy and bilioenteric anastomosis.

Biliary Colic and Pregnancy

Gallbladder disease is occasionally first noted or becomes more troublesome during pregnancy. The most common clinical presentations are worsening biliary colic and acute cholecystitis. Jaundice and acute pancreatitis as a result of choledocholithiasis are rare. Radiological evaluation of symptoms suggestive of biliary tract disease can nearly always be limited to ultrasonography. The potential teratogenic effects of conventional radiography and radionucleotide scanning make these techniques unjustified in the pregnant patient.

Therapeutic options for gallstone disease in pregnancy are limited. In the past, open cholecystectomy during pregnancy had been discouraged because of the fear of fetal loss. Complications such as spontaneous abortion and preterm labor were common in women who underwent surgery during the first and third trimesters of gestation, respectively. Similarly, concern regarding potential trocar injury to the uterus and the unknown effects of pneumoperitoneum on the fetal circulation initially made pregnancy an absolute contraindication to laparoscopic cholecystectomy. However, recent improvements in anesthesia and tocolytic agents have now rendered cholecystectomy safer during pregnancy. Several series have demonstrated that the laparoscopic removal of the gallbladder during all stages of pregnancy is safe, resulting in minimal fetal and maternal morbidity.[51–53]

Treatment

During the past three decades, a variety of options for the medical and surgical treatment of cholelithiasis have emerged. Whatever the treatment strategy employed, the goals of therapy include the elimination of biliary calculi and the prevention of recurrent stone-related symptoms. For approximately 100 years, open cholecystectomy has been the gold standard for the treatment of cholelithiasis, but the recent development of minimally invasive surgical techniques for the evaluation and treatment of biliary tract disease has revolutionized the approach to this condition. Randomized, controlled clinical trials comparing open versus laparoscopic removal of the gallbladder have clearly demonstrated that both approaches are safe and effective. Selecting among the different treatment options available, including dissolution and extracorporeal shock wave therapies, however, remains largely a matter of clinical judgment, the availability of the technology, and surgical expertise. As the collective world experience utilizing these various therapeutic options grows, one anticipates that the treatment of gallstone disease will continue to evolve.

Medical Treatments

Oral Dissolution

Gallstone dissolution was first reported in 1937 by a surgeon who noted the disappearance of stones in two of five patients ingesting a bile acid mixture.[54] This report went unconfirmed for several decades, until 1972 when gallstone dissolution using chenodeoxycholic acid was reported in both the United States and Europe.[55,56] In theory, biliary calculi, which specifically result from the cholesterol supersaturation of bile, should dissolve if the ratio of cholesterol to bile salts is reversed. In practice, this therapy is most effective for the treatment of small, noncalcified cholesterol stones in patients with a functioning gallbladder. Successful therapy in many patients can require upward of 6 to 12 months and necessitates periodic monitoring until the stones are dissolved. Approximately 50% to 60% of cholesterol stones measuring less than 10mm in diameter respond; however, the gallstones recur in one-half of these patients within 5 years. Considering the duration, expense, potential side effects, and lack of a durable cure, oral dissolution therapy should be reserved for those patients who either cannot risk or do not want an operation.

Contact Dissolution

Another approach to dissolving gallstones is to directly apply an agent that can solubilize cholesterol. There has been limited experience with this method of treatment, but the most commonly used contact dissolution agents are methyl tert-butyl ether and monooctanoin, both organic solvents. By pumping these solvents directly into the gallbladder, or into the common bile duct in the case of monooctanoin, cholesterol stones can be dissolved within hours to days.[57–59] While technically feasible, contact dissolution has at present a role limited to the treatment of cholelithiasis in patients who are not suitable for surgery.

Extracorporeal Shock Wave Lithotripsy

Introduced in the mid-1980s, extracorporeal shock wave lithotripsy (ESWL) utilizes high-energy sound (shock) waves to physically fragment gallstones into pieces small enough to be passed into the intestinal tract via the common bile duct. The potential advantages of ESWL include the noninvasive destruction of biliary calculi, decreased morbidity and mortality, shortened hospitalization, and the ability to treat patients who are poor candidates for a surgical procedure. Predicated on the results of early trials, a number of selection criteria were established, including a history of biliary colic, three or fewer gallstones that are noncalcified and less than 30mm in diameter, and a functioning gallbladder as determined by oral cholecystography. Given these inclusion criteria, it is estimated that approximately 15% to 20% of patients who are currently candidates for cholecystectomy would qualify for ESWL.

Although physicians in Germany have reported a success rate up to 91% for the treatment of solitary, noncalcified gallstones measuring less than 20mm in size,[60] the experience with ESWL in the United States remains experimental. In 1989, the Food and Drug administration voted for nonapproval of two lithotripters because of inadequate data and disappointing efficacy.[61] Shock wave lithotripsy has remained investigational to this day.

When this technology is employed, effective ESWL treatment begins with shock wave–induced fragmentation of the gallstones. In addition to stone fragmentation, bile acids are administered orally to aid in dissolving the resultant gallstone fragments. Virtually all biliary calculi that meet the selection criteria can be successfully fragmented using this technique. However, the long-term success of ESWL depends on clearing the remaining stone fragments from the biliary system, which requires weeks of litholytic treatment with adjuvant bile acids. In one study, fragment clearance occurred after 2 months in 30% of patients, within 4 months in 48%, and in 91% of patients after 12 to 18 months of adjuvant litholytic treatment.[60]

The long-term consequences of ESWL are not yet known, but the immediate complications include transient biliary colic as the stone fragments are passed into the gut (20%–40%), hemobilia or hematuria (8%–14%), and mild pancreatitis (1%–2%). Gallstones can recur because the lithogenic environment in which the gallstones initially formed is not altered by ESWL. Approximately one-third of patients developed recurrent gallstones within 5 years of stone clearance and cessation of bile acid therapy.[62] Although the probability of stone recurrence increased with time, fewer than 15% of patients experienced recurrent symptoms during the study period.

Surgical Treatments

Open Cholecystectomy

Karl Lugenbach of Germany is credited with performing the first elective cholecystectomy in 1882. For more than a century, open cholecystectomy has been the standard method for surgically treating calculous disease of the biliary system. In retrospective studies, 90% to 95% of patients undergoing cholecystectomy are substantially relieved or cured of their symptoms following surgery.[63]

Open cholecystectomy requires a general anesthetic, an incision in the anterior abdominal wall 12 to 20cm in length, a 4- to 7-day hospitalization, and a 4- to 6-week recuperation period. Under direct vision, the surgeon defines the extrahepatic biliary anatomy, resects the gallbladder and cystic duct, and when indicated explores the common bile duct to identify and remove all intraluminal calculi. This procedure is a safe and effective operation, with an overall morbidity of 2% to 8% and mortality of less than 2%. Thus, open cholecystectomy remains the time-honored standard against which newer therapies should be compared.[64–70]

The risk of open cholecystectomy has declined over the last half century. The overall mortality rate of cholecystectomy in 35,373 patients operated on before 1932 was 6.6%.[71] This rate decreased to 1.8% by 1952, and in 1993 was reported to be as low as 0.17%.[70] The mortality rate is severalfold lower in patients operated on electively as compared to the emergency setting of acute cholecystitis or when a common bile duct exploration is required. In addition, the mortality rate is directly proportional to age. In a report of the entire Danish experience with cholecystectomy from 1977 through 1981, patients under the age of 50 years had a risk of death from elective cholecystectomy of 0.03%[72]; the rate rose to 5.6% in patients over 80 years of age. Most of the deaths after open cholecystectomy are related to cardiovascular disease, in particular myocardial infarction.

The common postoperative complications following open cholecystectomy (Table 47.7) can be divided into biliary and nonbiliary complications. The most frequent complications are retained common bile duct stones, a bile leak or fistula, or a bile duct injury. The most feared of all complications during cholecystectomy is a major injury to the hepatic or common bile ducts. Such an injury can subsequently evolve into a benign stricture and may initiate a sequence of events that includes many corrective surgeries, secondary biliary cirrhosis, and liver failure. Fortunately, this complication occurs with an incidence of 0.08% to 0.3% and, as it is generally caused by an inadequate appreciation of the extrahepatic ductal anatomy, can be usually avoided.[73]

TABLE 47.7. Results of Open Cholecystectomy.

Length of stay (days)	5.4
Morbidity	0.17%
Biliary complications	
Retained stones	0.3%–4%
Bile leak/fistula	0.1%–0.4%
Bile duct injury	0.08%–0.3%
Pancreatitis	0.5%–1.0%
Nonbiliary complications	
Wound problems	1.1%–7.9%
Bleeding	0.2%–2.2%
Pulmonary problems	2.0%–5.3%
Deep venous thrombosis	0.6%–1.3%
Bowel obstruction	0.3%–0.7%
Pulmonary embolus	0.3%–1.0%
Stroke	0.8%
Mortality	0.17%–2.2%

Source: Data from references 64–70 and 138.

Postcholecystectomy Syndrome

Patients who return following cholecystectomy complaining of severe, episodic epigastric or right upper quadrant abdominal pain exemplify the postcholecystectomy pain syndrome. Although the majority of patients are symptomatically improved, it is not uncommon for patients to suffer minor gastrointestinal complaints after cholecystectomy. Indeed, following surgery up to 40% of patients may complain of excessive gas, bloating, abdominal pain, or dyspepsia. In a recent study, 14% of patients reported pain similar to their preoperative complaint, while another 16% noted pain of a distinctly different character.[74] For the majority of patients, the pain resolves altogether with time; however, for 2% to 5% the pain is of sufficient severity to necessitate further investigation and treatment.[75,76] First described in 1947 by Womack and Crider,[77] it is a challenge to determine the cause of the pain in these patients and then to identify that subgroup who will benefit from surgical or endoscopic intervention.

The failure of a cholecystectomy to resolve abdominal pain in selected patients may be the result of an initial misdiagnosis. Therefore, the first step in evaluating patients with postcholecystectomy syndrome is to search for a confounding nonbiliary diagnosis. Many of the signs and symptoms of gallbladder disease are relatively nonspecific and therefore overlap with those of other intraabdominal conditions (Table 47.8). Symptoms related to reflux esophagitis, peptic ulcers, chronic pancreatitis, diverticulosis, hepatitis, and irritable bowel syndrome are similar and would be ineffectively treated by removal of the gallbladder. Therefore, the diagnosis of symptomatic calculous disease must be predicated on more than the presence of gallstones, but must be the result of a detailed history, physical exam, and selected laboratory and radiological evaluations. Once the common nonbiliary causes of abdominal pain have been reasonably excluded, then the focus should return to the biliary system. The key issue in treating patients who return after cholecystectomy complaining of pain is the systematic evaluation and accurate diagnosis of their complaint. A thorough history, physical examination, screening laboratory evaluation, and endoscopic intervention as indicated are essential to the successful management of these complex patients.

The characteristic pain of the postcholecystectomy syndrome is episodic, located in the epigastrium or right upper quadrant, and unassociated with meals or specific types of food. The pain is usually colicky and intermittent, but it can be constant and last for 24 to 48h. Unless the patient is examined during an actual attack of pain, when the upper

TABLE 47.8. Differential Diagnosis of Postcholecystectomy Syndrome: Causes of Pain After Cholecystectomy.

Biliary	
	Choledocholithiasis
	Biliary stricture
	Cystic duct remnant
	Papillary stenosis
	Sphincter of Oddi dyskinesia
	Biliary tract malignancy
	Choledochocele
	Diverticular disease
Pancreatic	
	Pancreatitis
	Pancreatic pseudocyst
	Pancreatic malignancy
	Pancreas divisum
	Neurological disorders
	Herpes zoster infection
Other gastrointestinal disorders	
	Gastroesophageal reflux disease
	Esophageal motor disorders
	Peptic ulcer disease
	Mesenteric ischemia
	Intestinal adhesions
	Intestinal malignancy
	Irritable bowel syndrome
Extraintestinal disorders	
	Psychiatric disorder
	Coronary artery disease
	Intercostal neuritis
	Wound neuroma

abdomen may be tender, the abdominal examination is normal. The same applies to screening laboratory tests. During an attack, one may detect abnormal liver function tests or an elevated amylase or serum lipase; however, between attacks these values, along with other routine laboratory tests, are normal.

The exact etiology of the pain in postcholecystectomy syndrome is uncertain. However, it is most commonly ascribed to increased pressure within the ampulla of Vater. Elevated pressures within the biliary or pancreatic ducts secondary to intermittent obstruction of the choledochalduodenal sphincter of Oddi can be the result of either organic causes (e.g., calculi, ductal neoplasms, papillary fibrosis) or a functional abnormality of the sphincteric mechanism. Controversial causes of pain include the cystic stump syndrome, in which stones presumably form within a long cystic duct remnant and precipitate biliary colic, and cystic duct neuroma, in which transected nervous tissue is entrapped in scar and somehow produces pain. In both these cases, the mechanisms are unproved and speculative.

Biliary dyskinesia is a functional disorder of the choledochalduodenal sphincter that entails abnormal sphincter function in the absence of identifiable organic disease. Endoscopic transampullary biliary manometry is the most accurate method of measuring sphincteric pressure and overall function. Normal sphincter pressure is below 30 mmHg. When resting pressures greater than 40 mmHg are encountered, the sphincter is clearly abnormal, a result of either sphincteric stenosis or spasm. There is no effective medical therapy for biliary dyskinesia, although anecdotal success has been reported with the use of high-dose calcium channel blockers and nitrates. The mainstay of nonoperative treatment for biliary dyskinesia is endoscopic sphincterotomy. Of patients with elevated sphincter pressures, more than 90% report fair-to-good pain relief after sphincterotomy, as compared with only 25% of patients with normal pressures. Transduodenal sphincteroplasty remains an important therapeutic option because, when performed by experienced surgeons, the morbidity and mortality rates compare favorably with those of endoscopic sphincterotomy.[78]

Laparoscopic Cholecystectomy

Laparoscopic cholecystectomy has been a revolutionary advance in general surgery. It was first performed in 1987, and the subsequent decade has witnessed explosive growth in the performance of minimally invasive surgical procedures. Principally fueled by patient demand, laparoscopic techniques have dramatically reduced the inconvenience, morbidity, and overall costs of traditional gallbladder surgery.[79,80] Although open cholecystectomy necessitates a several-day hospitalization and an extended recuperation period, the laparoscopic equivalent is frequently performed on an outpatient basis, with patients returning to work within a few days of the procedure. It is now clear that much of the morbidity associated with open surgery results from the size of the incision required to gain access to the intraabdominal contents rather than from the direct manipulation of the involved organs.

Technique of Laparoscopic Cholecystectomy

Laparoscopic cholecystectomy is usually performed under general anesthesia with special attention paid to muscle relaxation. The operative team consists of a surgeon, assistant surgeon, circulating and scrub nurses, and an anesthesiologist. After induction of anesthesia, bladder and nasogastric tubes are placed for decompression. With the patient in the supine position, the abdomen is prepared with antiseptics and appropriately draped. Intravenous antibiotics are not routinely required for prophylaxis against wound infection in elective cases. Either sequential compression stockings or low-dose subcutaneous heparin are used in patients at high risk for deep venous thrombosis. The operating room setup is shown in Figure 47.15.

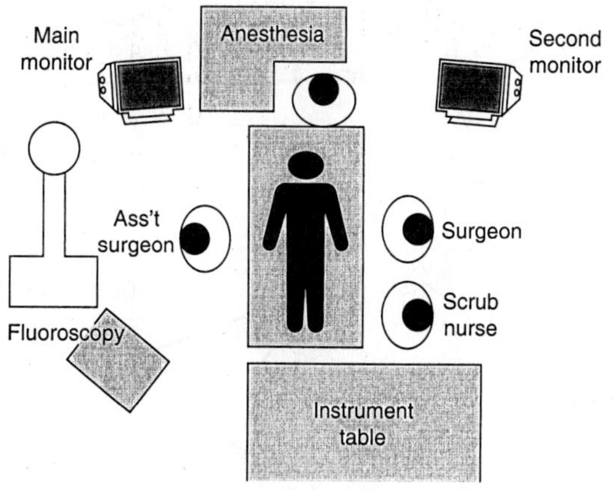

FIGURE 47.15. Operating room setup for laparoscopic cholecystectomy. (Reprinted with permission from *Seminars in Gastrointestinal Disease* 1994;5:122, W.B. Saunders Co.)

A pneumoperitoneum is created through a small umbilical incision with carbon dioxide to provide the space necessary to view the abdominal contents and manipulate instruments; this may be done with a special Verres needle or with a Hasson cannula. The latter technique is difficult in obese patients but adds an element of safety as the blind puncture of the abdomen is avoided. After satisfactory development of the pneumoperitoneum, a periumbilical trocar is placed for the laparoscope, and three additional trocars are placed in the right upper quadrant for exposure and dissecting instruments (Fig. 47.16). The assistant, standing on the patient's right side, elevates the gallbladder fundus toward the ipsilateral hemidiaphragm and retracts the infundibulum laterally, exposing the triangle of Calot. The surgeon, standing at the patient's left side, dissects the cystic artery and duct from the gallbladder wall down toward porta hepatis. This is a crucial step, and special care must be taken to avoid mistaking the common bile duct for the cystic duct. Once the anatomy is identified, a metallic clip is placed across the cystic duct at its gallbladder origin and a small incision is made in the cystic duct for placement of a cholangiogram catheter.

Cholangiography is performed in selected cases when it is necessary to both confirm the ductal anatomy and exclude the presence of gallstones in the common bile duct. Following completion of the cholangiogram, the cystic duct and artery are secured with metal clips and divided. The gallbladder is then dissected off the liver bed with electrocautery and delivered out the umbilical or epigastric trocar site. Care is taken during the procedure to avoid iatrogenic perforation of the gallbladder because the resultant spillage of bile or gallstones is associated with an increased risk of postoperative fever and intraabdominal abscess formation.[81,82]

Postoperative management is straightforward. The bladder and nasogastric catheters are removed at the end of the procedure, and a diet of clear liquids is offered the evening of surgery. Most patients require mild oral analgesics for several days; narcotic injections are rarely necessary to control pain. Patients are allowed to resume full physical activity within 1 week after surgery, although patients may return to sedentary employment before this time.

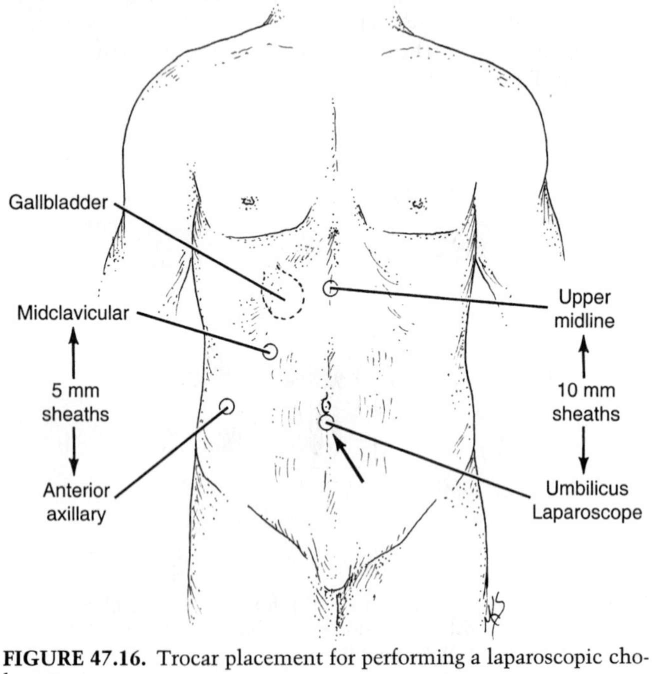

FIGURE 47.16. Trocar placement for performing a laparoscopic cholecystectomy.

Results of Laparoscopic Surgery

After little more than a decade of experience, many practitioners consider laparoscopic cholecystectomy to have replaced the open approach as the treatment of choice, if not the standard of care. The results of laparoscopic cholecystectomy have been reviewed, and the results of 14 series from around the world are summarized in Table 47.9.[81–96] Of the 79,401 patients reported, the cumulative operative morbidity was 7.2%, with an operative mortality of 0.12%. Bile duct injury occurred in 278 patients, for an overall injury rate of 0.35%. Patients spent on average less than 2 days in the hospital and returned to work or their normal daily activities after 6 days. Laparoscopic cholecystectomy is not only a safe and well-tolerated procedure but also has the attendant benefits of reduced perioperative morbidity and convalescence when compared to the standard open approach.[97–103]

While the indications for removal of the gallbladder are essentially identical regardless of the technical approach to be employed, *relative* contraindications to laparoscopy remain. These special circumstances include patients with prior abdominal surgery, acute cholecystitis, obesity, and pregnancy. None of the aforementioned conditions preclude a laparoscopic procedure, but each can represent an additional level of technical difficulty.[36,37,51]

The complications of laparoscopic cholecystectomy, like those of open surgery, can appropriately be divided into biliary and nonbiliary because the two procedures effectively achieve the same goal. However, the minimally invasive approach is associated with selected complications specific to laparoscopy and unique to performing an operation based on two-dimensional camera images, including trocar injuries, occult intraoperative bleeding, bowel perforations, and trocar site wound infections. Although relatively infrequent, there have been reports of major injuries resulting in significant morbidity and mortality.

No doubt the most serious biliary complication during laparoscopic cholecystectomy is injury to the bile duct (see Table 47.9). Immediately following the widespread introduction of this surgical technique, there was an alarming 5- to 10-fold increase in the incidence of bile duct injuries, rising from a prior rate of 0.08% to 0.3% to 0.6% to 1.2%.[104,105] In addition to increased frequency, the type of bile duct injuries also changed to include not only ligation but also in some cases the excision of large segments of the extrahepatic ductal system. This problem has warranted much attention, and subsequent analyses have underscored the absolute importance of defining the biliary anatomy with certainty before dividing any ductal structures.[106] Recent data suggest that the incidence of bile duct injury is equivalent between open versus laparoscopic cholecystectomy. At present, laparoscopic surgical technology continues to advance, providing clinicians and patients with an ever-improving option for the treatment of gallstone disease.

TABLE 47.9.
Global Results of Laparoscopic Cholecystectomy.

Reference	*n*	*Level of evidence*	*Mean OR time (min)*	*Conversion to open (%)*	*Mean LOS (days)*	*Mean return to work (days)*	*Morbidity (%)*	*Bile duct injury (%)*	*Mortality rate (%)*
Southern Surgeons 1991, United States[83]	1,518	III	90	4.7	1.2	—	5.1	0.46	0.07
Cuschieri et al. 1991, Europe[84]	1,236	III	50	3.6	3.0	11	1.6	0.30	0
Ferzli and Kloss 1991, New York[85]	111	III	57	2.7	1.4	7.0	0.9	0	0
Larson et al. 1992, United States[86]	1,983	III	—	4.4	—	—	2.1	0.25	0.10
Litwin et al. 1992, Canada[87]	2,201	III	—	4.3	—	—	—	0.14	—
Hugh et al. 1992, New South Wales[88]	97	III	88	10.3	3.0	7.0	15.5	0	1.03
Go et al. 1993, Netherlands[89]	6,076	III	70	6.8	4.5	—	4.3	0.86	0.12
Orlando et al. 1993, Connecticut[90]	4,640	III	—	6.9	3.0	—	8.6	0.32	0.13
Rubio 1993, Houston[91]	500	III	39	0.8	0.8	3–8	—	0.2	0
Dunn et al. 1994, England and Wales[92]	3,319	III	—	5.2	—	—	6.7	0.33	0.15
Savassi-Rocha et al. 1997, Brazil[93]	33,563	III	78	3.5	1.6	8	8.5	0.20	0.09
Ihasz et al. 1997, Hungary[94]	13,833	III	—	5.3	—	—	4.3	0.59	0.14
Hamour et al. 1998, Saudi Arabia[95]	150	III	100	4.0	3.0	—	6.0	0.67	0
Z'Graggen et al. 1998, Switzerland[96]	10,174	III	91	8.2	—	—	10.4	0.31	0.2
Totals	79,401	III	79	5.0	1.8	6.0	7.2	0.35	0.12

Neoplasms

Cancers of the gallbladder and biliary tree fortunately are uncommon because these malignancies are associated with an extremely poor prognosis. Despite recent advances in imaging technology, biliary cancers are clinically silent tumors that only become symptomatic when they reach an advanced stage of development and are difficult to treat. Surgery is the only curative therapy; chemotherapy and radiation therapies are largely experimental efforts or directed at palliation. Approximately 4000 deaths occur each year in the United States from biliary cancer, with half originating in the gallbladder and 25% in the extrahepatic bile ducts; the remaining tumors arise within the ampulla or are otherwise indeterminate. Despite a bleak history, selected innovations hold some promise for improved treatment rates, including gene therapy to render tumor cells more susceptible to both immunological and chemotherapeutic agents.

Gallbladder Cancer

Epidemiology

First described in 1771, carcinoma of the gallbladder is an uncommon but not rare tumor. It represents 1% of all cancers, is the most common biliary system malignancy, and is the fifth most common gastrointestinal tract cancer, with an overall incidence of 2 to 3 cases per 100,000 persons in the United States. Women outnumber men almost 3 to 1, with a mean age in the seventh decade of life. Interestingly, high-risk groups around the world for the development of gallbladder cancer include Native Americans (sixfold), Israelis, Chileans, Poles, Japanese, Bolivians, and Mexicans.

The etiology of this devastating disease is unknown but has been associated with cholelithiasis, chronic cholecystitis, exposure to specific industrial carcinogens, gallbladder adenomas, and inflammatory bowel disease. A frequently proposed pathogenic mechanism entails a multistage process in which persistent mucosal inflammation progresses first to mucosal hyperplasia, then metaplasia, dysplasia, and ultimately to frank carcinoma. There appears to be a relationship between cholelithiasis and gallbladder cancer, the exact nature of which has yet to be fully delineated. Approximately 80% of patients with gallbladder cancer have coincident gallstones, and the relative risk of this malignancy in patients with cholelithiasis is increased 3- to 20-fold compared to those without biliary calculi. The risk of gallbladder cancer is greater in patients with large gallstones.[107] These data, however, are far from proof of a causal relationship.

Even though the incidence of gallbladder cancer in people without gallstones is extremely low, the absolute risk of cancer in those with gallstones, albeit increased, is still not very great. In fact, only a small fraction of patients with cholelithiasis ever go on to develop cancer (0.5%–1.0%), leading some investigators to speculate that the same factors that predispose to gallstone formation may also contribute to the development of cancer, thereby yielding the appearance of a pathogenic relationship. Furthermore, 20% of cancer patients do not have identifiable gallstones.

In addition to gallstones, numerous clinical features of calculous disease have been identified as risk factors for gallbladder cancer. Diffuse calcification of the gallbladder wall, so-called porcelain gallbladder, can be readily seen on plain abdominal radiographs and carries a 15% to 60% incidence of concurrent cancer. Specific variations in biliary anatomy may also predispose to gallbladder cancer. Large gallbladder adenomas (>12 mm) may rarely degenerate into invasive carcinoma. Also, an anomalous union of the pancreaticobiliary duct that results in a long common channel may allow for continuous reflux of pancreatic juice into the biliary tree and thus serve as a carcinogenic factor.

Diagnosis

Cancer of the gallbladder is a difficult diagnosis to make as only 8% to 10% of these malignancies are diagnosed preoperatively. The diagnostic challenge is largely because there are no signs or symptoms specific to gallbladder cancer. As the condition most often mimics benign biliary disease, with a clinical course reminiscent of anything from biliary colic to chronic cholecystitis, the history and physical examination are insensitive diagnostic tools. Three-quarters of patients have had symptoms for more than 6 months before seeking medical attention. When they do present, the most common complaint is abdominal pain, followed by weight loss, jaundice, nausea, and a host of other nonspecific symptoms. As noted earlier, these tumors are clinically unrecognizable as cancer until the disease is quite advanced, by which time the disease is usually incurable.

Of the standard diagnostic studies for biliary tract disease, ultrasound is the most sensitive for detecting early-stage disease. Even though the sensitivity of abdominal ultrasound is greatly decreased in the presence of calculi, several patterns are suggestive of cancer, including a complex mass filling the gallbladder lumen, a marked thickening of the gallbladder wall, or the identification of a polypoid or fungating tumor. In practical terms, most gallbladder cancers are unexpectedly diagnosed in the operating room during cholecystectomy for gallstones. Thus, the practice of carefully examining the resected gallbladder following its removal is important. This is especially true when the patient is over 50 years of age as the incidence of cancer is 4% and steadily increases with advancing age.

Pathology and Staging

Of gallbladder cancers, 85% are adenocarcinomas (papillary and mucinous variants), with the remaining tumors either squamous cell (3%), adenosquamous (1.5%), or undifferentiated (7%) (Fig. 47.17). On rare occasions, the gallbladder can be the site of a melanoma, sarcoma, or carcinoid tumor. In 1976, Nevin et al. proposed a five-stage classification for

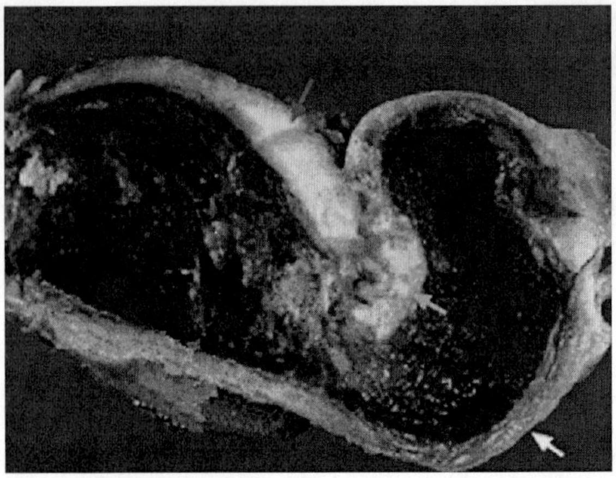

FIGURE 47.17. Gallbladder cancer. Hemisected gallbladder shown with a transmural carcinoma (arrow) located adjacent to a large pigmented gallstone.

cancer of the gallbladder predicated on the depth of tumor invasion into the gallbladder wall, presence of lymph node involvement, and invasion into adjacent or distant organs (Tables 47.10 and 47.11).[108] More recently, the standard TNM staging system has been applied to this cancer; this system principally differs from the Nevin classification by stratifying the depth of direct liver invasion by the tumor. As described here, this stratification dramatically affects the recommended surgical treatment. Regardless of staging classification, once the tumor is transmural, the chances of cure are remote (Table 47.12).[109]

Treatment

The prevailing opinion regarding the treatment of gallbladder cancer can best be summarized as futility. Given a cumulative survival of 3 to 6 months from initial diagnosis, a sense of medical nihilism is understandable. The relative rarity and rapidly fatal nature of gallbladder cancer render the disease difficult to study in a prospective, randomized fashion. However, data from numerous investigators suggest that a more aggressive approach than that reflected in the preceding statement may be warranted.[110–115] Unfortunately, it is difficult to summarize the results from these studies examining the benefit of radical resection in the treatment of gallbladder cancer because of the retrospective nature of the data, the application of different staging systems, and the inconsistent application of various surgical procedures. Regardless, the argument in support of a more radical surgical approach recognizes that surgery is the only chance for cure. In addition, the survival rates following resection are increased, especially for TNM stage II disease and the papillary variant of gallbladder adenocarcinoma (Table 47.13).[112,113,116]

Treatment recommendations are dependent on the stage of the disease (Fig. 47.18). When the cancer is limited to the mucosa and muscularis of the gallbladder (stage I), a simple cholecystectomy should prove curative. When the tumor is transmural and found to invade the subserosa (stage II), however, most authors favor a radical cholecystectomy, with resection of the gallbladder fossa and a regional lymphadenectomy. Even though a survival advantage has not been definitively proven, this recommendation reflects concern for an increased risk of lymphovascular spread and locoregional

TABLE 47.10. Nevin Gallbladder Cancer Staging System.

Nevin classification: *Nevin stage*	*Depth*	*5-Year survival (%)*
Stage I	Mucosa only	50–97%
Stage II	Muscularis, 57%–72%	
Stage III	All layers	0–25%
Stage IV	Lymph nodes	0–20%
Stage V	Liver invasion Adjacent organ Distant metastasis	0–15%

Source: Nevin JE, Moran TJ, Kay S, et al. (108), by permission of *Cancer (Phila).*

TABLE 47.11. Definition of TMN, Stage Grouping, Histopathologic Type, and Histologic Grade for Gallbladder Carcinoma.

Definition of TMN

Primary Tumor (T)

TX	Primary tumor cannot be assessed
T0	No evidence of primary tumor
Tis	Carcinoma *in situ*
T1	Tumor invades lamina propria or muscle layer
T1a	Tumor invades lamina propria
T1b	Tumor invades muscle layer
T2	Tumor invades the perimuscular connective tissue; no extension beyond the serosa or into liver
T3	Tumor perforates the serosa (visceral peritoneum) and/or directly invades the liver and/or other adjacent organ or structure, such as the stomach, duodenum, colon, or pancreas, omentum, or extrahepatic bile ducts
T4	Tumor invades main portal vein or hepatic artery or invades multiple extrahepatic organs or structures

Regional Lymph Nodes (N)

NX	Regional lymph nodes cannot be assessed
N0	No regional lymph node metastasis
N1	Regional lymph node metastasis

Distant Metastasis (M)

MX	Distant metastasis cannot be assessed
M0	No distant metastasis
M1	Distant metastasis

Stage Grouping

Stage 0	Tis	N0	M0
Stage IA	T1	N0	M0
Stage IB	T2	N0	M0
Stage IIA	T3	N0	M0
Stage IIB	T1	N1	M0
	T2	N1	M0
	T3	N1	M0
Stage III	T4	Any N	M0
Stage IV	Any T	Any N	M1

Source: Used with the permission of the American Joint Committee on Cancer (AJCC), Chicago, Illinois. The original source for this material is the *AJCC Cancer Staging Manual, Sixth Edition* (2002) published by Springer Science and Business Media LLC, www.springerlink.com.

TABLE 47.12. Survival Statistics for Gallbladder Cancer.

Stage of disease	*n*	*Median survival (months)*	*2-year survival (%)*
0	98	60	78
I	621	19	45
III	117	7	15
III	678	4	4
IV	936	2	2

Source: Modified from Henson et al.[116]

TABLE 47.13. Survival for Gallbladder Cancer by Tumor Type.

Tumor histology	*2-year survival (%)*	*Median survival (months)*
Adenocarcinoma	14	4
Papillary variant	47	20
Mucinous variant	12	4
Squamous cell	9	4
Adenosquamous	8	3
Undifferentiated	0	2

Source: From Henson et al.[116]

recurrence once the tumor extends beyond the muscular wall of the organ.

How to best treat stage III and IV tumors remains controversial, with the treatment recommendations ranging from major surgery (e.g., hepatic lobectomy, orthotopic liver transplantation) to palliative bilioenteric bypass, to adjuvant chemo- or radiotherapy. Opinions aside, at present there is no effective treatment for advanced gallbladder cancer. Trials examining various chemotherapeutic regimens have to date demonstrated little efficacy, while the use of radiotherapy has not been widely studied. Thus, any invasive therapeutic endeavor involving patients with stage III–IV cancer of the gallbladder should ideally be conducted within the structure of a clinical research activity.

Cholangiocarcinoma

Epidemiology

Approximately 2700 new cases of bile duct cancer are diagnosed annually in the United States. With an overall yearly incidence of 1 per 100,000 population, this tumor occurs less frequently than cancer of the gallbladder.[117] Interestingly, the epidemiology and proposed pathogenesis of cholangiocarcinoma are similar to that of gallbladder cancer, suggesting that these tumors may represent variants of the same disease process. As

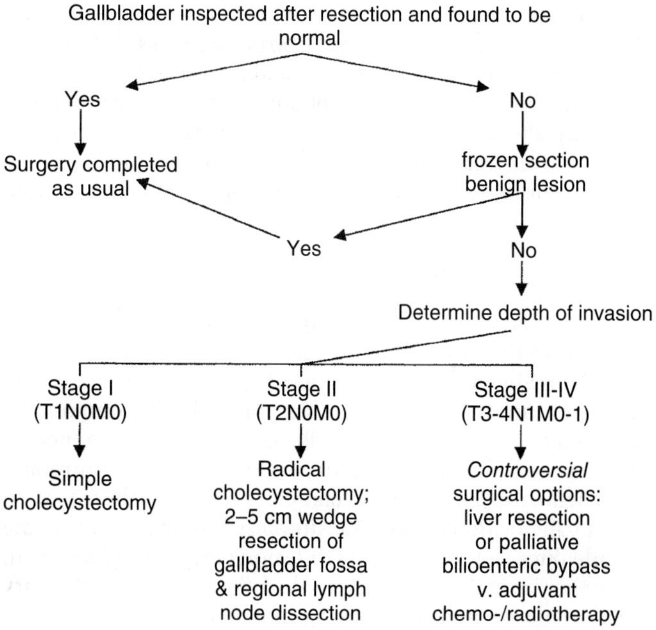

FIGURE 47.18. Treatment algorithm for cancer of the gallbladder.

with gallbladder cancer, the incidence increases with age. High-risk groups include Native Americans, Israelis, and Japanese. The etiology appears related to chronic inflammation, gallstones, and stasis within the biliary system. In contrast, bile duct tumors occur with equal frequency in men and women, are associated with several biliary tract diseases, and usually present with painless jaundice. Among the etiological risk factors for this cancer are ulcerative colitis, primary sclerosing cholangitis, hepatolithiasis, and choledochal cysts. Common to each of these factors is an element of biliary stasis, infection, and stones. Exactly how these elements yield a cancer are unknown, but as with gallbladder cancer it is thought to involve a sequence of chronic inflammation leading to mucosal dedifferentiation and neoplasia.

Diagnosis

The diagnosis is generally made when evaluating a patient with a case of gradually progressive, painless jaundice. More than 90% of patients present with this complaint, which may be accompanied by pruritus, weight loss, anorexia, fatigue, and other constitutional symptoms consistent with a malignancy. Cholangitis is rarely a presenting symptom, but may develop once the biliary system has been manipulated for diagnostic purposes because both percutaneous and endoscopic procedures result in some degree of bacterial contamination. Malignant obstruction of the common bile duct generally produces a marked elevation in the total serum bilirubin of more than 10mg/dL and an alkaline phosphatase that averages 500 to 600IU/L.[117]

Abdominal ultrasound or CT scan clearly identify the dilated intrahepatic ducts proximal to the obstruction but rarely visualize the tumor itself (Fig. 47.19A). Cholangiography remains the most sensitive and informative method for evaluating obstructing ductal masses (Fig. 47.19B). The level and nature of the lesion, along with the patient's overall medical condition, are the primary guidelines that dictate which approach is most appropriate. As previously noted, PTC is generally preferred when delineating a proximal ductal obstruction as it yields critical information regarding the most proximal extent of the tumor. In addition, depending on the nature and severity of the obstructing mass, ERCP may not be able to provide optimal visualization of the proximal lesion. It does enable one to obtain biopsies and brushings from any abnormal areas; however, these tissue samples are diagnostic in less than half of cases given the fibrotic, relatively acellular nature of this cancer. Angiography can be used to evaluate possible vascular invasion by tumor.

Pathology and Staging

Cholangiocarcinomas are classified according to their location within the biliary ductal system rather than their histology. These adenocarcinomas are typically very hard and sclerotic cancers with a paucity of cellular components against a background of dense fibrosis. Consequently, needle biopsies and intraoperative frozen sections are commonly nondiagnostic. There are several classification schemes used for cholangiocarcinomas. The simplest classification schema for bile duct cancers divides the lesions into those located in the upper, middle, or lower third of the extrahepatic biliary tree.[118] This method of stratifying cholangiocarcinomas proves useful with respect to their surgical management. The tumors are staged according to the TNM classification as either extrahepatic (Table 47.14) or intrahepatic (Table 47.15) bile duct cancers.[139]

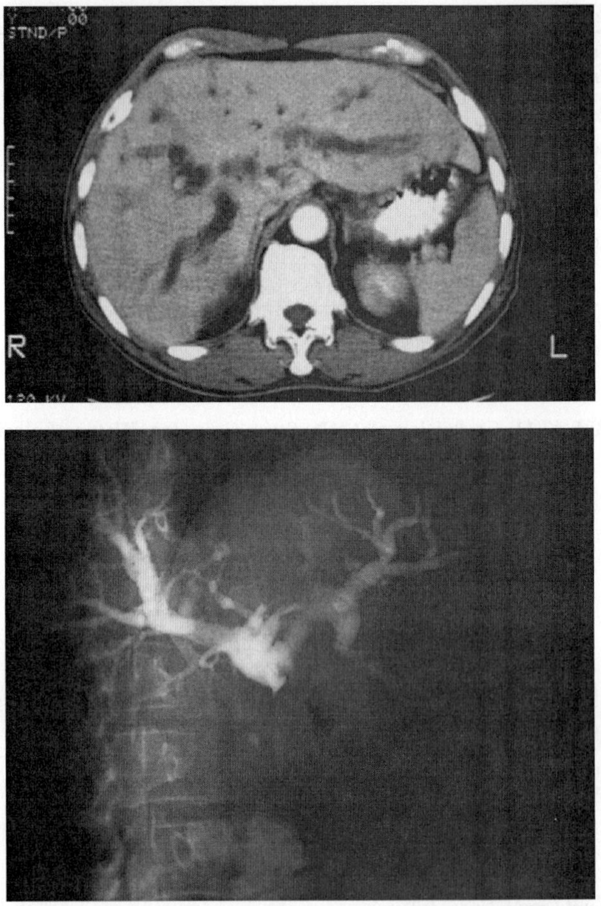

FIGURE 47.19. A. Computed tomographic image of dilated intrahepatic bile ducts. **B.** Percutaneous transhepatic cholangiogram demonstrating dilated intrahepatic bile ducts. (Figures courtesy of the UCSF Department of Radiology.)

Treatment

As with gallbladder cancer, surgery offers the only chance for cure when confronted with stage I and II tumors. Once there is lymph node, regional, or distant metastasis, the goal of intervention turns from cure to palliation. Therefore, when appropriately staged, resection is the treatment of choice. However, the technical challenges associated with bile duct surgery vary as a function of the tumor's exact location. When the lesion is situated within the middle third of the bile duct, resection with bilioenteric bypass is indicated. When the lesion is within the distal third of the bile duct, the appropriate operation is a pancreaticoduodenectomy (Whipple procedure). Tumors in these locations have a better collective prognosis than those located within the upper third, so-called hilar cholangiocarcinomas.

Hilar Cholangiocarcinomas

Bile duct cancers located within the hilum of the liver have been classified according to the pattern of right and left hepatic ductal involvement (Fig. 47.20).[119] There is consider-

TABLE 47.14. Definition of TMN, Stage Grouping, Histopathologic Type, and Histologic Grade for Extrahepatic Bile Duct Carcinoma.

Definition of TMN

Primary Tumor (T)

TX	Primary tumor cannot be assessed
T0	No evidence of primary tumor
Tis	Carcinoma *in situ*
T1	Tumor confined to the bile duct histologically
T2	Tumor invades beyond the wall of the bile duct
T3	Tumor invades the liver, gallbladder, pancreas, and/or unilateral branches of the portal vein (right or left) or hepatic artery (right or left)
T4	Tumor invades any of the following: main portal vein or its branches bilaterally, common hepatic artery, or other adjacent structures, such as the colon, stomach, duodenum, or abdominal wall

Regional Lymph Nodes (N)

NX	Regional lymph nodes cannot be assessed
N0	No regional lymph node metastasis
N1	Regional lymph node metastasis

Distant Metastasis (M)

MX	Distant metastasis cannot be assessed
M0	No distant metastasis
M1	Distant metastasis

Stage Grouping

Stage 0	Tis	N0	M0
Stage IA	T1	N0	M0
Stage IB	T2	N0	M0
Stage IIA	T3	N0	M0
Stage IIB	T1	N1	M0
	T2	N1	M0
	T3	N1	M0
Stage III	T4	Any N	M0
Stage IV	Any T	Any N	M1

Source: Used with the permission of the American Joint Committee on Cancer (AJCC), Chicago, Illinois. The original source for this material is the *AJCC Cancer Staging Manual, Sixth Edition* (2002) published by Springer Science and Business Media LLC, www.springerlink.com.

TABLE 47.15. Definition of TNM, Stage Grouping, Histopathologic Type, Histologic Grade, and Fibrosis Score for Intrahepatic Bile Duct Carcinoma.

Definition of TMN

Primary Tumor (T)

TX	Primary tumor cannot be assessed
T0	No evidence of primary tumor
T1	Solitary tumor without vascular invasion
T2	Solitary tumor with vascular invasion or multiple tumors, none more than 5 cm
T3	Multiple tumors more than 5 cm or tumor involving a major branch of the portal or hepatic vein(s)
T4	Tumor(s) with direct invasion of adjacent organs other than the gallbladder or with perforation of visceral peritoneum

Regional Lymph Nodes (N)

NX	Regional lymph nodes cannot be assessed
N0	No regional lymph node metastasis
N1	Regional lymph node metastasis

Distant Metastasis (M)

MX	Distant metastasis cannot be assessed
M0	No distant metastasis
M1	Distant metastasis

Stage Grouping

Stage I	T1	N0	M0
Stage II	T2	N0	M0
Stage IIIA	T3	N0	M0
IIIB	T4	N0	M0
IIIC	Any T	N1	M0
Stage IV	Any T	Any N	M1

Source: Used with the permission of the American Joint Committee on Cancer (AJCC), Chicago, Illinois. The original source for this material is the *AJCC Cancer Staging Manual, Sixth Edition* (2002) published by Springer Science and Business Media LLC, www.springerlink.com.

able controversy regarding the value of surgical versus nonsurgical treatment for hilar bile duct cancers (Klatskin tumors). First described in 1965 as a clinical entity,[120] these cancers are often considered unresectable and thus suitable only for palliative intervention. At the center of the debate is the 5-year survival of less than 10% for patients with these tumors regardless of intervention, and previous reports were of mortality rates greater than 20% following surgical resection. In contrast, there are several reported series of successful surgical resection of these cancers, with 30-day surgical mortality rates less than 4% and 5-year survival rates of 17% to 45% (Table 47.16).[119,121–123] As with cancer of the gallbladder, there are no randomized trials that compare the surgical versus nonsurgical management of similarly staged patients. Therefore, clinical decision making is predicated on the retrospective reports of experienced clinicians and personal judgment. While the debate cannot be resolved at present, it is useful to review the therapeutic options available for hilar cholangiocarcinomas.

Patients should be stratified on the basis of whether the disease appears to be surgically resectable and thus curable. Patients resected for cure have earlier staged disease and improved survival rates compared to those who undergo palliative surgery.[119,121–126] Because the determination of resectability often cannot be made preoperatively, all patients who are reasonable candidates for surgery deserve an exploratory operation. The criteria for unresectability are extensive vascular invasion of the portal vein or hepatic arteries, tumor involvement of secondary biliary radicals, evidence of metastatic disease, or carcinomatosis. As with gallbladder cancer, approximately 10% to 20% of patients can be resected for cure because most present with advanced disease.

Recently, there has been a trend throughout the world for surgeons to perform more extensive operations, resecting adjacent liver along with the hilar cholangiocarcinoma.[119,121–123] Although the goal of the more radical surgery is to decrease local recurrence and thus improve survival, the data thus far fail to conclusively demonstrate the superiority of this approach.

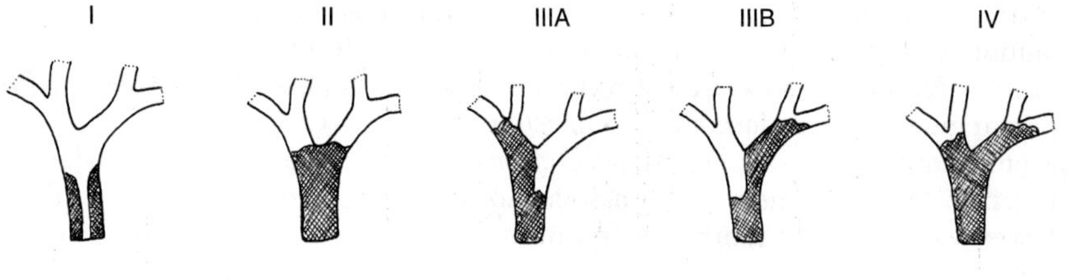

FIGURE 47.20. Modified Bismuth–Corlette classification of hilar cholangiocarcinomas. (From Bismuth et al.,[124] with permission.)

TABLE 47.16.
Results of Aggressive Surgical Resection of Hilar Cholangiocarcinoma (1996–1998).

Reference	*n*	*Study design*	*Level of evidence*	*Morbidity (%)*	*Mortality (%)*	*Mean survival (months)*	*5-year survival (%)*	*Findings/comments*
Nakeeb et al. 1996, Baltimore[119]	191	Retrospective	III	47	3.1	20	17	Classified tumors as intrahepatic, perihilar, and distal Survival was improved with resection and negative margins; poor prognosis associated with low serum albumin and postoperative sepsis
Miyazaki et al. 1998, Japan[122]	76	Retrospective	III	33	13	n/a	26	Rate of surgical curability was significantly higher in patients undergoing hepatic resection, but so was morbidity and mortality Stressed the importance of histologically negative resection margins to avoid recurrence
Burke et al. 1998, New York[121]	30	Retrospective	III	n/a	7	40	45	Stressed the poor ability of assessing node metastases preoperatively, which accounts for >50% of unresectability at laparotomy Mean and 5-year-survival figures are projected after median follow-up of 26 months Also emphasized importance of histologically negative resection margins for improved survival
Iwatsuki et al. 1998, Pittsburgh[123]	72	Retrospective	III	n/a	18	n/a	21	Categorical denial of orthotopic liver transplantation (OTL) not justifiable given that 27 patients underwent OTL with a 5-year survival of 36% Rate of histologically negative margins increased with the extent of surgical resection No 5-year survivors with lymph node metastasis

When compared, hilar versus hepatic resections each yield an operative mortality of approximately 8% to 15% and a 5-year survival ranging from 8% to 27%.[122,123,127–129] Experienced hepatobiliary surgeons should ideally perform these procedures because the operations are technically demanding, and the patients often have diminished physiological reserves.

For those patients with unresectable disease, opinions vary regarding the optimal method of palliation. At one end of the therapeutic spectrum are those who favor resection and intrahepatic bilioenteric bypass to palliate the obstructive jaundice, citing this as a durable and reasonably safe procedure.[130] At the other extreme are those who favor the use of percutaneously or endoscopically placed intraductal stents.[131] Stents require more frequent manipulation to maintain ductal patency, but their insertion is associated with significantly lower periprocedural morbidity and mortality rates.

Adjuvant radiation therapy has been given by means of several different methods, including intraoperative radiotherapy, charged-particle radiation, radioimmunotherapy, and external beam radiation to patients with hilar cholangiocarcinoma. The last has been the most extensively studied method; a dose of 45 to 60 Gy is generally administered. Unfortunately, radiation therapy has had no demonstrable effect on patient survival. The same conclusion currently applies to single and combination adjuvant chemotherapy.

Benign Neoplasms: Choledochal Cysts

Choledochal cysts are defined as localized or diffuse dilations of the biliary tract that can be either congenital or acquired and that predominantly affect women.[132,133] First reported in

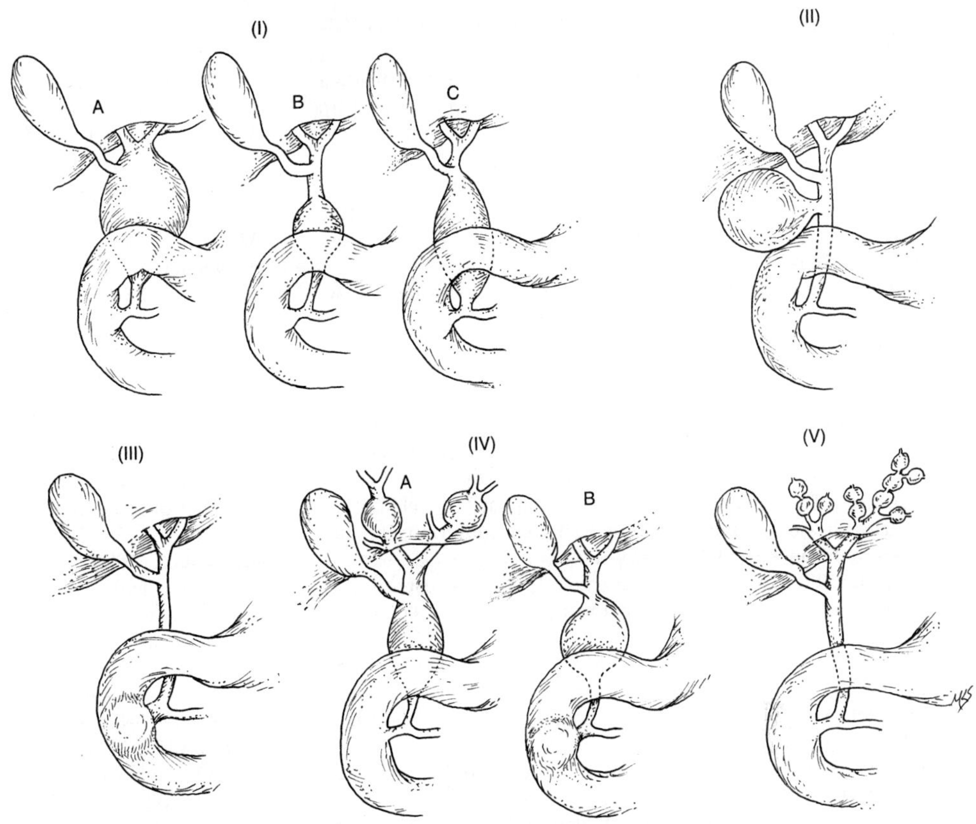

FIGURE 47.21. Todani classification of choledochal cysts. (From Todani et al.,[134] with permission.)

1723, more than 3000 cases of this relatively uncommon entity can be found throughout the world's literature. The etiology of choledochal cysts is unknown. As with cancer of the gallbladder and bile ducts, however, an anomalous junction of the common bile and pancreatic ducts and the attendant chronic reflux of biliopancreatic secretions has been postulated to cause this ductal abnormality. The clinical significance of choledochal cysts results from their propensity for complications, including cholangitis, biliary cirrhosis, portal hypertension, lithiasis, rupture, and malignant degeneration.

The signs and symptoms of a choledochal cyst depend on its location, size, and specific consequence. Frequently, they present as a right upper quadrant mass with associated jaundice and fever in up to 60% of patients. Other complaints include weight loss and back pain. The diagnosis can be confirmed through the use of various diagnostic modalities, including ultrasound, abdominal CT, biliary scintigraphy, and endoscopic cholangiography. Choledochal cysts have been classified according to their pattern of extra- and intrahepatic bile duct involvement (Fig. 47.21).[134]

Previous attempts to treat these cysts by internal cyst drainage via cystojejunostomy or cystoduodenostomy failed because of an unacceptably high rate of late complications, including cholangitis and the development of cholangiocarcinoma. Complete surgical excision and bilioenteric reconstruction constitute the current treatment of choice. However, when the cyst cannot be completely excised, as in the case of type IVA cysts, the patient remains at risk for recurrent cholangitis and the subsequent development of bile duct cancer.

References

1. Lindner HH. Embryology and anatomy of the biliary tree. In: Way LW, Pellegrini CA, eds. Surgery of the Gallbladder and Bile Ducts. Philadelphia: Saunders; 1987:3–15.
2. Thorek P. Gallbladder and Bile Ducts. 2nd ed. Philadelphia: Lippincott; 1962.
3. Adkins RB Jr, Chapman WC, Reddy VS. Embryology, anatomy and surgical applications of the extrahepatic biliary system. Surg Clin North Am 2000;363–379.
4. Moore KL. Clinically Oriented Anatomy. 2nd ed. Baltimore: Williams & Wilkins; 1980.
5. Nora PF. Gallbldder and Biliary Tract. 2nd ed. Philadelphia: Lea & Febiger; 1980.
6. Rathgaber S, Rex D. Right upper quadrant abdominal pain. Diagnosis in patients without evident gallstones. Postgrad Med 1993;94:159–161.
7. Adamek HE, Albert J, Weitz M, Breer H, Schilling D, Riemann JF. A prospective evaluation of magnetic resonance cholangiopancreatography in patients with suspected bile duct obstruction [see comments]. Gut 1998;43:680–683.
8. Davis LP, McCarroll K. Correlative imaging of the liver and hepatobiliary system. Semin Nucl Med 1994;24:208–218.
9. Admirand WH, Small DM. The physicochemical basis of cholesterol gallstone formation in man. J Clin Invest 1968;47:1043–1052.
10. Portincasa P, van de Meeberg P, van Erpecum KJ, Palasciano G, VanBerge-Henegouwen GP. An update on the pathogenesis and treatment of cholesterol gallstones. Scand J Gastroenterol Suppl 1997;223:60–69.
11. Strasberg SM. The pathogenesis of cholesterol gallstones, a review. J Gastrointest Surg 1998;2:109–125.
12. Konikoff FM, Laufer H, Messer G, Gilat T. Monitoring cholesterol crystallization from lithogenic model bile by time-lapse

density gradient ultracentrifugation. J Hepatol 1997;26:703–710.
13. Portincasa P, Di Ciaula A, Baldassarre G, et al. Gallbladder motor function in gallstone patients: sonographic and in vitro studies on the role of gallstones, smooth muscle function and gallbladder wall inflammation. J Hepatol 1994;21:430–440.
14. Pauletzki J, Althaus R, Holl J, Sackmann M, Paumgartner G. Gallbladder emptying and gallstone formation: a prospective study on gallstone recurrence [see comments]. Gastroenterology 1996;111:765–771.
15. Diehl AK. Epidemiology and natural history of gallstone disease. Gastroenterol Clin North Am 1991;20:1–19.
16. Williams CN, Johnston JL. Prevalence of gallstones and risk factors in Caucasian women in a rural Canadian community. Can Med Assoc J 1980;122:664–668.
17. Mellstrom D, Asztely M, Svanvik J. Gallstones and previous cholecystectomy in 77- to 78-year-old women in an urban population in Sweden. Scand J Gastroenterol 1988;23:1241–1244.
18. Jorgensen T. Gallstones in a Danish population. Relation to weight, physical activity, smoking, coffee consumption, and diabetes mellitus. Gut 1989;30:528–534.
19. Holzbach RT. Newer pathogenetic concepts in cholesterol gallstone formation: a unitary hypothesis. Digestion 1997;58:29–32.
20. Mok HY, Druffel ER, Rampone WM. Chronology of cholelithiasis. Dating gallstones from atmospheric radiocarbon produced by nuclear bomb explosions. N Engl J Med 1986;314:1075–1077.
21. Ko CW, Sekijima JH, Lee SP. Biliary sludge. Ann Intern Med 1999;130:301–311.
22. Messing B, Bories C, Kunstlinger F, Bernier JJ. Does total parenteral nutrition induce gallbladder sludge formation and lithiasis? Gastroenterology 1983;84:1012–1019.
23. Janowitz P, Kratzer W, Zemmler T, Tudyka J, Wechsler J. Gallbladder sludge: spontaneous course and incidence of complications in patients without stones. Hepatology 1994;20:291–294.
24. Lund J. Surgical indications in cholithiasis: prophylactic cholecystectomy elucidated on the basis of long-term follow up on 526 nonoperated cases. Ann Surg 1960;151:153–161.
25. Gracie WA, Ransohoff DF. The natural history of silent gallstones: the innocent gallstone is not a myth. N Engl J Med 1982;307:798–800.
26. McSherry CK, Ferstenberg H, Calhoun WF, Lahman E, Virshup M. The natural history of diagnosed gallstone disease in symptomatic and asymptomatic patients. Ann Surg 1985;202:59–63.
27. Friedman GD. Natural history of asymptomatic and symptomatic gallstones. Am J Surg 1993;165:399–404.
28. Ransohoff DF, Gracie WA, Wolfenson LB, Neuhauser D. Prophylactic cholecystectomy or expectant management for silent gallstones. A decision analysis to assess survival. Ann Intern Med 1983;99:199–204.
29. Del Favero G, Caroli A, Meggiato T, et al. Natural history of gallstones in noninsulin-dependent diabetes mellitus. A prospective 5-year follow-up. Dig Dis Sci 1994;39:1704–1707.
30. Linden Wvd, Sunzel H. Early versus delayed operation for acute cholecystitis. A controlled clinical trial. Am J Surg 1970;120:7–13.
31. McArthur P, Cuschieri A, Sells RA, Shields R. Controlled clinical trial comparing early with interval cholecystectomy for acute cholecystitis. Br J Surg 1975;62:850–852.
32. Lahtinen J, Alhava EM, Aukee S. Acute cholecystitis treated by early and delayed surgery. A controlled clinical trial. Scand J Gastroenterol 1978;13:673–678.
33. Jarvinen HJ, Hastbacka J. Early cholecystectomy for acute cholecystitis: a prospective randomized study. Ann Surg 1980; 191:501–505.
34. Norrby S, Herlin P, Holmin T, Sjodahl R, Tagesson C. Early or delayed cholecystectomy in acute cholecystitis? A clinical trial. Br J Surg 1983;70:163–165.
35. Sianesi M, Ghirarduzzi A, Percudani M, Dell'Anna B. Cholecystectomy for acute cholecystitis: timing of operation, bacteriologic aspects, and postoperative course. Am J Surg 1984;148:609–612.
36. Lo CM, Liu CL, Fan ST, Lai EC, Wong J. Prospective randomized study of early versus delayed laparoscopic cholecystectomy for acute cholecystitis [see comments]. Ann Surg 1998;227:461–467.
37. Lai PB, Kwong KH, Leung KL, et al. Randomized trial of early versus delayed laparoscopic cholecystectomy for acute cholecystitis. Br J Surg 1998;85:764–767.
38. Abboud PA, Malet PF, Berlin JA, et al. Predictors of common bile duct stones prior to cholecystectomy: a meta-analysis. Gastrointest Endosc 196;44:450–455.
39. Onken JE, Brazer SR, Eisen GM, et al. Predicting the presence of choledocholithiasis in patients with symptomatic cholelithiasis. Am J Gastroenterol 1996;91:762–767.
40. Leese T, Neoptolemos JP, Baker AR, Carr-Locke DL. Management of acute cholangitis and the impact of endoscopic sphincterotomy. Br J Surg 1986;73:988–992.
41. Lai EC, Mok FP, Tan ES, et al. Endoscopic biliary drainage for severe acute cholangitis [see comments]. N Engl J Med 1992;326:1582–1586.
42. Chijiiwa K, Kozaki N, Naito T, Kameoka N, Tanaka M. Treatment of choice for choledocholithiasis in patients with acute obstructive suppurative cholangitis and liver cirrhosis. Am J Surg 1995;170:356–360.
43. Sugiyama M, Atomi Y. Treatment of acute cholangitis due to choledocholithiasis in elderly and younger patients. Arch Surg 1997;132:1129–1133.
44. Acosta JM, Ledesma CL. Gallstone migration as a cause of acute pancreatitis. N Engl J Med 1974;290:484–487.
45. Kelly TR. Gallstone pancreatitis: pathophysiology. Surgery (St. Louis) 1976;80:488–492.
46. Barie P, Fischer E. Acute acalculous cholecystitis. J Am Coll Surg 1995;180:232–244.
47. Kalliafas S, Ziegler DW, Flancbaum L, Choban PS. Acute acalculous cholecystitis: incidence, risk factors, diagnosis, and outcome. Am Surg 1998;64:471–475.
48. Harris H, Kumwenda Z, Sheen-Chen S, Shah A, Schecter W. Recurrent pyogenic cholangitis. Am J Surg 1998;176:34–37.
49. Csendes A, Diaz JC, Burdiles P, Maluenda F, Nava O. Mirizzi syndrome and cholecystobiliary fistula: a unifying classification. Br J Surg 1989;76:1139–1143.
50. Pemberton M, Wells AD. The Mirizzi syndrome. Postgrad Med J 1997;73:487–490.
51. Glasgow RE, Visser BC, Harris HW, Patti MG, Kilpatrick SJ, Mulvihill SJ. Changing management of gallstone disease during pregnancy. Surg Endosc 1998;12:241–246.
52. Gouldman JW, Sticca RP, Rippon MB, McAlhany JC Jr. Laparoscopic cholecystectomy in pregnancy. Am Surg 1998;64:93–97; discussion 97–98.
53. Barone JE, Bears S, Chen S, Tsai J, Russell JC. Outcome study of cholecystectomy during pregnancy. Am J Surg 1999;177:232–236.
54. Rewbridge A. The disappearance of gallstone shadows following the prolonged administration of bile salts. Surgery (St. Louis) 1937;1:395–400.
55. Danzinger RG, Hofmann AF, Schoenfield LJ, Thistle JL. Dissolution of cholesterol gallstones by chenodeoxycholic acid. N Engl J Med 1972;286:1–8.
56. Bell GD, Whitney B, Dowling RH. Gallstone dissolution in man using chenodeoxycholic acid. Lancet 1972;2:1213–1216.
57. Palmer KR, Hofmann AF. Intraductal mono-octanoin for the direct dissolution of bile duct stones: experience in 343 patients. Gut 1986;27:196–202.
58. Brandon JC, Teplick SK, Haskin PH, et al. Common bile duct calculi: updated experience with dissolution with methyl tertiary butyl ether. Radiology 1988;166:665–667.

59. Hellstern A, Leuschner U, Benjaminov A, et al. Dissolution of gallbladder stones with methyl tert-butyl ether and stone recurrence: a European survey [published erratum appears in Dig Dis Sci 1998;43:2572]. Dig Dis Sci 1998;43:911–920.
60. Sackmann M, Delius M, Sauerbruch T, et al. Shock-wave lithotripsy of gallbladder stones. The first 175 patients. N Engl J Med 1988;318:393–397.
61. Katz S. Biliary lithotripsy: more questions than answers. The ACG Committee on FDA-Related Matters. Am J Gastroenterol 1990;85:497–509.
62. Pelletier G, Raymond JM, Capdeville R, Mosnier H, Caroli-Bosc FX. Gallstone recurrence after successful lithotripsy. J Hepatol 1995;23:420–423.
63. Gilliland TM, Traverso LW. Modern standards for comparison of cholecystectomy with alternative treatments for symptomatic cholelithiasis with emphasis on long-term relief of symptoms. Surg Gynecol Obstet 1990;170:39–44.
64. Glenn F, McSherry CK, Dineen P. Morbidity of surgical treatment for nonmalignant biliary tract disease. Surg Gynecol Obstet 1968;126:15–26.
65. Magee RB, MacDuffee RC. One thousand consecutive cholecystectomies. Arch Surg 1968;96:858–862.
66. Haff RC, Butcher HR Jr, Ballinger WFD. Biliary tract operations. A review of 1000 patients. Arch Surg 1969;98:428–434.
67. Arnold DJ. 28,621 cholecystectomies in Ohio. Results of a survey in Ohio hospitals by the Gallbladder Survey Committee, Ohio Chapter, American College of Surgeons. Am J Surg 1970;119:714–717.
68. McSherry CK, Glenn F. The incidence and causes of death following surgery for nonmalignant biliary tract disease. Ann Surg 1980;191:271–275.
69. Morgenstern L, Wong L, Berci G. Twelve hundred open cholecystectomies before the laparoscopic era. A standard for comparison. Arch Surg 1992;127:400–403.
70. Roslyn JJ, Binns GS, Hughes EF, Saunders-Kirkwood K, Zinner MJ, Cates JA. Open cholecystectomy. A contemporary analysis of 42,474 patients. Ann Surg 193;218:129–137.
71. Huer G. The factors leading to death in operations upon the gallbladder and bile ducts. Ann Surg 1934;99:881–885.
72. Bredesen J, Jorgensen T, Andersen TF, et al. Early postoperative mortality following cholecystectomy in the entire female population of Denmark, 1977–1981. World J Surg 1992;16:530–535.
73. Strasberg SM, Hertl M, Soper NJ. An analysis of the problem of biliary injury during laparoscopic cholecystectomy [see comments]. J Am Coll Surg 1995;180:101–125.
74. Gui GP, Cheruvu CV, West N, Sivaniah K, Fiennes AG. Is cholecystectomy effective treatment for symptomatic gallstones? Clinical outcome after long-term follow-up [see comments]. Ann R Coll Surg Engl 1998;80:25–32.
75. Lasson A. The postcholecystectomy syndrome: diagnostic and therapeutic strategy. Scand J Gastroenterol 1987;22:897–902.
76. Moody FG. Postcholecystectomy syndromes. Surg Annu 1987;19:205–220.
77. Womack NA, Crider RL. The persistence of symptoms following cholecystectomy. Ann Surg 1947;126:31–55.
78. Blumgart L, McCloy R. Postcholecystectomy syndrome. In: Way L, Pellegrini C, eds. Surgery of the Gallbladder and Bile Ducts. Philadelphia: Saunders; 1987:407–416.
79. de Pouvourville G, Ribet-Reinhart N, Fendrick M, Houry S, Testas P, Hugier M. A prospective comparison of costs and morbidity of laparoscopic versus open cholecystectomy. Hepatogastroenterology 1997;44:35–39.
80. Shea JA, Berlin JA, Bachwich DR, et al. Indications for and outcomes of cholecystectomy: a comparison of the pre- and post-laparoscopic eras. Ann Surg 1998;227:343–350.
81. Rice DC, Memon MA, Jamison RL, et al. Long-term consequences of intraoperative spillage of bile and gallstones during laparoscopic cholecystectomy. J Gastrointest Surg 1997;1:85–91.
82. Schafer M, Suter C, Klaiber C, Wehrli H, Frei E, Krahenbuhl L. Spilled gallstones after laparoscopic cholecystectomy. A relevant problem? A retrospective analysis of 10,174 laparoscopic cholecystectomies [see comments]. Surg Endosc 1998;12:305–309.
83. Southern Surgeons Club. A prospective analysis of 1518 laparoscopic cholecystectomies [published erratum appears in N Engl J Med 1991;325:1517–1518] [see comments]. N Engl J Med 191;324:1073–1078.
84. Cuschieri A, Dubois F, Mouiel J, et al. The European experience with laparoscopic cholecystectomy. Am J Surg 1991;161:385–387.
85. Ferzli G, Kloss DA. Laparoscopic cholecystectomy: 111 consecutive cases. Am J Gastroenterol 1991;86:1176–1178.
86. Larson GM, Vitale GC, Casey J, et al. Multipractice analysis of laparoscopic cholecystectomy in 1983 patients. Am J Surg 1992;163:221–226.
87. Litwin DE, Girotti MJ, Poulin EC, Mamazza J, Nagy AG. Laparoscopic cholecystectomy: trans-Canada experience with 2201 cases. Can J Surg 1992;35:291–296.
88. Hugh TB, Chen FC, Hugh TJ, Li B. Laparoscopic cholecystectomy. A prospective study of outcome in 100 unselected patients [see comments]. Med J Aust 1992;156:318–320.
89. Go PM, Schol F, Gouma DJ. Laparoscopic cholecystectomy in the Netherlands. Br J Surg 1993;80:1180–1183.
90. Orlando RD, Russell JC, Lynch J, Mattie A. Laparoscopic cholecystectomy. A statewide experience. The Connecticut Laparoscopic Cholecystectomy Registry. Arch Surg 1993;128:494–498; discussion 498–499.
91. Rubio PA. Laparoscopic cholecystectomy: experience in 500 consecutive cases. Int Surg 1993;78:277–279.
92. Dunn D, Nair R, Fowler S, McCloy R. Laparoscopic cholecystectomy in England and Wales: results of an audit by the Royal College of Surgeons of England [see comments]. Ann R Coll Surg Engl 1994;76:269–275.
93. Savassi-Rocha PR, Ferreira JT, Diniz MT, Sanches SR. Laparoscopic cholecystectomy in Brazil: analysis of 33,563 cases. Int Surg 1997;82:208–213.
94. Ihasz M, Hung CM, Regoly-Merei J, et al. Complications of laparoscopic cholecystectomy in Hungary: a multicentre study of 13,833 patients. Eur J Surg 1997;163:267–274.
95. Hamour OA, Kashgari RH, al-Harbi MA. Minimal invasive surgery: a district hospital experience. East Afr Med J 1998;75:274–278.
96. Z'Graggen K, Wehrli H, Metzger A, Buehler M, Frei E, Klaiber C. Complications of laparoscopic cholecystectomy in Switzerland. A prospective 3-year study of 10,174 patients. Swiss Association of Laparoscopic and Thoracoscopic Surgery. Surg Endosc 1998;12:1303–1310.
97. Attwood SE, Hill AD, Mealy K, Stephens RB. A prospective comparison of laparoscopic versus open cholecystectomy [see comments]. Ann R Coll Surg Engl 1992;74:397–400.
98. Farrow HC, Fletcher DR, Jones RM. The morbidity of surgical access: a study of open versus laparoscopic cholecystectomy. Aust N Z J Surg 1993;63:952–954.
99. Sanabria JR, Clavien PA, Cywes R, Strasberg SM. Laparoscopic versus open cholecystectomy: a matched study [see comments]. Can J Surg 193;36:330–336.
100. Barkun JS, Barkun AN, Meakins JL. Laparoscopic versus open cholecystectomy: the Canadian experience. The McGill Gallstone Treatment Group. Am J Surg 1993;165:455–458.
101. Williams LF Jr, Chapman WC, Bonau RA, McGee EC Jr, Boyd RW, Jacobs JK. Comparison of laparoscopic cholecystectomy with open cholecystectomy in a single center. Am J Surg 193;165:459–465.
102. Berggren U, Gordh T, Grama D, Haglund U, Rastad J, Arvidsson D. Laparoscopic versus open cholecystectomy: hospitalization, sick leave, analgesia and trauma responses [see comments]. Br J Surg 1994;81:1362–1365.

103. Stevens HP, van de Berg M, Ruseler CH, Wereldsma JC. Clinical and financial aspects of cholecystectomy: laparoscopic versus open technique. World J Surg 1997;21:91–96, discussion 96–97.
104. Savader SJ, Lillemoe KD, Prescott CA, et al. Laparoscopic cholecystectomy-related bile duct injuries: a health and financial disaster. Ann Surg 1997;225:268–273.
105. Bauer TW, Morris JB, Lowenstein A, Wolferth C, Rosato FE, Rosato EF. The consequences of a major bile duct injury during laparoscopic cholecystectomy. J Gastrointest Surg 1998;2:61–66.
106. Stewart L, Way LW. Bile duct injuries during laparoscopic cholecystectomy. Factors that influence the results of treatment. Arch Surg 1995;130:1123–1128; discussion 1129.
107. Diehl AK. Gallstone size and the risk of gallbladder cancer. JAMA 1983;250:2323–2326.
108. Nevin JE, Moran TJ, Kay S, King R. Carcinoma of the gallbladder: staging, treatment, and prognosis. Cancer (Phila) 1976;37:141–148.
109. Donohue JH, Stewart AK, Menck HR. The National Cancer Data Base report on carcinoma of the gallbladder, 1989–1995. Cancer (Phila) 1998;83:2618–2628.
110. Gall FP, Kockerling F, Scheele J, Schneider C, Hohenberger W. Radical operations for carcinoma of the gallbladder: present status in Germany. World J Surg 1991;15:328–336.
111. Shirai Y, Yoshida K, Tsukada K, Muto T, Watanabe H. Radical Surgery for gallbladder carcinoma. Long-term results. Ann Surg 1992;216:565–568.
112. Onoyama H, Yamamoto M, Tseng A, Ajiki T, Saitoh Y. Extended cholecystectomy for carcinoma of the gallbladder. World J Surg 1995;19:758–763.
113. Bartlett DL, Fong Y, Fortner JG, Brennan MF, Blumgart LH. Long-term results after resection for gallbladder cancer. Implications for staging and management. Ann Surg 1996;224:639–646.
114. Yamaguchi K, Chijiiwa K, Saiki S, et al. Retrospective analysis of 70 operations for gallbladder carcinoma. Br J Surg 197;84:200–204.
115. de Aretxabala XA, Roa IS, Burgos LA, Araya JC, Villaseca MA, Silva JA. Curative resection in potentially resectable tumours of the gallbladder. Eur J Surg 1997;163:419–426.
116. Henson DE, Albores-Saavedra J, Corle D. Carcinoma of the gallbladder. Histologic types, stage of disease, grade, and survival rates. Cancer (Phila) 1992;70:1493–1497.
117. Henson DE, Albores-Saavedra J, Corle D. Carcinoma of the extrahepatic bile ducts. Histologic types, stage of disease, grade, and survival rates. Cancer (Phila) 1992;70:1498–1501.
118. Langer JC, Langer B, Taylor BR, Zeldin R, Cummings B. Carcinoma of the extrahepatic bile ducts: results of an aggressive surgical approach. Surgery (St. Louis) 1985;98:752–759.
119. Nakeeb A, Pitt HA, Sohn TA, et al. Cholangiocarcinoma. A spectrum of intrahepatic, perihilar, and distal tumors. Ann Surg 1996;224:463–473; discussion 473–475.
120. Klatskin G. Adenocarcinoma of the hepatic duct at its bifurcation within the porta hepatis. An unusual tumor with distinctive clinical and pathological features. Am J Med 1965; 38:241–247.
121. Burke EC, Jarnagin WR, Hochwald SN, Pisters PW, Fong Y, Blumgart LH. Hilar cholangiocarcinoma: patterns of spread, the importance of hepatic resection for curative operation, and a presurgical clinical staging system. Ann Surg 1998;228:385–394.
122. Miyazaki M, Ito H, Nakagawa K, et al. Aggressive surgical approaches to hilar cholangiocarcinoma: hepatic or local resection? Surgery (St. Louis) 1998;123:131–136.
123. Iwatsuki S, Todo S, Marsh JW, et al. Treatment of hilar cholangiocarcinoma (Klatskin tumors) with hepatic resection or transplantation. J Am Coll Surg 1998;187:358–364.
124. Bismuth H, Nakache R, Diamond T. Management strategies in resection for hilar cholangiocarcinoma. Ann Surg 1992;215:31–38.
125. Su CH, Tsay SH, Wu CC, et al. Factors influencing postoperative morbidity, mortality, and survival after resection for hilar cholangiocarcinoma. Ann Surg 1996;223:384–394.
126. Strasberg SM. Resection of hilar cholangiocarcinoma. HPB Surg 1998;10:415–418.
127. Casavilla FA, Marsh JW, Iwatsuki S, et al. Hepatic resection and transplantation for peripheral cholangiocarcinoma. J Am Coll Surg 1997;185:429–436.
128. Madariaga JR, Iwatsuki S, Todo S, Lee RG, Irish W, Starzl TE. Liver resection for hilar and peripheral cholangiocarcinomas: a study of 62 cases. Ann Surg 1998;227:70–79.
129. Nagino M, Nimura Y, Kamiya J, et al. Segmental liver resections for hilar cholangiocarcinoma. Hepatogastroenterology 1998;45:7–13.
130. Jarnagin WR, Burke E, Powers C, Fong Y, Blumgart LH. Intrahepatic biliary enteric bypass provides effective palliation in selected patients with malignant obstruction at the hepatic duct confluence. Am J Surg 1998;175:453–460.
131. England RE, Martin DF. Endoscopic and percutaneous intervention in malignant obstructive jaundice. Cardiovasc Intervent Radiol 1996;19:381–387.
132. Fieber SS, Nance FC. Choledochal cyst and neoplasm: a comprehensive review of 106 cases and presentation of two original cases. Am Surg 1997;63:982–987.
133. Miyano T, Yamataka A. Choledochal cysts. Curr Opin Pediatr 1997;9:283–288.
134. Todani T, Watanabe Y, Narusue M, Tabuchi K, Okajima K. Congenital bile duct cysts: classification, operative procedures, and review of thirty-seven cases including cancer arising from choledochal cyst. Am J Surg 1977;134:263–269.
135. Thistle JL, Cleary PA, Lachin JM, Tyor MP, Hersh T. The natural history of cholelithiasis: the National Cooperative Gallstone Study. Ann Intern Med 1984;101:171–175.
136. Lamont JT, Carey MC. Cholesterol gallstone formation. 2. Pathobiology and pathomechanics. Prog Liver Dis 1992;10:165–191.
137. Alexander-Williams J. Bacteriology of biliary disease. In: Way L, Pellegrini C, eds. Surgery of the Gallbladder and Bile Ducts. Philadelphia: Saunders; 1987:93–102.
138. Harris H, Pellegrini C. Indications, operative technique, and complications of cholecystectomy (open)-cholecystostomy (open). In: Braasch J, Tompkins R, eds. Surgical Disease of the Biliary Tract and Pancreas—Multidisciplinary Management. St. Louis: Mosby-Year Book; 1994:129–143.
139. Beahrs O, Henson D, Hutter R, Kennedy B. American Joint Committee on Cancer: Manual for Staging Cancer. 4th ed. Philadelphia: Lippincott; 1992.
140. Braasch J, Tompkins R, eds. Surgical Disease of the Biliary Tract and Pancreas—Multidisciplinary Management. St. Louis: Mosby-Year Book; 1994.
141. Patten BM. Human Embryology. New York: McGraw-Hill; 1953.
142. Way LW, Pelligrini CA. Surgery of the Gallbladder and Bile Duct. Philadelphia: Saunders; 1987.

48

Liver

Courtney Scaife

Anatomy

The liver develops from a branching diverticular outpouching of the foregut in the fifth to seventh weeks of development. This gives rise to the hepatic cords, the secretory tubules of the liver, and the primary hepatic ducts. Fully developed, the liver is the largest parenchymal organ in the body and accounts for approximately 4% to 5% of the total body weight.

The liver receives a dual blood supply from the portal vein and the hepatic artery, which branch together with the bile duct within Glisson's sheath to form the portal triads. Glisson's sheath is a continuation of the visceral peritoneal capsule of the liver (Glisson's capsule). The portal vein, the hepatic artery, and the common hepatic duct form the portal pedicle, which divides at the portal confluence into right and left branches and then continues to branch to supply the liver in a segmental fashion. Venous drainage is via the right, middle, and left hepatic veins, which drain directly into the inferior vena cava. Surgical anatomy is based on this portal and hepatic venous (and biliary) segmental distribution.

The most commonly accepted anatomic description of the liver is based on the segmental anatomy described by Couinaud in 1957 (Fig. 48.1).[1] The hepatic veins run in the portal scissurae and divide the liver, medial to lateral, into four sectors. The sectors are in turn divided anterior to posterior by the portal pedicles running in the hepatic scissurae. The liver is therefore divided into the main right and left lobes by the middle hepatic vein, along Cantlie's line, anteroinferiorly to the gallbladder fossa (Fig. 48.1). The respective anteroposterior and inferosuperior sectors are divided by the portal triads and hepatic veins (Fig. 48.1).

Segmental anatomy becomes important in considering surgical resection when essentially any segment or combination of segments can be resected if attention is paid to maintaining vascular inflow and outflow and biliary continuity to remaining segments. Proper planning for surgical resection of the liver is dependent on the ability to assess the segmental anatomy based on modern radiographic imaging (Figs. 48.2 and Fig. 48.3). The ligaments of the liver include the falciform ligament, the coronary ligament, and the right and left triangular ligaments, as demonstrated in Figure 48.4.

Physiology

The liver has multiple complex functions, including the synthesis of glycogen, proteins, bile, and cholesterol; the clearance and transformation of waste products and toxins; and the storage of glycogen, fat-soluble vitamins, and minerals. Although the liver constitutes only 4% to 5% of body weight, it is responsible for 20% to 25% of body oxygen consumption and 20% of total energy expenditure. The liver receives a dual blood supply, with 75% of flow from the portal vein and 25% from the hepatic artery. Total blood flow to the liver is approximately $1.5\,L/min/1.73\,m^2$. Decreasing portal venous flow causes a subsequent increase in hepatic arterial flow; however, hepatic arterial flow cannot completely compensate. Decreasing flow in the hepatic artery does not cause a compensatory increase in flow in the portal vein.

Bile is formed at the canalicular membrane of the hepatocyte as well as in the bile ductules and is secreted by an active process that is relatively independent of blood flow. The main components of bile are the conjugated bile acids, cholesterol, phospholipid, bile pigments, and protein. Under normal conditions, 600 to 1000 mL of bile is produced per day.[2] Bilirubin, a product of heme catabolism, is removed from plasma by the hepatocytes, which then conjugate bilirubin with uridine diphosphate-glucuronyl transferase, which renders it more water soluble. Conjugated bilirubin is then eliminated in bile. The liver synthesizes many of the major human plasma proteins, including albumin, γ-globulin, and many of the coagulation proteins. Liver dysfunction can have a profound effect on coagulation by decreased production of coagulation proteins or, in the case of obstructive jaundice, decreased activity of factors II, V, VII, IX, and X secondary to a lack of vitamin K–dependent posttranslational modification. Reversal of coagulation abnormalities by exogenous administration of vitamin K differentiates between synthetic

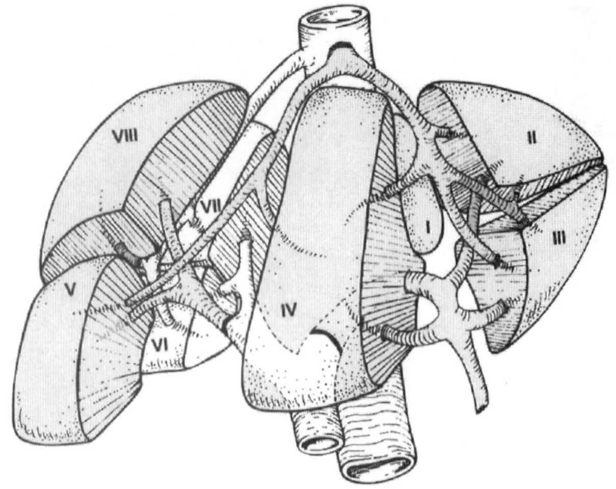

FIGURE 48.1. Diagrammatic representation of Couinaud's segmental anatomy of the liver. (From Blumgart,[194] with permission of Churchill Livingstone.)

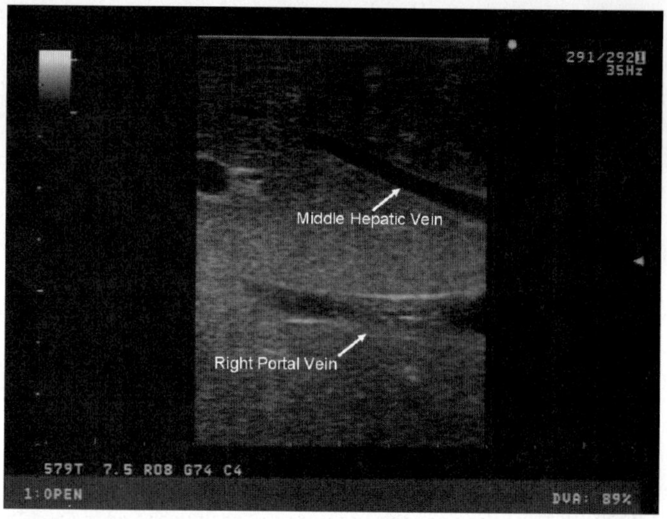

FIGURE 48.3. Intraoperative ultrasound of right portal vein and middle hepatic vein. Note hyperechoic image of portal vein due to Glisson's capsule versus middle hepatic vein.

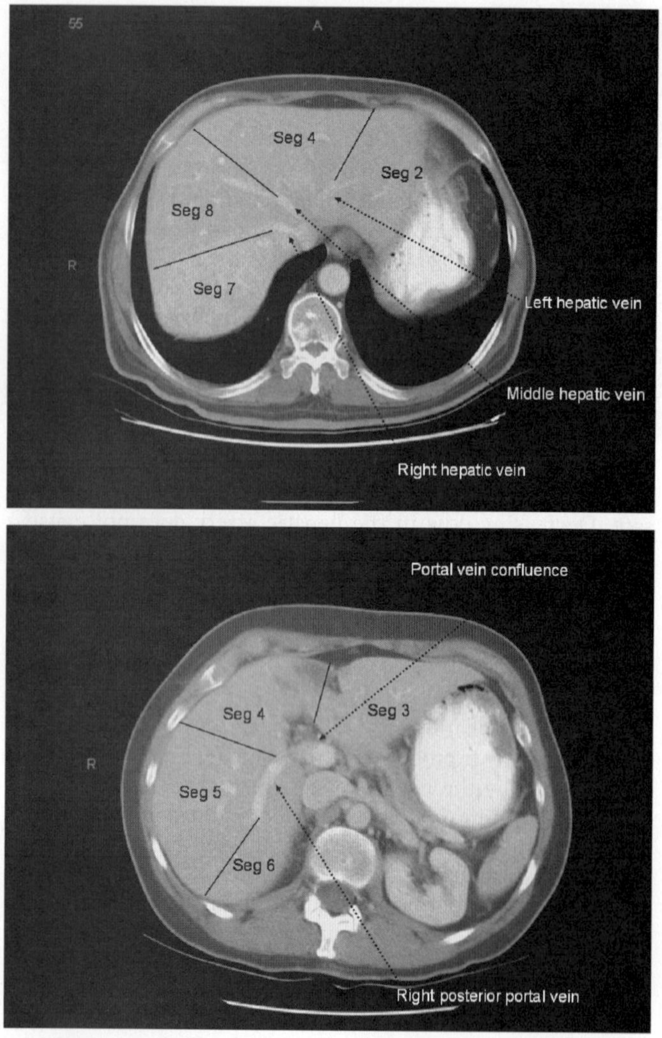

FIGURE 48.2. (A,B) Segmental anatomy of the liver relative to computed tomographic imaging.

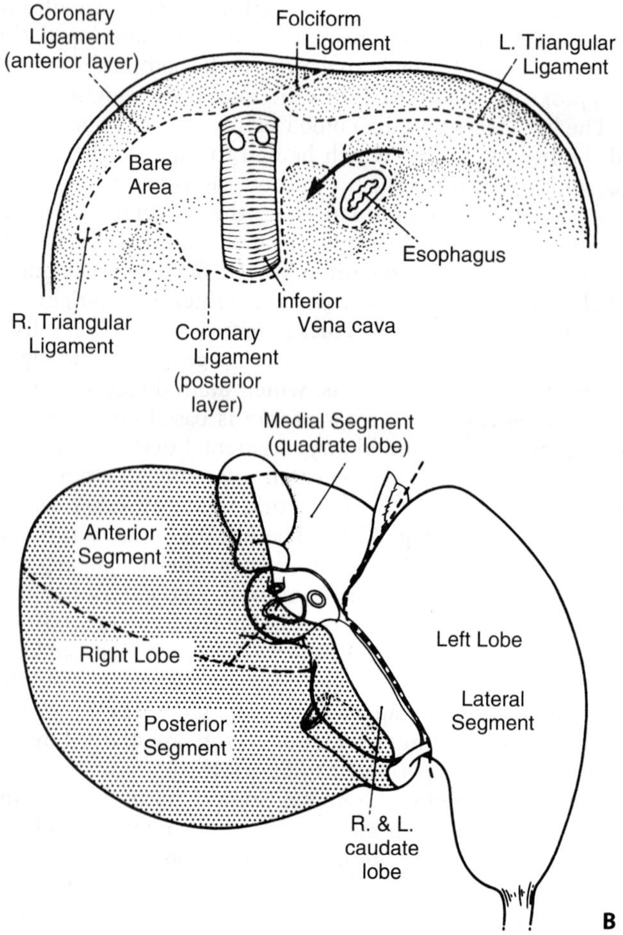

FIGURE 48.4. Diagrammatic representation of the ligaments of the liver. (A) anterior view (B) inferior view.

dysfunction and lack of vitamin K absorption secondary to obstructive jaundice.

Laboratory Studies

Liver function may be assessed by the laboratory evaluation of serum levels of hepatic transaminases, bilirubin levels, γ-glutamyl transaminase (GGT), alkaline phosphatase (AP), and ammonia. Hepatic transaminases AST (aspartate aminotransferase) and ALT (alanine aminotransferase) are produced within hepatocytes. Elevation of serum aminotransaminase levels may indicate hepatocyte dysfunction, although neither AST nor ALT is specific to the liver as the aminotransaminases are also produced in myocardium, skeletal muscle, pancreas, kidney, and red blood cells.

Alkaline phosphatase is a nonspecific hepatic marker, most commonly elevated in hepatic or bone disorders. The elevation of AP may result from biliary stasis or hepatic parenchymal disorders. An elevation of GGT, although also nonspecific, may be used to distinguish a hepatic etiology of an elevated AP as opposed to a bony source.

As mentioned, bilirubin is a product of heme catabolism excreted in bile. An elevation of serum bilirubin levels is indicative of defective bile formation or excretion. The measure of conjugated versus unconjugated serum bilirubin is a reflection of pre- or posthepatocyte dysfunction as an elevation of unconjugated bilirubin reflects an increase in heme metabolism or a failure of hepatocyte function, while an increase in conjugated bilirubin reflects bile stasis.

Ammonia is a nonspecific measure of hepatic dysfunction; its elevation is most commonly seen in disorders of portal hypertension, drug toxicity, and deficiency of urea metabolism. Ammonia levels are most commonly used to assess severity of and response to therapy for hepatic encephalopathy.

Benign Lesions

A variety of benign and usually asymptomatic lesions are found commonly in the liver. The use of abdominal computed tomographic (CT) imaging for diagnostics by primary care physicians leads to the detection of these incidental liver lesions. In most cases, a provisional diagnosis can be made by imaging characteristics with relative certainty without the need for biopsy (Table 48.1).

TABLE 48.1. Radiographic Imaging Characteristics of Benign Liver Lesions.

Lesion	*Ultrasound (accuracy %)*	*Nuclear medicine (accuracy %)*	*Computed tomography (accuracy %)*	*Magnetic resonance imaging (accuracy %)*
Hemangioma	Homogeneous, lobulated, hyperechoic mass (70%–80%) (Descottes et al. 2003)[177]	SPECT imaging (technetium-labeled red blood cells): Lesion fills on delayed images (85%–95% for lesions >3 cm only) (Biecker et al. 2003)[14]	IV contrast-enhanced study: Not visualized or peripheral enhancement in early phase, delayed phase contrast enhancement progression (Leslie et al. 1995)[188]	T1: hypointense T2: hyperintense—increases with time Gadolinium: enhancement (85%–95%) (Unal et al. 2002)[192]
Focal nodular hyperplasia	Not well imaged, variable intensity (Hussain et al. 2004)[182]	Technetium-sulfur-colloid: variable uptake (Kehagias et al. 2001)[184]	IV contrast-enhanced study: Hyperintense with central scar defect, delayed filling of central scar (85%–95%) (Brancatelli 2001)[175]	T1: hypointense central scar T2: hyperintense central scar Gadolinium: early enhancement (85%–95%) (Mortele et al. 2000)[191]
Adenoma	Variable, nonspecific appearance (Hung et al. 2001)[181]	Technetium-sulfur-colloid Variable uptake	IV contrast = enhanced study: Well-defined capsule, hypervascular, early enhancement, may have evidence of hemorrhage	T2: hypervascular, early enhancement, may have evidence of hemorrhage
Simple cyst	Hypoechoic, well circumscribed, no septations	Not visualized	IV contrast-enhanced study: Low attenuation, well circumscribed, no septations, 0–10 hounsfield units (Carrim and Murchison 2003)[18]	T1: hypointense T2: hyperintense, well circumscribed Gadolinium: enhancement Signal intensity parallels cerebrospinal fluid
Echinococcal cyst	Well circumscribed with distinct capsule (Caremani et al. 2003)[176]		Well circumscribed with distinct hypervascular capsule, may have calcifications (Haddad et al. 2001)[179]	T1: hypointense with rim evident T2: hyperintense with hypointense rim Gadolinium: Solid components of cyst may enhance (Kodama et al. 2003)[186]

Hemangiomas

Hepatic hemangiomas are the most common benign hepatic tumor, with incidences as high as 3%–20% in autopsy series, occurring most commonly in middle-aged women and with a 6:1 female-to-male ratio.[3–5] The majority of hemangiomas are small (<5 cm), often multiple, and asymptomatic.[5] The published Mayo Clinic experience confirms that fewer than 15% of hemangiomas less than 10 cm are symptomatic, while 90% of patients with hemangiomas larger than 10 cm have symptoms.[6] Hemangiomas are felt to arise from ectatic rather than hyperplastic vessels, with the blood supply arising from the hepatic artery.[7]

Hemangiomas are usually accurately diagnosed with radiologic imaging studies as there are characteristic features, summarized in Table 48.1. Percutaneous biopsy is avoided due to bleeding risk, and resection is rarely necessary (Fig. 48.5). Surgical resection or enucleation is indicated for rare cases in which symptoms are disabling; complications of rupture, thrombosis, necrosis, or disseminated intravascular coagulopathy occur; malignancy cannot be excluded.[8]

Focal Nodular Hyperplasia

Focal nodular hyperplasia (FNH), second in incidence of benign hepatic tumors, is a typically well-circumscribed lesion with a classical central stellate "scar" with radiating fibrous septae as seen in radiographic imaging (Table 48.1; Fig. 48.6). Although found in both males and females, FNH is more common in females of reproductive age (female-to-male ratio of 8:1).[5] The etiology of this lesion is not entirely clear, although in a classic morphometric study by Wanless et al. of 51 FNH cases it was shown that FNH is a hyperplastic response of the liver to a preexisting vascular abnormality.[9] There is limited evidence of an association of FNH development with the use of oral contraceptives.[10] Usually, FNH tumors are solitary, although at least 20% of individuals with FNH have multiple lesions.[11] The tumors of FNH can be safely observed without the need for biopsy or resection as there is no evidence of malignant potential, and they are most commonly asymptomatic. Spontaneous regression or growth can occur without concern. If the diagnosis is unclear, an FNH tumor may be biopsied if this can be done safely.

Adenoma

Hepatic adenomas are a benign proliferation of sheets of hepatocytes with no portal triads. Adenomas also arise predominantly in young women, with a female-to-male ratio of 4:1.[5] Of adenomas, 70% are solitary.[3] They are round, well-circumscribed, 5- to 15-cm lesions, often with a pseudocapsule (Fig. 48.7). Although these are benign tumors, there are isolated case reports of primary hepatocellular carcinomas (HCCs) developing within adenomas.[12] The incidence of hepatic adenomas has increased with the use of oral contraceptives, particularly in patients with long-term use of high-dose estrogen.[13] Patients with glycogen storage disorders also have an increased incidence of adenomas.[14]

Adenoma may be symptomatic with abdominal pain, or the sensation of a mass, in approximately 50% of patients secondary to frequent intratumoral hemorrhage or necrosis.

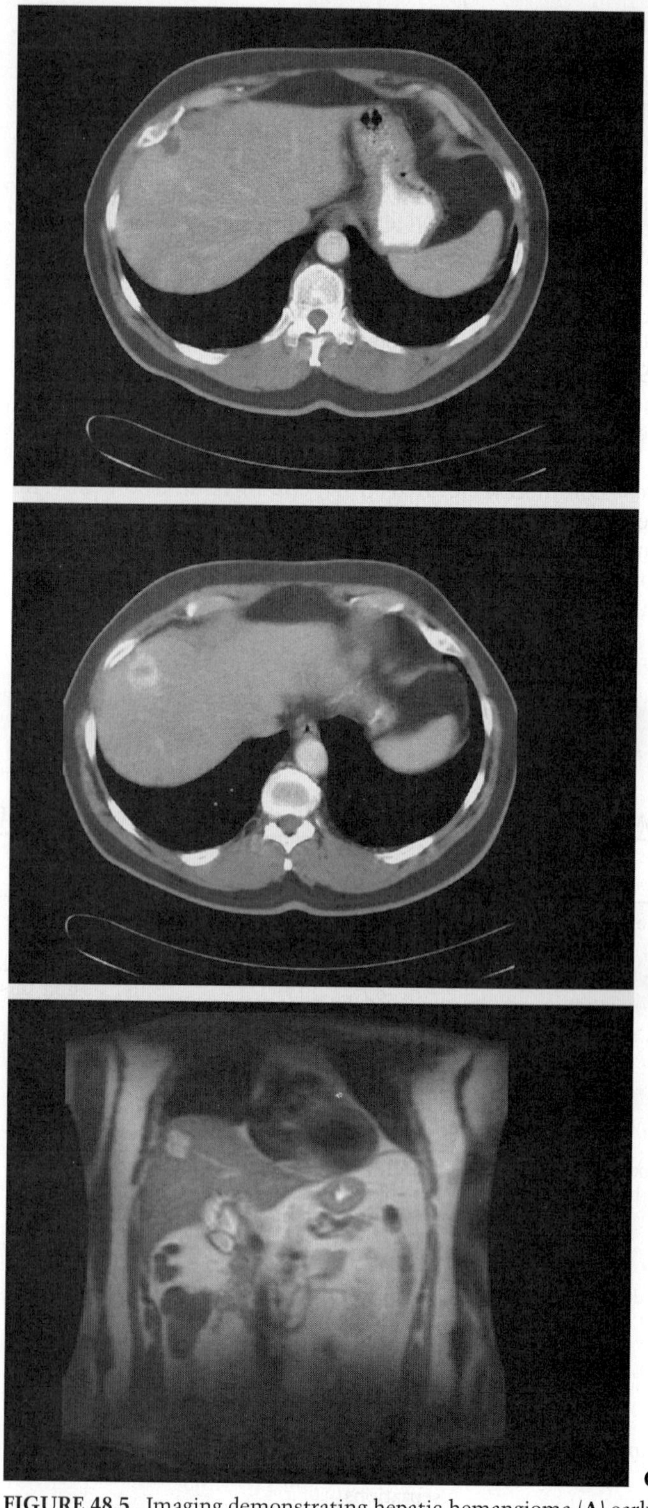

A

B

C

FIGURE 48.5. Imaging demonstrating hepatic hemangioma (**A**) early arterial phase image, (**B**) delayed image demonstrating delayed contrast enhancement, and (**C**) T2-phase, gadolinium-enhanced MRI demonstrating hepatic hemangioma.

Free intraperitoneal rupture, presenting with abdominal pain or signs of bleeding, occurs in 10% to 20% of cases, while the remainder of adenomas are found incidentally, either through imaging or at laparotomy. Diagnosis of adenoma is based on accurate imaging with CT and magnetic resonance imaging (MRI), reflecting the hypervascular and hemorrhagic nature

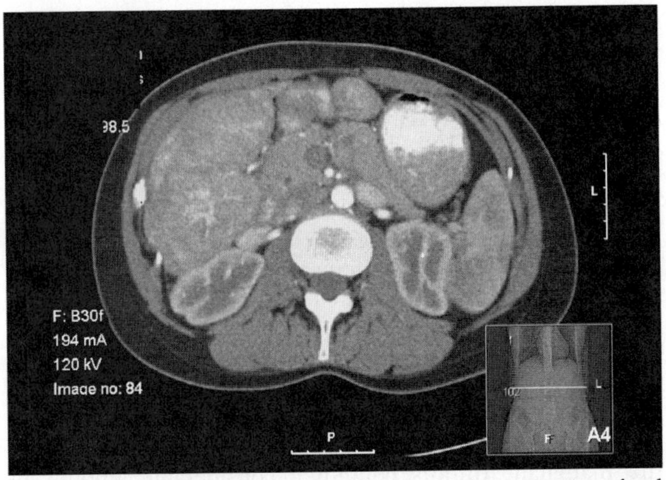

FIGURE 48.6. Computed tomographic scan demonstrating focal nodular hyperplasia.

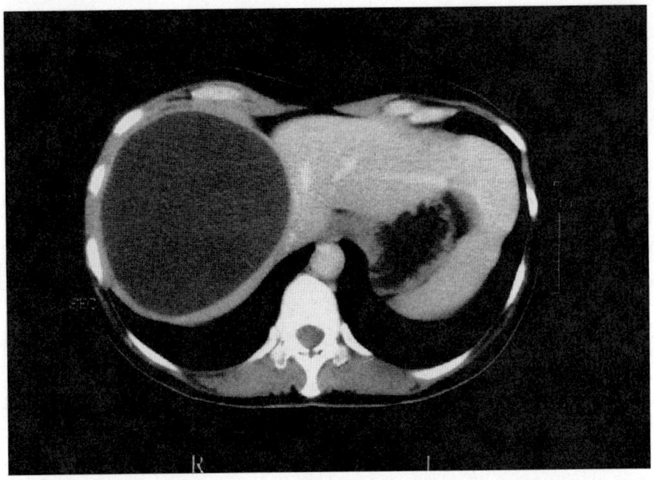

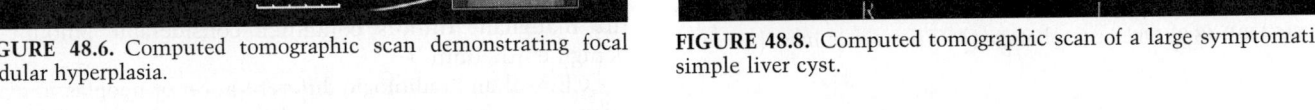

FIGURE 48.8. Computed tomographic scan of a large symptomatic simple liver cyst.

of these tumors (Table 48.1), so that percutaneous needle biopsy is rarely indicated.

Patients who present with a liver mass that on imaging is suspected to be an adenoma should stop use of oral contraceptives or anabolic steroids as regression of these lesions has been reported several months after steroid removal.[15] Adenomas have a risk of rupture or malignant transformation; therefore, all lesions that fail to regress should be resected or locally ablated to prevent life-threatening bleeding or progression to HCC.[16]

Liver Cysts

Liver cysts are frequently identified incidentally on radiographic imaging and at laparotomy (Fig. 48.8). The most common liver cyst encountered in Western society is the congenital or developmental cyst, which usually is solitary but may be associated with polycystic disease, which more often affects the kidneys alone but can affect both the kidneys and liver. Tumors of the liver are sometimes cystic as a result of degeneration, or they may have a primarily cystic component, as in cystadenoma or cystadenocarcinoma. Echinococcal disease is common in certain parts of the world and is the most common cystic lesion to require surgical treatment.

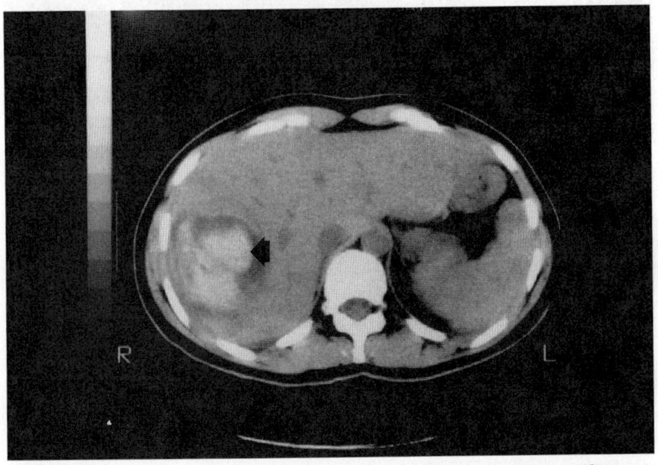

FIGURE 48.7. Computed tomographic scan demonstrating a hepatic adenoma with associated hemorrhage.

Congenital/Developmental Cysts

Solitary Cysts

Simple hepatic cysts are common incidental findings, seen in approximately 5% of hepatic radiographic studies, most commonly in the right lobe and most commonly in women.[17,18] Simple cysts are congenital and are felt to arise from abnormal embryologic bile duct differentiation and organization as the cysts are lined by cuboidal epithelium.[19] Congenital cysts are often diagnosed by ultrasound as having a thin wall and central fluid collection. These simple cysts are asymptomatic and require no treatment.

Polycystic Liver

Childhood polycystic disease is inherited in an autosomal recessive pattern and usually affects both the liver and the kidneys.[20] Hepatic cysts in childhood polycystic disease are usually asymptomatic, and the renal manifestations are of greater significance. Liver function is usually preserved throughout life, although fibrosis and portal hypertension can occur.[21,22]

Adult polycystic liver disease is inherited in an autosomal dominant pattern, with mutations in genes predisposing to renal and liver cysts (PKD1, PKD2, PRKCSH).[23,24] The liver is macroscopically diffusely cystic, although different patterns of disease, including unilobar cysts, are typical (Fig. 48.9). There is an increase in cyst development with progressing age, with hepatic cysts evident in 20% of affected individuals in their third decade of life, as opposed to 75% by the seventh decade of life.[25] Cysts may also be found in the kidney, spleen, pancreas, ovaries, and lungs. While polycystic liver disease may present independent of polycystic kidney disease, the incidence of association by autopsy series has been 50%–60%.[26]

The clinical presentation and complications of both adult polycystic liver disease and sporadic congenital cysts are similar.[27] Fewer than 15% of patients are symptomatic, and

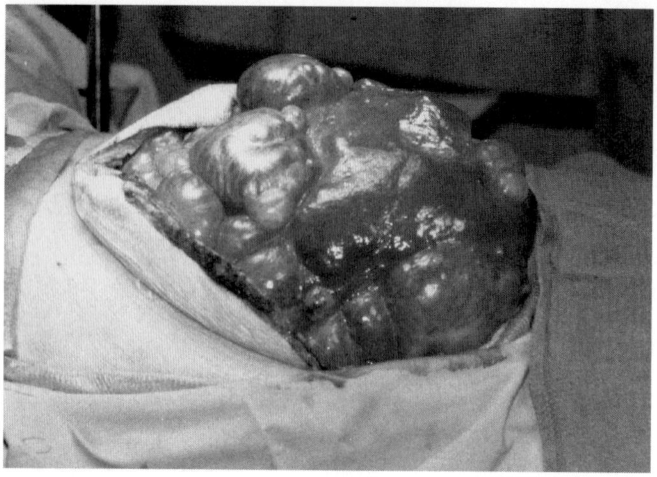

FIGURE 48.9. Operative photograph of polycystic liver disease.

most series suggest a preponderance of women presenting with symptomatic cysts. Symptoms are usually related to a mass effect, with abdominal fullness and mild pain, although portal hypertension and jaundice may result from mass effect in all forms of cystic liver disease. Perforation, infection, and hemorrhage occur rarely.[24,27]

Careful selection of only symptomatic or complicated cysts is important when deciding whether cystic lesions require treatment because outcomes are almost entirely dependent on successful decompression of large cysts for which pressure symptoms dominate the clinical picture. There is no medical treatment for polycystic liver disease. Simple aspiration of hepatic cysts is only of use for diagnostic purposes and occasionally as a provocative test before more definitive therapy because recurrence rates approach 100%. Percutaneous aspiration followed by injection of 95% ethanol or other sclerosants is now a well-accepted therapeutic modality, although recurrence rates vary widely.[24,27–29] Surgical unroofing and decompression of large hepatic cysts is an excellent and highly effective treatment.[30,31] Laparoscopic approaches, in which the cyst is decompressed and a large portion of the cyst wall is excised, are currently an attractive strategy because of low morbidity and high efficacy. In most cases, a large portion of the cyst is easily accessible laparoscopically, and the visible cyst wall and thinned-out liver are resected, leaving a shallow, epithelium-lined cavity.[32,33]

Traumatic Cysts

Hemorrhage into the liver parenchyma may occur with blunt or penetrating abdominal trauma. Bleeding is contained within the liver if the capsule is intact, and traumatic cysts containing blood, bile, and necrotic liver tissue may develop. Lack of a true epithelial lining denotes that traumatic cysts are in fact pseudocysts. Unless a traumatic cyst becomes infected secondarily, it is best treated expectantly. Arterial infarction of the liver or of biliary stricture secondary to bile duct transaction or periductal inflammation may result in ischemic necrosis or segmental atrophy and the development of hemorrhagic or bilious cysts.[34,35]

Cystadenoma and Adenocarcinoma

True neoplastic cysts of the liver are rare compared with congenital cysts. Cystadenomas account for fewer than 5% of hepatic cystic neoplasms and occur most commonly in women of middle age.[36] Grossly, the tumors are usually large, in the right lobe, and multilocular; they will have contrast enhancement of the septa on CT imaging, and they contain a clear, mucinous fluid[37] (Fig. 48.10). Bloody fluid occurs more often in malignant cysts. Microscopically, the diagnostic features include a multiloculated lesion lined by benign or malignant mucin-producing cells often showing polypoid papillary projections into the cyst. The surrounding stroma is typically dense. The tumors are thought to be congenital in origin and slow growing. It is believed that cystadenocarcinomas are derived from benign cystadenomas because most of the malignant tumors contain a considerable amount of benign epithelium.[38]

Clinical and radiologic differentiation of neoplastic cysts from congenital cysts may be difficult (Table 48.1). Features suggestive of neoplastic cysts on ultrasound and CT include papillary projections or irregularities in the cyst wall, complex multilocular cysts, and the presence of cyst contents of different densities in different parts of a multilocular cyst. Any cyst suspected of being a cystadenoma should be explored and completely excised either by the technique of enucleation or by liver resection.[39] Recurrence is rare if excision is complete, while incomplete resection yields a 90%–95% recurrence rate.[40] Cystadenocarcinoma requires liver resection, and if the cyst is nonmetastatic, the prognosis is excellent, with 5-year survivals near 100% and recurrence rates of less than 15%.[41]

Hydatid (Parasitic) Cysts

Hepatic hydatid cysts, the result of infection of the parasite *Echinococcus granulosus,* are common in rural areas where dogs are used for herding livestock and particularly in countries around the Mediterranean Sea and in South America and Australia. The ingested parasite embryo penetrates the wall of the intestine of the intermediate host, enters the portal circulation, and grows into a larva in the liver, forming a cystic structure.[42] Hydatid cysts of the liver are often

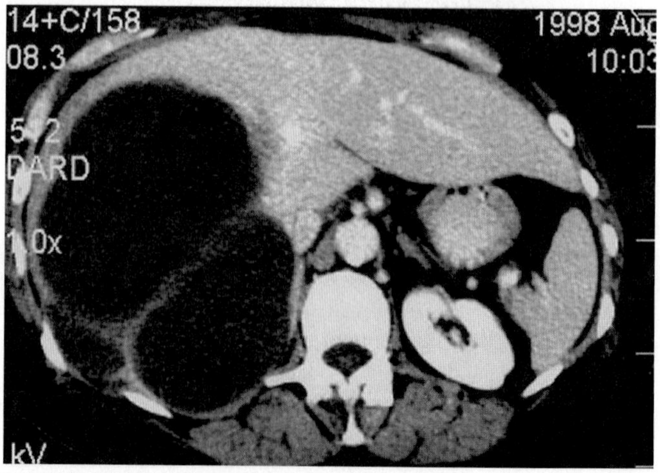

FIGURE 48.10. Computed tomographic scan demonstrating large, complex, thick-walled cystadenoma in right lobe of liver.

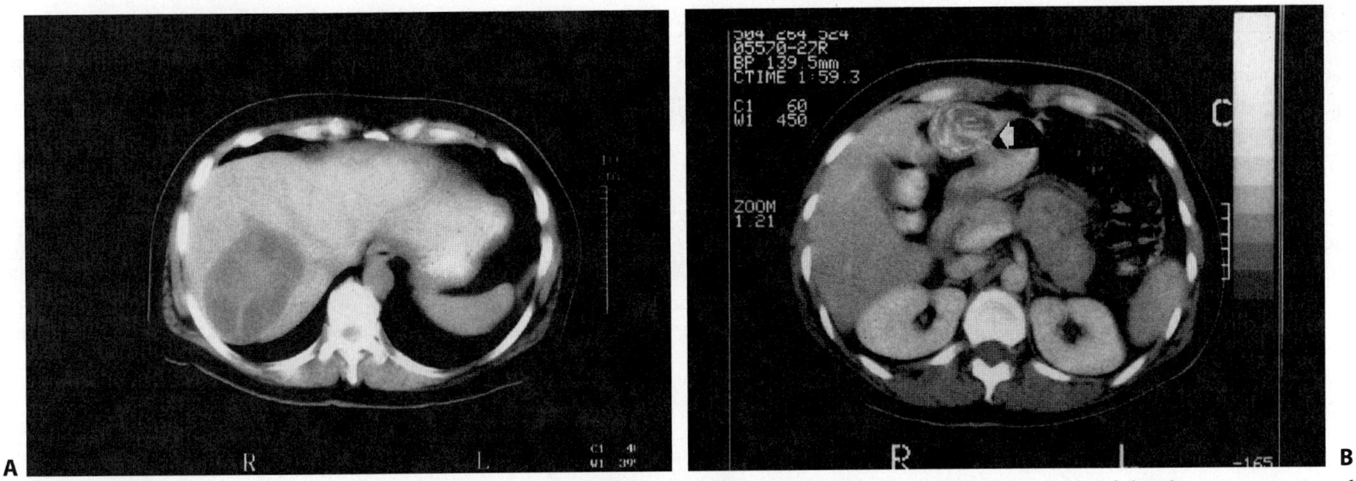

FIGURE 48.11. Hydatid cyst in right lobe (**A**) and in left lateral segment (**B**, *arrow*). Note thick-walled setations of daughter cysts in **A** and whorled calcifications in **B**.

asymptomatic and may remain so until they reach a large size. Cysts are found frequently as an incidental finding (82%) on ultrasound or CT studies (Fig. 48.11) or because of the onset of pain or jaundice. Expansion of cysts in the liver may cause localized pain, and a mild chronic inflammatory reaction around the cyst may cause pain associated with the adjacent parietal peritoneum. A cyst may become secondarily infected and produce pain and fever and behave clinically as a liver abscess or may develop a bile leak and produce jaundice.[43]

Hydatid cysts are diagnosed by radiographic findings (Table 48.1). The inflammation results in a hypervascular rim or halo around the cystic structure on CT scans and angiograms.[44,45] Calcification often occurs in the wall of the mature or dead cysts. In the jaundiced patient with hepatic hydatid disease, endoscopic retrograde cholangiopancreatography (ERCP) should also be performed to determine if the jaundice is the result of extrusion of cyst material into the bile duct or is merely a manifestation of cholangitis from the spill of infected fluid into the biliary tract.

Serological studies are currently the most reliable adjunct to imaging tests in confirming the diagnosis of echinococcosis of the liver, and a recent blinded, randomized trial compared six serum antigens, confirming 80%–82% diagnostic accuracy using three serum antigens (HCF, AgB, AgB8/1).[46] Although positive serological tests are helpful in diagnosis, their absence does not exclude the presence of echinococcosis. Percutaneous fine-needle aspiration may be necessary as a diagnostic test in the workup of the occasional complex liver cyst for which serology and imaging are nondiagnostic of hydatid disease.[47,48]

The treatment of hepatic hydatid disease requires control of the cyst and eradication of the parasite without host exposure to the severely antigenic cyst fluid. Systemic antihelminthic agents are generally not effective against human *Echinococcus*. Three randomized controlled trials comparing albendazole, mebendazole, and placebo all showed albendazole to be most effective, but complete eradication of cysts with drug therapy alone was rare.[49–51] Systemic drug therapy for cystic hydatid disease is considered an adjuvant to surgery in patients in whom accidental spillage of cyst fluid has occurred at operation, in patients with active disease who are unfit for surgery, and in patients who rupture hydatid cysts spontaneously into the peritoneal or pleural cavities.[52,53] The addition of the PAIR (percutaneous aspiration, injection with hypertonic saline, and reaspiration) technique in conjunction with systemic albendazole therapy has improved nonsurgical management of hydatid cysts with lower morbidity and mortality.[54,55] But, surgery remains the standard treatment approach, using aggressive resection versus fenestration approaches with an open or a laparoscopic approach.[56,57]

Malignant Lesions

Hepatocellular Carcinoma

Hepatocellular carcinoma (HCC) is the fifth most common cancer in the world, with more than 500,000 estimated annual cases each year.[58,59] With the disease on the rise in the United States, approximately 18,000 new cases are expected to occur in the United States in 2005.[60] The mean age at diagnosis is between 50 and 60 years.[60,61] Ninety-percent of HCC cases are associated with chronic liver disease, including principally due hepatitis B, hepatitis C, or alcoholic cirrhosis, which accounts for the high incidence in Southeast Asia and Africa, as well as the male-to-female ratio of 7:1 in these high-risk countries.[60,62–64] Expected survival times for HCC patients without treatment are 8 months for stage I, 2 months for stage II, and less than 1 month for stage III disease.[62]

Diagnosis

Most patients present with symptoms of tumor mass effect or progressive loss of hepatic function. Serum concentrations of α-fetoprotein (AFP) are elevated (>400 ng/mL) in 75% of patients with HCC, particularly those who are hepatitis B antibody positive.[65,66] Radiographic imaging, specifically gadolinium-enhanced MRI, may confirm the diagnosis of HCC in the setting of an elevated AFP. Imaging findings of HCC are summarized in Table 48.2 (Figs. 48.12 and 48.13). Histologic confirmation of HCC is not required in most cases if imaging and AFP levels are clinically conclusive, although percutaneous biopsy is feasible using CT or ultrasound guidance. Biopsy is rarely indicated in the diagnosis of HCC as it poses significant risks of hemorrhage in a cirrhotic patient as

TABLE 48.2. Radiographic Imaging Characteristics of Malignant Liver Lesions.

Lesion	*Ultrasound (accuracy %)*	*Nuclear medicine (accuracy %)*	*Computed tomography (accuracy %)*	*Magnetic resonance imaging (accuracy %)*
Hepatocellular carcinoma	Hypo, hyper, or isoechoic (Ding et al. 2001)[193]	PET imaging is poorly studied	Enhancement in arterial phase (Ding et al. 2001)[193]	Hyperintense on T2 images, enhanced with gadolinium (Ding et al. 2001)[193]
Colorectal liver metastases	Hypoechoic	Intense signal on PET imaging	Low signal in the venous phase (Fulcher and Sterling 2002)[178]	Hyperintense on T2 and with gadolinium (Fulcher and Sterling 2002)[178]
Other metastases	Hypoechoic	Usually increased PET signal	Enhancement in the arterial (hypervascular) or venous phase (hypovascular) (Fulcher and Sterling 2002)[178]	Hyperintense on T2 and with gadolinium (Fulcher and Sterling 2002)[178]

well as the risk of needle tract tumor implantation.[67] The 2004 National Comprehensive Cancer Network (NCCN) treatment guidelines recommend biopsy for a tumor associated with an AFP below 400 ng/mL or AFP less than 4000 ng/mL with a positive hepatitis B surface antigen.

The high incidence of HCC in countries in which chronic hepatitis B and C infection is endemic has led to HCC screening programs for these populations. Screening includes liver ultrasonography and evaluation of serum alkaline phosphatase, albumin, and AFP levels every 3–6 months.[68–71] These case series have shown that the annual incidence of HCC in these groups varies between 0.8% and 5.8% per year. Resectability rates of tumors found by screening vary from 7% to 66%.[72,73]

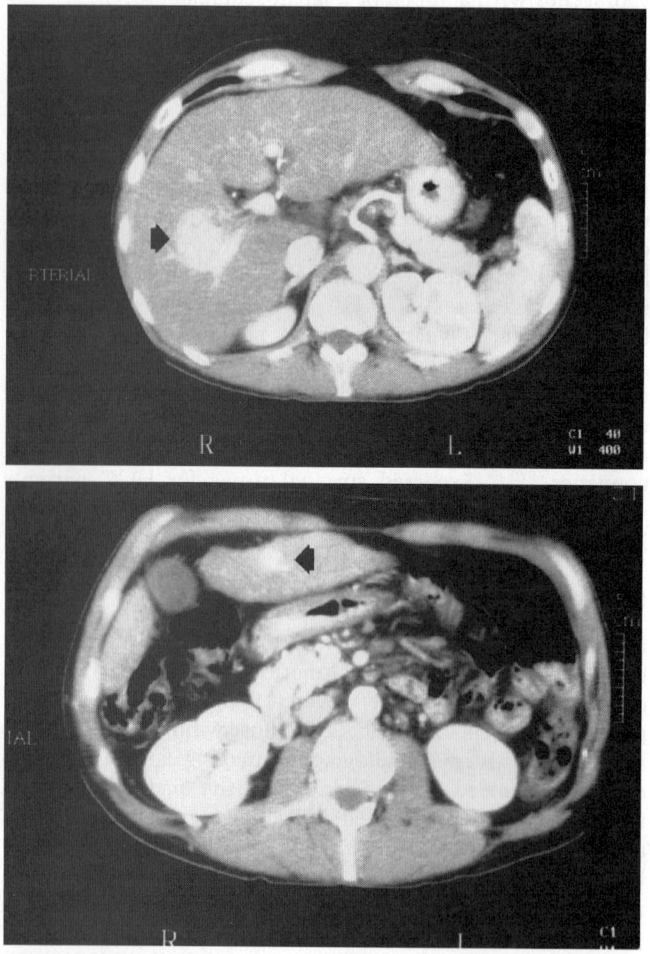

FIGURE 48.12. Computed tomographic scan demonstrating hypervascular hepatocellular carcinoma.

Staging

More than seven differing staging systems have been described for HCC.[74,75] The most well-described and most commonly used systems are the International Union Against Cancer (UICC)/American Joint Committee on Cancer (AJCC) standardized TNM approach, the CLIP (Cancer of Liver Italian Program) score, and the BCLC (Barcelona Clinic Liver Cancer) stage.[74,75] Table 48.3 compares these most commonly applied staging systems.

Treatment

Resection

Surgery, to include liver resection or transplantation, remains the only curative treatment for HCC.[76] Unfortunately, fewer

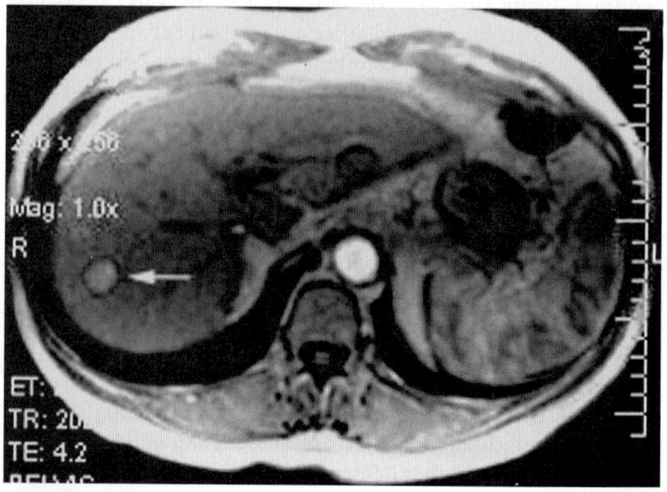

FIGURE 48.13. Magnetic resonance imaging scan demonstrating hepatocellular carcinoma.

TABLE 48.3. Staging Systems for Hepatocellular Carcinoma.

Staging system	*Staging criteria*				*Advantages of staging system*
TNM, 2002 #1 (Wildi et al. 2004; Marrero et al. 2005)[74,75]	T1 solitary lesion: No vascular invasion T2 solitary with vascular invasion or multiple <5 cm T3 multiple >5 cm or invades portal or hepatic veins T4 invasion of adjacent organs	N0 no nodal involvement N1 nodal metastases	M0 no distant metastases M1 distant metastases	Stage I T1 N0 M0 Stage II T2 N0 M0 Stage IIIA T3 N0 M0 Stage IIIB T4 N0 M0 Stage IIIC T any N1 M0 Stage IV T any N any M1	Does not include assessment of liver function Requires pathologic assessment for treatment planning
CLIP (Wildi et al. 2004; Marrero et al. 2005)[74,75]	Child-Pugh score A 0 B 1 C 2	Tumor morphology Uninodular 0 Multinodular 1 Extensive (>50%) 2	α-feto-protein (ng/dL) <400 0 ≥400 1	Portal vein thrombosis No 0 Yes 1	Most accurately predicts prognosis and survival
BCLC (Wildi et al. 2004; Marrero et al. 2005)[74,75]	Stage A Single tumor or <3 tumors all ≤ 3 cm Child-Pugh A-B	Stage B Multinodular Child-Pugh A-B	Stage C Vascular invasion Child-Pugh A-B	Stage D Child-Pugh C	Stratifies patients into treatment groups

than 30% of patients are resectable at the time of diagnosis.[62] The primary treatment of an isolated early lesion (resection vs. transplantation) remains controversial as negative surgical margin and poor baseline hepatic function are significant prognostic factors in multivariate analysis, favoring hepatic transplantation, but the limited number of available transplant organs leading to delayed time on the transplant list favors primary surgical resection.[62,77,78] The most recent case series reviewed at Memorial Sloan-Kettering Cancer Center indicates that hepatic resection in these early-stage (transplant-eligible) patients has equivalent outcomes to hepatic transplantation.[78] Five-year survival rates following surgical resection or transplantation range from 20% to 61%.[79,80] Unfortunately, nearly 80% of patients with HCC present with advanced, unresectable disease.

Factors that determine resectability of a primary HCC include general health of the patient, tumor stage, and functional capacity of the underlying liver. The AJCC stage IIIB or IV disease is considered to be incurable by resection. Other factors that are predictors of poor surgical cure rates include multiple tumors, large tumor size, vascular invasion, and decreased hepatic function that includes an elevated bilirubin and coagulopathy.[80,81] Primary hepatic resection for HCC has been shown to result in 5-year survivals of 30%–40%, with operative mortality rates of 10%.[80,82,83]

One of the most difficult aspects of assessment of resectability is determining functional reserve of the liver, that is, the ability of the cirrhotic patient not only to tolerate general anesthesia and an operative procedure but also to maintain adequate hepatic function after parenchymal and tumor resection. It is well known that this surgical risk is higher in cirrhotic than noncirrhotic patients.[84] While exact quantitative predictors of hepatic reserve are not available, techniques used include the Child-Turcotte-Pugh classification (Table 48.4), model for end-sage liver disease (MELD) criteria (MELD score = $0.957 \times \log \text{Cr} + 0.378 \times \log \text{Bilirubin} + 1.12 \times \log \text{INR} + 0.643$),[85] or imaging assessments of preoperative functional liver parenchyma including indocyanine green (ICG) clearance or the redox tolerance test.[86–88] More recently, an estimate of remaining functional liver volume relative to the planned hepatic resection is estimated by three-dimensional CT or MRI.[89–91]

The risk to patients with compromised liver function increases with the magnitude of resection planned; therefore, preoperative portal vein embolization of the lobe to be resected has been used to stimulate hepatic hypertrophy of the intended remaining lobe prior to surgery. Increases in liver volume from 44% to 90% have been reported.[91,92] The ideal margin for curative resection in HCC has not yet been defined. Many surgeons attempt to obtain a disease-free margin of 1 cm, yet multiple series have shown that simply a microscopically negative margin is adequate.[93–96]

The Milan criteria provide guidelines for liver transplantation for HCC. The use of the Milan criteria to select patients for transplantation has resulted in improved 5-year survival rates from 25% to nearly 61%.[79,95] The Milan criteria define a patient most likely to have a long-term survival following

TABLE 48.4. Child-Turcotte-Pugh Classification.

Measure	*Score 1 point*	*2 points*	*3 points*
Albumin (mg/L)	>35	28–35	<28
Ascites	None	Medically controlled	Refractory
Bilirubin (mg/dL)	<2	2–3	>3
Encephalopathy	None	Mild or medically controlled	Severe or refractory
INR	<1.7	1.7–2.2	>2.2

Class A = 5–6 points; class B = 7–9 points; class C = 10–15 points.

TABLE 48.5.
Review of Regional Therapies for Hepatic Neoplasms.

Author/Year	*Treatment*	*Study*	*Follow-up*	*No. of patients*	*Outcomes*
Machi et al.[190]/2005	RFA	HCC Case series	24 mo Mean	65	Disease-free survival 16 mo Overall survival mean 33 mo
Curley et al.[72]/2000	RFA	HCC Case series	19 mo median	110	Hepatic recurrence 45%
Livrhagi et al.[189]/2003	RFA	Colorectal metastases Case series	33 mo median	88	64% disease progression
Joosten et al.[183]/2005	RFA or CSA	Colorectal metastases Case series	25 mo median	58	2-year survival: RFA 75% CSA 61%
Lencioni et al.[187]/2003	RFA versus PEI	HCC Randomized trial	23 mo mean	102	2-year survival: RFA 96% PEI 88% 2-year recurrence-free survival: **RFA** 96% **PEI** 62%
Hori et al.[180]/2003	PEI	HCC Retrospective review		104	2-year local recurrence rate 15%
Koda et al.[185]/2001	TACE & PEI versus PEI	HCC Randomized trial	30 mo mean	53	3-year tumor recurrence: TACE-PEI 19% PEI 80%
Huang et al.[86]/1999	TACE versus observation	HCC Retrospective review		108	5-year survival: TACE 34% Observation 7%

CSA, cryosurgical ablation; HCC, hepatocellular carcinoma; PEI, percutaneous ethanol injection; RFA, radiofrequency ablation; TACE, transcatheter arterial chemoembolization.

liver transplantation. These criteria include a single lesion smaller than 5 cm, three or fewer lesions less than or equal to 3 cm in greatest dimension, and no evidence of vascular invasion.[97]

REGIONAL THERAPIES

Multiple regional, tumor-directed therapies have been developed in the treatment of HCC as many patients are poor surgical candidates based on primary liver function. These regional therapies include directed chemotherapy or chemoembolization therapy and ablative therapies.

Transcatheter arterial chemoembolization (TACE) is a regional therapy utilized based on vascular flow physiology; specifically, the hepatic artery provides 80% of the vascular supply to an HCC while it provides only 20% to the normal hepatic parenchyma. Using a catheter-directed arterial infusion of chemotherapy, usually therapy based on cisplatin and lipiodol (ethiodized oil, which helps to trap the chemotherapy in the treatment target region and facilitates vascular embolization). Following directed chemotherapy infusion, the arterial vascular supply to the lesion is embolized. Several case control series comparing TACE to supportive care have been published and showed little long-term survival benefit with TACE therapy. Yet, evidence of 1-year survival benefits are noted, showing only 32% of supportive care patients versus 57% of TACE patients achieving posttreatment 1-year survival.[98–101]

Other regional therapies include ablation techniques using cryotherapy, ethanol ablation, laser ablation, or radiofrequency ablation in an open surgical, laparoscopic, or percutaneous image-guided technique (Table 48.5) (Fig. 48.14). The experience with ablative therapies is limited to date, but several case series included patients with HCC and showed tumor responses up to 90% but had limited survival benefit.[102–104]

There is no evidence of a survival or palliative benefit to other treatment regimens, including systemic chemotherapy and radiation therapy.

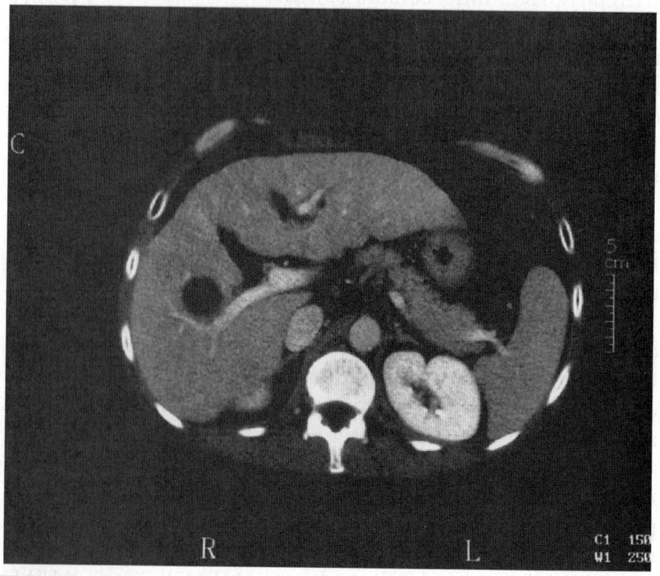

FIGURE 48.14. Computed tomographic scan following percutaneous ethanol ablation of hepatocellular carcinoma.

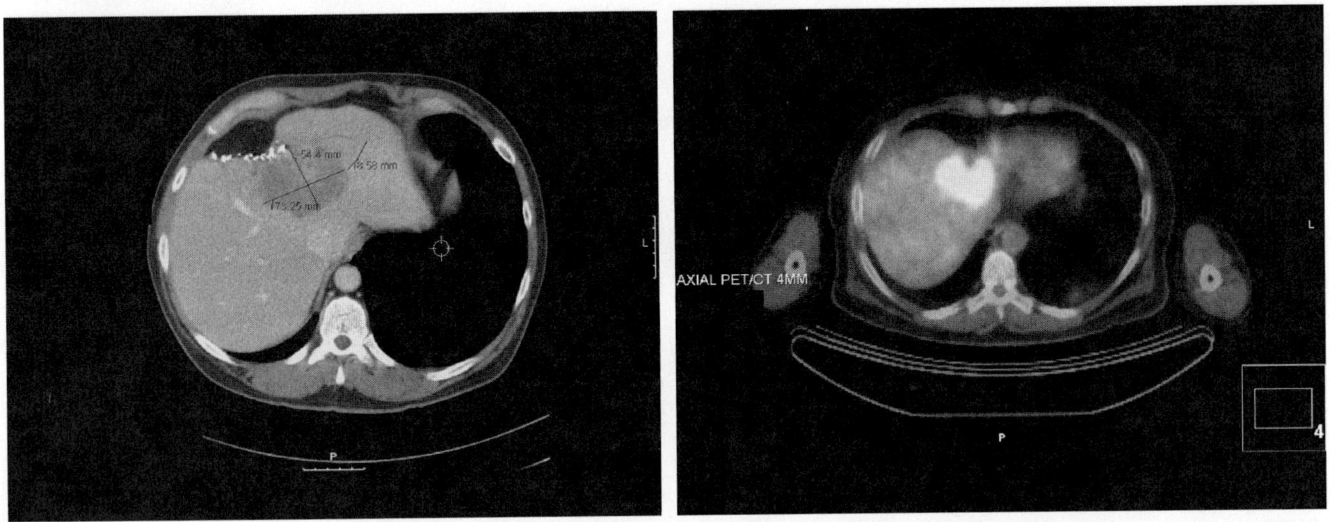

FIGURE 48.15. Colorectal cancer hepatic metastases (A) computed tomographic scan and (B) PET-CT imaging of colorectal hepatic metastases.

Colorectal Liver Metastases

Colorectal cancer is one of the most common cancers affecting men and women of the United States and the third most common cause of cancer deaths in the United States (Fig. 48.15). Approximately 50% of all patients diagnosed with colorectal cancer will develop liver metastases, with 15%–20% presenting with synchronous liver metastases.[105,106] Unfortunately, nearly 80% of those patients who develop liver metastases are not considered surgically resectable at the time of diagnosis.[82,107]

Diagnosis

Evaluation for colorectal liver metastases is most commonly performed with CT imaging, although more widespread use of positron emission tomographic (PET) imaging has led to frequent PET identification of colorectal hepatic metastases as well (Fig. 48.15; Table 48.2).[108] The NCCN staging guidelines for colorectal cancers includes an abdominal CT scan to evaluate for liver metastases. The NCCN guidelines for follow-up screening after treatment for primary colorectal cancer are less aggressive regarding liver imaging, but many practitioners follow a scheduled regimen of liver CT imaging given the more aggressive surgical approaches to liver metastases in the recent past.

Treatment

The primary treatment for colorectal liver metastases is surgical resection, but the recent application of combined modality therapy has improved 5-year survival following treatment for colorectal metastases. Improved outcomes with modern chemotherapy regimens have resulted in improved survival of patients with colorectal metastases and improved resection rates.[109]

Resection

Surgery for colorectal hepatic metastases requires complete margin-negative (R0) resection for improved survival benefit. Lobar or segmental anatomic resections have been shown to have improved margin-negative rates as well as improved survival and recurrence outcomes over nonanatomic wedge resections.[110] Most recent series confirmed that the factors most predictive of patient outcomes include negative margins and low operative morbidity.[110–112] Early resection case series showed a significant decrease in survival of patients with four or more lesions in the liver and therefore considered more than three lesions a contraindication to resection.[113,114] But, more recent series have confirmed the long-term survival of patients with four or more lesions if a margin-negative resection can be performed with low operative morbidity.[115]

A consensus statement established new guidelines for hepatic resection of colorectal metastases; it states that a patient is considered unresectable if the patient has extrahepatic disease, tumor involving more than 70% or six segments of the hepatic parenchyma, or is a poor surgical candidate.[116] Recent evidence also suggests that while complete resection of hepatic disease leads to improved survival, an anatomic resection with a minimum of a 1-cm margin further improves survival and recurrence rates.[110,117] While a very aggressive surgical approach has become the standard of care for isolated colorectal liver metastases, many surgeons recognize that liver metastases indicate a systemic disease and more often rely on a response to systemic chemotherapy prior to consideration of hepatic resection.

Local Therapy: Hepatic Artery Infusion, Radiofrequency Ablation, Chemoembolization, Perfusion

Local chemotherapy and ablative therapies are considered in the patient with surgically unresectable or multilobar disease as an adjunct to resection. While many local techniques have been applied, the literature is controversial, the experience remains premature, and no randomized trials compared the techniques. These local therapies include hepatic artery infusion chemotherapy, radiofrequency ablation therapy, chemoembolization, and hepatic chemotherapy perfusion techniques (Fig. 48.16). Table 48.5 summarizes the largest series of these local treatment techniques. Controversy regarding the efficacy of each of these techniques remains, and none should be

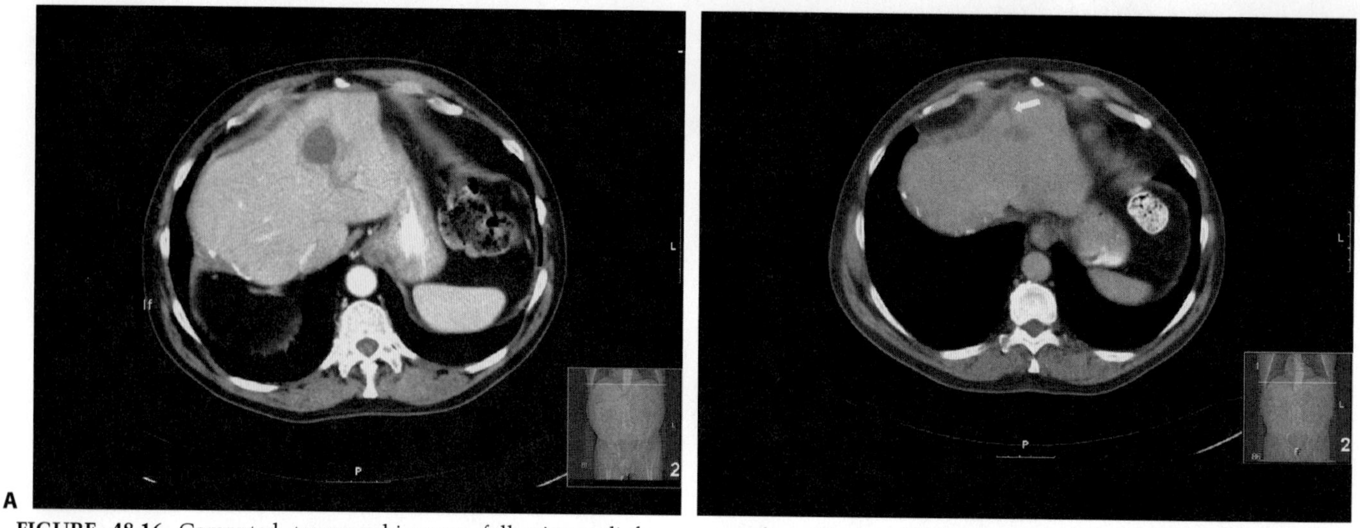

FIGURE 48.16. Computed tomographic scan following radiofrequency ablation of colorectal hepatic metastases: (A) CT scan 1 month following radiofrequency ablation with hyperemic ring surrounding ablation. (B) At 3 months postablation, with ablation of needle tract from steaming emission evident (*arrow*).

considered superior to surgical resection if resection is a feasible option for the treatment of a patient's disease.[118]

CHEMOTHERAPY

The incorporation of new chemotherapy agents, including oxaliplatin, irenotecan, bevacizumab, and capcitebene, in the treatment of colorectal metastases has significantly improved patient outcomes, with modern tumor partial response rates improving from 20% to near 60% using FOLFOX (5-fluorouracil [5FU], leucovorin, and oxaliplatin) and FOLFIRI (5FU, leucovorin, irinotecan) regimens.[119,120] Many institutions are promoting the use of a neoadjuvant chemotherapy approach to those with newly diagnosed colorectal hepatic metastases with evidence of improved rates of resectability in patients with evidence of tumor response to chemotherapy. Specifically, 13%–16% of patients judged to be unresectable prior to chemotherapy are rendered resectable following neoadjuvant therapy with no increase in perioperative morbidity rates.[109,121,122] While these modern chemotherapy regimens, in addition to newer trials including anti-VEGF (vascular endothelial growth factor) antibody therapy (bevacizumab), have shown significant promise, the optimal regimen remains to be defined.

RADIATION

Isolated radiation therapy is not effective for treatment of colorectal cancer hepatic metastases but may be used for symptom palliation. A phase I trial using stereotactic body radiation therapy found a maximum tolerated dose of 60 Gy without reaching maximum toxicity in 18 patients.[123] An ongoing phase II trial will further define the efficacy of stereotactic radiation for hepatic palliation.

Other Metastases

The treatment of noncolorectal, nonneuroendocrine metastases has been shown to have limited benefit in several series until recently. A review of noncolorectal, nonneuroendocrine metastases from Memorial Sloan-Kettering found a survival benefit of aggressive treatment of hepatic metastases of genitourinary primary malignancies, a negative resection margin, and patients with a disease-free interval of greater than 2 years.[124] Sixty-three percent of patients with reproductive tumors who underwent a margin-negative resection had 3-year disease-free survival.[124] There are an additional several case series that advocate aggressive resection of neuroendocrine metastases to the liver, concluding that overall symptom-free survival is improved if the primary disease is controlled, hepatic disease is less than 50% of the parenchyma, and low-morbidity resection is feasible. Cure rates remain low.[125–127] Treatment techniques for all noncolorectal metastases include resection, embolization, and ablative techniques.

Intrahepatic Cholangiocarcinoma

Intrahepatic cholangiocarcinoma is an unusual and rare form of cholangiocarcinoma and primary liver cancer. The most common form of cholangiocarcinoma is the perihilar (Klatskin tumor) lesion (see Biliary System Chapter 47), with intrahepatic cholangiocarcinoma representing fewer than 6% of cholangiocarcinomas.[128] Intrahepatic cholangiocarcinoma accounts for fewer than 4% of primary liver cancers, the remainder of which are HCC.[129]

Intrahepatic cholangiocarcinoma usually presents between the ages of 50 to 70 with painless jaundice and is most often diagnosed with CT, MRI, and cholangiogram imaging.[130–134] Intrahepatic cholangiocarcinomas are treated and staged as a HCC, and aggressive surgical resection remains the treatment of choice, with a negative margin and negative lymph nodes the greatest prognostic predictors.[135] There is little evidence of effective chemo- or radiation therapies for intrahepatic cholangiocarcinoma. Ablative and embolic therapies have been utilized for nonresection candidates, but little evidence of efficacy exists. The prognosis of intrahepatic cholangiocarcinomas is poor; aggressive resection yields a margin-negative resection in only 30% to 60% of patients, with a median postresection survival of 46 months and 3-year survival ranging from 40% to 55%.[111,136,137]

Portal Hypertension

Portal hypertension is an elevated venous pressure in the portal venous system and is defined as an increase in portal pressure greater than 5–10 mmHg (normal portal venous pressure ranges from 13 to 24 mmHg) or a pressure gradient of 12 mmHg or greater between the portal vein and the hepatic veins. Portal hypertension is often categorized as prehepatic, intrahepatic, or posthepatic regarding the etiology of the increased venous pressure. Prehepatic causes include portal vein thrombosis, portal vein compression, or increased flow states resulting from massive splenomegaly, arteriovenous malformations, or fistula. The most common intrahepatic cause of portal hypertension is cirrhosis. The posthepatic causes include right heart failure and Budd-Chiari syndrome. The most common cause of portal hypertension in North America is alcohol-related cirrhosis.

The clinically significant complications related to portal hypertension include venous varicosities that may lead to gastrointestinal bleeding, morbid ascites, and encephalopathy. Of these consequences, variceal bleeding is the most common indication for surgical consultation for venous decompression procedures.

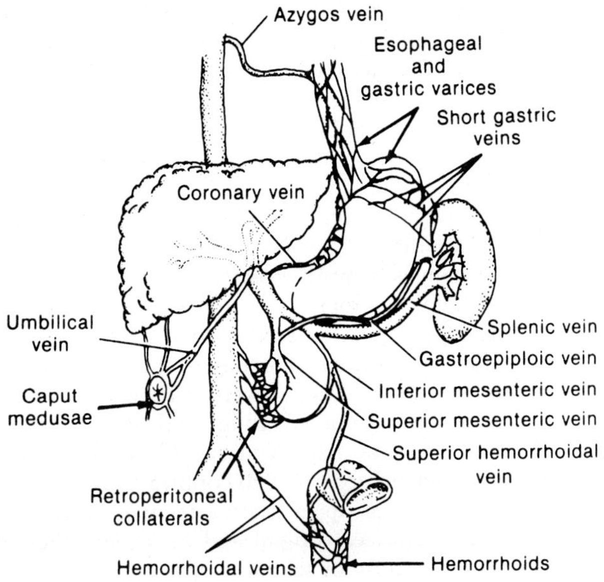

FIGURE 48.17. Diagrammatic representation of portal venous collateral circulation via the system venous pathway. (From Sabiston,[195] with permission.)

Anatomy

The portal vein is formed by the confluence of the splenic vein, the inferior mesenteric vein, and the superior mesenteric vein, which forms posterior to the neck of the pancreas and enters the porta hepatis lateral to the duodenum. The anatomy of this venous confluence is highly variable, with the inferior mesenteric vein entering the splenic vein, the superior mesenteric vein, or a triple confluence. In addition, the left gastric vein (coronary vein) also enters the portal vein, usually beyond the splenic vein insertion. The remnant umbilical vein often enters the left portal vein, within the hepatic parenchyma. These venous collaterals lead to the common venous varicosities in the face of portal hypertension, including gastric varices; esophageal varices; caput medusa, which is a result of canalization of the umbilical vein under increased portal pressure; and hemorrhoids. The collateral venous pathways are demonstrated in Figure 48.17.

Natural History

Nearly 50%–100% of patients with portal hypertension develop varices.[138] The risk of a severe gastrointestinal bleed in patients with varicosities from portal hypertension is related to the size of the varicosities. Of patients with large varicosities, 35% to 50% develop a clinically significant bleed, while 17% of those with small varices will bleed.[138,139] Death caused by uncontrolled bleeding occurs in 6%–8% of patients.[140] In case series of patients with viral hepatic cirrhosis, 20%–50% of patients develop severe ascites, 5%–30% develop a clinically significant gastrointestinal bleed, and 2%–5% develop hepatic encephalopathy.[141,142]

Treatment

The treatment of varicosities involves the prevention of initial bleeding, management of an acute variceal bleed, or prevention of bleeding recurrence. The first variceal bleeding episode is associated with a mortality rate of up to 50%, which has led to the use of prophylactic intervention for patients with known varicies.[143] Prophylactic measures are initiated in patients with medium-to-large varices. Primary prophylaxis includes endoscopic band ligation or pharmacologic therapy to reduce portal pressures by reducing cardiac output, heart rate, and portal resistance, including beta-blockade (noncardioselective agents such as propranolol or nadolol are used to achieve additional beta-2 blockade of splanchnic receptors) and octreotide therapy[140] Several randomized trials comparing band ligation to beta-blockade therapy have shown that band-ligation therapy is more effective than beta-blockade alone to prevent an initial bleed.[144–146] Yet, some trials continued to show no difference in bleeding prophylaxis between variceal banding and beta-blockade therapy.[147,148] Sclerotherapy has also been analyzed for use as prophylaxis for first variceal hemorrhage; this meta-analysis concluded that there may be a beneficial effect of sclerotherapy in the prevention of first bleeding in patients at high risk.[149] Even so, randomized trials comparing band ligation to sclerotherapy concluded that band ligation is a more effective prophylaxis for bleeding with lower morbidity.[150,151]

The prevention of recurrent bleeding is critical in the care of patients with varicosities as the incidence of recurrent bleeding is 60% in the year following the primary bleeding event, and the survival rate is 20%–30%.[152,153] The primary preventive therapy following a primary bleed is endoscopic band ligation.[154,155] Some randomized trials have shown beta-blockade (nadolol) and isosorbide therapy may be more effective for second bleed prevention than endoscopic variceal ligation and sclerotherapy,[156,157] while the combination of beta-blockade therapy with band ligation may further decrease the risk of primary bleed.[158]

Another series of randomized controlled trials suggested that transjugular-intrahepatic portosystemic shunting (TIPS) may further prevent the incidence of rebleeding when compared to endoscopic variceal band ligation, with rebleed rates reduced from 52%–60% with banding to 18%–21% with TIPS.[159–161] Yet, a meta-analysis of several prospective randomized controlled trials comparing TIPS endoscopic band ligation and sclerotherapy failed to show a survival advantage of TIPS despite the reduction in the rate of recurrent bleeding.[162] The TIPS procedure uses a minimally invasive, radiographically placed, percutaneous, transvascular, intrahepatic stent that creates a communication between the hepatic and portal veins (Fig. 48.18).

The initial management of a patient with an acute variceal bleed includes appropriate patient resuscitation and control of the bleeding. Intravascular volume resuscitation should be performed using blood products rather than crystalloid solutions as patients with cirrhosis risk the development of progressive ascites, edema, and fluid overload, resulting in increased portal pressure. Early endoscopic management is critical in acute bleeding episodes to confirm the etiology of the bleed (up to 60% of upper gastrointestinal bleeding in cirrhotics is of nonvariceal origin) and to initiate therapy, including variceal ligation or sclerotherapy.

Pharmacologic therapy should also be considered. Historically, vasopressin was utilized for vasoconstriction and portal decompression, but the associated decrease in cardiac output and myocardial blood flow leads to complicating myocardial infarctions, cardiac arrhythmias, and cerebrovascular accidents. Therefore, octreotide, which has equivalent efficacy to vasopressin in reducing portal pressures and aborting acute bleeding, has become the primary pharmacologic therapy.[163,164]

If endoscopic and pharmacologic management is unsuccessful, acute portal decompression should be considered using either TIPS or surgical shunting. As emergency portacaval shunts are associated with a mortality of at least 50%, TIPS is used more commonly in the emergency setting. The use of TIPS in the acute setting results in immediate control of bleeding in 88%–90% of cases, with 30-day mortality rates of 18%–20%.[165–167] Also, TIPS is used in the setting of severe refractory ascites and prevention of bleeding as a bridge to liver transplantation. Stenosis or thrombosis from TIPS has

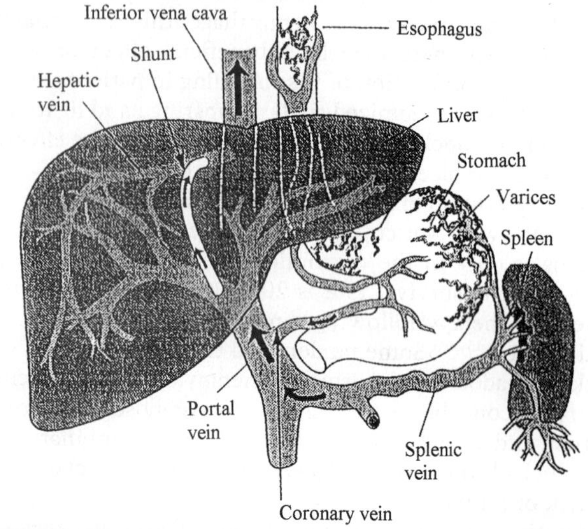

FIGURE 48.18. Diagram of transjugular intrahepatic portosystemic shunt demonstrating the communication between the hepatic portal and venous systems. (From Henderson et al.,[196] with permission of *Current Problems in Surgery.*)

been reported in 30% to 60% of cases, mandating repeat procedures, including stent dilations or the placement of parallel stents.[168,169]

Patients who are not candidates for TIPS in the acute setting or who fail initial management should be considered for surgical options, including portosystemic shunts or variceal devascularization (Sugiura procedure). Orthotopic liver transplantation is the only definitive therapy for patients with variceal bleeding secondary to intrahepatic portal hypertension, but TIPS or shunts may serve as a bridge to transplant. Operative shunts are classified as total or nonselective versus partial or selective depending on the resulting effect on portal flow. Nonselective shunts divert all portal flow into the systemic circulation via the inferior vena cava or one of its major branches, with a higher risk of hepatic encephalopathy. Nonselective shunts include the end-to-side portacaval shunt, in which the portal vein is divided at the bifurcation and anastomosed to the infrahepatic inferior vena cava. Other nonselective shunts are the functional side-to-side portocaval shunt, the proximal splenorenal shunt, and the mesocaval shunt. Selective portosystemic shunts include the Warren shunt (distal splenorenal shunt) and interposition portocaval (H-graft) or mesocaval shunts with limited diameters, between 8 and 10mm. The goal of partial shunts is to lower portal pressure to approximately 12mmHg while maintaining portal venous flow toward the liver with a lesser effect on hepatocellular function, thus reducing hepatic encephalopathy.

A review of six randomized trials comparing selective to nonselective shunts showed that half of these studies confirmed a significant reduction of the severity of hepatic encephalopathy with selective shunts, while three studies showed no long-term difference. There was no difference in rebleeding rates or overall survival between selective and nonselective portocaval shunts.[170] A randomized, controlled trial comparing TIPS to H-graft shunts showed that portal pressure reduction was equivalent, but TIPS was associated with significantly more complications, including thrombosis, hemorrhage, and need for repeat interventions, in addition to a higher mortality rate.[171] Many institutions consider TIPS for patients who are transplant candidates and selective shunts for noncandidates.

Esophageal transection and devascularization is performed for life-threatening refractory esophageal variceal bleeding. The most commonly utilized technique is a modified Sugiura procedure, which consists of splenectomy, proximal gastric devascularization, selective vagotomy, pyloroplasty, esophageal devascularization, and esophageal transection. The goal of devascularization procedures is to reduce inflow to the esophageal varices and therefore eliminate bleeding. Many series have reported successful termination of acute bleeding with moderate perioperative morbidity and mortality.[172–174]

References

1. Couinaud C. [Surgical anatomy of the liver. Several new aspects]. Chirurgie 1986;112:337–342.
2. Prandi D, Dumont M, et al. Influence of portacaval shunt on bile formation in the rat. Eur J Clin Invest 1975;4:197–200.
3. Ishak KG, Rabin L. Benign tumors of the liver. Med Clin North Am 1975;59:995–1013.
4. Mergo PJ, Ros PR. Benign lesions of the liver. Radiol Clin North Am 1998;36:319–331.

5. Trotter JF, Everson GT. Benign focal lesions of the liver. Clin Liver Dis 2001;5:17–42, v.
6. Nichols FC 3rd, van Heerden JA, et al. Benign liver tumors. Surg Clin North Am 1989;69:297–314.
7. Horton KM, Bluemke DA, et al. CT and MR imaging of benign hepatic and biliary tumors. Radiographics 1999;19:431–451.
8. Yoon SS, Charny CK, et al. Diagnosis, management, and outcomes of 115 patients with hepatic hemangioma. J Am Coll Surg 2003;197:392–402.
9. Wanless IR, Mawdsley C, et al. On the pathogenesis of focal nodular hyperplasia of the liver. Hepatology 1985;5:1194–1200.
10. Scalori A, Tavani A, et al. Oral contraceptives and the risk of focal nodular hyperplasia of the liver: a case-control study. Am J Obstet Gynecol 2002;186:195–197.
11. Vauthey JN. Liver imaging. A surgeon's perspective. Radiol Clin North Am 1998;36:445–457.
12. Janes CH, McGill DB, et al. Liver cell adenoma at the age of 3 years and transplantation 19 years later after development of carcinoma: a case report. Hepatology 1993;17:583–585.
13. Grazioli L, Federle MP, et al. Hepatic adenomas: imaging and pathologic findings. Radiographics 2001;21:877–892; discussion 892–894.
14. Biecker E, Fischer HP, et al. Benign hepatic tumours. Z Gastroenterol 2003;41:191–200.
15. Mortele KJ, Ros PR. Benign liver neoplasms. Clin Liver Dis 2002;6:119–145.
16. Tesluk H, Lawrie J. Hepatocellular adenoma. Its transformation to carcinoma in a user of oral contraceptives. Arch Pathol Lab Med 1981;105:296–299.
17. Coutsoftides T, Hermann RE. Nonparasitic cysts of the liver. Surg Gynecol Obstet 1974;138:906–910.
18. Carrim ZI, Murchison JT. The prevalence of simple renal and hepatic cysts detected by spiral computed tomography. Clin Radiol 2003;58:626–629.
19. Longmire WP Jr, WP, Jr, SA, Mandiola SA, et al. Congenital cystic disease of the liver and biliary system. Ann Surg 1971;174:711–726.
20. Dardik H, Glotzer P, et al. Congenital hepatic cyst causing jaundice: report of a case and analogies with respiratory malformations. Ann Surg 1964;159:585–592.
21. Campbell GS, Bick HD, et al. Bleeding esophageal varices with polycystic liver; report of three cases. N Engl J Med 1958;259:904–910.
22. Landing BH, Wells TR, et al. Morphometric analysis of liver lesions in cystic diseases of childhood. Hum Pathol 1980; 11(5 suppl):549–560.
23. Everson GT, Taylor MR. Management of polycystic liver disease. Curr Gastrointerol Rep 2005;7:19–25.
24. Li A, Davila S, et al. Mutations in PRKCSH cause isolated autosomal dominant polycystic liver disease. Am J Hum Genet 2003;72:691–703.
25. Gabow PA, Johnson AM, et al. Risk factors for the development of hepatic cysts in autosomal dominant polycystic kidney disease. Hepatology 1990;11:1033–1037.
26. Melnick PJ. Polycystic liver; analysis of 70 cases. AMA Arch Pathol 1955;59:162–172.
27. Everson GT, Taylor MR, et al. Polycystic disease of the liver. Hepatology 2004;40:774–782.
28. Montorsi M, Torzilli G, et al. Percutaneous alcohol sclerotherapy of simple hepatic cysts. Results from a multicentre survey in Italy. HPB Surg 1994;8:89–94.
29. Larssen TB, Jensen DK, et al. Single-session alcohol sclerotherapy in symptomatic benign hepatic cysts. Long-term results. Acta Radiol 1999;40:636–638.
30. Tocchi A, Mazzoni G, et al. Symptomatic nonparasitic hepatic cysts: options for and results of surgical management. Arch Surg 2002;137:154–158.
31. Yang GS, Li QG, et al. Combined hepatic resection with fenestration for highly symptomatic polycystic liver disease: a report on seven patients. World J Gastroenterol 2004;10:2598–2601.
32. Katkhouda N, Mavor E, et al. Laparoscopic management of benign cystic lesions of the liver. J Hepatobiliary Pancreat Surg 2000;7:212–217.
33. Gigot JF, Glineur D, et al. Laparoscopic liver resection for malignant liver tumors: preliminary results of a multicenter European study. Ann Surg 2002;236:90–97.
34. Chen BK, Gamagami RA, et al. Symptomatic post-traumatic cyst of the liver: treatment by laparoscopic surgery. J Laparoendosc Adv Surg Tech A 2001;11:41–42.
35. Kaushik S, Fulcher AS, et al. Segmental hepatic atrophy: a sequela of blunt intrahepatic bile duct injury. J Trauma 2003; 54:1225–1227.
36. Dixon E, Sutherland FR, et al. Cystadenomas of the liver: a spectrum of disease. Can J Surg 2001;44:371–376.
37. Korobkin M, Stephens DH, et al. Biliary cystadenoma and cystadenocarcinoma: CT and sonographic findings. AJR Am J Roentgenol 1989;153:507–511.
38. Devine P, Ucci AA. Biliary cystadenocarcinoma arising in a congenital cyst. Hum Pathol 1985;16:92–94.
39. Hansman MF, Ryan JA Jr, et al. Management and long-term follow-up of hepatic cysts. Am J Surg 2001;181:404–410.
40. Sanchez H, Gagner M, et al. Surgical management of nonparasitic cystic liver disease. Am J Surg 1991;161:113–118; discussion 118–119.
41. Lauffer JM, Baer HU, et al. Biliary cystadenocarcinoma of the liver: the need for complete resection. Eur J Cancer 1998;34:1845–1851.
42. Moro FL, Gonzalez AE, Gilman RH. Larval cestode infections. In: Cystic hydatid, disease. Hunter's Tropical Medicine. Philadelphia: Saunders; 1984;866.
43. Zaouche A, Haouet K, et al. Management of liver hydatid cysts with a large biliocystic fistula: multicenter retrospective study. Tunisian Surgical Association. World J Surg 2001;25:28–39.
44. Garti I, Deutsch V. The angiographic diagnosis of echinococcosis of the liver and spleen. Clin Radiol 1971;22:466–471.
45. Lewall DB. Hydatid disease: biology, pathology, imaging and classification. Clin Radiol 1998;53:863–874.
46. Lorenzo C, Ferreira HB, et al. Comparative analysis of the diagnostic performance of six major *Echinococcus granulosus* antigens assessed in a double-blind, randomized multicenter study. J Clin Microbiol 2005;43:2764–2770.
47. von Sinner WN, Nyman R, et al. Fine needle aspiration biopsy of hydatid cysts. Acta Radiol 1995;36:168–172.
48. Olcay L, Besim LA, et al. Hydatid cyst mimicking pulmonary hematoma in a patient with hemophilia A. Turk J Pediatr 1998;40:425–429.
49. Gil-Grande LA, Rodriguez-Caabeiro F, et al. Randomised controlled trial of efficacy of albendazole in intra-abdominal hydatid disease. Lancet 1993;342:1269–1272.
50. Franchi C, Di Vico B, et al. Long-term evaluation of patients with hydatidosis treated with benzimidazole carbamates. Clin Infect Dis 1999;29:304–309.
51. Keshmiri M, Baharvahdat H, et al. Albendazole versus placebo in treatment of echinococcosis. Trans R Soc Trop Med Hyg 2001;95:190–194.
52. Morris DL, Dykes PW, et al. Albendazole—objective evidence of response in human hydatid disease. JAMA 1985;253:2053–2057.
53. Nahmias J, Goldsmith R, et al. Three- to 7-year follow-up after albendazole treatment of 68 patients with cystic echinococcosis (hydatid disease). Ann Trop Med Parasitol 1994;88:295–304.
54. Khuroo MS, Wani NA, et al. Percutaneous drainage compared with surgery for hepatic hydatid cysts. N Engl J Med 1997;337: 881–887.

55. Smego RA Jr, Bhatti S, et al. Percutaneous aspiration-injection-reaspiration drainage plus albendazole or mebendazole for hepatic cystic echinococcosis: a meta-analysis. Clin Infect Dis 2003;37:1073–1083.
56. Emel'ianov SI, Khamidov MA. [Laparoscopic treatment of hydatid liver cysts]. Khirurgiia (Mosk) 2000;(11):32–34.
57. Dziri C, Haouet K, et al. Treatment of hydatid cyst of the liver: where is the evidence? World J Surg 2004;28:731–736.
58. Bosch FX, Ribes J, et al. Epidemiology of hepatocellular carcinoma. Clin Liver Dis 2005;9:191–211, v.
59. Merle P. [Epidemiology, natural history and pathogenesis of hepatocellular carcinoma.]. Cancer Radiother 2005;9:452–457.
60. Jemal A, Murray T, et al. Cancer statistics, 2005. CA Cancer J Clin 2005;55:10–30.
61. Jemal A, Ward E, et al. Trends in the leading causes of death in the United States, 1970–2002. JAMA 2005;294:1255–1259.
62. Okuda K, Ohtsuki T, et al. Natural history of hepatocellular carcinoma and prognosis in relation to treatment. Study of 850 patients. Cancer 1985;56:918–928.
63. Okuda K. Hepatocellular carcinoma: recent progress. Hepatology 1992;15:948–963.
64. Tsukuma H, Hiyama T, et al. Risk factors for hepatocellular carcinoma among patients with chronic liver disease. N Engl J Med 1993;328:1797–1801.
65. Kew MC. Tumour markers of hepatocellular carcinoma. J Gastroenterol Hepatol 1989;4:373–384.
66. McMahon BJ, London T. Workshop on screening for hepatocellular carcinoma. J Natl Cancer Inst 1991;83:916–919.
67. Wee A. Fine needle aspiration biopsy of the liver: algorithmic approach and current issues in the diagnosis of hepatocellular carcinoma. Cytojournal 2005;2:7.
68. Zoli M, Magalotti D, et al. Efficacy of a surveillance program for early detection of hepatocellular carcinoma. Cancer 1996;78:977–985.
69. El-Serag HB, Anand B, et al. Association between hepatitis C infection and other infectious diseases: a case for targeted screening? Am J Gastroenterol 2003;98:167–174.
70. Cusnir M, Patt YZ. Novel systemic therapy options for hepatocellular carcinoma. Cancer J 2004;10:97–103.
71. Sherman M. Screening for hepatocellular carcinoma. Best Pract Res Clin Gastroenterol 2005;19:101–118.
72. Curley SA, Izzo F, et al. Radiofrequency ablation of hepatocellular cancer in 110 patients with cirrhosis. Ann Surg 2000; 232:381–391.
73. Sherman M, Peltekian KM, et al. Screening for hepatocellular carcinoma in chronic carriers of hepatitis B virus: incidence and prevalence of hepatocellular carcinoma in a North American urban population. Hepatology 1995;22:432–438.
74. Wildi S, Pestalozzi BC, et al. Critical evaluation of the different staging systems for hepatocellular carcinoma. Br J Surg 2004; 91:400–408.
75. Marrero JA, Fontana RJ, et al. Prognosis of hepatocellular carcinoma: comparison of seven staging systems in an American cohort. Hepatology 2005;41:707–716.
76. Zhao WH, Ma ZM, et al. Prediction of recurrence and prognosis in patients with hepatocellular carcinoma after resection by use of CLIP score. World J Gastroenterol 2002;8:237–242.
77. Shabahang M, Franceschi D, et al. Comparison of hepatic resection and hepatic transplantation in the treatment of hepatocellular carcinoma among cirrhotic patients. Ann Surg Oncol 2002;9:881–886.
78. Cha CH, Ruo L, et al. Resection of hepatocellular carcinoma in patients otherwise eligible for transplantation. Ann Surg 2003;238:315–321; discussion 321–323.
79. Yoo HY, Patt CH, et al. The outcome of liver transplantation in patients with hepatocellular carcinoma in the United States between 1988 and 2001: 5-year survival has improved significantly with time. J Clin Oncol 2003;21:4329–4335.
80. Poon RT, Fan ST. Hepatectomy for hepatocellular carcinoma: patient selection and postoperative outcome. Liver Transpl 2004;10(2 suppl 1):S39–S45.
81. Schoniger-Hekele M, Muller C, et al. Hepatocellular carcinoma in Central Europe: prognostic features and survival. Gut 2001;48:103–109.
82. Fong Y, Blumgart LH. Hepatic colorectal metastasis: current status of surgical therapy. Oncology (Williston Park) 1998;12:1489–1498; discussion 1498–1500, 1503.
83. Poon RT, Fan ST, et al. Intrahepatic recurrence after curative resection of hepatocellular carcinoma: long-term results of treatment and prognostic factors. Ann Surg 1999;229:216–222.
84. Nagasue N, Yukaya H, et al. Clinical experience with 118 hepatic resections for hepatocellular carcinoma. Surgery 1986;99:694–701.
85. Kamath PS, Wiesner RH, et al. A model to predict survival in patients with end-stage liver disease. Hepatology 2001;33:464–470.
86. Huang YH, Wu JC, et al. Supportive treatment, resection and transcatheter arterial chemoembolization in resectable hepatocellular carcinoma: an analysis of survival in 419 patients. Eur J Gastroenterol Hepatol 1999;11:315–321.
87. Schneider PD. Preoperative assessment of liver function. Surg Clin North Am 2004;84:355–373.
88. Lao XM, Zhang YQ, et al. [Estimation of hepatic resection volume in hepatocellular carcinoma by ICG(R15) and its relation with postoperative liver failure]. Ai Zheng 2005;24:337–340.
89. Oldhafer KJ, Hogemann D, et al. [3-dimensional (3-D) visualization of the liver for planning extensive liver resections]. Chirurg 1999;70:233–238.
90. Lang H, Radtke A, et al. Extended left hepatectomy–modified operation planning based on three-dimensional visualization of liver anatomy. Langenbecks Arch Surg 2004;389: 306–310.
91. Madoff DC, Abdalla EK, et al. Portal vein embolization in preparation for major hepatic resection: evolution of a new standard of care. J Vasc Interv Radiol 2005;16:779–790.
92. Hemming AW, Reed AI, et al. Preoperative portal vein embolization for extended hepatectomy. Ann Surg 2003;237:686–691; discussion 691–693.
93. Lai EC, Ng IO, et al. Hepatic resection for small hepatocellular carcinoma: the Queen Mary Hospital experience. World J Surg 1991;15:654–659.
94. Poon RT, Fan ST, et al. Improving survival results after resection of hepatocellular carcinoma: a prospective study of 377 patients over 10 years. Ann Surg 2001;234:63–70.
95. Nagasue N, Ono T, et al. Prognostic factors and survival after hepatic resection for hepatocellular carcinoma without cirrhosis. Br J Surg 2001;88:515–522.
96. Yeh CN, Chen MF, et al. Prognostic factors of hepatic resection for hepatocellular carcinoma with cirrhosis: univariate and multivariate analysis. J Surg Oncol 2002;81:195–202.
97. Mazzaferro V, Regalia E, et al. Liver transplantation for the treatment of small hepatocellular carcinomas in patients with cirrhosis. N Engl J Med 1996;334:693–699.
98. Poon RT, Ngan H, et al. Transarterial chemoembolization for inoperable hepatocellular carcinoma and postresection intrahepatic recurrence. J Surg Oncol 2000;73:109–114.
99. Lo CM, Ngan H, et al. Randomized controlled trial of transarterial lipiodol chemoembolization for unresectable hepatocellular carcinoma. Hepatology 2002;35:1164–1171.
100. Camma C, Schepis F, et al. Transarterial chemoembolization for unresectable hepatocellular carcinoma: meta-analysis of randomized controlled trials. Radiology 2002;224:47–54.

101. Llovet JM, Bruix J. Systematic review of randomized trials for unresectable hepatocellular carcinoma: chemoembolization improves survival. Hepatology 2003;37:429–442.
102. Livraghi T, Giorgio A, et al. Hepatocellular carcinoma and cirrhosis in 746 patients: long-term results of percutaneous ethanol injection. Radiology 1995;197:101–108.
103. Livraghi T, Goldberg SN, et al. Hepatocellular carcinoma: radiofrequency ablation of medium and large lesions. Radiology 2000;214:761–768.
104. Yamamoto J, Okada S, et al. Treatment strategy for small hepatocellular carcinoma: comparison of long-term results after percutaneous ethanol injection therapy and surgical resection. Hepatology 2001;34(4 pt 1):707–713.
105. Jatzko G, Wette V, et al. Simultaneous resection of colorectal carcinoma and synchronous liver metastases in a district hospital. Int J Colorectal Dis 1991;6:111–114.
106. Scheele J, Stangl R, et al. Staging of resectable colorectal liver metastases. Surgery 1996;119:118–120.
107. Scheele J, Altendorf-Hofmann A, et al. [Resection of colorectal liver metastases. What prognostic factors determine patient selection?]. Chirurg 2001;72:547–560.
108. Fernandez FG, Drebin JA, et al. Five-year survival after resection of hepatic metastases from colorectal cancer in patients screened by positron emission tomography with F-18 fluorodeoxyglucose (FDG-PET). Ann Surg 2004;240:438–447; discussion 447–450.
109. Folprecht G, Grothey A, et al. Neoadjuvant treatment of unresectable colorectal liver metastases: correlation between tumour response and resection rates. Ann Oncol 2005;16:1311–1319.
110. DeMatteo RP, Palese C, et al. Anatomic segmental hepatic resection is superior to wedge resection as an oncologic operation for colorectal liver metastases. J Gastrointest Surg 2000;4:178–184.
111. Weber SM, Jarnagin WR, et al. Intrahepatic cholangiocarcinoma: resectability, recurrence pattern, and outcomes. J Am Coll Surg 2001;193:384–391.
112. Jarnagin WR, Gonen M, et al. Improvement in perioperative outcome after hepatic resection: analysis of 1803 consecutive cases over the past decade. Ann Surg 2002;236:397–406; discussion 406–407.
113. Ekberg H, Tranberg KG, et al. Determinants of survival in liver resection for colorectal secondaries. Br J Surg 1986;73:727–731.
114. Hughes KS, Simon R, et al. Resection of the liver for colorectal carcinoma metastases: a multi-institutional study of patterns of recurrence. Surgery 1986;100:278–284.
115. Weber SM, Jarnagin WR, et al. Survival after resection of multiple hepatic colorectal metastases. Ann Surg Oncol 2000;7:643–650.
116. Poston G, Adam, R, et al. OncoSurge: a strategy for improving resectability with curative intent in metastatic colorectal cancer. J Clinic Oncol 2005;23:7125–7134.
117. Wray CJ, Lowy AM, et al. The significance and clinical factors associated with a subcentimeter resection of colorectal liver metastases. Ann Surg Oncol 2005;12:374–380.
118. Curley SA, Marra P, et al. Early and late complications after radiofrequency ablation of malignant liver tumors in 608 patients. Ann Surg 2004;239:450–458.
119. Goldberg RM, Sargent DJ, et al. A randomized controlled trial of fluorouracil plus leucovorin, irinotecan, and oxaliplatin combinations in patients with previously untreated metastatic colorectal cancer. J Clin Oncol 2004;22:23–30.
120. Tournigand C, Andre T, et al. FOLFIRI followed by FOLFOX6 or the reverse sequence in advanced colorectal cancer: a randomized GERCOR study. J Clin Oncol 2004;22:229–237.
121. Adam R, Avisar E, et al. Five-year survival following hepatic resection after neoadjuvant therapy for nonresectable colorectal. Ann Surg Oncol 2001;8:347–353.
122. Delaunoit T, Alberts SR, et al. Chemotherapy permits resection of metastatic colorectal cancer: experience from Intergroup N9741. Ann Oncol 2005;16:425–429.
123. Schefter TE, Kavanagh BD, et al. A phase I trial of stereotactic body radiation therapy (SBRT) for liver metastases. Int J Radiat Oncol Biol Phys 2005;62:1371–1378.
124. Weitz J, Blumgart LH, et al. Partial hepatectomy for metastases from noncolorectal, nonneuroendocrine carcinoma. Ann Surg 2005;241:269–276.
125. Chamberlain RS, Canes D, et al. Hepatic neuroendocrine metastases: does intervention alter outcomes? J Am Coll Surg 2000;190: 432–445.
126. Sarmiento JM, Que FG. Hepatic surgery for metastases from neuroendocrine tumors. Surg Oncol Clin N Am 2003;12:231–242.
127. Gupta S, Johnson MM, et al. Hepatic arterial embolization and chemoembolization for the treatment of patients with metastatic neuroendocrine tumors. Cancer 2005;104:1590–1602.
128. Nakeeb A, Pitt HA, et al. Cholangiocarcinoma. A spectrum of intrahepatic, perihilar, and distal tumors. Ann Surg 1996;224:463–473; discussion 473–475.
129. Takayasu K, Choi B, et al. First International Symposium of Current Issues for Nationwide Survey of Primary Liver Cancer in Korea, Taiwan and Japan. Japanese J Clinic Oncol 2007; 37(3):233–240.
130. Sons HU, Borchard F. Carcinoma of the extrahepatic bile ducts: a postmortem study of 65 cases and review of the literature. J Surg Oncol 1987;34:6–12.
131. Pitt HA, Dooley WC, et al. Malignancies of the biliary tree. Curr Probl Surg 1995;32:1–90.
132. Yamashita Y, Takahashi M, et al. Parenchymal changes of the liver in cholangiocarcinoma: CT evaluation. Gastrointest Radiol 1992;17:161–166.
133. Wiersema MJ, Vilmann P, et al. Endosonography-guided fine-needle aspiration biopsy: diagnostic accuracy and complication assessment. Gastroenterology 1997;112:1087–1095.
134. Teefey SA, Hildeboldt CC, et al. Detection of primary hepatic malignancy in liver transplant candidates: prospective comparison of CT, MR imaging, US, and PET. Radiology 2003;226:533–542.
135. Nimura Y. Extended surgery in bilio-pancreatic cancer: the Japanese experience. Semin Oncol 2002;29(6 suppl 20):17–22.
136. Hanazaki K, Kajikawa S, et al. Prognostic factors of intrahepatic cholangiocarcinoma after hepatic resection: univariate and multivariate analysis. Hepatogastroenterology 2002;49:311–316.
137. Lang H, Sotiropoulos GC, et al. Extended hepatectomy for intrahepatic cholangiocellular carcinoma (ICC):when is it worthwhile? Single center experience with 27 resections in 50 patients over a 5-year period. Ann Surg 2005;241:134–143.
138. Boyer TD. Natural history of portal hypertension. Clin Liver Dis 1997;1:31–44, x.
139. Le Moine O, Hadengue A, et al. Relationship between portal pressure, esophageal varices, and variceal bleeding on the basis of the stage and cause of cirrhosis. Scand J Gastroenterol 1997;32:731–735.
140. de Franchis R, Dell'Era A, et al. Diagnosis and treatment of portal hypertension. Dig Liver Dis 2004;36:787–798.
141. Benvegnu L, Gios M, et al. Natural history of compensated viral cirrhosis: a prospective study on the incidence and hierarchy of major complications. Gut 2004;53:744–749.
142. Planas R, Balleste B, et al. Natural history of decompensated hepatitis C virus-related cirrhosis. A study of 200 patients. J Hepatol 2004;40:823–830.
143. Burroughs AK. The natural history of varices. J Hepatol 1993;17(suppl 2):S10–S13.
144. Sarin SK, Lamba GS, et al. Comparison of endoscopic ligation and propranolol for the primary prevention of variceal bleeding. N Engl J Med 1999;340:988–993.

145. Jutabha R, Jensen DM, et al. Randomized study comparing banding and propranolol to prevent initial variceal hemorrhage in cirrhotics with high-risk esophageal varices. Gastroenterology 2005;128:870–881.
146. Psilopoulos D, Galanis P, et al. Endoscopic variceal ligation versus propranolol for prevention of first variceal bleeding: a randomized controlled trial. Eur J Gastroenterol Hepatol 2005;17:1111–1117.
147. Thuluvath PJ, Maheshwari A, et al. A randomized controlled trial of beta-blockers versus endoscopic band ligation for primary prophylaxis: a large sample size is required to show a difference in bleeding rates. Dig Dis Sci 2005;50:407–410.
148. Schepke M, Kleber G, et al. Ligation versus propranolol for the primary prophylaxis of variceal bleeding in cirrhosis. Hepatology 2004;40:65–72.
149. D'Amico G, Pagliaro L, et al. The treatment of portal hypertension: a meta-analytic review. Hepatology 1995;22:332–354.
150. de la Pena J, Rivero M, et al. Variceal ligation compared with endoscopic sclerotherapy for variceal hemorrhage: prospective randomized trial. Gastrointest Endosc 1999;49(4 pt 1):417–423.
151. Zargar SA, Javid G, et al. Endoscopic ligation versus sclerotherapy in adults with extrahepatic portal venous obstruction: a prospective randomized study. Gastrointest Endosc 2005;61:58–66.
152. Patch D, Sabin CA, et al. A randomized, controlled trial of medical therapy versus endoscopic ligation for the prevention of variceal rebleeding in patients with cirrhosis. Gastroenterology 2002;123:1013–1019.
153. Bosch J, Garcia-Pagan JC. Prevention of variceal rebleeding. Lancet 2003;361:952–954.
154. Karsan HA, Morton SC, et al. Combination endoscopic band ligation and sclerotherapy compared with endoscopic band ligation alone for the secondary prophylaxis of esophageal variceal hemorrhage: a meta-analysis. Dig Dis Sci 2005;50:399–406.
155. Sarin SK, Wadhawan M, et al. Endoscopic variceal ligation plus propranolol versus endoscopic variceal ligation alone in primary prophylaxis of variceal bleeding. Am J Gastroenterol 2005; 100:797–804.
156. Villanueva C, Balanzo J, et al. Nadolol plus isosorbide mononitrate compared with sclerotherapy for the prevention of variceal rebleeding. N Engl J Med 1996;334:1624–1629.
157. Villanueva C, Minana J, et al. Endoscopic ligation compared with combined treatment with nadolol and isosorbide mononitrate to prevent recurrent variceal bleeding. N Engl J Med 2001;345:647–655.
158. de la Pena J, Brullet E, et al. Variceal ligation plus nadolol compared with ligation for prophylaxis of variceal rebleeding: a multicenter trial. Hepatology 2005;41:572–578.
159. Rossle M, Deibert P, et al. Randomised trial of transjugular-intrahepatic-portosystemic shunt versus endoscopy plus propranolol for prevention of variceal rebleeding. Lancet 1997;349: 1043–1049.
160. Pomier-Layrargues G, Villeneuve JP, et al. Transjugular intrahepatic portosystemic shunt (TIPS) versus endoscopic variceal ligation in the prevention of variceal rebleeding in patients with cirrhosis: a randomised trial. Gut 2001;48:390–396.
161. Tripathi D, Lui HF, et al. Randomised controlled trial of long term portographic follow up versus variceal band ligation following transjugular intrahepatic portosystemic stent shunt for preventing oesophageal variceal rebleeding. Gut 2004;53:431–437.
162. Burroughs AK, Vangeli M. Transjugular intrahepatic portosystemic shunt versus endoscopic therapy: randomized trials for secondary prophylaxis of variceal bleeding: an updated meta-analysis. Scand J Gastroenterol 2002;37:249–252.
163. Feu F, Ruiz del Arbol L, et al. Double-blind randomized controlled trial comparing terlipressin and somatostatin for acute variceal hemorrhage. Variceal Bleeding Study Group. Gastroenterology 1996;111:1291–1299.
164. Jenkins SA, Shields R, et al. A multicentre randomised trial comparing octreotide and injection sclerotherapy in the management and outcome of acute variceal haemorrhage. Gut 1997;41:526–533.
165. Encarnacion CE, Palmaz JC, et al. Transjugular intrahepatic portosystemic shunt placement for variceal bleeding: predictors of mortality. J Vasc Interv Radiol 1995;6:687–694.
166. Abujudeh H, Parikh D, et al. Emergency transjugular intrahepatic portosystemic shunt for uncontrolled variceal bleeding. Emerg Radiol 2005;11:183–185.
167. Molmenti EP, Segev DL, et al. The utility of TIPS in the management of Budd-Chiari syndrome. Ann Surg 2005;241:978–981; discussion 982–983.
168. Rossle M, Haag K, et al. The transjugular intrahepatic portosystemic stent-shunt procedure for variceal bleeding. N Engl J Med 1994;330:165–171.
169. Fillmore DJ, Miller FJ, et al. Transjugular intrahepatic portosystemic shunt: midterm clinical and angiographic follow-up. J Vasc Interv Radiol 1996;7:255–261.
170. Wolff M, Hirner A. Current state of portosystemic shunt surgery. Langenbecks Arch Surg 2003;388:141–149.
171. Rosemurgy AS, Serafini FM, et al. Transjugular intrahepatic portosystemic shunt versus small-diameter prosthetic H-graft portacaval shunt: extended follow-up of an expanded randomized prospective trial. J Gastrointest Surg 2000;4:589–597.
172. Mariette D, Smadja C, et al. The Sugiura procedure: a prospective experience. Surgery 1994;115:282–289.
173. Haciyanli M, Genc H, et al. Results of modified Sugiura operation in variceal bleeding in cirrhotic and noncirrhotic patients. Hepatogastroenterology 2003;50:784–788.
174. Ma YG, Li XS, et al. Modified Sugiura procedure for the management of 160 cirrhotic patients with portal hypertension. Hepatobiliary Pancreat Dis Int 2004;3:399–401.
175. Brancatelli G, Federle MP, et al. Focal nodular hyperplasia: CT findings with emphasis on multiphasic helical CT in 78 patients. Radiology 2001;219:61–68.
176. Caremani M, Lapini L, et al. Sonographic diagnosis of hydatidosis: the sign of the cyst wall. Eur J Ultrasound 2003;16:217–223.
177. Descottes B, Glineur D, et al. Laparoscopic liver resection of benign liver tumors. Surg Endosc 2003;17:23–30.
178. Fulcher AS, Sterling RK. Hepatic neoplasms: computed tomography and magnetic resonance features. J Clin Gastroenterol 2002;34:463–471.
179. Haddad MC, Birjawi GA, et al. Unilocular hepatic echinococcal cysts: sonography and computed tomography findings. Clin Radiol 2001;56:746–750.
180. Hori T, Nagata K, et al. Risk factors for the local recurrence of hepatocellular carcinoma after a single session of percutaneous radiofrequency ablation. J Gastroenterol 2003;38:977–981.
181. Hung CH, Changchien CS, et al. Sonographic features of hepatic adenomas with pathologic correlation. Abdom Imaging 2001; 26:500–506.
182. Hussain SM, Terkivatan T, et al. Focal nodular hyperplasia: findings at state-of-the-art MR imaging, US, CT, and pathologic analysis. Radiographics 2004;24:3–17; discussion 18–19.
183. Joosten J, Jager G, et al. Cryosurgery and radiofrequency ablation for unresectable colorectal liver metastases. Eur J Surg Oncol 2005;31:1152–1159.
184. Kehagias D, Moulopoulos L, et al. Focal nodular hyperplasia: imaging findings. Eur Radiol 2001;11:202–212.
185. Koda M, Murawaki Y, et al. Combination therapy with transcatheter arterial chemoembolization and percutaneous ethanol injection compared with percutaneous ethanol injection alone for patients with small hepatocellular carcinoma: a randomized control study. Cancer 2001;92:1516–1524.

186. Kodama Y, Fujita N, et al. Alveolar echinococcosis: MR findings in the liver. Radiology 2003;228:172–177.
187. Lencioni RA, Allgaier HP, et al. Small hepatocellular carcinoma in cirrhosis: randomized comparison of radio-frequency thermal ablation versus percutaneous ethanol injection. Radiology 2003;228:235–240.
188. Leslie DF, Johnson CD, et al. Single-pass CT of hepatic tumors: value of globular enhancement in distinguishing hemangiomas from hypervascular metastases. AJR Am J Roentgenol 1995;165:1403–1406.
189. Livraghi T, Solbiati L, et al. Percutaneous radiofrequency ablation of liver metastases in potential candidates for resection: the test-of-time approach. Cancer 2003;97:3027–3035.
190. Machi J, Bueno RS, et al. Long-term follow-up outcome of patients undergoing radiofrequency ablation for unresectable hepatocellular carcinoma. World J Surg 2005;29:1364–1373.
191. Mortele KJ, Praet M, et al. CT and MR imaging findings in focal nodular hyperplasia of the liver: radiologic-pathologic correlation. AJR Am J Roentgenol 2000;175:687–692.
192. Unal O, Sakarya ME, et al. Hepatic cavernous hemangiomas: patterns of contrast enhancement on MR fluoroscopy imaging. Clin Imaging 2002;26:39–42.
193. Ding H, Kudo M, et al. Sonographic diagnosis of pancreatic islet cell tumor: value of intermittent harmonic imaging. J Clin Ultrasound 2001;29:411–416.
194. Blumgart LH (ed.). Surgery of the Liver and Biliary Tract. New York: Churchill Livingstone; 1994.
195. Sabiston DE. Textbook of Surgery. 14th ed. Philadelphia: Saunders; 1991.
196. Henderson M, Barnes DS, Geisinger MA. Portal hypertension. Curr Probl Surg 1998;35:381–452.

49

Small Intestine

Richard A. Hodin and Jeffrey B. Matthews

The small intestine is a remarkably complex organ that is capable of digestion, vectorial transport (absorption and secretion), and endocrine function. In addition, the small intestine protects the internal environment against noxious ingested substances and against luminal bacteria and their toxins. It is increasingly appreciated that the mucosal immune system plays a critical role in mucosal defense, and that dysregulation of this function underlies the pathogenesis of a number of clinical disorders. The potential surface area available for digestion and absorption is amplified 600-fold by the presence of circular mucosal folds, villus mucosal architecture, and the microvillus surface of the small intestinal epithelium. Although specific properties (e.g., bile acid absorption) are confined to specific segments of the small bowel, a sizable fraction of the length of the small bowel can be removed without excessive morbidity. In fact, substantial compensatory adaptation of the remaining bowel can occur after massive resection.

This chapter begins with an overview of small bowel anatomy and physiology related to surgical disease. Small-bowel neoplasia, various inflammatory disorders, and short-bowel syndrome are then discussed in detail. Congenital anomalies, mesenteric vascular disease, peptic ulcer, trauma, and gastrointestinal hemorrhage are covered elsewhere in this volume.

Anatomy and Physiology

Gross and Histological Anatomy

General Considerations

The small bowel measures 12 to 20 feet in length from pylorus to ileocecal valve. The duodenum is mostly retroperitoneal and wraps in a C-shape around the head of the pancreas. Its first and second portions lie adjacent to the gallbladder and liver; thus, duodenal pathology may extend to involve these organs and vice versa. Pathology at the ampulla of Vater may produce obstructive jaundice or pancreatitis. The jejunum begins at the ligament of Treitz. The jejunum and ileum are suspended on a mobile mesentery covered by a visceral peritoneal lining that extends onto the external surface of the bowel to form the serosa. Adhesions caused by surgery or inflammation may limit the mobility of the loops and lead to obstruction or internal hernia. The jejunum and ileum comprise about two-fifths and three-fifths of the mobile portion of the small intestine, respectively. Circumferential mucosal folds (plicae circularis) are abundant in the jejunum but absent in proximal duodenum and distal ileum.

Blood Supply and Lymphatic Drainage

The proximal duodenum receives its blood supply from the celiac axis, but the remainder of the small intestine is supplied by the superior mesenteric artery (SMA). Although mesenteric arcades form a rich collateral network, occlusion of a major branch of the SMA may result in segmental intestinal infarction. Venous drainage is via the superior mesenteric vein, which then joins the splenic vein behind the neck of the pancreas to form the portal vein. Elliptical, approximately 2 cm, lymphoid aggregates (Peyer's patches) are present on the antimesenteric border along the distal ileum, and smaller follicles are evident throughout the remainder of the small intestine. Lymphatic drainage of the intestine is abundant. Regional lymph nodes follow vascular arcades and drain toward the cysterna chyli.

Layers of the Bowel Wall

The small bowel wall consists of the outermost serosa, followed by the muscularis, submucosa, and mucosa, the innermost (Fig. 49.1). The serosa is a single layer of flattened

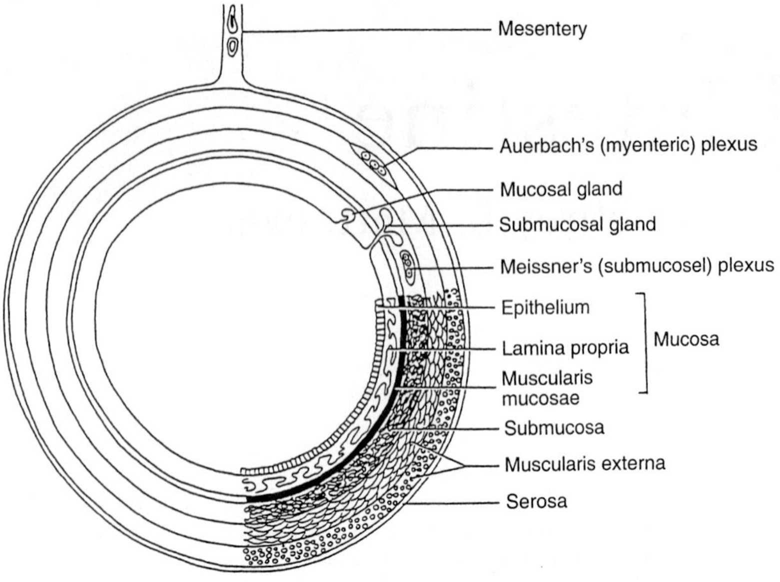

FIGURE 49.1. Layers of the intestinal wall. (From Dodd,[151] with permission.)

mesothelial cells that covers the jejunum and ileum but only the anterior surface of the duodenum. The muscularis consists of two layers of smooth muscle, a thicker inner circular layer and a thinner outer longitudinal layer. Specialized intercellular junctional structures called gap junctions electrically couple adjacent smooth muscle cells and allow efficient propagation of peristaltic signals. Ganglion cells and nerve fibers of Auerbach's myenteric plexus interdigitate between layers and communicate with smaller neural elements between cells. The submucosa is a dense connective tissue layer populated by diverse cell types, including fibroblasts, mast cells, lymphocytes, macrophages, eosinophils, and plasma cells. The submucosa is the strongest layer of the bowel wall, which should be taken into account when performing sutured anastomoses. Networks of arterioles, lymphatic and venous plexuses, and nerves crisscross through the submucosa. Meissner's submucosal neural plexus interconnects with neural elements from Auerbach's plexus in this region.

The mucosa is characterized by a villus architecture that, combined with circular folds, amplifies potential absorptive surface area 20-fold. The mucosa is subdivided into three layers. The muscularis mucosae consists of a thin sheet of smooth muscle cells. The lamina propria consists of connective tissue that extends from the base of the crypts up into the core of the intestinal villi. The innermost layer is made up of a continuous sheet of columnar epithelial cells composed of multiple cell types.

Intestinal Epithelium and Its Functions

General Considerations

Intestinal epithelial cells form the interface between the internal organism and an external environment and play a major role in the digestion and absorption of nutrients, in the absorption and secretion of water and electrolytes, and in intestinal immune function. Thus, it is not surprising that the intestinal epithelium is extraordinarily complex, composed of heterogeneous cell types that reside within a highly organized supporting tissue structure containing multiple regulatory elements (Fig. 49.2). Intestinal epithelial cells rest on a thin basement membrane overlying the lamina propria (Fig. 49.3). A central arteriole within the villus core is surrounded by a fenestrated capillary network that optimizes countercurrent exchange of oxygen and plasma solutes while providing an efficient pathway for absorption of nutrients. Mononuclear cells and neutrophils reside in or traffic into the lamina propria during normal or disease states. The secreted products of these cells may dramatically influence epithelial function.

There are two major compartments to the intestinal epithelium, the crypt and the villus, each with distinct function and cellular composition. The crypt compartment is populated by cells that are predominantly secretory and that derive from a pluripotent stem cell located several cell positions

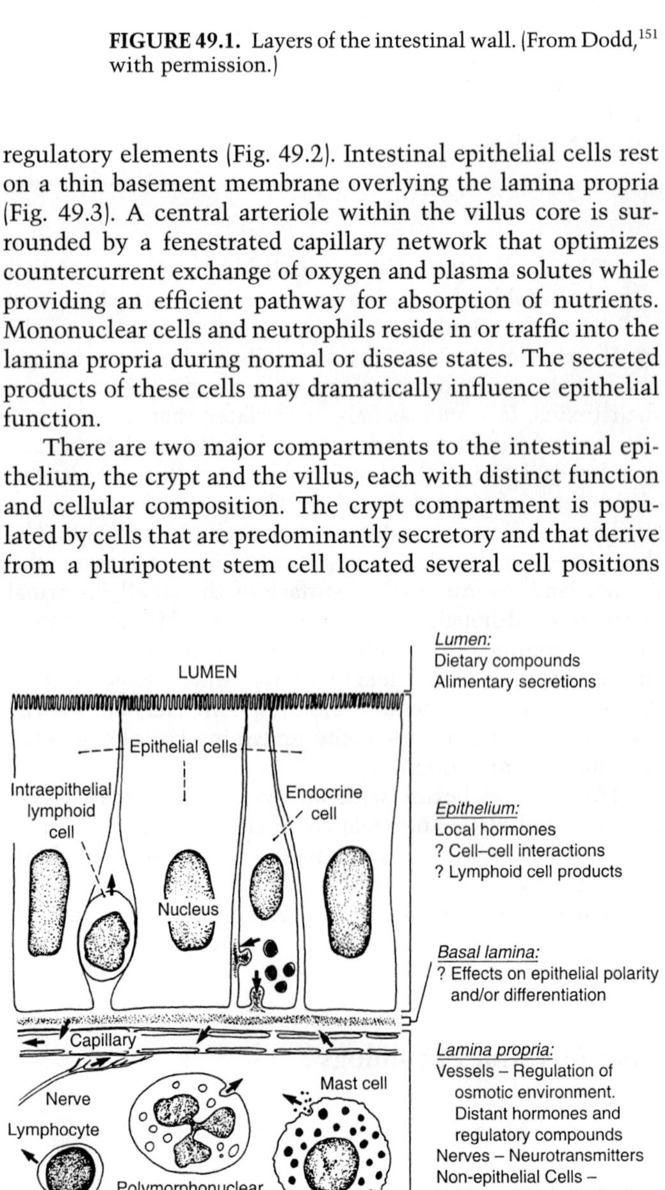

FIGURE 49.2. Schematic representation of various cell types and factors that may affect intestinal epithelial cell function. (From Schultz,[152] with permission.)

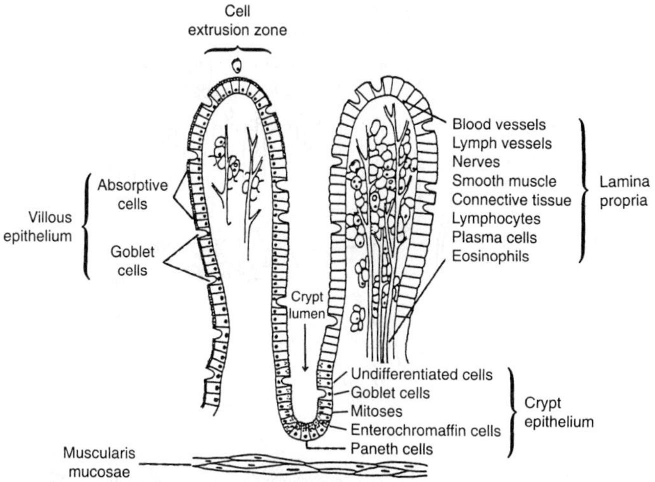

FIGURE 49.3. Schematic cross-sectional representation of two intestinal villi and an intervening crypt illustrating the structural architecture and relationship to supporting tissue structure. (From Sleisinger and Fordtran,[153] with permission.)

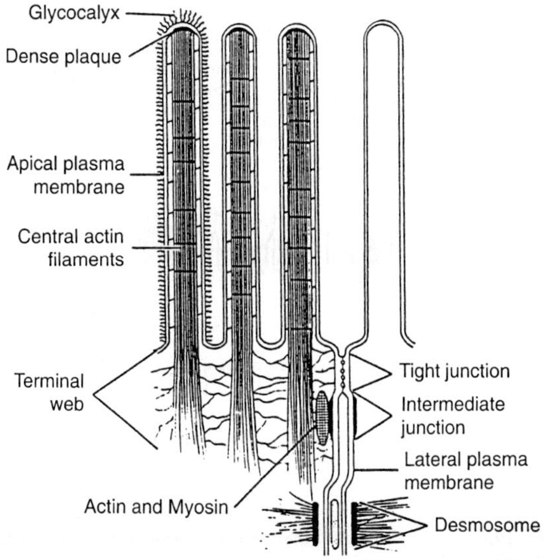

FIGURE 49.4. Schematic representation of the specialized apical plasma membrane and intercellular junctional complex of intestinal epithelial cells. Note that cytoskeletal actin forms the core of microvilli and interacts with the junctional complex to regulate paracellular permeability. (From Sleisinger and Fordtran,[153] by permission.)

above the base of the crypts of Lieberkuhn. Paneth cells reside at the base of the crypts and resemble zymogen-secreting cells of the pancreas. Except for Paneth cells, cells derived from the progenitor cell population migrate toward the villus surface. The majority of crypt cells are undifferentiated; some mature into mucus-secreting goblet cells and enteroendocrine cells, but most take on functional characteristics of absorptive enterocytes.[1,2] The life span of the enterocyte is 3 to 5 days.

The villus compartment is nonproliferative, and senescent enterocytes undergo apoptosis and are extruded.[3] Factors that influence enterocyte growth, differentiation, and apoptosis are incompletely defined but likely include growth factors (such as transforming growth factor-β), hormones (e.g., insulin, glucagon-like peptides), matrix proteins (e.g., collagens and laminins), and luminal nutrients (e.g., butyrate).[4–6]

Barrier Function

The intestinal epithelium selectively limits the permeation of potentially harmful luminal substances. The anatomical locus of this "barrier" is the intercellular junctional complex (Fig. 49.4),[7] a three-level structure that forms a circumferential seal between adjacent cells. The tight junction (zonula occludens) faces the lumen and is the site of membrane-to-membrane "kisses" that involve proteins such as ZO-1, ZO-2, and occludin. The intermediate or adherens junction (zonula adherens) lies deep to the tight junction, at which site the transmembrane protein E-cadherin interacts with cytoskeletally linked signaling elements. The desmosome is the innermost element of the junctional complex. Under a variety of pathological conditions, barrier function is perturbed.[8,9] Certain bacterial toxins (e.g., *Clostridium difficile*) directly perturb barrier function through disruption of cytoskeletal–junctional interactions, and various cytokines and proinflammatory mediators can also modulate junctional permeability. During critical illness, impairment of barrier function may result in enhanced systemic access of bacteria or bacterial products such as lipopolysaccharide and n-formylated peptides, resulting in a hyperdynamic, sepsis-like state associated with multiple organ failure.

Digestion and Absorption

The small intestine receives about 1 to 1.5 L/day of ingested fluid plus about 8 L of salivary, gastric, and pancreaticobiliary secretions. Most of this fluid is reabsorbed before reaching the colon. Water movement is driven by the active transcellular absorption of Na^+ and Cl^- and by the absorption of nutrients such as glucose and amino acids (Fig. 49.5). The energy for many of these transport processes derives from the activity of a basolateral Na^+-K^+ ATPase (adenosine triphosphatase), which maintains the low Na^+ internal environment that drives uptake via coupled ion exchangers (Na^+/H^+ and Cl^-/HCO_3^-) and Na^+-coupled nutrient transporters.

Digestion begins in the stomach with the action of gastric acid and pepsin. In the proximal duodenum, ingested foodstuffs are broken down by pancreatic proteases such as trypsin, elastase, chymotrypsin, and carboxypeptidases. The activity of brush border hydrolases and oligopeptidases then accomplishes terminal protein and carbohydrate digestion, and the

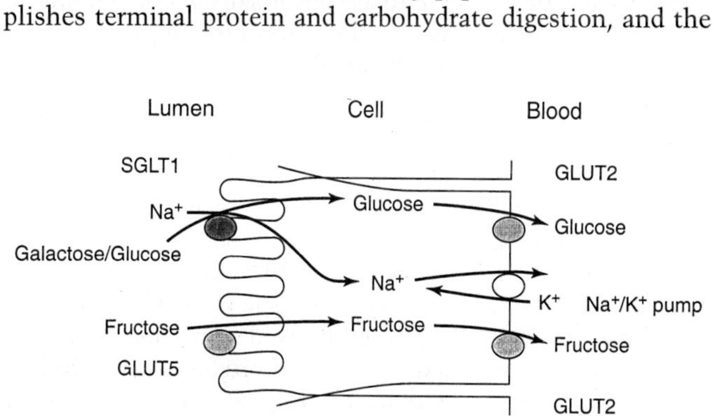

FIGURE 49.5. A model for sugar absorption by enterocytes. Glucose and galactose are absorbed across the brush border by SGLT1, a Na^+-glucose cotransporter, and then transported across the basolateral membrane into the systemic circulation down its concentration gradient by the GLUT2-facilitated glucose transporter. Fructose, in contrast, is absorbed entirely by facilitated transporters. (From Wright et al.,[154] by permission.)

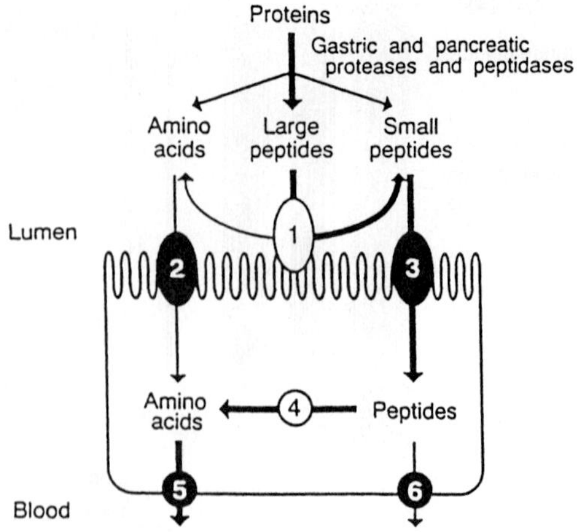

FIGURE 49.6. Digestion and absorption of peptides in the enterocyte by (1) brush border peptidases, (2) brush border amino acid transport systems, (3) brush border peptide transport systems, (4) cytoplasmic peptidases, (5) basolateral amino acid transport systems, and (6) basolateral peptide transport systems. (From Johnson,[155] by permission.)

resulting monosaccharides, amino acids, or di- and tripeptides then serve as substrates for Na^+- or H^+-coupled transporters in the apical membrane of absorptive enterocytes (Fig. 49.6). The apical membrane of these cells is well suited to the task of absorption by virtue of a microvillus brush border that amplifies absorptive area 30-fold.

Fat digestion and absorption occur in the proximal small intestine, where pancreatic lipase partially hydrolyzes triglycerides into two fatty acids plus a central fatty acid linked to glycerol (monoglyceride). These substances are solubilized by bile salts to form micelles or mixed micelles (which additionally contain phospholipids, cholesterol, and fat-soluble vitamins). Micelles diffuse into enterocytes through the overlying mucus and apical plasma membrane, releasing fatty acid and monoglyceride into the cell along the way (Fig. 49.7). Triglycerides are reformed intracellularly and are incorporated along with cellular protein, phospholipid, and cholesterol to form chylomicrons. Chylomicrons, which consist of an inner core of triglycerides and an outer coat of phospholipid and apoproteins, then exit the cell to be absorbed by the lymphatic system. Bile salts are resorbed into the enterohepatic circulation in the distal ileum by an ileal Na^+-coupled bile acid transporter.

Secretion

Intestinal crypt cells have the capacity to secrete an isotonic fluid through the active transcellular transport of Cl^-.[10] This process lubricates mucosal surfaces and facilitates the luminal extrusion of other secreted substances (e.g., secretory immunoglobulin [Ig] A and Paneth cell-derived cryptdins). Secretion of Cl^- may be stimulated by bacterial products (e.g., cholera toxin) as well as local mediator release. Clinical diarrhea results when secretion exceeds colonic absorptive capacity. The cellular basis for epithelial Cl^- secretion involves Cl^- uptake across the basolateral membrane via a Na^+-K^+-$2Cl^-$ cotransporter followed by Cl^- extrusion across the apical membrane via Cl^- channels, including the cystic fibrosis transmembrane conductance regulator (CFTR) (Fig. 49.8).

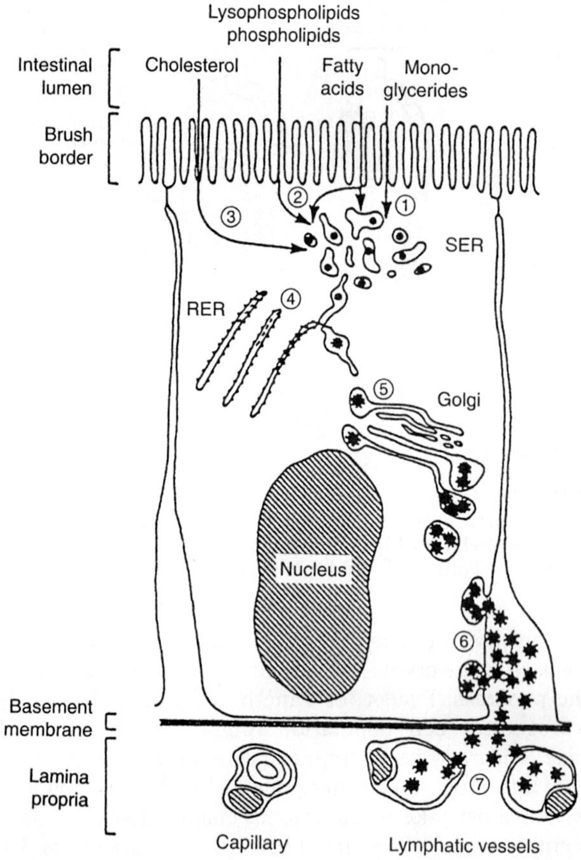

FIGURE 49.7. Pathway taken by lipids during passage through the enterocyte. Triglyceride and phospholipid are synthesized in the smooth endoplasmic reticulum and accumulate as dense droplets. Apolipoproteins assist in the formation of chylomicrons and very low density lipoproteins (asterisks), and these are transported from the Golgi, ultimately to be released across the basolateral membrane by exocytosis. (From Sleisinger and Fordtran,[153] by permission.)

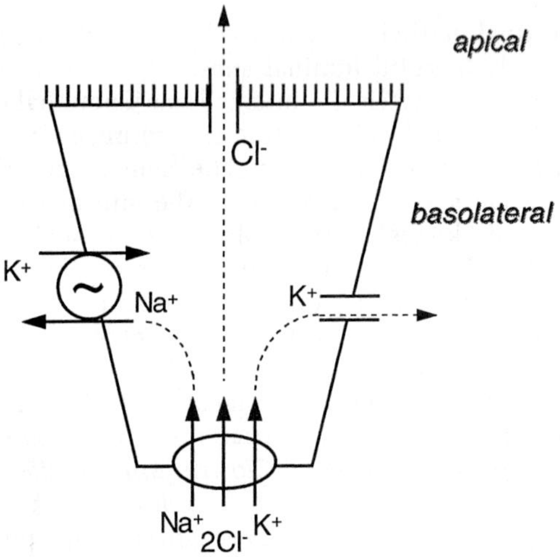

FIGURE 49.8. Model for active chloride secretion by crypt epithelial cells, the process underlying secretory diarrhea. Cl^2 accumulates intracellularly by the combined action of a basolateral Na^+-K^+-$2Cl^-$ cotransporter, coupled to the Na^+-K^+ ATPase pump and K^1 channels. Cl^- exits the cell across the apical membrane by regulated Cl^- channels, including the cystic fibrosis transmembrane conductance regulator (CFTR).

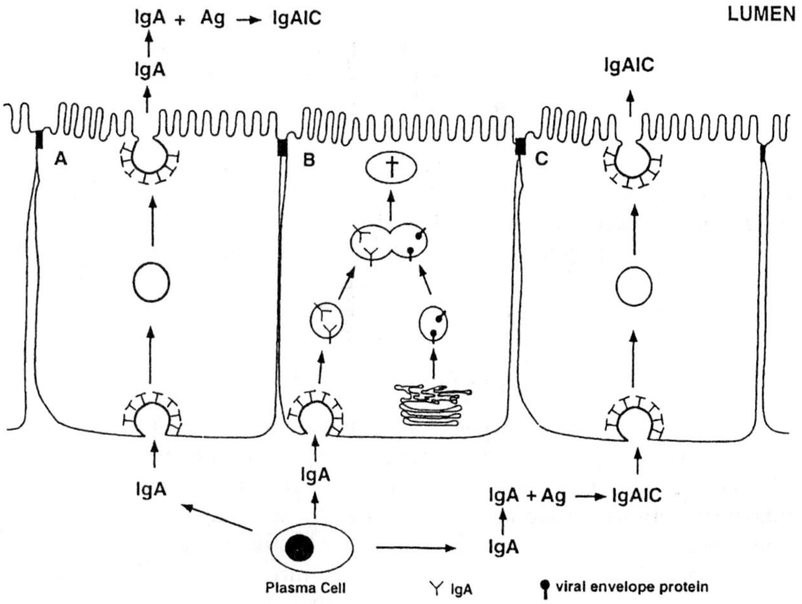

FIGURE 49.9. Compartments where IgA functions in relation to the intestinal epithelium. Plasma cells secrete IgA, which can be endocytosed, transcytosed, and secreted via the pIgR (*A*). The IgA can also interact with antigen directly internalized by the enterocyte (*B*). Also IgA may act subepithelially (*C*), and the immune complex may be transcytosed and exported. (From Lamm.[156] Used with permission of the American Physiological Society.)

Intestinal Immune Function

The mucosal immune system is critically important in defense against toxic and pathogenic threats from the luminal environment. The lamina propria contains numerous immune cells, including plasma cells, mast cells, and lymphocytes that produce not only immunoglobulins but also cytokine mediators.[11] Lamina propria plasma cells produce IgA in response to food antigens and microbes. Immunoglobulins A and M are secreted into the gut lumen by a mechanism that involves transcytosis through epithelial cells after binding to the polymeric immunoglobulin receptor (pIgR) on the basolateral membrane (Fig. 49.9).[12] Secretory IgA prevents microbial pathogens from penetrating the epithelial layer. The IgA–antigen interactions also occur within the intraepithelial and subepithelial compartments. In contrast to IgG, IgM, and IgE, antibodies of the IgA class evoke a much less proinflammatory (indeed, an antiinflammatory) response and thus contribute to the overall immunosuppressive tone of the mucosal immune system. Intestinal epithelial cells themselves may also contribute to the immune function of the gut.[11,12]

Specialized cells known as M cells are found overlying Peyer's patches (Fig. 49.10) and serve as the major portal of entry for foreign material. Specialized membrane invaginations in M cells create a pocket in which lymphocytes and macrophages gather. Luminal substances are immediately delivered to these professional antigen-processing cells, and this information is then directly conveyed to the underlying follicles. Antigen-specific lymphocyte proliferation occurs within Peyer's patches, and IgA-producing B cells migrate to regional lymph nodes and into the systemic circulation, from where they migrate back to diffusely populate the mucosa within the lamina propria.

Intraepithelial lymphocytes (IELs) are specialized T cells that reside in the paracellular space between absorptive enterocytes. A substantial fraction of IEL are immunosuppressive and express the $\gamma\delta$ T-cell receptor rather than the $\alpha\beta$ receptor that characterizes the more abundant T-cell lineage

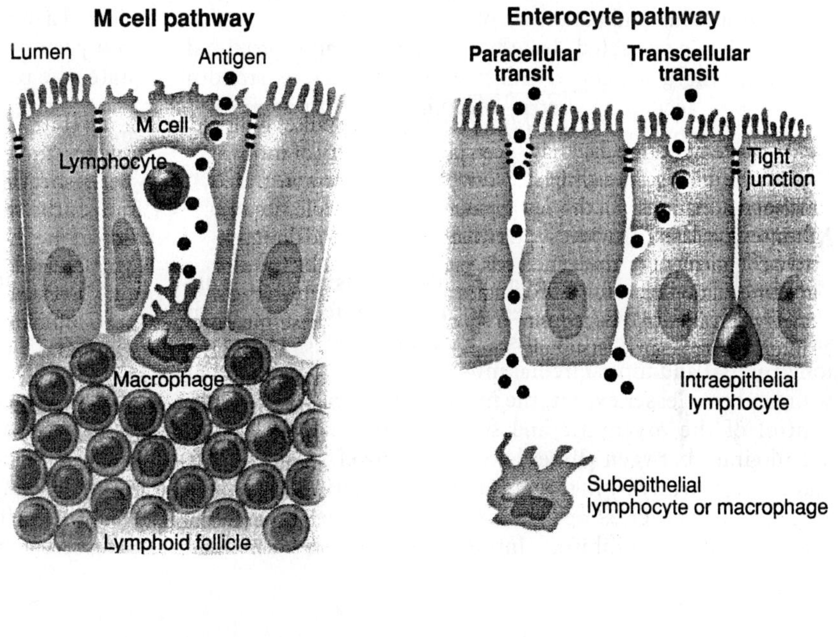

FIGURE 49.10. M cells and luminal pathways for antigen entry. Antigens can enter via M cells to deliver antigen directly to underlying immune cells. Alternatively, enterocytes may act as weak antigen-presenting cells. (From Madara, SCIENCE 277:910–911 [1997]. Illustration: K. Sutliff. Reprinted with permission from AAAS.)

populating most peripheral lymphoid sites. The precise role of IELs is uncertain, but they are thought to mediate cross talk between epithelial cells and the underlying immune and nonimmune cells of the lamina propria.

Within the lamina propria and submucosa, mature T cells, B cells, and macrophages carry out traditional cell-mediated immune responses, including phagocytosis, cell killing, and secretion of cytokines. Mucosal and connective tissue mast cells produce numerous mediators that contribute to overall immune responses and modulate the many functions of the epithelial cell layer.[13,14]

Intestinal Neuroendocrine Function

The intestine is a rich source of regulatory peptides that control various aspects of gut function. These substances, released in response to luminal or neural stimuli, exert their biological actions either at distant sites (by entering the bloodstream in classical hormone fashion) or locally (as paracrine factors or neurotransmitters). Those intestinal hormones with particular clinical relevance include secretin, cholecystokinin (CCK), somatostatin, and motilin.

Secretin is a 27-amino-acid peptide released by enteroendocrine cells in the proximal small bowel and functions to stimulate pancreatic ductal bicarbonate secretion and bile flow while inhibiting gastric acid secretion. Paradoxically, secretin stimulates rather than inhibits gastrin release in patients with gastrinoma, a phenomenon that forms the basis for the secretin infusion test in suspected Zollinger-Ellison syndrome.[15] Cholecystokinin is released by specialized small-bowel enteroendocrine cells in response to luminal amino acids and medium- to long-chain fatty acids. Two major targets of CCK that are of clinical importance are the gallbladder and the sphincter of Oddi, where it causes coordinated contraction and relaxation, respectively, to enhance luminal mixing of bile with ingested food.[16] In addition, CCK stimulates pancreatic enzyme secretion.

Somatostatin is a 14-amino-acid peptide that exerts a wide variety of inhibitory functions in the gastrointestinal tract. It is released from specialized enteroendocrine cells, where it acts in paracrine fashion to inhibit intestinal, gastric, and pancreaticobiliary secretion as well as cell growth. Synthetic forms of somatostatin are used clinically in patients with enterocutaneous and pancreaticobiliary fistulae.[17]

Motilin is secreted by the duodenum and proximal jejunum, where it acts to enhance contractility of smooth muscle and accelerate gastric emptying. Erythromycin is a motilin receptor agonist, which may explain its utility for certain forms of delayed gastric emptying.[18]

Motility of the Small Intestine

Intestinal motility consists of antegrade propulsion of luminal contents (peristalsis) combined with mixing action through segmentation. These functions are accomplished by the outer longitudinal and inner circular muscle layers of the intestinal wall, and to a lesser extent, the muscularis propria, under the control of the myenteric and submucosal nerve plexi that interdigitate between these layers. The bowel is also innervated extrinsically by both vagal and sympathetic fibers. Cholinergic sympathetic input is excitatory, while peptidergic input is probably inhibitory. Intestinal motility is also under positive control by local hormones such as motilin and CCK. Peristaltic waves are initiated by pacesetter potentials that originate in the duodenum. A nerve-related cell type known as the interstitial cell of Cajal appears to play a key role in the generation of pacemaker activity.[19]

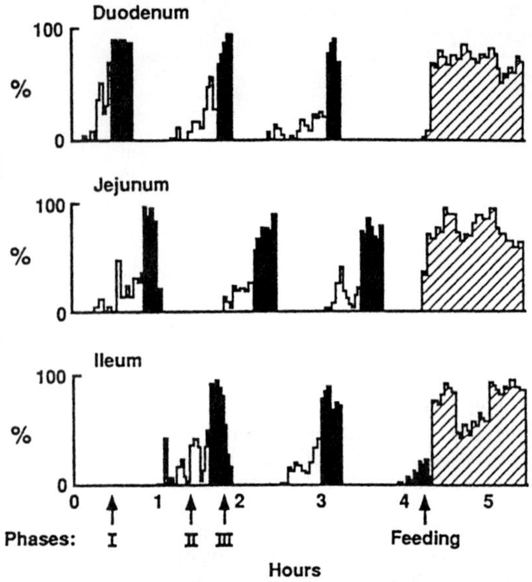

FIGURE 49.11. The migrating motor complex. Phases of intestinal motility during the fasting state are indicated (I, II, III). The periodicity of the fasted condition is interrupted by feeding, when activity rises to a more constant level. (From Sleisinger and Fordtran,[153] by permission.)

The intestinal wall undergoes two distinct forms of contraction. *Ring contractions* are circumferential indentations that propagate caudally and grossly appear as classical peristaltic waves, whereas *sleeve contractions* consist of a subtler shortening of the intestinal wall. Small-intestinal motility varies with the fasted and fed states (Fig. 49.11). During the interdigestive or fasting period between meals, a cyclical pattern of motor activity consisting of three phases is observed. Phase I is resting and occupies about 80% of the cycle. Phase II, about 15%, consists of random ring contractions of moderate amplitude. Phase III, about 5%, is a period of a series of brief high-pressure waves. This three-phase cycle, when viewed across the longitudinal axis of the small bowel, results in a pattern called the *migrating motor complex*. In the fed state, the pattern of contraction is more frequent and consistent over time. Rather than beginning from a proximal site and propagating distally, contractions in the fed state begin at all levels along the small bowel and spread distally for variable distances.

Mechanical Obstruction of the Intestine

Clinical Presentation and Diagnosis

Obstruction of the intestine occurs when there is impairment in the normal flow of luminal contents caused by an extrinsic or intrinsic encroachment on the lumen. Intestinal pseudoobstruction, or adynamic ileus, can mimic mechanical obstruction but differs in that the underlying problem is due to disordered motility. The key to management of small-

TABLE 49.1. Common Causes of Mechanical Obstruction of the Small Intestine as a Function of Age.

Neonate	*Infant*	*Young adult*	*Adult*
Atresia	Groin hernia	Adhesions	Adhesions
Midgut volvulus	Intussusception	Groin hernia	Groin hernia
Meconium ileus	Meckel's diverticulum		

intestinal obstruction is early diagnosis. Identification of those patients with strangulation is of critical importance because prompt surgical correction is needed to minimize morbidity and mortality. Numerous clinical and radiologic criteria can be helpful in distinguishing simple from strangulating obstruction, but this differentiation remains a challenge to even the most experienced clinicians.

Etiology

Intestinal obstruction has a variety of causes that differ as a function of age (Table 49.1). For example, in the neonate, congenital anomalies such as atresia, volvulus, and imperforate anus are common causes of obstruction, whereas infants are more likely to have strangulated hernias or intussusception. In contrast, small-intestinal obstruction in adults is primarily caused by either adhesive bands or groin hernias. Although strangulated hernias were the most common cause of small-bowel obstruction in the past, more recent series indicate that adhesive bands are now far more likely to be the etiology.

In 1900, Gibson reviewed the reports of 1000 patients with intestinal obstruction and found that 35% were on the basis of strangulated hernias, whereas only about 19% were caused by bands.[20] Similarly, Vick reviewed 6892 patients from Great Britain with acute obstruction between 1925 and 1930 and found that approximately 50% were due to strangulated hernias, whereas adhesions accounted for only 7% of the cases.[21] The increase in elective inguinal hernia repairs coupled with an increase in the number of laparotomies performed in recent decades likely account for a change in etiology of obstruction over time. In 1955, Wangenstein reviewed 1252 cases of obstruction and found only 10% to be due to hernias compared with 37% caused by adhesions.[22]

Clinical Presentation

In the setting of obstruction, the normal absorptive mechanisms of the small bowel are deranged such that excess fluid losses occur. Initially, there is vomitus, bowel wall edema, and transudative loss into the peritoneal cavity, but during the late stages of obstruction, venous pressure increases, with resultant hemorrhage into the lumen, worsening hypovolemia. The normal relatively sterile environment of the proximal small intestine is altered under obstructed conditions such that bacterial overgrowth occurs, most notably involving the anaerobes such as *Bacteroides*. The feculant vomiting seen in cases of long-standing distal small-bowel obstruction is the result of this bacterial overgrowth and is virtually pathognomonic for a high-grade or complete distal mechanical small-bowel obstruction. The importance of bacterial overgrowth in the morbidity and mortality of interstitial obstruction has been demonstrated in experimental animals; for example, germ-free dogs survive intestinal strangulation better than controls.[23] Thus, antibiotics may be of benefit in the setting of strangulation, although there is probably no role for antibiotics in patients with simple mechanical bowel obstruction.

The diagnosis of intestinal obstruction is usually made on clinical grounds with the symptoms of crampy abdominal pain, decreased or absent flatus and stool, nausea, or vomiting. A prior history of small-bowel obstruction should be sought because those patients with mechanical small-bowel obstruction caused by adhesions often experience recurrence. A history of other possible causes for small-bowel obstruction (e.g., Crohn's disease, radiation therapy) should be considered. The vomitus often contains occult blood and appears as "coffee grounds" in color, probably because of distension of the stomach with resultant mucosal hemorrhage. Evaluation of such patients for gastrointestinal bleeding will not be fruitful, however, and delays the diagnosis and treatment of the true problem. Reflex vomiting is common, and in cases of early or distal obstructions, the volume of the vomitus will be quite small because it takes some time for intestinal contents to back up to the stomach. The level of the obstruction is often suggested on the basis of the pattern of the pain, with proximal obstructions usually causing more frequent cramps.

The obstructed patient often displays signs of dehydration, with dry mouth and loss of skin turgor. The waves of abdominal pain, or colic, can actually be witnessed at the bedside and provide the strongest possible indication of a mechanically obstructed intestine. Occasionally, audible bowel sounds, or borborygmi, are present as a result of strong intestinal muscular contractions. Inspection of the abdomen usually reveals distension, although this may be absent in proximal obstruction. The degree of distension is greater with more distal or long-standing obstructions. Patients with large-bowel obstruction are especially distended because of the large capacitance of the colon. The presence of surgical scars should be noted, indicating the possibility of intraabdominal adhesions as the cause. An abdominal wall hernia might also be evident as the site of the obstruction. When hernia contents are soft and easily reducible in the obstructed patient, it is likely that an etiology other than the hernia exists. Any preexisting hernia tends to protrude in a patient who develops abdominal distension from a bowel obstruction.

Although mild diffuse tenderness is a common feature in patients with distension from a mechanical obstruction, involuntary guarding or other signs of peritoneal irritation are unusual and suggest the possibility of ischemia or infarction of the bowel, perhaps even with perforation. Rectal examination is important to detect mass lesions and to check for the presence of stool, which is usually absent in cases of mechanical bowel obstruction, especially of long-standing nature.

Diagnosis

Laboratory tests are not generally helpful in the diagnosis or management of patients with bowel obstruction. Routine blood counts reveal an elevated hematocrit indicative of intravascular volume depletion. Leukocytosis is sometimes present but is often the result of hemoconcentration and an acute stress response rather than underlying infection. A markedly elevated white blood cell count should raise the suspicion for strangulation. Elevated serum urea nitrogen and creatinine usually indicate hypovolemia with prerenal azotemia.

Plain x-rays of the abdomen are perhaps the most useful adjunctive test to confirm the diagnosis of bowel obstruction. Small-bowel obstruction leads to dilation of the small bowel with air–fluid levels on an upright film. Although the presence of air–fluid levels at different heights in the same loop of bowel have been considered an important finding suggesting a mechanical obstruction, Harlow et al.[24] found this sign to be present in only 52% of patients with proven mechanical obstruction. In addition, 29% of patients with adynamic ileus had this finding on plain radiographs. The presence of free air on a plain upright x-ray indicates perforation and the need for urgent operation. In small-bowel obstruction of long-standing nature, perhaps greater than 24 h, all the air and stool from the colon will have been evacuated, and this is evident on plain abdominal films. However, if the obstruction is in its early phase, or if it is only partial, then some air and stool are present within the colon, making distinction between an early complete and a partial small-bowel obstruction very difficult.

Computed tomography (CT) is often employed to evaluate patients with suspected bowel obstruction. The CT scan will generally identify dilated proximal and collapsed distal bowel, a feature that is aided by the administration of an oral contrast agent. The precise site and etiology of the obstruction may not be identified by CT, as in the case of adhesions, although in some instances an obstructing lesion can be seen. In a study of 90 cases of suspected small bowel obstruction, Frager et al.[25] noted that clinical findings along with plain x-rays led to the correct diagnosis of complete obstruction in only 46% of patients, whereas CT was found to be 100% sensitive in these cases. Also, CT was superior in cases of partial small-bowel obstruction. However, false-positive CT scans were obtained in 6 cases, suggesting that the radiologic criteria for small-bowel obstruction may have been too broad.

Based on these and other series in the literature, CT[26] has replaced the contrast small-bowel follow-through in many centers as the primary radiologic tool in suspected mechanical small-bowel obstruction. There are similar advantages of CT in large-bowel obstruction if tumor masses and pericolic inflammatory changes can be identified. Although ultrasound has been reported to be superior to plain films in detecting small-bowel obstruction, it is a highly operator-dependent technique and has a limited role in this clinical setting.

Treatment of Small-Bowel Obstruction

General Considerations

Among the most important distinctions in the patient with a mechanical bowel obstruction is whether the site is within the small or large intestine. This difference is usually evident on plain radiographs because the characteristic features of dilated colon are not present in patients with small-bowel obstruction. The differentiation between small- and large-bowel obstruction is critical in regard to both underlying cause (Table 49.2) and clinical management.

TABLE 49.2. Clinical Differences Between Small- and Large-Bowel Obstruction.

	Small-intestinal obstruction	*Large-intestinal obstruction*
Most common causes	Adhesions and groin hernias	Cancer and inflammatory diseases
Symptoms	Abdominal cramps and vomiting at regular/frequent intervals	Abdominal cramps and vomiting less prominent or frequent
Signs	Mild-to-moderate abdominal distension	Moderate-to-marked abdominal distension
Plain abdominal films	Dilated small-intestinal loops with air/fluid levels; paucity of air and stool distally	Dilated air-filled colon with or without small-bowel distension and air/fluid levels

Simple Versus Strangulating Obstruction

The most important issue to be addressed in patients with mechanical small-bowel obstruction is whether strangulation exists. Series that have compared mortality figures for simple versus strangulating obstruction have clearly demonstrated the importance of early recognition and treatment as mortality for strangulated cases is generally 2- to 10-fold higher than that for simple obstruction.[27] In those patients with strangulating groin hernias, the signs on physical exam are usually clear and include a firm, tender mass, sometimes with overlying erythema of the skin. In such situations, prompt surgical repair, usually with bowel resection, is mandatory.

However, in patients with obstruction on the basis of intraabdominal pathology, the identification of strangulation may be extremely difficult. Among the most common mechanisms for strangulating small-bowel obstruction is the "closed loop," which is usually due to adhesions and results in a twisting of a segment of intestine. Patients with closed-loop obstruction usually have severe pain early, and the fluid-filled loops of bowel are often not seen on plain abdominal radiographs. It is with this particular group of patients that the experienced clinician is called on to make a rapid and accurate diagnosis so that surgical intervention might prevent the sequelae of infarction and perforation.

The differentiation between simple and strangulating obstruction has been the subject of numerous studies designed to identify one or more key signs or symptoms that could reliably predict the presence of strangulation. Silen et al.[28] reviewed the case histories of 480 patients with mechanical small-bowel obstruction and were not able to easily differentiate simple from strangulating obstruction on the basis of clinical presentation. For example, although it has been generally taught that patients with strangulation have continuous pain whereas simple obstruction causes intermittent or colicky pain, this was not found to be the case in this series. Similar results were reported by Zollinger and Kinsey,[29] who found that constant pain was present in 18% of patients with simple obstruction and only 20% of those with strangulation. Tenderness to palpation is present in most (85%) patients with strangulation but is also present in a majority of patients with simple obstructions. A similar overlap has been documented in regard to other signs, such as fever, leukocytosis,

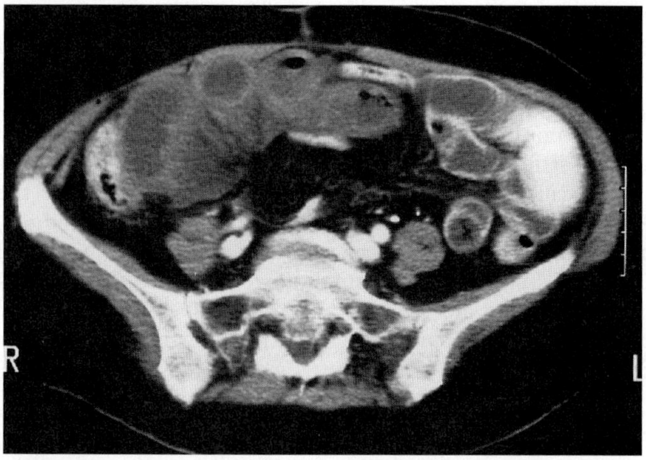

FIGURE 49.12. Computed tomographic scan of a patient with a strangulating small-bowel obstruction. Dilated proximal small intestine is seen to be filled with the oral contrast agent. More distal loops are fluid filled but without luminal contrast because the "closed loop" is completely obstructing. In addition, the bowel wall appears thickened, and there is evidence of streaky inflammatory changes in the adjacent mesentery.

and the presence of a mass. On the basis of these studies, as well as the anecdotal experience of numerous surgeons, it has generally been accepted that only short periods of observation (<24h) are appropriate for fear of missing an unsuspected strangulation in patients with apparent mechanical small-bowel obstruction.

Because clinical criteria are imperfect in terms of differentiating simple from strangulating obstructions, a variety of radiologic tests have been employed. It is clear that plain abdominal radiographs can be helpful in diagnosing a bowel obstruction, but normal x-rays can be seen in as many as 20% of those patients with strangulation. The presence of a single loop of dilated small bowel in the setting of acute, severe abdominal pain should raise the suspicion of a strangulated closed-loop obstruction. Abdominal CT has been reported to be useful in identifying strangulation, usually on the basis of bowel wall thickening, mesenteric edema, asymmetrical enhancement with contrast, pneumatosis, or portal venous gas. Figure 49.12 illustrates several features of strangulating obstruction detected by CT scan in a patient proven at operation to have a large segment of infarcted small intestine.

Frager et al. studied 60 patients with small-bowel obstruction and found CT to be 100% sensitive for the detection of ischemia, but there were 12 false positives (61% specificity).[30] Ogata et al.[31] reported that an akinetic loop seen on real-time ultrasonography had a high sensitivity (90%) and specificity (93%) for the presence of strangulation; however, the positive predictive value for strangulation was only 73%. These authors also found that the presence of peritoneal fluid was often an indicator of strangulation, a finding that has also been noted in studies using CT. It is clear, however, that the diagnosis of a strangulating obstruction remains difficult and requires a high degree of suspicion on the part of an experienced clinician.

Nonoperative Treatment

With improved surgical and anesthetic management, mortality from small-bowel obstruction has decreased during the past 50 to 60 years from approximately 25% to 5%. Initial therapy is directed at correction of intravascular fluid and electrolyte abnormalities. The patient should be given nothing by mouth. Nasogastric tube suction can provide symptomatic improvement for patients with emesis. Resolution of the obstruction may occur after adequate hydration and decompression via a nasogastric tube, avoiding the need for surgical intervention. This nonoperative approach is often successful in those patients with either partial obstruction from adhesions or obstructions related to impaction of food particles at the sites of luminal narrowing, such as a Crohn's stricture. In addition to standard nasogastric tubes, a variety of long intestinal tubes have been used in an attempt at optimizing luminal decompression. The tubes are generally weighted with a mercury-filled balloon and passed into the stomach, and the patient is placed in the right lateral decubitus position in the hope that peristalsis will carry the tube beyond the pylorus and into the more distal intestine. Fleshner et al. conducted a prospective, randomized trial in 55 patients with acute adhesive small-bowel obstruction and found no advantage of one tube type over the other.[32] This prospective study confirmed previous retrospective studies in the literature[33,34] that have shown no advantage of long intestinal tubes (Table 49.3).

Obstruction caused by incarcerated hernia can sometimes be relieved by reduction of the hernia, a procedure that should be performed cautiously and only by experienced clinicians. Excessive external pressure will lead to significant patient discomfort and, in rare circumstances, an inadvertent reduction "en masse" may occur, resulting in disappearance of the hernia bulge but with persistent bowel obstruction and possible strangulation within the constricting peritoneal sac.

Operative Treatment

Surgical intervention is indicated for those patients with a complete small-bowel obstruction who have any signs or symptoms indicative of strangulation or for those patients with simple obstruction that has not resolved within a reasonable period of nonoperative therapy, generally 24 to 48 h. Most clinicians would agree that constant or severe pain, especially associated with fever or signs of peritoneal irritation, are indications for urgent laparotomy.

The surgical approach to most patients with small-bowel obstruction is straightforward and includes laparotomy with adhesiolysis and resection of nonviable intestine. The determination of when and how much intestine to remove is usually simple and is based on the purple or black discoloration that occurs in severely ischemic or necrotic intestine.

TABLE 49.3.
Success Rates for Standard (Short) Versus Long Intestinal Tubes in Patients with Small-Bowel Obstruction.

		Required surgery		
Author	*Randomized*	*Short tube*	*Long tube*	*P value*
Fleshner[32]	Yes	38/28 (46%)	8/27 (30%)	NS
Brolin[33]	No	80/184 (44%)	83/145 (57%)	NS
Bizer[34]	No	48/91 (53%)	76/154 (49%)	NS

In addition to the normal pink coloration, viable intestine has mesenteric arterial pulsations and normal motility. In some cases of more limited ischemic damage, adhesiolysis should be followed by a 10- to 15-min period of observation to allow for possible improvement in the gross appearance of the involved segment.

Laser Doppler flowmetry has been advocated as an intraoperative method to assess bowel viability. Bulkley et al.[35] studied 71 ischemic bowel segments and found fluorescein ultraviolet fluorescence to be more accurate in determining bowel viability than either standard clinical judgment or Doppler blood flow measurements.

In making the judgment regarding the extent of resection, it should be kept in mind that a given marginally viable segment of intestine may survive in the short term, only to be followed weeks or months later by stricture formation that requires resection. As such, it is probably best to remove any segment that is not clearly viable by gross examination at the time of adhesiolysis. In most cases, all the adhesions should be lysed to ensure that the obstruction is relieved and perhaps to prevent future recurrences. When an obstructing lesion is identified, resection with primary anastomosis is performed.

Since the advent of minimally invasive surgical techniques in the 1980s, some surgeons have employed a laparoscopic approach to patients with small-bowel obstruction.[36] A single adhesive band may be lysed laparoscopically or a small laparotomy performed overlying the area of obstruction, thereby avoiding a long incision in the abdominal wall. Laparoscopy in the setting of a bowel obstruction can be performed safely, but the open technique is preferred to avoid the blind insertion of needles or trochars into the peritoneal cavity when distended loops of bowel are present.

Special Forms of Intestinal Obstruction

Stricture

Crohn's disease is among the most common etiologies for small intestinal stricture (Table 49.4). Certain drugs are known to cause mucosal ulceration and strictures, most notably enteric-coated potassium chloride preparations and the nonsteroidal antiinflammatory agents.[37,38] Radiation therapy for intraperitoneal malignancy can lead to stricture formation, especially in the patient who has undergone previous surgery such that adhesions may "fix" the loops of intestine, allowing for greater exposure to isolated segments. Because of problems with healing, obstructing segments of irradiated bowel either should be bypassed or, if a resection is performed, at least one end of an anastomosis should include nonirradiated bowel.[39] Mesenteric ischemia can also lead to stricture formation, with the distal ileum at greatest risk because the ileocolic artery is the last branch of the SMA.[40] Various neoplasms, including carcinoma, carcinoid, and lymphoma, can also cause strictures within the small intestine. In most cases of small-bowel stricture, the obstructive symptoms are chronic and progressive in nature, and the best surgical approach is resection whenever technically feasible.

TABLE 49.4. Etiologies of Small-Intestinal Strictures.

Trauma
Ischemia
Tumors
Drugs (KCl, nonsteroidal antiinflammatory drugs)
Anastomotic
Crohn's disease
Postinflammatory
Infectious (tuberculosis)
Radiation
Cystic fibrosis

Internal Hernias

Internal herniation can be related to abnormalities created by prior operations, as from adhesions or in the paracolic or paraileal spaces adjacent to end stomas. In addition, congenital defects causing hernias have been described in the mesenteries of the ileum, transverse colon, sigmoid colon, and that of a Meckel's diverticulum, as well as in the left paracolic gutter and within the falciform ligament.[41] The presentation is generally indistinguishable from other causes of intestinal obstruction, so that an accurate preoperative diagnosis is rarely made. Surgical repair of the defect should be performed along with resection of any nonviable bowel. If discovered incidentally at the time of laparotomy for other reasons, such defects should be repaired.[42] In addition to these intraperitoneal defects, retroperitoneal fossae can also be the site of internal herniation and bowel obstruction. The most common of these is the paraduodenal region, although they also occur in the ileocecal and sigmoid regions and are thought to arise as abnormalities in the gut rotation that occurs in utero.[43]

Gallstone Ileus

Gallstones account for approximately 1% to 2% of cases of intestinal obstruction, usually affecting patients older than 60 years.[44] To cause obstruction, the gallstone must be of large size (>.2.5 cm) and therefore can enter the intestinal tract only by a process of ulceration and fistulization. The most common site of entry is a cholecystoduodenal fistula, although stones may also erode into the stomach, jejunum, ileum, or colon or through the distal common bile duct into the duodenum. The gallstone causes obstruction in the distal ileum or rarely at other areas of intestinal narrowing.

The diagnosis is suggested by the concurrent radiologic features of intestinal obstruction along with air in the biliary tree. Often, the obstruction is described as "tumbling" as the stone passes distally.

Surgical treatment mandates removal of the stone via enterotomy or resection when the stone has become severely impacted in the wall of the bowel. Whether to perform a cholecystectomy at the time of laparotomy remains controversial, but as long as the gallbladder is emptied of all stones, the chances of recurrent intestinal obstruction are extremely low.

Kasahara et al. reviewed 112 cases of gallstone ileus and found a significant mortality (19%) in patients treated with a one-stage procedure (enterotomy plus cholecystectomy), whereas there was no mortality in those treated with enterolithotomy alone.[45] In contrast, Clavien et al. reviewed a series of 33 patients and concluded that a one-stage procedure was safe and effective for most patients.[46] Therefore, if the general condition of the patient is good and anatomical factors are propitious, a one-stage procedure can be recommended. In addition to gallstones, intraluminal foreign bodies including bezoars, worms, and swallowed objects can cause small-bowel obstruction.[47]

Early Postoperative Small-Bowel Obstruction

In the early postoperative period (within 3–4 weeks) following laparotomy for any cause, small-bowel obstruction occurs in approximately 1% of patients. The differentiation between obstruction and adynamic ileus can usually be made on clinical grounds because an ileus rarely persists for more than 5 to 6 days. Clearly, many patients thought to have a "prolonged ileus" really have some degree of mechanical small-intestinal obstruction.[48] The diagnosis of early postoperative obstruction can be made in those patients who initially experience return of bowel function, only subsequently to develop nausea, vomiting, and abdominal distension. Plain radiographs may distinguish adynamic ileus from obstruction because a predominance of small-bowel gaseous distension would not be seen in most cases of ileus. Frager et al. examined 36 patients with CT and reported 100% sensitivity and specificity in distinguishing mechanical small-bowel obstruction from paralytic ileus.[49]

It should be noted that the distinction between ileus and mechanical obstruction in the early postoperative period is rarely of clinical consequence because the treatment is usually nonoperative.[50] This is the case because in early postoperative obstruction the chances of nonoperative resolution appears to be higher and the incidence of strangulation lower than in other clinical settings. Soft, filmy, and broad-based adhesions form early after laparotomy, occasionally leading to some degree of luminal obstruction, a situation that resolves as the adhesions undergo their natural course of dissolution and reformation. The fact that the adhesions contain little scar tissue probably explains why the incidence of strangulation is so rare in the early postoperative setting. Many clinicians have suggested a relatively long trial of nonoperative therapy, perhaps 2 to 4 weeks, before considering surgical intervention. Clearly, there are some patients who have more severe forms of obstruction, for example, twisting of the mesentery, internal herniations, or bowel sutured in the abdominal closure, who will require prompt surgical correction, even in the early postoperative period.

Prevention

Adhesion formation can be reduced by avoiding excessive tissue ischemia, trauma, and manipulation. Because fibrin deposition is an initiating event in adhesion formation, anticoagulants (e.g., heparin and dextran) or thrombolytic agents (e.g., streptokinase and urokinase) have been used, but with minimal success. Several synthetic agents have been developed that may reduce the incidence of adhesions. Becker et al.[51] reported a prospective, randomized study using a bioresorbable membrane placed anterior to all bowel loops in patients undergoing colectomy–ileoanal pouch procedures with diverting loop ileostomies. At the time of ileostomy closure (8–12 weeks), laparoscopy was used to assess the degree of adhesion formation and showed that 51% of the patients treated with the membrane were free of adhesions, compared to only 5% of control patients. Whether the incidence of chronic adhesions and subsequent small-bowel obstruction will be lowered by using such treatments must be determined by further studies. A decrease in the incidence of adhesive small-bowel obstruction may be anticipated as laparoscopic operations replace formal laparotomies because it is well recognized that laparoscopy leads to minimal adhesion formation. In patients who are to receive postoperative pelvic radiotherapy, radiation-induced small-bowel strictures may be prevented by placement of a pelvic "sling" at the time of initial laparotomy, thereby restraining the small intestine in the upper abdomen and out of the radiation field.[52]

Crohn's Disease

In 1932, Crohn, Ginsberg, and Oppenheimer published their report of "regional ileitis," indicating that a cure for this disease could come only with complete surgical resection.[53] In fact, the authors reasoned that one of their patients who had presented with recurrent disease must have had an "incomplete" removal of the diseased bowel. Since that time, much has been learned regarding the natural history and pathophysiology of Crohn's disease. Although the etiology of Crohn's disease remains a mystery, a number of factors (e.g., environmental, genetic, and microbial) appear to play contributory roles.[54] The medical management of patients with Crohn's disease has focused primarily on the inflammatory process because activated T cells seem to be at the root of this disease. Indications for operation in Crohn's disease generally fall under the categories of (1) intractability, (2) luminal complications such as obstruction or hemorrhage, and (3) extraluminal complications such as perforation or fistula.

Intractibility

Elective operation in patients with Crohn's disease should be considered when nonoperative treatment has failed to control the symptoms. One must take into account side effects of medical therapy, notably steroid treatment, which can lead to excessive bone loss, diabetes, and weight gain, among other problems. Any discussion regarding elective surgery for Crohn's disease must include the issue of recurrent disease and the recognition that surgery rarely offers a permanent cure. Past experience shows that approximately 70% of patients with Crohn's disease ultimately come to operation at least once in their lifetime.[55]

Luminal Complications

Chronic inflammation with stricture formation can cause mechanical obstruction in some patients. The strictures may be either single or multiple with intervening "skip areas." In the setting of an acute small-bowel obstruction, a careful history often reveals some element of dietary indiscretion, for example, undigestible fiber products such as raw fruits or vegetables. Because luminal small-bowel obstruction related to Crohn's strictures does not lead to strangulation, initial nonoperative management is indicated and is usually successful. In Crohn's patients who have had prior surgery, however, the etiology for the obstruction could be an adhesive band, and in these cases a strangulating mechanism may exist.

Although most patients with acute small-bowel obstruction caused by a Crohn's stricture will improve, recurrent bouts of obstruction can be an indication for operation. Depending on the number, location, and length of the strictures, either resection or stricturoplasty should be performed. Stricturoplasty can be accomplished in several different ways, most notably the Heineke-Mickelicz and Finney methods. Interestingly, sites of stricturoplasty generally heal very nicely with a low incidence of suture line breakdown or recurrent stricture. For example, of 698 stricturoplasties in 162 patients reported from the Cleveland Clinic in 1996, the 5-year reoperative recurrence rate was 28%, but in only 5% of the patients was the new stricture at the previous stricturoplasty site. In other words, most reoperations were performed for "new" sites of disease. These same authors reported a significant decrease in the oral steroid dose following stricturoplasty, suggesting that this pharmacological therapy was often used for obstructive symptoms.[56] Clearly, stricturoplasty avoids the need for resection and subsequent loss of bowel mucosal surface area, which may be important for preventing the short-bowel syndrome that occurs in some patients with recurrent Crohn's disease. Interestingly, it is not known whether the mucosa at the site of a stricturoplasty functions normally in regard to nutrient digestion and absorption.

Although most Crohn's strictures are easily identified at the time of laparotomy, occasionally a luminal stricture can exist at a site that appears grossly normal from the serosal aspect and could therefore go unrecognized at the time of surgery. To prevent this problem, a balloon catheter can be inserted through one of the enterotomy sites and threaded along the entire length of the small bowel, thus ensuring that the lumen is widely patent throughout its entire course.

If a Crohn's stricture is too long to perform a stricturoplasty, for example, greater than 8 to 10 cm, or if there are separate strictures that are too close to allow for individual stricturoplasties to be performed, resection is indicated. Although Crohn and colleagues originally suggested that the resection must be carried at least 2 feet proximal to the site of disease, we now know that recurrence rates are unaffected by the presence of microscopic disease at resection margins. Fazio et al.[57] reported a randomized control trial comparing a limited (2-cm) versus extended (12-cm) margin in relation to the macroscopically involved area. In this series of 131 patients with a median follow-up of 56 months, the authors found no relationship between recurrence and resection margins. These prospective data confirmed earlier findings from retrospective analysis demonstrating no association between anastomotic recurrence and clinical or histological features at the time of the original resection.[58] As such, it appears that only grossly involved bowel needs to be resected.

The decision to operate for a Crohn's stricture should be based on clinical parameters and not on the radiologic picture. Goldberg et al.[59] reported the radiographic data from the National Cooperative Crohn's disease study. They reviewed barium studies from more than 400 patients and found little evidence of radiographic improvement during the study period and little correlation between the clinical response and evidence of radiologic improvement. Given the lack of correlation between radiographic findings and clinical symptoms, these authors concluded that the ritual use of x-ray to follow patients with Crohn's disease is unnecessary.

Endoscopic dilation has been used as an alternative to either resection or stricturoplasty in some patients with Crohn's strictures. This technique has generally been employed in patients with recurrent disease at an ileocolic anastomosis, a site that can be accessed at the time of colonoscopy. Although endoscopic dilation has been used successfully, relatively high failure rates have been reported along with significant risks of complications such as perforation.[60]

There is an increase in the incidence of carcinoma in Crohn's disease. Greenstein et al.[61] estimated the cancer risk in 589 patients with Crohn's disease and found an increased incidence of colon cancer, similar in magnitude to that found with left-sided ulcerative colitis but less than that found in universal ulcerative colitis. The incidence of small-bowel cancer in the Crohn's patients was greatly increased in the combined group of regional enteritis and ileocolitis (observed/expected [O/E] = 85.8) and even more so in the regional enteritis group alone (O/E = 114.5). The presence of a neoplasm may be suggested in a patient with long-standing Crohn's who develops an unresolving obstruction. If carcinoma is suggested by the clinical or radiolographic picture, then clearly surgical intervention is mandated, but in most patients with small-intestinal carcinoma complicating Crohn's disease the neoplasm is found incidentally. Massive hemorrhage is unusual in Crohn's disease but can be an indication for urgent operation. More common is the occurrence of occult bleeding, contributing to the chronic anemia associated with Crohn's disease. Because of the increased risk of small-bowel cancer in long-standing Crohn's disease, malignancy should be excluded by intraoperative biopsy at the time of stricturoplasty, especially if ulcerated mucosa is seen.

Extraluminal Complications

Patients who present with acute abdominal pain and evidence of localized peritonitis often have an extraluminal complication of their disease. Small perforations or "microperforations" are usually manifested by signs of infection, including pain, fever, and leukocytosis. Occasionally, an inflammatory mass can be palpated, and radiologic evaluation by CT will show evidence of extraluminal inflammatory changes. A frank abscess may be amenable to radiologically guided catheter drainage, leading to a more rapid resolution of the infection. Jawhari et al.[62] reviewed 27 drainage procedures in 24 Crohn's patients and found that surgery was avoided in approximately half these cases, a benefit that was maintained on long-term follow-up. These authors also reported a shorter hospital stay for those patients who were successfully drained percutaneously. Most patients with microperforation respond to bowel rest, intravenous hydration, and intravenous antibiotics. The use of steroids in this setting is controversial because of concern that inhibition of the immune response could lead to rapid deterioration in regard to the underlying infection. Rarely, a gross perforation from Crohn's disease leads to diffuse peritonitis and to mandatory, urgent laparotomy with resection of the involved segment.

The extraluminal component of Crohn's inflammation can lead to the development of fistulae, whether enteroenteric, enterocutaneous, enterovesicle, or enterovaginal. The existence of a fistula is not in itself an indication for operation. Rather, initial therapy should be focused on ensuring the absence of undrained or ongoing sepsis. Once the infectious process is controlled, operative intervention to alleviate symptoms that may be related to the underlying fistula may be appropriate.

Recurrence

In patients operated on for small-bowel Crohn's disease, the most common site for recurrence is the neoterminal ileum, with the inflammatory changes typically ending abruptly at the anastomotic line. In contrast, in patients who initially present with ileocolitis, a majority (approximately 65%) of the recurrences also involve the colon. The reported clinical recurrence rates in Crohn's disease have varied widely but are generally in the range of 35% at 5 years, 55% at 10 years, and approximately 75% by 15 years. The presence of a symptomatic recurrence, however, does not always mandate surgery, and the need for reoperation is approximately 10 percentage points lower at each of the intervals.

Rutgeerts and colleagues[63] employed colonoscopic surveillance in patients following restorative operations and found that within 1 year more than 70% of patients had developed recurrent endoscopic lesions, usually consisting of aphthous ulcers in the preanastomotic region. By 3 years following an operation, up to 85% of patients developed recurrent lesions as assessed by endoscopic surveillance. The subsequent clinical course could be predicted by the endoscopic findings in that patients having no or few lesions at 1 year tended to have more prolonged clinical remissions, whereas those with severe involvement had earlier clinical relapses. These reports of early endoscopic recurrences serve as an important reminder to clinicians that operation in patients with Crohn's disease should be reserved for those with significant complications because a "complete cure" is rarely attained. There is little evidence to support medical therapy as prophylaxis to prevent recurrence following resection (Table 49.5).

Occasionally, during operation for suspected acute appendicitis, acute ileitis is found. This entity is usually caused by an infectious process such as that caused by *Yersinia*.[64] Because it is rare for acute ileitis to progress into a chronic Crohn's disease, surgical resection is not indicated. The acute enteritis can generally be distinguished from Crohn's disease on the basis of the history and the findings at operation. In infectious ileitis, the serosal surface appears red in color with edema of the wall and perhaps with enlarged mesenteric lymph nodes, whereas Crohn's disease is usually associated with fibrosis, thickening of the mesentery, and creeping fat. Assuming the cecum itself is uninvolved, removal of the appendix at the time of surgery is indicated to avoid diagnostic dilemmas in the future. Crohn's disease of the appendix is quite rare and usually is not associated with synchronous or metachronous lesions in the bowel. Appendectomy is curative in approximately 90% to 95% of the cases.

TABLE 49.5. Drug Therapy to Prevent Postoperative Recurrence in Small-Intestinal Crohn's Disease.

Potentially beneficial	*No benefit*
Mesalamine (Asacol)	Sulfasalazine
Metronidazole	Prednisone

Perforative Versus Nonperforative Disease

Patients with Crohn's disease can be generally categorized into either "stricturing" or "fistulizing" groups. If a patient initially presents with fistulizing disease, that is, perforation or involvement of adjacent organs, then that patient's recurrent disease following operation will generally manifest in a similar way. In contrast, those patients with stricturing disease who initially present with signs and symptoms of obstruction tend to have recurrent strictures following an initial operation. Furthermore, Lautenbach et al.[65] examined risk factors for early postoperative recurrence in Crohn's disease and found that if the initial indication for resection was a perforation, then the risk of an early postoperative recurrence was increased. As our understanding of the genetic factors related to Crohn's disease improves, it is likely one day we will be able to predict one's clinical course or phenotype based on the individual's genetic profile.[66]

Laparoscopic Surgery for Crohn's Disease

A number of centers have reported early experiences with laparoscopic surgery for Crohn's disease. Unfortunately, the recurrent and inflammatory nature of Crohn's disease has limited the application of minimally invasive techniques. For example, those patients who have had multiple previous operations may have extensive adhesions throughout the peritoneal cavity, thereby precluding a laparoscopic approach. In addition, in some patients with marked thickening of the mesentery, including the presence of a mass or phlegmon, laparoscopic manipulation of the bowel can be difficult and even dangerous.

However, Wu et al.[67] reported on 46 laparoscopically assisted ileocolic resections, comparing those patients with an abscess or phlegmon and recurrent disease at previous anastomotic sites with patients having no previous operation and no phlegmon or abscess. All three laparoscopic groups compared favorably with a consecutive group of open ileocolic resections in regard to overall morbidity and hospital stay. In addition, these authors did not find that abscess, phlegmon, recurrent disease, or previous ileocolic anastomosis were contraindications to a successful laparoscopically assisted operation.

Laparoscopic Crohn's surgery generally involves an assisted technique in which the bowel is mobilized from its peritoneal attachments, and a small incision is then enlarged to deliver the intestine and perform an extracorporeal resection and anastomosis. The ideal candidate for such an approach would be a patient whose disease is limited to a segment of terminal ileum because mobilization of the distal small intestine and right colon can be easily accomplished using the laparoscopic approach. Reissman et al.[68] reported on 30 ileocolic resections with average length of stay of 5.2 days and a 10% morbidity. Importantly, the complications associated with these ileocolic resections were far less than in a series of patients with ulcerative colitis undergoing laparoscopically assisted total colectomies. The indications for a minimally invasive approach in Crohn's disease remain undefined. Clearly, if identical results regarding the bowel disease can be attained through a smaller incision and with less morbidity, then such approaches should be pursued.

Small-Bowel Fistula

A fistula is an abnormal communication between two epithelial-lined surfaces. The actual communication between the two surfaces can become completely epithelialized but in most cases is lined by simple granulation tissue. Internal fistulae can be surgically created (e.g., gastroenterostomy, cholodochojejunostomy), but internal fistulae can also occur as a complication of an underlying disease process and often require surgical correction. External fistulae, on the other hand, almost always require surgical intervention for physiological or psychosocial reasons.

Etiology

Almost all intestinal fistulae are acquired in the course of a disease process along with its associated operative interventions. Rarely, a patient vitelline duct produces a spontaneous umbilical fistula, indicating communication with the underlying ileum. To understand the principles of the management of patients with intestinal fistulae, it is important to recognize that most fistulae, regardless of location or etiology, will close spontaneously as long as the conditions are conducive to healing. If one or more of the following situations exist, however, then the fistula will not heal unless the underlying problem is addressed: distal obstruction, presence of a foreign body, malignancy, undrained associated abscess, radiation injury, or an underlying inflammatory process such as Crohn's disease (Table 49.6). The management of a patient with a fistula must first address the issues of fluid, electrolytes, and nutrition. This step should be followed by an assessment of the underlying process and a determination regarding whether the fistula is likely to heal spontaneously.

Nonoperative Management

Patients with intestinal fistulae often lose fluids and electrolytes in large amounts, especially when the site of involvement is the proximal gut. In these patients, adequate fluid and electrolyte replacement must be instituted and can ideally be accomplished via the enteral route, although parenteral supplementation may be required. In some cases, an attempt should be made to minimize fistula output, for example, by bowel rest and treatment with the long-acting somatostatin analog octreotide. Octreotide must be given parenterally and appears to be effective in reducing intestinal secretions. It is unclear, however, whether somatostatin treatment or the amount of fistula output actually affects the time to healing of the fistula.

Sitges-Sera et al. reported on a series of 27 patients with enterocutaneous fistulae treated with octreotide. They suggested that the drug was effective in reducing fistula output when compared with placebo, but compared with a historical series, the rate of spontaneous fistula closure was not modified by octreotide.[69] In two randomized studies, octreotide was not shown to be efficacious in patients with enterocutaneous fistulae. Scott et al. reported on 19 patients and found no difference in fistula output between patients given placebo or octreotide, and there was no benefit in terms of fistula closure rate.[70] Likewise, in a study of 31 patients with either intestinal or pancreatic fistulae, Sancho et al. found that treatment with octreotide did not alter the spontaneous fistula closure rate when compared to a placebo.[71] Based on these studies, if the situation is such that fistula healing is expected, it is likely that allowing enteral nutrition and avoiding the potential side effects of octreotide outweigh the potential benefits of bowel rest and octreotide.

Skin breakdown at the site of an external (enterocutaneous) fistula must be prevented. Activated enzymes within the intestinal lumen can cause significant maceration of the skin, leading to irritation, cellulitis, and even frank tissue loss. Simple measures using stoma appliances or topical agents can usually prevent these problems.

TABLE 49.6. Factors That Prevent Healing of Intestinal Fistulae.

Distal obstruction
Malignancy
Foreign body
Associated undrained infection
Radiation injury to tissues
Underlying inflammatory condition (e.g., Crohn's disease)

Radiologic Evaluation

Depending on the clinical scenario, the site of the fistula can often be predicted. In some cases, however, contrast studies with either oral agents or via direct injection through an external fistula opening are required to precisely determine the site of the problem. Abdominal CT scanning can often be useful in identifying both the fistula site and possibly the underlying disease process. The clinical and radiologic evaluation must be put in context of previous surgical procedures, including careful review of operative notes, to ascertain the proper diagnosis.

Surgical Treatment

The surgical approach involves takedown of the fistula and resection of the underlying involved/diseased bowel. Great care must be taken in the setting of irradiated bowel because healing can be impaired, and the risks of recurrent fistula formation are high. In the case of internal fistulae, the key principle is removal of the underlying diseased bowel. The "target" organ is generally intrinsically normal and therefore usually heals easily with minimal intervention. For example, simple suture closure and postoperative drainage of the bladder are usually sufficient in cases of enterovesicle fistula in Crohn's disease as long as the diseased bowel is completely dissected off the bladder and removed. Similarly, in patients with ileosigmoid fistulae related to Crohn's disease, the sigmoid colon is usually intrinsically normal and can be treated with simple suture closure. A preoperative sigmoidoscopic exam is important, however, to make sure that the colon is indeed free of Crohn's disease.

TABLE 49.7. Relative Frequency of Benign Neoplasms of the Small Intestine.

Type	*Relative frequency (%)*
Leiomyoma	30–35
Adenoma	20–25
Lipoma	15
Hemangioma	10
Fibroma	5
Other	15

TABLE 49.8. Relative Frequency and Prognosis of Malignant Neoplasms of the Small Bowel.

Type	*Frequency (%)*	*5-year survival (%)*
Adenocarcinoma	40	15–25
Carcinoid	25	50–60
Lymphoma	25	40–50
Sarcoma	10	35–50

Small-Bowel Neoplasms

General Considerations

Incidence and Pathogenesis

Although the small intestine represents 90% of the surface area of the gastrointestinal tract, tumors of this organ account for only 1% (0.6 to 1.4 per 100,000) of all gastrointestinal neoplasms and 0.3% of all tumors. A number of hypotheses have been put forth to explain the markedly lower incidence of small-bowel compared to colorectal cancer.[72,73]

Clinical Presentation

The most common modes of presentation are intestinal obstruction and occult gastrointestinal hemorrhage. Obstruction is often intermittent or partial and may be associated with diarrhea. Obstruction may involve intussusception, particularly for benign neoplasms in adults. Malignant tumors may cause obstruction by circumferential growth, growth into adjacent structures causing fixation and adhesive obstruction, or kinking due to longitudinal growth along the bowel wall. Occasionally, the presentation involves the development of a palpable but otherwise asymptomatic abdominal mass. Perforation and gross bleeding are rare. The clinical presentation is often vague, and a correct preoperative diagnosis is reached in only one-third of patients even in modern series.[74]

Pathology and Differential Diagnosis

Benign lesions include adenoma, leiomyoma, fibroma, hamartoma, lipoma, hemangioma, lymphangioma, myxoma, and neurogenic tumors. The most common malignant tumors are adenocarcinoma, leiomyosarcoma, lymphoma, and carcinoid. The relative incidence varies from series to series due to the rarity of small-bowel tumors in general (Tables 49.7 and 49.8). Small-bowel neoplasms are associated with a number of disease states.[75] Hamartomatous polyps of the small intestine (particularly the jejunum and ileum) occur as part of Peutz-Jeghers syndrome. Gardner's syndrome and familial polyposis coli predispose to small-bowel adenoma, whereas Crohn's disease of the small bowel and celiac disease predispose to adenocarcinoma. Celiac disease and Crohn's disease also predispose to small-bowel lymphoma, as do certain immunodeficiency states and autoimmune disorders. The differential diagnosis of neoplasms includes endometriosis, congenital pancreatic rest, splenosis, and duplication cysts.

Diagnosis

Delay in the diagnosis of small-bowel tumors is frequently the result of failure to obtain appropriate imaging studies or misinterpretation of such studies.[76] A variety of diagnostic tools are available in the setting of suspected small-bowel neoplasm (Table 49.9). Plain abdominal films may show obstruction but are nonspecific and usually unhelpful. Many tumors are within the reach of an upper endoscopy or simple upper gastrointestinal series. However, a more extended view of the small intestine is often necessary, such as small-bowel follow-through (SBFT) or enteroclysis.[77] Push endoscopy

TABLE 49.9. Comparison of Diagnostic Imaging Used in Evaluation of Suspected Small-Bowel Neoplasms.

	Advantage	*Disadvantage*
Plain abdominal film	May show obstruction	Nonspecific
UGI/SBFT	May show mass lesion, mucosal defect, or intussusception	No visualization outside lumen; not helpful in staging
Enteroclysis	More sensitive than conventional SBFT	Requires duodenal tube and additional technical skill
Computed tomography	Allows staging; may aid in diagnosis of tumor type	Lacks visualization of lumen or mucosal surface
Upper endoscopy	Direct visualization of mucosal surface of duodenum; allows for biopsy or polypectomy	Invasive; limited to duodenum and may miss submucosal lesions unless combined with endoscopic ultrasound
Push endoscopy	Extends visualization into proximal jejunum; allows for biopsy	Same as conventional endoscopy
Extended small-bowel endoscopy	Allows visualization of up to 70% of small bowel; more sensitive than enteroclysis	No biopsy capability; may take up to 8h to pass scope; increased patient discomfort

UGI/SBFT, upper gastrointestinal series/small-bowel follow-through.

utilizing a pediatric colonoscope allows extended visualization beyond the duodenum into the proximal jejunum and direct visualization of the mucosal surface as well as biopsy or polypectomy. Extended small-bowel enteroscopy, which requires a specialized endoscope and relies on peristalsis for instrument advancement, allows visualization of as much as 70% of the small-bowel surface. However, this approach may require 8h to pass the endoscope and is associated with substantial patient discomfort. Abdominal CT is frequently obtained during the course of evaluation of patients with vague abdominal complaints and may demonstrate a tumor mass. It may also be useful in preoperative staging because extraluminal spread and nodal or liver metastases may be detected. Capsule endoscopy is being increasingly used in the setting of chronic, low-grade small-bowel obstruction or bleeding and may detect a malignant lesion.[78]

Benign Neoplasms

Presentation and Management

Many benign lesions cause no symptoms and are discovered only incidentally. Adenomas are the most common, but leiomyomas are the most common lesions that cause symptoms. The presentation is usually obstruction or occult hemorrhage. Surgical excision is almost always indicated because of the obstruction or hemorrhage, the potential risk of complications, and the inherent impossibility of definitively confirming benign disease in the absence of full microscopic evaluation. Occasionally, small lesions may be simply excised via enterotomy. More commonly, segmental resection and primary anastomosis is appropriate. The entire small bowel must be carefully inspected to exclude additional lesions.

Adenoma

Three major histological subtypes are recognized: tubular adenoma, villous adenoma, and Brunner's gland adenoma. Tubular adenomas are often asymptomatic but may bleed or cause obstruction if large; they have low malignant potential. Villous adenomas have greater malignant potential. At least 30% harbor malignant foci on detailed microscopic evaluation.[79] Endoscopic polypectomy or submucosal resection may suffice if there is clearly no invasive carcinoma; however, segmental resection is more appropriate when technically feasible. Villous tumors of the duodenum are often periampullary and may necessitate pancreaticoduodenectomy,[80] although in selected patients local submucosal or full-thickness excision may achieve acceptable long-term results while avoiding the morbidity of more extensive extirpative surgery. Brunner's gland adenomas represent hyperplasia of the exocrine glands of the duodenum and have little malignant potential.

In the setting of familial polyposis syndromes such as adenomatous polyposis coli (APC), the duodenal surface and particularly the periampullary region may be carpeted with adenomatous growth, suggesting the presence of a more generalized field defect in terms of neoplastic susceptibility. For reasons that are not entirely clear, the stomach and proximal jejunum are usually relatively or completely spared of substantial polyp formation; this may reflect either an inherent increased susceptibility of duodenal mucosa to neoplastic change or, more likely, the adverse influence of high local concentrations of pancreaticobiliary fluid on susceptible tissue in this region. Progression of duodenal adenomas to invasive carcinoma is less frequent than of colonic adenomas in APC syndromes.[81] Indeed, some evidence suggests that selected patients may be monitored for the development of at least moderate dysplasia in these lesions (which may take years to occur if at all) before recommending aggressive resection. The logic of this conservative approach lies in the avoidance of resection and further digestive sequelae in patients who have already in most cases required total colectomy and for whom the risk of additional polyp formation in the remaining intestine cannot be eliminated.

Leiomyoma and Other Intestinal Stromal Tumors

Intestinal stromal tumors occur most frequently in the jejunum and may reach considerable size before diagnosis. Occasionally, these lesions present as a palpable, movable abdominal mass (Fig. 49.13). Symptoms may include obstruction caused by intraluminal tumor growth or pain and bleeding due to tumor necrosis. Many are asymptomatic and are found only incidentally. Hemorrhage is the most common indication for operation, and segmental resection is the recommended treatment. The cell of origin of a given tumor can generally be determined by immunohistochemical staining to characterize differentiation toward smooth muscle cells (leiomyoma), Schwann cells (schwannoma), enteric glial, or nerve cells. However, it may be difficult to confidently distinguish benign from malignant stromal tumors.

Tumor grade, which is based on mitotic activity and size, appears to correlate somewhat with prognosis. Lesions that harbor no more than five mitoses per 50 high-power fields and measure less than 5cm almost always follow a benign course. Lesions larger than 5cm, even with low mitotic index, behave malignantly, with about 50% of patients dead of recurrent disease within 3 years.[82]

A subset of mesenchymal tumors of the small bowel are gastrointestinal stromal tumors (GISTs), which are thought to derive from the interstitial cell of Cajal. About one-third of GISTs originate in the small bowel (the majority are found in the stomach). These tumors are associated with mutations

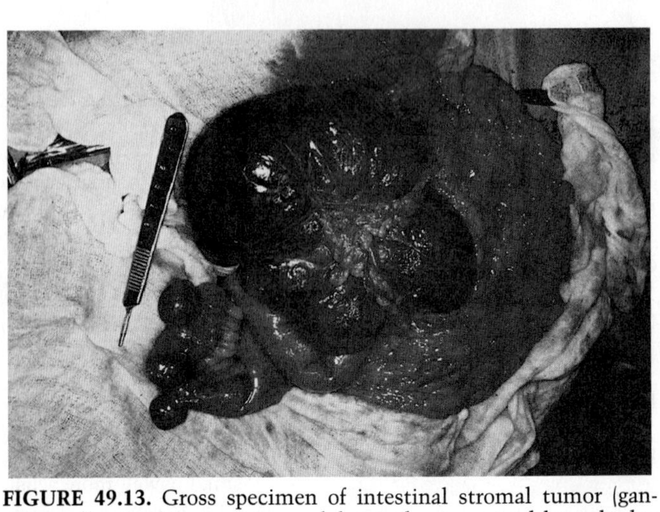

FIGURE 49.13. Gross specimen of intestinal stromal tumor (ganglion cell origin) presenting as abdominal pain caused by volvulus and tumor necrosis.

in the *c-kit* protooncogene and typically stain on immunohistochemistry for CD117 (the product of the *c-kit* gene). Up to two-thirds of GISTs are malignant.

Lipoma

Lipomas lesions occur most commonly in the ileum, have no malignant potential, and do not require removal unless symptomatic. A lipoma may form the lead point for intussusception. Bleeding may occur if the overlying mucosa becomes ulcerated. Computed tomography may distinguish lipomas of the small bowel from other lesions because of their characteristic low-attenuation appearance.

Peutz-Jeghers Syndrome

Peutz-Jeghers syndrome is an inherited disorder consisting of mucocutaneous melanotic pigmentation and gastrointestinal polyps. The syndrome is autosomal dominant with a high degree of penetrance. The polyps are hamartomatous and occur primarily in the jejunum and ileum; however, more than half of patients also have polyps in the colon or rectum, and 25% have gastric polyps. The pigmented lesions are small, 1- to 2-mm brown or black spots that occur singly or multiply in the oral cavity or in perioral or perianal areas. Lesions may also be evident on the palms or fingers, forearms, or soles of feet. Polyposis may develop in the absence of pigmentation lesions. Individual lesions may present with bleeding or obstruction, the latter often in the setting of intussusception.

Because of the diffuse involvement of the intestinal tract, surgical therapy should be confined to limited segments of bowel clearly producing symptoms. Occasionally, prophylactic subtotal colectomy may be indicated if there is a substantial colonic polyp burden and if the hamartomas reveal adenomatous changes. The risk of gastrointestinal cancer in Peutz-Jeghers syndrome is estimated at 18 times greater than that expected in the general population[83] Therefore, screening upper endoscopy and colonoscopy are recommended starting at age 20, followed by annual flexible sigmoidoscopy and by complete upper and lower examination every 3 years.

Malignant Neoplasms

Presentation and Management

Malignant neoplasms of the small intestine present much like benign lesions, typically with obstruction or occult bleeding. Delay in diagnosis is common, leading to advanced disease at presentation. Surgical resection is seldom curative for these advanced lesions.[84] Optimal treatment consists of wide resection, including regional lymph nodes. For duodenal neoplasms, pancreaticoduodenectomy is recommended unless the lesion is locally advanced, in which case palliative gastrojejunostomy is indicated. For malignant tumors of the small bowel, resection should be performed even if cure is not possible because possible complications of bleeding, obstruction, and perforation are prevented. If resection is not possible, side-to-side enteroenterostomy for bypass of the affected segment is recommended.

The relative incidence of various small-bowel malignancies varies from series to series. Some population-based studies, such as the Utah Cancer Registry,[73] indicated that carcinoid tumors are the most common small-bowel malignancy. However, in collected population-based series, adenocarcinoma is the most common, occurring in 3.9 per million people, followed by carcinoid (2.9 per million), lymphoma (1.6 per million), and sarcoma (1.2 per million).[85] Patients typically present in the sixth or seventh decade of life, with a slight male predominance. Overall survival after treatment appears to be greater in population- than hospital-based series (50% vs. 20% 5-year survival).[73,84,86]

Adenocarcinoma

Adenocarcinoma represents about half of all small-bowel malignancies in hospital-based series. These lesions are twice as common in men than women. Adenocarcinoma typically presents with weight loss, bleeding, anemia, obstruction, or (when periampullary) jaundice. The adenoma-to-carcinoma sequence appears to apply for the small bowel,[87] and activating mutations in codon 12 of the oncogene K-ras are as common in proximal small-bowel cancers (50% incidence) as in colorectal cancer.[88,89] Most lesions are located in the proximal bowel, except in the setting of Crohn's disease, in which most are ileal (Table 49.10).[90] Carcinoma should be suspected in patients with long-standing Crohn's disease who develop a change in their clinical status. Rarely, adenocarcinoma develops late (>20 years) after construction of an ileostomy, usually at the mucocutaneous junction.[91]

Resection is the best treatment for small-bowel adenocarcinoma. Pancreaticoduodenectomy is used for tumors involving the second or third portion of the duodenum.[92] Tumors of the fourth portion can usually be resected with sparing of the ampullary region[93]; a side-to-side duodenojejunostomy is simpler than an end-to-end reconstruction after this resection. Five-year survival for completely resected duodenal cancer ranges from 38% to 45% even in the presence of lymph node metastases.[94] Right colectomy is indicated for distal ileal lesions. Node-negative patients have a 5-year survival of 60% to 70%, but overall the prognosis is poor (15%–35% 5-year survival) because the majority of patients present late.[73,90] At present, there is no convincing evidence that adjuvant chemotherapy or radiation treatments are effective.[84]

Leiomyosarcoma and Malignant Stromal Tumors

Most small-bowel sarcomas are leiomyosarcomas, representing 10% to 20% of all malignant small-bowel tumors. These lesions may grow to considerable size before the development of symptoms. Leiomyosarcoma may spread by direct extension or may metastasize hematogenously to liver, lungs, or bone. As for other small-bowel neoplasms, wide en bloc resection with the associated mesentery is the treatment of choice. Extended lymphadenectomy is not indicated because lymphatic metastasis is rare. Five-year survival varies between

TABLE 49.10. Anatomical Distribution of Tumors (%).

	Carcinoid	*Adenocarcinoma*	*Lymphoma*	*Sarcoma*
Duodenum	6	50	12	16
Jejunum	20	28	40	26
Ileum	74	22	48	58

Source: DiSario et al.[73]

TABLE 49.11. Primary Intestinal Lymphoma.

	Adult Western	*Childhood*	*Immunoproliferative small-intestinal disease*	*Enteropathy-associated T-cell lymphoma*
Population	Nonspecific	Children	Low socioeconomic class; parasitic infestation	Celiac disease, malabsorption
Geography	Worldwide	Worldwide	Common in Middle East, Mediterranean	Common in Middle East
Peak incidence (decade of life)	Sixth	First	Second, third	Fourth, fifth
Signs and symptoms	Pain, perforation, obstruction, hemorrhage	Tender abdominal mass, acute intussusception	Pain, fever, diarrhea, steatorrhea, vomiting, wasting disease, circulating IgA-α heavy chain	Deterioration in chronic condition, malnutrition, acute abdomen, rising IgA titers
Location	Small intestine	Ileum	Jejunum, duodenum	Distal small bowel, disseminates early
Pathology	Large tumors, B cell in 75%, large-cell diffuse histology	Burkitt's type, small noncleaved B cell	Nodularity of long segments of small intestine, IgA-producing B cells	Villous atrophy, crypt hyperplasia, large T-cell origin
Prognosis	By stage	Very good for stages I and II, tumor bulk important factor	May undergo spontaneous regression but overall poor prognosis	Poor due to early disseminated disease
Therapy	Surgery, adjuvant chemotherapy and radiation	Surgery for early stage, chemotherapy major role	Antibiotics, aggressive chemotherapy	Chemotherapy, surgery only for complications

Source: Modified after Turowski and Basson. Am J Surg 1995;169:433–441.[159]

10% and 50%.[73] Criteria for malignancy include the number of mitoses (more than five per 50 high-power fields), nuclear atypia, the presence of necrosis, and cellularity. Tumor grade correlates with survival.[94] Low-grade lesions (fewer than 10 mitoses per 50 high-power fields) have an 80% disease-free survival rate at 8 years. High-grade lesions, however, have a median disease-free survival of less than 18 months. Palliative resections and bypass procedures are warranted because some of these tumors may be rather slow growing. There is no evidence that adjuvant chemotherapy or radiation therapy alone or in combination is effective.[84] The treatment of malignant GIST is primarily surgical. However, GIST tumors have been shown to be sensitive to the tyrosine kinase inhibitor imatinib, which inhibits the kinase activity of CD117. The use of imatinib in the adjuvant and possibly neoadjuvant setting has been the subject of recent study.[95]

Lymphoma

Lymphomas represent 10% to 20% of malignant small-bowel tumors. The ileum is the most common site of involvement because of the presence of the greatest amount of gut-associated lymphoid tissue. Primary small-bowel lymphoma is the most common extranodal form of lymphoma. Most are non-Hodgkin's lymphoma and predominantly B cell in origin,[96] although both Hodgkin's disease and plasma cell lymphoma have also been reported. Childhood abdominal lymphomas include Burkitt's lymphoma, undifferentiated non-Burkitt's lymphoma, and diffuse histiocytic lymphoma. Many patients with ostensibly primary small-bowel lymphoma in fact have disseminated disease.

Patients with small-bowel lymphoma commonly present with fatigue, weight loss, and abdominal pain.[97] A severe malabsorption syndrome is seen in about 10% of patients. Perforation, obstruction, bleeding, or intussusception are less-common modes of presentation.[98] Individuals infected with human immunodeficiency virus 1 (HIV-1) have a markedly greater risk of developing non-Hodgkin's lymphoma, usually high grade.[99]

A variant of small-bowel lymphoma referred to as immunoproliferative small-intestinal disease is characterized by involvement of long segments of proximal small intestine with a dense but diffuse lymphoplasmacytic infiltrate.[100] This syndrome is more common in younger patients from underdeveloped countries and presents with abdominal pain, diarrhea, malabsorption, and clubbing of the fingers.[101,102] Patients with long-standing celiac disease may develop a diffuse lymphoma caused by neoplastic proliferation of T-cell clones involved with the enteropathic process.[103] The differences among these entities are summarized in Table 49.11.

Intestinal lymphomas are staged according to a modification of the Ann Arbor system (Table 49.12). Treatment of primary small-bowel lymphoma (Western variety) is mainly surgical. Ideally, complete resection along with a wedge of

TABLE 49.12. Ann Arbor Classification of Primary Gastrointestinal Lymphoma.

Stage	*Subgroups description*
IE	Confined to single site
IIE	Confined below abdomen
IIE1	Regional (mesenteric or perigastric) nodes
IIE2	Distant (e.g., retroperitoneal) nodes
III	Involves organs on both sides of diaphragm
IV	Wide dissemination (liver, spleen)

Source: Modified after Musshoff and Schmidt-Vollmer.[158]

mesentery is accomplished. However, for patients with positive margins, adjuvant therapy is recommended. Survival for completely resected intestinal lymphoma is about 50%. A number of studies would suggest that the combination of surgery and adjuvant chemotherapy (typically CHOP [cyclophosphamide-hydroxydaunomycin-vincristine-prednisone] or a variant thereof) improves outcome stage for stage. Primary gastric lymphoma tends to fare better than primary intestinal lymphoma.[104–106]

Carcinoid Tumors

Carcinoid tumors of the gut represent about 20% to 40% of primary small-intestinal malignancies and are characterized by variable malignant potential and the secretion of multiple neurohormonal substances, notably serotonin and substance P. In population-based studies, carcinoid tumors are the most frequent of small-bowel neoplasms. The cell of origin is the Kulchitsky cell, an enterochromaffin or argentaffin cell located within the crypts of Lieberkuhn. The highest incidence of occurrence is in the sixth decade, although carcinoids have been reported in patients aged 20 to over 80.

Tumors are multicentric in 30% and frequently coexist with other cancers, particularly of the colon, stomach, and breast.[72,107] About 50% of intestinal carcinoids are located in the appendix. Of all nonappendiceal carcinoids, about half are present within the distal 2 feet of the ileum. The rectum is the third most common site. Carcinoids are the most common tumor found within Meckel's diverticula.[108] Grossly, carcinoids appear as firm submucosal nodules with a yellow, tan, or gray cut surface. The tumor may infiltrate the bowel wall and cause shortening and thickening of the mesentery due to an intense desmoplastic reaction. Microscopically, carcinoid tumors appear as solid nests of uniform small cells with round or oval nuclei and a varying amount of surrounding desmoplasia.

Carcinoid tumors often follow an indolent course, with median duration of symptoms up to 2 years before diagnosis. Symptoms tend to be nonspecific; like other small-bowel tumors, carcinoids may bleed, obstruct, or ulcerate. They may also present as segmental mesenteric ischemia associated with the mesenteric angiopathy that accompanies the intense desmoplasia surrounding the tumor. Intestinal obstruction may occur not only because of the primary tumor but also due to kinking of the mesentery from bulky nodal metastases or mesenteric fibrosis[109] (Fig. 49.14).

Radiologic findings may increase clinical suspicion of carcinoid tumors. Small-bowel follow-through examination typically reveals fixed loops of intestine, with angulation, luminal narrowing, or multiple filling defects. Mesenteric calcifications may be present. Computed tomography may show evidence of a fibrotic mesenteric reaction in the vicinity of a transition point between dilated proximal and distal collapsed small bowel (Fig. 49.14). Hepatic metastatic lesions are characteristically hypervascular and thus brightly enhance with intravenous contrast administration. Occasionally, mesenteric angiography performed during preoperative evaluation may reveal focal abnormalities in the mesenteric vasculature; these consist of narrowing of peripheral arterial branches and poor venous drainage. Ileal carcinoid is occasionally misdiagnosed and treated as Crohn's disease.[110,131]I-Metaiodobenzylguanidine (MIBG) scintigraphy may occasionally be useful to localize midgut carcinoid tumors, although the false-negative rate may be as high as 30%.[111]

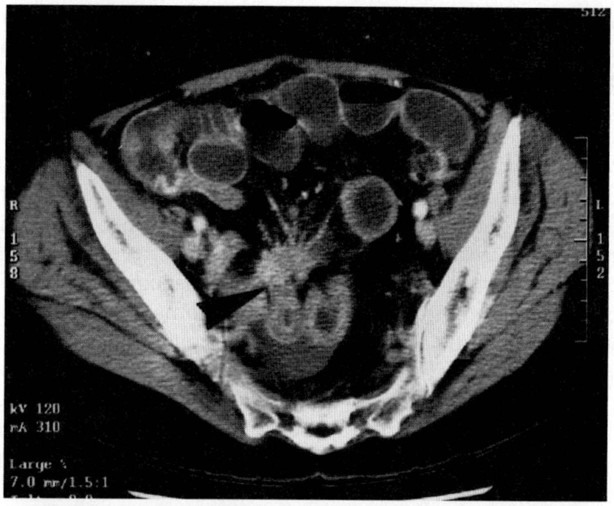

FIGURE 49.14. Intestinal carcinoid tumor (*arrow*), with characteristic surrounding desmoplasia, as demonstrated by CT scan, and intestinal obstruction by tumor deposits.

Metastatic disease is already present in as many as 60% of cases at the time of diagnosis.[112] The malignant potential of carcinoid tumors is related to location, size, depth of penetration, and pattern of growth. Metastasis from appendiceal and rectal carcinoid is uncommon (3%),[113] but in ileal carcinoids, metastatic spread occurs in approximately 35% of cases. It is rare for a carcinoid tumor of the appendix less than 1 cm in diameter to metastasize. Primary tumors of 1 to 2 cm metastasize in about 50% of cases, and tumors larger than 2 cm metastasize in up to 90%. Carcinoid tumors limited to the submucosa are rarely associated with metastases, whereas this is evident in at least two-thirds of lesions that show full-thickness penetration.

The pattern of growth appears to correlate somewhat with prognosis. Mixed insular plus glandular growth carries the best median survival (4.4 years), followed by insular (2.9 years), trabecular (2.5 years), and mixed insular plus trabecular (2.3 years). Glandular and undifferentiated growth patterns fare the worst, each with median survival of less than 1 year.[114] Overall, 5-year survival is approximately 30% to 50%.[115]

Treatment of carcinoid tumors of the small intestine is wide segmental resection. For tumors of the distal ileum, the cecum and right colon should be resected en bloc, and tumors involving the duodenum may require radical pancreaticoduodenectomy. Lesions without nodal metastases are almost always cured by resection. Palliative resections are probably worthwhile because most carcinoid tumors are slow growing.

Carcinoid tumors metastatic to the liver may produce the malignant carcinoid syndrome, which includes episodic diarrhea, flushing, abdominal cramps, and, later, right-sided valvular heart disease and asthma. It is estimated that fewer than 10% of patients with metastatic carcinoid tumors will develop the carcinoid syndrome. Carcinoid syndrome is usually associated with primary tumors of the foregut (lung, stomach, duodenum, pancreas) or the midgut (jejunum and ileum) and only rarely with carcinoids of the hindgut (appendix, colon, rectum).

The pathophysiology of the malignant carcinoid syndrome is largely attributable to elevated circulating levels of serotonin (5-hydroxytryptamine, 5-HT), which increases intestinal peristalsis and evokes intestinal fluid and electrolyte secretion, thereby producing diarrhea and intense abdominal cramping. Occasionally, the pain is quite severe and may reflect serotonin-induced mesenteric vasoconstriction and segmental bowel ischemia. Other symptoms of the carcinoid syndrome include flushing, which is frequently unrelated to diarrhea and may be caused by other mediators such as substance P, bradykinin, or prostaglandins of the E and F series. Elevated levels of serotonin probably induce the irreversible endocardial fibrotic reaction that accounts for the right-sided valvular heart disease seen in advanced cases. Another manifestation of the syndrome is asthma caused by bronchoconstriction induced by 5-HT, bradykinin, or substance P. Finally, carcinoid syndrome occasionally leads to malabsorption and pellagra (dementia, dermatitis, and diarrhea) caused by an acquired tryptophan deficiency.

Confirmation of malignant carcinoid syndrome is made by determination of urinary levels of 5-HIAA (5-hydroxyindolacetic acid), the inactive breakdown product of 5-HT produced by metabolism in the lung and liver. This assay may need to be repeated because a single determination may be normal; alternatively, provocative testing with intravenous pentagastrin, epinephrine, or calcium may be added. Patients with malignant carcinoid syndrome should avoid foods rich in 5-HT, including bananas, pineapples, tomatoes, and walnuts. Certain drugs, such as phenothiazines, glycerol guaicolate, and reserpine, are strongly contraindicated.

If possible, primary and metastatic lesions should be resected or at least debulked as this may produce substantial palliation of the symptoms of carcinoid syndrome. Hepatic artery embolization may be utilized when surgery is not possible and may produce dramatic, although frequently short-lived, relief of symptoms in about 90% of patients.[116] This treatment is not without complications, and a mortality of about 10% has been reported.[117] The long-acting somatostatin analog octreotide also appears to be of some benefit, particularly in patients with carcinoid diarrhea.[117] Some response to the combination of 5-fluorouracil and streptozotocin has been reported, although in general chemotherapy appears to be of limited usefulness. Median survival of patients with carcinoid tumors metastatic to the liver is 3 years, compared to 5 years in patients with nonresectable abdominal disease in the absence of liver metastases.

Other Tumors and Metastatic Lesions

Gastrinoma, somatostatinoma, paraganglioma, and undifferentiated neuroendocrine carcinomas of the small intestine have been reported. These tumors may present as a hormone-specific hyperfunctional state or as nonfunctioning mass lesions. The small bowel is the most common site of melanoma metastatic to the gastrointestinal tract. Primaries from the breast, lung, and kidney metastatic to the small bowel have also been described. Cervical, ovarian, and colonic tumors may involve the small bowel by direct extension. Treatment is, in general, palliative and consists of limited resection or bypass. In patients with small-bowel metastatic melanoma without a known primary, aggressive resection may improve the quality of life and disease-free survival.

Meckel's Diverticulum

In 1808, Johann Meckel described a diverticulum composed of a remnant of the duct between the intestinal tract and the yolk sac.[118] This embryological remnant was found to be the cause of an intussusception by Kuttner in 1898,[118] and in 1904 Salzer[119] described heterotopic gastric mucosa within the diverticulum. In 1907, Deet noted the association between aberrant gastric mucosa within the diverticulum and ulceration of the adjacent ileum.[120]

Based on autopsy series, Meckel's diverticulum is present in 0.3% to 2.5% of the population. The size and shape of the diverticulum can vary greatly, although it is usually between 3 and 5 cm long and is found 10 to 150 cm from the ileocecal valve. Meckel's diverticula contain a mesentery with an independent blood supply from the ileal vessels. There is an association between Meckel's diverticulum and a number of other congenital malformations, including exomphalos, esophageal or anorectal atresia, and various central nervous system or cardiovascular malformations. Although usually lined by mucosa similar to that seen in the adjacent ileum, heterotopic mucosa has been described, including that of gastric, duodenal, colonic, or pancreatic nature.

Mackey and Dineen[121] studied 140 Meckel's diverticula removed incidentally and found approximately 16% containing heterotopic mucosa. In 62 patients in whom the Meckel's was removed because of symptoms, however, the incidence of heterotopic mucosa was 34%, suggesting that the presence of these abnormal cells might be associated with eventual clinical sequelae.

Complications

Meckel's diverticula can be associated with various complications and often require surgical intervention. The presence of gastric mucosa with resultant acid production can lead to ulceration in the adjacent ileal mucosa, causing either hemorrhage or perforation. Perforation can also occur in the diverticulum itself, perhaps related to luminal obstruction from a foreign body. The resultant Meckel's diverticulitis presents with signs and symptoms that are generally indistinguishable from appendicitis. Meckel's diverticulum can also be associated with small-bowel obstruction from intussusception, volvulus, or an associated adhesive band. In rare instances, an umbilical sinus or fistula becomes evident, and even more uncommon is the presence of neoplasm within the diverticulum.

William[122] reviewed 1806 cases and found the incidence of complications as follows: hemorrhage, 31%; inflammation, 25%; bowel obstruction, 16%; bowel obstructions secondary to a band, 16%; intussusception, 11%; hernial involvement, 11%; umbilical sinus/fistula, 4%; and tumor, 2%. Soltero and Bill[123] estimated the chances of a Meckel's diverticulum causing one of these complications to be 4.2% in children, dropping to 3% in adults and almost 0% in the elderly. Special mention should be made of the extremely rare Littre's hernia, which refers to the presence of a Meckel's diverticulum within an inguinal hernia sac.

Diagnostic Studies

Meckel's diverticula are rarely demonstrated on routine barium studies. In the rare instance of an umbilical fistula, however, injection of contrast material directly into the external orifice demonstrates a communication with the underlying ileum, indicating a patent vitelline duct. Such a study will be able to differentiate the intestinal communication from a patent urachus that communicates with the urinary bladder. Technetium Tc 99m pertechnetate Meckel's scan detects the gastric mucosa within the Meckel's diverticulum and has been reported to be 90% accurate.[124] Meckel's diverticulum can also be detected angiographically, as shown by Mitchell et al.,[125] who reviewed angiograms in 16 patients and found that 69% had a persistent vitellointestinal artery; in another 4 patients, other angiographic abnormalities were seen, including a vascular blush, early venous return, and arterial irregularity. These authors concluded that angiography will detect a Meckel's diverticulum in most patients based primarily on the demonstration of a persistent vitellointestinal artery. However, because of the presence of overlying vessels, superselective catheterization of distal ileal arteries may be needed to detect this abnormality.

Surgical Treatment

When a Meckel's diverticulum causes symptoms or complications, resection is indicated. Either excision of the diverticulum alone or resection of the adjacent segment of ileum containing the diverticulum is acceptable. In most cases, simple excision is satisfactory as long as care is taken to avoid narrowing of the ileal lumen. Resection of the adjacent ileum should be performed in patients with peptic ulceration or if the base of the diverticulum is involved with an inflammatory process or neoplasm.

Whether to remove an asymptomatic Meckel's diverticulum found incidentally at the time of surgery is a matter of some debate. Cullen et al. performed an epidemiological, population-based study in Olmstead County, Minnesota, and concluded that Meckel's diverticula discovered incidentally at operation should be removed in most patients.[126] In contrast, Peoples et al.[127] reviewed their experience in 90 incidental diverticulectomies. Using a decision analysis, they reported that the conditional probabilities of producing morbidity or mortality in the adult population at risk by only resecting symptomatic diverticula are 0.2% and 0.04%, respectively. However, by resecting all incidentally discovered diverticula, the comparable respective risks were 4.6% and 0.2%. These authors therefore concluded that the practice of incidental diverticulectomy in adults should be abandoned.

Short-Bowel Syndrome

Maintenance of adequate nutrition is dependent on the normal digestive and absorptive function of the small-intestinal mucosa. A normal, healthy adult possesses an excess of gut mucosa, but depending on the amount of bowel removed and the specific level of resection, symptoms can

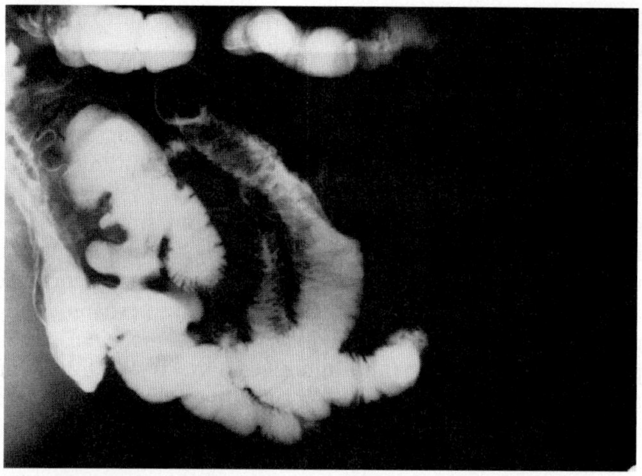

FIGURE 49.15. Radiographic appearance of short-bowel syndrome shown by a barium upper GI series and small-bowel follow-through. This patient underwent massive enterectomy because of mesenteric infarction. Note that barium has passed quickly from the stomach, through the shortened small intestine, and into the colon.

ensue following surgery, in some cases leading to a condition known as the *short-bowel syndrome* (Fig. 49.15). Because of the important functional capacities of the duodenum in regard to iron and calcium and of the distal ileum in regard to vitamin B_{12} and bile salts, resections of these specific regions tend to be poorly tolerated. In contrast, up to 40% of the mid-small bowel can be removed with only moderate clinical sequelae. As a general rule, resection of 50% of the small intestine produces significant malabsorption, and if 70% or more of the intestine is resected, survival is threatened. Clinical results in treating short-bowel syndrome have improved in recent decades, however, with a recognition of its pathophysiology, improved surgical techniques, and better enteral and parenteral nutritional support.

The most common etiology of short-bowel syndrome is a massive resection occurring in the setting of mesenteric thrombosis or embolus. In children, volvulus of the intestine caused by congenital malrotation can also result in the need for massive resection. Less commonly, patients with neoplasm, trauma, or recurrent Crohn's disease develop short-bowel syndrome. The jejunoileal anastomosis that was used in the past to treat intractable obesity and hypercholesterolemia can also result in severe malabsorption, similar to that seen in patients following massive resection.

The minimal amount of small intestine required to sustain life is variable. Prolonged survival has been recorded in isolated patients with as little as 1 foot of jejunum along with an intact duodenum, but in general survival is threatened in patients with less than 2 feet (60 cm) of intestine beyond the duodenum. An intact ileocecal valve is thought to be important in regard to improving function of the remaining small intestine, and clearly the colon is vitally important for preventing water loss. Patients with short-bowel syndrome have impairment in the absorption of water and electrolytes as well as that of all nutrients. Fluid losses can be greater than 5 to 10 L/day. As a result, patients with short bowel syndrome suffer weight loss, fatigue, calorie deprivation, electrolyte abnormalities, and vitamin deficiencies.

Important adaptive changes occur in the remaining intestine following massive resection. Postresectional adaptation has been extensively studied in experimental animals, demonstrating a significant increase in DNA synthesis and cellular number within the remaining gut. A variety of hormones and peptides have been shown to augment this adaptive response, most notably EGF (epidermal growth factor), IGF-1 (insulin-like growth factor-1), GLP-1 (glucagon-like peptide 1), IL-11 (interleukin-11), and neurotensin.[128] Postresectional adaptation response also appears to occur in humans, but this response has been less well documented. In addition to mucosal hyperplasia, there is generally seen to be an increase in the caliber of the remaining small intestine, perhaps adding to the increase in absorptive area. From a functional standpoint, the amount of fluid and electrolyte losses following massive resection decreases over time, whereas glucose absorption increases.

Short-bowel syndrome is associated with gastric hypersecretion, perhaps related to loss of the "ileal brake," a mechanism by which luminal fat within the distal small intestine inhibits gastric secretion. Loss of the terminal ileum also results in an impairment in the absorption of conjugated bile salts and fat. With limited ileal resections, an increase in the bile salt load to the colon can cause direct injury to the mucosa and resultant diarrhea. With more extensive (i.e., greater than 100 cm) ileal resections, there is a gradual loss in the total bile salt pool, eventually leading to impairment in fat absorption and the onset of steatorrhea. Ileal resections are also associated with lithogenic bile, such that gallstone formation is seen in approximately 30% of such patients. Thompson evaluated 50 adult patients with intestinal remnants of less than 180 cm over a 15-year period and found a significant risk of cholelithiasis (57% in those patients with benign conditions). He concluded that prophylactic cholecystectomy should be considered if long-term survival is anticipated.[129]

Treatment

Initial therapy involves maintenance of fluid and electrolyte balance. Total parenteral nutrition (TPN) is often indicated and, depending on the extent of resection, may be required throughout the lifetime of the patient. It is likely that even small amounts of enteral nutrition are beneficial, however, because the luminal nutrients appear to enhance the adaptive response of the remaining gut. Various antidiarrheal and stool-bulking agents have also been used with some benefit. Gastric hypersecretion should be treated with either H_2-blockers or proton pump inhibitors. Cholestyramine may be beneficial in patients with limited ileal resections, but if the bile salt pool has been depleted, then cholestyramine is contraindicated.[130]

Wilmore and colleagues have advocated intensive medical management, including maintenance of oral hydration, along with a combination of a high-fiber diet, growth hormone, and glutamine. This intestinal rehabilitation program has been reported to provide excellent results in a number of cases, including patients who previously were on chronic TPN and who could subsequently be maintained completely on enteral nutrition.[131]

The efficacy of this intestinal rehabilitation program, however, remains controversial. Scolapio et al.[132] conducted a randomized, double-blind, placebo-controlled crossover study in eight patients with short-bowel syndrome (average small-bowel length, 71 cm). Patients were treated according to the program described by Wilmore's group, and these authors did find a transient increase in body weight and in sodium and potassium absorption, as well as a decrease in gastric emptying. However, there was no change in small-bowel morphology, stool losses, or macronutrient absorption.

Surgical Approach

The surgical treatment of patients with short-bowel syndrome has been disappointing. In small numbers of patients, various procedures, including intestinal lengthening, reversal of short segments, and plication of excessively dilated bowel have been used.[133,134] Although some improvement has been seen in isolated cases, such operations have not become universally adopted. Panis et al. reported on 8 patients who underwent segmental reversal of the small bowel, and with a median follow-up of 35 months, they reported significant decreases in parenteral nutritional requirements in all 7 of the patients who are still alive.[135] Thompson and colleagues have extensive experience in the surgical approaches to patients with short-bowel syndrome. In a report of 45 patients who had undergone 49 surgical procedures, they reported reasonably good success in 14 of the patients with short remnants and dilated bowel who underwent intestinal lengthening procedures. In patients with very short remnants (<60 cm), however, intestinal transplantation was performed.[134]

The results of small-intestinal transplantation have been disappointing, primarily because of a high incidence of rejection. However, more recent experience with small-intestinal transplantation suggests that this may become a viable surgical alternative in patients with short-bowel syndrome. Abu-Elmagd et al.[136] reported on the University of Pittsburgh experience with intestinal transplantation. In 98 consecutive patients (59 children, 39 adults), 48% of the group survived and had grafts providing full (91%) or partial (9%) nutrition. Actuarial patient survival at 1 and 5 years was only 72% and 48%, respectively. Although survival was similar between intestinal and composite grafts, the loss rate of grafts from rejection was highest with the intestine alone, indicating that the liver was at least marginally protective in regard to the concomittantly engrafted intestine.

Malabsorption Syndromes

Clinical Aspects

Malabsorption results from the pathological disturbance of the normal sequence of digestion, absorption, and nutrient transport. Most disorders consist of defective absorption of multiple forms of nutrients, producing classical overt malabsorptive symptoms, whereas some involve the selective loss of one specific nutrient, producing a syndrome with a paucity of symptoms. Classically, malabsorption produces both intestinal and extraintestinal symptoms. Chronic diarrhea, consisting of watery, bulky, frequent stools, is common. Patients with steatorrhea may note pale, foul-smelling, greasy, floating stool. Anorexia, hyperphagia, nausea, vomiting, abdominal distention, gassiness, excessive flatus, or borborygmus are common symptoms. Pain is unusual. Several malabsorption syndromes are particularly relevant to surgical disease.[137]

Celiac disease, tropical sprue, and lactase deficiency are not considered further here.

Bile Acid Malabsorption

Bile salts are necessary for proper absorption of dietary fats and fat-soluble substances. Bile salts are synthesized in the liver, stored in the gallbladder between meals, and excreted into the duodenum in response to ingestion. Normally, more than 90% of excreted bile is reabsorbed in the small intestine as part of the enterohepatic circulation system. In the terminal 100 cm of ileum, bile salt absorption is mediated by a Na^+-coupled bile salt transporter. Primary or idiopathic bile salt malabsorption is unusual. More commonly, bile salt malabsorption is the result of resection of the terminal ileum, such as in Crohn's disease.[138,139] Some patients develop bile salt malabsorption after cholecystectomy or after vagotomy.[140] Bile salt malabsorption is manifest as diarrhea and is the consequence of excessive concentrations of bile salts (>3 mM) reaching the colon. Cholestyramine is effective in more than 90% of cases of bile salt diarrhea.[140]

Vitamin B_{12} Malabsorption

Inadequate absorption of vitamin B_{12} leads to macrocytic anemia. Vitamin B_{12} undergoes a complex process of absorption involving the salivary glands (protein R), the stomach (intrinsic factor), a pancreatic protease, and active absorption in the terminal ileum. As such, systemic absorption can be adversely affected by a number of surgical conditions, including extensive gastric resection, bacterial overgrowth syndrome, Crohn's disease, radiation enteritis, and ileal resection. Treatment is by periodic parenteral administration of vitamin B_{12} and, if relevant, the addition of specific therapy to reverse the underlying disorder.

Bacterial Overgrowth Syndrome

Bacterial overgrowth in poorly emptying or stagnant small-intestinal segments leads to a syndrome of diarrhea and steatorrhea accompanied by abdominal pain, weight loss, anemia (usually macrocytic), fat-soluble vitamin deficiencies, and, in late stages, neurological deficits.[141] This situation is sometimes referred to as the *blind-loop syndrome* but can occur in a variety of conditions not involving the presence of a self-filling, nonemptying intestinal segment. This syndrome is occasionally encountered after a side-to-side intestinal anastomosis that produces a recirculating loop,[142] and it may occur within the afferent jejunal limb after Bilroth II gastrectomy.[143] Bacterial overgrowth caused by stagnation of luminal contents may occur in the setting of chronic intestinal obstruction by stricture or in duodenal or jejunal diverticulosis. Gastrocolic or jejunocolic fistula may also produce bacterial overgrowth, as can small-bowel motility disorders associated with diabetes and intestinal pseudoobstruction. Gastric achlorhydria can predispose to overgrowth.

The pathophysiology of the syndrome involves excessive bacterial metabolism of vitamin B_{12}, leading to its insufficient availability for intestinal absorption. Furthermore, bile salt deconjugation by luminal bacteria leads to inadequate micellization of dietary fat and, consequently, steatorrhea. Deconjugated bile salts are toxic to enterocytes and may directly elicit diarrhea and further malabsorption of other nutrients. Medical treatment consists of intermittent oral antibiotic therapy. If feasible, the underlying anatomical arrangement favoring bacterial overgrowth should be surgically corrected.

Evaluation of Malabsorptive Conditions

The etiology of a malabsorptive condition is often suggested by a thorough history followed by inspection of the stool and an estimation of its volume. Specific testing may confirm the diagnosis, although in general specificity and sensitivity are suboptimal, and many specialized examinations are not routinely performed in many centers. Fat malabsorption is usually detectable by quantitative measurements of fecal fat content in a 24-h collection or by Sudan stain of feces. Breath tests utilizing ^{14}C-labeled carbohydrates are used to detect lactose intolerance or other syndromes of carbohydrate malabsorption. D-Xylose absorption and detection in either plasma or urine can be used as a general test of intestinal absorptive function.[144,145] There are currently no accurate tests to confirm or exclude bile salt malabsorption; the response to an empiric trial of bile salt-binding agents such as cholestyramine may be useful.

Vitamin B_{12} malabsorption is detected with 94% accuracy by dual-label Schilling test.[146] Pancreatic insufficiency leading to malabsorption and steatorrhea is usually suspected on clinical or radiologic grounds. A symptomatic response to pancreatic enzyme replacement therapy is useful supporting evidence, but occasionally detailed testing of pancreatic exocrine function is necessary. This testing usually involves breath tests after the ingestion of substances such as p-aminobanzoic acid (PABA), triolein, or pancreolauril.[147]

Bacterial overgrowth can be confirmed by quantitative culture of endoscopically aspirated small-bowel luminal contents or by ^{14}C-xylose breath testing.[148,149] However, the empiric response to antibiotic therapy using agents such as tetracycline or metronidazole is usually more helpful in establishing the presumptive diagnosis. A Schilling test that reverts to normal after a 3- to 5-day course of tetracycline but not after addition of exogenous intrinsic factor confirms the diagnosis.

Miscellaneous Conditions

Pneumatosis Intestinalis

Pneumatosis intestinalis refers to the presence of gas or air within the wall of the intestine, as seen either at the time of surgery or by a radiographic study. So-called benign pneumatosis is generally an incidental finding and does not imply an underlying intestinal pathology (i.e., intestinal perforation or sepsis). In contrast, when pneumatosis intestinalis occurs as a result of primary intestinal pathology, urgent surgery is usually required (Fig. 49.16). The intramural bowel gas can result from necrosis caused by ischemia, infarction, neutropenic colitis, volvulus, and, in children, necrotizing enterocolitis. Occasionally, trauma to the bowel can lead to pneumatosis, in some cases iatrogenic in nature, such as misplaced feeding tubes, stents, or endoscopic trauma. Immunocompromised patients are more likely to

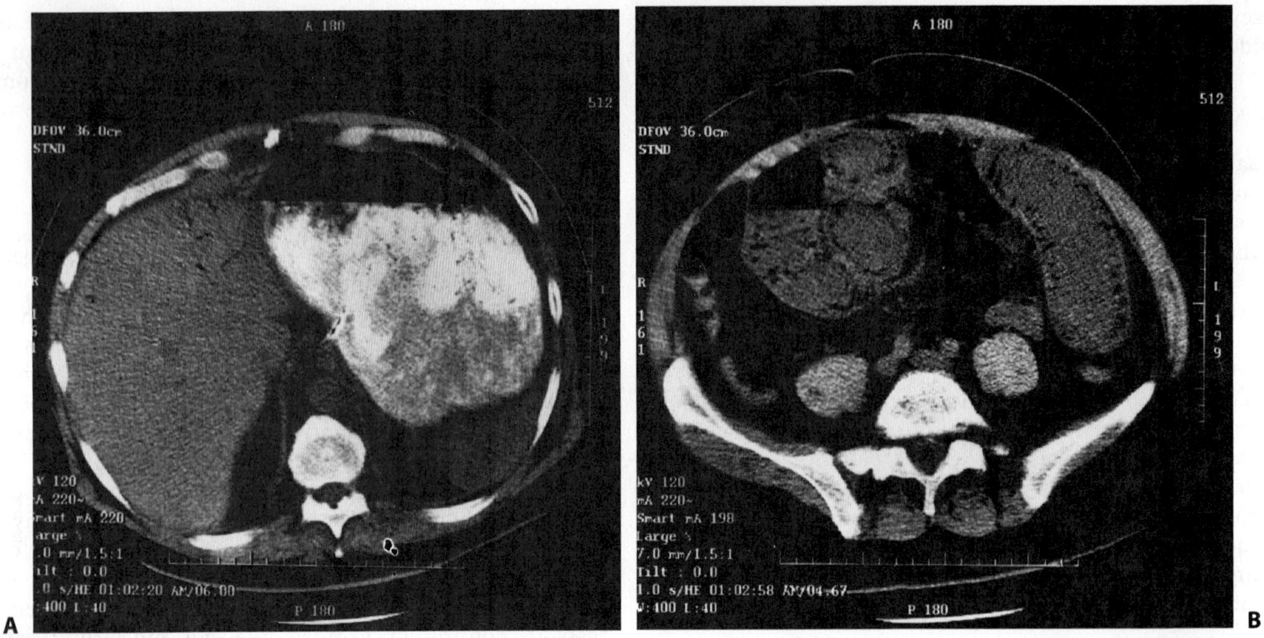

FIGURE 49.16. Pneumatosis intestinalis. **A.** Abdominal CT shows diffuse air within the small-bowel wall in this patient with a small-bowel obstruction caused by recurrent colon carcinoma involving the root of the mesentery. **B.** This patient also was noted to have air within the portal venous system, most evident in the left lobe of the liver.

develop pneumatosis, perhaps related to increased mucosal permeability.

Benign pneumatosis is often related to a pulmonary source in patients with chronic obstructive pulmonary disease (COPD), asthma, or cystic fibrosis. It can also occur secondary to barotrauma in patients on mechanical positive-pressure ventilation or after placement of chest tubes. The intrathoracic air can dissect via the retroperitoneum and into the intestinal wall. On rare occasions, the increased intrathoracic pressure leading to pneumatosis has been associated with severe retching and vomiting. In some cases, no cause for the pneumatosis is found.

Knechtle et al.[150] reported 27 patients with pneumatosis and concluded that patients with pneumatosis who had clinical evidence of either bowel obstruction or ischemia usually require urgent surgery, but the asymptomatic patient without sepsis can be safely treated nonoperatively. The presence of free air within the abdomen is not in itself an indication for surgery unless there are signs of peritonitis or sepsis. The presence of air within the bowel wall itself does not mandate resection, because the air may have tracked from another site within the bowel, such as a segment of ischemia with necrosis. In such a case, only the segment of bowel that is ischemic requires resection. Similarly, if the underlying etiology is inflammatory in nature, only resection of the involved bowel is indicated.

Small-Bowel Ulceration

Ulcerative lesions of the small bowel are most commonly the result of ingested medications such as enteric-coated potassium chloride, nonsteroidal antiinflammatory drugs, and corticosteroids. Less often, small-bowel ulcers are caused by segmental arterial or venous occlusion or vasculitis. Heterotopic gastric mucosa within a Meckel's diverticulum may lead to peptic ulceration of the small-bowel mucosa. Rarely, gastrinoma may be associated with small-bowel ulceration. Ulceration may develop in association with Crohn's disease and with small-bowel lymphoma. Finally, a number of infectious causes of small-bowel ulceration are recognized, including tuberculosis, syphilis, and typhoid fever. In a distinct minority of patients, no definable etiology of the small-bowel ulceration will be found. In this situation, the ulceration is usually single and located in the terminal ileum.

Small-bowel ulceration can present with obstruction or hemorrhage and less commonly with perforation. Preoperative localization and diagnosis can be problematic since lesions are usually not within the reach of an endoscope and are difficult to visualize on visceral angiography. They are frequently found by palpation of the small bowel at laparotomy or during intraoperative endoscopy. The treatment of a symptomatic small-bowel ulcer is surgical resection. Suture repair of perforated small-bowel ulceration is not recommended due to an unacceptably high rate of complications. Recurrence after resection is extremely unusual, particularly if the offending medication is stopped.

Foreign-Body Ingestion

Emergency department evaluation for the accidental or intentional ingestion of sharp or pointed foreign bodies, including fish bones, pins, toothpicks, and broken razor blades is not rare. Although there is a small potential for intestinal perforation, the vast majority of ingested foreign objects pass through the gastrointestinal tract without incident. Radiopaque objects may be followed by serial plain films of the abdomen. The development of abdominal pain associated with tenderness and leukocytosis strongly suggests that a contained local perforation has occurred, and surgical resection is indicated. Perforation after passage into the colon is rare because by that time the object generally has become safely embedded within solid fecal matter. Occasionally, larger objects such as whistles or coins may lead to intestinal obstruction if they become lodged, typically near the ileocecal valve.

References

1. Hermiston ML, Gordon JI. Organization of the crypt-villus axis and evolution of its stem cell hierarchy during intestinal development. Am J Physiol 1995;268:G813–G822.
2. Simon TC, Gordon JI. Intestinal epithelial cell differentiation: new insights from mice, flies and nematodes. Curr Opin Genet Dev 1995;5:577–586.
3. Potten C. Epithelial cell growth and differentiation. II. Intestinal apoptosis. Am J Physiol 1997;273:G253–G257.
4. Murphy MS. Growth factors and the gastrointestinal tract. Nutrition 1998;14:771–774.
5. Podolsky DK. Regulation of intestinal epithelial proliferation: a few answers, many questions. Am J Physiol 1993;264:G179–G186.
6. Hodin RA, Meng S, Archer S, Tang R. Cellular growth state differentially regulates enterocyte gene expression in butyrate-treated HT-29 cells. Cell Growth Differ 1996;7:647–653.
7. Mitic LL, Anderson JM. Molecular architecture of tight junctions. Annu Rev Physiol 1998;60:121–142.
8. Madara JL. Loosening tight junctions. Lessons from the intestine. J Clin Invest 1989;83:1089–1094.
9. Madara JL. Review article: Pathobiology of neutrophil interactions with intestinal epithelia. Aliment Pharmacol Ther 1997; 11(suppl 3):57–62; discussion 62–63.
10. Hansen MB, Skadhauge E. New aspects of the pathophysiology and treatment of secretory diarrhoea. Physiol Res 1995;44:61–78.
11. Mowat AM, Viney JL. The anatomical basis of intestinal immunity. Immunol Rev 1997;156:145–166.
12. Neutra MR. Current concepts in mucosal immunity. V. Role of M cells in transepithelial transport of antigens and pathogens to the mucosal immune system. Am J Physiol 1998;274:G785–G791.
13. Perdue MH, McKay DM. Integrative immunophysiology in the intestinal mucosa. Am J Physiol 1994;267:G151–G165.
14. Kraehenbuhl JP, Pringault E, Neutra MR. Review article: Intestinal epithelia and barrier functions. Aliment Pharmacol Ther 1997;11(suppl 3):3–8; discussion 8–9.
15. Geoghegan J, Pappas TN. Clinical uses of gut peptides. Ann Surg 1997;225:145–154.
16. Liddle RA. Regulation of cholecystokinin secretion by intraluminal releasing factors. Am J Physiol 1995;269:G319–G327.
17. Reichlin S. Somatostatin. N Engl J Med 1983;309:1495–1501.
18. Tonini M. Recent advances in the pharmacology of gastrointestinal prokinetics. Pharmacol Res 1996;33:217–226.
19. Der-Silaphet T, Malaysz J, Hagel S, Arsenault A, Huizinga J. Interstitial cells of Cajal direct normal propulsive contractile activity in mouse small intestine. Gastroenterology 1998;114:724–736.
20. Gibson C. A study of 1000 operations for acute intestinal obstruction. Ann Surg 1900;32:486.
21. Vick R. Statistics of acute intestinal obstruction. Br Med J 1932;2:546.
22. Wangenstein O. Intestinal Obstructions. Springfield: Thomas; 1955.
23. Yale C, Balish E. Intestinal obstruction in germ free and monocontaminated dogs. Arch Surg 1979;114:445.
24. Harlow C, Stears R, Zeligman B, Archer P. Diagnosis of bowel obstruction on plain abdominal radiographs: significance of air-fluid levels at different heights in the same loop of the bowel. AJR Am J Roentgenol 1993;161:291–295.
25. Frager D, Medwid S, Baer J, Mollinelli B, Friedman M. CT of small bowel obstruction: value in establishing the diagnosis and determining the degree and cause. AJR Am J Roentgenol 1994;162:37–41.
26. Balthazar E. CT of small bowel obstruction. AJR Am J Roentgenol 1994;162:225–261.
27. Maignot R. Maignot's abdominal operations. In: Shwartz SI, Ellis H, Husser WC, eds. East Norwalk CT: Appleton and Lange; 1989.
28. Silen W, Hein M, et al. Strangulation obstruction of the small intestine. Arch Surg 1962;85:12.
29. Zollinger R, Kinsey D. Diagnosis and management of intestinal obstruction. Am Surg 1964;30:1.
30. Frager D, Baer J, Medwid S, Rothpearl APB. Detection of intestinal ischemia in patients with acute small-bowel obstruction due to adhesions or hernia: efficacy of CT. AJR Am J Roentgenol 1996;166:67–71.
31. Ogata M, Imai S, Hosotani R, Aoyama H, Hayashi M, Ishikawa T. Abdominal ultrasonography for the diagnosis of strangulation in small bowel obstruction. Br J Surg 1994;81:421–424.
32. Fleshner P, Siegman M, Slater G, Brolin R, Chandler J, Aufses AJ. A prospective randomized trial of short versus long tubes in adhesive small bowel obstruction. Am J Surg 1995;170:366–370.
33. Brolin R, Krasna M, Mast B. Use of tubes and radiographs in the management of small bowel obstruction. Ann Surg 1987;206:126–133.
34. Bizer L, Leibling R, Delaney H, Gliedman M. Small bowel obstruction: the role of nonoperative treatment in simple intestinal obstruction and predictive criteria for strangulation obstruction. Surgery 1981;89:407–413.
35. Bulkley G, Zuidema G, Hamilton S, O'Mara C, Klacsmann P, Horna S. Intraoperative determination of small intestinal viability following ischemic injury: a prospective controlled trial of two adjuvant methods (Doppler and fluorescein) compared with standard clinical judgement. Ann Surg 1981;193:628–637.
36. Reissman P, Wexner S. Laparoscopic surgery for intestinal obstruction. Surg Endosc 1995;9:865–868.
37. Lee F. Drug-related pathological lesions of the intestinal tract. Histopathology 1994;25:303–308.
38. George C. Drugs causing intestinal obstruction: a review. J R Soc Med 1994;73:200.
39. Mann W. Surgical management of radiation enteropathy. Surg Clin North Am 1991;71:977–990.
40. Thaker P, Weingarten L, Friedman I. Stenosis of the small intestine due to nonconclusive ischemic disease. 1977;112:1216–1217.
41. Janin Y, Stone A, Wise L. Mesenteric hernia. Surg Gynecol Obstet 1980;150:747–754.
42. Meade H. Hernias through the mesentery of the ileocaecal junction. Ir J Med Sci 1942;6:103–108.
43. Hansmann G, Morton S. Intra-abdominal hernia report of a case and review of the literature. Arch Surg 1939;39:973–986.
44. Mclaughlin C, Raines M. Obstruction of the alimentary tract from gall stones. Am J Surg 1951;81:424.
45. Kasahara Y, Umemura H, Shiraha S, Kuyama T, Sakata K, Kubota H. Gallstone ileus review of 112 patients in the Japanese literature. Am J Surg 1980;140:437–440.
46. Clavien P, Richon J, Burgan S, Rohner A. Gallstone ileus. Br J Surg 1990;77:737–742.
47. Ward-McQuaid N. Intestinal obstruction due to food. Br Med J 1950;2:1106.
48. Silen W. Cope's Early Diagnosis of the Acute Abdomen. Oxford: Oxford University Press; 1996.
49. Frager D, Baer J, Rothpearl A, Bossart P. Distinction between postoperative ileus and mechanical small-bowel obstruction: value of CT compared with clinical and other radiographic findings. AJR Am J Roentgenol 1995;164:891–894.
50. Ludwig K, Condon R. Surgical Consultations. St. Louis: Mosby-Year Book; 1993.

51. Becker J, Dayton M, Fazio V, et al. Prevention of postoperative abdominal adhesions by a sodium hyaluronate-based bioresorbable membrane: a double-blind multicenter study. J Am Coll Surg 1996;183:297–306.
52. Rodier J, Janser J, Rodier D. Prevention of radiation enteritis and pelvic floor reconstruction by a polyglactin 910 (vicryl) mesh in gynecologic malignancies. Int J Oncol 1995;7:963.
53. Crohn B, Ginsburg L, Oppenheimer G. Regional ileitas: a pathologic and clinical entity. JAMA 1932;99:1232.
54. Fiocchi C. Inflammatory bowel disease: etiology and pathogenisis. Gastroenterology 1998;115:182–205.
55. Glotzer D. Surgical therapy for Crohn's disease. Gastroenterol Clin North Am 1995;24:577–596.
56. Ozuner G, Fazio VW, Lavery IC, et al. Reoperative rates for Crohn's disease following strictureplasty. Long term analysis. Dis Col Rectum 1996;39:1199–1203.
57. Fazio V, Marchette F, Church M, et al. Effect of resection margins on the recurrence of Crohn's disease in the small bowel. A randomized controlled trial. Ann Surg 1996;224:563–571.
58. Kotangi H, Kramer K, Fazio V, Petras R. Do microscopic abnormalities at resection margins correlate with increased anastomotic recurrence in Crohn's disease? Retrospective analysis of 100 cases. Dis Colon Rectum 1991;34:909–916.
59. Goldberg H, Caruthers SJ, Nelson J, Singleton J. Radiographic findings of the National Cooperative Crohn's Disease Study. Gastroenterology 1979;77:925–937.
60. Couckuyt H, Gevers A, Coremans G, Hiele M, Rutgeerts P. Efficacy and safety of hydrostatic balloon dilation of ileocolonic Crohn's strictures: a prospective long term analysis. 1995;36:577–580.
61. Greenstein A, Sachar D, Smith H, Janowitz H, Augses AJ. A comparison of cancer risk in Crohn's disease and ulcerative colitis. Cancer (Phila) 1981;48:2742–2745.
62. Jawhari A, Kamm M, Ong C, Forbes A, Bartram C, Hawley P. Intraabdominal and pelvic abscess in Crohn's disease: results of noninvasive and surgical management. Br J Surg 1998;85:367–391.
63. Rutgeerts P, Geboes K, Van Trappen G, Beyls J, Kerremans R, Hiele M. Predictability of the postoperative course of Crohn's disease. Gastroenterology 1990;99:956–963.
64. Persson S, Danielsson D, Kjellander J, Wallensten S. Studies on Crohn's disease. 1. The relationship between *Yersinia enterocolitica* infection and terminal ileitis. Acta Chir Scand 1976;142:84–90.
65. Lautenbach E, Berlin J, Lichtenstein G. Risk factors for early postoperative recurrence of Crohn's disease. Gastroenterology 1998;115:259–267.
66. Russell RK, Nimmo ER, and Satsangi J. Molecular genetics of Crohn's disease. Curr Opin Genet Dev. 2004;14:264–270.
67. Wu J, Birnbaum E, Kodner I, Fry R, Read T, Fleshman J. Laparoscopic-assisted ileocolic resections in patients with Crohn's disease: are abscesses, phlegmons, or recurrent disease contradictions? Surgery 1997;122:682–688.
68. Reissman P, Salky B, Pfeifer J, Edye M, Jagelman D, Wexner S. Laparoscopic surgery in the management of inflammatory bowel disease. Am J Surg 1996;171:47–51.
69. Sitges-Serra A, Guirao X, Pereira JA, et al. Treatment of gastrointestinal fistulas with Sandostatin. Digestion 1993;54(suppl 1):38–40.
70. Scott NA, Finnegan S, and Irving MH. Octreotide and postoperative entercutaneous fistula: a controlled prospective study. Acta Gastroenterol Belg 1993;56:266–270.
71. Sancho JJ, di Costanzo J, Nubiola P, et al. Randomized double-blind placebo-controlled trial of early octreotide in patients with postoperative enterocutaneous fistula. Br J Surg 1995; 82:1576.
72. Barclay TH, Schapira DV. Malignant tumors of the small intestine. Cancer (Phila) 1983;51:878–881.
73. DiSario JA, Burt RW, Vargas H, McWhorter WP. Small bowel cancer: epidemiological and clinical characteristics from a population-based registry. Am J Gastroenterol 1994;89:699–701.
74. Ashley SW, Wells SA Jr. Tumors of the small intestine. Semin Oncol 1988;15:116–128.
75. Nielsen SN, Wold LE. Adenocarcinoma of jejunum in association with nontropical sprue. Arch Pathol Lab Med 1986;110:822–824.
76. Maglinte DD, O'Connor K, Bessette J, Chernish SM, Kelvin FM. The role of the physician in the late diagnosis of primary malignant tumors of the small intestine. Am J Gastroenterol 1991; 86:304–308.
77. Bessette JR, Maglinte DD, Kelvin FM, Chernish SM. Primary malignant tumors in the small bowel: a comparison of the small-bowel enema and conventional follow-through examination. AJR Am J Roentgenol 1989;153:741–744.
78. Fireman Z, Kopelman Y. New frontiers in capsule endoscopy. J Gastroenterol Hepatol 2007;22:1174–1177.
79. Galandiuk S, Hermann RE, Jagelman DG, Fazio VW, Sivak MV. Villous tumors of the duodenum. Ann Surg 1988;207:234–239.
80. Seifert E, Schulte F, Stolte M. Adenoma and carcinoma of the duodenum and papilla of Vater: a clinicopathologic study. Am J Gastroenterol 1992;87:37–42.
81. Griffioen G, Bus PJ, Vasen HF, Verspaget HW, Lamers CB. Extracolonic manifestations of familial adenomatous polyposis: desmoid tumours, and upper gastrointestinal adenomas and carcinomas. Scand J Gastroenterol Suppl 1998;225:85–91.
82. Ma CK, De Peralta MN, Amin MB, et al. Small intestinal stromal tumors: a clinicopathologic study of 20 cases with immunohistochemical assessment of cell differentiation and the prognostic role of proliferation antigens. Am J Clin Pathol 1997;108:641–651.
83. Giardiello FM, Welsh SB, Hamilton SR, et al. Increased risk of cancer in the Peutz-Jeghers syndrome. N Engl J Med 1987; 316:1511–1514.
84. Cunningham JD, Aleali R, Aleali M, Brower ST, Aufses AH. Malignant small bowel neoplasms: histopathologic determinants of recurrence and survival. Ann Surg 1997;225:300–306.
85. Weiss NS, Yang CP. Incidence of histologic types of cancer of the small intestine. J Natl Cancer Inst 1987;78:653–656.
86. Minardi AJ Jr, Zibari GB, Aultman DF, McMillan RW, McDonald JC. Small-bowel tumors. J Am Coll Surg 1998;186:664–668.
87. Perzin KH, Bridge MF. Adenomas of the small intestine: a clinicopathologic review of 51 cases and a study of their relationship to carcinoma. Cancer (Phila) 1981;48:799–819.
88. Younes N, Fulton N, Tanaka R, Wayne J, Straus FH II, Kaplan EL. The presence of K-12 ras mutations in duodenal adenocarcinomas and the absence of ras mutations in other small bowel adenocarcinomas and carcinoid tumors. Cancer (Phila) 1997; 79:1804–1808.
89. Sutter T, Arber N, Moss SF, et al. Frequent K-ras mutations in small bowel adenocarcinomas. Dig Dis Sci 1996;41:115–118.
90. Ouriel K, Adams JT. Adenocarcinoma of the small intestine. Am J Surg 1984;147:66–71.
91. Starke J, Rodriguez-Bigas M, Marshall W, Sohrabi A, Petrelli NJ. Primary adenocarcinoma arising in an ileostomy. Surgery (St. Louis) 1993;114:125–128.
92. Jones BA, Langer B, Taylor BR, Girotti M. Periampullary tumors: which ones should be resected? Am J Surg 1985;149:46–52.
93. Lowell JA, Rossi RL. Munson JL, Braasch JW. Primary adenocarcinoma of third and fourth portions of duodenum. Favorable prognosis after resection. Arch Surg 1992;127:557–560.
94. Ricci A Jr, Ciccarelli O, Cartun RW, Newcomb P. A clinicopathologic and immunohistochemical study of 16 patients with small intestinal leiomyosarcoma. Limited utility of immunophenotyping. Cancer (Phila) 1987;60:1790–1799.

95. Eisenberg BL, Judson I. Surgery and imatinib in the management of GIST: emerging approaches to adjuvant and neoadjuvant therapy. Ann Surg Oncol 2004;11:465–475.
96. Radaszkiewicz T, Dragosics B, Bauer P. Gastrointestinal malignant lymphomas of the mucosa-associated lymphoid tissue: factors relevant to prognosis. Gastroenterology 1992;102:1628–1638.
97. Contreary K, Nance FC, Becker WF. Primary lymphoma of the gastrointestinal tract. Ann Surg 1980;191:593–598.
98. Beck P, Gill J, Sutherland L. HIV-associated non-Hodgkin's lymphoma of the gastrointestinal tract. Am J Gastroenterol 1996;91:2377–2381.
99. Gilinsky NH, Novis BH, Wright JP, Dent DM, King H, Marks IN. Immunoproliferative small-intestinal disease: clinical features and outcome in 30 cases. Medicine (Baltimore) 1987;66:438–446.
100. Al-Bahrani ZR, Al-Mondhiry H, Bakir F, Al-Saleem T. Clinical and pathologic subtypes of primary intestinal lymphoma. Experience with 132 patients over a 14-year period. Cancer (Phila) 1983;52:1666–1672.
101. Al-Mondhiry H. Primary lymphomas of the small intestine: east-west contrast. Am J Hematol 1986;22:89–105.
102. Murray A, Cuevas EC, Jones DB, Wright DH. Study of the immunohistochemistry and T cell clonality of enteropathy-associated T cell lymphoma. Am J Pathol 1995;146:509–519.
103. Loughran TP Jr, Kadin ME, Deeg HJ. T-cell intestinal lymphoma associated with celiac sprue. Ann Intern Med 1986;104:44–47.
104. ReMine SG, Braasch JW. Gastric and small bowel lymphoma. Surg Clin North Am 1986;66:713–722.
105. Amer MH, el-Akkad S. Gastrointestinal lymphoma in adults: clinical features and management of 300 cases. Gastroenterology 1994;106:846–858.
106. Ruskone-Fourmestraux A, Aegerter P, Delmer A, Brousse N, Galian A, Rambaud JC. Primary digestive tract lymphoma: a prospective multicentric study of 91 patients. Groupe d'Etude des Lymphomes Digestifs. Gastroenterology 1993;105:1662–1671.
107. Peck JJ, Shields AB, Boyden AM, Dworkin LA, Nadal JW. Carcinoid tumors of the ileum. Am J Surg 1983;146:124–132.
108. Moyana TN. Carcinoid tumors arising from Meckel's diverticulum. A clinical, morphologic, and immunohistochemical study. Am J Clin Pathol 1989;91:52–56.
109. Dawes L, Schulte WJ, Condon RE. Carcinoid tumors. Arch Surg 1984;119:375–378.
110. Hsu EY, Feldman JM, Lichtenstein GR. Ileal carcinoid tumors stimulating Crohn's disease: incidence among 176 consecutive cases of ileal carcinoid. Am J Gastroenterol 1997;92:2062–2065.
111. Hanson MW, Feldman JM, Blinder RA, Moore JO, Coleman RE. Carcinoid tumors: iodine-131 MIBG scintigraphy. Radiology 1989;172:699–703.
112. Stinner B, Kisker O, Zielke A, Rothmund M. Surgical management for carcinoid tumors of small bowel, appendix, colon, and rectum. World J Surg 1996;20:183–188.
113. Wareing TH, Sawyers JL. Carcinoids and the carcinoid syndrome. Am J Surg 1983;145:769–772.
114. Johnson LA, Lavin P, Moertel CG, et al. Carcinoids: the association of histologic growth pattern and survival. Cancer (Phila) 1983;51:882–889.
115. Strodel WE, Talpos G, Eckhauser F, Thompson N. Surgical therapy for small-bowel carcinoid tumors. Arch Surg 1983; 118:391–397.
116. Persson BG, Nobin A, Ahren B, Jeppsson B, Mansson B, Bengmark S. Repeated hepatic ischemia as a treatment for carcinoid liver metastases. World J Surg 1989;13:307–311; discussion 311–312.
117. Saslow SB, O'Brien MD, Camilleri M, et al. Octreotide inhibition of flushing and colonic motor dysfunction in carcinoid syndrome. Am J Gastroenterol 1997;92:2250–2256.
118. Kuttner H, Ileus durch intussusception eines. Meckelsche Divertikel. Beitr Klin Chir 1898;21:298.
119. Salzer H. Ueber das offene Meckelsche divertikel. Wien Klin Wochenschr 1904;17:614.
120. Deet E. Perforationsperitonitis von einem darmdivertikel mit Magenschleimhautbau ausgehend. Dtsch Z Chir 1907;88: 482.
121. Mackey W, Dineen P. A fifty year experience with Meckel's diverticulum. Surg Gynecol Obstet 1983;156:56–64.
122. William R. Management of Meckel's diverticulum. Br J Surg 1981;81:477–480.
123. Soltero M, Bill A. The natural history of Meckel's diverticulum and its relation to incidental removal. Am J Surg 1976;132:168.
124. Cooney D, Duszynski D, et al. The abdominal technetium scan (a decade of experience). J Pediatr Surg 1982;17:611.
125. Mitchell A, Spencer J, Allison D, Jackson J. Meckel's diverticulum: angiographic findings in 16 patients. AJR Am J Roentgenol 1998;170:1329–1333.
126. Cullen J, Kelly K, Moir C, Hodge D, Zinsmeister A, Melton LR. Surgical management of Meckel's diverticulum. An epidemiologic, population-based study. Ann Surg 1995;220:564–568.
127. Peoples J, Lichtenberger E, Dunn M. Incidental Meckel's diverticulectomy in adults. Surgery (St. Louis) 1995;118:649–652.
128. Fiore N, Lednickzky G, Liu Q, et al. Comparison of interleukin-11 and epidermal growth factor on residual small intestine after massive small bowel resection. J Pediatr Surg 1998;33:24–29.
129. Thompson J. The role of prophylactic cholecystectomy in the short-bowel syndrome. Arch Surg 1996;131:556–559.
130. Thompson J. Management of the short bowel syndrome. Gastroenterol Clin North Am 1994;23:403–420.
131. Byrne T, Persinger R, Young L, Ziegler T, Wilmore D. A new treatment for patients with short-bowel syndrome. Growth hormone, glutamine, and a modified diet. Ann Surg 1995;222:254–255.
132. Scolapio J, Carnilleri M, Fleming C, et al. Effect of growth hormone, glutamine, and diet on adaptation in short-bowel syndrome: a randomized, controlled study. Gastroenterology 1997;113:1074–1081.
133. Thompson J, Edgar J. Poth Memorial Lecture. Surgical aspects of the short-bowel syndrome. Am J Surg 1995;170:532–536.
134. Thompson J, Langnas A, Pinch L, Kaufman S, Quigley E, Vanderhoff J. Surgical approach to short-bowel syndrome. Experience in population of 160 patients. Ann Surg 1995;222:600–605.
135. Panis Y, Messing B, Rivet P, et al. Segmental reversal of the small bowel as an alternative to intestinal transplantation in patients with short bowel syndrome. Ann Surg 1997;255:401–407.
136. Abu-Elmagd K, Reyes J, Todo S, et al. Clinical intestinal transplantation: new perspectives and immunologic considerations. J Am Coll Surg 1998;186:512–525.
137. Brasitus TA, Sitrin MD. Intestinal malabsorption syndromes. Annu Rev Med 1990;41:339–347.
138. Fromm H, Malavolti M. Bile acid-induced diarrhoea. Clin Gastroenterol 1986;15:567–582.
139. Aldini R, Roda A, Festi D, et al. Bile acid malabsorption and bile acid diarrhea in intestinal resection. Dig Dis Sci 1982;27:495–502.
140. Sciarretta G, Furno A, Mazzoni M, Malaguti P. Post-cholecystectomy diarrhea: evidence of bile acid malabsorption assessed by SeHCAT test. Am J Gastroenterol 1992;87:1852–1854.
141. Mathias JR, Clench MH. Review: pathophysiology of diarrhea caused by bacterial overgrowth of the small intestine. Am J Med Sci 1985;289:243–248.
142. Schlegel DM, Maglinte DD. The blind pouch syndrome. Surg Gynecol Obstet 1982;155:541–544.

143. Armbrecht U, Lundell L, Lindstedt G, Stockbruegger RW. Causes of malabsorption after total gastrectomy with Roux-en-Y reconstruction. Acta Chir Scand 1988;154:37–41.
144. Romano TJ, Dobbins JW. Evaluation of the patient with suspected malabsorption. Gastroenterol Clin North Am 1989; 18:467–483.
145. King CE, Toskes PP. The use of breath tests in the study of malabsorption. Clin Gastroenterol 1983;12:591–610.
146. Domstad PA, Choy YC, Kim EE, DeLand FH. Reliability of the dual-isotope Schilling test for the diagnosis of pernicious anemia or malabsorption syndrome. Am J Clin Pathol 1981;75:723–726.
147. Goff JS. Two-stage triolein breath test differentiates pancreatic insufficiency from other causes of malabsorption. Gastroenterology 1982;83:44–46.
148. King CE, Toskes PP, Guilarte TR, Lorenz E, Welkos SL. Comparison of the one-gram d-[^{14}C]xylose breath test to the [^{14}C]bile acid breath test in patients with small-intestine bacterial overgrowth. Dig Dis Sci 1980;25:53–58.
149. King CE, Toskes PP. Comparison of the 1-g [^{14}C]xylose, 10-g lactulose-H_2, and 80-g glucose-H_2 breath tests in patients with small intestine bacterial overgrowth. Gastroenterology 1986; 91:1447–1451.
150. Knechtle SJ, Davidoff AM, Rice RP. Pneumatosis intestinalis surgical management and clinical outcome. Ann Surg 1990;212: 160–165.
151. Dodd EE. Atlas of Histology, New York: McGraw-Hill; 1979.
152. Schultz SG, ed. Handbook of Physiology: IV. The Gastrointestinal System. New York: Oxford University Press; 1991.
153. Sleisinger MH, Fordtran JS, eds. Gastrointestinal Disease. Philadelphia: Saunders; 1993.
154. Wright EM, et al. In: Johnson LR, ed. Physiology of the Digestive Tract. 3rd ed. Philadelphia: Lippincott Williams & Wilkins; 1994.
155. Johnson LR, ed. Physiology of the Digestive Tract. 3rd ed. Philadelphia: Lippincott Williams & Wilkins; 1994.
156. Lamm M. Current concepts in mucosal immunity: how epithelial transport of IgA antibodies relates to host defense. Am J Physiol 1998;274:G614–G617.
157. Madara JL. The chameleon within: improving antigen delivery. Science 1997;277:910–911.
158. Musshoff K, Schmidt-Vollmer H. Prognostic sequence of primary site after radiotherapy in non-Hodgkins lymphoma. Lancet 1975;31(suppl 2):425–434.
159. Turowski GA, Basson MD. Primary malignant lymphoma of the intestine. Am J Surg 1995;169:433–441.

50

Appendix

David Soybel

Historical Perspective

The vermiform appendix was recognized as an independent anatomical structure at the beginning of the 16th century.[1–3] The appendix was sketched in the anatomical notebooks of Leonardo Da Vinci (Fig. 50.1; ca. 1500) and was called an "orecchio" or ear. However, it appears to have been formally described in 1524 by Da Capri[4] and in 1543 by Vesalius.[5] In 1554, Fernel[6] described a case of a 7-year-old girl who was given a large quince as a remedy for diarrhea. The girl subsequently developed severe abdominal pain and ultimately died. At autopsy, the quince was found to have adhered to and obstructed the lumen of the appendix; the appendix had become necrotic and perforated. Until the 18th century, cases of appendicitis were described at autopsy.[1–3] Amyand is credited with the first recorded appendectomy (1736), performed when a boy presented with a fistula in a hernia.[7] Exploring the hernia, Amyand found the appendix in the scrotal sac. A calcified mass and fecal fistula had formed around the wall of the appendix where it had been perforated by a pin. Subsequently, in the mid-1800s, a number of cases of appendiceal abscess were recognized before death. Some were drained, with recovery of the patients.[1–3]

The modern era for recognizing and treating appendicitis began in the 1880s: In 1880, in London, Lawson Tait became the first surgeon to remove a gangrenous appendix[8] from deep within the peritoneal cavity and to have the patient recover. In 1886, Reginald Fitz,[9] professor of medicine at Harvard, described the natural history of the inflamed appendix and coined the term *appendicitis*. He proposed early operation and removal of the inflamed appendix as a life-saving decision. In 1889, Charles McBurney, professor of surgery at Columbia College of Physicians and Surgeons, reported a number of cases of acute appendicitis. In the first case, an acutely inflamed but unruptured appendix was removed from a 19-year-old man. This report[10] described the point of maximal tenderness that would bear his name: "very exactly between an inch and a half and two inches from the anterior spinous process of the ileum on a straight line drawn from that process to the umbilicus." McBurney's final comments about the case were as follows:

> This is, I believe the first recorded case where an acutely inflamed unruptured appendix has been removed full of pus. Who can doubt what the result would have been in this particular case had the cyst ruptured, and operation been delayed a few hours? Would not the opportunity for recovery have been lost had the advice so often and so recently given been followed—to delay operation until spreading peritonitis appeared?

Anatomy and Physiology

In the sixth week of human embryo development, the appendix and cecum appear as cone-shaped outpouchings from the caudal limb of the midgut loop. The tip of the appendix outpouching begins to elongate at about the fifth month to achieve the recognized vermiform (wormlike) shape. A transient, appendix-like structure, appearing during week 5, has been described[11]; it has been suggested that persistence of this structure may explain certain forms of duplication.[1] The appendix maintains its position at the tip of the cecum at birth. Subsequently, unequal enlargement of the lateral wall of the cecum causes the appendix to find its adult position on the posteromedial wall, just below the ileocecal valve. Figure 50.2 shows the relationship of the mouth of the appendix to the mouth of the ileocecal valve, as seen within the lumen by a colonoscope. In the adult,[1] the average length of the appendix is 9 cm. Its outside diameter varies between 3 and 8 mm, and the luminal diameter is between 1 and 3 mm. The tip of the appendix can be located anywhere in the right lower quadrant of the abdomen or pelvis (Fig. 50.3). The base of the appendix can be located by following the longitudinally oriented tenia coli to their confluence at the cecum.

The appendix receives its arterial supply from the appendicular branch of the ileocolic artery. This artery originates

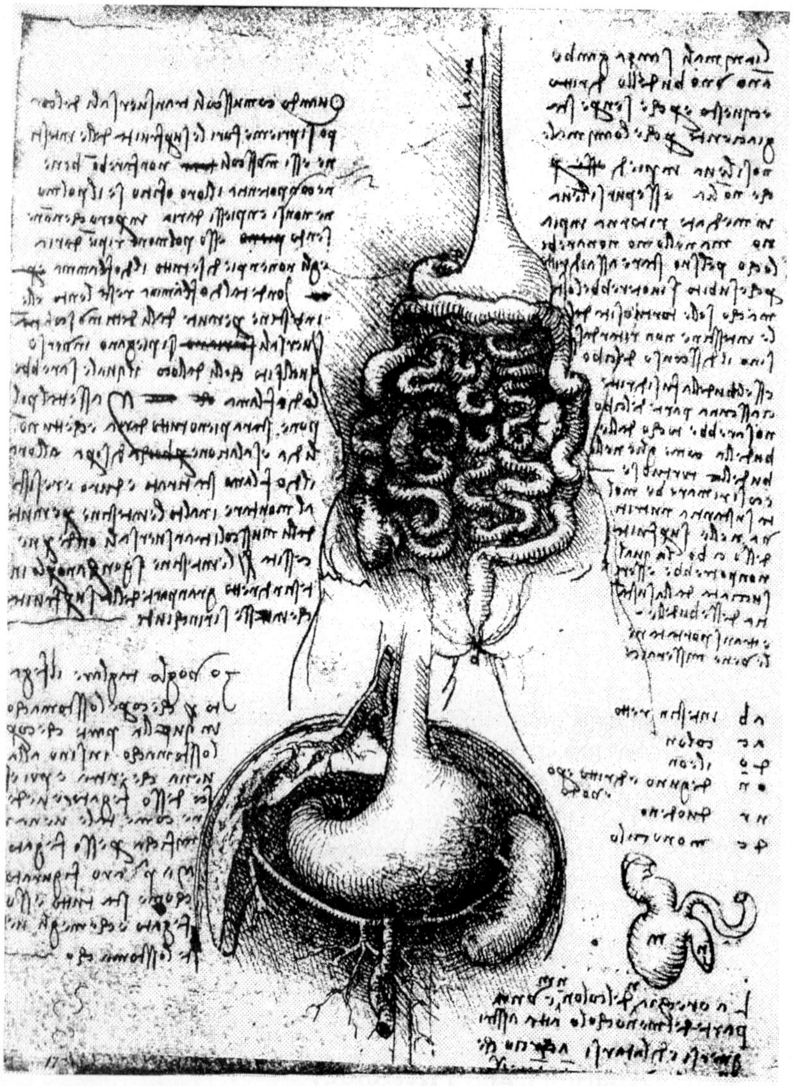

FIGURE 50.1. Reproduction of the original drawing by Leonardo Da Vinci of the alimentary tract. The cecum and appendix are shown in the *bottom right-hand corner* of the figure. Da Vinci's notes, characteristically, were handwritten in mirror image from right to left. (Reproduced from O'Malley and Saunders.[111])

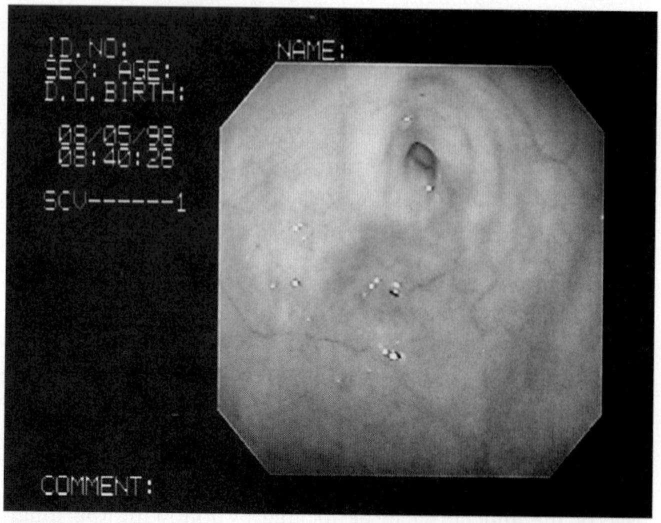

FIGURE 50.2. Endoscopic view of the appendix orifice from the inside of the cecum. The orifice usually is surrounded by whorls of mucosal fold but may present as a slit. (Photograph courtesy of Mary Lee Krinsky, MD, Division of Gastroenterology, West Roxbury VAMC, West Roxbury, MA.)

posterior to the terminal ileum, entering the mesoappendix close to the base of the appendix. A small arterial branch arises at this point that runs to the cecal artery. The arterial supply to the appendix is illustrated schematically in Figure 50.4. The lymphatic drainage of the appendix flows into lymph nodes that lie along the ileocolic artery. Innervation of the appendix is derived from sympathetic elements contributed by the superior mesenteric plexus (T10–L1), afferents from parasympathetic elements brought in via the vagus nerve.[12]

The histological features of the appendix include the following: First, the muscularis layers are not well defined and may be deficient in some locations.[1] Second, in the submucosa and mucosa, lymphoid aggregates occur with or without the typical structure of a germinal center. In the latter situation, the lymphoid follicular aggregate with a prominent germinal center seems to penetrate into the muscularis mucosa. Lymph vessels are prominent in regions underlying these lymphoid aggregates. Third, the mucosa is like that of the large intestine, except for the density of the lymphoid follicles. The crypts are irregularly sized and shaped, in contrast to the more uniform appearance of the crypts in the colon.

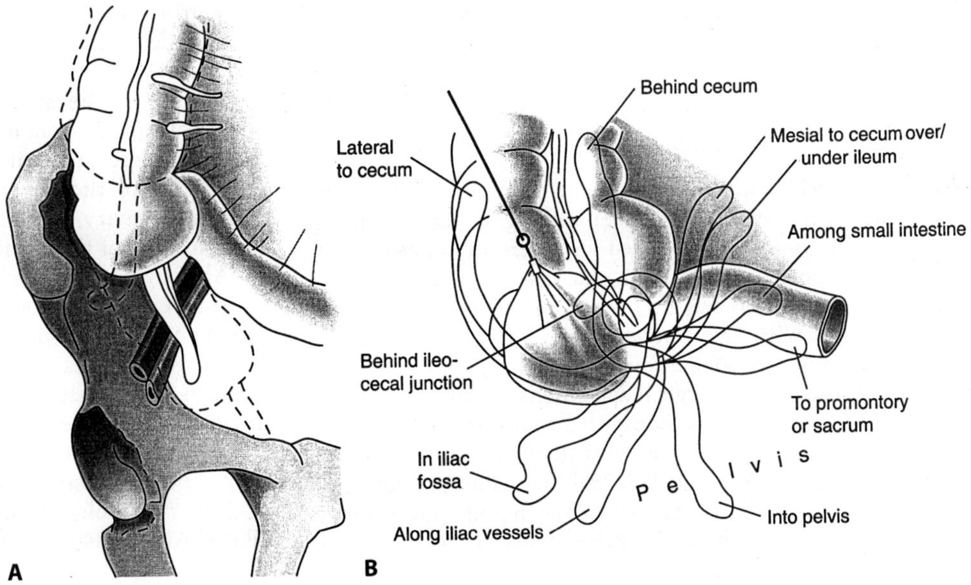

FIGURE 50.3. Variations in the normal position of the base (**A**) and the tip (**B**) of the vermiform appendix. (**A** redrawn from Silen[112]; **B** redrawn from Kelly and Hurdon.[11])

Neuroendocrine complexes composed of ganglion cells, Schwann cells, neural fibers, and neurosecretory cells are positioned just below the crypts. Serotonin is a prominent secretory product and has been implicated in mediating pain arising from the noninflamed appendix.[13,14] These complexes may be the source of carcinoid tumors, for which the appendix is known to be the most common site of origin.[1,14,15]

With regard to function, the widely held notion that the appendix is a vestigial organ is not consistent with the facts. Curiously, the appendix seems more highly developed in the higher primates, arguing against a vestigial role. Recent studies have focused on characterizing immune cell populations and their response to luminal antigens, offering the possibility that the appendix may play a role in immune surveillance.[16,17] Although the unique function of the appendix remains unclear, the mucosa of the appendix, like any mucosal layer, is capable of secreting fluid, mucin, and proteolytic enzymes.[1] In the 1930s, Dr. Owen Wangensteen at the University of Minnesota measured fluid output and intraluminal pressures generated within the normal human appendix.[18,19] Performing operations on patients with colorectal malignancies, Wangensteen brought the appendix out through the abdominal wall. He created an opening in the tip of the appendix that permitted insertion of a catheter, which allowed aspiration of fluid and measurement of intraluminal pressures. Very little fluid is required to generate substantial intraluminal pressure. When the outlet of the appendix was obstructed by a suture, Wangensteen found that specimens of normal appendix secreted fluid in the range of 0.25 to 2 mL/day and acutely generated pressures up to 125 cm H_2O (<100 mmHg).[19] He confirmed that no such fluid or pressures were generated when mucosa was atrophic.

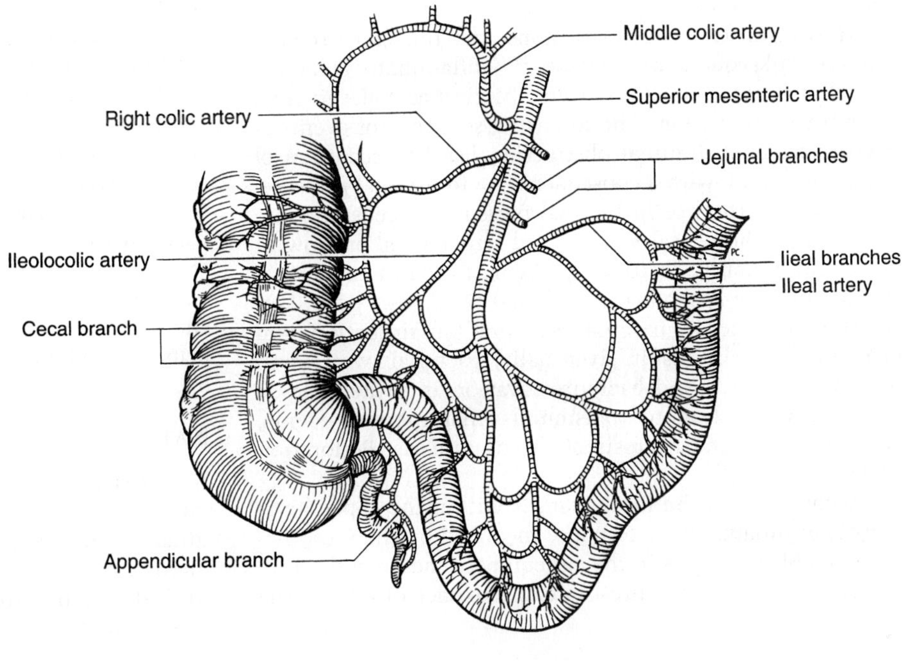

FIGURE 50.4. Details of the arterial blood supply to the terminal ileum, cecum, and appendix showing the normal divisions of the ileocolic artery. (After Keighley and Williams.[113])

Diseases of the Vermiform Appendix

Acute Appendicitis

Etiology and Pathogenesis

Early in the 1970s, Burkitt[20,21] proposed that the Western diet, notorious for its low levels of fiber and higher content of fat and refined sugar, was associated with certain conditions of the bowel. Appendicitis, diverticular disease, and colorectal carcinoma were observed with high frequency in peoples with such diet and with low frequency among peoples such as African bushmen who ate diets with much higher fiber content. In examining surgical specimens of patients undergoing colon resection for reasons other than appendicitis,[21] he noted that fecaliths were more prevalent in adults in developed countries such as Canada (32%) than adults in developing areas of South Africa (4%). He noted the general association of fecalith with acute appendicitis (52% in Canadian patients; 23% in South Africans). He proposed that low-fiber diets contribute to changes in motility, flora, or luminal conditions that predispose to development of fecaliths. Striking, however, was the confirmation of the observation that most patients with acute appendicitis do not have obvious fecalith or stone in either population group.

Role of Obstruction

Wangensteen conceptualized acute appendicitis as a closed-loop obstruction. He contended that obstruction could be demonstrated in about half of the cases, and that its cause was usually a fecalith.[18,19] In his earlier work, Wangensteen suggested that the outlet of the appendix to the cecum is susceptible to obstruction because of both the positioning of mucosal folds and a sphincter-like arrangement of muscularis fibers. More recently, it has become dogma that, in the absence of a fecalith, many cases of obstruction are caused by hyperplasia of lymphoid tissue in the mucosa and submucosa. In a very small percentage of cases, perhaps 2%, obstruction is caused by neoplasm (carcinoma or carcinoid tumor) or, very rarely, a foreign body.[22–24]

In Wangensteen's investigations and the experimental studies of subsequent investigators,[25–29] inflammatory changes typical of acute appendicitis were observed as consequences of luminal obstruction. The following sequence of events is envisioned: First, luminal obstruction leads to secretion of mucus and fluid, with a consequent rise in luminal pressure; second, when the rise in luminal pressure exceeds pressure within the submucosal venules and lymphatics, outflow of blood and lymph is obstructed, leading to increases in pressure within the appendiceal wall; and third, when capillary pressure is exceeded, mucosal ischemia, inflammation, and ulceration are the result. Eventually, bacterial overgrowth within the lumen and bacterial invasion into the mucosa and submucosa lead to transmural inflammation, edema, vascular stasis, and necrosis of the muscularis. Perforation ensues.

Accompanying the local changes within the appendix is a regional inflammatory response mediated by the mesothelium and blood vessels in the parietal peritoneum and serosa of nearby visceral structures. In one sequence of events, the outpouring of neutrophils and inflammatory mediators from these structures would lead to local inflammatory adhesions and walling-off of the inflammatory mass. In this sequence, perforation of the appendix would lead to formation of a walled-off, periappendiceal abscess. Alternatively, if surrounding structures fail to wall off the evolving phlegmon, perforation of the appendix would cause spillage into the peritoneal cavity, leading to spreading peritonitis, massive third-spacing of fluid, shock, prostration, and then death.

Although it is widely accepted that obstruction is the inciting event in most cases of acute appendicitis, it is worth pointing out some observations that are not consistent with this hypothesis. The first observation is that impacted fecaliths have been observed with no accompanying local inflammation or syndrome of appendicitis.[21] In addition, fecalith impaction or functional evidence of obstruction cannot be demonstrated in a substantial number, up to half, of cases.[26,27] In elegant studies of patients with acute appendicitis, Arnbjornsson and Bengmark repeated Wangensteen's earlier studies, using finer catheters to detect raised intraluminal pressure.[28,29] They could demonstrate such increases in pressure and evidence of obstruction to fluid infusion in only about 25% of cases of pathologically established, acute appendicitis. Thus, obstruction may be just one of many factors involved in the etiology and pathogenesis of acute appendicitis.

Role of Normal Colonic Flora

The flora of the inflamed appendix differ from that of the normal appendix. About 60% of aspirates of inflamed appendices have anaerobes, compared to 25% of aspirates from normal appendices.[30–32] Presumably, the lumen is the source of organisms that invade the mucosa when mucosal integrity is compromised by increased luminal pressure or intramural ischemia. Tissue specimens from the inflamed appendix wall (not luminal aspirates) virtually all culture out *Escherichia coli* and *Bacteroides* species.[31,32] There are about 10 isolates per tissue specimen. In addition to the other usual suspects (*Peptostreptococcus*, *Pseudomonas* spp., *Bacteroides splanchnicus*, *Bacteroides intermedius*, *Lactobacillus*), previously unreported fastidious gram-negative anaerobic bacilli have been encountered.[32] In a careful study by Pieper et al.,[31] serum antibody titers to polysaccharide regions in four of the *Bacteroides* species were found to be elevated in most patients with gangrenous or perforated appendicitis. These findings indicate that invasion of tissue by *Bacteroides* elicits specific humoral responses. Moreover, as is discussed next, in many cases in which acute appendicitis is highly likely, antibiotic therapy alone can reverse the evolving clinical syndrome and permit individuals to get well without an operation. Thus, the normal colonic flora play a key role in the evolution of acute appendicitis to gangrene and perforation.

Natural History and Complications

As classically conceptualized, acute appendicitis progresses inexorably, from obstruction to mucosal and then transmural inflammation, necrosis, and then gangrene with local inflammatory responses from the visceral and parietal peritoneum, to perforation with local abscess formation or spreading peritonitis. One time-honored observation has been that perforation is not common if symptoms have been present for less than 24h. In one study,[33] 95 consecutive adult patients with symptoms and signs of acute appendicitis were monitored prospectively. Fifteen patients ultimately were shown to have a perforation. Of these, 3 (20%) developed perforation earlier than 24h after onset of symptoms; in 1 patient, perforation occurred as early as 10h after the onset of symptoms. Average time from onset of symptoms to perforation was 64h.

Once necrotic or perforated, other complications can result. The great majority of patients with acute appendicitis present with symptoms and signs caused by inflammation of the appendix itself. The next most common complications involve abscess formation (with or without evidence of systemic sepsis) or spreading peritonitis. However, a small, but significant, number of patients present with symptoms and signs from complications other than local perforation and abscess formation or peritonitis. These rarer complications are listed in Table 50.1. What should be emphasized about such complications is that they are observed generally in the very young and the very old. In other words, these complications occur in patients who cannot speak for themselves or infirm patients who do not experience the acute lower abdominal symptoms that would ordinarily motivate the patient to see a physician more quickly. Appendicitis should be suspected with the appearance of intestinal obstruction in an elderly patient following what was thought to be a mild "viral" illness. It should be suspected in patients with acute systemic sepsis, but only rarely will it be the cause of a chronic fever of unknown origin (FUO).

Along with cholecystitis and diverticulitis, acute appendicitis is one of the main causes of pyogenic liver abscess and septic portal vein thrombosis (pylephlebitis). In pylephlebitis,[34,35] the portal vein has an infected clot and continuously seeds the liver and bloodstream with bacteria. This condition is characterized by high fever and jaundice. If the symptoms and signs of appendicitis are not prominent, as they often are not, then the patient appears to have cholangitis or biliary tract disease. This complication also occurs in the setting of acute cholecystitis or diverticulitis.

TABLE 50.1. Complications of Acute Appendicitis.

Complication	*Management*
Spreading peritonitis	Antibiotics, appendectomy
Abscess	Antibiotics, appendectomy
Abdominal	Percutaneous drainage reserved for poor surgical risk patients; interval appendectomy in 6 weeks recommended
Retroperitoneal	
Intestinal obstruction	Antibiotics, appendectomy
Bacteremia/systemic sepsis	Antibiotics, appendectomy, or percutaneous drainage of appendiceal abscess until acute episode resolves
Fistula	
Abdominal wall	Antibiotics until acute episode resolved, then bladder interval appendectomy and closure of fistula
Liver abscess	Broad-spectrum antibiotics; percutaneous drainage of liver and appendiceal abscess; interval appendectomy
Pyelophlebitis	Broad-spectrum antibiotics; systemic anticoagulation; percutaneous drainage of liver and appendiceal abscesses; interval appendectomy

Clinical Presentation

Symptoms

At the onset of the episode, the patient typically reports crampy (colicky) abdominal pain. This quality of the pain is attributable to the initial response of the muscularis of the appendix (or any hollow-lumen organ) to obstruction. The pain is described as diffuse or perhaps centered about the umbilicus; this is because the appendix arises from the midgut, an embryonic midline structure that derives its innervation from autonomic afferents related to the spinal cord centered around T10. Typically, this pain does not radiate, and the patients do not describe it as exacerbated by changes in body position, meals, urination, or defecation. As the response to luminal obstruction evolves to include luminal distension, intramural edema, and ischemia, the pain becomes constant. Vomiting is often reported by younger patients but is not a prominent symptom in mature adult and aged patients. In general, patients with appendicitis report nausea and loss of appetite; a patient reporting a normal appetite is very uncommon.

Signs

The invasion of bacteria with ensuing inflammatory response within the appendiceal wall and the surrounding visceral structures leads to appearance of pain and tenderness localized to the area of parietal peritoneum overlying the inflamed tissue (*phlegmon*). Fever above 100°F or 38.2°C rarely occurs early in the appendicitis syndrome and usually appears after the time when localizing tenderness appears. In many cases, the localized pain and tenderness are accompanied by peritoneal findings that are localized to the right lower quadrant of the abdomen. These symptoms include rebound tenderness, referred tenderness, and involuntary guarding in the area overlying the phlegmon. Although its predictive power is disputed,[36–38] McBurney's point is supposed to be the place where the appendix lies and therefore the place of maximum tenderness.[10,37] The visceral pain of distension and ischemia that is centered about the umbilicus does not necessarily go away, and it is probably not accurate to describe the pain as having "migrated."

When the inflamed portion of the appendix (usually the tip) is not located near the parietal peritoneum, the place of maximal tenderness is not necessarily in the right lower quadrant. In fact, there may be no localizing area of tenderness[38] when the appendix is located in a retroperitoneal or retroileal position or in the true pelvis. Although it is commonly held that a retrocecal position obscures localizing tenderness and peritoneal findings, there is evidence that this is not so.[38,39] Theoretically, an acutely inflamed appendix in the true pelvis can be suspected by means of rectal examination when the examiner elicits localized tenderness or palpates a mass. In one study,[40] rectal examination was useful in identifying a clinical picture of acute appendicitis; however, it was not an independent predictor if other abdominal peritoneal findings (i.e., rebound or localized tenderness) were absent.

Classic texts also recognize three diagnostic maneuvers: *Rovsing's sign* is positive when pressure applied in the left lower quadrant of the abdomen elicits pain on the right side, reflecting peritoneal irritation. The *psoas sign* is elicited by positioning the patient on the left side and extending the right hip. Pain produced with this maneuver reflects irritation of the right psoas muscle and indicates retrocecal and retroperitoneal irritation from a phlegmon or an abscess. The *obturator sign* is produced by positioning the patient supine and then rotating the flexed right thigh internally, from lateral to medial. Pain produced with this maneuver indicates inflammation near the obturator muscle in the true pelvis. It should be recognized that each of these "signs" is sought as a way of establishing the location of the inflamed or perforated appendix. It is only in the context of a characteristic history and examination that the diagnosis of appendicitis itself is made. These considerations emphasize that no one symptom or finding, observed at any single point in time, reliably establishes or excludes the diagnosis of acute appendicitis: it is the overall clinical picture that counts.

Laboratory Findings

Routine laboratory studies are helpful in diagnosing acute appendicitis, largely through exclusion of other conditions. Perhaps the only truly routine study is the leukocyte count. It is well recognized that the white blood cell (WBC) count is usually elevated in bona fide cases of appendicitis. However, a substantial number of patients have the diagnosis and a normal WBC count. Many times, in retrospect, a normal WBC count can be attributed to the early stage of the illness, and elevation might have been anticipated as the illness progressed. For this reason, serial measurements of the WBC count would undoubtedly improve the accuracy of the test, and this has been shown.[41]

Depending on the clinical circumstances, three other types of studies should be performed routinely. First, urine analysis with microscopic examination should be performed in all patients with suspected appendicitis.[42,43] The goal of performing the test is to exclude ureteral stones (hematuria) and to evaluate the possibility of urinary tract infection (UTI) (pyuria, bacteruria) as a cause of lower abdominal pain, particularly in elderly diabetic patients. Lower UTI is not infrequent among patients with acute appendicitis, especially women. The presence of UTI thus does not exclude acute appendicitis but does need to be identified. The newer "dipsticks" contain indicators for bacterial infection and can be used to supplant the microscopic examination.

Second, measurement of serum liver enzymes and amylase levels can be helpful in diagnosing liver, gallbladder, or pancreatic inflammation if the pain is described as more in the midabdomen or even right upper quadrant. Serum amylase levels are reported elevated in 3% to 10% of patients with acute appendicitis or acute lower abdominal pain not attributable to pancreatitis.[44,45] If pancreatitis is the cause, the pattern of amylase elevation is usually higher and is accompanied by elevations of serum lipase. Elevation of the latter, especially if it is more than threefold greater than normal, strongly indicates pancreatitis. Measurements of serum amylase are not recommended for all patients with abdominal pain but should be considered in patients with atypical clinical features.

Third, serum β-HCG (human chorionic gonadotropin) levels should be measured in women of childbearing years if there is any possibility of pregnancy. It is currently standard practice in many hospital emergency departments to use such tests to exclude the possibility of ectopic or concurrent pregnancy in patients with acute abdominal pain. This practice has not been systematically scrutinized for cost-effectiveness, but it makes sense because the stakes are so high if a pregnancy is not recognized before a fetus is exposed to ionizing radiation or the mother is explored under general anesthesia.

Imaging Studies

Four types of imaging studies may assist in the diagnosis of acute appendicitis (Table 50.2). Plain abdominal films have been used regularly in evaluation of patients with acute abdominal pain. The finding most commonly associated with acute appendicitis is the fecalith. Burkitt and associates[21] observed that fecaliths were quite commonly (about 30%) present in a group of Canadian patients who had undergone abdominal surgery for indications other than abdominal pain. When appendicitis was the indication for surgery, fecaliths were present in half of patients. Sarr and associates[27] performed a detailed review of their patients at the Mayo Clinic, noting that the prevalence of fecaliths or calculi was about 10% in adult patients with uncomplicated appendicitis, approximately 20% in adult patients with perforated appendicitis, and more than 40% in adult patients with appendiceal abscess. Of great interest, fecaliths or calculi were present in 7% of patients with clinically suspected appendicitis who ultimately had no appendicitis by pathological examination. In this series, only 2% of patients undergoing incidental appendectomy had fecaliths. Although these findings confirm the suspicion that fecaliths probably play a role in the etiology of acute appendicitis, it is difficult to formulate estimates of the sensitivity and specificity of the finding of a fecalith. It would appear, however, that in the setting of acute abdominal pain, the presence of fecalith is likely to be associated with acute appendicitis about 90% of the time. It may thus be regarded as a sensitive sign of acute appendicitis and predictive of a high likelihood of progression to perforation.

In older patients, for whom perforated viscus is a major part of the differential diagnosis, it is difficult to argue against

TABLE 50.2. Imaging Modalities in the Diagnosis of Acute Appendicitis.

Modality	*Key findings*	*Sensitivity (%)*	*Specificity (%)*
Plain abdominal film	Fecalith Loss of fat stripe Sentinel loop/ileus	30	50–80
Barium enema	Nonfilling of appendix; cecal wall irregularity/ mass effect	85	95
Ultrasound	"Target" sign abscess; loss of motility	80	90
CT scan	Phlegmon abscess	95	90

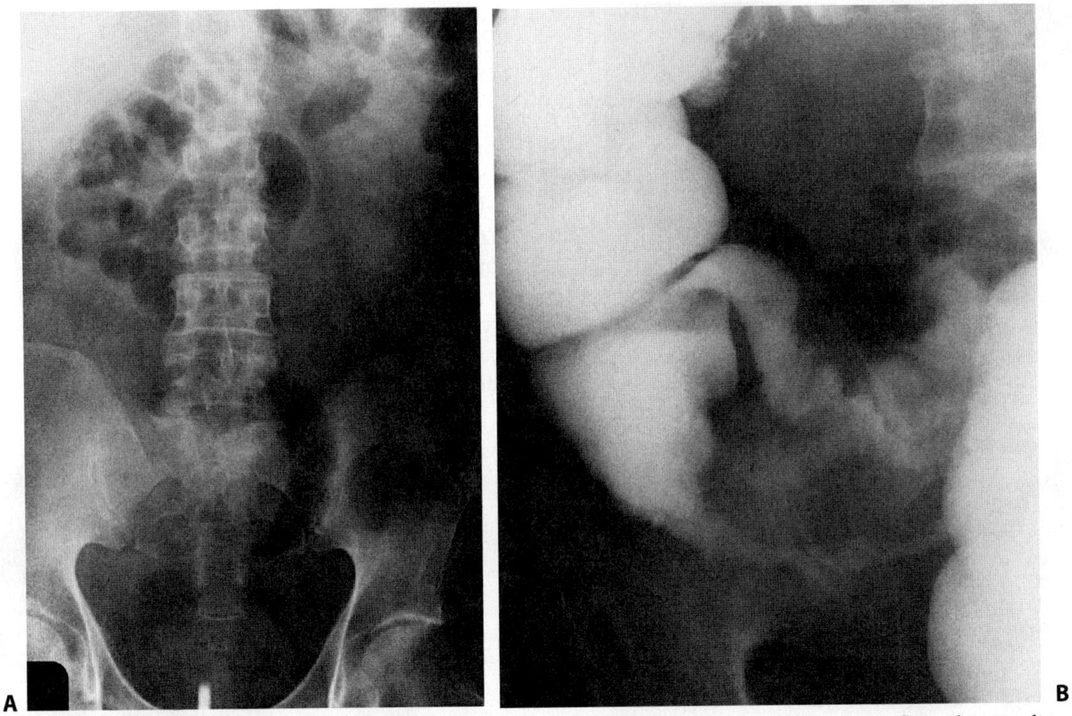

FIGURE 50.5. **A.** Plain abdominal radiograph in a 70-year-old man shows a mass effect, pushing bowel to the center of the abdomen. **B.** Barium enema in the same patient shows the mass effect on the medial cecal wall caused by the inflamed appendix and phlegmon. (Courtesy of Julian Gilliam, MD, Department of Radiology, West Roxbury VAMC, West Roxbury, MA.)

the plain film as the initial imaging study. In younger patients, the low likelihood of finding a fecalith suggests that obtaining plain films is not cost-effective. If such films are done, then it is best to obtain a complete series of plain films, including flat and upright views. A follow-up barium enema can be helpful (Fig. 50.5) but is not more helpful than other modalities.

Ultrasound examination of the abdomen has become increasingly popular in recent years. Key findings of this study include (1) thickening of the wall and loss of the normal layers ("target" sign); (2) loss of wall compressibility; (3) increased echogenicity of the surrounding fat; and (4) loculated pericecal fluid (Fig. 50.6). Although this test has a relatively low sensitivity level (80%), it has relatively high specificity (90%). This imaging modality is helpful in excluding other causes of abdominal pain in women, particularly those in their childbearing years. When gynecological causes of pain are difficult to exclude, vaginal ultrasound may be a useful adjunct in these patients.

Computerized tomography (CT) may be considered the gold standard for noninvasive imaging of acute appendicitis. The CT scan can detect and localize inflammatory mass and abscess (Fig. 50.7); if orally administered contrast fills the appendiceal lumen and no inflammatory changes are present, the diagnosis is essentially excluded. In addition, other abdominal pathology can be detected, including lesions in the pelvis. It has 95% sensitivity, 95% specificity, and 95% accuracy overall.[46,47]

A technique for focused helical CT of the appendix has also been introduced as a means of saving time and cost without reducing accuracy (Fig. 50.8). In 100 consecutive patients with clinically suspected appendicitis, Rao et al.[48] found that treatment plans were altered in 59. There were no false negatives in this study. Unnecessary appendectomy was prevented in 13 patients in whom exploration would otherwise have been done, and observation times in the hospital were reduced in 39 patients. Using the focused technique, the

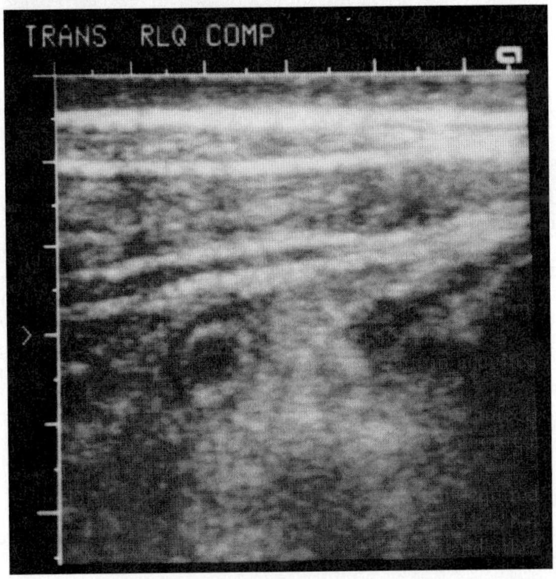

FIGURE 50.6. Sonographic detection of an acutely inflamed, unruptured appendix. A "target" sign is demonstrated just below the abdominal wall musculature. Edema (water density) in the wall separates the more dense mucosa and submucosa of the appendix from surrounding structures. (Courtesy of Fay Lang, MD, Department of Radiology, Brigham and Women's Hospital, Boston, MA.)

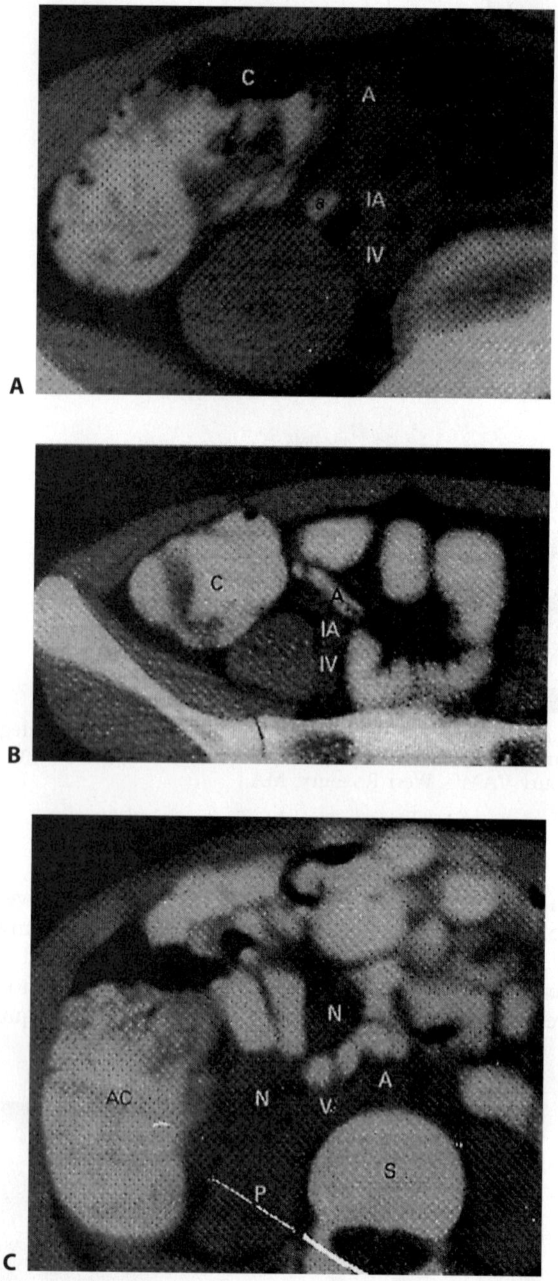

FIGURE 50.7. Computerized tomography of three patients with lower abdominal pain and suspected of having acute appendicitis. **A.** In a 17-year-old male, an unopacified appendix (*A*) and the appendicolith itself (*a*) are seen. Also visualized are the cecum (*C*), iliac artery (*IA*), and iliac vein (*IV*). **B.** In a 21-year-old woman, the opacified appendix (*A*) is normal. **C.** In an 8-year-old girl, enlarged lymph nodes (*N*) are seen at the level of the ascending colon (*AC*), consistent with a diagnosis of mesenteric adenitis. Also shown are the aorta (*A*), vena cava (*V*), and psoas muscle (*P*). (From Rao et al.,[48] with permission.)

authors estimated that, overall, the savings realized exceeded the cost of the scans by $447 per patient. It is not clear that such cost savings can be realized in institutions that do not have access to this technology and the support staff capable of providing round-the-clock coverage. However, these observations confirmed that CT is useful and potentially cost-effective in the correct clinical setting.

Evaluation and Management of the Patient with Suspected Appendicitis

Structured and History Examination

In his famous monograph, Sir Zachary Cope emphasized the importance of structuring the patient interview and examination so that each symptom and sign could be appraised in relation to others. Recently, it has been recognized that a structured approach to the patient with acute abdominal pain improves diagnostic accuracy and accelerates the initiation of the correct management plan.[49] Table 50.3 provides an example of a structured history, physical, and basic laboratory examination. Three points deserve repeat emphasis: First, the evolution of symptoms and signs is the key to correct

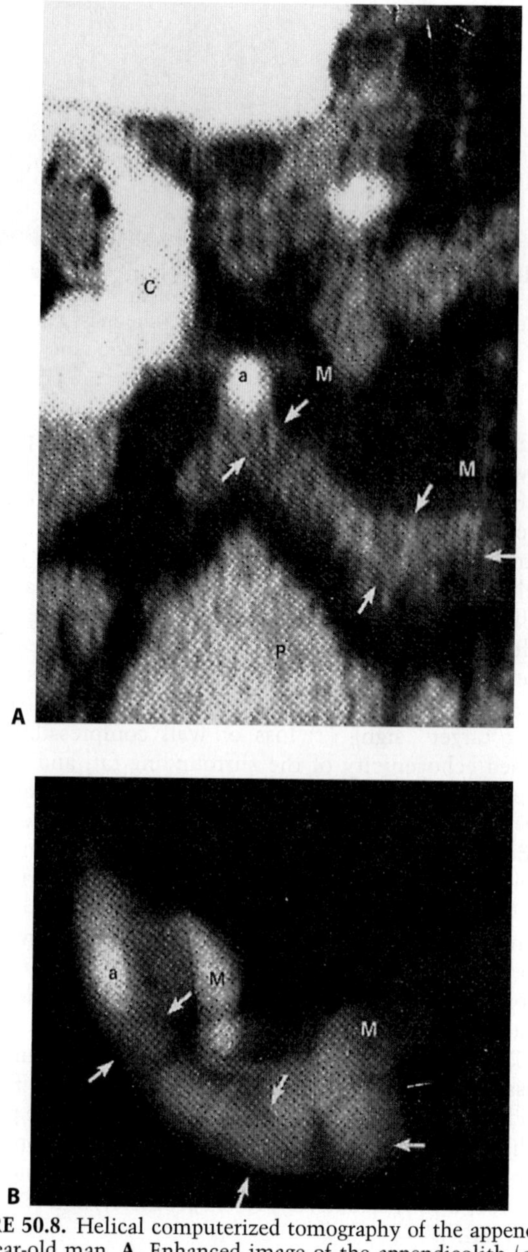

FIGURE 50.8. Helical computerized tomography of the appendix in a 30-year-old man. **A.** Enhanced image of the appendicolith (*a*), the inflamed unopacified appendix (*arrows*), and the hypodense appendiceal mesentery. Also seen are the cecum (*c*) and psoas muscle (*P*). **B.** Plain radiograph of the specimen after removal. (From Rao et al.,[48] with permission.)

TABLE 50.3. Structured Format for Diagnosis of Acute Appendicitis.

Patient identification		
History		
Previous laparotomy		
Previous right lower quadrant pain		
Other relevant medical problems		
First-degree relative with acute appendicitis		
Ob/gyn history and last menses (date)		
Clinical assessment		
Initial exam date/time/examiner/duration of illness		
Repeat exam date/time/examiner/duration of illness		
Symptoms/signs	***1st exam***	***2nd exam***
Classic history of pain (onset, quality, location, radiation, associated symptoms)		
Pain shift to right lower quadrant		
Pain with cough/movement		
Facial flush		
Tenderness at McBurney's point		
Guarding at McBurney's point		
Rectal exam: increased pain on right		
Pelvic exam: absence of discharge/adnexal tenderness		
Temperature		
Urinalysis		
Glucose		
WBCs		
RBCs		
β-HCG		
Blood test		
Hematocrit/hemoglobin		
WBC count		
Left shift?		
Indication for surgery		
Clear indications		
Uncertain indications		
Operation		
Date/time/surgeon		
Postoperative diagnosis		
Findings		
Operation performed		
Lessons learned:		

diagnosis, and one examination alone is not usually sufficient to render a diagnosis. Second, the examination is incomplete unless digital rectal and (in women) speculum/bimanual examinations of the pelvis are performed. Third, urine analysis and pregnancy test should be performed to avoid missing a diagnosis of urinary tract processes and pregnancy as well as to prevent unknowing exposure of an unborn fetus to x-ray radiation.

Differential Diagnosis

Causes of lower abdominal pain other than appendicitis are listed in Table 50.4, based on location. In young men, given the appropriate clinical setting, acute appendicitis is the likeliest cause of acute right lower quadrant pain. Inflammation of a Meckel's diverticulum is extremely uncommon but is not that different in pathogenesis or natural history from appendicitis.[50] Gastroenteritis may be suspected when gastrointestinal disturbances (vomiting, diarrhea) are prominent in the symptom complex; it should be suspected particularly when such symptoms precede the development of abdominal pain and when fever or leukocytosis occur very early in the course of the illness. Crohn's disease should also be considered with a chronic or relapsing history of pain, diarrhea, fever, or weight loss.

In middle-aged and older men, consideration must be given to inflammatory conditions such as perforating peptic ulcer with fluid tracking along the right colonic gutter, acute cholecystitis, and acute pancreatitis. These conditions are not commonly confused with acute appendicitis. More difficult to distinguish are episodes of acute diverticulitis, especially if the diverticulum is located in the cecum or ascending colon.[51] Cecal diverticuli are usually "true" diverticuli (i.e., encompassed by all layers of the bowel); the pathogenesis and presentation are similar to those of acute appendicitis. In contrast, diverticuli located in the sigmoid colon are outpouchings of mucosa and submucosa through the muscularis. When the sigmoid lies in the midline or in the right lower quadrant, a syndrome of acute diverticulitis may be characterized by pain, tenderness, and peritoneal findings. The key to suspecting acute sigmoid diverticulitis lies in its relatively more rapid evolution to localized or free peritonitis and a history of abdominal pain and changes in bowel habits before the current episode.

Malignancies must also be considered. Perforating carcinomas of the cecum or ascending colon may present with acute pain and peritoneal findings or abscess.[52] Rarely, a cecal carcinoma itself obstructs the lumen of the appendix, leading

TABLE 50.4. Differential Diagnosis of Acute Appendicitis.

A. When the appendix is located above the cecum:
Cholecystitis
Inflamed or perforated duodenal ulcer (fluid tracking down the right gutter)
Perinephric abscess
Hydronephrosis (acute or subacute)
Kidney/upper ureteral stone
Omental torsion
Pneumonia with pleurisy
Hepatitis
Pancreatitis

B. When appendix is in the iliac position:
Inflamed or perforated duodenal ulcer (fluid tracking down the right gutter)
Crohn's disease
Cecal carcinoma
Lymphoma
Ureteral stone
Yersinia, CMV, tuberculous infection
Inflamed Meckel's diverticulum
Psoas abscess (tuberculosis or other cause)
Rupture or hematoma of the rectus abdominis muscle
Cecal ulcer
Typhoid fever (*Salmonella typhi* or *Salmonella paratyphi*)

C. When the appendix is in the pelvic position:
Intestinal obstruction
Diverticulitis of the colon
Perforation of a typhoid ulcer
Gastroenteritis

D. In women:
Ectopic pregnancy
Ovarian cyst ruptured or twisted on its pedicle
Pelvic inflammatory disease (including rupture of pyosalpinx)
Ruptured ovarian follicle
Ruptured corpus luteum cyst

secondarily to an episode of acute appendicitis.[53] Lymphomas of the terminal ileum can also present with acute obstruction or perforation, mimicking an episode of complicated appendicitis. Most such abdominal malignancies, however, are usually accompanied by findings of guaiac-positive stool, anemia, history of weight loss, or chronic changes in bowel habits.

In young women, common causes of right lower quadrant pain include those mentioned for young men and the following problems: rupture of an ovarian follicle or cyst, torsion of an ovary, ectopic pregnancy, and acute salpingitis with or without tuboovarian abscess. In older but premenopausal women, endometriosis is a cause of chronic lower abdominal pain that, in very acute episodes, can sometimes be mistaken for appendicitis.[54] With regard to gynecological conditions, differentiation from acute appendicitis can usually be made based on gynecological history and association of the episode with the phases of the menstrual cycle. The relationship of the menstrual cycle to the presentation of appendicitis is complex. Arnbjornsson has reported that the illness develops more commonly in the luteal phase but has a higher complication rate when it appears in the follicular phase.[55] Others have noted that appendicitis is especially difficult to diagnose in the midphase of the menstrual cycle.

Initial Management

It is obvious, but necessary, to point out that patients with acute abdominal pain can be separated into those who are clearly sick and getting worse, those who are clearly not very sick and getting better, and those in whom the evolution of symptoms and signs is not certain. Those patients who are clearly sick require a management plan that includes the placement of intravenous access, initiation of intravenous fluid infusion to replace calculated losses and to anticipate future losses, and the inability to take fluids orally. In general, pain medication and antibiotic therapy should not be administered if the diagnosis is undecided. Although this point of management remains controversial, it should be emphasized that therapy can be initiated intelligently only when the diagnosis is known or when the failure to treat could result in unacceptable morbidity or mortality. When the diagnosis is not certain, it is my view that early use of pain medication and antibiotics can obscure and delay the diagnosis and initiation of appropriate therapy. On the other hand, if the diagnosis of appendicitis is decided, there are good reasons to make the patient comfortable and to initiate antibiotic therapy while awaiting definitive management. Such patients should be admitted to the care of the surgeon, who must then decide whether further diagnostic imaging is needed or whether the situation requires immediate operative exploration.

Patients who seem to be not very ill and getting better should be evaluated with the following question in mind: Is it possible that the apparent improvement of symptoms is only temporary? It is well recognized that perforation of a gangrenous appendix can temporarily be accompanied by relief of some aspects of the patient's discomfort. In this situation, however, such patients never quite lose their apprehensiveness, and the abdominal wall rigidity persists. In other circumstances, the perforation may be accompanied by formation of a walled-off abscess, which is associated with improvement in pain and tenderness and even a recovery in appetite. Such patients may return several days later with a mass that was not suspected at the initial evaluation. However, most such patients can be recognized by a rather slow progression of improvement. Most patients who present with acute abdominal pain that subsides within a few hours and is not accompanied by local tenderness, leukocytosis, anorexia, or signs of systemic illness can safely be assumed not to have appendicitis and can be discharged. All such patients should receive warnings to return for evaluation if their symptoms return.

The patient who is not clearly progressing in either direction requires a high level of vigilance. Intravenous access and fluids should be initiated. Pain medication and antibiotic therapy should not be started. It is a safe principle of management to admit all such patients to the hospital ward or to an observation ward in the emergency department. The progression of symptoms and signs, and perhaps the WBC count, should be evaluated over 6 to 24 h, preferably by the same examiner. In such cases, the progression of symptoms clarifies the diagnosis, and the interval of observation poses little real risk in terms of outcome.[56] Currently, and in most cases, it is preferable and cost-effective to obtain imaging studies early on.

Imaging

There is not a published consensus regarding the use of the different imaging modalities to evaluate patients with suspected appendicitis. In older patients, the decreased incidence of appendicitis relative to other diagnoses, particularly malignancy, makes it reasonable to consider the use of abdominal and pelvic CT to confirm the diagnosis and to exclude other processes. In some circumstances, CT can be used for directed interventions that avoid laparotomy in acutely ill patients or patients at very high risk for complications of general anesthesia.

In younger patients, particularly women in the childbearing years, ultrasound can be useful in excluding gynecological processes and in evaluating the appendix. Used in conjunction with a carefully obtained history and examination, it reduces the need for laparotomy and laparoscopy simply to establish a diagnosis. As it is generally an inexpensive test, it is our preferred modality in pediatric and young adult patients in whom the diagnosis is in doubt.

Although plain abdominal films have been included in the traditional evaluation of such patients,[57] it is difficult to justify their routine use unless there is concern for the possibility of a perforated viscus (e.g., duodenal ulcer or diverticulitis). When such lesions are seriously considered in the differential diagnosis, the ability of plain films to confirm the presence of free intraperitoneal air should result in quicker diagnosis. Except in unusual circumstances, barium enema would not be used to evaluate a patient in whom acute appendicitis is strongly suspected.

Indications for Operation

When the diagnosis of appendicitis has been made with a reasonable degree of certainty, operation is indicated except in unusual circumstances. One such circumstance involves the patient in whom the acute illness has passed but is now complicated by formation of a well-circumscribed abscess. Computed tomography is excellent at delineating such lesions. In some cases, antibiotic therapy alone can be used to help the mass resolve; in others, the use of CT directs a percutaneous approach to drainage.[58–60] In this situation, the base of the cecum and appendix are not recognizable in the inflammatory mass. A secure operative closure is not feasible, and operative intervention is not likely to accomplish much more than percutaneous drainage of the abscess. Drainage directed by CT drainage avoids laparotomy until definitive (so-called interval) appendectomy is performed some weeks later. This approach is particularly suited to the elderly, infirm patient who is at risk for more morbidity in the acutely ill and debilitated state. It should be emphasized that a nonoperative approach is employed most successfully when the acute illness is past or when the abscess is circumscribed. Most patients are better served by early operation once the diagnosis is made.[60]

It should be pointed out that a number of clinicians have also evaluated the possibility of treating acute appendicitis, in its early phases, using intravenous antibiotics alone. In one remarkable study, Eriksson and Granstrom[61] reported a randomized, controlled trial in 40 patients admitted with abdominal pain of less than 72h duration and a presumptive diagnosis of acute appendicitis. Twenty patients received 2 days of intravenous antibiotics followed by 8 days of oral antibiotics. Of these, 1 required early operation and 7 subsequently required appendectomy for recurrent appendicitis. In the 20 patients randomized to surgery, diagnostic accuracy was 85%, and there were no perioperative morbidities or mortalities.

In a recent study,[62] the use of antibiotics was evaluated as primary therapy for early appendicitis. The authors used 10 clinical criteria predicting the diagnosis of acute appendicitis[63] (Table 50.5) to select patients for no therapy (0 to 4 criteria), antibiotic therapy (5 to 7 criteria), or early surgery (8 to 10 criteria). Of the 42 patients selected for antibiotics only (with a predicted prevalence of acute appendicitis of 40% to 45%,[64] only 2 subsequently developed recurrent symptoms; in the entire group of 122 patients subjected to the protocol, there were two cases of delayed treatment associated with perforation. These data are not sufficiently conclusive for an endorsement of nonoperative management in cases that would otherwise be selected for observation or imaging. However, they do provide a rationale for design of prospective trials of antibiotic therapy versus operative management in cases of proven (i.e., ultrasound or CT-identified) and uncomplicated (i.e., nonperforated) appendicitis. Such studies should be designed with the power to evaluate the incidence of infrequent but highly morbid events and postoperative complications as well as costs and recurrence rates after nonoperative therapy. It would be difficult to argue that this nonoperative approach is a cost-effective approach in most clinical situations, but the data remain to be gathered.

TABLE 50.5. Modified Alvarado Scoring System for Predicting Clinical Diagnosis of Acute Appendicitis.

Localized tenderness in the right lower quadrant
Leukocytosis (WBC >10,500/mm^3)
Migration of pain after onset
Shift of differential count to the left
Fever >100.5°F
Nausea-vomiting
Anorexia
Ketones in urine
Rebound
Guarding
Predictions:
0 to 4 criteria: Low (~5%) likelihood of appendicitis—may be discharged with instructions to return if symptoms evolve
5 to 7 criteria: Intermediate (~40%–50%) likelihood of appendicitis—should be admitted for observation or imaging studies
8 to 10 criteria: High (>80%) likelihood of appendicitis—should be taken to the operating room

Preoperative Preparation

After a diagnosis is established and operative management is chosen, the patient should be made comfortable with pain medication. Fluid status should be monitored closely, using clinical indicators (pulse, blood pressure, urine output). If there is any doubt about the completeness of resuscitation, a Foley catheter is placed to monitor urine output. Patients with complex cardiac, renal, or respiratory conditions may require more invasive monitoring. If there is a short (less than 4-h) delay in getting to the operating room, this is more than offset by the increased safety of the entire operation if it results in full restoration of the intravascular volume. Electrolyte balance is not usually a problem unless the illness has been prolonged and other complications (i.e., bowel obstruction) have supervened. If such imbalances are detected in the admitting serum chemistry evaluation, they should also be addressed.

When the decision to operate has been made, antibiotic therapy is started, usually consisting of a second-generation cephalosporin alone or a combination regimen that includes broad-spectrum coverage of gram-negative aerobes (principally *E. coli*) and anaerobes (*Bacteroides* spp.).[65] It should be emphasized that, *ordinarily, the goal of antibiotic therapy is not to treat the appendicitis itself.* In uncomplicated cases, antibiotics are used to reduce the incidence of wound and deep peritoneal infections that may occur after the operation and to protect against the consequences of bacteremia. In cases complicated by abscess formation or bacteremia, antibiotics are used to treat the complications. The literature regarding antibiotic prophylaxis is complicated, but there does seem to be consensus about the following: (1) in uncomplicated cases, a second-generation cephalosporin is as effective in reducing wound complications as multiple-drug regimens; (2) antibiotics are most effective when given just before or at the time of surgery to obtain good tissue levels as the incision is made; and (3) in uncomplicated cases, one dose is enough, and additional doses after the operation do not further reduce infection rates.

Operative Decisions

The first decision to be made is whether the procedure will be performed through a traditional "open" approach or with the assistance of laparoscopy. Figures 50.9 and 50.10 illustrate a standard approach to open appendectomy through an incision in the right lower quadrant of the abdomen. Figure 50.11 illustrate an approach to laparoscopically assisted appendectomy. Numerous trials comparing open and laparoscopically assisted approaches have been performed since the technique was popularized in the early 1990s. A number of outcome–cost and meta-analyses have been published.[66–69] The most recently reported randomized trials[70–72] and analysis from the Cochrane Database of Systematic Reviews have also clarified the

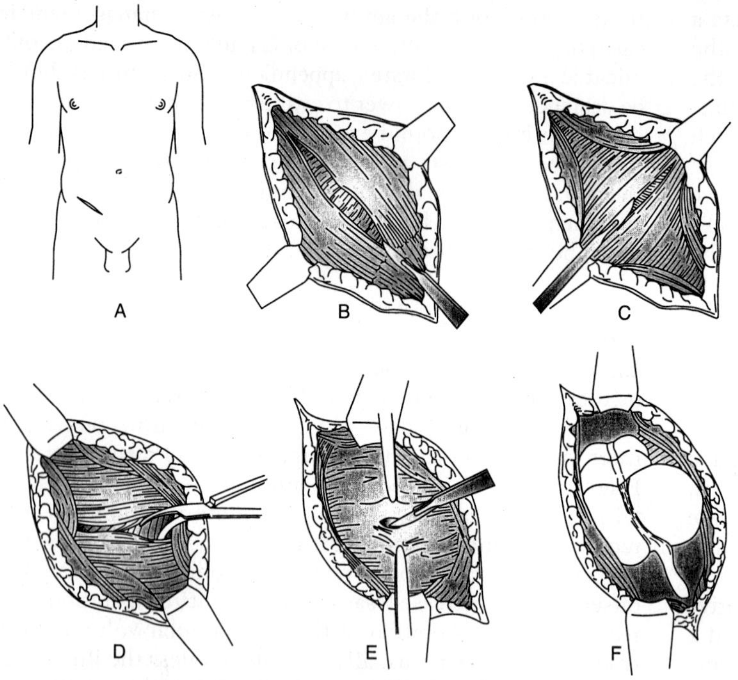

FIGURE 50.9. "McBurney" incision for appendectomy. **A.** Oblique McBurney incision through McBurney's point. **B.** Incision through the aponeurosis of the external oblique muscle. **C.** Incision through the fibers of the internal oblique muscle. **D.** Division of the fibers of the transversus abdominis muscle. **E, F.** Entry into the abdomen through the parietal peritoneum.

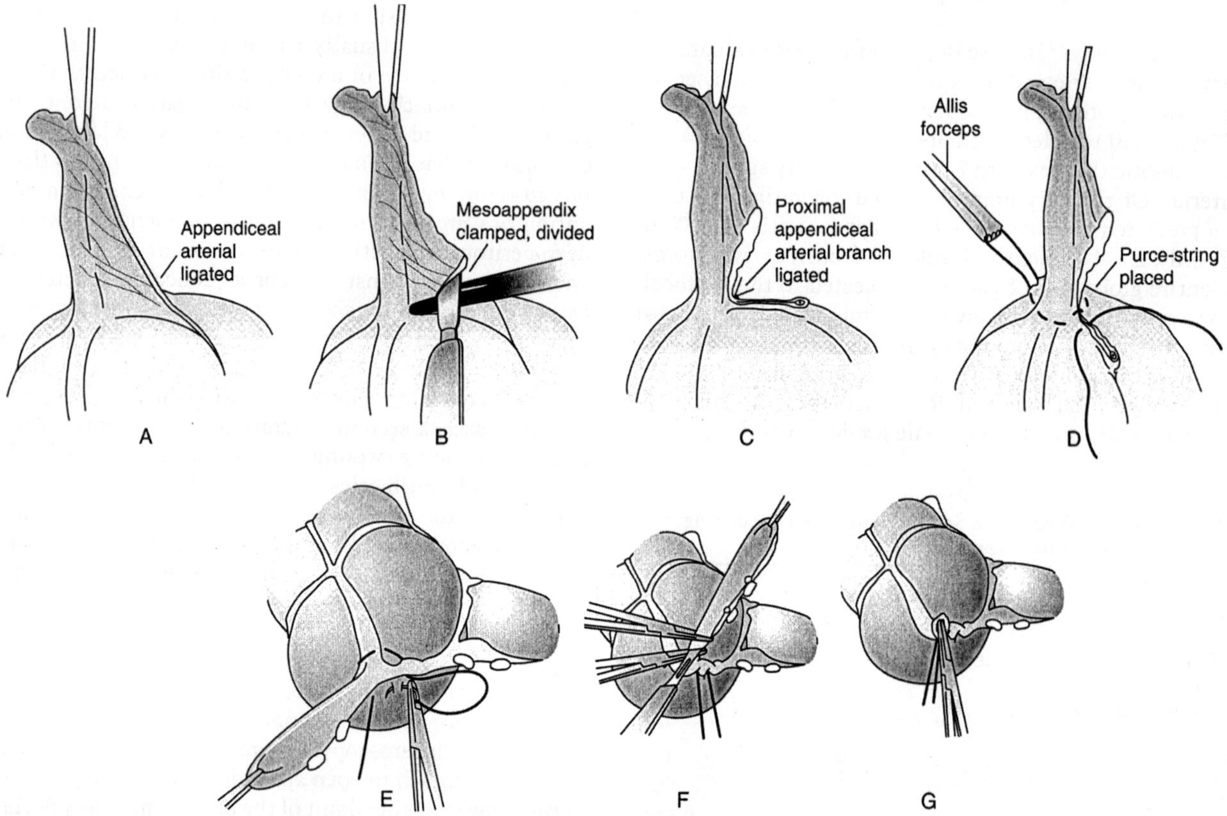

FIGURE 50.10. Appendectomy for uncomplicated acute appendicitis through the McBurney incision. **A.** The appendix is placed on stretch, allowing visualization of the mesoappendix. **B, C.** The appendiceal artery is ligated and divided between two ligatures. **D, E.** A purse-string suture is placed around the base of the appendix. **F.** The appendix is divided just above a clamp and tie placed close to the base. **G.** The clamp is used to maintain the position of the appendix as it is "dunked" below the purse-string suture. The appendix is now ligated and inverted into the lumen of the cecum.

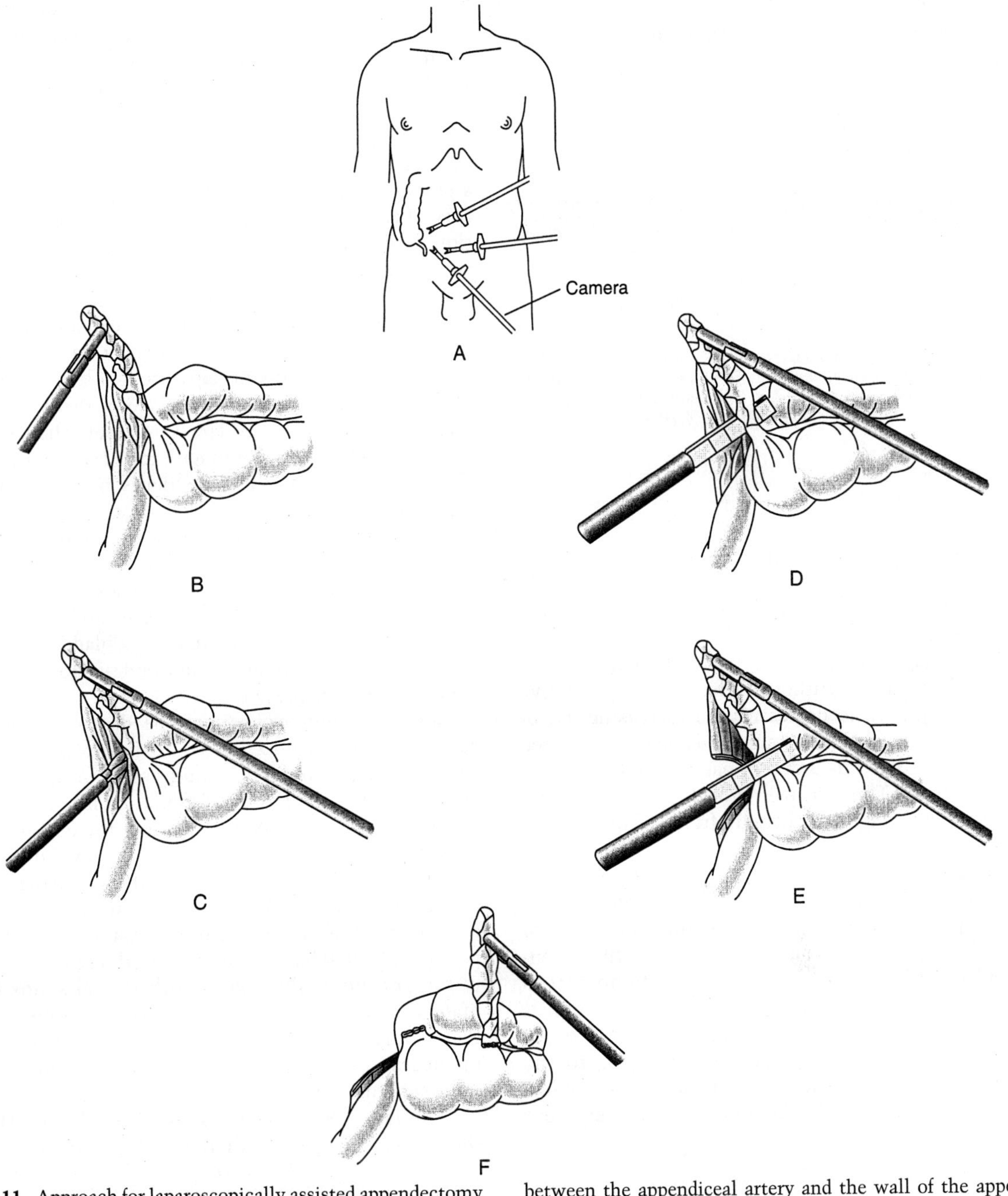

FIGURE 50.11. Approach for laparoscopically assisted appendectomy for uncomplicated acute appendicitis. **A.** Placement of ports, with the laparoscope repositioned from the umbilical port to the infraumbilical port. **B.** Retraction of the appendix. **C.** Dissection of the space between the appendiceal artery and the wall of the appendix itself. **D.** Division of the mesoappendix using a linear cutter-type stapling device. **E.** Division of the appendix at its base. **F.** The specimen is grasped and retrieved.

potential advantages and limitations of open and laparoscopic approaches in cases of early and uncomplicated appendicitis (Tables 50.6 and 50.7). Ideally, such trials would also have addressed: (1) outcomes associated with each approach in patients with appendicitis complicated by gangrene, free perforation, or abscess formation; and (2) outcomes associated with each approach in patients for whom the diagnosis is doubtful.

Based on the most recent information available, it seems clear that, in uncomplicated cases for which the diagnosis is secure, the laparoscopic approaches may offer a small reduction in pain scores, a mild reduction in hospital stay, and possibly a reduction in wound infection rates. Return to normal activity may also occur earlier. In these cases, however, the operating time and overall hospital costs of the laparoscopic approach are higher. Thus, in a cost analysis, the benefit of laparoscopically assisted appendectomy can only be realized if the patients routinely return to work and productive activity sooner than patients undergoing open procedures. This advantage has not yet been shown. Patients with complications of appendicitis have not yet been included in large enough numbers to reach conclusions about the relative advantages of either approach. In the meantime, the optimal choice for operative approach should be based on likelihood

TABLE 50.6.
Advantages of Laparoscopic Versus Conventional Open Appendectomy.

Laparoscopic	*Open*
Diagnosis of other conditions	Shorter time in operating room
Decreased wound infection	Operation less costly
Decrease in hospital stay	Overall decreased cost of hospital stay
Decrease in time for convalescence return to work or normal activity	Possibly less risk of intraabdominal abscess in perforated cases

Source: Data from meta-analysis and reviews of prior prospective controlled randomized trials (level I evidence), including Br J Surg 1997;84:1045–1050, Dis Colon Rectum 1998;41:398–403, J Am Coll Surg 1998;186:545–553; Cochrane Database of Systematic Reviews 2004;4:CD001546.

of diagnosis, complexity of the appendicitis, and severity of illness.

The one circumstance in which laparoscopic approach may offer a definite advantage is when the diagnosis is in doubt. The diagnosis is particularly difficult to make in young women. In this group, as many as 25% to 50% of patients explored for the diagnosis of acute appendicitis will actually have another disorder.[73,74] Although the rate of "negative exploration" is expected to decrease with increasing use of imaging modalities such as ultrasound and appendix-directed CT, it seems likely that this group of patients will continue to pose a challenge. Thus, it will probably turn out that patients in this subgroup will benefit from a laparoscopic approach.

At the time of the operation, the appendix is removed if it appears inflamed. A key point in the operation includes dissection of appendix to its true base at the confluence of the tenia on the cecal wall. Failure to fully dissect the appendix may lead to retention of an appendiceal stump that is sufficiently large to harbor recurring appendicitis. A number of such cases have been reported, occurring even many years later. Such cases should serve as a warning to the wary clinician: even when a patient reports a prior appendectomy and has a scar to prove it, there may yet be a recurrent appendicitis.

Once identified, the appendix is amputated close to the base. When the operation is performed open, it is customary to invert the appendiceal stump into the cecal lumen. However, there is no evidence that this reduces postoperative leak or fistula formation, either being exceedingly rare events in uncomplicated cases. When surgery is performed laparoscopically, the appendix is usually amputated at its base using a stapling device, and no inversion is performed. When the base of the appendix cannot be identified because inflammation or abscess formation precludes safe dissection, a closed suction drain may be placed into the cavity. If the lumen of the appendix has not been obliterated, the drain allows fecal contents to drain to the outside, thereby preventing accumulation of pus and fecal material inside the peritoneal cavity.

If the exploration or laparoscopy fails to reveal acute appendicitis, a search for the cause of the acute abdominal pain must be undertaken. The distal ileum should be followed at least 2 feet proximally to look for a Meckel's diverticulum or evidence of Crohn's disease, ileitis, or mesenteric adenitis. Especially in patients over the age of 40, the ileum, the cecum, and the sigmoid colon should be examined for evidence of malignancy or acute diverticulitis. The pelvic organs should be examined carefully in women to exclude ovarian, tubal, and uterine pathology. If possible, the hand or the laparoscope should be directed to evaluate the gallbladder and the duodenum, which is especially important if cloudy or purulent-appearing fluid is present.

If no other source of pain can be identified, it is reasonable to remove the appendix. There are three reasons for removing the appendix, even if it appears grossly normal: first, the presence of a scar and history of exploration for the diagnosis may lead future care providers to assume the appendix has been removed; second, if the pain recurs, removal of the appendix eliminates this diagnosis from the differential (with the caveat just noted); and third, even in grossly normal appendices, early intramural or serosal inflammatory changes (so-called periappendicitis) have been noted with regularity (25%–50%) in microscopic evaluation or with special stains for inflammatory cytokines.[75,76] These findings have been used to argue that failure to remove the appendix in these circumstances might lead to preventable recurrences in as many as 25% of such patients.

The last intraoperative decision is whether the wounds should be left open, with the risk of wound infection, or

TABLE 50.7.
Quantitative Comparison: Laparoscopic (L) Versus Conventional Open (O) Appendectomy: Summary of Information in the Cochrane Database of Systematic Reviews.

	Expected outcome[a]	*Form of comparison*	*Weighted result (min–max)*
Wound infection rate	5% to 10%	Odds ratio lap:open	0.45 (0.35 to 0.58)
Abdominal abscess	0.0% to 0.1%	Odds ratio lap:open	2.48 (1.45 to 4.21)
Operative time (incision to closure)	40 to 80 min	Difference in time (min)	11.5 (6.9 to 16.0)
Pain intensity (day 1)	Score 5	Differences in score (arbitrary)	–0.87 (–1.26 to +0.47) (arbitrary units)
Length of stay	2 d to 3 d	Difference in days	–1.0 (–1.5 to –0.6)
Return to normal activity	14 d to 28 d	Difference in days	–5.9 (–8.1 to –3.6)
Return to work	14 d to 28 d	Difference in days	0.0 (–2.0 to +2.0)

[a]Range of outcomes in studies included in the Cochrane Analysis.
Source: Data from summary analyses from Cochrane Database of Systematic Reviews 2004;4:CD001546.

whether they can be closed primarily. Although most authors recommend leaving the incisions open when there is gross contamination by pus and fecal material, there is increasing evidence that this may be no more unsafe and less cost-effective than closing all wounds (if it is feasible) and later treating any wound infections that result.[77] This decision should be individualized to each patient.

Postoperative Care

In uncomplicated cases, patients may take liquids and then solid food as soon as they feel able, and discharge should be anticipated within 24 to 48h. Postoperative antibiotics and nasogastric decompression are not indicated routinely in such patients. Patients with perforation, abscess, or other complications have a variable course. With established peritonitis or abscess formation, a longer course of antibiotics may be needed, from 5 to 7 days after surgery. Management decisions in this latter group are individualized on the basis of the complexity of the disease and severity of illness.

Special Considerations

Advanced Age

It is widely recognized that elderly patients with appendicitis present with less-acute symptoms, less-impressive clinical signs, and leukocytosis.[78–80] Up to 30% of elderly patients present more than 48h into the illness, and between 50% and 70% have a perforation at the time of surgery. In addition, the elderly are susceptible to malignancy and other processes that are in the differential diagnosis, making correct preoperative diagnosis of acute appendicitis more difficult. Perioperative complications and mortality of delayed intervention increase with age as well. However, timely intervention can result in very acceptable complication rates, even in the most elderly patients. In one series[80] of 100 patients over 80 years of age and undergoing exploration for a diagnosis of acute appendicitis, 31 did not have appendicitis. Negative exploration was associated with no mortality, compared with 21% mortality in the 49 patients who presented with perforation. These considerations argue that the risk of delay is higher than the risk of exploration. Therefore, in this age group, it is reasonable to be diagnostically aggressive (i.e., use CT scan) to establish the diagnosis or to identify other pathology and to move as quickly as possible to the appropriate intervention.

Pregnancy

The diagnosis of acute appendicitis during pregnancy is one of the most challenging of all clinical problems. The differential diagnosis includes pancreatitis, biliary tract disease, and processes involving the pelvic organs. Pregnancy itself, especially in the early stages, is associated with nausea, vomiting, and pain. In the first and early second trimester, the evolution of symptoms and signs is not different from that in nonpregnant women. After the fifth month, the cecum and appendix are shifted upward by the expanding uterus. In the last trimester, localized tenderness from the appendix may be found in the upper flank and right upper quadrant of the abdomen. Ultrasound is helpful in this setting as it may provide images of the appendix, gallbladder, uterus, and other pelvic organs.[81] Use of x-rays should be avoided if possible. However, there are highly individualized circumstances in which CT or other studies employing ionizing radiation truly may be necessary and in the best interest of the mother's health. In these circumstances, it should be remembered that the risk to the fetus, although never negligible, is thought to be less than the risks of spontaneous abortion or the likelihood of spontaneous birth defect.

When the diagnosis of appendicitis is considered likely, the patient should be explored. The following considerations should be borne in mind if the diagnosis is not certain[82–84]: (1) appendicitis is not more common in any of the three trimesters; (2) progression to perforation seems to be more common in the last trimester, presumably because of delays in seeking treatment and delays in recognition of the need for surgery; (3) fetal mortality is probably less than 5% if the appendix is removed before rupture and as high as 20% if the appendix is removed after rupture; and (4) maternal mortality is small (less than 1%) but has been reported almost exclusively in patients who had a ruptured appendix. On the other hand, patients and relatives need to be counseled about the risks of negative laparotomy to the fetus. Although this risk certainly appears to be less than when the patient has appendicitis, it has not been precisely quantitated and cannot be discounted. Overall, however, it would seem that, while the risk of preterm labor is increased, the actual harm to the fetus is not associated with increased perinatal mortality.[85,86] These considerations strongly argue for a proactive approach to exploration in doubtful cases and probably justify the higher negative laparotomy rates of 25% to 40% that have been reported.

One additional consideration is whether it is safe and appropriate to submit the pregnant patient to laparoscopic exploration and appendectomy. In the last trimester of pregnancy, it is technically too difficult for laparoscopic instruments to reach the appendix, which lies above or behind the uterus, and the procedure is most expeditiously performed using an open incision. In the first and early second trimester, however, it is feasible to perform laparoscopy and, if needed, appendectomy with laparoscopic assistance. Nevertheless, concerns have been raised regarding fetal responses to hypercarbia that might arise during insufflation of the abdomen with CO_2. In addition, increased abdominal pressure caused by insufflation may have adverse effects on uteroplacental blood flow. The safety of laparoscopic surgery in pregnancy remains a controversial subject, with some groups reporting no adverse events and some groups reporting higher than expected incidents of adverse fetal outcomes.[87–89] Although caution must certainly be exercised in using laparoscopy, it is useful for diagnosis of acute, worsening abdominal pain in the patient who is in the first or early second trimester of pregnancy. When the diagnosis of appendicitis seems likely, an open procedure is probably the most expeditious approach.

Immunocompromise

Immunocompromise alters responses of patients to localized infection and systemic stress as well as hinders normal processes of wound healing. Because appendicitis strikes patients in all age groups and walks of life, it must be considered in the differential diagnosis of acute abdominal pain of patients who have undergone organ transplantation, patients who have received chemotherapy for malignancy, patients with hematological malignancy or bone marrow failure, and patients who are infected with HIV or human T-lymphotrophic virus (HTLV). A comprehensive discussion of abdominal pain in the immunocompromised state is beyond the scope of this chapter. However, it is worth pointing out that the differential diagnosis is broad, including pancreatitis from medication or viral cytomegalovirus (CMV) infection, viral hepatitis, acalculous cholecystitis (viral, *Campylobacter*, ischemia), intraabdominal infection due to opportunistic organisms, secondary malignancies such as lymphoma, graft-versus-host disease, or neutropenic enterocolitis.

The patient with known HIV infection and AIDS may pose a particularly difficult diagnostic dilemma and therapeutic challenge. In recent years, however, several lessons have been learned. First, acute appendicitis should be suspected and managed as one would normally do in patients with HIV but who do not meet criteria for the diagnosis of AIDS. In this group of patients, appendicitis is the diagnosis in about 80% of patients who present with the appropriate clinical history, findings, and directed imaging studies. In the late 1980s, it appeared that the rate of perforation was close to 40%. Subsequent analysis has led to the conclusion that patient delays in seeking treatment and physician delays in recommending surgery probably contributed to the higher perforation rate in this group of patients. With early recognition and management, the perforation rate should be no different from that in the population without HIV infection.

When a patient with established AIDS and AIDS-related complications presents with an acute pain syndrome in the right lower quadrant of the abdomen, the differential diagnosis must specifically include infections by CMV, mycobacteria, or other opportunistic organisms such as cryptosporidia; it should also include neoplastic processes such as lymphoma and Kaposi's sarcoma. Indeed, the appendix may be inflamed, but in at least 30% of cases the cause of the inflammatory response may be an infective agent. The pain syndrome is frequently atypical, and delays in recognition and treatment are not uncommon. Expeditious use of CT is recommended, both to verify the diagnosis and to exclude other pathological processes. Morbidity and mortality rates from acute appendicitis were thought to be almost prohibitive; even now, it is clear that patients with AIDS may well have higher than expected complication and death rates after emergency laparotomy. However, early diagnosis and treatment are associated with excellent short-term survival and discharge. The presence of AIDS should not be viewed as a contraindication for aggressive diagnosis and operative intervention.[90–93]

Campylobacter Jejuni and Yersinia Enterocolitica

Campylobacter jejuni and *Yersinia enterocolitica* are responsible for a small percentage of cases of acute appendicitis.[94] In a prospective study[94] of 2861 patients undergoing appendectomy for suspected appendicitis, 3.6% had *Yersinia* (subtypes 03 and 09) as cultured from the specimen. In about 75% of cases, *Y. enterocolitica* was cultured from the stool, and mesenteric adenitis or terminal ileitis was observed in 62%. Acute suppurative appendicitis occurred in 1% of the *Yersinia*-positive patients; there were no instances of gangrene or perforation. The 03 strain is usually sensitive to ampicillin-clavulonic acid, cefoxitin, ciprofloxacin, and trimethoprim. Ampicillin alone is not effective treatment. Because of the generally self-limited nature of the illness, antibiotics are recommended only if fever and symptoms (diarrhea and cramping) are intense.

Campylobacter jejuni is cultured in about 2% of patients with suspected appendicitis. Pathology is usually limited to mucosal inflammation. Phlegmon, perforation, and abscess are rare, and terminal ileitis is observed in 50% of patients. Diarrhea is observed in about 80% of patients, in conjunction with the pain and often preceding it, and this may be the most distinctive symptom.[95] Blood in the stool is present in 50% of cases. Leukocytes and organisms with characteristic morphology (long, curved gram-negative bacilli) can be seen if the stool is collected for Gram stain. Fever is also common and occurs earlier in the course of the illness than it does in appendicitis. A prodrome of headache, myalgias, and malaise often precedes the onset of pain. Antibiotics are used only in cases that do not resolve quickly. Ultrasound may be helpful in these cases as it can show evidence of terminal ileitis.[96]

Chronic Appendicitis

Chronic right lower quadrant pain is sometimes attributed to chronic appendicitis. In careful reviews of individual cases, it has generally been possible to recognize an initial, acute episode that might have been recognized as acute appendicitis.[97,98] However, cases of chronic or recurrent acute appendicitis are now well documented. In addition, there are cases in which it is reasonable to explore or perform laparoscopy for selected patients with recurring pain and removing the appendix if no other lesion or source can be identified.[99]

Incidental Appendectomy

The term *incidental appendectomy* refers to the removal of the appendix when the laparotomy or laparoscopy is being performed to address an unrelated clinical problem. The stated goal of this practice is to prevent a later episode of acute appendicitis. In a review of elderly Medicare beneficiaries, Warren et al. estimated that 115 appendectomies would have to be performed without incident or complication to prevent one future instance of acute appendicitis, and 4472 such operations would be required to prevent a single future death from appendicitis.[100] It may be reasonable to perform incidental appendectomy in children and young adults, but it is difficult to justify the practice in patients over the age of 30 years. Incidental appendectomy should not be performed if, in the surgeon's judgment, there is a possibility that it would incur any additional morbidity.

Management of Acute Appendicitis as a Benchmark for Quality of Care and Education

As awareness of the costs of medical care have increased, so has the interest in using particular diagnoses and procedures to evaluate the quality of care and to track resource utilization. In this respect, few clinical problems have attracted as much attention as the diagnosis of acute appendicitis and the operation of appendectomy. Perforation rates, algorithms for use of laboratory tests and imaging modalities, utility and timing of perioperative antibiotic regimens, and the cost-effectiveness of wound management policies have all been scrutinized. Most strikingly, differences in patterns, based on insurance and socioeconomic status, of care have been discerned.[79] In addition, it has been suggested that the ability of surgical residents to process clinical information, develop an accurate diagnosis, and develop a management plan may be assessed using the clinical picture presented by acute appendicitis.[101]

For the individual student or resident, every case of suspected appendicitis should, when it has been resolved, provide an occasion for individual reflection: If the diagnosis was right and operation timely, what about the patient's presentation was atypical? If the diagnosis was right, but operation was delayed, what might have been done to get the patient to surgery sooner? If the diagnosis was not appendicitis and did not, in hindsight, require an operation, was there any piece of information or perspective that might have altered the decision to proceed to operation? The student of appendicitis should always remember that the decision for operation is based on the balance between the risk and cost of delay (rupture and complications) versus the risk and cost of negative laparotomy. In any individual case, when the diagnosis is not certain, the decision will generally favor operation. The quality of one's diagnostic acumen and care can only be assessed if all such cases are periodically reviewed and studied.

Neoplasms of the Appendix

Neoplasms are found in about 0.5% of appendices.[102,103] The major categories are primary adenocarcinoma, cystic neoplasms, carcinoid tumor, and metastatic tumors. Stromal tumors (leiomyoma, leiomyosarcoma, lipoma) have been reported also, but are extremely rare. Lymphoma has also been increasingly recognized, arising in patients with AIDS and causing significant complications.

Primary Adenocarcinoma

Primary adenocarcinoma of the appendix arises from the glandular epithelium of the mucosa.[104–106] Two major subtypes are recognized: mucinous and colonic. The diagnosis of malignancy is not uncommonly suspected before surgery as lymph node or distant metastases are observed in more than 50% of cases. However, the diagnosis of primary appendiceal adenocarcinoma is almost never suspected before surgery. The most common presentation is that of acute appendicitis or of carcinoma of the right colon. Associated with these tumors quite commonly are other primary malignancies, usually of the colon or the ovary (15%–30% of cases). The staging system for these lesions is similar to that for colon carcinoma. In a series reported by the Mayo Clinic,[103] Dukes stages A, B, C, and D were associated with 5-year survival rates of 100%, 67%, 50%, and 6%, respectively. Mucinous histology is associated with more favorable outcome than colonic histology, even when staging differences are taken into account. The optimal treatment is right hemicolectomy. When the lesion has been diagnosed by the pathologist in a simple appendectomy specimen, it is recommended that the patient undergo reexploration and formal hemicolectomy.[103,105]

Cystic Neoplasms and Pseudomyxoma Peritonei

On occasion, the appendix may be transformed into a cystic structure called a *mucocele*.[104,107] Various theories about the pathogenesis of these lesions have been advanced because they can harbor benign or neoplastic lesions. Perhaps the most persuasive explanation is that they represent secretion of mucus by hyperplastic or neoplastic lesions into the lumen of the appendix, which has been obliterated in such a way as to prevent decompression into the colonic lumen.[107] Neoplastic lesions (cystadenoma, cystadenocarcinoma) are found in approximately 75% to 85% of mucoceles, although most of these lesions are benign cystadenoma.[108] These lesions generally present as incidental findings on CT or as painless masses. Their walls may be calcified. On occasion they present with abdominal pain and peritoneal findings, being complicated by or simulating acute appendicitis. When the mucocele has ruptured, appendectomy is curative if the lesion is benign. If the lesion is malignant, however, cancer cells are spilled into the peritoneum and carcinomatosis may ensue.

Pseudomyxoma peritonei is caused by spillage and implantation of mucin-secreting cells into the peritoneal cavity.[109] Mucin secretion from these tumor cell implants leads to complications of recurrent inflammation, dense formation of adhesions with recurrent bowel obstruction, and fistula formation. Wide resection of the primary disease, if at all possible, is recommended. The natural history of such tumor implants is that of indolence, so that survival rates exceeding 50% at 5 years are expected. During this period, however, it is not uncommon for patients to be made miserable by repeated need for laparotomy and fistula management.

Carcinoid Tumors

Carcinoids represent the great majority of tumors found in the appendix, and the appendix is the most common site in the alimentary tract where carcinoids are found.[102,110] These tumors arise from the argentaffin cells lining the crypts of the glands. Some tumors are associated with mucocele formation, suggesting origin from stem cell lines that can differentiate into neuroendocrine and epithelial elements. About 50% of the time, these tumors are found incidentally at surgery, and about 50% of the time they present with acute appendicitis. About 75% of the time, the lesions are less than 1 cm in size; about 10% of the time they are more than 2 cm. Most lesions are found at the tip or in the distal third of the appendix. Lymph node and distant metastases have been reported almost exclusively when lesions are greater than 2 cm in size, although regional and distant spread have been reported in small tumors. It is very rare for the carcinoid syndrome to accompany an appendiceal carcinoid.

These lesions are best managed according to size. When less than 2 cm, simple appendectomy is sufficient because the likelihood of lymph node metastasis is low. When larger than 2 cm, right hemicolectomy is recommended to obviate the possibility of leaving diseased regional nodes undiagnosed. If the carcinoid is not recognized in the appendix specimen until after surgery, and it is more than 2 cm in size, it is probably best to reoperate and perform a right hemicolectomy, especially if the lesion is located near the base of the appendix. Patients with distant metastasis are treated by combination chemotherapy protocols used for carcinoid tumors in other regions. The metastases of these lesions grow slowly, so that 5-year survival rates are greater than 50% even when distant disease is present.

References

1. Williams RA, Myers P. Pathology of the Appendix. London: Chapman & Hall; 1994:1–7.
2. Meade RH. In: An Introduction to the History of General Surgery. Philadelphia: Saunders; 1968:291–304.
3. Richardson RG. The Surgeon's Tale. New York: Scribner's; 1958.
4. Da Capri JB. Commentaria cum Amplissimus Additionibus Super Anatomia Mundini Una cum Texta Ejusudem in Pristinum et Verum Nitorem Redanto [quoted in ref. 3]. Bolonial Imp. per H. Benedictus; 1521: 528 ff.
5. Vesalius A. Liber V. In: De Humani Corporis Fabrica. Basel: Johanes Oporinu; 1543:361–362.
6. Fernal JQiTC. In: Classic Description of Disease. Universa Medicina Springfield, 1932:614–615.
7. Amyand C. Of an inguinal rupture, with a pin in the appendix coeci, incrusted with stone, and some observations on wounds in the guts. Phil Trans R Soc Lond 1736;39:329–342.
8. Tait L. Surgical treatment of typhlitis. Birmingham Med Rev 1890;27:26–34.
9. Fitz RH. Perforating inflammation of the vermiform appendix; with special reference to its early diagnosis and treatment. Am J Med Sci 1886;92:321–346.
10. McBurney CM. Experience with early operative interference in cases of disease of the vermiform appendix. N Y Med J 1889; 50:676–684.
11. Kelly HA, Hurdon E. In: Anatomy of the Vermiform Appendix and Its Diseases. Philadelphia: Saunders; 1905:55–74.
12. Myers S, Miller TA. Acute abdominal pain: physiology of the acute abdomen. In: Miller TA, ed. The Physiological Basis of Modern Surgical Care. St. Louis: Quality Medical; 1998:641–667.
13. Dhillon AP, Rode J. Serotonin and its possible role in the painful non-inflamed appendix. Diagn Histopathol 1983;6:239–246.
14. Dhillon AP, Williams RA, Rode J. Age, site, and distribution of subepithelial neurosecretory cells in the appendix. Pathology 1992;24:56–59.
15. Rode J, et al., Neurosecretory cells of the lamina propria of the appendix, and their possible relationship to carcinoids. Histopathology 1982;6:69–73.
16. Bockman DE, Cooper MD. Early lymphoepithelial relationships in human appendix. Gastroenterology 1975;68:1160–1168.
17. Spencer J, Finn T, Isaacson PG. Gut-associated lymphoid tissue: a morphological and immunocytochemical study of the human appendix. Gut 1985;26:672–679.
18. Wangensteen OH, et al. Studies in the etiology of acute appendicitis: the significance of the structure and function of the vermiform appendix in the genesis of appendicitis. Ann Surg 1937;106:910–942.
19. Wangensteen OH, Dennis C. Experimental proof of the obstructive origin of appendicitis in man. Ann Surg 1939;119:629–647.
20. Burkitt DP. The aetiology of appendicitis. Br J Surg 1971;58:695–699.
21. Jones BA, et al. The prevalence of appendiceal fecaliths in patients with and without appendicitis. A comparative study from Canada and South Africa. Ann Surg 1985;202:80–82.
22. Peck JJ. Management of carcinoma discovered unexpectedly at operation for acute appendicitis. Am J Surg 1988;155:683–685.
23. Armstrong CP, et al., Appendicectomy and carcinoma of the cecum. Br J Surg 1989;76:1049–1053.
24. Klingler PJ, et al. Management of ingested foreign bodies within the appendix: a case report with review of the literature. Am J Gastroenterol 1997;92:2295–2298.
25. Pieper R, Kager L, Tidefeldt U. Obstruction of appendix vermiformis causing acute appendicitis. Acta Chir Scand 1982;148:63–72.
26. Sisson RG, Ahlvin RC, Hartlow MC. Superficial mucosal ulceration and the pathogenesis of acute appendicitis in childhood. Am J Surg 1971;122:378–380.
27. Nitecki S, Karmeli R, Sarr MG. Appendiceal calculi and fecaliths as indications for appendectomy. Surg Gynecol Obstet 1990; 171:185–188.
28. Arnbjornsson E, Bengmark S. Role of obstruction in pathogenesis of acute appendicitis. Acta Chir Scand 1983;149:789–791.
29. Arnbjornsson E, Bengmark S. Role of obstruction in pathogenesis of acute appendicitis. Am J Surg 1984;147:390–392.
30. Thadepalli H, et al. Bacteriology of the appendix and the ileum in health and in appendicitis. Am Surg 1991;57:317–322.
31. Pieper R, et al. The role of *Bacteroides fragilis* in acute appendicitis. Acta Chir Scand 1982;148:39–44.
32. Bennion RS, et al. The bacteriology of gangrenous and perforated appendicitis—revisited. Ann Surg 1990;211:165–171.
33. Temple CL, Huchcroft SA, Temple WJ. The natural history of appendicitis in adults: a prospective study. Ann Surg 1995; 221:278–281.
34. Saxena R, et al. Pylephlebitis: a case report and review of outcome in the antibiotic era. Am J Gastroenterol 1996;91:1251–1253.
35. Baril N, et al. The role of anticoagulation in pylephlebitis. Am J Surg 1996;172:449–452.
36. Ramsden WH, et al. Is the appendix where you think it is—and if not does it matter? Clin Radiol 1993;47:100–103.
37. Karim OM, Boothroyd AE, Wyllie JH. McBurney's point—fact or fiction? Ann R Coll Surg 1990;72:304–308.
38. Guidry SP, Poole GV. The anatomy of appendicitis. Am Surg 1994;60:68–71.
39. Shen GK, et al. Does the retrocecal position of the vermiform appendix alter the clinical course of acute appendicitis? A prospective analysis. Arch Surg 1991;126:569–570.
40. Dixon JM, et al. Rectal examination in patients with pain in the right lower quadrant of the abdomen. Br Med J 1991;302:386–388.
41. Thompson MM, et al. Role of sequential leucocyte counts and C-reactive protein measurements in acute appendicitis. Br J Surg 1992;79:822–824.
42. Scott JH, Amin M, Harty JI. Abnormal urinalysis in appendicitis. J Urol 1983;129:1015–1018.
43. Puskar D, et al. Urinalysis ultrasound analysis, and renal dynamic scintigraphy in acute appendicitis. Urology 1995;45:108–112.
44. Swensson EE, Maull KI. Clinical significance of elevated serum and urine amylase levels in patients with appendicitis. Am J Surg 1981;142:667–670.
45. Gumaste W, et al. Serum lipase levels in non-pancreatic abdominal pain. Am J Gastroenterol 1993;88:2051–2055.
46. Balthazar EJ, et al. Acute appendicitis: CT and US correlation in 100 patients. Radiology 1994;190:31–35.
47. Balthazar EJ, et al. Appendicitis: prospective evaluation with high resolution CT. Radiology 1991;180:21–24.
48. Rao PM, et al. Effect of computerized tomography of the appendix on treatment of patients and use of hospital resources. New Engl J Med 1998(338):141–146.
49. Korner H, et al. Structured data collection improves the diagnosis of appendicitis. Br J Surg 1998;85:341–344.
50. Cullen JJ, et al. Surgical management of Meckel's diverticulum: an epidemiologic, population-based study. Ann Surg 1994; 220:564–568.
51. Harada RN, Whelan TJ. Surgical management of cecal diverticulitis. Am J Surg 1993;166:666–669.
52. Soybel DI, Bliss DP, Wells SA. Colorectal carcinoma. Curr Probl Cancer 1987;11:259–356.
53. Bizer LS. Acute appendicitis is rarely the presentation of cecal cancer in the elderly patients. J Surg Oncol 1993;54:45–46.

54. Singh KK, et al. Presentation of endometriosis to general surgeons: a 10 year experience. Br J Surg 1995;82:1349–1351.
55. Arnbjornsson E. Influence of oral contraceptives on the frequency of acute appendicitis in different phases of the menstrual cycle. Surg Gynecol Obstet 1984;158:464–466.
56. Graff L, Radford MJ, Werne C. Probability of appendicitis before and after observation. Ann Emerg Med 1991;20:503–507.
57. Campbell JP, Gunn AA. Plain abdominal radiographs and acute abdominal pain. Br J Surg 1988;75:554–556.
58. Jeffrey RBJ, Federle MP, Tolentino CS. Periappendiceal inflammatory masses: CT-directed management and clinical outcome in 70 patients. Radiology 1988;167:13–16.
59. Hurme T, Nylamo E. Conservative versus operative treatment of appendicular abscess. Experience of 147 consecutive patients. Ann Chir Gynaecol 1995;84:33–36.
60. Gee D, Babineau TJ. The optimal management of adult patients presenting with appendiceal abscess: "conservative" versus immediate operative management. Curr Surg 2004;61:524–528.
61. Eriksson S, Granstrom L. Randomized controlled trial of appendectomy versus antibiotic therapy for acute appendicitis. Br J Surg 1995;82:166–169.
62. Winn RD, et al. Protocol-based approach to suspected appendicitis, incorporating the Alvarado score and outpatient antibiotics. Aust N Z J Surg 2004;74:324–329.
63. Alvarado A. A practical score for the early diagnosis of acute appendicitis. Ann Emerg Med 1986;15:1048–1049.
64. Douglas CD, et al. Randomised controlled trial of ultrasonography in diagnosis of acute appendicitis, incorporating the Alvarado score. Br Med J 2000;321:919–922.
65. Nichols RL. Surgical antibiotic prophylaxis. Surg Clin North Am 1995;79:509–522.
66. McCahill LE, et al. A clinical outcome and cost-analysis of laparoscopic versus open appendectomy. Am J Surg 1996;171:533–537.
67. McCall JL, Sharples K, Jadallah F. Systematic review of randomized controlled trials comparing laparoscopic with open appendectomy. Br J Surg 1997;84:1045–1050.
68. Minne L, et al. Laparoscopic vs. open appendectomy. Prospective randomized study of outcomes. Arch Surg 1997;132:708–711.
69. Golub R, Siddiqui F, Pohl D. Laparoscopic versus open appendectomy: a meta-analysis. J Am Coll Surg 1998;186:545–553.
70. Moberg AC, et al. Randomized clinical trial of laparoscopic versus open appendicectomy for confirmed appendicitis. Br J Surg 2005;92:298–304.
71. Katkhouda N, et al. Laparoscopic versus open appendectomy: a prospective randomized double-blind study. Ann Surg 2005;242:439–448.
72. Lau DH, et al. Comparison of needlescopic appendectomy versus conventional laparoscopic appendectomy: a randomized controlled trial. Surg Laparosc Endosc Percutan Tech 2005;15:75–79.
73. Cox MR, et al. Laparoscopic surgery in women with a clinical diagnosis of appendicitis. Med J Aust 1995;162:130–132.
74. Laine S, et al. Laparoscopic appendectomy—is it worthwhile? A prospective randomized study in young women. Surg Endosc 1997;11:95–97.
75. Fink AS, et al. Peri-appendicitis is a significant clinical finding. Am J Surg 1990;159:564–568.
76. Wang Y, Reen DJ, Puri P. Is a histologically normal appendix following emergency appendicectomy always normal? Lancet 1996;347:1076–1079.
77. Brasel KJ, Borgstorm DC, Weigelt JA. Cost-utility analysis of contaminated appendectomy wounds. J Am Coll Surg 1997;184:23–30.
78. Watters JM, et al. The influence of age on the severity of peritonitis. Can J Surg 1996;39:142–146.
79. Braveman P, et al. Insurance-related differences in the risk of ruptured appendix. New Engl J Med 1994;330:444–449.
80. Paajanen H, Kettunen J, Kostiainen S. Emergency appendectomy in patients over 80 years. Am Surg 1994;60:950–953.
81. Lim HK, Bae SH, Seo GS. Diagnosis of acute appendicitis in pregnant women: value of ultrasound. AJR Am J Roentgenol 1992;159:539–542.
82. Tamir IL, Bongard FS, Klein SR. Acute appendicitis in the pregnant patients. Am J Surg 1990;160:571–575.
83. To WW, Ngai CS, Ma HK. Pregnancies complicated by acute appendicitis. Aust N Z J Surg 1995;65:799–803.
84. Mahmoodian S. Appendicitis complicating pregnancy. South Med J 1992;85:19–24.
85. Kort B, Katz VL, Watson WJ. The effect of non-obstetric operation during pregnancy. Gynecol Obstet 1993;177:371–376.
86. Cohen-Kerem R, et al. Pregnancy outcome following non-obstetric surgical intervention. Am J Surg 2005;190:467–473.
87. Amos JD, et al. Laparoscopic surgery during pregnancy. Am J Surg 1996;171:435–437.
88. Gurbuz AT, Peetz ME. The acute abdomen in the pregnant patient. Is there a role for laparoscopy? Surg Endosc 1997;11:98–102.
89. Rollins MD, Chan KJ, Price RR. Laparoscopy for appendicitis and cholelithiasis during pregnancy: a new standard of care. Surg Endosc 2004;18:237–241.
90. Whitney TM, et al. Appendicitis in the acquired immunodeficiency syndrome. Am J Surg 1992;164:467–470.
91. Savioz D, et al. Acute right iliac fossa pain in acquired immunodeficiency. Br J Surg 1996;83:644–646.
92. Lowy AM, Barie PS. Laparotomy in patients infected with human immunodeficiency virus: indications and outcome. Br J Surg 1994;81:942–945.
93. Flum DR, et al. Appendicitis in patients with acquired immunodeficiency syndrome. J Am Coll Surg 1997;184:481–486.
94. Van Noyen R, et al. Causative role of *Yersinia* and other enteric pathogens in the appendicular syndrome. Eur J Clin Microbiol Infect Dis 1991;10:735–741.
95. van Spreeuwel JP, et al. *Campylobacter*-associated appendicitis: prevalence and clinicopathologic features. Pathol Annu 1987;22:55–65.
96. Puylaert JB, et al. *Campylobacter* ileocolitis mimicking acute appendicitis: differentiation with graded-compression US. Radiology 1988;166:737–740.
97. Mattei P, Sola JE, Yeo CJ. Chronic and recurrent appendicitis are uncommon entities often misdiagnosed. J Am Coll Surg 1994;178:385–389.
98. Barber MD, McLaren J, Rainey JB. Recurrent appendicitis. Br J Surg 1997;84:110–112.
99. Klingensmith ME, Soybel DI, Brooks DC. Laparoscopy for abdominal pain. Surg Endosc 1996;10:1085–1087.
100. Warren JL, et al. Appendectomy incidental to cholecystectomy among elderly Medicare beneficiaries. Surg Gynecol Obst 1993;177:288–294.
101. Anderson BO, et al. The development and evaluation of a clinical test of surgical resident proficiency. Surgery 1989;106:347–352.
102. Deans GT, Spence RA. Neoplastic lesions of the appendix. Br J Surg 1995;82:299–306.
103. Nitecki SS, et al. The natural history of surgically treated primary adenocarcinoma of the appendix. Ann Surg 1994;219:51–57.
104. Madwed D, Mindelzun R, Jeffrey RB. Mucocele of the appendix. AJR Am J Roentgenol 1993;159:69–72.
105. Cortina R, et al. Management and prognosis of adenocarcinoma of the appendix. Dis Colon Rectum 1995;38:848–852.
106. Carr NJ, McCarthy WF, Sobin LH. Epithelial noncarcinoid tumors and tumor-like lesions of the appendix. Cancer 1995;75:757–768.

107. Qizilbash AH. Mucoceles of the appendix: their relationship to hyperplastic polyps, mucinous cystadenomas, and cystadenocarcinomas. Arch Pathol 1995;99:548–555.
108. Misdraji J, et al. Appendiceal mucinous neoplasms: a clinicopathologic analysis of 107 cases. Am J Surg Pathol 2003;27:1089–1103.
109. Young RH. Pseudomyxoma peritonei and selected other aspects of the spread of appendiceal neoplasms. Semin Diagn Pathol 2004;21:134–150.
110. Modlin IM, et al. Current status of gastrointestinal carcinoids. Gastroenterology 2005;128:1717–1751.
111. O'Malley CD, Saunders JB de CM. Leonardo Da Vinci on the Human Body. New York: Schuman; 1952.
112. Silen W. Cope's Early Diagnosis of the Acute Abdomen. 16th ed. New York: Oxford University Press; 1983.
113. Keighley MRB, Williams NS. Surgery of the Anus, Rectum and Colon. London: Saunders; 1993.

51

Colon, Rectum, and Anus

Mark L. Welton, Andrew A. Shelton, George J. Chang, and Madhulika G. Varma

Anatomy and Physiology

Anatomy

Colonic Anatomy

The colon is one structural unit with two embryological origins. The cecum and right and midtransverse colons are of midgut origin and as such are supplied by the superior mesenteric artery (SMA). The distal transverse, splenic flexure, and descending and sigmoid colon are of hindgut origin and receive blood from the inferior mesenteric artery (IMA). The entire colon starts as a midline structure that rotates during development and attaches laterally to the right and left posterior peritoneum. The right and left colonic mesenteries are obliterated, fusing to the posterior peritoneum in these regions, leaving these portions of the colon covered by peritoneum on the lateral, anterior, and medial surfaces. The transverse and sigmoid colons, in contrast, are completely covered with peritoneum and are attached by long mesenteries, allowing for great variation in the location of these structures (Fig. 51.1).

Histology

Three layers form the mucosa of the colon: epithelium, lamina propria, and muscularis mucosa. The epithelium is columnar with crypts made of straight, nonbranching tubules (glands of Lieberkuhn). The cells around the crypts are simple columnar cells with occasional goblet cells. The crypts are mostly lined with goblet cells, except at the bases, where undifferentiated cells, amine precursor uptake and decarboxylation (APUD) cells, and enterochromaffin cells predominate. The lamina propria is connective tissue surrounding a network of capillaries. The muscularis mucosa is a thin sheet of muscle fibers containing a network of lymphatics. The submucosa is a layer of connective tissue containing vessels, lymphatics, and Meissner's plexus. The muscularis propria is composed of circular and longitudinal muscle. The inner circular muscle completely encompasses the entire colon and rectum, ending in the anus as the internal sphincter muscle. The myenteric plexus of Auerbach lies on the circular muscle. The longitudinal muscle is grouped into three dominant cables of muscle called taeniea coli that originate in the cecum and fuse together to form a circumferential coat at the junction of the sigmoid and rectum. The colon is covered with serosa on the intraperitoneal surfaces but not where it is attached to the retroperitoneum on the posterior aspects of the ascending and descending colon.

Arterial Supply

The blood supply to the colon is quite variable, but general patterns exist (Fig. 51.2). The ileocolic artery, a constant structure, is the terminal branch of the SMA. It commonly gives rise to cecal, appendiceal, ileal, and ascending branches, some of which anastomose with ileal and right colic vessels. The right colic artery may originate from the superior mesenteric, middle colic, or ileocolic vessels and is present in 10% to 98% of cases.[1,2] The middle colic artery arises from the SMA, branches early into the right and left branches, and anastomoses with the ascending branches of both the right and left colic arteries. The artery is present in 95% to 98% of cases.[2] The IMA originates from the aorta 3 to 4cm above the bifurcation.[3] It gives rise to the left colic artery and the sigmoid vessels and ends in the superior rectal artery. The left colic artery divides into ascending and descending branches. The ascending branch anastomoses with branches off the middle colic, and the descending branch anastomoses with the sigmoid vessels.

Collateral circulation between the vessels of superior mesenteric and inferior mesenteric arteries is through two named arteries: the marginal artery of Drummond and the "arc of Riolan" or "meandering mesenteric." The marginal artery of Drummond runs in the mesentery near the colon. It is essentially created by anastomoses between the terminal

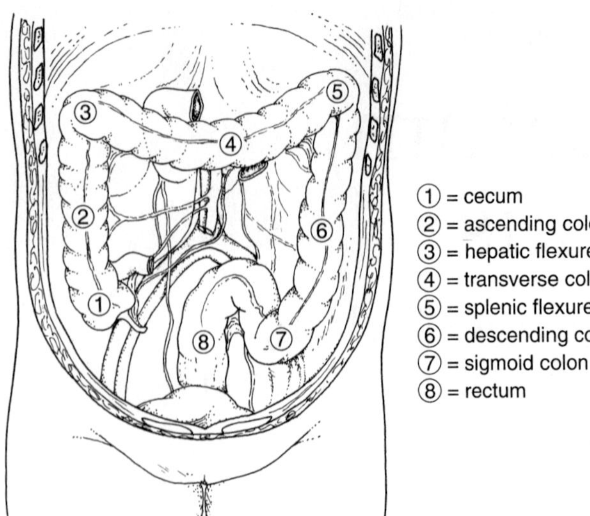

FIGURE 51.1. The posterior aspects of the ascending and descending colon are "extraperitoneal" as those surfaces are not covered with peritoneum, whereas the transverse and sigmoid colon are completely intraperitoneal as these segments are completely peritonealized and on mesenteries.

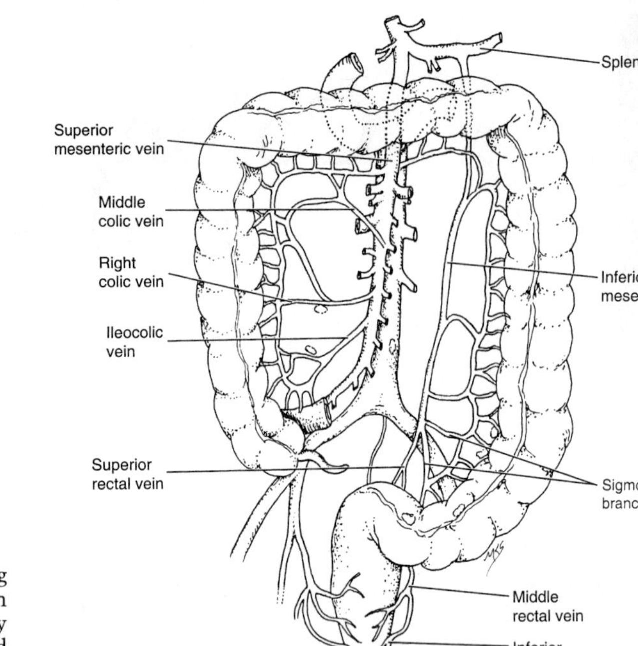

FIGURE 51.3. The venous drainage of the colon and rectum.

arcades of the ileocolic, right, middle, and left colic and sigmoid vessels. The arc of Riolan, present much less frequently, is found more centrally in the mesentery than the marginal artery and is generally a vessel connecting the left branch of the middle colic with the inferior mesenteric.[4]

Venous Drainage

The venous drainage (Fig. 51.3) of the colon is through veins that bear the same name as the arteries with which they run except for the inferior mesenteric vein (IMV) that runs above. Veins from the right and transverse colon form the superior mesenteric vein. It joins the splenic vein behind the head and neck of the pancreas to form the portal vein. Veins that drain the proximal anal canal, rectum, and left colon form the IMV. These tributaries course near their respective arteries, but the IMV travels separately from the IMA in the left colonic mesentery, passing just lateral to the ligament of Treitz and under the body of the pancreas, where it joins the splenic vein.

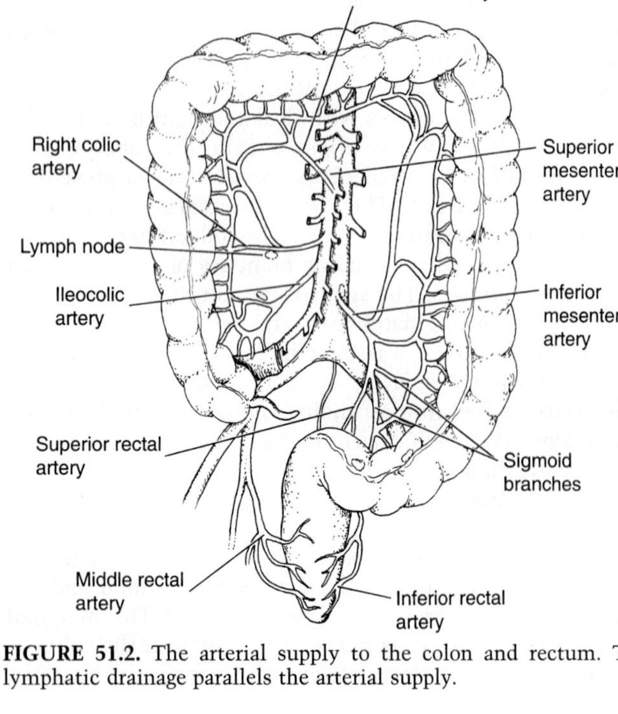

FIGURE 51.2. The arterial supply to the colon and rectum. The lymphatic drainage parallels the arterial supply.

Lymphatic Drainage

The lymphatic drainage of the colon starts as a network of vessels within the muscularis mucosa that drain into the extramural system. Small numbers of lymphatics actually exist in the lamina propria, but for practical purposes lymphatic drainage, and therefore the ability of malignancies to metastasize, begins once the tumor has invaded through the muscularis mucosa. The extramural lymphatic vessels and nodes follow along the arteries to their origins at the superior and inferior mesenteric vessels.

Innervation

The colon is innervated via the sympathetic and parasympathetic nervous systems. Sympathetic stimulation inhibits peristalsis, whereas it is promoted by the parasympathetic system. Controversy exists regarding which segments are involved in the origin of the sympathetic nerves, but there is agreement that at least the lower six thoracic segments give rise to fibers that join the paravertebral ganglia. The fibers leave these ganglia as the greater, lesser, least, and lumbar splanchnic nerves. They form the preaortic, celiac, and superior mesenteric ganglia, the superior hypogastric plexus, and eventually a pair of inferior hypogastric plexuses.

Parasympathetic innervation is from the vagus nerve and the sacral outflow. The vagus contributes to the preaortic plexus that sends fibers along the arteries to the cecum, ascending, and transverse colon. The nervi erigentes from the sacral outflow join the hypogastric plexuses and innervate the colon as high as the splenic flexure. The fibers synapse with the ganglia of the myenteric plexus of Auerbach and Meissner's plexus.

Anorectal Anatomy

The rectum is approximately 12 to 15 cm long. It extends from the rectosigmoid junction, marked by the fusion of the taenia, to the anal canal, marked by the passage of the bowel into the pelvic floor musculature. The rectum lies in the sacrum and forms three distinct curves, creating folds that when visualized endoscopically are known as the valves of Houston. The proximal and distal curves are convex to the left, and the middle curve is convex to the right. The middle curve roughly marks the anterior peritoneal reflection. The rectum gradually transitions from intraperitoneal to extraperitoneal, beginning posteriorly at 12 to 15 cm from the anus and becoming completely extraperitoneal at the anterior peritoneal reflection, 6 to 8 cm from the anus (Fig. 51.4). The rectum is "fixed" posteriorly, laterally, and anteriorly by the presacral or Waldeyer's fascia, the lateral ligaments, and Denonvillier's fascia, respectively[5–9] (Fig. 51.5).

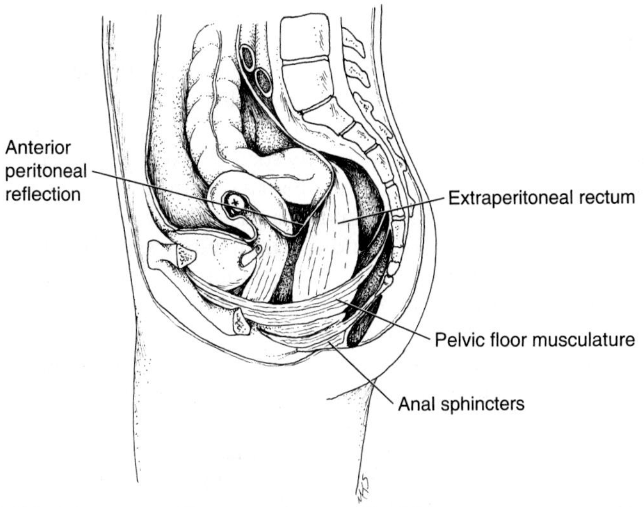

FIGURE 51.4. The rectum transitions from completely intraperitoneal to extraperitoneal as it passes into the pelvis. The point at which it becomes completely extraperitoneal is the anterior peritoneal reflection. The muscles of the pelvic floor create a broad sheet suspending the rectum.

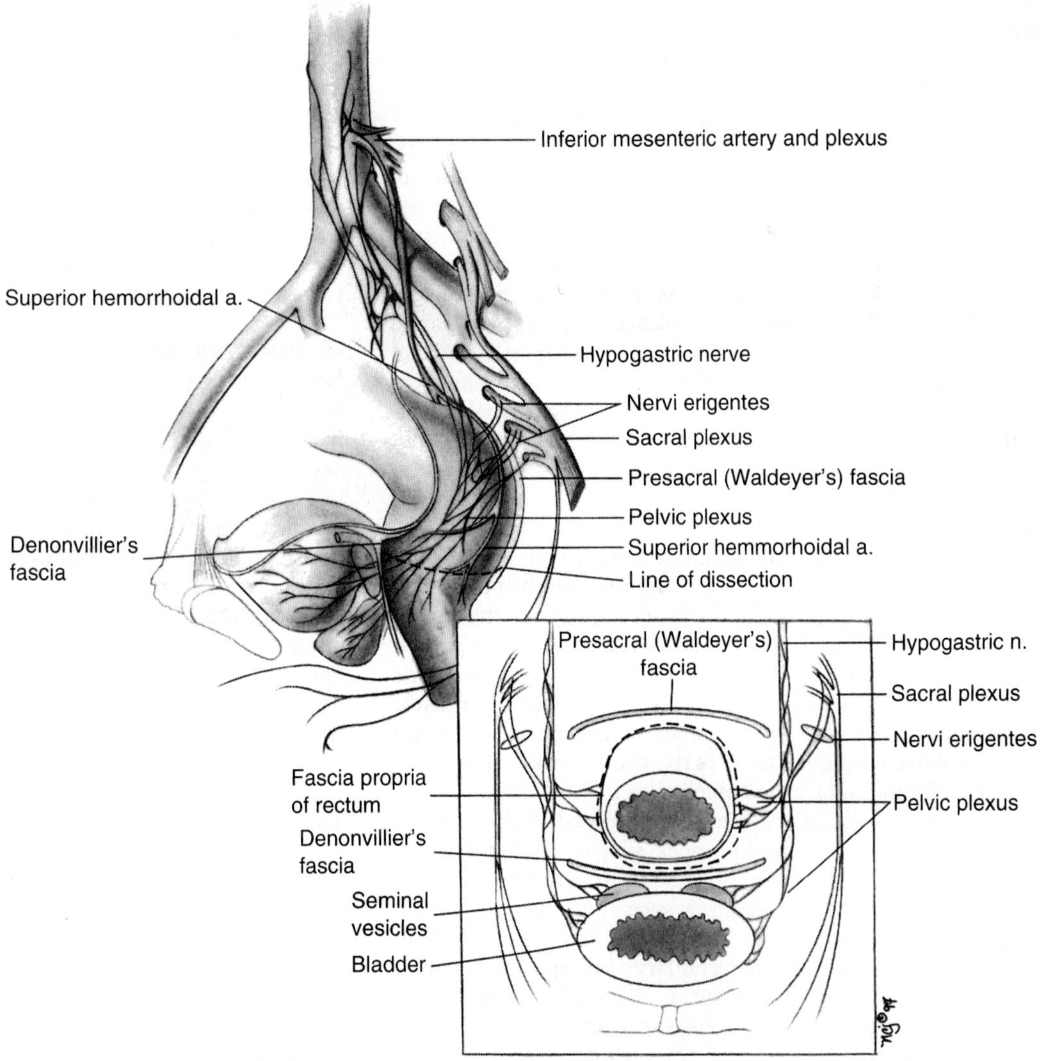

FIGURE 51.5. The supporting fascias of the rectum and adjacent nerve plexuses. (From Michelassi and Milsom,[644] with permission, © 1999, Springer-Verlag, New York.)

The anatomical anal canal starts at the dentate line and ends at the anal verge. However, a practical definition is the surgical anal canal, which extends from the termination of the muscular diaphragm of the pelvic floor to the anal verge.[7] It is a 3- to 4-cm long collapsed anteroposterior slit.[8] The anal verge is the junction of the highly specialized anoderm of the anal canal and the surrounding perianal skin. The anal canal is "supported" by the surrounding anal sphincter mechanism, composed of the internal and external sphincters. The internal sphincter is a specialized continuation of the circular muscle of the rectum. It is an involuntary muscle that is normally contracted at rest.

The structure and function of the external sphincter are controversial; however, current evidence suggests that the external sphincter is the spout on a funnel of one continuous circumferential functional muscle mass that includes the external sphincter caudally and extends cranially to the conical puborectalis and levator ani muscles.[9,10] The external sphincter is composed of voluntary striated muscle. The conjoined longitudinal muscle separates the internal and external sphincter. This intersphincteric plane is created by the continuation of the longitudinal muscle of the rectum, joined by fibers from the levator ani and puborectalis, forming the conjoined muscle.[11] Some fibers from this muscle become the corrugator cutis ani and insert on the perianal skin, creating rugal folds and a puckered appearance.[12] Other fibers traverse the internal sphincter and support the internal hemorrhoids as the mucosal suspensory ligaments.[13]

Hemorrhoids are found in the subepithelial tissue above and below the dentate line. These are cushions composed of vascular and connective tissues and supportive muscle fibers. Internal hemorrhoids originate above the dentate line and are lined with insensate rectal columnar and transitional mucosa. External hemorrhoids are similar vascular complexes except that they underlie the richly innervated anoderm rather than insensate rectal mucosa. As the rectum enters the narrow musculature of the pelvic floor and becomes the anal canal, the tissue is thrown into folds known as the columns of Morgagni. At the lower end of the columns lie small pockets called crypts, some of which communicate with anal glands lying in the intersphincteric plane.

Histology

The rectum is composed of an innermost layer of mucosa that lies over the submucosa; two continuous sheaths of muscle, the circular and longitudinal muscles; and in the upper rectum, serosa. The mucosa is subdivided into three layers: (1) epithelial cells, (2) lamina propria, and (3) muscularis mucosa. The muscularis mucosa is a fine sheet of muscle containing a network of lymphatics. Lymphatics are not present above this level, making the muscularis mucosa critical in defining metastatic potential of malignancies.

The epithelium of the canal is composed of three types: columnar epithelium in the upper anal canal, transitional (cuboidal) epithelium variably present for 6 to 12 mm above the dentate line, and anoderm, a specialized squamous epithelium, below the dentate line.[14] The anoderm is rich in nerve fibers but lacking in secondary skin appendages (hair follicles, sebaceous glands, or sweat glands). The dentate line marks the true mucocutaneous junction. The anal verge marks the junction of the anoderm with perianal skin.

Anal glands are lined with stratified columnar epithelium with interspersed mucus-secreting goblet cells. They communicate directly with crypts at the dentate line.

Arterial Supply

The arterial supply of the anorectum is via the superior, middle, and inferior rectal arteries.[15] The superior rectal artery is the terminal branch of the IMA and descends in the mesorectum. It supplies the upper and middle rectum. The middle rectal arteries generally arise from the internal pudendal artery but may come off the inferior gluteal or internal iliac arteries. They enter the rectum anterolaterally in the distal third of the rectum at the level of the pelvic floor musculature.[5,15] They supply the lower two-thirds of the rectum. The inferior rectal arteries, branches of the internal pudendal arteries, enter posterolaterally, do not anastomose extramurally with the blood supply to the rectum, and provide blood supply to the anal sphincters and epithelium. Although there is no evidence of extramural anastomosis, arteriography demonstrates extensive intramural anastomosis between the superior, middle, and inferior rectal arteries, and extramural collaterals exist between the middle and superior rectal arteries in hypertensive patients.[15,16]

Venous Drainage

The venous drainage of the anorectum is via the superior, middle, and inferior rectal veins draining into the portal and systemic systems. The superior rectal vein drains the upper and middle third of the rectum. It empties into the portal system via the IMV. The middle rectal veins drain the lower rectum and upper anal canal into the systemic system via the internal iliac veins. The inferior rectal veins drain the lower anal canal, communicating with the pudendal veins and draining into the internal iliac veins. There is communication between the venous systems, which allows low rectal cancers to spread via the portal and systemic systems.

Lymphatic Drainage

Lymphatic drainage of the upper and middle rectum is into the inferior mesenteric nodes. Lymph from the lower rectum may also drain into the inferior mesenteric system but may drain to the systems along the middle and inferior rectal arteries, posteriorly along the middle sacral artery, and anteriorly through channels in the retrovesical or rectovaginal septum. These drain to the iliac nodes and ultimately to the periaortic nodes. Lymphatics from the anal canal above the dentate line drain via the superior rectal lymphatics to the inferior mesenteric lymph nodes and laterally to the internal iliac nodes. Below the dentate line, drainage occurs primarily to the inguinal nodes but can occur to the inferior or superior rectal lymph nodes.

Innervation

The innervation of the rectum is via the sympathetic and parasympathetic nervous systems. The sympathetic nerves originate from the lumber segments L1–L3, form the inferior mesenteric plexus, travel through the superior hypogastric plexus, and descend as the hypogastric nerves to the pelvic plexus.[17]

The parasympathetic nerves arise from sacral roots S2–S4 and join the hypogastric nerves anterior and lateral to the rectum to form the pelvic plexus, from which fibers pass to form the periprostatic plexus.[17] Sympathetic and parasympathetic fibers pass from the pelvic and periprostatic plexi to the rectum and internal anal sphincter as well as the prostate, bladder, and penis. Injury to these nerves or plexi can lead to impotence, bladder dysfunction, and loss of normal defecatory mechanisms.[17]

The internal anal sphincter is innervated by the autonomic nervous system. It receives excitatory sympathetic innervation via the hypogastric nerves (L5) and inhibitory parasympathetic innervation by the pelvic splanchnic nerves S2–S4. The inferior rectal branch of the pudendal nerve S2–S4 innervates the external anal sphincter.

Sensations of noxious stimuli above the dentate line are conducted through afferent fibers of these parasympathetic nerves and experienced as an ill-defined dull sensation. Below the dentate line, the epithelium is exquisitely sensitive and richly innervated by somatic nerves. Cutaneous sensations of heat, cold, pain, and touch are conveyed through the inferior rectal and perineal branches of the pudendal nerve.

Pelvic Floor Anatomy

The pelvic floor is a consortium of funnel-shaped muscles that separate the pelvis and the perineum. It is composed of the levator ani and puborectalis muscles. The levator ani consists of two broad, thin, symmetrical muscular sheets that originate around the pelvic sidewall and in the sacrospinous ligament that forms the principal support of the pelvic viscera. The puborectalis muscle originates in the posterior aspect of the pubis, forms a sling around the rectum, and returns to the posterior aspect of the pubis. The fibers of the puborectalis are situated immediately adjacent to and below the innermost component of the levator ani muscle, where they are intimately associated with the upper posterolateral fibers of the deep external anal sphincter. Thus, the puborectalis serves as a bridge between the broad sheetlike component of the funnel created by the levators and the narrow spout of the funnel created by the external anal sphincter (Fig. 51.6). The puborectalis in the contracted state is responsible for the normal acute anorectal angle between the levators and the external sphincters. It is also responsible for the shelf that is normally palpable on digital exam as one passes from the distal narrow lumen of the "anus" to the more proximal capacious lumen of the "rectum."[18]

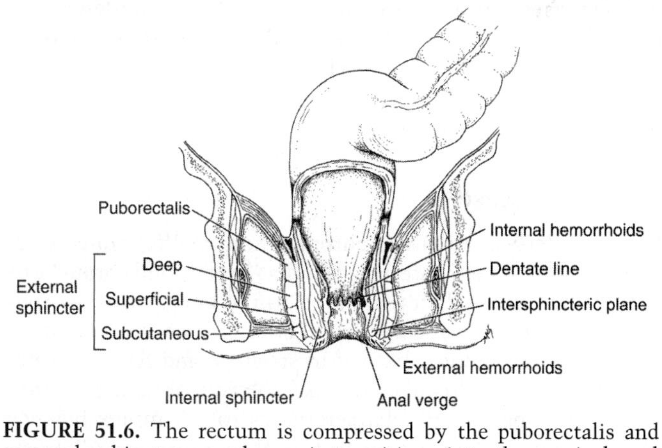

FIGURE 51.6. The rectum is compressed by the puborectalis and external sphincter complex as it transitions into the surgical anal canal.

Innervation of the pelvic floor is from branches of ventral nerve roots of S2–S4. These originate proximal to the formation of the sacral plexus and run on the inner surface of the levator ani muscles.[19]

Physiology

Colonic Physiology

The major functions of the colon are absorption, storage, propulsion, and digestion of the output of the proximal intestinal tract. Absorption of the salts and water of the ileal output is critical in the maintenance of normal fluid and electrolyte balance. It is regulated through a complex integrated neurohormonal pathway. In normal individuals, the ileum expels approximately 1500mL of fluid per day, of which 1350mL are absorbed by the colon. The right colon is more active in this process than the left. Water absorption is driven by active sodium absorption against concentration and electrical gradients.[20] An Na^+/K^+-ATPase (adenosine triphosphatase) pump at the basolateral membrane is responsible for the net absorption of Na^+ but does not account for the high concentrations of K^+ found in the stool. Colonic mucus, fecal bacteria, and desquamated cells may also be sources of the K^+ found in the stool.[21] Chloride is actively absorbed in exchange for bicarbonate. Urea is secreted into the lumen of the colon, metabolized by bacteria into ammonia, and absorbed passively in the nonionized form. The colon also actively secretes mucus that is high in K^+.

The propulsive and storage functions of the colon are difficult to study because of the nature of the luminal contents, the relative inaccessibility of the organ to intraluminal monitoring, and the paucity of "normal" controls. Radiographic studies have revealed three types of contractions: segmental nonpropulsive, retrograde, and anterograde propulsive mass movements. Segmental contractions occur primarily in the right colon and move contents over short distances distally or proximally. They may serve to slow colonic transit and mix contents, allowing for greater salt and water absorption. Retrograde contractions also mix the contents and slow transit, forcing the fluid into more proximal bowel and increasing absorption times. Mass movements move intraluminal contents rapidly over long distances. These mass movements are associated with spiking action potentials and sustained high-pressure contractions.[22,23] In contrast, most colonic motor activity is composed of low-amplitude short contractions, possibly associated with segmental contraction.[23]

The colon is extensively innervated with extrinsic and intrinsic nervous systems. The extrinsic system was mentioned earlier. The intrinsic or enteric nervous system is composed of sensory neurons, interneurons, and motor neurons. The sensory neurons are involved in feedback loops signaling the proximal bowel to contract and distal bowel to relax in response to distension. The motor neurons, both excitatory and inhibitory, are important in controlling colonic motility. The excitatory motor neurons innervate the circular and longitudinal muscle, and the cell bodies are located in the myenteric and submucosal plexuses. The inhibitory motor neuron cell bodies are located in the myenteric plexus, and they supply the circular muscle more than the longitudinal muscle. The list of transmitters is extensive and includes traditional neurotransmitter and regulatory peptides. Hormonal control of motility and secretion in the colon is incompletely understood.

Digestion is an underrecognized activity of the colon. Primarily anaerobic bacteria that ferment proteins, dietary fiber, and carbohydrates accomplish digestion. Carbohydrate fermentation produces short-chain fatty acids that are important mucosal fuels.[24] Their absorption is associated with sodium and water absorption and bicarbonate secretion.[25] The bacteria produce substances that the colon could not otherwise absorb, such as ammonia and vitamin K, and detoxify carcinogens.[26]

The microflora are important for proper electrolyte metabolism and nutritional support of the mucosa and influence the amount and nature of intestinal gas produced, which in the correct concentrations may be explosive if exposed to electrocautery.

Anorectal Physiology

The function of the pelvic floor is complex and poorly understood, partly because of the complexity of the interactions of the pelvic floor structures and partly because of the material passed per rectum, which compromises our ability to study function with intraluminal monitors as is done in the upper intestinal tract.

The levator ani muscles create a broad funnel cone suspending the rectum in a muscular sling that ends where the puborectalis pulls the rectum forward at the anorectal junction, creating an acute anorectal angle "at rest." The levators may contain sensory fibers that report pelvic fullness and therefore may be important in the sensation of the urge to defecate. The acuity of the angle created by the puborectalis is critical for maintaining continence. The puborectalis contracts, increasing the anorectal angle, during Valsalva maneuvers in which continence is maintained (coughing, straining) but relaxes, opening the angle, when a Valsalva is performed as part of normal defecation.

The internal sphincter, composed of smooth muscle, generates 85% of the resting tone. It is innervated with sympathetic and parasympathetic fibers. Both are inhibitory and keep the sphincter in a constant state of contraction.[27] The external sphincters are skeletal muscles innervated by the pudendal nerve with fibers that originate from S2–S4. The muscles provide 15% of the resting tone and 100% of the voluntary squeeze pressures. The external sphincter, pelvic floor, and cricopharyngeus are unique skeletal muscles because of their ability to maintain a state of tonic contraction. This tonic activity is increased with factors that increase intraabdominal pressure, such as erect posture, coughing, or Valsalva maneuver.[18] Voluntary contraction of the external sphincter should double the resting pressure but cannot be sustained longer than 3 min.[28,29]

Hemorrhoids are important participants in maintaining continence and minimizing trauma during defecation. They function as protective pillows that engorge with blood during the act of defecation, protecting the anal canal from direct trauma due to passage of stool.[30] They also seal the anal canal and prevent leakage of gas and stool. The internal and external sphincters alone cannot close the anal canal, but when combined with interdigitating internal hemorrhoidal cushions, continence is achieved.[31,32] Hemorrhoidal tissues engorge when intraabdominal pressure is increased, as occurs with obesity, pregnancy, lifting, and defecation.

The anal sphincters function as a unit in concert with the levator ani, the puborectalis, and the rectum through complex mechanisms not clearly understood, allowing appropriate defecation at socially acceptable times. Continence is maintained when intrarectal pressures are lower than the pressures generated by the resting internal and external sphincters. In the resting state, the rectum is not completely empty, but the contents are not sensed. Sensory fibers in the levators that initially signal the presence of pelvic fullness adapt, and the rectum accommodates (decreases muscle tone), allowing the contents to remain.

Periodically, the internal sphincter relaxes, allowing the rectal contents to drop down into the anal canal, where the contents can be sampled by the exquisitely sensitive anoderm. After sampling, the external sphincter contracts, and the contents are pushed back into the rectum. This *sampling reflex* or *rectoanal inhibitory reflex* also results from rectal distension, allowing the determination of rectal contents as the rectum fills. The sampling reflex occurs up to seven times per day.[23] Progressive distension of the rectum causes continuous inhibition of the internal sphincter and relaxation of the external sphincter, causing an urge to defecate.[33]

If solid waste is noted and one wishes to evacuate, a sitting or squatting position is assumed (straightening the anorectal angle), intraabdominal pressure is increased through a Valsalva, the puborectalis relaxes, and a reflex relaxation of the internal sphincter occurs as the contents enter the anal canal. As the puborectalis relaxes, the anorectal angle straightens, further shortening the anal canal and increasing the funnel shape of the musculature. Primarily the Valsalva maneuver then accomplishes evacuation. Thus, the act of normal defecation is complex, involving multiple steps for successful evacuation.

Inflammatory Bowel Disease

Inflammatory bowel disease (IBD) is a general term for a group of chronic, idiopathic inflammatory disorders of the gastrointestinal (GI) tract. Inflammatory bowel disease is divided into two major groups, Crohn's disease and ulcerative colitis (UC). Although similarities in the epidemiology of these disorders exist, and on occasion (10%–15%) the clinical distinction between these entities remains elusive, these disorders are in general distinct in terms of their clinical presentation, pathology and management. A growing body of evidence also supports a difference between these disorders in terms of their underlying pathogenesis.

Crohn's Disease

Crohn's disease causes a chronic, nonspecific, transmural inflammation of the intestine that has been found throughout the GI tract, from the oropharynx to the anus.[34] It was originally described in 1932 by Crohn et al.[35] as an inflammation of the terminal ileum that led to stricture and fistula formation. Since then, this disease has evolved from a description of the gross pathologic characteristics to a complex balance of numerous inflammatory factors that affect the GI tract. Crohn's disease also manifests itself in many extraintestinal symptoms of the eyes, skin, and joints.

The severity and relapsing nature of these symptoms severely affect a patient's quality of life and require dependence on long-term medical therapy. Surgical treatment is reserved for disease that is refractory to medical treatment and has produced severe complications, such as intestinal perforation or stricture. A subset of patients will have disease limited to the large intestine. In these people, Crohn's colitis is distinguished from UC on the basis of gross and microscopic pathology (Table 51.1). Approximately 10% to 15% of patients will be diagnosed

TABLE 51.1. Comparison of Ulcerative Colitis and Crohn's Colitis.

Manifestation	*Ulcerative colitis*	*Crohn's colitis*
Clinical features		
Bleeding per rectum	3+	1+
Diarrhea	3+	3+
Abdominal pain	1+	3+ Especially with involvement of ileum
Vomiting	R	3+
Fever	R	2+
Palpable abdominal mass	R	2+
Weight loss	+	3+
Clubbing	R	1+
Rectal involvement	4+	1+
Small-bowel involvement	0	4+
Anal and perianal involvement	R	4+
Risk of carcinoma	1+	1+
Clinical course	Relapses/remission	Slowly progressive
Radiologic		
Thumb printing sign on barium enema	R	1+
Endoscopic		
Distribution	Symmetric	Asymmetric
Continuous involvement	4+	1+
Rectal	4+	1+
Vascular architecture	Absent	1+
Friability	4+	1+
Erythema	3+	1+
Spontaneous petechiae	2+	R
Profuse bleeding	1+	R
Aphthous ulcer	0	4+
Serpiginous ulcer	R	4+
Deep longitudinal ulcer	0	4+
Cobblestoning	0	4+
Mucosa surrounding ulcer	Abnormal	Normal
Pseudopolyps	2+	2+
Bridging	R	1+
Gross appearance		
Thickened bowel wall	0	4+
Shortening of bowel	2+	R
Fat creeping onto serosa	0	4+
Segmental involvement	0	4+
Aphthous ulcer	R	4+
Linear ulcer	0	4+
Microscopic picture		
Depth of involvement	Mucosa and submucosa	Full thickness
Lymphoid aggregation	0	4+
Sarcoid-type granuloma	0	4+
Fissuring	0	2+
Goblet cell mucin depletion	4+	1+
Intramural sinuses	0	1+
Operative treatment		
Total proctocolectomy	Excellent option in selected patients	Indicated in total large bowel involvement
Segmental resection	R	Frequent
Ileal pouch procedure	"Gold standard"	Contraindicated
Prognosis		
Recurrence after total proctocolectomy	0	3+
Complications		
Internal fistula	R	4+
Intestinal obstruction (stricture or infection)	0	4+
Hemorrhage	1+	1+
Sclerosing cholangitis	1+	R
Cholelithiasis	0	2+
Nephrolithiasis	0	2+

R, rare; 0, not found; 1+, may be present; 2+, common; 3+, usual finding; 4+, characteristic (not necessarily common).

Source: From Nivatvongs[657] and Ogorek and Fisher.[658]

with indeterminate colitis and have features of both diseases.[36]

The incidence of Crohn's disease is variable, with the highest rates in Scandinavia, the British Isles, and North America. The incidence ranges from 0.30 to 10 per 100,000 population.[37] Since the 1950s, there has been an increase in the incidence that has continued to increase with time, with the highest concentration of cases occurring at increasing distances from the equator. The rates of Crohn's disease have now been recognized as rising at faster rates in Southeast Asia and China.[38,39] The prevalence is approximately 10 to 90 cases per 100,000 population. However, in Central Canada, the population prevalence has been reported to be as high as 2 per 1000 population, with some individual centers reporting 5 per 1000 population.[40]

There is a bimodal age distribution, with the first peak at age 15 to 30 years and the second at 55 to 80 years. Some studies have shown that women, Jewish people, cigarette smokers, urban dwellers, and oral contraceptive users are at increased risk.[41–44]

The etiology of Crohn's disease remains elusive and includes numerous hypotheses, such as infection with mycobacterium or measles, food allergy, intestinal permeability, and primary immune deficiency.[45] Crohn's disease has been noted in families, and a genetic predisposition to IBD clearly plays a role in disease causation. Loci containing IBD predisposition genes have been mapped to chromosomes 3, 6, 12, and 16.

The first IBD predisposition gene has been identified, nucleotide-binding oligomerization domain 2 (NOD2), on chromosome 16.[46] Activation of Toll-like receptors by pathogens and the NOD2 gene product activate NFK-β in response to bacterial lipopolysaccharide (LPS). Therefore, they play a key role in the innate immune response to gut bacteria.[47] Carriers of certain variants of the NOD2 gene are at risk for Crohn's. Heterozygotes have a relative risk for Crohn's disease of 2–6, while homozygotes have a relative risk for the disease of 10–30. The NOD2 allele carriers are at risk for Crohn's, but not UC. Since Crohn's disease and UC share many similarities, their etiology is thought also to be associated. A few theories for the etiology of IBD are reviewed in the UC section.

The presentation of Crohn's disease can be difficult to appreciate. Patients have a variety of symptoms that are directly related to the extent, character, and location of the inflammation. The disease occurs most commonly in the ileocolic region (30%–45%), followed by isolated small bowel (20%–40%) and colonic (16%–40%) disease.[48–51] Of patients, 5% will present with perianal disease and no evidence of other disease. Generally, 35% of patients with Crohn's will have some perianal involvement over their lifetime. For those with Crohn's disease limited to the colon, two of three will have total colonic involvement.[36] For those who develop disease in the small bowel or colon, the classic symptoms are abdominal pain; diarrhea, which can be bloody; and weight loss. Those who present with perianal disease may complain of anal pain, swelling, or drainage, which may be manifestations of a fissure, skin tag, or fistula. Other nonspecific signs and symptoms include fever, nausea, vomiting, anorexia, aphthous ulcerations of the mouth, cholelithiasis, and renal calculi.

The nature of Crohn's disease can be divided into three categories: inflammatory, stricturing, and fistulizing. Patients with an inflammatory presentation may have symptoms of malabsorption with its assorted sequelae. Those who have stricturing Crohn's disease may only present with symptoms of obstruction, whereas those with a fistula or abscess may have a more septic presentation, including fever, abdominal pain, and a palpable abdominal mass.

The evaluation for Crohn's disease verifies the diagnosis and assesses the severity and extent of the disease. Thus, although the initial workup may be targeted to the presumed focus of disease activity, assessment of the entire GI tract is necessary during the initial evaluation and periodically throughout the patient's life. Upper and lower endoscopy with directed and random biopsies and radiographic imaging, including computed tomographic (CT) scan, small-bowel follow-though, and enteroclysis, will help to elucidate the diagnosis. Stool cultures may find evidence of infectious enterocolitis that may mimic Crohn's disease.

Colonoscopy is the most sensitive test for identifying a patchy distribution of inflammation in the colon, terminal ileal involvement, and rectal sparing that are highly suggestive of Crohn's. Endoscopic findings include mucosal edema and erythema, aphthous or linear ulcerations, and fibrotic strictures. Biopsy is diagnostic when a sarcoid-type giant cell granuloma is found. However, these are seen only 15% to 36% of the time. More recently, capsule endoscopy has been used to diagnose lesions within the small intestine that are beyond the reach of a traditional endoscope and cannot be well visualized on a small-bowel contrast study. It has been suggested in a recent study that capsule endoscopy may be the most sensitive test to diagnose Crohn's disease when the diagnosis remains elusive.[52]

It is important to distinguish Crohn's colitis from UC so that appropriate medical or surgical therapy can be prescribed. Therefore, thorough evaluation of the remaining GI tract, which should be normal in UC, is critical. To evaluate the extent of Crohn's disease, an upper GI with small-bowel follow-through is imperative to find lesions of the stomach, duodenum, or small intestine, such as strictures or fistulas. A small-bowel enteroclysis may be more sensitive in detecting milder mucosal abnormalities. Terminal ileal disease, if not visualized colonoscopically, may be best evaluated with a barium enema (BE) that refluxes through the ileocecal valve. For patients with systemic signs of infection, a CT scan can reveal an abscess or phlegmon secondary to a fistula. In addition, a CT can delineate the extent of the disease by demonstrating the length of small-bowel or colonic thickening that is causing the symptoms of inflammation and any associated obstruction.

The most common symptoms found outside the GI tract involve the skin, eyes, and joints. Erythema nodosum and pyoderma gangrenosum are dermatological diseases that occur with both UC and Crohn's disease. Multiple subcutaneous nodules that are tender, red, raised, and microscopically composed of lymphocytes and histiocytes characterize erythema nodosum. Pyoderma gangrenosum develops from an erythematous lesion into a tender necrotizing ulcer. Most of these occur in the pretibial area, but they can also occur anywhere on the body. Treatment of both lesions is related to the treatment of intestinal disease, although there is no definite correlation.[53] Erythema nodosum is more likely related to an inflammatory reaction, whereas pyoderma, only found in IBD, is thought to be caused by an immunological process.

Ocular manifestations include uveitis, iritis, episcleritis, vasculitis, and conjunctivitis. These findings are more commonly associated with colonic disease and infrequently precede any intestinal symptoms. Arthritis, synovitis, ankylosing spondylitis, and sacroiliitis are all joint complications of UC and Crohn's disease. Although arthritis and synovitis may improve with treatment of intestinal disease, the last two can only be abated.

Similar to UC, in which the increased risk of colon cancer has been well documented, the incidence of carcinoma is increased in the setting of Crohn's disease and should be suspected in patients with a severe or chronic stricture. Multiple studies have shown that longer duration of disease is associated with an increased risk of colon cancer compared to the normal population.[54–57] The incidence of cancer in patients with colorectal strictures is 7% compared to 0.7% in those without strictures.[58] In addition, patients who have undergone surgery to bypass segments of bowel are at higher risk for cancer within that segment. Segmental resections may be adequate therapy for malignancy, although the extent of disease must be assessed.

The gross pathology in Crohn's disease has certain classic characteristics. The intestinal wall is generally thickened and hyperemic with a corkscrewing of the vessels. The mesentery is thickened and tends to wrap around the bowel wall as "creeping fat." Mesenteric lymph nodes can be quite enlarged. Involved segments of bowel are separated from each other by skip areas of normal bowel. The segment of intestine removed may contain an abscess cavity or direct fistulous communication to another loop of intestine or adjacent organ. The mucosal appearance is similar to that seen on endoscopy with patchy inflammation, deep ulcerations, inflammatory pseudopolyps, and cobblestoning. The microscopic characteristics include transmural inflammation with edema, lymphocyte and plasma cell infiltrates, and fibrosis. The granulomas specific for the disease are found in only 50% to 60% of resected specimens.

Medical Therapy

Crohn's disease is incurable, and the natural course of the disease is different for each patient. The exact clinical presentation of Crohn's disease largely reflects the anatomic location of the disease, the extent of the disease and its severity, and the phenotype the disease assumes. Symptoms are often intermittent. Patients will have episodes of disease exacerbation followed by periods of relative or complete remission. In a minority of patients, the disease is unrelenting, depending on the location and severity of the disease. Although the time course can be variable, at least 75% of patients will require surgery after 20 years with the disease.[59] Once that occurs, they will continue to be at a 10% increased risk per year for reoperative surgery.[60] Of those who do not proceed to surgery, the recurrence of significant symptoms after remission is as great as 60% at 2 years.[61] The primary treatment of Crohn's disease is medical. Surgery is indicated for those who do not respond adequately to medical therapy and who develop complications of the disease process.

Aminosalicylates

Sulfasalazine and mesalamine are the two aminosalicylates used for Crohn's disease. Sulfasalazine is a sulfapyridine linked to 5-aminosalicylic acid (5-ASA) by an azo bond. The sulfa component is what causes the side effects of nausea, headache, malaise, and anorexia. 5-Aminosalicylic acid differs from salicylic acid only by the addition of an amino group at the 5 (meta) position. However, this change produces a chemical entity with pharmacological properties different from conventional salicylates and appears to be necessary for treatment of IBD.

The primary antiinflammatory, antipyretic, and analgesic actions of salicylates such as aspirin are due to blockade of prostaglandin synthesis by inhibition of the cyclooxygenase 1 and 2 enzymes. However, aminosalicylates such as 5-ASA and sulfasalazine have highly variable effects on prostaglandin production. Thus, while modulation of prostaglandin metabolism in the inflamed gut may be a relevant antiinflammatory action of aminosalicylates, it is unlikely to be the sole therapeutic action since more potent inhibitors of cyclooxygenase, such as indomethacin, have no positive effect on or might even worsen IBD.

There is also evidence that these compounds scavenge oxygen free radicals that are destructive. Sulfasalazine works after the azo bond is cleaved in the colon, making the 5-ASA active component available. Thus, the drug is useful for patients with Crohn's colitis or ileocolitis.[62,63] For patients with isolated disease of the small intestine, it is less effective and has been shown in a large German trial to have no benefit 3 years after surgical intervention for maintenance therapy.[64] Mesalamine (unbound 5-ASA), however, is absorbed in the small intestine and is a first-line treatment for Crohn's disease.

Many preparations have been created to delay the release of the drug throughout the intestinal tract by coating the compound with resin or formulating it into slow-release microspheres. These are effective in maintaining remission in patients with mild-to-moderate diseases.[65,66] It has been noted that higher doses are required to treat Crohn's disease compared to UC. Mesalamine (5-ASA) delivered rectally in enema or suppository form allows direct topical therapy for rectal and descending colonic disease.

Corticosteroids

For patients with exacerbations leading to moderate or severe Crohn's disease, steroids are the primary therapy. However, they do not help to maintain remission and are detrimental when used for long-term treatment (more than 6–9 consecutive months). The synthetic analogs of cortisol have been developed with the primary goal of maximizing glucocorticoid activity while minimizing mineralocorticoid effects and decreasing the adverse effects of high quantities of systemically active glucocorticoid. Prednisone and prednisolone are the steroids most commonly used to treat IBD, and they have an intermediate duration of action that allows once-daily dosing.

A variety of high-glucocorticoid-potency, low-bioavailability synthetic molecules have been developed. Delayed-release oral preparations of these molecules, for example, controlled-ileal-release budesonide (Enterocort), allow topical delivery of the drug to the site of disease in IBD.

When present at supraphysiological amounts after exogenous administration, the glucocorticoids have pronounced antiinflammatory and immunosuppressive actions, mostly via binding of the cytosolic glucocorticoid receptor complex.

Effects of glucocorticoids that are well documented include inhibition of the production of proinflammatory cytokines such as tumor necrosis factor-α (TNF-α) and interleukin-1 (IL-1) and chemokines such as IL-8; repression of the transcription of the genes for certain enzymes such as inducible nitric oxide synthase, phospholipase A2, and cyclooxygenase 2; and blockade of adhesion molecule expression. These molecular actions of glucocorticoids result in a blockade of leukocyte migration and function and inhibit the effects of numerous important peptide and lipid-derived mediators of inflammation. Many of these activities are mediated through the inhibition of proinflammatory transcription factor nuclear factor kappa B (NF-κB) and the induction of transcription of its natural inhibitor, IkBa.

Corticosteroids can induce clinical remission in Crohn's disease, and in the National Cooperative Crohn's Disease trial had a 60% success rate compared to 30% placebo response.[63] They can be administered orally, rectally, and for severe cases, parenterally.[67] The side effects of corticosteroids are extensive and include osteonecrosis, osteoporosis, cataracts, glaucoma, hyperglycemia, hyperlipidemia, hypertension, psychosis, and skin changes.

For this reason, attempts have been made to create a synthetic drug that would have better mucosal absorption and fewer systemic side effects. One approach is rectal administration of the drug. Hydrocortisone enemas or foam are used in proctosigmoiditis to provide topical delivery of glucocorticoid directly to the diseased tissue, with good clinical results. Absorption of hydrocortisone enemas is less than after oral administration, but nevertheless bioavailability ranges from about 15% to 30%, sufficient to suppress adrenal steroid production.[68]

Budesonide is a synthetic analog of prednisolone that has proved to be therapeutically effective as oral delayed-release capsules in Crohn's disease of the ileum and right colon. This drug has high affinity for the glucocorticoid receptor, resulting in very high potency, and is subject to rapid inactivation in the liver, leading to low systemic bioavailability. The systemic bioavailability of oral budesonide capsules is approximately 10%, and the majority of absorption appears to occur in the distal small bowel.[69] However, even this degree of systemic exposure is sufficient to suppress adrenal steroid production. Budesonide has demonstrated efficacy in a few clinical trials[70–72] and was found to have remission rates comparable to prednisolone.[71] However, maintenance of remission has not been superior to placebo at 1 year.[73]

Antibiotics

Although antibiotics are not used to treat specific bacterial organisms, they have been found to be effective in the treatment of Crohn's disease, especially for the perianal area. Metronidazole is the most common agent employed, although ciprofloxacin has also been used. By decreasing the amount of bacterial flora in the intestinal lumen, they act to prevent the infectious complications of Crohn's disease, such as abscesses and fistulas. Clinical trials have shown their efficacy in inducing remission.[74,75] In one study comparing the use of metronidazole and ciprofloxacin to methylprednisolone in producing clinical remission, their results were comparable (46% vs. 63%).[76]

Immunomodulators

As increasing evidence points to an immunological etiology of IBD, efforts have been made to utilize various immunotherapies. The drugs most commonly used are azathioprine and its metabolite, 6-mercaptopurine (6-MP), antimetabolites that inhibit DNA synthesis. After administration of azathioprine or 6-MP, the 6-thioguanine nucleotides accumulate intracellularly and are believed to mediate the biological actions of these drugs.

Despite over 50 years of investigation, the precise molecular basis for the therapeutic effects of the purine analogs is not known. However, intracellular accumulation of 6-thioguanine nucleotides causes inhibition of the pathways of purine nucleotide metabolism and DNA synthesis and repair, resulting in inhibition of cell division and proliferation. It is plausible, but not proven, that antiproliferative or functionally inhibitory actions on cells of the immune system, such as lymphocytes, underlie the immunosuppressive actions of azathioprine and 6-MP. Their value was established in a study[77] that showed 67% of patients with a clinical response compared to 8% in the placebo group, although the effect was delayed by 3 to 6 months. In addition, 75% of patients were able to discontinue or reduce their steroid doses. A meta-analysis of nine trials found that azathioprine and 6-MP are effective in patients with active disease, but the adverse side effects approached 10%.[78]

Two categories of adverse effects to azathioprine and 6-MP have been described: allergic, occurring early during treatment; and dose-related, generally occurring later. Allergy to these drugs can manifest as pancreatitis, fever, rash, nausea, diarrhea, and an allergic hepatitis. Approximately 5% of the IBD population beginning treatment with azathioprine or 6-MP will experience an allergic reaction to the drug, which can be confirmed by rechallenge if necessary. Dose-related toxicities of azathioprine or 6-MP include bone marrow depression leading to leukopenia (10% cumulative risk), anemia, thrombocytopenia, and hepatic toxicity. If severe, leukopenia can potentially cause profound immune suppression and thus predispose to opportunistic infections or neoplasms. If leukopenia and a serious infection develop in a patient receiving azathioprine or 6-MP, reversal of bone marrow suppression is usually possible with granulocyte colony-stimulating factor. Decreases in the white blood cell (WBC) or elevations in liver function tests (LFTs) are common and generally respond to small dose reductions if needed, without discontinuation. The most important criteria for the success of azathioprine and 6-MP include adequate dosing and duration of treatment and individual metabolism of these drugs based on detectable thiopurine methyltransferase activity.[79] Withdrawal of drug has shown a 70% relapse rate.[78]

Methotrexate is a folate analog that inhibits purine and pyrimidine synthesis and has been shown in a number of trials to be effective in treating Crohn's disease.[80,81] The principal biochemical action of methotrexate, and the mechanism that is believed to be responsible for the drug's cytotoxic activity, is inhibition of dihydrofolate reductase. It has alternatively been proposed that the antiinflammatory action of methotrexate may be mediated by inhibition of cytokine release or by increased release of the endogenous antiinflammatory autocoid adenosine. Methotrexate may also have effects on activated T lymphocytes, a critical part of the inflammatory infiltrate in IBD. However, this drug has significant side effects, including hepatotoxicity and bone marrow suppression, and thus is reserved for patients with severe Crohn's that is refractory to other therapies.

Other drugs shown to be effective include cyclosporine, tacrolimus, and mycophenolate mofetil. Cyclosporine is a lipophilic peptide that inhibits the synthesis of IL-2 and interferon (IFN), thus exerting its immunologic effect. Although no clinical trial has shown a benefit in its use with active Crohn's disease, it has resulted in clinical improvement in patients with perianal fistulas.[67,82] Tacrolimus, a macrolide antibiotic, works in a similar fashion and has only been found effective in perianal Crohn's disease.[83]

Mycophenolate mofetil is an ester prodrug of mycophenolic acid, derived from penicillin. It exerts its effect by inhibiting monophosphate dehydrogenase, which inhibits lymphocyte proliferation. In a randomized trial comparing mycophenolate mofetil to azathioprine, it was found to be as effective and faster at inducing remission.[84] Its side effects include bone marrow suppression, nausea, diarrhea, and cramping abdominal pain.

The latest class of drugs that has resulted in huge advancements in the treatment of Crohn's disease are the anti-TNF agents. The chimeric mouse-human immunoglobulin G (IgG) antibody infliximab (Remicade) was created in the late 1980s and approved by the Food and Drug Administration for use in Crohn's disease at the end of the last decade. Levels of TNF-α are increased in Crohn's disease, and in a study of its efficacy, it was noted to produce fistula healing.

Present et al.[84] reported the results of a randomized, double-blind, multicenter trial in which 5 mg/kg of infliximab given at 0, 2, and 6 weeks were effective in reducing the number of fistulas by more than 50% in 68% of patients. Furthermore, 55% had complete closure of the fistulas. In the placebo group, 13% closed their fistulas, and 26% had a reduction of more than 50% of their fistulas. Remicade was also found to be effective against active Crohn's disease of the small intestine and colon.[85] However, with continued use of infliximab for maintenance therapy, acute and delayed hypersensitivity reactions and secondary loss of response to treatment have resulted in a need to look for other alternatives.

Adalimumab (Humira), a human IgG1 antibody that was commercially available for rheumatoid arthritis, is increasingly in use for Crohn's disease. A randomized placebo-controlled trial studying the dose-dependent efficacy of the drug for patients with active Crohn's disease demonstrated improvement in 36% of patients compared to 12% of controls at the highest dose.[86]

Other therapies currently under investigation include selective adhesion molecule-inhibiting agents such as natalizumab and MLN-02. The former drug has been shown to induce remission of Crohn's in 44% of patients versus 27% in the placebo group.[87] A phase III randomized controlled trial of 905 patients indicated that response is dependent on history of prior immunosuppression and elevation of C-reactive protein.[73] Antibodies to cytokines IL-12, IL-23, interferon-α, and CD-25, the IL-2 receptor, are currently in clinical trials.[86]

Surgical Therapy

As previously stated, the primary treatment of Crohn's disease is medical, and surgery is considered for patients with specific complications of the disease. However, some primary care physicians, gastroenterologists, and patients have translated this into a fear of surgeons and all surgical interventions. Crohn's disease cannot be cured by an operation, but surgery can help ameliorate certain situations rather than simply treat a life-threatening complication (Table 51.2). Therefore, the patient is best served by a team approach in which the surgeon, the patient, and the other care providers are involved in the long-term treatment plan rather than waiting for surgical crises.

The goal in the surgical management of Crohn's disease is to minimize the amount of healthy small bowel and colon resected and the amount of healthy perianal tissue divided while treating the complication that led to surgery. This goal can be achieved through sufficient preoperative assessment of disease and nutritional status, bowel rest, TPN (total parenteral nutrition), percutaneous drainage of abscesses, and maximal medical therapy to minimize the amount of inflammation in surrounding uninvolved normal tissue.

The three classic indications for surgery are stricture, bleeding, and perforation. Patients with symptoms of obstruction not responsive to medical treatment with radiographic evidence of a stricture, and without a predominant component of inflammation, require operative intervention for the stenotic diseases. Medical therapy may be adequate for fistulizing diseases of the perineum or between two loops of bowel, but if the fistulas result in undrained abscesses, either

TABLE 51.2. Indications for Surgical Treatment of Crohn's Disease.

Failure of medical treatment
Persistence of symptoms despite corticosteroid therapy for longer than 6 months
Recurrence of symptoms when high-dose corticosteroids tapered
Worsening symptoms or new onset of complications with maximal medical therapy
Occurrence of steroid-induced complications (Cushingoid features, cataracts, glaucoma, systemic hypertension, aseptic necrosis of the head of the femur, myopathy, or vertebral body fractures)
Obstruction
Intestinal obstruction (partial or complete)
Septic complications
Inflammatory mass or abscess (intraabdominal, pelvic, perineal)
Fistula if
—Drainage causes personal embarrassment (e.g., enterocutaneous, enterovaginal fistula, fistula-in-ano)
—Fistula communicates with the genitourinary system (e.g., entero- or colovesical fistula)
—Fistula produces functional or anatomic bypass of a major segment of intestine with consequent malabsorption or profuse diarrhea (e.g., duodenocolic or enterorectosigmoid fistula)
—Free perforation
Hemorrhage
Carcinoma
Growth retardation
Fulminant colitis with or without toxic megacolon

Source: From Michelassi and Milsom,[644] with permission, © 1999, Springer-Verlag, New York.

intraabdominal or perineal, or if they result in free perforation of the intestine, urgent surgical consultation is indicated. Finally, patients who are on maximal medical therapy but are continuing to have severe symptoms of bleeding, pain, or malabsorption may benefit from resection of the diseased segment.

Small-intestinal or ileocolic disease is treated by resection with primary anastomosis. Patients with disease of the small intestine often have a short segment involved, but when the disease is diffuse, care must be taken to be conservative. Only grossly involved intestine should be resected because wide resection or microscopically negative margins of resection have no impact on the recurrence rate of disease.[84] Endoscopic evidence of disease after resection has been reported to be as high as 73% at 1 year, but only 20% of patients reported symptoms.[88]

Rates of reoperation are higher in those with ileocolic disease compared to those with only small-bowel or colonic involvement.[59,89] Resection is also indicated for multiple chronic stenoses if they are closely grouped. The recurrence rate for reoperation after ileocolic resection approaches 50% at 10 years,[90–92] and these patients are at risk for short-gut syndrome if repeated operations with resection are required.

Although attempts to identify risk factors for recurrent operation have been made, only the number of intestinal sites, and younger age appear to be independently associated with reoperation.[91,93] Other potential factors include a greater extent of disease, smoking, postoperative complications, and perianal disease.[94] Many studies investigating the impact of surgical technique on recurrence have not definitely proven the superiority of stapled or hand-sewn techniques for anastomosis.

Strictureplasty should be considered for strictures widely separated by normal bowel and when multiple previous bowel resections have been performed. Strictureplasty was first utilized in the 1960s and gained popularity when it was discovered that it was as effective as resection in treating stenoses. The Heineke-Mikulicz technique is used for short strictures and the Finney-type closure for longer strictures (Fig. 51.7). Many studies have looked at the long-term follow-up of this technique, and the recurrence rate ranges from 10% to 40%[95] (Table 51.3). Reoperation and Crohn's disease recurrence rates were noted to be higher in patients undergoing a Heineke-Mikulicz technique for strictureplasties.[94]

Patients who present with fistulizing disease with either established fistulas or undrained sepsis require the greatest amount of judgment and caution. The surgical inclination is to operate urgently. However, percutaneous drainage of intra-abdominal abscesses, TPN, and bowel rest control sepsis and allow the inflammation of the uninvolved bowel and surrounding structures to resolve. This pause minimizes the risk of operative misadventures and maximizes the chances of a one-stage definitive procedure. Further, this time interval allows the surgeon and patient to become acquainted with the extent and severity of disease with radiologic imaging (CT scan or fistulogram) and endoscopy. When fistulas are established at the time of surgical consultation, attention should be directed to management of the fistula tract, minimizing the caustic effect of the intestinal contents on the skin. A thorough workup as outlined above may then ensue.

For isolated Crohn's colitis, a total proctocolectomy with ileostomy or total abdominal colectomy with ileorectal anastomosis or ileostomy and rectal stump are the primary therapies. The choice of operations is dependent on the extent of disease in the rectum and anus and the overall health of the patient. It may be prudent to perform a total colectomy and leave the rectal stump in the severely ill. In the 25% to 50% of patients with Crohn's who have rectal sparing, an ileorectal anastomosis may be created and an ileostomy avoided. Up to 70% of these patients will eventually develop significant disease in the residual rectum, and 50% will require completion proctectomy.[96] Thirty percent to 50% of patients with Crohn's do not have rectal sparing at initial evaluation and require proximal diversion or proctectomy.[97,98] Although a total proctocolectomy may avoid recurrent disease of the large intestine, this does not prevent recurrence of the small intestine, usually within 2 feet of the ileostomy.[99] Segmental colectomy for Crohn's disease results in much higher rates of recurrence and shorter time to recurrence compared to total proctocolectomy.[100] However, in select cases, they are performed for isolated segments of disease. One study reported 45% of patients did not require further surgery, and 86% avoided a stoma entirely after 14 years of follow-up.[53]

Perianal complications of Crohn's disease are common, and surgical management is controversial. Improved outcomes have defined a more prominent role for operative interventions, especially with respect to management of focal perineal sepsis and fistulas. Liberal placement of drainage catheters and noncutting Setons, advancement flap closure of perineal fistulas, and selective construction of diverting stomas have good results when combined with optimal medical therapy to induce remission of inflammation. Proctectomy can often be postponed for several years when complementary surgical and medical treatments are provided.

The manifestations of perianal Crohn's disease are multiple, including abscesses, fistulas, fissures, ulcers, strictures, and incontinence. Perianal disease is the first presentation of Crohn's disease in 8% of cases.[101] Estimates of the number of Crohn's patients who will develop perianal manifestations at some time range from 10% to 80%.[102] However, it is generally found to occur in about a third of patients.

Historically, surgeons were reluctant to operate on Crohn's perianal disease. Delayed wound healing was a cause for concern, as was compromised sphincter competence, a devastating complication in this patient population plagued by frequent loose stools. The prevailing sentiment among surgeons was expressed by Alexander-Williams in 1974[103]: "Fecal incontinence is the result of aggressive surgeons and not progressive disease."

In support of nonoperative therapy, surgical literature argued that perianal disease was well tolerated by patients.[104] These reports emphasized the physical rather than emotional well-being of patients. Improved operative outcomes today make it easier for surgeons to acknowledge the personal challenges of living with perineal disease. Success is attributed to improved preoperative medical management of perianal Crohn's disease, careful patient selection, and limited surgical intervention.

Although there continue to be features of Crohn's perianal disease that surgeons agree are best managed nonoperatively, a more active role for surgical intervention was defined in the late 1980s and remains the foundation for surgical management. As with Crohn's disease proximally, palliation of

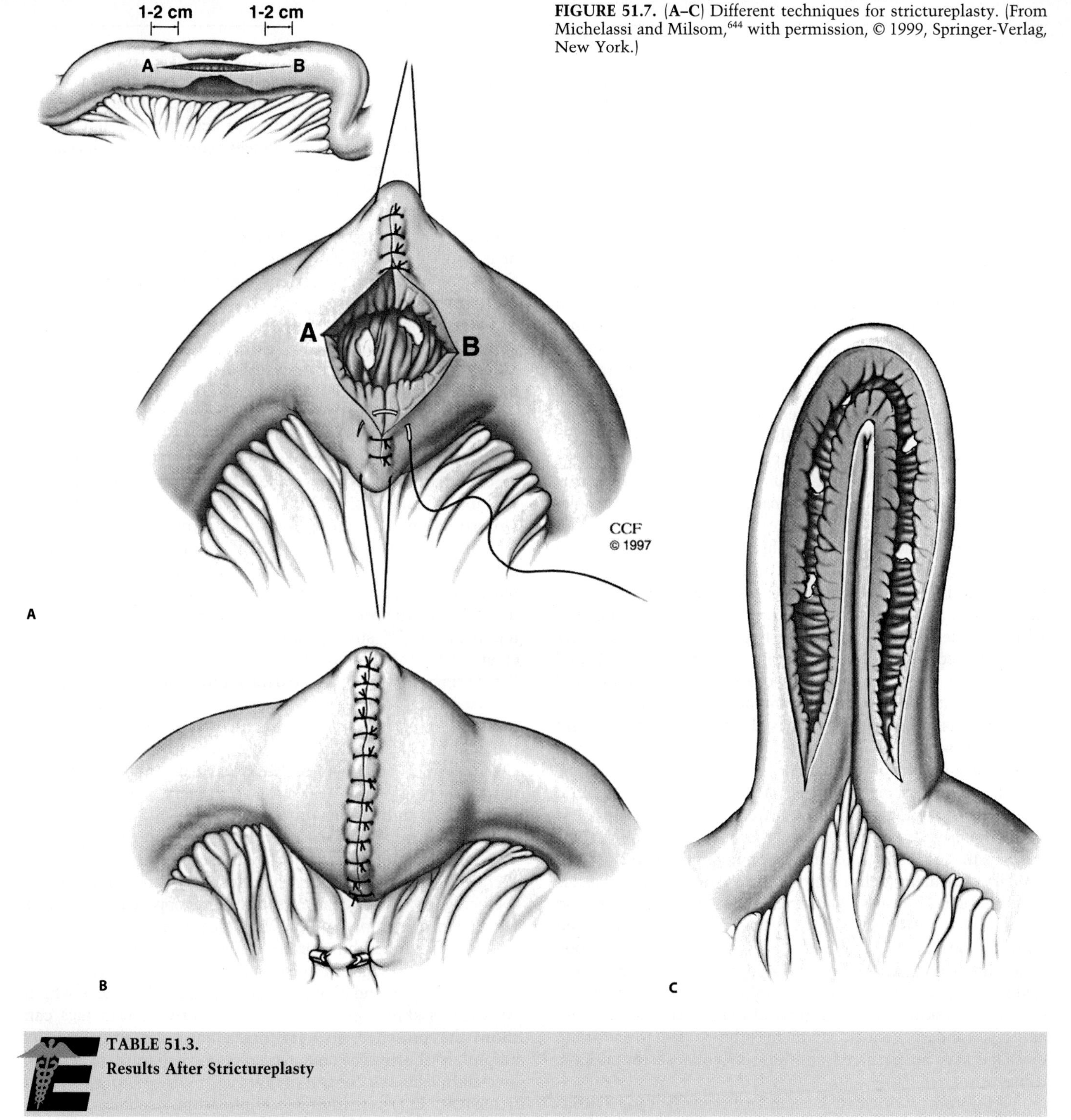

FIGURE 51.7. (A–C) Different techniques for strictureplasty. (From Michelassi and Milsom,[644] with permission, © 1999, Springer-Verlag, New York.)

TABLE 51.3.
Results After Strictureplasty

Author	*No. of patients*	*No. of procedures*	*Mortality*	*Complications: Overall (%)*	*Complications: Fistula/ leak (%)*	*Complications: Sepsis/ abscess (%)*	*Complications: Bleeding (%)*	*Follow-up (mo)*	*Further operation (%)*
Alexander-Williams[179] (1986)	57	146	0		8			36	14
Dehn et al.[180] (1989)	24	86	0		0			40	17
Spencer et al.[181] (1994)	35	71	0	14				36	17
Quandalle et al.[182] (1994)	22	107	0			5	5	36	22
Baba and Nakai[183] (1995)	69		0		0			37	17
Serra, Cohen, and McLeod[184] (1995)	43	154	0		2			54	33
Stebbing et al.[185] (1995)	52	241	0			4		50	36
Gardner, Kettlewell, and Mortensen[186] (1996)	52	241					8		
Ozuner et al.[187] (1996)	162	698				5		42	22

Source: Adapted from Gordon and Nivatvongs,[645] by permission of Taylor & Francis Group LLC.

symptoms and preservation of functional bowel are the priorities guiding surgical intervention. Likewise, the aim of therapy is the treatment of complications of disease rather than the disease itself. Two mandates clarify these principles with respect to perianal disease: (1) the management of a septic focus is an indication for surgery, and (2) the sphincter should be preserved as long as the patient is coping well.

As painful as Crohn's perineal lesions often appear, they are surprisingly well tolerated. In fact, the complaint of pain is indicative of an abscess, and surgical consultation should be arranged promptly. In contrast to the ordinary perianal or perirectal abscess, the septic focus in Crohn's disease is a smoldering process and rarely constitutes an emergency. Given the divergent clinical course of cryptoglandular and Crohn's abscesses, the pathogenesis is probably dissimilar. Cryptoglandular abscesses are thought to develop when an anal crypt occludes and bacteria proliferate in the associated impacted anal gland.[13] There should be no delay draining this type of abscess because infection can spread rapidly into adjacent tissue.

One theory about Crohn's abscesses is that they arise from fecal contamination of extraluminal tissue. Loss of bowel wall integrity as a feature of transmural inflammation may provide a route for contamination. Inflammatory changes, which are detrimental on the one hand, may simultaneously play a protective role. Inflammation of the bowel wall and surrounding tissue may help to localize focal infection and inhibit development of the disseminated soft tissue infection we know as necrotizing fasciitis. Hence, surgery to drain Crohn's abscesses can be scheduled urgently rather than emergently as long as the patient is not toxic.

Although perianal and perirectal abscesses are often treated in the office, our preference is to examine the patient in the operating room, where anesthesia enables a more thorough exam. Incision and drainage of acute abscesses are the primary treatment; delineation of the anatomy of any fistulas with the use of probes is reserved for subsequent operation unless an obvious tract is recognized or the process has been chronic. In these cases, a Seton, which can be a vessel loop or a silk suture, can be drawn through the fistula tract and tied in place. In some cases of horseshoe fistulas, a counterincision in the skin is required to avoid a large perianal incision, and a secondary Penrose drain may be placed to facilitate drainage via the incisions and help to collapse the abscess cavity.

Fistulotomy, which is the standard treatment for fistulas associated with cryptoglandular abscesses, is also the first-line treatment for Crohn's fistula-in-ano.[103,105] The danger of fistulotomy is sphincter injury and consequent incontinence. Two practices foster success. First, incise only superficial tracts that do not involve muscle; place a noncutting Seton if the sphincter is at risk. Second, fistulotomy at the anterior midline of the female perineum should not be done. The external sphincter is a thin loop of muscle anteriorly, making it especially vulnerable to injury. Another strategy for treating fistulas in this area is discussed in the section on advancement flaps.

The cutting Seton is associated with an unacceptable incontinence rate and should be avoided. The purpose of a noncutting Seton is to maintain a patent external opening to the fistulous tract and thereby control local sepsis in the patient who has recurrent abscesses. With free drainage of the tract, no abscess forms. The internal opening of the fistula persists because of Crohn's disease activity, and it will not close until medical therapy induces remission. Setons can be removed or downsized after initiation of medical therapy with evidence of clinical response in the anorectal area.

The rectal mucosal advancement flap is the optimal operation for management of rectovaginal and anterior perineal fistulas as well as perineal fistulas refractory to other therapy.[103] In the male patient, an anourethral or rectourethral fistula can similarly be closed with an advancement flap after diagnostic urethroscopy and proctoscopy have been performed. Advancement flap closure of fistulas can be undertaken when medical therapy has led to remission of rectal mucosal inflammation. Preoperatively, a standard bowel preparation is prescribed. A broad-based, myomucosal flap including rectal mucosa, submucosa, and a thin layer of internal sphincter is mobilized sharply and advanced caudad to cover the internal os of the fistula tract. A tension-free closure is made using 2-0 absorbable interrupted sutures. Unfortunately, flap failure occurs in up to 50% of patients who have Crohn's disease.[106,107] For this reason, other less-invasive techniques such as fibrin glue have also been tried, with even more dismal results. A new collagen plug has recently shown promise for anal fistulas, with an initial series reporting an 87% success rate.[108] However, no long-term data exist yet for this new technique, which essentially plugs the fistula tract, and there are no data yet in patients with Crohn's disease.

The creation of a diverting ileostomy or colostomy is typically unsuccessful when used alone to address perineal Crohn's disease. However, temporary diversion combined with (1) control of perineal sepsis, (2) advancement flap repair of fistulas, and (3) maximal medical therapy may allow sphincter preservation for 10 to 15 years.[109] In those patients who fail to have control of perianal disease with combination therapy, diverting ileostomy or colostomy can be regarded as a staging procedure; patients have the opportunity to live with a stoma and prepare psychologically for proctectomy.

Skin tags in Crohn's perineal disease have been described as "pseudo-skin tags" because they are usually inflamed skin between fissures and ulcers rather than redundant skin, which constitutes skin tags. Biopsy of these pseudo-skin tags can show the presence of granulomas and can, therefore, be helpful in securing the diagnosis of Crohn's disease. In general, local skin care and control of diarrhea are the cornerstones of treatment. Excision invites complications, such as delayed healing or chronic ulceration.[110]

Fissures that are off midline or are multiple may indicate the presence of Crohn's disease. However, because the majority of Crohn's-related fissures are on the midline, this diagnosis should be considered whenever a midline fissure fails to respond to conventional therapy.[109] Although lateral sphincterotomy is the standard operative treatment of routine anal fissures, it is to be avoided in the setting of Crohn's disease.

The anorectum that is stenosed as a result of inflammation but is still somewhat supple may be amenable to digital dilation with one finger. More commonly, the stricture that results from chronic inflammation is rigid and unyielding. Such strictures are unresponsive to dilation and are an indication for proctectomy when symptomatic.

When hemorrhoids are coincident with Crohn's disease, operative interventions are associated with a high rate of operative complications. Every effort should be made to avoid surgery. If surgery is necessary to treat a gangrenous, prolapsed hemorrhoid, a limited procedure is recommended, taking great care to avoid injury to the sphincter. These patients should be prepared preoperatively for the high probability of prolonged healing and possible incontinence.

Although the risk of developing squamous cell carcinoma of the anus is not increased in the Crohn's perineum, diagnosis may be delayed because of the presence of chronic inflammation. Failure of fissures to heal or persistence of painful ulcers should prompt consideration for biopsy of the lesion.[111]

Crohn's disease may increase the risk of adenocarcinoma of the rectum as it does for the colon. Chronic perineal disease can be a marker for more proximal active disease, which in turn may increase risk of malignancy. There is also a suggestion of increased risk of rectal adenocarcinoma in the rectal stump of patients with chronic Crohn's ileocolitis who have undergone partial colectomy and end ileostomy/colostomy. This concern parallels the observed increased risk of adenocarcinoma in bypassed segments of bowel proximally.[112] Therefore, patients with Crohn's disease and a rectal stump require cancer surveillance and should be considered for proctectomy when it is clear there is no chance for restoring intestinal continuity.

The majority of patients with a history of anorectal Crohn's disease never require proctectomy. In one study that reviewed outcomes between 10 and 20 years after initial consultation for perianal complications, only 17% of patients required proctectomy.[113,114] Typical indications for proctectomy include incontinence and stenosis or disabling recurrent abscesses and fistulas. However, many patients with complex perianal Crohn's disease are satisfied with their bowel function despite complications and are content to rely on medical management and local surgical treatment as required. Therefore, the patient should dictate the timing of proctectomy.

In preparation for surgery, the extent and severity of disease must be assessed. Enteroclysis studies, colonoscopy reports, and abdominal CT scans should be reviewed and repeated if necessary. When disease is confined to the rectum and perineum, proctectomy and end colostomy can be performed. This approach is justified by the observation that 5% of patients with this pattern of disease have no further evidence of Crohn's disease in follow-up.[101] They are essentially cured. If an end colostomy is performed in a patient with a history of diarrhea or multiple small-bowel resections, the stoma should be everted like an ileostomy rather than flush with the skin like a conventional colostomy. This method will allow liquid stool to flow into an appliance without contacting the skin.

When there is active small-bowel disease but relative sparing of the colon and rectum, the perineum may be an innocent bystander rather than the primary focus of the disease. Control of small-bowel disease may result in healing of the secondarily involved perineum, obviating the need for proctectomy. Every effort should be made to medically treat the small-bowel disease before recommending proctectomy. Conversely, those patients with severe perianal and rectal disease who have little inflammation in the rest of the GI tract may develop significant proximal colon or small-bowel disease after proctectomy.

Segmental involvement of the colon in addition to a history of small-bowel disease demands individualized treatment. The dictum "operate on complications of Crohn's disease, not Crohn's disease itself" applies. A segment of inflamed transverse colon, for example, would not be resected at the time of proctectomy unless there were an obstructing stricture or perforation.

For a proctectomy, dissection of the anus in the intersphincteric plane is recommended. The residual muscle will be incorporated into and strengthen the perineal closure. Any epithelialized (fistulous) tracts should be opened and curetted. Not surprisingly, patients with Crohn's disease have a higher rate of wound-healing complications; this may be a consequence of transecting fistulous tracts and granulomatous tissue during mobilization of the rectum. Drains are placed into the pelvis transabdominally. Transperineal drains do not seem to reduce the incidence of wound-healing complications. The pelvic floor fascia and subcutaneous tissues are reapproximated with 2-0 absorbable interrupted sutures, and the skin is left open to heal by secondary intention (Fig. 51.8). In some cases of severe fistulizing perianal disease that requires proctectomy with significant perineal tissue excision, rotational flap closure with rectus abdominus muscle or gluteus advancement flaps may be required.

Ulcerative Colitis

Ulcerative colitis (UC) is a mucosal inflammatory condition of the GI tract confined to the colon and rectum. Like Crohn's, it is considered a manifestation of IBD. Although the medical therapy is similar for Crohn's disease and UC, the surgical therapies for each differ radically, and it is imperative that a clear diagnosis is made whenever possible. The anatomical location and microscopic pathology of the two diseases helps to differentiate them. However, in about 15% of patients with IBD, a definitive diagnosis cannot be made. These patients are diagnosed with indeterminate colitis with features more consistent with UC or Crohn's but with elements suggestive of both diseases present on pathological evaluation. The treatment of these patients is complicated and individualized in consultation with a gastroenterologist, the patient, and the patient's support system.

The incidence of UC ranges from 2 to 15 per 100,000 population and has remained relatively constant for the past 20 years. Previously, the higher incidence appeared to correlate with northern countries and more developed nations, but the incidence in Asia has been increasing. A study of 15 regions of the United States showed the incidence to be 5.5 per 100,000 whites.[115] The prevalence of UC is 50 to 70 cases per 100,000 population per year. There is a bimodal age distribution, with the peak incidence occurring between 20 and 29 years of age and the second peak at 60 to 70 years.[116] No environmental or genetic factors have been found that are directly implicated in this disease, although smokers have a decreased incidence of UC, and a familial aggregation has been noted. Also, 20% to 30% of patients with UC have another family member with the disease.[117,118]

Our understanding of the immunologic basis for IBD has grown considerably in the last decade and has been crucial to the development of new medical therapies.[119,120] Both Crohn's

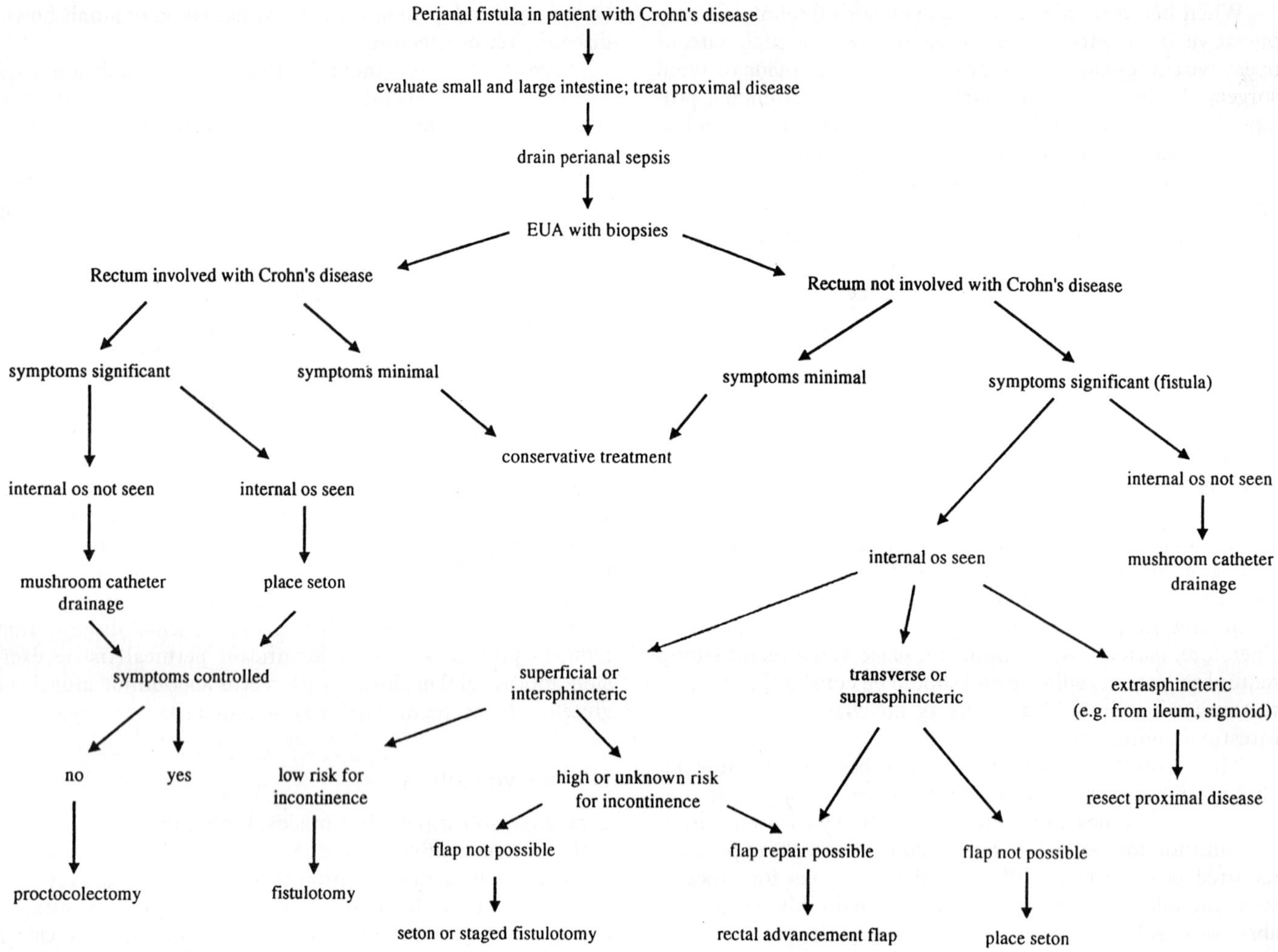

FIGURE 51.8. Algorithm for the treatment of abscesses and fistulas from perianal Crohn's disease. (From Michelassi and Milsom,[644] with permission, © 1999, Springer-Verlag, New York.)

disease and UC are characterized by a chronic inflammatory response, which may be incited by intraluminal pathogens that enter the bowel wall because of the increased permeability associated with a defective mucosal barrier.

The immune responses to this invasion are regulated by T cells, which elaborate proinflammatory and antiinflammatory cytokines and deliver activating and inhibitory signals through cell contact. This balance is facilitated by T-helper (TH) lymphocyte subsets, which are dysregulated in IBD. The TH1 cells regulate cell-mediated immune responses and subclasses of immunoglobulin that assist in opsonization and complement lysis of cellular targets. Crohn's disease results from an overabundance of this cell type in the gut mucosa. The TH2 cells mediate B-lymphocyte immunoglobulin synthesis and allergic reactions. Another subset, TH3, produced by TH2 cells, has been found to inhibit immune responses in mucosal tissues. Cytokines produced from these subsets all play a role in the pathogenesis of IBD.

The differentiation in these subsets is under genetic control and is a dynamic response. Elaboration of TH1 cells causes a decrease in TH2 cells and vice versa. Studies have shown that patients with Crohn's disease have selectively activated TH1 cells that produce IL-12 and IFN-α, both proinflammatory cytokines. The immunologic basis for UC is not as clear as for Crohn's; however, IL-13 production by natural killer (NK) cells is implicated.[121] Ulcerative colitis patients have selectively activated TH2 cells that produce certain antiinflammatory cytokines, such as IL-5, IL-6, and IL-10. The initiation of these cytokine cascades then results in an amplification of the inflammatory response, and the imbalance of these regulatory cells further exacerbates the diseases.

The clinical manifestations of UC vary with the severity of the disease. Patients may have active disease with intervening periods of quiescence. The most common symptom of UC is bloody diarrhea. Patients with mild disease may have occasional blood and mucus and a moderate number of stools. Frequent, explosive diarrhea with significant bleeding or discharge of mucus and pus manifests more severe disease. Massive hemorrhage from UC is rare. Severe disease may also be associated with fever, abdominal pain, tenesmus, malaise, anemia, or weight loss. Some may have fecal incontinence with severe disease activity. Most patients present with mild-to-moderate disease involving the rectum and a contiguous segment of the distal colon. About 25% of UC patients have proctitis alone, and 30% of UC patients have pancolitis.

The so-called toxic megacolon is a presentation of fulminant colitis with fever, abdominal pain, and leukocytosis that may or may not be associated with radiographic evidence of colonic dilation. Patients may require emergent operation for perforation or severe symptoms that are resistant to medical therapy. In the latter situation, superinfection with *Clostridium difficile* or cytomegalovirus (CMV) should always be checked prior to surgery in the event that medical treatment of these infections reverses the course of the disease.

Physical examination findings are dependent on the severity of the disease. In mild cases, the examination may be normal. In more severe cases, patients may have abdominal distension and tenderness or localized peritoneal signs. Digital rectal examination may reveal tenderness and blood, mucus, or pus in the rectal vault.

The diagnosis of UC is made endoscopically. For those patients with severe symptoms, a sigmoidoscopy may be preferrable to colonoscopy due to the risk of perforation when active disease is present. Enemas should not be given before the exam for the same reasons. For those with mild-to-moderate symptoms, however, a complete bowel prep and full colonoscopy can be performed to examine the entire colon and assess the extent of disease. There may be loss of the submucosal vascular pattern and edema with mild disease; a granular, hyperemic, and friable mucosa with moderate disease; and a deep-red, velvety appearance with more active disease. A mucopurulent exudate may obscure ulcerations. Pseudopolyps may also be seen.

Assessment of severity is important in choosing therapy. Multiple classifications have been developed to assess the severity, examine stool frequency, presence of bleeding, other symptoms, and endoscopic evaluation (Tables 51.4 and 51.5). Barium enema (BE) is generally not used to examine the colon for active disease. However, in long-standing disease, it may be superior to colonoscopy in demonstrating mild strictures or foreshortening of the colon. There is a loss of haustrations, and a rigid pipe appearance develops as the colon narrows and shortens. This test should not be performed in the setting of acute disease because of the risk of perforation. Strictures seen on BE should be considered malignant until proven otherwise.

Surveillance by colonoscopy in UC is important because of the increased risk of colorectal dysplasia and carcinoma. Patients at higher risk are those with colitis proximal to the splenic flexure and those with long-standing disease, at least 8 to 10 years.[122–126] Patients with ulcerative proctitis are not at increased risk for developing cancer. Other factors correlated with the risk of cancer are a positive family history of colorectal cancer and the presence of primary sclerosing cholangitis (PSC).[127,128] Although previous reports predicted the incidence of colorectal cancer in UC to be 60% at 30 years,[129] recent studies estimated the risk to be approximately 0.5% to 1.0% per year after 8 to 10 years of disease.[130,131]

For surveillance of these patients, dysplasia is used as a premalignant marker for carcinoma. As a result, the current recommendations are for patients with pancolitis to undergo colonoscopy every 1 to 2 years after the 8th year of disease and yearly after the 15th year. Biopsies should be taken at 10-cm intervals, resulting in a total of at least 30 biopsies. Pathological studies have confirmed that up to 33 biopsies may be required to have a 90% chance of detecting dysplasia.[132] In patients with left-sided colitis, yearly colonoscopy should be performed after the 15th year. Similar biopsies should be obtained as for pancolitis.

There are many difficulties with this surveillance regimen. Problems include sampling error, interobserver variability,[133] low negative predictive value, and the presence of cancer before detection of low-grade dysplasia. As many as 25% of colon cancers are not associated with dysplasia,[134] and in the setting of low-grade dysplasia, 20% of colectomy specimens will reveal a carcinoma. In the setting of a dysplasia-associated lesion or mass (DALM), 50% will have a colorectal cancer. Further, no randomized prospective trials have been performed to show the cost-effectiveness or benefit with this regimen.

Despite these shortcomings, multiple trials[134–138] have shown improved survival in patients surgically treated for

TABLE 51.4. Definition of Severity of Ulcerative Colitis Episode.

	Severity of attack[a]	
Symptoms	***Severe***	***Mild***
Diarrhea	Six or more stools daily	Four or fewer stools daily
Blood in stool	Large amount	Small amount
Fever	99.5°F or higher (evening)	None
Tachycardia	Heart rate 90 beats/min or more	None
Anemia	75% hemoglobin or less	None
Elevated erythrocyte sedimentation rate	30 mm/h or more	Normal

[a]Moderate = Intermediate between severe and mild.

Source: Modified from Truelove,[659] with permission of the Société Internationale de Chirurgie.

TABLE 51.5. Scoring System for Assessment of Ulcerative Colitis Disease Activity.

Stool frequency[a]	*Findings of flexible proctosigmoidoscopy*
0 = Normal number of stools for this patient	0 = Normal or inactive disease
1 = One to two stools more than normal	1 = Mild disease (erythema, decreased vascular pattern, mild friability)
2 = Three or more stools more than normal	2 = Moderate disease (marked erythema, absent vascular pattern, friability, erosions)
3 = Five or more stools more than normal	3 = Severe disease (spontaneous bleeding, ulceration)
Rectal bleeding[b]	***Physician's global assessment***[c]
0 = No blood seen	0 = Normal
1 = Streaks of blood with stool less than half the time	1 = Mild disease
2 = Obvious blood with stool most of the time	2 = Moderate disease
3 = Blood alone passed	3 = Severe disease

[a]Each patient served as his or her own control to establish the degree of abnormality of the stool frequency.

[b]The daily bleeding score represented the most severe bleeding of the day.

[c]The physician's global assessment acknowledged the three other criteria, the patient's daily record of abdominal discomfort and general sense of well-being, and other observations, such as physical findings and the patient's performance status.

Source: From Schroeder et al.,[660] © 1987, Massachusetts Medical Society. All rights reserved.

UC-associated cancers who had surveillance compared to their counterparts. Other premalignant markers with promise include flow cytometry of DNA content for aneuploidy, detection of abnormal mucins and glycoproteins, and evaluation of tumor suppressor genes such as p53.

The extraintestinal manifestations of UC are similar to those of Crohn's disease with the exception of hepatobiliary complications, which are more common and can be quite severe. Primary sclerosing cholangitis (PSC) is uncommon with Crohn's disease and occurs in 7.5% of patients with UC. Most patients are men under 40. Hepatobiliary symptoms may precede intestinal manifestations by as many as 7 years.[139] Symptoms include jaundice, pruritus, fatigue, abdominal pain, weight loss, and fever, but many patients are asymptomatic, with only biochemical abnormalities. Patients who progress to cirrhosis develop complications of severe liver disease, including bleeding varices, ascites, and encephalopathy. The only cure for this disease is liver transplant. For milder forms of the disease, antibiotics for cholangitis and cholestyramine for pruritus are used. Most immunosuppressive agents have not been shown to help. A small trial of methotrexate has shown promising results.[140] Ursodeoxycholic acid has also shown significant improvement in biochemical abnormalities and liver histology.[141,142] Treatment of the colonic disease with total proctocolectomy does not affect the clinical course of PSC but may reverse the fatty infiltration and liver function abnormalities seen with UC.[143]

Other manifestations of UC include involvement of the skin, eyes, and joints. These diseases are discussed in the Crohn's disease section of this chapter. Patients with UC have also been noted to have a higher risk of thromboembolic disease and vasculitis. The most significant extracolonic manifestations that can be reversed with surgical therapy are malnutrition and, in younger patients, growth retardation.

Unlike Crohn's disease, which has transmural inflammation, UC is a disease of the mucosa and submucosa. It starts in the rectum and extends proximally to include a variable amount of colon. The pathological characteristics vary depending on disease state (acute or chronic), severity, and presence of complications. Generally, the outer wall of the colon will look completely normal, or the serosa may have dilated blood vessels. However, in chronic cases, the bowel may be foreshortened secondary to a thickening and contraction of the muscularis mucosae. The mesentery remains normal, unlike the thickened mesocolon of Crohn's disease. The mucosa may be erythematous, thickened, friable, or granular and can have ulcerations, superficial fissures, or pseudopolyps. A mucopurulent exudate may be present on the mucosa. The mucosal inflammation always starts in the rectum and is continuous. If "skip lesions" with intervening normal mucosa are seen, Crohn's disease should be suspected. The rectal mucosa may appear less diseased or even normal if the patient has been treated with topical rectal therapy (enemas or suppositories).

In about 10% of patients with pancolitis, the distal ileum may appear inflamed and ulcerated. This finding is secondary to reflux of colonic contents through the ileocecal valve and is termed *backwash ileitis*. It should not be confused with Crohn's disease as this inflammation generally is contiguous with the rest of the inflammation of the colon.

Strictures of the colon associated with UC must be considered to be malignant or associated with Crohn's disease until proven otherwise. Most cancers occur in those with long-standing disease of at least 10 to 20 years, are proximal to the splenic flexure, and cause symptomatic large-bowel obstructions.[144]

Microscopic characteristics include the presence of polymorphonuclear leukocytes (PMNs) in the epithelium of the crypts of Lieberkuhn-forming crypt abscesses. Progression of the disease leads to coalescence of these crypts into broad-based ulcers eroding the mucosa. The residual normal mucosa that remains at the borders of these crypt abscesses is what projects into the lumen as a "pseudopolyp." The PMNs are also seen in the surface epithelium and lamina propria. The epithelial cells demonstrate mucin depletion, basophilic cytoplasm with hyperchromatic nuclei, and increased mitotic figures. Chronic features include distortion of crypt and gland architecture with branching and irregular size and spacing between glands. Lymphoid follicles can be seen in chronic UC, in the lamina propria and superficial submucosa, different in location to those seen with Crohn's disease, in which they may be found in the deeper submucosa, muscularis propria, and subserosa.

Medical Therapy

The medical therapy for UC overlaps significantly with those therapies used for Crohn's disease, discussed previously. However, certain drugs are more useful in the treatment of UC and are elaborated here.

Sulfasalazine (Azulfidine) was the first drug developed for the treatment of UC. This class of drugs, aminosalicylates, continues to be the most commonly prescribed therapy for mild-to-moderate UC. Sulfasalazine is a sulfapyridine linked to 5-ASA by an azo bond. The sulfa component is what causes the side effects of nausea, headache, malaise, and anorexia. The 5-ASA is the active agent inhibiting prostaglandin and leukotriene synthesis, which may directly inhibit inflammatory responses. There is also evidence that this compound scavenges destructive oxygen free radicals. Sulfasalazine is cleaved in the colon, making the active 5-ASA component available to act on the large intestine. A dosage of 4g/day can reduce the relapse rate at 1 year from 70% to 9%.[145]

Mesalamine (unbound 5-ASA) is absorbed in the small intestine and is not effective in UC. Preparations to delay the release of 5-ASA in the intestinal tract with resin, Asacol, or slow-release microspheres regulated by pH, Pentasa, are available. These therapies have been useful for maintaining remission and treating mild-to-moderate UC. In trials, both Asacol (0.8–1.6g/day) and Pentasa (4g/day) were found to maintain remission in 60% to 70% of patients compared to 30% to 40% of the placebo group.[146] Other sulfa-free aminosalicylates such as Olsalazine, two 5-ASA linked by an azo bond, and Balsalazide, 5-ASA linked to an inert carrier molecule, are also commonly used. Both drugs have shown benefit in maintaining remission of UC.[147,148] Unfortunately, most studies comparing the superiority of these agents over one another are limited by design flaws and the bioequivalence of all preparations of 5-ASA is not established.[149,150] Therefore, decisions regarding choice of 5-ASA drug should be based on other patient-related factors.[151]

Rowasa is a topical enema preparation of 5-ASA useful in the treatment of ulcerative proctitis. Topical preparations, used in conjunction with oral therapy, have been found to be more effective in maintaining remission than oral agents alone.[152]

Last, the use of 5-ASA drugs for chemoprevention has also been reported, although a Canadian study with a 2-year follow-up was unable to demonstrate a difference in reduction of colorectal cancer or dysplasia in IBD patients compared to controls.[153] A meta-analysis using pooled results of observational studies supports a protective association between 5-ASA and colorectal cancer/dysplasia.[154] It is postulated that treatment with 5-ASA resulting in milder inflammation of the colonic mucosa may correlate with lower rates of colorectal cancer.

For patients with moderate or severe exacerbations of UC, steroids exert an antiinflammatory effect. However, they do not help to maintain remission and are detrimental when used long-term. They act as an immunosuppressive agent by inhibiting the release of arachidonic acid, IL-1, and IL-2, causing lymphotoxicity and decreasing adherence and chemotaxis of neutrophils, eosinophils, and monocytes. Multiple trials have demonstrated that steroids have a response rate of 70% to 90%[63,155,156] with a dose response between 20 and 60mg. They can be administered orally or, for severe cases, parenterally.[67]

The side effects of corticosteroids are extensive and include osteonecrosis, osteoporosis, cataracts, glaucoma, hyperglycemia, hyperlipidemia, hypertension, psychosis, and skin changes. For this reason, attempts have been made to create a synthetic drug with better mucosal absorption and fewer systemic side effects. Budesonide (Enterocort) is a 17-α-substituted glucocorticoid that is rapidly metabolized and is effective in an enema preparation in ulcerative proctitis.[157,158] Only 10% to 15% of the drug is absorbed systemically. Oral budesonide is not useful for patients with distal disease as it is formulated to be released in the distal ileum.

As increasing evidence points to an immunological etiology of IBD, efforts have been made to utilize various immunotherapies. The most commonly used drugs are azathioprine and its metabolite 6-MP, antimetabolites that inhibit DNA synthesis. The mechanism of action of these drugs stems from their inhibition of T-cell clones. Remission rates exceed 50%–60%, and more than 70%–80% of responders will continue to respond over the next year.[79] The drugs continue to show a benefit with respect to maintenance of remission even after 4 years of continuous therapy. They are useful in managing steroid-dependent UC. Clinical response has been demonstrated with both drugs, with a decrease or elimination in steroid requirements[159–161]; they also maintain remission.[162,163] Adverse side effects include bone marrow suppression, pancreatitis, hepatitis, hypersensitivity reactions, increased infections, and potential risk of lymphoma.[164]

Other effective drugs with established efficacy in UC include cyclosporine and other monoclonal antibodies to cytokines. Cyclosporine is a lipophilic peptide that inhibits the synthesis of IL-2 and IFN, thus exerting its immunological effect. Controlled trials of intravenous cyclosporine used at a dose of 4mg/kg/day demonstrated an 80% response rate for patients with severe UC.[86,165,166] Oral cyclosporine has a variable intestinal absorption, but recent reports suggest efficacy.[167] Cyclosporine has many side effects, including nephrotoxicity, hypertension, seizures, gingival hyperplasia, hirsutism, tremors, headache, nausea, and opportunistic infections. The most common effect is dose-related renal insufficiency.[67]

Infliximab, a chimeric mouse-human monoclonal antibody to human TNF-α that has revolutionized the treatment of Crohn's disease has not been demonstrated to be as useful for UC. Nonetheless, a randomized, placebo-controlled trial of two different doses of infliximab reported remission rates of 25%–36% compared to 10% in the placebo group.[79] Visilizumab, a humanized antibody targeted to CD3 T cells, acts by inducing apoptosis and has been demonstrated to induce remission in 66% of patients. About 60% of patients developed cytokine release syndrome, with symptoms including nausea, emesis, chills, and arthralgias. However, all symptoms resolved quickly within hours.[168] Further clinical trials for this drug are underway.

The use of probiotics, porcine whipworm, and adsorptive leukocyte apheresis has also been reported to treat UC with promising results, although these more unusual treatments will require further study.[79]

Surgical Therapy

According to longitudinal studies, approximately 30% of all patients with UC ultimately have surgery. Within the first year of diagnosis, 10% require operative intervention, and the colectomy rate then is about 3% per year for the next 4 years and 1% per year thereafter.[169] The surgical treatment of UC involves removing the colon and the rectum. Segmental colectomies have a limited role in UC as the entire colon is at risk for subsequent problems. The indications for surgery depend on the severity and duration of the patient's disease.

For patients with active disease, emergency operation may be indicated for fulminant colitis unresponsive to medical therapy with bleeding, perforation, or toxic colitis. In these situations, the safest procedure is a total abdominal colectomy with end ileostomy, leaving the rectum in place. This allows an extremely ill patient to undergo a shorter, less-complicated procedure that does not prevent a subsequent restorative procedure. It is the preferred operation for those who require emergent surgery or are debilitated, malnourished, or receiving excessive doses of steroids or immunosuppressive agents. It is important to transect the bowel near the sacral promontory. This precaution prevents injury to important pelvic structures and allows for easy identification and mobilization of the rectal stump at future operations.

For patients with chronic active or quiescent disease, the indications for surgery include an inability to wean from steroids, extracolonic manifestations that may respond to colectomy, and the presence of dysplasia or carcinoma on colonoscopy for screening. Children with UC may require surgery to treat delayed growth and maturation secondary to medical therapy or malnutrition. For these patients, a number of surgical options may be entertained; these include total proctocolectomy with end ileostomy, continent ileostomy, or ileal pouch–anal anastomosis. Since UC generally begins in the rectum and extends proximally, a total proctocolectomy is performed because the disease in the rectum is severe enough to warrant excision.

Total proctocolectomy with end ileostomy produces the lowest morbidity and mortality for patients. Unfortunately, it relegates them to a permanent ileostomy and has largely been replaced by ileal pouch procedures. The abdominal portion is performed in a similar fashion as those performed in the acute setting except that the bowel is not divided at the sacral promontory, but rather the dissection is carried down into the pelvis to the level of the pelvic floor. The perineal portion is performed differently for UC and Crohn's disease than for malignancy. In IBD, an intersphincteric dissection of the anus allows for a less-vascular dissection and a smaller perineal defect. Once the proctocolectomy is performed, the end ileostomy is created. The advantage of a standard proctocolectomy is that all the disease is removed. The disadvantage, however, is that the patient is left with an "incontinent" end ileostomy that passes stool and flatus in an uncontrolled fashion. To remedy this, various continence-restoring procedures have been performed.

The continent ileostomy was introduced by Kock[170] in 1969. This method allowed patients with ileostomies to control elimination from the pouch by fashioning a "nipple" that maintained continence. The patient empties the pouch with a catheter and is not required to wear an appliance. Unfortunately, this procedure has a high rate of early and late complications and has been supplanted by the ileal pouch–anal procedure. It is still indicated for those patients who have end ileostomies and want conversion to a continent stoma. The complication rate is highest in the first 2 years; after that, pouch durability and patient satisfaction are high.[171]

The ileal pouch–anal anastomosis, developed in 1978 by Parks and Nicholls,[172] has become the standard operation for UC. The advantage of the procedure is that it allows the patient to evacuate stool through the anus, thus avoiding a stoma. The disadvantage is that the procedure is associated with significant morbidity, and the risk of cancer is not completely eliminated, as it is when a standard proctocolectomy is performed. Contraindications to this procedure are advanced age, preoperative fecal incontinence, possibility of Crohn's disease, previous significant small-bowel resection, and distal rectal cancer. Fulminant colitis and toxic colitis are relative contraindications because of the high rate of complications. Most of these procedures are performed with a proximal diverting loop ileostomy. However, in some centers, diversion is not performed for carefully selected patients.[173,174] The ileal pouch can be made as a J, S, or W, but the most common is a J-pouch, usually 12 to 15 cm in length (Fig. 51.9).

The ileal pouch anal anastomosis can be performed using a stapled technique or by performing a mucosectomy with a hand-sewn anastomosis. Proponents of the stapled technique, which include our institution, advocate dissection of the rectum down to the pelvic floor and stapling across the rectum within the surgical anal canal no more than 1 to 1.5 cm above the dentate line. A double-stapled anastomosis is then created between the ileal pouch and the anus with a circular stapler. Those in favor of mucosectomy will remove the mucosa starting at the dentate line so that the anal transition zone is also included in the removal of the rectal mucosa and then sew the pouch to the dentate line. Mucosectomy is generally considered to be a more critical factor when creating ileal pouches in patients with familial adenomatous polyposis (FAP) due to the possible cancer risk of leaving any rectal mucosa behind. Nonetheless, proponents of the mucosec-

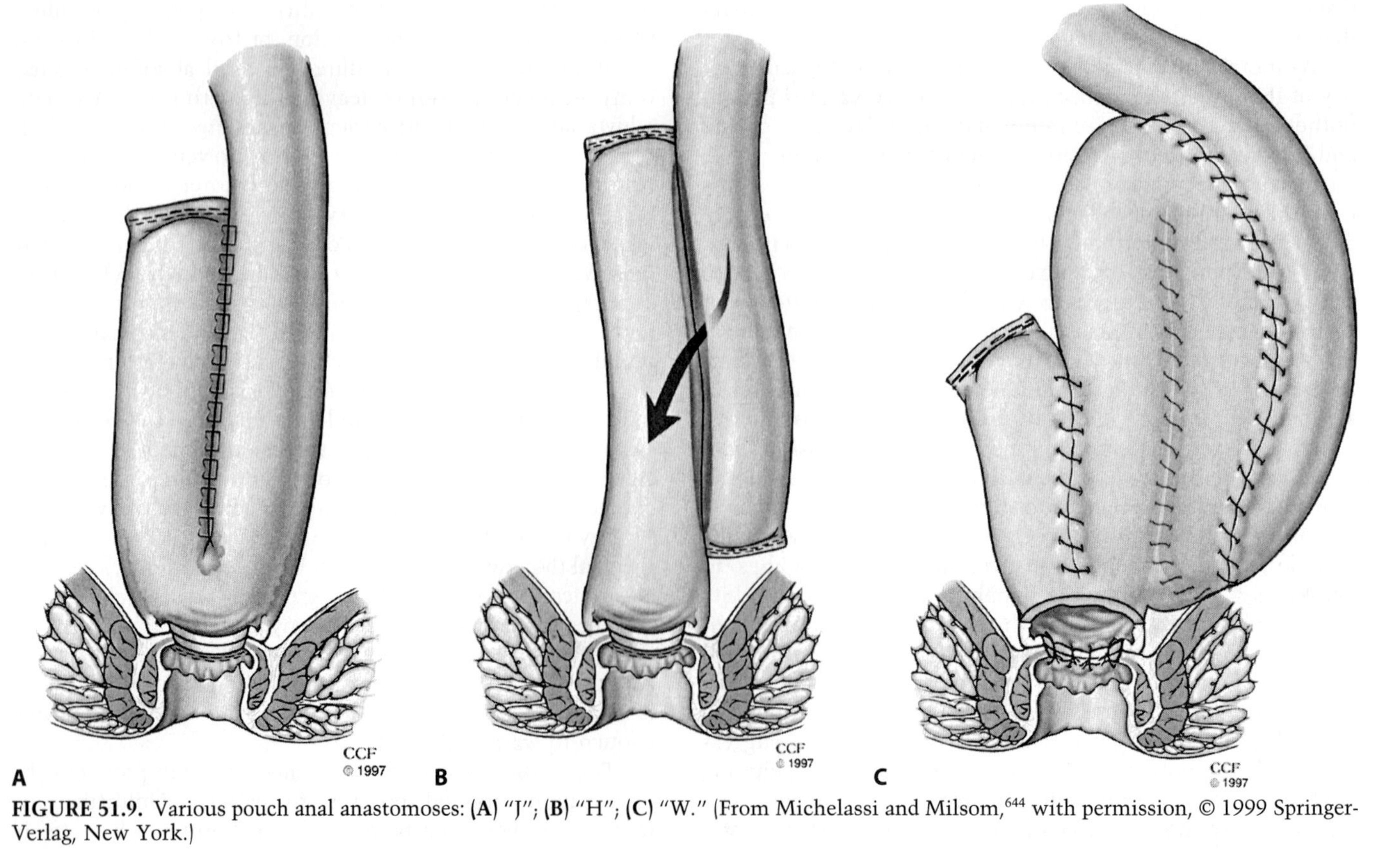

FIGURE 51.9. Various pouch anal anastomoses: (A) "J"; (B) "H"; (C) "W." (From Michelassi and Milsom,[644] with permission, © 1999 Springer-Verlag, New York.)

tomy for UC also feel that this last centimeter of mucosa is at risk for ongoing inflammatory disease and colitis-related cancer. The anastomosis may be created with a stapler after the mucosectomy by placing a purse string at the dentate line, but this is not widely done.

As stated, the issue of performing a mucosectomy relates to the subsequent risk of carcinoma or disease in the retained rectal mucosa. Studies have shown evidence of active disease or even dysplasia in specimens of stripped anorectal mucosa,[175] leading some authors to argue that a mucosectomy must always be performed. Others believe that the remnant mucosa is transitional mucosa (cuboidal epithelium) and does not represent true rectal mucosa at risk for malignancy or inflammation. Those who perform a stapled anastomosis often recommend yearly surveillance with anoscopy and digital exam of the residual mucosa. Cancer after ileopouch–anal anastomosis has only been reported after mucosectomy. The cancers presumably developed in residual mucosa that remained after mucosectomy and would therefore develop in tissue "outside" the anastomosis, making detection more difficult. Thus, mucosectomy may leave the patient and physicians with a false sense of security.

The mortality from this surgery is extremely low, less than 1%, especially when performed in an elective setting. In contrast, the morbidity is significant, even in an experienced surgeon's hands.[176] Despite this, the functional results are generally good. Complications such as ileus, wound infection, bleeding, and small-bowel obstructions are common to all abdominal surgery. Addisonian crisis (relative hypoadrenal state) may develop in any patient on high-dose maintenance therapy if exogenous steroid supplementation is not maintained. Urinary retention and sexual dysfunction are common to all pelvic operations. Complications specific to the procedure include the early complications of pelvic sepsis, pouch–anal anastomotic leak, and small-bowel obstruction at the loop ileostomy and the late complications of pouchitis, anal stricture, pouch fistula, bleeding, and excessive stools with dehydration or incontinence.

Pelvic abscess and pouch anastomotic leaks occur about 4% and 10% of the time, respectively. Those with diverting ileostomies are not prevented from developing these complications, but the systemic effects of the leak or abscess may be minimized by proximal diversion. In a patient who is not diverted, a localized pelvic abscess can be managed with percutaneous drainage. For major leaks, patients require reoperation with a diverting ileostomy. Leaks may be seen on radiographic study before closure of the loop ileostomy but may be missed and only become apparent after the ileostomy is closed. When the leak is documented before closure of the loop ileostomy, surgery is delayed. If the leak is detected after closure, drainage or drainage and diversion may be required.

Urinary retention and sexual dysfunction are related to injury or disruption of the presacral nerves during rectal dissection. Although these sequelae are reported to occur only about 1% to 3% of the time,[177,178] in an informal survey of patients who underwent an ileal pouch at our own institution, 30% of men and women reported some negative effect on their sexual function. Care should be taken to preserve the nerves of the pelvic plexus and in the presacral area.

Pouchitis is the most common late complication of this procedure. Up to 50% of these patients will have at least one episode of pouchitis, which is characterized by frequent loose stools, urgency, and tenesmus. At least 15% of patients will develop chronic pouchitis that requires ongoing treatment. The most commonly used drugs include metronidazole and ciprofloxacin. However, for refractory cases, other antibiotics, such as amoxicillin/clavulinic acid, rifaximin, budesonide, oral bismuth, or probiotics have been used.[79]

Other late complications include anal strictures, pouch fistulas, bleeding, and excessive stools with dehydration or incontinence. A small number of patients may require pouch excision or permanent ileostomy to treat these complications.

Diverticular Disease

Diverticular disease of the left colon is an acquired disease affecting primarily Western cultures (Fig. 51.10).[188] The incidence increases with age, with estimates of the incidence ranging from 5% in the fifth decade to 75% in the ninth decade of life.[189,190] Neither sex is more clearly affected, with conflicting reports of prevalence according to gender.[189–193] The etiology is not clearly understood, but the most accepted hypothesis is that diverticulosis occurs as a result of a highly refined, low-residue diet.[194] Increased dietary fiber results in softer stool directly and indirectly. Nonabsorbable dietary fibers bind water, leading to a softer formed stool. Further, a diet high in nonabsorbable fiber generates a bulky stool that stretches the colon wall, stimulating the intrinsic neural reflexes, resulting in distal circular muscle relaxation and proximal circular and longitudinal muscle contraction. The decreased transit time reduces the amount of time the stool is exposed to the mucosa, decreasing the amount of water absorbed. In contrast, diets low in fiber are less bulky, retain less water, and generate a more inspissated stool that is more difficult for the colon to pass.[195,196]

In this model of diverticular disease, a diverticulum develops along a weakness in the bowel wall that is created by a penetrating nutrient blood vessel.[197–199] A pulsion pseudodiverticulum develops when hypersegmentation of the descend-

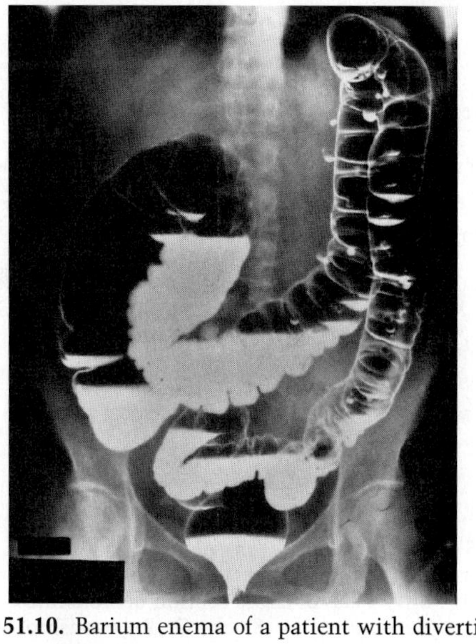

FIGURE 51.10. Barium enema of a patient with diverticulosis.

ing and sigmoid colon generates increased intraluminal pressures, forcing the mucosa of the bowel out through this weakness (Fig. 51.11). Hypersegmentation occurs because the bowel lumen is most narrow in this portion of the colon, and a low-residue stool allows the opposing walls to come into contact as waste is propelled distally. This creates a closed loop and generates markedly increased pressures. This model does not satisfactorily explain all the clinicopathological findings of diverticulosis and diverticulitis, leading some authors to propose two types of colonic diverticular disease[200]: relative distal obstruction at the rectosigmoid and a combination of wall weakness and increased pressures.[201]

Histopathological evaluation most consistently reveals thickened circular and longitudinal muscle and may also find a narrowed lumen, heaping up of the mucosa, and pericolic fibrosis.[193] Microscopic studies confirm a pseudodiverticulum composed of mucosa and serosa pouching through a neck of muscle. An adjacent artery and vein may be seen.

The thickening of the muscle has been attributed to hypertrophy, hyperplasia, and more recently elastosis.[199,202] Elastosis is a deposition of elastic tissue in the taeniae, resulting in an accordion-like colon with shortening of the colon and heaping up of the circular muscle and mucosa. These changes, limited to the sigmoid colon, occur before the development of diverticulosis and arguably are the cause of the hypersegmentation and increased intraluminal pressures that place a patient at risk for the development of diverticulosis.

Collagen composition changes may also be required for diverticular development. In autopsy studies of colons from patients with diverticulosis compared to specimens without diverticulosis,[203] the collagen quantity was unchanged, but the composition of the collagen was altered in the diverticulosis specimens.

Although diverticulosis is common, diverticulitis occurs in only 10%–25% of people with diverticulosis. Complications requiring surgery occur in only approximately 1% of patients with the disease, 30% of symptomatic patients,[189,204] and 15% to 30% of those who require hospital admission.[188,200] Although the incidence of diverticulosis increases with age, the risk of complications, other than bleeding, does not increase. In fact, the risk of complications related to perforation may be higher in the younger age groups.[189] Hospital admission and recurrent attacks increase the likelihood of significant complications and need for surgery. Medical treatment is less effective for recurrent attacks, and complications associated with the attack increase from 23% for the first attack to 58% after more than one attack. Patients who present with complicated diverticular disease (perforated diverticulum) fare even less well, and interval colectomy is often recommended after the initial hospitalization.

Fiber is the mainstay of the medical management of uncomplicated diverticulosis or mild diverticulitis. A high-fiber diet is believed to reduce intracolonic pressures, presumably eliminating the "cause" of diverticular disease. The fiber increases stool bulk and water content, generating a softer formed stool that requires the colon to generate less pressure to pass the stool in a shorter time.[205,206] Despite popular beliefs that dietary seeds may occlude a diverticulum, there is no evidence to suggest that patients with diverticulosis should avoid seeds.

While most cases of diverticulosis remain asymptomatic, complications of colonic diverticula that may require surgical consultation or intervention are hemorrhage or perforation of a diverticulum resulting in diverticulitis. Hemorrhage occurs in up to 20% of patients with diverticulosis. In 5%, the hemorrhage is massive.[207] The source of the bleeding is generally right sided, even though diverticula are predominantly present on the left.[208,209] The majority of patients (70%–82%) stop bleeding, but 12% to 30% continue to bleed and require intervention.[207,209,210] The cause of the hemorrhage appears to be an erosion into the vasa recta that courses along the diverticulum.[211]

Patients with GI hemorrhage need to be worked up and treated in a similar fashion no matter the cause. Initial assessment of the ABCs must be performed in all patients, with particular attention to the establishment of large-bore intravenous access. Six units of packed red blood cells should be typed and crossed. A nasogastric tube must be placed because the majority of GI hemorrhage is from a proximal gastroduodenal source. A Foley catheter is used to monitor adequacy of fluid resuscitation. Proctosigmoidoscopy may reveal a local source and may document the presence of blood and clots proximal to the rectum.

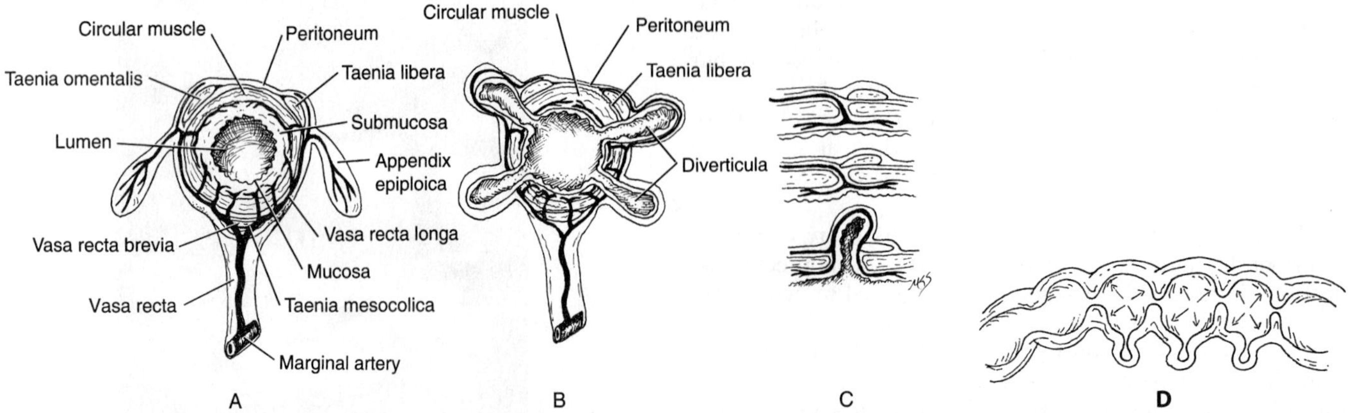

FIGURE 51.11. Pathogenesis of diverticular disease. **A.** Cross section of usual anatomical layers of colonic wall with special attention to course of vessels. **B.** Cross section demonstrating location of diverticula as determined by Slack. **C.** Relationship of vessels to diverticulum. (Adapted from Gordon and Nivatvongs,[645] by permission of Taylor & Francis Group LLC.) **D.** Hypersegmentation of bowel creating increased intraluminal pressures and diverticula. (Redrawn from Painter.[646])

Once resuscitation is underway, attention is directed toward localization of the source. If the nasogastric tube and proctosigmoidoscopic evaluation suggests a distal source, a nuclear medicine test is the preferred first step. Technetium-99 (^{99m}Tc) is used because it has a longer half-life and generates less background in the liver and spleen compared to sulfur colloid. A small aliquot of the patient's own blood is withdrawn, the red blood cells are labeled with ^{99m}Tc, and the blood is returned to the patient. Bleeding at a rate as low as 0.1 mL/min can be detected.[212] Success in localization is operator-dependent and varies widely between institutions, but sensitivities as high as 97% and specificities of 85% are reported from multiple centers.[213–215] Others have had less success,[216] but most centers require this before angiography because of the higher sensitivity of the nuclear medicine test compared to angiography, 0.1 mL/min versus 0.5 to 1.0 mL/min.

Angiographic localization is attempted in those with a positive nuclear medicine scan. This technique allows for confirmation of location and therapeutic intervention[209] with either microembolization of a terminal arcade (metal coils or gelatin sponges [Gelfoam])[217] or Pitressin infusion via the catheter positioned in a distal branch[218] (Fig. 51.12). Both techniques have a greater than 90% success rate. Pitressin infusion has significant cardiac toxicity and requires immobilization in an intensive care unit with a catheter in place; patients who have undergone embolization must be monitored for bowel ischemia.

Urgent colonoscopy after rapid bowel cleansing has been successfully performed as both a diagnostic and therapeutic technique in select institutions with dedicated teams, but this has not gained wide acceptance despite excellent results.[212,219,220]

The indications for surgery and the choice of operation remain controversial and require a good deal of clinical judgment. Efforts to localize the bleeding source are maximized to allow therapeutic intervention as mentioned and to direct the segmental resection if a colectomy is necessary. If the lesion is localized and hemorrhage controlled, then elective segmental colectomy may be carried out based on assessment of the patient's operative risks and risks of rebleeding.

An aggressive surgical approach is advocated by those who argue that these patients are often elderly[219] and tolerate rapid blood loss poorly because of medical comorbidities. However, the natural history of a bleeding source that has been controlled by Pitressin or embolization is undefined. It is doubtful that the same source bleeds as the vessel probably thromboses. Urgent segmental colectomy is indicated after localization (1) if the bleeding cannot be controlled with the aforementioned nonoperative measures or (2) if blood products are limited or unavailable while awaiting spontaneous cessation (for Jehovah's Witness or antibodies on cross match).

"Blind" segmental colectomy (right hemicolectomy or sigmoid colectomy in the absence of studies confirming the source of bleeding) is not recommended. Studies have shown a rebleeding rate of 35%–75% and a mortality rate of 20%–50% when blind segmental colectomy is performed for unlocalized lower GI hemorrhage.[221,222]

When emergent surgery is required to treat massive hemorrhage and the lesion cannot be localized preoperatively or with intraoperative techniques (enteroscopy/colonoscopy), total colectomy with an ileorectal anastomosis is the preferred surgical option.[221–223] Recurrent bleeding after total colectomy approaches zero,[6] but the morbidity of frequent loose bowel movements, in the elderly in particular, is not insignificant. An algorithm for treatment of lower GI hemorrhage is presented in Figure 51.13.

Diverticulitis is caused by perforation of a colonic diverticulum. In most cases, the perforation is microscopic, causing localized inflammation in the colonic wall or paracolic tissues. Acute diverticulitis can be classified into uncomplicated diverticulitis and complicated diverticulitis. Uncomplicated diverticulitis is a result of a microperforation of a colonic diverticulum, resulting in localized inflammation and infection of the pericolonic tissues. Complications of diverticulitis are generally a result of a larger, more severe perforation of the colon or repeated attacks of diverticulitis and include free perforation with generalized purulent or fecal peritonitis, abscess formation (mesocolic or pelvic), fistula formation (usually to the bladder or vagina), or stricture formation with colonic obstruction.

The average age at presentation is the early 60s; more than 90% of cases occur after 50 years of age. Fifty percent to 90% of cases in the United States occur in the left colon, particularly the sigmoid. However, among the Asian population,

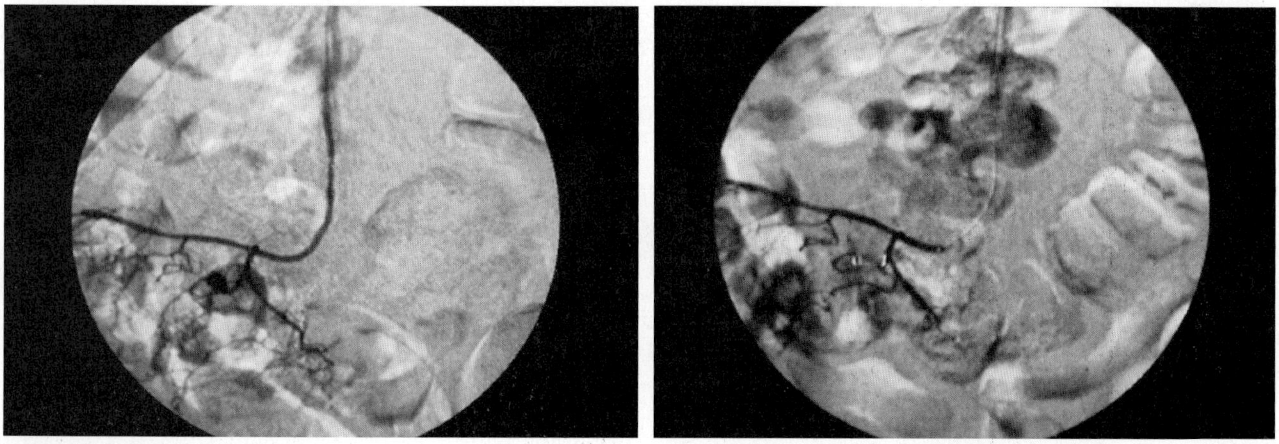

A B

FIGURE 51.12. Angiogram in a patient with gastrointestinal hemorrhage. Note the "blush" of extravasated intraluminal blood (**A**) and the coils in the terminal arcade postembolization (**B**).

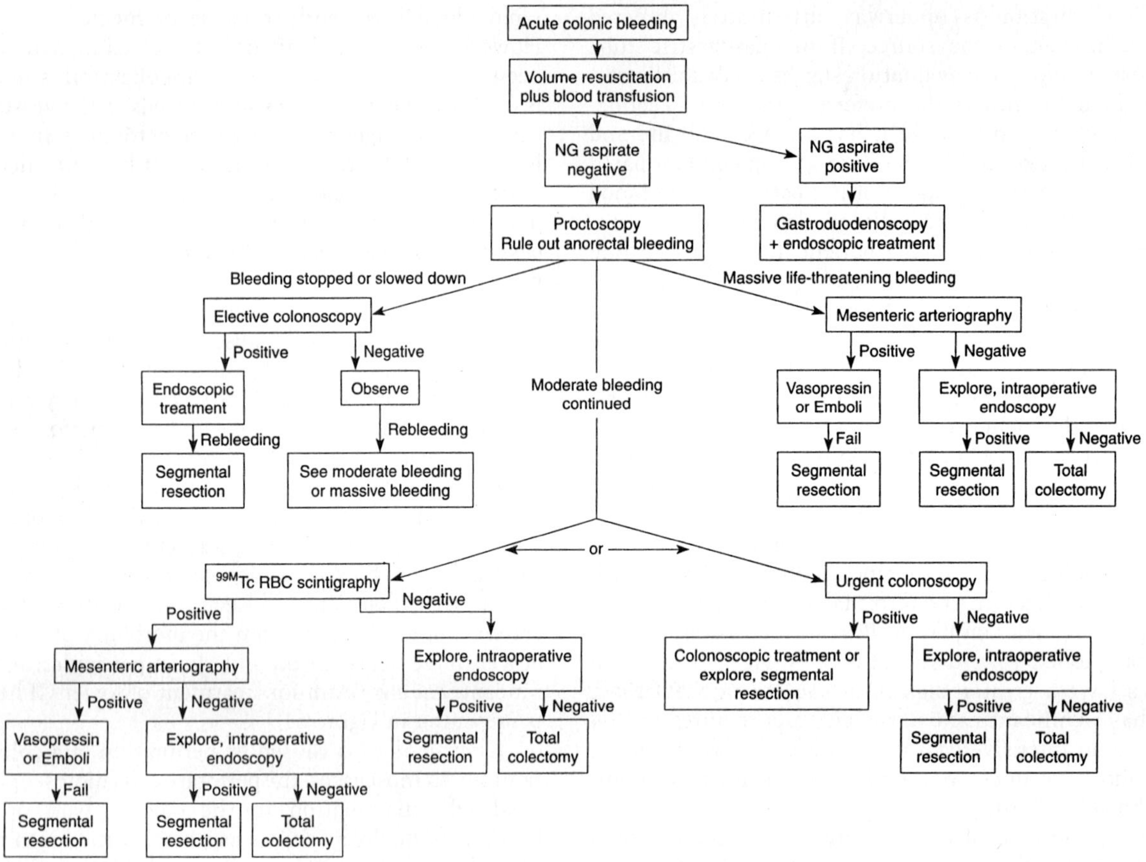

FIGURE 51.13. Algorithm for treatment of colonic hemorrhage.

up to 75% right-sided disease has been reported.[224–226] Fifty percent of patients have been symptomatic for less than 1 month before presentation; the duration of symptoms is inversely correlated with the severity of disease.

Patients with uncomplicated acute diverticulitis typically present with the gradual onset of left lower quadrant pain and low-grade fever. The pain is constant and does not radiate. The localized inflammatory process may lead to irritation of the contiguous small bowel, colon, and bladder, which may cause anorexia, nausea, vomiting, diarrhea, constipation, dysuria, frequency, or urgency. On physical examination, tenderness to palpation is usually present in the left lower quadrant or suprapubic region. In complicated cases, a mass suggestive of a peridiverticular abscess or phlegmon may also be palpable. Rectal examination may reveal a boggy mass anteriorly if a pelvic abscess is present. Unlike diverticulosis, acute diverticulitis is usually not associated with hemorrhage, but 30% to 40% of cases have guaiac-positive stool. With free perforation of a diverticulum, the patient presents with signs and symptoms of a perforated viscus with shock and generalized peritonitis. Pneumaturia or fecaluria suggest the presence of a colovesical fistula.

Laboratory studies are nonspecific and frequently unrevealing. Leukocytosis may be absent in up to half of cases. Urinalysis may be abnormal, with microscopic pyuria or hematuria. In elderly or immunocompromised patients, the presentation may be subtle, and immunocompromised patients are more likely to have complications of diverticulitis. The differential diagnosis is listed in Table 51.6.

Reliance on history and physical and laboratory findings to diagnose diverticulitis can be unreliable, with some series finding a correct diagnosis in only 43%–56% of cases.[227,228] In instances of suspected diverticulitis, CT scan of the abdomen and pelvis with intravenous, oral, and rectal contrast is the preferred test to confirm the diagnosis. Studies have shown CT to have a sensitivity of 97%–98% and a specificity of 99%–100% in cases of suspected diverticulitis.[227–230] Computed tomographic findings of acute diverticulitis include thickening of the wall of the colon, inflammatory changes in the pericolic fat, pericolonic or pelvic abscess, and extraluminal air.

TABLE 51.6. Differential Diagnosis of Acute Diverticulitis.

Appendicitis
Carcinoma
Colonic spasm
Gastroenteritis
Infectious colitis
Ischemia
Irritable bowel
Inflammatory bowel disease
Pelvic inflammatory disease
Perforated peptic ulcer
Foreign body perforation
Volvulus
Urosepsis
Pneumonia

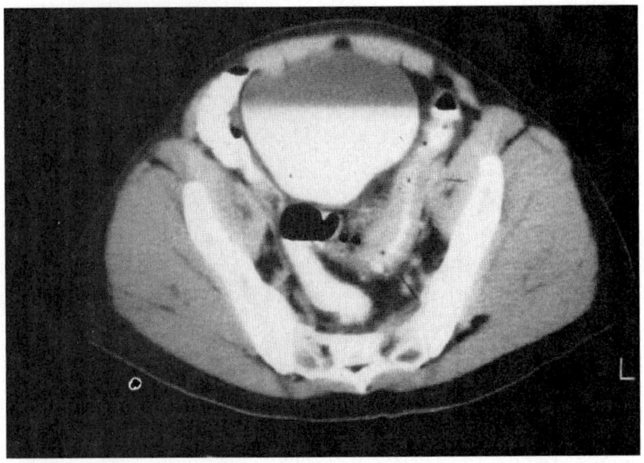

FIGURE 51.14. Computed tomographic scan of a patient with acute diverticulitis. Note the "streaking" of the fat characteristic of inflammation and the thickening of the sigmoid colon bowel wall.

Computed tomography is not useful in differentiating diverticulitis from cancer, which requires contrast study or preferably endoscopy and biopsy after resolution of the acute inflammation (Fig. 51.14).[231] It is superior to BE in that it can directly demonstrate extraluminal complications of the disease, such as abscess, phlegmon, free intraperitoneal air, or colovesical fistula and allows for therapeutic intervention with percutaneous drainage (Fig. 51.15). Interval contrast enema studies may be helpful in establishing the diagnosis in patients with mild disease and in ruling out adenocarcinoma of the proximal bowel when colonoscopy is incomplete. Barium should be avoided in the acute setting because of the risk of extravasation into the peritoneum, peritonitis, and vascular collapse. If an urgent contrast study must be done to evaluate for stricture or obstruction, water-soluble agents may be used.

Endoscopy is generally contraindicated in the setting of acute diverticulitis. It is hazardous and may aggravate a free perforation or convert a controlled perforation to a free perforation. Further, it is often difficult to visualize the involved segment because inflammation renders the bowel impassable, and the patient experiences pain as the lesion is approached. Limited examination with minimal or no air insufflation should be reserved for special situations when the diagnosis of diverticulitis is uncertain and other diagnoses, such as ischemic bowel, obstructing carcinoma, or colitis, are considered.

The treatment of uncomplicated diverticulitis is antibiotics effective against the gram-negative and anaerobic bacteria that make up the normal flora of the colon. Mild cases of acute diverticulitis in immunocompetent patients can be managed on an outpatient basis with clear liquids and oral antibiotics.[224] Ideal patients for outpatient management are those who are able to tolerate a diet, have no systemic symptoms or peritoneal signs, and are reliable with a reliable family. Immunocompromised patients, those on steroid therapy, and advanced age are contraindications to outpatient therapy. If outpatient therapy is elected, patients need to watch for systemic signs or progression of symptoms and should be instructed to return if these develop. Follow-up with the treating physician must occur within 48 to 72h after presentation.

Patients in whom any of the foregoing criteria are not met should be admitted to the hospital for total bowel rest, intravenous antibiotics for gram-negative organisms and anaerobes, serial exams, and further evaluation as indicated (Fig. 51.16). Conservative, nonoperative treatment of uncomplicated diverticulitis results in resolution of symptoms in 70%–100% of patients. If the patient worsens under observation or does not improve over a period of 48–72h and a CT was not done to confirm the diagnosis, a CT should be ordered to rule out the presence of an abscess (see treatment of complicated

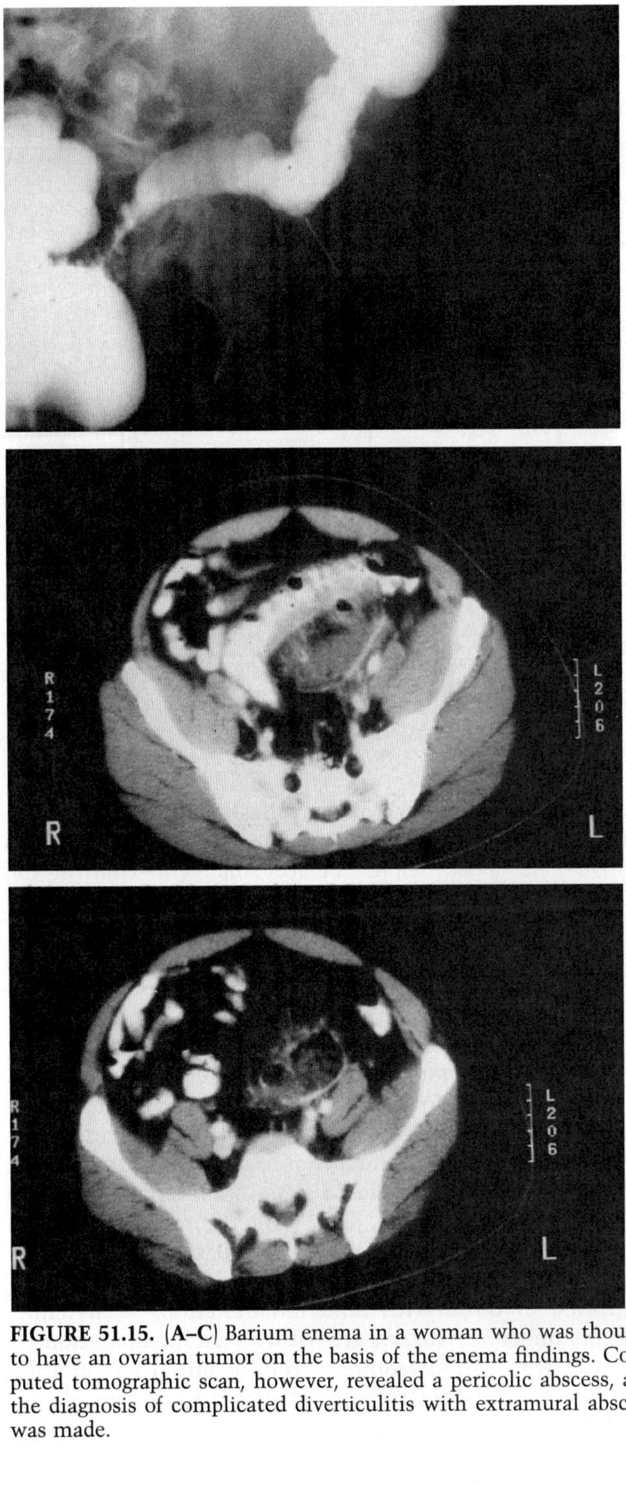

A

B

C

FIGURE 51.15. (A–C) Barium enema in a woman who was thought to have an ovarian tumor on the basis of the enema findings. Computed tomographic scan, however, revealed a pericolic abscess, and the diagnosis of complicated diverticulitis with extramural abscess was made.

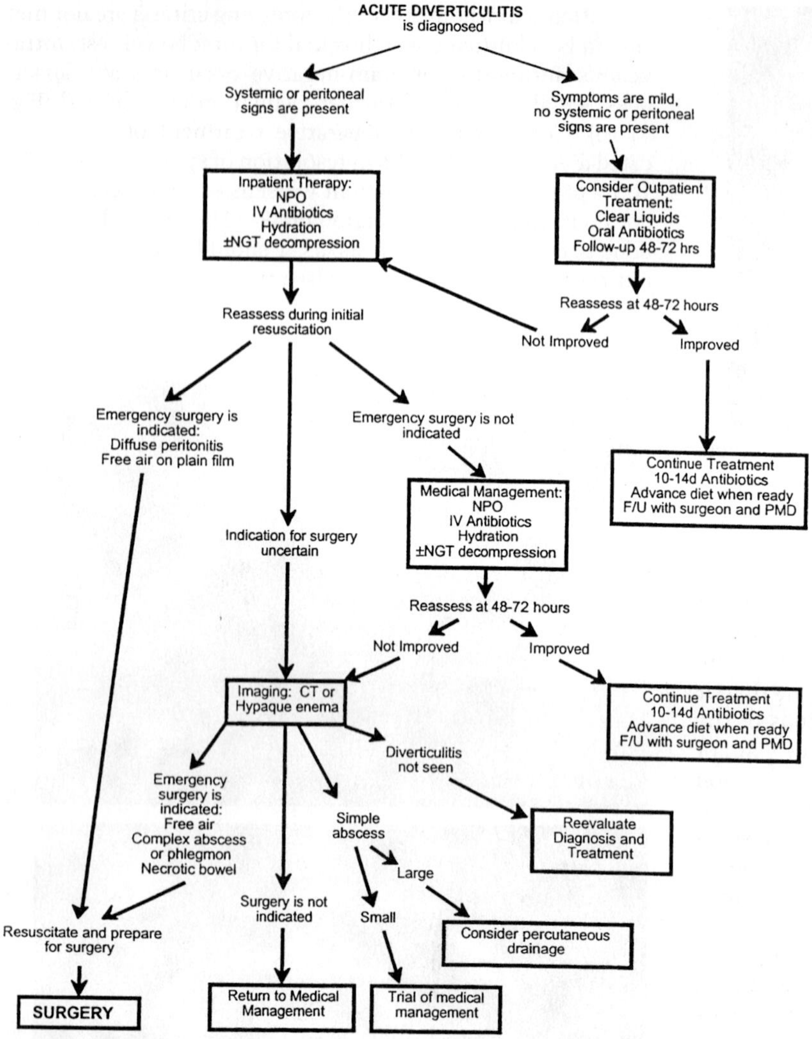

FIGURE 51.16. Algorithm for the management of acute diverticulitis.

diverticulitis). After the patient has recovered from the episode of diverticulitis and the acute inflammation has resolved, he or she should be reevaluated to confirm the initial diagnosis and rule out other colonic pathology, such as cancer or IBD. This is best done by colonoscopy although BE can also be done. Resumption of a high-fiber diet is recommended after resolution of the attack of diverticulitis and may be helpful in preventing future attacks.

It has been suggested that diverticulitis in patients under the age of 40 is more aggressive.[232] Patients present more frequently with perforation, and 77% proceed to surgery at the time of initial diagnosis. Others have noted an increased rate of recurrent attacks and therefore suggest colectomy after the first episode of diverticulitis.[233] Computerized tomography is useful in staging the disease and recommending operative versus nonoperative intervention. Patients with severe inflammation on CT have an increased rate of recurrence compared to those with mild inflammation.[234] Therefore, patients under 50 years of age with severe inflammation on CT scan who do not require surgery at initial presentation may benefit from elective surgery after the first episode has resolved.

Abscess or phlegmon, peritonitis, fistula, or bowel obstruction may complicate diverticulitis. Abscess or phlegmon is the most common complication of acute diverticulitis and may occur in the mesocolon, abdomen, pelvis, retroperitoneum, buttocks, or scrotum. A grading system for the degree of perforation has been developed by Hinchey et al. Stage I involves diverticulitis with a pericolic or mesocolic abscess; stage II, a pelvic abscess; stage III, perforation with purulent peritonitis; and stage IV, perforation with fecal peritonitis.[235] The location and size of the abscess dictate the clinical presentation and management. Small intramesenteric abscesses may resolve with conservative therapy and antibiotics alone, whereas larger intraabdominal or pelvic abscesses require further intervention.[226,236]

Patients with small abscesses contained in the mesentery may be treated with bowel rest and intravenous antibiotics and can be observed while undergoing a "gentle" bowel preparation in anticipation of a one-stage operation if nonoperative measures fail. If the patient improves, then surgical intervention may be individualized as long as there is no evidence of persistent abscess on repeat CT scan. If the patient worsens, fails to improve, or deteriorates under expectant management, then exploration is indicated. Primary anastomosis is preferred if the perforation is contained in the mesocolon and the proximal and distal bowel appear healthy.[237]

Most diverticular abscesses, whether pelvic or intra-abdominal, may be drained percutaneously by interventional radiology with CT or ultrasound guidance (Fig. 51.17).[238] Of patients with diverticular abscesses that are amenable to radiologic drainage, 70%–90% are successfully treated. The catheter should be left in place to rule out persistent communication with the colon. Most patients improve.

A pelvic abscess not amenable to CT guidance due to its location or lack of an available "window" may be drained transrectally in males or transvaginally in females. This approach has largely been replaced by CT-guided techniques, but its utility should not be underestimated. The major disadvantage to this approach is that it is performed in the operating room.

In rare cases, abscesses that cannot be drained by these techniques require abdominal exploration. In selected patients, bowel preparation may be accomplished preoperatively. The presence of an undrained abscess does not preclude primary anastomosis. In well-selected patients without significant comorbidities in whom the operation is otherwise uncomplicated and the proximal and distal margins of the bowel are healthy, a primary anastomosis may be performed (see below).

Fistulas occur as a complication of diverticulitis when an abscess spontaneously drains through an organ to which it has become adherent. The urinary bladder and vagina are the most common organs involved, with 68% of patients in one series having colovesical fistulas. Patients with diverticular fistulas are usually surprisingly well since the acute infectious process has already been drained. Presenting symptoms include pneumaturia (82%), fecaluria (43%); abdominal pain (25%); urinary symptoms such as frequency, urgency, and dysuria (23%); hematuria (21%); and fevers and chills (16%). Colovaginal fistulas account for 25% of diverticular fistulas and present with the passage of gas or stool per vagina, vaginal discharge, or recurrent bacterial vaginitis. In some cases, no antecedent history of acute diverticulitis can be obtained.

Fistulas develop in only 2% of patients with diverticulitis, but fistula is the indication for surgery in 20% of those undergoing surgery for diverticulitis and its associated complications (Fig. 51.18). Eight percent have multiple fistulas.[224] The incidence is greater in men than in women, presumably because the uterus separates the colon from the bladder, and the uterus, as a thick muscular structure, is resistant to fistula formation. Most women who develop fistulas have had a prior hysterectomy, but colouterine and colosalpingo fistulas have been reported. Colocutaneous fistulas generally develop in the postoperative setting as an anastomotic complication.[224]

A thorough preoperative evaluation, including abdominal–pelvic CT and colonoscopy to rule out colonic malignancy at the site of the fistula or in the proximal colon, is suggested. Fistulas are often hard to visualize on colonoscopy, BE, cystoscopy, or vaginogram. Triple-contrast CT is helpful and will diagnose colovesical fistulas more than 90% of the time.[224] Air in the bladder without a recent history of Foley catheterization is diagnostic of a colovesical fistula, and no further workup is necessary. Vaginal fistulas can be particularly elusive. A contrast enema with a tampon in place followed by radiographic evaluation of the tampon for contrast may document the presence of a fistula. Alternatively, a methylene blue enema with a tampon in the vagina may be performed.

Purulent or fecal peritonitis may develop secondary to rupture of a contained abscess or free perforation of a diverticulum. Most present with an acute abdomen and some degree of septic shock. Aggressive intravenous resuscitation, antibiotics, and surgery are recommended for patients who present in this fashion. The presentation in the immunosuppressed population may not be as clear, and abdominal films and a CT scan may be necessary to make the diagnosis.

Nonetheless, the treatment is the same. They are explored urgently, and a resection of the sigmoid colon is performed.[224,239] It is acceptable to drain the perforation and divert the fecal stream without a definitive resection in the rare patient who is too unstable to tolerate the procedure or when the operating team is unprepared or unable to dissect in the inflamed pelvis.[224,240] The reported mortality rates for purulent and fecal peritonitis are 6% and 35%, respectively.[224]

Diverticulitis is the cause of approximately 10% of all large-bowel obstructions.[224] The obstruction is usually partial, with complete obstruction occurring rarely. The obstruction is secondary to edema, spasm, and chronic inflammatory changes. The fibrosis from chronic inflammation will not

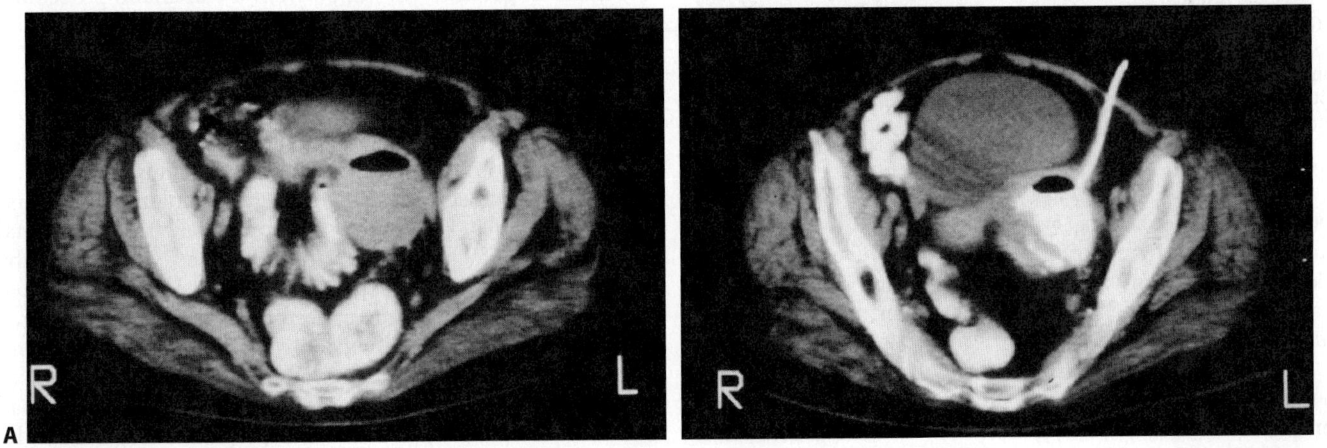

FIGURE 51.17. (A–B) Computed tomographic scan of patient pre- and postinterventional radiologic drainage of a pericolic abscess.

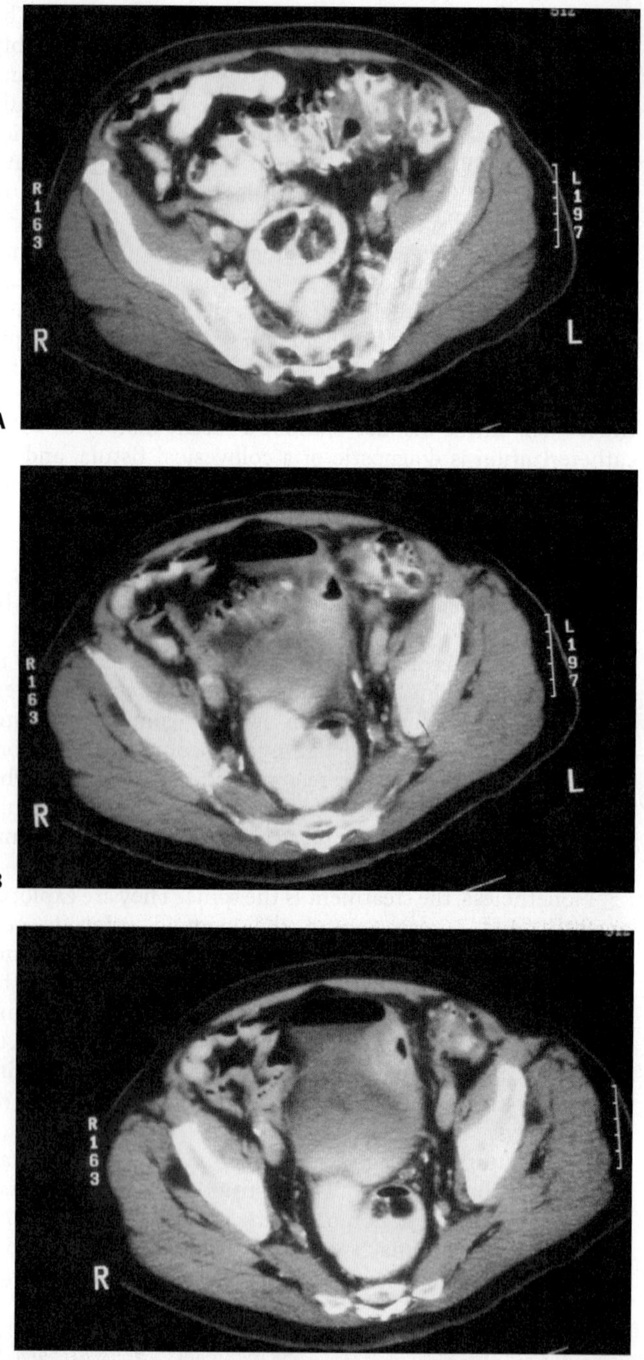

FIGURE 51.18. (A–B) Computed tomographic scan of a patient with a fistula to the bladder. Note the air collection outside the colon that can be traced down to the bladder on serial images. Air in the bladder without a history of recent catheterization is diagnostic of a communication with the gastrointestinal tract.

resolve, but the edema, spasm, and acute inflammatory changes will, allowing for elective management of this complication after a complete bowel preparation. The possibility that the obstruction is due to colon cancer must always be considered.

Indications for surgery for diverticulitis can be classified as emergent/urgent or elective. Regardless of the indication, some general principles apply. First and foremost, the entire sigmoid colon should be removed. The distal line of resection should be on normal rectum. Anatomically, the rectum is identified by its lack of the longitudinal taenae coli. When patients present with free perforation and generalized peritonitis, immediate surgical exploration is warranted. Not all diverticula-bearing colon need be removed, but all thickened, diseased bowel should be, sometimes necessitating removal of a portion of the distal descending colon.

Up to 20%–25% of patients present with free perforation, generalized peritonitis (Hinchy stage III and IV), or systemic complications requiring emergency surgery. At minimum, a sigmoid colectomy with end colostomy and oversewing of the rectal stump, the so-called Hartmann procedure, should be performed. The reported mortality rates after surgery for Hinchy stage III and IV diverticulitis are 6% and 35%, respectively.[215] A second operation to restore intestinal continuity is then required.

Although considered the standard treatment for emergent surgery for diverticulitis, the automatic need for a colostomy in this setting is being questioned in current practice for a number of reasons. The requirement for a stoma, even a temporary one, is often dreaded by the patient. In addition, reversal of a colostomy after a Hartmann procedure can be a difficult undertaking due to reoperation in previously violated tissue planes and adhesions from the prior peritoneal inflammation.

The anastomotic leak rate after Hartmann reversal has been reported to be as high as 30% (Underwood) and has a mortality between 0% and 14.3%.[241,242] Although initially constructed as a "temporary" colostomy, as many as 50%–60% of these stomas are never reversed due to age, comorbid medical problems, or a variety of other reasons and actually become permanent.[241,243]

In the setting of diverticulitis with peritonitis, a primary anastomosis can be performed with or without an on-table colonic lavage and with or without a defunctioning loop ileostomy. Although never studied in a prospective randomized trial, a recent meta-analysis of primary anastomosis versus Hartmann procedure for diverticulitis with peritonitis found no significant increase in morbidity or mortality when primary anastomosis was compared to Hartmann procedure plus colostomy takedown. Reported mortality rate was 18.8% for the Hartmann procedure, 0.8% for colostomy reversal, and 9.9% for sigmoid colectomy with a primary anastomosis. Anastomotic leaks occurred in 13.9% of patients after a primary anastomosis and in 4.3% of patients after colostomy reversal. Of patients who underwent a Hartmann procedure, 10.3% had complications directly related to their colostomy.[244]

In carefully selected, stable patients without serious medical comorbidities, a primary anastomosis can be an alternative in the setting of diverticulitis with peritonitis provided that a tension-free, well-vascularized anastomosis can be performed between soft, healthy, descending colon and rectum. In certain cases, a primary anastomosis with a proximal defunctioning loop ileostomy may be used, which has the advantage of avoiding reoperation in a previously inflamed pelvis when it comes time to restore intestinal continuity.

Most patients with diverticulitis and obstruction require urgent surgery after a brief period of nasogastric suction and intravenous hydration. In some cases, the obstruction may resolve, allowing for gentle bowel preparation and a single-stage resection with a primary anastomosis. Most patients, however, require sigmoid resection with a colostomy and closure of the rectum since the proximal bowel is frequently dilated, stool filled, and not suitable for a primary anastomosis. In carefully selected patients, the colon can be decompressed intraoperatively, an on-table colonic lavage performed, and a primary anastomosis created. The possibility that the obstruction is due to cancer rather than chronic diverticulitis should always be kept in mind.

The majority of patients with diverticulitis do not require urgent or emergent surgery and can be managed conservatively with antibiotics for uncomplicated diverticulitis or antibiotics and percutaneous CT-guided drainage for diverticulitis complicated by abscess with resolution of the acute event. Truly elective surgery for patients with successfully treated diverticulitis is done to prevent future attacks or to prevent future attacks that may be more severe and be associated with complications. Approximately one-third of patients successfully treated for uncomplicated diverticulitis will develop recurrent symptoms, usually within the first year. Fifty percent of recurrent attacks occur within the first year, and 90% occur within 5 years. A subset of patients develop chronic smoldering symptoms after an acute attack.

Often cited "indications" for elective surgery for diverticulitis are (1) two episodes of diverticulitis in a person aged 50 or older; (2) after the first attack of diverticulitis in a patient younger than 40 years old; (3) diverticulitis complicated by the development of an abscess requiring percutaneous drainage; (4) diverticulitis in immunocompromised patients. These should be viewed as guidelines and not rigid requirements that need be followed.

The decision of when and if to operate electively for diverticulitis should be individualized to the patient. Factors that should be taken into consideration should include the physiologic age of the patient, the number and severity of attacks, the rapidity and response to medical therapy, and the degree of persistent symptoms after medical treatment. The reported risk of recurrent diverticulitis after treatment of an episode of diverticulitis ranges from 7% to 45%. However, after each successive attack, patients are less likely to respond to medical therapy.

Younger patients and immunocompromised patients have been thought to be at higher risk for development of future severe complications after an episode of diverticulitis, but the literature supporting these views is contradictory; therefore, the actual risk is unclear.[245–247] Kidney transplant patients have been considered to be at increased risk because of an association between polycystic kidney disease and diverticulosis. Retrospective studies suggest that patients with an antecedent history of diverticulitis undergo a pretransplant colectomy. However, in a prospective study of transplant patients, no association between the preoperative finding of diverticulosis on sigmoidoscopy and posttransplant diverticulitis was found.[246]

Immunosuppression makes the abdominal exam less reliable, confounding the assessment and conservative management of the transplant patient. Early surgical intervention has been advised in the immunocompromised because an increase in morbidity and mortality has been associated with conservative management.[247] However, the high failure rate may be a reflection of the underassessment of disease severity secondary to immunosuppression. An aggressive approach that recognizes the limitations of the physical exam and proceeds with early CT imaging seems preferable to prophylactic colectomy or urgent laparotomy. Thus, a transplant patient with a pericolic abscess may be better treated with CT-guided drainage, bowel preparation, and primary anastomosis rather than urgent exploration and a Hartmann's procedure.

Diverticulitis is uncommon in younger patients, and it has been reported that diverticulitis in younger age groups is more virulent or follows a more aggressive course. A higher percentage of young patients with diverticulitis require urgent or emergent surgery at initial presentation (up to two-thirds in some series compared to less than one-third of older patients); however, the literature supporting a higher risk of future complications or more severe future attacks after successful medical management in young patients is unclear, with recent studies not finding this to be true.[248–250]

Diverticulitis complicated by abscess is a generally accepted indication for elective sigmoid colectomy after successful percutaneous drainage and treatment with antibiotics due to the severity of the initial attack. It is helpful to wait a period of 6 to 8 weeks after resolution of the abscess to allow the acute inflammation to resolve and to make surgery easier. Some surgeons have questioned whether surgery is necessary after every case of diverticulitis complicated by abscess. Although there is not enough evidence to universally support this, a study showed that up to half of patients with diverticular abscesses successfully treated nonoperatively do well without surgery. Patients with pelvic abscesses were more likely to eventually require surgery than those with mesocolic abscesses.[251]

Most patients with diverticular fistulas are symptomatic from the fistula and should be offered elective resection. Patients with colovesical fistulas can have symptoms of pneumaturia and fecaluria and are prone to recurrent urinary tract infections. Women with colovaginal fistulas note vaginal discharge and passage of gas or stool from the rectum. Patients are often minimally symptomatic from the diverticulitis itself, giving the surgeon time for a full preoperative evaluation prior to elective surgery. The possibility of a malignancy causing the fistula should be kept in mind since the operative approach for benign and malignant fistulas is different, with a malignant fistula requiring an en bloc resection of the secondarily affected organ.

Elective surgery for diverticulitis involves resection of the diseased sigmoid colon to normal, soft, healthy rectum distally and normal, soft, healthy descending colon proximally. "Recurrent" diverticulitis occurring after sigmoid colectomy is most often due to the distal margin of transection being at the level of the distal sigmoid colon rather than on the rectum.[252] Not infrequently, there is marked inflammation and fibrosis of the sigmoid colon and retroperitoneum, obliterating normal tissue planes and identification of vital retroperitoneal structures such as the ureter. If this is suspected preoperatively, cystoscopy and placement of bilateral ureteral catheters can aid identification of the ureters by palpation when dissection and direct visualization are difficult. It can be useful to begin mobilization of the bowel proximally where the planes are generally uninflamed and the ureters and gonadal vessels can be identified. The proximal bowel margin of resection must be uninflamed but need not be free of diverticula. In contrast, the distal margin must be free of both diverticula and inflammation because recurrent diverticulitis develops in the distal sigmoid colon.[252] Dissection onto the proximal third of the rectum is generally necessary to expose soft and pliable bowel distally. A phlegmon, abscess, or fistula is best approached with a combination of blunt, sharp, and circumferential dissection. It may be helpful to transect the proximal bowel early as this allows entry into a normal plane posteriorly. Once the bowel has been resected, fistulous communications to the bladder and vagina may be repaired, although this is not required for small cystotomies or vaginotomies. It is frequently necessary to fully mobilize the splenic flexure to provide a well-vascularized, tension-free anastomosis between the descending colon and rectum.

Infectious Colitides

Infections of the large bowel usually cause diarrhea and can produce fever or abdominal pain. Infectious colitis must be differentiated from other etiologies of colitis. It is critical to elicit a complete history from the patient, including recent travel, unusual ingestions suspect for food poisoning, similar illnesses among family members, recent hospitalizations, and treatment with antibiotics, sexual history, immunosuppression, and evidence of systemic disease. The pertinent positives of the history will help tailor the diagnostic workup. Patients often have physical signs of dehydration, such as decreased skin turgor, dry mucous membranes, tachycardia, or hypotension. In addition, the abdominal exam may reveal tenderness or local peritoneal signs. A rectal exam is done to check for blood and tenderness.

The diagnostic workup includes testing for fecal leukocytes and *Clostridium difficile* toxin and stool cultures for bacteria, ova, and parasites. Endoscopic evaluation may be useful in patients who require biopsy for diagnosis. It is important not to give enemas before testing or to use lubricants.[253] Occasionally, radiographic imaging is necessary to assess the degree of colonic involvement and to look for evidence of necrosis or perforation (Fig. 51.19). Once the source of colitis is found, the treatment depends on the severity of the patient's illness and the need for supportive care and antibiotics. Certain infections can result in fulminant colitis that is refractory to medical treatment and requires surgery.

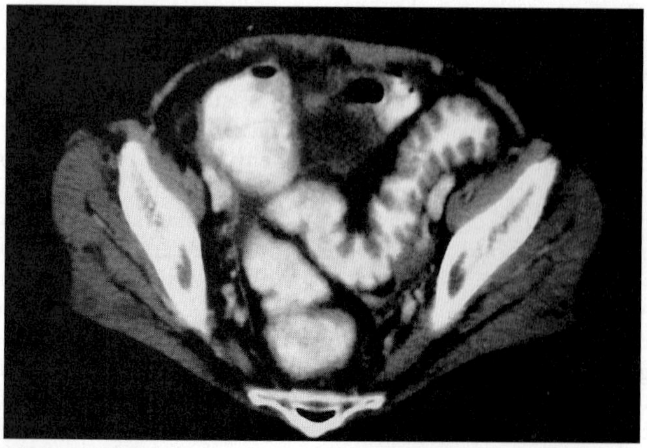

FIGURE 51.19. Computed tomographic scan demonstrating edema of the distal bowel from pseudomembranous colitis.

Bacterial Colitides

Clostridium Difficile

Most diarrhea that develops during antibiotic administration is not *C. difficile* colitis but rather is due to a change in the bacterial flora of the colon. This results in an osmotic diarrhea due an accumulation of complex carbohydrates, which are broken down by the normal colonic flora into short-chain fatty acids. This resolves spontaneously after cessation of therapy. However, a minority of patients on antibiotics will have a proliferation[254] of the toxin-producing strains of *C. difficile*, a gram-positive, anaerobic organism. The toxins produce mucosal damage and inflammation. *Clostridium difficile* exists within the GI tract in 3% to 5% of adults, 10% of hospitalized patients, and more than 50% of newborns.[255] However, children rarely develop *C. difficile* colitis. It most commonly occurs in elderly and debilitated patients and can even happen without antibiotic use. Although clindamycin was considered to be the primary culprit in producing this disease,[256,257] it is now known that any antibiotic can produce this colitis.

Humans transmit the organism in hospitals and nursing homes. The heat-resistant spores can persist in the environment for months and are transferred via an oral–fecal route. Careful hand washing is critical to preventing outbreaks because health care workers are the most common vectors of outbreaks. *Clostridium difficile* colitis is now one of the most common hospital-acquired infections.[255] Use of oral antibiotics during preoperative bowel preparation has been shown to increase the incidence of postoperative *C. difficile* colitis by nearly threefold (from 2.6% to 7.4%).[258]

Patients present with watery diarrhea, fever, and leukocytosis. Abdominal pain and tenderness are also common. Some patients develop toxic megacolon. Symptoms can occur both during antibiotic administration and weeks to months after cessation of treatment.

The gold standard test for *C. difficile* colitis is the cytotoxic assay. This has a sensitivity of 94%–100% and a specificity of 99%. However, the test can take several days to complete. The most commonly performed test is an enzyme-linked immunosorbant assay (ELISA) to toxin A produced by the *C. difficile* bacterium. This test has a sensitivity of 70%–90% and a specificity of 99% and can be rapidly done in a matter of hours. The false positives are due to the fact that some strains of *C. difficile* produce primarily toxin B or a mutant strain of toxin A.[255] If confirmation is needed, this tissue culture assay can be done using biopsies from a sigmoidoscopic or colonoscopic exam. The toxin binding to the bowel wall affects the mucosa. On endoscopic exam, the mucosa can look inflamed or develop plaque-like membranes, which is why it has been called "pseudomembranous" colitis (Fig. 51.20). These lesions can be diffuse or segmental, and if more proximal in the GI tract will be missed by sigmoidoscopy.[259] Fecal leukocytes, although not specific for *C. difficile* colitis, are present about 50% of the time. On CT scan, the colon wall is usually diffusely thickened.

The mainstay of therapy involves cessation of the antibiotics previously administered if the patient is still under treatment. In addition, oral vancomycin and metronidazole are very effective against *C. difficile*. Metronidazole (250 mg, four times a day) given for 10 days is the first line of therapy

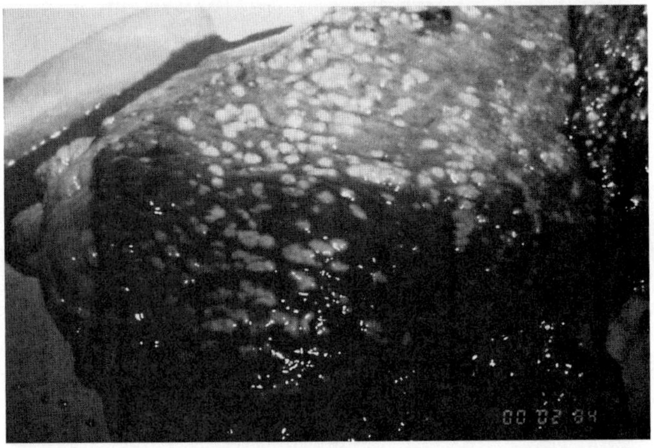

FIGURE 51.20. Colonic specimen with the yellow-white "plaque-like" membranes that led to the name pseudomembranous colitis.

because it is less expensive, and resistant organisms (such as vancomycin-resistant enterococcus) have not yet been described. Vancomycin (125 mg, four times a day) or even bacitracin (25,000 U, four times a day) can be administered if patients fail treatment with metronidazole. For those patients unable to tolerate an oral dose because of abdominal surgery or ileus, intravenous metronidazole is effective, with bactericidal levels of the drug in the stool. Vancomycin is only effective if delivered orally.[259,260]

Many patients have a relapse (10%–20%)[260,261] due to persistent infection as opposed to reinfection. The most common therapy in this situation is a tapering vancomycin dose,[261] which can be alternated with cholestyramine. Other treatments have attempted to reestablish normal bacterial flora with fecal and bacterial enemas.[262] Yogurt and yeast (*Saccharomyces boulardii*)[262] enemas have been tried with variable success.

Antidiarrheal agents should be avoided. Cholestyramine and colestipol are anion-exchange binding resins that can bind toxin but will also bind antibiotic. Therefore, they are generally effective for patients with mild colitis only. Patients who develop toxic megacolon may require emergent surgical therapy. The procedure of choice in this setting is a total abdominal colectomy with an end ileostomy, although use of segmental colectomy has been reported.[263,264] The mortality with emergent surgery is reported to be about 24% to 43%.[264]

Bacterial Colitis

Patients with bacterial colitis develop these infections from a fecal–oral route. Most patients have self-limiting infections and require only supportive care and rehydration. However, a minority of these patients develop toxic megacolon, bleeding, or perforation that requires surgery, with an associated high morbidity and mortality.

Shigella

Shigella is an invasive infection that is common in patients who have been traveling. The organism elaborates *Shigella* toxin, an enterotoxin that allows the bacteria to invade the bowel wall. Patients develop anorexia, cramping abdominal pain, fever, tenesmus, and multiple small bloody stools.[253] Typically, patients have 8–10 mucoid bloody bowel movement per day, but the frequency may be up to 100 per day. The severity of disease depends on the invading organism. The disease is self-limiting, lasting about 7 days.

Shigella has been associated with arthritis, hemolytic-uremic syndrome (HUS), and respiratory and neurological symptoms. Detecting fecal leukocytes suggests the diagnosis that is confirmed with stool cultures. Sigmoidoscopy shows nonspecific colitis. Rehydration is the mainstay of treatment, and in severe cases, ampicillin or trimethoprim-sulfamethoxazole can be given orally.

Campylobacter Jejuni

Campylobacter jejuni is one of the most common acute bacterial infections of the GI tract, transmitted by food products from infected animals. This organism also produces toxin that invades the colonic mucosa. The incubation period is approximately 2 to 5 days. Patients develop fever, myalgias, headaches, diarrhea, and colicky abdominal pain. Many patients are misdiagnosed with appendicitis.[265] The diagnosis can be made by stool culture. Endoscopic exam reveals inflammation and ulceration of the mucosa.

The disease is self-limited and treatment consists of supportive care with rehydration. If more aggressive treatment is required, erythromycin is the drug of choice.

Salmonella Enteritis

Nontyphoidal salmonellosis is the most common cause of bacterial food poisoning, most commonly through contaminated eggs, milk, and poultry. Other causes include *Staphylococcus aureus*, *Bacillus cereus*, and *Clostridium perfringens*. The organism is transmitted in contaminated food. Salmonella attacks the terminal ileum and to a lesser extent the colon. It invades bowel mucosa and proliferates in the lamina propria, causing fever, diarrhea, and even systemic illness. The incubation period is about 24 h. Patients develop headache, nausea, vomiting, cramping abdominal pain, and large-volume watery diarrhea that can last about 48 h.

The diagnosis is confirmed by stool culture, and on endoscopy the mucosa looks edematous and hyperemic. No treatment is necessary for the milder version of the disease. However, if symptoms are severe, ciprofloxacin or chloramphenicol can be used. Antidiarrheal agents should be avoided.

Escherichia Coli

Escherichia coli is a prominent component of the normal intestinal flora, and most strains are harmless. However, others are a significant cause of diarrhea. At least five different pathogenic strains have been identified, including enterotoxigenic *E. coli*, enteropathogenic *E. coli*, enterohemorrhagic *E. coli*, enteroinvasive *E. coli*, and enteroaggregative *E. coli*. *Escherichia coli* is the most common cause of travelers' diarrhea.

The organism elaborates enterotoxin and adheres to mucosa of the colon. Most strains cause watery diarrhea, nausea, and cramping abdominal pain. However, certain strains (enterohemorrhagic) of *E. coli* can cause severe hemorrhagic colitis. The incubation period is about 7 days. Ten percent of patients also develop HUS, most commonly after infection with *E. coli* O157:H7. Although the organism does not invade the bowel wall, it causes endothelial damage, microangiopathic hemolysis, and renal disease.[253] Patients develop diarrhea that progresses from watery, large-volume to grossly bloody stools. Cramping abdominal pain, nausea, and vomiting are common. Some patients have localized peritoneal signs.

The diagnosis is made from stool cultures and, if necessary, tests to confirm HUS. Endoscopic examination shows microulcerations, edema, and friable mucosa, but the biopsies are nonspecific. The treatment is supportive, with oral hydration using glucose-linked sodium absorption of water and electrolytes. Treatment with ciprofloxacin reduces the duration of diarrhea with enteroaggregative *E. coli*, but antibiotic treatment increases the risk of HUS so is contraindicated for the treatment of enterohemorrhagic *E. coli*. Rarely, some patients may develop toxic megacolon that requires surgical intervention.

Protozoal Colitides

Entamoeba Histolytica

Entamoeba histolytica is a water-borne organism that is transmitted by contaminated food or water. Its cysts are ingested, and the trophozoites released in the small intestine migrate to the colon, where they live in the lumen or bowel wall. They cause damage to the colonic mucosa. Many patients are asymptomatic, but the classic presentation includes chronic intermittent diarrhea, abdominal pain, weight loss, and flatulence. Very rarely, patients have a fulminant colitis that requires surgery.

Examination of the stool and identification of cysts or trophozoites confirms the diagnosis. Sigmoidoscopy will reveal mucosal thickening or flask-shaped ulcers[266] that are difficult to distinguish from UC. Patients can also be diagnosed with amebiasis by serological tests. The indirect hemagglutination test is the most sensitive. Metronidazole is the treatment of choice.

Giardia

Giardia comes from contaminated drinking water and is common in the western United States and eastern Europe. Beavers are the animal source that contaminates the water. The organism is also commonly found in daycare centers. Patients present with frequent diarrhea, mucus, steatorrhea, bloating, weight loss, and fatigue. Checking the stool for ova and parasites provides the diagnosis. As the diagnosis is sometimes difficult to make, patients are treated with metronidazole empirically when the disease is suspected.

Cryptosporidium Parvum

Cryptosporidiosis is a common cause of diarrhea in immunosuppressed patients and health care workers. Trophozoites attach firmly to the mucosa, causing an inflammatory cell infiltrate in the lamina propria. Patients present with fever, abdominal pain, and watery diarrhea. Colonic biopsy or acid-fast staining of the stool will reveal oocysts. The disease is self-limiting, lasting about 2 weeks. The treatment is supportive with rehydration. No medication is known to be effective.

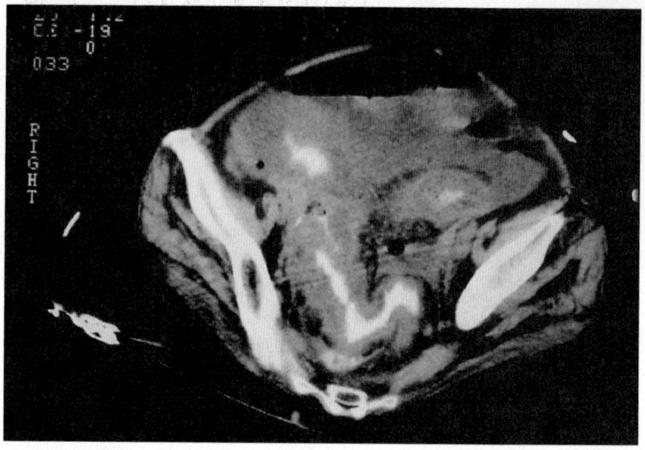

FIGURE 51.21. Cytomegalovirus (CMV) colitis with severe inflammation of the entire colon.

Viral Colitides

Cytomegalovirus

Immunocompromised patients frequently develop CMV infections (Fig. 51.21). Patients present with fever, abdominal pain, and weight loss. The stools are usually watery, but they can also be bloody. The presentation is commonly mistaken for appendicitis in the immunocompromised population. Diagnosis is made by tissue biopsy showing intranuclear viral inclusions. It is important to take biopsies from normal-appearing mucosa as the inclusion bodies are often detected in normal tissue. Endoscopically, the mucosa can show signs of diffuse colitis with ulcerations or hemorrhage. Treatment includes supportive care and the use of antiviral agents such as ganciclovir (DHPG) or foscarnet.

Herpes Simplex Virus

Herpes simplex virus (HSV) causes similar symptoms as CMV in this population. Patients are treated with acyclovir and require the same supportive care.

Ischemic Colitis

Ischemic colitis is the most common form of intestinal ischemia. It is thought to affect "watershed" areas of the colon where two blood supplies may incompletely overlap, that is, the splenic flexure supplied by the left branch of the middle colic (SMA origin) and the ascending left colic (IMA origin). It may result from vascular occlusion or a low-flow state. The severity of injury appears to be related to multiple factors, including duration of ischemia, vessel caliber, acuity of ischemia onset, collateral circulation, and virulence of intestinal bacteria. Of the cases of ischemic colitis, 70% affect the left colon.

Patients are often elderly, debilitated patients in the intensive care unit with multiple medical problems in which an inciting event is difficult to determine, although it has also been described in otherwise healthy patients after vigorous exercise and the use of drugs such as oral contraceptives, cyclooxygenase-2 (COX-2) inhibitors, and drugs used to treat irritable bowel syndrome.[267–270] The onset may be insidious, not recognized, or attributed to the medical comorbidities. The outcome depends as much on the reversibility of these comorbidities as it does on factors such as severity of disease and rapidity of disease onset.

Symptoms of ischemic colitis include abdominal pain, diarrhea, alteration in bowel function, and hematochezia.[271] Some have found that diarrhea and hematochezia are less common in patients with gangrenous colitis compared to those with milder forms of ischemic colitis. Physical exam may reveal abdominal distension and tenderness, particularly over the involved segment. In the gangrenous form, an abdominal catastrophe may be apparent, with septic shock and diffuse peritoneal signs (Table 51.7).[272]

TABLE 51.7. Etiological Factors for Colonic Ischemia.

- Idiopathic (spontaneous)
- Major vascular occlusion
  - Trauma
    - Thrombosis, embolization of mesenteric arteries
    - Arterial embolus
    - Cholesterol embolus
    - Aortography
    - Colectomy with inferior mesenteric artery ligation
    - Midgut ischemia
    - Postabdominal aortic reconstruction
  - Mesenteric venous thrombosis
  - Hypercoagulable states
    - Portal hypertension
    - Pancreatitis
- Small vessel disease
  - Diabetes mellitus
  - Rheumatoid arthritis
  - Amyloidosis
  - Radiation injury
  - Systemic vasculitis disorders
    - Systemic lupus erythematosus
    - Polyarteritis nodosa
    - Allergic granulomatosis
    - Scleroderma
    - Behçet's syndrome
    - Takayasu's arteritis
    - Thromboangiitis obliterans
    - Buerger's disease
- Shock
  - Cardiac failure
  - Hypovolemia
  - Sepsis
  - Neurogenic insult
  - Anaphylaxis
- Medications
  - Digitalis preparations
  - Diuretics
  - Catecholamines
  - Estrogens
  - Danazol
  - Gold
  - Nonsteroidal antiinflammatory drugs
  - Neuroleptics
- Colonic obstruction
  - Colon carcinoma
  - Adhesions
  - Stricture
  - Diverticular disease
  - Rectal prolapse
  - Fecal impaction
  - Volvulus
  - Strangulated hernia
  - Pseudoobstruction
- Hematologic disorders
  - Sickle-cell disease
  - Protein C deficiency
  - Protein S deficiency
  - Antithrombin III deficiency
- Cocaine abuse
- Long-distance running

Source: From Gandhi et al.,[272] with permission.

Ischemic colitis covers a wide clinical spectrum, from very mild to severe disease. It is classified by the degree of colonic injury.[273] It presents with two clinical patterns: gangrenous ischemic colitic, accounting for 15%–20% of cases, and nongangrenous colitis, accounting for 80%–85% of cases. In the nongangrenous cases, late complications of persistent colitis and stricture will develop in 20% and 10%, respectively.[272] In the transient form, the injury is localized primarily to the mucosa and submucosa. Superficial sloughing of the mucosa, submucosal hemorrhage, and edema generally resolve within 1 to 2 weeks without permanent sequelae. An ischemic stricture may develop if the injury extends beyond the submucosa into the muscular layers, and healing with fibrosis results in compromise of the lumen. Gangrenous ischemic colitis represents a full-thickness injury to the bowel wall and represents a surgical emergency. On initial presentation, these two subgroups cannot be distinguished unless the patient presents in extremis, in which case gangrene would be clearly suspected.

The workup of patients with suspected ischemic colitis should be focused on resuscitation and correction of the underlying medical conditions. Plain films of the abdomen may reveal the classic findings of "thumbprinting" of the bowel wall caused by the submucosal hemorrhages. Free air, pneumatosis, or portal venous gases all suggest gangrenous bowel and mandate emergent exploration. Computed tomographic scans may reveal nonspecific findings, such as thickening of the colon, but may also demonstrate associated occlusion of the IMA and unsuspected vascular disease.[274] Most abnormal laboratory values are nonspecific and occur late after the patient has declared clinically. Colonoscopy is the preferred diagnostic test. It should be done early and repeated if necessary to establish resolution or progression of disease.[272,275,276] Late changes suggestive of ischemic colitis are seen on BE as long, smooth narrowing with proximal dilation (Fig. 51.22). Similar late changes may be seen colonoscopically, by which granularity of the mucosa, loss of haustra, and stricture formation may be directly visualized.

The distribution of disease is classically thought to be at the "watershed" area, most specifically at the splenic flexure, where the marginal artery may be discontinuous.[277] This is known as *Griffith's point*. The marginal artery can be tenuous in this area and has been reported to be absent in 5% of people.[278] It has also been found that there is a 1.2- to 2.4-cm area at the splenic flexure that can be devoid of vasa recta, thereby predisposing the area to ischemia.[279] There is another watershed area at the junction of the rectum and sigmoid colon, Sudek's point, where the lowermost sigmoidal vessel usually communicates with the superior rectal artery, making this area prone to ischemia as well. However, reports in the literature do not uniformly support this belief. In one series of 1024 patients, the colonic distribution was right 8%, transverse 15%, splenic flexure 23%, descending 27%, and sigmoid 23%.[280] This classical distribution was found by others as well.[281,282] However, others have not found right-sided sparing in support of the watershed hypothesis and in fact have found

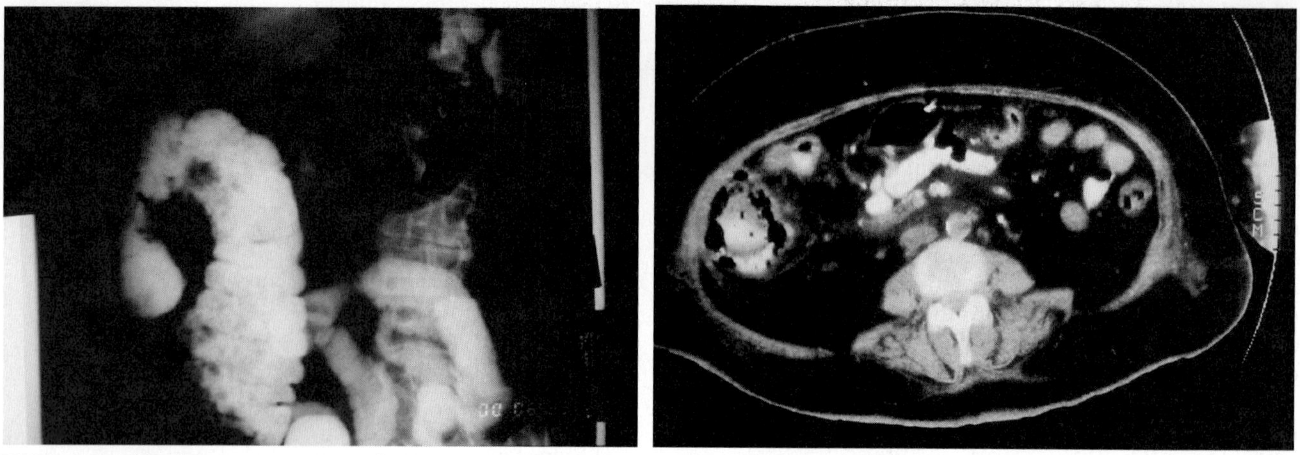

A B

FIGURE 51.22. (A–B) Barium enema and CT scan appearance of ischemic colitis. Note the long, narrow descending colon and proximal normal-appearing or somewhat dilated bowel seen on the barium enema. The CT scan demonstrates the clearly thickened ischemic section and thin-walled normal proximal transverse colon.

a predominance of disease in the well-vascularized right colon: right, 46%, splenic flexure, 4%, descending, 7%, rectosigmoid, 40%, and pancolitis, 8%.[275,280,283]

The differential diagnosis includes vascular catastrophes involving the remainder of the GI tract, bowel obstruction or perforation, peptic ulcer disease, volvulus, infectious colitis, pseudomembranous colitis, diverticulitis, and IBD.

The initial management of ischemic colitis is bowel rest, intravenous hydration, and intravenous antibiotics. Underlying medical conditions must be optimized and confounding medications discontinued when possible. Serial exams are mandatory. As noted above, most ischemic colitis resolves without long-term sequelae. Patients resume a diet when their pain, abdominal tenderness, and ileus resolve.

If the patient presents with an acute abdomen, worsens or fails to improve on maximal medical therapy, or develops refractory hemorrhage, surgery is indicated. At surgery, wide resection of all nonviable bowel should be carried out. Viability may be determined by antimesenteric continuous-wave Doppler, intravenous fluorescein, or intraoperative colonoscopy. An anastomosis is created or a stoma and mucous fistula or oversewing of the distal stump is performed.[284] A[285] second-look operation at 24 to 48 h may be indicated if there is concern for ongoing ischemia. Late stricture formation, if symptomatic, is an indication for segmental colectomy.

The prognosis for ischemic colitis is dependent on the medical comorbidities.[275,283] Overall, roughly 90% of the patients recover, and fewer than 5% progress to bowel infarction. However, with disease that mandates surgery, mortality is significantly increased and ranges from 29% to 88%.[275,283,286,287]

Volvulus

Intestinal volvulus is a closed-loop obstruction of the bowel resulting from an axial twist of the intestine on its mesentery of at least 180°; this results in luminal obstruction and progressive strangulation of the blood supply. Although it is rare in North America, the early diagnosis and treatment of volvulus is important to avoid intestinal ischemia or gangrene, which can lead to a high morbidity and mortality.

The incidence of colonic volvulus varies based on geographic and epidemiological factors. In other parts of the world, sigmoid volvulus causes up to 50% to 85% of all bowel obstructions. In the United States, however, it is responsible for only 5% of all intestinal obstructions and 10% of colonic obstructions. Sigmoid volvulus is the most common site (61%), followed by cecum/right colon (34%) and transverse colon (4%).[285]

The sigmoid colon is more predisposed to twisting when it is a long and floppy loop with a narrow mesenteric base, which can be congenital or the result of previous abdominal operations. When the colon becomes distended with air, the loop elongates and generally rotates in a counterclockwise direction. Intestinal volvulus has been associated with conditions that may result in a chronically dilated or elongated colon. Previous abdominal surgery, coarse high-fiber diets, chronic constipation, Parkinson's disease, neurological disorders, Hirschsprung's disease, diabetes, infectious and ischemic colitis, and pregnancy have all been implicated.[284,288–290] In a review of 16 series, advanced age, male gender, race (African American), and institutionalization predisposed patients to sigmoid volvulus.

Patients with sigmoid volvulus usually present with the triad of abdominal pain, distension, and obstipation. On questioning, one will often elicit a history of previous attacks. On exam, the abdomen will be dramatically distended, with high-pitched bowel sounds and tympany to percussion. The distension may be more prominent in the upper abdomen or significantly greater on one side. Minimal tenderness may be elicited in spite of this presentation. Patients with gangrene may present with a more fulminating picture of systemic illness and an acute abdomen. Younger patients often present in this fashion and are frequently diagnosed at exploratory laparotomy.[291] Interestingly, no correlation has been found with the length of history and the presence of gangrene or mortality. An algorithm for the workup of volvulus is given in Figure 51.23.

The diagnosis can be confirmed with a radiograph of the abdomen, which will show an extremely dilated sigmoid colon shaped as a "bent inner tube," with the apex extending up to the right upper quadrant (Fig. 51.24). The ends of the loop sit in the pelvis or left lower quadrant.[285] There can be

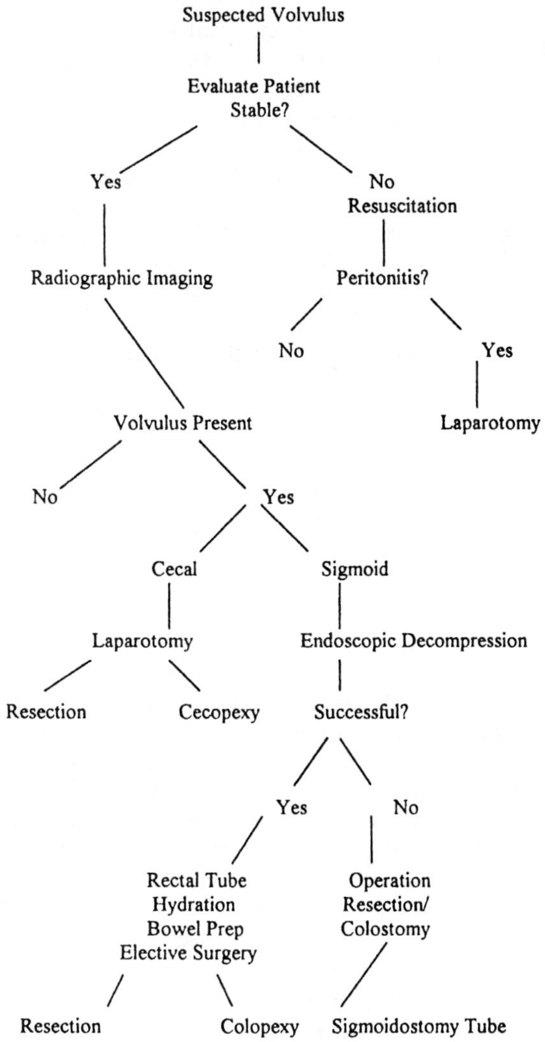

FIGURE 51.23. Algorithm for the workup of volvulus.

an air–fluid level in the two sides of the loop at different levels ("pair of scales"). Gastrografin enema will show a "bird's beak" or "ace of spades" at the point of the twist (Fig. 51.25). When the plain films or enema are nondiagnostic (30%–40%), CT scan can also be used; this will show a dilated sigmoid loop around a "whirl sign," mesenteric fat with engorged vessels converging toward the center (Fig. 51.26).[292]

The goals of treatment are to untwist and decompress the bowel before strangulation and to prevent recurrences. Those patients admitted with signs of sepsis indicative of gangrenous bowel must be aggressively resuscitated and taken emergently to the operating room. These patients will require resection of the gangrenous colonic segment with a primary anastomosis or colostomy and Hartman's pouch. If the bowel in question is simply ischemic, the bowel should be untwisted and observed. Doppler or Wood's lamp can further evaluate viability. The colon can be left untwisted, resected, or anchored in place. The mortality in patients with gangrenous bowel ranges from 40% to 80%.

When patients do not show signs of intestinal strangulation, the initial treatment of choice is endoscopic decompression; this allows the volvulus to reduce so that surgical treatment can be performed electively, after a full mechanical

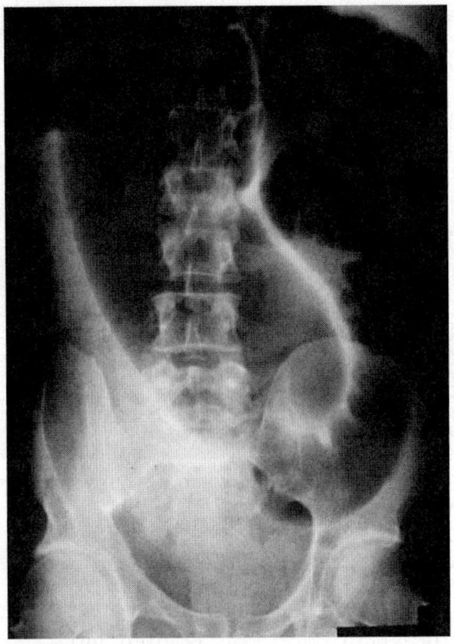

FIGURE 51.24. Classic sigmoid volvulus. Note that pelvis of kidney bean-shaped volvulus points to origin of volvulus.

bowel preparation, with lower morbidity and mortality. Rigid sigmoidoscopy can reduce and decompress the bowel, evaluate the rectal and colonic mucosa, and allow for the passage of a rectal tube to keep the bowel decompressed. However, the point of torsion may not be within reach of the rigid sigmoidoscope, and a flexible sigmoidoscope or colonoscope may be required. Generally, when the rectal tube or endoscope is passed through the twist, a rush of gas or stool will occur. The rectal tube should then be left in place for at least 48h. Endoscopic decompression is successful about 85% of the time.[290,293–296] If the patient cannot be reduced endoscopically, strangulation should be suspected and emergent laparotomy performed.

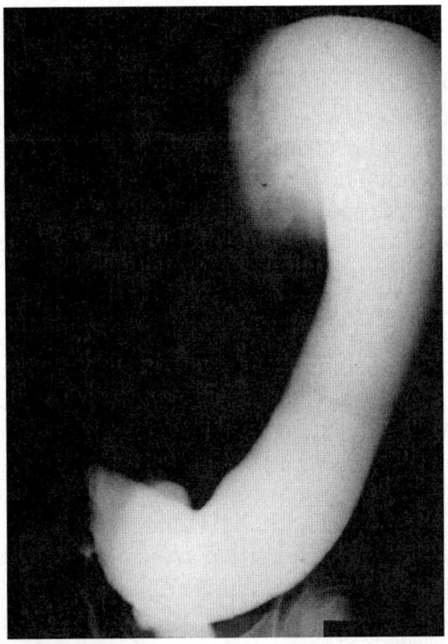

FIGURE 51.25. Barium enema with "bird's beak" deformity at site of volvulus.

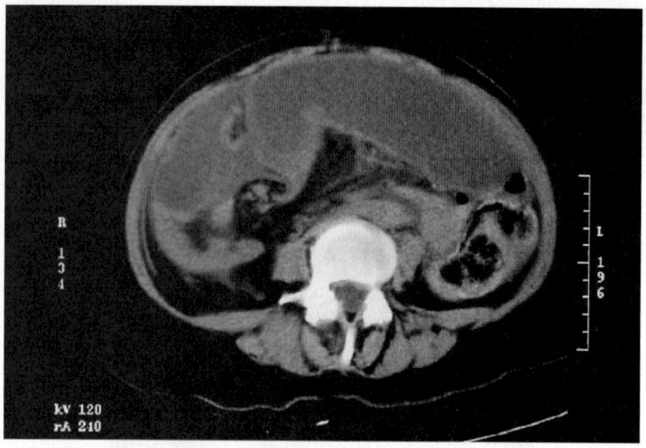

FIGURE 51.26. Computed tomographic scan with typical "whirl sign" of volvulus.

Although the mortality from this mode of therapy is low (5%–8%), the recurrence rate is high (40%–70%).[290,296–298] Therefore, once the patient is decompressed and can undergo a bowel prep, the most effective treatment is sigmoid resection; this results in a recurrence rate of less than 1% and a mortality of only 3%.[290] Much of the mortality for both endoscopic decompression and elective sigmoid resection can be ascribed to significant patient comorbidities. Other procedures that have been advocated for those too ill to undergo a sigmoid resection include colopexy, mesosigmoidoplasty, and sigmoidostomy tube placement. However, these procedures have higher recurrence rates.[288]

Cecal volvulus is the second most common type of volvulus, although it is the cause of only 1% of all intestinal obstructions. Most patients are younger, and there is a predominance of women. Anatomical considerations include incomplete peritoneal fixation of the cecum to the lateral abdominal wall that occurs normally in up to 25% of people. Other associations are similar to those that produce sigmoid volvulus. However, an important consideration that does not occur with sigmoid volvulus is distal obstruction resulting in proximal distension, which can occur in up to 50% of cases.[299]

Two types of volvulus can occur: an ileocolic twisting, generally in a clockwise direction, or a *cecal bascule*, which is an anterior and superior folding of the cecum over the ascending colon. The latter is much less common, occurring 10% of the time. Most patients present with symptoms of a small-bowel obstruction: nausea, vomiting, cramping abdominal pain, and distension. Abdominal plain films will show a markedly dilated cecum (coffee bean); it can be anywhere in the abdomen, but the "pelvis of the bean" will point to the colon segment of origin. Thus, for a cecal volvulus, a large, air-filled coffee bean will occupy the abdomen, and the pelvis of the bean will be facing the right lower quadrant. Gastrografin study can reveal a bird's beak, and CT may show a whirl sign.

These patients cannot be reduced endoscopically and require operation for definitive treatment. If the bowel is gangrenous, right hemicolectomy with ileostomy is the standard treatment. The mortality of this procedure ranges from 22% to 40%.[300,301] However, if no perforation is present and the patient is hemodynamically stable, then an ileocolectomy and primary anastomosis may be safely performed.[300–302] Reduction of the volvulus alone results in a high recurrence rate, 20%.[303] For those patients with viable bowel, the primary forms of treatment are resection, cecopexy, and cecostomy tube placement. The last has been abandoned because of the high complication and recurrence rate. Resection carries a higher morbidity and mortality, 0% to 22%,[300–302] than cecopexy. However, cecopexy has been shown to have a higher recurrence rate, 5% to 28%.[301,304,305] Recent studies have shown that patients undergoing more extensive fixation of the right colon have recurrence rates of less than 5%, and this has become the procedure of choice.

Volvulus of the transverse colon and splenic flexure do occur, although rarely. Generally, the fixation of the transverse colon by the hepatic and splenic flexure and the relatively short mesocolon keep it in place. Anatomical and acquired conditions can predispose patients to this problem. Patients present with symptoms similar to a small-bowel obstruction. These cases are generally treated by endoscopic decompression, followed by resection or colopexy.[306–309]

Colonic Inertia

Colonic inertia and obstructed defecation (discussed later) may lead to complaints of constipation. Constipation is a very common condition, and most patients with complaints of infrequent or difficult bowel movements do not require extensive workup after colorectal malignancy has been ruled out with either colonoscopy or BE and sigmoidoscopy. A thorough history often uncovers a change in diet, medication, or physical activity that is easily corrected. It will also establish the patient's definition of constipation.[310]

Patients and physicians alike often confuse constipation with straining at stool or firm bowel movements. Constipation is defined as two bowel movements per week or fewer than three per week in women or five per week in men while on a high-fiber diet (30 g dietary fiber/day). The nature of the complaint (infrequent bowel movements, firm bowel movements, or straining at stool) determines the tests required to establish the diagnosis.

The timing of onset of constipation and remedial methods used to correct the disorder are helpful as well. Patients who have suffered from constipation since early childhood may have congenital aganglionosis (Hirschsprung's disease), whereas those with later onset may have acquired a functional or mechanical obstruction. Prolonged or repeated straining at stool without result or sense of incomplete evacuation or digital anal–perianal maneuvers suggest a defecation disorder (discussed later under pelvic floor dysfunction).

There are many causes of constipation, including dietary factors, daily routine, structural and functional disorders, iatrogenic causes, extracolonic neurological diseases, psychiatric disorders, and endocrine diseases. These disorders are listed in Table 51.8, but a few bear special comment. Inadequate dietary fiber and fluid intake are common causes of constipation. Peristaltic movements are stimulated by distention of the intestine. Diets low in fiber move sluggishly because of insufficient distension. Because the stool is propelled slowly, more water may be absorbed from the already inspissated stool, confounding the problem. Cheese, choco-

TABLE 51.8. Common Causes of Constipation.

Faulty diets and habits
- Inadequate bulk (fiber)
- Excessive ingestion of foods that harden stools (e.g., cheese)
- Lack of exercise
- Ignoring call to stool
- Laxative abuse
- Environmental changes (e.g., hospitalization, vacation)

Structural or functional disorders
- Colonic obstruction
  - Neoplasm, volvulus, inflammation (diverticulitis), ameboma, tuberculosis, syphilis, lymphogranuloma venereum, ischemic colitis, anastomotic stricture, endometriosis, intussusception
- Diverticular disease
- Anorectal outlet obstruction
  - Anal obstruction (stenosis, fissure)
  - Rectocele
  - Rectal procidentia
  - Spastic pelvic floor syndrome (anismus)
- Descending perineum syndrome
- Visceral neuropathy or myopathy
  - Congenital aganglionosis (Hirschsprung's disease)
  - Acquired aganglionosis (Chagas' disease)
  - Slow-transit constipation (colonic inertia)
  - Megarectum (sometimes with megacolon)
  - Chronic intestinal pseudo-obstruction (Ogilvie's syndrome)
- Irritable bowel syndrome (visceral hypersensitivity)

Neurologic abnormalities (outside colon)
- Central nervous system (cerebral neoplasm, Parkinson's disease)
- Trauma
- Spinal cord (neoplasm, multiple sclerosis)
- Defective innervation (resection of nervi erigentes)

Psychiatric disorders
- Depression
- Psychoses
- Anorexia nervosa

Iatrogenic causes
- Medication (codeine, antidepressants, iron, anticholinergics)
- Immobilization

Endocrine and metabolic causes
- Hypothyroidism
- Hypercalcemia
- Pregnancy
- Diabetes mellitus
- Dehydration
- Hypokalemia
- Uremia
- Pheochromocytoma
- Hypopituitarism
- Lead poisoning
- Porphyria
- Mucoviscidosis

Source: From Gordon and Nivatvongs,[645] by permission of Taylor & Francis Group LLC.

late, and dehydration may create a hard stool that is difficult to pass.[311–314]

Irregular daily routines that do not allow for exercise or responding to a spontaneous call to stool may result in complaints of constipation. Exercise stimulates colonic contractility and decreases complaints of constipation. Repeatedly ignoring the call to stool because one is "too busy" may eventually result in desensitization of the rectum and subsequent complaints of constipation. Travel causes constipation through decreased opportunities for exercise; disruption of daily routines, which may force one to ignore the call to stool; and dehydration from air travel. Patients with complaints of constipation need to be counseled on these issues and made aware of the variability in the normal number of bowel movements per week (three per day to one every 3 days).

The initial management of the patient with constipation is directed toward ruling out structural (colorectal malignancy, stricture, volvulus) and systemic (hypothyroidism, diffuse dysmotility disorders, scleroderma, diabetes) diseases. Once these issues have been addressed, a trial of increased dietary fiber and water is instituted, with resolution of symptoms in most patients. Should symptoms persist, evaluation of colonic transit times and pelvic floor function are indicated. Pelvic floor function is assessed with defecography and anorectal manometry (discussed later). Colonic transit may be assessed with radiopaque markers that are ingested by the patient on day 0. Plain films of the abdomen are obtained on days 3 and 5; 80% of the markers should pass by day 5 if normal transit exists. Patients are prohibited from taking laxatives or promotility agents 48h before and during the study. If the patient has isolated colonic inertia without evidence of pelvic floor dysfunction or proximal dysmotility, then a total abdominal colectomy with ileorectal anastomosis may be considered in selected patients. Rare (disabled or institutionalized) patients with colonic inertia and either uncertain pelvic floor function or pelvic floor dysfunction may benefit from creation of an end ileostomy after total abdominal colectomy or total abdominal proctocolectomy.

Malignant Diseases: Colorectal Polyps and Cancer

The primary therapy for localized colorectal cancer is surgical resection. Operative mortality has diminished because of improved operative techniques, the availability of blood transfusions, appropriate antibiotic administration, better anesthesia care, and postoperative management.

Epidemiology

Colorectal cancer is the second leading cause of death by cancer in men and women in the United States (estimated at 10% of all malignancies) and the third leading cause of death from carcinoma in men and women when analyzed by sex (lung and prostate, and lung and breast, are first and second, in men and women, respectively). Approximately 54,000 deaths and 145,000 new cases were predicted[315] in 2005. Since 1985, there has been a decline in new cases as well as in deaths from colorectal cancer among the general population. Despite this recent decline, the probability of eventually developing a colorectal carcinoma in women is about 5.8% and in men about 6%.

The incidence and mortality from colorectal cancer shows a dramatic variation from one country to another. The highest mortality rates in the world occur in the Czech Republic (52 per 100,000), while the lowest rates are seen in Albania (4 per 100,000). The United States is in the middle with about 35 per 100,000. In general, countries of the Western world have the highest incidence of colorectal cancer. There is an increased risk in urban populations when compared to rural populations. Within the United States, African Americans have the highest incidence and mortality rates among all racial and ethnic groups. In fact, the incidence of colorectal cancer among African Americans has not changed since 1985, while it has declined 2.9%/year in white men and 1.7%/year in white women. The reasons for these differences are unknown but may be related to environmental, socioeconomic, and genetic factors. The US colon and rectal cancer mortality rates have decreased by 29% from 1950 through 1990. The colorectal mortality rate declined at a rate of 2.2% and 2.0% annually in white men and women, respectively, and 0.7% and 0.8% in African American men and women, respectively.[315]

Age

Carcinoma of the large intestine is predominantly a disease of older patients, with the peak incidence in the sixth and seventh decades. The mean age at onset is 65; however, it can occur at virtually any age. It has been estimated that only 5% of colorectal carcinomas occur in patients younger than 40 years of age.

Site

Cancers occur most commonly in the rectum and sigmoid colon, but over the past several decades there has been a shift in the location of carcinomas from the rectum and the left colon to the right colon.[316] Reasons for the shift are not entirely clear but may be related to better cancer screening. As a consequence, colorectal cancer screening should be directed at the entire colon rather than limited to the distal 25 cm of the large intestine.

Dietary and Environmental Risk Factors

A number of observational studies have demonstrated that the increased intake of fats and red meat along with the decreased intake of fruits and vegetables in the Western diet are associated with an increased risk for colorectal cancer. Furthermore, rather than the total fat intake, saturated animal fat appears to be a stronger risk factor, and polyunsaturated fats may be protective. The protective effects of fish oil may be inhibition of prostaglandin synthesis from arachidonic acid.[317–319]

Dietary fiber has a beneficial effect on colorectal cancer risk, and the mechanism by which dietary fiber is protective remains elusive. Effects of fiber on fecal bulk, water content, transit time, and pH have been proposed to be potential mechanisms.[320]

Physical Activity and Obesity

Both decreased physical activity and obesity have been related to an increased risk for colorectal cancer in both men and women.[321–323] The Canadian National Breast Screening Study of over 89,000 women between 40 and 59 years of age demonstrated[322] a hazard ratio of 1.88 (95% CI 1.24–2.86) for the risk of colorectal cancer in premenopausal women with a body mass index (BMI) above 30 kg/m^2.

Family History

There is a two- to threefold increased risk of colorectal carcinomas in first-order relatives of patients who have suffered from the disease.[324] Fuchs et al. found that the age-adjusted relative risk of colorectal carcinoma for men and women with affected first-degree relatives when compared with those without a family history of the disease was 1.72. This relative risk increased to 2.75 when two or more first-degree relatives were involved.[325] In individuals younger than 45 years who had one or more affected first-degree relatives, the risk was 5.37. The risk to first-degree relatives of patients diagnosed under the age of 45 was significantly increased (5.2 vs. 2.3). In addition, there are reports about an increased risk of pancreatic carcinoma (hazard ratio, 1.99), and bladder cancer (hazard ratio, 2.35) among patients with a family history of rectal carcinoma.

Inflammatory Bowel Disease

There is an increased risk of developing colorectal cancer with long-standing UC and Crohn's disease. Lennard-Jones et al. reported an increased risk for cancer development with long-standing UC of 3%, 5%, and 9% after 15, 20, and 25 years, respectively.[326] The risk is most significant with pancolitis versus left-sided disease alone (14.8% vs. 2.8%, respectively).[127] The incidence for colorectal cancer in Crohn's patients is 2.5 to 21 times greater than in the general population.[55]

Genetic Pathways

The majority of colorectal cancers develop through an orderly progression from normal mucosa to adenomas to carcinomas, the polyp–cancer sequence. The molecular events include the progressive accumulation of genetic mutations in regulatory genes that lead to uncontrolled cell growth. Three major categories of genes have been implicated in the development of colorectal cancer: oncogenes such as K-ras, tumor suppressor genes such as APC (adenomatous polyposis coli), DCC (deleted in colorectal carcinoma), p53, and MCC, and the mismatch repair genes hMSH2, hMLH1, hPMS, and hPMS2 (Table 51.9).

TABLE 51.9. Genes Commonly Altered in Colorectal Cancer.

Gene	*Chromosome*	*Gene class*	*Function*	*Comment*
APC	5q	Tumor suppressor	Adhesion and intercellular communication	Mutated in FAP, Gardner's, and Turcot's syndrome
DCC	18q	Oncogene	Cell–cell adhesion and interactions	Tumor growth, invasion, and metastasis
P53	17p	Tumor suppressor	Transcription factor for genes that inhibit tumor growth	>50% colon cancers have p53 mutation
K-ras	12p	Oncogene	Signal transduction	50% of colon cancers have K-*ras* activity
hMSH2, hMLH1, hPMS1, hPMS2	2p	Mismatch repair	Corrects DNA replication errors	HNPCC

A GENETIC MODEL FOR COLORECTAL TUMORGENESIS

Normal Epithelium		Chromosome	Alteration	Gene
⇓	⇐	5q	Mutation or Loss	FAP
Hyperproliferation Epithelium				
⇓				
Early Adenoma	⇐	DNA hypomethylation		
⇓	⇐	12p	Mutation	K-ras
Intermediate Adenoma				
⇓	⇐	18q	Loss	DCC
Late Adenoma				
⇓	⇐	17p	Loss	p53
Carcinoma				
⇓	⇐	Other Alteration		
Metastasis				

FIGURE 51.27. Multistep pathogenesis of colorectal malignancy. (From Fearon and Vogelstein.[327])

In 1990, Fearon and Vogelstein described a model for colorectal cancer (Fig. 51.27).[327] They postulated that at least five genes had to be mutated for cancer to develop. Further studies showed that in at least seven genes genetic alterations take place before the development of cancer. This multistep pathway, often referred as loss of heterozygosity (LOH), can be observed in inherited and sporadic colorectal cancer (Fig. 51.28).

A different pathway of cancer development consists of insertions or deletions of simple repeated sequences (microsatellite instability, MSI) and has been described by Loeb.[328] Carcinogenesis is initiated by defects within the mismatch repair genes. In that case, replication errors increase, leading to MSI and malfunction of the gene. These tumors are biologically different from those acquired through LOH, and this second pathway, also called RER (replication error), is found in the majority of hereditary nonpolyposis colorectal cancer (HNPCC) tumors and in approximately 10%–20% of sporadic cancers (Fig. 51.29). Thus, there are multiple factors that may act on a genetic predisposition or acquired defects, resulting in colorectal malignancy (Figs. 51.30–51.32).

LOH PATHWAY TO COLORECTAL CARCINOMA

APC gene mutation or 5q loss
(inherited mutation in adenomatous polyposis syndromes)

⇓

Hyperproliferation of crypt cells and clonal proliferation
of a stem cell results in small adenoma

⇓

Activation of K-*ras* oncogene within small
adenoma and proliferation of doubly mutated clone

⇓

Intermediate adenoma

⇓

Loss of *DCC* results in proliferation
of clone with multiple genetic alterations

⇓

Late adenoma with dysplasia

⇓

p53 loss or mutation results in proliferation of malignant clone

⇓

Invasive carcinoma

FIGURE 51.28. The LOH pathway to the development of colorectal cancer. (From Allen,[647] by permission of Thieme Medical Publishers, Inc.)

RER PATHWAY TO COLORECTAL CARCINOMA

Mutation or loss of mismatch repair genes
(inherited in HNPCC)

⇓

Accumulation of somatic mutations within microsatellites

⇓

Altered function of microsatellites

⇓

Altered function of genes that contain or are regulated
by microsatellites (type II *TGR*-β receptor gene)

⇓

Sequential accumulation of genetic changes
in carcinoma-related genes

⇓

Adenoma-carcinoma sequence
(usually does not involve *APC, MCC,* K-*ras, DCC, p53*)

FIGURE 51.29. Genetic alterations that appear to occur in a "preferred" sequence. (From Allen,[647] by permission of Thieme Medical Publishers, Inc.)

Adenomatous Polyposis Coli Gene

The APC (adenomatous polyposis coli) gene is located on the long arm of chromosome 5 (5q). It is mutated in FAP, including the variants Gardner's syndrome and Turcot's syndrome. The APC gene encodes for a 2843-amino-acid peptide of about 300 kDa that is expressed in most human tissues and

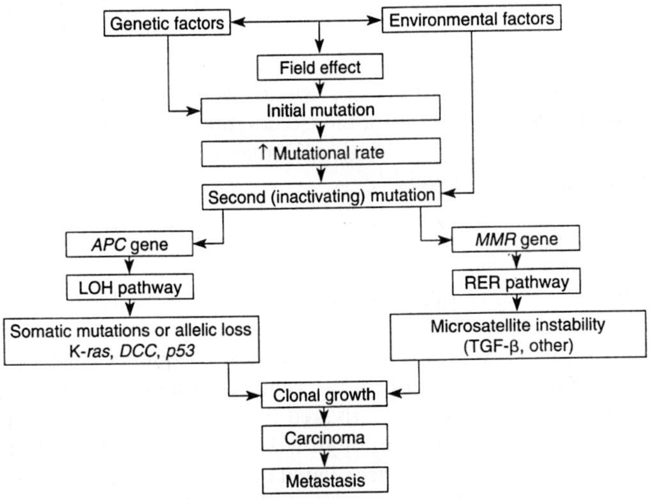

FIGURE 51.30. Molecular factors that appear related to the development of colorectal malignancy. "Genetic factors" may be inborn errors that initiate carcinogenesis or may result from environmental and field effect insults that lead to genetic alterations and carcinogenesis. APC, adenomatous polyposis coli; LOH, loss of heterozygosity; DCC, deleted in colon carcinoma; MMR, mismatch repair; RER, replication error; TGF, transforming growth factor. (From Allen,[647] by permission of Thieme Medical Publishers, Inc.)

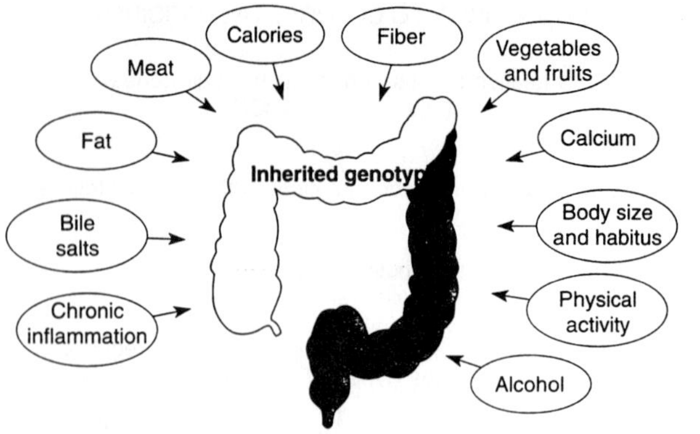

FIGURE 51.31. Environmental factors that may play a role in the development of colorectal malignancy by creating a "field effect" that increases the susceptibility of the tissue as a whole to genetic predisposition or other environmental insults, leading to the development of malignancy. (From Allen,[647] by permission of Thieme Medical Publishers, Inc.)

is a tumor suppressor gene involved in the regulation of β-catenin in cytoskeleton organization, apoptosis, cell cycle control, and cell adhesion. In FAP, genotype–phenotype relationships for specific sequence mutations have been characterized.

A mutated APC gene is found in the majority of colorectal tumors, being detectable in 80% of adenomas and carcinomas. The mutation is found in the adenoma and carcinoma but not in the surrounding tissues, indicating that this is a somatic mutation. Because APC is a tumor suppressor gene, inactivation of the second allele must occur for the cell to lose the tumor-suppressing activity of the APC gene. There is considerable evidence that APC mutations occur early and may be the first event in sporadic colorectal tumorigenesis.

DCC Gene

The DCC (deleted in colorectal carcinoma) gene is located on the long arm of chromosome 18 (18q). The gene product is involved in cell–cell adhesion and cell–matrix interactions, which may be important in preventing tumor growth, invasion, and metastases. In sporadic colorectal cancer, DCC gene expression is associated with a decreased risk for recurrence and improved survival.[329]

P53 Gene

The p53 gene is located on the short arm of chromosome 17p13.1. It is a tumor suppressor gene that is involved in cell cycle regulation, DNA replication, and apoptosis in response to DNA damage. As a tetramer, P53 binds sequences of DNA in the promoter region of other genes to enhance their transcription.[330] Most genes activated by P53 are thought to be involved in the inhibition of growth. Therefore, inactivation of P53 function allows unregulated cell growth. Mutations of P53 can be found in more than half of all human cancers, making it a component in biochemical pathways central to human carcinogenesis.[331] Approximately 30% of advanced adenomas and 75% of carcinomas will have a p53 mutation. The prognostic role of p53 expression in colorectal cancer remains unclear, but a number of prognostic studies are under way.[332,333]

K-ras Proto-oncogene

K-ras is an oncogene that acts in a classic transdominant fashion. It is located on the short arm of chromosome 12 (12p12.1). The K-ras protein interacts with putative effector molecules, conveying a growth response. This signal transduction process is perturbed with a mutant K-ras protein.[334] In sporadic colorectal tumors, K-ras mutations involving codons 12, 13, and 61 have been found in 47% of carcinomas and in 50% of large adenomas. The prognostic significance of K-ras mutations in colorectal cancer is unclear; however, a subset analysis of patients enrolled in the Intergroup Trial 0035 reported a hazard ratio for death of 4.5 (95% CI 1.7–12.1) in stage II patients with K-ras mutations compared to those with normal expression. Furthermore wild-type K-ras expression was associated with a hazard ratio for death of 0.4 (95% CI 0.2–0.8) in patients with stage III disease who received adjuvant therapy with 5-fluorouracil (5FU) and levamisole.[335]

Mismatch Repair Genes

Mismatch repair genes are needed for cells to repair DNA replication errors and spontaneous base repair loss. The four DNA mismatch repair genes found in humans are hMSH2 (chromosome 2p), hMLH1 (chromosome 3p21), hPMS1 (chromosome 2q31–33), and hPMS2 (chromosome 7p22) and hMSH6. Genetic alterations in these genes cause HNPCC syndrome, previously known as Lynch syndrome.[336]

Pyrimidine Metabolism

Thymidylate synthase (TS) and thymidine phosphorylase (TP) are enzymes involved in pyrimidine metabolism. Elevated levels of TS or TP within tumors are associated with a poor response to 5FU-based regimens in the setting of advanced disease.[337] Dihydropyrimidine dehydrogenase (DPD) is the rate-limiting enzyme in 5FU catabolism. Low expression of DPD correlates with susceptibility to toxicity with 5FU-based regimens.[338] Conversely, high expression of DPD within the tumor predicts a poor response to 5FU-based chemotherapy.[337]

Carcinoembryonic Antigen

Carcinoembryonic antigen (CEA) is a cell membrane glycoprotein that has been useful in prognosis and follow-up of patients with colorectal cancer. Serum CEA levels can be elevated in a variety of cancers, including those of colorectal, ovarian, breast, lung, pancreatic, and other GI origin, as well

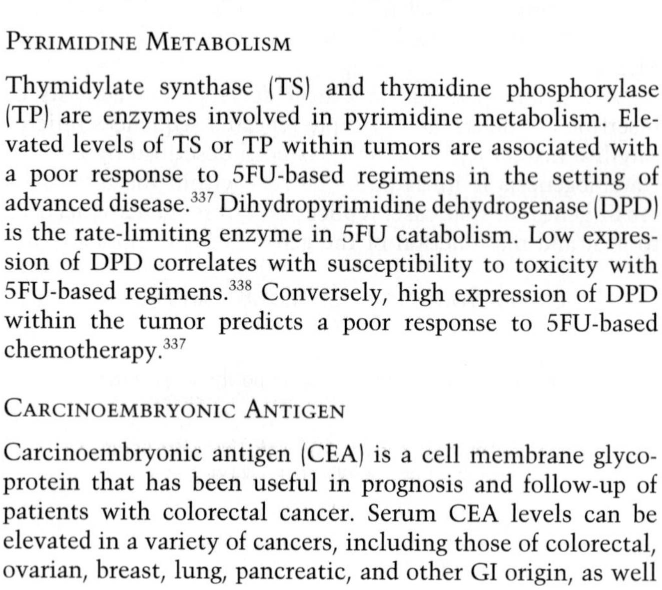

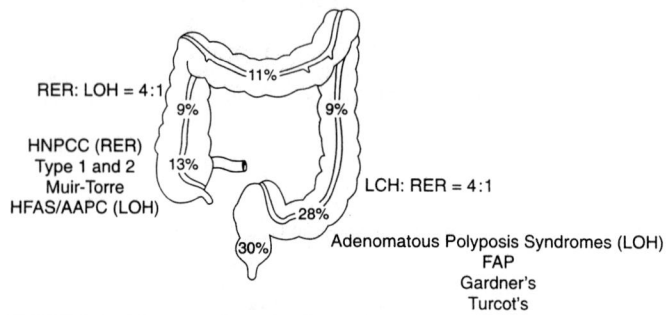

FIGURE 51.32. Distribution of neoplastic lesions and ratios of loss of heterozygosity (*LOH*) to replication error pathway (*RER*). (From Allen,[647] by permission of Thieme Medical Publishers, Inc.)

as nonmalignant conditions, including liver and renal dysfunction, bowel obstruction, and smoking. Not all colorectal cancers result in an elevated serum CEA, and the absolute value does not correlate with extent of disease.

Despite these limitations, CEA is a useful marker in the initial evaluation and follow-up of patients with colorectal cancer. Elevation of CEA has a positive predictive value of approximately 70%–80% for recurrent disease. Furthermore, CEA is often the first indicator of recurrent disease and is the first abnormal test in 38%–66% of cases. Approximately 30% of patients with colorectal cancer will have a normal CEA, and approximately 40% of patients with a normal preoperative CEA will have an elevated CEA at recurrence.[339] Monitoring of CEA detects recurrent disease sooner and leads to the identification of resectable recurrent disease in approximately 5% of patients. Although the advantages have not been dramatic, three meta-analyses of intensive follow-up that included serum CEA determination have demonstrated a survival advantage.[340–342] The American Society of Colon and Rectal Surgeons has recommended that serum CEA determinations be performed at a minimum of every 4-month intervals during the first 2 years after resection of stage II and III disease.

Screening and Surveillance

Cancer screening refers to the testing of a population of apparently asymptomatic individuals to determine the risk of developing colorectal cancer. To make screening effective in a large population, the following events must occur. The disease being screened must be a major health problem, effective therapy must be available if disease is found, a good screening test must be available that is both sensitive and specific, and the test must be cost-effective. The cost-effectiveness of colorectal cancer screening for asymptomatic patients has been established.[343]

Surveillance refers to the ongoing monitoring of individuals who have an increased risk for the development of a disease. For colorectal cancer, surveillance is reserved for patients with IBD; hereditary colorectal cancer syndromes, including FAP, HNPCC, mutant Y-homolog (MYH) polyposis, and as-of-yet uncharacterized familial colorectal cancers; and a previous history of colorectal cancer or colorectal adenomas. Current screening guidelines for colorectal cancer from the American Society of Colon and Rectal Surgeons are shown in Table 51.10.

Fecal Occult Blood Testing

Fecal occult blood testing (FOBT) of the stool was one of the first tests used in colorectal cancer screening. The advantage of fecal occult testing includes availability, convenience, good patient compliance, and low cost. Limitations include low sensitivity and low specificity. Sensitivity is affected by slide storage, ascorbic acid, lesions not bleeding at the time, and degradation of hemoglobin by colonic bacteria. Specificity

TABLE 51.10. Current Screening Guidelines for Colorectal Cancer from the American Society of Colon and Rectal Surgeons.

Risk	*Procedure*	*Onset (Age, year)*	*Frequency*
I. Low or average (65%–75% of people)	Digital rectal exam and one of the following:	50	Yearly
A. Asymptomatic: no risk factors	FOBT and flexible sigmoidoscopy	50	FOBT yearly, flexible sigmoidoscopy every 5 years
B. Colorectal cancer in none of first-degree relatives	Colonoscopy or DCBE and proctosigmoidoscopy	50	Every 5 to 10 years
II. Moderate risk (20% to 30% of people)			
A. Colorectal cancer in first-degree relative, age 55 or younger, or two or more first-degree relatives of any ages	Colonoscopy	40 or 10 years before the youngest case in the family, whichever is earlier	Every 5 years
B. Colorectal cancer in a first- degree relative over the age of 55	Colonoscopy	50, or 10 years before the age of the case, whichever is earlier	Every 5 to 10 years
C. Personal history of large (>1 cm) or multiple colorectal polyps of any size	Colonoscopy	One year after polypectomy	If recurrent polyps, 1 year; if normal, 5 years
D. Personal history of colorectal malignancy: surveillance after resection for curative intent	Colonoscopy	1 year after resection	If normal, 3 years; if still normal, 5 years; if abnormal, as above
III. High risk (6% to 8% of people)			
A. Family history of hereditary adenomatous polyposis	Flexible sigmoidoscopy; consider genetic counseling; consider genetic testing	12 to 14 (puberty)	Every 1 to 2 years
B. Family history of hereditary nonpolyposis colon cancer	Colonoscopy; consider genetic counseling; consider genetic testing	21 to 40 40	Every 2 years Every year
C. Inflammatory bowel disease	Colonoscopy	15th	Every 1 to 2 years
1. Left-side colitis	Colonoscopy	8th	Every 1 to 2 years
2. Pancolitis			

DCBE, double-contrast barium enema; FOBT, fecal occult blood testing.

Source: From the American Society of Colon and Rectal Surgeons. http://www.fascrs.org/displaycommon.cfm?an=1&subarticlenbr=229 (accessed 11/09/2007).

TABLE 51.11.
Impact of Fecal Occult Blood Testing on Mortality from Colorectal Malignancy.

Author	*Level of evidence*	*n*	*Design*	*Result*
Mandel[344]	I	46,551	Annual FOBT vs. biennial	Annual FOBT → 33% ↓ mortality, FOBT vs. usual care biennial no Δ
Hardcastle[345]	I	152,850	Biennial FOBT vs. usual care	Biennial FOBT → 15% ↓ mortality
Kronborg[346]	I	61,933	Biennial FOBT vs. usual care	Biennial FOBT → 18% ↓ mortality
Winawer[489]	I	21,756	Annual FOBT plus rigid sigmoidoscopy vs. annual rigid sigmoidoscopy alone	Annual FOBT → 43% ↓ mortality over rigid sigmoidoscopy alone
Kewenter[490]	I	21,347 initial and 19,991 at follow-up	FOBT initial evaluation and at 16–24 months	Mortality Δ pending but earlier stage tumors

is adversely affected by exogenous peroxidase activity by red meat and uncooked vegetables and medications that may induce bleeding from noncolonic sources such as aspirin and other nonsteroidal antiinflammatory drugs.

Three large randomized controlled trials of serial FOBTs conducted in Minnesota, the United Kingdom, and Denmark, involving more than 250,000 subjects followed for up to 18 years, have demonstrated that serial FOBT results in an increased detection of colorectal cancer in earlier stages and reduces colorectal cancer mortality from 15% to 33%, with the absolute risk reduction for colorectal cancer death ranging from 0.8 to 4.6 per 1000 person-years.[344–346] Although some authors have criticized the test, citing poor sensitivity for colorectal neoplasia, these studies suggest the test is effective in reducing the mortality of colorectal malignancy and is cost-effective when compared to treating an undetected malignancy.[343,347] When the test is repeated annually after the age of 50, the sensitivity is improved, and the malignancy is detected at an earlier stage than if no screening is performed (Table 51.11).

FLEXIBLE SIGMOIDOSCOPY

The benefit of proctosigmoidoscopy in screening programs has been suggested by several studies using the rigid sigmoidoscope. In one landmark study, rigid sigmoidoscopy screening was associated with a 59% reduction in colorectal cancer mortality (odds ratio 0.41; 95% confidence interval 0.25–0.69).[348] The advantages of the flexible sigmoidoscope over the rigid are improved patient comfort and that the 60-cm flexible sigmoidoscope allows the clinician to reach the descending colon or even the splenic flexure, suggesting more polyps and carcinomas would be identified with the flexible scope and the screening benefit enhanced. The National Cancer Institute (NCI)-funded Prostate, Lung, Colorectal, and Ovarian screening trial and the UK FlexiScope Trial are being performed with an anticipated 250,000 subjects to evaluate screening flexible sigmoidoscopy, but outcome data are not yet available.[349,350]

Both rigid and flexible sigmoidoscopies are inexpensive, require no conscious sedation, are relatively safe, and afford direct visualization and biopsy of polyps and cancers. The disadvantage is that the entire colon is not visualized with either procedure, and lesions may be missed in the proximal bowel. Three case-controlled studies suggest rigid sigmoidoscopy can effectively reduce the risk of death from sigmoid and rectal cancer (Table 51.12).[348,351,352] We believe flexible sigmoidoscopy is a safe (fewer than 1–2 perforations per 10,000) screening tool that may be repeated every 5 years. If adenomatous disease is found, full colonoscopy should be performed.

BARIUM ENEMA

Barium enema combined with sigmoidoscopy allows for visualization of the entire colon and rectum. Single-contrast BE is significantly less sensitive and specific than double-contrast barium enema (DCBE) and should not be used as a screening tool for colorectal malignancy. In contemporary multicenter audits, DCBE has an overall diagnosis rate of 85% (range 50%–100%) and an equivocal finding rate of 7%–8% (range 0%–35%)[353,354] (Fig. 51.33).

TABLE 51.12.
Impact of Sigmoidoscopy on Mortality from Colorectal Malignancy.

Author	*Level of evidence*	*n*	*Design*	*Result*	*Comments*
Selby[348]	III	1129	Case-control study of rigid sigmoidoscopy (261 case subjects)	59% ↓ in mortality	↓ in mortality only for portion of bowel visualized
Newcomb[352]	III	262	Case-control study of rigid sigmoidoscopy (66 case subjects)	80% ↓ in mortality	
Muller[351]	III	—	Case-control study of diagnostic procedures of the large bowel	59% ↓ in mortality	Greatest benefit with "tissue removal"

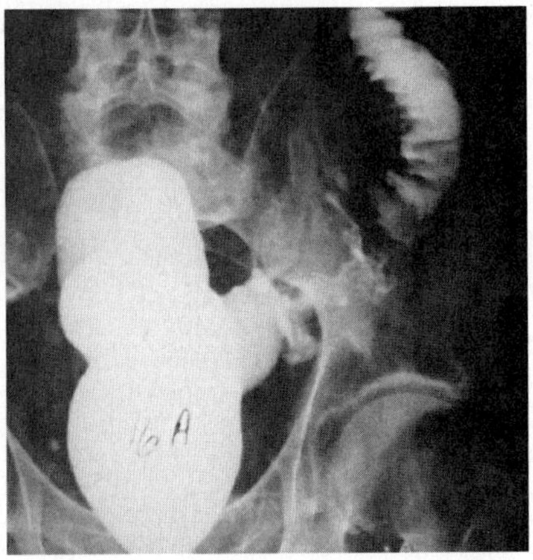

FIGURE 51.33. Barium enema from a patient with colorectal malignancy.

The rectum and distal sigmoid colon are better visualized with sigmoidoscopy, which should be performed if a DCBE is chosen to screen the bowel for colorectal malignancy. This approach results in a sensitivity of 98% and 99% for carcinomas and adenomas, respectively.[355] The most serious complication of DCBE, perforation, has recently been estimated to occur at a rate of 1 per 25,000 studies.[356]

Colonoscopy

Examination of the entire colon by colonoscopy is currently recommended for patients with any benign neoplasm found at the time of flexible sigmoidoscopy. When performed by experienced endoscopists, colonoscopy with polypectomy is a safe procedure, with a perforation incidence of 0.1% and overall major morbidity rate of 0.3% (hemorrhage, bleeding, cardiovascular complication); the cecum is visualized in over 97% of patients.[357,358]

A DCBE or CT colonography is required when the cecum is not reached. Detecting and removing polyps reduces the incidence of colorectal malignancy; detecting earlier lesions decreases disease-related mortality; and fewer carcinomas develop in patients who have colonoscopy and polypectomy.[359,360] Colonoscopy uncommonly misses lesions of 1 cm or more (6%), but can miss 13%–27% of smaller polyps.[361] However, colonoscopy has been shown to be superior to DCBE at detecting polyps and provides an opportunity for tissue diagnosis or therapeutic intervention at the time of initial evaluation.[362] Colonoscopy is better than flexible sigmoidoscopy and FOBT at detecting lesions because the entire colon may be directly visualized. In one study, a prevalence of 24% of new adenomas was found when 226 patients underwent colonoscopy within 1 year of flexible sigmoidoscopy. Advanced lesions proximal to the descending colon were found in 6% of these patients[363] (Table 51.13).

Computed Tomographic Colonography (Virtual Colonoscopy)

Computed tomographic colonography (also known as *virtual colonoscopy*) is a new technique that utilizes three-dimensional reconstruction of the air-distended colon. In a series of 1223 average-risk adults who subsequently underwent conventional (optical) colonoscopy, virtual colonoscopy was as good or better at detecting relevant lesions.[364] However, it may be less accurate in surveillance populations, and subsequent multiinstitutional studies have failed to confirm these excellent results.[365] Studies are ongoing to evaluate the efficacy of virtual colonoscopy in both screening and surveillance. Thus far, the major limitations include uncertain accuracy, the need for full-bowel preparation, and follow-up colonoscopy for tissue diagnosis of radiographic abnormalities. Because virtual colonoscopy is radiologist time- and labor-intensive, investigations into methods of automating the evaluation process are ongoing.

Future Directions

The utility of fecal DNA testing is currently under investigation. When compared to FOBT, fecal DNA testing in asymptomatic average-risk individuals resulted in an improved adenoma detection rate (18% vs. 11%); however, as a screening test it is less effective than colonoscopy.[366]

Signs and Symptoms

The presentation of large-bowel malignancy generally falls into three categories: insidious onset of chronic symptoms (77%–92%), acute onset of intestinal obstruction (6%–16%), or acute perforation with local or diffuse peritonitis (2%–7%).[367,368]

Bleeding is the most common symptom of colorectal malignancy. Twenty percent of patients over 40 years of age with rectal bleeding had colorectal neoplasia; 6% had colorectal adenocarcinoma, and 14% had polyps. Bleeding may be occult, or it may be seen as stool that is black, maroon, dark purple, or bright red, depending on the location of the malig-

TABLE 51.13. Summary of the Characteristics of Screening Tests for Colorectal Malignancy.

Screening test	*Overall performance*	*Complexity*	*Potential effectiveness*	*Evidence of effectiveness*	*Screening test risk*
FOBT	Intermediate for carcinomas, low for polyps	Lowest	Lowest	Strongest	Lowest
Flexible sigmoidoscopy	High for up to half of the colon	Intermediate	Intermediate	Intermediate	Intermediate
FOBT plus flexible sigmoidoscopy	Same as flexible sigmoidoscopy and FOBT	Intermediate	Intermediate	Intermediate	Intermediate
DCBE	High	High	High	Weakest	Intermediate
Colonoscopy	Highest	Highest	Highest	Weakest	Highest

DCBE, double-contrast barium enema; FOBT, fecal occult blood test.

Source: From Winawer et al.[661]

nancy. Occult bleeding may present with iron-deficiency anemia and associated fatigue.

Change in bowel habits is the second most common complaint, with patients noting either diarrhea or constipation. Constipation is more often associated with left-sided lesions because the diameter of the colon is smaller, and the stool is more formed than on the right side. Patients may report a gradual change in the caliber of the stool or may have diarrhea if the narrowing has progressed sufficiently to cause obstruction. Carcinomas of the right side of the colon do not typically present with changes in bowel habits, but large amounts of mucus generated by a tumor may cause diarrhea, and large right-sided lesions or lesions involving the ileocecal valve may cause obstruction.

Abdominal pain is as common a presentation as change in bowel habits.[369] Left-sided obstructing lesions may present with cramping abdominal pain associated with nausea and vomiting and relieved with bowel movements. Right-sided malignancies may result in vague pain that is difficult to localize. Rectal lesions may present with tenesmus, but pelvic pain is generally associated with advanced disease after the tumor has involved the sacral or sciatic nerves. Less-common symptoms include weight loss, malaise, fever, abdominal mass, and symptoms of urinary tract involvement (frequency, pneumaturia, and fecaluria). Bacteremia with *Streptococcus bovis* is highly suggestive of colorectal malignancy.[370]

Acute onset of intestinal obstruction was the presenting feature in up to 15% of cases. Physical exam is often unrevealing because the abdomen is distended, and masses, primary or metastatic, are not palpable. Tympany, ascites, and distension may be all that is noted on abdominal exam. Rectal exam will only rarely reveal an obstructing tumor. Colorectal malignancy should always be considered when patients present with large-bowel obstruction. The history, physical exam, and plain films of the abdomen may suggest the diagnosis. It may be confirmed with contrast enema, rigid or flexible endoscopy, or CT scans of the abdomen and pelvis.

Perforation is the third general class of presentation of colorectal malignancy. It may result in localized peritonitis or generalized peritonitis, or if walled off, it may present with obstruction or fistula to an adjacent structure such as the bladder. Concurrent obstruction and perforation occur in 12% to 19% of patients with obstruction.[361,362] When the perforation occurs proximal to the obstructing lesion, as with perforation of a dilated cecum proximal to an obstructing sigmoid carcinoma, the patients present with diffuse peritonitis and sepsis. Emergent surgical intervention after adequate fluid resuscitation is clearly indicated. However, in the case of perforation at the tumor, possibly secondary to tumor necrosis, the more indolent course may lead to confusion of the perforated tumor with inflammation associated with appendicitis, diverticulitis, or Crohn's disease.

Staging

Staging systems are important for predicting outcomes, selecting patients for various therapies, and comparing therapies for like patients across institutions. For a tumor to be considered as an invasive cancer and staged, it must penetrate through the muscularis mucosa. Malignant cells superficial to this layer are thought to lack metastatic potential because of a paucity of lymphatics, and their presence is considered high-grade dysplasia (previously carcinoma in situ).

TABLE 51.14. AJCC/TNM Staging System for Colorectal Carcinoma, Comparison to Dukes and Modified Aster-Coller Classification.*

Stage	*Depth*	*Nodal Status*	*Distant Metastasis*	*Dukes*	*MAC*
0	Tis	N0	M0		
I	T1	N0	M0	A	A
	T2				B1
IIA	T3	N0	M0	B	B2
IIB	T4				B3
IIIA	T1–2	N1	M0	C	C1
IIIB	T3–4	N1			C2/C3
IIIC	Any T	N2			C1/C2/C3
IV	Any T	Any N	M1	D	D

*See Table 93.1 for Colon and Rectum Carcinoma AJCC TNM and Stage Grouping.

In 1932, Dukes proposed a classification based on the extent of direct extension along with the presence or absence of regional lymphatic metastases for the staging of rectal cancer. Dukes A lesions are those in which the depth of penetration of the primary tumor is confined to the bowel wall. Dukes B tumors have primary tumor penetration through the full thickness of the bowel to include serosa or fat. Dukes C lesions have local (C1) or regional (C2) nodal involvement. Although not initially described, it became accepted as common practice to add a fourth category for distant spread (D) outside the resected specimen.

The Astler-Coller Modification divided the Dukes B and C cases depending on the depth of primary spread, with Dukes B1 including tumors with penetration confined to the bowel wall and B2 lesions including tumors that penetrate the bowel wall. If nodal disease is present, the tumor depth of penetration determines whether the lesion is C1 (B1 with nodal involvement) or C2 (B2 with nodal involvement).

The American Joint Committee on Cancer (AJCC) tumor/node/metastasis (TNM) staging system roughly correlates to the stages with Dukes classification: stage I equivalent to Dukes A; stage II equivalent to Dukes B; stage III equivalent to Dukes C; and stage IV equivalent to Dukes D. Stages II and III are further subclassified as IIA and IIB as well as IIIA, IIIB, and IIIC. A key distinction is made between stage II and stage III disease, which are defined by the status of the local-regional lymph nodes (Tables 51.14 and 51.15).

TABLE 51.15. Comparison of TNM System to Modified Dukes Classification.

Modified Dukes stage	*Tumor*	*Nodes*	*Distant disease*
A	Tis, T1	N0	M0
B1	T2	N0	M0
B2	T3–4	N0	M0
C1	T1–2	N1–2	M0
C2	T3–4	N1–2	M0
D	Any T	Any N	M1

TABLE 51.16. Preoperative Evaluation for Colorectal Malignancy.

Routine blood work	CBC, LFT, CEA
Colonoscopy	Tissue diagnosis, synchronous disease
Radiographs	Chest x-ray, select CT abdomen/pelvis
Ultrasound	Transrectal ultrasound

Classification of histological grade, cell type, lymphatic, venous or perineural invasion, tumor ploidy, CEA level, bowel perforation, and distal and radial margins allows for further subclassification of the tumors and improved prognostication. Although there were once many elaborate grading systems for adenocarcinomas of the colon and rectum, the AJCC has settled on two classifications, low grade (well and moderately differentiated) and high grade (poorly and undifferentiated). DNA ploidy assessment is the measurement of the quantum amount of DNA in cells. Diploidy is correlated with good prognoses; aneuploidy is correlated with poor prognoses.[363] Bowel perforation and elevated preoperative CEA are associated with poorer prognosis.

Preoperative Staging for Colorectal Cancer

The general physical examination remains a cornerstone in assessing a patient preoperatively to determine the extent of local disease, disclose distant metastases, and appraise the general operative risk. Special interest should be paid to weight loss, pallor as a sign of anemia, and signs of portal hypertension. In addition, a complete workup should include the investigations listed in Table 51.16.

Colonoscopy

Colonoscopy remains the single most important investigation in the evaluation of colonic diseases and may alter the operative procedure in approximately 30% of patients.[371,372] It allows assessment of tumor size and location within the colon and permits biopsy for histologic evaluation of the tumor. Finally, synchronous tumors are detected in 2% to 7% and synchronous polyps in 29.7%.[371,372]

Routine Laboratory Blood Work

A complete blood count (CBC) may reveal the presence of anemia. Liver function tests (LFTs) may be abnormal in the case of liver metastases, but abnormal LFTs are present in only approximately 15% of patients with liver metastases and may be elevated without liver metastases in up to 40%. Levels of CEA should be obtained as a baseline against which further values may be compared. Metastatic disease to the liver is often accompanied with very high levels of CEA, and elevated CEA levels are associated with an increased risk for disease failure independent of stage.[373]

Radiologic Evaluation

A chest x-ray is performed to evaluate for pulmonary metastasis and to provide a baseline evaluation of the patient's cardiac and pulmonary status. Although the routine use of CT in the preoperative evaluation of patients with colon cancer is controversial, it can provide valuable information on the extent of the primary tumor, involvement of contiguous organs, and distant metastatic sites (Fig. 51.34). Approximately 20% of patients will have synchronous liver metastasis at the time of diagnosis. The preoperative identification of liver metastasis is necessary for the surgical planning of combined resections of the primary tumor and the liver metastasis or for the treatment of tumors involving contiguous organs.

The improved sensitivity achieved with modern CT scanner technology may improve the sensitivity and utility of preoperative CT scanning in colorectal cancer. Furthermore, 15% to 20% of liver metastases will be nonpalpable at the time of surgery, leading to undertreated metastatic disease. Finally, data are emerging that routine preoperative CT scanning is cost-effective by improving treatment planning and altering therapy in approximately one-third of patients.[374,375]

Magnetic resonance imaging (MRI) may be helpful in circumstances when intravenous contrast-enhanced CT scanning is contraindicated. Transcutaneous abdominal ultrasound identifies liver metastases, ascites, and gross adenopathy but adds little to CT scanning as a screening exam. Positron emission tomography (PET) and now PET-CT have emerged as potentially important imaging modalities for colorectal cancer. The PET-CT technique utilizes the glucose analog

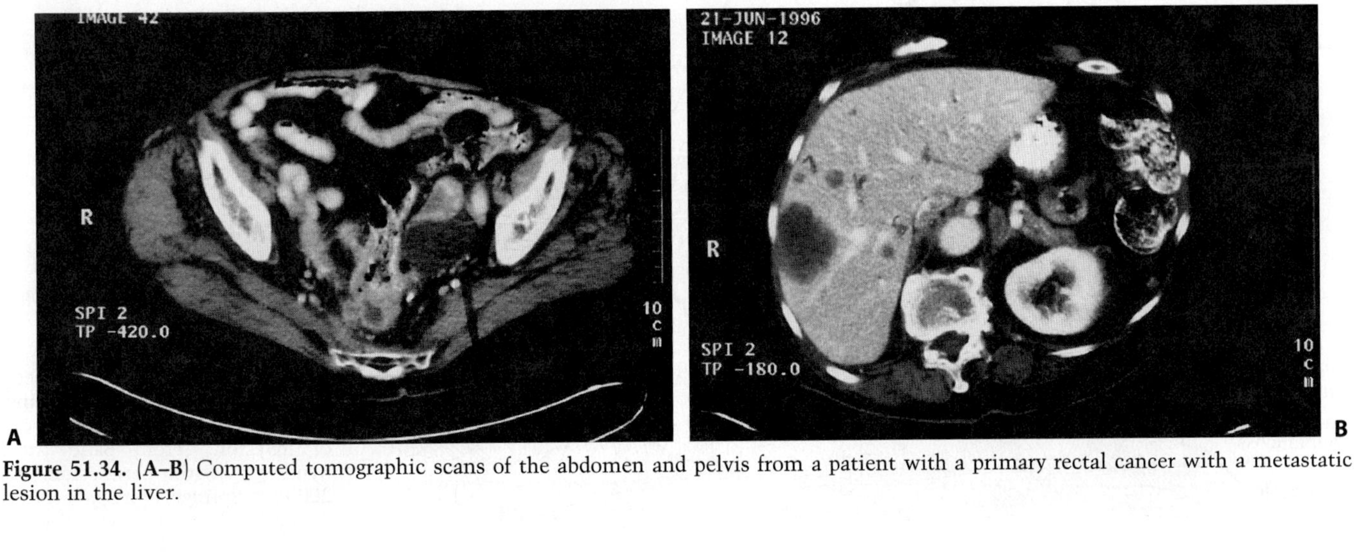

Figure 51.34. (A–B) Computed tomographic scans of the abdomen and pelvis from a patient with a primary rectal cancer with a metastatic lesion in the liver.

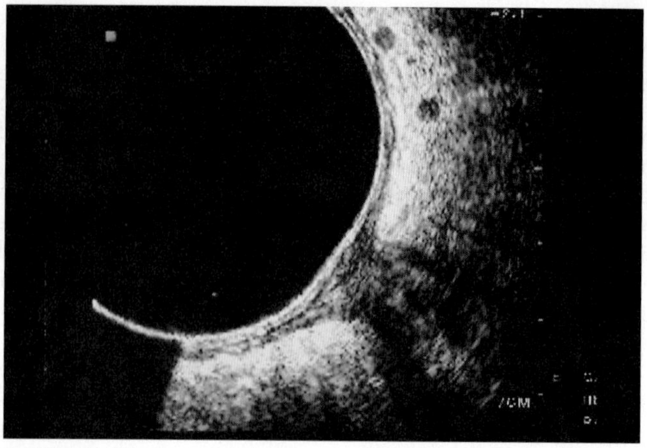

FIGURE 51.35. Transrectal ultrasound of a T3 N1 rectal adenocarcinoma.

fluorodeoxyglucose, which accumulates in metabolically active tissues. The standardized uptake value can provide a semiquantitative determination to help discriminate benign from malignant disease. Although potentially useful in recurrent cancer, it has not been helpful in the primary evaluation of patients with colon cancer due to false positives and high costs.

Endorectal Ultrasound

Endorectal ultrasound is an important diagnostic examination in the treatment of patients with rectal cancer and is performed by surgeons, gastroenterologists, or radiologists. The layers of the rectal wall can be identified and the depth of penetration determined. Sensitivity ranges from 55% to 100% and specificity from 24% to 100% in different studies. The status of lymph nodes also can be predicted in 73% to 85%[376] (Fig. 51.35). Depth of invasion and lymph node involvement are critical for planning operative and preoperative therapy.

Polyps: Colonic

Natural History

In healthy colonic epithelium, there is a normal, constant renewal of the surface epithelium approximately every 6 days by cellular proliferation and differentiation of crypt cells. The proliferation compartment is in the lower third of the crypt, characterized by mitoses and upward migration from anchored stem cells. As cells move up the crypt, differentiation and maturation occur, and the cells lose their capacity to divide again. Eventually, cells die and are shed into the colonic lumen. In the adenoma, this is markedly altered. There is continued mitosis and lack of differentiation of cells, so that the proliferative compartment may envelop the entire crypt. The persistent replication of cells near the crypt surface coupled with retarded cell maturation and extrusion result in an increased number of replicating surface cells.

A *colorectal polyp* is defined as a mass that protrudes into the lumen of the colon. These are classified histologically as adenomatous polyps (which may be benign or malignant), hyperplastic, inflammatory, or hamartomatous (including juvenile). It has previously been thought that only adenomatous polyps had malignant potential; however, more recent evidence suggests potential for alternative pathways of malignant transformation with hyperplastic polyps. These masses may either be sessile or pedunculated (Fig. 51.36).

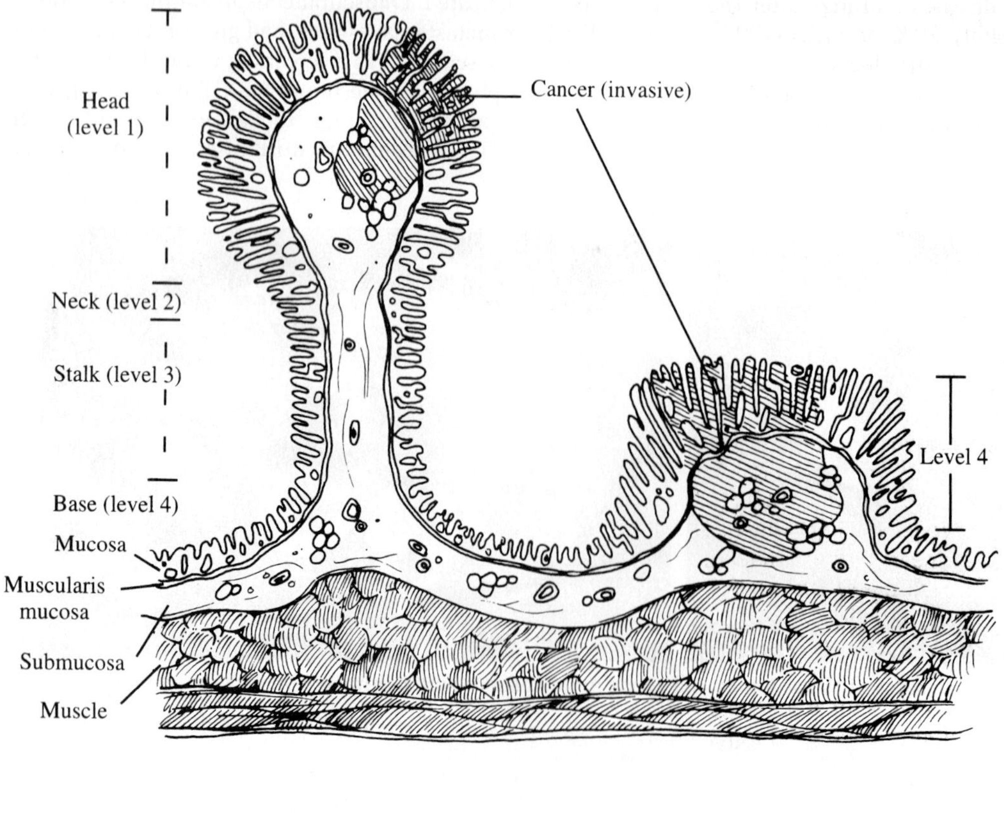

FIGURE 51.36. Sessile and pedunculated polyps illustrating Haggitt's classification of levels of invasion. (From Bailey and Synder,[648] with permission, © 2000, Springer-Verlag, New York.)

TABLE 51.17. Odds Ratio for High-Grade Dysplasia in Adenomas Based on Size and Villous Component.

Size, Villous component (%)	*<0.5 cm*	*0.5–1 cm*	*>1 cm*
0% (tubular)	1	3.1	7.3
<25% (tubular)	2.9	8.8	21.2
<75% (tubulovillous)	3.6	11	26.4
75%–100% (villous)	8.2	25.1	60

Odds ratio from a logistic model for the risk of high-grade dysplasia based on size and histology demonstrating that both have an effect on risk, based on data from the National Polyp Study.

Source: From O'Brien et al.[381]

Adenomatous polyps are found in approximately 33% of the general population by age 50 and in approximately 50% of the general population by age 70. Most lesions are less than 1 cm in size, with 60% of people having a single adenoma, and 40% having multiple lesions. Sixty percent of lesions will be located distal to the splenic flexure. Approximately 70% of colonoscopically removed polyps are adenomas. Their growth patterns as tubular, villous, or tubulovillous further classify adenomas.

Tubular adenomas are found with equal frequency throughout all segments of the bowel and consist of branching tubules lined by closely packed cells containing elongated nuclei parallel to the long axis of the cells and basophilic cytoplasm with reduced amounts of mucus. Fewer than 5% of tubular adenomas are malignant. Tubulovillous adenomas are also equally distributed throughout the bowel, and approximately 20% to 25% are malignant. Approximately 35% to 40% of villous adenomas are malignant. They are composed of elongated papillae, with villi classically extending in an uninterrupted manner from the muscularis mucosa to the luminal surface (Table 51.17). Overall, 87% are tubular, 8% are tubulovillous, and 5% are villous, as reported by the National Polyp Study.

The prevalence of sporadic colorectal adenomas increases with age and varies with country and lifestyle. In the United States and other countries with a high rate of colorectal adenocarcinomas, autopsy studies have shown an overall prevalence of adenomatous polyps in 30% to 50% of individuals. The prevalence is 30% at 50 years of age, 40% to 50% at 60 years, and 50% to 65% at 70 years of age. Endoscopic studies reveal lower rates, between 10% and 20%, in individuals, even though these studies are performed in populations with a high prevalence of adenomas.

Most colorectal cancers arise from polyps that are intermediate lesions in the genetic progression to invasive carcinoma. Accordingly, the National Polyp Study has shown that colonoscopic removal of adenomatous polyps significantly reduces the risk of developing colorectal cancer.[377] The overall risk of an adenoma progressing to cancer is between 2.5% and 8% over a 10-year period and increases with the size of the polyp.[378,379] After 20 years, the relative risk increases to 24%, and having multiple adenomas increases the risk for developing subsequent adenomas and adenocarcinomas.

After colonoscopy and polypectomy have been able to achieve "a clean colon," it takes about 5 years to develop an adenoma and about another 5 years to develop invasive cancer. Adenomas are further graded by the degree of epithelial dysplasia. Nuclei that are enlarged and hyperchromatic with minimal loss of polarity characterize mild dysplasia. There is a slight excess of mitotic figures, but the architecture is not disrupted. Moderate dysplasia is characterized by pleomorphic nuclei, which begin to stratify, and glands are more crowded. Severe dysplasia is characterized by increased pleomorphic nuclei, with marked stratification and loss of polarity. Further prominent nucleoli and increased nuclear-to-cytoplasmic ratios are seen. Crowded glands exhibit a back-to-back arrangement, mucin secretion is decreased, and mitotic figures are numerous.

Malignant Polyps

A malignant polyp is an adenoma in which carcinoma has invaded across the muscularis mucosa. A carcinoma that has not invaded the muscularis mucosa has no metastatic potential because of the absence of lymphatics in the colonic lamina propria except immediately above the muscularis mucosa. The relative risk of adenocarcinoma being present in a polyp is only 1.2 in polyps less than 1 cm in diameter, but this rises to 2.7 to 3.6 in polyps greater than 1 cm in diameter.[380] Only 1.3% of adenomas smaller than 1 cm harbor carcinoma, whereas this increases to 9.5% in adenomas between 1 and 2 cm and 46% in adenomas larger than 2 cm. Similarly, the degree of dysplasia predicts the presence of invasive cancer on complete polypectomy (5.7% of mild, 18% of moderate, and 34.5% of severe dysplasia).[381] Endoscopic polypectomy is curative in 99.7% of cases of pedunculated polyps, when the focus of malignancy is confined to the head of the polyp. In the case of incomplete resection, poor differentiation, lymphatic or vascular invasion, cure rates following endoscopic polypectomy decrease to 91%, and segmental colectomy may be indicated.

Overall, 8.5% to 25% of polyps harboring invasive carcinoma will metastasize to regional lymph nodes. Unfavorable pathologic features of malignant colorectal polyps increase the probability that regional lymph nodes will be involved with tumor and include (a) poor differentiation, (b) vascular or lymphatic invasion, (c) invasion below the submucosa, and (d) positive resection margin. Generally, the presence of one or more of these features is an indication for resection. Depth of invasion is an important prognostic factor for mesenteric lymph node involvement with invasive cancer arising in a polyp and has been characterized by Haggitt et al. (Table 51.18).[382] In a multivariate analysis, only invasion into the submucosa of the underlying bowel wall (level 4) was a significant prognostic factor. This is in keeping with previous pathologic studies that have shown that the lymphatic channels do not penetrate above the muscularis mucosa.

TABLE 51.18. Villous Adenoma Classification.

Classification	*Depth of invasion*
0	Carcinoma confined to the mucosa
1	Head of polyp
2	Neck of polyp
3	Stalk of polyp
4	Submucosa of the underlying colonic wall

An additional classification system for malignant colorectal polyps has been popularized in Japan and may be applicable to malignant sessile polyps; it was described by Kikuchi in 1995. It classifies invasive cancer as Sm1 (slight carcinoma invasion of the muscularis mucosa, 200–300μm), Sm2 (intermediate invasion), or Sm3 (deep submucosal invasion extending to the inner surface of the muscularis propria).[383] The Sm1 depth of invasion is associated with a low risk for local recurrence or lymph node metastasis. In one US study, Sm3 depth of invasion was associated with a 23% risk for lymph node metastasis.[384]

Endoscopic Management of Benign Adenomas

Most polyps throughout the colon can be removed through the colonoscope using the snare polypectomy technique. The polyp is visualized through the colonoscope; the snare wire is looped around the polyp and gently tightened while the electric current is applied. Whenever possible, the polyp is retrieved for histology. When performed by trained endoscopists, colonoscopy with polypectomy is a safe procedure, with a perforation incidence of 0.3% to 1% and a hemorrhage incidence of 0.7% to 2.5%.[379,380] A study by Macrae[382] of 5000 colonoscopies reported an overall hemorrhage rate of 1%, which all occurred in polyps larger than 2cm.

Two-channel endoscopes have become available. This technique allows safe endoscopic polypectomy of polyps larger than 2cm.[381] Endoscopic mucosal resection with submucosal elevation has improved the safety of endoscopic polypectomy. Laparoscopic-assisted colonoscopic polypectomy has also been described. Using this technique, the serosal surface of the colon can be monitored to detect any sign of perforation during endoscopic treatment.[382a]

Surgical Treatment of Colorectal Polyps

The majority of colorectal polyps found at endoscopy are suitable for diathermy snare excision via colonoscopy. However, because of location and size, some are deemed unsafe to treat in this manner and therefore require colectomy. Although surgical options, including segmental bowel resection as well as colotomy with open polypectomy, have been described, due to the uncertainty of harboring an occult malignancy, particularly with the larger polyps that are unable to be treated endoscopically, a formal oncologic resection is advocated. This may be performed using either conventional open or laparoscopic techniques.

Special problems arise with better understanding of the molecular changes in the development of colorectal cancer. The term *aggressive adenoma* was created because the adenoma–carcinoma sequence seems to be accelerated in patients with HNPCC. This theory is supported by the fact that in HNPCC patients only 2.8 polypectomies are performed to prevent one cancer, while 41 to 119 polypectomies are performed in the general population to prevent one cancer.[384] Patients with HNPCC but without invasive adenocarcinoma should undergo annual surveillance colonoscopy. The role for prophylactic colectomy for HNPCC in the absence of malignancy has not been established.

Approximately 7% of patients with polyps harbor a synchronous colorectal carcinoma, but about 29.7% of patients with carcinoma have synchronous polyps.[366] If the polyps are confined to the same anatomical region as the index carcinoma, the conventional cancer operation for that portion of the bowel is indicated. If the polyps are at different sites, a colonoscopic excision should be attempted. If one of the excised polyps contains a carcinoma or if the polyps are not suitable for colonoscopic resection, a colectomy to include the polyps and malignancy should be performed.[385]

Surgical Options for Rectal Polyps

Most rectal polyps are removed during colonoscopy or proctoscopy using different snaring devices. Most polyps up to 2cm can be removed with a single snare. Larger polyps may be removed by transanal excision. An endorectal ultrasound is an important component in the evaluation of large rectal polyps. If the tumor is not indurated or ulcerated and is less than 5cm in greatest dimension, the chance that it is benign is 90%.[386] Preoperative biopsies are unreliable as they have a false-negative rate up to 30%. The entire tumor is removed in one piece whenever possible to ensure adequate histological evaluation. The rectal wall defect may be closed transversely with absorbable sutures or left open.

Transanal endoscopic microsurgery (TEM) was introduced in 1983 by Buess, and it is used for local excision of benign and selected malignant tumors. The procedure is discussed more in detail in the section on local excision of malignant rectal tumors.

Cancer of the Colon

Natural History

Surgery remains the cornerstone of treatment for colorectal cancer but has inherent limitations imposed by the biology and stage of the tumor as well as its location. Ultimately, 50% of patients who undergo curative resection develop local, regional, or widespread recurrence; this presumably occurs as a result of progression of micrometastases present at the time of initial operation. Colorectal tumors are relatively slow-growing neoplasms, and metastases occur relatively late. The doubling time of about 2.5 years has been calculated for primaries and between 50 and 90 days for hepatic metastases.[387] The overall 5-year survival rates after colorectal cancer diagnosis in the United States have improved over time and are 63.5% and 64.7% in women and men, respectively. Five-year survival rates by stage are presented in Table 51.19.

Bowel Preparation

Mechanical bowel preparation has been a cornerstone in modern colorectal surgery. Mechanical cleansing may be accomplished by the use of vigorous laxatives along with repeated enemas until clearing. Oral lavage with a polyethylene glycol hypertonic electrolyte solution such as GoLYTELY or oral Phospho-Soda preparations are efficacious. Recently,

TABLE 51.19. The Stage-Dependent Relative 5-Year Survival Rate.

Location	*Stage 1 (% survival)*	*Stage 2 (% survival)*	*Stage 3 (% survival)*	*Stage 4 (% survival)*
Colon	70	60	44	7
Rectum	72	54	39	7

Source: From Beart et al.[369] and Jessup et al.[491]

the need for mechanical bowel preparation for elective colorectal surgery has been questioned. Several meta-analyses have suggested that mechanical bowel preparation is associated with an increased risk for complications when compared to no preparation.[388–390] However, large, multicenter, prospective randomized data are lacking, and bowel preparation remains common practice.

Antibiotic Administration

Although there is no question that preoperative antibiotic administration is beneficial in elective and emergency colorectal surgery, the route of administration and antibiotic combination have been debated. Most surgeons start antibiotic prophylaxis at the day of operation using a combination to cover gram-positive and gram-negative, aerobic and anaerobic bacteria. Whether the systemic antibiotic is given orally or intravenously does not appear to matter as long as the antibiotic is administered before skin incision. There is no evidence that antibiotic administration after the first postoperative day is beneficial.

Anastomotic Techniques in Colorectal Surgery

Hand-Sutured Techniques

The two-layer technique of hand-sutured bowel anastomosis has historically been considered the gold standard. An end-to-end anastomosis can be constructed after transecting the bowel between bowel clamps. When disparity in bowel size exists, a Cheadle incision along the antimesenteric aspect of the narrower bowel can be performed, equalizing the circumferences of each lumen. The two-layer technique is started as a posterior interrupted seromuscular layer, followed by a running inner-layer posterior suture, which is begun on one edge. The running full-thickness suture is continued around the anterior wall to the starting point. Then, a second interrupted anterior layer is added.

An alternative technique utilizes a one-layer anastomosis of interrupted 3-0 absorbable suture. This technique utilizes the technique of Gambee vertical mattress sutures, with a full-thickness bite on each side, but on the return bite only mucosa and submucosa are included. All sutures of the posterior wall are placed before tying; all knots are tied inside the lumen. An interrupted full-thickness suture with only mucosal inversion is used for the anterior wall.

Whether to use a single- or double-layer anastomosis is a matter of preference; both techniques are equally safe. Care must be taken not to narrow the lumen by inverting too much tissue. Using the two-layer technique, a slightly higher rate of stenosis is reported.

The resultant mesenteric defect, especially when small, should be closed with interrupted sutures to prevent bowel herniation and obstruction. When the defect is large, as is usually the case with proximal vascular ligation, it need not be closed as even if herniation of bowel occurs, it will not incarcerate.

Surgical Staplers in Colorectal Surgery

Surgical staplers have gained increasing popularity (Fig. 51.37). The general principles of anastomosis must be maintained: adequate blood supply, absence of tension, and accurate apposition of healthy tissue. Gastrointestinal anastomosis (GIA) staplers close the bowel with two rows of staples and divide the bowel between the staples at the same time. They may be used to resect bowel or perform the anastomosis, for which they create a side-to-side anastomosis. Transverse anastomosis (TA) staplers close the bowel transversely with a double row of staples. The instrument does not divide the bowel, but a knife is passed along the staple line, leaving one end of the bowel open. End-to-end anastomoses may be created in the rectum with the end-to-end anastomosis (EEA) stapler. The preference for the type of stapled technique may in part be determined by the resection performed and the availability of the remaining bowel for stapler access.

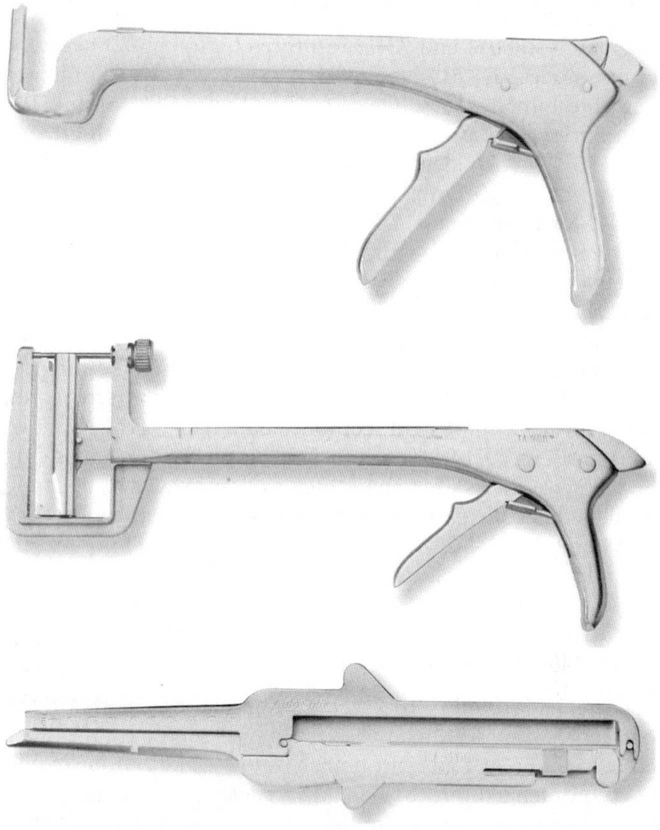
A B C

FIGURE 51.37. (A–C) Three kinds of surgical staplers. (Copyright © 2007 Covidien. All rights reserved. Reprinted with the permission of Covidien.)

Principles of Oncologic Resection

Radical surgery with curative intent is performed for the majority of colorectal cancers. The basic principles include complete abdominal exploration, gentle handling of the tumor, adequate tumor-free resection margins and level of mesenteric ligation to include the major vascular pedicles feeding the tumor along with its lymphatics, and en bloc resection of any organs or structures attached to the tumor.

Adequate lymphadenectomy has previously been defined as a minimum of 12 lymph nodes evaluated.[391] However, more recent evidence from the randomized trials of adjuvant chemotherapy for stage II and stage III colon cancer demonstrated improved survival associated with an increased number of lymph nodes evaluated. In the Intergroup 0089 trial of adjuvant 5FU and leucovorin, in stage II patients the identification of greater than 20 negative lymph nodes was associated with an 87% 5-year and 79% 10-year survival, compared to 80% and 73%, respectively, for 11–20 negative lymph nodes and 73% and 59%, respectively, for 10 or fewer negative lymph nodes. These compare with 90% 5- and 10-year survival, respectively, for stage III patients with greater than 40 lymph nodes evaluated and 74% and 64%, respectively, for 11–40 lymph nodes, and 67% and 56%, respectively, for fewer than 11 lymph nodes.[392] Clearly, improved survival is associated with improved lymph node evaluation, and adequate lymph node evaluation may require at least 14 to 20 lymph nodes in the resected specimen.[392–394]

Complete en bloc resection of involved adjacent structures is another important principle of cancer-directed surgery. It cannot be emphasized enough that organs and structures adherent to tumor will contain malignant tissue in the adhesions in over 40% of cases. If en bloc resection is not performed, the risk for recurrence and survival will be compromised.[395] This often requires preoperative preparation that may include a CT scan and determines the need for a multidisciplinary approach in the operating room.

Cancer of the Cecum, Ascending Colon, or Hepatic Flexure

For lesions located in the cecum or ascending colon, a right hemicolectomy to encompass the bowel served by the ileocolic, right colic, and right branch of the middle colic vessels is recommended (Fig. 51.38). After packing the small bowel toward the left side, the mobilization of the colon is begun by incising the parietal peritoneum from just below the terminal ileum toward the hepatic flexure. The right colon is elevated from the retroperitoneum and pulled medially and superiorly toward the left upper quadrant. Care is taken not to injure retroperitoneal structures such as the ureter, the gonadal vessels, the inferior vena cava, and the duodenum (Fig. 51.39).

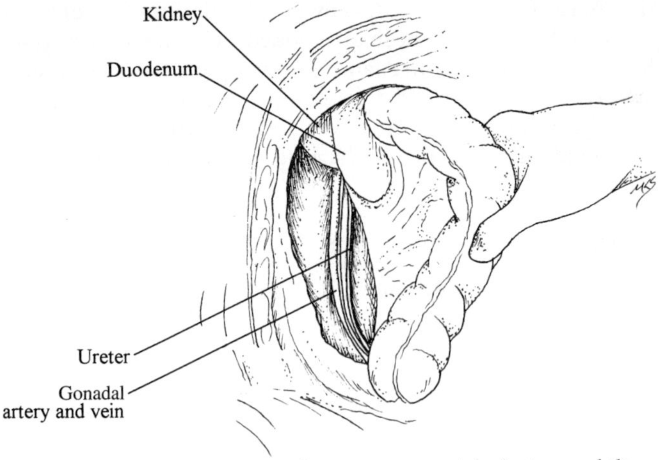

FIGURE 51.39. Retroperitoneal structures at risk during mobilization of the right colon. (Adapted from Gordon and Nivatvongs,[645] by permission of Taylor & Francis Group LLC.)

Peritoneal division is continued along the base of the small-bowel mesentery, around the hepatic flexure, and medially along the upper border of the transverse colon. Now, the stomach is pulled upward and the colon with the greater omentum downward so the lesser sac can be opened by dividing the gastrocolic ligament (Fig. 51.40). The medial aspect of the peritoneum is incised along the planned area of proximal and distal resection and across the top of the vessels to be transected such that they are displayed clearly. The greater omentum is divided vertically starting at the area of resection (Fig. 51.40). The vessels are divided after central ligation (Fig. 51.41). The small vessels adjacent to the small bowel and transverse colon at the level of the proposed transection are divided between clamps.

The two ends of bowel are now ready for division. The method of division depends on the planned anastomotic technique. Intestinal continuity can be established using staplers

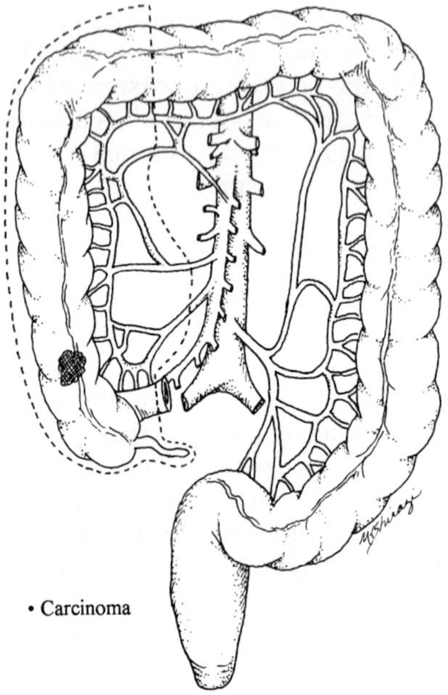

FIGURE 51.38. Extent of resection for cecal, ascending colon, or hepatic flexure carcinoma. (Adapted from Gordon and Nivatvongs,[645] by permission of Taylor & Francis Group LLC.)

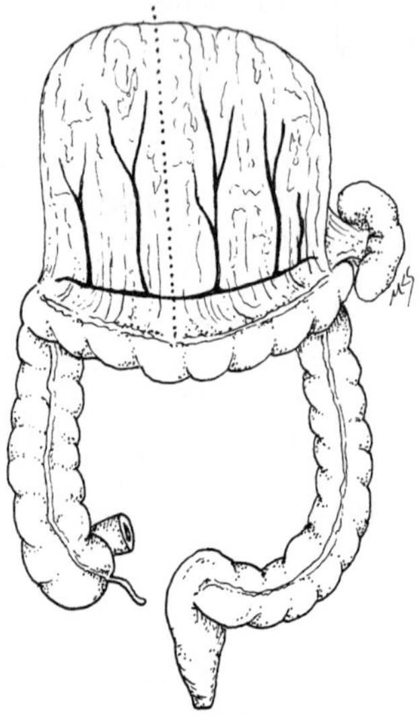

FIGURE 51.40. Division of the greater omentum along the axis of the colon for access to the lesser sac and transversely at the planned distal resection margin. (Adapted from Gordon and Nivatvongs,[645] by permission of Taylor & Francis Group LLC.)

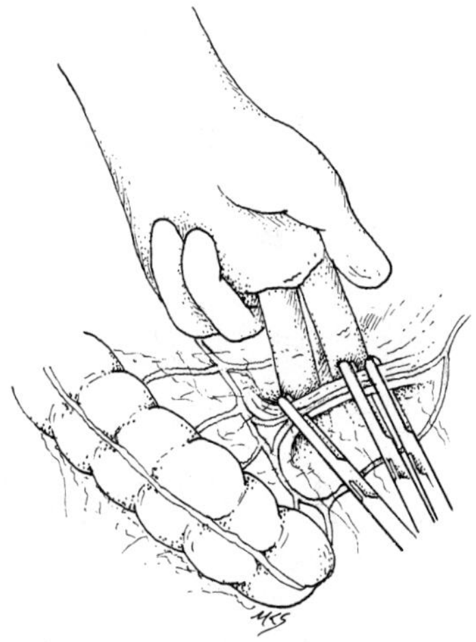

FIGURE 51.41. Division of the ileocolic vessels before transection of the bowel. (Adapted from Gordon and Nivatvongs,[645] by permission of Taylor & Francis Group LLC.)

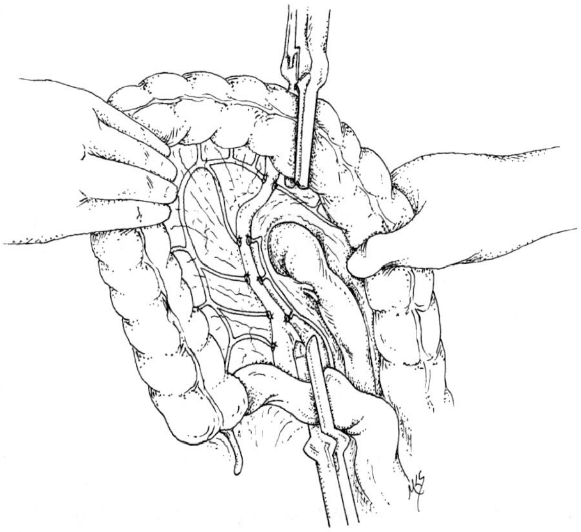

FIGURE 51.42. Division of the bowel with GIA staplers anticipating a stapled anastomosis. (Adapted from Gordon and Nivatvongs,[645] by permission of Taylor & Francis Group LLC.)

or a hand-suturing technique. Using either technique, a functional end-to-end anastomosis can be fashioned.

Staplers may be used to create a side-to-side functional end-to-end anastomosis. At each site of planned transection, the stapler is applied in the mesenteric antimesenteric plane, closed, and fired (Fig. 51.42). The staplers close and divide the bowel, allowing the specimen to be delivered without opening the intestines. The antimesenteric borders are aligned, and at each antimesenteric corner the staple line is excised, creating an enterotomy or colotomy adequate to insert the fork of a linear stapler. The instrument is inserted along the antimesenteric borders of the bowel to its full length to create a long anastomosis. After firing the instrument, the anastomosis is inspected for hemorrhage. The linear stapler is applied to hold the other staple lines in an open V position. By this maneuver, the area of anastomosis can be increased by as much as one-third. The instrument is fired, and excess tissue is cut away before release of the instrument to avoid injury to the anastomosis (Fig. 51.43). An alternative method utilizes two fires of the GIA stapler via enterotomies made within the specimen while it is in continuity with the remaining bowel.

The mesentery may be closed with running or interrupted sutures. With a large mesenteric defect typically associated with proximal bowel ligation, it is safe to leave the defect open. Some surgeons close the mesentery before construction of the anastomosis for ease and to decrease the chance of rotation of the ileum. The apex of the GIA staple line is reinforced with an absorbable suture to minimize tension at this point.

Using the staplers, an end-to-side anastomosis can be constructed by using an EEA circular stapler and one TA stapler. In that case, a purse-string instrument is applied on the terminal ileum next to a bowel clamp, and the bowel is divided between the two instruments. Alternatively, the bowel is divided between two bowel clamps, and a purse string is hand

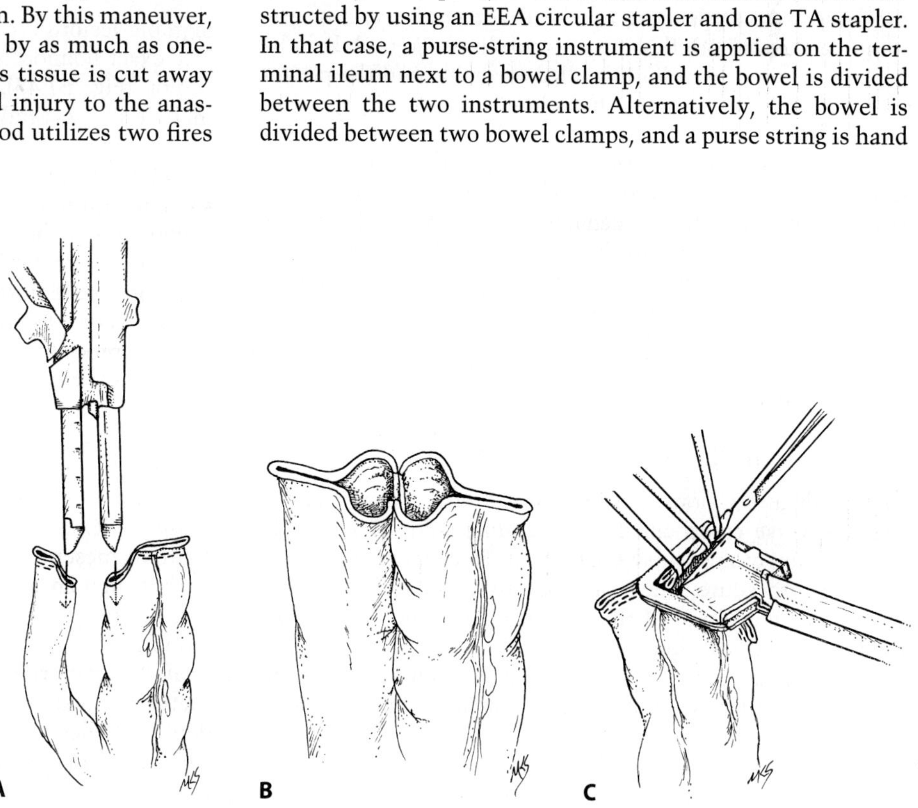

A B C

FIGURE 51.43. (A–C) Creation of a stapled anastomosis with the GIA and TA staplers. (Adapted from Gordon and Nivatvongs,[645] by permission of Taylor & Francis Group LLC.)

sewn in the proximal bowel. In either event, the detached anvil from the EEA stapler is inserted into the ileum, and the purse string is closed to avoid any spillage and to secure the anvil. The distal bowel is divided between two bowel clamps, and the specimen is removed. Now, the EEA stapler is inserted into the bowel lumen, and the central shaft is advanced through the medial taenia about 5 to 7 cm distal to the open end. The anvil is engaged and the anastomosis completed. The open end of the large bowel is then closed with a TA stapler. Again, the excess tissue is cut away before release of the instrument. The procedure is completed with closure of the mesentery.

For lesions involving the hepatic flexure, a more extended resection is indicated, including the right colon and proximal and midtransverse colon, including both branches of the middle colic artery (extended right hemicolectomy). Most of the time the procedure is started as a right hemicolectomy with the mobilization of the cecum, followed by mobilization of the ascending colon, hepatic flexure, transverse colon, and splenic flexure. Again, the method of bowel division depends on the preferred method of anastomoses.

Cancer of the Transverse Colon

Depending on the exact location of the tumor, the transverse colon is often resected, including either the hepatic or splenic flexure. As the resection needs to fulfill oncologic principles, the appropriate lymphatic drainage must be included. The lymphatic drainage may occur through the middle colic or the right or left colic branches. The general principle of all colon resections for cancer is to resect the tumor along with its two adjacent lymphovascular pedicles and associated bowel.

Generally, the operation is begun with division of the greater omentum from the greater curvature of the stomach, achieved by dividing the gastrocolic ligament and entering the lesser sac. Depending on the exact localization of the tumor, either or both flexures are mobilized. To mobilize the hepatic flexure, the colon is pulled medially, and the peritoneum is incised lateral to the colonic wall. As in the case of a right hemicolectomy, care must be taken not to injure the duodenum or the inferior vena cava. Mobilization of the splenic flexure is achieved by incising the lateral peritoneal attachments along the descending colon and mobilizing the colon out of the omentum that attaches to the colon and the spleen. The exact areas of transection are identified and freed circumferentially of mesentery and epiploic fat. The mesenteric vessels are identified and divided after ligation. The method of bowel division depends on the preferred method of anastomosis.

Cancer of the Splenic Flexure

Splenic flexure lesions require removal of the distal half of the transverse colon and the descending colon (Fig. 51.44). Mobilization of the transverse colon or descending colon may start this procedure. The gastrocolic ligament is divided, the colon is delivered out of the omentum, and the lateral peritoneum is incised along the descending colon. As in right colon mobilization, care is taken to avoid injury to the retroperitoneal structures (duodenum, splenic vein, pancreas, ureter, and gonadal vessels). After mobilization of the colon, the left colic artery is identified and ligated, and depending on the level of resection, the first sigmoidal vessels are divided as well. The left branch of the middle colic artery is usually not divided to ensure adequate blood supply to the remaining transverse colon. A tension-free anastomosis is performed between the transverse colon and the proximal sigmoid colon.

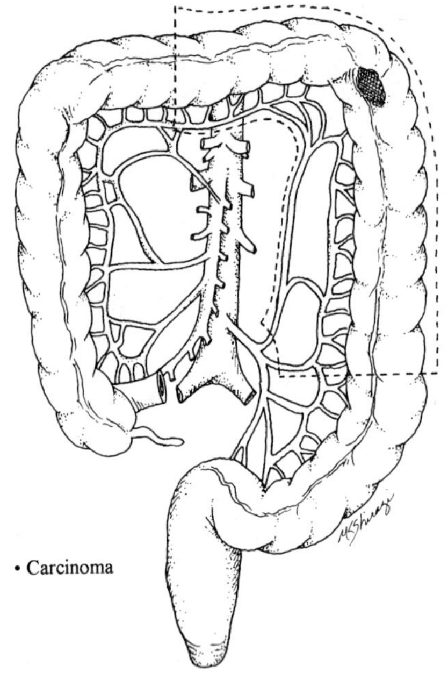

FIGURE 51.44. Extent of resection for a splenic flexure colon carcinoma. (Adapted from Gordon and Nivatvongs,[645] by permission of Taylor & Francis Group LLC.)

Cancer of the Sigmoid Colon

Sigmoid lesions are treated by removal of the sigmoid colon. The exact boundaries of resection depend on the level of the tumor (Fig. 51.45). Resections of higher sigmoid lesions include the descending–sigmoid junction, whereas resections for lower lesions include the recto–sigmoid junction.

The patient is placed in a modified lithotomy position so that simultaneous access can be obtained through the abdomen and the rectum. This access is necessary to allow the use of circular EEA stapling devices. Some surgeons, in addition to the normal bowel prep, perform irrigation of the rectum before the procedure at the time of surgery.

The procedure is started with packing the small bowel toward the right and upper abdomen. The sigmoid is pulled medially, and the peritoneum is incised along the lateral aspect of the colon from the pelvic rim to the splenic flexure. Releasing these attachments exposes the retroperitoneal structures such as the left ureter and the iliac and gonadal vessels. Next, the peritoneum over the medial aspect of the sigmoid mesentery is incised, exposing the underlying IMA with its branches. These are ligated just distal to the left colic origin. The distal line of resection is identified and mobilized circumferentially. Smaller vessels in the line of resection are ligated. Again, the method of bowel division depends on the method of anastomosis. However, many surgeons prefer the double-stapled technique to construct the lower anastomosis. This technique is described in detail under the topic of rectal cancer.

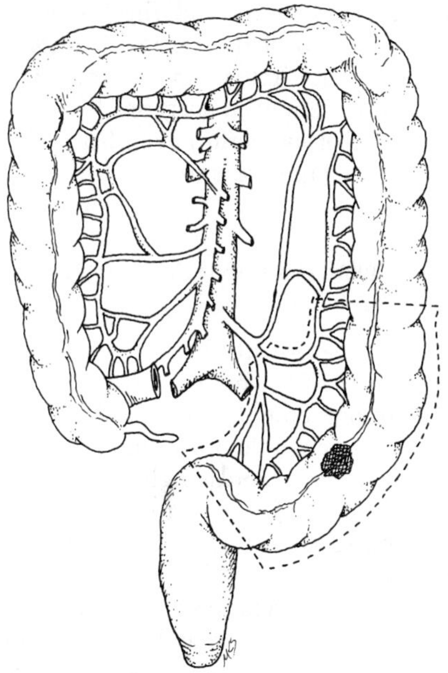

FIGURE 51.45. Extent of resection for sigmoid colon carcinoma. (Adapted from Gordon and Nivatvongs,[645] by permission of Taylor & Francis Group LLC.)

Total Abdominal Colectomy

The incidence of synchronous lesions (more than one carcinoma at different sites) is reported to be between 1.5% and 7.6%[396,397] (Fig. 51.46). Despite the presence of synchronous lesions, the overall prognosis is similar to patients with solitary lesions of the same stage as the worse of the two lesions (5-year survival by stage: 87% for stage I, 69% for stage II, 50% for stage III, and 14% for stage IV).[398] Depending on the distribution of the lesions, subtotal colectomy may be the treatment of choice for patients with synchronous lesions. If synchronous lesions are located in the same anatomical region, a conventional resection may be performed.

The patient is placed in a modified lithotomy position so that simultaneous access can be obtained through abdomen and rectum. The procedure is started as a right hemicolectomy, and the mobilization is continued to the hepatic flexure, transverse colon, splenic flexure, and descending and sigmoid colon. The rectum is not removed unless it has pathological lesions as well. When the rectum is removed, an ileoanal pouch procedure may be performed if intestinal continuity is to be restored.

Sentinel Lymph Node Mapping

Sentinel lymph node mapping has been successfully applied to the surgical management of malignant melanoma and breast cancer with a high sensitivity and specificity for identifying lymph nodes containing metastatic disease. However, although some authors have reported more than 90% success and 13% tumor upstaging with sentinel lymph node mapping for colorectal cancer, such good results have not been reproduced in a multiinstitutional trial sponsored by the Cancer and Leukemia Group B (CALGB) and other centers.[399–401] As a result, the technique remains investigational.

Laparoscopic Colectomy

Recent studies have confirmed that laparoscopy for colorectal carcinoma resection is technically feasible, is safe, and yields an equivalent number of resected lymph nodes and length of resected bowel when compared to open colectomy. Furthermore, it yields an equivalent oncologic result as open colectomy. The first adequately powered randomized trial was conducted in Barcelona, Spain. This trial randomized 219 patients to laparoscopic versus open colectomy for cancer and demonstrated oncologic equivalency and a trend toward improved oncologic outcomes in a small subset of stage III patients.[402]

The NCI-sponsored multicenter Clinical Outcomes of Surgical Therapy (COST) trial enrolled nearly 800 patients and definitively validated the oncologic safety and efficacy of laparoscopy for colon cancer. Laparoscopic-assisted colectomy for cancer was associated with equivalent recurrence-free and overall survival when compared to open surgery with no increase in wound recurrences.[403] Patient-related benefits included reduced length of hospital stay, decreased pain, faster resolution of ileus, improved cosmesis, and a small improvement in short-term quality of life.

The Medical Research Council-sponsored Conventional Versus Laparoscopic-Assisted Surgery in Patients With Colorectal Cancer (CLASICC) multicenter trial in the United Kingdom has finished accrual and has reported their short-term outcomes, which are oncologically equivalent for laparoscopic versus open colectomy for cancer.[404] Similar patient-related benefits as the COST trial were observed. The European multicenter Colon Carcinoma Laparoscopic or Open Resection (COLOR) trial is still ongoing.[405] An additional trial from Hong Kong demonstrated oncologic equiv-

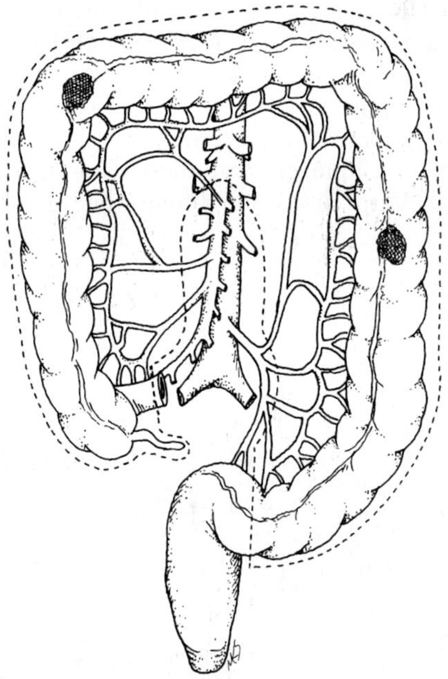

FIGURE 51.46. Total abdominal colectomy as might be performed for synchronous malignancies, colonic inertia, colonic Crohn's disease, or as a prophylactic measure for hereditary nonpolyposis colorectal cancer (HNPCC) or familial adenomatous polyposis (FAP) syndromes. (Adapted from Gordon and Nivatvongs,[645] by permission of Taylor & Francis Group LLC.)

alency with laparoscopy for sigmoid and rectosigmoid tumors.[406]

Laparoscopic-assisted approaches have consistently been associated with reductions in hospital stay, postoperative pain, and duration of postoperative ileus when compared to open surgery. However, the magnitude of these effects in randomized trials has been modest, approximately 20%–35%, and remains the subject of further investigation. Uncertain additional benefits of laparoscopy include potentially decreased morbidity, decreased convalescence, improved quality of life, and decreased costs.

Laparoscopic colectomy for colorectal cancer is one of the best examples of the use of a rigorous approach in the evaluation of the safety and efficacy of a new technique in the surgical literature. With data from the reported randomized control trials and the anticipated reports from additional large trials, laparoscopic colectomy for colorectal cancer has been validated and established as an important treatment modality for colorectal malignancies. It should be noted, however, that experienced surgeons who have demonstrated proficiency in laparoscopic colectomy for cancer obtained the results shown in these trials. However, to achieve these results, laparoscopic approaches to colon cancer must adhere to the same oncologic principles that guide open surgery and have been outlined above. The experience of the surgeon in both conventional open colorectal surgery and advanced laparoscopic techniques may be important variables in ensuring oncologic adequacy.

Cancer of the Rectum

Natural History

About 30% of all colorectal cancers occur in the rectum. In 2005, the American Cancer Society estimated 40,000 new cases in the United States. Historically, rectal cancer surgery has been associated with a high rate of local recurrence (30%–40%) due to a poor understanding of oncologic surgical techniques and the widespread use of conventional blunt dissection to mobilize the rectum. In 1982, Heald characterized the technique of total mesorectal excision, which emphasized sharp dissection along the avascular planes between the presacral fascia and the fascia propria of the mesorectum. In studies of the standardization of this technique, local recurrence rates have decreased to less than 10%.[407] However, experienced surgeons have always utilized the avascular plane of dissection even before Heald's formal description of the technique and had similar rates of local recurrence.[408]

Selection of Operation and Assessment of Resectability

Rectal cancer has historically been treated with abdominoperineal resection (APR), which removes the whole rectum and anus. With improvements in surgical technique and with advances in stapler technology, sphincter preservation with low anterior resection is increasingly performed. Abdominoperineal resection is now reserved for lesions of distal rectum that are too close to the dentate line to allow for coloanal reconstruction. (Fig. 51.47). In highly selected patients with well-differentiated superficial lesions without nodal involvement (uT1N0), local excision may be appropriate. Thus, preoperative staging is critical to the selection of the appropriate operation. General guidelines about staging were discussed earlier in this chapter.

Low Anterior Resection

For low anterior resection, the patient is placed in a modified lithotomy position so that simultaneous access can be obtained through abdomen and rectum. The operating table is set in a slight Trendelenburg position for better exposure of pelvic structures. After a lower midline incision, the small bowel is packed into the upper right abdomen, and the sigmoid colon is mobilized by incising the lateral peritoneal reflection. The sigmoid colon is elevated from its developmental attachments between the splenic flexure and the rectum without injuring the retroperitoneal structures, such as the ureter and the gonadal and iliac vessels. Further mobilization of the proximal bowel may become necessary to accomplish a tension-free anastomosis. The peritoneal dissection is continued distally parallel to the rectum until the cul-de-sac is reached.

Next, the peritoneum on the right side of the sigmoid mesentery is incised from the proximal resection margin to

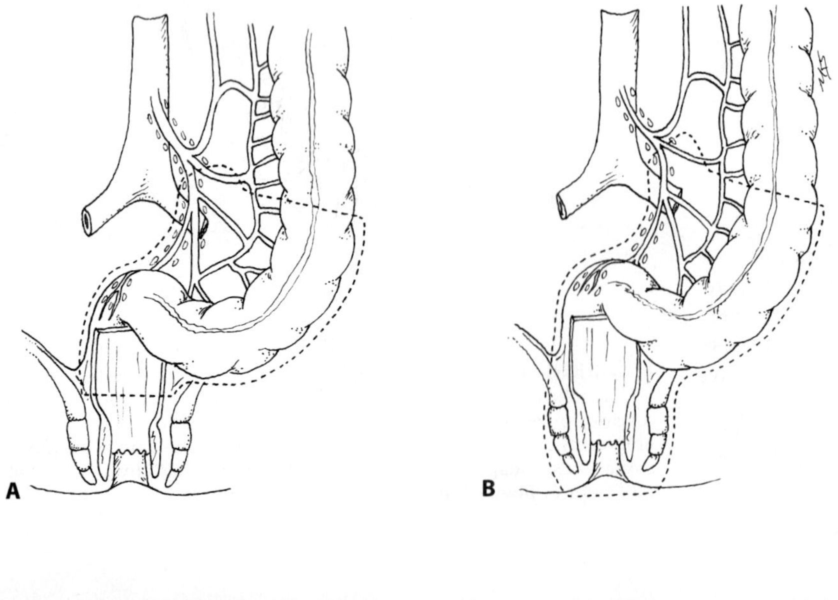

FIGURE 51.47. Extent of resection with either **(A)** low anterior resection of the rectum or **(B)** abdominal perineal resection for rectal adenocarcinoma. (Adapted from Gordon and Nivatvongs,[645] by permission of Taylor & Francis Group LLC.)

the distal resection margin in a fashion identical to the left side. The superior rectal artery is identified and ligated at its origin from the IMA just distal to the takeoff of the left colic artery. There is currently insufficient evidence to recommend routine high ligation of the IMA at its origin from the aorta; however, proximal ligation of the IMA and high ligation of the IMV at the inferior border of the pancreas may be necessary to obtain adequate bowel mobilization to perform a distal colorectal or coloanal anastomosis.

After ligation of the vessels, the colon may be divided proximally at the site of subsequent anastomosis (generally, the junction between the descending and sigmoid colon). The sigmoid and rectum are pulled taut anteriorly toward the symphysis pubis so the retrorectal space can be entered. This avascular space of areolar tissue between the presacral fascia and the fascia propria of the mesorectum (mesorectal plane) is entered just above the promontory of the sacrum without damaging the hypogastric nerve plexus and trunks. The plane should be further developed caudally and laterally sharply with electrocautery or scissors.

Anterior mobilization of the rectum is achieved in men by incising the rectovesical reflection, and further mobilization is continued in the plane between the seminal vesicles and Denonvilliers fascia behind the prostate (see Fig. 51.5). In women, the peritoneum over the rectovaginal reflection is incised and the rectum is separated from the vagina.

At this stage, the rectum is mobilized anteriorly away from the prostate and posteriorly to the tip of the coccyx. The rectum remains attached laterally by the lateral ligaments to the pelvis, which can then be divided easily with electrocautery at this stage. The lateral ligaments contain ascending branches of the middle rectal vessels, which are usually controlled with electrocautery or ligature. Care should be taken during the lateral dissection to avoid injury to the pelvic parasympathetic plexus containing the fibers of the nervi erigentes, which are important for erectile function. For more proximal lesions of the rectum, the distal mesorectum may be left in place.

When adequate mobilization has been achieved, the rectum is divided. The goal is to transect the rectum at least 2 cm inferior, and the mesorectum at least 5 cm inferior, to the lower end of the carcinoma. The mode of transection depends on the method of anastomosis, which is usually performed with the circular stapling device. For very distal rectal lesions, the rectum may be detached at the dentate line, preserving the internal sphincters, and a hand-sewn coloanal anastomosis may be performed. In experienced hands, this technique permits the restoration of intestinal continuity for selected lesions up to 2 cm from the dentate line.

Construction of a Double-Stapled Anastomosis

The proximal bowel end is cleared circumferentially of epiploic fat and mesentery for 1 cm at the proposed line of resection. A purse-string suture is applied using a specially designed fenestrated clamp, a fully automated disposable purse-string clamp, or hand sewing with monofilament suture. The bowel is divided with a knife. The anvil is detached from the EEA instrument and inserted into the proximal bowel, and the purse string is tied. The rectum is divided distal to the tumor with a TA stapler (Fig. 51.48). The instrument is fired, a right-angle bowel clamp is applied distal to the carcinoma, and the rectum is transected just proximal to the stapler, right along the TA instrument, with a knife. The EEA instrument is inserted into the anus and advanced to the TA staple line. The trocar is advanced through the staple line and engaged with the anvil in the proximal colon. The anvil is approximated to the cartridge, and the instrument is fired. Care must be taken not to entrap sponges, mesentery, bladder, vagina, or any other tissue. The instrument is opened slightly and removed carefully. The anastomosis is palpated and inspected with a rigid sigmoidoscope; air is insufflated via the rigid sigmoidoscope with the proximal bowel occluded, and the pelvis filled with saline in an attempt to identify an air leak.

In a slight modification of the double-stapled technique, a right-angle clamp is placed distal to the carcinoma, and the rectum is divided, leaving the stump open. A hand-sewn purse-string suture is then placed on the stump; this can be done transabdominally or transanally in very low lesions. The appropriate size of EEA instrument is inserted through the anus in the closed position and advanced until the cartridge is visualized. The central shaft is advanced, and the distal purse-string suture is tied. The anvil is engaged into the central shaft, and the instrument is closed and fired.

Abdominoperineal Resection

The APR is a combination of a very low anterior resection with a complete perineal excision of the anus and rectum. The procedure is often performed as a two-team or synchronous combined operation. In preparation for the procedure, the patient is positioned in the lithotomy position; the buttocks are retracted with tape laterally to permit better exposure of the perineum. In the male, the external genitalia also are retracted out of the way. The abdominal part is identical to the low anterior resection with the only exception that rectal mobilization is continued as low as possible, ideally down to the pelvic floor.

When the abdominal operator has confirmed that the rectum is resectable, an elliptical incision is made to encompass an adequate margin of tissue. The skin edges are then grasped, and the subcutaneous tissue is divided with cautery. The dissection is continued into the fat of the ischioanal fossa. The inferior rectal vessels on each side are either ligated or controlled with electrocautery.

Sharp dissection is carried deeper posteriorly toward the tip of the coccyx until it is reached. The levator ani muscle is divided just anterior to the coccyx to enter the presacral plane where the abdominal plane has led. This plane is continued laterally on each side. At this time, the specimen may be delivered into the perineal wound to improve exposure for the anterior dissection. In men, the plane between the rectum and the prostate is developed. This is often the most challenging part of the operation as great caution should be taken not to injure the male urethra or the prostate. In women, the plane between the vagina and the rectum is developed.

Once this dissection is completed, the diseased rectum can be completely removed. It is important to avoid the formation of a "waist" in the specimen at the level of the pelvic floor. The plane of dissection from the abdomen will direct the surgeon to bowel wall as the mesorectum tapers away. It is important to avoid the temptation to narrow the plane of dissection as it will increase the risk of compromising the radial margins. The levators should be divided widely, removing the perirectal tissue en bloc with the rectum.

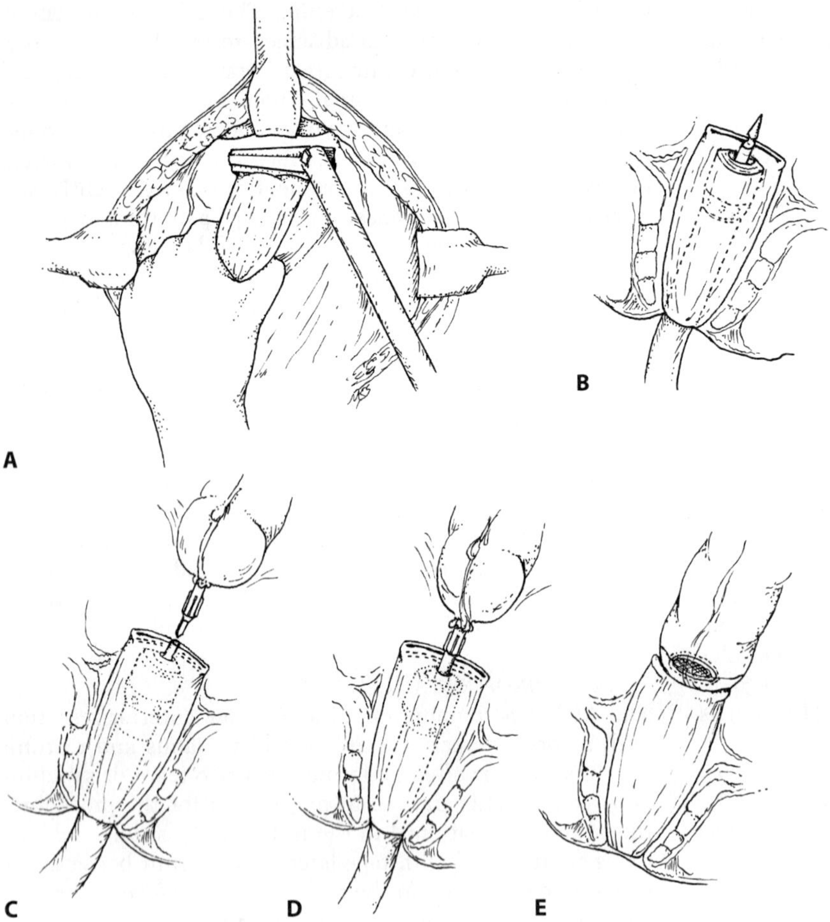

FIGURE 51.48A–E. (A–E) The rectum is divided with a TA stapler. The trocar of an EEA stapler is advanced through the staple line, the anvil is engaged, and the instrument is closed and fired. (Adapted from Gordon and Nivatvongs,[645] by permission of Taylor & Francis Group LLC.)

Hemostasis is secured, and the wound is irrigated copiously with saline. A suction catheter is placed in the pelvis and brought out through a separate stab wound on the abdominal wall. The pelvic floor musculature and ischioanal fat are approximated with interrupted sutures. The skin is closed loosely to allow small amounts of fluid to drain.

A disk of skin is excised at the premarked colostomy site, and the subcutaneous fat is divided with electrocautery. The anterior fascia is scored and notched in a cruciate fashion, the rectus muscle is separated, and the posterior fascia and the peritoneum are incised. The opening should admit two to three fingers loosely. The proximal sigmoid or descending colon, transected earlier with a GIA stapler or between bowel clamps at the site chosen for the colostomy, is brought through the opening. The colostomy is matured after closing the abdominal incision using interrupted absorbable suture through the full thickness of the bowel wall. A colostomy bag and skin barrier are placed around the stoma.

Local Excision

Generally, lesions within 8 cm of the anal verge that are less than 4 cm, mobile, not ulcerated, well differentiated, and are without evidence of nodal involvement are considered for transanal excision. Nodal involvement may be as high as 18% in T1 lesions and up to 37% in T2 lesions, leaving about 5% of rectal cancers suitable for attempt at cure with local excision alone[409] (Table 51.20). Furthermore, the risk for recurrence after local excision is high, 18% in a review of 16 published series in which local excision was used for tumors within 6 cm from the anal verge.[410] The role of local excision for T2 lesions followed by chemoradiation or radiation has been studied in two phase II multicenter trials as well as other, mostly retrospective, reports.

The CALGB trial evaluated 177 patients with a median 48 months of follow-up. Four of 59 patients with T1 lesions

TABLE 51.20.
Results for Selected Recent Series of Local Excision of Rectal Cancer Alone with Intent to Cure.

Author	*N*	*Stage*	*Recurrence*	*Survival (5-year actuarial)*	*Follow-up (months)*
Frazee[492]	25	T1	8%	100%[a]	30
Bleday[493]	22	T1	9%		40.5
Ishizaki[494]	15	T1 (13), T2 (2)	6.7%	85%[a]	36
Chakravarti[495]	52	T1 (44), T2 (8)	28%	66%[b]	51
Mellgren[496]	108	T1 (69), T2 (39)	18% T1, 45% T2	72% T1, 65% T2	53
Endreseth[497]	35	T1	12%	70%	24–97

[a]Survival at follow-up.
[b]Disease-free survival.

TABLE 51.21.
Results for Selected Recent Series of Local Excision of Rectal Cancer with Postoperative Adjuvant Therapy.

Author	*N*	*Stage*	*XRT*	*Chemotherapy*	*Recurrence*	*Survival (5-year actuarial)*	*Follow-up (months)*
Bailey[498]	24	T1, T2	45–50 Gy	None	8%	90%	44
Bleday[493]	26	T2 (21), T3 (5)	54 Gy	5FU	7.7%		40.5
Wagman[499]	39	T1 (6), T2 (25), T3 (8)	45–54 Gy	5FU (66%)	21%	77%	41
Steele[411]	51	T2	54 Gy	5FU	13.7%	85%[a]	48
Le Voyer[500]	35	T1 (15), T2 (15), T3 (4)	53 Gy (for >T1/poor histology)	5FU (40%)	11.4%	91%	46
Chakravarti[495]	47	T1 (14), T2 (33)	45–64.8 Gy	5FU (54%)	10%	74%	51
Russell[412]	51	T1 (13), T2 (25), T3 (13)	50–56 Gy (for >T1/poor histology)	5FU	13.7%	75%	73

XRT, external beam radiation therapy.
[a]Six-year actuarial.

(2 local, 1 local and distant, 1 distant) and 10 of 51 patients with T2 lesions (5 local, 2 local and distant, 3 distant) recurred. Overall and disease-free survival rates were 85% and 78%, respectively.[411] The Radiation Therapy Oncology Group (RTOG) protocol 89-02 utilized a similar strategy, with a median follow-up of 6.1 years in 52 patients with T1/T2 rectal cancers, and demonstrated a 4% local failure for T1 lesions and 16% local failure rate for T2 lesions. An additional 3 of 13 (23%) patients with T3 disease treated with local excision and chemoradiation were noted to have local failure.[412] We have reported a 45% local recurrence rate after local excision for T2 lesions without adjuvant chemoradiation with no recurrences noted after local excision for T2 lesions followed by adjuvant chemoradiation[413] (Table 51.21).

The patient is positioned in the prone jackknife position or lithotomy position for posterior lesions. A Foley catheter is placed into the bladder, and the anorectum is irrigated with diluted povidone iodine solution. A line of excision is marked with electrocautery around the lesion with at least a 1-cm grossly normal mucosa (Fig. 51.49). The incision is continued full thickness starting at the inferior end. This end is grasped with an Allis clamp, and the incision is continued all the way around, exposing the perirectal fat. The wound may be closed transversely using absorbable sutures or may be left open. No packing or drain is necessary. The specimen is carefully pinned on cardboard and handed to the pathologist for accurate staging.

Under active investigation is the role of local excision or observation in patients with T3 lesions who achieve a clinical

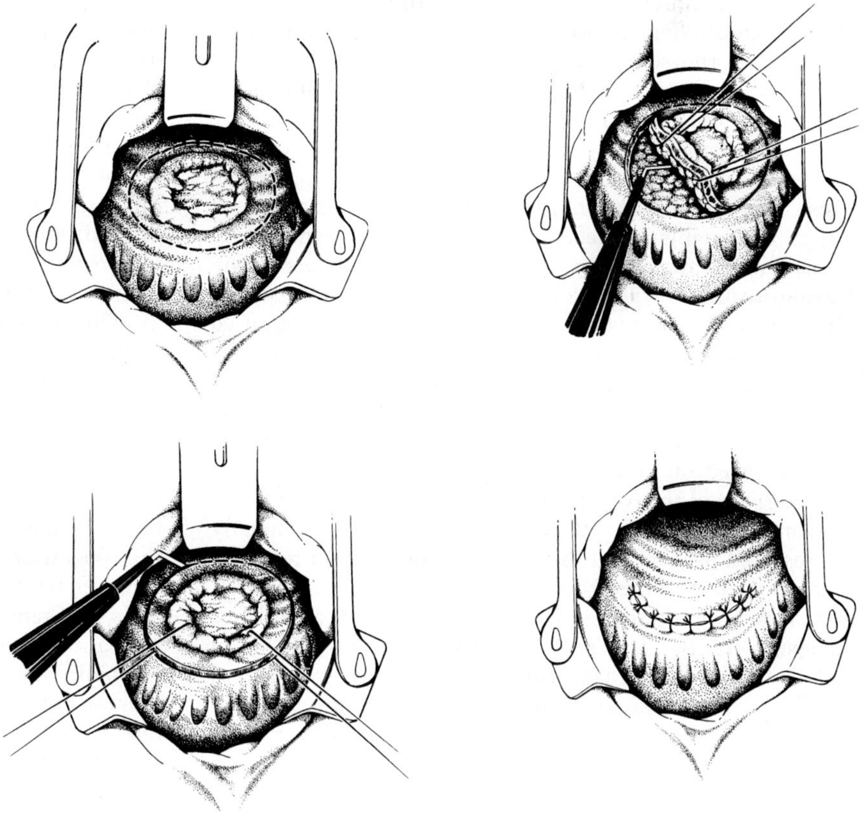

FIGURE 51.49. Local excision of rectal cancer with electrocautery. (From Bailey et al.,[498] with permission.)

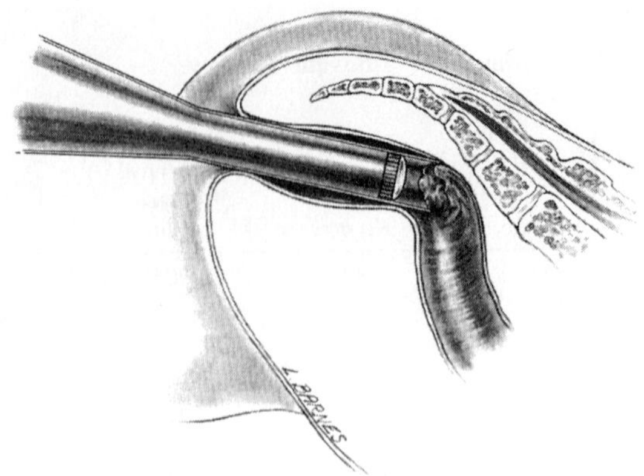

FIGURE 51.50. Endocavitary radiation for rectal tumors may be delivered as primary therapy and pre- or postexcision. We prefer postexcisional therapy because the tumor burden is minimal and the pathological staging is accurate. (From Corman,[649] with permission, © 1998, Lippincott, Williams and Wilkins.)

complete response to neoadjuvant chemoradiation. The difficulty arises in the insensitivity of the clinical examination in determining the presence of residual carcinoma and in the lack of the ability to evaluate the lymph nodes. Although good results have been reported in single-institution series, this strategy should only be performed under rigorous investigational protocols.[414,415]

Transanal destruction with electrocautery or contact radiation therapy may also be used for palliative control of the tumor within the pelvis. Papillon has popularized transanal endocavitary radiotherapy.[416] This treatment involves delivery of radiation via an endocavitary cone placed transanally directly onto the tumor. Two courses of 3000 cGy are delivered in this manner 3 weeks apart, and the pelvis is treated with 4500 cGy (Fig. 51.50). The radiation therapy may be delivered as the sole treatment or may be combined with excisional therapy as a means to maximize the radiation delivered to the tumor bed.

Transanal Endoscopic Microsurgery

Buess introduced TEM in 1983 for the local treatment of benign and malignant rectal tumors.[417] The system uses a special binocular rectoscope, which allows continuous carbon dioxide insufflation to keep the rectum open for exposure. The surgeon operates with instruments similar to those used in laparoscopic surgery. Vision is provided through a magnifying binocular optical system. The procedure is used for lesions in the upper, middle, and low rectum. The excision is done with electrocautery. The defect is closed with suture. Silver clips are used on either end instead of tying knots in the limited space of the rectum. Malignant lesions located above 8 cm anteriorly or higher than 12 cm posteriorly are generally not resected because full-thickness excision would result in leakage of gas into the abdominal cavity and loss of insufflation. However, these injuries may be repaired directly or transperitoneally. The principal advantages of TEM can include improved visualization and the ability to access lesions within the proximal rectum. Complication rates are low and are similar to those occurring with direct local excision.[418,419]

Special Situations in Colorectal Cancer

Obstructing Tumors

Colon cancer is the most common cause of large-bowel obstruction. This complication occurs as a presenting manifestation in up to 15% to 20% of patients with colorectal cancer.[420] The incidence of obstruction correlates with advancing patient age and is most commonly seen with left-sided colon cancer. In a study of 115 obstructing carcinomas, 37% were right-sided, and 63% were left-sided. Only 4% were Dukes A lesions; 15% already had distant metastases. Obstructing colon cancers are generally caused by larger tumors and have a poorer prognosis. This effect is also related to tumor location. Obstructing right-sided tumors were associated with a decreased disease-free survival, whereas obstructing left-sided tumors were not.[421] The treatment is dependent on the location of the obstruction. Primary resection and anastomosis generally treat right-sided and transverse tumors. A diverting colostomy or ileostomy is rarely needed. The anastomosis can be performed using either handsuturing or stapling techniques. The leak rate should not exceed 3% with either technique.

The treatment of descending and more distal tumors is more complex and controversial. Historically, there are three procedures: the three-stage procedure, the Hartmann's procedure, and the subtotal colectomy with primary anastomosis (Fig. 51.51). The three-stage operation with a transverse colostomy, as an initial procedure, followed by a resection and anastomosis and finally by closure of the colostomy, is generally of historical interest only. However, if the patient is too sick to tolerate a definitive procedure, this is certainly an option. Nonetheless, the procedure has a mortality rate of about 10% and a morbidity rate ranging between 20% and 37%. Complications related to the stoma range between 6% and 44%.[422,423]

The second, and more commonly utilized, option is resection of the colon and tumor, proximal colostomy, and oversewing of the distal bowel—commonly referred to as a Hartmann's procedure, which is incorrect because that procedure is for rectal cancer in particular. Alternatively, if the distal bowel is of adequate length, it may be brought up to the abdominal wall, opened, and sutured to the skin as a mucous fistula. Overall operative mortality is about 10%. Morbidity of 44% was reported in one series, with hospital stay ranging between 17 and 30 days.[422] Colostomy closure rates are approximately 60%.

The decision to perform an anastomosis in the setting of colonic obstruction is based on the intraoperative appearance of the bowel. An anastomosis should not be performed with markedly distended and dilated bowel.

Subtotal colectomy with primary anastomosis is a one-stage approach that has been validated by a prospective randomized trial comparing subtotal colectomy to on-table lavage for malignant left-sided obstructing tumors.[424] Although this operation seems more extensive, good results can be achieved with a single shorter hospitalization, no stoma problems, and removal of possible synchronous proximal lesions. Mortality rates are as low as 3% in experienced hands, and morbidity ranges between 6% and 31%, competitive with the more accepted resection and colostomy procedure. The leak rate ranges between 0% and 4.5%, and the hospital stay is considerably shorter than with a two-stage approach.[424] These

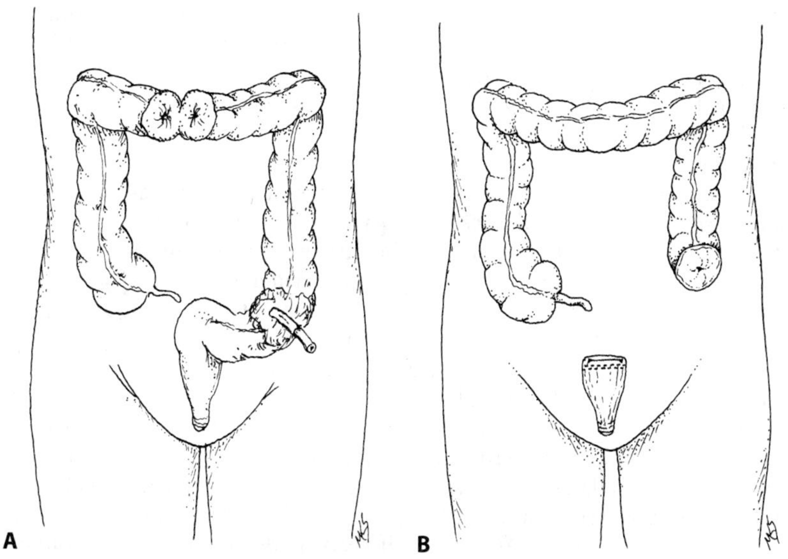

FIGURE 51.51. (A) The three-stage procedure for distal obstruction, whether it be for malignancy or inflammation, has largely been abandoned. The two most common procedures are the classic Hartmann's procedure (B) and subtotal colectomy and ileocolic or ileorectal anastomosis, depending on the level of obstruction. (Adapted from Gordon and Nivatvongs,[645] by permission of Taylor & Francis Group LLC.)

data all suggest that a subtotal colectomy and primary anastomosis is an excellent approach in the patient with an obstructing colon cancer on the left side.

Perforated Colon Cancer

Perforation of colorectal cancer is associated with a poor prognosis and a high recurrence rate. About 3% to 9% of patients with colorectal carcinoma present with a perforation as their initial manifestation. Two-thirds present with localized perforation and abscess, while about one-third present with free perforation and peritonitis. When patients with perforated colon cancers present with localized or diffuse peritonitis, the primary objective is resuscitation of the patient.

Once the patient has been stabilized, the tumor should be resected en bloc with involved adjacent structures utilizing the same surgical principles as for nonperforated tumors. The tumor itself may be perforated, or there may be a right-sided perforation with a left-sided tumor, and the perforated segment should be resected as well. If resection is not possible due to the inflammatory conditions or patient instability, proximal diversion with drainage of the perforation should be performed. Whenever possible, the perforated bowel segment should be resected at the initial operation.

Anastomosis is feasible in many patients and should be accompanied by a protective proximal stoma in most cases. If the patient has generalized peritonitis, colectomy, colostomy formation, and oversewing of the distal bowel or mucous fistula creation should be considered. In the case of a perforation remote from the diseased segment, a subtotal colectomy should be considered as the therapy of choice. In the event that definitive resection must be deferred, the drainage tract must be completely excised along with the primary tumor. Patients with perforated or incompletely resected tumors may benefit from adjuvant external beam radiation, and surgical clips should be placed in the tumor bed at the time of resection to help direct radiotherapy.[425]

Adjuvant Therapy: Colon Cancer

Most patients with colon cancer present with disease that appears localized and can be completely resected with surgery. However, almost 33% of patients undergoing curative resection will relapse with recurrent disease secondary to occult microscopic metastasis. Adjuvant therapy is administered to treat and hopefully eradicate this residual micrometastatic disease. Until recently, 5FU was the only effective agent for colon carcinoma, with response rates of 15% to 30% in patients with advanced disease. In the past 5 years, several new agents have shown excellent activity in colorectal cancer, including irinotecan, oxaliplatin, and various biologic agents.

Chemotherapy

The use of adjuvant chemotherapy for patients with high-risk colorectal cancer has been the subject of numerous investigations within the United States and around the world. A pilot prospective randomized study comparing 5FU/levamisole, levamisole, and surgery alone conducted by the North Central Cancer Treatment Group (NCCTG) and the Mayo Clinic was the first to demonstrate improved 5-year disease-free survival with 5FU and levamisole given for 1 year after curative resection for stage III colon cancer.[426] These results were confirmed by the landmark NCI-Intergroup protocol 0035, a larger study comparing the same treatment arms. At a median of 3 years after curative resection for stage III colon cancer, adjuvant treatment with 5FU and levamisole decreased the risk of cancer recurrence by 41% and the overall death rate by 36% compared to surgery alone or surgery and levamisole.[427] Based on these results, the National Institutes of Health Consensus Conference in 1990 recommended that all patients with stage III colon carcinoma receive adjuvant chemotherapy with 5FU and levamisole.

At the same time that 5FU and levamisole were being developed in the adjuvant setting, preclinical models suggested that leucovorin modulated the effects of 5FU, and this combination was being used in a number of regimens in the metastatic setting.[428] Initial efficacy of this combination in the adjuvant setting was demonstrated in two trials. The NSABP (National Surgical Adjuvant Breast and Bowel Project) C-04 trial compared 5-FU/LV (leucovorin) to 5FU/levamisole and 5FU/LV/levamisole. Duration of therapy for this trial was

1 year. The results showed that the 5FU/LV combination was superior to 5FU/levamisole, with disease-free survival of 65% versus 60% ($P = .04$) and a trend toward improved overall survival of 74% versus 69%, respectively ($P = .06$). The 5FU/LV/levamisole combination did not improve outcome but had marked increased toxicity.[429] The Intergroup protocol 0089 was a second trial that demonstrated a 30% improvement in 5-year survival when compared to surgery alone. Furthermore, this study showed that patients receiving 6 months of 5FU, leucovorin, and levamisole had a 5-year survival rate of 67% compared to 63% for those patients who received 5FU and levamisole for 12 months.[392]

A number of new agents have become available as important first-line agents for the adjuvant therapy of colon cancer. Capecitabine is a drug with rapid GI absorption that undergoes a three-step enzymatic conversion to 5FU in tumor tissue. When used in first-line treatment of metastatic colorectal cancer, it was associated with a better toxicity profile than 5FU. The phase III X-ACT trial investigated the use of capecitabine in the adjuvant setting for resected stage III colon cancer and noted an improved safety profile when compared to bolus 5FU and leucovorin with significantly less diarrhea, nausea/vomiting, stomatitis, and neutropenia. Capecitabine was associated with an increased risk for severe hand-and-foot syndrome.[430]

Irinotecan has shown significant activity in metastatic colorectal cancer, and its use in the adjuvant setting has been studied by several trials. The most important are the CALGB C89803 trial and European PETACC-3 trial. Addition of irinotecan has been associated with an increased 60-day mortality of 2.5% versus 0.8% with 5FU alone; therefore, irinotecan currently does not have a role in first-line adjuvant therapy for colon cancer.

Oxaliplatin, a new platinum derivative with activity against colorectal cancer, has shown impressive antitumor activity against advanced colorectal cancer. The multicenter international study of oxaliplatin, 5FU, and leucovorin in the adjuvant treatment of colon cancer (MOSAIC) trial has demonstrated that 3-year disease-free survival was significantly better with the addition of oxaliplatin ($85\,mg/m^2$) given every 2 weeks for 12 cycles versus 5FU/LV alone (78.2% vs. 72.9%, $P = .002$).

The monoclonal antibodies to the epidermal growth factor receptor (EGFR)-mediated pathways (cetuximab, panitumomab, and others) and to the vascular-endothelial growth factor (VEGF) family of glycoproteins (bevacizumab) have been effective in the metastatic setting and are under investigation in the adjuvant setting.

While adjuvant therapy has been proven to benefit patients with stage III disease, adjuvant therapy in patients with stage II disease remains controversial. While many of the adjuvant trials included patients with stage II disease, subgroup analysis showed trends toward benefit without reaching statistical significance. This issue has been addressed in three meta-analyses from NSABP, NCCTG, and IMPACT (International Multicenter Pooled Analysis of Colon Cancer Trials). All have suggested marginal improvements in disease-free and overall survival with 5FU and leucovorin in stage II colon cancer patients. Adjuvant chemotherapy in stage II patients provides a relative improvement in overall 5-year survival comparable to that of stage III patients (approximately 30% relative improvement). However, the absolute improvement in overall survival was only 2%–7%. Therefore, the routine use of adjuvant chemotherapy for stage II patients is still not recommended. Generally, patients with stage II disease are offered chemotherapy if adverse prognostic features such as lymphovascular invasion, T4 status, obstruction, or poor differentiation are present. The determination of molecular and genetic prognostic markers that will be useful in selecting those stage II patients who would benefit most from routine use of adjuvant therapy is an area of active investigation.

Adjuvant Therapy: Rectal Cancer

Adjuvant therapy for locally advanced rectal cancer is comprised of radiation to the pelvis and chemotherapy. Radiation therapy can reduce the risk for local failure, and concurrent chemotherapy is used to improve the radiation sensitivity of the tumor. Subsequent adjuvant chemotherapy completes the course of treatment and improves survival. It can be given preoperatively or postoperatively. Although there is general agreement that radiation therapy has an important role in the treatment of rectal cancer, the studies of these various modalities have noted wide variations in the technique of surgery and in the delivery of the radiotherapy. Currently, preoperative chemoradiation is indicated for lesions clinically staged T3–T4 or N1 either by preoperative endorectal ultrasound or cross-sectional imaging. Lesions located in the upper rectum are treated selectively with this approach.

The potential benefits of preoperative radiation are (1) large tumors may shrink, increasing resectability of the tumor; (2) radiation therapy works better in well-oxygenated tissues, and the postoperative tissue may be relatively hypoxic; (3) surgical complications may lead to a long delay in therapy; (4) preoperative radiation minimizes the risk of radiating the small bowel, which may be fixed in the pelvis after surgery; and (5) a healthy, nonirradiated neorectum is used for reconstruction. The disadvantages are possible overtreatment due to preoperative overstaging, loss of accurate pathological staging at the time of resection because of "downstaging," and risk of increased operative complications secondary to radiation injury.

The results for randomized trials of preoperative radiation and postoperative radiation are presented in Tables 51.22 and 51.23, respectively. There are two particularly notable European trials of preoperative radiotherapy. The Swedish Rectal Cancer Trial of short-course radiotherapy (25 Gy in five fractions, 1 week), followed by curative resection compared with curative surgery alone is the only study to show a significant survival advantage with the addition of radiotherapy.[431] The local recurrence rate and 9-year disease-specific survival were 11% and 74%, respectively, versus 27% and 65%, respectively, for the control group. A limitation of this study compared to more recent trials is the lack of surgical quality control, which is thought to be the reason for the high local recurrence rate in the control group. This was addressed in the Dutch Colorectal Cancer Group trial, in which over 1800 patients with rectal cancer located within 15 cm from the anal verge were randomized to receive preoperative short-course radiotherapy followed by TME versus TME alone. The local recurrence rate in the surgery-alone group was 8.2%. Preoperative radiotherapy improved this to 2.4%. However, there was no difference in overall survival. Also, subgroup analysis

TABLE 51.22.
Results of Randomized Trials of Preoperative Radiotherapy (Level I Evidence).

Overall Trial (author)	*No. of patients*	*Dose (Gy/Fractions)*	*Dukes stage C (%)*	*Local recurrence (%)*	*Distant metastases (%)*	*5-year survival (%)*
MRC 1[501] (1984)	824	Control	46	No difference	No difference	38
		5/1	45	41		
		20/10	36[a]			40
VASOG 2[502] (Higgins, Humphrey, and Dweight, 1986)	361	Control	41			42
		31.5/18	35			43
EORTC[503] (Gerard et al., 1988)	466	Control	59	30	39	59
		34.5/15	55	15[a]	39	69
Sao Paulo[504] (Reis Neto, Guilic, and Reis Neto, 1989)	68	Control	47	47	32	34
		40/20	26[a]	15[a]	15[a]	80[a]
Norway[505] (Dahl et al., 1990)	309	Control	28	21	21	58
		31.5/18	18[a]	15	23	57
ICRF[506] (Goldberg et al., 1994)	468	Control	No difference	24		40
		15/3		17[a]		39
Northwest Region[507] (Marsh, James, and Schofield, 1994)	284	Control	37	36	70	
		20/4		13[a]	43	70
Stockholm I[508] (Cedermark et al., 1995)	849	Control	28	28	37	36
		25/5–7	28	14[a]	30	36
Stockholm II[509] (Cedermark et al., 1996)	557	Control		21	26	56
		25/5		10[a]	19[a]	70[a]
SRCT[431] (1997)	1168	Control		27		48
		25/5		11		58[a]
Dutch TME[407]	1861	Control	36	8.2	16.8	81.8[b]
		25/5	33	2.4	14.8	82.0[b]

EORTC, European Organization for Research and Treatment of Cancer; ICRF, Imperial Cancer Research Foundation; MRC, Medical Research Council; SRCT, Swedish Rectal Cancer Trial; VASOG, Veterans' Administration Surgical Oncology Group Trial II.

[a]Statistically significant.

[b]Two-year survival data.

Source: From Gordon and Nivatvongs,[645] by permission of Taylor & Francis Group LLC.

TABLE 51.23.
Results of Randomized Trials of Postoperative Radiotherapy (Level I Evidence).

Overall Trial (authors)	*No. of patients*	*Dose (Gy/fractions)*	*Dukes stage*	*Local recurrence (%)*	*Distant metastases (%)*	*5-year survival (%)*
GITSG[432] (1985)	227	Operation alone	B_2 and C	24	34	43
		CT		27	27	57
		40–48 Gy/22–27		20	30	50
		CT140–44 Gy/22–24		11	26	59
Denmark[510] (Balslev et al., 1986)	494	Operation alone	B/C	18	14	Similar
		50 Gy/25		16	19	
NSABP[511] (Fisher et al., 1988)	555	Operation alone	B and C	25	27	43
		CT		21	24	53[a]
		46–47 Gy/26–27		16	31	50
Netherlands[512] (Treurniet-Donker et al., 1991)	172	Operation alone	B_2/C	33	26	57
		50 Gy/25		20	36	45
MRC3[513] (Gates et al., 1995)	469	Operation alone	B/C	34	35	38
		40 Gy/20		21[a]	31	41

CT, chemotherapy; GITSIG, Gastrointestinal Tumor Study Group; MRC, Medical Research Council; NSABP, National Surgical Adjuvant Breast and Bowel Project.

[a]Statistically significant.

Source: From Gordon and Nivatvongs,[645] by permission of Taylor & Francis Group LLC.

of data from this trial showed no significant benefit for irradiation of lesions located in the upper rectum greater than 10cm from the anal verge ($P = .17$). Regardless of the whether it is delivered preoperatively or postoperatively, radiation therapy appears to have a significant impact on local recurrence but probably has no impact on survival.

The addition of chemotherapy to radiation therapy has been used to enhance the radiation responsiveness of tumors and to have an impact on distant failure. Several studies have shown both improved local control and survival. The Gastrointestinal Tumor Study Group (GITSG) trial was an early four-arm study comparing surgery alone, postoperative chemotherapy, postoperative radiation, and postoperative radiation plus chemotherapy that demonstrated a decrease in pelvic failure with surgery and postoperative chemoradiation therapy (11% vs. 24% for surgery alone).[432] In addition, a statistically significant survival advantage was found at 7 years using the combination of resection, radiation, and chemotherapy.

The NCCTG subsequently conducted a trial randomizing 204 patients to radiotherapy (45–50.4Gy in 25–28 fractions) with or without concurrent chemotherapy (bolus 5FU). There was a significant decrease in pelvic recurrence (14% vs. 25%) and a significant decrease in cancer-related deaths for the group treated by resection, radiation, and chemotherapy compared with the group treated with resection and radiation therapy.[433] Protracted infusion 5FU has been compared to bolus 5FU by the NCCTG and has been demonstrated to result in improved local recurrence rates (8% vs. 11%) as well as improved disease-free (31% vs. 40%) and overall survival (60% vs. 70%).[434] Results of randomized trials of combined chemoradiation are presented in Table 51.24.

The findings from these studies prompted the publication of a clinical advisory by the NCI Consensus Conference in 1990 recommending adjuvant treatment for patients with Dukes B2 and C rectal carcinoma (T3–T4, N0; T3–T4, N1–N3, now stage II–III) consisting of six cycles of fluorouracil-based chemotherapy and concurrent radiation therapy to the pelvis. This regimen has remained the standard by which all current adjuvant rectal cancer protocols are compared. In the United States, postoperative chemoradiation has been the most common mode of delivering adjuvant therapy. This is usually given as a continuous infusion of 5FU and approximately 50.4Gy of irradiation delivered to the pelvis in 1.8- to 2.0-Gy fractions (6-week treatment). Although the trend in Europe is treatment with radiation therapy and no chemotherapy, the addition of chemotherapy in the United States has been shown to decrease the rate of distant metastases, something not attainable with radiation therapy alone. In addition, there has consistently been a 10% to 15% survival advantage when radiotherapy with chemotherapy is compared to radiotherapy alone. The NSABP R-2 and Intergroup 0114 trials have been designed to study the effects of different chemotherapeutic strategies and have established the role of 5FU as concurrent chemotherapeutic agent for pelvic radiation.

In recent years, practice in the United States has turned to an increasing use of preoperative rather than postoperative chemoradiation therapy due to the potential advantages of this approach. Two multicenter randomized trials have attempted to address the question of preoperative versus postoperative chemoradiation, but both have closed due to failure to accrue patients (RTOG 94-01 and NSABP R-03). The most definitive randomized data demonstrating the superiority of

TABLE 51.24.
Results of Randomized Trials of Combined Chemoradiation (Level I Evidence).

Overall Trial (authors)	*No. of patients*	*Dose (Gy/Fraction)*	*Local recurrence (%)*	*Distant metastases (%)*	*5-year survival (%)*
EORTC[514] (Boulis-Wassif et al., 1984)	247	Preop 34.5Gy/15.0	15	30	59
		Preop 34.5Gy/15.0 + 5FU	15	30	46
GITSG[432] (1985)	227	Operation alone	24	34	43
		CT	27	27	57
		Postop 40–48Gy/22–27	20	30	50
		CT140–44Gy/22–21	11	26	59
NCCTG[433] (Krook et al., 1991)	209	Postop 45Gy/25 + 5.4-Gy boost	23	46	38
		Postop 45Gy/25 + 5FU	14[a]	29[a]	53[a]
GITSG[515] (1992)	210	Postop 44.4Gy/23 + 5FU	15	25	44
		Postop 41.4Gy/23 + 5FU + Semustine	11	33	46
O'Connell et al.[434] (1994)	660	50.4/28Gy + CT bolus	11	40	60
		54Gy/30 + CT continuous	8	31	70[a]
NSABP[516] (Hyams et al., 1996)	741	MOF	14		66
		5FU-leucovorin			
		5FU + postop 46Gy (26.5)	9[a]		68
		5FU-leucovorin + postop 46Gy			

CT, Chemotherapy; EORTC, European Organization for Research and Treatment of Cancer; GITSG, Gastrointestinal Tumor Study Group; MOF, methyl CCNU, vincristine sulfate (Oncovin), 5FU; NCCTG, North Central Cancer Treatment Group; NSABP, National Surgical Adjuvant Breast and Bowel Project.

[a]Statistically significant.

Source: From Gordon and Nivatvongs,[645] by permission of Taylor & Francis Group LLC.

preoperative versus postoperative chemoradiation comes from the German Rectal Cancer Study Group. Patients (421) with tumors located within 16 cm from the anal verge were randomly assigned to preoperative long-course radiation (50.4 Gy in 28 fractions) with concurrent infusional 5FU (1000 mg/m^2/d) during weeks 1 and 5 followed by TME or to TME followed by postoperative radiation (45 Gy in 25 fractions) and concurrent infusional 5FU. All patients in the preoperative group and those patients with stage II or greater disease in the postoperative group also received four cycles of bolus 5FU in the adjuvant setting. Patients assigned to the preoperative arm had a lower 5-year cumulative risk of local failure (6% vs. 13%, $P = .006$) and decreased toxicity, both severe acute (27% vs. 40%, $P = .001$) and late (14% vs. 24%, $P = .01$). Moreover, improved sphincter preservation rates were noted in those patients who were initially deemed to require APR (39% vs. 19%, $P = .004$, preoperative versus postoperative, respectively.) Again, there was no difference in survival between the two arms.[435]

The main disadvantage of the preoperative regimens is that approximately 20% of patients with rectal cancer will be preoperatively overstaged and therefore will undergo unnecessary radiation and chemotherapy. In the German study, 20% of the patients randomized to the postoperative arm were noted to actually have stage I disease once the specimen was available for evaluation. These patients do not need adjuvant therapy and would have been overtreated if they were treated preoperatively. A number of groups have demonstrated efficacy of the oral fluoropyrimidine capecitabine as the chemotherapeutic radiation sensitizer in neoadjuvant regimens. Capecitabine has the advantages of convenient oral administration and reduced toxicity when compared to intravenous 5FU. The NSABP R-04 study hopes to address this issue in a multiinstitutional trial.

Therapy for Metastatic Colorectal Cancer

Recurrence of colorectal cancer occurs in approximately 50% of patients after curative resection. The most common sites of recurrence are the liver, lungs, regional lymph nodes, and peritoneum.[436] In women, the ovary is the site of recurrence in up to 8% of patients.[437] Brain and bone metastases are rare, but the incidence is rising as patients are living longer with improved control of disease within the liver or lung.

Up to 25% of patients present with liver metastases at their initial operation, and 15%–30% of patients undergoing apparently curative resection already have hepatic metastases that are not evident to the surgeon at the time of operation.[438]

Multiple agents and combination chemotherapeutic regimens now exist for metastatic colorectal cancer (Table 51.25). The past several years have witnessed the arrival of multiple new and effective regimens for metastatic colorectal cancer. Median survival for metastatic colorectal cancer treated with best supportive care only ranges from 6 to 9 months.[439] With 5FU-based regimens, median survival improved to 10–12 months, and the addition of irinotecan or oxaliplatin improved survival to 14–17 months.[440–444] These agents used in combination and in series as second- or third-line regimens can result in median survival of around 20 months.[445]

TABLE 51.25. Chemotherapeutic Agents and Regimens with Activity in Colorectal Cancer.

Single agents	***Mechanism of action***
5FU	Inhibition of DNA and RNA synthesis
Capecitabine	Metabolized to 5FU
Irinotecan	Topoisomerase I inhibitor
Oxaliplatin	Induction of DNA replication errors
Bevacizumab	Humanized monoclonal antibody to VEGF
Cetuximab	Chimeric monoclonal antibody to EGFR
Combination regimens	***Components***
Mayo, Roswell Park, de Garmont, AIO regimens	5FU Leucovorin
IFL, FOLFIRI	5FU Leucovorin Irinotecan
CapIri	Capecitabine Irinotecan
FOLFOX4, FOLFOX6, mFOLFOX6, FOLFOX7, FLOX, FUFOX, bFOL	5FU Leucovorin Oxaliplatin
XELOX, CapOx	Capecitabine Oxaliplatin
IROX	Irinotecan Oxaliplatin
IFL+ bev	5FU Leucovorin Irinotecan Bevacizumab
CB	Cetuximab Bevacizumab
CBI	Cetuximab Bevacizumab Irinotecan

EGFR, epidermal growth factor receptor; VEGF, vascular endothelial growth factor.

The most recent additions to the cytotoxic armamentarium have been the molecular-targeted agents, which are expected to further increase the median survival for patients with unresectable colorectal cancer. Bevacizumab is a humanized monoclonal antibody directed against VEGF. Cetuximab is a chimeric monoclonal antibody directed against the EGFR. The combination of bevacizumab with bolus 5FU, leucovorin, and irinotecan (IFL) resulted in a median survival of 20 months.[446] It is anticipated that the combination of bevacizumab with superior oxaliplatin-based regimens will yield even longer median survival times. Cetuximab has been extensively investigated as salvage therapy. Growing evidence suggests that it will also play an important role as part of first-line treatment.[447]

Liver

A spiral CT scan with intravenous contrast taken during both the arterial and the venous phases is currently the best preoperative imaging technique for delineating resectable colorectal liver metastases. Among those patients who develop liver metastases, the liver will be the only site of disease in approximately 20%.[448–450] Surgical resection of liver metastases remains the only potentially curative treatment for these patients. Five-year survival rates of 35%–58% have now been reported following curative resection of hepatic colorectal cancer metastases with low morbidity and mortality.[448,451–453] Furthermore, repeat resection has also been associated with good results of 32%–49% 5-year survival.[448,451–453] Radio frequency ablation with curative intent is an alternative strategy that has been associated with poorer long-term survival and higher rates of recurrence when compared to resection.[448] The resection of hepatic metastases in the presence of other lesions (which cannot be resected) is of no benefit.[454]

Patients with synchronous hepatic metastases can be treated with synchronous resections of the primary lesion as well as the metastasis. This approach has been shown to be safe in selected patients for whom a major colorectal resection is not combined with a major liver resection. When both a major hepatic resection and major colorectal resection are required for curative intent, resection of the primary is generally followed by resection of the liver metastasis after recovery from the first operation or after an interval of systemic chemotherapy. In some patients with metastatic disease outside a single anatomic distribution within the liver, a staged resection of liver metastases may be performed. Preoperative portal vein embolization is emerging as an important strategy to allow for hypertrophy of the retained liver segment and to permit a more extensive liver resection.[455]

Hepatic arterial infusion chemotherapy with floxuridine and dexamethasone in addition to systemic 5FU following liver resection has been associated with improved survival (median overall 68.4 months, 95% CI 55.2 to median survival not reached) when compared to monotherapy with systemic 5FU alone (median 58.8 months, 95% CI 42.0–85.2, $P = .10$). Ten-year survival rates were 41.1% and 27.2%, respectively. However, the German Cooperative study and another multicenter study in the United States failed to show a survival benefit when compared to surgery alone.[456–458]

Lung

Pulmonary metastases occur in 15%–20% of all patients with colorectal cancer. Pulmonary metastases alone are more common in patients with rectal primaries. However, with curative resection of pulmonary metastases, 5-year survival rates of 21%–62% and low operative mortality (<3%) have been demonstrated.[459–461] Resection of pulmonary metastases is indicated when complete resection of the metastases can be performed. Both wedge resections and lobectomy may provide similar long-term results, but some authors have advocated the importance of including a mediastinal lymph node dissection, both for prognosis and to guide the selection of subsequent chemotherapeutic regimens.

Peritoneal Disease

Peritoneal carcinomatosis carries a uniformly poor prognosis. In selected patients, cytoreductive surgery combined with intraperitoneal hyperthermic chemotherapy has been shown to improve survival.[462] The role of cytoreductive therapy for carcinomatosis from colorectal cancer is the subject of ongoing investigation.

Therapy for Local Recurrent Colorectal Cancer

Of colorectal recurrences, 70% occur within 2 years of operation.[463] Local recurrences vary between 1% and 20% for colon cancer and between 3% and 45% for rectal cancer.[464,465] Strict adherence to the oncologic principals of en bloc resection with adequate margins of resection and regional lymphadenectomy can minimize the risk for recurrence after curative resection of colorectal cancer.

Local recurrence after resection for colon cancer can be a difficult problem. Whenever possible, salvage surgery to yield a complete resection of the recurrence should be considered. Curative resection of local-regionally recurrent disease even in conjunction with resection of distant metastases has been shown to yield a median survival of 30 months.[466] For the recurrent unresectable tumor, relief of obstruction may also be possible with the use of an endoluminal stent with or without laser therapy.

Recurrent Rectal Cancer

Recurrent rectal cancer can vary significantly in its clinical presentation. For patients with localized recurrence, or selected patients with synchronous resectable metastases and resectable local recurrence, curative surgical resection is an important aspect of their treatment. Preoperative chemoradiation (50.4–54 Gy) followed by resection and intraoperative radiotherapy (IORT 10–20 Gy) when possible is the preferred approach. The Mayo Clinic has shown that such an approach results in a subsequent pelvic recurrence rate of 37% and a distant recurrence rate of 54%. The 5-year overall survival in their series was 25% and as high as 37% in patients in whom a negative margin of resection could be achieved.[467]

Patients who have previously undergone adjuvant radiotherapy for primary rectal cancer may still be candidates for reirradiation. Generally, an additional 30 Gy can be delivered over 2 weeks using intensity-modulated radiation therapy (IMRT). Use of IMRT may improve treatment tolerance in selected patients by reducing the dose to adjacent nontarget organs such as the small bowel. Patients with recurrent rectal cancer have safely undergone repeat irradiation with acceptable short-term toxicity.[468]

Palliative pelvic radiotherapy may delay progression of recurrent local disease in those who are not candidates for resection. Most commonly, it is performed for symptoms of pelvic pain. It has been associated with a widely variable symptom control rate of 32% to 92%, with a duration of symptom control of approximately 6 months.[469] There has been considerable interest in regional hyperthermia in conjunction with palliative radiation, with some investigators reporting improved rates of symptom control with regional hyperthermia.[470]

Polyposis Coli Syndromes

Familial Adenomatous Polyposis

Familial adenomatous polyposis (FAP) is an inherited, non-sex-linked, autosomal dominant disease characterized by the progressive development of hundreds of polyps. The mutated gene is found on the long arm of chromosome 5 and is called the APC gene. If the colorectal adenomas are left untreated, patients with FAP will develop colorectal cancer. Polyps occur at a mean age of 16 years, and almost all affected persons exhibit adenomas by age 35 years. Seven percent of untreated individuals have cancer by age 21, 50% by age 39, and 90% by the age of 45 years. In the milder phenotypic variant, attenuated FAP, colorectal polyps are less numerous, and colorectal carcinoma in general will occur in the early 50s. Because APC mutations can be detected in the germ line of the affected patients, genetic testing is recommended for affected individuals. If a mutation is known in the family, then individuals at risk can be tested for that mutation, and those in whom the mutation is detected can be spared intensive surveillance.

All first-degree relatives of an individual with newly diagnosed FAP should undergo colonoscopy to screen for the disease. In a family already known to have FAP, sigmoidoscopy screening in younger at-risk patients should begin between ages 10 to 12 years and be repeated every 1 to 2 years. If no adenomas have been identified by age 30, surveillance intervals can be increased to 2–3 years.[471]

Upper GI manifestations of FAP include gastric polyps in 50% to 100% of affected persons and duodenal polyps in 90% to 100%. Duodenal polyps are adenomatous polyps that also bear some malignant risk because a 10% to 12% lifetime occurrence of periampullary duodenal cancer has been reported. Extraintestinal manifestations of FAP include osteomas, soft tissue tumors of the skin, supernumerary teeth, desmoid tumors, and congenital hypertrophy of the retinal pigment epithelium (Gardner's syndrome).

The preferred operations are either a total colectomy with ileorectal anastomosis or a restorative proctocolectomy with an ileal J-pouch anal anastomosis. Both procedures have distinct advantages and disadvantages. The advantages of a total colectomy and ileorectal anastomosis are a lower complication rate, lower infertility rate, and normal continence. Patients selected for this procedure must have relative sparing of the rectum. They are followed with lifelong proctoscopy at 6-month intervals and annual proctoscopy and electrocautery destruction of new polyps in the operating room. The disadvantage of an ileorectal anastomosis is that diseased mucosa remains within the retained rectum, with the risk of subsequent carcinoma.[472] Proctectomy with ileal J-pouch restoration of intestinal continuity or end ileostomy is indicated if rectal cancer develops. The advantage of the ileal pouch procedure is eradication of all or nearly all mucosa at risk. In appropriately selected patients, quality of life after ileal J-pouch anal anastomosis has been shown to be similar to that after ileorectostomy.

MYH-Associated Polyposis

MYH-associated polyposis has recently been described but has not yet been fully characterized. It is caused by biallelic mutations in the base excision repair gene MYH, most commonly Y165C and G328D. Initially identified among a subgroup of patients with FAP in whom APC mutations had not been detected, MYH-associated polyposis results in the development of multiple adenomas and has an autosomal recessive pattern of inheritance.[473–476] The nature of the association between MYH-associated polyposis and the development of colorectal cancer is still under investigation.

Hamartomatous Polyposis

Genetic syndromes including juvenile polyposis syndrome (JPS), Peutz Jeghers syndrome (PJS), Cowden syndrome (CS), and Bannayan-Riley-Ruvalcaba syndrome all share the manifestations of intestinal juvenile polyps. Cowden syndrome has additional pathognomonic features of mucocutaneous lesions (facial trichilemmoma, oral fibromas, acral keratosis) and associated tumors of the thyroid, breast, and endometrium. Bannayan-Riley-Ruvalcaba syndrome is characterized by mental retardation, macrocephaly, lipomatosis, hemangiomas, and genital pigmentation.

Hundreds or even thousands of polyps may be distributed throughout the entire colon, rectum, stomach, and small bowel in juvenile polyposis. This condition is associated with hamartomatous polyps. Macroscopically, they are pink, smooth, round, and usually pedunculated. Although solitary hamartomatous polyps do not have malignant potential, an increased risk for intestinal malignancy has been demonstrated with JPS and PJS. Patients with PJS are also at risk for pancreas, breast, and uterine carcinoma as well as sex cord tumors, Sertoli cell tumors, and adenoma malignum of the cervix.[477–481]

Hereditary Nonpolyposis Coli Syndromes

Hereditary nonpolyposis colorectal cancer (HNPCC) is an autosomal dominant inherited disease characterized by early age onset of colorectal cancer, right-sided predominance, frequent synchronous and metachronous colorectal neoplasms, as well as extracolonic malignancies. In patients with HNPCC, the median age of onset of colorectal cancer is 45 years, and approximately 60% to 70% of cancers occur proximal to the splenic flexure. Despite its name, polyps are features of HNPCC as well in 8% to 17% of first-degree relatives. All first-degree relatives of patients with HNPCC have a 50% chance of carrying one of the deleterious genes. In a study with 130 HNPCC kindreds, the incidence for colorectal cancer was increased sevenfold in first-degree relatives.[482]

Patients with HNPCC are also at an increased risk for extracolonic malignancies such as endometrial cancer, small-bowel cancer, renal pelvis and ureter cancer, and skin lesions such as sebaceous adenomas, keratoacanthomas, and sebaceous carcinoma.[483] Endometrial cancer can be the index carcinoma in 35% of female patients.[484] Germ-line mutations in the mismatch repair genes (see mutator pathway) are responsible for the syndrome. MSH6 germ-line mutations have been associated with later-age onset of colorectal cancer and with predominant endometrial cancer families.[485]

The Amsterdam criteria are clinical criteria developed in 1990 to confirm the diagnosis of HNPCC: (1) at least three relatives with histologically verified colorectal carcinoma, one of whom should be a first-degree relative of the other two; (2) at least two successive generations should be affected; (3) in one of the relatives, colorectal carcinoma should have been diagnosed when the patient was younger than 50 years of age. The modified Amsterdam criteria include HNPCC-associated malignancies in addition to colorectal cancer.

Adenomas do occur in HNPCC. Currently, it is believed that once adenomas occur in HNPCC, they progress to carcinoma faster than in sporadic colorectal cancer patients.[486] Colonoscopy should be performed starting at age 21 with surveillance every 1 to 2 years until age 40 and annually thereafter. Close colonoscopic surveillance has been shown to decrease the colorectal cancer rate by 62% and decrease mortality by 65%.[487] Similar principles apply for genetic testing in HNPCC as in FAP. The role for screening for associated extracolonic malignancy has not been clearly established. Once colorectal cancer has been identified in a patient with HNPCC, the treatment should be individualized and may include a prophylactic total colectomy or a cancer-directed resection with close colonoscopic surveillance.[488]

Anus: Benign Diseases and Neoplasms

Benign Diseases

Anorectal Abscess and Fistula

Perirectal abscess fistulous disease not associated with a specific systemic disease is most commonly cryptoglandular in origin.[13] The anal canal has 6 to 14 glands that lie in or near the intersphincteric plane between the internal and external sphincters. Projections from the glands pass through the internal sphincters and drain into the crypts at the dentate line. Glands may become infected when a crypt is occluded, trapping stool and bacteria within the gland. This occlusion may occur secondary to impaction of vegetable matter or edema from trauma (firm stool or foreign body) or as a result of an adjacent inflammatory process. If the crypt does not decompress into the anal canal, an abscess may develop in the intersphincteric plane. Abscesses are classified by the space they invade (Fig. 51.52). The most difficult to treat is the abscess that tracts proximally or circumferentially within the intersphincteric plane (Fig. 51.53).

An abscess typically causes severe continuous throbbing anal pain that may worsen with ambulation and straining.[517] Swelling and discharge are noted less frequently. Occasionally, patients present with fever, urinary retention, and life-threatening sepsis, which is especially true in diabetics and the immunocompromised host. A patient with fistula-in-ano may report a history of severe pain, bloody purulent drainage associated with resolution of the pain, and subsequent chronic mucopurulent discharge.

Physical examination of the patient with an abscess reveals a tender perianal or perirectal mass. The size is often difficult to assess until the patient is provided adequate anesthesia. An apparently small abscess may extend high into the ischiorectal or supralevator space (Fig. 51.54). A fistula is present when an internal and external opening are identified. A firm connecting tract is often palpable.

No imaging studies are necessary in uncomplicated abscess fistulous disease, but imaging studies such as sinograms, transrectal ultrasound, CT, and MRI may be useful in the evaluation of complex or recurrent disease. Transrectal ultrasound can identify branching of fistulous tracts, persistent undrained sepsis, and extent of sphincter involvement[518]

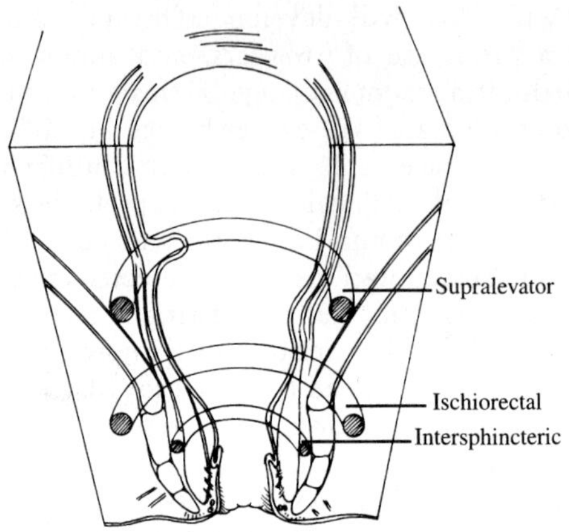

FIGURE 51.53. Planes through which infection may spread circumferentially. (From Parks,[651] with permission.)

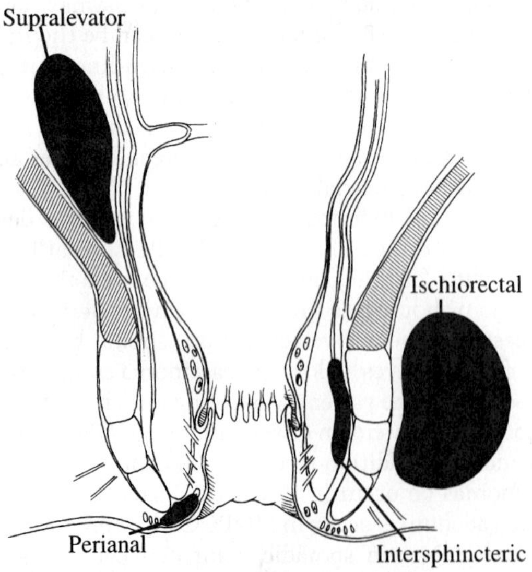

FIGURE 51.52. Abscesses are classified by location. (From Vasilevsky,[650] with permission, © 1992, McGraw-Hill.)

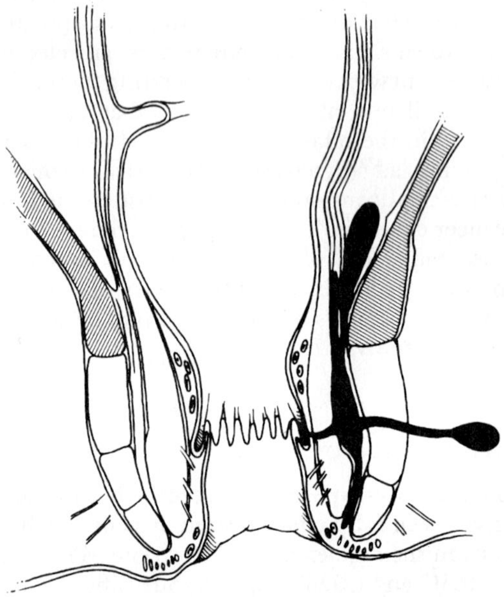

FIGURE 51.54. Supralevator extension of an apparent perianal abscess may be difficult to define in the conscious patient. The abscess may extend proximally or distally within the intersphincteric plane or across the sphincter. Extension of the apparent perianal abscess into the supralevator or ischiorectal space may be difficult to define in the conscious patient. (From Parks,[651] with permission.)

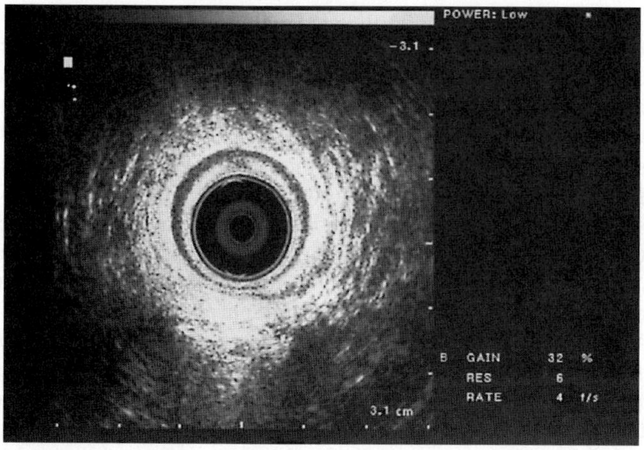

FIGURE 51.55. Utility of transrectal ultrasound in establishing the presence of abscess fistulous disease in the chronic recurrent setting.

(Fig. 51.55). Hydrogen peroxide injection of the tract may improve sensitivity.[519] Computed tomographic scanning may be helpful in finding the undiagnosed supralevator abscess. Recent reports for MRI and MRI with endorectal coil suggest MRI is better than transrectal ultrasound or preoperative physical exam for identifying and classifying fistulas.[520,521]

Abscess fistula disease of cryptoglandular origin must be differentiated from complications of Crohn's disease, pilonidal disease, hidradenitis suppurativa, tuberculosis, actinomycosis, trauma, fissures, carcinoma, radiation, chlamydia, local dermal processes, retrorectal tumors, diverticulitis, and ureteral injuries.

Five percent to 10% of patients with Crohn's disease present with anorectal abscess fistulous disease with no antecedent history of IBD. Tuberculosis may cause indolent, pale granulomatous perianal disease, but this is usually associated with a known history of tuberculosis. Hidradenitis suppurativa is considered in the patient with multiple, chronic, draining fistulas such as might be seen with undiagnosed horseshoe abscess fistula disease. Pilonidal disease may extend toward the perineum but may be distinguished from cryptoglandular disease by the presence of inspissated hairs, direction of the tract, and presence of other openings in the sacrococcygeal area. A colonic source may be suspected in a patient with known IBD or diverticular disease. Other less-common causes include tumors, radiation, infections, and urological injuries.

The complications of an undrained anorectal abscess may be severe. Antibiotics given while waiting for the abscess to mature are not helpful. The infection may spread rapidly, which may result in extensive tissue loss, sphincter injury, and even death. In contrast, a fistula-in-ano, which may develop when the abscess is drained, is not a surgical emergency. A chronic fistula may be associated with recurring perianal abscesses or rarely with occult malignancy; therefore, the fistula should be biopsied.

Abscesses should be drained surgically.[522] Patients often require drainage in the operating room, where anesthesia allows for adequate evaluation of the extent of the disease. Abscesses thought to be superficial in the office may extend above the levators. Intersphincteric abscesses are treated by internal sphincterotomy, which drains the abscess and destroys the crypt. Perirectal and ischiorectal abscesses should be drained by a catheter or with adequate excision of skin to prevent premature closure and reaccumulation of the abscess (Fig. 51.56). If the internal opening of the fistula is identified and significant external sphincter is not involved, a fistulotomy may be performed when the abscess is drained. However, the internal opening is often hard to find because of inflammation, and drainage is all that can be achieved. In this instance, we prefer catheter drainage to skin excision because the catheter (1) establishes drainage with a minimal disruption of normal perianal skin, (2) facilitates identification of the internal opening (present in approximately 50%) at subsequent evaluation, and (3) facilitates patient compliance by eliminating the need for packing or "wicking" the wound open.

Patients with a chronic or recurring abscess after apparent adequate surgical drainage often have an undrained deep postanal space abscess that communicates with the ischiorectal fossa via a horseshoe fistula. Treatment involves opening the deep postanal space and counterdraining the tract through the ischiorectal external opening[523] (Fig. 51.57). Once the postanal space heals, the counterdrain may be removed.

Immunocompromised patients are a particular challenge. In the moderately compromised host, such as the diabetic patient, urgent drainage in the operating room is required because these patients are more prone to necrotizing anorectal infections. In the severely compromised host, patients receiving chemotherapy, an infection may be present without an "abscess" due to neutropenia. In these patients, it is important to attempt to localize the process, establish "drainage," localize the internal opening, and biopsy the tissue for pathology and culture (to exclude hematologic malignancy and select antibiotics).

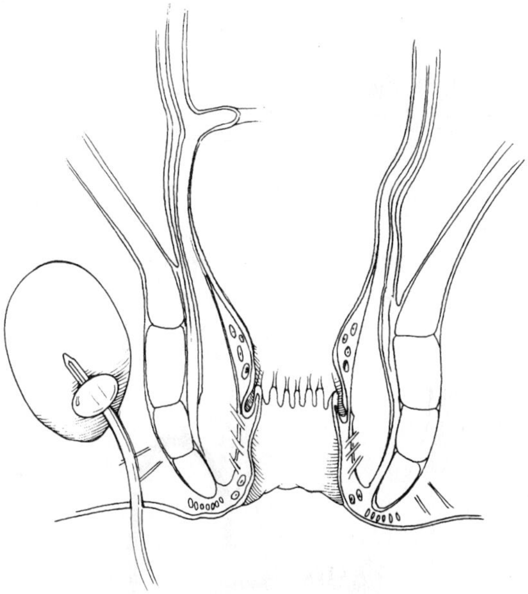

FIGURE 51.56. Catheter drainage of an ischiorectal abscess. The catheter is sewn to the skin with a 2-0 nylon that is cut after 1 week, and the "mushroom" anchors the tube in place. (From Bailey and Synder,[648] with permission, © 2000, Springer-Verlag, New York.)

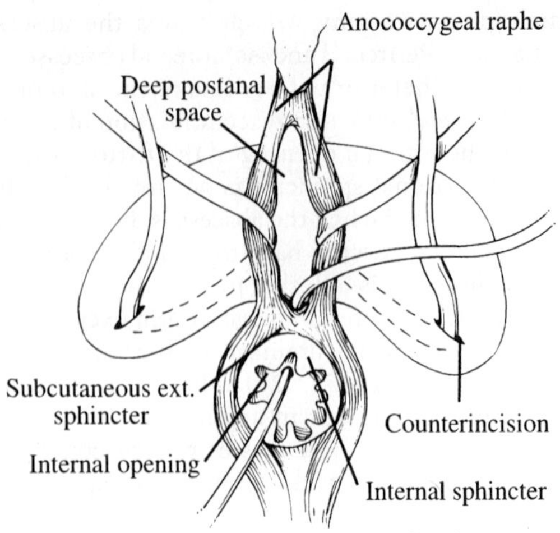

FIGURE 51.57. One method for drainage of a deep postanal space abscess. The Penrose drains may be replaced with mushroom catheters placed through small stab incisions so long as the deep postanal space is opened widely or marsupialized. (From Ustynoski,[652] with permission.)

The treatment of fistulas is dictated by the course of the fistula[522] (Fig. 51.58 and Table 51.26). If the tract passes superficially and does not involve sphincter muscle, then a simple incision of the tract with ablation of the gland and "saucerization" of the skin at the external opening is all that is necessary (Fig. 51.59). A fistula that involves a small amount of sphincter (except anterior midline in women) may be treated similarly. A tract that passes deep, or that involves an undetermined amount of muscle, is best treated with a mucosal advancement flap (Fig. 51.60). Immediate or delayed muscle division with a cutting Seton is associated with a high rate of incontinence, but a noncutting Seton may be used to control sepsis while preparing for definitive therapy of a complex fistula (Fig. 51.61). Anterior midline fistulas in women are best treated with advancement flap repair because the external sphincter is a particularly thin band of muscle in this location, and the risk of sphincter injury resulting in significant incontinence is increased.

Goodsall's rule assists in identifying the direction of the tract (Fig. 51.62) in fistulas with posterior external

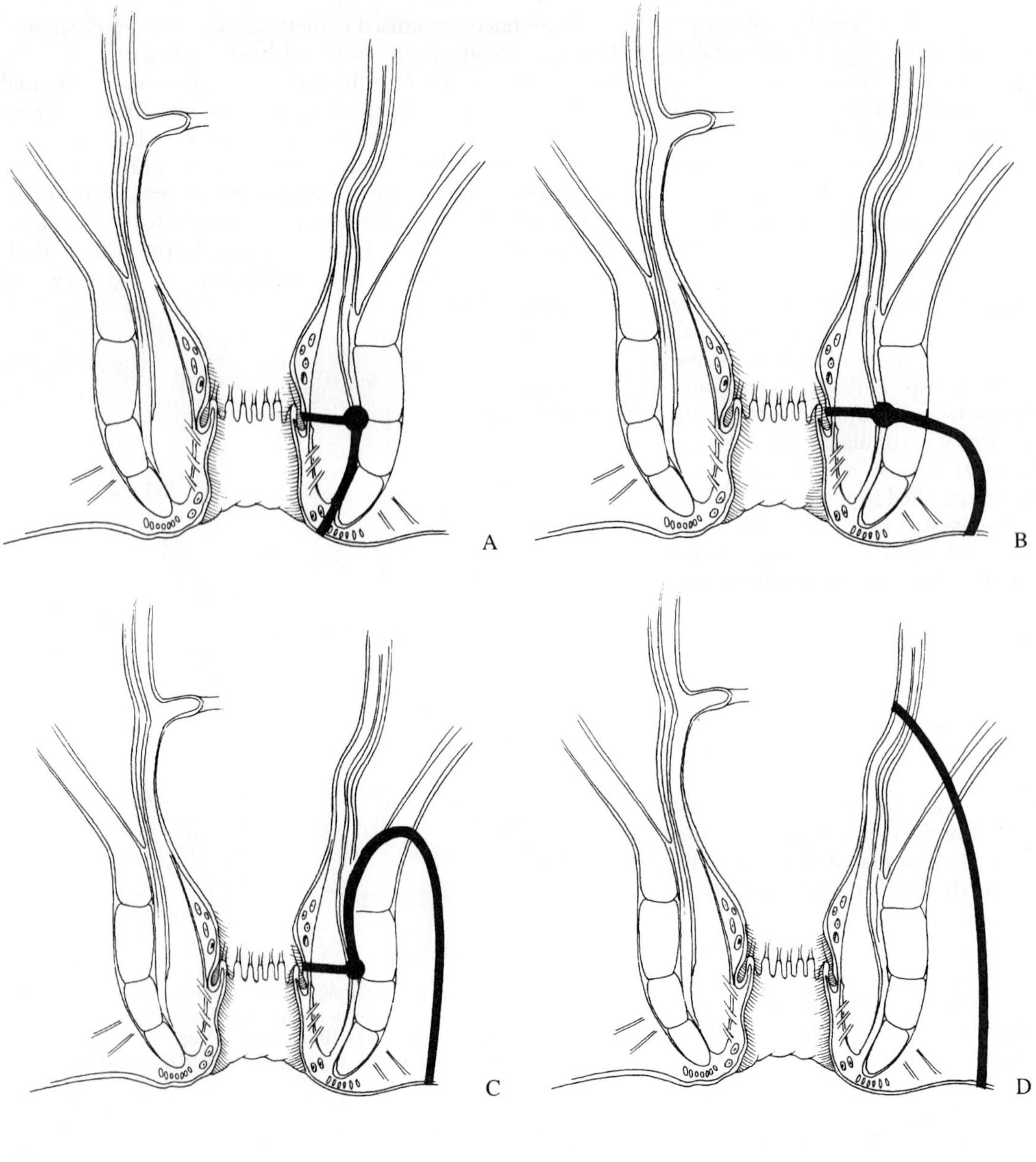

FIGURE 51.58. (A–D) Types of fistula-in-ano. The course of the fistulous tract and the amount and type of muscle involved determine operative intervention. (From Parks,[651] with permission.)

TABLE 51.26. Parks's Classification of Fistula-in-Ano.

Type 1. Intersphincteric fistula
a. Simple intersphincteric fistula
b. Intersphincteric fistula with a high blind tract
c. Intersphincteric fistula with a high tract opening into the lower rectum
d. High intersphincteric fistula without a perineal opening
e. High intersphincteric fistula with a pelvic extension
f. Intersphincteric fistula from pelvic disease
Type 2. Transsphincteric fistula
a. Uncomplicated
b. Transsphincteric fistula with a high blind tract
Type 3. Suprasphincteric fistula
Type 4. Extrasphincteric fistula
a. Extrasphincteric fistula secondary to a transsphincteric fistula
b. Extrasphincteric fistula due to trauma
c. Extrasphincteric fistula due to specific anorectal disease
d. Extrasphincteric fistula due to pelvic inflammation

Data from Parks et al.[651]

Source: From Bailey and Synder,[648] with permission, © 2000, Springer-Verlag, New York.

openings,[524] but reliability is decreased anteriorly and in particular as distance from the verge is increased.[525] In these reports, anterolateral openings were noted to communicate with anterior midline internal openings. In the case of recurrent or complex fistulas, these exceptions must be kept in mind.

The prognosis for cryptoglandular abscess fistula disease is excellent once the source of infection is identified. Fistulas persist when the source has not been identified or adequately drained, when the diagnosis is incorrect, or when postoperative care is insufficient.

Fissures

Anal Fissure/Ulcer

An anal *fissure* is a split in the anoderm. An *ulcer* is a chronic fissure. When mature, an ulcer is associated with a skin tag (sentinel pile) and a hypertrophied anal papilla. Fissures occur in the midline just distal to the dentate line. Two recent studies have called into question Goligher's rule that 90% are posterior, 10% are anterior, and fewer than 1% occur simultaneously in the anterior and posterior positions.[526,527] Both studies found anterior fissures to be more common than expected, but the fissures were still on the midline.

Fissures result from forceful dilation of the anal canal. The anoderm is disrupted, exposing the underlying internal sphincter muscle, leading to muscle spasm that fails to relax with the next dilation.[528,529] This leads to further tearing, deepening of the fissure, and increased muscle irritation and spasm.[529] The persistent muscle spasm leads to relative ischemia of the overlying anoderm and inhibits healing.[530] Ultraslow waves and low-frequency, high-amplitude pressure changes occur with increased frequency in patients with anal fissures and disappear with sphincterotomy and fissure healing.[529,531,532]

Classically, the initial insult is believed to be a firm bowel movement. The pain associated with the initial bowel movement is great, and the patient therefore ignores the urge to defecate for fear of experiencing the pain again. This delay allows a harder stool to form, which tears the anoderm more as it passes because of its size and the poor relaxation of the sphincter. A self-perpetuating cycle of pain, poor relaxation, and reinjury results. Factors that may predispose to fissure formation are previous anorectal surgery (hemorrhoidectomy, fistulotomy, destruction of condylomata), resulting in scarring of the anoderm and loss of elasticity, increasing the probability that the anoderm will tear.

Fissures cause pain and bleeding with defecation. The pain is often tearing or burning, worst during defecation, and subsides over a few hours. Blood is noted on tissue and on the stool but is not mixed in the stool or toilet water. Constipation may develop secondarily because of fear of recurrent pain. Although less common, fissures may present as painless nonhealing wounds that bleed intermittently.[526]

Physical examination by simple gentle traction on the buttocks will evert the anus sufficiently to reveal a disruption of the anoderm in the midline at the mucocutaneous junction. In the acute fissure, this may be all that is present. In the chronic fissure, a sentinel pile may be visualized at the inferior margin of the ulcer. Gentle, limited, digital examination will confirm internal sphincter spasm. Anoscopy and proctosigmoidoscopy should be deferred until healing occurs, or the procedure can be performed under anesthesia. Under anesthesia, the classic triad of a proximal hypertrophied anal papilla above a fissure with the sentinel pile at the anal verge may be identified.

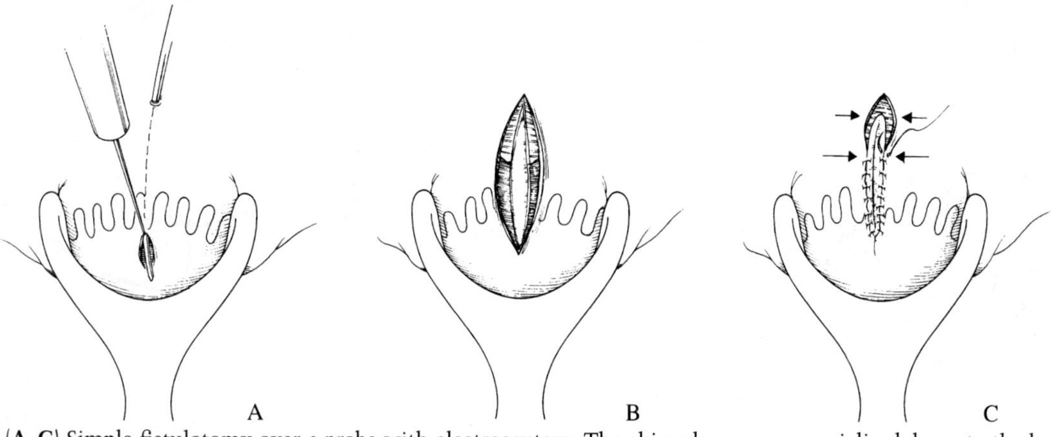

FIGURE 51.59. (A–C) Simple fistulotomy over a probe with electrocautery. The skin edges are marsupialized down to the base of the fistula tract edges. (From Vasilevsky,[650] with permission, © 1992, McGraw-Hill.)

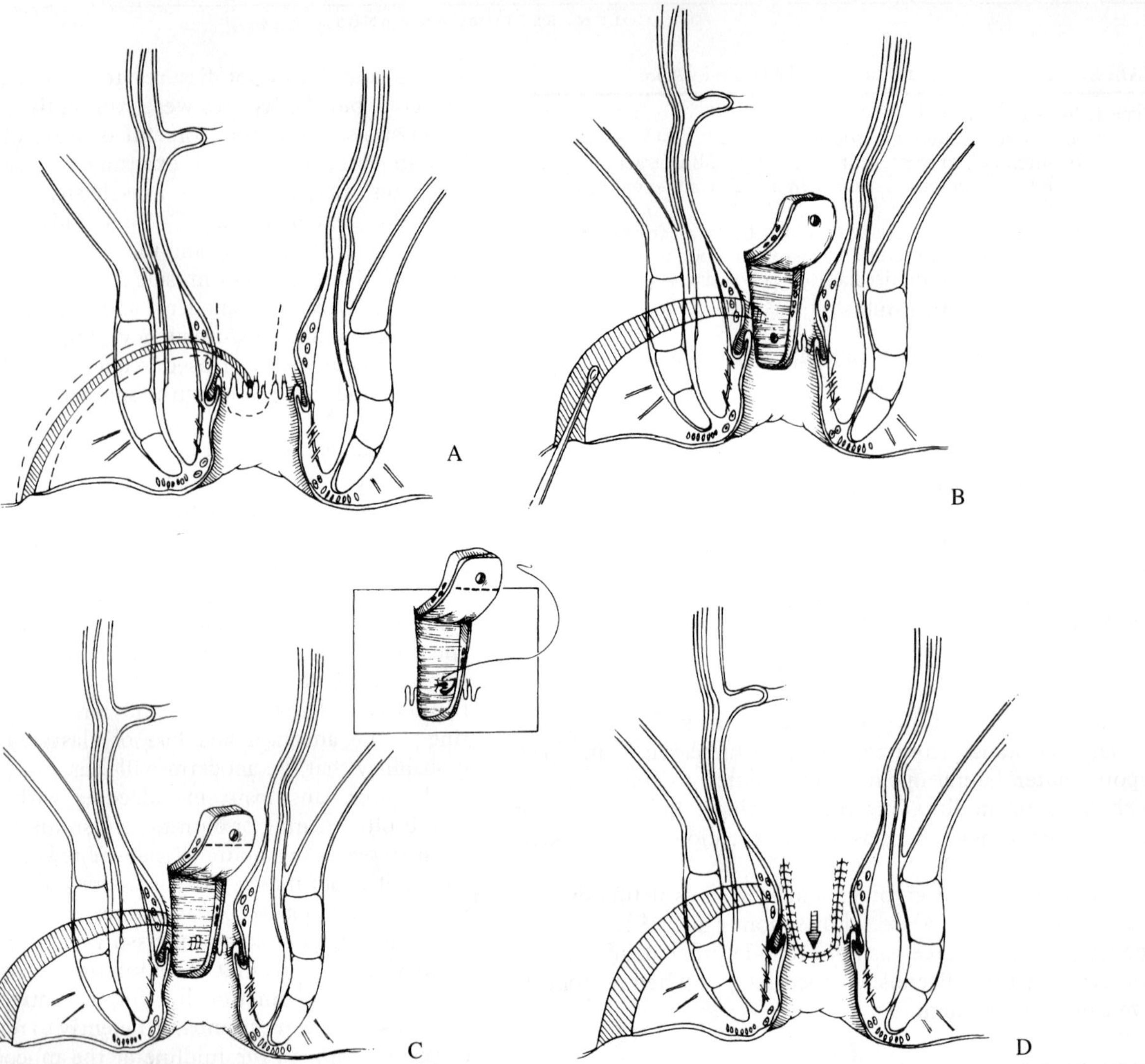

FIGURE 51.60. (A–D) Mucosal advancement flap procedure. A myomucosal flap ("just a little of the internal sphincter") is elevated with a broad base as in all flaps. The tract may be curetted and closed primarily or simply counterdrained with a mushroom-type catheter (present from the initial drainage procedure). The tip of the flap with the mucosal defect is excised and the flap sutured in place. This procedure may be used to treat anterior anovaginal fistulas from either Crohn's or cryptoglandular disease or when enough external sphincter is involved that division of the sphincter along the tract may result in incontinence. (From Reznick and Bailey,[653] with permission.)

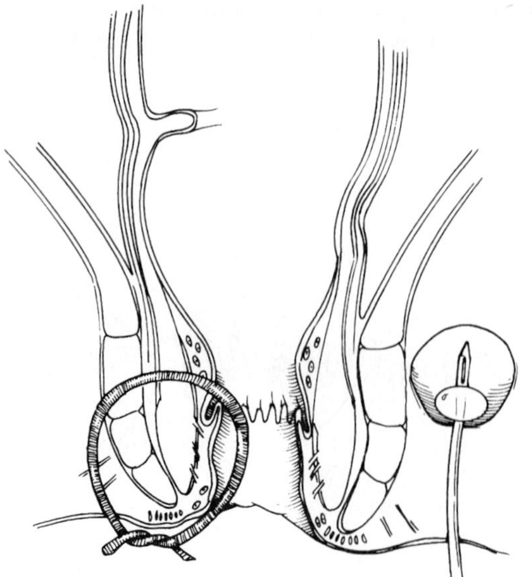

FIGURE 51.61. Control of perianal sepsis with a Seton and mushroom catheter for complex abscess fistulous disease or Crohn's disease. (From Bailey and Synder,[648] with permission, © 2000, Springer-Verlag, New York.)

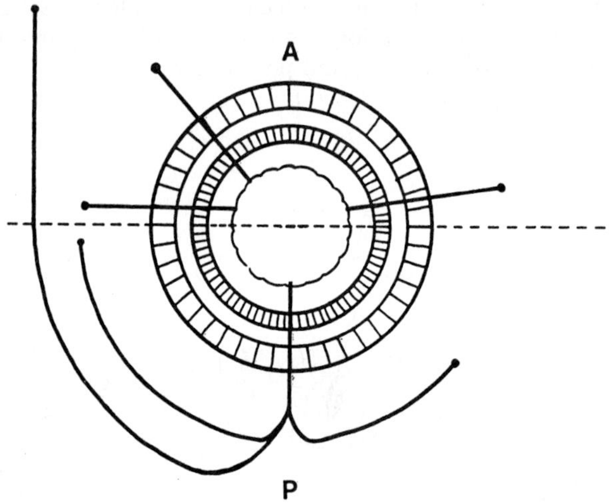

FIGURE 51.62. Goodsall's rule: External openings anterior to a line drawn between 3 and 9 o'clock will communicate with an internal opening along a straight line drawn toward the dentate line. Posterior external openings will communicate with the posterior midline in a nonlinear fashion. The exception may be an interior opening that is greater than 3 cm from the dentate line. (From Marti and Givel,[654] with permission, © 1999, Springer-Verlag, Heidelberg.)

Although anoscopy and proctosigmoidoscopy may not be performed in the initial evaluation of a patient with a fissure, they must be performed during a subsequent visit because the presence of associated anorectal malignancy or IBD must be excluded. If a midline fissure fails to heal, it must be biopsied to exclude Crohn's disease or malignancy. Anal manometry is unhelpful. Studies have shown increased pressures in patients with ulcers, but patients with high pressures have not been found to be at increased risk for fissure/ulcer disease.

Fissure/ulcer disease occurs in the anterior or posterior midline and involves the mucocutaneous junction. Ulcers occurring off the midline, or away from the mucocutaneous junction, are suspect. Crohn's disease, anal TB, anal malignancy, abscess/fistula disease, CMV, herpes, chlamydia, syphilis, AIDS, and some blood dyscrasias may all mimic certain aspects of fissure/ulcer disease. Initial manifestations of Crohn's disease are limited to the anal canal in 10% of patients. Anal TB will be associated with a prior or concomitant history of pulmonary TB. Anal cancer may present as a painless ulcer. Nonhealing ulcers must be biopsied to rule out malignancy. The complications are related to persistence of the disease and its associated pain, bleeding, and alteration in bowel habits. The ulcers do not become malignant.

Stool softeners, bulk agents, and sitz baths are successful in healing 90% of anal fissures. A second episode has a 60% to 80% chance of healing with this regimen. Sitz baths after painful bowel movements soothe the muscle spasm. Patients are instructed to soak in a hot bath and contract the sphincters to identify the muscle in spasm and then focus on relaxing that muscle. The effect is twofold; it decreases the pain associated with the spasm and improves blood flow to the fissure, allowing for improved healing. Stool softeners and bulk agents make the stool more malleable, decreasing the trauma of each successive bowel movement. Chronic (1-month history) or chronic recurrent ulcers should be considered for surgical excision and histopathologic evaluation.

Botulinum toxin (Botox) inhibits the release of acetylcholine from presynaptic nerve fibers, effecting a reversible paralysis that lasts several months. Many studies, including two randomized prospective trials comparing Botox to saline and nitroglycerin controls, have suggested that Botox infiltration into the internal sphincters is effective in the treatment of anal fissures.[533–535] In contrast, a Cochrane review and meta-analysis indicated that Botox is no better than placebo in healing anal fissures.[536]

Glyceryl trinitrate ointment is a nitric oxide source. Nitric oxide is an inhibitory neurotransmitter that causes relaxation of the internal sphincter and improved blood flow. Studies have suggested the efficacy of 0.2% glyceryl trinitrate in the treatment of anal fissures.[537–540] The major side effect, headache, is minimized at the lower doses of 0.2% and 0.3% but still occurs at a high enough rate to impair patient compliance and decrease effectiveness of this approach.[541] A Cochrane review and meta-analysis suggests glyceryl trinitrate and other similar compounds such as nifedipine and diltiazem are effective in relieving pain but are no better than placebo in healing anal fissures.[536]

Lateral internal anal sphincterotomy is the procedure of choice after conservative measures have failed.[542] This procedure may be performed "open," by which an incision is made in the skin and the hypertrophied distal one-third of the internal sphincter divided under direct vision (Fig. 51.63). It may also be done "closed," in which a scalpel is passed in the intersphincteric plane and swept medially, dividing the internal sphincter blindly (Fig. 51.64). Both techniques are associated with similar results, with a 90% to 95% success rate in treating chronic anal fissure/ulcer disease (Table 51.27). Fewer than 10% of patients so treated are incontinent to mucus and gas. Recurrence is less than 10%.

It is possible to disrupt the internal sphincter with a four-finger stretch, but this is an uncontrolled disruption of the internal sphincter and is associated with a higher rate of recurrence and incontinence and therefore not our preferred approach. A Cochrane review of surgical intervention has recommended abandonment of the stretch procedure and supports internal sphincterotomy whether done in an open or closed fashion.[542]

Hemorrhoids

Hemorrhoidal tissues are part of the normal anatomy of the distal rectum and anal canal. The disease state of "hemorrhoids" exists when the internal complex becomes chronically engorged or the tissue prolapses into the anal canal as the result of laxity of the surrounding connective tissue and dilation of the veins.[30] External hemorrhoids may thrombose, leading to acute onset of severe perianal pain. When the thrombosis resolves, the overlying skin may remain enlarged, creating a skin tag.

Internal hemorrhoids may have two main pathophysiological mechanisms seen in two distinct, but not exclusive, groups, older women and younger men.[543] In older women, the pathophysiological mechanism may be related to chronic straining, which leads to vascular engorgement and dilation, resulting in stretching and disruption of the supporting connective tissue surrounding the vascular channels.[30,544,545] The most common cause of prolonged straining is the act of defecation. Contrary to popular belief, the stool may be liquid or solid. There is no correlation between hemorrhoids and constipation (infrequent passage of stool)[31,546] or hemorrhoids and portal hypertension.[30,544,547,548] Hemorrhoids are not dilated vascular channels, varices, or vascular hyperplasias.[30] Another suggested pathological mechanism, and the one that may be more important in younger men, is that of increased resting pressures within the anal canal, leading to decreased venous return, venous engorgement, and disruption of the supporting tissues.[549–551]

Internal hemorrhoids are traditionally classified by the following scheme: first-degree hemorrhoids bleed; second-degree hemorrhoids bleed and prolapse, but reduce spontaneously; third-degree hemorrhoids bleed, prolapse, and require manual reduction; and fourth-degree hemorrhoids bleed, incarcerate, and cannot be reduced.

Internal hemorrhoids typically do *not* cause pain but rather bright-red bleeding per rectum, mucus discharge, and a sense of rectal fullness or discomfort. Infrequently, internal hemorrhoids will prolapse into the anal canal, incarcerate, thrombose, and necrose. In this instance, patients may complain of pain. Visual inspection of the perineum may reveal a normal-appearing perineum, edema near the involved hemorrhoid, a prolapsed hemorrhoid, or an edematous,

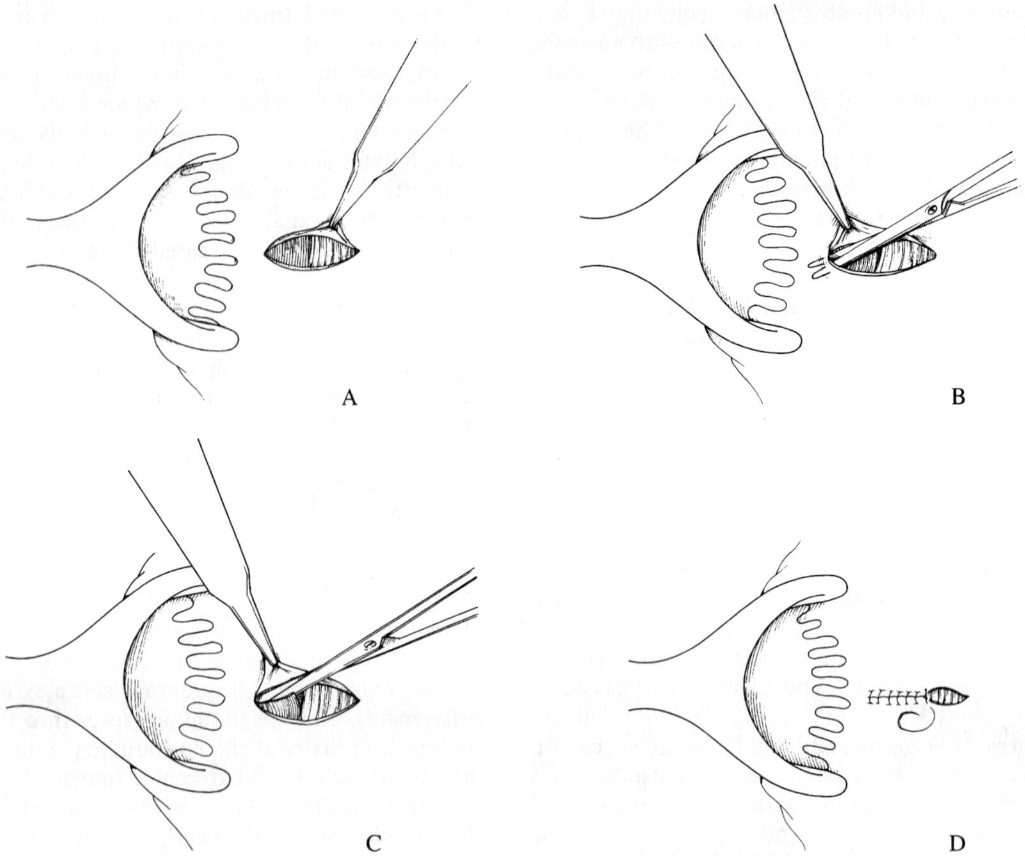

FIGURE 51.63. (A–D) Open lateral internal anal sphincterotomy. The skin edges are elevated to allow identification of the underlying internal and external sphincter. The internal sphincter is isolated with a clamp and divided with electrocautery or cut sharply with a knife or scissors. The skin may be closed or left open. (From Corman,[649] with permission, © 1998, Lippincott, Williams and Wilkins.)

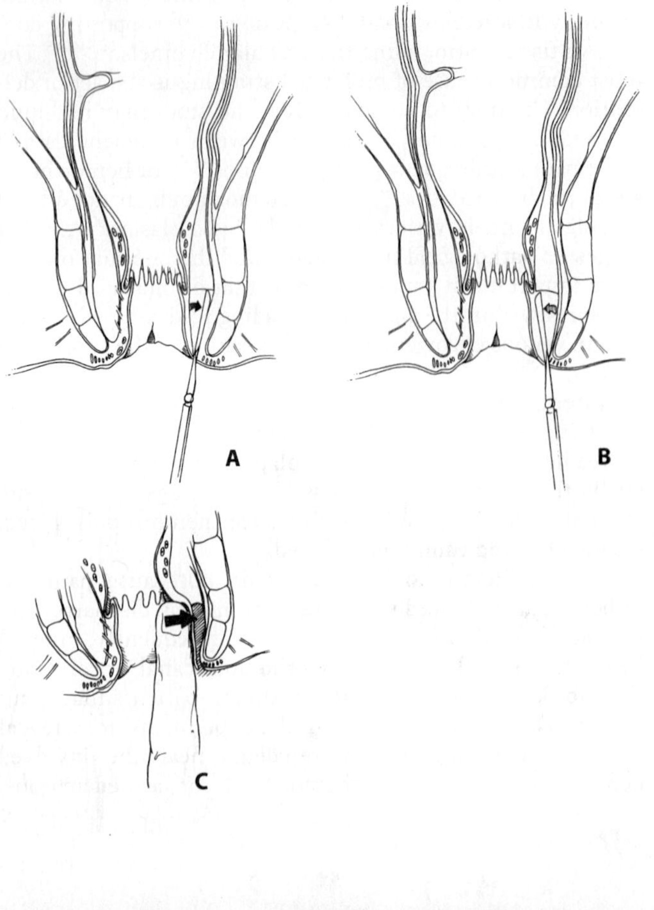

TABLE 51.27. Complications and Patient Satisfaction with Closed and Open Lateral Anal Sphincterotomy.

	Open (%)	*Closed (%)*	*P value*
Persistence of symptoms	3.4	5.3	.27
Fissure recurrence	10.9	11.7	.77
Need for reoperation	3.4	4	.70
Lack of control of gas	30.3	23.6	.06
Soiling underclothing	26.7	16.1	<.001
Accidental bowel movements	11.8	3.1	<.001
Very satisfied	49.7	64.4	NS
Satisfied	40.1	28.0	NS

NS, not specified.

Data from Garcia-Aguilar et al.[497a]

Source: From Bailey and Synder,[648] © 2000, Springer-Verlag, New York.

FIGURE 51.64. (A–C) Closed lateral internal anal sphincterotomy. The intersphincteric plane is palpated and an 11-blade scalpel is inserted in a vertical fashion. The blade is rotated 90° and swept inward, dividing the internal anal sphincter without injuring the external sphincter. (From Corman,[649] by permission, © 1998, Lippincott, Williams and Wilkins.)

gangrenous, incarcerated hemorrhoid. The perineum may be macerated from chronic mucus discharge, the resulting moisture, and local irritation. Anoscopy may reveal tissue with evidence of chronic venous dilation, friability, mobility, and squamous metaplasia. Proctosigmoidoscopy should be performed to rule out other disease of the distal colon and rectum.

External hemorrhoids may develop an acute intravascular thrombus, which is associated with acute onset of extreme perianal pain. No precipitating causes have been identified. The thrombus occasionally may cause ischemia and necrosis of the overlying anoderm, resulting in bleeding. The pain usually peaks within 48h. Repeated episodes of dilation and thrombosis may lead to enlargement of the overlying skin, which is seen as a skin tag on physical exam. The acutely thrombosed external hemorrhoid is seen as a purplish, edematous, tense subcutaneous perianal mass that is quite tender.

Chronic bleeding from internal hemorrhoids may cause anemia. However, until all other sources of blood loss have been ruled out, anemia must not be attributed to hemorrhoids regardless of the patient's age. Barium enema or colonoscopy are necessary to rule out malignancy and IBD. Defecography is helpful when obstructed defecation or rectal prolapse are suspected.

Patients with perianal pathology often present, or are referred, with a chief complaint of hemorrhoids. A thorough history frequently suggests the diagnosis. Those individuals with painless bleeding due to hemorrhoids must be distinguished from those with bleeding from colorectal malignancy, IBD, diverticular disease, and adenomatous polyps. Painful bleeding associated with a bowel movement is often due to an ulcer or fissure. Straining at stool may be attributed to hemorrhoids but is likely secondary to obstructed defecation. Similarly, rectal prolapse must be distinguished from hemorrhoids because it is safe to band a hemorrhoid but not a prolapsed rectum. Moisture or maceration may be secondary to hemorrhoids or condylomata acuminatum.

The complications of internal or external hemorrhoids are the indications for medical or surgical intervention; these are bleeding, pain, necrosis, mucus discharge, moisture, and, rarely, perianal sepsis. Initial medical management for all but the most advanced cases is recommended. Dietary alterations, including elimination of constipating foods (e.g., cheeses), addition of bulking agents, stool softeners, and increased intake of liquids are advised. Changing daily routines by adding exercise and decreasing time spent on the commode is often beneficial.

First- and second-degree hemorrhoids generally respond to medical management. Hemorrhoids that fail to respond to medical management may be treated with elastic band ligation, sclerosis, photocoagulation, cryosurgery, excisional hemorrhoidectomy, and many other local techniques that induce scarring and fixation of the hemorrhoids to the underlying tissues. The four most common techniques—elastic band ligation, sclerosis, excisional hemorrhoidectomy, and stapled hemorrhoidopexy—are discussed here.

Elastic band ligation is safe and effective in the treatment of first-, second-, third-, and selected fourth-degree hemorrhoids and is the preferred office-based treatment option.[552,553] Hemorrhoidal tissue 1 to 2cm above the dentate line is grasped and pulled into the barrel of an elastic band applicator, and two bands are placed at the base of the hemorrhoidal complex. After 7 to 10 days, the hemorrhoid itself sloughs, removing a portion of the offending redundant tissues, leaving a scar that inhibits further prolapse and bleeding of the remaining tissue. If the band is placed in the transitional zone or below, patients may experience sudden severe pain because this mucosa and skin are highly innervated. The band should be immediately removed. Immunocompromised patients[554] or those with unrecognized rectal prolapse have developed severe sepsis after banding. This complication is heralded by inordinate pain, fever, and urinary retention.[555] Treatment requires intravenous antibiotics, band removal, debridement of necrotic tissue, and observation.[556] Patients must avoid nonsteroidal antiinflammatory agents and aspirin for 10 days after ligation as significant bleeding may otherwise occur when the hemorrhoid sloughs.

Injection sclerotherapy is often tried for first-degree and second-degree hemorrhoids that continue to bleed despite medical measures. Sclerosant (1–2mL) is injected into the loose submucosal connective tissue above the hemorrhoidal complex, causing inflammation and scarring. This measure inhibits prolapse and bleeding of the remaining hemorrhoidal tissue. The depth of injection is critical because mucosal sloughing, infection, and full-thickness injury have been reported.

Excisional hemorrhoidectomy is reserved for the larger third- and fourth-degree hemorrhoids, mixed internal and external hemorrhoids not amenable to banding of the internal component, and incarcerated internal hemorrhoids requiring urgent intervention. The base of the hemorrhoid is visualized with an anoscope. The vascular pedicle is suture ligated with 3-0 chromic catgut. The hemorrhoidal tissue is excised using the "knife" (scalpel, scissors, cautery, laser, Harmonic Scalpel, Ligasure) preferred by the surgeon. Care must be taken to avoid the underlying internal sphincter while dissecting free the vascular cushion and overlying mucosa. The mucosal and skin defect may be left open, partially closed, or closed in a running fashion with the suture used for control of the vascular pedicle (Fig. 51.65). Severe pain, urinary retention, bleeding, and fecal impaction are the most common complications of excisional hemorrhoidectomy. The incidence of these complications can be minimized with improved postoperative pain control,[557] limited intraoperative intravenous fluid administration,[558] attention to surgical technique,[559] and stool bulking agents and stool softeners. Anal stenosis is a long-term complication that may be avoided by leaving adequate anoderm between excised hemorrhoidal complexes.

The procedure for prolapse and prolapsing hemorrhoids (PPH or stapled hemorrhoidectomy/hemorrhoidopexy) is a relatively new procedure in which the mucosa and submucosa of the rectum proximal to the hemorrhoidal complexes are excised with a modified circular stapling device, drawing the hemorrhoidal cushions up into the more proximal anal canal. As with any new procedure, there are many champions, and early results are promising. Randomized prospective trials comparing the procedure to excisional therapy have generally shown equal efficacy and less pain.[560–565] Rubber banding of symptomatic hemorrhoids is less expensive and results in less pain and fewer complications when compared to PPH, but there is a higher repeat procedure rate with the banding technique.[553,566] The long-term results are not known,

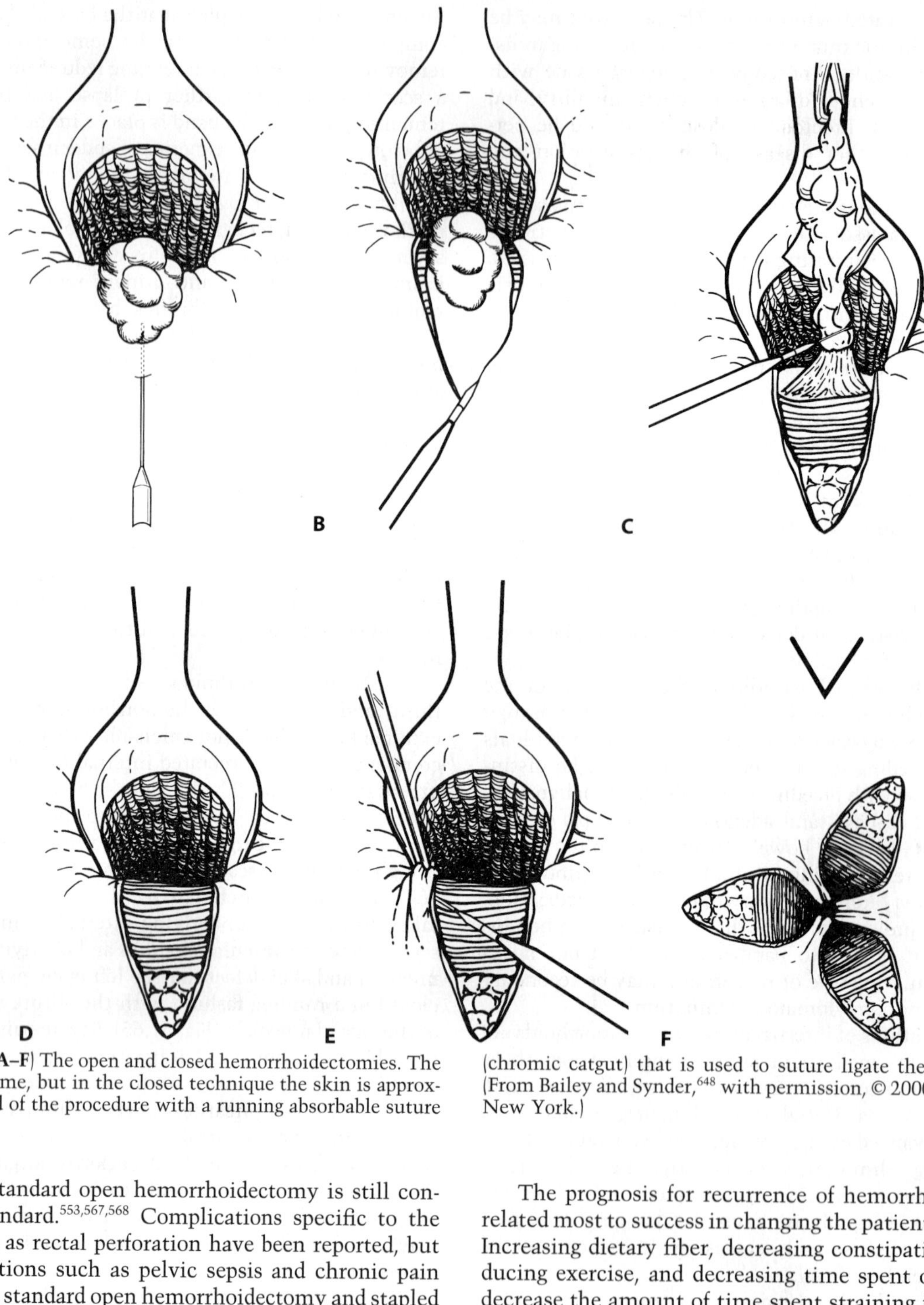

FIGURE 51.65. (A–F) The open and closed hemorrhoidectomies. The excision is the same, but in the closed technique the skin is approximated at the end of the procedure with a running absorbable suture (chromic catgut) that is used to suture ligate the vascular pedicle. (From Bailey and Synder,[648] with permission, © 2000, Springer-Verlag, New York.)

and therefore standard open hemorrhoidectomy is still considered the standard.[553,567,568] Complications specific to the procedure such as rectal perforation have been reported, but other complications such as pelvic sepsis and chronic pain may occur with standard open hemorrhoidectomy and stapled hemorrhoidectomy.[569]

The acutely thrombosed external hemorrhoid may be treated with excision of the hemorrhoid or clot evacuation if the patient presents within 48 h of onset of symptoms. Excision removes the clot and hemorrhoidal tissues, thereby decreasing the incidence of recurrence. However, many surgeons simply evacuate the thrombus, relieving the pressure and pain. If the patient presents more than 48 h after onset of symptoms, conservative management with warm sitz baths, high-fiber diet, stool softeners, and reassurance is advised. The thrombus has begun to organize, evacuation will not be successful, and excision will not reduce the amount or duration of anal pain.

The prognosis for recurrence of hemorrhoidal disease is related most to success in changing the patient's bowel habits. Increasing dietary fiber, decreasing constipating foods, introducing exercise, and decreasing time spent on the toilet all decrease the amount of time spent straining in the squatting position. These behavioral modifications are the most important steps in preventing recurrence.

Pilonidal Disease

The incidence of pilonidal disease is highest in Caucasian males (3 : 1 male : female ratio) between ages 15 and 40, with a peak incidence between 16 and 20 years of age.[570] It was once widely accepted that pilonidal disease is a congenital condition that develops along an epithelialized tract of the natal cleft.[570] However, more recently an acquired etiology has gained popularity. This theory suggests that a natal cleft hair follicle in a hirsute individual becomes distended, infected, obstructed, and ruptures into the subcutaneous tissues, forming a pilonidal abscess (Fig. 51.66).[571,572] Hair from the surrounding skin is sucked into the abscess cavity by the friction generated by the gluteal muscles during walking.

Patients with pilonidal disease may present with small midline pits or an abscess off the midline near the coccyx or sacrum. The patients are generally heavy, hirsute males. The workup is limited to a physical exam unless one suspects Crohn's disease, for which a more extensive evaluation may be necessary. The differential diagnosis includes abscess/fistulous disease of the anus, hidradenitis suppurativa, furuncle, and actinomycosis.

Pilonidal abscesses may be drained under local anesthesia. A probe may be inserted into the primary opening and the abscess unroofed. Granulation tissue and inspissated hair are curetted out, but definitive therapy is not required at the first procedure. Cure rates of 60% to 80% have been reported after primary unroofing.[573] For those who fail to heal after 3 months or develop a chronic draining sinus, definitive therapy is recommended. Nonoperative therapy with meticulous skin care (shaving of the natal cleft, perineal hygiene) and drainage of abscesses may significantly reduce the need for surgery.[574]

Excision with open packing, marsupialization, or primary closure with or without flaps have all been advocated for persistent disease. Open packing and marsupialization both leave the patient with painful wounds that are slow to heal, and marsupialization has a reported recurrence rate of 6% to 10%.[575] Limited excision and primary closure for both simple and complicated disease has recently been reported with excellent results, with recurrence rates of 0.9% in simple disease.[576,577] Others have advocated rotational flap closure over closed-suction drainage catheters, and this has been our preferred approach.[578]

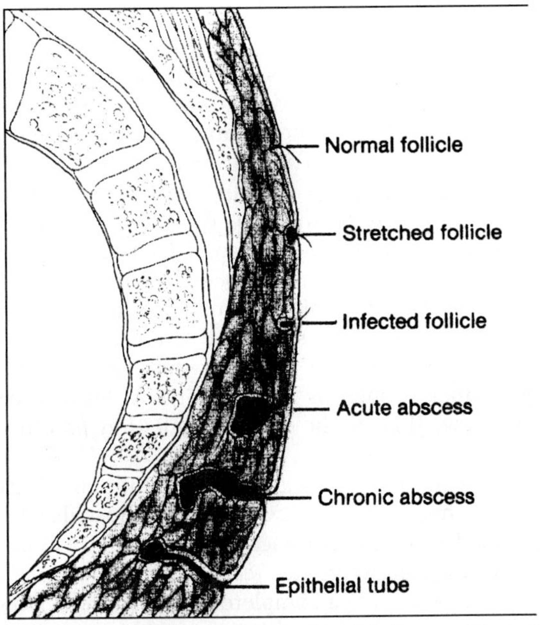

FIGURE 51.66. Pathophysiology of pilonidal disease. (From Gordon and Nivatvongs,[645] by permission of Taylor & Francis Group LLC.)

Pelvic Floor Dysfunction

Incontinence

Continence is maintained through a complex integrated pathway that involves rectal compliance, anorectal sensation, anorectal reflexes, and anal sphincter function.[28] Further, the nature and quantity of stool and colonic transit characteristics have an impact on assessment of continence. The incidence of fecal incontinence is difficult to assess because of underreporting and lack of standardization of what represents incontinence. What is perceived as incontinence in one patient may be perceived as normal staining in another. Of particular interest is the finding that although it is well accepted that incontinence is most commonly found in parous women, presumably secondary to obstetrical injuries, a high prevalence has been noted in men.[546,579]

Obstetrical trauma during delivery is the major cause of mechanical injury to the anal sphincter and potentially a cause of neurological injury.[580] There is an increased incidence of incontinence after third-degree perineal tears, multiple vaginal deliveries, and infection of an episiotomy repair.[581] The injury after prolonged labor may be twofold, with mechanical disruption of the sphincter and stretch of the pudendal nerve.

Incontinence may result from the treatment of cryptogenic abscess/fistula disease or perianal Crohn's disease, in which the external sphincter may be divided during a fistulotomy. In women, the external sphincter is a thin band of muscle anteriorly and therefore is especially susceptible to complete transection in this location. If it is surgically disrupted, or destroyed by chronic inflammation, continence is lost.

Neurogenic causes of incontinence include pudendal nerve stretch secondary to prolonged labor or multiple births or chronic history of straining to defecate.[580] Vaginal deliveries are associated with reversible pudendal nerve injury in 80% of primagravida births. The injury may be unilateral or bilateral. If the nerve injury is permanent or the insult is repeated multiple times, denervation and weakening of the external sphincter and pelvic floor result. A weakened pelvic floor is less able to withstand increased intraabdominal pressure, leading to further perineal descent and stretch injury. The neuropathy and sphincter dysfunction progress with time.[582] Chronic straining at stool and a sense of incomplete evacuation are common features of the descending perineum syndrome. Straining leads to descent of the pelvic floor and straightening of the anorectal angle; this may result in folding in or prolapse of the anterior rectal wall and further obstruction of defecation. The resultant increased straining and perineal descent leads to pudendal nerve injury as it is stretched over the ischial spine, leading to "idiopathic" fecal incontinence sometimes associated with internal rectal prolapse (intussusception).[583]

Other causes of incontinence include iatrogenic muscle disruption (anal dilation, internal sphincterotomy, hemorrhoidectomy); systemic diseases affecting either the muscular or neurological system (i.e., scleroderma, multiple sclerosis, dermatomyositis diabetes); and causes unrelated to the function of the sphincter itself (severe diarrhea, fecal impaction with overflow incontinence, radiation proctitis with fibrosis, tumors of the distal colon and rectum, low pelvic colorectal anastomoses).

Complete incontinence is lack of control of gas, liquid, and solid stool. Inability to control liquid and gas or gas alone is partial incontinence. Urgency, seepage, and soiling may occur regularly or intermittently depending on the nature of the stool presenting to the rectum. Elicitation of these symptoms is important in localizing the deficit. Patients who complain of soiling with urgency may have poor rectal compliance and normal sphincters, whereas those patients complaining of inability to sense stool until it has passed may have a neurological injury. The physical signs of incontinence may include a patulous anus, focal loss of corrugation of the anal verge, flattening and maceration of the perineum, exaggerated descent of the perineum with straining, decreased sphincter tone, diminished voluntary squeeze pressures, and loss of anal sensation.

Evaluation with anorectal manometry, transanal ultrasound, pudendal nerve latency studies, electromyography (EMG), and defecography may all be part of the evaluation of the incontinent patient. No particular study is diagnostic in all patients, and appropriate tests must be chosen based on history and physical examination.

Anorectal manometry is useful in defining the limits of the injury by measuring the maximum resting pressure, maximum squeeze pressure, sphincter length and symmetry, minimum sensory volume, presence or absence of the rectoanal inhibitory reflex, and coordinated relaxation of the puborectalis muscle. Normal maximal resting and maximal squeeze pressures have not been well standardized across laboratories, but within a lab standards of normal for men, nulliparous women, and parous women should be determined. These standard values will decrease with age.[584] The maximum squeeze pressure should be double the maximum resting pressure. The internal sphincter gives rise to 85% of the resting maximal pressure, while the external sphincter provides 15% of the resting pressure and 100% of the maximal squeeze pressures. The sphincter is typically 2.5 to 5 cm in length and asymmetrical (longer in back), and the whole complex is shorter in women.[8,584] The high-pressure zone also appears asymmetrical in that it is deeper within the body of the muscle posteriorly and more superficial anteriorly. The minimum sensory volume is usually 10 mL or less. The rectoanal inhibitory reflex is seen as a decrease in resting anal pressure when an air-filled balloon distends the rectum. The reflex is more pronounced in the proximal rectum, allowing for "sampling" of rectal contents by the anal canal while maintaining continence. At the completion of the anorectal manometry procedure, the patient is asked to pass a fully inflated 60-mL latex balloon. This task requires normal relaxation of the puborectalis and coordination of pelvic floor function.

Transrectal ultrasound provides clear anatomical images in the evaluation of internal and external anal sphincter defects.[585,586] Although EMG has been used for mapping sphincter defects, transrectal ultrasound has largely replaced the more painful and poorly tolerated EMG procedure (Fig. 51.67).[587] Good correlation between EMG changes and ultrasonographic evidence of sphincter injury have been documented.[588]

Pudendal nerve latency studies further define the nature of the injury in incontinent patients. If one or both nerves are injured, success in surgical or nonsurgical treatment of incontinence is diminished.[589] The study is performed by placing a gloved finger with a stimulating electrode at the tip of the finger in the rectum and stimulating the pudendal nerve as it traverses the ischial spine. An electrode at the base of the examining finger records the delay between stimulation and contraction of the external sphincter. A normal "delay" is 2.0 ± 0.2 s; this may be prolonged with age, after childbirth, in individuals with a history of excessive straining to defecate and perineal descent, and in certain systemic disease states such as diabetes and multiple sclerosis.

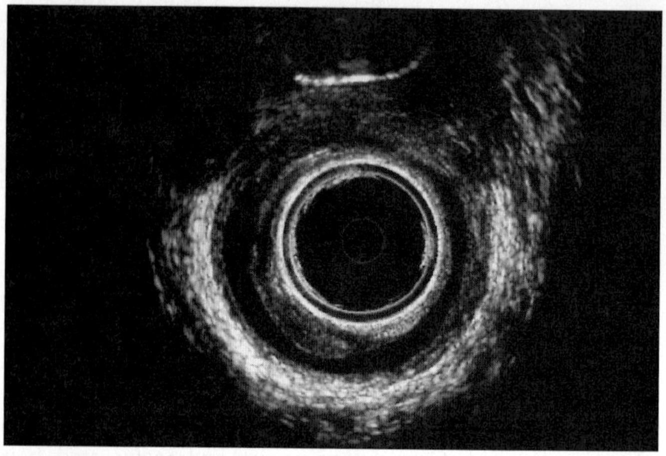

FIGURE 51.67. Transrectal ultrasound of the anal sphincters in a patient with an obstetrical injury to the external sphincter and fecal incontinence.

Defecography is useful in select patients with both constipation and incontinence as some patients with incontinence may be straining to defecate and intussuscept the rectum into itself, causing obstruction and apparent constipation, which is followed by uncontrolled release of liquid stool after the straining is stopped.

Obstructed defecation secondary to tumor or intussusception may lead to incontinence. Obstetrical injury from prolonged straining and pudendal nerve injury, disruption of the sphincter mechanism, or both, may cause varying degrees of incontinence. Incontinence may present immediately or after many years as the patient ages, sphincter tone decreases, and an occult injury is uncovered. Chronic straining during defecation stretches the pudendal nerve over the ischial spine, leading to idiopathic fecal incontinence in the elderly. An extreme of this example is seen in rectal prolapse, in which 30% of patients may be incontinent after repair because of stretch injury from chronic prolapse. Consideration of systemic diseases such as multiple sclerosis and diabetes mellitus is also necessary. Finally, incontinence may be unrelated to dysfunction of the anal sphincter mechanism but may be secondary to other diseases that overwhelm a normally functioning sphincter, such as severe diarrhea, fecal impaction with overflow, IBD of the rectum, radiation proctitis, and fibrosis.

An algorithm for the diagnosis and treatment of incontinence is summarized in Figure 51.68. If a muscular defect is limited and there is no neurological injury, surgical correction with an overlapping sphincter reconstruction restores continence by reestablishing a complete ring of muscle. However, if there is extensive loss of sphincter muscle or severe neurological injury, simple overlapping repair is not as successful,

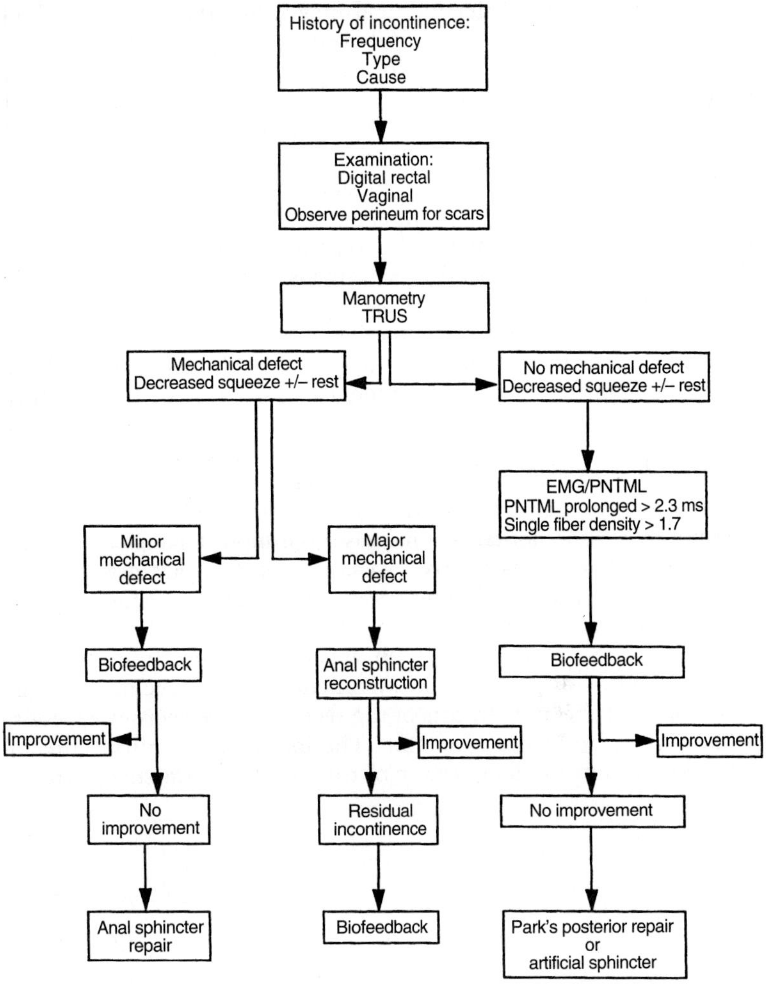

FIGURE 51.68. Algorithm for the workup and treatment of fecal incontinence. (From Shelton and Welton.[655])

and consideration must be given to muscle flap procedures or encirclement procedures. The stimulated gracilis, gracilis, and gluteal muscle flap procedures have been reserved for those patients with complete neurological injury or extensive muscle loss who wish to avoid a colostomy, but these are big operations, and results have been largely disappointing. Artificial sphincters have been evaluated in clinical trials with some success, but the explantation rate secondary to infection is 25%. Thus, artificial sphincters should be considered only in those patients with severe fecal incontinence with the only alternative being a permanent stoma.[590] New injectable agents are under trial for use in patients with complaints of seepage and leakage.[591]

Incontinence from muscular weakness or decreased sensation secondary to incomplete neurologic injury may respond to retraining with biofeedback.[592]

Anal encirclement procedures with foreign material have been reserved for the critically ill or patients with a short life expectancy. The anal canal is encircled with either a synthetic mesh or a silver wire. Patients are given daily enemas to evacuate the rectum, providing a form of continence with artificial obstruction and stimulated evacuation. The foreign body is prone to infection and erosion into the rectum, which often requires removal.

The incontinence associated with prolapse usually resolves after repair of the prolapse if there has not been significant nerve injury. The prolapsing segment often stimulates the rectoanal inhibitory reflex, decreasing internal sphincter pressure and fatiguing the external sphincter, leading to incontinence.

Obstructed Defecation

Obstructed defecation may result from anal stenosis, pelvic floor dysfunction, or abnormal rectal fixation. The most common cause of anal stenosis is scarring after anal surgery. In particular, inexpertly performed hemorrhoidectomies or the circumferential "Whitehead" hemorrhoidectomy lead to stenosis. Other causes include anal tumors, Crohn's disease, radiation injury, recurrent anal ulcers, infection, and trauma.

Patients with anal stenosis present with increasing difficulty and straining at defecation, thin and sometimes painful bowel movements, and bloating. Examination may reveal postsurgical changes and a stenotic anal canal. Digital exam may be quite painful or impossible.

Causes of anal pain that must be distinguished from anal stenosis include fissure, external hemorrhoids, perirectal abscess, malignancy, foreign body, and proctalgia fugax. Proctalgia fugax (levator syndrome), a diagnosis of exclusion, is suggested when a patient complains of pain that awakens them from sleep. The pain is generally left sided, short lived, and relieved by heat, dilation, or muscle relaxants. The patient often has a history of migraines and may report the occurrence of pain in relation to stressful events.

Mild anal stenosis may be treated successfully with gentle dilation and bulk agents. Severe anal stenosis is treated surgically if there is no evidence of active disease (i.e., Crohn's disease) and healthy tissue is available to perform the anoplasty; this can be achieved with an island or Y-V flap. Both procedures involve incision of the stenotic anus and incorporation of healthy tissue into the closure, relieving the stenosis (Fig. 51.69). The prognosis for anal stenosis is excellent if there is no evidence of active disease.

Pelvic floor dysfunction, alternatively referred to as nonrelaxing puborectalis syndrome, anismus, or paradoxical pelvic floor contraction, is a functional disorder in that the muscle is normal but control is dysfunctional. In health, the puborectalis is contracted "at rest," maintaining the anorectal angle. During defecation, the muscle relaxes, and evacuation occurs. In nonrelaxing puborectalis syndrome, the muscle does not relax and maintains or increases the anorectal angle. The patient therefore performs a Valsalva maneuver against an obstructed outlet, and elimination either does not occur or is significantly diminished (Fig. 51.70).

Patients who chronically strain at stool, whether from colonic inertia or pelvic floor dysfunction, may develop lengthening of the attachments of the rectum to the sacrum or descending perineum syndrome. The increased mobility that results from the lengthening of the sacral attachments allows for internal prolapse (intussusception), solitary rectal ulcer, and rectal procidentia. Intussusception causes outlet obstruction because the upper rectum moves away from the sacrum and telescopes into the more distal rectum.

Patients with nonrelaxing puborectalis syndrome may complain of straining and anal or pelvic pain, constipation, incomplete evacuation, or a need to perform digital maneuvers to evacuate rectal contents. Those who have developed internal intussusception complain of such but may also note mucus discharge, rectal bleeding, or tenesmus.

Digital examination of the patient with nonrelaxing puborectalis syndrome may reveal a tender pelvic muscular diaphragm. If asked to simulate a bowel movement by bearing down and relaxing the pelvic floor, they may not respond at all or may respond by contracting the pelvic musculature. Sigmoidoscopic examination may reveal a solitary rectal ulcer if intussusception has occurred chronically. The ulcer develops 4 to 12 cm from the anal verge, is anterior, and is the ischemic traumatized lead point of the internal intussusception.

Physical examination of the patient with intussusception may reveal a mass on digital exam. This is the lead point of the intussusceptum and may be mistaken for a malignancy. It may be a solitary rectal ulcer or may have progressed to colitis cystica profunda that develops as the healing solitary rectal ulcer entraps glands in the rectal submucosa. Biopsy reveals diffuse submucosal cysts that must be differentiated

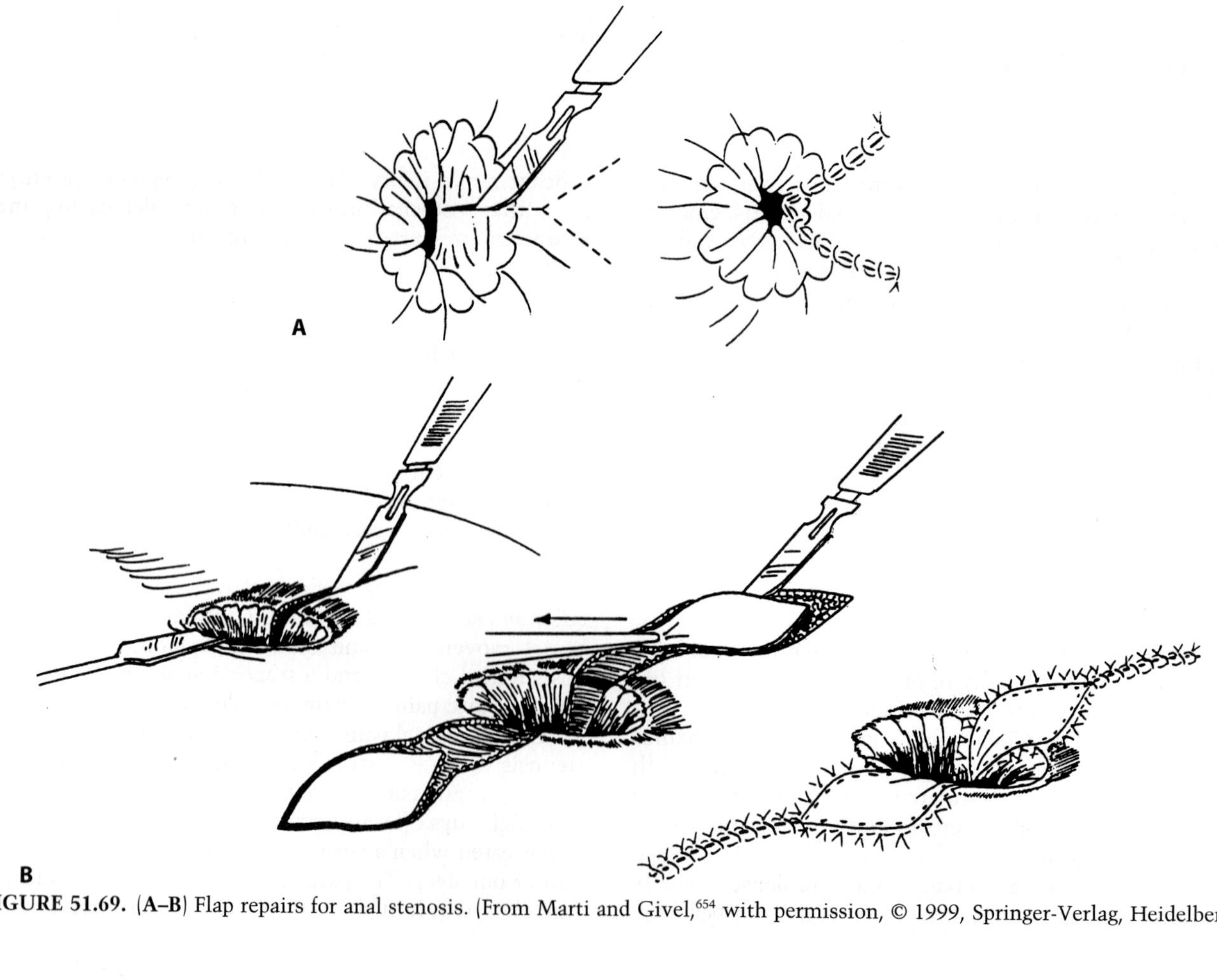

FIGURE 51.69. (A–B) Flap repairs for anal stenosis. (From Marti and Givel,[654] with permission, © 1999, Springer-Verlag, Heidelberg.)

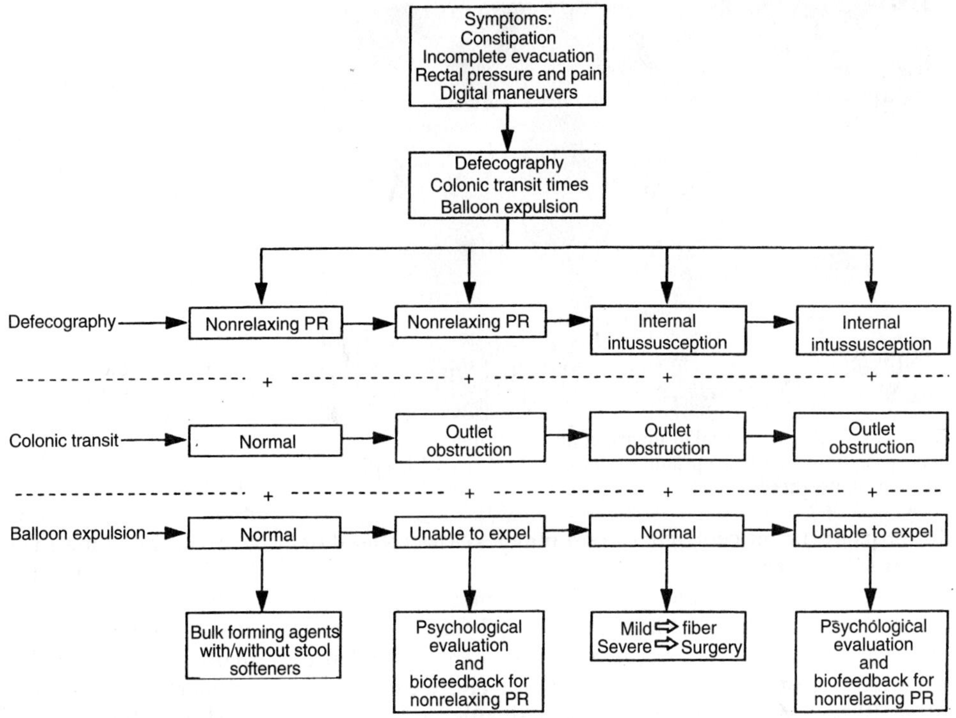

FIGURE 51.70. Algorithm for the workup of obstructed defecation. (From Shelton and Welton.[655])

from rectal cancer. Colitis cystica profunda may also be associated with radiation injury, postoperative changes, adenomatous polyps, malignancy, or IBD.

Patients with nonrelaxing puborectalis syndrome and intussusception may require defecography, colonic transit studies, anorectal manometry with the balloon expulsion test, and BE or colonoscopy to document the pathology suspected by history and physical examination. The patient with nonrelaxing puborectalis syndrome may demonstrate persistent anterior displacement of the rectum on the lateral view with cine defecography and may be unable to expel the balloon at the completion of anorectal manometric evaluation. The colon appears grossly normal with BE or colonoscopy. Colonic transit to the rectosigmoid will be normal.

In the patient with intussusception, colonic transit time will be normal to the rectosigmoid. Barium enema or colonoscopy will reveal a normal colon. Defecography will document the intussusception (Fig. 51.71). Those patients with intussusception secondary to nonrelaxing puborectalis will be unable to expel the latex balloon at the completion of the anorectal manometry.

Nonrelaxing puborectalis syndrome is best treated with biofeedback. The puborectalis is retrained to relax during the act of defecation, allowing the act to proceed without obstruction. Biofeedback results are excellent,[592] but patients may require occasional retraining before education is complete.

Mild-to-moderate intussception is treated with bulk agents, modification of bowel habits, and reassurance. The patient is instructed to stimulate a bowel movement in the morning and avoid the urge to defecate the remainder of the day because the fullness they sense is the proximal rectum intussuscepting into the distal rectum. With time, the urge to defecate resolves, as does the intussusception. Most patients with intussusception do quite well once they are reassured that there is an abnormality, and that the abnormality is not malignant. Severe intussusception with impending pudendal nerve damage is treated surgically, as follows.

Patients with rectal procidentia complain of mucus discharge, progressive incontinence, pain, and bleeding; on direct questioning, they may report their rectum "falls out." Physical examination of the patient who presents with an acute episode of rectal prolapse is not difficult. A large mass of prolapsed tissue with concentric mucosal rings will be apparent (Fig. 51.72). This finding is in contrast to the patient with prolapsed hemorrhoids, for whom physical exam reveals prolapsing tissue with deep radial grooves between areas of edematous tissue. However, the patient with a history of prolapse but without active prolapse may be more difficult. It may be necessary to give the patient an enema, allow the patient to evacuate, and then examine the perineum. This practice often induces prolapse, allowing confirmation of the

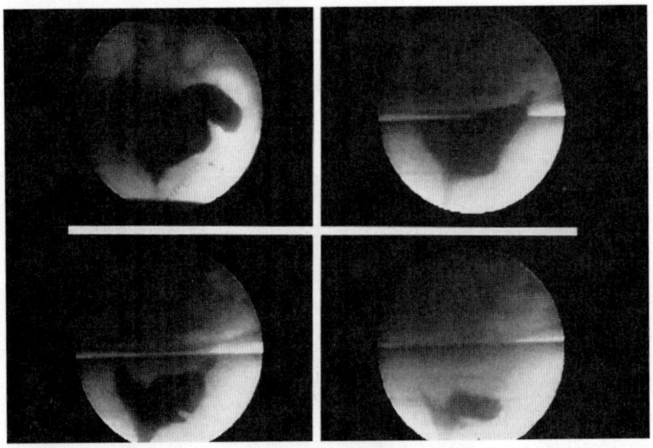

FIGURE 51.71. Defecography in a patient with intussusception.

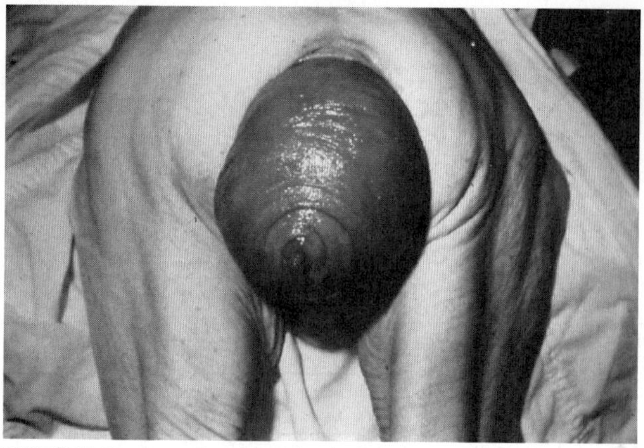

FIGURE 51.72. Rectal prolapse with concentric rings of mucosa, not masses of tissue with deep radial grooves as is seen with prolapsed internal hemorrhoids.

diagnosis in the office. Digital exam may reveal decreased or absent sphincter tone.

Patients with rectal prolapse may need anorectal manometry, EMG, pudendal nerve latency studies, defecography, and BE or colonoscopy. Defecography may document the prolapse if not clinically apparent. Evaluation of the entire colon with either BE or colonoscopy is necessary to rule out a malignancy. The surgical approach may be chosen based on the pudendal nerve latency studies and EMG.

There are two classes of operations for rectal prolapse, abdominal and perineal. The abdominal procedures have a lower recurrence rate and preserve the reservoir capacity of the rectum but submit the patients to a higher-risk intraabdominal procedure. The perineal procedures do not require an abdominal incision and do not have an intraabdominal anastomosis but do remove the rectum, eliminating the rectal reservoir. Thus, the abdominal procedures may be preferred over the perineal procedures in low-risk active patients less than 50 years of age and in patients who otherwise require an abdominal procedure.

The abdominal procedures for patients with severe intussusception or rectal prolapse with normal sphincter function are rectopexy with or without sigmoid resection. Either operation, rectopexy or resection rectopexy, requires complete mobilization of the entire rectum to the pelvic floor to avoid distal intussusception and may be performed either open or laparoscopically.

The rectopexy attempts to secure the rectum to the sacral hollow. It may be performed with sutures or prosthetic materials such as polypropylene mesh (Marlex), Gore-Tex, or polyglycolic acid or polygalactin mesh (Dexon or Vicryl). Many studies have suggested a higher complication rate with the prosthetics, a lower continence rate, and no difference in success rates, suggesting that suture rectopexy is preferable.[593–595] The suture rectopexy is performed with a heavy nonabsorbable suture attaching the rectum to the sacral hollow. The suture may be placed through the lateral ligaments or through the muscularis propria of the rectum. The addition of a sigmoid resection at the time of rectopexy lowers the recurrence rate and lowers the incidence of postoperative constipation but does not increase the morbidity of the surgery[593,596–601] (Table 51.28).

The perineal approaches to rectal prolapse include anal encirclement and the transanal Delorme procedure and Altemeier procedures. A complete mechanical bowel preparation is performed for all three procedures.

For those patients with prolapse who have prohibitively high operative risk or who have limited life expectancy, an anal encirclement procedure may be preferred. Thiersch originally described using a silver wire to encircle the external sphincter in the ischiorectal fat, but currently, synthetic mesh or silicone tubes are preferred. With any of these, an outlet obstruction is created, and laxatives or enemas are required for rectal evacuation. The encirclement procedures can be complicated by erosion of the foreign material into the rectum and infection. This procedure is utilized less frequently as the transanal approaches with the patient under spinal or epidural anesthesia have gained favor.

The Delorme procedure is essentially a mucosal proctectomy with imbrication of the prolapsing rectal wall (Fig. 51.73). The dissection is started 1 to 2 cm above the dentate line and carried to the apex of the prolapsing segment, where the mucosa is amputated. The muscle is reefed in with 4–8 heavy absorbable sutures, and the mucosa is reapproximated with suture (running or interrupted) or a circular stapler (Table 51.29).

The Altemeier procedure is a complete proctectomy and often partial sigmoidectomy. The apex of the prolapsing segment is delivered and placed on traction, and a full-thickness incision is made approximately 1 cm above the dentate line (Fig. 51.74). The rectum is everted. The dissection is carried into the deep cul-de-sac anteriorly, and posteriorly the

TABLE 51.28.
Results for Sigmoid Resection with Rectopexy for Rectal Prolapse.

Author	*No. of patients*	*Recurrence rate (%)*	*Mortality rate (%)*	*Morbidity rate (%)*	*Mean follow-up (years)*
Watts et al.[599] (1985)	102	1.9	0	4	4
Husa et al.[600] (1988)	48	9	2.1	0	4.3
Sayfan et al.[594] (1990)	13	0	0	23	
McKee et al.[598] (1992)	9	0	0	0	1.8
Luukkonen et al.[597] (1992)	15	0	6.7	20	
Canfrère et al.[601] (1996)	20	0	0	10	2.6
Huber et al.[596] (1995)	39	0	0	7.1	4.5

Source: Adapted from Gordon and Nivatvongs,[645] by permission of Taylor & Frances Group LLC.

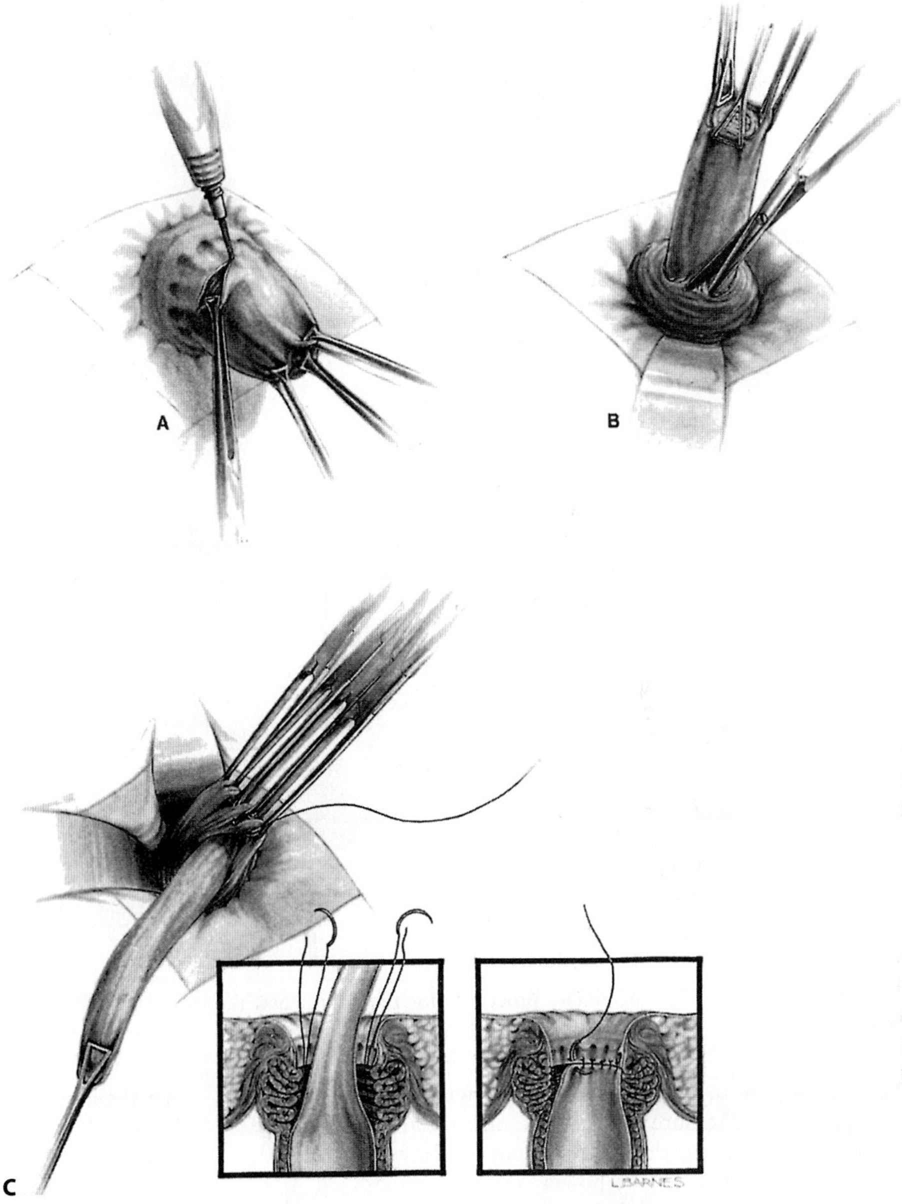

FIGURE 51.73. (**A–C**) The Delorme procedure for rectal prolapse. (Figures 51.73A and 51.73B from Corman,[649] with permission, © 1998, Lippincott, Williams and Wilkins. Figure 51.73C from Berman,[656] with permission.)

TABLE 51.29.
Results of the Delorme Procedure for Rectal Prolapse.

					Functional results			
Author	*No. of patients*	*Recurrence rate (%)*	*Mortality rate (%)*	*Morbidity rate (%)*	*Excellent*	*Satisfactory*	*Poor*	*Mean follow-up (months)*
Abulafi et al.[632] (1990)	22	5	0	14		Improved 75%		29
Graf et al.[633] (1992)	14	21	0	—		Improved 55%		18
White and Stitz[634] (1992)	17	17.6	0					24
Oliver et al.[635] (1994)	40	22	2.5	62.5[a]	61	29	10	48
Senapati et al.[636] (1994)	32	12.5	0	6.3		[b]		24
Tobin et al.[637] (1994)	43	25.6	0	12.2	53	21	26	20
Lechaux et al.[638c] (1995)	85	13.5	1.2	14	55	38	7	33
Plusa et al.[639] (1995)	104	25				[d]		28

[a]One major complication: anastomotic separation and bleeding.
[b]Incontinence improved in 46%.
[c]41 patients underwent modified Delorme.
[d]Of 13 patients, 4 incontinent preoperatively remained incontinent.
Source: Adapted from Gordon and Nivatvongs,[645] by permission of Taylor & Frances Group LLC.

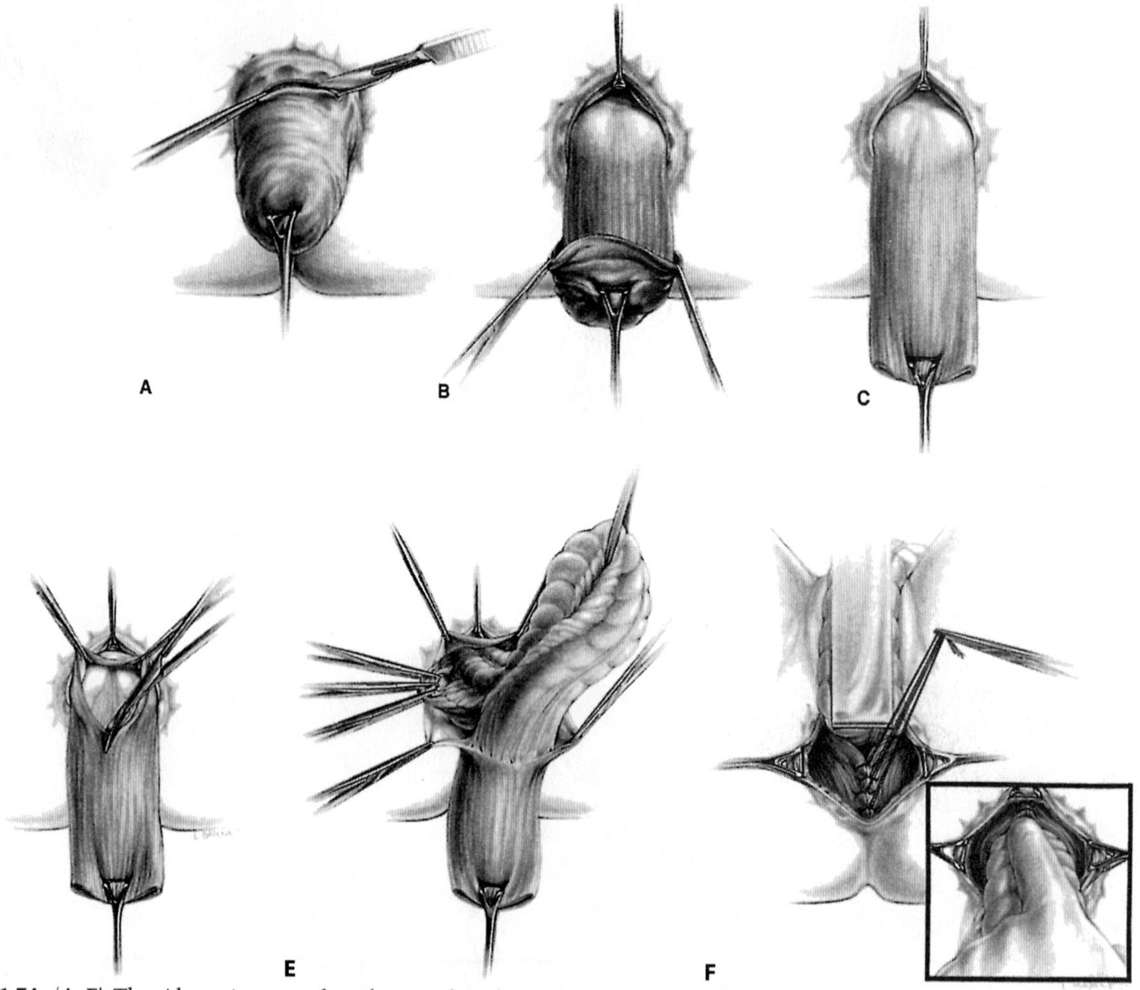

FIGURE 51.74. (A–F) The Altemeier procedure for rectal prolapse. (From Corman,[649] with permission, © 1998, Lippincott, Williams and Wilkins.)

vascular supply to the rectum is taken with electrocautery, clamps, or the Ligasure device. The dissection is carried up onto the midline mesorectum and sigmoid mesentery until the redundant segment of bowel has been mobilized. If a levatoroplasty is planned, it is most easily carried out at this time with heavy absorbable suture. A levatoroplasty plicates the pelvic floor musculature and adds to improved continence by increasing the anorectal angle. The bowel is transected proximally, encompassing the redundant bowel, and a hand-sewn (heavy absorbable suture) or stapled anastomosis may be performed (Table 51.30).

Of those patients with rectal prolapse and incontinence, 60% to 70% will have return of sphincter function. However, reliable means of identifying these patients do not exist. Those that do not have a return of sphincter function will not tolerate sigmoid resection. Therefore, perineal proctectomy and posterior sphincter enhancement are recommended in these patients. The posterior reconstruction may alter the angle of the rectum or obstruct the outlet sufficiently to allow for continence. Those individuals with severe intussusception and those who have rectal prolapse without sphincter dysfunction should do well.

TABLE 51.30.
Results for the Altemeier Procedure for Rectal Prolapse.

Author	*No. of patients*	*Recurrence rate (%)*	*Mortality rate (%)*	*Morbidity rate (%)*	*Mean follow-up (months)*
Altemeier et al.[640] (1971)	106	3	0	24	
Finlay and Aitchison[641] (1991)	17	6	6	18	24
Williams et al.[642] (1992)	114	11	0	12	3–90
Johansen et al.[643] (1993)	20	0	5	5	24

Source: Adapted from Gordon and Nivatvongs,[645] by permission of Taylor & Francis Group LLC.

Sexually Transmitted Diseases

Sexually transmitted diseases of the anorectum are found frequently in urban men who have sex with men,[602] but these diseases are not limited to this population. The anorectum appears more susceptible to certain infections, and it is therefore important to inquire, regardless of sex or overt evidence of sexual preference, into sexual practices. The external genitalia, oral cavity, and anorectum should be examined for evidence of infection. It should be remembered that the infections are often multiple, and the exact location, whether anus, perineum, or rectum, is helpful in making the pathological diagnosis. Herpes simplex virus type 2, *Treponema pallidum*, *Neisseria gonorrhoeae*, and *Chlamydia trachomatis* often cause proctitis. Anusitis or perineal infections suggest syphilis, chancroid, herpes, or lymphogranuloma venereum (LGV). Once a diagnosis is made, the patient should be counseled on safe sex practices and the partner or partners evaluated.

Herpes Proctitis

With herpes proctitis, patients may present early with anal pain and vesicles or later with ulcerations, discharge, rectal bleeding, tenesmus, constipation, fear of defecation, and even urinary retention secondary to severe pain.[603] Fever, generalized malaise, and adenopathy are often noted and are particularly prominent with primary infection. No history of anoreceptive intercourse is required as the disease may spread by extension from the vagina. Lesions appear as vesicles that rupture, forming ulcers that may become secondarily infected. Anoscopy may reveal single or confluent rectal ulcerations. Viral culture of the vesicle or biopsy of the ulcer makes the diagnosis. Confirmation of the diagnosis is made with a direct fluorescent monoclonal antibody. Herpes simplex type II is most common.

Herpes infections are self-limited, and if left untreated will resolve within 1 to 3 weeks. Oral acyclovir is the treatment of choice, but it is not curative.[604] It decreases the duration of outbreaks and viral shedding, however, and increases the interval between attacks. The first episode is associated with the most pain and longest duration of ulceration. Subsequent episodes are generally shorter and not as painful. Acyclovir or famciclovir may be used for suppressive therapy.

Anorectal Syphilis

The chancre, the primary lesion of syphilis, is an indurated ulcer at the site of inoculation whether it be rectal, perineal, or oral. Anal ulcers may be confused with fissures, but off-midline location and position relative to the dentate line (too proximal or distal) help to differentiate the two diseases. Lymphadenopathy may be prominent. Proctitis and pseudotumors may develop in individuals who practice anoreceptive intercourse, and these should be distinguished from lymphoma or neoplasms. Condylomata lata are contagious, hypertrophic, flat, pale papules associated with secondary syphilis.

Dark-field microscopy of exudate and serological testing are the preferred methods of diagnosis for *T. pallidum*.[603] Serological tests may initially be negative and should be repeated several months later. A long-acting preparation of penicillin is the preferred treatment.[604] The prognosis is good.

Gonococcal Proctitis

Gonococcal proctitis results from anoreceptive intercourse. Symptoms range from asymptomatic to anal itching and irritation or painful defecation. Rectal bleeding and discharge, perianal excoriation, and, rarely, fistulas may develop. Anoscopy reveals friable edematous, erythematous mucosa with pus expressing from crypts.[603]

Cultures of anus, vagina, urethra, and pharynx should be obtained and plated on a Thayer-Martin medium. Blind cultures of the anorectum or Gram stains from anoscopy are effective for diagnosis.[603] The gram-negative diplococcus *N. gonorrhoeae* is the causative agent.

A one-time dose of intramuscular Ceftriaxone plus 1 week of oral doxycycline is the treatment of choice.[603] Follow-up examination and cultures should be performed to confirm adequate therapy. The prognosis is excellent. Resistant strains are endemic and should be treated according to regional resistant antibiotic sensitivities.

Chlamydia Proctitis and Lymphogranuloma Venereum

Chlamydia is the most common sexually transmitted disease, with approximately 3 million new cases per year.[604] As in gonococcal proctitis, symptoms of chlamydia proctitis range from asymptomatic to rectal pain, bleeding, and discharge. The small shallow ulcer of LGV may be unnoticed, but the inguinal adenopathy may become quite marked. Biopsy reveals crypt abscesses and granulomas. Late findings include hemorrhagic proctitis, rectovaginal and rectovesical fistulas, and rectal stricture.

The causative agent, *C. trachomatis*, is an intracellular parasite that is spread by anal intercourse or direct extension through the lymphatics of the rectovaginal septum. Isolation of the organism from cell culture is the best method for identification. The diagnosis may also be made with the LGV complement fixation test, ELISA, or polymerase chain reaction (PCR).[605,606]

Twenty-one days of doxycycline is recommended, but one oral dose of azithromycin or erythromycin is an acceptable alternative.[604] Early strictures may be dilated. Although uncommon, strictures may cause bowel obstruction and require colostomy.

Chancroid

Haemophilus ducreyi causes a soft perianal ulcer that is painful, often multiple, and bleeds easily. Autoinoculation is common. Inguinal lymph nodes become fluctuant, rupture, and drain. Diagnosis is made by PCR.[606] Ciprofloxacin is the treatment of choice.[607]

Condylomata Acuminata

Human papilloma virus (HPV) is the cause of condylomata acuminatum. Multiple types have been identified. Types HPV-6 and HPV-11 are associated with the common "benign" genital wart, whereas HPV-16 and HPV-18 are associated with the development of high-grade dysplasia and anal cancer.[603] In the United States, condylomata acuminatum is the most common sexually transmitted viral disease. It is the most common anorectal infection within homosexual men and is particularly prominent in HIV-positive patients. However, the disease is not limited to men or women who practice anoreceptive intercourse. In women, the virus may tract down from the vagina, and in men, it may pool and tract from the base of the scrotum. Immunosuppression, either with drugs after kidney transplant or from HIV, has a significant impact on the incidence of condylomatous disease, with rates up to 4% and 86%, respectively.[613]

The most frequent complaint is that of a perianal growth. Pruritus, discharge, bleeding, odor, and anal pain are present to a lesser degree. Physical exam reveals the classic cauliflower-like lesion, which may be isolated, clustered, or coalescent. The warts tend to run in radial rows out from the anus. The lesions may be surprisingly large at the time of presentation.

Anoscopy and proctosigmoidoscopy are essential because the disease extends internally in more than three-fourths of patients, and 94% of homosexual men have intraanal disease. Cultures and serologies for other venereal diseases may be taken from the penis, anus, mouth, and vagina.

These lesions must be distinguished from condylomata lata and anal squamous cell carcinoma. Condylomata lata are the lesions of secondary syphilis. They are flatter, paler, and smoother than condylomata acuminata. Anal squamous cell carcinoma is generally painful and may be tender and ulcerated, whereas condylomata are not tender or ulcerated.

The extent of the disease or the risk of malignancy (dysplasia treatment is discussed later) determines the treatment. Minimal disease is treated in the office with topical agents such as bichloracetic acid or 25% podophyllin in tincture of benzoin.[603] The former is preferred because the latter must be washed off within 4 to 6h to limit pain, there are fewer complications (scarring), and warts respond promptly to therapy. Patients should be seen again at regular intervals until the treatment is complete. More extensive disease may require initial treatment under anesthesia in which random lesions may be excised for pathological evaluation to rule out dysplasia and the remainder coagulated. Electrocautery coagulates the lesions. Care is taken to spare the surrounding skin. Follow-up evaluation may reveal residual disease, but this is often easily treated with topical agents in the office. Laser therapy and infrared coagulation are other methods of condylomata destruction with acceptable recurrence rates.[603,608]

Refractory disease may respond to excision or destruction followed by intralesional interferon or autogenous vaccine created from excisional biopsies of the lesions.[609,610] Recurrence rates of only 4.6% have been reported for destruction and vaccination combined, but the preparation of the vaccine is tedious, and therefore this technique has not gained wide acceptance.[609] Recurrence rates for other treatments are listed in Table 51.31.

TABLE 51.31. Recurrence Rates After Various Forms of Therapy for Anal Condylomata.

Method	*Success rate (%)*	*Recurrence rate <6 months (%)*
Cryotherapy	83	28
Podophyllum resin	65	39
Trichloroacetic/bichloroacetic acid	81	36
CO_2 laser	89	8
Electrocautery	93	24
Excision	93	24
5-Fluorouracil	71	13
Interferon alfa	52	25

Source: From Mayeaux et al.,[662] with permission.

TABLE 51.32. Sexually Transmitted Diseases of the Anorectum and Their Treatments.

Organism	*Suggested treatment*
Neisseria gonorrhoeae	Ceftriaxone, 250mg, IM once plus doxycycline, 100mg, PO bid for 7 days
Chlamydia trachomatis	Doxycycline, 100mg, bid for 21 days, or azithromycin, 1g, PO as a single dose
Campylobacter spp.	Erythromycin, 500mg, qid for 7 days, or ciprofloxacin, 500mg, q 12h for 7 days
Shigella spp.	Trimethoprim-sulfamethoxazole double strength PO bid for 5 days
Haemophilus ducreyi	Azithromycin, 1g, PO as a single dose, or ceftriaxone, 250mg, IM one time
Donovania spp.	Tetracycline, 500mg, qid for 10 days
Treponema pallidum	Benzathine penicillin G, 2.4 million U, IM, or tetracycline, 500mg, qid for 30 days
Herpesvirus	Acyclovir, 200mg, 5 times a day for 5 days
Hepatitis virus	Symptomatic
Entamoeba histolytica	Metronidazole, 750mg, tid for 10 days, plus diloxanide furoate, 500mg, tid for 10 days
Giardia lamblia	Metronidazole, 250mg, PO tid for 7 days

Source: From Gordon and Nivatvongs,[645] by permission of Taylor & Francis Group LLC.

Human papilloma viruses 16 and 18 are causally associated with squamous cell carcinomas of the anal canal. This association has led to new screening techniques to evaluate high-risk patients for occult disease. These techniques are discussed in the anal cancer section. Representative biopsies of clinically apparent condylomata should be sent to pathology because unsuspected low- or high-grade dysplasia or squamous cell carcinoma of the anal canal may be found.

Buschke-Lowenstein tumors are giant condylomata acuminata that are locally aggressive and exhibit malignant behavior but benign histology. Radical excision is often the only therapeutic option for either palliation or cure, but wide local excision and even surgery with adjuvant chemotherapy and radiotherapy have been used with success.[609,611]

Other sexually transmitted diseases of the anorectum and their treatments are listed in Table 51.32.

Anal Neoplasms

Prediction of the biology and planning for treatment of tumors of the perianal region are dependent on precise localization of the tumor with respect to anal landmarks such as the dentate line, the anal verge, and the anal sphincters. These landmarks define two classes of perianal neoplasms: tumors of the anal margin and tumors of the anal canal. The Histologic Typing of Intestinal Tumors (adopted by the World Health Organization) defines the anal canal as extending from "the upper to the lower border of the internal anal sphincter (from the pelvic floor to the anal verge)."[612] The AJCC has agreed to this classification, and efforts are under way to classify tumors in this manner.

The anal margin extends from the anal verge (the junction of the highly specialized epithelium of the anoderm with the hair-bearing perianal skin) to 5 to 6 cm from this point. Historically, the anal canal has been defined as the region above the dentate line and the anal margin as the area below the dentate line, but recently some have suggested a system that clinicians across all specialties understand.[613] Squamous cell tumors of the anal margin are well-differentiated, keratinizing tumors that behave similarly to squamous cell tumors of the skin elsewhere. Tumors of the anal canal are aggressive high-grade tumors with significant risk for metastasis. The staging system for anal tumors is shown in Table 51.33.

Overall, anal cancers occur in 7 of 1 million men and 9 of 1 million women. In HIV-positive men who have sex with men, the rate is estimated at 35 of 100,000. In the immunocompromised (transplant recipients, HIV-positive individuals), this risk is considerably higher. In the HIV-positive men who have sex with men, the rate approaches 70 in 100,000.[613] There is a high incidence (15%) of anal dysplasias in the HIV-positive patients, and the rate of anal cancers may increase as lives are prolonged with highly active retroviral therapies.[614]

TABLE 51.33. Definition of TMN, Stage Grouping, Histopathologic Type, and Histologic Grade for Anal Carcinoma.

Definition of TMN

Primary Tumor (T)

TX	Primary tumor cannot be assessed
T0	No evidence of primary tumor
Tis	Carcinoma *in situ*
T1	Tumor 2 cm or less in greatest dimension
T2	Tumor more than 2 cm but not more than 5 cm in greatest dimension
T3	Tumor more than 5 cm in greatest dimension
T4	Tumor of any size invades adjacent organ(s), e.g., vagina, urethra, bladder*

**Note:* Direct invasion of the rectal wall, perirectal skin, subcutaneous tissue, or the sphincter muscle(s) is not classified as T4.

Regional Lymph Nodes (N)

NX	Regional lymph nodes cannot be assessed
N0	No regional lymph node metastasis
N1	Metastasis in perirectal lymph node(s)
N2	Metastasis in unilateral internal iliac and/or inguinal lymph node(s)
N3	Metastasis in perirectal and inguinal lymph nodes and/or bilateral internal iliac and/or inguinal lymph nodes

Distant Metastasis (M)

MX	Distant metastasis cannot be assessed
M0	No distant metastasis
M1	Distant metastasis

Stage Grouping

Stage 0	Tis	N0	M0
Stage I	T1	N0	M0
Stage II	T2	N0	M0
	T3	N0	M0
Stage IIIA	T1	N1	M0
	T2	N1	M0
	T3	N1	M0
	T4	N0	M0
Stage IIIB	T4	N1	M0
	Any T	N2	M0
	Any T	N3	M0
Stage IV	Any T	Any N	M1

Source: Used with the permission of the American Joint Committee on Cancer (AJCC), Chicago, Illinois. The original source for this material is the *AJCC Cancer Staging Manual, Sixth Edition* (2002) published by Springer Science and Business Media LLC, www.springerlink.com.

Human papilloma virus has been implicated as a causative agent in the development of anal cancer. As in the cervix, HPV types 16 and 18 appear causally related to the development of high-grade dysplasia and anal cancer, whereas types 6 and 11 cause common genital warts and low-grade dysplasia.[613,614]

These parallels to cervical disease have led investigators to explore the utility of anal Papanicolaou smears and high-resolution anoscopy (magnified examination of the anus with a culposcope or operating microscope) as a method of detecting and destroying high-grade lesions in high-risk patients before the development of cancer.[614] If high-grade disease is found, referral for surgical excision or ablation is recommended. In the operating room, the anus is painted with acetic acid and examined circumferentially with an operating microscope or culposcope. Vascular changes characteristic of severe dysplasia are noted, and the anus is "mapped" regarding the distribution of this disease. The anus is next painted with Lugol's solution and mapped again. The Lugol's solution is a concentrated (10%) iodine solution that stains glycogen stores in nondysplastic tissues a dark brown-black. Low-grade dysplasia stains partially, and high-grade disease does not take up the solution, leaving it mahogany in color. Representative biopsies are taken from the areas of severe dysplasia, and the surrounding severely dysplastic disease is destroyed with electrocautery.[614]

Tumors of the Anal Margin

Squamous Cell Carcinoma

Patients with squamous cell carcinomas of the anal margin frequently complain of a lump, bleeding, itching, pain, or tenesmus (complaints common to most lesions of this region). Typically, the lesions are large, centrally ulcerated with rolled everted edges and have been present for some time before the patient presents to a clinician. In contrast, patients followed closely because they are at increased risk for cancer often present with the more subtle findings of a submucosal nodule.

All chronic or nonhealing ulcers of the perineum should be biopsied to rule out squamous cell carcinoma. Small, well-differentiated lesions of 4 cm or less are treated by wide local excision.[615] Deep lesions that involve the sphincters may require an APR of the rectum. Chemoradiation is used for less-favorable lesions.[615,616] Spread is to the inguinal lymph nodes, which are generally included in the radiation fields. Treatment of inguinal disease is excision if palpable and symptomatic disease is identified. Disease recurring in the skin may be treated with reexcision or APR. The T stage determines survival, with reports of 5- and 10-year survival of 100% for T1 lesions compared to 60% and 40% for T2 lesions at 5 and 10 years, respectively.[616]

Basal Cell Carcinoma

Bleeding, itching, and pain are presenting symptoms of basal cell carcinoma. The lesions appear with raised edges and central ulceration. They are more frequent in men. As with squamous cell carcinoma of the margin, treatment is wide local excision.[617]

Bowen's Disease

Bowen's disease is squamous cell carcinoma in situ (high-grade squamous intraepithelial lesion) with a potential for progression to invasive squamous cell carcinoma in less than 10%. Patients often present with complaints of perianal burning, itching, or pain. Lesions are often found on routine histological evaluation of specimens acquired at unrelated procedures.[618] When grossly apparent, the lesions appear scaly, discrete, erythematous, and sometimes pigmented.

In immunocompromised (HIV-positive individuals, transplant recipient) patients, a Papanicolaou smear is a useful screening technique to detect evidence of dysplasia. If the Papanicolaou smear is positive, high-resolution anoscopy aided by acetic acid painting may reveal otherwise occult condylomata with dysplasia.

Historically, wide local excision with four quadrant biopsies to exclude occult disease has been advocated.[618,619] With this approach, local advancement flaps or skin grafts may be necessary, and in one series the recurrence rate was still almost 25% despite this radical approach.[619] We believe that there is no histological difference between Bowen's disease and a high-grade squamous intraepithelial lesion (high-grade dysplasia), and we have been treating dysplastic lesions with local excision or destruction for 10 years with minimal morbidity and no progression to invasive cancer in treated patients. Therefore, the need for radical excision and flap procedures is unclear.

Paget's Disease

In contrast to the three diseases just discussed, Paget's disease occurs predominantly in women. Patients are usually in the seventh or eighth decade. Severe intractable pruritus is characteristic. On physical examination, an erythematous, eczematoid rash is apparent. As before, biopsy of any nonhealing lesion should be taken to rule out this diagnosis. If Paget's disease is diagnosed, a thorough workup for an occult malignancy is indicated because 50% of patients have a coexistent carcinoma.[618]

Wide local excision with multiple perianal biopsies is the treatment of choice. An abdominal perineal resection may be indicated for advanced disease. Lymph node dissection should only be for palpable adenopathy. The role for chemoradiotherapy is less clear.[620] The prognosis is good unless there is metastatic disease or an underlying neoplasm, in which case patients do poorly.

Tumors of the Anal Canal

Epidermoid (Squamous, Basaloid, Mucoepidermoid) Carcinoma

Patients who present with epidermoid cancers of the anal canal generally have a long history of minor perianal complaints, such as bleeding, itching, or discomfort. A mass may or may not be associated with these symptoms. These cancers are more common in women and are caused by infection with oncogenic strains of HPV. Digital rectal exam and anoscopy are useful in determining depth of invasion, size, presence of pararectal nodes, and proximal extent of disease. The mass is biopsied to confirm the diagnosis. Both groins should be palpated for gross disease. Abdominal CT and chest radiographs evaluate the liver and chest for distant disease. Endorectal ultrasound can determine the depth of invasion and may identify pararectal nodes.

Early lesions that are small, mobile, confined to the submucosa, and well-differentiated may be treated with local excision. Overall, reported recurrence rates with local excision alone are high, with survival of 45% to 85% at 5 years.[621] However, in a series in which highly selected lesions were locally excised, recurrence was 8% and 5-year survival was 100%.[622] Radiation therapy or chemoradiotherapy are the preferred treatment options for larger lesions of the anal canal.[623–625]

Most centers within the United States give chemoradiation based on three randomized trials demonstrating improved local control and decreased risk of colostomy. However, there was no improvement in survival.[626–628] Nigro first introduced combined chemoradiotherapy initially as a measure to improve resectability of large anal cancers.[629] It worked so well that chemoradiotherapy became standard first-line therapy, and surgery is now only advised as a salvage procedure for persistent or recurrent disease. The combined regimen and dose of radiotherapy vary but are based on Nigro's protocol of 30 Gy to the primary tumor and pelvic and inguinal nodes with mitomycin C (15 mg/m^2 IV bolus) on day 1 of radiation therapy and 5FU (4-day infusion) on days 1 and 28. Sometimes, the planned second course of chemotherapy cannot be delivered because of toxicity, primarily related to the mitomycin C. The radiotherapy dose ranges from 30 to 59 Gy, but currently most centers provide the higher doses (50.4 to 54 Gy), with improved response rates.[624,629] Furthermore, the toxicity of mitomycin C may be eliminated by substituting it with cisplatin.

Failures of treatment are either local or at the regional lymph nodes. Patients with treatment failures should be offered salvage APR. Survival is related to extent of disease at the time of failure and is often poor.[630,631] Prophylactic groin dissection is not recommended, but the groins should be included in the radiation fields because of the 15% to 25% failure rates in those groins left untreated.[622,623]

There are reports of excellent 5- and 10-year survivals for T1–T3 node-negative disease of 88% and T1–T3 nonpositive disease of 52%.[613] Metastatic disease is more likely with increasing depth of invasion, size, and worsening histological grade.[622] Distant disease is uncommon at the time of diagnosis but most commonly involves the liver when present. Subsequent metastasis out of the pelvis is not uncommon.

References

1. Garcia-Ruiz, A., et al. Right colonic arterial anatomy. Implications for laparoscopic surgery. Dis Colon Rectum, 1996;39:906–11.
2. Michels, N.A., et al. Routes of collateral circulation of the gastrointestinal tract as ascertained in a dissection of 500 bodies. Int Surg, 1968;49:8–28.
3. Michels, N.A., et al. The variant blood supply to the descending colon, rectosigmoid and rectum based on 400 dissections. Its importance in regional resections: a review of medical literature. Dis Colon Rectum, 1965;49:251–78.
4. Moskowitz, M., H. Zimmerman, and B. Felson. The meandering mesenteric artery of the colon. Am J Roentgenol Radium Ther Nucl Med, 1964;92:1088–99.

5. Sato, K., and T. Sato. The vascular and neuronal composition of the lateral ligament of the rectum and the rectosacral fascia. Surg Radiol Anat, 1991;13:17–22.
6. Crapp, A.R., and A.M. Cuthbertson. William Waldeyer and the rectosacral fascia. Surg Gynecol Obstet, 1974;138:252–6.
7. Greene, F.L., et al., eds. AJCC Cancer Staging Manual. 6th ed. Springer: New York; 2002.
8. Nivatvongs, S., H.S. Stern, and D.S. Fryd, The length of the anal canal. Dis Colon Rectum, 1981;24:600–1.
9. Ayoub, S.F. Anatomy of the external anal sphincter in man. Acta Anat (Basel), 1979;105:25–36.
10. Nielsen, M.B., et al. Endosonography of the anal sphincter: findings in healthy volunteers. AJR Am J Roentgenol, 1991;157:1199–202.
11. Shafik, A. A new concept of the anatomy of the anal sphincter mechanism and the physiology of defecation. The external anal sphincter: a triple-loop system. Invest Urol, 1975;12:412–9.
12. Goligher, J.C., A.G. Leacock, and J.J. Brossy. The surgical anatomy of the anal canal. Br J Surg, 1955;43:51–61.
13. Parks, A.G. Pathogenesis and treatment of fistula-in-ano. Br Med J, 1961;5224:463–9.
14. Fenger, C. The anal transitional zone. Acta Pathol Microbiol Immunol Scand Suppl, 1987;289:1–42.
15. Ayoub, S.F. Arterial supply to the human rectum. Acta Anat (Basel), 1978;100:317–27.
16. Fisher, D.F., Jr., and W.J. Fry. Collateral mesenteric circulation. Surg Gynecol Obstet, 1987;164:487–92.
17. Havenga, K., et al. Anatomical basis of autonomic nerve-preserving total mesorectal excision for rectal cancer. Br J Surg, 1996;83:384–8.
18. Cherry, D.A., and D.A. Rothenberger. Pelvic floor physiology. Surg Clin North Am, 1988;68:1217–30.
19. Matzel, K.E., R.A. Schmidt, and E.A. Tanagho. Neuroanatomy of the striated muscular anal continence mechanism. Implications for the use of neurostimulation. Dis Colon Rectum, 1990;33:666–73.
20. Devroede, G.J., and S.F. Phillips. Conservation of sodium, chloride, and water by the human colon. Gastroenterology, 1969;56:101–9.
21. Giller, J., and S.F. Phillips. Electrolyte absorption and secretion in the human colon. Am J Dig Dis, 1972;17:1003–11.
22. Garcia, D., et al. Colonic motility: electric and manometric description of mass movement. Dis Colon Rectum, 1991;34:577–84.
23. Narducci, F., et al. Twenty four hour manometric recording of colonic motor activity in healthy man. Gut, 1987;28:17–25.
24. Latella, G., and R. Caprilli. Metabolism of large bowel mucosa in health and disease. Int J Colorectal Dis, 1991;6:127–32.
25. Gaginella, T.S. Absorption and secretion in the colon. Curr Opin Gastroenterol, 1995;11:2–8.
26. Bokkenheuser, V. The friendly anaerobes. Clin Infect Dis, 1993;16 Suppl 4:S427–34.
27. Henry, M.M., and J.P. Thomson. The anal sphincter. Scand J Gastroenterol Suppl, 1984;93:53–7.
28. Madoff, R.D., J.G. Williams, and P.F. Caushaj. Fecal incontinence. N Engl J Med, 1992;326:1002–7.
29. Parks, A.G., N.H. Porter, and J. Melzak. Experimental study of the reflex mechanism controlling the muscle of the pelvic floor. Dis Colon Rectum, 1962;5:407–14.
30. Thomson, W.H. The nature of haemorrhoids. Br J Surg, 1975;62:542–52.
31. Gibbons, C.P., et al. Role of anal cushions in maintaining continence. Lancet, 1986;1:886–8.
32. Loder, P.B., et al. Haemorrhoids: pathology, pathophysiology and aetiology. Br J Surg, 1994;81:946–54.
33. Miller, R., et al. Sensory discrimination and dynamic activity in the anorectum: evidence using a new ambulatory technique. Br J Surg, 1988;75:1003–7.
34. Janowitz, H.D. Crohn's disease—50 years later. N Engl J Med, 1981;304:1600–2.
35. Crohn, B.B., Ginzburg, L., and G.D., Oppenheimer. Regional ileitis. JAMA, 1932;99:1323–1329.
36. Nivatvongs, S., and P.H. Gordon. Crohn's disease In: Principles and Practice of Surgery for the Colon, Rectum, and Anus, P.H. Gordon and S. Nivatvongs, eds. St. Louis: Quality Medical; 1999:907–974.
37. Russel, M.G., and R.W. Stockbrugger. Epidemiology of inflammatory bowel disease: an update. Scand J Gastroenterol, 1996;31:417–27.
38. Leong, R.W., J.Y. Lau, and J.J. Sung. The epidemiology and phenotype of Crohn's disease in the Chinese population. Inflamm Bowel Dis, 2004;10:646–51.
39. Probert, C.S., et al. Diet of South Asians with inflammatory bowel disease. Arq Gastroenterol, 1996;33:132–5.
40. Bernstein, C.N., et al. Epidemiology of Crohn's disease and ulcerative colitis in a central Canadian province: a population-based study. Am J Epidemiol, 1999;149:916–24.
41. Odes, H.S., et al. Epidemiology of Crohn's disease in southern Israel. Am J Gastroenterol, 1994;89:1859–62.
42. Anseline, P.F. Crohn's disease in the Hunter Valley region of Australia. Aust N Z J Surg, 1995;65:564–9.
43. Katschinski, B., et al. Oral contraceptive use and cigarette smoking in Crohn's disease. Dig Dis Sci, 1993;38:1596–600.
44. Cottone, M., et al. Smoking habits and recurrence in Crohn's disease. Gastroenterology, 1994;106:643–8.
45. Korzenik, J.R. Past and current theories of etiology of IBD: toothpaste, worms, and refrigerators. J Clin Gastroenterol, 2005;39(4 suppl 2):S59–65.
46. Ogura, Y., et al. A frameshift mutation in NOD2 associated with susceptibility to Crohn's disease. Nature, 2001;411:603–6.
47. Cario, E. Bacterial interactions with cells of the intestinal mucosa: Toll-like receptors and NOD2. Gut, 2005;54:1182–93.
48. Farmer, R.G., W.A. Hawk, and R.B. Turnbull, Jr. Clinical patterns in Crohn's disease: a statistical study of 615 cases. Gastroenterology, 1975;68(4 pt 1):627–35.
49. Ritchie, J.K. The results of surgery for large bowel Crohn's disease. Ann R Coll Surg Engl, 1990;72:155–7.
50. Greenstein, A.J. The surgery of Crohn's disease. Surg Clin North Am, 1987;67:573–96.
51. Platell, C., et al. Anal pathology in patients with Crohn's disease. Aust N Z J Surg, 1996;66:5–9.
52. Marmo, R., et al. Capsule endoscopy versus enteroclysis in the detection of small-bowel involvement in Crohn's disease: a prospective trial. Clin Gastroenterol Hepatol, 2005;3:772–6.
53. Prabhakar, L.P., et al. Avoiding a stoma: role for segmental or abdominal colectomy in Crohn's colitis. Dis Colon Rectum, 1997;40:71–8.
54. Shorter, R.G. Risks of intestinal cancer in Crohn's disease. Dis Colon Rectum, 1983;26:686–9.
55. Ekbom, A., et al. Increased risk of large-bowel cancer in Crohn's disease with colonic involvement. Lancet, 1990;336:357–9.
56. Gillen, C.D., et al. Crohn's disease and colorectal cancer. Gut, 1994;35:651–5.
57. Savoca, P.E., G.H. Ballantyne, and C.E. Cahow. Gastrointestinal malignancies in Crohn's disease. A 20-year experience. Dis Colon Rectum, 1990;33:7–11.
58. Greenstein, A.J. Malignancy in Crohn's disease. Perspect Colon Rectal Surg, 1995;8:137–159.
59. Mekhjian, H.S., et al. National Cooperative Crohn's Disease Study: factors determining recurrence of Crohn's disease after surgery. Gastroenterology, 1979;77(4 pt 2):907–13.
60. Sachar, D.B. Maintenance strategies in Crohn's disease. Hospital Practice (office ed), 1996;31:99–106.
61. Stark, M.E., and W.J. Tremaine. Maintenance of symptomatic remission in patients with Crohn's disease. Mayo Clin Proc, 1993;68:1183–90.

62. Malchow, H., et al. European Cooperative Crohn's Disease Study (ECCDS): results of drug treatment. Gastroenterology, 1984;86:249–66.
63. Summers, R.W., et al. National Cooperative Crohn's Disease Study: results of drug treatment. Gastroenterology, 1979;77(4 pt 2):847–69.
64. Ewe, K., et al. Postoperative recurrence of Crohn's disease in relation to radicality of operation and sulfasalazine prophylaxis: a multicenter trial. Digestion, 1989;42:224–32.
65. Singleton, J.W., et al. Mesalamine capsules for the treatment of active Crohn's disease: results of a 16-week trial. Pentasa Crohn's Disease Study Group. Gastroenterology, 1993;104:1293–301.
66. Tremaine, W.J., et al. A randomized, double-blind, placebo-controlled trial of the oral mesalamine (5-ASA) preparation, Asacol, in the treatment of symptomatic Crohn's colitis and ileocolitis. J Clin Gastroenterol, 1994;19:278–82.
67. Hanauer, S.B. Inflammatory bowel disease. N Engl J Med, 1996;334:841–8.
68. Barlow, A.D., G.A. Clarke, and M.J. Kelly. Acute adrenal crisis in a patient treated with rectal steroids. Colorectal Dis, 2004;6:62–4.
69. Edsbacker, S., and T. Andersson. Pharmacokinetics of budesonide (Entocort EC) capsules for Crohn's disease. Clin Pharmacokinet, 2004;43:803–21.
70. Rutgeerts, P., et al. A comparison of budesonide with prednisolone for active Crohn's disease. N Engl J Med, 1994;331:842–5.
71. Greenberg, G.R., et al. Oral budesonide for active Crohn's disease. Canadian Inflammatory Bowel Disease Study Group. N Engl J Med, 1994;331:836–41.
72. Sachar, D.B. Budesonide for inflammatory bowel disease. It is a magic bullet? N Engl J Med, 1994;331:873–4.
73. Sandborn, W.J., et al. Natalizumab induction and maintenance therapy for Crohn's disease. N Engl J Med, 2005;353:1912–25.
74. Sutherland, L., et al. Double blind, placebo controlled trial of metronidazole in Crohn's disease. Gut, 1991;32:1071–5.
75. Brandt, L.J., et al. Metronidazole therapy for perineal Crohn's disease: a follow-up study. Gastroenterology, 1982;83:383–7.
76. Lobo, I.M., et al. Oral ciprofloxacin for treatment of severe infections. Int J Clin Pharmacol Res, 1993;13:81–5.
77. Present, D.H., et al. Treatment of Crohn's disease with 6-mercaptopurine. A long-term, randomized, double-blind study. N Engl J Med, 1980;302:981–7.
78. Pearson, D.C., et al. Azathioprine and 6-mercaptopurine in Crohn's disease. A meta-analysis. Ann Intern Med, 1995;123:132–42.
79. Katz, S. Update in medical therapy of ulcerative colitis: newer concepts and therapies. J Clin Gastroenterol, 2005;39:557–69.
80. Feagan, B.G., et al. Methotrexate for the treatment of Crohn's disease. The North American Crohn's Study Group Investigators. N Engl J Med, 1995;332:292–7.
81. Alfadhli, A.A.F., J.W.D. McDonald, and B.G. Feagan. Methotrexate for induction of remission in refractory Crohn's disease. Cochrane Database of Systematic Reviews, 2004, Issue 4. Art. No.: CD003459. DOI: 10.1002/14651858.CD003459.pub2.
82. Present, D.H., and S. Lichtiger. Efficacy of cyclosporine in treatment of fistula of Crohn's disease. Dig Dis Sci, 1994;39:374–80.
83. Lowry, P.W., et al. Combination therapy with oral tacrolimus (FK506) and azathioprine or 6-mercaptopurine for treatment-refractory Crohn's disease perianal fistulae. Inflamm Bowel Dis, 1999;5:239–45.
84. Present, D.H., et al. Infliximab for the treatment of fistulas in patients with Crohn's disease. N Engl J Med, 1999;340:1398–405.
85. Akobeng A.K., and M. Zachos. Tumor necrosis factor-alpha antibody for induction of remission in Crohn's disease. Cochrane Database of Systematic Reviews, 2003, Issue 4. Art. No.: CD003574. DOI: 10.1002/14651858.CD003574.pub2.
86. Van Assche, G., S. Vermeire, and P. Rutgeerts. Medical treatment of inflammatory bowel diseases. Curr Opin Gastroenterol, 2005;21:443–7.
87. Ghosh, S., et al. Natalizumab for active Crohn's disease. N Engl J Med, 2003;348:24–32.
88. Rutgeerts, P., et al. Natural history of recurrent Crohn's disease at the ileocolonic anastomosis after curative surgery. Gut, 1984;25:665–72.
89. Whelan, G., et al. Recurrence after surgery in Crohn's disease. Relationship to location of disease (clinical pattern) and surgical indication. Gastroenterology, 1985;88:1826–33.
90. Kim, N.K., et al. Long-term outcome after ileocecal resection for Crohn's disease. Am Surg, 1997;63:627–33.
91. Michelassi, F., et al. Primary and recurrent Crohn's disease. Experience with 1379 patients. Ann Surg, 1991;214:230–8; discussion 238–40.
92. Andrews, H.A., P. Lewis, and R.N. Allan. Prognosis after surgery for colonic Crohn's disease. Br J Surg, 1989;76:1184–90.
93. Griffiths, A.M., et al. Factors influencing postoperative recurrence of Crohn's disease in childhood. Gut, 1991;32:491–5.
94. Penner, R.M., K.L. Madsen, and R.N. Fedorak. Postoperative Crohn's disease. Inflamm Bowel Dis, 2005;11:765–77.
95. Sayfan, J., et al. Recurrence after strictureplasty or resection for Crohn's disease. Br J Surg, 1989;76:335–8.
96. Guillem, J.G., et al. Factors predictive of persistent or recurrent Crohn's disease in excluded rectal segments. Dis Colon Rectum, 1992;35:768–72.
97. Chevalier, J.M., et al. Colectomy and ileorectal anastomosis in patients with Crohn's disease. Br J Surg, 1994;81:1379–81.
98. Longo, W.E., et al. Outcome of ileorectal anastomosis for Crohn's colitis. Dis Colon Rectum, 1992;35:1066–71.
99. Scammell, B.E., et al. Results of proctocolectomy for Crohn's disease. Br J Surg, 1987;74:671–4.
100. Fichera, A., et al. Long-term outcome of surgically treated Crohn's colitis: a prospective study. Dis Colon Rectum, 2005;48:963–9.
101. Lockhart-Mummery, H.E. Symposium. Crohn's disease: anal lesions. Dis Colon Rectum, 1975;18:200–2.
102. Rankin, G.B., et al. National Cooperative Crohn's Disease Study: extraintestinal manifestations and perianal complications. Gastroenterology, 1979;77(4 Pt 2):914–20.
103. Williams, J.G., et al. Fistula-in-ano in Crohn's disease. Results of aggressive surgical treatment. Dis Colon Rectum, 1991;34:378–84.
104. Buchmann, P., et al. Natural history of perianal Crohn's disease. Ten year follow-up: a plea for conservatism. Am J Surg, 1980; 140:642–4.
105. Sangwan, Y.P., et al. Perianal Crohn's disease. Results of local surgical treatment. Dis Colon Rectum, 1996;39:529–35.
106. Sonoda, T., et al. Outcomes of primary repair of anorectal and rectovaginal fistulas using the endorectal advancement flap. Dis Colon Rectum, 2002;45:1622–8.
107. Mizrahi, N., et al. Endorectal advancement flap: are there predictors of failure? Dis Colon Rectum, 2002;45:1616–21.
108. Johnston, E., J. Gaw, and D. Armstrong. Efficacy of biodegradeable "collagen plug" versus fibrin glue in closure of anorectal fistulas. Dis Colon Rectum, 2005;48:631.
109. Levein, D.H., E.L., Gross, and W.S., Auriemma. Anal Crohn's disease. In: Surgery of the Colon, Rectum, and Anus, M.P. Mazier, Levein, D.H., et al., eds. Philadelphia: Saunders; 1995.
110. Cohen, Z., and R.S. McLeod. Perianal Crohn's disease. Gastroenterol Clin North Am, 1987;16:175–89.
111. Buchman, A.L., M.E. Ament, and J. Doty. Development of squamous cell carcinoma in chronic perineal sinus and wounds in Crohn's disease. Am J Gastroenterol, 1991;86:1829–32.

112. Nikias, G., et al. Crohn's disease and colorectal carcinoma: rectal cancer complicating longstanding active perianal disease. Am J Gastroenterol, 1995;90:216–9.
113. Wolff, B.G., et al. Anorectal Crohn's disease. A long-term perspective. Dis Colon Rectum, 1985;28:709–11.
114. Williamson, P.R., et al. Twenty-year review of the surgical management of perianal Crohn's disease. Dis Colon Rectum, 1995;38:389–92.
115. Garland, C.F., et al. Incidence rates of ulcerative colitis and Crohn's disease in 15 areas of the United States. Gastroenterology, 1981;81:1115–24.
116. Stewenius, J., et al. Ulcerative colitis and indeterminate colitis in the city of Malmo, Sweden. A 25-year incidence study. Scand J Gastroenterol, 1995;30:38–43.
117. Farmer, R.G., W.M. Michener, and E.A. Mortimer. Studies of family history among patients with inflammatory bowel disease. Clin Gastroenterol, 1980;9:271–7.
118. Lashner, B.A., et al. Prevalence and incidence of inflammatory bowel disease in family members. Gastroenterology, 1986;91: 1396–400.
119. Sartor, R.B. Pathogenesis and immune mechanisms of chronic inflammatory bowel diseases. Am J Gastroenterol, 1997;92(12 suppl):5S–11S.
120. Gordon, J.N., A. Di Sabatino, and T.T. Macdonald. The pathophysiologic rationale for biological therapies in inflammatory bowel disease. Curr Opin Gastroenterol, 2005;21:431–7.
121. Heller, F., et al. Oxazolone colitis, a Th2 colitis model resembling ulcerative colitis, is mediated by IL-13-producing NK-T cells. Immunity, 2002;17:629–38.
122. Willenbucher, R.F. Inflammatory bowel disease. Semin Gastrointest Dis, 1996;7:94–104.
123. Greenstein, A.J., et al. A comparison of cancer risk in Crohn's disease and ulcerative colitis. Cancer, 1981;48:2742–5.
124. Gyde, S.N., et al. Colorectal cancer in ulcerative colitis: a cohort study of primary referrals from three centres. Gut, 1988;29:206–17.
125. Sugita, A., et al. Colorectal cancer in ulcerative colitis. Influence of anatomical extent and age at onset on colitis-cancer interval. Gut, 1991;32:167–9.
126. Choi, P.M., and W.H. Kim. Colon cancer surveillance. Gastroenterol Clin North Am, 1995;24:671–87.
127. Ekbom, A., et al. Ulcerative colitis and colorectal cancer. A population-based study. N Engl J Med, 1990;323:1228–33.
128. Broome, U., G. Lindberg, and R. Lofberg, Primary sclerosing cholangitis in ulcerative colitis—a risk factor for the development of dysplasia and DNA aneuploidy? Gastroenterology, 1992;102:1877–80.
129. Devroede, G.J., et al. Cancer risk and life expectancy of children with ulcerative colitis. N Engl J Med, 1971;285:17–21.
130. Ransohoff, D.F., R.H. Riddell, and B. Levin. Ulcerative colitis and colonic cancer. Problems in assessing the diagnostic usefulness of mucosal dysplasia. Dis Colon Rectum, 1985;28:383–8.
131. Sachar, D.B., and A.J. Greenstein. Cancer in ulcerative colitis: good news and bad news. Ann Intern Med, 1981;95:642–4.
132. Rubin, C.E., et al. DNA aneuploidy in colonic biopsies predicts future development of dysplasia in ulcerative colitis. Gastroenterology, 1992;103:1611–20.
133. Melville, D.M., et al. Observer study of the grading of dysplasia in ulcerative colitis: comparison with clinical outcome. Hum Pathol, 1989;20:1008–14.
134. Connell, W.R., et al. Clinicopathological characteristics of colorectal carcinoma complicating ulcerative colitis. Gut, 1994; 35:1419–23.
135. Choi, P.M., et al. Colonoscopic surveillance reduces mortality from colorectal cancer in ulcerative colitis. Gastroenterology, 1993;105:418–24.
136. Rozen, P., et al. Low incidence of significant dysplasia in a successful endoscopic surveillance program of patients with ulcerative colitis. Gastroenterology, 1995;108:1361–70.
137. Giardiello, F.M., and T.M. Bayless. Colorectal cancer and ulcerative colitis. Radiology, 1996;199:28–30.
138. Lennard-Jones, J.E., et al. Cancer surveillance in ulcerative colitis. Experience over 15 years. Lancet, 1983;2:149–52.
139. Broome, U., et al. Subclinical time span of inflammatory bowel disease in patients with primary sclerosing cholangitis. Dis Colon Rectum, 1995;38:1301–5.
140. Knox, T.A., and M.M. Kaplan. Treatment of primary sclerosing cholangitis with oral methotrexate. Am J Gastroenterol, 1991; 86:546–52.
141. Beuers, U., et al. Ursodeoxycholic acid for treatment of primary sclerosing cholangitis: a placebo-controlled trial. Hepatology, 1992;16:707–14.
142. O'Brien, C.B., et al. Ursodeoxycholic acid for the treatment of primary sclerosing cholangitis: a 30-month pilot study. Hepatology, 1991;14:838–47.
143. Cangemi, J.R., et al. Effect of proctocolectomy for chronic ulcerative colitis on the natural history of primary sclerosing cholangitis. Gastroenterology, 1989;96:790–4.
144. Gumaste, V., D.B. Sachar, and A.J. Greenstein. Benign and malignant colorectal strictures in ulcerative colitis. Gut, 1992; 33:938–41.
145. Sutherland, L.R., G.R. May, and E.A. Shaffer. Sulfasalazine revisited: a meta-analysis of 5-aminosalicylic acid in the treatment of ulcerative colitis. Ann Intern Med, 1993;118: 540–9.
146. An oral preparation of mesalamine as long-term maintenance therapy for ulcerative colitis. A randomized, placebo-controlled trial. The Mesalamine Study Group. Ann Intern Med, 1996; 124:204–11.
147. Travis, S.P., et al. Optimum dose of olsalazine for maintaining remission in ulcerative colitis. Gut, 1994;35:1282–6.
148. Green, J.R., et al. Short report: comparison of two doses of balsalazide in maintaining ulcerative colitis in remission over 12 months. Aliment Pharmacol Ther, 1992;6:647–52.
149. Hanauer, S.B. Caution in the interpretation of safety and efficacy differences in clinical trials comparing aminosalicylates for ulcerative colitis. Am J Gastroenterol, 2003;98: 215–6.
150. Kane, S.V., and D.J. Bjorkman. The efficacy of oral 5-ASAs in the treatment of active ulcerative colitis: a systematic review. Rev Gastroenterol Disord, 2003;3:210–8.
151. Sandborn, W.J. Rational selection of oral 5-aminosalicylate formulations and prodrugs for the treatment of ulcerative colitis. Am J Gastroenterol, 2002;97:2939–41.
152. d'Albasio, G., et al. Combined therapy with 5-aminosalicylic acid tablets and enemas for maintaining remission in ulcerative colitis: a randomized double-blind study. Am J Gastroenterol, 1997;92:1143–7.
153. Bernstein, C.N., et al. Does the use of 5-aminosalicylates in inflammatory bowel disease prevent the development of colorectal cancer? Am J Gastroenterol, 2003;98:2784–8.
154. Velayos, F.S., J.P. Terdiman, and J.M. Walsh. Effect of 5-aminosalicylate use on colorectal cancer and dysplasia risk: a systematic review and metaanalysis of observational studies. Am J Gastroenterol, 2005;100:1345–53.
155. Margolin, M.L., et al. Clinical trials in ulcerative colitis: II. Historical review. Am J Gastroenterol, 1988;83:227–43.
156. Hanauer, S.B., and G. Stathopoulos. Risk-benefit assessment of drugs used in the treatment of inflammatory bowel disease. Drug Saf, 1991;6:192–219.
157. Hanauer, S.B., et al. Budesonide enema for the treatment of active, distal ulcerative colitis and proctitis: a dose-ranging study. US Budesonide Enema Study Group. Gastroenterology, 1998;115:525–32.

158. Lindgren, S., et al. Effect of budesonide enema on remission and relapse rate in distal ulcerative colitis and proctitis. Scand J Gastroenterol, 2002;37:705–10.
159. Adler, D.J., and B.I. Korelitz. The therapeutic efficacy of 6-mercaptopurine in refractory ulcerative colitis. Am J Gastroenterol, 1990;85:717–22.
160. Choi, P.M., and S.R. Targan. Immunomodulator therapy in inflammatory bowel disease. Dig Dis Sci, 1994;39:1885–92.
161. Gionchetti, P., et al. Standard treatment of ulcerative colitis. Dig Dis, 2003;21:157–67.
162. Ardizzone, S., et al. Guidelines for the treatment of ulcerative colitis in remission. Eur J Gastroenterol Hepatol, 1997;9:836–41.
163. George, J., et al. The long-term outcome of ulcerative colitis treated with 6-mercaptopurine. Am J Gastroenterol, 1996;91:1711–4.
164. Warman, J.I., et al. Cumulative experience with short- and long-term toxicity to 6-mercaptopurine in the treatment of Crohn's disease and ulcerative colitis. J Clin Gastroenterol, 2003;37:220–5.
165. Lichtiger, S., et al. Cyclosporine in severe ulcerative colitis refractory to steroid therapy. N Engl J Med, 1994;330:1841–5.
166. Message, L., et al. Efficacy of intravenous cyclosporin in moderately severe ulcerative colitis refractory to steroids. Gastroenterol Clin Biol, 2005;29:231–5.
167. de Saussure, P., et al. Low-dose oral microemulsion cyclosporin for severe, refractory ulcerative colitis. Aliment Pharmacol Ther, 2005;22:203–8.
168. Plevy, S., et al. A Phase I Study of Visilizumab, a Humanized Anti-CD3 Monoclonal Antibody, in Severe Steroid-Refractory Ulcerative Colitis. Results of a phase I study. Gastroenterology, 2004;126:A75.
169. Langholz, E., et al. Course of ulcerative colitis: analysis of changes in disease activity over years. Gastroenterology, 1994;107:3–11.
170. Kock, N.G. Intra-abdominal "reservoir" in patients with permanent ileostomy. Preliminary observations on a procedure resulting in fecal "continence" in five ileostomy patients. Arch Surg, 1969;99:223–31.
171. Litle, V.R., et al. The continent ileostomy: long-term durability and patient satisfaction. J Gastrointest Surg, 1999;3:625–32.
172. Parks, A.G., and R.J. Nicholls. Proctocolectomy without ileostomy for ulcerative colitis. Br Med J, 1978;2:85–8.
173. Gunnarsson, U., et al. Proctocolectomy and pelvic pouch—is a diverting stoma dangerous for the patient? Colorectal Dis, 2004;6:23–7.
174. Ky, A.J., T. Sonoda, and J.W. Milsom. One-stage laparoscopic restorative proctocolectomy: an alternative to the conventional approach? Dis Colon Rectum, 2002;45:207–10; discussion 210–1.
175. Gilchrist, K.W., B.A. Harms, and J.R. Starling. Abnormal rectal mucosa of the anal transitional zone in ulcerative colitis. Arch Surg, 1995;130:981–3.
176. Hurst, R.D., and F. Michelassi. Ileal-pouch anal restorative proctocolectomy for ulcerative colitis. Adv Surg, 2004;38:311–36.
177. Berndtsson, I., T. Oresland, and L. Hulten. Sexuality in patients with ulcerative colitis before and after restorative proctocolectomy: a prospective study. Scand J Gastroenterol, 2004;39:374–9.
178. Slors, F.J., P.P. van Zuijlen, and G.J. van Dijk. Sexual and bladder dysfunction after total mesorectal excision for benign diseases. Scand J Gastroenterol Suppl, 2000:48–51.
179. Alexander-Williams, J. The technique of intestinal strictureplasty. Int J Colorectal Dis, 1986;1:54–7.
180. Dehn, T.C., et al. Ten-year experience of strictureplasty for obstructive Crohn's disease. Br J Surg, 1989;76:339–41.
181. Spencer, M.P., et al. Strictureplasty for obstructive Crohn's disease: the Mayo experience. Mayo Clin Proc, 1994;69:33–6.
182. Quandalle, P., et al. Long-term follow-up of strictureplasty in Crohn's disease. Acta Gastroenterol Belg, 1994;57(5–6):314–9.
183. Baba, S., and K. Nakai, Strictureplasty for Crohn's disease in Japan. J Gastroenterol, 1995;30 Suppl 8:135–8.
184. Serra, J., Z. Cohen, and R.S. McLeod. Natural history of strictureplasty in Crohn's disease: 9-year experience. Can J Surg, 1995;38:481–5.
185. Stebbing, J.F., et al. Recurrence and reoperation after strictureplasty for obstructive Crohn's disease: long-term results [corrected]. Br J Surg, 1995;82:1471–4.
186. Gardiner, K.R., M.G. Kettlewell, and N.J. Mortensen. Intestinal haemorrhage after strictureplasty for Crohn's disease. Int J Colorectal Dis, 1996;11:180–2.
187. Ozuner, G., et al. How safe is strictureplasty in the management of Crohn's disease? Am J Surg, 1996;171:57–60; discussion 60–1.
188. Almy, T.P., and D.A. Howell. Medical progress. Diverticular disease of the colon. N Engl J Med, 1980;302:324–31.
189. Parks, T.G. Natural history of diverticular disease of the colon. Clin Gastroenterol, 1975;4:53–69.
190. Rodkey, G.V., and C.E. Welch. Changing patterns in the surgical treatment of diverticular disease. Ann Surg, 1984;200:466–78.
191. Eide, T.J., and H. Stalsberg. Diverticular disease of the large intestine in Northern Norway. Gut, 1979;20:609–15.
192. Hughes, L.E. Postmortem survey of diverticular disease of the colon. I. Diverticulosis and diverticulitis. Gut, 1969;10:336–44.
193. Morson, B.C. Pathology of diverticular disease of the colon. Clin Gastroenterol, 1975;4:37–52.
194. Painter, N.S. Diverticular disease of the colon. The first of the Western diseases shown to be due to a deficiency of dietary fibre. S Afr Med J, 1982;61:1016–20.
195. Painter, N.S. The cause of diverticular disease of the colon, its symptoms and its complications. Review and hypothesis. J R Coll Surg Edinb, 1985;30:118–22.
196. Painter, N.S., and D.P. Burkitt, Diverticular disease of the colon, a 20th century problem. Clin Gastroenterol, 1975;4:3–21.
197. Meyers, M.A., et al. The angioarchitecture of colonic diverticula. Significance in bleeding diverticulosis. Radiology, 1973;108:249–61.
198. Slack, W.W. The anatomy, pathology, and some clinical features of divericulitis of the colon. Br J Surg, 1962;50:185–90.
199. Whiteway, J., and B.C. Morson. Pathology of the ageing—diverticular disease. Clin Gastroenterol, 1985;14:829–46.
200. Ryan, P. Two kinds of diverticular disease. Ann R Coll Surg Engl, 1991;73:73–9.
201. Manousos, O.N. Diverticular disease of the colon. Dig Dis, 1989;7:86–103.
202. Whiteway, J., and B.C. Morson. Elastosis in diverticular disease of the sigmoid colon. Gut, 1985;26:258–66.
203. Wess, L., et al. Cross linking of collagen is increased in colonic diverticulosis. Gut, 1995;37:91–4.
204. Ulin, A.W., A.E. Pearce, and S.F. Weinstein. Diverticular disease of the colon: surgical perspectives in the past decade. Dis Colon Rectum, 1981;24:276–81.
205. Taylor, I., and H.L. Duthie. Bran tablets and diverticular disease. Br Med J, 1976;1:988–90.
206. Thompson, W.G., and D.G. Patel. Clinical picture of diverticular disease of the colon. Clin Gastroenterol, 1986;15:903–16.
207. McGuire, H.H., Jr., and B.W. Haynes, Jr. Massive hemorrhage for diverticulosis of the colon: guidelines for therapy based on bleeding patterns observed in 50 cases. Ann Surg, 1972;175:847–55.
208. Casarella, W.J., et al. "Lower" gastrointestinal tract hemorrhage: new concepts based on arteriography. Am J Roentgenol Radium Ther Nucl Med, 1974;121:357–68.
209. McGuire, H.H., Jr. Bleeding colonic diverticula. A reappraisal of natural history and management. Ann Surg, 1994;220:653–6.
210. Bokhari, M., et al. Diverticular hemorrhage in the elderly—is it well tolerated? Dis Colon Rectum, 1996;39:191–5.

211. Baer, J. Pathogenesis of bleeding colonic diverticulosis: new concepts. CRC Crit Rev Diagn Imaging, 1978;11:1–20.
212. Rossini, F.P., et al. Emergency colonoscopy. World J Surg, 1989;13:190–2.
213. Emslie, J.T., et al. Technetium-99m-labeled red blood cell scans in the investigation of gastrointestinal bleeding. Dis Colon Rectum, 1996;39:750–4.
214. Nicholson, M.L., et al. Localization of lower gastrointestinal bleeding using in vivo technetium-99m-labelled red blood cell scintigraphy. Br J Surg, 1989;76:358–61.
215. Suzman, M.S., et al. Accurate localization and surgical management of active lower gastrointestinal hemorrhage with technetium-labeled erythrocyte scintigraphy. Ann Surg, 1996; 224:29–36.
216. Hunter, J.M., and M.E. Pezim. Limited value of technetium 99m-labeled red cell scintigraphy in localization of lower gastrointestinal bleeding. Am J Surg, 1990;159:504–6.
217. Gordon, R.L., et al. Selective arterial embolization for the control of lower gastrointestinal bleeding. Am J Surg, 1997; 174:24–8.
218. Athanasoulis, C.A. Angiography in the management of patients with gastrointestinal bleeding. Adv Surg, 1983;16:1–23.
219. Gostout, C.J., et al. Acute gastrointestinal bleeding. Experience of a specialized management team. J Clin Gastroenterol, 1992; 14:260–7.
220. Jensen, D.M., and G.A. Machicado. Diagnosis and treatment of severe hematochezia. The role of urgent colonoscopy after purge. Gastroenterology, 1988;95:1569–74.
221. Eaton, A.C. Emergency surgery for acute colonic haemorrhage—a retrospective study. Br J Surg, 1981;68:109–12.
222. Drapanas, T., et al. Emergency subtotal colectomy: preferred approach to management of massively bleeding diverticular disease. Ann Surg, 1973;177:519–26.
223. Gianfrancisco, J.A., and H. Abcarian. Pitfalls in the treatment of massive lower gastrointestinal bleeding with "blind" subtotal colectomy. Dis Colon Rectum, 1982;25:441–5.
224. Rothenberger, D.A., and O. Wiltz. Surgery for complicated diverticulitis. Surg Clin North Am, 1993;73:975–92.
225. Schoetz, D.J., Jr. Uncomplicated diverticulitis. Indications for surgery and surgical management. Surg Clin North Am, 1993; 73:965–74.
226. Roberts, P., et al. Practice parameters for sigmoid diverticulitis. The Standards Task Force American Society of Colon and Rectal Surgeons. Dis Colon Rectum, 1995;38:125–32.
227. Rao, P.M., and J.T. Rhea. Colonic diverticulitis: evaluation of the arrowhead sign and the inflamed diverticulum for CT diagnosis. Radiology, 1998;209:775–9.
228. Werner, A., et al. Multi-slice spiral CT in routine diagnosis of suspected acute left-sided colonic diverticulitis: a prospective study of 120 patients. Eur Radiol, 2003;13:2596–603.
229. Ambrosetti, P., C. Becker, and F. Terrier. Colonic diverticulitis: impact of imaging on surgical management—a prospective study of 542 patients. Eur Radiol, 2002;12:1145–9.
230. Ambrosetti, P., et al. Computed tomography in acute left colonic diverticulitis. Br J Surg, 1997;84:532–4.
231. Montgomery, R.A., A.C. Venbrux, and G.B. Bulkley. Mesenteric vascular insufficiency. Curr Probl Surg, 1997;34:941–1025.
232. Freischlag, J., R.S. Bennion, and J.E. Thompson, Jr. Complications of diverticular disease of the colon in young people. Dis Colon Rectum, 1986;29:639–43.
233. Ambrosetti, P., et al. Acute left colonic diverticulitis in young patients. J Am Coll Surg, 1994;179:156–60.
234. Ambrosetti, P., et al. Prognostic factors from computed tomography in acute left colonic diverticulitis. Br J Surg, 1992;79:117–9.
235. Hinchey, E.J., P.G. Schaal, and G.K. Richards. Treatment of perforated diverticular disease of the colon. Adv Surg, 1978;12:85–109.
236. Detry, R., et al. Acute localized diverticulitis: optimum management requires accurate staging. Int J Colorectal Dis, 1992;7:38–42.
237. Ambrosetti, P., et al. Incidence, outcome, and proposed management of isolated abscesses complicating acute left-sided colonic diverticulitis. A prospective study of 140 patients. Dis Colon Rectum, 1992;35:1072–6.
238. Schechter, S., et al. Computerized tomographic scan-guided drainage of intra-abdominal abscesses. Preoperative and postoperative modalities in colon and rectal surgery. Dis Colon Rectum, 1994;37:984–8.
239. Smirniotis, V., et al. Perforated diverticulitis: a surgical dilemma. Int Surg, 1992;77:44–7.
240. Kronborg, O. Treatment of perforated sigmoid diverticulitis: a prospective randomized trial. Br J Surg, 1993;80:505–7.
241. Haas, P.A., and G.P. Haas. A critical evaluation of the Hartmann's procedure. Am Surg, 1988;54:380–5.
242. Ling, L., and T. Aberg. Hartmann procedure. Acta Chir Scand, 1984;150:413–7.
243. Belmonte, C., et al. The Hartmann procedure. First choice or last resort in diverticular disease? Arch Surg, 1996;131:612–5; discussion 616–7.
244. Salem, L., and D.R. Flum. Primary anastomosis or Hartmann's procedure for patients with diverticular peritonitis? A systematic review. Dis Colon Rectum, 2004;47:1953–64.
245. Tyau, E.S., et al. Acute diverticulitis. A complicated problem in the immunocompromised patient. Arch Surg, 1991;126:855–8; discussion 858–9.
246. McCune, T.R., et al. Colonic screening prior to renal transplantation and its impact on post-transplant colonic complications. Clin Transplant, 1992;6:91–6.
247. Soravia, C., et al. Acute colonic complications after kidney transplantation. Acta Chir Belg, 1995;95:157–61.
248. Guzzo, J., and N. Hyman. Diverticulitis in young patients: is resection after a single attack always warranted? Dis Colon Rectum, 2004;47:1187–90; discussion 1190–1.
249. Spivak, H., et al. Acute colonic diverticulitis in the young. Dis Colon Rectum, 1997;40:570–4.
250. Vignati, P.V., J.P. Welch, and J.L. Cohen. Long-term management of diverticulitis in young patients. Dis Colon Rectum, 1995;38:627–9.
251. Ambrosetti, P., et al. Long-term outcome of mesocolic and pelvic diverticular abscesses of the left colon: a prospective study of 73 cases. Dis Colon Rectum, 2005;48:787–91.
252. Benn, P.L., B.G. Wolff, and D.M. Ilstrup. Level of anastomosis and recurrent colonic diverticulitis. Am J Surg, 1986;151:269–71.
253. Schmitt, S.L., and S.D. Wexner. Bacterial, fungal, parasitic, and viral colitis. Surg Clin North Am, 1993;73:1055–62.
254. Bartlett, J.G., et al. Antibiotic-associated pseudomembranous colitis due to toxin-producing clostridia. N Engl J Med, 1978;298:531–4.
255. Kelly, C.P., C. Pothoulakis, and J.T. LaMont. Clostridium difficile colitis. N Engl J Med, 1994;330:257–62.
256. Keating, J.P., et al. Pseudomembranous colitis associated with ampicillin therapy. Am J Dis Child, 1974;128:369–70.
257. Tedesco, F.J., R.W. Barton, and D.H. Alpers. Clindamycin-associated colitis. A prospective study. Ann Intern Med, 1974;81:429–33.
258. Wren, S.M., et al. Preoperative oral antibiotics in colorectal surgery increase the rate of *Clostridium difficile* colitis. Arch Surg, 2005;140:752–6.
259. Tedesco, F.J., J.K. Corless, and R.E. Brownstein. Rectal sparing in antibiotic-associated pseudomembranous colitis: a prospective study. Gastroenterology, 1982;83:1259–60.
260. Kleinfeld, D.I., R.J. Sharpe, and S.T. Donta. Parenteral therapy for antibiotic-associated pseudomembranous colitis. J Infect Dis, 1988;157:389.

261. Young, G., and M. McDonald. Antibiotic-associated colitis: why do patients relapse? Gastroenterology, 1986;90:1098–9.
262. Tvede, M., and J. Rask-Madsen. Bacteriotherapy for chronic relapsing *Clostridium difficile* diarrhoea in six patients. Lancet, 1989;1:1156–60.
263. Longo, W.E., et al. Outcome after colectomy for *Clostridium difficile* colitis. Dis Colon Rectum, 2004;47:1620–6.
264. Jobe, B.A., et al. *Clostridium difficile* colitis: an increasing hospital-acquired illness. Am J Surg, 1995;169:480–3.
265. Vantrappen, G., et al. *Yersinia* enteritis and enterocolitis: gastroenterological aspects. Gastroenterology, 1977;72:220–7.
266. Ravdin, J.I., and R.L. Guerrant. A review of the parasite cellular mechanisms involved in the pathogenesis of amebiasis. Rev Infect Dis, 1982;4:1185–207.
267. Brinker, A.D., A.C. Mackey, and R. Prizont. Tegaserod and ischemic colitis. N Engl J Med, 2004;351:1361–4; discussion 1361–4.
268. Charles, J.A., et al. Ischemic colitis associated with naratriptan and oral contraceptive use. Headache, 2005;45:386–9.
269. DiBaise, J.K. Tegaserod-associated ischemic colitis. Pharmacotherapy, 2005;25:620–5.
270. Radaelli, F., et al. Ischemic colitis associated with rofecoxib. Dig Liver Dis, 2005;37:372–6.
271. Medina, C., et al. Outcome of patients with ischemic colitis: review of 53 cases. Dis Colon Rectum, 2004;47:180–4.
272. Gandhi, S.K., et al. Ischemic colitis. Dis Colon Rectum, 1996;39:88–100.
273. Marston, A., et al. Ischaemic colitis. Gut, 1966;7:1–15.
274. Philpotts, L.E., et al. Colitis: use of CT findings in differential diagnosis. Radiology, 1994;190:445–9.
275. Guttormson, N.L., and M.P. Bubrick. Mortality from ischemic colitis. Dis Colon Rectum, 1989;32:469–72.
276. Tada, M., F. Misaki, and K. Kawai. Analysis of the clinical features of ischemic colitis. Gastroenterol Jpn, 1983;18: 204–9.
277. Binns, J.C., and P. Isaacson. Age-related changes in the colonic blood supply: their relevance to ischaemic colitis. Gut, 1978; 19:384–90.
278. Baixauli, J., R.P. Kiran, and C.P. Delaney. Investigation and management of ischemic colitis. Cleve Clin J Med, 2003;70:920–1, 925–6, 928–30 passim.
279. Sierocinski, W. Arteries supplying the left colic flexure in man. Folia Morphol (Warsz), 1975;34:117–24.
280. Sakai, L., R. Keltner, and D. Kaminski. Spontaneous and shock-associated ischemic colitis. Am J Surg, 1980;140:755–60.
281. Welch, G.H., et al. Total colonic ischemia. Dis Colon Rectum, 1986;29:410–2.
282. West, B.R., J.E. Ray, and J.B. Gathright. Comparison of transient ischemic colitis with that requiring surgical treatment. Surg Gynecol Obstet, 1980;151:366–8.
283. Longo, W.E., G.H. Ballantyne, and R.J. Gusberg. Ischemic colitis: patterns and prognosis. Dis Colon Rectum, 1992;35:726–30.
284. Gama, A.H., et al. Volvulus of the sigmoid colon in Brazil: a report of 230 cases. Dis Colon Rectum, 1976;19:314–20.
285. Ballantyne, G.H. Review of sigmoid volvulus. Clinical patterns and pathogenesis. Dis Colon Rectum, 1982;25:823–30.
286. Abel, M.E., and T.R. Russell. Ischemic colitis. Comparison of surgical and nonoperative management. Dis Colon Rectum, 1983;26:113–5.
287. Parish, K.L., W.C. Chapman, and L.F. Williams, Jr. Ischemic colitis. An ever-changing spectrum? Am Surg, 1991;57:118–21.
288. Gibney, E.J. Volvulus of the sigmoid colon. Surg Gynecol Obstet, 1991;173:243–55.
289. String, S.T., and J.J. DeCosse. Sigmoid volvulus. An examination of the mortality. Am J Surg, 1971;121:293–7.
290. Shepherd, J.J. The epidemiology and clinical presentation of sigmoid volvulus. Br J Surg, 1969;56:353–9.
291. Mishra, S.B., and K.P. Sahoo. Primary resection and anastomosis for volvulus of sigmoid colon. J Indian Med Assoc, 1986;84: 265–8.
292. Catalano, O. Computed tomographic appearance of sigmoid volvulus. Abdom Imaging, 1996;21:314–7.
293. Biery, D.L., and S.M. Hoffman. Colonoscopic reduction of sigmoid volvulus. J Am Osteopath Assoc, 1978;77:543–5.
294. Drapanas, T., and J.D. Stewart. Acute sigmoid volvulus. Concepts in surgical treatment. Am J Surg, 1961;101:70–7.
295. Orchard, J.L., R. Mehta, and A.H. Khan. The use of colonoscopy in the treatment of colonic volvulus: three cases and review of the literature. Am J Gastroenterol, 1984;79:864–7.
296. Wertkin, M.G., and A.H. Aufses, Jr. Management of volvulus of the colon. Dis Colon Rectum, 1978;21:40–5.
297. Brothers, T.E., W.E. Strodel, and F.E. Eckhauser. Endoscopy in colonic volvulus. Ann Surg, 1987;206:1–4.
298. Mangiante, E.C., et al. Sigmoid volvulus. A four-decade experience. Am Surg, 1989;55:41–4.
299. Ritvo, M., G.E. Farrell, Jr., and I.A. Shauffer. The association of volvulus of the cecum and ascending colon with other obstructive colonic lesions. Am J Roentgenol Radium Ther Nucl Med, 1957;78:587–98.
300. Rabinovici, R., et al. Cecal volvulus. Dis Colon Rectum, 1990;33:765–9.
301. Todd, G.J., and K.A. Forde. Volvulus of the cecum: choice of operation. Am J Surg, 1979;138:632–4.
302. Burke, J.B., and G.H. Ballantyne. Cecal volvulus. Low mortality at a city hospital. Dis Colon Rectum, 1984;27:737–40.
303. Haskin, P.H., et al. Volvulus of the cecum and right colon. JAMA, 1981;245:2433–5.
304. Anderson, J.R., and G.H. Welch. Acute volvulus of the right colon: an analysis of 69 patients. World J Surg, 1986;10:336–42.
305. Tejler, G., and H. Jiborn. Volvulus of the cecum. Report of 26 cases and review of the literature. Dis Colon Rectum, 1988;31:445–9.
306. Fishman, E.K., et al. Transverse colon volvulus: diagnosis and treatment. South Med J, 1983;76:185–9.
307. Gumbs, M.A., et al. Volvulus of the transverse colon. Reports of cases and review of the literature. Dis Colon Rectum, 1983;26:825–8.
308. Kerry, R.L., and H.K. Ransom. Volvulus of the colon. Arch Surg, 1969;99:215–22.
309. Zinkin, L.D., L.D. Katz, and J.D. Rosin. Volvulus of the transverse colon: report of case and review of the literature. Dis Colon Rectum, 1979;22:492–6.
310. Moore-Gillon, V. Constipation: what does the patient mean? J R Soc Med, 1984;77:108–10.
311. Burkitt, D.P., A.R. Walker, and N.S. Painter. Effect of dietary fibre on stools and the transit-times, and its role in the causation of disease. Lancet, 1972;2:1408–12.
312. Burkitt, D.P., A.R. Walker, and N.S. Painter. Dietary fiber and disease. JAMA, 1974;229:1068–74.
313. Painter, N.S., and D.P. Burkitt. Diverticular disease of the colon: a deficiency disease of Western civilization. Br Med J, 1971;2:450–4.
314. Walker, A.R., B.F. Walker, and B.D. Richardson. Bowel transit times in Bantu populations. Br Med J, 1970;3:48–9.
315. Jemal, A., et al. Cancer statistics, 2005. CA Cancer J Clin, 2005;55:10–30.
316. Cucino, C., A.M. Buchner, and A. Sonnenberg. Continued rightward shift of colorectal cancer. Dis Colon Rectum, 2002;45:1035–40.
317. Caygill, C.P., A. Charlett, and M.J. Hill. Fat, fish, fish oil and cancer. Br J Cancer, 1996;74:159–64.
318. Rose, D.P., A.P. Boyar, and E.L. Wynder. International comparisons of mortality rates for cancer of the breast, ovary, prostate, and colon, and per capita food consumption. Cancer, 1986;58:2363–71.

319. Chao, A., et al. Meat consumption and risk of colorectal cancer. JAMA, 2005;293:172–82.
320. Kim, Y.I. AGA technical review: impact of dietary fiber on colon cancer occurrence. Gastroenterology, 2000;118:1235–57.
321. Giovannucci, E. Obesity, gender, and colon cancer. Gut, 2002;51:147.
322. Terry, P.D., A.B. Miller, and T.E. Rohan. Obesity and colorectal cancer risk in women. Gut, 2002;51:191–4.
323. Potter, J.D. Colorectal cancer: molecules and populations. J Natl Cancer Inst, 1999;91:916–32.
324. Burt, R.W. Colon cancer screening. Gastroenterology, 2000;119: 837–53.
325. Fuchs, C.S., et al. A prospective study of family history and the risk of colorectal cancer. N Engl J Med, 1994;331:1669–74.
326. Lennard-Jones, J.E., et al. Precancer and cancer in extensive ulcerative colitis: findings among 401 patients over 22 years. Gut, 1990;31:800–6.
327. Fearon, E.R., and B. Vogelstein. A genetic model for colorectal tumorigenesis. Cell, 1990;61:759–67.
328. Loeb, L.A. Microsatellite instability: marker of a mutator phenotype in cancer. Cancer Res, 1994;54:5059–63.
329. Shibata, D., et al. The DCC protein and prognosis in colorectal cancer. N Engl J Med, 1996;335:1727–32.
330. Vogelstein, B., and K.W. Kinzler. p53 function and dysfunction. Cell, 1992;70:523–6.
331. Greenblatt, M.S., et al. Mutations in the p53 tumor suppressor gene: clues to cancer etiology and molecular pathogenesis. Cancer Res, 1994;54:4855–78.
332. McLeod, H.L., and G.I. Murray. Tumour markers of prognosis in colorectal cancer. Br J Cancer, 1999;79:191–203.
333. Soong, R., et al. Prognostic significance of TP53 gene mutation in 995 cases of colorectal carcinoma. Influence of tumour site, stage, adjuvant chemotherapy and type of mutation. Eur J Cancer, 2000;36:2053–60.
334. Minamoto, T., M. Mai, and Z. Ronai. K-ras mutation: early detection in molecular diagnosis and risk assessment of colorectal, pancreas, and lung cancers—a review. Cancer Detect Prev, 2000;24:1–12.
335. Ahnen, D.J., et al. Ki-ras mutation and p53 overexpression predict the clinical behavior of colorectal cancer: a Southwest Oncology Group study. Cancer Res, 1998;58:1149–58.
336. Merg, A., et al. Hereditary colorectal cancer-part II. Curr Probl Surg, 2005;42:267–333.
337. Salonga, D., et al. Colorectal tumors responding to 5-fluorouracil have low gene expression levels of dihydropyrimidine dehydrogenase, thymidylate synthase, and thymidine phosphorylase. Clin Cancer Res, 2000;6:1322–7.
338. Diasio, R.B., T.L. Beavers, and J.T. Carpenter. Familial deficiency of dihydropyrimidine dehydrogenase. Biochemical basis for familial pyrimidinemia and severe 5-fluorouracil-induced toxicity. J Clin Invest, 1988;81:47–51.
339. Zeng, Z., A.M. Cohen, and C. Urmacher. Usefulness of carcinoembryonic antigen monitoring despite normal preoperative values in node-positive colon cancer patients. Dis Colon Rectum, 1993;36:1063–8.
340. Bruinvels, D.J., et al. Follow-up of patients with colorectal cancer. A meta-analysis. Ann Surg, 1994;219:174–82.
341. Renehan, A.G., et al. Impact on survival of intensive follow up after curative resection for colorectal cancer: systematic review and meta-analysis of randomised trials. BMJ, 2002;324:813.
342. Rosen, M., et al. Follow-up of colorectal cancer: a meta-analysis. Dis Colon Rectum, 1998;41:1116–26.
343. Pignone, M., et al. Cost-effectiveness analyses of colorectal cancer screening: a systematic review for the US Preventive Services Task Force. Ann Intern Med, 2002;137:96–104.
344. Mandel, J.S., et al. Reducing mortality from colorectal cancer by screening for fecal occult blood. Minnesota Colon Cancer Control Study. N Engl J Med, 1993;328:1365–71.
345. Hardcastle, J.D., et al. Randomised controlled trial of faecal-occult-blood screening for colorectal cancer. Lancet, 1996; 348:1472–7.
346. Kronborg, O., et al. Randomised study of screening for colorectal cancer with faecal-occult-blood test. Lancet, 1996;348:1467–71.
347. Towler, B.P., et al. Screening for colorectal cancer using the faecal occult blood test, hemoccult. Cochrane Database Syst Rev, 2000:CD001216.
348. Selby, J.V., et al. A case-control study of screening sigmoidoscopy and mortality from colorectal cancer. N Engl J Med, 1992;326:653–7.
349. Atkin, W.S., et al. Design of a multicentre randomised trial to evaluate flexible sigmoidoscopy in colorectal cancer screening. J Med Screen, 2001;8:137–44.
350. Prorok, P.C., et al. Design of the Prostate, Lung, Colorectal and Ovarian (PLCO) Cancer Screening Trial. Control Clin Trials, 2000;21(6 suppl):273S–309S.
351. Muller, A.D., and A. Sonnenberg. Protection by endoscopy against death from colorectal cancer. A case-control study among veterans. Arch Intern Med, 1995;155:1741–8.
352. Newcomb, P.A., et al. Screening sigmoidoscopy and colorectal cancer mortality. J Natl Cancer Inst, 1992;84:1572–5.
353. Thomas, R.D., J.J. Fairhurst, and R.A. Frost. Wessex regional radiology audit: barium enema in colo-rectal carcinoma. Clin Radiol, 1995;50:647–50.
354. Tawn, D.J., et al. National audit of the sensitivity of double-contrast barium enema for colorectal carcinoma, using control charts for the Royal College of Radiologists Clinical Radiology Audit Sub-Committee. Clin Radiol, 2005;60:558–64.
355. Kewenter, J., et al. The yield of flexible sigmoidoscopy and double-contrast barium enema in the diagnosis of neoplasms in the large bowel in patients with a positive Hemoccult test. Endoscopy, 1995;27:159–63.
356. Blakeborough, A., M.B. Sheridan, and A.H. Chapman. Complications of barium enema examinations: a survey of UK consultant radiologists 1992 to 1994. Clin Radiol, 1997;52:142–8.
357. Waye, J.D., B.S. Lewis, and S. Yessayan. Colonoscopy: a prospective report of complications. J Clin Gastroenterol, 1992;15:347–51.
358. Nelson, D.B., et al. Procedural success and complications of large-scale screening colonoscopy. Gastrointest Endosc, 2002; 55:307–14.
359. Winawer, S.J., and A.G. Zauber. Colonoscopic polypectomy and the incidence of colorectal cancer. Gut, 2001;48:753–4.
360. Winawer, S.J., and A.G. Zauber. The advanced adenoma as the primary target of screening. Gastrointest Endosc Clin N Am, 2002;12:1–9, v.
361. Rex, D.K., et al. Colonoscopic miss rates of adenomas determined by back-to-back colonoscopies. Gastroenterology, 1997; 112:24–8.
362. Winawer, S.J., et al. A comparison of colonoscopy and double-contrast barium enema for surveillance after polypectomy. National Polyp Study Work Group. N Engl J Med, 2000;342:1766–72.
363. Zarchy, T.M., and D. Ershoff. Do characteristics of adenomas on flexible sigmoidoscopy predict advanced lesions on baseline colonoscopy? Gastroenterology, 1994;106:1501–4.
364. Pickhardt, P.J., et al. Computed tomographic virtual colonoscopy to screen for colorectal neoplasia in asymptomatic adults. N Engl J Med, 2003;349:2191–200.
365. Cotton, P.B., et al. Computed tomographic colonography (virtual colonoscopy): a multicenter comparison with standard colonoscopy for detection of colorectal neoplasia. JAMA, 2004;291:1713–9.
366. Imperiale, T.F., et al. Fecal DNA versus fecal occult blood for colorectal-cancer screening in an average-risk population. N Engl J Med, 2004;351:2704–14.

367. Runkel, N.S., et al. Outcome after emergency surgery for cancer of the large intestine. Br J Surg, 1991;78:183–8.
368. Mandava, N., et al. Perforated colorectal carcinomas. Am J Surg, 1996;172:236–8.
369. Beart, R.W., et al. Management and survival of patients with adenocarcinoma of the colon and rectum: a national survey of the Commission on Cancer. J Am Coll Surg, 1995;181:225–36.
370. Gold, J.S., S. Bayar, and R.R. Salem. Association of Streptococcus bovis bacteremia with colonic neoplasia and extracolonic malignancy. Arch Surg, 2004;139:760–5.
371. Isler, J.T., et al. The role of preoperative colonoscopy in colorectal cancer. Dis Colon Rectum, 1987;30:435–9.
372. Slater, G., P. Fleshner, and A.H. Aufses, Jr. Colorectal cancer location and synchronous adenomas. Am J Gastroenterol, 1988; 83:832–6.
373. Compton, C., et al. American Joint Committee on Cancer Prognostic Factors Consensus Conference: Colorectal Working Group. Cancer, 2000;88:1739–57.
374. Mauchley, D.C., et al. Clinical utility and cost-effectiveness of routine preoperative computed tomography scanning in patients with colon cancer. Am J Surg, 2005;189:512–7; discussion 517.
375. Kerner, B.A., et al. Is preoperative computerized tomography useful in assessing patients with colorectal carcinoma? Dis Colon Rectum, 1993;36:1050–3.
376. Garcia-Aguilar, J., et al. Accuracy of endorectal ultrasonography in preoperative staging of rectal tumors. Dis Colon Rectum, 2002;45:10–5.
377. Winawer, S.J., et al. Prevention of colorectal cancer by colonoscopic polypectomy. The National Polyp Study Workgroup. N Engl J Med, 1993;329:1977–81.
378. Stryker, S.J., et al. Natural history of untreated colonic polyps. Gastroenterology, 1987;93:1009–13.
379. Winawer, S.J. Natural history of colorectal cancer. Am J Med, 1999;106(1A):3S–6S; discussion 50S–51S.
380. Atkin, W.S., B.C. Morson, and J. Cuzick. Long-term risk of colorectal cancer after excision of rectosigmoid adenomas. N Engl J Med, 1992;326:658–62.
381. O'Brien, M.J., et al. The National Polyp Study. Patient and polyp characteristics associated with high-grade dysplasia in colorectal adenomas. Gastroenterology, 1990;98:371–9.
382. Macrae, F.A., et al. Towards safer colonoscopy: a report on the complications of 5000 diagnostic or therapeutic colonoscopies. Gut, 1983;24:376–83.
382a. Franklin, M.E., et al. Laparoscopic-assisted colonoscopic polypectomy: the Texas Endosurgery Institute experience. Dis Col Rectum 2000;43:1246–9.
383. Kikuchi, R., et al. Management of early invasive colorectal cancer. Risk of recurrence and clinical guidelines. Dis Colon Rectum, 1995;38:1286–95.
384. Nascimbeni, R., et al. Risk of lymph node metastasis in T1 carcinoma of the colon and rectum. Dis Colon Rectum, 2002;45:200–6.
385. Nivatvongs, S. Surgical management of malignant colorectal polyps. Surg Clin North Am, 2002;82:959–66.
386. Nivatvongs, S., et al. Villous adenomas of the rectum: the accuracy of clinical assessment. Surgery, 1980;87:549–51.
387. Havelaar, I.J., et al. Rate of growth of intraabdominal metastases from colorectal cancer. Cancer, 1984;54:163–71.
388. Slim, K., et al. Meta-analysis of randomized clinical trials of colorectal surgery with or without mechanical bowel preparation. Br J Surg, 2004;91:1125–30.
389. Wille-Jorgensen, P., et al. Pre-operative mechanical bowel cleansing or not? An updated meta-analysis. Colorectal Dis, 2005;7:304–10.
390. Bucher, P., et al. Randomized clinical trial of mechanical bowel preparation versus no preparation before elective left-sided colorectal surgery. Br J Surg, 2005;92:409–14.
391. Nelson, H., et al. Guidelines 2000 for colon and rectal cancer surgery. J Natl Cancer Inst, 2001;93:583–96.
392. Le Voyer, T.E., et al. Colon cancer survival is associated with increasing number of lymph nodes analyzed: a secondary survey of intergroup trial INT-0089. J Clin Oncol, 2003;21:2912–9.
393. Goldstein, N.S. Lymph node recoveries from 2427 pT3 colorectal resection specimens spanning 45 years: recommendations for a minimum number of recovered lymph nodes based on predictive probabilities. Am J Surg Pathol, 2002;26:179–89.
394. Wong, J.H., et al. Number of nodes examined and staging accuracy in colorectal carcinoma. J Clin Oncol, 1999;17:2896–900.
395. Lopez, M.J., and W.W. Monafo. Role of extended resection in the initial treatment of locally advanced colorectal carcinoma. Surgery, 1993;113:365–72.
396. Keating, J., et al. The epidemiology of colorectal cancer: what can we learn from the New Zealand Cancer Registry? N Z Med J, 2003;116:U437.
397. Chu, D.Z., et al. The significance of synchronous carcinoma and polyps in the colon and rectum. Cancer, 1986;57:445–50.
398. Passman, M.A., R.F. Pommier, and J.T. Vetto. Synchronous colon primaries have the same prognosis as solitary colon cancers. Dis Colon Rectum, 1996;39:329–34.
399. Feig, B.W., et al. A caution regarding lymphatic mapping in patients with colon cancer. Am J Surg, 2001;182:707–12.
400. Bertagnolli, M., et al. Sentinel node staging of resectable colon cancer: results of a multicenter study. Ann Surg, 2004;240:624–8; discussion 628–30.
401. Saha, S., et al. Comparative analysis of nodal upstaging between colon and rectal cancers by sentinel lymph node mapping: a prospective trial. Dis Colon Rectum, 2004;47:1767–72.
402. Lacy, A.M., et al. Laparoscopy-assisted colectomy versus open colectomy for treatment of non-metastatic colon cancer: a randomised trial [see comment]. Lancet, 2002;359:2224–9.
403. A comparison of laparoscopically assisted and open colectomy for colon cancer. N Engl J Med, 2004;350:2050–9.
404. Guillou, P.J., et al. Short-term endpoints of conventional versus laparoscopic-assisted surgery in patients with colorectal cancer (MRC CLASICC trial): multicentre, randomised controlled trial. Lancet, 2005;365:1718–26.
405. Hazebroek, E.J., and G. Color Study. COLOR: a randomized clinical trial comparing laparoscopic and open resection for colon cancer. Surg Endosc, 2002;16:949–53.
406. Leung, K.L., et al. Laparoscopic resection of rectosigmoid carcinoma: prospective randomised trial. Lancet, 2004;363:1187–92.
407. Kapiteijn, E., et al. Preoperative radiotherapy combined with total mesorectal excision for resectable rectal cancer. N Engl J Med, 2001;345:638–46.
408. Wilson, S.M., and O.H. Beahrs. The curative treatment of carcinoma of the sigmoid, rectosigmoid, and rectum. Ann Surg, 1976;183:556–65.
409. Killingback, M. Local excision of carcinoma of the rectum: indications. World J Surg, 1992;16:437–46.
410. Graham, R.A., L. Garnsey, and J.M. Jessup. Local excision of rectal carcinoma. Am J Surg, 1990;160:306–12.
411. Steele, G.D., Jr., et al. Sphincter-sparing treatment for distal rectal adenocarcinoma. Ann Surg Oncol, 1999;6:433–41.
412. Russell, A.H., et al. Anal sphincter conservation for patients with adenocarcinoma of the distal rectum: long-term results of radiation therapy oncology group protocol 89-02. Int J Radiat Oncol Biol Phys, 2000;46:313–22.
413. Varma, M.G., et al. Local excision of rectal carcinoma. Arch Surg, 1999;134:863–7; discussion 867–8.
414. Habr-Gama, A., et al. Operative versus nonoperative treatment for stage 0 distal rectal cancer following chemoradiation therapy: long-term results. Ann Surg, 2004;240:711–7; discussion 717–8.
415. Bonnen, M., et al. Long-term results using local excision after preoperative chemoradiation among selected T3 rectal cancer patients. Int J Radiat Oncol Biol Phys, 2004;60:1098–105.

416. Papillon, J., and P. Berard. Endocavitary irradiation in the conservative treatment of adenocarcinoma of the low rectum. World J Surg, 1992;16:451–7.
417. Buess, G., et al. Technique of transanal endoscopic microsurgery. Surg Endosc, 1988;2:71–5.
418. Middleton, P.F., L.M. Sutherland, and G.J. Maddern. Transanal endoscopic microsurgery: a systematic review. Dis Colon Rectum, 2005;48:270–84.
419. Smith, L.E., et al. Transanal endoscopic microsurgery. Initial registry results. Dis Colon Rectum, 1996;39(10 suppl):S79–S84.
420. McGregor, J.R., and P.J. O'Dwyer. The surgical management of obstruction and perforation of the left colon. Surg Gynecol Obstet, 1993;177:203–8.
421. Wolmark, N., et al. The prognostic significance of tumor location and bowel obstruction in Dukes B and C colorectal cancer. Findings from the NSABP clinical trials. Ann Surg, 1983;198:743–52.
422. Deans, G.T., Z.H. Krukowski, and S.T. Irwin. Malignant obstruction of the left colon. Br J Surg, 1994;81:1270–6.
423. Stephenson, B.M., et al. Malignant left-sided large bowel obstruction managed by subtotal/total colectomy. Br J Surg, 1990; 77:1098–102.
424. Single-stage treatment for malignant left-sided colonic obstruction: a prospective randomized clinical trial comparing subtotal colectomy with segmental resection following intraoperative irrigation. The SCOTIA Study Group. Subtotal colectomy versus on-table irrigation and anastomosis. Br J Surg, 1995; 82:1622–7.
425. Willett, C.G., et al. Does postoperative irradiation play a role in the adjuvant therapy of stage T4 colon cancer? Cancer J Sci Am, 1999;5:242–7.
426. Laurie, J.A., et al. Surgical adjuvant therapy of large-bowel carcinoma: an evaluation of levamisole and the combination of levamisole and fluorouracil. The North Central Cancer Treatment Group and the Mayo Clinic. J Clin Oncol, 1989;7:1447–56.
427. Moertel, C.G., et al. Levamisole and fluorouracil for adjuvant therapy of resected colon carcinoma. N Engl J Med, 1990;322:352–8.
428. Rustum, Y.M., S. Cao, and Z. Zhang. Rationale for treatment design: biochemical modulation of 5-fluorouracil by leucovorin. Cancer J Sci Am, 1998;4:12–8.
429. Wolmark, N., L. Colangelo, and S. Wieand. National Surgical Adjuvant Breast and Bowel Project trials in colon cancer. Semin Oncol, 2001;28(1 suppl 1):9–13.
430. Scheithauer, W., et al. Oral capecitabine as an alternative to IV 5-fluorouracil-based adjuvant therapy for colon cancer: safety results of a randomized, phase III trial. Ann Oncol, 2003;14:1735–43.
431. Improved survival with preoperative radiotherapy in resectable rectal cancer. Swedish Rectal Cancer Trial. N Engl J Med, 1997;336:980–7.
432. Prolongation of the disease-free interval in surgically treated rectal carcinoma. Gastrointestinal Tumor Study Group. N Engl J Med, 1985;312:1465–72.
433. Krook, J.E., et al. Effective surgical adjuvant therapy for high-risk rectal carcinoma. N Engl J Med, 1991;324:709–15.
434. O'Connell, M.J., et al. Improving adjuvant therapy for rectal cancer by combining protracted-infusion fluorouracil with radiation therapy after curative surgery. N Engl J Med, 1994;331:502–7.
435. Sauer, R., et al. Preoperative versus postoperative chemoradiotherapy for rectal cancer. N Engl J Med, 2004;351:1731–40.
436. Galandiuk, S., et al. Patterns of recurrence after curative resection of carcinoma of the colon and rectum. Surg Gynecol Obstet, 1992;174:27–32.
437. Young-Fadok, T.M., et al. Prophylactic oophorectomy in colorectal carcinoma: preliminary results of a randomized, prospective trial. Dis Colon Rectum, 1998;41:277–83; discussion 283–5.
438. Scheele, J., and A. Altendorf-Hofmann. Resection of colorectal liver metastases. Langenbecks Arch Surg, 1999;384:313–27.
439. Scheithauer, W., et al. Randomised comparison of combination chemotherapy plus supportive care with supportive care alone in patients with metastatic colorectal cancer. BMJ, 1993;306:752–5.
440. Van Cutsem, E., et al. Oral capecitabine versus intravenous 5-fluorouracil and leucovorin: integrated efficacy data and novel analyses from two large, randomised, phase III trials. Br J Cancer, 2004;90:1190–7.
441. Douillard, J.Y., et al. Irinotecan combined with fluorouracil compared with fluorouracil alone as first-line treatment for metastatic colorectal cancer: a multicentre randomised trial. Lancet, 2000;355:1041–7.
442. Grothey, A., and R.M. Goldberg. A review of oxaliplatin and its clinical use in colorectal cancer. Expert Opin Pharmacother, 2004;5:2159–70.
443. Hoff, P.M., et al. Comparison of oral capecitabine versus intravenous fluorouracil plus leucovorin as first-line treatment in 605 patients with metastatic colorectal cancer: results of a randomized phase III study. J Clin Oncol, 2001;19:2282–92.
444. Douillard, J.Y., et al. Multicenter phase III study of uracil/tegafur and oral leucovorin versus fluorouracil and leucovorin in patients with previously untreated metastatic colorectal cancer. J Clin Oncol, 2002;20:3605–16.
445. Hurwitz, H., et al. Bevacizumab plus irinotecan, fluorouracil, and leucovorin for metastatic colorectal cancer. N Engl J Med, 2004;350:2335–42.
446. Cunningham, D., et al. Cetuximab monotherapy and cetuximab plus irinotecan in irinotecan-refractory metastatic colorectal cancer. N Engl J Med, 2004;351:337–45.
447. Scheele, J., et al. Indicators of prognosis after hepatic resection for colorectal secondaries. Surgery, 1991;110:13–29.
448. Abdalla, E.K., et al. Recurrence and outcomes following hepatic resection, radiofrequency ablation, and combined resection/ablation for colorectal liver metastases. Ann Surg, 2004;239:818–25; discussion 825–7.
449. Fong, Y., et al. Liver resection for colorectal metastases. J Clin Oncol, 1997;15:938–46.
450. Nadig, D.E., et al. Major hepatic resection. Indications and results in a national hospital system from 1988 to 1992. Arch Surg, 1997;132:115–9.
451. Sugawara, G., et al. Repeat hepatectomy for recurrent colorectal metastases. Surg Today, 2005;35:282–9.
452. Tuttle, T.M., S.A. Curley, and M.S. Roh. Repeat hepatic resection as effective treatment of recurrent colorectal liver metastases. Ann Surg Oncol, 1997;4:125–30.
453. Petrowsky, H., et al. Second liver resections are safe and effective treatment for recurrent hepatic metastases from colorectal cancer: a bi-institutional analysis. Ann Surg, 2002;235:863–71.
454. Wanebo, H.J., et al. Patient selection for hepatic resection of colorectal metastases. Arch Surg, 1996;131:322–9.
455. Madoff, D.C., E.K. Abdalla, and J.N. Vauthey. Portal vein embolization in preparation for major hepatic resection: evolution of a new standard of care. J Vasc Interv Radiol, 2005;16:779–90.
456. Lorenz, M., and H.H. Muller. Randomized, multicenter trial of fluorouracil plus leucovorin administered either via hepatic arterial or intravenous infusion versus fluorodeoxyuridine administered via hepatic arterial infusion in patients with nonresectable liver metastases from colorectal carcinoma. J Clin Oncol, 2000;18:243–54.
457. Kemeny, M.M., et al. Combined-modality treatment for resectable metastatic colorectal carcinoma to the liver: surgical resection of hepatic metastases in combination with continuous infusion of chemotherapy—an intergroup study. J Clin Oncol, 2002;20:1499–505.

458. Kemeny, N.E., and M. Gonen. Hepatic arterial infusion after liver resection. N Engl J Med, 2005;352:734–5.
459. Saito, Y., et al. Pulmonary metastasectomy for 165 patients with colorectal carcinoma: a prognostic assessment. J Thorac Cardiovasc Surg, 2002;124:1007–13.
460. Pfannschmidt, J., et al. Prognostic factors and survival after complete resection of pulmonary metastases from colorectal carcinoma: experiences in 167 patients. J Thorac Cardiovasc Surg, 2003;126:732–9.
461. Ike, H., et al. Results of aggressive resection of lung metastases from colorectal carcinoma detected by intensive follow-up. Dis Colon Rectum, 2002;45:468–73; discussion 473–5.
462. Verwaal, V.J., et al. Randomized trial of cytoreduction and hyperthermic intraperitoneal chemotherapy versus systemic chemotherapy and palliative surgery in patients with peritoneal carcinomatosis of colorectal cancer. J Clin Oncol, 2003;21:3737–43.
463. Russell, A.H., et al. Adenocarcinoma of the proximal colon. Sites of initial dissemination and patterns of recurrence following surgery alone. Cancer, 1984;53:360–7.
464. Gunderson, L.L., H. Sosin, and S. Levitt. Extrapelvic colon—areas of failure in a reoperation series: implications for adjuvant therapy. Int J Radiat Oncol Biol Phys, 1985;11:731–41.
465. Obrand, D.I., and P.H. Gordon. Incidence and patterns of recurrence following curative resection for colorectal carcinoma. Dis Colon Rectum, 1997;40:15–24.
466. Bowne, W.B., et al. Operative salvage for locoregional recurrent colon cancer after curative resection: an analysis of 100 cases. Dis Colon Rectum, 2005;48:897–909.
467. Hahnloser, D., et al. Curative potential of multimodality therapy for locally recurrent rectal cancer. Ann Surg, 2003;237:502–8.
468. Mohiuddin, M., G. Marks, and J. Marks. Long-term results of reirradiation for patients with recurrent rectal carcinoma. Cancer, 2002;95:1144–50.
469. Juffermans, J.H., et al. Reirradiation and hyperthermia in rectal carcinoma: a retrospective study on palliative effect. Cancer, 2003;98:1759–66.
470. van der Zee, J., et al. Comparison of radiotherapy alone with radiotherapy plus hyperthermia in locally advanced pelvic tumours: a prospective, randomised, multicentre trial. Dutch Deep Hyperthermia Group. Lancet, 2000;355:1119–25.
471. Church, J., A. Lowry, and C. Simmang. Practice parameters for the identification and testing of patients at risk for dominantly inherited colorectal cancer–supporting documentation. Dis Colon Rectum, 2001;44:1404–12.
472. Gingold, B.S., D. Jagelman, and R.B. Turnbull. Surgical management of familial polyposis and Gardner's syndrome. Am J Surg, 1979;137:54–6.
473. Sampson, J.R., et al. Autosomal recessive colorectal adenomatous polyposis due to inherited mutations of MYH. Lancet, 2003;362:39–41.
474. Sieber, O.M., et al. Multiple colorectal adenomas, classic adenomatous polyposis, and germ-line mutations in MYH. N Engl J Med, 2003;348:791–9.
475. Al-Tassan, N., et al. Inherited variants of MYH associated with somatic G:C→T:A mutations in colorectal tumors. Nat Genet, 2002;30:227–32.
476. Wang, L., et al. MYH mutations in patients with attenuated and classic polyposis and with young-onset colorectal cancer without polyps. Gastroenterology, 2004;127:9–16.
477. Giardiello, F.M., et al. Increased risk of cancer in the Peutz-Jeghers syndrome. N Engl J Med, 1987;316:1511–4.
478. Spigelman, A.D., V. Murday, and R.K. Phillips. Cancer and the Peutz-Jeghers syndrome. Gut, 1989;30:1588–90.
479. Wirtzfeld, D.A., N.J. Petrelli, and M.A. Rodriguez-Bigas. Hamartomatous polyposis syndromes: molecular genetics, neoplastic risk, and surveillance recommendations. Ann Surg Oncol, 2001;8:319–27.
480. Coburn, M.C., et al. Malignant potential in intestinal juvenile polyposis syndromes. Ann Surg Oncol, 1995;2:386–91.
481. Jass, J.R., et al. Juvenile polyposis—a precancerous condition. Histopathology, 1988;13:619–30.
482. Itoh, H., et al. Risk of cancer death in first-degree relatives of patients with hereditary non-polyposis cancer syndrome (Lynch type II): a study of 130 kindreds in the United Kingdom. Br J Surg, 1990;77:1367–70.
483. Lynch, H.T., and A. de la Chapelle. Genetic susceptibility to non-polyposis colorectal cancer. J Med Genet, 1999;36:801–18.
484. Aarnio, M., et al. Life-time risk of different cancers in hereditary non-polyposis colorectal cancer (HNPCC) syndrome. Int J Cancer, 1995;64:430–3.
485. Plaschke, J., et al. Lower incidence of colorectal cancer and later age of disease onset in 27 families with pathogenic MSH6 germline mutations compared with families with MLH1 or MSH2 mutations: the German Hereditary Nonpolyposis Colorectal Cancer Consortium. J Clin Oncol, 2004;22:4486–94.
486. Jass, J.R., et al. Pathology of hereditary non-polyposis colorectal cancer. Anticancer Res, 1994;14(4B):1631–4.
487. Winawer, S.J., et al. Risk of colorectal cancer in the families of patients with adenomatous polyps. National Polyp Study Workgroup. N Engl J Med, 1996;334:82–7.
488. Church, J., and C. Simmang. Practice parameters for the treatment of patients with dominantly inherited colorectal cancer (familial adenomatous polyposis and hereditary non-polyposis colorectal cancer). Dis Colon Rectum, 2003;46:1001–12.
489. Winawer, S.J., et al. Screening for colorectal cancer with fecal occult blood testing and sigmoidoscopy. J Natl Cancer Inst, 1993;85:1311–8.
490. Kewenter, J., et al. Results of screening, rescreening, and follow-up in a prospective randomized study for detection of colorectal cancer by fecal occult blood testing. Results for 68,308 subjects. Scand J Gastroenterol, 1994;29:468–73.
491. Jessup, J.M., et al. The National Cancer Data Base. Report on colon cancer. Cancer, 1996;78:918–26.
492. Frazee, R.C., et al. Transanal excision of rectal carcinoma. Am Surg, 1995;61:714–7.
493. Bleday, R., et al. Prospective evaluation of local excision for small rectal cancers. Dis Colon Rectum, 1997;40:388–92.
494. Ishizaki, Y., et al. Evaluation of local excision for sessile-type lower rectal tumors. Hepatogastroenterology, 1999;46:2329–32.
495. Chakravarti, A., et al. Long-term follow-up of patients with rectal cancer managed by local excision with and without adjuvant irradiation. Ann Surg, 1999;230:49–54.
496. Mellgren, A., et al. Is local excision adequate therapy for early rectal cancer? Dis Colon Rectum, 2000;43:1064–71; discussion 1071–4.
497. Endreseth, B.H., et al. Transanal excision versus major surgery for T1 rectal cancer. Dis Colon Rectum, 2005;48:1380–8.
497a. Garcia-Aguilar, J., et al. Open vs. closed sphincterotomy for chronic anal fissure: long-term results. Dis Colon Rectum, 1997;40:1439–42.
498. Bailey, H.R., et al. Local excision of carcinoma of the rectum for cure. Surgery, 1992;111:555–61.
499. Wagman, R., et al. Conservative management of rectal cancer with local excision and postoperative adjuvant therapy. Int J Radiat Oncol Biol Phys, 1999;44:841–6.
500. Le Voyer, T.E., et al. Local excision and chemoradiation for low rectal T1 and T2 cancers is an effective treatment. Am Surg, 1999;65:625–30; discussion 630–1.
501. The evaluation of low dose pre-operative x-ray therapy in the management of operable rectal cancer; results of a randomly controlled trial. Br J Surg, 1984;71:21–5.
502. Higgins, G.A., et al. Preoperative radiation and surgery for cancer of the rectum. Veterans Administration Surgical Oncology Group Trial II. Cancer, 1986;58:352–9.

503. Gerard, A., et al. Preoperative radiotherapy as adjuvant treatment in rectal cancer. Final results of a randomized study of the European Organization for Research and Treatment of Cancer (EORTC). Ann Surg, 1988;208:606–14.
504. Reis Neto, J.A., F.A. Quilici, and J.A. Reis, Jr. A comparison of nonoperative versus preoperative radiotherapy in rectal carcinoma. A 10-year randomized trial. Dis Colon Rectum, 1989; 32:702–10.
505. Dahl, O., et al. Low-dose preoperative radiation postpones recurrences in operable rectal cancer. Results of a randomized multicenter trial in western Norway. Cancer, 1990;66:2286–94.
506. Goldberg, P.A., et al. Long-term results of a randomised trial of short-course low-dose adjuvant pre-operative radiotherapy for rectal cancer: reduction in local treatment failure. Eur J Cancer, 1994;30A:1602–6.
507. Marsh, P.J., R.D. James, and P.F. Schofield. Adjuvant preoperative radiotherapy for locally advanced rectal carcinoma. Results of a prospective, randomized trial. Dis Colon Rectum, 1994; 37:1205–14.
508. Cedermark, B., et al. The Stockholm I trial of preoperative short term radiotherapy in operable rectal carcinoma. A prospective randomized trial. Stockholm Colorectal Cancer Study Group. Cancer, 1995;75:2269–75.
509. Randomized study on preoperative radiotherapy in rectal carcinoma. Stockholm Colorectal Cancer Study Group. Ann Surg Oncol, 1996;3:423–30.
510. Balslev, I., et al. Postoperative radiotherapy in Dukes' B and C carcinoma of the rectum and rectosigmoid. A randomized multicenter study. Cancer, 1986;58:22–8.
511. Fisher, B., et al. Postoperative adjuvant chemotherapy or radiation therapy for rectal cancer: results from NSABP protocol R-01. J Natl Cancer Inst, 1988;80:21–9.
512. Treurniet-Donker, A.D., et al. Postoperative radiation therapy for rectal cancer. An interim analysis of a prospective, randomized multicenter trial in The Netherlands. Cancer, 1991;67: 2042–8.
513. Randomised trial of surgery alone versus radiotherapy followed by surgery for potentially operable locally advanced rectal cancer. Medical Research Council Rectal Cancer Working Party. Lancet, 1996;348:1605–10.
514. Boulis-Wassif, S., et al. Final results of a randomized trial on the treatment of rectal cancer with preoperative radiotherapy alone or in combination with 5-fluorouracil, followed by radical surgery. Trial of the European Organization on Research and Treatment of Cancer Gastrointestinal Tract Cancer Cooperative Group. Cancer, 1984;53:1811–8.
515. Radiation therapy and fluorouracil with or without semustine for the treatment of patients with surgical adjuvant adenocarcinoma of the rectum. Gastrointestinal Tumor Study Group. J Clin Oncol, 1992;10:549–57.
516. Wolmark, N., et al. Randomized trial of postoperative adjuvant chemotherapy with or without radiotherapy for carcinoma of the rectum: National Surgical Adjuvant Breast and Bowel Project Protocol R-02. J Natl Cancer Inst, 2000;92:388–96.
517. Vasilevsky, C.A., and P.H. Gordon. The incidence of recurrent abscesses or fistula-in-ano following anorectal suppuration. Dis Colon Rectum, 1984;27:126–30.
518. Sudol-Szopinska, I., et al. Reliability of endosonography in evaluation of anal fistulae and abscesses. Acta Radiol, 2002;43:599–602.
519. Cheong, D.M., et al. Anal endosonography for recurrent anal fistulas: image enhancement with hydrogen peroxide. Dis Colon Rectum, 1993;36:1158–60.
520. Buchanan, G.N., et al. Clinical examination, endosonography, and MR imaging in preoperative assessment of fistula in ano: comparison with outcome-based reference standard. Radiology, 2004;233:674–81.
521. Hussain, S.M., et al. Fistula in ano: endoanal sonography versus endoanal MR imaging in classification. Radiology, 1996;200:475–81.
522. Whiteford, M.H., et al. Practice parameters for the treatment of perianal abscess and fistula-in-ano (revised). Dis Colon Rectum, 2005;48:1337–42.
523. Inceoglu, R., and R. Gencosmanoglu. Fistulotomy and drainage of deep postanal space abscess in the treatment of posterior horseshoe fistula. BMC Surg, 2003;3:10.
524. Cirocco, W.C., and J.C. Reilly. Challenging the predictive accuracy of Goodsall's rule for anal fistulas. Dis Colon Rectum, 1992;35:537–42.
525. Marks, C.G., and J.K. Ritchie. Anal fistulas at St Mark's Hospital. Br J Surg, 1977;64:84–91.
526. Hananel, N., and P.H. Gordon. Re-examination of clinical manifestations and response to therapy of fissure-in-ano. Dis Colon Rectum, 1997;40:229–33.
527. Petros, J.G., E.B. Rimm, and R.J. Robillard. Clinical presentation of chronic anal fissures. Am Surg, 1993;59:666–8.
528. Farouk, R., et al. Sustained internal sphincter hypertonia in patients with chronic anal fissure. Dis Colon Rectum, 1994; 37:424–9.
529. Keck, J.O., et al. Computer-generated profiles of the anal canal in patients with anal fissure. Dis Colon Rectum, 1995;38:72–9.
530. Schouten, W.R., et al. Ischaemic nature of anal fissure. Br J Surg, 1996;83:63–5.
531. Xynos, E., et al. Anal manometry in patients with fissure-in-ano before and after internal sphincterotomy. Int J Colorectal Dis, 1993;8:125–8.
532. Schouten, W.R., and J.D. Blankensteijn. Ultra slow wave pressure variations in the anal canal before and after lateral internal sphincterotomy. Int J Colorectal Dis, 1992;7:115–8.
533. Jost, W.H. One hundred cases of anal fissure treated with botulin toxin: early and long-term results. Dis Colon Rectum, 1997;40:1029–32.
534. Brisinda, G., et al. A comparison of injections of botulinum toxin and topical nitroglycerin ointment for the treatment of chronic anal fissure. N Engl J Med, 1999;341:65–9.
535. Maria, G., et al. A comparison of botulinum toxin and saline for the treatment of chronic anal fissure. N Engl J Med, 1998;338:217–20.
536. Nelson, R. A systematic review of medical therapy for anal fissure. Dis Colon Rectum, 2004;47:422–31.
537. Lund, J.N., and J.H. Scholefield. Aetiology and treatment of anal fissure. Br J Surg, 1996;83:1335–44.
538. Lund, J.N., and J.H. Scholefield. A randomised, prospective, double-blind, placebo-controlled trial of glyceryl trinitrate ointment in treatment of anal fissure. Lancet, 1997;349:11–4.
539. Lund, J.N., and J.H. Scholefield. Glyceryl trinitrate is an effective treatment for anal fissure. Dis Colon Rectum, 1997;40:468–70.
540. Oettle, G.J. Glyceryl trinitrate versus sphincterotomy for treatment of chronic fissure-in-ano: a randomized, controlled trial. Dis Colon Rectum, 1997;40:1318–20.
541. Hyman, N.H., and P.A. Cataldo. Nitroglycerin ointment for anal fissures: effective treatment or just a headache? Dis Colon Rectum, 1999;42:383–5.
542. Nelson, R. Operative procedures for fissure in ano. Cochrane Database Syst Rev, 2005:CD002199.
543. Graham-Stewart, C.W. What causes hemorrhoids?A new theory of etiology. Dis Colon Rectum, 1963;127:333–44.
544. Bernstein, W.C. What are hemorrhoids and what is their relationship to the portal venous system? Dis Colon Rectum, 1983;26:829–34.
545. Haas, P.A., T.A. Fox, Jr., and G.P. Haas. The pathogenesis of hemorrhoids. Dis Colon Rectum, 1984;27:442–50.
546. Johanson, J.F., and J. Lafferty. Epidemiology of fecal incontinence: the silent affliction. Am J Gastroenterol, 1996;91:33–6.

547. Hosking, S.W., et al. Anorectal varices, haemorrhoids, and portal hypertension. Lancet, 1989;1:349–52.
548. Wang, T.F., et al. Relationship of portal pressure, anorectal varices and hemorrhoids in cirrhotic patients. J Hepatol, 1992;15(1–2):170–3.
549. Hiltunen, K.M., and M. Matikainen. Anal manometric findings in symptomatic hemorrhoids. Dis Colon Rectum, 1985;28:807–9.
550. Sun, W.M., et al. Haemorrhoids are associated not with hypertrophy of the internal anal sphincter, but with hypertension of the anal cushions. Br J Surg, 1992;79:592–4.
551. Lin, J.K. Anal manometric studies in hemorrhoids and anal fissures. Dis Colon Rectum, 1989;32:839–42.
552. MacRae, H.M., and R.S. McLeod. Comparison of hemorrhoidal treatment modalities. A meta-analysis. Dis Colon Rectum, 1995;38:687–94.
553. Cataldo, P., et al. Practice parameters for the management of hemorrhoids (revised). Dis Colon Rectum, 2005;48:189–94.
554. Buchmann, P., and U. Seefeld. Rubber band ligation for piles can be disastrous in HIV-positive patients. Int J Colorectal Dis, 1989;4:57–8.
555. Shemesh, E.I., et al. Severe complication of rubber band ligation of internal hemorrhoids. Dis Colon Rectum, 1987;30:199–200.
556. Quevedo-Bonilla, G., et al. Septic complications of hemorrhoidal banding. Arch Surg, 1988;123:650–1.
557. O'Donovan, S., et al. Intraoperative use of Toradol facilitates outpatient hemorrhoidectomy. Dis Colon Rectum, 1994;37:793–9.
558. Hoff, S.D., et al. Ambulatory surgical hemorrhoidectomy—a solution to postoperative urinary retention? Dis Colon Rectum, 1994;37:1242–4.
559. Nivatvongs, S. Hemorrhoids. In: Principles and Practice of Surgery for the Colon, Rectum, and Anus, S. Nivatvongs and P.H. Gordon, eds. St. Louis: Quality Medical; 1999:193–216.
560. Basdanis, G., et al. Randomized clinical trial of stapled hemorrhoidectomy versus open with Ligasure for prolapsed piles. Surg Endosc, 2005;19:235–9.
561. Bikhchandani, J., et al. Randomized controlled trial to compare the early and mid-term results of stapled versus open hemorrhoidectomy. Am J Surg, 2005;189:56–60.
562. Cheetham, M.J., et al. A randomized, controlled trial of diathermy hemorrhoidectomy versus stapled hemorrhoidectomy in an intended day-care setting with longer-term follow-up. Dis Colon Rectum, 2003;46:491–7.
563. Chung, C.C., et al. Stapled hemorrhoidopexy versus Harmonic Scalpel hemorrhoidectomy: a randomized trial. Dis Colon Rectum, 2005;48:1213–9.
564. Gravie, J.F., et al. Stapled hemorrhoidopexy versus Milligan-Morgan hemorrhoidectomy: a prospective, randomized, multicenter trial with 2-year postoperative follow up. Ann Surg, 2005;242:29–35.
565. Senagore, A.J., et al. A prospective, randomized, controlled multicenter trial comparing stapled hemorrhoidopexy and Ferguson hemorrhoidectomy: perioperative and 1-year results. Dis Colon Rectum, 2004;47:1824–36.
566. Peng, B.C., D.G. Jayne, and Y.H. Ho. Randomized trial of rubber band ligation versus stapled hemorrhoidectomy for prolapsed piles. Dis Colon Rectum, 2003;46:291–7; discussion 296–7.
567. Lan, P., et al. The safety and efficacy of stapled hemorrhoidectomy in the treatment of hemorrhoids: a systematic review and meta-analysis of ten randomized control trials. Int J Colorectal Dis, 2005.
568. Nisar, P.J., et al. Stapled hemorrhoidopexy compared with conventional hemorrhoidectomy: systematic review of randomized, controlled trials. Dis Colon Rectum, 2004;47:1837–45.
569. Oughriss, M., R. Yver, and J.L. Faucheron, Complications of stapled hemorrhoidectomy: a French multicentric study. Gastroenterol Clin Biol, 2005;29:429–33.
570. Nivatvongs, S. Pilonidal disease. In: Principles and Practice of Surgery for the Colon, Rectum, and Anus, P.H. Gordon and S. Nivatvongs, eds. St. Louis: Quality Medical; 1999:287–302.
571. Bascom, J. Pilonidal disease: origin from follicles of hairs and results of follicle removal as treatment. Surgery, 1980;87:567–72.
572. Marks, J., et al. Pilonidal sinus excision—healing by open granulation. Br J Surg, 1985;72:637–40.
573. Jensen, S.L., and H. Harling. Prognosis after simple incision and drainage for a first-episode acute pilonidal abscess. Br J Surg, 1988;75:60–1.
574. Armstrong, J.H., and P.J. Barcia. Pilonidal sinus disease. The conservative approach. Arch Surg, 1994;129:914–7; discussion 917–9.
575. Allen-Mersh, T.G. Pilonidal sinus: finding the right track for treatment. Br J Surg, 1990;77:123–32.
576. Akinci, O.F. Limited separate ellyptical excision for complicated pilonidal disease. Colorectal Dis, 2005;7:424–5.
577. Akinci, O.F., A. Coskun, and A. Uzunkoy. Simple and effective surgical treatment of pilonidal sinus: asymmetric excision and primary closure using suction drain and subcuticular skin closure. Dis Colon Rectum, 2000;43:701–6; discussion 706–7.
578. Akca, T., et al. Randomized clinical trial comparing primary closure with the Limberg flap in the treatment of primary sacrococcygeal pilonidal disease. Br J Surg, 2005;92:1081–4.
579. Nelson, R., et al. Community-based prevalence of anal incontinence. JAMA, 1995;274:559–61.
580. Ryhammer, A.M., S. Laurberg, and A.P. Hermann. Long-term effect of vaginal deliveries on anorectal function in normal perimenopausal women. Dis Colon Rectum, 1996;39:852–9.
581. Gordon, P.H. Anal incontinence. In: Principles and Practice of Surgery for the Colon, Rectum, and Anus, S. Nivatvongs and P.H. Gordon, eds. St. Louis: Quality Medical; 1999:365–400.
582. Hill, J., A. Mumtaz, and E.S. Kiff. Pudendal neuropathy in patients with idiopathic faecal incontinence progresses with time. Br J Surg, 1994;81:1494–5.
583. Henry, M.M. Descending perineum syndrome. In: Coloproctology and the Pelvic Floor: Pathophysiology and Management, M.M. Henry and M. Swash, eds. London: Butterworths; 1985: 299–303.
584. Jameson, J.S., et al. Effect of age, sex and parity on anorectal function. Br J Surg, 1994;81:1689–92.
585. Sultan, A.H., et al. Endosonography of the anal sphincters: normal anatomy and comparison with manometry. Clin Radiol, 1994;49:368–74.
586. Falk, P.M., et al. Transanal ultrasound and manometry in the evaluation of fecal incontinence. Dis Colon Rectum, 1994;37:468–72.
587. Sangwan, Y.P., and J.A. Coller. Fecal incontinence. Surg Clin North Am, 1994;74:1377–98.
588. Cheong, D.M., et al. Electrodiagnostic evaluation of fecal incontinence. Muscle Nerve, 1995;18:612–9.
589. Shelton, A.A., and M.L. Welton. The pelvic floor in health and disease. West J Med, 1997;167:90–8.
590. Wong, W.D., et al. The safety and efficacy of the artificial bowel sphincter for fecal incontinence: results from a multicenter cohort study. Dis Colon Rectum, 2002;45:1139–53.
591. Tjandra, J.J., et al. Injectable silicone biomaterial for fecal incontinence caused by internal anal sphincter dysfunction is effective. Dis Colon Rectum, 2004;47:2138–46.
592. Ko, C.Y., et al. Biofeedback is effective therapy for fecal incontinence and constipation. Arch Surg, 1997;132:829–33; discussion 833–4.
593. Duthie, G.S., and D.C. Bartolo. Abdominal rectopexy for rectal prolapse: a comparison of techniques. Br J Surg, 1992;79:107–13.
594. Sayfan, J., et al. Sutured posterior abdominal rectopexy with sigmoidectomy compared with Marlex rectopexy for rectal prolapse. Br J Surg, 1990;77:143–5.

595. Athanasiadis, S., et al. The risk of infection of three synthetic materials used in rectopexy with or without colonic resection for rectal prolapse. Int J Colorectal Dis, 1996;11:42–4.
596. Huber, F.T., H. Stein, and J.R. Siewert. Functional results after treatment of rectal prolapse with rectopexy and sigmoid resection. World J Surg, 1995;19:138–43; discussion 143.
597. Luukkonen, P., U. Mikkonen, and H. Jarvinen. Abdominal rectopexy with sigmoidectomy versus rectopexy alone for rectal prolapse: a prospective, randomized study. Int J Colorectal Dis, 1992;7:219–22.
598. McKee, R.F., et al. A prospective randomized study of abdominal rectopexy with and without sigmoidectomy in rectal prolapse. Surg Gynecol Obstet, 1992;174:145–8.
599. Watts, J.D., et al. The management of procidentia. 30 years' experience. Dis Colon Rectum, 1985;28:96–102.
600. Husa, A., P. Sainio, and K. von Smitten. Abdominal rectopexy and sigmoid resection (Frykman-Goldberg operation) for rectal prolapse. Acta Chir Scand, 1988;154:221–4.
601. Lehur, P.A., et al. [Sacral rectopexy-sigmoidectomy in the treatment of rectal prolapse syndrome. Anatomical and functional results]. Gastroenterol Clin Biol, 1996;20:172–7.
602. Augenbraun, M.H., and W.M. McCormack. Sexually transmitted diseases in HIV-infected persons. Infect Dis Clin North Am, 1994;8:439–48.
603. Sexually transmitted diseases treatment guidelines 2002. Centers for Disease Control and Prevention. MMWR Recomm Rep, 2002;51(RR-6):1–78.
604. Workowski, K.A., and S.M. Berman. CDC sexually transmitted diseases treatment guidelines. Clin Infect Dis, 2002;35(suppl 2): S135–7.
605. Weinstock, H., D. Dean, and G. Bolan. *Chlamydia trachomatis* infections. Infect Dis Clin North Am, 1994;8:797–819.
606. Sturm, P.D., et al. Molecular diagnosis of lymphogranuloma venereum in patients with genital ulcer disease. J Clin Microbiol, 2005;43:2973–5.
607. Lewis, D.A. Chancroid: clinical manifestations, diagnosis, and management. Sex Transm Infect, 2003;79:68–71.
608. Goldstone, S.E., A.Z. Kawalek, and J.W. Huyett. Infrared coagulator: a useful tool for treating anal squamous intraepithelial lesions. Dis Colon Rectum, 2005;48:1042–54.
609. Wiltz, O.H., M. Torregrosa, and O. Wiltz. Autogenous vaccine: the best therapy for perianal condyloma acuminata? Dis Colon Rectum, 1995;38:838–41.
610. Fleshner, P.R., and M.I. Freilich. Adjuvant interferon for anal condyloma. A prospective, randomized trial. Dis Colon Rectum, 1994;37:1255–9.
611. Bjorck, M., L. Athlin, and B. Lundskog. Giant condyloma acuminatum (Buschke-Loewenstein tumour) of the anorectum with malignant transformation. Eur J Surg, 1995;161: 691–4.
612. Jass, J.R., and L.H. Sobin. Histologic Typing of Intestinal Tumors. New York: Springer-Verlag; 1989.
613. Welton, M.L., F.E. Sharkey, and M.S. Kahlenberg. The etiology and epidemiology of anal cancer. Surg Oncol Clin N Am, 2004;13:263–75.
614. Berry, J.M., J.M. Palefsky, and M.L. Welton. Anal cancer and its precursors in HIV-positive patients: perspectives and management. Surg Oncol Clin N Am, 2004;13:355–73.
615. Fuchshuber, P.R., et al. Anal canal and perianal epidermoid cancers. J Am Coll Surg, 1997;185:494–505.
616. Touboul, E., et al. Epidermoid carcinoma of the anal margin: 17 cases treated with curative-intent radiation therapy. Radiother Oncol, 1995;34:195–202.
617. Paterson, C.A., T.M. Young-Fadok, and R.R. Dozois. Basal cell carcinoma of the perianal region: 20-year experience. Dis Colon Rectum, 1999;42:1200–2.
618. Beck, D.E. Paget's disease and Bowen's disease of the anus. Semin Colon Rectal Surg, 1995;6:143–149.
619. Marchesa, P., et al. Perianal Bowen's disease: a clinicopathologic study of 47 patients. Dis Colon Rectum, 1997;40:1286–93.
620. McCarter, M.D., et al. Long-term outcome of perianal Paget's disease. Dis Colon Rectum, 2003;46:612–6.
621. Gordon, P.H. Current status—perianal and anal canal neoplasms. Dis Colon Rectum, 1990;33:799–808.
622. Boman, B.M., et al. Carcinoma of the anal canal. A clinical and pathologic study of 188 cases. Cancer, 1984;54:114–25.
623. Papillon, J., and J.F. Montbarbon. Epidermoid carcinoma of the anal canal. A series of 276 cases. Dis Colon Rectum, 1987;30:324–33.
624. Cummings, B.J., et al. Epidermoid anal cancer: treatment by radiation alone or by radiation and 5-fluorouracil with and without mitomycin C. Int J Radiat Oncol Biol Phys, 1991;21:1115–25.
625. Allal, A., et al. Chemoradiotherapy versus radiotherapy alone for anal cancer: a retrospective comparison. Int J Radiat Oncol Biol Phys, 1993;27:59–66.
626. Bartelink, H., et al. Concomitant radiotherapy and chemotherapy is superior to radiotherapy alone in the treatment of locally advanced anal cancer: results of a phase III randomized trial of the European Organization for Research and Treatment of Cancer Radiotherapy and Gastrointestinal Cooperative Groups. J Clin Oncol, 1997;15:2040–9.
627. Flam, M., et al. Role of mitomycin in combination with fluorouracil and radiotherapy, and of salvage chemoradiation in the definitive nonsurgical treatment of epidermoid carcinoma of the anal canal: results of a phase III randomized intergroup study. J Clin Oncol, 1996;14:2527–39.
628. Epidermoid anal cancer: results from the UKCCCR randomised trial of radiotherapy alone versus radiotherapy, 5-fluorouracil, and mitomycin. UKCCCR Anal Cancer Trial Working Party. UK Co-ordinating Committee on Cancer Research. Lancet, 1996;348:1049–54.
629. Nigro, N.D. Multidisciplinary management of cancer of the anus. World J Surg, 1987;11:446–51.
630. Nguyen, W.D., K.M. Mitchell, and D.E. Beck. Risk factors associated with requiring a stoma for the management of anal cancer. Dis Colon Rectum, 2004;47:843–6.
631. Ghouti, L., et al. Salvage abdominoperineal resection after failure of conservative treatment in anal epidermoid cancer. Dis Colon Rectum, 2005;48:16–22.
632. Abulafi, A.M., et al. Delorme's operation for rectal prolapse. Ann R Coll Surg Engl, 1990;72:382–5.
633. Graf, W., et al. Delorme's operation for rectal prolapse in elderly or unfit patients. Eur J Surg, 1992;158:555–7.
634. White, S., and R.W. Stitz, Rectal prolapse: Delorme or Ripstein repair. Aust N Z J Surg, 1992;62:193–5.
635. Oliver, G.C., et al. Delorme's procedure for complete rectal prolapse in severely debilitated patients. An analysis of 41 cases. Dis Colon Rectum, 1994;37:461–7.
636. Senapati, A., et al. Results of Delorme's procedure for rectal prolapse. Dis Colon Rectum, 1994;37:456–60.
637. Tobin, S.A., and I.H. Scott. Delorme operation for rectal prolapse. Br J Surg, 1994;81:1681–4.
638. Lechaux, J.P., D. Lechaux, and M. Perez. Results of Delorme's procedure for rectal prolapse. Advantages of a modified technique. Dis Colon Rectum, 1995;38:301–7.
639. Plusa, S.M., et al. Physiological changes after Delorme's procedure for full-thickness rectal prolapse. Br J Surg, 1995;82:1475–8.
640. Altemeier, W.A., et al. Nineteen years' experience with the one-stage perineal repair of rectal prolapse. Ann Surg, 1971;173:993–1006.
641. Finlay, I.G., and M. Aitchison. Perineal excision of the rectum for prolapse in the elderly. Br J Surg, 1991;78:687–9.
642. Williams, J.G., et al. Treatment of rectal prolapse in the elderly by perineal rectosigmoidectomy. Dis Colon Rectum, 1992;35: 830–4.

643. Johansen, O.B., et al. Perineal rectosigmoidectomy in the elderly. Dis Colon Rectum, 1993;36:767–72.
644. Michelassi, F., and J.W. Milsom, eds. Operative Strategies in Inflammatory Bowel Disease. New York: Springer-Verlag; 1999.
645. Gordon, P.H., and S. Nivatvongs, eds. Principles and Practice of Surgery for the Colon, Rectum, and Anus. St. Louis: Quality Medical; 1999.
646. Painter, N.S. Diverticular disease of the colon. Gastroenterol Clin North Am, 1975;4:3–21.
647. Allen, J.I. Molecular biology of colorectal cancer: a clinician's view. Perspect Colon Rectal Surg, 1995;8:181–202.
648. Bailey, H.R. and M.J. Synder, eds. Ambulatory Anorectal Surgery. New York: Springer-Verlag, 2000.
649. Corman, M.L., ed. Colon and Rectal Surgery. 4th ed. New York: Lippincott Williams & Wilkins; 1998.
650. Vasilevsky, C.A. Fistula-in-ano and abscess. In: Fundamentals of Anorectal Surgery, D.E. Beck and S.D. Wexner, eds. New York: McGraw-Hill; 1992.
651. Parks, A.G., P.H. Gordon, and J.D. Hardcastle. A classification of fistula-in-ano, Br J Surg, 1976;63:1–12.
652. Ustynoski, K. Horseshoe abscess fistula. Seton treatment. Dis Colon Rectum, 1990;33:602–605.
653. Reznick, R.K., and H.R. Bailey. Closure of internal opening for treatment of complex fistula-in-ano. Dis Colon Rectum 1988;31:116–118.
654. Marti M-C, and J.-C. Givel, eds. Surgical Management of Anorectal and Colonic Diseases. 2nd Ed. Heidelberg: Springer-Verlag; 1999.
655. Shelton, A.A., and M.L. Welton. The pelvic floor in health and disease. W J Med, 1997;167:90–8.
656. Berman, J.R. Delarme's transrectal incision for interanal rectal prolapse. Dis Colon Rectum 1990;33:573.
657. Nivatvongs, S. The colon, rectum, and anal canal. In: Basic Surgical Practice, E.C. James and R.J. Corry, and J.F. Perry, Jr., eds. Philadelphia: Hanley and Belfus; 1987:325.
658. Ogorek, C.P., and Fisher, R.S. Differentiation between Crohn's disease and ulcerative colitis. Med Clin North Am, 1994;78;1249–58.
659. Truelove, S.C. Medical management of ulcerative colitis and indications for colectomy. World J Surg, 1988;12:142–7.
660. Schroeder, K.W., W.J. Tremaine, and D.M. Ilstrup. Coated oral 5-aminosalicylic acid therapy for mildly to moderately active ulcerative colitis. A randomized study. N Engl J Med, 1987; 317:1625–9.
661. Winawer, S.J., Fletcher, H., Miller, L., et al. Colorectal cancer screening: clinical guidelines and rationale. Gastroenterology, 1997;112:594–642.
662. Mayeaux, E.J., et al. Noncervical human papillomavirus genital infections. Am Fam Physician, 1995;52:1137–46.

52

Spleen

Alan T. Lefor and Edward H. Phillips

The spleen has long been an organ of interest in popular as well as medical literature. Historically, the spleen has been associated with more functions than any other organ.[1] Of interest, the spleen had long been associated with the ability to run, with references in ancient literature to splenectomy being performed to allow men and horses to run faster. As recently as 1922, this myth was tested in the laboratory at Johns Hopkins University, where Macht and Finesilver observed that asplenic mice were able to run faster than mice with an intact spleen.[2] The ancient Greeks attributed the origin of black bile to the spleen. In the 16th century, Paracelsus (1490–1541) wrote that the spleen was a superfluous organ that should be excised when diseased. Vesalius (1514–1564) excised the spleens of many animals without adverse effects, supporting his contention that the spleen is not essential to life.[1] A number of experimental surgeons demonstrated in the next century that animals could live without their spleens. There are a number of "case reports" from the late 17th century in which successful partial splenectomies are described after traumatic prolapse of the spleen through penetrating wounds.

The first report of a splenectomy for disease is attributed to Quittenbaum in 1826, although the patient did not survive.[1] The first successful splenectomy is attributed to Pean in 1867, performed for a large splenic cyst. By 1877, there were more than 50 case reports of splenectomy for a wide range of indications. However, the overall mortality rate exceeded 70%, and most were performed for hematological diseases. The first splenectomy for trauma is attributed to a British naval surgeon, who excised the prolapsed spleen of an injured sailor. Splenectomy for blunt trauma was reported in 1892, on a patient who fell from a scaffold.

The indications for elective splenectomy became more defined through the 20th century, largely as a result of developments in hematology and oncology. This has been observed recently by Marble and coworkers,[3] who noted a decrease in the number of splenectomies for splenomegaly and Hodgkin's disease in 1986–1991 compared with 1979–1985. In contrast, more splenectomies were performed for hematological diseases (e.g., thrombocytopenia) during the later time period studied.

Since its 1991 introduction,[4] laparoscopic resection and partial resection of the spleen have become commonplace. Laparoscopic splenectomy (LS) is the gold standard for the surgical treatment of immune thrombocytopenia purpura.[5]

Embryology and Anatomy

The splenic primordium becomes evident during the fifth week of gestation as an outgrowth of the dorsal mesogastrium, which migrates to the left upper quadrant. A number of splenic conditions are easily related to the embryological development of the spleen, including congenital asplenia (complete absence of the spleen) and polysplenia (multiple splenic nodules). Accessory spleens are fairly common, reported in as many as 30% of patients. Although these are usually in the area of the splenic hilum, they can be located in a wide range of places, usually along the left gutter, and have been reported in the scrotum. In addition, they have been observed on the right side of the abdomen. In patients undergoing splenectomy for trauma or other nonhematological conditions, there is no indication to remove the accessory spleens. However, in patients with hematological or malignant diseases, it is important to carefully search for and excise accessory splenic tissue. The identification of accessory splenic tissue is enhanced during LS.[5] The last condition related to the embryological development of the spleen is wandering spleen, resulting from the absence of ligamentous attachments. Thus, the spleen can migrate throughout the abdomen, gradually lengthening its pedicle. The long, tortuous vessels that result are more prone to torsion, and thus wandering spleens are occasionally removed for infarction.

The gross appearance of the spleen is the result of its development from multiple anlage, resulting in an organ with multiple clefts. The normal spleen weighs 150 to 250 g and is located in the left upper quadrant, beneath the 9th, 10th, and

11th ribs. This location offers some protection to this fragile organ, but also explains why the spleen is the organ most commonly injured in blunt abdominal trauma. The parietal surface of the spleen is related to the diaphragm, and the visceral surface is related to the left colon, left kidney, tail of the pancreas, and stomach.[1] The capsule of the spleen is thin and consists of mesothelial cells. Many other species of mammals (e.g., dogs) have smooth muscle cells in the capsule that are absent in humans. Interestingly, this smooth muscle allows these animals to autotransfuse when they are hypotensive, necessitating splenectomy in experimental animals being used to study responses to hypovolemic shock.

The spleen receives its arterial supply from the splenic artery, which originates in the celiac axis. It is easy to identify on angiographic studies by its characteristic tortuous appearance. After its origin, the splenic artery courses along the superior edge of the pancreas, with multiple branches into the pancreatic parenchyma. The artery then gives off several branches into the spleen, the first being the superior polar artery (Fig. 52.1). There are other arterial vessels to the spleen from the left gastroepiploic artery and the short gastric artery. The splenic veins follow the arterial distribution closely, and the main splenic vein emerges from the spleen following a course to join the superior mesenteric vein, forming the portal vein. The veins are characteristically fragile, and avulsion results in annoying intraoperative bleeding, which must be especially avoided in the laparoscopic conduct of splenectomy. The tail of the pancreas is in close approximation to the splenic hilum. Great care must be taken to avoid injury to the pancreas during dissection in the region of the splenic hilum.

The spleen is held in place by a number of peritoneal attachments, which are commonly referred to as "ligaments":

Splenogastric ligament: also called the gastrosplenic omentum, contains the short gastric vessels.
Splenocolic ligament: A fold of peritoneum from the splenic flexure of the colon to the lower pole of the spleen.

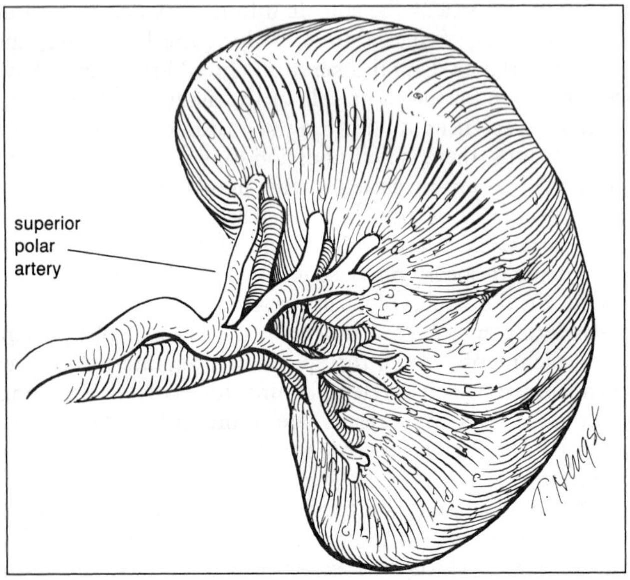

FIGURE 52.1. Anatomy of the splenic blood supply.

Splenorenal ligament: Posterior peritoneum that splits anterior to the underlying kidney to envelop the hilar vessels and tail of the pancreas.
Splenophrenic ligament: Usually very attenuated, from the superior pole of the spleen to the diaphragm.
Splenoomental ligament: A constant fold of peritoneum connecting the lower pole of the spleen to the omentum near the splenic flexure of the colon. Intraoperative traction on this structure is most commonly responsible for iatrogenic injuries to the lower pole.

There are occasionally other folds of peritoneum attached to the spleen, but those listed remain the most constant and are those with which the surgeon must be familiar at the time of splenic surgery.

Functions and Pathological Conditions of the Spleen

Circulation through the spleen is about 150 to 200 mL/min or about 5% of the cardiac output.[6] The spleen has traditionally been ascribed four functions: (1) filtration, (2) immunological, (3) reservoir, and (4) hematopoietic.[7] The filtration function is the most dominant splenic function in humans and refers to the removal of abnormal or senescent red blood cells from the circulation. Other particles removed include particulate antigens such as microorganisms or antigen–antibody complexes. The immunological functions of the spleen include trapping of antigens, homing of lymphocytes, antibody and lymphokine production, and macrophage activation. The spleen is the main site for immunoglobulin and antibody synthesis in the body and affects the capability of cellular populations in other lymphoid organs through largely unknown mechanisms.[6] Furthermore, the spleen can exert its impact on distinct populations of lymphoid cells at distant sites. The reservoir function refers to the fact that the spleen harbors about one-third of the total platelet mass and a large number of granulocytes. The hematopoietic functions are minimal in humans and much more prominent in other species. It is clear that a majority of pathological processes in the spleen are related to the filtration and immunological functions of the spleen.

Conditions associated with defective or absent splenic function are grouped together as conditions of *hyposplenism*. These conditions are characterized by the presence of Howell-Jolly bodies in the peripheral circulation. Conditions associated with *hypersplenism* remain the most frequent indication for elective splenectomy; these can be divided into those conditions in which the spleen is normal but increased destruction of abnormal blood elements causes hypersplenism, and those in which there is a primary disorder of the spleen that results in increased destruction of normal blood cells (Table 52.1).[7]

Splenic Rupture

The spleen can rupture from three underlying causes: trauma, spontaneous rupture, and pathological rupture. Traumatic rupture of the spleen remains the most frequent indication for splenectomy. Pathological causes of splenic rupture include infiltration of the spleen by reactive lymphoid cells

TABLE 52.1. Disorders Associated with Hypersplenism.

1. Disorders associated with sequestration of abnormal blood cells in an intrinsically normal spleen.
   A. Congenital disorders of erythrocytes
      1. Hereditary spherocytosis
      2. Hereditary elliptocytosis
      3. Hemoglobinopathies
   B. Acquired disorders of erythrocytes
      1. Autoimmune hemolytic anemia
      2. Parasitic diseases (e.g., malaria, babesiosis)
   C. Autoimmune thrombocytopenia
   D. Autoimmune neutropenia
2. Disorders of the spleen resulting in sequestration of normal blood cells
   A. Disorders of cordal macrophages: Banti's syndrome, storage diseases, parasitic diseases (e.g., kala-azar), Langerhan's cell histiocytosis, malignant histiocytosis
   B. Infiltrative disorders: leukemias, lymphomas, plasma cell dyscrasias, myeloid metaplasia, metastatic carcinoma
   C. Vascular abnormalities
   D. Splenic cysts
   E. Hamartomas
3. Miscellaneous conditions
   A. Hyperthyroidism
   B. Hypogammaglobulinemia
   C. Progressive multifocal leukoencephalopathy

Source: From Reiman.[7]

or by neoplastic cells. Most cases attributed to spontaneous rupture of the spleen are actually due to an undiagnosed pathological process.[7]

Benign Lesions of the Spleen

Hemangioma

Hemangioma is the most common benign primary neoplasm of the spleen and is frequently an incidental finding after splenectomy for other causes. Lesions can be solitary or multiple and are usually blue-red, well-circumscribed nodules. Microscopically, they usually appear as endothelium-lined spaces and are known as cavernous hemangiomas. The process can affect the entire spleen as a diffuse hemangiomatosis that can present with splenomegaly. Treatment of these lesions is usually splenectomy, although partial splenectomy may be indicated for isolated lesions.

Lymphangioma

Lymphangioma lesions are less common than hemangiomas and are usually subcapsular, appearing as soft, compressible, multicystic lesions on the splenic surface. When located within the parenchyma, they may be solitary or multiple. When large, they present with splenomegaly as an indication for resection. There are case reports of patients presenting with hypersplenic syndromes, consumptive coagulopathy, and even portal hypertension with these lesions.[8]

Peliosis

The rare peliosis lesions bear a superficial resemblance to vascular neoplasms of the spleen. They consist of blood-filled cysts distributed in patches or diffusely and can result in splenomegaly.[8] Intraperitoneal hemorrhage can result from the rupture of these lesions.[9]

Hemangioendothelioma

The rare hemangioendothelioma lesion is thought to be intermediate between hemangioma and angiosarcoma. These lesions usually contain cellular atypia, differentiating them from hemangiomas. The lesions may present with splenomegaly or rupture and should suggest the possibility of a malignant vascular neoplasm.[8]

Hamartomas

Hamartomas are focal developmental abnormalities within the normal spleen rather than true neoplasms. They consist of normal cellular elements in disarray and are usually found incidentally.

Other Benign Lesions

There are a number of other benign neoplasms, including hemangipericytoma, bacillary angiomatosis, inflammatory pseudotumors, and mycobacterial spindle cell pseudotumors. These are all extremely rare lesions and are rarely found except as incidental findings when the spleen is removed for other reasons.

Nonparasitic Cysts

Nonparasitic cysts have been reported in patients of all ages and are probably the result of a development anomaly. Patients with these benign lesions usually present with left upper quadrant pain. Evaluation of these patients usually reveals splenomegaly. A characteristic imaging study is shown in Figure 52.2. These lesions are round and well circumscribed on imaging studies. In general, cysts that are less than 4 cm in size and asymptomatic can be observed; those that are greater than 4 cm or are symptomatic should be resected.[8] Partial splenectomy is the preferred method of resection when possible.[10]

Parasitic Cysts

The only parasitic cyst of importance is the echinococcal cyst. This condition is endemic in the Near East, New Zealand, Australia, and the western United States. The

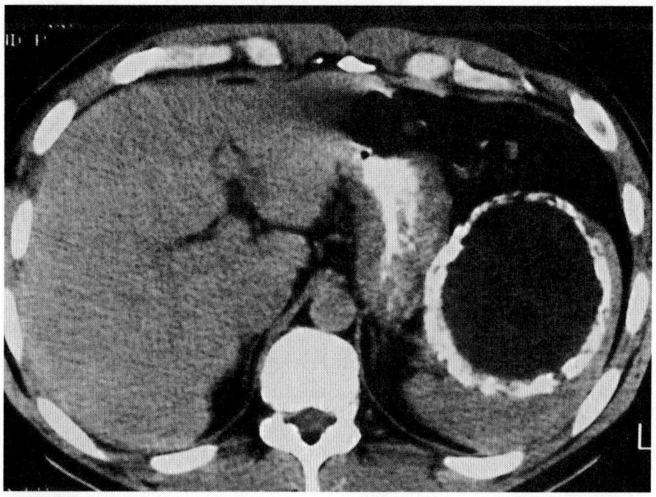

FIGURE 52.2. Epidermoid cyst of the spleen with peripheral calcification.

TABLE 52.2. Malignant Lesions of the Spleen.

I. Lymphoproliferative disorders
  A. Non-Hodgkin's lymphoma
  B. Hodgkin's disease
  C. Chronic lymphocytic leukemia
  D. Hairy cell leukemia
  E. Plasmacytoma
  F. Waldenström's macroglobulinemia
II. Myeloproliferative disorders
  A. Chronic myelogenous leukemia
  B. Polycythemia vera
  C. Myelofibrosis (agnogenic myeloid metaplasia)
  D. Essential thrombocythemia
III. Vascular tumors
  A. Hemangiosarcoma
  B. Lymphangiosarcoma
IV. Metastatic tumors: breast, lung, melanoma, etc.
V. Other lesions
  A. Sarcoma: fibrosarcoma, leiomyosarcoma, Kaposi's sarcoma

Source: Adapted from Giles and Lim.[11]

complement fixation test is used for diagnosis. The treatment of this condition is splenectomy.[8] During this procedure, wide exposure is necessary to help avoid intraoperative rupture of the cysts.

Malignant Lesions of the Spleen

There are many malignancies that affect the spleen. A list of these conditions is given in Table 52.2.[11]

Non-Hodgkin's Lymphoma

Non-Hodgkin's lymphoma is a diverse group of diseases with a wide range of biological behaviors. They may be very aggressive and rapidly fatal or may behave as one of the most indolent and well-tolerated malignancies afflicting humans.[12] As the clinical course is variable, the pattern of spread is also unpredictable. Non-Hodgkin's lymphoma is classified into low-, intermediate-, and high-grade pathological groups according to the National Cancer Institute (United States) working formulation. Each of these groups is further subdivided based on cell type (small cell, large cell, etc.). The therapy for these patients is still evolving, and surgical staging is generally reserved for the small minority of patients who will receive radiation therapy alone if the disease is localized.

The role of the surgeon in the care of patients with non-Hodgkin's lymphoma is almost always limited to the biopsy of a single peripheral lymph node to establish a tissue diagnosis. Abdominal surgery is rarely required except in the absence of peripheral lymphadenopathy, when laparotomy or laparoscopy may be necessary to obtain adequate tissue for diagnosis of intraabdominal disease. In non-Hodgkin's lymphoma, the precise definition of disease location, unlike Hodgkin's lymphoma, has less impact on therapeutic decision making.[13] In general, non-Hodgkin's lymphomas are systemic diseases at the time of diagnosis and require the use of systemic therapy (e.g., chemotherapy) rather than regional therapy (e.g., radiation) for treatment. This fact coupled with increasingly more sensitive and specific diagnostic tests have limited the number of operative staging procedures needed to assist in treatment planning.

Hodgkin's Disease

Hodgkin's lymphoma usually originates in a single nodal group and predictably proceeds in a stepwise progression from one contiguous node group to the next.[14] The disease originates above the diaphragm in 80% to 90% of patients[15] and is limited to the lymph nodes in 85% of cases.[16] Only 15% of patients initially present with extranodal disease as well as lymphatic involvement. Below the diaphragm, the spleen becomes involved by Hodgkin's lymphoma before proceeding along the periaortic lymph nodes to the iliac and inguinal nodal basins.[15] Rarely, the disease originates below the diaphragm and proceeds cephalad in reverse sequence.[15] The need for surgical staging has diminished significantly since the mid-1990's as a result of the increased use of chemotherapy, even in early stage disease. In addition, improved imaging technology has allowed the more accurate diagnosis of nodal disease without surgical exploration.

After the diagnosis is achieved with lymph node biopsy, patients are specifically questioned about "B" symptoms (night sweats, fevers, weight loss). A careful physical examination is undertaken to evaluate other lymph node–bearing areas. Laboratory studies include complete blood count (CBC), liver function tests, renal function tests, serum lactate dehydrogenase (LDH), and alkaline phosphatase. Radiologic studies include chest x-ray and chest and abdominal computed tomographic (CT) scan as well as bipedal lymphangiogram. Although bipedal lymphangiogram carries high sensitivity and specificity, it is unable to adequately visualize high celiac, splenic, portal, and mesenteric lymph nodes.[16] These nodes can be better evaluated by abdominal CT scan, which however lacks the sensitivity to accurately assess normal-size, lymphoma-bearing lymph nodes.[17] Thus, the combination of the tests is superior to either alone. The staging of Hodgkin's lymphoma takes into account the lymph node involvement above and below the diaphragm as well as the presence or absence of constitutional symptoms with the designations A or B.

Indications and techniques for the performance of the staging laparotomy, in attempts to influence the associated morbidity and mortality, have undergone considerable evolution during the past three decades. Although performed on up to 85% of patients with Hodgkin's disease in the past, since the mid-1990's the number of patients staged surgically has dramatically decreased.

Thus, at the present time, the role of the surgeon regarding patients with Hodgkin's lymphoma includes lymph node biopsy to establish a diagnosis and staging laparotomy in a very select group of patients. The surgeon should be in close consultation with the treating hematologist. Patients with obvious stage III or IV disease should rarely be subjected to staging laparotomy because they will be treated with chemotherapy. More recently, most patients with stage I and II disease are also treated with chemotherapy, thus obviating the need for laparotomy.[20]

If required, it is important to perform a thorough staging procedure that includes splenectomy, core needle biopsies from both left and right lobes of the liver, wedge biopsy of the liver (unless a specific lesion is visible), biopsy of right and left iliac and periaortic lymph nodes, and a bone marrow biopsy. For patients in whom it is indicated, a complete staging procedure can be performed laparoscopically, affording patients some of the same benefits seen with other laparoscopic procedures. Laparoscopic staging of abdominal lymphoma has been successfully performed by several groups.[21,22–25] The laparoscopic approach to this procedure follows the same principles as those delineated for the open procedure.[22] The indications, components, and the sequence of components should remain the same. There are no true contraindications to laparoscopic staging. Relative contraindications to laparoscopic staging include abdominal wall sepsis, gastrointestinal distension, intraabdominal sepsis, and extensive adhesions.[26] A comparison of laparoscopic and open staging of Hodgkin's disease has demonstrated equivalent oncological results and functionally superior results with laparoscopic staging.[22] These investigators found a slightly longer operative time (202 vs. 144 min) but significantly shortened postoperative ileus and postoperative hospitalization times. These data strongly support the use of laparoscopy for accurate staging of Hodgkin's disease when indicated.

Chronic Lymphocytic Leukemia

Chronic lymphocytic leukemia (CLL) is the most common of the chronic leukemias, usually found in patients over 60 years of age. It is usually of B-cell lineage and is characterized by an accumulation of incompetent lymphocytes.[27] CLL is incurable, but it is managed with a variety of chemotherapeutic agents and sometimes splenectomy. Splenectomy is indicated in those patients who progress despite chemotherapy, often with massive splenomegaly.

In one series, early splenectomy was advocated in certain patient subgroups.[28] These authors evaluated 77 consecutive patients with CLL seen between 1970 and 1994. They found that splenectomy significantly improved survival in selected subgroups of patients and advocated early splenectomy in patients with a hemoglobin (Hb) of 10 g/dL or platelet counts below 50,000/mm^3. They also observed that thrombocytopenia did not increase postoperative morbidity.

Hairy Cell Leukemia

Hairy cell leukemia is a rare lymphoproliferative disorder that affects middle-aged men; it presents with pancytopenia and splenomegaly and is characterized by the identification of "hairy cells" in the peripheral circulation. Splenectomy has long been the therapy of choice for this disease. In a large study of 194 patients with hairy cell leukemia, splenectomy provided rapid and predictable palliation and is recommended for patients with bone marrow cellularity less than 85%.[29] However, more recently, systemic chemotherapy employing 2-chloro-deoxyadenosine has been shown to induce remission in 80% to 90% of patients.[30] Splenectomy is thus reserved for patients who fail to respond to systemic chemotherapy or who have massive symptomatic splenomegaly.

Myeloproliferative Disorders

Myeloproliferative disorders include chronic myelogenous leukemia (CML), myelofibrosis (also called agnogenic myeloid metaplasia), polycythemia vera, and essential thrombocythemia. These diseases are often considered as existing along a spectrum with considerable overlap in clinical and laboratory findings. Chronic myelogenous leukemia accounts for 15% of all leukemias and presents at a median age of 49 years. The diagnosis is established by examination of the peripheral blood smear, which demonstrates leukocytosis with the full spectrum of myeloid differentiation. The Philadelphia chromosome is pathognomonic for this disease. Splenomegaly is the most common finding on physical examination, and the degree of splenomegaly is of prognostic importance.[11] Gross splenomegaly predicts a shorter time to blast crisis. The clinical course of this disease is usually divided into three phases: the chronic phase, the accelerated phase, and the terminal blast crisis.

Early splenectomy has not been shown to delay the onset of blast transformation or prolong survival. In the presence of splenomegaly, patients in the accelerated or blastic phases respond poorly to transfusions of blood products because of splenic sequestration.[31] The role of splenectomy remains controversial. Splenectomy can offer significant palliation to patients with CML. In a study of 53 patients with CML in accelerated or blastic phases from a single institution who underwent splenectomy, there were significantly fewer platelet and red blood cell transfusions in the 6 months after splenectomy than in the 6 months before splenectomy.[31] Furthermore, these authors observed that splenectomy can be performed with minimal morbidity and mortality, thus relieving symptomatic splenomegaly in addition to minimizing transfusion requirements.

Myelofibrosis is a rare disease, usually found in patients over 60 years of age. The disease is incurable, with a median survival of 5 years. Splenectomy is reserved for patients with massive splenomegaly and transfusion-dependent anemia.[11]

Primary Lymphoma of the Spleen

Primary lymphoma of the spleen is a subset of non-Hodgkin's lymphoma in which the disease begins in the spleen, and the bulk of disease is concentrated in the spleen with additional involvement of hilar lymph nodes.[32] Splenomegaly is a prominent feature of this disease, but peripheral adenopathy is absent. In a single institutional series, data suggested that patients with localized splenic and splenic hilar disease have the same prognosis as other patients with stage I non-Hodgkin's lymphoma, and that those patients with other sites of involvement have a similar prognosis as patients with similarly staged forms of non-Hodgkin's lymphoma.[32]

Hemangiosarcoma

Hemangiosarcoma is a rare primary tumor of the spleen in humans. Treatment is surgical, and no effective adjuvant therapies have been identified. Of interest is that this tumor is a common cause of death in certain breeds of dogs.

Indications for Splenectomy

There are two surgical procedures performed in reference to the spleen: partial splenectomy and splenectomy. Either of these can be conducted by conventional open technique (open splenectomy, OS) or by laparoscopic means (LS). The indications for splenectomy are unrelated to the technique that will be used to remove the spleen. There are some conditions for which OS is generally considered superior to LS, including trauma, some hematologic malignancies, splenic malignancy, parasitic splenomegaly, giant splenic cysts (>20 cm), and ruptured splenic artery aneurysm.[33] Of course, LS should only be performed by surgeons who are appropriately trained in this advanced laparoscopic procedure. Malignancies for which splenectomy is indicated have already been discussed.

Splenectomy for Trauma

The spleen is the organ most commonly injured in blunt abdominal trauma, and thus the majority of splenectomies in the United States are performed for trauma. At this time, it appears prudent that splenic surgery for trauma is conducted by OS techniques, although there may be rare instances when LS is a reasonable alternative and has been reported.[34] The treatment of iatrogenic trauma to the spleen is discussed in the section on incidental splenectomy.

Splenic injury is often suspected in the injured patient on the basis of mechanism of injury and the presence of associated injuries, such as left lower rib fractures. Some patients undergo CT scan of the abdomen, which reveals injuries such as those seen in Figure 52.3. Once splenic injury is identified, there are three options: nonoperative management, splenic salvage (repair of the injury or partial splenectomy), or splenectomy. There is no role for splenic salvage in the critically injured trauma patient with multiple intraabdominal injuries. In these patients, splenectomy is the only procedure to be considered.

Management of Splenic Injuries in Children

The nonoperative management of splenic injury has been applied primarily (and most uniformly) in children. Hemodynamic stability and transfusion requirement for less than 50% of the blood volume are essential to manage these injuries without surgery. Obviously, nonoperative management assumes no other intraabdominal injuries requiring exploration. Three factors form the basis for this approach: bleeding from splenic lacerations often ceases by the time of laparotomy; the spleen is immunologically important; and CT scanning permits accurate localization of intraabdominal solid organ injury. Delayed splenic rupture remains a possibility in patients managed nonoperatively. Those children who do require operative intervention usually do so within a median time of 2.3 h, and nearly all who needed operative intervention did so within 24 h.[35]

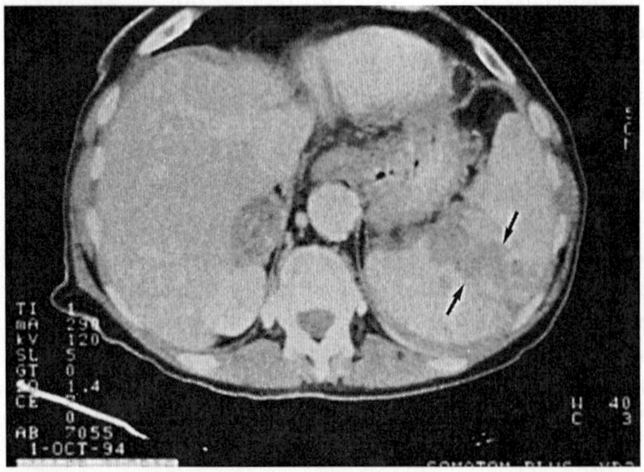

FIGURE 52.3. Splenic fracture (*arrows*). There is a small amount of fluid adjacent to the spleen posteriorly.

Guidelines for the nonoperative management of splenic injuries in children include documentation of splenic injury by imaging studies, admission to the intensive care unit with close observation, hemodynamic stability, serial hematocrit determination, absence of other intraabdominal injuries, transfusion requirements for less than 50% of total blood volume, and absence of neurotrauma permitting patient cooperation with serial history and physical examination. The operative management of splenic injuries in children is discussed further, including OS, partial splenectomy, and LS.

Management of Splenic Injuries in Adults

The nonoperative management of splenic injuries in adults is less established as a standard than in children. It is an evolving practice, with success rates reported from 27% to 100%. Patients are considered candidates for nonoperative management by meeting criteria such as hemodynamic stability, minimum transfusion requirement, absence of associated intraabdominal injury, and an ability to perform reliable serial abdominal examinations.[36] A stable defect on repeat imaging also supports this approach. Others have also advocated CT grading scales of splenic injury.

In a review of 135 patients with blunt splenic injury, 46 adults were treated nonoperatively,[36] which was successful in 24 (52%). These authors concluded that nonoperative management commonly fails in patients over 55 years of age (91% in this series), independent of other clinical and radiographic variables. More recently, nonoperative management of splenic injuries in patients over age 55 has been shown to be reasonable, especially in patients with lower-grade injuries and in the absence of free fluid in the pelvis on CT scan.[37] In this study, 55 patients over age 55 with blunt splenic injuries were treated, with successful nonoperative management in 62.5%. Patients treated without exploration should be carefully observed and undergo repeat CT scan at 3 weeks to assess stability of the defect. Selective splenic artery embolization has been reported to significantly increase the success of nonoperative management of blunt splenic injuries.[38,39]

The success rate for non-operative management of splenic injury varies widely in the literature.[40] Some of the factors associated with outcome are grade of splenic injury, degree of hemoperitoneum, and presence of associated injuries. The mortality rate of nonoperative management is greater in older patients when the nonoperative approach is not successful. Interestingly, the total mortality in patients with splenic injury has stayed nearly constant at 6%–7% because of the presence of associated injuries.[40]

An alternative is the use of splenic angiography in patients managed nonoperatively. In one study, by using a protocol for the management of patients investigated with angiography, investigators observed a decreased length of stay with higher therapeutic yield, and decreased use of hospital resources was observed.[41] A new imaging modality, contrast-enhanced sonography, has also shown promise in the evaluation of patients with splenic injury.[42] In a recent large series of patients with blunt splenic injury, a 15-year review showed improved splenic salvage rates without increased mortality by emphasizing splenic preservation and nonoperative management with greater use of splenic artery embolization.[43] Others have also observed the increased use of splenic preservation over time. In a study of 266 adult patients with blunt

TABLE 52.3. Grading of Traumatic Splenic Injuries.

I	Hematoma	Subcapsular, nonexpanding, <10% surface
	Laceration	Capsular tear, nonbleeding, <1 cm parenchymal depth
II	Hematoma	Subcapsular, nonexpanding, 10%–50% surface area
	Laceration	Capsular tear, active bleeding, 1–3 cm, not involving a trabecular vessel
III	Hematoma	Subcapsular, >50% surface area or expanding, ruptured subcapsular hematoma with active bleeding, intraparenchymal hematoma, <2 cm or expanding
	Laceration	>3 cm parenchymal depth or involving trabecular vessels
IV	Hematoma	Ruptured intraparenchymal hematoma with active bleeding
	Laceration	Laceration involving segmental or hilar vessel with major devascularization (>25%)
V	Laceration	Completely shattered spleen
	Vascular	Hilar vascular injury with devascularized spleen

Source: Adapted from Lipshy et al.[47]

splenic injury, the frequency of nonoperative management of splenic injuries significantly increased from 48.5% in 1992–1996 to 63.1% in 1997–2001 (P = .02).[44] They observed a similar mortality rate in both time periods.

The decision to embark on splenorrhaphy in the adult with a splenic injury is based on hemodynamic stability, presence of other injuries, and extent of splenic injury.[45] Adequate mobilization is essential. Grade I and II injuries (capsular avulsions and superficial parenchymal fractures) are managed by topical hemostatic agents. The argon beam coagulator may be helpful in the management of these lesions. Mattress sutures over Teflon pledgets may be useful to close deeper wounds. Grade III and IV splenic injury requires complete mobilization of the spleen to expose the hilum. Division of the short gastric vessels is required. Partial splenectomy may be indicated. Wrapping the spleen with absorbable mesh has also been employed to control extensive capsular avulsions.

There is a definite learning curve for the technique of splenorrhaphy. In a 10-year review of 314 patients with splenic injury,[45] there were 227 blunt injuries, 49 gunshot wounds (GSWs), and 38 stab wounds injuring the spleen. Splenorrhaphy was accomplished in 29% in the first year of the study and later rose to 63%. Splenorrhaphy was accomplished with hemostatic agents in 40%, debridement and suturing in 40%, splenic resection (partial) in 13%, and mesh bag in 7%. Treatment by grade included grade I, hemostatic agents alone; grade II, suturing/mesh bag in 43%, hemostatic agents; grade III, suture/mesh bag; grade IV, 88% required anatomical splenic resection; grade V, splenectomy. Of 63 splenectomies, 48 (76%) had grade V injuries. Other splenectomies were performed in patients with multisystem injuries. Most authors reported low incidence of reoperation (0%–2%) following splenic preservation. Not surprisingly, the laparoscopic control of splenic injury with splenic preservation has also been reported.[46]

The specific management of a patient with a splenic injury is guided by the overall stability of the injured patient, mechanism of injury, age, interval from time of injury, associated injuries, and preexisting medical conditions. Splenic injuries are graded by severity (Table 52.3). In a recent series of adults with splenic injuries, 18% were treated nonoperatively, 22% underwent splenorrhaphy, and 60% underwent splenectomy.[47]

Splenic Autotransplantation

Splenic autotransplantation is easy to carry out, but its efficacy is not really known. The concept is to preserve splenic function by transplanting fragments of the excised spleen elsewhere in the abdomen, usually within an omental pouch. It is possible to demonstrate function of such autotransplanted tissue with conventional ^{99}Tc scans, immunoglobulin (Ig) M levels, and examination of peripheral blood smears. At this time, the amount of splenic tissue needed to effectively prevent the complications of the asplenic state (especially overwhelming postsplenectomy infection, OPSI) is unknown; it has been estimated at 25% to 50%. The basis for this approach was the observation that splenosis was fairly common in adults following traumatic splenic rupture, and that OPSI was rare in adults. Thus, the idea of intentionally implanting splenic tissue was put forth.

There have been many reports of splenic autotransplantation. There is no consensus about the number, mass, or size of implants used. The only proven immunological result of replantation is the normal IgM levels. It is unclear whether lymphocyte function is normal. Overwhelming postsplenectomy infection has been reported in patients after autologous splenic transplantation. At this time, it appears that splenic salvage with preservation of an intact splenic vascular supply to even a small amount of spleen is a more effective method of preserving splenic function than autotransplantation.[48]

The method described by Moore involves transplantation of five fragments measuring 40 × 40 × 3 mm into omental pockets.[45] They are secured with silk sutures and marked with clips. After a period of necrosis, they regenerate. Uniform viability using this technique has been reported by Tc scan, IgM levels, and platelet count. Others have also noted the disappearance of Howell-Jolly bodies. At this time, splenic autotransplantation cannot be recommended.

Splenectomy for Hematological Disorders

Common indications for elective splenectomy are listed in Table 52.4. In a review of 727 splenectomies for hematological diseases from a single institution from 1958 to 1995, 30% were for idiopathic thrombocytopenia purpura (ITP), and 29%

TABLE 52.4. Indications for Elective Splenectomy.

ITP (idiopathic thrombocytopenia purpura)
Hereditary spherocytosis
Autoimmune hemolytic anemia
Staging for Hodgkin's disease
Lymphoma
Thrombocytopenic thrombotic purpura
AIDS-related thrombocytopenia
Leukemia
Splenic abscess
Gaucher's disease
Myelofibrosis
Splenic infarct

were for the staging of Hodgkin's disease.[49] The timing of the procedure requires judgment, and the decision to proceed with splenectomy is made after close consultation with the hematologists involved in the care of the patient.

In a review of 185 patients with hematological disorders who underwent splenectomy, the majority were performed for Hodgkin's disease, ITP, hereditary spherocytosis, and CML.[50] These authors identified 4 patients with significant pneumonia, 10 minor wound infections, and 4 patients requiring reoperation for hemorrhage. A total of 34 patients died in the late postoperative period, and 2 deaths were attributed to OPSI. These authors concluded that splenectomy is a procedure with a low morbidity in patients with hematological diseases.

Hereditary Spherocytosis

The clinically heterogeneous condition of hereditary spherocytosis is characterized by a deficiency in spectrin, resulting in a defective erythrocyte membrane that causes the cell to be less deformable and thus more susceptible to trapping within the spleen.[51] It is a congenital condition, transmitted in an autosomal dominant fashion, and is the most common hemolytic anemia for which splenectomy is performed. Patients with this condition present with anemia, splenomegaly, and jaundice. The diagnosis is established by examination of the peripheral blood smear. Therapy of this disease is splenectomy, with a nearly 100% response rate. Some of these patients have cholelithiasis due to hemolysis, resulting in pigmented stones, and cholecystectomy is recommended at the same time as splenectomy.[51,52] Because of the decreased risk of OPSI in older children, it is recommended that splenectomy be delayed until the fourth year of life.[49] Splenectomy results in decreased hemolysis and decreases the risk of developing pigmented gallstones.[51]

Thalassemia

Thalassemia is a disease of hemoglobin synthesis, transmitted in a dominant fashion, and common in people of Mediterranean descent. It presents as thalassemia major in patients with the homozygous trait and as thalassemia minor in those who are heterozygous. The diagnosis is established by examining the peripheral blood smear, which demonstrates target cells. Splenectomy is reserved for patients with symptomatic splenomegaly or pain from splenic infarcts.

Sickle Cell Anemia

Sickle cell anemia, a hereditary condition, is predominantly seen in African Americans. The peripheral blood smear demonstrates sickle-shaped erythrocytes, caused by abnormal Hb-S, which has replaced the normal Hb-A. Although splenomegaly may be present early in the course of this illness, ultimately the spleen infarcts, with resultant autosplenectomy. Splenectomy may benefit some patients in whom acute splenic sequestration of red blood cells is demonstrated.[52]

Idiopathic Autoimmune Hemolytic Anemia

This disease is characterized by hemolysis of normal erythrocytes after exposure to circulating antibodies. It is believed that the spleen serves as a source of antibody in this process. It generally occurs in older patients and is more common in women. Patients present with mild jaundice, and splenomegaly is common. The initial therapy is steroid administration, reserving splenectomy for patients in whom steroids are ineffective or contraindicated.

Idiopathic Thrombocytopenia Purpura

The most common indication for elective splenectomy in most series, ITP is an acquired disorder caused by the destruction of platelets exposed to IgG antiplatelet factors.[52] These factors are produced in the spleen, and the spleen also serves as the location for platelet sequestration and destruction. This is usually considered a diagnosis of exclusion, being reserved for the patient with thrombocytopenia with normal numbers of megakaryocytes in the bone marrow and in the absence of any systemic disease or medication that can cause thrombocytopenia. Also, ITP can occur as a result of HIV infection and is a component of systemic lupus erythematosis.

Patients with ITP present with ecchymoses, purpura, spontaneous bleeding from the gums, and occasionally gastrointestinal or urinary tract bleeding. Imaging studies demonstrate that these patients have normal-size spleens. Laboratory studies usually demonstrate a platelet count under 50,000/mm^3 or even lower. Patients usually have normal prothrombin and partial thromboplastin time, with a normal or prolonged bleeding time.

Therapy of this disease is usually begun with steroid administration. This protocol is often supplemented with intravenous immunoglobulin (IVIG), and these measures result in cure in about 15% to 20% of patients.[49] In children, ITP often follows a viral infection and is usually a self-limited condition with therapy. IVIG has been used successfully to treat ITP nonoperatively in these patients.[53] Failure of nonoperative therapy is usually followed by splenectomy, which results in a cure in about 85% of patients. A diligent search for accessory splenic tissue is essential at the time of splenectomy (see following). Following splenectomy, platelet counts will rise to more than 100,000/mm^3 in about 70% of patients. Therapeutic guidelines are identical in patients with HIV-associated ITP, and the response rates are similar. Patients who do not respond with normalization of platelet counts usually have no recurrences of petechiae and ecchymoses. Patients who do not respond to splenectomy or who relapse at a later date may have accessory splenic tissue that was not identified at the time of surgery (see following).

Thrombotic Thrombocytopenia Purpura

Thrombotic thrombocytopenia purpura (TPP) was first described in 1924 as an acute febrile illness with anemia and hyaline thrombosis of terminal capillaries and arterioles.[54] It is characterized by a pentad of clinical findings: microangiopathic hemolytic anemia, consumptive thrombocytopenia, central nervous system abnormalities, renal failure, and fever. Damage to the endothelium resulting in platelet aggregation and microvascular occlusion is central to the pathophysiology.[54]

Therapy for this illness includes plasmapheresis, steroids, splenectomy, dextran, antiplatelet agents, and vinca alkaloids.[55] Without treatment, the mortality rate is 80% to 90%. Currently, the first line of therapy is considered to be plasmapheresis and steroid administration. Patients who do not respond to this regimen or who relapse undergo splenectomy.[54] In a series of 15 patients, plasmapheresis was the initial therapy for 14 patients.[54] Nine patients were treated with medical therapy only, and 6 completely recovered, while 3 died. Six patients failed plasmapheresis and underwent splenectomy.

A similar treatment regimen has been described by others. Of 11 patients treated for TTP, 10 were initially treated with plasmapheresis.[55] Three responded completely, and 1 patient died. The remaining 6 patients had a transient partial response to plasmapheresis and then underwent splenectomy. Overall, durable remission was achieved in 91% of patients with minimal morbidity. In another series, 108 patients were treated with steroids or steroids plus plasmapheresis.[56] In 30 of these patients, steroids were the only therapy administered. Splenectomy was reserved for patients who relapsed after plasmapheresis and plasma exchange. The overall survival rate in this series was 91%. Splenectomy has a clear role in the treatment of this complex illness, but first-line therapy remains medical.

Felty's Syndrome

Felty's syndrome consists of rheumatoid arthritis, splenomegaly, and neutropenia. Patients are usually treated with steroids, but failure to respond to steroids may be an indication for splenectomy, which can reverse a profound neutropenia or at least permit a neutrophil response to infection.[49,52] Splenectomy is indicated for patients with serious or recurrent infections, anemia requiring repeated transfusions, and marked thrombocytopenia. The course of the arthritis is unaffected by splenectomy.

Other Conditions

Splenectomy may be indicated for some patients with a variety of diseases that result in hypersplenism or splenomegaly, including sarcoidosis, Gaucher's disease, porphyria erythropoietica, splenic cysts, splenic abscesses, Wiskott-Aldrich syndrome, Chediak-Higashi syndrome, iatrogenic injuries (see the incidental splenectomy section below) and systemic mast cell disease.[57]

Operative Approach to the Spleen

Patient Preparation

In preparation for splenectomy, patients should be immunized against *Pneumococcus*, *Haemophilus influenza* B, and *Meningococcus* at least 2 weeks before operation, if possible. Preoperative splenic artery embolization, used only in selected patients with splenomegaly or AIDS or in obese patients, should be performed on the day of surgery because patients may experience considerable pain after infarction of the spleen. Embolization with coils is preferred to embolization with cellulose or microspheres because the last two can embolize to unintended targets such as the pancreas.[58] A cephalosporin antibiotic is administered preoperatively to reduce the risk of wound infection. Platelets are not administered in the preoperative period for patients with ITP, regardless of the level of thrombocytopenia.[52] Platelet transfusions are withheld for patients with significant intraoperative bleeding until after removal of the spleen. Patients must be given a thorough discussion of OPSI before the procedure.

Open Splenectomy

The technique of OS has remained largely unchanged for many years. The patient is placed on the operating table in the supine position. The incision used is largely dependent on the preference of the operating surgeon as splenectomy can be performed with facility through a midline incision or a left subcostal incision. Some surgeons prefer to use the left subcostal incision when only a splenectomy is performed, reserving the midline incision for situations in which general exploration of the abdomen is required. A midline incision is always used for open staging procedures for Hodgkin's disease. Patients with massive splenomegaly may be approached through a midline incision, or by a chevron incision extending the left subcostal incision across the midline.

Patients with massive splenomegaly, defined as spleens greater than 1500g, present special problems. In a recent review of 47 patients with massive splenomegaly, these patients were more likely to have postoperative complications and mortality compared to patients with smaller spleens undergoing splenectomy.[59] However, when the study was controlled for diagnosis, complication rates and mortality were comparable in the two groups, suggesting that increasing age and underlying illness are the key factors, and that spleen size by itself is not a hazard.

The splenic artery can be managed in several ways. Some have suggested ligation of the artery in the lesser sac at the beginning of the procedure for patients with massive splenomegaly.[60] Others have suggested that patients should undergo preoperative splenic artery occlusion using radiologic techniques.[61] This is usually performed using coils and should be done on the day of surgery to minimize symptoms from splenic infarction. These authors reported excellent results with this technique, including no additional transfusion requirements and simplification of the technical aspects due to reduced splenic bulk. Another approach is ligation of the splenic artery along the border of the pancreas in the lesser sac. However, even in cases of splenomegaly, not all surgeons believe that it is necessary to approach the splenic artery before a routine splenectomy.

The surgeon stands on the patient's right side and places traction on the spleen to expose the splenorenal ligament (Fig. 52.4). Using electrocautery, the splenorenal, splenocolic, inferior gastrosplenic, and splenophrenic ligaments are divided. The short gastric vessels are identified along the greater curvature of the stomach and divided individually between clamps and ligated (Fig. 52.5). The hilar dissection is undertaken next, with care to avoid the tail of the pancreas. The splenic artery and vein at the hilum should be controlled and ligated individually. The artery is ligated doubly on the proximal side and singly on the specimen side. If there is considerable hemorrhage, often from a torn venous branch, then placement of a large atraumatic clamp across the entire pedicle allows dissection to proceed in a less bloody field. Mobilization then continues by dividing retroperitoneal attachments, and the spleen is delivered into the wound.

Following removal of the specimen, the left upper quadrant is irrigated with warm saline and inspected for adequacy of hemostasis. In particular, the region of the short gastric

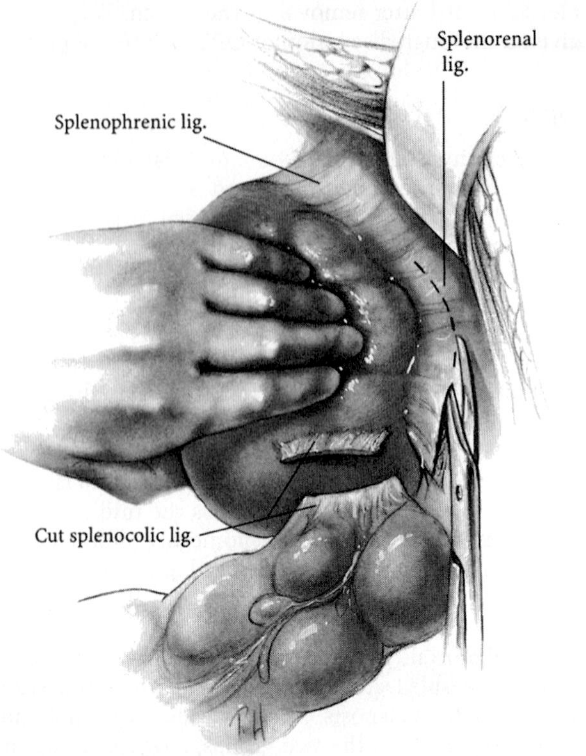

FIGURE 52.4. Exposure and division of the splenic ligaments.

vessels and hilum is carefully inspected, as well as the retroperitoneal attachments. A rolled laparotomy pad is placed in the deepest portion of the left upper quadrant and slowly unrolled, exposing areas of bleeding that are then controlled with ligatures or electrocautery as appropriate. Drains are not usually required, but when desired, closed-suction drains are employed. In those patients for whom splenectomy is performed for hematological diseases, a search for accessory splenic tissue is conducted. The wound is then closed in layers and routine postoperative care begun. Most surgeons leave a nasogastric tube in place for the first postoperative day.

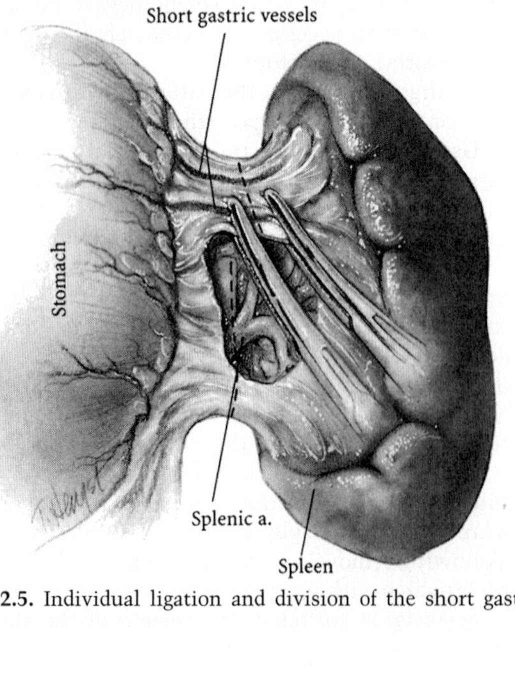

FIGURE 52.5. Individual ligation and division of the short gastric vessels.

Laparoscopic Splenectomy

In 1991, the LS technique was first described,[4,62] and it has become a well-accepted procedure. Initially, there was concern that the procedure would result in excessive blood loss, splenosis, and inaccurate pathological examination of the specimen. For the most part, these fears have been proven unwarranted. While splenomegaly remains a technical challenge, LS has become the preferred surgical technique for ITP and other diseases with normal spleen size. Furthermore, LS has been studied in the treatment of pediatric patients with hematologic diseases and shown to be safe and effective.[63]

An important element of the technique to optimize exposure of the spleen is the proper positioning of the patient on the operating table. Although the procedure was originally described with the patient in supine or lithotomy positions,[62,64] it was found that the lateral position[65] offered improved exposure of the splenic hilum (Fig. 52.6). Many still prefer the lateral approach for LS, but we use a double-access position. The patient is placed on a bean bag in a semilateral angle (45°), which allows for operating in both the supine and lateral positions. The supine position is preferred for initiating pneumoperitoneum, inserting trocars, exploring for accessory spleens, and ligating the splenic artery in the lesser sac, while

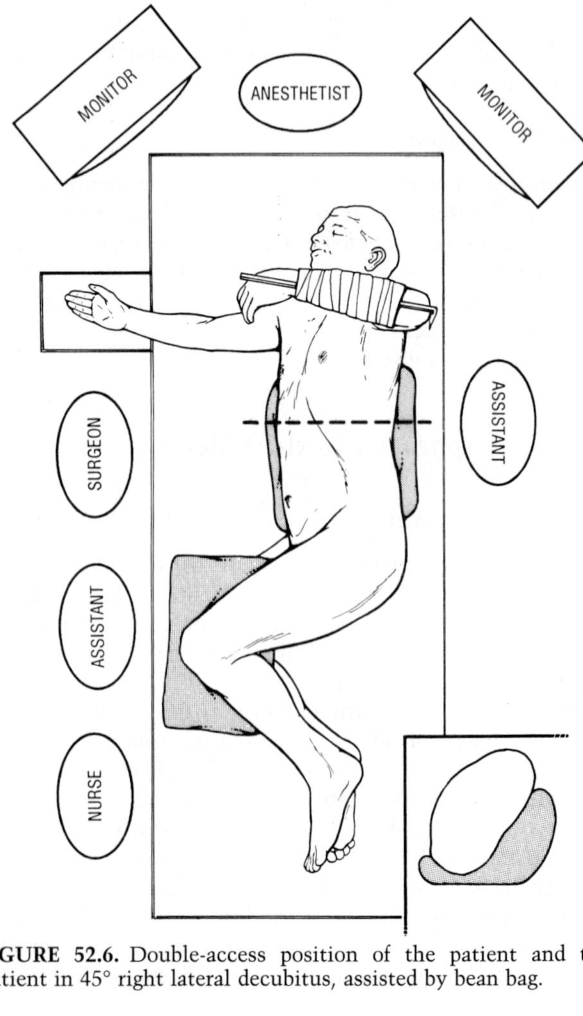

FIGURE 52.6. Double-access position of the patient and team. Patient in 45° right lateral decubitus, assisted by bean bag.

the lateral position offers excellent exposure of the hilum to facilitate dissection and vessel ligation.[66]

To minimize the risk of excessive intraoperative blood loss, Poulin initially advocated the use of routine preoperative splenic artery embolization.[58] We often perform operative ligation of the splenic artery in the lesser sac and reserve angioembolization for cases of splenomegaly, AIDS, and obesity. At present, preoperative embolization is used infrequently by most surgeons.

The sequence of splenic hilar dissection remains controversial. We advocate division of the splenocolic and splenorenal ligaments before hilar dissection,[67] while others recommend that the hilar vessels be dissected and divided first, leaving the lateral attachments to provide counteraction and elevation of the spleen.[65] The method of vessel ligation has also evolved. Initially, clips and sutures were used, but most surgeons now rely on endovascular cutting devices.

Increasing operative experience and technical refinements have produced good results relative to OS in terms of outcome, patient discomfort, length of hospitalization, and costs. It is anticipated that the procedure may have greatest benefit in patients at greatest risk of complications of laparotomy, including those with hypersplenism who are treated with steroids and other immunosuppressive regimens. Wound problems, infections, and pulmonary complications, which are particularly troublesome with conventional splenectomy techniques, may be avoided with LS.

The disease most commonly treated by LS is ITP, and the laparoscopic approach is ideal for two reasons. First, exposure and dissection of the normal-size spleen are simpler, and second, the specimen does not have to be delivered intact for pathological analysis. Instead, it can be morcellated and extracted through a port site, in contrast to patients with Hodgkin's lymphoma, from whom the spleen must be removed intact for histological examination. In our approach to laparoscopic staging for lymphomas, the splenectomy, liver, and upper abdominal lymph node specimens are dissected laparoscopically, and a Pfannenstiel incision is performed to dissect the aortic, iliac, and femoral nodes and to remove the upper abdominal specimens.

In patients with borderline-size spleens, body habitus and the volume of the spleen either allow or hinder adequate exposure. The laparoscopic approach is more difficult in obese patients. The massive omentum obscures the vasculature and makes dissection of the peritoneal attachments more challenging. Trocar locations and dissection sequences also must be modified for the enlarged spleen, which may rotate and obscure the hilar vessels, leaving insufficient space in which to elevate the organ. Nevertheless, the avoidance of a large incision and pulmonary complications in these patients justifies the extra effort required to complete the procedure laparoscopically.

Patient Positioning

Positioning is a crucial consideration (see Fig. 52.6). Three positions have been described, each with its advantages. The anterior position (patient supine) facilitates exploration of the abdomen for accessory spleens, which are present in 15% to 30% of the population.[68] The lateral position (patient right side down) has been called the "hanged spleen" technique.[65] In this position, the viscera fall away from the hilum when the spleen is elevated, providing better exposure of the vasculature. The "double-access" position (patient right side down, 45°, with a bean bag under the left flank) combines the advantages of the anterior and lateral positions. This technique allows for the creation of the pneumoperitoneum and abdominal exploration to be performed with the patient supine, while splenectomy is done in the lateral position.

Trocar Placement

Five trocars are used (Fig. 52.7). The camera port is placed first, except in some patients with prior abdominal surgery. Regardless of whether the pneumoperitoneum is created with a Veress needle or by open technique, the exact location of the first port varies with the body habitus of the patient. In average-size patients, the subumbilical region is preferred, but in large or tall patients, this port should be placed above and to the left of the umbilicus. A 10/11-mm or 5-mm port is placed in the subxiphoid area to accommodate instruments the surgeon uses with the left hand, and a 10/11-mm trocar is placed midway between the umbilicus and the subxiphoid trocar for instruments he or she uses with the right hand. The most lateral trocar (10/11-mm) is then placed in the left axillary line, halfway between the costal martin and the iliac crest. A 12-mm trocar used to accommodate the endovascular cutter is placed just lateral to the left rectus sheath, slightly above the level of the umbilicus between the optic and the most lateral trocar (Fig. 52.7). Infiltration with local anesthesia before insertion of each trocar helps to reduce postoperative pain and to confirm the precise location of each trocar site.

General Inspection

The procedure is initiated by tilting the table to the left so that the patient is supine. This position allows easier research for accessory spleens, which may be found in the splenic hilum, the splenic ligaments, the omentum, the small-bowel mesentery, and the pelvic viscera. All these areas must be

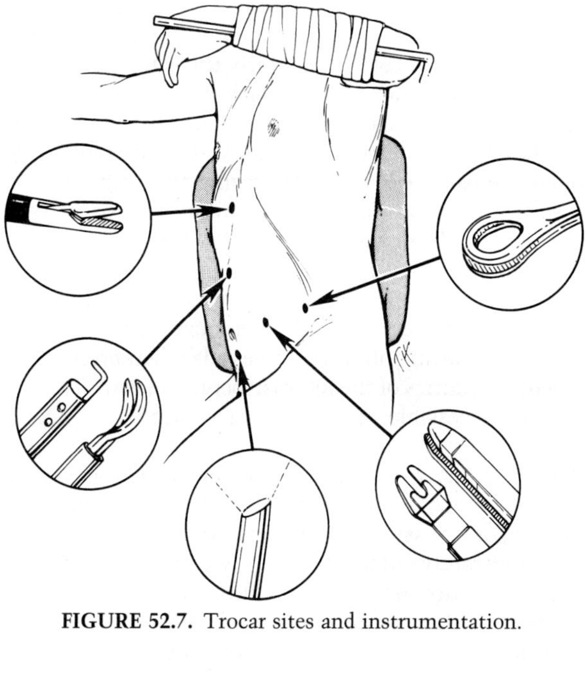

FIGURE 52.7. Trocar sites and instrumentation.

carefully inspected. We have identified an accessory spleen on the abdominal peritoneum in the right upper quadrant.

Ligation of the Splenic Artery

In most cases, the next step consists of ligation of the splenic artery in the lesser sac. Although this may seem unnecessary and time consuming in an uncomplicated splenectomy, it represents the safest course as hemorrhage during hilar dissection can occur in any situation. Access to the lesser sac is gained by elevating the stomach, using a grasper from the most lateral trocar, and placing inferior traction on the transverse colon with a grasper inserted via the left paramedian 12-mm trocar.

The surgeon's left hand (subxiphoid trocar) pierces, dissects, and coagulates the gastrocolic window using bipolar electrocautery or the harmonic scalpel (Ultracision; Ethicon Endosurgery, Cincinnati, OH). The lesser sac is entered, and the pancreas is identified and retracted posteriorly and slightly inferiorly with an atraumatic fan retractor inserted through the paramedian 12-mm trocar. The splenic artery or its pulsation should be visible just superior to the pancreas. Its tortuosity, location, and direction identify it as the splenic artery. The visceral peritoneum is opened with scissors. The artery is dissected free and occluded with a clip, but not divided.

In a study comparing 22 patients who underwent ligation of the splenic artery with 12 patients who did not, blood loss was significantly lower in the ligation group (161 mL) versus the nonligation group (292 mL), although the operative time was greater in the ligation group (155 min) compared to the nonligation group (140 min).[69]

Splenic Mobilization

The spleen is approached by rotating the table to the right so that the patient's left side is elevated into the lateral position. An element of head-up positioning may be needed, depending on the body habitus, to facilitate the division of the splenocolic ligament. This ligament is quite variable; it may be thin and avascular, covered by dense omentum, or obscured by the colon, which may even be adherent to the splenic capsule. Exposure is gained in part passively, as gravity causes the viscera to fall away from the spleen, and in part actively. The spleen is lifted gently, either with the surgeon's left-hand grasper (using it as a wand) or with a ring forcep or spleen grasper placed by the assistant through the most lateral trocar. The colon can be put on tension by the assistant's grasper through the paramedian trocar, freeing the surgeon's hands. The splenocolic ligament may be divided using scissors, a harmonic scalpel, or an electrocautery hook, taking care to avoid direct or remote electrocautery injury to the colon. The ligament must be divided so that the inferior pole of the spleen is completely visible. The next step is to divide the communicating inferior pole vessels when present. These are small tributaries of the left gastroepiploic vein. The hilum, now more accessible, is once again inspected for accessory spleens.

At this point, the surgeon must choose whether to mobilize the splenorenal ligament, allowing further elevation of the spleen, or to dissect and divide the hilar vessels. In normal-size or moderately enlarged spleens, we prefer to mobilize the splenic ligaments first as this facilitates the hilar dissection and vessel ligation. If bleeding is encountered during hilar dissection, it is much easier to control if the spleen has been mobilized. In addition, the endocutter can be inserted rapidly to divide the hilar vessels. In cases of splenomegaly, however, the splenic volume makes it more difficult, if not impossible, to mobilize the splenorenal ligament first. In these cases, the hilar vessels are divided first.

To dissect the splenorenal ligament, the spleen can be grasped with the atraumatic lung forceps or a ring clamp or elevated with a fan retractor. Specialized instruments for this purpose have been developed (Karl Storz Endoscopy, Tutlinger, Germany). Dissection proceeds from the inferior pole cephalad, progressing as high as possible. An electrocautery hook with suction and irrigation greatly facilitates this part of the procedure. The peritoneal attachment is divided, and a combination of electrocautery and blunt dissection with the hook cautery device is used. Often, limited exposure makes it necessary to divide some of the vessels to the inferior pole of the spleen before the splenophrenic ligament is reached; with this accomplished, the dissection can be restarted. In cases of splenomegaly, it is necessary to alternate dissection and ligation several times.

The key is that splenic elevation greatly facilitates division of the superior pole vessels and the short gastric vessels by putting them on stretch. Although some surgeons prefer to keep the spleen attached to the diaphragm to enable bag capture, we have not found that to be advantageous.

Hilar Dissection

The anatomy of the splenic artery and its branches supplying the spleen are of particular importance. Michel, in 1942, described two principal patterns.[70] The distributed type, present in 70% of the population, is characterized by a short splenic trunk with numerous long branches that enter 75% of the medial surface of the organ. The magistral type, present in 30%, is characterized by a long main splenic artery with short terminal branches that enter only 33% of the medial surface of the spleen. These patterns have important implications in dissection during splenectomy, with the distributed type offering an easier dissection.[71] There are as many as seven principal branches, including the superior terminal, inferior terminal, medial terminal, superior polar, inferior polar, left gastroepiploic, and short gastric arteries. The veins typically run posterior to the arteries.[71]

The hilar vessels are dissected with right-angled instruments and divided between clips and ligatures. The harmonic scalpel can be used for the short gastric vessels. We have found ligation and division of the vessels with the endocutters to be more secure and far quicker (Fig. 52.8). The cost of the endocutter (an issue of increasing importance in surgical decisions) is offset by the time savings. On several occasions, conversion to an open procedure has been avoided by using the endocutter to control hemorrhage. Clips can be used, but may become dislodged if handled during the dissection. A further disadvantage of clips is that they prevent complete closure of the endocutter and therefore limit its effectiveness in an emergency.

Once the spleen is detached, it is placed into a sturdy specimen bag (Cook Urologic, New Brunswick, NJ). This maneuver can be challenging and is accomplished by rolling the bag, grasping it with a Kelley clamp, and placing it into the abdomen through the 12-mm paramedian trocar site after the trocar has been removed. The bag is placed into the peritoneal cavity and unfurled in the splenic fossa. The

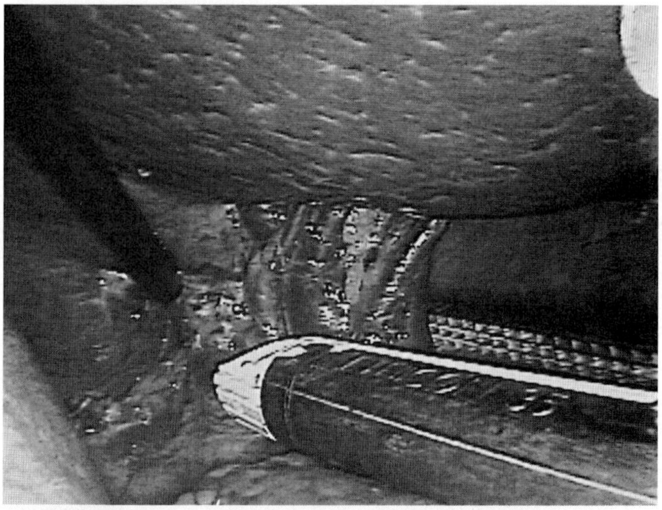

FIGURE 52.8. Division of the hilar vessels with the endovascular cutter device.

opening is triangulated with three graspers placed through the two upper midline trocars and the left lateral trocar. The spleen is grasped at its lower pole by the ring forceps placed through the paramedian trocar and then inserted into the bag (Fig. 52.9).

The specimen is extracted piecemeal by morcellation or intact via a small incision. In patients such as those with ITP for whom careful pathological analysis is not required, the specimen is morcellated in the bag using ring forceps or a tissue morcellator. It is most important to avoid spilling any fragments in the peritoneal cavity, which could result in splenosis and recurrent disease. To do this safely, the bag is pulled up into the abdominal wall defect at the 12-mm trocar site and is held up tightly against the abdominal wall while the specimen is morcellated manually under constant direct laparoscopic vision so the small bowel is not injured.

After morcellation, the 12-mm trocar is reinserted, and the splenic bed is inspected for hemostasis by placing the laparoscope in the 12-mm paramedian port. In patients such as those with Hodgkin's disease for whom an intact specimen is important for pathological analysis, one can extend the

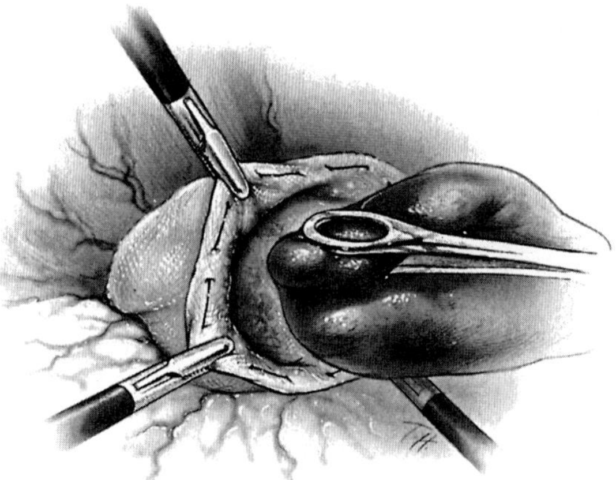

FIGURE 52.9. Placement of specimen into bag.

umbilical port into a lower midline incision or make a Pfannenstiel incision for extraction. The fascia of all trocar sites of 10mm or greater is closed with 0-polyglycolic acid suture.

Postoperative Care

The orogastric tube is removed before leaving the operating room. Oral feedings are begun the next day. Activity is unrestricted, and ambulation is encouraged. Parenteral analgesia is usually required the first night after surgery, while oral narcotic analgesics are adequate the next day. Platelets and hemoglobin are monitored as determined by the underlying disease and the clinical course.

Collected Experience

There are no prospective randomized trials recorded in the literature comparing OS with LS because for the most part the results are strongly in support of the laparoscopic approach. The establishment of this procedure as the gold standard has recently diminished the number of reports of large series of LS versus OS in the literature.

Retrospective comparative series of matched (Table 52.5) and unmatched (Table 52.6) adult patients undergoing LS

TABLE 52.5.
Adult Matched Retrospective Studies of Laparoscopic Versus Open Splenectomy for Disease (Level II Evidence).

Reference	*Procedure*	*n*	*Operating room time (min)*	*EBL (mL)*	*Spleen size (cm)*	*Major morbidity*	*Postoperative stay (days)*	*Total cost ($)*	*Operating room cost ($)*
Delaitre (1997)[106]	Lap	28	183			3	5.1		
	Open	28	127			8	8.6		
	Conversion	3 (%)							
Diaz (1997)[107]	Lap	15	196 ± 71	385 ± 168		1	2.3 ± 1.5	18,015 ± 2,550	12,827 ± 2,253
	Open	15	116 ± 64	359 ± 318		2	8.8 ± 6.8	16,362 ± 8,752	4,372 ± 2,038
Smith (1996)[108]	Lap	10	261 ± 31		17	0	3.0 ± 0.5	17,071 ± 1,849	8,400 ± 720
	Open	10	131 ± 12		14.5	2	5.8 ± 0.2	13,196 ± 1,418	3,627 ± 270
	Conversion	1 (%)							
Cogliandolo (2001)[109]	Lap	20	78 ± 15				3.95 ± 0.60		
	Open	24	74 ± 13				7.0 ± 1.68		

Lap, laparoscopy.

Data are mean ± SD.

Clinical studies are classified according to the design of the study and the quality of the resulting data. Class I, prospective randomized studies; class II, prospective nonrandomized studies or case-controlled retrospective studies; class III, retrospective analyses without case controls.

TABLE 52.6.
Adult Nonmatched Retrospective Studies.

Reference	Procedure	n	OR time (min)	EBL	Spleen size (g)	Major morbidity	Postop stay (days)	Days to liquids	Total cost ($)	OR cost ($)
Yuan	Lap	29	190.6 ± 79.4[a]	163.8 ± 110	9.6 ± 2.0 cm	0	4.1 ± 1.5	15.1 ± 6.8 h		
(1998)[110]	Open	22	113.9 ± 51.0[a]	210.5 ± 124	10.0 ± 2.5 cm	5	6.8 ± 1.5	52.6 ± 20.7 h		
	Conversion	1 (3%)								
Friedman	Lap	58	153 ± 80	259 ± 406	404 ± 750	3	3.5 ± 2.3	1.5 ± 0.7	7,300 ± 7,100	2,400 ± 1,400
(1997)[73]	Open	74	121 ± 64	437 ± 559	936 ± 1,226	9	6.7 ± 3.1	3.2 ± 1.9	9,400 ± 12,300	1,500 ± 600
	Conversion	5	171 ± 20	550 ± 260	727 ± 667	0	7.4 ± 4.8	2.8 ± 0.8	22,000 ± 15,800	2,100 ± 100
Glasgow	Lap	52	196 ± 8	320 ± 59	319 ± 87	5	4.8 ± 0.5		20,295 ± 3,482	
(1997)[111]	Open	28	156 ± 6	274 ± 56	157 ± 17	4	6.7 ± 0.5		17,876 ± 3,294	
	Conversion	6 (11%)								
Brunt	Lap	26	202 ± 55	222 ± 280	241 ± 250	3	2.5 ± 1.2			
(1996)[112]	Open	20	134 ± 43	376 ± 500	469 ± 410	3	5.8 ± 2.9			
Rege	Lap	10	187 ± 51	373 ± 271[a]	129 ± 90		2.5 ± 1.2			
(1996)[72]	Open	5	126 ± 25	330 ± 275[a]	432 ± 413		7.0 ± 1.0			
	Conversion	5 (33.3%)	131 ± 54	1,150 ± 370[a]	797 ± 837		6.4 ± 2.9			

n, number of patients; EBL, estimated blood loss.

TABLE 52.7.
Nonmatched Retrospective Study of Laparoscopic Splenectomy for Idiopathic Thrombocytopenia Purpura (LSI) Versus Laparoscopic Splenectomy for Other Diseases (LSO) (Level III Evidence).

Procedure	OR time (min)	Blood loss (mL)	Spleen weight (g)	Major morbidity	Postop stay (days)	Days to liquids	Direct cost ($)	OR cost ($)
LSI (n = 31)	113 ± 50	177 ± 160	156 ± 148	1	2.7 ± 1.3	1.2 ± 0.5	10,300 ± 500	2,700 ± 400
LSO (n = 23)	185 ± 88	314 ± 619	715 ± 1,089	1	7.4 ± 9.0	1.8 ± 0.7	18,500 ± 14,000	3,300 ± 100

TABLE 52.8.
Adult Matched Restrospective Study of Laparoscopic Versus Open Splenectomy for Idiopathic Thrombocytopenia Purpura (Level II Evidence).

Reference	Procedure	No.	OR time (min)	EBL (mL)	Spleen weight (g)	Major morbidity	Postoperative stay (days)	Days to liquids	Accessory	Platelet response
Marassi	Lap	14	140 (105–245)	150 (50–700)	181	1 (7.1%)	5 (3–7)	2 (1–3)	3 (21.4%)	13 (92.8%)
(1999)[113]	Open	15	75 (70–125)	200 (50–550)	203.1	2 (13%)	8 (5–15)	3 (2–4)	4 (26.6%)	12 (80%)
	Conversion	1 (7.1%)								

TABLE 52.9.
Adult Nonmatched Retrospective Studies of Laparoscopic Versus Open Splenectomy for Disease (Level III Evidence).

Reference	Procedure	n	OR time (min)	EBL (ml)	Spleen size (g)	Major morbidity	Postop stay (days)	Days to liquids	Accessory	Platelet response	Direct cost ($)	OR cost ($)
Tanoue	Lap	35	204.5 ± 79.9	154.4 ± 157	120.6 ± 116.4	4 (11.4%)	9.6 ± 3.2	1.3 ± 0.5	4 (11.4%)	31		
(1999)[114]	Open	41	99.8 ± 35.4	511.7 ± 375.1	121.9 ± 64.8	19 (46.3%)	20.1 ± 12.5	3.8 ± 1.9	5 (12.2%)	32		
Shimomatsuya	Lap	14	210 ± 81	560 ± 659	89 ± 52	3	8.9 ± 2.9		4 (29%)	13 (93%)		
(1999)[115]	Open	20	126 ± 52	321 ± 264	140 ± 95	3	15.2 ± 5.8		4 (20%)	13 (81%)		
Lozano-Salazar	Lap	22	4.5 ± 1		10 (7–15) cm	6	8.9 ± 2.9		2 (9%)	87%		
(1998)[116]	Open	27	2.7 ± 0.7		11 (8–15) cm	10	15.2 ± 5.8		3 (11%)	89%		
	Conversion	2 (9%)										
Watson	Lap	13	89 (48–140)			0	2 (1–3)		2 (15%)	12	2,238	1,478
(1997)[77]	Open	47	84 (50–165)			9 (19%)	10 (5–55)		3 (6%)	39	4,224	666
Friedman	Lap	29	122 ± 54	203 ± 155	184 ± 156	1	2.9 ± 1.3	1.2 ± 0.5	6 (21%)	27 (93%)	5,509 ± 3,636	2,762 ± 418
(1996)[5]	Open	18	103 ± 45	285 ± 196	167 ± 98	0	6.9 ± 3.0	3.2 ± 0.7	2 (11%)	15 (83%)	9,031 ± 1,2752	1,859 ± 380
	Conversion	2 (6%)										
Schlinkert	Lap	7	154			0	2.9 ± 1.3	0.7	0	7 (100%)		
(1997)[117]	Open	14	68			3	6.9 ± 3.0	2.6	2	11		

were compared. The majority were performed for ITP; other indications included hereditary spherocytosis, staging of Hodgkin's disease, autoimmune hemolytic anemia, TTP, abscess, and infarction (see the Indications section). Overall success rates for the procedures were better than 90%, with bleeding by far the most common reason for conversion. Comparing LS with OS, authors have reported significantly shorter postoperative hospital stay, no difference in blood loss (except as reported by Rege et al.[72]), earlier recovery of bowel function, but significantly greater operative times for LS (except as in Friedman et al.[73]).

It is inaccurate, however, to compare the results of LS to OS in a heterogeneous population. Most LS series contain patients with ITP primarily, while OS series include patients with trauma, splenectomy performed in conjunction with other procedures, and a greater number of patients with diseases other than ITP. To emphasize these issues, we first compared LS in ITP patients with LS in patients with other diseases and found that patients with ITP did indeed fare significantly better (Table 52.7). Those with ITP had significantly decreased operative times (113 vs. 185 min), time to oral intake (1.2 vs. 1.8 days), hospital stay (2.7 vs. 7.4 days), and total cost ($10,300 vs. $18,500).

Next, for an objective comparison, we analyzed our results of LS and OS in patients with ITP only and reviewed the matched (Table 52.8) and unmatched (Table 52.9) retrospective studies in the literature. Our data as well as those of others revealed that the size of the spleen did not differ significantly between the two groups. As this procedure has become established, it is difficult to find comparisons of OS versus LS in the literature.

More recently, investigators tried to identify factors that limit the performance of LS. In a direct comparison of outcomes based on splenic size, Heniford and colleagues found the operative time for LS to be significantly ($P < .05$) lower for patients with normal size spleens (127 min) compared to those with spleens over 500 g in weight (172 min).[74] They found no significant differences in other parameters such as conversion rate, length of stay, or rate of complications. In another study, Terrosu and coworkers similarly found that only operative time differed for normal-size spleens compared with spleens up to 2000 g.[75] They also found that for LS for spleens over 2000 g, patients had increased blood loss, more conversions, and a longer postoperative stay compared with those with spleens under 2000 g. The hand-assisted LS has also been evaluated, and shown to shorten operating time compared to LS, without increases in length of stay, morbidity, or mortality.[76]

The mean operative time was longer for LS than for OS except in the studies by Watson et al.[77] and Friedman et al.[73] Estimated blood loss appeared less in the laparoscopic group. Recovery of bowel function, measured as days to tolerance of oral liquids, was significantly earlier after LS. Hospital stay was also shorter, resulting in lower total costs, despite the fact that operating room costs were greater in the laparoscopic group. Accessory spleens were identified and removed in 0% to 29% of LS patients. Platelet response to LS was 87% to 100%, and none of the failures in this group was found to have residual splenic tissue on follow-up nuclear scan. Historically, platelet response to splenectomy has been approximately 80%,[78] and the response rate after OS in the reported series was 78% to 89%.

The pediatric literature has also recently exploded with comparative matched (Table 52.10) and unmatched (Table 52.11) retrospective studies that show the effectiveness of LS, mostly for ITP, in their patient population. There is only one unmatched retrospective study comparing LS to OS in splenomegaly (Table 52.12) reported in the literature. The results of this study are also in support of the laparoscopic approach. Laparoscopic splenectomy is considered to be the gold standard for splenectomy in children as well.[79]

A recent analysis of splenectomy performed for patients with benign and malignant diseases showed that while patients undergoing OS for malignant diseases have significantly higher complication and mortality rates compared to those undergoing OS for benign disease, these differences are eliminated in patients undergoing LS[80] (Table 52.13). These results further support the use of LS in patients with malignant diseases and establish a benefit for its use compared to OS.

Laparoscopic splenectomy is an established procedure. It is postulated that avoiding an upper abdominal incision and minimizing the operative trauma will decrease the incidence of pulmonary, thromboembolic, and wound complications associated with OS, and early reports seem to support this. As individual experience is gained with LS, operative times can be reduced to near those of the open procedure. Overall costs are lower with shorter hospital stays, and the patients benefit by having a shorter recovery period with an earlier return to normal activities.

Most LS procedures are now performed for ITP because the normal-size spleen is ideal for the laparoscopic procedure. Longer follow-up of these patients is necessary to determine whether accessory spleens will be missed more frequently and lead to increased rates of recurrence for the disease. Finally, further evolution of instrumentation and operative

TABLE 52.10.
Pediatric Matched Retrospective Study of Laparoscopic Versus Open Splenectomy for Disease (Level II Evidence).

Reference	*Procedure*	*n*	*OR time (min)*	*EBL (mL)*	*Major morbidity*	*Postop stay (days)*	*Direct cost ($)*	*OR cost ($)*
Curran (1998)[118]	Lap	7	147 (115–190)	41		2	10,899	3,195
	Open	7	86 (50–115)	34		4	8,276	1,751
Esposito (1997)[119]	Lap	8	170 (125–240)		1	3 (2–5)		
	Open	8	100 (50–155)		0	4.7 (3–9)		

TABLE 52.11.
Pediatric Nonmatched Retrospective Study of Laparoscopic Versus Open Splenectomy for Disease (Level III Evidence).

Reference	*Procedure*	*No.*	*OR time (min)*	*EBL (mL)*	*Spleen weight (g)*	*Major morbidity*	*Postoperative stay (days)*	*Accessory*	*Direct cost ($)*	*OR cost ($)*
Rescorla (1998)[124]	Lap	50	115 (60–210)	54.4		2	1.4 ± 0.97	9 (18%)	5,713	
	Open	32	83 (65–110)	49		0	2.5 ± 1.43	8 (25%)	6,564	
Farah (1997)[125]	Lap	16	3.9 (2.2–8.6)	74	218 (68–542)	5	3.6 (2–7)	0	13,410 (8,309–26,482)	5,020 (3,451–9,165)
	Open	20	2.3 (1.3–3.4)	78	360 (83–1279)	7	4.9 (3–9)	5 (25%)	14,405 (6,326–33,753)	2,873 (1,989–3,873)
	Conversion	1								
Janu (1996)[126]	Lap	14	187 (151–235)			1	3.57 (2–8)		7,008	4,167
	Open	47	81 (33–145)			12	2.70 (1–6)		5,221	1,248
	Conversion	1								
Hicks (1996)[127]	Lap	11	147	32		2	3.6			
	Open	10	112	86		3	5.3			
	Conversion	1 (9%)								
Yoshida (1995)[128]	Lap	8	226 ± 24	100 ± 39		0	6.8 ± 0.6			
	Open	11	101 ± 8	73 ± 11		0	10.4 ± 0.5			
	Conversion	2 (25%)								
Beanes (1995)[129]	Lap	7	221 (170–310)			1	3.6 (2–7)			
	Open	14	59 (40–85)			2	3.8 (2–5)			
	Conversion	1								

techniques will make the laparoscopic procedure more available for enlarged spleens and a wider range of indications.

Partial Splenectomy

The principal indication for partial splenectomy is trauma, for which one desires to maintain the splenic immune function to decrease the incidence of postoperative infectious complications. It is clear that this procedure is much more technically demanding than splenectomy. It is a particularly useful technique in children, for whom the risk of OPSI is greatest.

The first step in this procedure is to gain control of the splenic artery within the lesser sac using a vessel loop; this will allow control of splenic inflow during the dissection of the spleen. The spleen is then mobilized into the incision, being careful to do so in an atraumatic fashion. Care must be taken to avoid injury to the splenic capsule. Next, the surgeon must decide what is to be resected and to ligate the blood supply to that portion of the spleen. The vessel loop is then tightened, occluding inflow through the splenic artery, and transection is begun at least 1 cm on the cyanotic side of the line of demarcation.

Transection is performed using the "finger fracture" technique once the capsule is incised (Fig. 52.10). Control of the bleeding surface of transection can be achieved using individual ligatures, interrupted horizontal mattress sutures, continuous suture, surgical stapling devices, the argon beam coagulator, or a combination of these different techniques. The use of topical hemostatic agents may also be necessary to achieve hemostasis. In general, drains are not necessary. Laparoscopic partial splenectomy has been described and is obviously technically feasible.[81,82]

Accessory Splenic Tissue

Accessory splenic tissue is identified in 10% to 20% of patients undergoing splenectomy and remains an important issue in the operative management of these patients. The search for accessory splenic tissue remains an integral part of the procedure when performed for certain hematological conditions such as ITP because residual splenic tissue can hypertrophy and cause relapse of the disease, sometimes years after splenectomy.[83] Knowledge of the location of this tissue is important. Most commonly, accessory splenic tissue is located at or near the splenic hilum, but it has been reported along the left gutter and even into the left scrotum.

TABLE 52.12.
Nonmatched Retrospective Study of Laparoscopic Versus Open Splenectomy for Splenomegaly (Level III Evidence).

Reference	*Procedure*	*n*	*OR time (min)*	*Spleen weight (g)*	*Major morbidity*	*Postop stay (days)*	*Days to liquids*
Terrosu (1998)[120]	Lap	8	197 ± 65	1762 (500–3680)	1 (12.5%)	6 ± 3	2 ± 1
	Open	15	110 ± 21	2713 (800–3850)	5 (33%)	9 ± 3	4 ± 0.6

TABLE 52.13.
Nonmatched Retrospective Studies of Laparoscopy Performed for Benign and Malignant Diseases (Level III Evidence).

Reference	*Diagnosis*	*Number*	*Age (mean)*	*OR time (min)*	*Spleen weight (g, mean)*	*Conversion (%)*	*Complications (%)*	*Mortality (%)*	*LOS (days)*
Targona (2001)[121]	Benign	100	37	138	279	5	13	0	3.7
	Malignant	37	60[a]	161[a]	1210[a]	14	22	0	5[a]
Torelli (2002)[122]	ITP	23	42	122	300	0	4	0	4.8
	HA	5	25	173[a]	560	0	1	0	5.2
	Malignant	15	57	128	1270[a]	0	3	1	6.8
Rosen (2002) [123]	Benign	104	—	142	313	0	14	1	3.6
	Malignant	43	—	170*	822*	5*	19	0	4.3

HA, hemolytic anemia; ITP, idiopathic thrombocytopenia purpura; LOS, length of stay.
[a]Statistically significant difference ($P < .05$) between the two groups in that study.
Source: Adapted from Burch, Misra, and Phillips.[80]

A patient who presents with relapse of ITP should be assumed to have retained accessory splenic tissue until proven otherwise. The initial diagnostic test should be a technetium-99–sulfur colloid liver–spleen scan. If a focus of uptake is identified, then CT scan may be useful to locate the residual tissue. Long-term remission after excision of the accessory splenic tissue has been reported.[83]

The advent of LS has brought about new discussions of accessory splenic tissue. In an LS series, the incidence of accessory splenic tissue was similar to that previously reported after OS.[5,84] These authors believed that the magnification afforded by use of the laparoscope improves the ability to identify accessory spleens. However, a prospective clinical study reported that elective LS for hematological diseases may not allow complete detection of accessory splenic tissue.[85] This result points out the importance of a meticulous search for accessory splenic tissue.

When a patient presents with recurrent ITP, several authors have used a laparoscopic approach to identify and excise accessory splenic tissue.[86,87] One group used an intraoperative scintigraphic localization technique to identify the accessory spleen in the operating room.[76] The use of laparoscopic resection may afford these patients significantly shortened hospital stay compared to the open approach for resection of accessory spleens. The laparoscopic hand-assist device has been reported to help identify accessory splenic tissue not easily seen with conventional laparoscopy.[88]

Incidental Splenectomy

The spleen is easily injured during procedures in the upper abdomen involving the stomach, esophageal hiatus, vagus nerves, pancreas, left colon, and left kidney. Most commonly, this involves capsular tears, resulting in continuous bleeding. In a review of 981 consecutive splenectomies at a single institution, 18.9% were performed incidental to another procedure to facilitate exposure or because of capsular tears.[89] This was commonly associated with operations for peptic ulcer disease and more commonly associated with the use of midline incisions. Conversely, incidental splenectomy was noted in only 0.91% of all gastrectomies and 1.4% of all left colectomies at that institution. These authors believed that postoperative morbidity and mortality are increased by the incidental splenectomy. Most iatrogenic injuries involve capsular tears from excessive manipulation. When the splenic capsule is injured during the conduct of other procedures, attempts should be made at splenic salvage to minimize the necessity for incidental splenectomy.

Complications of Splenectomy

Splenic surgery, open or laparoscopic, can be associated with significant morbidity and mortality. Deaths and complications are the consequences of underlying diseases and their treatments as well as errors in technique and judgment. Expert training and proctoring, proper patient selection, precise anatomical dissection, and diligence in hemostasis will avoid most of the technical problems.

Published series of OS[78,90–93] reported morbidity rates that ranged from 15% to as high as 61%. Series of LS[5,66,94–97] reported morbidity rates of 0% to 14% (see Table 52.6). The mortality rates reported for OS ranged from 6% to 13% and those for LS from 0% to 5%. However, most series of OS

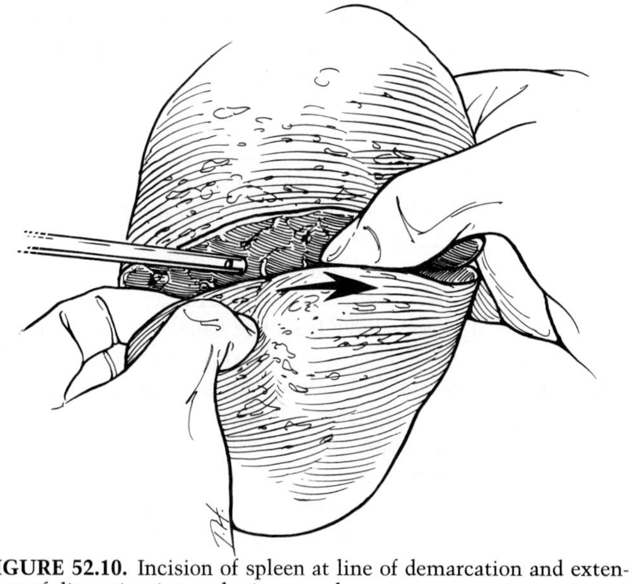

FIGURE 52.10. Incision of spleen at line of demarcation and extension of dissection into splenic parenchyma.

included splenectomies performed for trauma or iatrogenic operative injury, for which morbidity and mortality rates may be higher (36% and 16%, respectively).[91] Factors predisposing to complications include the underlying indication for the splenectomy, the patient's age, and associated diseases. For example, patients fared better if the splenectomy was performed for diagnostic purposes or primary hypersplenism (6.4% morbidity, 1% mortality).[91]

Operative Complications

Cardiovascular Effects of Pneumoperitoneum

Cardiovascular effects of pneumoperitoneum are minimal and rarely result in hypotension or arrhythmia.[98] Hemodynamic problems, usually during insufflation, occur in approximately 0.2% of patients and are associated with vasovagal reflex or decreased venous return. Most often, the problems are minor and can be corrected with administration of fluids or atropine. When significant rhythm disturbances occur, the pneumoperitoneum must be released immediately, and the specific arrhythmia must be treated. Cardiac disease and pacemakers are not contraindications.

Bowel Injury

Injury to the bowel is rare and usually occurs during creation of the pneumoperitoneum. Reported frequency, in the gynecology literature, is 0.16% to 0.27%.[99] Pneumoperitoneum may be administered by closed technique, using the Veress needle, or by open technique, using a blunt-tipped trocar (Hasson). Use of the open technique does not eliminate the risk of bowel injury, but it does facilitate immediate identification and repair. Patients who have had prior abdominal surgery are at increased risk of accidental enterotomy, regardless of the technique used. Prior abdominal surgery is a relative contraindication to LS.

Veress needle injury to the bowel rarely requires further intervention; such injuries can be managed with close observation. In contrast, intestinal trocar injuries require operative repair. The trocar should be left within the injured bowel so that the injury can be readily identified when the abdomen is opened. Although extensive injury to the left colon occasionally requires a diverting colostomy, most bowel injuries are treated by primary repair, either laparoscopic or open.

Vascular Injury

Injury to blood vessels may occur during Veress needle or trocar insertion. Use of the open technique eliminates the risk of injury to major intraabdominal vessels as a blunt-tipped trocar is inserted. While Veress needle injury to blood vessels rarely causes significant hemorrhage, trocar injuries to major blood vessels have been the cause of fatal bleeding. Major hemorrhage occurs with injury to the distal aorta or common iliac vessels, and mortality is as high as 15%. Major vascular injuries requiring further intervention occur in 0.64% of laparoscopic procedures.[99] Minor bleeding that causes abdominal wall hematomas may occasionally occur from trocar injuries to abdominal wall vessels. These areas should be identified by careful inspection of the trocar sites before the conclusion of the operation; simple ligation of the vessels usually contains the hemorrhage.

Hemorrhage

The most common intraoperative complication of splenectomy is hemorrhage, which occurs in roughly 5% of cases. In our LS series, it occurred in 6%. Hemorrhage was responsible for 75% of conversions to an open procedure. Defects of clotting factors and platelets cause bleeding from raw surfaces of the splenic bed, diaphragm, retroperitoneum, and less frequently from the pancreatic surface. Occasionally, topical hemostatic agents are necessary. The argon beam coagulator can be extremely useful when diffuse oozing complicates the mobilization of an adherent spleen. Bleeding from a single vessel caused by a dislodged or missing ligature may occur and can lead to reoperation. Meticulous hemostasis and accurate dissection can avoid this problem.

Hemorrhage may occur when the splenic vessels are being encircled.[64,71,95,100,101] Either the vessel being dissected or a posterior branch can be torn or punctured with a dissector. The risk is lessened by gentle dissection on both sides of the vessel, with a change in position of the laparoscopic viewing angle to visualize the sides and back of the vessel. If bleeding occurs, a grasper is used to apply pressure to the injured vessel until the field has been suctioned and the operative team has made a plan for ligation of the vessel. Additional trocars may be inserted for better exposure and control. Bleeding from a capsular tear of the spleen is best managed with hemostatic agents or with the argon beam coagulator. Minor bleeding from the splenic bed or ligated hilum can be controlled with pretied loop ligatures, electrocautery, or argon beam coagulation. The use of a cell saver autotransfusion device can minimize the need for transfusion of banked blood. While routine use is costly and unnecessary, the cell saver can be advantageous in patients with conditions that increase the risk for intraoperative hemorrhage, such as splenic abscess, AIDS, lymphoma, or coagulopathy.

Injury to Adjacent Organs

Injuries to structures adjacent to the spleen, reported in 1% to 3% of OS, have been rare during LS. The magnification of the laparoscopic technique seems to afford a better view of the organs and will probably decrease iatrogenic injuries.

Pancreas

Pancreatic injuries occur in 1% to 3% of OS[910] and in as many as 7% of patients with hemolytic malignancies.[92] Signs of pancreatic injury include abdominal tenderness, atelectasis, pleural effusion, and elevated serum amylase and lipase. Pancreatic injuries are avoided by adequate mobilization and elevation of the spleen in a bloodless field before dissection of the splenic pedicle and by ligation of the vessels close to the splenic parenchyma. If a pancreatic injury is suspected, a closed suction drain should be placed.

Stomach and Diaphragm

Gastric injuries occur in fewer than 1% of splenectomies.[91] These often are caused by direct trauma, but occasionally result from devascularization and may occur when dense adhesions, incomplete hemostasis, or splenomegaly hinder precise dissection. Excessive use of cautery or failure to identify the plane between the spleen and the stomach can lead to thermal or ischemic injuries. We injured the left hemidiaphragm while dissecting with scissors through dense adhesions caused by prior splenic infarcts. This type of injury may be more likely in the laparoscopic operation because manual blunt dissection cannot be used (except in laparoscopically facilitated technique). Atelectasis, pneumonia, or a subphrenic infection may indicate that one of these injuries exists.

Postoperative Complications

Respiratory

Respiratory complications affect 10% to 48% of patients after OS (atelectasis, 15%; pleural effusion, 11%; pneumonia, 7%–13%).[91] To avoid diaphragmatic irritation from blood and irrigant, the subphrenic space should be aspirated dry at the conclusion of the operation. These complications have been less frequent using the laparoscopic technique, which avoids a subcostal incision. In collected series of LS, atelectasis and pleural effusions occurred in fewer than 4% of cases, and there were no instances of pneumonia. However, ITP patients constitute the majority of cases in most series of LS, and these patients are at lower risk for respiratory complications than are patients in the open series.

Subphrenic Abscess

Subphrenic abscesses are reported to occur in 4% to 8% of OS[92,93] but to date have not been reported in the laparoscopic literature. No laparoscopic cases were performed for trauma, for which associated bowel injuries increase the risk of subphrenic infection.

Wound Problems

Wound complications such as hematoma, seroma, and infection occur because of impaired wound healing, coagulation abnormalities, steroid use, and immune defects. Wound infections occur in 3% of OS performed for diagnostic indications, in 6% performed for therapeutic indications, and in 11% of patients who require perioperative steroids.[78,102] Infections occasionally lead to incisional hernias and rarely to dehiscence. In our laparoscopic experience, wound complications were seen in only 2% of cases, and all were trivial.[66] However, trocar site hernias may occur, and bowel obstruction from incarceration has been reported following other laparoscopic procedures.

Ileus and Small-Bowel Obstruction

Postoperative ileus and small-bowel obstruction have been reported in 1% to 10% of OS for Hodgkin's disease, with a reoperation rate of 2% to 7%.[93] In the laparoscopic series, there is only one report of a prolonged postoperative ileus.[58]

Fever

Postoperative fever unrelated to any of the common postoperative causes has been reported in the OS literature. It is believed to be secondary to circulating leukoagglutinizing antibodies and is self-limited.[91] This complication has not been reported in the laparoscopic literature.

Thromboembolism

Thromboembolism complicates 2% to 11% of OS[91,93] and is more common in patients who have hypersplenism or myeloproliferative disorders. The presumed causes include eradication of splenic sequestration, removal of regulatory humoral factors produced by the spleen, altered platelet function, thrombocytosis, and thrombus extending from the splenic vein remnant secondary to intimal injury and stasis. Treatment with antiplatelet medication may be of some use if platelets exceed 500,000/mm^3, but no prospective studies have been performed. In addition, thrombolytic agents and anticoagulants may prove to be lifesaving.

Splenosis

Splenosis is defined as the autotransplantation of splenic tissue in an ectopic position and is usually seen following traumatic splenic rupture in children; the reported incidence is 48% to 66%.[103] This is worrisome to the laparoscopic surgeon because the ideal grasper for the spleen has not been developed, and fracture of the spleen may occur. Splenosis may also result from inadvertent spillage of fragments during morcellation of ITP patient spleens. Nevertheless, there have been no reports of splenosis following LS.

Overwhelming Postsplenectomy Infection

Overwhelming postsplenectomy infection (OPSI) follows 4% of splenectomies, with a mortality rate of 1.7%. This phenomenon was first discussed in the early 1950s.[104] It is important to apprise patients of their risks related to OPSI before surgery when possible. Splenectomy reduces phagocytosis and the clearance of microorganisms, the elaboration of specific immune responses, and the production of splenic opsonins.[104] More than 66% of these cases and 80% of deaths occur within the first 2 years of splenectomy. The incidence of this complication following LS should be the same as after OS.

Most important, patients who are to undergo elective splenectomy must be given appropriate vaccines as noted above (see Patient Preparation). Overwhelming postsplenectomy infection is a condition that occurs most commonly in young children. Other preventive measures include the use of prophylactic penicillin for all children younger than 2 years of age after splenectomy and providing adults with a prescription for penicillin to be filled at the first onset of symptoms. The role of prophylactic antibiotics appears somewhat controversial, especially in light of low documented compliance rates. Patients who undergo splenectomy after trauma should undergo vaccination immediately after surgery. Some physicians advise patients to wear a Medic-Alert bracelet.

The practice patterns among trauma surgeons for vaccination were recently studied by survey.[105] Practices vary widely, although 99.2% of surgeons do immunize patients undergoing splenectomy. Nearly all surgeons administer pneumococcal vaccine, 62.8% add the meningococcal vaccine, 72.4% add the *Haemophilus influenzae* vaccine, and 56.7% gave all three. Revaccination practices are extremely varied and show no consensus. Some surgeons administer vaccines after splenorrhaphy, and some also give them for patients with splenic injuries managed nonoperatively.

Acknowledgment. We gratefully acknowledge the assistance of Richard Friedman, MD, in the preparation of the text. All figures reprinted with permission from *Surgical Diseases of the Spleen,* edited by J.R. Hiatt, E.H. Phillips, and L. Morgenstern, © 1997 Springer-Verlag.

References

1. Morgenstern L. A history of splenectomy. In: Hiatt JR, Phillips EH, Morgenstern L, eds. Surgical Diseases of the Spleen. New York: Springer; 1997.
2. Macht DI, Finesilver EM. The effect of splenectomy on integration of muscular movements in the rat. Am J Physiol 1922; 62:525–530.
3. Marble KR, Deckers PJ, Kern KA. Changing role of splenectomy for hematologic disease. J Surg Oncol 1993;52:169–171.
4. Delaitre B, Maignien B. Splenectomy by the laparoscopic approach. Report of a case. Presse Med 1991;20:2263.
5. Friedman RL, Fallas MJ, Carroll BJ, et al. Laparoscopic splenectomy for ITP. The gold standard. Surg Endosc 1996;10:991–995.
6. Llende M, Santiago-Delpin EA, Lavergne J. Immunobiological consequences of splenectomy: a review. J Surg Res 1986;40:85–94.
7. Reiman RS. Pathology of the spleen. In: Hiatt JR, Phillips EH, Morgenstern L, eds. Surgical Diseases of the Spleen. New York: Springer; 1997.
8. Morgenstern L. Benign neoplasms of the spleen. In: Hiatt JR, Phillips EH, Morgenstern L, eds. Surgical Diseases of the Spleen. New York: Springer; 1997.
9. Kohr RM, Haendiges M, Taube RR. Peliosis of the spleen: a rare cause of spontaneous splenic rupture with surgical implications. Am Surg 1993;59:197–199.
10. Ehrlich P, Jamieson CG. Nonparasitic splenic cysts: a case report and review. Can J Surg 1990;33:306–308.
11. Giles FJ, Lim SW. Malignant splenic lesions. In: Hiatt JR. Phillips EH, Mogenstern L, eds. Surgical Diseases of the Spleen. New York: Springer; 1997.
12. Rosenberg SA. Non-Hodgkin's lymphoma—selection of treatment on the basis of histologic type. N Engl J Med 1979;301:924–928.
13. Longo DL, Devita VT, Jaffe ES, et al. Lymphocytic lymphomas. In: Devita VT, Hellman S, Rosenberg SA, eds. Cancer: Principles and Practice of Oncology. 4th ed. Philadelphia: Lippincott; 1993:1859–1937.
14. Rosenberg SA, Kaplan HS. Evidence for an orderly progression in the spread of Hodgkin's disease. Cancer Res 1966;26:1225–1231.
15. Moormeier JA, Williams SF, Golomb HM. The staging of Hodgkin's disease. Hematol Oncol Clin North Am 1989;3:237–251.
16. Williams SF, Golomb HM. Perspective on staging approaches in the malignant lymphomas. Surg Gynecol Obstet 1986;163:193–201.
17. Johna S, Lefor AT. Laparoscopic evaluation of lymphoma. Semin Surg Oncol 1998;15:176–182.
18. Bloomfield CD, DeCosse JJ. Staging laparotomy. Arch Surg 1978;113:1135–1142.
19. Urba WJ, Longo DL. Hodgkin's disease. N Engl J Med 1992; 326:678–687.
20. Moskowitz C. An update on the management of relapsed and primary refractory Hodgkin's disease. Semin Oncol 2004;31(2 suppl):54–59.
21. Lefor AT. Laparoscopic staging of abdominal lymphomas. In: Greene F, Rosin RD, eds. Minimal Access Surgical Oncology. New York: Radcliffe; 1995.
22. Baccarini U, Carroll BJ, Hiatt JR, et al. Comparison of laparoscopic and open staging in Hodgkin disease. Arch Surg 1998;133:517–522.
23. Carroll BJ, Phillips EH, Semel CJ, et al. Laparoscopic splenectomy. Surg Endosc 1992;6:183–185.
24. Tulman S, Holcomb GW, Karamanoukian HL, Reynhout J. Pediatric laparoscopic splenectomy. J Pediatr Surg 1993;28:689–692.
25. Lefor AT, Flowers JL, Heyman MR. Laparoscopic staging of Hodgkin's disease. Surg Oncol 1993;2:217–220.
26. Greene FL, Cooler AW. Laparoscopic evaluation of lymphomas. Semin Laparosc Surg 1994;1:13–17.
27. Thiruvengadam R, O'Brien S, Kantarjian H, et al. Splenectomy in advanced chronic lymphocytic leukemia. Leukemia 1990; 4:758–760.
28. Cusack JC, Seymour JF, Lerner S, et al. Role of splenectomy in chronic lymphocytic leukemia. J Am Coll Surg 1997;185:237–243.
29. Ratain MJ, Vardiman JW, Barker CM, Golomb HM. Prognostic variables in hairy cell leukemia after splenectomy as initial therapy. Cancer (Phila) 1988;62:2420–2424.
30. Tallman MS, Hakimian D, Variakojis D, et al. A single cycle of 2-chlorodeoxy-adenosine results in complete remission in the majority of patients with hairy cell leukemia. Blood 1992;2203–2209.
31. Bouvet M, Barbiera GV, Termuhlen PM, et al. Splenectomy in the accelerated or blastic phase of chronic myelogenous leukemia: a single-institution, 25 year experience. Surgery (St. Louis) 1997;122:20–25.
32. Kehoe J, Straus DJ. Primary lymphoma of the spleen. Cancer (Phila) 1988;62:1433–1438.
33. Morgenstern L. The remaining indications for open splenectomy. Probl Gen Surg 2002;19:9–15.
34. Mostafa G, Matthews BD, Sing RF, et al. Elective laparoscopic splenectomy for grade III splenic injury in an athlete. Surg Laparosc Endosc Percut Technol 2002;12:283–286.
35. Nance ML, Holmes JH, Wiebe DJ. Timeline to operative intervention for solid organ injuries in children. J Trauma 2006; 61:1389–1392.
36. Godley CD, Warren RL, Sheridan RL, McCabe CJ. Nonoperative management of blunt splenic injury in adults: age over 55 years as a powerful indicator for failure. J Am Coll Surg 1996; 183:133.
37. Albrecht RM, Schermer CR, Morris A. Non-operative management of blunt splenic injuries: factors influencing success in age > 55 years. Am Surg 2002;68:227–230.
38. Dent D, Alsabrook G, Erickson BA, et al. Blunt splenic injuries: high nonoperative management rate can be achieved with selective embolization. J Trauma-Injury Infect Crit Care 2004;56:1063–1067.
39. Haan JM, Biffl, Knudson MM, et al. Splenic embolization revisited: a multicenter review. J Trauma-Injury Infect Crit Care 2004;56:542–547.
40. Richardson JD. Changes in the management of injuries to the liver and spleen. J Am College Surg 2005;200:648–668.
41. Haan J, Ilahi ON, Kramer M, et al. Protocol-driven nonoperative management in patients with blunt splenic trauma and minimal associated injury decreases length of stay. J Trauma-Injury Infect Crit Care 2003;55:317–321.
42. Catalano O, Lobianco R, Sandomenico F, Siani A. Splenic trauma: evaluation with contrast-specific sonography and a second-generation contrast medium: preliminary experience. J Ultrasound Med 2003;22:467–477.
43. Rajani RR, Claridge JA, Yowler CJ, et al. Improved outcome of adult blunt splenic injury: a cohort analysis. Surgery 2006; 140:625–632.
44. Cadeddu M, Garnett A, Al-Anezi K, Farrokhyar F. Management of spleen injuries in the adult trauma population: a 10 year experience. Can J Surg 2006;49:386–390.

45. Pickhardt B, Moore EE, Moore FA, McCroskey BL, Moore GE. Operative splenic salvage in adults: a decade perspective. J Trauma 1989;29:1386–1393.
46. Rizk N, Chapault G, Boutelier P. Laparoscopic splenic salvage in blunt abdominal trauma. Acta Chir Belg 1995;95:202.
47. Lipshy KA, Shaffer DJ, Denning DA. An institutional review of the management of splenic trauma. Contemp Surg 1996; 48:330.
48. Holdsworth RJ. Regeneration of the spleen and splenic autotransplantation. Br J Surg 1991;78:270.
49. Schwartz SI. Role of splenectomy in hematologic disorders. World J Surg 1996;20:1156–1159.
50. Dawson AA, Jones PF, King DL. Splenectomy in the management of hematological disease. Br J Surg 1987;74:353–357.
51. Croom RD, McMillan CW, Sheldon GW, Orringer EP. Hereditary spherocytosis. Ann Surg 1986;203:34–39.
52. Schwartz SI. Splenectomy for hematologic disorders. In: Hiatt JR, Phillips EH, Morgenstern L, eds. Surgical Diseases of the Spleen. New York: Springer; 1997.
53. Lusher JM, Warrier I. Use of intravenous gamma globulin in children and adolescents with ITP and other immune thrombocytopenias. Am J Med 1987;83(suppl):10–15.
54. Winslow GA, Nelson EW. Thrombotic thrombocytopenic purpura: indications for and results of splenectomy. Am J Surg 1995; 170:558–563.
55. Schneider PA, Rayner AA, Linker CA, et al. The role of splenectomy in multimodality treatment of thrombotic thrombocytopenia purpura. Ann Surg 1985;202:318–322.
56. Bell WR, Braine HG, Ness PM, Kickler TS. Improved survival in thrombotic thrombocytopenic purpura-hemolytic uremic syndrome. N Engl J Med 1991;325:398–403.
57. Katz SC, Pachter HL. Indications for splenectomy. Am Surg 2006;72:565–580.
58. Poulin EC, Thibault C, Mamazza J. Laparoscopic splenectomy. Surg Endosc 1995;9:172–177.
59. McAneny D, LaMorte WW, Scott TE, et al. Is splenectomy more dangerous for massive spleens? Am J Surg 1998;175:102–107.
60. Hiatt JR, Allins A, Kong LR. Open splenectomy. In: Hiatt JR, Phillips EH, Morgenstern L, eds. Surgical Diseases of the Spleen. New York: Springer; 1997.
61. Fujitani RM, Johs SM, Cobb SR, et al. Preoperative splenic artery occlusion as an adjunct for high risk splenectomy. Am Surg 1988;54:602–608.
62. Carroll BJ, Phillips EH, Semel CJ, et al. Laparoscopic splenectomy. Surg Endosc 1992;6:183–185.
63. Sandoval C, Stringel G, Ozkaynak MF, et al. Laparoscopic splenectomy in pediatric patients with hematologic diseases. J Soc Laparosc Surg 2000;4:117–120.
64. Delaitre B, Maignien B. Laparoscopic splenectomy: technical aspects. Surg Endosc 1992;6:305–308.
65. Delaitre B. Laparoscopic splenectomy, the hanged spleen technique. Surg Endosc 1995;9:528–529.
66. Phillips EH, Carroll BJ, Fallas MJ. Laparoscopic splenectomy. Surg Endosc 1994;8:931–933.
67. Phillips EH, Caroll BJ, Rosenthal RJ. Laparoscopic splenectomy. In: Cameron JL, ed. Current Surgical Therapy. 5th ed. St. Louis: Mosby; 1995:1069–1072.
68. Sheldon GF, Croom RD, Meyer AA. The spleen. In: Sabiston DC, ed. Textbook of Surgery: The Biological Basis of Modern Surgical Practice. Philadelphia: Saunders; 1991:1108–1133.
69. Asoglu O, Ozmen V, Gorgun E, et al. Does the early ligation of the splenic artery reduce hemorrhage during laparoscopic splenectomy? Surg Laparosc Endosc Percutan Technol 2004;14:118–121.
70. Michel NA. The variational anatomy of the spleen and splenic artery. Am J Anat 1942;70:21–72.
71. Poulin EC, Thibault C. The anatomical basis for laparoscopic splenectomy. Can J Surg 1993;36:484–488.
72. Rege RV, Merriam LT, Joehl RJ. Laparoscopic splenectomy. Surg Clin North Am 1996;76:459–468.
73. Friedman RL, Hiatt JR, Korman JL, et al. Laparoscopic or open splenectomy for hematologic disease: which approach is superior? J Am Coll Surg 1997;185:49–54.
74. Heniford BT, Park A, Walsh RM, et al. Laparoscopic splenectomy in patients with normal-sized spleens versus splenomegaly: does size matter? Am Surg 2001;67:854–857.
75. Terrosu G, Baccarani U, Bresadola V, et al. The impact of splenic weight on laparoscopic splenectomy for splenomegaly.
76. Ailawadi G, Yahanda A, Dimick JB, et al. Hand-assisted laparoscopic splenectomy in patients with splenomegaly or prior upper abdominal operation. Surgery 2002;132:689–694.
77. Watson DI, Coventry BJ, Chin T, et al. Laparoscopic splenectomy for ITP. Surgery (St. Louis) 1997;121:18–22.
78. Musser G, Lazar G, Hocking W, Busuttil RW. Splenectomy for hematologic disease: the UCLA experience with 306 patients. Ann Surg 1984;200:40–45.
79. Rescorla FJ, Engum SA, West KW, et al. Laparoscopic splenectomy has become the gold standard in children. Am Surg 2002;68:297–301.
80. Burch M, Misra M, Phillips EH. Splenic malignancy: a minimally invasive approach. Cancer J 2005;11:36–42.
81. Poulin EC, Thibault C, DesCoteaux JG, Cote G. Partial laparoscopic splenectomy for trauma: technique and case report. Surg Laparosc Endosc 1995;5:306–310.
82. Uranues S, Grossman D, Ludwig L, Bergamaschi R. Laparoscopic partial splenectomy. Surg Endosc 2007;21:57–60.
83. Walters DN, Roberts JL, Votaw M. Accessory splenectomy in the management of recurrent immune thrombocytopenic purpura. Am Surg 1998;64:1077–1078.
84. Flowers JL, Lefor AT, Steers J, et al. Laparoscopic splenectomy in patients with hematologic diseases. Ann Surg 1996;224:19–28.
85. Gigot JF, Healy ML, Ferrant A, Michaux JL, Njinou B, Kestens PJ. Laparoscopic splenectomy for idiopathic thrombocytopenic purpura. Br J Surg 1994;81:1171–1172.
86. Coventry BJ, Watson DI, Tucker K, et al. Intraoperative scintigraphic localization and laparoscopic excision of accessory splenic tissue. Surg Endosc 1998;12:159–161.
87. Steers JA, Lefor AT, Flowers JL. Laparoscopic accessory splenectomy for recurrent thrombocytopenia. Surg Rounds 1994;17:477–481.
88. Kaban GK, Czerniach DR, Prugni RA, et al. Use of a laparoscopic hand assist device for accessory splenectomy. Surg Endosc 2004;18:1001.
89. Danforth DN, Thorbjarnarson B. Incidental splenectomy: a review of the literature and the New York Hospital experience. Ann Surg 1976;183:124–129.
90. Aksnes J, Abdelnoor M, Mathisen O. Risk factors associated with mortality and morbidity after elective splenectomy. Eur J Surg 1995;161:253–258.
91. Ellison EC, Fabri PJ. Complications of splenectomy: etiology, prevention and management. Surg Clin N Am 1983;63:1313–1330.
92. Horowitz J, Smith JL, Weber TK, Rodriguez-Bigas MA, Petrelli NJ. Postoperative complications after splenectomy for hematologic malignancies. Ann Surg 1996;223:290–296.
93. MacRae HM, Yakimets WW, Reynolds T. Perioperative complications of splenectomy for hematologic disease. Can J Surg 1992;35:432–436.
94. Gigot JF, Jamar F, Ferrant A, et al. Inadequate detection of accessory spleens and splenosis with laparoscopic splenectomy. Surg Endosc 1998;12:101–106.
95. Lefor AT, Melvin WS, Bailey RW, Flowers JL. Laparoscopic splenectomy in the management of immune thrombocytopenia purpura. Surgery (St. Louis) 1993;114:613–618.

96. Rhodes M, Rudd M, O'Rourke N, Nathanson L, Fielding G. Laparoscopic splenectomy and lymph node biopsy for hematologic disorders. Ann Surg 1995;222:43–46.
97. Yee LF, Carvajal SH, Lorimier A, Mulvihill SJ. Laparoscopic splenectomy: an initial experience at University of California, San Francisco. Arch Surg 1995;130:874–878.
98. Hanley ES. Anesthesia for laparoscopic surgery. Surg Clin North Am 1992;72:1013–1019.
99. Phillips JM. Laparoscopy. Baltimore: Williams & Wilkins; 1977: 220–246.
100. Cadiere GB, Verroken R, Himpens J, Bruyns J, Efira M, DeWitt S. Operative strategy in laparoscopic splenectomy. J Am Coll Surg 1994;179:668–672.
101. Cuschieri A, Shimi S, Banting S, Vander Velpen G. Technical aspects of laparoscopic splenectomy: hilar segemental devascularization and instrumentation. J R Coll Surg Edinb 1992;37:414–416.
102. Jockovich M, Mendenhall NP, Sombeck MD, Talbert JL, Copeland EM III, Bland KI. Long-term complications of laparotomy in Hodgkin's disease. Ann Surg 1994;219:615–624.
103. Mintz SJ, Petersen SR, Cheson B, Cordell LJ, Richards RC. Splenectomy for immune thrombocytopenic purpura. Arch Surg 1981;116:645–650.
104. Shaw JHF, Print CG. Postsplenectomy sepsis. Br J Surg 1989; 76:1074–1081.
105. Shatz DV. Vaccination practices among North American trauma surgeons in splenectomy for trauma. J Trauma-Injury Infect Crit Care 2002;53:950–956.
106. Delaitre B, Pitre J. Laparoscopic splenectomy versus open splenectomy: a comparative study. Hepatogastroenterology 1997;44:45–49.
107. Diaz J, Eisenstat M, Chung R. A case-controlled study of laparoscopic splenectomy. Am J Surg 1997;173:348–350.
108. Smith CD, Meyer TA, Goretsky MJ, et al. Laparoscopic splenectomy by the lateral approach. Surgery (St. Louis) 1996;120:789–794.
109. Cogliandolo A, Berland-Dai B, Pidoto RR, Marc OS. Results of laparoscopic and open splenectomy for nontraumatic diseases. Surg Laparosc Endosc Percut Technol 2001;11:256–261.
110. Yuan RH, Chen SB, Lee WJ, Yu SC. Advantages of laparoscopic splenectomy due to hematologic diseases. J Formosan Med Assoc 1998;97:485–489.
111. Glasgow RE, Yee LF, Mulvihill SJ. Laparoscopic splenectomy. The emerging standard. Surg Endosc 1997;11:108–112.
112. Brunt LM, Langer JC, Quasebarth MA, Whitman ED. Comparative analysis of laparoscopic versus open splenectomy. Am J Surg 1996;172:596–599.
113. Marassi A, Vignali A, Zuliani W, et al. Splenectomy for ITP: comparison of laparoscopic and conventional surgery. Surg Endosc 1999;13:17–20.
114. Tanoue K, Hashizume M, Akahoshi T, et al. Laparoscopic splenectomy: the latest modern technique. Hepatogastroenterology 1999;46:820–824.
115. Shimomatsuya T, Horiuchi T. Laparoscopic splenectomy for treatment of patients with ITP. Comparison with open splenectomy. Surg Endosc 1999;13:563–566.
116. Lozano-Salazar R, Herrera MF, Bezaury P, et al. Laparoscopic splenectomy in ITP. Rev Invest Clin 1998;50:127–132.
117. Schlinkert RT, Tsiotos G. Laparoscopic splenectomy for ITP. Arch Surg 1997;132:642–646.
118. Curran TJ, Foley MI, Swanstrom LL, Campbell TJ. Laparoscopy improves outcomes for pediatric splenectomy. J Pediatr Surg 1998;33:1498–1500.
119. Esposito C, Corcione F, Garipoli V, Ascione G. Pediatric laparoscopic splenectomy: are there real advantages in comparison with the traditional open approach? Pediatr Surg Int 1997;12:509–510.
120. Terrosu G, Donini A, Baccarani U, et al. Laparoscopic versus open splenectomy in the management of splenomegaly: our preliminary experience. Surgery (St. Louis) 1998;124:839–843.
121. Targarona EM, Cerdan G, Gracia E, et al. Results of laparoscopic splenectomy for treatment of malignant conditions. HPB Surg 2001;3:251–255.
122. Torelli P, Cavaliere D, Casaccia M, et al. Laparoscopic splenectomy for hematological diseases. Surg Endosc 2002;16:965–971.
123. Rosen M, Brody F, Walsh RM, et al. Outcome of laparoscopic splenectomy based on hematologic indication. Surg Endosc 2002;16:272–279.
124. Rescorla FJ, Breitfeld PP, West KW, et al. A case controlled comparison of open and laparoscopic splenectomy in children. Surgery (St. Louis) 1998;124:670–675.
125. Farah RA, Rogers ZR, Thompson WR, et al. Comparison of laparoscopic and open splenectomy in children with hematologic disorders. J Pediatr 1997;131:41–46.
126. Janu PG, Rogers DA, Lobe TE. A comparison of laparoscopic and traditional open splenectomy in childhood. J Pediatr Surg 1996;31:109–113.
127. Hicks BA, Thompson WR, Rogers ZR, Guzzetta PC. Laparoscopic splenectomy in childhood hematologic disorders. J Laparoendosc Surg 1996;1(suppl):S31–S34.
128. Yoshida K, Yamazaki Y, Mizuno R, et al. Laparoscopic splenectomy in children. Preliminary results and comparison with the open technique. Surg Endosc 1995;9:1279–1282.
129. Beanes S, Emil S, Kosi M, et al. A comparison of laparoscopic versus open splenectomy in children. Am Surg 1995;61:908–910.

53 Hernias and Abdominal Wall Defects

Daniel J. Scott and Daniel B. Jones

No disease of the human body, belonging to the province of the surgeon, requires in its treatment, a better combination of accurate, anatomical knowledge with surgical skill than Hernia in all its varieties.

Sir Astley Paston Cooper, *The Anatomy and Surgical Treatment of Inguinal and Congenital Hernia*, Cox, London, 1804

Groin Hernias

Definitions

A *hernia* is a protrusion of visceral contents through the abdominal wall. There are two key components of a hernia. The first is the defect itself, namely, the size and location of the defect. The second component is the hernia sac, which is a protrusion of peritoneum through the defect. The hernia sac may contain abdominal contents such as small intestine, colon, or bladder, or the sac may be empty.

A *sliding hernia* exists when a retroperitoneal organ, usually the sigmoid colon, cecum, bladder, or ureter, forms part of the wall of the sac; these organs may be injured during hernia repair. A *Richter's hernia* exists when the antimesenteric portion of intestine (not the complete circumference of bowel) protrudes into the hernia sac. A *Littre's hernia* exists when the sac contains a Meckel's diverticulum. If the sac and its contents can be returned to the abdominal cavity, a hernia is termed *reducible.* If it cannot be returned to the abdominal cavity, as is sometimes the case with a small fascial defect and a large hernia, the hernia is termed *irreducible* or *incarcerated.* If an irreducible hernia contains intestine or other viscera with blood supply that is compromised, the hernia is *strangulated.* This can lead to a life-threatening situation in which the hernia sac contains gangrenous bowel and requires emergent exploration.

Anatomy

Successful repair of a groin hernia requires thorough knowledge of the anatomy of the abdominal wall, inguinal canal, and femoral canal. The layers of the abdominal wall (Fig. 53.1), from superficial to deep, include skin, Camper's fascia, Scarpa's fascia, the external oblique aponeurosis and muscle, the internal oblique aponeurosis and muscle, the transversus abdominis aponeurosis and muscle, the transversalis fascia, the preperitoneal fat, and the peritoneum. These layers continue in the region of the groin as they form their insertions in the inguinal canal.

Inguinal Canal

Several structures course within the inguinal canal (Fig. 53.2) and require familiarity to avoid iatrogenic injury during herniorraphy. The canal contains the spermatic cord in males and the round ligament of the uterus in females. The canal lies obliquely between the internal or deep inguinal ring, derived from transversalis fascia, and the external or superficial inguinal ring, derived from external oblique aponeurosis.

The spermatic cord courses from the internal ring through the inguinal canal and exits through the external ring to join the testicle within the scrotum. The spermatic cord contains multiple structures (Table 53.1), including the superficial spermatic fascia, derived from Camper's and Scarpa's fascia; the external spermatic fascia, derived from external oblique muscle; a circumferential layer of cremaster muscle, derived from internal oblique muscle; the cremasteric or external spermatic artery; the internal spermatic fascia, derived from transversalis fascia; the vas deferens and arteries to the vas deferens; the testicular or internal spermatic artery, which arises from the aorta just inferior to the renal arteries; the pampiniform venous plexus, which coalesces into the testicular veins and drains into the inferior vena cava on the right and the renal vein on the left; the ilioinguinal nerve; the genital branch of the genitofemoral nerve; and sympathetic fibers from the hypogastric plexus.

The inguinal canal can be defined by its borders (Fig. 53.3). The inguinal canal is bound anteriorly by the external oblique aponeurosis, superiorly by internal oblique and transversus abdominis muscles and aponeuroses, and inferiorly by the inguinal and lacunar ligaments. The posterior wall or floor is formed by transversalis fascia. A defect in this layer may

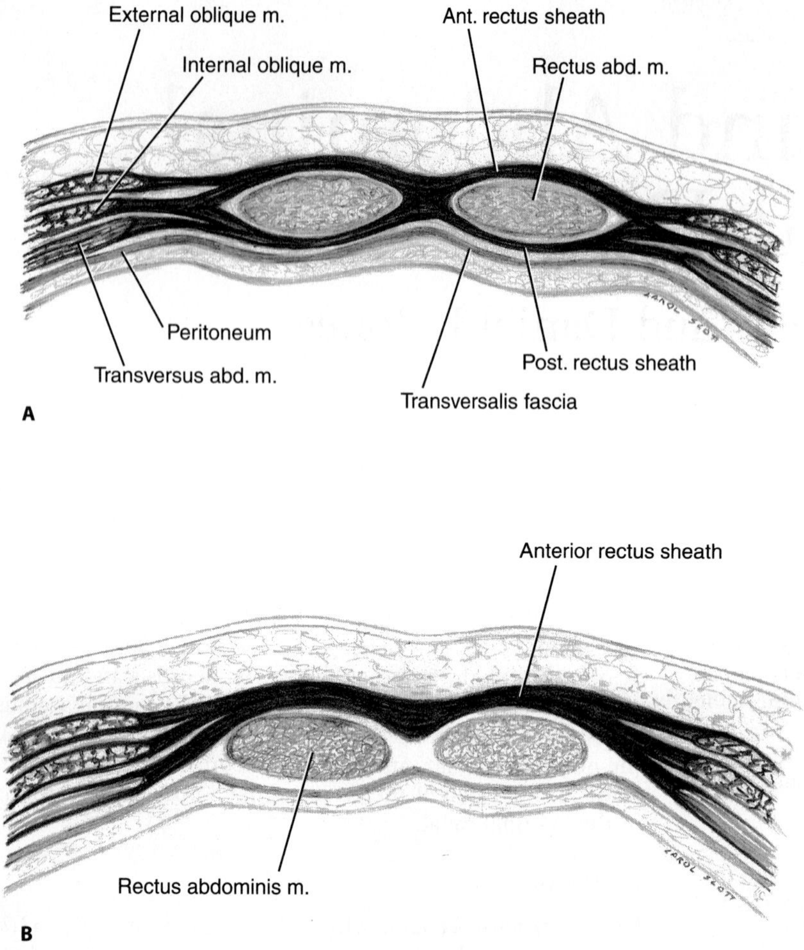

FIGURE 53.1. Abdominal wall layers (**A**), above the semicircular line of Douglas, and (**B**), below the semicircular line.

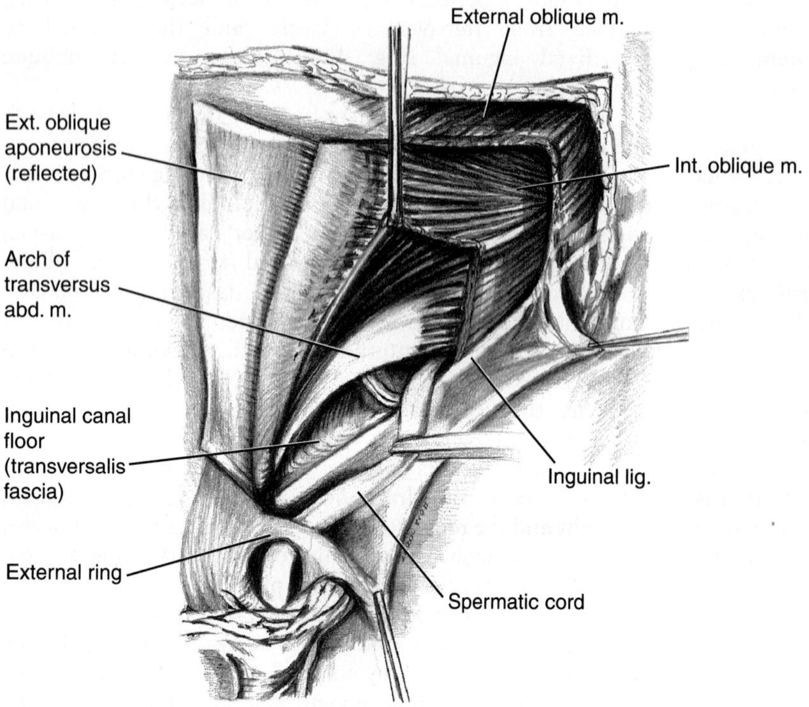

FIGURE 53.2. The inguinal canal with the external oblique aponeurosis incised and reflected.

TABLE 53.1. Spermatic Cord Contents.

Nerves
Ilioinguinal nerve
Genital branch of genitofemoral nerve
Sympathetic fibers
Arteries
Cremasteric (external spermatic) artery
Testicular (internal spermatic) artery
Arteries to vas deferens
Veins
Pampiniform plexus
Muscle
Cremaster muscle
Fascia
Superficial spermatic fascia
External spermatic fascia
Internal spermatic fascia
Vas deferens

allow peritoneum and the contents of the abdominal cavity to herniate. *Hesselbach's triangle* is formed by the inguinal ligament laterally, the rectus sheath medially, and the inferior epigastric vessels superiorly (Fig. 53.4). A direct hernia protrudes through the floor of the inguinal canal within this triangle (medial to the inferior epigastric vessels). Thus, a direct hernia is a protrusion of peritoneum through the transversalis fascia; it lies adjacent to (not within) the spermatic cord. The hernia sac exits the canal with the cord through the external ring into the scrotum. An indirect hernia forms lateral to the inferior epigastric vessels. An indirect hernia lies within the spermatic cord, and with the cord it passes through the internal ring. The hernia sac courses through the inguinal canal and can exit with the cord through the external ring into the scrotum. The sac of an indirect hernia is usually

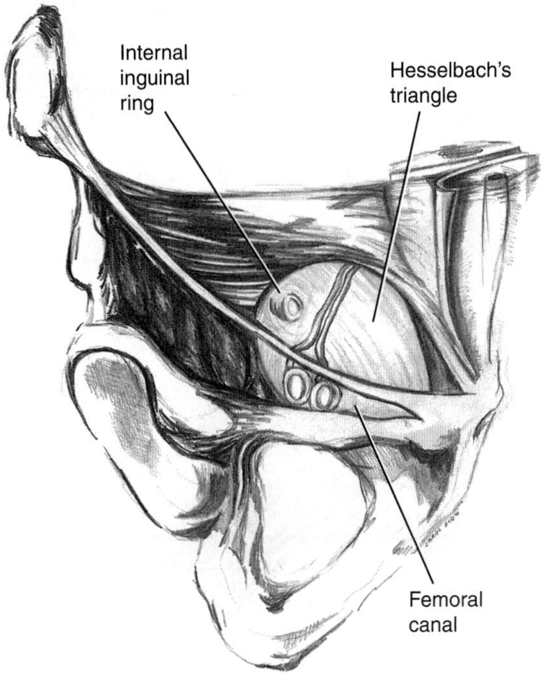

FIGURE 53.4. Indirect inguinal hernias occur through the internal ring. Direct inguinal hernias occur in Hesselbach's triangle, which lies between the inguinal ligament, the rectus sheath, and the inferior epigastric vessels. Femoral hernias occur through the femoral canal, which lies between the inguinal ligament, the lacunar ligament, Cooper's ligament, and the femoral vein. Fruchaud's myopectineal orifice refers to the entire musculoaponeurotic area through which inguinal and femoral hernias can occur.

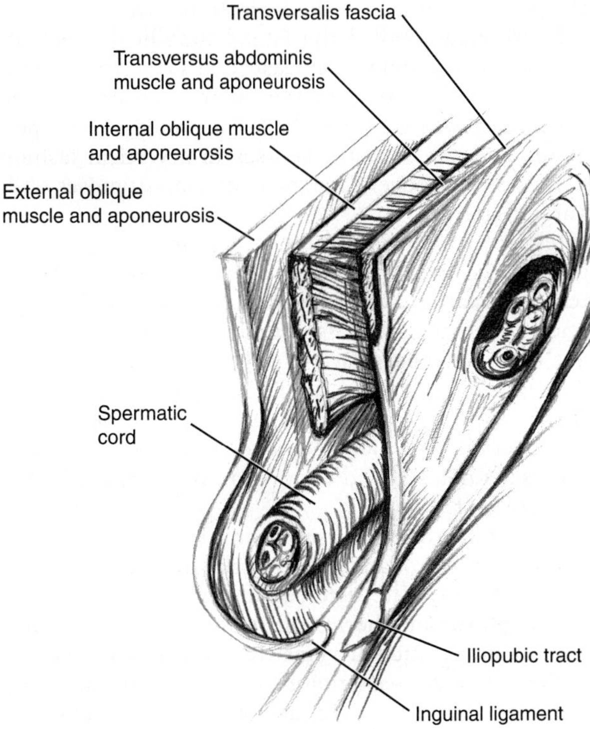

FIGURE 53.3. The inguinal canal in cross section.

found on the anteriomedial aspect of the cord. Hernias with both a direct and an indirect component are called *pantaloon hernias* since the two components drape over the inferior epigastric vessels like the legs of a pair of trousers.

Femoral Canal

A femoral hernia is a visceral protrusion through the femoral ring, which is bounded laterally by the femoral vein, anteriorly by the inguinal ligament, medially by the lacunar ligament, and posteriorly by Cooper's ligament. The femoral canal (Fig. 53.4) represents an extension of the femoral ring for approximately 2 cm inferior into the thigh. The femoral canal usually contains areolar tissue, lymphatic channels, and lymph nodes that drain the leg and perineum, the highest of which is named the Cloquet node (French) or Rosenmuller node (German). The femoral sheath is derived from transversalis fascia and contains the femoral artery, vein, and canal. The femoral triangle is bounded by the inguinal ligament, the sartorius muscle, and the adductor longus muscle and contains from lateral to medial the femoral nerve, artery, vein, "empty" space (femoral canal), and lymphatics (hence the pneumonic NAVEL).

Nerves

The nerves of the ilioinguinal region (Fig. 53.5) arise from the lumbar plexus, innervate the abdominal musculature, and provide sensation for the skin and parietal peritoneum. Entrapment usually causes severe pain, whereas transection results in numbness. Careful technique and anatomical

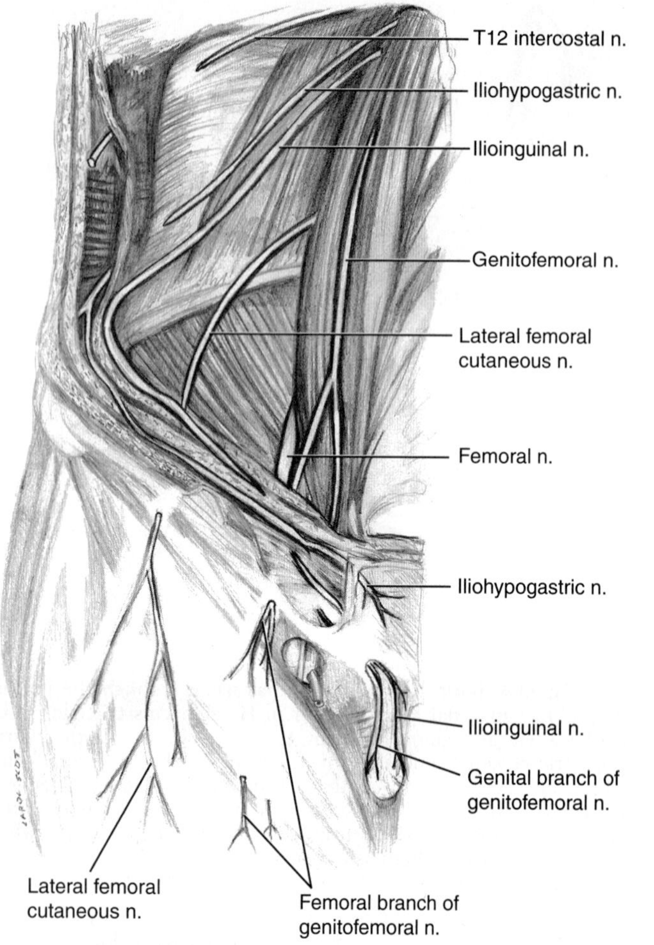

FIGURE 53.5. Nerves of the inguinal region.

knowledge are necessary to avoid nerve injury during herniorraphy.

The iliohypogastric nerve (T12, L1) emerges from the lateral edge of the psoas muscle and courses within the layers of the abdominal wall. It penetrates the external oblique muscle within 1–2 cm of the superiomedial aspect of the external ring, where it supplies the skin in the suprapubic region with sensory fibers. It also provides the afferent and efferent pathways for the abdominal reflex, by which stroking the skin in the suprapubic area produces contraction of the rectus abdominis musculature.

The ilioinguinal nerve (L1) courses with the iliohypogastric nerve and then joins the spermatic cord or round ligament through the internal and external inguinal rings to innervate the skin of the base of the penis or mons pubis, the scrotum or labia majora, and the medial aspect of the thigh. This nerve may be inadvertently cut during exposure of the inguinal canal or entrapped during closure of the external oblique aponeurosis.

The genitofemoral nerve (L1, L2) runs along the anterior aspect of the psoas muscle and divides before reaching the internal inguinal ring. The genital branch penetrates the iliopubic tract lateral to the internal inguinal ring and then enters the ring to join the cord. It supplies the anterior scrotum with sensory fibers and the cremaster muscle with motor fibers and is the efferent limb for the cremasteric reflex (stroking the inner thigh produces contraction of the cremaster muscle and elevation of the ipsilateral testicle). The femoral branch courses beneath the inguinal ligament to provide sensation to the anteriomedial thigh and is the afferent limb for the cremasteric reflex.

The lateral femoral cutaneous nerve (L2, L3) emerges at the lateral edge of the psoas muscle, courses along the iliac fossa, lateral to the iliac vessels, and beneath the iliopubic tract and inguinal ligament to provide sensation to the lateral thigh. Injury of this nerve may be common with inexperienced surgeons performing laparoscopic hernia repair.

The femoral nerve (L2–L4) emerges from the lateral aspect of the psoas muscle and courses beneath the inguinal ligament lateral to the femoral vessels and outside the femoral sheath to provide motor and sensory innervation for the thigh. Care must be taken to avoid femoral nerve injury during femoral hernia repair.

Blood Vessels

There are numerous blood vessels that course through the inguinal region and require familiarity to avoid iatrogenic injury and potentially devastating complications. The external iliac artery and vein lie on the medial aspect of the psoas muscle and course deep to the iliopubic tract to form the femoral artery and vein. The external iliac artery gives off two branches within its distal 2 cm. Laterally, it gives off the deep circumflex iliac artery, which courses along the iliacus muscle, deep to the iliopubic tract, making it at risk for injury during suturing or stapling. Medially, it gives off the inferior epigastric artery. The external iliac vein is medial and posterior to the artery and receives comparable branches. The inferior epigastric vein, however, is paired and joins the external iliac vein approximately 1 cm proximal to the takeoff of the inferior epigastric artery and is thus predisposed to injury.[1]

The inferior epigastric artery and vein cross over the iliopubic tract at the medial aspect of the internal ring and ascend along the posterior surface of the rectus muscles, invested in a fold of peritoneum called the lateral umbilical ligament. Near its takeoff, the inferior epigastric artery gives off two branches, the cremasteric and the pubic. The cremasteric branch penetrates the transversalis fascia and joins the spermatic cord. The pubic branch courses in a vertical fashion inferiorly, crossing Cooper's ligament, and anastomoses with the obturator artery.

The testicular vessels follow the ureter into the pelvis on its lateral border and then course along the lateral edge of the external iliac artery, cross the iliopubic tract, and join the spermatic cord at the lateral aspect of the internal ring. The testicular or internal spermatic artery arises from the aorta just below the renal arteries at the L2 level. Anastomoses between the testicular, deferential, and cremasteric arteries supply the testicle with rich collateral circulation.[2] The testicular veins drain into the inferior vena cava on the right and the renal vein on the left.

The deferential artery arises from the inferior vesicle artery, forming a microvascular network with the adventitia of the vas deferens. The deferential vein drains into the pampiniform plexus and the vesical plexus. The pampiniform plexus drains into testicular veins that course with the testicular artery. The cremasteric or external spermatic artery arises from the inferior epigastric artery. The cremasteric vein drains into the inferior epigastric vein.

Myopectineal Orifice

Fruchaud published in 1956 the idea that all hernias originate in a single weak area called the myopectineal orifice (Fig. 53.4).[3] This area is bounded superiorly by the internal oblique and transversus abdominis muscles, inferiorly by the superior pubic ramus, medially by the rectus muscle and sheath, and laterally by the iliopsoas muscle. Inguinal and femoral hernias occur within this area.

Inguinal Ligament

The inguinal ligament or Poupart's ligament forms from the thickened lateral inferior edge of the external oblique aponeurosis (Figs. 53.2 and 53.3). The ligament courses between the anterior superior iliac spine and the pubic tubercle.

Iliopubic Tract

The iliopubic tract is a thickened lateral extension of the transversalis fascia that runs from the superior pubic ramus to the iliopectineal arch (Fig. 53.3). It is anterior to Cooper's ligament and posterior to the inguinal ligament. Although intimately associated with the inguinal ligament, the iliopubic tract is a separate structure and serves a crucial anatomical role in preperitoneal hernia repairs as well as some anterior repairs.

Lacunar Ligament

The lacunar ligament or Gimbernat's ligament is the most inferior and posterior portion of the inguinal ligament. The ligament is triangular, and its fibers curve to meet Cooper's ligament as it inserts onto the pubic symphysis, forming the medial aspect of the femoral canal.

Cooper's Ligament

Cooper's ligament or the pectineal ligament is a condensation of transversalis fascia and periosteum of the superior pubic ramus lateral to the pubic tubercle. It is several millimeters thick, densely adherent to the pubic ramus, and joins the iliopubic tract and lacunar ligaments at their medial insertions. Cooper's ligament can be readily palpated as a thick strong fibrous band, and it is shiny when freed from surrounding fat and soft tissue.

Conjoined Tendon

The existence of this structure is debated or at least variable, but it is thought to be a fusion of the lower fibers of the internal oblique muscle and the aponeurosis of the transversus abdominis muscle at their insertions onto the pubic tubercle. This structure is largely indistinct from and confused with the falx inguinalis or ligament of Henle, which is derived from transversalis fascia as it forms the thickened lateral aspect of the rectus sheath at its insertion onto the pubic symphysis. Based on work from Hollinshead, Condon, and McVay, Skandalakis et al. concluded that the conjoined tendon and the falx inguinalis rarely exist and are usually mistaken for the lateral rectus sheath.[4]

Preperitoneal Space

Both in open and laparoscopic preperitoneal approaches to hernia repair, a sound understanding of the anatomical structures in the groin from a seemingly reversed perspective is necessary. The preperitoneal space (Fig. 53.6) is bounded internally by the peritoneum and externally by the transversalis fascia and contains fat, blood vessels, lymphatics, nerves, and the vas deferens. Some landmarks in this area are helpful in gaining a proper perspective. The peritoneum drapes over the deep aspect of the abdominal wall covering the remnant of the urachus, the obliterated umbilical arteries, and the inferior epigastric vessels to form the median, medial, and lateral umbilical ligaments, respectively. Between and in close proximity to the inferior aspect of medial umbilical folds lies the bladder. Arising from the seminal vesicle, the

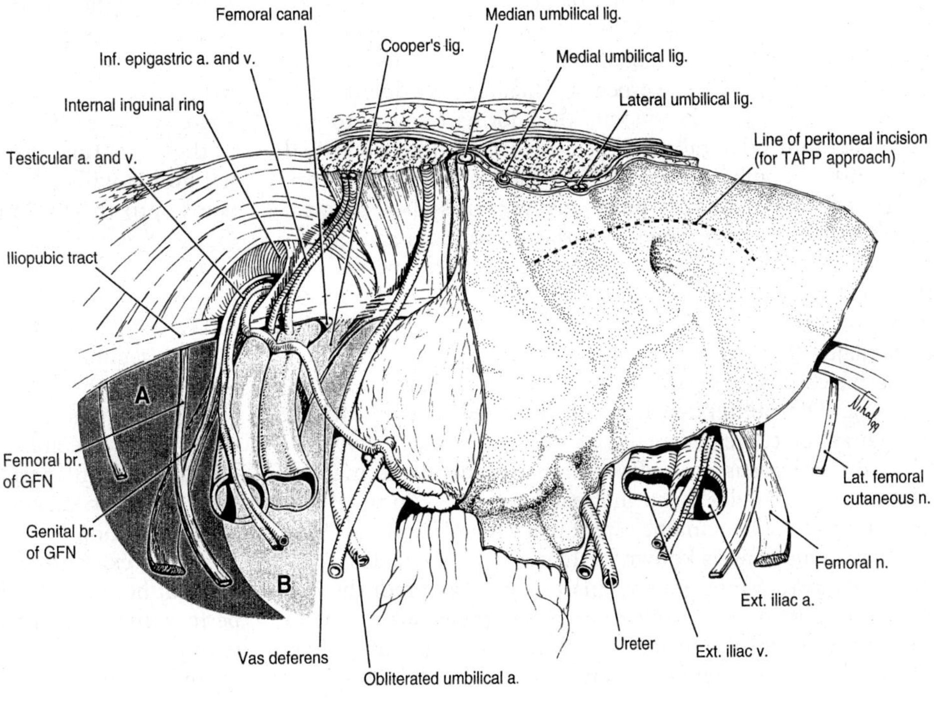

FIGURE 53.6. The preperitoneal space as viewed from within the abdomen. *Shaded area* **A** designates the triangle of pain. *Shaded area* **B** designates the triangle of doom. These areas contain nerves and blood vessels that are at risk of injury during hernia repair. GFN, genitofemoral nerve.

vas deferens courses laterally over Cooper's ligament, the external iliac vessels, and the iliopubic tract to enter the medial aspect of the internal ring and join the spermatic cord. Entering the internal ring laterally are the testicular vessels. The testicular vessels and the vas deferens at the internal ring form the apex of a theoretical triangle called the *triangle of doom*. Within this triangle lie the external iliac artery and vein, as well as the genital and femoral branches of the genitofemoral nerve, hidden under peritoneum and transversalis fascia, placing them at high risk of injury. The *triangle of pain* lies lateral to this, and its apex is formed inferomedially by the testicular vessels and superolaterally by the iliopubic tract. Within this triangle lie the femoral branch of the genitofemoral nerve, the femoral nerve, and the lateral cutaneous femoral nerve. Stapling of these structures during a laparoscopic hernia repair results in painful neuralgias and should be avoided.

Two eponyms refer to the preperitoneal space in the area of the bladder. The space of Retzius is retropubic and situated in front of and to the sides of the bladder. The space of Bogros is a lateral extension to the space of Retzius, bounded laterally by the iliac fascia, anteriorly by the transversalis fascia, and medially by the peritoneum.

A significant amount of preperitoneal fat may be present. If this fat herniates through the internal inguinal ring, it is known as a cord lipoma and may mimic an indirect hernia.

Etiology

There is no doubt that the first appearance of the mammal, with his unexplained need to push his testicles out of their proper home into the air, made a mess of the three layered abdominal wall that had done the reptiles well for 200 million years.

Sir Heneage Ogilvie, *Hernia*, Edward Arnold, London, 1959

Inguinal hernias may be caused by congenital factors, especially in children.[5] This necessitates an understanding of the embryology of the inguinal region for proper surgical management. The ligamentous gubernaculum descends on each side of the abdomen from the inferior pole of the gonad to the internal surface of the labial-scrotal swelling. The gubernaculum passes through the abdominal wall at the site of the future inguinal canal. The processus vaginalis is a diverticular evagination of the peritoneum that forms ventral to the gubernaculum bilaterally and passes through the abdominal wall with the gubernaculum. The testes are initially retroperitoneal, and with the processus vaginalis they descend through the inguinal canal into the scrotum as the gubernaculum contracts. The ovaries descend into the pelvis, and the inferior aspect of the gubernaculum becomes the round ligament, which passes through the internal ring into the labia majus. The processus vaginalis normally closes, obliterating this extension of the peritoneal cavity through the internal ring. The obliterated remnant attached to the testis is known as the tunica vaginalis.

If the processus vaginalis remains patent in the male, a variety of hydroceles or an indirect hernia may form. If the processus vaginalis remains patent in a female, it extends into the labia majus and is known as the canal of Nuck. The incidence of a patent processus vaginalis is 60% at 2 months and 40% at 2 years of age.[6] However, a patent processus vaginalis does not uniformly translate into having an inguinal hernia; the incidence of a patent processus vaginalis in adults without clinical appearance of a hernia is 20% to 30% in autopsy series.[5]

A variety of connective tissue abnormalities have also been demonstrated as associated with an increased incidence of hernias. Abnormal collagen structure and composition, as well as fibroblast dysfunction, have been noted in several studies.[7,8] Related to collagen formation, malnutrition and vitamin deficiencies have been implicated as contributing factors. Increased elastiolytic enzyme levels found in cigarette smokers and in patients with aortic aneurysms have been associated with groin hernias.[9] Connective tissue disorders such as Ehlers-Danlos syndrome and Marfan syndrome are also associated with an increased incidence of hernias.[10]

Increased intraabdominal pressure has also been associated with hernia formation. This is especially true with peritoneal dialysis and ascites.[11] Obesity and advanced age are also risk factors. Chronic cough in patients with chronic obstructive pulmonary disease, straining in patients with benign prostatic hypertrophy or chronic constipation, or strenuous labor may increase the wear-and-tear effect on the abdominal wall and increase the risk of hernia formation.[10]

Diagnosis

The gold standard for hernia diagnosis is a history and physical exam. Patients will usually complain of a persistent or intermittent bulge in the groin associated with some degree of discomfort, aggravated by physical exertion. If the hernia is reducible, the pain may wax and wane. A more persistent pain is typical of an incarcerated hernia. If fever, tachycardia, exquisite tenderness on palpation, erythema of the overlying skin, leukocytosis, and obstructive symptoms are present, an irreducible hernia is likely strangulated and warrants immediate operative intervention.

To examine a patient for a groin hernia, the physician is seated, and the disrobed patient stands and faces the examiner. First, the groin is visually inspected for evidence of a bulge and then palpated with the patient straining either by coughing or by performing a Valsalva maneuver. Next, this procedure is repeated with the examiner's gloved finger inserted into the redundant scrotal skin, reaching onto the abdominal wall and into the external inguinal ring, just lateral to the pubic tubercle. During the straining exercise, an inguinal hernia will be evident as a bulge or mass pushing downward onto the examiner's fingertip. The same examination can be performed on females by inserting the finger into the labia majus to gain access to the external ring. Although it has been claimed by some that it is possible to distinguish a direct hernia from an indirect one by physical exam, this is neither accurate nor necessary since the operative approach for either is the same.

A femoral hernia will appear as a mass below the inguinal ligament in the area medial to the femoral pulse and can be elicited by similar straining techniques. Femoral hernias may be difficult to diagnose, especially in obese patients, and a second opinion is frequently reassuring.

After examining the patient for both an inguinal and femoral hernia with the patient standing, the patient should be reexamined in a similar fashion in the supine position. It is important to note that both groins should be examined to exclude bilateral hernias. Masses other than hernias in this

TABLE 53.2. Differential Diagnosis of Groin Masses.

Inguinal hernia
Femoral hernia
Lipoma
Lymphadenitis
Lymphadenopathy
Abscess
Hematoma
Varicocele
Hydrocele
Testicular mass
Testicular torsion
Epididymitis
Ectopic testicle
Femoral aneurysm or pseudoaneurysm
Cyst
Seroma

area must be ruled out, and this can usually be done by physical exam (Table 53.2).

Herniography, by which a small amount of contrast material is injected into the peritoneal cavity and radiographs are taken during a Valsalva maneuver, has been advocated as a useful imaging study in patients with groin pain and no evidence of a hernia on physical exam.[12] Computed tomography (CT) and ultrasound scanning may help exclude other causes of groin masses.

Epidemiology and Classification

Approximately 680,000 inguinal hernia repairs are performed annually.[13] Greater than 90% are performed on males. Female patients undergo three times as many femoral repairs as males, although females undergo three times as many inguinal repairs as femoral repairs. In Rutledge's report of 1437 primary groin hernias, 60% were indirect, 36% direct, and 4% femoral.[14] In the Lichtenstein group's report of 4000 primary inguinal hernias, 44.4% were indirect, 43.1% direct, 12.5% pantaloon, 11.4% sliding, and 25% bilateral.[15] Indirect inguinal hernias are more common on the right side, possibly related to the later descent of the right testicle and delayed closure of the processus vaginalis. The true overall incidence of sliding hernias is only about 2% but rises with age. Multiple classification schemes have been developed; the most widely accepted is the Nyhus classification (Table 53.3).[16]

Management

Traditionally, hernias are electively repaired since the natural history of hernias dictates that they only become larger, do not resolve spontaneously, and can lead to intestinal obstruction or strangulation. However, several investigators have recently questioned the need to repair asymptomatic hernias, and a multicenter prospective randomized trial is underway comparing "watchful waiting" versus a Lichtenstein repair in this population of patients. Meanwhile, most surgeons agree that all symptomatic hernias should be repaired. The only exception to this dictum is in patients too debilitated to undergo repair or in patients whose operative risks are excessively high. In this instance, a truss, a device worn to compress the hernia, may offer some relief of symptoms. Otherwise, trusses are of little benefit and should not be offered as a treatment option. Trusses are contraindicated in femoral hernias due to a high risk of strangulation.[17] With the advent of highly successful local anesthetic techniques for hernia repair, most patients can undergo operative repair.

Generally, it is safe to attempt reduction of an incarcerated hernia in the absence of evidence of strangulation. Analgesics may be required, and Trendelenberg positioning may be helpful. In a chronically incarcerated hernia, a very small but real risk of en masse reduction exists, in which the hernia may be successfully reduced into the abdominal cavity but the contents of the sac remain incarcerated within a constricting fibrous band at the neck of the sac. This is usually manifested as continued obstructive symptoms and can lead to strangulation, bowel necrosis, and even patient death, warranting close follow-up after hernia reduction and immediate exploration if an en masse reduction is thought to have occurred.[18] Any hernia that is unable to be successfully reduced requires prompt operative intervention.

Repairs

Anterior Approaches

The goal of all repairs is to close the myofascial defect through which the hernia protrudes. This can be done from a number of approaches with or without placement of a prosthetic mesh. The classic tissue repairs use permanent suture to reinforce the internal inguinal ring and the floor of the inguinal canal and do not employ the use of a prosthesis. These include the Marcy, Bassini, Shouldice, and McVay repairs. The Lichtenstein repair employs prosthetic mesh, as does the plug technique. Common to all of these methods is the anterior dissection of the inguinal canal and hernia sac, followed by a myofascial repair, and closure of the canal. The basic technique of inguinal canal and sac dissection is the same for all anterior approaches, while the repair of the myofascial defect differs.

In an anterior repair, the groin is explored through an oblique incision parallel to the inguinal ligament in the lines of Langer and is carried down through Camper's and Scarpa's fascias to the external oblique aponeurosis. This aponeurosis is incised parallel to the axis of its fibers perpendicular to and through the external ring, taking care to preserve, if possible,

TABLE 53.3. Nyhus Classification of Groin Hernias.

Type 1.	Indirect inguinal hernia—normal internal inguinal ring
Type 2.	Indirect inguinal hernia—enlarged internal inguinal ring but intact inguinal canal floor
Type 3.	Posterior wall defect
	A. Direct inguinal hernia
	B. Indirect inguinal hernia—enlarged internal inguinal ring with destruction of adjacent inguinal canal floor (e.g., massive scrotal, sliding, or pantaloon hernias)
	C. Femoral hernias
Type 4.	Recurrent hernia
	A. Direct
	B. Indirect
	C. Femoral
	D. Combined

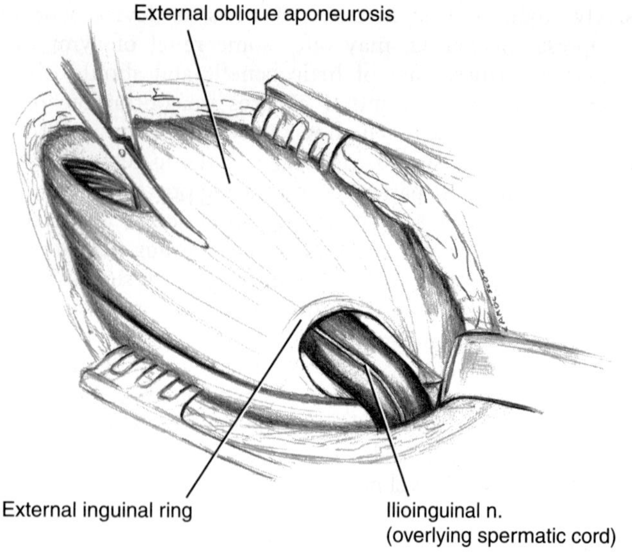

FIGURE 53.7. The external oblique aponeurosis is incised parallel to its fibers, taking care to avoid injury to the ilioinguinal and iliohypogastric nerves.

the underlying ilioinguinal and iliohypogastric nerves (Fig. 53.7). The incision is extended several centimeters lateral to the internal ring, exposing the entire inguinal canal.

The spermatic cord is isolated at the level of the pubic tubercle, completely encircled with a Penrose drain, and mobilized to the level of the internal ring (Fig. 53.8). The cord is then dissected by dividing cremasteric muscle fibers to identify an indirect sac, if present. The sac is usually found on the anteriomedial side of the cord and can be identified as a glistening white structure. During this dissection, great care must be taken to avoid injury to the cord structures. The sac is opened and its contents reduced back into the abdominal cavity. The sac is ligated at its base with a purse-string suture and amputated. If an indirect sac extends inferiorly beyond the pubic tubercle, the distal sac should simply be divided and left open. Dissection beyond the pubic tubercle results in increased trauma to the cord, disruption of collateral blood supply to the testicle, and an increased risk of ischemic orchitis.[2,19,20] An exception to this is a sliding hernia, in which case the sac is contiguous with a retroperitoneal organ and must be dissected free in its entirety and returned to the abdominal cavity. For similar reasons, other abnormalities in the inguinal canal and scrotum, such as hydroceles, must not be dealt with at the same time as a hernia repair for fear of damaging the spermatic cord.[2,19,20]

If a direct hernia sac is identified, it generally should not be opened but should be reduced bluntly back into the abdominal cavity and imbricated with one or more sutures placed superficially in the transversalis fascia. This effectively avoids injury to any organs such as the colon or bladder, which may form a sliding component in a direct hernia.

Marcy Repair

The Marcy repair was developed by Henry Marcy, first published in 1871, and refers to a high ligation of the sac and closure of the internal inguinal ring (Fig. 53.8). This technique can be used only to repair indirect inguinal hernias, and its main utility is in pediatric patients or in adults (especially women) with a small indirect hernia and minimal damage to the internal ring. Patients with a direct inguinal hernia require the addition of another type of repair.

The key point of this operation is adequate exposure of the internal ring, which may require division of the cremaster muscle from its internal oblique muscle origins, especially in adult men, for whom these fibers are well developed.[21] Once adequate exposure of the ring is obtained, the indirect hernia sac is opened, retracted into the wound, closed with a suture ligature or a purse-string suture under direct visualization, and allowed to retract back through the internal ring into the abdominal cavity. If a cord lipoma is present, it is ligated at its base and amputated. The internal ring, formed by transversalis fascia, is then closed along its medial aspect with multiple interrupted sutures, displacing the cord laterally. The reconstructed ring should be snug but still be large enough to admit the tip of a hemostat to avoid vascular compromise of the cord. In female patients, the ring can be completely closed after dividing the round ligament. The inguinal canal is closed by reapproximating the external oblique aponeurosis with a continuous suture, thereby reconstructing the external inguinal ring.

Bassini Repair

Edoardo Bassini published his technique in 1887. After a complete and deliberate dissection of the inguinal canal, the floor is reconstructed by approximating the internal oblique muscle, the transversus abdominis muscle, and the transversalis fascia (the Bassini triple layer) with the iliopubic tract and shelving edge of the inguinal ligament using interrupted sutures (Fig. 53.9). This repair may be used for both indirect and direct inguinal hernias.

First, dissection is carried out as for all anterior repairs, with exposure of the inguinal canal, mobilization of the cord,

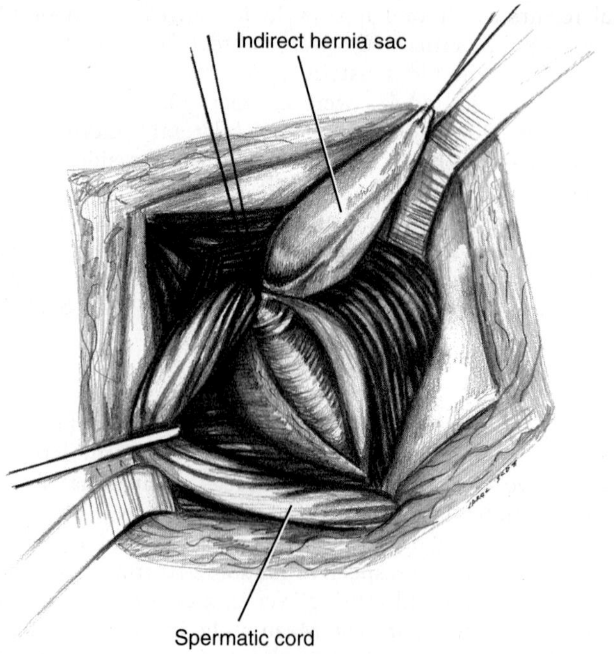

FIGURE 53.8. The spermatic cord is mobilized to the level of the internal ring, and a high ligation of the isolated hernia sac is performed.

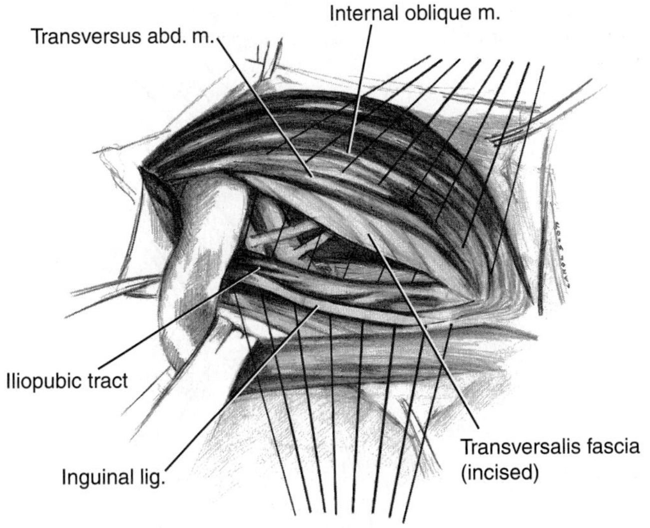

FIGURE 53.9. The Bassini repair reconstructs the canal floor using interrupted sutures to approximate the internal oblique muscle, the transversus abdominis muscle, and transversalis fascia (Bassini's triple layer) with the iliopubic tract and inguinal ligament.

and identification of the hernia sac(s). Next, the proximal cremasteric muscle fibers are divided, and a high ligation of the indirect sac is performed. The floor of the inguinal canal (i.e., the transversalis fascia) is then incised parallel and medial to the inguinal ligament, from the pubic tubercle medially to beyond the internal inguinal ring laterally. Care must be taken not to injure the inferior epigastric vessels. Cremasteric resection and transversalis division are essential steps of the true Bassini technique that are often omitted by surgeons in North America.[22] The spermatic cord is entirely freed, and exposure of the iliopubic tract and Cooper's ligament is facilitated. A direct hernia appears as a peritoneal evagination medial to the inferior epigastric vessels and can be held in a reduced position by several superficial sutures in the preperitoneal tissues to facilitate subsequent stages of repair. The femoral canal is inspected for evidence of a femoral hernia, which would necessitate additional repair. Interrupted sutures are then placed to approximate the triple layer (internal oblique muscle, transversus abdominis muscle, and transversalis fascia) with the iliopubic tract and inguinal ligament. Medially, the first suture includes the lateral edge of the rectus abdominis muscle near the pubic tubercle. Laterally, the sutures continue to the spermatic cord, and an internal ring is reconstructed snugly. The ring should be loose enough to admit the tip of a hemostat to avoid vascular compromise. The cord is then replaced to its native position, and the canal is closed by reapproximating the previously divided external oblique aponeurosis.

Shouldice Repair

Earle Shouldice published[23] his technique in 1953. More than 215,000 hernia repairs have been performed at the Shouldice hospital in Toronto, Canada, since its inception in 1945. This technique is remarkably similar to the Bassini operation in that the layers approximated to reconstruct the inguinal canal floor are the same for both. However, the Shouldice technique uses a series of running sutures to imbricate the reconstruction into several layers (Fig. 53.10).

As in the Bassini operation, the cord is mobilized, the cremaster muscle is divided, a high ligation of the sac is performed, and the transversalis fascia forming the floor of the inguinal canal is incised. The floor is reconstructed by placing a series of running sutures to approximate the lateral edge of the rectus abdominis muscle near the pubic tubercle, the internal oblique muscle, the transversus abdominis muscle, and the transversalis fascia to the iliopubic tract and the shelving edge of the inguinal ligament.

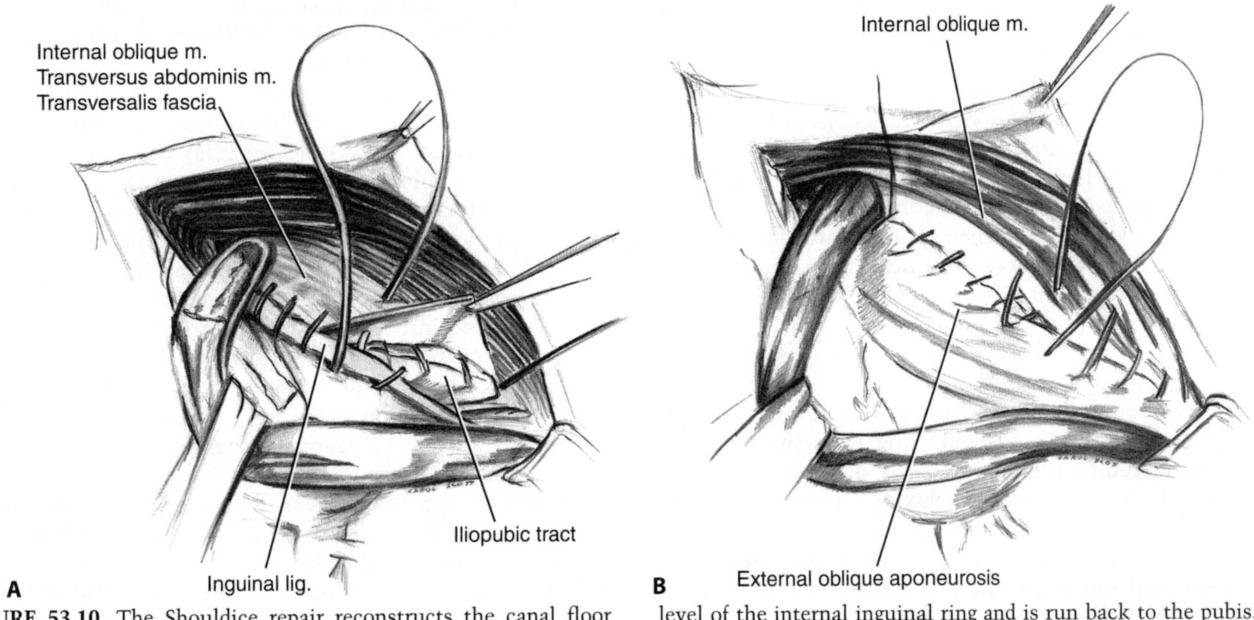

FIGURE 53.10. The Shouldice repair reconstructs the canal floor using a series of running sutures. **A.** The first suture is started at the pubis and is run laterally to approximate the internal oblique muscle, transversus abdominis muscle, and transversalis fascia with the iliopubic tract and inguinal ligament. The same suture is reversed at the level of the internal inguinal ring and is run back to the pubis. **B.** A second suture is started at the internal inguinal ring and is run medially to approximate the internal oblique muscle with the external oblique aponeurosis. The same suture is reversed at the pubis and is run back to the internal inguinal ring.

The Bassini and the Shouldice repairs are criticized for not addressing the femoral canal and for approximating tissue layers that are not normally in juxtaposition, yielding a nonanatomic reconstruction. However, proponents of both operations point out that postoperative femoral hernias occur very rarely (in 0.14% of cases),[24] and that a wealth of data supports the efficacy of these techniques.

Glassow published the largest series of Shouldice repairs in 1986 with outstanding results.[25] In 12,548 first-time repairs performed between 1954 and 1974, the recurrence rate was 1.1% over a 10-year follow-up period. In 1874 repairs of recurrent hernias, the recurrence rate was 3.3%. Likewise, Wantz published results of 5120 repairs with a recurrence rate of 1.3% for first-time hernias and 6.7% for recurrent hernias, with an overall complication rate of 1.9%.[26]

A multicenter prospective randomized controlled trial in France subsequently compared 1706 nonrecurrent hernia repairs in 1578 adult men using Bassini, Cooper's ligament, Shouldice with polypropylene suture, and Shouldice with stainless steel suture techniques.[27] Recurrence rates over 5.75-year median follow-up were 8.6% for Bassini, 11.2% for Cooper's ligament, 6.5% for Shouldice with polypropylene, and 5.9% for Shouldice with stainless steel. The difference in recurrence rates using different suture in the Shouldice groups was not statistically significant. Postoperative morbidity was comparable for all groups except for delayed ambulation in patients undergoing Cooper's ligament repairs. The authors concluded that the Shouldice repair should be the gold standard for inguinal hernia repair.

McGillicuddy reported the results of a prospective randomized trial comparing Shouldice and Lichtenstein repairs in 717 hernias in 672 patients.[28] Recurrence rates over 5-year mean follow-up were 2% for Shouldice and 0.5% for Lichtenstein repairs (not statistically different). Complications were comparable, and the author reported both procedures were comparable and effective, although he personally favored the Lichtenstein approach for its relative simplicity.

McVay (Cooper's Ligament) Repair

McVay popularized the use of Cooper's ligament in hernia repair after pointing out in 1939 that the normal insertion of the transversus abdominis muscle and the transversalis fascia was onto Cooper's ligament and not onto the inguinal ligament. Thus, its use in a groin reconstruction has a sound anatomic basis. The McVay repair approximates the transversus abdominis arch to Cooper's ligament, the iliopubic tract, and the inguinal ligament (Fig. 53.11). The McVay repair may be used for inguinal and femoral hernias.

The cord is mobilized and the transversalis fascia forming the canal floor incised. Cooper's ligament is dissected free, as is the anterior femoral fascia, which is derived from the iliopubic tract. Any vessels anastomosing with the obturator circulation, including the pubic vessels, are ligated to avoid their injury during the repair. A relaxing incision is made in the anterior rectus sheath from the pubic tubercle superiorly for about 10 to 15 cm. The proximal cremasteric muscle fibers and the external spermatic artery and the cord are retracted laterally. A high ligation of an indirect sac is performed. Direct hernia sacs are reduced into the abdominal cavity and imbricated under superficial sutures in the preperitoneal tissues. Femoral hernias are reduced from the femoral canal and converted to direct inguinal hernias and reduced. The reconstruction is then performed by placing interrupted sutures beginning at the pubic tubercle to approximate the transversus abdominis aponeurotic arch to Cooper's ligament. The placement of these sutures is carried laterally to the edge of the femoral vein. At this point, one or more transition sutures are placed between Cooper's ligament and the anterior femoral fascia to close the femoral canal. The repair is continued laterally, with sutures joining the transversus abdominis arch to the iliopubic tract and inguinal ligament, to the level of the cord. A reconstructed internal ring is fashioned to the appropriate snugness. The defect left by the relaxing incision is then closed with a mesh patch.

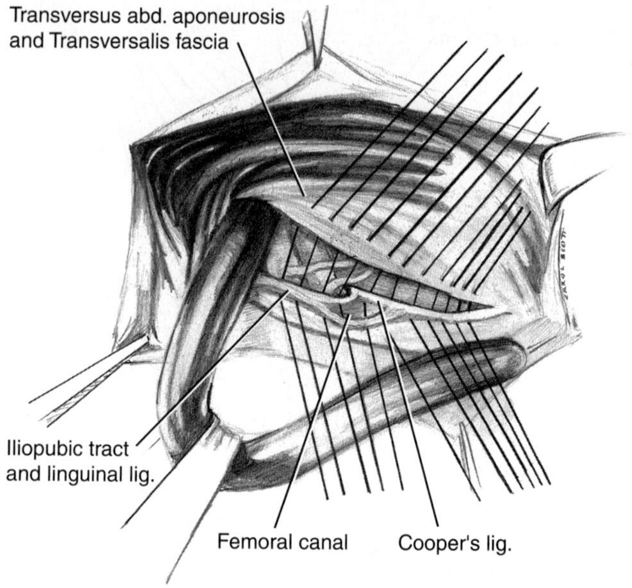

FIGURE 53.11. The McVay repair reconstructs the canal floor using interrupted sutures to approximate transversus abdominis aponeurosis and transversalis fascia with Cooper's ligament, the iliopubic tract, and the inguinal ligament. Transition sutures in Cooper's ligament and the anterior femoral fascia close the femoral canal.

Critics of this technique have pointed out that the extent of dissection is more extensive than in other repairs, and patients may have a slower convalescence. This is not a tension-free repair, necessitating a relaxing incision that may only partially relieve the tension. Vascular complications such as venous outflow obstruction or femoral vein injury may occur even with careful surgical technique.

Rutledge published results of 906 repairs in 747 patients over 9-year mean follow-up.[29] The recurrence rate was 2% (1.9% for first-time hernias and 2.4% for recurrent hernias). Although recurrence rates were low, 5% of patients developed testicular atrophy in this series.

Rutkow and Robbins reported a series of 2886 individuals undergoing a Cooper's ligament repair for primary and recurrent inguinal and femoral hernias; there was a 1.8% recurrence rate over 5.3-year mean follow-up.[30] They reported 4 (0.1%) cases of femoral vein compression and a 2.4% incidence of other complications, including infection (0.7%), urinary retention (0.6%), ischemic orchitis (0.7%), long-term pain (0.2%), and draining sinus tracts (0.2%).

Panos et al. presented a prospective randomized trial of the McVay versus Shouldice repairs performed at a teaching hospital.[31] The study included repairs of 308 direct inguinal hernias in 269 patients. Recurrence rates were 6.6% for McVay versus 8.8% for Shouldice (not statistically significant) over 36.4-month mean follow-up. Of note, bilateral hernias repaired simultaneously with either of these tension-creating methods produced a recurrence rate of 12.8% versus 5.6% for unilateral repairs ($P \leq .05$).

Lichtenstein Repair

Irving Lichtenstein has championed the tension-free approach to groin hernia repair since its introduction in 1986.[32] Lichtenstein emphasizes that classical repairs suture together tendinous structures that are not normally in apposition and thus create suture line tension, despite a relaxing incision. Suture line tension violates surgical principles and may be the ultimate cause of early recurrence.[33] Moreover, conventional repairs use attenuated fascial structures for the reconstruction, and impaired collagen metabolism leads to late failures.[34] The Lichtenstein approach alleviates these problems by using prosthetic mesh to reinforce the transversalis fascia forming the canal floor without attempting to use any attenuated native tissues in the repair (Fig. 53.12). Local anesthesia may be used, and several studies showed that this repair enables a quicker return to work, is associated with less postoperative pain, and has fewer recurrences than tissue repairs.[35] The Lichtenstein repair may be used for direct and indirect inguinal hernias but does not address femoral hernias.

Indirect sacs are opened, the femoral ring is palpated through this opening, and the sac is reduced back into the abdominal cavity without closure, which is claimed to cause more postoperative pain.[36] Direct sacs are reduced without opening them. The canal floor is reinforced by suturing a sheet of polypropylene mesh to the inguinal ligament laterally and the lateral edge of the rectus sheath and internal oblique muscle and aponeurosis medially, overlapping them by 2 cm. An 8 × 16 cm piece of mesh is used and trimmed to extend 4 cm lateral to the internal ring. Emphasis is placed on overlapping the mesh onto the pubic tubercle medially by 2 cm since failure of this step may lead to medial recurrences.[37] Emphasis is also placed on using a permanent monofilament suture (Prolene). Sutures to secure the mesh are placed to the level of the internal ring and not lateral to this point to avoid nerve entrapment. The internal ring is reconstructed by fitting tails around the cord. The tails are held in place on the inguinal ligament by a single suture and are tucked underneath the external oblique aponeurosis as it is closed.

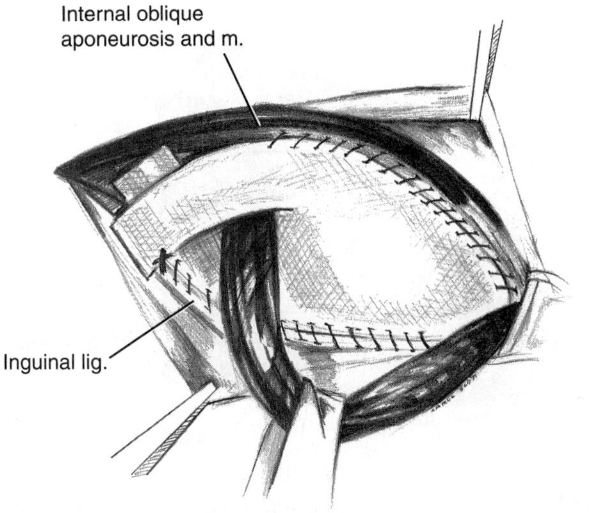

FIGURE 53.12. The Lichtenstein repair uses a mesh prosthesis to reinforce the canal floor. Tails are fashioned around the spermatic cord to reconstruct the internal inguinal ring.

Friis and Lindahl in Denmark reported a prospective randomized controlled study comparing the Lichtenstein repair to either a Marcy high ligation and ring plasty for indirect hernias or a McVay repair for direct or femoral hernias.[37] The study included 208 patients who underwent 102 Lichtenstein, 53 Marcy, and 53 McVay repairs of primary and recurrent hernias. There was 99% follow-up at 2 years. The recurrence rates were 0% for Lichtenstein and 3.8% for Marcy repairs of indirect hernias (no statistically significant difference). The recurrence rates were 8.6% for Lichtenstein and 26.4% for McVay repairs of direct or femoral hernias ($P = .014$). Complications occurred in 4.9% of Lichtenstein repairs and 5.3% of tissue repairs. There was no difference for discharge on day of operation or for time off from work. The authors admitted an unacceptably high recurrence rate in the tissue repair group and attributed it possibly to surgeon inexperience and lack of specialization in hernia repair per se.

Kark et al. reported a series of 3175 primary inguinal hernia repairs using the Lichtenstein technique combined with internal ring closure by suture or mesh plug insertion.[35] Over an 18-month to 5-year follow-up, their recurrence rate was 0.5%. Complications included hematomas, 2%; infections, 0.3%; testicular swelling, 1% (none progressed to testicular atrophy); and neuralgias, 1%. Mean time for return to work was 8 days.

The Lichtenstein group reported 4000 consecutive primary hernia repairs, with 87% follow-up for an average of 5.5 years, to include 3480 repairs in their analysis.[38] They had only 5 (0.1%) recurrences, 1 case of orchitis, and 1 case of neuralgia. Over 90% of their patients returned to work, including manual labor, within 2 weeks. Of note, the series included 1000 bilateral hernias that were repaired simultaneously under local anesthesia. No increase in complications or recurrences was associated with simultaneous repair of bilateral hernias using a tension-free technique. The authors attributed the recurrences to technical errors involving inadequate overlap of the mesh on the pubic bone and placement of mesh under tension. After correcting these mistakes, only one recurrence has been reported during the last 6 years.

The Lichtenstein group published another report, which summarized the results of five series at various institutions performing 3019 repairs for primary inguinal hernias.[34] In this report, results included recurrence, 0.2%; infection, 0.03%; and mesh rejection, 0%. In the Lichtenstein experience, rarely has mesh been removed for infection. Antibiotic therapy and drainage of the infection with wound granulation are usually sufficient.

The Lichtenstein repair has reshaped the way surgeons perform open herniorrhaphy. It has reduced patient discomfort and hernia recurrence rates dramatically. It has also reversed the notion that bilateral hernias should not be repaired simultaneously. The short- and long-term recurrence results seem better than the results previously achieved with tissue repairs. The procedure is readily reproducible by those who do not specialize in hernia repair, with comparable excellent results.[39]

Mesh Plug Repair

Various techniques have been developed that use a polypropylene mesh plug to fill the hernia defect and effect a repair. These techniques are championed as tension free and are becoming popular in combination with a mesh patch repair.

The Lichtenstein group reported using Marlex mesh tightly rolled into a cylindrical plug as their preferred repair method for recurrent direct and indirect inguinal hernias less than 3.5 cm in size and for all femoral hernias (Fig. 53.13).[40] A recurrent inguinal hernia larger than 3.5 cm requires a conventional patch Lichtenstein repair for adequate reinforcement. They cited that mesh darts or plugs that are not rolled tightly collapse and shrink over time, substantially diminishing their utility. In 1402 recurrent inguinal hernias treated with plug insertion, the recurrence rate was 1.6% with 3 to 21 years of follow-up in 91% of their patients; recurrence rate for femoral hernias was also under 2%.[41,42] The advantage of using a plug in recurrent hernias is that the cord may not need to be remobilized and may decrease the risk of ischemic orchitis.

Robbins and Rutkow[43] reported a technique that combines the insertion of a cone-shaped mesh plug (Fig. 53.14) into a direct, indirect, or femoral hernia defect and the sutureless placement of a mesh onlay graft on the floor of the inguinal canal, similar to a technique described by Gilbert.[44] They used a specially fabricated plug with a series of inner leaflets designed to maintain its conical shape and prevent collapse. They reported 2403 "plug-and-patch" repairs with less than 1% recurrence for primary hernias and 2% for recurrent hernias over 1.7 years mean follow-up.[30,43]

Wantz published information concerning 1252 primary inguinal hernia repairs combining the insertion of a mesh plug into indirect defects and a mesh onlay graft onto the floor of the inguinal canal, held in place by one suture medially and one laterally.[45] Over a follow-up of 1 to 6 years, the recurrence rate was 0.5%, and there were 15 (1.2%) complications, including 12 hematomas, 1 seroma, 1 infection, and 1 neuralgia. He noted that 0.5% is a lower recurrence rate than he had obtained in his previous experience with the Shouldice technique (1.3%) and emphasized the simplicity of this technique. He reserved the technique for men and preferred closure of the internal ring using sutures to repair primary indirect hernias in women. He also reserved this technique for primary hernias, preferring the open preperitoneal approach for recurrent hernias.

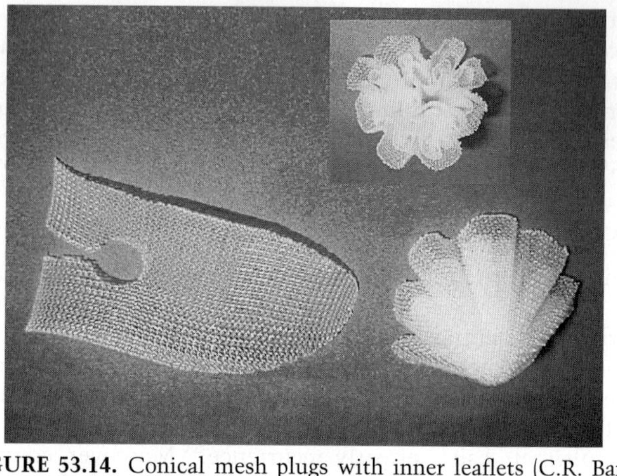

FIGURE 53.14. Conical mesh plugs with inner leaflets (C.R. Bard, Murray Hill NJ) are designed to minimize collapse and have recently become popular in combination with a mesh patch repair.

Open Preperitoneal Approach

In 1960, Nyhus introduced the open preperitoneal repair (Fig. 53.15).[46] He has championed this method for the repair of all recurrent and complicated groin hernias, namely, those involving incarcerated or strangulated intestine, as well as for femoral hernias. For the recurrent hernia, densely scarred tissue in the inguinal canal is avoided, possibly reducing the risk of nerve injury and cord damage.[19,20] In strangulated

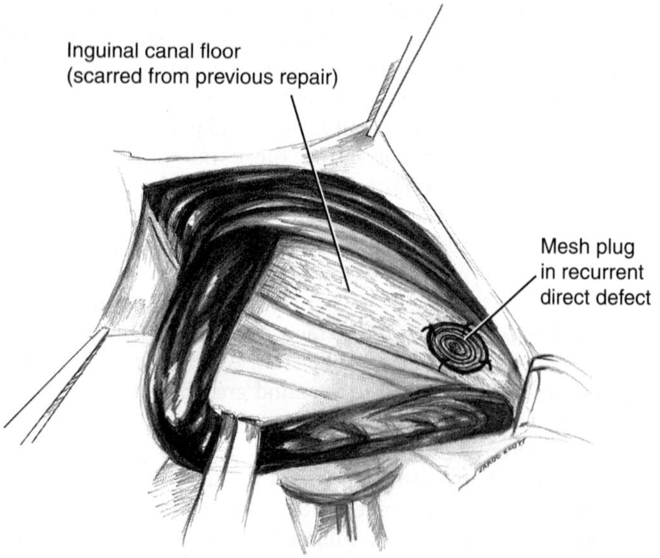

FIGURE 53.13. The Lichtenstein group uses a tightly rolled cylindrical mesh plug to repair recurrent inguinal hernias less than 3.5 cm in size.

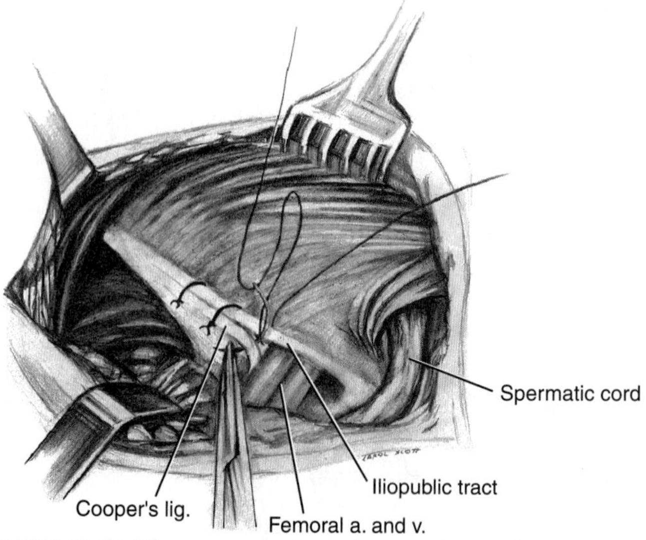

FIGURE 53.15. The open preperitoneal approach provides access to the abdominal cavity, if indicated, and exposure of inguinal and femoral hernias. A suture repair may be performed (shown here for a right-sided femoral hernia) or a mesh prosthesis may be used.

hernias, proximal unaffected intestine can be controlled, and necrotic intestine may be isolated prior to its reduction. The peritoneal cavity can be opened to perform an intestinal resection and anastomosis. Sliding hernias can also be readily reduced. For femoral hernias, ample access is afforded to reduce and repair the hernia without disturbing the floor of the inguinal canal, which is necessitated by anterior approaches. Preperitoneal repairs can be performed both with and without mesh. Although the use of mesh provides lower recurrence rates, contamination may preclude its use if bowel resection is necessary.

The repair is performed via a transverse incision positioned slightly higher than the standard anterior approach. The anterior rectus sheath is divided, and the rectus muscle is retracted toward the midline. The external oblique aponeurosis and internal oblique and transversus abdominis muscles are divided. The transversalis fascia is then exposed and is incised transversely, taking care not to enter the underlying peritoneum. Access to the preperitoneal space is thus obtained, and the preperitoneal fat and peritoneum are swept out of the pelvis bluntly, exposing any peritoneal projections through the posterior inguinal wall or femoral canal. The inferior epigastric vessels may be divided if necessary for greater exposure. Any projection (hernia) that is found is reduced by gentle traction. After high ligation of an indirect sac, the defect is closed by placing interrupted permanent monofilament sutures between the transversalis fascia and the iliopubic tract. Direct sacs are reduced into the peritoneal cavity without opening the sac. The defect is closed by suturing the transversalis fascia and transverse abdominis aponeurotic arch to the iliopubic tract. Femoral sacs are closed with a high ligation after inspecting and reducing sac contents. If incarcerated, the sac is released by incising the insertion of the iliopubic tract into Cooper's ligament at the medial margin of the femoral ring. The defect is closed by suturing the iliopubic tract to Cooper's ligament, obliterating the femoral canal medial to the femoral vein (Fig. 53.15).

Nyhus recommended buttressing the repair with polypropylene mesh for direct and large indirect primary hernias and for all recurrent inguinal hernias.[47] A 10 × 4 cm piece of mesh is sutured to Cooper's ligament and transversalis fascia. In the case of a recurrent indirect hernia, tails are fashioned to encircle the cord. The mesh is placed beyond the abdominal wall incision in the preperitoneal space to prevent incisional hernias. A relaxing incision through the anterior rectus sheath is made if there is any question of suture line tension.

Using a preperitoneal approach for 1200 nonrecurrent hernias without using a mesh buttress or relaxing incisions, Nyhus reported a recurrence rate of 3% for indirect, 6% for direct, and 1% for femoral hernias.[48] For 203 recurrent hernias repaired with a mesh reinforcement over a 10-year period, the rerecurrence rate was 1.7% compared to 5% if no mesh was used.[47] Complications included 2.5% infections, 0.5% hydrocele, and 1.5% incisional hernias (prior to incorporating mesh closure of the incision).

Hoffman reported a series of 152 primary and 52 recurrent hernias repaired using a preperitoneal approach with mesh.[49] No relaxing incisions were required. The recurrence rate was 0.5% over a 3.5-year mean follow-up. Complications included 1.5% wound infections, 4% hematomas, 1% seromas, 3% testicular pain, 12% long-term incisional pain, and 4% transient nerve irritation.

Giant Prosthetic Reinforcement of the Visceral Sac (Stoppa) Repair.

The first report of placing a giant prosthetic reinforcement of the visceral sac (GPRVS) in the preperitoneal space was by René Stoppa in 1969, using a large sheet of unsutured polyester mesh, and the repair is commonly referred to as the Stoppa repair (Fig. 53.16).[50] In contrast to other approaches, no attempt is made at repairing the musculofascial defect creating the hernia.[51] Instead, the transversalis fascia is functionally replaced by the insertion of a large chevron-shaped piece of mesh into the preperitoneal space after all hernias have been reduced. The transverse dimension of the mesh is equal to the distance between both anterior superior iliac spines minus 2 cm. The height is the distance between the umbilicus and the pubis, with an average mesh size of 24 × 16 cm. The mesh is placed through a midline or a Pfannenstiel incision and is oriented so that it stretches transversely. The mesh is held in place between the peritoneum and the inside of the abdominal wall initially by intra-abdominal pressure and later by connective tissue ingrowth. By adhering to the visceral sac, the mesh renders the peritoneum indistensible so that it cannot protrude through any abdominal wall defects. The mesh is large enough to extend far beyond the borders of the myopectineal orifice in all directions. The vas deferens and the testicular vessels are dissected from the parietal peritoneum to lie against the parietal wall of the pelvis (parietalization) so that a slit in the mesh for the cord is unnecessary. A single suture is placed superiorly at the midline to tack the mesh to the umbilical fascia. Mersiline mesh may be ideally suited for this repair because it is supple, elastic, freely conforms to the curvature of the visceral sac, has a grainy texture that adheres to the peritoneum, and induces prompt fibroblastic ingrowth.[52,53] Polypropylene mesh is semirigid and may not conform well; polytetrafluoroethylene (PTFE) is not quickly incorporated and may not adhere to the peritoneum.

The Stoppa repair can be useful in complex hernias, including recurrent and bilateral hernias and hernias at high

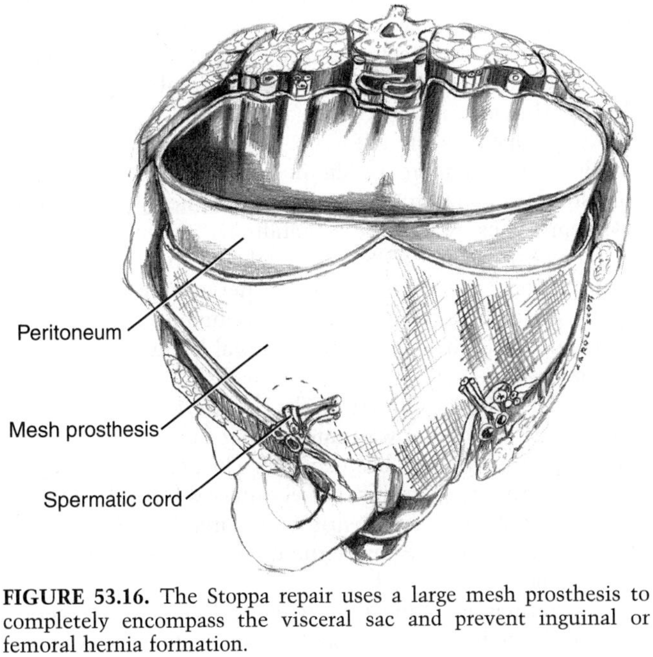

FIGURE 53.16. The Stoppa repair uses a large mesh prosthesis to completely encompass the visceral sac and prevent inguinal or femoral hernia formation.

risk for recurrence, such as in patients with connective tissue disorders, ascites, obesity, or advanced age. The Stoppa repair is contraindicated if contamination is present since risk of prosthetic infection is high.

In 1984, Stoppa published a series of 1223 GPRVS repairs with a recurrence rate of 1.4% and an incidence of complications comparable to conventional repairs.[52] In a subsequent report, the recurrence rate was less than 1% for primary hernias and 1.1% for recurrent hernias, with an overall complication rate of 3.3% for recurrent hernias.[54]

In 1997, Mathonnet reported 1048 GPRVS repairs of bilateral hernias using Dacron mesh with a 1.6% recurrence rate and an overall complication rate of 8.5%, including 2% hematoma, 1.6% infection (none required mesh removal), 9% pain, and 0.7% seroma.[55]

Wantz described a unilateral GPRVS repair using a 12 × 15 cm diamond-shaped piece of mesh inserted into a single groin through a transverse incision above the internal ring. Wantz reported in 1989 a series of 237 unilateral and bilateral GPRVS repairs using a variety of prosthetic materials for recurrent hernias and in patients at high risk for recurrences.[53] In 85 unilateral repairs, there were no recurrences. In 152 bilateral repairs, there were 9 (5.9%) recurrences. The overall recurrence rate was 3.7. More recently, Wantz published a series of GPRVS repairs of 15 primary and 54 recurrent femoral hernias with no recurrences.[56]

Laparoscopic Approaches

Considering all that is written about the radical treatment of the inguinal hernia up until now, it can be somewhat risky to try to publish more about this subject.

Edoardo Bassini, 1890

Since its introduction by Ger[57] in 1982 into the armamentarium of hernia repairs, laparoscopic repairs have undergone considerable evolution and have been the source of much controversy.[58] It was not until the 1990s with the tremendous success of laparoscopic cholecystectomies that the laparoscopic hernia repair received much attention. Early reports used a wide variety of techniques, initially met with high recurrence rates and numerous complications. Three techniques proved more effective and emerged as the most popular. These techniques are the transabdominal preperitoneal (TAPP), the intraperitoneal onlay mesh (IPOM), and the totally extraperitoneal (TEP).

These repairs approach the myopectineal orifice posteriorly, similar in anatomical perspective to the open preperitoneal approaches. A clear understanding of the anatomy from this perspective (Fig. 53.6) is crucial to avoid a number of complications, mainly vascular and nerve injuries. Laparoscopy provides a clear view of the entire myopectineal orifice, and repairs of both inguinal and femoral hernias can be performed.

In the TAPP procedure (Fig. 53.17), three trocars are placed through the abdominal wall into the peritoneal cavity after a pneumoperitoneum has been created. The peritoneum cephalad to the groin is then transversely incised from the median umbilical fold to several centimeters lateral to the internal ring, taking care not to injure the underlying inferior epigastric vessels.

The hernias are reduced using blunt dissection and gentle traction. Large indirect sacs can be divided after the contents are reduced, leaving the distal sac in situ. The preperitoneal tissues are broadly dissected beyond the midline and lateral to the internal ring, from below Cooper's ligament to above the transversus abdominis arch. The vas deferens and testicular vessels are parietalized by carefully freeing them from their proximal and lateral peritoneal attachments. The inferior epigastric vessels are defined but not completely skeletonized, which can lead to bleeding. Clear identification of Hesselbach's triangle, the femoral canal and vessels, and all anatomic landmarks is achieved.

A large piece of polypropylene mesh (12 × 15 cm) is then placed over the entire myopectineal orifice, with generous overlap of its borders, and secured in place with helical fasteners or staples. The fasteners are applied medially into the rectus muscle, superiorly to the transversus abdominis arch, inferiorly to Cooper's ligament up to the medial aspect of the external iliac vein, and laterally to the iliopubic tract. Alternatively, if a sufficiently large prosthesis is used, mesh fixation may not be required as excellent results can be obtained.

Some authors described placing a slit in the mesh, passing the cord through the slit, and tacking the tails in place with staples. Passing the cord through a slit and encircling the cord with mesh has been associated with chronic pain and seromas and may be unnecessary.[59–61]

The peritoneum is reapproximated using staples or sutures. Care must be taken to completely close the peritoneum without leaving gaps that can allow small-bowel entrapment or adherence to the mesh. Trocars are removed and the trocar fascial defects are closed to prevent incisional hernias.[62]

The IPOM repair uses an intraabdominal approach and places a large piece of mesh against the peritoneum after hernia contents have been reduced. The mesh is secured with staples placed into the same anatomic structures as in the TAPP repair but is placed in an intraperitoneal position instead of a preperitoneal position. Some authors described a minimal dissection of the peritoneum and clearly identifying Cooper's ligament to adequately secure the mesh and minimize recurrence.[63] To minimize the potential for adhesive complications, including bowel obstruction and fistulas, PTFE is favored over polypropylene mesh.[63,64]

The TEP technique (Fig. 53.18)[65] is now considered the ideal laparoscopic approach by many surgeons. The TEP operation avoids potential intraabdominal injuries by gaining access to the groin via a completely extraperitoneal approach. A small infraumbilical incision is made and carried down through the anterior rectus sheath. The rectus muscle is retracted away from the midline, and the anterior surface of the posterior rectus sheath is clearly visualized. A balloon dissector is placed along this surface, advanced inferiorly to the pubic bone, and is inflated with air or saline, creating a working space between the peritoneum and the abdominal wall. The balloon dissector is deflated and removed. Alternatively, the preperitoneal space can be dissected bluntly using an operating laparoscope or digitally; this technique may be slower and more tedious but can be more cost-effective.

After the preperitoneal working space has been developed, a cannula is inserted, and the preperitoneal space is insufflated. Two additional trocars are placed in the midline under direct visualization without violation of the peritoneum. The hernia is reduced using blunt dissection and gentle traction.

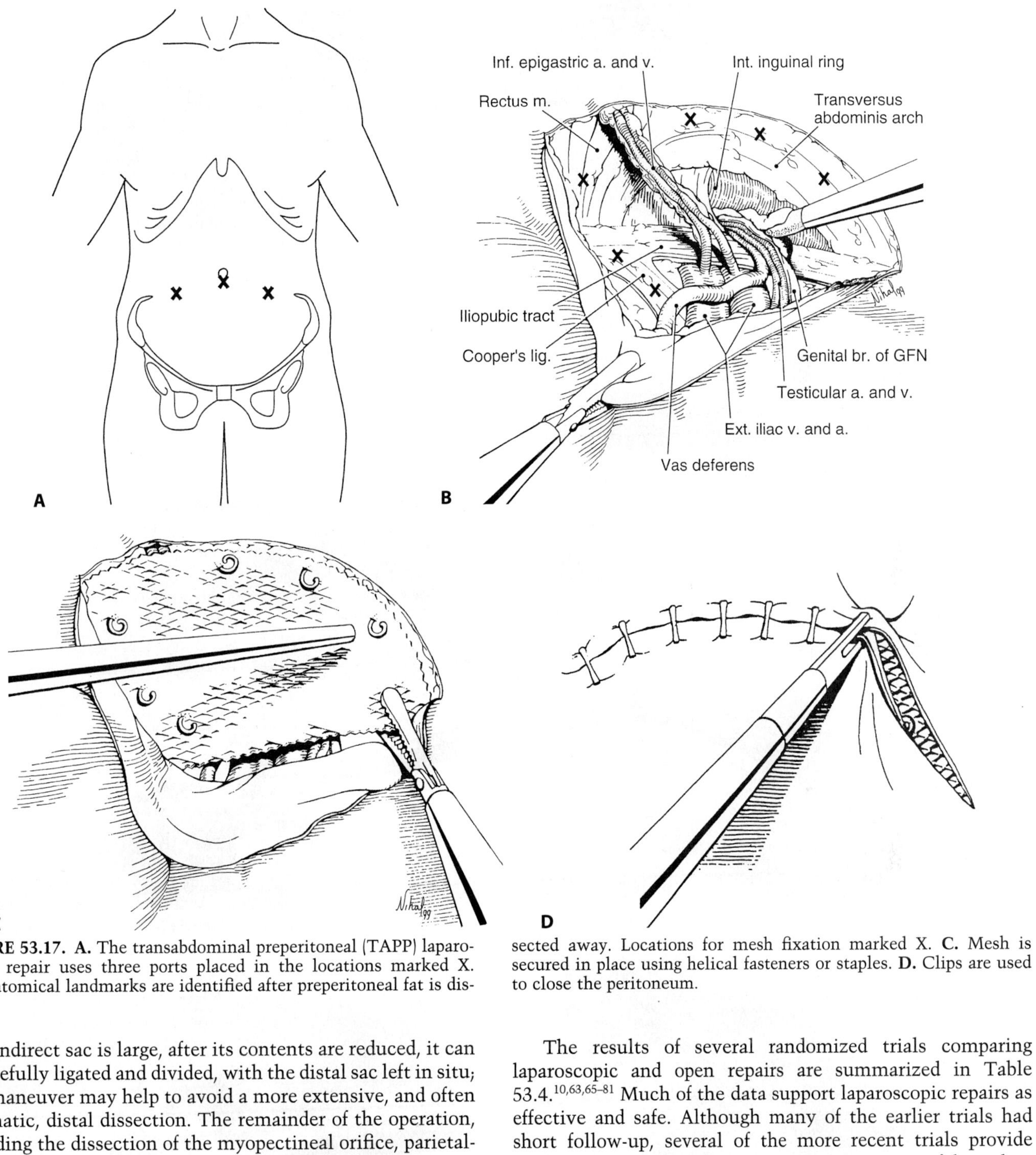

FIGURE 53.17. **A.** The transabdominal preperitoneal (TAPP) laparoscopic repair uses three ports placed in the locations marked X. **B.** Anatomical landmarks are identified after preperitoneal fat is dissected away. Locations for mesh fixation marked X. **C.** Mesh is secured in place using helical fasteners or staples. **D.** Clips are used to close the peritoneum.

If an indirect sac is large, after its contents are reduced, it can be carefully ligated and divided, with the distal sac left in situ; this maneuver may help to avoid a more extensive, and often traumatic, distal dissection. The remainder of the operation, including the dissection of the myopectineal orifice, parietalization of the cord and testicular vessels, and mesh placement, is identical to the TAPP procedure. Care during the TEP procedure must be taken to avoid violating the peritoneum, which results in a competing pneumoperitoneum and compromises exposure. Small peritoneal defects are usually well tolerated, and a Veress needle can be inserted into the peritoneal cavity as a vent. Alternatively, the intraabdominal gas can be evacuated through an incision at the umbilicus at the conclusion of the case. Large defects can severely compromise exposure and may require conversion to the TAPP or open repair. All defects should be closed, if possible, using endoloops, clips, or sutures to prevent possible bowel entrapment or adherence to the mesh.

The results of several randomized trials comparing laparoscopic and open repairs are summarized in Table 53.4.[10,63,65–81] Much of the data support laparoscopic repairs as effective and safe. Although many of the earlier trials had short follow-up, several of the more recent trials provide encouraging results, showing recurrence rates of less than 5% with lengthy follow-up intervals of 44, 60, and 70 months.[10,65–81] The incidence of complications associated with laparoscopic repairs is comparable to or better than that of open repairs, especially after the learning curve has been overcome.[67,73,75,76,81–83] Almost all of the trials show that laparoscopic repairs are associated with less postoperative pain and a decreased time for return to work but take longer to perform and cost more than conventional open repairs. Longer operative time and specialized equipment increase the costs, but interestingly, Kald et al. found that if the value of lost days of work was calculated into the total cost, laparoscopic repairs were more economical than open repairs.[69] Operative time

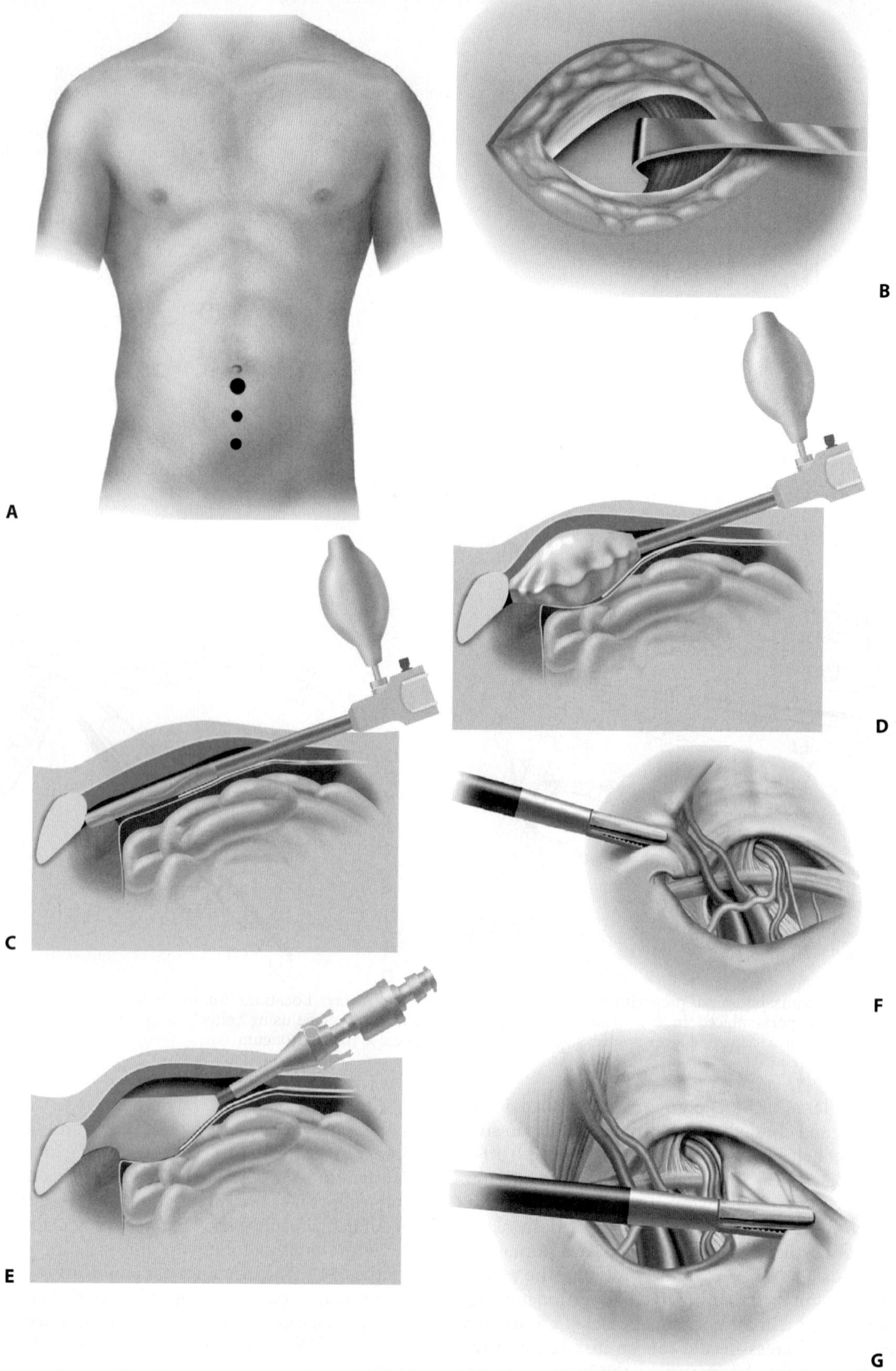

FIGURE 53.18. A. The totally extraperitoneal (TEP) laparoscopic repair uses three ports placed in the locations shown. **B.** Through the infraumbilical incision, the anterior rectus sheath is incised and the rectus muscle is retracted laterally. **C.** The balloon dissector is inserted into the preperitoneal space and advanced to the pubic symphysis. **D.** The balloon is then inflated to create a working space. **E.** The balloon is deflated, removed, and replaced with a Hasson or balloon-tip cannula. The preperitoneal working space is visualized with the laparoscope and other ports are placed. **F.** Blunt graspers and gentle traction are used to reduce indirect sacs as they course with the cord structures (gonadal vessels and vas deferens) through the internal inguinal ring. **G.** Similar techniques are used to reduce direct hernias within Hesselbach's triangle. Once all hernias are reduced, a mesh repair is performed in a similar fashion as shown for the TAPP procedure. (Reproduced with permission from Jones et al.[65])

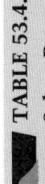

TABLE 53.4.
Select Prospective Randomized Trials Comparing Laparoscopic and Open Inguinal Hernia Repairs (Level I Evidence).

Reference	Study design	Average follow-up	No. of repairs	Complications (not including recurrences)	Recurrences	Operative time (min)	Cost	Postop pain	Return to work (days)	Conclusions/details
Neumayer, et al. 2004, United States (VA Trial)[75]	Lap (10% TAPP, 90% TEP) vs. Lichtenstein	24 mo	Lap: 862	386 (39%) total complications, 3 deaths (1 PE, 1 intestinal injury, 1 MI), 5% conversion to open	10.1%[a]	—	—	↓ pain score on POD 1–14[a]	4[a]	Intention-to-treat analysis. SF-36 outcomes similar to 2 years. Fewer perioperative and life-threatening complications for open repairs, but similar long-term complications. For recurrent hernias, recurrence rates were 10.0% for lap and 14.1% for open. For "highly experienced" surgeons (>250 cases), there was no difference in recurrence for primary hernias (5.1% lap vs. 4.1% open) but significantly fewer for recurrent hernias (3.6% lap vs. 17.4% open). "Open technique is superior."
			Licht: 834	332 (33.4%) total complications, 1 death (bowel obstruction in missed femoral hernia)	4.9%[a]	—	—	No difference at 3 mo	5[a]	
Liem et al. 2003, 1997, Netherlands[76]	TEP vs. open (Marcy, Lichtenstein, Bassini, Shouldice, McVay)	44 mo. (87% follow-up)	TEP: 487	24 (5%) conversion to TAPP or open, 54 (11%) total postop complications, 0 deep wound infection[a], 10 (2%) chronic pain[a], 7 (1%) seroma[a], 3 (1%) pneumoscrotum <1 day	4.9%[a]	45[a]	—	↓ pain score[a]	14[a]	71% of lap recurrences and 4% of open recurrences occur in the first postop year. 10 of 21 lap recurrences were by a single surgeon. Open repair associated with higher incidence of chronic pain. Bassini repair results in unacceptably high recurrence rates. TEP has more rapid recovery, fewer recurrences, and less chronic pain than open repairs, but takes slightly longer to perform.
			Open: 507	99 (19.5%) total postop complications, 6 (1%) deep wound infection[a], 70 (14%) chronic pain[a], 0 seroma[a]	10.0%[a]	40[a]	—		21[a]	

(continued)

TABLE 53.4. Select Prospective Randomized Trials Comparing Laparoscopic and Open Inguinal Hernia Repairs (Level I Evidence). (continued)

Reference	Study design	Average follow-up	No. of repairs	Complications (not including recurrences)	Recurrences	Operative time (min)	Cost	Postop pain	Return to work (days)	Conclusions/details
Bringman, et al., 2003, Sweden[77]	TEP vs. mesh plug vs. Lichtenstein	20 mo	TEP: 92	No conversions No perioperative complications, 12 (13%) total complications	2.1%	50	—	↓ pain score POD 0–1[a]	14[a]	Shorter operative time for mesh plug compared to TEP or Lichtenstein. Faster recovery for TEP compared to mesh-plug or Lichtenstein. No significant difference in complications. "Laparoscopic hernioplasty is superior to tension-free open herniorrhaphy in terms of postoperative pain and rehabilitation."
			Mesh plug: 104	No perioperative complications, 24 (23%) total complications	1.9%	36[a]	—		24.5	
			Lichtenstein: 103	No perioperative complications, 36 (35%) total complications	0	45	—		28.5	
Wright et al., 2002, United Kingdom[78]	TEP vs. open (Marcy, Lichtenstein, or Stoppa)	60 mo. (median)	TEP: 149	6% conversion to open No serious intraoperative or postoperative complications	2.0%	—	—	No difference in chronic pain	—	Single-surgeon experience as part of MRC trial with long-term follow-up. No recurrences for Lichtenstein repairs performed for primary hernias (all open recurrences were in Stoppa group). All laparoscopic recurrences occurred with large (>5 cm) direct defects; recommends 15 × 15 cm mesh to adequately repair these defects. Similar long-term outcomes for lap and open; both procedures have a role in hernia repair. Experience is very important for the laparoscopic repair.
			Open: 151	No serious intraoperative or postoperative complications	2.0%	—	—		—	

Leibl et al., 2000, Germany[79]	TAPP vs. Shouldice	70 mo. (median)	TAPP: 54	4 (7%) total complications	2.0%	65.0		↓ analgesia usage POD 1–2[a]	21[a]	Improved mobilization with lap repair. Greater long-term satisfaction with the lap repair. "TAPP is an effective alternative."
			Shouldice: 48	4 (8%) total complications	5.0%	47.5			38[a]	
MRC Hernia Group, 1999, United Kingdom[80]	Lap (23% TAPP, 77% TEP) vs. open (89% tension-free mesh)	12 mo. (n = 711)	Lap: 468	25 (5.6%) surgical complications (1 bladder, 1 LFCN/nerve, 1 common iliac artery)[a], 108 (29.9%) complications at 1 week[a], 6.6% conversion to open	1.9%[a]	58.4[a]	+£314	↓ groin pain at 1 year[a]	28[a]	SF-36 outcomes similar at 3 mo. 16/25 surgical complications were injury to inferior epigastric vessels. All serious complications and 2 trocar hernias happened in the TAPP group. Laparoscopic repairs offer advantages but potential for rare serious complications and recurrence support repairs being performed by specialist surgeons. "Open repair is the more appropriate option for the general surgeon."
			Open: 460	6 (1.4%) surgical complications (1 enterotomy)[a], 155 (43.5%) complications at 1 week[a]	0[a]	43.4[a]			42[a]	
Paganini et al., 1998, Italy[66]	TAPP vs. Lichtenstein	28 mo.	TAPP: 52	14 (26.9%) total complications, 4 (7.6%) hematoma, 1 (1.9%) hydrocele, 5 (9.6%) parasthesia, 4 (7.6%) seroma[a]	3.8%	66.6 unilateral primary[a] 71.1 unilateral recurrent 85.7 bilateral	$1249	↓ pain score at 48 h[a]	15	95% of Lichtenstein repairs performed under local anesthesia. TAPP had less postop pain. TAPP should not be adopted routinely unless its cost can be reduced.
			Licht.: 56	15 (26.7%) total complications, 8 (14.2%) hematoma, 2 (3.5%) hydrocele, 5 (8.9%) parasthesia, 0 seroma[a]	0	48.2 unilateral primary[a] 41.2 unilateral recurrent 75.9 bilateral	$306	↑ discomfort at 7 days, 3 mo	14	

(continued)

TABLE 53.4. Select Prospective Randomized Trials Comparing Laparoscopic and Open Inguinal Hernia Repairs (Level I Evidence). (continued)

Reference	Study design	Average follow-up	No. of repairs	Complications (not including recurrences)	Recurrences	Operative time (min)	Cost	Postop pain	Return to work (days)	Conclusions/details
Zieren et al., 1998, Germany[67]	TAPP vs. plug and patch vs. Shouldice	25 mo	TAPP: 80	2 (3%) intraop bleeding[a], 15 (19%) postop complications	0	61[a]	$1211		16	Plug and patch and TAPP cause less pain and have faster return to work than Shouldice; plug and patch cost less than TAPP and can be performed faster and under local anesthesia.
			Plug: 80	12 (15%) postop complications	0	36	$124		18	
			Shouldice: 80	13 (16%) postop complications	0	47	$69	↑ pain score[a]	26[a]	
Champault et al., 1997, France[68]	TEP vs. Stoppa	20.2 mo	TEP: 51	4% total complications[a], 3 (6%)conversions to open	6%	"Significantly longer"[a]	—	↓ pain score[a] ↓ meds[a]	17[a]	45% bilateral, 43% recurrent. Mesh for TEP was not fixed in place; mesh size increased from 6 × 11 cm to 12 × 15 cm due to early recurrences. Single piece of mesh for bilateral hernias felt to reduce recurrence rates. TEP has the same long-term recurrence rate as the Stoppa procedure but confers a real advantage in the early postop period.
			Stoppa: 49	20% total complications[a]	2%		—		35[a]	
Kald et al., 1997, Sweden[69]	TAPP vs. Shouldice	12 mo	TAPP: 122	8 (6.6%) total complications	0[a]	72[a]	+$483 direct cost	—	10[a]	TAPP had a faster recovery and return to work with comparable complication rates. TAPP is more cost-effective if indirect costs are compared (including income lost by a delay in return to work).
			Shouldice: 89	9 (10.1%) total complications	3.4%[a]	62[a]	+$1364 indirect cost	—	23[a]	
Bessell et al., 1996, Australia[70]	TEP vs. Shouldice	7.3 mo	TEP: 39	6 conversion to open, 3 conversion to TAPP, 4 (10%) postop complications	5.1%	87.5[a]	—	↓ pain score[a] ↓ meds[a]	30.5	Study biased because of large crossover to open group. Substantial conversion rate to open and TAPP repairs. TEP has significant decrease in pain, equivalent return to work, but longer operative time. TEP alleviates the inherent dangers associated with TAPP, but further studies are needed.
			Shouldice: 74	7 (9.5%) postop complications	0	50[a]	—		32	

Tschudi et al., 1996, Switzerland[72]	TAPP vs. Shouldice	6.7 mo	TAPP: 52	6 (12%) total complications	1.9%	87 unilateral[a] 124 bilateral	—	↓ pain score[a] ↓ meds[a]	25	Study biased because patients undergoing open repairs told not to resume activity for 4–6 weeks. Significantly less pain with TAPP, but longer OR time. Long-term follow-up is needed for analysis of recurrences.
			Shouldice: 56	9 (16%) total complications	3.5%	59 unilateral[a] 79 bilateral	—		48	
Barkun, et al., 1995, Canada[73]	TAPP or IPOM vs. open (Bassini, McVay, Shouldice, Lichtenstein, plug and patch)	14 mo	TAPP: 33 IPOM: 10	10 (22.5%) total complications	0	43	$1718	↓ meds[a]	9.6	Improved quality of life and decreased pain with laparoscopic repairs, but at increased cost. Laparoscopic repairs are feasible and comparable to open repairs.
			Open: 49	6 (11.9%) total complications	2%	49	$1224		10.9	
Vogt et al., 1995, United States[63]	IPOM (with meshed PTFE) vs. open (Bassini, McVay)	8 mo	IPOM: 30	5 (17%) total complications, 1 (3.3%) bladder perforation	3.3%	62.5	—	↓ meds	7.5	Less pain and faster return to work with IPOM, with comparable efficacy and morbidity. Longer follow-up needed. 2 patients had IPOM under local anesthesia.
			Open: 31	5 (16%) total complications	6.4%	80.9	—		18.5	
Stoker et al., 1994, United Kingdom[74]	TAPP vs. open (nylon darn plication)	7 mo	TAPP: 83	6 (8%) total complications[a], 1 deep wound infection, 3 persistent pain, 1 hematoma	0	50 unilateral[a] 92 bilateral	+$168	↓ pain score[a] ↓ meds[a]	14[a]	TAPP has less pain, faster return to work, and fewer complications, but increased operative time. Substantial economic savings in lost work days.
			Open: 84	16 (21%) total complications[a], 5 deep wound infection, 6 persistent pain, 3 hematoma	0	35 unilateral[a] 60 bilateral			28[a]	
Payne et al., 1994, United States[81]	TAPP vs. Lichtenstein	10 mo	TAPP: 48	6 (12%) total complications, 0 groin pain <1 mo, 2 (4%) conversions to open, 1 (2%) incarcerated omentum in peritoneal flap	0	68 unilateral 87 bilateral 67 recurrent	$3093[a]	—	9 unilateral[a] 7.5 bilateral 11.4 recurrent	TAPP can be performed with similar operative times and short-term recurrence rates, with faster return to work, but at an increased cost. 90% of Lichtensteins used local anesthesia. Biggest impact on faster return to work and increased ability to perform straight leg raises seen in manual labor population.[a]
			Licht.: 52	9 (18%) total complications, 4 (8%) groin pain <1 mo	0	56 unilateral 93 bilateral 73 recurrent	$2494[a]	—	17 unilateral[a] 25 bilateral 26 recurrent	

—, value was not measured; IPOM, intraperitoneal onlay mesh repair; TAPP, transabdominal preperitoneal approach; TEP, totally extraperitoneal approach.

[a]Statistical significance (all unmarked values are not statistically significant).

decreases with surgeon experience and the costs decrease as well.[84,85] In our own series comparing the cost of TEP versus Lichtenstein repairs (n = 60), TEP costs on average $778 more than Lichtenstein repairs.[86]

A steep learning curve for laparoscopic repairs exists and must be overcome to achieve reliably good outcomes in terms of both complications and recurrence rates.[76–78,80] The learning curve for TEP procedures has been estimated to be 30 cases or more.[76] Rare but serious complications such as visceral and vascular injury have been reported and highlight the need for adequate training. Fortunately, additional training outside the operating room using surgical simulators may shorten the learning curve and improve operative performance.[87] Nonetheless, the learning curve effect may account, to a large extent, for the great variability of reported results. For example, although surgeons enrolling patients in the recently reported Veterans Administration (VA) trial were required to have performed 25 laparoscopic procedures, the breakpoint for outcomes in this setting was over 250 cases. For these "highly experienced" surgeons, recurrences were similar for primary hernias (5.1% laparoscopic, 4.1% open) and improved for recurrent hernias (3.6% laparoscopic, 17.4% open) compared to the "less-experienced" surgeons, who had inferior results (10% recurrence) for laparoscopic but not open repairs. The learning curve for laparoscopic repairs in the VA trial seems much higher than that reported in other series, and some surgeons have questioned these results.[88] In any case, these data suggest that surgeon experience plays a major role in outcomes for laparoscopic hernia repairs. In the hands of experts, laparoscopic repairs may be performed faster than open repairs and with fewer complications.[83,89] Importantly, long-term data now support efficacy of laparoscopic repairs with acceptably low recurrence rates.[76,78,79]

Several studies have compared the various types of laparoscopic repairs and are summarized in Table 53.5.[78,90–92] The TEP approach avoids intraperitoneal dissection and the associated potential for visceral injury and postoperative adhesion formation.[78] In theory, it may avoid the cardiorespiratory alterations associated with creating a pneumoperitoneum, but there have been reports of respiratory acidosis associated with a pneumopreperitoneum.[93] It appears that TEP has the fewest complications, making it the preferred method.[78,90,91,94] Although rarely done, TEP repairs may be successfully performed using regional anesthesia.[90]

The disadvantage of the TEP approach is that it is technically more difficult since the working space is smaller, and the anatomic perspective is confusing until considerable experience is gained.[70,90,91] Moreover, previous lower abdominal surgery or irradiation is a relative contraindication to TEP since scars and peritoneal adhesions make this procedure dangerous and difficult, with a high rate of conversion to TAPP or open and a high rate of visceral injuries.[81,90,91] It is a difficult approach with incarcerated or large scrotal hernias, and some authors have recommended using the TAPP approach for these.[92] Others, however, have met with success using the TEP repair in large scrotal hernias, modifying their technique by routinely dividing the inferior epigastric vessels.[95] Although small peritoneal tears are usually well tolerated and can be sutured closed, large peritoneal breaches necessitate conversion to a TAPP procedure. The conversion rate in Liem's prospective trial of 487 TEP repairs was 5%, which is comparable to most large series.[10] Surgeons who use the TEP approach should therefore be proficient in the TAPP approach as well.[85]

The TAPP approach has several inherent dangers due to the violation of the peritoneal cavity. Abdominal organs and vasculature can be injured by trocar insertion.[92] The inferior epigastric vessels are especially at risk when lateral trocars are inserted medial to the edge of the rectus sheath. Injury of deeper structures can usually be avoided by placing trocars under direct visualization. Intraabdominal adhesions from prior abdominal operations can increase the risk of injury. The TAPP approach creates peritoneal flaps that must be completely closed. If a gap remains, bowel can be exposed to the mesh, allowing adhesions, erosions, or obstruction.[92] Bowel can also herniate through a peritoneal opening and become incarcerated.[81,96] Incisional hernias at trocar sites are more common after TAPP repairs, occurring in up to 1% of patients, necessitating fascial closure of all ports larger than 5 mm.[62] The advantage of the TAPP approach is a large working space, improved visualization, and an easier learning curve.[61,81] The approach facilitates easier reduction and repair of incarcerated and large scrotal hernias,[92] and it also allows other laparoscopic procedures to be performed simultaneously, which has been supported as a safe practice by limited data.[91]

Conceptually similar to laparoscopic ventral hernia repair, IPOM has appeal because of its simplicity and the lack of extensive preperitoneal dissection.[64] Although several trials have shown the efficacy and safety of this technique, many are skeptical of leaving a prosthetic in direct contact with the viscera, citing reports of bowel erosion and obstruction.[91] The prosthetic of choice in this circumstance has become PTFE, but structures under the peritoneum can also be obscured by placement of an opaque prosthesis, placing them at risk during mesh stapling. To overcome this problem, Vogt et al. meshed the PTFE graft with a skin graft mesher and reported favorable results.[63] Still, mesh cannot be fixated in the areas overlying the iliac vessels or the adjacent nerves. Although initial enthusiasm for this technique was fueled by its relatively simple nature, use of the IPOM repair has never become widespread.

As highlighted above, the optimal type of approach remains controversial. There is still some hesitancy in the surgical community to replace conventional hernia repairs with the laparoscopic approach. Multiple types of open repairs have long-standing and well-proven results, are associated with low morbidity and disability, and can be more easily performed under local anesthesia. It is difficult to endorse a new approach that is more difficult to learn, requires general anesthesia, costs more, and has the potential, although rare, of causing serious abdominal complications. There is currently a consensus that laparoscopic approaches are indicated in bilateral and recurrent hernias.[61,91,97,98] The laparoscopic approach provides access to both groins from the same approach with no additional incisions. The laparoscopic approach shares the same benefits as the open preperitoneal approach in recurrent hernia repair by avoiding scarred anterior tissue planes and potential cord injury.[63] Many surgeons also use the laparoscopic approach for unilateral nonrecurrent hernias, especially in individuals requiring a more rapid convalescence.

TABLE 53.5.
Trials Comparing Different Types of Laparoscopic Repairs.

Reference	*Study design*	*Average follow-up*	*No. of repairs*	*Complications (not including recurrences)*	*Recurrences*	*Operative time (min)*	*Return to work (days)*	*Conclusions/details*
Kald et al., 1997, Sweden[85]	Prospective nonrandomized TAPP vs. TEP	TAPP: 23 mo	TAPP: 393	0 conversions to open, 31 (7.8%) total complications, 2 bowel obstructions (at 12 and 19 weeks postop), 3 trocar hernias	1.8%	80	12[a]	High-quality hernia repairs can be performed with both TAPP and TEP. TEP is technically more difficult but results in fewer major complications and a faster return to work. TEP avoids the potential dangers of a transabdominal approach and may be the procedure of choice.
		TEP: 7 mo	TEP: 98	8 conversions to TAPP, 1 conversion to open, 7 (8.0%) total complications, 0 bowel obstructions, 0 trocar hernias	0	80	8[a]	
Ramshaw et al., 1996, United States[90]	Retrospective TAPP vs. TEP		TAPP: 300	2 conversions to open, 32 (10.6%) total complications, 1 enterotomy, 1 cystotomy, 1 trocar hernia, 6 parasthesia	2.0%			TAPP and TEP have acceptable complication and recurrence rates, but TEP has fewer.
			TEP: 300	2 conversions to open, 7 conversions to TAPP, 10 (3.3%) total complications, 2 enterotomies, 1 cystotomy, 0 trocar hernia, 1 parasthesia	0.3%			TEP has the advantage of staying out of the abdominal cavity and using epidural anesthesia (47 patients) and is the preferred technique. Previous lower abdominal surgery is a relative contraindication to TEP (all recurrences and visceral injuries occurred in these patients). TEP is more technically difficult.

(continued)

TABLE 53.5. Trials Comparing Different Types of Laparoscopic Repairs. (continued)

Reference	Study design	Average follow-up	No. of repairs	Complications (not including recurrences)	Recurrences	Operative time (min)	Return to work (days)	Conclusions/details
Fitzgibbons et al., 1995, United States[91]	Prospective nonrandomized TAPP vs. IPOM (with polypropylene mesh) vs. TEP	23 mo	TAPP: 562	Total complications: 2 bowel adhesions/obstructions, 5% neuralgias	5%	—	—	Laparoscopic hernia repair is effective with acceptable early recurrence rates. TAPP, IPOM, and TEP appear to be equally effective, although TEP is more difficult technically.
			IPOM: 217	12% neuralgias, 1 prosthetic infection (appendicitis vs. cecal erosion)	5.1%	—	—	
			TEP: 87	0% neuralgias	0	—	—	
			All 3 groups analyzed together	2 conversions to open, 29.2% total complications, 5 (0.7%) trocar hernias, 1 (0.1%) cystotomy, 1 (0.1%) enterotomy, 24 (3.5%) bleeding (2 requiring transfusion), 6 (0.87%) second abdominal procedure required (for bleeding, infection, adhesion, enterotomy, neuralgia)	4.5%	70 unilateral 90.6 bilateral	—	IPOM and TEP may be better suited for small indirect inguinal hernias, whereas TAPP may be better for complicated recurrent hernias. Other procedures can be safely performed at the same time as hernia repair (61 additional procedures performed with 1 associated complication). The incidence of neuralgias is disturbing but decreasing with increased surgeon experience. This series represents a very well done multicenter trial, but the total complication rate is disturbing. The authors stress the need for prospective randomized trials to further evaluate laparoscopic repairs.

Felix et al., 1995, United States[92]	Retrospective TAPP vs. TEP	TAPP: 24 mo	TAPP: 733	9 (1.2%) intraabdominal complications, 1 bowel obstruction, 2 enterotomies, 6 trocar hernias, 10% seroma, 7 hydroceles	0.3%	—	7 days for "normal activity" for TAPP and TEP	Time to return to work was the same in TAPP and TEP, but was 8 days for noncompensated patients vs. 16 days for compensated.
		TEP: 9 mo	TEP: 382	7 (1.8%) conversions to TAPP, 1 (1.2%) intraabdominal complication, 0 bowel obstructions, 0 enterotomies, 1 trocar hernia (in TAPP conversion), 10% seroma, 2 hydroceles	0.3%	—		TEP is less invasive, minimizes the risk of intraabdominal complications, and is the procedure of choice, except for incarcerated hernias and large scrotal hernias, which are more easily handled by TAPP. Slit in mesh associated with transient scrotal hyperesthesia. Parietalization of the cord more easily achieved in TEP, alleviating the need for a slit in the mesh. 50% of all repairs done with double-buttress technique. There were no recurrences, but all hydroceles occurred in this group.

—, value was not measured; IPOM, intraperitoneal onlay mesh repair; TAPP, transabdominal preperitoneal approach; TEP. totally extraperitoneal approach.

[a]Statistical significance (all unmarked values are not statistically significant).

Complications

There exists great variety in the methods and completeness by which complication rates are reported, and caution must be used not to draw premature conclusions from inadequate data. Generally complication rates decrease with increased surgeon experience, but a thorough knowledge of anatomy and of potential hazards is essential to hernia repair. Complication rates following open inguinal hernia repairs average 7% to 12%.[99] Reports on laparoscopic approaches are widely variable, but the rates of complications for both conventional and laparoscopic repairs is now thought to be comparable.[68,74,100,101]

Recurrence

Ten percent is reported as the average recurrence rate for groin hernias, although most surgeons boast to have rates well below the average.[13] Lichtenstein, for example, reports rates of less than 1%, with similar results reproduced by others using the same technique.[15,34] Recurrence rates following conventional repairs vary from 1% to 7% for indirect inguinal hernias, from 4% to 10% for direct inguinal hernias, from 1% to 7% for femoral hernias, and from 5% to 35% for recurrent hernia repair.[13,102] Lichtenstein noted that 50%of recurrences after anterior repairs first appear 5 years or more after the initial operation, and 75% of recurrences become evident within 10 years of the original operation.[103] In contrast, Stoppa noted that recurrences after a preperitoneal repair usually occur within the first postoperative year and are due to technical errors.[54] Failure to diagnose multiple hernias at the time of initial operation, failure to close an enlarged internal ring, and breakdown of the repair under tension have all been implicated in the causes of recurrences.[32,104] Elkberg showed an incidence of 6% for multiple ipsilateral hernias and 17% for bilateral hernias using herniography, suggesting missed hernias may account for recurrence.[105]

For laparoscopic repairs, the reasons for recurrence are surgeon inexperience, inadequate dissection, insufficient prosthesis size, insufficient prosthesis overlap of hernia defects, inadequate fixation, prosthesis folding or twisting, missed hernias or lipomas, and mesh dislodgment secondary to hematoma formation.[10,85,106–108] Recurrence is directly related to surgeon experience, with failures occurring much more frequently early in the surgeon's learning curve.[10,84,85] Incomplete dissection can result in missed indirect hernias and missed cord lipomas, especially in the TEP procedure and especially with inexperienced surgeons.[106,108,109] Inadequate dissection can also limit the size of mesh that can be used or result in incomplete fixation or folding. At least a 12 × 15 cm piece of mesh should be used to ensure a 2- to 3-cm overlap of all hernia defects and prevent technical causes for recurrence. Several investigators advocated that mesh fixation is unnecessary if the mesh is large enough, and the impressive results of Champault's series supports this practice.[68,84,107,110]

For laparoscopic repair of bilateral hernias, some advocate the use of a single piece of mesh to alleviate medial recurrence.[68,111] Using a slit to allow passage of the cord may increase recurrence.[109] Parietalization of the cord with alleviation of the need for a slit, or a slitted piece of mesh reinforced by a second nonslitted piece, the so-called double-buttress technique[112] may be used. Historically, Stoppa recommended not using a slit in the GPRVS to alleviate the possibility of recurrence through this defect.[52]

In contrast to conventional repairs, recurrences using laparoscopic repairs usually appear within the first postoperative year.[10,73,106] Tetik et al. published a multicenter retrospective analysis of 1514 laparoscopic repairs with a recurrence rate of 2.2% over an average follow-up of 13 months.[113] Recurrence rates were 22% for the plug and patch, 3% for simple ring closure, 2.2% for IPOM, 0.7% for TAPP, and 0.4% for TEP. Phillips et al. published a multicenter review of 3229 repairs with a recurrence rate of 1.6% over a mean follow-up of 22 months.[114] Felix et al. published a multicenter retrospective analysis of 10,053 TAPP and TEP repairs in 7661 patients; repairs were performed only by surgeons experienced in laparoscopic repairs. The recurrence rate was 0.4% over a mean follow-up of 36 months.[109] The rates in prospective randomized trials with up to 70-month follow-up vary widely, with most studies reporting less than 5%, but some documenting rates as high as 10% (Table 53.5).[10,63,66–73,81,85,90–92]

Nerve Entrapment

Nerve injury results in numbness, pain, and parasthesias in the distribution of the nerve; these results can be mild or incapacitating.[115] Complete nerve transection is likely to cause only numbness and little long-term morbidity, whereas partial transection or entrapment with a staple, suture, or subsequent encroachment by scar tissue is likely to cause neuroma formation and pain.[20,116] Symptoms usually appear immediately postoperatively and intensify over the first 2 weeks; most resolve within 8 weeks.[117] Treatment consists of rest and injections with local anesthetic and corticosteroids until symptoms resolve.[117] In a minority of patients, symptoms persist, necessitating exploration and entrapment release or neurectomy.[118]

The incidence of nerve injuries following conventional open repairs is less than 2%.[2,115,118] Cunningham et al. noted a disturbingly high incidence of postoperative pain in a prospective randomized trial comparing McVay, Bassini, and Shouldice repairs.[115] In 276 patients with 315 repairs performed, 62.9% had pain (11.9% moderate to severe) at 1 year, and 53.6% had pain (10.6% moderate to severe) at 2 years. The incidence of pain was not affected by the type of repair performed. Most often, the pain was associated with a ligamentous somatic etiology attributed to undue tightness of the inguinal ligament at its insertion on the pubic tubercle created by the repair. Only a minority of patients suffered from pain secondary to a neurologic etiology. The excellent results following tension-free repairs such as the Lichtenstein procedure support the conclusion that postoperative pain is due to tension created, with neuralgias occurring only rarely (well less than 1% in Lichtenstein's series).[15] The ilioinguinal, iliohypogastric, and genital branch of the genitofemoral nerve are most at risk during open repairs. The nerves are generally visible and can be avoided. If a nerve must be divided to perform the repair, complete nerve division is usually associated with minimal morbidity.[20,29,116,119]

Nerve entrapment can occur with any of the laparoscopic approaches but may be lowest with the TEP repair.[91] Tetik et al. reported nerve injury in less than 2% of 1514 repairs, with over 90% of these resolving with conservative therapy and only 2 patients requiring reexploration and staple removal.[113]

Phillips et al. reported a 1.6% incidence of neuralgias in 3229 repairs.[114] Other investigators have reported rates as high as 12%, with an increased incidence associated with the IPOM technique and with surgeon inexperience.[91]

Nerve injury typically occurs during laparoscopic repairs when staples are placed inferior to the iliopubic tract in the area lateral to the testicular vessels. The lateral femoral cutaneous nerve, femoral nerve, and femoral branch of the genitofemoral nerve are at risk. These nerves lie superficial to the internal oblique muscle and cannot be visualized. Careful attention to anatomical danger zones during mesh fixation is necessary to avoid entrapment. The triangle of pain and the triangle of doom (Fig. 53.6) designate areas that are anatomical danger zones that require avoidance. Seid combined the two triangles and extended their boundaries to the anterior superior iliac spine laterally, labeling this area the *trapezoid of disaster*.[117] MacFadyen noted that stapling or suturing that causes nerve entrapment will cause pain lasting 6 months or longer.[99] Some advocate not securing the mesh in place at all, which effectively alleviates this complication.[76]

Entrapment of the lateral femoral cutaneous nerve is the most common nerve injury encountered in laparoscopic repairs. It results in pain and numbness in the upper lateral thigh and is called *meralgia paraesthetica*.[120] Broin et al. carefully detailed its course in cadavers and found that it was a mean distance of 6.6cm from the inferior epigastric vessels and 5.6cm from the internal inguinal ring as it passes below the iliopubic tract.[121] They recommended avoiding entrapment of this nerve by staying above the iliopubic tract and not straying too far lateral to the internal inguinal ring when staples are placed.

Entrapment of the ilioinguinal, iliohypogastric, and genital branches of the genitofemoral nerve can occur during laparoscopic repairs if excessive pressure is applied externally during mesh fixation, compressing the muscles enough to allow the staples to reach the nerves.[117]

Ischemic Orchitis/Testicular Atrophy/Vas Deferens Injury

Wantz has extensively studied ischemic orchitis and its sequela testicular atrophy.[20,122] Ischemic orchitis is a potentially devastating but rare complication of hernia repair and is caused by surgical trauma to the veins of the spermatic cord. Anterior approaches are more apt to cause testicular atrophy than posterior approaches since they require more dissection and handling of the cord. It was once thought that the cause was insufficient arterial supply to the testicle secondary to overzealous tightening of the reconstructed internal inguinal ring. It is now known that the cause is venous thrombosis of the injured pampiniform plexus and disruption of collateral arterial and venous circulation by distal cord dissection.[19,20,122] This is more likely to occur in recurrent hernias, which involve scar tissue and a difficult dissection, or when the distal sac is dissected. The result is a swollen, hard cord, testicle, and epididymis. Fever and leukocytosis may occur, but infection is not part of the natural history of this phenomenon. The symptoms become apparent 2 to 5 days postoperatively. The pain usually lasts several weeks, but the swelling and induration may last 4 to 5 months.

Ischemic orchitis may resolve without sequelae or may cause the testicle to shrink, resulting in a completely atrophic testicle. There is no known treatment of ischemic orchitis that prevents progression to testicular atrophy. Only rarely does the testicle become necrotic or require removal. An atrophic testicle is painless, not prone to malignant degeneration, and does not diminish serum testosterone or fertility.[20]

Wantz made several recommendations to avoid ischemic orchitis: avoid dissection of the distal hernia sac except in sliding hernias, avoid dissection beyond the pubic tubercle, use a preperitoneal approach for all recurrent hernias or in patients with prior inguinal or scrotal surgery, and delay the repair of a contralateral hernia for at least 1 year in patients with ischemic orchitis.[20] Using this approach in over 6000 repairs, Wantz reduced the incidence of ischemic orchitis from 0.65% to 0.03% in primary hernias and from 2.25% to 0.97% in recurrent hernias when compared to his prior series.[122] Skandalakis et al. reported an incidence of testicular atrophy of 0.1% after 3010 cases of open hernia repairs.[2]

The incidence of ischemic orchitis following laparoscopic repair is not well documented but is thought to be sufficiently low since a minimum of cord handling and dissection are required, similar to the open preperitoneal approach.[2]

Direct injury to the vas deferens itself can result in infertility if the contralateral side is abnormal. Injury usually manifests as a painful spermatic granuloma, formed by highly antigenic spermatozoa once they have escaped the vas. Excision of the granuloma and microsurgical repair of the vas is treatment of choice.[81]

Bowel Obstruction and Intraabdominal Adhesive Complications

Unique to the laparoscopic approach is the potential for intraabdominal adhesions and intestinal obstruction. There have been multiple case reports of such occurrences, most of which followed TAPP repairs, but the overall incidence remains small, on the order of less than 1%.[60,81,96,98,123–125] The TAPP approach creates peritoneal flaps, which must be closed completely. If a gap remains, bowel can be exposed to the mesh, allowing adhesions, obstruction, erosions, and fistulas.[60,126–128] Bowel can herniate through a peritoneal opening and become incarcerated.[81,96]

The IPOM procedure places mesh in an intraperitoneal position with no protection between the mesh and bowel. Both polypropylene mesh and PTFE have been used, but proponents of PTFE cite its inertness and decreased adhesion formation as an advantage.[63,64] A porcine study compared meshed and unmeshed PTFE with Marlex placed by the TAPP and IPOM methods and noted equal rates of adhesion formation with both PTFE and Marlex but significantly fewer adhesions with the TAPP method.[129]

Others have also found a higher incidence of adhesion formation following the IPOM procedure in animal models.[130,131] Although several series support the efficacy and safety of the IPOM approach, many feel that a peritoneal covering over the prosthesis decreases the risk of complications.[91] Even though the TEP procedure avoids intraperitoneal dissection, there have been reports of intestinal obstruction following TEP repairs when bowel has herniated through peritoneal rents that were either not seen or not adequately repaired at the time of operation.[132,133]

Incisional hernias at trocar sites can occur after laparoscopic repairs and cause intestinal obstruction and strangulation.[62] They are more common after TAPP repairs, occurring in up to 1% of patients, necessitating fascial closure of all ports larger than 5 mm.[60,85] Alternatively, nonbladed and radially dilating trocars may obviate the need for fascial closure.[134] Preexisting umbilical hernias can substantially increase the risk of postoperative umbilical hernias, despite routine closure, and require additional attention.[132]

Some authors feel that the mere possibility of intestinal obstruction as a complication of hernia surgery is reason enough to completely abandon the laparoscopic approach. Others point out that the risk is minimal, especially with the TEP procedure, by following strict technical guidelines.

Vascular Injuries

In laparoscopic repairs, the inferior epigastric, external iliac, femoral, and testicular vessels are at risk. Injuries may result in intraoperative hemorrhage or may present as postoperative hematomas. The inferior epigastric vessels can be injured if trocars are placed medial to the lateral border of the rectus sheath. The pressure of insufflation during laparoscopic procedures can tamponade small venous injuries. After completion of the procedure, hemostasis should be verified with the insufflation pressure minimized. Injuries caused during trocar insertion may not be evident until trocars are removed, mandating careful inspection of these sites under camera visualization as trocars are removed.[101] The reported incidence of postoperative hematoma formation is 1% to 8%.[100] Laparoscopic repairs should be avoided in patients with uncorrected coagulopathies or in cirrhotics (especially with a history of varices) to minimize the risk of retroperitoneal bleeding, which has the potential to fill a very large volume prior to tamponading.

In open repairs, bleeding is not a common intraoperative problem, but the incidence of hematoma formation may be as high as 31%.[71] Meticulous efforts to achieve complete hemostasis should be made. Hematomas may be self-limited or may necessitate evacuation.

Visceral Injuries

At risk are the small intestine, colon, and bladder, and although rare, injuries to these structures can be the source of considerable morbidity, especially if their diagnosis and treatment are delayed.[101] Many of these injuries can occur if an attempt is made to open the sac of a direct sliding hernia. If direct sacs are not opened but are simply reduced and inverted, the risk of injury may be minimized.

In laparoscopic repairs, risk of injury may be minimized by bladder decompression with a Foley catheter, use of an open Hasson cannula technique, insertion of trocars under direct visualization, and thorough anatomical knowledge with cautious dissection.[135] Confining dissection to the area lateral to the medial umbilical ligament is helpful in avoiding bladder injury.[100] Entering the peritoneal cavity with the TAPP and IPOM techniques increases the potential for visceral injury.

Wound Infections

Hernia repair is regarded as a clean operation and as such should have an infection rate of less than 2%.[136] Antibiotic prophylaxis has been the area of controversy. For clean cases, prophylaxis is normally not indicated. However, implantation of a mesh prosthesis has been used as an indication, and some surgeons routinely give prophylactic antibiotics to all hernia repairs. Platt published a landmark study in 1990 that showed significant benefit to patients undergoing open hernia repairs who received antibiotics.[137] On the other hand, Taylor presented a randomized double-blinded prospective study of 619 open hernia repairs comparing antibiotic prophylaxis and no prophylaxis.[138] The study showed no benefit from antibiotic prophylaxis, but a high rate (8.9%) of wound infections occurred in both groups. Gilbert's prospective study comparing prophylaxis versus no prophylaxis and mesh versus no mesh in 2493 repairs confirmed these findings.[139] There was no difference in wound infections between patients who underwent repairs with mesh versus those without mesh, regardless of whether they had received antibiotics. The overall incidence for infection was less than 1%. There was a threefold increase in wound infections in patients over 60 years of age. The results of these studies continue to make antibiotic prophylaxis a controversial subject, and either point of view can be justified.

Of note, in repairs performed using mesh, deep wound infections very rarely, if ever, require removal of the prosthesis.[34,139] They can usually be managed with drainage and antibiotics, allowing the wound to granulate.

Special Considerations

Femoral Repairs

Femoral hernias are much less common than inguinal hernias but are more often associated with complicated presentations, with a 20% incidence of incarceration.[99] Some authors have suggested that the ideal way to repair femoral hernias is via a preperitoneal approach, either open or laparoscopic.[140] This facilitates control of hernia contents and avoids disruption of the inguinal floor mandated by an anterior approach and avoids the difficulty associated with approaching a femoral hernia through a thigh incision. The McVay repair has been used, however, with successful results.[29] Strangulated femoral hernias require proximal control, resection, and anastomosis of intestine and may best be approached through a preperitoneal incision or a midline laparotomy.

Complicated Groin Hernias

Approximately 10% of inguinal hernias and 20% of femoral hernias present incarcerated.[99] Incarcerated hernias can cause intestinal obstruction or strangulation and infarction, resulting in a high incidence of infection, hernia recurrence, and operative mortality, especially in elderly patients. The possibility of such complications has prompted the recommendation that all hernias be repaired electively and promptly as soon as the diagnosis is made.[141]

The laparoscopic approach in the repair of incarcerated hernias is controversial and may be contraindicated,[100] although successful reduction and repair have been reported.[142] The data on this indication are limited, and caution must be exercised, especially if there is any question of bowel viability, in which situation a resection would be required, and a mesh repair would be contraindicated for fear of infectious complications. The laparoscopic approach is, however, well suited for the repair of recurrent hernias.[61,75,91,97,98]

Many authors have advocated the open preperitoneal approach as the procedure of choice for recurrent and incarcerated hernias.[19,20] For recurrent hernias, dense scar tissue in the inguinal canal can be avoided, reducing the risk of nerve injury and cord damage. In strangulated hernias, proximal unaffected intestine can be controlled prior to the release of necrotic intestine. The peritoneal cavity can be opened without an additional incision, and an intestinal resection and anastomosis may be performed.

Pediatric Hernias

The incidence of inguinal hernias in children is between 10 and 20 per 1000 live births, with a 4:1 male-to-female ratio. The overall incidence, incidence of bilaterality, male predominance, and incidence of incarceration are higher in premature infants. The incidence of bilaterality is at least 10% in full-term infants and as high as 55% in premature infants. The incidence of inguinal hernia in cryptorchid infants approaches 65%. Approximately 55% to 70% of inguinal hernias in children are on the right side, and 1% have a direct component.[5] The higher incidence of right-sided hernias is thought to be due to the later descent of the right testicle and potentially delayed closure of the processus vaginalis. Incarceration occurs in 9% to 20% of cases, is more frequent in children younger than 6 months of age, and in the absence of signs of strangulation, can usually be managed by manual reduction followed by prompt elective repair. Elective repair is associated with a much lower incidence of complications compared to emergent operations, especially in low birth weight infants. Elective repair should be performed as soon as possible to avoid reincarceration, which occurs in up to 16% of cases.[143]

The most widely accepted repair of pediatric inguinal hernias is a high ligation of the sac (Fig. 53.8). This technique alone is usually sufficient since the vast majority of pediatric hernias are indirect with no laxity of the internal ring. If ring laxity exists, a few sutures can be placed in the transversalis fascia to approximate the tissues. Recurrence rates of less than 1% are reported.[5]

Considerable debate exists concerning routine contralateral groin exploration. Historically, this has been advocated, given the high incidence of bilaterality. The incidence of a patent contralateral processus vaginalis is higher in girls than in boys who present with a unilateral hernia. Development of a contralateral hernia following unilateral repair is also higher in infants presenting at less than 1 year of age and in infants who present initially with a left-sided unilateral hernia.

Surana and Puri reported the development of a contralateral hernia in only 10% of 116 patients following a unilateral repair and testicular damage in up to 10% of their patients; consequently, they viewed contralateral exploration as unnecessary and hazardous.[144] Jona prospectively analyzed 354 patients undergoing bilateral repairs or unilateral repairs with contralateral exploration and found bilateral involvement in 68% of patients younger than 1 year of age and 41% of patients 1 to 6 years of age, with no increased risk of complications.[145] Jona advocated routine contralateral exploration of all patients younger than 6 years old. Selective contralateral exploration on the basis of a laparoscopic evaluation for a patent processus vaginalis performed through the opened hernia sac decreases the number of negative explorations and may be the best option.[146]

Abdominal Wall Defects

Ventral Hernias

Approximately 90,000 ventral hernias are repaired in the United States each year.[147] Important to remember is the anatomical structure of the anterior abdominal wall, which above the semilunar line of Douglas consists of skin, subcutaneous fat, anterior rectus sheath, rectus muscle, posterior rectus sheath, and peritoneum. Below the semilunar line, the layers are the same except that there is no posterior rectus sheath. Laterally, the layers are skin, subcutaneous fat, external oblique aponeurosis and muscle, internal oblique aponeurosis and muscle, transversus abdominis aponeurosis and muscle, transversalis fascia, and peritoneum.

A *ventral hernia* is a defect in the abdominal wall. Ventral hernias present as a protrusion or bulge and may contain preperitoneal fat or intestinal contents. The size may range from very small to massive. Patients may or may not be symptomatic. The fascial edge along the circumference of the defect is usually palpable on exam. In obese patients, a CT scan or ultrasound examination may help confirm the diagnosis. As with groin hernias, ventral hernias may present with incarceration, strangulation, or bowel obstruction; elective repair is preferred to emergent repair.

Umbilical hernias are due to an error in the embryologic development of the abdominal wall. Umbilical hernias occur in 10% to 30% of live births but frequently close during the first few years of life. If larger than 2cm, the likelihood of the defect spontaneously closing is much less, and repair is not delayed. Otherwise, repair is usually postponed until the child reaches 4 years of age to allow time for spontaneous closure. Most infants are asymptomatic, and incarceration or strangulation is extremely rare.[5] Repair consists of simple fascial closure. Defects may persist, become evident in adulthood, and should be repaired. In cirrhotic patients with uncontrolled ascites, umbilical hernias may rupture, requiring emergent repair. In such instances, a herniorraphy combined with a peritoneal-venous shunt is effective, but mortality rates are high.

Epigastric hernias arise in the upper abdomen along the linea alba, and usually appear in adulthood, often in association with obesity or pregnancy. Epigastric hernias frequently present as small defects with incarcerated preperitoneal fat or omentum, causing pain and warranting repair. Diastasis recti is a condition in which the medial borders of the rectus muscles slowly spread apart, with thinning and stretching of the rectus sheath, resulting in a diffuse bulge in the upper midline abdomen. In contrast to epigastric hernias, diastasis recti is not a fascial defect or hernia per se and consequently presents no threat of complication. Diastasis recti is merely a cosmetic deformity. Excision of the thinned fascia and placement of a mesh prosthesis alleviate the deformity.

Incisional hernias occur in at least 2% to 11% of abdominal wound closures.[148–150] In a 10-year prospective trial of 337 laparotomy patients, Mudge showed that in 62 patients who developed hernias, 56% did so after the first postoperative year, and 35% did so after 5 years, demonstrating the wide variety in intervals between operation and hernia formation.[151] Approximately 17% present with incarceration,[152] and mortality rates for repair of complicated hernias is three times higher than for elective repairs.[153]

Many risk factors for developing an incisional hernia have been cited, including obesity, wound infection, advanced age, postoperative pulmonary complications, jaundice, abdominal distension, emergency operation, reuse of a previous incision, pregnancy, postoperative chemotherapy, steroids, malnutrition, ascites, and peritoneal dialysis. Most of these risk factors are associated with excessive strain on the incision or poor wound healing. Wound infection is the most important risk factor, with hernias four times more likely to occur after a wound infection.[154] Obesity has also been clearly established as a risk factor.[150,155]

Carlson showed that reuse of a previous midline incision in combination with a wound infection was associated with a 10-fold increase in risk of hernia formation.[149] Reuse of an incision has been shown to double the incidence of subsequent incisional hernias.[156] Incisional hernias occur more frequently after a vertical midline incision than after a transverse, subcostal, or paramedian incision.[149,157] This may be due to the fact that emergency operations are more likely to be performed through a midline incision for more complete and rapid exposure; the emergent nature of the operation, and not the type of incision, may be associated with a higher rate of postoperative hernias. This theory was supported by a trial conducted by Ellis, who found no difference in hernia incidence for different types of incisions in patients undergoing elective abdominal procedures.[158]

Suture technique has been extensively studied, with no difference in hernia incidence shown between continuous and interrupted suture techniques or layered versus mass wound closure.[148,159] The advantages of using a continuous suture are more rapid closure and decreased material costs with no increase in hernia or dehiscence rates.[154,160] Continuous sutures, at least theoretically, evenly distribute the tension and cause less tissue necrosis.[161] Permanent suture may be associated with suture sinus formation,[161] infection,[162] or late hernia formation due to gradual sawing of the suture through the fascia, resulting in a "buttonhole" hernia.[152,162]

Absorbable suture alleviates these problems, but must degrade slowly enough to provide sufficient tensile strength until adequate wound healing has occurred. Monofilament suture is preferred over braided suture, which has interstices that can harbor bacteria.[163] Polydioxanone (PDS) and polyglyconate (Maxon) are monofilament absorbable sutures that retain 70% to 75% of their tensile strength at 14 days, are completely absorbed by 180 to 210 days, and may be ideal for fascial closure.[159,162] Sutures that are more rapidly absorbed, such as polyglactin (Vicryl), may be associated with a higher incidence of incisional hernias.[159] Sutures should be placed at least 1 cm back from the fascial edge and no more than 1 cm apart to provide an adequate closure.[148] A suture-to-wound-length ratio of less than 4 is associated with an increased hernia incidence,[150] emphasizing the need to incorporate an adequate amount of tissue in the closure. Overtightening should be avoided, as tissue ischemia and necrosis can occur, predisposing to wound breakdown, dehiscence, and hernia formation.

Of note, the tremendous surge in laparoscopic procedures has spurred the birth of a new type of incisional hernia, the trocar hernia. Multiple reports of such hernias have appeared in the literature.[63] The overall incidence of trocar hernias following laparoscopic procedures is less than 1%.[164] All fascial defects larger than 5 mm should be closed with a fascial closure device to prevent this complication.[63] Recently, trocars that do not use traditional cutting obturators have been introduced to decrease the risk of hernia formation; some level I evidence suggests that these nonbladed and radially dilating trocars do not require closure.[134]

Repair Techniques

Various repair methods exist, and a prosthetic mesh may or may not be used. In open repairs, the hernia is approached through a skin incision placed directly over the fascial defect, usually incorporating the scar from the previous incision. The sac is dissected free from subcutaneous tissues and the fascial edges. The sac may be opened to facilitate lysis of adhesions and inspection and reduction of sac contents. If possible, the sac is not completely excised, so that there is a sufficient amount of sac to close over the intestinal contents. This provides protection against adhesive complications if mesh is to be used in the repair. The superficial and deep surfaces of the fascia are exposed several centimeters back from the hernia defect. Attenuated fascia is excised. A thorough search for concomitant hernias is performed. Depending on the type of repair, fascia may then be closed with or without placing a mesh buttress. Fascia should only be closed when it can be done so without tension. Closed suction drains may be placed in the dead space superficial to the fascia to minimize seroma formation.

In the case of very large hernias existing for a long period of time, most of the intestines and omentum reside in the hernia sac instead of the abdominal cavity. As a result, the abdominal cavity may no longer be large enough to accommodate the viscera when hernia repair is attempted. This can result in diaphragmatic dysfunction and intestinal circulatory congestion after contents are reduced.[54] In this case, the abdominal cavity can be enlarged preoperatively by creating a pneumoperitoneum.[165] The abdominal wall stretches as several liters of air are insufflated into the abdominal cavity over the course of 2 to 3 weeks. Because tension-free repairs can be performed using a mesh prosthesis, this technique is not routinely required.

Hernias recur on average 1.7 years after repair, according to a retrospective review by Leber of 200 hernias repaired with mesh followed for an average of 6.7 years.[157] Recurrence rates after incisional hernia repair vary widely but are disappointing at best, ranging from 20% to 63%, and are notably higher after primary repair than after mesh repairs.[148,157,166] Infection after hernia repair is a feared complication since infection is associated with a markedly higher rate of recurrence. Most infections can usually be managed with antibiotics and debridement and rarely necessitate mesh removal. Simultaneously performed intraabdominal procedures may increase the risk of infection and should be avoided.[167] Several repair techniques are worthy of detailed discussion.

Primary Repair

Ventral hernias may be repaired by primary closure as long as the repair can be performed in a tension-free fashion. The direction of closure is not important. Primary closure is the preferred technique for umbilical hernias in children and some small epigastric or umbilical hernias in adults. Permanent suture is used, and the fascial edges are approximated. Unfortunately, the results of primary repair in all but the smallest of incisional hernias are poor,[151,152] with failure rates as high as 49% to 63%.[166,168,169] This is likely due to the fact that patients with incisional hernias have fascia that is weakened and that does not have sufficient tensile strength to hold sutures when placed under mechanical stress. Multiple modifications of the primary repair technique have yielded widely variable results. The Mayo closure imbricates the fascia in two layers in a vest-over-pants fashion. Paul reported a recurrence rate of 54% in 114 patients who underwent Mayo repairs over a 5.7-year mean follow-up.[170]

Other variations of primary repair have met with better success. Shukla reported no recurrences over 52-month mean follow-up using a far-and-near suture technique in 50 patients with "small- and medium-" size incisional hernias.[171] Sitzmann reported a 2.5% recurrence rate over 42-month follow-up using internal retention sutures in 409 patients with massive incisional hernias (10 cm average defect size).[172] On the other hand, Luijendijk randomized patients with up to 6-cm midline defects to suture (continuous no. 1 polypropylene) versus mesh (polypropylene inlay) repairs and found significantly fewer recurrences for mesh repairs; recurrence rates were 63% over 75-month median follow-up for suture repairs versus 32% over 81-month follow-up for mesh repairs.[166] Thus, some surgeons would advocate mesh repairs for all hernia defects, except in extenuating circumstances such as emergency operations or in contaminated cases.

Mesh Onlay Repair

Significantly better results have been reliably achieved with mesh repairs, with rates of complications comparable to that of primary repairs.[173] Recurrence rates average 6% for mesh repairs according to a collected series of over 800 patients.[172] Several methods for mesh placement exist.

In the onlay method (Fig. 53.19), skin and subcutaneous tissues are elevated, and underlying adhesions are lysed to expose the fascial edges laterally for approximately 4 cm on both the superficial and deep surfaces. Horizontal mattress sutures are placed from within the peritoneal cavity along one-half of the defect, through the full thickness of fascia and muscle, at least 2 cm from the fascial edge. These sutures are passed through the mesh and tied. A second row of sutures is placed on the other half of the defect; sutures are individually clamped and held in moderate tension.

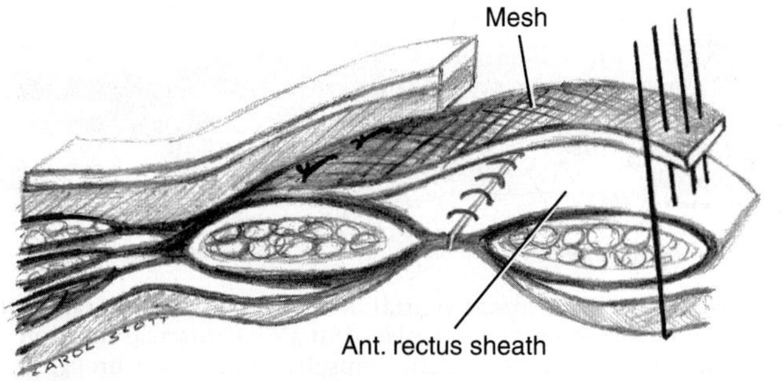

FIGURE 53.19. The mesh onlay technique uses a mesh prosthesis placed superficial to the anterior rectus sheath. The mesh is held in place by full-thickness horizontal mattress sutures.

To avoid risk of intestinal injury, all sutures are placed under direct visualization before the fascia is closed, as opposed to securing the mesh by blindly taking bites on the anterior fascial surface after the fascia has been closed. The latter practice is not only unsafe,[149] but also results in superficial bites that inadequately secure the mesh. After all of the sutures have been placed, the fascia is closed in a running fashion as long as it can be done in a tension-free fashion. This creates a barrier between the abdominal contents and the mesh to prevent adhesions and fistula formation. The clamped sutures are placed through the mesh and tied. If fascia cannot be reapproximated, hernia sac or peritoneum is closed at the midline, or omentum is interposed between the mesh and the intestinal contents to prevent bowel erosion. Alternatively, limited data suggest that placing an absorbable mesh on the intraperitoneal side of the repair may create an adequate barrier against adhesions.[174,175]

Molloy reported using Marlex mesh for the onlay technique in 50 patients with incisional hernias, 19 of which were recurrent.[176] Over a mean follow-up of 45 months, the recurrence rate was 8%. Recurrences were due to partial detachment of the mesh from the fascial edge. A generous overlap of mesh should therefore be used. Although not an advisable practice, in some patients mesh was placed in direct content with abdominal contents with no apparent complications. Complications included 8% wound infection, 4% seroma, and 12% wound sinus; no patients required mesh removal. Sugermann reported a 4% recurrence rate over 20-month mean follow-up using the onlay technique with polypropylene mesh in 98 patients.[155] Complications included 17% wound infection, 5% seroma, 3% hematoma, and 6% chronic pain; 1 patient required mesh removal.

Mesh Inlay and Patch Repairs

The inlay method of repair places a prosthetic mesh deep to the posterior rectus fascia. The mesh is placed in either an intraperitoneal or a preperitoneal position. Mattress sutures are placed from the deep aspect of the mesh through the abdominal wall. Once all sutures have been placed, they are tied on the anterior fascial surface. The patch method simply sutures the prosthesis to the fascial edge circumferentially. With either the inlay or patch technique, if the prosthesis is placed in an intraperitoneal position or if no tissue can be interposed between bowel and the prosthesis, the potential for adhesions and fistulization is created.

Multiple studies have looked at adhesion formation and the use of prostheses placed in an intraperitoneal position. Significant data from animal studies exist supporting the diminished adhesion formation associated with PTFE compared to polypropylene.[177,178] Clinical studies using PTFE with direct contact between abdominal contents and the prosthesis also support its use in this fashion.[169,179,180]

Bauer reported PTFE patch repairs in 28 patients with a recurrence rate of 11% over a 22.5-month mean follow-up.[179] Complications included wound infections in 2 patients (7.1%, both with stomas), and there were no erosions or bowel obstructions.

Sandwich and Cuffed Mesh Repairs

The sandwich or double-layer technique combines both the onlay and inlay techniques, theoretically providing reinforcement of attenuated fascial edges to prevent suture

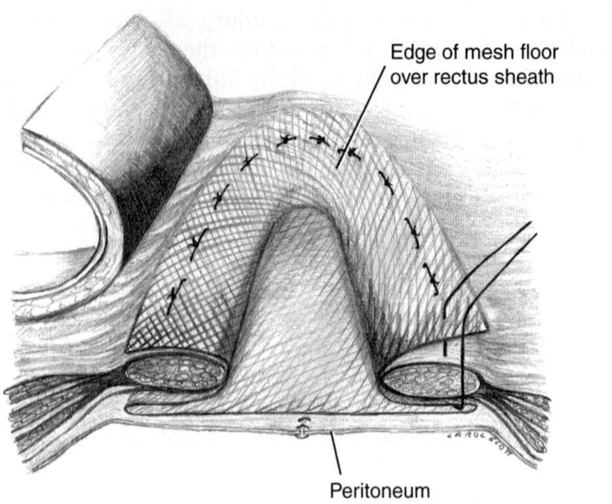

FIGURE 53.20. The "cuffed" technique uses a single piece of mesh and buttresses attenuated fascia by folding the mesh over the rectus sheath to prevent suture pull-through.

dislodgment and recurrence. This technique has been described in several varieties.

Condon described placing a PTFE inlay followed by a polypropylene onlay, using mattress sutures to hold both layers in place.[181] Rubio described using two pieces of Marlex mesh, suturing each piece in a cuffed manner to the anterior and posterior fascial surfaces, and then suturing the two pieces of mesh together in the midline.[182] More recently, Rubio described using two pieces of PTFE for this repair.[183] The disadvantage of two pieces of mesh may be entrapment of fluid between the layers and potential for infection. The surgical technique of using two pieces of mesh is also more cumbersome than using a single piece.

To alleviate the potential problems associated with using two pieces of mesh, McClelland described a modified sandwich approach using a single piece of mesh (Fig. 53.20).[184] A cuff of mesh is folded over the fascial edge for at least 2 cm and sutured into place circumferentially around the defect. McClelland noted that this approach is quicker and equally effective when compared to using two separate pieces of mesh. Although reinforcing the fascial edges by using a cuffed repair makes intuitive sense, trials using this method are lacking.

Stoppa Repair

Stoppa[54] and Wantz[185] have both described the use of a giant Mersilene mesh prosthesis in the repair of large (greater than 10-cm) incisional hernias (Fig. 53.21). This approach is similar to the inlay method but overlaps the defect by 8 to 10 cm and avoids raising extensive subcutaneous flaps by passing sutures through separate stab incisions. The hernia is reduced, and adhesiolysis is performed to widely expose the deep surface of the abdominal wall. Peritoneum is dissected free from the posterior rectus sheath, and the mesh is inserted in the preperitoneal space. Alternatively, the mesh may be inserted between the posterior rectus sheath and the rectus muscle. Prior to mesh insertion, peritoneum, hernia sac, or posterior rectus sheath is closed to prevent contact between abdominal contents and mesh to minimize potential adhesive complications. In the absence of sufficient autogenous tissue, Wantz suggested using an absorbable mesh to facilitate peritoneal or posterior rectus sheath closure as a barrier deep to the Mersilene repair. Others have suggested using PTFE for the definitive repair to lessen the risk of fistula formation.[167]

The repair is facilitated by placing mattress sutures from the deep aspect of the mesh, through the abdominal wall, and out through small stab incisions in the skin. A Reverdin needle facilitates suture placement. Alternatively, large double-arm retention sutures may be used. After sutures have been placed circumferentially around the defect, all sutures are tied on top of the anterior fascial surface through the stab incisions. The anterior rectus fascia is closed, which helps use intraabdominal pressure to hold the mesh in place until it becomes fully incorporated.[186] Making buttonholes in the anterior rectus fascia can release tension and facilitate closure of this layer at the midline. Alternatively, a sheet of absorbable mesh can be used. Closed-suction drains are place on top of the repair and brought out separate skin incisions.

Mersilene mesh may be associated with higher incidences of infection, fistula formation, and recurrence compared to polypropylene or PTFE.[157] However, Mersilene, polypropylene, and PTFE have all been used for this repair with good results. Stoppa reported 368 repairs using Mersilene with a 14.5% recurrence rate over 5.5-year mean follow-up; the overall complication rate was 14%, including 3.2% hematoma and 12% sepsis (none required mesh removal).[54]

McLanahan reported a 3.5% recurrence rate over 24-month follow-up in 106 patients who underwent this repair using polypropylene mesh.[187] Complications included an 18% incidence of wound problems, including one colocutaneous fistula. Five patients required removal of one or more anchoring sutures due to chronic pain. McLanahan noted, however, that suture removal was not necessary in any patient after his group switched to using absorbable sutures and stopped incorporating cartilage or rib in the repair.

Temudom reported no recurrences over 24-month follow-up in 50 patients using either polypropylene or PTFE prostheses.[167] Complications included a 22% incidence of wound problems (8% infections), including two deep infections

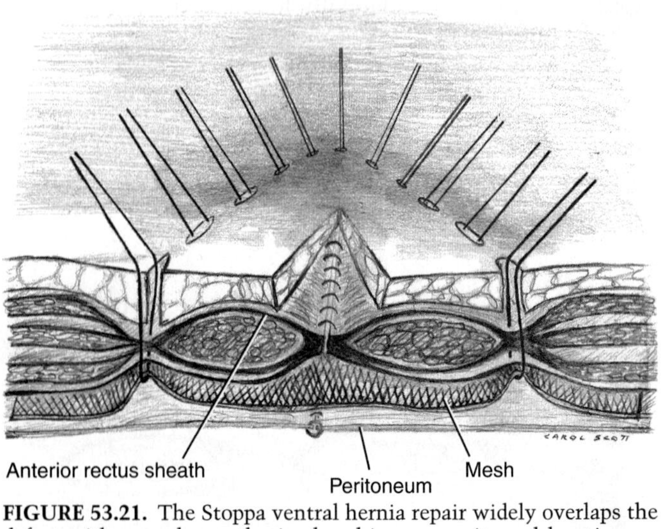

FIGURE 53.21. The Stoppa ventral hernia repair widely overlaps the defect with a mesh prosthesis placed in a preperitoneal location or, alternatively, deep to the rectus muscle. Sutures are brought out through separate stab incisions and tied on top of the anterior fascia.

requiring mesh removal (one patient who had undergone simultaneous gastric bypass, one who had an undetected enterotomy). Seven patients had chronic pain, which resolved without the need for suture removal.

Amid reported no recurrences in 54 patients (no follow-up interval specified) using polypropylene mesh, with the only complication being a seroma in 1 patient.[186] In 25 patients, mesh was secured with staples as opposed to anchoring sutures. Amid claimed that the stapling technique adequately holds the mesh in place until it is incorporated, is faster than suturing, and alleviates the cosmetically unappealing skin retractions at the stab incisions.

Laparoscopic Repair

Laparoscopy has gained considerable momentum in the area of ventral hernias, with standardized techniques becoming well established. Most often, a transabdominal approach is used by placing several trocars in an intraperitoneal position, reducing the hernia through sharp adhesiolysis and blunt manipulation, leaving the hernia sac in situ, and using a mesh prosthesis to close the defect. Mesh is sized externally to provide at least 3 cm of overlap on all sides of the defect. A suture is placed through each corner and tied, with tails left long. The skin is marked at the sites where the four corner sutures will exit, and small stab incisions are made. Mesh is then rolled and passed intraabdominally through a port, unfolded, and positioned over the defect.

A fascial closure device is passed through the skin stab incision and used to individually retrieve the tails of each corner suture. The tails are tied superficial to fascia in a subcutaneous position. Additional transfascial sutures are placed at 4- to 5-cm intervals. Helical fasteners or other similar fixation devices are used to secure the mesh to peritoneum and fascia at 1-cm intervals between the corner sutures, preventing herniation of bowel or omentum between the mesh and the abdominal wall.

The laparoscopic approach facilitates adhesiolysis and hernia repair with minimal access and without the need for a large subcutaneous dissection. Intraperitoneal mesh placement uses intraabdominal pressure to help hold the prosthesis in place. Intraperitoneal mesh placement does, however, create the potential for bowel adhesions and fistula formation. Polypropylene has been used successfully for this repair,[188] but most authors recommend PTFE[147,189,190] or several other newly available composite meshes to decrease the risks of adhesive complications. Recurrences are usually due to inadequate mesh overlap or fixation. Mesh security relies primarily on the transfascial sutures, and using only tacks for mesh fixation may be inadequate.[147] While some series have documented good results with tacks only,[191] most surgeons advocate routine use of sutures to prevent mesh migration.

With appropriate techniques, recurrence rates following laparoscopic repairs are generally about 4% with 4-year follow-up; conversion rates are about 4%. Although randomized controlled trials are still lacking, available data verify that this approach is safe and effective.[147,188,189] As shown in Table 53.6, numerous comparative trials suggest that the laparoscopic approach results in decreased overall complications, fewer wound infections, fewer recurrences, faster recovery, decreased overall cost, and less pain but is associated with an increased rate of seroma formation, more frequent bowel injuries, and longer operative times compared to the conventional open approaches (Table 53.6).[192–201] With 1- to 54-month (2 years on average) follow-up, these comparative trials documented recurrence rates of 0%–61% (13% average) for open repairs and 0%–13% (4% average) for laparoscopic repairs.

Several large cohort trials supported these results, as shown in Table 53.7. With up to 47-month follow-up, these trials documented an average conversion rate of 4.5% and, in studies that used both tacks and suture fixation, a recurrent rate of 3.9%.[147,191,202–210]

Importantly, there is a learning curve for the laparoscopic approach. Good surgical judgment, knowledge of the procedure, and great care must be taken to perform the repair correctly and safely. Special attention must be paid to identifying and repairing (laparoscopically or via a conversion to an open approach) enterotomies or other visceral injuries as they occur, such that missed injuries and postoperative abdominal sepsis may be avoided. By far, this is the most troubling pitfall regarding laparoscopic hernia procedures as missed injuries may lead to mortalities.[194,195,203,208] Whether to proceed with mesh placement in the setting of an adequately repaired enterotomy is controversial. Viable options include not placing mesh and performing a tissue repair or returning to the operating room after several days of antibiotic therapy.[203] Alternatively, if there is no spillage of enteric contents, several authors have successfully placed mesh during the initial operation, as planned, with good results.[203,204]

Since no effort is made to remove the hernia sac, seroma formation is a common occurrence following laparoscopic repairs. Depending on the definition used, seroma formation may occur as frequently as 43%,[197] but is self-limited in the vast majority of patients. While aspirating such seromas may be tempting, only the few (3%–18%) patients with persistent (>6 weeks) seromas should be decompressed since needle aspiration may be associated with subsequent mesh infection.[197,204] In addition, compression bandages or abdominal binders worn for 7–14 days following surgery may help minimize seromas.[210]

As previously mentioned, transfascial suture fixation seems important for repair durability. On the other hand, significant persistent pain may develop at these fixation sites in 1%–26% of cases. Some authors have suggested avoiding overzealous tightening of these sutures to avoid pain. Suture sites can be injected using a combination of steroid and local anesthetic, or sutures can be removed via a cut-down procedure if pain persists. Studies are currently underway investigating the use of absorbable sutures and the efficacy of repairs using nonsuture fixation strategies with a variety of prosthetic types.

Because of the advantages of fewer wound infections and recurrences and a faster recovery, laparoscopic approaches will likely continue playing a major role for ventral hernia repair.

Complex Abdominal Wall Closures and Biomaterials

Abdominal wall closure can be difficult and morbid in the emergency setting. Emergency closures are often required in the face of vigorous resuscitation with massive tissue edema

TABLE 53.6.
Trials Comparing Laparoscopic and Open Ventral Hernia Repairs.

Reference	*Study design*	*No. of repairs*	*Average follow-up*	*Complications (not including recurrences)*	*Recurrences*	*Operative time (min)*	*Length of hospitalization (days)*	*Cost*	*Postop pain*	*Conclusions/details*
McGreevy et al,. 2003, United States[192]	Prospective nonrandomized	Lap: 65	1 mo	Total: 8%[a] Mortality: 0 Wound infection: 0 Seroma: 3%	—	132[a]	1.1	—	—	This study provides perioperative data only with no further follow-up.
		Open: 71	1 mo	Total: 21%[a] Mortality: 0 Wound infection: 8% Seroma: 4%	—	102[a]	1.5	—	—	Reoperation was required for 2 mesh infections and 1 missed enterotomy in the laparoscopic group and 1 wound dehiscence and 1 intraperitoneal abscess in the open group.
Bencina et al., 2003, Italy[193]	Retrospective	Lap: 42	17 mo	Total: 26% Mortality: 0 Bowel injury: 5% Wound infection: 0[a] Seroma: 14%	0	108	5.0[a]	€3,091[a]	↓ medication requirements[a]	Defect size was significantly larger for open repairs (122 cm^2) compared to laparoscopic repairs (83 cm^2), which may have biased outcomes.
		Open: 49	18 mo	Total: 44% Mortality: 0 Bowel injury: 2% Wound infection: 12%[a] Seroma: 10%	6.0%	112	8.0[a]	€3,936[a]		
Salameh, et al., 2002, United States[194]	Retrospective	Lap: 25	13 mo	Total: 32% Mortality: 4% Wound infection: 8% Seroma: 12%	4.0%	173	2.3[a]	—	—	There was 1 death in the laparoscopic group due to a missed enterotomy.
		Open: 35	13 mo	Total: 37% Mortality: 0 Wound infection: 20% Seroma: 5%	8.5%	110	2.8[a]	—	—	

Wright et al., 2002, United States[195]	Retrospective	Lap: 86	24 mo	Total: 24%[a] Mortality: 1% Bowel injury: 6% (3/5 recognized) Wound infection: 4% Seroma/hematoma: 10.4%	1.1%	131[a]	1.5[a]	\$10,135[a]	—	Data in open group are given only for the subset of patients in this study who underwent open repairs *with* mesh. Defect size was significantly smaller for open repairs (79 cm²) compared to laparoscopic repairs (112 cm²) and significantly more recurrent hernias were repaired in the open (31%) vs. the laparoscopic (17%) groups, which may have biased outcomes. There were 2 missed enterotomies in the laparoscopic group, 1 of which resulted in death.
		Open: 90	24 mo	Total: 38%[a] Mortality: 0 Bowel injury: 1% Bladder injury: 1% Wound infection: 9% Seroma/hematoma: 16%	5.5%	102[a]	2.5[a]	\$6,567[a]	—	
Chari et al., 2000, United States[196]	Retrospective	Lap: 14	6–24 mo	Mortality: 0 Bowel Injury: 14%	0	124[a]	5.0	—	—	Very limited data provided by this study.
		Open: 14	6–24 mo	Mortality: 0 Bowel injury: 7%	0	78[a]	5.5	—	—	
DeMaria et al., 2000, United States[197]	Prospective nonrandomized	Lap: 21	12–24 mo	Mortality: 0 Bowel injury: 0 Wound infection: 10% Seroma: 43%	4.8%	—	0.8[a]	\$11,013	↓ at 6 and 24 h[a]	Significantly fewer recurrent hernias were repaired in the open (17%) vs. the laparoscopic (54%) groups, which may have biased outcomes.
		Open: 18	12–24 mo	Mortality: 0 Bowel injury: 0 Wound infection: 33% Seroma: 22%	0	—	4.4[a]	\$13,600		
Carbajo et al., 1999, Spain[198]	Prospective randomized	Lap: 30	27 mo	Mortality: 0 Bowel injury: 0 Wound infection: 0 Seroma/hematoma: 17%	0	87[a]	2.2[a]	—	—	This is a small but well-conducted study providing the only level I data available.
		Open: 30	27 mo	Mortality: 0 Bowel injury: 7% Wound infection: 10% Seroma/hematoma: 87%	6.7%	112[a]	9.1[a]	—	—	

(continued)

TABLE 53.6. Trials Comparing Laparoscopic and Open Ventral Hernia Repairs. (continued)

Reference	*Study design*	*No. of repairs*	*Average follow-up*	*Complications (not including recurrences)*	*Recurrences*	*Operative time (min)*	*Length of hospitalization (days)*	*Cost*	*Postop pain*	*Conclusions/details*
Ramshaw et al., 1999, United States[199]	Retrospective	Lap: 79	21 mo	Total: 19% Mortality: 0 Wound infection: 3% Seroma/hematoma: 3%	2.5%	58	1.7	—	—	There was 1 unrecognized bowel injury in each group; there was also a repair breakdown for a recognized bowel injury in the laparoscopic group. All cases required reoperation and mesh removal, but there were no deaths.
		Open: 174	21 mo	Total: 30%[a] Mortality: 0 Wound infection: 6% Seroma/hematoma: 7%	20.7%	82	2.8	—	—	
Park et al., 1998, United States[200]	Prospective lap, retrospective open	Lap: 56	24 mo on 45 patients	Total: 18%[a] Mortality: 0 Bowel injury: 0 Wound infection: 4% Seroma/hematoma: 4%	13.3%	95[a]	3.4[a]	—	—	Mean time to recurrence was 6 months for laparoscopic repairs and 10.5 months for open repairs.
		Open: 49	54 mo on 28 patients	Total: 37%[a] Mortality: 0 Bowel injury: 4% Wound infection: 8% Seroma/hematoma: 14%	60.7%	79[a]	6.5[a]	—	—	
Holzman, et al., 1997, United States[201]	Retrospective	Lap: 21	20 mo	Total: 23% Mortality: 0 Wound infection: 5% Seroma: 5%	9.5%	128	1.6	$4,395	—	The laparoscopic approach was less costly due to decreased shorter hospital stays and less-severe complications.
		Open: 16	19 mo	Total: 31%[a] Mortality: 0 Wound infection: 6% Seroma: 0%	12.5%	98	4.9	$7,299	—	

—, value was not measured.

[a]Statistical significance (all unmarked values are not statistically significant).

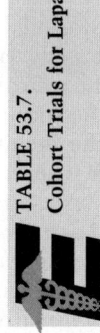

TABLE 53.7.
Cohort Trials for Laparoscopic Ventral Hernia Repair.

Reference	*Study design*	*No. of repairs*	*Average follow-up*	*Mesh/fixation*	*Conversion*	*Bowel injury (recognized/unrecognized)*	*Prolonged seroma*	*Persistent pain*	*Mortality*	*Recurrences*
Franklin et al., 2004, United States[202]	Retrospective	384	47 mo	Various/tacks and sutures	4%	1.3%/0	3%	3%	0	2.9%
Carbajo et al., 2003, Spain[191]	Prospective	270	44 mo	PTFE/tacks only	0.3%	3.3%/0	12%	7.4%	0	4.4%
Heniford et al., 2003, United States[203]	Prospective (85%) Retrospective (15%)	850	20 mo	PTFE/tacks and sutures	3.6%	1.7%/0.1%	2.6%	1.6%	0.1%	4.7%
LeBlanc et al., 2003, United States[204]	Retrospective	200	36 mo	PTFE/tacks and sutures	3.5%	4%/0	7.5%	1%	0	6.5%
Rosen et al., 2003, United States[205]	Retrospective	96	30 mo	Various/various	12.2%	2%/0	4%	—	0	17.7%
Bageacu et al., 2002, France[206]	Retrospective	159	49 mo	Various/tacks only	13.8%	6%/0	15.9%	26%	0	15.7%
Ben-Haim et al., 2002, Israel[207]	Retrospective	100	19 mo	PTFE/tacks and sutures	7.0%	4%/2%	11%	—	0	2.0%
Berger et al., 2002, Germany[208]	Prospective	150	15 mo	PTFE/tacks and sutures	0.6%	0.7%/1.3%	3.3%	—	0.7%	2.7%
Gillian et al., 2002, United States[209]	Retrospective	100	—	Composix/tacks	0	3%/0	3.0%	—	0	1.0%
Chowbey et al., 2000, India[210]	Retrospective	202	35 mo	Polypropylene/tacks	0.5%	0/0	18%	—	0	1.0%
Toy et al., 998, United States, Canada[147]	Prospective	144	7 mo	PTFE/tacks and sutures	0	1.3%/0	5.2%	—	0	4.4%

or, in the case of tissue loss secondary to trauma, surgical debridement for necrotizing infections, or resection of tumors. Such wounds may be heavily contaminated, and postoperative wound sepsis is common. Primary fascial approximation may create a closure under tension and result in abdominal compartment syndrome, dehiscence, evisceration, or fistula formation.[211,212] A prosthetic repair provides tension-free closure and is effective in alleviating evisceration and restoring abdominal wall continuity in the acute phase.[213]

Prosthetic repairs, however, can be fraught with long-term complications. Voyles reported nine of nine patients with Marlex mesh closures of contaminated abdominal wall defects followed by split-thickness skin grafting who either extruded their mesh or developed enteric fistulas.[213] Six of nine patients who underwent Marlex closures followed by wound healing by secondary intention without skin grafting developed fistulas or mesh extrusion. Voyles reported decreased complications if the Marlex closure was covered with full-thickness skin or tissue flaps.

In a review of 14 studies on polypropylene mesh closure emergency abdominal wall defects, Jones reported an overall complication rate of 55% in 128 patients, with enteric fistulization in 23%.[214] No fistulization or mesh extrusion occurred in wounds covered with full-thickness skin or muscle flaps. After polypropylene mesh closure followed by split-thickness skin grafting, Stone reported a mortality of 23% related to progressive wound sepsis.[212]

The use of absorbable mesh provides a lower incidence of fistulization and wound complications but universally leads to ventral hernias, which must be dealt with at a later date. The proponents of absorbable mesh note that it is effective in closing acute abdominal wall defects that are contaminated. Unlike permanent mesh, absorbable mesh does not chronically harbor infection. This allows complete clearance of infection prior to definitive ventral hernia repair, providing a better chance of a successful repair. It also provides no residual foreign body to complicate wound management should a fistula form.

Buck reported using polyglycolic acid (Dexon) mesh in 26 patients with no dehiscence or mesh infection and a fistula rate of 8%.[215] Greene reported a fistula rate of 12% using Dexon in 59 patients.[216] He noted that when polyglactin (Vicryl) was used as a substitute, it ripped with suturing and was too rapidly absorbed.

In 166 patients, Fabian reported an overall fistula rate of 8% and no wound-related deaths using a protocol that called for absorbable mesh repair of emergency defects, followed by mesh removal prior to wound coverage and planned repair of the ventral hernia at a later date.[211,217] Mesh was removed 2 to 3 weeks postinsertion (after granulation tissue developed) and split- or full-thickness skin grafts were placed 2 to 3 days later after wounds were packed to minimize bacterial contamination. Definitive hernia repairs were then performed 6 to 12 months later, after adhesions had matured to a filmy stage. Using this method, Fabian reported being able to perform primary fascial closure at the time of mesh removal in 22% of patients who originally received mesh closures for massive edema. These patients were spared a subsequent planned ventral hernia repair. Over a mean 24-month follow-up, only 5% of 73 patients who underwent planned delayed repair using a modified components separation (without mesh) developed recurrent hernias.

Complex cases, including intraabdominal abscesses, fistulas, mesh infections, abdomens originally closed by secondary intention, or recurrent hernias in the setting of hostile abdomens or previous skin grafts may be well suited for repair using autogenous tissue, namely, through methods of fascial partitioning. The so-called components separation technique, as described by Ramirez in 1990, involves adhesiolysis, reduction of the hernia (usually midline), and reconstruction of the abdominal wall using relaxing incisions that allow medial transposition of the muscular layers.[218] After widely undermining the subcutaneous tissue, parasagittal relaxing incisions are made in the external oblique aponeurosis and muscle about 2 cm lateral to its insertion into the rectus sheath starting at the groin and continuing 5 to 7 cm cephalad to the costal margin; the external oblique muscle is separated from the internal oblique muscle as far laterally as possible, and the linea alba is closed primarily. If tension exists, additional length can be gained by incising the rectus sheath and reflecting the fascia off the muscle toward the midline; alternatively, the transversus abdominis muscle may be incised via a transperitoneal approach to provide further medial mobilization. Defects as large as 20 cm at the umbilical level can be closed using these maneuvers.[219]

Mesh may also be used in conjunction with components separation, either for reinforcement of emaciated tissues or when inadequate autogenous tissue exists.[220] As an alternative to wide subcutaneous undermining, separate skin incisions can be used to mobilize the external oblique myoaponeurosis.

Recently, endoscopic techniques using balloon dissection and muscular transection under videoscopic control have been developed.[219] For massive hernias in patients with loss of domain, components separation may be combined with the use of tissue expanders to gain additional skin, muscle, and fascia laterally for subsequent midline mobilization.[221]

Shestak repaired 22 midline hernias up to 14 cm wide and 24 cm long using components separation (with mesh in only 1 patient) and reported a recurrence rate of 5% over 52-month mean follow-up.[222] De Vries Reilingh used components separation (primary running fascial closure without mesh) to repair complex midline hernias in 43 patients having a mean defect size of 18 cm long × 13 cm wide; the recurrence rate was 30% over 15.6-month mean follow-up.[219] While the recurrence rate in the latter series may seem high, 15 patients had simultaneous intestinal surgery (3 Hartmann's reversal, 2 ileostomy reversal, 4 enterocutaneous fistula repairs, 5 ostomy relocations, 2 other), and 35% of reconstructions were done under contaminated conditions. Thus, component separation may be quite useful in these settings with acceptable results; large series or comparative trials, however, are not yet available.

New biomaterials are now available that facilitate hernia repair through remodeling of native tissues and may be especially useful in the setting of contamination. Through tissue engineering, human or porcine specimens can be decellularized with maintenance of the architectural integrity, thus serving as a collagen matrix. Currently available materials made from porcine small intestine submucosa, porcine dermis, and human cadaveric dermis, when implanted, allow fibroblast ingrowth with subsequent collagen deposition and remodeling. The lack of a true foreign body has proven especially useful in complex abdominal wall reconstructions in the setting of contamination, but long-term documentation of efficacy for routine hernia repair is lacking. These prostheses are currently very expensive; are often available in only small sizes, requiring tedious suturing for creation of larger composite pieces; and some have difficult handling characteristics (very flimsy). Nonetheless, the recent introduction of these materials has fueled significant enthusiasm for their use.

Ueno repaired 18 ventral and 2 inguinal hernias in the setting of bacterial contamination using small intestinal submucosa (SIS; Surgisis, Cook Surgical, Bloomington, IN) and documented a 30% recurrence rate over 15.7-month mean follow-up.[223] Franklin repaired 58 hernias in 53 patients using SIS, including 34% with potential contamination and 22% with gross contamination, and reported no mesh-related complications and no recurrences over 19-month median follow-up.[224] Eid laparoscopically repaired 12 ventral hernias using SIS at the time of Roux-en-Y gastric bypass operations for morbid obesity and found no recurrences over 13-month mean follow-up.[225] These series documented no mesh reactions and good compatibility between the porcine-derived prosthetic and the human host. Moreover, SIS seems to withstand bacterial contamination relatively well. Porcine dermis (Permacol, Tissue Science Laboratories, Covington, GA) and human cadaveric dermis (Alloderm, LifeCell Corp., Branchburg, NJ) have recently been introduced, and although data are lacking, early reports suggest good utility of these biomaterials.[226,227]

Other Abdominal Hernias

Spigelian

The Spigelian or semilunar line marks the transition from muscle to aponeurosis of the transversus abdominis muscle. The Spigelian fascia lies between this line and the lateral border of the rectus sheath. A defect in this fascia results in a Spigelian hernia. Up to 90% are located 0 to 6 cm cranial to the interspinal plane (the horizontal plane through both anterior iliac spines).[228] The defect originates in the transversus abdominis muscle and may or may not involve the more superficial layers; hernia sac and contents often lie in an intramural location between the abdominal wall layers and may not be palpable. Consequently, patients often present with vague complaints of pain and nonspecific tenderness on exam. Computed tomography or ultrasound scanning may aid in the diagnosis. Ultimate diagnosis may not be made until the time of surgical exploration.

Exploration may be undertaken via an incision directly over the defect if palpable. If it is nonpalpable, exploration via a preperitoneal approach through a midline or paramedian incision avoids an extensive subcutaneous dissection. The defect is usually small and can be repaired primarily. Recently, success has been reported using laparoscopic approaches.[229,230]

Lumbar

Lumbar hernias occur spontaneously, posttraumatically, or as incisional hernias (such as following nephrectomy). They represent defects through the transversalis fascia and transversus abdominis muscle aponeurosis. Retroperitoneal fat or a peritoneum-lined sac may herniate through the defect. Patients present with a symptomatic posterior bulge but rarely with a strangulated hernia.

There are two lumbar triangles. The inferior or Petit's triangle is bordered by the latissimus dorsi muscle, the external oblique muscle, and the iliac crest; it is covered only by superficial fascia. The superior or Grynfeltt's triangle is bordered by the 12th rib, internal oblique muscle, and sacrospinalis muscle; it is covered by the lattissimus dorsi muscle.

Repair can be performed primarily if the defect is small, but a myofascial flap, such as a gluteus maximus fascial flap for inferior triangle hernias, or repair with mesh is necessary for larger defects. An oblique incision from the 12th rib medially to the iliac crest laterally provides adequate exposure. Recent reports documented success with laparoscopic repairs using mesh.[231]

Pelvic Floor Hernias

Pelvic floor hernias include (in decreasing frequency) obturator, perineal, and sciatic hernias. Obturator hernias occur when abdominal contents herniate through the obturator canal along the course of the obturator neurovascular bundle. The obturator membrane, which covers the obturator foramen and forms the canal, is indistensible, and herniated bowel often becomes incarcerated and strangulated. These hernias are most often seen in emaciated females in their eighth decade, almost always occurring on the right side. A preoperative diagnosis is difficult and infrequently made.

Patients usually present with partial or complete acute small-bowel obstruction without a palpable hernia. Rarely a mass may be palpable on the anteriomedial aspect of the thigh or on pelvic and rectal examinations. A Howship-Romberg sign (obturator neuralgia produced by compression of the obturator nerve by the hernia on extension and adduction followed by medial rotation of the ipsilateral thigh) may be present in up to 50% of cases. Computed tomography or abdominopelvic ultrasound scanning can confirm the diagnosis.

Exploration may be carried out via a number of incisions, but a lower midline provides the best exposure for resecting compromised bowel and adequate repair of the hernia defect.[232] The defect may be closed primarily, with mesh, or by advancing adductor longus muscle flap. Recently, success has also been reported using laparoscopic approaches.[233] Mortality rates may be as high as 75%, secondary to the advanced age and debilitated states of most patients and to delays in diagnosis. Therefore, prompt treatment should be rendered.[234]

Perineal hernias may occur spontaneously or as incisional hernias after procedures such as abdominoperineal resections or pelvic exenterations. These hernias occur anteriorly in women, involving the urogenital diaphragm and passing into the labia majora. Posterior perineal hernias are defects in the levator ani muscles and occur in the ischiorectal fossa between the bladder and the rectum. Patients present with soft reducible masses. A primary repair or a repair with mesh may be performed through either a perineal or an abdominal approach.[235]

Sciatic hernias are the rarest of all hernias and occur in the greater or lesser sciatic foramen through a defect in the piriformis muscle. Patients may be symptomatic with sciatic nerve palsy and a palpable mass or may simply present with intestinal obstruction. Repair can be performed via a gluteal approach or a transabdominal approach.[236]

Parastomal

Parastomal hernias occur through defects adjacent to ostomy sites. The incidence of paracolostomy hernias is 12% to 32% and for paraileostomy hernias is less than 10%.[237] Construction of the ostomy through an appropriately small fascial defect in the rectus sheath and not maturing the ostomy through the laparotomy incision decrease the risk of subsequent hernia formation. The majority of patients are asymptomatic. Patients may present with obstruction, incarceration, a poor-fitting appliance, or local pain and warrant repair. Options include primary fascial repair, prosthetic fascial repair, or stomal relocation. Local procedures can be technically demanding and pose infection risk if a prosthetic is used but avoid laparotomy and potentially extensive adhesiolysis. Formal laparotomy alleviates ostomy contamination of prosthetic material and provides access for repair or relocation.

No prospective randomized trials have been performed; Rubin published the largest study comparing repair techniques, which included a retrospective analysis of 68 repairs in 55 patients.[238] Hernias recurred in 63% of the 68 repairs, and complications occurred in 63% of the patients. Incisional hernias at the laparotomy site or at the old ostomy site occurred in 21%. In primary parastomal hernias, 76% of primary fascial repairs, 50% of prosthetic repairs, and 33% of stoma relocations failed. For recurrent parastomal hernias, 100% of primary fascial repairs, 33% of prosthetic repairs, and 71% of stomal relocations failed. Because parastomal hernias are generally well tolerated and all types of repair are associated with significant morbidity and high recurrence rates, repair should be avoided if possible.

Internal Hernias

Internal hernias occur when intraperitoneal contents prolapse through a normal or abnormal orifice. Normally existing orifices include the foramen of Winslow (known as the hernia of Blandin). Abnormally existing orifices are congenital peritoneal fossae and include left and right paraduodenal, pericecal, intersigmoid, paravascular, and supravesiclar and hernias inside the broad ligament of the uterus. These hernias account for up to 2% of all abdominal hernias.[239] Patients present with a closed-loop intestinal obstruction, and diagnosis is usually made at the time of operation.

The operation involves reduction of incarcerated bowel, resection of nonviable segments, and primary closure of the hernia orifice. In the case of left and right paraduodenal hernias, the orifices are intimately associated with the inferior and superior mesenteric vessels, respectively, and great care must be taken during reduction and repair to preserve these vessels.

Internal hernias may also be iatrogenic, occurring after a previous operation in which a defect in mesentery or omentum was not adequately closed. Frequently, these defects occur after loop or Roux-en-Y gastrojejunostomy formation either behind the afferent (known as a Petersen hernia) or efferent limbs. Retroanastomotic hernias are best avoided by closure of all mesenteric defects at the time of initial operation. If such a hernia occurs, reduction and closure are necessary at laparotomy.

Congenital Abdominal Wall Defects

Gastroschisis refers to herniation of the abdominal viscera without a sac and in the presence of an intact umbilical cord. It is now thought to be a separate entity from omphalocele. It is twice as common as omphalocele but associated with half as many anomalies. The most common associated anomaly is intestinal atresia, which is present in 10% of cases. The eviscerated intestine is edematous, matted with fibrinous adhesions, and shortened, resulting in intestinal absorptive and motility dysfunction.[240]

Repair can be performed by primary fascial closure or a staged procedure with closure of skin followed by subsequent fascial closure. Gentle stretching of the abdominal wall can enlarge the abdominal cavity and help facilitate repair. If visceroabdominal disproportion is severe, the eviscerated intestine is enclosed within a prosthetic silo attached at its base to the abdominal wall. As the edema diminishes, sequential compression of the top of the silo returns the herniated contents into the abdomen and allows fascial closure. Mortality is less than 10%.

Omphalocele refers to herniation of the abdominal viscera into the umbilical cord, resulting in a sac lined internally by peritoneum and externally by amnion. The size of the defect may range from small to massive. Pelvic involvement can result in cloacal extrophy. Structural and chromosomal anomalies are present in up to 50% of cases. Repair of the abdominal defect can be performed similar to the methods used for gastroschisis. The severity of associated anomalies largely determines long-term survival.

Congenital Diaphragmatic Hernias

Congenital diaphragmatic hernias occur in 1 of every 2100 pregnancies (including spontaneously aborted pregnancies) and 1 of every 4800 live births.[241] They can be characterized by their location. Bochdalek hernias are located posteriolaterally, and Morgagni hernias are located anteriorly.

Bochdalek hernias occur between the costal and spinal diaphragmatic attachments and account for the majority of congenital diaphragmatic hernias. The defect is the result of embryological failure of the pleuroperitoneal canal to close as the pleuroperitoneal membranes (laterally), the dorsal mesentery (posteriorly), and the septum transversum (anteriorly) fuse to form the diaphragm. The left side closes after the right; there is thus a 4:1 preponderance for left-sided hernias. Nonrotation of the intestine is usually associated with the defect. Hernia contents are enclosed within a sac in only 10% to 20% of cases. Because abdominal contents occupy the thoracic cavity during fetal development, pulmonary hypoplasia can be severe. Mortality rates are as high as 80% in the first month of life, despite advances in ionotropic therapy, ventilatory support, and extracorporeal membrane oxygenation (ECMO).[242]

Immediate repair at birth results in higher mortality rates and delaying repair to the first few days to weeks of life after pulmonary function has stabilized is advantageous.[242] Repair is via an abdominal approach and consists of reduction of hernia contents, sac excision, primary or prosthetic (usually PTFE) diaphragm repair, and a Ladd procedure. Occasionally,

Bochdalek hernias may be diagnosed in older children exhibiting only mild symptoms. Elective repair is indicated to avoid potential complications.

Morgagni hernias occur between the sternal and costal diaphragmatic attachments in a retrosternal or parasternal position. They result from failure of the septum transversum to fuse with the thoracic wall and account for 2% of congenital diaphragmatic hernias. Associated cardiac anomalies are frequent, and the defect may be part of the Cantrell pentalogy (defects in the abdominal wall, sternum, diaphragm, pericardium, and heart). Contents are usually enclosed within a sac, and 90% of hernias are right-sided. In infants, respiratory distress is usually present. When discovered in adults, symptoms are often mild or absent.

Repair is indicated in all cases to prevent incarceration. The repair can be performed via an abdominal or thoracic approach, similar to the repair of Bochdalek hernias. Recently, success in adult patients has been reported using laparoscopic approaches.[243]

References

1. Condon RE, Carilli S. The biology and anatomy of inguinofemoral hernia. Semin Laparosc Surg 1994;1:75–85.
2. Skandalakis JE, Skandalakis LJ, Colborn GL. Testicular atrophy and neuropathy in herniorrhaphy. Am Surg 1996;62:775–782.
3. Fruchaud H. Anatomie Chirurgicale des Hernies de l'Aine. Paris: Doin; 1956.
4. Skandalakis JE, Colborn GL, Androulakis JA, et al. Embryologic and anatomic basis of inguinal hernorrhaphy. Surg Clin North Am 1993;73:799–836.
5. Skinner MA, Grosfeld JL. Inguinal and umbilical hernia repair in infants and children. Surg Clin North Am 1993;73:439–449.
6. Rowe MI, Copelson LW, Clatworthy HW. The patent processus vaginalis and the inguinal hernia. J Pediatr Surg 1969;4:102–107.
7. Peacock EE, Madden JW. Studies on the biology and treatment of recurrent inguinal hernias: II. Morphologic changes. Ann Surg 1974;179:567–571.
8. Read RC. Attenuation of rectus sheath in inguinal herniation. Am J Surg 1970;120:610–614.
9. Read RC. A review: the role of protease-antiprotease imbalance in the pathogenesis of herniation and abdominal aortic aneurysm in certain smokers. Post Gen Surg 1992;4:161–165.
10. Liem MSL, Van Der Graff Y, Van Steensel CJ, et al. Comparison of conventional anterior surgery and laparoscopic surgery for inguinal-hernia repair. N Engl J Med 1997;336:1541–1547.
11. Hurst RD, Butler BN, Soybel DI, et al. Management of groin hernias in patients with ascites. Ann Surg 1992;216:696–700.
12. MacAthur DC, Grieve DC, Thompson AM, et al. Herniography for groin pain of uncertain origin. Br J Surg 1997;84:684–685.
13. Rutkow IM, Robbins AW. Demographic, classificatory, and socioeconomic aspects of hernia repair in the United States. Surg Clin North Am 1993;73:413–426.
14. Rutledge RH. Cooper's ligament repair. In: Nyhus LM, Baker RJ, Fischer JE, eds. Mastery of Surgery. Boston: Little Brown; 1997:1817–1825.
15. Amid PK, Shulman AG, Lichtenstein IL. Open "tension-free" repair of inguinal hernias: the Lichtenstein technique. Eur J Surg 1996;162:447–453.
16. Nyhus LM. Individualization of hernia repair: a new era. Surg 1993;114:1–2.
17. Cheek CM, Williams MH, Farndon JR. Trusses in the management of hernia today. Br J Surg 1995;82:1611–1613.
18. Sohrabi AK, Wille G, Guernsey J, et al. En masse reduction of hernia. Contemp Surg 1997;50:100–104.
19. Reid I, Devlin HB. Testicular atrophy as a consequence of inguinal hernia repair. Brit J Surg 1994;81:91–93.
20. Wantz GE. Testicular atrophy and chronic residual neuralgia as risks of inguinal hernioplasty. Surg Clin North Am 1993;73:571–582.
21. Griffith CA. The Marcy repair revisited. Surg Clin North Am 1984;64:215–227.
22. Wantz GE. The operation of Bassini as described by Attilio Catterina. Surg Gynecol Obstet 1989;168:67–80.
23. Shouldice EE. The treatment of hernia. Ontario Med Rev 1953;20:670–684.
24. Wantz GE. The Canadian repair: personal observations. World J Surg 1989;13:516–521.
25. Glassow F. The Shouldice hospital technique. Int Surg 1986;71: 148–153.
26. Wantz GE. Shouldice repair. Contemp Surg 1988;33:15–21.
27. Hay J, Boudet M, Fingerhut A, et al. Shouldice inguinal hernia repair in the male adult: the gold standard? A multicenter controlled trial in 1578 patients. Ann Surg 1995;222:719–727.
28. McGillicuddy JE. Prospective randomized comparison of the Shouldice and Lichtenstein hernia repair procedures. Arch Surg 1998;133:974–978.
29. Rutledge RH. A 25 year experience with a single technique for all groin hernias in adults. Surg 1988;103:1–10.
30. Rutkow IM, Robbins AW. "Tension-free" inguinal herniorrhaphy: a preliminary report on the mesh plug technique. Surg 1993;114:3–8.
31. Panos RG, Beck DE, Maresh JE, et al. Preliminary results of a prospective randomized study of Cooper's ligament versus Shouldice herniorrhaphy technique. Surg Gynecol Obstet 1992; 175:315–319.
32. Lichtenstein IL, Shulman AG. Ambulatory outpatient hernia surgery, including a new concept, introducing tension-free repair. Int Surg 1986;71:1–4.
33. Lichtenstein IL, Shulman AG, Amid PK, et al. The tension-free hernioplasty. Am J Surg 1989;157:188–193.
34. Shulman AG, Amid PK, Lichtenstein IL. The safety of mesh repair for primary inguinal hernias: results of 3019 operation from five diverse surgical sources. Am Surg 1992;58:255–257.
35. Kark AE, Kurzer MN, Belsham PA. Three thousand one hundred seventy-five primary inguinal hernia repairs: advantages of ambulatory open mesh repair using local anesthesia. J Am Coll Surg 1998;186:447–456.
36. Shulman AG, Amid PK, Lichtenstein IL. Ligation of hernia sac a needless step in adult hernioplasty. Int Surg 1993;78:152–153.
37. Friis E, Lindahl F. The tension-free hernioplasty in a randomized trial. Am J Surg 1996;172:315–319.
38. Burger JW, Luijendijk RW, Hop WC, et al. Long-term follow-up of a randomized controlled trial of suture versus mesh repair of incisional hernia. Ann Surg 2004;240:578–583.
39. Beecherl EE, Jones DB, Carrico CJ. McVay to Lichtenstein: evolution of inguinal herniorrhaphy at a teaching institution. Paper resented at: North Texas Chapter of American College of Surgeons; 1997.
40. Shulman AG, Amid PK, Lichtenstein IL. Patch or plug for groin hernia—which? Am J Surg 1994;167:331–336.
41. Shulman AG, Amid PK, Lichtenstein IL. The "plug" repair of 1402 recurrent inguinal hernias. Arch Surg 1990;125:265–267.
42. Shulman AG, Amid PK, Lichtenstein IL. Prosthetic mesh plug repair of femoral and recurrent inguinal hernias: the American experience. Ann R Coll Surg Engl 1992;74:97–99.
43. Rutkow IR, Robbins AW. Mesh plug hernia repair: a follow-up report. Surg 1995;117:597–598.
44. Gilbert AI. Sutureless repair of inguinal hernia. Am J Surg 1992;163:331–335.

45. Wantz GE. Experience with the tension-free hernioplasty for primary inguinal hernias in men. J Am Coll Surg 1996;183:351–356.
46. Nyhus LM, Condon RE, Harkins HN. Clinical experiences with the preperitoneal hernia repair for all types of hernia of the groin: with particular reference to the importance of transversalis fascia analogues. Am J Surg 1960;100:234–244.
47. Nyhus LM, Pollak R, Bombeck CT. The preperitoneal approach and prosthetic buttress repair for recurrent hernia: the evolution of a technique. Ann Surg 1988;208:733–737.
48. Nyhus LM. Iliopubic tract repair of inguinal and femoral hernia: the posterior (preperitoneal) approach. Surg Clin North Am 1993;73:487–499.
49. Hoffman HC, Traverso ALV. Preperitoneal prosthetic herniorrhaphy: one surgeon's successful technique. Arch Surg 1993;128: 964–970.
50. Stoppa RE, Quintyn M. Les deficiences de la paroi abdominale chez le suget age: colloque avec le praticien. Semin Hop Paris 1969;45:2182–2184.
51. Stoppa RE, Rives JL, Warlaumont CR, et al. The use of Dacron in the repair of hernias of the groin. Surg Clin North Am 1984;64:269–285.
52. Stoppa RE. The giant prosthesis for the reinforcement of the visceral sac in the repair of groin and incisional hernias. In: Nyhus LM, Baker RJ, Fischer JE, eds. Mastery of Surgery. Boston: Little Brown; 1997:1859–1869.
53. Wantz GE. Giant prosthetic reinforcement of the visceral sac. Surg Gynecol Obstet 1989;169:408–417.
54. Stoppa RE. The treatment of complicated groin and incisional hernias. World J Surg 1989;13:545–554.
55. Mathonnet M, Cubertafond, Gainant A. Bilateral inguinal hernias: giant prosthetic reinforcement of the visceral sac. Hernia 1997;1:93–95.
56. Munshi IA, Wantz GE. Management of recurrent and perivascular femoral hernias by the giant prosthetic reinforcement of the visceral sac. J Am Coll Surg 1996;182:417–422.
57. Ger R. The management of certain abdominal hernia by intra-abdominal closure of the neck of the sac. Ann R Coll Engl 1982:64:342–344.
58. Molmenti EP, Soper NJ. Inguinal hernias. In: Jones DB, Wu JS, Soper NJ, ed. Laparoscopic Surgery: Principles and Procedures. St. Louis: Quality Medical; 1997:233–246.
59. Korman JE, Hiatt JR, Feldmar D, et al. Mesh configurations in laparoscopic extraperitoneal herniorrhaphy. Surg Endosc 1997; 11:1102–1105.
60. Felix EL, Michas CA, Gonzalez MH. Laparoscopic hernioplasty: TAPP versus TEP. Surg Endosc 1995;9:984–989.
61. Swanstrom LL. Laparoscopic herniorraphy. Surg Clin North Am 1996;76:483–491.
62. Jones DB, Callery MP, Soper NJ. Strangulated incisional hernia at trocar site. Surg Laparosc Endosc 1996;6:152–154.
63. Vogt DM, Curet MJ, Pitcher DE, et al. Preliminary results of a prospective randomized trial of laparoscopic onlay versus conventional inguinal herniorrhaphy. Am J Surg 1995;169: 84–90.
64. Toy FK, Moskowitz M, Smoot RT, et al. Results of a prospective multicenter trial evaluating the ePTFE peritoneal onlay laparoscopic inguinal hernioplasty. J Laparoendosc Surg 1996;6:375–385.
65. Jones DB, Maithel SK, Schneider BE, eds. Atlas of Minimally Invasive Surgery. Cine-Med; Woodbury, CT, 2006.
66. Paganini AM, Lezoche E, Carle F, et al. A randomized, controlled, clinical study of laparoscopic versus open tension-free inguinal hernia repair. Surg Endosc 1998;12:979–986.
67. Zieren J, Zieren H, Jacobe CA, et al. Prospective randomized study comparing laparoscopic and open tension-free inguinal hernia repair with Shouldice's operation. Am J Surg 1998;175:330–333.
68. Champault G, Rizk N, Catheline JM, et al. Inguinal hernia repair: totally pre-peritoneal laparoscopic approach versus Stoppa operation, randomized trial: 100 cases. Hernia 1997;1: 31–36.
69. Kald A, Anderberg, Carlsson P, Park PO, et al. Surgical outcome and cost-minimization-analyses of laparoscopic and open hernia repair: a randomized prospective trial with 1 year follow-up. Eur J Surg 1997;163:505–510.
70. Bessell JR, Baxter P, Riddell P, et al. A randomized controlled trial of laparoscopic extraperitoneal hernia repair as a day surgical procedure. Surg Endosc 1996;10:495–500.
71. Wright DM, Kennedy A, Baxter JN, et al. Early outcome after open versus extraperitoneal endoscopic tension-free hernioplasty: a randomized clinical trial. Surg 1996;119:552–557.
72. Tschudi J, Wagner M, Klaiber C, et al. Controlled multicenter trial of laparoscopic transabdominal preperitoneal hernioplasty versus Shouldice herniorrhaphy. Surg Endosc 1996;10:845–847.
73. Barkun JS, Wexler MJ, Hinchey EJ, et al. Laparoscopic versus open inguinal herniorrhaphy: preliminary results of a randomized controlled trial. Surg 1995;118:703–710.
74. Stoker DL, Spiegelhalter DJ, Singh R, Wellwood JM. Laparoscopic versus open inguinal hernia repair: randomized prospective trial. Lancet 1994;343:1243–1245.
75. Neumayer L, Giobbie-Hurder A, Jonasson O, et al. Open mesh versus laparoscopic mesh repair of inguinal hernia. N Engl J Med 2004;350:1819–1827.
76. Liem MSL, Van Duyn EB, Van Der Graaf Y, Van Vroonhoven TJMV. Recurrences after conventional anterior and laparoscopic inguinal hernia repair: a randomized comparison. Ann Surg 2003;237:136–141.
77. Bringman S, Ramel S, Heikkinen T, et al. Tension-free inguinal hernia repair: TEP versus mesh-plug versus Lichtenstein: a prospective randomized controlled trial. Ann Surg 2003;237:142–147.
78. Wright D, Paterson C, Scott N, et al. Five-year follow-up of patients undergoing laparoscopic or open groin hernia repair: a randomized controlled trial. Ann Surg 2002;235:333–337.
79. Leibl BJ, Daubler P, Schmedt CG, et al. Long-term results of a randomized clinical trial between laparoscopic hernioplasty and Shouldice repair. Br J Surg 2000;87:780–783.
80. The MRC Laparoscopic Groin Hernia Trial Group. Laparoscopic versus open repair of groin hernia: a randomised comparison. Lancet 1999;354:183–188.
81. Payne JH, Grininger LM, Izawa MT, et al. Laparoscopic or open inguinal herniorrhaphy? A randomized prospective trial. Arch Surg 1994;129:973–981.
82. Schmedt CG, Sauerland S, Bittner R. Comparison of endoscopic procedures versus Lichtenstein and other open mesh techniques for inguinal hernia repair: a meta-analysis of randomized controlled trials. Surg Endosc 2005;19:188–199.
83. Memon MA, Cooper NJ, Memon B, et al. Meta-analysis of randomized clinical trials comparing open and laparoscopic inguinal hernia repair. Br J Surg 2003;90:1479–1492.
84. Liem MSL, Van Steensel CJ, Boelhouwer RU, et al. The learning curve for totally extraperitoneal laparoscopic inguinal hernia repair. Am J Surg 1996;171:281–285.
85. Kald A, Anderberg B, Smedh K, Karlsson M. Transperitoneal or totally extraperitoneal approach in laparoscopic hernia repair: results of 491 consecutive herniorrhaphies. Surg Laparosc Endosc 1997;7:86–89.
86. Schneider BE, Castillo JM, Villegas L, Scott DJ, Jones DB. Laparoscopic totally extraperitoneal versus Lichtenstein herniorrhaphy: cost comparison at teaching hospitals. Surg Laparosc Endosc Percutan Tech 2003;13:261–267.
87. Hamilton EC, Scott DJ, Kapoor A, et al. Improving operative performance using a laparoscopic hernia simulator. Am J Surg 2001;182:725–728.

88. Grunwaldt LJ, Schwaitzberg SD, Rattner DW, Jones DB. Is laparoscopic inguinal hernia repair an operation of the past? J Am Coll Surg 2005;200:616–620.
89. Winslow ER, Quasebarth M, Brunt LM. Perioperative outcomes and complications of open versus laparoscopic extraperitoneal inguinal hernia repair in a mature surgical practice. Surg Endosc 2004;18:211–217.
90. Ramshaw BJ, Tucker JG, Conner T, et al. A comparison of the approaches to laparoscopic herniorrhaphy. Surg Endosc 1996; 10:29–32.
91. Fitzgibbons RJ, Camps J, Cornet D, et al. Laparoscopic inguinal herniorrhaphy: results of a multicenter trial. Ann Surg 1995;221:3–13.
92. Felix EL, Michas CA, Gonzalez MH. Laparoscopic hernioplasty: TAPP versus TEP. Surg Endosc 1995;9:984–989.
93. Waisbren SJ, Herz BL, Ducheine Y, et al. Iatrogenic "respiratory acidosis" during laparoscopic preperitoneal hernia repair. J Laparoendosc Surg 1996;6:181–183.
94. Scott DJ, Jones DB. Hernia. In: McClelland RN, ed. Selected Readings in General Surgery. Vol. 26, No. 4, Issues 1 2, 1999.
95. Ferzli GS, Kiel T. The role of the endoscopic extraperitoneal approach in large inguinal scrotal hernias. Surg Endosc 1997;11: 299–302.
96. Hendrickse CW, Ewans DS. Intestinal obstruction following laparoscopic inguinal hernia repair. Br J Surg 1993;80:1432.
97. Neugebauer E, Troidl H, Kum Ck, et al. The EAES consensus development conferences on laparoscopic cholecystectomy, appendectomy, and hernia repair. Surg Endosc 1995;9:550–563.
98. Phillips EH, Arregui M, Carrol BJ, et al. Incidence of complications following laparoscopic hernioplasty. Surg Endosc 1995;9: 16–21.
99. MacFadyen BV, Mathis CR. Inguinal herniorraphy: complications and recurrences. Semin Laparosc Surg 1994:1:128–140.
100. Payne JH Jr. Complications of laparoscopic inguinal herniorrhaphy. Semin Laparosc Surg 1997;4:166–181.
101. Sayad P, Hallak A, Ferzli G. Laparoscopic herniorrhaphy: review of complications and recurrence. J Laparoendosc Surg 1998;8:3–10.
102. Condon RE, Nyhus LM. Complications of groin hernias. In: Nyhus LM, Condon RE, eds. Hernia. Philadelphia: Lippincott; 1995:269–282.
103. Lichtenstein IL, Shore JM. Exploding the myths of hernia repair. Am J Surg 1976;132:307.
104. LeBlanc KA, Booth WV. Avoiding complications with laparoscopic herniorrhaphy. Surg Laparosc Endosc 1993;3:420–424.
105. Elkberg O, Lasson A, Kesek P, et al. Ipsilateral multiple groin hernias. Surgery 1994;115:557–562.
106. Lowham AS, Filipi CJ, Fitzgibbons, et al. Mechanisms of hernia recurrence after preperitoneal mesh repair: traditional and laparoscopic. Ann Surg 1997;225:422–431.
107. Deans GT, Wilson MS, Royston CMS, et al. Recurrent inguinal hernia after laparoscopic repair: possible cause and prevention. Br J Surg 1995;82:539–541.
108. Phillips EP, Rosenthal R, Fallas MJ, et al. Reasons of early recurrences following laparoscopic hernioplasty. Surg Endosc 1995;9:140–145.
109. Felix E, Scott S, Crafton B, et al. Causes of recurrence after laparoscopic hernioplasty: a multicenter study. Surg Endosc 1998;12:226–231.
110. Van Steensel CJ, Weidema WF. Laparoscopic inguinal hernia repair without fixation of the prosthesis. In: Arregui MF, Nagan RF, eds. Inguinal Hernia, Advances or Controversies. Oxford: Radcliffe Medical Press; 1994:435–436.
111. Deans GT, Wilson MS, Royston CMS. Laparoscopic "bikini mesh" repair of bilateral inguinal hernia. Br J Surg 1995;82:1383–1385.
112. Felix EL, Michas C. Double-buttress laparoscopic herniorrhaphy. J Laparoendosc Surg 1993;3:1–8.
113. Tetik C, Arregui ME, Dulucq JL, et al. Complications and recurrences associated with laparoscopic repair of groin hernias. A multi-institutional retrospective analysis. Surg Endosc 1994;8: 1316–1323.
114. Phillips EH, Arregui M, Carrol BJ, et al. Incidence of complications following laparoscopic hernioplasty. Surg Endosc 1995;9: 16–21.
115. Cunningham J, Temple WJ, Mitchell P, et al. Cooperative hernia study: pain in the postrepair patient. Ann Surg 1996;224:598–602.
116. Sampath P, Yeo C, Campbell JN. Nerve injury associated with laparoscopic inguinal herniorrhaphy. Surg 1995;118:829–833.
117. Seid AS, Amos E. Entrapment neuropathy in laparoscopic herniorrhaphy. Surg Endosc 1994;8:1050–1053.
118. Choi PD, Nath R, Mackinnon SE. Iatrogenic injury to the ilioinguinal and iliohypogastric nerves in the groin: a case report, diagnosis, and management. Ann Plast Surg 1996;37:60–65.
119. Dittrick GW, Ridl K, Kuhn JA, McCarty TM. Routine ilioinguinal nerve excision in inguinal hernia repairs. Am J Surg 2004;188: 736–740.
120. Eubanks SE, Newman L, Goehring L, et al. Meralgia paraesthetica: a complication of laparoscopic herniorrhaphy. Surg Laparosc Endosc 1993;3:381–385.
121. Broin EO, Horner C, Mealy K, et al. Meralgia paraesthetica following laparoscopic inguinal hernia repair, an anatomical analysis. Surg Endosc 1995;9:76–78.
122. Fong Y, Wantz GE. Prevention of ischemic orchitis during inguinal hernioplasty. Surg Gynecol Obstet 1992;174:399–402.
123. Milkins R, Wedgwood K. Intestinal obstruction following laparoscopic inguinal hernia repair. Br J Surg 1994;81:471.
124. Spier LN, Lazzaro RS, Procaccino A, et al. Entrapment of small bowel after laparoscopic herniorrhaphy. Surg Endosc 1993;7:535–536.
125. Petersen TI, Qvist N, Wara P. Intestinal obstruction—a procedure-related complication of laparoscopic inguinal hernia repair. Surg Laparosc Endosc 1995;5:214–216.
126. Miller K, Junger W. Ileocutaneous fistula formation following laparoscopic polypropylene mesh hernia repair. Surg Endosc 1997;11:772–773.
127. Gray MR, Curtis JM, Elkington JS. Colovesical fistula after laparoscopic inguinal hernia repair. Br J Surg 1994;81:1213–1214.
128. Hume RH, Bour J. Mesh migration following laparoscopic inguinal hernia repair. J Laparoendosc Surg 1996;6:333–335.
129. Vader VL, Vogt DM, Zucker KA, et al. Adhesion formation in laparoscopic inguinal hernia repair. Surg Endosc 1997;11:825–829.
130. Rasim SM, Alzahrani MA, Sigman HH, et al. Comparison of adhesion formation and tensile strength after three laparoscopic herniorraphy techniques. Surg Lapar Endosc 1997;7: 133–136.
131. Schlechter B, Marks J, Shillingstad RB, et al. Intra-abdominal mesh prosthesis in a canine model. Surg Endosc 1994;8:127–129.
132. Azurin DJ, Schuricht AL, Stoldt HS, et al. Small bowel obstruction following endoscopic extraperitoneal-preperitoneal herniorrhaphy. J Laparoendosc Surg 1995;5:263–266.
133. Lodha K, Deans A, Bhattacharya P, et al. Obstructing internal hernia complication totally extraperitoneal inguinal hernia repair. J Laparoendosc Surg 1998;8:167–168.
134. Bhoyrul S, Payne J, Steffes B, Swanstrom L, Way LW. A randomized prospective study of radially expanding trocars in laparoscopic surgery. J Gastrointest Surg 2000;4:392–397.
135. Carter Sl, Jones DB. Complications of laparoscopic surgery. In: Jones DB, Wu JS, Soper NJ, eds. Laparoscopic Surgery: Principles and Procedures. St. Louis: Quality Medical; 1997:89–96.
136. Cruse PJE, Foord R. The epidemiology of wound infection. Surg Clin North Am 1980;60:27–40.

137. Platt R, Zaleznik DF, Hopkins CC, et al. Perioperative antibiotic prophylaxis for hernia and breast surgery. N Engl J Med 1990;322:153–160.
138. Taylor EW, Byrne DJ, Leaper DJ, et al. Antibiotic prophylaxis and open groin hernia repair. World J Surg 1997;21:811–815.
139. Gilbert AI, Felton LL. Infection in inguinal hernia repair considering biomaterials and antibiotics. Surg Gynecol Obstet 1993;177:126–130.
140. Condon RE. Surgical treatment of inguinal hernia, 1997 [editorial]. J Gastrointest Surg 1997;1:299–300.
141. Oishi SN, Page CP, Sxhwesinger WH. Complicated presentation of groin hernias. Am J Surg 1991;162:568–571.
142. Ishihara T, Kubota, Eda N, et al. Laparoscopic approach to incarcerated inguinal hernia. Surg Endosc 1996;10:1111–1113.
143. Gahukamble DB, Khamage AS. Early versus delayed repair of reduced incarcerated inguinal hernias in the pediatric population. J Ped Surg 1996;31:1218–1220.
144. Surana R, Puri P. Is contralateral exploration necessary in infants with unilateral inguinal hernia? J Pediatr Surg 1993;28:1026–1027.
145. Jona J. The incidence of positive contralateral inguinal exploration among preschool children—a retrospective and prospective study. J Pediatr Surg 1996;31:656–660.
146. Wulkan ML, Wiener ES, VanBalen N, et al. Laparoscopy through the open ipsilateral sac to evaluate presence of contralateral hernia. J Pediatr Surg 1996;31:1174–1177.
147. Toy FK, Bailey RW, Carey S, et al. Prospective, multicenter study of laparoscopic ventral hernioplasty: preliminary results. Surg Endosc 1998 12:955–959.
148. Santora TA, Roslyn JJ. Incisional hernia. Surg Clin North Am 1993;73:557–570.
149. Carlson MA, Ludqig KA, Condon RE. Ventral hernia and other complications of 1000 midline incisions. South Med J 1995;88: 450–453.
150. Israelsson LA, Jonsson T, Knutsson A. Suture technique and wound healing in midline laparotomy incisions. Eur J Surg 1996;162:605–609.
151. Mudge M, Hughes LE. Incisional hernia: a 10 year prospective study of incidence and attitudes. Br J Surg 1985;72:70–71.
152. Read RC, Yonder G. Recent trends in the management of incisional herniation. Arch Surg 1989;124:485–488.
153. Heydorn Wh, Velanovich V. A 5 year US army experience with 36,250 abdominal hernia repairs. Am Surg 1990;56:596–600.
154. Gislason H, Gronbech JE, Soreide O. Burst abdomen and incisional hernia after major gastrointestinal operations—comparison of three closure techniques. Eur J Surg 1995;161:349–354.
155. Sugerman HJ, Kellum JM, Reines D, et al. Greater risk of incisional hernia with morbidly obese than steroid-dependent patients and low recurrence with prefascial polypropylene mesh. Am J Surg 1996;171:80–84.
156. Lamont PM, Ellis H. Incisional hernia in re-opened abdominal incisions: an overlooked risk factor. Br J Surg 1988;75:374–376.
157. Leber GE, Garb JL, Alexander AI, et al. Long-term complications associated with prosthetic repair of incisional hernias. Arch Surg 1998;133:378–382.
158. Ellis H, Coleridge-Smith PD, Joyce AD. Abdominal incisions—vertical or transverse? Postgrad Med J 1984;60:407–410.
159. Trimbos JB, Smit IB, Holm JP, et al. A randomized clinical trial comparing two methods of fascia closure following midline laparotomy. Arch Surg 1992;127:1232–1234.
160. Sahlin S, Ahlberg J, Granström L, et al. Monofilament versus multifilament absorbable sutures for abdominal closure. Br J Surg 1993;80:322–324.
161. Wissing J, Van Vroonhoven TJMV, Schattenkerk ME, et al. Fascia closure after midline laparotomy: results of a randomized trial. Br J Surg 1987;74:738–741.
162. Krukowski ZH, Cusick EL, Engeset J, et al. Polydioxanone or polypropylene for closure of midline abdominal incisions: a prospective comparative clinical trial. Br J Surg 1987;74:828–830.
163. Chu CC, Williams DF. Effects of physical configuration and chemical structure of suture materials on bacterial adhesion. Am J Surg 1984;147:197–204.
164. Nezhat C, Nezhat F, Seidman DS, et al. Incisional hernias after operative laparoscopy. J Laparoendosc Surg 1997;7:111–115.
165. Caldizoni MW, Romano M, Bozza F, et al. Progressive pneumoperitoneum in the management of giant incisional hernias: a study of 41 patients. Br J Surg 1990;77:306–308.
166. Luijendijk RW, Hop WCJ, Van Den Tol P, et al. A comparison of suture repair with mesh repair for incisional hernia. N Engl J Med 2000;343:392–398.
167. Temudom T, Siadati M, Sarr MG. Repair of complex giant or recurrent ventral hernias by using tension-free intraparietal prosthetic mesh (Stoppa technique): lessons learned from initial experience (50 patients). Surg 1996;120:738–744.
168. Van Der Linden FTPM, Van Vroonhoven THJMV. Long-term results after correction of incisional hernia. Neth J Surg 1988;40: 127–129.
169. Koller R, Miholic J, Jakl RJ. Repair of incisional hernias with expanded polytetrafluoroethylene. Eur J Surg 1997;163:261–266.
170. Paul A, Korenkov M, Peters S, et al. Unacceptable results of the Mayo procedure for repair of abdominal incisional hernias. Eur J Surg 1998;164:361–367.
171. Shukla VK, Gupta A, Singh H, et al. Cardiff repair of incisional hernia: a university hospital experience. Eur J Surg 1998;164:271–274.
172. Sitzmann JV, McFadden DW. The internal retention repair of massive ventral hernia. Am Surg 1989;55:719–723.
173. George CD, Ellis H. The results of incisional hernia repair: a 12 year review. Ann R Coll Surg 1986;68:185–187.
174. Porter JM. A combination of Vicryl and Marlex mesh: a technique for abdominal wall closure in difficult cases. J Trauma 1995;39:1178–1180.
175. Naim JO, Pulley D, Scanlan K, et al. Reduction of postoperative adhesions to Marlex mesh using experimental adhesion barriers in rats. J Laparoendosc Surg 1993;3:187.
176. Molloy RG, Moran KT, Waldron RP, et al. Massive incisional hernia: abdominal wall replacement with Marlex mesh. Br J Surg 1991;78:242–244.
177. Brown LB, Richardson JD, Malangoni MA, et al. Comparison of prosthetic materials for abdominal wall reconstruction in the presence of contamination and infection. Ann Surg 1985;201:705–711.
178. Cristoforoni PM, Kim YB, Preys Z, et al. Adhesion formation after incisional hernia repair: a randomized porcine trial. Am Surg 1996;62:935–938.
179. Bauer JJ, Salky BA, Gelernt IM, et al. Repair of large abdominal wall defects with expanded polytetrafluoroethylene (PTFE). Ann Surg 1987;206:765–769.
180. Gillion JF, Begin GF, Marecos C, et al. Expanded polytetrafluoroethylene patches used in the intraperitoneal or extraperitoneal position for repair of incisional hernias of the anterolateral abdominal wall. Am J Surg 1997;174:16–19.
181. Condon RE. Incisional hernia. In: Nyhus LM, Condon RE, eds. Hernia. Philadelphia: Lippincott; 1995:319–336.
182. Rubio PA. New technique for repairing large ventral incisional hernias with Marlex mesh. Surg Gynecol Obstet 1986;162:275–276.
183. Rubio PA. Giant ventral hernias: a technical challenge. Int Surg 1994;79:166–168.
184. McClelland RN. Ventral hernia repair. Sel Readings Gen Surg 1993;20:38–47.
185. Wantz GE. Incisional hernioplasty with Mersiline. Surg Gynecol Obstet 1991;172:129–137.

186. Amid PK, Shulman AG, Lichtenstein IL. A simple stapling technique for prosthetic repair of massive incisional hernias. Am Surg 1994;60:934–937.
187. McLanahan D, King LT, Weems C, et al. Retrorectus prosthetic mesh repair of midline abdominal hernia. Am J Surg 1997;173: 445–449.
188. Holzman MD, Purut CM, Reintgen K, et al. Laparoscopic ventral and incisional hernioplasty. Surg Endosc 1997;11:32–35.
189. Park A, Gagner M, Pomp A. Laparoscopic repair of large incisional hernias. Surg Laparosc Endosc 1996;6:123–128.
190. LeBlanc KA, Booth WV, Whitaker JM. Laparoscopic repair of ventral hernias using an intraperitoneal onlay patch: report of current results. Contemp Surg 1994;45:211–214.
191. Carbajo MA, Martin del Olmo JC, Blanco JI, et al. Laparoscopic approach to incisional hernia: lessons learned from 270 patients over 8 years. Surg Endosc 2003;17:118–122.
192. McGreevy JM, Goodney PP, Birkmeyer CM, et al. A prospective study comparing the complication rates between laparoscopic and open ventral hernia repairs. Surg Endosc 2003;17:1778–1780.
193. Bencini L, Sanchez LJ, Boffi B, et al. Incisional hernia repair: retrospective comparison of laparoscopic and open techniques. Surg Endosc 2003;17:1546–1551.
194. Salameh JR, Sweeney JF, Graviss EA, et al. Laparoscopic ventral hernia repair during the learning curve. Hernia 2002;6:182–187.
195. Wright BE, Niskanen BD, Peterson DJ, et al. Laparoscopic ventral hernia repair: are there comparative advantages over traditional methods of repair? Am Surg 2002;68:291–296.
196. Chari R, Chari V, Eisenstat M, Chung R. A case controlled study of laparoscopic incisional hernia repair. Surg Endosc 2000;14:117–119.
197. DeMaria EJ, Moss JM, Sugerman HJ. Laparoscopic intraperitoneal polytetraflouroethylene (PTFE) prosthetic patch repair of ventral hernia: prospective comparison to open prefascial polypropylene mesh repair. Surg Endosc 2000;14:326–329.
198. Carbajo MA, Martin del Olmo JC, Blanco JI, et al. Laparoscopic treatment versus open surgery in the solution of major incisional and abdominal wall hernias with mesh. Surg Endosc 1999;13:250–252.
199. Ramshaw BJ, Esartia P, Schwab J, et al. Comparison of laparoscopic and open ventral herniorrhaphy. Am Surg 1999;65:827–832.
200. Park A, Birch DW, Lovrics P. Laparoscopic and open incisional hernia repair: a comparison study. Surgery 1998;124:816–822.
201. Holzman MD, Purut CM, Reintgen K, et al. Laparoscopic ventral and incisional hernioplasty. Surg Endosc 1997;11:32–35.
202. Franklin ME, Gonzalez JJ, Glass JL, Manjarrez A. Laparoscopic ventral and incisional hernia repair: an 11-year experience. Hernia 2004;8:23–27.
203. Heniford BT, Park AE, Ramshaw BJ, Voeller G. Laparoscopic repair of ventral hernias: 9 years' experience with 850 consecutive hernias. Ann Surg 2003;238:391–400.
204. LeBlanc KA, Whitaker JM, Bellanger DE, Rhynes VK. Laparoscopic incisional and ventral hernioplasty: lessns learned from 200 patients. Hernia 2003;7:118–124.
205. Rosen M, Brody F, Ponsky J, et al. Recurrence after laparoscopic ventral hernia repair: a 5-year experience. Surg Endosc 2003;17: 123–128.
206. Bageacu S, Blanc P, Breton C, et al. Laparoscopic repair of incisional hernia: a retrospective study of 159 patients. Surg Endosc 2002;16:345–348.
207. Ben-Haim M, Kuriansky J, Tal R, et al. Pitfalls and complications with laparoscopic intraperitoneal expanded polytetrafluoroethylene patch repair of postoperative ventral hernia: lessons from the first 100 consecutive cases. Surg Endosc 2002;16:785–788.
208. Berger D, Bientzle M, Muller A. Postoperative complications after laparoscopic incisional hernia repair: incidence and treatment. Surg Endosc 2002;16:1720–1723.
209. Gillian GK, Geis WP, Grover G. Laparoscopic incisional and ventral hernia repair (LIVH): an evolving outpatient technique. JSLS 2002;6:315–322.
210. Chowbey PK, Sharma A, Khullar R, et al. A. laparoscopic ventral hernia repair. J Laparoendosc Adv Surg Tech A 2000;10:79–84.
211. Fabian TC, Croce MA, Pritchard FE, et al. Planned ventral hernia: staged management for acute abdominal wall defects. Ann Surg 1994;219:643–653.
212. Stone HH, Fabian TC, Turkleson ML, et al. Management of acute full-thickness losses of the abdominal wall. Ann Surg 1981;193:612–618.
213. Voyles CR, Richardson JD, Bland KI, et al. Emergency abdominal wall reconstruction with polypropylene mesh: short-term benefits versus long-term complications. Ann Surg 1981;194:219–223.
214. Jones JW, Jurkovich GJ. Polypropylene mesh closure of infected abdominal wounds. Am Surg 1989;55:73–76.
215. Buck JR, Fath JJ, Chung SK, et al. Use of absorbable mesh as an aid in abdominal wall closure in the emergent setting. Am Surg 1995;61:655–658.
216. Greene MA, Mullins RJ, Malangoni MA, et al. Laparotomy wound closure with absorbable polyglycolic acid mesh. Surg Gynecol Obstet 1993;176:213–218.
217. Jernigan TW, Fabian TC, Croce MA, et al. Staged management of giant abdominal wall defects: acute and long-term results. Ann Surg 2003;238:349–357.
218. Ramirez OM, Ruas E, Dellon AL. "Components separation" method for closure of abdominal-wall defects: an anatomic and clinical study. Plast Recontr Surg 1990;86:519–526.
219. De Vries Reilingh TS, Van Goor H, Rosman C, et al. "Components separation technique" for the repair of large abdominal wall hernias. J Am Coll Surg 2003;196:32–37.
220. Hultman CS, Pratt B, Cairns BA, et al. Multidisciplinary approach to abdominal wall reconstruction after decompressive laparotomy for abdominal compartment syndrome. Ann Plast Surg 2005;54:269–275.
221. Admire AA, Dolich MO, Sisley AC, Samimi KJ. Massive ventral hernias: role of tissue expansion in abdominal wall restoration following abdominal compartment syndrome. Am Surg 2002;68: 491–496.
222. Shestak KC, Edington HJ, Johnson RR. The separation of anatomic components technique for the reconstruction of massive midline abdominal wall defects: anatomy, surgical technique, applications, and limitations revisited. Plast Reconstr Surg 2000;105:731–738.
223. Ueno T, Pickett LC, De La Fuente SG, et al. Clinical application of porcine small intestinal submucosa in the management of infected or potentially contaminated abdominal defects. J Gastrointest Surg 2004;8:109–112.
224. Franklin ME Jr, Gonzalez JJ Jr, Glass JL. Use of porcine small intestinal submucosa as a prosthetic device for laparoscopic repair of hernias in contaminated fields: 2-year follow-up. Hernia 2004;8:186–189.
225. Eid GM, Mattar SG, Hamad G, et al. Repair of ventral hernias in morbidly obese patients undergoing laparoscopic gastric bypass should not be deferred. Surg Endosc 2004;18:207–210.
226. Adedeji OA, Bailey CA. Varma JS. Porcine dermal collagen graft in abdominal-wall reconstruction. Br J Plast Surg 2002;55:85–86.
227. Buinewicz B, Rosen B. Acellular cadaveric dermis (AlloDerm): a new alternative for abdominal hernia repair. Ann Plast Surg 2004;52:188–194.
228. Spangen L. Spigelian hernia. Surg Clin N Am 1984;64:351–366.
229. Felix EL, Michas C. Laparoscopic repair of spigelian hernias. Surg Laparosc Endosc 1994;4:308–310.

230. Amendolara M. Videolaparoscopic treatment of spigelian hernias. Surg Laparosc Endosc 1998;8:136–139.
231. Heniford BT, Iannitti DA, Gagner M. Laparoscopic inferior and superior lumbar hernia repair. Arch Surg 1997;132:1141–1144.
232. Marchal F, Parent S, Tortuyaux JM, et al. Obturator hernias—report of seven cases. Hernia 1997;1:23–26.
233. Bryant TL, Umstot RK. Laparoscopic repair of an incarcerated obturator hernia. Surg Endosc 1996;10:437–438.
234. Ziegler D, Rhoads JE. Obturator hernia needs a laparotomy, not a diagnosis. Am J Surg 1995;170:67–68.
235. So JB, Palmer MT, Shellito PC. Postoperative perineal hernia. Dis Colon Rectum 1997;40:953–957.
236. Cali RL, Pitsch Rm, Blatchford GJ, et al. Rare pelvic floor hernias: report of a case and review of the literature. Dis Colon Rectum 1992;35:604–612.
237. Martin L, Foster G. Parasomal hernia. Ann R Coll Surg Engl 1996;78:81–84.
238. Rubin MS, Schoetz DJ, Matthews JB. Parastomal hernia: is relocation superior to fascial repair? Arch Surg 1994;129:413–419.
239. Armstrong O, Letessier E, Genier F, et al. Internal hernia: report of nine cases. Hernia 1997;1:143–145.
240. Langer JC. Gastroschisis and ophalocele. Semin Ped Surg 1996;5:124–128.
241. Heiss KF. Congenital diaphragmatic hernia in 1994: a hard look at the need for "emergency surgery." Semin Thor Cardiovasc Surg 1994;6:221–227.
242. West KWW, Bengston K, Rescorla FJ, et al. Delayed surgical repair and ECMO improves survival in congenital diaphragmatic hernia. Ann Surg 1992;216:454.
243. Orita M, Okino M, Yamashita K, et al. Laparoscopic repair of a diaphragmatic hernia through the foramen of Morgagni. Surg Endosc 1997;11:668–670.

SECTION FIVE

Endocrine Surgery

54

History of Endocrine Surgery

Jeffrey A. Norton

The science of endocrinology began relatively recently, at the beginning of the twentieth century. At that time, physiological theories were dominated by the Russian Ivan Pavlov, who argued that the nervous system primarily controlled all bodily activities. Because of this, few thought that ductless glands existed. However, in 1902 William Bayliss and Ernest Starling made a simple discovery that gave birth to the science of endocrinology. They demonstrated that acid in the gut stimulated the secretion of pancreatic juice when all connections from both organs to the nervous system were severed. They postulated that a "chemical" rather than a "nervous" substance is responsible for pancreatic secretion, and named the substance secretin.[1] This finding of secretin represented a whole new class of body messenger. In 1905 Starling proposed the term hormone from a Greek word meaning "to excite" for substances that mediate messages through the circulation.[2] Langerhans had previously attributed an endocrine function to the islets of the pancreas, and the science of endocrinology was born.

The science grew rapidly, and many who contributed to it won Nobel prizes for medicine. A surgeon named Theodor Kocher won the Nobel Prize for his observations on the physiology, pathology, and surgery of the thyroid gland. He noted that total thyroidectomy was associated with myxedema, which could be prevented by subtotal thyroidectomy. Kendall, a chemist at the Mayo Clinic, won the prize for isolating thyroxine from the thyroid gland. Banting and Best shared it for extraction of insulin from the pancreatic islets.

As the understanding of the interplay and interaction of various endocrine glands became clear, the notion of separation of the nervous and endocrine systems was challenged. Walter Cannon[3] noted that emotional stimuli caused secretion of the adrenal medulla, which he described as part of both the endocrine and the nervous systems. Further, in 1921, Loewi demonstrated that nerve transmission at the synapse was mediated by chemical substances. Subsequently, it was shown that secretory cells were present in the hypothalamus, with neurohormonal control over the pituitary, and that these secretions also controlled the hypothalamus itself through feedback mechanisms. Large neurohormonal systems such as Masson's Kulchitsky cells were identified involving neurons, enzymes, peptides, and amines. In 1960, Everson Pearse found that these systems shared a number of important characteristics, including the handling of amines and the production of peptides. He coined the term APUD, meaning amine precursor uptake and decarboxylation. Berson and Yalow greatly facilitated quantification of minute amounts of circulating hormones by the development of the radioimmunoassay (RIA), for which they received the Nobel Prize. This technique allowed precise diagnosis of endocrine conditions through measurement of hormonal levels within the circulation. Modern endocrine surgery was developed primarily to treat enlargements or tumors of the endocrine glands or conditions caused by excessive glandular secretion of hormones (Graves' disease, for example), whereas hormone replacement therapy was developed for conditions associated with decreased levels of hormones (Addison's disease, etc.). The history of surgical treatment for specific glandular conditions is described next.

Thyroid

In 952, a Moorish physician named Albucasis performed the first successful thyroidectomy (Table 54.1). Albucasis was truly ahead of his time, as he also introduced many other surgical interventions including the use of catgut and cotton suture. Unfortunately, his work was largely forgotten, and for many hundreds of years there was essentially no progress in thyroid surgery. In fact, in 1850 the mortality rate for thyroid surgery was prohibitively high in that 50% of patients died following thyroidectomy, usually from uncontrollable bleeding. This situation remained unchanged until Professor Kocher of Berne (Switzerland) made true progress. Iodine-deficient goiter was a common disease in mountainous regions, and Kocher performed approximately 4000 thyroidectomies for goiter. Kocher advocated precise, gentle, meticulous surgery that preserved the parathyroid glands and the

TABLE 54.1. Milestones of Endocrine Surgery.

Year	*Event*	*Year*	*Event*
952	Albucasis performs first thyroidectomy	1934	Albright describes parathyroid in renal failure
1835	Graves describes thyrotoxicosis	1935	Whipple describes insulinoma triad
1838	Rathke describes embryology of pituitary	1936	Young describes posterior approach to adrenal
1855	Addison describes adrenal insufficiency	1937	Kendall separates gluco- and mineralocorticoid
1856	Brown-Sequard shows adrenal essential for life	1943	Astwood uses thiouracil to treat Graves' disease
1869	Langerhans describes endocrine cells in the pancreas	1953	Rosenbaum and others describe carcinoid syndrome
1879	Sandstrom describes parathyroid glands in humans	1954	Conn describes aldosteronoma
1886	Felix describes pheochromocytoma	1954	Wermer describes inherited basis for MEN 1
1891	Gley notes that tetany is caused by parathyroidectomy	1955	Zollinger and Ellison describe syndrome
1897	Kulchitsky sees diffuse nature of gut endocrine cells	1958	Cope describes parathyroid hyperplasia
1902	Bayliss and Starling discover secretin	1958	Verner and Morrison describe syndrome
1903	Erdheim describes patient with MEN 1	1959	Aurbach isolates parathyroid hormone
1905	Starling proposes the term hormone	1959	Gregory extracts gastrin from ZE tumor
1905	Edkins discovers gastrin	1960	Pearse terms name APUDoma
1907	Oberndorfer describes carcinoid tumor	1961	Sipple describes syndrome
1909	Kocher wins Nobel Prize for thyroid surgery	1963	Berson and Yalow develop RIA
1909	Cushing removes pituitary tumor	1963	Unger describes glucagonoma
1911	Cannon notes emotions cause adrenal secretion	1968	Steiner describes MEN 2a
1912	Plummer describes toxic nodule	1968	Schimke describes MEN 2b
1921	Loewi notes synapse transmission by chemicals	1972	Said discovers vasoactive intestinal peptide
1922	Banting and Best discover insulin	1976	Computed tomography of the adrenal
1922	Murlin discovers glucagon	1976	Wells performs parathyroid transplant hyperplasia
1923	Crile introduces lateral approach to adrenal	1977	Larsson discovers somatostatin
1925	Mandl removes parathyroid tumor	1995	Chapius describes lapara roscopic adrenalectomy
1926	Roux removes a pheochromocytoma	1995	Santoro identifies that RET causes MEN 2a and MEN 2b
1929	Graham removes an insulinoma	1995	Wells does thyroidectomy based on gene mutations
1929	Barr and Bulger perform parathryoidectomy	1997	MEN 1 gene is identified and named MENIN
1929	Wilder describes parathyroid cancer	1999	NET imaged by somatostatin analogue

recurrent laryngeal nerve. With this technique, he was able to reduce the mortality of thyroidectomy from approximately 50% to 0.2%. Even more remarkable than his technical advances was his understanding that complete thyroidectomy resulted in a fatal condition called myxedema. We now know that myxedema is really hypothyroidism. Therefore, Kocher advocated subtotal thyroidectomy for the treatment of goiter, an operation that is still practiced today. As mentioned, for this finding he received the Nobel Prize in 1909. The American Halsted was a student of Kocher, and he evolved his own method of thyroidectomy that was instituted at Johns Hopkins Hospital in the United States. Subsequently, two other American surgeons founded institutes primarily to handle thyroid goiter: Charles Mayo of Rochester, Minnesota (Mayo Clinic) and George Crile of Cleveland, Ohio (Cleveland Clinic). At each of these institutions, thyroidectomy for goiter was practiced and taught such that morbidity and mortality rates of thyroid surgery became excellent throughout most of the United States.

The precise nature of thyrotoxicosis was unclear for many years. The condition is named after Graves, but he mistakenly thought that the thyroid enlargement was caused by overactivity of the heart.[4] The thyroid enlargement described by Graves was diffuse and symmetrical, involving the entire thyroid gland. Graves' hypothesis that the goiter was from a cardiac cause was inconsistent with the finding that thyroidectomy relieved the toxic features of the condition, including the protuberant eyes in some patients. Other types of thyrotoxicosis were subsequently described. In 1912, Henry Plummer at the Mayo Clinic described a solitary hot nodule that caused hyperthyroidism, and this was also described subsequently by Oliver Cope and given the name Plummer's disease.[5] Of importance to safe anesthesia and surgery for hyperthyroidism was the introduction of drugs that inhibit thyroid secretion, including thiouracil, and thiourea in 1943 by Astwood of Boston.[6] Surgery for thyrotoxicosis had a very high mortality rate, and preoperative preparation with these drugs allowed Francis Moore, Oliver Cope, and Howard Means to perform thyroidectomy safely in 35 consecutive patients with hyperthyroidism.[7] Similarly, in 1942 radioiodine was introduced for the treatment of Graves' disease and thyroid cancer. Finally, in 1960, preoperative preparation of hyperthyroid patients was modified to include beta-blockers to inhibit the effects of thyroid hormone on the heart, and it was demonstrated that surgery for this disorder could be performed safely with beta-blockade alone.[8]

Pituitary and Adrenal

In 1838, Rathke described the dual embryonic origin of the pituitary gland from both the entoderm and the neuroectoderm. Shortly after, in 1886 Marie described a patient with clinical features of acromegaly and a pituitary tumor.[9]

Schonemann recognized the glandular appearance of the pituitary in 1892 and first described that cells took up acid stain (acidophils), basic dye (basophils), or no stain at all (chromophobes).[10] In 1907 and 1908, investigators noted that the pituitary gland enlarges after pregnancy and castration. This awareness of the pituitary gland and its role in physiological and pathological processes led Harvey Cushing of Baltimore to correctly diagnose a pituitary tumor in a patient with acromegaly; this led him to develop the technique of hypophysectomy in dogs. In 1909, Cushing used these methods to remove a pituitary tumor from an acromegalic farmer from South Dakota.[11]

In 1909 Cushing introduced the terms hyperpituitism and hypopituitism to indicate hyper- and hypofunction, respectively, of the anterior lobe of the pituitary gland. Cushing recognized that hypopituitism caused loss of sexual activity and secondary sexual characteristics in adults. He regarded total absence of the anterior pituitary incompatible with life, a notion that was criticized by others. Cushing developed the use of stereoscopic X-ray films to improve the outcome of pituitary surgery.

Initially, Cushing used the transphenoidal approach to hypophysectomy. In 263 procedures, surgical mortality was 7% and meningitis rate was 2%.[12] Cushing later preferred the transfrontal approach because this procedure allowed removal of the supradiaphragmatic extension of tumor around the optic nerves and more complete recovery of vision. Amazingly, the operative mortality and meningitis rates were similar for this procedure despite the fact that antibiotics were not yet available. Subsequently, Guilot reawakened interest in the transsphenoidal technique that was greatly enhanced by the use of the operative microscope by Hardy.[13] Eventually, the use of antibiotics, cortisone, and vasopressin led to the high level of success seen with this operation today.

A Roman anatomist named Eustachius first described the adrenals in 1552. At the time he knew that the cortex was of mesodermal origin and the medulla was composed of sympathetic neural elements. In addition to the main glands, he described fragments of accessory adrenal tissue in the retroperitoneum, the most common of which was the organ of Zuckerkandl near the bifurcation of the aorta and to the left of the iliac artery. Endocrine tumors in this area were called paragangliomas. Today we know that these tumors were really extraadrenal pheochromocytomas. Surgery of the adrenal glands emerged as part of abdominal surgery toward the end of the nineteenth century. Operations on the adrenal cortex were facilitated and made safer by the introduction of cortisone in 1949, and operations for pheochromocytoma became safe when methods were developed to block catecholamines in the mid-1960s.

In 1855, Thomas Addison of London described 11 patients with anemia, debility, feebleness, a dark skin color, and a disease of the suprarenal glands.[14] At autopsy the adrenal glands were not visible; they were completely replaced by scrofula (tuberculosis) or cancer. Addison believed that the disease shed some light on the function of the adrenal glands. Following Addison's description, a Frenchman named Brown-Sequard demonstrated that the adrenals were essential for life by performing bilateral adrenalectomy in experimental animals.[15] Brown-Sequard noted that following adrenalectomy the animals developed a condition similar to that previously described by Addison and eventually died. Subsequently, it was demonstrated that cortical extracts could restore the health of patients with Addison's disease (hypocortisolism). In 1937, Edward Kendall, the chemist at the Mayo Clinic who had previously isolated thyroxine, separated the two critical components of adrenal cortical extract, mineralocorticoid and glucocorticoid. Eventually the mineralocorticoid was named aldosterone and the glucocorticoid was called cortisone. Glucocorticoid was subsequently found to be an effective treatment for rheumatoid arthritis. In 1950, Kendall and others won the Nobel Prize for their work separating the different hormonal components from adrenal cortical extract.

Measurement of adrenal steroids in the blood and urine became available for diagnosis of pituitary and adrenal tumors during the 1950s. Adrenal cortisol-secreting tumors were usually autonomous, whereas pituitary adrenocorticotropic hormone (ACTH)-secreting tumors remained responsive to hormonal control. This observation formed the basis for the dexamethasone suppression test and the metapyrone stimulation test for the diagnosis of either a pituitary ACTH-secreting tumor or an adrenal cortisol-secreting tumor as the cause of Cushing's syndrome. Radiology of the adrenal and pituitary was poor until 1975 when computed tomography (CT) became available to precisely image both glands.[16]

In 1954, 2 years after the discovery of aldosterone, Jerome Conn at the University of Michigan first described the syndrome of an adrenal tumor with excessive secretion of aldosterone (aldosteronoma).[17] The patient was a 34-year-old woman with severe muscle weakness, polyuria, polydipsia, and hypertension. She had increased serum levels of sodium and decreased levels of potassium. A 4-cm adenoma was removed from the right adrenal gland that weighed 15g and was chrome yellow in appearance. Assay of the tumor demonstrated very high levels of aldosterone. Subsequently, other patients were identified. In 1961, 7 years later, 108 patients with Conn's syndrome had been described.

Pheochromocytoma was the first adrenal tumor to be recognized. In 1886, Felix Frankel described a patient (Minna Roll) with a probable pheochromocytoma. This patient suffered intermittent attacks of headache, palpitations, nervousness, dizziness, nausea, and vomiting.[18] Similar tumors that were adrenal medullary in origin were identified and reported in autopsy studies. In 1926, Roux, a student of Kocher in Switzerland, removed a large right adrenal pheochromocytoma, and 1 year later, in the United States, Charles Mayo removed a left adrenal pheochromocytoma.[19] Both patients recovered. These events represent the first time that a pheochromocytoma was diagnosed preoperatively and the patient survived surgery. In 1926 adrenaline was extracted from a pheochromocytoma,[20] and norepinephrine was identified in another in 1949.[21]

The techniques of adrenalectomy developed slowly. The adrenal glands are located in the most superior aspect of the abdomen, nearly in the chest, and are not easily accessible to surgeons. Before CT, surgeons needed to explore both adrenals to be certain of the diagnosis and the location of the tumor. The anterior bilateral subcostal incision or midline incision is useful for exploring the entire abdomen and was the first incision used. In 1923, George Crile introduced the lateral or lumbar approach to expose the kidney and to remove adrenal tumors.[22] Hugh Young, a urologist from Baltimore, described the posterior approach to adrenalectomy, and this method was associated with less pain but limited exposure.[23] It became the incision of choice for small adrenal tumors. This technique has all changed recently with the development of endoscopic surgery. Laparoscopic approaches to the adrenal introduced by Chapius are now the method of choice for most tumors and hyperplasia,[24] primarily because less pain and a shorter convalescence are involved.

Parathyroid

In 1880, a Swedish student named Ivar Sandström first described the parathyroid glands in humans.[25] His finding went unnoticed for more than 10 years. In 1891, Gley again described the parathyroid glands and noted that their removal resulted in tetany.[26] MacCallum and Voegtlin subsequently noted that tetany associated with parathyroidectomy could be corrected with infusion of calcium.[27] Also in 1891, von Recklinghausen described the features of a specific bone disease associated with hyperparathyroidism. In 1903, Askanazy described a woman with severe bone disease and a large tumor lateral to the thyroid gland.[28] Scientists at the time incorrectly thought that the skeletal disease caused the parathyroid tumors. However, in 1915 Schagenhaufer correctly suggested that the parathyroid tumor was primary and the skeletal changes were secondary.[29] Mandl confirmed this hypothesis in 1925 when he removed a parathyroid tumor from a streetcar conductor and postoperatively serum calcium levels normalized and bone disease ameliorated. One year later at the Massachusetts General Hospital in Boston, a famous sea captain named Charles Martel underwent the first neck exploration for hyperparathyroidism in the United States. Unfortunately, the operation was unsuccessful and the patient was subsequently found to have a mediastinal parathyroid adenoma. Barr and Bulger of Saint Louis performed the first successful operation for parathyroid disease in 1929 at Barnes Hospital and coined the term hyperparathyroidism.[30]

The hypercalcemic effects of parathyroid hormone (PTH) were first identified in 1925 when it was extracted from parathyroid glands and infused into experimental animals. Subsequently, in 1959 Gerry Aurbach of Boston purified parathyroid hormone.[31] However, the precise diagnosis of hyperparathyroidism was impossible until 1963 when Berson et al. developed a specific radioimmunoassay to measure it in the bloodstream.[32] This technique allowed precise measurement of small amounts of PTH. With the widespread availability of precise diagnosis, surgery for hyperparathyroidism became more popular and surgeons discovered that most, but not all, cases were caused by an adenoma. In 1958, Oliver Cope described chief cell hyperplasia in 10% of patients with primary hyperparathyroidism and developed surgical procedures to treat it.[33] Most surgeons advocated subtotal parathyroidectomy, but Samuel A. Wells, Jr. suggested four-gland parathyroidectomy with transplantation of parathyroid tissue to the forearm.[34] Some of the parathyroid tissue could then be more easily removed if recurrent hypercalcemia developed. In 1929, Russell Wilder of the Mayo Clinic first described a malignant parathyroid tumor.[2] Malignant parathyroid tumors have been rare, occurring in approximately 0.5% of patients with primary hyperparathyroidism. Finally, in 1934 secondary hyperparathyroidism was recognized in patients with chronic renal failure.[35] The disorder resulted from low levels of calcium in the blood that stimulate secondary chief cell hyperplasia and parathyroid hormone secretion. The parathyroid condition appears to be compensatory in most cases, but in some patients it becomes autonomous with the development of severe bone disease. In these individuals with so-called tertiary hyperparathyroidism, subtotal or total parathyroidectomy with transplant may be indicated.

Pancreas and Endocrine Gut

The identification of secretin by Bayliss and Starling in 1902 first indicated that the gut is an endocrine organ. However, because of the more diffuse nature of endocrine cells in the gut, knowledge of the gastroenteropancreatic system developed slowly. In 1869, Paul Langerhans of Berlin discovered clumps of endocrine cells within the pancreas that subsequently were named the islets of Langerhans.[36] In 1870, Heidenhain of Prussia found enterochromaffin (EC) cells within the stomach,[37] and in 1887 Kulchitsky of Russia identified similar cells throughout the intestine.[38] In 1907, Oberndorfer of Munich noted the more benign course of chromaffin tumors of the intestine that resembled carcinoma and called them carcinoid ("karzinoide").[39]

Gastrin was discovered in 1905, insulin in 1922, and cholecystokinin in 1928. In 1952 it was demonstrated that the EC cells of the gut produced the hormone 5-hydroxytryptamine (5-HT). Subsequently, by 1977 it had been demonstrated that the pancreas produced multiple hormones including insulin, glucagon, somatostatin, pancreatic polypeptide, and vasoactive intestinal polypeptide. Hormone-producing cells were also identified throughout the gastrointestinal tract, including gastrin-secreting cells in the gastric antrum and duodenum and secretin-secreting and cholecystokinin-secreting cells in the small intestine.

Banting and Best discovered insulin in 1922. Endogenous hyperinsulism (insulinoma) was the first gastrointestinal hormonal syndrome to be discovered. Charles Mayo operated on the first patient with an insulinoma in 1926; however, the patient was found to have a malignant tumor with liver metastases so the tumor was not removed.[40] In 1929, Roscoe Graham successfully removed an insulinoma from a patient in Toronto.[41] In 1935, Alan Whipple, famous for the surgical procedure to remove the head of the pancreas and the duodenum, collected a series of 32 patients with insulinoma and identified the diagnostic triad of symptoms with fasting, low blood glucose levels, and relief of symptoms following glucose administration.[42]

The carcinoid syndrome was first described in 1953 simultaneously by two separate groups, Rosenbaum and others in Milwaukee[43] and Isler and Hedinger in Zurich.[44] They described two patients with flushing, cardiac failure, and liver metastases from an ileal carcinoid tumor. One year later Waldenstrom and Pernow identified 5-HT and histamine in the blood and urine of a patient with the carcinoid syndrome.[45] It subsequently became apparent that foregut carcinoid tumors may secrete 5-HT, histamine, 5-hydroxytryptophan, and kallikrein, an enzyme that releases bradykinin and prostaglandins in the blood. Foregut carcinoid tumors produced a different syndrome, the atypical carcinoid syndrome, because of the different hormones produced.

In 1905, John Edkins postulated a humoral mechanism for gastric acid secretion when it was observed that a denervated gastric pouch would secrete acid when food was placed in the main stomach.[46] He observed in dogs that extracts of pyloris mucous membrane would cause secretion of gastric juice when injected intravenously. He named the active substance gastrin for "gastric secretin." In 1948, Morton Grossman demonstrated that distension of an antral pouch caused acid secretion from a fundic pouch. In 1955 at the American Surgical Association meeting, Robert Zollinger and Ellison described two patients with recurrent stomal or jejunal ulceration, gastric acid hypersecretion, and a non-beta islet cell tumor of the pancreas.[47] In 1959, Gregory and Tracy extracted gastrin from an islet cell tumor in a patient with Zollinger–Ellison syndrome (ZES).[48] In 1964, Oberhelman first reported that the gastrinoma may also occur in the duodenum, which subsequently has been shown to be the most common primary site.[49] Zollinger recommended total gastrectomy for these patients because of the severe peptic ulcer disease, and it was the only procedure that could control the acid hypersecretion. This was the procedure of choice until 1979, when it was shown that gastric acid could be effectively controlled in all patients with ZES using the proton pump inhibitor omeprazole.[50] Subsequently, we have shown that surgery to remove the gastrinoma can cure approximately 40% of patients with sporadic ZES but few patients with ZES in the setting of multiple endocrine neoplasia type 1 (MEN 1).[51]

In 1958, Verner and Morrison of Durham, North Carolina, reported two patients who died of severe watery diarrhea, hypokalemia, and non-insulin-secreting islet cell tumor of the pancreas.[52] In 1970, a small peptide was isolated from an islet cell tumor in a similar patient by Sami Said; it was analyzed, synthesized, and named vasoactive intestinal polypeptide.[53]

In 1922, John Murlin of Rochester, New York, found that pancreatic extracts may cause a temporary rise in the blood glucose level, an effect opposite to that which is seen with insulin. He called the factor that increased blood glucose glucagon.[54] It was hypothesized to be secreted by the alpha cells in the pancreatic islets. In 1953, it was identified as a peptide and shown to be the antithesis of insulin. Glucagon is secreted in response to low concentrations of blood glucose; it stimulates glycogenolysis and gluconeogenesis and raises serum levels of glucose. In 1963, Roger Unger of Dallas recovered glucagon from extracts of four pancreatic islet cell tumors found at autopsy.[55] However, Malcom McGavran of St. Louis described the first patient with glucagonoma.[56] The patient had diabetes mellitus, anemia, a severe skin rash, and a pancreatic islet cell tumor with liver metastases. Hiram Polk performed surgery, and high levels of glucagon were assayed from the tumor and the plasma of the patient. The complete description of the glucagonoma syndrome was credited to Mallison of London, who had nine cases and also noted severe hypoaminoacidemia as part of the syndrome.[57]

In 1977, Larsson and colleagues first described somatostatin as an inhibitory pancreatic peptide.[58] Subsequently, Ganda and others described a patient who had had a cholecystectomy previously and currently needed a Whipple pancreaticoduodenectomy to remove an islet cell tumor in the head of the pancreas and several adjacent lymph node metastases.[59] The complete somatostatinoma syndrome was reported in 1979 by Guenter Krejs and others of Dallas, who described six patients with the triad of diabetes mellitus, steatorrhea, and cholelithiasis.[60]

Multiple Endocrine Neoplasia

Multiple endocrine tumors were first seen in 1903. Jakob Erdheim of Vienna, Austria, described the autopsy of a patient with acromegaly, a pituitary tumor, thyroid goiter, three large parathyroid glands, and pancreatic necrosis.[61] There were several case reports of patients with multiple endocrine tumors, but a true syndrome was not identified until 1953. Underdahl and others from the Mayo Clinic reported 8 patients with "multiple endocrine adenomas." All 8 had multiple parathyroid tumors; 2 also had acromegaly, and 3 had severe peptic ulcer disease (probable ZES). They coined the term multiple endocrine adenomas,[62] a term that initially was widely used but subsequently has been changed to multiple endocrine neoplasia because this name more clearly characterizes the pathology found. In 1954, Paul Wermer of New York proposed a genetic or inherited basis for the MEN 1 syndrome with autosomal dominance and high penetrance.[63] It became increasingly clear after the report of Zollinger and Ellison[47] that ZES was also prevalent in the MEN 1 syndrome. Wermer, for instance, noted that 19 of 20 patients from his previously reported family also had ZES. In addition, he noted that multiple lipomas and gastrointestinal carcinoid tumors may also be part of the syndrome. In 1964, Ballard and colleagues from Detroit analyzed 85 patients with MEN 1.[64] The commonest disorder was primary hyperparathyroidism (90%); pancreatic islet cell tumors were present in 80%, and pituitary tumors were found in 66%. Most recently, in 1997, the exact gene defect has been described in MEN 1 patients. It is located on chromosome 11 and is called Menin. Its exact function is unknown, but it is a tumor suppressor gene. It was discovered by Chandrasekharappa and a large team of others by a molecular biology technique called positional cloning.[65]

In 1961, John Sipple of Syracuse, New York, described a 33-year-old man with a large malignant tumor of the thyroid gland, bilateral adrenal pheochromocytomas, and enlarged parathyroid glands that were found at autopsy.[66] He identified 5 additional patients with thyroid cancer from a population of 537 patients with pheochromocytoma. The incidence was 1%, which was 14 times higher than expected in the general population. In 1963, Preston Manning at the Mayo Clinic correctly identified the type of thyroid cancer as medullary thyroid carcinoma on the basis of its amyloid stroma, and he noted that parathyroid disease can also be associated.[67] He referred to the condition as Sipple's syndrome, a name that persisted until 1968 when Alton Steiner described a kindred of 168 patients, many of whom were affected[68]; 25 patients had pheochromocytomas, 5 had medullary thyroid carcinoma, and 2 had parathyroid chief cell hyperplasia. He knew about MEN 1 and coined the term MEN 2. Also in that same year, Schimke and others reported similar but different patients with multiple neurofibromas, medullary thyroid carcinoma, and a characteristic appearance including bony abnormalities and marfanoid habitus.[69] Schimke said that these patients have MEN 3. Subsequently, as more patients with MEN 2 were recognized, Sizemore, Carney, and others from the Mayo Clinic called the patients with the phenotype MEN 2b, and the patients whom Steiner described were said to have MEN 2a. Both were inherited as autosomal dominant conditions. Calcitonin was found to be a very specific and sensitive serum and tumor marker for medullary thyroid carcinoma (MTC). Patients from kindreds with MEN 2a were screened for the presence of disease by measuring serum levels of calcitonin both in basal and following stimulation by calcium and pentagastrin. This technique correctly identified individuals with MTC before clinical evidence of tumor.[70] In 1995, Santoro and others identified the gene defect responsible for both MEN 2a and MEN 2b, an oncogene called RET. It is responsible for membrane tyrosine kinase activity and is located on chromosome 10. Missense mutations in RET are responsible for both the MEN 2a and MEN 2b clinical syndrome. Similar mutations also cause a familial medullary thyroid carcinoma syndrome in which only medullary thyroid carcinoma is inherited without other endocrine tumors. Once the exact mutation in a kindred with these inherited diseases is identified, family members at risk are identified by finding identical mutations in peripheral leukocytes. Because all patients with the inherited mutation will develop MTC, Wells has performed thyroidectomy based solely on identification of inherited mutations in individuals from kindreds with MEN 2a.[71] Each patient had either MTC or C-cell hyperplasia. This is the first instance in which a surgical procedure was performed based on identification of a gene defect. Eventually perhaps other conditions will be handled similarly, but currently only MEN 2a and MEN 2B are treated this way.

Conclusion

The history of endocrine surgery is relatively recent, with the discovery of glands and hormones at the beginning of the twentieth century. Theodore Kocher, an endocrine surgeon, won the Nobel Prize for the development of meticulous technique for thyroidectomy and the knowledge that subtotal thyroidectomy was necessary to prevent hypothyroidism. Most of the major endocrine glands were identified anatomically around 1900. The major hormones were identified by chemical extraction of the glands with subsequent purification and synthesis. The less focal diffuse gastrointestinal glandular system was not well characterized until the 1950s, when most of these hormones were described. Endocrine surgery was greatly facilitated in the 1960s by the development of the radioimmunoassay, which allowed precise measurement of very minute amounts of circulating hormones and thus enabled exact diagnosis of hormonal abnormalities. Surgeons and physicians have advanced endocrine surgery by careful description of unusual patients and families with endocrine syndromes; this helped to identify tumors and characterize the various functions of hormones. Surgeons have also improved techniques for preparation for surgery and methods such as laparoscopic surgery to remove endocrine tumors with less morbidity and mortality. Now, scientists are identifying the specific genetic changes that result in inherited endocrine syndromes and the development of endocrine tumors. These findings have already changed the indications for surgery in specific inherited conditions.

References

1. Bayliss WM, Starling EH. The mechanism of pancreatic secretion. J Physiol (Camb) 1902;28:325–353.
2. Welbourn RB. The History of Endocrine Surgery. New York: Praeger, 1990.
3. Cannon WB, Paz D. Emotional stimulation of adrenal secretion. Am J Physiol 1911;28:64–70.
4. Graves RJ. Newly observed affection of the thyroid gland in females. Lond Med J 1835;7:516.
5. Cope O, et al. Hyperfunctioning single adenoma of the thyroid. Surg Gynecol Obstet 1947;84:415–426.
6. Astwood EB. Treatment of hyperthyroidism with thiourea and thiouracil. JAMA 1943;122:78–81.
7. Moore FD, Cope O, Means JH, et al. Use of thiouracil in preparation of patients with hyperthyroidism for thyroidectomy. Ann Surg 1944;120:152–169.
8. Turner P, Granville-Grossman KL, Smart JV. Effect of adrenergic receptor blockade on the tachycardia of thyrotoxicosis. Lancet 1965;2:1316–1318.
9. Marie P. Sur deux les d'acromegalie. Rev Med (Paris) 1886;6:297.
10. Schonemann A. Hypophysis und thyreoidea. Arch Pathol Anat Physiol Klin Med 1892;129:310.
11. Cushing H. Partial hypophysectomy for acromegaly. Ann Surg 1909;50:1002.
12. Henderson WR. The pituitary adenomata. A follow-up study of the surgical results in 338 cases. Br J Surg 1926;811:1938–1939.
13. Hardy J, Wiger S. Transsphenoidal surgery of the pituitary fossa tumors with televised radiofluoroscopic control. J Neurosurg 1965;23:612.
14. Addison T. On the Constitutional and Local Effects of Disease of the Suprarenal Capsules. London: Samuel Highley, 1855.
15. Brown-Sequard E. Recherches experimentales sur la physiologie et la pathologie des capsules surrenales. Arch Gen Med (Paris) 1856;8:385–401.
16. Sheedy P, Stephens DH, et al. Computed tomography of the body. Am J Roentgenol 1976;127:23–51.
17. Conn JW. Primary alkdosteronism. J Lab Clin Med 1955;45:3–17.
18. Frankel F. Ein fall von doppelsetigen, vollig latent verlaufenen Nebenn ierentumor und zleichzeitizer Nephritis. Virchows Arch Pathol Anat Klin Med 1886;103:244–263.
19. Mayo CH. Paroxysmal hypertension with tumor of retroperitoneal nerve. JAMA 1927;89:1047–1050.
20. Rabin CB. Chromaffin cell tumor of the suprarenal medulla. Arch Pathol 1929;7:228–243.
21. Holton P. Noradrenaline in tumors of the adrenal medulla. J Physiol (Lond) 1949;108:525–529.
22. Crile GW. Clinical studies of adrenalectomy and sympathectomy. Ann Surg 1923;88:470–473.
23. Young HH. Techniques for simultaneous exposure and operation on the adrenals. Surg Gynecol Obstet 1936;63:179–188.
24. Chapius Y. Laparoscopic adrenalectomy: a report of 25 operations. Presse Med 1995;24:845–851.
25. Sandström I. On a new gland in man and several mammals. Upsula Lak Foren Forh 1879;15:441.
26. Gley E. Sur les functions du corps thyroide. CR Soc Biol 1891;43:841.
27. MacCallum WB, Voegtlin C. On the relation of tetany to the parathyroid glands and calcium metabolism. J Exp Med 1909;11:118.
28. Askanazy M. Uber ostitis deformans ohne osteoides gewebe. Arb Geb Pathol Anat Inst Tubingen 1903;4:398.
29. Schagenhaufer F. Zwei faller von parathyreoideatumoren. Wien Klin Wochenschr 1915;28:1362.
30. Barr DP, Bulger MA. The clinical syndrome of hyperparathyroidism. Ann J Med Sci 1930;179:449.

31. Aurbach GD. Isolation of parathyroid hormone after extraction with phenol. J Biol Chem 1959;234:3179.
32. Berson SA, Yalow RS, Aurbach GD, Potts JT. Immunoassay of bovine and human parathyroid hormone. Proc Natl Acad Sci U S A 1963;49:613.
33. Cope O, Keynes WM, Roth ST, Castleman B. Primary chief-cell hyperlasia of the parathyroid glands. Ann Surg 1958;148:375–388.
34. Wells SA, Ellis GJ, Gunnells JC, et al. Parathyroid autotransplantation in primary parathyroid hyperplasia. N Engl J Med 1976;295:57–62.
35. Albright F, Baird RC, Cope O, Bloomberg E. Physiology of the parathyroid glands. IV. Renal complications. Am J Med Sci 1934;287:49–65.
36. Langerhans P. Inaugural dissertation. Beitrage zur mikroskopischen Anatomie der Bauchspeicheldruse. Berlin: Bechdruckerei van Gustav Lange, Feb. 18, 1869:5–32.
37. Heidenhain RPH. Arch Mikrosk Anat 1870;6:368.
38. Kulchitsky N. Zur Frage uber den Bau des Darmkanals. Arch Mikrosk Anat 1897;49:7.
39. Oberndorfer S. Karcinoide: tumoren des duenndarmes. Frankf Z Pathol 1907;1:426.
40. Wilder RM, Allan FN, Power MH, Robertson HE. Carcinoma of the islets of the pancreas: hyperinsulinism and hypoglucemia. JAMA 1927;89:348–355.
41. Howland G, Campbell WR, Maltby EJ, Robinson WL. Dysinsulinism . . . due to islet cell tumor of the pancreas with operation and cure. JAMA 1929;93:674–679.
42. Whipple AO. The surgical therapy of hyperinsulinism. J Int Chir 1938;3:237.
43. Rosenbaum FF, Santer DG, Claudon DB. Essential telangiectasia, pulmonic and tricuspid stenosis and neoplastic liver disease. J Lab Clin Med 195;42:941–942.
44. Isler VP, Hedinger C. Metastasierendes Dunndaum carcinoid mit schweren, vorwiegend das rechte Herz. Schweiz Med Wochenschr 1953;83:4.
45. Pernow B, Waldenstrom J. Paroxysmal flushing and other symptoms caused by 5-hydroxytryptamine and histamine. Lancet 1954;2:951.
46. Edkins JS. The chemical mechanism of gastric secretion. Proc R Soc Lond Ser B 1905;76:376; J Physiol 1906;34:133.
47. Zollinger RM, Ellison EH. Primary peptic ulcerations of the jejunum association with islet cell tumors of the pancreas. Ann Surg 1955;142:709.
48. Gregory RA, Tracy HJ, French JM, Sircus W. Extraction of a gastrin-like substance from a pancreatic tumor. Lancet 1960;1:1045.
49. Oberhelman HA, Nelson TS. Surgical considerations on the management of ulcerogenic tumors. Am J Surg 1964;108:132–141.
50. Olbe L, Berglindh T, Elander B, et al. Properties of a new class of gastric acid inhibitors. Scand J Gastroenterol (Suppl) 1979; 14(55):131–35.
51. Norton JA, Fraker DL, Alexander HR, et al. Surgery to cure the Zollinger–Ellison syndrome. N Engl J Med 1999;341:635–644.
52. Verner JW, Morrison AB. Endocrine pancreatic islet disease with diarrhea. Arch Intern Med 1974;133:492–500.
53. Said ST, Mutt V. Potent peripheral and splanchnic vasodilator peptide from normal gut. Nature (Lond) 1970;225:863–864.
54. Murlin JR, Clough HD, Gibbs CBF, Stokes AM. Aqueous extracts of the pancreas. I. Influence on the carbohydrate metabolism of depancreatized animals. J Biol Chem 1923;56:253.
55. Unger RH, Eisentraut AM, Lochner J. Glucagon-producing tumors of the islets of Langerhans. J Clin Invest 1963;42:987.
56. McGavran MH, Unger RH, Polk HC, et al. A glucagon-secreting alpha-cell carcinoma of the pancreas. N Engl J Med 1966;274:1408.
57. Mallison CN, Bloom SR, Warin AP, et al. A glucagonoma syndrome. Lancet 1974;2:1.
58. Larsson LI, Ingamansson S, Rehfeld JF, et al. Pancreatic somatostatinoma. Lancet 1977;1:666.
59. Ganda OP, Ebeid AM, Reichlins S, et al. Somatostainoma. N Engl J Med 1977;296:963.
60. Krejs GJ, McCarthy DM, Unger RH, et al. Somatostatinoma syndrome. N Engl J Med 1979;301:285.
61. Erdheim J. Zur normalen und pathologischen Histologie der Glandula thyroidea, parathyroidea, und hypophysis. Beit Pathol Anat 1903;33:158–236.
62. Underdahl LO, Woolner LB, Black BM. Multiple endocrine adenomas. J Clin Endocrinol Metab 1953;13:20–47.
63. Wermer P. Endocrine adenomatosis: peptic ulcer in a large kindred. Am J Med 1963;35:205–212.
64. Ballard HS, Frame R, Hartsock RJ. Familial multiple endocrine adenoma-peptic ulcer complex. Medicine (Baltim) 1964;43:481–516.
65. Chandrasekharappa SG, Guru SC, Manickam P, et al. Positional cloning of the gene for multiple endocrine neoplasia type 1. Science 1997;276:404–407.
66. Sipple JH. The association of pheochromocytoma with carcinoma of the thyroid gland. Am J Med 1961;31:163–166.
67. Manning PC, Molnar GD, Black BM, Priestley JT, Woolner LB. Pheochromocytoma, hyperparathyroidism, and thyroid carcinoma occurring coincidentally. N Engl J Med 1963;268:68–72.
68. Steiner AL, Goodman AD, Powers SR. Studies of a kindred with pheochromocytoma, medullary thyroid carcinoma, primary hyperparathyroidism, and Cushing's disease: MEN-2. Medicine (Baltim) 1968;47:371–409.
69. Schimke RN, Hartmann WH, Prout T, Rimoin DL. Syndrome of bilateral pheochromocytomas, medullary thyroid carcinoma, and multiple neuromas. N Engl J Med 1968;279:1–7.
70. Wolfe HJ, Melvin KEW, Cervi-Skinner SJ, et al. C-cell hyperplasia preceding medullary thyroid carcinoma. N Engl J Med 1973;289:437–441.
71. Wells SA Jr, Chi DD, Toshima K, et al. Predictive DNA testing and prophylactic thyroidectomy in patients at risk for multiple endocrine neoplasia type 2A. Ann Surg 1994;220:237–247.

55

Parathyroid

Matthew B. Bloom and Jeffrey A. Norton

In their studies of anatomy, early pathologists failed to immediately recognize the distinct entities of the parathyroid glands. It was not until 1850 that the organ was first described during the necropsy of an Indian rhinoceros at the London Zoo.[1] Seventy-five years later, the first surgery for hyperparathyroidism was performed in Vienna by Dr. Felix Mandl on a trolley-car operator with severe osteitis fibrosa cystica known as "Albert J."[2–4] One enlarged gland was removed, and Albert had symptomatic improvement for about 6 years until his bone disease recurred. In 1926, a second parathyroid surgery was performed without any prior knowledge of Albert's case. This time, surgeons at the Massachusetts General Hospital explored the neck of Captain Charles Martell, a merchant marine who suffered severe back and leg pain, fractures of his arms and legs, kyphoscoliosis, urinary calculi, hypercalcemia, and hypophosphatemia.[5,6] The initial exploration and five subsequent operations revealed only normal parathyroid glands. Only during a seventh surgery was a large parathyroid adenoma identified in Captain Martell's mediastinum. Ninety percent of this enlarged gland was resected while a small remnant was intentionally left behind. Captain Martell later died of chronic renal failure from his long-standing parathyroid disease. Despite much improvement in our ability to diagnose and treat parathyroid disease, current therapies are still challenged by similar issues such as the recurrent hyperparathyroidism that was seen with "Albert," and the ectopic parathyroid adenoma and the difficulties of reoperative surgery, which were the case with Captain Martell.

However, there has been a great evolution in the surgical management of primary hyperparathyroidism as our experience has grown. The past decade, in particular, has seen a marked change in opinion regarding the best approach to the diagnosis and treatment of this disease. Because we are currently in the midst of a technological revolution, many of the former standard surgical procedures are being challenged by minimally invasive approaches. Present strategies for the surgical management of parathyroid disease have been made possible by innovative ways to identify aberrant pathology both before and during surgery. The conventional practice of identifying and evaluating all four parathyroid glands at the time of surgery, which had been purposely performed without preoperative imaging results, has been largely replaced by the practice of obtaining preoperative localization studies as part of the initial workup for primary hyperparathyroidism, followed by a targeted minimally invasive surgical approach when appropriate. This highly localized procedure ultimately provides a better operation for the patient, with resolution of primary hyperparathyroidism, less pain, and a quicker recovery.

Basic Science of Parathyroid Disease

Calcium Physiology

A detailed understanding of the homeostatic mechanisms of calcium is required for the optimal management of hyperparathyroidism, including the proper selection of patients for surgical treatment. The average daily dietary intake of calcium may range between 500 and 1000 mg/day.[7] However, despite marked dietary intake variations, the diurnal variation in the level of serum calcium is only 5% or less. This homeostasis is achieved by a careful balance between gastrointestinal absorption, bone deposition and release, and the urinary excretion of calcium. Absorption involves vitamin D metabolites, and occurs primarily in the duodenum and upper jejunum. In the kidney, approximately 99% of the filtered calcium is reabsorbed by the proximal tubule, but this amount varies inversely with the amount of dietary calcium intake. The absorption of calcium in the proximal tubule and loop of Henle is linked to sodium transport, whereas distal tubular absorption of calcium is influenced by parathyroid hormone and not sodium.[8] Calcium losses approximate 100 mg/day and 800 mg/day in perspiration and feces, respectively. By far, the body's single greatest reservoir of calcium is skeletal bone, which contains approximately 1000 g (99% of the body's calcium). Extracellular fluid, osteoblasts, and cells usually contain 1 g, 500 mg, and 11 g calcium, respectively[7] (Fig. 55.1).

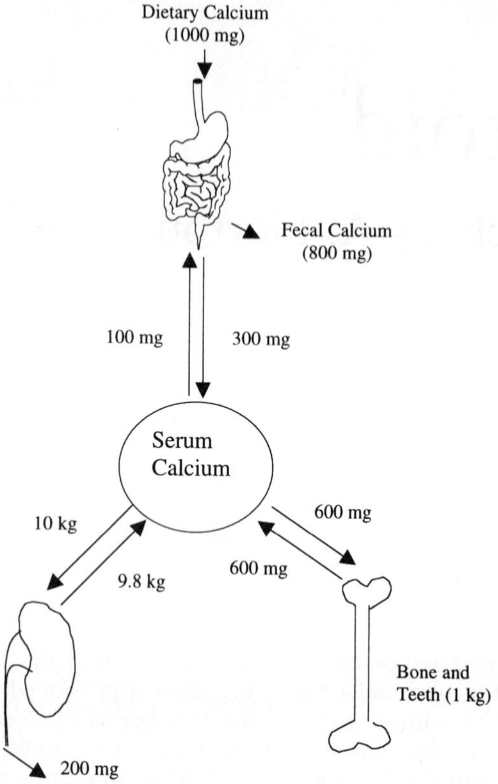

FIGURE 55.1. Diagram of the average distribution of calcium in the body. The average daily dietary calcium intake is approximately 1 g. A net of 200 mg is absorbed from the dietary calcium intake, and the rest is loss through feces. The largest calcium reservoir is the skeleton, which contains approximately 1 kg. The kidney contributes to calcium homeostasis with a net daily excretion of 200 mg calcium.

Calcium is the body's most abundant mineral, yet only its ionized form is physiologically active. Ionized calcium plays critical roles in signal transduction, nerve excitability, skeletal and cardiac muscle contractility, and bone matrix formation. Additionally, cell structure, function, and metabolism are regulated by calcium-dependent processes. Approximately 47% of calcium is in the ionized form in plasma; 45% is protein bound, and 8% is complexed to organic anions.[9] It is important to remember that in diseased states total serum calcium needs to be adjusted with plasma protein levels, particularly albumin. The following formula has been suggested to correct for adjustments in total serum calcium with respect to alterations in serum albumin levels:[9]

$$\text{Ca (adjusted)} = \text{Ca (total)} - 0.8 \times (\text{albumin} - 4.0)$$

However, ionized calcium can now be rapidly measured, making it the method of choice to measure calcium in the serum.

Serum calcium is regulated by a closely integrated interplay of three hormones: parathyroid hormone (PTH), vitamin D_3 (1,25-dihydroxycholecalciferol), and calcitonin (Fig. 55.2). The key target organs include the parathyroids, skeletal muscle, kidneys, and intestine. PTH is synthesized in the parathyroid glands as a larger molecule, pre-pro-PTH, which is cleaved into its inactive form, pre-PTH.[10] Pre-PTH is further cleaved into PTH, which is released into the circulation and rapidly broken down further into amino- and carboxyl-terminal fragments by the liver and kidney. Only the intact 84 amino acid long PTH molecule and the 1–34 amino-terminal fragment are physiologically active.[11] The double-antibody immunoradiometric assay (IRMA) is the current method of intact PTH detection[12]; it has greatly simplified the diagnosis of primary hyperparathyroidism.

PTH exerts its effect by activating membrane-bound adenylate cyclases, which in turn generate cyclic adenosine monophosphate (cAMP). PTH regulates serum calcium level by directly and indirectly affecting calcium exchange at the intestine, bone, and kidney. PTH directly increases serum calcium by inhibiting the synthetic function of osteoblasts and stimulating renal tubular calcium reabsorption. PTH indirectly contributes to calcium regulation by stimulating osteoclast maturation and inducing renal phosphate clearance and synthesis of calcitriol, which in turn promotes gastrointestinal absorption of calcium.

Vitamin D is another key regulator of bone mineral metabolism. Vitamin D synthesis begins with previtamin D_3 production via ultraviolet irradiation of 7-dihydroxycholesterol in the skin. Previtamin D_3 is then converted to vitamin D_3 (cholecalciferol), which is then 25-hyroxylated in the liver to produce 25-(OH)D_3 (calcifediol). Calcifediol undergoes 1a-hydroxylation in the kidneys to form calcitriol. Calcitriol is the major active form of vitamin D. It stimulates calcium-binding protein in the gut and enhances absorption of calcium and phosphorus; this in turn promotes deposition of hydroxyapatite in bone. On the other hand, calcitriol also inhibits pre-pro-PTH and induces calcium mobilization from bone.[10]

Calcitonin is produced by the parafollicular C cells of the thyroid. Calcitonin decreases bone resorption by antago-

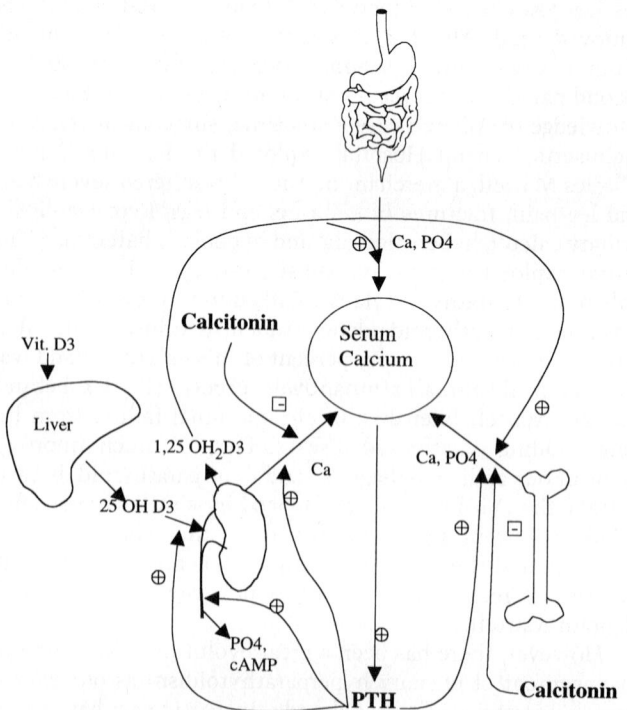

FIGURE 55.2. The interplay of parathyroid hormone (PTH), vitamin D, and calcitonin on calcium and phosphorus regulation at specific target organs. A decrease in serum calcium stimulates PTH secretion by the parathyroid glands. PTH directly and indirectly affects calcium exchange at the intestine, bone, and kidney to elevate the serum level of calcium. Calcitriol [1,25(OH)2D], the major active form of vitamin D, enhances calcium and phosphorus absorption in the intestine while inhibiting PTH. There is a negative feedback loop between serum calcium and calcitonin levels. An increase in serum calcium results in calcitonin secretion, which regulates bone and kidney to decrease serum calcium.

nizing the effects of PTH. Its physiological role has been implicated in minimizing calcium loss during development, pregnancy, and nursing.[13] Although calcitonin receptors are found in the kidneys, brain, and to a lesser extent throughout the body, neither the complete absence nor supernormal levels of calcitonin seem to have any significant clinical manifestations.

Embryology, Anatomy, and Pathophysiology

Facility in the identification of normal and abnormal parathyroid glands is essential for successful surgery. Parathyroid glands vary in their color from a light yellow to a reddish brown, with a consistency that is usually soft and pliable. A reddish color and a dense consistency reflect high parenchymal cell content (abnormal gland); a yellowish-white color is found with high fat content (normal gland).[14] Typically, four parathyroid glands are present, each measuring roughly 3 × 5 × 7 mm, although these glands can vary widely in their size and shape. Eighty-three percent are oval or bean shaped, 11% are elongated, 5% are bilobed, and 1% are multilobed (Fig. 55.3). Normal glands tend to be flat and ovoid; with enlargement, they become globular. The combined weight of the parathyroid glandular tissue ranges from 90 to 130 mg, with the inferior glands usually developing to a slightly larger size than the superior glands.[15] Most parathyroid glands are suspended by a small vascular pedicle and enveloped by a pad of fatty tissue.[16]

In one autopsy series, four glands were found in 91% of subjects, five glands in 4%, and three glands in 5%.[17] In examinations of serial sections of embryos, at least four parathyroid glands were found in every specimen.[18] In the approximately 4% to 5% of people who have supernumerary glands, this extra tissue is most commonly found within the thymus.[19]

Although gland distribution may deviate widely, the locations of the parathyroid glands are somewhat predictable from studies of embryology.[16] The parathyroid glands develop at approximately the fifth week of gestation. The upper parathyroid glands originate from the dorsal part of the fourth branchial pouches along with the lateral lobes of the thyroid and are commonly found along the upper two-thirds of its posterior surface (92%).[14] Often (40%) superior parathyroid gland

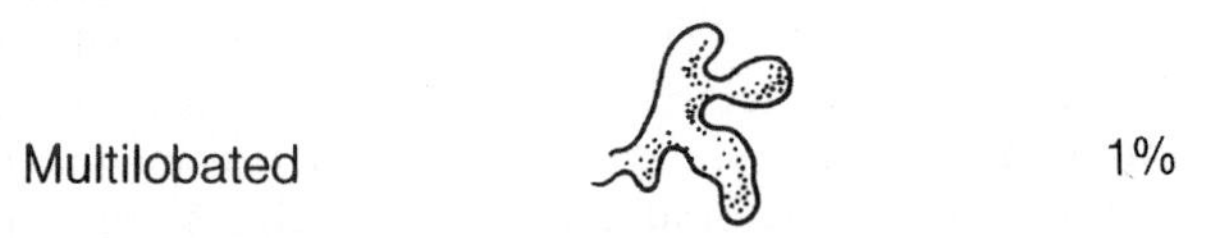
Oval, bean-shaped or spherical
83%
Elongated
11%
Bilobated
5%
Multilobated
1%

FIGURE 55.3. Recognition of the possible shapes of the parathyroid gland will assist in successful identification of the parathyroids during neck exploration. Represented here are some of the more common shapes encountered in a large autopsy series. (Data from Akerstrom G, Malmaeus J, Bergstrom R. Surgical anatomy of human parathyroid glands. Surgery (St. Louis) 1984;95(1):14–21.[14])

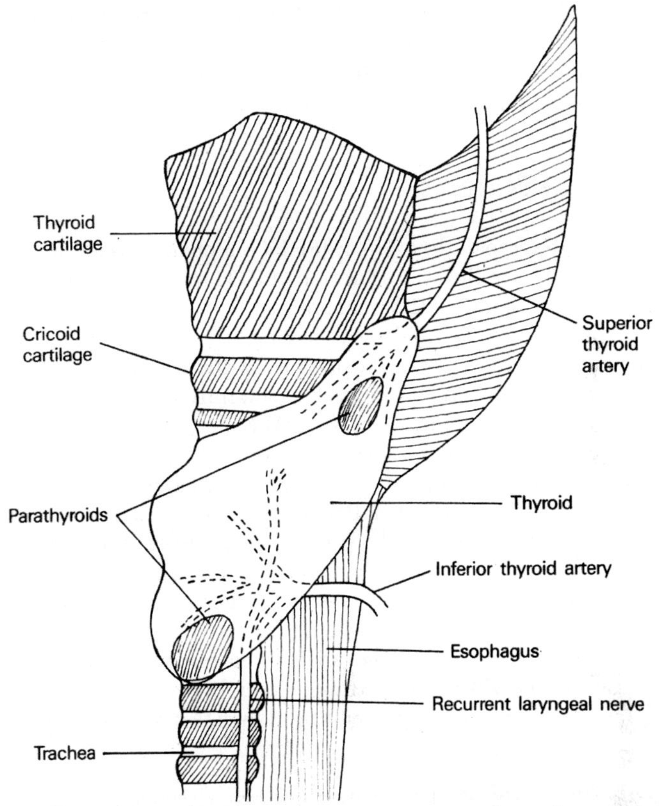

FIGURE 55.4. A lateral view of the anatomic relationship of the parathyroids to their arterial blood supply and the recurrent laryngeal nerve. The superior parathyroid glands are usually located in the upper portion of the lateral thyroid lobes and are supplied by the superior thyroid artery. The location of the inferior parathyroid glands is more variable but can usually be found in the lower pole of the thyroid. The inferior parathyroids are supplied by the inferior thyroid artery, which runs just lateral to the recurrent laryngeal nerve.

adenomas migrate further posteriorly, behind the inferior thyroid artery, to rest alongside the esophagus.[20] Division of the superior thyroid artery and mobilization of the superior thyroid pole are usually unnecessary to expose the superior parathyroid glands, but the fascia connecting the lateral portion of the thyroid lobe to the carotid sheath must be incised. As the location of the superior glands is relatively constant, these glands can usually be identified quickly and easily. Superior parathyroid gland adenomas may have a unique spatial relationship with the recurrent laryngeal nerve such that the nerve is embedded in the anterior medial portion of its capsule, or the gland is located at the spot where the recurrent nerve enters the larynx.

In contrast, the lower parathyroid glands develop from the dorsal part of the third branchial pouches along with the thymus. Their migratory path is longer, which helps account for their greater variability in final location. As the thymus descends, the lower parathyroid glands migrate until they reach the lower pole of the thyroid gland. Seventeen percent of inferior parathyroid glands touch the inferior border of the thyroid, 44% are within 1 cm of the inferior border of the thyroid (also known as the thyro-thymic ligament), 26% are within the superior horn of the thymus, and 2% are in the mediastinal thymus.[14,16] The remainder are most likely within the mass of the thyroid or are undescended in the upper portion of the neck near the carotid bifurcation.[21] (Fig. 55.4). The greater variability in location of the inferior glands makes their identification more difficult than the superior glands. Most commonly, however, they can be found bordered posteriorly and laterally by the recurrent laryngeal nerve, and lying inferior to the inferior thyroid artery.

Clinical Features

Primary hyperparathyroidism (PHPT) is characterized by an inappropriately elevated secretion of PTH relative to the level of serum calcium. PHPT accounts for 50% to 60% of hypercalcemia in the ambulatory setting, whereas malignancy accounts for 65% of hypercalcemia in the hospital setting[22] (Table 55.1) Certain factors such as a family history of PHPT or multiple endocrine neoplasia (MEN), childhood radiation to the head and neck, postmenopausal state, renal calculi, peptic ulcer, hypertension, or thiazide-induced hypercalcemia are more consistent with PHPT. Clinical presentations of primary hyperparathyroidism may be in one of three forms: (1) asymptomatic hypercalcemia; (2) nephrolithiasis; or (3) bone disease with more marked hypercalcemia, fatigue, general debility, bone pain, weight loss, pathological fractures, and even parathyroid crisis. The most common presentation, however, is asymptomatic hypercalcemia. The diagnosis of primary hyperparathyroidism is based on concurrent measurements of both elevated serum levels of intact parathyroid hormone (PTH)[23–26] and either total calcium[27,28] or ionized calcium.[29] Measurement of 24-h urinary calcium excretion, which is elevated in patients with PHPT, helps to distinguish against other entities such as familial hypocalciuric hypercalcemia (FHH) in which urine calcium is low.

TABLE 55.1. Differential Diagnosis of Hypercalcemia.[a]

Endocrine
Primary hyperparathyroidism
Thyrotoxicosis
Pheochromocytoma
Addison's disease
VIPomas
Malignancy
Solid tumors
Lytic bone metastasis
Parathyroid hormone-related protein
Lymphoma and leukemia
Granulomatous diseases
Sarcoidosis
Tuberculosis
Histoplasmosis
Coccidioidomycosis
Leprosy
Medication
Calcium
Vitamin A or D intoxication
Thiazides
Lithium
Estrogens and antiestrogens
Others
Milk alkali syndrome
Familial hypocalciuric hypercalcemia
Immobilization
Paget's disease
Renal insufficiency

[a]Malignancy is the most common cause of hypercalcemia in the inpatient setting; primary hyperparathyroidism is the most common cause in the outpatient setting.

Prognostic Indicators of Parathyroid Pathology

The possible causes of primary hyperparathyroidism are a single parathyroid adenoma (83%), multiple glandular parathyroid hyperplasia (10%–12%), double adenomas (1%–2%), or carcinoma (1%).[30] Some argue that "double adenomas" may represent missed cases of undetected hyperplasia. However, several authors believe that double adenomas are true entities and cite occurrence rates as high as 15%.[31–34] It has been observed that recurrent disease does not develop in patients with resected double adenomas even after long follow-up.

It is up to the operating surgeon to correctly diagnose the precise etiology of primary hyperparathyroidism. Certain patient history and physical examination findings may suggest particular types of parathyroid pathology. For example, a history of neck irradiation is associated with adenoma development.[15] Parathyroid adenoma is rarely ever palpable, but parathyroid carcinoma is palpable in a high percentage of cases.[35] Exceptionally high concentrations of serum PTH or calcium (>14 mg/dL) may also suggest parathyroid cancer.[36,37] A family history of parathyroid disease or other endocrine tumors is suggestive of hyperplasia. Parathyroid hyperplasia is often inherited in familial syndromes such as MEN I or MEN IIa.[38,39] However, because there is a wide variation in the size and appearance of the abnormal parathyroid glands in patients with MEN I, it is helpful for the surgeon to know preoperatively if an individual patient has a familial history of an inheritable syndrome.[40]

There are no findings upon physical examination that are characteristic of either MEN I or MEN IIa. Recent studies have identified the genetic defect in patients with MEN I as the MENIN mutation on chromosome 11q13[41] and in patients with MEN IIa as the RET proto-oncogene mutation on chromosome 10q11.2.[42] In contrast, patients with MEN IIb do not have primary hyperparathyroidism, and they are easier to identify because they may have a recognizable phenotype consisting of multiple neuromata on the tongue and buccal mucosa, prognathism, skeletal abnormalities, marfanoid body habitus, and ganglioneuromas of the colon.[39,43,44]

Familial hypocalciuric hypercalcemia (FHH) is an autosomal dominant trait presenting usually as asymptomatic mild hypercalcemia and relative hypocalciuria.[20,45] Mutations in the calcium-sensing receptor gene on chromosome 3 have been identified in its heterozygous form in benign FHH.[46] However, calcium-sensing receptor mutations could not be found in sporadic parathyroid tumors. In patients with FHH, the hypercalcemia is PTH-dependent and associated with mild parathyroid hyperplasia; however, subtotal parathyroidectomy is rarely successful in correcting hypercalcemia and is contraindicated. Without laboratory analyses, the only useful clue to this diagnosis is a family history of unsuccessful parathyroidectomy or of a relative with hypercalcemia recognized before the age of 10.[38] In such cases, measurement of urinary calcium excretion and detection of relative hypocalciuria (<100 mg/24 h) should lead to postponement of surgery and to testing for hypercalcemia in close relatives.

We have found that the yield from routine use of potential tumor markers for associated endocrine disease (MEN I or IIa) is too low to be indicated in all patients with primary hyperparathyroidism.[47–50] In MEN I patients, a circulating mitogenic factor has been shown to be associated with polyclonal hyperplasia of the parathyroid glands. Monoclonal parathyroid enlargement is attributed to loss of heterozygosity from chromosome 11. Similarly, in patients with sporadic parathyroid adenomas, there is a novel gene rearrangement involving the parathyroid hormone gene on chromosome 11 and a loss of heterozygosity of the PRAD1 gene on 11q13.[51] The initiation of parathyroid tumor growth apparently is heterogeneous and may be caused by deletion of a suppressor gene in a significant proportion of parathyroid tumors or by induction of an oncogene in a minority of tumors. Differential expression of gene products has been correlated with variations in clinical presentation.[52]

Hypercalcemic Crisis

Hypercalcemic crisis is an unusual state of progressive, marked primary hyperparathyroidism that produces accelerated bone resorption and an excessive elevation in serum and urinary levels of calcium. Clinical manifestations may include anorexia, vomiting, constipation, dehydration, acute pancreatitis, shortened QT interval, increased sensitivity to digitalis, polyuria, polydipsia, nephrocalcinosis, apathy, drowsiness, coma, and, if untreated, death.[53–56] The hypercalcemia may have been noted in the past but left untreated or inadequately treated. Often no apparent reason exists for sudden progression of hyperparathyroidism to the state of crisis, but some cases are apparently precipitated by the stress of bacterial or viral infection, trauma, or recent surgery. Serum levels of calcium should not be the only defining criteria for a hypercalcemic crisis because there have been reports of asymptomatic patients with serum calcium levels of 20 mg/dL and of patients in hypercalcemic crisis with serum calcium less than 14 mg/dL.[57] Acute severe hypercalcemia may also be caused by malignancy. Parathyroid carcinoma is in the differential diagnosis of patients who manifest severe hypercalcemia. PHPT is always diagnosed by increased serum levels of PTH, whereas nearly all patients with malignancy have low levels of PTH and either elevated serum levels of parathyroid hormone-related protein (PTHrP) or multiple bony metastases. Regardless of the source, the treatment of the hypercalcemia is similar.

The management of severe hypercalcemia in patients with parathyroid crisis centers on achieving four basic goals: (1) the correction of dehydration, (2) enhancement of renal excretion of calcium, (3) inhibition of accelerated bone resorption, and (4) treatment of the underlying disorder. The initial treatment is the administration of large volumes of saline to correct dehydration. Once fluid status is corrected, intravenous administration of saline followed by a loop diuretic (i.e., furosemide) is usually effective in reducing the hypercalcemia by inhibiting calcium reabsorption in the ascending limb of the loop of Henle. Thiazide diuretics are contraindicated because they enhance distal tubular reabsorption of calcium. In patients with a low serum concentration of phosphate, normal renal function, and moderate hypercalcemia, oral phosphate may also be used. If hydration and treatment with intravenous loop diuretics are not effective in reducing the hypercalcemia, then treatment with diphosphonates, mithramycin, calcitonin, or gallium should be started as necessary to normalize serum calcium levels.[55]

Preoperative and Intraoperative Localization Techniques

As mentioned in the introduction, the management of primary hyperparathyroidism has undergone a marked change in the last decade. Currently, to perform a maximally successful, minimally invasive parathyroidectomy (MIP), localization studies, which were once reserved only for reoperative cases, are now routinely employed both before and at the time of initial surgery (Table 55.2). When a single hyperfunctioning

TABLE 55.2.
Imaging Modalities Before Initial Operations for Primary Hyperparathyroidism (PHPT).[a]

References	*Level of evidence*[b]	*n*	*Sestamibi*	*Tech-thal*	*Ultrasound*	*CT*	*MRI*
Ammori 1998[180]	III	63	—	—	80/100	—	—
Norman 1998[137]	III	6331	91/99	—	—	—	—
Ishibashi 1998[181]	III	20	83/83	—	78/40	—	80/60
Sinha 1997[182]	III	60	90/—	63/—	—	—	—
Gofrit 1997[183]	II	52	—	—	83/100	—	—
Koslin 1997[184]	II	37	—	—	84/90	—	—
Light 1996[185]	II	21	87/44	—	57/24	—	—
Sofferman 1996[186]	III	34	91/97	—	—	—	—
Bugis 1995[187]	III	37	68/55	—	—	—	—
Mitchell 1992[188]	III	—	86/77–100	26–75/—	36–76/—	46–55/43–98	50–78/70–100
van Heerden 1991[189]	III	384	—	—	85/25	—	—

CT, computed tomography; MRI, magnetic resonance imaging.
[a]Imaging modalities: sensitivity/specificity (%).
[b]I, randomized prospective study; II, prospective study; III, retrospective study, review or anecdotal.

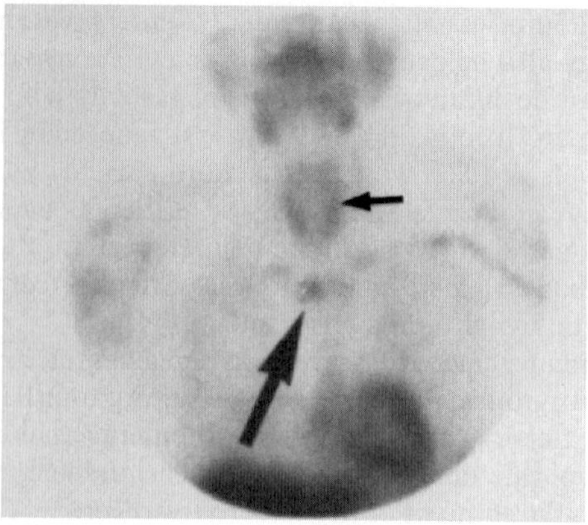

FIGURE 55.5. A positive sestamibi scan demonstrating an intrathymic parathyroid adenoma *(large arrow)* in the mediastinum. The *small arrow* points to the thyroid.

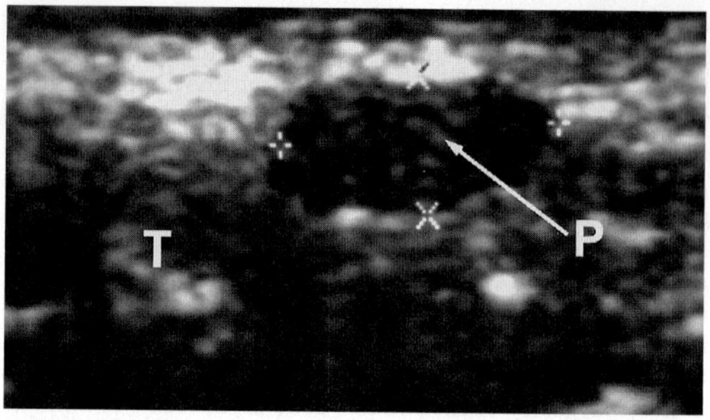

FIGURE 55.6. Ultrasound is best at identifying an intrathyroidal parathyroid adenoma. The hypoechoic mass *(P)* is an intrathyroidal parathyroid adenoma, and *(T)* is the more echogenic right superior thyroid lobe.

gland can be identified preoperatively, a highly minimally invasive surgery can be undertaken.

Localization Before Initial Parathyroidectomy

There is a general consensus that the best preoperative localization procedure for initial parathyroid operations is the combination of both ultrasound and sestamibi scanning. The single best study, however, is sestamibi, which has a sensitivity and specificity of 91% and 98%, respectively.[58] Sestamibi is a lipophilic monovalent cation that exhibits passive diffusion across the cell membrane and becomes concentrated in the mitochondria. It is preferentially taken up by hypercellular parathyroid glands because of their increased blood supply, higher metabolic activity, and an absence of *p*-glycoprotein on the cell membrane. Sestamibi scans may be performed as a preoperative outpatient procedure, or on the morning of surgery in combination with the use of the gamma probe in the operative room to guide the surgeon during the operation (Fig. 55.5).[59] High-resolution ultrasound with high-frequency transducers is also useful for preoperative parathyroid localization; it images the abnormal parathyroid gland as a sonolucent mass compared to the more echo-dense thyroid tissue (Fig. 55.6). It is highly specific, but is not as sensitive as a sestamibi study, with reported specificity of 98% and sensitivity of 66%.[60] If the sestamibi and ultrasound studies identify the same gland preoperatively, the minimally invasive parathyroidectomy will be facilitated.

Localization Before Reoperative Parathyroidectomy

In patients with persistent or recurrent hyperparathyroidism, the chance of successful repeat surgery is reduced[61,62] and the incidence of complications is greater.[63] Therefore, maximum effort at parathyroid gland localization is made, commencing with the noninvasive procedures [ultrasound (US), computed tomography (CT), magnetic resonance imaging (MRI), sestamibi] and proceeding (if necessary) to the more invasive studies (Fig. 55.7). Currently, noninvasive techniques localize

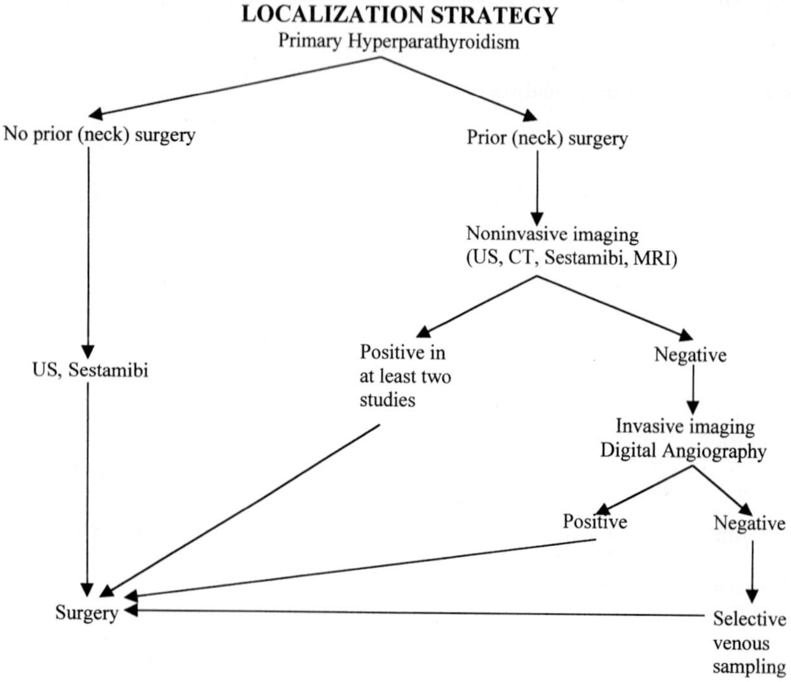

FIGURE 55.7. Flow diagram for localization strategy in unoperated and previously operated patients.

TABLE 55.3.
Imaging Modalities in Reoperative Parathyroidectomies: Overall Results.

References	*Level of evidence*[a]	*n*	*Sestamibi*	*Tech-thal*	*Ultrasound*	*CT*	*MRI*	*Angiography*	*Venous sampling*
Mariette 1998[190]	III	38	69/—	—	—	16/—	—	—	63/—
Peeler 1997[191]	III	25	74/—	—	45/—	68/—	—	—	—
Jaskowiak 1996[154]	II	227	67/0	42/8	48/21	52/16	48/14	59/9	76/4
Shen 1996[62]	III	102	77/—	68/—	57/—	42/—	77/—	—	77/—
MacFarlane 1994[192]	III	42	42/15	—	67/9	56/10	36/8	68/14	69/8
Rodriquez 1994[193]	III	152	70/0	60/16	53/16	42/12	69/12	—	69/15
Doherty 1992[194]	III	27/—	—	4/23	0/20	35/13	19/13	84/7	—

Imaging modalities: true-positive/false-positive (%).
[a]I, randomized prospective study; II, prospective study; III, retrospective study, review or anecdotal.
[b]Values represent sensitivities.

an abnormal gland in about 75% to 80% of patients requiring repeat surgery[64] whereas invasive studies help in the remainder (Table 55.3).[65]

Common Localization Studies

Ultrasound

Ultrasound (US) is the least expensive and least invasive technique used to image abnormal parathyroid glands. It is particularly effective in localizing enlarged parathyroid glands in the neck and can be used to identify 30% to 60% of the abnormal glands in patients requiring reoperation.[64] It clearly identifies juxtathyroidal parathyroid glands that appear sonolucent compared to the more echogenic thyroid (see Fig. 55.6).

US does have some relative disadvantages, however. It may fail to image posterior glands in the tracheoesophageal groove because its signal may be shielded by the air-filled trachea. Similarly, US may miss glands in the anterior mediastinum because the signal is shadowed by the sternum. In multiple gland hyperplasia, it generally demonstrates only the dominant gland. Finally, the quality of US examination is highly operator-dependent, and requires an ultrasonographer both knowledgeable and interested in locating abnormal parathyroid glands.

Sestamibi Scintigraphy

Sestamibi technetium 99m scans were first described as a means to identify parathyroid tissue by Coakely in 1989.[66] Sestamibi is sequestered in metabolically active tissue or in tissue with a high mitochondrial content. Both the thyroid and parathyroid glands will take up sestamibi, but its uptake will be stronger and the signal will persist longer in abnormal parathyroid glands (see Fig. 55.5). The combination of single-photon emission CT with sestamibi has improved the sensitivity to about 85%, especially for deep cervical and mediastinal parathyroid tumors.[67] Sestamibi technetium 99m scanning has superior resolution and sensitivity (80%–90%) to detect hypercellular parathyroid glands before reoperations.[68] The sensitivity of sestamibi scans to localize parathyroid tissue may be further improved by the suppression of thyroid function with thyroxin or liothyronine and worsened by patient use of calcium channel blockers.[69,70]

Sestamibi has been combined with the gamma probe for hand-held intraoperative localization of abnormal parathyroid glands.[71–73] Advocates suggest that this approach is less invasive and can be done as an outpatient procedure through a smaller incision, with less operating room time required.[74] However, most surgeons find it superfluous as the results of the preoperative imaging pinpoint the location of the abnormal gland. Sestamibi scans appear to facilitate the dissection and make the surgery easier, but they have not been shown to affect the outcome in previously unoperated patients. A recent study demonstrated that there was no significant difference in cure rates between patients who had preoperative sestamibi scans and those who did not (cure rates, 97.5% and 99%, respectively). However, there was a significant difference in cure rate between the negative sestamibi scan group (92.7%) and both the no-scan group (99.3%) and the positive-scan group (100%). Thus, the sestamibi scan can be used to identify those patients who are less likely to be cured.[75] Compared to ultrasound imaging, the nuclear medicine studies are less operator-dependent and subject to less variability in interpretation.

Computed Tomography

CT is particularly effective for identifying ectopic glands in the anterior mediastinum and enlarged glands in the tracheoesophageal groove, both areas where ultrasound scans may not visualize aberrant tissue. Mediastinal parathyroid adenomas often lie within the fat-replaced thymus, where even small adenomas can be readily visualized (Fig. 55.8). Ectopic glands in the tracheoesophageal groove are detected as a solid mass adjacent to the esophagus. Undescended glands near the carotid bifurcation can also be identified if the examination images at the level of the hyoid bone. On the other hand, CT is poor at detecting intrathyroid or juxtathyroid tumors and exposes the patient to the risks associated with contrast media and radiation.

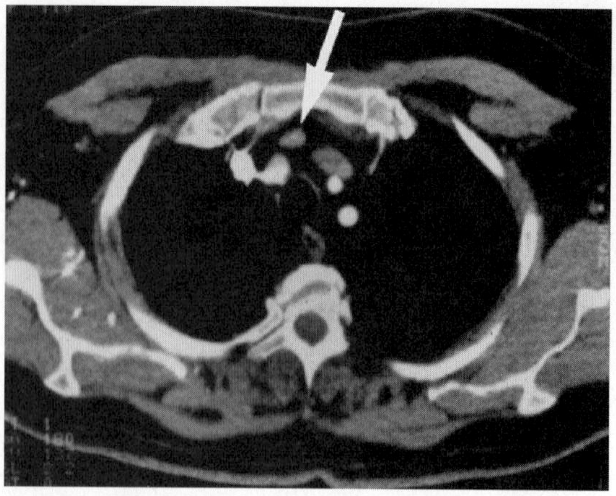

FIGURE 55.8. Computed tomography is the most useful imaging modality for identifying parathyroid adenomas located in the mediastinum.

Magnetic Resonance Imaging

Initial experience with MRI of abnormal parathyroid glands has been successful for large parathyroid adenomas, which on T_2-weighted or stir-pulse sequences produce a bright signal.[76] In the mediastinum this signal may be confused with fat, and a T_1-weighted image is required to specifically identify the pathology. With gadolinium-enhanced MRI and T_1- and T_2-weighted images, MRI can now provide higher sensitivity than CT for identifying ectopic parathyroid tumors. However, MRI is more expensive than CT and is less tolerable by patients.

Angiography

The potential for morbidity associated with angiographic procedures to localize parathyroid glands sharply limits its use to patients with persistent symptomatic or recurrent hyperparathyroidism requiring reoperation and the inability to detect the abnormal gland on other studies. Intraarterial digital techniques have greatly simplified angiographic localization of parathyroid pathology (Fig. 55.9). Because digital examination does not require highly selective catheter positioning, it can be accomplished more safely and expeditiously. The improved sensitivity of digital subtraction arteriography also makes it possible to significantly reduce the total dose of water-soluble contrast material, thereby decreasing adverse effects on the kidney in patients who may already have compromised renal function.

Selective Venous Sampling for Parathyroid Hormone

Selective venous sampling requires the greatest experience and is the most variably performed of all the localizing procedures. Contrast load, radiation exposure, and cost (15–20 PTH determinations), in addition to radiography costs, are all significant. Moreover, gradients determined by selective catheterization identify only the region of pathology (e.g., right side of the neck, mediastinum) but do not specifically image the missing abnormal gland. A new technique is to add the rapid PTH assay to selective venous sampling to provide a shorter turn-around time and allow the radiologist to obtain more selective samples in regions in which high concentrations of PTH are found. This combination of venous sampling and rapid PTH assay was shown to localize the abnormal parathyroid gland correctly in six of seven patients who had negative noninvasive imaging and required reoperation for prior unsuccessful parathyroid surgery.[77] It is indicated in only a small proportion of reoperative patients who have significant primary hyperparathyroidism and no apparent localizing information after completing all other noninvasive studies and angiography.

Summary of Localization Studies

Sestamibi and ultrasound should be used in patients undergoing initial exploration for primary hyperparathyroidism. Accurate preoperative localization studies allow for the performance of a minimally invasive parathyroidectomy that shortens hospital stay, minimizes scaring, and ensures a successful outcome. Further, in patients undergoing parathyroid reoperations, preoperative radiologic localization studies are essential to plan the reoperative surgical strategy (see Fig. 55.8). We recommend liberal use of each of the noninvasive imaging studies (US, sestamibi, CT, and MRI) as an initial imaging cluster. If two studies identify the abnormal parathyroid gland in the same location, we proceed with surgery. If the noninvasive studies are equivocal, we then perform digital arteriography. If that study is positive, we perform surgery; if negative, we recommend selective venous sampling for rapid PTH.[77]

Intraoperative Determination of Parathyroid Hormone

Intraoperative determination of PTH serum levels allows for the continuous monitoring of parathyroid function during

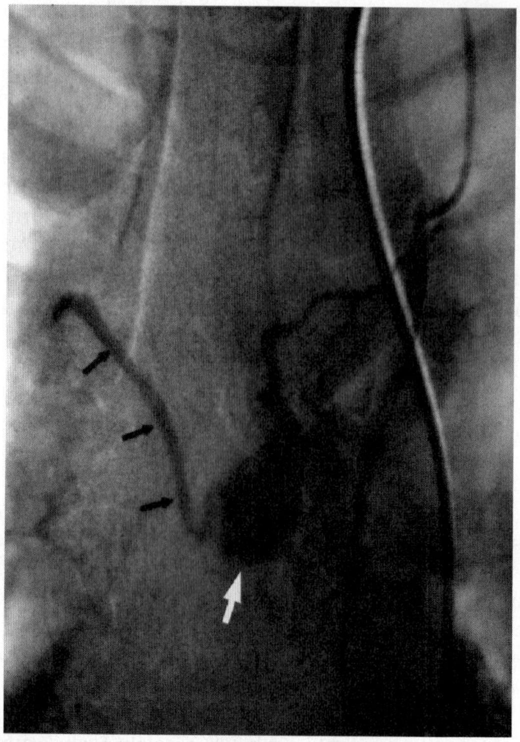

FIGURE 55.9. Angiogram demonstrating a large anterior mediastinal parathyroid adenoma (*large arrow*) with the right internal mammary artery (*small arrows*) as its blood supply.

surgery.[78–82] Generally, after successful removal of a single parathyroid adenoma or adequate resection of hyperplastic glands, serum PTH levels begin to fall immediately and reach either a 50% drop from the baseline level or normal range within 10 to 15 min.[83] Studies demonstrate that serum levels of intact PTH decline rapidly, only 10 min after resection of a parathyroid adenoma.[84,85] Furthermore, the rate of decline is less in patients with hyperplasia and may provide an additional intraoperative means of diagnosing hyperplasia.[86,87] A peripheral serum sample for PTH should be obtained just before surgery and after the induction of anesthesia. Repeated serum samples are obtained intraoperatively immediately following resection of an enlarged gland and then 10, 20, and 30 min later. This protocol has been designed to take into account the half-life of PTH, which is 1 to 4 min, and to avoid misleading results from a spike in concentration that may occur during handling and removal of the adenoma.[84] A 50% reduction in the PTH level from the median baseline level indicates a successful outcome.[85] The operation can be terminated based on this result without surgical identification of the other parathyroid glands.

This assay can also be used as a biologically specific method to identify a pathological sample without the need for histological examination of a specimen. A fine-needle aspiration (FNA) of a mass lesion can be diluted with heparinized saline and PTH levels measured. A high level of PTH has a specificity that approaches 100% for the identification of parathyroid tissue.[65,86,88,89] Although this technique can be performed as a preoperative study, it currently has its greatest utility as a method of intraoperative tissue identification.

Intraoperative determination of serum PTH levels appears to complement surgical skill and histopathological information and has the potential to provide additional guidance regarding the extent and degree of neck exploration.[90] However, false-negative results[84] or technical difficulties may be encountered, and this information may be difficult to interpret in the case of double adenoma, hyperplasia, or in the presence of secondary hyperparathyroidism.[91] Nevertheless, its use has greatly facilitated minimally invasive parathyroidectomy and it has reduced operative failure rates from 6% to 1.5% for initial operations[92] and for reoperations from 24% to 6%.[93]

Surgical Management of Parathyroid Disease

Primary Hyperparathyroidism

Indications for Surgery

In general, surgical exploration is indicated for all patients with clear biochemical evidence of primary hyperparathyroidism and documented signs or symptoms of the disease (Table 55.4).[94–97] Bone disease, evident as bone cysts, elevated serum levels of bony alkaline phosphatase, bone tumors, subperiosteal resorption, and decreased bone density (>2 standard deviations below normal), warrants parathyroidectomy. Nephrolithiasis, nephrocalcinosis, impaired renal function, pancreatitis, peptic ulcer, and parathyroid crisis are other indications for surgery. Additional indications for surgery include a serum calcium level greater than 12 mg/dL, a urinary calcium level greater than 400 mg/24 h, neuromuscular or musculoskeletal symptoms such as muscle weakness or fatigue, depression, and chondrocalcinosis with pseudogout.

TABLE 55.4. Symptomatic Manifestations of Primary Hyperparathyroidism that Warrant Surgery.

System	*Signs and symptoms*
Serum	Calcium level >12 mg/dL
Skeletal	Decreased bone density Pain Pathological fracture Bone cysts Brown tumors Osteitis fibrosa cystica Gout and pseudogout Nonspecific arthralgias
Renal	Urinary calcium >350 mg/24 h Renal colic Nephrocalcinosis Decreased creatinine clearance
Gastrointestinal	Peptic ulcer disease Pancreatitis
Neurological	Emotional lability Slow mentation Poor memory Depression Easy fatigability
Neuromuscular	Proximal muscular weakness Muscular atrophy
Other	Anemia

The best treatment for totally asymptomatic patients is still controversial.[94] As routine serum screening of patients became more widespread in the 1970s, the prevalence and incidence of primary hyperparathyroidism was recognized to be much higher than originally thought. Similarly, the clinical profile of the disease shifted from one with more overt physical manifestations to one with more subtle, or nearly asymptomatic, findings.[98,99] In 1991 the recommendations of the National Institutes of Health Consensus Conference on asymptomatic primary hyperparathyroidism were published, which identified several patient criteria including age, serum calcium levels, renal function, and bone mineral density.[94] These criteria were revisited in 2002 by a Consensus Development Workshop and made more inclusive by the further relaxation of abnormal serum calcium and bone mineral density values[98] (Table 55.5).

In apparently asymptomatic patients with primary hyperparathyroidism, surgery is indicated for younger patients (<50 years old) who have a low operative risk and the potential

TABLE 55.5. Current 2002 Consensus Panel Recommendations for Surgery in Asymptomatic Patients with Primary Hyperparathyroidism.

Serum calcium >1 mg/dL above upper limits of normal
24-h urinary calcium >400 mg
Creatinine clearance reduced more than 30% to age-matched controls
Bone density at lumbar spine, hip, or distal radius *t*-score <–2.5
Patient age <50 years
Patients for whom medical surveillance is not possible

Source: Bilezikian JP, Potts JT Jr, Fuleihan Gel H, et al.,[98] by permission of Journal of Clinical Endocrinology & Metabolism.

for a long temporal exposure to the disease. Symptoms will develop in a significant proportion of these patients with long-term follow-up.[100,101] Neuromuscular symptoms such as weakness occur in 20% to 60% of patients with apparently asymptomatic primary hyperparathyroidism, as well as other nonspecific somatic and neuropsychiatric symptoms, and successful surgery reverses these symptoms in most patients.[102–104] Similarly, osteopenia has been described in many studies of asymptomatic patients with hyperparathyroidism, and a marked improvement in bone mineral density can be seen after parathyroidectomy.[105–109] In apparently asymptomatic older patients, surgery is reserved for patients with evidence of progression and/or symptoms. Regular follow-up is indicated to avoid disease progression. Routine biannual screening of serum calcium and annual serum creatinine and bone density measurements are recommended.[98]

Before performing surgery for primary hyperparathyroidism, the surgeon must obtain informed consent, which requires careful discussion of the outcome and complications. A successful outcome is expected in approximately 97% of patients undergoing initial operations[15] and in 78% to 90% of reoperations.[110,111] Recurrent laryngeal nerve injury occurs in less than 1% of initial operations[15] and approximately 5% of repeat operations.[63] Fortunately, the symptoms in many of these nerve injuries are temporary, and full recovery may be seen at the 3- to 6-month follow-up. Hypoparathyroidism rarely occurs after initial explorations but may occur in 2.7% to 16% of reoperations.[110,111]

The Evolution of Surgical Procedures for PHPT

As mentioned in the introduction, the management of primary hyperparathyroidism has undergone a marked shift in the last decade. Classically, the standard operative procedure for primary PTH had long been the bilateral cervical exploration. With this technique, the correct identification of abnormal glandular tissue occurs in 95% of patients.[112–115] Documented complication rates are low, with recurrent laryngeal nerve injury rates of less than 1% at initial operation, and approximately 5% require repeat operations.[63,116] Some have suggested a role from intraoperative monitoring of recurrent laryngeal nerve function during surgery, especially in reoperative procedures, although such devices do not minimize the need for careful exploration and nerve identification.[117,118]

With the rare exception of cases of suspected parathyroid carcinoma, the driving reason to perform a bilateral four-gland cervical exploration was to identify and treat multiglandular disease.[119] The evolution of a more directed surgery began in the 1980s with Tibblin[120] publishing his results with unilateral exploration in conjunction with intraoperative histopathology to exclude the presence of multiglandular disease. A decade later, there were reports of successfully performed unilateral operations on patients who were preoperatively selected on the basis of a single site of scintigraphic hyperactivity, suggesting a single adenoma.[121]

The unilateral approach was based upon the idea that in patients with primary hyperthyroidism, if one can identify both an enlarged and a normal gland on a single side of the neck, then one may assume the enlarged gland to represent a single adenoma and the source of the hyperparathyroidism, and the surgery can be concluded without further dissection. Controversy exists surrounding these assumptions, including the true rates of double adenomas, missed extranumerary tissue, etc. but are countered by discussions of smaller scars, improved patient comfort, less perioperative hypoparathyroidism, and the absent risk of bilateral iatrogenic nerve injury.

In the past decade, surgical technology has allowed for an even more localized minimally invasive approach, which was the result of several important factors, including the availability of localization studies that could be performed in real time by the operating surgeon, and the ability to measure intraoperative PTH levels during surgery.

Minimally Invasive Parathyroidectomy for Adenoma

Minimally invasive parathyroid surgery has replaced standard bilateral neck exploration for primary hyperparathyroidism for adenoma (Table 55.6). This change is still controversial, and some recent studies suggest that standard bilateral neck exploration is just as good and less expensive.[122,123] However, most surgeons, endocrinologists, and patients now think that MIP is preferable because it is associated with similar excellent results, less pain, better cosmesis, and a more rapid recovery.[124–127] We recommend the use of intraoperative rapid PTH assay to assess outcomes intraoperatively without extensive exploration, but this has been controversial, as one group has demonstrated that this is unnecessary if sestamibi scan demonstrates a single abnormal gland.[128] General endotracheal anesthesia is used, although regional block anesthesia has been advocated by some and is equally effective.[129–131] Local anesthesia or regional block has been advocated for the elderly undergoing minimally invasive parathyroidectomy.[130] Intraoperative PTH assay is performed as described previously. The patient is positioned in a manner as for thyroid surgery. A transverse cervical incision less than or equal to 4 cm is made approximately 2 cm above the sternal notch in a skin crease. A focused approach to the abnormal parathyroid gland is made based on the preoperative imaging results. Some have advocated the use of perioperative administration of intravenous methylene blue dye as a method to stain parathyroid tissue during surgery and make it more visible to the surgeon.[132] Another variation combines the use of preoperative localization studies with the use of intraoperative surgeon-controlled ultrasound.[133,134] Alternatively, Norman and others recommend a radioguided approach based on a hand-held gamma probe to detect labeled radioactive sestamibi within the adenoma.[128,135,136] Because a high proportion (90%) of parathyroid adenomas are imaged by sestamibi scanning and are still radioemitting during surgery, this technique can be used to guide intraoperative localization of the abnormal gland with a hand-held gamma detector.[137] With this method, an incision is made in the area of highest radioactivity and dissection is focused on the abnormal "hot" adenoma. Intraoperative gamma localization may be combined with immediate parathyroid hormone assay to quickly determine whether all the abnormal parathyroid tissue has been removed. Because this method relies on radioactive detection and PTH measurement to guide surgery, rather than precise operative identification, it may be limited in the identification of multiple abnormal glands and glands adjacent to the thyroid that may also be hot.

TABLE 55.6.
Overall Results of Initial Operations for Primary Hyperparathyroidism.

References	n	Level of evidence[a]	Type of exploration[b]	Success (%)	RLN paresis	Permanent hypoparathyroidism	Wound complication	Persistent hypercalcemia	Recurrence	Mortality (%)
Ruda 2005[195]	20,225	meta	MIP radioguided	97	—	—	—	—	—	—
			MIP IOPTH	95	—	—	—	1.3%	—	—
Baliski 2005[196]	52	II	Unilateral	96	0	0	—	—	—	—
Grant 2005[119]	627	II	MIP IOPTH	97	—	0	—	1	—	—
	734	II	Bilateral	97	—	0	—	4	—	—
Carneiro 2004[197]	423	II	MIP IOPTH	97	—	—	—	3	6	0
Mortier 2004[198]	118	II	MIP IOPTH	92	—	—	—	2	10	
Sidiropoulos 2003[199]	31	II	MIP radioguided	97	6	—	—	—	—	0
	24	II	Bilateral	100	13	—	—	—	—	0
Goldstein 2003[128]	112	II	MIP radioguided	98	0	—	1	5	2	—
Shabtai 2003[200]	140	II	MIP radioguided	98	2	—	—	—	3	0
Bergenfelz 2002[201]	47	I	MIP IOPTH	96	2	3	0	—	2	—
	44	I	Bilateral	97	1	0	2	—	1	—
Schell 2003[122]	688	III	Bilateral methylene blue	98	0	—	0	—		0
Udelsman 2002[138]	329	II	Bilateral	98	0	—	2	—	2	—
	243	II	MIP IOPTH	99	1	—	1	—	1	—
Dillavou 2000[202]	90	III	Bilateral	97	0	—	3	3	1	0
Goldstein 2000[203]	20	III	MIP radioguided	100	0	—	0	0	—	0
	20	III	Uni + bilateral without radio	100	0	—	1	0	—	0
Flynn 2000[136]	36	II	MIP radioguided IOPTH methylene blue	100	2	—	3	0	—	0
Low 1998[204]	713	III	Bilateral	98	2	9	—	7	—	1
Summers 1996[205]	181	III	Bilateral	97	2	0	2	5	—	1
Worsey 1993[206]	246	III	Bilatreal	93	1	2	2	14	4	—
	125	III	Unilateral	99	0	0	1	1	4	0
van Heerden 1991[189]	384	III	Bilateral	99.5	3	1	4	2	2	.3
Tibblin 1991[207]	167	III	Bilateral	89	—	6	—	10	—	—
	50	III	Unilateral	96	—	1	—	1	—	—
Piemonte 1989[113]	71	III	Unilateral	94.4	1	—	—	8	1	—
Saaka 1988[208]	316	III	Bilateral	92	3	2	—	13	12	—
Russell 1982[209]	500	III	Bilateral	92	13	10	5	—	—	<1

MIP, minimally invasive parathyroidectomy; IOPTH, intraoperative parathyroid hormone; RLN, recurrent laryngeal nerve.
[a]I, randomized prospective study; II, prospective study; III, retrospective study, review or anecdotal.
[b]Bilateral exploration generally includes exploration of both sides of the neck with biopsy of at least one normal parathyroid gland or of all parathyroid glands found.

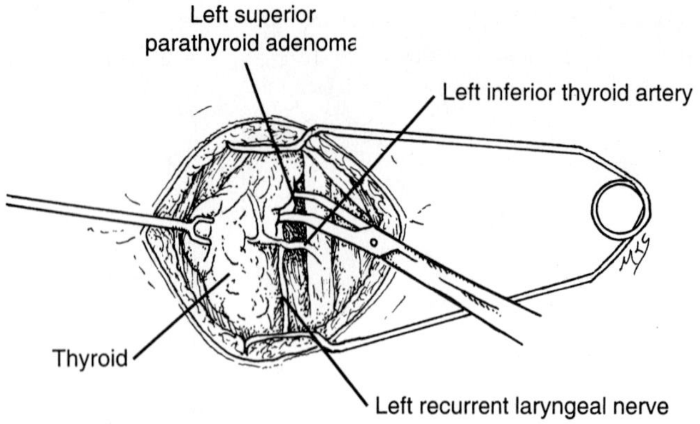

FIGURE 55.10. Identification of a left superior parathyroid adenoma. The thyroid gland is elevated with a Babcock clamp. The investing thyroid fascia is opened posterior to the upper pole of the left lobe. A left upper parathyroid adenoma is identified superior to the inferior thyroid artery and posterolateral to the recurrent laryngeal nerve. The left recurrent laryngeal nerve is shown in its usual location within the tracheoesophageal groove and posterior to the inferior thyroid artery.

In the minimally invasive parathyroidectomy, limited subplatysmal flaps are raised because the goal of surgery is to remove a solitary adenoma and not to perform a standard neck exploration. Because of this, there is limited mobilization of the thyroid gland and retraction of the strap muscles on the side of the dissection. Dissection is focused on the preoperative localization studies, and the abnormal parathyroid gland is removed. The surgeon should be aware of the relationship of the parathyroid glands to the recurrent laryngeal nerves and avoid injury to these nerves. The upper glands are posterior and lateral to the recurrent laryngeal nerve (Fig. 55.10), whereas the lower glands are anterior and medial to it (Fig. 55.11). The vascular pedicle is either ligated or clipped and the specimen is sent to pathology. The intraoperative PTH blood levels are measured while the wound is closed. The procedure is not terminated until the levels drop 50% from the median baseline level and/or into the normal range (<50 pg/mL). The success of MIP has been confirmed to be the same as bilateral standard neck exploration. For example, in 255 consecutive MIPs, the cure rate was 99% and the complication rate was 1.2%. MIP has been associated with a 50% reduction in operating room time and shorter hospitalization.[138] Further, MIP is associated with a cosmetically better scar, less pain, and more rapid return to health and normal activity. However, MIP may artificially increase the probability of finding only an adenoma and decrease the chance of detecting hyperplasia or multiple gland disease. Two recent studies documented that the rate of hyperplasia with MIP was lower than the expected rate of 15% for standard bilateral explorations.[139,140] If the intraoperative serum levels of PTH do not drop, or there is other evidence for hyperplasia, minimally invasive parathyroidectomy is abandoned and conventional bilateral neck exploration is performed.

Unsuccessful MIP

If focused minimally invasive parathyroidectomy is unsuccessful, bilateral neck exploration is recommended. Essentially this is the standard parathyroid exploration that was done previously with a consistently high probability of success and low complication rate. Any enlarged or abnormal glands are removed. The most useful indicator of normal or abnormal parathyroid tissue is the appearance of the gland. Pathologists may find it difficult to differentiate normal from hypercellular parathyroid tissue or hyperplasia from adenoma, but they can reliably confirm whether the biopsied tissue was parathyroid. Alternatively, the tissue in question can be heparinized and its PTH level measured.[89] If two glands are enlarged (double adenoma), both are removed. Long-term results with this method of management have been highly satisfactory.[15,34]

Hyperplasia

In generalized four-gland hyperplasia, the surgical management is more difficult and the results less satisfactory. Intraoperative PTH levels may help distinguish between adenoma and hyperplasia and help guide the amount of parathyroid resection. Abnormal parathyroid glands should be removed until the levels drop 50% from the median baseline preoperative level. Two possible surgical procedures designed for this diagnosis are the subtotal (3.5-gland) parathyroidectomy and the four-gland parathyroidectomy with immediate autografting. The cervical thymus should also be removed as supernumerary glands or fragments of parathyroid glands are commonly found within it. The results of subtotal parathyroidectomy have been variable, with a 13% incidence of persistent disease, a 15% incidence of recurrent disease, and a similar incidence of hypoparathyroidism. Moreover, in patients with MEN I, subtotal parathyroidectomy led to a recurrence rate of 50% at 12 years after surgery.[141] Similar data led others[142] to prefer total parathyroidectomy with autotransplantation over subtotal parathyroidectomy for patients with hyperplasia. Wells and colleagues reported results on 21 patients with hyperplasia who underwent this procedure.[143] Hypocalcemia developed in 20 of the 21 patients immediately postoperatively and necessitated vitamin D and calcium replacement. Within 2 months, 20 had a detectable PTH gradient between the grafted and nongrafted arm, indicative of normal parathyroid autograft function, and were able to discontinue vitamin D and calcium supplementation. However, recurrent disease developed in 2 of 10 patients with nonfamilial hyperplasia and 7 of 11 with familial hyperplasia.

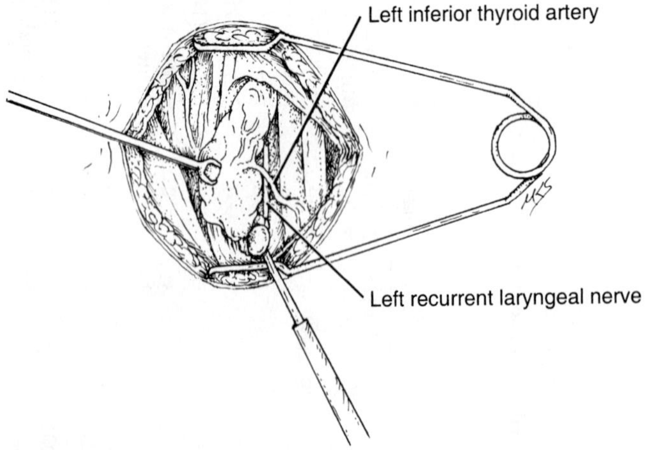

FIGURE 55.11. Identification of a left inferior parathyroid adenoma. The thyroid gland is elevated with a Babcock clamp. A left lower parathyroid adenoma is identified inferior to the inferior thyroid artery and anteromedial to the recurrent laryngeal nerve, which is the most common position for a left inferior parathyroid adenoma, although the inferior parathyroid gland can be located in other positions.

Four patients with recurrent disease underwent partial graft resection, and all 4 were again rendered normocalcemic.

Our approach to both familial and nonfamilial parathyroid hyperplasia is subtotal (3.5-gland) parathyroidectomy guided by intraoperative determination of PTH, with approximately 30 to 50 mg of the most normal-appearing parathyroid tissue left and marked with a surgical clip in the neck. The incidence of either persistent disease or hypoparathyroidism has been low, and we expect the rate of recurrent disease to be between 10% and 20%. We do not use four-gland resection with transplant because of an unacceptable incidence of hypoparathyroidism. In patients with recurrent disease after subtotal parathyroidectomy, total parathyroidectomy with cryopreservation of resected tissue is required. It is important to prove that all hyperplastic tissue has been removed before reimplantation.[144] Unfortunately, cryopreserved parathyroid autotransplantation appears to have a high incidence of failure inasmuch as only 70% of human cryopreserved autografts function normally.[145]

Mediastinal Exploration

If a patient undergoes an unsuccessful operation for hyperparathyroidism, reevaluation of the patient and localization procedures should be performed before performing additional surgery (see Fig. 55.7). Median sternotomy is indicated in only 1% to 2% of patients undergoing initial exploration. In our series of 33 patients who underwent median sternotomy as part of a reoperation for primary hyperparathyroidism, 30% did not have abnormal parathyroid tissue in the mediastinum.[146] Of the abnormal mediastinal glands found, most were discovered in the thymus (64%), and total thymectomy was always required. Wells and Cooper[147] have reported the ability to remove the entire thymus (including the mediastinal component) without dividing the sternum by using a special retractor to elevate the sternum. This procedure may be used to explore the anterior mediastinum less invasively. Video-assisted thoracoscopic surgery (VATS) techniques have been used to resect parathyroid tissue in the mediastinum, and the earlier described adjuncts of intraoperative PTH monitoring and gamma probes can be similarly employed.[148–150] Parathyroid adenomas have also been removed from the aortopulmonary window via the left chest and thoracoscopically, but this is even more rare.[151]

Reoperations for Primary Hyperparathyroidism

Reoperations for primary hyperparathyroidism should be classified as operations for either persistent disease or recurrent disease. Persistent disease means that hypercalcemia never resolved after the initial neck exploration. Recurrent disease means that hypercalcemia recurs after an initial period of hypocalcemia or normalization of serum calcium. The complexity of repeat neck surgery for primary hyperparathyroidism makes it imperative to confirm the diagnosis and presence of symptoms and to order preoperative localization studies (see Fig. 55.7).[64,65,111]

The prior operative report, pathology results, and localization studies are used to plan the re-exploration. For example, if two abnormal parathyroid glands were removed and the family history is positive for parathyroid disease, the working diagnosis is hyperplasia. A biopsy-proven normal gland found at the initial procedure and radiologic localization studies suggesting a mediastinal adenoma prompt a direct mediastinal approach. Designing the operation and the proper incision—right-sided, left-sided, median sternotomy, or any combination thereof—can be done only by putting all the information together. For reoperations, we prefer an alternative route in the neck along the medial border of the sternocleidomastoid muscle instead of between the strap muscles.[111] This technique requires a separate approach on each side of the neck. It is especially important to look for intrathyroid, intrathymic, and paraesophageal parathyroid adenomas because ectopic locations are more common in reoperations.

Another strategy for reoperations is the minimally invasive radioguided parathyroidectomy.[152] Norman and Denham reported their experience in 21 patients with primary hyperparathyroidism who had undergone previous neck exploration for parathyroid or thyroid disease.[137] The neck reexploration is guided by a hand-held gamma probe. Possible advantages of this technique include smaller incisions, less operative time, decreased risk of nerve injury and complications, outpatient surgery, and no frozen-section analysis. Others have advocated the use of intraoperative PTH level monitoring during the reoperative surgery to confirm the resection of metabolically active tissue.[93,153]

Finally, it should be remembered that even during reoperations for primary hyperparathyroidism, most abnormal glands can be removed through a cervical incision.[111] Abnormal parathyroid glands may be retroesophageal or posterior along the tracheoesophageal groove, which is the most common missed position.[154] They may also be intrathyroidal,[155] or they may be located in an undescended parathymic remnant high in the carotid sheath.[156] A missed adenoma may be located in pharyngeal or adjacent structures such as the vagus nerve.[157] If these abnormal glands are not in the neck, they may be in the thymus. Slow, meticulous exploration in a bloodless field is generally necessary to find these "ectopic" glands (Fig. 55.12).

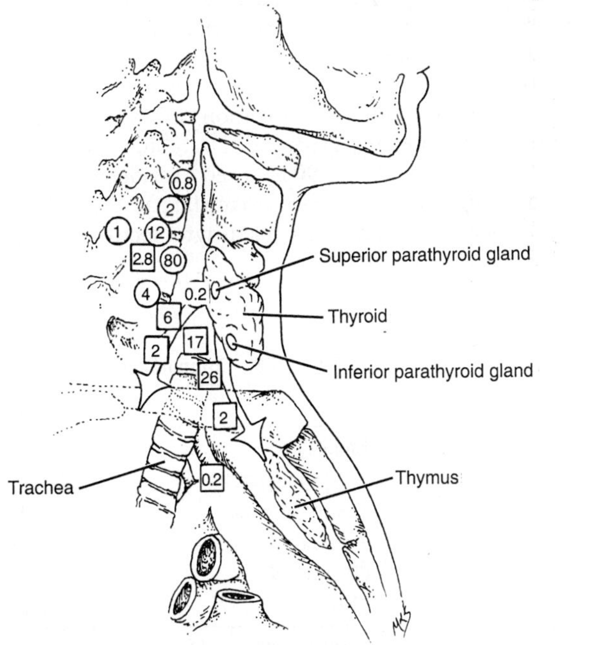

FIGURE 55.12. Diagram of potential locations of superior and inferior parathyroid glands. *Numbers* refer to the percentage of glands found at each location. (Data from Akerstrom G, Malmaeus J, Bergstrom R. Surgical anatomy of human parathyroid glands. Surgery (St. Louis) 1984;95(1):14–21.[14])

TABLE 55.7.
Surgical Outcome for Reoperative Surgery.

References	*n*	*Level of evidence*[a]	*Success (%)*	*RLN paresis*	*RLN paralysis*	*Permanent hypocalcemia*	*Transient hypocalcemia*	*Wound infection*	*Mortality (%)*
Mariette 1998[190]	38	III	92	—	3	2	—	—	—
Jaskowiak 1996[154]	222	II	97	6	3	12	49	0	0
Shen 1996[62]	102	III	95	1	1	1	6	—	—
Rodriquez 1994[193]	152	III	93	1	0	1	6	—	—
Weber 1994[215]	51	III	92	1	0	1	11	1	2
Carty 1991[61]	206	III	95	12	1	17	—	—	0.5
Jarhult 1993[216]	93	III	82	—	9	15	—	—	—
Rothmund 1990[217]	70	III	96	—	4	19	—	—	—
Cheung 1989[218]	83	III	86	2	1	8	10	1	1.2
Grant 1986[110]	157	III	89	13	6	20	27	—	0

[a]I, randomized prospective study; II, prospective study; III, retrospective study, review or anecdotal.

Cryopreservation of removed parathyroid tissue during reoperations is indicated. One cannot predict from prior records whether normal parathyroid tissue remains in the neck. In our experience with reoperations on 175 patients, 35% left the hospital taking vitamin D medication and 43% were taking supplemental calcium.[61,111] Twenty-two patients (12%) were ultimately found to be permanently hypoparathyroid and required cryopreserved autologous parathyroid grafts. This outcome agrees well with other published reports in which the rate of hypoparathyroidism after reoperative parathyroid surgery is between 2.7% and 16%. Cryopreservation with delayed autografting is a standard approach, although the overall success rate with cryopreserved grafts is only approximately 50% to 60%; this rate appears to be less than for fresh grafts, which have a 75% to 100% success rate.[145]

Reoperative parathyroid surgery remains a major challenge. It is clear that operative risk increases with each succeeding reexploration. With careful attention, however, to confirmation of the diagnosis, prior operative records, judicious use of preoperative localization, and postoperative cryopreserved autografting, a successful outcome may be achieved in approximately 80% to 90% of reoperations (Table 55.7).[111] Economically, when compared to initial parathyroidectomies, most aspects of reoperative parathyroidectomies are more costly (Table 55.8).

Secondary and Tertiary Hyperparathyroidism

Almost all patients with advanced renal failure who are maintained by chronic dialysis have evidence of bone disease secondary to hyperparathyroidism and elevated serum levels of PTH. Secondary hyperparathyroidism should be suppressed in these individuals by measures that normalize serum levels of calcium and phosphorus. These methods include the use of a dialysate calcium concentration of 3.5 mEq/L, oral calcium supplementation, dietary restriction of phosphorus (<600 mg/day), phosphate-binding antacids, and vitamin D analogues to promote intestinal absorption of calcium.[158] Failure of these strategies occurs in a minority of individuals, and tertiary hyperparathyroidism is diagnosed when serum levels of ionized calcium and intact PTH are elevated. Subtotal parathyroidectomy is then used to decrease the mass of hyperplastic parathyroid tissue.

Potential indications for subtotal parathyroidectomy in these patients include (1) hypercalcemia in prospective renal transplant patients; (2) pathological fractures secondary to renal osteodystrophy; (3) symptoms such as pruritus, bone pain, and extensive soft tissue calcification and calciphylaxis; (4) hypercalcemia in patients with well-functioning renal transplants; and (5) a calcium times phosphate product greater than 70.[159,160] Improvements in medical management have

TABLE 55.8. Comparison of Costs Between Initial and Reoperative Parathyroidectomy.

	Initial operation[a]	*Reoperation*[a]	*P value*[b]
Radiology	43 (0–912)	3,378 (1,130–3,856)	<0.001
Ultrasonography	0 (0–191)	279 (0–293)	<0.001
Operating room	1,317 (840–2,858)	1,703 (1,234–3,055)	<0.05
Surgical pathology	732 (345–1,229)	320 (179–1,503)	<0.03
Chemistry	66 (27–174)	159 (51–1,049)	<0.006
Total	3,948 (2,215–9,747)	8,383 (5,051–26,241)	<0.001

[a]Median (range) in U.S. dollars.

[b]Mann–Whitney test. The cost of reoperation is significantly higher in all categories.

Source: Doherty GM, Weber B, Norton JA. Cost of unsuccessful surgery for primary hyperparathyroidism. Surgery (St. Louis) 1994;116(6):954–957; discussion 957–958.[214] Reprinted with permission.

TABLE 55.9.
Overall Results of Initial Operations for Secondary Hyperparathyroidism.

References	*n*	*Level of evidence*[a]	*Technique*	*Recurrence (%)*	*Improvement of bone pain (%)*	*Improvement of pruritus (%)*	*Hypocalcemia (%)*	*Mortality (%)*
Punch 1995[210]	91	III	Subtotal	5	—	—	—	3
Rothmund 1991[211]	20	II	Subtotal	20	68	45	5	—
	20	II	Total	0	87	100	5	—
Niederle 1989[212]	35	III	Total	—	97	—	3	—
Leapman 1989[213]	47	III	Subtotal	5	—	—	—	—
	9	III	Total	22	—	—	—	—

[a]I, randomized prospective study; II, prospective study; III, retrospective study; 4, review or anecdotal.

reduced the need for surgery. Successful parathyroid surgery plus appropriate supplementation with vitamin D and calcium has provided a marked increase in lumbar bone marrow density and a modest increase in radial bone marrow density in renal failure patients with secondary HPT.[161]

Controversy exists about whether to perform subtotal parathyroidectomy,[158] total parathyroidectomy without an autograft,[162] or total parathyroidectomy with an immediate autograft[163] in this patient population (Table 55.9). We recommend subtotal parathyroidectomy for the treatment of secondary and tertiary hyperparathyroidism. Subtotal ($3\frac{1}{2}$ gland) parathyroidectomy ensures a high probability of a durable successful outcome with a low probability of hypoparathyroidism. It is particularly important to avoid permanent hypoparathyroidism in these patients because of the increased likelihood of aluminum-related bone disease.[159]

Parathyroid Carcinoma

Parathyroid carcinoma should be considered in the working diagnosis of patients with primary hyperparathyroidism when the serum level of calcium is very high (>14 mg/dL), in patients with vocal cord paralysis, in patients with evidence of local recurrence of an abnormal gland after resection, or when a palpable neck mass is present.[36,164]

It is difficult to accurately assess the spectrum of clinical manifestations, degree of malignancy, and prognosis of parathyroid carcinoma. The incidence is very low, and the malignancy appears to be diagnosed at an earlier stage as a result of earlier detection of hypercalcemia. A major problem is failure to properly identify the correct pathological diagnosis during the operation and, therefore, failure to perform adequate resection of the malignant parathyroid tissue along with the ipsilateral lobe of the thyroid.[36,165] Unequivocal pathological features of parathyroid carcinoma include the identification of mitoses in several high-power microscopic fields, fibrous bands or desmoplasia, and evidence of distant metastases or direct local invasion of the capsule, adjacent structures, and blood vessels.[166] However, not all patients with parathyroid carcinoma have all these features, so the diagnosis must be ascertained from clinical as well as pathological evidence. Furthermore, the natural history of patients with parathyroid cancer appears to be variable. Some tumors disseminate rapidly and have a poor prognosis,[167] whereas others tend to recur locally and have a long disease-free interval.[36]

Literature reports involving single cases tend to emphasize more serious tumors, either intrinsically malignant or long-standing, with clear evidence of extraglandular spread at the initial operation. Typically the cancer invades along the tracheoesophageal groove, and the patient may have hoarseness secondary to a recurrent laryngeal nerve injury. At neck exploration, the carcinomatous tissue appears gray with a thick, hard capsule. We recommend, based on suspicion (e.g., mass, local recurrence, vocal cord paralysis, high serum level of calcium), a wide excision including thyroid lobectomy in continuity with the tumor.[36,165,166] If one has doubt about the diagnosis, biopsy of tumor extrinsic from the main tumor mass either within lymph nodes or invading local strap muscle should provide evidence of cancer. Recurrent laryngeal nerve injury, either from the tumor itself or from the surgeon attempting to completely resect the tumor mass with the ipsilateral thyroid lobe, is possible and occurs in a significant proportion of patients. Locally recurrent benign parathyroid adenomas may occur and be confused with parathyroid carcinomas. Recurrent adenomas generally have a longer disease-free interval, a lower serum level of calcium, and a history of either incomplete resection or spillage of tumor at the time of initial surgery.[36] Nevertheless, both locally recurrent parathyroid adenoma and cancer appear to respond favorably to aggressive local reresection, and most patients can be rendered either hypocalcemic or normocalcemic for a reasonable period.[36] Once disease has spread to distant sites, surgery is less effective. Resection of pulmonary metastases has been performed without clear benefit.[167] In patients with distant metastases, DTIC chemotherapy has been effective in some instances.[166] Medical therapy is directed at controlling the severe hypercalcemia.

Parathyroid Autotransplantation

Halsted performed the first experimental parathyroid transplant in 1909. Since then, many successful transplants in laboratory animals and humans have been reported.[142,143,168,169] Parathyroid glands have been successfully cryopreserved for long periods and then transplanted back into humans.[170] Parathyroid tissue has been successfully allografted into immunosuppressed human hosts.[171] The clinical indications for parathyroid autotransplantation are primary or secondary parathyroid hyperplasia, reexploration for persistent or recurrent hyperparathyroidism, and total thyroidectomy.

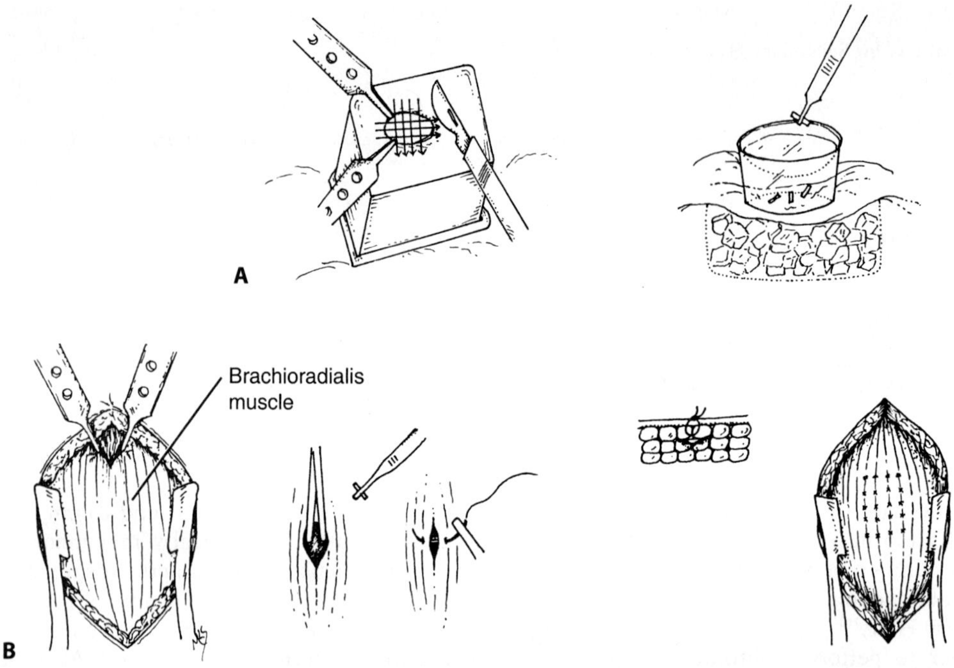

FIGURE 55.13. Operative method of cryopreservation and transplantation of abnormal hyperplastic parathyroid tissue. **A.** The abnormal gland is sliced into small fragments (1–2 mm) and kept in iced saline. **B.** Twenty fragments are grafted into small pockets in the nondominant brachioradialis muscle of the forearm. Each graft is marked with a suture to facilitate future identification of the grafted site.

The function of immediate (stored in the operating room in iced saline) parathyroid autografts is between 75% and 100%.[145,172] The function of delayed cryopreserved autografts varies from 54%[172] to 83%.[143] Immediate autografts of either adenoma or hyperplasia may lead to recurrent hypercalcemia and may require partial reexcision. Cryopreserved abnormal parathyroid tissue has not resulted in recurrent hypercalcemia but has a higher likelihood of poor function. Our procedure for parathyroid transplantation and cryopreservation is as follows: maintain the tissue on the operating table chilled in sterile saline, and slice the tissue into slivers 1 × 1 × 3 mm in size (Fig. 55.13). For immediate autografting, 20 pieces are implanted into the sternocleidomastoid muscle of the neck (only normal parathyroid tissue during thyroidectomy) or the brachioradialis muscle of the forearm (abnormal hyperplastic parathyroid tissue during total parathyroidectomy). Care is taken to not induce bleeding, and each implantation site is closed with 6-0 silk suture. Should graft-dependent hyperparathyroidism subsequently develop, a portion of the graft can be removed under local anesthesia. For cryopreservation, the parathyroid slivers are put into 3-mL glass vials, 10 pieces each, with 1.5 mL solution containing 10% dimethyl sulfoxide, 10% autologous serum, and 80% tissue culture medium. The vials are immediately placed in an automated freezing chamber and the temperature programmed to decrease 1°C/min to 80°C. The vials are then stored in a liquid nitrogen freezer at 190°C.

Postoperative Hypocalcemia

Most patients who have undergone successful surgery for primary hyperparathyroidism have some (albeit mild) symptoms of hypocalcemia, and a positive Trosseau or Chvostek sign. These symptoms should initiate measurement of the serum levels of calcium and phosphorus. Treatment is directed at maintaining a serum level of calcium above 8.0 mg/dL. Initially, dietary calcium is employed. However, dietary calcium, typically milk products, is associated with a large phosphate load and may result in hyperphosphatemia. If this complication occurs, elemental calcium may be given in the usual oral doses of 1 to 2 g/day. It has been shown that early postoperative testing of PTH level can be predictive of postoperative hypocalcemia, but this is not routinely employed.[173] When parathyroidectomy is performed as an outpatient procedure, patients are simply given prescriptions for oral calcium and calcitriol to minimize hypocalcemia and its symptoms. This practice has resulted in shorter hospitalizations and fewer symptoms of tetany. It is thought that a minimally invasive surgical approach may lessen the severity of postoperative hypocalcemia.[174]

If the symptoms of hypocalcemia are severe and the patient appears to be on the verge of tetany (occurring most frequently in patients with "hungry bone syndrome"), the clinician may need to treat with intravenous calcium. These symptoms can usually be rapidly corrected by the infusion of 2 mg/kg elemental calcium over a 15-min period. Symptoms return unless a longer infusion is used. Approximately 15 mg/kg elemental calcium is then infused over a 24-h period, with half the total amount administered in the initial 6 h. Serum levels of calcium should be monitored closely during the infusion, and infusion rates and amounts may be adjusted accordingly. Only approximately 13% of patients have severe symptoms of hypoparathyroidism after surgery. These patients appear to be older; have higher preoperative serum levels of calcium, PTH, alkaline phosphatase, and urea nitrogen; and have large adenomas removed at surgery[57] and typically require intravenous calcium. Most patients do not need this type of calcium replacement.

When hypocalcemia persists despite maximal oral replacement doses and hyperphosphatemia develops, $1,25(OH)_2D_3$ (calcitriol) is initiated.[175] This drug is recommended because of rapid onset of action and short duration of use. The usual initial dose of calcitriol is 0.25 to 1.0 g/day given on a twice-daily schedule. The dose can be increased to a maximum of 2.0 g/day, depending on the response in terms of serum levels of calcium and phosphorus. In general, the lowest possible dose that produces low normal serum levels and no hypocalcemic symptoms should be used. Serum levels of calcium should be monitored weekly after discharge to further adjust oral calcium and calcitriol doses.

Some patients with severe forms of primary hyperparathyroidism, including altered renal function and bone resorption, may demonstrate worsening kidney function in the postoperative period.[176] The exact cause is not known, but the complication appears temporarily, and kidney function reverses within several days. Renal insensitivity to PTH may be a cause of elevation of PTH levels after successful surgery for primary hyperparathyroidism.[177] Specific joint complaints may also occur in a small proportion of patients following successful parathyroidectomy. Pseudogout develops in approximately 5% of individuals, and examination of joint fluid demonstrates calcium phosphate crystals.[178,179] These patients usually respond to a short course of indomethacin. Bone remineralization following parathyroid surgery may cause a significant reduction in serum levels of magnesium. Patients with serum magnesium levels less than 1.1 mEq/L should be treated with both intravenous magnesium and calcium. The usual dose of magnesium is approximately 50 mmol/day in divided doses. Hypomagnesemia may contribute to the development of tetany in patients following parathyroidectomy. It inhibits secretion of PTH by the remaining parathyroid glands, and it exacerbates symptoms of hypocalcemia.

References

1. Owen R. On the anatomy of the Indian rhinoceros. Trans Zool Soc Lond 1862;4:31–58.
2. Thompson NW. The history of hyperparathyroidism. Acta Chir Scand 1990;156(1):5–21.
3. Chaouat Y, Chaouat D. [Primary hyperparathyroidism. History.] Rev Rhum Mal Osteoartic 1988;55(7):475–478.
4. Niederle BE, Schmidt G, Organ CH, Niederle B. Albert J and his surgeon: a historical reevaluation of the first parathyroidectomy. J Am Coll Surg 2006;202(1):181–190.
5. Bauer W, Federman DD. Hyperparathyroidism epitomized: the case of Captain Charles E. Martell. Metabolism 1962;11:21–29.
6. Spence HM. The life and death of Captain Charles Martell and kidney stone disease. J Urol 1984;132(6):1204–1207.
7. Mallette LE. Regulation of blood calcium in humans. Endocrinol Metab Clin N Am 1989;18(3):601–610.
8. Agus ZS, Goldfarb S, Wasserstein A. Calcium transport in the kidney. Rev Physiol Biochem Pharmacol 1981;90:155–169.
9. Marcus R. Laboratory diagnosis of primary hyperparathyroidism. Endocrinol Metab Clin N Am 1989;18(3):647–658.
10. Pocotte SL, Ehrenstein G, Fitzpatrick LA. Regulation of parathyroid hormone secretion. Endocr Rev 1991;12(3):291–301.
11. Mihai R, Farndon JR. Parathyroid disease and calcium metabolism. Br J Anaesth 2000;85(1):29–43.
12. Kao PC, van Heerden JA, Grant CS, Klee GG, Khosla S. Clinical performance of parathyroid hormone immunometric assays. Mayo Clin Proc 1992;67(7):637–645.
13. McDermott MT, Perloff JJ, Kidd GS. Effects of mild asymptomatic primary hyperparathyroidism on bone mass in women with and without estrogen replacement therapy. J Bone Miner Res 1994;9(4):509–514.
14. Akerstrom G, Malmaeus J, Bergstrom R. Surgical anatomy of human parathyroid glands. Surgery (St. Louis) 1984;95(1):14–21.
15. Wells SA Jr, Leight GS, Ross AJ III. Primary hyperparathyroidism. Curr Probl Surg 1980;17(8):398–463.
16. Wang C. The anatomic basis of parathyroid surgery. Ann Surg 1976;183(3):271–275.
17. Alveryd A. Parathyroid glands in thyroid surgery. I. Anatomy of parathyroid glands. II. Postoperative hypoparathyroidism: identification and autotransplantation of parathyroid glands. Acta Chir Scand 1968;389:1–120.
18. Norris E. The parathyroid glands and the lateral thyroid in man: their morphogenesis, histogenesis, topographic anatomy and prenatal growth. Contrib Embryol 1937;26:247.
19. Wang C, Mahaffey JE, Axelrod L, Perlman JA. Hyperfunctioning supernumerary parathyroid glands. Surg Gynecol Obstet 1979;148(5):711–714.
20. Levin KE, Clark OH. The reasons for failure in parathyroid operations. Arch Surg 1989;124(8):911–914; discussion 914–915.
21. Edis AJ, Purnell DC, van Heerden JA. The undescended "parathymus." An occasional cause of failed neck exploration for hyperparathyroidism. Ann Surg 1979;190(1):64–68.
22. Lafferty FW. Differential diagnosis of hypercalcemia. J Bone Miner Res 1991;6(suppl 2):S51–S59; discussion S61.
23. Papapoulos SE, Manning RM, Hendy GN, Lewin IG, O'Riordan JL. Studies of circulating parathyroid hormone in man using a homologous amino-terminal specific immunoradiometric assay. Clin Endocrinol (Oxf) 1980;13(1):57–67.
24. Mallette LE, Tuma SN, Berger RE, Kirkland JL. Radioimmunoassay for the middle region of human parathyroid hormone using an homologous antiserum with a carboxy-terminal fragment of bovine parathyroid hormone as radioligand. J Clin Endocrinol Metab 1982;54(5):1017–1024.
25. Hitzler W, Schmidt-Gayk H, Spiropoulos P, Raue F, Hufner M. Homologous radioimmunoassay for human parathyrin (residues 53–84). Clin Chem 1982;28(8):1749–1753.
26. Lindall AW, Elting J, Ells J, Roos BA. Estimation of biologically active intact parathyroid hormone in normal and hyperparathyroid sera by sequential N-terminal immunoextraction and midregion radioimmunoassay. J Clin Endocrinol Metab 1983;57(5):1007–1014.
27. Christensson T, Hellstrom K, Wengle B. Hypercalcemia and primary hyperparathyroidism. Prevalence in patients receiving thiazides as detected in a health screen. Arch Intern Med 1977;137(9):1138–1142.
28. Christensson T, Hellstrom K, Wengle B, Alveryd A, Wikland B. Prevalence of hypercalcaemia in a health screening in Stockholm. Acta Med Scand 1976;200(1–2):131–137.
29. Ladenson JH, Lewis JW, McDonald JM, Slatopolsky E, Boyd JC. Relationship of free and total calcium in hypercalcemic conditions. J Clin Endocrinol Metab 1979;48(3):393–397.
30. Thompson NW, Eckhauser FE, Harness JK. The anatomy of primary hyperparathyroidism. Surgery (St. Louis) 1982;92(5):814–821.
31. Abboud B, Sleilaty G, Helou E, et al. Existence and anatomic distribution of double parathyroid adenoma. Laryngoscope 2005;115(6):1128–1131.
32. Bergson EJ, Heller KS. The clinical significance and anatomic distribution of parathyroid double adenomas. J Am Coll Surg 2004;198(2):185–189.
33. Attie JN, Bock G, Auguste LJ. Multiple parathyroid adenomas: report of thirty-three cases. Surgery (St. Louis) 1990;108(6):1014–1019; discussion 1019–1020.
34. Roses DF, Karp NS, Sudarsky LA, Valensi QJ, Rosen RJ, Blum M. Primary hyperparathyroidism associated with two enlarged parathyroid glands. Arch Surg 1989;124(11):1261–1265.
35. Shane E, Bilezikian JP. Parathyroid carcinoma: a review of 62 patients. Endocr Rev 1982;3(2):218–226.

36. Fraker DL, Travis WD, Merendino JJ Jr, et al. Locally recurrent parathyroid neoplasms as a cause for recurrent and persistent primary hyperparathyroidism. Ann Surg 1991;213(1):58–65.
37. Robert JH, Trombetti A, Garcia A, et al. Primary hyperparathyroidism: can parathyroid carcinoma be anticipated on clinical and biochemical grounds? Report of nine cases and review of the literature. Ann Surg Oncol 2005;12(7):526–532.
38. Rizzoli R, Green J III, Marx SJ. Primary hyperparathyroidism in familial multiple endocrine neoplasia type I. Long-term follow-up of serum calcium levels after parathyroidectomy. Am J Med 1985;78(3):467–474.
39. Keiser HR, Beaven MA, Doppman J, Wells S Jr, Buja LM. Sipple's syndrome: medullary thyroid carcinoma, pheochromocytoma, and parathyroid disease. Studies in a large family. NIH conference. Ann Intern Med 1973;78(4):561–579.
40. Marx SJ, Menczel J, Campbell G, Aurbach GD, Spiegel AM, Norton JA. Heterogeneous size of the parathyroid glands in familial multiple endocrine neoplasia type 1. Clin Endocrinol (Oxf) 1991;35(6):521–526.
41. The search for the MEN1 gene. The European Consortium on MEN-1. J Intern Med 1998;243(6):441–446.
42. Lairmore TC, Howe JR, Korte JA, et al. Familial medullary thyroid carcinoma and multiple endocrine neoplasia type 2B map to the same region of chromosome 10 as multiple endocrine neoplasia type 2A. Genomics 1991;9(1):181–192.
43. Carney JA, Roth SI, Heath H III, Sizemore GW, Hayles AB. The parathyroid glands in multiple endocrine neoplasia type 2b. Am J Pathol 1980;99(2):387–398.
44. Norton JA, Froome LC, Farrell RE, Wells SA Jr. Multiple endocrine neoplasia type IIb: the most aggressive form of medullary thyroid carcinoma. Surg Clin N Am 1979;59(1):109–118.
45. Marx SJ, Stock JL, Attie MF, et al. Familial hypocalciuric hypercalcemia: recognition among patients referred after unsuccessful parathyroid exploration. Ann Intern Med 1980;92(3):351–356.
46. Marx SJ, Fraser D, Rapoport A. Familial hypocalciuric hypercalcemia. Mild expression of the gene in heterozygotes and severe expression in homozygotes. Am J Med 1985;78(1):15–22.
47. Muhr C, Ljunghall S, Akerstrom G, et al. Screening for multiple endocrine neoplasia syndrome (type 1) in patients with primary hyperparathyroidism. Clin Endocrinol (Oxf) 1984;20(2):153–162.
48. Primrose JN, Joffe SN. Hyperparathyroidism and hypergastrinemia revisited. Surgery (St. Louis) 1984;96(6):1144–1150.
49. Raymond JP, Isaac R, Merceron RE, Wahbe F. Comparison between the plasma concentrations of prolactin and parathyroid hormone in normal subjects and in patients with hyperparathyroidism or hyperprolactinemia. J Clin Endocrinol Metab 1982;55(6):1222–1225.
50. Oberg K, Walinder O, Bostrom H, Lundqvist G, Wide L. Peptide hormone markers in screening for endocrine tumors in multiple endocrine adenomatosis type I. Am J Med 1982;73(5):619–630.
51. Friedman E, Bale AE, Marx SJ, et al. Genetic abnormalities in sporadic parathyroid adenomas. J Clin Endocrinol Metab 1990;71(2):293–297.
52. Rosen JE, Costouros NG, Lorang D, et al. Gland size is associated with changes in gene expression profiles in sporadic parathyroid adenomas. Ann Surg Oncol 2005;12(5):412–416.
53. Maselly MJ, Lawrence AM, Brooks M, et al. Hyperparathyroid crisis. Successful treatment of ten comatose patients. Surgery (St. Louis) 1981;90(4):741–746.
54. MacLeod WA, Holloway CK. Hyperparathyroid crisis. A collective review. Ann Surg 1967;166(6):1012–1015.
55. Bilezikian JP. Management of acute hypercalcemia. N Engl J Med 1992;326(18):1196–1203.
56. Fitzpatrick LA, Bilezikian JP. Acute primary hyperparathyroidism. Am J Med 1987;82(2):275–282.
57. Brasier AR, Nussbaum SR. Hungry bone syndrome: clinical and biochemical predictors of its occurrence after parathyroid surgery. Am J Med 1988;84(4):654–660.
58. Denham DW, Norman J. Cost-effectiveness of preoperative sestamibi scan for primary hyperparathyroidism is dependent solely upon the surgeon's choice of operative procedure. J Am Coll Surg 1998;186(3):293–305.
59. Sosa JA, Udelsman R. Minimally invasive parathyroidectomy. Surg Oncol 2003;12(2):125–134.
60. Purcell GP, Dirbas FM, Jeffrey RB, et al. Parathyroid localization with high-resolution ultrasound and technetium Tc 99m sestamibi. Arch Surg 1999;134(8):824–828; discussion 828–830.
61. Carty SE, Norton JA. Management of patients with persistent or recurrent primary hyperparathyroidism. World J Surg 1991;15(6):716–723.
62. Shen W, Duren M, Morita E, et al. Reoperation for persistent or recurrent primary hyperparathyroidism. Arch Surg 1996;131(8):861–867; discussion 867–869.
63. Patow CA, Norton JA, Brennan MF. Vocal cord paralysis and reoperative parathyroidectomy. A prospective study. Ann Surg 1986;203(3):282–285.
64. Miller DL, Doppman JL, Shawker TH, et al. Localization of parathyroid adenomas in patients who have undergone surgery. Part I. Noninvasive imaging methods. Radiology 1987;162(1 pt 1):133–137.
65. Miller DL. Pre-operative localization and interventional treatment of parathyroid tumors: when and how? World J Surg 1991;15(6):706–715.
66. Coakley AJ, Kettle AG, Wells CP, O'Doherty MJ, Collins RE. 99Tcm sestamibi: a new agent for parathyroid imaging. Nucl Med Commun 1989;10(11):791–794.
67. McBiles M, Lambert AT, Cote MG, Kim SY. Sestamibi parathyroid imaging. Semin Nucl Med 1995;25(3):221–234.
68. Wei JP, Burke GJ, Mansberger AR Jr. Preoperative imaging of abnormal parathyroid glands in patients with hyperparathyroid disease using combination Tc-99m-pertechnetate and Tc-99m-sestamibi radionuclide scans. Ann Surg 1994;219(5):568–572; discussion 572–563.
69. Royal RE, Delpassand ES, Shapiro SE, et al. Improving the yield of preoperative parathyroid localization: technetium Tc 99m-sestamibi imaging after thyroid suppression. Surgery (St. Louis) 2002;132(6):968–974; discussion 974–965.
70. Friedman K, Somervell H, Patel P, et al. Effect of calcium channel blockers on the sensitivity of preoperative 99mTc-MIBI SPECT for hyperparathyroidism. Surgery (ST. Louis) 2004;136(6):1199–1204.
71. Norman J, Chheda H, Farrell C. Minimally invasive parathyroidectomy for primary hyperparathyroidism: decreasing operative time and potential complications while improving cosmetic results. Am Surg 1998;64(5):391–395; discussion 395–396.
72. Berland T, Smith SL, Huguet KL. Occult fifth gland intrathyroid parathyroid adenoma identified by gamma probe. Am Surg 2005;71(3):264–266.
73. Takeyama H, Shioya H, Mori Y, et al. Usefulness of radio-guided surgery using technetium-99m methoxyisobutylisonitrile for primary and secondary hyperparathyroidism. World J Surg 2004;28(6):576–582.
74. Hutchinson JR, Yandell DW, Bumpous JM, Fleming MM, Flynn MB. Three-year financial analysis of minimally invasive radio-guided parathyroidectomy. Am Surg 2004;70(12):1112–1115.
75. Allendorf J, Kim L, Chabot J, DiGiorgi M, Spanknebel K, LoGerfo P. The impact of sestamibi scanning on the outcome of parathyroid surgery. J Clin Endocrinol Metab 2003;88(7):3015–3018.
76. Auffermann W, Gooding GA, Okerlund MD, et al. Diagnosis of recurrent hyperparathyroidism: comparison of MR imaging and other imaging techniques. AJR Am J Roentgenol 1988;150(5):1027–1033.

77. Udelsman R, Aruny JE, Donovan PI, et al. Rapid parathyroid hormone analysis during venous localization. Ann Surg 2003;237(5):714–719; discussion 719–721.
78. Patel PC, Pellitteri PK, Patel NM, Fleetwood MK. Use of a rapid intraoperative parathyroid hormone assay in the surgical management of parathyroid disease. Arch Otolaryngol Head Neck Surg 1998;124(5):559–562.
79. Nussbaum SR, Thompson AR, Hutcheson KA, Gaz RD, Wang CA. Intraoperative measurement of parathyroid hormone in the surgical management of hyperparathyroidism. Surgery (St. Louis) 1988;104(6):1121–1127.
80. Chen H, Mack E, Starling JR. A comprehensive evaluation of perioperative adjuncts during minimally invasive parathyroidectomy: which is most reliable? Ann Surg 2005;242(3):375–383.
81. Inabnet WB. Intraoperative parathyroid hormone monitoring. World J Surg 2004;28(12):1212–1215.
82. Carneiro DM, Solorzano CC, Nader MC, Ramirez M, Irvin GL III. Comparison of intraoperative iPTH assay (QPTH) criteria in guiding parathyroidectomy: which criterion is the most accurate? Surgery (St. Louis) 2003;134(6):973–979; discussion 979–981.
83. Bergenfelz A, Isaksson A, Lindblom P, Westerdahl J, Tibblin S. Measurement of parathyroid hormone in patients with primary hyperparathyroidism undergoing first and reoperative surgery. Br J Surg 1998;85(8):1129–1132.
84. Yang GP, Levine S, Weigel RJ. A spike in parathyroid hormone during neck exploration may cause a false-negative intraoperative assay result. Arch Surg 2001;136(8):945–949.
85. Garner SC, Leight GS Jr. Initial experience with intraoperative PTH determinations in the surgical management of 130 consecutive cases of primary hyperparathyroidism. Surgery (St. Louis) 1999;126(6):1132–1137; discussion 1137–1138.
86. Westra WH, Pritchett DD, Udelsman R. Intraoperative confirmation of parathyroid tissue during parathyroid exploration: a retrospective evaluation of the frozen section. Am J Surg Pathol 1998;22(5):538–544.
87. Gauger PG, Mullan MH, Thompson NW, Doherty GM, Matz KA, England BG. An alternative analysis of intraoperative parathyroid hormone data may improve the ability to detect multiglandular disease. Arch Surg 2004;139(2):164–169.
88. Doppman JL, Krudy AG, Marx SJ, et al. Aspiration of enlarged parathyroid glands for parathyroid hormone assay. Radiology 1983;148(1):31–35.
89. Chan RK, Ibrahim SI, Pil P, Tanasijevic M, Moore FD. Validation of a method to replace frozen section during parathyroid exploration by using the rapid parathyroid hormone assay on parathyroid aspirates. Arch Surg 2005;140(4):371–373.
90. Arciero CA, Peoples GE, Stojadinovic A, Shriver CD. The utility of a rapid parathyroid assay for uniglandular, multiglandular, and recurrent parathyroid disease. Am Surg 2004;70(7):588–592.
91. Kaczirek K, Riss P, Wunderer G, et al. Quick PTH assay cannot predict incomplete parathyroidectomy in patients with renal hyperparathyroidism. Surgery (St. Louis) 2005;137(4):431–435.
92. Boggs JE, Irvin GL III, Carneiro DM, Molinari AS. The evolution of parathyroidectomy failures. Surgery (St. Louis) 1999;126(6):998–1002; discussion 1002–1003.
93. Irvin GL III, Molinari AS, Figueroa C, Carneiro DM. Improved success rate in reoperative parathyroidectomy with intraoperative PTH assay. Ann Surg 1999;229(6):874–878; discussion 878–879.
94. NIH conference. Diagnosis and management of asymptomatic primary hyperparathyroidism: consensus development conference statement, April 1, 1991. Bethesda: National Institutes of Health, 1991.
95. Norton JA. Controversies and advances in primary hyperparathyroidism. Ann Surg 1992;215(4):297–299.
96. Sheldon DG, Lee FT, Neil NJ, Ryan JA Jr. Surgical treatment of hyperparathyroidism improves health-related quality of life. Arch Surg 2002;137(9):1022–1026; discussion 1026–1028.
97. Quiros RM, Alef MJ, Wilhelm SM, Djuricin G, Loviscek K, Prinz RA. Health-related quality of life in hyperparathyroidism measurably improves after parathyroidectomy. Surgery (St. Louis) 2003;134(4):675–681; discussion 681–683.
98. Bilezikian JP, Potts JT Jr, Fuleihan Gel H, et al. Summary statement from a workshop on asymptomatic primary hyperparathyroidism: a perspective for the 21st century. J Clin Endocrinol Metab 2002;87(12):5353–5361.
99. Bilezikian JP, Potts JT Jr, Fuleihan Gel H, et al. Summary statement from a workshop on asymptomatic primary hyperparathyroidism: a perspective for the 21st century. J Bone Miner Res 2002;17(suppl 2):N2–N11.
100. Scholz DA, Purnell DC. Asymptomatic primary hyperparathyroidism: 10-year prospective study. Mayo Clin Proc 1981;56(8):473–478.
101. Silverberg SJ, Brown I, Bilezikian JP. Age as a criterion for surgery in primary hyperparathyroidism. Am J Med 2002;113(8):681–684.
102. Delbridge LW, Marshman D, Reeve TS, Crummer P, Posen S. Neuromuscular symptoms in elderly patients with hyperparathyroidism: improvement with parathyroid surgery. Med J Aust 1988;149(2):74–76.
103. Sywak MS, Knowlton ST, Pasieka JL, Parsons LL, Jones J. Do the National Institutes of Health consensus guidelines for parathyroidectomy predict symptom severity and surgical outcome in patients with primary hyperparathyroidism? Surgery (St. Louis) 2002;132(6):1013–1019; discussion 1019–1020.
104. Eigelberger MS, Cheah WK, Ituarte PH, Streja L, Duh QY, Clark OH. The NIH criteria for parathyroidectomy in asymptomatic primary hyperparathyroidism: are they too limited? Ann Surg 2004;239(4):528–535.
105. Elvius M, Lagrelius A, Nygren A, Alveryd A, Christensson TA, Nordenstrom J. Seventeen year follow-up study of bone mass in patients with mild asymptomatic hyperparathyroidism some of whom were operated on. Eur J Surg 1995;161(12):863–869.
106. Almqvist EG, Becker C, Bondeson AG, Bondeson L, Svensson J. Early parathyroidectomy increases bone mineral density in patients with mild primary hyperparathyroidism: a prospective and randomized study. Surgery (St. Louis) 2004;136(6):1281–1288.
107. Sitges-Serra A, Girvent M, Pereira JA, et al. Bone mineral density in menopausal women with primary hyperparathyroidism before and after parathyroidectomy. World J Surg 2004;28(11):1148–1152.
108. Nomura R, Sugimoto T, Tsukamoto T, et al. Marked and sustained increase in bone mineral density after parathyroidectomy in patients with primary hyperparathyroidism: a six-year longitudinal study with or without parathyroidectomy in a Japanese population. Clin Endocrinol (Oxf) 2004;60(3):335–342.
109. Heaney RP. The basis for the post-parathyroidectomy increase in bone mass. J Bone Miner Res 2002;17(suppl 2):N154–N157.
110. Grant CS, van Heerden JA, Charboneau JW, James EM, Reading CC. Clinical management of persistent and/or recurrent primary hyperparathyroidism. World J Surg 1986;10(4):555–565.
111. Brennan MF, Norton JA. Reoperation for persistent and recurrent hyperparathyroidism. Ann Surg 1985;201(1):40–44.
112. Tibblin S, Bondeson AG, Bondeson L, Ljungberg O. Surgical strategy in hyperparathyroidism due to solitary adenoma. Ann Surg 1984;200(6):776–784.
113. Piemonte M, Miani P, Bacchi G. Parathyroid surgery in primary hyperparathyroidism: an update. Arch Otorhinolaryngol 1989;246(5):324–327.
114. Poole GV Jr, Albertson DA, Myers RT. Causes of the failed cervical exploration for primary hyperparathyroidism. Am Surg 1988;54(9):553–557.

115. Rudberg C, Akerstrom G, Palmer M, et al. Late results of operation for primary hyperparathyroidism in 441 patients. Surgery (St. Louis) 1986;99(6):643–651.
116. Cowie AG. Morbidity in adult parathyroid surgery. J R Soc Med 1982;75(12):942–945.
117. Brennan J, Moore EJ, Shuler KJ. Prospective analysis of the efficacy of continuous intraoperative nerve monitoring during thyroidectomy, parathyroidectomy, and parotidectomy. Otolaryngol Head Neck Surg 2001;124(5):537–543.
118. Yarbrough DE, Thompson GB, Kasperbauer JL, Harper CM, Grant CS. Intraoperative electromyographic monitoring of the recurrent laryngeal nerve in reoperative thyroid and parathyroid surgery. Surgery (St. Louis) 2004;136(6):1107–1115.
119. Grant CS, Thompson G, Farley D, van Heerden J. Primary hyperparathyroidism surgical management since the introduction of minimally invasive parathyroidectomy: Mayo Clinic experience. Arch Surg 2005;140(5):472–478; discussion 478–479.
120. Tibblin S, Bondeson AG, Ljungberg O. Unilateral parathyroidectomy in hyperparathyroidism due to single adenoma. Ann Surg 1982;195(3):245–252.
121. Russell CF, Laird JD, Ferguson WR. Scan-directed unilateral cervical exploration for parathyroid adenoma: a legitimate approach? World J Surg 1990;14(3):406–409.
122. Schell SR, Dudley NE. Clinical outcomes and fiscal consequences of bilateral neck exploration for primary idiopathic hyperparathyroidism without preoperative radionuclide imaging or minimally invasive techniques. Surgery (St. Louis) 2003; 133(1):32–39.
123. Siperstein A, Berber E, Mackey R, Alghoul M, Wagner K, Milas M. Prospective evaluation of sestamibi scan, ultrasonography, and rapid PTH to predict the success of limited exploration for sporadic primary hyperparathyroidism. Surgery (St. Louis) 2004;136(4):872–880.
124. Burkey SH, Snyder WH III, Nwariaku F, Watumull L, Mathews D. Directed parathyroidectomy: feasibility and performance in 100 consecutive patients with primary hyperparathyroidism. Arch Surg 2003;138(6):604–608; discussion 608–609.
125. Udelsman R, Donovan PI, Sokoll LJ. One hundred consecutive minimally invasive parathyroid explorations. Ann Surg 2000;232(3):331–339.
126. Inabnet WB, Fulla Y, Richard B, Bonnichon P, Icard P, Chapuis Y. Unilateral neck exploration under local anesthesia: the approach of choice for asymptomatic primary hyperparathyroidism. Surgery (St. Louis) 1999;126(6):1004–1009; discussion 1009–1010.
127. Gallagher SF, Denham DW, Murr MM, Norman JG. The impact of minimally invasive parathyroidectomy on the way endocrinologists treat primary hyperparathyroidism. Surgery (St. Louis) 2003;134(6):910–917; discussion 917.
128. Goldstein RE, Billheimer D, Martin WH, Richards K. Sestamibi scanning and minimally invasive radioguided parathyroidectomy without intraoperative parathyroid hormone measurement. Ann Surg 2003;237(5):722–730; discussion 730–731.
129. Saxe AW, Brown E, Hamburger SW. Thyroid and parathyroid surgery performed with patient under regional anesthesia. Surgery (St. Louis) 1988;103(4):415–420.
130. Biertho L, Chu C, Inabnet WB. Image-directed parathyroidectomy under local anaesthesia in the elderly. Br J Surg 2003;90(6):738–742.
131. Ditkoff BA, Chabot J, Feind C, Lo Gerfo P. Parathyroid surgery using monitored anesthesia care as an alternative to general anesthesia. Am J Surg 1996;172(6):698–700.
132. Kuriloff DB, Sanborn KV. Rapid intraoperative localization of parathyroid glands utilizing methylene blue infusion. Otolaryngol Head Neck Surg 2004;131(5):616–622.
133. Solorzano CC, Lee TM, Ramirez MC, Carneiro DM, Irvin GL. Surgeon-performed ultrasound improves localization of abnormal parathyroid glands. Am Surg 2005;71(7):557–562; discussion 562–563.
134. Kell MR, Sweeney KJ, Moran CJ, Flanagan F, Kerin MJ, Gorey TF. Minimally invasive parathyroidectomy with operative ultrasound localization of the adenoma. Surg Endosc 2004;18(7):1097–1098.
135. Norman J, Chheda H. Minimally invasive parathyroidectomy facilitated by intraoperative nuclear mapping. Surgery (St. Louis) 1997;122(6):998–1003; discussion 1003–1004.
136. Flynn MB, Bumpous JM, Schill K, McMasters KM. Minimally invasive radioguided parathyroidectomy. J Am Coll Surg 2000;191(1):24–31.
137. Norman J, Denham D. Minimally invasive radioguided parathyroidectomy in the reoperative neck. Surgery (St. Louis) 1998;124(6):1088–1092; discussion 1092–1083.
138. Udelsman R. Six hundred fifty-six consecutive explorations for primary hyperparathyroidism. Ann Surg 2002;235(5):665–670; discussion 670–672.
139. Genc H, Morita E, Perrier ND, et al. Differing histologic findings after bilateral and focused parathyroidectomy. J Am Coll Surg 2003;196(4):535–540.
140. Lee NC, Norton JA. Multiple-gland disease in primary hyperparathyroidism: a function of operative approach? Arch Surg 2002;137(8):896–899; discussion 899–900.
141. Lamers CB, Froeling PG. Clinical significance of hyperparathyroidism in familial multiple endocrine adenomatosis type I (MEA I). Am J Med 1979;66(3):422–424.
142. Wells SA Jr, Ellis GJ, Gunnells JC, Schneider AB, Sherwood LM. Parathyroid autotransplantation in primary parathyroid hyperplasia. N Engl J Med 1976;295(2):57–62.
143. Wells SA Jr, Farndon JR, Dale JK, Leight GS, Dilley WG. Long-term evaluation of patients with primary parathyroid hyperplasia managed by total parathyroidectomy and heterotopic autotransplantation. Ann Surg 1980;192(4):451–458.
144. Saxe AW, Brennan MF. Reoperative parathyroid surgery for primary hyperparathyroidism caused by multiple-gland disease: total parathyroidectomy and autotransplantation with cryopreserved tissue. Surgery (St. Louis) 1982;91(6):616–621.
145. Senapati A, Young AE. Parathyroid autotransplantation. Br J Surg 1990;77(10):1171–1174.
146. Norton JA, Schneider PD, Brennan MF. Median sternotomy in reoperations for primary hyperparathyroidism. World J Surg 1985;9(5):807–813.
147. Wells SA Jr, Cooper JD. Closed mediastinal exploration in patients with persistent hyperparathyroidism. Ann Surg 1991; 214(5):555–561.
148. Medrano C, Hazelrigg SR, Landreneau RJ, Boley TM, Shawgo T, Grasch A. Thoracoscopic resection of ectopic parathyroid glands. Ann Thorac Surg 2000;69(1):221–223.
149. Quiros RM, Warren W, Prinz RA. Excision of a mediastinal parathyroid gland with use of video-assisted thoracoscopy, intraoperative ^{99m}Tc-sestamibi scanning, and intraoperative monitoring of intact parathyroid hormone. Endocr Pract 2004; 10(1):45–48.
150. Tovar EA. Minimally invasive resection of mediastinal parathyroid adenomas. Ann Thorac Surg 2001;71(1):402–403.
151. Prinz RA, Lonchyna V, Carnaille B, Wurtz A, Proye C. Thoracoscopic excision of enlarged mediastinal parathyroid glands. Surgery (St. Louis) 1994;116(6):999–1004; discussion 1004–1005.
152. Rossi HL, Ali A, Prinz RA. Intraoperative sestamibi scanning in reoperative parathyroidectomy. Surgery (St. Louis) 2000; 128(4):744–750.
153. Thompson GB, Grant CS, Perrier ND, et al. Reoperative parathyroid surgery in the era of sestamibi scanning and intraoperative parathyroid hormone monitoring. Arch Surg 1999; 134(7):699–704; discussion 704–695.

154. Jaskowiak N, Norton JA, Alexander HR, et al. A prospective trial evaluating a standard approach to reoperation for missed parathyroid adenoma. Ann Surg 1996;224(3):308–320; discussion 320–321.
155. Wang C, Gaz RD, Moncure AC. Mediastinal parathyroid exploration: a clinical and pathologic study of 47 cases. World J Surg 1986;10(4):687–695.
156. Fraker DL, Doppman JL, Shawker TH, Marx SJ, Spiegel AM, Norton JA. Undescended parathyroid adenoma: an important etiology for failed operations for primary hyperparathyroidism. World J Surg 1990;14(3):342–348.
157. Chan TJ, Libutti SK, McCart JA, et al. Persistent primary hyperparathyroidism caused by adenomas identified in pharyngeal or adjacent structures. World J Surg 2003;27(6):675–679.
158. Johnson WJ, McCarthy JT, van Heerden JA, Sterioff S, Grant CS, Kao PC. Results of subtotal parathyroidectomy in hemodialysis patients. Am J Med 1988;84(1):23–32.
159. Andress DL, Ott SM, Maloney NA, Sherrard DJ. Effect of parathyroidectomy on bone aluminum accumulation in chronic renal failure. N Engl J Med 1985;312(8):468–473.
160. Clark OH. Secondary hyperparathyroidism. In: Clark OH, ed. Endocrine Surgery of the Thyroid and Parathyroid Glands. St. Louis: Mosby, 1985.
161. Yano S, Sugimoto T, Tsukamoto T, et al. Effect of parathyroidectomy on bone mineral density in hemodialysis patients with secondary hyperparathyroidism: possible usefulness of preoperative determination of parathyroid hormone level for prediction of bone regain. Horm Metab Res 2003;35(4):259–264.
162. de Francisco AL, Fresnedo GF, Rodrigo E, Pinera C, Amado JA, Arias M. Parathyroidectomy in dialysis patients. Kidney Int Suppl 2002(80):161–166.
163. Baumann DS, Wells SA Jr. Parathyroid autotransplantation. Surgery (St. Louis) 1993;113(2):130–133.
164. Wang CA, Gaz RD. Natural history of parathyroid carcinoma. Diagnosis, treatment, and results. Am J Surg 1985;149(4):522–527.
165. Cohn K, Silverman M, Corrado J, Sedgewick C. Parathyroid carcinoma: the Lahey Clinic experience. Surgery (St. Louis) 1985;98(6):1095–1100.
166. Calandra DB, Chejfec G, Foy BK, Lawrence AM, Paloyan E. Parathyroid carcinoma: biochemical and pathologic response to DTIC. Surgery (St. Louis) 1984;96(6):1132–1137.
167. Flye MW, Brennan MF. Surgical resection of metastatic parathyroid carcinoma. Ann Surg 1981;193(4):425–435.
168. Palazzo FF, Sywak MS, Sidhu SB, Barraclough BH, Delbridge LW. Parathyroid autotransplantation during total thyroidectomy: does the number of glands transplanted affect outcome? World J Surg 2005;29(5):629–631.
169. El-Sharaky MI, Kahalil MR, Sharaky O, et al. Assessment of parathyroid autotransplantation for preservation of parathyroid function after total thyroidectomy. Head Neck 2003;25(10):799–807.
170. Leight GS, Parker GA, Sears HF, Marx SJ, Terrill RE. Experimental cryopreservation and autotransplantation of parathyroid glands: technique and demonstration of function. Ann Surg 1978;188(1):16–21.
171. Wells SA Jr, Burdick JF, Hattler BG, et al. The allografted parathyroid gland: evaluation of function in the immunosuppressed host. Ann Surg 1974;180(6):805–813.
172. Niederle B, Roka R, Brennan MF. The transplantation of parathyroid tissue in man: development, indications, technique, and results. Endocr Rev 1982;3(3):245–279.
173. Lombardi CP, Raffaelli M, Princi P, et al. Early prediction of postthyroidectomy hypocalcemia by one single iPTH measurement. Surgery (St. Louis) 2004;136(6):1236–1241.
174. Bergenfelz A, Kanngiesser V, Zielke A, Nies C, Rothmund M. Conventional bilateral cervical exploration versus open minimally invasive parathyroidectomy under local anaesthesia for primary hyperparathyroidism. Br J Surg 2005;92(2):190–197.
175. Reichel H, Koeffler HP, Norman AW. The role of the vitamin D endocrine system in health and disease. N Engl J Med 1989;320(15):980–991.
176. Mallette LE, Bilezikian JP, Heath DA, Aurbach GD. Primary hyperparathyroidism: clinical and biochemical features. Medicine (Baltim) 1974;53(2):127–146.
177. Yamashita H, Noguchi S, Moriyama T, et al. Reelevation of parathyroid hormone level after parathyroidectomy in patients with primary hyperparathyroidism: importance of decreased renal parathyroid hormone sensitivity. Surgery (St. Louis) 2005;137(4):419–425.
178. O'Duffy JD. Pseudogout syndrome in hospital patients. JAMA 1973;226(1):42–44.
179. Bilezikian JP, Connor TB, Aptekar R, et al. Pseudogout after parathyroidectomy. Lancet 1973;1(7801):445–446.
180. Ammori BJ, Madan M, Gopichandran TD, et al. Ultrasound-guided unilateral neck exploration for sporadic primary hyperparathyroidism: is it worthwhile? Ann R Coll Surg Engl 1998;80(6):433–437.
181. Ishibashi M, Nishida H, Hiromatsu Y, Kojima K, Tabuchi E, Hayabuchi N. Comparison of technetium-99m-MIBI, technetium-99m-tetrofosmin, ultrasound and MRI for localization of abnormal parathyroid glands. J Nucl Med 1998;39(2):320–324.
182. Sinha CK, Hamaker R, Hamaker RC, Freeman SB, Borrowdale RW, Huntley TC. Utility of preoperative radionuclide scanning for primary hyperparathyroidism. Laryngoscope 1997;107(6):753–758.
183. Gofrit ON, Lebensart PD, Pikarsky A, Lackstein D, Gross DJ, Shiloni E. High-resolution ultrasonography: highly sensitive, specific technique for preoperative localization of parathyroid adenoma in the absence of multinodular thyroid disease. World J Surg 1997;21(3):287–290; discussion 290–291.
184. Koslin DB, Adams J, Andersen P, Everts E, Cohen J. Preoperative evaluation of patients with primary hyperparathyroidism: role of high-resolution ultrasound. Laryngoscope 1997;107(9):1249–1253.
185. Light VL, McHenry CR, Jarjoura D, Sodee DB, Miron SD. Prospective comparison of dual-phase technetium-99m-sestamibi scintigraphy and high resolution ultrasonography in the evaluation of abnormal parathyroid glands. Am Surg 1996;62(7):562–567; discussion 567–568.
186. Sofferman RA, Nathan MH, Fairbank JT, Foster RS Jr, Krag DN. Preoperative technetium Tc 99m sestamibi imaging. Paving the way to minimal-access parathyroid surgery. Arch Otolaryngol Head Neck Surg 1996;122(4):369–374.
187. Bugis SP, Berno E, Rusnak CH, Chu D. Technetium 99m-sestamibi scanning before initial neck exploration in patients with primary hyperparathyroidism. Eur Arch Otorhinolaryngol 1995;252(3):149–152.
188. Mitchell LS. Re: Diagnosis and management of parathyroid diseases. Surgery (St. Louis) 1992;112(3):611.
189. van Heerden JA, Grant CS. Surgical treatment of primary hyperparathyroidism: an institutional perspective. World J Surg 1991;15(6):688–692.
190. Mariette C, Pellissier L, Combemale F, Quievreux JL, Carnaille B, Proye C. Reoperation for persistent or recurrent primary hyperparathyroidism. Langenbecks Arch Surg 1998;383(2):174–179.
191. Peeler BB, Martin WH, Sandler MP, Goldstein RE. Sestamibi parathyroid scanning and preoperative localization studies for patients with recurrent/persistent hyperparathyroidism or significant comorbid conditions: development of an optimal localization strategy. Am Surg 1997;63(1):37–46.
192. MacFarlane MP, Fraker DL, Shawker TH, et al. Use of preoperative fine-needle aspiration in patients undergoing reoperation

for primary hyperparathyroidism. Surgery (St. Louis) 1994;116(6):959–964; discussion 964–965.
193. Rodriquez JM, Tezelman S, Siperstein AE, et al. Localization procedures in patients with persistent or recurrent hyperparathyroidism. Arch Surg 1994;129(8):870–875.
194. Doherty GM, Doppman JL, Miller DL, et al. Results of a multidisciplinary strategy for management of mediastinal parathyroid adenoma as a cause of persistent primary hyperparathyroidism. Ann Surg 1992;215(2):101–106.
195. Ruda JM, Hollenbeak CS, Stack BC Jr. A systematic review of the diagnosis and treatment of primary hyperparathyroidism from 1995 to 2003. Otolaryngol Head Neck Surg 2005;132(3):359–372.
196. Baliski CR, Stewart JK, Anderson DW, Wiseman SM, Bugis SP. Selective unilateral parathyroid exploration: an effective treatment for primary hyperparathyroidism. Am J Surg 2005; 189(5):596–600; discussion 600.
197. Carneiro DM, Solorzano CC, Irvin GL III. Recurrent disease after limited parathyroidectomy for sporadic primary hyperparathyroidism. J Am Coll Surg 2004;199(6):849–853; discussion 853–855.
198. Mortier PE, Mozzon MM, Fouquet OP, et al. Unilateral surgery for hyperparathyroidism: indications, limits, and late results: new philosophy or expensive selection without improvement of surgical results? World J Surg 2004;28(12):1298–1304.
199. Sidiropoulos N, Vento J, Malchoff C, Whalen G. Radioguided tumorectomy in the management of parathyroid adenomas. Arch Surg 2003;138(7):716–720.
200. Shabtai M, Ben-Haim M, Muntz Y, et al. 140 consecutive cases of minimally invasive, radio-guided parathyroidectomy: lessons learned and long-term results. Surg Endosc 2003;17(5):688–691.
201. Bergenfelz A, Lindblom P, Tibblin S, Westerdahl J. Unilateral versus bilateral neck exploration for primary hyperparathyroidism: a prospective randomized controlled trial. Ann Surg 2002;236(5):543–551.
202. Dillavou ED, Jenoff JS, Intenzo CM, Cohn HE. The utility of sestamibi scanning in the operative management of patients with primary hyperparathyroidism. J Am Coll Surg 2000; 190(5):540–545.
203. Goldstein RE, Blevins L, Delbeke D, Martin WH. Effect of minimally invasive radioguided parathyroidectomy on efficacy, length of stay, and costs in the management of primary hyperparathyroidism. Ann Surg 2000;231(5):732–742.
204. Low RA, Katz AD. Parathyroidectomy via bilateral cervical exploration: a retrospective review of 866 cases. Head Neck 1998;20(7):583–587.
205. Summers GW. Parathyroid update: a review of 220 cases. Ear Nose Throat J 1996;75(7):434–439.
206. Worsey MJ, Carty SE, Watson CG. Success of unilateral neck exploration for sporadic primary hyperparathyroidism. Surgery (St. Louis) 1993;114(6):1024–1029; discussion 1029–1030.
207. Tibblin S, Bizard JP, Bondeson AG, et al. Primary hyperparathyroidism due to solitary adenoma. A comparative multicentre study of early and long-term results of different surgical regimens. Eur J Surg 1991;157(9):511–515.
208. Saaka MB, Sellke FW, Kelly TR. Primary hyperparathyroidism. Surg Gynecol Obstet 1988;166(4):333–337.
209. Russell CF, Edis AJ. Surgery for primary hyperparathyroidism: experience with 500 consecutive cases and evaluation of the role of surgery in the asymptomatic patient. Br J Surg 1982;69(5):244–247.
210. Punch JD, Thompson NW, Merion RM. Subtotal parathyroidectomy in dialysis-dependent and post-renal transplant patients. A 25-year single-center experience. Arch Surg 1995;130(5):538–542; discussion 542–543.
211. Rothmund M, Wagner PK, Schark C. Subtotal parathyroidectomy versus total parathyroidectomy and autotransplantation in secondary hyperparathyroidism: a randomized trial. World J Surg 1991;15(6):745–750.
212. Niederle B, Horandner H, Roka R, Woloszczuk W. [Parathyroidectomy and autotransplantation in renal hyperparathyroidism. I. Clinical and chemical laboratory studies following tissue selection.] Chirurg 1989;60(10):665–670.
213. Leapman SB, Filo RS, Thomalla JV, King D. Secondary hyperparathyroidism. The role of surgery. Am Surg 1989;55(6):359–365.
214. Doherty GM, Weber B, Norton JA. Cost of unsuccessful surgery for primary hyperparathyroidism. Surgery (St. Louis) 1994; 116(6):954–957; discussion 957–958.
215. Weber CJ, Sewell CW, McGarity WC. Persistent and recurrent sporadic primary hyperparathyroidism: histopathology, complications, and results of reoperation. Surgery (St. Louis) 1994; 116(6):991–998.
216. Jarhult J, Nordenstrom J, Perbeck L. Reoperation for suspected primary hyperparathyroidism. Br J Surg 1993;80(4):453–456.
217. Rothmund M, Wagner PK, Seesko H, Zielke A. [Lessons from reoperations in 55 patients with primary hyperparathyroidism.] Dtsch Med Wochenschr 1990;115(42):1579–1585.
218. Cheung PS, Borgstrom A, Thompson NW. Strategy in reoperative surgery for hyperparathyroidism. Arch Surg 1989;124(6):676–680.

56

Thyroid

Ronald J. Weigel

Anatomy and Physiology

The common indications for thyroidectomy include a suspicion of cancer, local symptoms of a large neck mass (e.g., difficulty breathing or swallowing), and abnormal thyroid function (e.g., hyperthyroidism). Surgical management of thyroid problems requires a thorough understanding of the anatomy and pathophysiology of the thyroid gland.

Surgical Approach

The normal thyroid weighs approximately 20 g and is situated anterior and slightly inferior to the thyroid cartilage. Figure 56.1 depicts the relevant anatomy and surgical approach to the thyroid. The thyroid is highly vascular and derives its blood supply from paired superior and inferior thyroid arteries. The superior thyroid artery is a branch of the external carotid artery, and the inferior thyroid artery is derived from the thyrocervical trunk. Thyroid ima vessels are branches directly from the aorta and enter the gland inferiorly. The recurrent laryngeal nerve ascends from the superior mediastinum and runs in the tracheoesophageal groove. The nerve courses directly posterior to the thyroid lobe and passes through the cricopharyngeus to innervate the intrinsic muscles of the larynx. The location of the parathyroid glands is variable but the glands are usually found lateral and posterior to the thyroid. The identification of these structures is critical during neck exploration.

Thyroid Function Tests and Thyroid Imaging

The thyroid synthesizes thyroid hormone, which is necessary for normal metabolism. The secretion of thyroid hormone is precisely regulated, as depicted in Figure 56.2. The hypothalamus secretes thyrotropin-releasing hormone (TRH), which induces the anterior pituitary to secrete thyroid-stimulating hormone (TSH). TSH stimulates growth and function of the follicle cells of the thyroid. In response to TSH, the thyroid concentrates iodine and synthesizes the thyroid hormones thyroxine (T4) and the more metabolically active form of thyroxine, T3. Free thyroxine is the active form of the hormone and exerts a negative feedback on the pituitary and probably the hypothalamus. The plasma concentrations of these hormones provides the clinician with a reliable means of assessing thyroid physiological function. The half-lives of T4 and T3 are approximately 7 and 3 days, respectively. For this reason, thyroid tests are commonly examined 4 to 6 weeks after altering dosages of thyroid medications.

The commonly employed thyroid function tests are listed in Table 56.1. TSH is the single best test for diagnosis of hyper- and hypothyroidism. In hyperthyroid states, TSH is suppressed. In mild cases of hyperthyroidism, the TSH may be suppressed although thyroid hormone levels remain in the normal range. However, in most cases all three parameters of thyroxine measurement [free T4 (FT4), total T4, and total T3] are increased simultaneously. Additionally, there are cases of hyperthyroidism in which only T3 is measurably increased (T3 thyrotoxicosis). In hypothyroid states, TSH is elevated and the thyroxine parameters are below normal. In instances of mild hypothyroidism, TSH is elevated with normal thyroxine parameters. Under certain physiological conditions, such as pregnancy, patients on thyroid hormone replacement require increased thyroid hormone dosage, as can be evidenced by a measured increase in TSH.

Thyroid scan using ^{123}I is a useful test to help diagnose diseases of the thyroid involving abnormal thyroid function. The thyroid scan has limited usefulness in the setting of a suspicion of thyroid malignancy. The common findings of thyroid scans include cold nodules, hot nodules (solitary or multiple), and Graves' disease. Examples of these pathological states as identified by thyroid scan are shown in Figure 56.3.

Hyperthyroidism

Hyperthyroidism is caused by thyroid hormone excess. The usual pathological states causing hyperthyroidism are toxic nodule, toxic multinodular goiter, Graves' disease, and the

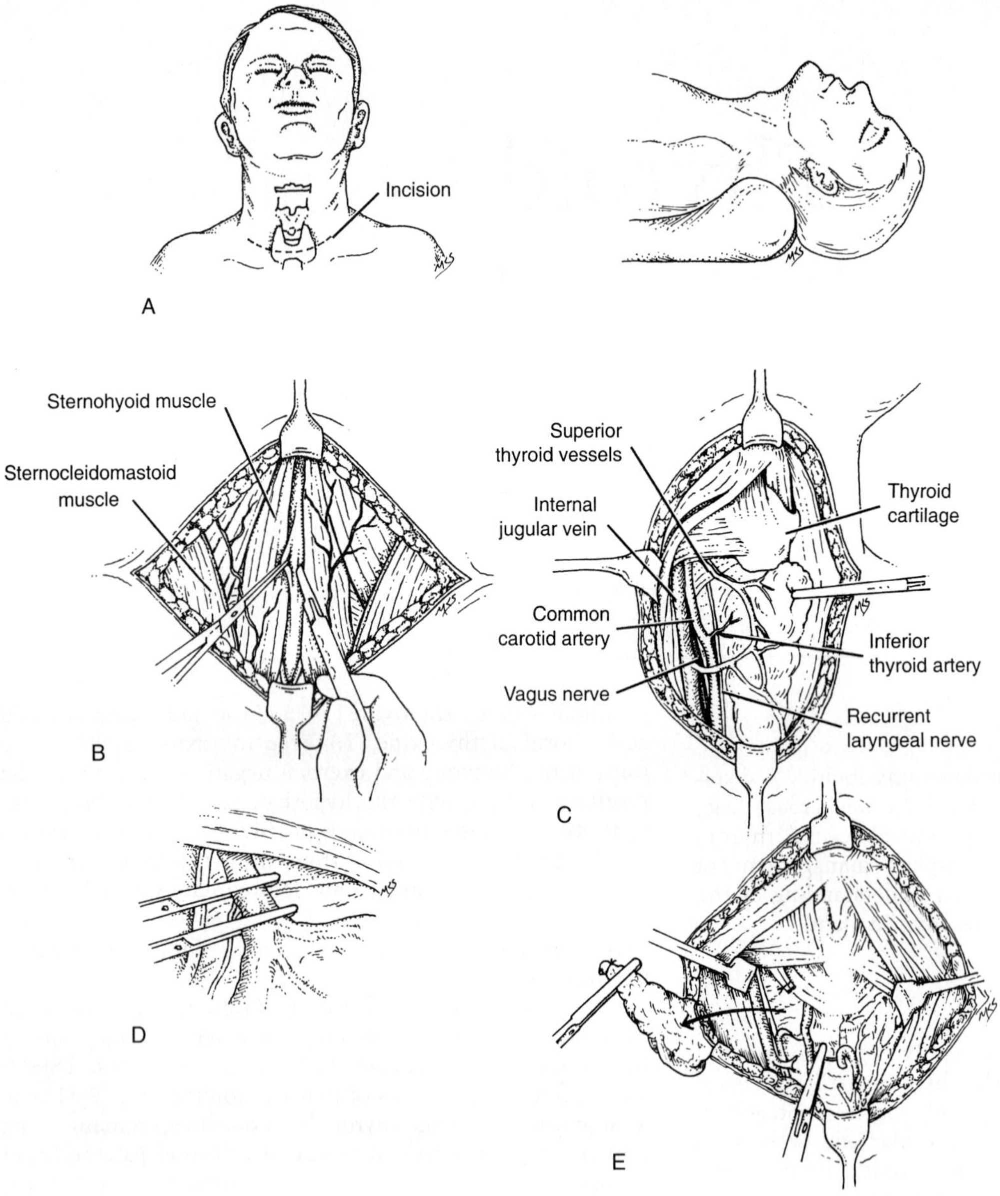

FIGURE 56.1. Thyroidectomy. **A.** The patient is placed with the neck in extension. The thyroid is approached through a Kocher collar incision, which is commonly made approximately 2.0 cm superior to the sternal notch. **B.** The strap muscles are divided in the midline to expose the thyroid gland. **C.** The strap muscles are retracted laterally and the thyroid is retracted medially, exposing the structures of the midneck. The recurrent laryngeal nerve can be seen lying within the tracheoesophageal groove. **D.** The superior pole vessels are individually clamped and ligated as they enter the thyroid gland. Inferior thyroid vessels, as well as the vessels of the thyroid (ima), are individually suture ligated. **E.** The dissection is completed by dissection of the thyroid gland off the trachea. The isthmus is then transected and can be oversewn with a suture for hemostasis. (Redrawn with permission from Macdonald J, Haller D, Weigel R. Endocrine system. In: Abeloff MD, ed. Clinical Oncology. New York: Churchill Livingstone, 1995:1051.)

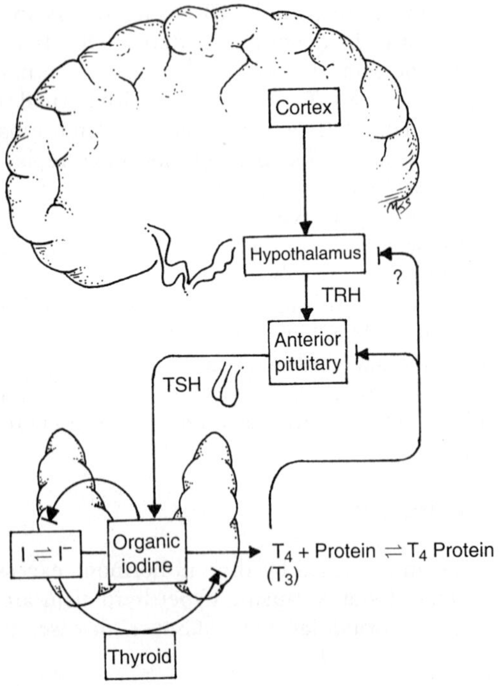

FIGURE 56.2. Schema of the homeostatic regulation of thyroid function. Thyroid-stimulating hormone (TSH) stimulates release of thyroid hormone. Secretion of TSH is regulated by a negative feedback mechanism acting directly on the pituitary gland and is normally inversely related to the concentration of unbound hormone in the blood. Release of TSH is induced by the thyrotropin-releasing hormone (TRH). Factors regulating secretion of TRH are uncertain but may include the free hormone in the blood and stimuli from higher centers. (Redrawn with permission from Ingbar SH, Woeber KA. The thyroid gland. In: Williams RH, ed. Textbook of Endocrinology, 6th ed. Philadephia: Saunders, 1981:134.)

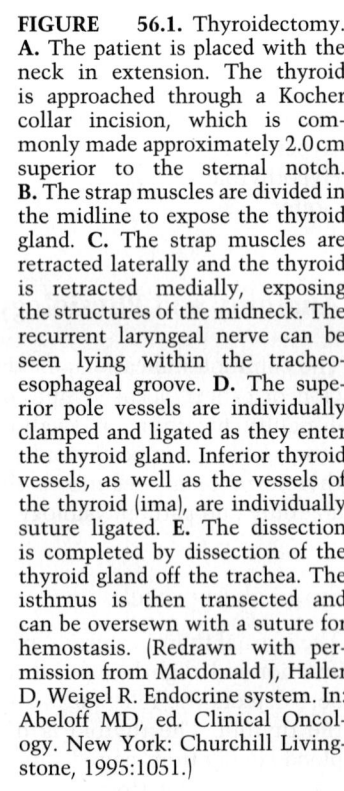

TABLE 56.1. Laboratory Evaluation of the Thyroid Patient.

Test	*Normal values*
Free T4	0.73–2.01 ng/dL
Thyroid-stimulating hormone	0.4–4.0 mIU/mL
T3, total	100–190 ng/dL
T4, total	6.2–11.8 mg/dL
Thyroglobulin	With thyroid gland: <20 ng/mL Athyreotic on T4: <2 ng/mL Athyreotic off T4: <5 ng/mL
Antithyroid microsomal	Negative: <0.3 U/mL
24-h ^{131}I uptake	5%–30%

early stage of subacute thyroiditis. Iatrogenic thyrotoxicosis can be caused by an inappropriate dosage of thyroid hormone replacement. Symptoms associated with hyperthyroidism include heat intolerance, sweating, weight loss, tremulousness, palpitations, restlessness, emotional instability, and insomnia. Atrial fibrillation is a common finding in older patients. A severe form of hyperthyroidism called thyroid storm can be precipitated by surgery, sepsis, or trauma in patients with untreated or incompletely treated Graves' disease.[1,2] Storm can have mortality rates of 20% to 30% and is characterized by fever, hypotension, congestive heart failure (CHF), and circulatory collapse. Treatment involves initial resuscitation with IV fluids and cooling blankets. Potassium iodine is given to suppress thyroid synthesis, and steroids are given to treat associated adrenal insufficiency. Administration of β-blockade, usually propranolol, is helpful in managing the cardiac manifestations. Propylthiouracil (PTU) is used to suppress thyroid hormone synthesis and also blocks the peripheral conversion of T4 to the more active metabolite T3.

Graves' Disease

Graves' disease is characterized by hyperthyroidism, goiter, and exophthalmos. These features may occur singly or in any combination; approximately one-third of patients have manifestations of thyrotoxicosis and eye findings with initial presentation. The pathophysiology of Graves' disease is attributable to thyroid autoantibodies that recognize and stimulate the TSH receptor.[3] These antibodies stimulate growth of the thyroid and increase synthesis of hormone. However, there can be disparity between gland size and degree of hyperthyroidism, suggesting that there may be different subsets of antibodies affecting thyroid growth and thyroid function.[3] Antithyroid antibodies also infiltrate the eye muscles and periorbital tissues, accounting for the eye manifestations. Graves' ophthalmopathy presents a significant clinical problem in approximately one-third of patients with Graves' disease.[4]

The thyroid in Graves' disease is diffusely enlarged, although the enlargement can be asymmetrical. Distinct nodules are unusual and should raise the suspicion of malignancy. Thyroid carcinoma has been reported to occur in 5% to 7% of patients undergoing surgery for Graves' disease.[5–7] There have also been reports in the literature suggesting that thyroid-stimulating antibodies may increase aggressiveness of thyroid carcinomas occurring in the setting of Graves' disease.[8] Thyroid function tests should be used to confirm the diagnosis of hyperthyroidism. Normally, patients present with a suppressed TSH and elevated FT4. Thyroid uptake is increased, with 50% to 90% of administered iodine dose localized to the thyroid. The thyroid scan is used to confirm the diagnosis of Graves' disease and demonstrates diffuse uptake, lacking nodularity (see Fig. 56.3). The presence of a cold nodule noted on radioiodine scan should raise the suspicion of malignancy and is an indication for thyroidectomy.[9]

The initial treatment of Graves' disease is aimed at establishing a euthyroid state. In the United States, the two commonly used antithyroid medications are PTU and methimazole (Tapazole). These drugs inhibit thyroid hormone synthesis by interfering with organification of iodine in the thyroid. Additionally, PTU inhibits peripheral conversion of T4 to T3. Side effects include allergic reactions characterized by skin rash, fever, and polyarteritis. More serious side effects are agranulocytosis and aplastic anemia. Patients treated with these

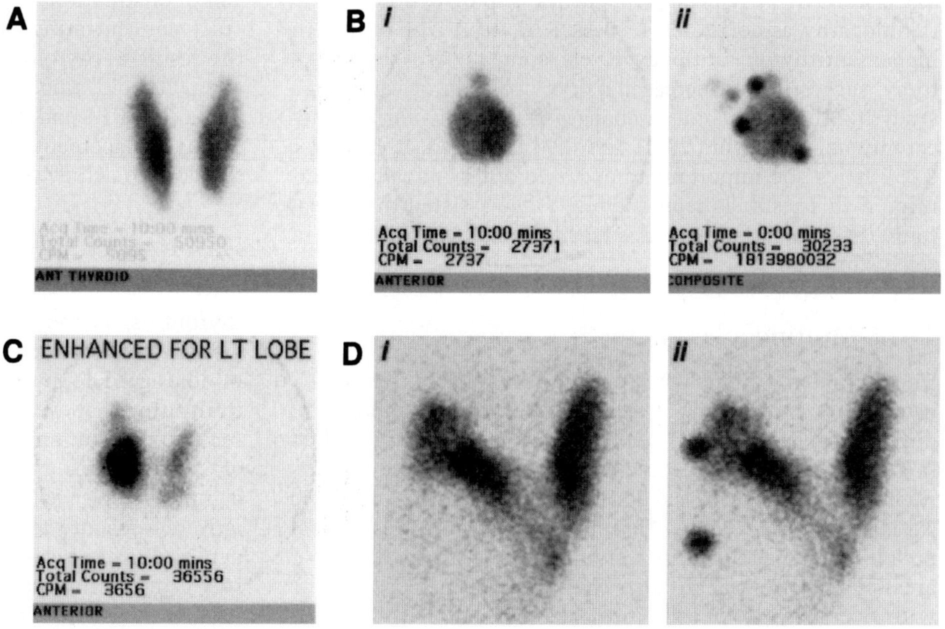

FIGURE 56.3. Radioiodine scan of thyroid pathology. **A.** Graves' disease. Diffuse uptake of radioactive iodine. Total uptake is elevated at 24 h (65%). **B.** Toxic nodule with contralateral thyroid suppression: *i*, thyroid scan showing toxic nodule of right lobe of the thyroid with suppression of the contralateral lobe; *ii*, toxic nodule corresponds to palpable abnormality. **C.** Toxic nodule, right lobe of the thyroid, with partial suppression of the contralateral thyroid lobe. **D.** Cold nodule, right lobe of the thyroid: *i*, cold nodule, right lobe of the thyroid with normal remaining thyroid uptake; *ii*, palpable nodule corresponds to cold defect.

medications should have periodic evaluation of their CBC and should be instructed to seek evaluation if symptoms of a fever or sore throat develops. Following medical treatment, most patients achieve a euthyroid state in approximately 6 weeks. For patients with cardiac manifestations associated with thyrotoxicosis, a beta-blocker such as propranolol may be added until a euthyroid state is achieved.

Although some clinicians treat patients with long-term medical therapy, definitive treatment of Graves' disease is accomplished with either radioactive iodine (RAI) or surgery. In the United States, RAI treatment has become the preferred treatment option.[10,11] The thyroid gland in Graves' disease is extremely sensitive to RAI. Small doses of ^{131}I, less than 10 mCi in most cases, can be used to reduce the thyroid mass with the intent of making the patient euthyroid. An alternate approach utilizes ^{131}I doses in the range of 10 to 15 mCi, which will produce hypothyroidism in the majority of patients. Patients are subsequently treated with thyroxine to attain a euthyroid state. Using this approach, thyrotoxicosis can be cured in 80% to 90% of patients. In some instances, retreatment or surgery is required. Contraindications to the use of RAI include pregnancy and a suspicion of thyroid malignancy.

Thyroidectomy is an alternative treatment option for Graves' disease. A number of recent series report low complication rates with negligible recurrence of hyperthyroidism.[12–15] There are two basic approaches to surgical treatment. Some surgeons perform a lobectomy on one side and a subtotal thyroidectomy on the contralateral lobe, leaving approximately 4 g tissue. The intent of this approach is to render the patients euthyroid without the need for medication. The bilateral subtotal approach is associated with a significant increase in recurrent hyperthyroidism and is not suggested.[16] There is a reported incidence of recurrent hyperthyroidism of 2% to 15% in patients treated by subtotal thyroidectomy.[13,16,17] An alternative approach is to perform a total or near-total thyroidectomy and treat patients with thyroxine replacement postoperatively. Total thyroidectomy has a lower recurrence rate and has been shown to result in lower antithyroid antibodies compared to subtotal thyroidectomy.[13] There is also some suggestion that surgical treatment of Graves' disease is associated with a decreased incidence of progression of ophthalmopathy as compared to RAI. RAI treatment results in higher antithyroid antibody levels compared to thyroidectomy, suggesting an increased risk of ophthalmopathy.[14] In a study by Abe et al.,[18] mean changes in proptosis for thyroidectomy and RAI were 20.01 and 0.93 mm, respectively ($P < 0.05$). It will be important to examine other series to determine if this result is reproducible. Video-assisted thyroidectomy has recently been described for Graves' disease in selected patients.[19]

Toxic Multinodular Goiter

The thyroid in patients with toxic multinodular goiter (MNG) usually contains several palpable nodules. Local symptoms of difficulty in breathing or swallowing are more common than in Graves' disease. Thyroid function tests indicate hyperthyroidism with a suppressed TSH, although a normal FT4 and T3 is a common finding. Thyroid scan demonstrates several nodules that usually have varying degrees of uptake. Cold areas noted on scan are also commonly seen. For patients with overt thyrotoxicosis, medical treatment with antithyroid medications is the initial treatment.

Definitive treatment for toxic MNG can be accomplished with RAI or surgery. The dose of ^{131}I is calculated based upon the size of the gland and iodine uptake. The doses needed to treat toxic MNG are generally much larger than for Graves' disease, and approximately 10% of patients require doses in the range of 150 to 200 mCi.[20] In the series reported by Erickson et al.,[21] 20% of patients treated by RAI required a second treatment. Heterogeneous uptake on scan and the need for large doses of RAI often make surgery the preferable treatment, especially in patients with large goiters who develop local symptoms of difficulty swallowing or breathing. Compared to RAI, thyroidectomy has been shown to render patients euthyroid sooner.[21] Total thyroidectomy is the preferred surgical procedure for toxic MNG because it is more likely to cure hyperthyroidism compared to subtotal thyroidectomy or thyroid lobectomy.[21]

Toxic Nodule

A solitary hot nodule is usually caused by a follicular adenoma, although in children hot nodules may be malignant. Nodules larger than 3 cm often cause overt thyrotoxicosis. Thyroid scan demonstrates a hot nodule with partial or complete suppression of the remaining thyroid (see Fig. 56.3B,C). After the patient is rendered euthyroid, definitive treatment can be accomplished with RAI or surgery (most often lobectomy). RAI doses required for treatment depend on the size of the nodule. The rates of persistent hyperthyroidism and post-treatment hypothyroidism after RAI are both approximately 10%.[20] RAI treatment may also result in persistent nodularity.[22] Surgical treatment is a reasonable option for toxic nodules occurring in young patients, during pregnancy or lactation, in patients who require a rapid correction of thyrotoxicosis, or in cases where malignancy is suspected.

Hypothyroidism

Hypothyroidism is the result of a deficiency of thyroid hormone and is characterized by cold intolerance, weight gain, constipation, dry skin, brittle hair, hoarse voice, difficulty concentrating, and fatigue. Hypothyroidism is usually the result of thyroiditis or the result of surgery or RAI ablation. Thyroid function tests demonstrate an increased TSH and a low FT4 and T3. Hypothyroidism is treated with thyroxine replacement starting with a low dose and increasing the dose to achieve a euthyroid state.

Hashimoto's Thyroiditis

Hashimoto's thyroiditis, also known as chronic lymphocytic thyroiditis, is the most common form of thyroiditis. The disease occurs almost exclusively in women, usually in middle age. The thyroid gland is involved with a lymphocytic infiltration that eventually results in a fibrotic gland. Nodules may be present, and some patients develop local symptoms of compression. Usually, however, patients have no local symptoms and lack the thyroid tenderness that is characteristic of subacute thyroiditis. Antithyroid antibodies can be detected in the serum of patients with Hashimoto's thyroiditis. Antimicrosomal and antithyroglobulin antibodies are usually measured. Treatment involves supplementation with thyroxine. Surgery is rarely indicated and is reserved for patients with local compression or in cases in which malignancy is suspected.

Subacute Thyroiditis

Subacute thyroiditis is characterized by a tender swelling of the thyroid that usually lasts for 2 to 4 months. The initial presentation may be associated with hyperthyroidism. Treatment during this stage of the disease relies on nonsteroidal antiinflammatory drugs to treat local symptoms. Steroids have been used but may be associated with a protracted course. Several months following initial presentation, patients may develop hypothyroidism. The disease is characterized by recurrence but is usually self-limited. Surgery is rarely indicated, and patients are treated with thyroid replacement.

Goiter

Goiter is a term commonly used to refer to a benign enlargement of the thyroid gland. Goiters can be diffuse or multinodular. Iodine deficiency has been shown to cause goiters. These patients also demonstrate an elevated TSH that is likely to be the etiology of thyroid enlargement in this condition. However, iodine deficiency is a rare cause of goiter in the United States today, although there are areas of the world that are endemic for goiter. The etiology of goiters is multifactorial and probably involves genetic influences and environmental exposures to goitrogens. In most cases, thyroid function is normal, and there is little to be gained from treatment with thyroxine.

Goiters often cause symptoms from local compression. These large glands concentrate iodine poorly as compared to their size. Therefore, RAI is not effective in treating goiters that occur in the euthyroid setting. Surgical resection is indicated in most cases because of local compression. Malignancy may also be a consideration, particularly with nodular goiter. Total or subtotal thyroidectomy through a Kocher collar incision is effective in relieving symptoms. However, with long-term follow-up, subtotal thyroidectomy has been shown to have a recurrence rate of 40% to 50%.[23] A more extensive thyroidectomy has been reported to result in a lower recurrence rate,[24] thus avoiding the increased morbidity of reoperative surgery.

Substernal goiters deserve special mention. These goiters can cause problems by local compression of mediastinal structures.[25,26] Patients may present with engorged neck veins caused by venous compression. Airway obstruction and difficulty swallowing are common symptoms that are often exacerbated by recumbency. Mechanical trauma to the recurrent laryngeal nerve or sympathetic chain can cause hoarseness or Horner's syndrome, respectively. The mediastinal location of the goiter precludes diagnostic evaluation with fine-needle aspiration (FNA). The optimal treatment of substernal goiters is surgical removal.[27,28] In most instances, substernal goiters can be removed through cervical incisions.[25–28] However, primary intrathoracic goiters that have no cervical component require a median sternotomy. Postoperatively, patients should be treated with thyroid hormone replacement.

Evaluation of the Thyroid Nodule

Thyroid nodules are common in the general population, and their occurrence increases with age.[29] Most thyroid cancers present as a thyroid nodule in patients who have normal

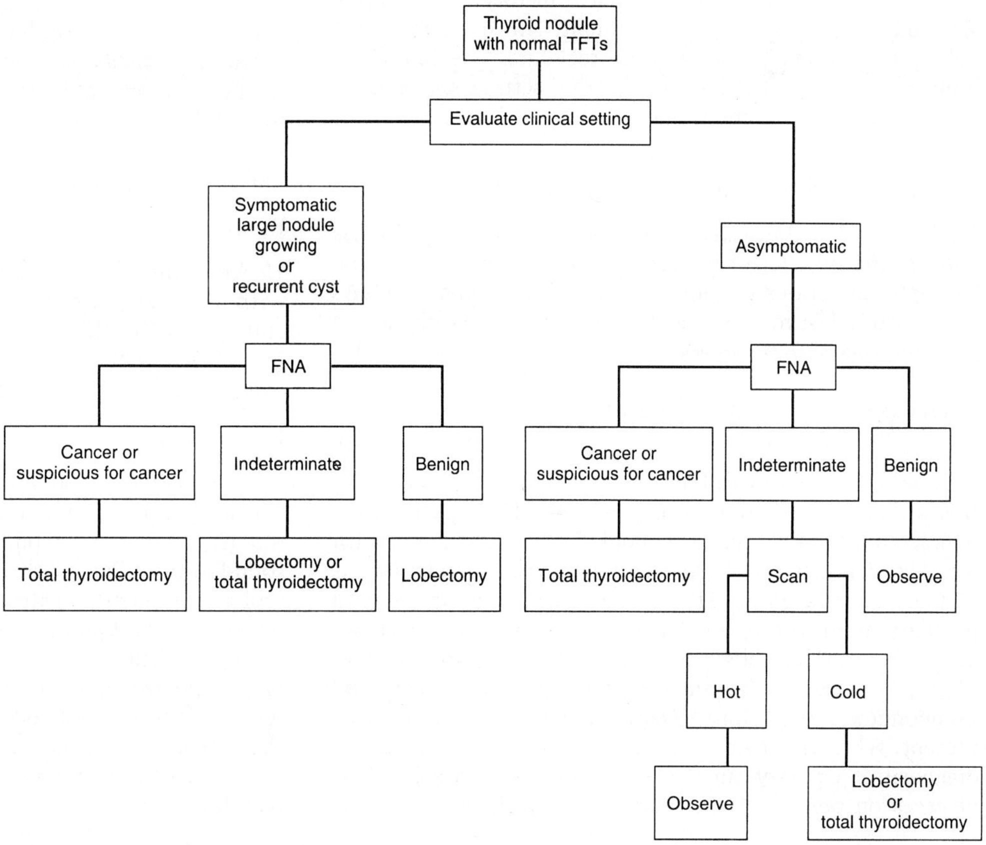

FIGURE 56.4. Flow diagram for evaluation of thyroid nodule in patients with normal thyroid function tests (TFTs).

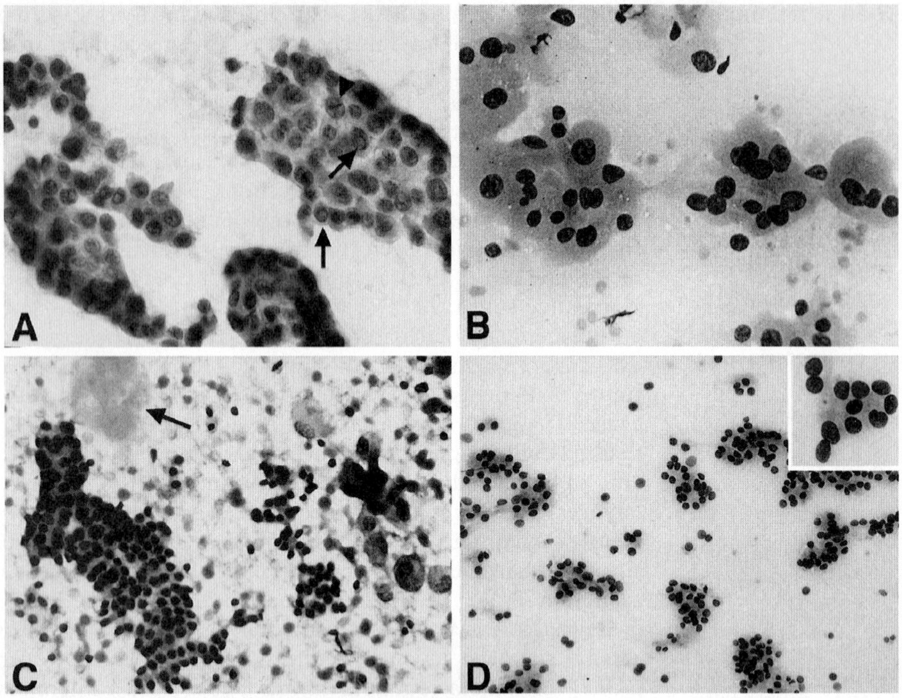

FIGURE 56.5. Fine-needle aspiration (FNA) of thyroid nodules. **A.** Papillary thyroid carcinoma with classic features of pseudonuclear inclusions (*arrow*) and nuclear grooves (*arrowhead*). **B.** Hürthle cell neoplasm with enlarged cells demonstrating large nucleus with prominent nucleoli and granular cytoplasm. **C.** Benign thyroid aspirate shows sheets of benign follicular cells, colloid (*arrow*), multinucleated giant cells, and macrophages. **D.** Indeterminate FNA with microfollicular neoplasm shows repetitive microfollicles (see *inset*).

thyroid function. Figure 56.4 outlines one approach to the evaluation of thyroid nodules. Determining the clinical setting is the first step of evaluation. The treatment of asymptomatic nodules is largely dependent upon the results of FNA.[29,30] The use of radioiodine scan has limited value in the evaluation of thyroid nodules.[29–31] Nodules that are symptomatic, causing difficulty swallowing or breathing, usually require surgery. The occurrences of large nodules (>5 cm), recurrent cysts, or nodules with a clear history of growth are also indications for surgical treatment. However, FNA can help guide the choice of surgical procedure. The finding of lymphoma or anaplastic cancer in this setting also significantly alters the treatment plan.

Fine-Needle Aspiration

Most thyroid nodules are benign, and the use of FNA has reduced the number of patients requiring surgical excision. Examples of various cytological findings from thyroid FNAs are shown in Figure 56.5. Results from FNA can be characterized into one of four categories.[29,30]

Papillary Cancer or Suspicious for Papillary Cancer

A number of cytological criteria are present in papillary thyroid cancer (PTC) (see Fig. 56.5A). The specimen is hypercellular with minimal colloid. Colloid associated with papillary cancer has a dense appearance and is referred to as "bubble gum" colloid. The cells may form groups with a papillary architecture, although the vascular core is classically absent. The cells demonstrate large squamoid cytoplasm, and nuclear features include nuclear grooves and pseudonuclear inclusions. Psammoma bodies may also be present. When the majority of these features are present, the diagnosis of papillary cancer is made and is confirmed in 98% of cases on permanent sections.[32] A suspicious FNA lacks several classic features and has a 50% to 75% chance of papillary cancer.[32]

Indeterminate

The finding of indeterminate FNA refers to follicular neoplasms (see Fig. 56.5D) that are either follicular adenoma (FA) or follicular thyroid carcinoma (FTC). Hürthle cell neoplasms are also included in this category (see Fig. 56.5B). The distinction between the benign and malignant entities requires the determination of vascular or capsular invasion, features that cannot be reliably determined by FNA. FNA results of these nodules demonstrate a hypercellular aspirate with a repetitive microfollicular pattern of a predominant single cell type. Approximately 20% of indeterminate FNAs are found to be malignant on permanent section.[33]

Benign

FNA of benign thyroid nodules demonstrates abundant colloid with a mixed cell type including sheets of benign follicular epithelium, Hürthle cells, macrophages, or lymphocytes (see Fig. 56.5C). The chance that a thyroid cancer will yield a benign result on FNA is approximately 4%.[32,33]

Inadequate

The category designated inadequate indicates a poor aspirate and should be repeated. Usual findings are hypocellular specimens, often with blood. The use of high-resolution ultrasound to guide FNA of thyroid lesion has proven to be a useful tool to complement palpation-guided FNA. Ultrasound FNA (USFNA) is particularly useful for the evaluation of nonpalpable or difficult-to-palpate nodules, for previously failed FNA, and for incidentally identified nodules. In a recent review of 497 thyroid nodules, USFNA was shown to decrease the incidence of inadequate biopsies and to provide a higher incidence of correct cancer diagnosis on significantly smaller nodules.[34]

Frozen-Section Evaluation of Thyroid Nodules

There is some debate as to the role of frozen-section evaluation at the time of surgery to aid in determining the extent of operation. This discussion assumes that most surgeons would treat benign lesions with lobectomy and malignant lesions with total or near-total thyroidectomy (see following discussion). Most studies agree that when a FNA result is diagnostic for papillary cancer, a definitive cancer operation can be performed without the need for frozen-section confirmation.[35–37] However, indeterminate FNA of follicular neoplasms poses a particular dilemma. Several studies have reported that frozen-section diagnosis of follicular lesions was not helpful and in some cases was misleading.[38–42] Some studies recommend the use of clinical parameters to aid in decisions regarding definitive resection. In patients more than 50 years of age[43] or if nodules are larger than 4 cm,[44] the occurrence of malignancy is increased. However, some investigators have advocated the use of frozen section in this setting, concluding that frozen section can reliably discriminate benign from malignant follicular lesions. One study from the Mayo Clinic of 1023 patients reported that sensitivity, specificity, positive predictive value, negative predictive value, and accuracy for frozen section diagnosis of malignant follicular lesions were 78%, 99%, 90%, and 98%, respectively.[45] Other studies have not been able to replicate these excellent results and recommend that permanent section be obtained before performing definitive resection.[38,40]

Thyroid Cancer

There are approximately 17,000 new cases of thyroid cancer annually in the United States.[46] However, the annual mortality from thyroid malignancies is only 1,200, indicating that most patients with thyroid cancer have an excellent prognosis. The male-to-female ratio of thyroid cancer incidence is 1:2.7, but the ratio of cancer-associated mortality is 1:2, indicating that the tumors may be slightly more aggressive in men. Table 56.2 summarizes the common histological types of thyroid malignancies, and Figure 56.6 illustrates their histological findings. The majority of thyroid cancers are well-differentiated tumors that are derived from thyroid follicular epithelium. Anaplastic cancer is also derived from follicular epithelial cells and may represent a more malignant transformation of well-differentiated tumors. Medullary thyroid cancer (MTC) is derived from the calcitonin-secreting C-cells or parafollicular cells of the thyroid. Thyroid lymphomas and metastases to the thyroid account for 5% to 6% of thyroid malignancies.

TABLE 56.2. Types of Thyroid Cancers.

Tumor histology	*Incidence (%)*
Well-differentiated	85
Papillary (80%–90%) (papillary and follicular variant)	
Follicular (10%–20%) (micro- and macroinvasion, Hürthle)	
Medullary	6–8
Anaplastic	2–4
Lymphoma	4–5
Metastatic	<1

Radiation-Associated Thyroid Cancer

Ionizing radiation exposure increases the incidence of benign and malignant thyroid nodules. Most of the radiation-induced thyroid malignancies are PTC. Laboratory studies have demonstrated thyroid-induced malignancies in rats exposed to ionizing radiation that can be increased in the setting of elevated TSH.[47] Radiation exposures in humans have resulted in an increased incidence of thyroid cancer caused by radiation from medical treatment for benign and malignant conditions or by exposures from nuclear weapons or nuclear reactor accidents.[48] A study of 1,787 patients, of whom 1,730 received radiotherapy for Hodgkin's disease, demonstrated a 20-fold increase in Graves' disease and a 16-fold increase in thyroid cancer compared to expected risk.[49] A study of 2,657 infants irradiated for a purported enlarged thymus demonstrated a linear dose–response relationship with a relative risk for thyroid cancer of 10 times normal at a dose of 1 Gy.[50] Thyroid cancer rates were also found to be elevated for low-dose exposure in the range of 0 to 0.3 Gy. In addition, there was noted to be an increased risk of thyroid cancer even so long as 45 years after exposure. The risk of thyroid cancer and radiation exposure is also dependent upon age of exposure, with an increased risk with exposure at an earlier age. In a study of 10,834 children in Israel who received radiotherapy to the scalp for ringworm, there was a fourfold increase in the incidence of malignant thyroid tumors with exposures of 9 cGy compared to a matched population.[51] These studies also demonstrated an age association, with children exposed when younger than 5 years being more likely to develop tumors than older children. Increased incidence of thyroid malignancies has also been reported from exposures resulting from nuclear detonations. The most significant exposures from atomic bomb explosions are from the Hiroshima and Nagasaki detonations in 1945 and nuclear tests in the Marshall Islands in 1954 and at the Nevada test site in the mid-1950s.[48,52]

Internal radiation exposure, usually in the form of iodine radioisotopes, may also be an etiological factor in thyroid carcinomas. Animal models have demonstrated the occurrence of thyroid tumors in rats exposed to ^{131}I under conditions designed to elevate TSH.[53] The best evidence for internal radiation-associated cancers in humans derives from exposures caused by nuclear fallout containing short-lived iodine isotopes. Significant increases in thyroid cancer has been reported as a result of the Chernobyl nuclear disaster in 1986.[48] Particularly interesting is the rapid increase of thyroid malignancies, which were noted as early as 3 years after exposure. The short-lived iodine isotopes of ^{132}I, ^{133}I, and ^{135}I have been implicated in these malignancies. There is considerable debate as to whether exposure to ^{131}I in doses commonly used to treat Graves' disease is associated with an increased incidence of thyroid malignancy.[54–56] The natural history of thyroid cancer occurring after ^{131}I therapy appears to be identical to that of sporadic cancers.[57]

Molecular Genetics of Thyroid Cancer

One of the earliest observations indicating a genetic basis for thyroid cancer was the recognition of the association between

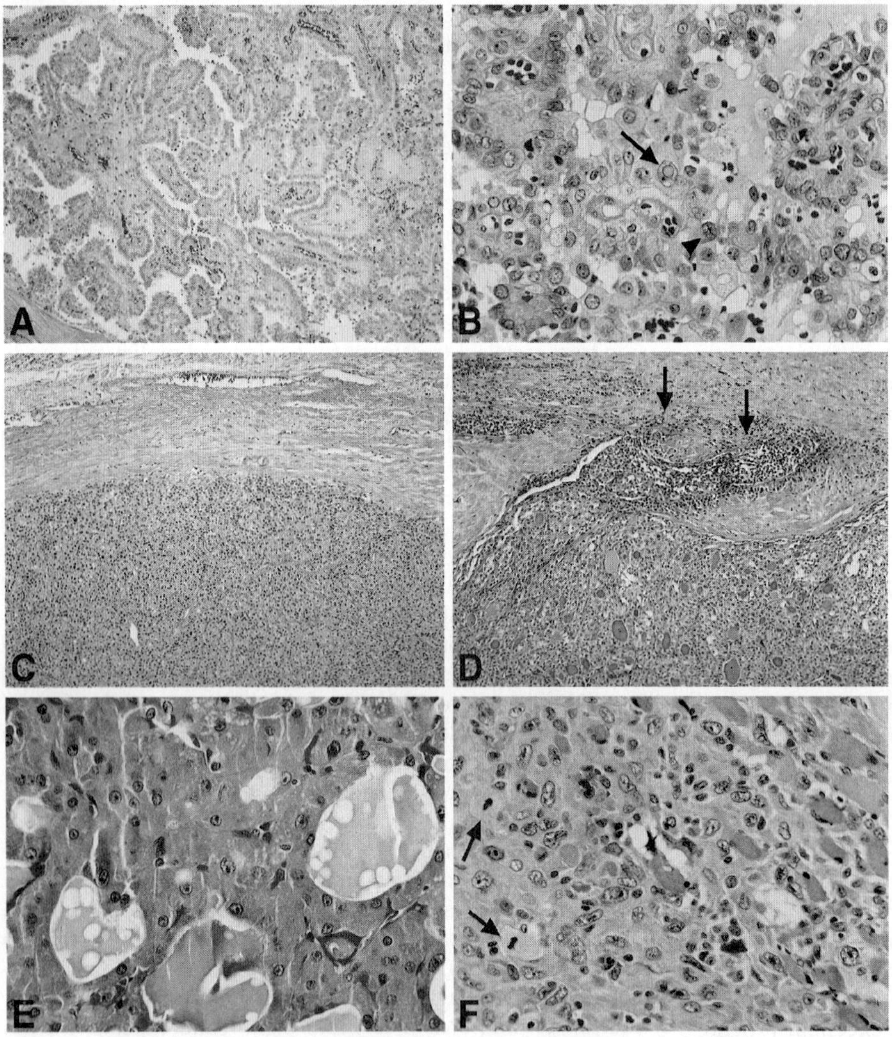

FIGURE 56.6. Common histology of thyroid neoplasms. **A.** Papillary thyroid carcinoma showing common papillary architecture. **B.** Nuclear features of papillary thyroid carcinoma with pseudonuclear inclusions and nuclear grooves (*arrow*). Nuclei show nuclear clearing with molding of adjacent nuclei. **C.** Follicular adenoma demonstrating capsule. **D.** Follicular carcinoma demonstrating capsular invasion (*arrows*). **E.** Hürthle cell neoplasm. **F.** Anaplastic carcinoma with invasion in muscle shows numerous mitotic figures (*arrow*).

familial adenomatous polyposis (FAP) and the development of PTC.[58] Inheritance of a mutation of the adenomatous polyposis coli (APC) gene results in predisposition to FAP. The increased incidence of PTC in FAP patients implies a role for APC mutations in thyroid oncogenesis. The APC gene is expressed in normal and malignant thyroid tissues. In a study of 80 thyroid neoplasms, loss of heterozygosity (LOH) of the APC locus was detected in only two benign thyroid nodules.[59] Mutation and allelic loss were also demonstrated in two anaplastic carcinoma cell lines. Although this study did not suggest a role for APC in sporadic thyroid carcinomas, it would be interesting to examine LOH of the APC locus in thyroid cancers arising in FAP patients to determine if a higher rate of LOH occurs in this setting compared to sporadic PTC.

There is a familial form of PTC that occurs independent of FAP. As with other familial cancers, these tumors demonstrate vertical transmission in consecutive generations.[60] Although the cancers do not appear to occur at an earlier age, they are more often multifocal and bilateral. The gene responsible for familial PTC has not been identified but has been localized to chromosome 2q21.[61]

The *ret* proto-oncogene is a receptor tyrosine kinase that has been identified as the gene responsible for inheritance of multiple endocrine neoplasia (MEN)2A, MEN2B, and familial MTC.[62–64] Ret mutations in MEN2A and familial MTC target one of five cysteine residues in the extracellular domain, and mutation of Cys634 to Arg carries a greater risk of parathyroid hyperplasia.[65] In MEN2B, mutations are targeted to the tyrosine kinase catalytic domain of the protein.[64]

Ret mutations have also been examined in PTC.[66] Three chromosomal rearrangements have been reported between *ret* and one of three loci designated PTC1, PTC2, and PTC3.[67–70] These rearrangements result in overexpression of ret chimeric proteins. There is evidence that oligomerization by virtue of a coiled-coil domain in the fusion protein results in *ret* proto-oncogene activation.[68] The expression of ret fusion proteins has been observed in approximately 30% of PTC tumors.[70] Other chromosomal abnormalities have been consistently observed in thyroid cancers.[71] Most extensively reported are chromosomal translocations involving 19q13[72,73] and LOH of 3p[74] in FTC. The 19q13 translocation has also been described in FAP, indicating that a gene at this locus may be involved in early steps of oncogenesis in FTC.[73]

N-*ras* activation has been examined in thyroid cancer.[74,75] In a study of 91 PTC tumors, N-*ras* activation was demonstrated in 4.8% of class I, 4.5% of class II, 15.8% of class III, and 27.8% of class IV carcinomas.[75] In all tumors, activation involved a missense mutation at codon 61. N-*ras* activation was also shown to be an independent prognostic factor for increased mortality. Other data, however, have suggested a role for *ras* activation in early thyroid tumorigenesis.[76] These data suggest that thyroid carcinomas with *ras* mutations may have a different clinical phenotype than tumors developing independent of the *ras* pathway.

The p53 tumor suppressor gene is targeted in many different human malignancies. In a study of 57 well-differentiated thyroid cancers, p53 overexpression was found in 7 (12%) of these tumors.[77] Overexpression was confirmed to be caused by a p53 point mutation in exon 8. All patients with tumors overexpressing p53 had metastatic disease or dedifferentiated tumors. A study of anaplastic cancers occurring within PTC demonstrated p53 overexpression in 50% of the anaplastic components but was not found in the adjacent PTC components.[78] Clinical studies have demonstrated that p53 overexpression is an independent prognostic factor for survival of patients with thyroid cancer.[79] These studies support the hypothesis that p53 mutation in thyroid cancer plays a role in progression to a more aggressive phenotype.

Well-Differentiated Thyroid Cancer

Papillary thyroid cancer (PTC) accounts for 80% to 90% of well-differentiated thyroid cancers. Within the past decade, it has become recognized that there is a follicular variant of papillary cancer that lacks the normal papillary architecture. The follicular variant is recognized by cytological features shared with other PTC, and the clinical course of this tumor is consistent with the papillary phenotype.[80] Occult papillary carcinoma (OPC) of the thyroid has been reported in a significant percentage of the population. OPC has histological features that are indistinguishable from clinically evident PTC; however, OPC is less than 10mm and is generally considered to be a benign entity because it is found incidentally in thyroid specimens or at autopsy in approximately 20% of the general population.[81] However, some studies have reported deaths resulting from lesions that otherwise would have been considered OPC.[82]

Extent of Surgery

There has been long-standing controversy concerning the appropriate extent of surgical resection for well-differentiated thyroid cancer.[83,84] Studies examining the outcome of thyroidectomy for patients with thyroid cancer are all retrospective. The relatively good prognosis for thyroid cancer patients makes it difficult to design a prospective trial. To detect a modest (10%) improvement in mortality comparing treatment groups would require enrollment of a minimum of 8000 patients who would need to be followed for three decades.[85] Therefore, treatment decisions have been based upon retrospective evaluations of patients who in many cases have had varied treatment regimens. Several earlier reviews have addressed the arguments for lobectomy versus total thyroidectomy.[83,84]

Proponents of Less Than Total Thyroidectomy

Several recent series have provided an argument for limited resections for thyroid carcinoma. These studies are summarized in Table 56.3. The basis for this position is that there is insignificant improvement of recurrence or mortality to

TABLE 56.3.
Proponents Supporting Less Than Total Thyroidectomy (Level II Evidence).

Authors	*Total patients*	*Risk stratification (basis)*	*Mean follow-up (years)*	*Outcome*	*Conclusions*
Nguyen and Dilawari 1995[92]	155	(AMES) 141 low	9	Mortality TT vs. <TT; 2.3% vs. 1.85% (NS)	For low-risk patients, conservative resection is adequate
Shaha et al.1997[93]	1,038	(AMES) 465 low	20	Local recurrence, Lob vs. <Lob; 27% vs. 4% (*P* = 0.005) Local recurrence, TT vs. Lob; 1% vs. 4% (*P* = 0.1) Overall failure, TT vs. Lob; 8% vs. 13% (*P* = 0.06)	Avoid less than lobectomy; for low-risk patients, no advantage in recurrence or survival for total thyroidectomy vs. lobectomy
Sanders and Cady 1988[94]	1,019	(AMES) 790 low	13	Recurrence TT vs. Lob: Low risk; 5% vs. 5% High risk; 29% vs. 34% (NS)	For low-risk (AMES) patients, lobectomy is adequate
Wanebo et al.1998[95]	347	(AGE) 216 low, 103 intermediate, 28 high		10-year mortality TT vs. Lob: Low; 16.5% vs. 12.4% (NS) Intermediate; 75.4% vs. 33.5 (NS) High; 65% vs. 20% (NS)	No benefit of total thyroidectomy in any risk group
Kim et al.[96] 2004[1]	727	(AMES)	14.5	Survival, TT vs. Lob; No survival in low-risk group advantage in 100% vs. 97% at 20 years low-risk group	

AMES, age, metastasis, extent, size; TT, total thyroidectomy; Lob, lobectomy; NS, not significant.

justify the potential risk of recurrent laryngeal nerve injury or permanent hypoparathyroidism for performing more than a lobectomy in most cases. The reported incidence of recurrent nerve injury (0%–7%) and permanent hypoparathyroidism (0%–8%) varies with the extent of operation, the history of previous neck surgery, and the experience and training of the surgeon.[83,86–90] The majority of studies advocating lobectomy have focused on the low-risk group [based upon AMES (age, metastasis, extent, size) criteria].[91] For low-risk patients, lobectomy appears to be adequate.[92–96] The study by Shaha et al.[93] reported a significant improvement in outcome for lobectomy compared to lesser procedures. There was no significant improvement in recurrence or mortality comparing lobectomy with total thyroidectomy. However, there was a trend for better outcome with total thyroidectomy, and a larger series may have reached statistical significance. The study by Wanebo et al.[95] stratified patients by risk based on age. These data were striking in that no differences were observed comparing extent of surgery in any risk group. However, the small number of patients in the high-risk group weakens this argument. The study by Kim et al.[96] found no difference in outcome in the low-risk group, but older patients had a survival benefit with total thyroidectomy.

Proponents of Total Thyroidectomy

A number of considerations argue in favor of treating thyroid cancer patients with a total thyroidectomy. First, patients with thyroid cancer are usually treated with thyroid hormone replacement to suppress TSH, so there is no functional reason to preserve a thyroid lobe. Second, thyroid cancer is multifocal in 10% to 30% of cases, and resecting the contralateral lobe removes foci of cancer that might otherwise metastasize. It has been shown that cancer multifocality in a resected lobe predicts the occurrence of cancer in the contralateral lobe.[97] Third, total thyroidectomy facilitates treatment with radioactive iodine (RAI) because it removes normal thyroid tissue that would take up iodine and also allows treatment under a hypothyroid protocol. Fourth, patients treated with total thyroidectomy and RAI often have undetectable or very low thyroglobulin (Tg) levels, thus facilitating the use of this test as a screen for recurrence. Fifth, there is evidence that total thyroidectomy results in fewer recurrences and less mortality compared to lesser procedures. Table 56.4 summarizes the results of recent retrospective studies[98–101] that have demonstrated favorable outcome with more extensive surgery. The study by Degroot et al.[98] demonstrated improved recurrence and survival for tumors greater than 1 cm with near-total or total thyroidectomy compared to lesser resections. Samaan et al.[99] showed a significant improvement in mortality with more extensive surgical resection in patients not treated with RAI. In the study by Mazzaferri and Jhiang,[100] near-total or total thyroidectomy resulted in improved 30-year recurrence and survival compared to lesser resections in patients with class II and III tumors. These data (Fig. 56.7) demonstrate improved survival for all time points after initial resection. Although Kim et al.[96] showed that the extent of surgery had no effect in low-risk paients, older patients had a survival advantage with total thyroidectomy. Given the low complication rate for thyroidectomy among most endocrine surgeons, total thyroidectomy has been advocated as the treatment of choice for well-differentiated thyroid cancer.[102]

Radioactive Iodine

RAI has been successfully used for many years to ablate normal thyroid remnants and residual carcinoma following

TABLE 56.4.
Proponents Supporting Total Thyroidectomy (Level II Evidence).

Authors	*Total patients*	*Risk stratification (basis)*	*Mean follow-up (years)*	*Outcome*	*Conclusions*
DeGroot et al. 1990[98]	269	I: 128, II: 89, III: 29, IV: 20 (class)	12	Recurrence TT/NT vs. ST/Lob; ($P < 0.016$) 20-year mortality TT/NT vs. ST/Lob; 10% vs. 20% ($P < 0.004$) (tumors >1.0 cm)	Decreased risk of recurrence for TT/NT vs. ST/Lob Decreased mortality for tumors >1.0 cm for TT/NT vs. ST/Lob
Samaan et al. 1992[99]	1,599	I: 670, II: 563, III: 271, IV: 95 (class)	11	Mortality TT vs. Lob vs. <Lob; 9% vs. 15% vs. 19% ($P < 0.003$)	In patients not receiving RAI, decreased recurrence and mortality for TT Trend for improved outcome with TT for patients receiving RAI
Mazzafferi and Jhiang 1994[100]	1,355	I: 170, II: 948, III: 204, IV: 33 (class)	15.7	30-year recurrence (class II, III) TT vs. Lob; 26% vs. 40% ($P < 0.002$) 30-year mortality TT vs. Lob; 6% vs. 9% ($P = 0.02$)	Total thyroidectomy results in lower recurrence and mortality compared to lesser resections
Loh et al. 1997[101]	700	I: 516, II: 57, III: 104, IV: 23 (TNM)	11.3	10-year recurrence TT vs. Lob; 23% vs. 46% ($P < 0.0001$) 10-year mortality TT vs. Lob; 5% vs. 11% ($P < 0.01$)	Patients undergoing less than total thyroidectomy had higher recurrence and mortality
Kim et al.[96] 2004[1]	727	(AMES)	14.5	Survival TT vs. Lob; at 20 years in older patients 55% vs. 25%	Improved survival for older patients treated with TT

TT, total thyroidectomy; Lob, lobectomy; ST/Lob, subtotal thyroid lobectomy; NT, near-total thyoidectomy; RAI, radioactive iodine.

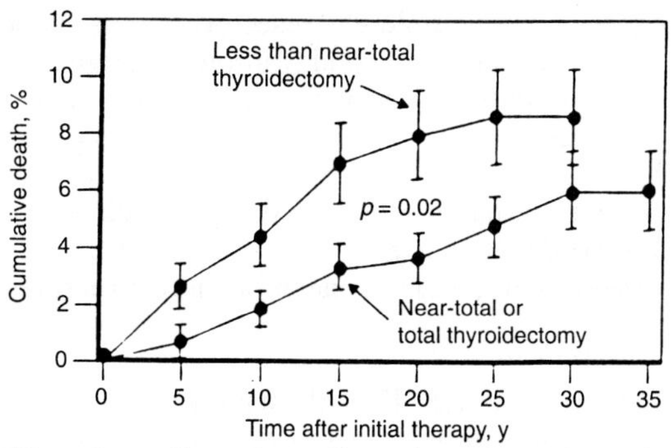

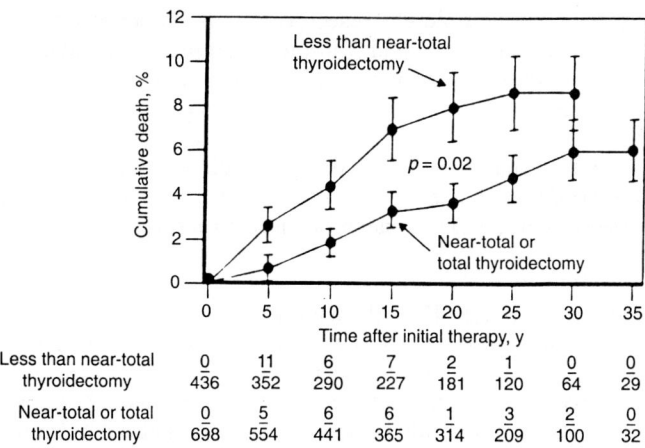

	0	5	10	15	20	25	30	35
Less than near-total thyroidectomy	0/436	11/352	6/290	7/227	2/181	1/120	0/64	0/29
Near-total or total thyroidectomy	0/698	5/554	6/441	6/365	1/314	3/209	2/100	0/32

FIGURE 56.7. Cancer deaths for well-differentiated thyroid cancer comparing near-total or total thyroidectomy with lesser resections. (From Mazzaferri and Jhiang,[100] with permission.)

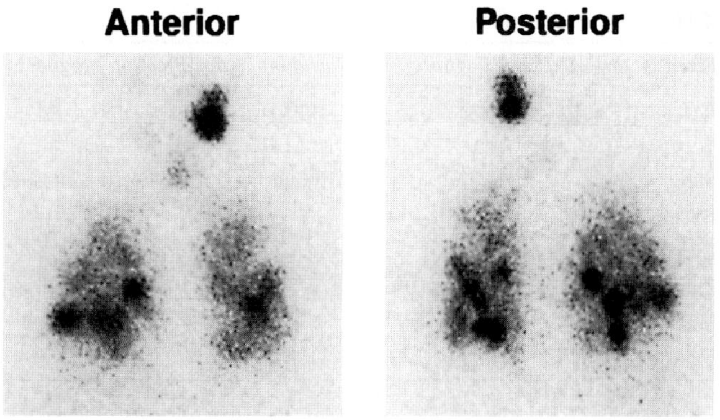

FIGURE 56.8. Metastatic papillary thyroid carcinoma detected by ^{131}I scan. Diffuse pulmonary metastases are noted with foci of lymph node metastases in the left neck.

surgical resection. The usual protocol after thyroidectomy withholds thyroid hormone replacement for 4 to 6 weeks to induce a hypothyroid state. The elevation in TSH stimulates iodine uptake in residual thyroid tissue and thyroid carcinoma. In the face of elevated TSH, an increase in Tg levels is also usually evident. Often a test dose of 2 mCi ^{131}I is administered and the uptake used to estimate the therapeutic dose of ^{131}I. There has been some debate as to whether a test dose of ^{131}I "stuns" the tumor cells, thereby decreasing effectiveness of the therapy dose.[103,104] Usual therapy doses employed are in the range of 50 to 200 mCi. Although some authors advocate the empiric treatment of thyroid cancer patients even in the absence of uptake,[105] other physicians elect not to treat patients in the absence of uptake on thyroid scan.[106]

There is evidence that the ability to ablate the thyroid remnant is dependent on the extent of surgical resection. Several studies have demonstrated increased success of ablation following total thyroidectomy as compared to subtotal resections.[107,108] Some recent attempts have been made to ablate an entire lobe in a patient treated by lobectomy.[109] RAI is also commonly employed to treat distant metastases. An example of a patient with pulmonary metastases detected with radioiodine scan is shown in Figure 56.8. Treatment of pulmonary metastases is more effective than bone metastases.[110] The rates of complications from RAI treatment, which include radiation thyroiditis, chronic sialoadenitis, odynophagia, and facial edema, are low. Complication rates and the need for repeated treatments are higher with less extensive surgery.[109–111] RAI does not appear to have adverse effects on female fertility,[112] but at least one study indicated an association with transient impairment of testicular function.[113]

A number of retrospective studies have reported improved recurrence and survival rates for patients treated with RAI.[99,100,114] Samaan et al.[99] identified RAI treatment as the single most significant indicator of improved recurrence and survival. Similarly, Mazzaferri and Jhiang[100] reported improved recurrence and survival in patients treated with RAI. These results are even more impressive when one considers that patients selected for ^{131}I treatment had more aggressive tumors with a higher predicted recurrence and mortality (Fig. 56.9). However, some studies have failed to demonstrate a benefit for patients without evidence of locoregional[115] or distant[96,116]spread. A recent study by Morris et al.[116] demonstrated a trend for improved survival with RAI

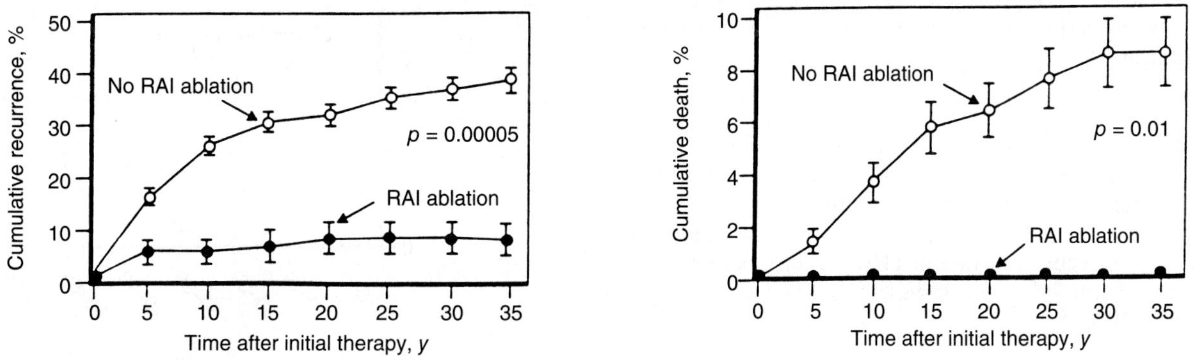

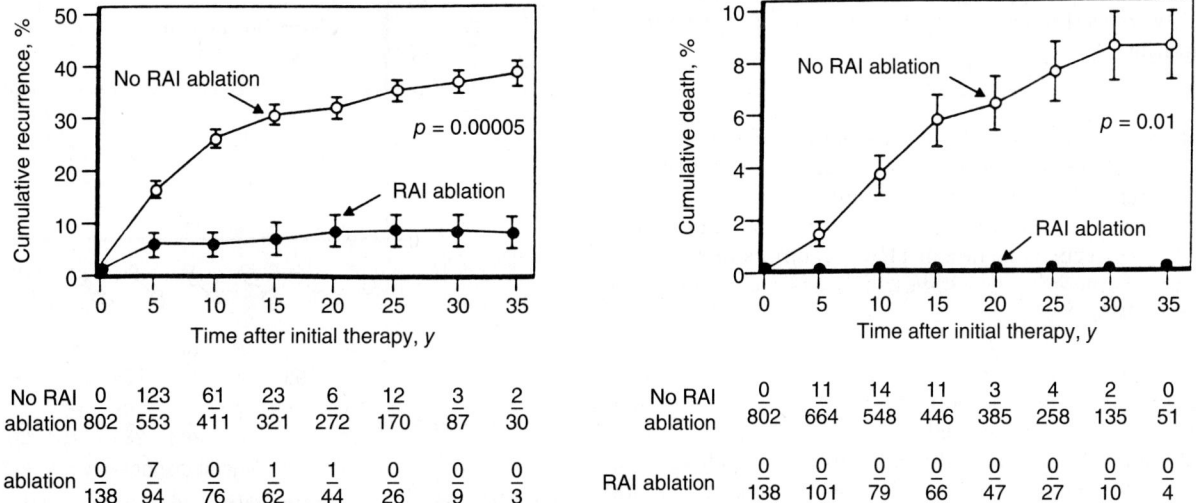

	0	5	10	15	20	25	30	35
No RAI ablation	0/802	123/553	61/411	23/321	6/272	12/170	3/87	2/30
RAI ablation	0/138	7/94	0/76	1/62	1/44	0/26	0/9	0/3

	0	5	10	15	20	25	30	35
No RAI ablation	0/802	11/664	14/548	11/446	3/385	4/258	2/135	0/51
RAI ablation	0/138	0/101	0/79	0/66	0/47	0/27	0/10	0/4

FIGURE 56.9. Cancer recurrence and mortality comparing patients treated with ^{131}I radioiodine (*RAI*) ablation and those without RAI ablation. (From Mazzaferri and Jhiang,[100] with permission.)

TABLE 56.5. Prognosis.

Fixed factors affecting prognosis	*Variable factors affecting prognosis*
Age of patient	Extent of thyroidectomy
Clinical stage of primary	Use of RAI
Size	Time from diagnosis to treatment
Extension	
Lymph node metastasis	
Distant metastasis	
Histology	
Gender	

in patients with disease confined to the neck, but these data failed to reach statistical significance.

The use of recombinant human TSH (rhTSH) has been investigated as an alternate protocol in preparation for RAI treatment.[117,118] Patients treated with rhTSH demonstrate similar physiological response with respect to Tg stimulation and increased iodine uptake compared to treatment with thyroxine withdrawal.[117] Although rhTSH avoids the symptoms of hypothyroidism, this protocol is less sensitive in the detection of residual disease than withdrawal of thyroid hormone.[118]

Prognosis of Well-Differentiated Thyroid Cancer

A number of variables that have been shown to influence prognosis for well-differentiated thyroid cancer are listed in Table 56.5. Fixed characteristics are based on clinical parameters that are present at the time of diagnosis. Variable characteristics can be influenced by treatment and may give clinicians an opportunity to improve outcomes in patients.

Age

Age of a patient at diagnosis has a profound effect on prognosis in well-differentiated thyroid cancer.[91,95,98,100] Some series have demonstrated that age is the single most significant variable affecting mortality.[91,95] Interestingly, recurrence has a bimodal distribution with age (Fig. 56.10). Although recurrence rates are higher in younger patients, mortality remains relatively low.[100,119] By contrast, recurrence in patients over the age of 45 is a poor prognostic indicator, and overall mortality rates increase linearly with age of patients at presentation.

Size

Size of the primary tumor is an important prognostic criterion.[98,100,101] There is a nearly linear increase in mortality with the diameter of the primary tumor at presentation.[100] Tumors less than 1 to 1.5 cm have negligible cancer-related mortality and a 30-year recurrence rate of 11%.[100] Tumors more than 3 to 4 cm in diameter have a 30-year disease-specific mortality of 20% to 30%.[98,100]

Extent of Tumor Invasion

Extrathyroidal tumor invasion carries a worse prognosis than tumors that are intrathyroidal or have minor capsular invasion. Tumors that invade adjacent structures such as strap muscles or trachea are associated with high recurrence and mortality.[91,98,100,101] Related to the extent of invasion is the ability to completely excise the tumor. As may be expected, inability to completely resect tumor is associated with a worse outcome,[98,120] and completely resecting disease can improve outcome even in the presence of local invasion.[120] For this reason, locally invasive cancers should be resected as completely as possible. Strap muscles can be resected en bloc with minimal morbidity. Wedge or circumferential sleeve resections of the trachea or esophagus can be performed in cases of carcinoma invasion of these structures.[121–123]

Metastasis

Patients over age 45 with distant metastatic disease at presentation have 15-year and 30-year mortality rates of 50% to 65% and 65% to 70%, respectively.[98,100] Papillary cancer frequently metastasizes to lung, and this is exclusively the site of metastasis in children. Bone metastasis is also common in older patients and in patients with follicular cancer. Other less common sites of metastasis include brain and liver.[99]

Lymph node metastasis is common in well-differentiated thyroid cancer. However, lymph node involvement has a modest effect on prognosis. In patients with T1–T3 primary tumors, the 30-year mortality rates for patients with nodal involvement is 4% to 6% compared to 0% to 1% without nodal metastasis.[100,124] Nodal metastasis has been found to influence prognosis except in cases of T4 tumors (extrathyroidal invasion), supporting the role of lymphadenectomy as part of the initial surgical treatment.[124]

Histology

Many studies have demonstrated prognostic differences between papillary and follicular cancers.[125–127] The Mayo Clinic reported the 20-year cancer-specific mortality for FTC to be approximately 70% compared to 90% to 95% for papillary cancer.[127] FTC and Hürthle cell cancers tend to occur in older patients. However, at least one study that corrected for stage at presentation did not find FTC to have a worse prognosis compared to PTC.[100] FTCs with widely invasive and poorly differentiated histology have a worse prognosis than microinvasive FTCs.[127,128] Hürthle cell cancers have a prognosis similar to pure FTCs.[128] Hürthle cell tumors tend not to take up radioactive iodine as well as other FTCs, and this may

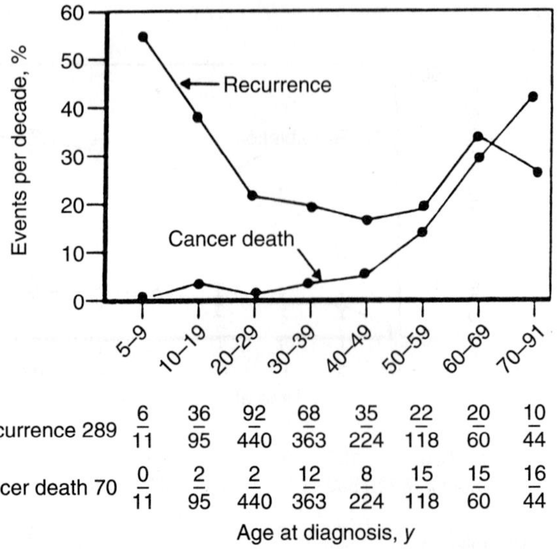

FIGURE 56.10. Recurrence rate and cancer death for well-differentiated thyroid cancer as a function of patient age at diagnosis. (From Mazzaferri and Jhiang,[100] with permission.)

account for differences in outcome in some series. Certain subtypes of papillary cancer demonstrate a propensity for local invasion and carry a worse prognosis, including tall cell, diffuse sclerosing, and oxyphilic variants.[129–131]

Gender

Women with well-differentiated thyroid cancer tend to demonstrate an improved prognosis compared to men.[100,132] The 30-year mortality for women and men with thyroid cancer was reported to be 7% and 11%, respectively ($P < 0.01$).[100] However, other large series have not demonstrated a significant difference.[98]

Treatment Variables

A number of retrospective studies have reported that treatment modalities can influence the prognosis of thyroid cancer. As noted earlier, extent of surgery and use of RAI have been reported to improve recurrence and mortality from thyroid cancer. Time from first recorded tumor manifestation to initial treatment has been reported to have a significant effect on outcome. In a study of 1355 patients, those who died of cancer had a mean delay of 18 months compared to 4 months for those who survived ($P < 0.001$).[100]

Tumor Staging

Based upon the variables determined to affect prognosis, several staging systems have been devised for thyroid cancer. The AMES (Age, Metastasis, Extent, Size)[91] and AGES (Age, Grade, Extent, Size)[133] systems use similar categories and have been shown to be predictive of high- and low-risk patients. Clinical class has been applied with good success and is based on tumor spread: class I, intrathyroidal disease; class II, lymph node metastases; class III, extrathyroidal invasion; class IV, distant metastases.[98] The TNM system[134] has been developed and can be used to assess tumor stage as shown in Table 56.6. The approximate 30-year mortality rates for stages I, II, III, and IV are 0% to 1%, 6%, 10% to 15%, and 65% to 80%, respectively.[98,100,135]

Follow-Up for Patients with Thyroid Cancer

After initial treatment for thyroid cancer, patients are followed for tumor recurrence at 6-month intervals for the first 3 years and yearly thereafter.[30] The plan for following patients is influenced by the suspicion of possible recurrence based on prognostic factors. Patients are usually treated with suppressive doses of thyroxine. The goal of thyroid suppression is to

TABLE 56.6. Definition of TMN, Stage Grouping, and Histopathologic Type for Thyroid Carcinoma.

Definition of TMN

Primary Tumor (T)

Note: All categories may be subdivided: (a) solitary tumor, (b) multifocal tumor (the largest determines the classification).

TX	Primary tumor cannot be assessed
T0	No evidence of primary tumor
T1	Tumor 2 cm or less in greatest dimension limited to the thyroid
T2	Tumor more than 2 cm but not more than 4 cm in greatest dimension limited to the thyroid
T3	Tumor more than 4 cm in greatest dimension limited to the thyroid or any tumor with minimal extrathyroid extension (e.g., extension to sternothyroid muscle or perithyroid soft tissues)
T4a	Tumor of any size extending beyond the thyroid capsule to invade subcutaneous soft tissues, larynx, trachea, esophagus, or recurrent laryngeal nerve
T4b	Tumor invades prevertebral fascia or encases carotid artery or mediastinal vessels

All anaplastic carcinomas are considered T4 tumors.

T4a	Intrathyroidal anaplastic carcinoma—surgically resectable
T4b	Extrathyroidal anaplastic carcinoma—surgically unresectable

Regional Lymph Nodes (N)

Regional lymph nodes are the central compartment, lateral cervical, and upper mediastinal lymph nodes.

NX	Regional lymph nodes cannot be assessed
N0	No regional lymph node metatasis
N1	Regional lymph nodal metastasis
N1a	Metastasis to level VI (pretracheal, paratracheal, and prelaryngeal/Delphian lymph nodes)
N1b	Metastasis to unilateral, bilateral, or contralateral cervical or superior mediastinal lymph nodes

Distant Metastasis (M)

MX	Distant metastasis cannot be assessed
M0	No distant metastasis
M1	Distant metastasis

Stage Grouping

Separate stage groupings are recommended for papillary of follicular, medullary, and anaplastic (undifferentiated) carcinoma.

	Papillary or Follicular		
	Under 45 years		
Stage I	Any T	Any N	M0
Stage II	Any T	Any N	M1
	Papillary or Follicular		
	45 years and older		
Stage I	T1	N0	M0
Stage II	T2	N0	M0
Stage III	T3	N0	M0
	T1	N1a	M0
	T2	N1a	M0
	T3	N1a	M0
Stage IVA	T4a	N0	M0
	T4a	N1a	M0
	T1	N1b	M0
	T2	N1b	M0
	T3	N1b	M0
	T4a	N1b	M0
Stage IVB	T4b	Any N	M0
Stage IVC	Any T	Any N	M1
	Medullary Carcinoma		
Stage I	T1	N0	M0
Stage II	T2	N0	M0
Stage III	T3	N0	M0
	T1	N1a	M0
	T2	N1a	M0
	T3	N1a	M0
Stage IVA	T4a	N0	M0
	T4a	N1a	M0
	T1	N1b	M0
	T2	N1b	M0
	T3	N1b	M0
	T4a	N1b	M0
Stage IVB	T4b	Any N	M0
Stage IVC	Any T	Any N	M1
	Anaplastic Carcinoma		
All anaplastic carcinomas are considered Stage IV			
Stage IVA	T4a	Any N	M0
Stage IVB	T4b	Any N	M0
Stage IVC	Any T	Any N	M1

Source: Used with the permission of the American Joint Committee on Cancer (AJCC), Chicago, Illinois. The original source for this material is the *AJCC Cancer Staging Manual, Sixth Edition* (2002) published by Springer Science and Business Media LLC, www.springerlink.com.

have TSH levels at the lower limit of normal or slightly below normal without signs or symptoms of hyperthyroidism. Thyroglobulin (Tg) levels are a useful means to detect tumor recurrence.[30,136,137] Tg is synthesized by normal thyroid cells and also by most well-differentiated cancers. Interpretation of Tg levels is simplified after total thyroidectomy and RAI ablation. Normally, Tg levels are undetectable after such treatment.[137] It is also important to check for the presence of antithyroglobulin antibodies that can falsely lower the measured Tg level.[136] In the setting of a rising Tg level, patients should have thyroid replacement withheld and a thyroid scan performed. As a general guideline, recurrences detected by scan alone can be treated with RAI. Recurrences that can be detected clinically by either physical examination or imaging [ultrasound, computed tomography (CT), or magnetic resonance imaging (MRI)] should undergo surgical resection followed by RAI.[138] It is important to obtain cytological confirmation of thyroid cancer before subjecting a patient to exploration. Ultrasound-guided biopsy is a particularly useful technique to confirm the presence of local recurrence.[34] Recent imaging modalities with real-time MRI using a split magnet have also been successful for biopsy of potential recurrence not accessible with ultrasound (Fig. 56.11).

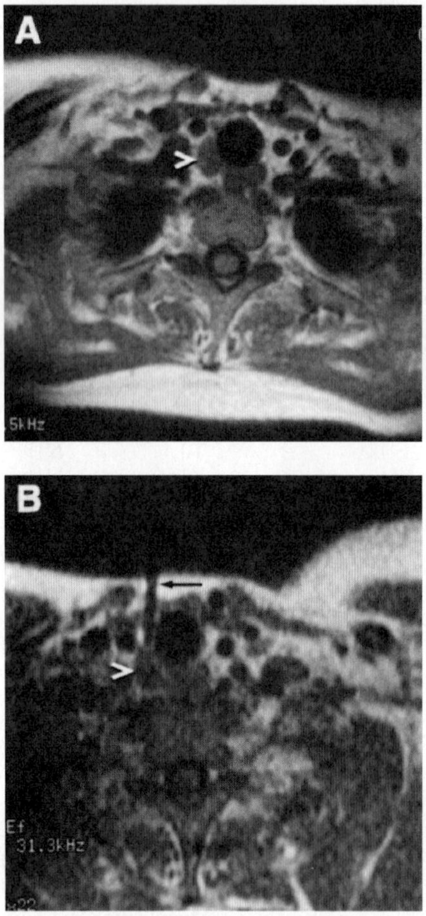

FIGURE 56.11. Biopsy of recurrent papillary cancer with real-time magnetic resonance imaging (MRI). **A.** MRI scan showing mass in right neck lateral to trachea and esophagus (*white arrowhead*). **B.** Needle biopsy of neck mass using real-time MRI with mass (*white arrowhead*); needle can be seen entering mass (*black arrow*). Mass was determined to be recurrent papillary thyroid carcinoma by cytology from this needle aspiration.

One particularly difficult clinical problem is patients who present with elevated Tg levels but have negative radioiodine scan, presumably caused by recurrence of thyroid cancer that has lost the ability to take up iodine. In these cases, the effectiveness of RAI treatment is questionable.[106] An alternative approach is to attempt localization of tumor with technetium 99-m sestamibi or positron emission tomography (PET) scan. CT and MRI scans of the neck and chest are useful for detecting metastasis or for confirming the anatomic location of recurrence detected by scan. If possible, surgical resection should be performed after cytological confirmation. High-resolution ultrasound has been shown to be particularly helpful in the evaluation and surgical exploration of patients with recurrent cancer that does not trap iodine.[139] Intraoperative ultrasound is particularly helpful for identifying nonpalpable, locoregional recurrences in patients who had previous external beam radiotherapy and in the identification of tumor nodules of 20 mm or less that were invasive or adherent to the airway.[140] External-beam therapy has also been reported for the treatment of thyroid cancer[141,142] and is a useful adjuvant for tumors that have lost the ability to concentrate iodine.

Medullary Thyroid Cancer

Medullary thyroid cancer (MTC) is derived from the calcitonin-secreting C-cells or parafollicular cells of the thyroid. Because MTC can occur in association with familial cancer syndromes (MEN2A, MEN2B, and familial MTC), family members should be screened for the presence of *ret* mutations.[143] Surgical treatment at a young age, before the development of carcinoma, can be performed safely and will likely cure patients of an otherwise incurable disease.[144] Patients with MTC should also be screened for pheochromocytoma because this tumor occurs in approximately 40% of MEN2 patients.[145]

Primary surgical treatment for MTC is a total thyroidectomy and central node dissection.[143,146] Patients with pheochromocytoma should undergo adrenalectomy first, although combination procedures have been described with excellent results. Mortality for patients with MTC is influenced by patient age, the extent of local disease (tumor size and local invasion), and the presence of distant metastases.[147,148] The cancer-specific mortality for MTC at 5 and 10 years is approximately 30% and 40%, respectively.[148,149]

Calcitonin levels are an extremely sensitive assay for the detection of persistent and recurrent tumor. High levels of calcitonin can be associated with systemic symptoms, most commonly diarrhea. Carcinoembryonic antigen (CEA) levels can be elevated and have also been used to follow patients with MTC for recurrence. High-resolution ultrasound, CT scan, and MRI are useful for localizing locoregional and distant metastasis. Because MTC is a neuroendocrine tumor, octreotide scans may be effective in localization.[150,151] Labeled anti-CEA monoclonal antibodies have also been shown to localize tumor recurrence.[152]

To avoid local complications of tumor invasion, patients with clinically apparent recurrence in the central neck should undergo resection. Palliative operations for symptomatic metastases have also been advocated.[153] Several studies have attempted to address the role of neck exploration in asymptomatic patients whose only evidence of disease is a persistent elevation of calcitonin. Several studies have suggested improved outcome with bilateral radical neck dissections to remove all lymph node metastases.[154] These patients must first have a complete evaluation for metastatic disease, including laparoscopy to detect small liver metastases.[155] Approximately one-third of patients undergoing extensive neck dissection subsequently display normalized calcitonin levels. It is still not clear if this approach will significantly improve survival. It is possible that the improved outcome in patients with normalized calcitonin levels after extensive neck dissections represents those patients who have minimal disease and would have done as well without reoperation.

Anaplastic Thyroid Cancer

Patients with anaplastic thyroid cancer (ATC) usually present with a rapidly enlarging neck mass, often associated with dysphagia or airway obstruction. ATC has the worst prognosis of all thyroid malignancies, with 5-year survival rates of approximately 10%.[156] The goal of surgical treatment is to maintain a patent airway and, if possible, clear the neck of disease. Surgery has a limited role in the primary treatment. Once the diagnosis is established, patients should be treated with hyperfractionated radiotherapy and doxorubicin-based chemotherapy.[157]

References

1. Tietgens ST, Leinung MC. Thyroid storm. Med Clin North Am 1995;79:169–184.
2. Yoshida D. Thyroid storm precipitated by trauma. J Emerg Med 1996;14:697–701.
3. Brown RS. Editorial: Immunoglobulins affecting thyroid growth: a continuing controversy. J Clin Endocrinol Metab 1996;80:1506–1508.
4. Bartley GB, Fatourechi V, Kadrmas EF, et al. Long-term follow-up of Graves ophthalmopathy in an incidence cohort. Ophthalmology 1996;103:958–962.
5. Razack MS, Lore JM, Lippes HA, Schaefer DP, Rassael H. Total thyroidectomy for Graves' disease. Head Neck 1997;19:378–383.
6. Linos DA, Karakitsos D, Pappademetriou J. Should the primary treatment of hyperthyroidism be surgical? Eur J Surg 1997; 163:651–657.
7. Gerenova J, Buysschaert M, de Burbure CY, Daumerie C. Prevalence of thyroid cancer in Graves' disease: a retrospective study of a cohort of 103 patients treated surgically. Eur J Intern Med 2003;14:321–325.
8. Belfiore A, Garofalo MR, Giuffrida D, et al. Increased aggressiveness of thyroid cancer in patients with Graves' disease. J Clin Endocrinol Metab 1990;70:830–835.
9. Joseph UA, Jhingran SG. Graves' disease and concurrent thyroid carcinoma: the importance of thyroid scintigraphy in Graves' disease. Clin Nucl Med 1995;20:416–418.
10. Levy EG. Treatment of Graves' disease: the American way. Bailliere's Clin Endocrinol Metab 1997;11:585–595.
11. American Association of Clinical Endocrinologists medical guidelines for clinical practice for the evaluation and treatment of hyperthyroidism and hypothyroidism. Endocr Pract 2002; 8:457–469.
12. Witte J, Goretzki PE, Roher HD. Surgery for Graves disease in childhood and adolescence. Exp Clin Endocrinol Diabetes 1997; 105:58–60.
13. Miccoli P, Vitti P, Rago T, et al. Surgical treatment of Graves' disease: subtotal or total thyroidectomy? Surgery (St. Louis) 1996;11:1020–1025.
14. Torring O, Tallstedt L, Wallin G, et al. Graves' hyperthyroidism: treatment with antithyroid drugs, surgery, or radioiodine—a prospective, randomized study. J Clin Endocrinol Metab 1996; 81:2986–2993.
15. Rudberg C, Johansson H, Akerstrom G, Tuvemo T, Karlsson FA. Graves' disease in children and adolescents. Late results of surgical treatment. Eur J Endocrinol 1996;134:710–215.
16. Chi SY, Hsei KC, Sheen-Chen SM, Chou FF. A prospective randomized comparison of bilateral subtotal thyroidectomy versus unilateral total and contralateral subtotal thyroidectomy for Graves' disease. World J Surg 2005;18:18.
17. Sugino K, Mimura T, Ozaki O, et al. Management of recurrent hyperthyroidism in patients with Graves' disease treated by subtotal thyroidectomy. J Endocrinol Invest 1995;18:415–419.
18. Abe Y, Sato H, Noguchi M, et al. Effect of subtotal thyroidectomy on natural history of ophthalmopathy in Graves' disease. World J Surg 1998;22:714–717.
19. Berti P, Materazzi G, Galleri D, Donatini G, Minuto M, Miccoli P. Video-assisted thyroidectomy for Graves' disease: report of a preliminary experience. Surg Endosc 2004;18:1208–1210.
20. Siegel RD, Lee SL. Toxic nodular goiter. Endocrinol Metab Clin N Am 1998;27:151–168.
21. Erickson D, Gharib H, Li H, vanHeerden JA. Treatment of patients with toxic multinodular goiter. Thyroid 1998;8:277–282.
22. David E, Rosen IB, Bain J, James J, Kirsh JC. Management of the hot thyroid nodule. Am J Surg 1995;170:481–483.
23. Rojdmark J, Jarhult J. High long term recurrence rate after subtotal thyroidectomy for nodular goitre. Eur J Surg 1995; 161:725.
24. Seiler CA, Glaser C, Wagner HE. Thyroid gland surgery in an endemic region. World J Surg 1996;20:593–597.
25. Mack E. Management of patients with substernal goiters. Endocr Surg 1995;75:377–394.
26. Newman E, Shaha AR. Substernal goiter. J Surg Oncol 1995; 60:207–212.
27. Allo MD, Thompson NW. Rationale for the operative management of substernal goiters. Surgery (St. Louis) 1983;94:969–977.
28. Torre G, Borgonovo G, Amato A, et al. Surgical management of substernal goiter: analysis of 237 patients. Am Surg 1995;61:826–831.
29. Mazzaferri EL. Management of a solitary thyroid nodule. N Engl J Med 1993;328:553–559.
30. Singer PA, Cooper DS, Daniels GH, et al. Treatment guidelines for patients with thyroid nodules and well-differentiated thyroid cancer. Arch Intern Med 1996;156:2165–2172.
31. Sabel MS, Staren ED, Gianakakis LM, Dwarakanathan S, Prinz RA. Effectiveness of the thyroid scan in evaluation of the solitary thyroid nodule. Am Surg 1997;63:660–664.
32. Agrawal S. Diagnostic accuracy and role of fine needle aspiration cytology in management of thyroid nodules. J Surg Oncol 1995;58:168–172.
33. Woeber KA. Cost-effective evaluation of the patient with a thyroid nodule. Endocr Surg 1995;75:357–363.
34. Carmeci C, Jeffrey RB, McDougall IR, Nowels KW, Weigel RJ. Ultrasound-guided fine-needle aspiration biopsy of thyroid masses. Thyroid 1998;8:283–289.
35. Rodriquez JM, Parrilla P, Sola S, et al. Comparison between preoperative cytology and intraoperative frozen-section biopsy in the diagnosis of thyroid nodules. Br J Surg 1994;81:1151–1154.
36. Chen H, Zeiger MA, Clark DP, Westra WH, Udelsman R. Papillary carcinoma of the thyroid: can operative management be based solely on fine-needle aspiration? J Am Coll Surg 1997;184:605–610.
37. Aguilar-Diosdado M, Contreras A, Gavilan I, et al. Thyroid nodules: role of fine needle aspiration and intraoperative frozen section examination. Acta Cytol 1997;41:677–682.

38. Chen H, Nicol TL, Udelsman R. Follicular lesions of the thyroid: does frozen section evaluation alter operative management? Ann Surg 1995;222:101–106.
39. McHenry CR, Raeburn C, Strickland T, Marty JJ. The utility of routine frozen section examination for intraoperative diagnosis of thyroid cancer. Am J Surg 1996;172:658–661.
40. Hamming JF, Vriens MR, Goslings BM, Songun I, Fleuren GJ, VanDeVelde CJH. Role of fine-needle aspiration biopsy and frozen section examination in determining the extent of thyroidectomy. World J Surg 1998;22:575–580.
41. Rios Zambudio A, Rodriguez Gonzalez JM, Sola Perez J, et al. Utility of frozen-section examination for diagnosis of malignancy associated with multinodular goiter. Thyroid 2004;14:600–604.
42. Callcut RA, Selvaggi SM, Mack E, Ozgul O, Warner T, Chen H. The utility of frozen section evaluation for follicular thyroid lesions. Ann Surg Oncol 2004;11:94–98.
43. Tyler DS, Winchester DJ, Caraway NP, Hickey RC, Evans DB. Indeterminate fine-needle aspiration biopsy of the thyroid: identification of subgroups at high risk for invasive carcinoma. Surgery (St. Louis) 1994;116:1054–1060.
44. Chen H, Nicol TL, Zeiger MA, et al. Hurthle cell neoplasms of the thyroid. Ann Surg 1998;227:542–546.
45. Paphavasit A, Thompson GB, Hay ID, et al. Follicular and Hurthle cell thyroid neoplasms. Arch Surg 1997;132:674–679.
46. Landis SH, Murray T, Bolden S, Wingo PA. Cancer statistics, 1998. CA Cancer J Clin 1998;48:6–30.
47. Doniach I. Carcinogenic effect of 100, 250 and 500 rad x-rays on the rat thyroid gland. Br J Cancer 1974;30:487–495.
48. Fraker DL. Radiation exposure and other factors that predispose to human thyroid neoplasia. Endocr Surg 1995;75:365–375.
49. Hancock SL, Cox RS, McDougall IR. Thyroid diseases after treatment of Hodgkin's disease. N Engl J Med 1991;325:599–605.
50. Shore RE, Hildreth N, Dvoretsky P, Andresen E, Moseson M, Pasternack B. Thyroid cancer among persons given x-ray treatment in infancy for an enlarged thymus gland. Am J Epidemiol 1993;137:1068–1080.
51. Ron E, Modan B, Preston D, et al. Thyroid neoplasias following low-dose radiation in childhood. Radiat Res 1989;120:516–531.
52. Nagataki S, Shibata Y, Inoue S, Yokoyama N, Izumi M, Shimaoka K. Thyroid diseases among atomic bomb survivors in Nagasaki. JAMA 1994;272:384–370.
53. Doniach I. Experimental induction of tumours of the thyroid by radiation. Br Med J 1958;14:181–183.
54. McDougall LR, ed. Thyroid Disease in Clinical Practice. London: Chapman & Hall, 1992:304–324.
55. Tezelman S, Grossman RF, Siperstein AE, Clark OH. Radioiodine-associated thyroid cancers. World J Surg 1994;18:522–528.
56. Holm L-E, Hall P, Wiklund K, et al. Cancer risk after iodine-131 therapy for hyperthyroidism. J Natl Cancer Inst 1991;83:1072–1077.
57. Dobyns BM, Sheline GE, Workman JB, Tompkins EA, McConahey WM, Becker DV. Malignant and benign neoplasms of the thyroid in patients treated for hyperthyroidism: a report of the cooperative thyrotoxicosis therapy follow-up study. J Clin Endocrinol Metab 1974;38:976–998.
58. Smith WG, Kern BB. The nature of the mutation in familial multiple polyposis: papillary carcinoma of the thyroid, brain tumors, and familial multiple polyposis. Dis Colon Rectum 1973;16:264–271.
59. Zeki K, Spambalg D, Sharifi N, Gonsky R, Fagin JA. Mutations of the adenomatous polyposis coli gene in sporadic thyroid neoplasms. J Clin Endocrinol Metab 1994;79:1317–1321.
60. Grossman RF, Tu S-H, Duh Q-Y, Siperstein AE, Novosolov F, Clark OH. Familial nonmedullary thyroid cancer. Arch Surg 1995;130:892–897.
61. McKay JD, Lesueur F, Jonard L, et al. Localization of a susceptibility gene for familial nonmedullary thyroid carcinoma to chromosome 2q21. Am J Hum Genet 2001;69:440–446.
62. Mulligan LM, Kwok JBJ, Healey CS, et al. Germ-line mutations of the *RET* proto-oncogene in multiple endocrine neoplasia type 2A. Nature (Lond) 1993;363:458–460.
63. Donis-Keller H, Dou S, Chi D, et al. Mutations in the RET proto-oncogene are associated with MEN 2A and FMTC. Hum Mol Genet 1993;2:851–856.
64. Eng C, Smith DP, Mulligan LM, et al. Point mutation within the tyrosine kinase domain of the *RET* proto-oncogene in multiple endocrine neoplasia type 2B and related sporadic tumours. Hum Mol Genet 1994;3:237–241.
65. Mulligan LM, Eng C, Healey CS, et al. Specific mutations of the *RET* proto-oncogene are related to disease phenotype of MEN 2A and FMTC. Nat Genet 1994;6:70–74.
66. Santoro M, Carlomagno F, Hay ID, et al. Ret oncogene activation in human thyroid neoplasms is restricted to the papillary cancer subtype. J Clin Invest 1992;89:1517–1522.
67. Pierotti MA, Santoro M, Jenkins RB, et al. Characterization of an inversion on the long arm of chromosome 10 juxtaposing *D10S170* and *RET* and creating the oncogenic sequence *RET*/PET. Med Sci 1992;89:1616–1620.
68. Tong Q, Li Y, Smanik PA, Fithian LJ, Xing S, Mazzaferri EL, Jhiang SM. Characterization of the promoter region and oligomerization domain of H4 (D10S170), a gene frequently rearranged with the *ret* proto-oncogene. Oncogene 1995; 10:1781–1787.
69. Sozzi G, Bongarzone I, Miozzo M, et al. A t(10;17) translocation creates the *RET/PTC2* chimeric transforming sequence in papillary thyroid carcinoma. Genes Chromosomes Cancer 1994;9:244–250.
70. Bongarzone I, Butti MG, Coronelli S, et al. Frequent activation of *ret* protooncogene by fusion with a new activating gene in papillary thyroid carcinomas. Cancer Res 1994;54:2979–2985.
71. Teyssier J-R, Liautaud-Roger F, Ferre D, Patey M, Dufer J. Chromosomal changes in thyroid tumors: relation with DNA content, karyotypic features, and clinical data. Cancer Genet Cytogenet 1990;50:249–263.
72. Belge G, Thode B, Bullerdiek J, Bartnitzke S. Aberrations of chromosome 19. Cancer Genet Cytogenet 1992;60:23–26.
73. DalCin P, Sneyers W, Aly MS, et al. Involvement of 19q13 in follicular thyroid adenoma. Cancer Genet Cytogenet 1992;60:99–101.
74. Farid NR, Shi Y, Zou M. Molecular basis of thyroid cancer. Endocr Rev 1994;15:202–232.
75. Hara H, Fulton N, Yashiro T, Ito K, DeGroot LJ, Kaplan EL. N-*ras* mutation: an independent prognostic factor for aggressiveness of papillary thyroid carcinoma. Surgery (St. Louis) 1994;116:1010–1016.
76. Namba H, Rubin SA, Fagin JA. Point mutations of *ras* oncogenes are an early event in thyroid tumorigenesis. Mol Endocrinol 1990;4:1474–1479.
77. Simon D, Goretzki PE, Gorelev V, et al. Significance of p53 in human thyroid tumors. World J Surg 1994;18:535–541.
78. Matias-Guiu X, Cuatrecasas M, Musulen E, Prat J. p53 expression in anaplastic carcinomas arising from thyroid papillary carcinomas. J Clin Pathol 1994;47:337–339.
79. Nishida T, Nakao K, Hamaji M, Nakahara M-A, Tsujimoto M. Overexpression of p53 protein and DNA content are important biologic prognostic factors for thyroid cancer. Surgery (St. Louis) 1996;119:568–575.
80. Grebe SKG, Hay ID. Follicular thyroid cancer. Endocrinol Metab Clin N Am 1995;24:761–801.
81. Martinez-Tello FJ, Martinez-Cabruja R, Fernandez-Martin J, Lasso-Oria C, Ballestin-Carcavilla C. Occult carcinoma of the thyroid. Cancer (Phila) 1993;71:4022–4029.

82. Allo MD, Christianson W, Koivunen D. Not all "occult" papillary carcinomas are "minimal." Surgery (St. Louis) 1988;104:971–976.
83. Patwardhan N, Cataldo T, Braverman LE. Surgical management of the patient with papillary cancer. Surg Clin N Am 1995;75:449–464.
84. Soh EY, Clark OH. Surgical considerations and approach to thyroid cancer. Endocrinol Metab Clin N Am 1996;25:115–139.
85. Wong JB, Kaplan MM, Meyer K, Pauker SG. Ablative radioactive iodine therapy for apparently localized thyroid carcinoma. Endocrinol Metab Clin N Am 1990;19:741–760.
86. Stephenson BM, Wheeler MH, Clark OH. The role of total thyroidectomy in the management of differentiated thyroid cancer. Curr Opin Gen Surg 1994;53–59.
87. Harness JK, Thompson NW, McLeod MK, Pasieka JL, Fukuuchi A. Differentiated thyroid carcinoma in children and adolescents. World J Surg 1992;16:547–554.
88. Hoelting T, Buhr HJ, Herfarth C. Intraoperative tumour classification in papillary thyroid cancer—a diagnostic dilemma. Eur J Surg Oncol 1995;21:353–356.
89. Liu Q, Djuricin G, Prinz RA. Total thyroidectomy for benign thyroid disease. Surgery (St. Louis) 1998;123:2–7.
90. Burge MR, Zeise T-M, Johnsen MW, Conway MJ, Qualls CR. Risks of complication following thyroidectomy. J Gen Intern Med 1998;13:24–31.
91. Cady B, Rossi R. An expanded view of risk-group definition in differentiated thyroid carcinoma. Surgery (St. Louis) 1988;104:947–953.
92. Nguyen KV, Dilawari RA. Predictive value of AMES scoring system in selection of extent of surgery in well differentiated carcinoma of thyroid. Am Surg 1995;61:151–155.
93. Shaha AR, Shah JP, Loree TR. Low-risk differentiated thyroid cancer: the need for selective treatment. Ann Surg Oncol 1997;4:328–333.
94. Sanders LE, Cady B. Differentiated thyroid cancer: reexamination of risk groups and outcome of treatment. Arch Surg 1988;133:419–425.
95. Wanebo H, Coburn M, Teates D, Cole B. Total thyroidectomy does not enhance disease control or survival even in high-risk patients with differentiated thyroid cancer. Ann Surg 1998;227:912–921.
96. Kim S, Wei JP, Braveman JM, Brams DM. Predicting outcome and directing therapy for papillary thyroid carcinoma. Arch Surg 2004;139:390–394; discussion 393–394.
97. Kim ES, Kim TY, Koh JM, et al. Completion thyroidectomy in patients with thyroid cancer who initially underwent unilateral operation. Clin Endocrinol (Oxf) 2004;61:145–148.
98. DeGroot LJ, Kaplan EL, McCormick M, Straus FH. Natural history, treatment and course of papillary thyroid carcinoma. J Clin Endocrinol Metab 1990;71:414–424.
99. Samaan NA, Schultz PN, Hickey RC, et al. The results of various modalities of treatment of well differentiated thyroid carcinoma: a retrospective review of 1599 patients. J Clin Endocrinol Metab 1992;75:714–720.
100. Mazzaferri EL, Jhiang SM. Long-term impact of initial surgical and medical therapy on papillary and follicular thyroid cancer. Am J Med 1994;97:418–428.
101. Loh K-C, Greenspan FS, Gee L, Miller TR, Yeo PPB. Pathological tumor-node-metastasis (pTNM) staging for papillary and follicular thyroid carcinomas: a retrospective analysis of 700 patients. J Clin Endocrinol Metab 1997;82:3553–3562.
102. Weigel RJ. Advances in the diagnosis and management of well-differentiated thyroid cancers. Curr Opin Oncol 1996;8:37–43.
103. Park HM, Park YH, Zhou XH. Detection of thyroid remnant/metastasis without stunning: an ongoing dilemma. Thyroid 1997;7:277–280.
104. McDougall IR. 74 MBq radioiodine ^{131}I does not prevent uptake of therapeutic doses of ^{131}I (i.e., it does not cause stunning) in differentiated thyroid cancer. Nucl Med Commun 1997;18:505–512.
105. Pineda JD, Lee T, Ain K, Reynolds JC, Robbins J. Iodine-131 therapy for thyroid cancer patients with elevated thyroglobulin and negative diagnostic scan. J Clin Endocrinol Metab 1995;80:1488–1492.
106. McDougall IR. ^{131}I treatment of ^{131}I negative whole body scan, and positive thyroglobulin in differentiated thyroid carcinoma: what is being treated? Thyroid 1997;7:669–672.
107. Arad E, O'Mara RE, Wilson GA. Ablation of remaining functioning thyroid lobe with radioiodine after hemithyroidectomy for carcinoma. Clin Nucl Med 1993;18:662–663.
108. Samuel AM, Rajashekharrao B. Radioiodine therapy for well-differentiated thyroid cancer: a quantitative dosimetric evaluation for remnant thyroid ablation after surgery. J Nucl Med 1994;35:1944–1950.
109. Hoyes KP, Owens SE, Millns MM, Allan E. Differentiated thyroid cancer: radioiodine following lobectomy—a clinical feasibility study. Nucl Med Commun 2004;25:245–251.
110. Lin J-D, Kao P-F, Chao T-C. The effects of radioactive iodine in thyroid remnant ablation and treatment of well differentiated thyroid carcinoma. Br J Radiol 1998;71:307–313.
111. DiRusso G, Kern KA. Comparative analysis of complications from I-131 radioablation for well-differentiated thyroid cancer. Surgery (St. Louis) 1994;116:1024–1030.
112. Dottorini ME, Lomuscio G, Mazzucchelli L, Vignati A, Colombo L. Assessment of female fertility and carcinogenesis after iodine-131 therapy for differentiated thyroid carcinoma. J Nucl Med 1995;36:21–27.
113. Pacini F, Gasperi M, Fugazzola L, et al. Testicular function in patients with differentiated thyroid carcinoma treated with radioiodine. J Nucl Med 1994;35:1418–1422.
114. Pacini F, Cetani F, Miccoli P, et al. Outcome of 309 patients with metastatic differentiated thyroid carcinoma treated with radioiodine. World J Surg 1994;18:600–604.
115. McHenry C, Jarosz H, Davis M, Barbato AL, Lawrence AM, Paloyan E. Selective postoperative radioactive iodine treatment of thyroid carcinoma. Surgery (St. Louis) 1989;106:956–959.
116. Morris DM, Boyle PJ, Stidley CA, Altobelli KK, Parnell T, Key C. Localized well-differentiated thyroid carcinoma: survival analysis of prognostic factors and ^{131}I therapy. Ann Surg Oncol 1998;5:329–337.
117. Meier CA, Braverman LE, Ebner SA, et al. Diagnostic use of recombinant human thyrotropin in patients with thyroid carcinoma (phase I/II study). J Clin Endocrinol Metab 1994;78:188–196.
118. Ladenson PW, Braverman LE, Mazzaferri EL, et al. Comparison of administration of recombinant human thyrotropin with withdrawal of thyroid hormone for radioactive iodine scanning in patients with thyroid carcinoma. N Engl J Med 1997;337:888–896.
119. Newman KD, Black T, Heller G, et al. Differentiated thyroid cancer: determinants of disease progression in patients less than 21 years of age at diagnosis. Ann Surg 1998;227:533–541.
120. Andersen PE, Kinsella J, Loree TR, Shaha AR, Shah JP. Differentiated carcinoma of the thyroid with extrathyroidal extension. Am J Surg 1995;170:467–470.
121. Melliere DJM, Yahia NEB, Becquemin JP, Lange F, Boulahdour H. Thyroid carcinoma with tracheal or esophageal involvement: limited or maximal surgery? Surgery (St. Louis) 1993;113:166–172.
122. Ozaki O, Sugino K, Mimura T, Ito K. Surgery for patients with thyroid carcinoma invading the trachea: circumferential sleeve resection followed by end-to-end anastomosis. Surgery (St. Louis) 1995;117:268–271.

123. Ballantyne AJ. Resections of the upper aerodigestive tract for locally invasive thyroid cancer. Am J Surg 1994;168:636–639.
124. Scheumann GFW, Gimm O, Wegener G, Hundeshagen H, Dralle H. Prognostic significance and surgical management of locoregional lymph node metastases in papillary thyroid cancer. World J Surg 1994;18:559–568.
125. DeGroot LJ, Kaplan EL, Shukla MS, Salti G, Straus FH. Morbidity and mortality in follicular thyroid cancer. J Clin Endocrinol Metab 1995;80:2946–2953.
126. Schlumberger MJ. Papillary and follicular thyroid carcinoma. N Engl J Med 1998;338:297–305.
127. Brennan MD, Bergstralh EJ, van Heerden JA, McConahey WM. Follicular thyroid cancer treated at the Mayo Clinic, 1946 through 1970: initial manifestations, pathologic findings, therapy, and outcome. Mayo Clin Proc 1991;66:11–22.
128. Grant CS. Operative and postoperative management of the patient with follicular and Hurthle cell carcinoma. Surg Clin N Am 1995;75:395–403.
129. Terry JH, St. John SA, Karkowski FJ, et al. Tall cell papillary thyroid cancer: incidence and prognosis. Am J Surg 1994;168:459–461.
130. Moreno-Egea A, Rodriguez-Gonzalez JM, Sola-Perez J, Soria-Cogollos T, Parrilla-Paricio P. Multivariate analysis of histopathological features as prognostic factors in patients with papillary thyroid carcinoma. Br J Surg 1995;82:1092–1094.
131. Segal K, Fridental R, Lubin E, Shvero J, Sulkes J, Feinmesser R. Papillary carcinoma of the thyroid. Otolaryngol Head Neck Surg 1995;113:356–363.
132. Ruiz de Almodovar JM, Ruiz-Garcia J, Olea N, Villalobos M, Pedraza V. Analysis of risk of death from differentiated thyroid cancer. Radiother Oncol 1994;31:207–212.
133. Hay ID, Grant CS, Taylor WF, McConahey WM. Ipsilateral lobectomy versus bilateral lobar resection in papillary thyroid carcinoma: a retrospective analysis of surgical outcome using a novel prognostic scoring system. Surgery (St. Louis) 1987;102:1088–1095.
134. Thyroid gland. In: Beahrs OH, Myers MH, eds. Manual for Staging of Cancer. Philadelphia: Lippincott, 1988:55–60.
135. Noguchi S, Murakami N, Kawamoto H. Classification of papillary cancer of the thyroid based on prognosis. World J Surg 1994;18:552–558.
136. Ladenson PW. Optimal laboratory testing for diagnosis and monitoring of thyroid nodules, goiter, and thyroid cancer. Clin Chem 1996;42:183–187.
137. Ozata M, Suzuki S, Takahide M, et al. Serum thyroglobulin in the follow-up of patients with treated differentiated thyroid cancer. J Clin Endocrinol Metab 1994;79:98–105.
138. Coburn M, Teates D, Wanebo H. Recurrent thyroid cancer. Ann Surg 1994;291:587–595.
139. Desai D, Jeffrey RB, McDougall IR, Weigel RJ. Intraoperative ultrasonography for localization of recurrent thyroid cancer. Surgery (St. Louis) 2001;129:498–500.
140. Karwowski JK, Jeffrey RB, McDougall IR, Weigel RJ. Intraoperative ultrasonography improves identification of recurrent thyroid cancer. Surgery (St. Louis) 2002;132:924–928; discussion 928–929.
141. Farahati J, Reiners C, Stuschke M, et al. Differentiated thyroid cancer: impact of adjuvant external radiotherapy in patients with perithyroidal tumor infiltration (stage pT4). Cancer (Phila) 1996;77:172–180.
142. Tsang RW, Brierley JD, Simpson WJ, Panzarella T, Gospodarowicz MK, Sutcliffe SB. The effects of surgery, radioiodine, and external radiation therapy on the clinical outcome of patients with differentiated thyroid carcinoma. Cancer (Phila) 1998;82:375–388.
143. Moley JF. Medullary thyroid cancer. Surg Clin N Am 1995;75:405–420.
144. Wells SA, Chi DD, Toshima K, et al. Predictive DNA testing and prophylactic thyroidectomy in patients at risk for multiple endocrine neoplasia type 2A. Ann Surg 1994;220:237–250.
145. Howe JR, Norton JA, Wells SA. Prevalence of pheochromocytoma and hyperparathyroidism in multiple endocrine neoplasia type 2A: results of long-term follow-up. Surgery (St. Louis) 1993;114:1070–1077.
146. Kallinowski F, Buhr HJ, Meybier H, Eberhardt M, Herfarth C. Medullary carcinoma of the thyroid—therapeutic strategy derived from fifteen years of experience. Surgery (St. Louis) 1993;114:491–496.
147. Brierley J, Tsang R, Simpson WJ, Gospodarowicz M, Sutcliffe S, Panzarella T. Medullary thyroid cancer: analyses of survival and prognostic factors and the role of radiation therapy in local control. Thyroid 1996;6:305–310.
148. Dottorini ME, Assi A, Sironi M, Sangalli G, Spreafico G, Colombo L. Multivarate analysis of patients with medullary thyroid carcinoma. Cancer (Phila) 1996;77:1556–1565.
149. Hoie J, Jorgensen OG, Stenwig AE, Langmark F. Medullary thyroid cancer in Norway. Acta Chir Scand 1988;154:339–343.
150. Baudin E, Lumbroso J, Schlumberg M, et al. Comparison of octreotide scintigraphy and conventional imaging in medullary thyroid carcinoma. J Nucl Med 1996;37:912–916.
151. Dorr U, Sautter-Bihl M-L, Bihl H. The contribution of somatostatin receptor scintigraphy to the diagnosis of recurrent medullary carcinoma of the thyroid. Semin Oncol 1994;21:42–45.
152. Juweid M, Sharkey RM, Swayne LC, Goldenberg DM. Improved selection of patients for reoperation for medullary thyroid cancer by imaging with radiolabeled anticarcinoembryonic antigen antibodies. Surgery (St. Louis) 1997;122:1156–1165.
153. Chen H, Roberts JR, Ball DW, et al. Effective long-term palliation of symptomatic, incurable metastatic medullary thyroid cancer by operative resection. Ann Surg 1998;227:887–895.
154. Moley JF, Debenedetti MK, Dilley WG, Tisell LE, Wells SA. Surgical management of patients with persistent or recurrent medullary thyroid cancer. J Intern Med 1998;243:521–526.
155. Tung WS, Vesely TM, Moley JF. Laparoscopic detection of hepatic metastases in patients with residual or recurrent medullary thyroid cancer. Surgery (St. Louis) 1995;118:1024–1030.
156. Tan RK, Robert K, Finley I, et al. Anaplastic carcinoma of the thyroid: a 24-year experience. Head Neck 1995;17:41–48.
157. Tennvall J, Lundell G, Hallquist A, Wahlberg P, Wallin G, Tibblin S. Combined doxorubicin, hyperfractionated radiotherapy, and surgery in anaplastic thyroid carcinoma. Cancer (Phila) 1994;74:1348–1354.

57

Adrenal

Robert Udelsman

Anatomy

The adrenal glands were first described and illustrated by the Roman anatomist Bartholomaeus Eustachius in 1552.[1] These glands are paired retroperitoneal organs located in close contact to the superior surface of either kidney. They are surrounded by a loose layer of areolar connective tissue and have multiple fibrous bands and vascular attachments through which they are associated with the superior poles of the kidneys. They are recognizable by their firm texture and chromate yellow color, which is distinctly darker than the pale retroperitoneal fat. The normal adrenal gland is slightly nodular and generally weighs between 4 and 5g in the adult.[2] The presence of adrenal nodules is not uncommon, and their frequency increases with age.[3]

The anatomic relationships of the adrenal glands are important and have significant surgical ramifications. The computed tomography (CT) findings of the normal adrenal glands (Fig. 57.1) are easily visualized on most CT scans, and the width of each adrenal gland limb is similar to that of the nearby diaphragm. Their anatomic relationships have been summarized by Mihai and Farndon[2] (Table 57.1). The location of the adrenal gland deep in the retroperitoneum has in the past made it relatively inaccessible. However, laparoscopic adrenalectomy has dramatically changed the surgical management of adrenal tumors. It is therefore important to appreciate their anatomic position and their relationship to the arterial supply and venous drainage.

Each adrenal gland is supplied by small arterial branches that originate from three distinct sources. The major supplying vessels are the inferior phrenic artery, the aorta, and the ipsilateral renal artery. Occasional additional sources include the intercostal and ovarian vessels. The arterial branches ramify over the capsule of the gland and form a subcapsular plexus.[2,4] The microcirculation of the adrenal gland has received extensive interest because of its physiological implications. Vessels arising from the subcapsular plexus perfuse the zona glomerulosa and then run longitudinally along the cells of the zona fasciculata and terminate in a larger sinusoidal network in the zona reticularis.[4] The blood supply to the adrenal medulla appears to arise from two sources. A direct supply to the adrenal medulla was described as early as 1990 by Flint.[5] However, the major source of adrenal medullary blood appears to be via the adrenal cortex from which blood rich in glucocorticoids flows from the cortical layers into the medulla.[4] This intraadrenal "portal venous" circulation has significant physiological ramifications. The final pathway for the catecholamine epinephrine requires the enzyme phenylethanolamine *N*-methyltransferase (PNMT), and glucocorticoids are required for this final step.[6] Thus, there is significant functional interaction between the adrenal medulla and cortex.

The venous drainage of the adrenal gland is more constant than the arterial supply. The right adrenal gland usually drains by one short vein, which empties directly into the vena cava. Accessory adrenal veins are not infrequently present and have significant ramifications for laparoscopic adrenalectomy. In addition, the short right adrenal vein is at risk as at times it can be difficult to control. The left major adrenal vein is often joined by the inferior phrenic vein, which drains into the left renal vein. There may be associated small additional veins. Lymphatic drainage from the adrenal glands drains directly into adjacent periaortic and paracaval nodes. These structures are important when operating for malignant adrenal lesions.[4]

Physiology

The adrenal gland is composed of two distinct organs, the adrenal cortex and the adrenal medulla. The cortex is divided into three functional zones: the outer glomerulosa, the inter-

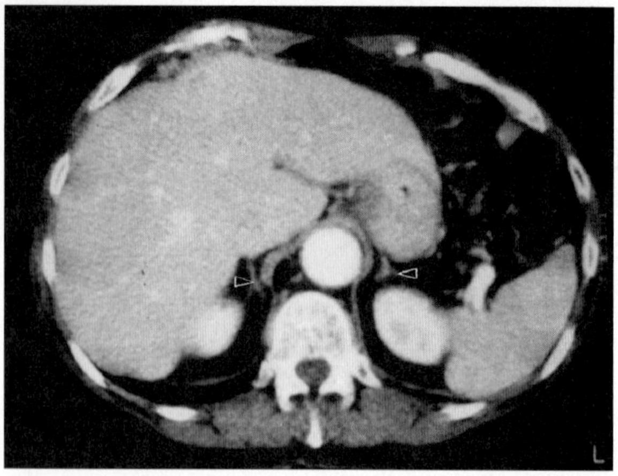

FIGURE 57.1. Computed tomography (CT) scan demonstrating normal adrenal glands (*arrowheads*). (From Sosa JA, Udelsman R. Imaging of the adrenal gland. In: Kurtzman S, ed. Surgical Oncology Clinics of North America. Philadelphia: Saunders, 1998;109–127, with permission.)

mediate fasciculata, and the inner reticularis. These three zones are associated with the production of mineralocorticoids, glucocorticoids, and sex steroids, respectively. The biochemical pathways for the predominant examples of each of these hormone classes are shown in Figure 57.2. Of these three hormone classes, the only one absolutely required for life is glucocorticoids.

Glucocorticoids were initially described as a family of steroids that have glucose-regulating properties. However, this definition is far too restrictive because glucocorticoids exert a myriad of effects on essentially every tissue in the body. A partial list of the effects of glucocorticoids is presented in Table 57.2. A more useful definition for glucocorticoids is a class of steroids that bind to glucocorticoid receptors. Cortisol is the major glucocorticoid in humans. The rate-limiting step in adrenal steroid synthesis, which is controlled by adrenocorticotropic hormone (ACTH), is the cleavage of the cholesterol side chain to yield pregnenolone.[7,8] This mitochondrial reaction is cytochrome P-450-dependent and occurs in response to elevated levels of cyclic AMP.[9] Glucocorticoids are secreted directly into the circulation immediately upon their synthesis. Cortisol circulates in both the bound form (95%) and in a free unbound state (5%). The free form passes into target cells by diffusion and binds to cytosolic receptors. All physiological actions of glucocorticoids are mediated through binding to steroid receptors, which are present in virtually every nucleated cell.[10] The actions of glucocorticoids are both "permissive," allowing other hormones to function in the basal state, as well as "regulatory," which are observed under stress-induced conditions.[11]

The autonomic nervous system develops in parallel to the hypothalamic–pituitary–adrenal (HPA) axis. The autonomic nervous system regulates moment-to-moment arousal, activation, and physiological responses. It has been divided into the anatomically, chemically, and functionally distinct sympathetic and parasympathetic systems. The major transmitter of the preganglionic autonomic nervous system is acetylcholine. The neurotransmitter for most postganglionic sympathetic nerve fibers is norepinephrine, although a few postganglionic fibers also use acetylcholine.[12] The adrenal medulla is embryologically analogous to a peripheral sympathetic ganglia. The medullary chromaffin cells have rudimentary nerve fibers and the ability to synthesize, store, and secrete catecholamines.[13] The primary secretory product of the adrenal medulla is epinephrine. The proximity of the adrenal medulla and the adrenal cortex results in a unique site of catecholamine–glucocorticoid interactions.[14,15]

The biosynthetic pathway for catecholamines as originally described by Blaschko is demonstrated in Figure 57.3.[16] The rate-limiting step is the formation of dopa from tyrosine via the enzyme tyrosine hydroxylase.[17] Activity of this enzyme is dependent on both ACTH and sympathetic activity.[14] Although norepinephrine is the principal end product of catecholamine synthesis in peripheral nerve terminals, in the adrenal medulla the additional enzyme, phenylethanolamine-*N*-methyltransferase (PNMT), is present and converts norepinephrine to epinephrine. Therefore, epinephrine constitutes approximately 80% of adrenal medullary secretion[12] (see Fig. 57.3). Catecholamine synthesis is dynamic, and long-term stimulation results in elevated levels of tyrosine hydroxylase, dopamine-beta hydroxylase, and PNMT.[14,17] Catecholamines exert their effects through interactions with a large family of transmembrane-signaling molecules termed adenoreceptors.

TABLE 57.1. Anatomic Relationships of the Adrenal Glands.

Surface	*Area*	*Description*
Right adrenal		
Anterior	Medial area	Not covered by peritoneum; posterior to the inferior vena cava
	Lateral area	Upper part in contact with the inferomedial angle of bare area of liver; lower part may be covered by peritoneum, reflected onto it from the inferior layer of the coronary ligament
Posterior	Upper area	Rests against the diaphragm
	Lower area	In contact with the superior pole and the adjacent anterior surface of right kidney
Medial border		Right celiac ganglion Right inferior phrenic artery
Left adrenal		
Anterior	Superior area	Covered with peritoneum of the omental bursa, which separates it from the cardia
	Inferior area	Not covered by peritoneum; in direct contact with the tail of pancreas and splenic artery
Posterior	Medial part	In contact with left crus of diaphragm
	Lateral part	Close to the kidney
Medial border		Left celiac ganglion Left inferior phrenic artery Left gastric arteries

Source: Modified from Mihai R, Farndon JR. Surgical embryology and anatomy of the adrenal glands. In: Clark OH, Duh QY, eds. Textbook of Endocrine Surgery. Philadelphia: Saunders, 1997:452, reprinted with permission.

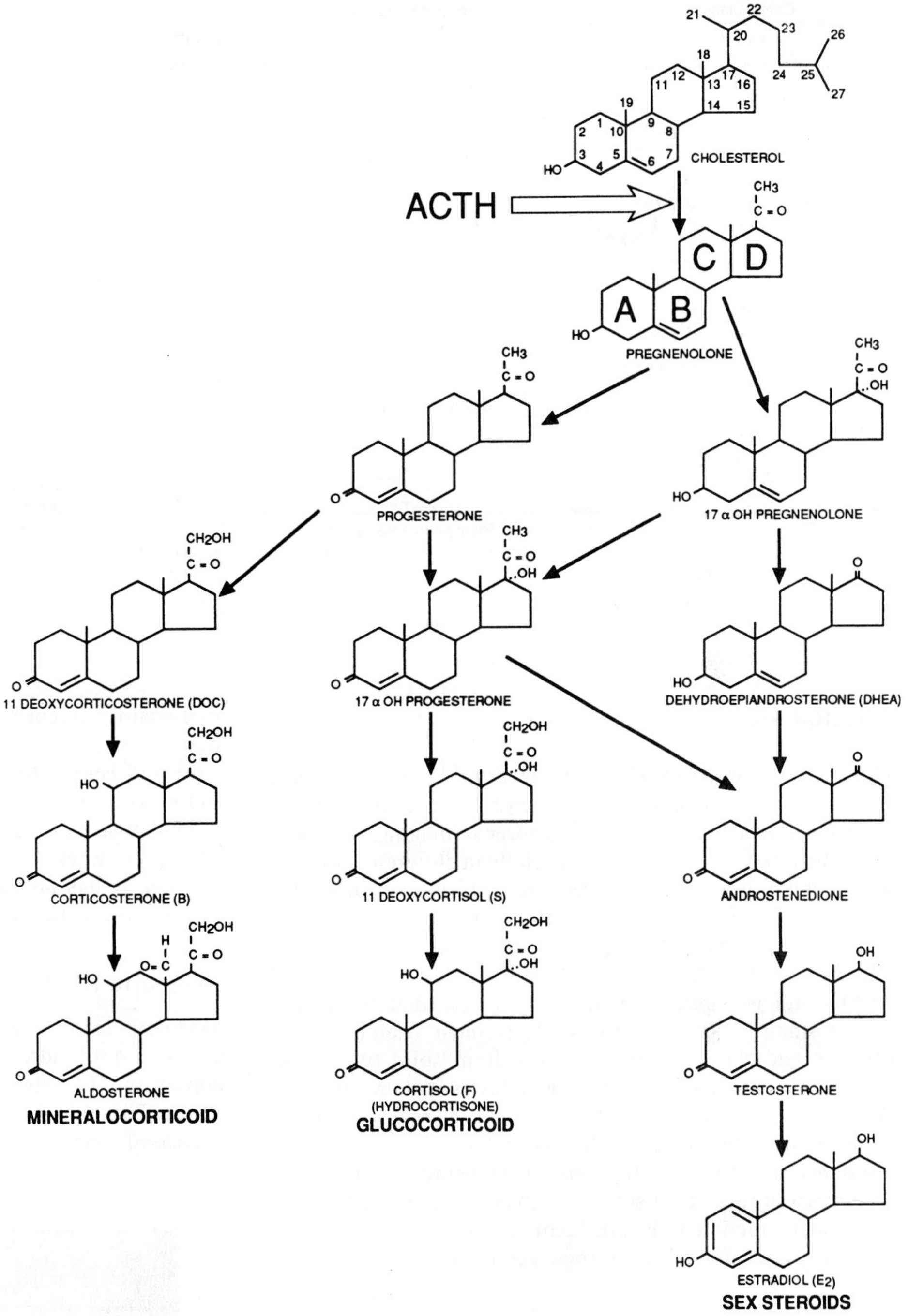

FIGURE 57.2. Major biochemical pathways for adrenal steroidogenesis. *ACTH*, adrenocorticotropic hormone. (From Udelsman R, Holbrook NJ. Endocrine and molecular responses to surgical stress. Curr Probl Surg 1994;31:653–728, with permission.)

TABLE 57.2. Glucocorticoid Actions.

Area	*Increase*	*Decrease*
Liver	Gluconeogenesis, glycogenesis, protein synthesis	Glycogenolysis
Muscle	Lactate release	Protein synthesis
Peripheral tissues		Glucose uptake and use (increased insulin levels)
Adipose tissue	Lipolysis, redistribution of body fat	
Bone	Osteoporosis, osteoclast activity, PTH	Intestinal absorption of calcium, renal reabsorption of calcium
Cardiovascular	Vascular tone, binding to mineralocorticoid receptor, catecholamine synthesis	
Immunological	Immunosuppression Leukocyte distribution	Production and activity of prostaglandins, kinins, and histamine Leukocyte movement, antigen processing
Wound healing		Collagen formation, glycosaminoglycan, and fibroblast function
CNS	Behavior and mood effects	

CNS, central nervous system; PTH, parathyroid hormone.

Source: Udelsman R, Holbrook NJ. Endocrine and molecular responses to surgical stress. Curr Probl Surg 1994;8:653–728, with permission.

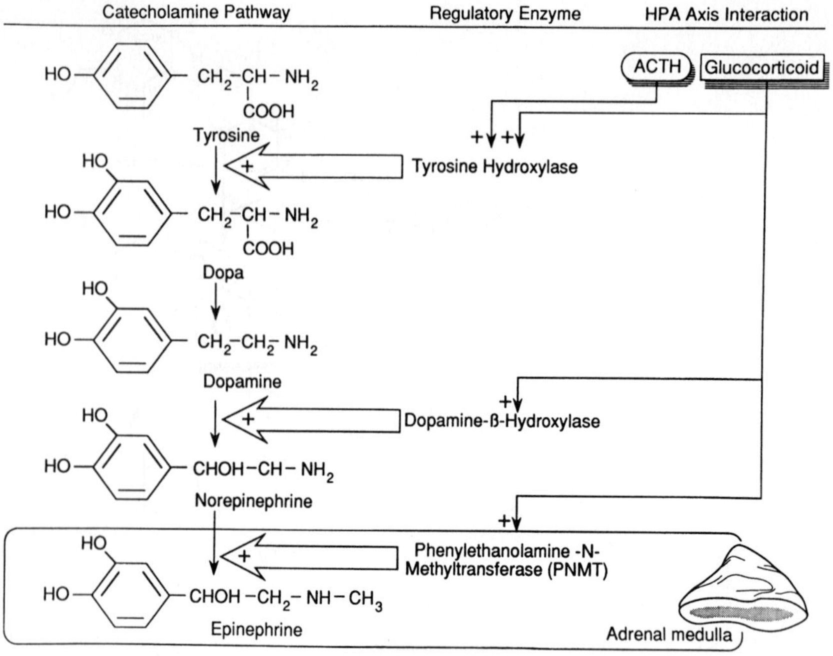

FIGURE 57.3. Biosynthetic pathway for catecholamines, their regulatory enzymes, and interactions with the hypothalamic–pituitary–adrenal (*HPA*) axis. *ACTH*, adrenocorticotropic hormone. (From Udelsman R, Holbrook NJ. Endocrine and molecular responses to surgical stress. Curr Probl Surg 1994;31:653–728, with permission.)

Adrenal Imaging

The adrenal glands are relatively inaccessible retroperitoneal organs that are surrounded by perinephric fat. Plain abdominal films have a very limited role in adrenal imaging. However, they can detect calcifications, especially in children who have had neonatal hemorrhage or have neuroblastoma. In adults, calcifications of the adrenal glands are highly suggestive of granulomatous disease including tuberculosis, histoplasmosis, and sarcoidosis. Ultrasonography can detect adrenal lesions and is a relatively inexpensive method to serially follow small adrenal adenomas. It is most useful in thin patients and can differentiate cystic from solid tumors. In addition, it can demonstrate liver metastases. Adrenal ultrasound has a limited role for diagnostic purposes and is largely supplemented by computed tomography (CT) or magnetic resonance imaging (MRI) scans. Intraoperative ultrasound performed during laparoscopic adrenalectomy has proven to be a useful modality. It can identify the location of small adrenal glands and delineate their vasculature.[18]

Computed Tomography Scans

Computed tomography scanning of the adrenal gland has proven to be the diagnostic procedure of choice for most patients. Simple cysts and myelolipomas can be diagnosed with virtual certainty based on their CT characteristics (Fig. 57.4). Standard CT techniques employ continuous 1-cm sections through the entire gland, although 5-mm or 1.5-mm sections may be used when small lesions are expected, especially in patients with suspected aldosteronomas. Intravenous contrast is generally not required, and a low attenuation value on an unenhanced CT scan can help differentiate benign (low density) from malignant lesions as well as metastases, which generally have a higher density.[19–21] Lesions with low Hounsfield units (HU) are most likely benign, whereas lesions that have a HU density greater than 20 are more likely to be malignant.[22] Accordingly, it has been suggested that a cutoff point of 30 HU should be accepted for discriminating malignant and benign lesions.[23] However, CT scans have limitations with reference to their specificity. In spite of the foregoing suggestions, they cannot consistently differentiate among an adrenal adenoma, carcinoma, and a pheochromocytoma. It has also been recently suggested that CT scans underestimate the size of many adrenal tumors.[24,25]

Magnetic Resonance Imaging Scan

Magnetic resonance imaging has a significant role in the evaluation of adrenal tumors. Nonfunctioning adenomas appear on T_2-weighted images similar to normal adrenal tissue. Functional adenomas tend to demonstrate a slightly increased signal intensity, whereas adrenal metastases or

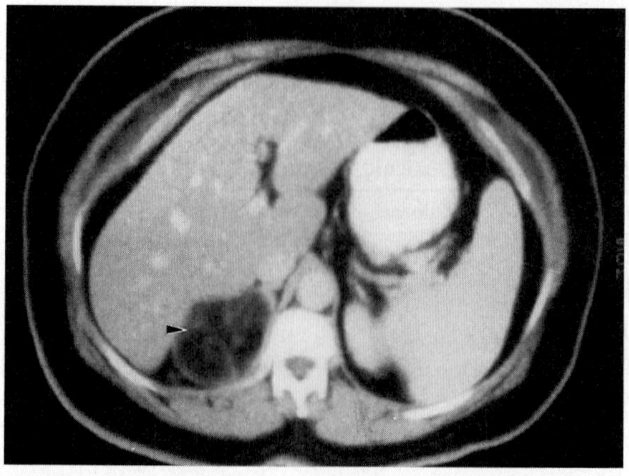

FIGURE 57.4. CT scan demonstrating a right adrenal myelolipoma (*arrowhead*). The characteristic fatty elements are diagnostic. (From Sosa JA, Udelsman R. Imaging of the adrenal gland. In: Kurtzman S, ed. Surgical Clinics of North America. Philadelphia: Saunders, 1998, with permission.)

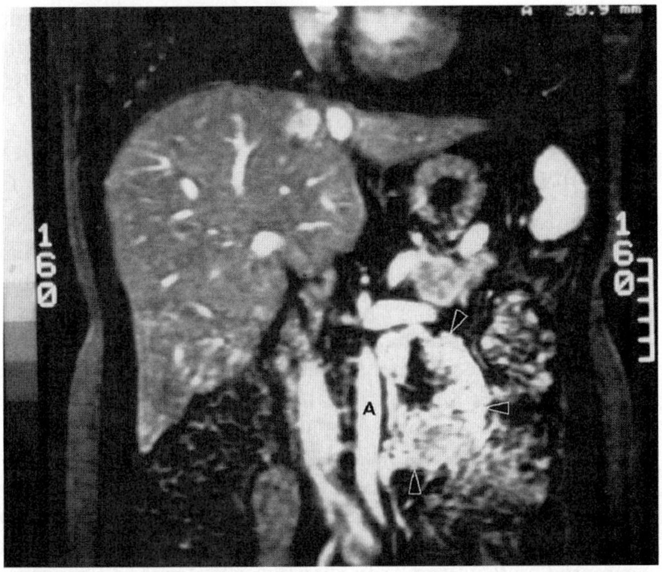

FIGURE 57.5. Magnetic resonance imaging (MRI) angiogram demonstrates a large ectopic pheochomocytoma (*arrowheads*). Note the distinct plane between the tumor and the aorta (*A*).

primary adrenal cortical carcinomas tend to be relatively bright. Enhancement on T_2-weighted images is particularly useful for pheochromocytomas, and therefore MRI appears to be the imaging study of choice in patients with suspected pheochromocytomas. A variety of investigators have employed chemical-shift imaging in MRI scans. Chemical-shift imaging can discriminate between the resonance frequencies of the protons in water and triglyceride molecules and can therefore identify adrenal adenomas because they contain abundant lipid.[26] It has been suggested that chemical-shift imaging with a lesion-to-spleen ratio less than 70 indicates a benign adrenaloma, whereas a ratio greater than 70 suggests metastatic disease.[22,26] MRI scans also play a useful role in large invasive pheochromocytomas as well as extraadrenal pheochromocytomas. In such circumstances MRI angiograms can delineate the arterial and venous anatomy and thereby avoid the use of IV contrast material (Fig. 57.5).

Radioisotope Scan

Iodocholesterol-labeled agents including ^{131}I-6-β-iodomethyl-19-norcholesterol (NP59) are incorporated into steroidogenesis pathways in the form of intracellular cholesterol and therefore have the ability to visualize functional adrenal cortical lesions.[27] These scans are particularly useful in patients who are undergoing an aldosteronoma workup because the primary lesions are often quite small. However, NP59 is not readily available at most institutions, and dexamethasone pretreatment is required.[28] These two factors limit its clinical utility.

Meta-iodobenzylguanidine (MIBG) is frequently used for the evaluation of pheochromocytoma as well as neuroblastoma. ^{131}I-MIBG and ^{123}I-MIBG are concentrated in catecholamine storage vesicles and therefore are useful in suspected cases of pheochromocytoma.[29,30] A ^{131}I-MIBG scan and its corresponding CT scan of a patient with a large right retrocaval pheochromocytoma are shown in Figure 57.6. A subset of patients have negative MRI and MIBG scans in the setting of biochemical evidence for pheochromocytoma or have extraadrenal disease, which has a lower propensity for MIBG uptake. In this case, positron emission tomography (PET) utilizing 2-fluorine-18-fluoro-2-deoxy-D-glucose (FDG) may be useful.[31]

Angiography

Angiography and venography were at one time more commonly employed for the evaluation of adrenal tumors. These procedures have been largely replaced by noninvasive imaging. For occasional patients, however, particularly those with small aldosteronomas, venous sampling is required. In this situation, one is attempting to demonstrate an aldosterone gradient in the venous effluent from the affected adrenal gland.[32] Each adrenal vein and a peripheral vein is simultaneously catheterized, and levels of aldosterone and cortisol are measured before and after ACTH administration. Aldosteronomas secrete aldosterone in response to ACTH.[32] It should be noted that adrenal venous sampling is cumbersome because

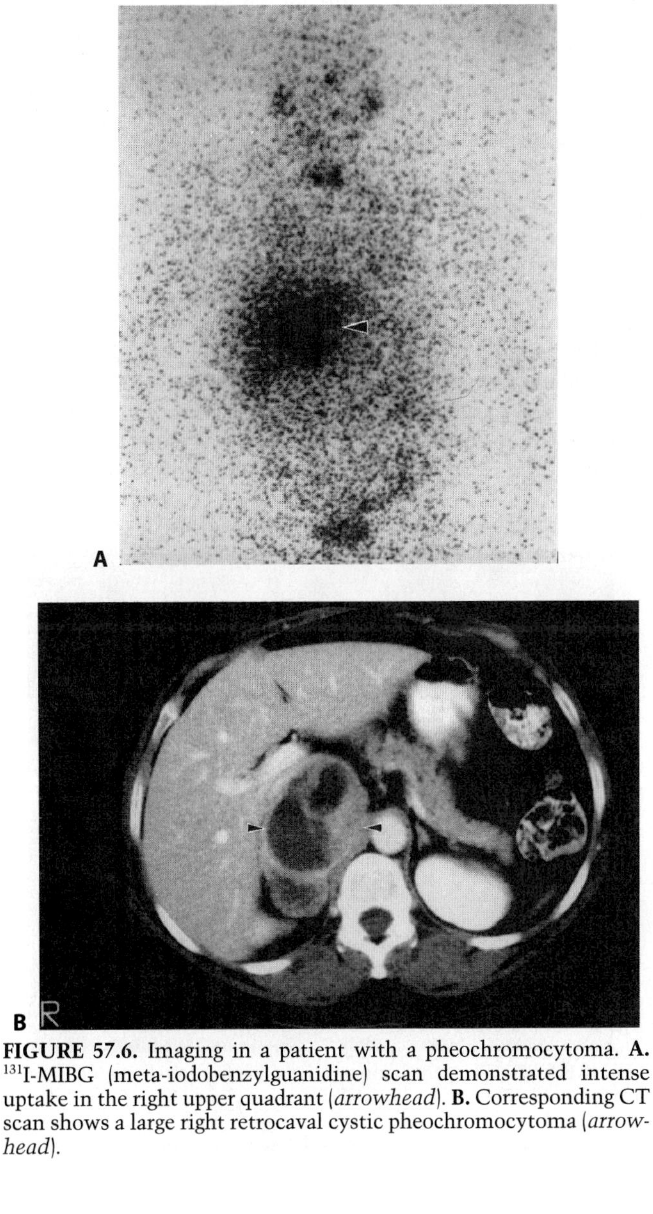

FIGURE 57.6. Imaging in a patient with a pheochromocytoma. **A.** ^{131}I-MIBG (meta-iodobenzylguanidine) scan demonstrated intense uptake in the right upper quadrant (*arrowhead*). **B.** Corresponding CT scan shows a large right retrocaval cystic pheochromocytoma (*arrowhead*).

even experienced angiographers find catheterization of the right adrenal vein difficult.

Percutaneous Biopsy

Percutaneous biopsy of the adrenal gland can be performed under either CT or ultrasound guidance. However, there are very few appropriate indications for this procedure. A percutaneous biopsy cannot reliably distinguish between an adrenal adenoma and an adrenal carcinoma.[33] The most common indication is in the setting of suspected metastatic disease to the adrenal gland. In such a case, when a fine-needle aspiration demonstrates nonadrenal malignant tissue, the diagnosis of metastasis is confirmed. This procedure should never be performed in a patient until a biochemical workup has been completed to rule out a pheochromocytoma because sudden death has been reported following biopsy of unsuspected pheochromocytoma.

Incidentaloma

Adrenal "incidentalomas" are adrenal tumors discovered on an imaging study that has been obtained for indications exclusive of adrenal-related conditions. The frequent use of CT scans, which can detect adrenal lesions greater than 1 cm, has resulted in their detection in 0.35% to 5% of studies.[3] However, the prevalence of occult adrenal adenomas is even higher, as autopsy series demonstrate adrenocortical neoplasms in 6.5% to 8.7% of adults.[34,35] A typical incidentaloma is shown in Figure 57.7. The evaluation and decision paradigm for an incidentaloma hinges on three issues: (1) Is it functional? (2) Is it likely to be a malignant adrenal tumor? (3) Is it metastatic?

The adrenal gland, although a relatively small gland, has the highest blood flow of any endocrine organ on a gram per flow basis.[36] In addition, because glucocorticoids are synthesized in the adrenal cortex, it may represent a relatively immunosuppressed organ. It is therefore not surprising that metastatic disease, particularly from lung, esophageal, and breast cancer, not uncommonly occurs in the adrenal gland. The evaluation is focused on answering each of the foregoing questions.

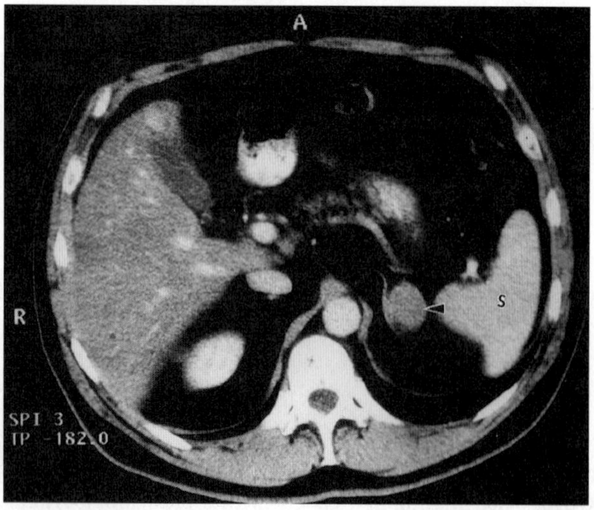

FIGURE 57.7. CT scan demonstrating a left adrenal incidentaloma (*arrowhead*). The spleen (*S*) is also shown. (From Sosa JA, Udelsman R. In: Kurtzman S, ed. Surgical Oncology Clinics of North America. Philadelphia: Saunders, 1998:109–127, with permission.)

Hormone Evaluation

All evaluations begin with a detailed history and physical examination. If symptoms or signs suggesting a functional adrenal neoplasm are detected, then, in addition to a routine screening evaluation, specific hormone studies are indicated. However, most patients are asymptomatic. The CT findings of a specific subset of adrenal masses including simple adrenal cysts and myelolipomas can be pathognomonic. In these instances, hormonal screening studies are not required.[37,38]

Screening studies are directed at three specific syndromes: pheochromocytoma, aldosteronoma, and Cushing's syndrome. Pheochromocytomas are rare; the prevalence in a series of 40,078 autopsies was 0.13%.[39] However, it has been estimated by Ross and Aron that the prevalence of pheochromocytomas in the population who have an incidentaloma should be 50 times higher (6.5%).[38] Because the risk of complications associated with an occult pheochromocytoma is significant, virtually all investigators agree that all incidentaloma patients should be screened for catecholamine hypersecretion.[38,40,41] Most commonly, urinary collections over 24 h are obtained in bottles containing acid. These collections are analyzed for metanephrines, vanillylmandelic acid (VMA), or fractionated catecholamines.

The screen for aldosteronoma in the setting of an incidentaloma is often limited. If the patient is normotensive and not receiving hypertension or diuretic therapy and has a normal serum potassium (>3.5 mEq/L), then an aldosteronoma is very unlikely. If the patient does not satisfy these criteria, then an aldosteronoma evaluation is performed as delineated later in this chapter.

Cushing's syndrome is important to consider in all patients with adrenal tumors. Patients with advanced Cushing's syndrome present with classic symptoms and signs of glucocorticoid excess and are therefore not difficult to diagnose. However, patients not uncommonly present with subtle stigmata of Cushing's syndrome or with occult or "subclinical" disease. In this situation the patient has an adrenal adenoma that has attained functional autonomy in its ability to secrete glucocorticoids but has not yet manifest findings of Cushing's syndrome.[42] This silent but subtle hypercortisolism occurs in approximately 15% of patients with incidentalomas.[42] Other series have suggested that 50% to 75% of such patients have subtle abnormalities indicating mild hypercortisolism.[43,44] It is important to rule out subclinical Cushing's syndrome for two reasons: (1) if one elects not to perform an adrenalectomy, then the endocrinopathy will continue and deleterious effects will occur, and (2) if one does perform an adrenalectomy, the contralateral adrenal will be suppressed, and if perioperative glucocorticoids are not administered the patient will be at risk for Addisonian crisis.

It is important to recognize that an incidentaloma may represent a metastatic lesion in the adrenal gland. The majority of patients with metastatic disease to one or both adrenal glands have both a history of malignant disease and metastases to multiple additional sites. In the setting of widespread metastatic disease, the adrenal disease is not treated directly

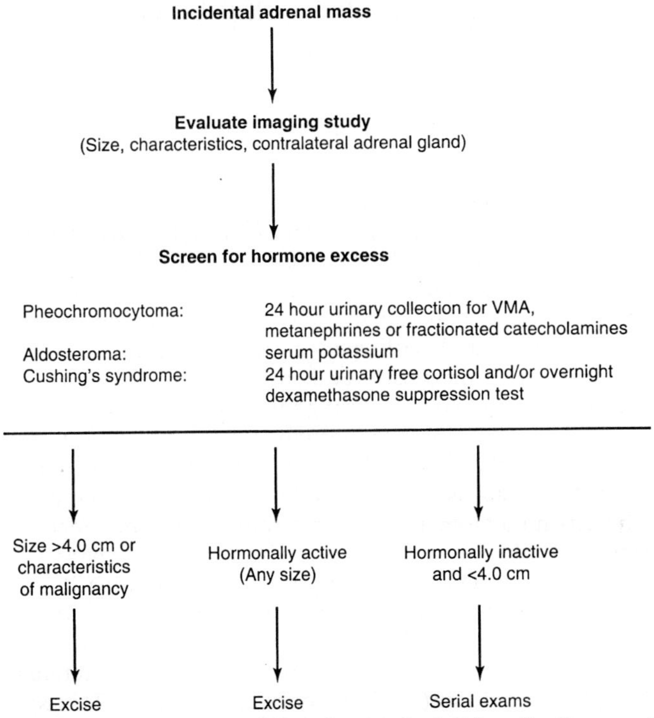

FIGURE 57.8. Recommended evaluation for incidentally discovered adrenal mass. *VMA*, vanillylmandelic acid.

as it represents only a small focus of total tumor burden. Patients with bilateral adrenal metastases are at some risk for adrenal insufficiency.

Patients with isolated adrenal metastases pose a diagnostic dilemma. In this setting a tissue diagnosis may affect subsequent care or an adrenalectomy might be indicated. Some experienced surgeons and endocrinologists have suggested that fine-needle aspiration (FNA) biopsy is an important diagnostic tool in the evaluation of most incidentaloma patients.[45,46] However, this recommendation appears ill advised for most incidentaloma patients. It is well recognized that FNA cannot distinguish an adrenal adenoma from an adrenal carcinoma.[33] Therefore, the only situation in which adrenal FNA appears indicated is when metastatic disease is not only likely but its detection would also alter patient management.[47] It must also be emphasized that adrenal FNA should never be undertaken until an occult pheochromocytoma has been ruled out.[48] Some investigators have utilized ^{131}I-6-β-iodomethyl-norcholesterol (NP59) to help determine the functional significance of an incidentaloma.[49] This agent can be helpful in select patients; however, it is not available in most centers in the United States.

An important and unresolved issue in the management of incidentalomas is the determination of what size of adrenal tumor is in itself an indication for extirpation. In the absence of scientific trials an empiric approach has been employed. Virtually all experts agree that any lesion greater than 5 cm on initial presentation should be excised because of the risk of malignancy. Lesions less than 3 cm are generally followed with serial imaging studies. Several experienced investigators have recommended excision of all adrenal tumors greater than 4 cm.[50,51]

A recent multicenter retrospective study of 210 patients confirmed that tumor diameter correlated with cancer. A cutoff of 5 cm discriminated between benign and malignant adrenal cortical lesions with a sensitivity of 93% and a specificity of 64%.[52] However, only 44% of the patients underwent adrenalectomy, and of those not explored 12-month follow-up data were available for only 41 of 95 patients. Therefore, this 5-cm cutoff recommendation must be interpreted with caution. Furthermore, in many series small (<5 cm) adrenocortical carcinomas have been reported.[52,53] Laparoscopic adrenalectomy is likely to cause a subtle downward shift in the size recommendations, and a cutoff of 4 cm appears reasonable. If one elects not to excise an incidentaloma, then a follow-up imaging study should be obtained at a relatively short interval (approximately 3 months) to determine if serial growth has occurred. Lesions that grow should be excised.

An algorithm for the evaluation of incidentally discovered adrenal masses is depicted in Figure 57.8. It is based upon a systematic literature review and the acceptance of 4.0 cm as a size that is in itself an indication for adrenalectomy.

Hyperaldosteronism

Excessive secretion of aldosterone results in hypertension and hypokalemia. It may be caused by primary aldosteronism, an intrinistic abnormality of one or both adrenal glands. It can also be caused by excessive renin secretion, which results from a low effective arterial blood volume, in which case it is termed secondary aldosteronism.[54] Primary aldosteronism is rare, with a prevalence among hypertensive patients estimated to range between 0.05% and 2%.[55] This section is focused on primary aldosteronism, with emphasis on the most common and surgically correctable etiology, aldosteronoma.

The six recognized causes of primary aldosteronism and their relative frequencies are summarized in Table 57.3.[56] The most common etiology, an aldosterone-producing adrenocortical adenoma (APA), and curative treatment by unilateral adrenalectomy were first reported by Conn in 1955.[57] Aldosteronomas occur in approximately 65% of patients with primary aldosteronism. They are almost always unilateral and are often less than 2 cm in size (Fig. 57.9, top).

It is extremely important to distinguish a unilateral aldosteronoma from idiopathic hyperaldosteronism (IHA), which occurs in 25% of patients with primary aldosteronism and is caused by bilateral adrenal hyperplasia. In this case, both adrenal glands contain multiple macro- and microscopic nodules, as shown in Figure 57.9 (bottom). Importantly, unilateral adrenalectomy in the setting of IHA is not curative.

TABLE 57.3. Primary Aldosteronism.

Etiology	*Percent*
Solitary aldosterone-producing adrenocortical adenoma (APA)	65%
Idiopathic hyperaldosteronism (IHA) with bilateral adrenal hyperplasia	25%
Primary adrenal hyperplasia	5%
Renin-responsive aldosterone-producing adenoma	5%
Glucocorticoid-remedial aldosteronism	Rare
Adrenocortical carcinoma	Rare

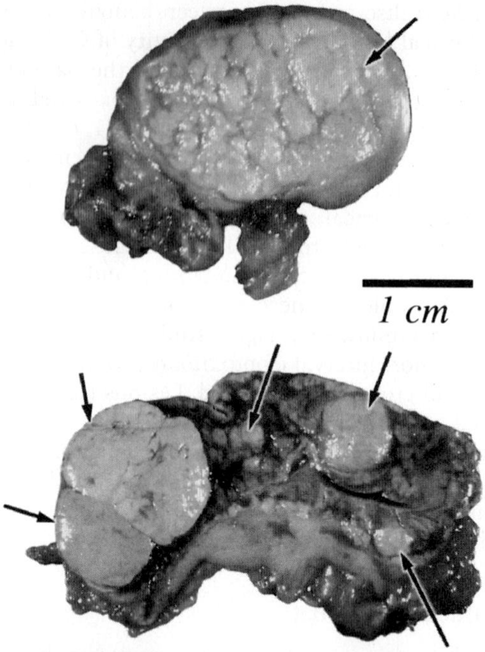

FIGURE 57.9. Primary aldosteronism. *Top:* The upper adrenal gland demonstrates a unilateral aldosterone-producing adrenocortical adenoma (APA) (*arrow*). *Bottom:* The lower adrenal gland demonstrates idiopathic hyperaldosteronism (IHA); it contains multiple hyperplastic nodules (*arrows*).

Unfortunately, the distinction between APA and IHA can be difficult. This distinction is further complicated as some authors have suggested that micronodules and macronodules can occur in association with a so-called single adenoma in a significant proportion of patients.[58]

Additional, but less common, surgically correctable causes of primary aldosteronism include primary adrenal hyperplasia and renin-response aldosterone-producing adenoma (see Table 57.3). Primary adrenal hyperplasia may be unilateral or bilateral, and the glands appear histologically like those seen in patients with IHA. The biochemical profile, however, is similar to that seen in an APA and unilateral adrenalectomy appears to be beneficial in patients with unilateral lesions.[56,59] Renin-responsive aldosterone-producing adenomas appear biochemically similar to IHA, and they also respond to surgical resection.[56,60] Adrenal cortical aldosterone-producing carcinoma is extremely rare and represents another surgically treatable form of primary aldosteronism.[61]

Clinical Presentation

The signs and symptoms of primary aldosteronism are nonspecific and include hypertension and hypokalemia. The mean age at presentation ranges from 30 to 50 years, and it is twice as common in women.[58,62] The hypertension is generally indistinguishable from that seen in the population with essential hypertension. The hypokalemia may result in the characteristic symptoms of polydipsia, polyuria, headaches, muscle weakness, cramping, and periodic paralysis.[63]

There are three major steps in the evaluation of patients who are likely to have primary aldosteronism: (1) screen the individual and establish a clear diagnosis of primary aldosteronism; (2) discriminate between the different causes of primary aldosteronism; and (3) localize the site of an APA if present.

Screening for Primary Aldosteronism

The presence of spontaneous hypokalemia in a hypertensive individual strongly suggests the diagnosis. Unfortunately, the common use of diuretics, as well as antihypertensive agents including angiotension-converting enzyme inhibitors and spironolactone, interfere with the ability to establish the diagnosis.[64,65] Most endocrinologists recommend discontinuation of all diuretic and antihypertensive therapy for at least 4 weeks before a diagnostic evaluation. If the patient's blood pressure requires control during this interval, prazosin can be used as it will not interfere with the workup.[64] A wide variety of biochemical tests have been recommended, but there is no clear consensus as to which tests are the most appropriate. There is no argument that the serum potassium concentration should be measured in virtually all hypertensive patients.[66] However, a single potassium determination can miss the diagnosis as the result of momentary as well as circadian variations.[67] Furthermore, Bravo et al. reported that nearly 30% of patients with proven primary aldosteronism had plasma potassium values above 3.5 mmol/L.[68] Therefore, hypokalemia, although highly suggestive of the diagnosis, should not be considered as a necessary criterion.[69]

Plasma Aldosterone/Renin Ratio

Excess autonomous secretion of aldosterone results in salt retention, hypertension, and suppression of plasma renin activity. However, single isolated measurements of either plasma renin or aldosterone are of limited diagnostic value.[67,69,70] Simultaneous measurements of both plasma renin activity and aldosterone was proposed by Hiramatsu et al. as a means to increase diagnostic sensitivity.[70] Because primary aldosteronism results in elevated aldosterone and suppressed plasma renin levels, this determination appears more useful and is less affected by physiological or pharmacological variables.[71,72]

Saline Infusion Test

The saline infusion test is used to demonstrate autonomous aldosterone secretion that does not decrease appropriately following sodium loading.[72–74] Recent reviews have addressed the limitations of the study.[69,72] A frequently used protocol requires measurement of plasma aldosterone at baseline and 4 h after lying in the supine position and receiving 2 L intravenous normal saline solution. Failure to suppress plasma aldosterone below 8.5 mg/dL is considered diagnostic of primary aldosteronism.[74]

Distinction Between Aldostrone-Producing Adrenocortical Adenoma (APA) and Idiopathic Hyperaldosteronism (IHA)

The majority of cases of primary aldosteronism are caused by either an APA (65%) or IHA (25%). It is important to discriminate between these as an APA is treated by unilateral adrenalectomy, whereas IHA is generally treated with spironolactone.[75] A variety of biochemical and imaging studies are available to make this distinction (Table 57.4). Postural

TABLE 57.4. Aldosteronoma Screening Studies.

Test	*Results*
Aldosterone-producing adenoma (APA)	
Plasma aldosterone after postural stimulation	Decrease or <30% increase
18-Hydroxycorticosterone	>100 ng/dL
Computed tomography scan	Unilateral mass
Iodocholesterol scan	Localization
Adrenal venous sampling	Localization
Idiopathic aldosteronism	
Plasma aldosterone after postural stimulation	>30% increase
18-Hydroxycorticosterone	<100 ng/dL
Computed tomography scan	? Bilateral masses
Iodocholesterol scan	Bilateral uptake
Adrenal venous sampling	No localization

Source: Udelsman R. Tumors of the adrenal cortex. In: Cameron JL, ed. Current Surgical Therapy, 6th ed. St. Louis: Mosby, 1998:577–580, with permission.

stimulation is performed by measuring a morning plasma aldosterone level 4h after assuming an upright posture. A postural response with suppression or a minimal increase in aldosterone is suggestive of an APA, whereas a marked increase in aldosterone is characteristic of IHA.[76] Unfortunately, the accuracy of this test was only 85% in a large collected series reported by Young et al. in 1990.[77]

The aldosterone precursor 18-hydroxycorticosterone (18-OH-B) has also been measured to help discriminate between an APA and IHA.[78] A plasma value of 100 ng/dL or greater is highly suggestive of an APA. Patients with IHA usually have values less than 100 ng/dL. Although this assay is not universally available, it is relatively straightforward and can be a useful part of the diagnostic evaluation.[79]

Localization

Once the biochemical criteria for an APA have been satisfied, the next step is tumor localization. High-quality CT scans have simplified this workup for the majority of patients. If a unilateral adrenal mass is detected and the contralateral adrenal gland is normal, then proceeding directly to unilateral adrenalectomy appears reasonable.[56,65,80] In the past several authors have recommended routine use of NP-59 studies as well as adrenal vein sampling.[81,82] The argument for obtaining these studies is to minimize the risk of removing a nonfunctional adrenal adenoma and leaving behind an occult (usually less than 1 cm) aldosteronoma in the contralateral adrenal gland that appeared "normal" on CT scan. In addition, subtle cases of asymmetrical IHA could appear like a unilateral APA. However, NP-59 is most sensitive for larger tumors and it is also likely to miss small aldosteronomas. Furthermore, accurate adrenal vein sampling is cumbersome, expensive, and not available at many centers. The consensus has now shifted, and most adrenal experts recommend selective use of adrenal vein sampling for equivocal cases in which the imaging studies are ambiguous.[56,65]

Treatment

There is an ever-expanding body of literature to suggest that laparoscopic adrenalectomy is the procedure of choice for aldosteronomas.[83–85] This technique results in improvement in length of stay, morbidity, and costs. In addition, the patient is able to return to normal activity in a much shorter interval.[18,86] The traditional surgical treatment has required a unilateral total adrenalectomy. Recently, aldosteronoma enucleation or subtotal adrenalectomy has been suggested as an equally effective technique.[87,88]

Results

The surgical treatment of APA results in correction of hypokalemia in almost all cases.[89] Hypertension is usually improved, but may persist, particularly if the patient has long-standing hypertension at the time of surgery.[89] The incidence of persistent hypertension is approximately 30%.[90] Risk factors associated with persistent hypertension include age greater than 50 at the time of surgery, male sex, and the presence of "multiple adenomas" or inappropriately diagnosed IHA.[58]

Cushing's Syndrome

Harvey Cushing described eight patients in 1932 with moon facies, truncal obesity, hypertension, polyphagia, polydipsia, polycythemia, and pulmonary infections. Pituitary basophil adenomas were noted in autopsy in four of these patients, and he correctly associated this syndrome with pituitary adenomas.[91] The most common cause of Cushing syndrome is iatrogenic administration of glucocorticoids. Endogenous Cushing syndrome is, for the most part, either ACTH-dependent or ACTH-independent (Table 57.5). The most common cause of endogenous Cushing's syndrome, accounting for nearly 85% of all cases, is Cushing's disease, glucocorticoid excess caused by a pituitary adenoma. The other cause of ACTH-dependent Cushing's syndrome is the rare ectopic ACTH syndrome. The majority of ACTH-independent causes of Cushing's syndrome are adrenal in origin, consisting of adrenal adenoma and rare adrenal carcinomas. Recently, a new source of ACTH-independent Cushing's syndrome has been appreciated, termed primary pigmented nodular adrenal dysplasia (PPNAD).[92] In addition, macronodular adrenal hyperplasia (MAH) has also been described (Fig. 57.10).[93] In most cases, MAH appears to be ACTH-independent, but there is a wide spectrum of ACTH levels in patients with MAH.[92] The management of ACTH-dependent Cushing's syndrome requires accurate tumor identification and extirpation whenever possible. In some circumstances, pituitary surgery is unsuccessful or the source of the ectopic ACTH secretion cannot be identified. In this situation, bilateral adrenalectomy may be required to alleviate the sequela of life-threatening glucocorticoid excess.

TABLE 57.5. Endogenous Causes of Cushing's Syndrome.

ACTH-dependent
Cushing's disease (pituitary adenoma)
Ectopic ACTH syndrome
ACTH-independent
Adrenal adenoma
Adrenal carcinoma
Primary pigmented nodular adrenal dysplasia (PPNAD)
ACTH-variable
Macronodular adrenal hyperplasia

The treatment of choice of ACTH-independent Cushing's syndrome is surgical resection. Patients with endogenous Cushing's syndrome caused by a unilateral adrenal tumor will have an elevated 24-h urinary free cortisol and 17-hydroxycorticosteroid levels. Because these tumors produce glucocorticoids in the absence of ACTH stimulation, the normal pituitary secretion of ACTH is suppressed. Therefore, an elevated plasma ACTH level in this setting is inconsistent with the diagnosis. The dexamethasone suppression test can be extremely useful in discriminating between ACTH-dependent and ACTH-independent causes of Cushing's syndrome. It is also crucial to carefully evaluate the imaging studies. In the setting of an adrenal adenoma, one anticipates unilateral adrenal enlargement and a contralateral normal or slightly suppressed adrenal gland. In the setting of adrenocortical carcinoma, the ipsilateral adrenal gland should be significantly enlarged and may be associated with local tumor invasion (Fig. 57.11). The contralateral adrenal gland should be normal in size. In addition, in the setting of an adrenal carcinoma one is likely to find elevated levels of adrenal androgens.[94]

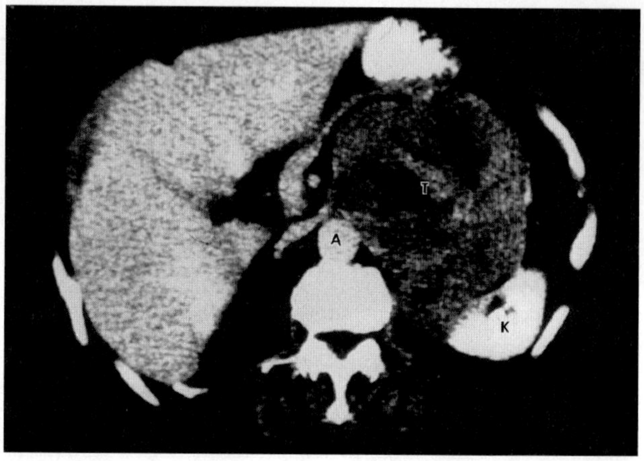

FIGURE 57.11. CT scan demonstrates a large left adrenocortical carcinoma that caused ACTH-independent Cushing's syndrome. The tumor (*T*) invaded the kidney (*K*), aorta (*A*), and diaphragm. (From Sosa JA, Udelsman R. Imaging of the adrenal gland. In: Kurtzman S, ed. Surgical Oncology Clinics of North America. Philadelphia: Saunders, 1998:109–127, with permission.)

Surgical treatment of adrenal causes of Cushing's syndrome has undergone significant changes.[95] Adrenal surgery can be performed safely with low morbidity and operative mortality in the 2% to 3% range. The recent advent of laparoscopic adrenalectomy has dramatically changed the management of these patients.[18,84] Unilateral adrenalectomy is the treatment of choice for most patients with a tumor causing ACTH-independent endogenous Cushing's syndrome.

Bilateral Adrenalectomy

Bilateral adrenalectomy will continue to play a small but significant role in the management of selected patients with Cushing's disease.[96] In spite of the best neurosurgical series, there may be failures following pituitary resection. These patients often develop life-threatening hypercortisolism and require definitive treatment. The natural history of untreated Cushing's syndrome results in a mortality rate of approximately 50% at 5 years.[97] Patients with ectopic ACTH syndrome not uncommonly present with explosive Cushing's syndrome, and it is often difficult or impossible to locate the source of the ACTH production.[98] In addition, patients with primary pigmented nodular adrenal dysplasia as occurs in the Carney complex require bilateral adrenalectomy.[99] A subset of patients with MAH may respond to a variety of receptor blockers.[100] However, it appears that the majority of patients with MAH who develop Cushing's syndrome require bilateral adrenalectomy. The role of bilateral adrenalectomy in this setting has been reviewed by Favia et al. in 1994, who recommended a posterior approach.[96] A more recent publication by Chapuis et al. in 1996 reported their experience with bilateral adrenalectomy in 82 patients during a 15-year period.[101] The operative mortality rate was 2.4%, and complications tended to occur in patients with more advanced disease. We and others have performed bilateral adrenalectomy for persistent Cushing's disease and MAH using a laparoscopic approach.[18]

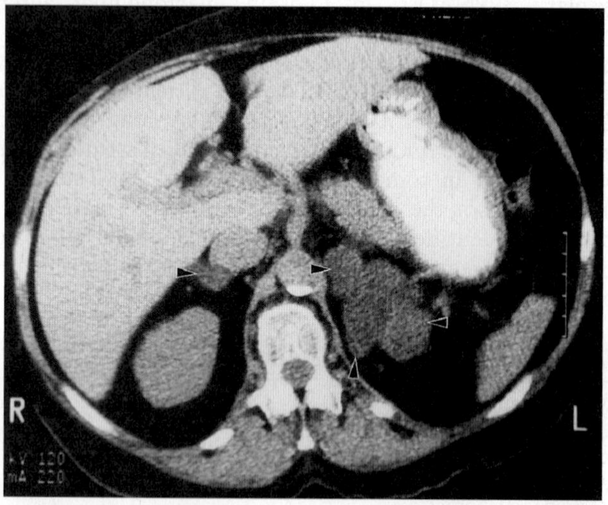

FIGURE 57.10. CT scan demonstrates macronodular adrenal hyperplasia (MAH) in a patient with ACTH-independent severe Cushing's syndrome. Multiple macronodules were present in both adrenal glands (*arrowheads*). Bilateral laparoscopic adrenalectomy was performed.

Bilateral adrenalectomy is associated with significant long-term morbidity. These patients require lifelong replacement with both mineralocorticoids and glucocorticoids. Occult adrenal insufficiency may occur and can be life-threatening.[102] It is also important to note that even patients who undergo unilateral adrenalectomy for ACTH-independent causes of Cushing's syndrome will have contralateral adrenal gland suppression, and there may be a prolonged interval until endogenous glucocorticoid production is sufficient.[103] It is clear, however, that laparoscopic adrenalectomy is appropriate and does pose significant advantages in the management of these patients.[18,84,104,105] The laparoscopic approach minimizes tissue trauma, which is especially useful in patients who have advanced manifestations of Cushing's syndrome.

Pheochromocytoma

Pheochromocytomas are rare tumors that arise from the neuroectodermally derived chromaffin cells. The majority of pathologists believe that all pheochromocytomas are of

TABLE 57.6. Extraadrenal Pheochromocytoma Locations.

Organ of Zuckerkandl
Urinary bladder
Liver hilum
Renal hilum
Posterior mediastinum
Intrapericardial
Neck

adrenal origin, and they refer to extraadrenal chromaffin tumors as paragangliomas, which may or may not be functional. However, most clinicians designate catecholamine-secreting tumors as either adrenal or extraadrenal pheochromocytomas.[106]

The majority of pheochromocytomas (90%) in adults are located in the adrenal gland. However, in children the incidence of extraadrenal pheochromocytomas is much higher (35%).[106] Extraadrenal pheochromocytomas sites are listed in Table 57.6. Most pheochromocytomas (90%) are unilateral. However, the incidence of synchronous or metachronous pheochromocytomas are more common in patients with familial forms of pheochromocytomas. These syndromes and their associated findings are listed in Table 57.7. The majority of pheochromocytomas (90%) are thought to be benign. However, because the criteria for malignancy require the demonstration of distant metastasis or direct invasion into surrounding organs, it is possible that surgical extirpation of a subset of presumptively benign pheochromocytomas results in excision of a malignant lesion that has not yet satisfied the requisite malignant criteria.

Functional pheochromocytomas secrete a variety of vasoactive compounds either continually or episodically. Norepinephrine is the most common. Occasional tumors secrete only epinephrine, but the majority secrete a combination of norepinephrine, epinephrine, and dopamine.[106] Occasionally pheochromocytomas secrete additional active peptides including adrenocorticotropic hormone (ACTH), vasoactive intestinal polypeptide (VIP), encephalins, and serotonin.[106,107]

TABLE 57.7. Genetic Syndromes Associated with Pheochromocytoma.

Syndrome	*Findings*
MEN2A (Sipple's syndrome)	Medullary carcinoma of the thyroid Pheochromocytoma Hyperparathyroidism
MEN 2B	Medullary carcinoma of the thyroid Pheochromocytoma Mucosal neuroma Marfanoid habitus Ganglioneuromas of the gastrointestinal tract
Neurofibromatosis (von Recklinghausen's disease)	Café-au-lait spots Axillary freckling Multiple freckling Multiple neurofibromas Pheochromocytoma
Von Hippel–Lindau disease	Retinal hemanagiomatosis Cerebellar hemangioblastoma Pheochromocytoma Renal cell tumors

MEN, multiple endocrine neoplasia.

TABLE 57.8. Symptoms of Paroxysmal Attacks in Adults with Pheochromocytoma.

Symptom	*Mean (%)*
Headache	60
Diaphoresis	53
Palpitations	51
Pallor	43
Nausea	34
Tremor	31
Anxiety	29
Abdominal pain	24
Chest pain	21
Weakness	20
Dyspnea	18
Flushing	13
Visual disturbance	13

Source: Gifford RW Jr, Manager WM, Bravo EL. Pheochromocytoma. Endocrinol Metab Clin North Am 1994;23:387–404, with permission.

Clinical Manifestations

The classic presentation of a symptomatic pheochromocytoma is episodic attacks of headaches, diaphoresis, and palpitations.[106,108] The duration of an individual attack can range from 30 s to 1 week, but most last about 15 min.[106] The episodes may be infrequent (every other month) or they may occur multiple times in a single 24-h period. Although hypertension is commonly present during an attack, it is important to remember that between attacks approximately 50% of affected individuals are normotensive. A list of the more common symptoms elicited during paroxysmal attacks compiled from two large series is presented in Table 57.8. The hypertension can result in stroke, renal insufficiency, and cardiac failure.[109]

Diagnosis

The diagnosis of pheochromocytoma is dependent upon the ability to demonstrate elevated levels of catecholamines or their metabolites in plasma or urine. Gifford et al. have suggested 10 clinical situations in which it is appropriate to screen for a pheochromocytoma (Table 57.9).[106]

TABLE 57.9. Indication for Pheochromocytoma Screening.

Symptomatic episodes, especially when paroxysmal and accompanied by hypertension
Refractory hypertension
Accelerated hypertension
Paradoxical hypertensive response to beta-blockers
Hypertensive paroxysms during anesthesia, surgery, parturition, or angiography
Family screening in recognized families
Hypertension coexistent with associated conditions (neurofibromatosis, von Hippel–Lindau disease, Cushing's syndrome)
Marked labile hypertension
Orthostatic hypotension in the absence of antihypertension therapy
Incidentally discovered adrenal tumor

TABLE 57.10. Sensitivity and Specificity of Various Biochemical Tests in the Diagnosis of Pheochromocytoma.

Biochemical test	*Reference value*[a]	*Sensitivity (% range)*[b]	*Specificity (% range)*[b]
Plasma NE1E	>950 pg/ml	88–100	93–101
Urinary NMN1MN	>1.8 mg/24 h	67–91	83–103
Urinary VMA	>11 mg/24 h	28–56	98–102

NE1E, norepinephrine plus epinephrine; NMN1MN, normetanephrine plus metanephrine. VMA, vanillymandelic acid.

[a]Upper 95% confidence limits obtained from essential hypertension subjects under basal conditions.

[b]Values are expressed as 62 SE.

Source: Gifford RW Jr, Manger WM, Bravo EL. Pheochromocytoma. Endocrinol Metab Clin North Am 1994;23:387–404, with permission.[106]

The most commonly employed biochemical screening tests require 24-h urinary collections for the measurement of vanillylmandelic acid (VMA), metanephrines, or fractionated catecholamines.[108] It is important to note that multiple medications and some foods can interfere with these assays, and at times 24-h urinary collections can be difficult to obtain. Although some experts[106,108] have recommended measuring plasma catecholamines, this practice has not been widely accepted. However, recent studies indicate that plasma levels of metanephrine and normetanephrine are sensitive and specific for pheochromocytoma. The relative sensitivity and specificity of various biochemical tests in the diagnosis of pheochromocytoma have been summarized by Gifford et al.[106] (Table 57.10).

In select circumstances, additional pharmacological tests are required to yield an unequivocal biochemical diagnosis.[110] However, the clonidine suppression test and the glucagon stimulation test are not routinely required.[106,108,110,111]

Imaging

Once the diagnosis of a pheochromocytoma has been made, the next step is tumor localization using imaging studies including ultrasound, CT, MRI, and MIBG scans. MRI scans have several unique characteristics that make them the imaging study of choice. The MRI scan will enhance on T_2-weighted images, and administration of IV contrast agents is not required (see Adrenal Imaging).

Preoperative Pharmacological Treatment

Because of chronic hypersecretion of catecholamines, patients with pheochromocytomas are often severely volume-contracted. In the past, when these patients underwent general anesthesia, it was not uncommon for them to experience severe hemodynamic instability. Accordingly, it is necessary to initiate a 1- to 4-week period of preoperative alpha-adrenergic receptor blockade. The most commonly used agent is the selective alpha-1-adrenergic receptor blocker phenoxybenzamine. It is usually started at a dose of 10 to 20 mg, two to four times a day, and the dose is escalated, often until the patient experiences orthostatic hypotension.[112] Occasional patients who do not tolerate phenoxybenzamine can be treated with the tyrosine hydroxylase inhibitor metyrosine.[113] Prazosin (2–5 mg twice daily) can also be used preoperatively.[108] Others have suggested that a combination regimen of phenoxybenzamine and metyrosine results in improved intraoperative hemodynamic control.[114] Occasional patients will also require beta-adrenergic receptor blockade because of breakthrough tachycardia. However, beta-receptor blockade should not be administered in the absence of prior alpha-receptor blockade because of the risk of unapposed alpha receptor-induced malignant hypertension.[106,112] Even the combined alpha- and beta-adrenergic receptor blocking agent, labetolol, has been reported to induce paradoxical hypertension.[115] Although the majority of centers employ preoperative blockage, the Cleveland Clinic group has demonstrated that pheochromocytoma patients can undergo successful surgical treatment without preoperative preparation with long-lasting alpha-adrenergic blockade.[116]

The anesthetic and surgical care of these patients is critical and requires a concerted effort. Patients may experience both hypertension and hypotension (following tumor removal), and the anesthesiologist must be prepared to treat precipitous changes in blood pressure. Infusions of phentolamine and sodium nitroprusside are often required.[106] In addition, anesthetic agents that lower the threshold of catecholamine-induced arrhythmias (halothane) or histamine release (morphine) should be avoided.[117]

Surgical treatment in the past required an open laparotomy with early control of the main adrenal vein and bilateral as well as extraadrenal exploration. This practice has been changed by the exquisite sensitivity of current imaging techniques and the use of laparoscopic adrenalectomy. At many institutions, laparoscopic adrenalectomy has become the procedure of choice.[18] Patients with large pheochromocytomas that appear to be malignant or difficult to control should be explored by an open technique.[18,84]

Postoperative management may require liberal volume replacement as the result of hypotension. This need does not appear to occur when adequate preoperative alpha-receptor blockade and its resultant volume expansion have been performed. Patients will also require glucocorticoid replacement if they undergo bilateral adrenalectomy. Hypoglycemia can also occur, and plasma glucose should be monitored in the early postoperative period.[118]

Malignant Pheochromocytoma

Complete surgical excision is the only potentially curative therapy for malignant pheochromocytoma.[108,109] Accordingly, aggressive surgical resection is indicated in all patients who can tolerate the procedure. However, the criteria for malignancy, invasion into adjacent tissue or distant metastases, are not always demonstrable at the time of surgery or on pathological review of the specimen. Long-term follow-up has demonstrated that patients with apparently benign, completely excised, well-encapsulated tumors can develop distant metastases.[119,120] It is for this reason that initial total tumor extirpation as well as long-term follow-up are essential.

Patients with malignant pheochromocytomas, even in the setting of metastatic disease, can have prolonged survival. The mean 5-year survival ranges from 30% to 40%.[121] Surgical resection is indicated whenever feasible. The most effective chemotherapeutic regimen includes cyclophosphamide, vincristine, and dacarbazine.[122] Although pheochromocytomas are not generally radiosensitive,[106] treatment with ^{131}I-MIBG has been shown to be of benefit in selected patients.[123,124]

Familial Pheochromocytoma

Pheochromocytomas occur in association with several genetic syndromes including multiple endocrine neoplasia (MEN)2, von Hippel–Lindau disease, and von Recklinghausen's disease (see Table 57.7). When individuals from an affected family are identified, they should undergo screening. If they are found to have biochemical evidence of catecholamine excess, localization procedures are indicated. Bilateral adrenalectomy has been generally recommended in familial patients because at the time of biochemical abnormalities at least bilateral adrenal medullary hyperplasia has already developed.[125,126]

A recent publication by Lairmore et al. questioned this practice in MEN2 patients.[127] They followed 23 patients who underwent resection of a unilateral pheochromocytoma, with the macroscopically normal contralateral adrenal gland being left in situ. A pheochromocytoma developed in the residual gland in 52% of the patients at a mean of 12 years after initial surgery. Furthermore, 48% of the patients retained normal adrenal function and did not develop a contralateral pheochromocytoma during a mean interval of 5 years. Addisonian crisis or acute adrenal insufficiency occurred in 23% of the patients who had undergone bilateral adrenalectomy. It therefore seems prudent to perform a unilateral adrenalectomy for macroscopically normal glands in the setting of familial pheochromocytomas. Serial follow-up is required to detect and treat subsequent pheochromocytomas, which will develop in a significant number of these patients.

Adrenocortical Carcinoma

Adrenocortical carcinoma is rare, with an incidence of 0.6 to 2 cases per million individuals per year.[128–130] The prognosis is poor, and most series report a 5-year mortality between 55% and 90%.[131,132] It accounts for approximately 0.2% of cancer deaths.[133] Because of its rare incidence, controlled clinical trials have not addressed major issues in the diagnosis or treatment of this disease. The largest series are retrospective and generally report the experience of individual institutions over decades.

Presentation

The majority of patients (68%–80%) present with an endocrinopathy, most commonly Cushing's syndrome.[94,129] An even higher percentage have endocrine abnormalities detected after undergoing a diagnostic evaluation. Other endocrinopathies include virilization and feminization. Hyperaldosternism can occur but is much less common.[130,131]

Patients often have advanced disease at the time of presentation, with almost 40% presenting with metastatic disease.[129] The most common sites of distant metastases are the liver, lung, bone, and brain.[129,131] However, local invasion into adjacent organs including the kidney, liver, diaphragm, spleen, pancreas, and vena cava are common at the time of diagnostics (see Fig. 57.11).[75] A female predominance of at least 2:1 is noted in most series,[94,132,134] and the mean age at presentation ranges from 30 to 50 years.[94,130–132] The staging criteria for adrenocortical carcinoma are shown in Table 57.11. The majority of patients present with tumors greater than 5 cm in size with local invasion into adjacent organs with or without distant metastases (stage II or III).[75]

TABLE 57.11. Staging Criteria for Adrenocortical Carcinoma.

T_1	Less than 5 cm, no local invasion
T_2	More than 5 cm, no local invasion
T_3	Any size, local invasion
N_0	No positive lymph nodes
N_1	Positive lymph nodes
M_0	No distant metastasis
M_1	Distant metastasis
Stage	
I	T_1, N_0, M_0
II	T_2, N_0, M_0
III	T_1, or T_2, N_1, M_0, or T_3, N_0, M_0
IV	Any T, any NM_1, or T_3, N_1, M_0

Source: Udelsman R. Tumors of the adrenal cortex. In: Cameron JL, ed. Current Surgical Therapy, 6th ed. St. Louis: Mosby, 1998:579.

Surgery is the mainstay of therapy and remains the only potential for cure. Aggressive local resection is indicated whenever feasible. Adjacent organs including lymph nodes, kidney, spleen, diaphragm, distal pancreas, liver, and vena cava are often resected in continuity with the primary tumor. MRI scans, especially MRI "angiograms," are used when there is a suspicion of major vascular involvement. Conventional angiography is rarely required.

The role of adjuvant chemotherapy is somewhat controversial.[94] The single most effective agent, mitotane (*o,p'*-DDD or 1,1-dichlorodiphenyldichloroethane), has been used since 1960[135] with moderate success. In spite of the absence of a randomized-prospective placebo-controlled trial, its use has been adopted by most centers as standard adjuvant therapy.[94,129,130,133,134] It is the only agent associated with long-term remissions and regression of metastases.[94,132–134] Toxicity is dose-dependent and often rate-limiting in the ability to escalate the dose beyond 6g per day. The major side effects are gastrointestinal (anorexia, nausea, and vomiting) and neurological (ataxia, speech difficulty, somnolence, vertigo, and lethargy).[94] Additional side effects include gynecomastia and dermatitis.[94,130] Because this agent is adrenolytic, patients may become adrenal-insufficient, and replacement doses of glucocorticoids are recommended.[130]

The overall prognosis for adrenal cortical carcinoma remains poor. Mean survival rates are approximately 22 to 47 months.[94,132,133] However, long-term survival can occur. Patients who develop locally recurrent disease can benefit from reoperative surgery. The Italian National Registry for Adrenal Carcinoma reported the mean survival in 20 patients who underwent reoperations was significantly higher (15.85 ± 14.9 months) than those not resected (3.2 ± 2.9 months).[136]

Laparoscopic Adrenalectomy

There are multiple surgical approaches to the adrenal gland, including anterior transabdominal, flank, thoracoabdominal,

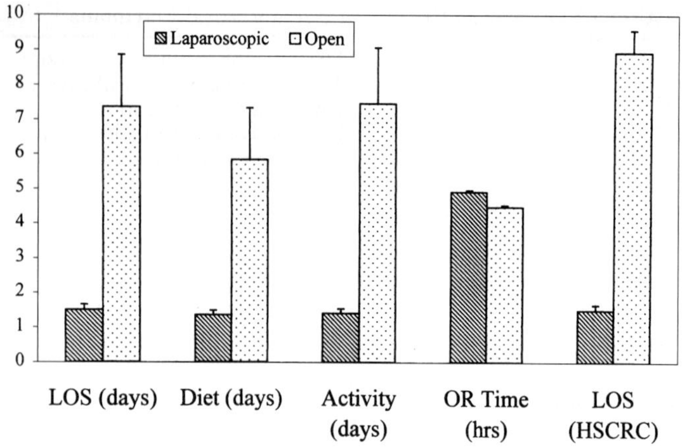

FIGURE 57.12. Comparison of laparoscopic (*hatched*) and open (*stippled*) adrenalectomy. LOS (length of stay) is HSCRC (health services cost review commission); this reflects a statewide database in Maryland, USA. (From Shell SR, Talamini MA, Udelsman R. Laparoscopic adrenalectomy for nonmalignant disease: improved safety, morbidity, and cost-effectiveness. Surg Endosc 1998;13:30–34, with permission.)

supracostal, posterior, and the newer laparoscopic techniques via a transperitoneal or retroperitoneal approach. The traditional techniques of adrenalectomy are well described and are beyond the scope of this review.[137–140] Laparoscopic adrenalectomy has already had a major impact on the management of adrenal neoplasms.

The successful application of laparoscopic adrenalectomy was reported by Gagner and colleagues in 1992.[141] They described an anterior transabdominal approach in patients with Cushing's syndrome and pheochromocytoma. Since that time, the techniques and indications have been refined and in many institutions it has become the standard technique employed for adrenalectomy. The indications for laparoscopic adrenalectomy have expanded, and in skilled hands this technique is appropriate for virtually all nonmalignant adrenal tumors. Most, but not all, endocrine surgeons agree that large tumors and clearly malignant tumors should be excised using an open technique.[18,105,142,143]

Laparoscopic adrenalectomy appears to have distinct advantages compared to traditional open techniques. Avoidance of large incisions and decreased tissue trauma appears to decrease morbidity and mortality.[18,144–147] Interestingly, even pheochromocytomas have been successfully managed with this technique.[18,147–150]

Several investigations have compared various anatomic approaches with laparoscopic adrenalectomy.[18,105,151–154] It is now clear that in skilled hands laparoscopic adrenalectomy can be performed safely, resulting in decreased hospital stays, increased patient comfort, and a shorter interval until the resumption of normal activity.[152,153] The result obtained in a recent study by Shell et al. compared the results of laparoscopic and open transabdominal adrenalectomy.[18] The results (Fig. 57.12) demonstrated a marked improvement in length of stay and time until resumption of normal diet and activity. In addition, when the length of stay was compared to statewide data, the improvement was even more pronounced. The decreased length of stay resulted in significant cost savings when the results of laparoscopic adrenalectomy were compared to statewide data.[18]

There are no randomized prospective trials comparing the results of laparoscopic and open adrenalectomy. The results obtained in several retrospective case-controlled studies are presented in Table 57.12. These data demonstrate that laparoscopic adrenalectomy is consistently associated

TABLE 57.12.
Laparoscopic Versus Open Adrenalectomy.

Study	*Laparoscopic*	*Open anterior*	*Level of evidence*[a]
Prinz 1995[105]			
n:	10	11	II
OR time (min):	212	174	
Postoperative stay (days):	2.1	6.4	
Guazzoni et al. 1995[155]			
n:	20	20	II
OR time (min):	170	145	
Postoperative stay (days):	3.4	9	
Return to work activity (days):	9.7	16	
Brunt et al. 1996[143]			
n:	24	25	II
OR time (min):	183	242	
Postoperative stay (days):	3.2	8.7	
Resumption of regular diet (days):	1.6	6.0	
MacGillivray et al. 1996[156]			
n:	14	9	II
OR time (min):	289	201	
Postoperative stay (days):	3.0	7.9	
Resumption of regular activity (days):	8.9	14.6	
Vargas et al. 1997[157]			
n:	20	20	II
OR time (min):	193	178	
Postoperative stay (days):	3.1	7.2	
Convalescence (weeks):	3	7	
Korman et al. 1997[158]			
n:	10	10	II
OR time (min):	164	124	
Postoperative stay (days):	4.1	5.9	
Direct charges:	$3,645	$5,752	
Linos et al. 1997[159]			
n:	18	86	II
OR time (min):	116	155	
Postoperative stay (days):	2.2	8	
Winfield et al. 1998[160]			
n:	21	17	II
OR time (min):	309	233	
Postoperative stay (days):	2.7	6.2	
Resumption of regular diet (days):	1.7	4.6	
Shell et al. 1998[18]			
n:	22	17	II
OR time (min):	267	257	
Postoperative stay (days):	1.7	7.8	
Resumption of regular diet (days):	1.6	6.1	
Resumption of independent activity (days):	1.6	7.9	
Hospital charges:	$8,698	$12,610	

[a]Clinical studies are classified according to the design of study and the quality of the resulting data: class I, prospective randomized studies; class II, prospective, nonrandomized or case-controlled retrospective studies; class III, retrospective analyses without case controls.

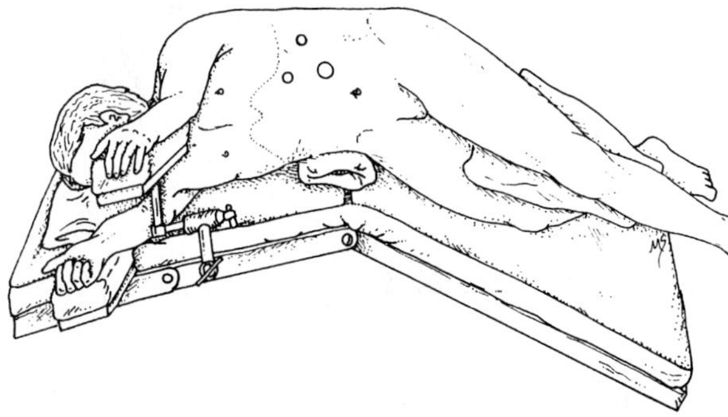

FIGURE 57.13. Patient position and port sites for left laparoscopic adrenalectomy. A 10-mm port is inserted midway between the umbilicus and the left costal margin, and a 30° side-viewing telescope is inserted. Two additional 5-mm ports are placed through which the harmonic scalpel, coagulation scissors, or grasping forceps are utilized. Note the careful positioning of the patient to pad all extremities and the head.

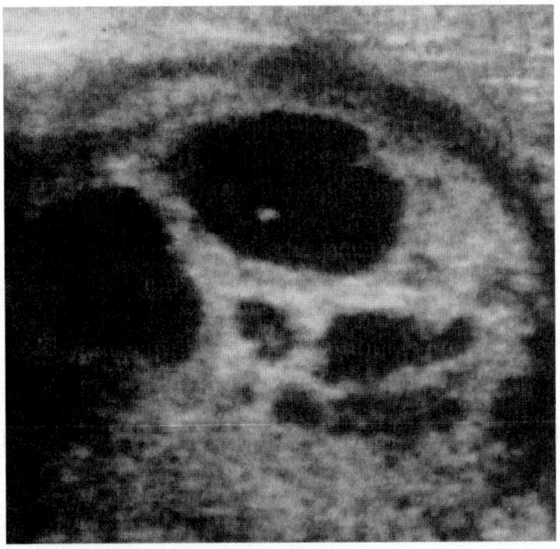

FIGURE 57.15. Intraoperative laparoscopic ultrasound image shows a cystic left-sided pheochromocytoma.

with marked decreases in the postoperative length of stay and the interval until resumption of normal diet and activity.

The majority of surgeons have adopted the transperitoneal flank approach when performing laparoscopic adrenalectomy. A posterior retroperitoneal approach has also been successfully employed.[88] This technique may have select advantages in patients who have had previous intraabdominal surgery.

Laparoscopic adrenalectomy has already become the standard of care in several institutions.[18,149,154–161] This technique is technically demanding, and requires special equipment, experienced surgeons, and mature judgment.

Technique of Laparoscopic Adrenalectomy

The techniques for both left and right laparoscopic adrenalectomy are briefly illustrated. For left adrenal tumors, the patient is placed in a lateral decubitus position with the left side elevated. The operating table is flexed to increase the space between the costal margin and the iliac crest. The patient is carefully padded to protect all extremities as well as the head. For routine left-sided cases, three port sites are utilized (Fig. 57.13). The first port is inserted midway between the umbilicus and the costal margin, and a 10-mm port is utilized for a 30° side-viewing telescope. Two additional working ports (5 mm) are employed for either coagulation scissors or the harmonic scalpel in conjunction with a pair of grasping forceps. Mobilization of the colon and spleen is demonstrated in Figure 57.14. The colon is displaced inferiorly and the spleen is displaced medially, allowing access to the superior pole of the left kidney. Occasionally it is difficult to locate the left adrenal gland in the retroperitoneal fat. In such cases, intraoperative ultrasound (Fig. 57.15) can be utilized through a 10-mm port. Once the spleen has been mobilized, the harmonic scalpel is utilized to transect the soft tissues in Gerota's fascia to mobilize the adrenal gland from its superior, lateral, and posterior attachments (Fig. 57.16). The left

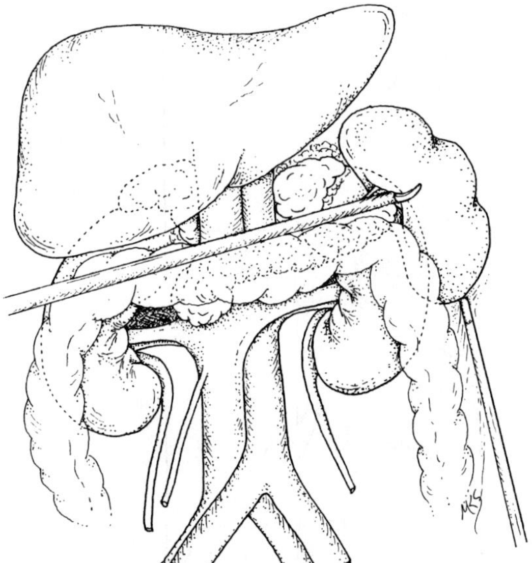

FIGURE 57.14. The lateral attachments to the splenic flexure of the colon are mobilized. The colon is displaced inferiorly, and the spleen is mobilized from its posterior attachments, allowing it to be displaced medially.

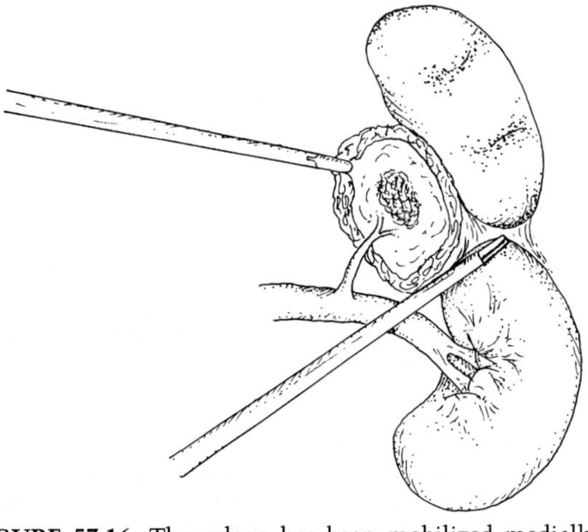

FIGURE 57.16. The spleen has been mobilized medially, and the colon has been displaced inferiorly. The harmonic scalpel is used to transect the tissues at the superior pole of the kidney, thereby allowing the adrenal gland to be mobilized. A rim of fat is mobilized in continuity with the adrenal gland.

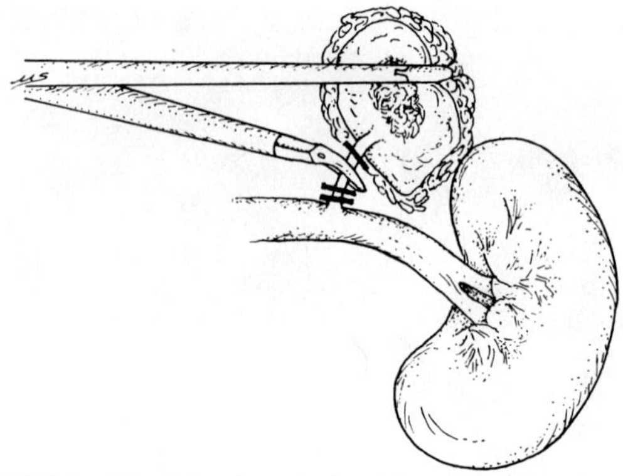

FIGURE 57.17. The left adrenal gland has been completely mobilized. The main left adrenal vein is identified and transected between metal clips.

adrenal vein is visualized, clips are placed, and it is transected as demonstrated in Figure 57.17. The adrenal gland and its surrounding fat are inserted into an extraction pouch and removed via the 10-mm port. A 5-mm camera must be inserted into one of the 5-mm ports to accomplish this task.

The position for a right-sided laparoscopic adrenalectomy via the lateral transperitoneal approach is demonstrated in Figure 57.18. On the right side, because of the liver, four ports are utilized. The first port (10mm) is placed midway between the umbilicus and the costal margin, and a 30° side-viewing telescope is utilized. A second 10-mm port is required in a subcostal position to elevate the liver with a laparoscopic retractor. Through two additional 5-mm ports, the harmonic scalpel, a grasping forceps, or a coagulation scissors is utilized. In performing a right adrenalectomy it is important to completely mobilize the right lobe of the liver from its lateral and posterior attachments, allowing access to the inferior vena cava (Fig. 57.19). Once the liver has been mobilized, it is elevated superiorly with a liver retractor, and the adrenal gland is identified with its dominant vein draining into the inferior vena cava. Accessory veins are occasionally encountered. The main adrenal vein is identified, clipped, and transected (Fig. 57.20). The retroperitoneal soft tissues and Gerota's fascia are transected with a harmonic scalpel. The gland and surrounding fat are then removed via an extraction pouch (Fig. 57.21).

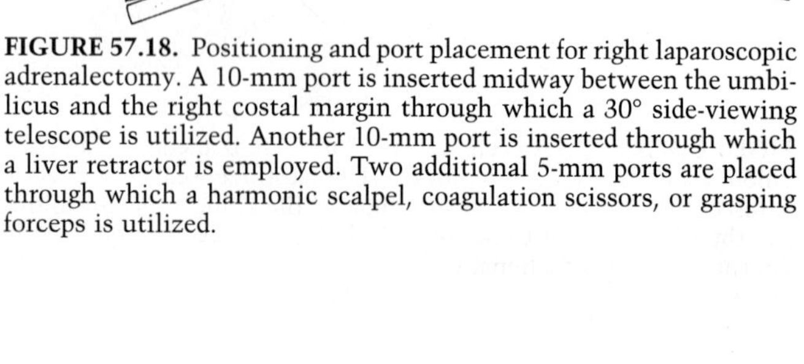

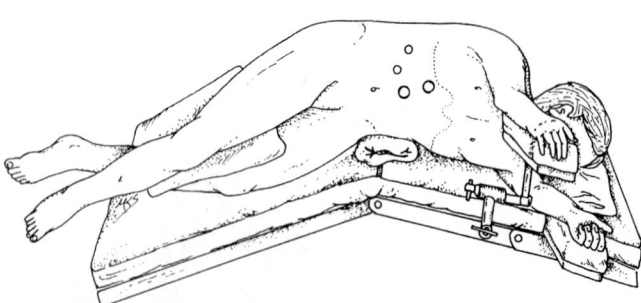

FIGURE 57.18. Positioning and port placement for right laparoscopic adrenalectomy. A 10-mm port is inserted midway between the umbilicus and the right costal margin through which a 30° side-viewing telescope is utilized. Another 10-mm port is inserted through which a liver retractor is employed. Two additional 5-mm ports are placed through which a harmonic scalpel, coagulation scissors, or grasping forceps is utilized.

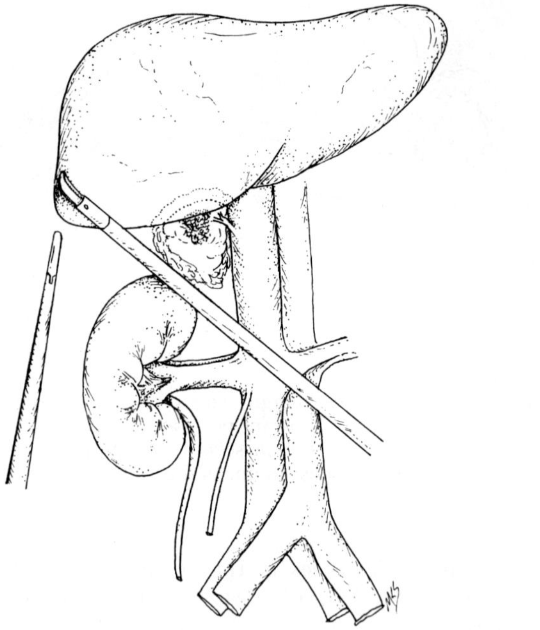

FIGURE 57.19. The lateral attachments of the liver are mobilized to elevate the liver and pull it medially, allowing exposure of the retrocaval adrenal gland.

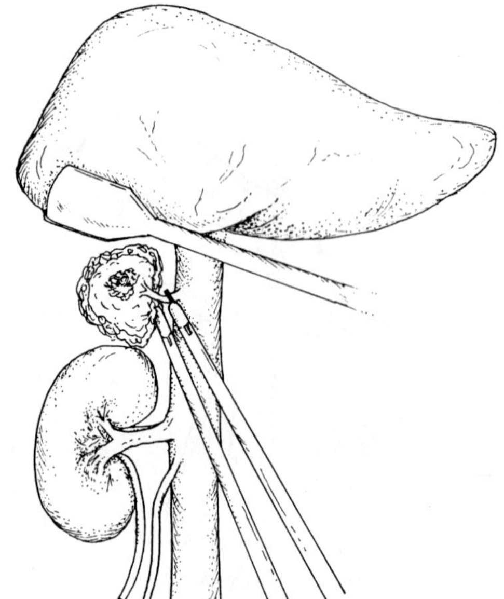

FIGURE 57.20. The liver is retracted superiorly and the adrenal gland is identified. The main adrenal vein is clipped and transected.

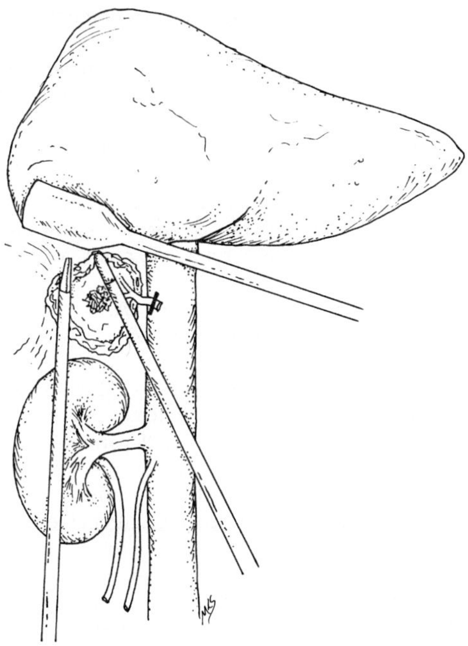

FIGURE 57.21. The retroperitoneal soft tissues and Gerota's fascia are transected with the harmonic scalpel.

Adrenal Insufficiency

Patients with overt or occult adrenal insufficiency pose significant management issues that have not yet been resolved. Primary adrenal insufficiency occurs when there is direct destruction of the adrenal glands, which occurs most commonly from autoimmune adrenal atrophy (Addison's disease) and infectious diseases (tuberculosis, histoplasmosis), as well as following adrenal hemorrhage, metastasis, and surgical resection. Secondary adrenal insufficiency occurs when there is an impairment of ACTH secretion at either the pituitary or hypothalamic level. The most common cause of adrenal insufficiency is iatrogenic administration of glucocorticoids, which results in suppression of ACTH. This population of adrenal-insufficient patients poses significant surgical ramifications.

It was estimated that in 1971 more than 5 million patients in the United States received glucocorticoids at doses sufficient to cause adrenal suppression.[162] This population includes individuals with rheumatological disease and inflammatory bowel disease and immunosuppressed transplant recipients, all of whom are likely to be referred for surgical intervention.[163,164] Because of the known deleterious effects of adrenal cortical crisis, it had become the standard of care to administer large doses of perioperative glucocorticoids to obviate hemodynamic inability in this population. However, a series of clinical studies published in the 1970s suggested that physiological rather than pharmacological glucocorticoid supplementation may be sufficient for patients with adrenal insufficiency who require surgical intervention.[165–167] Substantial evidence to support this concept was obtained in a primate stress model in which adrenal-insufficient monkeys successfully underwent general anesthesia and surgery when given glucocorticoids at a dose equivalent to their normal (unstressed) production rate.[168] There was no hemodynamic advantage to pharmacological glucocorticoid administration. This evidence-based study suggests that the perioperative pharmacological doses that are often administered to adrenal-insufficient patients far exceed their physiological requirements.

References

1. Eustachius B. In: Lancisius B, ed. Tabulae Anatomicae Clarissimi Viri Bartholomeai Eustachii. Amsterdam: 1722.
2. Mihai R, Farndon JR. Surgical embryology and anatomy of the adrenal glands. In: Clark OH, Duh QY, eds. Textbook of Endocrine Surgery. Philadelphia: Saunders, 1997:447–459.
3. Kloss RT, Gross MD, Francis IR, et al. Incidentally discovered adrenal masses. Endocr Rev 1995;16(4):460–484.
4. Hamaji M, Harrison TS. Blood vessels and lymphatics of the adrenal gland. In: Blood Vessels and Lymphatics in Organ Systems. New York: Academic Press, 1984:280–295.
5. Flint JM. The blood supply, angiogenesis, organogenesis, reticulum and histology of the adrenal. Johns Hopkins Hosp Rep 1990;4:154–229.
6. Pohorecky L, Wortman R. Adrenocortical control of epinephrine synthesis. Pharmacol Rev 1971;2:1–35.
7. Hayashi K, Sala G, Catt KJ, et al. Regulation of steroidogenesis by adrenocorticotrophic hormone in isolated adrenal cells. J Biol Chem 1979;154:6678–6683.
8. Gill GN. ACTH regulation of the adrenal cortex. In: Gill GN, ed. Pharmacology of Adrenal Cortical Hormones. New York: Pergamon, 1979:35.
9. Privalle CT, Crivello JF, Jefcoate CR. Regulation of intramitochondrial cholesterol transfer to side-chain cleavage cytochrome P-450 in rat adrenal gland. Proc Natl Acad Sci U S A 1983;80:702–706.
10. Udelsman R, Holbrook NJ. Endocrine and molecular responses to surgical stress. Curr Probl Surg 1994;31:653–728.
11. Munck A, Guyre PM, Holbrook NJ. Physiological functions of glucocorticoids in stress and their relation to pharmacological actions. Endocr Rev 1984;5:25–44.
12. Lefkowitz RJ, Hoffman BB, Taylor P. Neurohumoral transmission: the autonomic and somatic motor nervous systems. In: Gilman AG, Rall TW, Nies AS, et al, eds. Goodman and Gilman's: The Pharmacological Basis of Therapeutics, 8th ed. New York: Pergamon Press, 1990:84–121.
13. Cryer PE. Physiology and pathophysiology of the human sympathoadrenal neuroendocrine system. N Engl J Med 1980;303:436–444.
14. Axelrod J, Weinshilboum R. Catecholamines. N Engl J Med 1972;287:237–242.
15. Badder EM, Santen R, Sasmojlik E, et al. Adrenal medullary epinephrine secretion: effects of cortisol alone and combined with aminoglutethimide. J Lab Med 1980;96:815–821.
16. Blaschko H. The specific action of L-dopa decarboxylase. J Physiol 1939;96:50P–51P.
17. Weiner N. Control of the biosynthesis of adrenal catecholamines by the adrenal medulla. In: Blaschko H, Sayers G, Smith AD, eds. Adrenal Gland: Endocrinology. Washington, DC: American Physiology Society, 1975:357–366.
18. Shell SR, Talamini MA, Udelsman R. Laparoscopic adrenalectomy for non-malignant disease: improved safety, morbidity and cost-effectiveness. Surg Endosc 1998;13:30–34.
19. Korobkin M, Brodeur FJ, Yutzy GG, et al. Differentiation of adrenal adenomas from nonadenomas using CT attenuation values. Am J Roentgenol 1996;166:531–536.
20. Lee MJ, Hahn PF, Papanicolaou N, et al. Benign and malignant adrenal masses: CT distinction with attenuation coefficients, size, and observer analysis. Radiology 1991;79:415–418.
21. Singer AA, Obuchowski NA, Einstein DM, et al. Metastasis or adenoma? Computed tomographic evaluation of the adrenal mass. Clevel Clin J Med 1994;18:432–438.

22. McNicholas MMJ, Lee MJ, Mayo-Smith WW, et al. An imaging algorithm for the differential diagnosis of adrenal adenomas and metastases. Am J Roentgenol 1995;165:1453–1459.
23. Boland GW, Hahn PF, Pena C, et al. Adrenal masses: characterization with delayed contrast-enhanced CT. Radiology 1997; 202:693–696.
24. Cerfolio RJ, Vaughan ED Jr, Brennan TG Jr, et al. Accuracy of computed tomography in predicting adrenal tumor size. Surg Gynecol Obstet 1993;176(4):307–309.
25. Linos DA, Sylopoulos N. How accurate is computed tomography in predicting the real size of adrenal tumors? A retrospective study. Arch Surg 1997;32:740–743.
26. Bilbey JH, McLoughlin RF, Kurkjian PS, et al. MR imaging of adrenal masses: value of chemical-shift imaging for distinguishing adenomas from other tumors. Am J Roentgenol 1995;164:637–642.
27. Thrall JH, Freitas JE, Beierwaltes WH. Adrenal scintigraphy. Semin Nucl Med 1978;8(1):23–41.
28. Herd GW, Semple PF, Parker D, et al. False localization of an aldosteronoma by dexamethasone-suppressed adrenal scintigraphy. Clin Endocrinol 1987;26(2):699–705.
29. Ackery DM, Tippett P, Condon B, et al. New approach to the localization of pheochromocytoma: imaging with 131-I-MIBG. Br Med J 1984;288:1587–1599.
30. Sisson JC, Frager MS, Balk TW, et al. Scintigraphic localization of pheochromocytoma. N Engl J Med 1981;305:12–17.
31. Arnold DR, Villemagne VI, Civelek AC, et al. FDG-PET scan: a sensitive tool for the localization of MIBG negative pelvic pheochromocytomas. Endocrinologist 1998;8:295–298.
32. Doppman JL, Gill JR Jr. Hyperaldostronism: sampling the adrenal veins. Radiology 1996;198:309–312.
33. Sosano H, Shizawa S, Nagura H. Adrenocortical cytopathology. Am J Clin Pathol 1995;104:161–166.
34. Abecassis M, McLoughlin MJ, Langer B, et al. Serendipitous adrenal masses: prevalence, significance and management. Am J Surg 1985;149:783–788.
35. Hedeland H, Ostberg G, Hokfelt B. On the prevalence of adrenocortical adenomas in autopsy material in relation to hypertension and diabetes. Acta Med Scand 1968;184:211–214.
36. Willis RA. Metastatic tumors in the thyroid gland. Am J Pathol 1931;7:187–208.
37. Moulton JS. CT of the adrenal glands. Semin Roentgenol 1988;23:288–303.
38. Ross NS, Aron DC. Hormonal evaluation of the patient with an incidentally discovered adrenal mass. New Engl J Med 1990;323:1401–1405.
39. Sutton MG, Sheps SG, Lie JT. Prevalence of clinically unsuspected pheochromocytoma: a review of a 50-year autopsy series. Mayo Clin Proc 1981;56:354–360.
40. Osella G, Terzol M, Borretta G, et al. Endocrine evaluation of incidentally discovered adrenal masses (incidentalomas). J Clin Endocrinol Metab 1994;79:1532–1539.
41. Staren ED, Prinz RA. Selection of patients with adrenal incidentalomas for operation. Surg Clin N Am 1995;75:499–509.
42. Terzolo M, Osella G, Ali A, et al. Subclinical Cushing's syndrome in adrenal incidentaloma. Clin Endocrinol 1998;48:89–97.
43. Kobayashi S, Seki T, Nonomura K, et al. Clinical experience of incidentally discovered adrenal tumor with particular reference to cortical function. J Urol 1993;150:8–12.
44. Ambrosi B, Peverelli S, Passini E, et al. Abnormalities of endocrine function in patients with clinically "silent" adrenal masses. Eur J Endocrinol 1995;132:422–428.
45. Siren JE, Haapiainen RK, Huikuri KT, et al. Incidentalomas of the adrenal gland: 36 operated patients and review of the literature. World J Surg 1993;17:634–639.
46. Cook DM, Loriaux DL. The incidental adrenal mass. Am J Med 1996;101:88–94.
47. Lee JE, Evans DB, Hickey RC, et al. Unknown primary cancer presenting as an adrenal mass: implications for FNA of adrenal incidentalomas. Surgery (St. Louis) 1998;124:1115–1122.
48. Gajraj H, Young AE. Adrenal incidentaloma. Br J Surg 1993;80:422–426.
49. Kloos RT, Gross MD, Shapiro B, et al. Diagnostic dilemma of small incidentally discovered adrenal masses: role for 131-I-6-β-iodomethyl-norcholesterol scintigraphy. World J Surg 1997; 21:36–40.
50. Herrera MF, Grant CS, van Heerden JA, et al. Incidentally discovered adrenal tumors: an institutional perspective. Surgery (St. Louis) 1991;110:1014–1021.
51. Kasperlik-Zaluska AA, Roslonowska E, Slowinska-Srzednicka J, et al. Incidentally discovered adrenal mass (incidentaloma): investigation and management of 208 patients. Clin Endocrinol 1997;46:29–37.
52. Terzolo M, Ali A, Osella G, et al. Prevalence of adrenal carcinoma among incidentally discovered adrenal masses. Arch Surg 1997;132:914–919.
53. Linos DA, Stylopoulos N, Raptis SA. Adrenaloma: a call for more aggressive management. World J Surg 1996;20:788–793.
54. Corry DB, Tuck ML. Secondary aldosteronism. Endocrinol Metab Clin N Am 1995;24:511–528.
55. Gröndal S, Hamberger B. Primary aldosteronism. Br J Surg 1992;79:484–485.
56. Blevins LS Jr, Wand GC. Primary aldosteronism: an endocrine perspective. Radiology 1992;184:599–600.
57. Conn JW. Primary aldosteronism: a new clinical syndrome. J Lab Clin Med 1955;45:3–17.
58. Obara T, Ito Y, Okamato T, et al. Risk factors associated with postoperative persistent hypertension in patients with primary aldosteronism. Surgery (St. Louis) 1992;112:987–993.
59. Biglieri EG, Irony I, Kater CE. Identification and implications of new types of mineralocorticoid hypertension. J Steroid Biochem 1989;32:199–204.
60. Irony I, Kater CE, Biglieri EG, et al. Correctable subsets of primary aldosteronism: primary adrenal hyperplasia and renin responsive adenoma. Am J Hypertens 1990;3:576–582.
61. Taylor W, Carroll D, Bethwaite P. Adrenal carcinoma presenting as Conn's syndrome. Aust NZ J Med 1997;27:201–202.
62. Grant C, Carpenter P, van Heerden JA, et al. Primary aldosteronism. Clinical management. Arch Surg 1984;119:585–590.
63. Obara T, Ito Y, Fujimoto Y. Hyperaldosteronism. In: Clark OH, Duh QY, eds. Textbook of Endocrine Surgery. Philadelphia: Saunders, 1997;483–489.
64. Young WF Jr, Klee GG. Primary aldosteronism: diagnostic evaluation. Endocrinol Metab Clin N Am 1988;14:367–395.
65. Young WF Jr. Primary aldosteronism: update on diagnosis and treatment. Endocrinologist 1997;7:213–221.
66. Holland OB. Primary aldosteronism. Semin Nephrol 1995;15:116–125.
67. Kem DC, Weinberger MH, Gomez-Sanchez CE, et al. Circadian rhythms of plasma aldosterone concentration in normal subjects and patients with primary aldosteronism. J Clin Invest 1973; 52:2272–2277.
68. Bravo EL, Trazi RC, Dustan HP, et al. The changing clinical spectrum of primary aldosteronism. Am J Med 1983;74:641–651.
69. Vallotton MB. Primary aldosteronism. Part I. Diagnosis of primary hyperaldosteronism. Clin Endocrinol 1996;45:47–52.
70. Hiramatsu K, Yamada T, Yukimura Y, et al. A screening test to identify aldosterone-producing adenoma by measuring plasma renin activity. Results in hypertensive patients. Arch Intern Med 1981;141:1589–1593.
71. Gordon RD. Primary aldosteronism. J Endocrinol Invest 1995;18:495–511.

72. Gomez-Sanchez CE. Primary aldosteronism and its variants. Cardiovasc Res 1998;37:8–13.
73. Holland O, Brown H, Kuhnert L, et al. Further evaluation of saline infusion for the diagnosis of primary aldosteronism. Hypertension 1984;6:717–723.
74. Streeten DHP, Tomyez N, Anderson GH. Reliability of screening methods for the diagnosis of primary aldosteronism. Am J Med 1979;67:403–413.
75. Udelsman R. Tumors of the adrenal cortex. In: Cameron JL, ed. Current Surgical Therapy, 6th ed. St. Louis: Mosby, 1998:577–580.
76. Ganguly A, Melada GA, Luetscher JA, et al. Control of plasma aldosterone in primary aldosteronism: distinction between adenoma and hyperplasia. J Clin Endocrinol Metab 1973;37:765–775.
77. Young WF Jr, Hogan MJ, Klee GG, et al. Primary aldosteronism: diagnosis and treatment. Mayo Clin Proc 1990;65:96–110.
78. Biglieri EG, Schambelan M, Hirai J, et al. The significance of elevated levels of plasma 18-hydroxycorticosterone in patients with primary aldosteronism. J Clin Endocrinol Metab 1979;49:87–91.
79. Vallotton MB. Primary aldosteronism. Part II. Differential diagnosis of primary hyperaldosteronism and pseudoaldosteronism. Clin Endocrinol 1996;45:53–60.
80. Dunnick NR, Leight GS, Roubidoux MA, et al. CT in the diagnosis of primary aldosteronism: sensitivity in 29 patients. Am J Radiol 1993;160:321–324.
81. Doppman JL, Gill JR Jr, Miller DL, et al. Distinction between hyperaldosteronism due to bilateral hyperplasia and unilateral aldosteronoma: Reliability of CT. Radiology 1992;184:677–682.
82. Young WF Jr, Stanson AW, Grant CS, et al. Primary aldosteronism: adrenal venous sampling. Surgery (St. Louis) 1996;120:913–920.
83. Go H, Takeda M, Takahashi H, et al. Laparoscopic adrenalectomy for primary aldosteronism: a new operative method. J Laparoendosc Surg 1993;3:455–459.
84. Gagner M, Lacroix A, Prinz RA, et al. Early experience with laparoscopic approach for adrenalectomy. Surgery (St. Louis) 1993;114:1120–1125.
85. Takeda M, Go H, Imai T, et al. Laparoscopic adrenalectomy for primary aldosteronism: report of initial ten cases. Surgery (St. Louis) 1994;115:621–625.
86. Horgan S, Sinanan M, Helton S, et al. Use of laparoscopic techniques improves outcome from adrenalectomy. Am J Surg 1997;173:371–374.
87. Nakada T, Kobota Y, Sasagawa I, et al. Therapeutic outcome of primary aldosteronism: adrenalectomy versus enucleation of aldosterone-producing adenoma. J Urol 1995;153:1775–1780.
88. Walz MK, Peitgen K, Saller B, et al. Subtotal adrenalectomy by the posterior retroperitoneoscopic approach. World J Surg 1998;22:621–627.
89. Lo CY, Tam PC, Kung AWC, et al. Primary aldosteronism: results of surgical treatment. Ann Surg 1996;224:125–130.
90. Favia G, Lumachi F, Scarpa V, et al. Adrenalectomy in primary aldosteronism: a long-term follow-up study in 52 patients. World J Surg 1992;16:680–684.
91. Cushing H. The basophil adenomas of the pituitary body and their clinical manifestations (pituitary basophilism). Bull Johns Hopkins Hosp 1932;50:137–195.
92. Samuels MH, Loriaux DL. Cushing's syndrome and the nodular adrenal gland. Endocrinol Metab Clin N Am 1994;23:555–569.
93. Kirschner MA, Powell RD, Lipsett MB. Cushing's syndrome: nodular cortical hyperplasia of adrenal glands with clinical and pathological features suggesting adrenocortical tumor. J Clin Endocrinol 1964;24:947–955.
94. Luton JP, Cerdas S, Billaud L, et al. Clinical features of adrenocortical carcinoma, prognostic factors, and the effect of mitotane therapy. N Engl J Med 1990;322:1195–1201.
95. Van Heerden JA, Young WF Jr, Grant CS, et al. Adrenal surgery for hypercortisolism—surgical aspects. Surgery (St. Louis) 1995;117:466–472.
96. Favia G, Boscaro M, Lumachi F, et al. Role of bilateral adrenalectomy in Cushing's disease. World J Surg 1994;18:462–466.
97. Plotz CM, Knowlton Al, Ragan C. Natural history of Cushing's syndrome. Am J Med 1952;13:597–614.
98. Zeiger MA, Pass HI, Doppman JD, et al. Surgical strategy in the management of non-small cell ectopic adrenocorticotropic hormone syndrome. Surgery (St. Louis) 1992;112:994–1000.
99. Carney JA, Gordon H, Carpenter PC, et al. The complex of myxomas, spotty pigmentation, and endocrine activity. Medicine (Baltim) 1985;64:270–283.
100. Lacroix A, Tremblay J, Rousseau G, et al. Propranolol therapy for ectopic beta-adrenergic receptors in adrenal Cushing's syndrome. N Engl J Med 1997;337:1429–1434.
101. Chapuis Y, Pitre J, Conti F, et al. Role of operative risk of bilateral adrenalectomy in hypercorticalism. World J Surg 1996; 20:775–780.
102. O'Riordain DS, Farley DR, Young WF Jr, et al. Long-term outcome of bilateral adrenalectomy in patients with Cushing's syndrome. Surgery (St. Louis) 1994;116:1088–1094.
103. Valimaki M, Pelkonen R, Porkka L. Long-term results of adrenal surgery in patients with Cushing's syndrome due to adrenocortical adenoma. Clin Endocrinol 1984;20:229–236.
104. Norton JA. Invited commentary. World J Surg 1996;20:786–787.
105. Prinz RA. A comparison of laparoscopic and open adrenalectomies. Arch Surg 1995;130:489–494.
106. Gifford RW Jr, Manger WM, Bravo EL. Pheochromocytoma. Endocrinol Metab Clin N Am 1994;23:387–404.
107. Chen H, Doppman JL, Chrousos GP, et al. Adrenocorticotropic hormone-secreting pheochromocytoma: the exception to the rule. Surgery (St. Louis) 1995;118:988–995.
108. Bravo EL, Gifford RW Jr. Pheochromocytoma: diagnosis, localization and management. N Engl J Med 1984;311:1298–1303.
109. Shapiro B, Gross MD. Pheochromocytoma. Crit Care Clin 1991;7:1–20.
110. Grossman E, Goldstein DS, Hoffman A, et al. Glucagon and clonidine testing in the diagnosis of pheochromocytoma. Hypertension 1991;17:733–741.
111. Sioberg RJ, Simcic KJ, Kidd GS. The clonidine suppression test for pheochromocytoma: a review of its utility and pitfalls. Arch Intern Med 1992;152:1193–1197.
112. Malone MJ, Liberetino JA, Tsapatsaris NP, et al. Preoperative and surgical management of pheochromocytoma. Urol Clin N Am 1989;6:567–582.
113. Sheps SS, Jiang NS, Klee GG, et al. Recent developments in the diagnosis and treatment of pheochromocytoma. Mayo Clin Proc 1990;65:88–95.
114. Perry RR, Keiser HR, Norton JA, et al. Surgical management of pheochromocytoma with the use of metyrosine. Ann Surg 1990;212:621–628.
115. Briggs RSJ, Birtwell AJ, Pohl JEF. Hypertensive response to labetalol in phaeochromocytoma. Lancet 1978;1:1045–1046.
116. Boutros AR, Bravo EL, Zanettin G. Perioperative management of 63 patients with pheochromocytoma. Clevel Clin J Med 1990;57:613–617.
117. Jovenich JJ. Anesthesia in adrenal surgery. Urol Clin N Am 1998;16:583–587.
118. Wilkins GE, Schmidt N, Doll WA. Hypoglycemia following excision of pheochromocytoma. Can Med Assoc J 1977;116:367–368.
119. Van Heerden JA, Roland CF, Carney JA, et al. Long-term evaluation following resection of apparently benign pheochromocytoma(s)/paraganglioma(s). World J Surg 1990;4:325–329.
120. Thompson NW. Malignant pheochromocytoma. Acta Chir Aust 1993;4:235–239.

121. Grant CS. Pheochromoytoma. In: Clark OH, Duh QY, eds. Textbook of Endocrine Surgery. Philadelphia: Saunders, 1997;513–522.
122. Averbuch SD, Steakley CS, Young RC, et al. Malignant pheochromocytoma: effective treatment with a combination of cyclophosphamine, vincristine, and dacarbazine. Ann Intern Med 1988;109:267–273.
123. Thompson NW, Allo MD, Shapiro B, et al. Extra-adrenal and metastatic pheochromocytoma: the role of 131I betaiodobenzylguanidine (131I MIBG) in localization and management. World J Surg 1984;8:605–611.
124. Krempf M, Lumbroso J, Mornex R, et al. Use of m-[^{131}]iodobenzylguanidine in the treatment of malignant pheochromocytoma. J Clin Endocrinol Metab 1991;72:455–461.
125. Webb TA, Sheps SG, Carney JA. Differences between sporadic pheochromocytoma and pheochromocytoma in multiple endocrine neoplasia, type 2. Am J Surg Pathol 1980;4:121–126.
126. Van Heerden JA, Sizemore GW, Carney JA, et al. Surgical management of the adrenal glands in the multiple endocrine neoplasia type II syndrome. World J Surg 1984;8:612–621.
127. Lairmore TC, Bull DW, Baylin SB, et al. Management of pheochromocytoma in patients with multiple endocrine neoplasia type 2 syndrome. Ann Surg 1993;217:595–603.
128. Ross N, Aron D. Hormonal evaluation of the patient with an incidentally discovered adrenal mass. N Engl J Med 1990; 323:1401–1405.
129. Gicquel C, Audin E, Lebove Y, et al. Adrenocortical carcinoma. Ann Oncol 1997;8:423–427.
130. Schteingart DE. Treating adrenal cancer. Endocrinologist 1992;2:149–157.
131. King DR, Lack EE. Adrenal cortical carcinoma: a clinical and pathologic study in 49 cases. Cancer (Phila) 1979;44:239–244.
132. Icard P, Louvel A, Chapuis Y. Survival rates and prognostic factors in adrenocortical carcinoma. World J Surg 1992;16:753–758.
133. Schteingart DE, Motazedi A, Noonan RA, et al. Treatment of adrenal carcinomas. Arch Surg 1982;17:1142–1146.
134. Kasperlik-Zahuska AA, Migdalska BM, Zgliczynski S. Adrenocortical carcinoma: a clinical study and treatment results in 52 patients. Cancer (Phila) 1995;75:2587–2591.
135. Bergenstal DM, Hertz R, Lipsett MB, et al. Chemotherapy of adrenocortical cancer with *o,p*-DDD. Ann Intern Med 1960; 53:672–682.
136. Bellantone R, Ferrante A, Boscherini M, et al. Role of reoperation in recurrence of adrenal cortical carcinoma: results from 188 cases collected in the Italian National Registry for adrenal cortical carcinoma. Surgery (St. Louis) 1997;122:1212–1218.
137. Guz BV, Straffon RA, Novick AC. Operative approaches to the adrenal gland. Urol Clin North Am 1989;16:527–534.
138. Gonzalez-Serva L, Glenn JF. Adrenal surgical techniques. Urol Clin N Am 1977;4:327–336.
139. Raynor RW, Del Guercio LRM. The eleventh rib transcostal incision: an extrapleural, transperitoneal approach to the upper abdomen. Surgery (St. Louis) 1985;99:95–100.
140. Vaughan ED Jr, Phillips H. Modified posterior approach for right adrenalectomy. Surg Gynecol Obstet 1987;165:453–455.
141. Gagner M, Lacroix A, Bolte E. Laparoscopic adrenalectomy in Cushing's syndrome and pheochromocytoma [letter]. N Engl J Med 1992;327:1033.
142. Gagner M. Laparoscopic adrenalectomy. Surg Clin N Am 1996;76(3):523–537.
143. Brunt LM, Doherty Gm, Norton JA, et al. Laparoscopic adrenalectomy compared to open adrenalectomy for benign adrenal neoplasms [see comments]. J Am Coll Surg 1996;183(1):1–10.
144. Takeda M, Go H, Imai T, Komeyama T, et al. Experience with 17 cases of laparoscopic adrenalectomy: use of ultrasonic aspirator and argon beam coagulator. J Urol 1994;152(3):902–905.
145. Go H, Takeda M, Imai T. Laparoscopic adrenalectomy for Cushing's syndrome: comparison with primary aldosteronism. Surgery (St. Louis) 1995;117:11–17.
146. Fletcher DR, Beiles CB, Hardy KJ. Laparoscopic adrenalectomy. Aust N Z J Surg 1994;64(6):427–430.
147. Gagner M, Lacroix A, Bolte E, et al. Laparoscopic adrenalectomy. The importance of a flank approach in the lateral decubitus position. Surg Endosc 1994;8(2):135–138.
148. Miccoli P, Iacconi P, Conte M, et al. Laparoscopic adrenalectomy. J Laparoendosc Surg 1995;5(4):221–226.
149. Ganger M, Pomp A, Heniford BT. Laparoscopic adrenalectomy. Ann Surg 1997;226:238–247.
150. Fernandez-Cruz L, Taura P, Saenz A, et al. Laparoscopic approach to pheochromocytoma: hemodynamic changes and catecholamine secretion. World J Surg 1996;20:762–768.
151. Duh QY, Siperstein AE, Clark OH, et al. Laparoscopic adrenalectomy. Comparison of the lateral and posterior approaches. Arch Surg 1996;13(8):870–875.
152. Guazzoni G, Montorsi F, Bergamaschi F, et al. Effectiveness and safety of laparoscopic adrenalectomy. J Urol 1994;152(5 pt 1): 1375–1378.
153. Rutherford JC, Stowasser M, Tunny TJ, et al. Laparoscopic adrenalectomy. World J Surg 1996;20(7):758–760; discussion 761.
154. Thompson GB, Grant CS, can Heerden JA, et al. Laparoscopic versus open posterior adrenalectomy: a case-controlled study in 100 patients. Surgery (St. Louis) 1997;122:1132–1136.
155. Guazzoni G, Montorsi F, Bocciardi A, et al. Transperitoneal laparoscopic versus open adrenalectomy for benign hyperfunctioning adrenal tumors: a comparative study. J Urol 1995; 153:1597–1600.
156. MacGillivray DC, Shichman SJ, Ferrer SJ, et al. A comparison of open vs. laparoscopic adrenalectomy. Surg Endosc 1996;10:987–990.
157. Vargas HI, Kavoussi LR, Bartlett DL, et al. Laparoscopic adrenalectomy: a new standard of care. Urology 1997;49:673–678.
158. Korman JE, Ho T, Hiatt JR, et al. Comparison of laparoscopic and open adrenalectomy. Am Surg 1997;63:908–912.
159. Linos DA, Stylopoulos N, Boukis M, et al. Anterior, posterior, or laparoscopic approach for the management of adrenal diseases? Am J Surg 1997;173:120–125.
160. Winfeld HN, Hamilton BD, Brovo EL, et al. Laparoscopic adrenalectomy: the preferred choice? A comparison to open adrenalectomy. Am J Urol 1998;160:325–329.
161. Jacobs JK, Goldstein RE, Geer RJ. Laparoscopic adrenalectomy: a new standard of care. Ann Surg 1997;225:495–502.
162. Christy NP. Iatrogenic Cushing's syndrome. In: Christy NP, ed. The Human Adrenal Cortex. New York: Harper & Row, 1971:395–425.
163. Prohaska JV, Dragstedt LR, Thompson RG. Ulcerative colitis: surgical problems in corticosteroid treated patients. Ann Surg 1961;154:408–416.
164. Melby JC. Systemic corticosteroid therapy: pharmacology and endocrinologic considerations. Ann Intern Med 1974;81:505–512.
165. Kehlet H, Binder C. Adrenocortical function and clinical course during and after surgery in unsupplemented glucocorticoid treated patients. Br J Anaesth 1973;45:1043–1048.
166. Kehlet H. A rational approach to dosage and preparation of parenteral glucocorticoid substitution therapy during surgical procedures. Acta Anaesthesiol Scand 1975;19:260–264.
167. Symreng T, Karlberg E, Kageldal B, et al. Physiological cortisol substitution of long-term steroid-treated patients undergoing major surgery. Br J Anaesth 1981;53:949–953.
168. Udelsman R, Ramp J, Gallucci WT, et al. Adaptation during surgical stress: a reevaluation of the role of glucocorticoids. J Clin Invest 1986;77:1377–1378.

58

Neuroendocrine Tumors of the Pancreas and Gastrointestinal Tract and Carcinoid Disease

David A. Peterson, James P. Dolan, and Jeffrey A. Norton

The neuroendocrine, or islet cell, and carcinoid tumors of the pancreas and gastrointestinal tract are a group of similar neoplasms that, despite several differences in clinical and biochemical behavior, share many common features. Although originally thought to be of neural crest origin, these cells are now considered to originate from embryonic endoderm.[1] They are capable of taking up and decarboxylating aromatic amines or their precursors, giving rise to the term APUD (amine precursor uptake and decarboxylation) cells or *apudomas*. This term has been replaced by their designation as neuroendocrine neoplasms of the gastrointestinal tract.[2] Although largely concentrated in the stomach, midgut, and pancreas, neuroendocrine cells share a number of histochemical and ultrastructural characteristics with other endocrine cell types such as chromaffin cells of the adrenal medulla, melanotrophs and corticotrophs of the pituitary, parafollicular (C) cells of the thyroid, and neuroendocrine cells of the sympathetic ganglia and carotid body. They also share a similarity with carcinoid tumors.[3,4] Histologically, these tumors are composed of monotonous sheets of small round cells with a uniform nucleus and cytoplasm and a general lack of mitotic figures.[5,6] In general, they are well vascularized and tend to have a similar pattern of metastatic spread, involving primarily the regional lymph nodes and liver, although widespread metastases to lung, bone, and brain can also occur.[7]

Neuroendocrine tumors may differ in their clinical manifestations and biological behavior. Except for insulinomas, each is a slow-growing malignancy in 60% to 100% of cases. Each tumor may also be classified as either functional or nonfunctional, depending on the presence or absence of a clinical syndrome resulting from unregulated hormone secretion.[3] In addition, there appears to be a correlation between tumor size and malignant potential. Insulinomas tend to be small and benign, whereas glucagonomas, gastrinomas, somatostatinomas, and the other rare islet cell tumors are generally large and malignant. They usually occur in a sporadic form (noninherited) but in 5% to 25% of cases they may be inherited as part of multiple endocrine neoplasia type 1 (MEN 1).[5] In the setting of MEN 1, approximately 80% of patients will develop an islet cell tumor.[5,8] Neuroendocrine tumors may also be found in other inherited disorders such as von Hipple–Lindau disease, von Recklinghausen's disease, and tuberous sclerosis.[5]

Epidemiology

Neuroendocrine tumors of the gastrointestinal tract are uncommon. Functional tumors are reported to have a prevalence of 10 per million population.[9] The incidence of clinically significant neuroendocrine tumors is around 3.6 to 4 per

TABLE 58.1. Incidence, Location, and Pathology of Gastrointestinal Neuroendocrine Tumors.

		Location (%)[a]					
Name	*Incidence*	*Pancreas*	*Duodenum*	*Other*	*Malignant (%)*[a]	*MEN 1 (%)*[a]	*Found at surgery (%)*[a]
Insulinoma	4 in 5 million	>99			5–11	5	95
Gastrinoma	2 in 5 million	21–65[b]	6–35[b]	1–26[b]	60	18–24	52–87
Glucagonoma	Rare	>99			>70	Occasional	98–100
VIPoma	Rare	85–90	10–15		50	Occasional	100
Somatostatinoma	Very rare	50	50		90	—	100
Nonfunctioning	1 in 5 million	>99			>50	—	100
Carcinoids	2.8–21 in 1 million	<1	3	>97	2–50	Occasional	>95

MEN, multiple endocrine neoplasia.
[a]Data from Norton (1998)[5]; Norton et al. (1993).[24]
[b]Data from Weber et al. (1995).[52]
[c]Data from Jensen (1995).[3]

million population per year.[3,9] Nonfunctional tumors are reported to account for 15% to 30% of all neuroendocrine tumors.[10] Insulinoma is the most common islet cell tumor, with an approximate prevalence of 4 per 5 million population per year,[5] while gastrinoma or PPomas are the most common malignant islet cell tumors. The incidence of gastrinomas is estimated to be 0.1 to 3 persons per million each year.[8,11] The remaining neuroendocrine tumors occur less frequently (Table 58.1).

Embryology and Anatomy

The gut and its associated organs develop between the third and eighth week of embryonic life.[12] During this period, the three germ layers undergo differentiation and give rise to the tissues and organ systems unique to each. During the fourth week of development, when the body of the developing embryo folds, the somatic mesoderm expands ventrally to form the intraembryonic coelomic cavity. Suspended within this cavity by the dorsal mesentery is the endodermal-lined primitive gut. This endoderm forms the epithelial lining of the digestive tract as well as giving rise to the liver and pancreas.

The duodenum is formed from the terminal part of the foregut and cephalic part of the midgut. As the primitive stomach and midgut rotate, the duodenum is rotated to the right and takes the form of a C-shaped loop before coming to rest in a retroperitoneal position. The pancreas, in turn, arises from two outgrowths of the endodermal lining of the duodenum. The dorsal pancreatic bud is located on the right side of the duodenum within the dorsal mesentery, whereas the ventral pancreatic bud is derived from endoderm on the left side of the developing duodenum in an area that is also associated with the origin of the common bile duct. During the rotation of the duodenum into its final position, the dorsal pancreatic bud maintains a constant connection with the duodenum. The ventral pancreatic bud, however, migrates posteriorly around the duodenum and comes to lie immediately below and behind the dorsal bud (Fig. 58.1). Eventually,

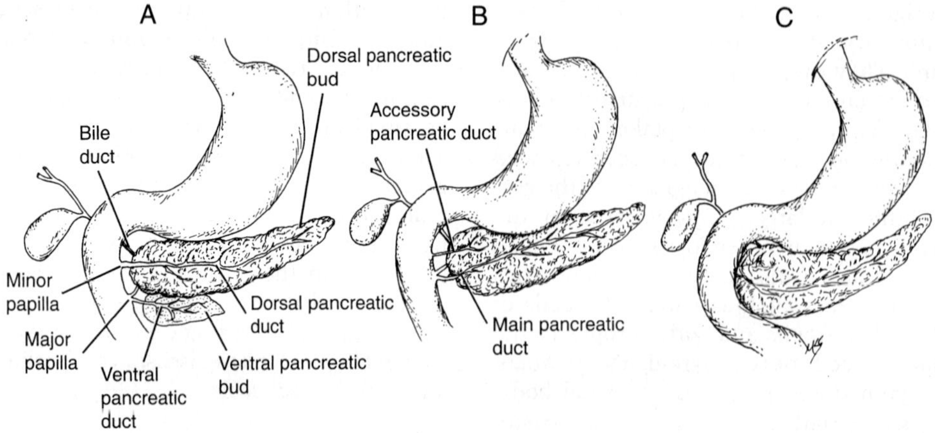

FIGURE 58.1. In utero development of the pancreas. **A.** During the sixth week of development, the ventral pancreatic bud (*lower*), in close association with the common bile duct, rotates posteriorly to come into close contact with the dorsal pancreatic bud (*upper*). **B.** This close association allows fusion of the two buds into the adult pancreas (**C**). In **B**, the ventral pancreatic duct fuses with the dorsal pancreatic duct to form the main pancreatic duct that enters the duodenum in association with the common bile duct at the major duodenal papilla (ampulla of Vater). The proximal remnant of the dorsal bud duct is usually obliterated but may persist as the accessory pancreatic duct (of Santorini) to enter the duodenum at the minor duodenal papilla. In about 10% of individuals, the two duct systems fail to fuse and the original double-duct system persists.

the parenchyma and duct systems of the closely opposed pancreatic buds fuse, forming one gland around which the duodenum is draped. In the adult organ, the uncinate process and inferior part of the head is derived from the ventral pancreatic bud, while the remainder of the gland is derived from the dorsal bud. The main pancreatic duct is formed by the fusion of the distal portion of the dorsal pancreatic duct with the entire ventral pancreatic duct. The proximal portion of the dorsal pancreatic duct is obliterated or persists as the accessory pancreatic duct. In about 10% of individuals, the two duct systems fail to fuse and the original double-duct system persists.

The embryonic epithelium of the pancreatic ducts contains the basic cell types for the development of the cells of the endocrine pancreas. During the 12th to 16th week of development, endocrine glands migrate from the ductal system and aggregate around capillaries to form isolated clumps of cells scattered throughout the exocrine glandular tissue. These collections are known as the *islets of Langerhans* and contain at least five different types of secretory cells, namely, *alpha, beta, delta, F,* and *enterochomaffin cells,* which secrete glucagon, insulin, somatostatin, pancreatic polypeptide, and serotonin, respectively. Histochemically, islet cells stain positive for chromogranin A and neuron-specific enolase. In addition, islet cell tumors have been reported to contain an argyrophilic cell (one lacking the ability to reduce silver stains unless exogenous reducing substances are added). It has been postulated that this cell may be the precursor for both normal and neoplastic islet cells.[13] The epithelium of the primitive gut also gives rise to a number of other neuroendocrine-secreting cells that have a varied distribution within the adult gastrointestinal tract (Table 58.2). Because gastrin-producing G cells are not normally present in the adult pancreas, it has been proposed that pancreatic gastrinomas are ectopic and that gastrinomas arising in the duodenum or jejunum, areas where gastrin-producing cells are normally found, are entopic.[14]

The eventual adult anatomy of the duodenum, pancreas, and midgut is a result of the close anatomic relationship of these organs during embryological development. Likewise, blood supply to these organs is closely related. Because the foregut is supplied by the celiac artery and the midgut by the superior mesenteric artery, the duodenum and pancreas are supplied by branches of both arteries. The main arterial blood supply of the body and tail of the pancreas is derived from branches of the splenic artery, which include the dorsal or superior pancreatic artery and the great pancreatic artery, both of which communicate by means of the inferior or transverse pancreatic artery. The transverse pancreatic artery also communicates with the superior mesenteric artery. The pancreatic head and uncinate process share a common blood supply with the duodenum, a fact that underlies the need for a pancreaticoduodenectomy for a tumor involving this area. Both are supplied by branches of the anterior and posterior pancreaticoduodenal artery, which originate as superior branches from the gastroduodenal artery and common hepatic artery and as inferior branches from the superior mesenteric artery. The supraduodenal artery, the first branch of the gastroduodenal artery, provides additional arterial supply to the first part of the duodenum.

Physiology of the Duodenum, Pancreas, and Small Intestine

The organs and glands of the foregut and midgut have evolved in close association to facilitate digestion and absorption of ingested foods. As such, most gastrointestinal activities are under both neural and hormonal control and result in a number of exocrine and endocrine products (see Table 58.2). Moreover, these products may produce significant symptoms and signs if they are elaborated in an unregulated or ectopic manner (Table 58.3). Individual pancreatic islet cells may produce more than one hormone, and they may also produce hormones such as gastrin, adrenocorticotrophin (ACTH), vasoactive intestinal polypeptide (VIP), and growth hormone-releasing hormone (GRH) that are not normally present in the pancreas.[15] Neuroendocrine cells are also found in the proximal portion of the duodenum as well as the antrum of the stomach, where they produce gastrin and somatostatin. Although each functional neuroendocrine tumor may produce clinical symptoms, it is those produced by gastrinoma, insulinoma, glucagonoma, and VIPoma that are the most clinically recognized and best studied.

Neuroendocrine Tumors and the MEN 1 Syndrome

The multiple endocrine neoplasia syndromes (MEN) are a fascinating group of endocrine syndromes first reported by Wermer in 1963.[16] In his study of a large kindred, he described the occurrence of multiple endocrine tumors or hyperplasia of the parathyroid, pituitary, and pancreas and expanded the syndrome to include the observation of frequent occurrence of peptic ulceration in these patients. This work, combined with the previous reports of Zollinger and Ellison in identifying jejunal peptic ulceration associated with gastric acid hypersecretion and pancreatic islet cell tumors in two patients,[17] unified the concept of an endocrine system malignancy syndrome.

MEN 1 (Wermer's syndrome) describes a wide range of pathology including parathyroid hyperplasia, pituitary adenoma, and endocrine tumors of the duodenum and pancreas. MEN 1 patients may also develop multiple subcutaneous lipomas, adenomas of the thyroid gland, and adrenocortical adenomas or carcinomas (Table 58.4). This familial disease has an autosomal dominant mode of transmission with incomplete penetrance. The genetic basis for the syndrome has been ascribed to a mutation in the MEN 1 or *menin* gene that maps to the long arm of chromosome 11.[18,19] The finding of deletions or translocations of one or both copies of the menin gene in cases of parathyroid hyperplasia and other endocrine tumors points to its function as a tumor suppressor gene. Although up to 80% of patients with MEN 1 have an associated islet cell tumor,[5,8,19] islet cell tumors are associated with MEN 1 in only 5% to 25% of cases.[5] Of these patients, approximately 54% have gastrinomas, 20% to 30% have insulinomas, and less than 15% have glucagonoma, somatostatinoma, or one of the less common neuroendocrine tumors.[19–21] The initial manifestation of MEN 1 is primarily hyperparathyroidism, but one study[22] reported that gastrinomas may be the initial manifestation of the syndrome. For

TABLE 58.2. Distribution and Actions of the Common Neuroendocrine Cells and Enteric Neuropeptides Involved in Neuroendocrine Pathology.

Designation[a]	*Cell type*	*Distribution*	*Active Product(s)*	*Target product*	*Organs*	*Actions*
B	β cell	Pancreas	Insulin	51aa polypeptide	Muscle Liver Other	Stimulates glucose uptake by muscle cells Stimulates hepatic glycogenesis Stimulates muscle protein synthesis Stimulates triglyceride deposition Inhibits hepatic gluconeogenesis
G IG	G cell	Stomach Duodenum Jejunum	Gastrin (? ACTH, met-enkephalin, GH)	17aa "little" and 34aa "big" polypeptide	Stomach Pancreas (small effect)	Stimulates parietal cell H^1 secretion, pepsinogen secretion, gastric mucosal growth
	α cell	Pancreas	Glucagon	Linear polypeptide	Liver Pancreas Heart	Stimulates gluconeogenesis, glycogenolysis, lipolysis and ketogenesis; increases blood glucose Stimulates growth hormone ***and insulin secretion and*** positive cardiac inotropy
D_1	? δ cell	Small bowel Colon Pancreas Gallbladder CNS	VIP	28aa polypeptide	GI tract Vasculature	Stimulates intestinal, pancreatic and bilary secretion GI smooth muscle relaxation Splanchnic vasodilatation
D	δ cells	Pancreas Pylorus Duodenum	Somatostatin	14aa and 28aa polypeptide		Inhibition of gastrin release, blockade of glucagon action on jejunum Inhibition of release of most GI and pancreatic hormones
$EC_{1,2,n}$	Enterochromaffin cells	Stomach Small bowel Large bowel CNS	Serotonin Substance P ? Leuenkephalin ? Others	Neuropeptide ? Polypeptide	Smooth muscle Nerve cells	Vasomotor disturbance (flushing, diarrhea, nausea, and vomiting) Bronchospasm Right-sided valvular endocardial fibrosis
PP	F cells ? Other islet cells	Pancreas	Pancreatic polypeptide	36aa polypeptide	Pancreas	Inhibits pancreatic exocrine secretion
N	N cells	Ileum Jejunum Duodenum Colon CNS	Neurotensin	Tridecapeptide	? GI tract	? Inhibition of gastric secretion ? Modulation of GI tract motility
PYY	?	Terminal ileum Colon Rectum	Peptide YY	36aa polypeptide	GI tract Pancreas	Inhibits autonomic neuro-transmission in GI tract and prolongs small bowel transit time Inhibits pancreatic exocrine secretion
L	L cell	Small intestine Large intestine	Enteroglucagon	Variety of peptides	? Liver ? Pancreas	? Compete with, and have similar actions to, glucagon
X	? Islet cell	Pancreas Lung Small intestines	Growth hormone-releasing factor (GRF)	Polypeptide	Bone Muscle Other	Stimulation of growth hormone release
	? Islet cell	Pancreas ? Other	ACTH	39aa polypeptide	Adrenal	Stimulation of release of glucocorticoids, mineralo-corticoids and androgenic steroids from adrenal cortex

aa, amino acid.

TABLE 58.3. Common Symptoms and Signs of the Main Neuroendocrine Tumor Syndromes.

Tumor	*Syndrome*	*Main hormone(s)*	*Symptoms*	*Signs*	*Diagnostic study*	*Diagnostic criteria*
Insulinoma	Insulinoma	Insulin	Neuroglycopenic	Somnolence Seizures Coma Diaphoresis Tremulousness	Supervised 72-h fast	Serum glucose <45 mg/dL Serum insulin >5 μU/mL C-peptide >1.2 ng/mL Proinsulin >25%
Gastrinoma	Zollinger–Ellison	Gastrin	Heartburn Dysphagia Diarrhea	Peptic ulceration Esophagitis or strictures Weight loss	Serum gastrin Basal acid output (BAO) Secretin stimulation test	Serum gastrin >100 pg/mL BAO >15 mEq/h (>5 mEq/h if prior operation for peptic ulcers) >200 pg/mL increase in gastrin levels after secretin stimulation
Glucagonoma	Glucagonoma	Glucagon	Skin rash Diarrhea Abdominal pain	Diabetes mellitus type II Weight loss/cachexia Venous thrombosis Pulmonary emboli	Fasting plasma glucagon Plasma amino acids	Plasma glucagon >500 pg/mL Decreased plasma amino acids
VIPoma	Verner–Morrison Pancreatic cholera Endocrine cholera WDHA	Vasoactive intestinal peptide (VIP)	Secretory diarrhea Abdominal colic Flushing	Hypokalemia Dehydration Weight loss	Serum potassium Fasting plasma VIP	Plasma VIP >500 pg/mL (potassium <2.5 mmol/L)
Somatostatinoma	Somatostatinoma	Somatostatin	Diarrhea Abdominal pain	Diabetes mellitus type II Cholelithiasis Steatorrhea Weight loss Hypochlorhydria	Fasting plasma somatostatin	Elevated plasma somatostatin
GRFoma	GRFoma	Growth hormone-releasing factor (GRF)		Acromegaly	Fasting Plasma GRF	Elevated plasma GRF
ACTHoma	Cushing's	Adrenocorticotropic hormone (ACTH)	Easy bruisability Atrophied skin	Hypertension Centripetal obesity Skin/mucosal pigmentation	Urinary free cortisol Plasma ACTH Dexamethasone suppression test	Elevated urinary cortisol Elevated plasma ACTH Failure to suppress with dexamethasone
Neurotensinoma	Neurotensinoma	Neurotensin	Tachycardia Flushing Diarrhea	Hypotension Malabsorption Weight loss Cyanosis Diabetes mellitus	Fasting plasma neurotensin	Elevated plasma neurotensin
PTH-RPoma	PTH-RPoma	Parathyroid hormone-related peptide (PTH-RP)	Bone pain Renal colic Weakness	Decreased bone density Pathological fractures Nephrolithiasis Pseudogout Peptic ulcers Pancreatitis	Serum calcium Serum PTH Serum PTH-related peptide	Elevated serum calcium Low or nondetectable serum PTH Elevated serum PTH-related peptide
Nonfunctional	None	Neuron-specific enolase Pancreatic polypeptide Chromogranin A	Abdominal pain Weakness Palpated mass	Bowel obstruction Gastrointestinal bleeding/anemia jaundice	None	Radiologic imaging
Carcinoid	Carcinoid	5-HT 5-HTP	Diarrhea Flushing Wheezing Pain	Flushing rash Anemia Bowel obstruction Recurrent pneumonia Heart failure Pellagra	Urinary 5-HIAA Urinary 5-HT Platelet 5-HT	Elevated urinary 5-HIAA Elevated urinary 5-HT Increased platelet 5-HT

Sources: Norton (1998)[5]; Meko and Norton (1994)[8]; Feldman (1989)[136]; Norheim et al. (1987)[170]; Thorson (1958).[180]

TABLE 58.4. Usual Components of the Multiple Endocrine Neoplasia Type 1 (MEN 1) Syndrome.

Mutation in *menin* gene on chromosome 11
Parathyroid hyperplasia
Pituitary adenoma (rarely, hyperplasia)
Multiple neuroendocrine tumors involving the pancreas and duodenum
Adrenocortical adenoma or carcinoma (rare)
Thyroid adenoma
Carcinoid tumors of foregut and midgut
Multiple lipomas

this reason, in patients diagnosed with neuroendocrine tumors, it is important to consider the diagnosis of MEN 1, particularly if the individual has primary hyperparathyroidism and nephrolithiasis or a family history suspicious for multiple endocrine neoplasia. Further, there is a relationship between the signs and symptoms of primary hyperparathyroidism (HPT) and Zollinger–Ellison syndrome (ZES). Surgery to correct the manifestations of primary HPT (usually 3.5-gland parathyroidectomy or 4-gland parathyroidectomy with autotransplantation) will clearly improve the signs and symptoms of ZES.[11,23] In this case, in MEN 1 patients with both primary HPT and ZES, surgery to correct the HPT is recommended before surgery to resect an islet cell tumor.

Neuroendocrine tumors in patients with MEN 1 are characteristically multiple and often small.[5,19,24] Depending on the particular tumor, they may also have an increased propensity to occur at extrapancreatic sites and may be difficult to localize radiologically. The management of neuroendocrine tumors in the setting of MEN 1 is dependent on the clinical syndrome that results from hormone overproduction.[19] For insulinomas, tumors do not occur outside the pancreas, and there is little controversy over management because surgical resection is the treatment of choice. Gastrinomas, however, because of their malignant potential and tendency to originate in the duodenum, have generated some controversy over the years.[20,25] With the introduction of histamine H_2-receptor antagonists and proton pump inhibitors, the management of these patients has changed considerably over the past decade[19,20] and continues to evolve. In patients with MEN 1 and ZES, because surgical resection is seldom curative, it is usually directed toward larger tumors (>2–3 cm) to remove any other potentially malignant neuroendocrine neoplasm. In patients with MEN 1 and glucagonomas or VIPomas, management is similar to that of insulinomas, with surgery appearing to be the treatment of choice.[19] Nonfunctioning neuroendocrine tumors, which produce no symptoms, are generally treated surgically only in situations where the tumor is clearly imaged (2–3 cm) or if complications such as obstruction arise. Overall, the surgical treatment of a given tumor, when it occurs in the MEN 1 setting, is less successful than treatment of the same tumor when it occurs sporadically.[19]

Neuroendocrine Tumors

Insulinoma

Insulinoma is the most common pancreatic islet cell tumor and was first recognized by Whipple in the 1930s.[26] It is generally a small tumor of the pancreas and is malignant in 5% to 11% of cases.[27] In the sporadic form, solitary tumors are generally evenly distributed throughout the entire pancreas (Fig. 58.2). Tumors may be multiple in the setting of MEN 1.[24] Although it may occur at any age, the mean age of patients with insulinoma is 45 years and the female-to-male ratio is around 1.5 to 2:1.[3,28] It generally occurs at a younger age in the context of MEN 1, in which patients usually present in the third decade of life. The excessive production of insulin deprives the brain of glucose and produces neuroglycopenic symptoms including sleepiness, seizures, and loss of consciousness.

Tumor Characteristics

Approximately 80% to 90% of insulinomas are small (roughly 2 cm), solitary, benign tumors distributed with equal probability among the head, body, and tail of the pancreas (see Fig. 58.2). Approximately 5% to 10% occur as multiple islet cell tumors in the setting of MEN 1.[5,20] A similar proportion are malignant as determined by the detection of lymph node or liver metastases. The presence of diffuse microadenomatosis, in which multiple small nonencapsulated tumors or nodules are distributed throughout the pancreas (nesidioblastosis), may occur in the neonatal and infant setting and cause neonatal hypoglycemia. This entity is largely absent in adults, although some may dispute this contention.[28–30]

Most benign insulinomas are between 0.5 and 2 cm in diameter. Tumors appear reddish brown in color as a consequence of increased vascularity. Microscopic examination cannot distinguish between benign and malignant insulinomas, although malignant lesions tend to be larger with an average size of 6.2 cm. The diagnosis of malignancy is made at the time of surgery by the identification of either lymph node or liver metastases. When insulinomas arise in the setting of MEN 1, multiple tumors are generally found.[5,19,24] However, even in this instance, the functional insulinoma is usually a large dominant tumor that can be removed for amelioration of hypoglycemia. Pathological analysis of resected pancreatic specimens from these patients has demonstrated that multiple other neuroendocrine tumors are present that generally do not secrete insulin.

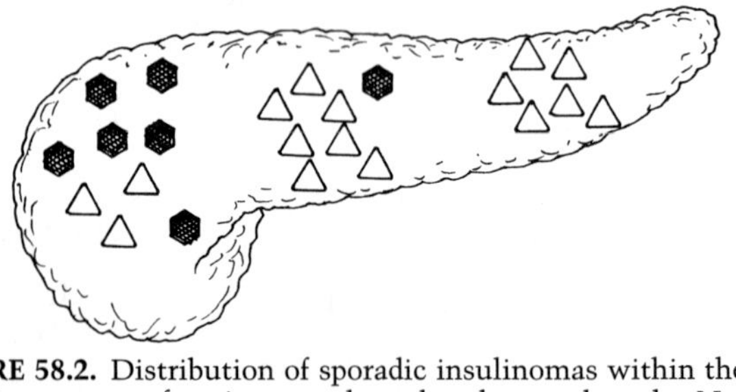

FIGURE 58.2. Distribution of sporadic insulinomas within the pancreas in a group of patients evaluated and treated at the National Institutes of Health.[95] In the sporadic form, tumors are generally evenly distributed throughout the entire pancreas. The *open triangles* indicate tumors that were palpable and imageable by intraoperative ultrasound (IOUS); the *dark hexagons* indicate nonpalpable tumors that were found only with the use of IOUS. Note how the majority of nonpalpable tumors are located in the head of the pancreas.

Presenting Symptoms and Signs

In almost all cases, patients with insulinoma have symptoms that are caused by hypoglycemia, with rare cases causing symptoms because of the size of the tumor itself (see Table 58.3). Most commonly, patients have neuroglycopenic symptoms that include seizures, difficulty awakening, visual disturbances, confusion, lethargy, weakness, or transient motor deficits.[5,24] Hypoglycemia also causes catecholamine release with subsequent sympathetic discharge resulting in sweating, anxiety, and palpitations.[5] Erroneous psychiatric or neurological diagnoses are common and, on average, it may take up to 2 years before the correct diagnosis is made.[24,31] In one study, 33% of patients were initially treated for primary neuropsychiatric disorders before diagnosis of insulinoma was made.[32] Symptoms tend to occur early in the morning after an overnight fast or during periods of fasting for religious or other observances. Patients come to learn that food relieves or avoids symptoms and thus most gain weight. A family history of hypoglycemia or other endocrine abnormalities should be sought to exclude the presence of MEN 1.

Diagnosis

The measurement of severe hypoglycemia and inappropriately elevated levels of insulin is essential for the diagnosis (see Table 58.3). Before the development of laboratory techniques to measure serum insulin levels, Whipple proposed the diagnostic triad of symptomatic hypoglycemia induced by fasting, a blood glucose level less than 45 mg/dL, and prompt relief of symptoms following administration of glucose.[26] Since that time, the development of a sensitive radioimmunoassay for serum insulin as well as several suppression and stimulation tests have simplified the diagnosis of insulinoma.[24,33] Stimulation tests include measuring plasma levels of insulin after administration of any of a number of different agents including tolbutamide, calcium, and glucagon.[24,33] Suppression tests involve the administration of exogenous insulin derived from porcine, fish, or recombinant human sources that suppress insulin and C-peptide levels in normal individuals but not those with insulin-secreting tumors. However, the diagnostic test of choice is a 72-h fast during which serum levels of glucose and insulin are measured every 6 h.[27,34] The fast is terminated at 72 h or when the patient develops neuroglycopenic symptoms. At that point serum levels of glucose, insulin, C-peptide, and proinsulin are measured and intravenous glucose administered. Intravenous glucose is administered and the neuroglycopenic symptoms are ameliorated.

Most patients with insulinoma develop neuroglycopenic symptoms within 12 to 24 h and few, if any, will fast for 72 h. Administration of the test requires hospitalization, and completion of the diagnostic fast without symptoms excludes insulinoma as a cause for hypoglycemia. During the fast, careful observation is necessary to avoid any complications of hypoglycemia and to exclude the use of either insulin or oral hypoglycemic drugs that produce factitious hypoglycemia, a condition that can closely mimic insulinoma.[34] Patients with factitious hypoglycemia are typically young women who are associated with the healthcare profession or are relatives of individuals with diabetes mellitus.[34] These patients surreptitiously take either insulin injections or oral hypoglycemic drugs. Urinary levels of sulfonylurea are also measured by gas chromatography mass spectroscopy to help exclude the use of oral hypoglycemic drugs.

The diagnosis of insulinoma is made based primarily on the fast results. It is important that patients develop neuroglycopenic symptoms at the time the samples are drawn. The diagnosis is established by a serum glucose level less than 45 mg/dL and a concomitant insulin level greater than 5 mU/mL at the time symptoms develop. In interpreting laboratory results it is important to understand the usual components of insulin secretion (Fig. 58.3). Insulin is secreted from cells in secretory granules that contain both the inactive, or proinsulin, form of the hormone as well as a protease that cleaves the terminal C-peptide sequence of the molecule. This cleavage yields both active insulin as well as inactive C-peptide fragments in equimolar amounts. Although some proinsulin may be released from cells without proteolytic activation, it is usually less than 25% of the total serum insulin concentration. Thus, patients with an insulinoma have an immunoreactive insulin-to-glucose ratio greater than 0.3 and an elevated serum level of proinsulin. These values are not found in normal individuals or in patients with factitious hypoglycemia. A ratio of proinsulin to insulin greater than 25% is consistent with insulinoma, and C-peptide levels are also elevated.[5] If factitious hypoglycemia is caused by the administration of exogenous insulin, appreciable amounts of C-peptide will not be detected and the proinsu-

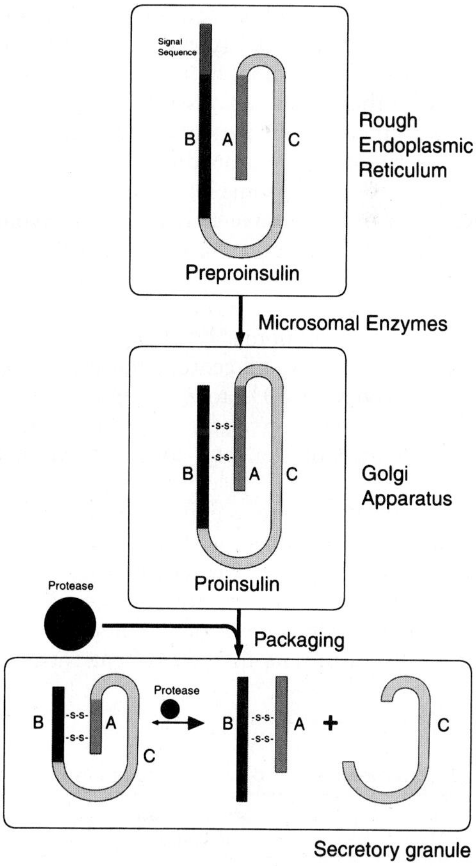

FIGURE 58.3. Diagrammatic illustration of the insulin secretion pathway in pancreatic beta cells or insulinomas. The secretory granules contain both active insulin as well as inactive C-peptide fragments in equimolar amounts.

lin-to-insulin ratio is generally low. If factitious hypoglycemia is caused by bovine or porcine insulin, antibodies to insulin may be detected.[35] Thus, patients with insulinoma develop neuroglycopenic symptoms during a monitored fast with serum glucose levels less than 45 mg/dL and insulin levels greater than 5 mU/mL. In addition, the diagnosis is confirmed with the findings of a glucose-to-insulin ratio greater than 0.3, a proinsulin level greater than 25%, or a C-peptide level greater than 1.2 ng/mL. Urinary sulfonylurea and serum insulin antibodies should not be detectable (Table 58.5).

Radiologic Localization

Because insulinomas are usually small and lack a high density of somatostatin receptors, the results of conventional, noninvasive, radiographic imaging studies are poor (Table 58.6). Computed tomography, magnetic resonance imaging, and ultrasound identify only 17% to 26% of tumors in some studies.[28,36,37] However, either MR or CT should be obtained to exclude liver metastases or the presence of a large malignant primary tumor. In this case, helical CT with pancreatic protocol should be performed with intravenous contrast to optimize the study. On MR, most insulinomas and other neuroendocrine tumors appear bright on T_2-weighted, short-time inversion recovery (STIR), and weighted spin-echo sequences.[31,38] Somatostatin receptor scintigraphy (SRS) utilizing [^{111}In-diethylenetriamine pentacetic acid (DTPA)-D-phe1]-octreotide is also poor at imaging insulinomas because these tumors do not have a high density of type 2 somatostatin receptors (SSTR2 subtype). Although some investigators have reported localization of up to 53% of insulinomas using this modality,[39] other studies reported that SRS failed to localize any tumors in any of the patients studied.[5,7,40]

Because of the inability of preoperative studies to accurately localize insulinoma, some have recommended surgical exploration with intraoperative ultrasound and avoidance of other costly invasive preoperative imaging techniques.[24,41,42] However, other studies may be useful. Endoscopic ultrasound (EUS), for instance, appears to be one of the best preoperative studies to identify insulinoma.[8,43,44] EUS is observer-dependent and is not available in all centers, but it has been found to have a sensitivity of 80% to 85% and a specificity of 95% in identifying intrapancreatic neuroendocrine tumors.[8] However, EUS cannot reliably localize extrapancreatic disease.[8,43]

Because insulinomas are evenly distributed throughout the pancreas, regional localization to determine the area with the tumor may be helpful. In this regard, portal venous sampling (PVS) for insulin is an older invasive procedure that can locate tumor in, on average, 75% of patients.[5,45] In one study, it actually localized tumors in 100% of patients.[46] PVS can localize tumors to a particular region of the pancreas and thus facilitate surgical resection, but its disadvantages include the need for expertise as well as cost, pain, and other complications related to the procedure.[47] Intraarterial calcium angiogram, which has largely supplanted PVS, provides similar localization information in that up to 80% of tumors are localized in a similar number of patients with less cost and fewer complications.[5,48] If provocative calcium injection is used (calcium angiogram), 90% to 100% of tumors can be localized. It also has the potential to image tumor based on a characteristic vascular "blush" (Fig. 58.4). In general, if the surgeon wants confirmation of the pancreatic region within which the insulinoma is contained, calcium angiogram is the preoperative invasive study of choice.[34,48]

The single best modality in localizing insulinomas during surgery, even when preoperative imaging studies are equivocal, is intraoperative ultrasound (IOUS).[45,49] It is now apparent that surgical exploration with exposure and palpation of the pancreas combined with the use of IOUS is the most cost-effective therapy for insulinomas, even when other preoperative studies are negative (see Table 58.6).

Gastrinoma

It was Zollinger and Ellison who first reported the unusual occurrence of jejunal peptic ulcer disease in association with gastric acid hypersecretion and islet cell tumors of the pancreas.[17] Following conventional acid-reduction surgery, the patients ultimately developed recurrent peptic ulceration that required total gastrectomy for control of symptoms. Zollinger and Ellison postulated that the pancreatic tumor was the cause of the severe peptic ulcer disease. We now know that the Zollinger–Ellison syndrome (ZES) is caused by a pancreatic or duodenal neuroendocrine tumor called a *gastrinoma* that elaborates excessive and unregulated amounts of the hormone gastrin, which stimulates excessive gastric acid secretion, leading to peptic ulcer disease.

ZES is a functional neuroendocrine tumor syndrome. In 80% of cases it occurs in a sporadic form, whereas the familial or inherited form occurs in 20% of cases.[11,49] The familial form is associated with the multiple endocrine neoplasia type 1 (MEN 1) syndrome and, within this setting, most functional neuroendocrine tumors are gastrinomas.[19] ZES is the underlying cause in approximately 0.1% to 1% of patients with peptic ulcer disease.[50]

Gastrinomas are slow growing but approximately 60% are malignant, with patients having lymph node, liver, or distant metastatic disease at diagnosis.[51] In 25% of cases, the tumor may pursue a particularly aggressive course.[52] Currently, it is thought that, as screening for hypergastrinemia has become more common, a larger proportion of tumors are being discovered and referred for surgical treatment.

TABLE 58.5. Interpretation of Biochemical Studies in the Diagnosis of Insulinoma.

Patient type	*Serum glucose (mg/dL)*	*Serum insulin (mU/mL)*	*Proinsulin (%)*	*C-peptide (ng/mL)*	*Antibodies to insulin*	*Sulfonylurea (blood or urine)*
Normal	80–100	2–10	12–20	0.5–1	Absent	Absent
Insulinoma	<45	>5	>25	>1.2	Absent	Absent
Factitious hypoglycemia	<45	>5	12–20	≤0.5	Present	Present

TABLE 58.6.
Outcome of Various Preoperative Localization Studies for Neuroendocrine Tumors.

				True positive/total (%)									
Reference	*Level of evidence*[a]	n	*MEN*	*US*	*CT*	*MRI*	*SRS*	*PVS*	*Angiography*	*Provocative angiography*	*EUS*	*IOUS*	*Palpation*
Insulinoma													
Norton et al. (1992)[99]	II	8	0									6/8 (75)	5/8 (63)
Böttger et al. (1990)[41]	III	43	1	13/21 (62)	11/15 (73)			10/13 (77)	20/30 (67)			12/16 (75)	40/42 (95)
Norton et al. (1990)[45]	II	12	0					9/12 (75)				10/125/12 (42) (83)	
Doherty et al. (1991)[95]	II	25	0	6/22 (27)	4/22 (18)	2/22 (9)		17/22 (77)	9/22 (41)			22/24 (92)	16/24 (67)
Kisker et al. (1997)[40]	II	6	0	4/6 (67)	4/6 (67)		0/6 (0)						
Lo et al. (1997)[32]	II	27	1	2/6 (33)	11/25 (44)			2/3 (67)	11/21 (52)	7/7 (100)	1/3 (33)	17/17 (100)	22/27 (81)
Boukhman et al. (1998)[21]	III	67	11	4/6 (67)	13/35 (37)	6/14 (43)		7/10 (70)	14/30 (47)			9/11 (82)	42/56 (75)
Gastrinoma													
Norton et al. (1988)[73]	II	39	0									29/35 (83)	33/35 (94)
Kisker et al. (1997)[40]	II	17	NR	7/17 (41)	7/17 (41)		9/17 (53)						15/17 (88)
Krausz et al. (1998)[89]	II	5	0		2/5 (40)		4/5 (80)						
Alexander et al. (1998)[68]	II	37	4	6/37 (16)	18/37 (49)	21/37 (57)	29/37 (78)		21/37 (57)				
Kisker et al. (1998)[71]	II	25	2	11/25(44)	14/25 (56)	1/4 (25)	9/17 (53)		1/10 (10)		4/6 (67)	14/15 (93)	24/25 (96)
Other NETs													
Krausz et al. (1998)[89]	II	6	NR		4/6 (67)		5/6 (83)						
Carcinoid													
Kisker et al. (1997)[40]	II	22	NR	8/22 (36)	12/22 (55)		9/22 (41)						11/11 (100)
Krausz et al. (1998)[89]	II	23	0		4/9 (44)		3/9 (33)						

[a]I, prospective, randomized; II, prospective; III, retrospective, review or anecdotal; NR, not reported.
Other NETs (neuroendocrine tumors): glucagonoma (n53), somatostatinoma (n51), VIPoma (n51); PTH-RPoma (n51).

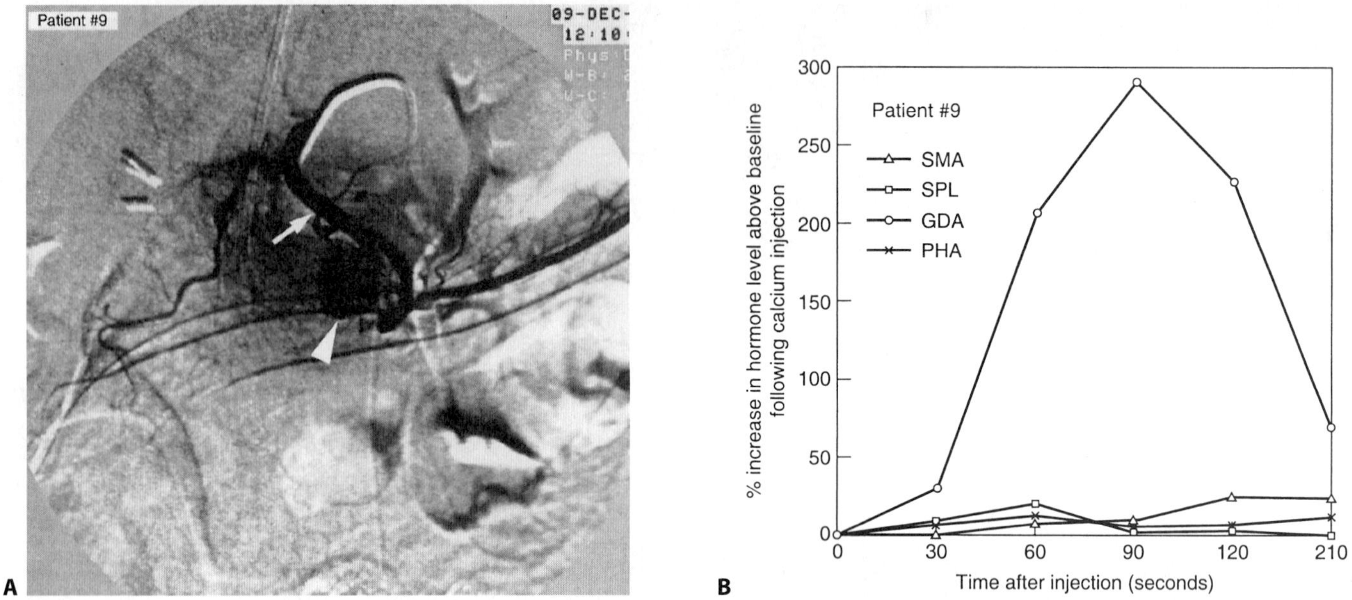

FIGURE 58.4. Provocative (calcium) angiogram identifying an insulinoma in the head of the pancreas. **A.** Standard arteriogram shows a hypervascular blush (*white arrowhead*) after injection of the gastroduodenal artery (*white arrow*). In **B**, the same patient (patient 9) shows a significant increase in insulin sampled from the hepatic vein 90s after calcium is injected into the gastroduodenal artery (GDA) during the angiogram outlined in **A.** In **B**, concurrent sampling of the superior mesenteric artery (SMA), splenic artery (SPL), or proper hepatic artery (PHA) shows no significant increase in hepatic vein insulin levels.

Tumor Characteristics

Gastrinomas may be single or multiple and may range in size from less than 1 cm to more than 3 cm. Multiple duodenal or pancreatic tumors are found in patients with the MEN 1 syndrome.[53,54] Although it has been suggested that the tumors found in MEN 1 patients may have a lower potential for metastases, they appear to metastasize with a similar frequency to their sporadic counterparts when evaluated in long-term follow-up.

Approximately 80% of gastrinomas are found within the *gastrinoma triangle*, an area that includes the first, second, and third portion of the duodenum and the head of the pancreas.[55] Although rare, primary gastrinomas have also been found in the jejunum, stomach, liver, spleen, mesentery, ovary, and heart.[56,57] In addition, patients have been reported to be cured of ZES after excision of solitary gastrinomas that appear to have arisen within a lymph node, and this has given rise to the idea of a lymph node primary gastrinoma.[51,58] Gastrinomas of the duodenum and pancreas appear to have a similar incidence of overall metastases. However, pancreatic gastrinomas appear to have a higher incidence of liver metastases as compared with duodenal tumors, which have a higher incidence of lymph node metastases. Because liver metastases have a direct influence on survival, pancreatic gastrinomas have decreased long-term survival compared to duodenal primary tumors.[52]

Presenting Symptoms and Signs

The mean age at diagnosis of ZES is 50 years, although children as young as 7 years and adults as old as 90 have been reported. There is a slight male preponderance with a male-to-female ratio of approximately 2:1. In patients with the MEN 1 syndrome, ZES is usually diagnosed in the third decade of life.[51] Clinical manifestations of the syndrome are related to the excessive secretion of gastric acid (see Table 58.3). The most common symptoms are epigastric pain, heartburn, diarrhea, and dysphagia. Approximately 90% of patients with ZES are found to have peptic ulceration, with the proximal duodenum as the most commonly involved site.[59] However, some patients still have multiple peptic ulcers or ulcers in unusual locations such as the distal duodenum (14%) and jejunum (11%), and a minority have recurrent ulceration following surgery.[51,59,60] In 7% to 10% of patients, a perforated peptic ulcer may be the initial sign of the disease.[61] Gastric acid hypersecretion also leads to a secretory diarrhea, which is seen in up to 40% of patients with ZES, and may be the sole presenting complaint in 20% of individuals.[51] In those with diarrhea, malabsorption may manifest itself as weight loss and malnutrition. In approximately 10% of patients, endoscopy shows evidence of lower esophageal inflammation and even stricture if the reflux symptoms are long-standing and severe. As the tumor develops and metastases occur, symptoms may be related to the size of the tumor itself.

Diagnosis

In most cases, the diagnosis of ZES is not immediately considered. Many series report a mean period of 6 years from presentation of symptoms to diagnosis.[11] This delay may be the consequence of a number of factors. First, hypergastrinemia may also occur as a manifestation of other diseases or conditions, most of which do not lead to excessive gastric acid secretion and ulcer formation (Table 58.7). Second, because

TABLE 58.7. Differential Diagnoses of Hypergastrinemia.

With excessive gastric acid secretion (ulcerogenic):
ZES (Zollinger–Ellison syndrome)
Gastric outlet obstruction
Retained gastric antrum (after Bilroth II reconstruction)
G-cell hyperplasia
Medications for peptic ulcers or GERD (H_2-receptor antagonists or proton pump inhibitors)
No excessive gastric acid secretion (nonulcerogenic):
Pernicious anemia
Atrophic gastritis
Renal failure
Postvagotomy
Short gut syndrome (after significant intestinal resection)

ZES is rare and few clinicians have seen many cases, there may be a failure to consider the diagnosis of ZES initially. ZES should be considered in all patients who present with one or more symptoms referable to the upper gastrointestinal tract, or in those with peptic ulcer disease and primary hyperparathyroidism and nephrolithiasis or a family history suspicious for multiple endocrine neoplasia (see Table 58.4).

ZES can be accurately diagnosed in all patients by measurement of an elevated fasting serum level of gastrin and an elevated basal acid output (BAO) (see Table 58.3). Patients should be off all antisecretory medications (H_2-receptor antagonists and proton pump inhibitors) for 3 to 7 days before the determination because medications that reduce gastric acid secretion cause a false elevation of serum gastrin levels. The diagnosis can be confirmed by the addition of a secretin test. Measurement of the fasting serum level of gastrin is the initial study to diagnose ZES, and 100% of patients with ZES have a fasting serum gastrin level greater than 100pg/mL.[51] It should also be noted that fasting serum gastrin levels increase in individuals with renal failure, pernicious anemia, or atrophic gastritis and in those taking acid-reduction medications. Therefore, measurement of BAO is necessary to ascertain the diagnosis of ZES. A BAO greater than 15mEq/h in most patients and above 5mEq/h in patients with prior acid-reduction operations, in conjunction with an elevated fasting gastrin level, unequivocally establishes the diagnosis. When a working diagnosis of ZES is made, confirmatory provocative testing should be undertaken. The secretin stimulation test is the test of choice as it has a sensitivity of 85% or greater.[62] Using this test, a 2U/kg bolus of secretin is given intravenously, and serum levels of gastrin are measured before and at 2, 5, 10, and 15min after administration. An increase of 200pg/mL in the serum gastrin level, following secretin administration, is consistent with a diagnosis of ZES. This test may be of particular utility in patients who have undergone prior operations to reduce acid output. These patients may have a minimally or moderately elevated gastrin level and BAO.

Radiologic Localization

Because of the nature of the tumor, preoperative localization of gastrinoma may prove difficult or, in some cases, unreliable. No single imaging or localization study alone can clearly identify total tumor extent (see Table 58.6). Noninvasive, preoperative imaging includes ultrasound (US), computed tomography (CT), magnetic resonance imaging (MRI), and selective angiography. More invasive studies, including portal venous sampling for gastrin levels or intraarterial secretin (IAS) with hepatic venous sampling for gastrin levels, provide functional localization to a region of the pancreas. Current noninvasive localization studies may fail to detect tumor in approximately 20% of patients with ZES.[63]

As a first-line study, ultrasound has a sensitivity no greater than 30% but its specificity approaches 92%.[64] The accuracy of CT scanning is dependent on the size of the gastrinoma.[51,65] Tumors less than 1cm in size are rarely visualized, even with current advanced helical sequences, but 30% of those between 1 and 3cm are seen. However, CT can detect all primary and metastatic lesions greater than 3cm in size. Overall, CT imaging can identify approximately 80% of pancreatic and 35% of extrahepatic gastrinomas.[65] MRI is expensive and, on the basis of most studies, images only about 25% of primary gastrinomas.[64] It has utility, however, in identifying small lesions and, in particular, liver metastases. It is also useful in distinguishing metastatic lesions from benign hemangiomas.

Somatostatin receptor scintigraphy (SRS), which was first evaluated in 1993,[66] is the accepted standard for localizing both primary and metastatic gastrinomas (Fig. 58.5). The radiolabeled somatostatin analogue has a high affinity for the type 2 somatostatin receptor, which is expressed in up to 80% of gastrinomas;[40] overall, 90% of tumors can be imaged by this modality with a specificity approaching 100%.[67] In the setting of ZES, when clinical suspicion of gastrinoma is high, it has a positive predictive value of 100% and can have a sensitivity exceeding all other imaging studies combined.[67,68] However, it still may be unable to identify small primary duodenal gastrinomas.

Endoscopic ultrasound (EUS) is a fairly recent method utilized to localize gastrinomas. It is relatively invasive and attempts to detect small tumors by endoscopically placing an

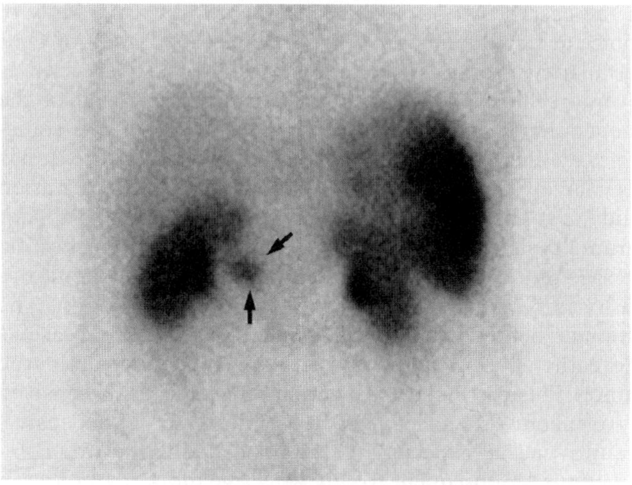

FIGURE 58.5. Somatostatin receptor scintigraphy (SRS) in a patient with Zollinger–Ellison syndrome (ZES) shows signal uptake in a lesion that is consistent with a gastrinoma (*arrows*) within the area of the gastrinoma triangle. On exploration, the lesion was found in the wall of the duodenum.

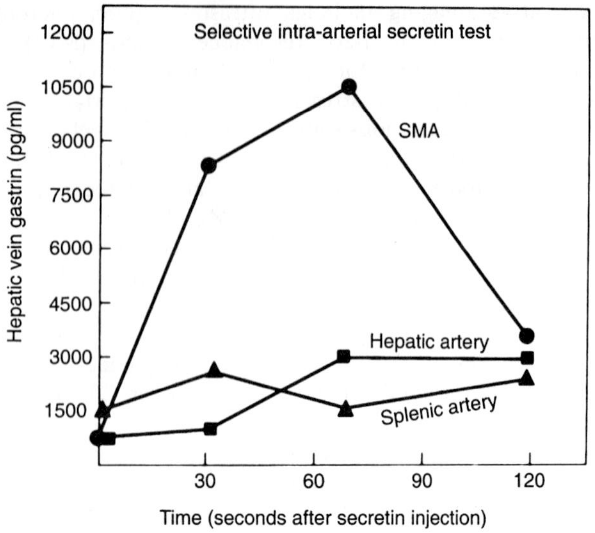

FIGURE 58.6. Provocative intraarterial secretin test in a patient with ZES shows a significant (>50%) increase in hepatic vein gastrin levels approximately 70s after injection of secretin into the superior mesenteric artery (SMA). Injection of the hepatic and splenic arteries showed no effective increase in sampled gastrin levels. This finding effectively localizes the gastrinoma to the area of the uncinate process, inferior portion of the head of the pancreas, or third or fourth part of the duodenum.

ultrasonic transducer in the vicinity of the gastrinoma triangle and the liver. It has been used to successfully image pancreatic islet cell tumors such as insulinomas,[69] but it is operator-dependent and has not been able to reliably identify small duodenal tumors. In addition, EUS may have difficulty differentiating normal lymph nodes from those containing tumor because the sonographic appearance is similar. One study found the sensitivity of EUS to be 50% to 75% for duodenal, 75% for pancreatic, and 63% for lymph node gastrinomas.[70]

To aid in gastrinoma localization, invasive imaging and regional localization studies have also been used extensively. In the past, selective angiography was the imaging study of choice and could identify 60% of tumors. As a result of their vascularity, primary or metastatic gastrinomas were seen as a tumor "blush" within the liver, pancreas, or wall of the duodenum. This study required arterial puncture and, sometimes, delivery of a significant volume of contrast dye. It has been largely supplanted by SRS. Another invasive localization study that has been used is portal venous sampling (PVS) for serum levels of gastrin[47]; this is performed by transhepatic passage of a catheter into the portal vein and its tributaries with sampling of gastrin levels along this distribution. The rationale behind the study is that gastrin levels increase as the catheter is moved into selective veins that drain the tumor. This particular localization procedure had a sensitivity of about 80%. However, it is cumbersome, expensive, requires special expertise, and is associated with some complications.[47] Subsequent to this, selective infusion of secretin was combined with angiography in an attempt to identify the region of the pancreas that contains the gastrinoma. This approach is popular because it avoids the need for transhepatic portal venous sampling. In this study, secretin is selectively injected into arteries supplying specific regions of the pancreas and liver, and gastrin levels are measured in the hepatic vein. A 50% increase in hepatic vein gastrin levels localizes the gastrinoma to the area supplied by the injected artery (Fig. 58.6). However, occult gastrinomas are most commonly located in the gastrinoma triangle,[51,71] and this limits the new information that can be obtained by this study.

Intraoperative studies have been used to localize gastrinomas, particularly those not imaged preoperatively, or to confirm preoperative findings. In these instances, intraoperative ultrasound (IOUS) and intraoperative endoscopy (IOE) with and without transillumination have proven utility.[72] IOUS images gastrinomas within the pancreas as sonolucent masses and facilitates removal of these tumors by showing the real-time relationship of the tumor to the pancreatic duct and other structures. IOUS has not been effective in imaging duodenal gastrinomas.[73] For this reason, intraoperative endoscopy (IOE) with duodenal transillumination was developed. With transillumination, duodenal wall tumors appear as a photopaque mass. Once identified, the tumor can be marked with a suture and removed with a small margin of normal duodenal tissue (Fig. 58.7).

Other Neuroendocrine Tumors

Glucagonoma

Glucagonoma is a malignant pancreatic islet cell tumor that usually presents during the fifth or sixth decade of life; 16% of cases may occur in those less than 40 years old.[74] Patients have a characteristic raised red pruritic rash called necrolytic migratory erythema (NME) (Fig. 58.8), which was first described by Wilkinson in 1973.[75] It typically involves the pretibial, perioral, and intertriginous areas, and it is initially erythematous and scaly but can progress to bullous lesions that slough. It is seen in approximately 64% to 90% of patients. Patients also have severe hypoaminoacidemia, weight loss, type 2 diabetes mellitus, and marked muscle wasting or cachexia (see Table 58.3). Patients with glucagonoma are at increased risk of deep venous thrombosis and pulmonary embolism, and these entities may be seen in up to 24% and 11% of patients, respectively.[74,76]

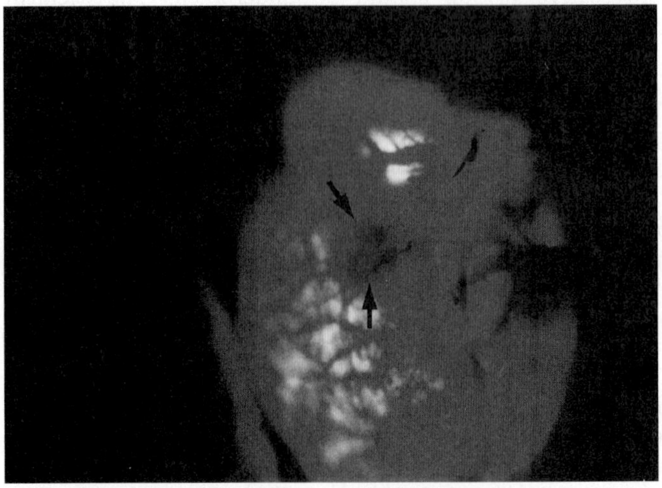

FIGURE 58.7. Transillumination of the duodenum using intraoperative endoscopy showing a duodenal wall gastrinoma (*arrows*).

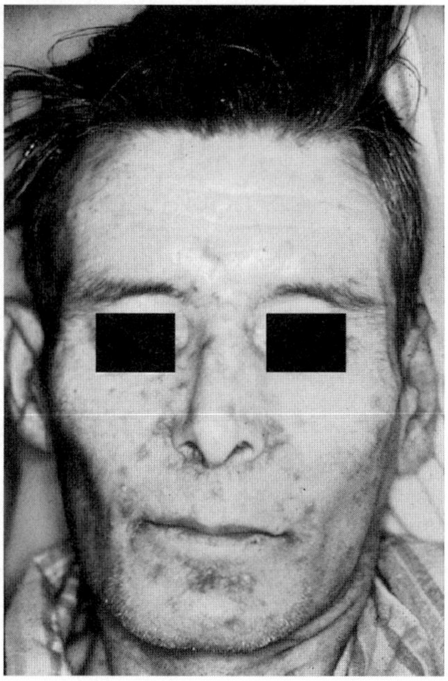

FIGURE 58.8. Usual appearance of the characteristic necrolytic migratory erythema (NME) rash in a patient with glucagonoma.

NME can precede diagnosis or suspicion of a glucagonoma for many years, leading to patients being treated for dermatological findings. The biochemical diagnosis of glucagonoma is made by measuring elevated plasma levels of glucagon (>500 pg/mL) and decreased plasma levels of amino acids (see Table 58.3). Most patients with glucagonoma have plasma glucagon levels greater than 1000 pg/mL. Because the cachexia is so severe, most patients are initially managed by total parenteral nutrition (TPN) with supplemental zinc, trace metals, and insulin. This intervention improves the hypoaminoacidemia, malnutrition, NME, and immune status in preparation for surgery. Long-term management of patients with metastatic glucagonoma has relied on the use of octreotide, which can reduce circulating plasma levels of glucagon and improve the rash and malnutrition.[77] At the time of diagnosis, most tumors are large (average size, 5–10 cm) and either locally advanced or metastatic and unresectable. For this reason, surgery for glucagonoma is seldom curative.[76]

Vasoactive Intestinal Peptide Tumor

The vasoactive intestinal peptide tumor (VIPoma) syndrome was first reported by Verner and Morrison in 1958[78] and came to bear their names. Because of the associated severe diarrhea, it is also referred to as the pancreatic cholera syndrome,[79] endocrine cholera syndrome,[80] or WHDA (watery diarrhea, hypokalemia, and achlorhydria) syndrome.[81] The mean age at diagnosis is 50 years, and there is a slight female preponderance.[80,82]

VIPomas induce a severe secretory diarrhea, a form of diarrhea that is defined by persistence despite abstaining from oral intake; this leads to hypokalemia, hypochlorhydria, hypovolemia, and dehydration (see Table 58.3). Patients with VIPoma commonly have 5 to 10 L of stool output per day and report abdominal cramping and flushing. Persistent hypokalemia causes a generalized weakness that may be severe, and patients may also have hypercalcemia. Approximately 85% to 90% of VIPomas arise within the pancreas, but extrapancreatic duodenal VIPomas have also been described.[24,83] Elevated serum levels of pancreatic polypeptide have been used to distinguish pancreatic VIPomas from extrapancreatic tumors.[82] In children, a ganglioneuroma or ganglioneuroblastoma may also produce the syndrome.[83] The diagnosis of VIPoma is made when fasting plasma levels of VIP are above 500 pg/mL in the presence of secretory diarrhea (Table 58.3).

Because of the severe dehydration and electrolyte abnormalities, it is necessary to correct these abnormalities before surgery. Before the use of octreotide, patients required large amounts of fluid, potassium, and chloride. Octreotide dramatically reduces serum VIP levels and secretory diarrhea in more than 80% of patients and greatly simplifies fluid and electrolyte resuscitation before surgery.[77,80] Although these tumors are malignant, surgery is often effective.

Somatostatinoma

Somatostatinomas, which were first described fully in 1977,[84] and are very rare malignant neuroendocrine tumors that arise in either the duodenum or pancreas. Pancreatic tumors are seen in about 50% of cases, and duodenal tumors may be associated with von Recklinghausen's disease. The somatostatinoma syndrome includes steatorrhea, cholelithiasis, diabetes mellitus type 2, and hypochlorhydria (see Table 58.3). The mean age at presentation is 52 years.[85] Some patients present with colicky abdominal pain secondary to the cholelithiasis, and somatostatinoma may be diagnosed incidentally at the time of cholecystectomy or during CT scanning of the abdomen for nonspecific complaints. Somatostatin-like activity can be measured by immunological assays and is the key to the diagnosis (Table 58.3). Most patients have unresectable metastatic tumor at the time of diagnosis.

Nonfunctioning Islet Cell Tumors

Nonfunctioning islet cell tumors or pancreatic polypeptide-producing tumors (PPomas) do not have a clinical syndrome related to the excessive hormone secretion.[5] These tumors are usually present during the fourth or fifth decade of life.[85] They are usually malignant and large at the time of clinical diagnosis and produce symptoms secondary to the mass effects of the tumor. Some patients with MEN 1 may undergo CT scanning for islet cell tumors because an elevated serum level of pancreatic polypeptide (PP) has been measured as a screening marker (Table 58.3). Large tumors may cause symptoms of extrahepatic bile duct obstruction, bleeding, or intestinal obstruction[5] (Table 58.3). Patients may also have hepatic metastases in association with large tumor volumes. Most of these tumors are resectable but often require pancreaticoduodenectomy (Whipple resection) or subtotal pancreatectomy.[86]

Rare Islet Cell Tumors

Islet cell tumors can produce a variety of unusual hormones, including growth hormone–releasing factor (GRF), adrenocorticotropic hormone (ACTH), parathyroid hormone-related peptide (PTH-RP), neurotensin, and serotonin. Islet cell tumors have been found to cause severe hypercalcemia secondary to parathyroid hormone-related peptide, Cushing's syndrome secondary to ectopic ACTH production, and acromegaly secondary to GRF production. Cushing's syndrome has been reported in a small number of ZES patients as the result of concomitant elaboration of ACTH.[87] Rarely, neurotensinomas, once regarded as nonfunctional tumors,[88] produce neurotensin that causes diarrhea, hypotension, flushing, and cyanosis.

Radiologic Localization of Rare Islet Cell Tumors

Radiologic localization of the less frequent islet cell tumors such as somatostatinoma, VIPoma, glucagonoma, PPoma, and nonfunctional tumors is relatively simple. In contrast to insulinomas or gastrinomas, virtually all these tumors are visible with current CT imaging. Some studies have demonstrated that MRI is better able to detect liver metastases than CT.[31] However, CT may be superior at imaging the primary tumor because CT images have clearer anatomic resolution than MR. Further, CT is less expensive than MRI. SRS should also be used for these patients to detect occult distant metastases and to determine if the tumor has functional somatostatin receptors.[40] Approximately 80% to 90% of these rare islet cell tumors image on octreoscan.[31,40,89] If an individual tumor can be detected by this modality, the hormonal syndrome will usually respond to octreotide. Some preliminary studies suggest that the long-term use of octreotide in patients with unresectable rare neuroendocrine tumors may prolong survival.[77]

TABLE 58.8. Medical and Preoperative Treatment Modalities for Neuroendocrine Tumors.

Tumor	*Treatment*
Insulinoma	Frequent small meals Cornstarch Diazoxide Verapamil Octreotide Propanolol Phenytoin
Gastrinoma	Omeprazole or lansoprazole H_2-receptor antagonists
Glucagonoma	Octreotide Total parenteral nutrition with added trace elements Diabetes control
VIPoma	Octreotide
Somatostatinoma	Octreotide Fluids Diabetes control
PTH-RPoma	Fluids Lasix Mitramycin Diphosphonates
ACTHoma	Ketoconazole Aminoglutethimide Mifepristone
GRFoma	Octreotide
Carcinoid	Octreotide

Treatment of Neuroendocrine Tumors

Insulinoma

Medical Management

Medical management is the initial treatment of patients diagnosed with insulinoma (Table 58.8). This approach allows for stabilization of symptoms and time to localize the tumor, if possible, and plan for surgical resection. Initial management includes dietary adjustment to include more frequent as well as nighttime meals. Cornstarch can be added to the diet at bedtime to slow the absorption of food from the intestines.[33,34] Diazoxide, an antihypertensive agent, can successfully suppress insulin secretion in approximately 60% of patients.[33,90] It appears to act through stimulation of islet cell α-adrenergic receptors and may have peripheral glycogenolytic effects by inhibition of cAMP phosphodiesterase.[27,33] Side effects, particularly nausea and sodium retention, may be problematical.[27,33] Treatment is usually started at a dose of 150 to 200 mg/day in divided doses to a maximum of 800 mg/day.[27,33] Because diazoxide has been associated with life-threatening hypotension on induction of anesthesia, it should be discontinued at least 7 days before the planned operation.[91] Calcium channel blockers such as verapamil may also function by reducing insulin secretion and may be of utility in selected patients who do not tolerate diazoxide.[92] Likewise, the β-adrenergic antagonist propanolol and the antiepilepsy drug phenytoin have also been used to control symptoms in a small number of patients, as have prednisone and glucagon.[27] Octreotide, the long-acting somatostatin analogue, in contrast to its lack of utility for localization of insulinomas, has been used extensively to treat infants with hypoglycemia caused by nesidioblastosis.[34] In adults, it can control symptoms of hypoglycemia in approximately 40% of patients and is generally well tolerated at a dose of 100 to 1500 μg/day administered subcutaneously in divided doses.[93,94] If it is effective, it can be converted to somatostatin-LAR 30 mg IM every 3 weeks. If medical management is successful in controlling symptoms, then the surgeon is under less pressure to find and remove the tumor. However, if the patient cannot tolerate drug therapy, the outcome of exploration is more critical. In this instance, a preoperative calcium angiogram can be used to locate the precise region of the pancreas that contains the tumor.

Surgical Management

Surgery is the only curative treatment for patients with an insulinoma.[21,28,45,95] Often, medical control of the hypoglycemia is unsatisfactory, placing more emphasis on a successful surgical outcome. The presence of MEN 1 should be excluded by testing for other components of the syndrome, which may include primary hyperparathyroidism, nephrolithiasis, and the presence of other endocrine or pituitary tumors.[23]

Enucleation is the preferred surgical treatment for insulinoma[49] because most tumors are solitary and benign. IOUS is critical during surgery for insulinoma as it facilitates both identification and removal of these tumors. Occasionally, the surgeon is unable to remove these tumors by enucleation because of the relationship to the pancreatic duct or other

TABLE 58.9.
Outcome of Surgical Management of Insulinoma and Gastrinoma and Survival After Gastrinoma Resection.

Reference	*Level of evidence*[a]	*n*	*With MEN (n)*	*With malignancy (n)*	*Tumor resected (%)*	*Cured (%)*	*Cured with malignancy (%)*	*Operative complications (%)*	*Mortality (%)*
Insulinoma									
Norton et al. (1990)[45]	II	23	0	0	92	92	N/A	17	0
Doherty et al. (1991)[95]	II	25	0	0	96	96	N/A	16	0
Lo et al. (1997)[32]	II	27	1	11	100	93	33	33	3.7
Boukhman et al. (1998)[21]	III	54	11	13	93	84	86	43	3.7
Gastrinoma									
MacFarlane et al. (1995)[103]	II	10	10	60	70	0	0	NR	0
McArthur et al. (1996)[63]	II	22	3	44	41	14	75	NR	0
Jaskowiak et al. (1996)[101]	II	17	2	94	100	29	31	11	6
Kisker et al. (1998)[71]	II	25	2	48	92	44	42	16	0
Norton et al. (1999)[54]	II	151	28	46	93	48	NR	NR	

Long-term survival			*5-year (localized disease) (%)*	*5-year (metastatic disease) (%)*	*10-year (overall) (%)*
Norton et al. (1988)[102]	II	73	95	95	NR
McArthur et al. (1996)[63]	II	22	100	75	81
Kisker et al. (1998)[71]	II	25	100	28	NR
Norton et al. (1999)[54]	II	151		40	34

[a]I, prospective, randomized; II, prospective; III, retrospective, review or anecdotal; NR, not reported.

vital structures. In this case, lesions are resected by either distal pancreatectomy or Whipple pancreaticoduodenectomy. Blind distal pancreatectomy, a procedure that was formerly recommended, is no longer indicated because studies have reported that occult tumors are usually found within the head of the pancreas, an area which is difficult to palpate but is relatively accessible to IOUS (see Fig. 58.2).[32,34,45] Many large series from different institutions have demonstrated that more than 90% of patients can have successful surgery and complete correction of the hypoglycemia[32,45,95] (Table 58.9). Further, because as much of the normal pancreatic architecture as possible is preserved, there is a low risk for the development of diabetes mellitus postoperatively. Patients with MEN 1 and insulinoma are treated in the same manner. In these patients, however, a dominant large islet cell tumor is usually identified and resected, leading to control of hypoglycemia. The complications of insulinoma excision are primarily those associated with pancreatic resection and include abscess, fistula, pseudocyst formation, or wound infection. Drainage of the pancreatic enzymes by closed-suction drains usually minimizes these complications.

Gastrinoma

Medical Management

Originally, total gastrectomy was the only procedure that effectively controlled gastric acid hypersecretion in patients with gastrinoma, but it is no longer necessary.[51,96] With the advent of histamine H_2-receptor antagonists and, more importantly, proton pump inhibitors, all patients can experience control of acid hypersecretion and complete relief of symptoms (see Table 58.8). Omeprazole and lansoprazole block gastric acid secretion by inhibiting the parietal cell apical H^+–K^--ATPase. The usual dose is 20 to 40mg twice daily.[51] H_2-receptor antagonists are also effective, but progressively higher doses may be required to control symptoms. They may be associated with a long-term failure rate, making proton pump inhibitors the current drugs of choice.

Measurement of BAO, following initiation of drug therapy, is necessary to adjust the dose of medication for effective medical treatment because relief of symptoms is not a reliable indicator of effective acid control.[51,96] To allow healing of ulceration and to prevent recurrences, gastric acid secretion should be maintained below 10mEq/h; it should be maintained below 5mEq/h if prior ulcer surgery has been performed[96] or in patients with reflux esophagitis and ZES.[51] Effective acid control reduces the need for esophageal dilatation in these patients.[51] However, with long-term medical control of ZES, there may exist associated risks. Animal studies originally raised the concern of gastric malignancy in the setting of long-term acid suppression,[97] and there have been cases of MEN 1 patients who have developed diffuse malignant gastric carcinoid tumors after prolonged treatment with omeprazole.[51] Therefore, periodic gastric surveillance endoscopy should be performed on all patients treated with proton pump inhibitors for long periods.

Surgical Management

Medical control of acid hypersecretion allows time for localization and surgical treatment of the gastrinoma and obviates the need for total gastrectomy.[51,96] Based on the results of a number of long-term studies, the malignant potential of the tumor itself is the main determinant of long-term survival.[55,98,99] Because of this, all patients with sporadic gastrinomas are candidates for tumor localization and surgery for attempted cure to prolong survival.[54] The management of patients with MEN 1 and ZES is controversial and more complex. In patients with the MEN 1 and primary hyperparathyroidism (HPT), the usual parathyroid pathology is multigland hyperplasia. It has been shown that successful neck exploration for resection of parathyroid hyperplasia can significantly lessen the end-organ effects of hypergastrinemia. Therefore, in patients with MEN 1 who have HPT in conjunction with ZES, neck exploration and subtotal or four-gland parathyroidectomy with autotransplantation should be performed before attempting gastrinoma resection[23] (Fig. 58.9). Overall, however, removal of pancreatic and duodenal tumors seldom cures patients of ZES[54,61] (see Table 58.9). It has been shown that resection of primary gastrinomas decreases the likelihood of liver metastases, which are the main determinant of survival in these patients.[52] Therefore, the goals of surgical management are resection of the primary tumor for potential cure and to prevent malignant progression. This latter goal is the same whether the patient has a sporadic gastrinoma or gastrinoma in the setting of the MEN 1 syndrome. The operative management of patients with MEN 1 and gastrinoma is complicated by the fact that the tumors tend to be multiple, small (4–6mm), and usually involve the duodenum[53,54] more often than the pancreas. In these patients, the controversy has centered on the fact that surgery is seldom curative yet it may be effective to decrease or prevent the development of liver metastases.[19,53]

We recommend surgery when the duodenal or pancreatic tumor is 2cm or larger on CT[51] because the risk of liver metastases increases with tumor size. Overall, 4% of patients with gastrinomas less than 1cm, 28% with tumors between 1 and 3cm, and 61% with tumors greater than 3cm have liver metastases.[51,52] After review of current data, it seems prudent to operate on MEN 1 patients with much smaller pancreatic and duodenal gastrinomas because resection may decrease the risk of developing hepatic metastases. In one study of 124 patients without evidence of hepatic metastases, 98 patients (15 with MEN 1) had primary gastrinomas resected while 26 patients (9 with MEN 1) refused surgery and were managed medically. After a mean follow-up of 8.5 years, hepatic metastases were detected in 23% of the patients who had been managed medically and 3% of the patients who had undergone surgery.[100] Thus, surgical resection of the primary gastrinoma significantly reduced the probability of liver metastases.

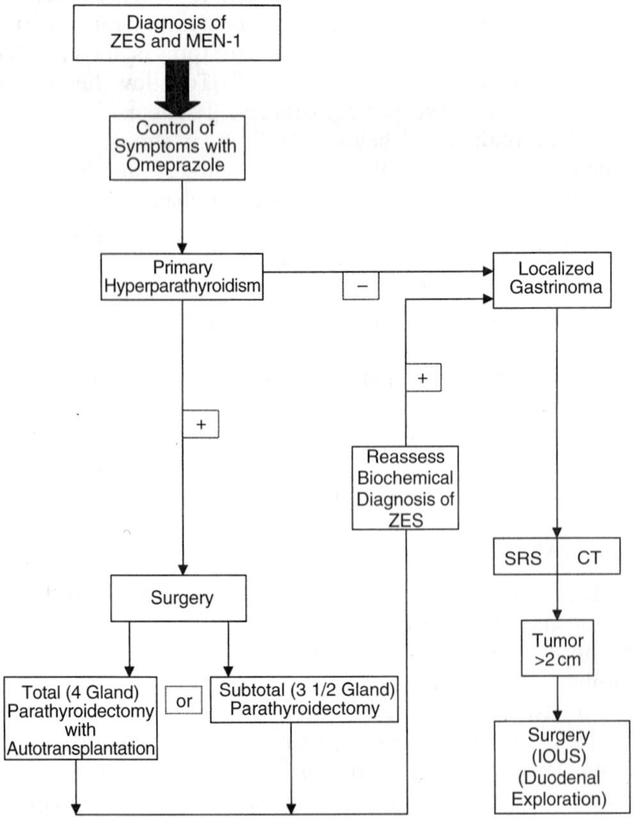

FIGURE 58.9. Flow diagram for the management of ZES in the setting of multiple endocrine neoplasia (MEN 1).

At surgery, a tumor is found in approximately 78% of sporadic gastrinoma patients, and 14% to 58% of patients are cured immediately following resection.[19,73] The long-term cure rate, with surgery, is 34% to 81% depending on the series (see Table 58.9). Surgery is also effective treatment for localized metastatic gastrinoma, as it appears to prolong survival and cures approximately one-third of patients.[101,102] In patients with MEN 1 and gastrinoma, the identification of all tumor foci is imprecise, and surgery results in a significantly lower cure rate.[54,103] Paradoxically, although patients with gastrinoma and MEN 1 may present earlier, have multiple small extrapancreatic islet cell tumors, and may undergo abdominal exploration without surgical cure, there is evidence that they will develop liver metastases at a lesser rate following surgery for resection of tumor. This finding suggests that the tumor biology of gastrinomas found in MEN 1 patients is similar to that found in sporadic patients.

In patients with ZES, the development of intraoperative imaging techniques has greatly facilitated tumor identification and resection; this is particularly true for small duodenal tumors that are difficult to locate. With improvement in intraoperative localization methods such as ultrasound and endoscopy with transillumination and duodenotomy, as well as increased awareness of duodenal tumors, some studies have reported that gastrinomas can be found and resected in nearly 100% of patients with MEN 1 and ZES.[54] In a series of 143 patients, undergoing routine duodenotomy in ZES was associated with increased short- and long-term cure rates.[104] In addition, the experience of the surgeon appears to be another factor in achieving a good surgical outcome.[11]

In general, in MEN 1 patients, if tumors are clearly imaged on preoperative studies, laparotomy is indicated. In sporadic patients with ZES who have no clearly imaged disease, laparotomy is still indicated as recent series suggest that tumors will still be found in nearly all patients.[51] In this instance, the gastrinoma is invariably located in the duodenum.[51,54] All regional lymph nodes should be removed for histological examination. Enucleation of pancreatic head tumors is usually sufficient, whereas distal or even subtotal pancreatectomy may be necessary for tumors of the body and tail. A careful examination of the duodenum is critical in all patients with ZES, as occult tumors are nearly always located here.

Other Islet Cell Tumors

Medical Management

Medical therapy may be used to control the signs and symptoms of excessive hormonal secretion, but it will seldom control the tumoral process (see Table 58.8). Medical therapy is not curative, but at best it can provide symptomatic relief, although it is not effective as an antitumor treatment and will not prolong survival.[5,77] Glucagonoma patients often need intense medical management before surgery. They have severe malnutrition, hypoaminoacidemia, and type 2 diabetes mellitus, which can be corrected by total (glucose, fat, and amino acids) parenteral nutrition with added trace elements (particularly zinc) and insulin. Octreotide may also be of benefit in alleviating symptoms.[77] Interestingly, we have previously demonstrated that correction of the hypoaminoacidemia with total parental nutrition corrects the NME rash.[3] Because of the risk of deep venous thrombosis and pulmonary embolism, vena cava interruption filter placement after anticoagulation with heparin is often recommended.

Somatostatinoma patients invariably develop symptomatic cholelithiasis, and cholecystectomy is recommended as part of the overall treatment. Cholycystectomy is also indicated for any patient requiring long-term treatment with octreotide. Diabetes control with insulin and proper hydration is also important. In these patients, octreotide has been reported to show objective response in up to 11% of individuals.[94] Similarly, VIPoma patients usually have severe dehydration and electrolyte abnormalities that must be corrected before surgery. Large amounts of intravenous fluid, with potassium supplementation, were necessary in the past and most patients responded poorly. Currently, octreotide effectively controls the secretion of VIP in nearly every patient, and the management of fluid and electrolytes has been dramatically simplified.[77,80]

Severe hypercalcemia secondary to PTH-RP-producing neuroendocrine tumors must be controlled by the use of intravenous saline solution, lasix, mithramycin, and diphosphonates (Table 58.8). Cushing's syndrome, caused by ectopic ACTH-producing islet cell tumors, should be controlled by agents such as ketoconazole, aminoglutethimide, and mifepristone (RU 486). Octreotide has largely been ineffective for the treatment of ectopic ACTH secretion.[77] Medical control of the severe hypercortisolism is often inadequate, and patients usually require bilateral adrenalectomy if complete resection of the ACTH-producing islet cell tumor is not possible.[105] Serotonin-producing islet cell tumors require octreotide as a premedication at the time of surgery to prevent a life-threatening carcinoid crisis while under anaesthesia.[106]

Surgical Management

Overall, surgical resection is the only potentially curative therapy for patients with islet cell tumors.[5,24] However, surgical therapy is dependent on a variety of factors including the type of tumor, extent of disease, presence of MEN 1, and ability to control hormonal symptoms medically, as well as the overall operative risk of the patient. In general, surgery is indicated for all patients with islet cell tumors in whom all tumors can be imaged and removed with acceptable morbidity and mortality. This procedure is necessary because, despite considerable variability, any type of neuroendocrine tumor can be malignant. Debulking surgery may also be indicated in any patient with a large tumor burden or metastatic disease in whom medical treatment does not control hormonal symptoms.[8] Similarly, other procedures such as bilateral adrenalectomy may be indicated because of the inability to effectively treat symptoms.[105]

In patients with MEN 1 and concomitant neuroendocrine tumors, resection should be pursued if the tumors are larger than 2 cm because size correlates with increased malignant potential. Further, MEN 1 patients should undergo surgery in an attempt to control the signs and symptoms of excessive hormone secretion by an islet cell tumor. The major consideration in dealing with the tumors found in the setting of MEN 1 is that these tumors are usually multiple and it may be unclear which exact tumor is responsible for the excessive hormone production.[20] However, most patients have a large dominant tumor that may be responsible for most, if not all, the symptoms.[49] These tumors, with the exception of gastrinomas, are usually radiologically apparent. Therefore, in MEN 1 patients, surgery should be attempted for all large pancreatic islet cell tumors that are detected by conventional studies.

The rare pancreatic islet cell tumors are generally easily identified on preoperative CT. Once identified, the tumor and its metastases, if present, are resected by either pancreaticoduodenectomy or subtotal pancreatectomy-splenectomy, depending on the location to remove the largest identifiable tumor.[49] Secondary liver metastases are removed, either by multiple wedge resections or lobectomy, depending on the size and location of the metastasis. Resection of both pancreatic and hepatic disease is indicated if the operative procedure planned can remove all gross disease, again, with acceptable mortality and morbidity.[24] Resection of all identifiable tumor appears to improve survival and may even produce biochemical cure in a subset of patients. It is important to remember that, even with liver metastases, patients still have, on average, a long-term (10-year) survival of more than 20%.

Surgery is also an important therapeutic option in ameliorating the signs and symptoms of excessive hormone secretion in patients who do not respond adequately to optimal medical management; this is particularly true in patients with VIPoma and glucagonoma who fail to respond to octreotide or patients with metastatic insulinoma who do not respond to octreotide, verapamil, diazoxide, or frequent feedings. Reduction of tumor mass reduces the circulating concentrations of hormones and subsequently reduces intensity and severity of symptoms,[49] as well as the dosage of medications necessary to achieve symptomatic control. In the case of an ACTH-secreting islet cell tumor, surgical resection of the target organs may substantially improve the quality and duration of life. Surgery may also be indicated in nonfunctional islet cell tumors that develop serious or life-threatening symptoms such as gastrointestinal hemorrhage and biliary or intestinal obstruction. In these instances, the tumor may either be resected or bypassed to relieve the symptoms.

Metastatic Disease

Malignant Insulinoma

Surgery in patients with malignant insulinoma may still be curative, but this is only accomplished if all tumor can be completely removed.[49,107] Depending on the tumor location, either Whipple pancreaticoduodenectomy or subtotal pancreatectomy with splenectomy may be necessary. Multiple wedge resections, radiofrequency ablation, or lobectomy can then be used to treat secondary liver metastases. Resection of all identifiable tumors appears to improve survival and may even cure a subset of patients. Another indication for debulking surgery or radiofrequency ablation in combination with debulking is to lessen the signs and symptoms of hypoglycemia, especially in patients who do not respond adequately to medical management with octreotide, verapamil, diazoxide, or frequent feedings. Aggressive surgery may also be indicated in instances in which the tumor causes gastrointestinal hemorrhage or biliary or intestinal obstruction.

Chemotherapy for metastatic insulinoma has been largely ineffective. Single-agent therapy is based on streptozotocin with combination therapy of streptozotocin plus 5-fluorouracil or streptozotocin plus doxorubicin, producing transient responses in 45% and 69% of patients, respectively,[108] with no complete responses identified; thus, this may translate into a minimal (1- to 2-year) survival advantage for responders.[108] Chemoembolization, a combination of simultaneous hepatic artery occlusion and chemotherapy, has had some significant antitumor responses and may also be used to ameliorate symptoms.[109] Using this approach, symptoms and hormone levels have improved in nearly every patient. However, side effects and complications may occur, including life-threatening liver abscesses. Alcohol injection, radiofrequency ablation, and cryotherapy have also been used in the treatment of metastatic insulinoma without clear benefit.

Malignant Gastrinoma

With successful control of gastric acid hypersecretion and the indolent growth pattern of the gastrinoma, distant metastatic disease becomes the most important determinant of mortality. In the past, about 60% of patients had metastatic disease, but with current biochemical testing and workup, only between 25% and 33% of patients now have metastasis at the time of diagnosis.[52] The 5-year survival for patients with metastatic disease is, on average, approximately 40%.[51] In addition, 20% of these patients experience accelerated tumor growth, which ultimately results in more rapid demise. Although the exact mechanism underlying this more aggressive tumor behavior has yet to be understood, it is associated with high serum levels of gastrin, tumor production of multiple hormones (especially ACTH), and the presence of bilobar liver or bone metastases.[98] It has been suggested that gastrinomas in patients with the MEN 1 syndrome appear to behave less aggressively than those found in patients with sporadic disease, although both have an equal rate of lymph node metastasis.[103] Duodenal gastrinomas have a similar rate of lymph node metastases but a lower rate of liver metastases than pancreatic tumors.

Chemotherapy has been utilized in the treatment of metastatic gastrinomas but does not prolong survival. A combination of doxorubicin, 5-fluorouracil, and streptozotocin provides a 40% partial response rate but no survival benefit or complete responses.[110] Similarly, hepatic artery chemoembolization has minimal, and transient, efficacy and the use of octreotide or alpha-interferon as antitumor agents has also shown little effect on the malignant process.[111]

Surgery remains the major effective treatment for metastatic gastrinoma. Originally, Zollinger and associates reported good results in the postoperative course of a series of selected patients who had undergone resection of metastatic disease, including those with liver metastases.[112] Patients with localized lymph node metastases seem to benefit most from surgery, with up to 30% showing biochemical cure,[51] whereas patients with resected localized metastatic liver disease have on average an 85% 5-year survival[63,99,101] (see Table 58.9). Aggressive surgery in appropriate patients with hepatic metastases seems to demonstrate a survival advantage. In one study in which 17 patients underwent resection of hepatic metastases, there was a 79% 5-year survival. In contrast to this, a similar group of 25 patients with unresectable hepatic disease had a 28% 5-year survival.[113] Although studies are ongoing, it appears that, even in those patients with unresectable disease, hepatic cryosurgery or radiofrequency ablation may serve to reduce symptoms and prolong survival.

Other Islet Cell Tumors

Chemotherapy has been used in the treatment of metastatic islet cell tumors, with 40% partial but few documented complete responses.[110] Again, the usual agents include doxorubicin, 5-fluorouracil, and streptozotocin. These drugs have been used individually and in combination, with the combination therapy providing more responses. One recent study found that the combination of decarbazine, 5-fluorouracil, and leucovorin produced objective response in 44% of patients with neuroendocrine tumors.[114] In Sweden, α-interferon has had similar response rates in patients who have failed chemotherapy.[115] Recent studies have investigated the use of long-acting analogues of somatostatin as antitumor agents to slow tumor growth and metastatic rate. These hormonal therapies appear to be effective in controlling medical signs and symptoms of hormonal excess and are indicated for that purpose, but the antitumor effects are less clear.

Recently, chemoembolization, with simultaneous hepatic artery occlusion and doxorubicin infusion, has had dramatic antitumor responses in individuals with large hepatic tumor volumes.[109] Symptoms have improved in nearly every patient, and hormonal levels have significantly decreased in approximately 80% of individuals, suggesting that this may have a real benefit in those with a significant disease burden. However, side effects have been reported, and complications may occur. Intralesional alcohol injection and cryotherapy have been also been used in a few patients without clear benefit.

Surgical Techniques

Enucleation of Insulinoma

Because insulinomas are usually benign, small, and uniformly distributed throughout the pancreas, the goal of surgery is precise localization of tumor and excision with preservation of normal pancreas and spleen. At the time of surgery, the pancreas is fully exposed to allow complete palpation and inspection of the gland (Fig. 58.10). After dividing the gastro-

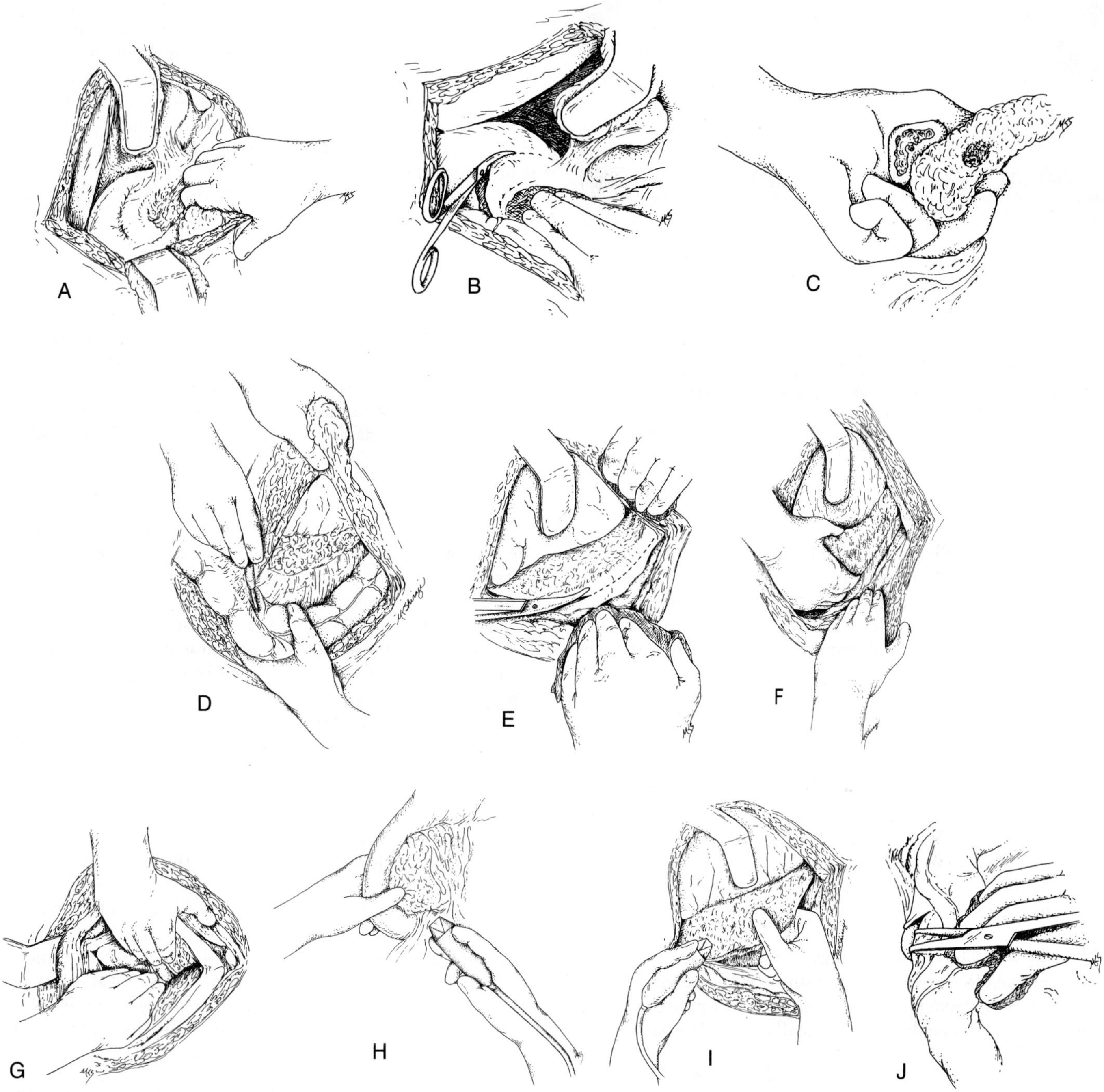

FIGURE 58.10. Surgical approach for the resection of an insulinoma or other neuroendocrine tumor. In the obese patient (not uncommon in the case of an insulinoma), a bilateral subcostal incision may be necessary. Otherwise, a generous upper midline incision may be preferred. The abdomen is then entered and carefully explored. Next (**A**), the head and neck of the pancreas are exposed anteriorly by reflecting the omentum and hepatic flexure of the colon to the left. The lateral peritoneal attachments of the duodenum are then incised (**B**), and the duodenum is freed from the underlying aorta and vena cava by blunt and sharp dissection (Kocher maneuver). It should now be possible to palpate the duodenum, as well as the head and uncinate process of the pancreas, between fingers and thumb as shown in **C**. The *dark area* within the pancreas shown in **C** represents a small insulinoma. If the uncinate process is still poorly palpated, complete mobilization of the right colon medially (Cattell maneuver) should allow for complete palpation. Next, the body and tail of the pancreas are exposed by first dividing the gastrocolic ligament (**D**), and the peritoneum along the inferior border of the body and tail of the pancreas is then incised (**E**). Once the peritoneum is divided, the areolar tissue deep to the pancreas may be opened by blunt dissection (**F**), until the whole gland is mobilized from its retroperitoneal attachments (**G**); this allows for a complete palpation and ultrasound examination of the head (**H**), as well as the body and tail of the gland (**I**), using the ultrasound transducer. After a complete ultrasound and manual examination, the tumor is located and enucleated (**J**), in this case from the posterior aspect of the head of the pancreas.

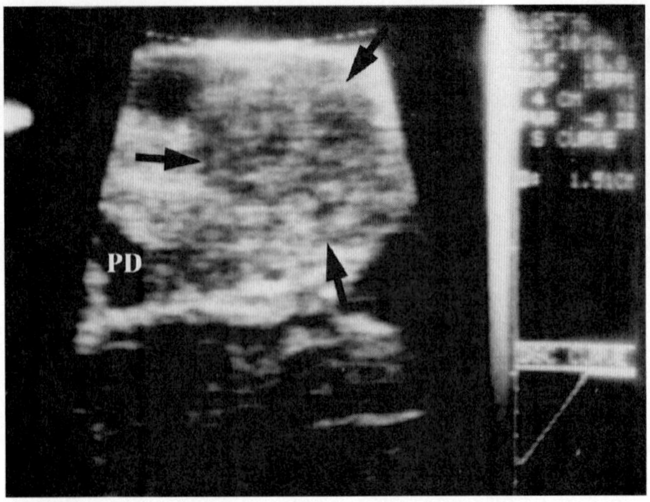

FIGURE 58.11. Intraoperative ultrasound (IOUS) shows the echogenic characteristics of a 2-cm gastrinoma within the head of the pancreas (*arrows*). *PD*, pancreatic duct.

colic ligament, a wide extended Kocher maneuver is performed that includes mobilization of the right colon. In some instances, the lateral peritoneal attachments of the spleen are divided to elevate the spleen and the tail of the pancreas to facilitate identification of any small tumor that may be located within the tail. The peritoneum along the inferior border of the gland is incised to allow palpation between the thumb and forefinger. At this stage, IOUS is performed with a high-resolution real-time transducer (7.5–10 MHz). Doppler flow capabilities allow for more accurate discrimination between the tumor, ducts, arteries, and veins. Insulinomas appear sonolucent compared to the more echo-dense normal pancreas (Fig. 58.11). Masses or tumors are always imaged in two directions to visualize their three-dimensional extent. Further, IOUS can be used to precisely identify the relationships of the tumor to other vital structures such as the pancreatic duct, bile duct, arteries, and veins to allow safe excision. IOUS has been useful in facilitating the enucleation of nonpalpable insulinomas within the pancreatic head. Recent reports have also suggested that insulinoma resection can be accomplished laparoscopically.[116,117] The surgeon is positioned between the legs of the patient as is done for a Nissen fundoplication. The pancreas is exposed using the harmonic scalpel to divide the gastrocolic ligament. Laparoscopic ultrasound is then performed and used to localize the tumor, which is enucleated using ultrasound for guidance. The procedure is performed in an identical fashion to the open procedure, and formal laparotomy should be done if the tumor is not identified.

Duodenotomy for Gastrinoma

During surgery for a gastrinoma, it is important to remember that these tumors can occur in extrapancreatic locations, particularly the duodenum. The operation itself requires a careful exploration of the abdomen and its contents, as has been previously described.[24,72] It is important to explore and palpate the liver, stomach, small bowel, and mesentery as well as the pancreas and pelvis. The uterus, fallopian tubes, and ovaries should be inspected and palpated in female patients. Again, an extended Kocher maneuver should be performed to mobilize the duodenum and pancreatic head. The pancreatic body and tail may be better visualized by opening the gastrocolic ligament and dividing along the inferior border of the pancreas. Once this has been accomplished, the duodenum and pancreas can be fully palpated and examined by IOUS (Fig. 58.12). IOUS should also be used to image the liver. A 7.5- to 10-mHz near-field transducer is necessary for studying the pancreas, whereas the 2.5- to 5-mHz wide-angle transducer is best for the liver. Tumors appear sonolucent and should be imaged in two dimensions. The duodenum can then be palpated between thumb and forefinger for the presence of mass lesions (Fig. 58.12). IOE with duodenal transillumination may also be performed. A duodenal gastrinoma appears as a photopaque mass lesion within the wall of the duodenum upon transillumination (see Fig. 58.7). The endoscopist may occasionally also visualize the tumor as a raised mucosal defect (Fig. 58.13).

Once duodenal lesions are identified, they can be marked with suture and included within the confines of a modest longitudinal duodenotomy (Fig. 58.14). It should be remembered that, regardless of the results of IOUS or IOE, a duodenotomy is indicated in all cases. This procedure allows for visualization as well as a more careful palpation of the entire

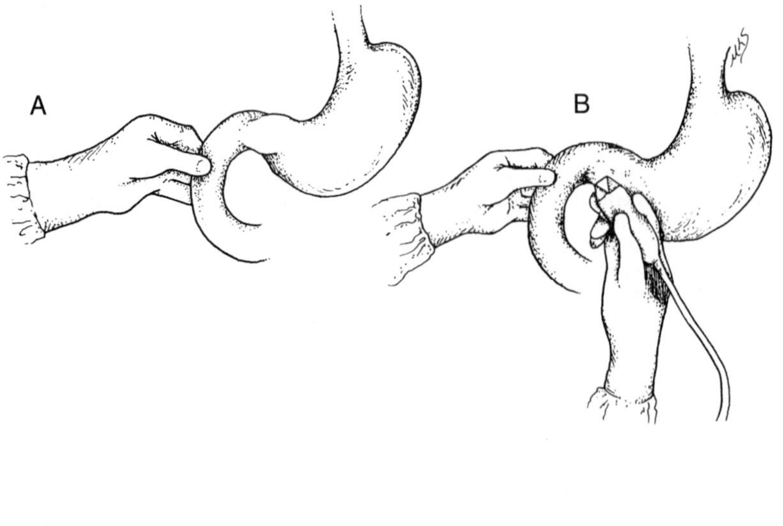

FIGURE 58.12. Palpation of the duodenum between thumb and forefinger (**A**) and use of ultrasound (**B**) in attempting to locate a duodenal gastrinoma intraoperatively.

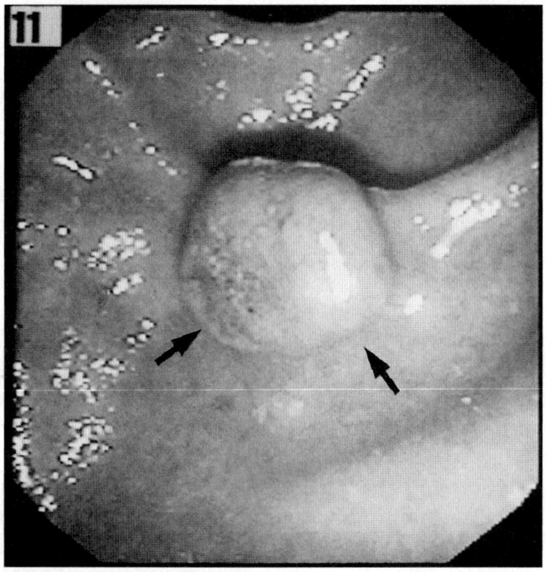

FIGURE 58.13. Endoscopic view of a duodenal gastrinoma, here seen as a submucosal mass (*arrows*).

duodenal wall, particularly its medial portion. Starting the incision at the junction between the first and second parts of the duodenum allows examination of an area where a large proportion of duodenal gastrinomas have been found (Fig. 58.15). Suspicious nodules on the medial wall should not be excised until a catheter is passed through the ampulla of Vater to mark its location. On occasion, this may have to be accomplished by passing the catheter through the common bile duct and into the duodenum. Finally, the duodenum is closed transversely in two layers to minimize the risk of leakage or obstruction (Fig. 58.16). If a long duodenotomy is necessary, longitudinal closure is indicated. Peripancreatic, bile duct, and celiac axis lymph nodes should also be excised for histological review. Reoperation for recurrent localized gastrinoma is also indicated if the tumor is imageable and the patient is a suitable candidate for surgery. Reoperation can result in elimination of all tumor in nearly every patient and complete remission in 30%.[110]

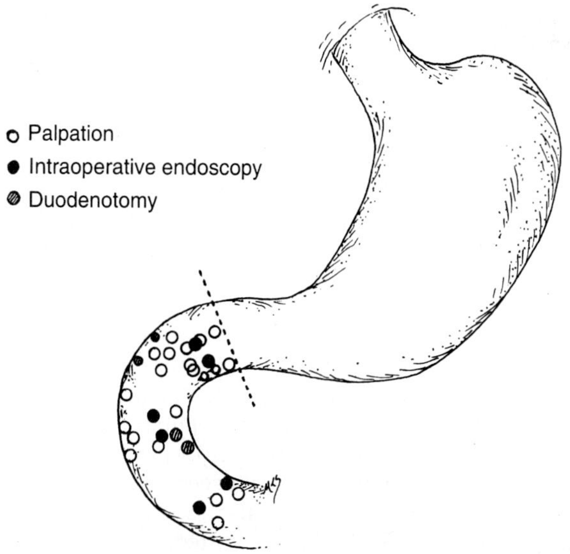

FIGURE 58.15. Illustration of the location of a series of duodenal gastrinomas as determined by palpation (*open circles*), intraoperative endoscopy (*solid circles*), or duodenotomy (*shaded circles*). Most lesions were located in the first or second portion of the duodenum with a surprising number located just beyond the distal border of the pylorus (*dotted line*), highlighting the need for beginning a duodenotomy incision in this region to allow for proper palpation and examination of this area. Also, note that the tumors found by duodenotomy were located on the medial wall of the duodenum.

Carcinoid Disease

Carcinoid tumors are derived from neoplastic outgrowth of certain cells of the diffuse neuroendocrine system[2] and continue to be regarded by some as an enigmatic and controversial tumor.[118] The term *carcinoid* was first coined by Oberndorfer in 1907[119] to describe the atypical pathological features of a tumor that was first identified by Ranson, more than a decade earlier, as a carcinoma of the ileum.[120] The origin of these carcinoma-like cells was not elucidated until 1928 when Masson identified a carcinoid originating from the chromaffin cells at the base of the crypts of Lieberkuhn in a specimen of appendix.[121] He found that the carcinoid cells took up and reduced silver and termed them argentaffin cell tumors, after the histochemical reaction that now bears his name. However, it was not until the early 1950s that Lembech first described the presence of serotonin

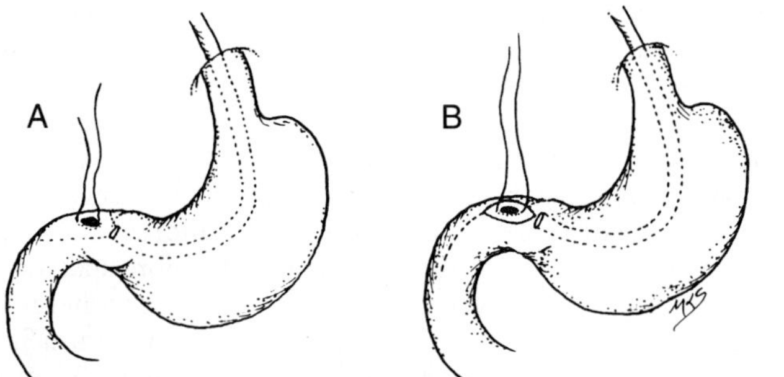

FIGURE 58.14. Illustration of how intraoperative endoscopy allows for the transillumination of a duodenal wall gastrinoma. Once located, a suture may be placed around the tumor to mark it (**A**) and the lesion removed by inclusion in the duodenotomy incision (**B**).

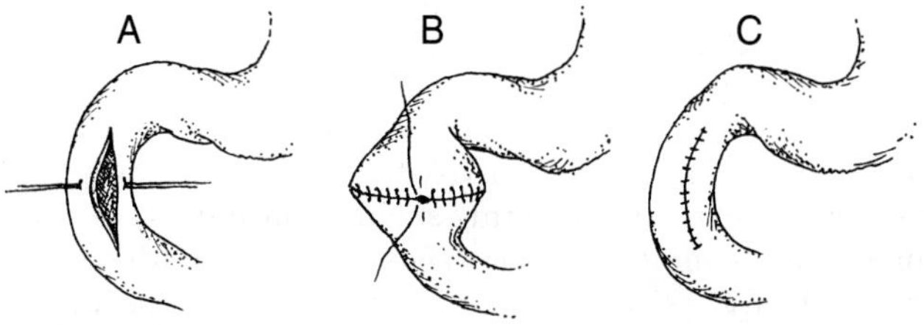

FIGURE 58.16. Illustration of the closure of a duodenotomy after examination and palpation for the presence of a duodenal gastrinoma. The duodenotomy (**A**), which is usually started at the junction of the first and second portion of the duodenum, is normally closed transversely (**B**) in two layers to minimize the risk of leakage or narrowing. In the case of a long duodenotomy, it may be necessary to close the incision longitudinally (**C**).

(5-hydroxytryptamine, 5-HT) in carcinoid cells[122] and Page detected increased levels of the serotonin metabolite 5-hydroxyindoleacetic acid (5-HIAA) in the urine of patients with carcinoid syndrome.[123]

Epidemiology

The exact incidence of carcinoid disease is unknown because it differs considerably in different populations and with different study types. This variation probably reflects the presence of subclinical disease, which is supported by autopsy studies, as well as the different occurrence rates at distinct anatomical sites and in different age groups and populations (see Table 58.1). Overall, the estimated incidence is thought to be 1.5 per 100,000 of the general population.[124] In Europe, the incidence is approximately 0.7 to 0.9 per 100,000 population,[125–127] with even higher incidence seen in certain regions.[128] The incidence in Scandinavia is also reported to be approximately 0.7 per 100,000.[129] In the United States, others have reported an incidence of 0.28 per 100,000 population for intestinal carcinoids.[130]

Autopsy studies have suggested a higher incidence of carcinoid tumors in the general population. Data from the Mayo Clinic have reported the incidence of carcinoids to be 65 per 100,000 cases.[131,132] The majority of these tumors were found in the appendix and small intestine. Based on these data, approximately 1 in every 200 to 300 resected appendiceal specimens contains a carcinoid tumor.[131–133] Others have reported a lower incidence of 2.1 per 100,000 cases per year.[134]

The incidence of carcinoid disease also seems to vary with regard to age and gender. The age of patients ranges from 8 to 93 years,[127,135–138] with a mean age at presentation of 55 to 60 years in different study groups.[127,136–138] Interestingly, a lower incidence is reported in younger age groups, particularly males,[135,136] and tumors at certain anatomic sites, such as the rectum, may also present at a younger age.[139] The incidence in women seems to be, overall, slightly higher than in men, with an incidence of 0.8 to 0.9 per 100,000 population in certain groups.[125] This same study also found that, for women aged 15 to 19, the female-to-male ratio was as high as 7:1. Others report a significant incidence of carcinoid tumors in girls under the age of 15,[135] whereas the incidence is similar in women and men beyond age 15.[125]

Classification and Tumor Characteristics

Carcinoid tumors are derived from chromaffin or Kulchitsky cells,[121] which are ubiquitous throughout the gastrointestinal and urogenital tract as well as the bronchial epithelium.[140,141] This finding explains the occurrence of carcinoids in a wide range of anatomic sites. Embryologically, their origin is in the endoderm and neuroectoderm,[1] and they are capable of taking up aromatic amines or their precursors and decarboxylating them, thus classifying them as *apudomas*. As such, they share cytochemical and histological features with other neuroendocrine tumors as well as with pheochromocytomas, medullary carcinomas of the thyroid, and melanomas.[3] Because of their close similarities to the endocrine tumors of the pancreas, some authors have proposed naming carcinoids neuroendocrine tumors to facilitate better classification of this diverse neoplasm.[2,142]

Carcinoid tumors may be classified along histological, cytochemical, and anatomic lines. Each classification system, by itself, is imprecise, and pathologists and surgeons must rely on a composite of information in correctly identifying a carcinoid tumor.[2,6] More importantly, malignancy cannot be identified on the basis of histology or cytochemical findings alone and, as with other neuroendocrine tumors, remains a clinical diagnosis after the finding of lymph node or distant metastases.

From a histological standpoint, carcinoid tumors generally cannot be differentiated from other neuroendocrine tumors when viewed under the light microscope with the usual stains. They are composed of homogeneous sheets of small round cells with uniform cytoplasm and nuclei and rare mitotic figures.[4,6,143] An experienced pathologist may be able to tentatively identify the tumor as a carcinoid, but true identification and characterization relies on histological and cytochemical staining patterns of intracellular reactions, secreted products, and intracellular proteins.[4,6] The original, and still most important, stain is that of the cell's reaction with silver salts.[2,121,143] Characteristically, carcinoid tumors may take up and reduce silver salts (argentaffin reaction of Masson) or may take up, but not reduce, silver unless exogenous reducing substances are added (argyrophilic reaction). This argentaffin or argyrophilic staining pattern is seen in carcinoids, generally, as a function of anatomic location[6] and serotonin content.[144] The histochemical diagnosis of the tumor may be complemented by the use of monoclonal antibodies to serotonin.[4,6] Some authors have recognized certain histological and histochemical characteristics of carcinoid tumors and have proposed classifying the tumor on the basis of these findings.[4,6,142,145] Under this classification system, carcinoid tumors may be grouped according to specific growth patterns into nodular, trabecular, glandular, undifferentiated, or mixed. Further, some authors have proposed that these different histological types may have different prognosis for survival, with a mixed histology showing the longest median survival (4.4 years) and an undifferentiated histology showing the least (0.5 years).[146]

Ultrastructurally, it is now recognized that the cells of carcinoid tumors contain numerous dense secretory granules of 80 to 200 nm or larger,[2] all of which contain active products synthesized by the cell. These granules, and other organelles, have been shown to contain a wide range of substances including 5-hydroxytryptamine, 5-hydroxytryptophan (5-HTP), chromogranin A and C, neuron-specific enolase, and synaptophysin as well as other peptides such as growth hormone, growth hormone-releasing hormone, gastrin, calcitonin, substance P, insulin, neurotensin, and various tachykinins as well as growth factors.[2,4,6,147] Recently, cytochemical localization of chromogranin A, neuron-specific enolase, and synaptophysin has been used to further identify and classify carcinoids, particularly with regard to anatomic regions.[2,4,146,148] Chromogranin A, in particular, seems to be more specific for carcinoids than the silver stains because it detects other intracellular proteins.[6,147] Chromogranin A levels in serum have also been useful as a marker for carcinoid tumors. They are elevated in approximately 90% of patients. The level correlates with extent of tumor burden. However, neuron-specific enolase is present in the cytoplasm of most neuroendocrine cells and may be detected in the cells of other neoplasms such as fibroadenomas of the breast or certain lymphomas.[2,6]

In the early 1960s, Williams and Sandler proposed a classification system based on the carcinoid tumor anatomic site of origin.[149] This system proposed that tumors be classified into foregut (including respiratory tract and thymus), midgut, and hindgut carcinoids. This classification has become useful to the pathologist and surgeon, particularly in light of recent advances in histocytochemistry, because carcinoid tumors from these areas show differences in histology, cytochemistry, secretory products, and clinical manifestations. Foregut carcinoids are derived from the respiratory tract, stomach, proximal duodenum, and pancreas. They are generally argentaffin-negative but argyrophilic, and contain low levels of 5-HT and small cytoplasmic granules (180nm). They occasionally secrete 5-HTP or ACTH and other hormones, are associated with an atypical carcinoid syndrome, and have the potential to metastasize to bone.[149] In addition, thymic carcinoids may be associated with the MEN 1 syndrome.[150] Midgut carcinoids (jejunum, ileum, and right colon) are argentaffin-positive, have a high 5-HT content, and larger (230-nm) cytoplasmic granules. They rarely secrete 5-HTP or ACTH but do release 5-HT and tachykinins and do cause the classic carcinoid syndrome with metastasis. They rarely metastasize to bone.[149]

Hindgut (transverse colon, left colon, and anorectum) carcinoid tumors form another distinct group. These tumors are described as being argentaffin negative, but often argyrophilic, rarely contain 5-HT, and possess round (190-nm) cytoplasmic granules of variable density. They hardly ever secrete 5-HTP or ACTH, but can contain numerous gastrointestinal hormones and rarely cause a classic carcinoid syndrome. Similar to midgut carcinoids, they rarely metastasize to bone.[149] Foregut carcinoids frequently display a mixed growth pattern, whereas midgut carcinoids display the most typical morphology of insular or glandular tumor cells. Hindgut carcinoid tumors usually show a solid or trabecular histology.[4,6,143,145] Recently, others have proposed an updated classification system, incorporating both histological and clinical data such as tumor size, local invasion, or presence of metastasis.[142]

Tumor Biology

The exact factors involved in carcinoid tumorigenesis are largely unknown, although some suggestions have been made. Molecular mechanisms involving mutations or alterations in proto-oncogenes or tumor suppressor genes have been investigated using a transgenic mouse model.[151] In these studies, activation of the nuclear oncogenes n-*myc* and c-*jun* were correlated with the development of bowel carcinoids. Similarly, studies of bronchial carcinoids have detected a high level of the proto-oncogenes c-*fos*, c-*jun*, c-*met*, and c-*myc* in tumors.[152] The HER-2/*neu* proto-oncogene has also been reported to be overexpressed in a proportion of carcinoid tumors.[153] Putative tumor suppressor genes have been mapped to chromosome 9 and 16 in mice,[154] but p53 gene mutations, or overexpression of p53 protein, have not been implicated in the development of carcinoid tumors in humans.[155–157] Some investigators have suggested that conditions promoting elevated gastrin levels and achlorhydria (see Table 58.7) also promote gastric carcinoid development[158] and that those patients with MEN 1 and ZES are at higher risk for the development of these tumors.[159–161] These observations appear to have some clinical validity.

Although diverse in their site of origin, most carcinoid tumors are found in the jejunoileum, appendix, bronchus, rectum, and stomach although carcinoids of the larynx, thymus, ovary, testis, urethra, and gallbladder have also been described or reviewed.[162–167] Tumors at each of these sites present different biochemical profiles, clinical behavior, and malignant potential. As a general rule, carcinoids synthesize, store, and secrete a wide range of substances,[2,4,6,147] which tends to complicate classification and diagnosis as well as treatment.[148] The presence of the classic carcinoid syndrome, the clinical manifestation of carcinoid disease, is directly related to tumor size, secretion of products into the systemic circulation, and presence of metastases.[132,168]

Carcinoid tumors are generally slow-growing neoplasms, and clinical manifestation of the disease tends to increase with tumor size and metastatic behavior.[132,168] However, not all carcinoid tumors possess the same potential to metastasize and produce symptoms. The most frequent site of occurrence is the appendix, where up to 40% of tumors are found[169]; these are usually small and frequently asymptomatic. Appendiceal carcinoids are usually benign. The next most common sites are the small intestine, rectum, and bronchus.[169] Small intestine carcinoids, especially those in the jejunoileum, seem to manifest the most aggressive clinical behavior.[131,132,137] They may be multiple; 87% are present in the ileum and, although generally small, up to 35% metastasize to regional lymph nodes and liver.[132,169] Because of this, one report found that they account for up to 87% of cases of the carcinoid syndrome, primarily by metastases to liver, whereas foregut and hindgut tumors account for up to 1% and 8%, respectively.[170] Occasionally midgut carcinoids with retroperitoneal invasion, ovarian and testicular carcinoids, or carcinoids of the lung, pancreas, and stomach cause the carcinoid syndrome after gaining access to systemic circulation, sometimes without local extension.[168,171] Foregut carcinoids, particularly those of the stomach and duodenum, are usually found on endoscopy,[172,173] although anemia may be an associated finding.[161] Occasionally, cough, hemoptysis, and recurrent respiratory tract infections are associated symptoms.[141] These carcinoids, in contrast to those found at other sites, may be more likely to produce a variety of enteropeptides as well as the usual amine derivatives. In addition, some authors have proposed three different subtypes of gastric carcinoids based on their review of 191 tumors.[174] Two of these subtypes were associated with a hypergastrinemic state and manifested different pathological behavior than the 27 other cases with no specific association. Other authors report that gastric carcinoids may not be so rare as once thought and may constitute up to 30% of carcinoid tumors.[118] To date, *Heliobacter pylori* has not been implicated in their pathogenesis. Duodenal carcinoids or neuroendocrine tumors are also associated with the ZES syndrome.[3] Rectal carcinoids may also be asymptomatic and discovered only on a routine screening examination, although occasionally they may cause a distal bowel obstruction. Bronchial and thymic carcinoids are asymptomatic in some, whereas approximately one-third of cases[175] have pneumonia, hemoptysis, cough, or an abnormal chest radiograph. Gonadal carcinoids are usually detected as masses on physical or ultrasound examination.

The release of 5-HT into the systemic circulation has long been thought to be responsible for the symptoms of the carcinoid syndrome, and numerous studies have documented

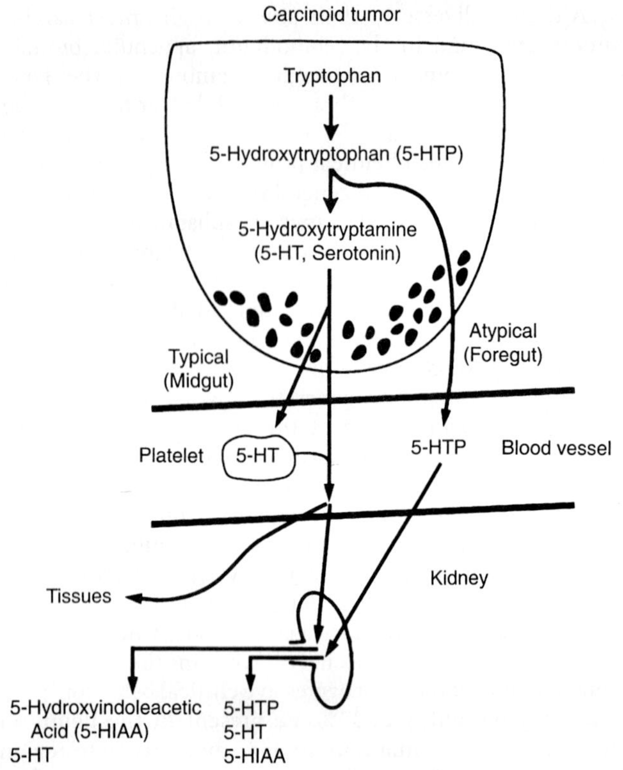

FIGURE 58.17. Illustration of the typical (*left*) and atypical (*right*) serotonergic pathway in carcinoid tumors.

both an increase in serum and platelet serotonin levels as well as urinary levels of the serotonin metabolite 5-HIAA. In these reports, 18% to 84% of individuals were found to have elevated 5-HT serum levels[136,168] while up to 88% of individuals in another study had elevated urinary levels of 5-HIAA.[170] Platelet 5-HT levels were also elevated, particularly in cases of midgut carcinoids.[176] The classic carcinoid syndrome consists of signs and symptoms including facial flushing, diarrhea, diaphoresis, weight loss, right-sided cardiac valvular disease, and bronchoconstriction,[3,131,138,168,177] usually a consequence of disseminated midgut carcinoids. Foregut carcinoids, on the other hand, rarely cause the classic syndrome but may manifest an atypical carcinoid syndrome, mainly comprising a generalized flushing, headache, cutaneous edema, lacrimation, and bronchoconstriction.[136] The manifestation of a typical as opposed to atypical carcinoid syndrome is thought to be a consequence of a derangement in the serotonergic pathway of the carcinoid cell (Fig. 58.17). Typically, tryptophan is converted to 5-HT during a sequential two-step reaction involving the enzymes tryptophan hydroxylase and dopa decarboxylase. The final product, 5-HT, is then released into the blood where it is taken up by tissues and platelets. 5-HT is then excreted by the kidneys in the form of 5-HIAA, its principal metabolite, after the action of tissue and blood monoamine oxidase or aldehyde dehydrogenase.

In certain carcinoid tumors, there is a deficiency in dopa decarboxylase, leading to an inability to convert the intermediate 5-hydroxytryptophan (5-HTP) to the final products, 5-HT. In this case, 5-HTP is released into the circulation and is eliminated unchanged in the urine. Blood 5-HT levels are usually normal in patients with atypical carcinoid syndrome, but urine levels are usually elevated because some of the 5-HTP is converted to 5-HT by renal DOPA decarboxylase. Thus, patients with an atypical carcinoid syndrome usually have significantly increased urinary levels of 5-HT and 5-HTP but normal or only slightly elevated levels of 5-HIAA.[136] However, there remains an inconsistent relationship between elevated 5-HT or 5-HTP levels and symptoms caused by carcinoid disease. A number of reports have found that between 44% and 88% of individuals have symptoms of the carcinoid syndrome, such as flushing or diarrhea, whereas the majority may have elevated 5-HT levels.[136] Elaboration of other products such as pancreatic polypeptide (PP), motilin, gastrin, or various prostaglandins has not, as yet, been associated with any clinical symptoms,[178] although elaboration of growth hormone-releasing factor and ACTH by foregut carcinoids have been documented as causes of acromegaly and Cushing's syndrome, respectively.[136,179] Small cell carcinoma of the lung and medullary thyroid carcinoma have been reported as rare causes of the carcinoid syndrome.

Signs and Symptoms

Approximately 40% to 60% of carcinoid tumors can be asymptomatic[131,138] and are only diagnosed after investigation of nonspecific complaints or after appendectomy. Up to 20% may be discovered at autopsy.[130] In those that are symptomatic, the presentation varies considerably according to tumor location. As previously mentioned, foregut carcinoids are usually asymptomatic or present with upper respiratory signs and symptoms. Gastric carcinoids may present with epigastric pain or anemia, whereas midgut carcinoids, the most common location for clinical significance,[132,136,137] may show signs of the carcinoid syndrome, vague abdominal pain, intestinal obstruction, or venous infarction. Occasionally, they may present with intestinal volvulus, abdominal mass, pellagra, asthma, or right-sided heart failure. The most dramatic presentation is that of the carcinoid syndrome itself, and it is usually a consequence of tumor factors gaining access to the systemic circulation, thus circumventing metabolism in the portal or pulmonary arterial circulation. Again, this depends on the primary tumor's anatomic location (such as gonads), regional extension (such as retroperitoneal or peripancreatic), and degree of metastatic spread (usually to the liver).

As a general rule, patients with the classic syndrome present with diarrhea, flushing, localized, or generalized pain and right-sided endocardial involvement, ultimately producing valvular heart disease and heart failure (Tables 58.3, 58.10). Most components of the syndrome have been extensively investigated. Flushing occurs in approximately 74% of cases,[180] and appears as a deep-red erythema on the face and

TABLE 58.10. Usual Presenting Symptoms in Patients with Classic Carcinoid Syndrome.

Symptom	*Presenting (%)*
Diarrhea	32–68
Flushing	23–74
Reactive airway disease	4–18
Heart disease	41
Pain	10
Pellagra	5

Sources: Norheim et al. (1987)[170]; Thorson (1958).[180]

neck accompanied by a subjective feeling of warmth, and sometimes accompanied by pruritis, palpitations, and diarrhea. It may occur spontaneously or be precipitated by alcohol or cheese ingestion, stress, catecholamines, or exercise.[137,168,178] Flushing is more common with midgut carcinoids, and the episode is usually brief initially but may become prolonged as the disease progresses. The atypical flushing associated with foregut carcinoids, especially bronchial, is usually more severe. In this case, it is more prolonged, extensive, and associated with lacrimation, subcutaneous edema, diaphoresis, and diarrhea.[136] Over time, patients with atypical flushing caused by bronchial carcinoids may develop a constant reddish-blue discoloration in addition to finger clubbing.[132] Gastric carcinoids may also be associated with a flushing that is pruritic but also manifests wheals and involves the arms.[136,181]

The exact mechanism underlying the flushing reaction is still a matter of much debate,[182,183] although it does appear that the different manifestations are dependent on the tumor type and location. Overproduction of serotonin does not appear to be involved because antagonists do not appear to abrogate the symptoms.[182–184] Likewise, 5-HTP infusion or administration of antagonists seem to have no major effect on flushing.[182] In foregut carcinoids, the flushing pattern has been attributed to histamine or histamine metabolites because this type of flushing can be prevented by the administration of H_1- or H_2-receptor blockade.[185] In midgut carcinoids, numerous substances including 5-HT, neuropeptide K, substance P, gastrointestinal peptides, and prostaglandins have been studied.[178,184] Although prostaglandins have not been proven to play a role, elevated levels of substance P and neuropeptide K, both tachykinins, may play a minor role in the genesis of the classic carcinoid flush, although this remains controversial.[178,186] Some reports have found that these substances were elevated in patients with carcinoid tumors, especially with pentagastrin stimulation, but that somatostatin relieved pentagastrin-induced flushing without significantly affecting substance P levels in all patients.[148,187] Several investigations of gastrointestinal peptides have shown no elevation of these factors during flushing episodes.[188,189] Still others have proposed a role for vasodilation secondary to nitric oxide liberation during platelet activation.[190]

Diarrhea is another finding in a majority of patients with the carcinoid syndrome (see Table 58.10). Usually, it is described as watery, can occur up to 30 times per day,[136] and is usually associated with flushing episodes. Persistent diarrhea may lead to steathorrhea and weight loss. Occasionally, it may be accompanied by abdominal colic. 5-HT and its metabolites are thought to be predominantly responsible for the diarrhea, as it has known effects on gastrointestinal motility, and 5-HT receptor antagonists (especially 5-HT_3 antagonists) have been shown to alleviate the symptoms.[191,192]

Heart disease is seen in up to 41% of patients with carcinoid disease, although some studies have found a higher percentage.[193] The basic pathology remains poorly understood but is thought to involve 5-HT.[136,184] The hallmark of carcinoid heart disease is endocardial fibrosis, which predominantly involves the right side of the heart.[193,194] In particular, the ventricular aspect of tricuspid valve and chordae, more so than the pulmonary valve, are involved. Fibrotic constriction ultimately leads to tricuspid regurgitation and pulmonary stenosis, which precipitates cardiac failure. Significant cardiac failure was evident in up to 80% of individuals with carcinoid heart disease in some reports.[180,193] In some instances, systemic fibrosis may occur leading to retroperitoneal or intraabdominal fibrosis, sexual dysfunction in men, or even occlusion of mesenteric arteries and veins.[136]

Other symptoms, such as reactive airway disease, pellagra, and nonspecific abdominal pain, may also be associated with carcinoid disease. Asthma, seen in up to 18% of patients (see Table 58.10), is thought to be caused by the actions of both 5-HT[195] and histamine as well as local inflammatory mediators. The pathophysiology of pellagra is more interesting. In this case, usurption of tryptophan by the tumor cells to effect the formation of 5-HT leads to a depletion in the total body pool of endogenous niacin, which in turn leads to the manifestation of pellagra.[196] In most cases, this manifests as a sharply demarcated dermatitis involving areas exposed to chronic irritation or sunlight such as the face, hands, wrists, elbows, or knees that may progress to hyperkeratosis and scaling. The dementia component, which is rare, is usually a consequence of long-standing disease and results from degeneration in neurons of the central nervous system.

Diagnosis

The presumptive diagnosis of carcinoid disease can be suspected in all patients with clinical symptoms or signs suggestive of a carcinoid tumor or carcinoid syndrome. However, the characteristic clinical presentation may not always be apparent, and symptoms such as flushing or diarrhea can also be seen in menopausal individuals, or those taking certain medications or food products, or in those with various intestinal diseases or other neuroendocrine tumors.[197] Because of nonspecific symptoms, the diagnosis of small intestinal carcinoids may be frequently delayed, sometimes with a median time from presentation to diagnosis of approximately 2 years.[132] Simlarly, vague upper respiratory complaints referable to a bronchial carcinoid may be treated until repeated presentations force a more intensive search for the cause. Biochemical testing remains the cornerstone of diagnosis for symptomatic carcinoid tumors (see Table 58.3). The most widespread and inexpensive tests rely on the measurements of serotonin or its metabolites in urine. In this regard, the measurement of the serotonin metabolite 5-HIAA in a 24-h urine sample is commonly used.[198] Patients with carcinoid tumors have increased urinary 5-HIAA excretion, in the range of 8 to 30 mg per day, but false-positive results can be seen in individuals eating certain foods, such as fruits or nuts, that have a high serotonin content,[199] or in individuals taking certain analgesics or cough-suppressing medications. When used alone, urinary 5-HIAA levels have a sensitivity of around 73% and a specificity of 88% to 100%.[135,178,198] Some authors also recommend measuring platelet and urine 5-HT levels because this may help with biochemical diagnosis and may not be affected by diet. One study found an increased sensitivity of this method over conventional urinary 5-HIAA determinations.[176] This same study also found that urinary 5-HT levels had sensitivities of 55%, 82%, and 60% for foregut, midgut, and hindgut carcinoid tumors, respectively.[176] It should be remembered that, in patients with an atypical carcinoid syndrome, urinary 5-HIAA levels may not be significantly elevated because the principal metabolite in this case is 5-HTP. In this case, measurement of urinary 5-HT, platelet serotonin levels, or urinary levels of tryptophan metabolites will contribute to the diagnosis.[200]

There have been numerous investigations into identifying serum factors that would aid in the diagnosis of carcinoid tumors.[136,147,178,201] Most research has focused on neurotensin, substance P, and the chromogranins (A, B, and C) because these factors are usually found within tumor cells and assist in histochemical diagnosis. Most results seem to indicate that substance P and neurotensin have a sensitivity as a plasma marker for carcinoid disease of no more than 50%. Use of the chromogranins seems to have more diagnostic application. In one study of 44 patients with carcinoid tumors, 100% had elevated chromogranin A levels, 86% had elevated chromogranin B levels, and 5% had elevated chromogranin C levels.[202] However, use of these factors as markers for carcinoid disease is limited by their specificity because they may also be found in association with other neuroendocrine tumors.[9,123,202]

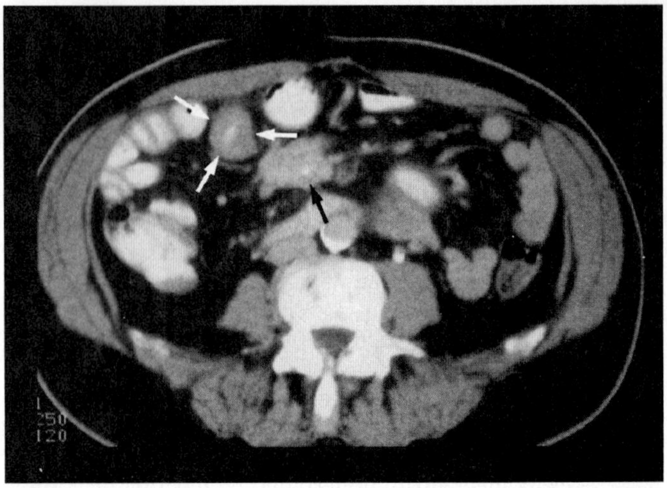

FIGURE 58.18. Computed tomography (CT) scan demonstrates the finding of a circumferential small bowel carcinoid tumor (*white arrows*). Regional nodal disease was read as being present (*black arrow*).

Localization

Tumor localization is of great importance in identifying the primary tumor and its site of origin, determining presence or extent of metastatic disease, and contributing to preoperative strategy or follow-up after surgery or chemotherapy. Virtually all radiologic techniques have been used, or are currently used, in attempts to localize and treat carcinoid disease.[203] The utility of each different modality is dependent on the tumor location and size, and up to 40% of primary and metastatic disease may not be visualized by the usual techniques.[204] Chest radiography is usually the first imaging modality to detect bronchial carcinoids and is usually performed to investigate nonspecific respiratory complaints.[136,175] As the tumors are slow-growing, they may compress airways and induce an obstructive pneumonia or atelectasis and may appear as opacities with notched margins.[205] CT scanning then allows for greater resolution of the lesion, and tissue for diagnosis may be obtained by bronchoscopy if the lesion is proximal in the respiratory tree. Gastric carcinoids are also usually asymptomatic and are usually diagnosed on endoscopy. Upper gastrointestinal barium contrast studies are generally nonspecific or fail to visualize the lesion.[161,206] Similarly, lower gastrointestinal contrast studies have poor sensitivity and specificity for hindgut carcinoid tumors[207] but are more successful in localizing those in the cecum and ascending colon.[137,207]

Ultrasonography has received renewed interest in recent years in the localization of primary as well as metastatic disease. Transabdominal US can identify about 36% of small bowel carcinoids (see Table 58.6) and 67% or more of liver metastases.[40] Others have reaffirmed these results and reported a higher percentage of positive results.[208] Ultrasound may also be useful in guiding percutaneous liver biopsies of suspected lesions.[209] Endoscopic ultrasound has become increasingly important in the localization of tumors, particularly colorectal carcinoids. One study has reported a 75% to 90% accuracy for depth of invasion in colorectal lesions,[210] thus assisting in staging of the primary tumor for treatment. EUS may also be valuable in identifying local nodal involvement.[211]

The localization of midgut carcinoid disease remains a problem. The tumors are usually small and asymptomatic, or are larger and have metastasized at the time of symptomatic presentation. Usually barium studies fail to localize these lesions.[212] CT scanning has been used extensively in the localization of carcinoid tumors (Fig. 58.18) but images only about 44% to 55% of the primary lesions, with some studies reporting an 82% localization rate[213] and others only 2%.[212] Its greatest utility, and that of MR imaging, lies in the detection of metastatic disease and in monitoring medical therapy.[214] Some authors have found angiography to be more sensitive than CT in localizing liver metastases.[136,212,215] SRS imaging has also been applied to carcinoid localization. Some investigations have reported that up to 88% of carcinoid tumors possess receptors (SSTR-1 to -3) that have moderate to high affinity for somatostatin and its analogues.[216] On average, SRS images 33% to 89% of carcinoid tumors.[39,89,204] In some studies, it has been reported to image up to 16% of lesions not previously seen with other modalities.[213] Still others have found it to have a specificity and positive predictive value of 100% with an overall accuracy of 83%.[217] Because of its sensitivity, as well as the ability to image the whole body, many regard SRS as the initial imaging procedure of choice for localizing carcinoid tumors. Beyond CT and SRS, whole body ^{11}C-5-hydroxytryptophan positron emission tomography has demonstrated superior sensitivity for neuroendocrine tumors, although this modality is not widely available.[218]

Another scintigraphic technique utilizes iodine-131 metaiodobenzylguanidine (^{131}I-MIBG) to image tumors. This agent is concentrated by a sodium-dependent membrane pump in both pheochromocytomas and carcinoids. This modality localizes about 68% of midgut and 38% of foregut carcinoids[218] and has an average sensitivity of about 70% with a specificity of 95%[66] when using the iodine-123 isotope. The utility of ^{131}I-MIBG scanning seems to lie in its ability to localize metastatic tumor rather than as a first-line imaging modality.[219] Technetium-99m bone scanning appears to be superior to other isotopic studies at imaging bony metastases.[219]

Metastatic Disease and Survival

Carcinoid tumors are malignant, and the presence of metastasis directly influences survival. In one multivariate analysis of gastrointestinal carcinoids, gender and the presence of local or distant metastases were independently predictive of death.[220] A number of factors have been found to have an influence on the development of metastatic disease, the most important being the size and location of the primary tumor as well as its histological stage.[131,207,220–222]

The metastatic potential of gastric carcinoids may be influenced by their particular subtype, as proposed by Rindi et al.[174] Although 54% to 66% of patients with sporadic gastric carcinoid develop metastases, advanced disease occurs in only about 9% of individuals with carcinoids and hypergastrinemia[160,168,174] (Table 58.11). Tumor size is also associated with metastases. Sporadic gastric carcinoids tend to be large, single lesions with atypical histology while those found in the setting of hypergastrinemia tend to be small and multiple. Duodenal carcinoids are seldom suspected before the diagnosis is made by endoscopy.[135] In one review of 99 cases,[172] there were no metastases in tumors less than 1 cm whereas 33% of those more than 2 cm in size had metastasized at the time of diagnosis. In addition, invasion into the muscularis propria was also found to be a strong predictor of metastatic spread. Bronchial or lung carcinoids have been found to metastasize in up to 20% of cases,[168] and aggressive behavior is also dependent on the histological classification of the tumor.[174,223] In the case of jejunoileal carcinoids, if the tumor is less than 1 cm, metastases are usually found in 15% to 18% of cases, although one study reported a rate of 29% with these small lesions.[224] Tumors between 1 and 2 cm metastasize in 60% to 80% of cases,[131] and metastases are usually present with tumors larger than 2 cm at the time of diagnosis. Most appendiceal carcinoids are less than 1 cm in size and very rarely metastasize (0%–2%),[131] but tumors between 1 and 2 cm may have metastatic spread in up to 50% of cases.[207] The metastatic rate of colon and rectal carcinoids is particularly dependent on size. Most of these tumors are confined to the sigmoid colon and rectum. Metastatic disease can occur in 10% to 70% of patients with colon carcinoid tumors[168,225] and in virtually all when the tumor is 2 cm or greater in size. Overall, about 15% of patients with rectal carcinoids have metastatic disease.[168,226] Rectal tumors less than 1 cm metastasize in 0% to 20% of cases[226] while those greater than 2 cm are metastatic in virtually every case (see Table 58.11).

In addition to the location of the primary tumor and presence of metastatic disease, prognosis and long-term survival may also be influenced by a number of other factors. The presence of the carcinoid syndrome is usually associated with underlying advanced disease, and the majority of patients manifesting it have distant metastases. In the past, decreased survival was associated with the onset of symptoms, and the median survival was no better than 8.5 years.[167] Current medical therapy, as well as aggressive debulking surgery, have made it possible for individuals with advanced metastatic disease to remain active for a longer period of time. In one analysis of a large number of cases of carcinoid disease,[223] favorable prognosis was suggested by female gender, incidentally discovered tumors, absence of symptoms, small size, minimal histological tumor invasion, and absence of local or distant metastases.

Overall survival rates are dependent on tumor location and size and vary among studies (see Table 58.11). One analysis of more than 2500 cases reported a 94% 5-year survival with local disease and an 18% 5-year survival with distant metastases if all sites are considered.[169] In this study, appendiceal lesions showed the most favorable prognosis, with 99% to 100% 5-year survival, even with regional metastases, and 27% 5-year survival with distant involvement. Others have reported a 76% to 100% 5-year survival for apendiceal carcinoids.[131,227,228] Jejunoileal tumors have been reported to have

TABLE 58.11.
Incidence, Metastatic Disease, and 5-Year Survival for Carcinoid Tumors at Different Anatomic Sites.

Site	*Reference*	*Level of evidence*[a]	*Incidence (%)*	*Metastatic disease* <1 cm	1–2 cm	>2 cm	Overall	*Carcinoid syndrome (%)*	*Overall 5-year survival (%)*
Foregut									
Bronchus/lung	168	III	12	—	—	—	20	13	87
Thymus	168	III	2	—	—	—	25	—	85
Gastric	168	III	2	—	—	—	22	10	52
Sporadic	160	III	—	—	—	—	66	11	—
Hypergastrinemia[b]	160	III	—	—	—	—	9	11	—
Duodenum	168	III	3	—	—	—	20	3	—
	172	II	—	0	8	33	21	1	58
Midgut									
Jejunum	168	III	1	—	—	—	35	9	54
Ileum	168	III	23	—	—	—	35	9	54
Jejunum, ileum	131	III	—	16	70	90	—	—	—
Appendix	168	III	38				2	1	83
	131	III	—	0–2	50	—	—	—	—
	130	III	—	—	—	33	—	—	—
Hindgut									
Colon	168	III	2	—	—	—	60	5	52
	224	II	3.6	10	70	99	53		
Rectum	168	III	13	—	—	—	15	3	83
	225	III	—	0–20	—	99	—	—	—

[a]I, prospective, randomized; II, prospective; III, retrospective, review or anecdotal.
[b]Hypergastrinemia indicates tumors arising in the setting of hypergastrinemia.

a 5-year survival ranging between 19% and 77% depending upon the presence of local disease or distant metastases at the time of diagnosis, with overall survival for all stages being 54%.[131,169] Colon tumors have been reported to have an overall 5-year survival of 52% and rectal carcinoids an 83% overall 5-year survival.[169] However, only 7% to 44% of patients with rectal disease will survive 5 years if there is evidence of nodal or hepatic metastases, compared with 92% 5-year survival in those found to have only local disease. In the case of bronchial tumors, 5-year survival has been reported to be 96% for local disease and 11% with distant spread (overall, 87%).[169] Carcinoids of the stomach have an overall 5-year survival of 52% for all stages. Individual survival ranged from 0% to 93%, depending on the presence of distant metastases or local disease at the time of diagnosis.

Treatment of Carcinoid Disease

Medical Management and Chemotherapy

Medical management of carcinoid disease involves treatment of carcinoid syndrome caused by stress, dietary elements, anesthesia, chemotherapy or spontaneous occurrence. Carcinoid crisis can be life-threatening and is marked by varying degrees of intense flushing, diarrhea, abdominal pain, altered mental status, and cardiovascular derangements, particularly hypertension or hypotension.[229]

Although a variety of agents have been employed to treat the carcinoid syndrome or crisis, octreotide is the only current agent with broad utility in treatment and prevention.[229–232] In one report, only 7% of patients failed to respond in any way to octreotide.[132] Its specificity for the type-2 somatostatin receptor (SSTR-2), which is expressed in a large proportion of carcinoid tumors, leads to a reduction in peripheral serotonin levels and a reduction in gut motility.[230] In addition, it has been shown to reduce the risk of a carcinoid crisis intraoperatively.[23,105] When administered subcutaneously every 6 to 12h at a starting dose of 150µg, one large trial found up to a 50% improvement in diarrhea and an 82% improvement in flushing for at least 1 year.[233] The most common side effects are mild elevations in blood glucose levels and steatorrhea and are usually only seen with higher treatment doses. Gallstone formation is also a complication of long-term octreotide administration, and cholecystectomy is indicated in any patient with the malignant carcinoid syndrome. Next-generation somatostatin analogues, including SOM230, target additional somatostatin receptors and are undergoing clinical trials.[234]

Interferon-α is another treatment for carcinoid syndrome and metastatic disease. Initial reports described striking responses in postoperative patients.[235,236] However, long-term follow-up has reported an objective response rate on the order of 12% to 48%.[237,238] The usual dosing range was 1.5 to 7mU, three to seven times per week. In studies using a higher dosage (24mU/m^2/day), 39% of patients had a decrease in 5-HIAA secretion, a 33% improvement in diarrhea, and a 65% improvement in flushing, but responses were transient.[239] Combinations of interferon-α and interferon-γ have been found to elicit clinical improvement in 6 of 12 patients in one study, but side effects were common, including skin lesions and profound fatigue.[240] The adverse side effects of interferon therapy, unlike those of octreotide, have limited its use. Pruritis, hair loss, fatigue, nausea, and myalgia have all been reported, and circulating antibodies to interferon-α have been detected in the blood of patients on long-term treatment.[241] At present, interferon therapy has utility in patients who have failed octreotide treatment, or in combination with hepatic embolization or certain chemotherapy regimens.

Other agents are used to control the symptoms of carcinoid syndrome. Antidiarrheal agents such as loperamide, selective bronchodilators, and diuretics have all been employed to control diarrhea, wheezing, or heart failure seen with advanced disease. 5-HT receptor antagonists such as ketanserin, methylsergide, and cyproheptadine have also been used to treat carcinoid syndrome with some success.[242] In one report, ketanserin reduced flushing episodes in 68% of 31 patients and diarrhea in 75% of 29 patients.[243] α-Methyldopa, which blocks the conversion of 5-HTP to serotonin, has occasionally relieved flushing in a small number of patients without any appreciable effect on gastrointestinal symptoms. Other 5-HT receptor antagonists such as ondansetron and tropisetron, as well as the α-adrenergic antagonist clonidine, have some benefit in controlling gastrointestinal symptoms.[244]

The type and timing of chemotherapy for malignant carcinoid tumors remains controversial. Given the indolent growth pattern of the tumor, the generally poor efficacy of chemical agents, and the ability to control symptoms of the carcinoid syndrome with octreotide or interferon, chemotherapy is usually reserved for advanced tumors. Chemotherapy for metastatic carcinoid tumors has generally had poor results, with single-agent regimens producing no more than a 30% transient response rate.[245] Streptozotocin (STZ), dacarbazine (DTIC), or 5-fluorouracil (5-FU) showed the largest response.[231,245]

Interferon monotherapy decreases tumor size in up to 22% of patients but does not have lasting antitumor effects. One study, however, found it to prolong survival in a group of patients with metastatic disease as compared with STX + 5-FU.[246] Similarly, octreotide has been shown to have poor tumoricidal effect and has shown benefit in only approximately 17% of patients.[232] Combination chemotherapy has also been investigated in a large number of studies. The most common combinations of STZ + 5-FU, STX + cyclophosphamide, or STZ + doxorubicin have produced only a 2% to 40% response rate[232,247,248] and offer no apparent improvement over the use of single agents alone. The combination of these agents with interferon-α has been the subject of some recent studies. Here again, however, the results have been disappointing, with interferon-α in combination with STZ and doxorubicin or interferon-α with 5-FU showing no superiority over the individual agents alone.[249,250] The combination of interferon-α and octreotide has produced no objective tumor responses.[251,252]

The introduction of hepatic artery embolization has allowed for the application of more aggressive multimodality therapy. Hepatic artery embolization relies on the fact that hepatic carcinoid metastases derive their blood supply from branches of the hepatic artery, and it was initially found that metastases showed a significant response to ligation of branches of the hepatic artery.[251,252] However, ligation of the hepatic artery alone had transient response because of the fairly rapid development of collateral circulation. The development of minimally invasive transcatheter embolization has circumvented this problem by occluding more distal intrahepatic vessels and has become the standard for palliation in symptomatic individuals who have become refractory to octreotide or interferon treatments and who have a hepatic tumor burden that is not amenable to surgery. Numerous studies[253–257] have evaluated selected embolization using both oil emulsions and gelfoam and found overall favorable biochemical (5-HIAA) and symptom response. In one study,[257] 61% of patients were free of carcinoid symptoms 1 year after the procedure. Other studies have reported symptomatic and biochemical improvement in all patients treated,[253,255] but no significant increase in survival.[254] Embolization can have significant side effects in up to 12% of patients, including nausea, abscess formation, abdominal pain, fever, and ileus. Moreover, the mortality rate may be as high as 3%.[256] Embolization is usually contraindicated in patients with obstructive jaundice or cases of portal vein occlusion by tumor.

Multimodality therapy using hepatic embolization and chemotherapy (chemoembolization) has received much attention in recent years. This aggressive approach has combined the use of gelfoam embolization with 5-FU, doxorubicin, STZ or dacarbazine (DTIC), and/or interferon-α. A number of large studies have documented improvement of carcinoid symptoms in virtually all patients with objective response, in terms of reduction in tumor size, seen in 35% to 100% of individuals.[132,258–260] In one study, 47% of patients with advanced disease survived 2 years after embolization and doxorubicin treatment.[259] Other authors have reported that chemoembolization significantly increased the duration of the tumor response over embolization alone (18 months versus 4 months), although both therapies induced a similar initial tumor response (69% versus 67%).[258]

Radiation therapy is usually reserved for cases of advanced metastatic and unresectable carcinoid tumors whose symptoms have become resistant to maximal medical management. In a retrospective review of a 16-year experience, the authors concluded that radiation therapy was of benefit in achieving palliation in patients with significantly advanced disease.[261] Currently, radiation is particularly helpful in controlling symptomatic bone metastases.

Surgical Management

Surgery remains the only potentially curative treatment for patients with carcinoid disease.[262–265] However, surgery for cure is mainly dependent on the location and size of the primary tumor because these elements largely influence the potential for metastatic spread.[207,222–224] In addition, even with regional lymph node metastases, surgery may still be curative in some patients,[263] and there is still a role for more aggressive surgical therapy in select patients with advanced disease.[264]

Appendiceal carcinoids are the most frequently encountered carcinoid,[131–133] and they are mostly asymptomatic and usually incidental findings in pathology review of resected appendectomy specimens. In most cases, the lesions are less than 1 cm in diameter and appendectomy is curative.[132,263] In one report, 103 patients were followed after appendectomy during which small carcinoid tumors were removed.[133] At 5 years, there was no evidence of recurrent or metastatic disease in any patient. For tumors between 1 and 2 cm, where metastatic potential may be greater,[207] the surgical approach is less well defined in the literature. Some, with considerable experience, advocate appendectomy alone with periodic surveillance[132,262] whereas others advocate more aggressive surgery, such as cecectomy or right hemicolectomy, in cases where the tumor is located at the base of the appendix.[207] Clearly, in cases of mesoappendix invasion, the more radical approach is favored.[207] One group has also advocated right hemicolectomy for tumors containing mucin-producing cells.[266] For tumors of 2 cm or larger, a formal right hemicolectomy with removal of regional lymph nodes is the procedure of choice.[262,263] With carcinoids of the jejunum and ileum that are less than 1 cm, there is controversy as to the extent of operation. Although uncommon, some studies have reported metastatic rates of 29% to 69% with ileal tumors of less than 1 cm,[224,267] although most series report a range from 15% to 20%. These former findings have led some to speculate that midgut carcinoids manifest a malignant potential that is independent of size. Depth of tumor penetration through the bowel wall may also be an important consideration.[132] Nevertheless, given the available data, many surgeons recommend a wide resection with extensive mesenteric lymph node resection for small tumors and an extended (full-scale) cancer operation for tumors of 2 cm or larger.[132,207,263]

In the case of colorectal carcinoids, outcomes after surgery are clearly defined by the size of the lesion. For rectal carcinoids less than 1 cm in diameter, local excision is adequate for cure.[225,268] For tumors between 1 and 2 cm, where metastasis may be present 11% of the time,[268] local, full-thickness resection is advocated as the initial procedure, with abdominoperineal or low anterior resection reserved for cases displaying invasion of the muscularis propria.[260,268] In cases in which tumors exceed 2 cm in size, and metastatic disease is usually present, abdominoperineal or low anterior resection is usually performed although this form of aggressive surgery is sometimes questioned over local resection alone. In one study,[268] all patients with tumors greater than 2 cm died less than 1 year after abdominoperineal or low anterior resection of metastatic disease.

Carcinoid tumors of the foregut, particularly the stomach and duodenum, may be locally advanced at the time of diagnosis, and this fact complicates surgical management for favorable outcome. In the case of gastric carcinoids, the difference in opinion regarding management may be considerable among different surgeons. The malignant behavior of these tumors is influenced not only by size, but also by histology and the presence of hypergastrinemia. Gastric carcinoids that develop in the presence of hypergastrinemia are not only smaller and multiple but also tend to metastasize in a lower percentage of patients than their sporadic counterparts.[161,169,174] In the past, it was recommended that tumors less than 1 cm be removed locally or endoscopically[206,207] while those showing local invasion or more than 2 cm in size be treated with partial or total gastrectomy depending on location.[207] Others suggested that large tumors without local invasion could be treated by local resection alone.[206] More recently, the classification of gastric carcinoids[174] has allowed for the stratification of treatment,[161] which has allowed for histologically typical carcinoids of less than 2 cm, in the setting of hypergastrinemia, to be resected endoscopically with routine follow-up surveillance. Tumors greater than 2 cm with atypical histology, and with or without hypergastrinemia, are usually treated with partial or total gastrectomy with regional node excision. Small duodenal carcinoids of less than 1 cm rarely metastasize and are treated by endoscopic excision, although larger lesions, up to one-third of which have metastasis at diagnosis, are usually managed by open resection. Lung or bronchial carcinoids are usually resected, if this is possible, either for attempted cure or for control of symptoms. In the case of MEN 1/ZES, surgical excision is recommended to prevent symptoms and control metatstatic spread to the liver.[269] One group reported a 35-year experience revealing low disease-related mortality but frequent recurrences in patients with MEN 1 and pancreatoduodenal neuroendocrine tumors managed with surgery.[270]

Surgery has a role in the treatment of metastatic carcinoid disease. Resection of regional metastases may be curative in some patients,[261,262] and resection of hepatic metastases may provide considerable benefit in most patients and cure in a few.[256,260,261] One group, with considerable experience, reported a clear benefit to resection of hepatic metastases for alleviation of symptoms if more than 90% of the tumor mass can be removed.[271] Another report documents a mean of 5 years of survival in 10 patients who underwent resection of isolated hepatic metastasis.[132] Finally, an additional series demontrated an actuarial survival of 82% in patients with carcinoids and pancreatic neuroendocrine tumors.[272] In cases of hepatic resection, the primary tumor should be removed, although in certain cases this may be difficult. This aggressive debulking surgery is also advocated by a number of authors as having a role in the treatment of advanced carcinoid disease.[262,263,266] In a number of studies, it has been shown that debulking mesenteric metastases and removing compromised segments of bowel, even without resection of liver metastases, has provided considerable symptomatic relief to a large number of individuals.[263,266]

Partial hepatectomy and liver transplantation are described approaches to managing malignant carcinoid disease.[273] The role for hepatectomy has yet to be clearly defined, with one study reporting symptomatic improvement in 60% of 47 patients and a mean survival of slightly more than 6 years.[273] Orthotopic liver transplantation, as a general rule, is contraindicated when there is unresectable extrahepatic disease. It is usually not performed because immunosuppressive drugs needed to prevent graft rejection may stimulate tumor growth.[274] In the case of carcinoid heart disease, tricuspid valve replacement may be therapeutic, but this method carries significant mortality risk. Although they remain investigational, cryoreductive surgery and radiofrequency ablation in hepatic disease hold promise for the future.

References

1. LeDouarin NM. The Embryological Origin of Cells Associated with the Digestive Tract. Edinburgh: Churchill Livingstone, 1978.
2. Kloppel G, Heitz PU. Classification of normal and neoplastic neuroendocrine cells. Ann N Y Acad Sci 1994;733:18–24.
3. Jensen RT, Norton JA. Endocrine tumors of the pancreas. In: Yamada T, Alpers DH, Owyang C, Powell DW, Silverstein FE, eds. Textbook of Gastroenterology, 2nd ed. Philadelphia: Lippincott, 1995.
4. Wilander E, Scheibenpflug L, Ericksson B, Oberg K. Diagnostic criteria of classical carcinoids. Acta Oncol 1991;30:469–476.
5. Norton JA. Pancreatic Islet Cell Tumors Excluding Gastrinomas. St. Louis: Mosby, 1998.
6. Wilander E. Diagnostic pathology of gastrointestinal and pancreatic neuroendocrine tumors. Acta Oncol 1989;28: 363.
7. Meko JB, Doherty GM, Siegel BA, Norton JA. Evaluation of somatostatin-receptor scintigraphy for detecting neuroendocrine tumors. Surgery (St. Louis) 1996;120(6):975–983; discussion 983–984.
8. Meko JB, Norton JA. Endocrine tumors of the pancreas. Curr Opin Gen Surg 1994:186–194.
9. Metz DC. Diagnosis and treatment of pancreatic neuroendocrine tumors. Semin Gastrointest Dis 1995;6:67–74.
10. Dent RB. Nonfunctioning islet cell tumors. Ann Surg 1981;193:185–189.
11. Meko JB, Norton JA. Management of patients with Zollinger–Ellison syndrome. Annu Rev Med 1995;46:395–411.
12. Sadler TW. Digestive System, 6th ed. Baltimore: Williams & Wilkins, 1990.
13. Creutzfeldt W, Arnold R, Creutzfeld C. Pathomorphological, biochemical and diagnostic aspects of gastrinomas (Zollinger–Ellison syndrome). Hum Pathol 1975;6:47–53.
14. Friesen SR. Tumors of the endocrine pancreas. N Engl J Med 1982;306:580–585.
15. Kloppel G, Schroder S, Heitz PU. Histopathology and immunopathology of pancreatic endocrine tumors. In: Mignon M, Jensen RT, eds. Endocrine Tumors of the Pancreas: Recent Advances in Research and Management. Basel: Karger, 1995:120–129.
16. Wermer P. Endocrine adenomatosis and peptic ulcer in a large kindred: inherited multiple tumors and mosaic pleiotropism in man. Am J Med 1963;35:205.
17. Zollinger RM, Ellison EH. Primary peptic ulceration of the jejunum associated with islet cell tumors of the pancreas. Ann Surg 1955;142:709–728.
18. Chan FK. Differential diagnosis, causes, and management of hypercalcemia. Curr Probl Surg 1997;34(6):445–523.
19. Veldhuis JD, Norton JA, Wells SA Jr, Vinik AI, Perry RR. Surgical versus medical management of multiple endocrine neoplasia (MEN) type I. J Clin Endocrinol Metab 1997;82(2):357–364.
20. Sheppard BC, Norton JA, Doppman JL, Maton PN, Gardner JD, Jensen RT. Management of islet cell tumors in patients with multiple endocrine neoplasia: a prospective study. Surgery (St. Louis) 1989;106(6):1108–1117; discussion 1117–1118.
21. Boukhman MP, Karam JH, Shaver J, Siperstein AE, Duh QY, Clark OH. Insulinoma—experience from 1950 to 1995. West J Med 1998;169(2):98–104.
22. Benya RV, Metc DC, Venzon DJ, et al. Zollinger-Ellison syndrome can be the initial endocrine manifestation in patients with multiple endocrine neoplasia-type I. Am J Med 1994;97:436–444.
23. Norton JA, Cornelius MJ, Doppman JL, Maton PN, Gardner JD, Jensen RT. Effect of parathyroidectomy in patients with hyperparathyroidism, Zollinger–Ellison syndrome, and multiple endocrine neoplasia type I: a prospective study. Surgery (St. Louis) 1987;102(6):958–966.
24. Norton JA, Doherty GM, Fraker DL. Surgery for Endocrine Tumors of the Pancreas, 2nd ed. New York: Raven Press, 1993.
25. Pipeleers-Marichal M, Somers G, Willems G, et al. Gastrinomas in the duodenum of patients with multiple endocrine neoplasia type 1 and the Zollinger–Ellison syndrome. N Engl J Med 1990;322:723–727.
26. Whipple AO. The surgical therapy of hyperinsulinism. J Int Chir 1938;3:237.
27. Fajans SS, Vinik AI. Insulin-producing islet cell tumors. Endocrinol Metab Clin N Am 1989;18(1):45–74.
28. Pasieka JL, McLeod MK, Thompson NW, Burney RE. Surgical approach to insulinomas. Assessing the need for preoperative localization. Arch Surg 1992;127(4):442–447.

29. Harrison TS, Fajans SS, Floyd JC, et al. Prevalence of diffuse pancreatic beta islet cell disease with hyperinsulin problems in recognition and management. World J Surg 1984;8:583–589.
30. Stovroff MC, Norton JA. Invited commentary. World J Surg 1988;12:608–609.
31. Modlin IM, Tang LH. Approaches to the diagnosis of gut neuroendocrine tumors: the last word (today). Gastroenterology 1997;112(2):583–590.
32. Lo CY, Lam KY, Kung AW, Lam KS, Tung PH, Fan ST. Pancreatic insulinomas. A 15-year experience. Arch Surg 1997;132(8):926–930.
33. Comi RJ, Gorden P, Doppman JL, Norton JA. Insulinoma. New York: Raven Press, 1986.
34. Norton JA, Whitman ED. Insulinoma. Endocrinologist 1993; 3(4):258–267.
35. Grunberger G, Weiner JL, Silverman R, Taylor S, Gorden P. Factitious hypoglycemia due to surreptitious administration of insulin. Diagnosis, treatment, and long-term follow-up. Ann Intern Med 1988;108(2):252–257.
36. Fraker DL, Norton JA. Localization and resection of insulinomas and gastrinomas [clinical conference]. JAMA 1988;259(24):3601–3605.
37. Doppman JL, Miller DL, Chang R, Shawker TH, Gorden P, Norton JA. Insulinomas: localization with selective intraarterial injection of calcium [published erratum appears in Radiology 1993;187(3):880]. Radiology 1991;178(1):237–241.
38. Moore NR, Rogers CE, Britton BJ. Magnetic resonance imaging of endocrine tumours of the pancreas. Br J Radiol 1995;68(808):341–347.
39. Krenning EP, Kwekkeboom DJ, Oei HY, et al. Somatostatin-receptor scintigraphy in gastroenteropancreatic tumors. An overview of European results. Ann N Y Acad Sci 1994;733:416–424.
40. Kisker O, Bartsch D, Weinel RJ, et al. The value of somatostatin-receptor scintigraphy in newly diagnosed endocrine gastroenteropancreatic tumors. J Am Coll Surg 1997;184(5):487–492.
41. Böttger TC, Weber W, Beyer J, Junginger T. Value of tumor localization in patients with insulinoma. World J Surg 1990;14(1):107–112; discussion 112–114.
42. Daggett PR, Goodburn EA, Kurtz AB, et al. Is preoperative localisation of insulinomas necessary? Lancet 1981;1(8218):483–486.
43. Palazzo L, Roseau G, Salmeron M. Endoscopic ultrasonography in the preoperative localization of pancreatic endocrine tumors. Endoscopy 1992;24(suppl 1):350–353.
44. Rëosch T, Lightdale CJ, Botet JF, et al. Localization of pancreatic endocrine tumors by endoscopic ultrasonography [see comments]. N Engl J Med 1992;326(26):1721–1726.
45. Norton JA, Shawker TH, Doppman JL, et al. Localization and surgical treatment of occult insulinomas [see comments]. Ann Surg 1990;212(5):615–620.
46. Vinik AI, Delbridge L, Moattari R, Cho K, Thompson N. Transhepatic portal vein catheterization for localization of insulinomas: a ten-year experience [see comments]. Surgery (St. Louis) 1991;109(1):1–11; discussion 111.
47. Miller DL, Doppman JL, Metz DC, Maton PN, Norton JA, Jensen RT. Zollinger–Ellison syndrome: technique, results, and complications of portal venous sampling. Radiology 1992;182(1):235–241.
48. Doppman JL, Chang R, Fraker DL, et al. Localization of insulinomas to regions of the pancreas by intra-arterial stimulation with calcium [see comments] [published erratum appears in Ann Intern Med 1995;123(9):734]. Ann Intern Med 1995;123(4):269–273.
49. Norton JA. Surgical treatment of islet cell tumors with special emphasis on operative ultrasound. In: Mignon M, Jensen RT, eds. Endocrine Tumors of the Pancreas: Recent Advances in Research and Management. Basel: Krager, 1995;309–332.
50. Isenberg JI, Walsh JH, Grossman MI. Zollinger–Ellison syndrome. Gastroenterology 1973;65(1):140–165.
51. Norton JA. Gastrinoma: advances in localization and treatment. Surg Oncol Clin N Am 1998;7(4):845–861.
52. Weber HC, Venzon DJ, Lin JT, et al. Determinants of metastatic rate and survival in patients with Zollinger–Ellison syndrome: a prospective long-term study. Gastroenterology 1995;108(6): 1637–1649.
53. Thompson NW. Surgical treatment of the endocrine pancreas and Zollinger–Ellison syndrome in the MEN 1 syndrome. Henry Ford Hosp Med J 1992;40(3–4):195–198.
54. Norton JA, Fraker DL, Alexander HR, et al. Surgery for the cure of the Zollinger–Ellison Syndrome. N Engl J Med 1999;341:635–644.
55. Stabile BE, Morrow DJ, Passaro E Jr. The gastrinoma triangle: operative implications. Am J Surg 1984;147(1):25–31.
56. Gibril F, Curtis LT, Termanini B, et al. Primary cardiac gastrinoma causing Zollinger–Ellison syndrome. Gastroenterology 1997;112(2):567–574.
57. Maton PN, Mackem SM, Norton JA, Gardner JD, O'Dorisio TM, Jensen RT. Ovarian carcinoma as a cause of Zollinger–Ellison syndrome. Natural history, secretory products, and response to provocative tests. Gastroenterology 1989;97(2):468–471.
58. Arnold WS, Fraker DL, Alexander HR, Weber HC, Norton JA, Jensen RT. Apparent lymph node primary gastrinoma. Surgery (St. Louis) 1994;116(6):1123–1129; discussion 1129–1130.
59. Deveney CW, Deveney KE. Zollinger–Ellison syndrome (gastrinoma). Current diagnosis and treatment. Surg Clin N Am 1987;67(2):411–422.
60. Stage JG, Stadil F. The clinical diagnosis of the Zollinger–Ellison syndrome. Scand J Gastroenterol Suppl 1979;53:79–91.
61. Norton JA. Advances in the management of Zollinger–Ellison syndrome. Adv Surg 1994;27:129–159.
62. Slaff JL, Howard JM, Maton PN, et al. Prospective assessment of provocative gastrin tests in 81 consecutive patients with Zollinger–Ellison syndrome. Gastroenterology 1986;90:1637–1643.
63. McArthur KE, Richardson CT, Barnett CC, et al. Laparotomy and proximal gastric vagotomy in Zollinger–Ellison syndrome: results of a 16-year prospective study [see comments]. Am J Gastroenterol 1996;91(6):1104–1111.
64. Frucht H, Doppman JL, Norton JA, et al. Gastrinomas: comparison of MR imaging with CT, angiography, and US. Radiology 1989;171(3):713–717.
65. Wank SA, Doppman JL, Miller DL, et al. Prospective study of the ability of computed axial tomography to localize gastrinomas in patients with Zollinger–Ellison syndrome. Gastroenterology 1987;92(4):905–912.
66. Krenning EP, Kwekkeboom DJ, Bakker WH, et al. Somatostatin receptor scintigraphy with [^{111}In-DTPA-D-Phe1]- and [^{123}I-Tyr3]-octreotide: the Rotterdam experience with more than 1000 patients. Eur J Nucl Med 1993;20(8):716–731.
67. Gibril F, Reynolds JC, Doppman JL, et al. Somatostatin receptor scintigraphy: its sensitivity compared with that of other imaging methods in detecting primary and metastatic gastrinomas. A prospective study [see comments]. Ann Intern Med 1996;125(1):26–34.
68. Alexander HR, Fraker DL, Norton JA, et al. Prospective study of somatostatin receptor scintigraphy and its effect on operative outcome in patients with Zollinger–Ellison syndrome. Ann Surg 1998;228(2):228–238.
69. Thompson NW, Czako PF, Fritts LL, et al. Role of endoscopic ultrasonography in the localization of insulinomas and gastrinomas. Surgery (St. Louis) 1994;116(6):1131–1138.
70. Ruszniewski P, Amouyal P, Amouyal G, et al. Localization of gastrinomas by endoscopic ultrasonography in patients with Zollinger–Ellison syndrome. Surgery (St. Louis) 1995;117(6):629–635.

71. Kisker O, Bastian D, Bartsch D, Nies C, Rothmund M. Localization, malignant potential, and surgical management of gastrinomas. World J Surg 1998;22(7):651–657; discussion 657–658.
72. Sugg SL, Norton JA, Fraker DL, et al. A prospective study of intraoperative methods to diagnose and resect duodenal gastrinomas. Ann Surg 1993;218(2):138–144.
73. Norton JA, Cromack DT, Shawker TH, et al. Intraoperative ultrasonographic localization of the islet cell tumors. A prospective comparison to palpation. Ann Surg 1988;207(2):160–168.
74. Stacpoole PW. The glucagonoma syndrome: clinical features, diagnosis, and treatment. Endocr Rev 1981;2(3):347–361.
75. Wilkinson DS. Necrolytic migratory erythema with carcinoma of the pancreas. Trans St Johns Hosp Dermatol Soc 1973;59(2):244–250.
76. Guillausseau PJ, Guillausseau-Scholer C. Glucagonomas: Clinical Presentation, Diagnosis, and Advances in Management. Basel: Karger, 1995.
77. Maton PN. Use of octreotide acetate for control of symptoms in patients with islet cell tumors. World J Surg 1993;17(4):504–510.
78. Verner JV, Morrison AB. Islet cell tumor and a syndrome of refractory water diarrhea and hypokalemia. Am J Med 1958;29:529–533.
79. Matsumoto KK, Perer JB, Schultze RG, et al. Watery diarrhea and hypokalemia associated with a pancreatic islet cell adenoma. Gastroenterology 1967:52:695–699.
80. Matuchansky C, Rambaud JC. VIPomas and Endocrine Cholera: Clinical Presentation, Diagnosis, and Advances in Management. Basel: Karger, 1995.
81. Verner JV, Morrison AB. Non-B islet tumors and the syndrome of watery diarrhea, hypokalemia, and hypochlorhydria. Clin Gastroenterol 1974;3:595–600.
82. Mekhjian HS, O'Dorisio TM. VIPoma syndrome. Semin Oncol 1987;14(3):282–291.
83. Long RG, Bryant MG, Mitchell SJ, Adrian TE, Polak JM, Bloom SR. Clinicopathological study of pancreatic and ganglioneuroblastoma tumours secreting vasoactive intestinal polypeptide (vipomas). Br Med J (Clin Res Ed) 1981;282(6278):1767–1771.
84. Ganda OP, Weir GC, Soeldner JS, et al. "Somatostatinoma": a somatostatin-containing tumor of the endocrine pancreas. N Engl J Med 1977;296(17):963–967.
85. Vinik AI, Strodel WE, Eckhauser FE, Moattari AR, Lloyd R. Somatostatinomas, PPomas, neurotensinomas. Semin Oncol 1987;14(3):263–281.
86. Kent RB 3rd, van Heerden JA, Weiland LH. Nonfunctioning islet cell tumors. Ann Surg 1981;193(2):185–190.
87. Maton PN, Gardner JD, Jensen RT. The incidence and etiology of Cushing's syndrome in patients with the Zollinger-Ellison syndrome. N Engl J Med 1986;315(1):1–5.
88. Chiang HC, O'Dorisio TM, Huang SC, Maton PN, Gardner JD, Jensen RT. Multiple hormone elevations in Zollinger–Ellison syndrome. Prospective study of clinical significance and of the development of a second symptomatic pancreatic endocrine tumor syndrome. Gastroenterology 1990;99(6):1565–1575.
89. Krausz Y, Bar-Ziv J, de Jong RB, et al. Somatostatin-receptor scintigraphy in the management of gastroenteropancreatic tumors. Am J Gastroenterol 1998;93(1):66–70.
90. Boden G. Insulinoma and glucagonoma. Semin Oncol 1987; 14:253–262.
91. Burch PG, McLeskey CH. Anesthesia for patients with insulinoma treatment with oral diazoxide. Anesthesiology 1981; 55(4):472–475.
92. Murakami K, Taniguchi H, Kobayshi T, Seki M, Olmon M, Baba S. Suppression of insulin release by calcium antagonist in human insulinoma in vivo and in vitro: its possible role for clinical use. Kobe J Med Sci 1979;25:237–247.
93. Comi RJ, Gorden P, Doppman JL. Insulinoma. New York: Raven, 1993.
94. Maton PN. The use of the long-acting somatostatin analogue, octreotide acetate, in patients with islet cell tumors. Gastroenterol Clin N Am 1989;18(4):897–922.
95. Doherty GM, Doppman JL, Shawker TH, et al. Results of a prospective strategy to diagnose, localize, and resect insulinomas. Surgery (St. Louis) 1991;110(6):989–996; discussion 996–997.
96. Maton PN, Frucht H, Vinayek R, et al. Medical management of patients with Zollinger–Ellison syndrome. Gastroenterology 1988;94:294–299.
97. Larsson H, Carlsson E, Matsson H. Plasma gastrin and gastric enterochromaffin cell activation and proliferation—studies with omeprazole and ranitidine in intact and adrenalectomized rats. Gastroenterology 1986;90:391–399.
98. Sutliff VE, Doppman JL, Gibril F, et al. Growth of newly diagnosed, untreated metastatic gastrinomas and predictors of growth patterns. J Clin Oncol 1997;15(6):2420–2431.
99. Norton JA, Doppman JL, Jensen RT. Curative resection in Zollinger–Ellison syndrome. Results of a 10-year prospective study. Ann Surg 1992;215(1):8–18.
100. Fraker DL, Norton JA, Alexander HR, Venzon DJ, Jensen RT. Surgery in Zollinger–Ellison syndrome alters the natural history of gastrinoma. Ann Surg 1994;220(3):320–328; discussion 328–330.
101. Jaskowiak NT, Fraker DL, Alexander HR, Norton JA, Doppman JL, Jensen RT. Is reoperation for gastrinoma excision indicated in Zollinger–Ellison syndrome? Surgery (St. Louis) 1996; 120(6):1055–1062; discussion 1062–1063.
102. Norton JA, Doherty GM, Fraker DL, et al. Surgical treatment of localized gastrinoma within the liver: a prospective study. Surgery (St. Louis) 1998;124(6):1145–1152.
103. MacFarlane MP, Fraker DL, Alexander HR, Norton JA, Lubensky I, Jensen RT. Prospective study of surgical resection of duodenal and pancreatic gastrinomas in multiple endocrine neoplasia type 1. Surgery (St. Louis) 1995;118(6):973–979; discussion 979–980.
104. Norton JA, Alexander HR, Fraker DL, Venzon DL, Gibril F, Jensen RT. Does the use of routine duodenectomy (DUODX) affect rates of cure, development of liver metastases, or survival in patients with Zollinger–Ellison syndrome? Ann Surg 2004;239(5):617–625.
105. Norton JA. Neuroendocrine tumors of the pancreas and duodenum. Curr Probl Surg 1994;31(2):77–156.
106. Roy RC, Carter RF, Wright KD. Somatostatin, anesthesia and the carcinoid syndrome. Perioperative administration of a somatostatin analogue to suppress carcinoid tumor activity. Anaesthesia 1987;42:627.
107. Fraker DL, Norton JA. The role of surgery in the management of islet cell tumors. Gastroenterol Clin N Am 1989;18(4):805–830.
108. Moertel CG, Lefkopoulo M, Lipsitz S, Hahn RG, Klaassen D. Streptozocin-doxorubicin, streptozocin-fluorouracil or chlorozotocin in the treatment of advanced islet-cell carcinoma [see comments]. N Engl J Med 1992;326(8):519–523.
109. Berwaerts J, Verhelst J, Hubens H, et al. Role of hepatic arterial embolisation in the treatment for metastatic insulinoma. Report of two cases and review of the literature. Acta Clin Belg 1997;52(5):263–274.
110. von Schrenck T, Howard JM, Doppman JL, et al. Prospective study of chemotherapy in patients with metastatic gastrinoma. Gastroenterology 1988;94:1326–1331.
111. Creutzfeldt W, Bartsch HH, Jacubaschke U, St Ëockmann F. Treatment of gastrointestinal endocrine tumours with interferon-alpha and octreotide. Acta Oncol 1991;30(4):529–535.
112. Zollinger RM, Martin EW Jr, Carey LC, Sparks J, Minton JP. Observations on the postoperative tumor growth behavior of certain islet cell tumors. Ann Surg 1976;184(4):525–530.

113. Carty SE, Jensen RT, Norton JA. Prospective study of aggressive resection of metastatic pancreatic endocrine tumors. Surgery (St. Louis) 1992;112(6):1024–1031; discussion 1031–1032.
114. Ollivier S, Fonck M, Becouarn Y, Brunet R. Dacarbazine, fluorouracil, and leucovorin in patients with advanced neuroendocrine tumors: a phase II trial. Am J Clin Oncol 1998;21(3): 237–240.
115. Eriksson B, Oberg K. Interferon therapy of malignant endocrine pancreatic tumors. Basel: Krager, 1995.
116. Sussman LA, Christie R, Whittle DE. Laparoscopic excision of distal pancreas including insulinoma. Aust N Z J Surg 1996;66(6):414–416.
117. Gagner M, Pomp A, Herrera MF. Early experience with laparoscopic resections of islet cell tumors. Surgery (St. Louis) 1996;120(6):1051–1054.
118. Gilligan CJ, Lawton GP, Tang LW, West AB, Modlin IM. Gastric carcinoid tumors: the biology and therapy of an enigmatic and controversial lesion. Am J Gastroenterol 1995;90(3):338–352.
119. Oberndorfer S. Uber die "kleinen dunndarm carcinome." Verh Dtsch Ges Pathol 1907;11:113–116.
120. Ranson WB. Case of primary carcinoma of the ileum. Lancet 1890;2:1020–1023.
121. Masson P. Carcinoids (argentaffin-cell tumors) and nerve hyperplasia of appendicular mucosa. Am J Pathol 1928;4:181–212.
122. Lembech F. 5-Hydroxytryptamine in carcinoid tumor. Nature (Lond) [Letter] 1953;172:910–911.
123. Page IH, Corcoran AC, Vollenfrend S, et al. Argentaffinoma as an endocrine tumor. Lancet 1955;1:198–199.
124. Buchanan KD, Johnston CF, O'Hare MM, et al. Neuroendocrine tumors. A European view. Am J Med 1986;81(6B):14–22.
125. Newton JN, Swerdlow AJ, dos Santos Silva IM, et al. The epidemiology of carcinoid tumours in England and Scotland. Br J Cancer 1994;70(5):939–942.
126. Lu Cortez L, Clemente C, Puig V, Mirada A. [Carcinoid tumor. An analysis of 131 cases]. Rev Clin Esp 1994;194(4):291–293.
127. Woods HF, Bax ND, Ainsworth I. Abdominal carcinoid tumours in Sheffield. Digestion 1990;45(suppl 1):17–22.
128. Watson RG, Johnston CF, O'Hare MM, et al. The frequency of gastrointestinal endocrine tumours in a well-defined population—Northern Ireland 1970–1985. Q J Med 1989;72(267):647–657.
129. Eriksson B. Recent advances in the diagnosis and management of endocrine pancreatic tumors. Acta Univer Ups 1988;160.
130. Weiss NS, Yang CP. Incidence of histologic types of cancer of the small intestine. J Natl Cancer Inst 1987;78:653.
131. Moertel CG, Suer WG, Docherty MG, et al. Life history of the carcinoid tumor of the small intestine. Cancer (Phila) 1961;14:901–905.
132. Moertel CG. Karnofsky memorial lecture. An odyssey in the land of small tumors. J Clin Oncol 1987;5(10):1502–1522.
133. Moertel CG, Docherty MB, Judd ES. Carcinoid tumors of the veriform appendix. Cancer (Phila) 1968;21:270.
134. Berge T, Linell F. Carcinoid tumours. Frequency in a defined population during a 12-year period. Acta Pathol Microbiol Scand A Pathol 1976;84(4):322–330.
135. Parkes SE, Muir KR, al Sheyyab M, et al. Carcinoid tumours of the appendix in children 1957–1986: incidence, treatment and outcome [see comments]. Br J Surg 1993;80(4):502–504.
136. Feldman JM. Carcinoid tumors and the carcinoid syndrome. Curr Probl Surg 1989;26(12):835–885.
137. Vinik AI, McLeod MK, Fig LM, Shapiro B, Lloyd RV, Cho K. Clinical features, diagnosis, and localization of carcinoid tumors and their management. Gastroenterol Clin N Am 1989;18(4):865–896.
138. Eller R, Frazee R, Roberts J. Gastrointestinal carcinoid tumors. Am Surg 1991;57(7):434–437.
139. Matsui K, Iwase T, Kitagawa M. Small, polypoid-appearing carcinoid tumors of the rectum: clinicopathologic study of 16 cases and effectiveness of endoscopic treatment. Am J Gastroenterol 1993;88(11):1949–1953.
140. Zeitels J, Naunheim K, Kaplan EL, Straus F. Carcinoid tumors: a 37-year experience. Arch Surg 1982;117:732–737.
141. Todd TR, Cooper JD, Weissberg D, Delarue NC, Peason FG. Bronchial carcinoid tumors: twenty years experience. J Thorac Cardiovasc Surg 1980;71:532–536.
142. Kloppel G, Heitz PU, Capella C, Solcia E. Pathology and nomenclature of human gastrointestinal neuroendocrine (carcinoid) tumors and related lesions. World J Surg 1996;20:132–141.
143. Creutzfeldt W. Historical background and natural history of carcinoids. Digestion 1994;55:3–12.
144. Pentilla IA. Histochemical reactions of the enterochromaffin cells and the 5-hydroxytryptamine content of the mammalian duodenum. Acta Physiol Scand 1966;74(suppl):218.
145. Soga J, Tazawa K. Pathologic analysis of carcinoids: histologic reevaluation of 62 cases. Cancer (Phila) 1971;28:990–998.
146. Johnson KA, Lavin PT, Moertel CG, et al. Carcinoids: the prognostic effect of primary site histologic variations. J Surg Oncol 1986;33:81–86.
147. Eriksson B, Oberg K. Peptide hormones as tumor markers in neuroendocrine gastrointestinal tumors. Acta Oncol 1991;30:477–485.
148. Creutzfeldt W. Carcinoid tumors: development of our knowledge. World J Surg 1996;20:126–131.
149. Williams ED, Sandler M. The classification of carcinoid tumors. Lancet 1963;1:238–239.
150. Zeiger MA, Swartz SE, MacGillvray DC, Linnoila I, Shakir M. Thymic carcinoid in association with MEN syndromes. Am Surg 1992;58:430–434.
151. Sagara M, Sugiyama F, Horiguchi H, et al. Activation of the nuclear oncogenes N-*myc* and c-*jun* in carcinoid tumors of transgenic mice carrying the human genome adenovirus type 12 E1 region gene. DNA Cell Biol 1995;14:95–101.
152. Kogan EA, Shtabskii AB, Sekamova SM, Sukhova NM, Mazurenko NN. Expression and co-expression of cellular oncogenes in the course of tumor progression in the course of neuroendocrine lung tumors. Arkh Patol 1994;56:16–21.
153. Wiedenmann B, Ahnert-Hilger G, Kvols KL, Riecken EO. New molecular aspects for the diagnosis and treatment of neuroendocrine gastroenteropancreatic tumors. Ann N Y Acad Sci 1994;733:515–522.
154. Dietrich WF, Radany EH, Smith JS, Bishop JM, Hanahan D, Lander ES. Genome-wide search for loss of heterozygosity in transgenic mouse tumors reveals candidate tumor suppressor genes on chromosomes 9 and 16. Proc Natl Acad Sci USA 1994;91:9451–9455.
155. Lohmann DR, Fesseler B, Putz B, et al. Infrequent mutation in the p53 gene in pulmonary carcinoid tumors. Cancer Res 1993; 53:5797–5801.
156. Wang DG, Johnston CF, Anderson N, Sloan JM, Buchanan KD. Overexpression of the tumor suppressor gene p53 is not implicated in neuroendocrine tumor carcinogenesis. J Pathol 1995;175:397–402.
157. O'Dowd G, Gosney JR. Absence of overexpression of p53 protein by intestinal carcinoid tumors. J Pathol 1995;175:403–404.
158. Freston JW. Omeprazole, hypergastrinemia, and gastric carcinoid tumors. Ann Intern Med 1994;121:232.
159. Jensen RT. Gastrinoma as a model for prolonged hypergastrinemia in man. In: Walsh JH, ed. Gastrin. New York: Raven Press, 1993:373.
160. Cadiot G, Laurent-Puig P, Thuille B, Lehy T, Mignon M, Olschwang S. Is the multiple endocrine neoplasia type 1 gene a suppressor for fundic argyrophil tumors in the Zollinger–Ellison syndrome? Gastroenterology 1993;105:579.
161. Gough DB, Thompson GB, Crotty TB, et al. Diverse clinical and pathologic features of gastric carcinoid and the relevance of hypergastrinemia. World J Surg 1994;18:473–478.

162. Goldman NC, Hood CI, Singleton GT. Carcinoid of the larynx. Arch Otolaryngol 1969;90:64–67.
163. Hughes JP, Ancalmo N, Leonard GL, Ochsner JL. Carcinoid tumor of the thymus gland: report of a case. Thorax 1975;30:470–475.
164. Robboy SJ, Norris HJ, Scully RE. Insular carcinoid primary in the ovary: a clinicopathologic analysis of 48 cases. Cancer (Phila) 1975;36:404–418.
165. Yalla SV, Yalla SS, Morgan JW, Eberhart CA, Olley JE. Primary argentaffinoma of the testis: a case report and survey of the literature. J Urol 1974;111:50–52.
166. Sylora HO, Diamond HM, Kaufman M, Straus F, Lyons ES. Primary carcinoid tumor of the urethra. J Urol 1975;114:150–153.
167. Porter JM, Kalloo AN, Abernathy EC, Yeo CJ. Carcinoid tumor of the gallbladder: laparoscopic resection and review of the literature. Surgery (St. Louis) 1992;112:100–105.
168. Davis Z, Moertel CG, McIlrath DC. The malignant carcinoid syndrome. Surg Gynecol Obstet 1973;137:637–642.
169. Godwin JD. Carcinoid tumors: an analysis of 2837 cases. Cancer (Phila) 1975;36:560–565.
170. Norheim I, Oberg K, Theodorsson-Norheim E, et al. Malignant carcinoid tumors. Ann Surg 1987;206:373–378.
171. Haq AU, Yook CR, Hiremath V, Kasimis BS. Carcinoid syndrome in the absence of liver metastasis: a case report and review of literature. Med Pediatr Oncol 1992;20:221–226.
172. Ahlman H, Dahlstrom A, Enerback L, et al. Two cases of gastric carcinoids; diagnostic and therapeutic aspects. World J Surg 1988;12:356–361.
173. Burke AH, Sobin LH, Federspiel BH, Shekitka KM, Helwing EB. Carcinoid tumor of the duodenum. Arch Pathol Lab Med 1990;114:700–705.
174. Rindi G, Luinetti O, Cornaggia M, Capella C, Solcia E. Three subtypes of the gastric argyrophil carcinoid and the gastric neuroendocrine carcinoma: a clinicopathologic study. Gastroenterology 1993;104:994–999.
175. Dusmet M, McNeally MF. Bronchial and thymic carcinoid tumors: a review. Digestion 1994;55:70–75.
176. Kema IP, deVries GE, Sloof MJH, Biesma B, Muskiet FAJ. Serotonin, catecholamines, histamine, and their metabolites in urine, platelets, and tumor tissue of patients with carcinoid tumors. Clin Chem 1994;40:86–91.
177. Rosenberg JC. Carcinoid and other amine-producing tumors. Prog Clin Cancer 1966;2:297–308.
178. Feldman JM. Carcinoid tumors and syndrome. Semin Oncol 1987;14:237.
179. Becker M, Aron DC. Ectopic ACTH syndrome and CRH-mediated Cushing's syndrome. Endocrinol Metab Clin N Am 1994;23:585.
180. Thorson AH. Studies on carcinoid disease. Acta Med Scand 1958;334:81–85.
181. Oates JA, Sjoerdsma A. A unique syndrome associated with secretion of 5-hydroxytryptophan by metastatic gastric carinoids. Am J Med 1962;32:333–339.
182. Grahame-Smith DG. What is the cause of the carcinoid flush? Gut 1987;28:1413–1416.
183. Matuchansky C, Luanay JM. Serotonin, catecholamines, and spontaneous midgut carcinoid flush: plasma studies from flushing and nonflushing sites. Gastroenterology 1995;108(3):743–751.
184. Creutzfeldt W, Stockman F. The carcinoid syndrome. Am J Med 1987;82(suppl 58):4.
185. Roberts LJ, Marney SRj, Oates JA. Blockade of the flush associated with metastatic gastric carcinoid by combined H1 and H2 receptor antagonists: evidence for an important role of H2 receptors in human vasculature. N Engl J Med 1979;300:236–238.
186. Oates JA. The carcinoid syndrome. N Engl J Med 1986;315:702–707.
187. Vinik AI, Gonin J, England BG, Jackson T, McLeod MK, Cho K. Plasma substance-P in neuroendocrine tumors and idiopathic flushing: the value of pentagastrin stimulation tests and the effects of the somatostatin analog. J Clin Endocrinol Metab 1990;70:172–179.
188. Lucas KJ, Feldman JM. Flushing in the carcinoid syndrome and plasma kallikrein. Cancer (Phila) 1986;58:2290–2293.
189. Gustafsen J, Boesby S, Nielsen F, Giese J. Bradykinin in carcinoid syndrome. Gut 1987;28:1417–1419.
190. Furchgott RF, Zawadski JV. The obligatory role of endothelial cells in the relaxation of arterial smooth muscle by acetylcholine. Nature (Lond) 1980;288:373–376.
191. Feldman JM, Plank JW. Gastrointestinal and metabolic function in patients with the carcinoid syndrome. Am J Med Sci 1977;273:43.
192. Schworer H, Munke H, Stockman F, Ramadori G. Treatment of diarrhea in carcinoid syndrome with ondansetron, topisetron, and clonidine. Am J Gastroenterol 1995;56:645–652.
193. Pelikka PA, Tajik J, Khandheria BK, et al. Carcinoid heart disease: clinical and echocardiographic spectrum in 74 patients. Circulation 1993;87:1188.
194. Lundin L. Carcinoid heart disease. Acta Oncol 1991;30:499–503.
195. Herxheimer H. Influence of 5-hydroxytryptamine on bronchial function. J Physiol 1953;122:49.
196. Cotran RS, Kumar V, Robbins SL. Nutritional disease. In: Cotran RS, Kumar V, Robbins SL, eds. Robbins Pathologic Basis of Disease, 4th ed. Philadelphia: Saunders, 1989:435–467.
197. Wilkin JK. Flushing reactions: consequences and mechanisms. Ann Intern Med 1981;95:468.
198. Tormey WP, Fitzgerald RJ. The clinical and laboratory correlates of an increased urinary 5-hydroxyindoleactic acid. Postgrad Med J 1995;71:542–545.
199. Feldman JM, Lee EM. Serotonin content of foods: effect on urinary excretion of 5-hydroxyindoleacetic acid. Am J Clin Nutr 1985;42:639–643.
200. Feldman JM. Urinary serotonin in the diagnosis of carcinoid tumors. Clin Chem 1986;32:840–845.
201. Feldman JM, O'Dorisio TM. The role of neuropeptides and serotonin in the diagnosis of carcinoid tumors. Am J Med 1986;81:41.
202. Stridsberg M, Oberg K, Li Q, Engstrom U, Lundqvist G. Measurements of chromagranin A, chromagranin B (secretogranin I), chromagranin C (secretogranin II) and pancreastatin in plasma and urine from patients with carcinoid tumours and endocrine pancreatic tumors. J Endocrinol 1995;114:49.
203. Wallace S, Agani JA, Charnsangavej C, et al. Carcinoid tumor: images, procedures and interventional radiology. World J Surg 1996;20:147–156.
204. Kisker O, Weinel RJ, Geks J, Zacara F, Joseph K, Rothmund M. Value of somatostatin receptor scintigraphy for preoperative localization of carcinoids. World J Surg 1996;20:162–167.
205. Nessi R, Ricci D, Ricci SB, Bosco M, Blanc M. Bronchial carcinoid tumors: radiologic observations in 49 cases. J Thorac Imaging 1991;6:47–52.
206. Davies MG, O'Dowd GO, McEntee GP, Hennessey TPJ. Primary gastric carcinoid tumors: a view on management. Br J Surg 1990;77:1013.
207. Thompson GB, van Heerden JA, Martin JK, et al. Carcinoid tumors of the gastrointestinal tract: presentation, management and prognosis. Surgery (St. Louis) 1985;98:1054–1059.
208. Rioux M, Langis P, Naud F. Sonographic appearance of small bowel carcinoid tumor. Abdom Imaging 1995;20:37–43.
209. Andersson T, Eriksson B, Lindgren PG, Wilander E, Oberg K. Percutaneous ultrasonography-guided cutting biopsy from liver metastases of endocrine gastrointestinal tumors. Ann Surg 1987;206:728–732.

210. Yoshida M, Tsukamoto Y, Niwa Y, et al. Endoscopic assessment of invasion of colorectal tumors with a new high frequency ultrasound probe. Gastrointest Endosc 1995;41:587–592.
211. Yoshikane H, Tsukamoto Y, Niwa Y, et al. Carcinoid tumors of the gastrointestinal tract: evaluation with endoscopic ultrasonography. Gastrointest Endosc 1993;39:375–383.
212. Sugimoto E, Lorelius LE, Eriksson B, Oberg K. Midgut carcinoid tumors. Acta Radiol 1995;36:367–374.
213. Westlin JE, Janson ET, Arnberg H, Ahlstrom H, Oberg K, Nilsson S. Somatostatin receptor scintigraphy of carcinoid tumors using the [^{111}In-DTPA-D-Phe^{1}]-octreotide. Acta Oncol 1993;32:783.
214. Makridis C, Oberg K, Juhlin C, et al. Surgical treatment of midgut carcinoid tumors. World J Surg 1990;14:377–383.
215. Collatz L, Stage JG, Henriksen FW. Angiography in the diagnosis of carcinoid syndrome. Scand J Gastroenterol 1979;53:111–116.
216. Reubi JC, Laissue J, Waser B, Horisberger U, Schaer JC. Expression of somatostatin receptors in normal, inflamed, and neoplastic human gastrointestinal tissue. Ann N Y Acad Sci 1994;733:122.
217. Modlin IM, Cornelius E, Lawton GP. Use of an isotopic somatostatin probe to image gut endocrine tumors. Arch Surg 1995;130:367–373.
218. Orlefors H, Sundin A, Garske U, et al. Whole-body (11)C-5-hydroxytryptophan positron emission tomography as a universal imaging technique for neuroendocrine tumors: comparison with somatostatin receptor scintigraphy and computed tomography. J Clin Endocrinol Metab 2005;90:3392–3400.
219. Hanson MW, Feldman JM, Blinder RH, Moore JO, Coleman RE. Carcinoid tumors: iodine^{131}I MIBG scintigraphy. Radiology 1989;172:699.
220. Feldman JM, Plunk JW. ^{99m}Tc-pyrophosphate bone scans in patients with metastatic carcinoid tumors. J Med 1977;8:71.
221. McDermott EWM, Guduric B, Brennan MF. Prognostic variables in patients with gastrointestinal carcinoid tumors. Br J Surg 1994;81:1007–1009.
222. Agranovich AL, Anderson GH, Manji M, Acker BD, MacDonald WC, Threlfall WJ. Carcinoid tumor of the gastrointestinal tract: prognostic factors and disease outcome. J Surg Oncol 1991;47:45.
223. MacGillivary DG, Snyder DA, Druker W, Remine SR. Carcinoid tumors: the relationship between clinical presentation and the extent of disease. Surgery (St. Louis) 1991;110:68.
224. Haselton PS. Histopathology and prognostic factors in bronchial carcinoid tumours. Thorax 1994;49:S56.
225. Strodel WE, Talpos G, Eckhauser F, Thompson N. Surgical therapy for small bowel carcinoid tumors. Arch Surg 1983;118:391–397.
226. Federspiel BH, Burke AP, Sokin LH, Shekitka KM. Rectal and colonic carcinoids. Cancer (Phila) 1990;65:135–139.
227. Caldarola VT, Jackman RJ, Moertel CG. Carcinoid tumors of the rectum. Am J Surg 1964;107:844–848.
228. Deans GT, Spence RA. Neoplastic lesions of the appendix. Br J Surg 1995;82:299–306.
229. Warner RRP, Mani S, Profeta J, Grunstein E. Octreotide treatment of carcinoid hypertensive crisis. Mt Sinai Med J 1994;61:349–355.
230. Reichlin S. Somatostatin. N Engl J Med 1983;309:1495–1501.
231. Kvols LK, Martin JK, Marsh HM, Moertel CG. Rapid reversal of carcinoid crisis with a somatostatin analog [letter]. N Engl J Med 1985;313:1229.
232. Kvols LK. Therapy of malignant carcinoid syndrome. Endocrinol Metab Clin N Am 1989;18:557.
233. Arnold R, Frank M, Kajdan U. Management of gastroenteropancreatic endocrine tumors: the place of somatostatin analogues. Digestion 1994;55:107.
234. Oberg K. Neuroendocrine tumors of the gastrointestinal tract: recent advances in molecular genetics, diagnosis and treatment. Curr Opin Oncol 2005;17(4):386–391.
235. Oberg K, Funa K, Alm G. Effects of leukocyte interferon on clinical symptoms and hormone levels in patients with midgut carcinoid tumors and the carcinoid syndrome. N Engl J Med 1983;309:129–133.
236. Hanssen LE, Schrumpf E, Klobenstiedt AN, Tausjo J, Dolva LO. Treatment of metastatic midgut carcinoid tumors with recombinant human alpha 2b interferon with or without prior hepatic artery embolization. Scand J Gastroenterol 1989;24:787–795.
237. Oberg K, Norheim I, Lind E, et al. The treatment of malignant carcinoid tumors with human leukocyte interferon: long term results. Cancer Treat 1986;70:1297–1304.
238. Norbin A, Lindblom A, Mansson B, Sundbert M. Interferon treatment in patients with malignant carcinoids. Acta Oncol 1989;28:445–449.
239. Ramage JK, Catnach SM, Williams R. Overview: the management of metastatic carcinoid tumors. Liver Transplant Surg 1995;1:107.
240. Janson ET, Kauppinen HL, Oberg K. Combined alpha and gamma interferon therapy for malignant midgut carcinoids: a phase II trial. Acta Oncol 1993;32:231–233.
241. Ahren B, Engman K, Lindblom A. Tolerance to long-term treatment of malignant midgut carcinoid with a highly purified human leukocyte alpha-interferon. Anticancer Res 1992;12:881–884.
242. Gregor M. Therapeutic principles in the management of metastasising carcinoid tumors: drugs for symptomatic treatment. Digestion 1994;55:60.
243. Robertson JIS. Carcinoid syndrome and serotonin: therapeutic effect of ketanserin. Cardiovasc Drugs Therapy 1990;4:53–56.
244. Schworer H, Munke H, Stockmann F, Ramadori G. Treatment of diarrhea in carcinoid syndrome with ondansetron, tropisetron and clonidine. Am J Gastroenterol 1995;90:645–648.
245. Maton PN, Hodgson HJF. Carcinoid tumours and the carcinoid syndrome. In: Bouchier IAD, Allan RN, Hodgson HJF, Keighly MRB, eds. Textbook of Gastroenterology. London: Balliere-Tindall, 1984:620.
246. Oberg K, Erikson B. The role of interferons in the management of carcinoid tumors. Acta Oncol 1991;30:519.
247. Moertel CG, Hanley JA. Combination chemotherapy trials in metastatic carcinoid and malignant carcinoid syndrome. Cancer Clin Trials 1979;2:327–330.
248. Kelsen DG, Cheng E, Kemeny N, Magill GB, Yagoda A. Streptozotocin and adriamycin in the treatment of APUD tumors (carcinoid, islet cell and medullary thyroid). Proc Am Assoc Cancer Res 1982;23:433.
249. Janson ET, Ronnblom L, Ahlstrom H, et al. Treatment with alpha interferon versus alpha interferon in combination with streptozocin and doxorubicin in patients with malignant carcinoid tumors: a randomized trial. Ann Oncol 1992;3:635–638.
250. Saltz L, Kemeny N, Schwartz G, Kelsen D. A phase II trial of alpha interferon and 5-fluorouracil in patients with advanced carcinoid and islet cell tumors. Cancer (Phila) 1994;74:958–961.
251. Khoury GA, Devine J, Bolt DE. Complete liver dearterialisation and the carcinoid syndrome. Br J Surg 1979;66:253–256.
252. McDermott WV, Hersle TW. Metastatic carcinoid to the liver treated by hepatic dearterialisation. Ann Surg 1974;180:305–308.
253. Winkelbauer FW, Niederle B, Pietschmann F, et al. Hepatic artery embolectomy of hepatic metastases from carcinoid tumors: value of using a cranacrylate and ethiodized oil. Am J Roentgenol 1995;165:323–327.

254. Maton PN, Camilleri M, Griffin G, Allison DJ, Hodgson HJ, Chadwick VS. Role of hepatic artery embolization in the carcinoid syndrome. Br Med J 1983;287:932–935.
255. Mitty HA, Warner RR, Newman LH, Train J, Parnes IH. Control of carcinoid syndrome with hepatic artery embolization. Radiology 1985;155:623–626.
256. Marlink RG, Lakich JJ, Robins JR, Clouse ME. Hepatic arterial embolization for metastatic hormone secreting tumors. Cancer (Phila) 1991;65:2227–2231.
257. Norbin A, Mansson B, Lunderquist A. Evaluation of temporary liver dearterialization and embolization in patients with metastatic carcinoid tumors. Acta Oncol 1989;28:419.
258. Moertel CG, Johnson CM, McKusick MA, et al. The management of patients with advanced carcinoid tumors and islet cell carcinomas. Ann Intern Med 1994;120:302.
259. Stokes KR, Stuart K, Clouse ME. Hepatic arterial chemoembolization for metastatic endocrine tumors. J Vasc Intervent Radiol 1993;4:341.
260. Therasse E, Breittmayer F, Roche A, et al. Transcatheter chemoembolization of progressive carcinoid liver metastasis. Radiology 1993;189:541.
261. Chakravarthy A, Abrams RA. Radiation therapy in the management of patients with malignant carcinoid tumors. Cancer (Phila) 1995;75:1386–1390.
262. Loftus JP, van Heerden JA. Surgical management of gastrointestinal carcinoid tumors. Adv Surg 1995;28:317–336.
263. Rothmund M, Kister O. Surgical treatment of carcinoid tumors of the small bowel, appendix, colon and rectum. Digestion 1995;55:86.
264. Norton JA. Surgical management of carcinoid tumors: role of debulking and surgery in patients with advanced disease. Digestion 1995;55(suppl 3):98–103.
265. Stinner B, Kisker O, Zielke A, Rothmund M. Surgical management of carcinoid tumor of small bowel, appendix, colon and rectum. World J Surg 1996;20:183–188.
266. Sauven P, Ridge JE, Quan SH, Siguardson ER. Anorectal carcinoid tumors: is aggressive surgery warranted? Ann Surg 1990;211:67–71.
267. Makridis C, Oberg K, Juhlin C, et al. Surgical treatment of midgut carcinoid tumors. World J Surg 1990;14:377.
268. Naunheim KS, Zeitel J, Kaplan EL, et al. Rectal carcinoid tumors: treatment and prognosis. Surgery (St. Louis) 1983;94: 670.
269. Norton JA, Melcher ML, Gibril F, Jensen RT. Gastric carcinoid tumors in multiple endocrine neoplasia-1 patients with Zollinger–Ellison syndrome can be symptomatic, demonstrate aggressive growth, and require surgical treatment. Surgery (St. Louis) 2004;136(6):1267–1274.
270. Hausman MS Jr, Thompson NW, Gauger PG, Doherty GM. The surgical management of MEN 1 pancreatoduodenal neuroendocrine disease. Surgery (St. Louis) 2004;136:1205–1211.
271. Foster JH, Berman MM. Solid liver tumors. Major Probl Surg 1977;22:1–342.
272. Norton JA, Warren RS, Kelly MG, Zuraek MB, Jensen RT. Aggressive surgery for metstatic liver neuroendocrine tumors. Surgery (St. Louis) 2003;134(6):1057–1063.
273. Nagorney DM, Que FG. Cytoreductive hepatic surgery for metastatic gastrointestinal neuroendocrine tumors. In: Mignon M, Jensen RT, eds. Endocrine Tumors of the Pancreas: Recent Advances in Research and Management. Basel: Karger, 1995:416.
274. Frilling A, Rogiers X, Knofel WT, Broelsch CE. Liver transplantation for metastatic carcinoid tumors. Digestion 1994;55(suppl 3):104–106.

59

Multiple Endocrine Neoplasia

Terry C. Lairmore

Cancer Genetics

Cancer is a genetic disease. Neoplastic transformation is characterized by a stepwise accumulation of genetic damage within a cell that results in the acquisition of increasingly more aggressive and uncontrolled growth properties. Most sporadic cancers result from the chance occurrence of multiple *somatic* mutations within an individual cell. Patients with one of the rare familial cancer syndromes have a predisposition to tumor development that is conferred by the inheritance of a cancer-associated mutation in the *germline* DNA.

Genetic alterations in one of three broad categories of genes are associated with neoplastic transformation: these include proto-oncogenes, tumor suppressor genes, and DNA mismatch repair genes. Mutation in one allele of a proto-oncogene, the normal cellular copy of the gene, results in an oncogene that encodes a protein product with abnormal function or inappropriate expression. Mutations in proto-oncogenes result in a *gain-of-function* that confers oncogenic potential in a dominant fashion. In contrast, tumor suppressor genes encode proteins that normally exert a negative control on cellular growth. A combination of gene mutation and/or chromosome deletion resulting in the inactivation of both copies of the tumor suppressor gene results in a *loss-of-function* that leads to unregulated cellular growth and division and neoplastic transformation. *Loss-of-function* mutations in a third category of genes that normally function in DNA damage recognition and repair (DNA mismatch repair genes) have also been described.

Hereditary Cancer Syndromes

Cancers that arise in association with a familial cancer syndrome are characterized by an early age at onset, the occurrence of multiple tumors in a single organ, and the simultaneous development of tumors in multiple target tissues. Importantly, understanding the molecular mechanisms responsible for cancer predisposition in the relatively rare hereditary cancer syndromes sheds important light on the common genetic defects that are responsible for the development of sporadic tumors in the same tissues. For example, somatic *ret* mutations are present in a subset of sporadic medullary thyroid carcinomas (MTCs),[1,2] and mutations in the multiple endocrine neoplasia type 1 (*MEN1*) gene are responsible for the development of some sporadic parathyroid adenomas.[3]

Advances in our understanding of the molecular oncogenesis of familial endocrine neoplasms have had a measurable impact on the clinical management of patients with the multiple endocrine neoplasia syndromes. The identification of mutations in the *ret* proto-oncogene in patients with multiple endocrine neoplasia types 2A and 2B has allowed the development of direct DNA testing for at-risk individuals. Patients who have inherited a *ret* mutation may be treated by early thyroidectomy at an age when the MTC is confined to the thyroid gland and therefore curable[4]. The identification of the *MEN1* gene has allowed the development of direct genetic testing for family members at risk for MEN 1. The ability to make an early genetic diagnosis places new emphasis on optimal cancer surveillance, biochemical screening, and early surgical intervention for the neuroendocrine tumors of the pancreas and duodenum that are responsible for most of the disease-related morbidity and mortality.

Multiple Endocrine Neoplasia Type 1

Clinical Features

Multiple endocrine neoplasia type 1 is characterized by the development of parathyroid neoplasms, neuroendocrine tumors of the pancreas and duodenum, and pituitary adenomas. In addition, bronchial and thymic carcinoids, benign thyroid tumors, benign and malignant adrenocortical tumors, lipomas, ependymomas of the central nervous system (CNS),[5] and cutaneous angiofibromas[6] occur with increased frequency in patients with MEN 1. Clinically, MEN 1 is usually defined as the occurrence of neoplasms in at least two endocrine tissues (parathyroid, endocrine pancreas, pituitary) in an individual, and familial MEN 1 is defined as the occurrence of at least one tumor type in a first-degree relative.

Hyperparathyroidism

More than 98% of individuals with MEN 1 ultimately develop primary hyperparathyroidism (HPT) as a result of multiglandular parathyroid disease. Genetically, the parathyroid tumors are most accurately defined as multiple adenomas, resulting from the occurrence of "two hits" in a parathyroid cell.[7,8] The clinical features of HPT in patients with MEN 1 include a prolonged early phase of asymptomatic hypercalcemia, generally low morbidity, and the infrequent development of severe renal or bone disease. When compared to sporadic HPT, patients with MEN 1 generally develop hypercalcemia at a markedly earlier age. The cumulative age-related penetrance for expression of MEN 1 (with HPT being the most consistent feature) has been estimated to be 7% at age less than 10 years, 52% at age 20 years, and 87% at age 30 years.[9] Recently, prospective biochemical screening of genetically positive patients has demonstrated that the onset of hypercalcemia occurs as early as age 11 to 14 years.[10] Owing to the autosomal dominant pattern of inheritance for MEN 1, males and females are affected nearly equally.

The parathyroid gland enlargement in patients with MEN 1 is typically asymmetrical,[8,11] and it is not uncommon to find only two or three enlarged glands with the remaining parathyroid glands grossly normal in appearance. This morphological pattern likely reflects the metachronous development of "second hits," with the resulting cellular expansion leading to a parathyroid neoplasm. In a strict genetic sense, these neoplasms are best defined as multiple adenomas.[8]

Neuroendocrine Tumors of the Pancreas and Duodenum

Depending on the method of study, 35% to 75% of patients with MEN 1 develop clinically evident neuroendocrine tumors (NET) of the pancreas and duodenum, but microscopic islet cell neoplasia is evident in essentially 100% of patients at necropsy.[12] These tumors cause symptoms as a result of either hormone oversecretion or the mass effects from tumor growth itself. The NET of the pancreas and duodenum, along with the malignant intrathoracic carcinoids, cause most of the disease-related mortality in patients with MEN 1.[13,14]

Gastrinoma

Gastrinoma is the most common functional NET associated with the MEN 1 syndrome (Table 59.1). Gastrinomas in patients with MEN 1 are located within the "gastrinoma triangle"[15] and are frequently extrapancreatic, occurring either in the wall of the duodenum[16–18] or within peripancreatic lymph nodes. There is controversy about the development of "primary gastrinoma" within lymph nodes.[19–21] Although occasional patients have been biochemically cured after resection of gastrinomas within lymph nodes,[19–22] it is unclear whether an occult gastrinoma primary was missed within the pancreas or wall of the duodenum.[16,18]

TABLE 59.1. Endocrine Tumors Expressed in 130 Patients with Multiple Endocrine Neoplasia Type 1 Admitted to the National Institutes of Health[a]

Tumor	*Patients, n (%)*
Tumor in principal MEN 1-related organ	
Parathyroid tumor	129 (99)
Enteropancreatic neuroendocrine tumor	86 (66)
Gastrinoma	61 (47)
Insulinoma	15 (12)
Nonfunctioning tumor[b]	5 (4)
Other[c]	5 (4)
Pituitary tumor	61 (47)
Prolactinoma	34 (26)
Nonfunctioning tumor	14 (11)
Corticotropinoma	9 (7)
Somatotropinoma	4 (3)
Tumor in organ possibly related to MEN 1	
Carcinoid	21 (16)
Bronchial	11 (8)
Gastric	9 (7)
Thymic	1 (1)
Adrenocortical tumor	21 (16)
Nonfunctioning	14 (11)
Functioning	7 (5)
Thyroid tumor	16 (12)
Follicular adenoma	10 (8)
Papillary carcinoma	6 (5)

MEN 1, multiple endocrine neoplasia type 1.
[a]Each tumor type was scored only once per patient.
[b]Excludes multiple "nonfunctioning" islet tumors that were encountered incidental to each pancreatic operation for MEN 1.
[c]Other, glucagonoma, somatostatinoma, and VIP (vasoactive intestinal peptide)oma.
Source: Reproduced with permission from Marx et al.[42]

The diagnosis of Zollinger–Ellison syndrome is made by the finding of an inappropriately elevated fasting serum gastrin level in association with gastric acid hypersecretion. The diagnostic criteria for gastric acid hypersecretion include a basal acid output (BAO) of greater than 15 mEq/h in patients with no history of gastric surgery or greater than 5 mEq/h in patients with prior gastric surgery for peptic ulcer disease, and an elevated serum gastrin level (>100 pg/mL). The diagnosis may be confirmed by an abnormal secretin stimulation test. A positive test is present when serum levels of gastrin rise more than 200 pg/mL following the intravenous administration of secretin (2 U/kg). Patients with Zollinger–Ellison syndrome frequently present with pain in the epigastrium,[18,23,24] reflux esophagitis,[25,26] weight loss, and secretory diarrhea. Although some degree of peptic ulcer disease is identifiable in approximately 70% to 80% of patients, a severe ulcer diathesis is infrequent in the current era. Control of the acid hypersecretion is usually achievable with medical treatment either with potent H_2-receptor antagonists or proton pump inhibitors. The acid output should be maintained at levels less than 5 mEq/h at all times. Very high doses of antisecretory medicines may be required to eliminate the gastric acid hypersecretion in patients with ZES.

Approximately 15% to 50% of patients with gastrinoma have liver metastases at the time of diagnosis.[27] A cross-sectional imaging test such as computed tomography (CT) scanning or magnetic resonance imaging (MRI) should be performed to rule out obvious liver metastases. Gastrinomas within the duodenal wall or pancreas may be occult and difficult to localize by radiographic imaging tests. Noninvasive imaging tests such as ultrasound, CT, MRI, and somatostatin receptor scintigraphy (SRS; octreotide scanning) have a relatively low sensitivity for imaging primary gastrinomas. However, SRS has been demonstrated to be as sensitive as all other imaging studies combined and is the imaging study of choice for gastrinoma in MEN 1. Pancreaticoduodenal angiography with selective intraarterial injection of secretin and measurement of the gastrin gradient in the hepatic veins has been reported to be a very accurate method to regionally localize gastrinoma.[28] Endoscopic ultrasonography is also an excellent imaging modality for localizing small gastrinomas within the duodenal wall or head of the pancreas, but the success of this test is dependent on the skill and experience of the operator.

The indications for and efficacy of surgical treatment for gastrinoma in patients with MEN 1 are controversial. Owing to the multiplicity and occult nature of gastrinomas in patients with MEN 1, localized surgical resection rarely results in long-term normalization of gastrin levels.[29–31] Weber and coworkers suggested a relationship between the size of the primary gastrinoma and the frequency of lymph node and hepatic metastases.[32] However, a study of all neuroendocrine tumors arising in patients with MEN 1 failed to show any relationship between the diameter of the largest tumor and the presence of metastases.[33] The availability of proton pump inhibitors allows effective medical therapy for patients with unresectable gastrinoma or extensive metastatic disease. However, careful observation of the stomach by repeated endoscopy is necessary because long-term administration of proton pump inhibitors to patients with MEN 1 and ZES has been associated with the development of gastric carcinoid tumors.[34]

Although most evidence indicates that patients with ZES and MEN 1 are rarely cured biochemically by surgery,[35] localized resection of a potentially malignant neuroendocrine tumor may be indicated in an attempt to control the tumoral process and prevent subsequent malignant dissemination. The more recent recognition that gastrinomas occur frequently in the duodenal wall combined with a focused surgical approach[36] to localize and remove these occult tumors, as well as the performance of an extended regional lymphadenectomy, may improve the success rate of surgery for ZES. Total gastrectomy is rarely indicated currently for patients with gastrinoma, because medical management effectively controls all symptoms related to acid hypersecretion.

Insulinoma

The second most common functional pancreatic neuroendocrine tumor in patients with MEN 1 is insulinoma (see Table 59.1). The clinical elements needed for making the diagnosis of insulinoma are the signs and symptoms of neuroglycopenia during fasting (anxiety, tremor, confusion, sweating, seizure, syncope), profound hypoglycemia, and alleviation of symptoms after the administration of glucose. These bizarre complaints may initially be attributed to malingering or psychiatric illness unless the association with fasting is recognized. Patients with insulinoma commonly gain weight. Factitious hypoglycemia (intentional exogenous insulin administration) and postprandial reactive hypoglycemia must be excluded.

The biochemical diagnosis of insulinoma is best established during a supervised fast with the measurement of plasma levels of glucose, insulin, proinsulin, and C-peptide. Patients with insulinoma develop neuroglycopenic symptoms and have inappropriately elevated plasma insulin (greater than 5 μU/mL) associated with profound hypoglycemia (glucose <40 mg/dL). Sulfonylureas should also be measured to exclude the surreptitious administration of oral hypoglycemic drugs. The finding of elevated C-peptide at the termination of the fast also supports the presence of abnormal insulin secretion from an endogenous source. Preoperative regional localization of insulinoma within the pancreas can be accomplished by selective catheterization of the arteries supplying the pancreas, injection of an insulin secretagogue (calcium gluconate) and measurement of insulin gradients in a hepatic vein.[37,38] Intraoperative ultrasound greatly facilitates the identification of small tumors, especially within the pancreatic head or uncinate process.[39–41] The treatment for insulinomas is accurate localization and resection to control the potentially life-threatening hyperinsulinemia.

Neuroendocrine tumors that secrete vasoactive intestinal peptide (VIP), glucagon, or somatostatin occur less frequently. These tumors produce characteristic syndromes depending on the specific hormone produced.

Extrapancreatic Carcinoid Tumors

Bronchial carcinoid tumors occur in approximately 8% of patients with MEN 1.[42] An increased representation of foregut carcinoids has been described in patients with MEN 1 as compared with the distribution of sporadic carcinoids.[43] The malignant enteropancreatic tumors and intrathoracic tumors account for the majority of the disease-related morbidity and mortality in *MEN1* mutation carriers.[13,14]

Pituitary Tumors

Adenomas of the anterior pituitary gland occur in 16% to 65% of patients with MEN 1.[42] The most frequent pituitary tumor in patients with MEN 1 is prolactinoma. Medical treatment with bromocriptine or cabergoline is effective in controlling the hyperprolactinemia in most patients. Transphenoidal pituitary microsurgery is indicated infrequently for rapidly enlarging macroadenomas that are unresponsive to medical therapy or result in local compressive symptoms owing to their mass effect. Cushing's disease caused by an ACTH-producing pituitary tumor may also occur in the MEN 1 syndrome.

Other Features

Other tumors that occur with increased frequency in patients with MEN 1 include benign and malignant tumors of the thyroid, macronodular adrenocortical hyperplasia, multiple subcutaneous lipomas, facial angiofibromas, collagenomas of the skin, and ependymomas of the CNS[42] (see Table 59.1).

Genetics of MEN 1

MEN1 Tumor Suppressor Gene

The recently identified *MEN1* tumor suppressor gene is located on human chromosome 11 and encodes a predicted

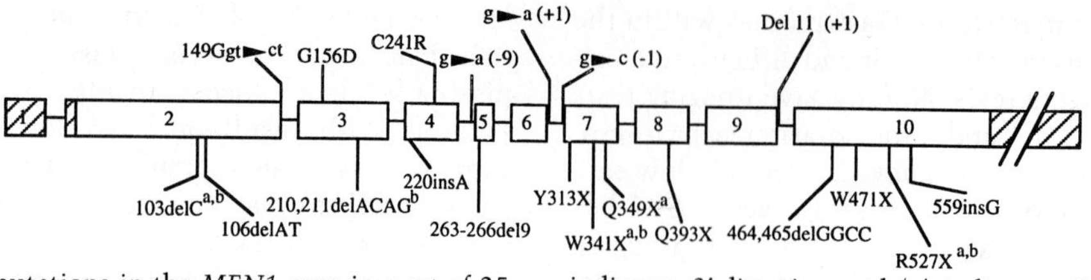

FIGURE 59.1. Germline mutations in the *MEN1* gene in a set of 25 independent kindreds. The mutations are distributed throughout the nine coding exons of the gene. Five splicing defects and two missense mutations are depicted above the *MEN1* gene, and seven nonsense and six frameshift mutations are depicted below the *MEN1* gene. The position of the mutation is reported as the codon in which it occurs relative to the open reading frame. The position of the splicing defects are reported as the number of bases 3′ or 5′ to the nearest exon [(+) indicates 3′-direction and (−) indicates 5′-direction relative to the exon]. For the deletions, insertions, and splicing defects, *uppercase letters* refer to exon nucleotides and *lowercase letters* refer to intron nucleotides. a, Previously reported mutations; b, mutations that occur in more than one family. (Reproduced with permission from Mutch et al.[46] Reprinted with permission of Wiley-Liss, Inc., a subsidiary of John Wiley & Sons, Inc.)

610-amino-acid protein product termed menin.[44] The *MEN1* RNA transcript is ubiquitously expressed in lymphocytes, thymus, pancreas, thyroid, the gonads, and other tissues. Menin has no significant sequence similarity to other known proteins. As is true for the products of most previously described tumor suppressor genes, evidence has been provided that menin is a nuclear protein.[45] There are two nuclear localization signals (NLSs) in the 3′-portion of menin that are believed to be responsible for the translocation of the protein to its appropriate subcellular localization in the nucleus of the cell.

The diverse array of *MEN1* mutations includes missense, nonsense, frameshift, and mRNA splicing defects that are distributed throughout the nine coding exons[46] (Fig. 59.1). Approximately two-thirds of the reported mutations in the *MEN1* gene result in truncation of the C-terminal portion of the menin protein and loss of one or more of the putative NLSs. No specific genotype–phenotype correlations have been established to date.[47,48]

Cellular Biology of Menin Protein Product

MEN 1 is caused by the functional loss of the tumor suppressor protein menin. The protein sequence has no significant homology to known consensus motifs. In vitro studies have shown physical binding of menin to various proteins including JunD, Pem, Smad3, NF-kappaB, and nm23H1.[49–54] However, none of these binding studies has led to a convincing theory of how loss of menin leads to neoplasia.

Agarwal and coworkers[49] have identified the transcription factor JunD as a protein that interacts directly with menin. Several previously described *MEN1* missense mutations were shown to disrupt menin interaction with JunD. These observations suggest that the menin tumor suppressor function involves inhibition of JunD-activated transcription.

Evaluation and Management of Endocrine Neoplasia in Patients with MEN 1

Hyperparathyroidism

The ideal surgical treatment for hyperparathyroidism in patients with MEN 1 results in the lowest incidence of recurrent hypercalcemia, while minimizing the complication of permanent hypocalcemia. Because patients with MEN 1 have multiple gland involvement of the parathyroids, there is a significantly higher rate of recurrent or persistent hyperparathyroidism[55–59] after parathyroidectomy when compared to the results for the treatment of sporadic parathyroid adenoma. The appropriate initial surgical procedure for patients with MEN 1 is either total four-gland parathyroidectomy with intramuscular autotransplantation of parathyroid tissue to an accessible site in the forearm, or subtotal three-and-one-half gland parathyroidectomy leaving the parathyroid tissue remnant in situ in the neck. Series of subtotal parathyroidectomies for HPT in MEN 1 report persistent or recurrent HPT in 22% to 61% of cases and permanent hypoparathyroidism in 10% to 23%.[55,57–60] Series of total parathyroidectomies report recurrent HPT in 20% to 57% of cases and permanent hypoparathyroidism in up to 30%.[56,57] In one study the incidence of hypoparathyroidism following total parathyroidectomy and autotransplantation was 46%,[60] although this number is an outlier from other studies. Currently, either procedure produces acceptable results and may be practiced as standard of care by expert endocrine surgeons. Direct comparison of these two accepted surgical treatments awaits the performance of a prospective, randomized study. Most surgeons also perform a transcervical thymectomy to exclude an ectopic or supernumerary parathyroid gland within the cranial horns of the thymus. In general, preoperative imaging tests are not useful for patients with MEN 1, because appropriate treatment requires bilateral neck exploration and identification of all four glands.

MEN 1 patients with persistent or recurrent hyperparathyroidism following initial neck exploration may have one or more missed hyperplastic glands in the neck or an ectopic gland located in the mediastinum in association with the thymus. Noninvasive imaging tests such as sestamibi scanning and ultrasound may be useful for parathyroid localization before reoperative surgery.

Pancreaticoduodenal Neuroendocrine Tumors

The optimal management of the neuroendocrine tumors of the pancreas and duodenum in patients with MEN 1 remains the most important clinical controversy. The controversy is a reflection of the lack of agreement on the most useful methods for early diagnosis of these tumors, the optimal timing for intervention, and the most appropriate operative procedure to perform once the tumors are identified. Some are reluctant to advocate routine pancreatic exploration in young, otherwise healthy patients for small tumors that are potentially clinically insignificant. On the other

Greater than 95% of patients with MEN 2A have a missense germline *ret* mutation involving one of five codons in either exon 10 or 11 (codons 609, 611, 618, 620, 634), each of which specifies a highly conserved cysteine residue in the extracellular portion of the molecule immediately adjacent to the transmembrane domain. The mutations result in replacement of a cysteine residue with one of several other amino acids. The MEN 2A-associated mutations involving one of these conserved cysteine codons have been shown to result in receptor dimerization and autophosphorylation of the protein with ligand-independent activation of the intracellular tyrosine kinase.[84] These studies have confirmed that mutated *ret* can act as a dominantly transforming oncogene in vitro.

A study of the relationship between genotype and phenotype[85] has established a correlation between mutations involving *ret* codon 634 and the development of pheochromocytomas. In addition, the specific mutation TGC < CGC (cysteine to arginine) at codon 634 is significantly related to the development of parathyroid disease in patients with MEN 2A.[85,86]

Virtually all patients with MEN 2B have been shown to harbor an identical mutation at codon 918 in the tyrosine kinase catalytic domain of *ret*, which results in substitution of a threonine for a methionine[1,87] (see Fig. 59.3). The *ret-MEN2B* mutation is postulated to result in altered catalytic properties or substrate specificity of the tyrosine kinase domain of *ret*.[84] Recently, two patients without a codon 918 mutation, but with clinical features indistinguishable from MEN 2B, were found to have a mutation in codon 883 resulting in the substitution of phenylalanine for alanine.[88] The *ret* codon 918 mutation in patients with de novo MEN 2B arises virtually exclusively on the paternally derived allele and is associated with advanced paternal age.[89] These findings suggest that a *ret* allele may be more susceptible to mutation when inherited from a father as opposed to from a mother.

Familial medullary thyroid carcinoma (FMTC) may be associated with germline mutations in one of the same conserved cysteine codons mutated in some families with MEN 2A, or may be associated with unique mutations in exons 13 or 14 within the intracellular portions of *ret*[90,91] (see Fig. 59.3).

Evaluation and Management of Endocrine Neoplasia in MEN 2

Calcitonin as a Tumor Marker for MTC

Medullary thyroid carcinoma (MTC) arises from the parafollicular C-cells of the thyroid gland, which are derived embryologically from the neural crest. Calcitonin (CT), the hormone secreted by the thyroid C-cells, serves as a sensitive plasma tumor marker for the detection of MTC or C-cell hyperplasia.[92] Before the advent of direct genetic testing, measurement of the stimulated levels of plasma CT at timed intervals after the sequential intravenous injection of calcium gluconate and pentagastrin was the gold standard test for early detection of MTC.[93] However, this provocative test will only be positive after a C-cell neoplasm has developed. Furthermore, the test needs to be performed annually and is associated with transient unpleasant side effects. Calcium/pentagastrin stimulation remains the most sensitive method for the detection of persistent or recurrent MTC following thyroidectomy. The basal plasma calcitonin level is related to the extent of MTC and the frequency of regional and distant metastases[94] (Table 59.3).

TABLE 59.3. Plasma Calcitonin (CT) Levels and Prognosis.

Group	*Preoperative CT (pg/mL)*	*RLNM* (%)*	*Postoperative CT* (%) (>300 pg/mL)*	*DM (%)*	*Death (%)*
1	250–1,000 (*n* = 25)	1 (4)	1 (4)	0	0
2	1,000–5,000 (*n* = 36)	3 (8.3)	6 (16.7)	0	0
3	5,000–10,000 (*n* = 8)	2 (25)	1 (12.5)	0	0
4	>10,000 (*n* = 23)	13 (57)	14 (61)	4 (17)	2 (8.7)

Preoperative CT, preoperative stimulated plasma calcitonin level; Postoperative CT, postoperative stimulated plasma CT level; RLNM, regional lymph node metastases; DM, distant metastases.

*Group 1 or group 2 vs. group 4, $P < 0.001$.

Source: Reproduced with permission from Wells et al.[94]

Early Thyroidectomy for Medullary Thyroid Carcinoma Based on Genetic Testing

Medullary thyroid carcinoma (MTC) is the malignant feature of the MEN 2 syndromes that is responsible for almost all of the disease-related morbidity and mortality. Therefore, early detection and effective treatment of the MTC is the key to improving outcome in patients with the MEN 2 syndromes. Total thyroidectomy before regional or distant metastases of MTC is the preferred treatment, because MTC is not significantly responsive to either radiation therapy or chemotherapeutic agents.[95–97] The ability to detect germline *ret* mutations in patients at risk for the MEN 2 syndromes represents a unique model for directed surgical intervention based on the results of a molecular diagnostic test.[4,98] Patients who are determined to have inherited a *ret* mutation by DNA testing may undergo early surgical extirpation of the target organ with the intent of complete removal of macro- or microscopic C-cell neoplasms while they are still confined to the thyroid gland and therefore likely curable.

Total thyroidectomy may be safely performed in the first decade of life with very low morbidity and no mortality.[4,99,100] The preferred operation for patients diagnosed by genetic testing is total thyroidectomy with a lymphadenectomy in the central compartment of the neck. When early thyroidectomy is performed on the basis of genetic testing in patients with MEN 2, pathological examination of the thyroid gland typically reveals microscopic C-cell carcinoma or small gross foci of invasive MTC.[4] However, microscopic cervical lymph node metastases occur infrequently, even in the absence of elevated stimulated CT levels[101] (Table 59.4). These findings constitute the strongest argument for thyroidectomy in the first decade of life in patients with an MEN 2A-associated mutation. Patients with MEN 2B should undergo thyroidectomy as soon as the disease is recognized owing to the early onset and aggressive nature of the MTC in this syndrome. Long-term follow-up of a large cohort of MEN 2A patients undergoing early thyroidectomy based on genetic testing was

TABLE 59.4. Results of Early Thyroidectomy in Patients Inheriting a Mutation in the *Ret* Proto-Oncogene.

	Number of patients	*MTC/C-cell disorder*	*Lymph node metastases*	*Normal postoperative stimulated CT*	*Complications*
Normal preoperative stimulated CT	16	16/16	1/16	16/16	0/16
Elevated preoperative stimulated CT	12	12/12	0/12	12/12	0/12
Totals	28	28/28	1/28	28/28	0/28

MTC, medullary thyroid carcinoma; CT, calcitonin.

Source: Reproduced with permission from Lairmore et al.[101]

reported by Dr. Samuel Wells group.[102] A total of 50 patients underwent total thyroidectomy, central zone lymphadenectomy, and parathyroid autotransplantation based on mutational testing. A follow-up of 100% of patients 5–10 years (mean 7 yrs) following surgery was achieved. A rigorous definition of "cure" was employed, namely an undetectable stimulated calcitonin level. In this study, 44/50 (88%) of patients had undetectable stimulated calcitonin levels, 4/50 (8%) had stimulated levels within normal range, 2/50 (4%) had elevated stimulated calcitonin levels 5–10 years after prophylactic thyroidectomy.

A modified lateral lymph node dissection is indicated when clinically suspicious nodes are palpable on either the ipsilateral or contralateral side of the neck. In patients with MTC who present with a palpable thyroid mass, the risk of more extensive nodal metastatic disease is markedly increased. Moley and coworkers demonstrated lymph node metastases in over 75% of patients with a palpable MTC.[103] In the absence of effective non-surgical treatment for lymph node metastases in these patients, an ipsilateral functional (modified radical) lymphadenectomy has been recommended. Patients who demonstrate elevated calcitonin levels following primary surgery have evidence of residual or recurrent MTC. Because there is no established efficacy for chemotherapy or radiation therapy in these patients, reoperation and meticulous cervical and anterior mediastinal lymph node clearance can be performed with curative or palliative intent.[104,105]

Pheochromocytoma

Patients with MEN 2 are diagnosed with pheochromocytoma based on the findings of signs and symptoms of catecholamine excess, elevated plasma metanephrines or 24-h urinary catecholamine excretion, and unilateral or bilateral adrenal masses on cross-sectional imaging tests. It is imperative that the presence of pheochromocytomas is excluded before performing thyroidectomy for MTC because of the anesthetic risks of unsuspected catecholamine excess.

Controversy exists concerning the optimal surgical management of the adrenal glands in patients with the MEN 2 syndromes. Understanding the natural history and clinical significance of pheochromocytomas in patients with these disorders is essential to adopting a rational surgical approach. Preneoplastic (adrenal medullary hyperplasia) and neoplastic change of the adrenal medulla in patients with MEN 2A or MEN 2B are nearly always bilateral at the histopathological level.[106,107] For this reason, some experts have advocated routine bilateral adrenalectomy for patients with MEN 2A or MEN 2B, whether or not both adrenal glands contain a pheochromocytoma.[107–110] The rationale for total adrenalectomy is based on the arguments that (1) adrenal medullary disease in patients with the MEN type 2 syndromes is frequently bilateral, (2) there is a high likelihood of subsequent development of another pheochromocytoma in the contralateral gland if it is not removed at the initial operation, (3) the pheochromocytoma may rarely malignant, and (4) the permanent Addisonian state resulting from bilateral adrenalectomy is infrequently associated with complications.

Our group and others have recommended a selective approach[111,112] with excision only of those adrenal glands containing a grossly evident pheochromocytoma at the time of intervention. The proponents of a selective approach emphasize that the risk of developing a pheochromocytoma in the opposite gland must be weighed against the risk of producing a lifelong Addisonian state by the performance of bilateral adrenalectomies. Tibblin and coworkers[111] in 1983 reported 13 patients with MEN 2A who were followed for a mean of 7.4 years after a unilateral adrenalectomy for pheochromocytoma. Four patients (31%) subsequently developed a pheochromocytoma in the opposite gland at 1, 2, 4, and 10 years following the primary adrenalectomy. The remaining 9 (69%) patients had no evidence of pheochromocytoma during the follow-up period. Our group reported the results of unilateral or bilateral adrenalectomy in a series of 58 patients with pheochromocytomas arising in patients with MEN 2A or MEN 2B.[112] Twenty-three patients with a unilateral pheochromocytoma and a grossly normal contralateral gland were treated by unilateral adrenalectomy. A pheochromocytoma developed in the remaining gland a mean of 11.9 years after the primary adrenalectomy in 12 (52%) patients. Conversely, 11 (48%) patients did not develop a second pheochromocytoma during a mean follow-up period of 5.2 years (Table 59.5). No patient treated by unilateral adrenalectomy experienced a hypertensive crisis or other complication related to an unrecognized functioning pheochromocytoma, including several patients who underwent childbirth or general anesthesia. Conversely, almost 25% of the patients undergoing total adrenectomy experienced at least one episode of Addisonian crisis requiring hospital admission and treatment with intravenous saline and corticosteroids. Therefore, the argument in favor of a selective approach includes the observation that approximately half these patients will not develop a pheochromocytoma in the opposite adrenal gland for at least

TABLE 59.5.
Development of a Contralateral Pheochromocytoma After Unilateral Adrenalectomy (Level II Evidence).

	Number of patients (%)	*Mean follow-up (years)*
No contralateral pheochromocytoma	11 (48)	5.2 ± 1.9
Contralateral pheochromocytoma	12 (52)	11.9 ± 2.0
Total	23	9.4 ± 1.0

Source: Reproduced with permission from Lairmore et al.[112]

TABLE 59.6.
Results of Operation for Hyperparathyroidism in Patients with MEN 2A (Level II Evidence).

Author	*Year*	*No. of MEN 2A patients*	*Type of resection*	*Persistent or recurrent HPT (%)*	*Permanent hypocalcemia (%)*	*Cure–initial/ follow-up*	*Follow-up (years)*
van Heerden et al.	1983[59]	9	Subtotal/selective[a]	13[a]	13[a]	93/87	3.6 (mean)[a]
Kraimps et al.	1992[58]	4	Selective	0	25	100/100	8.0 (median)[b]
O'Riordian et al.	1993[120]	18	Overall	0	22	100/100	5.8 (median)
Raue et al.	1995[121]	67	Overall	15	13	97/85	8.0 (median)
		49	Selective/subtotal	16	16	96/84	
		11	Total PTX/AT	18	9	100/82	
Herfarth et al.	1996[86]	35	Overall	23	23	91/77	14.7 (mean)
		29	Selective/subtotal	28	17	72	14.4 (mean)
		5	Total PTX/AT	0	20	100/100	16.3 (mean)

HPT, hyperparathyroidism; PTX, parathyroidectomy; AT, autotransplantation.
[a]Thirty-six MEN 1 and 9 MEN 2A patients combined.
[b]Follow-up combined with 38 MEN 1 patients.
Source: Reproduced with permission from Herfarth et al.[86]

10 years, and perhaps many never will. The development of a second pheochromocytoma is readily detectable by clinical, biochemical, and radiographic evaluation. Finally, in our experience unnecessary bilateral adrenalectomy is associated with substantial morbidity.

Although some studies have reported the occurrence of malignant pheochromocytomas in patients with MEN 2,[107] other series suggest that malignancy is very infrequent in this setting.[108,109,111,112] However, the risk of a malignant pheochromocytoma should not be totally dismissed, and bilateral adrenalectomy may be appropriate for members of families with a clear history of malignant pheochromocytoma.

Patients with pheochromocytoma are prepared preoperatively with an alpha-adrenergic blocker to control hypertension and permit reexpansion of intravascular volume. Typically, phenoxybenzamine is initiated at a dose of 10mg orally BID and increased to 20 to 40mg orally BID over 5 to 10 days preoperatively with concomitant rehydration. The development of postural hypotension is the desired and expected endpoint. In addition, adequately prepared patients will have correction of their mild lactic acidosis. Patients may undergo alpha blockade in the outpatient setting, and should be instructed to take oral fluids liberally and watch for the expected postural changes.

Laparoscopic adrenalectomy is now the standard of care for removal of benign, functional adrenal tumors.[113–117] Patients with MEN 2A and 2B may be ideally suited to laparoscopic adrenalectomy because the pheochromocytomas arising in these syndromes are rarely malignant and are almost never extraadrenal.[112] Unilateral or bilateral laparoscopic adrenalectomies are appropriate treatment provided the adrenal tumor(s) are small, confined to the adrenal gland, accurately localized preoperatively by CT or MRI scanning, and the patient is adequately prepared pharmacologically. Laparoscopic adrenalectomy is associated with a shorter hospital stay, decreased postoperative pain, and more rapid recovery when compared with open adrenalectomy.[116,118,119] Contraindications to the laparoscopic approach include large benign tumors (>8cm), malignant pheochromocytomas, and existing contraindications to laparoscopy.

Hyperparathyroidism

The appropriate management of the parathyroid glands in MEN 2 patients undergoing thyroidectomy for inherited MTC remains controversial. Our group has recommended total parathryoidectomy and autotransplantation of parathyroid tissue into the forearm muscle, especially in patients undergoing early thyroidectomy based on genetic testing.[56,86] The rationale for performing total parathyroidectomy and autotransplantation is to minimize permanent postoperative hypoparathyroidism (the blood supply to the parathyroid glands may be inadvertently compromised during radical total thyroidectomy) and to prevent the need for neck reexploration, which carries substantial morbidity, in the small subset of patients who develop hyperparathyroidism during the lifetime period of risk. Other experts argue that selective parathyroidectomy is effective in almost all patients and that routine total parathyroidectomy with autotransplantation results in an increased rate of permanent postoperative hypoparathyroidism (Table 59.6).[120,121]

Conclusion

Germline genetic alterations in oncogenes, tumor suppressor genes, and DNA mismatch repair genes are associated with the development of familial cancer syndromes. The unraveling of the basic genetic defects responsible for the development of multiple endocrine tumors in the familial endocrine neoplasia syndromes has provided insight into the common mechanisms of tumorigenesis in more common sporadic neoplasms that arise in the same endocrine tissues.

The endocrine neoplasms that develop in patients with the MEN types 1 and 2 syndromes are generally managed by surgical intervention. Because neoplasms that arise in the setting of a familial cancer syndrome are characterized by multifocality and an earlier age of onset when compared with their sporadic counterparts, the approach to diagnosis and treatment of these tumors requires special considerations.

Direct DNA testing for mutations in the *MEN1* tumor suppressor gene allows for a genetic test in patients at risk. The principal clinical challenge in the management of patients with an *MEN1* mutation will be to develop effective cancer surveillance and screening programs and to implement optimal early surgical intervention for the pancreatic and duodenal neuroendocrine tumors that are responsible for the majority of the disease-related morbidity and mortality. Early thyroidectomy based on genetic testing for patients at risk for one of the MEN 2 syndromes is now the standard of clinical care. This goal of this operation is to remove the end organ at a time when hereditary MTC is generally confined to the thyroid gland and therefore amenable to cure by surgical resection.

References

1. Hofstra RMW, Landsvater RM, Ceccherini I, et al. A mutation in the *RET* proto-oncogene associated with multiple endocrine neoplasia type 2B and sporadic medullary thyroid carcinoma. Nature (Lond) 1994;367:375–376.
2. Blaugrund JE, Johns MM Jr, Eby YJ, et al. RET proto-oncogene mutations in inherited and sporadic medullary thyroid cancer. Hum Mol Genet 1994;3:1895–1897.
3. Heppner C, Kester MB, Agarwal SK, et al. Somatic mutation of the *MEN1* gene in parathyroid tumours. Nat Gen 1997;16:375–378.
4. Wells SA, Jr., Chi D, Toshima K, et al. Predictive DNA testing and prophylactic thyroidectomy in patients at risk for multiple endocrine neoplasia type 2A. Ann Surg 1994;220:237–250.
5. Kato H, Uchimura I, Morohoshi M, et al. Multiple endocrine neoplasia type 1 associated with spinal ependymoma. Intern Med 1996;35(4):285–289.
6. Darling TN, Skarulis MC, Steinberg SM, et al. Multiple facial angiofibromas and collagenomas in patients with multiple endocrine neoplasia type 1. Arch Dermatol 1997;133:853–857.
7. Knudson AG Jr, Hethcote HW, Brown BW. Mutation and childhood cancer: a probabilistic model for the incidence of retinoblastoma. Proc Natl Acad Sci U S A 1975;72:5116–5120.
8. Doherty GM, Lairmore TC, DeBenedetti MK. Multiple endocrine neoplasia type 1 parathyroid adenoma development over time. World J Surg 2004;28(11):1139–1142.
9. Bassett JHD, Forbes SA, Pannett AAJ, et al. Characterization of mutations in patients with multiple endocrine neoplasia type 1. Am J Hum Genet 1998;62:232–244.
10. Lairmore TC, Piersall LD, DeBenedetti MK, et al. Clinical genetic testing and early surgical intervention in patients with multiple endocrine neoplasia type 1 (MEN 1). Ann Surg 2004;239(5):637–645; discussion 645–647.
11. Marx SJ, Menczel J, Campbell S, et al. Heterogeneous size of the parathyroid glands in familial multiple endocrine neoplasia type 1. Clin Endocrinol 1991;35:521–526.
12. Majewski JT, Wilson SD. The MEA-I syndrome: An all or none phenomenon. Surgery (St. Louis) 1979;86:475–484.
13. Wilkinson S, Teh BT, Davey KR, et al. Cause of death in multiple endocrine neoplasia type 1. Arch Surg 1993;128:683.
14. Doherty GM, Olson JA, Frisella MM, et al. Lethality of multiple endocrine neoplasia type I. World J Surg 1998;22(6):581–586; discussion 586–587.
15. Stabile BE, Morrow DJ, Passaro EJ. The gastrinoma triangle: operative indications. Am J Surg 1984;147:25–32.
16. Thompson NW, Vinik AI, Eckhauser FE. Microgastrinomas of the duodenum. Ann Surg 1989;209:396–404.
17. Delcore RJ, Cheung LY, Friesen SR. Characteristics of duodenal wall gastrinomas. Am J Surg 1990;160:621–624.
18. Norton JA, Doppman JL, Jensen RT. Curative resection in Zollinger–Ellison syndrome: results of a 10 year prospective study. Ann Surg 1992;215:8–18.
19. Friesen SR. Are "aberrant nodal gastrinomas" pathogenetically similar to "lateral aberrant thyroid" nodules? Surgery (St. Louis) 1990;107:236–238.
20. Wolfe MM, Alexander RW, McGuigan JE. Extrapancreatic, extraintestinal gastrinoma: effective treatment by surgery. N Engl J Med 1982;306:1533–1536.
21. Delcore RJ, Cheung LY, Friesen SR. Outcome of lymph node involvement in patients with Zollinger–Ellison syndrome. Ann Surg 1988;206:291–298.
22. Norton JA, Alexander HR, Fraker DL, et al. Possible primary lymph node gastrinoma: occurrence, natural history, and predictive factors: a prospective study. Ann Surg 2003;237(5):650–657; discussion 657–659.
23. Friesen SR. Treatment of the Zollinger–Ellison syndrome. Am J Surg 1982;143:331–338.
24. Cameron AJ, Hoffman HN. Zollinger–Ellison syndrome: clinical features and long-term follow-up. Mayo Clin Proc 1974;49:44–51.
25. Bondeson AG, Bondeson L, Thompson NW. Stricture and perforation of the esophagus: overlooked threats in Zollinger–Ellison syndrome. World J Surg 1990;14:361–364.
26. Miller LS, Vinayek R, Frucht H, et al. Reflux esophagitis in patients with Zollinger–Ellison syndrome. Gastroenterology 1990;98:341–346.
27. Norton JA. Neuroendocrine tumors of the pancreas and duodenum. Curr Probl Surg 1994;31:77–156.
28. Doppman JL, Miller DL, Chang R, et al. Gastrinomas: localization by means of selective intraarterial injection of secretin. Radiology 1990;174:25–29.
29. van Heerden JA, Smith SL, Miller LJ. Management of the Zollinger–Ellison syndrome in patients with multiple endocrine neoplasia type I. Surgery (St. Louis) 1986;100:971–977.
30. Wolfe MM, Jensen RT. Zollinger–Ellison syndrome: current concepts in diagnosis and management. N Engl J Med 1987;317:1200–1209.
31. Sheppard BC, Norton JA, Doppman JL, et al. Management of islet cell tumors in patients with multiple endocrine neoplasia: a prospective study. Surgery (St. Louis) 1989;106:1108–1118.
32. Weber HC, Venzon DJ, Lin J-T, et al. Determinants of metastatic rate and survival in patients with Zollinger–Ellison syndrome: a prospective long-term study. Gastroenterology 1995;108:1637–1649.
33. Lowney JK, Frisella MM, Lairmore TC, Doherty GM. Pancreatic islet cell tumor metastasis in multiple endocrine neoplasia type 1: correlation with primary tumor size. Surgery (St. Louis) 1998;124:1043–1049.
34. Norton JA, Melcher ML, Gibril F, Jensen RT. Gastric carcinoid tumors in multiple endocrine neoplasia-1 patients with Zollinger–Ellison syndrome can be symptomatic, demonstrate aggressive growth, and require surgical treatment. Surgery (St. Louis) 2004;136(6):1267–1274.
35. Norton JA, Fraker DL, Alexander R, et al. Surgery to cure the Zollinger–Ellison syndrome. N Engl J Med 1999;341:635–644.
36. Norton JA, Alexander HR, Fraker DL, et al. Does the use of routine duodenotomy (DUODX) affect rate of cure, development of liver metastases, or survival in patients with Zollinger–Ellison syndrome? Ann Surg 2004;239(5):617–625; discussion 626.
37. Doppman JL, Miller DL, Chang R, et al. Insulinomas: localization with selective intraarterial injection of calcium. Radiology 1991;178:237–241.
38. Cohen MS, Picus D, Lairmore TC, et al. Prospective study of provocative angiograms to localize functional islet cell tumors of the pancreas. Surgery (St. Louis) 1997;122:1091–1100.

39. Grant CS, van Heerden J, Charboneau JW, et al. Insulinoma: the value of intraoperative ultrasonography. Arch Surg 1988;123:843–848.
40. Norton JA, Cromack DT, Shawker TH, et al. Intraoperative ultrasonographic localization of islet cell tumors. Ann Surg 1988;207:160–168.
41. Doherty GM, Doppman JL, Shawker TH, et al. Results of a prospective strategy to diagnose, localize, and resect insulinomas. Surgery (St. Louis) 1991;110:989–996.
42. Marx S, Spiegel AM, Skarulis MC, et al. Multiple endocrine neoplasia type 1: clinical and genetic topics. Ann Intern Med 1998;129:484–494.
43. Duh Q-Y. Carcinoids associated with multiple endocrine neoplasia syndromes. Am J Surg 1987;154:142–148.
44. Chandrasekharappa SC, Guru SC, Manickamp P, et al. Positional cloning of the gene for multiple endocrine neoplasia-type 1. Science 1997;276:404–407.
45. Guru SC, Goldsmith PK, Burns AL, et al. Menin, the product of the *MEN1* gene, is a nuclear protein. Proc Natl Acad Sci U S A 1998;95:1630–1634.
46. Mutch MG, Dilley WG, Sanjurjo F, et al. Germline mutations in the multiple endocrine neoplasia type 1 gene: evidence for frequent splicing defects. Hum Mutat 1999;13(3):175–185.
47. Olufemi SE, Green JS, Manickam P, et al. Common ancestral mutation in the *MEN1* gene is likely responsible for the prolactinoma variant of MEN 1 (MEN1 Burin) in four kindreds from Newfoundland. Hum Mutat 1998;11:264–269.
48. Kassem M, Kruse TA, Wong FK, et al. Familial isolated hyperparathyroidism as a variant of multiple endocrine neoplasia type 1 in a large Danish pedigree. J Clin Endocrinol Metab 2000; 85:165–167.
49. Agarwal SK, Guru SC, Heppner C, et al. Menin interacts with the AP1 transcription factor JunD and represses JunD-activated transcription. Cell 1999;96:143–152.
50. Gobl AE, Berg M, Lopez-Egido JR, et al. Menin represses JunD-activated transcription by a histone deacetylase-dependent mechanism. Biochim Biophys Acta 1999;1447(1):51–56.
51. Lemmens IH, Forsberg L, Pannett AA, et al. Menin interacts directly with the homeobox-containing protein Pem. Biochem Biophys Res Commun 2001;286(2):426–431.
52. Heppner C, Bilimoria KY, Agarwal SK, et al. The tumor suppressor protein menin interacts with NF-kappaB proteins and inhibits NF-kappaB-mediated transactivation. Oncogene 2001; 20(36):4917–4925.
53. Kaji H, Canaff L, Lebrun JJ, et al. Inactivation of menin, a Smad3-interacting protein, blocks transforming growth factor type beta signaling. Proc Natl Acad Sci U S A 2001;98(7):3837–3842.
54. Ohkura N, Kishi M, Tsukada T, Yamaguchi K. Menin, a gene product responsible for multiple endocrine neoplasia type 1, interacts with the putative tumor metastasis protein nm23. Biochim Biophys Res Commun 2001;282(5):1206–1210.
55. Rizzoli R, Green J, Marx SJ. Long-term follow-up of serum calcium levels after parathyroidectomy. Am J Med 1985;78:467–473.
56. Wells SA Jr, Farndon JR, Dale JK, et al. Long term evaluation of patients with primary parathyroid hyperplasia managed by total parathyroidectomy and heterotopic autotransplantation. Ann Surg 1980;192:451–458.
57. Hellman P, Skogseid B, Juhlin C, et al. Findings and long term results of parathyroid surgery in multiple endocrine neoplasia type 1. World J Surg 1992;16:718–723.
58. Kraimps JL, Duh Q-Y, Demeure M, Clark OH. Hyperparathyroidism in multiple endocrine neoplasia syndrome. Surgery (St. Louis) 1992;112:1080–1088.
59. van Heerden JA, Kent RB, Sizemore GW, et al. Primary hyperparathyroidism in patients with multiple endocrine neoplasia syndromes: surgical experience. Arch Surg 1983;118:533–536.
60. Elaraj DM, Skarulis MC, Libutti SK, et al. Results of initial operation for hyperparathyroidism in patients with multiple endocrine neoplasia type 1. Surgery (St. Louis) 2003;134(6):858–864; discussion 864–865.
61. Lairmore TC, Chen VY, DeBenedetti MK, et al. Duodenopancreatic resections in patients with multiple endocrine neoplasia type 1. Ann Surg 2000;231:909–918.
62. Thompson NW, Lloyd RV, Nishiyama RH, et al. MEN I pancreas: a histological and immunohistochemical study. World J Surg 1984;8:561–574.
63. Skogseid B, Eriksson B, Lundqvist G, et al. Multiple endocrine neoplasia type 1: a 10-year prospective screening study in four kindreds. J Clin Endocrinol Metab 1991;73:281–287.
64. Skogseid B, Grama D, Rastad J, et al. Operative tumour yield obviates preoperative pancreatic tumour localization in multiple endocrine neoplasia type 1. J Intern Med 1995;238:281–288.
65. Skogseid B, Öberg K. Experience with multiple endocrine neoplasia type 1 screening. J Intern Med 1995;238:255–261.
66. Doppman JL. Multiple endocrine neoplasia syndromes. A nightmare for the endocrinologic radiologist. Semin Roentgenol 1985;20:7–16.
67. Skogseid B, Öberg K, Benson L, et al. A standardized meal stimulation test of the endocrine pancreas for early detection of pancreatic endocrine tumors in multiple endocrine neoplasia type 1 syndrome: Five years experience. J Clin Endocrinol Metab 1987;64:1233–1240.
68. Lairmore TC. Complications in endocrine pancreatic surgery. In: Mulholland M, Doherty G, eds. Complications in Surgery. Philadelphia: Lippincott Williams & Wilkins, 2005.
69. Sipple JH. The association of pheochromocytoma with carcinoma of the thyroid gland. Am J Med 1961;31:163–166.
70. Steiner AL, Goodman AD, Powers SR. Study of a kindred with pheochromocytoma, medullary thyroid carcinoma, hyperparathyroidism and Cushing's disease: multiple endocrine neoplasia type 2. Medicine (Baltim) 1968;47:371–409.
71. Howe JR, Norton JA, Wells SA Jr. Prevalence of pheochromocytoma and hyperparathyroidism in multiple endocrine neoplasia type 2A: results of long-term follow-up. Surgery (St. Louis) 1993;114:1070–1077.
72. Williams ED, Pollack DJ. Multiple mucosal neuromata with endocrine tumours: a syndrome allied to von Recklinghausen's disease. J Pathol Bacteriol 1966;91:71–80.
73. Schimke RN, Hartmann WH, Prout TE, Rimoin DL. Syndrome of bilateral pheochromocytoma, medullary thyroid carcinoma and multiple neuromas. N Engl J Med 1968;279:1–7.
74. Farndon JR, Leight GS, Dilley WG, et al. Familial medullary thyroid carcinoma without associated endocrinopathies: a distinct clinical entity. Br J Surg 1986;73:278–281.
75. Trupp M, Arenas E, Fainzilber M, et al. Functional receptor for GDNF encoded by the c-*ret* proto-oncogene. Nature (Lond) 1996;381:785–789.
76. Durbec P, Macos-Gutierrez CV, Kilkenny C, et al. GDNF signalling through the Ret receptor tyrosine kinase. Nature (Lond) 1996;381:789–793.
77. Jing S, Wen D, Yu Y, et al. GDNF-induced activation of the ret protein tyrosine kinase is mediated by GDNFR-a, a novel receptor for GDNF. Cell 1996;85:1113–1124.
78. Pachnis V, Mankoo B, Costantini F. Expression of the *c-ret* proto-oncogene during mouse embryogenesis. Development (Cambr) 1993;119:1005–1017.
79. Avantaggiato V, Dathan NA, Grieco M, et al. Developmental expression of the RET protooncogene. Cell Growth Differ 1994;5:305–311.
80. Schuchardt A, D'Agati V, Larsson-Blomberg L, et al. Defects in the kidney and enteric nervous system of mice lacking the tyrosine kinase receptor Ret. Nature (Lond) 1994;367:380–383.

81. Edery P, Lyonnet S, Mulligan LM, et al. Mutations of the *RET* proto-oncogene in Hirschsprung's disease. Nature (Lond) 1994;367:378–380.
82. Romeo G, Ronchetto P, Luo Y, et al. Point mutations affecting the tyrosine kinase domain of the *RET* proto-oncogene in Hirschsprung's disease. Nature (Lond) 1994;367:377–378.
83. Pasini B, Borrello MG, Greco A, et al. Loss of function effect of *RET* mutations causing Hirschsprung disease. Nat Genet 1995;10:35–40.
84. Santoro M, Carlomagno F, Romano A, et al. Activation of *RET* as a dominantly transforming gene by germline mutations of MEN2A and MEN2B. Science 1995;267:381–383.
85. Mulligan LM, Eng C, Healey CS, et al. Specific mutations of the *RET* proto-oncogene are related to disease phenotype in MEN 2A and FMTC. Nat Genet 1994;6:70–74.
86. Herfarth KK-F, Bartsch D, Doherty GM, et al. Surgical management of hyperparathyroidism in patients with multiple endocrine neoplasia type 2A. Surgery (St. Louis) 1996;120:966–974.
87. Carlson KM, Dou S, Chi D, et al. Single missense mutation in the tyrosine kinase catalytic domain of the *RET* proto-oncogene is associated with multiple endocrine neoplasia type 2B. Proc Natl Acad Sci U S A 1994;91:1579–1583.
88. Smith DP, Houghton C, Ponder BAJ. Germline mutation of *RET* codon 883 in two cases of *de novo* MEN 2B. Oncogene 1997;15:1213–1217.
89. Carlson KM, Bracamontes J, Jackson CE, et al. Parent-of-origin effects in multiple endocrine neoplasia type 2B. Am J Hum Genet 1994;55:1076–1082.
90. Eng C, Smith DP, Mulligan LM, et al. A novel point mutation in the tyrosine kinase domain of the *RET* proto-oncogene in sporadic medullary thyroid carcinoma and in a family with FMTC. Oncogene 1995;10:509–513.
91. Bolino A, Schuffenecker I, Luo Y, et al. *RET* mutations in exons 13 and 14 of FMTC patients. Oncogene 1995;10:2415–2419.
92. Tashjian AH Jr, Howland BG, Melvin KEW, Hill CS Jr. Immunoassay of human calcitonin: clinical measurement, relation to serum calcium and studies in patients with medullary carcinoma. N Engl J Med 1970;283:890–895.
93. Wells SA Jr, Baylin SB, Linehan WM, et al. Provocative agents and the diagnosis of medullary carcinoma of the thyroid gland. Ann Surg 1978;188:139–141.
94. Wells SA, Jr., Baylin SB, Leight GS, et al. The importance of early diagnosis in patients with hereditary medullary thyroid carcinoma. Ann Surg 1982;195:595–599.
95. Gottlieb JA, Hill CS. Chemotherapy of thyroid cancer with Adriamycin. N Engl J Med 1974;290:193–197.
96. Steinfeld AD. The role of radiation therapy in medullary carcinoma of the thyroid. Radiology 1977;123:745–746.
97. Tubiani M. External radiotherapy and radioiodine in the treatment of thyroid cancer. World J Surg 1981;1981:75–84.
98. Lips CJM, Landsvater RM, Höppener JWM, et al. Clinical screening as compared with DNA analysis in families with multiple endocrine neoplasia type 2A. N Engl J Med 1994;331:828–835.
99. Skinner MA, DeBenedetti MK, Moley JF, et al. Medullary thyroid carcinoma in children with multiple endocrine neoplasia types 2A and 2B. J Pediatr Surg 1996;31:177–182.
100. Lairmore TC, Frisella MM, Wells SA Jr. Genetic testing and early thyroidectomy for inherited medullary thyroid carcinoma. Ann Med 1996;28(5):401–406.
101. Lairmore TC, Frisella MM, Wells SAJ. Genetic testing and early thyroidectomy for inherited medullary thyroid carcinoma. Ann Med 1996;28:401–406.
102. Skinner MA, Moley JF, Dilley WG, Owzar K, DeBenedetti MK, Wells SA Jr. Prophylactic thyroidectomy in multiple endocrine neoplasia type 2A. NEJM 2005;353:1105–1113.
103. Moley JF, DeBenedetti MK. Patterns of nodal metastases in palpable medullary thyroid carcinoma: recommendations for extent of node dissection. Ann Surg 1999;229(6):880–887; discussion 887–888.
104. Moley JF, Dilley WG, DeBenedetti MK. Improved results of cervical reoperation for medullary thyroid carcinoma. Ann Surg 1997;225:734–743.
105. Tisell LE, Hansson G, Jansson S, Salander H. Reoperation in the treatment of asymptomatic metastasizing medullary thyroid carcinoma. Surgery (St. Louis) 1986;99:60–66.
106. Carney JA, Sizemore GW, Tyce GM. Bilateral adrenal medullary hyperplasia in multiple endocrine neoplasia, type 2: the precursor of bilateral pheochromocytoma. Mayo Clin Proc 1975;50:3–10.
107. Carney JA, Sizemore GW, Sheps SG. Adrenal medullary disease in multiple endocrine neoplasia, type 2: pheochromocytoma and its precursors. Am J Clin Pathol 1976;66:279–290.
108. Freier DT, Thompson NW, Sisson JC, et al. Dilemmas in the early diagnosis and treatment of multiple endocrine adenomatosis, type II. Surgery (St. Louis) 1977;82:407–413.
109. Lips KJM, van der Sluys Veer J, Struyvenberg A, et al. Bilateral occurrence of pheochromocytoma in patients with the multiple endocrine neoplasia syndrome type 2A (Sipple's syndrome). Am J Med 1981;70:1051–1060.
110. van Heerden JA, Sizemore GW, Carney JA, et al. Surgical management of the adrenal glands in the multiple endocrine neoplasia type II syndrome. World J Surg 1984;8:612–621.
111. Tibblin S, Dymling J-F, Ingemansson S, Telenius-Berg M. Unilateral versus bilateral adrenalectomy in multiple endocrine neoplasia IIA. World J Surg 1983;7:201–208.
112. Lairmore TC, Ball DW, Baylin SB, Wells SA Jr. Management of pheochromocytomas in patients with multiple endocrine neoplasia type 2 syndromes. Ann Surg 1993;217:595–603.
113. Gagner M, Lacroix A, Prinz RA, et al. Early experience with laparoscopic approach for adrenalectomy. Surgery (St. Louis) 1993;114:1120–1125.
114. Gagner M, Lacroix A, Bolte E, Pomp A. Laparoscopic adrenalectomy: the importance of a flank approach in the lateral decubitus position. Surg Endosc 1994;8:135–138.
115. Lepsien G, Neufang T, Ludtke FE. Laparoscopic resection of pheochromocytoma. Surg Endosc 1994;8:906–909.
116. Brunt LM, Doherty GM, Norton JA, et al. Laparoscopic adrenalectomy compared to open adrenalectomy for benign adrenal neoplasms. J Am Coll Surg 1996;183:1–10.
117. Brunt LM, Lairmore TC, Doherty GM, et al. Adrenalectomy for familial pheochromocytoma in the laparoscopic era. Ann Surg 2002;235(5):713–720; discussion 720–721.
118. Guazzoni G, Montorsi F, Bocciardi A, et al. Transperitoneal laparoscopic versus open adrenalectomy for benign hyperfunctioning adrenal tumors. J Urol 1995;153:1597–1600.
119. Prinz RA. A comparison of laparoscopic and open adrenalectomies. Arch Surg 1995;130:489–494.
120. O'Riordain DS, O'Brien T, Grant CS, et al. Surgical management of primary hyperparathyroidism in multiple endocrine neoplasia types 1 and 2. Surgery (St. Louis) 1993;114:1031–1039.
121. Raue F, Kraimps JL, Dralle H, et al. Primary hyperparathyroidism in multiple endocrine neoplasia type 2A. J Intern Med 1995;238:369–373.
122. Phan GQ, Yeo CJ, Cameron JL, et al. Pancreaticoduodenectomy for selected periampullary neuroendocrine tumors: fifty patients. Surgery (St. Louis) 1997;122:989–997.
123. Park BJ, Alexander R, Libutti SK, et al. Operative management of islet cell tumors arising in the head of the pancreas. Surgery (St. Louis) 1998;124:1056–1062.
124. Guo SS, Sawicki MP. Molecular and genetic mechanisms of tumorigenesis in multiple endocrine neoplasia type-1. Mol Endocrinol 2001;15(10):1653–1664.
125. Lairmore TC, Moley JF. The multiple endocrine neoplasia syndromes. In: Townsend CM, Beauchamp DR, Evers BM, Mattox KL eds. Sabiston Textbook of Surgery: The Biological Basis of Modern Surgical Practice, 17th ed. Philadelphia: Saunders, 2004;1071–1087.

SECTION SIX

Vascular Surgery

60

History of Vascular Surgery

Jesse E. Thompson

The past 50 years have witnessed the most spectacular period of growth and development of vascular surgery during its long and fascinating history. As in all matters, the basis for today's modern vascular surgery rests on achievements from the past. As Thomas Carlyle said, "History is the essence of innumerable biographies."

Vascular surgery has a number of supporting pillars: these include anesthesia, antisepsis, asepsis, antibiotics, blood transfusion, anticoagulants, angiography, vascular sutures, and vascular grafts. Vascular surgery itself comprises many elements. Many nationalities have been involved as well as numerous individuals. Developments in industrial and technical fields outside medicine have also played important roles. In this chapter, because of constraints of space, the author has been selective and many contributions of necessity have been omitted. The reader interested in more historical details may consult the writings of Barker, DeBakey, Friedman, Haimovici, Rob, Shumacker, Smith, and others.[1–11]

The Ancients

Studies of Egyptian mummies have revealed that atherosclerosis and arterial calcification were prevalent 3500 years ago. Marc Armand Ruffer in 1911 published his findings, in Egyptian mummies of the period 1580 BC to AD 525, that atherosclerotic lesions, similar to present-day lesions, were relatively common.[12] The Ebers Papyrus is among the earliest medical writings, thought to have been prepared around 2000 BC. The writer has clearly identified arterial aneurysms, probably peripheral aneurysms, and recommends the following treatment: "treat it with a knife and burn it with a fire so that it bleeds not too much."[13]

Antyllus, who lived in the second century AD, mentioned the ligature, although the ligature was not brought to light again until resurrected by Ambroise Paré in the sixteenth century. Antyllus treated aneurysms by applying ligatures to the arteries entering and leaving the aneurysm, cutting into the sac, and packing the cavity. Although bleeding was common, this method held until the time of John Hunter in the eighteenth century.[14]

The Renaissance

Very few advances were made in the treatment of aneurysms during the ensuing millenium. Ambroise Paré (1510–1590) was the greatest surgeon of the Renaissance. In 1536 he discontinued the use of boiling oil and cautery in stopping hemorrhage. Although he did not invent the ligature, he was a staunch advocate of its use and by 1552 was applying it to control hemorrhage in extremity amputations. To Paré is owed the famous remark made when he was congratulated on the cure of a difficult case: "I treated him, God cured him." His work on gunshot and other wounds published in 1545 is an important contribution. Paré advocated the application of a proximal ligature to aneurysms, but did not believe the sac should be opened because of the danger of severe and fatal hemorrhage. Paré also described a ruptured aneurysm of the thoracic aorta and stated, "The aneurismaes which happened in the internale parts are uncurable."[1,13,15]

Another giant of the Renaissance was Andreas Vesalius (1514–1564). On the basis of work in the anatomy dissection room, he threw over the superstitions regarding anatomy and put the field once and for all on a scientific basis. His magnificent book, *De Fabrica Humani Corporis*, published in 1543 when he was 29 years old, is one of the great medical books of all times. Vesalius was the first to diagnose and describe, in 1555, aneurysms of the abdominal and thoracic aorta.[16]

Matheus Purmann operated on an antecubital space aneurysm in 1680, ligated the artery above and below the aneurysm, and removed the sac. In medieval times the antecubital fossa aneurysm was quite common as a complication of blood letting by puncture of the median basilic vein.[1]

An important problem needing solution was circulation of the blood. It was the genius of William Harvey (1578–1657) that completed the answer to this problem. His book, *De Motu Cordis*, was published in 1628.[16]

Eighteenth and Nineteenth Centuries

The first of the great surgeons of this era was John Hunter (1728–1793), a Scotsman who went to London in 1748. He was one of the great surgeons of all time, the founder of scientific surgery based on anatomy and physiology. His contributions to vascular surgery were basic. In addition to his clinical observations, he studied the development of collateral circulation when main arteries were occluded, which led to his method of treating aneurysms. On December 12, 1785, he ligated the superficial femoral artery high in the thigh in the area known as Hunter's canal to treat a popliteal aneurysm. The patient did well, the aneurysm shrunk down to a hard knot, and the limb survived. The specimen of Hunter's first case is in the Hunterian Museum in London. Hunter's method was the first major innovation in the treatment of popliteal aneurysms since the Antyllus operation of the second century, a lapse of 1600 years. His method lasted for another 100 years until the method of Rudolph Matas was developed in 1888.

Hunter had angina pectoris and said, "My life is in the hands of any rascal who chooses to annoy and tease me." During a heated argument at a board meeting of St. George's Hospital in London on October 14, 1793, Hunter had a fatal heart attack, dying at the age of 65.[17]

Astley Cooper (1768–1841) was one of the great English surgeons of the late eighteenth and first half of the nineteenth century. Cooper made contributions in many fields of surgery, but his name is permanently linked to advances in vascular surgery (Fig. 60.1). In 1817 he was called to see a man in extremis who had a leaking iliac aneurysm. He decided that the only possible treatment was to ligate the aorta above the aneurysm. Through a small transperitoneal incision he managed to get his finger around the aorta, and then with an aneurysm needle passed a single ligature around the vessel, which was then tied. The patient's right leg remained viable, but the left leg was totally ischemic, livid, and cold, and the patient died 40 h later. This was the first recorded case of ligation of the aorta for aneurysm. The specimen of Cooper's operation is preserved in the Department of Surgery at St. Thomas's Hospital in London.[18]

Valentine Mott (1785–1865), of New York City, was one of the most outstanding American surgeons during the first half of the nineteenth century. He has been called by Rutkow the "father of American vascular surgery." He was best known for his contributions to vascular surgery, which at that time consisted largely of arterial ligations and amputations.[19,20] In the ligation of arteries Valentine Mott was without peer. In all, he performed 138 ligations of the great vessels for treat-

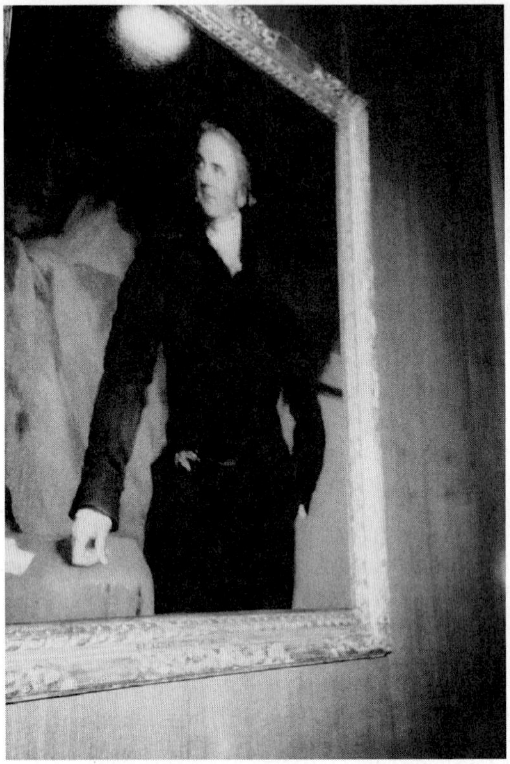

FIGURE 60.1. Sir Astley Cooper.

ment of aneurysms. The operation that thrust Valentine Mott into prominence was the first ligation of the innominate artery on May 11, 1818, for a traumatic subclavian aneurysm. Although the patient did well at first, he died of infection on the 26th postoperative day. The first successful ligation of the innominate artery for subclavian aneurysm was performed by Andrew Woods Smyth at the Charity Hospital in New Orleans on May 15, 1864, 46 years later.[1] Another spectacular operation performed by Mott was the first successful ligation of the common iliac artery for a traumatic aneurysm of the right external iliac artery on March 15, 1827, performed through a retroperitoneal approach.[20]

Suture of Blood Vessels

Arterial repair was slow to develop. In 1759 Hallowell, at the suggestion of Richard Lambert, in treating a brachial artery injured during phlebotomy, closed the laceration by running a short steel pin through the edges of the wound and passing a figure-of-eight ligature around it to approximate the wound edges. Later Asman attempted to repeat the procedure in animals, without success. Arterial repair was not used again for about 100 years. It was left for Jassinowsky in 1891 to report success in suturing arteries. His sutures avoided penetrating the intima. Dörfler in 1899 modified Jassinowsky's method by passing the suture through all areas of the artery wall. He was the first to note that penetration of the intima did no harm, did not lead to thrombosis, and was soon covered by a glistening membrane. In 1896, Jaboulay and Briau described successful end-to-end anastomosis of the carotid using an inverted U-shaped suture.[1,4–6,8,21]

J.B. Murphy of Chicago, after a series of animal experiments on arterial and venous repair, on October 7, 1896 successfully united the ends of the femoral artery injured by a gunshot wound. He excised the damaged section of the artery, invaginated the proximal end into the distal vessel, and held it in place with sutures, the first successful circular suture in a human.[21]

The individual who established the modern technique of suturing blood vessels in the opening days of the twentieth century was Alexis Carrel. A Frenchman, he came to the United States in 1905, worked first in Chicago with C.C. Guthrie, and then from 1906 to 1939 at the Rockefeller Institute for Medical Research in New York City. He revolutionized the surgery of the vascular system with a meticulous technique in which he triangulated the arteries and sutured them end to end with fine needles and suture materials. From end-to-end anastomosis, he advanced to grafting of arteries using a vein, and then he proceeded to the transplantation of organs from animal to animal. He developed the patch graft technique of reconstruction. Carrel also pioneered in the preservation of blood vessels in cold storage so that such preserved arteries could be used days or weeks after harvesting from the donor animals.[22]

Alexis Carrel developed a very close friendship with Charles Lindbergh because Carrel was attempting to devise a pump for organ perfusion. Charles Lindbergh became his collaborator and devised a pump that was used for a number of years at the Rockefeller Institute for preserving organs. This device may be considered to be the first pump oxygenator or mechanical heart.[22]

Following the technical lead of Carrel, José Goyanes, a Spaniard, in 1906 performed the first successful vein graft for treatment of popliteal aneurysms. His graft was a venous autograft of in situ popliteal vein adjacent to the diseased artery. Circulation to the extremity was preserved.[23]

Some 6 months later in 1907, Eric Lexer in Germany repaired a large traumatic false aneurysm in the axilla with a segment of the greater saphenous vein removed from the patient's leg. The patient died 5 days later of delirium tremens with a patent graft. Lexer later repeated the operation successfully many times.[24]

In Scotland, J. Hogarth Pringle in 1913 reported two successful vein grafts for popliteal and brachial aneurysms.[25] In the United States, Bertram Bernheim of the Johns Hopkins Hospital in 1913 published a monograph on vascular surgical techniques. In 1915 he removed a popliteal aneurysm and replaced it with a 12-cm segment of saphenous vein, probably the first American to perform this procedure successfully.[26]

William S. Halsted and his group at Johns Hopkins had a long and abiding interest in vascular problems, especially vascular trauma and aneurysms. Halsted devised an apparatus for metallic banding of arteries to produce gradual occlusion, a method that failed, usually because of hemorrhage.[27]

Aortic Aneurysms: Early Experience

During the 100 years after Cooper, several attempts were made to ligate the aorta but all the patients died, until April 9, 1923, when Rudolph Matas (1860–1957) successfully ligated the abdominal aorta in the treatment of an abdominal aneurysm. The patient survived the operation but died 18 months later of pulmonary tuberculosis.[28] By 1940 Dan Elkin was able to identify only 24 recorded cases of ligation in the world literature, to which he added 1 of his own, and in only 5 cases was the operation a success.[29]

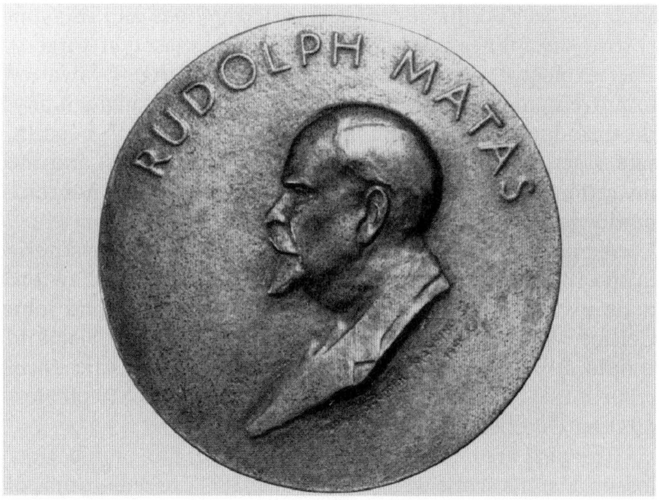

FIGURE 60.2. Rudolph Matas. (From the collection of Dr. Isidore Cohn.)

Rudolph Matas of New Orleans was a pioneer in vascular surgery. He made many contributions to all areas of surgery, but in vascular surgery he is best remembered for his operation of endoaneurysmorrhaphy (Fig. 60.2), which he first performed on May 6, 1888, for a large traumatic brachial artery aneurysm of the left arm. Following ligation of the proximal and distal arteries, an incision was made into the aneurysm and the clot removed. The orifices of the blood vessels entering the sac were then sutured from within, thus preserving the collateral blood supply to the extremity. This operation reduced markedly the incidence of gangrene and amputation that followed in a high percentage of patients undergoing the Hunterian ligation for popliteal aneurysm. This principle is still employed.[30] William Osler, in his 16 years at the Johns Hopkins Hospital from 1889 to 1904, saw only 17 cases of abdominal aortic aneurysm, an average of 1 per year.[31]

Over the years a number of methods have been used in an effort to treat aortic aneurysms. These techniques, designed either to cause thrombosis of the aneurysm or to fibrose the wall to prevent rupture, included needling, wiring, proximal banding, ligation, and cellophane wrapping, to mention a few.

C.H. Moore, a British surgeon from Middlesex Hospital, in 1864 introduced wiring of aneurysms by inserting either silver, iron, steel, or copper wire in an effort to thrombose the aneurysm. Corradi from Pavia in 1879 attached Moore's wires to a battery in an attempt to induce coagulation. Results were dismal, with only an occasional reported cure.[3,31] The principle persisted, however, and was brought to its culmination by Arthur Blakemore of New York, who advocated progressive constrictive occlusion of the abdominal aorta with a rubber band wrapped with polythene film proximal to the aneurysm, followed by insertion of wire and electrothermic coagulation with 100 V direct current. Blakemore's final major presentation of this method was given in 1952.[32]

Basic Supports to Vascular Surgery

Thus, shortly after the end of the nineteenth century, all the techniques necessary for suturing, anastomosing, and grafting arterial vessels had been developed. Clearly, technical advances had outdistanced diagnostic methods and the supporting disciplines necessary for successful vascular surgery. The explosive development of vascular surgery awaited improvements in anesthesia, the evolution of angiography, the introduction of suitable anticoagulants, especially heparin, safe blood transfusion, the discovery of antibiotics, and the invention of satisfactory arterial substitutes and nontraumatic instruments and suture materials.

A major pillar was the discovery of inhalation anesthesia in the 1840s, so named by Oliver Wendell Holmes. Crawford Long in Georgia, William Thomas Green Morton and John Collins Warren in Boston, and Horace Wells of Hartford should all be mentioned. The first public demonstration of ether anesthesia was made at the Massachusetts General Hospital on October 16, 1846.[33]

The next great influence was the elimination of infection. Joseph Lister's work was published in 1867, based on that of Louis Pasteur. Finally came the discovery and development of antibiotics by Fleming, Chain, and Florey, for which they shared the Nobel Prize in 1945.[34]

Another pillar supporting modern vascular surgery is the transfusion of blood. It remained for Karl Landsteiner and his group at the Rockefeller Institute to distinguish, in 1901and 1902, the four human blood groups. Landsteiner received the Nobel Prize in 1930.[16] Methods of administering blood have also evolved in a most interesting manner. Early on, a direct transfusion from one individual to another was the usual method. One of the pioneers in direct transfusion was the American Dr. George Crile of Cleveland, who in 1906 described his method.[35] Another important pillar was the use of anticoagulants, especially heparin. Howell, McLean, and Gordon Murray in the years between 1916 and 1940 were involved with the discovery, extraction, and clinical application of heparin.[1,3]

If the topics just mentioned are the pillars of vascular surgery, then its cornerstone is arteriography. Wilhelm Konrad Roentgen on November 8, 1895, first observed the new rays that were to bear his name and become the basis of our diagnostic armamentarium. Roentgen won the Nobel Prize for this discovery in 1901.[36]

In 1923, Barney Brooks of Nashville initiated clinical angiography by injecting sodium iodide and studied the femoropopliteal system.[37] Egas Móníz of Portugal first performed cerebral arteriography in 1927. Another Portuguese physician, Reynaldo Dos Santos, in 1929 first reported translumbar aortography.[36] In 1953, Seldinger reported the technique of retrograde femoral catheter injection to visualize the vessels using local anesthesia. These pioneering achievements have evolved into today's sophisticated methods of visualizing all the vessels in the body.[38]

The development of satisfactory arterial conduits was basic for progress in vascular surgery. Veins had been substituted for arteries as early as 1906. It was in the 1940s and early 1950s that methods of graft preservation were perfected and artery banks established, based on the early work of Carrel and Guthrie and of Gross and associates.[1,39]

A number of important breakthroughs had already occurred before 1950. On August 26, 1938, Robert Gross (Fig. 60.3) of Boston performed the first successful ligation of a patent ductus arteriosus.[40] On October 19, 1944, Crafoord and Nylin in Sweden reported the first successful end-to-end anastomosis of the aorta after resection of an aortic coarctation.[41]

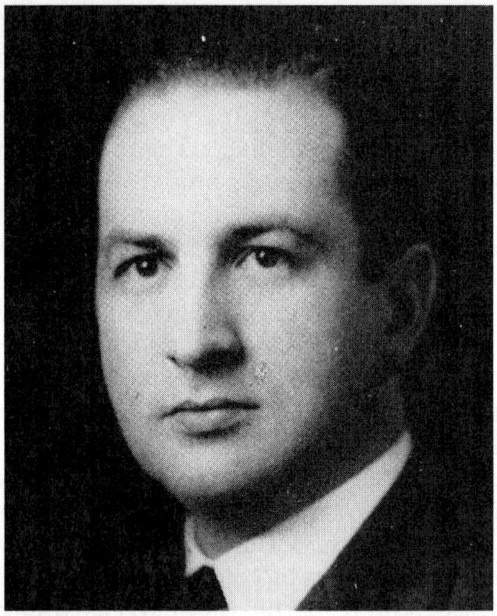

FIGURE 60.3. Robert E. Gross. (Reprinted with permission from Thompson JE. The founding fathers. J Vasc Surg 1996;23:1027, 1028, 1029, 1030.)

Gross performed his first successful coarctation resection and anastomosis on July 6, 1945.[42,43] Alfred Blalock of Johns Hopkins, on November 30, 1944, performed the first successful anastomosis of the subclavian artery to the pulmonary artery on a blue baby for the relief of tetralogy of Fallot.[44] On May 24, 1948, Gross successfully replaced a long segment of a resected coarctation with a preserved arterial homograft. The stage was set for the rapid developments that were to follow.

Aortic Aneurysms: Recent Experience

The modern method of treating abdominal aortic aneurysms began in 1951. On March 2, 1951, Schafer and Hardin resected an abdominal aortic aneurysm using a bypass shunt and replaced the aorta with a human homograft. The patient survived the operation but died 29 days later of hemorrhage from a leak in the native aortic wall.[45]

The first *successful* resection of an abdominal aortic aneurysm with graft replacement was done on March 29, 1951, by Charles Dubost in Paris, France (Fig. 60.4). Dubost used an extraperitoneal thoracoabdominal approach with resection of the 11th rib. The graft used was the thoracic aorta taken 3 weeks previously from a 20-year-old girl (Figure 60.5). The patient's left common iliac artery was then anastomosed to a side of the graft.[46]

Following Dubost's landmark procedure, reports of successful operations appeared in quick succession by Julian,[47] Brock,[48] DeBakey and Cooley,[49] Bahnson,[50] and Szilagyi[11] (Figs. 60.6, 60.7). Following Dubost's report the abdominal aortic aneurysm sac was completely removed before the graft was placed, but this technique was sometimes difficult and hazardous. In 1966, therefore, Oscar Creech combined the endoaneurysmorrhaphy technique of Matas with graft replacement leaving the aneurysm sac in place. This single step has greatly simplified aneurysm surgery by reducing the incidence of venous injury and is the technique employed at the present time.[51]

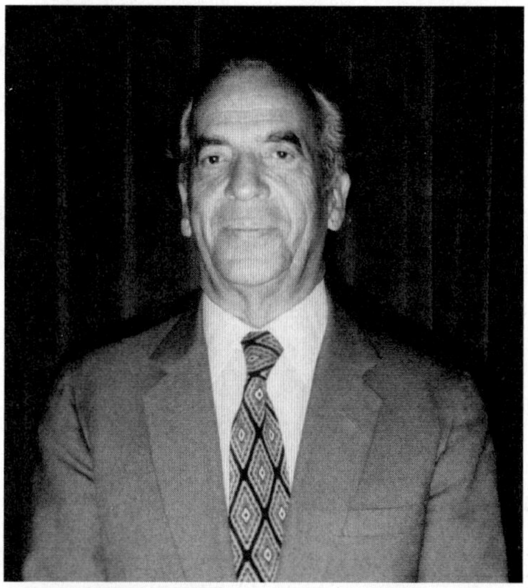

FIGURE 60.4. Charles Dubost.

Vascular Prostheses

The arterial homografts were a great step forward, but problems of procurement and availability were major limiting factors. In 1952, Voorhees, Jaretski, and Blakemore of New York reported that a tube of vinyon-N cloth as a plastic arterial substitute would remain open in a dog's aorta (Fig. 60.8). This observation was soon confirmed, and although vinyon-N did not prove to be a satisfactory material, the principle was established.[52] In 1955, Sterling Edwards reported the development of nylon prostheses and with associate J.S. Tapp devised the technique of crimping prosthetic grafts. Nylon did not hold up, but Teflon grafts soon followed.[53]

Beginning in 1954, DeBakey and his group were working on various materials for grafts. They collaborated with Professor Thomas Edman, a Philadelphia textile engineer, to build a new knitting machine to make seamless Dacron grafts of all sizes, shapes, and configurations. A number of companies have since entered the graft field. Various refinements have been made in these prosthetic grafts, culminating in the standard Dacron and Teflon grafts in use today.[2] Emerick Szilagyi played an important role in the development of vascular grafts with his introduction of the elasticized woven Dacron graft

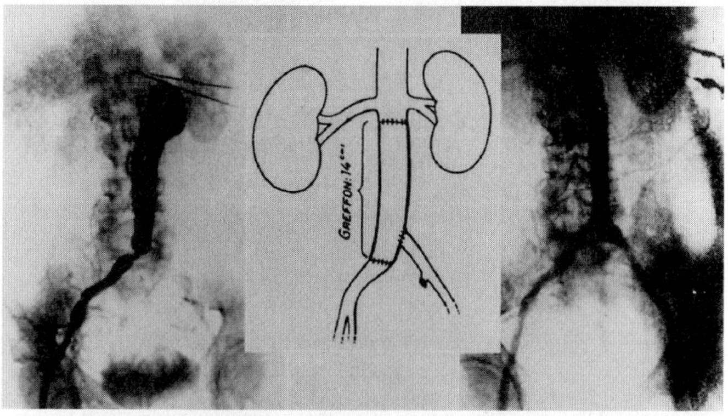

FIGURE 60.5. Diagram of Dubost's operative procedure for the first successful abdominal aortic aneurysm resection with graft replacement. (From Dubost C, Allary M, Oeconomos N. Arch Surg 1952;64:405–408. Copyright: 1952, American Medical Association. Used by permission.)[46]

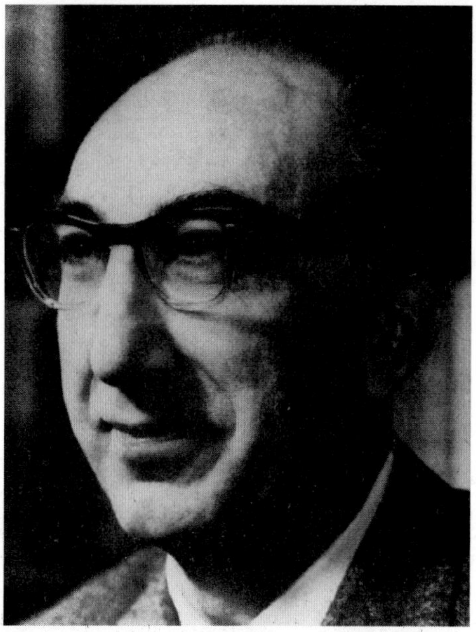

FIGURE 60.6. Michael E. DeBakey. (Reprinted with permission from Thompson JE. The founding fathers. J Vasc Surg 1996;23:1027, 1028, 1029, 1030.)

bearing his name. His follow-up reports on aortic aneurysm surgery have been landmark contributions, as have been his reports on the biological fate of saphenous vein grafts implanted in the infrainguinal region.[54,55] A number of investigators have been involved in developing vascular grafts, including Cooley, Deterling, Julian, Shumacker, and Von Liebig.[7,56] More recently, prosthetic grafts of polytetrafluoroethylene (PTFE) have been introduced and have found increasing application, especially in the femoropopliteal position.[7]

Ruptured Aneurysms

Following successful elective treatment of abdominal aortic aneurysms, ruptured aneurysms were subjected to resection and repair. Henry Bahnson is credited with the first successful

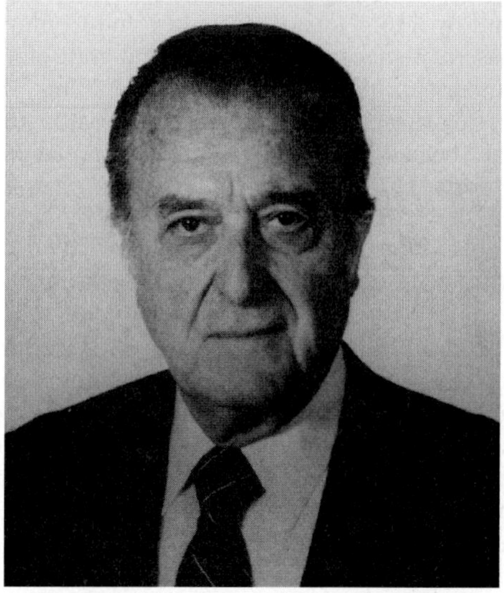

FIGURE 60.7. D. Emerick Szilagyi.

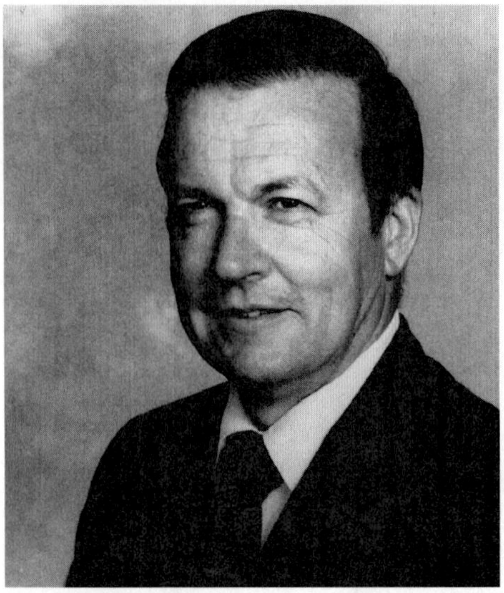

FIGURE 60.8. Arthur B. Voorhees, Jr.

repair of a ruptured aortic aneurysm, done March 13, 1953.[57] Other early successful cases were reported by Gerbode, Cooley and DeBakey, and Javid et al.[58–60]

Thoracic Aneurysms

Thoracic aneurysms have presented a challenge to surgeons for many years. These aneurysms can be saccular, fusiform, or associated with coarctation of the aorta. Following the lead of Moore in 1864, they were treated by wiring until more definitive measures were developed.[31] Among lesions associated with coarctation, John Alexander in Ann Arbor in 1941 simply resected the aneurysm and the coarctation and sewed off the ends without doing an anastomosis or using a graft.[61] Henry Swan, on June 28, 1949, apparently was the first to resect an aneurysm associated with a coarctation and replace the resected area with a homograft.[62] In 1951, Gross reported five cases of aneurysm associated with coarctation treated by resection and graft.[63] Bahnson[50] and Cooley and DeBakey[64] in the early 1950s resected saccular aneurysms and repaired the arterial wall by lateral suture. DeBakey and Cooley reported the first case of a successful resection and graft of a fusiform thoracic aneurysm, done January 5, 1953.[65] Since that time, all sections of the thoracic aorta from the arch to the diaphragm have been successfully resected and replaced by grafts of various sorts.

Thoracoabdominal Aneurysms

Thoracoabdominal aneurysms have presented an even greater challenge. A forgotten pioneer in vascular surgery is the Austrian surgeon, Ernst Jeger, who died at age 30 in World War I. Jeger was a brilliant investigator who devised many vascular and cardiac procedures, including one for complicated thoracoabdominal aneurysms.[66] Etheredge described resection of this lesion in 1955. He used a temporary shunt from the distal thoracic aorta to the distal abdominal aorta. A homograft was then inserted and the visceral vessels implanted into the homograft.[67] DeBakey described a similar technique in 1956 using a temporary bypass shunt.[68] Shumacker (Fig. 60.9) modified this technique by employing the homograft shunt as the permanent conduit and implanting the visceral vessels into it, then excising the aneurysm.[69] Stanley Crawford reported his experience in 1974. The earliest cases consisted of inserting a Dacron graft and reattaching consecutively involved branches to side-arm tube grafts arising from the bypass. In the later cases, the graft was inserted inside the aneurysm with reattachment of visceral branch origins directly to an opening in the graft wall—the inclusion technique, as used today.[70] Peripheral aneurysms (e.g., popliteal) may be managed by either resection and graft or bypass techniques.

Arterial Occlusive Disease

René Leriche (1879–1955) first published his observations on obliteration of the terminal aorta in 1923, and stated that the ideal treatment would be resection of the area and reestablishment of patency. In 1940, he published a detailed description of the syndrome that now bears his name. He recommended resection of the terminal aorta and common iliac arteries together with bilateral lumbar sympathectomy through a retroperitoneal approach. Results of this procedure were variable, depending on the preoperative status of the patient. When Jacques Oudot resected the terminal aorta and replaced it with a preserved homologous aortic graft in 1950, the Leriche procedure became obsolete.[71]

A direct attack on occluded vessels was made by J. Cid Dos Santos of Portugal in 1946. He performed the first successful thromboendarterectomy for peripheral occlusive disease and established this as a feasible procedure. His first operation was performed August 27, 1946, on a left femoral artery and his second operation on December 12, 1946, on a subclavian artery. Both of these cases were successful so far as patency was concerned. He termed this operation disobliteration, but it came to be known as thromboendarterectomy, or just endarterectomy.[72] By 1948 Bazy in France had performed endarterectomy on 12 abdominal aortic occlusion

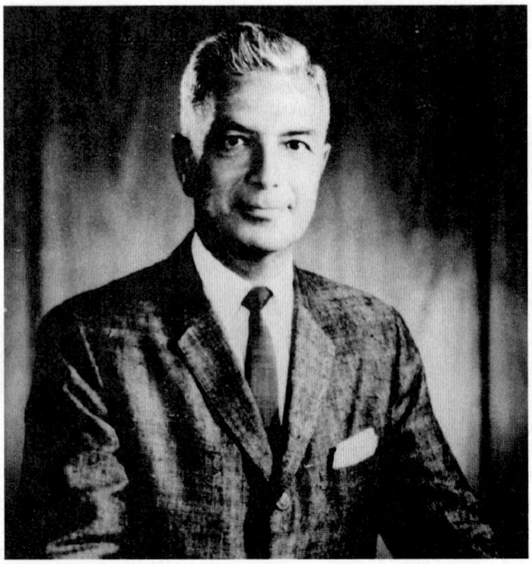

FIGURE 60.9. Harris B. Shumacker, Jr. (Reprinted with permission from Thompson JE. The founding fathers. J Vasc Surg 1996;23:1027, 1028, 1029, 1030.)

cases, and Kunlin in Leriche's clinic had also carried out the procedure in a number of patients.[1]

In 1951, aortic endarterectomy was introduced into the United States (Fig. 60.10) by E. Jack Wylie of San Francisco.[73] Wiley Barker and Jack Cannon of Los Angeles were pioneers in the use of endarterectomy for femoral occlusive disease.[74] Endarterectomy has gradually given way to bypass grafting, except for the carotid area and certain localized obstructions in other large vessels.[75]

A giant step forward in the treatment of aortic occlusive disease was made November 14, 1950 when Jacques Oudot, another Frenchman, was the first to resect the terminal aorta for the Leriche syndrome and replace it with a preserved homologous aortic graft 24 days old using end-to-end anastomoses. Six months later, because of thrombosis of the right iliac limb of the graft, he placed a crossover graft from the left distal external iliac to the right distal external iliac, the first extraanatomical bypass. Oudot, a French mountaineer, lost his life in an automobile accident at the age of 40.[1,76] Resection of the aortoiliac segment with graft replacement gave way first to endarterectomy and then gradually to aortoiliac or aortofemoral bypass, leaving the native vessels in situ.

The principle of bypass surgery had been suggested by Ernst Jager,[66] but it remained for a French surgeon, Jean Kunlin, working in Leriche's clinic, to perform the first long bypass graft of the femoral artery with a reversed saphenous vein on June 3, 1948, using end-to-side anastomoses both proximally and distally.[77] The first patient treated by Kunlin was a 54-year-old man who had previously had an arteriectomy of the superficial femoral artery, the Leriche operation. His ischemia was not relieved, and Kunlin decided to do a venous graft with end-to-end anastomoses; however, exposure of the previous operative sites was difficult because of a tremendous fibrotic reaction and end-to-end anastomoses could not be done. Kunlin had no other choice but to do end-to-side implantations of the venous graft into the femoral artery above and below. Thus, the bypass procedure was born by serendipity.[1] The femoropopliteal bypass has become a standard vascular operation for the treatment of infrainguinal atherosclerotic occlusive disease. It was popularized by Robert Linton (Fig. 60.11) of Boston, among others.[55,78,79]

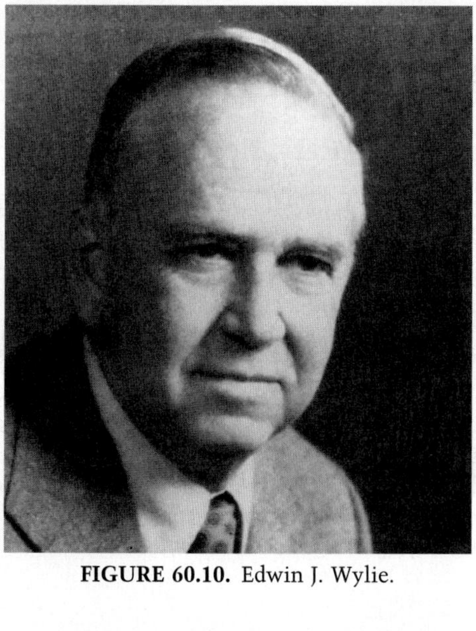

FIGURE 60.10. Edwin J. Wylie.

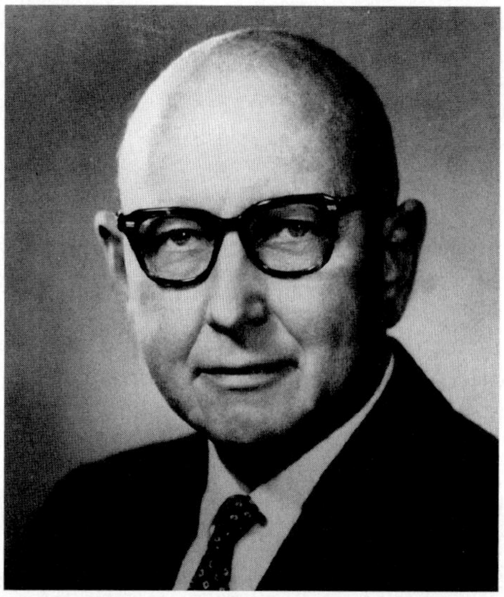

FIGURE 60.11. Robert R. Linton. (Reprinted with permission from Thompson JE. The founding fathers. J Vasc Surg 1996;23:1027, 1028, 1029, 1030.)

In Situ Saphenous Bypass

A variation of the femoropopliteal bypass technique was introduced by K.V. Hall in 1962, the nonreversed in situ saphenous vein bypass after obliterating the venous valves.[80] The technique was recommended by Connolly in 1964, but the operation was slow to gain acceptance.[81] Leather, in the 1970s, resurrected the concept and improved the method of rendering the venous valves incompetent.[82] Since then the procedure has been widely used with distal extension of the bypass to the lower leg, ankle, and foot for limb salvage.[83]

The bypass principle was extended to the aorta by Frank Cockett of London, who probably did the first aortic bypass in 1955 for treatment of aortic thrombosis without removing the aorta.[1] This operation was another step forward and was less demanding than aortoiliofemoral endarterectomy. An important feature critical to the success of aortofemoral bypass is proper handling of the profunda femoris artery, the orifice of which must be endarterectomized to allow for maximum distal runoff. Aortofemoral bypass has become the standard procedure for treatment of aortoiliac occlusive disease.[84,85]

Fluids

In the early days of aortic surgery, one of the major problems besetting surgeons was proper fluid management during the operative procedure and immediately postoperative. At first surgeons followed the recommendations current at that time, avoiding salt solutions and using almost exclusively limited quantities of dextrose in water. With this regimen there was a high incidence of shock, oliguria, hypotension, and renal shutdown, especially when the aorta was declamped.[86]

In the 1960s surgeons began to follow the recommendations of Shires et al.[87] and give fairly large quantities of dextrose in lactated Ringer's solution to keep the perioperative urine output above 125 mL/h. These large quantities compensated for the sequestration of extracellular fluid to maintain an effective circulating blood volume. With this regimen, hypotensive and renal complications of elective aortic surgery largely disappeared.[88]

Embolectomy

Arterial embolism has long been a problem for vascular surgeons. Embolectomy, a direct arterial procedure, was first performed successfully on the femoral artery by Labey in 1911 and reported by Mosny and Dumont.[89] The first successful aortic embolectomy by direct aortotomy was reported by Bauer in 1913.[90] Results were less than ideal until heparin was introduced to aid in the prevention of distal thrombosis. The most significant advance, however, was the introduction of the balloon catheter by Fogarty (Fig. 60.12) and associates in 1963, which has improved not only the management of embolism but vascular surgery in general.[91]

Sympathectomy

Periarterial sympathectomy was first reported by Jaboulay in 1899 and was later championed by Rene Leriche.[92] Lumbar sympathectomy was first performed by Royle in Australia on September 1, 1923, for spastic paralysis.[93] Independently, it was carried out by Julio Diez in Buenos Aires on July 24, 1924, for peripheral occlusive disease.[94] Stellate ganglionectomy was reported by Jonnesco and by Bruning in 1923.[92] In the 1930s and 1940s, thoracolumbar splanchnicectomy for essential hypertension was carried out by a number of surgeons, especially Reginald Smithwick (Fig. 60.13) in Boston.[95] With the advent of antihypertensive drugs, the use of thoracolumbar splanchnicectomy was no longer necessary. Similarly, with the advent of direct arterial surgery, sympathectomy is now reserved for the treatment of causalgia and related pain syndromes, hyperhidrosis, and vascular disorders when vasomotor instability is a major component. Smithwick and Geza DeTakats were leading proponents of sympathectomy in the early days for treatment of peripheral vasospastic and occlusive disorders.[95,96]

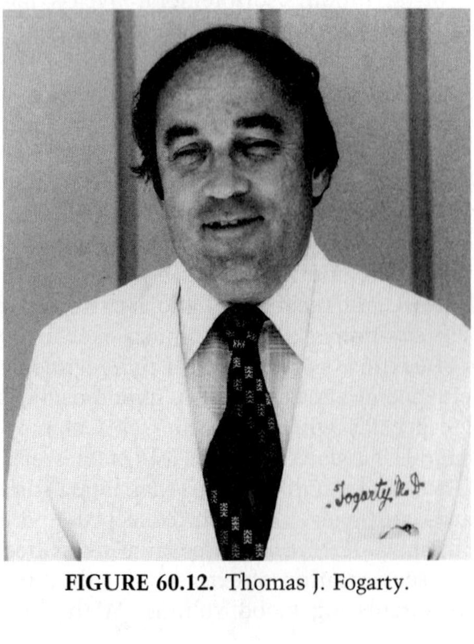

FIGURE 60.12. Thomas J. Fogarty.

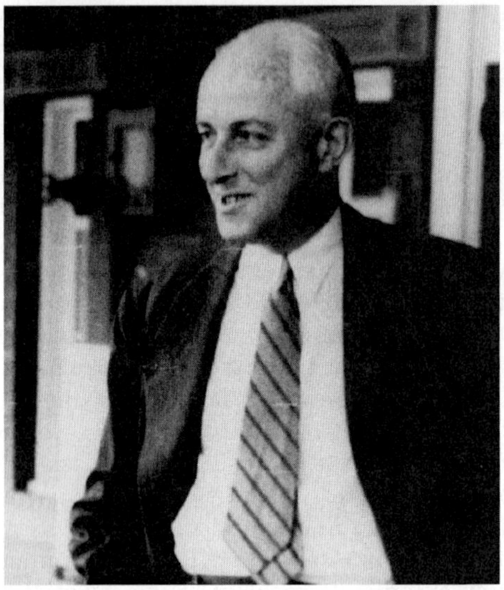

FIGURE 60.13. Reginald H. Smithwick. (Reprinted with permission from Thompson JE. The founding fathers. J Vasc Surg 1996;23:1027, 1028, 1029, 1030.)

Extraanatomic Procedures

Oudot in 1951 had performed a crossover graft from the left distal external iliac to the right distal iliac artery.[76] Norman Freeman in San Francisco, in 1952, performed the first crossover femoral graft using an endarterectomized segment of the left femoral artery to crossover and revascularize successfully the right leg.[97] In 1962, Vetto reported 10 transabdominal subcutaneous femorofemoral graft operations to bypass iliac occlusive disease in high-risk patients.[98] Femorofemoral crossover graft is now a useful standard procedure.

In 1959, Lewis resected an abdominal aortic aneurysm and was forced to reconstruct with a nylon graft from the subclavian artery subcutaneously into the abdomen for anastomosis to a homograft replacement.[99] In 1961, Blaisdell et al. performed an extraperitoneal thoracic aorta to femoral bypass graft using Dacron as replacement for an infected aortic bifurcation prosthesis. The following year, on March 25, 1962, Blaisdell and Hall performed a bypass procedure for aortoiliac occlusion using a Dacron graft carried from the axillary artery subcutaneously to the femoral artery.[100] At about the same time, the same procedure was performed by Louw in South Africa.[101] Such were the beginnings of extraanatomical bypass procedures.

Renal and Mesenteric Lesions

Renal artery lesions have been treated surgically in the management of renovascular hypertension, renal insufficiency, and aneurysms. In 1951 splenorenal arterial anastomosis was first used, although unsuccessfully, in the treatment of hypertension.[102] It was later applied successfully by De Camp et al. in 1957.[103] Since then a number of techniques have been used for renal artery lesions, the most common being aortorenal bypass, but also including splenorenal and hepatorenal bypass. Transaortic endarterectomy has also been successfully employed by Stoney and associates.[104] Endarterectomy and bypass techniques have also been applied successfully in the management of mesenteric vascular lesions.[104]

Cerebrovascular Disease

Increasing awareness, in the past 45 years, of the extracranial location and segmental nature of atherosclerotic occlusive disease in a large proportion of patients with cerebrovascular insufficiency was followed by the development and use of appropriate vascular surgical techniques for removing or bypassing offending plaques, thus increasing cerebral blood flow or eliminating sources of cerebral emboli.[9]

The word carotid is derived from the Greek term *karotids* or *karos*, meaning to stupefy or plunge into a deep sleep. According to Rufus of Ephesus (circa AD 100), the term was applied to the arteries of the neck because compression of these vessels produced stupor or sleep.[105] The ancient Greeks were aware of the significance of the carotid artery; the 31st metope from the south side of the Parthenon in Athens depicts a centaur applying left carotid compression to the neck of a Lapith warrior (Fig. 60.14).

With the advent of Hippocrates (460–370 BC), ancient descriptive neurology was born. He described paralysis of the right arm with loss of speech in what is probably the first written description of aphasia.[105] Galen (AD 131–201) was aware that hemiplegia resulted from a lesion in the opposite side of the brain as a cause of apoplexy.[105] With Galen as the authority, European medicine remained at a dead level for nearly 14 centuries until the time of Vesalius, who in 1543, with the publication of *De Fabrica Humani Corporis*, threw overboard Galenical traditions.[16]

Ambroise Paré, in the sixteenth century, was familiar with the carotid phenomenon and stated, "The two branches they call carotides or soporales, the sleepy arteries, because they being obstructed or any way stopt we presently fall asleep."[15] The seventeenth century saw the work of Thomas Willis and Richard Lower in connection with the circle of arteries at the base of the brain.[9]

The first operations on the carotid artery were quite naturally ligation procedures for trauma or hemorrhage. Hebenstreit of Germany, in his translation of Benjamin Bell's *Surgery* in 1793, mentions a case in which the carotid artery was injured during operative removal of a scirrhous tumor. The surgeon ligated the vessel to stop hemorrhage, and the patient lived for many years. This is thought to be the first case on record of ligature of the carotid.[106–108]

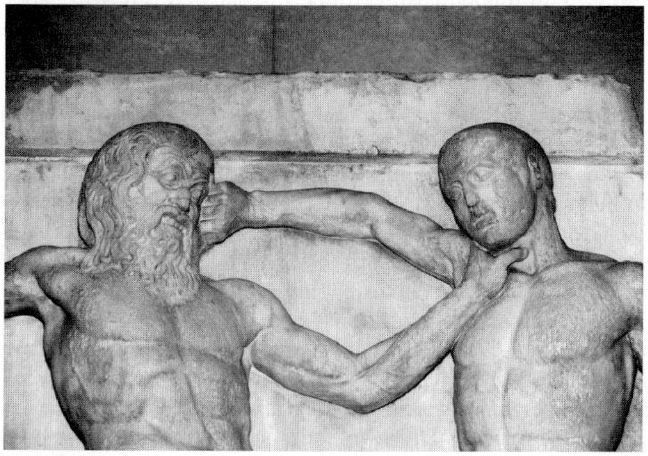

FIGURE 60.14. The 31st metope from the south side of the Parthenon in Athens.

John Abernethy of London, a pupil of John Hunter, in 1804 reported a case of carotid ligation performed some years previously, probably in 1798. The patient, a man, was gored in the neck by the horn of a cow, and hemorrhage was profuse. Compression controlled the bleeding temporarily only to have it recur when pressure was released. Abernethy was compelled to ligate the common carotid artery. Hemorrhage was controlled, and the patient appeared well. However, the man died 30h later of cerebral causes, and Abernethy abandoned the procedure.[106,108–110]

With the beginning of the nineteenth century, the history of carotid surgery becomes more accurate. The first successful ligation of a carotid artery was performed by David Fleming on October 17, 1803. Fleming was a young naval surgeon aboard His Majesty's ship *Tonnant* during the Napoleonic era. Mark Jackson, a servant, attempted to commit suicide by cutting his throat on October 9, 1803. The knife had grazed the outer and muscular coats of the carotid artery but left the artery intact. Eight days later, on October 17, the carotid ruptured. Fleming cut down on the artery proximal to the rupture and ligated it. He had not done this before, nor had he heard of Abernethy's case. The patient survived and made an uninterrupted recovery. This was the first authentic successful case of ligation of the carotid artery on record.[111,112]

The first successful ligation of the carotid artery in the United States was performed by Amos Twitchell of Keene, New Hampshire, on October 18, 1807. John Taggart, a cavalry soldier of age 20, during a mock fight at a regimental review was accidentally wounded in the neck by a pistol shot on October 8, 1807. The wound was treated by simple dressings, although Dr. Twitchell commented, "There was a good deal of arterial excitement." Taggart, however, improved rapidly until the 10th day when the internal carotid artery ruptured. Twitchell stopped the hemorrhage by compression, then made an incision lower in the neck and ligated the common carotid artery with the patient's mother acting as his assistant. He then packed the wound with dry sponges. The patient made an uneventful recovery.[106,113]

Sir Astley Cooper in London was the first to attempt ligation of a carotid artery for cervical aneurysm on November 1, 1805. The patient died of sepsis on the 21st day with a left hemiparesis. Cooper repeated the operation on June 22, 1808, at Guy's Hospital. The patient was 55 years of age and had a pulsating tumor the size of an egg at the angle of the jaw. Two ligatures were applied to the artery, which was divided. The patient made a perfect recovery with no untoward symptoms and lived until 1821. This was the first successful case of ligature of the carotid artery for aneurysm.[114,115]

Benjamin Travers, on May 23, 1809, first successfully ligated the left carotid for carotid-cavernous fistula, with disappearance of signs and symptoms. In 1885 Victor Horsley first successfully ligated the carotid in the neck for an intracranial aneurysm. The patient was well 5 years later. By 1868, Pilz was able to collect 600 recorded cases of carotid ligation for cervical aneurysm or hemorrhage with a mortality rate of 43%.[9,110]

Until fairly recently, the prevailing notion held by most physicians was that strokes were caused by intracranial vascular disease. William Osler, in his 1909 textbook, attributed apoplectic stroke largely to cerebral hemorrhage. No mention is made of extracranial occlusive disease, and emphasis is on blockage of intracranial vessels.[31] This is somewhat curious in view of the fact that several authors had already described occlusive lesions in the extracranial segments of the main arteries supplying the brain and noted their association with symptoms of cerebral ischemia. These authorities included Heberden, Gull, Savory, Virchow, Broadbent, Penzoldt, and Chiari.[9]

A landmark article was that publised by J. Ramsay Hunt of New York City in 1914, who called attention to the importance of extracranial occlusions in cerebrovascular disease, and even used the term "cerebral intermittent claudication" to describe transient ischemic attacks (TIAs).[116] The next significant contribution was the report of Egas Móniz of Portugal, who in 1927 first described the technique of cerebral arteriography for the study of cerebral tumors, using sodium iodide as the contrast medium, and thus laid the groundwork of a practical method for the diagnosis of occlusive lesions.[117] The first report of carotid thrombosis demonstrated by arteriography was that of Sjöqvist in 1936.[118] The following year, 1937, Móniz, Lima, and de Lacerda reported four patients with occlusion of the cervical portion of the internal carotid artery in whom the diagnosis had been established by arteriography.[119] Egas Móniz won a Nobel Prize in 1949, not for cerebral arteriography but for his work on prefrontal lobotomy. By 1951 Johnson and Walker were able to collect 107 instances of carotid thrombosis, all diagnosed by arteriography.[120]

In two important articles published in 1951 and 1954, C. Miller Fisher, working in Montreal and later in Boston, reemphasized the relationship between and frequency of disease of the carotid artery in the neck and cerebrovascular insufficiency. He observed that with severe stenosis of the carotid bifurcation, the distal vessels could be entirely free of disease. He stated, "It is even conceivable that some day vascular surgery will find a way to bypass the occluded portion of the artery during the period of ominous fleeting symptoms. Anastomosis of the external carotid artery or one of its branches with the internal carotid artery above the area of narrowing should be feasible."[121,122]

In 1952, John Conley of New York reported anastomosing the distal ends of the internal carotid artery and external carotid artery to restore flow to the brain after tumor resection, a procedure previously reported by LeFevre in France in 1918. In 1953, Conley reported 11 cases in which the superficial femoral or saphenous vein had been used as an interposition graft to reconstruct a resected cervical carotid artery after tumor surgery.[123,124] Dos Santos in 1946 had introduced thromboendarterectomy for restoring flow in peripheral vessels.[72] In 1951, E.J. Wylie introduced into the United States thromboendarterectomy for the removal of atherosclerotic plaques from the aortoiliac segments, but this technique had not been used on the carotid artery.[73]

Fisher's prophecy of surgical reconstruction of the carotid artery in the neck as therapy for occlusive disease was soon fulfilled. The first successful reconstruction of the carotid artery was performed by Carrea, Molins, and Murphy in Buenos Aires in 1951, after they read Fisher's article, and was reported in 1955 (Fig. 60.15). A 41-year-old male patient had recurring symptoms of right hemiparesis, aphasia, and left amaurosis over a 6-month period. A left percutaneous arteriogram demonstrated an atherosclerotic plaque with severe stenosis in the internal carotid artery. On October 20, 1951, Molins, a vascular surgeon, and Carrea performed an end-to-end anastomosis between the left external carotid and distal internal carotid arteries after partial resection of the stenosed area, together with cervical sympathectomy. The patient made an uneventful recovery and died 23 years later of myocardial infarction. His neurological status was normal except for loss of vision in the left eye.[125]

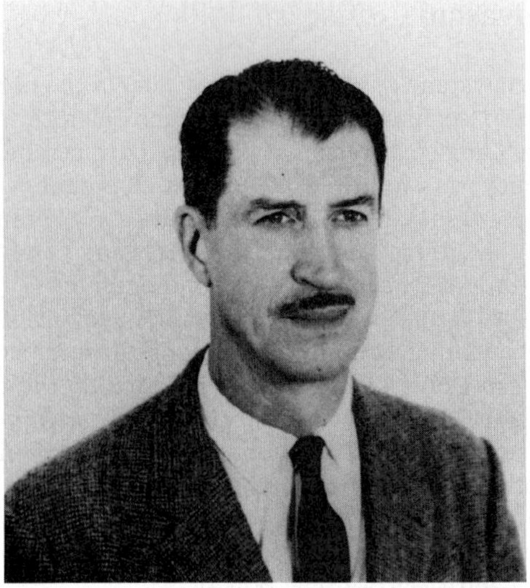

FIGURE 60.15. Mahelz Molins. (Reprinted with permission from Friedman SG. A History of Vascular Surgery. Mount Kisco, NY: Futura, 1989:167.[3])

On January 28, 1953, Strully, Hurwitt, and Blankenberg in New York operated on a patient with a frank stroke and a totally occluded internal carotid artery. They performed a thrombectomy but were unable to obtain retrograde flow; consequently, a section of the internal carotid was removed. They suggested that thromboendarterectomy should be feasible in such cases when the distal vasculature was patent.[126]

The first successful carotid endarterectomy was performed by Michael DeBakey on August 7, 1953. A 53-year-old schoolbus driver gave a history of recurring episodes of transient right hemiparesis and dysphasia during a 2-year period. On examination, he had a mild residual right hemiparesis and a weak pulsation in his left carotid artery. No preoperative arteriogram was performed. During surgery, a severely stenotic atherosclerotic plaque with superimposed fresh clot completely occluding the left internal carotid artery was found. Thromboendarterectomy was carried out with good retrograde flow from both internal and external carotid arteries. An arteriogram performed postoperatively on the operating table showed the internal carotid to be patent in both its extracranial and intracranial portions. The patient made a good recovery and lived for 19 years without having further strokes. He died of complications of coronary artery disease on August 17, 1972.[127]

The operation that gave the greatest impetus to the development of surgery for carotid occlusive disease was that performed by Eastcott, Pickering, and Rob on May 19, 1954, at St. Mary's Hospital in London (Figs. 60.16, 60.17). In this case, a 66-year-old housewife who had suffered 33 transient episodes of right hemiparesis, aphasia, and left amaurosis over a 5-month period was found to have a severe stenosis of the left carotid bifurcation after a percutaneous left carotid arteriogram. With the patient under general anesthesia and with hypothermia to 28°C (82.4°F) by means of ice bags for cerebral

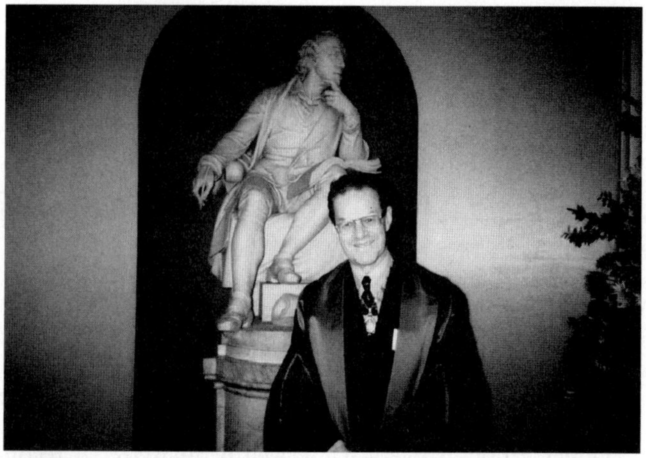

FIGURE 60.16. H.H.G. Eastcott, in front of a statue of John Hunter.

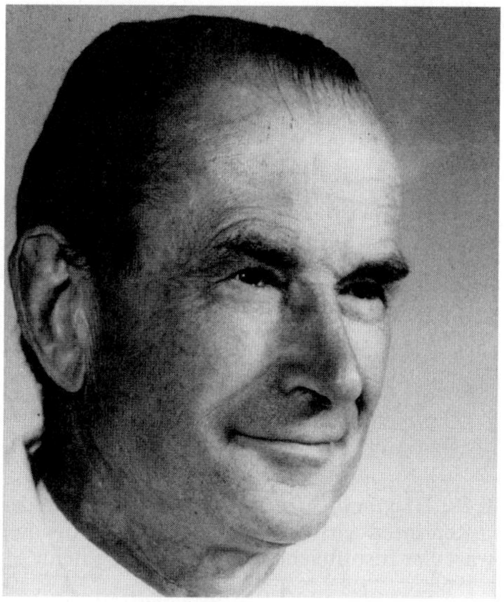

FIGURE 60.17. Charles G. Rob.

protection, the bifurcation was resected and blood flow restored by end-to-end anastomosis between the common carotid and distal internal carotid arteries. The patient was completely relieved of her symptoms and was alive and well at the age of 86.[128]

Following these landmark cases, a number of different methods of carotid reconstruction were reported. Table 60.1 lists in chronological order some early procedures performed.[125–133] With increasing experience, the various procedures listed were abandoned with the exception of endarterectomy, which has become the standard operation (Fig. 60.18). At first an external shunt was used for cerebral protection, but this gave way to the intraluminal shunt, which is now used either routinely or selectively when the carotid is occluded during endarterectomy.[9]

A variant of the standard endarterectomy technique is eversion endarterectomy, introduced by DeBakey's group in 1959.[134] It has been used infrequently over the years, but recently it has been employed more often by a number of surgeons in an effort to reduce the incidence of long-term recurrent carotid stenosis.[135]

Surgical treatment of occlusive lesions of the great vessels arising from the aortic arch did not lag far behind that of the carotid artery in the neck. Gordon Murray of Toronto in 1950 successfully restored, by means of a probe and instrumentation, circulation in a left common carotid artery totally occluded at the aortic arch.[136] On March 20, 1954, Davis, Grove, and Julian performed the first innominate endarterectomy. On January 4, 1957, DeBakey and his group constructed a bypass graft from the innominate to the distal subclavian and carotid arteries and shortly thereafter successfully performed subclavian endarterectomy. Bypass procedures including extrathoracic bypass such as carotid–subclavian bypass and endarterectomy remain the usual standard operations today for lesions of the aortic arch vessels.[137,138]

TABLE 60.1.
First Carotid Reconstructions for Cerebrovascular Insufficiency in Chronological Order.

Author	*Date of operation*	*Degree of stenosis*	*Procedure of flow*	*Restoration*
Carrea, Molins, and Murphy[125]	October 20, 1951	Partial	End-to-end anastomosis, external carotid to internal carotid	Yes
Strully, Hurwitt, and Blankenberg[126]	January 28, 1953	Total	Thromboendarterectomy followed by ligation and resection	No
DeBakey[127]	August 7, 1953	Total	Thromboendarterectomy	Yes
Eastcott, Pickering, and Rob[128]	May 19, 1954	Partial	End-to-end anastomosis, common carotid to internal carotid	Yes
	June 1954	Partial	Thromboendarterectomy	Yes
Denman, Ehni, and Duty[129]	July 14, 1954	Total	Resection with homograft	Yes
Lin, Javid, and Doyle[130]	December, 1955	Partial	Resection with saphenous vein graft	Yes
Murphey and Miller[131]	February 6, 1956	Total	Thromboendarterectomy	Yes
	February 24, 1956	Partial	Thromboendarterectomy	Yes
Cooley, Al-Naaman, and Carton[132]	March 8, 1956	Partial	Endarterectomy	Yes
Lyons and Galbraith[133]	August 9, 1956	Partial	Subclavian–carotid nylon bypass graft	Yes

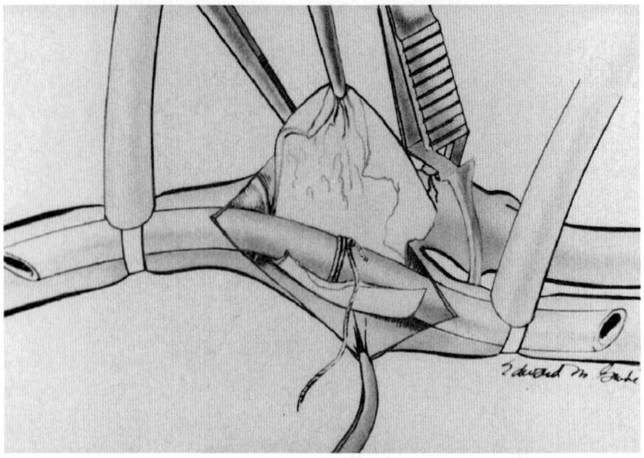

FIGURE 60.18. Diagram of technique of carotid endarterectomy with shunt. (Reprinted with permission from Thompson JE. Surgery for Cerebrovascular Insufficiency (Stroke). Spring-field, MA: Charles C. Thomas, 1968:32.[138])

As a result of studies by Hutchinson and Yates in 1956 directing attention to the importance of occlusive lesions in the cervical portion of the vertebral arteries, reconstructive operations on the vertebral vessels were developed.[139] On September 7, 1957, Cate and Scott in Nashville carried out successful endarterectomy of the left subclavian and left vertebral arteries. In 1958, Crawford, DeBakey, and Fields described treatment of vertebral-basilar insufficiency by means of vertebral endarterectomy in one case and bypass graft from the subclavian to the distal patent vertebral in another.[137,138] Newer techniques have enlarged the scope of vertebral surgery. Edwards et al. have been foremost in promoting subclavian and vertebral transpositions into the common carotid artery.[140] Berguer has devised innovative procedures on the distal vertebral artery near the base of the skull.[141] On the basis of microsurgical techniques developed in the 1960s, Yasargil, et al. carried out extracranial to intracranial bypass procedures hoping for improvement in patients with strokes who had occluded cervical internal carotid arteries.[142] In 1977, a randomized trial was initiated. Unfortunately, the trial failed to demonstrate significant benefit from the surgery, and the operation is no longer performed except in occasional situations, in which it may be quite beneficial.[143]

Venous Surgery

Venous problems, similar to arterial diseases, have been present since ancient times. As early as 1550 BC, varicose veins were mentioned in the Ebers Papyrus.[144] In 500 BC, Hippocrates recommended compression treatment of varices. Galen advocated removal of varices with a hook. Aegineta (AD 625–690) performed ligation and division followed by bandaging.[3,145]

Ambroise Paré treated varicose veins and varicose ulcers. For varices, he recommended ligation and excision. He treated ulcers by means of bed rest, elevation, and pressure dressing over the ulcer and wrapped the legs with a roller bandage of linen, much like present-day therapy. In the late 1800s Trendelenburg popularized ligation of varices. In 1884 Madelung of Germany removed varicose saphenous veins through a long incision in the leg similar to that used today for removal of a vein for bypass procedures. There were many complications of Madelung's procedure.[3,15,145] The plaster boot was introduced by Unna of Germany in 1896.[3]

In 1905 Keller in the United States first reported stripping by tying the vein to a wire and then pulling it out. Also in 1905, Babcock devised his rigid intraluminal stripper. In 1906 Mayo introduced the extraluminal straight stripper. Homans, in 1916, emphasized the importance of ligation at the saphenofemoral junction and removed varicose veins by radical excision and stripping. In 1938 Linton advocated ligation, stripping, and extensive removal of segments. In 1947, T.T. Myers of the Mayo Clinic developed a flexible intraluminal stripper that greatly facilitated the removal of both small and large varices.[145] All modern-day strippers are modifications of these older strippers. Sclerotherapy has also been used in conjunction with or instead of ligation and stripping.

Direct venous surgery has lagged behind arterial reconstruction operations. Eck, in 1877, performed the first successful venovenous anastomosis between the portal vein and the vena cava. In 1902, Alexis Carrel and C.C. Guthrie published their results of arterial and venous anastomosis and transplantation of organs using their meticulous technical methods. Payr in 1904 devised a method of uniting divided vessels by using cylinders of magnesium. Exner in 1903 made the first attempt at vein grafting by transplanting autologous segments of jugular veins into the opposite side of the neck in two dogs, using the magnesium prosthesis of Payr. The results were poor, and thus little was done during the next 40 years.[146] With the flowering of arterial reconstructive surgery during the past 50 years, much investigation has gone on in the field of venous surgery.

A great step forward occurred in 1923 when Berberich and Hirsch first performed radiography following intravenous injection of strontium bromide, thus introducing venography. In 1929, McPheeters and Rice used lipiodol as the contrast medium, and in 1934 Edwards and Biguria used diodone (an iodine base), a much safer medium. Both ascending and descending venography followed introduction of the procedure.[147]

Management of deep venous thrombosis with prevention and treatment of pulmonary embolism has been a major problem for physicians for years. John Homans (Fig. 60.19) is credited with using femoral vein ligation in 1934 to prevent fatal pulmonary embolism. In 1944 the inferior vena cava was first ligated for the prevention of pulmonary embolism. By 1958, 468 cases had been reported in the United States.[148,149] Numerous devices have been used to prevent pulmonary embolism, including plication of the vena cava, vena cava clips for partial occlusion, vena caval umbrellas, and vena caval filters of various sorts. The most popular filter, that of Lazar Greenfield, has been very effective and can be inserted readily from the neck or the groin.[150–153]

In the 1940s a series of patients at the Massachusetts General Hospital were subjected to bilateral superficial femoral vein ligation under local anesthesia in a study aimed at prevention of fatal and nonfatal pulmonary embolism. Several hundred cases were operated upon with minimal complications. Compared with other methods of therapy, it could not be shown that this operation reduced significantly the incidence of pulmonary embolism. The operation was therefore abandoned as routine treatment.[154] Linton devised an operation of extensive subfascial division of incompetent perforating veins for the treatment of severe symptoms of chronic postphlebitic syndrome.[155]

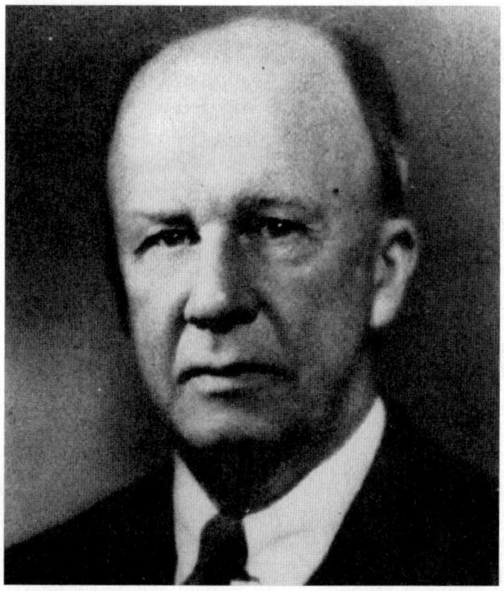

FIGURE 60.19. John Homans. (Reprinted with permission from Thompson JE. The founding fathers. J Vasc Surg 1996;23:1027, 1028, 1029, 1030.)

Since midcentury, a number of noninvasive tests have been developed in an effort to study deep venous thrombosis, including Doppler ultrasonography, impedance plethysmography, and phleborheography. A major breakthrough came when it was demonstrated that B-mode ultrasonography could be used to diagnose deep venous thrombosis. Duplex scanning was found to have major advantages. At the present time, color-flow duplex scanning is the method of choice.[156]

Surgical procedures have been developed to bypass obstructions in the iliac veins using a crossover graft as the conduit or the distally divided saphenous vein from the opposite leg, the Palma procedure, reported first in 1958.[157] Bypass of obstruction in the lower leg can relieve problems at the lower level as well; this is the saphenopopliteal bypass or Husni operation.[158]

Techniques have been developed to repair or replace incompetent valves in the veins of the lower extremity in certain selected patients with chronic venous insufficiency. These procedures include valvuloplasty, internal or external, and various vein transfers.[144,159,160] Balloon angioplasty has been introduced to dilate venous obstructions, and stents have been placed in the venous system. Results have been less satisfactory than when these techniques are used for arterial lesions.

Vascular Injuries

Over the years vascular injuries have been treated in a variety of ways. Antyllus used ligation to stop bleeding and packed his wounds. Galen, who was very influential, used ligatures and cautery to control hemorrhage. There was very little progress in treatment of vascular injuries during the next 1300 years, the main elements of therapy being amputation, boiling oil, cautery, and the ligature and packing of wounds.[3]

It was left for Ambroise Paré to bring some improvement in wound management. The story is that in a battle Paré ran out of boiling oil and applied nonirritating simple dressings to bleeding areas; much to his astonishment, the patients improved and progressed much better than when boiling oil and cautery were used. Paré thus used ligation and a simple dressings and amputations as necessary.[3] The work of Hallowell, Murphy, Carrel, and Guthrie, and others on direct arterial suture has already been described.[21]

Over the centuries, wars have provided a fruitful source of vascular injuries, which were first treated by boiling oil, cautery, ligation, packing, and amputation, until vascular repair began to be carried out on the battlefield. Battlefield repair was done in the Balkan wars before World War I by a Serbian army surgeon named V. Soubbotitch, who initiated a program whereby injured blood vessels were treated by direct repair rather than primary amputation. In 1914 he reported his results with 185 operations for vascular injuries. His work was largely ignored until the 1950s.[3]

Ligation remained the primary method of treating vascular injuries during World War I. Allied military surgeons believed that battlefield repair of injured arteries was not practicable and that controlling hemorrhage by ligation was sufficient. The Germans did make some effort to repair blood vessels. Ernst Jeger even attempted to use fresh arterial and venous homografts from limbs severed in battle to replace wounded arteries. Most of these grafts thrombosed, however, and Jeger's idea was never culminated.[3,66]

Despite a number of supportive innovations such as the availability of blood and antibiotics, these aids did not advance vascular surgery in World War II, which still consisted largely of ligation and amputation. DeBakey and Simeone reported on 2471 arterial wounds in World War II. They found only 81 instances of suture repair, with an amputation rate of 36%. Amputation rate following ligation was nearly 50%. Based on sound considerations, DeBakey and Simeone did not believe that battlefield repair was practical or realistic, mainly because of the great delay between wounding and surgical treatment.[161] Those soldiers with vascular injuries whose limbs survived and who were evacuated to the Zone of the Interior received subsequent repair of false aneurysms and arteriovenous fistulas by ligation and excision when collateral circulation was deemed adequate, and these did very well.

When the Korean War broke out, a new policy was soon inaugurated, the restoration of vascular continuity in injured vessels by direct anastomosis, lateral repair, or graft replacement, either arterial or venous, in an effort to improve amputation rates. The use of the helicopter to reduce the time between wounding and repair was invaluable. Repairs were done in Mobile Army Surgical Hospitals (MASH). The first 130 cases were performed with an 89% limb salvage rate, and a new era in vascular surgery had begun. Ligation of major arteries in World War II had given an amputation rate of 49%. In the Korean War, in contrast, the eventual amputation rate was 13%.[3,162]

The war in Vietnam provided an opportunity to corroborate the lessons learned in the Korean War about management of vascular injuries. A Vietnam Vascular Registry was begun under the direction of Carl Hughes and Norman Rich to analyze all vascular injuries treated in army hospitals in Vietnam. Data from the Registry showed a limb salvage rate of 87%.[3,162,163]

Techniques for the management of civilian vascular injuries since midcentury have paralleled the explosive development of the techniques used for treatment of aneurysmal and occlusive vascular diseases. Appropriate management for injuries in all areas of the body has been developed by a number of surgeons. These techniques have involved the proper use of angiography, direct vascular repair, bypass procedures, and the use of arterial and venous autografts, homografts, and prosthetic grafts of various sorts.[162–165]

Vascular Disorders

A number of vascular disorders, such as dissection, dissecting aneurysms,[166] aortoenteric fistulas, and aortocaval fistulas, can now be managed satisfactorily with modern vascular surgical techniques. The retroperitoneal approach to the aorta first advocated by Astley Cooper in 1817 has found increasing usefulness. Dilatation of stenoses by balloon angioplasty techniques, introduced by Dotter and Gruentzig, has been shown to be helpful, especially when accompanied by implantation of stents.[3,167] Clagett et al. have recently replaced infected aortic prostheses in situ with deep and superficial veins from the lower extremity.[168]

Most recently, an exciting new era of endovascular grafting has opened up avenues of therapy with techniques of lesser magnitude, hopefully lowering the morbidity and mortality of current techniques and extending the field of vascular surgery to areas not previously available.

Thus, at the beginning of the twentieth century, basic vascular techniques were available but the supporting pillars were lacking. By midcentury all necessary items had fallen into place, resulting in the spectacular development of vascular surgery as we know it today.

References

1. Barker WF. Clio: The Arteries. Austin: Landes, 1992:2–502.
2. DeBakey ME. The development of vascular surgery. Am J Surg 1979;137:697–738.
3. Friedman SG. A history of vascular surgery. Mount Kisco, NY: Futura, 1989.
4. Haimovici H. Landmarks in vascular surgery. Contemp Surg 1982;21:63–84.
5. Rob CG. A history of arterial surgery. Arch Surg 1972;105:821–823.
6. Shumacker HB Jr, Muhm HY. Arterial suture techniques and grafts: past, present and future. Surgery (St. Louis) 1969;66:419–433.
7. Smith RB III. The foundations of modern aortic surgery. J Vasc Surg 1998;27:7–15.
8. Thompson JE. Vascular surgical techniques: historical perspective. In: Bergan JJ, Yao JST, eds. Techniques in Arterial Surgery. Philadelphia: Saunders, 1990:3–13.
9. Thompson JE. The evolution of surgery for the treatment and prevention of stroke. Stroke 1996;27:1427–1434.
10. Thompson JE. Early history of aortic surgery. J Vasc Surg 1998;28:746–752.
11. Dale WA. In: Johnson G Jr, DeWeese JA, eds. Band of Brothers: Creators of Modern Vascular Surgery. Pittsboro: Kachergis, 1996.
12. Ruffer MA. On arterial lesions found in Egyptian mummies (1580 BC–525 AD). J Pathol Bacteriol 1911;15:453–462.
13. Slaney G. A history of aneurysm surgery. In: Greenhalgh RM, Mannick JA, Powell JT, eds. The Cause and Management of Aneurysms. London: Saunders, 1990:1–18.
14. Crowe SJ. Halsted of Johns Hopkins: The Man and His Men. Springfield: Thomas, 1957:210–218.
15. Paré A. The Workes of That Famous Chirurgion Ambrose Parey. (Translated from Latin and compared with French by T. Johnson. From the first English edition, London, 1634. Reprinted, New York: Milford House, 1968.)
16. Garrison FH. An Introduction to the History of Medicine. Philadelphia: Saunders, 1929:217–221.
17. Perry MO. John Hunter—triumph and tragedy. J Vasc Surg 1993;17:7–14.
18. Brock RC. The Life and Work of Astley Cooper. Edinburgh: Livingstone, 1952:1–174.
19. Rutkow IM. Valentine Mott (1785–1865) the father of American vascular surgery: a historical prospective. Surgery (St. Louis) 1979;85:441–450.
20. Thompson JE. Valentine Mott. Pioneer American vascular surgeon. In: Veith FJ, ed. Current Critical Problems in Vascular Surgery, vol 7. St. Louis: Quality Medical, 1996:540–543.
21. Yao JST. Historical perspectives: the 100th anniversary of the first arterial anastomosis in a human. In: Yao JST, Pearce WH, eds. Techniques in Vascular and Endovascular Surgery. Stamford: Appleton & Lange, 1998:xxxiii–xl.
22. Edwards ES, Edwards PD. Alexis Carrel, Visionary Surgeon. Springfield: Thomas, 1974.
23. Goyanes J. Nuevos trabajos de cirugia vascular, substitucion plastica de las arterias por la vena o arterioplastia venosa aplicada como nuevo metodo del tratamiento de los aneurismas. El Siglo Medico 1906;53:546–561.
24. Lexer E. Die ideale operation des arteriellen und des arteriellenvenosen aneurysma. Arch Klin Chir 1907;83:459–477.
25. Pringle JH. Two cases of vein grafting for the maintenance of a direct arterial circulation. Lancet 1913;1:1795–1796.
26. Bernheim BM. The ideal operation for aneurisms of the extremity. Bull Johns Hopkins Hosp 1916;27:93–97.
27. Cameron JL. William Stewart Halsted. Our surgical heritage. Ann Surg 1997;225:445–458.
28. Matas R. Ligation of the abdominal aorta. Ann Surg 1925;81:457–464.
29. Elkin DC. Aneurysm of the abdominal aorta. Treatment by ligation. Ann Surg 1940;112:895–908.
30. Matas R. Traumatic aneurysm of the left brachial artery. Incision and partial excision of the sac—recovery. Med News NY 1888;53:462–466.
31. Osler W. The Principles and Practice of Medicine, 7th ed. New York: Appleton, 1909:862–863.
32. Blakemore AH. Progressive constrictive occlusion of the aorta with wiring and electrothermic coagulation for the treatment of arteriosclerotic aneurysms of the abdominal aorta. Trans South Surg Assoc 1952;64:202–219.
33. Rutledge RH. America's greatest medical discovery: 150 years later, who gets the credit? J Am Coll Surg 1996;183:625–636.
34. Wangensteen OH, Wangensteen SD. The rise of surgery. From empiric craft to scientific discipline. Minneapolis: University of Minnesota Press, 1978:516–518.
35. Crile GW. Technique of direct transfusion of blood. Ann Surg 1907;46:329–332.
36. Foster JH. Arteriography. Cornerstone of vascular surgery. Arch Surg 1974;109:605–611.
37. Brooks B. Intra-arterial injection of sodium iodide. Preliminary report. JAMA 1924;82:1016–1019.
38. Seldinger SI. Catheter replacement of the needle in the percutaneous angiography; a new technique. Acta Radiol 1953;39:368–376.
39. Gross RE, Bill AH Jr, Peirce EC II. Methods for preservation and transplantation of arterial grafts; observations on arterial grafts in dogs. Report of transplantation of preserved arterial grafts in 9 human cases. Surg Gynecol Obstet 1949;88:689–701.

40. Gross RE. Surgical ligation of a patent ductus arteriosus: report of first successful case. JAMA 1939;112:729–731.
41. Crafoord C, Nylin G. Congenital coarctation of the aorta and its surgical treatment. J Thorac Surg 1945;14:347–361.
42. Gross RE. Surgical correction for coarctation of the aorta. Surgery (St. Louis) 1945;18:673–678.
43. Gross RE, Hufnagel CA. Coarctation of the aorta: experimental studies regarding its surgical correction. N Engl J Med 1945;233: 287–293.
44. Blalock A, Taussig H. Surgical treatment of malformations of the heart in which there is pulmonary stenosis or atresia. JAMA 1945;128:189–202.
45. Schafer PW, Hardin CA. The use of temporary polythene shunts to permit occlusion, resection and frozen homologous graft replacement of vital vessel segments. Surgery (St. Louis) 1952;31: 186–193.
46. Dubost C, Allary M, Oeconomos N. Resection of an aneurysm of the abdominal aorta. Arch Surg 1952;64:405–408.
47. Julian OC, Grove WJ, Dye WS, et al. Direct surgery of arteriosclerosis. Ann Surg 1953;138:387–403.
48. Brock RC. Discussion on reconstructive arterial surgery. Proc R Soc Med 1953;46:115–130.
49. DeBakey ME, Cooley DA. Surgical treatment of aneurysm of abdominal aorta by resection and restoration of continuity with homograft. Surg Gynecol Obstet 1953;97:257–266.
50. Bahnson HT. Considerations in the excision of aortic aneurysms. Ann Surg 1953;138:377–386.
51. Creech O. Endoaneurysmorrhaphy. Treatment of aortic aneurysm. Ann Surg 1966;164:935–946.
52. Voorhees AB Jr, Jaretski A IV, Blakemore AH. The use of tubes constructed from Vinyon-"N" cloth in bridging arterial defects. Ann Surg 1952;135:332–336.
53. Edwards WS, Tapp JS. Chemically treated Nylon tubes as arterial grafts. Surgery (St. Louis) 1955;38:61–70.
54. Szilagyi DE, Smith RF, Derusso RJ, et al. Contribution of abdominal aortic aneurysmectomy to prolongation of life. Ann Surg 1966;164:678–698.
55. Szilagyi DE, Elliott JP, Hageman JG, et al. Biologic fate of autogenous vein implants as arterial substitutes: clinical, angiographic and histopathologic observations in femoro-popliteal operations for atherosclerosis. Ann Surg 1973;178:232–246.
56. DeBakey ME, Cooley DA, Crawford ES, Morris GC Jr. Clinical application of a new flexible knitted dacron arterial substitute. Am Surg 1958;24:862–869.
57. Bahnson HT. Treatment of abdominal aortic aneurysms by excision and replacement by homograft. Circulation 1954;9:494–503.
58. Gerbode F. Ruptured aortic aneurysm—a surgical emergency. Surg Gynecol Obstet 1954;98:579.
59. Cooley DA, DeBakey ME. Ruptured aneurysm of abdominal aorta—excision and homograft replacement. Postgrad Med 1954;16:334–342.
60. Javid H, Dye WS, Grove WJ, Julian OC. Resection of ruptured aneurysm of the abdominal aorta. Ann Surg 1955;142:613–623.
61. Alexander J, Byron FX. Aortectomy for thoracic aneurysm. JAMA 1944;126:1139–1145.
62. Swan H, Maaske C, Johnson M, Groves R. Arterial homografts. Resection of thoracic aortic aneurysm using a stored human arterial transplant. Arch Surg 1950;61:732–737.
63. Gross RE. Treatment of certain aortic coarctations by homologous grafts. A report of 19 cases. Ann Surg 1951;134:753–768.
64. Cooley DA, DeBakey ME. Surgical considerations of intrathoracic aneurysms of the aorta and great vessels. Ann Surg 1952;135:660–680.
65. DeBakey ME, Cooley DA. Successful resection of aneurysm of thoracic aorta and replacement by graft. JAMA 1953;152:673–676.
66. Nunn DB, Bunzendahl H, Handy JR. Ernst Jeger: a forgotten pioneer in cardiovascular surgery. Surgery (St. Louis) 1994;116:569–575.
67. Etheredge SN, Yee JY, Smith JV, Schonberger S, Goldman MJ. Successful resection of a large aneurysm of the upper abdominal aorta and replacement with homograft. Surgery (St. Louis) 1955;38:1071–1081.
68. DeBakey ME, Creech O, Morris GC. Aneurysm of thoracoabdominal aorta involving the celiac, mesenteric and renal arteries. Report of four cases treated by resection and homograft replacement. Ann Surg 1956;144:549–573.
69. Shumacker HB Jr. Innovation in the operative management of the thoracoabdominal aneurysms. Surg Gynecol Obstet 1973;136:793–794.
70. Crawford ES. Thoraco-abdominal aortic aneurysms involving renal, superior mesenteric and celiac arteries. Ann Surg 1974;179: 763–772.
71. Leriche R, Morel A. The syndrome of thrombotic obliteration of the aortic bifurcation. Ann Surg 1948;127:193–206.
72. Dos Santos JC. Sur la désobstruction des thromboses arterielles anciennes. Mem Acad Chir 1947;73:409–411.
73. Wylie EJ, Kerr E, Davies O. Experimental and clinical experiences with the use of fascia lata applied as a graft about major arteries after thromboendarterectomy and aneurysmorrhaphy. Surg Gynecol Obstet 1951;93:257–272.
74. Barker WF, Cannon JA. An evaluation of endarterectomy. Arch Surg 1953;66:488–495.
75. Inahara T. Endarterectomy: the beginning of modern vascular surgery. Am J Surg 1991;162:94–98.
76. Oudot J. La greffe vasculaire dans les thromboses du carrefour aortique. Presse Med 1951;59:234–236.
77. Kunlin J. Le traitement de l'ischemic arteritique par la greffe veineuse longue. Rev Chir Paris 1951;70:206–236.
78. Darling RC, Linton RR, Razzuk MA. Saphenous vein bypass grafts for femoro-popliteal occlusive disease: a reappraisal. Surgery (St. Louis) 1967;61:31–40.
79. Cutler BS, Robert R, Linton MD. A legacy of "Doing it right." J Vasc Surg 1994;19:951–963.
80. Hall KV. The great saphenous vein used in situ as an arterial shunt after extirpation of the vein valves. Surgery (St. Louis) 1962;51:492–495.
81. Connolly JE, Harris EJ, Mills W Jr. Autogenous in situ saphenous vein for bypass of femoral-popliteal obliterative disease. Surgery (St. Louis) 1964;55:144–153.
82. Leather RP, Powers SR, Karmody AM. A reappraisal of the *in situ* saphenous vein arterial bypass: its use in limb salvage. Surgery (St. Louis) 1976;86:453–461.
83. Donaldson MC, Mannick JA, Whittemore AD. Femoral-distal bypass with *in situ* greater saphenous vein. Long term results using the Mills valvulotome. Ann Surg 1991;213:457–465.
84. Morris GC Jr, Edwards WH, DeBakey ME. Surgical importance of the profunda femoris. Analysis of 102 cases. Arch Surg 1961;82:32–37.
85. Martin P, Renwick S, Stephenson C. On the surgery of the profunda femoris artery. Br J Surg 1968;55:539–543.
86. Porter JM, McGregor F Jr, Acinapura AJ, Silver D. Renal function following abdominal aortic aneurysmectomy. Surg Gynecol Obstet 1966;123:819–825.
87. Shires T, Williams J, Brown F. Acute change in extracellular fluids associated with major surgical procedures. Ann Surg 1961;154:803–810.
88. Thompson JE, Vollman RW, Austin DJ, Kartchner MM. Prevention of hypotensive and renal complications of aortic surgery using balanced salt solution: thirteen-year experience with 670 cases. Ann Surg 1968;167:767–778.
89. Labey G (case reported by Mosny M, Dumon MJ). Embolic femorala au cours d'un retrecissement mitral pur arterotomie. Bull Acad Med 1911;66:358–361.

90. Bauer F. Fall von embolus aortae abdominalis operation heilung. Zentralbl Chir 1913:40;1945–1946.
91. Fogarty TJ, Cranley JJ, Krause RJ, et al. A method for extraction of arterial emboli and thrombi. Surg Gynecol Obstet 1963;116:241–244.
92. White JC, Smithwick RH, Simeone FA. The Autonomic Nervous System. New York: Macmillan, 1952.
93. Royle ND. A new operative procedure in the treatment of spastic paralysis and its experimental basis. Med J Aust 1924; 1:77–81.
94. Diez J. Le traitement des affections trophiques et gangreneuses des membres inferieurs par la resection du sympathetique lombre-sacre. Rev Neurol 1926;33:184–187.
95. Smithwick RH. Sympathectomy, splanchnicectomy and vagotomy. Rev Surg 1973;30:153–173.
96. DeTakats G. Place of sympathectomy in the treatment of occlusive arterial disease. Arch Surg 1958;77:656–676.
97. Freeman NE, Leeds FH. Operations on large arteries. Application of recent advances. Calif Med 1952;77:229–233.
98. Vetto RM. The treatment of unilateral iliac artery obstruction with a transabdominal subcutaneous femorofemoral graft. Surgery (St. Louis) 1962;52:342–345.
99. Lewis CD. A subclavian artery as the means of blood supply to the lower half of the body. Br J Surg 1961;48:574–575.
100. Blaisdell FW, Hall AD. Axillary femoral bypass for lower extremity ischemia. Surgery (St. Louis) 1962;54:563–565.
101. Louw JH. Splenic-to-femoral and axillary-to-femoral bypass grafts in diffuse atherosclerotic occlusive disease. Lancet 1963;1:1401–1402.
102. Thompson JE, Smithwick RH. Human hypertension due to unilateral renal disease which special reference to renal artery lesions. Angiology 1952;3:493–505.
103. De Camp PT, Snyder CH, Bost RB. Severe hypertension due to congenital stenosis of artery to solitary kidney: correction by splenorenal arterial anastomosis. Arch Surg 1957;75:1023–1026.
104. Stoney RJ, Wylie EJ. Surgical management of arterial lesions of the thoraco-abdominal aorta. Arch Surg 1973;126:157–163.
105. Garrison FH. History of Neurology. (Revised and enlarged by McHenry LC, Jr.) Springfield: Thomas, 1969.
106. Cutter IS: Ligation of the common carotid—Amos Twitchell. Surg Gynecol Obstet Intern Abst Surg 1929;48:1–3.
107. Hebenstreit EBG. Zusatze Zu Benj. Bell's Abhandlung von den Geschwuren und deren Behandlung. Germany, 1793.
108. Wood JR. Early history of the operation of ligature of the primitive carotid artery. NY J Med 1857;July:1–59.
109. Abernethy J. Surgical observations. Surgical Works (London) 1804;2:193–209.
110. Hamby WB. Intracranial Aneurysms. Springfield: Thomas, 1952.
111. Coley RW. Case of rupture of the carotid artery, and wounds of several of its branches, successfully treated by tying the common trunk of the carotid itself. Med Chir J Rev 1817;3(13):1–4.
112. Keevil JJ. David Fleming and the operation for ligation of the carotid artery. Br J Surg 1949;37:92–95.
113. Twitchell A. Gun-shot wound of the face and neck. Ligature of the carotid artery. New Engl Q J Med Surg 1842;1(2):188–193.
114. Cooper A. Second case of carotid aneurysm. Med Chir Trans 1809;1:222–233.
115. Cooper A. Account of the first successful operation performed on the common carotid artery for aneurysm in the year 1808 with the postmortem examination in the year 1821. Guy's Hosp Rep 1836;1:53–59.
116. Hunt JR. The role of the carotid arteries in the causation of vascular lesions of the brain, with remarks on certain special features of the symptomatology. Am J Med Sci 1914;147:704–713.
117. Móniz E. L'encephalographic artérielle son importance dan la localization des tumeurs cerebrales. Rev Neurol (Paris) 1927; 2:72–90.
118. Sjöqvist O. Uber intrakrenielle aneurysmen der arteria carotis und deren beziehung zur ophthalmoplegischen migraine. Nervenarzt 1936;9:233–241.
119. Móniz E, Lima A, de Lacerda R. Hemiplegies par thrombose de la carotide interne. Presse Med 1937;45:977–980.
120. Johnson HC, Walker AE. The angiographic diagnosis of spontaneous thrombosis of the internal and common carotid arteries. J Neurosurg 1951;8:631–659.
121. Fisher M. Occlusion of the internal carotid artery. Arch Neurol Psychiatry 1951;65:346–377.
122. Fisher M. Occlusion of the carotid arteries. Arch Neurol Psychiatry 1954;72:187–204.
123. LeFevre M. Concerning a case involving a wound of the carotid bulb caused by a bullet, treated by ligature of the common carotid and end-to-end anastomosis of the external carotid with the internal carotid. Bull Mem Soc Chir 1918;44:923–925.
124. Conley JJ. Free autogenous vein graft to the internal and common carotid arteries in the treatment of tumors in the neck. Ann Surg 1953;137:205–214.
125. Carrea R, Molins M, Murphy G. Surgical treatment of spontaneous thrombosis of the internal carotid artery in the neck. Carotid-carotideal anastomosis. Report of a case. Acta Neurol Latinoam 1955;1:71–78.
126. Strully KJ, Hurwitt ES, Blankenberg HW. Thromboendarterectomy for thrombosis of the internal carotid artery in the neck. J Neurosurg 1953;10:474–482.
127. DeBakey ME. Successful carotid endarterectomy for cerebrovascular insufficiency. JAMA 1975;233:1083–1085.
128. Eastcott HHG, Pickering GW, Rob CG. Reconstruction of internal carotid artery in a patient with intermittent attacks of hemiplegia. Lancet 1954;2:994–996.
129. Denman FR, Ehni G, Duty WS. Insidious thrombotic occlusion of cervical arteries treated by arterial graft; a case report. Surgery (St. Louis) 1955;38:569–577.
130. Lin PM, Javid H, Doyle EJ. Partial internal carotid artery occlusion treated by primary resection and vein graft. J Neurosurg 1956;13:650–655.
131. Murphey F, Miller JH. Carotid insufficiency—diagnosis and surgical treatment. J Neurosurg 1959;16:1–23.
132. Cooley DA, Al-Naaman YD, Carton CA. Surgical treatment of arteriosclerotic occlusion of common carotid artery. J Neurosurg 1956;13:500–506.
133. Lyons C, Galbraith JG. Surgical treatment of atherosclerotic occlusion of the internal carotid artery. Ann Surg 1957;146:487–496.
134. Crawford ES, DeBakey ME, Fields WS, et al. Surgical considerations in the treatment of cerebral arterial insufficiency. Postgrad Med 1959;26:227–237.
135. Darling RC III, Paty PSK, Shah DM, et al. Eversion endarterectomy of the internal carotid artery: technique and results in 449 procedures. Surgery (St. Louis) 1996;120:635–640.
136. Ross RS, McKusick VA. Aortic arch syndromes: diminished or absent pulses in arteries arising from the aortic arch. Arch Intern Med 1953;92:701–740.
137. Fields WS, Lemak NA. A history of stroke. New York: Oxford University Press, 1989.
138. Thompson JE. Surgery for Cerebrovascular Insufficiency (Stroke). Springfield: Thomas, 1968.
139. Hutchinson EC, Yates PO. Cervical portion of vertebral artery: clinico-pathological study. Brain 1956;79:319–331.
140. Edwards WH Jr, Tapper SS, Edwards WH Sr, et al. Subclavian revascularization: a quarter century experience. Ann Surg 1994;219:673–678.

141. Berguer R. Advances in vertebral artery surgery. In: Veith FJ, ed. Current Critical Problems in Vascular Surgery. St. Louis: Quality Medical, 1991:404–408.
142. Yasargil MG, Krayenbuhl HA, Jacobson JH II. Microneurosurgical arterial reconstruction. Surgery (St. Louis) 1970;67:222–233.
143. EC/IC Bypass Study Group. Failure of extracranial-intracranial arterial bypass to reduce the risk of ischemic stroke. N Engl J Med 1985;313:1191–1200.
144. Bergan JJ, Kistner RL. Atlas of Venous Surgery. Philadelphia: Saunders, 1992.
145. Lofgren KA. Varicose veins. In: Fairbairn JF II, Juergens JL, Spittell JA Jr, eds. Peripheral Vascular Diseases, 4th ed. Philadelphia: Saunders, 1972:601–622.
146. Haimovici H. History of vascular surgery. In: Haimovici H, ed. Vascular Surgery: Principles and Techniques, 2nd ed. Norwalk: Appleton-Century-Crofts, 1984:3–18.
147. Thomas ML, Browse NL. Venography of the lower extremity. In: Neiman HL, Yao JST, eds. Angiography of Vascular Disease. New York: Churchill Livingstone, 1985:421–480.
148. Homans J. Thrombosis of deep veins of lower leg, causing pulmonary embolism. N Engl J Med 1934;211:993–997.
149. Cranley JJ. Vascular Surgery, vol II. Peripheral Venous Diseases. Hagerstown: Harper & Row, 1975.
150. Miles RM, Richardson RR, Wayne L, et al. Long-term results with the serrated Teflon vena caval clip in the prevention of pulmonary embolism. Ann Surg 1969;169:881–888.
151. Mobin-Uddin K, McLean R, Bolooki H, et al. Caval interruption for prevention of pulmonary embolism. Long-term results of a new method. Arch Surg 1969;99:711–715.
152. Greenfield LJ, Proctor MC. Twenty-year clinical experience with the Greenfield filter. Cardiovasc Surg 1995;3(2):199–205.
153. Golueke PJ, Garrett WV, Thompson JE, et al. Interruption of the vena cava by means of the Greenfield filter: expanding the indications. Surgery (St. Louis) 1988;103:111–117.
154. Linton RR. Venous interruption in thromboembolic disease [editorial]. Surgery (St. Louis) 1946;19:434–436.
155. Linton RR. The communicating veins of the lower leg and the operative treatment for their ligation. Ann Surg 1938;107:582–593.
156. Sumner DS. Diagnosis of deep venous thrombosis. In: Rutherford RB, ed. Vascular Surgery, 4th ed. Philadelphia: Saunders, 1995:1698–1743.
157. Palma EC, Esperon R. Vein transplants and grafts in the surgical treatment of the post phlebitic syndrome. J Cardiovasc Surg (Torino) 1960;1:94–107.
158. Husni EA. In situ saphenopopliteal bypass graft for incompetence of the femoral and popliteal veins. Surg Gynecol Obstet 1970;120:279–284.
159. Raju S. Operative management of chronic venous insufficiency. In: Rutherford RB, ed. Vascular Surgery, 4th ed. Philadelphia: Saunders, 1995:1851–1862.
160. Rodriguez AA, O'Donnell TF Jr. Surgical management of chronic venous insufficiency. In: Ernst CB, Stanley JC, eds. Current Therapy in Vascular Surgery. St. Louis: Mosby-Yearbook, 1995:914–919.
161. DeBakey ME, Simeone FA. Battle injuries of the arteries in World War II: an analysis of 2471 cases. Ann Surg 1946;123:534–578.
162. Rich NM. Penetrating arterial injuries in the extremities. In: Ernst CB, Stanley JC, eds. Current Therapy in Vascular Surgery. St. Louis: Mosby-Yearbook, 1995:617–619.
163. Rich NM, Spencer FC. Vascular Trauma. Philadelphia: Saunders, 1978.
164. Mattox KL, Feliciano DV, Burch J, et al. Five thousand seven hundred sixty cardiovascular injuries in 4459 patients: epidemiologic evolution 1958 to 1987. Ann Surg 1989;209:698–707.
165. Thal ER, Snyder WH IV, Perry MO. Vascular injuries of the extremities. In: Rutherford RB, ed. Vascular Surgery, 4th ed. Philadelphia: Saunders, 1995:713–735.
166. DeBakey ME, McCollum CH, Crawford ES, et al. Dissection and dissecting aneurysms of the aorta: twenty-year follow-up of five hundred twenty-seven patients treated surgically. Surgery (St. Louis) 1982;92:1118–1134.
167. Johnston KW, Rae M, Hogg-Johnston MA, et al. Five year results of a prospective study of percutaneous transluminal angioplasty. Ann Surg 1987;206:403–413.
168. Clagett GP, Bowers BL, Lopez-Viego MA, et al. Creation of a neo-aortoiliac system from lower extremity deep and superficial veins. Ann Surg 1993;218:239–249.

61

Pathobiology of Vascular Disease

Bryan W. Tillman and Randolph L. Geary

Normal Artery Wall Structure and Function

Knowledge of the structure and function of the circulatory system and the consequences of temporary or permanent disruption of regional blood flow is imperative in surgery because operative procedures by their very nature disrupt tissues and their blood supply. Moreover, reconstruction of blood vessels is often necessary as they fail from disease or trauma. Repair or replacement requires an understanding of vascular anatomy, vessel wall structure, hemodynamics, and the healing properties of vessels and grafts. This chapter focuses on the arterial system, providing an overview of its origin, structure, and function. The pathobiology of common artery wall diseases is then considered. Subsequent chapters focus on contemporary evidence-based management of regional artery wall pathology.

Vasculogenesis, Angiogenesis, and Collateral Formation

The cardiovascular system is the first to function in the developing embryo, with blood flow and heartbeat beginning in the third week of gestation. At that point the circulation becomes a sophisticated system for delivering nutrients, removing wastes, and routing biochemical signals throughout the body. The primordial vasculature arises from mesoderm formed at gastrulation in the first few days of gestation through processes of vasculogenesis and angiogensis.[1–3] Vasculogenesis refers to de novo vessel formation from stem cells. Within daysof conception a subset of stem cells differentitate into angioblasts, which in turn provide endothelial cell precursors. Angioblasts set the pattern of the vasculature by coalescing into strands that later become endothelial tubes (Fig. 61.1).

The first blood vessels form in the yolk sac where hemopoietic precursor cells become enveloped by angioblasts, creating blood islands, which eventually merge to form vitelline vessels.[2,3] A parallel process occurs within the embryo proper, where strands of angioblasts first coalesce along the lateral somite edges to form the nascent dorsal aortae.[2,3] Endothelial cells then recruit adjacent mural cells to the developing artery wall that differentiate into smooth muscle cells or fibroblasts, giving rise to the tunica media and tunica adventitia, respectively.[1–3]

Angiogenesis is the second major process contributing to the development of the nascent vasculature and involves the sprouting from existing vessels of new vessels, which then invade surrounding tissues (see Fig. 61.1).[1,2,4] Angiogenesis plays a greater role in later stages of development when organs and tissues become fully vascularized by angiogenic ingrowth from the primordial circulation. This is also the major mechanism of new capillary formation after birth and plays a vital role in wound healing and tissue regeneration. Perhaps as important, dysregulation of angiogenesis contributes to the pathogenesis of common diseases including cancer, arthritis, and retinopathy.[4]

A third process critical in maintaining and regulating tissue perfusion is the growth of collateral blood vessels through collateralization or arteriogenesis.[5] Blood flow via collaterals can preserve limbs and organs that lose their primary arterial inflow from occlusion or injury. This process involves remodeling and enlargement of existing arterioles that bridge the microcirculation proximal and distal to a site of occlusion. Arteriogenesis is mediated by fluid mechanical and biochemical signals generated as a result of occlusion and resulting invasion by (but not incorporation of) bone marrow-derived cells and proliferation of existing endothelial and smooth muscle cells.[5] Arterial occlusion lowers the pressure beyond proximal arterioles, creating a pressure gradient that increases flow through preexisting collaterals. Increased shear stress then activates endothelial cells to upregulate adhesion molecules and mitogens that in turn promote cell growth and leukocyte invasion required for vessel enlargement and remodeling. Resulting increases in lumen diameter and wall thickness normalize wall stresses to terminate further enlarge-

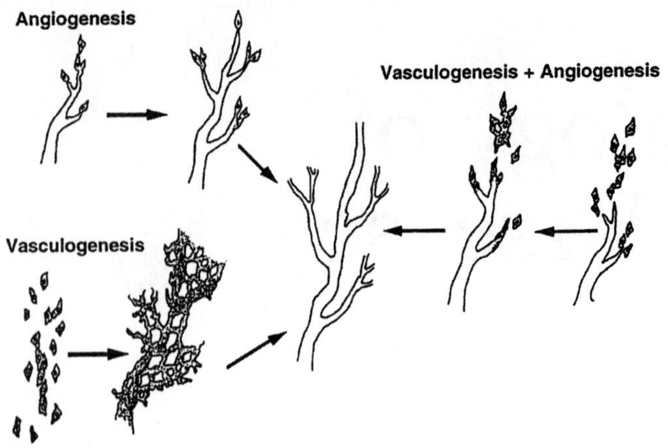

FIGURE 61.1. Illustration of vasculogenesis, a coalescence of precursor cells (angioblasts) into capillary tubes, and angiogenesis, the sprouting of new capillaries from established blood vessels. Both mechanisms are critical to blood vessel formation in fetal development, whereas angiogenesis is the sole mechanism of new blood vessel formation after birth. (Reprinted from Baldwin HS.[2] Early embryonic vascular development. Cardiovascular Research 1996;31: E34–E35, with permission from Elsevier Science.)

ment. Although often adequate to maintain tissue homeostasis, collaterals can generally deliver no more than 40% of normal flow.[5]

Regulation of Cell Growth and Differentiation

The pattern of molecular signals that determines whether a progenitor differentiates into an endothelial cell, smooth muscle cell, or adventitial fibroblast is incompletely defined. However, a number of factors have been identified that are important for specific steps of blood vessel formation during embryogenesis.[1–4,6,7] The impact of these and other factors on smooth muscle cell and endothelial cell behavior have also been explored extensively in culture and in animal models of angiogenesis and arterial injury in which a fetal pattern of gene expression is often recapitulated.[6–9] New techniques in molecular biology have enabled mapping of expression of specific genes during the course of development, and genes can now be added or deleted from small animals to study their effects in isolation (i.e., transgenic or knockout mice). Families of genes vital for normal blood vessel development include: transcription factors, growth factors and their receptors, adhesion molecules, and extracellular matrix components.[1,4,6–9]

Gradients of growth factors likely direct the recruitment and differentiation of locally derived mesodermal cells into smooth muscle cells and fibroblasts.[1–4] Growth factors bind receptors on target cells to activate intracellular signaling pathways that in turn activate specific genes. The resulting pattern of gene expression determines cell phenotype (e.g., smooth muscle alpha-actin, myosin heavy chain, and SM-22 alpha) and behavior (e.g., replication, migration, and extracellular matrix synthesis).[1,7] Secreted proteins may act on the cell of origin to induce autocrine effects or, on adjacent cells, signaling in a paracrine mechanism. Some remain bound to the cell surface, signaling adjacent cells through direct cell–cell interactions, and many growth factors target more than one cell type. Most induce a spectrum of responses, some of which are unique, such as inducing gastrulation, differentiation, and capillary tube formation, and others are more generic, such as proliferation and migration.

Although cell proliferation, migration, and differentiation are central to vasculogenesis and angiogenesis, the mature artery wall normally exists in a quiescent state in which replication of smooth muscle cells has been estimated to be less than 0.06% per day[10,11]; this means that cells in the artery wall exist in a state of chronic growth inhibition and may take months or years to turn over. Inhibition is lost transiently after mechanical injury (e.g., endarterectomy or angioplasty)[11] and chronically in diseases such as atherosclerosis and hypertension.[9,12] An understanding of normal vascular cell growth regulation is thus central to our consideration of artery wall pathology and its prevention and treatment.

A review of the embryology of vessels provides some clues to adult angiogenesis. While the patterning of venous, arterial and lymphatic cell types from primordial angioblasts remains a complex system, several key effectors of this transition have been identified. At the outset, expression of basic FGF signals the onset of gastrulation and is required for commitment of mesoderm to vascular primordia.[1–3] FGF is also a potent endothelial cell and smooth muscle cell mitogen in developed arteries and induces angiogenesis in a number of experimental models.[13,14] Basic fibroblast growth factor (bFGF) lacks a signal sequence for secretion and is released through a poorly defined mechanism or by cell disruption.[12,13] Growth factors involved in collateral vessel formation also belong to the FGF family, which induce signaling via the Ras/Raf and the Rho cascades.[5] The angioblast precursor expresses one of the first markers of vasculogenesis, VEGFR2, also known as flk1. These precursors are capable of developing into an array of endothelial, smooth muscle and hematopoetic precursors.[14A] Vascular endothelial growth factor (VEGF) is expressed at the onset of vasculogenesis and binds its receptors, VEGFR-2, on angioblasts to induce endothelial tube and blood island formation.[1–3] Absence of either the flk1 receptor or its ligand VEGF-A is a lethal mutant. Even before circulation begins in the embryo, these precursors have been assigned to an arterial or venous fate. The Notch signaling pathway, in particular, is pivotal in the determination of arterial versus venous assignment. Specifically, absence of Notch expression results in a venous phenotype.[14A] Downstream, the angiopoietin (Ang) family of endothelial cell growth factors is also vital in early vessel patterning.[1–3] Both ang-1 and ang-2 bind Tie-2, a receptor tyrosine kinase that signals endothelial cell growth and maturation. Tie-1, a related receptor tyrosine kinase, is also important in vasculogenesis, but its ligand has not been identified.[1] The importance of these and other growth factors and their receptors is underscored by the effect of knocking out genes in mice, each of which is lethal early in embryonic development as the result of defective blood vessel formation.[1] For example, platelet-derived growth factors (PDGF) and their receptors are critical in recruitment of smooth muscle cells to nascent endothelial cell tubes. Loss of the genes for PDGF or their receptors is lethal to the developing fetus, where a smooth muscle cell coat fails to form, resulting in friable vessels and hemmorhage.[1] In a similar fashion, lymphatics are transdifferentiated from venous precursors by expression of the transcription factor Prox-1. Deletion of this gene results in failure of lymphatic budding from the early veins.[14B] Also implicated in lymphatic development is the receptor VEGFR-3. While initially expressed on all early vascular cell progenitors, VEGFR3 ultimately becomes limited to mostly lymphatic endothelium.

Cell-surface adhesion molecules and integrins are also critical in regulating vascular cell growth and differentiation and cell–cell and cell–matrix interactions.[1,6,8,15] Each adhesion molecule or integrin binds a specific cell type or matrix component, and the pattern of expression determines the binding options. Vascular cell–cell adhesion is mediated by a number of receptors including platelet-endothelial cell adhesion molecule (PECAM-1), vascular endothelial cadherin (VE-cadherin), and CD34 expressed by angioblasts and hemopoietic precursors.[1–3] PECAM-1 binding may induce the expression of a specific pattern of endothelial cell integrins. By directing integrin upregulation, PECAM and other factors induce receptors appropriate for the early matrix environment of the embryo.

Integrins exist as dimers of one alpha- and one beta-subunit; there are many of these dimers, and combinations determine matrix ligand specificity.[6,8,16] Fibronectin is a key matrix component in the developing vessel wall, and its $\alpha_5\beta_1$ integrin receptor is expressed on both endothelial cells and smooth muscle.[1,6] Knockout of α_5 integrin or fibronectin genes result in lethal defects in blood vessel formation.[1] Vitronectin is also prominent in the matrix surrounding endothelium during angiogenesis, and its $\alpha_v\beta_3$ integrin receptor is required for tumor angiogenesis.[4,5] Antibodies to $\alpha_v\beta_3$ disrupt normal fetal angiogenesis and prevent tumor angiogenesis in adults.[4,6] Binding initiates intracellular signaling while providing structural integrity to forming vessels, and certain adhesive interactions are required for cell survival at specific times during development. In their absence, cells undergo apoptosis (programmed cell death), which is an important mechanism for remodeling the developing vascular circuit.[4,17,18] In fact, most blood vessels formed within the developing embryo and fetus involute before birth.

Organization of the Artery Wall

The innermost layer of the artery wall is the tunica intima bounded by the lumen and the internal elastic lamina (IEL) (Fig. 61.2). In its simplest form the intima is composed of a single cell layer, the endothelium. Smooth muscle cells may accumulate beneath the endothelium to form intimal pads at branches and curves within the arterial tree. Intimal pads are present at birth and represent an adaptation to the altered hemodynamic forces that occur at these sites.[19,20]

Endothelial cells create a monolayer that lines the entire inner surface of the vasculature. This unique location requires a repertoire of specialized functions including inhibition of intravascular coagulation and regulation of hemostasis; control of inflammation and leukocyte diapedesis out from the circulation; tissue nutrient and waste exchange; regulation of intravascular oncotic pressure; and control of vasomotor tone. Endothelial cells secrete a number of anticoagulant molecules, including heparan sulfates that increase antithrombin III activity; thrombomodulin, which binds thrombin to activate protein C; nitric oxide, which inhibits platelet aggregation and adhesion; tissue factor pathway inhibitor, which blocks Factor Xa formation from tissue factor; and prostaglandin I_2 and tissue plasminogen activator (tPA), important in fibrinolysis.[21] When unactivated, the endothelium does not express platelet or leukocyte adhesion molecules, but various inflammatory stimuli result in expression of specific ligands on the cell surface that correspond to specific platelet and leukocyte receptors.[22] Adhesion molecules then selectively recruit neutrophils, monocytes, or lymphocytes into surrounding tissues and platelets to sites requiring hemostasis.

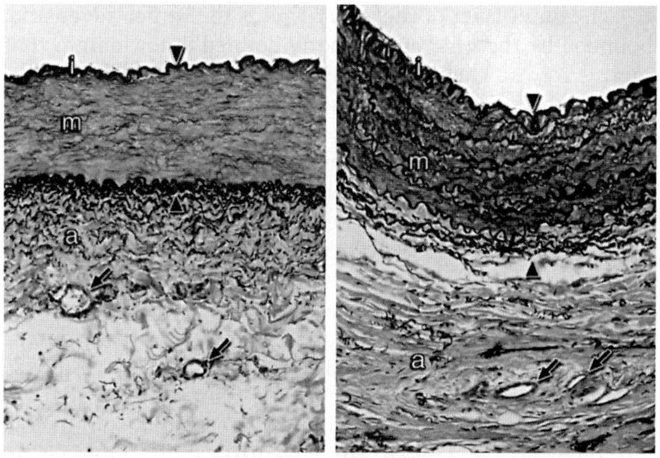

FIGURE 61.2. Micrographs of normal muscular and elastic arteries. The lumen is at *top*, with the adjacent intima (*i*) composed of an endothelial cell monolayer overlying the internal elastic lamina (*arrowhead*). The media (*m*) is bounded by the internal and external elastic laminae (*arrowheads*). The elastic artery (*right*) has well-defined lamellae of medial smooth muscle cells between sheets of elastin, whereas the muscular artery (*left*) has a single lamella. The adventitia is composed of loose collagen and elastin fibers, fibroblasts, leukocytes, and microvessels termed vasa vasorum (*arrows*).

The endothelium also senses and responds to altered fluid mechanical forces by changing shape to align in the direction of flow, which decreases effective resistance and by secreting vasoactive molecules, which cause medial smooth muscle cells to relax (e.g., nitric oxide, PGI_2, and PGE_2) or constrict (endothelin-1), regulating lumen diameter.[23,24] In addition to regulating medial tone, the endothelium likely helps maintain a state of smooth muscle cell growth inhibition as a number of endothelial products inhibit growth [heparan sulfate, NO, transforming growth factor-beta (TGF-β)].

Surrounding the intima is the tunica media bounded by the IEL and the external elastic lamina (EEL). The media is composed of layers of smooth muscle cells and extracellular matrix separated into lamellae by thin sheets of elastic fibers (see Fig. 61.2). There can be multiple lamellae, as in large elastic arteries such as the aorta and its branches, or a single well-defined lamella, as in medium and small muscular arteries such as the coronary and femoral arteries (see Fig. 61.2). The number of lamellae appears to be set at birth, so artery wall growth occurs by medial smooth muscle cell hyperplasia and extracellular matrix production rather than by an increase in the number of medial layers.[25] The media and the elastic lamellae provide most of the structural integrity of the artery wall, evenly distributing the tension transmitted from intraluminal pressure.[26] Medial smooth muscle cells of small arteries and arterioles regulate systemic blood pressure and the distribution of blood flow by contracting or relaxing in response to endothelial cell factors (NO), circulating factors (angiotensin II, catecholamines, etc.), and autonomic innervation.

The outer layer of the artery wall is the tunica adventitia, bounded by the EEL, and a poorly defined outer margin that merges into surrounding tissues (see Fig. 61.2). Although the outer boundary of the adventitia can be histologically indistinct, it is obvious at surgery, providing a clear plane of dissection. The adventitia is composed of loose connective tissue fibers rich in collagen and elastin with interspersed fibroblasts, microvessels, nerves, and lymphatics. Autonomic innervation regulates central vasomotor responses and contributes to basal tone. Microvessels in the adventitia of medium and large arteries create a rich plexus called the vasa vasorum.[27] Vasa originate from artery branches and provide nutrient flow to the outer artery wall.[28,29] The vasa also provide access into the adventitia to leukocytes, which are normally absent from the underlying intima and media. Although poorly defined, the adventitia likely provides an important immune function to the artery wall.

To maintain blood pressure and flow at the tissue level requires a sophisticated balance among artery wall diameter and thickness, compliance, and branching frequency. This balance achieves adequate capillary perfusion with the most efficient energy expenditure by the heart. As arteries branch, changes in flow patterns, wall compliance, and caliber result in energy losses to flowing blood. Sudden changes in wall compliance at these sites reflect pressure waves back toward the heart that add to the pressure wave generated during each contraction of the left ventricle. Energy may be stored as compliant arteries distend during systole then rebound in diastole to augment pressure and flow. Peripheral resistance is largely regulated in the microcirculation by changes in postcapillary venule and precapillary arteriolar tone, whereas muscular arteries constrict or dilate to redistribute blood flow among various vascular beds. Aging of the arterial circuit leads to a gradual loss of wall compliance and increased resistance from stenoses, occlusions, and autonomic dysfunction. The result is an imbalance in the work required to maintain capillary perfusion pressure and dysregulation of the regional distribution of flow.

Artery Wall Remodeling

Adaptive changes in artery wall geometry are termed remodeling. As we grow, tissues and organs enlarge with proportional demands for increases in blood pressure, flow, and oxygen delivery. The artery wall is remarkably plastic and will remodel (enlarge and thicken) to accommodate these needs. Changes in flow and pressure cause associated changes in wall shear stress and tension, respectively. Shear stress, the frictional force on endothelium from flowing blood, is proportional to blood flow velocity. As volume flow increases, velocity and shear stress are increased, prompting the artery wall to dilate to increase lumen area.[30,31]

Altered shear stress leads to endothelial cell deformation, ion channel activation with changes in intracellular calcium, G-protein signaling, and activation of pathways linked to the cytoskeleton via integrins and other receptor tyrosine kinases[32,33]; this in turn leads to altered release of vasoactive molecules such as NO that signals medial smooth muscle cell relaxation. The result is altered lumen diameter and a return of blood flow velocity and shear stress to a normal physiological range. Wall tension decreases in proportion to wall thickness and increases to the fourth power of changes in wall diameter. As an artery dilates to accommodate increased flow, radial wall tension increases disproportionately.[31,34] The media must thicken to redistribute the radial stress and bring it back within a favorable physiological range. Pathological medial thickening occurs in a number of diseases, the most important being hypertension, in which chronic increases in blood pressure and wall tension lead to medial thickening and inward remodeling of resistance vessels that impair wall function.[34]

A number of smooth muscle and endothelial cell genes contain promoter sequences that are activated by altered cell stretch and shear stress.[24] Thus, fluid mechanical forces are transduced into biochemical signals, which in turn regulate wall thickness and caliber. Although sudden changes in flow and shear stress result in nearly instantaneous vasomotor responses (dilation or relaxation), chronic changes in flow produce a true restructuring of the artery wall, resulting in a new caliber setpoint from which subsequent vasomotor responses occur.[30] Remodeling is a consequence of cell and extracellular matrix turnover and reorganization. It is not surprising, then, that genes regulated by shear stress include growth factors such as TGF-β, PDGF-A and -B, and endothelin-1 and growth inhibitors (NO).[24,35]

Atherosclerosis

The atherosclerotic plaque is the consequence of focal accumulation of leukocytes and smooth muscle cells within the intima of the artery wall. Plaques enlarge by an expansion of these cells, accumulation of extracellular matrix, and deposition of lipid and debris.[36] As plaques grow, the artery wall attempts to accommodate by remodeling, enlarging to maintain lumen caliber.[37,38] If the remodeling process fails, or if the plaque becomes unstable and ruptures, blood flow is compromised and ischemia ensues.

Prevalence and Impact on Public Health

Atherosclerosis has long been viewed as an inevitable consequence of aging. Although this premise has recently been challenged, atherosclerosis and its complications (myocardial infarction, stroke, and gangrene of the extremities) remain the most common cause of death and disability worldwide. The World Health Organization estimates that 25% more healthy life years will be lost to cardiovascular disease globally by 2020, and that worldwide 12 million lives are lost to vascular diseases.[38A] One million deaths per year are attributed to vascular diseases; this figure represents 38% of all deaths in the United States and an average of 1 death every 33 s.[39] Women, commonly perceived to be protected from atherosclerosis, have surpassed men in atherosclerosis-related deaths each year since 1995.[39] Atherosclerosis is a disease of the aged, as 85% of related deaths occur in individuals 65 and older. Our population is aging, so the problem is growing, with more individuals living to suffer from ischemic syndromes.

Lesions often develop for decades before causing symptoms because of the tremendous plasticity of the artery wall.[36–38] In the early and intermediate stages of plaque development, lesions may regress with intensive risk factor modification and lipid-lowering therapy.[40] However, this approach can take years to measurably diminish lesion size, and treatment of acute ischemia often requires an invasive procedure to rapidly reopen the lumen and restore blood flow (angioplasty, stenting, endarterectomy, thromboembolectomy, and bypass grafting). More than 3 million revascularization procedures are performed in the United States each year, underscoring the magnitude of the problem and the enormous cost to society.[39]

Pathogenesis

The sequence of events initiating lesion formation is incompletely defined. A leading theory is the "reaction to injury hypothesis" first proposed by Ross and Glomset in 1976 and subsequently modified to incorporate new information emerging from basic and clinical research (Fig. 61.3).[36,41] In his last update, Ross suggested that atherosclerosis results from chronic endothelial cell dysfunction (rather than a denuding injury as originally proposed) that leads to very specific cellular and molecular events best described as an "inflammatory disease."[36] Although the response may be highly specific, causes of endothelial injury and dysfunction vary widely, and atherosclerosis is truly a multifactorial disease with many genetic, cultural, and environmental risk factors contributing to lesion initiation and progression.[42–44]

Once perturbed, the endothelium loses many of its protective properties.[36,42–44] Activated endothelial cells express leukocyte adhesion molecules (selectins) including intracellular adhesion molecule 1 (ICAM-1), vascular cell adhesion molecule (VCAM-1), and PECAM. They also release the cytokines monocyte colony-stimulating factor (M-CSF) and monocyte chemoattractant protein 1 (MCP-1). These and other molecules attract leukocytes and coordinate their attachment, rolling, spreading, and diapedesis into the subendothelial space. Leukocytes accumulating within the intima are predominantly monocyte-derived macrophages and T lymphocytes.[36] Early in the pathogenesis, the intimal macrophages accumulate lipid to become foam cells that form fatty streaks, one of the earliest manifestations of this disease process. These fatty streaks, seen as early as childhood, are a reversible change, in contrast to mature plaques that are not reversible to any significant degree. In particular the regression of fatty streaks is highlighted in animal models with both diet and pharmacologic intervention as well as review of human specimens.[44A,44B] Once in the intima, leukocytes replicate and release growth factors and cytokines including PDGF, IL-1, bFGF, epidermal growth factor (EGF), and TGF-β, which induce smooth muscle cells in the preexisting intima or adjacent tunica media to replicate, migrate toward their source, and produce extracellular matrix. The result is plaque expan-

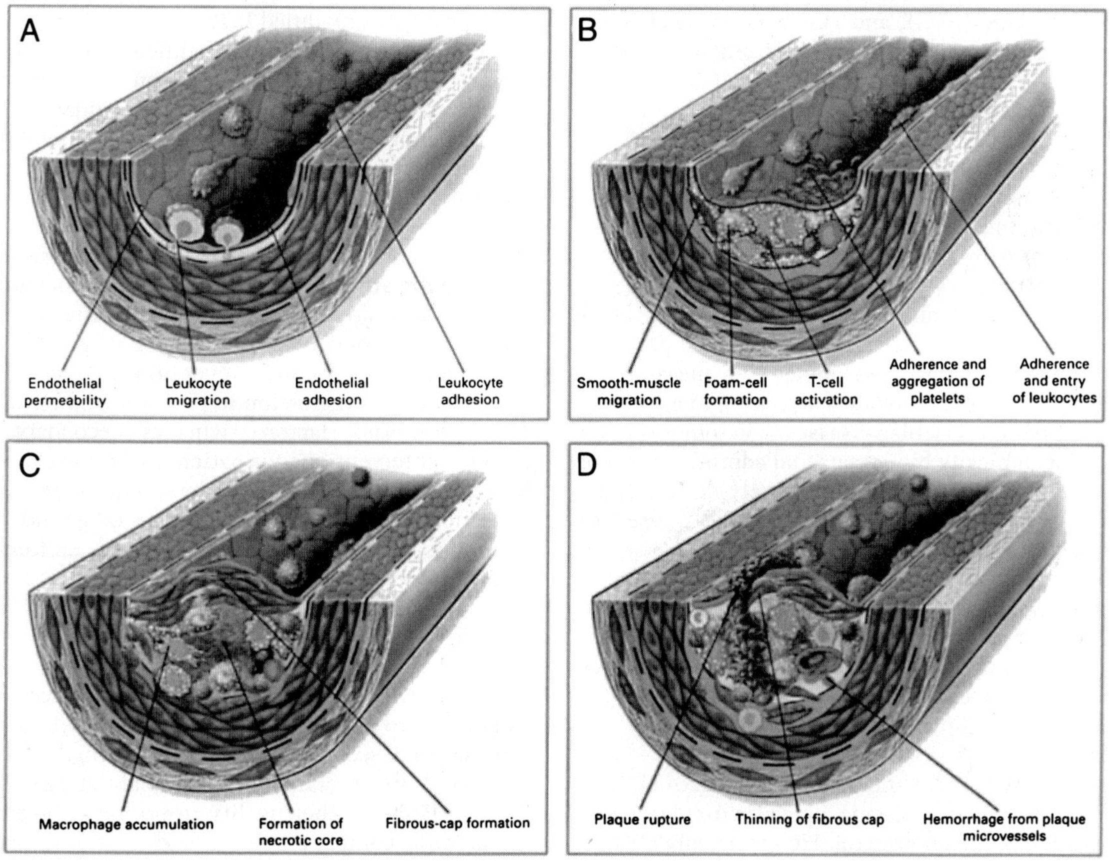

FIGURE 61.3. Illustration of the sequence of lesion progression in atherosclerosis. **A.** Plaque is initiated by endothelial cell activation with leukocyte recruitment. **B.** A fatty streak progresses to a fibrofatty lesion as macrophage foam cells accumulate beneath the endothelium and recruit smooth muscle cells from the adjacent artery wall. **C.** A mature fibrous plaque results from further accumulation of smooth mucle cell and matrix. Plaques become complicated, forming a necrotic core of foam cells, lipid, and cellular debris. **D.** Ischemic symptoms result from lumen encroachment or from plaque rupture and thrombosis. (Reproduced with permission from R. Ross.[36] Atherosclerosis: an inflammatory disease. N Engl J Med 1999;340:115–126. Copyright © 1999 Massachusetts Medical Society. All rights reserved.)

sion, adding a fibrous component to the lesion. Platelet and endothelial cell factors and autocrine release of factors from smooth muscle cells also help recruit additional cells into the diseased intima. T lymphocytes release the cytokine gamma interferon (IFN-γ), which activates macrophages and smooth muscle cells, leading to expression of the transplant antigen HLA-DR. INF-γ can induce smooth muscle cell apoptosis and alters collagen metabolism.[44] Activation of macrophages causes an increased production of cytokines, growth factors, and oxidative free radicals. The result is further endothelial cell injury and leukocyte and smooth muscle cell accumulation with elaboration of extracellular matrix.[36]

Dysfunctional endothelium may lose anticoagulant activity with diminished expression of NO and increased expression of adhesion molecules, leading to platelet adhesion and aggregation. Coagulation is further promoted by the expression of tissue factor and platelet-activating factor, shifting the balance toward a procoagulant state. Tissue factor activates Factor VII, which in turn activates Factor X and the coagulation cascade leading to fibrin formation on the endothelial surface. If the endothelium is denuded, collagen, von Willebrand factor (vWF), and other matrix components are exposed while endothelial disruption releases intracellular stores of vWF from Weibel–Palade bodies. These molecules function as ligands for platelet receptors and clotting proteins. Adherent platelets may then degranulate, releasing contents of alpha granules including smooth muscle cell growth factors PDGF, EGF, and TGF-β. Clotting proteins such as thrombin are also mitogenic for smooth muscle cells.[12,36,42–44]

Endothelial dysfunction also impairs vasodilation and directly and indirectly promotes vasoconstriction.[33,36,42–45] This effect is from decreased basal expression of endothelial nitric oxide synthase (eNOS or NOS-III), which converts L-arginine into NO and citrulline. Activation also leads to expression of endothelin-1 and growth factors such as PDGF with constrictor activity,[12,46,47] and adherent platelets release the vasoconstrictors thromboxane and serotonin.[12,36] It is important to note that endothelial cell dysfunction precedes and then accompanies lesion development, so measures of vasomotor dysfunction may provide a screening tool to identify patients at risk for vascular diseases.[47] Vasomotion can be studied angiographically by intraarterial administration of vasodilators and constrictors, or noninvasively in superficial vessels such as the brachial artery. Ultrasound is used to measure changes in artery wall diameter in response to increased forearm blood flow from hyperemia. The normal response is flow-mediated dilation, whereas endothelial cell dysfunction will impair dilation or cause paradoxical vasoconstriction. Screening for abnormal endothelial responses may prove useful in documenting treatment effects of risk factor modification and lipid-lowering therapy.[47]

Well-established risk factors, identified from basic research, large observational studies, and randomized clinical trials,[36,39,48] include elevated plasma lipids, particularly low density lipoprotein (LDL) cholesterol. However, only 50% to 60% of persons who develop atherosclerosis have hypercholesterolemia or hypertriglyceridemia. Other important risk factors include family history, age, menopause, smoking, hypertension, diabetes, obesity, and sedentary lifestyle. The sum of these and other risk factors determine an individual's susceptibility to atherosclerosis, and each factor contributes directly or indirectly to endothelial cell dysfunction. Acquired and environmental risks vary significantly over time, and transient exposures may have little permanent impact. However, even brief exposure to a potent risk could precipitate lesion progression if exposure comes at a susceptible time in lesion development.

Hypercholesterolemia is a potent risk factor, and more than half of the population have an elevated total plasma cholesterol level (>200 mg/dL).[36,39,48] Lipid accumulation is a prominent feature in advanced atherosclerotic lesions, and lipid accumulation appears to precede the recruitment of leukocytes into the intima.[36] Ingested lipid gives macrophage cytoplasm a foamy appearance and thus the term foam cell. Cholesterol, particularly LDL, binds to matrix proteoglycans within the intima, where it becomes trapped and can then undergo modification by oxidation or glycation into more damaging and proatherogenic forms.[49]

Oxidative products can come from many sources including leukocyte and smooth muscle cell metabolism and free radicals generated by smoking.[42,49] Glycation results from hyperglycemia, most commonly associated with diabetes mellitus.[50] A popular hypothesis is that LDLs modified by oxidation or glycation are toxic to endothelium, directly causing denudation or inducing M-CSF, MCP-1, and tissue factor expression, and that oxidation and glycation may create antigenic epitopes and an antibody response against LDL trapped within the intima.[36,42,49] Macrophages then attempt to clear modified LDL from the intima using scavenger receptors for its uptake. Modified LDLs are toxic to macrophages, causing further activation, cytokine release, and cell death. Although popular, the "oxidation hypothesis" remains controversial as large prospective randomized trials of antioxidant therapy have failed to provide clear evidence for improvement in atherosclerosis risk.[51] The natural antioxidants, vitamins A, C, and E, have received the most attention, and none has been shown to consistently reduce the risk for atherosclerosis and its complications. Current Level I data do not support prescribing antioxidants in primary or secondary prevention of atherosclerosis and its complications.[51] Primary prevention includes prevention of atherosclerotic progression in patients who have defined cardiovascular risk factors, whereas secondary prevention involves interventions for patients who have already manisfested an adverse cardiovascular event, such as myocardial infarction or stroke. The definition of *cardiovascular risk factors* is in constant evolution but uniformly include smoking, hypertension, elevated LDL cholesterol, sedentary lifestyle, diabetes, age, and family history.[48,51A] Risk factor modifications in lifestyle that include weight management, physical activity, smoking cessation, diabetic management and blood pressure control have been endorsed by consensus statements to preclude atherosclerotic complications in both a primary and secondary prevention setting.[48,51A–E] In the pharmacologic arena, statins and antiplatelet agents have been demonstrated for their utility in primary prevention of atherosclerotic complications in high risk populations (Table 61.1).[48,51F]

For secondary prevention of coronary events in postmenopausal women, the use of hormone replacement therapy has not been shown to be effective.[51G] Similar to primary prevention, a variety of pharmacologics have demonstrated their effectiveness in the secondary prevention of subsequent car-

TABLE 61.1.
Primary prevention of atherosclerosis in high risk patients (Level 1 evidence).

Intervention	*Criteria for Intervention**
Statins ± Niacin	LDL-C is >160 mg/dL if ≤1 cardiovascular risk factor LDL-C is >130 mg/dL if ≥2 risk factors and 10 year risk is <20% LDL-C is >100 mg/dL if ≥2 risk factors and 10 year risk is ≥20% or diabetic Triglycerides >200, use therapy to reduce non-HDL-C
Aspirin	Patients with 10 year CHD risk ≥10%, unless contraindicated
Blood pressure management	>140/90 in all patients >130/80 if patient is a diabetic
Smoking cessation	All patients
Diabetes management	Fasting plasma glucose >110 HbA1c >7%
Dietary management	Saturated fat intake >10% of total calories Cholesterol >300 mg per day
Physical activity	All patients with under 30 minutes moderate intensity activity most days of the week

CHD, coronary heart disease; LDL-C, low density lipoprotein cholesterol; HDL-C, high density lipoprotein cholesterol.

*The degree of risk is determined by the number of risk factors and may vary the intensity of therapy.

Source: Data from references 48 and 51A.

diovascular events (Table 61.2) including lipid lowering agents such as niacin therapy and statins as well as angiotensin converting enzyme inhibitors.[51H–K]

Additional genetic and acquired risk factors for atherosclerosis have been identified, including homocysteine and infections. Homocysteine is an intermediary in the metabolism of the amino acid methionine, and elevated plasma levels are strongly associated with atherosclerosis and thrombosis.[52,53] Homocysteine is toxic to endothelial cells in culture and leads to endothelial cell injury, denudation, tissue factor expression, and platelet activation in animal models.[52,53] Severe increases in plasma homocysteine occur in individuals with rare defects in genes encoding cystathionine beta-synthase, homocysteine methyl transferase, and methylene tetrahydrofolate reductase. These individuals develop severe atherosclerosis in childhood and thrombotic and ischemic events as young adults. Mild elevation of plasma homocysteine is common, and clinical studies have demonstrated a significant association between these variants of homocysteinemia and complications of atherosclerosis.[53–55] For instance, in patients presenting with peripheral vascular disease, an elevated plasma homocysteine level (>14 mmol/L) doubles the risk of cardiac morbidity and mortality compared to well-matched controls at 3 years follow-up.[55] Homocysteinemia is an attractive therapeutic target because plasma levels can be normalized in the majority of patients by simple dietary supplementation with folate and vitamins B_6 and B_{12}.[56] Whether lowering plasma homocysteine will actually reduce the risk of vascular disease has not been established, but folate is inexpensive, with few side effects, and treatment of high-risk patients seems justified.[57] However, type I evidence does not support treatment of homocysteine.[57A]

Microorganisms represent another potential source of endothelial cell dysfunction and atherosclerotic plaque progression.[58] Herpesvirus infections in avian species result in a profound arteriopathy resembling atherosclerosis. *Chlamydia* infection accelerates lesion formation in the artery wall of cholesterol-fed rabbits, and antibiotics block the effect, providing evidence for causality. *Chlamydia* and cytomegalovirus have been localized within human atherosclerotic plaques using molecular probes, and circulating antibodies to these and other microorganisms (e.g., *Helicobacter pylori*) are present more often in patients with complications of atherosclerosis.[59] In a recent study, patients seropositive for *Chlamydia* with carotid atherosclerosis were treated with macrolide antibiotics in an attempt to reduce the risk of lesion growth and stroke. A transient reduction in lesion thickness was noted but then lost after 2 years' follow-up, and stroke risk was not significantly altered. Data such as these support a role for infection in lesion progression but indicate that transient antibiotic therapy may have a limited role in preventing complications of atherosclerosis over the long term.[60] At present meta-analysis of antibiotic treatment of *Chlamydia* does not support effectiveness of antibiotics in patients with coronary vascular disease.[60A]

Just as there is variability in extent of atherosclerosis between individuals, there is regional variability in the distribution of plaques within the arterial tree. The earliest recognizable form of intimal thickening is present at birth and represents a normal adaptive response.[20,61,62] Smooth muscle

TABLE 61.2.
Secondary prevention of atherosclerosis in patients with established atherosclerotic vascular disease (Level 1 evidence).

Intervention	*Criteria for Intervention**
Lipid lowering	A) Dietary therapy: reduction of saturated fats (to <7% of total calories), trans-fatty acids and cholesterol (to <200 mg/dL) B) LDL-C should be kept <100 mg/dL, employing statins as a primary pharmacologic with ezetimibe, bile acid sequestrant or niacin as needed C) For triglycerides 200–499 mg/dL, non-HDL should be less than 130 mg/dL
Physical Activity	After a physical activity assessment, 30–60 minutes of moderate intensity aerobic activity on most days of the week.
Diabetic management	Maintain HbA1c <7%, vigorous reduction of other risk factors
ACE-inhibitors and/or Beta-blockers	Patients with hypertension ≥140/90 mm Hg
Weight management	BMI >24.9 kg/m^2, waist >40 inches in men, >35 inches in women

LDL-C, low density lipoprotein cholesterol; ACE-inhibitors, angiotensin-converting enzyme inhibitors.

*Includes patients with established coronary, carotid or peripheral vascular disease.

Source: Data from reference 51K.

cells accumulate beneath the endothelium at branch points and bend in response to blood flow disturbances present at these locations. Atherosclerosis often appears first within intimal pads, suggesting that normal intima provides the "soil" for lesion growth.[19] Alternatively, disturbed blood flow at these sites (i.e., low shear stress) may result in chronic endothelial cell activation, predisposing to leukocyte adhesion and lesion initiation (Fig. 61.4).[33,63] Examples include the carotid bulb, where flow separation at the outer wall results in low shear stress and early onset of atherosclerosis. The medial wall of the carotid bulb, the flow divider, experiences higher shear and is relatively protected from early lesions. Similar associations exist for ostia of coronary and intercostal arteries.

A number of endothelial cell factors implicated in atherogenesis are induced by altered shear stress (see Fig. 61.4). For instance, endothelium downstream of aortic branches (sites of low shear) in hypercholesterolemic rabbits expresses the adhesion molecule VCAM-1 in a pattern that colocalizes with monocyte foam cell accumulation in the intima.[63] Lowering shear stress in the rat carotid artery to levels found in the human carotid bulb results in increased expression of PDGF-A and -B chains and endothelial cell turnover.[35] In addition to increased growth factor expression, low shear inhibits release of vasodilators such as NO, which are anti-atherogenic, releasing the normal state of chronic growth inhibition in the artery wall.

Regional predilection to lesion formation could also stem from regional differences in the origin of vascular smooth muscle cells. During vasculogenesis, endothelium is derived from a common pool of mesodermal angioblasts, whereas smooth muscle cells are recruited into the artery wall from regionally derived mesenchyme.[1–3,7] Smooth muscle cells in the atherosclerosis-prone coronary artery arise from the pro-epicardioal organ whereas in the aortic arch and proximal thoracic aorta they arise from neural crest and in the abdominal aorta from local mesenchyme. Differences in smooth muscle cell lineage may contribute to regional differences in artherogenesis.[19,36]

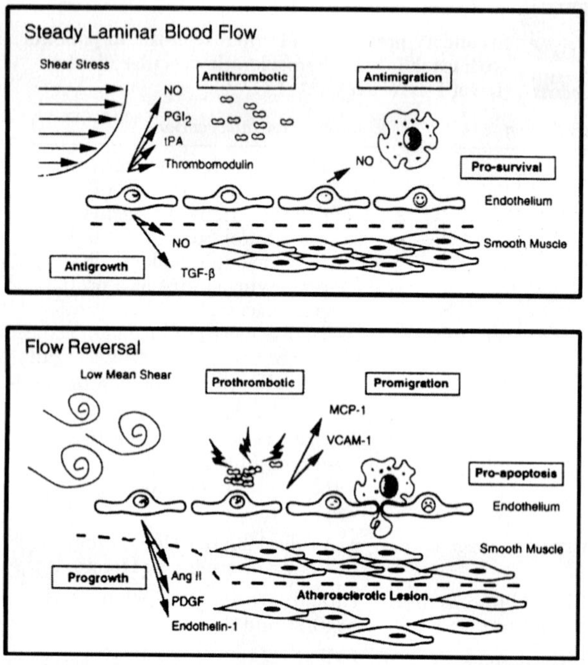

FIGURE 61.4. Illustration of the atheroprotective effects of laminar blood flow and physiological shear stress (*top*) and the atherogenic effects of turbulent blood flow and low shear stress (*bottom*). (Reproduced by permission of American Heart Association. O. Traub and B.C. Berk, Arteriosclerosis Thrombosis Vascular Biology 1998;18:677–685.[33])

Sequence of Lesion Progression

Progression of human atherosclerosis has been extensively characterized in histological studies of arteries removed at autopsy.[37,38,42,43,64] Atherosclerosis has also been modeled in animals where a more controlled analysis of lesion progression can be undertaken.[38] From these studies and others have come a comprehensive description of the stages of lesion progression to ischemic syndromes.

The earliest recognizable atherosclerotic lesion is the "fatty streak," composed largely of monocytes that have emigrated beneath the endothelium to become lipid-laden foam cells (see Fig. 61.3). Fatty streaks may be present in children and are often seen in young adults.[36,64] They may regress, or persist and progress to the next stage of lesion development. Accumulation of smooth muscle cells and extracellular matrix adds a fibrous component to the enlarging lesion, giving rise to the early "fibrofatty" plaque. Further lesion coalescence and progression in size and complexity lead to formation of the mature "fibrous plaque" (see Fig. 61.3).

Aging of the advanced fibrous plaque typically leads to development of complicating features with direct implications for the initiation of ischemic events.[36,43] A core develops within the intima of advanced plaques that is filled with foam cells, extracellular lipid, cholesterol crystals, and amorphous debris from dead cells—thus the terms lipid core and necrotic core (see Fig. 44.3).[65] Core components are highly thrombogenic and must be excluded from flowing blood by an overlying fibrous "cap" of smooth muscle cells in a collagenous matrix. As discussed next, cap thickness and size of the necrotic core are important determinants of plaque stability. Ulcers occasionally form in plaques that have ruptured and emptied the necrotic core. Other complicating features include plaque microvessels. A rich plexus of capillaries forms by angiogenic invasion inward from the adventitial vasa vasorum in response to poorly defined signals (possibly VEGF, bFGF, or hypoxia). Plaque vasa provide nutrient flow to the inner lesion and a source for leukocyte trafficking into and out from the lesion.[66] Vasa also deliver endothelial and plasma-derived growth factors and cytokines. Rupture of vasa leads to intraplaque hemorrhage and, if extensive, acute lesion expansion. Plaque microvessels have also been linked experimentally to atherosclerosis progression in mice.[67] Hemorrhage leads to acute inflammation within the plaque and late fibrosis. Plaque mineralization is another complicating feature and tends to correspond to plaque size.[68] Calcification may arise in areas of necrosis but also appears to be actively deposited by specific cell populations in response to unique molecular cues.[68,69] Although the role of mineralization in lesion progression is unclear, it corresponds to more advanced lesions and clinical syndromes.

Ischemic Syndromes

The clinical significance of atherosclerosis is the risk of plaque progression and complications resulting in decreased blood flow with end-organ ischemia, infarction, and death. This result occurs by three basic mechanisms: stenosis, thrombosis, and embolization. Each is discussed separately here, but it is important to realize that all may occur in the same lesion over time or in separate lesions within the same artery.

Stenosis

Fixed stenoses account for the majority of chronic ischemic syndromes such as exertional angina and lower-extremity claudication. As a lesion progresses, the lumen may eventually narrow to a point where resistance to flow is so severe that tissue oxygenation is impaired at rest. This impairment leads to ischemic rest pain in the extremities, unstable angina in the coronary bed, and may progress to infarction and necrosis. The degree of ischemia is determined in part by the extent to which a collateral circulation develops around the stenosis.[5] Chronic progression is more likely to result in well-developed collaterals than a rapid course, minimizing the potential for profound ischemia.

Most atherosclerotic lesions do not cause hemodynamically significant stenoses (i.e., >50% reduction in lumen diameter) because the artery wall normally enlarges in response to atherosclerosis, remodeling to accommodate even extensive plaque growth and thereby preserving lumen caliber (Fig. 61.5). Remodeling has been extensively characterized in human arteries at autopsy and in animal models of atherosclerosis.[37,38] In a landmark paper, Glagov et al. showed that human coronary arteries typically enlarge as plaques enlarge, resulting, on average, in slight lumen dilation.[37] Stenosis does occur, however, so this compensatory remodeling is not always successful. Glagov suggested that stenosis develops when the capacity of the artery wall to remodel is overcome by plaque growth and suggested that a threshold existed for

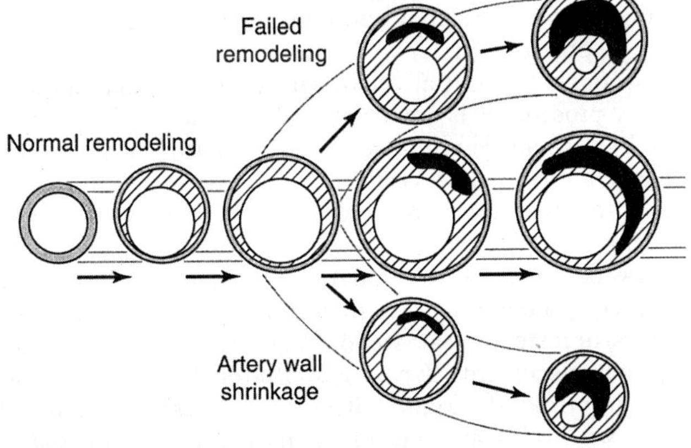

FIGURE 61.5. Normal and abnormal artery wall remodeling in response to atherosclerotic plaque growth. Most often the artery wall compensates (or overcompensates) for plaque growth by enlarging. If the wall fails to enlarge, or actively shrinks, further plaque growth encroaches upon the lumen, creating a stenosis. Intimal plaque, *cross-hatching*; necrotic core, *solid black*; lumen, *white*.

artery wall dilation. Although stenosis does represent failed remodeling, the "threshold hypothesis" is flawed because it attributes all stenoses to a fixed limit of wall enlargement when in fact the artery wall may stop enlarging prematurely or actively shrink to cause stenosis (see Fig. 61.5).

Evidence is accruing that each of these scenarios occurs. Imaging of arteries in living patients using intravascular ultrasound has demonstrated that plaque size is often no greater at a focal stenosis than at an adjacent nonstenotic segment of the same artery.[70,71] Thus, stenosis is not just excessive plaque growth but a combination of plaque growth and failed remodeling with some artery wall segments actually shrinking. The cellular and molecular events that precipitate a focal failure of remodeling have not been defined. More than likely artery wall shrinkage or constriction involves an imbalance in matrix production and degradation, fibrosis, and tissue contraction.

Plaque Rupture

A second major cause of ischemia is erosion or rupture of the fibrous cap, creating a fissure into the necrotic core and exposing tissue factor, macrophage foam cells, oxidized LDL, collagen, vWF, and necrotic debris to blood with resulting thrombosis (Fig. 61.6).[44,72,73] Thrombosis may also occur in the absence of an identifiable rupture or stenosis, leading to speculation about erosion of the lumen surface.[74] The unstable plaque is probably the cause of most acute ischemic syndromes including unstable angina, myocardial infarction, sudden death, crescendo transient ischemic attack (TIA), and thrombotic mesenteric and extremity ischemia. Acute ischemia may be profound, with infarction, or waxing and waning, as in unstable angina. The latter may result from a nonocclusive thrombus formed at the site of plaque errosion or rupture that contracts and expands from endogenous thrombolysis and thrombosis, respectively. The benefit of antiplatelet therapy with aspirin or clopidogrel in preventing ischemic events results in part from prevention of thrombosis at these sites. Of importance, more than one-half of unstable lesions have not progressed to a critical stenosis before rupture[75]; this means that dangerous lesions cannot be identified by traditional angiographic imaging to allow intervention before symptoms occur.[44,72,76]

Triggers of plaque rupture are not well defined, and thus treatment strategies to stabilize lesions are poorly developed. Careful histological evaluation of plaques removed from patients who died of sudden cardiac death have provided clues, however, and confirmed the presence of fissures and erosion of lesions underlying acute coronary thrombosis.[73] Culprit lesions, when compared to stable plaques, have larger necrotic cores; thinner fibrous caps; increased cap inflammation, particularly in the shoulder regions; and an imbalance between extracellular matrix production and degradation, particularly fibrillar collagen (see Fig. 61.6).[44,72,73,76]

Fibrous cap composition may also play a pivotal role in rupture, as proposed by Libby and others.[44,72] If smooth muscle cells and collagen provide strength to the cap, loss of either may increase the risk of erosion and fissures. Collagen production by smooth muscle cells increases in response to TGF-β and other growth factors but may be impaired by specific cytokines, including INF-γ produced by plaque T cells. INF-γ

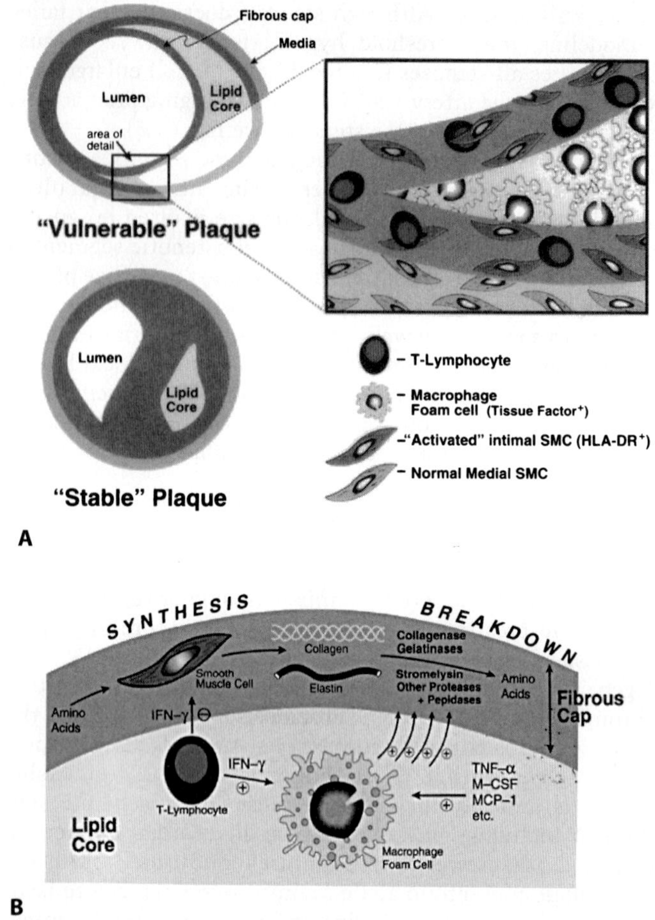

FIGURE 61.6. The unstable plaque is a major source of acute ischemic symptoms. **A.** Stable versus unstable plaques. Large lipid core, thin fibrous cap, and plaque inflammation predispose to cap rupture. **B.** Suggested molecular mechanisms of cap degeneration with altered matrix production and degradation and loss of smooth muscle cells (refer to text). (Reproduced by permission of American Heart Association. P. Libby, Circulation 1995;91:2844–2850.)

also activates macrophages and induces smooth muscle cell apoptosis in vitro.[44] Macrophage activation leads to increased expression of metalloproteinases (MMPs) including interstitial collagenase or MMP-1 and the gelatinases MMP-2 and MMP-9. Cap inflammation then may lead to loss of smooth muscle cells and increased degradation of collagen and other matrix components, further tipping the balance toward loss of cap integrity (see Fig. 61.6).

Embolization

A third major cause of ischemia in atherosclerosis is embolization from one of two basic mechanisms. Thrombus forming over an unstable lesion may break free to embolize distally, or plaque rupture may release the contents of the necrotic core. Thromboembolism may arise from nonocclusive lesions in large vessels such as the aorta or at the time of a complete thrombotic occlusion. For example, 15% of patients suffer an embolic stroke or TIA at the time of acute carotid artery thrombosis,[77] and a similar scenario may also occur in the extremities with distal emboli resulting from thrombosis of iliac and femoral artery lesions. Small emboli that lodge in the digital arteries result in toe ischemia and cyanosis, coined the "blue toe syndrome." Large emboli from the aorta may occlude branch vessels with profound regional ischemia of the abdominal viscera or extremities, although most commonly the source is from an intracardiac thrombus rather than an atherosclerotic lesion per se.

Microemboli from plaque rupture include cholesterol crystals, lipid, and necrotic debris and are referred to as atheroemboli or cholesterol emboli.[78] Plaque debris may also be released at the time of surgical manipulation of large arteries or dislodged by catheters and devices during arteriography and endovascular procedures. The aorta and its branches are the most common source, and the small size and content of the material leads to a constellation of ischemic symptoms and signs referred to as the "cholesterol emboli syndrome."[78] The presentation may include levido reticularis, a lacy mottling of the skin from cutaneous microembolization, and severe pain and cyanosis of the toes from digital artery occlusion that may progress to gangrene. Muscle emboli cause pain and occasionally progress to myonecrosis. The syndrome varies, however, depending on the site of the culprit lesion and tissue beds involved. Cholesterol emboli from carotid plaques cause strokes or TIAs, and cholesterol crystals (Hollenhorst plaques) can be seen lodged in branches of the ipsilateral retinal artery on fundoscopic evaluation. Emboli to abdominal viscera may present as bowel ischemia or acute tubular necrosis from renal artery emboli with lipid and eosinophils in the urine sediment.[78]

Intimal Hyperplasia and Restenosis

Failure of Arterial Reconstruction

Injured and diseased arteries frequently require reconstruction to restore function and correct ischemia. Despite a continuous search for less invasive techniques, virtually all forms of reconstruction are mechanical. Whether surgical (bypass grafting and endarterectomy) or endovascular (angioplasty, atherectomy, and stenting), each method causes substantial injury to the treated artery wall, resulting in a thrombogenic surface and setting into motion a specific healing response that may subsequently contribute to failure of the reconstruction.

Although the initial technical success in appropriately selected procedures is greater than 90%, late results are tempered by substantial numbers of intermediate (within 2 years) and late (more than 2 years) failures. Acute failures result from thrombosis and often indicate an underlying technical problem, as thrombosis is otherwise unusual given the effectiveness of modern anticoagulation. Intermediate failures are a frequent problem and are most often caused by recurrent stenosis, or restenosis, at sites of endarterectomy, angioplasty, and stent placement. Bypass grafts often fail in this period from neointimal thickening. Restenosis rates vary from 15% to 80% within 2 years, depending on the intervention and the site of treatment.[79] For example, coronary angioplasty carries a 30% to 60% restenosis rate, often accompanied by recurrent symptoms of ischemia,[80,81] whereas carotid endarterectomy carries a 15% to 20% restenosis rate that is usually clinically silent.[82,83] Late failures are also a significant problem and usually indicate progression or recurrence of the underlying

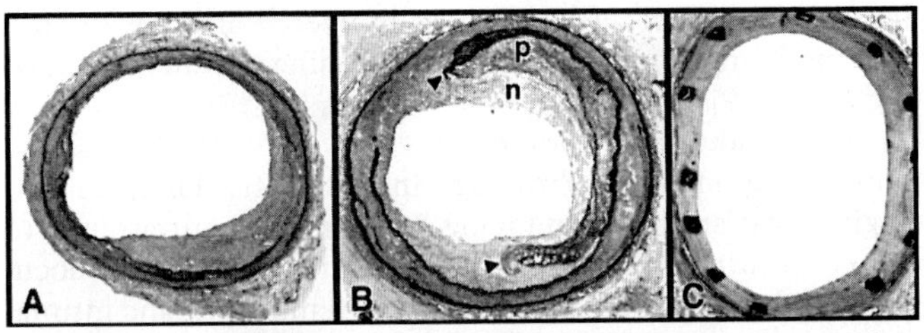

FIGURE 61.7. Composite micrograph of an atherosclerotic iliac artery (**A**) in a cynomolgus monkey before angioplasty. One month after angioplasty (**B**) and stenting (**C**) of the contralateral iliac artery, significant neointima (*n*) has developed at the site of plaque (*p*) fracture (*arrowhead*) and within the stent struts. Angioplasty without stenting resulted in artery wall shrinkage (negative remodeling) with lumen narrowing (restenosis). Stents prevent wall shrinkage and overcome negative remodeling. (Reproduced by permission of American Heart Association. J.S. Deitch et al., Arteriosclerosis Thrombosis Vascular Biology 1998;18:1730–1737.)

pathology, typically atherosclerosis, in contiguous vessel segments. Atherosclerotic degeneration also accounts for late vein graft failures, particularly after coronary artery bypass grafting, where only 40% to 50% of vein grafts remain patent after 10 years. In contrast, 89% of internal mammary artery grafts remain patent in patients surviving 20 years after coronary artery bypass.

Restenosis

Restenosis is simply a recurrent lumen narrowing at the site of a prior arterial reconstruction for occlusive disease. In contrast to atherosclerosis, restenosis has few well-established risk factors to provide insight into its underlying molecular mechanisms. Traditional risk factors for atherosclerosis have not consistently correlated with restenosis after angioplasty, suggesting that mechanisms governing smooth muscle cell growth and artery wall remodeling after acute mechanical trauma are distinct from those in chronic endothelial dysfunction and atherosclerosis. Despite decades of intensive research, few strategies have emerged to significantly reduce restenosis rates after angioplasty. The first major advance was the intraarterial stent used to physically support the artery wall after angioplasty (Fig. 61.7).[84,85] New treatment strategies to prevent restenosis are emerging, including intraarterial radiation and drug-eluting stents coated within the immunosupressant sirolimus or the cytoskeletal inhibitor taxol.[86–88]

Intimal Hyperplasia

Just as endothelial cell dysfunction and atherosclerosis result from a wide variety of risk factors, intimal hyperplasia is the common response to virtually all forms of mechanical artery wall injury, leading to accumulation of smooth muscle cells and matrix to form a neointima. This new tissue represents an adaptive response in many ways analogous to wound healing.[89] Because of its location, excessive neointima formation can encroach into the lumen, leading to restenosis or bypass graft stenosis (Fig. 61.7, 61.8).

Intimal hyperplasia has been characterized extensively in animal models. The prototype is the rat carotid balloon injury model characterized by Clowes and colleagues and subsequently used worldwide in studies of intimal formation.[12,90] Balloon catheter denudation removes the endothelium and stretches the artery wall, killing approximately 25% of medial smooth muscle cells. Platelets adhere to exposed subendothelial matrix and degranulation releases growth factors PDGF, EGF, bFGF, and TGF-β while disrupted medial smooth muscle cells release intracellular stores of bFGF. The result is medial smooth muscle cell replication, driven in part by bFGF, which peaks at 48 h. This reaction is followed by migration of smooth muscle cells from the media into the intima 4 to 7 days after injury, driven in part by PDGF released from smooth muscle cells and platelets.[91,92] Once across the IEL, cells replicate further within the intima before becoming quiescent after 4 weeks. The neointima continues to thicken up to 6 weeks from accumulation of extracellular matrix. The rat lesion has then matured and may actually regress slightly with further observation.

Intimal hyperplasia with neointima formation at sites of injury appeared, from these studies and others, to be the primary mechanism of restenosis after injury. This result prompted a search for compounds to inhibit smooth muscle cell replication as a means of controlling neointimal accumulation and restenosis. Many agents have been identified, including the prototypes heparin and angiotensin-converting enzyme inhibitors,[90,93] but when studied in human angioplasty restenosis trials their effects have been uniformly disappointing.[94,95]

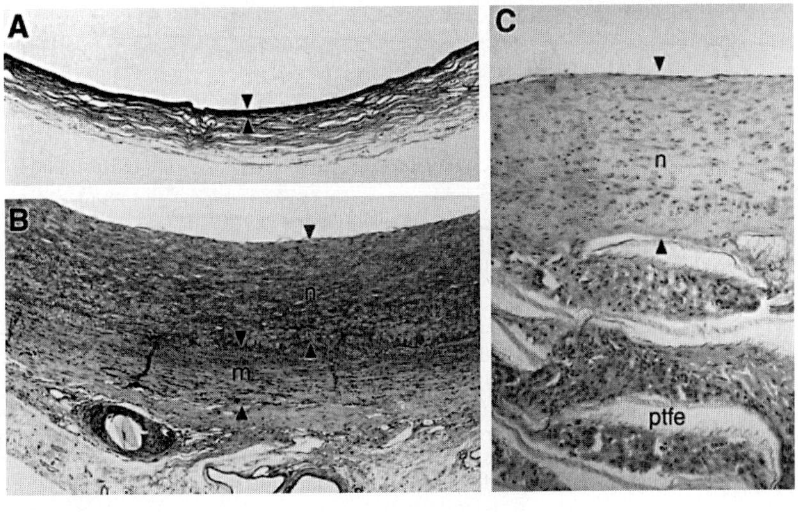

FIGURE 61.8. Micrographs of baboon internal jugular vein before (**A**) and 1 month after (**B**) grafting into the carotid artery circulation. Note thin vein media (*arrowheads*) before implantation and the significant neointimal (*n*) and medial (*m*) thickening in response to arterialization. **C.** Polytetrafluoroethylene (*ptfe*) bypass graft removed from the same animal 1 month after implantation. Note the neointimal accumulation (*n*) overlying the PTFE graft material.

Failure of animal models to predict effective therapies for human restenosis raised many questions and led to a critical reappraisal of animal models of artery wall pathology. Key questions include these: Are there significant species differences in the regulation of smooth muscle cell growth? Is intimal hyperplasia the only important mechanism of restenosis? and Have animal models accurately represented the contribution of the advanced human atherosclerotic plaque to the injury response and restenosis? The answers to these questions appear to be yes, sometimes, and probably not, respectively (see following).

Remodeling

Remodeling is a normal physiological process by which arteries change their geometry to maintain optimal wall stress and lumen caliber. As discussed for atherosclerosis,[37,38] remodeling is an important adaptation to pathology as well, allowing the artery wall to enlarge and thus compensate for atherosclerotic plaque growth to maintain lumen caliber (see Fig. 61.5). As alternative mechanisms for restenosis were explored, it was discovered that changes in artery wall geometry contributed substantially to loss of lumen caliber following injury.[96–101]

A recently established restenosis model in nonhuman primates with complex preexisting atherosclerosis specifically addresses the three questions just raised.[89,100,101] In this model, species differences in regulation of smooth muscle cell growth are minimized and complex atherosclerotic lesions more closely depict the human plaque leading to reconstruction. Iliac artery angioplasty increases lumen size by fracturing the atherosclerotic plaque and stretching or tearing the surrounding media. The artery wall injury is transmural and results in intimal hyperplasia and adventitial fibrosis. Damage leads to acute inflammation with monocytes invading a thin thrombus covering fractured plaques (days 2–7). Following a brief wave of proliferation, smooth muscle cells and myofibroblasts move into the lesion to form a neointima (days 7–14). Inflammation then resolves, and neointima replaces the thrombus and enlarges from further accumulation of cells and extracellular matrix (days 14–28). As a result, the artery wall defect heals in a process that is in many ways analogous to wound healing (see Fig. 61.7).[89] Despite the accumulation of neointima, restenosis in this model is not caused by increased lesion size but rather by changes in overall artery wall size, or remodeling, with wall shrinkage leading to lumen narrowing (Fig. 61.9).[101]

Two additional lines of evidence support the role of remodeling and wall shrinkage in restenosis. First, clinical angioplasty studies employing intravascular ultrasound to image the artery wall over time after angioplasty have documented the contribution of artery wall remodeling and intimal hyperplasia to restenosis.[99] The relative change in lumen caliber accounted for by remodeling has been estimated at 60% to 80%, with new wall mass contributing only 20% to 40%. The second line of evidence comes from stent studies in which angioplasty is followed by placement of a rigid metal scaffolding inside the artery lumen. Stents resist artery wall constriction and shrinkage, thus overcoming any impact of remodeling (see Fig. 61.7). Stents placed at the time of coronary and iliac angioplasty have reduced restenosis rates by about 15% despite the fact that stents increase the amount of neointima formed; this occurs because stents maintain significantly more of the initial gain in lumen caliber after angioplasty, preventing wall contraction and constrictive remodeling.[102]

The cellular and molecular determinants of remodeling are unknown, and strategies to prevent wall shrinkage (other than stenting) do not exist at present. However, experimental data suggest that tissue reorganization analogous to wound healing may play a role. Wounds mend by tissue regeneration and contraction mediated by adhesive interactions among cells and extracellular matrix molecules. These interactions use cell-surface receptors including integrins, and the pattern of receptor expression is altered by injury.[89] Matrix contraction can be blocked in vitro with integrin-blocking antibodies or by altering the composition of extracellular matrix. If healing results in variable tissue contraction, inhibiting cell–matrix interactions may minimize restenosis by shifting the balance away from artery wall shrinkage.

In summary, then, restenosis is caused by a combination of intimal hyperplasia and constrictive remodeling, or new tissue ingrowth and artery wall shrinkage, respectively. Not surprizingly then, the only effective inhibitor of postangioplasty restenosis to date combines a treatment for constrictive remodeling (a stent) with a treatment to prevent intimal hyperplasia (drugs such as sirolimus) in the form of drug-eluting stents.[87,88] Drug-eluting stents do not prevent the

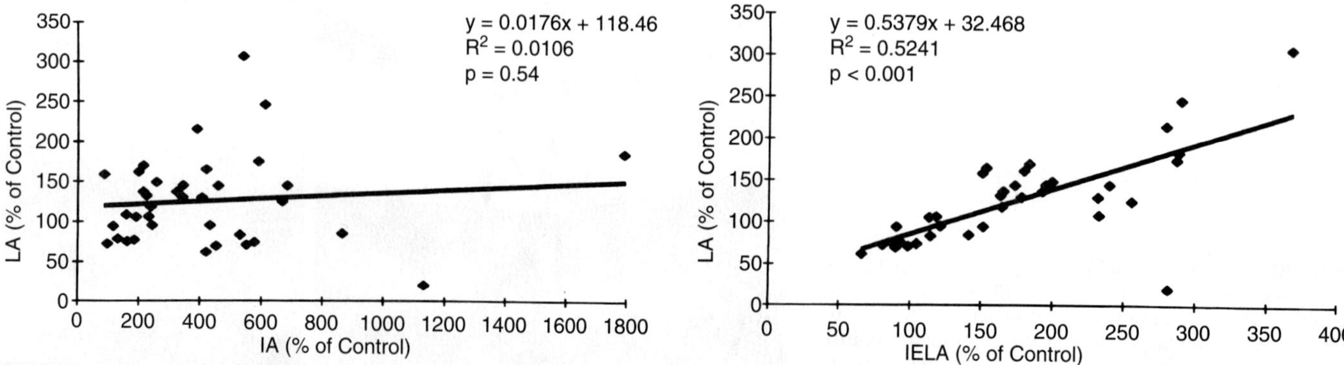

FIGURE 61.9. Scattergrams demonstrate the relationship between changes in lumen area (*LA*) after angioplasty and changes in intimal area (*IA*; *left panel*) or changes in artery wall size (*IELA*; *right panel*). Changes in plaque size (intimal hyperplasia) after angioplasty do not correlate with lumen size. Rather, changes in overall artery wall size (remodeling) predict lumen caliber and restenosis. (Reproduced with permission from JS Mondy et al. Journal of Vascular Surgery 1997;26:875–883.[101])

problem for all patients, nor in all vascular beds but remarkable data from clinical studies in coronary angioplasty have shown conclusive benefits in the context of the SIRIUS and RAVEL trials for sirolimus eluting stents and the TAXUS trials for paclitaxel eluting stents.[88A] While effectively precluding restenosis, these stents have been associated with an increased risk of thrombosis, the magnitude of which is still under investigation. In contrast to their clear advantage in prevention of restenosis in the coronary vasculature, a similar approach of drug eluting stents in the peripheral vessels, such as extremity atherosclerotic lesions, has not proven to confer any advantage over traditional bare metal stents, as shown in the SIROCCO trial.[88B] Similarly, preliminary data for drug eluting stents applied towards renal atherosclerotic lesions appears not to reduce restenosis over bare metal stents, but randomized trial results of this have yet to be published. It is interesting to note the difference in restenosis rates for DES depending on their placement in either the coronary and peripheral vascular beds.

Vein Graft Arterialization

Intimal hyperplasia has long been recognized in both synthetic and autologous conduits placed into the arterial circulation (see Fig. 61.8). Carrel and Guthrie were the first investigators to describe vein wall thickening after implantation.[103] Areas adjacent to anastomoses developed a smooth, white "scar-like appearance" and the process was termed "arterialization." Initially this was believed to be a normal adaptation to the stress of arterial hemodynamics and a repair process necessary for anastomotic healing and restoration of a nonthrombogenic lumen surface. It is now recognized that, at times, intimal hyperplasia is poorly regulated and can cause lumen encroachment, produce atherosclerotic lesions, and lead to graft thrombosis.[104]

In human beings, the intimal hyperplastic response is difficult to characterize because grafts are unavailable for serial pathological examination. However, fragmentary evidence available from human specimens has been largely corroborated by animal studies. In a rabbit jugular vein to carotid artery graft model, there is acute patchy loss of endothelium throughout the graft because of surgical trauma.[105,106] Denuded areas are quickly covered with platelet thrombi and leukocytes, and the underlying media develops regions of hemorrhage, swelling, and smooth muscle necrosis.[105,106] The acute injury can be limited with meticulous technique in dissecting, clamping, and valvulotomy and by avoiding graft overdistension. Although the contribution of these factors to acute graft failure is undeniable, long-term consequences are less clear.

Reendothelialization is complete within 2 weeks of implantation, at which point platelets and leukocytes are again excluded from the graft luminal surface. Intimal thickening begins very early and is characterized by smooth muscle cell replication, migration, and extracellular matrix deposition. Proliferation is maximal at 1 week and returns to baseline within 1 month, whereas the intima continues to thicken from further extracellular matrix production for up to 12 weeks. The structure of grafts at later times is similar to grafts at 12 weeks, but degenerative changes occur.[105,106] One year after implantation there is increased endothelial cell permeability, red blood cell and fibrin deposition in the graft wall, and macrophage foam cell accumulation in the intima. These changes are not unlike early atherosclerotic lesions and are the precursors to degenerative lesions seen in human vein grafts. Hypercholesterolemia (200–600 mg/dL) accelerates atherosclerotic degeneration of vein grafts in this model, increasing intimal thickening at 3 and 6 months from deposition of foam cells.[106]

Hemodynamic factors also modify the intimal thickening response in vein grafts because wall thickness and luminal area adjust to changes in pressure (tangential wall stress) and flow (shear stress).[105,107,108] A number of factors have been shown to inhibit intimal hyperplasia in experimental vein grafts, including NO donors,[109] inhibitors of growth factors,[110] angiotensin-converting enzyme (ACE),[111] and cell cycle, but none has yet proven effective at improving human vein graft patency. However, antiplatelet therapy and anticoagulation[112,113] are useful in preventing perioperative graft thrombosis and help prevent late graft thrombosis in selected patients. This action probably relates to the thrombogenic surface caused by graft denudation in the perioperative period and by endothelial cell dysfunction with increased tissue factor expression at later times.[114]

Prosthetic Graft Failure

The development of synthetic vascular grafts, particularly Dacron and expanded polytetrafluoroethylene (PTFE), was a milestone in the history of vascular surgery. These prostheses are invaluable in large vessel reconstructions and provide an alternative in medium and small artery reconstruction when autogenous vein is not available. Despite a relative inertness, prosthetic grafts are thrombogenic and develop lesions similar in composition and equally as detrimental to those described for vein grafts (see Fig. 61.8). As prosthetic grafts are fairly rigid and do not remodel, lumen encroachment is usually a function of thrombosis or neointimal formation. The magnitude of this problem is underscored by high failure rates of prosthetic grafts used for infrainguinal reconstructions. For example, a randomized trial of PTFE versus saphenous vein for femoral to popliteal bypass grafting reported a 5-year primary patency rate in PTFE of 38% compared to 68% for vein grafts,[115] in contrast to the 70% to 85% patency of prosthetic grafts in the aortofemoral position.

Intimal hyperplasia inside prosthetic grafts is limited to the first few millimeters adjacent to anastomoses (see Fig. 61.8), beyond which the lumen is incompletely endothelialized and lacks a true cellular intima. A pseudointima forms on the lumen surface from platelet and fibrin deposition, which remains slightly thrombogenic. In conventional low-porosity PTFE grafts (30-mm internodal distance), cells healing the anastomoses grow onto the graft lumen surface from the cut arterial edge. Smooth muscle cells replicate and migrate inward beneath an advancing endothelium, in contrast to intimal hyperplasia after arterial injury where the endothelium plays an inhibitory role.[116] Anastomotic neointima thickens as cells and extracellular matrix accumulate and, when excessive, stenosis occurs. Strategies to reduce graft thrombogenicity and inhibit anastomotic intimal hyperplasia, such as seeding the graft lumen surface with endothelial cells before implantation, have been largely unsuccessful.[117]

Resulting neointimal lesions resemble those in vein grafts and injured arteries (see Fig. 61.8) and are regulated in part by hemodynamic forces. Shear stress at anastomoses is affected by the angle of the anastomosis, graft caliber, and volume flow required to supply the distal vascular bed. Low shear increases intimal hyperplasia. The effects of shear have been dramatically illustrated in a baboon model of PTFE grafting in which high shear is induced by creating a distal arteriovenous fistula.[118,119] The result is limited smooth muscle cell accumulation beneath the endothelium. Subsequent fistula ligation normalizes shear and induces smooth muscle cell proliferation, with a fivefold increase in neointimal area within 1 month.[119] In this model, endothelial cell expression of eNOS and NO production are increased by high shear, contributing in part to inhibition of smooth muscle cell growth.[120] Reducing shear stress to normal levels decreases eNOS expression and NO production, whereas expression of the growth factors PDGF-A and -B increase significantly in the endothelium and underlying smooth muscle.[121] Increased neointima formation and thrombosis are two important contributors to graft failure when prosthetic grafts are used in extremities with low flow as a consequence of poor runoff.

Aneurysmal Degeneration

Incidence and Impact on Public Health

True aneurysms represent a degeneration of the artery wall with loss of structural integrity leading to gradual dilation of all artery wall layers. Aneurysms have been reported in virtually all segments of the arterial tree, but the majority localize to the aorta, iliac, femoral, and popliteal segments, and more than 90% involve the abdominal aorta below the renal arteries. Aneurysms are most commonly diagnosed in the sixth and seventh decades of life, and the incidence has been rising for unknown reasons. Most occur in patients with concomitant atherosclerosis, and men are affected three to four times more often than women.[123,124] The prevalence of abdominal aortic aneurysms (AAAs) in ultrasound screening programs approximates 2,000 per 100,000 population for adult white males and 10,000 per 100,000 for men more than 70 years of age.[124] A familial tendency is reported in 6% to 15% of AAA patients, indicating a genetic contribution to the underlying pathobiology. However, the majority of patients lack this history and, as in atherosclerosis, there are multiple associated genetic and acquired risk factors.[125]

Aneurysms are often unsuspected in the absence of deliberate screening by physical examination or ultrasound imaging because they do not typically cause symptoms before sudden rupture, thrombosis, or embolization. Some are diagnosed incidentally on radiographs or ultrasound studies obtained for unrelated medical problems, but patients often present emergently with poor outcomes, as underscored by the 60% to 90% mortality associated with rupture of an AAA compared to the 2% to 7% mortality with elective repair.[124] Unfortunately, the sequence of molecular and cellular events initiating aneurysmal degeneration is incompletely defined and thus preventive therapies have not been established. Treatment remains surgical with interposition grafting, endografting, or bypass and exclusion techniques, as described in subsequent chapters.

Pathogenesis

Basic Mechanisms

The major features of aneurysmal degeneration are loss of collagen, elastin, and cells from the tunica media.[126,127] The loss of structural integrity accompanies gradual dilation of the artery wall, with increases in wall tensile stress that predispose to rupture. Mural thrombus forms within the aneurysm sac and can lead to thrombotic occlusion or embolization, particularly in aneurysms of peripheral arteries such as in the popliteal. Association of aneurysms with atherosclerosis has led to speculation about shared risk factors and common mechanisms of disease.[125] Structural changes within the aneurysmal artery wall, however, are distinct from the atherosclerotic lesion and probably do not simply represent one end of the spectrum of atherosclerotic wall degeneration (Fig. 61.10).[126,127]

Just as in atherosclerosis, rare inherited disorders have provided insight into basic mechanisms of aneurysm pathobiology. Patients with inborn errors in connective tissue metabolism, specifically collagen and elastin, have an extraordinary risk of aneurysm formation in the absence of atherosclerosis; these include individuals with Ehlers–Danlos syndrome type IV from a defect in the gene encoding type III procollagen and those with Marfan syndrome from a defect in the gene encoding fibrillin-1, a protein required for elastin fiber formation. In the more common familial clustering of aneurysms, a variety of genetic abnormalities have been identified, including polymorphisms in the genes encoding type III procollagen, haptoglobin, alpha-1-antitrypsin, and cholesterol ester transfer protein.[127] Many of the associated gene variants or defects suggest abnormal extracellular matrix production, or turnover, as key factors in the pathogenesis of aneurysms. However, more than 80% of aneurysms have no

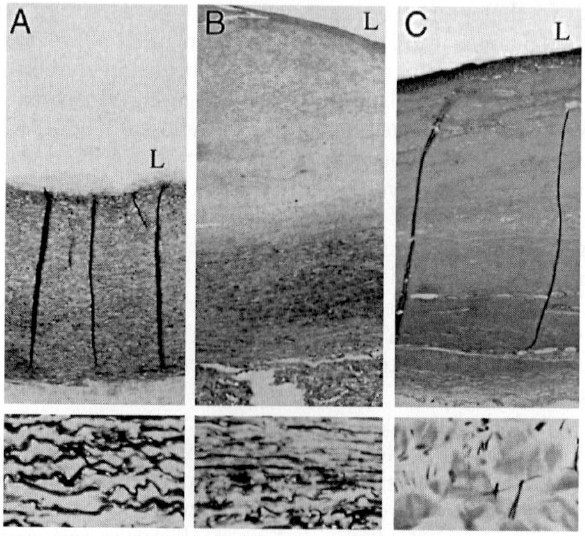

FIGURE 61.10. Micrographs demonstrate the differences in medial elastin content of normal aorta (**A**), atherosclerotic aorta (**B**), and aneurysmal aorta (**C**). Lumen is at *top* (*L*). Atherosclerosis is largely an intimal disease with reasonably intact medial elastic fibers. In contrast, the aneurysmal media is characterized by loss of elastin, smooth muscle cells, and collagen. (Reproduced with permission from DR Holmes et al., Journal of Vascular Surgery 1995;21:761–772.)

clear pattern of inheritance, and it has been suggested that a spectrum of genetic factors predispose individuals to loss of extracellular matrix in the presence of acquired and environmental risk factors such as smoking, atherosclerosis, hypertension, and infection.[125,127,128]

The association of aneurysms with rare disorders of matrix metabolism, and the loss of collagen and elastin noted in the media of atherosclerotic aneurysms (see Fig. 61.10), have prompted investigators to explore an imbalance between matrix production and degradation as the etiology of this disease.[127–129] Collagen and elastin are produced in proforms that require posttranslational modification and cleavage to produce components of fibrillar collagens and elastin.[130,131] Further processing occurs outside the cell to create structural load-bearing collagen and elastin fibers. Matrix production is tightly regulated in smooth muscle cells and adventitial fibroblasts, increasing substantially with artery wall injury and atherosclerosis, in response to associated growth factors TGF-β, EGF, and others. Growth inhibitors that maintain normal artery wall quiescence may inhibit matrix production. Other factors, such as IFN-γ from plaque T cells, inhibit collagen production in the atherosclerotic artery wall and may play a similar role in aneurysms. An alternative mechanism for decreased matrix production may simply be smooth muscle cell death.[126] In fact, medial cell loss is a prominent histological feature of the aneurysmal tunica media and is associated with markers of apoptosis such as fragmented DNA and increased expression of p53, a mediator of cell-cycle arrest and programmed cell death.[126] Pregnancy is unique condition where the process of aneurysmal degeneration of pre-existing aneurysms appears accelerated, perhaps as a result of the extensive remodeling that is necessary in the pregnant condition. Pathologic evidence of changes in the vessel media layer as well as expression of matrix metalloproteinases in pregnancy that are already implicated in aneurysmal disease may provide further clues to the aneurysm disease process.[131A–C]

Artery wall cells produce a wide variety of matrix-degrading proteases, and matrix turnover is tightly regulated in the normal artery wall. Protease activity increases in the artery wall in response to inflammation associated with aneurysms and atherosclerosis.[127] Some, such as the plasminogen activators, have broad substrate specificities and others, including serine elastases and members of the large family of matrix metalloproteinases (MMPs), are more selective. Aneurysmal arteries have increased expression of the interstitial collagenase MMP-1 and the elastases MMP-2 and MMP-9.[127,132] MMP-9 is more prominent in aneurysms than in atherosclerotic lesions whereas MMP-2 is increased in both. MMP-1 expression localizes to endothelial and connective tissue cells within the adventitia of the aneurysmal aorta, and MMP-9 is expressed primarily by inflammatory cells (macrophages) within the wall. MMP-2 localizes to both macrophages and smooth muscle cells.

Although protease expression increases within the diseased artery wall, regulation of protease activity is complex and dependent upon a number of factors. For example, MMPs are secreted as proenzymes requiring cleavage for activation. Activation is inhibited by a family of tissue inhibitors of metalloproteinases (TIMPs) that bind MMPs to prevent their cleavage.[127] MMP-9 may be secreted bound to its TIMP-1 inhibitor and MMP-2 to TIMP-2. In fact, expression of TIMPs may actually increase within the aneurysmal artery wall.[127] However, the balance between expression and inhibition is tipped in favor of activity, as documented by substrate gel zymography. In this assay, protein extracts from the aneurysmal artery wall are run onto gels impregnated with protein substrates (e.g., gelatin). Clear lytic bands at the appropriate molecular weight indicate active enzyme. Activity of both MMP-2 and MMP-9 is increased in aneurysm samples compared to those of normal wall.[127]

Expression of MMPs and other proteases increases in response to inflammatory cytokines including interleukin-1β and tumor necrosis factor (TNF-α) present in the diseased artery wall. Others, such as INF-γ and IL-4, may be inhibitory. Macrophages are a prominent source of proteases, and increased inflammation is associated with both atherosclerosis and aneurysmal degeneration.[133] As mentioned earlier for atherosclerosis, microvessels invade the diseased artery wall and provide a mechanism for increased leukocyte trafficking. Medial microvessel ingrowth has been documented in aneurysms, and their number increases 15 fold over the normal aortic media and 3 fold over the atherosclerotic media. Microvessels colocalize with medial elastin destruction and macrophages, in support of a pathogenic role.[127]

In summary, aneurysms are a significant and growing public health problem with no current preventative therapy. The etiology appears to be medial degeneration from cell apoptosis, decreased structural matrix production, and increased matrix degradation.[127] Degradation of elastin and collagens is most prominent and appears to result in large part from protease expression (e.g., MMPs) in response to chronic inflammation.[133] Although specific inciting events are not well defined, recent studies have suggested a number of inflammatory stimuli, including those common to atherosclerosis; to autoantigens against matrix components as popularized by Tilson and colleagues[134]; or to low-grade infection of the artery wall from viruses or bacteria.[135]

Inflammatory Aneurysms

Three percent to 10% of AAAs present with a peculiar pattern of retroperitoneal inflammation referred to as the inflammatory aneurysm.[123] The triad of a thickened aneurysm wall, retroperitoneal fibrosis, and adhesion of the aneurysm to adjacent intraabdominal structures (e.g., duodenum) defines this variant, which presents on average one decade earlier than a bland aortic aneurysm. In contrast to the bland aneurysm, symptoms are common in inflammatory aneurysms, with 65% to 95% of patients presenting with abdominal pain, weight loss, or anorexia. Nonspecific markers of inflammation (e.g., increased sedimentation rate and C-reactive protein) are also more common.[123] Risk factors more prominent for inflammatory aneurysms than for bland aneurysms include male sex and smoking, and in some series a greater familial tendency has been reported.[123] Other risks appear to be common to all AAAs, as described in the previous section.

The cicatrix overlying the aneurysm may involve other retroperitoneal structures (e.g., ureters), and the duodenum is nearly always densely adhered to the aneurysm. These attributes present the surgeon with a unique challenge during aneurysmorrhaphy. No pharmacological therapy has been shown to improve the situation before surgery, in part because the etiology of the inflammation is unknown. It has been suggested that the inflammatory aneurysm is just one end of a spectrum because all aneurysms have varying degrees of wall inflammation. Other hypotheses are that inflammation is caused by blood leaking into the retroperitoneum, by lymphatic obstruction, by infection, or by the development of autoantigens against specific aortic wall components.[123] Unfortunately, little evidence exists for bleeding or lymphatic obstruction in inflammatory aneurysms, and the other theories add little to those proposed for aneurysms in general. Evidence that the process is distinct from a bland aneurysm is that the inflammatory process and cicatrix subside after repair, in contrast to the process of aneurysmal degeneration, which is known to progress in contiguous aortic segments.

Infected (Mycotic) Aneurysms

Mycotic aneurysms are the result of artery wall infections that often begin in normal caliber vessels leading to subsequent aneurysmal degeneration.[136] Infections may also begin within preexisting aneurysms, and both are associated with rapid degeneration of the artery wall, dilation, and rupture. Historically, infections were most often associated with valvular heart disease and endocarditis. Bacteremia or septic emboli seeded the artery wall, most commonly the aorta (more than 30% of cases), causing focal infectious arteritis. In the preantibiotic era, infected aneurysms were uniformly fatal. Currently, about 80% of infected aneurysms are the result of inoculation from contiguous tissues, direct artery wall trauma, or hematogenous seeding of preexisting atherosclerotic plaques and aneurysms.[136] In contemporary series, outcomes have improved significantly as the result of refined antimicrobial therapy and surgical techniques, including prosthetic grafts for extraanatomic reconstruction remote from the site of infection and in situ reconstruction with deep vein.[137] However, morbidity and mortality remain high.

The most common organisms in historical series were streptococcal and staphylococcal species, or, in the case of syphilitic aortitis, *Treponema pallidum*. Modern series are composed largely of bacterial or fungal infections, and *Staphylococcus aureus* and species of *Salmonella* are the most common agents. *Salmonella* infections appear to have a predilection for diseased atherosclerotic arteries. A number of less common organisms have also been reported in each of the small contemporary series, and their representation is likely increasing because of the greater numbers of immunocompromised hosts.

It is of some interest that many AAAs contain microorganisms that can be cultured at the time of elective repair. Positive cultures can be obtained from aneurysmal contents in 14% to 37% of routine AAA cases, and most bacteria grown represent normal skin flora. The number of aneurysms harboring microorganisms may be higher as many organisms are difficult to isolate routinely. Newer techniques using DNA profiles are beginning to identify some of these other culprit pathogens.[137A] Despite a positive culture, a postoperative graft or aortic infection occurs in less than 2% of cases.[138] The significance of bacteria in the absence of gross infection is unclear and is difficult to reconcile with the fulminant course of the less common infected aneurysm. As suggested for atherosclerosis and for aneurysms, microorganisms likely play an etiological role in their pathogenesis by inducing chronic artery wall inflammation that in turn results in atherosclerotic or aneurysmal wall degeneration. However, artery wall destruction from a suppurative infection is a distinct entity, with entirely different prognostic and treatment implications.

References

1. Jain RK. Molecular regulation of vessel maturation. Nat Med 2003;9:685–693.
2. Baldwin HS. Early embryonic vascular development. Cardiovasc Res 1996;31(suppl S):E34–E45.
3. Risau W, Flamme I. Vasculogenesis. Annu Rev Cell Biol 1995;11:73–91.
4. Folkman J. Fundamental concepts of the angiogenic process. Curr Mol Med 2003;3(7):643–651.
5. Heil M, Schaper W. Influence of mechanical, cellular, and molecular factors on collateral artery growth (arteriogenesis). Circ Res 2004;95:449–458.
6. Friedlander M, Brooks PC, Shaffer RW, Kincaid CM, Varner JA, Cheresh DA. Definition of two angiogenic pathways by distinct alpha v integrins. Science 1995;270:1500–1502.
7. Owens GK. Regulation of differentiation of vascular smooth muscle cells. Physiol Rev 1995;75:487–517.
8. Bischoff J. Cell adhesion and angiogenesis. J Clin Invest 1997;99:373–376.
9. Schwartz SM, Heimark RL, Majesky MW. Developmental mechanisms underlying pathology of arteries. Physiol Rev 1990;70:1177–1210.
10. Schwartz SM, Benditt EP. Clustering of replicating cells in aortic endothelium. Proc Natl Acad Sci USA 1976;73:651–653.
11. Clowes AW, Reidy MA, Clowes MM. Kinetics of cellular proliferation after arterial injury. I. Smooth muscle growth in the absence of endothelium. Lab Invest 1983;49:327–333.
12. Raines EW, Ross R. Multiple growth factors are associated with lesions of atherosclerosis: specificity or redundancy? BioEssays 1996;18:271–282.
13. Lindner V, Lappi DA, Baird A, Majack RA, Reidy MA. Role of basic fibroblast growth factor in vascular lesion formation. Circ Res 1991;68:106–113.
14. Friesel RE, Maciag T. Molecular mechanisms of angiogenesis: fibroblast growth factor signal transduction. FASEB J 1995;9:919–925.

14A. Coultas L, Chawengsaksophak K, Rossant J. Endothelial cells and VEGF in vascular development. Nature 2005;438:937–945.

14B. Wigle JT, Harvey N, Detmar M, et al. An essential role for Prox1 in the induction of the lymphatic endothelial cell phenotype. EMBO J 2002;21:1505–1513.

15. Vernon RB, Sage EH. Between molecules and morphology—extracellular matrix and creation of vascular form. Am J Pathol 1995;147:873–883.
16. Ruoslahti E, Engvall E. Integrins and vascular extracellular matrix assembly. J Clin Invest 1997;99:1149–1152.
17. Ruoslahti E, Reed JC. Anchorage dependence, integrins, and apoptosis. Cell 1994;77:477–478.
18. Stromblad S, Becker JC, Yebra M, Brooks PC, Cheresh DA. Suppression of p53 activity and p21WAF1/CIP1 expression by vascular cell integrin alpha$_v$beta$_3$ during angiogenesis. J Clin Invest 1996;98:426–433.
19. Schwartz SM, DeBlois D, O'Brien ERM. The intima—soil for atherosclerosis and restenosis. Circ Res 1995;77:445–465.
20. Friedman MH, Hutchins GM, Bargeron CB, Deters OJ, Mark FF. Correlation between intimal thickness and fluid shear in human arteries. Atherosclerosis 1981;39:425–436.
21. Wu KK, Thiagarajan P. Role of endothelium in thrombosis and hemostasis. Annu Rev Med 1996;47:315–331.
22. Zimmerman GA, McIntyre TM, Prescott SM. Adhesion and signaling in vascular cell–cell interactions. J Clin Invest 1996;98:1699–1702.

23. Gimbrone MA, Nagel T, Topper JN. Biomechanical activation: an emerging paradigm in endothelial adhesion biology. J Clin Invest 1997;99:1809–1813.
24. Resnick N, Gimbrone MA Jr. Hemodynamic forces are complex regulators of endothelial gene expression. FASEB J 1995;9:874–882.
25. Wolinsky H, Glagov S. A lamellar unit of aortic medial structure and function in mammals. Circ Res 1967;20:99–111.
26. Fung YC, Liu SQ. Determination of the mechanical properties of the different layers of blood vessels in vivo. Proc Natl Acad Sci USA 1995;92:2169–2173.
27. Clarke JA. An x-ray microscopic study of the postnatal development of the vasa vasorum in the human aorta. J Anat 1965;99:877–889.
28. Williams JK, Heistad DD. Structure and function of vasa vasorum. Trends Cardiovasc Med 1996;6:53–57.
29. Bo WJ, McKinney WM, Bowden RL. The origin and distribution of vasa vasorum at the bifurcation of the common carotid artery with atherosclerosis. Stroke 1989;20:1484–1487.
30. Langille BL, O'Donnell F. Reductions in arterial diameter produced by chronic decreases in blood flow are endothelium-dependent. Science 1986;231:405–407.
31. Langille BL. Remodeling of developing and mature arteries: endothelium, smooth muscle, and matrix. J Cardiovasc Pharmacol 1993;21(suppl 1):S11–S17.
32. Davies PF. Flow-mediated endothelial mechanotransduction. Physiol Rev 1995;75:519–560.
33. Traub O, Berk BC. Laminar shear stress. Mechanisms by which endothelial cells transduce an atheroprotective force. Arterioscler Thromb Vasc Biol 1998;18:677–685.
34. Mulvany MJ. Resistance vessel growth and remodelling: cause or consequence in cardiovascular disease. J Hum Hypertens 1995;9:479–485.
35. Mondy JS, Lindner V, Miyashiro J, Berk BC, Dean RH, Geary RL. Platelet-derived growth factor ligand and receptor expression in response to altered blood flow in vivo. Circ Res 1997;81:320–327.
36. Ross R. Atherosclerosis. An inflammatory disease. N Engl J Med 1999;340:115–125.
37. Glagov S, Weisenberg E, Zarins CK, Stankunavicius R, Kollettis GJ. Compensatory enlargement of human atherosclerotic coronary arteries. N Engl J Med 1987;316:1371–1375.
38. Clarkson TB, Prichard RW, Morgan TM, Petrick GS, Klein KP. Remodeling of coronary arteries in human and nonhuman primates. JAMA 1994;271:289–294.
38A. http://www.who.int/mediacentre/news/releases/pr83/en/ 17 October 2002.
39. American Heart Association. Heart Disease and Stroke Statistics: 2005 Update. Dallas: American Heart Association, 2005.
40. Jensen LO, Thayssen P, Pedersen KE, Stender S, Haghfelt T. Regression of coronary atherosclerosis by simvastatin: a serial intravascular ultrasound study. Circulation 2004;110(3):265–270.
41. Ross R, Glomset JA. The pathogenesis of atherosclerosis. N Engl J Med 1976;295:369–377, 420–425.
42. Navab M, Ananthramaiah GM, Reddy ST, et al. The oxidation hypothesis of atherogenesis: the role of oxidized phospholipids and HDL. J Lipid Res 2004;45:993–1007.
43. Lusis AJ, Fogelman AM, Fonarow GC. Genetic basis of atherosclerosis: part I: new genes and pathways. Circulation 2004;110:1868–1873.
44. Aikawa M, Libby P. The vulnerable atherosclerotic plaque: pathogenesis and therapeutic approach. Cardiovasc Pathol 2004;13:125–138.
44A. Pitman WA, Osgood DP, Smith D, et al. The effects of diet and lovastatin on regression of fatty streak lesions and on hepatic and intestinal mRNA levels for the LDL receptor and HMG CoA reductase in F1B hamsters. Atherosclerosis 1998;138(1):43–52.
44B. Stein Y, Stein O. Does therapeutic intervention achieve slowing of progression or bona fide regression of atherosclerotic lesions? *Arterioscler Thromb Vasc Biol* 2001;21:183–188.
45. McLenachan JM, Williams JK, Fish RD, Ganz P, Selwyn AP. Loss of flow-mediated endothelium-dependent dilation occurs early in the development of atherosclerosis. Circulation 1991;84:1273–1278.
46. Berk BC, Alexander RW, Brock TA, Gimbrone MA Jr, Webb RC. Vasoconstriction: a new activity for platelet-derived growth factor. Science 1986;232:87–90.
47. Lerman A, Holmes DR Jr, Bell MR, Garratt KN, Nishimura RA, Burnett JC. Endothelin in coronary endothelial dysfunction and early atherosclerosis in humans. Circulation 1995;92:2426–2431.
48. Pearson TA, Blair SN, Daniels SR, et al. AHA Guidelines for Primary Prevention of Cardiovascular Disease and Stroke: 2002 Update. Consensus Panel Guide to Comprehensive Risk Reduction for Adult Patients Without Coronary or Other Atherosclerotic Vascular Diseases. American Heart Association Science Advisory and Coordinating Committee. Circulation 2002;106:388–391.
49. Berliner JA, Navab M, Fogelman AM, et al. Atherosclerosis. Basic mechanisms: oxidation, inflammation, and genetics. Circulation 1995;91:2488–2496.
50. Basta G, Schmidt AM, De Caterina R. Advanced glycation end products and vascular inflammation: implications for accelerated atherosclerosis in diabetes. Cardiovasc Res 2004;63(4):582–592.
51. Gotto AM. Antioxidants, statins, and atherosclerosis. J Am Coll Cardiol 2003;41:1205–1210.
51A. Napoli C, Lerman LO, de Nigris F, et al. Rethinking primary prevention of atherosclerosis-related diseases. Circulation 2006;114(23):2517–2527.
51B. Stampfer MJ, Hu FB, Manson JE, et al. Primary prevention of coronary heart disease in women through diet and lifestyle. N Engl J Med 2000;343:16–22.
51C. Willigendael EM, Teijink JAW, Bartelink MEL, et al. Influence of smoking on incidence and prevalence of peripheral arterial disease. J Vasc Surg 2004;40:1158–1165.
51D. The Diabetes Control and Complications Trial Research Group. The effect of intensive treatment of diabetes on the development and progression of long-term complication in insulin-dependent diabetes mellitus. N Engl J Med 1993;329:977–986.
51E. Adler AI, Stevens RJ, Neil A, et al. UKPDS 59: hyperglycemia and other potentially modifiable risk factors for peripheral vascular disease in type 2 diabetes. Diabetes Care 2002;25:894–899.
51F. Heart Protection Study Collaborative Group. MRC/BHF Heart Protection Study of cholesterol lowering with simvastatine in 20,536 high-risk individuals: a randomised placebo-controlled trial. Lancet 2002;360:7–22.
51G. Hulley S, Grady D, Bush T, et al. Randomized trial of estrogen plus progestin for secondary prevention of coronary heart disease in postmenopausal women. Heart and Estrogen/progestin Replacement Study (HERS) Research Group. JAMA 1998;280:605–613.
51H. S. Yusuf P, Sleight J, Pogue O, et al. Heart Outcomes Prevention Evaluation Study Investigators, effects of an angiotensin-converting-enzyme inhibitor, ramipril, on death from cardiovascular causes. N Engl J Med 2000;342:145–153.
51I. Roberts DH, Tsao Y, McLoughlin GA, et al. Placebo-controlled comparison of captopril, atenolol, labetolol, and pindolol in hypertension complicated by intermittent claudication. Lancet 1987;2(8560):650–653.
51J. Elam MB, Hunninghake DB, Davis KB, et al. Effect of niacin on lipid and lipoprotein levels and glycemic control in patients with diabetes and peripheral arterial disease. The ADMIT Study: a randomized trial. JAMA 2000;284:1263–1270.

51K. Smith SC, Allen J, Blair SN, et al. AHA/ACC guidelines for secondary prevention for patients with coronary and other atherosclerotic vascular disease: 2006 update. Circulation 2006;113(19):2363–2372.
52. Pearson TA. New tools for coronary risk assessment: what are their advantages and limitations? Circulation 2002;105:886–892.
53. Welch GN, Loscalzo J. Homocysteine and atherothrombosis. N Engl J Med 1998;338:1042–1050.
54. Nygard O, Nordrehaug JE, Refsum H, Ueland PM, Farstad M, Vollset SE. Plasma homocysteine levels and mortality in patients with coronary artery disease. N Engl J Med 1997;337:230–236.
55. Taylor LM, Moneta GL, Sexton GJ, Schuff RA, Porter JM. The Homocyseine and Progression of Atherosclerosis Study Investigators. Prospective blinded study of the relationship between plasma homocysteine and progression of symptomatic peripheral arterial disease. J Vasc Surg 1999;29:8–21.
56. Malinow MR, Duell PB, Hess DL, et al. Reduction of plasma homocyst(e)ine levels by breakfast cereal fortified with folic acid in patients with coronary heart disease. N Engl J Med 1998;338:1009–1015.
57. Malinow MR, Bostom AG, Krauss RM. Homocyst(e)ine, diet, and cardiovascular diseases: a statement for healthcare professionals from the Nutrition Committee, American Heart Association. Circulation 1999;99:178–182.
57A. Kaul S, Zadeh AA, Shah PK. Homocysteine hypothesis for atherothrombotic cardiovascular disease: not validated. J Am Coll Cardiol 2006;48(5):914–923.
58. Etminan M, Carleton B, Delaney JA, Padwal R. Macrolide therapy for *Chlamydia pneumoniae* in the secondary prevention of coronary artery disease: a meta-analysis of randomized controlled trials. Pharmacotherapy 2004;24:338–343.
59. Campbell LA, O'Brien ER, Cappuccio AL, et al. Detection of *Chlamydia pneumoniae* TWAR in human coronary atherectomy tissues. J Infect Dis 1995;172:585–588.
60. Sander D, Winbeck K, Klingelhofer J, Etgen T, Conrad B. Progression of early carotid atherosclerosis is only temporarily reduced after antibiotic treatment of *Chlamydia pneumoniae* seropositivity. Circulation 2004;109:1010–1015.
60A. Andraws R, Berger JS, Brown DL. Effects of antibiotic therapy on outcomes of patients with coronary artery disease: A Meta-analysis of randomized controlled trials. *JAMA* 2005;293:2641–2647.
61. McMillan DE. Blood flow and the localization of atherosclerotic plaques. Stroke 1985;16:582–587.
62. Stary HC, Blankenhorn DH, Chandler AB, et al. A definition of the intima of human arteries and of its atherosclerosis-prone regions: a report from the committee on vascular lesions of the council on arteriosclerosis, American Heart Association. Arterioscler Thromb 1992;12:120–134.
63. Truskey GA, Herrmann RA, Kait J, Barber KM. Focal increases in vascular cell adhesion molecule-1 and intimal macrophages at atherosclerosis-susceptible sites in rabbit aorta after short-term cholesterol feeding. Arterioscler Thromb Vasc Biol 1999;19:393–401.
64. Stary HC. Evolution and progression of atherosclerotic lesions in coronary arteries of children and young adults. Atherosclerosis 1989;9(1 suppl):119–132.
65. Guyton JR, Klemp KF. Development of the lipid-rich core in human atherosclerosis. Arterioscler Thromb Vasc Biol 1996;16:4–11.
66. O'Brien KD, McDonald TO, Chait A, Allen MD, Alpers CE. Neovascular expression of E-selectin, intercellular adhesion molecule-1, and vascular cell adhesion molecule-1 in human atherosclerosis and their relation to intimal leukocyte content. Circulation 1996;93:672–682.
67. Moulton KS, Vakili K, Zurakowski D, et al. Inhibition of plaque neovascularization reduces macrophage accumulation and progression of advanced atherosclerosis. Proc Natl Acad Sci U S A 2003;100:4736–4741.
68. Abedin M, Tintut Y, Demer LL. Vascular calcification: mechanisms and clinical ramifications. Arterioscler Thromb Vasc Biol 2004;24:1161–1170.
69. Luo G, Ducy P, McKee M, et al. Spontaneous calcification of arteries and cartilage in mice lacking matrix GLA protein. Nature (Lond) 1997;385:78–81.
70. Losordo DW, Rosenfield K, Kaufman J, Pieczek A, Isner JM. Focal compensatory enlargement of human arteries in response to progressive atherosclerosis: in vivo documentation using intravascular ultrasound. Circulation 1994;89:2570–2577.
71. Pasterkamp G, Borst C, Post MJ, et al. Atherosclerotic arterial remodeling in the superficial femoral artery—individual variation in local compensatory enlargement response. Circulation 1996;93:1818–1825.
72. Falk E, Shah PK, Fuster V. Coronary plaque disruption. Circulation 1995;92:657–671.
73. Davies MJ, Thomas AC. Plaque fissuring: the cause of acute myocardial infarction, sudden death, and crescendo angina. Br Heart J 1985;53:363–373.
74. Farb A, Burke AP, Tang AL, et al. Coronary plaque erosion without rupture into a lipid core. A frequent cause of coronary thrombosis in sudden coronary death. Circulation 1996;93:1354–1363.
75. Mann JM, Davies MJ. Vulnerable plaque—relation of characteristics to degree of stenosis in human coronary arteries. Circulation 1996;94:928–931.
76. Burke AP, Farb A, Malcom GT, Liang YH, Smialek J, Virmani R. Coronary risk factors and plaque morphology in men with coronary disease who died suddenly. N Engl J Med 1997;336:1276–1282.
77. Nicholls SC, Kohler TR, Bergelin RO, Primozich JF, Lawrence RL, Strandness DE Jr. Carotid artery occlusion: natural history. J Vasc Surg 1986;4:479–485.
78. Pai RG, Heywood JT. Atheroembolism. N Engl M Med 1995; 333:852.
79. Moliterno DJ, Topol EJ. Restenosis: epidemiology and treatment. In: Topol EJ, ed. Textbook of Cardiovascular Medicine, 2nd ed. Philadelphia: Lippincott-Raven, 2002.
80. Weintraub WS, Ghazzal ZMB, Douglas JS, et al. Long-term clinical follow-up in patients with angiographic restudy after successful angioplasty. Circulation 1993;87:831–840.
81. Nobuyoshi M, Kimura T, Nosaka H, et al. Restenosis after successful percutaneous transluminal coronary angioplasty: serial angiographic follow-up of 229 patients. J Am Coll Cardiol 1988;12:616–623.
82. Carballo RE, Towne JB, Seabrook GR, Freischlag JA, Cambria RA. An outcome analysis of carotid endarterectomy: the incidence and natural history of recurrent stenosis. J Vasc Surg 1996;23:749–753.
83. Healy DA, Zierler RE, Nicholls SC, et al. Long-term follow-up and clinical outcome of carotid restenosis. J Vasc Surg 1989;10:662–669.
84. Kimura T, Yokoi H, Nakagawa Y, et al. Three-year follow-up after implantation of metallic coronary-artery stents. N Engl J Med 1996;334:561–566.
85. Serruys PW, De Jaegere P, Kiemeneij F, et al. A comparison of balloon-expandable-stent implantation with balloon angioplasty in patients with coronary artery disease. N Engl J Med 1994;331:489–495.
86. Sheppard R, Eisenberg MJ, Donath D, Meerkin D. Intracoronary brachytherapy for the prevention of restenosis after percutaneous coronary revascularization. Am Heart J 2003;146:775–786.
87. Moses JW, Leon MB, Popma JJ, et al. SIRIUS Investigators. Sirolimus-eluting stents versus standard stents in patients with stenosis in a native coronary artery. N Engl J Med 2003;349: 1315–1323.

88. Colombo A, Drzewiecki J, Banning A, et al. TAXUS II Study Group. Randomized study to assess the effectiveness of slow- and moderate-release polymer-based paclitaxel-eluting stents for coronary artery lesions. Circulation 2003;108:788–794.
88A. Slavin L, Chhabra A, Tobis J. Drug-eluting stents: Preventing restenosis. Cardiol Rev 2007;15(1):1–12.
88B. Duda, SH, Bosiers M, Lammer J, et al. Sirolimus-eluting versus bare nitinol stent for obstructive superficial femoral artery disease: the SIROCCO II trial. J Vasc Interv Radiol 2005;16(3):331–338.
89. Geary RL, Nikkari ST, Wagner WD, Williams JK, Adams MR, Dean RH. Wound healing: a paradigm for lumen narrowing following arterial reconstruction. J Vasc Surg 1997;27:96–108.
90. Clowes AW, Karnovsky MJ. Suppression by heparin of smooth muscle cell proliferation in injured arteries. Nature (Lond) 1977;265:625–626.
91. Jawien A, Bowen-Pope DF, Lindner V, Schwartz SM, Clowes AW. Platelet-derived growth factor promotes smooth muscle migration and intimal thickening in a rat model of balloon angioplasty. J Clin Invest 1992;89:507–511.
92. Ferns GAA, Raines EW, Sprugel KH, Motani AS, Reidy MA, Ross R. Inhibition of neointimal smooth muscle accumulation after angioplasty by an antibody to PDGF. Science 1991;253:1129–1132.
93. Powell JS, Clozel JP, Muller RKM, et al. Inhibitors of angiotensin-converting enzyme prevent myointimal proliferation after vascular injury. Science 1989;245:186–188.
94. Faxon DP, Spiro TE, Minor S, et al. Low molecular weight heparin in prevention of restenosis after angioplasty: results of enoxaparin restenosis (ERA) trial. Circulation 1994;90:908–914.
95. Faxon DP. Effect of high dose angiotensin-converting enzyme inhibition on restenosis: final results of the MARCATOR study, a multicenter, double-blind, placebo-controlled trial of cilazapril. J Am Coll Cardiol 1995;25:362–369.
96. Kakuta T, Currier JW, Haudenschild CC, Ryan TJ, Faxon DP. Differences in compensatory vessel enlargement, not intimal formation, account for restenosis after angioplasty in the hypercholesterolemic rabbit model. Circulation 1994;89:2809–2815.
97. Post MJ, Borst C, Kuntz RE. The relative importance of arterial remodeling compared with intimal hyperplasia in lumen renarrowing after balloon angioplasty: a study in the normal rabbit and the hypercholesterolemic Yucatan micropig. Circulation 1994;89:2816–2821.
98. Lafont A, Guzman LA, Whitlow PL, Goormastic M, Cornhill JF, Chisolm GM. Restenosis after experimental angioplasty: intimal, medial, and adventitial changes associated with constrictive remodeling. Circ Res 1995;76:996–1002.
99. Mintz GS, Popma JJ, Pichard AD, et al. Arterial remodeling after coronary angioplasty. A serial intravascular ultrasound study. Circulation 1996;94:35–43.
100. Geary RL, Williams JK, Golden D, Brown DG, Benjamin ME, Adams MR. Time course of cellular proliferation, intimal hyperplasia, and remodeling following angioplasty in monkeys with established atherosclerosis: a nonhuman primate model of restenosis. Arterioscler Thromb Vasc Biol 1996;16:34–43.
101. Mondy JS, Williams JK, Adams MR, Dean RH, Geary RL. Structural determinants of lumen narrowing following angioplasty in atherosclerotic nonhuman primates. J Vasc Surg 1997;26:875–883.
102. Post MJ, Borst C, Pasterkamp G, Haudenschild CC. Arterial remodeling in atherosclerosis and restenosis: a vague concept of a distinct phenomenon. Atherosclerosis 1995;118(suppl):S115–S123.
103. Carrel A, Guthrie CC. Uniterminal and biterminal venous transplantations. Surg Gynecol Obstet 1906;2:266–286.
104. Bourassa MG, Fisher LD, Campeau L, Gillespie MJ, McConney M, Lesperance J. Long-term fate of bypass grafts: the coronary artery surgery study (CASS) and Montreal Heart Institute experiences. Circulation 1985;72:V-71–V-78.
105. Zwolak RM, Adams MC, Clowes AW. Kinetics of vein graft hyperplasia: association with tangential stress. J Vasc Surg 1987;5:126–136.
106. Zwolak RM, Kirkman TR, Clowes AW. Atherosclerosis in rabbit vein grafts. Arteriosclerosis 1989;9:374–379.
107. Dobrin PB, Littooy FN, Endean ED. Mechanical factors predisposing to intimal hyperplasia and medial thickening in autogenous vein grafts. Surgery (St. Louis) 1989;105:393–400.
108. Galt SW, Zwolak RM, Wagner RJ, Gilbertson JJ. Differential response of arteries and vein grafts to blood flow reduction. J Vasc Surg 1993;17:563–570.
109. Davies MG, Dalen H, Kim JH, Barber L, Svendsen E, Hagen PO. Control of accelerated vein graft atheroma with the nitric oxide precursor: L-arginine. J Surg Res 1995;59:35–42.
110. Mann MJ, Gibbons GH, Kernoff RS, et al. Genetic engineering of vein grafts resistant to atherosclerosis. Proc Natl Acad Sci U S A 1995;92:4502–4506.
111. O'Donohoe MK, Schwartz LB, Radic ZS, Mikat EM, McCann RL, Hagen P-O. Chronic ACE inhibition reduces intimal hyperplasia in experimental vein grafts. Ann Surg 1991;214:727–732.
112. Goldman S, Copeland J, Moritz T, et al. Improvement in early saphenous vein graft patency after coronary artery bypass surgery with antiplatelet therapy: results of a Veterans Administration Cooperative Study. Circulation 1988;77:1324–1332.
113. McCollum C, Alexander C, Dip N, Kenchington G, Franks PJ, Greenhalgh R. Antiplatelet drugs in femoropopliteal vein bypasses: a multicenter trial. J Vasc Surg 1991;13:150–162.
114. Muluk SC, Vorp DA, Severyn DA, Gleixner S, Johnson PC, Webster MW. Enchancement of tissue factor expression by vein segments exposed to coronary arterial hemodynamics. J Vasc Surg 1998;27:521–527.
115. DeWeese JA, Leather R, Porter J. Practice guidelines: lower extremity revascularization. J Vasc Surg 1993;18:280–294.
116. Clowes AW, Gown AM, Hanson SR, Reidy MA. Mechanisms of arterial graft failure. I. Role of cellular proliferation in early healing of PTFE prostheses. Am J Pathol 1985;118:43–54.
117. Herring M, Smith J, Dalsing M, et al. Endothelial seeding of polytetrafluoroethylene femoral popliteal bypasses: the failure of low-density seeding to improve patency. J Vasc Surg 1994;20:650–655.
118. Kohler TR, Kirkman TR, Kraiss LW, Zierler BK, Clowes AW. Increased blood flow inhibits neointimal hyperplasia in endothelialized vascular grafts. Circ Res 1991;69:1557–1565.
119. Geary RL, Kohler TR, Vergel S, Kirkman TR, Clowes AW. Time course of flow-induced smooth muscle cell proliferation and intimal thickening in endothelialized baboon vascular grafts. Circ Res 1994;74:14–23.
120. Mattson EJR, Geary RL, Kraiss LW, et al. Is smooth muscle growth in primate arteries regulated by endothelial nitric oxide synthase? J Vasc Surg 1998;28:514–521.
121. Kraiss LW, Geary RL, Mattsson EJR, Vergel S, Au YPT, Clowes AW. Acute reduction in blood flow and shear stress induce PDGF-A expression in baboon prosthetic grafts. Circ Res 1996;79:45–53.
122. Hart CE, Kraiss LW, Vergel S, et al. PDGFb receptor blockade inhibits intimal hyperplasia in the baboon. Circ Res 1999;99:564–569.
123. Rasmussen TE, Hallett JW. Inflammatory aortic aneurysms. A clinical review with new perspectives in pathogenesis. Ann Surg 1997;225:155–164.
124. Scott RAP, Tisi PV, Ashton HA, Allen DR. Abdominal aortic aneurysm rupture rates: a 7-year follow-up of the entire abdominal aortic aneurysm population detected by screening. J Vasc Surg 1998;28:124–128.
125. Alcorn HG, Wolfson SW, Sutton-Tyrell K, Kuller LH, O'Leary D. Risk factors for abdominal aortic aneurysms in older adults

enrolled in the Cardiovascular Health Study. Arterioscler Thromb Vasc Biol 1996;16:963–970.
126. Lopez-Candales A, Holmes DR, Liao S, Scott MJ, Wickline SA, Thompson RW. Decreased vascular smooth muscle cell density in medial degeneration of human abdominal aortic aneurysms. Am J Pathol 1997;150:993–1007.
127. Thompson RW, Geraghty PJ, Lee JK. Abdominal aortic aneurysms: basic mechanisms and clinical implications. Curr Probl Surg 2002;39:110–230.
128. Newman KM, Malon AM, Shin RD, Scholes JV, Ramey WG, Tilson MD. Matrix metalloproteinases in abdominal aortic aneurysm: characterization, purification, and their possible sources. Connect Tissue Res 1994;30:265–276.
129. Irizarry E, Newman KM, Gandhi RH, et al. Demonstration of interstitial collagenase in abdominal aortic aneurysm disease. J Surg Res 1993;54:571–574.
130. Prockop DJ, Kivirikko KI. Collagens: molecular biology, diseases, and potentials for therapy. Annu Rev Biochem 1995;64:403–434.
131. Rosenbloom J, Abrams WR, Mecham R. Extracellular matrix 4: the elastic fiber. FASEB J 1993;7:1208–1218.
131A. Kelly BA, Bond BC, Poston L. Aortic adaptation to pregnancy: elevated expression of matrix metalloproteinases-2 and -3 in rat gestation. Molecular Human Reproduction 2004;10(5):331–337.
131B. Manallo-Estrella P and Barker AE. Histopathologic findings in human aortic media associated with pregnancy. Arch Pathol 1967;83:336–341.
131C. Hunsaker DM, Turner S, Hunsaker JC. Sudden and unexpected death resulting from splenic artery aneurysm rupture: two case reports of pregnancy-related fatal rupture of splenic artery aneurysm. Am J Forensic Med Pathol 2002;23(4):338–341.
132. Knox JB, Sukhova GK, Whittemore AD, Libby P. Evidence for altered balance between matrix metalloproteinases and their inhibitors in human aortic diseases. Circulation 1997;95:205–212.
133. Curci JA, Thompson RW. Adaptive cellular immunity in aortic aneurysms: cause, consequence, or context? J Clin Invest 2004;114:168–171.
134. Hirose H, Ozsvath KJ, Xia S, Gaetz HP, Tilson MD. Immunoreactivity of adventitial matrix fibrils of normal and aneurysmal abdominal aorta with antibodies against vitronectin and fibrinogen. Pathobiology 1998;66:1–4.
135. Kuo CC, Gown AM, Benditt EP, Grayston JT. Detection of *Chlamidia pneumoniae* in aortic lesions of atherosclerosis by immunohistochemical stain. Arterioscler Thromb 1993;13:1501–1504.
136. Gomes MN, Choyke PL, Wallace RB. Infected aortic aneurysms. A changing entity. Ann Surg 1992;215:435–442.
137. Valentine RJ, Clagett GP. Aortic graft infections: replacement with autogenous vein. Cardiovasc Surg 2001;9:419–425.
137A. Marques da Silva R, Caugant DA, Eribe ER, et al. Bacterial diversity in aortic aneurysms determined by 16S ribosomal RNA gene analysis. J Vasc Surg 2006;44(5):1055–1060.
138. Farkas J, Fichelle J, Laurian C, et al. Long-term follow-up of positive cultures in 500 abdominal aortic aneurysms. Arch Surg 1993;128:284–288.

62

Cerebrovascular Disease

Peter L. Faries, Sheela T. Patel, and K. Craig Kent

Stroke is the third leading cause of death in the United States. Approximately 500,000 people develop new strokes each year, making stroke the leading cause of neurological disability. Survivors of stroke account for $29 billion annually in healthcare costs and lost productivity. Despite this enormous clinical problem, during the past 50 years there has been tremendous progress in reducing mortality from stroke. This success in part is related to the evolution of the surgical treatment of extracranial cerebrovascular disease. Carotid endarterectomy (CEA) is the primary treatment used, and the frequency with which this procedure is performed has steadily increased since the early 1990s. Currently, CEA is the most commonly performed peripheral vascular operation in the United States. In this chapter, the anatomy, pathophysiology, diagnosis, and treatment of cerebrovascular disease are reviewed.

Anatomy

Anterior Circulation

The brain is supplied anteriorly by paired internal carotid arteries, which provide approximately 80% to 90% of the total cerebral blood flow. The left common carotid artery originates directly from the aortic arch, whereas the right common carotid artery originates from the innominate artery. The common carotid arteries bifurcate at the angle of the mandible into external and internal branches. The external carotid artery has many divisions, several of which supply the cerebral circulation through collaterals. The internal carotid artery can be divided into the cervical (or extracranial), intrapetrosal, intracavernous, and supraclinoid segments. The cervical, intrapetrosal, and intracavernous portions of the internal carotid artery have no branches. The supraclinoid segment gives rise to the opthalmic and the posterior communicating arteries before bifurcating into its terminal branches, the anterior and middle cerebral arteries. The intracavernous and supraclinoid segments of the internal carotid artery are referred to as the carotid siphon.

Posterior Circulation

The vertebral arteries supply 10% to 20% of the total cerebral circulation. Both vertebral arteries originate from the first portion of their respective subclavian arteries and then enter the vertebral canal at the transverse foramina of the sixth cervical vertebra. The vertebral arteries unite to form the basilar artery, which then branches into the right and left posterior cerebral arteries. The posterior circulation supplies the brainstem, cranial nerves, cerebellum, and the occipital and temporal lobes of the cerebrum.

Circle of Willis

The anterior communicating artery connects the two anterior cerebral arteries. The posterior communicating artery connects the internal carotid arteries (anterior circulation) to the posterior cerebral arteries (posterior circulation). This interconnecting network, which is termed the circle of Willis, is completely intact in 20% to 40% of individuals and allows for collateral flow between the hemispheres and the anterior and posterior circulations (Fig. 62.1).

Clinical Presentation and Pathophysiology

Atherosclerosis is the pathological process most often responsible for cerebrovascular insufficiency. The carotid bifurcation is the predominant location for atherosclerotic disease. Low shear stress in well-defined regions of the carotid bulb appears to stimulate the formation of atherosclerotic plaque.

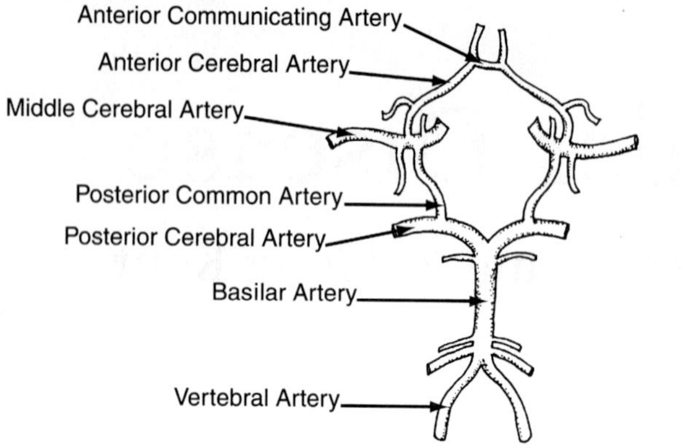

FIGURE 62.1. Configuration of the terminal branches of the vertebral and internal carotid arteries and their interconnections to form the circle of Willis.

Symptoms of cerebrovascular disease may be the consequence of distal embolization from an atherosclerotic plaque or hypoperfusion related to a flow-limiting lesion. The most common cause of a cerebral ischemic event, however, is embolization. Platelets accumulate on the thrombogenic surface of an irregular or ulcerated plaque. Symptoms are produced when these platelet and cholesterol aggregates embolize and obstruct the more distal circulation. Plaque hemorrhage with rupture and extrusion of thrombus into the arterial lumen is another mechanism by which embolization can occur. Although an ulcerated atherosclerotic lesion can embolize even if there is no luminal encroachment, highly stenotic plaques are more often ulcerated and thus more likely to produce emboli.

Hypoperfusion related to carotid artery stenosis is a less common source of symptoms because extensive collateral circulation is provided by the contralateral carotid and vertebral arteries via the circle of Willis and by the external carotid artery via transcranial connections. The fact that 90% to 95% of patients undergoing CEA do not develop cerebral insufficiency during clamping of the carotid artery confirms that, in the majority of individuals with progressive atherosclerotic disease, this collateral network is adequate to prevent cerebral ischemia.

Symptoms of cerebrovascular disease include hemispheric transient ischemic attacks (TIAs), amaurosis fugax, and stroke. A TIA is defined as an acute loss of cerebral function that persists for less than 24h, although most events are brief, lasting 15min or less. The specific clinical presentation depends on the anatomic location of the area of cerebral ischemia. Symptoms associated with anterior or carotid bifurcation disease include sensory or motor deficits affecting the contralateral face, arms, or legs, aphasia (if the dominant hemisphere is affected), or alterations in higher cortical dysfunction. Patients with posterior or vertebrobasilar ischemia may present with vertigo, dizziness, gait ataxia, dysarthria, nystagmus, diplopia, bilateral visual loss, drop attacks (collapse caused by loss of control of extremities without loss of consciousness), as well as bilateral or alternating motor or sensory impairment. Nonfocal symptoms such as syncope, confusion, and "light-headedness" are rarely the result of cerebrovascular disease. Reversible ischemic neurological deficits (RINDs) are cerebral vascular symptoms that persist for more than 24h but less than 7 days. Although the definitions can vary, deficits that persist more than 7 days are usually considered strokes. A stroke may or may not be associated with an obvious infarct identified by computed tomography (CT) or magnetic resonance imaging (MRI).

Transient unilateral loss of vision is referred to as amaurosis fugax. This symptom is classically described as the sensation of a shade coming down over the entire, half, or a quadrant of one eye. This event is the consequence of a microembolus lodging in the opthalmic artery or one of its retinal branches. A cholesterol crystal (Hollenhorst plaque) is occasionally observed on funduscopic examination as a bright refractile body in a branch of the retinal artery. Although amaurosis fugax is a temporary event, retinal artery occlusion may lead to permanent blindness.

There are several symptoms that suggest instability of a carotid lesion and the potential of an imminent stroke. The term crescendo TIAs is used to describe a series of transient neurological events that occur with increasing frequency, duration, or severity. A stroke-in-evolution is a neurological deficit that progressively worsens through a series of discrete exacerbations without intervening periods of normal neurological function. A patient may experience a "waxing-and-waning" neurological deficit if the symptoms fluctuate between mild and severe over a period of several hours. Patients with these clinical presentations should be treated with anticoagulation if there is no radiologic evidence of hemorrhage and then urgent CEA so long as the neurological deficit is not severe.[1] Although no randomized data are available, the outcome of urgent operation appears to be superior to the natural history of this disease process.[2,3]

Indications for Carotid Endarterectomy

Although CEA is now a well-accepted intervention for carotid bifurcation disease, in the 1980s, because of the frequent and at times indiscriminate use of this procedure, the efficacy and indications for CEA were questioned.[4,5] Consequently, several prospective randomized trials were designed to test the efficacy of CEA relative to best medical management for patients with both symptomatic and asymptomatic carotid stenosis.

Symptomatic Carotid Artery Disease

The North American Symptomatic Carotid Endarterectomy Trial (NASCET) was a large prospective randomized trial designed to test the efficacy of CEA in patients with symptomatic carotid stenosis.[6] From 50 centers in the United States and Canada, 659 patients with greater than 70% symptomatic carotid stenosis were randomized to CEA or best medical management. This study was initially designed as a 5-year trial. However, after only 18 months, a markedly significant benefit for CEA was found. The 30-day mortality and stroke morbidity was 5.8% in patients randomized to carotid endarterectomy. The cumulative 2-year risk of ipsilateral stroke was 26% in patients treated medically and 9% in patients treated with carotid endarterectomy, representing an absolute risk reduction of 17% and a relative risk reduction of 65%. Patients in this study who had surgical correction of high-grade carotid stenoses gained a durable benefit from their operation that persisted for at least 8 years.[7] In subset analysis, it was found that the degree of stenosis, clinical presentation, and the presence or absence of ulceration affected the efficacy of CEA. The benefit of CEA increased with the degree of carotid stenosis. Medically treated patients with stenoses of 70% to 79%, 80% to 89%, and 90% to 99% had a 2-year risk of stroke of 19.9%, 28.5%, and 34.6%, respectively. The 2-year risk of stroke in patients treated with CEA was 9% regardless of the degree of stenosis. The largest benefit for CEA was observed in those patients who experienced a prior stroke, and the least benefit was found in patients who presented with amaurosis fugax.[8] The presence of ulceration dramatically increased the incidence of stroke in patients treated medically; ulceration also increased the risk of CEA but to a much lesser degree.[9] Interestingly, the existence of comorbidities, such as diabetes, coronary artery disease, or hypertension, increased the incidence of stroke in medically treated patients.[6] However, the stroke rate was constant at 9% in the surgical group regardless of the number of comorbidities. These findings challenge the frequently expressed notion that patients with multiple comorbidities benefit less from surgical intervention.

A second cohort of patients, those with symptomatic 30% to 69% stenoses, were also studied as part of NASCET.[7] These patients were divided into two subsets: those with carotid stenoses of 50% to 69% and those with stenoses of 30% to 49%. For patients with 50% to 69% stenoses, the risk of ipsilateral stroke at 5 years was 22.2% with medical treatment versus 15.7% with surgery, yielding a statistically significant absolute risk reduction of 6.5%. For patients with carotid stenoses less than 50%, the 5-year risk of ipsilateral stroke was 18.7% with medical treatment versus 14.9% with surgery, yielding a nonsignificant absolute risk reduction of only 3.8%. Although patients with symptomatic moderate 50% to 69% stenoses benefit less from carotid endarterectomy than those with 70% to 99% lesions, in both groups surgery provided a more durable long-term benefit than did treatment with the best medical therapy. Thus, carotid endarterectomy has been shown in prospective randomized trials to be effective in treating symptomatic patients with greater than 50% carotid artery stenosis.

Asymptomatic Carotid Disease

The Asymptomatic Carotid Atherosclerosis Study (ACAS) is the largest available randomized trial of patients with asymptomatic carotid stenosis.[10] In this study, 1662 asymptomatic patients with 60% to 99% carotid stenoses were randomized to receive CEA or medical management. The 5-year risk of stroke was 5.1% in patients treated surgically and 11% in patients treated medically, yielding a statistically significant 5.9% absolute risk reduction. This beneficial effect of surgery in asymptomatic carotid disease was in large part the result of a low 30-day operative risk (2.3%) for CEA. Interestingly, only one-half of strokes were related to the surgical procedure, whereas the remainder followed contrast arteriography. Because of the smaller number of events, subset analysis was not as revealing for ACAS. The effect of degree of stenosis on the efficacy of CEA in asymptomatic patients was not adequately addressed by ACAS. Because preoperative contrast arteriography was not uniformly obtained, the number of patients in whom the degree of stenosis was accurately defined was too small to allow an analysis to be performed. Several nonrandomized studies, however, have demonstrated an association in asymptomatic patients between increasing degrees of stenosis and the benefit of CEA.[11,12] The 5-year risk reduction provided by CEA was 66% in men and only 17% in women, although this difference was not statistically different. A higher rate of perioperative stroke in women (3.6% for women versus 1.7% in men) partially explains this finding. Although not examined in ACAS, the rate of disease progression and the presence or absence of ulceration have been found to influence the risk of stroke in asymptomatic patients who are treated nonoperatively. Roederer et al.[13] found, in asymptomatic patients, that progression of carotid stenosis to greater than 80% was associated with a 46% chance of a neurological event; neurological deficits developed in only 1.5% of patients in whom disease did not progress. Dixon et al.[14] observed annual stroke rates of 0.9%, 4.5%, and 7.5%, respectively, in asymptomatic patients with small, medium, and large complex ulcerated lesions.

Although a statistical benefit for CEA in asymptomatic patients with 60% to 99% carotid stenoses was demonstrated by ACAS, skeptics argue that 17 operations were required to prevent one stroke over 5 years. This observation raised questions about the cost-effectiveness as well as the sensibility of treating asymptomatic patients with CEA.[15,16] Two recent analyses, however, have demonstrated that CEA in the cohort of asymptomatic patients defined by ACAS is indeed cost-effective.[17,18] The authors of these studies made several interesting observations. First, longevity of a patient is an important criterion when selecting asymptomatic candidates for CEA because the benefit demonstrated by ACAS can only be achieved in patients who are expected to live at least an additional 5 years. Accordingly, CEA is rarely cost effective in individuals above the age of 80. Degree of stenosis may also be an important factor in patient selection. Several studies have shown an increased risk of stroke in medically managed patients with stenoses greater than 80%. Thus, patients with high-grade stenoses may comprise a subgroup of patients in whom CEA provides greater benefit. Although the indications for carotid endarterectomy in the asymptomatic patient are still not completely defined, many surgeons have adopted a policy of treating patients with high-grade stenoses who have a reasonable life expectancy and in whom a low operative morbidity and mortality can be achieved.

Tandem Lesions/Contralateral Carotid Occlusion/"String Sign"

The carotid siphon is the second most common location for cerebrovascular atherosclerotic disease. Thus, the coexistence of tandem lesions in the carotid siphon and the ipsilateral carotid bifurcation is not unusual. Several retrospective studies have addressed the question of whether a carotid siphon lesion adversely affects the perioperative risk as well as the long-term benefit of CEA.[19–22] Schuler et al.[22] found no difference in early or late stroke rates in patients with bifurcation stenoses versus those with a bifurcation lesion and a tandem, greater than 20% siphon stenosis. Lord et al.[21] reported no significant difference in the perioperative stroke rate in patients with extracranial carotid stenoses and no siphon disease versus those with tandem 50% to 80% siphon stenoses. It has been suggested that atherosclerotic plaques in the carotid siphon are less ulcerated and more stable than lesions of the carotid bifurcation. Thus, under most circumstances, CEA is still indicated in patients with tandem siphon stenoses.

CEA can be performed contralateral to an occluded carotid artery with acceptable safety. Although some studies suggest that CEA in these patients is associated with an increased incidence of stroke, in many other studies the rate of stroke is equivalent to that of patients without contralateral disease.[23–26] Patients may present with a carotid "string sign" in which arteriography reveals only minimal flow in the internal carotid artery. The presence of a string sign may imply markedly diminished flow through a highly stenotic proximal carotid stenosis. In these patients urgent CEA can be performed with the usual morbidity and mortality.[27] A string sign may also be associated with a diffusely diseased and fibrotic carotid artery that is technically challenging to reconstruct.[28] The rate of stroke with CEA is increased under this circumstance.

Timing of Carotid Endarterectomy

The timing of CEA after an acute stroke is a critical issue that has been studied in some detail. Early reperfusion following endarterectomy of a large recently infarcted region of the brain can lead to cerebral hemorrhage and potentially devastating consequences. This observation led to the traditional dictum that CEA should be delayed a minimum of 4 to 6 weeks in patients presenting with completed strokes.[29] Unfortunately, if this policy is rigidly followed, some patients, because of instability of their carotid artery disease, will be vulnerable to a second stroke that occurs during this 4- to 6-week interval.[30] It has since been shown that, in patients with small fixed deficits or small infarcts seen by CT or MRI, the risk of early CEA is not increased.[31,32] Thus, patients with small strokes and significant carotid stenosis should be considered for early operative intervention.

Patients scheduled for elective coronary artery bypass grafting (CABG) may harbor significant carotid disease. Reports estimate that 4% to 12% of patients awaiting elective CABG will have, by duplex ultrasound, a carotid artery stenosis greater than 80%.[33] Conversely, up to 35% of patients with carotid disease will have significant coexisting coronary artery disease.[34] The appropriate treatment of patients with surgical lesions of both the carotid and coronary arteries remains controversial. Options include initial CEA followed by CABG, initial CABG followed by CEA, or simultaneous CEA and CABG. CEA performed without correcting severe coronary artery disease may be associated with an increased incidence of myocardial infarction. Alternatively, CABG performed without correction of severe symptomatic carotid artery stenosis may be associated with an increased risk of stroke. In a prospective, randomized trial, Hertzer et al.[35] compared simultaneous CEA/CABG and CABG followed by delayed CEA in patients with unilateral asymptomatic carotid stenosis. Patients undergoing CABG with interval CEA had an increased incidence of perioperative stroke (13.8%) compared to patients undergoing simultaneous procedures (2.8%). Unfortunately, only a small number of patients were enrolled in this study, and statistical significance was lacking. Brener et al.[36] performed a meta-analysis of more than 30 studies in which this question was addressed and calculated the following mortality and stroke rates: CEA before CABG (9.4%, 5.3%), CABG before CEA (3.6%, 10%), and simultaneous CABG and CEA (5.6%, 6.2%). Until further data are available, the timing of CEA in patients requiring CABG should be individualized with consideration given to the severity of symptoms. Initial CEA followed by interval CABG should be utilized in patients with recent or unstable neurological symptoms whose coronary artery disease is clinically stable. The strategy of CABG before CEA should be considered in those patients with unstable angina, left main disease, or those requiring an intraaortic balloon pump whose carotid disease is clinically stable. All other subsets of patients should be at least considered for simultaneous CEA and CABG.

Preoperative Studies

Contrast Arteriography

Contrast arteriography is the traditional method for evaluating the carotid bifurcation before CEA. Angiography can provide complete and detailed images of the proximal (aortic arch and branches) and distal (intracranial) circulation as well as the carotid bifurcation. Unfortunately, the incidence of stroke associated with arteriography is not insignificant, and this morbidity must be included when calculating the overall risk of intervention for carotid artery disease. In ACAS, the combined perioperative stroke and death rate associated with carotid endarterectomy was 2.3%.[10] However, there was a 1.2% rate of stroke associated with arteriography. Contrast arteriography is also associated with insertion site complications, renal dysfunction, and contrast reactions as well as ionizing radiation. Furthermore, the cost of arteriography is significant. All these issues have led to an increasing interest in the use of noninvasive modalities for the preoperative imaging of carotid artery disease. Magnetic resonance angiography and duplex ultrasonography are the two noninvasive methods that have received the greatest attention, although spiral CT angiography is currently under evaluation at a number of institutions.[37]

Duplex Ultrasonography

Duplex ultrasound (DU) can be an accurate, noninvasive preoperative method of imaging the carotid bifurcation. Peak systolic and end-diastolic velocities measured in the common and internal carotid arteries are used to determine the degree of stenosis. Accuracies for DU in the 90% range have been obtained in laboratories with appropriate expertise.[38] There are, however, several limitations to DU. The accuracy of this test is dependent upon the experience, skill, and dedication of the technologist and interpreter of this study. Moreover, the anatomy of the intracranial or intrathoracic circulation cannot be accurately defined with DU. Differentiation between a high-grade stenosis and occlusion with DU has also been problematic. The false diagnosis of an occlusion can be made if the internal carotid artery courses medially, or an occlusion can be missed if a branch of the external carotid artery is mistaken for the internal carotid artery. Artifacts originating from calcified plaque can compromise the quality of DU. Because DU is based on flow velocities for the determination of lesion severity, hyperdynamic states can lead to an overestimation of the degree of stenosis. Thus, validation of the accuracy of DU in individual laboratories is essential before DU can be used as the sole imaging modality before

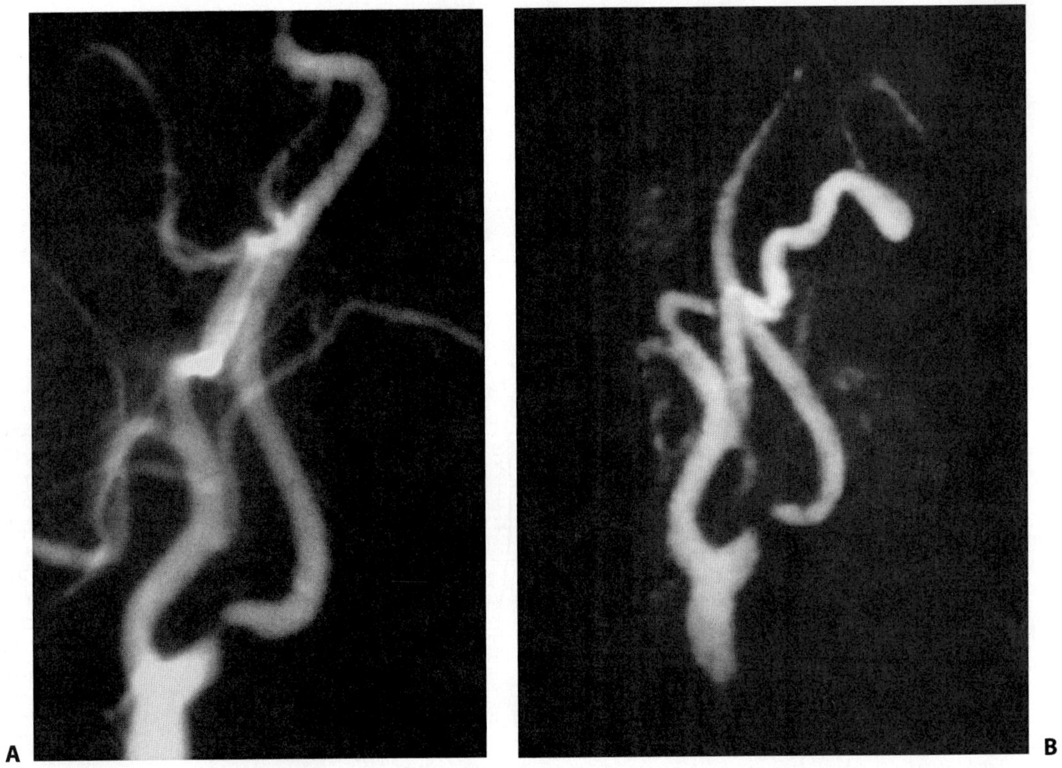

FIGURE 62.2. Contrast arteriogram (A) and (B) magnetic resonance angiography (MRA) of the carotid bifurcation. MRA can provide a precise anatomic depiction of carotid bifurcation disease.

carotid endarterectomy. Despite these limitations, the practice of performing CEA with DU has become increasingly common.[39–42] In a recent survey, 73% of respondents agreed that carotid endarterectomy could be performed using duplex ultrasound as the sole preoperative test.[43]

Magnetic Resonance Angiography

Magnetic resonance angiography (MRA) is a variant of magnetic resonance imaging (MRI) that has been used increasingly in the evaluation of patients with cerebrovascular occlusive disease. The carotid bifurcation, because of its straight-line configuration and rapid blood flow, is especially well suited for evaluation by MRA. An appealing advantage of MRA over DU is that it anatomically displays the intracranial and extracranial circulation in a format strikingly similar to that of a conventional arteriogram (Figs. 62.2, 62.3). MRA can be performed in conjunction with MRI of the brain with only a small increase in examination time and therefore cost.

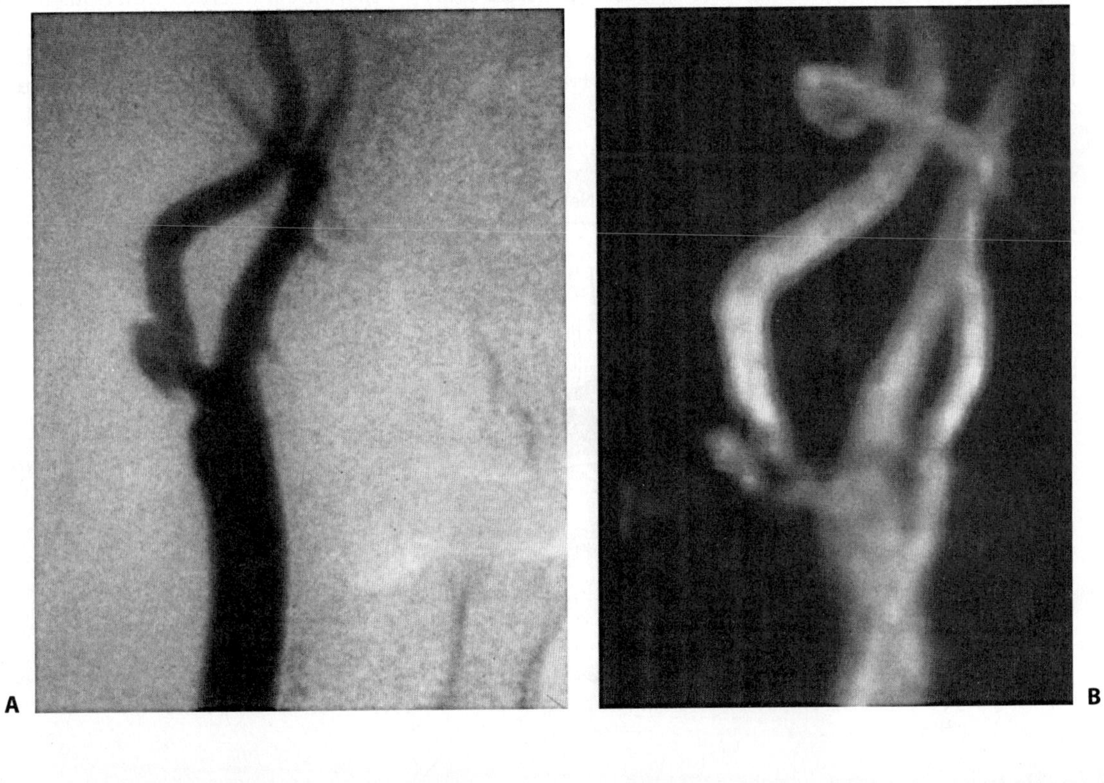

FIGURE 62.3. Carotid contrast arteriogram reveals type C ulceration at the origin of the internal carotid artery (A). Because of three-dimensional imaging, MRA in this circumstance provides a more accurate depiction of this ulcer (B).

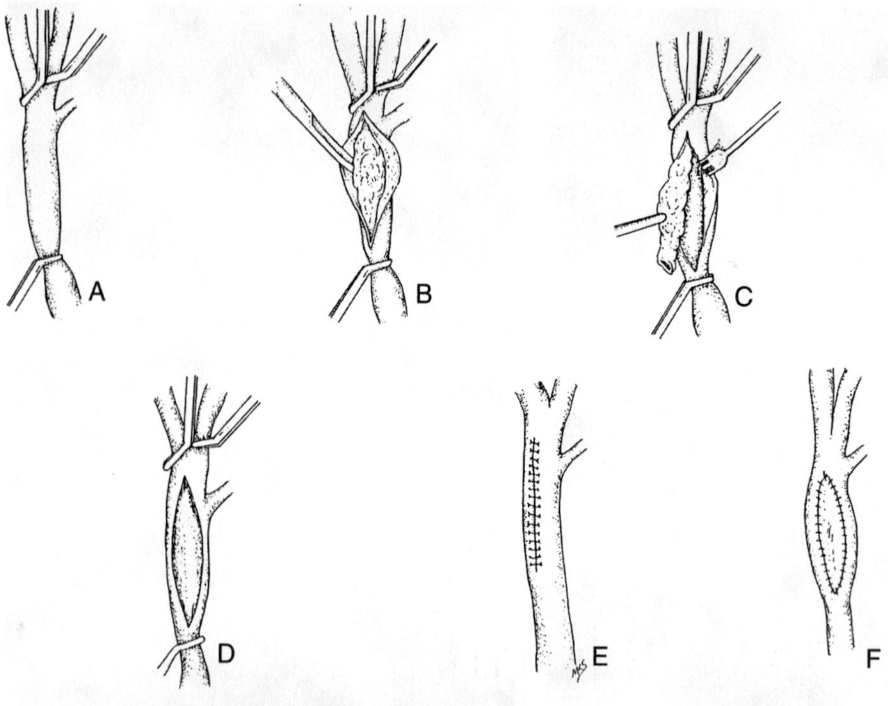

FIGURE 62.4. Technique of standard carotid endarterectomy. After adequate exposure is achieved, the internal, external, and common carotid arteries are clamped (**A**). A plane of dissection is created between the arterial wall and the atheromatous process (**B**). After the plaque is transected proximally, it can be reflected upward to aid in the distal portion of the endarterectomy (**C**). After completion of the endarterectomy, any remaining loose pieces of atheroma or strands of media are removed (**D**). The arteriotomy is closed primarily (**E**) or with a patch graft (**F**).

The MRA technique most often used for evaluation of the carotid bifurcation is referred to as time-of-flight (TOF). The TOF sequence can be acquired in either a two-dimensional (2-D) or as a three-dimensional (3-D) mode; 2-D TOF is more accurate in differentiating between a high-grade stenosis and occlusion, and 3-D TOF has better spatial resolution and provides a more accurate estimation of the degree of stenosis. Thus, when imaging the carotid bifurcation, both studies should be routinely performed.

DU and MRA can be complementary techniques for evaluating carotid artery disease; when there is agreement between both studies, contrast arteriography is rarely necessary.[44–46] In a large study in which both techniques were evaluated, the accuracy of DU and MRA in predicting a greater than 70% carotid stenosis (86% and 88%, respectively) increased to 94% when the results of these two tests were combined.[45]

Carotid Endarterectomy

Since its introduction by DeBakey in 1953, CEA has undergone a number of technical modifications that have increased its efficacy. Although CEA is a conceptually simple operation, precision and attention to technical detail are required to achieve a low rate of stroke (Fig. 62.4). It has been demonstrated that the outcome of CEA is directly related to the frequency with which this operation is performed. Accordingly, it has been advised that CEA be performed by surgeons who perform 12 to 15 or more CEAs per year.[47–49] Although there are numerous variations in the technique of performing CEA, multiple different approaches have produced equally favorable results. The most critical factor appears to be the experience and expertise of the surgeon, who must perform a technically flawless procedure.

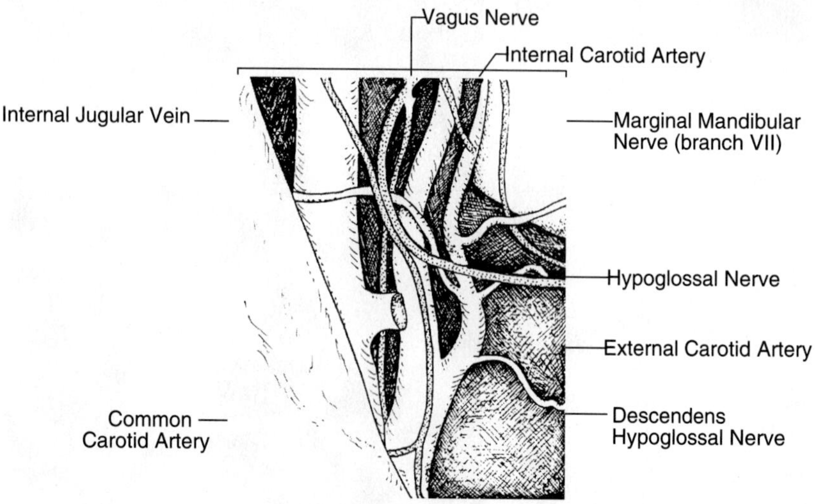

FIGURE 62.5. The anatomic relationship between the carotid bifurcation and the cranial nerves in the neck.

TABLE 62.1.
Influence of the Technique of Carotid Endarterectomy on Rates of Perioperative Stroke/Death and Restenosis.

		Standard endarterectomy				*Eversion endarterectomy*			
Author	*Year*	*CEAs*	*Stroke/death (%)*	*Restenosis (%)*	*F/U (months)*	*CEAs*	*Stroke/death (%)*	*Restenosis (%)*	*F/U (months)*
Ballotta et al.[51]	1999	167[a]	4.2*	4.9*	34	169	0*	0*	34
Shah et al.[52]	1998	474	4.2	1	18	2249	1.9	0.3	18
Cao et al.[53]	1998	675	1.3	4.1	14.9	678	1.3	2.4	14.9
Entz et al.[54]	1997	715[a]	4.0*			739	1.4*		
Vanmaele et al.[55]	1994	98[a]	6.1	2	12	102	2.9	1	12
Kieny et al.[56]	1993	156[b]		13.5	44	212	2.4	1.9	27.1

CEA, carotid endarterectomy; F/U, mean follow-up time.
[a]All CEAs performed with patch closure.
[b]All CEAs performed with primary closure.
**P* value, 0.05 (standard versus eversion endarterectomy).

Technique of Carotid Endarterectomy

The supine patient is prepared with his head extended and turned away from the side of the operation. The incision can be longitudinal along the anterior border of the sternocleidomastoid muscle or oblique along skin creases. The former provides greater exposure whereas the latter is more cosmetically appealing, although neither incision appears to affect the outcome of CEA.[50] Exposure of the carotid bifurcation is facilitated by dividing the common facial vein, a tributary of the internal jugular vein. The common, external, and internal carotid arteries are identified. Division of the posterior belly of the digastric muscle or mandibular subluxation may be needed if the carotid bifurcation is high or if there is distal plaque that cannot be accessed by conventional means. Undiseased segments of the carotid vessels are dissected and controlled so as to decrease the potential for embolization while the arteries are being mobilized. The classical dictum that "the patient should be dissected away from the carotid artery" emphasizes the need for careful technique during exposure. The surgeon must be aware of the mandibular branch of the facial nerve, and the hypoglossal and vagus nerves, although visualization of these nerves is not mandatory (Fig. 62.5). Following systemic heparinization, the distal internal, common, and external carotid arteries are clamped. A longitudinal arteriotomy is made in the common carotid artery, and this incision is extended into the internal carotid artery beyond the distal extent of the plaque. A decision as to whether to shunt is made at this stage, based upon criteria that are discussed later. A dissector is used to begin the endarterectomy in the common carotid artery, and the plaque is transected transversely, creating a proximal endpoint. An eversion endarterectomy of the external carotid artery is performed. The endarterectomy is continued into the internal carotid artery where the distal plaque usually "feathers" away from the remaining arterial wall. If an endpoint is not achieved, the plaque is transected and tacked with fine suture. All loose intimal fragments are removed from the base of the endarterectomized lumen. The arteriotomy is closed primarily or with a patch. Flow is restored first to the external carotid and then to the internal carotid artery to avoid cerebral embolization.

In recent years, the technique of eversion endarterectomy has been popularized (Table 62.1[51–56]). The internal carotid artery is transected obliquely from the common carotid artery (Fig. 62.6). The internal carotid artery wall is everted over the atheromatous core until a distal endpoint is directly visualized. After the internal carotid artery has been completely endarterectomized, significant disease in the common and external carotid arteries is removed. The internal carotid artery is then reanastomosed to the common carotid artery. This technique avoids the need for a suture line in the distal internal carotid artery where the luminal diameter is small. As such, it has been suggested that eversion endarterectomy reduces the incidence of occlusion and restenosis compared to the more conventional endarterectomy techniques.

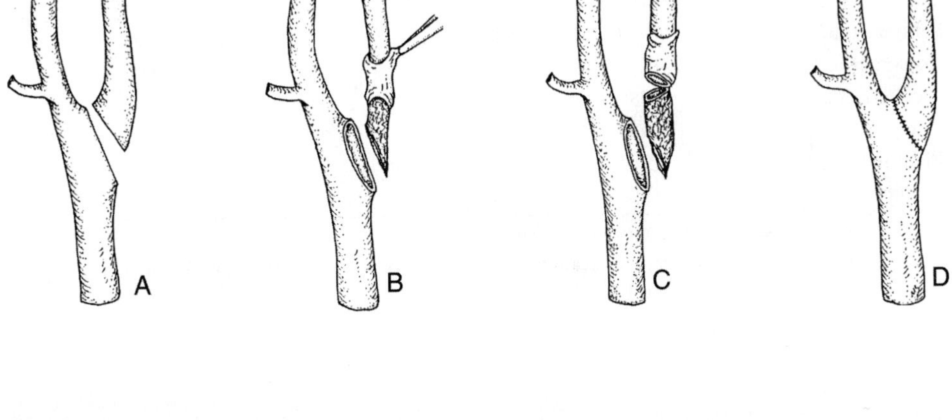

FIGURE 62.6. Technique of eversion carotid endarterectomy. Internal carotid artery is transected obliquely at the carotid bifurcation (**A**). Medial and adventitial layers of the internal carotid artery are everted over the atheromatous core (**B**). Completion of endarterectomy with the distal endpoint directly visualized (**C**). Internal carotid artery is reanastomosed to the common carotid artery (**D**).

Type of Anesthesia

Carotid endarterectomy may be performed under either general or regional anesthesia. The choice of anesthetic technique has been the subject of intense debate (Table 62.2[57–71]). Although both alternatives have been studied and compared on numerous occasions, no consistent benefit has been found with either approach. An advantage of regional anesthesia is the precision by which cerebral ischemia can be detected during cross-clamping of the carotid artery. There is no need for electroencephalography (EEG), monitoring, transcranial Doppler, or stump pressures because the patient is awake and communicative and neurological changes can be immediately identified. The need for shunting is less than when general anesthesia is used, and consequently the risk of shunt-related complications is reduced. A disadvantage associated with regional anesthesia is the need for the patient to remain quiet and still for the duration of the operative procedure. Patient agitation or swallowing can make operation technically difficult, and intubation, if urgently necessary, can be disruptive and technically challenging. Despite the advantages and disadvantages of both techniques, in experienced hands either general or regional anesthesia can be associated with minimal morbidity and mortality.

Prevention of Cerebral Ischemia

Several mechanisms are currently employed to prevent cerebral ischemia during carotid endarterectomy. Options include routine shunting of all patients versus selective shunting, based upon measures of cerebral ischemia such as stump pressures, EEG, or awake monitoring. Although numerous authors have reported a diminution in the rate of stroke when routine shunting is employed, it is argued that such a policy requires the unnecessary placement of shunts in the 85% to 95% of patients who already have adequate collateral circulation. Disadvantages of routine shunting include the potential for cerebral embolization and intimal damage related to shunt placement as well as increased technical difficulty of performing the endarterectomy when a shunt is in place. For surgeons who selectively shunt, there is no unanimity as to the optimal method of identifying cerebral ischemia. Regional anesthesia with placement of a shunt in those patients who develop symptoms is the most reliable method for detecting cerebral ischemia.[72] Other mechanisms for evaluating cerebral ischemia have been devised for patients under general anesthesia. Measurement of internal carotid artery stump pressures is one such method. Occluding vascular clamps are placed across the external and the proximal common carotid arteries. Pressure is transduced through a needle placed into the common carotid artery distal to the proximal clamp. The back-pressure transmitted down the internal carotid artery is measured; this pressure reflects the adequacy of the collateral circulation to the ipsilateral hemisphere. Stump pressures of 40 to 50 mmHg have been proposed as thresholds above which cerebral perfusion is considered adequate.[73,74] Electroencephalographic monitoring during CEA is another valuable guide for detecting intraoperative cerebral ischemia.[75–77] EEG is, however, the most costly of all techniques for cerebral protection and requires sophisticated equipment and an experienced technologist. Despite these limitations, EEG is used routinely with excellent results by many surgeons who perform endarterectomy. Transcranial doppler and somatosensory evoked potentials have been advocated as alternative methods for

TABLE 62.2.
Influence of Anesthetic Technique on Perioperative Complications in Patients Undergoing CEA.

		General anesthesia			*Regional anesthesia*		
Author	*Year*	*CEAs*	*Stroke/death (%)*	*MI*	*CEAs*	*Stroke/death (%)*	*MI*
Fiorani et al.[57]	1997	337	5.0*	0.6	683	2.0*	0.3
Ombrellaro et al.[58]	1996	126	4.8	0.8	140	2.1	2.1
Rockman et al.[59]	1996	349	4.1*	1.2	1414	2.1*	0.6
Shah et al.[60]	1994	419	1.9		654	2.0	
Allen et al.[61]	1994	361	3.9	2.5	318	2.5	0.6
Becquemin et al.[62]	1991	242	5.4	4.1*	145	4.1	0*
Bergeron et al.[63]	1991	250[a]	4.4*		114	1.8*	0
Forssell et al.[64]	1989	55[a]	3.6	1.8	56[a]	5.4	3.6
Godin et al.[65]	1989	50	2.0		50[a]	0	
Palmer et al.[66]	1989	37[a]	2.0	5.4	184[a]	1.5	1.6
Corson et al.[67]	1987	242	2.9*	0.8	157	1.3*	1.3
Muskett et al.[68]	1986	45[a]	0	6.7	30[a]	3.3	0
Gabelman et al.[69]	1983	46[a]	6.5	2.2	54[a]	3.7	0
Pietzman et al.[70]	1982	53	5.7		226	3.1	
Andersen et al.[71]	1980	189	3.1		232	4.8	

CEA, carotid endarterectomy; MI, myocardial infarction.
[a]Number of patients undergoing carotid endarterectomy (number of procedures performed not indicated).
*P value, 0.05 (general versus regional anesthesia).

cerebral monitoring; however, studies thus far have not proven a definite advantage of either of these techniques over other more well-established measurements of cerebral ischemia.[78,79] No method of cerebral protection has been proven to be superior. Maintainence of adequate cerebral flow, however, is an essential part of CEA because strokes related to hypoperfusion are usually major and devastating.

Patch Angioplasty

Although CEA has become a well-established and commonly performed procedure, there remains controversy as to the appropriate method of closing the arteriotomy (Table 62.3[80–98]). Primary closure is the most expeditious. Alternatively, patch angioplasty with autogenous or prosthetic material serves to increase the luminal diameter of the endarterectomized vessel. Proponents of carotid patch angioplasty argue that this technique reduces the incidence of perioperative thrombosis and carotid occlusion. Hertzer et al.,[97] reporting the results of 917 patients undergoing CEA at the Cleveland Clinic, found that in 483 patients receiving primary closure the perioperative stroke rate was 3.1%, whereas the 434 patients who underwent patch closure had a stroke rate of 0.7%. AbuRahma et al.[81] also demonstrated a significant reduction in acute neurological complications with patch angioplasty compared with primary closure. It is also argued that the incidence of recurrent carotid stenosis may be significantly reduced with patch closure. Katz et al.[95] in a prospective study observed that primary closure was associated with an eightfold higher incidence of restenosis when compared to patch angioplasty.

Advantages of primary closure include its simplicity, technical ease, and a reduction in operative time. Moreover, primary closure does not involve complications inherent to patch angioplasty, such as vein patch "blowout," pseudoaneurysm formation, and prosthetic graft infection. Interestingly, a number of authors report no advantage in terms of either perioperative stroke or late restenosis rates in patients treated with patch angioplasty versus primary closure.[80,86,87,89,93] Rosenthal et al.[93] studied 1000 consecutive CEAs and compared four groups: primary closure, PTFE patch closure, Dacron patch closure, and vein patch closure. The incidence of early postoperative neurological events and long-term restenosis was similar in all four groups.

When primary closure is used, technique is paramount and the closure must be performed with precision. Patient selection may also be a critical factor. The incidence of perioperative complications and restenosis may be increased if small carotid arteries are not closed with a patch. Both approaches, patch angioplasty and primary closure, have been associated with excellent short- and long-term outcomes following CEA. Surgeon experience and preference is the primary determinant of which technique is used.

Verification of Technical Result

Many surgeons have recommended intraoperative imaging of the reconstructed carotid artery with the presumption that immediate recognition of technical defects will decrease the incidence of postoperative stroke and late restenosis.[99–103] Scott et al.[103] were able to reduce their incidence of perioperative stroke from 6.8% to 3.6% using intraoperative arteriography. Others have found a similar relationship between defects found intraoperatively and recurrent stenosis.[104–107] Opponents of intraoperative arteriography argue that this technique is invasive and may result in embolization or the creation of new intraluminal defects. There are no randomized studies available that address this question, nor is there a consensus. Currently, most surgeons evaluate the adequacy of CEA using a Doppler probe and palpation of the distal internal carotid artery pulse.

Postoperative Care

Current practice standards dictate that patients following CEA can be discharged to the ward after a brief stay in the recovery room if they are neurologically intact and hemodynamically stable. Only a small percentage of patients actually require intensive care unit monitoring.[108] Moreover, most patients can be discharged safely to home on the first postoperative day. These approaches, which have been successfully employed in many centers, substantially reduce the hospital cost of CEA and are well accepted by patients.[109–111]

Postoperative Complications

The most devastating consequence of CEA is stroke. Causes of intra- or postoperative stroke include (1) embolization that occurs during dissection of the carotid artery, (2) inadequate cerebral protection during carotid cross-clamping, (3) postoperative thrombosis, and (4) intracerebral hemorrhage (reperfusion syndrome). Before leaving the operating room, the patient is fully awakened and assessed for neurological deficits. The finding of a major neurological deficit warrants immediate reexploration with intraoperative imaging of the carotid reconstruction. A neurological deficit that occurs within the first 24h should likewise lead to either an urgent duplex ultrasound or surgical reexploration. A hemorrhagic stroke may develop 3 to 7 days postoperatively as a consequence of a hyperperfusion syndrome. This syndrome occurs more frequently in patients who initially present with recent large strokes, critical stenoses, and cerebral hypoperfusion.[112,113] Chronic hypoperfusion leads to loss of autoregulation in the cerebral vessels; the lack of appropriate vasoconstriction may lead to edema or hemorrhage once normal circulation is restored. The initial symptom may be a severe unilateral throbbing headache. There is usually associated hypertension. Seizures may then occur, followed by a permanent neurological deficit that is usually associated with intracranial hemorrhage. Early recognition is essential and should be rapidly followed by precise blood pressure control, avoidance of anticoagulation, and anticonvulsants as necessary. If cerebral hemorrhage occurs, placement of an intraventricular pressure monitor or craniotomy with evacuation of the hematoma may be lifesaving, although the outcome once hemorrhage has developed is usually poor.[112–114]

Other than stroke, myocardial infarction is the most common major complication following CEA. Because of the frequent coexistence of coronary artery disease in patients with carotid stenosis, preoperative cardiac evaluation of patients scheduled for CEA is appropriate in some patients. Alternatively, it is important to realize that this procedure, which requires only a brief general or regional anesthetic, can be safely performed in patients with mild to moderate cardiac

TABLE 62.3.
Influence of Method of Arteriotomy Closure on Perioperative Complications and Restenosis in Patients Undergoing CEA.

		Primary closure				*Vein patch closure*				*Prosthetic patch closure*			
Author	*Year*	*CEAs*	*Stroke/ death (%)*	*Restenosis (%)*	*F/U (months)*	*CEAs*	*Stroke/ death (%)*	*Restenosis (%)*	*F/U (months)*	*CEAs*	*Stroke/ death*	*Restenosis*	*F/U (months)*
Nene et al.[80]	1999	75	0	1.3	18					67	1.5	0	18
AbuRahma et al.[81]	1998	135	5.9*	34*	30	130	1.5*	9*	30	134	0.7*	2*	30
Desiron et al.[82]	1997	837		13*	69	1320		4.8*	35				
Allen et al.[83]	1997					287	1.7	1.0	29.3	110	4.5	2.7	27.6
Katz SG and Kohl[84]	1996					100	1.0	0	19	107	2.8	0.9	19
Goldman et al.[85]	1995					184	2.2	4.2	16.1	91	1.1	7.9	9.3
Katz D et al.[86]	1994	51	3.9	3.9	29.2					49	2.0	0	29.2
Myers et al.[87]	1994	64	1.6	7.8	57	61	0	14.8	59				
Gonzales-Fajardo et al.[88]	1994					45	0	0	29	50	4	4	29
Treiman et al.[89]	1993	1173	2.7			240	4.6			266	2.3		
Ranaboldo et al.[90]	1993	104	2.9	16.3*	12	109b	2.8	5.5*	12				
De Letter et al.[91]	1993	62	6.5	27.4*	60	67	4.5	11.9*	60				
Whereatt et al.[92]	1990					75	4.0	5.3	29.3	16	12.5	6.3	29.3
Rosenthal et al.[93a]	1990	250	1.6	4.1	37.8	250	0	0.9	37.8	500	1.8	4.8	37.8
Lord et al.[94]	1989	50	2	19.1*	<1	43	0	0*	<1	47	0	0*	<1
Katz MM et al.[95]	1987	47	4.3	19.1*	6-24	42	0	2.4*	6-24				
Ouriel and Green[96a]	1987	82C	3.7	28.6*	17.2					70§	0	5.7*	16
Hertzer et al.[97a]	1987	483	3.3*	14*	21	434	0.9*	4.8*	21				
Fode et al.[98]	1986	2714	6.6*			266	2.3*			257	7		

CEA, carotid endarterectomy; F/U, mean follow-up time.

[a]Only stroke rates given; death rates not specified.

[b]Patched group includes 52 vein and 56 prosthetic patches; rates not stratified although authors state that there was no significant difference between vein and prosthetic subgroups with respect to neurological complications or restenosis rates.

[c]Number of patients undergoing CEA (number of procedures performed not indicated).

*P value < 0.05 (primary versus patch closure).

disease. Postoperative fluctuations in blood pressure, either hyper- or hypotension, develop in 20% to 60% of patients.[115,116] Severe hypertension should be controlled with sodium nitroprusside and hypotension with fluid administration or phenylephrine. These fluctuations may be related to carotid sinus manipulation. The reactive nature of the carotid sinus can be diminished by the injection of 1% lidocaine at the time of initial surgical dissection. Cranial nerve injury can complicate CEA, particularly if the carotid bifurcation is high and more cephalad exposure is required.[117–119] In NASCET, the overall incidence of cranial nerve injury was 7.6%.[6] The most commonly injured nerves are the mandibular branch of the facial nerve (ipsilateral drooping of corner of mouth, drooling of saliva), hypoglossal nerve (deviation of tongue toward side of injury, difficulty with speech and swallowing), recurrent laryngeal nerve (vocal cord paralysis, hoarseness, loss of effective cough mechanism), superior laryngeal nerve (easy fatigability of voice, inability to phonate high-pitched notes), and the great auricular nerve (numbness or painful paresthesias of the earlobe and scalp). Glossopharyngeal (difficulty swallowing) and spinal accessory nerve (winging of scapula, difficulty raising the shoulder) injuries are occasionally observed. Bilateral recurrent laryngeal nerve injury may lead to airway obstruction requiring emergency tracheostomy. Thus, when staged CEAs are planned, interval assessment of the vocal cords by indirect laryngoscopy is advisable. Most injuries result from traction rather than inadvertent division of the nerve and resolve completely within a few weeks. A wound hematoma is unusual, but if large may compromise either the arterial repair or a patient's airway. An early postoperative hematoma deserves close monitoring and urgent surgical evacuation if there is suspicion of airway compromise.

Postoperative Surveillance

CEA is a durable procedure; however, restenosis and occasionally recurrent symptoms may develop. Restenosis is the result of either myointimal hyperplasia, which tends to develop within the first 2 years following CEA, or recurrent atherosclerosis, which is most predominant after 2 years. Thus, depending on the time interval after operation, recurrent plaque may have differing morphological characteristics.[120] Symptoms are relatively rare in patients who develop intimal hyperplasia because these lesions are smooth, nonulcerated, and do not act as a nidus for cholesterol or platelets. Beyond 2 years, symptoms are more frequent and are related to embolization from atherosclerotic plaque. Recurrent stenosis and symptoms are more frequent in women, in patients with atherosclerotic risk factors such as cigarette smoking and hypercholesterolemia, or if residual disease remains following the initial endarterectomy.[104,121,122] Postoperative surveillance protocols using duplex ultrasound are frequently employed in patients following CEA. Recurrent stenoses of greater than 50% are identified in 12% to 36% of endarterectomized vessels. However, the incidence of stenosis greater than 80% is only 2% per year and the incidence of recurrent symptoms is even less.[123] It has been argued that because high-grade stenoses and recurrent symptoms are infrequent routine duplex ultrasound surveillance following CEA is not essential.[124–127] Although there is variation with regard to the appropriate frequency, postoperative surveillance is still employed by most surgeons.

Although controversial, many authors have reported an increased rate of complication following CEA in patients with recurrent disease. Thus, "redo" CEA is usually reserved for symptomatic patients or those without symptoms who have preocclusive lesions. Patch angioplasty rather than endarterectomy is indicated in patients in whom intimal hyperplasia is the pathological lesion because a precise endarterectomy plane cannot usually be identified.

Carotid Angioplasty and Stenting

Recently, carotid angioplasty and stenting (CAS) has been proposed as an alternative treatment to prevent stroke in patients with carotid artery occlusive disease[128,129] (Table 62.4, Fig. 62.7). CAS has been evaluated for the treatment of patients considered to be at increased risk for conventional carotid endarterectomy. Patients may be considered high risk for anatomic as well as physiological reasons. Anatomic high-risk categories have included prior carotid endarterectomy, prior neck dissection, cervical irradiation, surgically inaccessible distal carotid lesions, contralateral recurrent laryngeal nerve palsy, and ostial conditions that prohibit neck extension and rotation. Physiological high-risk conditions including significant coronary and pulmonary disease have been used for indications for CAS. In addition, contralateral carotid occlusion and age over 80 years have been considered as potential inclusion criteria for CAS.

The results of several clinical trials have recently been published or presented. The SAPPHIRE trial evaluated 310 patients considered to be at increased risk for CEA. Patients were randomized to receive either CEA (151) or CAS (159). Both symptomatic and asymptomatic patients were included in the study. Analysis of the combined stroke/death/myocardial infarction rate within 1 year demonstrated a significant advantage for CAS over CEA in these high-risk patients (12.0% vs. 20.1%, $P = 0.053$). In addition, the need for subsequent reintervention was significantly lower in patients treated with CAS as compared with CEA (0.6 vs. 4.3%, $P = 0.04$). The individual rates of stroke, myocardial infarction and death within one year were not statistically different between the groups (CAS: 5.8, 2.5, 7.0 vs. CEA: 7.7, 8.1, 12.9, P = NS).[130] Carotid angioplasty and stenting has also been evaluated in several additional registry trials including the CABERNET, MAVErIC, BEACH, and ARCHeR trials. Results for the ARCHeR trial have demonstrated a 30-day combined stroke/death/myocardial infarction rate of 8.3% in symptomatic and asymptomatic patients considered to be at high risk for CEA.[131] These results compared favorably with weighted historical controls in the study. The 30 combined stroke/death/myocardial infarction rate for the MAVErIC trial was 7.3% whereas the rate was 3.8% in the CABERNET trial. Again, comparison with historical controls was considered favorable.

Cerebral Protection

Each of these clinical trials utilized cerebral protection to minimize the risk of cerebrovascular accident during the CAS procedure. Interestingly, in the ARCHeR trial no significant decrease in ipsilateral procedural stroke rate was observed for patients treated with cerebral protection as compared to those

TABLE 62.4.
Series of Carotid Angioplasty and Stenting (Level II Evidence).

Author	*Year*	*Center*	*Carotids (number)*	*Asx (%)*	*Immediate technical success (%)*	*Stroke/ death (%)*	*Restenosis (%)*	*F/U (months)*
Meta-analysis								
Wholey et al.[167]	1998	24 centers in Europe, S. and N. America	2048	34	98.6	5.8	4.8	6
Single-center studies								
Henry et al.[168]	1998	Polyclinique, Essey-les-Nancy, France	174	65	99.4	2.9	2.3	12.7
Jordan et al.[169]	1998	University of Alabama, Birmingham	312	63		8.7		
Naylor et al.[170]	1998	Leicester Royal Infirmary, UK	7	0	100	71.4		
Tietelbaum et al.[171]	1998	University of Southern California	26	32	96.2	27.3	14.3	5.9
Wholey et al.[172]	1998	Pittsburgh Vascular Institute	206		96	5.3	3.9	6
Beyssen et al.[173]	1998	Broussais Hospital, Paris, France	15	34	100	6.7	0	7.2
Criado et al.[174]	1997	Union Memorial Hospital, Baltimore, MD	33	27	100	0	3	8
Vozzi et al.[175]	1997	Hemodinamia Instituto, Rosario, Argentina	24	55	95.8	8.3	8.3	6.3
Mathias et al.[176]	1997	Stadtische Kliniken, Dortmund, Germany	428		99.3	2.3	11	60
Jagic et al.[177]	1997	Clinical Hospital, Kragujevac, Yugoslavia	36	0	97.2	0	5.6	
Yadav et al.[178]	1997	University of Alabama, Birmingham	126	42	99.2	7.9	4.9	6
Diethrich et al.[179]	1996	Arizona Heart Center, Phoenix	117	72	99.1	6.8	3.4	7.6
Bergeron et al.[180]	1996	St. Joseph Hospital, Marseilles, France	20		90	0	0	8

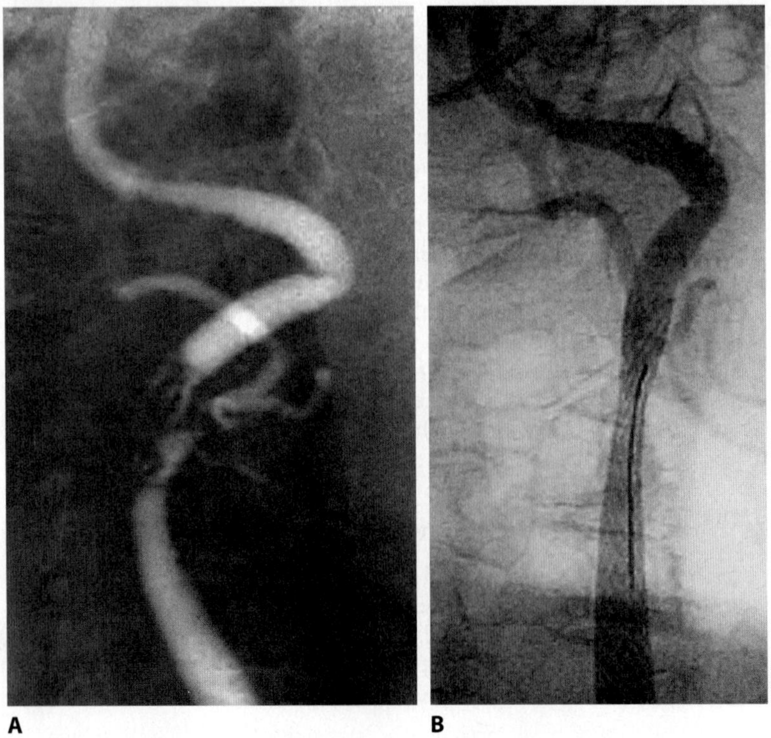

A B

FIGURE 62.7. Carotid angioplasty and stenting with cerebral protection. **A.** Digital subtraction angiogram of the carotid artery demonstrates a high-grade, heavily calcified stenosis at the level of the carotid bifurcation. **B.** The cerebral protective filter is withdrawn after the angioplasty and stenting procedure resolved the stenosis.

treated without cerebral protection. In the lead-in phase of the CREST trial, which is designed to compare CAS with CEA for standard-risk patients, a trend in improved stroke rates was seen with the use of cerebral protection.[132] However, this trend failed to achieve statistical significance. Similarly, in the feasibility and CASCADE trials utilizing the angioguard cerebral protection device, a trend toward lower procedural stroke rates was observed that again did not reach statistical significance. It is important to note that these studies have not been powered to demonstrate a difference between CAS with and CAS without cerebral protection. The potential for specific lesions to generate emboli during treatment should also be considered. In particular, intimal hyperplastic stenoses occurring after prior CEA appear to generate little particulate matter during CAS and therefore may not require the use of a cerebral protection device. In general, three mechanisms of cerebral protection have been developed for use during CAS: these are (1) microporous filter deployed in the internal carotid artery, (2) temporary occlusion of the internal carotid artery, and (3) reversal of flow in the internal carotid artery.

Microporous Filters

Microporous filters are positioned in the internal carotid artery distal to the target lesion. The filter is constrained within a delivery sheath to enable the carotid stenosis to be crossed. Once in position in the internal carotid, the delivery sheath is withdrawn to deploy the filter. Antegrade cerebral flow is maintained through the filter during the CAS procedure. Particulate matter dislodged during the procedure is trapped within the filter. Upon completion of CAS, the filter is recaptured and withdrawn. The filter devices currently being evaluated include the Cordis Angioguard, the Boston Scientific Filter Wire, the Guidant Accunet, the Medtronic Interceptor, the eV3 Spider and Intraguard, the Abbott Neuroshield, the Rubicon, and the Scipro. Most of these devices, including the Angioguard, EPI Filter Wire, Accunet, and Interceptor incorporate the filter as a component of the angiographic wire itself. Other filters, including the Neuroshield and Spider, are deployed separately over an angiographic wire. Microporous filters offer the advantage of continued cerebral perfusion in patients whose intracranial collateral circulation does not allow them to tolerate temporary carotid occlusion. Their delivery systems are significantly larger that those of occlusion balloons, ranging up to 4 Fr. in diameter, which may result in difficulty in crossing severe carotid stenoses. Difficulty in advancing the filter delivery system through tortuous vessels may also be encountered because of the stiffness of the filter and its delivery system. The potential exists for embolization to occur before or during advancement of the filter across the carotid lesion as well.

Occlusion Balloons

Occlusion balloons provide cerebral protection by temporarily occluding the internal carotid artery during the CAS procedure. The occlusion balloon is a component of an angiographic wire and is inflated through the hollow core of the wire. It is passed through the carotid stenosis and then inflated in the distal internal carotid. The carotid angioplasty and stenting is then performed, and the standing column of blood containing any dislodged particulate debris is evacuated through an export catheter. The balloon is then deflated and flow restored to the cerebral circulation. Occlusion balloon protection devices include the Medtronic Percusurge and the Abbott Guardian. Occlusion balloons offer the advantage of lower device crossing profiles and easier maneuverability for positioning in tortuous vessels. However, they still require crossing the carotid stenosis before deployment of the protection device. In addition, because they require interruption of cerebral perfusion, they may lead to cerebral intolerance.

Flow Reversal

Two devices that provide cerebral protection by reversing flow in the internal carotid artery are currently being evaluated. These devices occlude flow in the common and external carotid arteries. The resulting pressure gradient causes reversal of flow in the internal carotid artery. This flow is passed through a filter and returned to the circulation via a femoral vein puncture. The Parodi device and the MoMa device utilize internal carotid flow reversal during CAS. The devices are somewhat cumbersome in their current formulations; however, they provide cerebral protection before crossing the carotid lesion. Because flow is reversed in the internal carotid, a proportion of patients may be expected to experience cerebral intolerance.

Cerebral protection appears to be of benefit in preventing stroke during the performance of carotid angioplasty and stenting. A wide array of devices is currently being evaluated in large-scale clinical trials. Each type of device offers specific advantages and disadvantages. The decision regarding which specific device should be utilized must take into account factors including the severity of the stenosis, the tortuousity of the common and internal carotid arteries, the likelihood of generating emboli in trying to advance a device across the stenosis, and the degree of intracranial collateral flow to allow temporary interruption of antegrade carotid flow.

A multicenter prospective, randomized trial, the Carotid Revascularization Endarterectomy versus Stent Trial (CREST), has been instituted to evaluate the safety and efficacy of carotid angioplasty and stenting compared to carotid endarterectomy in normal-risk patients.[132] This study will provide the most valid and accurate data regarding the relative morbidity and mortality of these two interventions. Preliminary results from the lead-in registry component of the study have indicated increasing levels of periprocedural complications for patients with increasing age. As a consequence, the CREST study has stopped enrolling patients over the age of 80 years. Ultimately the indication for carotid stenting and for the use of specific cerebral protection devices will be determined by the results of prospective clinical trials.

Vertebrobasilar Ischemia

Posterior ischemic symptoms may result from atherosclerotic disease involving the vertebral or proximal subclavian arteries. Symptoms of vertebrobasilar ischemia usually result from hypoperfusion and only rarely from embolization. A systemic process that decreases blood pressure, such as orthostatic hypotension, overaggressive treatment with antihypertensives, anemia, or arrhythmias, can precipitate symptoms. Symptoms may also be prompted by rotation of the neck if osteophytes arising from the cervical vertebrae compress the vertebral artery as it passes through the vertebral canal. Hypoperfusion-related vertebrobasilar ischemia seldom results in cerebral infarction but can produce functional disability. Because the vertebral arteries unite to form the basilar artery, occlusive disease involving both vertebral arteries is required for symptoms of hypoperfusion to develop. The exception to this rule is in patients with subclavian steal.

There is little role for surgery in the treatment of asymptomatic vertebrobasilar insufficiency. It can be assumed that these patients are receiving adequate collateral flow from either the anterior circulation and/or the contralateral vertebral artery. In patients who have concomitant carotid and vertebral lesions, correction of the anterior circulation lesion should be the initial treatment and is usually effective in alleviating symptoms.

Vertebral artery reconstructions can be divided into proximal (vertebral artery from its origin to the cervical canal) and distal (cervical canal and intracranial). The most common lesion affecting the vertebral artery is an atherosclerotic plaque arising at its origin from the subclavian artery. Proximal lesions are best treated with transposition of the proximal vertebral artery to the common carotid artery. Berguer[133] recently reported treatment of 140 patients with unilateral proximal vertebral artery reconstructions with no strokes or deaths. Cure or substantial improvement of symptoms was achieved in 83% of patients. The second most common lesion of the vertebral artery is a stenosis or occlusion as this artery courses through the vertebral canal. For distal vertebral reconstructions, the treatment of choice is a vein bypass between the common carotid and distal vertebral arteries. For these reconstructions, Berguer et al.[134] noted a higher mortality rate (4%) and a higher incidence of graft thrombosis compared with proximal vertebral interventions. However, cure or substantial improvement was noted in 87% of patients.

Subclavian steal syndrome is a more frequent cause of vertebrobasilar insufficiency. A proximal stenosis or occlusion of the subclavian artery can produce reversal of flow in the ipsilateral vertebral artery. The resultant "stealing" of blood from the vertebral artery to the arm may result in a diminution in cerebral perfusion. If symptoms of posterior ischemia develop, relief can be gained by subclavian artery angioplasty, carotid–subclavian bypass, or subclavian-to-carotid transposition.[135–137]

Carotid Artery Occlusion

The extracranial internal carotid artery has no branches. Thus, if a lesion at the origin of the internal carotid artery leads to occlusion, clot propagates distally to the next collateral, which is either the opthalmic or the middle cerebral arteries. Unless urgently addressed, this clot cannot be removed. Thus, CEA is not an option in patients with chronic internal carotid artery occlusion. If symptoms develop in a patient with chronic carotid artery occlusion, they may be related to hypoperfusion, embolization through external carotid artery collaterals, or embolization from the stump of the occluded carotid artery. The rate of stroke associated with carotid occlusion is as high as 5% per year.[138,139] Although treatment of symptomatic patients with carotid artery occlusion is usually with coumadin or antiplatelet agents, there are several surgical options that should be considered. If there is severe disease of the contralateral carotid artery, contralateral CEA should be performed. Extracranial–intracranial bypass was developed for the treatment of symptomatic patients with internal carotid occlusion and involves the anastomosis, through a craniotomy, of the superficial temporal artery branch of the external carotid artery to the ipsilateral middle cerebral artery. This procedure achieved great popularity at a time when it was assumed that hypoperfusion rather than embolization was the cause of infarction in patients with cerebrovascular disease. After a prospective randomized trial in 1985 demonstrated that extracranial–intracranial bypass was ineffective in preventing long-term stroke, enthusiasm for this procedure markedly diminished.[140] There has recently been a renewed interest in this technique. Patients with moyamoya disease, a disease characterized by progressive stenosis of the supraclinoid internal carotid artery, have been found to benefit from extracranial–intracranial bypass.[141] Modalities that test cranial perfusion, such as transcranial Doppler ultrasound, positron emission tomography, single-photon emission computed tomography, and zenon computed tomography, have been able to identify subgroups of patients with carotid occlusion who have cerebral hypoperfusion.[142,143] It has been postulated that these patients may benefit from extracranial–intracranial bypass, although further studies are necessary to prove this hypothesis.

The external carotid artery can become an important source of collateral blood flow when the ipsilateral internal carotid artery is occluded. If patients with internal carotid artery occlusion develop ipsilateral amaurosis fugax, transient ischemic attacks, or stroke, the culprit may be hypoperfusion or emboli related to an atherosclerotic lesion involving the origin of the external carotid artery. External carotid endarterectomy may alleviate these symptoms and can be performed using a number of techniques. In one such technique, the occluded internal carotid artery is divided flush with the common carotid artery. The resultant opening in the common carotid artery is extended into the external carotid artery, and an endarterectomy is performed. The arteriotomy is then closed with a patch. In a collective review of 23 reports that included 218 patients treated with external CEA, symptoms resolved in 83% and an additional 7% were improved.[144] The procedure was associated with a perioperative mortality of 3% and an overall neurological complication rate of 5%. As might be anticipated, the best results were obtained when operation was performed to relieve specific hemispheric or retinal symptoms rather than nonspecific neurological complaints.

Extracranial Carotid Artery Aneurysms

Extracranial carotid artery aneurysms are uncommon lesions, accounting for less than 2% of all carotid interventions. Atherosclerosis, trauma, previous carotid surgery, dissection, and fibromuscular dysplasia are the usual etiologies. Patients may present with an asymptomatic pulsatile neck or pharyngeal mass or with symptoms, including neck pain, hoarseness, or dysphagia (the latter two related to compression of the vagus or glossopharyngeal nerves). TIAs or strokes are also common presenting symptoms and most often result from the distal embolization of atheromatous debris from the aneurysmal sac.[145,146] Rupture of carotid artery aneurysms is rare.

The distinction between carotid aneurysm and physiological dilation of the carotid bulb has not been clearly defined. de Jong et al.[145] proposed that a carotid aneurysm be defined as a bulb dilation greater than 200% of the diameter of the internal carotid artery or 150% of the diameter of the common carotid artery. All aneurysms of the carotid artery should be repaired regardless of symptoms.[147] Resection of the aneurysm and restoration of arterial continuity is the procedure of choice.[148] For carotid artery aneurysms located close to the base of the skull where reconstruction is technically formidable, a reasonable alternative is carotid ligation with or without extracranial–intracranial bypass. There has also been recent interest in treating aneurysms in this location using endovascular techniques.[149]

Nonatherosclerotic Cerebrovascular Disease

Carotid Body Tumors

The carotid body is a highly vascular chemoreceptor located in the adventitial layer of the carotid bifurcation. Carotid body tumors (or carotid paragangliomas) present as painless, pulsatile but not expansile, usually asymptomatic neck masses that are found just below the angle of the mandible. They lie between the internal and external carotid arteries, just cephalad to the carotid bifurcation, and may extend to the base of the skull. Symptoms occasionally develop (related to pressure on the adjacent cranial nerves or local structures) and include neck or ear pain, dysphagia, hoarseness, tinnitus, or dizziness. Although duplex ultrasound can be used to identify carotid body tumors, MRI/MRA, CT, and/or arteriography are usually necessary for diagnosis and preoperative planning. Typical arteriographic features include splaying of the internal and external carotid arteries by a vascular mass (Fig. 62.8). The blood supply to the tumor is derived predominantly from the external carotid artery. Needle or open biopsy of these masses should be avoided.

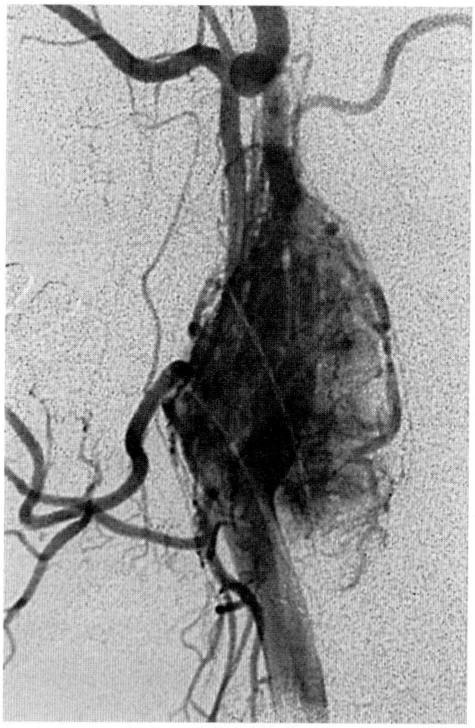

FIGURE 62.8. Carotid arteriogram shows carotid body tumor with extensive vascularization and splaying of the internal and external carotid arteries.

The recommended treatment for a carotid body tumor is surgical excision.[150–152] Even small asymptomatic carotid body tumors should be resected. If left untreated, these lesions slowly enlarge and gradually encase the carotid artery and adjacent cranial nerves. Although most tumors are benign, distant metastases have been reported. Neurovascular complications increase with the size of the carotid body tumor, and therefore surgery is best performed early. Several perioperative and operative techniques have been used to facilitate surgical treatment. Nasotracheal intubation with general anesthesia is preferable because subluxation of the mandible may be necessary for adequate exposure. Cranial nerve injury (particularly the vagus and hypoglossal) is avoided by identification and meticulous mobilization of the major nerves away from the tumor. For large tumors, the external carotid artery may be ligated to reduce bleeding and facilitate dissection. A saphenous vein donor site should be prepared in the event that carotid reconstruction with an interposition graft is required. Preoperative angiographic embolization performed by experienced interventional radiologists may be helpful in reducing the vascularity and the size of the tumor.[153] Carotid body tumors can be resected with a low incidence of stroke; however, cranial nerve injury is the most common complication and may occur in up to 40% of cases.[152] This complication is particularly common when large tumors are resected.

Fibromuscular Dysplasia of the Extracranial Carotid Artery

Fibromuscular arterial dysplasia is an uncommon disorder that primarily affects the renal and carotid arteries of young women. There are four histological subtypes: intimal fibroplasia, medial fibroplasia, medial hyperplasia, and perimedial dysplasia. The most frequently encountered form in the extracranial carotid artery is medial fibroplasia. Morphologically, lesions present as alternating stenoses and regions of dilatation involving the internal carotid artery distal to the bifurcation. Angiographically, this appears as a "string of beads," a finding that is pathognomonic for fibromuscular dysplasia. Associated intracranial aneurysms are found in 10% of patients.[154] Fibromuscular dysplasia has also been associated with spontaneous carotid dissection. The pathogenesis of fibromuscular dysplasia is unknown. Although natural history data are lacking, patients with asymptomatic lesions should probably be treated with antiplatelet agents and carefully observed. Intervention should be reserved for patients with symptoms.[155,156] Open surgery with graduated intraluminal dilatation is the most widely used procedure for treating fibromuscular dysplasia. Other treatment options include percutaneous carotid angioplasty (although experience with this technique is limited) and resection with primary anastomosis or an interposition bypass.

Carotid Coils and Kinks

Coils (circular or exaggerated S-shape configurations) and kinks (sharp angulations) of the carotid artery may be congenital or acquired. Congenital lesions develop if the heart and great vessels do not descend properly into the mediastinum during embryogenesis. Acquired lesions develop with aging when the internal carotid artery, which is fixed between the skull base and the thoracic inlet, loses its elasticity and elongates.

The most common symptomatic lesion is the carotid kink. Atherosclerotic plaques are frequently found at the site of kinks and may be responsible for embolic symptoms. Turning of the head or twisting of the neck may accentuate a kink and also produce symptoms related to hypoperfusion. Operation should be considered only in patients with symptoms.[157–160] Options for treatment include patch angioplasty, resection of the redundant segment of the carotid artery with primary end-to-end anastomosis, resection of a segment of the common carotid artery with reduction of the kink and primary reanastomosis, or detachment of the internal carotid artery at its origin with translocation to a more proximal location on the common carotid artery.

Stenotic atherosclerotic carotid bifurcation disease is often associated with distal internal carotid artery redundancy. During endarterectomy, removal of plaque with primary closure may create a redundant segment that can kink and predispose to postoperative thrombosis or restenosis. Patch angioplasty or resection of the redundant carotid artery is necessary to prevent this complication.

Carotid Dissection

Carotid dissection is increasingly recognized as a major cause of cerebral infarction in young adults. An intimal tear or a ruptured vasa vasorum allows blood to penetrate and dissect into the arterial wall. This process may result in narrowing or occlusion of the arterial lumen. Carotid artery dissection may be either spontaneous or traumatic. Most traumatic carotid artery dissections result from blunt trauma and are related to abrupt flexion, extension, and rotation of the neck. Even trivial trauma, such as coughing, vomiting, or nose-blowing, can produce a dissection.[161] The most commonly reported symptom is an abrupt neurological deficit preceded by a sudden, severe, ipsilateral headache or neck–face pain.[162] Patients may also develop an incomplete Horner's syndrome (ptosis and miosis without facial sweating) or a lower cranial nerve palsy, secondary to nerve compression by an intramural hematoma.[163]

Because prodromal symptoms are common, prompt recognition and timely treatment is of the utmost importance.[164,165] Systemic anticoagulation is the initial treatment for carotid dissection and is administered to patients who do not have radiographic evidence of intracranial bleeding or massive infarction. In the majority of patients, there is gradual restoration of the arterial lumen over time.[166] Anticoagulation is thought to reduce the risk of embolization and to prevent extension of thrombus and is usually continued for 3 to 6 months or until the carotid artery recanalizes.[167] Surgical treatment, such as carotid resection with graft interposition or carotid ligation with or without extracranial–intracranial bypass, is indicated only in patients who develop progressive or recurrent neurological symptoms despite adequate anticoagulation.

Arteriopathies Affecting the Carotid Vessels

Takayasu's Arteritis

Takayasu's disease is an arteriopathy of unknown etiology that affects the major branches of the aorta and the pulmonary artery. Patients are typically young to middle-aged females, often of Asian descent. The early phase of Takayasu's disease is characterized by nonspecific symptoms such as headache, malaise, myalgia, and fever. As the disease progresses, segmental stenoses or occlusions occur in the arteries branching from the aortic arch. When subclavian arteries are involved, extremity pulses may be absent. When the common carotid arteries are affected, cerebral ischemia may result.

It is generally agreed that corticosteroids should be administered as the initial therapy for symptomatic disease. One-third of symptomatic patients require surgery for ischemic complications. Bypass is considered the procedure of choice. Percutaneous transluminal stenting has been useful in treating selected patients but the long-term durability needs to be understood before elective stenting is applied indiscriminately to young patients.[168]

Temporal Arteritis

Temporal arteritis, also known as giant cell arteritis, is a disease of unknown etiology affecting predominantly older women. Symptoms associated with temporal arteritis result from the gradual occlusion of the branches of the carotid and vertebral arteries. In the early stages of the disease, there is low-grade fever, malaise, myalgia, and headache. After 1 to 3 weeks, jaw claudication and tenderness or erythema of the temporal artery develop. Approximately 50% of patients have polymyalgia rheumatica with pain and stiffness involving the pectoral and pelvic muscles. The most serious complication of temporal arteritis is loss of vision. The erythrocyte sedimentation rate is almost always elevated and provides an accurate measure of disease activity. Once the diagnosis of temporal arteritis is made, usually by temporal artery biopsy, steroids should be immediately administered. Unlike Takayasu's disease, steroids are highly effective in treating the complications of temporal arteritis and surgical intervention is almost never required.

Radiation-Induced Arteritis

Patients who have received irradiation for treatment of malignancies are at risk for the later development of radiation-induced carotid artery occlusive disease.[169] Lesions related to a radiation injury are morphologically indistinguishable from those of atherosclerosis and are frequently associated with cerebrovascular symptoms. It is unclear whether irradiation induces atherosclerosis or accelerates its formation in susceptible individuals. Lesions are limited to the irradiated areas and, in contrast to atherosclerotic disease, frequently are isolated to the common carotid artery.

Extensive changes occur in the entire arterial wall, particularly if the radiation injury is more than 5 years old. As such, it may be difficult to establish a plane in the vessel wall, thereby precluding endarterectomy. Radiation injury can cause extensive skin changes or atrophy, resulting in wound complications following CEA. Despite these concerns, in a recent large series of patients treated for radiation-induced carotid stenoses, 20 of 26 carotid arteries were successfully treated with CEA; only 2 patients required bypass grafting. There were no strokes or wound complications in this series.[165] Thus, although technically more demanding, CEA has been successfully used to treat irradiated stenotic carotid arteries.[170,171]

Conclusion

A wide spectrum of pathology including atherosclerosis, aneurysmal disease, dysplasias, and arteriopathies can affect the cerebrovascular circulation. Atherosclerosis of the carotid bifurcation, however, is the most common lesion that produces symptoms. Carotid endarterectomy remains the most effective treatment. However, carotid angioplasty and stenting have demonstrated favorable results, particularly in patients considered to be at increased risk for endarterectomy. The success of each procedure is dependent on many variables but most importantly on the technical expertise of the surgeon performing the operation. The evolution of the surgical treatment of carotid artery stenosis has substantially reduced the enormous burden of stroke upon society.

References

1. Wilson SE, Mayberg MR, Yatsu F, et al. Crescendo transient ischemic attacks: a surgical imperative. J Vasc Surg 1993;17:249–256.
2. Gertler JP, Blankensteijn JD, Brewster DC, et al. Carotid endarterectomy for unstable and compelling neurologic conditions: do results justify an aggressive approach? J Vasc Surg 1994;19:32–42.
3. Mentzer RM Jr, Finkelmeier BA, Crosby IK, et al. Emergency carotid endarterectomy for fluctuating neurologic deficits. Surgery (St. Louis) 1981;89:60–66.
4. Barnett HJ, Plum F, Walton JN. Carotid endarterectomy: an expression of concern. Stroke 1984;15:941–943.
5. Winslow CM, Solomon DH, Chassin MR, et al. The appropriateness of carotid endarterectomy. N Engl J Med 1988;318:721–727.
6. North American Symptomatic Carotid Endarterectomy Trial Collaborators. Beneficial effect of carotid endarterectomy in symptomatic patients with high-grade carotid stenosis. N Engl J Med 1991;325:445–453.
7. Barnett HJ, Taylor DW, Eliasziw M, et al. Benefit of carotid endarterectomy in patients with symptomatic moderate or severe stenosis. North American Symptomatic Carotid Endarterectomy Trial Collaborators. N Engl J Med 1998;339:1415–1425.
8. Streifler JY, Eliasziw M, Benavente OR, et al. The risk of stroke in patients with first-ever retinal vs. hemispheric transient ischemic attacks and high-grade carotid stenosis. Arch Neurol 1995;52:246–249.
9. Eliasziw M, Streifler JY, Fox AJ, et al. Significance of plaque ulceration in symptomatic patients with high-grade carotid stenosis. Stroke 1994;25:304–308.
10. Executive Committee for the Asymptomatic Carotid Atherosclerosis Study. Endarterectomy for asymptomatic carotid artery stenosis. JAMA 1995;273:1421–1428.
11. Norris JW, Zhu CZ, Bornstein NM, et al. Vascular risks of asymptomatic carotid stenosis. Stroke 1991;22:1485–1490.
12. Moore DJ, Miles RD, Gooley NA, et al. Noninvasive assessment of stroke risk in asymptomatic and nonhemispheric patients with suspected carotid disease: five-year follow-up of 294 unoperated and 81 operated patients. Ann Surg 1985;202:491–504.
13. Roederer GO, Langlois YE, Jager KA, et al. The natural history of carotid arterial disease in asymptomatic patients with cervical bruits. Stroke 1984;15:605–613.
14. Dixon S, Pais SO, Raviola C, et al. Natural history of nonstenotic, asymptomatic ulcerative lesions of the carotid artery: a further analysis. Arch Surg 1982;117:1493–1498.
15. Perry JR, Szalai JP, Norris JW. Consensus against both endarterectomy and routine screening for asymptomatic carotid artery stenosis. Arch Neurol 1997;54:25–28.
16. Barnett HJM, Meldrum HE, Eliasziw M. The dilemma of surgical treatment for patients with asymptomatic carotid disease. Ann Intern Med 1995;123:723–725.
17. Cronenwett JL, Birkmeyer JD, Nackman GB, et al. Cost-effectiveness of carotid endarterectomy in asymptomatic patients. J Vasc Surg 1997;25:298–311.
18. Kuntz KM, Kent KC. Is carotid endarterectomy cost-effective? An analysis of symptomatic and asymptomatic patients. Circulation 1996;94:II-194–II-198.
19. Mattos MA, van Bemmelen PS, Hodgson KJ, et al. The influence of carotid siphon stenosis on short- and long-term outcome after carotid endarterectomy. J Vasc Surg 1993;17:902–911.
20. Mackey WC, O'Donnell TF Jr, Callow AD. Carotid endarterectomy in patients with intracranial vascular disease: short-term risk and long-term outcome. J Vasc Surg 1989;10:432–438.
21. Lord RS, Raj TB, Graham AR. Carotid endarterectomy, siphon stenosis, collateral hemispheric pressure, and perioperative cerebral infarction. J Vasc Surg 1987;6:391–397.
22. Schuler JJ, Flanigan DP, Lim LT, et al. The effect of carotid siphon stenosis on stroke rate, death, and relief of symptoms following elective carotid endarterectomy. Surgery (St. Louis) 1982;92:1058–1067.
23. Mackey WC, O'Donnell TF, Callow AD. Carotid endarterectomy contralateral to an occluded carotid artery: perioperative risk and late results. J Vasc Surg 1990;11:778–785.
24. Perler BA, Burdick JF, Williams GM. Does contralateral internal carotid artery occlusion increase the risk of carotid endarterectomy? J Vasc Surg 1992;16:347–353.
25. Aungst M, Gahtan V, Berkowitz H, et al. Carotid endarterectomy outcome is not affected in patients with a contralateral carotid artery occlusion. Am J Surg 1998;176:30–33.
26. Mattos MA, Barkmeier LD, Hodgson KJ, et al. Internal carotid artery occlusion: operative risks and long-term stroke rates after contralateral carotid endarterectomy. Surgery (St. Louis) 1992;112:670–680.
27. Morgenstern LB, Fox AJ, Sharpe BL, et al. The risks and benefits of carotid endarterectomy in patients with near occlusion of the carotid artery. Neurology 1997;48:911–915.
28. Archie JP Jr. Carotid endarterectomy when the distal internal carotid artery is small or poorly visualized. J Vasc Surg 1994;19:23–31.
29. Giordano JM, Trout HH III, Kozloff L, et al. Timing of carotid artery endarterectomy after stroke. J Vasc Surg 1985;2:250–255.
30. Dosick SM, Whalen RC, Gale SS, et al. Carotid endarterectomy in the stroke patient: computerized axial tomography to determine timing. J Vasc Surg 1985;2:214–219.
31. Whittemore AD, Mannick JA. Surgical treatment of carotid disease in patients with neurologic deficits. J Vasc Surg 1987;5:910–913.
32. Piotrowski JJ, Bernhard VM, Rubin JR, et al. Timing of carotid endarterectomy after acute stroke. J Vasc Surg 1990;11:45–52.

33. Salasidis GC, Latter DA, Steinmetz OK, et al. Carotid artery duplex scanning in preoperative assessment for coronary artery revascularization: the association between peripheral vascular disease, carotid artery stenosis, and stroke. J Vasc Surg 1995;21:154–162.
34. Hertzer NR, Beven EG, Young JR, et al. Coronary artery disease in peripheral vascular patients: a classification of 1000 coronary angiograms and results of surgical management. Ann Surg 1984;199:223–333.
35. Hertzer NR, Loop FD, Beven EG, et al. Surgical staging for simultaneous coronary and carotid disease: a study including prospective randomization. J Vasc Surg 1989;9:455–463.
36. Brener BJ, Hermans H, Eisenbud D, et al. The management of patients requiring coronary bypass and carotid endarterectomy. In: Moore WS, ed. Surgery for Cerebrovascular Disease. Philadelphia: Saunders 1996:278–287.
37. Cinat M, Lane CT, Pham H, et al. Helical CT angiography in the preoperative evaluation of carotid artery stenosis. J Vasc Surg 1998;28:290–300.
38. Fillinger MF, Baker RJ Jr, Zwolak RM, et al. Carotid duplex criteria for a 60% or greater angiographic stenosis: variation according to equipment. J Vasc Surg 1996;24:856–864.
39. Nicholas GG, Osborne MA, Jaffe JW, et al. Carotid artery stenosis: preoperative noninvasive evaluation in a community hospital. J Vasc Surg 1995;22:9–16.
40. Dawson DL, Zierler RE, Strandness DE, et al. The role of duplex scanning and arteriography before carotid endarterectomy: a prospective study. J Vasc Surg 1993;18:673–683.
41. Muto PM, Welch HJ, Mackey WC, et al. Evaluation of carotid artery stenosis: is duplex ultrasonography sufficient? J Vasc Surg 1996;24:17–24.
42. Goodson SF, Flanigan P, Bishara RA, et al. Can carotid duplex scanning supplant arteriography in patients with focal carotid territory symptoms? J Vasc Surg 1987;5:551–557.
43. Dawson DL, Roseberry CA, Fujitani RM. Preoperative testing before carotid endarterectomy: a survey of vascular surgeons' attitudes. Ann Vasc Surg 1997;11:264–272.
44. Turnipseed WD, Kennell TW, Turski PA, et al. Combined use of duplex imaging and magnetic resonance angiography for evaluation of patients with symptomatic ipsilateral high-grade carotid stenosis. J Vasc Surg 1993;17:832–840.
45. Patel MR, Kuntz KM, Klufas RA, et al. Preoperative assessment of the carotid bifurcation: can magnetic resonance angiography and duplex ultrasonography replace contrast arteriography? Stroke 1995;26:1753–1758.
46. Kent KC, Kuntz KM, Patel MR, et al. Perioperative imaging strategies for carotid endarterectomy: an analysis of morbidity and cost-effectiveness in symptomatic patients. JAMA 1995;274: 888–893.
47. Kucey DS, Bowyer B, Iron K, et al. Determinants of outcome after carotid endarterectomy. J Vasc Surg 1998;28:1051–1058.
48. Rubin JR, Pitluk HC, King TA, et al. Carotid endarterectomy in a metropolitan community: the early results after 8535 operations. J Vasc Surg 1988;7:256–260.
49. Mattos MA, Modi JR, Mansour AM, et al. Evolution of carotid endarterectomy in two community hospitals: Springfield revisited—seventeen years and 2243 operations later. J Vasc Surg 1995;21:719–728.
50. Skillman JJ, Kent KC, Anninos E. Do neck incisions influence nerve deficits after carotid endarterectomy? Arch Surg 1994;129: 748–752.
51. Ballotta E, Da Giau G, Saladini M, et al. Carotid endarterectomy with patch closure versus carotid eversion endarterectomy and reimplantation: a prospective randomized study. Surgery (St. Louis) 1999;125:271–279.
52. Shah DM, Darling RC, Chang BB, et al. Carotid endarterectomy by eversion technique: its safety and durability. Ann Surg 1998;228:471–478.
53. Cao P, Giordano G, De Rango P, et al. A randomized study on eversion versus standard carotid endarterectomy: study design and preliminary results: the Everest Trial. J Vasc Surg 1998; 27:595–605.
54. Entz L, Jaranyi Z, Nemes A. Comparison of perioperative results obtained with carotid eversion endarterectomy and with conventional patch plasty. Cardiovasc Surg 1997;5: 16–20.
55. Vanmaele RG, Van Schil PE, DeMaeseneer MG, et al. Division-endarterectomy-anastomosis of the internal carotid artery: a prospective randomized comparative study. Cardiovasc Surg 1994;2:573–581.
56. Kieny R, Hirsch D, Seiller C, et al. Does carotid eversion endarterectomy and reimplantation reduce the risk of restenosis? Ann Vasc Surg 1993;7:407–413.
57. Fiorani P, Sbarigia E, Speziale F, et al. General anaesthesia versus cervical block and perioperative complications in carotid artery surgery. Eur J Vasc Endovasc Surg 1997;13:37–42.
58. Ombrellaro MP, Freeman MB, Stevens SL, et al. Effect of anesthetic technique on cardiac morbidity following carotid artery surgery. Am J Surg 1996;171:387–390.
59. Rockman CB, Riles TS, Gold M, et al. A comparison of regional and general anesthesia in patients undergoing carotid endarterectomy. J Vasc Surg 1996;24:946–956.
60. Shah DM, Darling RC, Chang BB, et al. Carotid endarterectomy in awake patients: its safety, acceptability, and outcome. J Vasc Surg 1994;19:1015–1020.
61. Allen BT, Anderson CB, Rubin BG, et al. The influence of anesthetic technique on perioperative complications after carotid endarterectomy. J Vasc Surg 1994;19:834–843.
62. Becquemin JP, Paris E, Valverde A, et al. Carotid surgery: is regional anesthesia always appropriate? J Cardiovasc Surg 1991;32:592–598.
63. Bergeron P, Benichou H, Rudondy P, et al. Stroke prevention during carotid surgery in high risk patients (value of transcranial Doppler and local anesthesia). J Cardiovasc Surg 1991;32:713–719.
64. Forssell C, Takolander R, Bergqvist D, et al. Local versus general anaesthesia in carotid surgery: a prospective, randomized study. Eur J Vasc Surg 1989;3:503–509.
65. Godin MS, Bell WH, Schwedler M, et al. Cost-effectiveness of regional anesthesia in carotid endarterectomy. Am Surg 1989;55:656–659.
66. Palmer MA. Comparison of regional and general anesthesia for carotid endarterectomy. Am J Surg 1989;157:329–330.
67. Corson JD, Chang BB, Shah DM, et al. The influence of anesthetic choice on carotid endarterectomy outcome. Arch Surg 1987;122:807–812.
68. Muskett A, McGreevy J, Miller M. Detailed comparison of regional and general anesthesia for carotid endarterectomy. Am J Surg 1986;691–694.
69. Gabelman CG, Gann DS, Ashworth CJ, et al. One hundred carotid reconstructions: local versus general anesthesia. Am J Surg 1983;145:477–482.
70. Peitzman AB, Webster MW, Loubeau J, et al. Carotid endarterectomy under regional (conductive) anesthesia. Ann Surg 1982;196:59–64.
71. Andersen CA, Rich NM, Collins GJ, et al. Carotid endarterectomy: regional versus general anesthesia. Am Surg 1980;48:323–327.
72. Hafner CD, Evans WE. Carotid endarterectomy with local anesthesia: results and advantages. J Vasc Surg 1988;7:232–239.
73. Moore WS, Yee JM, Hall AD. Collateral cerebral blood pressure: an index of tolerance to temporary carotid occlusion. Arch Surg 1973;106:521–523.
74. Baker WH, Littooy FN, Hayes AC, et al. Carotid endarterectomy without a shunt: the control series. J Vasc Surg 1984;1: 50–56.

75. Whittemore AD, Kauffman JL, Kohler TR, et al. Routine electroencephalographic (EEG) monitoring during carotid endarterectomy. Ann Surg 1983;197:707–713.
76. Plestis KA, Loubser P, Mizrahi EM, et al. Continuous electroencephalographic monitoring and selective shunting reduces neurologic morbidity rates in carotid endarterectomy. J Vasc Surg 1997;25:620–628.
77. Evans WE, Hayes JP, Waltke EA, et al. Optimal cerebral monitoring during carotid endarterectomy: neurologic response under local anesthesia. J Vasc Surg 1985;2:775–777.
78. Cao P, Giordano G, Zannetti S, et al. Transcranial doppler monitoring during carotid endarterectomy: is it appropriate for selecting patients in need of a shunt? J Vasc Surg 1997;26:973–980.
79. Kearse LA Jr, Brown EN, McPeck K. Somatosensory evoked potentials sensitivity relative to electroencephalography for cerebral ischemia during carotid endarterectomy. Stroke 1992;23:498–505.
80. Nene S, Moore W. The role of patch angioplasty in prevention of early recurrent carotid stenosis. Ann Vasc Surg 1999;13:169–171.
81. AbuRahma AF, Robinson PA, Saiedy S, et al. Prospective randomized trial of carotid endarterectomy with primary closure and patch angioplasty with saphenous vein, jugular vein, and polytetrafluoroethylene: long-term follow-up. J Vasc Surg 1998;27:222–234.
82. Desiron Q, Detry O, Van Damme H, et al. Comparison of results of carotid artery surgery after either direct closure or use of a vein patch. Cardiovasc Surg 1997;5:295–303.
83. Allen PJ, Jackson MR, O'Donnell SD, et al. Saphenous vein versus polytetrafluoroethylene carotid patch angioplasty. Am J Surg 1997;174:115–117.
84. Katz SG, Kohl RD. Does the choice of material influence early morbidity in patients undergoing carotid patch angioplasty? Surgery (St. Louis) 1996;119:297–301.
85. Goldman KA, Su WT, Riles TS, et al. A comparative study of saphenous vein, internal jugular vein, and knitted Dacron patches for carotid artery endarterectomy. Ann Vasc Surg 1995;9:71–79.
86. Katz D, Snyder SO, Gandhi RH, et al. Long-term follow-up for recurrent stenosis: a prospective randomized study of expanded polytetrafluoroethylene patch angioplasty versus primary closure after carotid endarterectomy. J Vasc Surg 1994;19:198–205.
87. Myers SI, Valentine RJ, Chervu A, et al. Saphenous vein patch versus primary closure for carotid endarterectomy: long-term assessment of a randomized prospective study. J Vasc Surg 1994;19:15–22.
88. Gonzalez-Fajardo JA, Perez JL, Mateo AM. Saphenous vein patch versus polytetrafluoroethylene patch after carotid endarterectomy. J Cardiovasc Surg 1994;35:523–528.
89. Treiman RL, Foran RF, Wagner WH, et al. Does routine patch angioplasty after carotid endarterectomy lessen the risk of perioperative stroke? Ann Vasc Surg 1993;7:317–319.
90. Ranaboldo CJ, Barros D'Sa AAB, Bell PRF, et al. Randomized controlled trial of patch angioplasty for carotid endarterectomy. Br J Surg 1993;80:1528–1530.
91. De Letter JAM, Moll FL, Welten RJT, et al. Benefits of carotid patching: a prospective randomized study with long-term follow-up. Ann Vasc Surg 1993;8:54–58.
92. Whereatt N, Burke K, Littooy FN, et al. An evaluation of external jugular vein patch angioplasty after carotid endarterectomy. Am Surg 1990;56:455–459.
93. Rosenthal D, Archie JP, Garcia-Rinaldi R, et al. Carotid patch angioplasty: immediate and long-term results. J Vasc Surg 1990;12:326–333.
94. Lord RSA, Raj TB, Stary DL, et al. Comparison of saphenous vein patch, polytetrafluoroethylene patch, and direct arteriotomy closure after carotid endarterectomy. Part I: perioperative results. J Vasc Surg 1989;9:521–529.
95. Katz MM, Jones GT, Degenhardt J, et al. The use of patch angioplasty to alter the incidence of carotid restenosis following thromboendarterectomy. J Cardiovasc Surg 1987;28:2–8.
96. Ouriel K, Green RM. Clinical and technical factors influencing recurrent carotid stenosis and occlusion after endarterectomy. J Vasc Surg 1987;5:702–706.
97. Hertzer NR, Beven EG, O'Hara PJ, et al. A prospective study of vein patch angioplasty during carotid endarterectomy: three-year results for 801 patients and 917 operations. Ann Surg 1987;206:628–635.
98. Fode NC, Sundt TM, Robertson JT, et al. Multicenter retrospective review of results and complications of carotid endarterectomy in 1981. Stroke 1986;17:370–376.
99. Courbier R, Jausseran J, Reggi M, et al. Routine intraoperative carotid angiography: its impact on operative morbidity and carotid restenosis. J Vasc Surg 1986;3:343–350.
100. Donaldson MC, Ivarsson BL, Mannick JA, et al. Impact of completion angiography on operative conduct and results of carotid endarterectomy. Ann Surg 1993;217:682–687.
101. Baker WH, Koustas G, Burke K, et al. Intraoperative duplex scanning and late carotid artery stenosis. J Vasc Surg 1994;19:829–833.
102. Westerband A, Mills JL, Berman SS, et al. The influence of routine completion arteriography on outcome following carotid endarterectomy. Ann Vasc Surg 1997;11:14–19.
103. Scott SM, Sethi GK, Bridgman AH. Perioperative stroke during carotid endarterectomy: the value of intraoperative angiography. J Cardiovasc Surg (Torino) 1982;23:353–358.
104. Barnes RW, Nix ML, Wingo JP, et al. Recurrent versus residual carotid stenosis: incidence detected by doppler ultrasound. Ann Surg 1986;203:652–660.
105. Sanders EACM, Hoeneveld H, Eikelboom BC, et al. Residual lesions and early recurrent stenosis after carotid endarterectomy: a serial follow-up study with duplex scanning and intravenous digital subtraction angiography. J Vasc Surg 1987;5:731–737.
106. Bandyk DF, Kaebnick HW, Adams MB, et al. Turbulence occurring after carotid bifurcation endarterectomy: a harbinger of residual and recurrent carotid stenosis. J Vasc Surg 1988;7:261–274.
107. Kinney EV, Seabrook GR, Kinney LY, et al. The importance of intraoperative detection of residual flow abnormalities after carotid artery endarterectomy. J Vasc Surg 1993;17:912–923.
108. O'Brien MS, Ricotta JJ. Conserving resources after carotid endarterectomy: selective use of the intensive care unit. J Vasc Surg 1991;14:796–802.
109. Hirko MK, Morasch MD, Burke K, et al. The changing face of carotid endarterectomy. J Vasc Surg 1996;23:622–627.
110. Kraiss LW, Kilberg L, Critch S, et al. Short-stay carotid endarterectomy is safe and cost-effective. Am J Surg 1995;169:512–515.
111. Back MR, Harward TRS, Huber TS, et al. Improving the cost-effectiveness of carotid endarterectomy. J Vasc Surg 1997;26:456–464.
112. Ouriel K, Shortell CK, Illig KA, et al. Intracerebral hemorrhage after carotid endarterectomy: incidence, contribution to neurologic morbidity, and predictive factors. J Vasc Surg 1999;29:82–89.
113. Hafner DH, Smith RB III, King OW, et al. Massive intracerebral hemorrhage following carotid endarterectomy. Arch Surg 1987;122:305–307.
114. Pomposelli FB, Lamparello PJ, Riles TS, et al. Intracranial hemorrhage after carotid endarterectomy. J Vasc Surg 1988;7:248–255.

115. Skydell JL, Machleder HI, Baker JD, et al. Incidence and mechanism of post-carotid endarterectomy hypertension. Arch Surg 1987;122:1153–1155.
116. Wong JH, Findlay JM, Suarez-Almazor ME. Hemodynamic instability after carotid endarterectomy: risk factors and associations with operative complications. Neurosurgery 1997;41:35–43.
117. Schauber MD, Fontenelle LJ, Solomon JW, et al. Cranial/cervical nerve dysfunction after carotid endarterectomy. J Vasc Surg 1997;25:481–487.
118. Zannetti S, Parente B, De Rango P, et al. Role of surgical techniques and operative findings in cranial and cervical nerve injuries during carotid endarterectomy. Eur J Vasc Endovasc Surg 1998;15:528–531.
119. Ballotta E, Da Giau G, Renon L, et al. Cranial and cervical nerve injuries after carotid endarterectomy: a prospective study. Surgery (St. Louis) 1999;125:85–91.
120. Clagett GP, Robinowitz M, Youkey JR, et al. Morphogenesis and clinicopathologic characteristics of recurrent carotid disease. J Vasc Surg 1986;3:10–23.
121. Clagett GP, Rich NM, McDonald PT, et al. Etiologic factors for recurrent carotid artery stenosis. Surgery (St. Louis) 1983;93:313–318.
122. Reilly LM, Okuhn SP, Rapp JH, et al. Recurrent carotid stenosis: a consequence of local or systemic factors? The influence of unrepaired defects. J Vasc Surg 1990;11:448–460.
123. Ouriel K, Green RM. Appropriate frequency of carotid duplex testing following carotid endarterectomy. Am J Surg 1995; 170:144–147.
124. Golledge J, Cuming R, Ellis M, et al. Clinical follow-up rather than duplex surveillance after carotid endarterectomy. J Vasc Surg 1997;25:55–63.
125. Patel ST, Kuntz KM, Kent KC. Is routine duplex ultrasound surveillance after carotid endarterectomy cost-effective? Surgery (St. Louis) 1998;124:343–352.
126. Cook JM, Thompson BW, Barnes RW, et al. Is routine duplex examination after carotid endarterectomy justified? J Vasc Surg 1990;12:334–340.
127. Mattos MA, van Bemmelen PS, Barkmeier LD, et al. Routine surveillance after carotid endarterectomy: does it affect clinical management? J Vasc Surg 1993;17:819–831.
128. Roubin GS, New G, Iyer SS, et al. Immediate and late clinical outcomes of carotid artery stenting in patients with symptomatic and asymptomatic carotid artery stenosis: a 5-year prospective analysis. Circulation 2001;103:532–538.
129. Wholey MH, Al-Mubarek N, Wholey MH. Updated review of the global carotid artery stent registry. Catheter Cardiovasc Interv 2003;60:259–260.
130. Yadev JS, Wholey MH, Kuntz RE, et al, for the SAPPHIRE trial investigators. Protected carotid-artery stenting versus endarterectomy in high risk patients. N Engl J Med 2004;351:1493–1501.
131. Gray WA for the ARCHeR Executive Committee. Prospective clinical trials for carotid stenting with embolic protection in high surgical risk patients. Am Coll Cardiol 2004.
132. Hobson RW II for the CREST investigators. Update on the carotid revascularization endoarterectomy versus stent trial (CREST) protocol. J Am Coll Surg 2002;194 (I suppl):S9–14.
133. Berguer R. Long-term results of reconstructions of the vertebral artery. In: Yao JST, Pearce WH, eds. Long-Term Results in Vascular Surgery. Norwalk: Appleton & Lange, 1993:69–80.
134. Berguer R, Morasch MD, Kline RA. A review of 100 consecutive reconstructions of the distal vertebral artery for embolic and hemodynamic disease. J Vasc Surg 1998;27:852–859.
135. Perler BA, Williams GM. Carotid-subclavian bypass: a decade of experience. J Vasc Surg 1990;12:716–723.
136. Edwards WH Jr, Tapper SS, Edwards WH Sr, et al. Subclavian revascularization: a quarter century experience. Ann Surg 1994;219:673–678.
137. Burke DR, Gordon RL, Mishkin JD, et al. Percutaneous transluminal angioplasty of subclavian arteries. Radiology 1987;164:699–704.
138. Cote R, Barnett HJ, Taylor DW. Internal carotid occlusion: a prospective study. Stroke 1983;14:898–902.
139. Nicholls SC, Kohler TR, Bergelin RO, et al. Carotid artery occlusion: natural history. J Vasc Surg 1986;4:479–485.
140. The EC/IC Bypass Study Group. Failure of extracranial-intracranial arterial bypass to reduce the risk of ischemic stroke: results of an international randomized trial. N Engl J Med 1985;313:1191–1200.
141. Okada Y, Shima T, Nishida M, et al. Effectiveness of superficial temporal artery-middle cerebral artery anastomosis in adult moyamoya disease: cerebral hemodynamics and clinical course in ischemic and hemorrhagic varieties. Stroke 1998;29:625–630.
142. Grubb RL Jr, Derdeyn CP, Fritsch SM, et al. Importance of hemodynamic factors in the prognosis of symptomatic carotid occlusion. JAMA 1998;280:1055–1060.
143. Klijn CJ, Kappelle LJ, Tulleken CA, et al. Symptomatic carotid artery occlusion: a reappraisal of hemodynamic factors. Stroke 1997;28:2084–2093.
144. Gertler JP, Cambria RP. The role of external carotid endarterectomy in the treatment of ipsilateral internal carotid occlusion: collective review. J Vasc Surg 1987;6:158–167.
145. de Jong KP, Zondervan PE, van Urk H. Extracranial carotid artery aneurysms. Eur J Vasc Surg 1989;3:557–562.
146. Painter TA, Hertzer NR, Beven EG, et al. Extracranial carotid aneurysms: report of six cases and review of the literature. J Vasc Surg 1985;2:312–318.
147. Zwolak RM, Whitehouse WM Jr, Knake JE, et al. Atherosclerotic extracranial carotid artery aneurysms. J Vasc Surg 1984;1:415–422.
148. Faggioli G, Freyrie A, Stella A, et al. Extracranial internal carotid artery aneurysms: results of a surgical series with long-term follow-up. J Vasc Surg 1996;23:587–595.
149. May J, White GH, Waugh R, et al. Endoluminal repair of internal carotid artery aneurysm: a feasible but hazardous procedure. J Vasc Surg 1997;26:1055–1060.
150. Westerband A, Hunter GC, Cintora I, et al. Current trends in the detection and management of carotid body tumors. J Vasc Surg 1998;28:84–93.
151. Muhm M, Polterauer P, Gstottner W, et al. Diagnostic and therapeutic approaches to carotid body tumors: review of 24 patients. Arch Surg 1997;132:279–284.
152. Hallett JW, Nora JD, Hollier LH, et al. Trends in neurovascular complications of surgical management for carotid body and cervical paragangliomas: a fifty-year experience with 153 tumors. J Vasc Surg 1988;7:284–291.
153. LaMuraglia GM, Fabian RL, Brewster DC, et al. The current surgical management of carotid body paragangliomas. J Vasc Surg 1992;15:1038–1045.
154. Cloft HJ, Kallmes DF, Kallmes MH, et al. Prevalence of cerebral aneurysms in patients with fibromuscular dysplasia: a reassessment. J Neurosurg 1998;88:436–440.
155. Moreau P, Albat B, Thevenet A. Fibromuscular dysplasia of the internal carotid artery: long-term surgical results. J Cardiovasc Surg 1993;34:465–472.
156. Effeney DJ, Ehrenfeld WK, Stoney RJ, et al. Why operate on carotid fibromuscular dysplasia? Arch Surg 1980;115:1261–1265.
157. Ballotta E, Abbruzzese E, Thiene G, et al. The elongation of the internal carotid artery: early and long-term results of patients having surgery compared with unoperated controls. Ann Vasc Surg 1997;11:120–128.
158. Fearn SJ, McCollum CN. Shortening and reimplantation for tortuous internal carotid arteries. J Vasc Surg 1998;27:936–939.

159. Poindexter JM, Patel KR, Clauss RH. Management of kinked extracranial cerebral arteries. J Vasc Surg 1987;6:127–133.
160. Coyle KA, Smith RB, Chapman RL, et al. Carotid artery shortening: a safe adjunct to carotid endarterectomy. J Vasc Surg 1995;22:257–263.
161. Kumar SD, Kumar V, Kaye W. Bilateral internal carotid artery dissection from vomiting. Am J Emerg Med 1998;16:669–670.
162. Silbert PL, Mokri B, Schievink WI. Headache and neck pain in spontaneous internal carotid and vertebral artery dissections. Neurology 1995;45:1517–1522.
163. Mokri B, Silbert PL, Schievink WI, et al. Cranial nerve palsy in spontaneous dissection of the extracranial internal carotid artery. Neurology 1996;46:356–359.
164. Biousse V, D'Anglejan-Chatillon J, Touboul PJ, et al. Time course of symptoms in extracranial carotid artery dissections: a series of 80 patients. Stroke 1995;26:235–239.
165. Sturzenegger M. Spontaneous internal carotid artery dissection: early diagnosis and management in 44 patients. J Neurol 1995; 242:231–238.
166. Treiman GS, Treiman RL, Foran RF, et al. Spontaneous dissection of the internal carotid artery: a nineteen-year clinical experience. J Vasc Surg 1996;24:597–607.
167. Lucas C, Moulin T, Deplanque D, et al. Stroke patterns of internal carotid artery dissection in 40 patients. Stroke 1998;29:2646–2648.
168. Sharma S, Bahl VK, Saxena A, et al. Stenosis in the aorta caused by non-specific aortitis: results of treatment by percutaneous stent placement. Clin Radiol 1999;54:46–50.
169. Moritz MW, Higgins RF, Jacobs JR. Duplex imaging and incidence of carotid radiation injury after high-dose radiotherapy for tumors of the head and neck. Arch Surg 1990;125:1181–1183.
170. Kashyap VS, Moore WS, Quinones-Baldrich WJ. Carotid artery repair for radiation-associated atherosclerosis is a safe and durable procedure. J Vasc Surg 1999;29:90–99.
171. Rockman CB, Riles TS, Fisher FS, et al. The surgical management of carotid artery stenosis in patients with previous neck irradiation. Am J Surg 1996;172:191–195.

63

Diseases of the Thoracic Aorta

Marineh Yagubian and Thoralf M. Sundt

Acute Aortic Syndromes

Advances in imaging technologies have revealed an entire spectrum of aortic disease where previously we saw only aortic dissection. The moniker "acute aortic syndrome" is now applied to aortic dissection, intramural hematoma (IMH), and penetrating atherosclerotic ulcer of the aorta (PAU).[1] Collectively, acute aortic syndromes remain highly lethal conditions for which medical therapy is imperfect and for which surgical treatment carries significant risk.

Aortic Dissection

Acute aortic dissection is the most common catastrophe of the thoracic aorta, occurring with an incidence of 10 to 20 per 1,000,000 population, exceeding rupture of abdominal aortic aneurysms as a cause of death by as much as twofold.[2] Acute onset of severe pain and potentially rapid progression of the disease to fatal rupture or visceral malperfusion dominates the clinical picture. Prompt diagnosis and aggressive institution of medical or surgical therapy are critical.

Etiology

Despite its common occurrence, little is known with certainty of the factors responsible for aortic dissection. Degenerative changes in collagen and elastin are commonly observed in dissected aorta, although their causal relationship has been questioned as such changes are normal with aging.[3,4] Biochemical analysis of age-matched aortic specimens has demonstrated abnormalities in elastin and collagen deposition among dissected aortas, suggesting that alterations in mechanical properties may play a role.[5] In vitro analysis of aneurysmal aorta has confirmed increasing stiffness and loss of residual strain.[6]

Genetic factors such as Marfan syndrome may play a role in predisposing to acute dissection. Dissections may occur in as many as one-third of Marfan's patients, even in the absence of significant aneurysmal dilatation,[7] and at a much younger age than that for non-Marfan's patients.[8] Unfortunately, data defining the risk of dissection at a given aortic diameter are lacking.[9] The genetic basis of the condition is, in most instances, one of more than 100 mutations of the fibrillin-1 gene on the short arm of chromosome 15,[10,11] although a phenotype indistinguishable from Marfan syndrome, dubbed MFS-2,[12] has been traced to mutation in the gene for transforming growth factor-beta (TGF-β) receptor type II.[13] This discovery confirms the central role of abnormal cell signaling in these conditions. Traditional thinking had focused on the structural role of fibrillin-1 in elastin deposition and engagement with adjacent endothelial or smooth muscle cells, which is necessary for maintaining the architecture of the wall and allowing for coordinated contractile and elastic functions. Indeed, without normal elastin structure, smooth muscle cells shift from a contractile to synthetic state,[14] producing matrix metalloproteinase 9 (MMP), which exacerbates thinning and fragmentation of elastic fibers as does the inflammatory cellular response that follows.[15] Further elastolysis of the wall leads to architectural collapse, and smooth muscle cell apoptosis, triggered by peroxisome proliferator-activated receptor-γ (PPAR-γ) upregulation, ensues.[16] Studies in the murine model of Marfan syndrome, however, have uncovered another mechanism whereby abnormal fibrillin may impact the extracellular matrix; in addition to a structural role, fibrillin plays a regulatory role in TGF-β signaling, with an excess of this cytokine present in Marfan tissues.[17,18] Increased hyaluronan and impaired progenitor cell recruitment as well as directional migration in association with increased TGF-β expression has been demonstrated in tissue from Marfan patients, suggesting a possible mechanism to explain the fragile tissues observed.[19]

Other heritable conditions associated with dissection include autosomal dominant Ehlers–Danlos syndrome type IV, a condition caused by a defect in procollagen III,[20] congenital contracural arachnodactyly, Noonan's syndrome, and Turner's syndrome.[21] Familial dissection without known collagen–vascular conditions is also well documented, with at least three genetic loci identified thusfar.[22–24] Bicuspid aortic valve,[25] aortic coarctation,[26] and pregnancy[21] also predispose to dissection. Given the increased number of diagnostic and therapeutic vascular and cardiac procedures, iatrogenic aortic dissection now accounts for as many as 5% of cases.[27] Unfortunately, iatrogenic type B dissections have a significantly higher mortality rate than spontaneous type B dissection, perhaps attributable to the comorbidities of those patients most susceptible to this complication.

Pathophysiology

Pathologically, aortic dissection is defined by the presence of blood within the layers of the tunica media. There is, however, uncertainty about the initiating event. An obvious intimal disruption is present in most instances,[28] leading to the hypothesis that an intimal tear occurs first, permitting entry of blood into the diseased media. The alternative hypothesis is that rupture of the vasa vasora into a diseased media is the primary event, with progression to free rupture into the lumen in the majority of patients. Containment of such a hematoma without intimal rupture explains the entity intramural hematoma discussed next.

In the acute phase, dissection is thought to rapidly progress distally from the site of intimal disruption, ending either in a blind pouch or with a reentry tear into the true lumen. The process may be limited to the ascending or descending aorta only, or may involve both. Two schemes for the classification of aortic dissections are in common use (Fig. 63.1). The more descriptive and hence complex one is that proposed by DeBakey et al. in 1965.[29] Type I dissection, which is most common, is considered most often to originate from a tear in the ascending aorta with progression through the arch into the descending thoracoabdominal aorta. There is recent evidence that the site of intimal disruption is more variable, with the most proximal tears identifiable in the arch in one-third of such cases and in the descending aorta in 7%.[30] DeBakey type II dissection is limited to the ascending aorta and is the least common, whereas type III is limited to the descending thoracic or thoracoabdominal aorta. The alternative Stanford classification is based on the natural history of the disease and the treatment strategies that have evolved.[31] Those dissections involving the ascending aorta, whether DeBakey type I or II, are designated type A, whereas those limited to the descending aorta are type B. Unusual dissections involving the arch and descending aorta, but not the ascending aorta, are designated type A.[32]

Clinical Presentation

Intense pain, often described as tearing or ripping, which is abrupt in onset occurs in 85% of patients, although occasional patients present with chronic dissection without history of such an episode.[33] The pain may be migratory, typically anterior when the ascending aorta is involved and moving to the back as the dissection progresses distally. Syncope was a presenting symptom in 13% of patients in the International Registry of Acute Dissection (IRAD) database.[34] These patients often had cardiac tamponade or stroke and more often experienced complications or death. Occasionally dissection occurs without an identifiable history of pain, a condition curiously associated with an increased mortality risk.[35]

On examination, among those with type A dissection, one-fourth of patients are hypertensive and another one-fourth hypotensive. Hypertension is present in 70% of those with type B pathology.[33] Extremity blood pressures may be quite disparate, and peripheral pulses may be absent as the false lumen compresses the true lumen. Pulses may reappear as distal reentry restores flow via the false lumen. Pulse deficit is more common with type A dissection, and portends a worse prognosis, with hospital mortality almost triple that of patients without such a deficit.[36] Malperfusion may also result in stroke, intestinal ischemia, or rarely paraplegia. Renal failure is a particularly ominous finding, with an almost fivefold increased risk of death in the IRAD database.[37] Auscultation of the heart may reveal aortic regurgitation which, if known to be acute in onset, is a highly reliable sign present in almost half of patients with type A dissection.[33]

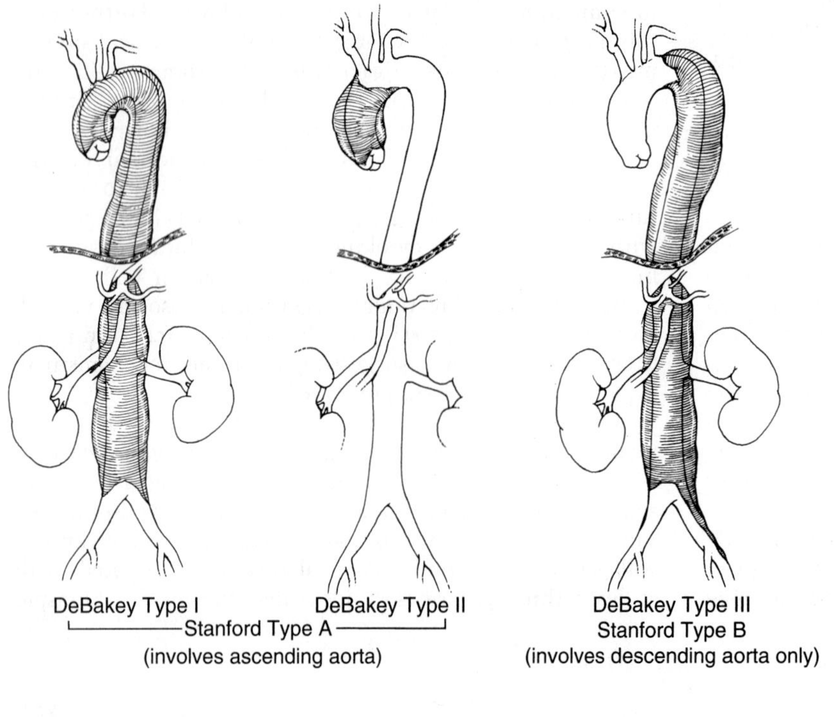

FIGURE 63.1. Two classification schemes are commonly applied to describe the extent of aortic dissection. The first, proposed by Debakey,[29] is more descriptive yet more complex. It has largely given way to the Stanford classification, which simply distinguished between those that do or do not involve the ascending aorta.[31]

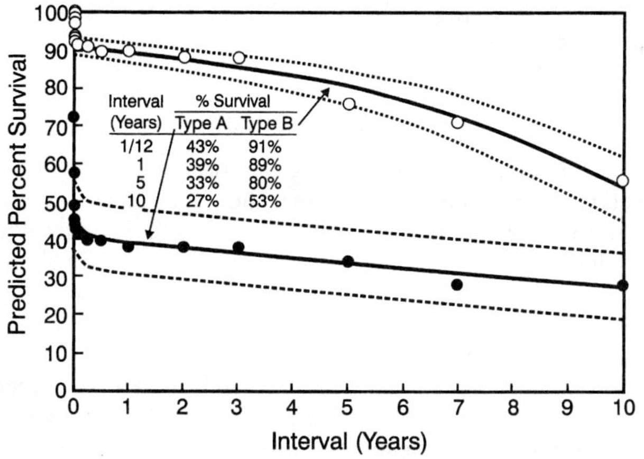

FIGURE 63.2. The natural history of acute aortic dissection involving the ascending aorta (type A) or limited to the descending aorta (type B). (Adapted from Kirklin JW, Barratt-Boyes BG. Cardiac Surgery, 2nd ed. New York: Churchill Livingstone, 1993.)

The natural history of acute dissection is dismal without treatment (Fig. 63.2). Early studies demonstrated mortality of one-third of patients within 24h and 80% within 1 week when the ascending aorta was involved leading to the mortality rule "one percent per hour."[38] Those with distal dissection have a more favorable natural history, with three-quarters surviving more than 1 month from the acute event. Rupture of the aorta into the pleural or pericardial space is responsible for three-quarters of mortalities,[31] with free rupture occurring most often adjacent to the intimal tear.[39] Myocardial infarction may occur secondary to involvement of the right coronary sinus with compression of the right coronary artery. Distal progression may create a malperfusion syndrome in as many as 30% of patients by compression of the true lumen by the false lumen.[40] The mortality rate for patients with stroke or visceral infarction secondary to malperfusion is particularly high, whether treated surgically or medically.[41]

Diagnostic Evaluation

Chest radiography will demonstrate a widened mediastinum in only one-third of patients.[33] Additionally, a left pleural effusion or enlarged cardiomediastinal silhouette may be evident. Electrocardiography may show left ventricular hypertrophy or acute inferior myocardial ischemia but is normal in up to a third of patients.[33] Unfortunately, when electrocardiography (EKG) abnormalities are present, the diagnosis of dissection may be mistaken for myocardial infarction.

The definitive diagnosis of acute aortic dissection relies on advanced imaging techniques.[42] Aortography, the traditional mode of diagnosis in the past, can demonstrate the origins of important branches and their perfusion by the true or false lumen. As such it remains particularly useful in the evaluation of the candidate for endovascular stenting or fenestration; however, it may miss conditions such as intramural hematoma and has a reported false negative rate as high as 5% to 15%.[43] As an initial diagnostic test, it has been supplanted by transesophageal echocardiography (TEE), computerized axial tomography (CT), and magnetic resonance imaging (MRI). Among these modalities, TEE is minimally invasive, highly sensitive, and provides important information regarding ventricular function and aortic valve function.[44,45] It is operator dependent, however, and requires on-site cardiology support. Because of its widespread availability, CT scanning is commonly employed as it is both more rapid and less operator dependent than other modalities. With proper image acquisition, sensitivity approaches 100% for spiral CT.[46,47] The diagnosis may be made by visualization of a dissection flap in several images, although streak artifact may be mistaken for the same (Fig. 63.3) Displacement of

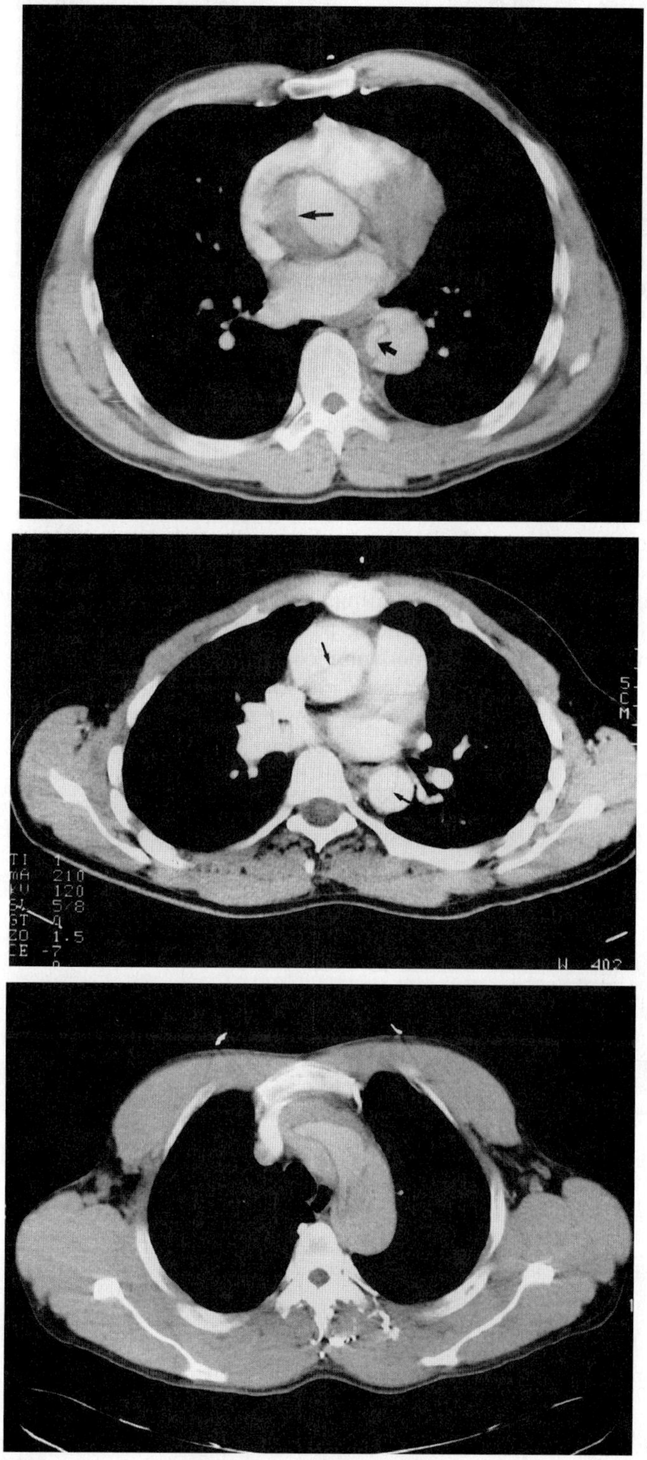

A
B
C

FIGURE 63.3. Computerized tomography of acute dissection. **A.** Thrombosis of the false lumen in the ascending aorta (*thin arrow*) and compression of the true lumen in the descending aorta (*thick arrow*). **B.** Patency of true and false lumen with an intimal flap visible in both the ascending and descending aorta (*arrows*). **C.** Complex dissection involving the arch.

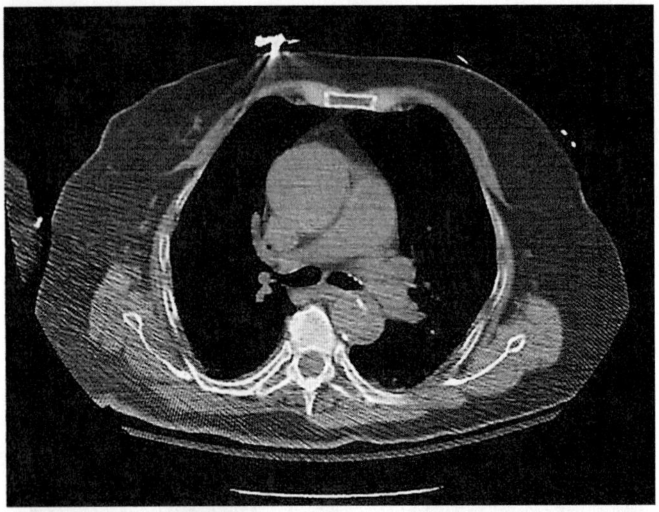

FIGURE 63.4. Displacement of intimal calcium by eccentric intramural hematoma (IMH).

intimal calcium and compression of the true lumen are helpful additional clues (Fig. 63.4).

Magnetic resonance imaging (MRI) can provide enhanced definition over CT scanning in some instances and may be better able to distinguish between blood and other fluid in and around the dissected aorta. Sagittal reconstructions of the aorta can easily be obtained as well, and the technique can provide information regarding aortic valve function; however, it is time-consuming. Its principal application is in ruling out dissection among patients with complex aortic anatomy who are hemodynamically stable. Choice among these modalities depends on the technology and expertise locally available.

Despite general interest in diagnostic biomarkers today, only a few have been explored in the setting of dissection. Serum smooth muscle myosin heavy chain is thought to have a sensitivity of 90% and specificity of 83% in differentiating between dissection and myocardial infarction.[48] Serum D-dimers are of negative predictive value, being elevated in aortic dissection but only one-third of controls.[49] Given the advances in imaging technology, however, these tests will likely have limited application.

Medical and Surgical Management

The cornerstone of pharmacological intervention in aortic dissection is the reduction of both the mean blood pressure and the rate of rise of the pulse wave (*dp*/*dt*). Therapy with beta-blockers to reduce the heart rate to 60 beats/min should be instituted as soon as the diagnosis of acute dissection is suspected. Additional blood pressure control may require nitroprusside or other vasodilators.

Immediate surgical intervention is indicated if the ascending aorta is involved. As shown in Table 63.1, although the operative risk is significant, the mortality rate for nonoperative treatment of type A dissection is even higher. There has been some recent debate over the exclusion of some subsets of particularly high-risk patients from operative treatment, such as those in shock or those with malperfusion syndrome.[37,41] Such patients are candidates for an integrated hybrid approach with endovascular stenting of branch vessels and subsequent open repair.[50,51] Although operative risk is clearly highest in these patients, with operative risk reportedly increased threefold to fivefold for those in shock preoperatively,[52,53] others have reported outstanding results with a policy of treating all acute type A dissections surgically.[54] Preoperative coronary angiography, advocated in the past,[55] has been abandoned by most surgeons today because of concern about the delay in treatment imposed.[56] Operative mortality may range from 10% to 35% depending on experience of the surgical staff and comorbidities of the patient.[33,37,57] Preoperative predictors of operative risk derived from the IRAD database include age greater than 70 years, prior cardiac surgery, hypotension or shock at presentation, migrating pain, cardiac tamponade, and evidence of malperfusion by pulse deficit, or electrocardiographic evidence of cardiac ischemia.[57]

The principal objective of surgical repair is replacement of the fragile ascending aorta, the region at greatest risk of rupture. If the aortic root and valve are significantly involved, full root replacement as described below is indicated. The

TABLE 63.1.
Management of Acute Aortic Syndromes.

			Mortality	
Entity Author	*Year*	*No. Patients*	*Medical*	*Surgical*
Acute dissection				
Ehrlich[54]	2000	124		15.3% (type A)
Hagan[33]	2000	464	58% (type A)	26% (type A)
			10.7% (type B)	31.4% (type B)
Long[53]	2003	70		18.6% (type A)
Hata[68]	2003	79	2% at 1 month (type B)	
Trimarchi[162]	2005	526		25.1% (type A)
Intramural hematoma				
Maraj (meta-analysis)[85]	2000	143	36% (type A)	14% (type A)
			14% (type B)	20% (type B)
Song[88]	2002	41 (type A)	7%	
		83 (type B)	1%	
Suzuki[163]	2003	384 (type B)	13%	
Penetrating atherosclerotic ulcer				
Cho[81]	2004	104 (type B)	4%	21%

extent of distal resection required is debatable. In the interest of extirpating as much of the diseased aorta as possible, the current trend is toward construction of an open anastomosis immediately below the innominate artery or hemiarch replacement under circulatory arrest. Resection of the entry site, even if present in the arch, in the interest of promoting thrombosis of the false lumen and improved late outcomes,[58] has long been held as an important component of the operation. Although there is logic to this approach, there is, so far, no hard evidence of improved long-term outcomes with the more radical approach.[53,59–61] Open distal anastomosis requires interruption of cerebral blood flow for at least a portion of the repair. Cerebral protection has been enhanced of late via use of retrograde cerebral perfusion (RCP)[62] or early antegrade perfusion.[63] Other recent technical modifications include use of the axillary artery for pump inflow,[64] although its superiority over femoral cannulation continues to be debated.[65]

There is general agreement that the initial management of distal dissection (DeBakey type III or Stanford B) is nonoperative. Recurrent pain suggestive of ongoing dissection, malperfusion syndrome, uncontrollable hypertension, or rupture are indications for surgical intervention. Although no prospectively randomized trials have been or are likely to be conducted,[60] early analyses of well-matched patients demonstrated no difference in acute mortality rates among surgical versus medical patients. The Duke/Stanford cooperative study included 136 patients with acute (n = 89) or chronic type B dissections treated between 1975 and 1988 at either institution.[66] At Duke, surgery was restricted to those with complications whereas earlier surgical intervention was the norm at Stanford. Fifty-six patients (63%) with acute type B dissection were treated medically while the remainder underwent acute operative procedures. Of the total 89 patients with acute type B dissection, 30 were identified who had no complications mandating surgery and in whom there was neither severe cardiac or renal disease (i.e. "good surgical risk"). Of these 30, 11 underwent surgery and 19 were treated medically. Among these patients, only age was a predictor of death. One-year survival was 94% in the medical group and 90% in the surgical group (P = NS). Cox model multivariable analysis of the entire study group identified aortic rupture, complications of dissection, increasing age, and cardiac disease—but not medical versus surgical therapy—as predictors of mortality. These data may be criticized as among unmatched patient cohorts; mortality rates may be higher among surgical patients, in part because of the distribution of high-risk patients failing medical therapy or presenting with complications who fall to this treatment group (see Table 63.1). Subsequent retrospective studies, however, have confirmed these findings using propensity analysis.[67]

Careful long-term follow-up with intervention in the chronic phase if significant aortic dilatation (more than 6.0 to 6.5 cm) occurs is critical to the late survival of these patients.[68,69] Chronic dissections, by definition those more than 14 days from the index event, should be monitored by periodic (annual or semiannual) imaging studies, with surgery indicated on the basis of the onset of symptoms or size criteria identical to those for chronic degenerative aneurysms of the descending thoracic and thoracoabdominal aorta (see following). The role of endovascular stent grafting in acute[70–73] and chronic dissection[74] is being explored currently, although apart from complicated dissection with malperfusion, there is currently no indication for such therapy in this condition.

Intramural Hematoma and Penetrating Atherosclerotic Ulcer

In addition to acute dissection, the advances of high-resolution imaging techniques have demonstrated intramural hematoma (IMH) and penetrating atherosclerotic ulcer (PAU) as causes of acute aortic syndrome. The clinical profile is similar for all these conditions, with patients presenting typically with severe, acute chest pain and, frequently, hemodynamic instability. A history of hypertension is frequent albeit not universal. These entities are linked insofar as one may lead to another, with PAU progressing to IMH and, in some instances, frank dissection as intraluminal blood is provided entry into a diseased media. Similarly, IMH can progress to dissection, although this is not always the case. Importantly, these entities may also be found incidentally in an asymptomatic patient during workup of a related or unrelated condition. These entities are classified by their timing as acute or chronic, and by their location in a manner analogous to dissection as Stanford type A or type B, depending on the involvement of the ascending aorta.

Etiology

Intramural hematoma is likely the more accurate diagnosis in 5% to 20% of patients admitted with a diagnosis of acute dissection.[75–78] The distinction depends on high-resolution imaging showing a circumferential or eccentric intramural hemorrhage in the aortic wall without intimal disruption. The latter, of course, is difficult to prove ante mortem, however.

Patients with IMH tend to be somewhat older than those with classic dissection, supporting the notion that degenerative changes in the media are of particular importance.[79] This variant is also far more often observed in the descending than ascending aorta, again in contrast to typical dissection.[78]

By definition, a PAU is an ulceration in the intima extending into the media that is frequently, but not invariably, associated with IMH.[80] Similar to IMH, PAU is more frequently observed in the descending thoracic aorta and is typically observed in the elderly patient with advanced atherosclerotic disease.[81,82] Although the true incidence of PAU is unclear, ulcers were identifiable retrospectively among 7.6% of patients admitted with a diagnosis of acute dissection in a study from the Yale University database, leading to the suggestion that they are far more commonly the cause of dissection than is currently recognized.[79]

Pathophysiogy

The most commonly cited explanation for IMH is rupture of vasa vasora with intramural hemorrhage. In those patients in whom IMH appears to progress to dissection, the intimal flap is assumed to rupture into the lumen. Among patients with PAU and IMH, the former is assumed to have led to the latter. Progression of such a complicated ulcer to contained rupture may occur secondary to disintegration of overlying medial layers.[83] Ulcers are often multiple, are relatively evenly distributed along the entire thoracic aorta, and may range in size from 2 to 25 mm in diameter and 4 to 30 mm in depth.[84] Some PAUs do not have associated IMH. Presumably medial fibrosis secondary to chronic atherosclerotic disease prevents propagation of the hematoma. PAU may lead to saccular pseudoaneurysm of the aorta.

Clinical Presentation

Clinically, patients with IMH or PAU may be indistinguishable from those with dissection. Acute, severe back pain is typical, although asymptomatic cases are identified on occasion. Malperfusion and pulse deficit are decidedly rare, however.[79] There is debate over the natural history of these entities. Although some view IMH and PAU as less malignant than dissection when the descending aorta is involved,[75,78,81,85,86] this view is not universally held.[82] Complete resolution of type B IMH in 50% to 70% of patients is well documented.[87–89] Progression to frank dissection or late aneurysm is also well documented,[83,90] however, making prediction the challenge.

Diagnostic Evaluation

The characteristic finding of IMH on axial imaging studies is a hyperdense, crescentic, or circumferential thickening of the wall with a smooth wall distinguishing it from intraluminal thrombus or atherosclerotic disease.[46] Intimal displacement of calcium also helps distinguish intramural thickening from intraluminal clot. No dissection flap or contrast enhancement should be seen. Distinguishing between IMH and acute dissection with thrombosis of the false lumen, however, may be challenging, with eccentric or circumferential thickening of the wall absent contrast enhancement and a visible dissection flap. The extent and thickness of the IMH is important for comparison with subsequent studies.

A penetrating ulcer may appear as an ulcer-like projection into the media, often with an associated pseudoaneurysm.[46] The diagnosis of PAU may be obtained through the demonstration of a contrast-filled aortic wall outpouching. Extensive aortic atherosclerosis is often obvious during the study with calcifications noted throughout the aorta. TEE of the PAU shows a crater-like ulcer with jagged edges. Angiography is not a first-choice examination for diagnosis of PAU as the ulcer may not be obvious, depending on the projection of the image obtained. Associated pleural effusion or mediastinal widening may also be apparent.

Medical and Surgical Management

Most Western authors agree that patients with type A IMH are at high risk of death without surgical intervention[83,91–93] (Fig. 63.5). In the recently published IRAD study, the acute mortality rate of IMH involving the ascending aorta was more than fourfold that for IMH involving the arch and descending thoracic aorta (42% vs. 8%).[75] Curiously, some authors from the Far East have reported excellent results with nonoperative or, at a minimum, expectant treatment of ascending IMH.[94–96] A maximum diameter less than 5.0 cm appears predictive of successful nonoperative treatment.[87,94]

There is more agreement on the management of type B IMH (see Table 63.1) Progression to dissection, aneurysm, or

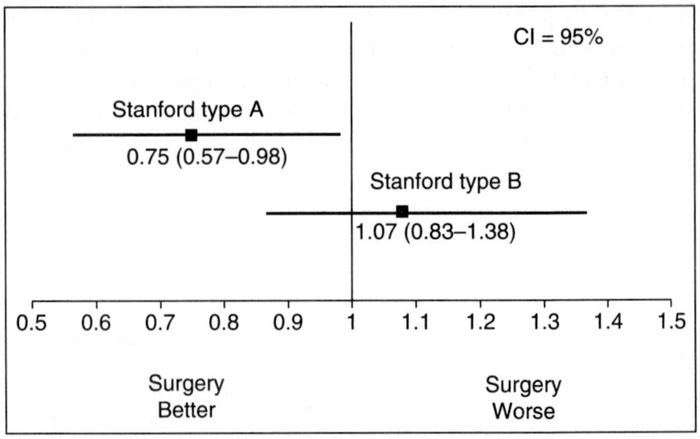

FIGURE 63.5. Outcome of surgical versus medical management of IMH. (Adapted from Maraj R, Rerkpattanapipat P, Jacobs LE, et al.,[85] by permission of American Journal of Cardiology.)

contained rupture may occur; therefore, long-term follow-up is recommended.[82,83] In-hospital mortality rates, however, are generally as low or lower than those reported for type B dissection.[75,78,92] Predictors of resolution include aortic diameter less than 4.0 to 4.5 cm,[75,87] thickness of the hematoma less than 1 cm,[75,83,97] and postoperative beta-blocker use.[83] Some authors have identified presence of a PAU as a predictor of progression as well.[76] Resolution of ulcer-associated hematoma has been reported in 85% of patients, however, in one study.[81]

Indications for surgical intervention on type B IMH include recurring, refractory chest pain and evidence of increasing extent or diameter of the hematoma. Patients should be followed over time to assure that the injured aorta does not become frankly aneurysmal. Operative repair consists of graft replacement of the involved aorta. Of particular note, when a PAU is identified, it must be included in the resection. As PAU may occur anywhere in the thoracic aorta, one must be prepared to replace the mid- and distal aorta as well as the proximal portion more typically replaced when repairing type B dissection.[98]

The role of endovascular stent grafts in the repair of IMH and PAU is in evolution. Success in the treatment of IMH and dissection has been reported.[70,71] Arguably, PAU should be the ideal entity for such treatment,[72,99–101] although extensive atherosclerotic disease may make access challenging. Unfortunately it is unclear whether this will truly impact long-term survival of these very ill patients.[73]

Degenerative Aneurysmal Disease

Etiology

Histologically, disruption of the elastic lamellae with thinning of the media and loss of smooth muscle cells is typically present in aneurysms of degenerative origin. Degradation of elastin is likely central to the development of degenerative aneurysms, although its biochemical basis remains incompletely defined. Increased levels of elastases have been identified in abdominal aortic aneurysms, as have serine proteases,[102] and more recently matrix metalloproteinases and plasminogen activators.[103,104] Smooth muscle cell apoptosis as well as dedifferentiation with increased synthetic capacity also contribute to the degenerative changes.[14,15]

Intense production of reactive oxygen species in thoracoabdominal aneurysms compared to control aortas, especially in regions of increased inflammatory cell infiltration, have been demonstrated, with expression of NADH/NADPH oxidase p22^{phox}, overlapping with the areas of increased metalloproteinase activity.[105] The biomechanical consequence of these changes is increased vessel wall stiffness and reduced residual strain.[6]

As is true for aortic dissection, the association between hypertension and degenerative aneurysmal disease is clear but the mechanism is not. Genetic factors likely play a significant role here as well. Apart from the recognized collagen vascular diseases such as Marfan syndrome and Ehlers–Danlos syndrome, familial clustering has been recognized,[106] and linked to at least three genetic loci.[12,22,23,107] Conversely, a family history of aneurysmal disease is present in 10% to 15% of patients with abdominal[108,109] and thoracic aortic aneurysms.[110] Abnormalities in type II procollagen have been identified in some of these cases[20] as has mutation in TGF-receptor type II.[13]

Pathophysiology

Degenerative aneurysms are heterogeneous in their location and gross appearance. Aneurysms of the ascending aorta may produce insufficiency of the aortic valve despite structurally normal valve leaflets because of loss of central leaflet coaptation. Alternatively, the ascending aorta and arch may be spared with dilatation only of the descending thoracic aorta. Crawford established a classification scheme for thoracoabdominal aortic aneurysms (Fig. 63.6).

The natural history of thoracic aortic aneurysmal disease is grave, with progressive dilatation to eventual rupture is common for thoracic aneurysms.[111,112] Aneurysms exceeding 6cm in diameter are particularly prone to rupture, with the annual risk of rupture or dissection approximately 7% at this dimension.[112–117] Other factors, however, including patient age, history of pain, and chronic obstructive pulmonary disease, as well as maximum aortic diameter, increase the risk of rupture.[118] The critical diameter for the ascending aorta appears somewhat less than that for the ascending aorta, perhaps because of differences in hemodynamic stress.[115] Once symptoms occur, the mean interval to rupture is 2 years.[111] The majority of degenerative aneurysms are fusiform, but saccular aneurysms do occur, and are probably at higher risk of rupture, as are those caused by chronic dissection.[69]

Clinical Presentation

Degenerative aneurysms are often asymptomatic, being discovered incidentally during an imaging study performed for another purpose. Rapid expansion, particularly of the thoracoabdominal aorta, may produce pain that may be mistaken for arthritic symptoms. Involvement of the aortic root with resultant aortic regurgitation may result in heart failure. Distal embolization with the resulting "blue toe syndrome" may also occur. Physical examination may reveal aortic regurgitation, a palpable pulsatile abdominal mass, or abdominal bruits. Most often, however, the diagnosis is made via advanced imaging modalities.

Diagnostic Evaluation

Chest radiography often offers the first clue to the presence of a thoracic aortic aneurysm. A widened mediastinum or apparent mass may lead to other studies that make the diagnosis. Calcification of the wall of aneurysm occasionally makes the diagnosis clear on the basis of the plain film alone.

Aortography is less often the initial diagnostic test today than it was previously, although it continues to provide useful information, particularly in the preoperative evaluation of thoracoabdominal aneurysmal disease. Transesophageal echo is diagnostic when aneurysmal dilatation of the ascending aorta is questioned, but is less useful in the assessment of descending thoracic aneurysms and those involving the aortic arch. Axial imaging techniques offer a complete view of the pathology and may also rule out other intrathoracic pathology; furthermore, these may identify other aneurysms, which are present in 25% of patients with thoracic aneurysms and 10% of those with abdominal aneurysms.[119] Computerized tomography (with contrast) will define the external size, the longitudinal extent, the presence of intraluminal thrombus, ulceration, or atheroma. As is the case for acute dissection, MRI can provide excellent detail in any plane but is limited by its time-consuming nature. Its utility is greatest in evaluating complex anatomy in detail.

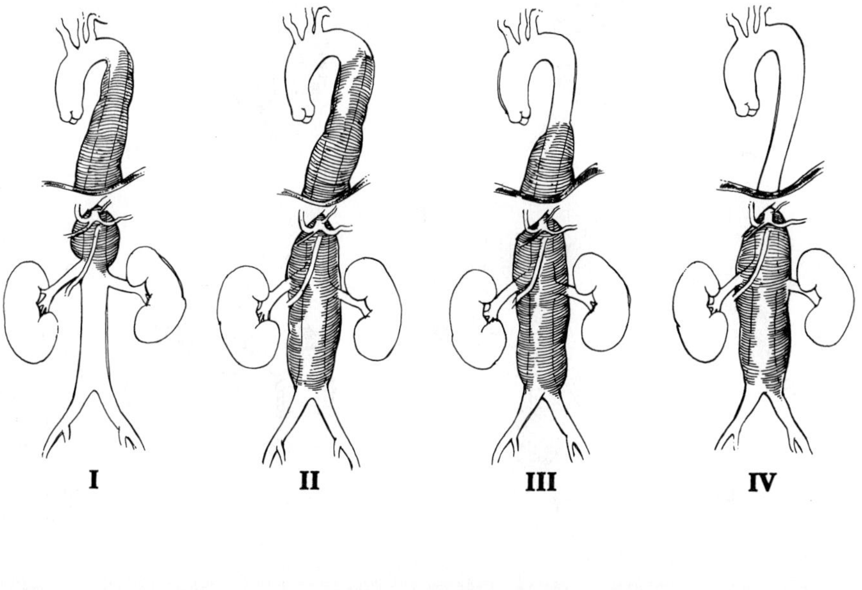

FIGURE 63.6. The Crawford Classification for thoracoabdominal aortic aneurysms.

Medical and Surgical Management

Medical therapy of aneurysms of degenerative etiology is focused on aggressive antihypertensive therapy and beta-blockade. Prophylactic beta-blockers have been shown to reduce aortic events in patients with Marfan syndrome in a prospectively randomized study and have been convincingly shown to reduce late expansion of the chronically dissected aorta[120] or aorta injured by intramural hematoma.[83] Beyond this, the emphasis of nonoperative treatment is on the close monitoring of aneurysm size.

Surgical intervention is indicated in most circumstances for aneurysms of the ascending aorta exceeding 5 to 5.5 cm in maximum diameter.[115] The relatively low risk associated with repair of ascending aortic aneurysms in the current era[121,122] supports this practice. Repair of aneurysms of the descending thoracic and thoracoabdominal aorta is usually recommended at 6.0 to 6.5 cm in diameter,[115] although age and comorbidities impact this decision in terms of both risk of surgery and risk of rupture.[118]

Surgical Techniques for Repair of Aneurysms of the Thoracic Aorta

From a technical standpoint, methods of aortic repair are similar regardless of etiology. The approach is primarily dependent upon the region of the aorta to be replaced. Accordingly, we address repair of the ascending aorta and root, the aortic arch, and the descending thoracic and thoracoabdominal aorta in order.

Aneurysms of the Ascending Aorta

Preoperative Evaluation

Once aneurysmal disease of the ascending aorta requiring surgical intervention has been identified, the extent of aortic involvement proximally and distally and the presence of coexisting cardiac valve disease or coronary artery disease requiring concomitant correction must be determined. An exception is acute dissection, in which preoperative coronary arteriography has largely been abandoned.[56] The extent of aortic pathology affects the technical approach as well as the preoperative assessment of risk. Diagnostic studies revealing involvement of the aortic arch may dictate the use of profound hypothermic cardiopulmonary bypass and circulatory arrest. Proximal involvement of the aortic root may mandate root replacement with a valved conduit or tissue valve root prosthesis such as a human allograft or stentless xenograft.

Surgical Technique

The ascending aorta is most conveniently approached via median sternotomy. Arterial cannulation for cardiopulmonary bypass is via the femoral or axillary artery in the setting of acute dissection. In degenerative disease, cannulation of the aortic arch or even the aneurysm itself may be performed, although the trend is increasingly toward axillary artery cannulation.[64] If the disease is limited to the ascending aorta with sufficient room to cross-clamp the aorta below the innominate artery, the operation can be performed with only mild hypothermia (28°–32°C) or even normothermic cardiopulmonary bypass. If the aneurysm extends to the innominate artery, an episode of circulatory arrest under profound hypothermia (13°–18°c) may be required to perform the distal anastomosis. Liberal use of circulatory arrest in cases of acute dissection is also gaining popularity.[123] Reconstructive options are shown in Figure 63.7.

Aneurysms of the Aortic Arch

Preoperative Evaluation

The use of profound hypothermia and circulatory arrest in acute dissection permits open distal anastomosis and provides an opportunity for direct inspection of the aortic arch for intimal disruption intraoperatively. This approach lessens

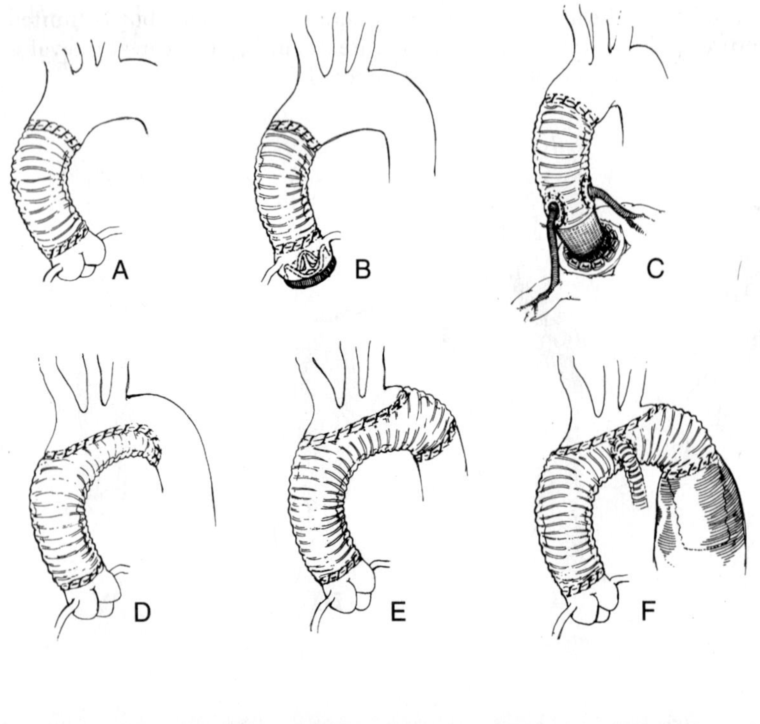

FIGURE 63.7. Options for repair of ascending and arch aneurysms include supracoronary tube graft (**A**), separate tube graft and aortic valve replacement when the sinuses are normal (**B**), composite graft repair with reimplantation of the coronary arteries when the sinuses are diseased (**C**), hemiarch replacement (**D**), total arch replacement (**E**), and elephant trunk arch replacement (**F**).

the importance of excessive preoperative imaging studies in this potentially unstable subset of patients. Patients with chronic dissection or degenerative disease that appears to involve the arch are most often adequately imaged today with CT scanning or MRI. Attention should be paid to the brachiocephalic anatomy, including the presence of a separate origin of the left vertebral artery from the arch. The presence of concomitant coronary artery disease and valvular heart disease should be investigated so that corrective intervention may be performed during the same operation.

Surgical Technique

Repair of aneurysms of the aortic arch continues to represent a major surgical challenge. Neurological function must be preserved by moderate hypothermia and selective antegrade cerebral perfusion or profound hypothermia permitting cerebral circulatory arrest while arch reconstruction is underway. At temperatures of 13°–18°C, 30 to 45 min of circulatory arrest is likely safe.[124] Retrograde cerebral perfusion with oxygenated blood via the superior vena cava during circulatory arrest has been advocated as a means of prolonging the safe period although its effectiveness has never been proven.[62] The current trend is toward early antegrade perfusion.[63,125]

Arch replacement may be accomplished via a variety of techniques, depending on the extent of disease proximally and distally (see Fig. 63.7). Subtotal or hemiarch replacement is most often employed when ascending aneurysmal disease extends to involve the proximal arch or when an intimal tear is present in acute dissection. Total arch replacement entails separate suture lines to the proximal descending thoracic aorta and to the brachiocephalic vessels. Most recently grafts with separate branches for each brachiocephalic vessel have been developed.[126] The additional complexity of the procedure translates into the prolonged circulatory arrest time and, in most cases, higher operative risk.

When the aorta distal to the left subclavian is also diseased and it is anticipated that a subsequent resection of the thoracic or thoracoabdominal aorta will be required, the elephant trunk procedure may be performed. Performance of the distal anastomosis to the proximal descending thoracic aorta with the graft folded onto itself and invaginated into the distal aorta results in a distal tail or "trunk" of graft, dangling intraluminally. Subsequently, control of the graft may be obtained from the left chest, opening the native aorta distal to the previous suture line, avoiding adhesions. This procedure can be performed safely, but once again entails greater risk because of its greater complexity.[127–129] Alternatively, a single-stage procedure with resection of the ascending aorta, arch, and descending thoracic aorta may be performed via transverse thoracosternotomy.[130]

Aneurysms of the Descending Thoracic and Thoracoabdominal Aorta

Preoperative Evaluation

Thoracic and thoracoabdominal aortic repair are major operative procedures taxing the patient's cardiovascular, pulmonary, and renal reserves. Accordingly, preoperative evaluation should include assessment of these systems as well as the anatomic extent of the disease. The presence of ischemic heart disease before elective procedures may be sought noninvasively by thallium-201 scintigraphy[131–133] or by using echocardiography with dobutamine infusion.[134] Contrast coronary arteriography, however, is the definitive test, and one that should be seriously considered in any patient over the age of 45. The risks of this test today are low, particularly in light of the magnitude of the planned surgical procedure. The advent of 64- and 128-detector CT scanning may obviate the need for angiography of the coronary arteries in the near future just as more conventional scanners have all but eliminated the need for visceral angiography. Preoperative echocardiography will reveal impaired ventricular function or aortic regurgitation, either of which would discourage the use of circulatory arrest because subendocardial myocardial perfusion may be impaired once ventricular fibrillation ensues.

Pulmonary dysfunction is a common complication; therefore, pulmonary function tests may be helpful in the estimation of operative risk. History of smoking and chronic obstructive pulmonary disease are independent predictors of prolonged ventilatory support following thoracoabdominal aortic aneurysm repair. Renal function should be optimized postoperatively, as acute perioperative renal failure is a risk factor for paraplegia and postoperative death.[135–138]

Surgical Techniques

Surgical procedures on thoracic and thoracoabdominal aneurysms continue to carry significant risk of death and complications. In addition to risks of renal and respiratory failure, paraplegia may occur because of the tenuous blood supply to the anterior spinal cord. Enormous efforts have been directed toward the development of techniques to reduce the incidence of this devastating complication. Although a variety of surgical approaches to such aneurysms have been championed, none has proven clearly superior (Table 63.2).

Simple "clamp and sew" has been advocated by some authors, and is supported for the treatment of aneurysms limited to the thoracic aorta by the work of Coselli and colleagues.[139] Even in this series, however, the risk of paraplegia rises with cross-clamp time, making the technique critically dependent upon the technical expertise of the surgeon and the vicissitudes of complications and intraoperative factors. Based upon the recognized neuroprotective effects of hypothermia, Cambria et al.[140] have advocated the addition of topical spinal cord cooling via an epidural catheter to the "clamp and run" technique. Review of their 5-year results and those of others reveals an apparent reduction in the incidence of postoperative spinal cord ischemic events to 7% (paraplegia, 2%–4%) compared to the predicted rate of 18.5%.[140,141] Others have focused on the maintenance of spinal cord blood flow via distal perfusion with a left atrial to femoral bypass circuit, often combined with cerebrospinal fluid drainage to reduce intrathecal pressure to promote blood flow to the spinal cord.[142,143] Profound hypothermia and circulatory arrest is an alternative protective strategy.[123] Recently attention has been drawn to postoperative hypotension as a contributor to delayed paraplegia.[144,145] The comparison of all such techniques is inherently complicated by the recognized differences in risk associated with aneurysms of different extent. Few authors separate their results according to Crawford classification. The relative rarity of Crawford type I and II aneurysms, for which the incidence of postoperative paraplegia is highest, is an obstacle to defining the optimal approach to avoid this complication.

TABLE 63.2.
Prevention of Spinal Cord Infarction During Thoracic and Thoracoabdominal Aortic Aneurysm Repair.

Author	*Year published*	*Adjuncts*	*No. patients*	*Surgical mortality*	*Paraplegia/Paraparesis*
Borst[164]	1994	Left heart bypass Intercostal reimplantaton	132	3%	2.3%
Cambria[165]	2002	Epidural cooling in 57%	337	8.3%	11.4%
Kouchoukos[166]	2001	Hypothermic circulatory arrest	161	6.2%	3.2%
Galla[167]	1999	Left heart bypass PHCA Somatosensory evoked potentials	100 49	 8.7%	 6.0%
Safi[142]	2003	Left heart bypass Spinal drainage	741 (of 1004)	14%	2.4%
Coselli[139a]	2004	Clamp and sew (thoracic only)	387	4.4%	2.6%
Coselli[168b]	2002	Left heart bypass CSF drainage No CSF drainage	 76 69	 5.3% 2.9%	 2.6% 13%

CSF, cerebrospinal fluid; PHCA, profound hypothermia and circulatory arrest.
[a]Distal perfusion used in 11.9%.
[b]Prospectively randomized trial.

Stimulated by the success seen in endovascular treatment of abdominal aortic disease, endovascular approaches to thoracic aortic pathology have been explored. The results of several large studies are currently available. In the European Collaborators on Stent-Graft Techniques for Thoracic Aortic Aneurysm and Dissection Repair (EUROSTAR) and United Kingdom Thoracic Endograft Registries, 443 patients were treated for a variety of conditions including degenerative disease in 249, dissection in 131, and false anastomotic aneurysm in 13 or traumatic pseudoaneurysm in 50.[146] Primary technical success approached 90%, with paraplegia in 4% and a mortality rate of 10% among those with degenerative aneurysm. Late mortality was 10% as well, with endoleaks in 4.2%, aneurysm sac expansion in 14.6%, and reintervention in 5.2%. Remarkably similar results were reported by Criado et al. among 186 patients undergoing stent-graft repair of thoracic aortic pathology for degenerative disease or dissection.[147] The perioperative mortality rate was 4.7% and paraplegia rate was 4.3%. Survival was 62.5% at 40 months' mean follow-up for those with degenerative aneurysms. In the WL Gore Phase II pivotal U.S. clinical trial, comparable results were reported among 142 patients.[148] The 30-day mortality rate was 2%, the incidence of stroke, 4%, and paraplegia, 3%. Major adverse events occurred in 32% of patients.

Posttraumatic Thoracic Aortic Aneurysms

Acute aortic transection is the most common traumatic process resulting in aneurysmal dilatation or, more properly, pseudoaneurysm formation of the thoracic aorta. While the management of acute transaction is considered elsewhere, chronic posttraumatic aneurysms are often seen in an elective setting for repair. Often the traumatic episode is in the distant past with the chronic pseudoaneurysm apparent on chest X-ray or CT scan performed for an unrelated reason. Frequently such aneurysms are calcified (Fig. 63.8). Occasional airway or esophageal compression may be noted. Despite the proximity of the recurrent laryngeal nerve, hoarseness is uncommon.

Such pseudoaneurysms are often calcified, and accordingly there is some debate over their need for repair. Early studies[149–151] suggested that such aneurysms should be repaired once identified. However, a number of authors have argued in favor of serial imaging studies, reserving surgery for those with symptoms or evidence of enlargement.[152,153] The advent of intraluminal stents may push many of these issues aside as both acute and chronic transections may be readily correctable with this technology.[154] The long-term durability in this

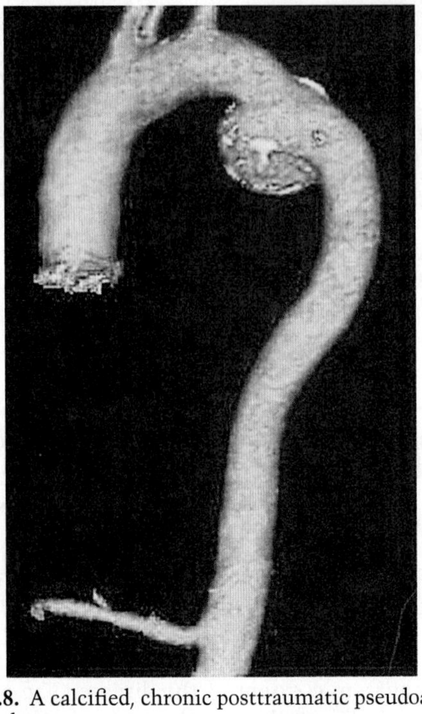

FIGURE 63.8. A calcified, chronic posttraumatic pseudoaneurysm of the aortic isthmus.

setting is yet to be defined, and it is equally arguable that, under elective circumstances the otherwise good-risk patient is best served with an open procedure.[155,156] Surgical repair is performed with left heart partial bypass or circulatory arrest, as previously described.

Congenital Abnormalities

Coarctation of the Aorta

The most common congenital anomaly of the aorta is coarctation, occurring in 40 to 50 of 100,000 live births.[26] The majority of such lesions are identified and treated in infancy and childhood. As such their diagnosis and treatment fall within the purview of the pediatric cardiac surgeon. Occasionally, however, coarctation or even aortic interruption remains undetected until adulthood during evaluation of hypertension, when delayed or diminished femoral pulsation is found, or a routine chest X-ray demonstrates rib notching or an abnormal cardiomediastinal silhouette.

The natural history of coarctation is well established. Left untreated, 80% of adults will die of complications of proximal hypertension, most often in the second, third, or fourth decades of life.[157,158] Correction is indicated when the condition is diagnosed. Even with late repair, postoperative normotension or only mild hypertension can be anticipated in the majority of patients.[159] Subclavian flap angioplasty and aortic mobilization with primary anastomosis are the methods of choice in children and infants but may be difficult in adults. Insertion of an interposition graft provides excellent long-term results,[160] as does extraanatomic bypass.[158] Recently, balloon dilatation has been applied to adolescents and adults, as it is in infants.[161] Long-term postoperative follow-up is indicated, as ascending and descending aortic complications may occur as well as reflections of associated inherent abnormalities of the aorta.[157]

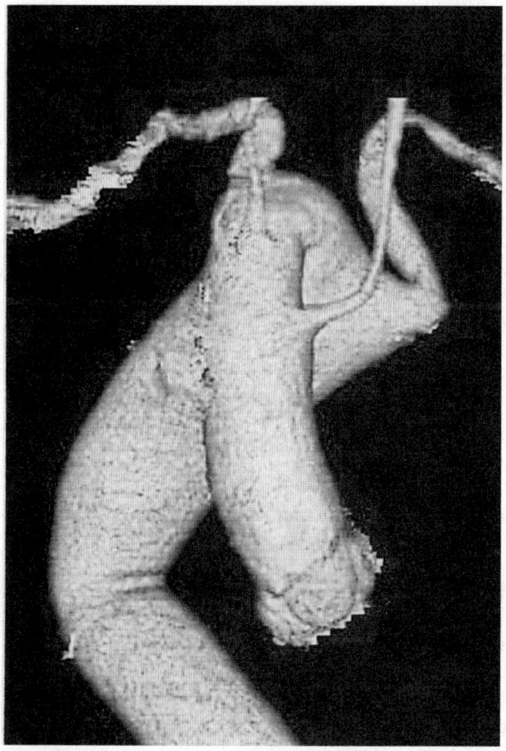

FIGURE 63.9. Three-dimensional reconstruction of computerized tomographic image of a patient with right aortic arch and an aberrant left subclavian artery with aneurysmal dilatation of the origin or "diverticulum of Kommerell."

Aberrant Subclavian Artery

As in coarctation, the majority of clinically significant congenital abnormalities related to aortic arch development, such as double aortic arch with vascular ring, become apparent in infancy and childhood. Occasionally, however, adults may present with dysphagia secondary to an aberrant right subclavian artery from a left-sided arch, or an aberrant left subclavian artery from a right-sided arch. The origin of the aberrant vessel is usually dilated and is known as a Kommerell's diverticulum (Fig. 63.9). This anomaly results in compression of surrounding structures, most often the esophagus behind which the aberrant vessel most often passes. Diagnostic evaluation may begin with CT or MRI scanning. These studies often provide all the required information, although aortography may also be helpful. Surgical correction can be accomplished simply by carotid–subclavian bypass and oversewing of the origin of the aberrant vessel, most often via a left thoracotomy.

References

1. Vilacosta I, Roman JA. Acute aortic syndrome. Heart 2001;85(4):365–368.
2. Ponraj P, Pepper J. Aortic dissection. Br J Clin Pract 1992;46:127–131.
3. Schlatmann TJ, Becker AE. Pathogenesis of dissecting aneursym of the aorta: comparative histopathologic study of significance of medial changes. Am J Cardiol 1977;39(1):21–26.
4. Schlatmann TJM, Becker AE. Histologic changes in the normal aging aorta: implications for dissecting aortic aneursym. Am J Cardiol 1977;39:13–20.
5. Cattell MA, Hasleton PS, Anderson JC. Increased elastin content and decreased elastin concentration may be predisposing factors in dissecting aneurysms of human thoracic aorta. Cardiovasc Res 1993;27(2):176–181.
6. Okamoto RJ, Xu H, Kouchoukos NT, et al. The influence of mechanical properties on wall stress and distensibility of the dilated ascending aorta. J Thorac Cardiovasc Surg 2003;126(3):842–850.
7. Marsalese DL, Moodie DS, Vacante M, et al. Marfan's syndrome: natural history and long-term follow-up of cardiovascular involvement. J Am Coll Cardiol 1989;14:422–428.
8. Murdoch JL, Walker BA, Halpern BL, et al. Life expectancy and causes of death in the Marfan syndrome. N Engl J Med 1972;286(15):804–808.
9. Kim SY, Martin N, Hsia EC, et al. Management of aortic disease in Marfan syndrome: a decision analysis. Arch Intern Med 2005;165(7):749–755.
10. Kainulainen K, Pulkkinen L, Savolainen A, et al. Location on chromosome 15 of the gene defect causing Marfan syndrome. N Engl J Med 1990;323(14):935–939.
11. Dietz HC, Cutting GR, Pyeritz RE, et al. Marfan syndrome caused by a recurrent de novo missense mutation in the fibrillin gene. Nature (Lond) 1991;352(6333):337–339.
12. Collod G, Babron MC, Jondeau G, et al. A second locus for Marfan syndrome maps to chromosome 3p24.2-p25. Nat Genet 1994;8(3):264–268.
13. Pannu H, Fadulu VT, Chang J, et al. Mutations in transforming growth factor-beta receptor type II cause familial thoracic aortic

aneurysms and dissections. Circulation 2005;112(4):513–520.
14. Lesauskaite V, Tanganelli P, Sassi C, et al. Smooth muscle cells of the media in the dilatative pathology of ascending thoracic aorta: morphology, immunoreactivity for osteopontin, matrix metalloproteinases, and their inhibitors. Hum Pathol 2001;32(9): 1003–1011.
15. Bunton TE, Biery NJ, Myers L, et al. Phenotypic alteration of vascular smooth muscle cells precedes elastolysis in a mouse model of Marfan syndrome. Circ Res 2001;88(1):37–43.
16. Sakomura Y, Nagashima H, Aoka Y, et al. Expression of peroxisome proliferator-activated receptor-gamma in vascular smooth muscle cells is upregulated in cystic medial degeneration of annuloaortic ectasia in Marfan syndrome. Circulation 2002;106(12 suppl 1):I259–I263.
17. Neptune ER, Frischmeyer PA, Arking DE, et al. Dysregulation of TGF-beta activation contributes to pathogenesis in Marfan syndrome. Nat Genet 2003;33(3):407–411.
18. Habashi JP, Judge DP, Holm TM, et al. Losartan, an AT1 antagonist, prevents aortic aneurysm in a mouse model of Marfan syndrome. Science 2006;312(5770):117–121.
19. Nataatmadja M, West J, West M. Overexpression of transforming growth factor-beta is associated with increased hyaluronan content and impairment of repair in Marfan syndrome aortic aneurysm. Circulation 2006;114(1 suppl):I371–I377.
20. Kontusaari S, Tromp G, Kuivaniemi H, et al. A mutation in the gene for type III procollagen (COL3A1) in a family with aortic aneurysms. J Clin Invest 1990;86:1465–1473.
21. Svensson LG, Crawford ES. Aortic dissection and aortic aneurysm surgery: clinical observations, experimental investigations, and statistical analyses. Part II. Curr Probl Surg 1992;29:915–1057.
22. Hasham SN, Willing MC, Guo DC, et al. Mapping a locus for familial thoracic aortic aneurysms and dissections (TAAD2) to 3p24-25. Circulation 2003;107(25):3184–3190.
23. Vaughan CJ, Casey M, He J, et al. Identification of a chromosome 11q23.2-q24 locus for familial aortic aneurysm disease, a genetically heterogeneous disorder. Circulation 2001;103(20): 2469–2475.
24. Kakko S, Raisanen T, Tamminen M, et al. Candidate locus analysis of familial ascending aortic aneurysms and dissections confirms the linkage to the chromosome 5q13-14 in Finnish families. J Thorac Cardiovasc Surg 2003;126(1):106–113.
25. Edwards WD, Leaf DS, Edwards JE. Dissecting aortic aneurysm associated with congenital bicuspid aortic valve. Circulation 1978;57:1022–1025.
26. Abbott ME. Coarctation of the aorta of the adult type, II. Am Heart J 1928;3:574–618.
27. Januzzi JL, Sabatine MS, Eagle KA, et al. Iatrogenic aortic dissection. Am J Cardiol 2002;89(5):623–626.
28. Hirst AE Jr, Johns VJ Jr, Kime SW. Dissecting aneurysm of the aorta: a review of 505 cases. Medicine (Baltim) 1958;37:217–279.
29. DeBakey ME, Henly WS, Cooley DA, et al. Surgical management of dissecting aneurysms of the aorta. J Thorac Cardiovasc Surg 1965;49:130–149.
30. Lansman SL, Galla JD, Schor JS, et al. Subtypes of acute aortic dissection. J Card Surg 1994;9(6):729–733.
31. Daily PO, Trueblood HW, Stinson EB, et al. Management of acute aortic dissections. Ann Thorac Surg 1970;10(3):237–247.
32. Miller DC, Mitchell RS, Oyer PE, et al. Independent determinants of operative mortality for patients with aortic dissections. Circulation 1984;70(suppl I):I153–I164.
33. Hagan PG, Nienaber CA, Isselbacher EM, et al. The International Registry of Acute Aortic Dissection (IRAD): new insights into an old disease. JAMA 2000;283(7):897–903.
34. Nallamothu BK, Mehta RH, Saint S, et al. Syncope in acute aortic dissection: diagnostic, prognostic, and clinical implications. Am J Med 2002;113(6):468–471.
35. Park SW, Hutchison S, Mehta RH, et al. Association of painless acute aortic dissection with increased mortality. Mayo Clin Proc 2004;79(10):1252–1257.
36. Bossone E, Rampoldi V, Nienaber CA, et al. Usefulness of pulse deficit to predict in-hospital complications and mortality in patients with acute type A aortic dissection. Am J Cardiol 2002;89(7):851–855.
37. Mehta RH, Suzuki T, Hagan PG, et al. Predicting death in patients with acute type A aortic dissection. Circulation 2002; 105(2):200–206.
38. Lindsay J Jr, Hurst JW. Clinical features and prognosis in dissecting aneurysms of the aorta: a re-appraisal. Circulation 1967;35: 880–888.
39. Ergin MA, Griepp RB. Dissections of the aorta. In: Baue AE, Geha AS, Hammond GL, et al, eds. Glenn's Thoracic and Cardiovascular Surgery. Stamford: Appleton & Lange, 1996:2273–2298.
40. Fann JI, Sarris GE, Mitchell RS, et al. Treatment of patients with aortic dissection presenting with peripheral vascular complications. Ann Surg 1990;212:705.
41. Deeb GM, Williams DM, Bolling SF, et al. Surgical delay for acute type A dissection with malperfusion. Ann Thorac Surg 1997;64(6):1669–1675.
42. Nienaber CA, von Kodolitsch Y, Nicolas V, et al. The diagnosis of thoracic aortic dissection by noninvasive imaging procedures. N Engl J Med 1993;328(1):1–9.
43. Bansal RC, Chandrasekaran K, Ayala K, Smith DC. Frequency and explanation of false negative diagnosis of aortic dissection by aortography and transesophageal echocardiography. J Am Coll Cardiol 1995;25(6):1393–1401.
44. Evangelista A, Garcia-del-Castillo H, Gonzalez-Alujas T, et al. Diagnosis of ascending aortic dissection by transesophageal echocardiography: utility of M-mode in recognizing artifacts. J Am Coll Cardiol 1996;27(1):102–107.
45. Movsowitz HD, Levine RA, Hilgenberg AD, Isselbacher EM. Transesophageal echocardiographic description of the mechanisms of aortic regurgitation in acute type A aortic dissection: implications for aortic valve repair. J Am Coll Cardiol 2000;36(3):884–890.
46. Ledbetter S, Stuk JL, Kaufman JA. Helical (spiral) CT in the evaluation of emergent thoracic aortic syndromes. Traumatic aortic rupture, aortic aneurysm, aortic dissection, intramural hematoma, and penetrating atherosclerotic ulcer. Radiol Clin N Am 1999;37(3):575–589.
47. Zeman RK, Berman PM, Silverman PM, et al. Diagnosis of aortic dissection: value of helical CT with multiplanar reformation and three-dimensional rendering. AJR Am J Roentgenol 1995;164(6): 1375–1380.
48. Suzuki T, Katoh H, Tsuchio Y, et al. Diagnostic implications of elevated levels of smooth-muscle myosin heavy-chain protein in acute aortic dissection. The smooth muscle myosin heavy chain study. Ann Intern Med 2000;133(7):537–541.
49. Weber T, Hogler S, Auer J, et al. D-dimer in acute aortic dissection. Chest 2003;123(5):1375–1378.
50. Bavaria JE, Brinster DR, Gorman RC, et al. Advances in the treatment of acute type A dissection: an integrated approach. Ann Thorac Surg 2002;74(5):S1848–S1852; discussion S1857–S1863.
51. Vedantham S, Picus D, Sanchez LA, et al. Percutaneous management of ischemic complications in patients with type B aortic dissection. J Vasc Intervent Radiol 2003;14(2 pt 1):181–194.
52. Hata M, Shiono M, Inoue T, et al. Preoperative cardiopulmonary resuscitation is the only predictor for operative mortality of type A acute aortic dissection: a recent 8-year experience. Ann Thorac Cardiovasc Surg 2004;10(2):101–105.
53. Long SM, Tribble CG, Raymond DP, et al. Preoperative shock determines outcome for acute type A aortic dissection. Ann Thorac Surg 2003;75(2):520–524.

54. Ehrlich MP, Ergin MA, McCullough JN, et al. Results of immediate surgical treatment of all acute type A dissections. Circulation 2000;102(19 suppl 3):III248–III252.
55. Creswell LL, Kouchoukos NT, Cox JL, Rosenbloom M. Coronary artery disease in patients with type A aortic dissection. Ann Thorac Surg 1995;59(3):585–590.
56. Motallebzadeh R, Batas D, Valencia O, et al. The role of coronary angiography in acute type A aortic dissection. Eur J Cardiothorac Surg 2004;25(2):231–235.
57. Rampoldi V, Trimarchi S, Eagle KA, et al. Simple risk models to predict surgical mortality in acute type A aortic dissection: the International Registry of Acute Aortic Dissection score. Ann Thorac Surg 2007;83(1):55–61.
58. Ergin MA, Phillips RA, Galla JD, et al. Significance of distal false lumen after type A dissection repair. Ann Thorac Surg 1994;57(4):820–824; discussion 825.
59. Moon MR, Sundt TM III, Pasque MK, et al. Does the extent of proximal or distal resection influence outcome for type A dissections? Ann Thorac Surg 2001;71(4):1244–1249; discussion 1249–1250.
60. Myrmel T, Lai DT, Miller DC. Can the principles of evidence-based medicine be applied to the treatment of aortic dissections? Eur J Cardio-Thorac Surg 2004;25(2):236–242; discussion 242–245.
61. Lai DT, Robbins RC, Mitchell RS, et al. Does profound hypothermic circulatory arrest improve survival in patients with acute type A aortic dissection? Circulation 2002;106(12 suppl 1):I218–I228.
62. Deeb GM, Jenkins E, Bolling SF, et al. Retrograde cerebral perfusion during hypothermic circulatory arrest reduces neurologic morbidity. J Thorac Cardiovasc Surg 1995;109(2):259–268.
63. Strauch JT, Spielvogel D, Lauten A, et al. Technical advances in total aortic arch replacement. Ann Thorac Surg 2004;77(2):581–589; discussion 589–590.
64. Sabik JF, Nemeh H, Lytle BW, et al. Cannulation of the axillary artery with a side graft reduces morbidity. Ann Thorac Surg 2004;77(4):1315–1320.
65. Fusco DS, Shaw RK, Tranquilli M, et al. Femoral cannulation is safe for type A dissection repair. Ann Thorac Surg 2004;78(4):1285–1289; discussion 1285–1289.
66. Glower DD, Fann JI, Speier RH, et al. Comparison of medical and surgical therapy for uncomplicated descending aortic dissection. Circulation 1990;82(5 suppl):IV39–IV46.
67. Umana JP, Lai DT, Mitchell RS, et al. Is medical therapy still the optimal treatment strategy for patients with acute type B aortic dissections? J Thorac Cardiovasc Surg 2002;124(5):896–910.
68. Hata M, Shiono M, Inoue T, et al. Optimal treatment of type B acute aortic dissection: long-term medical follow-up results. Ann Thorac Surg 2003;75(6):1781–1784.
69. Juvonen T, Ergin MA, Galla JD, et al. Risk factors for rupture of chronic type B dissections. J Thorac Cardiovasc Surg 1999;117(4):776–786.
70. Dake MD, Kato N, Mitchell RS, et al. Endovascular stent-graft placement for the treatment of acute aortic dissection. N Engl J Med 1999;340(20):1546–1552.
71. Grabenwoger M, Fleck T, Czerny M, et al. Endovascular stent graft placement in patients with acute thoracic aortic syndromes. Eur J Cardio-Thorac Surg 2003;23(5):788–793; discussion 793.
72. Sailer J, Peloschek P, Rand T, et al. Endovascular treatment of aortic type B dissection and penetrating ulcer using commercially available stent-grafts. AJR Am J Roentgenol 2001; 177(6):1365–1369.
73. Umana JP, Miller DC, Mitchell RS. What is the best treatment for patients with acute type B aortic dissections: medical, surgical, or endovascular stent-grafting? Ann Thorac Surg 2002;74(5): S1840–S1843; discussion S1857–S1863.
74. Shimono T, Kato N, Yasuda F, et al. Transluminal stent-graft placements for the treatments of acute onset and chronic aortic dissections. Circulation 2002;106(12 suppl 1):I241–I247.
75. Evangelista A, Mukherjee D, Mehta RH, et al. Acute intramural hematoma of the aorta. A mystery in evolution. Circulation 2005;111:1063–1070.
76. Ganaha F, Miller DC, Sugimoto K, et al. Prognosis of aortic intramural hematoma with and without penetrating atherosclerotic ulcer: a clinical and radiological analysis. Circulation 2002;106(3):342–348.
77. Nienaber CA, Eagle KA. Aortic dissection: new frontiers in diagnosis and management. Part I: from etiology to diagnostic strategies. Circulation 2003;108(5):628–635.
78. Shimizu H, Yoshino H, Udagawa H, et al. Prognosis of aortic intramural hemorrhage compared with classic aortic dissection. Am J Cardiol 2000;85(6):792–795.
79. Coady MA, Rizzo JA, Elefteriades JA. Pathologic variants of thoracic aortic dissections. Penetrating atherosclerotic ulcers and intramural hematomas. Cardiol Clin 1999;17(4):637–657.
80. Stanson AW, Kazmier FJ, Hollier LH, et al. Penetrating atherosclerotic ulcers of the thoracic aorta: natural history and clinicopathologic correlations. Ann Vasc Surg 1986;1(1):15–23.
81. Cho KR, Stanson AW, Potter DD, et al. Penetrating atherosclerotic ulcer of the descending thoracic aorta and arch. J Thorac Cardiovasc Surg 2004;127(5):1393–1399; discussion 1399–1401.
82. Tittle SL, Lynch RJ, Cole PE, et al. Midterm follow-up of penetrating ulcer and intramural hematoma of the aorta. J Thorac Cardiovasc Surg 2002;123(6):1051–1059.
83. von Kodolitsch Y, Csosz SK, Koschyk DH, et al. Intramural hematoma of the aorta: predictors of progression to dissection and rupture. Long-term prognosis of patients with type A aortic intramural hematoma. Circulation 2003;107(8):1158–1163.
84. Troxler M, Mavor AI, Homer-Vanniasinkam S. Penetrating atherosclerotic ulcers of the aorta. Br J Surg 2001;88(9):1169–1177.
85. Maraj R, Rerkpattanapipat P, Jacobs LE, et al. Meta-analysis of 143 reported cases of aortic intramural hematoma. Am J Cardiol 2000;86(6):664–668.
86. Kaji S, Akasaka T, Katayama M, et al. Long-term prognosis of patients with type B aortic intramural hematoma. Circulation 2003;108(1):9.
87. Nishigami K, Tsuchiya T, Shono H, et al. Disappearance of aortic intramural hematoma and its significance to the prognosis. Circulation 2000;102(19 suppl 3):III243–III247.
88. Song JK, Kang DH, Lim TH, et al. Different remodeling of descending thoracic aorta after acute event in aortic intramural hemorrhage versus aortic dissection. Am J Cardiol 1999;83(6):937–941.
89. Song JK, Kim HS, Song JM, et al. Outcomes of medically treated patients with aortic intramural hematoma. Am J Med 2002; 113(3):181–187.
90. Evangelista A, Dominguez R, Sebastia C, et al. Long-term follow-up of aortic intramural hematoma: predictors of outcome. Circulation 2003;108(5):583–589.
91. Vilacosta I, San Roman JA, Ferreiros J, et al. Natural history and serial morphology of aortic intramural hematoma: a novel variant of aortic dissection. Am Heart J 1997;134(3):495–507.
92. Harris KM, Braverman AC, Gutierrez FR, et al. Transesophageal echocardiographic and clinical features of aortic intramural hematoma. J Thorac Cardiovasc Surg 1997;114(4):619–626.
93. Robbins RC, McManus RP, Mitchell RS, et al. Management of patients with intramural hematoma of the thoracic aorta. Circulation 1993;88(suppl II):II1–II10.
94. Kaji S, Nishigami K, Akasaka T, et al. Prediction of progression or regression of type A aortic intramural hematoma by computed tomography. Circulation 1999;100(19 suppl):II281–II286.
95. Moizumi Y, Komatsu T, Motoyoshi N, Tabayashi K. Management of patients with intramural hematoma involving the ascending aorta. J Thorac Cardiovasc Surg 2002;124(5):918–924.

96. Sohn DW, Jung JW, Oh BH, et al. Should ascending aortic intramural hematoma be treated surgically? Am J Cardiol 2001; 87(8):1024–1026; A5.
97. Sueyoshi E, Imada T, Sakamoto I, et al. Analysis of predictive factors for progression of type B aortic intramural hematoma with computed tomography. J Vasc Surg 2002;35(6):1179–1183.
98. Mohiaddin RH, McCrohon J, Francis JM, et al. Contrast-enhanced magnetic resonance angiogram of penetrating aortic ulcer. Circulation 2001;103(4):E18–E19.
99. Demers P, Miller DC, Mitchell RS, et al. Stent-graft repair of penetrating atherosclerotic ulcers in the descending thoracic aorta: mid-term results. Ann Thorac Surg 2004;77(1):81–86.
100. Eggebrecht H, Baumgart D, Schmermund A, et al. Endovascular stent-graft repair for penetrating atherosclerotic ulcer of the descending aorta. Am J Cardiol 2003;91(9):1150–1153.
101. Schoder M, Grabenwoger M, Holzenbein T, et al. Endovascular stent-graft repair of complicated penetrating atherosclerotic ulcers of the descending thoracic aorta. J Vasc Surg 2002;36(4):720–726.
102. Cohen JR, Mandell C, Wise L. Characterization of human aortic elastase found in patients with abdominal aortic aneurysms. Surg Gynecol Obstet 1987;165(4):301–304.
103. Reilly JM, Sicard GA, Lucore CL. Abnormal expression of plasminogen activators in aortic aneurysmal and occlusive disease. J Vasc Surg 1994;19(5):865–872.
104. Schneiderman J, Bordin GM, Engelberg I, et al. Expression of fibrinolytic genes in atherosclerotic abdominal aortic aneurysm wall. A possible mechanism for aneurysm expansion. J Clin Invest 1995;96(1):639–645.
105. Ejiri J, Inoue N, Tsukube T, et al. Oxidative stress in the pathogenesis of thoracic aortic aneurysm: protective role of statin and angiotensin II type 1 receptor blocker. Cardiovasc Res 2003; 59(4):988–996.
106. Clifton MA. Familial abdominal aortic aneurysm. Br J Surg 1977;64:765–766.
107. Guo D, Hasham S, Kuang SQ, et al. Familial thoracic aortic aneurysms and dissections: genetic heterogeneity with a major locus mapping to 5q13-14. Circulation 2001;103(20):2461–2468.
108. Bengtsson H, Norrgard O, Angquist KA, et al. Ultrasonographic screening of the abdominal aorta among siblings of patients with abdominal aortic aneurysms. Br J Surg 1989;76:589–591.
109. Majumber PP, St. Jean PL, Ferrell RE, et al. On the inheritance of abdominal aortic aneurysm. Am J Hum Genet 1991;48:164–170.
110. Milewicz DM, Chen H, Park ES, et al. Reduced penetrance and variable expressivity of familial thoracic aortic aneurysms/dissections. Am J Cardiol 1998;82(4):474–479.
111. Bickerstaff LK, Pairolero PC, Hollier LH, et al. Thoracic aortic aneurysms: a population-based study. Surgery (St. Louis) 1982;92:1103–1109.
112. Clouse WD, Hallett JW Jr, Schaff HV, et al. Improved prognosis of thoracic aortic aneurysms: a population-based study. JAMA 1998;280(22):1926–1929.
113. McNamara JJ, Pressler VM. Natural history of arteriosclerotic thoracic aortic aneurysms. Ann Thorac Surg 1978;26:468–473.
114. Perko MJ, Norgaard M, Herzog TM, et al. Unoperated aortic aneurysm: a survey of 170 patients. Ann Thorac Surg 1995; 59(5):1204–1209.
115. Coady MA, Rizzo JA, Hammond GL, et al. Surgical intervention criteria for thoracic aortic aneurysms: a study of growth rates and complications. Ann Thorac Surg 1999;67(6):1922–1926; discussion 1953–1958.
116. Coady MA, Rizzo JA, Hammond GL, et al. What is the appropriate size criterion for resection of thoracic aortic aneurysms? J Thorac Cardiovasc Surg 1997;113(3):476–491; discussion 489–491.
117. Davies RR, Goldstein LJ, Coady MA, et al. Yearly rupture or dissection rates for thoracic aortic aneurysms: simple prediction based on size. Ann Thorac Surg 2002;73(1):17–27; discussion 27–28.
118. Juvonen T, Ergin MA, Galla JD, et al. Prospective study of the natural history of thoracic aortic aneurysms. Ann Thorac Surg 1997;63(6):1533–1545.
119. Crawford ES, Cohen ES. Aortic aneurysm: a multifocal disease. Presidential address. Arch Surg 1982;117(11):1393–1400.
120. Genoni M, Paul M, Tavakoli R, et al. Predictors of complications in acute type B aortic dissection. Eur J Cardio-Thorac Surg 2002;22(1):59–63.
121. Kouchoukos NT, Wareing TH, Murphy SF, Perrillo JB. Sixteen-year experience with aortic root replacement. Results of 172 operations. Ann Surg 1991;214(3):308–318; discussion 318–320.
122. Gott VL, Cameron DE, Alejo DE, et al. Aortic root replacement in 271 Marfan patients: a 24-year experience. Ann Thorac Surg 2002;73(2):438–443.
123. Kouchoukos NT, Masetti P, Rokkas CK, Murphy SF. Hypothermic cardiopulmonary bypass and circulatory arrest for operations on the descending thoracic and thoracoabdominal aorta. Ann Thorac Surg 2002;74(5):S1885–S1887; discussion S1892–S1898.
124. Ergin MA, Galla JD, Lansman L, et al. Hypothermic circulatory arrest in operations on the thoracic aorta. Determinants of operative mortality and neurologic outcome. J Thorac Cardiovasc Surg 1994;107(3):788–797; discussion 797–799.
125. Kouchoukos NT, Masetti P, Rokkas CK, Murphy SF. Single-stage reoperative repair of chronic type A aortic dissection using the arch-first technique. Ann Thorac Surg 2002;74(5):S1800–S1802; discussion S1825–S1832.
126. Kouchoukos NT, Masetti P. Total aortic arch replacement with a branched graft and limited circulatory arrest of the brain. J Thorac Cardiovasc Surg 2004;128(2):233–237.
127. Heinemann MK, Buehner B, Jurmann MJ, Borst HG. Use of the "elephant trunk technique" in aortic surgery. Ann Thorac Surg 1995;60(1):2–6; discussion 7.
128. Svensson LG, Kim KH, Blackstone EH, et al. Elephant trunk procedure: newer indications and uses. Ann Thorac Surg 2004;78(1):109–116; discussion 109–116.
129. Svensson LG. Rationale and technique for replacement of the ascending aorta, arch, and distal aorta using a modified elephant trunk procedure. J Cardiovasc Surg 1992;7(4):301–312.
130. Kouchoukos NT, Masetti P, Rokkas CK. Single-stage replacement of the thoracic aorta. Ann Thorac Surg 2002;74(4):1292; author reply 1293.
131. Eagle KA, Coley CM, Newell JB, et al. Combining clinical and thallium data optimizes preoperative assessment of cardiac risk before major vascular surgery. Ann Intern Med 1989;110:859–866.
132. Cutler BS, Leppo JA. Dipyridamole thallium 201 scintigraphy to detect coronary artery disease before abdominal aortic surgery. J Vasc Surg 1987;5:91–100.
133. Boucher CA, Brewster DC, Darling RC, et al. Determination of cardiac risk by dipyridamole-thallium imagining before peripheral vascular surgery. N Engl J Med 1985;1312:389–394.
134. Lalka SG, Sawada SG, Dalsing MC, et al. Dobutamine stress echocardiography as a predictor of cardiac events associated with aortic surgery. J Vasc Surg 1992;15:831–842.
135. Coselli JS, LeMaire SA, Conklin LD, et al. Morbidity and mortality after extent II thoracoabdominal aortic aneurysm repair. Ann Thorac Surg 2002;73(4):1107–1115; discussion 1115–1116.
136. Coselli JS, LeMaire SA, Miller CC III, et al. Mortality and paraplegia after thoracoabdominal aortic aneurysm repair: a risk factor analysis. Ann Thorac Surg 2000;69(2):409–414.
137. LeMaire SA, Miller CC III, Conklin LD, et al. Estimating group mortality and paraplegia rates after thoracoabdominal aortic aneurysm repair. Ann Thorac Surg 2003;75(2):508–513.

138. Miller CC III, Porat EE, Estrera AL, et al. Analysis of short-term multivariate competing risks data following thoracic and thoracoabdominal aortic repair. Eur J Cardiothorac Surg 2003;23(6):1023–1027; discussion 1027.
139. Coselli JS, LeMaire SA, Conklin LD, Adams GJ. Left heart bypass during descending thoracic aortic aneurysm repair does not reduce the incidence of paraplegia. Ann Thorac Surg 2004;77(4):1298–1303; discussion 1303.
140. Cambria RP, Davison JK, Carter C, et al. Epidural cooling for spinal cord protection during thoracoabdominal aneurysm repair: A five-year experience. J Vasc Surg 2000;31(6):1093–1102.
141. Motoyoshi N, Takahashi G, Sakurai M, et al. Safety and efficacy of epidural cooling for regional spinal cord hypothermia during thoracoabdominal aneurysm repair. Eur J Cardiothorac Surg 2004;25(1):139–141.
142. Safi HJ, Miller CC III, Huynh TT, et al. Distal aortic perfusion and cerebrospinal fluid drainage for thoracoabdominal and descending thoracic aortic repair: ten years of organ protection. Ann Surg 2003;238(3):372–380; discussion 380–381.
143. Hamilton IN Jr, Hollier LH. Adjunctive therapy for spinal cord protection during thoracoabdominal aortic aneurysm repair. Semin Thorac Cardiovasc Surg 1998;10(1):35–39.
144. Maniar HS, Sundt TM III, Prasad SM, et al. Delayed paraplegia after thoracic and thoracoabdominal aneurysm repair: a continuing risk. Ann Thorac Surg 2003;75(1):113–119; discussions 119–120.
145. Estrera AL, Miller CC III, Huynh TT, et al. Preoperative and operative predictors of delayed neurologic deficit following repair of thoracoabdominal aortic aneurysm. J Thorac Cardiovasc Surg 2003;126(5):1288–1294.
146. Leurs LJ, Bell R, Degrieck Y, et al. Endovascular treatment of thoracic aortic diseases: combined experience from the EUROSTAR and United Kingdom Thoracic Endograft registries. J Vasc Surg 2004;40(4):670–679; discussion 679–680.
147. Criado FJ, Abul-Khoudoud OR, Domer GS, et al. Endovascular repair of the thoracic aorta: lessons learned. Ann Thorac Surg 2005;80(3):857–863; discussion 863.
148. Makaroun MS, Dillavou ED, Kee ST, et al. Endovascular treatment of thoracic aortic aneurysms: results of the phase II multicenter trial of the GORE TAG thoracic endoprosthesis. J Vasc Surg 2005;41(1):1–9.
149. Bennett DE, Cherry JK. The natural history of traumatic aneurysms of the aorta. Surgery (St. Louis) 1967;61:516–523.
150. McCollum CH, Graham JM, Noon GP, et al. Chronic traumatic aneurysms of the thoracic aorta: an analysis of 50 patients. J Trauma 1979;19:248–252.
151. Finkelmeier BA, Mentzer RM, Kaiser DL, et al. Chronic traumatic thoracic aneurysm. Influence of operative treatment on natural history: an analysis of reported cases, 1950–1980. J Thorac Cardiovasc Surg 1982;84:257–266.
152. Bacharach JM, Garratt KN, Rooke TW. Chronic traumatic thoracic aneurysm: report of two cases with the question of timing for surgical intervention. J Vasc Surg 1993;17(4):780–783.
153. Katsumata T, Shinfeld A, Westaby S. Operation for chronic traumatic aortic aneurysm: when and how? Ann Thorac Surg 1998;66:774–778.
154. Semba CP, Kato N, Kee ST, et al. Acute rupture of the descending thoracic aorta: repair with use of endovascular stent-grafts. J Vasc Intervent Radiol 1997;8(3):337–342.
155. Demers P, Miller C, Scott Mitchell R, et al. Chronic traumatic aneurysms of the descending thoracic aorta: mid-term results of endovascular repair using first and second-generation stent-grafts. Eur J Cardiothorac Surg 2004;25(3):394–400.
156. Demers P, Miller DC, Mitchell RS, et al. Midterm results of endovascular repair of descending thoracic aortic aneurysms with first-generation stent grafts. J Thorac Cardiovasc Surg 2004;127(3):664–673.
157. Warnes CA. Bicuspid aortic valve and coarctation: two villains part of a diffuse problem. Heart (Br Cardiac Soc) 2003;89(9):965–966.
158. Connolly HM, Schaff HV, Izhar U, et al. Posterior pericardial ascending-to-descending aortic bypass: an alternative surgical approach for complex coarctation of the aorta. Circulation 2001;104(12 suppl 1):I133–I137.
159. Lawrie GM, DeBakey ME, Morris GC Jr, et al. Late repair of coarctation of the descending thoracic aorta in 190 patients. Results up to 30 years after operation. Arch Surg 1981;116(12):1557–1560.
160. Rokkas CK, Murphy SF, Kouchoukos NT. Aortic coarctation in the adult: management of complications and coexisting arterial abnormalities with hypothermic cardiopulmonary bypass and circulatory arrest. J Thorac Cardiovasc Surg 2002;124(1):155–161.
161. Fawzy ME, Sivanandam V, Pieters F, et al. Long-term effects of balloon angioplasty on systemic hypertension in adolescent and adult patients with coarctation of the aorta. Eur Heart J 1999;20(11):827–832.
162. Trimarchi S, Nienaber CA, Rampoldi V, et al. Contemporary results of surgery in acute type A aortic dissection: The International Registry of Acute Aortic Dissection experience. J Thorac Cardiovasc Surg 2005;129(1):112–122.
163. Suzuki T, Mehta RH, Ince H, et al. Clinical profiles and outcomes of acute type B aortic dissection in the current era: lessons from the International Registry of Aortic Dissection (IRAD). Circulation 2003;108(1):9.
164. Borst HG, Jurmann M, Buhner B, Laas J. Risk of replacement of descending aorta with a standardized left heart bypass technique. J Thorac Cardiovasc Surg 1994;107(1):126–132; discussion 132–133.
165. Cambria RP, Clouse WD, Davison JK, et al. Thoracoabdominal aneurysm repair: results with 337 operations performed over a 15-year interval. Ann Surg 2002;236(4):471–479; discussion 479.
166. Kouchoukos NT, Masetti P, Rokkas CK, et al. Safety and efficacy of hypothermic cardiopulmonary bypass and circulatory arrest for operations on the descending thoracic and thoracoabdominal aorta. Ann Thorac Surg 2001;72(3):699–707; discussion 707–708.
167. Galla JD, Ergin MA, Lansman SL, et al. Use of somatosensory evoked potentials for thoracic and thoracoabdominal aortic resections. Ann Thorac Surg 1999;67(6):1947–1952; discussion 1953–1958.
168. Coselli JS, Lemaire SA, Koksoy C, et al. Cerebrospinal fluid drainage reduces paraplegia after thoracoabdominal aortic aneurysm repair: results of a randomized clinical trial. J Vasc Surg 2002;35(4):631–639.

64

Diseases of the Great Vessels and the Thoracic Outlet

Spencer J. Melby and Robert W. Thompson

Occlusive Diseases of the Aortic Arch Branches

Atherosclerosis

Etiology and Pathophysiology

The aortic arch and its branches are a common location for the development of atherosclerosis. Similar to atherosclerosis in other areas of the arterial tree, the pathology ranges from mild, nonocclusive intimal thickening to complex atheromata. Complex atheromatous plaques may evolve to a size large enough to encroach upon the lumen, thereby restricting flow, or they may be complicated by intraplaque hemorrhage, ulceration and discharge of atheromatous debris, and surface thrombosis. Well-established clinical risk factors for atherosclerosis include family history, aging, cigarette smoking, hypertension, hyperlipidemia, and diabetes.

Clinical Presentation and Diagnosis

Symptoms caused by atherosclerotic lesions of the innominate artery may be either acute or chronic. Acute symptoms include either stroke or transient ischemic attacks, caused by atheroembolization to the internal carotid circulation, or acute atheroembolism to the right upper extremity, which can cause hand ischemia, digital infarction, and necrosis. With gradual occlusion, innominate lesions may lead to chronic or intermittent ischemia of the arm, particularly during active use or when the arm is used in an overhead position, with symptoms analogous to intermittent calf claudication caused by lower extremity occlusive disease. Isolated innominate artery disease is an unusual cause of chronic cerebrovascular symptoms, which usually suggest the presence of additional atherosclerotic lesions affecting other vessels.

Occlusive lesions of the proximal subclavian artery are responsible for the "subclavian steal" syndrome. In this situation, low flow to the upper extremity is compensated by collateral flow through the intracranial circulation via the ipsilateral vertebral artery. When exacerbated by arm exercise, retrograde flow in the vertebral artery may transiently lower perfusion pressure in the posterior vertebrobasilar circuit, leading to sudden episodes know as "drop attacks." These episodes are characterized by a near loss of consciousness and collapse, without antecedent cortical symptoms; typically, consciousness is quickly regained without sequelae. Drop attacks caused by subclavian steal are therefore usually easy to distinguish from true syncope or transient ischemic attacks (TIAs) arising from the anterior circulation.

Surgical Management

The medical management of atherosclerosis is discussed in more detail elsewhere. In general, this consists of lifestyle modifications and medical control of risk factors such as diabetes and hypertension. Treatment for symptomatic atherosclerotic lesions may include regular administration of aspirin or other platelet antagonists; in some circumstances, anticoagulation is also used. These approaches are of limited value, however, in preventing the cerebrovascular or limb-threatening complications of complex atheromatous plaques in this location. Thus, surgical or endoluminal interventions remain the mainstay of treatment for atherosclerotic lesions affecting the aortic arch branches. The specific operative approaches to be used vary with the precise location of the atherosclerotic lesions to be treated and individual variations in anatomy, as well as the preferential use of certain routes for reconstruction based an accumulated clinical experience.

Innominate Artery Reconstruction

Symptomatic lesions of the innominate artery may be treated by either innominate thromboendarterectomy (TEA) or bypass grafting. The surgical approach for either of these options requires direct exposure through a median sternotomy (Fig. 64.1). For endarterectomy, the innominate artery is isolated from its origin on the aortic arch to its bifurcation, with separate control of the subclavian and common carotid arteries.

It is necessary to recognize that orificial lesions of the innominate artery represent an extension of atherosclerosis arising in the aortic arch; thus, effective removal of the plaque requires access to a disease-free segment along the superior aspect of the arch, which can be safely controlled with a partial occlusion clamp. Another consideration in exposure of the proximal innominate artery is the location of the left common carotid artery origin, as it is necessary to avoid occlusion of this branch during clamp control of the innominate origin. In some cases, the common carotid artery arises from a common origin with the innominate artery, precluding safe isolation of the innominate; endarterectomy cannot be undertaken in this circumstance, requiring an alternative approach to innominate reconstruction. Following satisfactory isolation of the innominate artery and systemic anticoagulation, a longitudinal arteriotomy is performed; this typically extends from the level of the arch to the innominate bifurcation, but may be advanced into either the subclavian or right common carotid artery if necessary. It is notable that, because of the abundance of collateral circulation in this region, shunting to protect the cerebral circulation is usually not needed. The atherosclerotic lesion is then removed by standard endarterectomy techniques, and the vessel is closed primarily.

Innominate artery bypass is also performed through a median sternotomy (Fig. 64.1B). The lateral aspect of the intrapericardial ascending aorta is often free of significant atherosclerosis; thus, this area usually offers an optimal site for the origin of a prosthetic bypass graft. The distal innominate artery is exposed and controlled, and the ascending aorta is controlled with a partial occlusion clamp. An oblique end-to-side anastomosis is created between the aorta and the trunk of an 8- to 10-mm-diameter Dacron graft, and the aortic clamp is removed; for short innominate lesions, a straight bypass graft may be used with the distal anastomoses placed in an end-to-end fashion to the innominate bifurcation. For disease extending into the right subclavian or common carotid arteries, a short bifurcation graft originating from the aorta can be used with end-to-end anastomoses to each of the target vessels. In more difficult circumstances where a previous median sternotomy has been performed, innominate reconstruction may also be accomplished by alternative approaches,

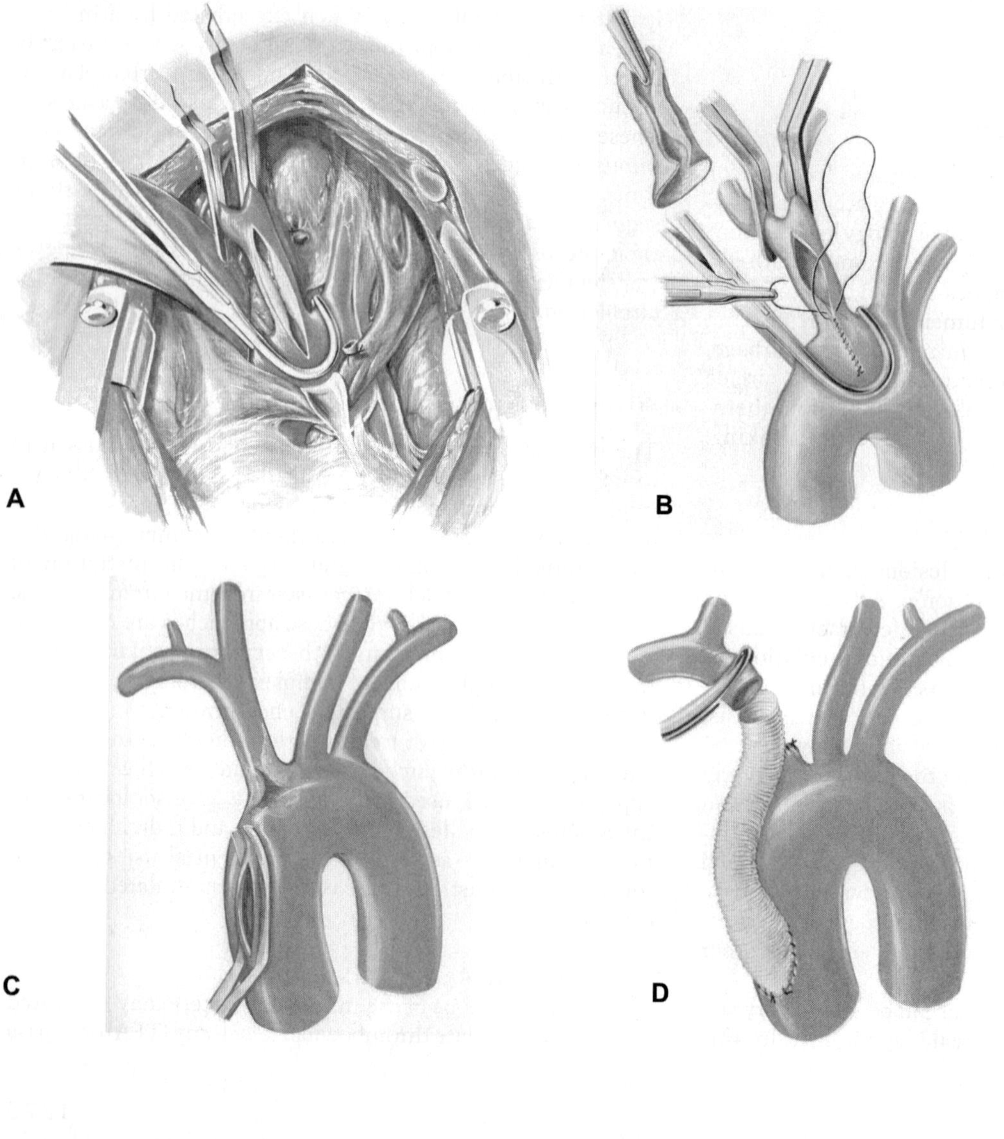

FIGURE 64.1. Direct innominate artery reconstruction. **A.** Median sternotomy is required to control the origin of the innominate artery. Endarterectomy is performed by isolating the innominate origin with a partial-occlusion J-clamp, taking care to include the aortic origin of the plaque. Arterial shunting is normally not required in this location. **B.** Primary closure of the innominate arteriotomy following endarterectomy, which in this case is extended into the right subclavian artery. **C.** Innominate artery bypass is performed by isolating a disease-free area along the lateral aspect of the ascending aorta to serve as the origin for a prosthetic graft, using a partial-occlusion (Satinsky) clamp. **D.** Straight prosthetic tube graft repair is placed end-to-end to the distal innominate artery. Alternatively, a bifurcation graft may be used if disease extends into the proximal right subclavian and/or common carotid arteries, with use of two separate distal anastomoses. (From Stoney RJ, Effeney DJ, eds. Wylie's Atlas of Vascular Surgery. Extracranial Cerebrovascular Disease. Philadelphia: Lippincott, 1993, with permission.)

TABLE 64.1.
Results of Innominate Artery Reconstruction (Level III Evidence).

Source	*Patients (n)*	*TEA/BPG/Ex*	*Mortality (%)*	*Neurological Cx (%)*	*Patency (f/u)*
Reul et al. 1991[10]	54	11/27/16	0	1.8	92.6 (10)
Kieffer et al. 1995[9]	148	32/116	5.4	5.4	96.3 (10)
Berguer et al. 1998[8]	100	8/92	8	8	88% (10)
Azakie et al. 1998[7]	94	72/22	3	6	97% (10)
Totals	396	123/257	2.8	5.8	93.8

TEA, thromobendartercetomy; BPG, innominate artery bypass graft; Ex, extrathoracic reconstruction; Cx, complications; f/u, years follow-up.

such as extrathoracic carotid–carotid or axillary–axillary bypass grafting.

Although no prospective clinical studies are available, a number of clinical trials have demonstrated that excellent results can be achieved by direct innominate artery reconstruction with either thromboendarterectomy or prosthetic bypass grafting.[1–6] In addition, four particularly large studies have been published in the past decade that offer detailed analysis of perioperative and long-term results for a total of nearly 400 patients (Table 64.1).[7–10] Operative mortality rates in these series ranged from 0% to 8% (mean, 2.8%), with the majority of deaths due to cardiac causes, and perioperative neurological complications occurred in 1.8% to 8% of patients (mean, 5.8%). The 10-year patency rates for innominate reconstruction were 88% to 97%, with similar figures reported for long-term relief of symptoms. These results demonstrate that direct innominate artery reconstruction is safe and durable when either endarterectomy or prosthetic bypass is used. The experience reported by Azakie et al.[7] indicates that anatomic variations and the distribution of disease permit the use of innominate endarterectomy for most patients, which can be extended safely to outflow and adjacent vessels. As emphasized by Berguer et al.,[8] direct innominate artery reconstruction should be reserved for symptomatic patients, whereas lower-risk alternatives (i.e., cervical extraanatomic bypass or endovascular approaches) should be considered for those with asymptomatic lesions, particularly in patients with significant concomitant conditions.

Subclavian-to-Carotid Artery Transposition

Atherosclerotic lesions of the proximal subclavian artery were previously treated by direct endarterectomy. However, this approach requires adequate exposure of the subclavian artery at its origin, and this can present a particular challenge on the left side, where a thoracotomy is required to isolate the subclavian origin at the level of the distal aortic arch. By avoiding the morbidity of median sternotomy or thoracotomy, extrathoracic approaches have superseded the use of endarterectomy for subclavian reconstruction. The most widely utilized approach to subclavian reconstruction is direct transposition of the subclavian artery to the side of the common carotid artery (Fig. 64.2A). This repair can be accomplished

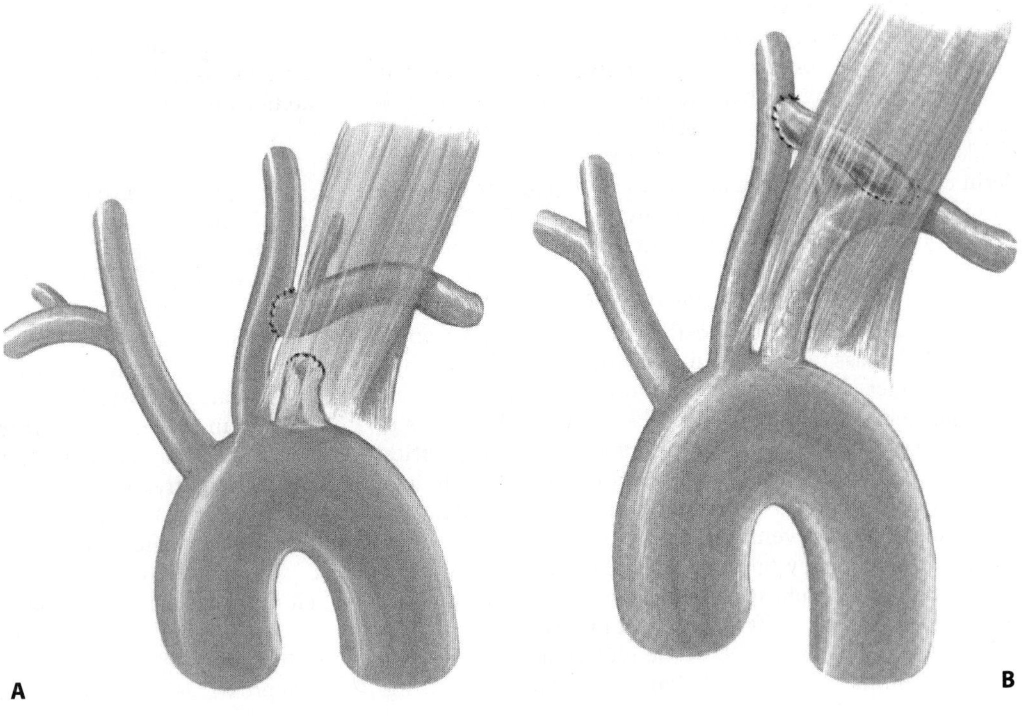
A B

FIGURE 64.2. Subclavian artery reconstruction. Proximal atherosclerosis of the subclavian artery is usually managed by extrathoracic forms of arterial reconstruction. The midportion of the subclavian artery is approached through a supraclavicular cervical incision, with reflection of the scalene fat pad and division of the anterior scalene muscle (not shown). **A.** Subclavian-to-carotid transposition. **B.** Carotid-to-subclavian bypass. (From Stoney RJ, Effeney DJ, eds. Wylie's Atlas of Vascular Surgery. Extracranial Cerebrovascular Disease. Philadelphia: Lippincott, 1993, with permission.)

with relative ease on either side using a supraclavicular incision. After dissection of the scalene fat pad and division of the anterior scalene muscle, the subclavian artery is exposed proximal to the vertebral artery origin. It is important to point out that the subclavian artery in this region can be very delicate, and it is essential to avoid tears in the arterial wall. After clamp occlusion and ligation of the proximal subclavian artery, the vessel is mobilized to the side of the adjacent common carotid artery. The carotid artery is then clamped and an arteriotomy is created on the lateral wall, and an end-to-side anastomosis is created with the subclavian artery.

Carotid-to-Subclavian Artery Bypass

Carotid–subclavian bypass is also commonly utilized for symptomatic lesions of the proximal subclavian artery. This procedure is performed through a supraclavicular exposure similar to that described for subclavian artery transposition. It is not necessary to achieve the extent of subclavian exposure required for transposition, as the bypass graft is usually placed upon the superior aspect of the vessel just distal to the origin of the vertebral artery (Fig. 64.2B). Once the subclavian and common carotid arteries have been satisfactorily controlled, a short 8- to 10-mm prosthetic graft is interposed between the vessels using end-to-side anastomoses. Prosthetic grafts are preferred in this circumstance, as they tend to be less prone than reversed saphenous vein grafts to kinking or twisting caused by the oblique angle of the reconstruction, and because they have been demonstrated to have a higher long-term patency rate in this location than autologous conduits.

Clinical experience demonstrates excellent long-term results for extraanatomic subclavian artery reconstruction.[11–17] In one of the largest series reported to date, Edwards et al.[12] described a 4-year patency rate of 99.4% for 178 patients undergoing carotid–subclavian transposition, with an operative mortality rate of 1.1%. Schardey et al.[15] reported no deaths in 108 patients undergoing transposition procedures, with 100% patency at a mean follow-up of 6 years. The tendency to favor transposition over bypass is further supported by two retrospective comparative series. Thus, van der Vliet et al.[17] found that the patency rate of 21 carotid–subclavian transpositions was 100% at 10 years, compared to 52.2% for 21 patients undergoing carotid–subclavian bypass. Deriu et al.[11] compared the outcomes of 40 patients undergoing either transposition ($n = 20$) or bypass ($n = 20$). Operative mortality rates (5%) were equivalent in each group; however, at 6-year follow-up the patency rate of carotid–subclavian transpositions was 100% while that of carotid–subclavian bypasses was 66%. As noted earlier, it is generally accepted that, when bypass procedures are performed, prosthetic grafts have a distinct advantage over autologous vein grafts in this position. Thus, Law et al.[13] reported a series of 60 patients in which the patency rate for carotid–subclavian transposition was 100%, whereas it was 95.2% for polytetrafluoroethylene (PTFE) bypass grafts, 83.9% for Dacron bypass grafts, and 64.9% for saphenous vein grafts.

In addition to symptomatic atherosclerotic occlusive disease, two new indications have emerged over the past decade specifically for left-sided carotid-to-subclavian reconstruction. The first is related to the prevalent use of the left internal mammary artery (LIMA) in coronary bypass grafting, where left subclavian artery stenosis may diminish perfusion pressure in a LIMA that provides critical coronary flow. Patients who are dependent on a LIMA–coronary bypass graft may thereby exhibit "coronary-subclavian steal syndrome" in the presence of left subclavian artery occlusion, in which upper extremity exercise results in acute angina symptoms.[18–20] Increasing recognition of this syndrome has led to efforts to identify and revascularize left subclavian artery lesions before coronary bypass operations; conversely, the development of this syndrome following successful coronary revascularization represents an important indication for either endovascular or extraanatomic left subclavian artery reconstruction. A second new indication for left subclavian artery reconstruction has emerged with the increasing use of endovascular stent-grafts in the treatment of thoracic aortic aneurysms and dissections.[21–23] Placement of these stent-grafts requires a suitable proximal site of attachment, which may not be present within the descending thoracic aorta distal to the origin of the left subclavian artery. In these situations it has become commonplace to accept obstruction of the left subclavian artery origin to achieve a firm proximal stent-graft attachment site. Although this may be well tolerated by many individuals, extrathoracic subclavian artery reconstruction is indicated when stent-graft obstruction of the left subclavian artery has resulted in upper extremity symptoms.

Subclavian-to-Carotid Artery Bypass

Subclavian-to-carotid artery reconstructions represent another extraanatomic (cervical) approach that may be used for the treatment of isolated common carotid artery lesions, when the subclavian artery is suitably free of disease to serve as an inflow source. These procedures are performed in the same fashion as for lesions of the proximal subclavian artery, using either transposition of the common carotid artery to the subclavian artery or short bypass grafts from the subclavian to the common carotid. In situations in which the entire common carotid artery is occluded, or when concomitant carotid bifurcation endarterectomy is also indicated, a prosthetic bypass graft arising from the subclavian artery may be extended to the carotid bifurcation.

Axillary-to-Axillary Artery Bypass

Axillo-axillary artery crossover bypass offers another alternative for extraanatomic revascularization of the aortic arch branch vessels. The axillary arteries are approached through bilateral infraclavicular incisions, splitting the pectoralis major muscle fibers. The axillary arteries are exposed medial to the pectoralis minor muscle on each side, and a crossover bypass graft is passed in the subcutaneous plane in front of the sternum. Like other extraanatomic reconstructions, externally reinforced prosthetic grafts are preferred to reduce the chances of extrinsic graft compression. As summarized in a comprehensive review by Lowell and Mills,[24] operative mortality and complication rates for axillo-axillary artery bypass are generally less than 2%, in contrast to other approaches that may involve thoracotomy, sternotomy, or carotid dissection and clamping. One of the most common complications of this procedure is transient brachial plexopathy, occurring in approximately 3.5% of patients; graft infection or skin erosion occurred in about 1.6%. The long-term patency rate is approximately 90%. A recent report suggests that axillo-axillary bypass grafting may be particularly valuable as a surgical alternative to transthoracic anatomic reconstructions for innominate lesions, long stenoses of the subclavian artery, and short subclavian artery stenoses associated with ipsilateral carotid artery lesions.[25]

ENDOVASCULAR REPAIR

Although endovascular techniques for arterial reconstruction are considered in detail elsewhere, recent advances in endovascular technology have provided an alternative means of therapy for the treatment of occlusive lesions in the innominate and proximal subclavian arteries. Innovations in imaging, guidewire, catheter, balloon, and stent technology now allow one to obtain percutaneous access and perform therapeutic procedures in a relatively safe manner. Despite the appeal of these less invasive techniques, the morbidity, mortality, and durability of such novel treatments for disease of the aortic arch branches remain largely unknown.[26] Nonetheless, it can be expected that endovascular approaches will continue to assume an increasingly prominent role in the management of these lesions.

Large Vessel Arteritides

A number of inflammatory disorders have a predilection for affecting the thoracic aorta and its branches. The most important of these conditions are giant cell (temporal) arteritis and Takayasu's arteritis, each of which is much less common than atherosclerosis (Table 64.2). These conditions tend to affect patients with substantially different clinical characteristics, and their existence is often suspected on the basis of clinical history. Although the etiology of large vessel arteritides is largely unknown and specific diagnosis may be difficult, clinical recognition of these conditions is important because they usually require alternative approaches to treatment than those used for occlusive atherosclerosis.[27,28]

ETIOLOGY AND PATHOPHYSIOLOGY

The etiology of large vessel vasculitides is unknown, but each of these disorders appears to be characterized by cell-mediated immune or inflammatory responses localized to the arterial wall. Both giant cell arteritis and Takayasu's arteritis exhibit arterial infiltration by T- and B lymphocytes, mononuclear phagocytes, and macrophages (multinucleated "giant cells" being a particularly common feature in temporal arteritis). The histological findings of these two diseases therefore appear quite similar, and they are distinguished to a greater extent by the size and location of the arteries involved.[29] Large vessel vasculitides are suspected to involve an immune response specifically targeted against arterial wall antigens, but the specific antigens that might be involved remain to be identified. It is possible that certain antigens are involved in the initial pathogenesis of disease and that the immune response is amplified to include secondary antigens as the disease progresses (a phenomenon known as "epitope spreading"). There is accumulating evidence that large vessel vasculitides are associated with specific HLA class I antigens, which may vary in different ethnic populations or geographic groups consistent with the clinical patterns exhibited by these conditions, regardless of the initiating factors. It is clear that chronic vascular wall inflammation can amplify the pathological inflammatory response through neovascularization and increased expression of vascular adhesion molecules. In turn, soluble factors released by inflammatory cells are thought to play a significant role in thrombosis, vessel occlusion, and ischemic complications.[30]

TABLE 64.2. Features Distinguishing Temporal Arteritis and Takayasu's Arteritis.

	Giant cell (temporal) arteritis	*Takayasu's arteritis*
Prevalence	Common	Rare
Age/gender	Elderly women	Young women
Descent	Caucasian	South American, Asian, Indian
Vessels	Small and medium	Large
Definitive diagnosis	Histology	Arteriography
Steroids	Curative	Palliative (active phase)
Surgery	Diagnosis	Definitive (quiescent phase)

GIANT CELL (TEMPORAL) ARTERITIS

CLINICAL PRESENTATION AND DIAGNOSIS

Giant cell arteritis is a disorder of small and medium-sized blood vessels that commonly presents in elderly Caucasian women.[31] It may occur in association with polymyalgia rheumatica or as isolated temporal arteritis, but both types are thought to represent variants of the same disease. The annual incidence of giant cell arteritis is 7 per 100,000, but this rises to approximately 15 per 100,000 in populations over 50 years of age.[32,33] It is rare before the age of 50 and typically occurs between 65 and 75 years of age; there is a 2:1 predominance of women over men. Giant cell arteritis appears to have a unique predilection for the temporal and ophthalmic arteries, and it only rarely involves the aortic arch or carotid arteries. Symptoms typically occur with rapid onset (within 1 month). Some patients exhibit only nonspecific symptoms, including weight loss, fever, sweats, fatigue, and anorexia. Patients with polymyalgia rheumatica typically complain of muscle tenderness in the shoulder and pelvic girdles, with morning stiffness and difficulty rising from bed. The classical symptoms of temporal arteritis are headache, scalp and temporal tenderness, visual symptoms, and jaw claudication.[34] Ocular symptoms may include blurred vision, diplopia, visual hallucinations, or amaurosis fugax. These symptoms are particularly important because failure to promptly initiate treatment may lead to permanent loss of vision.[35]

The erythrocyte sedimentation rate (ESR) is almost always markedly elevated in patients with giant cell arteritis, as a reflection of a systemic acute-phase response.[36,37] Elevated levels of C-reactive protein and interleukin 6 have also been reported.[37,38] Some patients have abnormal liver function tests with elevations in alkaline phosphatase, transaminases, and G-glutamyl transferase, but muscle enzymes (creatine phosphokinase) are not elevated. Some patients with giant cell arteritis have anticardiolipin antibodies, an alteration associated with vascular complications.[39,40]

TABLE 64.3. Diagnostic Criteria for Giant Cell (Temporal) Arteritis.

1.	Age at onset more than 50 years
2.	New onset of localized headache
3.	Temporal artery abnormality (tenderness or reduced pulsation) unrelated to arteriosclerosis
4.	Erythrocyte sedimentation rate (ESR) greater than 50 mm in first hour
5.	Abnormal arterial biopsy

At least three of five features are required for diagnosis.
Source: American College of Rheumatology.[41]

The diagnosis of giant cell arteritis is usually suggested by a characteristic clinical history and supplemented by physical findings, but it can only be confirmed by a positive tissue biopsy. Problems are encountered when the history is atypical or the biopsy is negative; thus, the American College of Rheumatology has outlined a series of five diagnostic criteria when the diagnosis of giant cell arteritis is in question (Table 64.3).[41] The typical histological features of temporal arteritis include a patchy chronic inflammatory infiltrate consisting of multinucleated giant cells, often focused upon the internal elastic lamina (Fig. 64.3). There may also be a mixed inflammatory response with no giant cells, and the arteritis may occur in a transmural distribution. There is often marked intimal thickening and narrowing or occlusion of the arterial lumen. Importantly, the absence of pathological changes in a particular biopsy specimen does not completely exclude the diagnosis of giant cell arteritis, and in individual patients, the histological findings must always be placed in the context of other clinical features.

Medical Management

Large vessel vasculitides often respond favorably to treatment with glucocorticosteroids. Prompt steroid treatment is particularly important in temporal arteritis, because the response is often rapid and dramatic, and because early intervention may prevent the progression to loss of vision. Because of the risk of rapidly progressive (and irreversible) ophthalmic artery disease, steroid treatment is started as soon as the diagnosis of temporal arteritis is suspected. Prednisone is most commonly used at initial doses of 40 to 80 mg/day, with the aim of abolishing symptoms within several days or weeks.[42,43] Treatment is also guided by a fall in the ESR, and once a clinical response has been obtained, the dose of prednisone is reduced and then slowly tapered off over a period of 2 to 5 years.[44] When prednisone does not produce sufficient relief of clinical symptoms, or if steroid toxicity limits further treatment, azathioprine or methotrexate have been advocated as alternative immunosuppressant approaches. These approaches to the treatment of temporal arteritis have proven to be highly effective, with a low rate of recurrence in long-term follow-up.

Surgical Management

There is no direct role for surgical treatment in giant cell (temporal) arteritis other than that of obtaining appropriate biopsy material. Nonetheless, this is an important consideration in diagnosis, and the proper conduct of temporal artery biopsy may have a significant influence on medical treatment. Symptomatic patients with temporal arteritis often respond quickly to the initiation of steroid therapy, as prompt treatment may prevent irreversible loss of vision by halting the rapid progression of changes in the ophthalmic arteries. Confirmation of the diagnosis requires histological study, and high-dose steroid therapy may be unwelcome in elderly patients for whom the diagnosis is in question. Thus, surgeons are often requested to perform temporal artery biopsy on a semiurgent basis even for patients without visual symptoms. For patients with visual symptoms in whom there are contraindications to steroid treatment (in the absence of a firm diagnosis), temporal artery biopsy may be a justifiable emergency. Although medical therapy should be started before biopsy when necessary, treatment with steroids may decrease the histological changes of arteritis within a few days, thereby reducing the yield of positive biopsies from 80% to less than 60% within 1 week. After 1 week of treatment, the positive biopsy rate falls further, to 20%. Thus, in the event that early temporal artery biopsy does not support the diagnosis of arteritis, steroid treatment can be discontinued without a significant chance of complications. On the other hand, failure to expeditiously obtain biopsy material often commits the patient to a full course of steroid therapy without the certainty of diagnosis.

Temporal artery biopsy is performed over the site of any localized tenderness or nodularity, or on the side where the patient's dominant symptoms appear to be localized. Although selection of a temporal artery with palpable abnormalities is

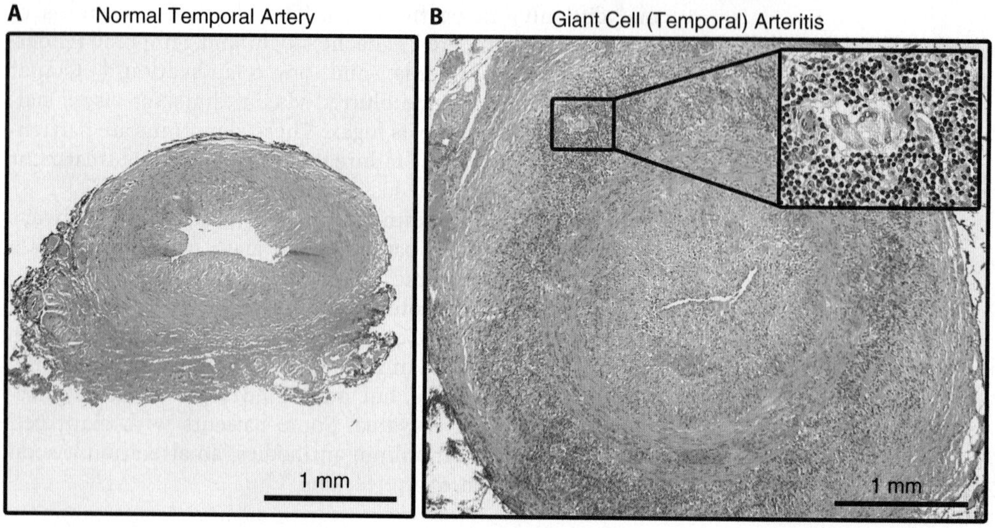

FIGURE 64.3. Histopathology of giant cell (temporal) arteritis. **A.** Normal temporal artery biopsy. **B.** Temporal artery biopsy from a patient with active arteritis, illustrating arterial thickening and obstruction, transmural inflammation, and polymorphonuclear neutrophils interspersed with focal clusters of multinucleated giant cells (*inset*). Hematoxylin and eosin. *Bar* 1 mm.

TABLE 64.4. Diagnostic Criteria for Takayasu's Arteritis.

Ishikawa criteria[50]: Age less than 40 years plus two major or one major/two minor or four minor criteria
- Major criteria: (1) left midsubclavian artery lesion; (2) right midsubclavian artery lesion
- Minor criteria: (1) elevated ESR; (2) carotid artery tenderness; (3) hypertension; (4) aortic regurgitation or annuloaortic ectasia; (5) pulmonary artery lesion; (6) left midcommon carotid artery lesion; (7) distal brachiocephalic lesion; (8) descending thoracic aortic lesion; (9) abdominal aortic lesion

American College of Rheumatology[51]: at least three of six features are required for diagnosis
1. Age at onset less than 40 years
2. Extremity claudication
3. Reduced brachial artery pressure
4. More than 10 mmHg difference in systolic blood pressure between arms
5. Subclavian or aortic bruit
6. Abnormal arteriogram

usually accurate for diagnostic material, some advocate bilateral temporal artery biopsies when there are no local findings or when the diagnosis remains in significant doubt. Biopsy is performed under local anesthesia using an incision placed along the path of the hairline. The temporal artery is easily identified in the subcuticular tissue and is then exposed over a length of 2 to 3 cm, and the intervening segment is removed after simple ligature of each end. Because the inflammatory changes in temporal arteritis often occur in a patchy distribution, it is important to procure a sufficiently long segment of the vessel for study. In some instances, unilateral temporal artery biopsy may not reflect active arteritis even when the disease is present, and a follow-up biopsy of the contralateral side may be indicated if it can be performed within the first week of starting steroid treatment.

Takayasu's Arteritis (Pulseless Disease)

Clinical Presentation and Diagnosis

Takayasu's arteritis exhibits a more varied and nonspecific pattern of clinical presentation than temporal arteritis.[45,46] Although it remains a rare disorder, it is most commonly seen in young women from South America, India, or Asia.[47–49] The inflammatory occlusive aspects of the disease can affect the thoracic or abdominal aorta, the brachiocephalic vessels, or other aortic branches and their tributaries. Symptoms and clinical findings of Takayasu's arteritis are most often related to cerebrovascular disease, brachiocephalic occlusions, or renovascular hypertension; although ophthalmological manifestations may also occur, they are usually seen only late in the course of the disease. There is a distinct female predominance at a ratio of 5:1, and the onset is usually at 15 to 40 years of age. The condition is characterized by a biphasic illness, with an initial inflammatory phase and a late stage when vascular stenosis and occlusion predominate. Systemic features often predominate in the inflammatory phase, consisting of fever, malaise, and other nonspecific symptoms. Some patients are asymptomatic during this phase. Symptoms localize in the late phase according to the specific pattern of vessel involvement; symptoms may therefore include headache, limb fatigability, dizziness, palpitations, dyspnea, or visual disturbances. In contrast to giant cell (temporal) arteritis, arterial wall biopsies play little role in the diagnosis or management of Takayasu's arteritis. There have been a number of attempts to establish diagnostic criteria for this disease (Table 64.4), with the most widely used criteria known as the Ishikawa classification.[50] The major criteria required for diagnosis include age less than 40 years, left and/or right midsubclavian artery lesions, and characteristic signs and symptoms of at least 1 month in duration. There are nine minor criteria, including an elevated erythrocyte sedimentation rate; carotid artery tenderness; hypertension; aortic regurgitation or annuloaortic ectasia; pulmonary artery stenosis; left midcommon carotid lesion; distal brachiocephalic trunk lesion; descending thoracic aortic lesion; abdominal aortic lesion; and coronary artery lesion. A high probability is associated with the presence of two major criteria, one major criterion and two minor criteria, or four minor criteria. This system was found to have a diagnostic sensitivity of 92.5% and a specificity of 95% when applied to a series of 106 patients with angiographically proven Takayasu's arteritis. A similar classification system has been established by the American College of Rheumatology (see Table 64.4).[51]

It is notable that arteriography plays a major role in the diagnosis of Takayasu's arteritis (Fig. 64.4). In addition to the clinical criteria just discussed, angiography provides specific information on the location and extent of occlusive or aneurysmal lesions, and it is especially helpful in planning treatment. In some instances, arteriographic interventions may also be utilized as the primary form of treatment.

Medical Management

In Takayasu's arteritis, steroid therapy is usually considered only palliative for active phases of disease. Clinical symptoms, ESR, and angiographic findings are the means most commonly used to assess clinical activity. Prednisone is ini-

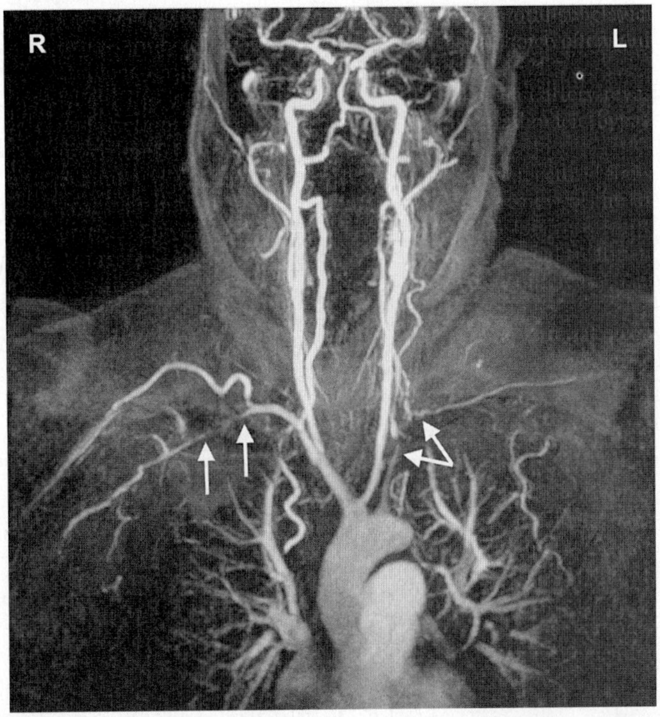

FIGURE 64.4. Takayasu's arteritis. Contrast-enhanced magnetic resonance arteriogram (MRA) in a 40 year-old patient with a 10-year history of Takayasu's arteritis treated with corticosteroids. There are segmental occlusions of the midportion of the right subclavian artery and of the proximal left subclavian artery (*arrows*), which had resulted in symptoms of bilateral arm claudication.

tially administered at high doses, then as prolonged therapy at lower maintenance dose schedules to prevent flares of disease. If possible, steroid therapy is tapered over 3 to 5 years using the ESR as a guide. For patients refractory to steroids, additional treatment options include cyclophosphamide or methotrexate. For patients with renovascular hypertension, treatment with angiotensin-converting enzyme (ACE) inhibitors may be deleterious.

SURGICAL MANAGEMENT

Interventional techniques may be used in patients with symptoms related to specific occlusive lesions caused by Takayasu's arteritis, but they have a high rate of recurrence and are usually considered only a secondary or temporizing method of treatment for this disease. Surgical reconstruction is therefore the preferred method for managing symptomatic occlusive or aneurysmal lesions in patients who have had remission into an inactive phase of the disease.[52–60] Surgical reconstruction for Takayasu's arteritis consists of various forms of bypass procedures, as thromboendarterectomy is precluded by the obliterative or aneurysmal nature of the disease process. Bypass procedures are generally performed to circumvent the specific region affected, with grafts originating from and terminating in arterial segments free of disease. Surgical reconstruction is reserved for patients in an inactive phase of the disease to limit the risk of graft occlusion by disease progression. The most common locations of disease requiring surgical reconstruction are cerebrovascular lesions, brachiocephalic lesions, and those causing renovascular hypertension. The conduct of these procedures is essentially the same as that described earlier for atherosclerotic occlusive disease.

Disorders of the Thoracic Outlet

The thoracic outlet encompasses a unique region dominated by the first rib, the anterior and middle scalene muscles, and their associated neurovascular structures (Fig. 64.5). The sub-

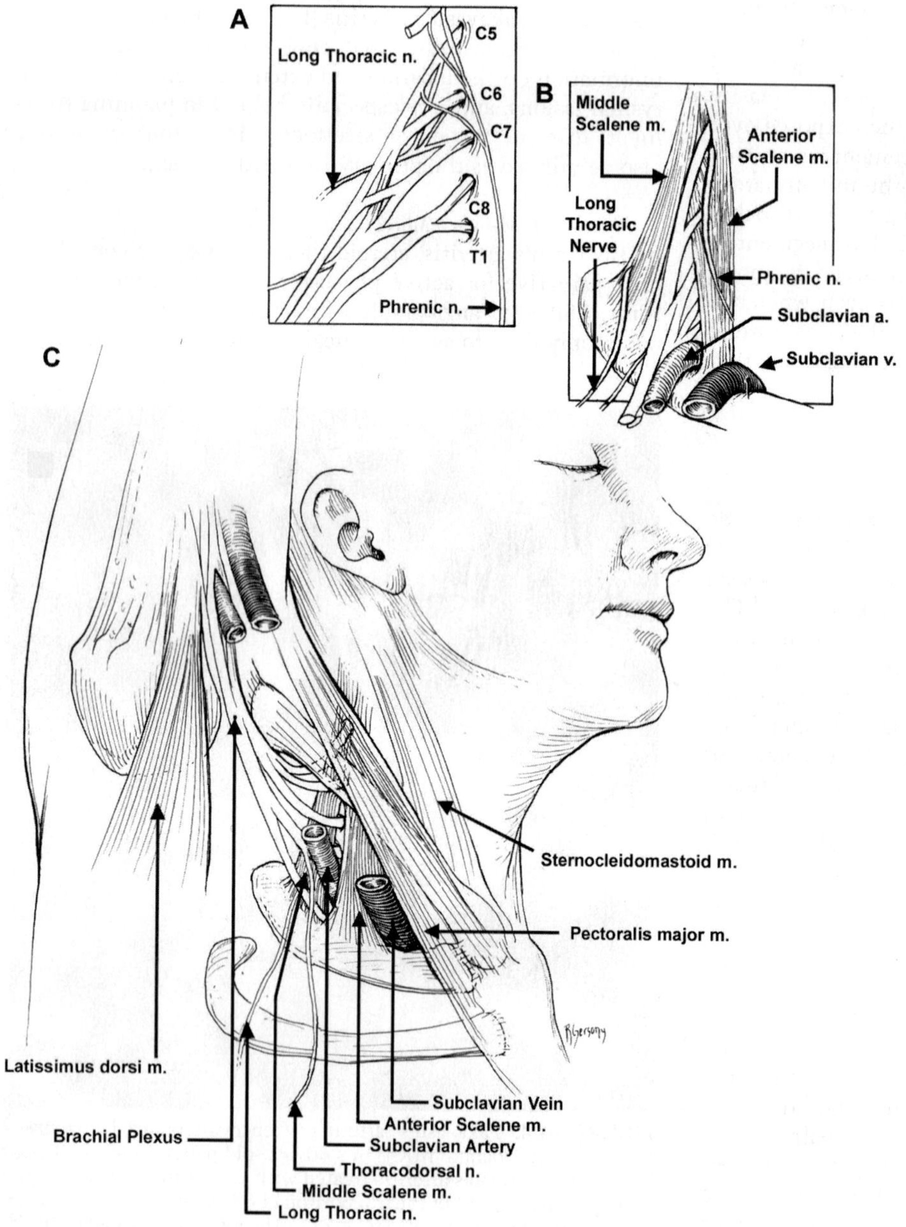

FIGURE 64.5. Surgical anatomy of the thoracic outlet. **A.** The brachial plexus arises from cervical nerve roots C5, C6, C7, C8, and T1, which begin to merge into the trunks and cords of the plexus as they exit the scalene triangle, crossing over the first rib posterior to the clavicle. The phrenic nerve arises from the upper cervical nerve roots with a contribution from C5, passing vertically upon the surface of the anterior scalene muscle before entering the mediastinum. **B.** The thoracic outlet is conceptualized as a triangle bordered by anterior scalene muscle, the middle scalene muscle, and the first rib. The nerve roots of the brachial plexus and the subclavian artery course through this triangle, whereas the subclavian vein crosses the first rib just in front of the anterior scalene muscle before joining with the internal jugular vein to form the innominate vein. Each of these structures is potentially subject to extrinsic compression at several different levels by the musculoskeletal components of the scalene triangle. **C.** The anatomy of the thoracic outlet as viewed from underneath the clavicle with the arm elevated. This position places greater strain on the neurovascular structures passing through the scalene triangle, thereby exacerbating symptoms of thoracic outlet syndrome (TOS). The long thoracic and thoracodorsal nerves pass vertically along the lateral chest wall, where they may be readily identified during transaxillary exposures. The second intercostal brachial cutaneous nerve courses in a transverse orientation through the midportion of the axilla (not shown). (From Thompson and Bartoli,[93] with permission.)

clavian artery, the subclavian vein, and the five nerve roots of the brachial plexus are all potentially subject to extrinsic compression within this relatively confined space; thus, thoracic outlet syndrome (TOS) represents a complex array of clinical conditions characterized by one or more of the following: occlusive or aneurysmal lesions of the subclavian artery (arterial TOS), "effort thrombosis" of the subclavian vein (venous TOS), or symptoms related to compression and irritation of the brachial plexus nerve roots (neurogenic TOS). Because the nerve roots comprising the brachial plexus innervate the entire upper extremity, sensory and/or motor symptoms may occur in a spectrum of patterns (Table 64.5).[61,62]

Classification and Diagnosis

Although vascular lesions associated with thoracic outlet compression typically give rise to easily recognized syndromes, the diagnosis of neurogenic TOS often remains difficult, confusing, and elusive. Uncertainties in diagnosis and disappointing results of treatment have led some to question the existence of neurogenic TOS, adding to the many controversies surrounding this condition.[63,64] Nonetheless, recognition of this condition is important in that approximately 80% of patients with TOS suffer from neurogenic symptoms rather than vascular pathology.

Neurogenic TOS

Patients with TOS frequently describe previous trauma to the head, neck, or upper extremity, followed by a variable interval before the onset of progressively disabling upper extremity symptoms.[61,62] The interval between traumatic injury and the onset of symptoms may range from days to weeks, or even several years. It is thought that scalene muscle injury leads to muscle spasm and persistent inflammation that can lead to delayed healing, with fibrosis and nerve root irritation that eventually result in compressive neurological symptoms. Even low-grade repetitive trauma can contribute to this disorder, such as prolonged work at computer consoles. Conversely, not all patients with TOS have their condition brought on by a specific traumatic event or activity. In these situations, it is postulated that extrinsic neural compression is caused by age-related changes in posture superimposed upon congenital variations of scalene musculature.

Symptoms of TOS include hand or arm pain, dysesthesias, numbness, and weakness. The symptoms may be bilateral, but they most commonly have their greatest effect on the dominant upper extremity. The distribution of symptoms does not follow typical patterns referable to a single nerve root or peripheral nerve, a factor allowing TOS to be distinguished from compressive conditions affecting specific nerve roots (cervical disc disease or arthritis), the ulnar nerve at the

TABLE 64.5. Brachial Plexus Innervation of the Upper Extremity Muscles.

Muscle	*Nerve root(s)*	*Trunk or cord*	*Peripheral nerve*
Rhomboids	C5	C5 root	Dorsal scapular
Supraspinatus	C5, C6	Upper trunk	Suprascapular
Deltoid	C5, C6	Posterior cord	Axillary
Latissimus dorsi	C6, C7, C8	Posterior cord	Thoracodorsal
Serratus anterior	C5, C6, C7	C5–C7 roots	Long thoracic
Subscapularis	C5, C6	Upper trunk	Subscapular
Biceps brachii	C5, C6	Lateral cord	Musculocutaneous
Brachialis	C5, C6	Lateral cord	Musculocutaneous
Brachioradialis	C6, C5	Posterior cord	Radial
Triceps brachii	C5, C6, C7, C8, T1	Posterior cord	Radial
ECRL	C6, C7	Posterior cord	Radial
EDC	C6, C7, C8	Posterior cord	Radial
ECU	C7, C6	Posterior cord	Radial
Pronator teres	C7, C6	Lateral cord	Median
FCR	C7, C6	Lateral cord	Median
FCU	C8, C7	Medial cord	Ulnar
FDP, 2 and 3	C8, C7	Medial cord	Median
FDP, 4 and 5	C8, C7	Medial cord	Ulnar
Intrinsic muscles[a]	T1, C8, C7, C6	Medial cord	Ulnar, median

LC, lateral cord; MC, medial cord; PC, posterior cord; UT, upper trunk; ECRL, extensor carpi radialis longus; EDC, extensor digitorum communis; ECU, extensor carpi ulnaris; FCR, flexor carpi radialis; FCU, flexor carpi ulnaris; FDP, flexor digitorum profundus.

The brachial plexus arises from cervical nerve roots C5, C6, C7, C8, and T1, which subsequently interdigitate to form the trunks, cords, and peripheral nerves that innervate the upper extremity. The upper trunk arises from the junction of the C5 and C6 nerve roots, the middle trunk from the C7 nerve root, and the lower trunk arises from the junction of the C8 and T1 nerve roots. Below this, the lateral cord arises from the anterior divisions of the upper and middle trunks, the medial cord arises from the anterior division of the lower trunk, and the posterior cord arises from the posterior divisions of all three trunks.

[a]Includes dorsal interossei, palmar interossei, lumbricals, and thenar and hypothenar muscles.

Source: Wheeless' Textbook of Orthopaedics. www.wheelessonline.com

elbow (cubital compression syndrome), the median nerve at the wrist (carpal tunnel syndrome), or other related disorders. Occipital headache is a common complaint associated with TOS, most likely caused by secondary spasm within the trapezius and paraspinous muscles. Symptoms of TOS are typically reproduced or exacerbated by activity requiring elevation or sustained use of the arms or hands, such as reaching for objects overhead, lifting, carrying, prolonged work at keyboards, driving, speaking on handheld phones, shaving, or combing or brushing the hair. Positional complaints may also be brought on by lying supine, resulting in pain and difficulty sleeping. Many patients with TOS are affected to a mild and tolerable degree, yet the majority of patients consulting the surgeon have developed progressively disabling symptoms that effectively prevent them from working or carrying out simple daily activities. In some cases, the symptoms of TOS may have progressed to resemble those of causalgia (reflex sympathetic dystrophy), with persistent vasospasm, disuse edema, and hypersensitivity. The acuity of these symptoms often leads to avoidance and withdrawal from even light touch of the affected extremity. The clinical course of patients with neurogenic TOS is often accompanied by multiple physician consultations and numerous partial or ineffective treatments.

Physical examination is directed toward eliciting the degree of neurogenic disability and particular factors that exacerbate hand and arm complaints. A thorough peripheral nerve examination is performed to exclude ulnar nerve entrapment, carpal tunnel syndrome, and other etiologies. The neck is examined to identify the extent of local muscle spasm and to localize areas where focal digital compression reproduces the individual patient's symptom pattern. The presence of "trigger points" over the scalene triangle serves to reinforce the diagnosis of TOS. The Adson maneuver is used to identify any degree of subclavian artery compression, by detecting ablation of the radial pulse when the patient elevates the arm, inspires deeply, and turns the neck away from the affected extremity. Although this maneuver does not specifically reveal nerve root compression, positive findings are often associated with neurogenic TOS. Because a positive Adson sign is also quite common in the asymptomatic general population, this maneuver (or similar tests in the noninvasive vascular laboratory) only serves to support, but not prove, the diagnosis of TOS; similarly, negative findings of arterial compression do not exclude a diagnosis of neurogenic TOS. Perhaps the most useful component of physical examination is the 3-min elevated arm stress test ("EAST"), in which the patient is asked to repetitively open and close the fists with the arms elevated in a "surrender" position. Most patients with neurogenic TOS report the rapid reproduction of upper extremity symptoms with EAST, often being unable to complete the exercise beyond 30 to 60 s.

There are no specific diagnostic tests or imaging studies that can replace the clinical diagnosis of neurogenic TOS, but plain radiographs of the neck are helpful in determining if an osseous cervical rib is present. Although cervical ribs are relatively uncommon (an incidence of approximately 0.25% in the general population), they are quite often present in patients with arterial TOS and occur in approximately 10% of patients with the venous or neurogenic types of TOS (Fig. 64.6). The results of computed tomography, magnetic resonance imaging, electromyography and nerve conduction

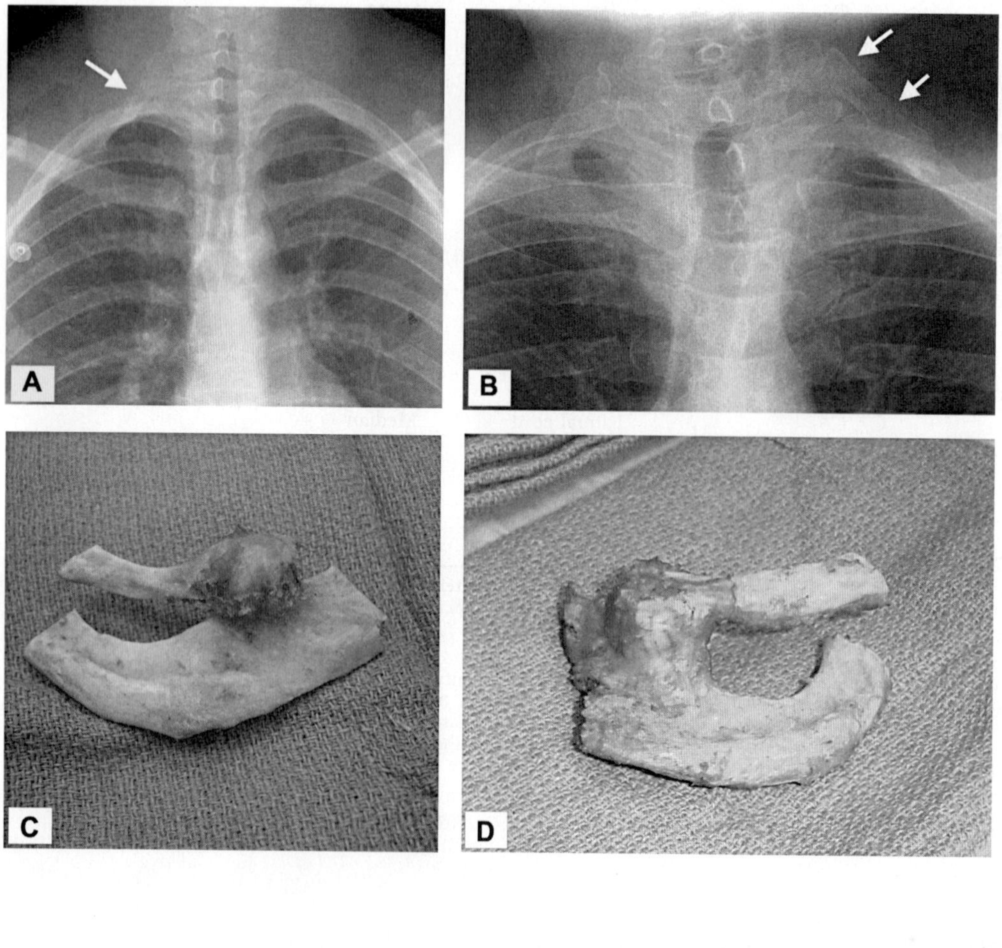

FIGURE 64.6. Congenital cervical ribs. **A.** Plain radiograph of the neck illustrating a right-sided cervical rib anomaly (*arrow*) that had contributed to TOS. **B.** Radiograph depicting a left-sided cervical rib (*arrows*). **C.** Operative specimen excised during supraclavicular thoracic outlet decompression, illustrating a right-sided cervical rib with fibrous attachment to the midportion of the first rib. **D.** Operative specimen of a thick left-sided cervical rib excised during supraclavicular exploration, which was fused to the midportion of the first rib at a site of a large exostosis.

studies are frequently negative or nondiagnostic, even in patients with pronounced disability. Nonetheless, inclusion of these tests is important in the overall evaluation to exclude other conditions considered in the differential diagnosis, such as degenerative cervical spine or disc disease, neoplasms or other masses, intracranial pathology, and specific peripheral neuropathies (Table 64.6). Anesthetic blockade of the anterior scalene muscle has attracted increasing attention in the diagnosis of neurogenic TOS, as well as in predicting which patients are most likely to benefit from surgical treatment.[65] Patients experiencing relief of neurogenic symptoms following scalene blockade, even if temporary, are thought to be more likely to have a form or stage of neurogenic TOS that will respond well to thoracic outlet decompression. Although scalene muscle injection with botulinum toxin has also been reported in the treatment of neurogenic TOS, early experience suggested that this can be associated with substantial complications (dysphagia). Better results have been reported when scalene muscle injection of botulinum toxin is used in conjunction with electrophysiologically and fluoroscopically guided injection, but this approach does not produce definitive treatment and is still not widely advocated.[66]

Arterial TOS

Extrinsic compression of the subclavian artery may occur between the anterior scalene muscle and the first rib and is often associated with the presence of a congenital cervical rib. Sustained compression of the subclavian artery leads to pathological changes in the arterial wall, which may include intimal thickening with atherosclerotic plaque formation or the development of flow-related ("poststenotic") subclavian artery aneurysms. In either case, the complications of subclavian artery pathology that cause the most concern are those related to development of mural thrombus and acute thromboembolism to the upper extremity. In some cases, complete occlusion of the subclavian artery may also result in chronic arterial insufficiency; however, because subclavian occlusions associated with TOS occur distal to the origin of the vertebral artery, TOS is not associated with the subclavian steal syndrome.

TABLE 64.6. Differential Diagnosis of Neurogenic Thoracic Outlet Syndrome (TOS).

Condition	*Differentiating features*
Carpal tunnel syndrome	Hand pain and paresthesia in median nerve distribution; positive findings on nerve conduction studies.
Ulnar nerve compression	Hand pain and paresthesia in ulnar nerve distribution; positive findings on nerve conduction studies.
Rotator cuff tendonitis	Localized pain and tenderness over biceps tendon and shoulder pain on abduction; positive findings on MRI; relief from NSAIDs, local steroid injections, or arthroscopic surgery.
Cervical spine strain/sprain	Posttraumatic neck pain and stiffness localized posteriorly along cervical spine; paraspinal tenderness; relief with conservative measures over weeks to months.
Fibromyositis	Posttraumatic inflammation of trapezius and parascapular muscles; tenderness, spasm and palpable nodules over affected muscles; may coexist with TOS and persist after surgery.
Cervical disc disease	Neck pain and stiffness, arm weakness, and paresthesia involving thumb and index finger (C5–C6 disc);symptom improvement with arm elevation; positive findings on CT or MRI.
Cervical arthritis	Neck pain and stiffness; arm or hand paresthesia infrequent; degenerative rather than posttraumatic; positive findings on spine radiographs.
Brachial plexus injury	Caused by direct injury or stretch; arm pain and weakness, hand paresthesias; symptoms constant not intermittent or positional; positive findings on neurophysiological studies.

Patients with arterial TOS may present with acute ischemia of the hand or digits, with pain, paresthesias, and weakness of the affected upper extremity. The brachial and axillary artery pulses may be absent with extensive thromboembolism; however, palpable pulses suggest a proximal source of atheroembolism. One should also seek additional evidence of arterial compromise to the upper extremity, such as sympathetic overactivity with vasospasm, digital or hand ischemia, cutaneous ulceration or emboli, forearm claudication, or the pulsatile supraclavicular mass or bruit characteristic of a subclavian artery aneurysm. Because the anatomic abnormalities underlying TOS are often bilateral, it may also be informative to examine the contralateral extremity for evidence of subclavian artery compression, occlusion, or aneurysm. In cases where acute intervention is necessary to restore flow to the brachial artery and its branches, the diagnosis of arterial TOS may be entertained after initial thrombectomy or thrombolysis has allowed more definitive evaluation by contrast arteriography. A subset of patients present with chronic symptoms related to subclavian artery compression, including hand or arm weakness, early fatigue with use, and digital ulcerations or periodic discoloration reminiscent of Raynaud's phenomenon. In these cases, compression of the subclavian artery is often incomplete, with total occlusion being apparent only with positional maneuvers (i.e., the Adson test).

Patients with features suggesting arterial TOS may be evaluated by positional noninvasive vascular laboratory studies (segmental arterial pressures, waveform analysis, and duplex imaging), but it is often difficult to visualize the subclavian artery behind the clavicle. The definitive examination necessary to completely exclude or prove the existence of a fixed arterial lesion is provided by contrast arteriography; this may be accomplished by traditional catheter-based arteriography, or in recent years by contrast-enhanced (gadolinium) magnetic resonance imaging techniques (Fig. 64.7). In these examinations it is important to specifically alert the vascular radiologist to the potential need for positional maneuvers during radiographic examination and to consider bilateral studies even in the absence of contralateral symptoms.

Venous TOS

Venous TOS is caused by compression of the subclavian vein immediately anterior to the anterior scalene muscle. This condition typically occurs in young, otherwise healthy patients, who are often involved in vigorous occupational or recreational use of the upper extremity. This habit is thought to cause repetitive venous trauma between the first rib and clavicle, resulting in the evolution of fibrosis and encasement

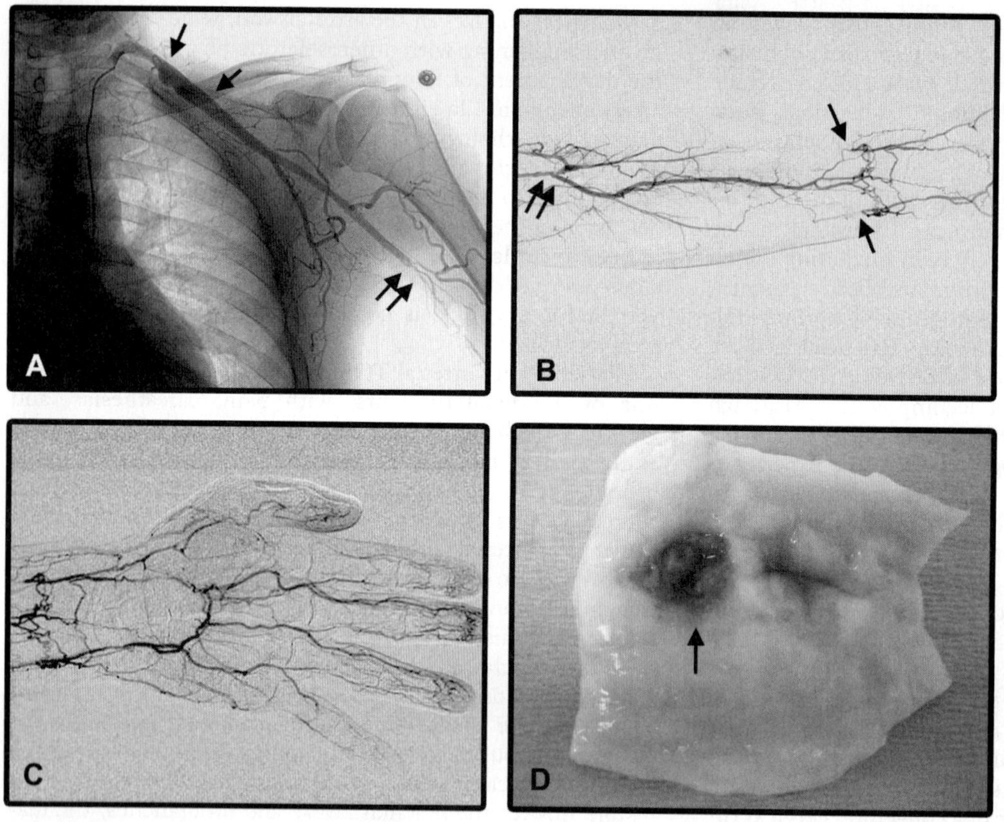

FIGURE 64.7. Subclavian artery aneurysm. **A.** Contrast arteriogram illustrating a left subclavian artery aneurysm at the level of the thoracic outlet (*arrows*), which had caused distal thromboembolism to the brachial circulation and hand. Occlusion of the proximal brachial artery is present (*double arrow*). **B.** The distal brachial artery is reconstituted through collaterals (*double arrow*), but there is occlusion of the radial and ulnar arteries throughout the forearm. Flow is provided primarily through the interosseous artery, with reconstitution of the radial and ulnar arteries just above the wrist (*arrows*). **C.** The palmar arch is incomplete and there are multiple branch vessel occlusions from previous thromboembolism. **D.** Opened operative specimen of subclavian artery aneurysm excised during supraclavicular thoracic outlet decompression, illustrating intraluminal ulceration with thrombus (*arrow*).

of the vein by scar tissue, as well as eventual venous thrombosis. Patients with venous TOS most commonly present with the "effort thrombosis" syndrome, an acute event characterized by the sudden development of hand and arm edema, upper extremity cyanosis, enlarged subcutaneous collateral veins, and early forearm fatigue in the absence of arterial compromise. Although this condition may occur in the setting of an acute strain to the upper extremity, it frequently appears to develop as an unprovoked spontaneous event in the absence of a specific traumatic injury; it is also important to distinguish "effort thrombosis" from subclavian vein occlusion caused by indwelling central venous catheters, tumors, or other forms of intrathoracic pathology. Some patients with venous TOS may exhibit a low-grade, chronic form of subclavian venous compression, with or without a superimposed effort thrombosis event.

Patients in whom venous TOS is suspected should be studied promptly by contrast venography, particularly in the context of an effort thrombosis event (Fig. 64.8A). Focal occlusion of the subclavian vein at the angle between the first rib and clavicle is characteristic of venous TOS; in some cases, the absence of venous branches may give the appearance of segmental venous thrombosis. Following thrombolysis or spontaneous recanalization of the subclavian vein, the vein may appear patent with the exception of a focal stenosis in the expected location (Fig. 64.8B). With or without complete occlusion, a dense network of cervical collaterals is typically present, providing a route for venous drainage from the affected extremity; this also reflects the chronic nature of venous TOS. As in arterial TOS, it is frequently necessary to conduct these studies with positional maneuvers to detect subclavian vein occlusion at the level of the first rib, and it is often helpful to examine the contralateral side to detect evidence of symmetrical abnormalities.

Treatment

Initial Management

Neurogenic TOS

Conservative approaches serve as the initial treatment for neurogenic TOS.[67–69] These therapeutic efforts are focused on relaxing and stretching the scalene muscles and strengthening the muscles of posture through physical therapy, combined with hydrotherapy and massage. Pain medications, nonsteroidal antiinflammatory agents, and muscle relaxants are often useful adjuncts in treatment. Many patients (about 30%–60%) will experience considerable relief of symptoms following 4 to 6 weeks of physical therapy, thereafter requiring only further conservative measures for maintenance. Physical therapy provides insufficient benefit in a subset of patients, and for some may even exacerbate the condition. These individuals are then considered for surgical treatment.

Arterial TOS

The initial treatment of arterial TOS is focused on revascularization for acute ischemia, if necessary. This step is typically performed via brachial artery thromboembolectomy, with the hope of restoring sufficient inflow to the hand and digits to permit salvage. If not performed before surgical intervention, or when arterial TOS is suspected in the absence of an acute thromboembolic complication, arteriography is necessary to help define the proximal source of pathology. The demonstration of a fixed arterial lesion, either occlusive

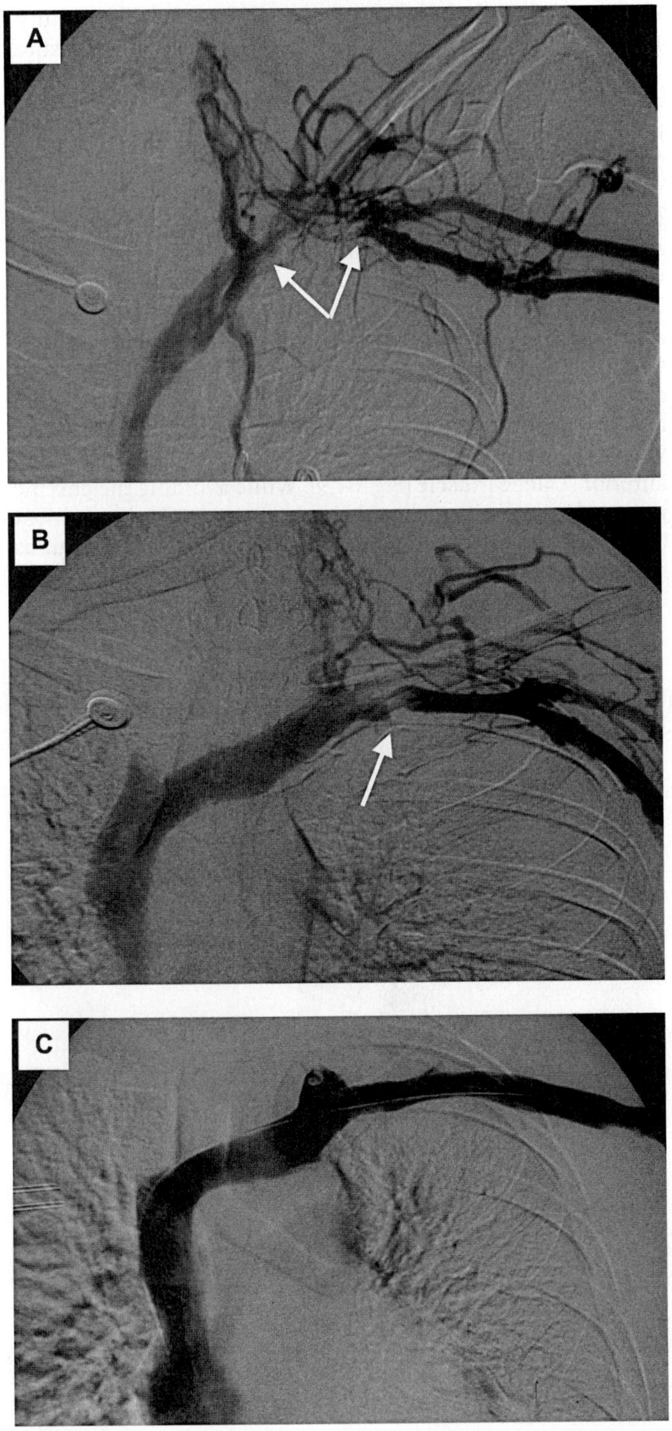

FIGURE 64.8. Effort thrombosis of the subclavian vein. **A.** Contrast venogram depicting left subclavian vein thrombosis at the level of the first rib (*arrows*). **B.** Venographic appearance following successful catheter-directed thrombolytic therapy, illustrating return of patency to the subclavian vein with a high-grade residual stenosis at the level of the first rib (*arrow*). **C.** Venographic appearance several weeks following thoracic outlet decompression and external venolysis, demonstrating a widely patent subclavian vein without residual stenosis in the absence of the first rib.

or aneurysmal in nature, is an indication for surgical reconstruction. Given that these lesions occur secondary to extrinsic compression rather than atherosclerosis or other forms or intrinsic arterial disease, there is no significant role for endovascular approaches to their management.

Venous TOS

As discussed earlier, the initial treatment of effort thrombosis generally involves contrast venography and catheter-directed thrombolytic therapy. In recent years, the addition of catheter-based mechanical methods to achieve dissolution of thrombus ("mechano-rheologic" therapy), often coupled with "pulse-spray" local delivery of thrombolytic agents, has added greater flexibility and speed in accomplishing this initial step in treatment. Prompt thrombolysis for venous TOS frequently results in restoration of venous drainage through the subclavian vein and cervical collaterals and early resolution of the acute symptoms. Although intraluminal balloon angioplasty of the subclavian vein is sometimes used at this stage of management, it is frequently difficult to achieve satisfactory results because of the fibroelastic nature of the venous lesion; moreover, even successful balloon angioplasty is viewed as a temporizing maneuver that does not alter the recommendation for surgical decompression. Following interventional management, patients are maintained on intravenous heparin and converted to subcutaneous heparin therapy (Lovenox) or to oral anticoagulation with warfarin. Although in some cases anticoagulation may be used for 3 to 6 months to assess the individual patient's needs for further treatment, there is some risk that another effort thrombosis event will occur during this interval. Most patients with venous TOS are candidates for surgical decompression, and it is now clear that this can be safely performed during the same hospitalization as the initial effort thrombosis event. It is also necessary to emphasize that interventional approaches with placement of indwelling venous stents can be particularly deleterious in this condition, as extrinsic compression of the stented vein predictably leads to stent occlusion and rethrombosis despite the appearance of early technical success. In contrast, transluminal balloon angioplasty may be of value in some patients with residual venous stenosis, once surgical decompression has been accomplished.

Surgical Strategies

Several surgical operations have been devised to provide relief from neurovascular compression in the thoracic outlet, as well as arterial and venous reconstruction. These procedures have undergone considerable evolution over the past four decades, consistent with changing pathophysiological concepts regarding the various forms of TOS. It is now generally accepted that neurogenic TOS may arise from compression of the brachial plexus nerve roots at several different levels and by different etiological factors, not solely as a consequence of bony deformation by the first rib. Indeed, numerous soft tissue anomalies within the thoracic outlet have been described and classified, each of which can give rise to symptomatic neural compression.[70,71] Significant factors playing a role in this process appear to include scalene muscle injury with spasm, scarring, and fibrotic inflammatory reactions surrounding the brachial plexus nerve roots, which may also be associated with pathologic changes in the scalene musculature.[72,73] Current approaches to surgical treatment take each of these potential contributing factors into account in selecting the optimal treatment for individual patients.

Transaxillary First Rib Resection

Transaxillary first rib resection has been the mainstay of surgical treatment for TOS for many years.[74–77] The primary advantages of transaxillary first rib resection include a relatively limited field of operative dissection, a cosmetically placed skin incision, and sufficient exposure to reliably accomplish resection of the anterolateral first rib. This approach also makes it possible to achieve at least partial resection of the anterior scalene muscle, as well as identification and removal of most anomalous ligaments and fibrous bands that may be associated with TOS. The disadvantages of the transaxillary approach include incomplete exposure of the structures comprising the scalene triangle, difficulty achieving complete anterior and middle scalenectomy or brachial plexus neurolysis, and the necessity for first rib resection in all cases. This approach is also limited when vascular reconstruction is needed, requiring the addition of a separate incision or repositioning of the patient.

This procedure is performed under general anesthesia, with a transverse skin incision made at the lower border of the axillary hairline.[62] The arm is prepped circumferentially and held by a reliable, flexible, and sturdy assistant. The incision is carried to the chest wall, and blunt dissection is used to establish a plane extending to the apex of the axilla. The long thoracic, thoracodorsal, and second intercostal brachial nerves are identified near the chest wall to avoid direct injury. Excess elevation of the arm (unique to transaxillary exposure) is an additional mechanism of injury to the second intercostal brachial cutaneous nerve, which can result in troublesome postoperative pain and numbness along the medial aspect of the arm. The first rib is exposed in the upper aspect of the wound by retracting the subcutaneous tissues and axillary contents away from the chest wall; it is necessary to lift the arm carefully to facilitate this exposure, and it is essential that the operating surgeon use a fiberoptic headlight to properly illuminate the operative field. It is important that the surgeon be constantly aware of how the retractors are positioned with respect to the nerve roots and blood vessels to avoid serious injury. Periodic reinspection of the retractors and relief for the assistants is recommended. The subclavian vein and artery are identified, along with the intervening anterior scalene muscle (Fig. 64.9). While avoiding the phrenic nerve, the anterior scalene muscle tendon is encircled just above its insertion upon the first rib and divided as high as feasible. The importance of resecting a portion of the scalene muscle, rather than simply dividing it at the level of the first

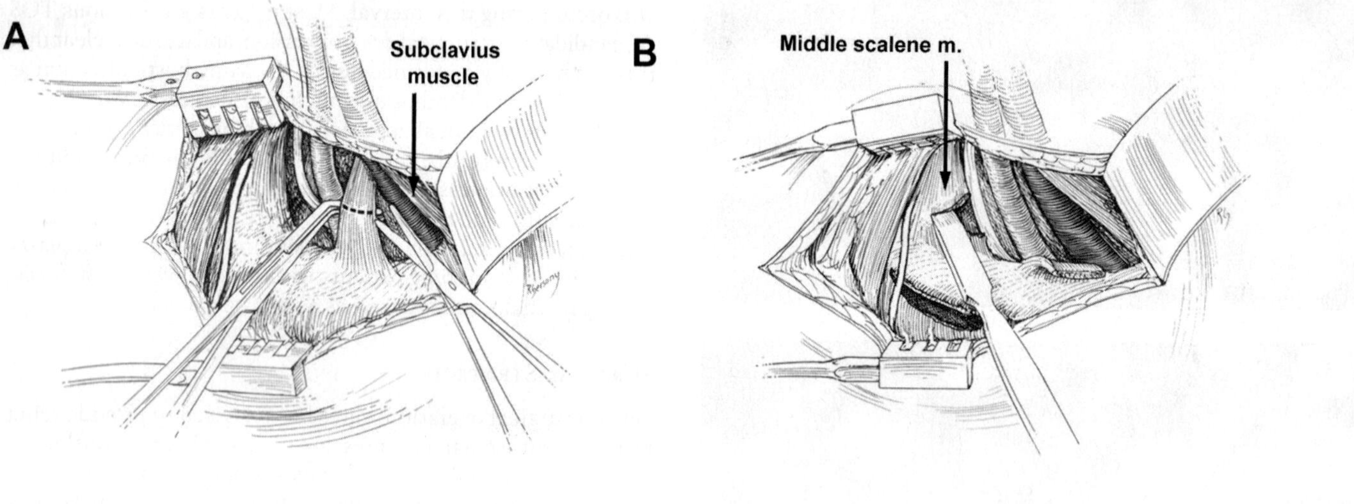

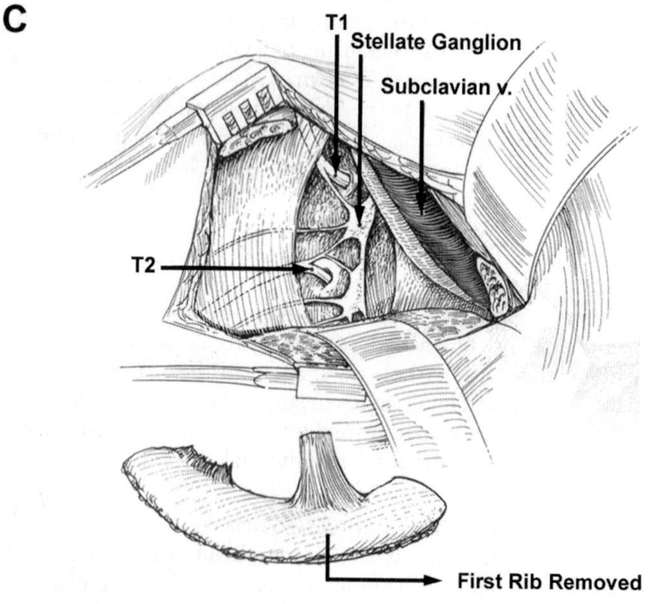

FIGURE 64.9. Transaxillary first rib resection, illustrated from the surgeon's view for a right-sided procedure. **A.** Division of the anterior scalene muscle. With the arm elevated, the first rib is exposed and the neurovascular structures are protected from injury. The tendinous insertion of the anterior scalene muscle is elevated with a right-angle clamp just above the first rib. The anterior scalene muscle is divided several centimeters above the rib, leaving the distal portion attached to the bone. Injury to the underlying nerves is meticulously avoided. **B.** The middle scalene muscle is detached from its insertion onto the top of the first rib, protecting the long thoracic nerve from injury. The intercostal muscle attachments are similarly divided along the inferior margin of the first rib. **C.** The first rib is removed. The operative specimen includes a portion of the resected anterior scalene muscle and the site of attachment of the middle scalene muscle as shown. When an adjunctive sympathectomy is indicated (patients with TOS complicated by reflex sympathetic dystrophy), the cervical sympathetic chain is identified behind the extrapleural tissues at the level of the posterior second rib. It is subsequently resected from the lower edge of the stellate ganglion to the level of the third rib. (From Thompson and Bartoli,[93] with permission.)

rib itself, has been underscored by analysis of the factors causing recurrent neurogenic TOS.[78] The intercostal muscles are divided along with the middle and posterior scalene muscles, preventing injury to the long thoracic nerve to avoid serratus anterior muscle weakness, which results in a "winged scapula." The rib is then fully detached and removed from the field. The exposure can be used to perform adjunctive cervical sympathectomy for patients with symptoms of reflex sympathetic dystrophy. Any additional soft tissue bands crossing the brachial plexus nerve roots are sought and carefully divided, particularly those that may insert upon the thickened pleural surface at the apex (Sibson's fascia). Potential complications include injury to the brachial plexus nerve roots, dysfunction of the phrenic or long thoracic nerves, and hemothorax or pneumothorax.

SUPRACLAVICULAR EXPLORATION

Treatment of TOS often requires a more versatile and comprehensive surgical approach than that afforded by the transaxillary route alone.[62,79] Initial efforts to overcome these limitations led to the introduction of combined approaches, in which transaxillary first rib resection was performed concomitantly with supraclavicular exploration.[80] Experience with this strategy subsequently led many groups to adopt the supraclavicular approach as the predominant treatment, because supraclavicular exploration carries the advantages of wider exposure of all anatomic structures associated with thoracic outlet compression.[81–83] This approach allows complete resection of the anterior and middle scalene muscles to be achieved, as well as brachial plexus neurolysis with direct visualization of all five nerve roots. In many cases symptomatic relief of neurogenic TOS can be achieved by extended scalenectomy without the need for first rib resection, an option permitted by the supraclavicular approach. This approach also allows for resection of cervical ribs, anomalous first ribs, or the normal first rib. A further advantage is that all forms of vascular reconstruction can also be accomplished through supraclavicular exposure; although removal of the anteromedial portion of the first rib and distal control of the vessels may require addition of a second infraclavicular incision, this is performed without the need for repositioning the patient. The balance of advantages and disadvantages between these two operative approaches has now led many groups to prefer the supraclavicular approach to TOS, with some adopting a highly selective approach in which resection of the first rib is reserved solely for patients with vascular complications.[84,85] Thoracic outlet decompression through supraclavicular exploration is currently indicated for all appropriately selected patients with neurogenic, arterial, or venous forms of TOS, or any combination of these clinical syndromes, as well as for patients undergoing reoperation.[86–88]

A transverse skin incision is made two fingerbreadths above the clavicle, beginning at the lateral border of the sternocleidomastoid muscle (Fig. 64.10A). The incision is carried through the platysma muscle layer and the scalene fat pad is mobilized from medial to lateral to expose the anterior surface of the anterior scalene muscle, where the phrenic nerve is found coursing within the investing fascia (superolateral to inferomedial). With further reflection of the scalene fat pad, the subclavian artery and the underlying roots of the brachial plexus are exposed as they emerge from behind the anterior scalene muscle (Fig. 64.10B). Taking care to avoid excessive traction on the phrenic nerve, the anterior scalene muscle is then mobilized circumferentially to its attachment upon the first rib and sharply divided (Fig. 64.10C). The anterior scalene muscle is elevated and dissected superiorly to the level of its origin on the transverse process of the sixth cervical vertebra, from where it is divided and removed (Fig. 64.10D). There may also be additional slips of muscle or tendon that must be divided more posteriorly, including direct connections between the anterior scalene muscle and the thickened extrapleural fascia underneath the first rib, the subclavian artery, or the brachial plexus nerve roots. It is also common to observe a scalene minimus muscle as an additional source of neural compression. This is an anomaly characterized by fibers originating behind the C5 and C6 nerve roots in the plane of the middle scalene muscle, which pass across the lower nerve roots to join the plane of the anterior scalene muscle. Laboratory studies show that a high proportion of TOS patients exhibit significant myopathic changes in the anterior scalene muscle, including fiber type redistribution, fibrous thickening of the endomysium, and even mitochondrial abnormalities.[72,73] Each of the nerve roots contributing to the brachial plexus is then identified and meticulously dissected free of inflammatory scar tissue by external neurolysis (Fig. 64.10E). A moderate to dense fibrotic tissue reaction encasing these nerve roots is not uncommon in patients with neurogenic TOS, and it is especially apparent in those undergoing reoperations. Relief of this source of nerve compression requires adequate visualization of the posterior first rib to effect complete nerve root mobility, particularly of T1. The attachment of the middle scalene muscle is next divided from the first rib using a periosteal elevator; the separation between the middle and posterior scalene muscles is defined by the oblique course of the long thoracic nerve, which is preserved (Fig. 64.10F). If a truncated cervical rib is present it is readily encountered and exposed at this stage of the procedure, because congenital cervical ribs arise within the same tissue plane as the middle scalene muscle. Once a thorough scalenectomy has been completed and the brachial plexus nerve roots are fully mobilized (Fig. 64.10G), the intercostal muscles attached to the first rib are divided (Fig. 64.10H). A segment of the first rib is then removed as a single specimen, extending from the scalene tubercle anteriorly to a level even with the transverse process of the spine posteriorly, with the surgeon directly protecting the T1 nerve root (Fig. 64.10I). Although some surgeons consider retaining the first rib following scalenectomy, we prefer to excise the first rib in any situation where it might contribute to residual neurovascular compression, as well as in all patients with arterial or venous TOS. In rare situations in which the first rib is particularly enlarged and cannot be removed through the supraclavicular exposure alone (e.g., a previous rib fracture with a large callus), a second transaxillary incision may be added to accomplish this step. Finally, in some patients with neurogenic TOS there is evidence of brachial plexus compression at the level of the pectoralis minor muscle, determined on physical examination by focal tenderness in the lateral infraclavicular space on direct palpation. In these situations the pectoralis minor muscle tendon may be divided, through a short vertical inci-

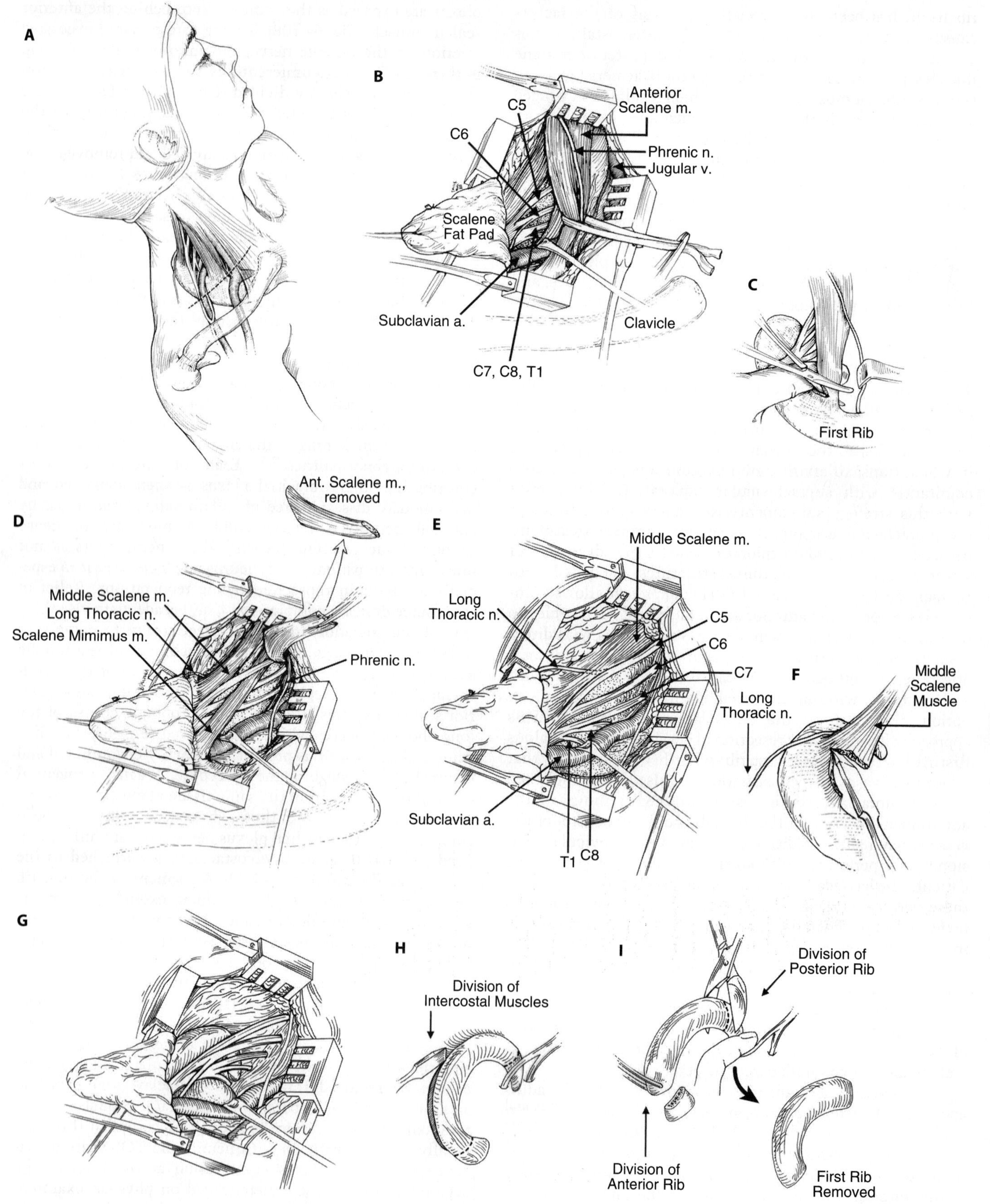
A
B
Anterior Scalene m.
C5
C6
Phrenic n.
Jugular v.
Scalene Fat Pad
Subclavian a.
Clavicle
C7, C8, T1
C
First Rib
Ant. Scalene m., removed
D
Middle Scalene m.
Long Thoracic n.
Scalene Mimimus m.
Phrenic n.
E
Middle Scalene m.
Long Thoracic n.
C5
C6
C7
Subclavian a.
T1
C8
F
Long Thoracic n.
Middle Scalene Muscle
G
H
Division of Intercostal Muscles
I
Division of Posterior Rib
Division of Anterior Rib
First Rib Removed

sion in the deltopectoral groove, just inferior to the acromion process.

Arterial Reconstruction

First rib resection and subclavian artery reconstruction are required for any degree of aneurysmal degeneration, particularly if the patient has had preoperative symptoms of digital thromboembolism, as well as for persistent occlusive lesions of the arterial wall that are still evident after scalenectomy. Proximal exposure of the subclavian artery is generally quite adequate given the degree of dissection typically accomplished during routine supraclavicular exploration, and subclavian artery replacement is readily accomplished by interposition bypass grafting with end-to-end anastomoses. If additional exposure is necessary to control the distal subclavian or axillary artery, this is accomplished through a second incision placed parallel to the clavicle in the deltopectoral groove, to permit exposure of the axillary artery at the level of the pectoralis minor muscle. Although prosthetic materials such as ringed PTFE or Dacron may be used for subclavian artery reconstruction, autologous conduits are preferable for use in young active patients, because they will require an unusually durable reconstruction that is subject to considerable motion with use of the arm. Reversed greater saphenous vein harvested from the thigh may be of adequate caliber for this purpose, but it often is too small for replacement of the subclavian artery. In this case, creation of a saphenous vein panel graft may provide a suitable alternative. In these unique situations, it is also beneficial to consider use of autologous arterial conduits, such as the proximal internal iliac artery or the external iliac artery. When this approach is used to replace the subclavian artery, a short segment of appropriately sized prosthetic graft material is used to replace the iliac artery after its transfer to the subclavian position.

Cervical Sympathectomy

Patients with disabling neurogenic or arterial TOS may present with symptoms characteristic of sympathetic overactivity resulting in painful vasospasm, delayed healing of digital skin lesions, and, at times, even reflex sympathetic dystrophy. In these situations, cervical sympathectomy is a useful adjunct to thoracic outlet decompression, helping to alleviate vasospastic complaints and to facilitate healing of digital lesions caused by atheroemboli or ischemic injury. Through either the transaxillary or supraclavicular approaches, the cervical sympathetic chain is identified by palpation as a rubber band-like structure that passes vertically over the neck of the first or second rib in the extrapleural space. The sympathetic chain is exposed, elevated, and divided sharply at the level of the third rib distally. The rami connecting to each ganglion are sharply divided as the chain is dissected proximally. To reduce the incidence of Horner's syndrome, the proximal extent of sympathetic resection is marked by the lower half of the stellate ganglion, which is observed just above the level of the first rib.

Venous Decompression

Thoracic outlet decompression for venous TOS involves several additional considerations to the standard supraclavicular exploration for neurogenic TOS.[89,90] Although the initial steps of the procedure are conducted as described (anterior and middle scalenectomy and brachial plexus neurolysis), resection of the first rib is always indicated for venous TOS. Two additional aspects of the procedure are then specifically directed toward the venous problem: circumferential venolysis and resection of the medial first rib. The subclavian vein in effort thrombosis is typically compressed between the medial first rib and the overlying clavicular head. Repeated compression and previous episodes of venous thrombosis also incite a substantial local inflammatory response. This response is frequently characterized by dense fibrosis encasing the subclavian vein, evident throughout the operative field during supraclavicular exposure. Despite the venographic appearance of persistent venous thrombosis, the subclavian vein itself may be patent without permanent obstructive changes; for this reason, relief of the encasing scar tissue usually results in some redistension of the vein to a normal caliber. Furthermore, once the vein has been circumferentially exposed, it is often found to be soft, compressible, and free of residual intraluminal obstruction or thrombus. The subclavian vein is therefore dissected in its entirety before considering the need for other forms of venous reconstruction.

It is important to note that complete first rib resection, particularly the medial aspect where it contributes most to venous compression, cannot be performed through supraclavicular exposure alone. To accomplish this component of venous decompression, an additional incision is made over the medial infraclavicular space parallel to the clavicle. The sternal attachment of the first rib is identified by palpation and exposed on its anterior surface using cautery. With downward pressure applied to the remaining segment of first rib

FIGURE 64.10. Supraclavicular thoracic outlet decompression, illustrated from the surgeon's view for a right-sided procedure. **A.** Transverse supraclavicular incision. **B.** The scalene fat pad is mobilized from medial to lateral, followed by circumferential dissection of the anterior scalene muscle away from the underlying subclavian artery and roots of the brachial plexus. **C.** While the surgeon displaces and protects the neurovascular structures with a finger, the tendinous insertion of the anterior scalene muscle upon the first rib is sharply divided with scissors. **D.** The cut end of the anterior scalene muscle is reflected superiorly and dissected away from the underlying nerve roots, then divided at the level of its origin on the transverse process of the C6 vertebra and removed. In many cases, a scalene minimus muscle anomaly is also found, passing between the roots of the brachial plexus. **E.** Complete dissection of the brachial plexus nerve roots is accomplished along with resection of any surrounding inflammatory scar tissue and/or fibrous bands, to achieve thorough visualization and mobilization of each nerve root from C5 to T1. The middle scalene muscle is exposed posterior to the nerve roots, and the long thoracic nerve is identified where it emerges from the midportion of the middle scalene muscle. **F.** The middle scalene muscle is detached from the first rib using a periosteal elevator. **G.** The first rib is exposed and its potential role in neurovascular compression is assessed in different arm positions. **H.** The intercostal muscles attached to the first rib are divided. **I.** First rib resection is accomplished with direct visualization and protection of the T1 nerve root. The bone is cut posteriorly at a level nearly even with the transverse process of the spine; anteriorly, the rib is cut at a level just medial to the scalene tubercle (the site of bony attachment of the anterior scalene muscle). Additional bony resection can be accomplished piecemeal with a rongeur, then the ends of the bone are made smooth before sealing with wax. (From Thompson et al.,[86] with permission.)

through the supraclavicular incision, the medial portion of the rib is dissected from its soft tissue attachments through the infraclavicular incision. The remaining portion of the first rib is then removed by detaching it from the sternum, and any residual scar tissue encasing the proximal subclavian vein is divided into the upper mediastinum as visualized through the supraclavicular incision.

In situations where external venolysis and paraclavicular first rib resection has been insufficient to relieve venous obstruction, additional venous reconstruction may be required. A number of techniques have been described for this purpose, including direct venous patch angioplasty, segmental interposition bypass grafting, or the use of the internal jugular vein as a "turn-down" bypass. In the latter procedure, the internal jugular vein is ligated and divided high in the neck, and its cephalad end is brought down to an end-to-side anastomosis with the distal subclavian or axillary vein. All patients undergoing operation for venous TOS are maintained on anticoagulation for at least 6 to 12 weeks in the postoperative period.

Postoperative Care

Postoperative care includes continued use of pain medications, muscle relaxants, and antiinflammatory agents. The expected recovery from thoracic outlet decompression is approximately 3 days in the hospital and 4 to 6 weeks at home, during which physical therapy remains an important component of treatment. Patients with venous TOS may undergo predischarge contrast venography, both to assess the adequacy of venous decompression on the operative side and, if not previously determined, to assess the possibility that symmetrical venous compression may exist on the contralateral side. Any residual venous stenosis may be safely treated at this time by transluminal balloon angioplasty, a therapeutic option that is contraindicated before surgical decompression. In patients with bilateral TOS, it is essential to ensure that any degree of phrenic nerve paresis has completely resolved before undertaking a second operation on the contralateral side.

Results of Treatment

The overall results of surgical treatment for neurogenic TOS remain difficult to define. Assessment of results for TOS depends on functional evaluation of symptoms and the subjective perception of the degree of disability. Because this is also dependent on the extent of disability before operation, results vary considerably for those with differing degrees or duration of preexisting symptoms. Published reports also vary widely in how outcomes for surgical treatment of TOS are defined, with most authors dividing results into separate categories such as "excellent" (complete relief of all symptoms), "good" (relief of major symptoms but some persistent symptoms), "fair" (partial relief but persistence of some major symptoms), or "poor" (no improvement). Finally, interpretation of outcomes may be complicated by the type of operation performed; however, no single operative strategy has been adopted by all those who perform operations for neurogenic TOS, and the operations performed by some may have changed over time. Moreover, some reports do not distinguish between patients undergoing operation for neurogenic TOS versus arterial or venous TOS, making it impossible to separate the results for treatment of neurogenic TOS alone.

Transaxillary first rib resection has been one of the most frequently performed operations for neurogenic TOS since its introduction by Roos in 1966.[74] By 1989, more than 3000 of these operations were reported in 21 separate publications. The largest of these series included 1315 patients, with a successful outcome in 92% and a failure rate of 8%. As summarized in Table 64.7, the overall rate of good outcomes for transaxillary first rib resection has ranged from 37% to 100% (mean, 80%), with fair outcomes in 0% to 14% (mean, 6%) and failure of operation in 0% to 41% (mean, 15%). Supraclavicular exploration, including first rib resection coupled with anterior and middle scalenectomy, has become more commonly performed over the past two decades. Table 64.8 summarizes results of operation from seven different publications including a total of 1222 patients), the largest being the series reported by Hempel et al. (770 operations).[87] Overall, the results for supraclavicular decompression were good in 59% to 91% (mean, 77%), fair in 5% to 33% (mean, 15%), and poor in 3% to 18% (mean, 8%). In the most comprehensive analysis of results for neurogenic TOS, Sanders used the life-table method to compare outcomes for different operative procedures.[61,79,91,92] In a comparison of patients undergoing transaxillary first rib resection (n = 112), anterior and middle scalenectomy (n = 286), or supraclavicular scalenectomy with

TABLE 64.7.
Results for Transaxillary First Rib Resection (Level III Evidence).

First author	*Year*	*No. operations*	*Outcomes reported (%)* Good	Fair	Failed
Sanders[94]	1968	69	90	0	10
Roeder[95]	1973	26	92	4	4
Hoofer[96]	1973	135	100	0	0
Dale[97]	1975	49	94	0	6
Kremer[98]	1975	48	86	0	14
McGough[99]	1979	113	80	13	7
Youmans[100]	1980	258	75	16	9
Roos[101]	1982	1315	92	0	8
Batt[102]	1983	94	80	0	20
Sallstrom[103]	1983	72	81	12	7
Heughan[104]	1984	44	75	0	25
Qvarfordt[80]	1984	97	79	0	21
Narakas[105]	1986	43	77	0	23
Tagaki[106]	1987	48	79	0	21
Davies[107]	1988	115	89	0	11
Selke[108]	1988	460	79	14	7
Stanton[109]	1988	87	85	4	11
Wood[110]	1988	54	89	9	2
Cikrit[111]	1989	30	63	0	37
Lindgren[112]	1989	175	59	0	41
Lepantalo[113]	1989	112	52	25	23
Jamieson[114]	1996	380	53	25	22
Totals		3824	80%	6%	15%

TABLE 64.8.
Results for Supraclavicular Scalenectomy/First Rib Resection (Level III Evidence).

First author	*Year*	*No. operations*	*Outcomes reported (%)* Good	Fair	Failed
Graham[115]	1973	78	91	5	4
Thompson[116]	1979	15	87	0	13
Thomas[117]	1983	128	83	13	4
Reilly[83]	1988	39	59	33	8
Loh[118]	1989	22	68	23	9
Hempel[87]	1996	770	86	13	1
Axelrod[119]	2001	170	65	17	18
Totals		1222	77%	15%	8%

first rib resection (n = 249), there was no difference in the initial success rate between these three procedures (91%, 93%, and 93%, respectively). The proportion of patients with successful outcomes also declined over time with all three procedures. Although the long-term success with supraclavicular scalenectomy and first rib resection appeared somewhat better at 10 to 15 years (71%) than the results with either anterior scalenectomy (66%) or transaxillary first rib resection (64%), there was no statistically significant difference between these operations. It must therefore be concluded that at the present time there is no demonstrable difference in either short- or long-term outcomes among these three operative approaches as applied to neurogenic TOS.

References

1. Carlson RE, Ehrenfeld WK, Stoney RJ, Wylie EJ. Innominate artery endarterectomy: a 16-year experience. Arch Surg 1977;112:1389–1393.
2. Brewster DC, Moncure AC, Darling RC, et al. Innominate artery lesions: problems encountered and lessons learned. J Vasc Surg 1985;2:99–112.
3. Cherry KJ, Jr., McCullough JL, Hallett JW Jr, et al. Technical principles of direct innominate artery revascularization: a comparison of endarterectomy and bypass grafts. J Vasc Surg 1989;9:718–723.
4. Crawford ES, Stowe CL, Powers RW Jr. Occlusion of the innominate, common carotid, and subclavian arteries: long-term results of surgical treatment. Surgery (St. Louis) 1983;94:781–791.
5. Vogt DP, Hertzer NR, O'Hara PJ, Beven EG. Brachiocephalic arterial reconstruction. Ann Surg 1982;196:541–552.
6. Zelenock GB, Cronenwett JL, Graham LM, et al. Brachiocephalic arterial occlusions and stenoses. Manifestations and management of complex lesions. Arch Surg 1985;120:370–376.
7. Azakie A, McElhinney DB, Higashima R, et al. Innominate artery reconstruction: over 3 decades of experience. Ann Surg 1998;228:402–410.
8. Berguer R, Morasch MD, Kline RA. Transthoracic repair of innominate and common carotid artery disease: immediate and long-term outcome for 100 consecutive surgical reconstructions. J Vasc Surg 1998;27:34–41.
9. Kieffer E, Sabatier J, Koskas F, Bahnini A. Atherosclerotic innominate artery occlusive disease: early and long-term results of surgical reconstruction. J Vasc Surg 1995;21:326–336.
10. Reul GJ, Jacobs MJ, Gregoric ID, et al. Innominate artery occlusive disease: surgical approach and long-term results. J Vasc Surg 1991;14:405–412.
11. Deriu GP, Milite D, Verlato F, et al. Surgical treatment of atherosclerotic lesions of subclavian artery: carotid-subclavian bypass versus subclavian-carotid transposition. J Cardiovasc Surg (Torino) 1998;39:729–734.
12. Edwards WH Jr, Tapper SS, Edwards WH Sr, et al. Subclavian revascularization: a quarter century experience. Ann Surg 1994;219:673–677.
13. Law MM, Colburn MD, Moore WS, et al. Carotid-subclavian bypass for brachiocephalic occlusive disease. Choice of conduit and long-term follow-up. Stroke 1995;26:1565–1571.
14. Salam TA, Lumsden AB, Smith RB III. Subclavian artery revascularization: a decade of experience with extrathoracic bypass procedures. J Surg Res 1994;56:387–392.
15. Schardey HM, Meyer G, Rau HG, et al. Subclavian carotid transposition: an analysis of a clinical series and a review of the literature. Eur J Vasc Endovasc Surg 1996;12:431–436.
16. Toursarkissian B, Rubin BG, Reilly JM, et al. Surgical treatment of patients with symptomatic vertebrobasilar insufficiency. Ann Vasc Surg 1998;12:28–33.
17. van der Vliet JA, Palamba HW, Scharn DM, et al. Arterial reconstruction for subclavian obstructive disease: a comparison of extrathoracic procedures. Eur J Vasc Endovasc Surg 1995;9:454–458.
18. Tarazi RY, O'Hara PJ, Loop FD. Symptomatic coronary-subclavian steal corrected by carotid-subclavian bypass. J Vasc Surg 1986;3:669–672.
19. Norsa A, Gamba G, Ivic N, et al. The coronary subclavian steal syndrome: an uncommon sequel to internal mammary-coronary artery bypass surgery. Thorac Cardiovasc Surg 1994;42:351–354.
20. Lobato EB, Kern KB, Bauder-Heit J, et al. Incidence of coronary-subclavian steal syndrome in patients undergoing noncardiac surgery. J Cardiothorac Vasc Anesth 2001;15:689–692.
21. Yano OJ, Faries PL, Morrissey N, et al. Ancillary techniques to facilitate endovascular repair of aortic aneurysms. J Vasc Surg 2001;34:69–75.
22. Tiesenhausen K, Hausegger KA, Oberwalder P, et al. Left subclavian artery management in endovascular repair of thoracic aortic aneurysms and aortic dissections. J Cardiovasc Surg 2003;18:429–435.
23. Peterson BG, Eskandari MK, Gleason TG, Morasch MD. Utility of left subclavian artery revascularization in association with endoluminal repair of acute and chronic thoracic aortic pathology. J Vasc Surg 2006;43:433–439.
24. Lowell RC, Mills JL. Critical evaluation of axilloaxillary artery bypass for surgical management of symptomatic subclavian and innominate artery occlusive disease. Cardiovasc Surg 1993;1:530–535.
25. Mingoli A, Sapienza P, Feldhaus RJ, et al. Long-term results and outcomes of crossover axilloaxillary bypass grafting: a 24-year experience. J Vasc Surg 1999;29:894–901.
26. Greenberg RK, Waldman D. Endovascular and open surgical treatment of brachiocephalic arterial disease. Semin Vasc Surg 1998;11:77–90.
27. Cid MC, Font C, Coll-Vinent B, Grau JM. Large vessel vasculitides. Curr Opin Rheumatol 1998;10:18–28.
28. Giordano JM. Takayasu's disease and temporal arteritis. Semin Vasc Surg 1995;8:335–341.
29. Lie JT. Histopathologic specificity of systemic vasculitis. Rheum Dis Clin N Am 1995;21:883–909.
30. Weyand CM, Goronzy JJ. Molecular approaches toward pathologic mechanisms in giant cell arteritis and Takayasu's arteritis. Curr Opin Rheumatol 1995;7:30–36.
31. AbuRrahma AF, Thaxton L. Temporal arteritis: diagnostic and therapeutic considerations. Am Surg 1996;62:449–451.

32. Huston KA, Hunder GG, Lie JT, et al. Temporal arteritis: a 25-year epidemiologic, clinical, and pathologic study. Ann Intern Med 1978;88:162–167.
33. Nordborg E, Bengtsson BA. Epidemiology of biopsy-proven giant cell arteritis (GCA). J Intern Med 1990;227:233–236.
34. Desmet GD, Knockaert DC, Bobbaers HJ. Temporal arteritis: the silent presentation and delay in diagnosis. J Intern Med 1990;227:237–240.
35. Clearkin LG, Watts MT. Ocular involvement in giant cell arteritis. Br J Hosp Med 1990;43:373–376.
36. Andersson R, Malmvall BE, Bengtsson BA. Acute phase reactants in the initial phase of giant cell arteritis. Acta Med Scand 1986;220:365–367.
37. Kyle V, Cawston TE, Hazleman BL. Erythrocyte sedimentation rate and C reactive protein in the assessment of polymyalgia rheumatica/giant cell arteritis on presentation and during follow-up. Ann Rheum Dis 1989;48:667–671.
38. Dasgupta B, Panayi GS. Interleukin-6 in serum of patients with polymyalgia rheumatica and giant cell arteritis. Br J Rheumatol 1990;29:456–458.
39. Espinoza LR, Jara LJ, Silveira LH, et al. Anticardiolipin antibodies in polymyalgia rheumatica-giant cell arteritis: association with severe vascular complications. Am J Med 1991;90:474–478.
40. McHugh NJ, James IE, Plant GT. Anticardiolipin and antineutrophil antibodies in giant cell arteritis. J Rheumatol 1990;17:916–922.
41. Hunder GG, Bloch DA, Michel BA, et al. The American College of Rheumatology 1990 criteria for the classification of giant cell arteritis. Arthritis Rheum 1990;33:1122–1128.
42. Kyle V, Hazleman BL. Treatment of polymyalgia rheumatica and giant cell arteritis. II. Relation between steroid dose and steroid associated side effects. Ann Rheum Dis 1989;48:662–666.
43. Kyle V, Hazleman BL. Treatment of polymyalgia rheumatica and giant cell arteritis. I. Steroid regimens in the first two months. Ann Rheum Dis 1989;48:658–661.
44. Kyle V, Hazelman BL. Stopping steroids in polymyalgia rheumatica and giant cell arteritis. Br Med J 1990;300:344–345.
45. Pariser KM. Takayasu's arteritis. Curr Opin Cardiol 1994;9:575–580.
46. Procter CD, Hollier LH. Takayasu's arteritis and temporal arteritis. Ann Vasc Surg 1992;6:195–198.
47. Kerr G. Takayasu's arteritis. Curr Opin Rheumatol 1994;6:32–38.
48. Moriwaki R, Noda M, Yajima M, et al. Clinical manifestations of Takayasu arteritis in India and Japan: new classification of angiographic findings. Angiology 1997;48:369–379.
49. Robles M, Reyes PA. Takayasu's arteritis in Mexico: a clinical review of 44 consecutive cases. Clin Exp Rheumatol 1994;12:381–388.
50. Ishikawa K. Diagnostic approach and proposed criteria for the clinical diagnosis of Takayasu's arteriopathy. J Am Coll Cardiol 1988;12:964–972.
51. Arend WP, Michel BA, Bloch DA, et al. The American College of Rheumatology 1990 criteria for the classification of Takayasu arteritis. Arthritis Rheum 1990;33:1129–1134.
52. Giordano JM, Leavitt RY, Hoffman G, Fauci AS. Experience with surgical treatment of Takayasu's disease. Surgery (St. Louis) 1991;109(3 pt 1):252–258.
53. Hoffman GS. Takayasu arteritis: lessons from the American National Institutes of Health experience. Int J Cardiol 1996; 54(suppl):S99–S102.
54. Kieffer E, Piquois A, Bertal A, et al. Reconstructive surgery of the renal arteries in Takayasu's disease. Ann Vasc Surg 1990;4: 156–165.
55. Miyata T, Sato O, Deguchi J, et al. Anastomotic aneurysms after surgical treatment of Takayasu's arteritis: a 40-year experience. J Vasc Surg 1998;27:438–445.
56. Robbs JV, Abdool-Carrim AT, Kadwa AM. Arterial reconstruction for non-specific arteritis (Takayasu's disease): medium to long term results. Eur J Vasc Surg 1994;8:401–407.
57. Sharma S, Rajani M, Kaul U, et al. Initial experience with percutaneous transluminal angioplasty in the management of Takayasu's arteritis. Br J Radiol 1990;63:517–522.
58. Takagi A, Tada Y, Sato O, Miyata T. Surgical treatment for Takayasu's arteritis. A long-term follow-up study. J Cardiovasc Surg (Torino) 1989;30:553–558.
59. Weaver FA, Yellin AE, Campen DH, et al. Surgical procedures in the management of Takayasu's arteritis. J Vasc Surg 1990;12:429–437.
60. Giordano JM. Surgical treatment of Takayasu's arteritis. Int J Cardiol 2000;75(suppl 1):S123–S128.
61. Sanders RJ. Thoracic Outlet Syndrome: A Common Sequelae of Neck Injuries. Philadelphia: Lippincott, 1991.
62. Thompson RW, Petrinec D. Surgical treatment of thoracic outlet compression syndromes. I. Diagnostic considerations and transaxillary first rib resection. Ann Vasc Surg 1997;11:315–323.
63. Wilbourn AJ. Thoracic outlet syndromes: a plea for conservatism. Neurosurg Clin N Am 1991;2:235–245.
64. Wilbourn AJ. Thoracic outlet syndrome is overdiagnosed. Muscle Nerve 1999;22:130–136.
65. Jordan SE, Machleder HI. Diagnosis of thoracic outlet syndrome using electrophysiologically guided anterior scalene blocks. Ann Vasc Surg 1998;12:260–264.
66. Jordan SE, Ahn SS, Freischlag JA, et al. Selective botulinum chemodenervation of the scalene muscles for treatment of neurogenic thoracic outlet syndrome. Ann Vasc Surg 2000;14:365–369.
67. Walsh MT. Therapist management of thoracic outlet syndrome. J Hand Ther 1994;7:131–144.
68. Novak CB. Conservative management of thoracic outlet syndrome. Semin Thorac Cardiovasc Surg 1996;8:201–207.
69. Aligne C, Barral X. Rehabilitation of patients with thoracic outlet syndrome. Ann Vasc Surg 1992;6:381–389.
70. Roos DB. Congenital anomalies associated with thoracic outlet syndrome. Am J Surg 1976;132:771–778.
71. Juvonen T, Satta J, Laitala P, et al. Anomalies at the thoracic outlet are frequent in the general population. Am J Surg 1995;170:33–37.
72. Machleder HI, Moll F, Verity MA. The anterior scalene muscle in thoracic outlet compression syndrome: histochemical and morphometric studies. Arch Surg 1986;121:1141–1144.
73. Sanders RJ, Jackson CG, Banchero N, Pearce WH. Scalene muscle abnormalities in traumatic thoracic outlet syndrome. Am J Surg 1990;159:231–236.
74. Roos DB. Transaxillary approach for first rib resection to relieve thoracic outlet syndrome. Ann Surg 1966;163:354–358.
75. Roos DB. Experience with first rib resection for thoracic outlet syndrome. Ann Surg 1971;173:429–442.
76. Machleder HI. Transaxillary operative management of thoracic outlet syndrome. In: Ernst CB, Stanley JC, eds. Current Therapy in Vascular Surgery, 2nd ed. Philadelphia: Decker, 1991:227–230.
77. Urschel HC Jr. The transaxillary approach for treatment of thoracic outlet syndromes. Semin Thorac Cardiovasc Surg 1996;8:214–220.
78. Sanders RJ, Monsour JW, Gerber WJ. Recurrent thoracic outlet syndrome following first rib resection. Vasc Surg 1979;13:325–330.
79. Sanders RJ, Monsour JW, Gerber FG, et al. Scalenectomy versus first rib resection for treatment of the thoracic outlet syndrome. Surgery (St. Louis) 1979;85:109–121.

80. Qvarfordt PG, Ehrenfeld WK, Stoney RJ. Supraclavicular radical scalenectomy and transaxillary first rib resection for the thoracic outlet syndrome: a combined approach. Am J Surg 1984;148:111–116.
81. Hempel GK, Rusher AH Jr, Wheeler CG, et al. Supraclavicular resection of the first rib for thoracic outlet syndrome. Am J Surg 1981;141:213–215.
82. Sanders RJ, Raymer S. The supraclavicular approach to scalenectomy and first rib resection: description of technique. J Vasc Surg 1985;2:751–756.
83. Reilly LM, Stoney RJ. Supraclavicular approach for thoracic outlet decompression. J Vasc Surg 1988;8:329–334.
84. Cheng SW, Reilly LM, Nelken NA, et al. Neurogenic thoracic outlet decompression: rationale for sparing the first rib. Cardiovasc Surg 1995;3:617–623.
85. Fantini GA. Reserving supraclavicular first rib resection for vascular complications of thoracic outlet syndrome. Am J Surg 1996;172:200–204.
86. Thompson RW, Petrinec D, Toursarkissian B. Surgical treatment of thoracic outlet compression syndromes. II. Supraclavicular exploration and vascular reconstruction. Ann Vasc Surg 1997;11:442–451.
87. Hempel GK, Shutze WP, Anderson JF, Bukhari HI. 770 consecutive supraclavicular first rib resections for thoracic outlet syndrome. Ann Vasc Surg 1996;10:456–463.
88. Sanders RJ, Haug CE, Pearce WH. Recurrent thoracic outlet syndrome. J Vasc Surg 1990;12:390–398.
89. Thompson RW, Schneider PA, Nelken NA, et al. Circumferential venolysis and paraclavicular thoracic outlet decompression for "effort thrombosis" of the subclavian vein. J Vasc Surg 1992;16:723–732.
90. Azakie A, McElhinney DB, Thompson RW, et al. Surgical management of subclavian vein "effort" thrombosis secondary to thoracic outlet compression. J Vasc Surg 1998;28:777–786.
91. Sanders RJ, Pearce WH. The treatment of thoracic outlet syndrome: a comparison of different operations. J Vasc Surg 1989;10:626–634.
92. Sanders RJ. Results of the surgical treatment for thoracic outlet syndrome. Semin Thorac Cardiovasc Surg 1996;8:221–228.
93. Thompson RW, Bartoli MA. Neurogenic thoracic outlet syndrome. In: Rutherford RB, ed. Vascular Surgery, 6th ed. Philadelphia: Elsevier Saunders, 2005:1347–1365.
94. Sanders RJ, Monsour JW, Baer SB. Transaxillary first rib resection for the thoracic outlet syndrome. Arch Surg 1968;97:1014–1023.
95. Roeder DK, Mills M, McHale JJ, et al. First rib resection in the treatment of thoracic outlet syndrome: transaxillary and posterior thoracoplasty approaches. Ann Surg 1973;178:49–52.
96. Hoofer WD, Burnett AD. Thoracic outlet relief. J Kansas Med Soc 1973;74:329–331.
97. Dale WA. Management of thoracic outlet syndrome. Ann Surg 1975;181:575–585.
98. Kremer RM, Ahlquist REJ. Thoracic outlet compression syndrome. Am J Surg 1975;130:612–616.
99. McGough EC, Pearce MB, Byrne JP. Management of thoracic outlet syndrome. J Ther Card Med 1979;77:169–174.
100. Youmans CRJ, Smiley RH. Thoracic outlet syndrome with negative Adson's and hyperabduction maneuvers. Vasc Surg 1980;14:318–329.
101. Roos DB. The place for scalenectomy and first-rib resection in thoracic outlet syndrome. Surgery (St. Louis) 1982;92:1077–1085.
102. Batt M, Griffet J, Scotti L, LeBas P. Le syndrome de la transversee cervico-brachiale: a propos de 112 cas: vers une attitude tactique plus nuancee. J Chir (Paris) 1983;120:687–691.
103. Sallstrom J, Gjores JE. Surgical treatment of the thoracic outlet syndrome. Acta Chir Scand 1983;149:555–560.
104. Heughan C. Thoracic outlet syndrome. Can J Surg 1984;27:35–36.
105. Narakas A, Bonnard C, Egloff DV. The cervico-thoracic outlet syndrome. Ann Chir Main 1986;5:185–207.
106. Takagi K, Yamaga M, Morisawa K, Kitagawa T. Management of thoracic outlet syndrome. Arch Orthop Trauma Surg 1987;106:78–81.
107. Davies AL, Messerschmidt W. Thoracic outlet syndrome: a therapeutic approach based on 115 consecutive cases. Del Med J 1988;60:307–310.
108. Sellke FW, Kelly TR. Thoracic outlet syndrome. Am J Surg 1988;156:54–57.
109. Stanton PEJ, Vo NM, Haley T, et al. Thoracic outlet syndrome: a comprehensive evaluation. Am Surg 1988;54:129–133.
110. Wood VE, Twito R, Verska JM. Thoracic outlet syndrome: the results of first rib resection in 100 patients. Orthop Clin N Am 1988;19:131–146.
111. Cikrit DF, Haefner R, Nichols WK, Silver D. Transaxillary or supraclavicular decompression for the thoracic outlet syndrome: a comparison of the risks and benefits. Am Surg 1989;55:347–352.
112. Lindgren SHS, Ribbe EB, Norgren LEH. Two-year follow-up of patients operated on for thoracic outlet syndrome: effects on sick-leave incidence. Eur J Vasc Surg 1989;3:411–415.
113. Lepantalo M, Lindgren KA, Leino E, et al. Long term outcome after resection of the first rib for thoracic outlet syndrome. Br J Surg 1989;76:1255–1256.
114. Jamieson WG, Chinnick B. Thoracic outlet syndrome: fact or fancy? A review of 409 consecutive patients who underwent operation. Can J Surg 1996;39:321–326.
115. Graham GG, Lincoln BM. Anterior resection of the first rib for thoracic outlet syndrome. Am J Surg 1973;126:803–806.
116. Thompson JB, Hernandez IA. The thoracic outlet syndrome: a second look. Am J Surg 1979;138:251–253.
117. Thomas GI, Jones TW, Stavney LS, Manhas DR. The middle scalene muscle and its contribution to the TOS. Am J Surg 1983;145:589–592.
118. Loh CS, Wu AVO, Stevenson IM. Surgical decompression for thoracic outlet syndrome. J R Coll Surg Edinb 1989;34:66–68.
119. Axelrod DA, Proctor MC, Geisser ME, et al. Outcomes after surgery for thoracic outlet syndrome. J Vasc Surg 2001;33:1220–1225.

65

Abdominal Aortic Aneurysms

B. Timothy Baxter and Brad A. Winterstein

Definition, Prevalence, and Significance

The standard definition of an arterial aneurysm is a permanent, localized dilation of an artery with at least a 50% increase in diameter when compared to the normal expected diameter of the vessel.[1] The diameter of the infrarenal aorta, the most common extracranial location for arterial aneurysms, is normally less than 2 cm. Thus, most studies use an aortic diameter of 3 cm or greater to define the presence of an abdominal aortic aneurysm (AAA). Data from multiple screening studies using this definition have determined the prevalence of AAA to range from 4% to 8% in elderly individuals.[2,3]

Although embolization, compression, fistula formation, and occlusion can occur, rupture is the gravest and most common complication of AAA. AAA rupture is thought to be responsible for more than 9000 deaths per year,[4] making it one of the leading causes of death in the elderly population of the United States. In addition to mortality, the health care costs associated with AAA are substantial. In the United States alone, where more than 40,000 procedures are performed each year for AAA, the overall hospital charges for the year 2001 were estimated to exceed $950 million.[5]

Pathogenesis, Risk Factors, Expansion, and Rupture Risk

During the past 20 years, both clinical and basic science researchers have begun to unravel the underlying pathogenesis of AAAs.[6] Once thought to be simply an end-stage complication of atherosclerosis, the AAA is now beginning to be recognized as a unique pathological entity. Current research is focused on four main areas: (1) the genetics of aneurysm inheritance and formation; (2) the role of inflammation and the immune system in aneurysm development; (3) the enzymatic degradation of the aorta connective tissue structure during aneurysm formation; and (4) the biomechanical aspects of aneurysm initiation and progression.[7] The ultimate goals of this basic research are twofold: (1) the development of genetic or biochemical tests to identify aneurysms earlier and (2) finding pharmacological targets and developing medical therapies to prevent and/or retard aneurysm formation.

The clinical risk factors for AAA are similar to those associated with atherosclerosis. Advanced age, male gender, another affected family member, and smoking are the characteristics most strongly correlated with the presence of AAA.[8] Other risk factors include hyperlipidemia and hypertension.[9,10] Interestingly, diabetes mellitus, one of the chief risk factors for atherosclerosis, appears to be negatively associated with AAA.[8]

The natural history of AAA is that of progressive expansion to the point of eventual rupture. Imaging studies have followed the expansion rates of AAAs and have found the mean expansion rate to be approximately 0.3 cm/year.[11] Importantly, many of these studies have shown that the expansion rate increases as the size of the aneurysm increases. There is also a consistent relationship between aneurysm size and risk of rupture.[12] Although aneurysms smaller than 5.5 cm have a 1-year risk of rupture of only 0.6%,[11] aneurysms with diameters measuring 5.5 to 5.9 cm, 6.0 to 6.9 cm, and greater than 7.0 cm have yearly rupture rates of 9.4%, 10.2%, and 32.5%, respectively.[13] These findings are explained, in part, by increases in aortic wall stress described by the law of Laplace, which states that wall stress is directly proportional to the aortic diameter.

Diagnosis and Screening

A large majority of intact AAAs are asymptomatic. A family history of aneurysm disease is a major risk factor for AAA and should prompt an increased awareness and a search for

TABLE 65.1.
Randomized Controlled Trials of Ultrasound Screening for Abdominal Aortic Aneurysm (AAA).

Reference	*Year*	*Randomized groups*	*Intervention*	*Follow-up*	*Outcomes*	*Comments*
Norman[17]	2004	41,000 men 65–83 years old randomized	Abdominal ultrasound	43-month median	No significant difference in AAA-related deaths	Subgroup analysis shows men ages 65–74 benefit most from screening
Lindholt[16]	2002	12,658 men greater than 65 years old randomized	Abdominal ultrasound	5.1 years	68% reduction in inpatient AAA-related deaths in screened group	
Ashton[18]	2002	67,800 men 65–74 years old randomized	Abdominal ultrasound Elective operation if AAA > 5.5 cm	4.1-year mean follow-up	42% reduction in AAA-related death in screened group	6% 30-day mortality with elective surgery, 37% mortality with emergent surgery No difference in all-cause mortality
Scott[15]	1995	15,775 men and women 65–80 years old randomized	Abdominal ultrasound Elective operation if AAA > 6 cm, symptomatic, or rapid increase in size	5 years	42% reduction in AAA-related deaths in screened group (not statistically significant)	50% decrease in ruptured AAAs

an AAA in older individuals. A careful physical examination of the abdomen is useful and can detect 76% of aneurysms greater than 5 cm.[14] Unfortunately, physical examination is not very sensitive in detecting aneurysms of smaller size, and the problem of obesity can obscure even larger aneurysms. As such, most aneurysms are discovered incidentally during radiologic examinations for other purposes, or through screening.

Radiologic screening, primarily using ultrasonography, has been suggested as a means to identify AAAs before rupture, and a number of prospective randomized trials have been performed (Table 65.1).[15–18] Data from these studies suggest that screening a target population, defined as men between the ages of 65 and 73, who also have a history of smoking, may be the most cost-effective screening strategy.[19] Because of the evidence demonstrating decreased mortality in some of these screened populations, the United States Preventive Services Task Force has endorsed one-time screening for men between the ages of 65 and 75 who have a history of smoking.[20]

Treatment

Patients with symptoms referable to an AAA should undergo urgent repair of the aneurysm. The indication for elective repair of an asymptomatic AAA is based on the risk of rupture, the operative risk, and the life expectancy of each patient. Because aneurysm size is a critical factor in determining rupture risk, the diameter of an aneurysm is often the most important factor in deciding when to operate. Two randomized trials have shown that the survival benefit of open, elective AAA repair is limited to those with aneurysms that are 5.5 cm or greater (Table 65.2).[11,21] This diameter is based on balancing the risk of rupture with the operative risk as determined by the populations sampled in these two large-scale trials. Because endovascular aneurysm repair (EVAR) is associated with decreased morbidity and mortality, clinical trials are planned to assess the risks and benefits of EVAR for AAAs with diameters less than 5.5 cm.

Open Operative Treatment

The goal of treatment for an AAA is the exclusion of the aneurysm with prevention of rupture and its associated consequences. The current gold standard therapy is open interposition grafting of the aorta. The first successful treatment of AAA dates back to 1951 when Dubost et al. removed an AAA and replaced it with a homograft.[22] Since that time, operations for AAA have become commonplace, with progressively improving outcomes for elective repair. Currently the mortality rates for the open operation range from 2% to 6%, with the best results found in high-volume hospitals with experienced surgeons.[11,21,23] Complications following open AAA repair include myocardial infarction, renal failure, colonic ischemia, and postoperative sexual dysfunction in men.

Endovascular Treatment

Since Parodi's pioneering work in 1991 using stented grafts for aneurysm exclusion,[24] endovascular aneurysm repair has

TABLE 65.2.
Randomized Controlled Trials of AAA Intervention.

Reference	*Year*	*Randomized groups*	*Intervention*	*Follow-up*	*Outcomes*	*Comments*
Open AAA Repair						
Lederle[11]	2002	1136 men with 4- to 5.4-cm aneurysms randomized to immediate elective repair versus surveillance	Open AAA repair or radiologic surveillance every 6 months	4.9-year mean follow-up	Aneurysm-related mortality: 2.6% in surveillance group; 3% in immediate repair group	Operative mortality rate 2.1%
21	2002	1090 men and women aged 60–76 years with 4- to 5.5-cm aneurysms randomized to early elective repair versus surveillance	Open AAA repair or radiologic surveillance every 6 months	8-year mean follow-up	Overall 5 year survival: 62% in surveillance group; 71% in early surgery group – No statistical difference	Overall all-cause mortality: 45% survival in surveillance group; 53% survival in early surgery group (statistically significant) Operative mortality rate 5.5% Fourfold higher rupture rate for women
Endovascular AAA repair						
Greenhalgh[26]	2004	1082 patients randomized to open repair or endovascular aneurysm repair (EVAR)	Open repair or EVAR	30 days	30-day mortality: 1.7% EVAR group; 4.6% open repair group	
Prinssen[25]	2004	345 patients randomized to open repair or EVAR	Open repair or EVAR	30 days	30-day mortality: 1.2% EVAR group; 4.6% open repair group	Systemic complications: EVAR 11%; open repair 26%; Local complications: EVAR 26%; Open repair 8%

gained in popularity. A number of different devices and techniques have been employed with varying degrees of success for carefully selected patients. Although randomized trials comparing open repair and EVAR are ongoing, the short-term results of EVAR appear promising (see Table 65.2).[25,26] Currently, data favor EVAR over the open repair when based solely upon the short-term morbidity and mortality comparisons, primarily because many of the complications associated with the open operation are eliminated using the minimally invasive endovascular methods. The long-term durability of the endovascular repairs and optimal patient selection remain in question, however, and await additional data.[27] The treatment of EVAR complications, mainly endoleaks, is another issue that requires additional study.

Treatment of the ruptured AAA remains a difficult problem. Despite advances in intensive care and the evolution of endovascular therapy, the overall mortality of a ruptured AAA remains near 80%.[28] Even for those who make it to the hospital alive, the operative mortality is at least 40% to 50%.[29] These facts underscore the importance of optimizing methods of detecting and managing aneurysms before rupture. These methods may soon include widespread screening of those at risk for the disease,[30] developing pharmacological therapies to slow or stop aneurysm progression,[31] and additional refinements to existing techniques for our operative and interventional therapies.

Visceral and Renal Artery Aneurysms

As with AAA, visceral artery aneurysms may also cause death by rupture. Most are asymptomatic and detected as incidental findings on imaging studies. Table 65.3 summarizes the features of each of the more common types of visceral artery aneurysms.[32] Because these aneurysms are rare, the only data available upon which to base treatment decisions are from retrospective reviews and case reports.[33–40] Surgical intervention is usually the best approach, although the aneurysm location, size, and patient comorbidities may warrant observation in some cases. Repair typically involves interposition grafting, although operative ligation is another option depending on the location of the aneurysm and presence of collaterals. Endovascular repairs, using transluminal embolization[41] or stent grafting,[42] have also been used in certain situations and are likely to become more popular as catheter-based treatments become more widely used.

Table 65.3. Characteristics of Visceral and Renal Artery Aneurysms.

Location	*Percentage of visceral aneurysms*	*Pathogenesis*	*Risk factors*	*Signs/symptoms*	*Diagnosis*	*Treatment*
Splenic artery	60%	Medial degeneration	Multiple pregnancies, portal hypertension, splenomegaly, local inflammation from pancreatitis, local trauma 1:4 male:female	Asymptomatic Epigastric pain	Calcified aneurysm wall on plain films CT, US, angiography	If symptomatic, of childbearing age or more than 3 cm: • Resection • Ligation • Catheter embolization Splenectomy not required
Hepatic artery	20%	Medial degeneration Infection Iatrogenic injury	2:1 male:female	Asymptomatic RUQ pain	CT, US, angiography	• Resection • Ligation • Bypass • Catheter embolization
Superior mesenteric artery	5%	Infection Medial degeneration	Subacute bacterial endocarditis	90% symptomatic Progressive abdominal pain	CT, US, angiography	• Resection if infected • Ligation • Rarely bypass
Celiac artery	4%	Medial degeneration	Men > women	Asymptomatic	CT, US, angiography	• Resection • Ligation • Bypass
Renal artery	0.09% estimated prevalence	Fibrodysplasia	Female > male	Asymptomatic 70%–80% hypertensive	CT, US, angiography	• Resection with revascularization • Ex vivo repair • Catheter embolization, stent graft placement

CT, computed tomography; US, ultrasound; RUQ, right upper quadrant.

Aortoiliac Occlusive Disease

Pathophysiology

The risk factors for aortoiliac occlusive disease (AOD) are the same as those for generalized atherosclerosis. Smoking, hypertension, hyperlipidemia, and hyperhomocysteinemia are all associated with AOD.[43] Diabetes is a significant risk factor, although it is has a stronger association with the development of infrainguinal atherosclerotic occlusive disease.[44] Patients presenting with AOD are also, on the average, 10 to 20 years younger than those presenting with infrainguinal occlusive disease.[45] Women appear to have a similar prevalence of AOD when compared to men.[46]

Atherosclerosis commonly begins and progresses in regions of turbulent blood flow. Normal laminar flow is disrupted at arterial bifurcations and in areas of vessel fixation, and these sites are the most frequent locations for disease development.[47] The natural history of atherosclerotic lesions is that of progressively increasing size and complexity, ultimately resulting in signs or symptoms related to stenosis, thrombosis, or embolism. Although atherosclerosis is a diffuse process, its severity typically is greater in the infrarenal aorta, and the severity decreases at or above the renal arteries. This consideration is important in the operative treatment of AOD because adequate inflow can usually be obtained just below the renal arteries, eliminating concerns about renal ischemia during surgery.

As atherosclerotic obstructions persist and progress, increasing chronic ischemia induces collateral arterial pathways to enlarge, naturally bypassing the obstructions. The development of collateral pathways is critical to maintaining viability of the lower extremities in advanced AOD. Important collateral pathways include (1) the internal mammary artery to the inferior epigastric artery, (2) the hypogastric and gluteal branch arteries to the common femoral and profunda branches, (3) the superior mesenteric and inferior mesenteric arteries to the middle and inferior hemorrhoidal arteries, and (4) the lumbar artery branches to the circumflex iliac and internal iliac arteries. Importantly, an artery without an obstructing lesion will not develop enhanced collateralization. Hence, the acute occlusion of a minimally stenotic vessel will rapidly cause limb-threatening ischemia.

Clinical Manifestations

The initial manifestation of moderate AOD is lower extremity ischemia. The first symptom is often exertional pain in the muscle groups of the thigh, hip, and buttock region, also known as intermittent claudication. Symptoms may also occur in the calf; however, calf pain is usually caused by multilevel disease involving the infrainguinal vasculature. This cramping-type pain of intermittent claudication is characterized by its appearance after a fixed amount of activity, such as walking a specific distance, and its disappearance with rest. Men may also experience erectile dysfunction, and the combination of bilateral lower extremity claudication, impotence, and absent femoral pulses is referred to as Leriche's syndrome.[48]

Patients with focal AOD rarely progress to limb-threatening ischemia with rest pain or ischemic tissue loss. When these manifestations occur, it is usually the result of multilevel disease involving both the aortoiliac and infrainguinal vessels. Limb-threatening ischemia may also result from thromboembolic complications involving aortoiliac atherosclerotic plaque. "Blue toe syndrome" describes the digital ischemia and gangrene resulting from downstream embolization of debris from ulcerated atheromatous plaque.[49]

Diagnosis and Evaluation

The diagnosis of AOD is usually straightforward. However, the complaint of intermittent claudication may sometimes be confused with the pain associated with spinal stenosis or intervertebral disk herniation. These other processes can be distinguished from ischemic claudication because their symptoms are produced while standing rather than walking and are only relieved by sitting. This neurogenic pain is also present in the distribution of the sciatic nerve, although in some cases it may be difficult for patients to localize.

A wealth of information may be gained by a careful physical examination. Inspection of the legs may be normal or reveal slight atrophy. Trophic changes, such as loss of hair on the legs and toes, may also be present. A marked decrease or absence of palpable femoral pulses is a good indication of aortoiliac-level disease. However, the presence of normal pulses does not rule out the possibility of significant obstruction, as exercise may unmask hemodynamically important lesions to produce symptoms.[50]

Noninvasive assessment of ischemic disease of the lower extremities starts with determination of ankle brachial indices (ABIs), which measure the systolic blood pressures at the ankles compared to those of the brachial arteries. A ratio of 1.0 to 1.2 is normal. Ratios less than 1.0 signify atherosclerotic disease of the arteries of the lower extremities. A ratio of 1.0 may be obtained at rest if there is focal disease at the aortic bifurcation because of the rich collateral network that forms around the stenosis. If this is the case, ABIs obtained after exercise may expose the lesion, as pressures will decrease when the metabolic demand increases beyond the capacity of the collateral network to provide adequate blood flow.

Duplex ultrasonography may provide additional information regarding disease location and severity. Duplex ultrasonography allows direct evaluation of AOD by identifying areas of disturbed flow, seen as increases in peak systolic velocity. Duplex scanning has been shown to have 95% sensitivity and 80% specificity in predicting significant aortoiliac disease when compared to angiography.[51] Although duplex ultrasonography may allow visualization of diseased arteries, direct imaging of the diseased aortoiliac segment can be challenging because of obesity and the presence of overlying bowel gas.

Computed tomographic (CT) angiography is being used more frequently to image the aortoiliac segment as technological advances have greatly improved the speed and image quality of the exams. Multidetector row CT (MDCT) angiography compares favorably with magnetic resonance angiography (MRA) and conventional arteriography in characterizing AOD.[52] It also has the ability to image distal runoff vessels that may be absent on conventional arteriography.[53] Small prospective studies comparing MDCT angiography to conventional digital subtraction angiography have demonstrated sensitivities and specificities exceeding 90%.[54,55] Advantages of MDCT angiography compared to MRA include higher resolution and the ability to perform the test on patients with implanted devices, such as pacemakers and defibrillators. A major disadvantage is the requirement of nephrotoxic contrast material.[53]

The other noninvasive imaging option gaining in popularity is MRA. Three-dimensional MRA using gadolinium enhancement is able to accurately visualize the entire lower extremity arterial tree. For detecting occlusions and stenoses greater than 50% in the aortoiliac segment, multiple studies have demonstrated sensitivities ranging from 80% to 100% and specificities ranging from 92% to 100%.[56] Currently, its primary use is in planning arterial reconstructions as opposed to screening, and its use should be limited to those patients for whom interventional therapy is warranted. Important advantages of MRA compared to arteriography are its noninvasive nature and its use of nonnephrotoxic contrast material. As this technology has improved, MRA is replacing conventional arteriography for planning lower extremity arterial reconstructions in some institutions.

Conventional angiography is reserved for patients with signs and symptoms severe enough to require intervention. The goal of angiography is not only to diagnose and determine the significance of lesions but also to plan therapy and in many cases to perform a definitive endovascular procedure. The procedure is invasive, with the potential for both puncture site complications and contrast-related nephrotoxicity.

Angiography is usually performed in a retrograde fashion through the common femoral artery. Translumbar or transaxillary approaches can also be used if the femoral artery is inaccessible. Views should be obtained in the anteroposterior and oblique projections. Images should include the renal arteries proximally to the pedal circulation distally to assess the adequacy of both the inflow and outflow vessels before surgery. If angiography does not conclusively show a significant stenosis, a measurement of the pressure gradient across any potentially stenotic areas can be measured. This measurement is performed while pulling the angiography catheter back from the aorta, across the stenotic lesion, to the femoral artery. A mean pressure gradient of 7 to 10 mmHg at rest is considered a hemodynamically significant obstruction.[57–60] After instilling papaverine to induce hyperemia in the lower extremity, a mean pressure gradient greater or equal to 30 mmHg is also considered significant.[60]

Treatment

There are several options available to treat AOD. All patients should be counseled regarding risk factor modification. Smoking cessation, along with evaluation and treatment of hypertension, hyperlipidemia, hyperhomocysteinemia, and diabetes, are essential. Treatment with a platelet inhibitor, such as aspirin, is standard therapy. Other options for conservative management may include medications such as cilostazol, and exercise programs. Absolute indications for operative or endovascular intervention include ischemic rest pain and tissue loss. Claudication is a relative indication,

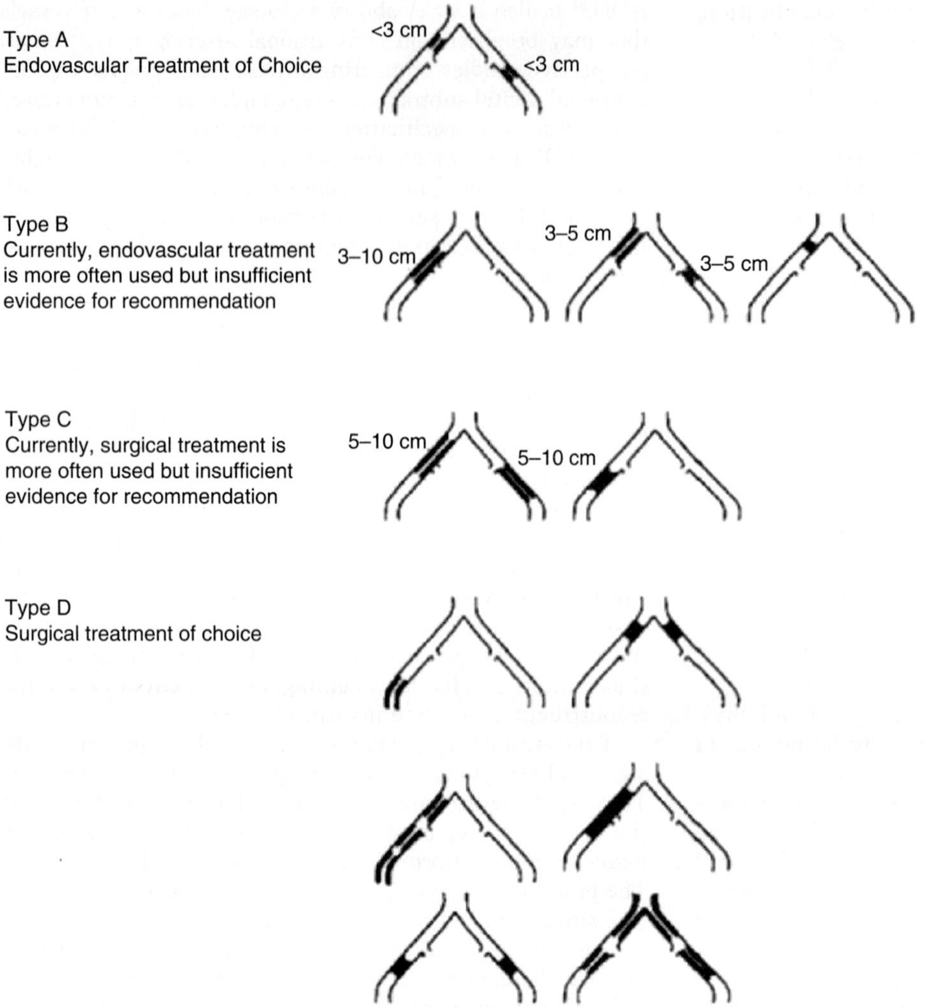

FIGURE 65.1. Preferred options for interventional management of iliac lesions. (From Dormandy JA, Rutherford RB,[57] by permission of Journal of Vascular Sugery.)

with intervention typically reserved for those patients with severe, lifestyle-limiting claudication who have failed conservative management.

The choice of intervention for AOD depends on the morphology and location of the lesion(s), as well as the comorbid conditions of the patient. Figure 65.1 demonstrates the preferred options for intervention in AOD as determined by the TransAtlantic Inter-Society Consensus (TASC) Group. Table 65.4 shows the patency rate ranges for the various treatment options.[57] It must be remembered that patency rates and outcomes depend not only on the selected procedure but also on the indication for the procedure and the health status of the patient. Thus, a procedure performed for claudication in healthy patients will have improved patency rates and fewer complications when compared with the same procedure performed for limb-threatening ischemia in sick patients.

Aortic Reconstruction

The current gold standard treatment for AOD is aortobifemoral bypass. The proximal anastomosis can be end-to-end or end-to-side. The end-to-end anastomosis is clearly indicated in patients with aneurysmal disease or complete aortic occlusion and is preferable in most other cases because of a slightly better long-term patency. The end-to-side anastomosis is indicated when retrograde flow from the femoral arteries would not provide adequate flow to the internal iliac arteries or a large inferior mesenteric artery. The site for the distal anastomosis is usually the femoral arteries. Although extending a bypass graft below the inguinal canal can lead to such complications as lymphatic leaks, infection, and anastomotic aneurysms, it addresses the need for providing adequate outflow, as the severity of external iliac disease is often underestimated by arteriography. The operative mortality for an aortobifemoral bypass ranges between 1% and 3%.[61,62]

TABLE 65.4. Patency Rates for Aortoiliac Occlusive Disease (AOD) Interventions.

Procedure	*5-Year patency (%)*
Aortobifemoral bypass	81–98
Aortoiliac endarterectomy	60–94
Femoral–femoral bypass	55–92
Axillofemoral bypass	30–85
Angioplasty	54–78
Angioplasty and stenting	72

Extraanatomic Bypass

The role for extraanatomic bypasses has been debated because patency rates are slightly compromised in favor of less morbidity with the operative procedure. The use of a femoral–femoral bypass in unilateral iliac disease is an accepted alternative to an intraabdominal procedure. Axillounifemoral and axillobifemoral bypasses are two other procedures that can be used for limb-threatening ischemia associated with AOD. The use of these procedures should be limited to those individuals in whom a transabdominal approach places them at an increased risk. This group typically includes patients with significant comorbid disease or those with the so-called hostile abdomen, in which infection or dense adhesions are anticipated. Although improvements in techniques and the use of prosthetic ringed grafts are associated with improved patency rates, these bypasses are still inferior to aortobifemoral bypass. Thoracofemoral bypass is another useful consideration when faced with a hostile abdomen.

Endovascular Treatment

The use of endovascular techniques, such as percutaneous transluminal angioplasty (PTA), with or without stent placement, has become an important component in the management of AOD. Short, focal stenoses in patients with good distal runoff appear most amenable to endovascular treatment. PTA involves inflating a pressurized balloon across a lesion, which fractures the atherosclerotic plaque and expands the lumen of the vessel. The angiographic appearance of the lesion and measured pressure gradient across the lesion are the factors that determine the technical success or failure of the procedure. Following vessel dilation, a stent may be placed. Although routine stent placement after PTA is advocated by some, the general consensus is that the indications for stent placement in AOD are (1) failure to achieve an adequate post-PTA angiographic lesion appearance or (2) persistence of a pressure gradient greater than 10mmHg across the lesion.[57,58] Five-year follow-up results in patients randomized to primary iliac stent placement versus primary angioplasty with selective stent placement revealed no differences in the numbers of reinterventions or outcomes between the two groups.[63] Although the current literature does not show that routine stenting of stenotic lesions is superior to angioplasty alone, lesions that are eccentric, calcified, and near bifurcations may be best served with stent placement.

Mesenteric Ischemia

Anatomy/Pathophysiology

During fetal development, multiple segmental arteries branch from the aorta to supply the primitive foregut, midgut, and hindgut. As normal development proceeds, all but three of these vessels regress, leaving the celiac, superior mesenteric, and inferior mesenteric arteries to dominate the blood supply to the gut. These three mature arteries connect through rich vascular anastomoses found throughout the mesentery.[64] These interconnections become clinically important in the presence of long-standing atherosclerotic occlusive disease, whereby abundant networks of collaterals form and have the capacity to maintain bowel viability even when all three major named aortic branches are occluded.

Approximately 20% of the resting cardiac output supplies the bowel, with most of this nourishing the mucosa. In addition to intrinsic autoregulation, this blood flow is regulated by both humoral and neural factors. Catecholamines, vasopressin, and angiotensin II are examples of humoral factors that are able to cause intense vasoconstriction of the visceral circulation. Endogenous humoral mediators such as these, along with adrenergic innervation of the arterial system, may be responsible for the intense vasospasm seen in cases of nonocclusive mesenteric ischemia.[65]

Bowel ischemia may cause a wide spectrum of bowel injury, ranging from focal areas of mucosal damage to global transmural necrosis. Accompanying ischemic bowel injury may be a systemic inflammatory response; This may progress to sepsis as mucosal integrity is lost and bacterial translocation occurs.[66] These processes do not necessarily subside when perfusion is restored. With the return of blood flow, the reintroduction of oxygen to ischemic areas can result in the production of harmful free radicals that can injure tissues locally and cause deleterious effects systemically. This reperfusion injury can lead to complications such as cardiac arrest, or amplification of the systemic inflammatory response resulting in multiorgan failure.[67]

The clinical and pathological syndromes of mesenteric ischemia can be broadly divided into two categories: (1) acute mesenteric ischemia and (2) chronic mesenteric ischemia. Both the acute and chronic forms of the disease offer difficult and challenging problems in both diagnosis and treatment. Regardless of the etiology, the mortality associated with mesenteric ischemia is high and is directly related to the extent of bowel infarction. Delays in diagnosis are common and usually result from failure to consider mesenteric ischemia in the differential diagnosis of abdominal pain. As such, having a high index of suspicion for the presence of mesenteric ischemia in at-risk patients with abdominal pain is of utmost importance.

Acute Mesenteric Ischemia

Clinical Manifestations

Table 65.5 outlines the characteristics of each of the most common causes of acute mesenteric ischemia.[68–70] Most cases involve elderly patients with preexisting generalized atherosclerosis. The sudden onset of abdominal pain is the most common presenting complaint, although patients with thrombotic etiologies may have pain with a more insidious course. A prior history of an embolic event, usually secondary to atrial fibrillation or hypokinetic, infarcted areas of myocardium, is present in up to one-half of patients with acute mesenteric ischemia of embolic etiology.[69] Nonocclusive mesenteric ischemia, sometimes referred to as "low-flow" mesenteric ischemia, is found predominately in patients who are critically ill.

The physical examination of the abdomen may appear relatively benign until late in the disease course. Once perforation has occurred, distension, rigidity, and tenderness may all be present. Early on, however, there are few, if any, signs to suggest the grave nature of the disease process, giving rise

TABLE 65.5. Etiologies and Characteristics of Acute Mesenteric Ischemia.

Etiology	*Frequency*	*Pathogenesis*	*History/risk factors*	*Diagnosis*	*Treatment*	*Mortality*
Embolic	50%	Cardiac embolism to superior mesenteric artery	Acute onset of abdominal pain Prior history of embolic event Atrial fibrillation	Arteriography	Anticoagulation Exploratory laparotomy • Embolectomy • ± necrotic bowel resection • Second-look procedure if questionably viable bowel	70%
Thrombotic	25%	Ostial atherosclerotic plaque rupture and obstruction	Prior history of abdominal pain Food fear New-onset acute abdominal pain Atherosclerosis	Arteriography	Anticoagulation Exploratory laparotomy • Bypass • Endarterectomy • ± necrotic bowel resection • Second-look procedure if questionably viable bowel	87%
Nonocclusive	20%	Hypotension/ vasospasm of splanchnic vessels	Critically ill patients with impaired splanchnic blood flow	Arteriography	Correction of underlying condition Hemodynamic optimization Catheter-directed vasodilator infusion Surgery reserved for infarcted/perforated bowel	80%
Mesenteric venous thrombosis	5%	Thrombosis of superior mesenteric vein/ portal vein	Hypercoaguable state Abdominal pain	CT scan	Anticoagulation Surgery reserved for infarcted/perforated bowel	44%

to the classic description of "pain out of proportion" to the physical findings.

Diagnosis

Having a high index of suspicion for the presence of mesenteric ischemia is the key to making the diagnosis. The presence of fever, leukocytosis, acidosis, and other associated laboratory findings are all nonspecific and frequently appear only late in the course of the disease. Because of this, the confirmation of the diagnosis depends on the radiologic evaluation.

Abdominal computed tomography (CT) may give clues to the diagnosis, but for most cases of intestinal ischemia, it has been neither sensitive nor specific. Thickened bowel wall and dilated, fluid-filled loops of bowel are common, but nonspecific, findings. Pneumatosis and portal venous gas are relatively specific but are late manifestations.[71] The use of multidetector row CT angiography with three-dimensional imaging can provide information about both vessel patency and tissue perfusion.[72] Future comparison to angiography will be needed to determine the sensitivity and specificity of this method. The ability of contrast-enhanced CT to reliably detect instances of mesenteric venous thrombosis makes it the diagnostic study of choice for this subset of patients.[73]

Arteriography is the gold standard for making the diagnosis of acute mesenteric ischemia resulting from arterial embolism, arterial thrombosis, and nonocclusive etiologies. In at-risk patients with severe, persistent, abdominal pain and peritoneal signs, arteriography should be avoided in lieu of an urgent exploratory laparotomy.[74] In all other patients, arteriography is indicated to confirm the diagnosis of intestinal ischemia. Initial films should include a lateral aortogram to view the ostia of the superior mesenteric and celiac arteries. By selectively injecting contrast into these vessels, emboli can be seen and nonocclusive ischemia can be identified by pruning of the distal vessels. In some situations, catheters may also be used therapeutically by infusing vasodilators, thrombolytics,[75] or anticoagulants.

Treatment

Once the diagnosis is made, fluid resuscitation and systemic anticoagulation are instituted. Any underlying medical problems that may have caused, or exacerbated, the mesenteric ischemia are corrected. The administration of broad-spectrum antibiotics is advocated by some because of concerns of bacterial translocation and sepsis. Definitive therapy may consist of either operative or nonoperative management, depending on the patient's condition and the suspected etiology of the acute ischemia.[74]

Nonoperative Therapy

Nonoperative therapy with the infusion of vasodilators, such as papaverine, into the affected arterial tree, is the mainstay of treatment for nonocclusive mesenteric ischemia.[74] The preferred treatment for mesenteric venous thrombosis is also nonoperative, consisting of systemic anticoagulation, with the occasional use of catheter-directed thrombolytics, to help speed resolution of the ischemia.[73] Many of these patients also require testing for hypercoaguability and frequently need to be maintained on long-term warfarin therapy. Localized thrombolytic therapy has been used for acute embolic occlusion of the superior mesenteric artery;[76] however, even with the successful nonoperative restoration of blood flow to the gut, operative exploration is often indicated to examine the bowel and to resect necrotic segments of intestine.

Operative Therapy

There are several clear indications for surgical intervention: (1) mesenteric embolization requiring embolectomy, (2) thrombotic occlusion requiring revascularization, (3) peritonitis, and (4) other clinical signs suggestive of bowel infarction. The goals of surgery are to restore blood flow when possible and to resect any bowel that is obviously necrotic. Because the appearance of ischemic bowel may improve dramatically when flow is restored, it should be observed for 30 min after reperfusion before resection. Adjunctive measures to help determine the viability of ischemic bowel include hand-held Doppler assessment of antimesenteric bowel wall blood flow and visualization of the bowel under ultraviolet light after the intravenous injection of fluorescein.[77,78] When there are extensive areas of questionable bowel, it may be preferable to resect only areas that are clearly necrotic and plan a "second-look" operation within 24 h in hopes that there may be some recovery. A planned second-look operation should never be abandoned because of improving clinical status, as a temporary improvement in clinical status does not exclude progression to infarction.

There are several surgical options for the restoration of blood flow.[79] Performing a simple thrombectomy usually leads to reocclusion. Revascularization with bypass or endarterectomy is required for thrombotic occlusion. Complete revascularization of both celiac and superior mesenteric arteries with saphenous vein or prosthetic grafts is the most common procedure and is recommended to prevent bowel infarction in case of future thrombosis of one graft.[80] Superior mesenteric artery thromboembolectomy will restore flow in cases of embolization.

Chronic Mesenteric Ischemia

Clinical Manifestations

Chronic mesenteric ischemia, also known as "intestinal angina," is a rare condition. The typical patient is elderly and vasculopathic, usually having undergone multiple procedures for coronary, cerebral, and peripheral vascular disease. Patients with chronic mesenteric ischemia typically complain of postprandial abdominal pain that persists for 1 to 3 h. Because of this pain, they often develop food fear, which leads to weight loss in approximately 70% to 85% of patients.[81,82]

Diagnosis

Duplex ultrasound is the preferred initial screening test when this diagnosis is suspected. This test can usually demonstrate occlusion or stenosis of the ostia along with collateral flow patterns. Adding additional stress to the bowel, such as feeding, has been suggested as a way to improve the diagnostic accuracy of ultrasound. When duplex studies are positive or equivocal, arteriography should be performed in anticipation of identifying occlusion or stenosis of the mesenteric vessels.

Treatment

Nonoperative Therapy

If the patient has extensive comorbidities and is not a surgical candidate, mesenteric angioplasty with or without stenting can be performed. High rates of initial success and relief of symptoms occur in a majority of patients.[83,84] Disease recurrence is common, however, with up to a third of patients experiencing recurrent symptoms.[85] Close follow-up with duplex surveillance and repeat angioplasty can be used to enhance results in nonsurgical candidates, with assisted clinical success rates as high as 96%.[83]

Operative Therapy

Surgical revascularization is the treatment of choice for chronic mesenteric ischemia. Saphenous vein or prosthetic grafts may be used for the restoration of blood flow. When the infrarenal aorta is to be replaced because of extensive atherosclerosis or aneurysmal disease, the new aortic conduit is used as the graft inflow for mesenteric revascularization. Because of excellent long-term patency rates, an antegrade bypass from the supraceliac aorta is the optimal procedure in those patients not requiring infrarenal aortic reconstruction. Retrospective reviews document 79% to 92% of patients to be symptom-free at 5 years following operative intervention.[81,82] Transaortic endarterectomy is also an acceptable alternative to bypass procedures.

Renal Artery Occlusive Disease

Renal artery occlusive disease can be associated with both hypertension and ischemic nephropathy. Renovascular hypertension is the most common form of surgically correctable hypertension, responsible for approximately 1% to 5% of all cases of hypertension in the general population.[86] Ischemic nephropathy is the other major complication of renal artery stenosis and may be present even in the absence of hypertension. Atherosclerotic renal artery occlusive disease is estimated to contribute to up to 15% of end-stage renal disease in elderly patients each year.[87] The diagnosis of renal artery stenosis has become more common as a consequence of improved diagnostic techniques, an expanding at-risk population, and an increased awareness of the disease and its associated syndromes.

Pathophysiology and Pathology

The seminal experiments that described the relationship between renal artery occlusion and hypertension were performed more than 70 years ago by Goldblatt et al.[88] These canine experiments showed that hypertension can be caused by narrowing of the renal arteries. Later studies have demonstrated that this hypertensive effect is mediated through the activation of the renin-angiotensin system.[89] Activation occurs when decreases in renal perfusion are sensed by the juxtaglomerular apparatus, stimulating the secretion of renin from the kidney. Renin is a proteolytic enzyme that acts on circulating angiotensinogen to produce angiotensin I. Angiotensin I then travels to the lung where it is converted to angiotensin II by angiotensin-converting enzyme (ACE). Angiotensin II has properties that affect both the acute phase, and the chronic phase, of hypertension. The acute phase is caused by the direct, potent vasoconstrictive properties of angiotensin II. The chronic phase involves the activation of the adrenal cortex by angiotensin II, increasing aldosterone secretion. This, in turn, increases sodium retention and intravascular volume. Angiotensin II normally exerts a negative feedback on renin release by increasing blood pressure. With severe renal artery stenosis, however, renal perfusion will not increase appropriately, resulting in a perpetuation of renin release and systemic hypertension.

There are several potential pathological causes of renal artery stenosis. Atherosclerosis is by far the most common etiology. Fibrodysplasia of the arterial wall is the other major cause frequently seen.[90] The characteristics associated with renal artery stenosis resulting from atherosclerosis and fibrodysplasia are shown in Table 65.6. Congenital aortic malformations, arterial dissections, renal artery emboli, and extrinsic masses may also impede flow through the renal arteries but are only rarely encountered.

Clinical Manifestations

Because most cases of renal artery stenosis are caused by atherosclerosis, elderly patients with known preexisting atherosclerosis and patients with major risk factors for atherosclerosis are most at risk. Oftentimes, renovascular hypertension may be superimposed upon essential hypertension, making the diagnosis less apparent. The sudden worsening of previously controlled hypertension, hypertension refractory to three or more antihypertensive medications, and new-onset hypertension in a patient over the age of 55 are all situations that should trigger an evaluation for renal artery stenosis. In addition, an acute worsening of renal function, and congestive heart failure or pulmonary edema without an easily explained cause, may also be associated with stenoses of the renal arteries.[91] In young female patients and children with hypertension, fibrodysplasia of the renal arteries should be considered and addressed. The physical examination in patients with renal artery stenosis may be unrevealing. Findings on the physical examination supporting the diagnosis include the presence of atherosclerosis in other vascular territories and abdominal bruits.[92]

TABLE 65.6. Characteristics of Atherosclerotic and Fibrodysplastic Renal Artery Stenosis.

Atherosclerosis	*Fibrodysplasia*
90% of cases of renal artery stenosis	5%–10% of cases of renal artery stenosis
More common in men	Three types:
Ostia/proximal one-third of artery	1. Medial fibroplasia • 85% of dysplastic renal artery stenoses • More common in women • Middle/distal one-third of renal artery • "String of beads" appearance on arteriography
Lesions are progressive	
May cause hypertension and ischemic nephropathy	
Poor response to percutaneous transluminal angioplasty (PTA)	2. Perimedial dysplasia • 10% of dysplastic renal artery stenoses • More common in women • Middle/distal one-third of renal artery • "String of beads" appearance on arteriography
	3. Intimal fibroplasia • 5% of dysplastic renal artery stenoses • Children and adolescents • Distal renal artery
	May cause hypertension, but rarely results in ischemic nephropathy
	Responds well to PTA

Diagnosis

Both functional studies and anatomical imaging may be used to help make the diagnosis of renal artery stenosis. Although there are many tests currently available, arteriography remains the gold standard. However, because of the risks associated with the procedure, such as contrast-induced nephropathy and atheroembolization, it is not often chosen as the initial screening study. Duplex ultrasonography, magnetic resonance angiography (MRA), and computed tomographic angiography (CTA) are the radiologic tests most frequently used to detect the presence of renal artery occlusive disease.

Renal artery duplex scanning can provide information about kidney size and blood flow through the renal arteries. A peak systolic velocity greater than 200 cm/s is a reliable predictor of a stenotic lesion greater than 60% in the renal artery.[93] In addition, measurement of the renal resistance index [1 − (end-diastolic velocity ÷ maximal systolic velocity) × 100] using duplex ultrasonography has been shown to predict the outcome of treatment for renal artery stenosis. In one study, patients with a renal resistance index greater than 80 failed to show improvement in blood pressure, renal function, or kidney survival following renal revascularization.[94] The overall reported sensitivities and specificities of renal artery duplex scanning range from 75%–98% and 90%–100%, respectively.[95,96] Because it is highly operator dependent and technically difficult, duplex scanning is time intensive and has a failure rate of 10% to 25%.[97]

Gadolinium-enhanced MRA and CTA are also useful for detecting disease in the renal arteries. A 2001 meta-analysis demonstrated the superiority of MRA and CTA at identifying renal artery stenosis when compared to ultrasonography, captopril renal scintigraphy, and the captopril test.[98] The reported sensitivities and specificities of MRA and CTA typically exceed 90%. However, a recent prospective, multicenter trial comparing CTA and MRA to arteriography found that the sensitivities and specificities were 64% and 92% for CTA and 62% and 84% for MRA.[99] Nevertheless, the superior anatomic detail and noninvasive nature of these studies make them attractive initial screening tests for renal artery stenosis. MRA has the additional benefits of being able to measure physiological functions of the kidney, such as the glomerular filtration rate,[100] and does not require the use of nephrotoxic contrast agents in comparison to CTA.

Several functional studies are available to assess whether hypertension is caused by renovascular disease. Captopril renal scintigraphy involves obtaining a baseline radionucleotide renogram, followed by the administration of an ACE inhibitor, and then another subsequent renogram. The ACE inhibitor decreases the activity of the intrarenal renin-angiotensin system and its vasoconstrictive effect on the efferent arterioles, causing a decrease in GFR and less uptake of radionucleotide by the affected kidney. The reported sensitivity and specificity ranges for detecting renal artery stenosis are 83%–96% and 87%–100%, respectively.[101] This test is less accurate when patients have bilateral disease and preexisting renal insufficiency. Measurement of renin from the renal veins is a less frequently used functional study but may be particularly useful in lateralizing the disease when bilateral stenoses are present.

Treatment

Several options are available to treat renovascular disease, including medical therapy, endovascular therapy, and operative revascularization. The primary goals of treatment are blood pressure reduction and prevention of ischemic nephropathy. The decision to progress to invasive therapy depends on the patient's comorbidities, the suspected pathology of the disease, the disease severity, and the patient's response to conservative measures. At this time, there have been five prospective randomized trials comparing medical therapy, percutaneous angioplasty (PTA), PTA with stenting, and surgery.[102–106] A summary of these trials is provided in Table 65.7.

Nonoperative Therapy

For the majority of patients with renal artery stenosis, the disease is of atherosclerotic origin, and risk factor assessment and modification is an important first step in management.

TABLE 65.7.
Randomized Trials of Renal Artery Stenosis Treatment Options.

Reference	*Year*	*Randomized groups*	*Intervention*	*Follow-up*	*Outcomes*	*Comments*
van Jaarsveld[102]	2000	106 hypertensive patients with atherosclerotic renal artery stenosis randomized to angioplasty versus medical treatment	Renal artery angioplasty or medical therapy	12 months	No significant differences in blood pressure measurements or daily blood pressure medication doses at 3 and 12 months	No significant differences in renal function
van de Ven[103]	1999	85 hypertensive patients with ostial atherosclerotic renal artery stenosis randomized to angioplasty alone versus angioplasty with stent placement	Renal artery angioplasty or angioplasty with stent placement	6 months	Primary patency: PTA 29% Stent 75% Secondary patency: PTA 51% Stent 80%	No significant difference in renal function or blood pressure between groups
Webster[105]	1998	55 hypertensive patients with atherosclerotic renal artery stenosis randomized to angioplasty versus medical treatment	Renal artery angioplasty or medical therapy	6 months	Blood pressure improved in patients with bilateral stenoses Equivalent in patients with unilateral stenosis	No difference in renal function
Plouin[104]	1998	49 hypertensive patients with unilateral atherosclerotic renal artery stenosis randomized to angioplasty versus medical treatment	Renal artery angioplasty or medical therapy	6 months	No differences in blood pressure	
Weibull[106]	1993	58 patients, age greater than 70 years with severe hypertension and unilateral atherosclerotic renal artery stenosis randomized to open repair versus angioplasty	Open reconstruction versus percutaneous transluminal angioplasty (PTA)	24 months	Primary patency: PTA 75% Surgery 96% Secondary patency: PTA 90% Surgery 97%	Hypertension cured or improved: PTA 90% Surgery 86% Renal function improved or unchanged: PTA 83% Surgery 72%

Smoking cessation, lipid management, and antiplatelet therapy are all required to reduce these patients' overall risk of morbidity and mortality associated with atherosclerotic cardiovascular disease. With the availability of multiple classes of potent antihypertensive medications, medical management of renovascular hypertension is often adequate. The most effective medications for the treatment of renovascular hypertension are the ACE inhibitors and angiotensin II receptor blockers.[90] However, these drugs must be used with caution as they may cause deterioration in renal function, especially in those patients with a high degree of stenosis, bilateral disease, or a solitary kidney.[107]

A recent meta-analysis of the three prospective, randomized controlled trials comparing medical therapy to PTA concluded that PTA gives only a modest improvement in blood pressure in patients with atherosclerotic renal artery stenosis and shows no discernible effect on renal function.[108] Further analysis of these trials has concluded that there is insufficient evidence to conclude that PTA is superior to drug therapy and that the beneficial effect of PTA may be limited to those patients with hypertension refractory to pharmacological treatment.[109]

Endovascular Therapy

When medical management has failed for atherosclerotic renal artery stenosis, or the disease etiology is suspected to be fibrodysplasia, interventional treatment is warranted. PTA is considered by many to be the first-line revascularization therapy for renal artery stenosis. This recommendation is based on the only prospective, randomized trial comparing surgical revascularization to PTA, published in 1993.[106] In this study of 58 highly selected patients with unilateral renal artery stenosis, there were no significant differences in blood pressure control or renal function between the groups at 2 years after treatment. The study also demonstrated similar secondary patency rates at 2 years, although primary patency rates were better for the surgical group.

Fibromuscular disease responds well to PTA alone, with an 87% predicted patency rate at 10 years.[110] In addition, hypertension is cured in up to one-half of all patients with fibromuscular dysplasia undergoing PTA. Atherosclerotic disease responds less favorably to PTA. In a prospective randomized trial comparing PTA to PTA with stenting in patients with ostial atherosclerotic renal artery disease, the 6-month primary patency rate was 29% for the PTA group versus 75% for the PTA with stent group.[103] Thus, it appears that if endovascular therapy is chosen to treat ostial atherosclerotic renal artery stenosis, it should include stenting. Larger clinical trials are currently underway to determine the effects of endovascular therapy compared to medical therapy on the progression of ischemic nephropathy in patients with atherosclerotic renal artery stenosis.[111]

Complications related to the endovascular treatment of renal artery stenosis commonly include arterial puncture site problems, such as hematomas and pseudoaneurysms. Rarely, more serious complications such as atheroembolization, renal artery rupture, or renal artery dissection occur, which may lead to kidney loss.[112] Contrast-related nephrotoxicity may be reduced by maintaining adequate hydration along with the administration of renoprotective agents, such as acetylcysteine.[113]

Operative Treatment

Failure of medical therapy and progression of ischemic nephropathy, in association with renal artery lesions not amenable to PTA, are the indications often cited for surgical therapy. Ostial atherosclerotic lesions and stenoses involving branches of the renal arteries are both thought to be better treated with surgery. Before an operation, patients should be thoroughly evaluated for the presence of extrarenal vascular disease and managed appropriately.

The most common surgical procedure for revascularization of the renal artery is aortorenal bypass with saphenous vein graft. Dacron or polytetrafluoroethylene (PTFE) can also be used, and these conduits are preferable in younger patients where vein graft aneurysm formation is problematical. One large series demonstrated 1- and 5-year patency rates of 98% and 96%, respectively, following prosthetic renal artery reconstruction.[114]

Nonanatomic renal artery revascularization can also be performed with excellent results. Splenorenal and hepatorenal bypasses are the two most common procedures. Assessment of the celiac and superior mesenteric arteries, to ensure they are free of occlusive disease, is essential before performing these bypasses. Occasionally, in patients with compromised renal artery flow from aortic dissection, the iliac artery may be the best inflow source for bypass.

Endarterectomy with or without a vein patch, provides good results for atherosclerotic lesions of the proximal renal arteries. An axial aortotomy may be performed for diffuse disease of the aorta and for bilateral disease. The incision is made from the superior mesenteric artery to the infrarenal aorta. Superior mesenteric artery stenosis can also be treated at this time. Arteriotomy of the renal artery may be performed for more focal lesions of the artery. The arteriotomy may be closed with or without a patch graft. The adequacy of the revascularization should be documented by intraoperative ultrasonography, especially when blind endarterectomy is performed.

Ex vivo reconstruction of the renal arteries can be performed for more complicated disease in the hilar areas. The downside of this procedure is the need for cold ischemia, long operative time, and most importantly, the loss of established collateral networks, which may be critical if revascularization fails.

Results of surgical revascularization for renovascular hypertension vary with the underlying etiology of the disease. Cure rates for the surgical treatment of fibrodysplasia are superior to those for treating atherosclerosis. Long-term results of surgical revascularization show a beneficial effect in the treatment of both renovascular hypertension and renal dysfunction. In 2002, Cherr et al. published a 12-year institutional review of 500 patients with atherosclerotic renovascular hypertension treated with surgery.[115] The operative mortality in this series was 4.6%, with 85% showing improvement (73%) or cure (12%) of hypertension. Just as important, 43% of patients demonstrated improved postoperative renal function when compared to their preoperative evaluation, including 28 patients who were able to be permanently removed from dialysis. Thus, although many patients with renal artery stenosis may be successfully treated with medications or endovascular therapy, there remains a place for surgical revascularization in properly selected patients.

References

1. Johnston KW, et al. Suggested standards for reporting on arterial aneurysms. Subcommittee on Reporting Standards for Arterial Aneurysms, Ad Hoc Committee on Reporting Standards, Society for Vascular Surgery and North American Chapter, International Society for Cardiovascular Surgery. J Vasc Surg 1991;13(3):452–458.
2. Lederle, FA, et al. Prevalence and associations of abdominal aortic aneurysm detected through screening. Aneurysm Detection and Management (ADAM) Veterans Affairs Cooperative Study Group. Ann Intern Med 1997;126(6):441–449.
3. Singh K, et al. Prevalence of and risk factors for abdominal aortic aneurysms in a population-based study: The Tromso Study. Am J Epidemiol 2001;154(3):236–244.
4. Gillum RF. Epidemiology of aortic aneurysm in the United States. J Clin Epidemiol 1995;48(11):1289–1298.
5. Lee WA, et al. Perioperative outcomes after open and endovascular repair of intact abdominal aortic aneurysms in the United States during 2001. J Vasc Surg 2004;39(3):491–496.
6. Thompson RW, Geraghty PJ, Lee JK. Abdominal aortic aneurysms: basic mechanisms and clinical implications. Curr Probl Surg 2002;39(2):110–230.
7. Wassef M, et al. Pathogenesis of abdominal aortic aneurysms: a multidisciplinary research program supported by the National Heart, Lung, and Blood Institute. J Vasc Surg 2001;34(4):730–738.
8. Lederle FA, et al. The aneurysm detection and management study screening program: validation cohort and final results. Aneurysm Detection and Management Veterans Affairs Cooperative Study Investigators. Arch Intern Med 2000;160(10):1425–1430.
9. Rodin MB, et al. Middle age cardiovascular risk factors and abdominal aortic aneurysm in older age. Hypertension 2003;42(1):61–68.
10. Alcorn HG, et al. Risk factors for abdominal aortic aneurysms in older adults enrolled in The Cardiovascular Health Study. Arterioscler Thromb Vasc Biol 1996;16(8):963–970.
11. Lederle FA, et al. Immediate repair compared with surveillance of small abdominal aortic aneurysms. N Engl J Med 2002; 346(19):1437–1444.
12. Cronenwett JL. Variables that affect the expansion rate and rupture of abdominal aortic aneurysms. Ann N Y Acad Sci 1996;800:56–67.
13. Lederle FA, et al. Rupture rate of large abdominal aortic aneurysms in patients refusing or unfit for elective repair. JAMA 2002;287(22):2968–2972.
14. Lederle FA, Simel DL. The rational clinical examination. Does this patient have abdominal aortic aneurysm? JAMA 1999;281(1):77–82.
15. Scott RA, et al. Influence of screening on the incidence of ruptured abdominal aortic aneurysm: 5-year results of a randomized controlled study. Br J Surg 1995;82(8):1066–1070.
16. Lindholt JS, et al. Hospital costs and benefits of screening for abdominal aortic aneurysms. Results from a randomised population screening trial. Eur J Vasc Endovasc Surg 2002;23(1):55–60.
17. Norman PE, et al. Population based randomised controlled trial on impact of screening on mortality from abdominal aortic aneurysm. BMJ 2004;329(7477):1259.
18. Ashton HA, et al. The Multicentre Aneurysm Screening Study (MASS) into the effect of abdominal aortic aneurysm screening on mortality in men: a randomised controlled trial. Lancet 2002;360(9345):1531–1539.
19. Lederle FA. Ultrasonographic screening for abdominal aortic aneurysms. Ann Intern Med 2003;139(6):516–522.
20. Screening for Abdominal Aortic Aneurysms. U.S.P.S.T. Force, ed. 2005.
21. United Kingdom Small Aneurysm Trial Participants. Long-term outcomes of immediate repair compared with surveillance of small abdominal aortic aneurysms. N Engl J Med 2002;346(19): 1445–1452.
22. Dubost C, Allary M, Oeconomos N. Resection of an aneurysm of the abdominal aorta: reestablishment of the continuity by a preserved human arterial graft, with result after five months. AMA Arch Surg 1952;64(3):405–408.
23. Birkmeyer JD, et al. Surgeon volume and operative mortality in the United States. N Engl J Med 2003;349(22):2117–2127.
24. Parodi JC, Palmaz JC, Barone HD. Transfemoral intraluminal graft implantation for abdominal aortic aneurysms. Ann Vasc Surg 1991;5(6):491–499.
25. Prinssen M, et al. A randomized trial comparing conventional and endovascular repair of abdominal aortic aneurysms. N Engl J Med 2004;351(16):1607–1618.
26. Greenhalgh RM, et al. Comparison of endovascular aneurysm repair with open repair in patients with abdominal aortic aneurysm (EVAR trial 1), 30-day operative mortality results: randomised controlled trial. Lancet 2004;364(9437):843–848.
27. Lederle FA. Abdominal aortic aneurysm: open versus endovascular repair. N Engl J Med 2004;351(16):1677–1679.
28. Heikkinen M, Salenius JP, Auvinen O. Ruptured abdominal aortic aneurysm in a well-defined geographic area. J Vasc Surg 2002;36(2):291–296.
29. Bown MJ, et al. A meta-analysis of 50 years of ruptured abdominal aortic aneurysm repair. Br J Surg 2002;89(6):714–730.
30. Kent KC, et al. Screening for abdominal aortic aneurysm: a consensus statement. J Vasc Surg 2004;39(1):267–269.
31. Baxter BT. Could medical intervention work for aortic aneurysms? Am J Surg 2004;188(6):628–632.
32. Messina LM, Shanley CJ. Visceral artery aneurysms. Surg Clin N Am 1997;77(2):425–442.
33. English WP, et al. Surgical management of renal artery aneurysms. J Vasc Surg 2004;40(1):53–60.
34. Abbas MA, et al. Hepatic artery aneurysm: factors that predict complications. J Vasc Surg 2003;38(1):41–45.
35. Abbas MA, et al. Splenic artery aneurysms: two decades experience at Mayo Cclinic. Ann Vasc Surg 2002;16(4):442–449.
36. Stone WM, et al. Superior mesenteric artery aneurysms: is presence an indication for intervention? J Vasc Surg 2002;36(2):234–237; discussion 237.
37. Stone WM, et al. Celiac arterial aneurysms: a critical reappraisal of a rare entity. Arch Surg 2002;137(6):670–674.
38. Carr SC, et al. Visceral artery aneurysm rupture. J Vasc Surg 2001;33(4):806–811.
39. Henke PK, et al. Renal artery aneurysms: a 35-year clinical experience with 252 aneurysms in 168 patients. Ann Surg 2001;234(4):454–462; discussion 462–463.
40. Carr SC, et al. Current management of visceral artery aneurysms. Surgery (St. Louis) 1996;120(4):627–633; discussion 633–634.
41. Schmittling ZC, McLafferty R. Transcatheter embolization of a splenic artery aneurysm. J Vasc Surg 2004;40(5):1049.
42. Larson RA, Solomon J, Carpenter JP. Stent graft repair of visceral artery aneurysms. J Vasc Surg 2002;36(6):1260–1263.
43. Cacoub P, Godeau P. Risk factors for atherosclerotic aortoiliac occlusive disease. Ann Vasc Surg 1993;7(4):394–405.
44. Haimovici H. Patterns of arteriosclerotic lesions of the lower extremity. Arch Surg 1967;95(6):918–933.
45. Friedman SA, Holling HE, Roberts B. Etiologic factors in aortoiliac and femoropopliteal vascular disease. The Leriche syndrome. N Engl J Med 1964;271:1382–1385.
46. Brewster DC, Darling RC. Optimal methods of aortoiliac reconstruction. Surgery (St. Louis) 1978;84(6):739–748.
47. Texon M, Imparato AM, Helpern M. The role of vascular dynamics in the development of atherosclerosis. JAMA 1965;194(11): 1226–1230.

48. Leriche R, Morel A. The syndrome of thrombotic obliteration of the aortic bifurcation. Ann Surg 1948;127:193.
49. Karmody AM, et al. "Blue toe" syndrome. An indication for limb salvage surgery. Arch Surg 1976;111(11):1263–1268.
50. Sobinsky KR, et al. Is femoral pulse palpation accurate in assessing the hemodynamic significance of aortoiliac occlusive disease? Am J Surg 1984;148(2):214–216.
51. Sensier Y, Bell PR, London NJ. The ability of qualitative assessment of the common femoral Doppler waveform to screen for significant aortoiliac disease. Eur J Vasc Endovasc Surg 1998;15(4):357–364.
52. Willmann JK, et al. Aortoiliac and renal arteries: prospective intraindividual comparison of contrast-enhanced three-dimensional MR angiography and multi-detector row CT angiography. Radiology 2003;226(3):798–811.
53. Rubin GD, et al. Multi-detector row CT angiography of lower extremity arterial inflow and runoff: initial experience. Radiology 2001;221(1):146–158.
54. Catalano C, et al. Infrarenal aortic and lower-extremity arterial disease: diagnostic performance of multi-detector row CT angiography. Radiology 2004;231(2):555–563.
55. Martin ML, et al. Multidetector CT angiography of the aortoiliac system and lower extremities: a prospective comparison with digital subtraction angiography. AJR Am J Roentgenol 2003;180(4):1085–1091.
56. Koelemay MJ, et al. Magnetic resonance angiography for the evaluation of lower extremity arterial disease: a meta-analysis. JAMA 2001;285(10):1338–1345.
57. Dormandy JA, Rutherford RB. Management of peripheral arterial disease (PAD). TASC Working Group. TransAtlantic Inter-Society Consensus (TASC). J Vasc Surg 2000;31(1 pt 2):S1–S296.
58. Tetteroo E, et al. Randomised comparison of primary stent placement versus primary angioplasty followed by selective stent placement in patients with iliac-artery occlusive disease. Dutch Iliac Stent Trial Study Group. Lancet 1998;351(9110):1153–1159.
59. Bonn J. Percutaneous vascular intervention: value of hemodynamic measurements. Radiology 1996;201(1):18–20.
60. Archie JP Jr. Analysis and comparison of pressure gradients and ratios for predicting iliac stenosis. Ann Vasc Surg 1994;8(3):271–280.
61. Dimick JB, et al. Hospital volume-related differences in aorto-bifemoral bypass operative mortality in the United States. J Vasc Surg 2003;37(5):970–975.
62. Ballard JL, et al. Aortoiliac stent deployment versus surgical reconstruction: analysis of outcome and cost. J Vasc Surg 1998;28(1):94–101; discussion 101–103.
63. Klein WM, et al. Long-term cardiovascular morbidity, mortality, and reintervention after endovascular treatment in patients with iliac artery disease: The Dutch Iliac Stent Trial Study. Radiology 2004;232(2):491–498.
64. Lin PH, Chaikof EL. Embryology, anatomy, and surgical exposure of the great abdominal vessels. Surg Clin N Am 2000;80(1):417–433, xiv.
65. Bradbury AW, et al. Mesenteric ischaemia: a multidisciplinary approach. Br J Surg 1995;82(11):1446–1459.
66. Pastores SM, Katz DP, Kvetan V. Splanchnic ischemia and gut mucosal injury in sepsis and the multiple organ dysfunction syndrome. Am J Gastroenterol 1996;91(9):1697–1710.
67. Montgomery RA, Venbrux AC, Bulkley GB. Mesenteric vascular insufficiency. Curr Probl Surg 1997;34(12):941–1025.
68. Schoots IG, et al. Systematic review of survival after acute mesenteric ischaemia according to disease aetiology. Br J Surg 2004;91(1):17–27.
69. Stanley JC. Mesenteric arterial occlusive and aneurysmal disease. Cardiol Clin 2002;20(4):611–622, vii.
70. Stoney RJ, Cunningham CG. Acute mesenteric ischemia. Surgery (St. Louis) 1993;114(3):489–490.
71. Wiesner W, et al. CT of acute bowel ischemia. Radiology 2003;226(3):635–650.
72. Horton KM, Fishman EK. Multi-detector row CT of mesenteric ischemia: can it be done? Radiographics 2001;21(6):1463–1473.
73. Kumar S, Sarr MG, Kamath PS. Mesenteric venous thrombosis. N Engl J Med 2001;345(23):1683–1688.
74. Brandt LJ, Boley SJ. AGA technical review on intestinal ischemia. American Gastrointestinal Association. Gastroenterology 2000;118(5):954–968.
75. Train JS, et al. Mesenteric venous thrombosis: successful treatment by intraarterial lytic therapy. J Vasc Intervent Radiol 1998;9(3):461–464.
76. Savassi-Rocha PR, Veloso LF. Treatment of superior mesenteric artery embolism with a fibrinolytic agent: case report and literature review. Hepatogastroenterology 2002;49(47):1307–1310.
77. Ballard JL, et al. A critical analysis of adjuvant techniques used to assess bowel viability in acute mesenteric ischemia. Am Surg 1993;59(5):309–311.
78. Bulkley GB, et al. Intraoperative determination of small intestinal viability following ischemic injury: a prospective, controlled trial of two adjuvant methods (Doppler and fluorescein) compared with standard clinical judgment. Ann Surg 1981;193(5):628–637.
79. Mansour MA. Management of acute mesenteric ischemia. Arch Surg 1999;134(3):328–330; discussion 331.
80. Johnston KW, et al. Mesenteric arterial bypass grafts: early and late results and suggested surgical approach for chronic and acute mesenteric ischemia. Surgery (St. Louis) 1995;118(1):1–7.
81. Cho JS, et al. Long-term outcome after mesenteric artery reconstruction: a 37-year experience. J Vasc Surg 2002;35(3):453–460.
82. Park WM, et al. Current results of open revascularization for chronic mesenteric ischemia: a standard for comparison. J Vasc Surg 2002;35(5):853–859.
83. Matsumoto AH, et al. Percutaneous transluminal angioplasty and stenting in the treatment of chronic mesenteric ischemia: results and long-term follow up. J Am Coll Surg 2002;194(1 suppl):S22–S31.
84. Allen RC, et al. Mesenteric angioplasty in the treatment of chronic intestinal ischemia. J Vasc Surg 1996;24(3):415–421; discussion 421–423.
85. Kasirajan, K, et al. Chronic mesenteric ischemia: open surgery versus percutaneous angioplasty and stenting. J Vasc Surg 2001;33(1):63–71.
86. Derkx FH, Schalekamp MA. Renal artery stenosis and hypertension. Lancet 1994;344(8917):237–239.
87. Rimmer JM, Gennari FJ. Atherosclerotic renovascular disease and progressive renal failure. Ann Intern Med 1993;118(9):712–719.
88. Goldblatt H, Lynch J, Hanzal RE, Summerville WW. Studies on experimental hypertension. I. The production of persistent elevation of systolic blood pressure by means of renal ischemia. J Exp Med 1934;59:347–379.
89. Welch WJ. The pathophysiology of renin release in renovascular hypertension. Semin Nephrol 2000;20(5):394–401.
90. Safian RD, Textor SC. Renal-artery stenosis. N Engl J Med 2001;344(6):431–442.
91. Zucchelli PC. Hypertension and atherosclerotic renal artery stenosis: diagnostic approach. J Am Soc Nephrol 2002;13(suppl 3):S184–S186.
92. Krijnen P, et al. A clinical prediction rule for renal artery stenosis. Ann Intern Med 1998;129(9):705–711.
93. Motew SJ, et al. Renal duplex sonography: main renal artery versus hilar analysis. J Vasc Surg 2000;32(3):462–469; 469–471.

94. Radermacher J, et al. Use of Doppler ultrasonography to predict the outcome of therapy for renal-artery stenosis. N Engl J Med 2001;344(6):410–417.
95. Olin JW, et al. The utility of duplex ultrasound scanning of the renal arteries for diagnosing significant renal artery stenosis. Ann Intern Med 1995;122(11):833–838.
96. Hansen KJ, et al. Renal duplex sonography: evaluation of clinical utility. J Vasc Surg 1990;12(3):227–236.
97. Lee HY, Grant EG. Sonography in renovascular hypertension. J Ultrasound Med 2002;21(4):431–441.
98. Vasbinder GB, et al. Diagnostic tests for renal artery stenosis in patients suspected of having renovascular hypertension: a meta-analysis. Ann Intern Med 2001;135(6):401–411.
99. Vasbinder GB, et al. Accuracy of computed tomographic angiography and magnetic resonance angiography for diagnosing renal artery stenosis. Ann Intern Med 2004;141(9):674–682; discussion 682.
100. Ros PR, et al. Diagnosis of renal artery stenosis: feasibility of combining MR angiography, MR renography, and gadopentetate-based measurements of glomerular filtration rate. AJR Am J Roentgenol 1995;165(6):1447–1451.
101. Taylor A. Functional testing: ACEI renography. Semin Nephrol 2000;20(5):437–444.
102. van Jaarsveld BC, et al. The effect of balloon angioplasty on hypertension in atherosclerotic renal-artery stenosis. Dutch Renal Artery Stenosis Intervention Cooperative Study Group. N Engl J Med 2000;342(14):1007–1014.
103. van de Ven PJ, et al. Arterial stenting and balloon angioplasty in ostial atherosclerotic renovascular disease: a randomised trial. Lancet 1999;353(9149):282–286.
104. Plouin PF, et al. Blood pressure outcome of angioplasty in atherosclerotic renal artery stenosis: a randomized trial. Essai Multicentrique Medicaments vs. Angioplastie (EMMA) Study Group. Hypertension 1998;31(3):823–829.
105. Webster J, et al. Randomised comparison of percutaneous angioplasty vs. continued medical therapy for hypertensive patients with atheromatous renal artery stenosis. Scottish and Newcastle Renal Artery Stenosis Collaborative Group. J Hum Hypertens 1998;12(5):329–335.
106. Weibull H, et al. Percutaneous transluminal renal angioplasty versus surgical reconstruction of atherosclerotic renal artery stenosis: a prospective randomized study. J Vasc Surg 1993;18(5):841–850; discussion 850–852.
107. Textor SC, Wilcox CS. Renal artery stenosis: a common, treatable cause of renal failure? Annu Rev Med 2001;52:421–442.
108. Nordmann AJ, et al. Balloon angioplasty or medical therapy for hypertensive patients with atherosclerotic renal artery stenosis? A meta-analysis of randomized controlled trials. Am J Med 2003;114(1):44–50.
109. Nordmann AJ, Logan AG. Balloon angioplasty versus medical therapy for hypertensive patients with renal artery obstruction. Cochrane Database Syst Rev 2003(3):CD002944.
110. Tegtmeyer CJ, et al. Results and complications of angioplasty in fibromuscular disease. Circulation 1991;83(2 suppl):I155–I161.
111. Bax L, et al. The benefit of stent placement and blood pressure and lipid-lowering for the prevention of progression of renal dysfunction caused by atherosclerotic ostial stenosis of the renal artery. The STAR study: rationale and study design. J Nephrol 2003;16(6):807–812.
112. Wong JM, et al. Surgery after failed percutaneous renal artery angioplasty. J Vasc Surg 1999;30(3):468–482.
113. Bagshaw SM, Ghali WA. Acetylcysteine for prevention of contrast-induced nephropathy after intravascular angiography: a systematic review and meta-analysis. BMC Med 2004;2(1):38.
114. Paty PS, et al. Is prosthetic renal artery reconstruction a durable procedure? An analysis of 489 bypass grafts. J Vasc Surg 2001;34(1):127–132.
115. Cherr GS, et al. Surgical management of atherosclerotic renovascular disease. J Vasc Surg 2002;35(2):236–245.

66

Arterial Disease of the Lower Extremity

Michael A. Golden

The overwhelming majority of vascular disease of the lower extremities is secondary to atherosclerosis. Depending on the severity of the vascular lesions and the existing collateral circulation, symptoms generally follow a continuum ranging from claudication to rest pain to frank gangrene with tissue loss. A primary goal of the vascular surgeon is the preservation of limb function by risk factor management and appropriate timing of vascular reconstruction.

The term claudication is from the Latin word *claudico*, meaning to limp. Claudication is defined as a reproducible pain in a muscle group, usually in the calf or thigh, depending on the level of vascular disease. The pain is brought on by exercise; usually a specific distance walked is enough to elicit the pain, which is generally relieved by a brief period of rest.

Epidemiological studies suggest that up to 5% of men and 2.5% of women over 60 years of age have symptoms of claudication.[1,2] Fortunately, the natural history of claudication is that of a generally benign course, with 70% of patients reporting no change in symptoms over 5 to 10 years, with 20% to 30% eventually progressing to require some form of intervention, and less than 10% eventually requiring amputation.[3,4] However, it is important to recall that intermittent claudication reflects systemic vascular disease, with affected patients carrying a threefold increase in cardiovascular mortality.[1,2]

Rest pain is not merely claudication while at rest; rather, it is pain, usually in the forefoot, that occurs at rest, is often made worse by limb elevation, and is often relieved by dependency of the affected limb. Rest pain indicates inadequate perfusion of the extremity even at rest and portends eventual progression to frank tissue loss.

Nonhealing ischemic ulcers or gangrene indicate insufficient perfusion to maintain viability of the affected limb, and progression to limb loss in the absence of intervention is almost certain.

Epidemiology of Lower-Extremity Ischemia

Prevalence

The prevalence of vascular disease is dependent on the definition used. Lower-extremity arterial disease can be classified as (1) asymptomatic, (2) symptomatic disease presenting as intermittent claudication confirmed by noninvasive testing, and (3) critical leg ischemia, as described by the Ad Hoc Committee on Reporting Standards, Society for Vascular Surgery/North American Chapter, International Society for Cardiovascular Surgery. The reader is referred to this report to read in its entirety.[5]

Asymptomatic arterial insufficiency is defined by a low ankle–brachial index (ABI). This index is acquired by comparing Doppler occlusion pressures of the lower extremity and comparing this to an upper-extremity occlusion pressure as a fraction. A normal ABI is approximately 1.1; a low ABI is generally defined as below 0.9. When this value is used as a standard, the incidence of asymptomatic lower-extremity arterial disease is about 10% in the 55- to 74-year-old age group.[6]

Epidemiological studies in which questionnaires were used to evaluate the prevalence of symptomatic vascular disease revealed a 4.6% prevalence in the 55- to 74-year-old age group.[6] The rate of development of intermittent claudication during a 2-year period in individuals older than 50 was 0.7% for men and 0.4% for women, with the predominance in men diminishing after age 70.[7,8] Population-based studies using the ABI less than 0.9 as a reference standard revealed a

17% prevalence of lower-extremity arterial disease in individuals 55 to 74 years of age.

It is estimated that 15% to 20% of patients with lower-extremity arterial disease will progress from intermittent claudication to critical leg ischemia over time.[2,9] If the prevalence of intermittent claudication is about 15% for patients older than 50,[6,8] about 1% of this population has critical limb ischemia.

To summarize the available data for patients older than 50, approximately 15% to 20% have some form of lower-extremity arterial disease. Of these, 20% to 30% eventually require some intervention, with 10% eventually requiring amputation. Alternatively, a full 70% of patients with lower-extremity arterial disease will not experience a significant progression of their disease.

Risk Factors

Age

For males younger than 50, the prevalence of intermit claudication is 1% to 2%, rising to 5% for those over 50 years of age.[9,10] This trend is similar in women as well.

Male Gender

The prevalence of intermittent claudication in women over 50 is about half that of males; however, by age 70, the rates are similar.[10]

Diabetes

Diabetics have constituted up to 25% of patients in series of lower-extremity revascularization.[11] The amputation rate in diabetics is about seven times that of nondiabetics.[12]

Smoking

The association between smoking and peripheral vascular disease has been well documented.[13] Additionally, smokers are diagnosed with peripheral vascular disease a full decade earlier than nonsmokers.[14]

Hypertension

Hypertension seems to have a greater impact on females than males, with a relative risk ratio of approximately 4 in female hypertensives and 2 in males.[15]

Hyperlipidemia

A fasting cholesterol level greater than 270 mg/dL has been associated with a doubled incidence of intermittent claudication.[16]

Patient Evaluation

Patient evaluation should begin with a complete history, focusing on the symptoms and risk factors just described. The physical examination should be thorough, with a focused vascular exam. This latter should include a complete assessment of the pulses, as well as evaluation for pallor, cyanosis, dependent rubor, ulceration, gangrene, atrophy, infection, temperature, and trophic changes such as thickened nails and loss of hair on dorsum of foot. Ischemic ulcers are generally painful, do not bleed, and are located on the heel, toes, or forefoot, in distinction from venous ulcers, which are usually not painful, may bleed, and are located above the medial malleolus. A careful neurological exam is important as well, particularly because occasionally symptoms of neurological origin may mimic vascular insufficiency.

The most common conflicting diagnosis is that of neurogenic leg pain. As this condition can occur concomitantly with vascular occlusion, the absence of distal pulses does not rule it out. Symptoms that begin with a change in position and are relieved only by assuming the recumbent position must be suspected to be of spinal origin.[17] Additionally, a normal systolic pressure response to exercise, despite the occurrence of symptoms with exercise, effectively excludes vascular claudication.[17] Further studies to evaluate patients with atypical symptoms thought likely neurogenic in origin include lumbosacral spine films, electromyography, lumbosacral spinal magnetic resonance imaging (MRI) or computed tomography (CT), and myelography. In addition, patients in whom symptoms do not resolve following revascularization should be evaluated for a neurogenic process.

Patients with signs and symptoms suggestive of vascular disease should first undergo noninvasive testing of the arterial system. Two simple tests include the measurement of segmental systolic pressures and the ankle–brachial index (ABI). Normally, Doppler segmental pressures increase 20 mmHg from the brachial artery to the proximal femoral artery. Any change less than a 20 mmHg increase suggests aortoiliac disease. A pressure drop of more than 30 mmHg between any two successive cuffs normally placed at the arm, proximal thigh, distal thigh, proximal calf, and distal calf signifies a significant arterial obstruction.[18] The ABI is also a helpful test that can be performed at the bedside. The ABI is the ratio of the ankle blood pressure to the brachial blood pressure. An ABI greater than 0.9 is considered normal. An ABI between 0.5 and 0.85 suggests the degree of arterial obstruction often associated with claudication, and an ABI less than 0.50 suggests severe arterial obstruction often associated with critical ischemia.[18]

A more rigid objective determination of claudication severity utilizes exercise testing. The standard exercise test is a treadmill test for 5 min at 2 mph on a 12% incline. Severe claudication can be defined as an inability to complete the treadmill exercise because of leg symptoms and ankle pressures less than 50 mmHg following exercise.[19] Often exercise testing is required in patients with a convincing history and physical examination but with normal resting ankle pressures. In these patients, segmental Doppler pressures and ABIs performed both before and after exercise may unmask the severity and location of the obstruction. Although angiography remains the gold standard for anatomic evaluation of vascular lesions, its use should be limited to only those patients who are to undergo intervention.

Toe Systolic Pressure Index

The prevalence of peripheral disease has been reported to be as much as 20 fold higher in diabetics than in age- and sex-matched controls.[20] In diabetics, calcification of the media often makes their vessels noncompressible, leading to artifactually high ankle pressures. However, this medial calcification generally does not extend into the digital arteries. Therefore, it is possible to measure toe pressure using a strain-gauge sensor or photoplethysmograph.[21] Toe systolic pressure can then be used with the pressure recorded from the arm as a ratio, thereby generating the toe systolic pressure index (TSPI). This value is normally greater than 0.60. If the absolute toe systolic pressure is less than 30 mmHg, healing without intervention is unlikely.[21]

Duplex Ultrasound

Duplex ultrasound is the combination of B-mode imaging and Doppler ultrasound. It was not until relatively recently that technology developed sufficiently to allow duplex imaging of the lower extremities with their multiple vessels at varying depths to become feasible. Although B-mode imaging can demonstrate a stenotic vessel segment, the degree of stenosis cannot be accurately measured. Doppler ultrasound, however, allows accurate measurement of blood velocity. In normal volunteers, the normal peak systolic velocity is 100 ± 20 cm/s in the aorta, 119 ± 22 cm/s in the external iliac artery, and 69 ± 14 cm/s in the popliteal artery. In general, a 20% to 49% stenosis is indicated by an increase in peak systolic velocity more than 30% but less than 100% from the preceding vessel segment. A critical (50%–99%) stenosis is indicated by an increase in peak systolic velocity greater than 100%. No flow, obviously, indicates occlusion.[22] Duplex scanning has been reported to be able to detect significant stenoses with an average 82% sensitivity and 92% specificity, depending on the vessels studied.[23]

Angiography

Magnetic resonance angiography (MRA) is becoming increasingly popular in the evaluation of lower-extremity ischemia, particularly for patients who have a contraindication to standard contrast angiography. Its safe use as a replacement for angiography requires careful evaluation and significant experience with MRA.[24]

Computed tomographic angiography (CTA) is also increasing in popularity for evaluation of lower-extremity arterial occlusive disease and aneurysmal disease. Although this modality avoids the arterial puncture and intraarterial catheter and guidewire manipulation, it still involves the use of iodinated contrast with its associated allergic risk and renal toxicity. CTA also uses ionizing radiation. In experienced hands, it can be quite useful and may obviate the use of contrast arteriography.[25]

Contrast angiography should be reserved for patients without a contraindication who are expected to undergo revascularization. Currently, angiography remains the gold standard in the evaluation of lower-extremity ischemia. A complete study of the aorta, iliac, femoral, popliteal, and runoff vessels is usually performed on both the affected and contralateral sides because atherosclerotic disease is most commonly bilateral and occurs at multiple levels.

Lower-Extremity Occlusive Disease

As discussed, the large majority of lower-extremity occlusive disease is caused by the lesions of atherosclerosis. As lesions become hemodynamically significant, the resulting relative ischemia produces symptoms of claudication and rest pain, as well as potential tissue loss.

Natural History

The natural history of claudication makes the distinction of incapacitating symptoms very important. Investigators who have had the opportunity to follow claudication patients without intervention have demonstrated that only 7% at 5 years and 12% at 10 years will go on to require amputation.[26] This finding was revisited by Imparato and colleagues, who determined that of patients with claudication followed for a mean of 2.5 years and up to 8 years, 79% remained stable or improved, with only 21% worsening; only 5.8% had progression to gangrene and required an amputation. Of the patients who remained stable, 19% eventually underwent elective operation with immediate relief of their symptoms. A key finding in this classic study was that five of the six patients who required amputation were in the most severe category of less than one block claudication.[3] These studies have established the safety of treating most patients with claudication nonoperatively with programs of exercise, risk management, including smoking cessation and control of lipid, glucose, and blood pressure levels, medication with antiplatelet and rheological agents, and meticulous care of the lower extremity. These studies have also provided the basis for considering claudication as only a relative indication for revascularization, warranting careful selection of low-risk patients with disabling symptoms for such procedures. It has also been reported that toe pressures less than 40 mmHg in patients with intermittent claudication portend clinical deterioration and that these patients should be followed very closely.[27] It is well accepted that ischemic rest pain and certainly tissue loss are signs of limb-threatening ischemia, the natural history of which is progression to amputation unless intervention with improvement of arterial perfusion occurs.

Aortoiliac Occlusive Disease

Atherosclerotic lesions in the aortoiliac location generally begin at the bifurcation of the aorta or the common iliac arteries and can progress in either direction. In general, patients complaining of claudication as a result of isolated aortoiliac disease tend to be younger than those whose claudication is caused by disease of the femoropopliteal system. Additionally, the fact that lesions of the aortoiliac system are less likely to cause symptoms is a tribute to the excellent collateral system in this area. However, because of the larger number of muscle groups directly perfused by these vessels, claudication as a result of aortoiliac disease may result in greater disability. In addition, lesions of the aortoiliac system, regardless of lumen diameter, are at risk for distal embolization. It is for these reasons, as well as the excellent long-term results obtained with invasive therapy in this patient population, that a more aggressive approach to claudication is taken as a result of aortoiliac disease.

In their study evaluating functional outcome after surgical treatment for intermittent claudication, Zannetti and colleagues reported that 62% of the procedures performed for claudication were inflow procedures, the great majority of which were for aortoiliac disease. Primary unassisted patency at 4 years for this group was 92% ± 4% with no operative deaths.[28]

It must be stressed, however, that to continue to achieve excellent functional and survival results, we must be careful in selecting good-risk patients with disabling symptoms for revascularization if the only indication is claudication.

Operative Alternatives for Patients with Aortoiliac Occlusive Disease

A number of surgical options are available for the treatment of aortoiliac disease. In recent years, however, percutaneous techniques have become more frequently employed. Such procedures, including percutaneous transluminal angiography (PTA) and stenting, are discussed later in this chapter.

In recent years, the aortofemoral bypass graft, having achieved perioperative mortality rates well under 5%, has become the preferred method of open operative treatment of symptomatic aortoiliac occlusive disease in good-risk patients who cannot be successfully treated with catheter-based techniques. In general, approximately one-fourth to one-third of aortofemoral bypass grafts are performed for limb salvage with the remainder performed for severe claudication. Overall 5-year cumulative patency rates approach 88%, with 10-year rates approaching 75%.[29] In their evaluation of 1000 consecutive cases of aortofemoral bypass, Poulias and colleagues had similar overall patency rates. However, when further categorized by the severity of disease, cumulative patency rates of aortofemoral bypass grafts in patients with rest pain or gangrenous tissue loss were 78% and 63%, respectively, at 5 years, and 63% and 49%, respectively, at 10 years.[30] In situations in which extensive superficial femoral artery disease coexists with aortoiliac disease, the deep femoral artery has been shown to provide a durable outflow tract for an aortofemoral graft.[31]

Aortoiliac endarterectomy is utilized far less commonly than in the past. This procedure may still be considered in situations when localized disease occurs in young patients in whom a higher incidence of graft-related problems might be anticipated or when a theoretical improvement in sexual potency is an issue. Endarterectomy is utilized for localized disease of the distal aorta, aortic bifurcation, or common iliac arteries. In such patients, excellent long-term patency can be achieved.[32] Aortoiliac endarterectomy is contraindicated when disease is extensive, extends superiorly close to the renal arteries, or if any evidence of aneurysmal degeneration of involved vessels is noted. Currently, endarterectomy is used relatively rarely because endovascular techniques may be applied to that patient population.

Ileofemoral bypass is an option when unilateral iliac disease not amenable to a less invasive percutaneous angioplasty or stenting is present. Some authorities suggest aortobifemoral bypass, particularly in younger, good-risk patients with primarily unilateral iliac disease, because progression of contralateral disease requiring reoperation has been cited to be as high as 30% to 40%.[33] However, other reports suggest this occurs in only about 10% of patients, warranting a unilateral approach when there is little evidence of contralateral disease.[34]

In high-risk patients, the axillobifemoral bypass graft offers a reasonable alternative. Because neither the thoracic nor the abdominal cavity is violated in performing an axillofemoral graft, the procedure usually does not interfere with the patient's ability to breathe, cough, or take oral feedings. In addition, it is possible to perform the procedure under local anesthesia in particularly poor-risk patients. Cumulative graft patency of 70% at 5 years has been obtained with this procedure.[35] These results are inferior to results for aortofemoral bypass, and therefore axillofemoral bypass grafting is usually reserved for high-risk patients with limb-threatening ischemia and is not performed for claudication alone. In one of the largest series of axillofemoral grafting published, the authors reported life-table primary patency, limb salvage, and survival rates at 5 years of 71%, 92%, and 52%, respectively.[36] For patients with unilateral iliac occlusive disease, and whose aorta and contralateral iliac artery are free of disease, unilateral iliofemoral or femorofemoral bypass are useful options. Femorofemoral bypass is particularly useful in high-risk patients, in that it can be performed under regional or local anesthesia. Cumulative 5-year patency rates greater than 80% can be achieved.[35]

Another alternative for aortoiliac reconstruction in adequate-risk patients is the descending thoracic aorta-to-iliofemoral bypass. Criado and colleagues reviewed the procedure and documented a 6.4% combined operative mortality rate with a primary patency rate of 98% at 1 year, 88% at 2 years, and 70.4% at 5 years.[37] Care must be taken in selecting the procedure with the best combination of durability and operative risk in treating patients with aortoiliac disease.

Additionally, excellent short-term results have been reported with the use of endoluminal stented grafts for aortoiliac occlusive disease.[38] As experience with endoluminal devices increases, the population of patients who can be treated with less invasive techniques should broaden as well. Techniques such as PTA and stenting are discussed later in this chapter.

Infrainguinal Arterial Occlusive Disease

Atherosclerotic lesions often affect the major arteries below the inguinal ligament. The most common lesion is a short-segment occlusion of the distal superficial femoral artery, especially in the region of Hunter's canal. Other vessels commonly involved include the above- and below-knee popliteal artery, the anterior and posterior tibial arteries, and the peroneal artery. The common and deep femoral arteries may be affected as well. Evidence of disease is probably present in early adult life and progresses gradually until becoming symptomatic. Because of the large potential for collateral flow, a single lesion is often asymptomatic or at least not limb-threatening. In general, to produce significantly severe symptoms or limb-threatening ischemia, lesions at multiple levels must be present; this then is called combined segment disease and involves any combination of aortoiliac, femoropopliteal, and infrapopliteal lesions.

As discussed earlier, the great majority of patients complaining of intermittent calf claudication can be safely observed until symptoms of critical ischemia provide an absolute indication for revascularization. However, it is quite reasonable to consider a good-risk patient with incapacitating claudication for revascularization as well.

In 1980, Donaldson and Mannick reviewed their experience with 51 femoropopliteal reconstructions to relieve disabling claudication.[39] This report represented 17% of the infrainguinal procedures performed during that time period. In this group, all patients experienced relief of their symptoms after surgery. Cumulative graft patency was 93% at 2 years and 88% at 5 years, with no operative mortality. These patency rates are clearly superior to collective results of femoropopliteal graft patency performed for limb salvage.[40] More recently, Zannetti and colleagues reported their results of infrainguinal revascularization for intermittent claudication. At a mean follow-up of 4.5 years, 96% of surviving patients had a patent graft, with a primary unassisted patency at 4 years of 81% ± 6%. In this series, there were no operative deaths or early or late amputations.[28] Also recently, Conte and colleagues reviewed their results of 57 femorotibial bypass procedures for claudication.[41] This group represented only 5% of all infrainguinal vein reconstructions performed at their institution over a 16-year period. There were no operative deaths. Overall 5-year survival was 54% ± 15%; no major amputations were performed. Cumulative primary and secondary graft patency rates at 5 years were 81% ± 6% and 86% ± 5%, respectively. These rates were equivalent to those achieved with femoropopliteal bypass for claudication and were significantly better than their rates for limb salvage.

Although these reports demonstrate that revascularization for claudication at any level can lead to excellent, durable results with a high degree of patient satisfaction, the importance of careful patient selection cannot be overemphasized.

Open Surgical Alternatives for Patients with Limb-Threatening Ischemia and Infrainguinal Occlusive Disease

Femoropopliteal bypass is indicated when the superficial femoral artery or proximal popliteal artery is occluded and the patent popliteal artery has luminal continuity on arteriogram with any of its three terminal branches. In the case of a popliteal occlusion, bypass to an isolated segment of popliteal artery is effective if the segment is more than 7 cm long. If the isolated popliteal segment is less than 7 cm, or if there is severe gangrene of the foot, a sequential bypass to the popliteal and then to a more distal vessel should be considered.[42] Femoropopliteal bypass grafts are categorized as either above knee or below knee (Tables 66.1, 66.2). A review of series published since 1981 reported primary above-knee femoropopliteal graft patency rates as 84% and 69% at 1 and 4 years, respectively, with reversed saphenous vein as the conduit, and 79% and 60% at 1 and 4 years, respectively, using polytetrafluoroethylene (PTFE).[40] In the below-knee position, performed specifically for limb salvage, cumulative patency with reversed saphenous vein is 90% and 75% at 1 and 4 years, respectively, with similar results for in situ bypass. Secondary patency for PTFE grafts in the below-knee position for all indications is 68% and 40% at 1 and 4 years, respectively.[40] Based on these data, prosthetic material is avoided whenever possible for infrageniculate bypass.

TABLE 66.1.
Above-Knee Femoropopliteal Grafts.

	Primary patency		
	1 Year	*3 Years*	*4 Years*
Autologous vein[41,94–99]	84%		69%
Polytetrafluoroethylene (PTFE)[43,95–97,99–101]	79%	57%	60%
Dacron[100]		62%	

Source: McCann RL.[5] Peripheral artery aneurysms. In: Porter JM, Taylor LM Jr, eds. Basic Data Underlying Clinical Decision Making in Vascular Surgery. St. Louis: Quality Medical, 1994:137–140.

TABLE 66.2.
Below-Knee Femoropopliteal Grafts.

	Primary patency/ secondary patency	
	1 Year	*4 Years*
Autologous vein[43,94–99,102–106]	82%/96%72%/81%	
PTFE (secondary patency only)[95–97,99–101,103]	68%	40%
Limb salvage (autologous vein only)[44, 94,102]	92%	75%

Source: McCann RL.[5] Peripheral artery aneurysms. In: Porter JM, Taylor LM Jr, eds. Basic Data Underlying Clinical Decision Making in Vascular Surgery. St. Louis: Quality Medical, 1994:137–140.

The use of PTFE in the above-knee position is a far more viable alternative. Proponents of its use as the material of choice in the above-knee position cite early patency rates similar to those for autologous vein,[43] and the frequent need of saphenous vein for future coronary bypass or more distal peripheral arterial bypass revision. Several more recent studies address this issue specifically. In a retrospective analysis of their 20-year experience, Berlakovich and colleagues determined that the need for secondary below-knee repair was only 7%, a probability that did not support the routine use of PTFE when adequate saphenous vein was available.[44] Wilson and colleagues report similar requirements of vein for secondary procedures, and report an amputation rate following graft occlusion of 12% in the vein group and 26% in the PTFE group. In addition, the level of the amputation site was significantly different in that only 20% of amputations following graft occlusion were above knee in the vein bypass group and 80% of amputations were above knee in the PTFE group.[45] These authors advocate the preferential use of vein for above-knee bypass grafting based on their data. It must be remembered, however, that in these retrospective studies PTFE was used in patients who, for whatever reason, did not have available autologous vein, which could clearly skew patency and amputation data. However, the argument for future vein requirements does not appear justified. A policy of the preferential use of autologous vein graft in any position is followed by most vascular surgeons.

Infrapopliteal bypass should be performed only in situations of lower-extremity ischemia in which femoropopliteal bypass is not feasible (Table 66.3). A review of the series of infrapopliteal grafting published since 1981 reports primary patency rates for all indications with reversed saphenous vein graft of 77% and 62% at 1 and 4 years, respectively, and secondary patency rates with PTFE as the conduit of 68% and

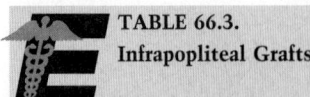

TABLE 66.3.
Infrapopliteal Grafts.

	1 Year	*4 Years*
Primary patency		
Reverse saphenous vein[43,94–96,102,103,107–114]	76%	62%
In situ vein bypass[97,104–107]	81%	68%
Secondary patency		
Reverse saphenous vein[94,107,108,111,113]	83%	76%
In situ vein bypass[105–107]	87%	81%
PTFE[43,96,107,112,114]	47%	21%
Limb salvage		
Reverse saphenous vein[43,103,109–112,115]	85%	82%
In situ vein bypass[104,116]	91%	83%
PTFE[43,103,112]	68%	48%

Source: McCann RL.[5] Peripheral artery aneurysms. In: Porter JM, Taylor LM Jr, eds. Basic Data Underlying Clinical Decision Making in Vascular Surgery. St. Louis: Quality Medical, 1994:137–140.

48% at 1 and 4 years, respectively.[5] When performed for limb salvage, cumulative patency rates for reversed saphenous vein grafts were 85% and 82% at 1 and 4 years, respectively, and 68% and 48%, respectively, for PTFE. These data are the basis for the avoidance of the use of prosthetic material to bypass to infrapopliteal arteries if at all possible.

The selection of the posterior tibial artery, the anterior tibial artery, or the peroneal artery for the infrapopliteal anastomosis is important. The peroneal artery is not directly continuous with the pedal arteries, and the question has been raised as to whether bypass to this artery might produce an inferior result. Raftery and colleagues addressed this question with a retrospective review of 118 infrainguinal vein grafts of which 98 were evenly distributed among the peroneal, anterior tibial, and posterior tibial vessels; the remaining 20 were to the popliteal vessels. The authors report no difference in hemodynamic parameters among the four different outflow groups.[46] The choice of outflow vessel should be based on the overall quality of the vessel. If two vessels of excellent quality are available, the preference probably should go to the vessel with the greatest degree of direct continuity with the foot.

One of many unanswered questions in vascular surgery is which operation is best for infrapopliteal reconstruction. There is general agreement that autologous vein is currently the best conduit. However, this can be used as a reversed graft, requiring complete excision from its bed, or left in situ, requiring ablation of all valves, and side-branch ligation but allowing the vein to remain, for the most part, in its bed, theoretically preventing ischemic damage to the vein graft wall and avoiding significant size mismatch at the proximal and distal anastomoses. In a prospective, randomized comparison of reversed and in situ vein grafts, Harris and colleagues demonstrated no significant difference between the types of bypass, particularly when the veins were greater than 3.5mm in diameter.[47] For veins of 3.5cm in diameter, there was a trend toward improved results in the in situ group.

In a situation where extensive disease involves multiple levels of the lower extremity, a long bypass from groin to ankle may be required. In a study of in situ grafts for this situation, Shah et al. demonstrated a 73% cumulative patency rate at 5 years with an 89% limb salvage rate.[48]

Commonly conduit is limited, and severe infrapopliteal disease creates limb-threatening ischemia. In a report of their 12-year experience with popliteal to distal artery bypass, Wengerter and colleagues demonstrated 55% and 60% primary and secondary patency at 5 years and 73% limb salvage. The authors noted that moderate amounts of disease in the superficial femoral artery or proximal popliteal artery, or the performance of preoperative angioplasty on these vessels, did not adversely affect graft patency or limb salvage.[49] Factors that were noted to be associated with a decrease in graft patency included small-diameter grafts, a dorsalis pedis outflow site, and poor-quality outflow.

Similarly, Ballard and colleagues, in a 5-year review of popliteal–tibial bypass grafts, reported primary graft patency and limb salvage rates at 1, 3, and 5 years were 73%, 59%, and 59%, and 87%, 57%, and 57%, respectively. These authors did not note significant disease progression proximally that would have warranted a more proximal graft origin. They also conclude that a short graft originating from the popliteal artery is a durable graft in limb salvage situations.[50]

Finally, bypass to inframalleolar sites such as the dorsalis pedis artery has proven to be a durable procedure. When compared to peroneal bypass in a large series, no significant differences were found, with 5-year secondary patency rates of 76% and 68% in the peroneal and dorsalis pedis arteries, respectively. Limb salvage rates in the same groups were 93% and 87%, respectively, at 5 years.[51] In a series of nearly 3000 operations during a 7-year period on diabetic patients, LoGerfo and colleagues demonstrated a marked decline in amputation rates, which correlated precisely with an increased rate of dorsalis pedis bypasses.[52]

Clearly all forms of bypass benefit when good-quality, large-diameter autologous greater saphenous vein is available. However, that is often not the case. As a rule of thumb, the shortest graft between adequate inflow and outflow vessels is advisable. One should not hesitate to use the dorsalis pedis or plantar arteries when adequate outflow above the ankle is not available, particularly in the diabetic patient.

Use of the Deep Femoral Artery in Limb Salvage

Profundaplasty is a procedure consisting of endarterectomy of the origin and proximal portion of the deep femoral artery. It is most useful when combined with an inflow procedure such as an aortobifemoral bypass or axillofemoral bypass. On occasion it is performed as an isolated procedure, usually following graft failure, in attempt to achieve limb salvage by less than maximal improvement in limb perfusion. On occasion the deep femoral artery is required as an inflow vessel for distal bypass. Indications for this approach include inadequate vein length, need for a concomitant extended profundaplasty, and desire to avoid groin scarring from previous reconstruction or infection. In a series of 56 bypass procedures in which the graft originated from the middle or distal deep femoral artery, primary and secondary patency rates at 3 years were 78% and 96%, respectively. These rates did not differ significantly from those grafts originating from the common or superficial femoral artery or the popliteal artery. The authors concluded that, in appropriately selected patients, use of the deep femoral artery as a site of inflow increases the versatility of lower-extremity bypass grafting without sacrificing durability.[53]

Axillopopliteal bypass is generally used as a final effort to prevent amputation. It is usually performed in a situation in which the usual options are not available, whether this is the result of groin infection with or without graft infection, extensive operative scarring, or extensive involvement of the iliac and femoral systems.

Postoperative Graft Surveillance

There are three major causes of graft failure. Failure in the immediate postoperative period (<30 days) is most often caused by technical or judgmental error. Other causes include inadequate inflow or outflow, poor conduit, infection, or an unrecognized hypercoagulable state. Failure between 30 days and 2 years is most often the result of myointimal hyperplasia within the vein graft or at anastomotic sites. Late graft failure is usually caused by the natural progression of atherosclerotic disease. It is estimated that strictures develop in 20% to 30% of infrainguinal vein bypasses during the first year.[54] Careful surveillance is justified in that intervention based on a duplex surveillance protocol has resulted in 5-year assisted patency rates of 82% to 93% for all infrainguinal grafts studied, significantly higher than the 30% to 50% secondary patency rates of thrombosed vein grafts. A typical surveillance protocol would include duplex ultrasonography to measure flow velocity and the velocity ratio across a stenosis. Further workup would be indicated in vein grafts with flow velocity less than 45 cm/s and a velocity ratio greater than 3.5 across a stenosis. In addition, ABIs can be easily measured, with decrease more than 0.15 between examinations considered significant. Examinations should be performed perioperatively and at 6 weeks, at 3-month intervals for 2 years, and every 6 months thereafter.

Considerable progress has been made during the past 10 to 20 years in the treatment of limb-threatening ischemia, particularly with the success of distal bypass grafts. Patients with limb-threatening ischemia are most likely to do well if they receive an aggressive approach of graft surveillance with revision if indicated.

A typical scenario consists of elevated velocities detected on routine surveillance suggesting a graft stenosis. This finding should generally be followed up with biplanar angiography to delineate the lesion more specifically. If a stenotic area is detected, there are a variety of ways to address it. Short lesions may be treated by percutaneous balloon angioplasty at the time of diagnosis. Longer lesions or those that fail angioplasty may require operative intervention in the form of a patch angioplasty at the site of the lesion, or a segmental jump graft with reversed vein to bypass the stenotic area.

The Role of Endovascular Therapy in the Management of Lower-Extremity Occlusive Disease

Percutaneous Transluminal Balloon Angioplasty

Since the earliest reports in 1964,[55] percutaneous transluminal balloon angioplasty (PTA) has become an important tool in the management of patients with lower-extremity occlusive disease (Table 66.4). More recently, the use of intravascular stents has increased the number of lesions amenable to endovascular therapy and has been shown to improve on results of PTA alone.[56] The more common indications for iliac PTA are focal concentric stenosis of the common and/or external iliac arteries, to increase flow (1) in patients with claudication from aortoiliac disease, (2) in patients in whom either PTA or surgical bypass is considered for infrainguinal arterial occlusive disease, and to increase flow for limb salvage (3) in the patient with severe infrainguinal arterial disease. Relative contraindications include combined aneurysmal and occlusive disease, diffuse iliac artery stenoses, and heavily calcified lesions or popcorn lesions.

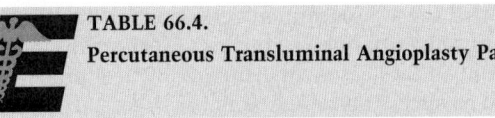

TABLE 66.4.
Percutaneous Transluminal Angioplasty Patency.

	1 Year	*4 Years*
Aortoiliac[58,117–119]	88%	75%
Femoropopliteal[58,117,118,120]	81%	63%

Source: Wilson SE, Sheppard B.[57] Results of percutaneous transluminal angioplasty for peripheral vascular occlusive disease. In: Porter JM, Taylor LM Jr, eds. Basic Data Underlying Clinical Decision Making in Vascular Surgery. St. Louis: Quality Medical, 1994:144–148.

Current indications for iliac artery stent placement include atherosclerotic stenosis with ulcerated plaques, iliac artery occlusion, post-PTA arterial dissection, failure of balloon angioplasty (defined as a residual stenosis of 30% or greater or a pressure gradient greater than 5 mmHg), and recurrent stenosis following PTA.

A review of reports with sufficient long-term follow-up reveals that 3-year patency rates of iliac PTA are comparable to surgical reconstruction, although technical failure rates are higher with PTA.[57] A recent meta-analysis revealed 4-year primary patency rates of iliac PTA to range from 58% to 87% and after stent placement to range from 41% to 86%.[56] The authors noted, however, that these numbers do not take into account disease severity and selection for stenting. A summary of this meta-analysis revealed 4-year primary patency rates of 65% for stenoses and 54% for occlusion after PTA for claudication, and 53% for stenoses and 44% for occlusions after PTA for critical ischemia. Following stent placement, 4-year primary patency rates were 77% for stenoses and 61% for occlusions in treating patients with claudication, and 67% for stenoses and 53% for occlusion in the treatment of critical ischemia. This meta-analysis suggests that the risk of long-term failure was reduced 39% after stent placement compared with PTA alone.[56] Factors that appear to be associated with success of PTA include common iliac site, good runoff, short lesions, and a stenosis versus an occlusion.

It should be noted that in recent years the indications for iliac PTA and stenting have liberalized significantly. In addition to acceptable results with a less-invasive procedure, compared to open surgery, PTA and stenting rarely interfere with subsequent open surgical revascularization if needed.

Johnston and colleagues prospectively evaluated the use of PTA in the femoropopliteal vessels over a 5-year period.[58] In their series, 26% of PTAs were of the femoropopliteal vessels; 80% of these procedures were for claudication and 20% for limb-threatening ischemia. Technical failures occurred in only 4% of cases. At 1 month, 89% of procedures were defined as successful. Predictors of success at 1 month included PTA of a stenosis as opposed to an occlusion and PTA for claudication as opposed to limb salvage. Variables that were not related to success at 1 month included site of PTA, runoff, diabetes, age, sex, limb, number of lesions dilated, and predilation ABI.

Late success rates were 63% at 1 year, with progressively lower results to 38% at 5 years. Predictors of improved long-term success included PTA for claudication as opposed to limb salvage, an ABI above 0.57, stenosis versus occlusion, and good runoff. Factors that did not seem to significantly affect late results included site of PTA, diabetes, number of sites treated, and pressure gradient across the lesion. Overall, the best results seem to have been in stenotic lesions with good runoff. Occlusions with poor runoff were associated with a 16% success rate at 5 years. PTA is a satisfactory option for lower-extremity revascularization, particularly in patients at high risk for surgery with good runoff and stenotic lesions.

Other Endovascular Interventions

Recent experience with newer technologies has led to an increased use of endovascular interventions for infrainguinal arterial occlusive disease in certain instances. In addition to angioplasty with possible stenting, these include drug-eluting stents, brachytherapy, subintimal angioplasty, excimer laser-assisted angioplasty, atherectomy and thrombectomy, cutting balloon angioplasty, covered stents, biodegradeable stents, and cryoplasty. Some of these interventions are still experimental and the others are approved only for limited applications. There are varied degrees of success and of durability for these methods, which leave them as not standard first-line treatments.[59]

Lumbar Sympathectomy

In a small number of cases, reconstructive arterial surgery is not feasible in a patient with severe lower-extremity ischemia. Lumbar sympathectomy may be a reasonable alternative to improve rest pain and avoid amputation. In a review of 60 consecutive patients undergoing lumbar sympathectomy, van Driel and colleagues reported a zero mortality rate and minimal morbidity.[60] At 6 months, 14% of the patients with rest pain only and 45% of those with gangrene had required major amputation. Importantly, all the limbs with an ABI less than 0.30 required major amputations, although an ABI greater than 0.30 did not guarantee a satisfactory result. The authors concluded that lumbar sympathectomy is a useful procedure in patients with lower-extremity ischemia presenting only as rest pain without gangrenous changes and having an ABI greater than 0.30.

In an effort to evaluate the role of lumbar sympathectomy for patients with nonreconstructable disease and focal superficial ulcers, Johnson and associates[61] reviewed 29 sympathectomies for focal necrosis, with long-term follow-up in 10 patients. All patients had ABIs greater than 0.30, as well as transcutaneous oxygen tension levels below 30 mmHg. The authors noted that clinical improvement was associated with a mean increase in oxygen tension of 29 mmHg, whereas the mean increase in oxygen tension in those that showed no healing of their foot ulcers was 5 mmHg. The authors noted further that those patients who demonstrated an increase in transcutaneous oxygen levels of greater than 15 mmHg with dependency of the involved limb had a greater chance of responding favorably to sympathectomy. Johnson and associates suggested lumbar sympathectomy may be useful in patients with nonreconstructable disease and focal tissue loss, with an ABI greater than 0.03, but with transcutaneous oxygen tensions less than 30 mmHg that increase by more than 20 mmHg with limb dependency. Endoscopic approaches to lumbar sympathectomy have also been reported.[62]

Amputation

Fortunately, most patients presenting with even critical ischemia can be offered a reasonable attempt at limb salvage. However, there are situations in which the best option remains primary amputation. In cases in which gangrene extends into the deeper tissues of the tarsal region of the foot, primary amputation at the below-knee level is indicated. If the patient was previously reasonably healthy, a well-fitting prosthesis will provide excellent functionality.

Some specific indications of lower-extremity amputation include nonsalvageable dry or wet gangrene, unremitting and unreconstructable rest pain, nonhealing ulcers, chronic infection, neuroma, frostbite, malignancy, chronic pain, congenital deformity, and unsalvageable venous insufficiency. Amputation in the setting of lower-extremity trauma is discussed more specifically in the section on trauma.

The selection of amputation levels should consider the objectives of removing all nonviable tissue while ensuring primary wound healing and an acceptable functional result. The outcome following below-knee amputation is far better than that following amputation at the ankle despite the higher level. In cases where the patient has severe depression of mental status such that he or she is unable to ambulate, communicate, or provide self-care, an above-knee primary amputation should be considered. Severe, long-standing contractures can occur with below-knee amputations in this bedridden patient group, and often local trauma may make the below-knee amputation less likely to heal than an amputation at the more proximal level.

Clearly, therefore, selection of the correct level of amputation is critical to ensure maximum rehabilitation potential and avoid multiple procedures. In one published series that retrospectively analyzed healing of amputations in 214 patients wherein the amputation level was determined by nonobjective criteria, 8.9% of above-knee amputations and 25% of below-knee amputations had to be revised to a higher level.[63] Multiple noninvasive techniques have been developed in an effort to create more sensitive and objective means of selecting amputation level. Some of these techniques include Doppler ankle and calf systolic pressures and pulse volume recordings, xenon-133 skin blood flow studies, digital or transmetatarsal photoplesthmographic pressure, transcutaneous oxygen determination, skin fluorescence after intravenous dye, laser Doppler skin blood flow, pertechnetate skin blood pressure studies, and photoelectrically measured skin color changes. It is beyond the scope of this chapter to discuss these methods in any detail; however, it is clear that some objective data should be used in planning an amputation level and that those means will depend on available equipment and experience. A useful algorithm is described by Dwars and colleagues.[64] The authors analyzed a series of 85 lower-extremity amputations and determined that the presence of a palpable pulse immediately above the level of amputation correlated well with primary wound healing and a 100% negative predictive value. The absence of palpable pulses was of no use in selecting an amputation level. They found a skin perfusion pressure greater than 20 mmHg to be highly predictive of primary amputation healing, with a positive predictive value of 89% and a negative predictive value of 99%. The authors suggest if there is no palpable pulse immediately proximal to the level of amputation, and the skin perfusion pressure at that level is less than 20 mmHg, a higher amputation level should be selected.

The indications for toe amputation include gangrene, infection, ulceration, or osteomyelitis confined to the mid- or distal phalanx. If gangrene is dry, consideration can be made toward expectant management allowing autoamputation as this would allow for maximal retention of viable tissue. The downside to this approach is that it could take months for autoamputation to be complete. Contraindications to toe amputation include cellulitis proximal to the site, presence of dependent rubor, forefoot infection, and involvement of the metatarsalphalangeal joint or distal metatarsal head. Technique should avoid disarticulation, but rather employ transection through the proximal phalanx. Skin flaps should be reapproximated without tension; 100% rehabilitation potential should be expected. It has been reported that as many as three-quarters of patients undergoing toe amputation will eventually require more proximal amputation.[65]

If gangrene or infection approaches the phalangeal–metatarsal crease or involves the metatarsal head, a partial distal forefoot amputation in the form of a ray amputation can be performed by extending the toe amputation to include the distal metatarsal shaft and head. As in toe amputations, infection or gangrene proximal to the involved site is a contraindication to ray amputation. Again, with the proper postoperative footwear, 100% rehabilitation should be expected.

Transmetatarsal amputation is indicated when gangrene or infection involves multiple toes. It is contraindicated when deep forefoot infection, cellulitis, lymphangitis, or dependent rubor involve the dorsal forefoot proximal to the metatarsal–phalangeal crease. If gangrene involves even a small portion of the plantar surface of the foot proximal to the metatarsal–phalangeal crease, this amputation is contraindicated. The technique is based on formation of a plantar flap that is folded over anteriorly after division of each metatarsal shaft with an oscillating saw. If the wound heals successfully, transmetatarsal amputation affords an excellent functional result, particularly with proper shoe modification.

The Syme's amputation involves disarticulation at the ankle. It has generally fallen into disfavor in that it is technically demanding and, more importantly, it is more difficult to create a well-fitting prosthetic for a Syme's amputation than for a below-knee amputation. Additionally, newer below-knee prosthetics are more aesthetic than the device required to make a Syme's amputation functional.

The below-knee amputation is a commonly performed procedure indicated when gangrene, infection, or ischemic lesions are present that preclude a more distal amputation. If objective criteria are used, primary healing of below-knee amputations should approach 95%. Contraindications to below-knee amputation include situations wherein the gangrenous or infectious process extends to involve the anterior portion of the lower extremity within 4 or 5 cm of the tibial tuberosity or would involve the posterior skin flap, a flexion contracture greater than 20°, or neurological dysfunction creating muscle spasticity or rigidity on the affected side. The technique involves an anterior incision several inches below the tibial tuberosity, with division of the tibia at least 1 cm proximal to that and division of the fibula another centimeter even more proximal. A posterior flap of appropriate thickness is then reflected anteriorly and sutured in place with minimal trauma to the soft tissues. Usually a cast or posterior splint is used in the immediate postoperative period to prevent flexion contractures, minimize edema, and protect the healing stump. The energy requirement for a unilateral below-knee amputee is increased approximately 40% to 60% compared to normal. Most patients who were ambulatory before hospitalization can expect to have a reasonable degree of function with a well-fitted below-knee prosthesis.

An above-knee amputation is indicated when a more distal amputation is contraindicated, or in an elderly or disabled patient who is not expected to be ambulatory or stand and pivot. The most common contraindication is extension of infection or gangrene to the level of the planned above-knee amputation. Surgical technique involves creation of equal-length anterior and posterior flaps with transection of the femur 2 to 3 cm proximal to the level of skin incision at approximately midthigh. Primary healing is usually excellent. Energy expenditure is increased 80% to 120%, and only 40% to 50% of patients can be expected to ambulate after above-knee amputation.

Lower-extremity amputation should not be regarded as a minor procedure as it is often performed on high-risk patients and complications can be significant. These sequelae include primary nonhealing, pain, stump infection, flexion contractures, deep venous thrombosis, and death. Success requires careful preoperative selection, meticulous technique with gentle handling of wound edges, fastidious protection of the healing stump postoperatively, properly fitted prosthetics, and a dedicated rehabilitation team.

Acute Arterial Obstruction

The manifestations of acute arterial occlusion vary greatly, depending on the level and severity of the obstruction, timing from onset to presentation, and degree of chronic vascular disease and collateral circulation. The classic signs and symptoms of acute arterial occlusion include pain, pallor, pulselessness, paresthesias, and paralysis.

Cutaneous manifestations are among the earliest in an acute occlusion. Pallor is seen initially and occurs with the loss of pulses. With progression of ischemia, pallor is replaced by mottling. If the mottled area blanches with pressure, the capillary bed is still patent. With further progression, the mottled area does not blanch, which is evidence of capillary sludging and portends early gangrene. If timely revascularization does not take place, blistering of the skin may develop, followed by frank gangrene.

Sensorimotor manifestations are among the most common symptoms in acute ischemia. Pain is noted early in the course of events; however, this may progress to numbness, which should not be mistaken as improvement. As ischemia progresses, nerve dysfunction may lead to sensory loss, followed by paralysis and muscle destruction resulting in paralysis; a late manifestation of ischemia in muscle is rigor, suggesting muscle death.

The quality of pulses in the contralateral extremity can be very informative. It is uncommon for a patient with chronic vascular disease in one extremity to have full, strong, distal pulses in the other. A normal pulse examination in the contralateral leg suggests that the patient has had an acute event in the absence of chronic disease. This patient is unlikely to have developed significant collaterals, and expediency in obtaining revascularization is vital.

The two major causes of acute arterial occlusion are emboli and thrombosis. An embolic source accounts for 80% of cases. Sources of emboli include the heart, usually in patients with a history of atrial fibrillation or myocardial infarction or valvular heart disease. A proximal arterial source, usually an atherosclerotic plaque or aneurysm, or a paradoxical emboli, in which venous emboli cross a patent foramen ovale to embolize in the arterial tree, are also common sources of an occlusive embolus. The most common sites in the lower extremity for emboli to become lodged are, in descending order, the femoral, iliac, aorta, and popliteal arteries.

Acute thrombosis, usually of a previously stenotic area in the setting of atherosclerosis, is the second most common cause of acute arterial occlusion. Thrombosis may also occur in the setting of low flow states such as congestive heart failure or hypotension, in hypercoagulable states, and in vascular grafts.

In one series of acute lower-extremity ischemia, 82% presented with severely threatened limb viability, and 18% had major irreversible ischemic limb changes.[66] In this series, patient survival at 1 month was 85%, with 51% patient survival at 3 years. If ischemia was severe but reversible, 1-month mortality was 8%, which increased to 46% if irreversible ischemia was present. Results of revascularization included a primary patency rate of approximately 80% at 3 years and a cumulative limb salvage rate of 68% at 3 years.

The management of the patient with acute lower-extremity ischemia includes a thorough but expeditious history and physical, followed by optimization of hemodynamics and fluid balance. Unless a contraindication exists, most patients are heparinized. If the patient is thought to have potentially viable extremities, the lesion can be further delineated with arteriography. Arteriographic criteria suggesting an embolism as opposed to thrombosis include arterial bifurcation defects, meniscus sign, and multiple occlusion sites.

At this point a decision is made whether to treat the patient operatively or with an attempt at thrombolysis. If open surgery is chosen, the most common procedure is a catheter embolectomy, usually via a cutdown at the femoral or below-knee popliteal location. Alternatively, particularly in the setting of a thrombosed bypass graft, bypass reconstruction may be necessary. In an analysis of multiple series, the mortality and limb salvage rates were 12.6% and 78%, respectively, for the use of heparin alone in the setting of acute ischemia, 17% and 84% for thromboembolectomy alone, and 10.2% and 92% when the combination of perioperative heparin and catheter embolectomy was used.[67] Postoperatively one should consider long-term anticoagulation as it may reduce the incidence of recurrent embolization from 21% to 7%.[67]

The comparison of lytic therapy and surgical therapy in the initial management of acute lower-extremity ischemia has been carefully studied in several multiinstitutional studies. In 1994, the Surgery versus Thrombolysis for Ischemia of the Lower Extremity (STILE) trial prospectively randomized patients with nonembolic acute lower-extremity ischemia to an optimal surgical procedure, or catheter-directed thrombolysis with urokinase. This study was stopped early as there was a significantly increased number of major adverse events in the thrombolysis group at 1 month as compared to the surgery-alone group. However, when patients were stratified to duration of ischemia, there were clear trends in favor of lysis in patients whose onset of ischemic symptoms was less than 14 days before presentation.[68]

This study was followed up by prospective randomized trials of patients with ischemia of less than 14 days duration only. In the phase I TOPAS trial, the safety and efficacy of thrombolysis was established, and a significant decrease in the frequency and magnitude of surgery was noted in the lytic therapy group.[69] The phase II TOPAS trial, published in 1998, reconfirmed that the use of thrombolysis in the acute setting could significantly reduce the number and magnitude of operations required with no significant difference in mortality. There was, however, a significantly higher incidence of bleeding complications in the lytic therapy group.[70] An optimal situation in the setting of acute ischemia would be that of a patient with evidence of an acute thrombotic event who undergoes thrombolysis that clears the thrombus and reestablishes flow nonoperatively and also uncovers a culpable lesion which would be angioplastied or surgically reconstructed electively.

Other principles of management of the patient with acute lower-extremity ischemia include careful monitoring postoperatively for metabolic derangements related to reperfusion such as acidosis and hyperkalemia, evaluation of the urine for myoglobin, and, if present, treatment with hydration, manitol, and bicarbonate to induce an alkaline diuresis. Additionally, if a limb has been ischemic for a significant time or develops elevated compartment pressures, one should have a low threshold for performing fasciotomy. In one series of acute lower-extremity ischemia, the incidence of fasciotomy requirement was 13.5%, 80% of those patients achieving limb salvage.[66]

Embolic events can also take the form of atheroemboli as atherosclerotic debris in a proximal artery dislodges and occludes distal arteries. The most common manifestation of this event is the blue toe syndrome. Blue toe syndrome consists of the sudden appearance of a cool, painful, cyanotic toe or forefoot in the often-perplexing presence of strong pedal pulses and a warm foot. Other manifestations of atheroembolism include peripheral gangrene, renal failure, and mesenteric ischemia. By far the most common source is the distal aorta, but atheromatous debris can embolize from anywhere along the aorta as well as from peripheral arteries such as the femoral or popliteal. Occasionally, biopsies of the involved area are required to distinguish atheroemboli from systemic vasculitis. These episodes portend both similar and more severe episodes in the future. Therefore, location and eradication of the embolic source are usually indicated.[71] The use of anticoagulation in this setting is somewhat controversial for fear of theoretically unroofing plaques and in fact potentially promoting an atheroembolic event; however, its safety has been documented in randomized trials.[72]

Lower-Extremity Aneurysms

Aneurysms of the lower extremity are not uncommon, and share similar risk factors with their abdominal counterparts, as discussed elsewhere. It is clear that patients with aneurysmal disease have a propensity for aneurysmal degeneration in other locations.

Although quite rare, femoral artery aneurysms are important for reasons of their propensity to thrombose or rupture. Additionally, femoral artery aneurysm serves as a marker for aneurysmal disease elsewhere in the body. In a series of 100 patients with femoral artery aneurysms, 72% of patients had a contralateral femoral artery aneurysm, 85% had a concomitant aortoiliac aneurysm, and 44% had a concurrent popliteal aneurysm.[73] Conversely, a patient with an abdominal aortic aneurysm (AAA) has a 3% chance of a concomitant femoral artery aneurysm. There is a strong predilection of peripheral artery aneurysms in males as compared to females.

In recent times, the majority of femoral artery aneurysms present while asymptomatic. However, these lesions can present with a variety of symptoms. Acute thrombosis, which occurs approximately 8% of the time, is manifest as sudden onset of ischemic symptoms such as coolness, hypesthesia, and pain. Chronic thrombosis, which occurs about 8% of the time, is similar in presentation to the more common occlusion of the superficial femoral artery (SFA), causing calf claudication or ischemic rest pain. In both the acute and chronic situation, the presence of a mass at the level of the femoral artery should help distinguish the diagnoses. An aneurysm of the femoral artery can cause symptoms secondary to local compression. The structures most commonly affected include the femoral vein, which can produce signs of unilateral edema, or compression of the femoral nerve, which produces symptoms of pain or numbness in the medial thigh. Material from within the aneurysm can embolize distally, presenting as mottling or infarction of the skin or toes. Of the symptoms creating complications, rupture is the rarest, accounting for fewer than 5%. Rupture in this location causes a painful expanding mass, which eventually develops into a large inguinal and thigh ecchymosis.[74]

Femoral artery aneurysms can be classified according to vessel involvement. Type 1 lesions are confined to the common femoral artery. Lesions are classified as type 2 when the deep femoral artery originates from the aneurysm. Although both types occur with relatively equal frequency, type 2 aneurysms require more complex reconstruction. Isolated aneurysm of the SFA or profunda accounts for only 5% of femoral artery aneurysms.[75]

The natural history of femoral artery aneurysm is difficult to analyze, largely because of the rarity of the problem. In a series of 100 patients with femoral artery aneurysms, serious limb-threatening complications were seen in only 2.9% of the 172 aneurysms followed nonoperatively. Additionally, the size of the aneurysms did not appear to correlate with any propensity for causing serious complications.[73] In general, it is recommended that asymptomatic femoral artery aneurysms greater than two times the diameter of the external iliac artery be repaired in good-risk patients. Additionally, all symptomatic femoral artery aneurysms should be considered for repair.

If treatment is elective, most patients should undergo preoperative angiography, and all should have a search for other aneurysms, particularly in the aortic and popliteal locations. Additionally, preoperative lower extremity arterial noninvasive studies may help establish a baseline. If the SFA is patent, type 1 aneurysms are best treated with a short interposition graft of PTFE or Dacron. Smaller aneurysms may be excised; however, larger aneurysms are best repaired from within the sac, using an endoaneurysmorrhaphy technique similar to repair of AAAs, mainly to avoid injury of adherent nerve or vein. If the SFA is occluded, the interposition graft can be the inflow for a femoral popliteal or tibial bypass. For type 2 aneurysms, one could either implant the origin of the deep femoral artery to the interposition graft or place a second graft to the profunda. If the SFA is occluded, the surgeon can place the interposition graft directly to the profunda and use this as the origin for a distal bypass. If performing concomitant repair of other aneurysms, it is important not to place any proximal or distal anastomoses near the aneurysmal segment, but rather place the femoral interposition graft first and then use this graft as the site of inflow or outflow. This method is suggested to avoid pseudoaneurysm formation.

Results are largely dependent on distal runoff. In general, excellent results should be expected in 80% of asymptomatic patients and satisfactory results in 68% of those presenting with lower-extremity ischemia.[73] It is important to remember that all patients treated for femoral artery aneurysms need to be followed for life for aneurysms in other locations. Successful cases of management of femoral artery aneurysms with endoluminally placed covered stents have been reported.[76,77]

The popliteal artery is the most common site for peripheral aneurysmal disease. Similar to femoral artery aneurysms, the danger of popliteal artery aneurysms is their propensity to thrombose, embolize, or rupture. A patient with a unilateral popliteal artery aneurysm has an approximately 50% chance of a contralateral aneurysm and a greater than 30% chance of having an AAA. As with most peripheral artery aneurysms, most popliteal artery aneurysms occur in men. The average age at time of diagnosis is between 50 and 70 years.

Approximately half of popliteal artery aneurysms are detected while asymptomatic. As popliteal pulses are generally somewhat difficult to appreciate, a very easily felt or generous popliteal pulse should raise suspicion regarding potential aneurysmal degeneration. If it is thought that the vessel is aneurysmal, the diagnosis can be confirmed with duplex ultrasound. If confirmed, a thorough search with ultrasound for aneurysmal disease in the aortoiliac system and femoral artery as well as the contralateral popliteal artery should be made. A popliteal artery is considered aneurysmal if its diameter exceeds 2 cm or is 1.5 times the diameter of the proximal nonaneurysmal arterial segment.[78] In general, patients should undergo arteriography to evaluate the proximal and distal vasculature before reconstruction.

Additionally, preoperative lower extremity arterial noninvasive studies may provide useful information regarding the patient's baseline vascular status. The complications of acute thrombosis, distal embolization, or rupture can be severe.[79] Such complications can occur in 50% to 70% of cases, with associated amputation rates as high as 20%. In one series, aneurysm rupture only occurred in 7% of cases but carried a 50% rate of amputation.[80] In a review of their 25-year experience with popliteal artery aneurysms, Shortell and colleagues reported a 69% cumulative patency rate at 1 year for reconstructions in patients who presented with limb-threatening ischemia as compared to a 100% rate in patients undergoing elective repair.[81] In another series, a subgroup of seven patients were described who presented with thrombosis of their aneurysm and all runoff vessels and were treated with preoperative thrombolytic therapy. Clearing of at least two runoff vessels was accomplished in all patients. The patients in this group had significantly better graft patency ($P < 0.005$) and limb salvage ($P < 0.01$) than comparable patients treated with emergency operations.[82]

Based on the available data, it is recommended to repair all popliteal aneurysms electively in good-risk patients. Additionally, patients presenting with popliteal artery aneurysm and limb-threatening ischemia secondary to thrombosis or distal emboli should be treated with initial angiography and lytic therapy before surgical revascularization. Endoluminal repair of popliteal artery aneurysms with covered stents has been reported.[83]

Pseudoaneurysms

The majority of pseudoaneurysms encountered by the vascular surgeon are the result of percutaneous catheterization procedures. In a large series of cardiac catheterizations, the incidence of vascular injury requiring repair was approximately 1%.[84] Most complications of catheterization involve some degree of extravasation of blood, leading to eccymosis and hematoma formation. The majority of these resolve without surgical intervention. However, if a large amount of blood accumulates to the point that the thigh becomes tense, painful, or blistered, operative intervention with evacuation of the hematoma and repair of the affected vessel should be considered. In some cases where the puncture site fails to heal, a cavity lined by thrombus and soft tissue may form. If blood flow persists within this cavity, it is considered a pseudoaneurysm. In general, small pseudoaneurysms less than 2 to 3 cm in diameter may resolve spontaneously. If a pseudoaneurysm persists, increases in size, or is more than 3 cm in diameter, some form of obliteration is indicated. The conventional approach is operative exploration of the site of injury with suture repair of the defect. More recently, reasonable success with ultrasound-guided compression therapy has been reported. One series of ultrasound-guided compression therapy demonstrated a 73% success rate, with failures attributed to advanced age of the pseudoaneurysms and operator inexperience.[85] Additionally, the injection of thrombin in the pseudoaneurysm sac under ultrasound guidance has produced impressive results.[86] Based on these experiences, it would seem appropriate to attempt thrombosis of pseudoaneurysms via ultrasound-guided techniques, if experienced personnel are available, reserving operative repair for pseudoaneurysms that are particularly large or have large necks.

Unfortunately, femoral artery pseudoaneurysms also occur as a result of drug abuse. Intravenous drug abusers who have run out of venous sites may turn to the femoral artery as means of access. The patient usually presents with a painful groin mass, which is pulsatile only half the time. A major error would be to treat this as merely an abscess and attempt blind incision and drainage. The most frequently recovered organism is *Staphylococcus aureus*. Angiography should be obtained in most patients with a history of self-injection and a groin mass and will distinguish pseudoaneurysm from simple abscess. Duplex ultrasound can also confirm the presence of a pseudoaneurysm, but the use of compression techniques in this setting is not advisable.

The definitive treatment of an infected pseudoaneurysm relies on principles of debridement of all affected tissue including artery to healthy vessel, proximal ligation, and distal revascularization if needed. Revascularization should be attempted with autologous tissue if possible and should be tunneled in such a way to avoid contact with potentially infected sites. This restriction becomes even more vital if the use of prosthetic conduit is unavoidable.

Popliteal Entrapment Syndrome

Popliteal entrapment usually occurs because of an abnormal relationship between the popliteal artery and the medial head of the gastrocnemius muscle. The normal position of the popliteal artery is in the popliteal fossa, running between the medial and lateral heads of the gastrocnemius muscle. The most common anatomic abnormality is that of medial deviation of the popliteal artery around the medial head of the gastrocnemius. The second most common variant occurs when the popliteal artery passes medial to the medial head of the gastrocnemius muscle, but the actual medial deviation of the artery is not as dramatic. Other anatomic configurations leading to potential popliteal entrapment include an accessory slip of gastrocnemius muscle or fibrous band crossing the popliteal artery.[87] On occasion, the popliteal vein can follow the artery in its medial course around the medial head of the gastrocnemius.

Patients are most commonly male, presenting before the age of 40 years. In the absence of acute thrombosis or occlusion, the most common presentation is that of intermittent claudication, which often occurs with walking, more so than with running. The differential diagnosis in young adults presenting with claudication includes premature atherosclerosis, medial cystic degenerative occlusive disease, vasculitis associated with underlying collagen vascular disease, chronic exertional compartment syndrome, or popliteal entrapment.[88] The diagnosis of popliteal entrapment is suggested by disappearance or weakening of tibial pulses with forced plantar flexion and knee extension. Additionally, pulse volume recordings performed with the foot in both the neutral position and with the foot plantar flexed may show significant attenuation in the latter position. If suspected on the basis of history and physical and initial noninvasive studies, the best study to evaluate for popliteal entrapment syndrome is an MRI. Additionally, duplex imaging may demonstrate popliteal artery impingement with plantar flexion. On occasion, overly trained athletes and soldiers may be affected by functional popliteal entrapment without a particular anatomic variant.

Surgical treatment is almost always indicated for patients with intermittent claudication with evidence of popliteal entrapment. Additionally, if the anatomic variant is detected incidentally, asymptomatic cases of popliteal entrapment should be surgically correlated as well to help prevent secondary vascular complications such as embolism or acute thrombosis. The approach is usually posterior, involving resection or division of muscle segments or fibrous bands causing popliteal impingement. If stenotic or aneurysmal lesions are identified, arterial reconstruction may be necessary.

Patients with symptomatic functional popliteal entrapment should be treated with the main goal of minimizing alteration of function and time of rehabilitation, as these patients are often competitive athletes. A medial approach is used with the goal of incising any fibrous band of fascia that may be impinging on the neurovascular bundle. Surgical correction of asymptomatic functional entrapment is generally not warranted.

Adventitial Cystic Disease of the Popliteal Artery

Adventitial cystic disease almost always affects the popliteal artery. This entity is relatively rare, but must be considered, particularly in cases of young males presenting with intermittent claudication. Additionally, patients with this disorder are generally nonsmokers and have no other evidence of atherosclerotic disease.

The lesions, in contrast to those of atherosclerosis, develop within the adventitial layer of the arterial wall. The lesions are cystic, either single or multiloculated, and consist of a viscid, gel-like fluid rich in mucopolysaccharides.[89] The fluid is remarkably similar to that contained in ganglion cysts.

Patients presenting with intermittent claudication as a result of adventitial cystic disease generally have diminished or absent pedal pulses on the affected side, with normal contralateral pulses. Full flexion of the knee may reduce the pedal pulse of patients with this disorder. In contrast, patients with popliteal entrapment syndrome often have normal pulses at rest and reduction in pedal pulse elicited by knee extension and plantar flexion.

Before the advent of noninvasive and cross-sectional imaging studies, adventitial cystic disease of the popliteal artery was confirmed by biplanar arteriography. The typical finding is that of extrinsic compression creating a smooth eccentric luminal narrowing. If occlusion is present, the correct diagnosis is more difficult to ascertain by angiography, but findings suggestive of adventitial cystic disease include location of the occlusion distal to the adductor hiatus and absence of other atherosclerotic disease in a young patient. Currently, CT and MRI provide excellent views of the popliteal fossa and can accurately evaluate sources of extrinsic compression of the popliteal artery.

If the correct diagnosis can be confirmed preoperatively, most cases can be corrected via a posterior approach to the popliteal fossa. Surgical correction generally involves evacuation of the cyst contents and excision of the wall.[90] In cases of complete occlusion, resection of the involved popliteal artery followed by vein interposition grafting is warranted. Successful thrombolysis of an acute occlusion followed by nonresectional cystotomy has been reported.[91]

A variety of hypercoagulable states and local and systemic vasculidities may cause lower-extremity ischemia, the extent of which is beyond the scope of this chapter. Although uncommon, cases of Buerger's disease are encountered by most surgeons, and it is worthy of further discussion. Buerger's disease, or thromboangiitis obliterans, is an inflammatory, occlusive vascular disease that involves both small and medium-sized arteries and veins. This process usually affects both the upper and lower extremities. Buerger's disease most commonly affects male smokers under the age of 40. The pathological lesions run a course of initial polymorphonuclear infiltrate with thrombus being subsequently replaced by monocytes and giant cells. A chronic stage of perivascular fibrosis and recanalization of the thrombus follows.[92]

Most often patients present with intermittent claudication, but 90% eventually develop upper-extremity manifestations as well. Progression to tissue loss and amputation is very common. Arteriographic findings of smooth tapered segmental narrowing of peripheral arteries without evidence of more proximal atherosclerotic disease may suggest the diagnosis.[93]

Although bypass of larger vessels is possible, treatment depends almost completely on cessation of smoking, with potential for a remarkable recovery. Unfortunately, a large number of patients are unable to quit smoking, and their prognosis is one of continuing tissue loss and multiple amputations.

References

1. Reunanen A, Takkunen H, Aromaa A. Prevalence of intermittent claudication and its effect on mortality. Acta Med Scand 1982;211:249–256.
2. Jelnes R, Gaardsting O, Hougaard Jensen K, Baekgaard N, Tonnesen KH, Schroeder T. Fate in intermittent claudication: outcome and risk factors. Br Med J (Clin Res Ed) 1986;293:1137–1140.
3. Imparato AM, Kim GE, Davidson T, Crowley JG. Intermittent claudication: its natural course. Surgery (St. Louis) 1975;78:795–799.
4. Cronenwett JL, Warner KG, Zelenock GB, et al. Intermittent claudication. Current results of nonoperative management. Arch Surg 1984;119:430–436.
5. McCann RL. Peripheral artery aneurysms. In: Porter JM, Taylor LM Jr, eds. Basic Data Underlying Clinical Decision Making in Vascular Surgery. St. Louis: Quality Medical, 1994:137–140.
6. Fowkes FG, Housley E, Cawood EH, Macintyre CC, Ruckley CV, Prescott RJ. Edinburgh Artery Study: prevalence of asymptomatic and symptomatic peripheral arterial disease in the general population. Int J Epidemiol 1991;20:384–392.
7. Kannel WB, McGee DL. Update on some epidemiologic features of intermittent claudication: the Framingham Study. J Am Geriatr Soc 1985;33:13–18.
8. Schroll M, Munck O. Estimation of peripheral arteriosclerotic disease by ankle blood pressure measurements in a population study of 60-year-old men and women. J Chronic Dis 1981;34:261–269.
9. Dormandy J, Mahir M, Ascady G, et al. Fate of the patient with chronic leg ischaemia. A review article. J Cardiovasc Surg 1989;30:50–57.

10. Vogt MT, Wolfson SK, Kuller LH. Lower extremity arterial disease and the aging process: a review. J Clin Epidemiol 1992;45:529–542.
11. Farkouh ME, Rihal CS, Gersh BJ, et al. Influence of coronary heart disease on morbidity and mortality after lower extremity revascularization surgery: a population-based study in Olmsted County, Minnesota (1970–1987). J Am Coll Cardiol 1994;24:1290–1296.
12. Jonason T, Ringqvist I. Factors of prognostic importance for subsequent rest pain in patients with intermittent claudication. Acta Med Scand 1985;218:27–33.
13. Gordon T, Kannel WB. Predisposition to atherosclerosis in the head, heart, and legs. The Framingham study. JAMA 1972;221:661–666.
14. Kannel WB, Shurtleff D. The Framingham Study. Cigarettes and the development of intermittent claudication. Geriatrics 1973;28:61–68.
15. Hughson WG, Mann JI, Garrod A. Intermittent claudication: prevalence and risk factors. Br Med J 1978;1:1379–1381.
16. Kannel WB, Skinner JJ Jr, Schwartz MJ, Shurtleff D. Intermittent claudication. Incidence in the Framingham Study. Circulation 1970;41:875–883.
17. Goodreau JJ, Creasy JK, Flanigan P, et al. Rational approach to the differentiation of vascular and neurogenic claudication. Surgery (St. Louis) 1978;84:749–757.
18. Barnes RW. Noninvasive diagnostic assessment of peripheral vascular disease. Circulation 1991;83(suppl):I20–I27.
19. Anonymous. Suggested standards for reports dealing with lower extremity ischemia. Prepared by the Ad Hoc Committee on Reporting Standards, Society for Vascular Surgery/North American Chapter, International Society for Cardiovascular Surgery [published erratum appears in J Vasc Surg 1986;4(4):350]. J Vasc Surg 1986;4:80–94.
20. Beach KW, Brunzell JD, Strandness DE Jr. Prevalence of severe arteriosclerosis obliterans in patients with diabetes mellitus. Relation to smoking and form of therapy. Arteriosclerosis 1982;2:275–280.
21. Orchard TJ, Strandness DE Jr. Assessment of peripheral vascular disease in diabetes. Report and recommendations of an international workshop sponsored by the American Diabetes Association and the American Heart Association September 18–20, 1992, New Orleans, Louisiana [see comments]. Circulation 1993;88:819–828.
22. Strandness DE Jr. Peripheral arterial system. In: Duplex Scanning in Vascular Disorders. New York: Raven Press, 1993:159–195.
23. Kohler TR, Nance DR, Cramer MM, Vandenburghe N, Strandness DE Jr. Duplex scanning for diagnosis of aortoiliac and femoropopliteal disease: a prospective study. Circulation 1987;76: 1074–1080.
24. Auerbach EG, Martin ET. Magnetic resonance imaging of the peripheral vasculature. Am Heart J 2004;148(5):755–763.
25. Romano M, Mainenti PP, Imbriaco M, et al. Multidetector row CT angiography of the abdominal aorta and lower extremities in patients with peripheral arterial occlusive disease. Diagnostic accuracy and interobserver agreement. Eur J Radiol 2004;50:303–308.
26. Boyd AM. The natural course of arteriosclerosis of the lower extremities. Proc R Soc Med 1962;55:591–593.
27. Bowers BL, Valentine RJ, Myers SI, Chervu A, Clagett GP. The natural history of patients with claudication with toe pressures of 40mmHg or less. J Vasc Surg 1993;18:506–511.
28. Zannetti S, L'Italien GJ, Cambria RP. Functional outcome after surgical treatment for intermittent claudication. J Vasc Surg 1996;24:65–73.
29. Abbott WM, Kwolek CJ. Aortofemoral bypass for atherosclerotic aortoiliac occlusive disease. In: Ernst CB, Stanley JC, eds. Current Therapy in Vascular Surgery. St. Louis: Mosby-Year Book, 1995:355–359.
30. Poulias GE, Doundoulakis N, Prombonas E, et al. Aorto-femoral bypass and determinants of early success and late favourable outcome. Experience with 1000 consecutive cases. J Cardiovasc Surg 1992;33:664–678.
31. Prendiville EJ, Burke PE, Colgan MP, Wee BL, Moore DJ, Shanik DG. The profunda femoris: a durable outflow vessel in aortofemoral surgery. J Vasc Surg 1992;16:23–29.
32. Brewster DC, Darling RC. Optimal methods of aortoiliac reconstruction. Surgery (St. Louis) 1978;84:739–748.
33. Piotrowski JJ, Pearce WH, Jones DN, et al. Aortobifemoral bypass: the operation of choice for unilateral iliac occlusion? [see comments]. J Vasc Surg 1988;8:211–218.
34. van der Vliet JA, Scharn DM, de Waard JW, Roumen RM, van Roye SF, Buskens FG. Unilateral vascular reconstruction for iliac obstructive disease. J Vasc Surg 1994;19:610–614.
35. Mannick JA, Whittemore AD. Aortoiliac occlusive disease. In: Moore WS, ed. Vascular Surgery: A Comprehensive Review. Philadelphia: Saunders, 1991:350–363.
36. Taylor LM Jr, Moneta GL, McConnell D, Yeager RA, Edwards JM, Porter JM. Axillofemoral grafting with externally supported polytetrafluoroethylene. Arch Surg 1994;129:588–594; discussion 594–595.
37. Criado E, Johnson G Jr, Burnham SJ, Buehrer J, Keagy BA. Descending thoracic aorta-to-iliofemoral artery bypass as an alternative to aortoiliac reconstruction. J Vasc Surg 1992;15:550–557.
38. Sanchez LA, Wain RA, Veith FJ, Cynamon J, Lyon RT, Ohki T. Endovascular grafting for aortoiliac occlusive disease. Semin Vasc Surg 1997;10:297–309.
39. Donaldson MC, Mannick JA. Femoropopliteal bypass grafting for intermittent claudication: is pessimism warranted? Arch Surg 1980;115:724–727.
40. Dalman RL, Taylor LM Jr. Infrainguinal revascularization procedures. In: Porter JM, Taylor LM Jr, eds. Basic Data Underlying Clinical Decision Making in Vascular Surgery. St. Louis: Quality Medical, 1994:141–143.
41. Conte MS, Belkin M, Donaldson MC, Baum P, Mannick JA, Whittemore AD. Femorotibial bypass for claudication: do results justify an aggressive approach? J Vasc Surg 1995;21:873–880.
42. Veith FJ, Gupta SK, Wengerter KR, Rivers SP. Femoral-popliteal-tibial occlusive disease. In: Moore WS, ed. Vascular Surgery: A Comprehensive Review. Philadelphia: Saunders, 1991:364–389.
43. Veith FJ, Gupta SK, Ascer E, et al. Six-year prospective multicenter randomized comparison of autologous saphenous vein and expanded polytetrafluoroethylene grafts in infrainguinal arterial reconstructions. J Vasc Surg 1986;3:104–114.
44. Berlakovich GA, Herbst F, Mittlbock M, Kretschmer G. The choice of material for above-knee femoropopliteal bypass. A 20-year experience. Arch Surg 1994;129:297–302.
45. Currie IC, Wilson YG, Baird RN, Lamont PM. Treatment of intermittent claudication: the impact on quality of life. Eur J Vasc Endovasc Surg 1995;10:356–361.
46. Raftery KB, Belkin M, Mackey WC, O'Donnell TF. Are peroneal artery bypass grafts hemodynamically inferior to other tibial artery bypass grafts? J Vasc Surg 1994;19:964–968; discussion 968–969.
47. Harris PL, Veith FJ, Shanik GD, Nott D, Wengerter KR, Moore DJ. Prospective randomized comparison of in situ and reversed infrapopliteal vein grafts [see comments]. Br J Surg 1993;80:173–176.
48. Shah DM, Darling RC III, Chang BB, Kalufman JL, Fitzgerald KM, Leather RP. Is long vein bypass from groin to ankle a durable procedure? An analysis of a ten-year experience. J Vasc Surg 1992;15:402–407; discussion 407–408.
49. Wengerter KR, Yang PM, Veith FJ, Gupta SK, Panetta TF. A twelve-year experience with the popliteal-to-distal artery bypass:

the significance and management of proximal disease. J Vasc Surg 1992;15:143–149; discussion 150–151.
50. Ballard JL, Killeen JD, Smith LL. Popliteal-tibial bypass grafts in the management of limb-threatening ischemia. Arch Surg 1993;128:976–980; discussion 980–981.
51. Darling RC III, Chang BB, Shah DM, Leather RP. Choice of peroneal or dorsalis pedis artery bypass for limb salvage. Semin Vasc Surg 1997;10:17–22.
52. LoGerfo FW, Gibbons GW, Pomposelli FB Jr, et al. Trends in the care of the diabetic foot. Expanded role of arterial reconstruction. Arch Surg 1992;127:617–620; discussion 620–621.
53. Mills JL, Taylor SM, Fujitani RM. The role of the deep femoral artery as an inflow site for infrainguinal revascularization. J Vasc Surg 1993;18:416–423.
54. Bandyk DF. Surveillance of lower extremity bypass grafts. In: Ernst CB, Stanley JC, eds. Current Therapy in Vascular Surgery. St. Louis: Mosby-Year Book, 1995:492–499.
55. Dotter CT, Judkins MP. Transluminal treatment of arteriosclerotic obstruction. Description of a technique and a preliminary report of its application. Circulation 1964;30:654–670.
56. Bosch JL, Hunink MG. Meta-analysis of the results of percutaneous transluminal angioplasty and stent placement for aortoiliac occlusive disease [published erratum appears in Radiology 1997;205(2):584]. Radiology 1997;204:87–96.
57. Wilson SE, Sheppard B. Results of percutaneous transluminal angioplasty for peripheral vascular occlusive disease. In: Porter JM, Taylor LM Jr, eds. Basic Data Underlying Clinical Decision Making in Vascular Surgery. St. Louis: Quality Medical, 1994:144–148.
58. Johnston KW, Rae M, Hogg-Johnston SA, et al. 5-Year results of a prospective study of percutaneous transluminal angioplasty. Ann Surg 1987;206:403–413.
59. Ruef J, Hofmann M, Haase J. Endovascular interventions in iliac and infrainguinal occlusive artery disease. J Intervent Cardiol 2004;17(6):427–435.
60. Johnson WC, Watkins MT, Baldwin D, Hamilton J. Foot $TcPO_2$ response to lumbar sympathectomy in patients with focal ischemic necrosis. Ann Vasc Surg 1998;12:70–74.
61. Van Driel OJR, van Bockel JH, Schilfgaarde R. Lumbar sympathectomy for severe lower limb ischemia: results and analysis. J Cardiovasc Surg 1988;29:310–314.
62. Hourlay P, Vangertruyden G, Verduyckt F, Trimpeneers F, Hendrickx J. Endoscopic extraperitoneal lumbar sympathectomy. Surg Endosc 1995;9:530–533.
63. Robbs JV, Ray R. Clinical predictors of below-knee stump healing following amputation for ischaemia. South Afr J Surgery 1982;20:305–310.
64. Dwars BJ, van den Broek TA, Rauwerda JA, Bakker FC. Criteria for reliable selection of the lowest level of amputation in peripheral vascular disease. J Vasc Surg 1992;15:536–542.
65. Little JM, Stephen MS, Zylstra PL. Amputation of the toes for vascular disease: fate of the affected leg. Lancet 1976;2:1318–1319.
66. Yeager RA, Moneta GL, Taylor LM Jr, Hamre DW, McConnell DB, Porter JM. Surgical management of severe acute lower extremity ischemia. J Vasc Surg 1992;15:385–391; discussion 392–393.
67. Mills JL, Porter JM. Acute limb ischemia. In: Porter JM, Taylor LM Jr, eds. Basic Data Underlying Clinical Decision Making in Vascular Surgery. St. Louis: Quality Medical, 1994:134–136.
68. Anonymous. Results of a prospective randomized trial evaluating surgery versus thrombolysis for ischemia of the lower extremity. The STILE trial. Ann Surg 1994;220:251–266; discussion 266–268.
69. Ouriel K, Veith FJ, Sasahara AA. Thrombolysis or peripheral arterial surgery: phase I results. TOPAS Investigators [see comments]. J Vasc Surg 1996;23:64–73; discussion 74–75.
70. Ouriel K, Veith FJ, Sasahara AA. A comparison of recombinant urokinase with vascular surgery as initial treatment for acute arterial occlusion of the legs. Thrombolysis or Peripheral Arterial Surgery (TOPAS) Investigators [see comments]. N Engl J Med 1998;338:1105–1111.
71. Karmody AM, Powers SR, Monaco VJ, Leather RP. "Blue toe" syndrome. An indication for limb salvage surgery. Arch Surg 1976;111:1263–1268.
72. Blackshear JL, Zabalgoitia M, Pennock G, et al. Warfarin safety and efficacy in patients with thoracic aortic plaque and atrial fibrillation. SPAF TEE Investigators: Stroke Prevention and Atrial Fibrillation; Transesophageal Echocardiography. Am J Cardiol 1999;83:453–455; A9.
73. Graham LM, Zelenock GB, Whitehouse WM Jr, et al. Clinical significance of arteriosclerotic femoral artery aneurysms. Arch Surg 1980;115:502–507.
74. Cutler BS. Arteriosclerotic femoral artery aneurysm. In: Ernst CB, Stanley JC, eds. Current Therapy in Vascular Surgery. St. Louis: Mosby, 1995:315–318.
75. Cutler BS, Darling RC. Surgical management of arteriosclerotic femoral aneurysms. Surgery (St. Louis) 1973;74:764–773.
76. Michel C, Laffy PY, Leblanc G, et al. Percutaneous treatment of a superficial femoral artery aneurysm using an intravascular stent-prosthesis (in French). J Radiol 1999;80:473–476.
77. Schneider PA. Abcarian PW, Leduc JR, Ogawa DY. Stent-graft repair of mycotic superficial femoral artery aneurysm using a Palmaz stent and autologous saphenous vein. Ann Vasc Surg 1998;12:282–285.
78. Szilagyi DE, Schwartz RL, Reddy DJ. Popliteal arterial aneurysms. Their natural history and management. Arch Surg 1981;116:724–728.
79. Reilly MK, Abbott WM, Darling RC. Aggressive surgical management of popliteal artery aneurysms. Am J Surg 1983;145:498–502.
80. Evans WE, Vermilion BD. Popliteal aneurysms. In: Bergan JJ, Yao JST, eds. Aneurysms: Diagnosis and Treatment. New York: Grune & Stratton, 1982:487.
81. Shortell C, DeWeese JA, Ouriel K, Green RM. Popliteal artery aneurysms: a 25-year surgical experience. J Vasc Surg 1991;14:771–776; discussion 776–779.
82. Carpenter JP, Barker CF, Roberts B, Berkowitz HD, Lusk EJ, Perloff LJ. Popliteal artery aneurysms: current management and outcome [see comments]. J Vasc Surg 1994;19:65–72; discussion 72–73.
83. Kudelko PE Jr, Alfaro-Franco C, Diethrich EB, Krajcer Z. Successful endoluminal repair of a popliteal artery aneurysm using the Wallgraft endoprosthesis. J Endovasc Surg 1998;5:373–377.
84. McCann RL, Schwartz LB, Pieper KS. Vascular complications of cardiac catheterization. J Vasc Surg 1991;14:375–381.
85. Weatherford DA, Taylor SM, Langan EM, Coffey CB, Alfieri MA. Ultrasound-guided compression for the treatment of iatrogenic femoral pseudoaneurysms. South Med J 1997;90:223–226.
86. Liau CS, Ho FM, Chen MF, Lee YT. Treatment of iatrogenic femoral artery pseudoaneurysm with percutaneous thrombin injection. J Vasc Surg 1997;26:18–23.
87. Rich NM, Collins GJ Jr, McDonald PT, Kozloff L, Clagett GP, Collins JT. Popliteal vascular entrapment. Its increasing interest. Arch Surg 1979;114:1377–1384.
88. Turnipseed WD. Popliteal vascular entrapment syndrome. In: Ernst CB, Stanley JC, eds. Current Therapy in Vascular Surgery. St. Louis: Mosby, 1995:504–508.
89. Jay GD, Ross FL, Mason RA, Giron F. Clinical and chemical characterization of an adventitial popliteal cyst. J Vasc Surg 1989;9:448–451.
90. Melliere D, Ecollan P, Kassab M, Becqemin JP. Adventitial cystic disease of the popliteal artery: treatment by cyst removal. J Vasc Surg 1988;8:638–642.

91. Samson RH, Willis PD. Popliteal artery occlusion caused by cystic adventitial disease: successful treatment by urokinase followed by nonresectional cystotomy. J Vasc Surg 1990;12:591–593.
92. McKusick VA. Buerger's disease: a distinct clinical and pathological entity. JAMA 1962;181:5–12.
93. Rivera R. Roentgenographic diagnosis of Buerger's disease. J Cardiovasc Surg 1973;14:40–46.
94. Taylor LM Jr, Edwards JM, Porter JM. Present status of reversed vein bypass grafting: five-year results of a modern series. J Vasc Surg 1990;11:193–205.
95. Bergan JJ, Veith FJ, Bernhard VM, et al. Randomization of autogenous vein and polytetrafluorethylene grafts in femoral-distal reconstruction. Surgery (St. Louis) 1982;92:921–930.
96. Rutherford RB, Jones DN, Bergentz SE, et al. Factors affecting the patency of infrainguinal bypass. J Vasc Surg 1988;8:236–246.
97. Kent KC, Whittemore AD, Mannick JA. Short-term and midterm results of an all-autogenous tissue policy for infrainguinal reconstruction. J Vasc Surg 1989;9:107–114.
98. Brewster DC, LaSalle AJ, Darling RC. Comparison of above-knee and below-knee anastomosis in femoropopliteal bypass grafts. Arch Surg 1981;116:1013–1018.
99. Hall RG, Coupland GA, Lane R, Delbridge L, Appleberg M. Vein, Gore-Tex or a composite graft for femoropopliteal bypass. Surg Gynecol Obstet 1985;161:308–312.
100. Davies MG, Dalen H, Svendsen E, Hagen PO. The functional and morphological consequences of balloon catheter injury in veins. J Surg Res 1994;57:122–132.
101. Quinones-Baldrich WJ, Busuttil RW, Baker JD, et al. Is the preferential use of polytetrafluoroethylene grafts for femoropopliteal bypass justified? [see comments]. J Vasc Surg 1988;8:219–228.
102. Anonymous. Comparative evaluation of prosthetic, reversed, and in situ vein bypass grafts in distal popliteal and tibial-peroneal revascularization. Veterans Administration Cooperative Study Group 141. Arch Surg 1988;123:434–438.
103. Hobson RW Jr, Lynch TG, Jamil Z, et al. Results of revascularization and amputation in severe lower extremity ischemia: a five-year clinical experience. J Vasc Surg 1985;2:174–185.
104. Harris RW, Andros G, Dulawa LB, Oblath RW, Apyan R, Salles-Cunha S. The transition to "in situ" vein bypass grafts. Surg Gynecol Obstet 1986;163:21–28.
105. Leather RP, Shah DM, Chang BB, Kaufman JL. Resurrection of the in situ saphenous vein bypass. 1000 cases later [see comments]. Ann Surg 1988;208:435–442.
106. Bandyk DF, Kaebnick HW, Stewart GW, Towne JB. Durability of the in situ saphenous vein arterial bypass: a comparison of primary and secondary patency. J Vasc Surg 1987;5:256–268.
107. Varty K, Allen KE, Jones L, Sayers RD, Bell PR, London NJ. Influence of Losartan, an angiotensin receptor antagonist, on neointimal proliferation in cultured human saphenous vein. Br J Surg 1994;81:819–822.
108. Barry R, Satiani B, Mohan B, Smead WL, Vaccaro PS. Prognostic indicators in femoropopliteal and distal bypass grafts. Surg Gynecol Obstet 1985;161:129–132.
109. Cantelmo NL, Snow JR, Menzoian JO, LoGerfo FW. Successful vein bypass in patients with an ischemic limb and a palpable popliteal pulse. Arch Surg 1986;121:217–220.
110. Schuler JJ, Flanigan DP, Williams LR, Ryan TJ, Castronuovo JJ. Early experience with popliteal to infrapopliteal bypass for limb salvage. Arch Surg 1983;118:472–476.
111. Berkowitz HD, Greenstein SM. Improved patency in reversed femoral-infrapopliteal autogenous vein grafts by early detection and treatment of the failing graft. J Vasc Surg 1987;5:755–761.
112. Dalsing MC, White JV, Yao JS, Podrazik R, Flinn WR, Bergan JJ. Infrapopliteal bypass for established gangrene of the forefoot or toes. J Vasc Surg 1985;2:669–677.
113. Rosenbloom MS, Walsh JJ, Schuler JJ, et al. Long-term results of infragenicular bypasses with autogenous vein originating from the distal superficial femoral and popliteal arteries. J Vasc Surg 1988;7:691–696.
114. Flinn WR, Rohrer MJ, Yao JS, McCarthy WJ III, Fahey VA, Bergan JJ. Improved long-term patency of infragenicular polytetrafluoroethylene grafts. J Vasc Surg 1988;7:685–690.
115. Taylor LM Jr, Edwards JM, Brant B, Phinney ES, Porter JM. Autogenous reversed vein bypass for lower extremity ischemia in patients with absent or inadequate greater saphenous vein. Am J Surg 1987;153:505–510.
116. Leather RP, Shan DM, Karmody AM. Infrapopliteal arterial bypass for limb salvage: increased patency and utilization of the saphenous vein used "in situ." Surgery (St. Louis) 1981;90:1000–1008.
117. Gallino A, Mahler F, Probst P, Nachbur B. Percutaneous transluminal angioplasty of the arteries of the lower limbs: a 5 year follow-up. Circulation 1984;70:619–623.
118. Hewes RC, White RI Jr, Murray RR, et al. Long-term results of superficial femoral artery angioplasty. AJR Am J Roentgenol 1986;146:1025–1029.
119. Spence RK, Freiman DB, Gatenby R, et al. Long-term results of transluminal angioplasty of the iliac and femoral arteries. Arch Surg 1981;116:1377–1386.
120. Krepel VM, van Andel GJ, van Erp WF, Breslau PJ. Percutaneous transluminal angioplasty of the femoropopliteal artery: initial and long-term results. Radiology 1985;156:325–328.

67

Venous Disease and Pulmonary Embolism

Gregory L. Moneta and Mathew I. Foley

Venous Thromboembolism

Epidemiology

Venous thromboembolism (VTE) is an important cause of preventable morbidity and mortality in the United States. Although precise figures are difficult to obtain as a consequence of undiagnosed cases, the annual incidence of VTE has been estimated at 71 and 117 per 100,000 by two different recent retrospective population-based studies (Worcester and Olmstead Counties).[1,2] Their reported annual incidences for deep venous thrombosis were nearly identical (48 per 100,000), but for pulmonary embolus (PE) there was great disparity (23 versus 69 per 100,000). This difference was believed to be secondary to the threefold higher rate of autopsy acquisition in Olmstead County as compared to the U.S. average.[2] In-hospital case-fatality rates were also different, 12% versus 28%, respectively. Based on the Worcester data, Anderson and Wheeler have estimated the prevalence of clinically significant VTE at 600,000 cases per year, with as many as two-thirds of these being undiagnosed.[3] Deep venous thrombosis (DVT) poses not only the immediate threat of pulmonary embolus (PE) but chronic disability secondary to venous insufficiency as well. PE is estimated to be responsible for the deaths of 50,000 to 100,000 persons per year in U.S. hospitals who would not otherwise be expected to die of their underlying disease process.[4–6] Despite this awareness and evidence for the efficacy of various forms of prophylaxis, attention toward prevention remains inadequate.[7]

Pathophysiology

The complexities of the coagulation system are beyond the scope of this chapter and are detailed elsewhere. Suffice it to say the coagulation system exists in a state of homeostasis. Its objectives are to maintain a constant flow of blood and repair damage incurred to the vascular endothelium. Unbalance in this system may result in thrombus formation. Rudolf Virchow, a pathologist, identified three conditions that tended toward thrombosis. His well-known triad consists of intimal injury, stasis of blood flow, and a hypercoagulable state. All risk factors relate back to one of the conditions described by Virchow.

Risk Factors

Most studies that have examined risk factors for VTE have been in hospital-based populations. Data from the Worcester study showed that multiple risk factors for VTE were present in 74% of hospitalized patients and that the average number of risk factors increased with age.[8] Among patients with a diagnosis of VTE, at least 95% had multiple risk factors.[1] As these authors have pointed out, it is difficult to identify independent risk factors, despite multivariate analysis, because some risk factors are very closely related.[9] Table 67.1 lists the risk factors that are discussed.

History of VTE

In earlier studies, a previous history of VTE was shown to increase the risk of postoperative thrombosis.[10,11] These studies used radiofibrinogen leg scanning to make the diagnosis of venous thrombosis. In a population-based study from Malmo, Sweden, 26% of patients with DVT confirmed by phlebography had a history of DVT.[12] Additionally, 6% developed new DVT within 3 years of follow-up. A previous DVT is probably the greatest risk factor for a new DVT. The SIRIUS study in France determined a previous history of VTE was the strongest "intrinsic factor" contributing to a new objectively determined DVT with an odds ratio of 7.9 [95% confidence interval (CI), 4.4–14.19].[13]

Age

Increased age is consistently associated with increased incidence of VTE. U.S. population-based studies demonstrate dramatic increases after age 40 that continue exponentially until death (Fig. 67.1).[1,2] However, the number of risk factors does also increase with age.

Major Surgery

In 1988 Clagett and Reisch performed a meta-analysis of trials analyzing the use of VTE prophylaxis in general surgery

TABLE 67.1. Risk Factors for Venous Thromboembolism (VTE).

History of VTE
Age
Major surgery
Malignancy
Obesity
Trauma
Varicose veins/superficial thrombophlebitis
Cardiac disease
Hormones
Prolonged immobilization/paralysis
Pregnancy
Central venous catheterization
Hypercoagulable states

patients over age 40.[14] Although most patients were undergoing abdominal and/or pelvic procedures, there were exceptions. The overall incidence of DVT determined by the radioactive fibrinogen uptake test (FUT) was found to be 25%. However, in studies in which FUT was verified by phlebography, the incidence dropped to 19.1%. Incidences are even higher in major lower-extremity joint replacement operations. A prospective study of 517 patients who underwent 638 total knee replacements (TKAs) demonstrated that, despite prophylaxis, 57% of patients developed DVT in the ipsilateral extremity[15]; 11% were in the proximal veins (popliteal or above). The rate for total hip replacement (THA) is also high but somewhat lower than that for TKA.[16] It is important to note that patients undergoing vascular surgical procedures during which they are systemically anticoagulated are not exempt from VTE.[17–19] The incidence rate of venogram-positive DVT in 50 consecutive patients undergoing abdominal aortic aneurysm repair was 18% (4% at or proximal to the popliteal vein) when studied prospectively.[17]

Malignancy

Trousseau is generally credited with recognizing the association of malignancy and VTE in 1868.[20] Since that time, numerous studies have shown an increase in postoperative VTE in patients with malignancy.[21,22] The meta-analysis of general surgery patients by Clagett and Reisch distinguished patients with malignancy in 16 studies and found a 4% higher incidence of VTE. At least 2 prospective studies have shown an increased incidence of occult malignant neoplasm in patients with DVT.[23,24]

Goldberg et al.[23] compared 370 patients with DVT diagnosed by impedance plethysmography (IPG) to 1073 patients with negative IPG results and found a relative risk of developing cancer within 5 years of 19.0 (95% CI, 2.2–168) for patients with DVT who were less than 50 years old. Prandoni et al.[24] compared 153 patients with venography-proven idiopathic venous thrombosis to 107 patients with secondary thrombosis and found there was a significant increase in the subsequent finding of cancer [odds ratio (OR), 2.3; 95% CI, 1.0–5.2] over the next 2 years. Furthermore, in patients with a recurrent idiopathic venous thrombosis, the risk was much greater (OR, 9.8; 95% CI, 1.8–52.2). Cancer also substantially adds to the risk of VTE in patients with a thrombophilia, especially those with Factor V Leiden mutation or a prothrombin gene mutation, with the risk being especially high in patients with hematological malignancies (odds ratio, 28.0; 95% CI, 4.0 to 200).[25]

Obesity

Obesity has traditionally been regarded as a risk factor for VTE. Using univariate analysis, Kakkar et al.[11] initially found almost twice as many obese postoperative patients to have DVT. However, Nicolaides and Irving,[10] when using multivariate analysis, did not find obesity to be an independent risk factor. Interestingly, an increased body mass index was found to be an independent risk factor for VTE in women using oral contraceptives.[26] When specifically assessing obesity as a risk factor for VTE, it seems at worst to provide only a small incremental risk of VTE.[27]

Trauma

In an autopsy study done in 1959, Sevitt and Gallagher[28] were the first to demonstrate a high incidence of VTE in injured and burned patients. The risk factors for VTE in trauma patients have been difficult to discern secondary to the variety of injury patterns. Geerts et al.[29] performed a prospective study of 716 consecutive trauma patients admitted to a regional trauma unit with an Injury Severity Score (ISS) of at least 9; none of these patients received any form of prophylaxis. Of the 716, 349 had adequate venographic studies performed during their admission; 58% had DVT, of which 18% were in a proximal location. These authors identified five independent risk factors by multivariate analysis (Table 67.2). Surprisingly, less than 2% of patients with DVT confirmed by venography had clinical symptoms. Another study performed during the same time period in which 84% of 177 "high-risk" patients were receiving some form of prophylaxis showed only a 7% incidence of DVT.[30] However, DVT was initially diagnosed by IPG (confirmed by venography), and patients considered "low-risk" had diagnostic studies performed as directed by symptoms only, potentially underesti-

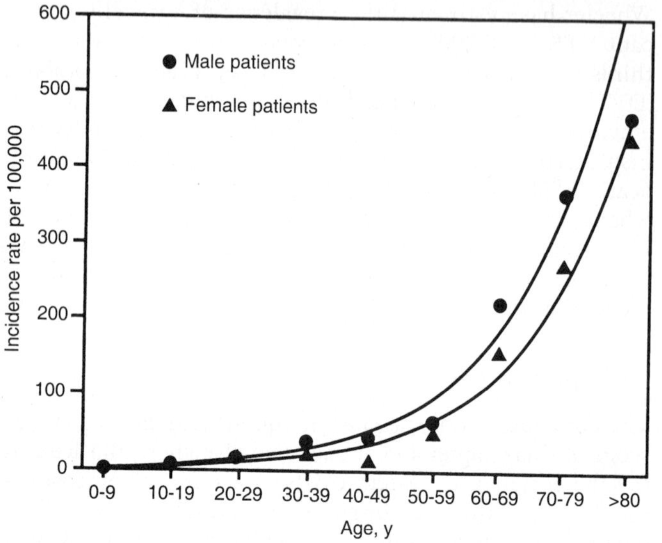

FIGURE 67.1. Incidence rate of clinically recognized deep vein thrombosis and/or pulmonary embolism per 100,000 population. The increase in rates for both male and female patients is well approximated by an exponential function of age. (From Anderson FA, Wheeler HB, Goldberg RJ, et al.,[1] with permission.)

TABLE 67.2. Risk Factors for Venous Thromboembolism in 349 Trauma Patients.

Risk factor	*Odds ratio (95% confidence interval)*
Age (each 1-year increment)	1.05 (1.03–1.06)
Blood transfusion	1.74 (1.03–2.93)
Surgery	2.30 (1.08–4.89)
Fracture of femur or tibia	4.82 (2.79–8.33)
Spinal cord injury	8.59 (2.92–25.28)

Determined by multivariate logistic regression.

Source: Geerts WH, Code KI, Jay RM, et al.,[29] with permission.

mating the true prevalence of DVT. A retrospective review of 9721 trauma patients from the same institution identified 36 patients with objectively confirmed PE, 80% of which were receiving prophylaxis.[31] The authors identified four patterns of injury that were independent predictors of PE (Table 67.3) compared to a control group who had neither PE nor inferior vena cava (IVC) filters placed.

Varicose Veins/Superficial Thrombophlebitis

Varicose veins (VVs) appear to be an associated but not an independent risk factor for VTE. May[32] reported an exceeding low rate of fatal PE in a large series of patients who underwent surgical intervention for VVs. However, in a recent prospective study of 44 consecutive patients with superficial thrombophlebitis,[33] 23% were found to have DVT by duplex ultrasound (DUS), of which 40% was in proximal veins.

Cardiac Disease

Patients with cardiac disease are likely to have associated risk factors for DVT (i.e., age, immobilization). Older studies looking for DVT in patients with acute myocardial infarction using radiofibrinogen leg scanning showed an incidence as high as 40%.[34,35] It has been shown that this rate can be reduced using low-dose heparin as prophylaxis.[36,37]

Hormones

Today there are numerous oral contraceptives (OCs) on the market, and their formulations have changed since their introduction in 1960. There has been controversy regarding the risks of VTE with OC use. A recent multicenter international study found an increased risk of VTE in OC users with OR 4.15 (95% CI, 3.09–5.57) in Europe and 3.25 (95% CI, 2.59–4.08) in "developing" countries.[26] The risk was greatest when third-generation progestagens were used. Fewer than half their cases were confirmed objectively; the case-fatality rate was 1% to 2%. There does seem to be some increased risk that must be weighed against the benefits of OC use. Initially estrogen replacement therapy was not felt to carry an increased risk of VTE.[38,39] More recent studies indicate increased risk of VTE in postmenopausal woman using equine-derived estrogens with addition of progestin to the formulation.[40,41]

Prolonged Immobilization/Paralysis

Gibbs reported an autopsy series in 1957 in which patients who were at bed rest for more than 1 week had an 80% incidence of thrombosis compared to an incidence of 15% in those at bed rest less than 1 week.[42] More recently, a study using data from the National Spinal Cord Injury Statistical Center discovered an incidence of 14.5% for DVT and 4.6% for PE in patients with acute spinal cord injury.[43] These risks seem to diminish with time.[44,45] Long-haul air travel (travel-related DVT) is also a potential risk factor, although most patients with travel-associated DVT have additional, well-recognized risk factors for DVT.

Pregnancy

There are two recent cohort studies examining venous thrombosis during pregnancy.[46,47] Both examined a series of consecutive patients with clinically suspected DVT. Ginsberg et al.[46] only studied patients with objectively determined DVT. They found that 58 of 60 women had isolated left leg thrombosis, 2 had bilateral, and the peak incidence was in the second trimester. Hull et al.[47] reported a series of 152 consecutive pregnant women and confirmed proximal DVT in 11 (7%); all were confined to the left leg. These series also emphasize that DVT can occur during any trimester and the immediate postpartum period. Suggestive symptoms in the first trimester are likely to be confirmed as DVT, and the left leg is by far most often involved.

Central Venous Catheterization

The incidence of central venous catheter (CVC)-associated DVT and its sequelae are probably underappreciated. Because patients with indwelling central venous catheters are not healthy to begin with, many have a poor short- and intermediate-term prognosis. Pulmonary emboli may be detected in these patients, although PE originating from an upper-extremity DVT as a sole cause of death is unusual, but not unheard of. Monreal et al.[48] did ventilation-perfusion (V/Q) scanning in 86 consecutive patients with upper-extremity CVC-associated DVT within 24h of diagnosis and found 13 patients with PE; only 4 were symptomatic, and 2 died of PE despite treatment. The incidence of CVC-associated DVT has also been demonstrated in children requiring long-term access for parenteral nutrition.[49] CVC-associated DVT is more common at the femoral site. A prospective trial randomized 45 patients to receive either an upper-extremity or lower-extremity (femoral) CVC.[50] Thirteen of 24 (54%) of the lower-extremity group had either a positive (6) or nondiagnostic (7) DUS compared to none in the upper-extremity group (mean duration

TABLE 67.3. Pattern of Injury Analysis: Pulmonary Embolus (PE) Versus Control.

Injury pattern	*Number*	*Number (%) of pulmonary emboli*	*Odds ratio*
Head + spinal cord injury	195	3 (1.5)	4.5*
Head + long bone fracture	471	11 (2.3)	8.8%
Severe pelvis + long bone fracture	106	4 (3.8)	12*
Multiple long bone fracture	275	8 (2.9)	10*

*$P < 0.05$ compared with control group.

Source: Winchell RJ, Hoyt DB, Walsh JC, et al.,[31] with permission.

TABLE 67.4. Hypercoagulable States.

Antiphospholipid syndrome
Activated protein C resistance (Factor V Leiden)
Sticky platelet syndrome
Protein S defects
Protein C defects
Antithrombin defects
Heparin cofactor II defects
Plasminogen defects
Tissue plasminogen activator defects
Plasminogen activator inhibitor defects
Factor XII defects
Dysfibrinogenemia
Homocystinemia

Source: Bick RL, Kaplan H,[53] with permission.

of catheterization, 3.8 versus 4.2 days) at $P = 0.02$. Femoral CVCs have also been shown to promote ipsilateral iliofemoral DVT when used even for short-term access (<1 day) in trauma patients[51] and lead to a 10% IVC thrombosis rate when used in children for more than 6 days' duration.[52]

Hypercoagulable States

Numerous blood protein and platelet defects have been implicated in venous thrombosis (Table 67.4).[53] The most prevalent appears to be resistance to activated protein C.[54]

Natural History

DVT and PE are not pathologically distinct entities; they lie along the continuum of VTE. Since Barritt and Jordan convincingly showed improved survival in patients diagnosed with PE treated with anticoagulation compared to no treatment,[55] the natural history of VTE has been obscured by intervention. What information exists is largely based on trials in which patients were undertreated.

It has been shown in a recent large study using duplex ultrasound that patients who present with symptomatic DVT may have a thrombus located anywhere within the deep system (even within the contralateral leg).[56] However, symptomatic isolated calf vein thrombosis was less common (9%).[56] Despite this, both radioactive fibrinogen uptake and venography have demonstrated that the majority of causes of DVT originate in the infrapopliteal veins or muscular sinuses of the calf.[57,58]

Philbrick and Becker, in 1988, reviewed the published studies of calf vein DVT (CDVT) and assigned a "strength of evidence rating" based on a set of standard criteria to each study.[59] They cited two studies (rated moderately strong) of postoperative patients in whom anticoagulants were not used. These studies demonstrated proximal propagation in 23% and 5.6% of cases using radioactive fibrinogen uptake and venography, respectively.[57,60] The incidence of PE was not objectively determined but was only suspected in cases where proximal propagation had occurred.[59] Two additional studies (rated as weak) in which short-term intravenous (IV) heparin was used (1–2 weeks) showed a 10% incidence of propagation[61] in one and a 29% recurrence rate[62] in the other, both determined by venogram. Finally, they examined studies in which short- and longer-term anticoagulants were used; three (two rated highest strength) showed minimal proximal propagation,[63–65] five (variable ratings) showed a combined 8 PEs in 180 patients evaluated (no case fatalities),[62–64,66,67] and four showed minimal recurrence of CDVT when treated with anticoagulation.[62,63,68,69] Based upon their review, Philbrick and Becker recommended either anticoagulation or surveillance for proximal propagation of CDVT, depending on the clinical situation.[59]

Using sequential ultrasound studies, Lohr et al. showed that 15% of 75 patients with CDVT propagated into the proximal veins.[70] In addition, 5% of these patients had high-probability ventilation/perfusion (V/Q) scans on presentation (all 75 had scans). Passman et al.[71] obtained V/Q scans in 26 patients with DUS-documented isolated CDVT and respiratory symptoms and found that 35% had high-probability V/Q scans whereas 100% (5/5) of patients who later developed symptoms developed high-probability V/Q scans. None of the latter group had evidence of CDVT progression by repeat DUS.

Because they are virtually always treated, little is really known about the natural history of proximal vein DVT (PDVT). Some information has been gained from three randomized trials that have compared different pharmacological regimens for treatment of objectively diagnosed DVT.[72–74] Hull et al. compared IV versus subcutaneous (SQ) heparin and found DVT recurrence rates of 5.2% versus 19.3% ($P = 0.024$), respectively.[72] Most recurrences occurred in patients whose anticoagulation was subtherapeutic. Brandjes et al. terminated their study early secondary to a significant difference ($P < 0.001$) in DVT extension rates in patients receiving acenocoumarol and heparin (8.2%) versus acenocoumarol alone (39.6%).[73] Most recently, Schulman et al. performed a multicenter trial of 6 weeks versus 6 months of oral anticoagulant therapy and found the odds ratio for recurrence in the 6-weeks group to be 2.1 (95% CI, 1.4–3.1).[74] In addition, recurrent disease was nearly twice as common in patients with PDVT compared to CDVT.

Two recent studies found that between 40% and 50% of patients with venographically proven DVT and no respiratory symptoms had high-probability V/Q scans for PE at presentation.[75,76] However, Nielson et al.[76] chose to randomize their ambulatory population to receive or not to receive anticoagulant therapy and found no difference in progression of PE or development of PE symptoms at 2 months. These authors noted a low incidence of severe underlying disorders in addition to active early mobilization as separating their population from others.

Resolution of DVT by DUS 6 months after diagnosis occurs in 70% for all lower-extremity veins affected by DVT, with damage to the vessel wall or valves occurring in 44% of patients by this time.[77] Chronic venous insufficiency can eventually be demonstrated in a large percentage of persons with a history of DVT and is discussed later in this chapter.

Since the study of Barritt and Jordan,[55] information gathered about the natural history of symptomatic PE has been from treated patients. The greatest risk of death from PE and incidence of recurrent PE appears to be within the first few hours[78] to weeks of the initial event. Beyond this period, most patients who die do so of their underlying illnesses. Carson et al. followed 399 patients with PE and found at 1 year the majority of the 95 deaths were caused by either cancer (34.7%), infection (22.1%), or cardiac disease (16.8%).[79]

TABLE 67.5. Risk of Venous Thromboembolism.

Event	*Low risk (uncomplicated surgery in patients age <40 with no other risk factors)*	*Moderate risk (major surgery in patients age >40 with no other clinical risk factors)*	*High risk (major surgery in patients age >40 with additional risk factors)*	*Very high risk (major surgery in patients age >40 with previous VTE, cancer or orthopedic surgery, hip fracture, stroke, or spinal cord injury)*
Calf vein thrombosis (%)	2	10–20	20–40	40–80
Proximal vein thrombosis (%)	0.4	2–4	4–8	10–20
Clinical pulmonary embolism (%)	0.2	1–2	2–4	4–10
Fatal pulmonary embolism (%)	0.002	0.1–0.4	0.4–1.0	1–5

Source: Salzman EW, Hirsh J,[82] with permission.

Similar to DVT, PE has been objectively shown to resolve. Dalen et al. demonstrated that pulmonary artery pressures begin to decline within 2 to 3 weeks of an acute PE.[80] The Urokinase Pulmonary Embolism Trial (UPET) demonstrated 73% resolution of lung scan defects at 3 months with little change beyond this period.[81]

Prophylaxis

The primary goal of prophylaxis is to prevent the morbidity and mortality of VTE. DVT is frequently asymptomatic, so the first evidence of VTE may be a life-threatening PE.

The first issue is to determine who is at risk. Salzman and Hirsh[82] have estimated the risk of thromboembolism in patients undergoing surgery based on risk factors from published data (Table 67.5). The second issue is to pick an appropriate prophylactic method that is efficacious without unacceptable levels of side effects. Clagett et al.[83] reviewed the medical literature through 1992 and estimated the incidence of DVT in patients undergoing various surgical procedures without prophylaxis, as well as the effect of various prophylactic modalities (Table 67.6). The high incidence of VTE without prophylaxis and the ability to significantly reduce this incidence with treatment speaks strongly in favor of prophylaxis.

The general surgery population has been the most extensively studied. A meta-analysis by Clagett and Reisch[14] of studies using radioactive fibrinogen uptake for diagnosis of DVT found low-dose heparin (LDH) with or without dihydroergotamine (DHE), low molecular weight heparin (LMWH), warfarin, intermittent pneumatic compression (IPC), and elastic stockings (ES) all to reduce the incidence of DVT from 25% to 10% or less. In this meta-analysis there was a trend toward greater efficacy for LMWH over LDH. In more recent, randomized, prospective studies LMWH is shown to be at least as efficacious as LDH with perhaps a lower incidence of major bleeding complications, although this finding is not consistent.[84–86]

Elective hip replacement and hip fracture have similar incidences of DVT (40%–50%) when evaluated by venography (see Table 67.5). Geerts et al.[87] found adjusted-dose heparin, LMWH, and oral anticoagulants to all reduce the incidence below 20% (IPC reduced DVT to 21% in hip replacement procedures). In a meta-analysis of studies with venogram-proven DVTs by Mohr et al.,[88] LMWH was consistently found to perform better than all other agents as prophylaxis in elective hip surgery. Although warfarin and IPC performed similarly in a prospective, randomized trial in total hip arthroplasty (incidence of DVT, 31% versus 27%, respectively), proximal DVT was found significantly less often with warfarin (3% versus 12%; $P = 0.012$).[89] Total knee arthroplasty has similar prophylaxis data, but IPC has been found to be more effective (close to LMWH) in knee surgery.[90,91] Although LDH was found to be safe and effective in one study,[92] neurosurgeons seem to prefer IPC (also effective; see Table 67.6) as prophylaxis in neurosurgical procedures, presumably to avoid potential intracranial hemorrhagic complications.

As discussed earlier, the incidence of DVT is high in patients with traumatic injuries. Prophylaxis is more complicated in these patients given the heterogeneous nature of

TABLE 67.6. Incidence of Venous Thromboembolism Without Prophylaxis and Relative Risk Reduction (%) with Selected Methods of Prophylaxis.

Condition	*DVT (%)*	*LDH*[a]	*LDH + DHE*[b]	*LMWH*[c]	*Warfarin*	*Dextran*	*ASA*[d]	*IPC*[e]	*ES*[f]
General surgery	25	68	64	86	59	38	19	61	63
Hip replacement	50	32	26	68	63	41	11	60	25
Hip fracture	43	9	17	74	43	32	6	n/a	n/a
Neurosurgery	24	75	n/a[g]	n/a	n/a	n/a	n/a	73	64

[a]Low-dose heparin.
[b]Dihydroergotamine.
[c]Low molecular weight heparin.
[d]Aspirin.
[e]Intermittent pneumatic compression.
[f]Elastic stockings.
[g]Not available.
Source: Clagett GP, Anderson FA Jr, Levine MN, et al.,[83] with permission.

injuries and contraindications to various prophylactic modalities. In a study using venous Doppler surveillance, Dennis et al.[93] showed that prophylaxis, primarily with IPC, can be effective. LMWH was shown to be superior to LDH by Geerts et al.[94] (PDVT, 6% versus 15%), but only approximately 30% of patients were eligible for LMWH, and the overall incidence of DVT remained high (31%).

There is some evidence that prophylactic insertion of IVC filters may be beneficial in high-risk trauma patients compared to historical controls.[95] However, there is a potentially significant morbidity and mortality associated with vena cava filter placement.[96] A high rate of phlegmasia (24%) has been seen in patients receiving IVC filters that could not be concurrently anticoagulated.[97] Patients with acute spinal cord injury are also known to have a high incidence of DVT, but these have not been extensively studied. One small prospective, randomized study has shown LMWH to be significantly better that LDH in preventing thrombotic events with fewer bleeding complications.[45] There is now intense interest in placement of retrievable vena cava filters in patients, including those with significant trauma, who may be at temporary high risk for pulmonary embolism. Unfortunately many so-called temporary vena cava filters are never removed either because of patient condition or patient or physician failure to follow up for filter removal.[98]

It should be noted that the risk of VTE does not disappear at the time of hospital discharge and that perhaps some patients should continue to receive prophylaxis at home. In a retrospective study, Huber et al.[99] discovered the rate of postoperative PE increased by 30% when including PEs that occurred within 30 days of discharge from a digestive surgery hospital. Specific risk factors for postdischarge DVT were not identified. After discharge from THA, the incidence of PDVT may be as high as 10.5%.[100] However, this rate was not significantly reduced by LMWH versus placebo in a prospective randomized trial although the overall rate of DVT was significantly reduced, 7.1% versus 19.3% ($P = 0.018$).[101] Further trials are necessary before definite conclusions can be drawn.

Finally, cost-effectiveness must be a concern. Based on data from the Worcester DVT Study, Anderson et al.[8] have estimated that $59 to $118 million spent on VTE prophylaxis in 1.18 million major abdominal surgery patients over age 40 would save $59.3 to $118.5 million in DVT diagnosis and treatment and $60 to $120 million on fatal PEs each year.

Recommendations for VTE prophylaxis based on available evidence have been made by the American College of Chest Physicians (ACCP) Consensus statement of 2004. (87) These are summarized in Table 67.7.

Diagnosis of Deep Venous Thrombosis

Signs and symptoms of deep venous thrombosis (DVT) include swelling, pain, tenderness, warmth, discoloration, and a palpable cord. In extreme cases, phlegmasia alba dolens (pain, pitting edema, and blanching) or phlegmasia cerulea dolens (loss of sensory and motor function) may occur. In the Worcester study, leg swelling was the most common presentation

TABLE 67.7.
Recommendations for Venous Thromboembolism Prophylaxis.

Condition	*International Consensus Statement (1997)*	*ACCP[a] Consensus Statement (1995)*
Low-risk general surgery (minor surgery, age less than 40, no risk factors)	None suggested	Early ambulation
Moderate-risk general surgery (major surgery, age less than 40, no risk factors)	One of the following: LDH[b], LMWH[c], dextran, aspirin, elastic stockings, IPC[d]	One of the following: elastic stockings, LDH, IPC
High-risk general surgery (major surgery, age less than 60, or additional risk factors)	LDH or LMWH + elastic stockings or IPC	LDH, LMWH, or dextran + IPC warfarin in selected patients
Neurosurgery	IPC	IPC ± elastic stockings; LDH may be acceptable
Hip replacement	One of the following: LDH, LMWH, or therapeutic warfarin (INR[e] 2–3)	One of the following: LMWH, therapeutic warfarin, or adjusted dose UFH[f]
Knee replacement	IPC, LMWH	IPC, LMWH
Hip fracture	UFH, LMWH, heparinoid, IPC, foot impulse	LMWH or therapeutic warfarin
Acute spinal cord injury	None made	UFH or LMWH; warfarin may be effective
Multiple trauma	None made	IPC; warfarin or LMWH if feasible

[a]American College of Chest Physicians.
[b]Low-dose unfractionated heparin.
[c]Low molecular weight heparin.
[d]Intermittent pneumatic compression.
[e]International normalized ratio.
[f]Adjusted-dose unfractionated heparin.
Sources: International Consensus Statement. Prevention of thromboembolism. Int Angiol 1997;16:3; and Clagett GP, Anderson FA, Heit J, et al. Prevention of venous thromboembolism: fourth ACCP consensus conference on antithrombotic therapy. Chest 1995;108S:312.

(88%).[1] Unfortunately, signs and symptoms of DVT are not reliable for diagnosis. In large studies using either DUS or venography, DVT was found in 50% or less of patients in whom it was clinically suspected.[56,58] However, these signs and symptoms cannot be ignored and generally merit consideration for the presence of DVT.

Contrast Venography

Contrast venography is considered the "gold standard" for the diagnosis of DVT. The procedure involves placement of a needle in the dorsum of the foot and injection of a radioopaque contrast medium. X-rays are then obtained in at least two projections. Studies are determined to be positive when a persistent filling defect is present (Fig. 67.2). Hull et al. followed 160 patients suspected of having DVT with an initial normal venogram over 3 months, and only 2 patients (1.3%) developed subsequent DVT.[102]

Not all patients are candidates for venography based on previous history of contrast reactions or renal insufficiency. The test is also expensive, and the use of high osmolar ionic contrast has been associated with an incidence of postvenogram DVT of 9% to 31%.[103] However, newer, nonionic contrast agents have reduced the incidence of postphlebography DVT to 3% or less.[104,105] AbuRahma et al. prospectively studied 102 patients undergoing contrast venography for DVT evaluation with nonionic contrast and found no cases of postphlebographic DVT by DUS and a low incidence (7%) of minor complications.[106] Despite this apparent improvement, contrast venography has largely been replaced by noninvasive techniques.

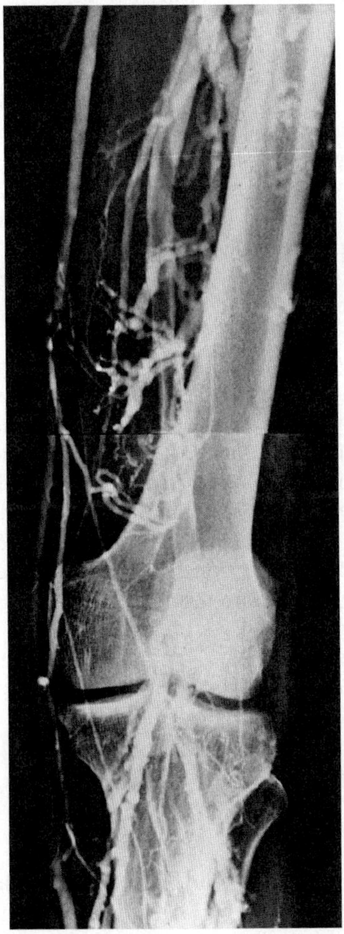

FIGURE 67.2. Contrast venogram of the left lower extremity demonstrates thrombus in the superficial femoral and popliteal veins.

Iodine-125 Fibrinogen Uptake (FUT)

Iodine-125 fibrinogen uptake (FUT) is based on the idea that by radiolabeling fibrinogen and injecting it into a peripheral vein, DVT can be identified by scanning the legs for "hot spots." Hot spots represent fibrinogen being incorporated into fibrin clots. Most of the studies pertaining to DVT prophylaxis in general surgery patients reviewed by Clagett and Reisch[14] used FUT for DVT diagnosis. When comparing FUT studies to phlebography, they found phlebography to detect 6% fewer DVTs (19.1% versus 25%). In agreement with this finding, Comerota et al. found FUT to have a specificity of 71% (sensitivity, 73%) for DVT in a prospective study of symptomatic and asymptomatic patients.[107] This study and at least one other have shown minimal improvement in sensitivity by combining FUT with IPG in DVT screening.[107,108] FUT has, however, been replaced by other diagnostic tests. Its primary disadvantage is that the I-125-labeled fibrinogen must be circulating at the time the DVT is forming.

Impedance Plethysmography (IPG)

Impedance plethysmography (IPG) involves obstructing the venous outflow of the leg with some external device, removing the device, and then quantifying changes in electrical resistance resulting from changes in calf blood volume. Serial IPG has been shown as safe when applied to an outpatient or inpatient population suspected of having DVT, with a venogram-documented positive predictive value of approximately 90% and a low incidence of subsequent clinical DVT or PE in patients with serially negative IPG exams.[109–111] More recently, the sensitivity of IPG has been called into question. Using phlebography, Comerota et al. confirmed a low sensitivity of IPG for CDVT (8%).[107] Although the sensitivity of IPG for PDVT was moderate in symptomatic patients (83%), it was poor when used as surveillance (32%).[107] This finding has also been consistently reported in prospective studies of prophylaxis in hip surgery patients in which IPG with or without FUT was used as surveillance. Sensitivities of IPG alone for all DVTs ranged from 12% to 19% and improved to approximately 50% with the addition of FUT.[107,112,113] It would appear that IPG with or without FUT is not acceptable for the purpose of surveillance of high-risk asymptomatic patients. Finally, Anderson et al. showed an IPG sensitivity of only 66% for venogram-confirmed symptomatic PDVT in their population (university-based tertiary care medical center associated with a cancer clinic).[114]

Duplex Ultrasound (DUS)

Duplex ultrasound (DUS) is now considered by many to be the new "gold standard" for diagnosing PDVT. DUS combines real-time B-mode ultrasound (US) with pulsed Doppler capability. This combination allows determination of vein compressibility as well as flow characteristics. Veins that are incompressible with firm pressure applied by the ultrasound scanhead are considered to be thrombosed. Normal lower-extremity venous flow is phasic, decreasing with inspiration.

It can also be increased by leg elevation or compression and decreased by increasing intraabdominal pressure (Valsalva maneuver). Prospective studies comparing B-mode US to venography using lack of vein compression as the sole determinant of a positive ultrasound study show sensitivities of at least 91% and specificities of 97% or better.[115–119] In addition, Lensing et al. developed and tested flow criteria for PDVT and found a sensitivity of 91% and specificity of 99% in patients with venogram-confirmed DVT.[120] Detection of CDVT is generally regarded as poor but may be improved with the addition of duplex scanning in which flowing blood is color coded on the gray-scale B-mode image (color flow). In symptomatic inpatients who could undergo venogram (80%), Heijboer et al. showed comparable results with both IPG and DUS for detection of PDVT with sensitivities of 96% versus 97%, specificities of 83% and 86%, positive predictive values (PPV) of 82% and 87%, and negative predictive values (NPV) of 97% and 97%, respectively.[121] They performed a similar study on symptomatic outpatients and found a higher PPV for DUS versus IPG (94% versus 83%).[122] DUS is reliable, noninvasive, and portable but does require experienced personnel to obtain results similar to those reported. Less than 15% of duplex ultrasound examinations performed for evaluation of DVT are positive. The "yield" may be increased by combining clinical assessment and evaluation of D-dimer levels (see below) with selective use of venous duplex ultrasound examinations.[123–125]

D-Dimer

The most studied serological marker for VTE is the D-dimer (DD). There are many available D-dimer assays, each with differing sensitivities and specificities. DD is a specific derivative of cross-linked fibrin that is released when fibrin is lysed by plasmin. It is indicative of thrombosis but can be falsely elevated postoperatively and in the setting of sepsis, acute respiratory distress syndrome (ARDS), and myocardial infarction. It may be helpful as a screening examination in outpatients suspected of having DVT, as the sensitivity of a positive DD assay was found to be 93% for PDVT and 70% for CDVT in 214 consecutive patients using venography as the standard.[126] Adding IPG, the NPV and PPV for all DVT became 97% and 93%, respectively, when the studies were concordant; discordant results were obtained in 28% of patients.[126] A negative D-dimer test may permit elimination of evaluation of calf veins with duplex ultrasound in patients with negative examinations of their proximal lower extremity veins.[123]

Diagnosis of Pulmonary Embolism

Signs and symptoms of pulmonary embolism (PE) include dyspnea, tachypnea, chest pain, tachycardia, cyanosis, hemoptysis, hypotension, syncope, evidence of right-sided heart failure, and a pleural rub or rales. Investigators involved in the Prospective Investigation of Pulmonary Embolism Diagnosis (PIOPED) trial found that 90% of patients without a history of cardiac or pulmonary disease and who had a PE confirmed by pulmonary angiography (PA) had either dyspnea or tachycardia.[127] However, there were no statistically significant differences in signs and symptoms between patients who did or did not subsequently have PE diagnosed by PA.[127] Patients with PE may also present with coexisting signs and symptoms of DVT.

Nonspecific Tests

An arterial blood gas (ABG), chest X-ray (CXR), and electrocardiogram (EKG) are usually obtained in cases in which the diagnosis of PE is considered. Characteristic early ABG findings include respiratory alkalosis, decreased CO_2, and decreased O_2, which results in an increased alveolar–arterial gradient (A-a). However, in patients in the PIOPED study on room air without preexisting cardiac or pulmonary disease and angiographically confirmed PE, the O_2 was normal (80 mmHg or greater) and the A-a was normal (less than 20 mmHg) in 26% and 14%, respectively.[127] In more severe cases, or during progression of PE, acidosis and worsening hypoxia may develop.

Suggestive CXR findings of PE include Westermark's sign (prominent central pulmonary artery and decreased pulmonary vascularity) and a pleural-based, wedge-shaped pulmonary density. These findings are, however, infrequent and present in both patients with and without PE. Nonspecific abnormalities on CXR are more prevalent in patients with PE compared to those without symptoms similar to those present in PE[128] but are not diagnostic. The most common EKG findings in the PIOPED trial in patients with PE were nonspecific ST segment or T-wave changes.[127] The importance of these nonspecific tests is to rule out other pathological processes with signs and symptoms similar to PE.

Pulmonary Angiography

Pulmonary angiography was introduced in 1964.[129] The test is still considered the gold standard for diagnosis of pulmonary embolism but is infrequently used in modern practice, having been initially surplanted by ventilation/perfusion scanning and now by computed tomography angiography (CTA). In pulmonary angiography a catheter is placed into the pulmonary artery, usually via a femoral vein puncture, and a contrast agent is injected into both lungs. Either complete obstruction of, or filling defects within, the vessels are the basis for diagnosis (Fig. 67.3). Major complications may include death, respiratory distress, arrhythmias, contrast reactions (allergy and renal failure), and hematomas. Death occurred in 5 of 1111 patients (0.5%) who underwent PA in the PIOPED trial; 2 of these patients were considered unstable before the procedure.[128] An additional 9 patients (1%) had major nonfatal complications, and 60 patients (5%) had minor, less significant complications.[128] The death rate is comparable to large, previously reported series.[130,131] Nondiagnostic angiograms are uncommon (5% or less),[128,132] and a negative PA effectively rules out a PE. There is no standard for comparison, but in the PIOPED trial only 6 of 380 patients (1.6%) who had a negative angiogram and received no anticoagulants developed PE within the following year. Five of these patients had a history of thrombophlebitis or DVT.[133]

Ventilation/Perfusion (V/Q) Scanning

Perfusion scans involve injection of radiolabeled colloid through a peripheral vein followed by lung scanning in several views. Although perfusion scans alone are sensitive for PE, they lack specificity because many conditions other than PE

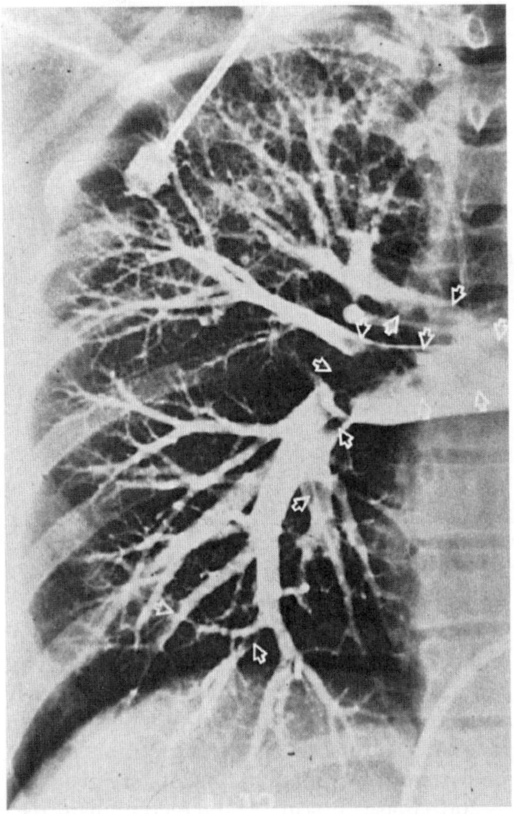

FIGURE 67.3. Pulmonary angiogram demonstrates thrombus in the distal right main pulmonary artery extending into the lobar branches.

cause perfusion defects [pneumonia, bronchospasm, chronic obstructive pulmonary disease (COPD), cancer]. In an attempt to improve specificity, ventilation studies (using radiolabeled aerosol) have been added, producing the V/Q scan. In the presence of PE, a perfusion defect should be present without a corresponding ventilation defect (V/Q mismatch). The PIOPED trial was a landmark study in determining the role of the V/Q scan in the diagnosis of acute PE.[134] This multicenter, prospective study compared V/Q scans to pulmonary angiograms in 755 patients. There were well-defined V/Q scan interpretation criteria defining five categories (Table 67.8). The categories consisted of high probability, intermediate probability, low probability, very low probability, and normal scans. Combining scans of high, intermediate, and low probability, the V/Q scan had a sensitivity of 98%, but specificity was only 10% for diagnosis of PE. A high-probability scan was quite specific (97%) but missed more than half of PA-determined PE (sensitivity, 41%). V/Q scans were diagnostic in only 27% of patients (either high probability or normal/near normal). When clinical judgment was also considered, high- and low-probability V/Q scans were much more accurate in the diagnosis or exclusion of PE. A supporting clinical judgment improved both the PPV of a high-probability scan and the NPV of a low-probability scan to 96%. Overall, a high-probability scan in a suspicious clinical setting is highly suggestive of PE. Low-probability V/Q scans combined with low clinical suspicion or normal/near-normal scans effectively ruled out PE. These results are obtained, however, in a minority of patients, frequently necessitating additional diagnostic studies. The diagnostic utility of V/Q scanning in the PIOPED study was not altered by the presence of preexisting cardiac or pulmonary disease.[135]

D-Dimer

D-Dimers (DDs) can be used for the detection of PE as well as DVT. They are most useful as a screening test in the outpatient setting. Bounameaux et al. found, in 171 consecutive patients presenting to an emergency room with suspected PE, that a positive DD by enzyme-linked immunosorbent assay (ELISA) (500 μg/L or greater) had a sensitivity of 98% and specificity of 39% for the diagnosis of PE using V/Q scanning or PA as the reference study.[136] Similarly, Turkstra et al. showed a high sensitivity for a newer, rapid assay for both PE and DVT.[137]

Additional Noninvasive Testing

When V/Q scanning is nondiagnostic, some investigators have evaluated the lower-extremity veins where the majority

TABLE 67.8.
PIOPED[a] Central Scan Interpretation Categories and Criteria.

High probability
Two or more large (>75% of a segment) segmental perfusion defects without corresponding ventilation or roentgenographic abnormalities or substantially larger than either matching ventilation or chest roentgenogram abnormalities
Two or more moderate segmental (25% or more and 75% or less of a segment) perfusion defects without matching ventilation or chest roentgenogram abnormalities and one large mismatched segmental defect
Four or more moderate segmental perfusion defects without ventilation or chest roentgenogram abnormalities
Intermediate probability (indeterminate)
Not falling into normal, very low, low-, or high-probability categories
Borderline high or borderline low
Difficult to categorize as high or low
Low probability
Nonsegmental perfusion defects (e.g., very small effusion causing blunting of the costophrenic angle, cardiomegaly, enlarged aorta, hila and mediastinum, and elevated diaphragm)
Single moderate mismatched segmental perfusion defect with normal chest roentgenogram
Any perfusion defect with a substantially larger chest roentgenogram abnormality
Large or moderated segmental perfusion defects involving no more than four segments in 1 lung and no more than three segments in one lung region with matching ventilation defects either equal to or larger in size and chest roentgenogram either normal or with abnormalities substantially smaller than perfusion defects
Three or more small segmental perfusion defects (less than 25% of a segment) with a normal chest roentgenogram
Very low probability
Three or fewer small segmental perfusion defects with a normal chest roentgenogram
Normal
No perfusion defects seen
Perfusion outlines exactly the shape of the lungs as seen on the chest roentgenogram (hilar and aortic impressions may be seen, chest roentgenogram and/or ventilation study may be abnormal)

[a]Prospective Investigation of Pulmonary Embolism Diagnosis.
Source: The PIOPED Investigators,[134] with permission.

of PEs are believed to originate. A small study examined 41 patients who underwent V/Q scanning, duplex ultrasound of the lower-extremity veins, and pulmonary angiography and found the combination of V/Q scanning and DUS yielded only a sensitivity of 62% and a specificity of 78% for diagnosing PE using PIOPED criteria.[138] Hull et al. also have previously shown that only 50% of patients with high-probability V/Q scans had DVT diagnosed by venography.[139] However, more recently, Kruit et al. found 93% of patients with high-probability V/Q scans had DVT by venography, 30% of which were CDVT only.[140] Of 62 patients with abnormal V/Q scans and normal venography who received no anticoagulant therapy, only 1 (1.6%) had documented VTE (DVT) within the next year.[140] MR angiography has similarly been shown to miss small peripheral PEs.[141]

CT Angiography (CTA)

CT angiography (CTA) has now become the test of choice for initial evaluation of possible pulmonary embolism. Extremely fast, multidetector CT scanners are now available in most hospitals. A large prospective study of 824 patients recently established accuracy of CTA for detection of pulmonary embolism. The test was inconclusive in about 10% of patients because of poor-quality images. However, with good images, CTA had a 90% sensitivity and a 95% specificity for diagnosis of pulmonary embolism.[142]

Treatment

Once the diagnosis of VTE has been made, treatment should begin. If the clinical suspicion is high, it is prudent to begin treatment before an objective diagnosis is made.

Thrombolytic Therapy

Ideally, treatment of DVT would result in early dissolution of thrombus, thereby eliminating the risk of PE and theoretically reducing the incidence of the postphlebitic syndrome. Early thrombolysis of PE could also potentially reverse the hemodynamic consequences of PE and be lifesaving. Unfortunately, only a minority of patients with VTE are candidates for thrombolytic therapy. Two recent studies investigating the role of thrombolytic therapy in DVT found that less than 10% of patients were eligible for thrombolysis.[143,144] Contraindications to lytic therapy are listed in Table 67.9.

Three potential thrombolytic agents are available (Table 67.10): streptokinase, urokinase, and recombinant tissue plasminogen activator (rtPA). All convert plasminogen to plasmin. Streptokinase, discovered in 1933, is isolated from beta-hemolytic streptococci.[145] It is antigenic, can induce allergic reactions, and can be inactivated by circulating antibodies. It is not specific for fibrin-bound plasminogen and requires plasminogen as a cofactor. Urokinase was originally isolated from urine in 1947.[146] It is now produced by human fetal renal cell culture. It is not antigenic but is still nonspecific and can produce febrile reactions. rtPA is found in all human tissues and was first isolated in 1979[147]; it has the advantage of being more specific for fibrin-bound plasminogen compared to the other agents but has not been shown to be superior in terms

TABLE 67.9. Contraindications to Systemic Lytic Therapy.

Absolute:
- Active internal bleeding
- Recent (<2 months) cerebrovascular accident
- Intracranial pathology

Relatively major:
- Recent (<10 days) major surgery, obstetrical delivery, or organ biopsy
- Active peptic ulcer or gastrointestinal pathology
- Recent major trauma
- Uncontrolled hypertension

Relatively minor:
- Minor surgery or trauma
- Recent cardiopulmonary resuscitation
- High likelihood of left heart thrombus (i.e., atrial fibrillation with mitral valve disease)
- Bacterial endocarditis
- Hemostatic defects (i.e., renal or liver disease)
- Pregnancy
- Diabetic hemorrhagic retinopathy

Source: Quinones-Baldrich,[331] with permission.

TABLE 67.10. Thrombolytic Agents.

	Streptokinase	*Urokinase*	*Tissue plasminogen activator*
Source	Beta-hemolytic *Streptococcus*	Fetal renal cell culture	Recombinant DNA technology
Mechanism	Streptokinase–plasminogen complex	Direct plasminogen activator	Direct plasminogen activator
Metabolism	Liver	Liver	Liver
Advantages	Low cost	Direct activator; no allergic reaction	Fibrin-selective direct activator; no allergic reaction
Disadvantages	Affected by antistreptococcus A,B; allergic reactions; complex mechanism of action	High cost	High cost
Systemic dosage	250,000 units i.v. over 30 min loading; 100,000 units i.v./h	2,000 units/lb i.v. over 10 min loading; 2,000 units/lb i.v./h	50 mg i.v. over 2 h; may repeat 30–50 mg i.v. over 4–6 h
Regional dosage	Low dose: 5,000–10,000 units/h High dose: 30,000–60,000 units/h	30,000–50,000 units/h 2,000–4,000 units/min for 1–2 h, then 1,000–2,000 units/min	0.05–0.1 units/kg/h

Source: Quinones-Bladrich,[331] with permission.

of ultimate thrombolysis of documented thrombi or reducing bleeding complications of thrombolytic therapy.

Several studies comparing streptokinase and heparin in the treatment of DVT were performed before 1980. Goldhaber et al.[148] reviewed 11 such studies and analyzed 6 that were randomized.[149–154] All 6 used venography for DVT diagnosis and to assess the effects of thrombolysis. Thrombolytic agents were administered systemically. Some degree of thrombolysis was achieved 3.7 times more often with streptokinase compared to heparin alone ($P < 0.0001$; 95% CI, 2.5, 3.7).[148] In the 3 studies with adequate data for comparison,[149–151] however, major bleeding complications were 2.9 times more common in the streptokinase group ($P = 0.04$; 95% CI, 1.1, 8.1).[148] Data regarding subsequent incidence of PE and long-term follow-up are not available.

Subsequently, Goldhaber et al., in an attempt to reduce major bleeding complications, have compared urokinase boluses to heparin alone with conflicting results.[144,155] An additional prospective study followed 153 patients with venographically proven DVT for 2 years. There was no difference in venous insufficiency (by foot volumetry) between patients who received thrombolysis versus heparin alone.[156]

Currently, there is no clear benefit for thrombolytic therapy in the large majority of patients with DVT. Nevertheless, thrombolytic therapy for DVT may be appropriate in highly selected cases of massive iliofemoral DVT. Thrombolytic therapy delivered by catheter-directed techniques may provide more effective thrombolysis with decreased bleeding complications compared to systemically delivered thrombolysis.[157,158] In such cases, lytic agents are delivered directly into the thrombus via percutaneously placed catheters.[157] Additional procedures may be required to maintain patency once established.[158]

The largest study investigating thrombolytics in acute PE was the Urokinase Pulmonary Embolism Trial (UPET).[81,159] In phase I of UPET, patients with acute PE were randomized to receive either a 12-h peripheral infusion of urokinase followed by heparin or heparin alone.[81] Although pulmonary angiography demonstrated accelerated thrombolysis and decreased pulmonary resistance in the urokinase group, there were no differences in mortality and recurrence rates.[81] In addition, there were more bleeding complications in the urokinase group (45% versus 27%).[81] Phase II failed to demonstrate significant differences between 12-h and 24-h infusions of urokinase or streptokinase.[159] Based on these data, an NIH Consensus Development Conference in 1980 believed that thrombolytic therapy followed by heparin resulted in a more rapid normalization of the hemodynamic consequences of PE compared to heparin alone.[160] Since this time, smaller U.S. and European trials have shown rtPA to have similar short-term benefits.[161–164] Goldhaber et al. randomized 46 hemodynamically stable patients with PE to rtPA (100mg over 2h) followed by heparin to heparin alone and found significant improvements in pulmonary perfusion scans and right ventricular wall motion by echocardiography at 24h in patients treated with rtPA.[165] rtPA has been shown to be as effective when given through a peripheral vein as when given directly through the pulmonary artery.[166] A large prospective randomized trial to determine PE recurrence, death, and chronic pulmonary hypertension is necessary before definite recommendations are possible.

Heparin

Unfractionated heparin (UFH) has been the initial pharmacological treatment of choice for VTE since it was first found by Barritt and Jordan to be efficacious in reducing death in cases of PE.[55] UFH functions by two mechanisms: (1) it binds to antithrombin III (ATIII) and amplifies the inhibition of thrombin and activated Factor X by ATIII, and (2) it catalyzes the inhibition of thrombin by heparin cofactor II. The half-life of UFH is approximately 90min. The level of anticoagulation produced by the administration of UFH can be monitored by the activated prothrombin time (aPTT), which is usually evaluated at 6-h intervals until a steady state has been reached.

As the mortality associated with VTE is highest within the first few hours of presentation, it is important to rapidly establish therapeutic heparin levels, which is accomplished with an intravenous (IV) bolus of heparin followed by a continuous infusion. The lower limit for the aPTT when treating VTE is 1.5 times control. The incidence of both recurrence and extension have been shown to be unacceptably high when either levels are subtherapeutic (as with subcutaneous heparin)[72] or when oral anticoagulation is initiated alone.[70] In contrast, there does not appear to be an increased risk of hemorrhagic complications in patients with supratherapeutic levels (aPTT 2.5).[167]

It is best to dose UFH according to a nomogram. Raschke et al. randomized 115 patients who required anticoagulation to receive UFH by either a weight-based or a standard care nomogram.[168] Significantly more patients assigned to the weight-based nomogram were therapeutic within the first 24h (97% versus 77%; $P < 0.002$).[168] Treatment typically is continued until the patient has become therapeutic on oral anticoagulation. Hull et al. showed no difference in objectively documented recurrent VTE during the following 3 months in patients who received 5 versus 10 days of intravenous heparin for initial DVT treatment.[169]

In addition to hemorrhage, heparin also has unique complications. Heparin-induced thrombocytopenia (HIT) is estimated to occur in approximately 2% to 5% of patients receiving heparin.[170,171] HIT is believed to be secondary to antibodies directed against platelets complexed with heparin.[172,173] Although assays for HIT antibodies are available, the diagnosis is initially clinical and all forms of heparin should be withheld once the diagnosis is considered. The most feared complication of HIT, which may occur in as many as 35% of patients affected, is venous or arterial thrombosis.[174] Another less well understood complication in patients on long-term heparin therapy is heparin-associated osteoporosis (HAO).[175]

Warfarin

Dicumarol was isolated from sweet clover by Link at the University of Wisconsin in 1939.[176] The sweet clover was believed to be causing hemorrhage in cattle that consumed it. Link later developed warfarin from dicumarol (initially used as rat poison).[177] It has been used as an anticoagulant in humans since the early 1950s. Warfarin acts by interfering with the production of both the procoagulant (II, VII, IX, X) and anticoagulant (proteins C and S) vitamin K-dependent cofactors. Patient response to warfarin is variable depending on liver function, diet, age, and concomitant medications. The level of anticoagulation produced by warfarin can be monitored with prothrombin time (PT). The PT is determined using commercially available thromboplastin reagents. Secondary to a wide variability of thromboplastin reagents used, the International Normalized Ratio was created (INR). An INR of 2.0 to 3.0 is generally accepted to be therapeutic in most patients with VTE.[178] INR must be closely monitored in all patients on warfarin.

It was initially thought that several days of heparin were necessary before initiating warfarin therapy. However, several prospective randomized trials have shown that starting warfarin therapy in addition to heparin within the first few days of VTE diagnosis is safe, effective, and permits earlier discharge from the hospital.[169,179,180] Patients should not be started on warfarin if any invasive procedures are planned. Warfarin has a long half-life and must be withheld for several days for the INR to normalize. Fresh-frozen plasma may be administered to provide vitamin K-dependent cofactors when rapid reversal is necessary.

Warfarin has been shown to reduce the recurrence of VTE after an initial event.[181,182] What has been less clear is how long to treat a patient with warfarin after an initial event or recurrence. Schulman et al. randomized 20 patients with an initial DVT and a "temporary risk factor" to either 6 weeks or 3 months of therapy; 40 patients with an initial DVT and a "permanent risk factor" received 3 or 6 months of therapy.[183] No differences in DVT recurrence were found between these small groups at 1 year of follow-up using IPG for surveillance of recurrence.[183] Holmgren et al. found no difference in symptomatic recurrence of DVT in medical patients who were randomized to receive either 1 or 6 months of warfarin therapy after an initial DVT.[184] However, these patients had few "temporary risk factors," and the recurrence rate in both groups was high (17%).[184] In contrast, a large multicenter trial (DURAC) demonstrated a significant difference in the number of symptomatic recurrences between patients randomized to either 6 weeks or 6 months of warfarin treatment (18.1% versus 9.5%, respectively; $P < 0.001$) after initial VTE.[185] This difference was limited to the first 6 months after the initial event; thereafter, both groups had an equivalent recurrence rate of 5% to 6% per year.[185] If patients with "temporary risk factors" were considered separately, there was no statistical significance between the groups.[185] An additional trial (DURAC II) randomized patients with a second episode of VTE to either 6 months or indefinite warfarin treatment and again found a significant difference of symptomatic recurrence (20.7% versus 2.6%, respectively; $P < 0.001$).[186] There were more major hemorrhages in the indefinitely treated group, but this was not statistically significant; no difference in mortality was found between the groups.[186]

Recent studies suggest DVT secondary to a nonreversible risk factor, such as a thrombophilic disorder, should be treated for at least 6 months with the INR maintained between 2 and 3 following a first time unprovoked episode of VTE.[187] Assessment of D-dimer or thrombin generation at the end of oral anticoagulant therapy may also help guide the duration of antiocoagulation.[188–190] Patients with a recurrence of so-called idiopathic VTE should very likely be treated indefinitely.

Low Molecular Weight Heparins (LMWHs)

Perhaps the most notable advance in the treatment of DVT in the past several decades has been the use of low molecular weight heparins (LMWHs). LMWHs are derived from UFH using depolymerization techniques. LMWHs have been shown to differ from UFH in significant ways. LMWHs have increased bioavailability, greater than 90% after a subcutaneous injection.[191,192] They have a much longer half-life than UFH[191,193] and predictable elimination rates,[194] allowing once- or twice-daily dosing. LMWHs also have a predictable anticoagulant effect based upon body weight, so that laboratory monitoring is unnecessary.[195] It has also been hoped that LMWHs would lack some of the complications seen with UFH such as hemorrhage, HIT, and osteoporosis. It is important to note that the different LMWHs differ in their anti-X_a and anti-II_a activities. For this reason, data from one LMWH may not be extrapolated to another. Early trials using LMWHs were necessary to establish dosages for each of the compounds. These early trials suggested LMWHs may be as effective as UFH.

Several randomized trials of different LMWHs versus UFH in the initial treatment of DVT have now been completed (Table 67.11).[196–199] All these studies used venography to establish the diagnosis, and all but one[199] repeated venography within the first 10 days. Follow-up varied between 3 and 6 months, and recurrences were objectively documented. Two of these studies showed no statistically significant differences in VTE recurrence or major bleeding.[196,197] The study by Simmonneau et al. found significant differences between

TABLE 67.11.
Randomized Trials of LMWH[a] versus UFH[b] for Treatment of Deep Venous Thrombosis (DVT) (Level I Evidence).

Agent	*Dose*	*Recurrent DVT (%): LMWH vs. UFH*	*Major bleeding (%): LMWH vs. UFH*
Fraxiparine[196]	<55 kg 12,500 XaI U[c] >55 kg <80 kg 15,000 XaI U >80 kg 17,500 XaI U (q 12 h)	7 vs. 14 (P = NS)	1 vs. 4 (P = NS)
Dalteparin[197]	200 XaI U/kg (q 24 h)	5 vs. 3 (P = NS)	None, either group
Enoxaparin[198]	100 XaI U/kg (q 12 h)	1 vs. 10 ($P < 0.02$)	None, either group
Logiparin[199]	175 XaI U/kg (q 24 h)	3 vs. 7 ($P = 0.07$)	0.5 vs. 5 ($P = 0.06$)

[a]Low molecular weight heparin.
[b]Adjusted dose unfractionated heparin.
[c]Factor Xa inhibitory units.

venography appearances and recurrent VTE 10 days after enrollment favoring LMWH ($P < 0.002$ for both), but there were no significant differences in death, recurrent VTE, and bleeding complications during 3 months of follow-up.[198] Hull et al. found fewer VTE recurrences approaching significance ($P < 0.07$) and fewer major hemorrhages ($P = 0.006$) in patients initially receiving LMWH.[199] Based on these trials, it can be concluded that LMWHs are at least as effective and as safe as UFH. The benefits of once- to twice-daily administration, lack of need for laboratory monitoring, and potential for home administration make LMWH appealing as initial primary therapy for VTE.

At least two prospective, randomized trials have shown LMWHs can be safe and efficacious in the outpatient treatment of DVT in selected patients.[200,201] Major exclusion criteria included suspicion of PE, need for hospitalization, and poor candidacy for outpatient treatment. Between one-third and one-half of patients were treated entirely at home.

As stated, there does not appear to be a significant difference in the incidence of major hemorrhage between LMWHs and UFH, although there is a trend favoring LMWHs. HIT is seen in approximately 2% to 3% of patients on LMWHs, similar to UFH.[200,202] Animal studies suggest heparin-associated osteoporosis is less pronounced with the LMWHs,[203–205] but this has not been demonstrated conclusively in humans.

Inferior Vena Cava (IVC) Filters

Interruption of the inferior vena cava (IVC) for treatment of lower-extremity DVT was first suggested by Trousseau in 1868. As this procedure carries an inherent morbidity, transvenous devices have been designed to filter emboli while allowing continuous flow through the IVC. The Kimray–Greenfield filter was introduced in the United States in 1973.[206] Numerous different IVC filters are available today. Filters that may be placed temporarily are now also available. A contraindication to, or a failure of anticoagulation, are the main indications for IVC filter placement in the treatment of lower-extremity DVT.

The early filters were placed surgically, but percutaneous techniques now allow placement via percutaneous venotomy, usually through the right femoral vein. As the technology has evolved, smaller delivery sheaths have decreased the incidence of insertion site thrombosis.[207] Other nonfatal potential complications include technical difficulties during placement, filter migration, erosion into the IVC wall, and IVC obstruction.[208]

Level I evidence for the efficacy of IVC filters is scarce. There are no randomized, prospective trials. Becker et al.[208] reviewed the data on IVC filters in 1992 and found the incidence of death from PE to be 0.7% in trials placing a Greenfield filter in consecutive patients. However, some of these patients had filters placed for prophylaxis rather than treatment. The incidence of fatal complications from all trials was low (0.12%).[208]

There is no perfect filter. Some filters offer advantages in certain situations depending upon the extent of thrombus or the anatomy. Temporary, or retrievable filters, allow the filter to be removed once a contraindication of anticoagulation has resolved. The Bird's Nest filter has been shown in vitro to have the highest clot-trapping capacity,[209] but it also has the highest incidence of IVC thrombosis in vivo.[210] Because the data on IVC filter efficacy are poor and the data on medical treatment are well established, the role of the IVC filter in the treatment of DVT should be limited to cases in which anticoagulation is contraindicated or has failed or the patient has very marginal cardiopulmonary reserve. The ability to retrieve filters may be leading to increased filter placement for prophylactic purposes.

Surgical Treatment

Lohr et al.[211] have recommended greater saphenous vein (GSV) ligation in cases of GSV thrombosis within 3 cm of the saphenofemoral junction. This recommendation was based on the high likelihood of propagation into the common femoral vein and potential cost savings compared to patients treated with anticoagulation.[211] In contrast, Ascer et al.[212] treated 20 patients with GSV thrombosis with anticoagulants and found no PE, recurrent thrombosis, or complications at 14 months' follow-up; 40% of patients had concurrent DVT.[212]

Results of early surgical management of iliofemoral DVT were poor, with high rates of rethrombosis and complications.[213] Modern techniques include venous thrombectomy and creation of a temporary arteriovenous fistula in the affected leg, as well as use of endoluminal stents. A recent French study followed 77 limbs after venous thrombectomy for acute iliofemoral DVT for a mean of 8.5 years.[214] There were 12 early failures (16%), but valvular competence in early successes was 80% at 5 years and 56% at 10 years.[214] More than 90% of patients had minimal or no symptoms of the postphlebitic syndrome.[214] These results are better than historic controls,[215] but randomized data are lacking.

Survival rates for surgical pulmonary embolectomy improved markedly with the addition of cardiopulmonary bypass. The procedure has largely been reserved for patients with massive PE who have failed thrombolysis or have contraindications to thrombolytics. Modern series report between 20% and 40% mortality for the procedure.[216–218] One retrospective study found the results of thrombolysis to be satisfactory when cardiopulmonary bypass was not available for patients with massive PE.[218]

Greenfield et al.[219] reported results of transvenous catheter pulmonary embolectomy for massive PE over 22 years from multiple institutions using evolving techniques. Emboli were extracted in 76% (35/46), and 30-day survival was 70%.[219] Patients with chronic PE were less likely to benefit.[219] Randomized trials comparing thrombolytics to catheter or surgical pulmonary embolectomy would be of value but are not likely forthcoming.

Chronic Venous Insufficiency/Venous Ulceration

Twenty-seven percent of the adult U.S. population has some form of detectable lower-extremity venous abnormality,[210] usually superficial varicosities and/or telangiectasis. As many as 1.5% of European adults develop venous stasis ulceration at some point.[211]

Symptoms of chronic venous insufficiency (CVI) include leg fatigue, discomfort, and heaviness. Signs include venous telangiectasias and varicose veins as well as lipodermatosclerosis and venous ulceration. Risk factors associated with varicose veins may include prolonged standing,[220] heredity,[222] female sex,[222,223] parity,[224] and history of phlebitis.[223]

Risk factors for venous ulceration are different. The prevalence of venous disease increases with age, and many risk factors for venous ulceration are associated with older age. The median age for patients with venous ulcers may be as high as 70 to 77 years.[225,226] Estimated incidence of venous ulcer in patients over 45 years of age is 3.5 per thousand per year.[227] Multivariant analysis suggests, in addition to age, the primary risk factors for venous ulceration are a history of deep venous thrombosis, a history of severe lower-extremity trauma, male sex, and obesity.[223]

Patients with venous ulceration have a severely impaired quality of life. Feelings of anger, depression, isolation, and/or diminished self-image are present in nearly 70%, and 80% have decreased mobility.[228] Moderate to severe limitation of leisure activities results in more than 40% of patients with venous ulcer, and 40% of employed patients with venous ulceration have decreased earning capacity directly attributable to the presence of the venous ulcer.[229] As many as 2 million workdays are lost per year in the United States secondary to venous ulceration,[230] and 5% of patients with venous ulcers lose jobs as a result of their venous ulcer.[229]

A postal survey in Edinburgh, Scotland, emphasized the chronicity of problems associated with venous ulceration.[231] In this community, 1477 patients were noted to be receiving treatment for lower-extremity ulceration, and 76% of ulcerated limbs were classified as having a venous etiology. Thirty-five percent of ulcerated limbs had four or more recurrences and 45% of patients had lower-extremity ulceration for more than 10 years. The cost of treatment for venous ulceration alone is staggering, with annual healthcare costs estimated at $1 billion in the United States.[232]

Pathophysiology

Macrocirculation

Venous reflux, venous obstruction, and calf muscle pump dysfunction contribute singularly or in combination to the signs and symptoms of chronic venous insufficiency. Of these, reflux is probably the most important. Venous reflux can be described as primary or secondary and results from abnormalities of the venous valve. Primary valvular reflux (incompetence) is diagnosed when there is no known underlying etiology of valvular dysfunction. Most cases of what clinically appears to be isolated superficial venous insufficiency are secondary to primary venous incompetence.[233] Such cases may develop from a loss of elasticity of the venous wall.[234] Loss of venous elasticity precedes development of reflux in patients with apparent primary venous incompetence.[235]

An obvious identifiable antecedent condition is required for valvular incompetence to be described as secondary. Most frequently, this is a deep venous thrombosis (DVT). The presence of thrombus within the vein is thought to have led to destruction or dysfunction of the venous valves.

Evaluation of Venous Insufficiency

Evaluation of the macrocirculation in chronic venous insufficiency initially utilized invasive measurements of ambulatory venous pressure and venous recovery times. The test depends on the fact that pressures measured in the dorsal veins of the foot reflect those in the deep veins of the calf. A needle is inserted in a dorsal foot vein and connected to a pressure transducer. The patient is then asked to perform 10 tiptoe exercises. Initially there is often a slight upward deflection of pressure with the onset of exercise. With each subsequent tiptoe maneuver the measured pressure should, however, decrease. After about 10 tiptoes the measured pressure stabilizes and reflects a balance of venous inflow and outflow. The pressure at this point is called the ambulatory venous pressure (AVP) (measured in mmHg). The patient is then asked to stop exercising and the venous pressure is allowed to recover. The time required for venous pressure to return from the ambulatory venous pressure level to 90% of the baseline pressure is known as the venous recovery time (VRT).

Ambulatory venous pressure measurements indicate that the presence of venous hypertension is strongly associated with chronic venous insufficiency. Extremities with ambulatory venous pressures less than 40 mmHg have a trivial incidence of venous ulceration.[236] However, in patients with an ambulatory venous pressure greater than 80 mmHg there is an 80% incidence of venous ulceration.[236]

Photoplethysmography (PPG) is a noninvasive alternative to the performance of direct ambulatory venous pressure measurements. A light-emitting diode is placed just above the medial malleolus and the patient asked to perform a series of tiptoe maneuvers. The device is calibrated in such a fashion that light transmitted into the skin and reflected back to the light-sensitive diode is displayed in a tracing similar to that of an ambulatory venous pressure measurement. Although it is clear that the maximum negative displacement of the photoplethysmographic curve cannot be used to noninvasively determine ambulatory venous pressures, the recovery portion of the curve does provide an excellent noninvasive alternative to the measurement of invasively determined venous recovery times. Venous recovery times reflect the time required for refilling of the calf veins after their emptying in response to the tiptoe maneuvers. In limbs with venous insufficiency, the calf veins will refill from capillary inflow as well as from axial reflux. In such extremities, the venous recovery time is shortened compared to normals. In most vascular laboratories, a PPG VRT less than 17 to 20 s is considered to indicate the presence of venous reflux in that extremity. Most cases of venous ulceration are associated with VRTs of less than 10 s.

Unfortunately, invasive measurements of AVP and its noninvasive alternative, PPG VRT, do not completely characterize the function of the lower-extremity venous system. Although AVP elevations are associated with increased incidences of venous ulceration, AVP measurements may not reflect the patient's symptoms.[237] In a study of ambulatory venous pressure measurements in 207 limbs, 52 were determined to have severe ambulatory venous hypertension. Of these 52 limbs, 25 (48%) were only mildly symptomatic or asymptomatic.[238]

It is also important to note that invasively determined AVP measurements, and VRT determined invasively or with photoplethysmography, measure overall function of the lower-extremity venous system. These tests do not distinguish the combined effects of reflux and obstruction, localize the site of reflux, or evaluate the role of the calf muscle pump in venous insufficiency.

The air plethysmograph (APG) theoretically permits assessment of calf muscle pump function, venous reflux, and overall lower-extremity venous function. Both measured and calculated values are obtained with the instrument. A polyvinyl chloride pressure bladder is placed between the knee and the ankle of the lower extremity to be examined. The patient is then placed supine, the leg is elevated, and the baseline volume of venous blood is recorded. The patient is then asked to assume an upright position with the examined leg non-weight-bearing. The venous volume of the leg is then determined when the plethysmographic curve reaches a maximum plateau; this is termed the venous volume (VV). The time required to reach 90% of the VV is termed the venous filling index (VFI). VFI is a measure of reflux. The patient is then asked to perform a single tiptoe maneuver. The change between the recorded volume before and after the tiptoe maneuver is termed the ejection fraction (EF) and is a measure of calf muscle pump function. The veins of the leg are then allowed to refill until the venous volume is again achieved. The patient is then asked to perform 10 tiptoe maneuvers, and the volume then recorded is termed the residual volume. The residual volume divided by the venous volume is the residual volume fraction (RVF), a measure of overall venous function. A tracing of these maneuvers is shown in Figure 67.4.

Abnormalities in RVF correlate with ambulatory venous pressures and reflect inadequate calf muscle pump action (decreased EF), the presence of valvular reflux (increased VFI), or a combination of both. When corrected for location and magnitude of lower-extremity venous reflux, calf muscle pump function as measured by APG appears to have an independent effect on the severity of chronic venous insufficiency.[239] Studies of ankle range of motion correlated with measurements of EF and RVF indicate calf muscle function impairment, and decreased ankle range of motion is associated with deterioration and increased clinical severity of chronic venous insufficiency.[240]

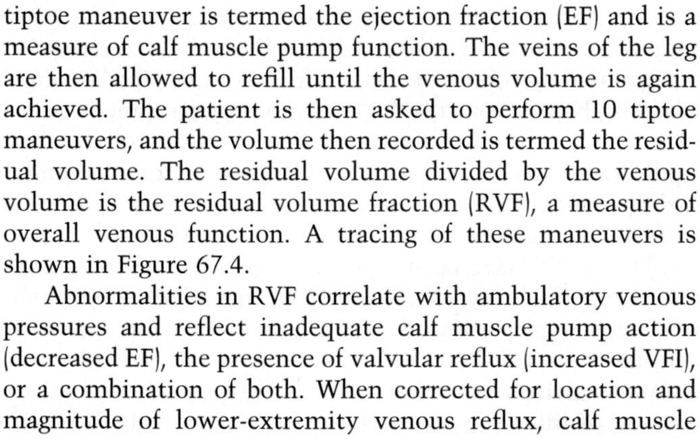

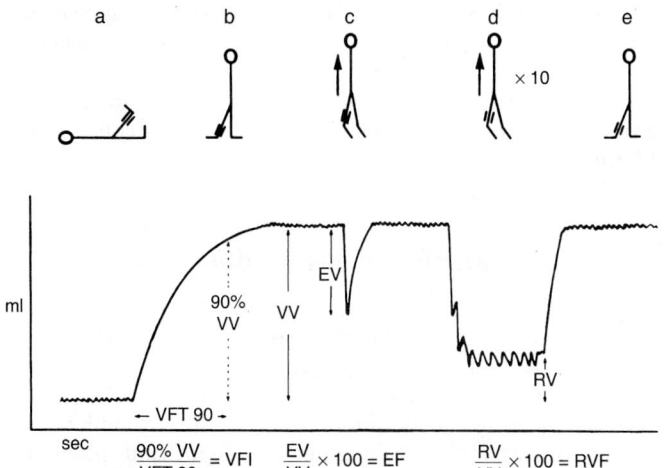

FIGURE 67.4. Typical recording of volume changes during a standard sequence of postural changes and exercise: patient in a supine position with the legs elevated 45° (*a*); patient standing with weight on the nonexamined leg (*b*); patient performing a single tiptoe movement (*c*); patient performing 10 tiptoe movements (*d*); patient again standing with weight on the nonexamined leg (*e*). *VV*, functional venous volume; *VFT*, venous filling time; *VFI*, venous filling index; *EV*, ejected volume; *EF*, ejected fraction; *RVF*, residual volume fraction. (From Christopoulos DG, Nicolaides AN, Szendro G, et al.,[332] with permission.)

Information obtained from the APG may allow for more precise preoperative assessment of patients before deep venous reconstruction or ablative superficial vein procedures. Patients with normal VFIs and diminished EFs would seem unlikely to benefit from antireflux surgery, while those patients with increased VFIs and normal EFs would appear to be appropriate candidates for antireflux procedures.

Duplex ultrasound has also now achieved considerable importance in the evaluation of patients with chronic venous insufficiency. In addition to ruling out the presence of acute venous thrombosis, duplex ultrasound can be used to evaluate venous reflux in individual venous segments of the lower extremity. The examination is performed with the patient upright and the leg to be studied non-weight-bearing. Pneumatic cuffs are placed about the thigh, calf, and around the foot. The width of the cuff and the pressure to which it is inflated are determined by the cuff location. The venous segment to be examined is insonated just below the appropriate pneumatic cuff. The cuff is then inflated and then rapidly deflated. With inflation of the cuff venous flow ceases, and with deflation of the cuff a short period of reflux is observed. The duplex technique allows determination of reproducible values for venous valve closure times, peak reflux velocities, and calculated volume flow at peak reflux in specific locations in both the deep and superficial veins. Ninety-five percent of normal venous valves close within 0.5 s of cuff deflation.[241] Determination of duplex valve closure times allows individual venous segments to be assessed. Knowledge of the relative contribution of individual venous segments to overall venous reflux may prove to be useful in planning venous reconstructive procedures.

Clearly, location of venous reflux is important. Reflux in popliteal and infrapopliteal veins is more significant than more proximal reflux in the development of skin changes and ulcers associated with severe venous insufficiency.[242–244] Venous ulceration can, however, also occur with reflux isolated to the superficial veins.[245,246] Up to 17% of patients with venous ulceration have reflux isolated to the superficial veins alone.[242–246]

The relative importance of communicating vein incompetence to the development of lipodermatosclerosis and venous ulceration is controversial. Communicating veins have long been thought to be important in the development of venous ulceration. There has, however, been little proof other than "guilt by association." Recent data derived from duplex studies of communicating veins in the region of venous ulcers indicate communicating vein incompetence is present in the communicating veins in the region of a venous ulcer in up to 86% of cases.[247] Recurrence of varicose veins after vein stripping procedures may also be related to the presence of communicating vein incompetence.[249]

Approximately 60% to 80% of patients have symptoms of lower-extremity pain, swelling, or both 3 to 10 years following an episode of acute deep venous thrombosis.[211,249,250] However, less than 5% of limbs initially involved with the deep venous thrombosis develop a venous ulcer.[211,249,250] Currently, one of the most intense areas of investigation related to chronic venous insufficiency (CVI) is the relationship between the development of CVI symptoms and the location of valvular dysfunction with respect to extent and location of thrombus following an acute episode of deep venous thrombosis. Using duplex ultrasound, detailed follow-up studies of the development of venous reflux have been performed in patients with an acute deep venous thrombosis. These studies indicate that some degree of recanalization of thrombosed veins occurs by 3 months in almost all lower extremities involved with deep venous thrombosis and treated with standard intravenous heparin and follow-up warfarin therapy.[211,249,250] In fact, by 90 days approximately half the lower extremities involved with deep venous thrombosis show recanalization of all segments initially noted to be thrombosed.[250] Interestingly, valvular incompetence in patients with deep venous thrombosis develops not only in venous segments involved with venous thrombi but also in segments never noted to be involved with the thrombotic process.[251] Incorporation of venous valves in the thrombotic process may therefore not be the only etiology of venous reflux following acute deep venous thrombosis.

As noted, an estimated 50% of above-knee deep venous thrombi and the great majority of isolated calf vein thrombi are asymptomatic.[62] This fact, combined with the fact that many patients who clearly have venous insufficiency have never had a documented episode of deep venous thrombosis,[242–246] suggests that subclinical venous thrombi may play a role in the development of chronic venous insufficiency. This involvement seems particularly likely because distal valvular incompetence appears more important in the development of clinical symptoms[242–244] and distal leg thrombi are much more likely to be clinically asymptomatic than proximal thrombi.[62] In addition, because valvular incompetence occurs in venous segments never involved with venous thrombi,[250] it may be that mechanisms other than simple valvular destruction by acute venous thrombus are also responsible for the development of venous incompetence. Valvular incompetence may, in some instances, arise secondary to venous distension resulting from proximal obstruction. Several months of unrelenting distension may result in permanent valvular incompetence.[252]

Microcirculatory Considerations

Skin and subcutaneous tissue are the end organs of chronic venous insufficiency. Functional and morphological abnormalities of the cutaneous capillaries and lymphatics characterize advanced chronic venous insufficiency. Several theories seek to link these abnormalities with venous reflux.

Microcirculatory capillary endothelial cells are functionally and morphologically altered in chronic venous insufficiency. Such cells demonstrate increased production of inflammatory mediator interleukin-1 and intracellular adhesion molecule (ICAM) and have increased pinocytotic vesicles and a widening of the interendothelial space.[253–256] Mononuclear cells, normally required for wound healing, have diminished function in chronic venous insufficiency, suggesting diminished capacity for cellular proliferation and repair.[257] This loss may explain in part the difficulty of healing a venous ulcer. Dermal fibroblasts in extremities with chronic insufficiency also have a decreased response to cytokines and growth associated with normal wound healing.[258]

Studies using video microscopic systems reveal tortuous perimalleolar capillaries in patients with chronic venous insufficiency. Such studies also reveal areas of capillary microthrombosis and abnormal cutaneous lymphatics in lipodermatosclerotic skin,[259] as well as reductions in capillary numbers in areas of prior ulceration (atrophie blanche).[260] Such data suggest destruction of the components of the cutaneous microcirculation may contribute to venous ulceration.

A major theory of venous ulcer pathogenesis depends in large part on the presence of postulated cutaneous capillary diffusion abnormalities; this is the so-called fibrin cuff theory.[261] Semiocclusive pericapillary cuffs may result from leakage of fibrinogen and other matrix proteins into the interstitium. This leakage occurs secondary to increased pressure within the venous end of the cutaneous microcirculation. The cuffs are postulated to act as a barrier to oxygen and nutrient diffusion to cutaneous skin cells and interstitial tissues. Materials contained within the fibrin cuffs may also act as potent chemoattractants as well as leukocyte and platelet activators and thereby provide a basis for the chronic inflammatory response of chronic venous insufficiency. Studies have also demonstrated less fibrinolytic activity in patients with chronic venous insufficiency and lipodermatosclerosis than in controls.[262,263] Skin biopsy specimens from patients with chronic venous insufficiency demonstrate pericapillary fibrin deposition.[264] Thus, the presence of fibrin cuffs in chronic venous insufficiency is well documented. Although biochemical markers of ischemia[265] and diminished tissue PO_2 levels[266–268] have been reported in patients with chronic venous insufficiency, conclusive evidence that these cuffs produce tissue hypoxia or localized cellular malnutrition is lacking.

Another theory of venous ulceration currently attracting widespread interest suggests that white blood cells become trapped in the microcirculation of patients with chronic venous insufficiency, resulting in microvascular congestion and thrombosis. The trapped white cells then migrate into the interstitium and release tissue-destruction lysosomal enzymes. Approximately 20% of white blood cells, predominately monocytes, are lost in lower-extremity venous effluent after 40 min of dependency, suggesting limb dependency results in microcirculatory white cell trapping or leakage into the interstitium.[269] Venous hypertension also appears to result in upregulation and expression of leukocyte adhesion molecules.[270] It is postulated this permits adherence of the white cells to the capillary endothelial cells as an initial step in trapping of the white cells within the cutaneous microcirculation.

Therapy for Chronic Venous Insufficiency

Nonoperative therapy has long been the basic treatment for venous ulceration and chronic venous insufficiency. It is highly effective in controlling symptoms of chronic venous insufficiency and promoting healing of venous ulcers. However, healing can be prolonged and painful, and recurrence of ulceration post healing is a significant problem. Although lower-extremity elevation (feet above the thighs when sitting and above the heart when supine) is very effective treatment, enforced inactivity is impractical for most patients. Ideally, nonoperative therapy for chronic venous insufficiency should control symptoms while promoting healing of existing ulcers and preventing recurrence of ulceration. At the same time, the patient should be allowed to maintain a normal ambulatory status.

Compression Therapy

Compression therapy is the primary treatment for chronic venous insufficiency and remains so despite progress in both ablative[271] and reconstructive venous surgery (see following).[237,272] Compression therapy is usually delivered in the form of elastic stockings, paste boots, or elastic wraps. Results obtained with elastic wraps in general have, however, been inferior to those achieved with elastic stockings or paste boots.[273–276]

The benefit of elastic compression stockings in the treatment of chronic venous insufficiency and venous ulceration is well documented.[277–279] At the authors' institution venous ulcers are primarily treated with local wound care and compression therapy. Patients with venous ulcers may initially be prescribed a short period of bed rest to resolve lower-extremity edema. If cellulitis is present it is treated with local wound care (dry gauze dressings changed every 12h) and with short-term courses of intravenous or oral antibiotics. When the cellulitis and edema are resolved, patients are then fitted with below-knee compression (30–40mm) stockings. Patients wear the stockings at all times when ambulatory and remove them on going to bed. Wound care consists only of dry gauze dressings and soap and water washing of the ulcer. Topical cortical steroids are applied to surrounding areas of stasis dermatitis but not to the ulcer itself. No other topical agents are used. The ulcer is covered with a dry gauze dressing held in place by the compression stockings. The patient continues ambulatory compression therapy indefinitely after the ulcer has healed.

We treated 113 patients over a 15-year period using the treatment regimen outlined above[280]; 102 patients (90%) were compliant with stocking use, and 105 (93%) had complete ulcer healing. Mean healing time was 5.3 months. Total ulcer recurrence in patients who were compliant with long-term therapy was 16%. Recurrence was 100% in patients who were noncompliant with long-term use of elastic stockings.

There are problems with compression therapy. Most noteworthy is patient compliance.[281] Patients may be initially intolerant of the sensation of compression. Frequently, stockings can initially be worn only for brief periods. At the beginning of therapy, patients need to be instructed to wear elastic stockings only for so long as tolerable and then increase gradually the time wearing the stockings. Patients also may initially need to be fitted with lesser strength of compression (20–30mmHg).

Many elderly, weak, or arthritic patients cannot apply elastic stockings. In one study of elderly (mean age, 72 years) and predominately female patients (69%), 15% of patients were incapable of applying stockings and 26% could only put them on with significant difficulty.[282] A number of aids have therefore been developed to assist in the application of elastic stockings. With open-toed stockings, an inner silk sleeve can be placed over the patient's forefoot to allow the stocking to slide smoothly during application. The sleeve is removed through the toe opening after the stocking has been placed. Another device allows the patient to load the stocking onto a wire frame (Fig. 67.5). The patient then steps into the stocking and pulls the device upward, applying the stocking to the leg.

Paste gauze compression dressings were developed by the German dermatologist Unna in 1896.[283] The current Unna's boot consists of dome paste dressing containing calamine, zinc oxide, glycerine, sorbitol, gelatin, and magnesium aluminum silicate. This dressing provides both compression and topical therapy and is preferentially applied by trained personnel. The dome paste gauze bandage is first applied with graded compression from the forefoot to the knee. A second layer consists of a 4-inch-wide continuous gauze dressing. The final layer is an elastic wrap applied with graded compression. The bandage stiffens with drying and is generally changed weekly. Studies evaluating the effectiveness of Unna boot therapy indicate about 70% of ulcers can be healed with Unna boot treatment.[284–286] After healing, lifetime compression therapy with elastic compression stockings is required to minimize recurrence.

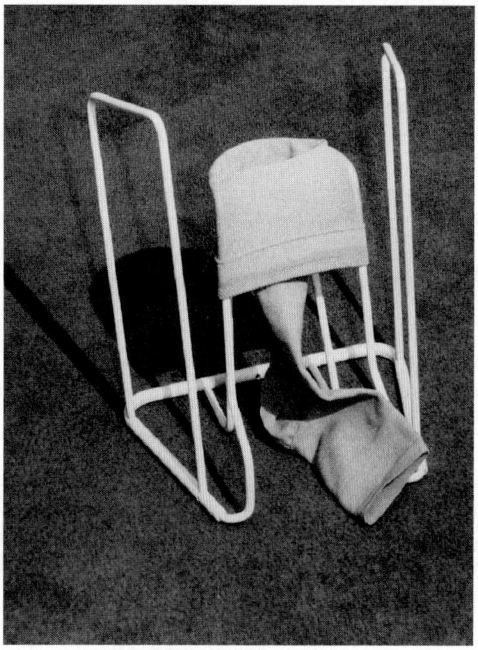

FIGURE 67.5. The Butler device.

Circ-Aid is a legging orthosis consisting of multiple pliable, rigid, adjustable compression bands.[287] These bands wrap around the leg from the ankle to the knee and are held in place with Velcro. The device provides rigid compression similar to an Unna boot with increased ease of application. Because the bands are adjustable, the orthosis can be tailored to the individual as limb edema decreases. The orthosis appears effective in promoting resolution of edema and is especially useful in patients who for various reasons are either unable or unwilling to wear compression stockings. A preliminary study suggests this legging orthosis may be superior to elastic stockings in preventing limb swelling in patients with advanced venous insufficiency.[288]

External pneumatic compression devices can serve as adjunctive measures in the treatment of lower-extremity lymphedema, venous ulceration, or both. These devices may be particularly applicable to patients who have severe edema or morbid obesity. Relative contraindications to external pneumatic compression are arterial insufficiency and uncontrolled congestive heart failure.

Pneumatic compression devices that provide sequential gradient intermittent pneumatic compression (IPC) have received the most attention. Results with these devices suggest improvement in ulcer healing, but must be qualified by the fact pump patients may also elevate their legs longer each day than nonpump patients. Despite the results of the few available studies indicating pneumatic compression may be useful in treatment of venous ulcers, especially those refractory to previous ambulatory compression alone,[288,290] the use of the adjuvant intermittent compression has not gained widespread acceptance.

Pharmacological Therapy

There are multiple pharmacological strategies to treat lipodermatosclerosis and venous ulceration. With the exception of diuretics, these agents are relatively unknown in the United States. Diuretics have, in fact, little role in the treatment of chronic venous insufficiency. They may be appropriate for short periods in patients with severe edema but must be used judiciously. Diuretic use in elderly patients without chronic intravascular volume overload can lead to hypovolemia and metabolic complications.

Other pharmacological agents for treatment of chronic venous insufficiency are widely used in Europe. In 1993, a German study indicated that 11% of people in Germany 15 years of age and older received a medication for venous disease in the previous 12 months.[291]

Zinc

It has been noted that patients with venous ulcers may have depressed serum zinc levels.[292,293] However, in a double-blind trial of patients with venous ulceration that compared zinc therapy and compression bandage use with compression bandage use alone, zinc did not increase ulcer healing.[294] Two other studies of zinc therapy in patients with venous ulcers have also shown no benefit.[295,296]

Fibrinolytic Agents

Despite the attractiveness of the fibrin cuff theory of venous ulceration, use of fibrinolytic agents, such as the anabolic steroid stanozol, has not demonstrated major benefits in patients with chronic venous insufficiency.[297–299] Oxypentifylline is a cytokine antagonist with profibrinolytic activity. Although the drug may have some benefit in ulcer healing,[300] it has significant side effects, including edema, dyspepsia, depression, and diarrhea, that make its widespread use impractical.

Phlebotrophic Agents

Studies of hydroxyutosides (flavonoid drugs derived from plant glycosides) in the treatment of patients with chronic venous insufficiency without ulceration suggest marginal subjective improvement in symptoms of pain, night cramps, and restless legs. Studies also suggests that these drugs appear mildly beneficial in controlling lower-extremity edema,[301–303] but they have not been demonstrated to improve healing of venous ulcers.[304] Calcium 2,5-dihydroxybenzene sulfonate increases lymphatic flow and proteolysis mediated by macrophages. The net effect is edema reduction,[305–307] but no convincing evidence exists that this medication improves venous ulcer healing.

Hemorrheological Agents

Pentoxifylline, in addition to its well-known hemorrheological effects, reduces white blood cell adhesiveness and decreases release of supraoxide free radicals, as well as inhibiting cytokine-mediated neutrophil activation.[308] A multicenter trial of pentoxifylline and compression stockings versus compression stockings alone in patients with venous ulcers demonstrated a significant reduction in ulcer size after 6 months in patients treated with the combination of pentoxifylline and compression stockings compared to those treated with compression alone.

An increased rate of venous ulcer healing has also been reported with aspirin therapy.[309] It is speculated aspirin may promote ulcer healing by inhibiting platelet function or decreasing associated inflammation.[310]

Prostaglandins

Prostaglandin E_1 (PGE_1) reduces white blood cell activation, decreases small vessel vasodilatation, and inhibits platelet aggregation.[311] This drug, administered intravenously, has been used in treatment of venous ulcers with significant improvement in edema and ulcer healing.[312] Horse chestnut seed extract stimulates release of prostaglandins from the PGF series. PGFs mediate vasoconstriction. A randomized trial found horse chestnut seed extract to be superior to placebo and equivalent to compression stockings in reducing leg edema with minimal adverse effects.[313]

Topical Therapies

Without evidence of invasive infection, wound bacteriology appears to have little impact on healing of venous ulcers.[314] Use of topical antibiotics on a routine basis is therefore not recommended. Application of antiseptics is also counterproductive to wound healing. Povidone-iodine, acetic acid, hydrogen peroxide, and sodium hypochlorite are all 100% cytotoxic to cultured fibroblasts.[315]

The serotonin II antagonist ketanserin increases fibroblast collagen synthesis. A double-blind study of venous ulcers comparing the use of topical 2% ketanserin and compressive bandage use with bandage use alone indicated a 91% improvement in the ketanserin-treated group compared with 50% of controls.[316]

Hydrocolloid occlusive dressings (DuoDERM) maintain a moist wound environment. Such dressings are often comfortable for the patient and may produce more rapid epithelialization of granulating wounds.[317] However, although occlusive dressings are comfortable, they have not been conclusively demonstrated to produce more rapid healing and may lead to an increased number of local infectious complications.[285]

Skin Substitutes

Advances in biotechnology have led to development of human skin substitutes to promote permanent closure of open wounds. These products vary from simple acellular skin substitutes to complete living bioengineered, bilayered human skin equivalents with allogenic epidermal and dermal layers. They may possibly serve as delivery vehicles for various growth factors and cytokines important in wound healing.

Apligraf is a bioengineered product consisting of keratinocyte-containing epidermis and a dermal layer of fibroblasts in a collagen matrix.[318] The two layers are separated by a basement membrane. Both the keratinocytes and fibroblasts are derived from human neonatal foreskin. The epidermal and dermal layers secrete collagen and other matrix elements and are mitotically active. In a randomized trial of Apligraf versus multilayered compression therapy, Apligraf was shown effective in promoting healing of venous ulcers. Long-standing ulcers (more than 12 months) and large ulcers (>6cm) demonstrated the greatest benefit with Apligraf skin substitute treatment.[319]

Surgical Therapy

Procedures designed to treat chronic venous insufficiency can be classified as ablative or reconstructive. Ablative procedures are generally applicable only to disease of the superficial veins. Reconstructive procedures are designed to treat either reflux or obstruction of the deep veins.

Venous Sclerotherapy

Venous sclerotherapy is the most widespread method for treatment of venous telangiectasias and small superficial varicose veins. Both telangiectatic vessels and small varicose veins may be associated with symptoms of leg heaviness, as well as localized pain or burning sensation. Many, of course, are asymptomatic and are treated primarily for cosmetic purposes.

Telangiectatic vessels are frequently associated with subdermal reticular veins. Subdermal reticular veins lie just below the dermis and usually transverse the lateral thigh and calf in a longitudinal fashion. When present, they should be treated before treatment of telangiectatic vessels.

There are many reported techniques for sclerotherapy treatment of different-sized varicosities and telangiectatic vessels. Although the specifics of these techniques vary, there are a number of underlying principles. The first is treatment of larger varicosities initially, followed by treatment of smaller varicosities, and then reticular veins, and finally telangiectatic veins. Varicosities greater than 4 to 5mm in size with the patient in the upright position generally respond poorly to sclerotherapy and should be treated by a direct surgical approach (see following).

Treatment of superficial varicosities by injection sclerotherapy begins with the patient in the upright position. First, 1-mL syringes of sclerosant are attached to 23-gauge butterfly needles. The needles are placed in the varicosities approximately every 5 to 7cm and held in place with adhesive tape. The patient is then placed supine and the varicosities are injected. A tight compressive bandage is then placed on the leg, and the patient is instructed to wear this bandage for approximately 5 to 7 days. There is often considerable cutaneous discoloration after removal of the bandage, and this may require months to completely resolve. In a minority of patients, the light-brown hyperpigmentation associated with injection sclerotherapy never resolves completely. A number of solutions may be used for injection sclerotherapy of small varicose veins: these include 0.5% to 1% sodium tetradecyl sulfate, 0.5% to 1% polidoconal (POL) (not FDA-approved), and dextrose sclerodex.

Reticular veins are treated with the patient recumbent. These bluish-green veins are easily seen and cannulated with 30-gauge needles using 1- to 3-mL syringes. Between 0.5 and 1 mL injectate is injected at each site. Some of the sclerosing solutions utilized for treatment of reticular veins include 23.4% hypertonic saline (not FDA-approved for varicose vein treatments), 0.5% to 1% POL (not FDA-approved), and 0.2% to 0.5% sodium tetradecyl sulfate.

Telangiectatic vessels are also treated with the patient supine. Appropriate sclerosing solutions for such vessels include 0.1% to 0.2% sodium tetradecyl sulfate, 0.1% to 0.2% POL (not FDA-approved), or 11.7% to 23.4% hypertonic saline (not FDA-approved). Sclerosing solutions are placed in 1-mL syringes, and the telangiectatic vessels are accessed with 30-gauge needles with the needle bent 10° to 30° with bevel up. Post procedure, the patient's leg is placed in a tight compressive bandage left in place for 5 days.

There are a number of complications associated with sclerotherapy. Initially the patient may experience pain at the time of injection, most frequently with hypertonic saline solutions. Allergic reactions, including anaphylaxis, have been reported with the use of sclerosing solutions. Deep vein thrombosis is a rare complication of superficial vein sclerotherapy. Hyperpigmentation occurs frequently after sclerotherapy of telangiectatic and reticular veins. Generally this resolves over several months but may on occasion be permanent. If the injectate is placed into the subcutaneous tissue rather than into the vein, patients may develop a small ulcer at the site of the injection. Another complication is so-called venous matting, the recurrence of additional telangiectatic vessels in the areas of previous injection. It is thought to be related to insufficient compressive bandaging after the initial procedure.

Vein Stripping and Venous Ablative Proceedurees

Varicose veins not suitable for treatment by injection sclerotherapy may be treated by surgical removal or endovenous ablation using laser or radiofrequency energy. The minimally invasive techniques of laser or radiofrequency ablation are generally applied to either the long or short saphaenous vein with branch varicosities treated either with sclerotherapy or phlbectomy. The so-called stab-avulsion technique is the technique of choice for phlebectomy of branch varicosities. In this technique, tiny, no more than 2-mm, incisions are made directly over branch varicosities. The varicosity is teased away from surrounding subcutaneous tissue as far proximally and distally as possible through the small incision. The vein is then avulsed, and no attempt is made to ligate the vessel. If the patient has significant greater saphenous reflux, the greater saphenous vein should also be removed or ablated with an endovascular technique (see above). With surgical removal, the greater saphenous vein is "stripped" from the level of the saphenous bulb to just below the knee. Stripping to the ankle is not necessary and is associated with a greater incidence of saphenous nerve injury and a resulting burning paraesthesia pain in the instep of the foot. Specific complications associated with removal of superficial varicosities by surgery include bleeding, deep venous thrombosis, and injury to the nerves or arteries of the lower extremity. Complications should be very infrequent, and surgical removal of varicose veins is very well tolerated and effective. Ednovenous ablation either with laser or radiofrequency energey involes percutaneous access to the long or short saphenous vein and delivery of heat to the luminal surface of the vein at sufficient intensity to induce thrombosis and subsequent obliteration of the vein.

Perforator Ligation

Linton and others before him observed that incompetence of the perforating veins connecting the superficial and deep venous systems of the lower extremities may play a role in the development of venous ulceration.[320–323] Linton described a procedure involving ligation of these perforating veins for treatment of CVI.[323] However, this procedure had a high incidence of wound complications. In addition, isolated perforating vein incompetence is uncommon. A newer technique, subfascial endoscopic perforator vein surgery (SEPS), has evolved with the advent of the endoscope. A registry of cases performed using SEPS was the basis of a retrospective analysis of 155 procedures that demonstrated ulcer healing in 88% of ulcers (75 of 85).[324] The procedure was shown to be safe, but follow-up was only 5.4 months on average and concomitant venous procedures, primarily stripping of superficial veins, were performed in 72% of patients. Thus far, the ability of SEPS in improving healing of venous ulcers has not been conclusively demonstrated, althought it may reduce recurrence over time.

Venous Reconstruction

In the absence of deep venous valvular incompetence, saphenous vein stripping and perforator ligation can be effective in treating CVI. Sottiurai has shown, however, that in patients with a combination of superficial and deep venous valvular incompetence, the addition of deep venous valve correction improved the ulcer healing rate from 43% (14 of 33) to 79% (34 of 43) during an average 43 months of follow-up.[325]

Numerous techniques of deep venous valve correction exist for treatment of CVI. These techniques consist of repair of existing valves, transplant of venous segments from the arm, and transposition of an incompetent vein onto an adjacent competent vein. Kistner was the first to perform venous valve repair in 1968[326] and reported a series of valve reconstructions in 1975.[327] Numerous series of venous valve reconstructions by internal suture repair report successful long-term outcomes in the range of 60% to 80%.[237,325,328] However, in patients who initially had ulceration, 40% to 50% had persistence or recurrence of ulcers in the long term.[237,328] In these series, adjunctive venous procedures such as vein stripping and perforator ligation were performed at the discretion of the surgeons involved.

Venous valve transplant involves replacing a segment of superficial femoral vein (SFV) or popliteal vein (PV) where valvular incompetence is present with an axillary vein containing competent valves. Early results of transplant to the SFV are comparable to valve reconstruction,[237,325,328] but long-term results suggest development of valvular incompetence in the transplanted segments with successful outcomes in only 40% to 50%.[237,328] This result may be secondary to the fact that more patients who received valve transplant had CVI secondary to the postthrombotic syndrome rather than primary valve insufficiency.[328] Early reports by Taheri et al.[329] suggest that venous valve transplant to the popliteal segment may be more durable. Venous transposition has successful long-term outcomes in less than 50% of patients, similar to valvular transplant.[330]

Summary

Venous thromboembolism (VTE) continues to be a concern in surgical patients. Specific risk factors for VTE have been identified. Efficacious methods for VTE prophylaxis are available but continue to be underutilized. The diagnosis of VTE can be made noninvasively in a large proportion of patients. Thrombolytic therapy has a limited role in the treatment of VTE but deserves consideration. LMWHs now allow increasing numbers of patients with acute venous thrombosis to be treated as outpatients. Length of treatment for VTE should be at least 3 months for an initial episode and probably indefinite for recurrence.

Chronic venous insufficiency (CVI) results from the postthrombotic state and from primary valvular incompetence. Most patients with CVI can be managed nonoperatively. Surgical repair may have a role in patients with refractory CVI, but these techniques as well as their indications need better definition.

References

1. Anderson FA Jr, Wheeler HB, Goldberg RJ, et al. A population-based perspective of the hospital incidence and case-fatality rates of deep venous thrombosis and pulmonary embolus. Arch Intern Med 1991;151:933–938.
2. Silverstein MD, Heit JA, Mohr DN, Petterson TM, O'Fallon WM, Melton LJ III. Trends in the incidence of deep vein thrombosis and pulmonary embolism; a 25-year population-based study. Arch Intern Med 1998;158:585–593.
3. Anderson FA Jr, Wheeler HB. Venous thromboembolism, risk factors and prophylaxis. Clin Chest Med 1995;16(2):235–251.
4. Dalen JE, Albert JS. Natural history of pulmonary embolism. Prog Cardiovasc Dis 1975;17:257–270.
5. Dismuke SE, Wagner EH. Pulmonary embolism as a cause of death; the changing mortality in hospitalized patients. JAMA 1986;255(15):2039–2042.
6. Salzman EW, Hirsh J. The epidemiology, pathogenesis, and natural history of venous thromboembolism. In: Colman RW, Hirsh J, Marder VJ, Salzman EW, eds. Hemostasis and Thrombosis. Philadelphia: Lippincott, 1994:1275–1296.
7. Anderson FA Jr, Wheeler HB. Physician practices in the management of venous thromboembolism: a community wide survey. J Vasc Surg 1992;16:707–714.
8. Anderson FA Jr, Wheeler HB, Goldberg RJ, Hosner DW, Forcier A. The prevalence of risk factors for venous thromboembolism among hospital patients. Arch Intern Med 1992;152:1660–1664.
9. Carter CJ, Anderson FA Jr, Wheeler HB. Epidemiology and pathophysiology of venous thromboembolism. In: Hull RD, Raskob GE, Pineo GF, eds. Venous Thromboembolism: An Evidence-Based Atlas. Armonk: Futura, 1996:3–27.
10. Nicolaides AN, Irving D. Clinical factors and the risk of deep venous thrombosis. In: Nicolaides AN, eds. Thromboembolism: Aetiology, Advances in Prevention and Management. Lancaster: MTP Press, 1975:193–204.
11. Kakkar VV, Howe CT, Nicolaides AN, Renney JTG, Clarke MB. Deep venous thrombosis of the leg. Is there a "high risk" group? Am J Surg 1970;120:527–530.
12. Nordstrom M, Lindblad B, Bergquist D, Jellstrom T. A prospective study of the incidence of deep-vein thrombosis within a defined urban population. J Intern Med 1992;232:155–160.

13. Samama MM, Simmoneau G, Wainstein JP, et al. SIRIUS study: epidemiology of risk factors of deep venous thrombosis of the lower limbs in community practice. Thromb Haemostasis 1993;69(6):763.
14. Clagett GP, Reisch JS. Prevention of venous thromboembolism in general surgical patients; results of meta-analysis. Ann Surg 1988;208(2):227–240.
15. Stulberg BN, Insall JN, Williams GW, Ghelman B. Deep-vein thrombosis following total knee replacement. J Bone Joint Surg 1984;66A(2):194–201.
16. Hull RD, Raskob GE. Current concepts review; prophylaxis of venous thromboembolic disease following hip and knee surgery. J Bone Joint Surg 1986;68A(1):146–150.
17. Olin JW, Graor RA, O'Hara P, Young JR. The incidence of deep venous thrombosis in patients undergoing abdominal aortic aneurysm resection. J Vasc Surg 1993;18:1037–1041.
18. Gillinov AM, Davis EA, Alberg AJ, et al. Pulmonary embolism in the cardiac surgical patient. Ann Thorac Surg 1992;53:988–991.
19. Reis SE, Polak JF, Hirsch DR, et al. Frequency of deep venous thrombosis in asymptomatic patients with coronary artery bypass grafts. Am Heart J 1991;122:478.
20. Phlegmasia alba dolens. In: Trousseau A. Lectures on Clinical Medicine, Delivered at the Hotel-Dieu, Paris [Cormack JR, transl.]. London: New Syndenham Society, 1872:281–295.
21. Walsh JJ, Bonnar J, Wright FW. A study of pulmonary embolism and deep vein thrombosis after major gynaecological surgery using labeled fibrinogen-phlebography and lung scanning. J Obstet Gynaecol Br Commonw 1974;81:311–316.
22. Sue-Ling HM, Johnston D, McMahon MJ, et al. Preoperative identification of patients at high risk for deep venous thrombosis after elective major abdominal surgery. Lancet 1986;1:1173–1176.
23. Goldberg RJ, Seneff M, Gore JM, et al. Occult malignant neoplasm in patients with deep venous thrombosis. Arch Intern Med 1987;147:251–253.
24. Prandoni P, Lensing AWA, Buller HR, et al. Deep-vein thrombosis and the incidence of subsequent cancer. N Engl J Med 1992;327:1128–1133.
25. Bloom JW, Doggen CJM, Osmoto S, et al. Malignancies, prothrombotic mutatios, and the risk of venous thrombosis. JAMA 2005;293:715–722.
26. WHO Collaborative Study of Cardiovascular Disease and Steroid Hormone Contraception. Venous thromboembolic disease and combined oral contraceptives: results of international multicentre case-control study. Lancet 1995;346:1575–1582.
27. Priten KJ, Miller EV, Mason E, et al. Venous thrombosis in the morbidly obese. Surg Gynecol Obstet 1978;147:63–64.
28. Sevitt S, Gallagher N. Venous thrombosis and pulmonary embolism: a clinico-pathological study in injured and burned patients. Br J Surg 1961;48:475–489.
29. Geerts WH, Code KI, Jay RM, et al. A prospective study of venous thromboembolism after major trauma. N Engl J Med 1994;331:1601–1606.
30. Shackford SR, Davis JW, Hollingsworth-Fridlund P, et al. Venous thromboembolism in patients with major trauma. Am J Surg 1990;159:365–369.
31. Winchell RJ, Hoyt DB, Walsh JC, et al. Risk factors associated with pulmonary embolism despite routine prophylaxis: implications for improved protection. J Trauma 1994;37(4):600–606.
32. May R. Varicose veins. In: May R, ed. Surgery of the Veins of the Leg and Pelvis. Stuttgart: Theime, 1979.
33. Jorgensen JO, Hanel KC, Morgan AM, Hunt JM. The incidence of deep venous thrombosis in patients with superficial thrombophlebitis of the lower limbs. J Vasc Surg 1993;18:70–73.
34. Mauer BJ, Wray R, Shillingford JP. Frequency of venous thrombosis after myocardial infarction. Lancet 1971;ii:1385–1387.
35. Kotilainen M, Ristola P, Ikkala E, Pyorala K. Leg vein thrombosis diagnosed by ^{125}I-fibrinogen test after acute myocardial infarction. Ann Clin Res 1973;5:365–368.
36. Handley AJ, Emerson PA, Fleming PR. Heparin in the prevention of deep vein thrombosis after myocardial infarction. Br Med J 1972;2:436–438.
37. Warlow C, Terry G, Kenmure ACF, et al. A double-blind trial of low-dose subcutaneous heparin in the prevention of deep vein thrombosis after myocardial infarction. Lancet 1973;2:934–937.
38. Devor M, Barrett-Connor E, Renvall M, et al. Estrogen replacement therapy and the risk of venous thrombosis. Am J Med 1991;92:275–282.
39. Boston Collaborative Drug Surveillance Program. Surgically confirmed gall bladder disease, venous thromboembolism, and breast tumours in relation to post-menopausal estrogen therapy. N Engl J Med 1974;290:15–19.
40. Cushman M, and the Woman's Health Initiative Investigators. Estrogen plus progestin and the risk of venous thrombosis. JAMA 2004;292:1573–1580.
41. Smith NL, Heckbert SR, Lemaitre RN, et al. Esterfied estrogens and conjugated equine estrogens and the risk of venous thrombosis. JAMA 2004;292;1581–1587.
42. Gibbs NM. Venous thrombosis of the lower limbs with particular reference to bedrest. Br J Surg 1957;45:209–236.
43. Waring WP, Karunas RS. Acute spinal cord injuries and the incidence of clinically occuring thromboembolic disease. Paraplegia 1991;29:8–16.
44. Green D, Lee Y, Ito VY, et al. Fixed- vs adjusted-dose heparin in the prophylaxis of thromboembolism in spinal cord injury. JAMA 1988;260:1255–1258.
45. Green D, Lee MY, Lim AC, et al. Prevention of thromboembolism after spinal cord injury using low-molecular weight heparin. Ann Intern Med 1990;113:571–574.
46. Ginsberg JS, Brill-Edwards P, Burrows RF, et al. Venous thrombosis during pregnancy: leg and trimester of presentation. Thromb Haemostasis 1992;67(5):519–520.
47. Hull RD, Raskob GE, Carter CJ. Serial impedance plethysmography in pregnant patients with clinically suspected deep venous thrombosis. Ann Intern Med 1990;112:663–667.
48. Monreal M, Raventos A, Lerma R, et al. Pulmonary embolus in patients with upper extremity DVT associated to venous central lines: a prospective study. Thromb Haemostasis 1994;72(4):548–550.
49. Dollery CM, Sullivan ID, Bauraind O, et al. Thrombosis and embolism in long-term central venous access for parenteral nutrition. Lancet 1994;344:1043–1045.
50. Trottier SJ, Veremakis C, O'Brien J, Auer AI. Femoral deep vein thrombosis associated with central venous catheterization: results from a prospective randomized trial. Crit Care Med 1995;23(1):52–59.
51. Meredith JW, Young JS, O'Neil EA, et al. Femoral catheters and deep venous thrombosis: a prospective evaluation with venous duplex sonography. J Trauma 1993;35(2):187–191.
52. Shefler A, Gillis J, Lam A, et al. Inferior vena cava thrombosis as a complication of femoral vein catheterisation. Arch Dis Child 1995;72:343–345.
53. Bick RL, Kaplan H. Syndromes of thrombosis and hypercoagulability, congenital and acquired causes of thrombosis. Med Clin N Am 1998;82(3):409–458.
54. Svensson PJ, Dahlback B. Resistance to activated protein C as a basis for thrombosis. N Engl J Med 1994;330:517–522.
55. Barritt DW, Jordan SC. Anticoagulant drugs in the treatment of pulmonary embolism: a controlled trial. Lancet 1960;1:1309–1312.
56. Markel A, Manzo RA, Bergelin RO, Strandness DE Jr. Pattern and distribution of thrombi in acute venous thrombosis. Arch Surg 1992;127:305–309.

57. Kakkar VV, Howe CT, Franc C, Clarke MB. Natural history of postoperative deep venous thrombosis. Lancet 1969;2:230–232.
58. Nicolaides AN, Kakkar VV, Field ES, Renney JTG. The origin of deep venous thrombosis: a venographic study. Br J Radiol 1971;44:653–663.
59. Philbrik JT, Becker DM. Calf deep venous thrombosis; a wolf in sheep's clothing. Arch Intern Med 1988;148:2131–2138.
60. Doouss TW. The clinical significance of venous thrombosis of the calf. Br J Surg 1976;63:377–378.
61. Kakkar VV, Lawrence D. Hemodynamic and clinical assessment after therapy for deep vein thrombosis: a prospective study. Am J Surg 1985;150(4A):54–63.
62. Langerstedt CI, Olsson CG, Fagher BO, et al. Need for longterm anticoagulant treatment in symptomatic calf-vein thrombosis. Lancet 1985;2:515–518.
63. Hull R, Delmore T, Genton E, et al. Warfarin sodium versus low-dose heparin in the long-term treatment of venous thrombosis. N Engl J Med 1979;301:855–858.
64. Bentley PG, Kakkar VV, Scully MF, et al. An objective study of alternative methods of heparin administration. Thromb Res 1980;18:177–187.
65. Schulman S, Granqvist S, Juhlin-Danfelt A, et al. Long-term sequelae of calf vein thrombosis treated with heparin or low-dose streptokinase. Acta Med Scand 1986;219:349–357.
66. Kistner RL, Ball JJ, Nordyke RA, et al. Incidence of pulmonary embolism in the course of thrombophlebitis of the lower extremities. Am J Surg 1972;124:169–176.
67. Menzoian JO, Sequeira JC, Doyle JE, et al. Therapeutic and clinical course of deep vein thrombosis. Am J Surg 1983;146:581–585.
68. Holmgren K, Andersson G, Fagrell B, et al. One-month versus six-month therapy with oral anticoagulants after symptomatic deep venous thrombosis. Acta Med Scand 1985;218:279–284.
69. Schulman S, Lockner D, Juhlin-Dannfelt A. The duration of oral anticoagulation after deep vein thrombosis: a randomized study. Acta Med Scand 1985;217:547–552.
70. Lohr JM, Kerr TM, Lutter KS, et al. Lower extremity calf thrombosis: to treat or not to treat. J Vasc Surg 1991;14:618–623.
71. Passman MA, Moneta GL, Taylor LM, et al. Pulmonary embolism is associated with the combination of isolated calf vein thrombosis and respiratory symptoms. J Vasc Surg 1997;25:39–45.
72. Hull RD, Raskob GE, Hirsh J, et al. Continuous intravenous heparin compared with intermittent subcutaneous heparin in the initial treatment of proximal-vein thrombosis. N Engl J Med 1986;315:1109–1114.
73. Brandjes DPM, Heijboer H, Buller HR, et al. Acenocoumarol and heparin compared with acenocoumarol alone in the initial treatment of proximal-vein thrombosis. N Engl J Med 1992;327:1485–1489.
74. Schulman S, Rhedin AS, Lindmarker P, et al. A comparison of six weeks with six months of oral anticoagulant therapy after a first episode of venous thromboembolism. N Engl J Med 1995;332:1661–1665.
75. Moser KM, Fedullo PF, LitteJohn JK, Crawford R. Frequent asymptomatic pulmonary embolism in patients with deep venous thrombosis. JAMA 1994;271:223–225.
76. Nielsen HK, Husted SE, Kursell LR, et al. Silent pulmonary embolism in patients with deep venous thrombosis. Incidence and fate in a randomized, controlled trial of anticoagulation versus no anticoagulation. J Intern Med 1994;235:457–461.
77. Caprinin JA, Arcelus JI, Hoffman KN, et al. Venous duplex imaging follow-up of acute symptomatic deep vein thrombosis of the leg. J Vasc Surg 1995;21:472–476.
78. Donaldson GA, Williams C, Scannel JG, et al. A reappraisal of the application of the Trendelenburg operation to massive fatal embolism: report of a successful pulmonary-artery thrombectomy using cardiopulmonary bypass. N Engl J Med 1963;268:171–174.
79. Carson JL, Kelley MA, Duff A, et al. The clinical course of pulmonary embolism. N Engl J Med 1992;326:1240–1245.
80. Dalen JE, Banas JS Jr, Brooks HL, et al. Resolution rate of acute pulmonary embolus in man. N Engl J Med 1992;280:1194–1199.
81. National Heart, Lung and Blood Institute. Urokinase Pulmonary Embolism Trial: phase I results. JAMA 1970;214:2163–2172.
82. Salzman EW, Hirsh J. Prevention of venous thromboembolism. In: Colman RW, Hirsh J, Marder VJ, Salzman EW, eds. Hemostasis and Thrombosis: Basic Principles and Clinical Practice. Philadelphia: Lippincott, 1987:1253.
83. Clagett GP, Anderson FA Jr, Levine MN, et al. Prevention of venous thromboembolism. Chest 1992;4:391S–407S.
84. Kakkar VV, Cohen AT, Edmonson RA, et al. Low molecular weight versus standard heparin for prevention of venous thromboembolism after major abdominal surgery. Lancet 1993;341:259–265.
85. Nurmohamed MT, Verhaeghe R, Haas S, et al. A comparative trial of a low molecular weight heparin (enoxaparin) versus standard heparin for the prophylaxis of postoperative deep vein thrombosis in general surgery. Am J Surg 1995;169:567–571.
86. Koppenhagen K, Adolf J, Matthes M, et al. Low molecular weight heparin and prevention of postoperative thrombosis in abdominal surgery. Thromb Haemostasis 1992;67(6):627–630.
87. Geerts WH, Pineo, GF, Heit JA, et al. Prevention of venous thromboembolism: the 7th ACCP conference on antithrombotic and thrombolytic therapy. Chest 2004;126:388S–400S.
88. Mohr DN, Silverstein MD, Murtaugh PA, Harrison JM. Prophylactic agents for venous thrombosis in elective hip surgery; meta-analysis of studies using venographic assessment. Arch Intern Med 1993;153:2221–2228.
89. Francis CW, Pellegrini VD, Marder VJ, et al. Comparison of warfarin and external pneumatic compression in prevention of venous thrombosis after total hip replacement. JAMA 1992;267: 2911–2915.
90. Hull R, Delmore TJ, Hirsh J, et al. Effectiveness of intermittent pulsatile stockings for prevention of calf and thigh vein thrombosis in patients undergoing elective knee surgery. Thromb Res 1979;16:37–45.
91. McKenna R, Galante J, Bachman F, et al. Prevention of venous thromboembolism after total knee replacement using high-dose aspirin or intermittent calf and thigh compression. Br Med J 1980;1:514–517.
92. Cerrato D, Ariano C, Fiacchino F. Deep vein thrombosis and low-dose heparin prophylaxis in neurosurgical patients. J Neurosurg 1978;137:378–381.
93. Dennis JW, Menawat S, Von Thron J, et al. Efficacy of deep venous thrombosis prophylaxis in trauma patients and identification of high-risk groups. J Trauma 1993;35(1):132–139.
94. Geerts WH, Jay RM, Code KI, et al. A comparison of low-dose heparin with low molecular weight heparin as prophylaxis against venous thromboembolism after major trauma. N Engl J Med 1996;355:701–707.
95. Rogers FB, Shackford SR, Ricci MA, et al. Routine prophylactic vena cava filter insertion in severely injured trauma patients decreases the incidence of pulmonary embolism. J Am Coll Surg 1995;180(6):641–647.
96. Alexander JJ, Yuhas JP, Piotrowski JJ. Is the increasing use of prophylactic percutaneous IVC filters justified. Am J Surg 1994;168:102–106.
97. Harris EJ Jr, Kinney EV, Harris EJ Sr, et al. Phlegmasia complicating prophylactic inferior vena caval interruption: a work of caution. J Vasc Surg 1995;22:606–611.
98. Ray CE, Mitchell EL, Zipser S, et al. Outcomes with retrievable vena cava filters: a multicenter study. J Vasc Intervent Radiol 2006;17:1595–1604.

99. Huber O, Bounameaux H, Borst F, Rohner A. Postoperative pulmonary embolism after hospital discharge; an undetermined risk. Arch Surg 1992;127:310–313.
100. Trowbridge A, Boese CK, Woodruff B, et al. Incidence of posthospital proximal deep venous thrombosis after total hip arthroplasty; a pilot study. Clin Orthop Res 1994;299:203–208.
101. Planes A, Vochelle N, Darmon J, et al. Risk of deep-venous thrombosis after hospital discharge in patients having undergone total hip replacement: double-blind randomised comparison of enoxaparin versus placebo. Lancet 1996;348:224–228.
102. Hull RD, Hirsh J, Sackett DL, et al. Clinical validity of a negative venogram in patients with a clinically suspected venous thrombosis. Circulation 1981;64:622–625.
103. Bettmann MA, Salzman EW, Rosenthal D, et al. Reduction of venous thrombosis complicating phlebography. Am J Roentgenol 1980;134:1169–1172.
104. Walters HL, Clemenson J, Browse NL, Lea TM. ^{125}I-Fibrinogen uptake following phlebography of the leg: comparison of ionic and nonionic contrast media. Radiology 1980;135:619–621.
105. Laerum F, Holm HA. Post-phlebographic thrombosis. Radiology 1981;140:651–654.
106. AbuRahma AF, Powell M, Robinson PA. Prospective study of safety of lower extremity phlebography with nonionic contrast medium. Am J Surg 1996;171:255–257.
107. Comerota AJ, Katz ML, Grossi RJ, et al. The comparative value of noninvasive testing for diagnosis and surveillance of deep vein thrombosis. J Vasc Surg 1988;7:40–49.
108. Cruickshank MK, Levine MN, Hirsh J, et al. An evaluation of impedance plethysmography and 125I-fibrinogen leg scanning in patients following hip surgery. Thromb Haemostasis 1989;62(3): 830–834.
109. Hull RD, Hirsh J, Carter CJ, et al. Diagnostic efficacy of impedance plethysmography for clinically suspected deep-vein thrombosis; a randomized trial. Ann Intern Med 1985;102:21–28.
110. Huisman MV, Buller HR, ten Cate JW, Vreeken J. Serial impedance plethysmography for suspected deep venous thrombosis in outpatients; the Amsterdam general practitioner study. N Engl J Med 1986;314:823–828.
111. Huisman MV, Buller HR, ten Cate JW, et al. Management of clinically suspected acute venous thrombosis in outpatients with serial impedance plethysmography in a community hospital setting. Arch Intern Med 1989;149:511–513.
112. Agnelli G, Cosmi B, Ranucci V, et al. Impedance plethysmography in the diagnosis of asymptomatic deep vein thrombosis in hip surgery; a venography-controlled study. Ann Intern Med 1991;151:2167–2171.
113. Paiement G, Wessinger SJ, Waltman AC, et al. Surveillance of deep vein thrombosis in asymptomatic total hip replacement patients; impedance phlebography and fibrinogen scanning versus roentgenographic phlebography. Am J Surg 1988;155:400–404.
114. Anderson DR, Lensing AWA, Wells PS, et al. Limitations of impedance plethysmography in the diagnosis of clinically suspected deep-vein thrombosis. Ann Intern Med 1993;118:25–30.
115. Lensing AWA, Prandoni P, Brandjes D, et al. Detection of deep-vein thrombosis by real-time B-mode ultrasonography. N Engl J Med 1989;320:342–345.
116. Cronan JJ, Dorfman GS, Scola FH, et al. Deep venous thrombosis: US assessment using vein compression. Radiology 1987;162:191–194.
117. Appelman PT, De Jong TE, Lampmann LE. Deep venous thrombosis of the leg: US findings. Radiology 1987;163:743–746.
118. Vogel P, Laing FC, Jeffrey RB Jr, Wing VW. Deep venous thrombosis of the lower extremity: US evaluation. Radiology 1987; 163:747–751.
119. O'Leary DH, Kane RA, Chase BM. A prospective study of the efficacy of B-scan sonography in the detection of deep venous thrombosis in the lower extremities. J Clin Ultrasound 1988;16:1–8.
120. Lensing AWA, Levi MM, Buller HR, et al. Diagnosis of deep vein thrombosis using an objective doppler method. Ann Intern Med 1990;113:9–13.
121. Heijboer H, Cogo A, Buller HR, et al. Detection of deep vein thrombosis with impedance plethysmography and real-time compression ultrasonography in hospitalized patients. Arch Intern Med 1992;152:1901–1903.
122. Heijboer H, Buller HR, Lensing AWA, et al. A randomized comparison of the clinical utility of real-time compression ultrasonography versus impedance plethysmography in the diagnosis of deep-vein thrombosis in symptomatic outpatients. N Engl J Med 1993;329:1365–1369.
123. Kearou C, Ginsberg JS, Donketis JS, et al. A randomized trial of diagnostic strategies after normal proximal vein ultrasonography for suspected deep venous thrombosis; D-dimer testing compared with repeated ultrasonography. Ann Intern Med 2005;142:490–496.
124. Vermeer HJ, Ypma P, van Strijen MJL, et al. Exclusion of venous thromboembolism: evaluation of D-dimer PLUS for the quantitative determination of D-dimer. Thromb Res 2005;115:381–386.
125. Constams J, Boutinet C, Salmi LR, et al. Comparison of four clinical prediction scores for the diagnosis of lower limb venous thrombosis in outpatients. Am J Med 2003;115:436–440.
126. Wells PS, Brill-Edwards P, Stevens P, et al. A novel and rapid whole-blood assay for D-dimer in patients with clinically suspected deep vein thrombosis. Circulation 1995;91:2184–2187.
127. Stein PD, Terrin ML, Hales CA, et al. Clinical, laboratory, roentgenographic, and electrographic findings in patients with acute pulmonary embolism and no pre-existing cardiac or pulmonary disease. Chest 1991;100:598–603.
128. Stein PD, Athanasoulis C, Alavi A, et al. Complications and validity of pulmonary angiography in acute pulmonary embolism. Circulation 1992;85:462–468.
129. Sasahara AA, Stein M, Simon M, Littmann D. Pulmonary angiography in the diagnosis of thromboembolic disease. N Engl J Med 1964;270:1075–1081.
130. The Urokinase Pulmonary Embolism trial: a national cooperative study. Circulation 1973;47(suppl II):II-1–II-108.
131. Mills SR, Jackson DC, Older RA, et al. The incidence, etiologies, and avoidance of complications of pulmonary angiography in a large series. Radiology 1980;136:295–299.
132. Dalen JE, Brooks HL, Johnson LW, et al. Pulmonary angiography in acute pulmonary embolism; indications, techniques, and results in 367 patients. Am Heart J 1971;81:175–185.
133. Henry JW, Relyea B, Stein PD. Continuing risk of thromboemboli among patients with normal pulmonary angiograms. Chest 1995;107:1375–1378.
134. The PIOPED Investigators. Value of the ventilation/perfusion scan in acute pulmonary embolism; results of the prospective investigation of pulmonary embolism diagnosis (PIOPED). JAMA 1990;263:2753–2759.
135. Stein PD, Coleman RE, Gottschalk A, et al. Diagnostic utility of ventilation/perfusion lung scans in acute pulmonary embolism is not diminished by pre-existing cardiac or pulmonary disease. Chest 1991;100:604–606.
136. Bounameaux H, Cirafici P, DeMoerloose P, et al. Measurement of D-dimer in plasma as diagnostic aid in suspected pulmonary embolism. Lancet 1991;337:196–200.
137. Turkstra F, van Beek EJR, ten Cate JW, Buller HR. Reliable rapid blood test for the exclusion of venous thromboembolism in symptomatic outpatients. Thromb Haemostasis 1996;76(1):9–11.
138. Killewich LA, Nunnelee JD, Auer AI. Value of lower extremity venous duplex examination in the diagnosis of pulmonary embolism. J Vasc Surg 1993;17:934–939.

139. Hull RD, Hirsh J, Carter CJ, et al. Pulmonary angiography, ventilation lung scanning and venography for clinically suspected pulmonary embolism with abnormal perfusion lung scan. Ann Intern Med 1983;98:891–899.
140. Kruit WHJ, DeBoer AC, Sing AK, Van Roon F. The significance of venography in the management of patients with clinically suspected pulmonary embolism. J Intern Med 1991;230:333–339.
141. Schiebler ML, Holland GA, Hatabu H, et al. Suspected pulmonary embolism: prospective evaluation with pulmonary MR angiography. Radiology 1993;189:125–131.
142. Stein PD, Fowler SE, Goodman LR, et al. Multidetector computed tomography for acute pulmonary embolism. N Engl J Med 2006;354:2317–2327.
143. Markel A, Manzo RA, Standness DE. The potential role of thrombolytic therapy in venous thrombosis. Arch Intern Med 1992;152:1265–1267.
144. Goldhaber SZ, Hirsch DR, MacDougall RC, et al. Bolus recombinant urokinase versus heparin in deep venous thrombosis: a randomized controlled trial. Am Heart J 1996;132:314–318.
145. Tiller WS, Garner RL. The fibrinolytic activity of hemolytic streptococci. J Exp Med 1933;58:485.
146. MacFarlane RG, Pilling J. Fibrinolytic activity of normal urine. Nature (Lond) 1947;159:779.
147. Rijken DC, Wijngaards G, Zaal-DeJong M, et al. Purification and partial characterization of plasminogen activator from human uterine tissue. Biochim Biophys Acta 1979;580:140.
148. Goldhaber SZ, Buring JE, Lipnik RJ, Hennekens CH. Pooled analyses of randomized trials of streptokinase and heparin in phlebographically documented acute deep venous thrombosis. Am J Med 1984;76:393–397.
149. Robertson BR, Nilsson IM, Nylander G. Value of streptokinase and heparin in treatment of acute deep venous thrombosis: a coded investigation. Acta Chir Scand 1968;134:203–208.
150. Porter JM, Seaman AJ, Common HH, et al. Comparison of heparin and streptokinase in the treatment of venous thrombosis. Am Surg 1975;41:511–519.
151. Elliot MS, Immelman EJ, Jeffery P, et al. A comparative randomized trial of heparin versus streptokinase in the treatment of acute proximal venous thrombosis; an interim report of a prospective trial. Br J Surg 1979;66:838–843.
152. Kakkar VV, Flanc C, Howe CT, et al. Treatment of deep vein thrombosis: a trial of heparin, streptokinase, and arvin. Br Med J 1969;1:806–810.
153. Robertson BR, Nilsson IM, Nylander G. Thrombolytic effect of streptokinase as evaluated by phlebography of deep venous thrombi of the leg. Acta Chir Scand 1970;136:173–180.
154. Tsapogas MJ, Peabody RA, Wu KT, et al. Controlled study of thrombolytic therapy in deep vein thrombosis. Surgery (St. Louis) 1973;74:973–984.
155. Goldhaber SZ, Polak JF, Feldstein ML, et al. Efficacy and safety of repeated boluses of urokinase in the treatment of deep venous thrombosis. Am J Cardiol 1994;73:75–79.
156. Kakkar VV, Lawrence D. Hemodynamic and clinical assessment after therapy for acute deep vein thrombosis; a prospective study. Am J Surg 1985:54–63.
157. Comerota AJ, Aldridge SC, Cohen G, et al. A strategy of aggressive regional therapy for acute iliofemoral venous thrombosis with contemporary venous thrombectomy or catheter-directed thrombolysis. J Vasc Surg 1994;20:244–254.
158. Molina JE, Hunter D, Yedlicka JW. Thrombolytic therapy for iliofemoral venous thrombosis. Vasc Surg 1992;26:630–637.
159. National Heart and Lung Institute Cooperative Study Group: Urokinase-Streptokinase Embolism Trial: Phase II results. JAMA 1974;229:1606–1613.
160. NIH Consensus Development Conference: thrombolytic therapy in treatment. Br Med J 1980;1:1585.
161. Goldhaber SZ, Vaughan DE, Markis JE, et al. Acute pulmonary embolus treated with tissue plasminogen activator. Lancet 1986;ii:886–889.
162. Goldhaber SZ, Kessler CM, Heit J, et al. Randomised controlled trial of recombinant tissue plasminogen activator versus urokinase in the treatment of acute pulmonary embolism. Lancet 1988;ii:293–298.
163. Dalla-Volta S, Palla A, Santolicandro A, et al. PAIMS 2: altepase combined with heparin versus heparin in the treatment of acute pulmonary embolism. Plasminogen activator Italian multicenter study 2. J Am Coll Cardiol 1992;20:520–526.
164. Meyer G, Sors H, Charbonnier B, et al. Effects of intravenous urokinase versus alteplase on total pulmonary resistance in acute massive pulmonary embolism: a European multicenter double-blind trial. J Am Coll Cardiol 1992;19:239–245.
165. Goldhaber SZ, Haire WD, Feldstein ML, et al. Alteplase versus heparin in acute pulmonary embolism: randomised trial assessing right-ventricular function and pulmonary perfusion. Lancet 1993;341:507–511.
166. Verstraete M, Miller GAH, Bounameaus H, et al. Intravenous and intrapulmonary recombinant tissue-type plasminogen activator in the treatment of acute massive pulmonary embolism. Circulation 1988;77:353–360.
167. Hull RD, Raskob GE, Rosenbloom D, et al. Optimal therapeutic level of heparin therapy in patients with venous thrombosis. Arch Intern Med 1992;152:1589–1595.
168. Raschke RA, Reilly BM, Guidry JR, et al. The weight-based heparin dosing nomogram compared with a "standard care" nomogram: a randomized controlled trial. Ann Intern Med 1993;119:874–881.
169. Hull RD, Raskob GE, Rosenbloom D, et al. Heparin for 5 days as compared with 10 days in the initial treatment of proximal venous thrombosis. N Engl J Med 1990;322:1260–1264.
170. Warkentin TE, Kelton JG. Heparin and platelets. Hematol Oncol Clin N Am 1990;4:243.
171. Warkentin TE, Levine MN, Hirsh J, et al. Heparin-induced thrombocytopenia in patients treated with low-molecular-weight heparin of unfractionated heparin. N Engl J Med 1995;332:1330.
172. Amiral J, Bridey F, Dreyfus M, et al. Platelet factor 4 complexed to heparin is the target for antibodies generated in heparin-induced thrombocytopenia. Thromb Haemostasis 1992;68:95.
173. Aster RH. Heparin-induced thrombocytopenia and thrombosis. N Engl J Med 1995;332:1374.
174. Wallis DE, Lewis BE, Pifarre R, et al. Active surveillance for heparin-induced thrombocytopenia or thromboembolism. Chest 106;1994:106:120S.
175. Hirsch J, Raschke R, Warkentin TE, et al. Heparin: mechanism of action, pharmacokinetics, dosing considerations, monitoring, efficacy and safety. Chest 1995;108(suppl):258–275.
176. Link KP. The discovery of dicumarol and its sequels. Circulation 1959;19:97–107.
177. Link KP. The anticoagulant from spoiled sweet clover hay. Harvey Lect 1944;34:162–216.
178. Hirsh J, Dalen JE, Deykin D, et al. Oral anticogulants: mechanism of action, clinical effectiveness, and optimal therapeutic range. Chest 1995;108(suppl 4):231–465.
179. Mohiuddin SM, Hilleman DE, Destache CJ, et al. Efficacy and safety of early versus late initiation of warfarin during therapy in acute thromboembolism. Am Heart J 1992;123:729–732.
180. Safety and efficacy of warfarin started early after submassive venous thrombosis of pulmonary embolism. Lancet 1986;ii:1293–1296.
181. Coon WW, Willis PW III, Symons MJ. Assessment of anticoagulant treatment of venous thromboembolism. Ann Surg 1969;170:559–568.

182. Hull R, Delmore T, Genton E, et al. Warfarin versus low-dose heparin in the long-term treatment of venous thrombosis. N Engl J Med 1979;301:855–858.
183. Schulman S, Lockner D, Juhlin-Dannfelt A. The duration of anticoagulation after deep vein thrombosis: a randomized study. Acta Med Scand 1985;217:547–552.
184. Holmgren K, Andersson G, Fagrell B, et al. One-month versus six-month therapy with oral anticoagulants after symptomatic deep vein thrombosis. Acta Med Scand 1985;218:279–284.
185. Schulman S, Rhedin AS, Lindmarker P, et al. A comparison of six weeks with six months of oral anticoagulant therapy after a first episode of venous thromboembolism. N Engl J Med 1995;332:1661–1665.
186. Schulman S, Granqvist S, Holmstrom M, et al. The duration of oral anticoagulant therapy after a second episode of venous thromboembolism. N Engl J Med 1997;336:393–398.
187. Kearon C, Ginsberg JS, Kovacs MJ, et al. Comparison of low-intensity warfarin therapy with conventional intensity warfarin therapy for long-term prevention of recurrent venous thromboembolism. N Engl J Med 2003;349:631–639.
188. Eichinger S, Minar E, Bialouczyk KC, et al. D-Dimer levels and risk of recurrent venous thromboembolism. JAMA 2003;290:1071–1074.
189. Palareti G, Cosmi B, Legnani C, et al. D-Dimer testing to determine the duration of anticoagulation therapy. N Engl J Med 2006;355:1780–1789.
190. Hron G, Kollars N, Binden BR, et al. Identification of patients at low risk for recurrent venous thromboembolism by measuring thrombin generation. JAMA 2006;296:397–402.
191. Anderson LO, Barrowcliffe TW, Holmer E, et al. Molecular weight dependency of the heparin potentiated inhibition of thrombin and activated factor X: effect of heparin neutralization in plasma. Thromb Res 1979;115:531–538.
192. Fareed J, Walenga JM, Racanelli A, et al. Validity of the newly established low molecular weight heparin standard in cross referencing low molecular weight heparins. Haemostasis 1988;3(suppl):33–47.
193. Fareed J, Walenga JM, Hoppensteadt D, et al. Comparative study on the in vitro and in vivo activities of seven low-molecular weight heparins. Haemostasis 1988;18(suppl):3–15.
194. Boneu B, Caranobe C, Cadroy Y, et al. Pharmacokinetic studies of standard unfractionated heparin, and low molecular weight heparins in the rabbit. Semin Thromb Hemostasis 1988;14:18–27.
195. Matzsch T, Bergqvist D, Hedner U, et al. Effects of low molecular weight heparin and unfragmented heparin on induction of osteoporosis in rats. Thromb Haemostasis 1990;63:505–509.
196. Prandoni P, Lensing AWA, Buller HR, et al. Comparison of subcutaneous low-molecular-weight heparin with intravenous standard heparin in proximal deep-vein thrombosis. Lancet 1992;339:441–445.
197. Lindmarker P, Holstrom M, Granqvist S, et al. Comparison of once-daily subcutaneous fragmin with continuous intravenous unfractionated heparin in the treatment of deep vein thrombosis. Thromb Haemostasis 1994;72(2):186–190.
198. Simmonneau G, Charbonnier B, Decousus H, et al. Subcutaneous low-molecular-weight heparin compared with continuous intravenous unfractionated heparin in the treatment of proximal deep vein thrombosis. Arch Intern Med 1993;153:1541–1546.
199. Hull RD, Raskob GE, Pineo GF, et al. Subcutaneous low-molecular-weight heparin compared with continuous intravenous heparin in the treatment of proximal-vein thrombosis. N Engl J Med 1992;326:975–982.
200. Koopman MMW, Prandoni P, Piovella F, et al. Treatment of venous thrombosis with intravenous unfractionated heparin in the hospital as compared with subcutaneous low-molecular-weight heparin administered at home. N Engl J Med 1996;334:682–687.
201. Levine M, Gent M, Hirsh J, et al. A comparison of low-molecular-weight heparin administered primarily at home with unfractionated heparin administered in the hospital for proximal deep-vein thrombosis. N Engl J Med 1996;334:677–681.
202. Hull RD, Raskob GE, Pineo GF, et al. A comparison of subcutaneous low-molecular-weight heparin with warfarin sodium for prophylaxis against deep-vein thrombosis after hip or knee implantation. N Engl J Med 1993;329:1370–1376.
203. Muir JM, Hirsh J, Weitz JI, et al. A histomorphometric comparison of the effects of heparin and low-molecular-weight heparin on cancellous bone in rats. Blood 1997;89:3236–3242.
204. Murray WJ, Lindo VS, Kakkar VV, et al. Long term administration of heparin and heparin fractions and osteoporosis in experimental animals. Blood Coagul Fibrinolysis 1995;6:113–118.
205. Shaughnessy SG, Young E, Deschamps P, et al. The effects of low molecular weight and standard heparin on calcium loss from fetal rat calvaria. Blood 1995;86:1368–1373.
206. Kanter B, Moser KM. The Greenfield vena cava filter. Chest 1988;93:170–175.
207. Molgaard CP, Yucel EK, Geller SC, et al. Access-site thrombosis after placement of inferior vena cava filters with 12–14 Fr delivery sheaths. Radiology 1992;185:257–261.
208. Becker DM, Philbrick JT, Selby JB. Inferior vena cava filters; indications, safety, effectiveness. Arch Intern Med 1992;152:1985–1994.
209. Hammer FD, Rousseau HP, Joffre FG, et al. In vitro evaluation of vena cava filters. J Vasc Intervent Radiol 1994;5:869–876.
210. Mohan CR, Hoballah JJ, Sharp WJ, et al. Comparative efficacy and complications of vena cava filters. J Vasc Surg 1995;21:235–246.
211. Lohr JM, McDevitt DT, Lutter KS, et al. Operative management of greater saphenous thrombophlebitis involving the saphenofemoral junction. Am J Surg 1992;164:269–275.
212. Ascer E, Lorensen E, Pollina RM, et al. Preliminary results of a nonoperative approach to saphenofemoral junction thrombophlebitis. J Vasc Surg 1995;22:616–621.
213. Lansing AM, Davis WM. Five-year follow-up study of iliofemoral venous thrombectomy. Ann Surg 1968;168:620–628.
214. Juhan CM, Alimi YS, Barthelemy PJ, et al. Late results of iliofemoral venous thrombectomy. J Vasc Surg 1997;25:417–422.
215. Lindner DJ, Edwards JM, Phinney ES, et al. Long-term hemodynamic and clinical sequelae of lower extremity deep venous thrombosis. J Vasc Surg 1986;4:436–442.
206. Schmid C, Zietlow S, Wagner TOF, et al. Fulminant pulmonary embolism: symptoms, diagnostics, operative techniques and results. Ann Thorac Surg 1991;52:402–407.
207. Kieny R, Charpentier A, Kieny MT. What is the place of pulmonary embolectomy today? J Cardiovasc Surg 1991;32:549–554.
208. Gulba DC, Schmid C, Borst H-B, et al. Medical compared with surgical treatment for massive pulmonary embolism. Lancet 1994;343:576–577.
209. Greenfield LJ, Proctor MC, Williams DM, Wakefield TW. Long-term experience with transvenous catheter pulmonary embolectomy. J Vasc Surg 1993;18:450–458.
220. Brand FN, Dannenberg AL, Abbott RD, Kannel WB. The epidemiology of varicose veins: the Framingham study. Am J Prev Med 1988;4:96.
221. Madar G, Widmer LK, Zemp E, Maggs M. Varicose veins and chronic venous insufficiency—a disorder or disease? A critical epidemiological review. Vasa 1986;15:126.
222. Jamieson WG. State of the art of venous investigation and treatment. Can J Surg 1993;36:119.
223. Scott TE, La Morte WW, Gorin DR, et al. Risk factors for chronic venous insufficiency: a dual case-control study. J Vasc Surg 1995;22:622.
224. Criado E, Johnson G Jr. Venous disease. Curr Probl 1991;28:339.

225. Baker SR, Stacey MC, Jopp-McKay AG, et al. Ulcers. Br J Surg 1991;78:864.
226. Cornwall JV, Dore CJ, Lewis JD. Leg ulcers: epidemiology and aetiology. Br J Surg 1986;73:693.
227. Lees TA, Lambert D. Prevalence of lower limb ulcers in an urban health district. Br J Surg 1992;79:1032.
228. Phillips T, Stanton B, Provan A, et al. A study of the impact of leg ulcers on quality of life: financial, social, and psychologic implications. J Am Acad Dermatol 1994;31:49.
229. Callam MJ, Harper DR, Dale JJ, Ruckley CV. Chronic leg ulceration: socioeconomic aspects. Scott Med J 1988;33: 358.
230. Browse NL, Burnand KG, Thomas ML. Diseases of the Veins. Pathology, Diagnosis and Treatment. London: Hodder and Stoughton, 1988.
231. Callam MJ, Harper DR, Dale JJ, Ruckley CV. Chronic ulcer of the leg: clinical history. Br Med J 1987;294:1389.
232. Abenhaim L, Kurx X, VEINES Study Collaborators. The VEINES Study: an international cohort study on chronic venous disorders of the leg. Angiology 1997;48:59.
233. Clarke H, Smith SR, Vasdekis SN, et al. Role of venous elasticity in the development of varicose veins. Br J Surg 1989;76:577.
234. Clarke GH. Venous elasticity. Doctoral thesis. London: University of London, 1989.
235. Clarke GH, Vasdekis SN, Hobbs JT, Nicolaides AN. Venous wall function in the pathogenesis of varicose veins. Surgery (St. Louis) 1992;111:402.
236. Nicolaides AN, Zukowski AJ. The value of dynamic pressure measurements. World J Surg 1986;10:919.
237. Raju S, Fredericks R. Valve reconstruction procedures for non-obstructive venous insufficiency: rationale, techniques, and results in 107 procedures with two- to eight-year followup. J Vasc Surg 1988;7:301.
238. Randhawa GK, Dhillon JS, Kistner RL, Ferries EB. Assessment of chronic venous insufficiency using dynamic venous pressure studies. Am J Surg 1984;148:203.
239. Araki CT, Back TL, Padberg FT, et al. The significance of calf muscle pump function in venous ulceration. J Vasc Surg 1994;20:872.
240. Back TL, Padberg FT, Araki CT, et al. Limited range of motion is a significant factor in venous ulceration. J Vasc Surg 1995;22:519.
241. van Bemmelen PS, Bedford G, Beach K, Strandness DE. Quantitative segmental evaluation of venous valvular reflux with duplex ultrasound scanning. J Vasc Surg 1989;10:425.
242. Rosfors S, Lamke LO, Nordstrom E, Bygdeman S. Severity and location of venous valvular insufficiency: the importance of distal valve function. Acta Chir Scand 1990;156:689.
243. Hanrahan LM, Araki CT, Rodriguez AA, et al. Distribution of valvular incompetence in patients with venous stasis ulceration. J Vasc Surg 1991;13:805.
244. Moore DJ, Himmel PD, Summer DS. Distribution of venous valvular incompetence in patients with the postphlebitic syndrome. J Vasc Surg 1986;3:49.
245. Sethia KK, Darke SG. Long saphenous incompetence as a cause of venous ulceration. Br J Surg 1984;71:754.
246. Hoare MC, Nicolaides AN, Miles CR, et al. The role of primary varicose veins in venous ulceration. Surgery (St. Louis) 1982; 92:450.
247. Labropoulos N, Giannoukas AD, Nicolaides AN, et al. New insights into the pathophysiologic condition of venous ulceration with color-flow duplex imaging: implications for treatment? J Vasc Surg 1995;22:45.
248. Linton RR, Hardy IB. Postthrombotic syndrome of the lower extremity: treatment by interruption of the superficial femoral vein and ligation and stripping of the long and short saphenous veins. Surgery (St. Louis) 1948;24:452–468.
249. Strandness DE, Langlois Y, Cramer M, et al: Long-term sequelae of acute venous thrombosis. JAMA 1983;250:1289.
250. Killewich LA, Bedford GR, Beach KW, Strandness DE. Spontaneous lysis of deep venous thrombi: rate and outcome. J Vasc Surg 1989;9:89.
251. Caps MT, Manzo RA, Bergelin RO, et al. Venous valvular reflux in veins not involved at the time of acute deep venous thrombosis. J Vasc Surg 1995;22:524.
252. van Bemmelen PS. Venous Valvular Incompetence: An Experimental Study in the Rat. Alblasserdam: Offsetdrukkerij Kaners BV, 1984.
253. Leu HJ. Morphology of chronic venous insufficiency: light and electron microscopic examinations. Vasa 1991;20:330.
254. Wenner A, Leu HJ, Spycher M, et al. Ultrastructural changes of capillaries in chronic venous insufficiency. Exp Cell Biol 1980;48:1.
255. Coleridge Smith PD. The role of white cell trapping in the pathogenesis of venous ulceration. Phlebol Dig 1992;4:4.
256. Veraart JCJM, Verhaegh MEJM, Neumann HAM, et al. Adhesion molecule expression in venous leg ulcers. Vasa 1993;2:243.
257. Pappas PJ, Teehan EP, Fallek SR, et al. Diminished mononuclear cell function is associated with chronic venous insufficiency. J Vasc Surg 1995;22:580.
258. Hasan A, Murata H, Falabella A, et al. Dermal fibroblasts from venous ulcers are unresponsive to the action of transforming growth factor-β. J Dermatol Sci 1997;16:59.
259. Bollinger A, Leu AJ. Evidence for microvascular thrombosis obtained by intravital fluorescence videomicroscopy. Vasa 1991;20:252.
260. Leu AJ, Leu H-J, Franzeck UK, et al. Microvascular changes in chronic venous insufficiency: a review. Cardiovasc Surg 1995;3:237.
261. Burnand KG, Whimster I, Naidoo A, Browse NL. Pericapillary fibrin in the ulcer-bearing skin of the leg: the cause of lipodermatosclerosis and venous ulceration. Br Med J 1982; 285:1071.
262. Wolf JH, Morland M, Browse NL. The fibrinolytic activity of varicose veins. Br J Surg 1979;66:185.
263. Lotti T, Chimenti M, Bianchini G, et al. Cutaneous and plasmatic fibrinolytic activity in the subject of stasis dermatitis. Ital Gen Rev Dermatol 1983;20:9.
264. Vanscheidt W, Laaf H. Wokalck H, et al. Pericapillary fibrin cuff: a histologic sign of venous ulceration. J Cutan Pathol 1990; 17:266.
265. Taheri SA, Pollack L, Loomis R. P-13-NMR studies of muscle in patients with venous insufficiency. Int Angiol 1987;6:95.
266. Clyne CA, Ramsden WH, Chant AD, Webster JH. Oxygen tension on the skin of the gaiter area of limbs with venous disease. Br J Surg 1985;72:644.
267. Mani R, White JE, Barrett DF, Weaver PW. Tissue oxygenation, venous ulcers and fibrin cuffs. J R Soc Med 1989;82:345.
268. Franzeck UK, Bollinger A, Huch R, Huch A. Transcutaneous oxygen tension and capillary morphology characteristics and density in patients with chronic venous incompetence. Circulation 1984;70:806.
269. Moyses C, Cederholm-Williams SA, Michel CC. Haemoconcentration and accumulation of white cells in the feet during venous stasis. Int J Microcirc Clin Exp 1987;5:311.
270. Thomas PR, Nash GB, Dormandy JA. White cell accumulation in dependent legs of patients with venous hypertension: a possible mechanism for trophic changes in the skin. Br Med J 1988;290:1693.
271. Cikrit DF, Nichols WK, Silver D. Surgical management of refractory venous stasis ulceration. J Vasc Surg 1988;7:473.
272. Bergan JJ, Yao JST, Flinn WR, McCarthy WJ. Surgical treatment of venous obstruction and insufficiency. J Vasc Surg 1986; 3:174.

273. Stewart AJ, Leaper DJ. Treatment of chronic leg ulcers in the community: a comparative trial of Scherisorb and Iodosorb. Phlebology 1987;2:115.
274. Ormiston MC, Seymour MT, Venn GE, et al. Controlled trial of Iodosorb in chronic venous ulcers. Br Med J 1985;291:308.
275. Ryan TJ, Biven HF, Murphy JJ, et al. The use of a new occlusive dressing in the management of venous stasis ulceration. In: Ryan TJ, ed. An Environment for Healing: The Role of Occlusion. London: Royal Society of Medicine, 1984:99–103.
276. Eriksson G. Comparative study of hydrocolloid dressing and double layer bandage in treatment of venous stasis ulceration. In: Ryan TJ, ed. An Environment for Healing: The Role of Occlusion. London: Royal Society of Medicine, 1984:111–113.
277. Wright AD. The treatment of indolent ulcer of the leg. Lancet 1931;1:457.
278. Anning ST. Leg ulcers—the results of treatment. Angiology 1956;7:505.
279. Kitahama A, Elliot LF, Kerstein MD, Menendez CV. Leg ulcer: conservative management or surgical treatment? JAMA 1982;247:197.
280. Mayberry JC, Moneta GL, Taylor LM, Porter JM. Fifteen-year results of ambulatory compression therapy for chronic venous ulcers. Surgery (St. Louis) 1991;109:575.
281. Chant AD, Davies LJ, Pike JM, Sparks MJ. Support stockings in practical management of varicose veins. Phlebology 1989; 4:167.
282. Franks PJ, Oldroyd MI, Dickson D, et al. Risk factors for leg ulcer recurrence: a randomized trial of two types of compression stockings. Age Aging 1994;24:490–494.
283. Unna PG. Ueber Paraplaste, eine neue Form medikamentoser Pflaster. Wien Med Wochenschr 1896;43:1854.
284. Rubin JR, Alexander J, Plecha EJ, Marman C. Unna's boots vs. polyurethane foam dressings for the treatment of venous ulceration. Arch Surg 1990;125:489.
285. Kitka MJ, Schuler JJ, Meyer JP, et al. A prospective, randomized trial of Unna's boots versus hydroactive dressing in the treatment of venous stasis ulcers. J Vasc Surg 1988;7:478.
286. Cordts PR, Hanrahan LM, Rodriguez AA, et al. A prospective, randomized trial of Unna's boot versus DuoDERM CGF hydroactive dressing plus compression in the management of venous leg ulcers. J Vasc Surg 1992;15:480.
287. Vernick SH, Shapiro D, Shaw FD. Legging orthosis for venous and lymphatic insufficiency. Arch Phys Med Rehabil 1987;68: 459.
288. Spence RK, Cahall E. Inelastic versus elastic leg compression in chronic venous insufficiency: a comparison of limb size and venous hemodynamics. J Vasc Surg 1996;24:783–787.
289. Pekanmaki K, Kolari PJ, Kiistala U. Intermittent pneumatic compression treatment for postthrombotic leg ulcers. Clin Exp Dermatol 1987;12:350.
290. Coleridge Smith P, Sarin S, Hasty J, Scurr JH. Sequential gradient pneumatic compression enhances venous ulcer healing: a randomized trial. Surgery (St. Louis) 1990;108:871.
291. Uber A. The socioeconomic profile of patients treated by phlebotropic drugs in Germany. Angiology 1997;48:595–607.
292. Graves MW, Boyde TR. Plasma zinc concentrations in patients with psoriasis, other dermatoses, and venous leg ulceration. Lancet 1967;2:1019.
293. Withers AF, Baker H, Musa M, Dormandy TL. Plasma zinc in psoriasis. Lancet 1968;2:278.
293. Hallbook T, Lanner E. Serum-zinc and healing of venous leg ulcers. Lancet 1972;2:780.
295. Myers MB, Cherry G. Zinc and the healing of chronic ulcers. Am J Surg 1970;120:77.
296. Phillips A, Davidson M, Greaves MW. Venous leg ulceration: evaluation of zinc treatment, serum zinc and rate of healing. Clin Exp Dermatol 1977;2:395.
297. Burnand K, Lemenson G, Morland M, et al. Venous lipodermatosclerosis: treatment by fibrinolytic enhancement and elastic compression. Br Med J 1980;280:7.
298. McMullin GM, Watkin GT, Coleridge Smith PD, Scurr JH. The efficacy of fibrinolytic enhancement with stanozolol in the treatment of venous insufficiency. Aust N Z J Surg 1991;61: 306.
299. Layer GT, Stacey MC, Burnand KG. Stanozolol and the treatment of venous ulceration: an interim report. Phlebology 1986;1:197.
300. Colgan M, Dormandy JA, Jones PW, et al. Oxpentifylline treatment of venous ulcers of the leg. Br Med J 1990;300:972–975.
301. Balmer A, Limoni C. A double-blind placebo-controlled trial of venorutin on the symptoms and signs of chronic venous insufficiency. Vasa 1980;9:76.
302. Pulvertaft TB. Paroven in the treatment of chronic venous insufficiency. Practitioner 1979;223:838.
303. Pulvertaft TB. General practice treatment of symptoms of venous insufficiency with oxyrutins. Results of a 660 patient multicenter study in the UK. Vasa 1983;12:373.
304. Mann RJ. A double-blind trial of oral O. B-hydroxy-ethyl rutosides for stasis leg ulcers. Br J Clin Pract 1981;35:79.
305. Casley-Smith JR, Casley-Smith JR. The effects of calcium dobesilate on acute lymphoedema (with and without macrophages) and on burn edema. Lymphology 1985;18:37.
306. Casley-Smith JR. The effect of variations in tissue protein concentration and tissue hydrostatic pressure on fluid and protein uptake by the initial lymphatics, and the action of calcium dobesilate. Microcirc Endothelium Lymphatics 1985;2:385.
307. Casley-Smith JR. A double-blind trial of calcium dobesilate in chronic venous insufficiency. Angiology 1988;39:853–857.
308. Sullivan GW, Carper HT, Novick WJ, Mandell GL. Inhibition of the inflammatory action of interleukin-1 and tumor necrosis factor (alpha) on neutrophil function by pentoxifylline. Infect Immunol 1988;56:1722.
309. Layton AM, Ibbotson SH, Davies JA, et al. The effect of oral aspirin in the treatment of chronic venous leg ulcers. Lancet 1994;344:164–165.
310. Ibbotsen SH, Layton AM, Davies JA, et al. The effect of aspirin on haemostatic activity in the treatment of chronic venous leg ulceration. Br J Dermatol 1995;132:422–426.
311. Sinzinger H, Virgolini I, Fitscha P. Pathomechanisms of atherosclerosis beneficially affected by prostaglandin E_1 (PGE_1): an update. Vasa 1989;28(suppl):6.
312. Rudofsky G. Intravenous prostaglandin E_1 in the treatment of venous ulcers: a double-blind, placebo controlled trial. Vasa 1989;28(suppl):39.
313. Diehm C, Trampisch HJ, Lange S, et al. Comparison of leg compression stockings and oral chest-horsenut seed extract in patients with chronic venous insufficiency. Lancet 1996;347:292–294.
314. Gilchrist B, Reed C. The bacteriology of chronic venous ulcers treated with occlusive hydrocolloid dressings. Br J Dermatol 1989;121:337.
315. Lineaweaver W, Howard R, Souey D, et al. Topical antimicrobial toxicity. Arch Surg 1985;120:267.
316. Roelens P. Double-blind placebo-controlled study with topical 2% ketanserin ointment in the treatment of venous ulcers. Dermatologica 1989;178:98.
317. Alvarez OM, Mertz PM, Eaglstein WH. The effect of occlusive dressings on collagen synthesis and re-epithelialization in superficial wounds. J Surg Res 1983;35:142.
318. Wilkins LM, Watson SR, Prosky SJ, et al. Development of a bilayered living skin construct for clinical applications. Biotechnol Bioeng 1994;43:747–756.
319. Falanga V, Margolis D, Alvarez O, et al. Rapid healing of venous ulcers and lack of clinical rejection with an allogenic cultured human skin equivalent. Arch Dermatol 1998;134(3):293–300.

320. Linton RR. The communicating veins of the lower leg and the operative technique for their ligation. Ann Surg 1938;107:582–593.
321. Gay J. Lettsonian Lectures 1867. Varicose Disease of the Lower Extremities. London: Churchill, 1868.
322. Homans J. The operative treatment of varicose veins and ulcers, based upon a classification of these lesions. Surg Gynecol Obstet 1916;22:143–158.
323. Linton RR. The post-thrombotic ulceration of the lower extremity: its etiology and surgical treatment. Ann Surg 1953;138:415–432.
324. Gloviczki P, Bergan JJ, Menawat SS, et al. Safety, feasibility, and early efficacy of subfascial endoscopic perforator surgery: a preliminary report from the North American registry. J Vasc Surg 1997;25:94–105.
325. Sottiurai VS. Surgical correction of recurrent venous ulcer. J Cardiovasc Surg 1991;32:104–109.
326. Kistner RL. Surgical repair of venous valve. Straub Clin Proc 1968;34:41–43.
327. Kistner RL. Surgical repair of the incompetent femoral vein valve. Arch Surg 1975;110:1336–1342.
328. Masuda EM, Kistner RL. Long-term results of venous valve reconstruction: a four- to twenty-one-year follow-up. J Vasc Surg 1994;19:391–403.
329. Taheri SA, Pendergast DR, Lazar E, et al. Vein valve transplantation. Am J Surg 1985;150:201–202.
330. Kistner RL. Methods for reconstruction of deep venous reflux: long-term results. Vasc Surg 1997;31(3):268–269.
331. Quinones-Baldrich WT. Thrombolytic therapy for vascular disease. In: Moore WS, ed. Vascular Surgery: A Comprehensive Review. Philadelphia: Saunders, 1998:361–389.
332. Christopoulos DG, Nicolaides AN, Szendro G, et al. Air-plethysmography and the effect of elastic compression on venous hemodynamics of the leg. J Vasc Surg 1987;5:148. In: Rutherford RB, ed. Vascular Surgery. Philadelphia: Saunders, 1995:1838.

68

Vascular Access for Dialysis, Chemotherapy, and Nutritional Support

R. Randal Bollinger and Stuart J. Knechtle

The success of many modern medical therapies is intimately tied to the success of vascular access. Hemodialysis for renal failure, chemotherapy for cancer, hyperalimentation for nutritional support, plasmapheresis for autoimmune disease, central pressure monitoring for the patient in intensive care, and blood replacement for the trauma victim are examples of therapies that depend on effective and reliable vascular access. The importance of angioaccess is so great that entire monographs have been written on vascular access in general,[1] catheter access to the central veins,[2] and vascular access specifically for dialysis,[3] chemotherapy,[4] and nutritional support.[5] The evolution of vascular access has a long and interesting but somewhat disjointed history.

Historical Development of Vascular Access

Following William Harvey's description of the circulatory system in 1628, Sir Christopher Wren used a goose quill attached to a porcine bladder to infuse a mixture of opium, wine, and ale intravenously into dogs.[6,7] Richard Lower performed a series of infusions and transfusions in animals,[8,9] culminating in the first reports of blood transfusions from animals to men in England[10] and in France.[11] These early experiments were soon curtailed, not only because of technical limitations, but also because of frequent, severe, often fatal transfusion reactions. Three hundred years later, Werner Forssmann experimented on himself to develop the technique of central venous catheterization in 1929. Andre Cournand and Dickinson Richards applied the technique to cardiac catheterization in 1936.[12] These three early investigators of central venous access shared the Nobel Prize for Medicine in 1956.

The development of hemodialysis by William Kolff[13] and others in the 1940s and 1950s made possible artificial kidney support for patients in acute renal failure. However, because of the need to cannulate arteries and veins directly, therapy could only be applied to patients in acute renal failure. Early attempts at chronic hemodialysis were thwarted by the failure of vascular access, which had to be surgically and repeatedly established for each session of dialysis. The situation improved significantly when Scribner, Dillard, and Quinton developed first Teflon, then inert Silastic, indwelling arteriovenous shunts for long-term hemodialysis access.[14] Catheter tips were placed into an artery and vein, usually at the wrist, and Silastic tubes brought out through small skin incisions were joined outside the body with a Teflon connector. The arteriovenous shunt was opened for connection to the dialysis machine before each hemodialysis, then reconnected after dialysis, and protected under an arm dressing until the next treatment. However, infection and thrombosis of these external shunts remained significant problems until Brescia, Cimino, Appel, and Hurwich developed the totally internal radial artery-to-cephalic vein arteriovenous fistula.[15] Needle puncture of the fistula for each dialysis session provided a high-flow, largely complication-free route of reliable, repeated vascular access for treatment of chronic renal failure. For those patients without suitable vessels for a Brescia–Cimino fistula, a large vessel shunt attached to the side of the femoral artery and vein was devised by Thomas.[16] The subsequent development of saphenous vein grafts as well as the use of bovine grafts and expanded polytetrafluoroethylene (PTFE) grafts were later efforts. Because of their availability and durability, PTFE grafts have been adopted as the standard prosthetic material when a Brescia–Cimino fistula is not technically feasible.

The demonstration by Dudrick, Wilmore, Vars, and Rhoads in 1969 that a child could grow normally with intravenous feeding as its sole means of nutritional support produced a new demand for stable vascular access.[17] Early hyperalimentation catheters were stiff, thrombogenic, and easily infected. Broviac developed a more flexible catheter of silicone tubing which, together with placement of the catheter tip at the junction of the vena cava and right atrium, reduced thrombosis.[18] The addition of a Dacron cuff in a subcutaneous tunnel as an infection barrier led to safe and reliable indwelling vascular access for long-term nutritional support. However, the demands of cancer treatment, requiring not only alimentation, but also transfusion, blood sampling, and intravenous chemotherapy, often exceeded the capabilities of feeding catheters. Hickman developed a stronger catheter with a thicker wall, a larger internal diameter, and, subsequently, one, two, or three parallel lumens that provided effective, multipurpose vascular access to facilitate treatment of leukemia with chemotherapy, transfusion, and bone marrow transplant.[19] Totally implantable subcutaneous ports for cancer treatment were developed subsequently.[20]

Indications for Vascular Access

Central venous catheters are in place for the infusion of drugs and fluids during 54% of patient-days in U.S. intensive care units, a total of 9.7 million catheter-days each year.[21] The incidence rate of treated end-stage renal disease in the United States is 180 per million and is increasing.[22] More than 260,000 renal failure patients in the United States require vascular access for hemodialysis.[23] Moreover, as the population ages and the number of diabetics increases, the hemodialysis population is growing at a rate of 5.5% each year. The cost of creating and maintaining vascular access for dialysis exceeds $1 billion annually in the United State alone. In addition to the large numbers of patients requiring vascular access for intensive care and hemodialysis, many others need reliable access for cancer chemotherapy, total parenteral nutrition, antibiotic administration, continuous vasodilator drug infusions, blood sampling, plasmapheresis, and blood or blood product transfusion, for example, in hemophilia.[24] Whenever a high-flow system is needed, an irritating or sclerosing intravenous medication must be given, frequent blood draws are required, or recurrent parenteral treatments are necessary, then placement of one of the several types of catheter, fistula, or graft for vascular access should be considered.

Types and Techniques of Vascular Access

There is much overlap in the uses of vascular access devices, a fact that is well demonstrated by the several techniques of dialysis access for acute and chronic renal failure patients. The key steps of the most important surgical procedures for chronic dialysis access have been illustrated well and described succinctly.[25]

Acute Vascular Access for Short Periods of Time

An estimated 2% to 5% of hospitalized patients develop acute renal failure, which most often resolves.[26] However, the mortality in critically ill patients with acute renal failure remains high, at 40% to 70%.[27] Such patients often require renal replacement therapy, either with hemodialysis or with continuous therapies such as slow continuous ultrafiltration, continuous venovenous hemofiltration, or continuous venovenous hemodialfiltration. Temporary dialysis access for replacement therapy of this nature is obtained most easily by insertion of a dual-lumen catheter into the subclavian, external jugular, internal jugular, or femoral vein. These percutaneously placed, nontunneled polyurethane or Silastic catheters may be inserted through a break-away sheath using sterile technique at the patient's bedside. The double-lumen dialysis catheters allow blood to be withdrawn from a proximal port and reinfused through a distal port such that admixture of blood from the two ports is minimized. Insertion of percutaneous dialysis catheters follows the principles of central catheter placement and currently depends on the use of a modified Seldinger technique. A central vein is cannulated with a needle, a wire is threaded through the needle, the needle is removed, and a dilator and pull-away sheath are passed over the wire. The dialysis catheter is then passed through the sheath, which is then removed. An X-ray is used to confirm good catheter placement. Placement of dual-lumen dialysis catheters can be complicated by pneumothorax, hemothorax, nerve injury, arteriovenous (AV) fistula, and air embolism (see section on "Complications," following). They are ideal for single dialysis sessions and may be left in place for a few days in patients requiring acute, frequent, but temporary hemodialysis. If they are left in place for longer periods, not only is there danger of site infection, catheter sepsis, catheter thrombosis, central venous thrombosis, and dislodgement, but also they may make construction of permanent vascular access impossible. Almost 50% of subclavian veins and 10% of internal jugular veins have a significant stenosis after temporary dialysis catheters have been in place for 2 weeks. Subsequently, when a native vessel or prosthetic graft AV fistula is created distal to the stenosis, the obstruction may cause clotting of the fistula and/or a swollen arm. Moreover, the stenosis may not be clinically evident until the fistula is created, the patient begins dialysis, and the increased blood flow causes an abnormally high venous pressure. A venogram or duplex Doppler ultrasound study should be considered to document the patency of the central veins before an AV access is placed distal to the site of a long-dwelling central venous catheter.

In patients requiring acute dialysis access for whom percutaneous placement of a dual lumen catheter into the femoral, jugular, or subclavian vein is not possible, the assistance of interventional radiology to achieve translumbar, transhepatic, or ileofemoral placement into the inferior vena cava may be lifesaving. Other alternatives include a cut down on smaller, tributary veins such as the cephalic vein at the shoulder or the saphenous vein in the leg; placement of an external Scribner shunt at the wrist; or insertion of a Tenckhoff catheter through the abdominal wall for peritoneal dialysis.

Temporary Vascular Access for Longer Periods of Time

A patient who will require longer-term access should be given a cuffed, tunneled catheter that is bound strongly to the surrounding body wall by ingrowth of connective tissue that

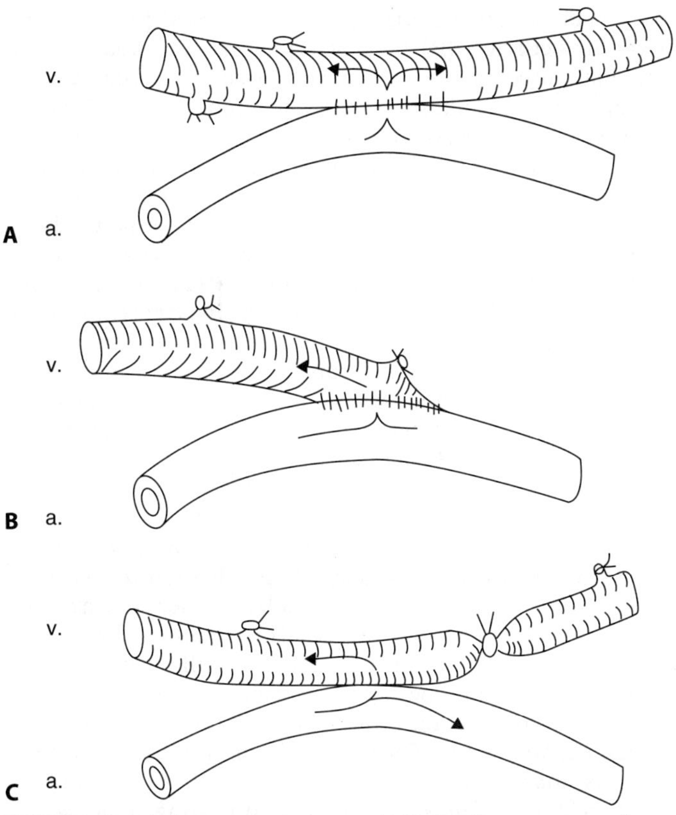

FIGURE 68.1. Primary arteriovenous (AV) fistulas are most often created between the cephalic vein and the radial artery at the wrist or the deep, posterior branch of the radial artery in the anatomic snuff box of the hand using a side-to-side (**A**) or an end-to-side (**B**) configuration. An end-to-end anastomosis is possible but little used because of the lower flow rate that predisposes it to thrombosis. The distal limb of the vein may be ligated (**C**), particularly if swelling of the hand from venous hypertension becomes a problem.

prevents catheter dislodgement and reduces the incidence of infection. The insertion technique is a modified Seldinger method, resembling that described earlier for the temporary dialysis catheter except for the addition of a subcutaneous tunnel several centimeters in length from the vein entry site to a separate skin exit site. The soft, silicone rubber catheters may have two lumens in a single unit or may have separate inflow and outflow catheters that are placed through two separate needle sticks.[28] When their tips are placed into or near the right atrium, these catheters can achieve blood flows of more than 400 mL/min without significant recirculation or thrombosis. Totally implantable ports have been reported to have comparable performance to these cuffed, tunneled catheters but with even fewer thrombotic and infectious complications.[29] However, they are more expensive, more likely to hemorrhage, and less frequently used.

Those patients with inadequate vessels or physiology for creation of an AV fistula may undergo hemodialysis for many months through their tunneled, Silastic "temporary" access catheters. Approximately 50% of soft, cuffed, tunneled catheters placed in the right subclavian position survive for 1 year.[30] Similarly, the survival rate of PermCaths was 74% at 1 year and 43% at 2 years.[31] However, despite routine postdialysis flushing, these long-indwelling catheters often become occluded by clots or internal sheaths of fibrin (for treatment, see "Complications," following).

Chronic Vascular Access Through Autogenous Fistulas

Successful long-term hemodialysis is best achieved using a primary AV fistula (Fig. 68.1), which has a 3-year patency rate of approximately 70%.[32] Autogenous tissue is less likely to cause thrombosis or become infected than any type of prosthetic material. The Brescia–Cimino fistula utilizing autogenous vein and artery has a lower complication rate than fistulas involving prosthetic material (Table 68.1).[33] To avoid distal ischemia after diversion of radial artery blood flow through the AV fistula, an Allen test is performed preoperatively to ensure adequate ulnar artery collateral flow to the hand. Under local anesthesia, the artery and vein are isolated through a longitudinal incision, preferably on the nondominant side. The superficial branch of the radial nerve is avoided. The small vessels may be dilated with coronary dilators to improve blood flow during the initial period when the risk of thrombosis is greatest. The principal limitation of a Brescia–Cimino fistula is that many patients, especially those with chronic illness, have had numerous percutaneous venous catheters and blood draws and do not have a patent cephalic vein. In addition, some cephalic veins are of inadequate size to permit enough flow for technically successful hemodialysis. The radial artery to cephalic vein side-to-side anastomosis (see Fig. 68.1A) or the end-to-side anastomosis (see Fig. 68.1B) is an optimal choice, because the flow is adequate to maintain patency but the small size of the radial artery limits flow enough to avoid the problem of high-output cardiac failure. This fistula requires 4 to 6 weeks to mature, meaning that the cephalic vein enlarges, thickens, and arterializes, permitting safe cannulation. An end-to-end anastomosis is used infrequently because the lesser outflow predisposes to early thrombosis. A more-proximal AV fistula between the brachial artery and basilic vein or cephalic vein is much more likely to develop such a large flow that high-output cardiac failure develops, requiring fistula takedown. Even a side-to-side Brescia–Cimino fistula at the wrist may, however, result in venous hypertension in the hand, requiring ligation of the cephalic vein between the AV fistula and the hand (see Fig. 68.1C). Aneurysm formation may also become problematical and, if very unsightly or symptomatic, may require takedown

TABLE 68.1.
Vascular Access for Hemodialysis: Complication-Free Function (Level III Evidence).

Time since implant (years)	*Brescia–Cimino fistula (%)*	*Bovine heterograft (%)*	*PTFE prosthetic graft (%)*
1	88	54	61
2	77	30	37
3	67	16	22
4	59	9	14
5	51	5	8

Based on assumption of exponential distribution of interval between two complications.

Source: Mehta S. 1991.[33] Statistical summary of clinical results of vascular access procedures for hemodialysis. In: Sommer B, Henry M, eds. Vascular Access for Hemodialysis, vol II. WL Gore Associates, Inc.: Precept Press, pp 145–157.

of the fistula. A relative disadvantage of the Brescia–Cimino fistula is the need to wait for the fistula to mature before it can be used for dialysis.

Several other types of upper extremity AV fistula have been described and given standardized definitions.[22] Some of these require relocation, that is, transposition, of a deep artery or vein to a more superficial position so that the vein, once mature, is readily accessible for dialysis: examples include the autogenous ulnar-cephalic forearm transposition and the autogenous brachial-basilic upper arm transposition. The basilic vein transposition AV fistula requires dissection of the peripheral upper arm basilic vein and its transfer to a superficial position on the medial portion of the upper extremity before anastomosis to the brachial artery above the elbow.[34] The durability and cumulative functional patency of transposed AV fistulas compare favorably to nontransposed ones.[35] Primary functional patency of transposed AV fistulas at 1 and 2 years were 76.2% and 67.7%, compared to 53.3% and 34.4%, respectively, for nontransposed fistulas ($P < 0.001$) Whenever possible, the patient's own vessels should be used to create an entirely autogenous AV fistula before resorting to prosthetic materials for dialysis access.[36] Use of autogenous vessels is especially important for infection-prone immunosuppressed transplant, cancer, and acquired immunodeficiency syndrome (AIDS) patients. If the patient lacks a suitable vein in the upper extremity for an autogenous AV fistula, then one of the saphenous veins in a lower extremity may be used as a looped transposition to the ipsilateral superficial femoral artery.[37] Alternatively, the saphenous vein may be used for a translocation access by disconnecting it proximally and distally then inserting it in a remote position, for example, the upper extremity, with both new arterial and new venous anastomoses.

The National Kidney Foundation's Dialysis Outcome Quality Initiative (DOQI) Guidelines pointed out that native vessel AV fistulas have the best long-term patency rates and require fewer interventions than other types of vascular access.[38] The updated DOQI Guidelines point out that the quality of life and overall outcomes for hemodialysis patients could be improved significantly by increasing the placement of native AV fistulas and by detecting access dysfunction before access thrombosis.[36] Based on the evidence regarding patient evaluation, monitoring, prevention of problems, and management of complications for vascular access, the current goals are to construct primary AV fistulas in at least 50% of new hemodialysis patients and to maintain less than 10% of chronic hemodialysis patients on catheters as their permanent vascular access. To achieve a high rate of patent autogenous AV fistulas, Doppler ultrasound mapping can be used to locate suitable vessels.[39] The inflow artery should be 2mm or more in diameter and the outflow vein 2.5mm or more in diameter to create a functional fistula. Furthermore, venous mapping may improve success rates in difficult access patients such as diabetics[40] and those who have had multiple previous access procedures, including the placement of prosthetic grafts.[41]

Chronic Vascular Access Through Prosthetic Grafts

For long-term hemodialysis patients with inadequate arteries, poor peripheral veins, or failed previous fistulas, placement of an autogenous AV fistula may not be possible, and a forearm loop graft of a prosthetic material such as expanded polytetrafluoroethylene (PTFE) may be the next best choice. Other materials used in the past such as Dacron, bovine carotid artery, or human umbilical vein were prone to thrombosis or aneurysmal dilatation after the frequent punctures and continuous arterial pressure that are required for dialysis fistulas. However, a newer, more durable bovine mesenteric vein bioprosthesis has recently become available. It is particularly useful as a conduit for patients who already have failed multiple synthetic vascular access grafts.[42] PTFE is used most commonly because it is a relatively inexpensive, easily sutured, biocompatible material that resists aneurysm formation by ingrowth of the surrounding connective tissue into the graft interstices and lessens thrombosis by the rapid formation of an autogenous pseudointima. A PTFE graft 6mm in diameter is often used because puncture with large dialysis needles is easy, adequate flow is achieved with this diameter, and high-output cardiac failure is not a risk. Common locations for a PTFE graft are the forearm (65%), upper arm (30%), and the thigh (5%) (Fig. 68.2a–g).[33] When these sites have been exhausted or are otherwise unavailable, then the axillary vessels may be used for chest wall loop grafts and necklace grafts (Fig. 68.2h,i). In extreme cases, an axillary artery PTFE graft may even be connected to the ipsilateral internal jugular vein, iliac vein, femoral vein, the right atrium, or the contralateral axillary artery. The total number of possible AV graft sites is maximized by starting as distal as possible in the nondominant upper extremity and moving as necessary to more centrally located sites. Successful placement of a

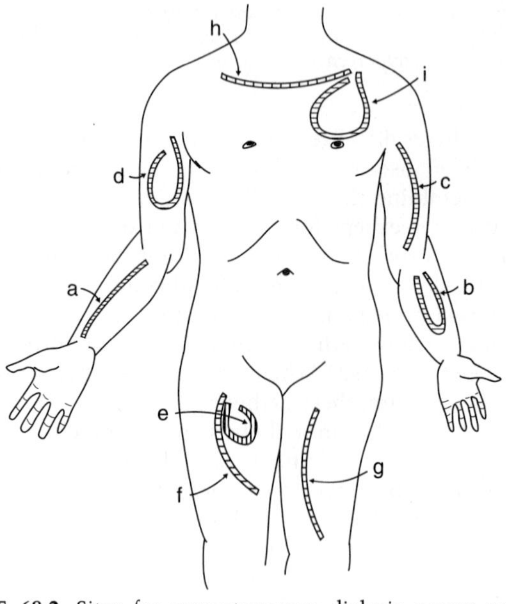

FIGURE 68.2. Sites for nonautogenous dialysis access grafts are found throughout the body. They are named by their arterial inflow site followed by a hyphen and then the venous outflow site.[22] Shown here are the prosthetic (**a**) radial-median cubital forearm straight access, (**b**) brachial-antecubital forearm loop access, (**c**) brachial-axillary upper arm straight access, (**d**) axillary-axillary upper arm loop access, (**e**) superficial femoral-femoral inguinal loop access, (**f**) superficial femoral-saphenous midthigh access, (**g**) popliteal-deep saphenous thigh access, (**h**) axillary-axillary chest straight access, and (**i**) axillary-axillary chest loop access. Not shown are the less common femoral-femoral suprainguinal straight access, axillary-femoral body wall straight access, and axillary-internal jugular chest loop access.

prosthetic AV fistula requires not only excellent arterial inflow but also unobstructed venous outflow. In the patient who has already had multiple intravenous lines for fluids and drugs, finding a suitable vein may require prior Doppler ultrasound mapping to avoid a proximal stenosis. The graft must be placed carefully into its tunnel to avoid rotation or kinking and should be allowed to seal to the tissue of the tunnel wall for up to 4 weeks before use. Although a new prosthetic AV access may be used immediately in urgent circumstances, there is danger of hemorrhage from the graft puncture site into the subcutaneous tunnel, which may lead to arm swelling, distal ischemia, graft thrombosis, and tunnel infection. Some extremity swelling is seen after placement of every AV graft in response to surgical trauma and venous hypertension; however, in contrast to a large perigraft hematoma, this swelling resolves in a short time with simple elevation of the extremity. Lower extremity prosthetic AV access grafts (see Fig. 68.2e–g) are less successful than upper extremity grafts[43] and have higher rates of infection and limb amputation.[44,45] They should be avoided in patients with significant peripheral vascular disease, such as elderly diabetics. However, with improved surgical techniques and careful, aseptic needle puncture for dialysis, PTFE grafts may be placed in the groin with results approximating those achieved in the upper extremity.[46]

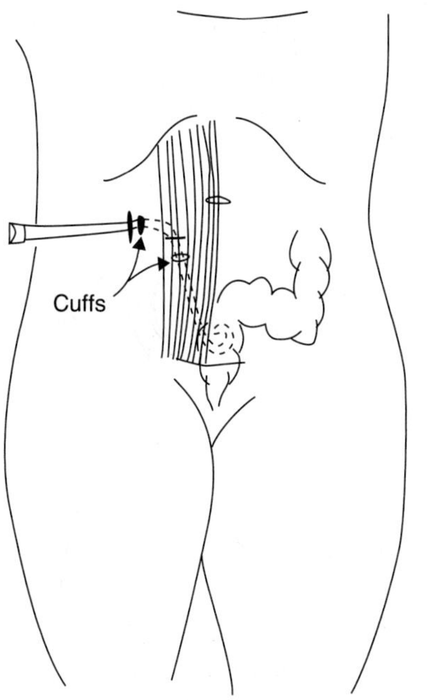

FIGURE 68.3. The Tenckhoff peritoneal dialysis catheter is placed through the rectus muscle of the abdominal wall and into the deep pelvis just anterior to the rectum. The catheter is fixed and leakage prevented by tissue ingrowth into the Dacron cuffs beneath the rectus fascia and in the subcutaneous tunnel beneath the skin.[25]

Alternatives to Vascular Access for Dialysis

The primary alternative available to renal failure patients who will not or cannot undergo hemodialysis is peritoneal dialysis. The catheter devised by Striker and Tenckhoff for this purpose in 1971 is still in use today.[47] Patients with cardiovascular instability, lack of vascular access sites, or clotting disorders are candidates for dialysis through a peritoneal catheter. Approximately 10% of patients with end-stage renal failure are on peritoneal dialysis in the United States.[48] Chronic ambulatory peritoneal dialysis (CAPD) provides a better quality of life compared to hemodialysis, although relatively less efficient dialysis. On one hand, CAPD patients have more independence, avoid anticoagulation, can eat largely what they wish, and are generally more satisfied than hemodialysis patients. On the other hand, CAPD is less effective in removing small waste molecules than is hemodialysis.[49] Patients must be able to care for their dialysis catheters adequately and to perform the exchanges themselves or with available assistance. Catheter insertion can be performed under local anesthesia using either an infraumbilical or supraumbilical incision, inserting the catheter into the pelvis, and tunneling the catheter subcutaneously to an exit site on the abdominal wall (Fig. 68.3). Laparoscopic insertion of the CAPD catheter[50] avoids the most common reasons for mechanical malfunction of the catheter, and the laparoscopically inserted catheter can be used immediately, but the laparoscopic insertion procedure requires general anesthesia.[25] CAPD catheters exist in several configurations including straight, curved, shower-head, and pig-tail. In a prospective, randomized study, the curled Tenckoff dialysis catheter was found to be superior to the straight one in terms of catheter survival at 12 months (77% for curled vs. 36% for straight).[51] The catheter may have one or two Dacron cuffs to prevent fluid leaks, infection, and inadvertent removal. Patients who develop catheter sepsis can be treated with antibiotics, both systemically and through the peritoneal dialysis catheter; however, fungal catheter infections and bacterial infections not responsive to antibiotics generally require catheter removal. Culturing of enteric organisms, especially more than one enteric organism, should raise suspicion of perforation of the gastrointestinal (GI) tract. The early and late complications of peritoneal dialysis catheters, including their diagnosis, management, and prevention, have been reviewed.[52]

Vascular Access for Chemotherapy and Nutritional Support

Vascular access for infusion chemotherapy, nutritional support, and blood products, as well as blood sampling and central pressure monitoring, is most often obtained by inserting a catheter into the vena cava or right atrium through either a central or a peripheral vein entry site. The subclavian vein[53] or the internal jugular vein[54] is used most commonly for central placement (Fig. 68.4) and the cephalic vein or basilic vein for peripheral entry. Guidance with ultrasound or fluoroscopy facilitates entry into the central veins and proper placement of the catheter tip at the superior vena cava–right atrial junction. When high flow rates are needed for hemodialysis or pheresis, the tip is best located within the right atrium.[55] Difficult cases such as those patients with multiple stenosed or thrombosed veins from prior indwelling access catheters may require referral to interventional radiology for venography, thrombectomy, dilatation, stenting, and/or placement of the access catheters through the less commonly used translumbar or transhepatic routes. Alternate sites and techniques have been described for insertion of central venous

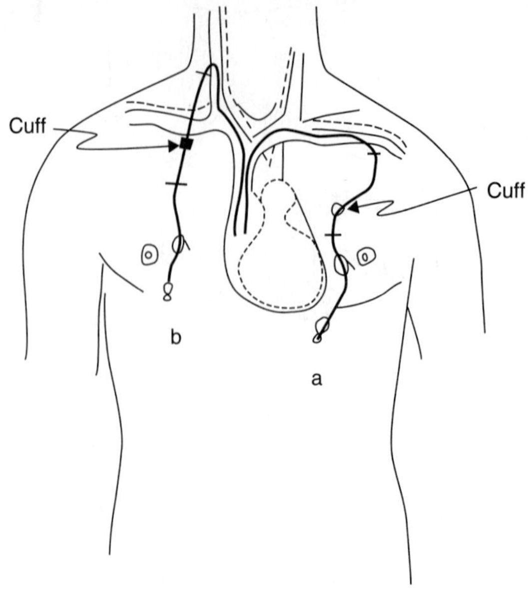

FIGURE 68.4. The two most common sites of entry for cuffed, tunneled central venous catheters are the subclavian vein (**a**) and the internal jugular vein (**b**). In most cases the tip should lie near the junction of the superior vena cava with the right atrium. When high flow rates are needed for hemodialysis or pheresis, the tip is best located within the right atrium.[55] The Dacron cuff that prevents infection and inadvertent removal of the catheter is positioned in the subcutaneous tunnel 2cm from the skin exit site in (**a**) and a somewhat longer distance in (**b**).

catheters into the azygous vein, superior vena cava, right atrium, saphenous vein, femoral vein, inferior epigastric vein, gonadal vein, and the inferior vena cava.[56] On the other hand, a patient with large, high-quality, unused arm veins often may have a PICC line (i.e., peripherally inserted central catheter) placed through a peripheral arm vein using sterile technique under local anesthesia at the patient's bedside.[57]

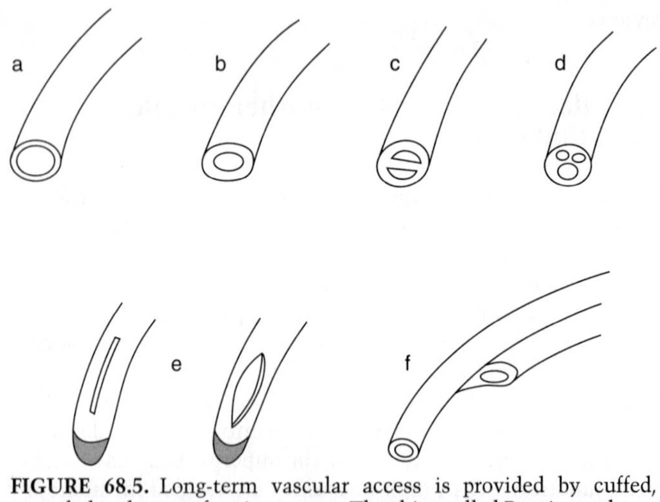

FIGURE 68.5. Long-term vascular access is provided by cuffed, tunneled catheters of various types. The thin-walled Broviac catheter (**a**) is excellent for total parenteral nutrition. The thicker-walled Hickman catheter, which comes with one (**b**), two (**c**), or three (**d**) lumens permits blood sampling, blood product infusion, and chemotherapy, as well as nutritional support. The slit valve in the tip of the Groshong catheter (**e**) is closed when not in use but opens with negative or positive pressure in the catheter lumen. Those patients with renal failure benefit from a catheter with the proximal blood removal port separated from the distal blood return port to prevent recirculation during hemodialysis (**f**).

Catheters currently in use[58] that exit externally onto the chest wall are named for their inventors and include the thin-walled silicone rubber catheter described by Broviac et al.[18] (Fig. 68.5a), the thicker-walled catheter described by Hickman et al.,[19] which comes with one, two, or three lumens (Fig. 68.5b–d), and the valve-tipped catheter attributed to Groshong (Fig. 68.5e).[59] The Groshong valve (see left panel, Fig. 68.5e) prevents passive blood flow into the catheter between uses to reduce clotting within the lumen. When positive pressure is applied to the catheter lumen (see right panel) or when negative pressure is applied to withdraw blood through the catheter, the valve opens to allow flow. The Port-A-Cath and the Infus-A-Port add single- or double-lumen implantable reservoirs that make them entirely internal to the skin.[60] The reservoirs are accessed by puncture through their self-sealing membranes with special, noncoring Huber needles, and must be flushed free of blood after each use or periods of disuse.

Complications of Vascular Access

Complications of **central venous catheters** may be immediate or delayed. *Immediate complications* at the time of catheter placement include pneumothorax, hemothorax, great vessel injury, nerve injury, thoracic duct injury, arteriovenous (AV) fistula, mechanical problems, and air embolism. *Air embolism* most commonly occurs through the introducer sheath during insertion of a tunneled catheter.[61] Air embolism is often asymptomatic but may be fatal if massive. Placing the patient in Trendelenburg position, occluding the sheath lumen digitally before inserting the catheter, and having the patient perform a Valsalva maneuver while at maximum inspiration during insertion of the catheter through the breakaway sheath will prevent the problem. Supplemental oxygen, with hyperbaric pressure if available, is used to treat it. On the postprocedure chest X-ray taken to document catheter position and localize the catheter tip, a collapsed lung with air or blood in the pleural space indicates a *pneumothorax* or *hemothorax* (1%–4% incidence), which should be treated with a chest tube if the patient becomes symptomatic or the pneumothorax is enlarging.[62] A widened mediastinum indicates a *great vessel injury* (<1% incidence), which may require surgical repair. *Mechanical problems* are common and may prevent placement of the catheter into a usable position. Congenital malformations, anatomic variations, pathological processes, or previous catheters may have caused stenosis, thrombosis, or obliteration of the target vein. Ultrasound guidance has proven helpful in clarifying difficult anatomic situations and will lead to a high rate of success in cannulating the central veins.[63] Malpositioned catheters that will not permit blood withdrawal or fluid infusion may be kinked, wedged into small branches, forced into extravascular positions, or pinched between the clavicle and first rib. They should be promptly repositioned under fluoroscopic control or removed to avoid shearing of the catheter or thrombosis of the vein. Despite proper placement, subclavian catheters may also cause *subclavian vein stenosis and thrombosis*, causing arm swelling or compromising the patency of an ipsilateral arm AV fistula needed for chronic hemodialysis.

Later complications of long-term catheter use include catheter thrombosis, central vein thrombosis, and catheter sepsis. Despite flushing after each use or period of disuse, *thrombosis* of the catheter, heralded by inability to withdraw blood, is a frequent problem seen in 4% to 10% of patients. Thrombosis is caused by mechanical problems, as noted previously, irritating infusion solutions, endothelial damage from the catheter itself, failure to flush the catheter adequately after use, or a hypercoagulable state in the patient. Tissue plasminogen activator (tPA) instilled into the catheter is a safe and nonallergenic way of removing fibrin sheaths to keep catheters open. Infusion of 2.5 mg recombinant tPA (rtPA) in 50 mL saline over 3 h produced a 100% immediate technical success rate but a 30-day probability of patency of only 0.67.[64] Another, cheaper alternative is to fill the occluded catheter with 5,000 IU urokinase for 1 h. If the catheter remains blocked and a second static treatment with urokinase also fails, then infusion with 60,000 IU urokinase per hour over 4 h may prove successful in reopening it. In a prospective, randomized trial comparing transcatheter urokinase infusion to percutaneous fibrin sheath stripping, the median duration of additional function was 32 days for stripping and 42 days for urokinase (difference, NS).[65] No matter which alternative is chosen to reopen a patient's occluded temporary dialysis catheter, alternative vascular access should be planned. If not just the catheter but also the surrounding central vein has become thrombosed, then the catheter should be removed and systemic anticoagulation instituted. Endovascular thrombectomy, angioplasty, and stenting may be necessary before that central vein is used again for vascular access. Angioplasty proved to be an effective treatment for central vein stenosis in 17 of 22 patients who developed the stenosis after having subclavian vein catheters.[66] Stents placed after angioplasties are useful for maintaining the patency of large, central veins without confluences.[67]

Catheter *infections* are less common but more devastating complications than thrombosis. Epidemiological data establish firmly that a major risk for vascular access infections is the type of access used.[68] Tunneled catheters are less likely to become infected than temporary catheters but more likely than AV grafts. An autogenous AV fistula is the access least likely to become infected. Infections may occur at any time after placement of the catheter, either from the skin exit site or from the bloodstream. They occur at a rate of 0.5 to 3.9 infections per 1000 catheter-days[69] and are commonly caused by *Staphylococcus epidermidis* or *S. aureus* from the skin. They occasionally lead to severe secondary infections such as septic arthritis, osteomyelitis, and bacterial endocarditis. They occur frequently in patients who are already immunosuppressed by cancer, malnutrition, AIDS, or other diseases, so diagnosis may prove difficult. Inflammation and purulent drainage from the exit site or over the subcutaneous tunnel suggest the diagnosis. In the absence of local signs, the best alternative is removal of the catheter for semiquantitative culture and Gram stain of the catheter tip.[62] Alternatively, differential colony counts from blood cultures taken simultaneously from the catheter and a peripheral vein may indicate that the catheter is the source of an infection. A multilumen catheter is more likely to become infected than a single-lumen one.[70] A femoral vein catheter is associated with a greater risk of infectious and thrombotic complications than is a subclavian vein catheter. A prospective, randomized trial in intensive care unit patients demonstrated higher rates of infection (19.8% vs. 4.5%, $P < 0.001$), catheter thrombosis (21.5% vs. 1.9%, $P < 0.001$), and vein thrombosis (6% vs. 0%, $P = 0.01$) in the femoral catheter group.[71] A catheter infection is best treated by removal of the catheter. However, if the exit site and tunnel are free of inflammation, then the catheter may be exchanged over a guidewire.[72]

The best way to combat catheter infections is to prevent them. Catheters impregnated with antibiotics or antiseptics on their external and internal surfaces are less likely to become infected.[73,74] Similarly, antibiotic ointment or disks at the exit site covered by a barrier dressing may reduce infection by local skin flora. The U.S. Centers for Disease Control and Prevention (CDC) National Nosocomial Infections Surveillance System found that intensive care units of all types had catheter infection rates of 1.8 to 5.2 per 1000 catheter-days[75] and recommended evidence-based procedures to reduce that high rate. The interventions judged by the CDC to have the greatest potential effects and lowest barriers to implementation were hand scrubbing before catheter insertion, chlorhexidine skin preparation before catheter insertion, full barrier precautions during catheter insertion, preferential use of the subclavian vein for catheter insertion, and removal of all unnecessary catheters.[76] A prospective study in 103 Michigan intensive care units over 18 months demonstrated that these five interventions reduced the median rate of catheter-related bloodstream infection per 1000 catheter-days from 2.7 (mean, 7.7) to 0 (mean, 1.4), $P < 0.002$.[77] The five components of the intervention have been recommended strongly for adoption in all intensive care units.[21]

Autogenous AV fistulas may cause several complications of which failure to mature is the most common and failure of the heart is the most severe. [34] Other common complications are stenosis of the venous outflow (48% of late complications), thrombosis (9%), aneurysms (7%), infection (<3%), and arterial steal syndrome (1.6%). *Maturation failure*, often caused by vessels that are too small or too scarred from prior use to dilate properly, results in inadequate size and flow for successful hemodialysis. Many end-stage renal disease (ESRD) patients have cardiac disease, which is their most common cause of death. When an ESRD patient with borderline cardiac function receives a new AV fistula, his heart may be unable to compensate for the additional flow of 0.5 to 1.0 L/min. The resulting *heart failure* may require banding of the fistula to reduce flow, its ligation, and placement of a central venous catheter for hemodialysis access or conversion to peritoneal dialysis (see foregoing for "Alternatives to Vascular Access for Dialysis"). *Aneurysms*, which occur from weakening of the vessel wall at the site of repeated needle punctures, can be prevented by rotating the entry sites. The *arterial steal syndrome*, which causes distal limb ischemia, is rare with wrist fistulas but common with more-proximal, larger, higher-flow upper arm fistulas.[78] The steal syndrome of distal limb pain, pallor, coolness, numbness, weakness, atrophy, and eventually ischemic necrosis is caused by blood flowing preferentially from the anastomosed artery to the low-resistance vein rather than to the distal extremity. Not only does arterial blood flow antegrade through the fistula but also blood from the distal artery flows retrograde through it, a physiological alteration of AV fistulas demonstrated well by intraoperative flow measurements.[79] Ligation of the fistula solves the problem. *Venous hypertension*, which causes swelling, hyperpigmentation, and skin breakdown of the hand and extremity distal to the AV fistula, is another manifestation of the high AV flow, usually in association with a proximal stenosis of the vein.[78] If a side-to-side anastomosis has been created, then ligation of the distal venous limb may solve the problem (see Fig. 68.1C). However, any proximal stenosis in the draining vein should be identified, perhaps by Doppler ultrasound, and corrected at the time of the distal limb ligation to prevent thrombosis from low proximal flow.

Complications of **prosthetic AV grafts** include edema of the involved limb and higher rates of hemorrhage, thrombosis, and infection compared to autogenous AV fistulas. False aneurysms of the graft at needle-stick sites may be bypassed with interposition grafts. Venous hypertension, congestive heart failure, and vascular access neuropathy are treated by graft ligation or banding. In addition, patients with peripheral vascular disease, most typically diabetics, the elderly, and smokers, may develop a significant *arterial steal syndrome* from a PTFE graft. The arterial steal is manifested in an arm graft by distal paresthesias, numbness, and pain. If severe, the graft may require banding to reduce the diameter of the graft or graft ligation. If not done soon enough, permanent neurological injury to the hand can result. Tapered grafts with a 4-mm arterial anastomosis and a 7-mm venous anastomosis provide lower but adequate flow for hemodialysis and are helpful in patients at risk for steal syndrome. Another useful alternative that preserves a functional dialysis access graft is to bypass it with a reversed saphenous vein graft. After the vein is anastomosed to the artery both above and below the takeoff of the prosthetic graft, the artery is ligated between the graft and the distal vein anastomosis; this increases flow to the distal extremity, preserves flow through the graft, and relieves all symptoms in the majority of patients.[80]

Hemorrhage early after placement of the graft is usually from an anastomosis or an unligated vessel in the graft tunnel. Surgical repair is indicated, not only to stop the bleeding but also to evacuate the large perigraft hematoma that develops. Hemorrhage at later times is usually from needle puncture sites and may cease with direct pressure until the anticoagulant effects of heparin have been reversed. If the needle has lacerated the graft, then closure with fine monofilament suture may be necessary. *Infections* are a serious problem for prosthetic dialysis grafts but PTFE grafts do not always have to be removed when they become infected.[81] Infections involving a midsegment of a PTFE graft away from the anastomotic suture lines can be managed with local drainage and antibiotics, with debridement and coverage by a skin flap, or with excision of the infected portion of the graft and oversewing of both ends. In the latter case, the wound is left open to granulate, and the patient is temporarily dialyzed via a percutaneous catheter. Once the wound has healed, a jump graft of 6-mm PTFE is placed after removing thrombus from the remaining graft ends. If these measures fail, if the graft thromboses, if the suture line is involved, or if the tunnel is infected, the graft should be removed. Thrombosed PTFE grafts may become a source of infection in the future so should be removed in cases of unexplained sepsis.[82] Graft infections are particularly likely in intravenous drug abusers and immunosuppressed AIDS patients.[83,84]

Early *thrombosis* of a new PTFE graft may be caused by anastomotic stricture, stenosis of the arterial inflow or venous outflow, kinking in the tunnel, excessive external pressure on the graft while tamponading needle holes after dialysis, patient hypotension, and/or a hypercoagulable state. If the thrombosis occurred because of transient obstruction, then simple thrombectomy or instillation of thrombolytic urokinase may be sufficient to remedy the problem. If no anatomic reason can be found for early or frequent thrombosis of the graft, then a coagulation workup should be done and the appropriate chemical intervention instituted.[85] The principal reason for late thrombosis of a PTFE graft is neointimal hyperplasia at the venous anastomosis. This complication can often be managed with longitudinal opening of the graft and vein followed by patch venoplasty using a PTFE patch, but may require more extensive revision with an interposition graft to normal vein.

Endovascular techniques for extraction of clot, chemical thrombolysis, and balloon angioplasty of stenotic areas have become increasingly sophisticated.[86,87] For example, cutting balloons may be effective against hyperplastic intimal lesions.[88] There is general agreement that if impending thrombosis from developing stenosis can be detected before the graft is occluded, then endovascular balloon angioplasty has the best chance of prolonging graft function. Surgical salvage procedures have been less successful with each repetition: 65% success after the first attempt, 53% after the second, and 44% after the third.[89] However, some interventional radiologists have achieved equally good initial patency results after each of several sequential angioplasty attempts.[90] Furthermore, lesions not amenable to percutaneous angioplasty may be identified angiographically and then rectified surgically. Measurements of venous pressure within the graft on multiple occasions under standardized conditions has led to early detection of stenosis, preemptive angioplasty, and reduction in graft thrombosis.[91] Doppler ultrasound scanning, recirculation measurements, and physical examination for a palpable thrill also have been used to detect AV graft dysfunction before occlusion. Once thrombosis occurs, the optimal management is more controversial.[92] Most evidence is Level III reporting of experience with either surgical or radiologic approaches, and the outcomes largely favor the reporting group. As shown in Table 68.2, comparing surgical to endovascular management of stenosis or thrombosis of dialysis access grafts, the outcomes of prospective, randomized trials (Level I data) either show no difference or favor surgery slightly. A meta-analysis of 479 patients in seven acceptable studies showed surgery to be superior in terms of graft patency at 30, 60, 90, and 365 days.[93] However, endovascular techniques are more easily repeated, often more available as outpatient procedures, do not use up more vessel, and do not require temporary central venous catheters for dialysis. Consequently, there is an important place for each technique in dealing with the stenotic and thrombotic complications of dialysis access grafts. For example, stent deployment can salvage thrombosed dialysis grafts but sustained patency is infrequent.[94] The results of endovascular stenting are better in the axillary area of the upper arm whereas surgical repair is most straightforward lower in the arm. A team approach that provides the ESRD patient with the best of all available surgical and endovascular techniques will likely maximize the survival of his vascular access.

TABLE 68.2.
Trials Comparing Surgical to Endovascular Management of Stenosis or Thrombosis of Dialysis Access Grafts.

Author	*Year*	*Level of evidence*	*Number of subjects (n)*	*Surgical (S): early success*	*Endovascular (EV): early success*
1 Brooks et al.[98]	1987	I	43	18/19 (95%)	19/24 (76%)
2 Schuman et al.[99]	1994	I	31	94%	67%
3 Schwartz et al.[100]	1995	III	48	87%	88%
4 Uflacker et al.[101]	1996	I	37	83%	89%
5 Vesely et al.[102]	1996	I	20	80%	70%
6 Marston et al.[103]	1997	I	115	83%	72%
7 Dougherty et al.[104]	1999	I	80	Cost $1512	Cost $2945
8 Vesely et al.[105]	1999	I	153	79%	73%
9 Lombardi et al.[106]	2002	II	41	N/A	N/A
10 Uflacker et al.[107]	2004	I	174	73.4%	79.2%

Surgical late patency	*Endovascular late patency*	*Comment*
1 6/19 (32%) at 2 years Median = 12 months	0/24 (0%) at 2 years Median = 4 months	An early trial, $P < 0.01$
2 Mean = 147 days	Mean = 120 days	Increasing rate of complications with EV (53%) vs. S (6%), P = NS
3 Mean = 4.5 months	Mean = 5.4 months	Historical surgical control group, P = NS
4 77% at 30 days	68% at 30 days	EV: angioplasty in 18 and stent in 6, P = NS
5 Mean = 93.9 days	Mean = 81.6 days	EV: thrombolysis and angioplasty, P = NS
6 36% at 6 months 25% at 12 months	11% at 6 months 9% at 12 months	Early P = NS, late $P < 0.05$ S: revision in 78%
7 Mean = 7 months	Mean = 6 months	Crossover: 11 EV to S and 2 S to EV; cost $P < 0.001$; patency P = NS
8 41% at 1 months, 32% at 2 months, 26% at 3 months	32% at 1 months, 21% at 2 months, 15% at 3 months	Early P = NS; late $P = 0.053$, which approaches statistical significance
9 78% at 3 months, 78% at 6 months, 54% at 12 months	59% at 3 months, 48% at 6 months, 32% at 12 months	Axillary vein stenosis; case-matched S controls for EV patients, $P = 0.13$
10 73% at 30 days, 68% at 90 days	79% at 30 days, 75% at 90 days	Reenrollment after 90-day trial increased n to 74 (S) and 140 (EV), P = NS

Source: Data based on references 98–107.

Outcomes of Vascular Access

Central venous access devices come in so many different forms, are placed in such varied sites by such different techniques, and are used for so many different purposes that direct comparisons among them are all but impossible. However, the evidence supports some conclusions. The most serious complications of long-term vascular access are infection and thrombosis. Infectious complications are more common with double-lumen than single-lumen catheters.[70] The mean time to infection was 78 days for double-lumen catheters compared to 213 days for single-lumen ones ($P < 0.02$). The total complication rates were similar (33% and 31%), so the needs of the patient should determine the catheter selected. However, a double-lumen catheter should not be placed when a single-lumen catheter will suffice. Complications requiring removal of the access are more common with external devices than with internal ports.[95] The time to removal for complications was 501 days for external catheters compared to 1450 days for ports ($P < 0.005$). Moreover, the external catheters are subject to inadvertent removal, particularly in the first 2 weeks after placement, whereas the ports are not. However, the ports cost more, require surgery for removal, require needle puncture for access, and may extravasate subcutaneously during drug infusion. Consequently, although they are cosmetically superior and better accepted by patients, ports are best reserved for patients who require vascular access for 6 months or more.

The actuarial patency rates for various types of access for chronic hemodialysis are shown in Table 68.3. The cumulative, total time of graft function until ultimate failure is shown (Table 68.3) regardless of whether intervening surgical or endovascular procedures were required to achieve that function. Although the cumulative patency of PTFE AV grafts is 79% at 1 year and 69% at 2 years, the primary patency without intervention for PTFE AV grafts is much less, for example, 44% at 1 year in 632 patients[96] and 37% at 2 years in 1477 patients.[97] In general, high-flow vascular access has better initial success than low-flow access. Nonautogenous AV grafts are lost more rapidly than autogenous AV fistulas. In fact, bovine artery heterografts are no longer used because of their poor long-term function, although the new bovine mesenteric vein graft appears to be useful in patients who have experienced multiple PTFE graft failures. The

TABLE 68.3.
Patency Rates of Various Types of Vascular Access for Chronic Hemodialysis (Level III Data).

Type of access	*Number*	*Patency at 1 year*	*Patency at 2 years*
Radial-cephalic (Brescia–Cimino)	1476	65%	63%
Posterior radial-cephalic (snuff-box)	493	76%	73%
Brachial-cephalic	150	70%	67%
Brachial-basilic	275	78%	75%
PTFE prosthetic graft	1719	79%	69%
Bovine artery heterograft	1454	54%	43%

PTFE, polytetrafluoroethylene.

Based on data from Marx A, Landmann J, Harder F. 1990. Surgery for vascular access. Curr Probl Surg 27:1–48.[34]

short-term disadvantage and long-term advantage of autogenous distal AV fistulas is illustrated by the experience at University Hospital, Basel. The patency rates after 1, 2, and 3 years of 216 snuff-box fistulas were 74%, 67%, and 64% and of 148 Brescia–Cimino fistulas were 65%, 61%, and 60%, respectively. On the other hand, the patency of 43 prosthetic AV grafts declined from 74% after 1 year to only 57% after 2 years.[34] Prosthetic grafts are rarely functional for 3 or more years. The high-flow, autogenous brachiobasilic AV fistula had a 1-year patency rate of 78% and, after 2 years, 74% of them were still patent.

Several principles of successful vascular access may be derived from the available evidence. Optimum short- and long-term vascular access demands (1) strictly aseptic insertion and maintenance, (2) careful attention to the details of placement, (3) use of autogenous before nonautogenous conduits, (4) use of distal before proximal sites of insertion, and (5) prompt removal when a catheter or device is no longer in use. Above all, the physician must endeavor to protect the forearm veins of those patients with renal insufficiency and the central veins of those with cancer because those patients may need reliable vascular access in the future. Recognition of the requirements, knowledge of the techniques, and awareness of the complications make vascular access a surmountable challenge for the clinician and a lifesaving therapy for the patient.

References

1. Wilson SE. Vascular Access: Principles and Practice, 4th ed. St. Louis: Mosby, 2002.
2. Ray CE Jr. Central Venous Access. Philadelphia: Lippincott Williams & Wilkins, 2001.
3. Sommer BG, Henry ML. Vascular Access for Hemodialysis. Los Angeles: Pluribus Press, 1989.
4. Alexander HR. Vascular Access in the Cancer Patient: Devices, Insertion Techniques, Maintenance, and Prevention and Management of Complications. Philadelphia: Lippincott, 1994.
5. Peters JL. A Manual of Central Venous Catheterization and Parenteral Nutrition. Bristol: John Wright and Sons, 1983.
6. Wren C. An account of the rise and attempts, of a way to conveigh liquors immediately into the mass of the blood. Philos Trans R Soc Lond 1665;1:128–130.
7. Dudrick S, Rhoads J. New horizons for intravenous feeding. JAMA 1971;215(6):939–949.
8. Lower R. The method observed in transfusing the blood out of one animal into another. Philos Trans R Soc Lond 1666;1:353–358.
9. Lower R. An account of the experiment of transfusion practised upon man in London. Philos Trans R Soc Lond 1667;2:557–559.
10. Lower R. Tractatus de Corde. In: Franklin KJ, ed. Early Science in Oxford, 1932 ed. London: Oxford Press, 1667.
11. Denis J. A letter concerning a new way of curing sundry diseases by transfusion of blood. Philos Trans R Soc Lond 1667;2:489–504.
12. Cournand A. Cardiac catheterization. Development of the technique, its contributions to experimental medicine, and its initial application in man. Acta Med Scand 1975;(suppl):7–32.
13. Kolff W. The first clinical experience with the artificial kidney. Ann Intern Med 1965;62(3):608–619.
14. Quinton W, Dillard D, Scribner B. Cannulation of blood vessels for prolonged hemodialysis. Trans Am Soc Artif Intern Organs 1960;6:104–113.
15. Brescia M, Cimino J, Appel K, Hurwich B. Chronic hemodialysis using venipuncture and a surgically created arteriovenous fistula. N Engl J Med 1966;275(20):1089–1092.
16. Thomas G. A large-vessel applique A-V shunt for hemodialysis. Trans Am Soc Artif Intern Organs 1969;15:288–292.
17. Dudrick S, Wilmore D, Vars H, Rhoads J. Can intravenous feeding as the sole means of nutrition support growth in the child and restore weight loss in an adult? An affirmative answer. Ann Surg 1969;169(6):974–984.
18. Broviac J, Cole J, Scribner B. A silicone rubber atrial catheter for prolonged parenteral alimentation. Surg Gynecol Obstet 1973;136(4):602–606.
19. Hickman R, Buckner C, Clift R, Sanders J, Stewart P, Thomas E. A modified right atrial catheter for access to the venous system in marrow transplant recipients. Surg Gynecol Obst 1979;148(6):871–875.
20. Niederhuber J, Ensminger W, Gyves J, Lipeman M, Doan K, Cozzi E. Totally implanted venous and arterial access system to replace external catheters in cancer treatment. Surg Gynecol Obstet 1982;92:706–712.
21. Wenzel RP, Edmond MB. Team-based prevention of catheter-related infections [comment]. N Engl J Med 2006;355(26):2781–2783.
22. Sidawy A, Gray R, Besarab A, et al. Recommended standards for reports dealing with arteriovenous hemodialysis accesses. J Vasc Surg 2002;35(3):603–610.
23. Roy-Chaudhury P, Kelly B, Melhem M, et al. Vascular access in hemodialysis: Issues, management and emerging concepts. Cardiol Clin 2005;23(3):249–273.
24. Valentino L, Ewenstein B, Navikis R, Wilkes M. Central venous access devices for haemophilia. Haemophilia 2004;10(2):134–146.
25. Khwaja K. Dialysis access procedures. In: Humar A, Matas A, Payne W, eds. Atlas of Organ Transplantation. London: Springer, 2006:35–58.
26. Thadhani R, Pascual M, Bonventre J. Acute renal failure. N Engl J Med 1996;334:1448–1460.
27. Manns M, Sigler M, Techan B. Continuous renal replacement therapies: an update. Am J Kidney Dis 1998;32:185–207.
28. Tesio F, Baz HD, Panarello G, et al. Double catheterization of the internal jugular vein for hemodialysis: indications, techniques, and clinical results. Artif Organs 1994;18(4):301–304.
29. Sandhu J. Dialysis ports: a new totally implantable option for hemodialysis access. Tech Vasc Intervent Radiol 2002;5(2):108–113.
30. McLaughlin K, Jones B, Mactier R, Porteus C. Long-term vascular access for hemodialysis using silicon dual-lumen catheters

with guidewire replacement of catheters for technique salvage. Am J Kidney Dis 1997;29(4):553–559.
31. Mosquera DA, Gibson SP, Goldman MD. Vascular access surgery: a 2-year study and comparison with the Permcath. Nephrol Dial Transplant 1992;7(11):1111–1115.
32. Williams R, Hollander L, Benyon R, et al. Principles of vascular access surgery. In: Wilson S, Veith F, Hobson R, Williams R, eds. Vascular Surgery: Principles and Practice. New York: McGraw-Hill, 1987:857–872.
33. Mehta S. Statistical summary of clinical results of vascular access procedures for hemodialysis. In: Sommer B, Henry M, eds. Vascular Access for Hemodialysis, vol II. Los Angeles: WL Gore Associates and Precept Press, 1991:145–157.
34. Marx A, Landmann J, Harder F. Surgery for vascular access. Curr Probl Surg 1990;27:1–48.
35. Choi H, Lal B, Cerveira J, et al. Durability and cumulative functional patency of transposed and nontransposed arteriovenous fistulas. J Vasc Surg 2003;38(6):1206–2003.
36. National Kidney Foundation. K/DOQI Clinical Practice Guidelines for Vascular Access: Update 2000. Am J Kidney Dis 2001;37(1 suppl 1):S137–S181.
37. Gorski T, Nguyen H, Gorski Y, Chung H, Jamal A, Muney J. Lower-extremity saphenous vein transposition arteriovenous fistula: an alternative for hemodialysis access in AIDS patients. Am Surg 1998;64:338–340.
38. National Kidney Foundation. NKF-DOQI Clinical Practice Guidelines for Vascular Access. National Kidney Foundation-Dialysis Outcomes Quality Initiative. Am J Kidney Dis 1997;30(4 suppl 3):S150–S191.
39. Silva M Jr, Hopson R, Pappas P, et al. A strategy for increasing use of autogenous hemodialysis access procedures: impact of preoperative, noninvasive evaluation. J Vasc Surg 1998;27:302–308.
40. Allon M, Robbin M. Increasing arteriovenous fistulas in hemodialysis patients: Problems and solutions. Kidney Int 2002;62: 1109–1124.
41. Parmley M, Broughan T, Jennings W. Vascular ultrasonography prior to dialysis access surgery. Am J Surg 2002;184:568–572.
42. Katzman HE, Glickman MH, Schild AF, Fujitani RM, Lawson JH. Multicenter evaluation of the bovine mesenteric vein bioprosthesis for hemodialysis access in patients with an earlier failed prosthetic graft. J Am Coll Surg 2005;201(2):223–230.
43. Taylor S, Eaves G, Weatherford D. Results and complications of arteriovenous access dialysis grafts in the lower extremity: a five-year review. Am Surg 1996;62:188–191.
44. Mandel S, McDougal E. Popliteal artery to saphenous vein vascular access for hemodialysis. Surg Gynecol Obstet 1985;160:358–359.
45. Connolly J, Brownell D, Levine E, et al. Complications of renal dialysis access procedures. Arch Surg 1984;119:1325–1328.
46. Tashjian D, Lipkowitz G, Madden R, et al. Safety and efficacy of femoral-based hemodialysis. J Vasc Surg 2002;35(4):691–693.
47. Striker G, Tenckoff H. A transcutaneous prosthesis for prolonged access to the peritoneal cavity. Surgery (St. Louis) 1971;69(1):70–74.
48. USRDS. 1997 Annual Report. In: US Renal Data System Annual Report. Bethesda, MD: The National Institutes of Health, National Institute of Diabetes and Digestive and Kidney Disease, 1997.
49. Nolph K. Comparison of continuous ambulatory peritoneal dialysis and hemodialysis. Kidney Int 1988;24(suppl):S123–S131.
50. Crabtree J, Fishman A. A laparoscopic method for optimal peritoneal dialysis access. Am Surg 2005;71(2):135–143.
51. Nielsen P, Hemmingsen C, Friis S, Ladefoged J, Olgaard K. Comparison of straight and curled Tenckhoff peritoneal dialysis catheters implanted by percutaneous technique: a prospective, randomized study. Perit Dial Int 1995;15(1):18–21.
52. Diaz-Buxo J. Complications of peritoneal dialysis catheters: early and late. Int J Artif Organs 2006;29(1):50–58.
53. Alexander H. Insertion technique for long-term venous access catheters: percutaneous subclavian vein catheterization. In: Alexander H, ed. Vascular Access in the Cancer Patient. Philadelphia: Lippincott, 1994:37–55.
54. Steinhaus E. Long-term access via internal jugular vein cutdown. In: Alexander H, ed. Vascular Access in the Cancer Patient. Philadelphia: Lippincott, 1994:57–66.
55. Vesely T. Central venous catheter tip position: a continuing controversy. J Vasc Intervent Radiol 2003;14(5):527–534.
56. Torosian M. Difficult vascular access: alternate sites and techniques of insertion. In: Alexander H, ed. Vascular Access for the Cancer Patient. Philadelphia: Lippincott, 1994:67–88.
57. Brown J. Peripherally inserted central catheters: use in home care. J Intraven Nurs 1989;12:144–150.
58. Alexander H, Lucas A. Long-term venous access catheters and implantable ports. In: Alexander H, ed. Vascular Access in the Cancer Patient: Devices, Insertion Techniques, Maintenance and Prevention and Management of Complications. Philadelphia: Lippincott, 1994:2–16.
59. Malviya V, Deppe G, Gove N, Malone JJ. Vascular access in gynecologic cancer using the Groshong right atrial catheter. Gynecol Cancer 1989;33(3):313–316.
60. Strum S, McDermid J, Korn A, Joseph C. Improved methods for venous access: the Port-A-Cath, a totally implanted catheter system. J Clin Oncol 1986;4:596–603.
61. Vesely T. Air embolism during insertion of central venous catheters. J Vasc Intervent Radiol 2001;12(11):1291–1295.
62. Whitman E. Complications associated with the use of central venous access devices. Curr Probl Surg 1996;33:309–378.
63. Denys B, Uretsky B, Reddy P. Ultrasound-assisted cannulation of the internal jugular vein: a prospective comparison to the external landmark-guided technique. Circulation 1993;87:1557–1562.
64. Savader S, Haikal L, Karen O, Porter D, Oteham A. Hemodialysis catheter-associated fibrin sheaths: treatment with a low-dose rtPA infusion. J Vasc Intervent Radiol 2000;11:1131–1136.
65. Gray R, Levitin A, Buck D, et al. Percutaneous fibrin sheath stripping versus transcatheter urokinase infusion for malfunctioning well-positioned tunneled central venous dialysis catheters: a prospective, randomized trial. J Vasc Intervent Radiol 2000;11(9):1121–1129.
66. Lumsden A, McDonald M, Isiklar H, et al. Central venous stenosis in the hemodialysis patient: incidence and efficacy of endovascular treatment. Cardiovasc Surg 1997;5:504–509.
67. Vesely T, Hovsepian D, Pilgram T. Upper extremity central venous obstruction in hemodialysis patients: treatment with Wallstents. Radiology 1997;204:343–348.
68. Stevenson KB, Hannah EL, Lowder CA, et al. Epidemiology of hemodialysis vascular access infections from longitudinal infection surveillance data: predicting the impact of NKF-DOQI clinical practice guidelines for vascular access. Am J Kidney Dis 2002;39(3):549–555.
69. Marr K, Sexton D, Conlon P, et al. Catheter-related bacteremia and outcome of attempted catheter salvage in patients undergoing hemodialysis. Ann Intern Med 1997;125:275–280.
70. Early T, Gregory R, Wheeler J, Snyder S, Gayle R. Increased infection rate in double-lumen versus single-lumen Hickman catheters in cancer patients. South Med J 1990;83:34–36.
71. Merrer J, DeJonghe B, Golliot F, et al. Complications of femoral and subclavian venous catheterization in critically ill patients: a randomized controlled trial. JAMA 2001;286(6):700–707.
72. Bethard G. Management of bacteremia associated with tunneled-cuffed hemodialysis catheters. J Am Soc Nephrol 1999;10:1045–1049.
73. Darouiche R, Raad I, Heard S, et al. A comparison of two antimicrobial-impregnated central venous catheters. N Engl J Med 1999;340:1–8.

74. Rupp M, Lisco S, Lipsett P, et al. Effect of a second-generation venous catheter impregnated with chlorhexidine and silver sulfadiazine on central-catheter-related infections: a randomized clinical trial. Ann Intern Med 2005;143(8):570–580.
75. NNIS System. NNIS Report, data summary from January 1992 through October 2004, issued October 2004. Am J Infect Control 2004;32:470–485.
76. Mermel L. Prevention of intravascular catheter-related infections. Ann Intern Med 2000;132:391–402.
77. Pronovost P, Needham D, Berenholtz S, et al. An intervention to decrease catheter-related bloodstream infections in the ICU. N Engl J Med 2006;355(26):2725–2732.
78. Haimov M, Baez A, Neff M, et al. Complications of arteriovenous fistulas for hemodialysis. Arch Surg 1975;110:708–712.
79. Anderson C, Allen B, Sicard G. Physiology and hemodynamics of vascular access. In: Sommer B, Henry M, eds. Vascular Access for Hemodialysis. Los Angeles: WL Gore and Associates and Pluribus Press, 1989:17–31.
80. Katz S, Kohl R. The treatment of hand ischemia by arterial ligation and upper extremity bypass after angioacess surgery. J Am Coll Surg 1996;183:239–242.
81. Ryan S, Calligaro K, Dougherty M. Management of hemodialysis access infections. Semin Vasc Surg 2004;17(1):40–44.
82. Nasser G, Ayus J. Infectious complications of the hemodialysis access. Kidney Int 2001;60:1–13.
83. Brock J, Sussman M, Wamsley M, et al. The influence of human immunodeficiency virus infection and intravenous drug abuse on complications of hemodialysis access surgery. J Vasc Surg 1992;16:904–912.
84. Nannery W, Stoldt H, Fares LG Jr, et al. Hemodialysis access operations performed upon patients with human immunodeficiency virus. Surg Gynecol Obstet 1991;173:387–390.
85. O'Shea S, Lawson J, Reddan D, Murphy M, Ortel T. Hypercoagulable states and antithrombotic strategies in recurrent vascular access site thrombosis. J Vasc Surg 2003;38(3):541–548.
86. Barth K, Gosnell M, Palestrant A, et al. Hydrodynamic thrombectomy system versus pulse-spray thrombolysis for thrombosed hemodialysis grafts: a multicenter prospective randomized comparison. Radiology 2000;217(3):678–684.
87. Vesely T. Mechanical thrombectomy devices to treat thrombosed hemodialysis grafts. Tech Vasc Intervent Radiol 2003 6(1):35–41.
88. Vesely T, Siegel J. Use of the peripheral cutting balloon to treat hemodialysis-related stenosis. J Vasc Intervent Radiol 2005; 16(12):1593–1603.
89. Etheridge E, Haid S, Maesner M, et al. Salvage operations for malfunctioning polytetrafluoroethylene hemodialysis access grafts. Surgery (St. Louis) 1983;96:464–470.
90. Bethard G. Percutaneous transvenous angioplasty in the treatment of vascular access stenosis. Kidney Int 1992;42:1390–1397.
91. Schwab S, Raymond J, Saeed M, Newman G, Dennis P, Bollinger R. Prevention of hemodialysis fistula thrombosis. Early detection of venous stenosis. Kidney Int 1989;36:707–711.
92. Konner K. Interventional strategies for haemodialysis fistulae and grafts: interventional radiology or surgery? Nephrol Dial Transplant 2000;15:1922–1923.
93. Green L, Lee D, Kucey D. A metaanalysis comparing surgical thrombectomy, mechanical thrombectomy, and pharmacomechanical thrombolysis for thrombosed dialysis grafts. J Vasc Surg 2002;36:939–945.
94. Kolakowski S, Dougherty M, Calligaro K. Salvaging prosthetic dialysis fistulas with stents: forearm versus upper arm grafts. J Vasc Surg 2003;38(4):719–723.
95. Stanislav GV, Fitzgibbons RJ Jr, Malliard J, Johnson S, Feole J. Reliability of implanted central venous access devices in patients with cancer. Arch Surg 1987;122:1280–1283.
96. Schuman E, Standage B, Ragsdale J, Gross G. Reinforced versus nonreinforced polytetrafluoroethylene grafts for hemodialysis access. Am J Surg 1997;173(5):407–410.
97. Kennedy M, Quinton H, Bubolz T, Wennberg J, Wilson S. An analysis of the patency of vascular access grafts for hemodialysis using the Medicare Part B database. Semin Vasc Surg 1996;9(3):262–265.
98. Brooks J, Sigley R, May K, Mack R. Transluminal angioplasty versus surgical repair for stenosis of hemodialysis grafts. Am J Surg 1987;153:530–531.
99. Schuman E, Quinn S, Standage B, Cross G. Thombolysis versus thrombectomy for occluded hemodialysis grafts. Am J Surg 1994;167(5):473–476.
100. Schwartz C, McBrayer C, Sloan J, Menesis P, Ennis W. Thrombosed dialysis grafts: comparison of treatment with transluminal angioplasty and surgical revision. Radiology 1995;194(2):337–341.
101. Uflacker R, Rajagopalan P, Vujic I, Stutley J. Treatment of thrombosed dialysis access grafts: randomized trial of surgical thrombectomy versus mechanical thrombectomy with the Amplatz device. J Vasc Intervent Radiol 1996;7(2):185–192.
102. Vesely T, Idso M, Audrain J, Windus D, Lowell J. Thrombolysis versus surgical thrombectomy for the treatment of dialysis graft thrombosis: pilot study comparing costs. J Vasc Intervent Radiol 1996;7(4):507–512.
103. Marston W, Criado E, Jaques P, Mauro M, Burnham S, Keagy B. Prospective randomized comparison of surgical versus endovascular management of thrombosed dialysis access grafts. J Vasc Surg 1997;26:373–381.
104. Dougherty M, Calligaro K, Schindler N, Raviola C, Ntoso A. Endovascular versus surgical treatment for thrombosed hemodialysis grafts: a prospective randomized study. J Vasc Surg 1999;30(6):1016–1023.
105. Vesely T, Williams D, Weiss M, et al. Comparison of the Angiojet rheolytic catheter to surgical thrombectomy for the treatment of thrombosed hemodialysis grafts. J Vasc Intervent Radiol 1999;10(9):1195–1205.
106. Lombardi J, Dougherty M, Veitia N, Somal J, Calligaro K. A comparison of patch angioplasty and stenting for axillary venous stenoses of thrombosed hemodialysis grafts. Vasc Endovasc Surg 2002;36(3):223–229.
107. Uflacker R, Rajagopolan P, Selby J, Hannegan C. Thrombosed dialysis access grafts: randomized comparison of the Amplatz thrombectomy device and surgical thromboembolectomy. Eur Radiol 2004;14(11):2009–2014.

SECTION SEVEN

Thoracic Surgery

69 History of Cardiac Surgery

Larry W. Stephenson

After the development of general anesthetics such as ether and chloroform during the middle of the nineteenth century, investigators began to study techniques to repair heart wounds in the animal laboratory. Soon, simple operations in humans for heart wounds were reported.

Heart Wounds

On July 10, 1893, Dr. Daniel Hale Williams, a surgeon from Chicago, successfully operated on a 24-year-old man who had been stabbed in the heart during a fight.[1] Initially, the wound was thought to be superficial, but during the night there was persistent bleeding, pain, and pronounced symptoms of shock. Williams opened the patient's chest and tied off an artery and vein that had been injured inside the chest wall, likely causing the blood loss. Then he noticed a tear in the pericardium and a puncture wound to the heart, "about one-tenth of an inch in length." The wound itself in the right ventricle was not bleeding, so Williams did not place a stitch through the heart wound. He did, however, stitch closed the hole in the pericardium. The patient recovered. Williams reported this case 4 years later. This operation, which is frequently referred to, is probably the first successful surgery where a documented stab wound to the heart was identified. At the time, Williams' surgery was considered bold and daring, and although he did not actually place a stitch through the wound in the heart, his treatment seems to have been appropriate. Under the circumstances, he most likely saved the patient's life.

Dr. Ludwig Rehn, a surgeon in Frankfurt, Germany, performed what many consider the first successful heart operation. On September 9, 1896, he operated on a 22-year-old man who had been stabbed 2 days before, and the patient appeared moribund. He opened the patient's chest; the mammary artery was not injured. He noticed continuous bleeding from a hole in the pericardium. He enlarged the opening and exposed the heart. He emptied out a blood clot and found a 1.5-cm right ventricular wound. He controlled the bleeding with finger pressure and placed three silk sutures to close the wound. The patient recovered. In Rehn's report in a medical journal, he stated that, "This proves the feasibility of cardiac suture repair without a doubt! I hope this will lead to more investigation regarding surgery of the heart. This may save many lives."[2]

Dr. Luther Hill was the first American to report the successful repair of a cardiac wound. He operated on a 13-year-old boy with multiple stab wounds to the chest in 1902.[3] The surgery took place on the patient's kitchen table in a rundown shack during the middle of the night. Lighting was provided by two kerosene lamps borrowed from the neighbors. The stab wound to the left ventricle was repaired with two catgut sutures. The postoperative course was stormy, but the patient recovered.

Another milestone in cardiac surgery for trauma occurred during World War II when Dwight Harken, then a U.S. Army surgeon, removed 134 missiles from the mediastinum, including 55 from the pericardium and 13 from cardiac chambers, without a death.[4] At the time, the battle wounds were sustained on the Continent and the U.S. Army thoracic specialty hospital was back in England, so these were highly selective patients. Nonetheless, it is hard to imagine this type of elective (and semielective) surgery taking place without sophisticated monitoring equipment. Rapid blood infusion consisted of pumping air into glass bottles of blood.

Operative Management of Pulmonary Emboli

Frederic Trendelenburg, in 1908, was the first to attempt a pulmonary embolectomy. The patient did not survive the procedure, nor did his next two cases.[5] Martin Kirschner, however, Trendelenburg's student, reported the first patient who fully recovered after undergoing a pulmonary embolectomy in 1924.[6] In 1937, John Gibbon estimated that 9 of 142 patients who had undergone the Trendelenburg Procedure worldwide left the hospital alive.[7] These dismal results were an impetus for Gibbon to start working on a pump oxygenator that could maintain the circulation during pulmonary embolectomy. Sharp, in 1962 was the first to perform a pulmonary embolectomy using cardiopulmonary bypass.[8]

Surgery of the Pericardium

Pericardial resection for constrictive pericarditis was introduced independently by Rehn and Sauerbruch, both from Germany, in 1913.[9,10] Since Rehn's report there have been few advances in the surgical treatment of pericarditis. Some operations are now performed with the aid of cardiopulmonary bypass. In many situations, radical pericardectomy is performed, which includes most of the pericardium posterior to the phrenic nerve.

Catheterization of the Heart

Although cardiac catheterization is not considered heart surgery, it is an invasive procedure, and some catheter procedures have replaced heart operations. Warner Forssmann is credited with the first heart catheterizations in 1929. He performed the procedure on himself and reported it in *Kleinische Wochenschrift*.[11] In 1956, Forssmann shared the Nobel Prize in Physiology or Medicine with Andre F. Cournand and Dickenson W. Richards, Jr., for using a catheter to chart the heart's interior and study circulatory changes.

Heart Valve Surgery Before the Era of Cardiopulmonary Bypass

There were isolated cases of heart valve dilatation reported between 1912 and Charles Bailey's 1949 paper entitled "The Surgical Treatment of Mitral Stenosis."[12] Only the fifth operation, done on June 10, 1948, of the five cases Bailey reported in that paper was successful. One week later, Bailey brought the patient by train 1000 miles to Chicago where he presented the woman to the American College of Chest Physicians. A few days after Bailey's success, on June 16, in Boston, Dr. Dwight Harken successfully performed his first valvulotomy for mitral stenosis.[13] Bailey and Harken dilated the valve blindly by passing a finger or instrument through the valve from the left atrial appendage. The first successful pulmonary valvulotomy was performed by Thomas Holmes Sellors on December 4, 1947. Sellors used a tenotomy knife, which he passed through the right ventricle, to perform the valvulotomy.[14]

In the early 1950s, Charles Hufnagel developed and implanted artificial valves in the descending aorta. The valves consisted of a mobile ball inside a Lucite case. Hufnagel et al. reported a series of 23 patients starting September 1952 who had this operation for aortic insufficiency.[15] There were 4 deaths among the first 10 patients and 2 deaths among the next 13. Hufnagel's caged ball valve was the only surgical treatment for aortic valvular incompetence until the advent of cardiopulmonary bypass and heart valves that could be sewn into the aortic annulus position.

Congenital Cardiac Surgery: Pre-Heart-Lung Machine Era

On August 16, 1938, Robert Gross, at Boston Children's Hospital, successfully ligated a ductus in a 7-year-old girl with dyspnea after moderate exercise.[16] The patient made a good recovery.

Dr. Clarence Crafoord, in Stockholm, Sweden, successfully resected a coarctation of the aorta in a 12-year-old boy on October 19, 1944.[17] Twelve days later he successfully resected the coarctation of a 27-year-old patient. In 1945, Dr. Gross reported the first successful case of surgical relief for tracheal obstruction from a vascular ring.[18] In the 5 years that followed Gross's first successful vascular ring operation, he reported 40 more cases.[19]

The famous Blalock–Taussig operation also was reported in 1945. The first patient was a 15-month-old girl with a clinical diagnosis of tetralogy of Fallot. The operation was performed by Dr. Alfred Blalock at Johns Hopkins University on November 29, 1944.[20] The left subclavian artery was anastomosed to the left pulmonary artery in an end-to-side fashion. Thus, within a 7-year period, three congenital cardiovascular defects—patent ductus arteriosus, coarctation of the aorta, and vascular ring—were attacked surgically and treated successfully. However, the introduction of the Blalock–Taussig shunt was probably the most powerful stimulus to the development of cardiac surgery, because this operation palliated a complex intracardiac lesion and focused attention on the pathophysiology of cardiac disease.

Anomalous coronary artery in which the left coronary artery communicates with the pulmonary artery was the next surgical conquest. The surgery was performed on July 22, 1946, and was reported by Gunnar Biorck and Clarence Crafoord.[21] Muller reported successful surgical treatment of transposition of the pulmonary veins in 1951, but the operation addressed a partial form of the anomaly.[22] Later, in the 1950s, Gott, Varco, Lillehei, and Cooley reported successful operative variations for anomalous pulmonary veins.

Another of Gross' pioneering surgical procedures was the surgical closure of an aortopulmonary window.[23] The operation was carried out on May 22, 1948. Cooley et al. were the first to report the use of cardiopulmonary bypass to repair this defect and converted a difficult and hazardous procedure into a relatively straightforward one.[24]

Glenn reported the first successful clinical application in the United States in 1958 for what has been termed the Glenn shunt.[25] Similar work was done in Russia during the 1950s by several investigators. In 1956 and 1957, Russian surgeons Meshalkin, Vishnevsky, and Galankin used this procedure clinically to treat patients with tetralogy of Fallot and tricuspid atresia.[26]

The Development of Cardiopulmonary Bypass

John Gibbon contributed more to the success of the development of the heart machine than anyone else. His interest began as a young doctor one night in 1930 in Boston "during an all-night vigil by the side of a patient with a massive embolus . . ." The patient did not survive an attempted pulmonary embolectomy.[27]

Gibbon's work on the heart-lung machine took place over the next 25 years, in laboratories at the Massachusetts General Hospital, the University of Pennsylvania, and Thomas Jefferson University. In 1937, Gibbon reported the first successful demonstration that life could be maintained by an artificial heart and lung and that the native heart and lungs could resume function. Unfortunately, only three animals recovered adequate cardiorespiratory function after total pulmonary artery occlusion and bypass, and even they died a few hours later.[28] Gibbon's work was interrupted by World War II; afterward, he resumed his work at the Thomas Jefferson Medical College in Philadelphia. Meanwhile, other groups, including Clarence Crafoord in Stockholm, Sweden, J. Youngblood at the University of Utrecht in Holland, Clarence Dennis at the University of Minnesota, Mario Dogliotti and coworkers at the University of Turino in Italy, and Forest Dodrill at Harper Hospital in Detroit also worked on a heart-lung machine. Clarence Dennis' first clinical attempt at open heart surgery was in a 6-year-old girl with end-stage cardiac disease. Although the heart-lung machine functioned well, the patient did not survive, probably because of a combination of blood loss and surgically induced tricuspid stenosis.[29]

In August 1951, Mario Dogliotti[30] used his heart-lung machine to partially support the circulation at the flow of 1 L/min in a 49-year-old patient during resection of a large mediastinal tumor.

Forest Dodrill and colleagues used the mechanical blood pump they developed with General Motors on a 41-year-old man. The machine was used to substitute for the left ventricle for 50 min while a surgical procedure was carried out to repair the mitral valve; the patient's own lungs were used to oxygenate the blood. This, the first clinically successful total left-sided heart bypass in a human, was done July 3, 1952, and followed from Dodrill's experimental work with a mechanical pump for univentricular, biventricular, or cardiopulmonary bypass. Later, on October 21, 1952, Dodrill used the machine in a 16-year-old boy with congenital pulmonary stenosis to perform a pulmonary valvuloplasty under direct vision; this was the first successful right-sided heart bypass. Between July 1952 and December 1954, Dodrill performed approximately 13 clinical operations on the heart and thoracic aorta using the Dodrill-General Motors machine with at least 5 hospital survivors. Although he used this machine with an oxygenator in the animal laboratory, he did not start using an oxygenator with the Dodrill-General Motors mechanical heart clinically until early 1955.[31,32]

John Lewis closed an atrial septal defect in a 5-year-old girl on September 2, 1952, using a hypothermic technique. She was anesthetized and the trachea was intubated.[33] She was then wrapped in refrigerated blankets until, after a period of 2 h and 10 min, her rectal temperature had fallen to 28°C. At this point, the chest was entered and the cardiac inflow occluded for a total of 5.5 min. During this time the septal defect was closed under direct vision. The patient was rewarmed by placing her in hot water kept at 45°C and, after 35 min, her rectal temperature had risen to 36°C, at which time she was removed from the bath. Recovery from the anesthesia was prompt, and her subsequent postoperative convalescence was uneventful.

Shortly after, Swan et al. reported successful results in 13 clinical cases using a similar technique.[34] However, use of systemic hypothermia for open intracardiac surgery was relatively short-lived. After the heart-lung machine was introduced clinically, it appeared the deep hypothermia was obsolete. However, during the 1960s, it became apparent that operative results in infants under 1 year of age using cardiopulmonary bypass were poor. In 1967, Hikasa et al., from Kyoto, Japan, published an article that reintroduced profound hypothermia for cardiac surgery in infants and used the heart-lung machine for rewarming.[35] Their technique involved surface cooling to 20°C, cardiac surgery during circulatory arrest for 15 to 75 min, and rewarming with cardiopulmonary bypass. Soon, other groups reported using profound hypothermia with circulatory arrest in infants with the heart-lung machine for cooling and rewarming. Results were much improved, and subsequently the technique also was applied for resection of aortic arch aneurysms.

After World War II, John Gibbon resumed his research. Gibbon used a new machine built with the help of International Business Machine (IBM) Corporation engineers. In 1949, Gibbon's early mortality in dogs was 80%, but it gradually improved. Gibbon operated on a 15-month-old girl with severe congestive heart failure in February 1952. The preoperative diagnosis was atrial septal defect, but at operation, none was found. She died, and a huge patent ductus was found at autopsy. The next patient was an 18-year-old girl with congestive heart failure caused by an atrial septal defect. This defect was closed successfully on May 6, 1953, with the Gibbon-IBM heart-lung machine.[36] The patient recovered, and several months later the defect was confirmed closed at cardiac catheterization. She was the first patient to undergo successful heart surgery in which a heart-lung machine was used. Unfortunately, Gibbon's next two patients did not survive intracardiac procedures when the heart-lung machine was used. These failures distressed Dr. Gibbon, who declared a 1-year moratorium for the heart-lung machine until more work could be done to solve the problems causing the deaths.

During this period, C. Walton Lillehei and colleagues at the University of Minnesota studied a technique called controlled cross-circulation. With this technique the circulation of one dog was temporarily used to support that of a second dog while the second dog's heart was temporarily stopped and opened. After a simulated repair in the second dog, the animals were disconnected and allowed to recover. Lillehei et al. used this technique at the University of Minnesota to correct a ventricular septal defect (VSD) in a 12-month-old infant on March 26, 1954. The patient made an uneventful recovery until death on the 11th postoperative day from a rapidly progressing tracheal bronchitis. At autopsy, the VSD was closed, and the respiratory infection was confirmed as the cause of death. Two weeks later, the second and third patients had VSDs closed by the same technique 3 days apart. Both remained long-term survivors with normal hemodynamics confirmed by cardiac catheterization. By July 1955, the blood

TABLE 69.1.
First Year of Successful Intracardiac Repairs Using Cardiopulmonary Bypass or Cross-Circulation.

Lesion	*Surgeon*	*Year*	*Comment*	*Reference*
Atrial septal defect	Gibbon	1953	May 6, 1953	36
Ventricular septal defect	Lillehei	1953	Cross-circulation	86
Complete atrioventricular canal	Lillehei	1954	Cross-circulation	87
Tetralogy of Fallot	Lillehei	1954	Cross-circulation	86
Tetralogy of Fallot	Kirklin	1955	Cardiopulmonary bypass (CPB)	88
Total anomalous pulmonary veins	Kirklin	1956		89
Congenital aneurysm sinus of Valsalva	Kirklin	1956		90
Congenital aortic stenosis	Kirklin	1956	First direct visual correction	91
Aortopulmonary window	Cooley	1957	First closure using CPB	92
Double outlet right ventricle	Kirklin	1957	Extemporarily devised correction	93
Corrected transposition great arteries	Lillehei	1957		94
Transposition great arteries: atrial switch	Senning	1959	Physiological total correction	95
Coronary arteriovenous fistula	Swan	1959		96
Ebstein's anomaly	Hardy	1964	Repair of atrialized tricuspid valve	97
Tetralogy with pulmonary atresia	Ross	1966	Used aortic allograft	98
Truncus arteriosus	McGoon	1967	Used aortic allograft	99
Tricuspid atresia	Fontan	1968	Physiological correction	100
Single ventricle	Horiuchi	1970		101
Subaortic tunnel stenosis	Konno	1975		102
Transposition great arteries: arterial switch	Jatene	1975	Anatomic correction	103
Hypoplastic left heart syndrome	Norwood	1983	Two-stage operation	104
Pediatric heart transplantation	Bailey	1985		105

pump used for systemic cross-circulation by Lillehei et al. was coupled with a bubble oxygenator developed by Drs. DeWall and Lillehei, and cross-circulation was abandoned after use in 45 patients during 1954 and 1955.[37] Although its clinical use was short-lived, cross-circulation was an important stepping stone in the development of cardiac surgery. Meanwhile, at the Mayo Clinic only 90 miles away, John W. Kirklin and colleagues launched their open heart program on March 5, 1955. They used a heart-lung machine based on the Gibbon-IBM machine, but with their own modifications. Four of Kirklin's 8 patients survived.[38] The Mayo team was able to claim the first successful series of cases (i.e., more than 1) using the heart-lung machine. By the end of 1956, many university groups around the world had launched into open heart programs.

Evolution of Congenital Cardiac Surgery During the Era of Cardiopulmonary Bypass

With the advent of cardiopulmonary bypass using either the cross-circulation technique of Lillehei et al. or the version of the mechanical heart-lung machine used by Kirklin et al., the two groups led the way for intracardiac repairs for many of the commonly occurring congenital heart defects (Table 69.1).

Valvular Surgery: Cardiopulmonary Bypass Era

Cardiac valve repair or replacement under direct vision awaited the development of the heart-lung machine. The first successful aortic valve replacement in the subcoronary position was performed by Dr. Dwight Harken and colleagues.[39] A caged ball valve was used. Many of the techniques described in Harken's 1960 report are similar to those used today for aortic valve replacement. That same year, Starr successfully replaced the mitral valve using a caged ball valve of his own team's design.[40] By 1967, nearly 2000 Starr–Edwards valves had been implanted, and the cage ball valve prosthesis was established as the standard against which all other mechanical prostheses would be compared.

Cartwright et al., on November 1, 1961, were first to successfully replace both the aortic and mitral valves with ball-valve prostheses that they had developed.[41] In 1964, Starr and associates reported 13 patients who had undergone multiple valve replacement.[42] One patient had the aortic, mitral, and tricuspid valves replaced on February 21, 1963. Knott-Craig et al., from the Mayo Clinic, in 1992 reported successful replacement of all four heart valves in a patient with carcinoid involvement.[43]

In 1961, Andrew Morrow and Edwin Brockenbrough reported the treatment for idiopathic hypertrophic subaortic stenosis by resecting a portion of the thickened ventricular septum.[44] They referred to this as subaortic ventriculomyotomy. They gave credit to William Cleland and H.H. Bentall in London, who had earlier encountered this condition unexpectedly at operation and resected a small portion of the ventricular mass. The patient improved, but no postoperative hemodynamic studies had been reported. The subaortic ventriculomyotomy became the standard surgical treatment for this cardiac anomaly, although patients with systolic anterior motion (SAM) of the anterior leaflet of the mitral valve require mitral valve replacement with a low-profile mechanical valve. An aortic homograft valve was used clinically for the first time by Heimbecker and associates in Toronto for replacement of the mitral valve in one patient and an aortic valve in another.[45] Survival was short, 1 day in one patient and 1 month in the other. Donald Ross reported on the first successful aortic valve replacement with an aortic valve homograft.[46] The technique of aortic valve replacement with a pulmonary autograft initially described by Ross in 1967 is advocated by some groups for younger patients who require aortic valve replacement. An aortic or pulmonary valve homograft is used to replace the pulmonary valve that has been transferred to the aortic position.[47,48] Other autogenous materials that have been used to manufacture valve prostheses include pericardium, fasciae latae, and dura mater. In the 1960s, Binet et al. began to develop and test tissue valves. In 1964, Duran and Gunning in England replaced an aortic valve in a patient using a xenograft porcine aortic valve. Early results with formaldehyde-fixed xenografts were good, but in a few years these valves began to fail because of tissue degeneration and calcification.[49] Carpentier and associates revitalized interest in xenograft valves by fixating porcine valves with gluteraldehyde. Carpentier–Edwards porcine valves and Hancock and Angell–Shiley bioprostheses became popular and have been implanted in large numbers of patients.[50,51]

Coronary Artery Surgery

Selective coronary angiography developed by Sones and Shirey, at the Cleveland Clinic, was reported in their 1962 classic paper "Cine Coronary Arteriography."[52] They used a catheter to inject contrast material directly into the coronary artery ostia. This technique gave a major impetus to direct revascularization of obstructed coronary arteries.

In the early 1960s, several sporadic instances of coronary grafting have subsequently been reported. All were isolated cases and, for uncertain reasons, were not reproduced. None had an impact on the development of coronary surgery. Dr. Robert H. Goetz performed what appears to be the first clearly documented coronary artery bypass operation in a human, which was successful.[53] The surgery took place at Van Etten Hospital in New York City on May 2, 1960. He operated on a 38-year-old man who was severely symptomatic and used a nonsuture technique to connect the right internal mammary artery to a right coronary artery. It took him 17 second to join the two arteries using a hollow metal tube. The internal mammary artery (IMA)–coronary artery connection was confirmed patent by angiography performed on the 14th postoperative day. The patient remained asymptomatic for about a year, when he developed recurrent angina and died of a myocardial infarction on June 23, 1961. Goetz was severely criticized by his medical and surgical colleagues for this procedure, although he had performed it successfully many times in the animal laboratory. He never attempted another coronary bypass operation in a human.

Another example involved a case of autogenous saphenous vein bypass grafting performed on November 23, 1964, in a 42-year-old man who was scheduled to have endarterectomy of his left coronary.[54] Because the lesion involved the entire bifurcation, endarterectomy with venous patch graft was abandoned as too hazardous. The anterior descending coronary artery was softer distal to the bifurcation. An autogenous saphenous vein graft was therefore placed from the aorta to the left anterior descending. This was probably the first clinical case of successful coronary artery bypass surgery using saphenous vein. The authors, Garrett, Dennis, and DeBakey, however, did not report this case until 1973. The patient was alive at that time, and angiograms showed the vein graft to be patent.

As early as 1952, Vladimir Demikhov, the renowned Soviet surgeon, was anastomosing the internal mammary artery to the left coronary artery in dogs.[55] In 1967, at the height of the Cold War, a Soviet surgeon, V.I. Kolessov, from Leningrad, reported his experience in an American surgical journal with mammary artery–coronary artery anastomoses for treatment of angina pectoris in six patients.[56] The first patient in that series was done in 1964. Operations were performed through a left thoracotomy without extracorporeal circulation or preoperative coronary angiography. The following year, Green et al. and Bailey and Hirose separately published reports in which the internal mammary artery was used for coronary artery bypass in patients.[57,58] Bailey and Hirose carried out the anastomosis on the beating heart and advocated using loupes for magnification. Green et al. advocated using cardiopulmonary bypass, fibrillating the vented heart, cross-clamping the aorta, and washing all blood from the coronary system while performing the anastomosis.

Rene Favalaro from the Cleveland Clinic used saphenous vein for bypassing coronary obstructions. Favalaro's 1968 article focused on 15 patients.[59] An interpositional graft of the saphenous vein was placed between the ascending aorta and the right coronary artery distal to the blockage. The right coronary was divided, and the vein graft was anastomosed end-to-end. Favalaro states that this procedure was done because of the unfavorable results with pericardial patch reconstruction of the coronary artery. In an addendum to that paper, 55 cases were added, 52 for segmental occlusion of the right coronary and 3 others for circumflex disease.

The contributions by Favalaro, Kolessov, Green et al., and Bailey and Hirose were all important, but arguably the official start date of coronary artery bypass surgery as we know it today happened in 1969 when W. Dudley Johnson and his colleagues from Milwaukee reported their series of 301 patients who had undergone various operations for coronary artery disease since February 1967.[60] Johnson reported these results, covering a 19-month period, at the annual meeting of the American Surgical Association. Most importantly, he showed that multiple vein grafts could be placed to all three coronary artery systems and their major branches. He recommended using end-to-side anastomosis for the saphenous vein–coronary anastomosis, and he advocated working in a dry, quiet field. He said that the grafts did not need to be limited to the proximal portions of the large arteries, and he recommended, if possible, not placing the graft in the diseased portion of the artery but to go to a more distal normal area to place the graft.

The direct anastomosis between the internal mammary artery and the coronary artery was not initially as popular as the vein graft technique; however, because of the persistence of Drs. Green, Loop, Grondin, and others, internal mammary artery grafts eventually became the conduit of choice when their superior long-term patency became known.

Denton Cooley and colleagues made two important contributions to the surgery for ischemic heart disease. In 1956, with the use of cardiopulmonary bypass, they were the first to repair a ruptured interventricular septum following acute myocardial infarction.[61] The patient initially did well but died from complications 6 weeks after the operation. Cooley et al. also were the first to report the resection of a left ventricular aneurysm with the use of cardiopulmonary bypass.[62]

Dysrhythmia Surgery

Sealy and colleagues at Duke University developed the first successful surgical treatment for cardiac arrhythmias.[63] A 32-year-old fisherman was referred for symptomatic episodes of atrial tachycardia that caused congestive heart failure. On May 2, 1968, after epicardial mapping, a 5- to 6-cm cut was made extending from the base of the right atrial appendage to the right border of the right atrium during cardiopulmonary bypass. The incision transected the conducted pathway between the atrium and ventricle. Ross et al., in Sydney, Australia, and Cox et al., in St. Louis, Missouri, used cryosurgical treatment of atrial ventricular node reentry tachycardia.[64,65] Subsequently, Cox, after years of laboratory research, developed the maze operation for atrial fibrillation. Subsequent epicardial mapping indicated eradication of the pathway.[66]

Guiraudon et al., from Paris, France, reported their results with an encircling endomyocardial ventriculotomy for the treatment of malignant ventricular arrhythmias.[67] The following year, in 1979 Josephson et al. described a more specific procedure for treatment of malignant ventricular arrhythmias.[68] After endocardial mapping, the endocardial source of the arrhythmia was excised. Although the Guiraudon technique usually isolated the source of the arrhythmia, the incision also devascularized healthy myocardium and was associated with high mortality. Endocardial resection was safer and more efficacious and became the basis of all approaches for the treatment of ischemic ventricular tachycardia.

Surgery for ventricular arrhythmia, however, became much less common after development of the implantable defibrillator. Stimulated by the death of a close personal friend from ventricular arrhythmias, Dr. Mirowski developed a prototype implantable defibrillator over a 3-month period in 1969. In 1980, Mirowski et al. described three successful cases using their implantable myocardial defibrillator at Johns Hopkins.[69]

Paul Zoll is given credit for ushering in the clinical era of cardiac pacemakers.[70] In 1952, he reported on two patients suffering from recurring ventricular standstill whom he treated with an external pacemaker. The first patient was a 75-year-old man with complete heart block who had been revived with 34 intracardiac injections of epinephrine over a 4-h period. Zoll applied electric shocks 2 ms in duration that were transmitted through the chest wall at frequencies from 25 to 60 per minute and increased the intensity of the shock until ventricular responses were observed. The next step came when Lillehei and associates reported a series of patients during the 1950s who had external pacing after open heart surgery for surgically induced heart block.[71] The major difference between Zoll's pacing and that of Lillehei et al. was that Zoll used external electrodes placed on the chest wall whereas Lillehei et al. attached electrodes directly to the heart at operation. Lillehei et al. used a relatively small external pacemaker to stimulate the heart and much less electric current. This form of heart pacing was better tolerated by the patient and was a more efficient way to stimulate the heart.

Elmquist and Senning developed a totally implantable pacemaker.[72] They implanted the unit in a patient with atrioventricular block in 1958. The first pacemaker that was implanted functioned only 8 h; the second pacemaker implanted in the same patient had better success. The patient had many additional pacemakers and survived until January 2002.

Heart and Heart-Lung Transplantation

Richard Lower and Norman Shumway established the technique for heart transplantation as it is performed today.[73] Preservation of the cuff of recipient left and right atria with part of the atrial septum was described earlier by Brock in England and Demikhov in the Soviet Union, but it became popular only after Shumway and Lower reported it in their 1960 paper.[74,75]

The first human-to-human heart transplant occurred on December 3, 1967, at the Groote Schuur Hospital in Capetown, South Africa.[76] The surgical team, headed by Christiaan Barnard, transplanted the heart of a donor who had been certified dead after the electrocardiogram showed no activity for 5 min into a 54-year-old man whose heart was irreparably damaged by repeated myocardial infarctions. Barnard's patient, Lewis Washkansky, died on the 18th postoperative day. At autopsy, the heart appeared normal, and there was no evidence of chronic liver congestion, but bilateral pneumonia, possibly caused by severe myeloid depression from immunosuppression, was present. On January 2, 1968, Barnard performed a second heart transplant on Phillip Blaiberg, 12 days after Washkansky's death. Blaiberg was discharged from the hospital and became a celebrity during the several months he lived after the transplant.[77] Blaiberg's procedure indicated that a heart transplant was an option for humans suffering from end-stage heart disease. Within a year of Barnard's first heart transplant, 99 heart transplants had been performed by cardiac surgeons around the world. However, by the end of 1968, most groups abandoned heart transplantation because of the extremely high mortality related to rejection. Shumway and Lower, Barnard, and a few others, persevered both clinically and in the laboratory. Their efforts in the discovery of better drugs for immunosuppression eventually established heart transplantation as we know it today.

A clinical trial of heart-lung transplantation was commenced at Stanford University in 1981 by Reitz et al.[78] Their first patient was treated with a combination of cyclosporine and azothioprine. The patient was discharged from the hospital in good condition and was well more than 5 years after the transplant. The current success with heart, heart-lung, and lung transplantation is in part related to the discovery of cyclosporine by workers at Sandoz Laboratory in Basel, Switzerland, in 1970. In December 1980, cyclosporine was introduced at Stanford for cardiac transplantation. The incidence of rejections was not reduced, nor was the incidence of infection. However, these two major complications of cardiac transplantation were less severe when cyclosporine was used. Availability of cyclosporine stimulated the development of many new transplant programs across the United States in the mid-1980s.

Heart Assist and Artificial Hearts

In 1963, Kantrowitz and associates reported the first use of the intraaortic balloon pump in three patients. All were in cardiogenic shock but improved during balloon pumping. One survived to leave the hospital.[79]

Akutsu and Kolff reported the development and first application of a totally artificial heart in an animal model at the Cleveland Clinic in 1957. The authors implanted a totally artificial heart in a dog that survived for 90 min with the mechanical heart.[80]

In 1966, DeBakey used a left ventricular assist device in a woman who could not be weaned from cardiopulmonary bypass after double valve replacement.[81] After 10 days of circulatory assistance, the patient was weaned successfully from the device and recovered. This woman was probably the first patient to be weaned from an assist device and to leave the hospital.

The first human application of a totally artificial heart was by Denton Cooley and colleagues as a "bridge" to transplantation.[82] They implanted a totally artificial heart in a patient who could not be weaned from cardiopulmonary bypass. After 64 h of artificial heart support, heart transplantation was performed, but the patient died of *Pseudomonas* pneumonia after transplantation. The first two patients successfully bridged to transplantation were reported at almost the same time and in the same location by different groups. On September 5, 1984, in San Francisco, Donald Hill implanted a Pierce–Donachy left ventricular assist device in a patient in cardiogenic shock.[83] The patient was transplanted successfully 2 days later and was later discharged. Phillip Oyer and associates at Stanford University placed an electrically driven Novacor left ventricular assist device in a patient in cardiogenic shock on September 7, 1984.[84] The patient was transplanted successfully and survived beyond 3 years. The first implantation of a permanent totally artificial heart (Jarvik-7) was performed by DeVries and colleagues at the University of Utah in 1982. By 1985, they had implanted the Jarvik in four patients, and one survived for 620 days after implantation.[85]

Summary

The history of cardiac surgery continues and will continue indefinitely so long as heart disease shortens lives. In the early days after the introduction of cardiopulmonary bypass, the pace of advance was torrid but, in a way, narrowly focused. Now, thousands of clinicians, scientists, and engineers are involved in a broad and deep effort to develop new and safer operations and procedures, new valves, new revascularization techniques, new biomaterials, new heart substitutes, new life-support systems, and new methods to control cardiac arrhythmias and ventricular remodeling after injury. This research and development is supported by a vigorous infrastructure of basic science in biology and medicine, chemistry and pharmacology, and engineering and computer technology.

References

1. Williams DH. Stab wound of the heart, pericardium—suture of the pericardium—recovery—patient alive three years afterward. Med Rec 1897;51:1–8.
2. Rehn L. On penetrating cardiac injuries and cardiac suturing. Arch Klin Chir 1897;55:315.
3. Hill LL. A report of a case of successful suturing of the heart, and table of thirty seven other cases of suturing by different operators with various terminations, and the conclusions drawn. Med Rec 1902;2:846.
4. Harken DE. Foreign bodies in and in relation to the thoracic blood vessels and heart: I. Techniques for approaching and removing foreign bodies from the chambers of the heart. Surg Gynecol Obstet 1946;83:117.
5. Trendelenburg F. Operative management of pulmonary emboli. Verh Dtsch Ges Chir 1908;37:89.
6. Kirschner M. Ein durch die Trendelenburgische operation geheiter fall von embolie der art. pulmonalis. Arch Klin Chir 1924;133:312.
7. Gibbon JH. Artificial maintenance of circulation during experimental occlusion of pulmonary artery. Arch Surg 1937; 34:1105.
8. Sharp EH. Pulmonary embolectomy: successful removal of a massive pulmonary embolus with the support of cardiopulmonary bypass. Case report. Ann Surg 1962;156:1.
9. Rehn I. Zur experimentellen pathologie des herzbeutels. Verh Dtsch Ges Chir 1913;42:339.
10. Sauerbruch R. Die Chirurgie der Brustorgane, vol II. Berlin: Springer, 1925.
11. Forssmann W. Catheterization of the right heart. Klin Wochenshr 1929;8:2085.
12. Bailey CP. The surgical treatment of mitral stenosis. Dis Chest 1949;15:377.
13. Naef AP. The Story of Thoracic Surgery. New York: Hogrefe & Huber, 1990:94.
14. Sellors TH. Surgery of pulmonary stenosis: a case in which the pulmonary valve was successfully divided. Lancet 1948;1: 988.
15. Hufnagel CA, Harvey WP, Rabil PJ, et al. Surgical correction of aortic insufficiency. Surgery (St. Louis) 1954;35:673.
16. Gross RE, Hubbard JH. Surgical ligation of a patent ductus arteriosus: report of first successful case. JAMA 1939;112:729.
17. Crafoord C, Nylin G. Congenital coarctation of the aorta and its surgical treatment. J Thorac Cardiovasc Surg 1945;14:347.
18. Gross RE. Surgical relief for tracheal obstruction from a vascular ring. N Engl J Med 1945;233:586.
19. Gross RE, Neuhauser EBD. Compression of the trachea or esophagus by vascular anomalies: surgical therapy in 40 cases. Pediatrics 1951;7:69.
20. Blalock A, Taussig HB. The surgical treatment of malformations of the heart in which there is pulmonary stenosis or pulmonary atresia. JAMA 1945;128:189.
21. Biorck G, Crafoord C. Arteriovenous aneurysm on the pulmonary artery simulating patent ductus arteriosus botalli. Thorax 1947;2:65.
22. Muller WH Jr. The surgical treatment of the transposition of the pulmonary veins. Ann Surg 1951;134:683.
23. Gross RE. Surgical closure of an aortic septal defect. Circulation 1952;5:858.
24. Cooley DA, McNamara DR, Latson JR. Aorticopulmonary septal defect: diagnosis and surgical treatment. Surgery (St. Louis) 1957;42:101.
25. Glenn WWL. Circulatory bypass of the right side of the hearts: IV. Shunt between superior vena cava and distal right pulmonary artery—report of clinical application. N Engl J Med 1958; 259:117.

26. Konstantinov IE, Alexi-Meskishvilli VV. Cavo-pulmonary shunt: from the first experiments to clinical patients. Ann Thorac Surg 1999;68:1100–1161.
27. Gibbon JH Jr. The gestation and birth of an idea. Phila Med 1963;59:913.
28. Gibbon JH Jr. Artificial maintenance of circulation during experimental occlusion of the pulmonary artery. Arch Surg 1937;34:1105.
29. Dennis C, Spreng DS, Nelson GE, et al. Development of a pump oxygenator to replace the heart and lungs: an apparatus applicable to human patients, and application to one case. Ann Surg 1951;134:709.
30. Digliotti AM. Clinical use of the artificial circulation with a note on intra-arterial transfusion. Bull Johns Hopkins Hosp 1952;90:131.
31. Stephenson LW, Arbulu A, Bassett JS, Silbergleit A, Hughes CA. The Michigan heart: the world's first successful open heart operation? part I. J Card Surg 2002;17:238–246.
32. Stephenson LW, Arbulu A, Bassett JS, Silbergleit A, Hughes CA. Forest Dewey Dodrill: heart surgery pioneer. Michigan heart, part II. J Card Surg 2002;17:247–257.
33. Lewis FJ, Taufic M. Closure of atrial septal defects with the aid of hypothermia: experimental accomplishments and the report of one successful case. Surgery (St. Louis) 1953;33:52.
34. Swan H, Zeavin I, Blount SG Jr, Virtue RW. Surgery by direct vision in the open heart during hypothermia. JAMA 1953; 153:1081.
35. Hikasa Y, Shirotani H, Satomura K, et al. Open heart surgery in infants with the aid of hypothermic anesthesia. Arch Jpn Chir 1967;36:495.
36. Gibbon JH Jr. Application of a mechanical heart and lung apparatus to cardiac surgery. Minn Med 1954;37:171.
37. Lillehei CW. Historical development of cardiopulmonary bypass. Cardiopulmon Bypass 1993;1:26.
38. Kirklin JW, DuShane JW, Patrick RT, et al. Intracardiac surgery with the aid of a mechanical pump-oxygenator system (Gibbon type): report of eight cases. Mayo Clin Proc 1955;30:201.
39. Harken DE, Soroff HS, Taylor WJ, et al. Partial and complete prostheses in aortic insufficiency. J Thorac Cardiovasc Surg 1960;40:744.
40. Starr A, Edwards ML. Mitral replacement: clinical experience with a ball-valve prosthesis. Ann Surg 1961;154:726.
41. Cartwright RS, Giacobine JW, Ratan RS, et al. Combined aortic and mitral valve replacement. J Thorac Cardiovasc Surg 1963; 45:35.
42. Starr A, Edwards LM, McCord CW, et al. Multiple valve replacement. Circulation 1964;29:30.
43. Knott-Craig CJ, Schaff HV, Mullany CJ, et al. Carcinoid disease of the heart: surgical management of ten patients. J Thorac Cardiovasc Surg 1992;104:475.
44. Morrow AG, Brockenbrough EC. Surgical treatment of idiopathic hypertrophic subaortic stenosis: technic and hemodynamic results of subaortic ventriculomyotomy. Ann Surg 1961;154:181.
45. Heimbecker RO, Baird RJ, Lajos RJ, et al. Homograft replacement of the human valve: a preliminary report. Can Med Assoc J 1962;86:805.
46. Ross DN. Homograft replacement of the aortic valve. Lancet 1962;2:487.
47. Ross DN. Replacement of aortic and mitral valves with a pulmonary autograft. Lancet 1967;2:956.
48. Gerosa G, McKay R, Davies J, et al. Comparison of the aortic homograft and the pulmonary autograft for aortic valve or root replacement in children. J Thorac Cardiovasc Surg 1991;102:51.
49. Binet JP, Carpentier A, Langlois J, et al. Implantation de valves heterogenes dans le traitment des cardiopathies aortiques. C R Acad Sci Paris 1965;261:5733.
50. Carpentier A. Principles of tissue valve transplantation. In: Ionescu MI, Ross DN, Wooler GH, eds. Biological Tissue in Heart Valve Replacement. London: Butterworth, 1971:49.
51. Kaiser GA, Hancock WD, Lukban SB, Litwak RS. Clinical use of a new design stented xenograft heart valve prosthesis. Surg Forum 1969;20:137.
52. Sones FM, Shirey EK. Cine coronary arteriography. Mod Concepts Cardiovasc Dis 1962;31:735.
53. Konstantinov IE. Robert H. Goetz: the surgeon who performed the first successful clinical coronary artery bypass operation. Ann Thorac Surg 2000;69;1966–1972.
54. Garrett EH, Dennis EW, DeBakey ME. Aortocoronary bypass with saphenous vein grafts: seven-year follow-up. JAMA 1973; 223:792.
55. Demikhov VP. Experimental Transplantation of Vital Organs. [Authorized translation from the Russian by Basil Haigh.] New York: Consultants Bureau, 1962.
56. Kolessov VI. Mammary artery–coronary artery anastomosis as a method of treatment for angina pectoris. J Thorac Cardiovasc Surg 1967;54:535.
57. Green GE, Stertzer SH, Reppert EH. Coronary arterial bypass grafts. Ann Thorac Surg 1968;5:443.
58. Bailey CP, Hirose T. Successful internal mammary–coronary arterial anastomosis using a minivascular suturing technic. Int Surg 1968;49:416.
59. Favalaro RG. Saphenous vein autograft replacement of severe segmental coronary artery occlusion. Ann Thorac Surg 1968; 5:334.
60. Johnson WD, Flemma RJ, Lepley D Jr, Ellison EH. Extended treatment of severe coronary artery disease: a total surgical approach. Ann Surg 1969;171:460.
61. Cooley DA, Belmonte BA, Zeis LB, Schnur S. Surgical repair of ruptured interventricular septum following acute myocardial infarction. Surgery (St. Louis) 1957;41:930.
62. Cooley DA, Henly WS, Amad KH, Chapman DW. Ventricular aneurysm following myocardial infarction: results of surgical treatment. Ann Surg 1959;150:595.
63. Cobb FR, Blumenshein SD, Sealy WC, et al. Successful surgery interruption of the bundle of Kent in a patient with Wolff–Parkinson–White syndrome. Circulation 1968;38:1018.
64. Ross DL, Johnson DC, Denniss AR, et al. Curative surgery for atrioventricular junctional (AV node) reentrant tachycardia. J Am Coll Cardiol 1985;6:1383.
65. Cox JL, Holman WL, Cain ME. Cryosurgical treatment of atrioventricular node reentrant tachycardia. Circulation 1987;76: 1329.
66. Cox JL. The surgical treatment of atrial fibrillation: IV. Surgical technique. J Thorac Cardiovasc Surg 1991;101:584.
67. Guiraudon G, Fontaine G, Frank R, et al. Encircling endocardial ventriculotomy: a new surgical treatment for life-threatening ventricular tachycardias resistant to medical treatment following myocardial infarction. Ann Thorac Surg 1978;26:438.
68. Josephson ME, Harken AH, Horowitz LN. Endocardial excision: a new surgical technique for the treatment of recurrent ventricular tachycardia. Circulation 1979;60:1430.
69. Mirowski M, Reid PR, Mower MM, et al. Termination of malignant ventricular arrhythmias with an implanted automatic defibrillator in human beings. N Engl J Med 1980;303:322.
70. Zoll PM. Resuscitation of the heart in ventricular standstill by external electrical stimulation. N Engl J Med 1952;247: 768.
71. Lillehei CW, Gott VL, Hodges PC Jr, et al. Transistor pacemaker for treatment of complete atrioventricular dissociation. JAMA 1960;172:2006.
72. Elmquist R, Senning A. Implantable pacemaker for the heart. In: Smyth CN, ed. Medical Electronics: Proceedings of the Second International Conference on Medical Electronics, Paris, June, 1959. London: Iliffe & Sons, 1960.

73. Lower RR, Shumway NE. Studies on orthotopic homotransplantations of the canine heart. Surg Forum 1960;11:18.
74. Brock R. Heart excision and replacement. Guys Hosp Rep 1959;108:285.
75. Demikhov VP. Experimental Transplantation of Vital Organs. [Authorized translation from the Russian by Basil Haigh.] New York: Consultants Bureau, 1962.
76. Barnard CN. A human cardiac transplant: An interim report of a successful operation performed at Groote Schuur Hospital, Cape Town. S Afr Med J 1967;41:1271.
77. Ruggiero R. Commentary on Barnard CN. A human cardiac transplant: an interim report of a successful operation performed at Groote Schuur Hospital, Cape Town. S Afr Med J 1967;41:1271. In: Stephenson LW, Ruggiero R, eds. Heart Surgery Classics. Boston: Adams, 1994:327.
78. Reitz BA, Wallwork JL, Hunt SA, et al. Heart-lung transplantation: successful therapy for patients with pulmonary vascular disease. N Engl J Med 1982;306:557.
79. Kantrowitz A, Tjonneland S, Freed PS, et al. Initial clinical experience with intraaortic balloon pumping in cardiogenic shock. JAMA 1968;203:135.
80. Akutsu T, Kolff WJ. Permanent substitutes for valves and hearts. Trans ASAIO 1958;4:230.
81. DeBakey ME. Left ventricular heart assist devices. In: Heart Surgery Classics. Boston: Adams, 1994.
82. Cooley DA, Liotta D, Hallman GL, et al. Orthotopic cardiac prosthesis for two-staged cardiac replacement. Am J Cardiol 1969;24:723.
83. Hill JD, Farrar DJ, Hershon JJ, et al. Use of a prosthetic ventricle as a bridge to cardiac transplantation for postinfarction cardiogenic shock. N Engl J Med 1986;314:626.
84. Starnes VA, Oyer PE, Portner PM, et al. Isolated left ventricular assist as bridge to cardiac transplantation. J Thorac Cardiovasc Surg 1988;96:62.
85. DeVries WC, Anderson JL, Joyce LD, et al. Clinical use of total artificial heart. N Engl J Med 1984;310:273.
86. Lillehei CW, Cohen M, Warden HE, et al. The results of direct vision closure of ventricular septal defects in eight patients by means of controlled cross circulation. Surg Gynecol Obstet 1955;101:446.
87. Lillehei CW, Cohen M, Warden HE, et al. The direct vision intracardiac correction of congenital anomalies by controlled cross circulation. Surgery (St. Louis) 1955;38:11.
88. Kirklin JW, DuShane JW, Patrick RT, et al. Intracardiac surgery with the aid of a mechanical pump-oxygenator system (Gibbon type): report of eight cases. Mayo Clin Proc 1955;30:201.
89. Burroughs JT, Kirklin JW. Complete correction of total anomalous pulmonary venous correction: report of three cases. Mayo Clin Proc 1956;31:182.
90. McGoon DC, Edwards JE, Kirklin JW. Surgical treatment of ruptured aneurysm of aortic sinus. Ann Surg 1958;147:387.
91. Ellis FH Jr, Kirklin JW. Congenital valvular aortic stenosis: anatomic findings and surgical techniques. J Thorac Cardiovasc Surg 1962;43:199.
92. Cooley DA, McNamara DG, Jatson JR. Aortico-pulmonary septal defect: diagnosis and surgical treatment. Surgery (St. Louis) 1957;42:101.
93. Kirklin JW, Harp RA, McGoon DC. Surgical treatment of origin of both vessels from right ventricle including cases of pulmonary stenosis. J Thorac Cardiovasc Surg 1964;48:1026.
94. Anderson RC, Lillehei CW, Jester RG. Corrected transposition of the great vessels of the heart. Pediatrics 1957;20:626.
95. Senning A. Surgical correction of transposition of the great vessels. Surgery (St. Louis) 1959;45:966.
96. Swan H, Wilson JH, Woodwork G, Blount SE. Surgical obliteration of a coronary artery fistula to the right ventricle. Arch Surg 1959;79:820.
97. Hardy KL, May IA, Webster CA, Kimball KG. Ebstein's anomaly: a functional concept and successful definitive repair. J Thorac Cardiovasc Surg 1964;48:927.
98. Ross DN, Somerville J. Correction of pulmonary atresia with a homograft aortic valve. Lancet 1966;2:1446.
99. McGoon DC, Rastelli GC, Ongley PA. An operation for the correction of truncus arteriosus. JAMA 1968;205:59.
100. Fontan F, Baudet E. Surgical repair of tricuspid atresia. Thorax 1971;26:240.
101. Horiuchi T, Abe T, Okada Y, et al: Feasibility of total correction for single ventricle: A report of total correction in a six-year-old girl. Jpn J Thorac Surg 1970;23:434 (in Japanese).
102. Konno S, Iami Y, Iida Y, et al. A new method for prosthetic valve replacement in congenital aortic stenosis associated with hypoplasia of the aortic valve ring. J Thorac Cardiovasc Surg 1975;70:909.
103. Jatene AD, Fontes VF, Paulista PP, et al. Anatomic correction of transposition of the great vessel. J Thorac Cardiovasc Surg 1976;72:364.
104. Norwood WI, Lang P, Hansen DD. Physiologic repair of aortic atresia-hypoplastic left heart syndrome. N Engl J Med 1983; 308:23.
105. Bailey LL, Gundry SR, Razzouk AJ, et al. Bless the babies: one hundred fifteen late survivors of heart transplantation during the first year of life. J Thorac Cardiovasc Surg 1993;105:805.

70 Preoperative and Postoperative Care of the Thoracic Surgery Patient

Jessica Scott Donington

Major pulmonary and esophageal procedures place tremendous physiological stress on patients. Over the past three decades, the morbidity and mortality associated with thoracic surgical procedures has dropped significantly. This increase in safety is attributable to a shift in disease process from infectious to malignant, and advances in anesthetic techniques, surgical precision, patient selection, and perioperative care. The process of patient selection includes better preoperative staging of malignancy and physiological assessment and evaluation of fitness for operation. Today, a grand majority of general thoracic operations are performed for malignancy; we treat far fewer infectious processes than our predecessors. Our patients in general are better fit for surgery and their expectation for full functional recovery is much higher. We review some significant points in perioperative care of thoracic surgery patients including preoperative cardiac and pulmonary assessment, perioperative antibiotic use, pain management, chest tube management, and the use of postoperative anticoagulants and antiarrhythmics.

Preoperative Cardiac Assessment and Reduction of Risk

Cardiovascular disease and pulmonary disease share common origins and symptoms and frequently coexist. Uncertainty still exists as to when it is appropriate to investigate cardiac disease preoperatively, which tests are most accurate, and what type of cardiac intervention is appropriate in the perioperative setting.

The combined effects of surgery and anesthesia on the heart are complex but relate to a balance between increased sympathetic activity caused by the stress of surgery and the cardiodepressant effects of anesthesia. These two forces combine to create a window of maximum cardiac risk between 8 and 24h after surgery.

Chronic obstructive pulmonary disease (COPD) is well recognized as an important risk marker for arteriosclerosis. Even modest reductions in forced expiratory volume in 1 second (FEV_1) result in a large increase in the hazard ratio for ischemic heart disease independent of age, sex, cigarette use, blood pressure, cholesterol, body mass index, or social class.[1] FEV_1 is equivalent to cholesterol in predicting risk for cardiac ischemia.[1] Pathogenesis of this connection is related to the commonality of disease origin and other endogenous factors. A low level of inflammation from the airway can act as a trigger for parallel inflammatory changes in the coronary arteries.[2] Inhaled beta-agonist agents, such as albuterol, have also been linked to elevated risk for cardiac ischemia.[3] Patients with COPD have evidence of abnormal endogenous sympathetic tone. Patients with COPD had depressed global heart rate variability in response to sympathetic and vagal stimuli compared to age-matched controls.[4]

The American Heart Association rates thoracic surgery as an intermediate cardiac risk, defined as an estimated risk rate of less than 5%, which is consistent with an estimated overall mortality of 5%.[5] Data relating specifically to the cardiovascular risk of thoracic surgery are limited; however, most investigators assessing risk in noncardiac surgery have studied patients undergoing major vascular surgery. At least 10 multivariate studies have been published analyzing cardiac risk in noncardiac surgery. Goldman's cardiac risk index was published in 1977 and has been used extensively.[6] After several modifications of this system and the publication of several other systems, a consensus panel from the American Heart Association and the American College of Cardiology was formed in 1996. This committee collated the existing evidence into a set of guidelines[7]; these are reviewed annually and were updated most recently in 2002.[8] The consensus

TABLE 70.1. Clinical Predictors of Increased Perioperative Cardiovascular Risk.

Major	Unstable coronary syndrome, recent or acute (<30 days) myocardial infarct (MI), unstable angina (class III or IV)
	Decompensated heart failure
	Significant arrhythmias, high-grade AV block, symptomatic ventricular arrhythmia, supraventricular arrhythmias with uncontrolled ventricular rate
	Severe valvular disease
Intermediate	Mild angina pectoris (class I or II)
	Previous MI by history or Q wave
	Compensated heart failure
	Diabetes mellitus (insulin-dependent)
	Renal insufficiency
Minor	Advanced age
	Abnormal EKG: left bundle branch block of left ventricular hypertrophy
	Rhythm other than sinus–atrial fibrillation
	Low functional capacity
	History of stroke
	Uncontrolled systemic hypertension

offered a stepwise algorithm for the management of preoperative cardiac risk. It combines clinical predictors derived from multivariate analysis (Table 70.1), estimated functional capacity, and surgery-specific risk. The guidelines are designed to address when further invasive or noninvasive testing would be helpful in assessing perioperative risk.

Common cardiovascular tests such as 12-lead EKG or echocardiography offer little in the way of further information on perioperative risk.[9] In contrast, exercise or pharmacological testing allows for early detection and localization of ischemia. Kertai[10] performed a meta-analysis of the accuracy of different tests for predicting perioperative cardiac risk and found that dobutamine stress-echo had the optimal sensitivity (85%) and specificity (70%) for predicting perioperative events.

Implicit in the determination of perioperative risk is the assumption that the risk can be attenuated by appropriately targeted interventions, be that revascularization or medical therapy. The fact that a patient is scheduled to undergo elective surgery does not alter the indications for bypass surgery (left main stem and/or multivessel disease). The long-term efficacy of bypass surgery is well established, but the procedure is associated with significant risk and should not be used simply to reduce perioperative risk. Percutaneous interventions (PCIs) have lower risk and represent more of a gray area. There is widespread acceptance that inducible ischemia in an artery with angiographically significant stenosis should be treated before elective surgery, but the choice of intervention is a dilemma. Although healing after simple balloon angioplasty is relatively short, perhaps 1 week, implantation of a bare metal stent must be accompanied by 4 weeks of potent antiplatelet therapy. Implantation of a drug-eluting stent warrants a minimum of 3 to 6 months of antiplatelet treatment. This obligatory delay to surgery needs to be incorporated into preoperative decision making.

The benefits of preoperative medical interventions for patients with elevated cardiac risk have been better studied and are more established. Two randomized placebo-controlled trials have examined the impact of perioperative beta-blockade on patients with increased cardiac risk (Table 70.2). Mangano et al.[11] randomized 200 patients to atenolol or placebo; overall mortality at discharge and at 2 years was significantly lower in the atenolol-treated patients. Poldermans et al.[12] randomized 173 patients with positive dobutamine echocardiography to bisoprolol or standard care and saw a significant decrease in cardiac deaths and nonfatal myocardial infarction. The ability of these trials to achieve statistical significance with small numbers of patients suggests a potent protective effect for beta-blockade in postoperative period for patients with elevated cardiac risk.

It could be argued that that the applicability of beta-blocker studies in thoracic surgery patients is limited by the presence of COPD, which traditionally precluded the use of these medications. Recent studies have demonstrated that there is little to no downside to the use of cardioselective beta-blockers in patients with COPD.[13] Cardioselective agents produce no significant change in FEV_1 or respiratory symptoms compared to placebo and do not significantly affect pulmonary response to beta-2 agonist treatments.[14] Gottlieb et al. have demonstrated that overall risk of perioperative cardiac events is reduced by the use of beta-blockade in COPD patients at a rate similar to the general population.[15]

Pulmonary Physiological Assessment

Pulmonary complications occur frequently after major thoracic operations. Their occurrence is related to the type of operation performed, the surgical approach, and the underlying condition of the patient. The ability to predict which patients are at higher risk for postoperative complications allows us to appropriately select patients for surgery and accurately discuss relative risks.

Many patients who undergo thoracic surgery have poor underlying pulmonary function, in large part caused by long-term tobacco use. It is the responsibility of the thoracic surgeon to accurately assess the pulmonary function of a

TABLE 70.2.
Randomized Controlled Trials Examining the Impact of Perioperative Beta-Blockade on Patients with Cardiac Risk Ractors.

Author	*Year*	*Number of patients*	*Treatment arms*	*Two-year mortality*	*Cardiac death*	*Nonfatal MI*	P
Mangano[11]	1996	200	Atenolol vs. placebo	10% vs. 21%	N/R	N/R	0.019
Poldermans[12]	1999	173	Bisprolol vs. standard care	NR	3.4% vs. 17%	0% vs. 17%	0.02 < 0.001

NR, not reported.

potentially operable patient. The assessment provides an objective risk profile for the planned procedure, should help to define morbidity and mortality and may lead the surgeon to recommend alternative therapies.

Preoperative pulmonary history should include investigation into tobacco usage, including current use, total number of pack-years, and time since cessation. Active use of tobacco is associated with a variety of postoperative pulmonary complications.[16,17] These complications are related to the increased production of sputum and decreased sputum clearance in the perioperative period, which can result in significant atelectasis, pneumonia, and respiratory insufficiency. Prolonged tobacco exposure may also suggest significant paranchymal disease and occult COPD. Other important pulmonary history that needs to be elicited includes history of prior thoracic surgery, history of paranchymal lung disease, or active pulmonary infection. The patient's preoperative activity level needs to be assessed. Patients with suboptimal performance on objective exercise testing are at increased risk for perioperative cardiopulmonary complications.[18–21] Self-reported poor exercise tolerance has also been shown to be associated with increased operative risk.[22]

Spirometry is a simple, inexpensive, and readily available test for the evaluation of pulmonary function. For the majority of patients, spirometry along with history and physical examination are an adequate preoperative pulmonary evaluation, and it should be the starting point for evaluation of all patients. Spirometry should be performed on a patient in stable condition, with and without the use of bronchodilators. A bronchodilator response greater than 15% is considered significant and indicates reactive airway disease. FEV_1 is the most commonly used parameter for the assessment of surgical risk. Many large series have outlined different FEV_1 criteria for safe pulmonary resection. FEV_1 greater than 1.5 L is proposed as safe for a lobectomy and FEV_1 greater than 2.0 L as being safe for a pneumonectomy.[23–25] These absolute values provide a good yet crude set of selection criteria as they do not take into account gender or body size. Therefore, FEV_1 expressed as a percent of predicted is thought to be more accurate. FEV_1 greater than 80% of predicted is associated with a low risk of perioperative complications following major pulmonary resection. Patients with a FEV_1 greater than 80% of predicted usually require no further pulmonary testing.[26]

The diffusion capacity in the lung for carbon dioxide (DLCO) has been identified as the most important predictor of perioperative morbidity and mortality in thoracic surgery patients. In a large meta-analysis by Ferguson et al.,[27] preoperative DLCO less than 60% of predicted was associated with increased mortality. Other studies have substantiated the importance of DLCO in the risk assessment for thoracic surgery, with little correlation with FEV_1 or maximum oxygen consumption (VO_{2max}).[28,29]

If preoperative pulmonary assessment is suboptimal with FEV_1 or DLCO less than 80% of what was predicted, further evaluation is warranted. Predicted postoperative values for FEV_1 and DLCO ($ppoFEV_1$ and ppoDLCO) should be calculated. Predicted postoperative FEV_1 historically needed to be greater than 800 mL.[30] Recent studies indicate that $ppoFEV_1$ less than 40% is associated with a significant increase in morbidity and mortality.[31–34] Similarly, ppoDLCO less than 40% is strongly predictive of postoperative complications and death.[28]

The most common methods for calculating $ppoFEV_1$ and ppoDLCO are nuclear medicine ventilation-perfusion (V/Q) scanning, quantitative computed tomography (CT) scan, or segment counting. Nuclear medicine V/Q scanning and quantitative CT provide the relative contribution of each region of the lung to the overall pulmonary function. The $ppoFEV_1$ and ppoDLCO are calculated by subtracting the percent perfusion to the resected segment from the preoperativeFEV_1. These tests are very useful when all lung segments are not contributing or functioning equally secondary to obstruction, infection, or intrinsic disease.

An alternative method of calculating $ppoFEV_1$ without a quantitative perfusion scan involves accounting for the anticipated number of resected segments as a percentage of the total number of segments in both lungs.[35] There are 19 segments, each accounting for roughly 5.26% of overall lung function. Therefore:

$$ppoFEV_1 = \text{preoperative } FEV_1 \times [1 - (\text{number segments resected} \times 5.26)/100]$$

This relatively simple calculation obviates the need for expensive nuclear medicine testing in patients without anticipated functional differences between segments.

Patients considered high risk for thoracic surgery based on standard spirometry and estimation of $ppoFEV_1$ and ppoDLCO should undergo exercise testing. The purpose of this testing is to identify those patients with marginal pulmonary function who can still tolerate a resection. The simplest form of exercise testing is stair climbing. The height climbed is inversely related to the rate of postoperative complications. The old rule of thumb was that patients who could climb one flight can tolerate a lobectomy and those who can climb two flights can tolerate a pneumonectomy. Different investigators have identified increased morbidity and mortality when patient can climb less than three flights,[36,37] two flights,[38,39] 12 m,[40] or 44 steps.[41] The 6-min walk test is a more formalized evaluation that provides objective evidence of a patient's functional ability. The test measures the distance that a patient can walk on a hard flat surface during 6 min. The test is self-paced and does not represent maximal exercise capacity. Achieved distances greater than 1000 feet have been associated with improved survival following lung resection.[41] A variation on the 6-min walk test is the shuttle test, in which patients ambulate between two cones placed 10 m apart and the patient's pace is increased each minute. The inability to complete 25 shuttles (250 m) suggests poor function and VO_{2max} less than 10 mL/kg/min.[42]

The most formal type of exercise testing is determination of VO_{2max}, which denotes a plateau above which further work does not result in greater oxygen consumption. The test is usually performed on a treadmill or bicycle with incremental increases in work. Preoperative VO_{2max} greater than 20 mL/kg/min is associated with a low risk for perioperative complications.[43,44] Many studies suggest that VO_{2max} greater than 15 mL/kg/min as a cutoff for respectability.[45,46] Bolliger et al. demonstrated that $ppoVO_{2max}$ less than 10 mL/kg/min is associated with 100% operative mortality.[46]

In 2001 the British Thoracic Society and the Cardiothoracic Surgeons of Great Britain and Ireland Working Party reviewed the available literature and made evidence-based recommendations on the preoperative pulmonary evaluation

TABLE 70.3. Summary of Recommendations for Preoperative Pulmonary Assessment by the British Thoracic Society and the Cardiothoracic Surgeons of Great Britain and Ireland Working Party, 2001.[47]

Step 1	Patients with $FEV_1 > 1.5$ L undergoing a lobectomy, or $FEV_1 > 2.0$ L undergoing a pneumonectomy, without shortness of breath, require no further testing.
Step 2	All patients not operable based on spirometry alone should undergo full pulmonary function tests, measurement of oxygen saturation at room air, and a quantitative perfusion scan if a pneumonectomy is being considered
	$ppoFEV_1$ and ppoDLCO should be calculated
	$ppoFEV_1 > 40\%$, ppoDLCO $< 40\%$, and room air oxygen saturation $>90\%$, average operative risk
	$ppoFEV_1 < 40\%$, ppoDLCO $< 40\%$, high operative risk
	All other combinations: risk of resection is unclear and referral to exercise testing is recommended
Step 3	Best distance on a two-shuttle test <25 shuttles (250 m), high operative risk
	Other patients should be referred for formal cardiopulmonary exercise testing
	$VO_{2peak} > 15$ mL/kg/min, average operative risk
	$VO_{2peak} < 15$ mL/kg/min, high operative risk
Step 4	The management of high-risk patients should be discussed in a multidisciplinary setting for consideration of limited resection or nonoperative therapy

for thoracic surgery.[47] The algorithm shown in Table 70.3 is based upon their recommendations.

Perioperative Antibiotic Use

The introduction of antisepsis greatly increased the safety and utility of elective thoracic procedures. Strict attention and asepsis and meticulous surgical technique are the most important factors in decreasing the incidence of postoperative infections. Perioperative antibiotics should be seen as an adjunct to meticulous surgical care. The goal of the use of prophylactic perioperative antibiotics is not to sterilize tissue but rather to decrease the bacteria load to a level that does not overwhelm the host. In general thoracic surgery, three types of perioperative infections account for the majority of infection issues: surgical wound infections, bronchopneumonias, and empyemas. One of these three infections is seen in 12% to 40% of patients following a pulmonary resection.[48,49]

The use of prophylactic antibiotics in general thoracic surgery is well established. Without proof of preexisting infection, the majority of general thoracic surgery procedures are considered "clean contaminated" because of the bronchial opening during the operation. There are numerous randomized trials supporting the use of prophylactic antibiotics to decrease the incidence of surgical wound infection, but much controversy still exists as to the recommended length of prophylaxis and the ideal agents. There remains little such proof demonstrating the benefit of antibiotics in the reduction of postoperative bronchopneumonia and empyema (Table 70.4).

Kvale et al.[48] reported the first randomized trial on the topic of prophylactic antibiotics in thoracic surgery in 1977. They randomized 77 patients to cephazolin or placebo and found a significant decrease in the rate of wound infections, pneumonias and empyema. Truesdale[49] and Cameron[50] performed similar placebo-randomized trials but were unable to detect a decrease in infections with the prophylactic use of first generation cephalosporins. A large trial by the Toronto group, published in 1981, supported the finding of Kvale, with a statistically significant decrease in wound infections, and a lesser decrease in the rate of empyema and pneumonia.[51] The policy of the Toronto general thoracic surgical group was to "employ prophylactic perioperative antibiotic coverage in clean-contaminated general thoracic cases."

The question of single-dose or prolonged postoperative prophylaxis was examined by Olak et al.[53] They randomized 208 patients to receive a single preoperative dose of cephazolin or the induction dose plus five postoperative doses. They found no difference in the rate of wound infections or deep infections and concluded there was no benefit from prolonged

TABLE 70.4.
Prospective Randomized Double-Blind Trials Addressing the Use of Prophylactic Antibiotics in Elective Pulmonary Resections.

Author	*Year*	*Agents*	*Number of patients*	*Wound infection*	*Pneumonia*	*Empyema*
Kvale[48]	1977	Cefazolin vs. placebo	77	Decreased	Decreased	Decreased
Truesdale[49]	1979	Cefazolin vs. placebo	57	No difference	No difference	No difference
Cameron[50]	1981	Cephalothin vs. placebo	171	No difference	No difference	No difference
Ilves[52]	1981	Cephalothin vs. placebo	211	Decreased	No difference	No difference
Frimodt-Moller[97]	1982	Penicillin G vs. placebo	101	Decreased	No difference	No difference
Tarkka[98]	1987	Doxycycline vs. cefuroxime	120	No difference	No difference	No difference
Aznar[99]	1991	Cefazolin vs. placebo	127	Decreased	No difference	Decreased
Olak[53]	1991	Cefazolin 1 vs. 6 doses	199	No difference	No difference	No difference
Krasnick[100]	1991	Penicillin G vs. cefuroxime	94	No difference	No difference	No difference
Wertzel[54]	1992	Ampicillin/sulbactam 1 vs. 3 doses	60	No difference	No difference	No difference
Bernard[55]	1994	Cefuroxime vs. placebo	203	No difference	Decreased by CXR	Decreased
Boldt[101]	1999	Ampicillin/sulbactam vs. cefazolin	120	NR	Decreased	NR
Turna[102]	2003	Cefuroxime vs. cefepime	102	No difference	No difference	No difference

perioperative antibiotic use. Wertzle et al.[54] further confirmed the use of a single dose of antibiotics in their randomized trial of one versus three doses of ampicillin/sulbactam (Unasyn). They also found no difference in wound or deep tissue infection rates.

The data are convincing that a short course of antibiotics is effective in decreasing the rate of surgical wound infections in general thoracic surgery. Unfortunately, the data are far less clear for the effectiveness of prophylactic antibiotics to decrease the rate of pneumonia or empyema following thoracic surgery. Of the 14 randomized-placebo trials presented here, only 3 demonstrated a significant decrease in the risk of pneumonia or empyema. The trial by Bernard et al.,[55] which demonstrated a decrease in empyemas in patients prophylaxed with cefuroxime. This trial was complicated by a high rate of bronchial fistulas in the control group. These fistulas were the likely cause of the empyemas, and the development of a fistula was most likely a result of local factors and surgical technique and unrelated to antibiotic use. Their conclusions that 48h of antibiotic prophylaxis decreases the rate of deep infections following thoracic surgery may be mistaken. At present, data from the literature remain conflicting, and therefore the use of prophylactic antibiotics for the prevention of pneumonias and empyemas remains nonuniform throughout thoracic surgery.

Pain Management

Pain relief is an important aspect to the postoperative care of thoracic surgery patients, not only because all patients deserve to be pain-free, but more importantly because pain is one of the leading reason for noncompliance with pulmonary rehabilitation in the postoperative setting. Deep breathing, coughing, and ambulation in the early postoperative period help to prevent unwanted pulmonary complications. Mild to moderate pain can generally be managed with opioids via patient-controlled analgesia (PCA) or by continuous or intermittent intravenous administration.[56–58] PCA provides more stable plasma drug levels, better pain relief, and greater patient satisfaction.[59] Potential side effects include sedation and respiratory depression, both of which can be exaggerated in the elderly. Although systemic opioids alone may provide adequate analgesia following a video-assisted thoracoscopic surgical (VATS) procedure or median sternotomy, they typically do not provide adequate analgesia for postthoracotomy patients.[60] Epidural analgesia with local anesthetics, opioids, or a combination of the two provides excellent pain control with fewer side effects.[61] The major factor limiting the use of local anesthetics in the epidural is systemic hypotension. Patients receiving epidermal opioid analgesia for postthoracotomy pain management have better pulmonary function and greater comfort than those receiving systemic opioids.[62]

The epidural catheter is typically inserted into an awake patient, preoperatively in either the lumbar or thoracic location. Only the lumbar position should be considered if the catheter is inserted into a patient who is already asleep, as may occur when a VATS procedure is converted to an open thoracotomy. Contraindications to epidural placement include an active systemic infection and anticoagulation.

Nonsteroidal antiinflammatory drugs (NSAIDs), alone or as adjuncts, may improve pain relief and pulmonary function while reducing the amount and side effects of opioids.[63–67] Gastrointestinal bleeding and renal and platelet dysfunction are potential concerns. Routine laboratory values should be followed during their use.

Chest Tube Management

Chest tubes are used to drain pleural fluid and to maintain lung expansion. Surgeons have a variety of choices with regard to the type and number of chest tubes used and to the collection system available. The goal of chest tube positioning is to allow for the drainage of air while the patient is upright and fluid while the patient is supine. For standard lung resections, traditionally surgeons have placed two tubes: these can be positioned either with one anterior and one posterior, both to the apex, or with one posteriorly to the apex and the other at the base. A single tube placed posteriorly to the apex is now gaining popularity for standard resections. There are no strong clinical data supporting any one of these choices. In general, more tubes (up to three) are advocated for decortications or excessively bloody procedures.

Chest tubes are attached to a drainage system. Typically, a three-chamber system is used, which allows for one-way drainage of fluid and air. Until recently, chest tubes were placed to $-20\,cmH_2O$ in the operating room and left to suction until air leaks resolved. It was thought that the apposition of the lung to the chest wall was vital to the healing of air leaks; this was done, despite a clear lack of supporting data. The advent of lung volume reduction surgery (LVRS) brought much sicker patients with compromised pulmonary parenchyma into the surgical arena. Surgeons quickly recognized that these patients could not be managed with their chest tubes to suction because of the large volume of their air leaks. When surgeons switched the postoperative management of the chest tubes from suction to water seal, the morbidity and mortality associated with LVRS were greatly reduced.[33,68] On the basis of the LVRS experience, surgeons began to recognize that the application of suction may be counterproductive to the healing of air leaks in all patients. Prospective randomized trials from Marshall et al.[69] and Cerfolio et al.[70] have recently demonstrated that early placement of chest tubes to water seal despite the status of air leaks resulted in faster healing of air leaks and decreased chest tube time following standard pulmonary resections (Table 70.5).

Regardless of whether suction is used, chest tubes must be assessed at least daily to determine patency, output, and air leaks. Obstructions can occur secondary to kinking of the tube or clots within the tubing and are recognized by the lack of respiratory variation within the drainage system. "Stripping" the tubes can clear small obstructions. Air leaks are assessed by observing the water seal chamber. There are several systems for grading air leaks, but in general they are described by the amount of force necessary to produce bubbling in the chamber. Drainage should be recorded daily, and the character along with the volume should be noted. Change from sanguineous to serous is generally considered good. When contemplating chest tube removal, the volume of drainage must be at a tolerable level. As a rule of thumb,

TABLE 70.5.
Prospective Randomized Trials Comparing Suction to Water Seal Following Pulmonary Resections.

Author	*Year*	*Level of evidence*	*n*	*Intervention*	*Endpoint*	*Interpretation*	*P*
Cerfolio[70]	2001	IB	140	Suction vs. water seal, postoperative day (POD) 2	Percent with air leak on POD 3	93% vs. 37%	0.001
Marshall[69]	2002	IB	68	Suction vs. water seal, recovery room	Number of air leak days	3.27 vs. 1.50	0.05

3 mL/kg/24 h is acceptable; in an average patient, this would represent 240 to 300 mL/day.[71,72]

Postoperative Anticoagulation

Deep venous thrombosis (DVT) and pulmonary embolism (PE) represent a significant postoperative concern. Thoracic surgery patients frequently have several risk factors for the development of DVT, including advanced age, malignancy, and a history of smoking. Despite the high level of concern over postoperative DVT and PE, there is little written regarding their incidence in patients undergoing thoracotomy. There is only one prospective series considering the incidence of PE in the thoracic surgery population,[73] which found a DVT in 19% of patients and PE in 5%.

Guidelines from the Seventh American College of Chest Physicians Conference on Antithrombotic and Thrombotic Therapy were published in 2004[74] and do not specifically address prophylactic recommendations for thoracic procedures; guidelines from the general surgery population may be appropriate.

The greatest risk factor for the development of a PE is the need for a major surgical procedure. Patients undergoing major surgery have a sixfold increase in the risk for PE. The presence of malignancy also increases the risk for PE nearly sixfold.[75] A retrospective review of autopsies demonstrated that 25% of patients dying with lung cancer had a PE, and the PE was the cause of death in half those patients.[76] Advancing age and a history of smoking are also common risk factors for thrombotic disease found in the thoracic surgery population.[73]

There are three large published series on the risk and prophylaxis for PE in thoracic surgery patients (Table 70.6). Ziomek et al.[73] published the only prospective series on the subject. They performed preoperative venous Doppler studies and perfusion scans on 77 patients before to elective thoracic operations. Early ambulation was the only routine DVT prophylaxis used. There was a 14% incidence of pulmonary embolism and 6% incidence of PE in the postoperative period. Advancing age, cancer (compared to benign process), primary lung cancer (compared to metastatic lesion), and adenocarcinoma were all identified as risk factors for the development of a DVT. Kalweit et al.[76] reported on 1735 patients undergoing pulmonary resections for malignancy. PE prophylaxis included intravenous heparin, starting on the first postoperative day, transitioning to subcutaneous heparin with ambulation. Compression stockings were only used on patients with varicose veins or a prior history of DVT. There were 27 massive PEs, (1.6%), resulting in mortality in 25 of the 27 patients. PE-related mortality was 1.4%. The incidence of DVT and nonmassive PE was not reported. The most recent of these series is by Nagahiro et al.,[77] who retrospectively reviewed 706 thoracic surgery patients comparing pneumatic compression devices versus no intervention for perioperative DVT prophylaxis. There were 7 postoperative PEs in the patients without prophylaxis and none in the patients with compression devices, with a statistical difference. They found no correlation with age, sex, or time to ambulation.

Postoperative Antiarrhythmics

Atrial tachyarrhythmias, predominantly atrial fibrillation, are the most common complication following general thoracic surgery. The reported incidence of atrial tachyarrhythmia varies between 10% and 33% following lung resections[78] and between 13% and 60% following esophagectomy.[79] They are associated with an increased risk for an acute cardiac event, infection, or cerebral vascular accident and with a 33% increase in the length of hospital stays.[80] Major causative factors include increases in pulmonary vascular resistance,

TABLE 70.6.
Trials Evaluating Incidence and Prophylaxis for Deep Venous Thrombosis (DVT) in Thoracic Surgery Patients.

Author	*Year*	*Type of trial*	*Number of patients*	*Prophylaxis*	*DVT rate*	*Pulmonary embolism (PE) rate*	*PE mortality*
Ziomek[73]	1993	Prospective	77	Early ambulation	14%	6%	0.01%
Kalweit[76]	1996	Retrospective	1735	IV heparin POD 1, SQ heparin with ambulation	NR	1.6%	1.4%
Nagahiro[77]	2004	Retrospective	706	Nothing (344), Compression devices (362)	NR	2% 0%	0.005 0%

TABLE 70.7.
Randomized Trials with Placebo Control for the Prophylactic Use of Medication for the Prevention of Postoperative Atrial Fibrillation in General Thoracic Surgery Patients.

Author	*Year*	*Number of patients*	*Atrial tachyarrhythmia (%)*		*Hypotension (%)*		*Bradycardia (%)*		*Pulmonary (%)*		*Mortality (%)*	
			Med	*Placebo*	*Med*	*Placebo*	*Med*	*Placebo*	*Med*	*Placebo*	*Med*	*Placebo*
Calcium channel blockers:												
Amar[103]	2000	330	15	24	0.04	<0.01	n/a	n/a	2	2	0.6	2
Lindgren[104]	1991	25	0	31	0	0	0	0	0	0	0	0
Van Mieghem[91]	1994	96	0	22	9	3	0	0	0	0	9	3
Van Mieghem[105]	1996	199	8	15	14	0	9	0	4	3	4	3
Beta-blockers:												
Bayliff[86]	1999	99	6	4	48	26	24	2	16	8	4	2
Jakobsen[82]	1997	30	20	47	n/a	n/a	n/a	n/a	7	0	n/a	n/a
Magnesium:												
Terzi[106]	1996	200	11	27	0	0	0	0	n/a	n/a	1	1
Digitalis:												
Kaiser[89]	1994	65	33	11	n/a	n/a	20	0	n/a	n/a	n/a	n/a
Ritchie[79,87]	1993	80	31	22	n/a	n/a	n/a	n/a	n/a	n/a	8	5
Ritchie[88,90]	1992	140	29	23	n/a	n/a	6	3	n/a	n/a	n/a	n/a
Flecainide:												
Borgeat[107]	1989	30	0	19	57	0	0	0	0	0	0	0
Amiodarone:												
Van Mieghem[91]	1994	96	3	22	3	3	3	0	9	0	6	0

electrolyte disturbances, acid–base abnormalities, hypoxia, anemia, volume shifts, myocardial ischemia, and increased sympathetic tone.[81–84] A review of more than 2500 thoracic surgery procedures at MD Anderson Cancer Center identified risk factors for the development of postoperative atrial tachyarrhythmia that include advanced age, male sex, a history of congestive heart failure, or arrhythmias, peripheral vascular disease, the extent of procedure performed, and the use of intraoperative transfusion.[85] The treatment and prophylaxis for these arrhythmias remains a very important topic in the perioperative care of thoracic surgery patients.

Table 70.7 outlines the randomized, placebo-control trials evaluating pharmacological prophylaxis for atrial fibrillation following general thoracic surgery procedures. The trials are all small and single-institution studies, but they provide our best evidence-based information on the topic. Calcium channel blockers, beta-blockers, and magnesium have all been found to reduce the risk of atrial tachyarrhythmia. Both calcium channel blockers and beta-blockers are associated with increased rates of bradycardia and hypotension, which is temporary and resolves after discontinuation of medication. One trial noted an association between the use of beta-blockers and increased pulmonary edema.[86] All trials evaluating digitalis demonstrate an increase in the risk of arrhythmia compared to placebo and an associated significant increase in the risk of bradycardic events.[79,87–90] Although the use of amiodarone resulted in a significant reduction in atrial tachyarrhythmias, it was also associated with three cases of acute respiratory distress syndrome (ARDS), resulting in two deaths.[91] There remains little evidence to support the use of this agent for prophylaxis in the general thoracic surgery population. Calcium channel blocker and beta-blocker prophylaxis seem reasonable in high-risk patients, but a multicenter trial is warranted.

The peak incidence for the development of atrial tachyarrhythmias is between postoperative days 2 and 4. Even though most postoperative episodes resolve spontaneously after 24 to 48 h, treatment is indicated. Patients with resulting hemodynamic instability require synchronized cardioversion.[92] In hemodynamically stable patients, pharmacological treatment for rate control is indicated. Options for treatment include adenosine, amiodarone, beta-blockade, calcium channel blockers, and digoxin.[93–95] After 48 h in atrial fibrillation, the risk for stroke increases,[96] so anticoagulation should be considered and weighed against the potential risk of postoperative bleeding.

References

1. Hole DJ, Watt GC, Davey-Smith G, Hart CL, Gillis CR, Hawthorne VM. Impaired lung function and mortality risk in men and women: findings from the Renfrew and Paisley prospective population study. BMJ 1996;313(7059):711–715.
2. Ridker PM, Rifai N, Rose L, Buring JE, Cook NR. Comparison of C-reactive protein and low-density lipoprotein cholesterol levels in the prediction of first cardiovascular events. N Engl J Med 2002;347(20):1557–1565.
3. Au DH, Lemaitre RN, Curtis JR, Smith NL, Psaty BM. The risk of myocardial infarction associated with inhaled beta-adrenoceptor agonists. Am J Respir Crit Care Med 2000;161(3 pt 1):827–830.
4. Volterrani M, Scalvini S, Mazzuero G, et al. Decreased heart rate variability in patients with chronic obstructive pulmonary disease. Chest 1994;106(5):1432–1437.

5. The Society of Thoracic Surgeons. General Thoracic Surgery Procedure Database. Chicago: The Society of Thoracic Surgeons, 2005.
6. Goldman L, Caldera DL, Nussbaum SR, et al. Multifactorial index of cardiac risk in noncardiac surgical procedures. N Engl J Med 1977;297(16):845–850.
7. Eagle KA, Brundage BH, Chaitman BR, et al. Guidelines for perioperative cardiovascular evaluation for noncardiac surgery. Report of the American College of Cardiology/American Heart Association Task Force on Practice Guidelines (Committee on Perioperative Cardiovascular Evaluation for Noncardiac Surgery). J Am Coll Cardiol 1996;27(4):910–948.
8. Eagle KA, Berger PB, Calkins H, et al. ACC/AHA guideline update for perioperative cardiovascular evaluation for noncardiac surgery. Executive summary: a report of the American College of Cardiology/American Heart Association Task Force on Practice Guidelines (Committee to Update the 1996 Guidelines on Perioperative Cardiovascular Evaluation for Noncardiac Surgery). Circulation 2002;105(10):1257–1267.
9. Ashley EA, Raxwal VK, Froelicher VF. The prevalence and prognostic significance of electrocardiographic abnormalities. Curr Probl Cardiol 2000;25(1):1–72.
10. Kertai MD, Boersma E, Bax JJ, et al. A meta-analysis comparing the prognostic accuracy of six diagnostic tests for predicting perioperative cardiac risk in patients undergoing major vascular surgery. Heart 2003;89:1327–1334.
11. Mangano DT, Layug EL, Wallace A, Tateo I. Effect of atenolol on mortality and cardiovascular morbidity after noncardiac surgery. Multicenter Study of Perioperative Ischemia Research Group. N Engl J Med 1996;335(23):1713–1720.
12. Poldermans D, Boersma E, Bax JJ, et al. The effect of bisoprolol on perioperative mortality and myocardial infarction in high-risk patients undergoing vascular surgery. Dutch Echocardiographic Cardiac Risk Evaluation Applying Stress Echocardiography Study Group. N Engl J Med 1999;341(24):1789–1794.
13. Andrus MR, Holloway KP, Clark DB. Use of beta-blockers in patients with COPD. Ann Pharmacother 2004;38(1):142–145.
14. Salpeter SR, Ormiston TM, Salpeter EE, Poole PJ, Cates CJ. Cardioselective beta-blockers for chronic obstructive pulmonary disease: a meta-analysis. Respir Med 2003;97(10):1094–1101.
15. Gottlieb SS, McCarter RJ, Vogel RA. Effect of beta-blockade on mortality among high-risk and low-risk patients after myocardial infarction. N Engl J Med 1998;339(8):489–497.
16. Myrdal G, Gustafsson G, Lambe M, Horte LG, Stahle E. Outcome after lung cancer surgery. Factors predicting early mortality and major morbidity. Eur J Cardiothorac Surg 2001;20(4):694–699.
17. Moores LK. Smoking and postoperative pulmonary complications. An evidence-based review of the recent literature. Clin Chest Med 2000;21(1):139–146.
18. Matsuoka H, Nishio W, Sakamoto T, Harada H, Tsubota N. Prediction of morbidity after lung resection with risk factors using treadmill exercise test. Eur J Cardiothorac Surg 2004; 26(3):480–482.
19. Gerson MC, Hurst JM, Hertzberg VS, Baughman R, Rouan GW, Ellis K. Prediction of cardiac and pulmonary complications related to elective abdominal and noncardiac thoracic surgery in geriatric patients. Am J Med 1990;88(2):101–107.
20. Epstein SK, Faling LJ, Daly BD, Celli BR. Predicting complications after pulmonary resection. Preoperative exercise testing vs. a multifactorial cardiopulmonary risk index. Chest 1993; 104(3):694–700.
21. Epstein SK, Faling LJ, Daly BD, Celli BR. Inability to perform bicycle ergometry predicts increased morbidity and mortality after lung resection. Chest 1995;107(2):311–316.
22. Reilly DF, McNeely MJ, Doerner D, et al. Self-reported exercise tolerance and the risk of serious perioperative complications. Arch Intern Med 1999;159(18):2185–2192.
23. Boushy SF, Billig DM, North LB, Helgason AH. Clinical course related to preoperative and postoperative pulmonary function in patients with bronchogenic carcinoma. Chest 1971;59(4):383–391.
24. Miller JI Jr. Physiologic evaluation of pulmonary function in the candidate for lung resection. J Thorac Cardiovasc Surg 1993;105(2):347–351.
25. Wernly JA, DeMeester TR, Kirchner PT, Myerowitz PD, Oxford DE, Golomb HM. Clinical value of quantitative ventilation-perfusion lung scans in the surgical management of bronchogenic carcinoma. J Thorac Cardiovasc Surg 1980;80(4):535–543.
26. Wyser C, Stultz P, Soler M, et al. Prospective evaluation of an algorithm for the functional assessment of lung resection candidates. Am J Resp Crit Care Med 1999:159(5.1):1450–1456.
27. Ferguson MK, Little L, Rizzo L, et al. Diffusing capacity predicts morbidity and mortality after pulmonary resection. J Thorac Cardiovasc Surg 1988;96(6):894–900.
28. Ferguson MK, Reeder LB, Mick R. Optimizing selection of patients for major lung resection. J Thorac Cardiovasc Surg 1995;109(2):275–281.
29. Wang J, Olak J, Ultmann RE, Ferguson MK. Assessment of pulmonary complications after lung resection. Ann Thorac Surg 1999;67(5):1444–1447.
30. Olsen GN, Block AJ, Swenson EW, Castle JR, Wynne JW. Pulmonary function evaluation of the lung resection candidate: a prospective study. Am Rev Respir Dis 1975;111(4):379–387.
31. Kearney DJ, Lee TH, Reilly JJ, DeCamp MM, Sugarbaker DJ. Assessment of operative risk in patients undergoing lung resection. Importance of predicted pulmonary function. Chest 1994;105(3):753–759.
32. Putnam JB Jr, Lammermeier DE, Colon R, McMurtrey MJ, Ali MK, Roth JA. Predicted pulmonary function and survival after pneumonectomy for primary lung carcinoma. Ann Thorac Surg 1990;49(6):909–914.
33. Cooper JD, Patterson GA, Sundaresan RS, et al. Results of 150 consecutive bilateral lung volume reduction procedures in patients with severe emphysema. J Thorac Cardiovasc Surg 1996;112(5):1319–1329.
34. Wahi R, McMurtrey MJ, DeCaro LF, et al. Determinants of perioperative morbidity and mortality after pneumonectomy. Ann Thorac Surg 1989;48(1):33–37.
35. Juhl B, Frost N. A comparison between measured and calculated changes in the lung function after operation for pulmonary cancer. Acta Anaesthesiol Scand Suppl 1975;57:39–45.
36. Olsen GN, Bolton JW, Weiman DS, Hornung CA. Stair climbing as an exercise test to predict the postoperative complications of lung resection. Two years' experience. Chest 1991;993):587–590.
37. Pate P, Tenholder MF, Griffin JP, Eastridge CE, Weiman DS. Preoperative assessment of the high-risk patient for lung resection. Ann Thorac Surg 1996;61(5):1494–1500.
38. Van Nostrand D, Kjelsberg MO, Humphrey EW. Preresectional evaluation of risk from pneumonectomy. Surg Gynecol Obstet 1968;127(2):306–312.
39. Girish M, Trayner E Jr, Dammann O, Pinto-Plata V, Celli B. Symptom-limited stair climbing as a predictor of postoperative cardiopulmonary complications after high-risk surgery. Chest 2001;120(4):1147–1151.
40. Brunelli A, Al Refai M, Monteverde M, Borri A, Salati M, Fianchini A. Stair climbing test predicts cardiopulmonary complications after lung resection. Chest 2002;121(4):1106–1110.
41. Holden DA, Rice TW, Stelmach K, Meeker DP. Exercise testing, 6-min walk, and stair climb in the evaluation of patients at high risk for pulmonary resection. Chest 1992;102(6):1774–1779.
42. Singh SJ, Morgan MD, Hardman AE, Rowe C, Bardsley PA. Comparison of oxygen uptake during a conventional treadmill

test and the shuttle walking test in chronic airflow limitation. Eur Respir J 1994;7(11):2016–2020.
43. Abbott RD, Levy D, Kannel WB, et al. Cardiovascular risk factors and graded treadmill exercise endurance in healthy adults: The Framingham Offspring Study. Am J Cardiol 1989;63(5):342–346.
44. Morice RC, Peters EJ, Ryan MB, Putnam JB, Ali MK, Roth JA. Exercise testing in the evaluation of patients at high risk for complications from lung resection. Chest 1992;101(2):356–361.
45. Olsen GN, Weiman DS, Bolton JW, et al. Submaximal invasive exercise testing and quantitative lung scanning in the evaluation for tolerance of lung resection. Chest 1989;95(2):267–273.
46. Bolliger CT, Wyser C, Roser H, Soler M, Perruchoud AP. Lung scanning and exercise testing for the prediction of postoperative performance in lung resection candidates at increased risk for complications. Chest 1995;108(2):341–348.
47. British Thoracic Society, Society of Cardiothoracic Surgeons of Great Britain, Ireland Working Party. Guidelines on the selection of patients with lung cancer. Thorax 2001;56:89–108.
48. Kvale P, Ranga V, Kopacz M, Cox F, Magalligan D, Davila J. Pulmonary resection. South Med J 1977;70(Suppl 1):64–69.
49. Truesdale R, D'Alessandri R, Manuel V, Daicoff G, Kluge RM. Antimicrobial vs. placebo prophylaxis in noncardiac thoracic surgery. JAMA 1979;241(12):1254–1256.
50. Cameron JL, Imbembo A, Kieffer RF, Spray S, Baker RR. Prospective clinical-trial of antibiotics for pulmonary resections. Surg Gynecol Obstet 1981;152(2):156–158.
51. Lancon JP, Caillard B, Coulon C, Beaulieu C, Viard H. Postoperative complications of pulmonary surgery. Lyon Chirurg 1986;82(1):14–17.
52. Ilves R, Cooper JD, Todd TRJ, Pearson FG. Prospective, randomized, double-blind study using prophylactic cephalothin for major, elective, general thoracic operations. J Thorac Cardiovasc Surg 1981;81(6):813–817.
53. Olak J, Jeyasingham K, Forrester-Wood C, Hutter J, al-Zeerah M, Brown E. Randomized trial of one-dose versus six-dose cefazolin prophylaxis in elective general thoracic surgery. Ann Thor Surg 1991;51(6):956–958.
54. Wertzel H, Swoboda L, Jooswurtemberger A, Frank U, Hasse J. Perioperative antibiotic-prophylaxis in general thoracic-surgery. Thorac and Cardiovas Surg 1992;40(6):326–329.
55. Bernard A, Pillet M, Goudet P, Viard H. Antibiotic-Prophylaxis in pulmonary surgery: a prospective randomized double-blind trial of flash cefuroxime versus 48-hour cefuroxime. J Thorac Cardiovas Surg 1994;107(3):896–900.
56. Boulanger A, Choiniere M, Roy D, et al. Comparison between patient-controlled analgesia and intramuscular meperidine after thoracotomy. Can J Anaesth 1993;40(5 pt 1):409–415.
57. Etches RC, Gammer TL, Cornish R. Patient-controlled epidural analgesia after thoracotomy: a comparison of meperidine with and without bupivacaine. Anesth Analg 1996;83(1):81–86.
58. Grant RP, Dolman JF, Harper JA, et al. Patient-controlled lumbar epidural fentanyl compared with patient-controlled intravenous fentanyl for post-thoracotomy pain. Can J Anaesth 1992;39(3):214–219.
59. Smythe M. Patient-controlled analgesia: a review. Phamacotherapy 1992;12(2):132–143.
60. Senturk M, Ozcan PE, Talu GK, et al. The effects of three different analgesia techniques on long-term postthoracotomy pain. Anesth Analg 2002;94(1):11–15, table.
61. Sandler AN. Post-thoracotomy analgesia and perioperative outcome. Minerva Anestesiol 1999;65(5):267–274.
62. Gray JR, Fromme GA, Nauss LA, Wang JK, Ilstrup DM. Intrathecal morphine for post-thoracotomy pain. Anesth Analg 1986;65(8):873–876.
63. Alexander R, El Moalem HE, Gan TJ. Comparison of the morphine-sparing effects of diclofenac sodium and ketorolac tromethamine after major orthopedic surgery. J Clin Anesth 2002;14(3):187–192.
64. Perttunen K, Nilsson E, Kalso E. IV diclofenac and ketorolac for pain after thoracoscopic surgery. Br J Anaesth 1999;82(2):221–227.
65. Singh H, Bossard RF, White PF, Yeatts RW. Effects of ketorolac versus bupivacaine coadministration during patient-controlled hydromorphone epidural analgesia after thoracotomy procedures. Anesth Analg 1997;84(3):564–569.
66. Rhodes M, Conacher I, Morritt G, Hilton C. Nonsteroidal antiinflammatory drugs for postthoracotomy pain. A prospective controlled trial after lateral thoracotomy. J Thorac Cardiovasc Surg 1992;103(1):17–20.
67. Perttunen K, Kalso E, Heinonen J, Salo J. IV diclofenac in postthoracotomy pain. Br J Anaesth 1992;68(5):474–480.
68. Cooper JD, Patterson GA. Lung-volume reduction surgery for severe emphysema. Chest Surg Clin N Am 1995;5:815–831.
69. Marshall MB, Deeb ME, Bleier JIS, et al. Suction vs. waterseal after pulmonary resection. Chest 2002;121(3):831–835.
70. Cerfolio RJ, Bass C, Katholi CR. Prospective randomized trial compares suction versus water seal for air leaks. Ann Thorac Surg 2001;71(5):1613–1617.
71. Zehr KJ, Dawson PB, Yang SC, Heitmiller RF. Standardized clinical care pathways for major thoracic cases reduce hospital costs. Ann Thorac Surg 1998;66(3):914–919.
72. Wright CD, Wain JC, Grillo HC, Moncure AC, Macaluso SM, Mathisen DJ. Pulmonary lobectomy patient care pathway: a model to control cost and maintain quality. Ann Thorac Surg 1997;64(2):299–302.
73. Ziomek S, Read RC, Tobler HG, Harrell JE, Gocio JC, Fink LM, et al. Thromboembolism in patients undergoing thoracotomy. Ann Thorac Surg 1993;56(2):223–227.
74. Schunemann HJ, Cook D, Grimshaw J, et al. Antithrombotic and thrombolytic therapy: from evidence to application: the seventh ACCP conference on antithrombotic and thrombolytic therapy. Chest 2004;126(3S):688S–696S.
75. Heit JA, Petterson TM, Marks RS, Bailey KR, Melton LJ. The risk of venous thromboembolism (VTE) among cancer patients by tumor site: a population-based study. Blood 2004;104(11):711A.
76. Kalweit G, Huwer H, Volkmer I, Petzold T, Gams E. Pulmonary embolism: a frequent cause of acute fatality after lung resection. Eur J Cardiothorac Surg 1996;10(4):242–246.
77. Nagahiro I, Andou A, Aoe M, Sano Y, Date H, Shimizu N. Intermittent pneumatic compression is effective in preventing symptomatic pulmonary embolism after thoracic surgery. Surg Today 2004;34(1):6–10.
78. Amar D, Burt M, Reinsel RA, Leung DH. Relationship of early postoperative dysrhythmias and long-term outcome after resection of non-small cell lung cancer. Chest 1996;110(2):437–439.
79. Ritchie AJ, Whiteside M, Tolan M, McGuigan JA. Cardiac dysrhythmia in total thoracic oesophagectomy. A prospective study. Eur J Cardiothorac Surg 1993;7(8):420–422.
80. Polanczyk CA, Goldman L, Marcantonio ER, Orav EJ, Lee TH. Supraventricular arrhythmia in patients having noncardiac surgery: clinical correlates and effect on length of stay. Ann Intern Med 1998;129(4):279–285.
81. Todd TRJ, Ralph-Edwards AC. Perioperative management. In: Pearson FG, Cooper JD, Deslauries J, Ginsberg RJ, Hiebert CA, Patterson GA, eds. Thoracic Surgery. New York: Livingstone, 2002.
82. Jakobsen CJ, Bille S, Ahlburg P, Rybro L, Hjortholm K, Andresen EB. Perioperative metoprolol reduces the frequency of atrial fibrillation after thoracotomy for lung resection. J Cardiothorac Vasc Anesth 1997;11(6):746–751.

83. Amar D, Roistacher N, Burt M, Reinsel RA, Ginsberg RJ, Wilson RS. Clinical and echocardiographic correlates of symptomatic tachydysrhythmias after noncardiac thoracic surgery. Chest 1995;108(2):349–354.
84. Backlund M, Laasonen L, Lepantalo M, Metsarinne K, Tikkanen I, Lindgren L. Effect of oxygen on pulmonary hemodynamics and incidence of atrial fibrillation after noncardiac thoracotomy. J Cardiothorac Vasc Anesth 1998;12(4):422–428.
85. Vaporciyan AA, Correa AM, Rice DC, et al. Risk factors associated with atrial fibrillation after noncardiac thoracic surgery: analysis of 2588 patients. J Thorac Cardiovasc Surg 2004;127(3):779–786.
86. Bayliff CD, Massel DR, Inculet RI, et al. Propranolol for the prevention of postoperative arrhythmias in general thoracic surgery. Ann Thorac Surg 1999;67(1):182–186.
87. Ritchie AJ, Tolan M, Whiteside M, McGuigan JA, Gibbons JR. Prophylactic digitalization fails to control dysrhythmia in thoracic esophageal operations. Ann Thorac Surg 1993;55(1):86–88.
88. Ritchie AJ, Bowe P, Gibbons JR. Prophylactic digitalization for thoracotomy: a reassessment. Ann Thorac Surg 1990;50(1):86–88.
89. Kaiser A, Zund G, Weder W, Largiader F. Preventive digitalis therapy in open thoracotomy. Helv Chir Acta 1994;60(6):913–917.
90. Ritchie AJ, Danton M, Gibbons JR. Prophylactic digitalisation in pulmonary surgery. Thorax 1992;47(1):41–43.
91. Van Mieghem W, Coolen L, Malysse I, Lacquet LM, Deneffe GJ, Demedts MG. Amiodarone and the development of ARDS after lung surgery. Chest 1994;105(6):1642–1645.
92. Chung MK. Cardiac surgery: postoperative arrhythmias. Crit Care Med 2000;28(10 suppl):N136–N144.
93. Basta M, Klein GJ, Yee R, Krahn A, Lee J. Current role of pharmacologic therapy for patients with paroxysmal supraventricular tachycardia. Cardiol Clin 1997;15(4):587–597.
94. Ferguson JD, DiMarco JP. Contemporary management of paroxysmal supraventricular tachycardia. Circulation 2003;107(8):1096–1099.
95. Solomon AJ. Treatment of postoperative atrial fibrillation: a nonsurgical perspective. Semin Thorac Cardiovasc Surg 1999;11(4):320–324.
96. Kannel WB, Wolf PA, Benjamin EJ, Levy D. Prevalence, incidence, prognosis, and predisposing conditions for atrial fibrillation: population-based estimates. Am J Cardiol 1998;82(8A):2N–9N.
97. Frimodt Moller N, Ostri P, Pedersen IK, Poulsen SR. Antibiotic-prophylaxis in pulmonary surgery: a double-blind study of penicillin versus placebo. Ann Surg 1982;195(4):444–450.
98. Tarkka M, Pokela R, Lepojarvi M, Nissinen J, Karkola P. Infection prophylaxis in pulmonary surgery: a randomized prospective study. Ann Thorac Surg 1987;44(5):508–513.
99. Anzar R, Mateu M, Miro J. Antibiotic prophylaxis in non-cardiac thoracic surgery: cefazolin versus placebo. Eur J Cardiothorac Surg 1991;5:515–518.
100. Krasnik M, Thiis J, Frimodtmoller N. Antibiotic prophylaxis in noncardiac thoracic surgery: a double-blind study of penicillin vs. cefuroxime. Scand J Thorac Cardiovasc Surg 1991;25(1):73–76.
101. Boldt J, Piper S, Uphus D, Fussle R, Hempelmann G. Preoperative microbiologic screening and antibiotic prophylaxis in pulmonary resection operations. Ann Thorac Surg 1999;68(1):208–211.
102. Turna A, Kutlu CA, Ozalp T, Karamustafaoglu A, Mulazimoglu L, Bedirhan MA. Antibiotic prophylaxis in elective thoracic surgery: cefuroxime vs. cefepime. Thorac Cardiovasc Surg 2003;51(2):84–88.
103. Amar D, Roistacher N, Rusch VW, et al. Effects of diltiazem prophylaxis on the incidence and clinical outcome of atrial arrhythmias after thoracic surgery. J Thorac Cardiovasc Surg 2000;120(4):790–798.
104. Lindgren L, Lepantalo M, von Knorring J, Rosenberg P, Orko R, Scheinin B. Effect of verapamil on right ventricular pressure and atrial tachyarrhythmia after thoracotomy. Br J Anaesth 1991;66(2):205–211.
105. Van Mieghem W, Tits G, Demuynck K, et al. Verapamil as prophylactic treatment for atrial fibrillation after lung operations. Ann Thorac Surg 1996;61(4):1083–1085.
106. Terzi A, Furlan G, Chiavacci P, Dal Corso B, Luzzani A, Dalla VS. Prevention of atrial tachyarrhythmias after non-cardiac thoracic surgery by infusion of magnesium sulfate. Thorac Cardiovasc Surg 1996;44(6):300–303.
107. Borgeat A, Biollaz J, Bayer-Berger M, Kappenberger L, Chapuis G, Chiolero R. Prevention of arrhythmias by flecainide after noncardiac thoracic surgery. Ann Thorac Surg 1989;48(2):232–234.

71

Lung Neoplasms

Frank C. Detterbeck, Scott N. Gettinger, and Mark A. Socinski

General Background

Lung cancer is the leading cause of cancer deaths in men and in women in both the United States and the world.[1] In fact, lung cancer accounts for more cancer deaths than the next four leading causes of cancer deaths combined (Fig. 71.1). Although the incidence of cancer deaths in men has been decreasing since 1990 and has begun to level off in women, lung cancer will continue to be the leading cause of cancer deaths for at least the next 30 years based on the current trends.[2,3]

Much progress has been made in the management and treatment of patients with lung cancer during the last 40 years. Survival rates have nearly doubled during this time.[4] However, lung cancer is still associated with much pessimism, which is not surprising considering how much progress still needs to be made (overall 5-year survival for all patients is 15%).[1] There are many reasons for the high mortality of lung cancer. One reason is the fact that in almost half of patients with non-small cell lung cancer (NSCLC) and the majority of patients with small cell lung cancer (SCLC), the disease is already systemic when it is diagnosed. Notably, screening for lung cancer is not an established intervention, in contrast to breast, colon, and prostate cancer. Another factor in the high mortality is the fact that untreated lung cancer is rapidly fatal.[4–7] This is true even for stage I NSCLC.[4–7] However, nihilism and lack of referral of patients for appropriate treatment also contribute to the poor survival.[8–12]

Lung cancer is clearly associated with smoking. However, currently almost half of those diagnosed with lung cancer are people who quit smoking many years earlier.[13–15] The accumulated risk of developing lung cancer does not diminish after cessation of smoking, although it does not continue to climb as it does in people who do not quit smoking.[16,17] These facts are a strong argument against the tendency of patients, physicians, and the public to blame the patients for bringing the disease on themselves by smoking. This attitude of guilt promotes nihilism and a lack of motivation to treat the disease optimally. These responses however, are unjustified, as evidenced by the data presented in this chapter.

Classification

Histologic Classification

Lung neoplasms can be classified into a variety of histologic types. From a clinical standpoint, however, these can be broadly grouped into three categories: SCLC, NSCLC, and low-grade tumors (see Table 71.1). In addition, one can distinguish several specific histologic types of NSCLC that have a somewhat distinct behavior and thus deserve special consideration. Some of these special types are best considered variants of the broader groups, such as mixed SCLC/NSCLC tumors, atypical carcinoid tumors, and large cell neuroendocrine (LCNEC) tumors. Other, relatively rare tumors have sufficiently unusual behavior to be viewed individually rather than by extrapolating from other lung cancers. These include pure bronchioloalveolar carcinoma (BAC) and primary pulmonary sarcomas. It is recognized that this categorization is somewhat arbitrary and does not reflect official histologic classification schemes. However, it represents a practical way of grouping tumors based on clinical management considerations.

Non-small cell lung cancer accounts for approximately 80%–85% of cases. This group is divided largely into adenocarcinoma, squamous cell carcinoma, and large cell carcinoma. Other rare subtypes of NSCLC include adenosquamous and basaloid cancers. The differences in clinical characteristics and prognosis between these tumor subtypes are minor. The treatment is driven by the anatomic characteristics and

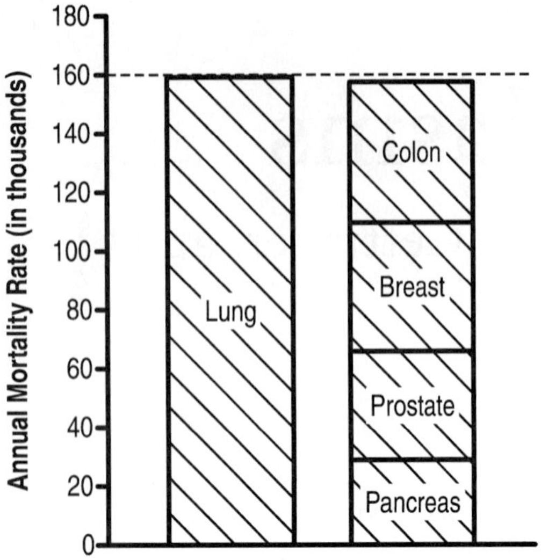

FIGURE 71.1. Mortality of lung cancer compared with next four leading causes of cancer deaths. (Data from Landis et al.[307])

stage of the tumor and is not significantly influenced by the histologic subtype. Therefore, the NSCLC subtypes are generally considered together as one group. Many adenocarcinomas have peripheral features of BAC; in this case, they are considered simply as an adenocarcinoma, consistent with the published survival data.[18,19]

Small cell lung cancer is characterized clinically by rapid growth and a frequent incidence of extrathoracic metastases. Radiographically, there is bulky mediastinal involvement in the vast majority of patients, often without an obvious parenchymal primary tumor. Microscopically, these tumor cells contain neurosecretory granules. These granules are a characteristic that SCLC has in common with carcinoid and LCNEC tumors, but the presentation and biologic behavior of SCLC have nothing in common with carcinoid tumors. Almost all patients with SCLC have a significant history of smoking.

Low-grade tumors of the lung include typical carcinoid tumors, mucoepidermoid tumors, and adenoid cystic tumors. These tumors are characterized by slow growth and relatively late spread to extrathoracic sites. Nevertheless, they all do exhibit the characteristic features of malignant tumors, namely, the ability to invade other tissues and metastasize. Therefore, they are all classified as malignant tumors, even typical carcinoid tumors. These tumors are also characterized by arising in the tracheobronchial tree, although a minority of carcinoid tumors present as a peripheral parenchymal mass.

Several subtypes of lung cancer have some peculiar characteristics and deserve to be considered somewhat separately. Bronchioloalveolar carcinoma is characterized by palisading cells that spread along the alveolar membrane. These tumors are usually classified among NSCLC, but they have a somewhat better prognosis. They involve lymph nodes less frequently than other types of NSCLC. Most important, the majority of recurrences are within the lung parenchyma and do not involve distant sites. Atypical carcinoid tumors clearly have a worse prognosis than typical carcinoid tumors, with more frequent involvement of lymph nodes and distant sites. The overall prognosis is slightly better than that of NSCLC. The LCNEC cells have a similar appearance to NSCLC microscopically but also contain neurosecretory granules. These tumors have very aggressive behavior, almost as aggressive as SCLC.

Stage Classification

The staging system used for NSCLC is the TNM system, most recently defined in 1997 by the AJCC (American Joint Commission for Cancer) and UICC (Union Internationale Contre le Cancer).[20] The definitions of the TNM descriptors and the stage groupings are shown in Table 71.2. Thus, the stage is determined by the anatomic extent of the tumor by standard microscopy. These stage groupings are based primarily on survival statistics from a large registry of patients, primarily with NSCLC, treated by a variety of modalities. It is possible that in the future stage will be redefined to include other characteristics of prognostic value, such as molecular oncologic characteristics or the presence of occult tumor cells by sensitive molecular detection methods.

Staging of SCLC is by a two-stage system as either limited stage (LS) or extensive stage (ES). *Limited stage* is defined as tumor confined to the thorax and mediastinum. It is somewhat controversial whether LS should include patients with involvement of contralateral hilar nodes, supraclavicular nodes (especially contralateral), an ipsilateral pleural effusion, or a tumor that is greater than 50% of the diameter of the thorax. *Extensive stage* is the presence of distant metastases or intrathoracic tumor that is beyond the definition of limited disease as outlined above.

Carcinoid and mucoepidermoid tumors are usually classified using the TNM system as defined for NSCLC. Tumors such as BAC, atypical carcinoid tumors, and LCNEC tumors are also classified using the TNM system. There is no well-accepted staging system for adenoid cystic carcinoma of the tracheobronchial tree.

TABLE 71.1. Major Histologic Types of Lung Neoplasms.

Category	*Histologic types*	*Types with special features*
Small cell	Oat cell	Mixed SCLC/NSCLC
Non-small cell	Adenocarcinoma Squamous cell carcinoma Large cell Adenosquamous carcinoma	Adenocarcinoma with BAC features LCNEC Atypical carcinoid
Low-grade tumors	Adenoid cystic carcinoma Mucoepidermoid tumor Typical carcinoid	High-grade mucoepidermoid tumor
Special types	Bronchioloalveolar carcinoma Sarcoma, carcinosarcoma	

BAC, bronchioloalveolar carcinoma; LCNEC, large cell neuroendocrine carcinoma; NSCLC, non-small cell lung cancer; SCLC, small cell lung cancer.

TABLE 71.2. Definition of TMN, Stage Grouping, Histopathologic Type, and Histologic Grade for Lung Cancer.

Definition of TMN

Primary Tumor (T)

TX	Primary tumor cannot be assessed, or tumor proven by the presence of malignant cells in sputum or bronchial washings but not visualized by imaging or bronchoscopy
T0	No evidence of primary tumor
Tis	Carcinoma in situ
T1	Tumor 3 cm or less in greatest dimension, surrounded by lung or visceral pleura, without bronchoscopic evidence of invasion more proximal than the lobar bronchus,* (i.e., not in the main bronchus)
T2	Tumor with any of the following features of size or extent: More than 3 cm in greatest dimension Involves main bronchus, 2 cm or more distal to the carina Invades the visceral pleura Associated with atelectasis or obstructive pneumonitis that extends to the hilar region but does not involve the entire lung
T3	Tumor of any size that directly invades any of the following: chest wall (including superior sulcus tumors), diaphragm, mediastinal pleura, parietal pericardium; or tumor in the main bronchus less than 2 cm distal to the carina, but without involvement of the carina; or associated atelectasis or obstructive pneumonitis of the entire lung
T4	Tumor of any size that invades any of the following: mediastinum, heart, great vessels, trachea, esophagus, vertebral body, carina; or separate tumor nodules in the same lobe; or tumor with malignant pleural effusion**

**Note:* The uncommon superficial tumor of any size with its invasive component limited to the bronchial wall, which may extend proximal to the main bronchus, is also classified T1.

***Note:* Most pleural effusions associated with lung cancer are due to tumor. However, there are a few patients in whom multiple cytopathologic examinations of pleural fluid are negative for tumor. In these cases, fluid is nonbloody and is not an exudate. Such patients may be further evaluated by videothoracoscopy (VATS) and direct pleural biopsies. When these elements and clinical judgment dictate that the effusion is not related to the tumor, the effusion should be excluded as a staging element and the patient should be staged T1, T2, or T3.

Regional Lymph Nodes (N)

NX	Regional lymph nodes cannot be assessed
N0	No regional lymph node metastasis
N1	Metastasis to ipsilateral peribronchial and/or ipsilateral hilar lymph nodes, and intrapulmonary nodes including involvement by direct extension of the primary tumor
N2	Metastasis to ipsilateral mediastinal and/or subcarinal lymph nodes(s)
N3	Metastasis to contralateral mediastinal, contralateral hilar, ipsilateral or contralateral scalene, or supraclavicular lymph nodes(s)

Distant Metastasis (M)

MX	Distant metastasis cannot be assessed
M0	No distant metastasis
M1	Distant metastasis present

Note: M1 includes separate tumor nodule(s) in a different lobe (ipsilateral or contralateral).

Stage Grouping			
Occult Carcinoma	TX	N0	M0
Stage 0	Tis	N0	M0
Stage IA	T1	N0	M0
Stage IB	T2	N0	M0
Stage IIA	T1	N1	M0
Stage IIB	T2	N1	M0
	T3	N0	M0
Stage IIIA	T1	N2	M0
	T2	N2	M0
	T3	N1	M0
	T3	N2	M0
Stage IIIB	Any T	N3	M0
	T4	Any N	M0
Stage IV	Any T	Any N	M1

Source: Used with the permission of the American Joint Committee on Cancer (AJCC), Chicago, Illinois. The original source for this material is the *AJCC Cancer Staging Manual, Sixth Edition* (2002) published by Springer Science and Business Media LLC, www.springerlink.com

Presentation and Evaluation of NSCLC

Presentation

The median age of patients who present with lung cancer is between 65 and 70 years in population-based series.[8,21,22] The risk of lung cancer increases with age, independent of smoking,[4] and lung cancer is relatively uncommon in patients younger than 40 unless there is a family history.[23] Fewer than 10% of patients with lung cancer are asymptomatic, consistent with the fact that no screening test for lung cancer is routinely used.[23,24] Approximately half of the patients present with local symptoms related to intrathoracic tumor (cough, dyspnea, chest pain, hemoptysis, hoarseness).[24–27] Approximately one-third of patients have symptoms related to metastatic disease at the time of presentation (primarily weight loss, fatigue, anorexia, bone pain, headache).[25–27] This is consistent with the finding that 30% to 40% of patients with NSCLC have stage IV disease, and 30% to 40% have stage III tumors.[23,28] Approximately two-thirds of lung cancers develop in the upper lobes, with a fairly equal distribution between central and peripheral locations.[29–31] The common perception that central tumors are primarily squamous cancers and peripheral tumors are adenocarcinoma is no longer true,[30] possibly reflective of changes in the composition and design of cigarettes.[4]

Evaluation

General Approach

The likelihood of lung cancer is determined primarily by assessment of risk factors for lung cancer, a compatible clinical presentation, and the radiographic appearance on a chest computed tomographic (CT) scan. *Independent risk factors* for lung cancer include smoking, a family history of lung cancer, the presence of significant chronic obstructive pulmonary disease, and a prior history of a smoking-related malignancy. Continued smoking is associated with an approximately 2000% increased risk compared with a lifelong nonsmoker, but a 200%–300% increased risk remains 20 years after cessation of smoking.[4] A first-degree relative with lung cancer or the presence of COPD imparts a 400% increased risk (corrected for other factors, such as second-hand smoke

TABLE 71.3. Approach to Diagnosis and Staging of Patients with Probable Lung Cancer.

Clinical scenario	*Clinical evaluation*	*Confirmation of extrathoracic stage*	*Confirmation of intrathoracic stage*	*Confirmation of diagnosis*
NSCLC				
Peripheral cI	Neg (FN 5%)	None	CT (FN < 10%)	Surgical resection
cII, central cI	Neg (FN 5%?)[a]	None (PET?)	Med (FN < 10%)[b]	Surgical resection
cIII, discrete N2,3 enlargement	Neg (FN 30%)	PET, brain MRI	Med (FN < 10%) or FNA (FN 10%–30%)	Mediastinal node biopsy
cIII, diffuse infiltration	Neg (FN 30%)	PET, brain MRI	CT	Easiest site[c]
cIV	Pos (FP 50%)	PET, brain MRI	Not needed	Easiest site if multiple typical metastases[c] Biopsy of suspected site if solitary potential metastasis
SCLC				
Any	Any	Radiographic[d]	CT	Easiest site[c]

cI, clinical stage I; cII, clinical stage II; cIII, clinical stage III; cIV, clinical stage IV; CT, computed tomographic scan; FNA, fine-needle aspiration (transbronchial, esophageal, or transthoracic); Med, Mediastinoscopy; Neg, negative; NSCLC, non-small cell lung cancer; MRI, magnetic resonance imaging scan; PET, positron emission tomography; SCLC, small cell lung cancer; TTNA, transthoracic needle aspiration; FN, false negative rate; FP, false positive rate.

[a]Rate not specifically defined for stage II (defined for stage I and II combined). FN rate may be up to 15% using PET scan.

[b]FNA carries FN rate of about 30% in most series.

[c]For example, sputum, bronchoscopy, FNA of supraclavicular node, TTNA.

[d]Bone scan and abdominal CT, and brain CT or MRI.

exposure).[4] The risk is increased approximately 50% in women (corrected for other factors), whereas secondhand smoke increases the risk approximately 20%–40% (up to 75% at the highest levels of exposure).[4] More important, the risk increases substantially with age (corrected for other factors). A previous, successfully treated lung cancer imparts a very high risk of a new lung cancer (approximately 2% per year).[32] *Radiographic factors* include the rapidity of appearance of the lesion as well as the border characteristics. A spiculated lesion carries approximately an 80% chance of malignancy, a lobulated lesion approximately 60%, whereas a lesion with indistinct borders is more typical of an inflammatory process.[4]

In many patients, a high likelihood (>80%) of cancer can be predicted from the clinical and radiographic features. Although tissue confirmation of the diagnosis is necessary, the further evaluation is directed by staging considerations. In patients with a low or intermediate likelihood of cancer, a positron emission tomographic (PET) scan can be useful for diagnosis, provided the lesion is larger than 1 cm.[33] In lesions smaller than 1 cm, the false-negative (FN) rate for PET is high (about 30%), as it is for transthoracic needle aspiration (TTNA) or bronchoscopy.[23,33] Therefore, the only realistic options for most of these smaller lesions is either clinical follow-up or a thoracoscopic excisional biopsy.[33]

Patients who are suspected of having a lung cancer almost always have had a chest radiograph and a chest CT scan by the time they are referred to a specialist for further evaluation. The approach to the patient at this point starts with a clinical evaluation (assessment of risk factors, clinical presentation and symptoms, physical examination) and a review of the radiographic characteristics of the pulmonary abnormality. This generally allows a presumptive diagnosis to be made (including a presumptive classification of SCLC vs. NSCLC), as well as determination of the presumptive clinical stage if it is thought to be lung cancer. If there is a high degree of suspicion of lung cancer, it is usually best not to pursue a tissue biopsy as the next step but to first evaluate the reliability of the clinical stage (with regard to both extrathoracic disease and intrathoracic or mediastinal staging). Often, further testing is needed to define the stage more accurately; this is often a test that results in a tissue confirmation of the diagnosis as well. It is generally best to consider whether further tests of possible distant disease are needed first and to consider further assessment of the mediastinum when there is confidence that no systemic disease is present. This general approach to patients with a high suspicion of lung cancer is summarized in Table 71.3.

Extrathoracic Staging

Patients with stage IV NSCLC usually present with either constitutional symptoms (fatigue, anorexia, weight loss) or organ-specific symptoms suggestive of distant metastases (neurologic symptoms, bone pain).[34] Laboratory studies (calcium, liver function tests) have often been obtained as well, although data demonstrate there is essentially no value to this practice in NSCLC.[34] The high false-positive (FP) rate of such symptoms (70%) necessitates further investigation.[34] Traditionally, this has involved a bone scan, a CT of the liver and adrenals, and brain magnetic resonance imaging (MRI) or CT, but a PET scan (in addition to a brain MRI) is now recommended when this is available.[35] Radiographic evidence of metastases on such imaging tests is generally accepted as accurate in patients with SCLC or patients with NSCLC and a typical presentation and radiographic appearance consistent with metastatic disease.[36] If there is a solitary site suspicious of being a metastasis, tissue confirmation from this site is usually needed because of the high FP rate of imaging tests (10%–15%) alone in this situation.[34,36–38]

The need for extrathoracic imaging in the face of a negative clinical evaluation has been controversial. Closer examination of the data, however, discloses that the intrathoracic tumor stage defines the need for such imaging. In patients with clinical stage I NSCLC and a negative clinical evaluation for systemic symptoms, conventional imaging detects distant metastases in fewer than 5%,[34,39,40] and similarly PET detects such metastases in about 5% of stage cI patients.[35,41–45] In fact, a distant site suspicious of metastasis on PET in stage cI patients is more likely to be an FP finding than a metastasis.[44] On the other hand, asymptomatic patients with stage cIII disease have about a 30% incidence of distant metastases when subjected to either conventional [34,40,46,47] or PET imaging.[35,41,42,48] In patients with stage II NSCLC, conventional imaging has rarely detected metastases, and the role of PET scanning for distant metastases is still relatively undefined. Thus, imaging for distant metastases (preferably with PET and a brain MRI) is indicated in asymptomatic patients with stage III disease, not indicated in patients with stage cI disease, and the role is limited and poorly defined in patients with stage II disease.

Intrathoracic Staging

The initial assessment of intrathoracic stage is based on the chest CT scan. Of course, this matters only when distant metastases have been reasonably excluded. Four different situations can be distinguished (Fig. 71.2a–71.2d): (1) a peripheral stage cI tumor with no evidence of N1 or N2,3 nodal enlargement (peripheral cI); (2) a central tumor or a tumor with N1 nodal enlargement but without N2,3 enlargement (cII or central cI); (3) enlargement of discrete N2,3 nodes (cIII); and (4) mediastinal infiltration by tumor, such that discrete nodes can no longer be distinguished (cIII).[49] A *central tumor* is defined as a tumor within the proximal third of the lung. The accepted criterion for nodal enlargement is a short-axis measurement of 1 cm or more on a transverse CT image. Nodes smaller than 1 cm are considered normal radiographically.

A large amount of data is available comparing the sensitivity and specificity of CT versus PET imaging.[50] However,

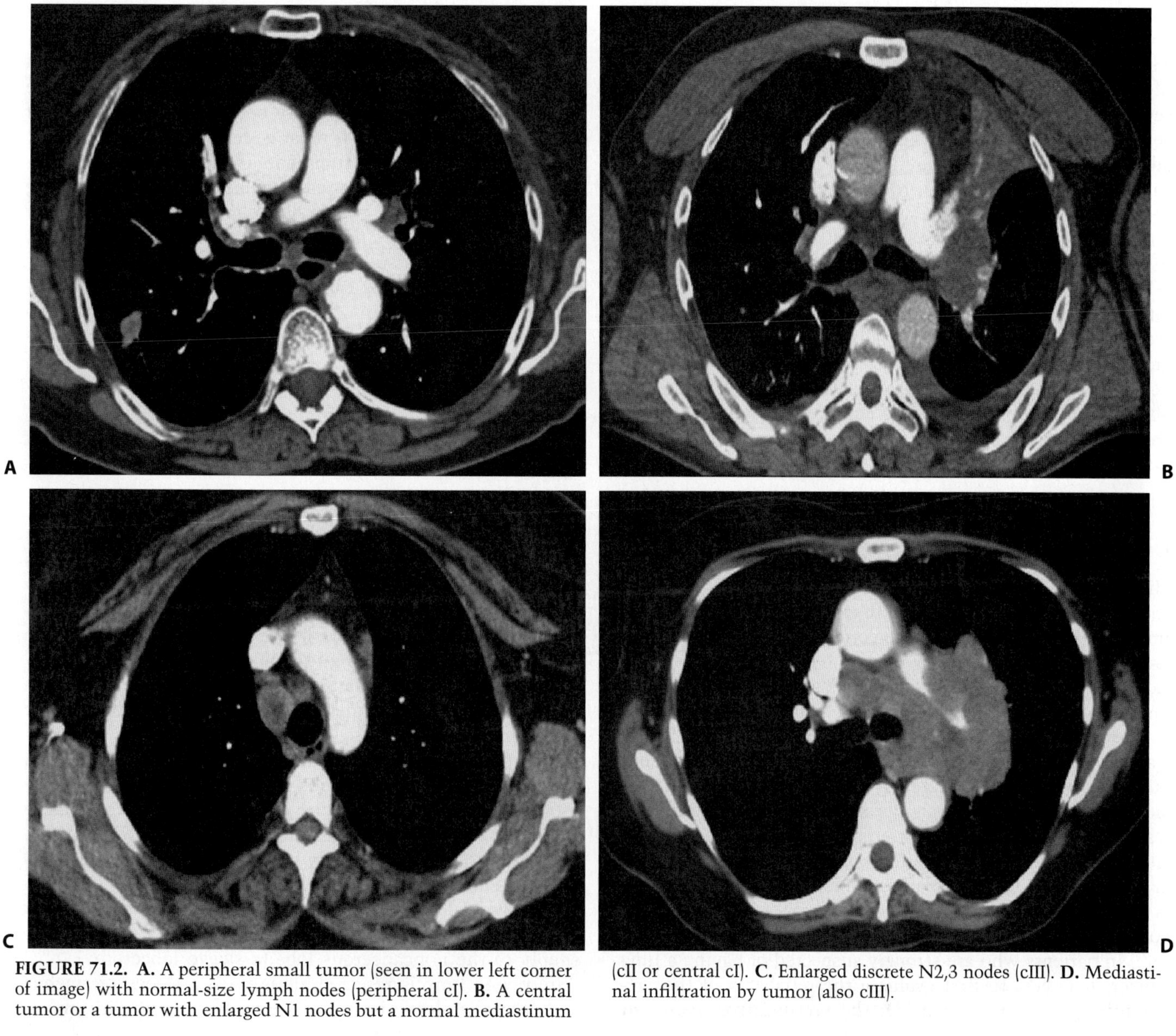

FIGURE 71.2. **A.** A peripheral small tumor (seen in lower left corner of image) with normal-size lymph nodes (peripheral cI). **B.** A central tumor or a tumor with enlarged N1 nodes but a normal mediastinum (cII or central cI). **C.** Enlarged discrete N2,3 nodes (cIII). **D.** Mediastinal infiltration by tumor (also cIII).

this is of questionable relevance because CT alone for mediastinal staging is notoriously inaccurate for many patient cohorts, and appropriate staging involves CT *with confirmation* by mediastinoscopy for normal-size nodes or by either mediastinoscopy or needle aspiration (via bronchoscopy, esophageal ultrasound, or transthoracic) for enlarged nodes.[51,52] Furthermore, sensitivity and specificity cannot be used in interpretation of test results in an individual patient. This requires knowledge of the probability of an FN or FP test result (the FN or FP rate, also known as the negative predictive value or positive predictive value). Finally, choosing the optimum method of confirming the mediastinal stage is complicated by the need to achieve histologic confirmation of the diagnosis—often an invasive method of mediastinal staging is the most efficient way to confirm both the diagnosis and the stage, and a PET scan will not yield a tissue confirmation of malignancy.[35]

In patients with a peripheral cI tumor, the FN rate of CT is low enough that further confirmation of the lack of mediastinal involvement is not deemed necessary (Table 71.3).[53] Imaging by PET adds little in this situation.[35] On the other hand, 20%–25% of patients with a central tumor or cII disease harbor mediastinal node involvement despite a negative CT. The traditional confirmatory test is mediastinoscopy because of a high FN rate for needle aspiration techniques in the setting of normal-size nodes.[51] The FN rate of PET in this setting appears to be around 20%, although data specifically addressing this situation are limited. [35,54–56] A positive PET in the mediastinum, however, requires a biopsy because of an FP rate of 15%–25%.[35,56–58] CT evidence of discrete N2,3 node enlargement has a very high FP rate (40%).[53] The data for PET in such patients suggest that both the FN and FP rates are relatively high, mandating confirmatory invasive staging either way.[35,57] Either mediastinoscopy or a needle aspiration technique is acceptable.[51] Finally, diffuse infiltration or encasement of mediastinal structures on CT has generally been accepted as adequate evidence of stage III disease, although data to prove this are lacking. The role of PET in this situation is solely to detect possible distant metastatic disease.

Diagnosis

Histologic or cytologic confirmation of the diagnosis of lung cancer is generally required before treatment with either chemotherapy or radiation. Tissue confirmation of lung cancer is often not needed prior to surgical resection, however. For example, in patients with a high probability of cancer based on radiologic characteristics and risk factors and a resectable early-stage lesion, intraoperative confirmation of the diagnosis by excisional biopsy is typically preferred. The argument is based on the high FN rates (about 30%) of other, nonexcisional diagnostic methods (bronchoscopy for peripheral lesions or TTNA), which led to the recommendation of excision whether these investigations are positive for malignancy or not. In many instances, a tissue biopsy of a particular site is necessary for confirmation of the stage, which will, of course, provide confirmation of the diagnosis as well. Therefore, in patients who are strongly suspected of having a lung cancer, it is best to first evaluate the reliability of the presumptive stage and to consider the presumptive treatment approach rather than to immediately pursue a tissue biopsy of the primary lesion.[36]

In patients who have a presumed SCLC or who have signs and symptoms of obvious advanced lung cancer (either SCLC or NSCLC), confirmation of the diagnosis is generally obtained from whatever site and method is easiest (Table 71.3). This may involve needle aspiration of a supraclavicular node or a pleural effusion, sputum analysis, bronchoscopy, or TTNA. If there is a solitary site suspicious of being a metastasis, tissue confirmation from this site is usually needed. In patients with clinical stage III NSCLC (enlarged discrete mediastinal nodes and no evidence of distant metastases), the diagnosis is obtained at the time of confirmation of the mediastinal node involvement (by either a needle aspiration technique or mediastinoscopy). In patients with clinical stage I or II NSCLC who are candidates for resection, the diagnosis is usually obtained at the time of resection.

Sputum cytology has a diagnostic yield of about 70% and 40% for central and peripheral lesions, provided multiple samples are obtained in centers with a formal program for the acquisition, handling, and interpretation of such samples.[23,36] Bronchoscopy has a yield respectively of about 85%, 70%, and 30% for central lesions, for large peripheral lesions under optimal conditions (e.g., fluoroscopy, multiple samples) and for small peripheral lesions (≤2 cm).[23,36] A transthoracic needle biopsy of a peripheral pulmonary nodule has a sensitivity of about 90%.[23,36] However, it must be remembered that the FN rate of bronchoscopy or transthoracic needle biopsy is high (average about 30%), making these unreliable tests for *ruling out* lung cancer.[23,36] Although the FN rate for lung cancer may be lower when a *specific* benign diagnosis is achieved, the chance of making a specific benign diagnosis in patients suspected of having a lung cancer is low (1%).[59] Needle biopsy primarily plays a role in confirming a suspected benign diagnosis when it is thought highly likely that the patient does not have lung cancer.

Treatment of NSCLC

General Aspects of Surgical Resection

Surgical resection is the main treatment for NSCLC tumors that appear to be localized to the lung. These are generally stage I or stage II tumors that involve one lobe (most commonly one of the upper lobes). The most common procedure is a lobectomy, accounting for approximately 75% of resections.[24,60–62] Lobectomy can be accomplished by either a traditional open thoracotomy incision or a minimally invasive approach using thoracoscopy. Comparison of series of thoracoscopic resection in experienced centers to those of open resection suggests that there is no difference in perioperative mortality or in long-term survival.[60,63–69] Occasionally (approximately 10% of cases), a central tumor will involve the airway or vascular supply of the whole lung, necessitating a pneumonectomy.[24,60–62] In some instances, a lobe can be removed along with a portion of the main bronchus or artery with reconstruction of the bronchus or vascular supply of the noncancerous lobe (a sleeve lobectomy).[24,70–72] Rarely, one lung is resected along with a sleeve of trachea and carina (a sleeve pneumonectomy).[73] In some instances, a small peripheral tumor is resected with a sublobar resection (either a nonanatomic wedge resection or a formal segmentectomy). The results of sublobar resection are discussed in detail.

Some pulmonary resections involve excision of adjacent structures that have become involved with tumor.[74] Most commonly, this entails removal of a portion of the ribs en bloc with the tumor (T3). Resection of the diaphragm, pericardium, and phrenic nerve (also T3 structures) is easily accomplished as well.[74] Resection of other mediastinal structures such as the superior vena cava (SVC), left atrium, aorta, or vertebral column (all T4 structures) can also be performed but requires expertise in techniques of reconstruction of these structures.[73]

The standard of care is to perform a systematic sampling of all ipsilateral mediastinal node stations at the time of resection (exploration and biopsy of each ipsilateral and midline mediastinal node station).[75] This provides more accurate staging information than a selective node sampling (biopsy of suspicious nodes only)[76–78] or, worse yet, than no node sampling at all. Stage classification is the same after systematic mediastinal node sampling versus a formal lymph node dissection (LND; complete excision of all ipsilateral and midline mediastinal node-bearing tissues).[62,76,79]

The average perioperative mortality of surgical resection for lung cancer in larger series is 4%.[80] Pneumonia combined with respiratory failure is the most common cause of perioperative death (41%), followed by myocardial infarction (14%) and empyema (11%).[80] The mortality is greater after a pneumonectomy (9%), especially on the right, than after lobectomy (3%) or wedge resection (2%).[80] Extended resection (lung parenchyma plus adjacent contiguous structures) carries an average mortality of 12% in larger series.[80] The perioperative mortality is lower when performed by thoracic surgeons versus general surgeons,[81] when resection is performed in a teaching institution,[82] or in high-volume hospitals,[82–85] even when case mix or comorbidity is taken into account. Mortality increases slightly with increasing age for lobectomy (2%, 5%, 6%, and 8% for ages below 60, 60–69, 70–79, and ≥80, respectively) but increases dramatically with age for pneumonectomy (7%, 16%, 28% for ages below 70, 70–79, and ≥80, respectively).[80]

Selection of appropriate patients for surgical resection is crucial in order to avoid excessive morbidity or mortality. Attention has been directed primarily toward assessment of pulmonary reserve. The pulmonary function test (PFT) used most commonly is spirometry, specifically the forced expiratory volume in 1 s (FEV_1). Additional tests include the diffusion capacity of lung for carbon monoxide (DLCO) and the maximal oxygen consumption during exercise (VO_{2max}).

Four concepts are crucial in appropriately applying the available data. First, a distinction must be made between a conventional resection (lobectomy or pneumonectomy via a thoracotomy) and a sublobar resection. When liberal use is made of sublobar resection, multiple studies have shown that the mortality is remarkably low (~5%), even in high-risk patients with limited pulmonary reserve.[86] Furthermore, the mortality of a lobectomy via video-assisted thoracic surgery (VATS) in high-risk patients has not been defined, although one might surmise it would be lower than following resection via thoracotomy.

The second crucial concept is that the values used for the assessment should be "normalized" to the individual patient and the planned conventional resection. The absolute value of the preoperative FEV_1 is of limited value; when it is expressed relative to what would be predicted for a normal person of the same gender, height, race, and age (% predicted), it is much more useful. Furthermore, it stands to reason that the preoperative value that is safe is different whether the patient will undergo a lobectomy, pneumonectomy, or segmentectomy. The size of the resection is taken into account by calculating the projected postoperative FEV_1 (ppo-FEV_1) as follows: ppo-FEV_1 % = Preoperative FEV_1 % × Number of lung segments remaining ÷ Total amount of lung segments (18 segments). Actual measured postoperative FEV_1 correlates remarkably well with the calculated ppo-FEV_1 in multiple studies.[86] A ppo-FEV_1 of 40% or higher carries a consistently low operative mortality (~5%) in multiple studies.[86] These calculations to normalize results to body size and extent of resection can be applied equally to other pulmonary function parameters.

The third crucial concept is that the major issue for patients with limited pulmonary reserve is the perioperative mortality and not long-term functional status. This may seem counterintuitive until one considers the dramatic decrease in PFTs immediately after pulmonary resection, which then gradually improve over many months. The patients who would have such little long-term function that they would be severely functionally limited can be expected to have such poor short-term pulmonary function that they are unlikely to survive the first few weeks. Furthermore, those patients that do have long-term functional limitations experience complications that appear to be due to random events (e.g., acute respiratory distress syndrome, ARDS) not predicted by preoperative variables.[87,88] Whether long-term functional capacity correlates with preoperative pulmonary reserve is unclear. Most studies have found that the majority of patients with limited pulmonary reserve who survive the short term have acceptable long-term survival and functional capacity.[89–92] However, a few studies have found that long-term functional impairment and survival were associated with preoperative limited pulmonary reserve.[61,93]

A fourth important concept in the evaluation of PFTs is that perioperative risk is not simply a binary acceptable/prohibitive issue, but the actual magnitude of risk should be weighed against the magnitude of benefit (chance of cure of cancer) for an individual patient. Widely cited PFT thresholds define levels *above* which patients generally do well but do not as clearly define the *magnitude* of risk for patients who fall below the threshold. Only limited data exist for such patients. The largest amount of data pertains to patients with a ppo-FEV_1 below 40%, in which 26% of 87 such patients died.[94–99] A ppo-DLCO below 50% (corrected for alveolar volume) carried a 24% mortality among 33 such patients,[94,95,100] and a mortality of 16% was observed among 94 patients with a VO_{2max} of less than 15 mL/kg min.[94–96,100–103] These mortality figures pertain to studies in which the majority of patients underwent conventional resection. Furthermore, it is important to note that the patients with a VO_{2max} of less than 15 mL/kg min who underwent surgery did not also have a low FEV_1 but were probably selected for surgery because their risk appeared to be low by other criteria. These data form the basis for the algorithm shown in Figure 71.3.

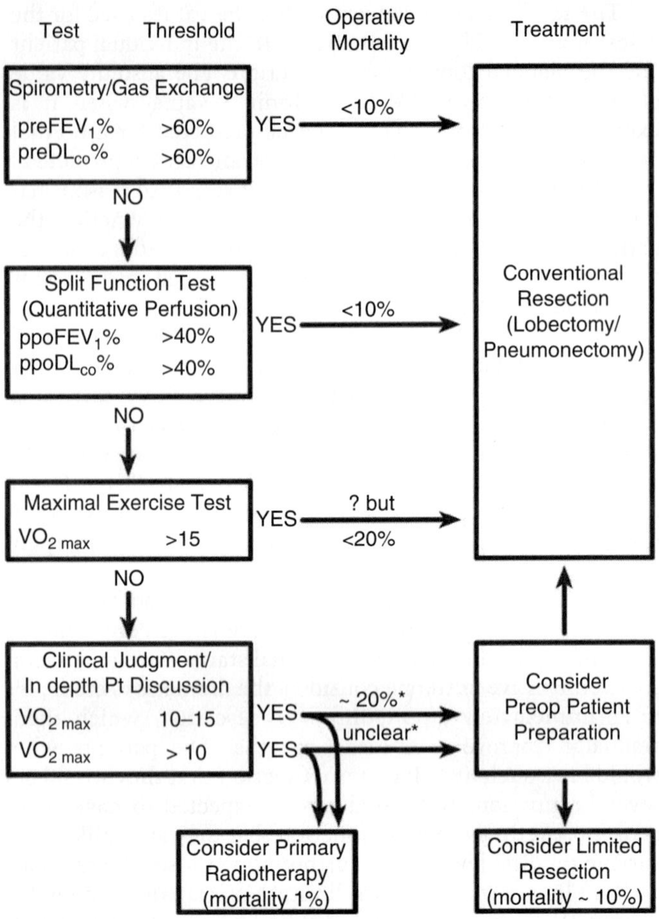

FIGURE 71.3. Suggested algorithm for evaluation of patients for pulmonary resection. *Operative mortality estimated from limited amounts of data. (From Martinolich and Rivera.[86])

Stages I and II

Surgery Alone

Surgery involving a lobectomy or pneumonectomy has been the mainstay of treatment for early-stage (stages I, II) NSCLC for the past 50 years. Survival by clinical (preoperative) stage is probably the clinically more relevant statistic for new patients and demonstrates 5-year survival rates of 51% and 30% for stages I and II, respectively (Table 71.4). Most reports have focused on the pathologic (postoperative) stage, with an average 5-year survival of 63% and 42% for stages I and II, respectively (Table 71.4). The results are fairly consistent, with variability most likely due to the accuracy of the stage classification, reflecting the extent of intraoperative nodal biopsy and evaluation. The standard of care calls for at least systematic sampling of mediastinal nodes (exploration and biopsy of at least one node per ipsilateral node station) as well as systematic investigation of resected intralobar nodes by the pathologist,[75] but this is not always done consistently. The survival statistics must be viewed with the knowledge that recurrence of the lung cancer accounts for only a little more than 50% of deaths for stage I tumors.[60] Thus, the disease-free survival after resection of lung cancer is approximately 80% and 60% for stages pI and pII, respectively.

Among stage I and II patients, survival is approximately 15% better with T1 tumors compared with T2 lesions. Analyses based on size alone of stage I NSCLC have generally found a continuum of worsening survival as tumor size increases,[104–107] with some exceptions.[108] There is little difference in survival based on histologic type, especially for stage I NSCLC, although the prognosis tends to be slightly better for squamous cancers as compared with adenocarcinoma.[60,70,109] Among stage I NSCLC, well-differentiated tumors appear to have a better prognosis than moderately or poorly differentiated tumors (by multivariate analysis) in most studies (5-year survival approximately 90% vs. 70% vs. 50%, respectively).[110–113] Nodal factors appear to have prognostic significance in stage II tumors. Survival is better for patients with involvement of a single N1 node versus multiple nodes[114–116] and with involvement of lobar or segmental nodes versus hilar N1 nodes in most[116–123] but not all studies,[115,124,125] whereas involvement by direct extension to nodes versus discontinuous spread does not appear to matter.[116,119,121,124] The prognostic value of molecular markers continues to be unclear and probably awaits the results of large-scale studies and gene array technology.[126]

TABLE 71.4. Survival of Patients with Stage I or II NSCLC Undergoing Resection.

5-year survival	*Subgroup*	*No. of pts (total)*	*No. of studies*	*Average (%)*	*Range (%)*
Clinical (preresection) stage					
I		1692	3	51	37–67
Ia		1686	5	70	61–77
Ib		1835	3	47	38–54
II		900	3	30	24–34
Pathologic (postresection) stage					
I		6818	16	63	43–75
T1N0		8953	17	71	54–82
T2N0		9628	17	55	38–68
II		2286	9	42	32–49
T1N1		2036	8	52	33–65
T2N1		3175	10	40	33–49
Histologic subtype					
pI	Squamous	4830	10	66	51–83
pI	Adenocarcinoma	4867	10	61	42–74
pII	Squamous	1418	6	46	41–53
pII	Adenocarcinoma	1154	6	30	18–40

Inclusion criteria: reported series from 1980 to 2004 with 100 or more patients (total) except for pathologic stage I (≤250 patients).[24,60,69,70,108,117,126,128]

Recurrence of lung cancer occurs in approximately 33% and 50% of patients with stages I and II NSCLC, respectively, after surgical resection.[60,70,116] The majority of recurrences (approximately 70%–75%) involve systemic sites.[60,70,127] There is controversy whether a radical mediastinal LND provides any therapeutic benefit.[78,128–130] Two randomized studies have found no differences in recurrence rates or survival in patients undergoing LND versus systematic lymph node sampling (in 115 patients with 2-cm or smaller stage pI NSCLC tumors and 182 cI–IIIa patients).[129,130] Another randomized study found a benefit to LND as compared with selective sampling, although this was potentially confounded by better staging after LND.[78] Finally, two retrospective studies have found conflicting results.[128,131] The results of the completed American College of Surgeons Oncology Group randomized trial of mediastinal node dissection (ACOSOG Z0030) are not yet available.

Sleeve resection is a viable alternative to a pneumonectomy for patients with tumors at or surrounding the lobar structures, although there is debate whether the type of resection affects survival.[132,133] The average survival is 58% for stage I tumors, 45% for stage II, and 33% for stage IIIa.[70] This is comparable to other resections, particularly given the fact that these series include very few T1 tumors. The average perioperative mortality is 3%.[70] A local recurrence is seen in only about 17% of cases.[70] A margin of at least 0.5 cm should be sought intraoperatively.[70] Sleeve resection appears reasonable whether this is due to bronchial involvement or due to peribronchial nodal involvement,[70] although a positive peribronchial nodal margin carries a worse prognosis than a positive bronchial margin.[134,135] Resection involving a sleeve of both the bronchus and the pulmonary artery can be accomplished with good outcomes.[136–138]

Role of Limited Resection

A *limited resection* is defined as removal of less than a lobe of the lung. It is important to distinguish between different types of limited resections and different clinical situations. A *segmentectomy* involves complete removal of an anatomic lung segment with isolation of the segmental bronchus, artery, and vein. An *open wedge resection* involves removal of a portion of lung, not respecting the segmental anatomic planes, through a thoracotomy. A *thoracoscopic wedge resection* is a nonanatomic removal of a portion of lung with the added limited ability to manipulate the lung and palpate the lesion that is associated with a thoracoscopic approach. In addition, it is important to distinguish between a limited resection carried out as an optional alternative in patients who would be able to tolerate a lobectomy and a limited resection carried out as a compromise in poor-risk patients.

The only prospective, randomized trial of lobectomy versus limited resection demonstrated better survival in the lobectomy group (5-year survival 73% vs. 56%; $P = .06$).[139,140] The recurrence-free survival was also significantly better in the lobectomy group ($P = .04$). This study involved a highly select group of 247 patients with T1N0 tumors who underwent careful segmental, lobar, hilar, and mediastinal lymph node staging and who were all fit enough to tolerate a lobectomy (see Fig. 71.4). The limited resection involved a formal segmentectomy in approximately two-thirds of the patients and a wedge with at least a 2-cm margin in the remainder.

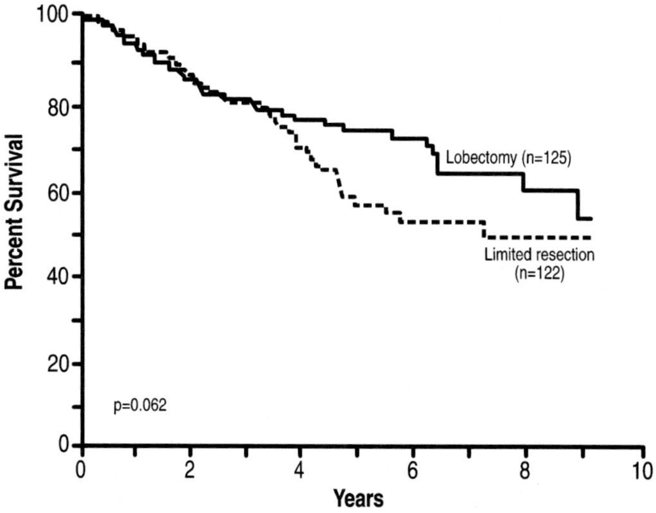

FIGURE 71.4. Survival of 247 T1N0 patients randomized to lobectomy or limited resection. $P = .062$, one-tailed log rank test. (From Rubinstein and Ginsberg.[140])

The rate of distant recurrences was the same in both groups, but the limited resection patients experienced a threefold higher rate of locoregional recurrence (5.4% vs. 1.9% per person per year, $P = .009$).[140]

Several nonrandomized studies have generally corroborated the findings of the randomized trial. Overall survival is generally worse,[104,141–144] although in some studies the difference was minimal.[112,145,146] A two- to fourfold higher local recurrence rate was seen in all five nonrandomized trials that evaluated recurrence patterns.[104,112,141,143,146]

The average 5-year survival is 65% for patients undergoing an optional limited resection (segmentectomy in almost all).[60] The average 5-year survival is 47% for patients undergoing limited resection as a compromise (open wedge resection in most), although there is a fair amount of variation among studies.[60] The reported rate of non-cancer-related deaths has varied from 0% to 50%, but at an average of 22%[139,143,144,146–148] it is similar to that of resected stage I patients in general.[60] Local recurrence is reported to occur in 15% (range 6%–24%) of all patients[104,139,143,146–150] and accounts for at least half of all recurrences in most studies,[104,139,143,146] with only two exceptions.[147,149] Of the patients who experience a local recurrence, consistently fewer than one-third are able to undergo a second resection.[112,141,146,150]

There are some special situations in which a limited resection may be justified. A wedge resection appears to be adequate in patients with a solitary focus of bronchioloalveolar cancer.[151] The difficulty, of course, is in reliably establishing this diagnosis prior to resection. Several authors have noted that lesions that have a ground glass or nonsolid appearance are more likely to be a BAC and be appropriate for limited resection.[18,152–155] It is important to note, however, that size is not an adequate criterion. Many studies have found that nodal metastases are present in 10%–20% of patients with small (<2 cm) T1N0 lesions.[152,156,157] This is applicable even to lesions found on a screening CT. Thus, while a wedge resection may be an appropriate way to establish a diagnosis, it is not an appropriate treatment for most patients with NSCLC, who should ideally undergo a lobectomy.[139,140]

Radiotherapy Alone

Radiotherapy (RT) is the most commonly chosen alternative to surgical resection for stage cI,II NSCLC. Pulmonary comorbidity is the reason for selecting RT in about 50%, cardiac reasons in 25%, and age and patient preferences in most of the remainder.[158] The average age is 70 years, but only about 17% have a performance status (PS) of 60 or lower.[158] Typically, doses of approximately 60 Gy have been given, and most centers have included irradiation of the mediastinum despite the clinical stage of I or II.[158] The overall 5-year survival is 15% on average, even in those studies involving only stage cI patients.[159–165] Because patients treated with RT are only clinically staged, their survival must be compared to clinically staged patients undergoing resection (50% and 30% for cI and cII, respectively). The 5-year survival is about 25% for cT1N0 tumors and 15% for cT2N0 tumors.[159,160,163,166–169] Cancer-specific survival is 25%, and cancer is the cause of death in approximately 75% of patients.[158] Freedom from local recurrence is achieved in about 50% of patients.[158] There are few data that higher doses of RT result in better local control or survival,[160–162,166,170] but there is only limited experience with substantially higher doses.[158] Hyperfractionated RT (69.6 Gy) may result in slightly better outcomes according to two studies.[167,171]

Surgery and Radiotherapy

Surgery and postoperative RT were evaluated in several randomized trials (see Table 71.5) These trials have generally included a mixture of stage I–IIIa patients, although some trials have focused specifically on stage III or stage I patients. Survival does not appear to be improved by the addition of RT. The only trial to show a significant difference found worse survival after RT,[172] with the rest showing no difference and no consistent trends. On the other hand, local control was better after postoperative RT in most studies, with the difference being statistically significant in a little less than half. Given that most recurrences after resection are distant, it is not surprising that the addition of a second local modality results in better local control without a survival benefit. However, RT can be harmful due to toxicity. A metaanalysis[173] of randomized trials of adjuvant RT published in 1998 found worse survival with the addition of RT, which occurred primarily in the stage I patients, in whom the recurrence rate and thus the potential benefit is quite low.

The available data regarding adjuvant RT have been criticized for not involving technological advances in RT equipment, although the studies have involved patients treated in the 1980s and 1990s. Better targeting of potential tumor-bearing tissues with three-dimensional (3D) conformal treatment planning is becoming more widely available, and higher doses of RT may be more effective. Furthermore, as systemic treatment improves, the impact of better local control may change. There is little interest in investigating adjuvant RT for stage I patients. There continues to be controversy regarding stage IIIa patients,[174] although subset analyses of randomized studies do not suggest a survival benefit in stage IIIa patients.[172,173,175,176]

Surgery and Adjuvant Chemotherapy

Treatment with surgery and adjuvant (postoperative) chemotherapy has become standard in stage II and resected stage IIIa NSCLC. This is based on data showing a 13% reduction in the rate of death. Translated to absolute survival, there is about a 4% improvement in 5-year survival with resection and adjuvant chemotherapy compared with surgery alone. This was clearly demonstrated ($P < .0001$) by a metaanalysis of randomized adjuvant chemotherapy trials (Fig. 71.5). Most of these trials used platin-based chemotherapy regimens. When the metaanalysis was conducted using only platin-based chemotherapy trials, the result is consistent, with a hazard ratio (HR) of 0.89 (95% CI 0.82–0.96, $P = .003$).[177] Further analysis did not reveal evidence of heterogeneity among the studies or evidence of publication bias.[177]

Since the metaanalysis mentioned in the previous paragraph was conducted, the results of three additional trials have been presented in abstracts. The study with the most dramatic difference (NCIC JBR10) involved 482 patients with stage Ib,II tumors.[178] A 31% reduction in the risk of death was noted ($P = .011$).[178] The largest study (Adjuvant Navelbine International Trialist Association, ANITA) involved 840 stage I–IIIa patients, half of whom were given adjuvant navalbine and cisplatin. Again, about a 30% reduction in the risk of death was found.[179] A third study involved 344 patients with stage Ib (T2N0) tumors only (Cancer and Leukemia Group B

TABLE 71.5.
Surgery and Adjuvant Radiotherapy.

Trial	*Year*	*Level of evidence*	*N*	*Design*	*Local recurrence*	*Overall survival*	*Comments*
Dautzenberg[172]	1999	I	728	Rand	(Lower)	Worse	
Stephens[175]	1996	I	308	Rand	(Lower)	(Better)	
Lung Cancer Study Group[309]	1986	I	210	Rand	Lower	No difference	Only squamous cell
Mayer[310]	1997	I	155	Rand	Lower	(Better)	
Van Houtte[311]	1980	I	175	Rand	Lower	(Worse)	All N0, 8% SCLC
Lafitte[312]	1996	I	132	Rand	No difference	(Worse)	Only T2N0
Debevec[313]	1996	I	74	Rand	(Higher)	(Better)	Only N2

Rand, randomized; SCLC, small cell lung cancer.
Results in parentheses indicate trends that are not statistically significant.

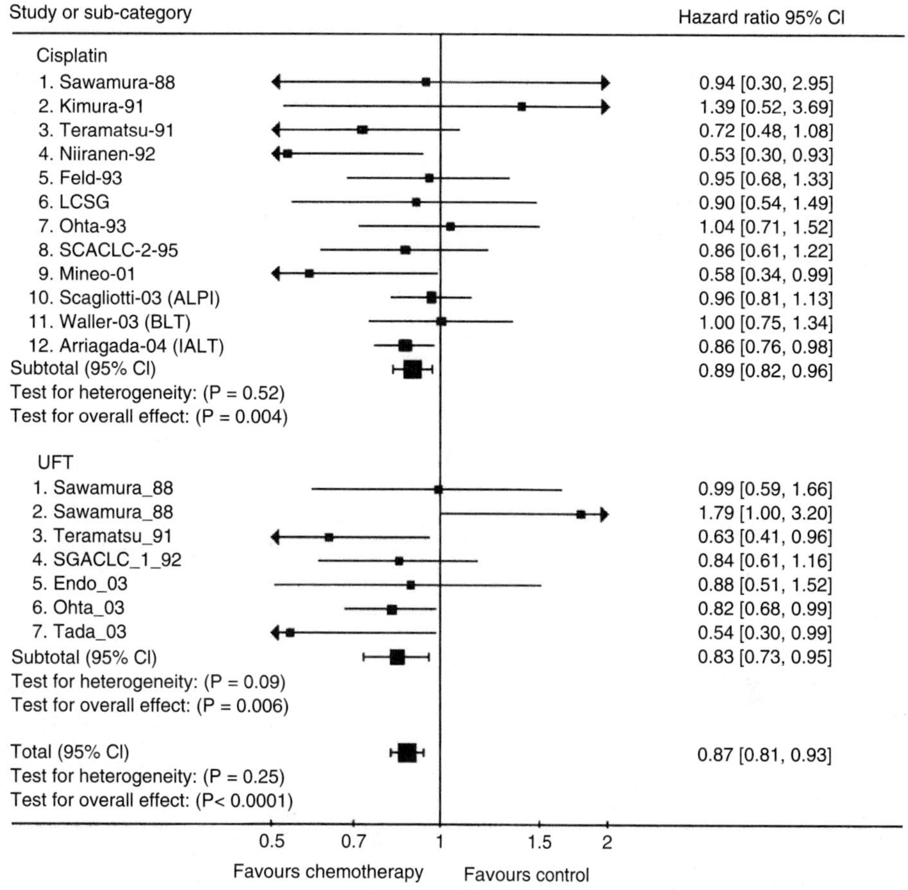

FIGURE 71.5. Metaanalysis of postoperative chemotherapy for NSCLC. The horizontal axis is based on a log scale for hazard ratio (HR). The black boxes and lines correspond to HR estimates and 95% CI for individual studies. (From Sedrakyan et al.[177])

[CALGB] 9633).[180] A preliminary report of this trial suggested a 38% reduction in the risk of death was found, with an absolute survival increase of 12% ($P < .028$).[180] However, more mature results found only better disease-free survival (HR 0.74, $P = .03$) and a nonsignificant trend in overall survival with chemotherapy (HR 0.8, $P = .1$).[181]

Therefore, although these additional studies further strengthen the conclusion that adjuvant chemotherapy results in improved survival, it is unclear whether this is true for patients with stage I disease. There is general agreement that adjuvant chemotherapy is not indicated in patients with stage Ia tumors and should not be given routinely in patients with stage Ib disease.[181] A subset analysis of the CALGB trial suggested that patients with stage Ib tumors that are larger than 4 cm have a significant benefit to adjuvant chemotherapy,[49] but it must be acknowledged that this is based on an unplanned subset analysis.

Individual studies of adjuvant platin-based chemotherapy are shown in Table 71.6. Many of the individual studies have only demonstrated a nonsignificant trend to improved survival. However, it must be noted that a study with an 80% power of detecting a 5% improvement in survival for stage I,II NSCLC would have to involve approximately 3,000 randomized patients.[176] Thus, all of the trials conducted to date have been underpowered, and it is not surprising that it takes a metaanalysis to demonstrate the actual effect of adjuvant chemotherapy.

The relatively small improvement in absolute survival with adjuvant platin-based chemotherapy is consistent with results in other cancer types. Adjuvant chemotherapy results in a 6% survival benefit in breast cancer ($P = .00001$ by metaanalysis)[182] and a 5% benefit in colon cancer.[183]

Toxicity associated with adjuvant platin-based chemotherapy has been relatively low. The incidence of specific toxicities among these studies is low: 14% grade 4 neutropenia, 2% grade 4 thrombocytopenia, 2% grade 3 or higher nephrotoxicity, and 10% grade 3 or higher nausea and vomiting.[184] The mortality due to adjuvant chemotherapy was 0.6% in 10 trials involving 2,559 patients.[184]

In Japan, the approach to adjuvant chemotherapy has involved prolonged daily administration (usually at least 2 years) of an oral agent, UFT (uracil/tegafur), in many trials. A metaanalysis of these results also demonstrated a survival benefit (HR 0.83, CI 0.73–0.95, $P = .006$; Fig. 71.5).[177] The results of individual trials involving this agent are shown in Table 71.7. Most of these studies have demonstrated either improved survival or a trend to improved survival. The toxicity associated with this approach has been low: 0.7% grade 3 or higher nausea and vomiting, 0.2% grade 3 or higher diarrhea, 0.2% grade 3 or higher hepatic toxicity.[184]

The oral agent UFT is available only in Asia, and trials involving this drug are limited to Japan. Most of these patients had stage I adenocarcinoma, and survival rates on the observation-only arms were notably higher than reported in Western populations. The approach of prolonged oral administration is a different strategy from the short course of cytotoxic chemotherapy administered at maximally tolerated doses than is practiced in the United States. Furthermore, the objective response rate to UFT in patients with advanced stage NSCLC is only 6%.[185] These points leave questions about the reason

TABLE 71.6.
Surgery and Platin-Based Chemotherapy.

Trial	*Year*	*Level of evidence*	*N*	*Design*	*Median F/U (mo)*	*Chemo mort (%)*	*Overall survival*	*Comments*
Arriagada[314+]	2004	I	1867	Rand	56	0.8	Better	RT given to both arms
Scagliotti[315+]	2003	I	1209	Rand	65	—	No diff	
Douillard[179+]	2004	I	840	Rand	>70	1	Better	RT given to both arms
Winton[178+]	2004	I	482	Rand	—	0.8	Better	
Strauss[180−]	2004	I	344	Rand	34	0	Better	
Waller[316+]	2003	I	381	Rand	35	1.6	No diff	
Keller[317+]	1999	I	358	Rand	63	0.4	No diff	RT given to both arms
Dautzenberg[318+]	1995	I	267	Rand	—	—	(Better)	RT given to both arms
Imaizumi[319−]	1995	I	309	Rand	—	0	(Better)	Significant difference when corrected for pN imbalance
Feld[320−]	1993	I	269	Rand	46	0.7	No diff	
Wada[321−]	1999	I	225	Rand	—	0	(Better)	
Wada[322−]	1996	I	207	Rand	—	0	(Better)	
Ohta[323+]	1993	I	181	Rand	31	0	(Better)	
Lad[324+]	1988	I	164	Rand	18	0	(Better)	RT given to both arms
Wolf[325+]	2001	I	150	Rand	—	—	No diff	RT given to both arms
Holmes[326,327+]	1993	I	130	Rand	—	0	(Better)	
Tada[328+]	2004	I	119	Rand	—	0	No diff	
Niiranen[329−]	1992	I	110	Rand	—	—	Better	
Imaizumi[330−]	2003	I	100	Rand	78	—	Better	
Tada[331+]	2002	I	95	Rand	—	—	No diff	
Ichinose[332−]	1991	I	86	Rand	53	0	No diff	
Pisters[333+]	1994	I	72	Rand	—	2.7	(Worse)	RT given to both arms
Xu[334+]	2000	I	70	Rand	—	0	(Better)	
Kimura[335+]	1996	I	69	Rand	—	—	Better	
Mineo[336−]	2001	I	66	Rand	62	0	Better	
Park[337+]	1999	I	57	Rand	42	0	(Better)	RT only in those not receiving chemotherapy

Chemo mort, chemotherapy-related mortality; diff, difference; F/U, follow-up; Rand, randomized; RT, radiotherapy; SCLC, small cell lung cancer.
+Primarily node-positive (N1,2) patients.
−Primarily node-negative patients.

TABLE 71.7.
Surgery and UFT-Based Chemotherapy.

Trial	*Year*	*Level of evidence*	*N*	*Design*	*Median F/U (mo)*	*Chemo mort (%)*	*Overall survival*	*Comments*
Kato[338−]	2004	I	979	Rand	73		Better	
Nakagawa[339−]	2005	I	331	Rand	76	0	(Better)	
Endo[340−]	2003	I	221	Rand	64	0	(Better)	
Wada[322−]	1996	I	208	Rand	—	0	Better	
Imaizumi[330−]	2003	I	100	Rand	78	—	No diff	For UFT-only group; significantly better for CVUft.

Chemo mort, chemotherapy-related mortality; CVUft, cisplatin, vindesine, UFT; F/U, follow-up; UFT, uracil/tegafur; diff, difference; Rand, randomized.
−Primarily node-negative patients.

for the apparent benefit of UFT and the applicability of UFT to populations outside Asia or to patients with resected stage II or IIIa disease.

Preoperative Chemotherapy Followed by Surgery

Few of the studies of induction chemotherapy have included many patients who had stage I or II NSCLC. A prospective phase II study of 94 patients with stage Ib, IIa,b and T3N1 disease, known as the Bimodality Lung Oncology Team (BLOT) trial,[186] involved preoperative and postoperative treatment with carboplatin and paclitaxel. The radiographic response rate to two cycles of induction chemotherapy was 56%, disease progression was seen in 3%, and 86% of all patients underwent a complete resection. The planned induction therapy could be given in 96% of the patients, whereas only 64% of those eligible for postoperative chemotherapy received the planned treatment. The 5-year survival rate was 46%. The encouraging results of the BLOT trial led to a randomized clinical trial (Southwest Oncology Group [SWOG] 9900) comparing induction therapy with paclitaxel and carboplatin versus surgery alone. This trial was closed prematurely after a survival benefit was reported in adjuvant chemotherapy trials. Preliminary progression-free and overall survival of the 354 patients enrolled (median follow-up 28 months) have shown trends toward improvement but have not reached statistical significance.[187]

A French trial randomized 355 stage Ib–IIIa patients (53% were stage I or II) to surgery alone versus induction chemotherapy and surgery (two cycles of mitomycin, ifosfamide, and cisplatin).[188] Postoperatively, two additional cycles of chemotherapy were given to responding patients (as well as RT for stage IIIa patients). A trend toward improved survival with induction chemotherapy was seen for the entire group (median survival, 36 vs. 26 months; $P = .09$). This study had sufficient power to reliably detect only an increase of more than 15% in median survival. Furthermore, a slight maldistribution of N2 patients favoring the surgery-alone arm occurred (N2 patients, 33% for surgery vs. 40% for induction therapy). When corrected for stage using multivariate analysis, induction chemotherapy was found to be a statistically significant independent factor associated with better survival. Although better survival with induction therapy was seen in both the stage Ib-II and IIIa subgroups, subset analysis suggested that the early-stage patients (Ib-II) experienced a greater survival benefit (Fig. 71.6).

Induction chemotherapy for early-stage NSCLC remains an investigational approach. Four ongoing European randomized trials (LU22, CHEST, CLINCH, NATCH) continue to evaluate the role of preoperative chemotherapy.

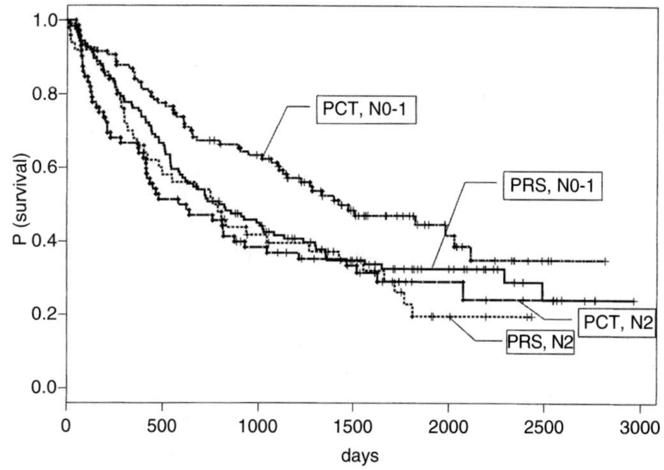

FIGURE 71.6. Overall survival of patients with stage Ib, IIa,b, and IIIa non-small cell lung cancer, randomized to induction chemotherapy and surgery versus surgery alone. PCT, preoperative chemotherapy; PRS, primary surgery. (From Pisters et al.[187])

Stage III

Definition of Subgroups

Stage III NSCLC constitute a heterogeneous group, which makes interpretation of data across studies difficult. The heterogeneity stems primarily from differences in the extent of staging and the resultant accuracy of the designation as stage III. It is extensively demonstrated that about 30% of patients with stage III NSCLC harbor distant metastases even though they have no signs or symptoms suggestive of this (see previous evaluation section). Thus, imaging that demonstrates the absence of distant metastases is imperative. The accuracy of mediastinal nodal staging is an equally large source of confusion (see previous evaluation section). Radiographic staging by CT is notoriously inaccurate when discrete nodal enlargement is seen. Even mediastinal staging by PET carries a 15% FP rate. In these situations, classification of patients as stage III without a corroborative biopsy is often inaccurate. Mediastinal staging by radiographic imaging alone is accepted as accurate only when there is diffuse tumor infiltration and encasement of the mediastinum (discrete nodes cannot be discerned). The accuracy of the staging must be kept in mind when interpreting published reports.

However, stage III NSCLC remain a heterogeneous group even if thorough staging has been carried out. The vast majority of patients have involvement of ipsilateral (N2, IIIa) or contralateral (N3, IIIb) mediastinal nodes. However, stage III also includes patients without mediastinal node involvement, most notably those with direct involvement of mediastinal structures such as the mainstem bronchi, carina, or SVC (T4N0,1), and Pancoast tumors (T3,4N0,1) and those with involvement of less-crucial mediastinal or chest wall structures (pericardium, ribs) with N1 involvement (T3N1). Surgery has a much greater role in the treatment of these patients than in those with N2,3 nodal involvement, and these subgroups are discussed in greater detail in the following section. Stage III NSCLC also includes (by strict definition) some patients who are generally viewed as having a disease course more similar to patients with stage IV disease, namely, those with supraclavicular node involvement or a malignant pleural effusion. These patients are usually grouped with stage IV patients regarding treatment and outcomes despite the stage classification.

Even among stage III patients with mediastinal nodal involvement, there is controversy about differences related to the extent of involvement. Retrospective data define differences in survival after surgical resection of patients with single nodal station versus multiple nodal station involvement, extracapsular versus intranodal involvement.[189] However, these characteristics cannot be used easily to select patients because they are not available until after a resection. Furthermore, the survival data for these cohorts exclude the substantial number of patients who were unable to be completely resected. Patients who are staged preoperatively as N0,1 but are found after resection to have N2 involvement ("incidental" N2) have a 5-year survival of 14%–31%.[190–194] Again, while this defines a special subgroup of patients, the criteria cannot be used to select patients for surgical therapy. Patient cohorts who are identified as having N2 disease preoperatively uniformly have poor survival (9%–15%) after resection, even when carefully selected,[195–197] making it fairly clear that primary surgical therapy for preoperatively defined N2 disease is not justified.

Treatment of Specific Subgroups

T4N0,1

Most patients with involvement of T4 structures have mediastinal node involvement as well. These patients should be treated with chemoradiotherapy (ChRT), as is generally recommended for patients with stage IIIb NSCLC.[198] However, very selected patients with T4 involvement but without mediastinal node involvement can be viewed as candidates for surgery.[199] Patients should be selected carefully and should undergo imaging for potential distant metastases even if asymptomatic for distant disease.[199] Furthermore, a mediastinoscopy should be performed even if the mediastinal nodes appear normal in patients with T4 tumors being considered for a surgical approach.[199] This argument is based on the fact that CT evaluation of the mediastinum in central tumors has a high FN rate and the lack of data defining the reliability of PET for this cohort.[35]

Although many reports have demonstrated the technical feasibility of resection of T4 structures, fewer series have provided long-term survival data (Table 71.8). The largest experience of resection for T4 involvement involves carinal resections, usually together with a right pneumonectomy (722 patients in whom long-term survival data was reported). A moderate experience is available with SVC (182 patients) or left atrial involvement (104 patients). The fact that so few patients have been reported with long-term survival statistics underscores the fact that patients who are candidates for a surgical approach are extremely rare and highly selected. In a fairly large series from Japan involving an aggressive approach to T4 tumors, approximately one-third of patients were able to undergo complete (R_0) resection, one-third a microscopically incomplete resection (R_1), and one-third a grossly incomplete (R_2) resection (5-year survival 22%, 18%, and 0%, respectively).[200]

The data regarding the outcome after resection in patients with carinal involvement show an average 5-year survival of 28%. However, the survival comes at a price of an average operative mortality of 17% (range 7%–29%). It should be noted, however, that the survival statistics have included all operative deaths as well. The fact that the best reported 5-year survival (44%) comes from the largest series,[201] which also reported an operative mortality of only 7%, can be interpreted to suggest that such resections should only be undertaken in experienced centers. In general, the survival of patients with involvement of other T4 structures has been similar to that reported for patients with carinal involvement (Table 71.8).

Preoperative chemotherapy or ChRT in patients with T4 tumors has been reported in several trials. A 5-year survival of 20% was reported among all patients in the largest trial (57 patients, 62% of whom underwent complete resection).[202] By comparison, 5-year survival results for ChRT without surgery in patients with stage IIIa,b tumors have been approximately 9% and 14% in large randomized trials involving sequential or concurrent ChRT trials, respectively.[203] However, these series have included both stage IIIa and IIIb patients and have not reported data separately or reported any data specifically in patients with T4N0,1 tumors. A retrospective analysis of the SWOG experience suggested that patients with T4N0,1M0 tumors benefited from preoperative ChRT and surgery compared to ChRT alone (2-year survival of 64% vs. 33%, respectively).[204]

Pancoast

A Pancoast tumor is a lung cancer arising in the apex of the lung that involves structures of the apical chest wall, whether or not the classic Pancoast syndrome is present (pain radiating down the arm due to involvement of the lower roots of the brachial plexus and Horner's syndrome due to involvement of the stellate ganglion).[205] Tumors arising at or below the level of the second rib should not be included. The invasion of apical chest structures (brachial plexus, stellate ganglion,

TABLE 71.8.
Results of Resection of Patients with T4 Involvement from NSCLC.

				5-year survival (%)		
Structure	*No. of studies*	*No. of patients*	*Hospital mortality*	*Average*	*Highest*	*Lowest*
Any[200]	1	101	13	13	23 (R_0)	0 (R_2)
Carina[341–348,201,349–351]	12	722	17	28	44	13
Superior vena cava[342,352–360]	6	182	6	24	31	15
Left atrium[200,352,357–359]	6	104	7	9	22	0
Vertebral bodies[361–363]	3	48	0	42	—	—
Aorta[200,352,364,365]	3	60	13	27	37	17
Esophagus[357]	1	7	—	14	—	—
Main pulmonary artery[200]	1	7	—	0	—	—

R_0, complete resection; R_2, incomplete resection with gross residual disease. Inclusion criteria: studies reporting actuarial 5-year survival after resection of T4 tumors.

Inclusion criteria: studies reporting actuarial 5-year survival after resection of T4 tumors.

subclavian vessels, ribs, vertebral bodies) creates characteristic technical issues that make treatment of this entity difficult.[205] These patients should be seen in an experienced center for consideration of resection and undergo imaging for extrathoracic metastases and mediastinoscopy.[199] An MRI and cervical ultrasound are useful to define the extent of tumor involvement.[206]

Preoperative concurrent chemotherapy and radiation is the current standard approach.[199,205] This is based on phase II data that consistently demonstrated a higher rate of complete resection, better local control, and better survival than the traditional approach of preoperative radiation.[205,207,208] Typically, the approach consists of two cycles of cisplatin and etoposide and 45 Gy of RT. Surgical resection is accomplished through one of several anterior approaches or the traditional high-posterior approach.[205] The anterior approaches offer better ability to perform a complete resection of tumors that are invading structures such as the subclavian vessels, vertebral bodies, or those of the thoracic inlet.[205] Adequate surgical experience is important to avoid an incomplete resection, which offers no benefit.[205,209] The resection should consist of an en bloc lobectomy and chest wall resection because a simple wedge resection of the lung is associated with worse survival.[199,210] Extensive resections involving the vertebral bodies or neural foramina can be carried out with reasonable 5-year survival rates (20%) in highly specialized centers.[205]

Incidental N2

About 15% of patients who are thought to have stage I or II NSCLC are found after resection to have unanticipated N2 node involvement despite a thorough evaluation of the mediastinum preoperatively. This is known as *incidental N2* involvement. Usually, this involves a small focus of malignant involvement in normal-size lymph nodes. The average 5-year survival of such patients after resection is 23% (range 14%–31%) in multiple series.[190–194] This provides reasonable justification for proceeding with resection if N2 disease is discovered intraoperatively despite a thorough preoperative mediastinal evaluation. Many of the patients in these series had undergone mediastinoscopy. Postoperative RT was given in about half of these series, although the data demonstrated only improved local control but no difference in survival. No data specifically proved the value of adjuvant chemotherapy for incidental N2 patients, but this treatment can be generally recommended for resected patients with a significant chance of recurrence (see section on surgery and adjuvant chemotherapy).

These data cannot be used to justify avoidance of mediastinal node biopsy in patients with a single enlarged mediastinal lymph node. A few series have reported results of resection of highly selected patients in whom N2 disease was found before resection. These were generally patients with small foci of cancer in a single nodal station. Despite being highly selected, the overall 5-year survival is only 10%–15%.[190,196,197] Thus, there appears to be a difference between preoperatively identified "minimal N2" and patients with incidental N2 involvement. The survival is better when subgroups of patients are culled out retrospectively, but this cannot be used to justify resection in preoperatively identified N2 patients because these subgroups cannot be identified preoperatively. Therefore, patients should undergo thorough evaluation and should not undergo surgery as the primary therapy if N2 disease is suspected or found. On the other hand, true incidental N2 involvement discovered intraoperatively or postoperatively carries a reasonable expectation of survival. The conventional wisdom dictated from the aforementioned adjuvant studies at this time is for these patients to receive postoperative chemotherapy.

Stage III N2,3

Approximately 40% of patients with NSCLC have N2,3 node involvement, which is generally readily apparent on CT and can be easily confirmed by appropriate staging tests. For these patients, treatment options consist primarily of either traditional ChRT or a more aggressive approach with ChRT combined with surgery or with more aggressive ChRT alone. The data for each of these approaches are discussed in the following sections.

Traditional Chemoradiotherapy

The role of combined-modality therapy using ChRT in unresectable stage IIIa,b was initially defined in a number of phase III trials evaluating both sequential (typically chemotherapy followed by RT) and concurrent approaches (Table 71.9). One of the early landmark trials randomized 155 stage IIIA/B NSCLC patients to either standard RT (60 Gy) or a brief course of induction chemotherapy with cisplatin and vinblastine followed by the same course of RT.[211] The median and long-term survival were significantly increased for the combined-modality arm (median survival 14 vs. 10 months; 5-year survival 17% vs. 6%; $P = .012$). This observation was confirmed in a number of subsequent randomized trials (Table 71.9). This survival benefit was further supported by two metaanalyses.[212,213]

As noted, both sequential and concurrent strategies have improved survival in randomized phase III trials. Table 71.10 briefly summarizes the randomized trials that have directly compared the sequential versus concurrent approach in unresectable stage III NSCLC. The two largest trials were performed by the West Japan Group[214] and the Radiation Therapy Oncology Group (RTOG)[215] and yielded identical results in favor of the concurrent approach. It should be noted that although the concurrent approach yields improved survival rates, there is an increased risk of severe toxicity, particularly esophagitis and myelosuppression.

Although concurrent ChRT has been largely accepted as the standard approach to patients with unresectable stage III disease, there still exists much controversy regarding the optimal concurrent regimen. Commonly used chemotherapy regimens in the United States include both systemic dose chemotherapy, as utilized by the SWOG, and low dose, primarily radiosensitizing chemotherapy. Phase III trials comparing these approaches are needed. Another question being addressed by ongoing randomized trials is if additional chemotherapy is beneficial, either before the concurrent ChRT (CALGB 39801) or afterward (SWOG 0023, Hoosier Oncology Group). The answer may be different for regimens using standard versus low doses of concurrent chemotherapy.

Induction Therapy and Surgery

Many prospective phase II studies conducted throughout the last 20 years involved induction chemotherapy or ChRT fol-

TABLE 71.9.
Results of Traditional Chemoradiotherapy for Stage III NSCLC.

Trial	*Year*	*Level of evidence*	*N*	*Design*	*Median follow-up (months)*	*Local control*	*Overall survival*
Sequential chemoradiotherapy versus radiotherapy alone							
Sause[237,366]	1995, 2000	I	450	Random	60 (min)	—	Better
Cullen[367]	1999	I	446	Random	31	—	(Better)[a]
LeChevalier[368,369]	1991, 1992	I	353	Random	61 (mean)	(Better)[a]	Better
Brodin[402]	1996	I	327	Random	>60 (act)	(Better)[a]	No improvement
Mattson[370b]	1988	I	238	Random	—	No improvement	No improvement
Dillman[211]	1996	I	155	Random	>74	Better	Better
Kim[371]	2002		89	Random	—	—	(Better)[a]
Gregor[372]	1993	I	72	Random	—	—	No improvement
Planting[373]	1996	I	70	Random	—	—	No improvement
Crino[374]	1993	I	61	Random	72 (act)	No improvement	(Better)[a]
VanHoutte[375]	1988	I	59	Random	—		No improvement
Concurrent chemoradiotherapy versus radiotherapy alone							
Schaake-Koning[376]	1992	I	331	Random	22 (min)	Better	Better
Ansari[377,378]	1991, 1995	I	215	Random	52m	No improvement	No improvement
Cakir[379]	2004	I	176	Random	36 (min)	Better	Better
Trovo[380]	1992	I	167	Random	6 (min)	(Better)[a]	No improvement
Groen[381c]	2004	I	160	Random	—	No improvement	No improvement
Jeremic[382c,d]	1996	I	131	Random	—	Better	Better
Soresi[383]	1988	I	95	Random	12	(Better)[a]	(Better)[a]

act, actuarial follow-up; mean, mean follow-up; min, minimum follow-up.
[a]Nonsignificant trend toward improvement with chemotherapy.
[b]Includes stages I,II (defined as inoperable) and III.
[c]Carboplatin based.
[d]Hyperfractionated radiotherapy used in both arms.

lowed by surgical resection. These trials typically involved patients with bulky N2,3 node involvement and who had pathologic confirmation of N2,3 node involvement.[216] Only a few trials included some patients with T3N0 tumors or did not require invasive mediastinal staging. Approximately half of the trials were restricted to patients with IIIa tumors, but in the rest approximately half of the patients had stage IIIb tumors (due to either N3 or T4 involvement).[216] The average patient age of 57 years in these studies was somewhat younger than for most patients with NSCLC.[216]

The phase II studies clearly demonstrated that induction therapy and resection were feasible. The average treatment-related mortality was about 7%, with an induction-related mortality of about 3% (of all patients).[216] There was no clear difference in induction mortality whether chemotherapy was given alone or concurrently with RT.[216] The subsequent surgical mortality averaged about 6% (of patients undergoing surgery).[216] For comparison, the average surgical mortality for lobectomy is 3%, but it is 9% for a pneumonectomy and 12% for an extended resection.[80] Many of the patients undergoing

TABLE 71.10.
Randomized Trial of Sequential Versus Concurrent Chemoradiotherapy for Stage III NSCLC.

Trial	*Year*	*Level of evidence*	*N*	*Design*	*Median follow-up (yr)*	*PFS concurrent: Sequential*	*MS concurrent: Sequential*
Curran[215]	2003	I	595	Random	4[a]	—	Better
Furuse[214]	1999	I	314	Random	5	No difference	Better
Fournel[384]	2005	I	205	Random	4.8	(Better)[b]	(Better)[b]
Belani[385]	2005	II[c]	183	Random	3.3	No difference	(Better)[b]
Zatloukal[386]	2004	II[c]	102	Random	3.25	Better	Better

MS, median survival; PFS, progression-free survival.
[a]Minimum follow-up 4 years with maximum potential follow-up of 6 years.
[b]Nonsignificant ($P > .05$) trend to improvement.
[c]Randomized phase II trials.

resection for stage IIIa,b NSCLC underwent pneumonectomy or extended resection. Several other studies have suggested that surgical mortality was not significantly altered by induction therapy,[188,217–223] with one exception.[224]

Induction therapy results in a radiographic response in approximately two-thirds of patients.[216] Approximately 7% of patients have evidence of disease progression during the induction therapy.[216] Approximately 50%–60% of all patients are able to be completely resected. Furthermore, a pathologic complete response (pCR) is seen in approximately 16% of operated patients, and absence of any residual tumor in mediastinal lymph nodes is seen in nearly 50% of operated patients following induction therapy.[216] There was no clear difference in any of these rates whether induction chemotherapy or ChRT was given. Furthermore, no substantial difference was demonstrated in an interim report of a randomized study of induction chemotherapy and postoperative RT versus induction ChRT (concurrent hyperfractionated RT).[225]

Survival in the phase II studies has been encouraging, with an average 5-year survival rate of about 25% of all patients intended to be treated.[216] By comparison, the survival rate for traditional ChRT alone for patients with IIIa,b tumors is approximately 15%.[203] However, a real comparison is only possible in a randomized study due to potential differences in patient selection for phase II studies.

One randomized study has been reported comparing induction therapy and surgery versus traditional ChRT.[226] The induction therapy consisted of two cycles of cisplatin and etoposide concurrent with 45 Gy of RT prior to resection, while the ChRT consisted of two cycles of cisplatin and etoposide concurrent with 61 Gy of RT, with consolidation therapy of another two cycles of cisplatin and etoposide given to both groups.[226] A total of 429 pathologically confirmed IIIa (N2) patients were enrolled. The median survival and the 3-year overall survival were the same, as shown in Figure 71.7 (Median survival 22 vs. 22 months, 3-year survival 38% vs. 33% in the induction therapy and surgery arm vs. the ChRT arm, respectively). There was also no difference in the patterns of failure.[226] Progression-free survival, however, was superior for the surgical arm (median 14 vs. 12 months, 3-year survival 29% vs. 19%, respectively; $P = .02$). This is explained by the fact that fewer patients in the surgical arm experienced

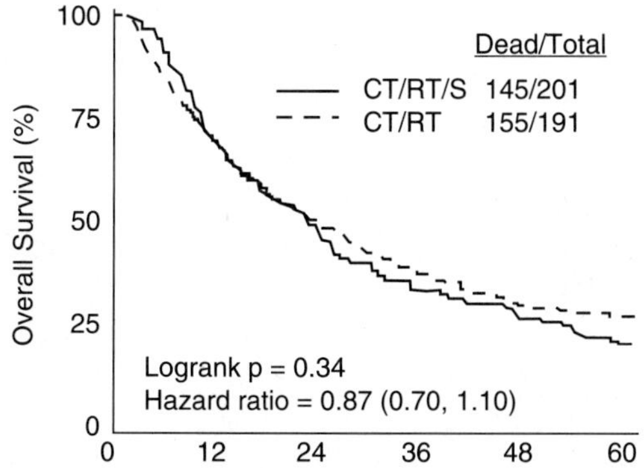

FIGURE 71.7. Overall survival of patients with stage IIIa non-small cell lung cancer by treatment arm in the INT 0139 study. CT, chemotherapy; RT, radiotherapy. (From West and Albain.[226])

death or recurrence from lung cancer. This benefit was offset by the higher treatment-related mortality (7% vs. 2%) in the surgical arm.

Thus, induction therapy and surgery cannot be recommended as the standard approach, although it is a reasonable alternative to traditional ChRT alone. It is possible that a benefit to surgical resection can be realized in patients and centers that are more carefully selected to minimize the perioperative mortality. However, the other alternative approach of more aggressive ChRT for stage III patients should also be considered.

Aggressive RT with or Without Chemotherapy

Efforts to improve on the results over traditional ChRT have also involved not only trimodality treatment but also more aggressive RT, mostly in combination with chemotherapy. The traditional RT dose of 60 Gy dates to the 1970s[227,228] and has been consistently found to result in poor local control in these bulky stage III tumors.[228–230] A reluctance to escalate the RT above 60 Gy stemmed in part from a fear of increasing toxicity. Modern RT techniques have resulted in a number of factors that improve the ratio of benefit to toxicity. Higher energy radiation sources create beams that penetrate deeper. The advent of 3D treatment planning has allowed exploration of dose escalation in stage I–III NSCLC. The 3D treatment planning allows for enhanced tumor targeting using CT-based imaging as well as limitation of excessive dose to normal tissues, thereby reducing toxicity.[231,232]

One of the first trials showing benefit to more intense RT evaluated the approach of continuous hyperfractionated accelerated RT (CHART).[233,234] This approach gives multiple smaller fractions daily, achieving the intended dose in an accelerated fashion. In this phase III trial, 563 patients were randomized to the standard arm of 60 Gy over 6 weeks or CHART at a dose of 1.5 Gy three times a day to a total dose of 54 Gy delivered over 12 consecutive days. This trial included not only stage III disease but also approximately 40% inoperable stage I/II patients, and the vast majority of patients had squamous cell histology. No chemotherapy was employed. There was a significant survival advantage in favor of the CHART-treated patients, with a 2-year survival rate of 29% versus 20% for the standard treatment ($P = .004$).[233,234] There was also a locoregional advantage as well as a reduction in the rate of distant metastases in the CHART-treated patients. A confirmatory trial was attempted in the United States that added induction chemotherapy prior to a randomization between conventional RT versus hyperfractionated accelerated RT.[235] This trial was closed early due to poor accrual (141 patients), but the survival experience mirrored that of the original CHART trial. Other trials have been reported evaluating hyperfractionated approaches and have been negative.[236,237] This may be related to the differences in RT strategies employed.

Several investigators have evaluated the feasibility of more aggressive RT in combination with chemotherapy in phase I and II trials. Two key concepts underlie these more aggressive RT approaches: the use of 3D planning and limiting the overall size of the RT volume. A series of phase I and II studies at the University of North Carolina and affiliated institutions explored dose escalation of RT to 74 Gy concurrent with chemotherapy[238] and to 90 Gy sequentially after induction chemotherapy.[239] These doses of RT (74 and 90 Gy) were found to be feasible with concurrent and sequential chemotherapy. The major acute toxicity was esophagitis, with grade 3 and higher rates of 8% at 74 Gy and 16% at 90 Gy. Late toxicity was due primarily to bronchial issues, which appeared to be significant with higher doses and longer survival.[240] Survival results (nonrandomized comparisons) have been promising. Other centers have explored similar approaches with similar results.[241–243] However, when this approach was tried in a broader context of CALGB institutions, it became clear that there was a learning curve.[244] Although these phase I/II trials establish the feasibility of delivering higher thoracic RT (TRT) doses, the affect on local control and overall survival await phase III trials.

Targeted therapies such as erlotinib (anti-epidermal growth factor receptor, EGFR); cetuximab (anti-EGFR); and bevacizumab (anti-vascular endothelial growth factor, VEGF) have also been shown to have radiosensitizing properties[245] and may, in combination with TRT, be a strategy to enhance local control and perhaps survival. Other radiotherapeutic techniques such as intensity-modulated RT, respiratory gating, and image-guided RT are being explored.

TABLE 71.11. Definition of Performance Status Scales.

Zubrod scale	*Karnofsky scale*	
0 Asymptomatic	100	Asymptomatic
1 Symptomatic, but ambulatory (able to work)	90	Normal activity, minor symptoms
	80	Normal activity, some symptoms
2 In bed < 50% of day (unable to work, but able to live at home with some assistance)	70	Unable to work, care for self
	60	Occasional assistance with needs
3 In bed > 50% of day (unable to care for self)	50	Considerable assistance
	40	Disabled, full assistance needed
4 Bedridden	30	Needs some active supportive care
	20	Very sick, hospitalization needed
	10	Moribund
	0	Dead

Source: From Detterbeck and Rivera.[23]

Stage IV

First-Line Therapy

Approximately 40% of patients with NSCLC present with either stage IV or advanced stage IIIB disease with malignant pleural/pericardial effusions or supraclavicular adenopathy. These patients are not appropriate for an aggressive, potentially curative approach. The most important prognostic factor remains the PS of the patient (Table 71.11). Patients with a good PS (Eastern Cooperative Oncology Group [ECOG] PS 0–1 or Karnofsky > 70%) should be considered for chemotherapy, while those with a poor PS (ECOG PS 3–4 or Karnofsky < 50%) have generally been excluded from trials evaluating the role of chemotherapy and are not known to benefit from treatment. The optimal approach to the patient with a borderline PS (ECOG PS 2 or Karnofsky 50%–70%) remains controversial.

The true impact of chemotherapy in advanced NSCLC is best judged by trials comparing active treatment strategies to best supportive care (BSC). Table 71.12 compares such trials in chemonaïve as well as previously treated advanced NSCLC

TABLE 71.12.
Randomized Trials of Chemotherapy Versus Basic Supportive Care in Advanced NSCLC.

Trial	*Year*	*Level of evidence*	*N*	*Design*	*Median follow-up (mo)*	*QOL: Chemo vs. BSC*	*Median survival*
Platin-based chemotherapy							
Spiro[246]	2004	I	725	Random	23	(No difference)[a]	Longer
Cullen[367]	1999	I	351	Random	26	Better	Better
Thongprasert[387]	1999	I	287	Random	—	Better	Better
Woods[388]	1990	I	188	Random	—	No difference	(Better)[b]
Rapp[389]	1988	I	137	Random	—	—	Better
Cellerino[390]	1991	I	123	Random	30	—	(Better)[b]
Cartei[391]	1993	I	102	Random	—	—	Better
Kaasa[392]	1991	I	87	Random	—	—	(Better)[b]
Ganz[393]	1989	I	48	Random	—	—	(Better)[b]
Helsing[394]	1998	I	48	Random[c]	40	Better	Better
Non-platin-based monotherapy							
Anderson[395]	2000	I	300	Random	25	Better	No difference
Roszkowski[396]	2000	I	207	Random	—	Better	Longer
Ranson[397]	2000	I	157	Random	—	Better	Longer
ELVIS[277,398]	1999, 2001	I	154	Random	14	Better	Longer
Cormier[399]	1982	I	37	Random	—	—	Longer

BSC, basic supportive care; chemo, — chemotherapy; ELVIS, Elderly Lung Cancer Vinorelbine Italian Study Group; QOL, quality of life.

Platin based refers to cisplatin combination chemotherapy unless otherwise stated.

[a]QOL data incomplete; no difference in subset analysis of 273 patients.

[b]Nonsignificant ($P = .05$) trend to improved survival with chemotherapy.

[c]Carboplatin based.

patients. In the first-line setting, a number of platinum-based combination regimens as well as active single agents have improved survival over BSC. A 1995 metaanalysis found significantly improved survival with platin-based chemotherapy compared with BSC alone (1190 patients).[212] The difference in median survival was approximately 2 months (HR = 0.73, $P < .0001$) with a 10% improvement in the 1-year survival rate. This observation was confirmed in a subsequent prospective randomized phase III trial known as the Big Lung Trial (BLT) and involving 725 patients.[246]

Most of the trials comparing chemotherapy with BSC have used second-generation agents (etoposide, ifosfamide, mitomycin, vindesine, vinblastine, and others) combined with cisplatin. During the 1990s, several new third-generation agents were identified with significant single-agent activity in advanced NSCLC. These included paclitaxel, docetaxel, gemcitabine, irinotecan, and vinorelbine, all of which could be combined safely with either cisplatin or carboplatin (a less-toxic and more conveniently administered platinum analogue). Trials comparing the second- and third-generation regimens have yielded mixed results, but two metaanalyses suggested a modest survival advantage with the use of the third-generation regimens.[247,248] However, trials comparing different third-generation regimens to one another have generally suggested equivalent efficacy, with a median survival of 8–11 months and 1-year survival rate of 30%–40%.[249–253] The toxicity patterns of these regimens vary depending on the combination, but in general most are well tolerated. Thus, a number of platinum-based doublets are reasonable choices for first-line treatment of advanced NSCLC (Table 71.13). If a platinum is contraindicated, a third-generation combination such as gemcitabine/paclitaxel may be substituted with similar efficacy.[254]

The duration of first-line therapy has been evaluated in several phase III trials comparing brief (three or four cycles) to more prolonged courses of therapy (six or more cycles) with platinum-based doublets.[255–257] The results of these trials have been consistent and demonstrated no benefit to continuing chemotherapy beyond three or four cycles. Furthermore, with more prolonged therapy, the risk of cumulative toxicities increases, potentially decreasing the palliative benefit of therapy.

In efforts to improve the efficacy of first-line combination chemotherapy in NSCLC, numerous trials have evaluated the addition of a novel "targeted" agent. Four phase III trials have combined daily dosing of standard platinum-based doublet regimens with either gefitinib or erlotinib (small molecule tyrosine kinase inhibitors of the EGFR).[258–261] All have failed to show a survival advantage and presently are not recommended. Different dosing schemes are being evaluated. In contrast, bevacizumab (Avastin), a monoclonal antibody to VEGF, has shown benefit in combination with chemotherapy in a phase III trial of 878 previously untreated patients with advanced nonsquamous NSCLC (overall response rate 27% vs. 10%, $P < .0001$; median survival 13 vs. 10 months, $P = .0075$; 1-year survival 58% vs. 22%).[262] Fatal hemoptysis occurred in 5 patients, and bevacizumab must be avoided in patients with an increased risk of bleeding.

Salvage Therapy

Prior to 1999, there was no accepted therapy for patients who progressed following platinum-based first-line treatment (essentially all patients). Since many patients have disease progression documented radiographically before a significant detriment in PS occurs, they remain candidates for subsequent therapy. More recently, better survival with second-line therapy compared to BSC has been demonstrated for several agents. A randomized trial comparing docetaxel to BSC yielded improved survival (median survival 7 vs. 5 months, $P = .047$; 1-year survival 37% vs. 11%, $P = .003$).[263] Quality of life (QOL) was also improved in the treated patients.[264] A second trial comparing docetaxel to a control arm of either vinorelbine or ifosfamide showed a survival advantage for docetaxel.[265] Docetaxel was subsequently compared to pemetrexed in a phase III multicenter trial and was found to have similar efficacy with less toxicity.[266] However, pemetrexed was better tolerated with less hematologic toxicity, particularly neutropenia and rates of febrile neutropenia, and less alopecia.

TABLE 71.13. Commonly Used First-Line Chemotherapy Regimens for Advanced NSCLC.

Gemcitabine plus cisplatin Gemcitabine 1000 mg/m^2 d1,8,15 Cisplatin 100 mg/m^2 d1 4-week cycle[250]	***Vinorelbine plus cisplatin*** Vinorelbine 25 mg/m^2 d1,8,15,22 Cisplatin 100 mg/m^2 d1 4-week cycle[253,401]
Gemcitabine 1,250 mg/m^2 d1,8 Cisplatin 75 mg/m^2 d2 3-week cycle[253,400,249]	Vinorelbine 25 mg/m^2 d1,8 Cisplatin 80 mg/m^2 d1 3-week cycle[400]
Docetaxel plus cisplatin Docetaxel 75 mg/m^2 d1 Cisplatin 75 mg/m^2 d1 3-week cycle[250]	***Paclitaxel plus cisplatin*** Paclitaxel 135 mg/m^2 d1 Cisplatin 75 mg/m^2 d2(1) 3-week schedule[249,250]
Irinotecan plus cisplatin Irinotecan 60 mg/m^2 d1,8,15 Cisplatin 80 mg/m^2 d1 Every 4 weeks[400]	***Gemcitabine plus paclitaxel*** Gemcitabine 1250 mg/m^2 d1,8 Paclitaxel 175 mg/m^2 d1 3-week cycle[249]
Paclitaxel plus carboplatin Paclitaxel 225 (200) mg/m^2 over 3 h d1 Carboplatin AUC 6 mg/mL/min d1 3-week cycle[250,400]	***Docetaxel plus carboplatin*** Docetaxel 75 mg/m^2 d1 Carboplatin AUC 6 mg/mL/min d1 3-week cycle[251]

AUC, area under the curve; d, day.

Erlotinib (a tyrosine kinase inhibitor of EGFR) also has significant activity in advanced, previously treated NSCLC patients and has been shown to be superior to BSC in this setting (731 patients; median survival 7 vs. 5 months; HR 0.70, $P < .001$; 1-year survival 31% vs. 21%).[267] Quality-of-life analysis also found significant improvements in cough, dyspnea, and pain with erlotinib versus placebo ($P < .05$). Erlotinib was generally well tolerated, with primary toxicities consisting of rash and diarrhea. As in previous phase II trials, response to erlotinib was associated with certain clinical characteristics: female sex, nonsmoking history, adenocarcinoma histology, and Asian origin. However, EGFR mutations were not found to be significant predictors of response or survival. Currently, docetaxel, pemetrexed and erlotinib are the only treatment options approved by the Food and Drug Administration (FDA) for patients who have received one or two prior regimens for advanced NSCLC.

Borderline Performance Status and Elderly Patients

The optimal management of the poor PS patient (ECOG 2 or Karnofsky PS 50%–70%) with advanced NSCLC remains controversial. No randomized trials specific to the poor PS have been performed against BSC, but trials have established responsiveness and tolerability of chemotherapy in such patients.[268,269] Although single-agent therapy is currently recommended by both American and European expert panels,[254,270] some patients may benefit from combination chemotherapy. In a subset analysis of a larger trial, the PS 2 patients receiving combination therapy had higher response rates and overall survival without any obvious detriment in QOL (99 PS 2 patients; paclitaxel and carboplatin vs. paclitaxel alone).[268] However, patient selection is crucial because there is a great deal of heterogenicity among poor PS patients in general (e.g., aggressive disease vs. comorbidities).

The elderly also deserve special comment. Although the definition of elderly varies among trials, most define the elderly as 70 years or greater. Several retrospective subset analyses of elderly patients have found similar response and survival rates compared with younger patients using various platinum-based therapies.[271–277] A randomized study of patients 70 years and older found a 20% response rate to vinorelbine alone as well as a significant survival advantage compared to BSC (median survival 28 vs. 21 weeks, $P = .03$; 1-year survival 32% vs. 14%).[277] There were also fewer lung cancer-related symptoms and better QOL in those receiving chemotherapy. A subsequent trial of combination therapy found greater toxicity with no improvement in survival compared with single-agent therapy (vinorelbine plus gemcitabine vs. vinorelbine alone or gemcitabine alone).[278] Based on these data, the American Society of Clinical Oncologists (ASCO) currently recommends single-agent therapy for the elderly.[254] Some trials have suggested the elderly experience more severe toxicity (particularly with cisplatin, perhaps not with carboplatin-based regimens).[271,276] Like the PS 2 group, the elderly are a heterogeneous group of patients. Some are quite fit and appropriately managed with platinum-based therapies, while others are more compromised and cautiously approached with single agents. Furthermore, the currently published experience is almost universally restricted to patients under the age of 80. Few data are available on older patients regarding the activity and tolerance of chemotherapy.

Specific Groups (Limited M1)

Patients with metastatic disease limited to the brain should be considered for aggressive therapy with curative intent.[199,279] This may involve either a synchronous or a metachronous presentation of the lung primary disease and the brain metastasis. In patients with a synchronous presentation, it seems clear that a thorough search for other metastatic sites should be undertaken, and that patients with extracranial metastases be excluded from a resection with curative intent.[199,279] Patients should be considered for resection only if all of the tumor (at both the primary and any metastatic sites) can be completely resected.[280] The presence of more than one brain metastasis is probably not significant provided the number of metastases is small (i.e., ≤3) and provided that all metastases can be completely resected with confidence and with acceptable morbidity.[280] The patient must also be fit enough to tolerate both operations. The histologic subtype is not important.[280] A preoperative mediastinoscopy should be carried out to rule out N2,3 node involvement, although the data supporting the hypothesis that the presence of mediastinal node involvement precludes a good outcome are unclear.[199,279,280] Patients with a metachronous presentation should also undergo a careful search for other distant metastases, preferably with a PET scan.[199,279]

The outlook is likely to be more optimistic for patients who are younger and female and have a metachronous presentation.[279] The outlook may also be better in patients with supratentorial lesions and those with brain metastases smaller than 3 cm. In patients with a metachronous presentation, the outlook may be better with a longer disease-free interval.[279] However, these considerations are relative and should not necessarily exclude patients who are otherwise fit and in whom a complete resection is likely to be achieved.

The 5-year survival of patients undergoing surgical resection of brain metastases is 15%.[279] The survival is 21% in patients undergoing a complete resection, and this appears to be the most important prognostic factor.[279,280] The operative mortality of resection of the brain metastasis is 2%.[279] An alternative to surgical resection is radiosurgery (RS), which involves tumor ablation using a highly focused beam of radiation. The outcomes are equal following resection or RS for brain metastases. Technical considerations guide the choice of which is more appropriate, and these modalities should be viewed as complementary.[279] Typically, whole-brain RT is given after resection or RS of the brain metastases, although the data are conflicting and unclear whether this is worthwhile.[199] The role of adjuvant chemotherapy is undefined.[199]

In patients in whom cure is not feasible, palliative resection or RS of brain metastasis is still indicated for some patients. This is because of randomized data showing better survival and QOL after such aggressive palliative treatment compared with either steroids or whole-brain RT.[37,279,281,282] This benefit is realized in patients with stable extracranial disease and with a good PS (PS 0–1). The 2-year survival after palliative resection of a brain metastasis is 20%.[279] Furthermore, repeat craniotomy is indicated for recurrence of a brain metastasis in selected patients, with several studies consistently reporting a 5-year survival of approximately 15% in this situation.[279]

Resection of all sites of disease with intent to cure is also indicated in patients with isolated adrenal metastases.[199,279] A careful search should be undertaken to rule out other sites of metastases, and mediastinoscopy should be done for patients with a synchronous presentation to rule out mediastinal node involvement.[199] The 5-year survival after resection of an adrenal metastasis is 10%–23%.[199,279] Resection of an isolated adrenal metastasis may also be of palliative benefit.[279]

Patients with a metastasis to the vertebral column may benefit from resection and spine stabilization.[283] A randomized study has shown better maintenance of functional status with surgery as compared with RT alone.[283]

Small Cell Lung Cancer

Presentation and Evaluation

Recent data suggest that SCLC comprises approximately 13% of new cases of lung cancer.[284] Approximately one-third of these cases have limited-stage (LS) disease,[34] defined as disease confined to one hemithorax and that can be encompassed within a "reasonable" radiation port.[285] Although somewhat arbitrary, this typically includes the primary tumor volume and ipsilateral mediastinal and supraclavicular lymph nodes as well as contralateral mediastinal lymph nodes.[285] Areas of controversy include the contralateral hilar and supraclavicular lymph nodes as well as pleural disease.[285] The typical radiographic findings include a hilar or central mass with bulky mediastinal adenopathy. LS-SCLC rarely presents as a peripheral nodule. The presenting symptoms are usually related to the presence of bulky intrathoracic disease and include cough, dyspnea, hemoptysis, chest pain, and hoarseness.

Extensive-stage (ES) SCLC accounts for approximately two-thirds of the cases at the time of presentation.[34] Typical sites of metastases include the liver, bones, brain, lymph nodes, pleura, and the contralateral lung.[34] The presenting symptoms are related to bulky disease within the chest or to distant metastases. These symptoms may be organ specific (bone pain, right upper quadrant pain with liver metastases, headache with brain metastases, etc.) or nonspecific (weight loss, anorexia, and fatigue). Small cell lung cancer is also characterized by a high incidence of paraneoplastic syndromes, with the most common ones the syndrome of inappropriate antidiuretic hormone (SIADH) release, Cushing's syndrome, and the Lambert-Eaton myasthenic syndrome.

Once the diagnosis is suspected, a staging chest CT should be obtained to evaluate the intrathoracic contents as well as the liver and adrenal glands. Further evaluation of the brain (by CT or MRI) and bones should be performed unless distant disease is identified. The role of additional staging once distant or extensive disease is documented is controversial and should be symptom directed. However, brain imaging is reasonable as intracranial metastases are common in SCLC, and detection of brain metastases may alter the therapeutic approach. Although the data with PET scanning are substantially less robust than the data in NSCLC, PET scanning appears to have utility in the initial evaluation of SCLC.[35]

Treatment

Limited Stage

With combined-modality therapy, LS-SCLC is a potentially curable disease. Local modalities alone (surgery or RT) should generally not be offered to LS-SCLC patients because this is considered a systemic disease at the time of diagnosis. Thirteen randomized trials have addressed the added benefit of RT to combination chemotherapy.[285] The data from these trials have been conflicting, with approximately half of them statistically negative. However, many of these trials had insufficient statistical power to detect small but clinically meaningful survival differences. Almost all of these trials did show an improvement in locoregional control, with an approximate doubling of the local control rate. Two metaanalyses evaluating the role of RT and combination chemotherapy compared with chemotherapy alone have been reported.[286,287] Warde and Payne analyzed the results of 11 randomized trials and found a statistically significant survival advantage in those patients receiving combined-modality therapy.[286] There was a 53% greater likelihood of surviving 2 years with the addition of RT, which translated into an absolute difference in 2-year survival of 5% ($P < .05$). Local control at 2 years was improved by 25%. This benefit was associated with a 1.2% increased treatment-related mortality. The second metaanalysis included 13 trials (10 common to both metaanalyses) and essentially confirmed the results noted above. These metaanalyses together show a consistent benefit in favor of combined-modality therapy compared to chemotherapy alone, both for survival and local control.

Although the paradigm of combined-modality therapy is embraced by most, the optimal sequence, timing, and the RT dose and fractionation remain controversial. Historically, relatively conservative RT dosing schedules were used (generally ≤ 50 Gy).[285] However, escalating total RT dose with newer technologies is presently being explored. One CALGB phase II trial has already established the feasibility of TRT to 70 Gy (once-daily fractions with concurrent cisplatin-based chemotherapy).[288] Accelerated hyperfractionated RT has also been investigated in a series of randomized trials. A landmark trial compared once- versus twice-daily RT (total dose on both arms was 45 Gy) with cisplatin and etoposide. Thoracic RT was initiated with the first cycle of chemotherapy. The LS-SCLC patients receiving twice-daily RT had better survival (median survival 23 vs. 19 months, $P = .04$; 5-year survival 26% vs. 16%) but significantly worse grade III esophagitis (27% vs. 11%, $P < .001$). Although this trial established the role of accelerated hyperfractionated RT in LS-SCLC, it is still unclear if daily RT to doses of 50–60 Gy is a reasonable alternative with concurrent chemotherapy.

The timing of RT in relation to the initiation of chemotherapy is another area of controversy. A metaanalysis found a survival benefit at 2 years for early versus late RT (risk ratio 1.17, $P = .03$; seven randomized trials, including 1524 patients with LS-SCLC).[289] Subset analyses suggested that the benefit of early RT was limited to those patients treated with hyperfractionated RT (relative risk [RR] 1.44 and 1.39 at 2 and 3 years, respectively) or platinum-based chemotherapy (RR 1.30 and 1.35 at 2 and 3 years, respectively).[289] These data taken in total suggest that more aggressive approaches (early and more intense RT) in LS-SCLC patients with a good PS improve survival.

There are a large number of chemotherapeutic agents with substantial single-agent activity in both LS- as well as ES-SCLC.[285] There was a suggestion from several older phase II and III trials that combination chemotherapy is superior to single agents.[285] The optimal regimen remains elusive, but the data currently support the combination of etoposide and cisplatin (EP) as the standard regimen, particularly given its ability to be safely combined with TRT.[290–293] Four to six cycles of chemotherapy are generally offered because maintenance chemotherapy has not been shown to improve survival.[285]

Based on the above-mentioned studies, the standard approach to LS-SCLC presently involves initiation of concurrent twice-daily RT in 1.5-Gy fractions (45Gy total) during the first or second of four to six cycles of chemotherapy with cisplatin and etoposide. However, as delivering twice-daily RT can be time consuming and expensive, once-daily RT in 1.8- or 2-Gy fractions to higher doses (50–60Gy) with concurrent chemotherapy is often substituted.

Prophylactic Cranial Irradiation

Patients with LS-SCLC who experience a complete response to initial therapy have a 50%–67% risk of developing brain metastases.[294,295] The role of prophylactic cranial irradiation (PCI) has been investigated but had inconsistent results in underpowered trials. A metaanalysis was performed that included seven randomized trials and 967 patients.[296] There was a significant reduction in the risk of death in the treated patients (HR = 0.84, $P = .01$) and an absolute 3-year survival advantage of 5.4%. The risk of brain metastases was reduced by 45%. Two of the largest trials also performed serial neuropsychologic testing, which failed to show any negative impact of PCI.[294,295]

Taken together, the individual studies and subsequent metaanalysis have established the role of PCI in the treatment of LS-SCLC, and perhaps ES-SCLC, after complete response to therapy, with a clear reduction in the incidence of brain metastases and a suggestion of a 5% overall survival advantage. The optimal dose (total and daily) and schedule of PCI are still the subject of ongoing randomized clinical trials, with most trials employing between 30 and 36Gy given in daily fractions of no greater than 2Gy. With these doses, it appears that PCI does not negatively affect short-term neurocognitive ability. Longer follow-up, which is often limited by subsequent relapse and death, is needed to fully assess the protracted effects of PCI.

Extensive Stage

Extensive-stage SCLC is not curable, and the goal of therapy is to maximize survival and palliate disease-related symptoms. There are many combination chemotherapy regimens that have clear activity in ES-SCLC. The most commonly employed regimen includes a platinum (cisplatin or carboplatin) with etoposide.[297] The response rates to combination chemotherapy are over 50%; however, median survival and 1-year survival rates remain at 8–10 months and 20%–30%, respectively.[297] Recent phase III strategies tested in ES-SCLC include the addition of a third or fourth agent such as paclitaxel or ifosfamide, increasing chemotherapy dose intensity and dose density, and extending treatment beyond four to six cycles. These approaches have not significantly changed the survival outlook for patients with ES-SCLC and were all associated with increased risk of severe and lethal toxicities.[298–302] One encouraging Japanese phase III trial substituted irinotecan for etoposide in a cisplatin doublet.[303] This small trial was stopped early due to a significant survival advantage of irinotecan-cisplatin (IP) over EP (median survival 13 vs. 9 months, $P = .002$). However, this benefit was not found in a randomized U.S. trial employing a modified weekly regimen of IP compared to EP.[304] The results of a larger randomized SWOG trial comparing EP to the IP regimen employed in the Japanese trial are awaited.

All patients with ES-SCLC and the majority with LS-SCLC will eventually experience disease recurrence or progression. Relapses of SCLC have been divided into sensitive versus refractory categories based on the response to initial therapy (complete/partial response vs. stable/progressive disease) as well as the durability of the response (progression-free interval of at least 2–3 months). In the sensitive-relapse patient, decreased toxicity, better relief of certain disease-related symptoms, and equivalent survival were achieved with topotecan compared with cyclophosphamide, adriamycin, vincristine (CAV).[305] No therapeutic approach has yielded encouraging results in the truly refractory patients, who are best managed with BSC or investigational therapies.

Role of Surgery

The role of surgery in LS-SCLC is restricted to patients in whom the diagnosis is either unknown or in doubt, as well as to patients who have failed nonsurgical treatment but remain resectable. If the accuracy of a diagnosis of SCLC is in doubt, there should not be hesitation in proceeding with resection.[285] On the other hand, if the diagnosis is secure, there is little role for surgery in general. Rarely, patients with SCLC present with a peripheral stage I,II tumor for whom surgical resection might be considered. Primary chemotherapy followed by surgical resection as adjuvant treatment in patients with SCLC have been investigated in a number of prospective phase II studies.[285] Approximately 80% of patients entered in studies of adjuvant surgical resection have undergone surgery, and a complete resection (R_0) was achieved in approximately 90% of these.[285] Although the stage-specific survival is encouraging, it is impossible to assess the impact of surgery without a randomized trial. One such trial has been conducted and did not suggest a benefit in survival or local control with chemotherapy and surgery (and postoperative RT) compared with ChRT alone.[306]

Those select patients who fail to respond to ChRT or who experience a relapse but have resectable tumors should undergo surgery. There is a fairly high probability that these patients have a NSCLC component to their tumor, and there is compelling, albeit limited, data suggesting that a substantial number of these patients can be cured by resection.[285]

Conclusion

The treatment of lung cancer has become a very complex field with a solid scientific basis and a vast amount of data regarding the relative value of different approaches. There is solid evidence that treatment according to the results of current phase II and III trials results in better outcomes than more traditional approaches. Unfortunately, it is still too common to see these patients cared for by suboptimal approaches, stemming from an incomplete understanding of the current literature. This is probably partially explained by the nihilism that is associated with lung cancer and the extent and complexity of the data that are available. Furthermore, because much of the treatment of lung cancer involves multimodality treatment, a fully informed approach requires familiarity with data contributed by many disciplines. It is important for surgeons to be knowledgeable about the data and to use a thoughtful and evidence-based approach. This knowledge must extend beyond the field of surgery, as has been summarized in this chapter. Much progress has been made over the last decades, and the level of understanding is increasing rapidly, leaving little doubt that outcomes will continue to improve significantly in the coming years.

References

1. Jemal, A., et al. Cancer statistics, 2005. CA Cancer J Clin 2005. 55:10–30.
2. Brown, C.C., and L.G. Kessler. Projections of lung cancer mortality in the United States: 1985–2025. J Natl Cancer Inst 1988. 80:43–51.
3. U.S. Department of Health and Human Services. Cigarette smoking among high school students—11 states, 1991–1997. MMWR Morb Mortal Wkly Rep 1998. 48:686–692.
4. Rivera, M.P., F.C. Detterbeck, and D.P. Loomis. Epidemiology and classification of lung cancer, in Diagnosis and Treatment of Lung Cancer: An Evidence-Based Guide for the Practicing Clinician, F.C. Detterbeck, et al., eds. Philadelphia: Saunders; 2001:25–44.
5. Flehinger, B.J., M. Kimmel, and M.R. Melamed. The effect of surgical treatment on survival from early lung cancer: implications for screening. Chest 1992. 101:1013–1018.
6. Vrdoljak, E., et al. Survival analysis of untreated patients with non-small-cell lung cancer. Chest 1994. 106:1797–1800.
7. Kyasa, M.J., and A.R. Jazieh. Characteristics and outcomes of patients with unresected early-stage non-small cell lung cancer. South Med J 2002. 95:1149–1152.
8. Fry, W.A., H.R. Menck, and D.P. Winchester. The National Cancer Data Base report on lung cancer. Cancer 1996. 77:1947–1955.
9. Bach, P.B., et al. Racial differences in the treatment of early-stage lung cancer. N Engl J Med 1999. 341:1198–1205.
10. Potosky, A.L., et al. Population variations in the initial treatment of non-small-cell lung cancer. J Clin Oncol 2004. 22:3261–3268.
11. Janssen-Heijnen, M.L., et al. Effect of comorbidity on the treatment and prognosis of elderly patients with non-small cell lung cancer. Thorax 2004. 59:602–607.
12. Ramsey, S.D., et al. Chemotherapy use, outcomes, and costs for older persons with advanced non-small-cell lung cancer: evidence from surveillance, epidemiology and end results—Medicare. J Clin Oncol 2004. 22:4971–4978.
13. Visbal, A.L., et al. Gender differences in non-small-cell lung cancer survival: an analysis of 4618 patients diagnosed between 1997 and 2002. Ann Thorac Surg 2004. 78:209–215; discussion 215.
14. Garces, Y.I., et al. The relationship between cigarette smoking and quality of life after lung cancer diagnosis. Chest 2004. 126:1733–1741.
15. Tong, L., et al. Lung carcinoma in former smokers. Cancer 1996. 78:1004–1010.
16. Centers for Disease Control. Public Health Service, U.S. Department of Health and Human Services, The health benefits of smoking cessation. DHHS Publication No. (CDC)90–8416. Washington, DC: U.S. Government Printing Office.
17. Halpern, M.T., B.W. Gillespie, and K.E. Warner. Patterns of absolute risk of lung cancer mortality in former smokers. J Natl Cancer Inst 1993. 85:457–464.
18. Ikeda, N., et al. A clinicopathological study of resected adenocarcinoma 2 cm or less in diameter. Ann Thorac Surg 2004. 78:1011–1016.
19. Ebright, M.I., et al. Clinical pattern and pathologic stage but not histologic features predict outcome for bronchioloalveolar carcinoma. Ann Thorac Surg 2002. 74:1640–1647.
20. Mountain, C.F. Revisions in the International System for Staging Lung Cancer. Chest 1997. 111:1710–1717.
21. Janssen-Heijnen, M.L.G., et al. Prevalence of co-morbidity in lung cancer patients and its relationship with treatment: a population-based study. Lung Cancer 1998. 21:105–113.
22. Malmberg, R., et al. Lung cancer in West Sweden 1976–1985. Acta Oncologica 1996. 35:185–192.
23. Detterbeck, F.C., and M.P. Rivera. Clinical presentation and diagnosis, in Diagnosis and Treatment of Lung Cancer: An Evidence-Based Guide for the Practicing Clinician, F.C. Detterbeck, et al., eds. Philadelphia: Saunders; 2001:45–72.
24. Fang, D., et al. Results of surgical resection of patients with primary lung cancer: a retrospective analysis of 1905 cases. Ann Thorac Surg 2001. 72:1155–1159.
25. Chute, C.G., et al. Presenting conditions of 1539 population-based lung cancer patients by cell type and stage in New Hampshire and Vermont. Cancer 1985. 56:2107–2111.
26. Huhti, E., et al. Lung cancer in a defined geographical area: history and histological types. Thorax 1980. 35:660–667.
27. Ferguson, M.K. Diagnosing and staging of non-small cell lung cancer. Hematol/Oncol Clin N Am 1990. 4:1053–1068.
28. Bülzebruck, H., et al. New aspects in the staging of lung cancer: prospective validation of the International Union Against Cancer TNM classification. Cancer 1992. 70:1102–1110.
29. Byers, T.E., J.E. Vena, and T.F. Rzepka. Predilection of lung cancer for the upper lobes: an epidemiologic inquiry. J Natl Cancer Inst 1984. 72:1271–1275.
30. Quinn, D., A. Gianlupi, and S. Broste. The changing radiographic presentation of bronchogenic carcinoma with reference to cell types. Chest 1996. 110:1474–1479.
31. Quekel, L.G.B.A., et al. Miss rate of lung cancer on the chest radiograph in clinical practice. Chest 1999. 115:720–724.
32. Detterbeck, F.C., D.R. Jones, and W.K. Funkhouser Jr. Satellite nodules and multiple primary cancers, in Diagnosis and Treatment of Lung Cancer: An Evidence-Based Guide for the Practicing Clinician, F.C. Detterbeck, et al., eds. Philadelphia: Saunders; 2001:437–449.
33. Detterbeck, F., et al. Seeking a home for a PET, Part 1: Defining the appropriate place for positron emission tomography imaging in the diagnosis of pulmonary nodules or masses. Chest 2004. 125:2294–2299.
34. Detterbeck, F.C., D.R. Jones, and P.L. Molina. Extrathoracic staging, in Diagnosis and Treatment of Lung Cancer: An Evidence-Based Guide for the Practicing Clinician, F.C. Detterbeck, et al., eds. Philadelphia: Saunders; 2001:94–110.
35. Detterbeck, F., et al. Seeking a home for a PET, Part 2: Defining the appropriate place for positron emission tomography imaging in the staging of patients with suspected lung cancer. Chest 2004. 125:2300–2308.
36. Rivera, M.P., F. Detterbeck, and A.C. Mehta. Diagnosis of lung cancer: the guidelines. Chest 2003. 123:129S–136S.
37. Patchell, R.A., et al. A randomized trial of surgery in the treatment of single metastases to the brain. N Engl J Med 1990. 322:494–500.

38. Jacobson, A.F., et al. Bone scans with one or two new abnormalities in cancer patients with no known metastases: frequency and serial scintigraphic behavior of benign and malignant lesions. Radiology 1990. 175:229–232.
39. Ichinose, Y., et al. Preoperative examination to detect distant metastasis is not advocated for asymptomatic patients with stages 1 and 2 non-small cell lung cancer: preoperative examination for lung cancer. Chest 1989. 96:1104–1109.
40. Grant, D., D. Edwards, and P. Goldstraw. Computed tomography of the brain, chest, and abdomen in the postoperative assessment of non-small cell lung cancer. Thorax 1988. 43:883–886.
41. MacManus, M.P., et al. High rate of detection of unsuspected distant metastases by PET in apparent stage III non-small-cell lung cancer: implications for radical radiation therapy. Int J Radiation Oncology Biol Phys 2001. 50:287–293.
42. Weder, W., et al. Detection of extrathoracic metastases by positron emission tomography in lung cancer. Ann Thorac Surg 1998. 66:886–893.
43. Viney, R.C., et al. Randomized controlled trial of the role of positron emission tomography in the management of stage I and II non-small-cell lung cancer. J Clin Oncol 2004. 22:2357–2362.
44. Reed, C., et al. Results of the American College of Surgeons Oncology Group Z0050 Trial: the utility of positron emission tomography in staging potentially operable non-small cell lung cancer. J Thorac Cardiovasc Surg 2003. 126:1943–1951.
45. Farrell, M.A., et al. Non-small cell lung cancer: FDG PET for nodal staging in patients with stage I disease. Radiology 2000. 215:886–890.
46. Salvatierra, A., et al. Extrathoracic staging of bronchogenic carcinoma. Chest 1990. 97:1052–1058.
47. Quinn, D.L., et al. Staging of non-small cell bronchogenic carcinoma: relationship of the clinical evaluation to organ scans. Chest 1986. 89:270–275.
48. Eschmann, S.M., et al. FDG PET for staging of advanced non-small cell lung cancer prior to neoadjuvant radio-chemotherapy. Eur J Nucl Med Mol Imaging 2002. 29:804–808.
49. Strauss GM, Herndon JE, Maddaus MA, et al. Adjuvant chemotherapy in stage IB non-small cell lung cancer: update of Cancer and Leukemia Group B protocol 9633. J Clin Oncol 2006 ASCO Ann Mtg Proc 2006;24(18S):7007.
50. Birim, O., et al. Meta-analysis of positron emission tomographic and computed tomographic imaging in detecting mediastinal lymph node metastases in nonsmall cell lung cancer. Ann Thorac Surg 2005. 79:375–382.
51. Detterbeck, F.C., et al. Invasive staging: the guidelines. Chest 2003. 123:167S–175S.
52. Silvestri, G.A., et al. The noninvasive staging of non-small cell lung cancer. Chest 2003. 123:147S–156S.
53. Detterbeck, F.C., D.R. Jones, and L.A. Parker Jr. Intrathoracic staging, in Diagnosis and Treatment of Lung Cancer: An Evidence-Based Guide for the Practicing Clinician, F.C. Detterbeck, et al., eds. Philadelphia: Saunders; 2001:73–93.
54. Verhagen, A.F.T., et al. FDG-PET in staging lung cancer: how does it change the algorithm? Lung Cancer 2004. 44:175–181.
55. Serra, M., et al. Routine positron tomography (PET) and selective mediastinoscopy is as good as routine mediastinoscopy to rule out N2 disease in non-small cell lung cancer (NSCLC). J Clin Oncol 2006. 24(18S), pt 1 of II:371s.
56. Gould, M.K., et al. Test performance of positron emission tomography and computed tomography for mediastinal staging in patients with non-small-cell lung cancer: a meta-analysis. Ann Intern Med 2003. 139:879–892.
57. Dietlein, M., et al. Cost-effectiveness of FDG-PET for the management of potentially operable non-small cell lung cancer; priority for a PET-based strategy after nodal-negative CT results. Eur J Nucl Med 2000. 27:1598–1609.
58. Toloza, E.M., et al. Invasive staging of non-small cell lung cancer: a review of the current evidence. Chest 2003. 123:157S–166S.
59. Rolston, K.V.I., et al. Pulmonary infections mimicking cancer: a retrospective, 3-year review. Support Care Cancer 1997. 5:90–93.
60. Jones, D.R., and F.C. Detterbeck. Surgery for stage I non-small cell lung cancer, in Diagnosis and Treatment of Lung Cancer: An Evidence-Based Guide for the Practicing Clinician, F.C. Detterbeck, et al., eds. Philadelphia: Saunders; 2001:177–190.
61. Handy, J.R., Jr., et al. What happens to patients undergoing lung cancer surgery? Outcomes and quality of life before and after surgery. Chest 2002. 122:21–30.
62. Allen, M.S., et al. Morbidity and mortality of major pulmonary resections in patients with early-stage lung cancer: initial results of the randomized, prospective ACOSOG Z0030 Trial 10.1016/j.athoracsur.2005.06.066. Ann Thorac Surg 2006. 81:1013–1020.
63. McKenna, R.J., Jr., et al. Video-assisted thoracic surgery (VATS) lobectomy for bronchogenic carcinoma. Semin Thorac Cardiovasc Surg 1998. 10:321–325.
64. Kaseda, S., T. Aoki, and N. Hangai. Video-assisted thoracic surgery (VATS) lobectomy: the Japanese experience. Semin Thorac Cardiovasc Surg 1998. 10:300–304.
65. Walker, W.S. Video-assisted thoracic surgery (VATS) lobectomy: the Edinburgh experience. Semin Thorac Cardiovasc Surg 1998. 10:291–299.
66. Iwasaki, A., et al. Results of video-assisted thoracic surgery for stage I/II non-small cell lung cancer. Eur J Cardiothorac Surg 2004. 26:158–164.
67. Solaini, L., et al. Long-term results of video-assisted thoracic surgery lobectomy for stage I non-small cell lung cancer: a single-centre study of 104 cases. Interact Cardiovasc Thorac Surg 2004. 3:57–62.
68. Roviaro, G., et al. Long-term survival after videothoracoscopic lobectomy for stage I lung cancer. Chest 2004. 126:725–732.
69. Thomas, P., et al. Stage I non-small cell lung cancer: a pragmatic approach to prognosis after complete resection. Ann Thorac Surg 2002. 73:1065–1070.
70. Detterbeck, F.C., and T.M. Egan. Surgery for stage II non-small cell lung cancer, in Diagnosis and Treatment of Lung Cancer: An Evidence-Based Guide for the Practicing Clinician, F.C. Detterbeck, et al., eds. Philadelphia: Saunders; 2001:191–197.
71. Van Schil, P.E., et al. TNM staging and long-term follow-up after sleeve resection for bronchogenic tumors. Ann Thorac Surg 1991. 52:1096–1101.
72. Okada, M., et al. Survival related to lymph node involvement in lung cancer after sleeve lobectomy compared with pneumonectomy. J Thorac Cardiovasc Surg 2000. 119:814–819.
73. Detterbeck, F.C., and D.R. Jones. Surgery for stage IIIb non-small cell lung cancer, in Diagnosis and Treatment of Lung Cancer: An Evidence-Based Guide for the Practicing Clinician, F.C. Detterbeck, et al., eds. Philadelphia: Saunders; 2001:283–289.
74. Detterbeck, F.C., and A.C. Kiser. T3 non-small cell lung cancer (stage IIb-IIIa), in Diagnosis and Treatment of Lung Cancer: An Evidence-Based Guide for the Practicing Clinician, F.C. Detterbeck, et al., eds. Philadelphia: Saunders; 2001:223–232.
75. Smythe, W.R. Treatment of stage I non-small cell lung carcinoma. Chest 2003. 123(1 suppl):181S–187S.
76. Bollen, E.C.M., et al. Mediastinal lymph node dissection in resected lung cancer: morbidity and accuracy of staging. Ann Thorac Surg 1993. 55:961–966.
77. Gaer, J.A.R., and P. Goldstraw. Intraoperative assessment of nodal staging at thoracotomy for carcinoma of the bronchus. Eur J Cardiothorac Surg, 1990. 4:207–210.
78. Wu, Y., et al. A randomized trial of systematic nodal dissection in resectable non-small cell lung cancer. Lung Cancer 2002. 36:1–6.

79. Izbicki, J.R., et al. Impact on radical systematic mediastinal lymphadenectomy on tumor staging in lung cancer. Ann Thorac Surg 1995. 59:209–214.
80. Kiser, A.C., and F.C. Detterbeck. General aspects of surgical treatment, in Diagnosis and Treatment of Lung Cancer: An Evidence-Based Guide for the Practicing Clinician, F.C. Detterbeck, et al., eds. Philadelphia: Saunders; 2001:133–147.
81. Silvestri, G.A., et al. Specialists achieve better outcomes than generalists for lung cancer surgery. Chest 1998. 114:675–680.
82. Romano, P.S., and D.H. Mark. Patient and hospital characteristics related to in-hospital mortality after lung cancer resection. Chest 1992. 101:1332–1337.
83. Hillner, B.E., T.J. Smith, and C.E. Desch. Hospital and physician volume or specialization and outcomes in cancer treatment: importance in quality of cancer care. J Clin Oncol 2000. 18:2327–40.
84. Begg, C.B., et al. Impact of hospital volume on operative mortality for major cancer surgery. JAMA, 1998. 280:1747–1751.
85. Birkmeyer, J.D., et al. Surgeon volume and operative mortality in the United States. N Engl J Med 2003. 349:2117–2127.
86. Martinolich, D., and M.P. Rivera. Pulmonary assessment and treatment, in Diagnosis and Treatment of Lung Cancer: An Evidence-Based Guide for the Practicing Clinician, F.C. Detterbeck, et al., eds. Philadelphia: Saunders; 2001:113–132.
87. Kohman, L.J., et al., Random versus predictable risks of mortality after thoracotomy for lung cancer. J Thorac Cardiovasc Surg 1986. 91:551–554.
88. Lopez-Encuentra, A., et al. Surgical lung cancer. Risk operative analysis. Lung Cancer 2004. 44:327–337.
89. Wang, J., et al. Assessment of pulmonary complications after lung resection. Ann Thorac Surg 1999. 67:1444–1447.
90. Boysen, P.G., J.O. Harris, and A.J. Block. Prospective evaluation for pneumonectomy using perfusion scanning: follow-up beyond 1 year. Chest 1981. 80:163–166.
91. Dales, R.E., et al. Quality-of-life following thoracotomy for lung cancer. J Clin Epidemiol 1994. 47:1443–1449.
92. Zieren, H.U., et al. Quality of life after surgical therapy of bronchogenic carcinoma. Eur J Cardiothorac Surg 1996. 10:233–237.
93. Myrdal, G., et al. Quality of life following lung cancer surgery. Thorax 2003. 58:194–197.
94. Markos, J., et al. Preoperative assessment as a predictor of mortality and morbidity after lung resection. Am Rev Respir Dis 1989. 139:902–910.
95. Holden, D.A., T.W. Rice, and K. Stelmach. Exercise testing, 6-min walk, and stair climb in the evaluation of patients at high risk for pulmonary resection. Chest 1992. 102:1774–1779.
96. Pierce, R., et al. Preoperative risk evaluation for lung cancer resection: predicted postoperative product as a predictor of surgical mortality. Am J Respir Crit Care Med 1994. 150:947–955.
97. Wahi, R., et al. Determinants of perioperative morbidity and mortality after pneumonectomy. Ann Thorac Surg 1989. 48:33–37.
98. Nakagawa, K., K. Nakahara, and S. Miyoshi. Oxygen transport during incremental exercise load as a predictor of operative risk in lung cancer patients. Chest 1992. 101:1369–1375.
99. Nakahara, K., et al. A method for predicting postoperative lung function and its relation to postoperative complications in patients with lung cancer. Ann Thorac Surg 1985. 39:260–265.
100. Bolliger, C.T., et al. Lung scanning and exercise testing for the prediction of postoperative performance in lung resection candidates at increased risk for complications. Chest 1995. 108:341–348.
101. Bolliger, C.T., P. Jordan, and M. Soler. Exercise capacity as a predictor of postoperative complications in lung resection candidates. Am J Respir Crit Care Med 1995. 151:1472–1480.
102. Bechard, D., and L. Wetstein. Assessment of exercise oxygen consumption as preoperative criterion for lung resection. Ann Thorac Surg 1987. 44:344–349.
103. Smith, T.P., et al. Exercise capacity as a predictor of post-thoracotomy morbidity. Am Rev Respir Dis 1984. 129:730–734.
104. Martini, N., et al. Incidence of local recurrence and second primary tumors in resected stage I lung cancer. J Thorac Cardiovasc Surg 1995. 109:120–129.
105. Padilla, J., et al. Surgical results and prognostic factors in early non-small cell lung cancer. Ann Thorac Surg 1997. 63:324–326.
106. Sobue, T., et al. Screening for lung cancer with low-dose helical computed tomography: anti-lung cancer association project. J Clin Oncol 2002. 20:911–920.
107. Okada, M., et al. Prognostic significance of perioperative serum carcinoembryonic antigen in non-small cell lung cancer: analysis of 1000 consecutive resections for clinical stage I disease. Ann Thorac Surg 2004. 78:216–221.
108. Patz, E.F., Jr., et al. Correlation of tumor size and survival in patients with stage IA non-small cell lung cancer. Chest 2000. 117:1568–1571.
109. Padilla, J., et al. Survival and risk model for stage IB non-small cell lung cancer. Lung Cancer 2002. 36:43–48.
110. Ichinose, Y., et al. Prognostic factors obtained by a pathologic examination in completely resected non-small-cell lung cancer: an analysis in each pathologic stage. J Thorac Cardiovasc Surg 1995. 110:601–605.
111. Takizawa, T., et al. Lymph node metastasis in small peripheral adenocarcinoma of the lung. J Thorac Cardiovasc Surg 1998. 116:276–280.
112. Harpole, D.H., Jr., et al. Stage I nonsmall cell lung cancer: a multivariate analysis of treatment methods and patterns of recurrence. Cancer 1995. 76:787–796.
113. Chung, C.K., et al. Carcinoma of the lung: evaluation of histological grade and factors influencing prognosis. Ann Thorac Surg 1982. 33:599–604.
114. Martini, N., et al. Survival after resection of stage II non-small cell lung cancer. Ann Thorac Surg 1992. 54:460–466.
115. Osaki, T., et al. Survival and characteristics of lymph node involvement in patients with N1 non-small cell lung cancer. Lung Cancer 2004. 43:151–157.
116. Marra, A., et al. Pathologic N1 non-small cell lung cancer: correlation between pattern of lymphatic spread and prognosis. J Thorac Cardiovasc Surg 2003. 125:543–553.
117. Yano, T., et al. Surgical results and prognostic factors of pathologic N1 disease in non-small-cell carcinoma of the lung—significance of N1 level: lobar or hilar nodes. J Thorac Cardiovasc Surg 1994. 107:1398–1402.
118. van Velzen, E., et al. Type of lymph node involvement influences survival rates in T1N1M0 non-small cell lung carcinoma. Chest 1996. 110:1469–1473.
119. Riquet, M., et al. Prognostic significance of surgical-pathologic N1 disease in non-small cell carcinoma of the lung. Ann Thorac Surg 1999. 67:1572–1576.
120. Sawyer, T.E., et al. Factors predicting patterns of recurrence after resection of N1 non-small cell lung carcinoma. Ann Thorac Surg 1999. 68:1171–1176.
121. van Velzen, E., et al. Lymph node type as a prognostic factor for survival in T2 N1 M0 non-small cell lung carcinoma. Ann Thorac Surg 1997. 63:1436–1440.
122. Yoshino, I., et al. Unfavorable prognosis of patients with stage II non-small cell lung cancer associated with macroscopic nodal metastases. Chest 1999. 116:144–149.
123. Tanaka, F., et al. Prognostic factors in patients with resected pathologic (p-) T1-2N1M0 non-small cell lung cancer (NSCLC). Eur J Cardiothorac Surg 2001. 19:555–561.
124. Khan, O.A., et al. Histological determinants of survival in completely resected T1-2N1M0 nonsmall cell cancer of the lung. Ann Thorac Surg 2004. 77:1173–1178.

125. Luzzi, L., et al. Pneumonectomy versus lobectomy in the treatment of pathologic N1 NSCLC: could the type of surgical resection dictate survival? J Cardiovasc Surg 2003. 44:119–123.
126. Iyengar, P., and M.S. Tsao. Clinical relevance of molecular markers in lung cancer. Surg Oncol 2002. 11:167–179.
127. Rena, O., et al. Stage I non-small cell lung carcinoma: really an early stage? Eur J Cardiothorac Surg 2002. 21:514–519.
128. Keller, S.M., et al. Mediastinal lymph node dissection improves survival in patients with stages II and IIIa non-small cell lung cancer; from the Eastern Cooperative Oncology Group. Ann Thorac Surg 2000. 70:358–365.
129. Sugi, K., et al. Systematic lymph node dissection for clinically diagnosed peripheral non-small-cell lung cancer less than 2 cm in diameter. World J Surg 1998. 22:290–294.
130. Izbicki, J.R., et al. Radical systematic mediastinal lymphadenectomy in non-small cell lung cancer: a randomized controlled trial. Br J Surg 1994. 81:229–235.
131. Funatsu, T., et al. Preoperative mediastinoscopic assessment of N factors and the need for mediastinal lymph node dissection in T1 lung cancer. J Thorac Cardiovasc Surg 1994. 108:321–328.
132. Martin-Ucar, A.E., et al. Can pneumonectomy for non-small cell lung cancer be avoided? An audit of parenchymal sparing lung surgery. Eur J Cardiothorac Surg 2002. 21:601–605.
133. Deslauriers, J., et al. Sleeve lobectomy versus pneumonectomy for lung cancer: a comparative analysis of survival and sites or recurrences. Ann Thorac Surg 2004. 77:1152–1156; discussion 1156.
134. Kaiser, L.R., et al. Significance of extramucosal residual tumor at the bronchial resection margin. Ann Thorac Surg 1989. 47:265–269.
135. Gaissert, H.A., et al. Survival and function after sleeve lobectomy for lung cancer. J Thorac Cardiovasc Surg 1996. 111:948–953.
136. Naruke, T. Bronchoplastic and bronchovascular procedures of the tracheobronchial tree in the management of primary lung cancer. Chest 1989. 96:53S–56S.
137. Vogt-Moykopf, I., et al. Bronchoplastic and angioplastic operation in bronchial carcinoma: long-term results of a retrospective analysis from 1973 to 1983. Intern Surg 1986. 71:211–220.
138. Rendina, E.A., F. Venuta, and T. De Giacomo. Sleeve resection and prosthetic reconstruction of the pulmonary artery for lung cancer. Ann Thorac Surg 1999. 68:995–1002.
139. Ginsberg, R.J., L.V. Rubinstein, and the Lung Cancer Study Group. Randomized trial of lobectomy versus limited resection for T1 N0 non-small cell lung cancer. Ann Thorac Surg 1995. 60:615–623.
140. Rubinstein, L.V., and R.J. Ginsberg. Reply to "Randomized trial of lobectomy versus limited resection for T1 N0 non-small cell lung cancer," 1995 article by the Lung Cancer Study Group. Ann Thorac Surg 1996. 62:1249–1250.
141. Warren, W.H., and L.P. Faber. Segmentectomy versus lobectomy in patients with stage I pulmonary carcinoma. J Thorac Cardiovasc Surg 1994. 107:1087–1094.
142. Strauss, G., et al. Extent of surgical resection influences survival in stage IA non-small cell lung cancer (NSCLC). Proc ASCO, 1998. 17:462a.
143. Landreneau, R.J., et al. Wedge resection versus lobectomy for stage I (T1 N0 M0) non-small-cell lung cancer. J Thorac Cardiovasc Surg 1997. 113:691–700.
144. Errett, L.E., et al. Wedge resection as an alternative procedure for peripheral bronchogenic carcinoma in poor-risk patients. J Thorac Cardiovasc Surg 1985. 90:656–661.
145. Pastorino, U., et al. Limited resection for stage I lung cancer. Eur J Surg Oncol 1991. 17:42–46.
146. Kodama, K., et al. Intentional limited resection for selected patients with T1 N0 M0 non-small-cell lung cancer: a single-institution study. J Thorac Cardiovasc Surg 1997. 114:347–353.
147. Crabbe, M.M., G.A. Patrissi, and L.J. Fontenelle. Minimal resection for bronchogenic carcinoma: should this be standard therapy? Chest 1989. 95:968–971.
148. Yano, T., et al. Results of a limited resection for compromised or poor-risk patients with clinical stage I non-small cell carcinoma of the lung. J Am Coll Surg 1995. 181:33–37.
149. Miller, J.I., and C.R. Hatcher Jr. Limited resection of bronchogenic carcinoma in the patient with marked impairment of pulmonary function. Ann Thorac Surg 1987. 44:340–343.
150. Jensik, R.J. The extent of resection for localized lung cancer: segmental resection, in Current Controversies in Thoracic Surgery, C.F. Kittle, ed. Philadelphia: Saunders; 1986:175–182.
151. Detterbeck, F.C., D.R. Jones, and W.K. Funkhouser Jr. Bronchioloalveolar carcinoma, in Diagnosis and Treatment of Lung Cancer: An Evidence-Based Guide for the Practicing Clinician, F.C. Detterbeck, et al., eds. Philadelphia: Saunders; 2001:394–407.
152. Sakao, Y., et al. Predictive factors for survival in surgically resected clinical IA peripheral adenocarcinoma of the lung. Ann Thorac Surg 2004. 77:1157–1161; discussion 1161–1162.
153. Kondo, T., et al. Radiologic-prognostic correlation in patients with small pulmonary adenocarcinomas. Lung Cancer 2002. 36:49–57.
154. Matsuguma, H., et al. Objective definition and measurement method of ground-glass opacity for planning limited resection in patients with clinical stage IA adenocarcinoma of the lung. Eur J Cardiothorac Surg 2004. 25:1102–1106.
155. Yoshida, J., et al. Limited resection trial for pulmonary ground-glass opacity nodules: 50-case experience. J Thorac Cardiovasc Surg 2005. 129:991–996.
156. Suzuki, K., et al. Predictors of lymph node and intrapulmonary metastasis in clinical stage IA non-small cell lung carcinoma. Ann Thorac Surg 2001. 72:352–356.
157. Koike, T., et al. Clinical analysis of small-sized peripheral lung cancer. J Thorac Cardiovasc Surg 1998. 115:1015–1020.
158. Johnson, H., and J.S. Halle. Radiotherapy for stage I, II non-small cell lung cancer, in Diagnosis and Treatment of Lung Cancer: An Evidence-Based Guide for the Practicing Clinician, F.C. Detterbeck, et al., eds. Philadelphia: Saunders; 2001:198–205.
159. Gauden, S., J. Ramsay, and L. Tripcony. The curative treatment by radiotherapy alone of stage I non-small cell carcinoma of the lung. Chest 1995. 108:1278–1282.
160. Morita, K., et al. Radical radiotherapy for medically inoperable non-small cell lung cancer in clinical stage I: a retrospective analysis of 149 patients. Radiother Oncol 1997. 42:31–36.
161. Sibley, G.S., et al. Radiotherapy alone for medically inoperable stage I non-small-cell lung cancer: the Duke experience. Int J Radiation Oncology Biol Phys 1998. 40:149–154.
162. Krol, A.D.G., et al. Local irradiation alone for peripheral stage I lung cancer: could we omit the elective regional nodal irradiation? Int J Radiat Oncol Biol Phys 1996. 34:297–302.
163. Graham, P.H., V.J. Gebski, and A.O. Langlands. Radical radiotherapy for early nonsmall cell lung cancer. Int J Radiat Oncol Biol Phys 1994. 31:261–266.
164. Sandler, H.M., W.J. Curran Jr., and A.T. Turrisi III. The influence of tumor size and pre-treatment staging on outcome following radiation therapy alone for stage I non-small cell lung cancer. Int J Radiat Oncol Biol Phys 1990. 19:9–13.
165. Kaskowitz, L., et al. Radiation therapy alone for stage I non-small cell lung cancer. Int J Radiat Oncol Biol Phys 1993. 27:517–523.
166. Hayakawa, K., et al. High-dose radiation therapy for inoperable non-small cell lung cancer without mediastinal involvement (clinical stage N0, N1). Strahlenther Onkol 1996. 172:489–495.

167. Jeremic, B., et al. Hyperfractionated radiotherapy for clinical stage II non-small cell lung cancer. Radiother Oncol 1999. 51:141–145.
168. Rosenthal, S.A., et al. Clinical stage II non-small cell lung cancer treated with radiation therapy alone: the significance of clinically staged ipsilateral hilar adenopathy (N1 disease). Cancer 1992. 70:2410–2417.
169. Noordijk, E.M., et al. Radiotherapy as an alternative to surgery in elderly patients with resectable lung cancer. Radiother Oncol 1988. 13:83–89.
170. Dosoretz, D.E., et al. Radiation therapy in the management of medically inoperable carcinoma of the lung: results and implications for future treatment strategies. Int J Radiat Oncol Biol Phys 1992. 24:3–9.
171. Jeremic, B., et al. Hyperfractionated radiotherapy alone for clinical stage I nonsmall cell lung cancer. Int J Radiat Oncol Biol Phys 1997. 38:521–525.
172. Dautzenberg, B., et al., and the Groupe d'Etude et de Traitement des Cancers Bronchiques. A controlled study of postoperative radiotherapy for patients with complete resected nonsmall cell lung carcinoma. Cancer 1999. 86:265–273.
173. PORT Meta-analysis Trialists Group. Postoperative radiotherapy in non-small-cell lung cancer: systemic review and meta-analysis of individual patient data from nine randomised controlled trials. Lancet 1998. 352:257–263.
174. Sawyer, T.E., et al. Effectiveness of postoperative irradiation in stage IIIA non-small cell lung cancer according to regression tree analyses of recurrence risks. Ann Thorac Surg 1997. 64:1402–1408.
175. Stephens, R.J., et al. The role of post-operative radiotherapy in non-small-cell lung cancer: a multicentre randomised trial in patients with pathologically staged T1-2, N1-2, M0 disease. Br J Cancer 1996. 74:632–639.
176. Socinski, M.A., F.C. Detterbeck, and J.G. Rosenman. Adjuvant therapy of resected non-small cell lung cancer, in Diagnosis and Treatment of Lung Cancer: An Evidence-Based Guide for the Practicing Clinician, F.C. Detterbeck, et al., eds. Philadelphia: Saunders; 2001:206–219.
177. Sedrakyan, A., et al. Postoperative chemotherapy for non-small cell lung cancer: a systematic review and meta-analysis. J Thorac Cardiovasc Surg 2004. 128:414–419.
178. Winton, T.L., et al. A prospective randomised trial of adjuvant venorelbine (VIN) and cisplatin (CIS) in completely resected stage 1B and II non small cell lung cancer (NSCLC) Intergroup JBR.10 [abstract]. J Clin Oncol 2004 ASCO Annu Mtg Proc 2004. 22(14S):7018.
179. Douillard, J., Rosell, R, Delena, M, et al. ANITA: Phase III adjuvant vinorelbine (N) and cisplatin (P) versus observation (OBS) in completely resected (stage I-III) non-small-cell lung cancer (NSCLC) patients (pts): final results after 70-month median follow-up. On behalf of the Adjuvant Navelbine International Trialist Association. Proc Am Soc Clin Oncol 2004. 23:615a.
180. Strauss, G.M., et al. Randomized clinical trial of adjuvant chemotherapy with paclitaxel and carboplatin following resection in Stage IB non-small cell lung cancer (NSCLC): report of Cancer and Leukemia Group B (CALGB) Protocol 9633 [abstract]. J Clin Oncol 2004 ASCO Annu Mtg Proc 2004. 22(14S):7019.
181. Scott, W.J., J. Howington, S. Feigenberg, et al. Treatment of Non-small Cell Lung Cancer—Stage I and II: ACCP Evidence-Based Clinical Practice Guideline. 2nd ed. Chest 2007;132:234–242.
182. Early Breast Cancer Trialists' Collaborative Group. Systemic treatment of early breast cancer by hormonal, cytotoxic, or immune therapy. Lancet 1992. 339:71–85.
183. International Multicentre Pooled Analysis of Colon Cancer Trials (IMPACT). Efficacy of adjuvant fluorouracil and folinic acid in colon cancer. Lancet 1995. 356:939–944.
184. Hotta, K., et al. Role of adjuvant chemotherapy in patients with resected non-small-cell lung cancer: reappraisal with a meta-analysis of randomized controlled trials. J Clin Oncol 2004. 22:3860–3867.
185. Keicho, N., et al. Phase II study of UFT in patients with advanced non-small cell lung cancer. Jpn J Clin Oncol 1986. 16:143–146.
186. Pisters, K.M.W., et al., Induction chemotherapy before surgery for early-stage lung cancer: a novel approach. J Thorac Cardiovasc Surg 2000. 119:429–439.
187. Pisters K.V., P. Bunn, et al. S9900: a phase III trial of surgery alone or surgery plus preoperative (preop) paclitaxel/carboplatin (PC) chemotherapy in early stage non-small cell lung cancer (NSCLC): preliminary results. ASCO Mtg Abstracts 2005. June 1:7012.
188. Depierre, A., et al. Preoperative chemotherapy followed by surgery compared with primary surgery in resectable stage I (exept T1N0), II, and IIIa non-small-cell lung cancer. J Clin Oncol 2002. 20:247–253.
189. Detterbeck, F.C., and D.R. Jones. Surgical treatment of stage IIIa (N2) non-small cell lung cancer, in Diagnosis and Treatment of Lung Cancer: An Evidence-Based Guide for the Practicing Clinician, F.C. Detterbeck, et al., edis. Philadelphia: Saunders; 2001:244–256.
190. Cybulsky, I.J., et al. Prognostic significance of computed tomography in resected N2 lung cancer. Ann Thorac Surg 1992. 54:533–537.
191. Maggi, G., et al. Results of surgical resection of Stage IIIA (N2) non small cell lung cancer, according to the site of the mediastinal metastases. Intern Surg 1993. 78:213–217.
192. Mountain, C.F. Surgery for stage IIIa-N2 non-small cell lung cancer. Cancer 1994. 73:2589–2598.
193. Goldstraw, P., et al. Surgical management of non-small-cell lung cancer with ipsilateral mediastinal node metastasis (N2 disease). J Thorac Cardiovasc Surg 1994. 107:19–28.
194. Daly, B.D.T., et al. N2 lung cancer: outcome in patients with false-negative computed tomographic scans of the chest. J Thorac Cardiovasc Surg 1993. 105:904–911.
195. Coughlin, M., et al. Role of mediastinoscopy in pretreatment staging of patients with primary lung cancer. Ann Thorac Surg 1985. 40:556–560.
196. Pearson, F.G., et al. Significance of positive superior mediastinal nodes identified at mediastinoscopy in patients with resectable cancer of the lung. J Thorac Cardiovasc Surg 1982. 83:1–11.
197. Vansteenkiste, J.F., et al. Survival and prognostic factors in resected N2 non-small cell lung cancer: a study of 140 cases. Ann Thorac Surg 1997. 63:1441–1450.
198. Jett, J.R., et al. Guidelines on treatment of stage IIIB non-small cell lung cancer. Chest 2003. 123(1 suppl):221S–225S.
199. Detterbeck, F.C., et al. Special treatment issues. Chest 2003. 123:244S–258S.
200. Tsuchiya, R., et al. Extended resection of the left atrium, great vessels, or both for lung cancer. Ann Thorac Surg 1994. 57:960–965.
201. de Perrot, M., et al. Long-term results after carinal resection for carcinoma: does the benefit warrant the risk? J Thorac Cardiovasc Surg 2006. 131:81–89.
202. Rendina, E.A., et al. Induction chemotherapy for T4 centrally located non-small cell lung cancer. J Thorac Cardiovasc Surg 1999. 117:225–233.
203. Hensing, T.A., J.S. Halle, and M.A. Socinki. Chemoradiotherapy for stage IIIa,b non-small cell lung cancer, in Diagnosis and Treatment of Lung Cancer: An Evidence-Based Guide for the Practicing Clinician, F.C. Detterbeck, et al., eds. Philadelphia: Saunders; 2001:291–303.
204. Albain, K.S., et al. Concurrent cisplatin/etoposide plus radiotherapy (PE + RT) for pathologic stage (pathTN) IIIB non-small cell lung cancer (NSCLC): a Southwest Oncology Group (SWOG) phase II study (S9019) [abstract]. Proc ASCO 1997. 16:446a.
205. Detterbeck, F.C. Changes in the treatment of Pancoast tumors. Ann Thorac Surg 2003. 75:1990–1997.

206. Macchiarini, P. Resection of superior sulcus carcinomas (anterior approach). Thorac Surg Clin 2004. 14:229–240.
207. Rusch, V.W., et al. Induction chemoradiation and surgical resection for non-small cell lung carcinomas of the superior sulcus: initial results of Southwest Oncology Group Trial 9416 (Intergroup Trial 0160). J Thorac Cardiovasc Surg 2001. 121:472–483.
208. Wright, C.D., et al. Induction chemoradiation compared with induction radiation for lung cancer involving the superior sulcus. Ann Thorac Surg 2002. 73:1541–1544.
209. Detterbeck, F.C. Pancoast (superior sulcus) tumors. Ann Thorac Surg 1997. 63:1810–1818.
210. Ginsberg, R.J., et al. Influence of surgical resection and brachytherapy in the management of superior sulcus tumor. Ann Thorac Surg 1994. 57:1440–1445.
211. Dillman, R.O., et al. Improved survival in stage III non-small-cell lung cancer: 7-year follow-up of Cancer and Leukemia Group B (CALGB) 8433 trial. J Natl Cancer Inst 1996. 88:1210–1215.
212. The Non-small Cell Lung Cancer Collaborative Group. Chemotherapy in non-small cell lung cancer: a meta-analysis using updated data on individual patients from 52 randomised clinical trials. Br Med J 1995. 311:899–909.
213. Marino, P., A. Preatoni, and A. Cantoni. Randomized trials of radiotherapy alone versus combined chemotherapy and radiotherapy in Stages IIIa and IIIb nonsmall cell lung cancer: a meta-analysis. Cancer 1995. 76:593–601.
214. Furuse, K., et al. and for the West Japan Lung Cancer Group, Phase III study of concurrent versus sequential thoracic radiotherapy in combination with mitomycin, vindesine, and cisplatin in unresectable stage III non-small-cell lung cancer. J Clin Oncol 1999. 17:2692–2699.
215. Curran, W.J., et al. Long-term benefit is observed in a phase III comparison of sequential versus concurrent chemo-radiation for patients with unresected stage III non small cell lung cancer: RTOG 9410. Proc Am Soc Clin Oncol 2003. 22:621a.
216. Detterbeck, F.C., and M.A. Socinski. Induction therapy and surgery for I-IIIa,b non-small cell lung cancer, in Diagnosis and Treatment of Lung Cancer: An Evidence-Based Guide for the Practicing Clinician, F.C. Detterbeck, et al., eds. Philadelphia: Saunders; 2001:257–266.
217. Siegenthaler, M.P., et al. Preoperative chemotherapy for lung cancer does not increase surgical morbidity. Ann Thorac Surg 2001. 71:1105–1112.
218. Veronesi, G., et al. Low morbidity of bronchoplastic procedures after chemotherapy for lung cancer. Lung Cancer 2002. 36:91–97.
219. Novoa, N., G. Varela, and M. Jimenez. Morbidity after surgery for non small cell lung carcinoma is not related to neoadjuvant chemotherapy. Eur J Cardiothorac Surg 2001. 20:700–704.
220. Rosell, R., et al. A randomized trial comparing preoperative chemotherapy plus surgery with surgery alone in patients with non-small-cell lung cancer. N Engl J Med 1994. 330:153–158.
221. Roth, J.A., et al. A randomized trial comparing perioperative chemotherapy and surgery with surgery alone in resectable stage IIIA non-small-cell lung cancer. J Natl Cancer Inst 1994. 86:673–680.
222. Wagner, H., Jr., S. Piantadosi, and J.C. Ruckdeschel. Randomized phase II evaluation of preoperative radiation therapy and preoperative chemotherapy with mitomycin, vinblastine, and cisplatin in patients with technically unresectable stage IIIA and IIIB non-small cell cancer of the lung (Lung Cancer Study Group 881). Chest 1994. 106(suppl):348S–354S.
223. Sonett, J.R., et al. Pulmonary resection after curative intent radiotherapy (>59 Gy) and concurrent chemotherapy in non-small-cell lung cancer. Ann Thorac Surg 2004. 78:1200–1205; discussion 1206.
224. Roberts, J., et al. Induction chemotherapy increases perioperative complications in patients undergoing resection for non-small cell lung cancer. Ann Thor Surg, 2001. 72:885–888.
225. Semik, M., et al. Preoperative chemotherapy with and without additional radiochemotherapy: benefit and risk for surgery of stage III non-small cell lung cancer. Eur J Cardiothorac Surg 2004. 26:1205–1210.
226. West, H and Albain, K. Current standards and ongoing controversies in the management of locally advanced non-small cell lung cancer. Semin Oncol 2005. 32:284–292.
227. Perez, C.A., et al. A prospective randomized study of various irradiation doses and fractionation schedules in the treatment of inoperable non-oat-cell carcinoma of the lung: preliminary report by the Radiation Therapy Oncology Group. Cancer 1980. 45:2744–2753.
228. Perez, C.A., et al. Long-term observations of the patterns of failure in patients with unresectable non-oat cell carcinoma of the lung treated with definitive radiotherapy: report by the Radiation Therapy Oncology Group. Cancer 1987. 59:1874–1881.
229. Arriagada, R., et al. ASTRO Plenary: effect of chemotherapy on locally advanced non-small cell lung carcinoma: a randomized study of 353 patients. Int J Radiat Oncol Biol Phys 1991. 20:1183–1190.
230. Clark, J.A., J.G. Rosenman, and F.C. Detterbeck. Radiotherapy alone for stage IIIa,b non-small cell lung cancer, in Diagnosis and Treatment of Lung Cancer: An Evidence-Based Guide for the Practicing Clinician, F.C. Detterbeck, et al., eds. Philadelphia: Saunders; 2001:257–266.
231. Rosenman, J.G., et al. Image registration: an essential part of radiation therapy treatment planning. Int J Radiat Oncol Biol Phys 1998. 40:197–205.
232. Rosenman, J., M.B. Hazuka, and M.K. Martel. Three-dimensional treatment planning in lung cancer radiotherapy, in Lung Cancer: Principles and Practice, Pass, H.I., ed. Philadelphia: Lippincott-Raven; 1996:685–696.
233. Saunders, M., et al. Continuous, hyperfractionated, accelerated radiotherapy (CHART) versus conventional radiotherapy in non-small cell lung cancer: mature data from the randomised multicentre trial. Radiother Oncol 1999. 52:137–148.
234. Saunders, M., et al. Continuous hyperfractionated accelerated radiotherapy (CHART) versus conventional radiotherapy in non-small-cell lung cancer: a randomised multicentre trial. Lancet 1997. 350:161–165.
235. Belani, C.P., et al. Phase III study of the Eastern Cooperative Oncology Group (ECOG 2597): induction chemotherapy followed by either standard thoracic radiotherapy or hyperfractionated accelerated radiotherapy for patients with unresectable stage IIIA and B non-small-cell lung cancer 10.1200/JCO.2005.09.108. J Clin Oncol 2005. 23:3760–3767.
236. Komaki, R., et al. Induction cisplatin/vinblastine and irradiation versus irradiation in unresectable squamous cell lung cancer: failure patterns by cell type in RTOG 88-08/ECOG 4588. Int J Radiat Oncol Biol Phys 1997. 39:537–544.
237. Sause, W., et al. Final results of phase III trial in regionally advanced unresectable non-small cell lung cancer (Radiation Therapy Oncology Group, Eastern Cooperative Oncology Group, and Southwest Oncology Group). Chest 2000. 117:358–364.
238. Socinski, M.A., et al. Dose-escalating conformal thoracic radiation therapy with induction and concurrent carboplatin/paclitaxel in unresectable stage IIIA/B nonsmall cell lung carcinoma. Cancer 2001. 92:1213–1223.
239. Socinski, M.A., et al. Induction and concurrent chemotherapy with high-dose thoracic conformal radiation therapy in unresectable stage IIIA and IIIB non-small-cell lung cancer: a dose-escalation phase I trial. J Clin Oncol 2004. 22:4341–4350.
240. Miller, K.L., et al. Bronchial stenosis: an underreported complication of high-dose external beam radiotherapy for lung cancer? Int J Radiat Oncol Biol Phys 2005. 61:64–69.

241. Marks, L.B., et al. Carboplatin/paclitaxel or carboplatin/vinorelbine followed by accelerated hyperfractionated conformal radiation therapy: report of a prospective phase I dose escalation trial from the Carolina Conformal Therapy Consortium. J Clin Oncol 2004. 22:4329–4340.
242. Hayman, J.A., et al. Dose escalation in non-small-cell lung cancer using three-dimensional conformal radiation therapy: update of a phase I trial. J Clin Oncol 2001. 19:127–136.
243. Wu, K.-L., et al. Three-dimensional conformal radiation therapy for non-small-cell lung cancer: a phase I/II dose escalation clinical trial. Int J Radiat Oncol Biol Phys 2003. 57:1336–1344.
244. Blackstock, A.W., et al. Induction (Ind) plus concurrent (Con) chemotherapy with high-dose (74 Gy) three-dimensional (3-D) thoracic radiotherapy (TRT) in stage III non-small cell lung cancer (NSCLC): preliminary report of Cancer and Leukemia Group B (CALGB) 30105. J Clin Oncol 2006 ASCO Annu Mtg Proc Part I 2006. 24(18S):7042.
245. O'Reilly, M. Radiation combined with antiangiogenic and antivascular agents. Semin Radiat Oncol 2006. 16:45–50.
246. Spiro, S.G., et al. Chemotherapy versus supportive care in advanced non-small cell lung cancer: improved survival without detriment to quality of life. Thorax 2004. 59:828–836.
247. Chu, Q., et al. Taxanes as first-line therapy for advanced non-small cell lung cancer: a systematic review and practice guideline. Lung Cancer 2005. 50:355–374.
248. Le Chevalier, T., et al. Efficacy of gemcitabine plus platinum chemotherapy compared with other platinum containing regimens in advanced non-small-cell lung cancer: a meta-analysis of survival outcomes. Lung Cancer 2005. 47:69–80.
249. Smit, E.F., et al. Three-arm randomized study of two cisplatin-based regimens and paclitaxel plus gemcitabine in advanced non-small-cell lung cancer: a phase III trial of the European Organization for Research and Treatment of Cancer Lung Cancer Group—EORTC 08975 10.1200/JCO.2003.03.195. J Clin Oncol 2003. 21:3909–3917.
250. Schiller, J.H., et al. Comparison of four chemotherapy regimens for advanced non-small-cell lung cancer 10.1056/NEJMoa011954. N Engl J Med 2002. 346:92–98.
251. Fossella, F., et al. Randomized, multinational, phase III study of docetaxel plus platinum combinations versus vinorelbine plus cisplatin for advanced non-small-cell lung cancer: the TAX 326 Study Group 10.1200/JCO.2003.12.046. J Clin Oncol 2003. 21:3016–3024.
252. Kelly, K., et al. Randomized phase III trial of paclitaxel plus carboplatin versus vinorelbine plus cisplatin in the treatment of patients with advanced non-small-cell lung cancer: a Southwest Oncology Group Trial. J Clin Oncol 2001. 19:3210–3218.
253. Scagliotti, G.V., et al. Phase III randomized trial comparing three platinum-based doublets in advanced non-small-cell lung cancer 10.1200/JCO.2002.02.068. J Clin Oncol 2002. 20:4285–4291.
254. Pfister, D.G., et al. American Society of Clinical Oncology Treatment of Unresectable Non-Small-Cell Lung Cancer Guideline: update 2003 10.1200/JCO.2004.09.053. J Clin Oncol 2004. 22:330–353.
255. Westeel, V., et al. Randomized study of maintenance vinorelbine in responders with advanced non-small-cell lung cancer 10.1093/jnci/dji096. J Natl Cancer Inst 2005. 97:499–506.
256. Smith, I.E., et al. Duration of chemotherapy in advanced non-small-cell lung cancer: a randomized trial of three versus six courses of mitomycin, vinblastine, and cisplatin. J Clin Oncol 2001. 19:1336–1343.
257. Socinski, M.A., et al. Phase III trial comparing a defined duration of therapy versus continuous therapy followed by second-line therapy in advanced-stage IIIB/IV non-small-cell lung cancer 10.1200/JCO.20.5.1335. J Clin Oncol 2002. 20:1335–1343.
258. Gatzemeier, U., et al. Results of a phase III trial of erlotinib (OSI-774) combined with cisplatin and gemcitabine (GC) chemotherapy in advanced non-small cell lung cancer (NSCLC). Proc Am Soc Clin Oncol 2004. 22:14S [abstract 7010].
259. Herbst, R.S., et al. Gefitinib in combination with paclitaxel and carboplatin in advanced non-small-cell lung cancer: a phase III trial—INTACT 2 10.1200/JCO.2004.07.215. J Clin Oncol 2004. 22:785–794.
260. Herbst, R.S., et al. TRIBUTE: a phase III trial of erlotinib hydrochloride (OSI-774) combined with carboplatin and paclitaxel chemotherapy in advanced non-small-cell lung cancer 10.1200/JCO.2005.02.840. J Clin Oncol 2005. 23:5892–5899.
261. Giaccone, G., et al. Gefitinib in combination with gemcitabine and cisplatin in advanced non-small-cell lung cancer: a phase III trial—INTACT 1 10.1200/JCO.2004.08.001. J Clin Oncol 2004. 22:777–784.
262. Sandler, A.B., et al. Randomized phase II/III trial of paclitaxel (P) plus carboplatin (C) with or without bevacizumab (NSC 704865) in patients with advanced non-squamous non-small cell lung cancer (NSCLC): an Eastern Cooperative Oncology Group (ECOG) trial— E4599. J Clin Oncol 2005 ASCO Annu Mtg Proc 2005. 23(16S), part I of II (June 1 supplement):4.
263. Shepherd, F.A., et al. Prospective randomized trial of docetaxel versus best supportive care in patients with non-small-cell lung cancer previously treated with platinum-based chemotherapy. J Clin Oncol 2000. 18:2095–2103.
264. Dancey, J., et al. Quality of life assessment of second-line docetaxel versus best supportive care in patients with non-small-cell lung cancer previously treated with platinum-based chemotherapy: results of a prospective, randomized phase III trial. Lung Cancer 2004. 43:183–194.
265. Fossella, F.V., et al. Randomized phase III trial of docetaxel versus vinorelbine or ifosfamide in patients with advanced non-small-cell lung cancer previously treated with platinum-containing chemotherapy regimens. J Clin Oncol 2000. 18:2354–2362.
266. Hanna, N., et al. Randomized phase III trial of pemetrexed versus docetaxel in patients with non-small-cell lung cancer previously treated with chemotherapy 10.1200/JCO.2004.08.163. J Clin Oncol 2004. 22:1589–1597.
267. Shepherd, F.A., et al. Erlotinib in previously treated non-small-cell lung cancer 10.1056/NEJMoa050753. N Engl J Med 2005. 353:123–132.
268. Lilenbaum, R.C., et al. Single-agent versus combination chemotherapy in advanced non-small-cell lung cancer: the cancer and leukemia group B (study 9730). J Clin Oncol 2005. 23:190–196.
269. Langer, C.J., et al. O-52 ECOG 1599: randomized phase II study of paclitaxel/carboplatin versus cisplatin/gemcitabine in performance status (PS) 2 patients with treatment-naive advanced NSCLC. Lung Cancer 2003. 41(suppl. 2):S18.
270. Gridelli, C., et al. Treatment of advanced non-small-cell lung cancer patients with ECOG performance status 2: results of an European Experts Panel 10.1093/annonc/mdh087. Ann Oncol 2004. 15:419–426.
271. Kelly, K., et al. Should older patients (Pts) receive combination chemotherapy for advanced stage non-small cell lung cancer (NSCLC)? An analysis of Southwest Oncology Trials 9509 and 9308. Proc Am Soc Clin Oncol 2001. 20:329a [abstract 1313].
272. Ramalingam, S., et al. Treatment of elderly non-small cell lung cancer (NSCLC) patients with three different schedules of weekly paclitaxel in combination with carboplatin: sub-analysis of a randomized trial. Proc Am Soc Clin Oncol 2003. 22:670 [abstract 2693].
273. Langer, C.J., et al. Age-specific subanalysis of ECOG 1594: fit elderly patients (70–80 years) with NSCLC do as well as younger patients (<70). Proc Am Soc Clin Oncol 2003. 22:639 [abstract 2571].
274. Rocha Lima, C.M.S., et al. Therapy choices among older patients with lung carcinoma. Cancer 2002. 94:181–187.

275. Kosty, M.P., et al. Cisplatin, vinblastine, and hydrazine sulfate in advanced, non-small-cell lung cancer: a randomized placebo-controlled, double-blind phase III study of the Cancer and Leukemia Group B. J Clin Oncol 1994. 12:1113–1120.
276. Langer, C.J., et al. Cisplatin-based therapy for elderly patients with advanced non-small-cell lung cancer: implications of Eastern Cooperative Oncology Group 5592, a randomized trial 10.1093/jnci/94.3.173. J Natl Cancer Inst 2002. 94:173–181.
277. The Elderly Lung Cancer Vinorelbine Italian Study Group. Effects of vinorelbine on quality of life and survival in elderly patients with advanced non-small-cell lung cancer. J Natl Cancer Inst 1999. 91:66–72.
278. Gridelli, C., et al. Chemotherapy for elderly patients with advanced non-small-cell lung cancer: the Multicenter Italian Lung Cancer in the Elderly Study (MILES) phase III randomized trial 10.1093/jnci/95.5.362. J Natl Cancer Inst 2003. 95:362–372.
279. Detterbeck, F.C., M.S. Bleiweis, and M.G. Ewend. Surgical treatment of stage IV non-small cell lung cancer, in Diagnosis and Treatment of Lung Cancer: An Evidence-Based Guide for the Practicing Clinician, F.C. Detterbeck, et al., eds. Philadelphia: Saunders; 2001:326–338.
280. Wronski, M., et al. Survival after surgical treatment of brain metastases from lung cancer: a follow-up study of 231 patients treated between 1976 and 1991. J Neurosurg 1995. 83:605–616.
281. Vecht, C.J., et al. Treatment of single brain metastasis: radiotherapy alone or combined with neurosurgery? Ann Neurol 1993. 33:583–590.
282. Mintz, A.H., et al. A randomized trial to assess the efficacy of surgery in addition to radiotherapy in patients with a single cerebral metastasis. Cancer 1996. 78:1470–1476.
283. Patchell, R.A., et al. Direct decompressive surgical resection in the treatment of spinal cord compression caused by metastatic cancer: a randomised trial. Lancet 2005. 366:643–648.
284. American Cancer Society. Cancer Facts and Figures 2006. Atlanta: American Cancer Society; 2006.
285. Morris, D.E., M.A. Socinski, and F.C. Detterbeck. Limited stage small cell lung cancer, in Diagnosis and Treatment of Lung Cancer: An Evidence-Based Guide for the Practicing Clinician, F.C. Detterbeck, et al., eds. Philadelphia: Saunders; 2001:341–359.
286. Warde, P., and D. Payne. Does thoracic irradiation improve survival and local control in limited-stage small cell carcinoma of the lung? A meta-analysis. J Clin Oncol 1992. 10:890–895.
287. Pignon, J.P., R. Arriagada, and D.C. Ihde. A meta-analysis of thoracic radiotherapy for small-cell lung cancer. N Engl J Med 1992. 327:1618–1624.
288. Bogart, J., J.E. Herndon, 2nd, A.P. Lyss, et al. 70 Gy thoracic radiotherapy is feasible concurrent with chemotherapy for limited-stage small-cell lung cancer: analysis of Cancer and Leukemia Group B study 39808. Int J Radiat Oncol Biol Phys 2004. 59:460.
289. Fried, D., et al. Systematic review evaluating the timing of thoracic radiation therapy in combined modality therapy for limited-stage small-cell lung cancer. J Clin Oncol 2004. 22:4785–4793.
290. Turrisi, A., et al. Twice-daily compared with once-daily thoracic radiotherapy in limited small-cell lung cancer treated concurrently with cisplatin and etoposide. N Engl J Med 1999. 340:265–271.
291. Takada M., F.M., M. Kawahara, et al. Phase III study of concurrent versus sequential thoracic radiotherapy in combination with cisplatin and etoposide for limited-stage small-cell lung cancer: results of the Japan Clinical Oncology Group study 9104. J Clin Oncol 2002. 20:3054–3060.
292. Sundstrom, S., et al. Cisplatin and etoposide regimen is superior to cyclophosphamide, epirubicin, and vincristine regimen in small-cell lung cancer: results from a randomized phase III trial with 5 years' follow-up. J Clin Oncol 2002. 20:4665.
293. Mascaux, C., et al. A systematic review of the role of etoposide and cisplatin in the chemotherapy of small cell lung cancer with methodology assessment and meta-analysis. European Lung Cancer Working Party (ELCWP). Lung Cancer 2000. 30:23–36.
294. Arriagada, R., et al. Prophylactic cranial irradiation for patients with small-cell lung cancer in complete remission. J Natl Cancer Inst 1995. 87:183–190.
295. Gregor, A., et al. Prophylactic cranial irradiation is indicated following complete response to induction therapy in small cell lung cancer: results of a multicentre randomised trial. United Kingdom Coordinating Committee for Cancer Research (UKCCCR) and the European Organization for Research and Treatment of Cancer (EORTC). Eur J Cancer 1997. 33:1717–1719.
296. Aupérin, A., et al. Prophylactic cranial irradiation for patients with small-cell lung cancer in complete remission. N Engl J Med 1999. 341:476–484.
297. Gillenwater, H.H., and M.A. Socinski. Extensive stage small cell lung cancer, in Diagnosis and Treatment of Lung Cancer: An Evidence-Based Guide for the Practicing Clinician, F.C. Detterbeck et al., eds. Philadelphia: Saunders; 2001:360–375.
298. Murray, N., et al. Randomized study of CODE versus alternating CAV/EP for extensive-stage small-cell lung cancer: an intergroup study of the National Cancer Institute of Canada Clinical Trials Group and the Southwest Oncology Group. J Clin Oncol 1999. 17:2300.
299. Loehrer, P.J., et al. Cisplatin plus etoposide with and without ifosfamide in extensive small-cell lung cancer: a Hoosier Oncology Group study. J Clin Oncol 1995. 13:2594–2599.
300. Niell, H.B., et al. Randomized phase III intergroup trial of etoposide and cisplatin with or without paclitaxel and granulocyte colony-stimulating factor in patients with extensive-stage small-cell lung cancer: Cancer and Leukemia Group B Trial 9732 10.1200/JCO.2005.09.071. J Clin Oncol 2005. 23:3752–3759.
301. Sculier, J.P., M. Paesmans, and J. Lecomte. A three-arm phase III randomised trial assessing, in patients with extensive-disease small-cell lung cancer, accelerated chemotherapy with support of haematological growth factor or oral antibiotics. Br J Cancer 2001. 85:1444–1451.
302. Thatcher, N., et al. Ifosfamide, carboplatin, and etoposide with midcycle vincristine versus standard chemotherapy in patients with small-cell lung cancer and good performance status: clinical and quality-of-life results of the British Medical Research Council Multicenter Randomized LU21 Trial 10.1200/JCO.2004.00.9969. J Clin Oncol 2005. 23:8371–8379.
303. Noda, K., Nishiwaki, Y, Kawahara, M, et al. Irinotecan plus cisplatin compared with etoposide plus cisplatin for extensive small-cell lung cancer. N Engl J Med 2002. 346:85.
304. Hanna, N., L. Einhorn, A. Sandler, et al. Randomized, phase III trial comparing irinotecan/cisplatin (IP) with etoposide/cisplatin (EP) in patients (pts) with previously untreated, extensive-stage (ES) small cell lung cancer (SCLC) [abstract]. J Clin Oncol 2005. 23:622s.
305. von Pawel, J., et al. Topotecan versus cyclophosphamide, doxorubicin, and vincristine for the treatment of recurrent small-cell lung cancer. J Clin Oncol 1999. 17:658–667.
306. Lad, T., et al. A prospective randomized trial to determine the benefit of surgical resection of residual disease following response of small cell lung cancer to combination chemotherapy. Chest 1994. 106(suppl):320S–323S.
307. Landis, S.H., et al. Cancer statistics 1999. CA-Cancer J Clinicians 1999. 49:8–31.
308. AJCC Cancer Stagina Manual, 6th ed. New York: Springer-Verlag; 2002. www.springer.ny.com.
309. Weisenburger, T.H., M. Gail, and The Lung Cancer Study Group. Effects of postoperative mediastinal radiation on completely resected stage II and stage III epidermoid cancer of the lung. N Engl J Med 1986. 315:1377–1381.

310. Mayer, R., et al. Postoperative radiotherapy in radically resected non-small cell lung cancer. Chest 1997. 112:954–959.
311. Van Houtte, P., et al. Postoperative radiation therapy in lung cancer: a controlled trial after resection of curative design. Int J Radiat Oncol Biol Phys 1980. 6:983–986.
312. Lafitte, J.J., et al. Postresection irradiation for T2 N0 M0 non-small cell carcinoma: a prospective, randomized study. Ann Thorac Surg 1996. 62:830–834.
313. Debevec, M., et al. Postoperative radiotherapy for radically resected N2 non-small-cell cancer (NSCLC): randomised clinical study 1988–1992. Lung Cancer 1996. 14:99–107.
314. Arriagada, R., et al. Cisplatin-based adjuvant chemotherapy in patients with completely resected non-small-cell lung cancer. N Engl J Med 2004. 350:351–360.
315. Scagliotti, G.V., et al. Randomized study of adjuvant chemotherapy for completely resected stage I, II, or IIIA non-small-cell Lung cancer. J Natl Cancer Inst 2003. 95:1453–1461.
316. Waller, D., et al. The Big Lung Trial (BLT): determining the value of cisplatin-based chemotherapy for all patients with non-small cell lung cancer (NSCLC). Preliminary results in the surgical setting [abstract]. Proc ASCO 2003. 22:632.
317. Keller, S.M., et al. A randomized trial of postoperative adjuvant therapy in patients with completely resected stage II or IIIa non-small-cell lung cancer. N Engl J Med 2000. 343:1217–1222.
318. Dautzenberg, B., et al. Adjuvant radiotherapy versus combined sequential chemotherapy followed by radiotherapy in the treatment of resected nonsmall cell lung carcinoma: a randomized trial of 267 patients. Cancer 1995. 76:779–786.
319. Imaizumi, M., et al., for the Study Group of Adjuvant Chemotherapy for Lung Cancer (Chubu, Japan). A randomized trial of postoperative adjuvant chemotherapy in non-small cell lung cancer (the second cooperative study). Eur J Surg Oncol 1995. 21:69–77.
320. Feld, R., et al. Adjuvant chemotherapy with cyclophosphamide, doxorubicin, and cisplatin in patients with completely resected stage I non-small-cell lung cancer (LCSG 801). J Natl Cancer Inst 1993. 85:299–306.
321. Wada, H., et al., and the West Japan Study Group for Lung Cancer Surgery (WJSG). Postoperative adjuvant chemotherapy with PVM (cisplatin + mitomycin C) and UFT (uracil + tegaful) in resected stage I–II NSCLC (non-small cell lung cancer): a randomized clinical trial. Eur J Cardiothorac Surg 1999. 15:438–443.
322. Wada, H., et al. Adjuvant chemotherapy after complete resection in non-small-cell lung cancer. J Clin Oncol 1996. 14:1048–1054.
323. Ohta, M., et al. Adjuvant chemotherapy for completely resected stage III non-small-cell lung cancer: results of a randomized prospective study. J Thorac Cardiovasc Surg 1993. 106:703–708.
324. Lad, T., et al. The benefit of adjuvant treatment for resected locally advanced non-small-cell lung cancer. J Clin Oncol 1988. 6:9–17.
325. Wolf, M., et al. Randomized phase III trial of adjuvant radiotherapy versus adjuvant chemotherapy followed by radiotherapy in patients with N2 positive non small cell lung cancer (NSCLC) [abstract]. Proc ASCO 2001. 20:31.
326. Holmes, E.C., et al. for the Lung Cancer Study Group, Surgical adjuvant therapy for stage II and stage III adenocarcinoma and large-cell undifferentiated carcinoma. J Clin Oncol 1986. 4:710–715.
327. Holmes, E.C. Postoperative chemotherapy for non-small-cell lung cancer. Chest 1993. 103:30S–34S.
328. Tada, H., et al. A randomized trial comparing adjuvant chemotherapy versus surgery alone for completely resected pN2 non-small cell lung cancer (JCOG9304). Lung Cancer 2004. 43: 167–173.
329. Niiranen, A., et al. Adjuvant chemotherapy after radical surgery for non-small cell lung cancer: a randomized study. J Clin Oncol 1992. 10:1927–1932.
330. Imaizumi, M. A randomized trial of postoperative adjuvant chemotherapy for p-stage I non-small cell lung cancer (fourth cooperative study) [abstract]. Lung Cancer 2003. 41 (suppl 2): S54.
331. Tada, H., et al. Randomized study of adjuvant chemotherapy for completely resected non-small cell lung cancer: lack of prognostic significance in DNA ploidy pattern at adjuvant setting [abstract]. Proc Am Soc Clin Oncol 2002. 21:313a.
332. Ichinose, Y., et al. Postoperative adjuvant chemotherapy in non-small cell lung cancer: prognostic value of DNA ploidy and postrecurrent survival. J Surg Oncol 1991. 46:15–20.
333. Pisters, K.M.W., et al. Randomized trial comparing postoperative chemotherapy with vindesine and cisplatin plus thoracic irradiation with irradiation alone in stage III (N2) non-small cell lung cancer. J Surg Oncol 1994. 56:236–241.
334. Xu, G., T. Rong, and P. Lin. Adjuvant chemotherapy following radical surgery for non-small-cell lung cancer: a randomized study on 70 patients. Chin Med J (Engl) 2000. 113:617–620.
335. Kimura, H., and Y. Yamaguchi. Adjuvant chemo-immunotherapy after curative resection of stage II and IIIA primary lung cancer. Lung Cancer 1996. 14:301–314.
336. Mineo, T.C., et al. Postoperative adjuvant therapy for stage IB non-small-cell lung cancer. Eur J Cardiothorac Surg 2001. 20:378–384.
337. Park, J.H., et al. Postoperative adjuvant therapy for stage II non-small-cell lung cancer. Ann Thorac Surg 1999. 68:1821–1826.
338. Kato, H., et al. A randomized trial of adjuvant chemotherapy with uracil-tegafur for adenocarcinoma of the lung. N Engl J Med 2004. 350:1713–1721.
339. Nakagawa, M., et al. A randomized phase III trial of adjuvant chemotherapy with UFT for completely resected pathological stage I non-small-cell lung cancer: the West Japan Study Group for Lung Cancer Surgery (WJSG)—the fourth study 10.1093/annonc/mdi008. Ann Oncol 2005. 16:75–80.
340. Endo, C., et al. A randomized trial of postoperative UFT therapy in p stage I, II non-small cell lung cancer: North-east Japan Study Group for Lung Cancer Surgery. Lung Cancer 2003. 40:181–186.
341. Vogt-Moykopf, I., et al. Bronchoplastic techniques for lung resection, in Glenn's Thoracic and Cardiovascular Surgery, G.A. Baue et al., eds. East Norwalk, CT: Appleton-Lange; 1991:403–417.
342. Dartevelle, P.G. Extended operations for the treatment of lung cancer. Ann Thorac Surg 1997. 63:12–19.
343. Deslauriers, J., M. Beaulieu, and A. McClish. Tracheal sleeve pneumonectomy, in General Thoracic Surgery, Shields TW, ed. Philadelphia: Lea and Febiger; 1989:382–387.
344. Mathisen, D.J., and H.C. Grillo. Carinal resection for bronchogenic cancer. J Thorac Cardiovasc Surg 1991. 102:16–23.
345. Jensik, R.J., et al. Survival in patients undergoing tracheal sleeve pneumonectomy for bronchogenic carcinoma. J Thorac Cardiovasc Surg 1982. 84:489–496.
346. Maeda, M., et al. Operative approaches for left-sided carinoplasty. Ann Thorac Surg 1993. 56:441–446.
347. Roviaro, G.C., F. Varoli, and C. Rebuffat. Tracheal sleeve pneumonectomy for bronchogenic carcinoma. J Thorac Cardiovasc Surg 1994. 107:13–18.
348. Tsuchiya, R., et al. Resection of tracheal carina for lung cancer. J Thorac Cardiovasc Surg 1990. 99:779–787.
349. Mitchell, J.D., et al. Resection for bronchogenic carcinoma involving the carina: long-term results and effect of nodal status on outcome. J Thorac Cardiovasc Surg 2001. 121:465–471.
350. Porhanov, V.A., et al. Indications and results of sleeve carinal resection. Eur J Cardiothorac Surg 2002. 22:685–694.

351. Regnard, J.-F., et al. Resection for tumors with carinal involvement: technical aspects, results, and prognostic factors. Ann Thorac Surg 2005. 80:1841–1846.
352. Fukuse, T., H. Wada, and S. Hitomi. Extended operation for non-small cell lung cancer invading great vessels and left atrium. Eur J Cardiothorac Surg 1997. 11:664–669.
353. Thomas, P., et al. Extended operation for lung cancer invading the superior vena cava. Eur J Cardiothorac Surg 1994. 8:177–182.
354. Spaggiari, L., et al. Extended resections for bronchogenic carcinoma invading the superior vena cava system. Ann Thorac Surg 2000. 69:233–236.
355. Spaggiari, L., et al. Results of superior vena cava resection for lung cancer. Analysis of prognostic factors. Lung Cancer 2004. 44:339–346.
356. Bernard, A., et al. Pneumonectomy for malignant disease: factors affecting early morbidity and mortality. J Thorac Cardiovasc Surg 2001. 121:1076–1082.
357. Burt, M.E., et al. Results of surgical treatment of stage III lung cancer invading the mediastinum. Surg Clin N Am, 1987. 67:987–1000.
358. Shirakusa, T., and M. Kimura. Partial atrial resection in advanced lung carcinoma with and without cardiopulmonary bypass. Thorax 1991. 46:484–487.
359. Sellman, M., A. Henze, and A. Peterffy. Extended intrathoracic resection for lung cancer: follow-up of 49 cases. Scand J Thorac Cardiovasc Surg 1987. 21:69–72.
360. Ratto, G.B., et al. Twelve-year experience with left atrial resection in the treatment of non-small cell lung cancer. Ann Thorac Surg 2004. 78:234–237.
361. DeMeester, T.R., et al. Management of tumor adherent to the vertebral column. J Thorac Cardiovasc Surg 1989. 97:373–378.
362. Grunenwald, D.H., et al. Radical en bloc resection for lung cancer invading the spine. J Thorac Cardiovasc Surg 2002. 123:271–279.
363. Gandhi, S., et al. A multidisciplinary surgical approach to superior sulcus tumors with vertebral invasion. Ann Thorac Surg 1999. 68:1778–1785.
364. Ohta, M., et al. Surgical resection for lung cancer with infiltration of the thoracic aorta. J Thorac Cardiovasc Surg 2005. 129:804–808.
365. Shiraishi, T., et al. Extended resection of T4 lung cancer with invasion of the aorta: is it justified? Thorac Cardiovasc Surg 2005:375–379.
366. Sause, W.T., et al. Radiation Therapy Oncology Group (RTOG) 88-08 and Eastern Cooperative Oncology Group (ECOG) 4588: preliminary results of a phase III trial in regionally advanced, unresectable non-small-cell lung cancer. J Natl Cancer Inst 1995. 87:198–205.
367. Cullen, M.H., et al. Mitomycin, ifosfamide, and cisplatin in unresectable non-small-cell lung cancer: effects on survival and quality of life. J Clin Oncol 1999. 17:3188–3194.
368. Le Chevalier, T., et al. Radiotherapy alone versus combined chemotherapy and radiotherapy in nonresectable non-small-cell lung cancer: first analysis of a randomized trial in 353 patients. J Natl Cancer Inst 1991. 83:417–423.
369. Le Chevalier, T., et al. Significant effect of adjuvant chemotherapy on survival in locally advanced non-small-cell lung carcinoma. J Natl Cancer Inst, 1992. 84:58.
370. Mattson, K., et al. Inoperable non-small cell lung cancer: radiation with or without chemotherapy. Eur J Cancer Clin Oncol 1988. 24:477–482.
371. Kim, T.-Y.M.D.Y., H. Sung Hyun, S.H. Lee, et al. A phase III randomized trial of combined chemoradiotherapy versus radiotherapy alone in locally advanced non-small-cell lung cancer. Am J Clin Oncol 2002. 25:238–243.
372. Gregor, A., et al. Radical radiotherapy and chemotherapy in localized inoperable non-small-cell lung cancer: a randomized trial. J Natl Cancer Inst 1993. 85:997–999.
373. Planting, A., et al. A randomized study of high-dose split course radiotherapy preceded by high-dose chemotherapy versus high-dose radiotherapy only in locally advanced non-small-cell lung cancer: An EORTC Lung Cancer Cooperative Group trial. Ann Oncol 1996. 7:139–144.
374. Crino, L., et al. Induction chemotherapy plus high-dose radiotherapy versus radiotherapy alone in locally advanced unresectable non-small-cell lung cancer. Ann Oncol 1993. 4:847–851.
375. Van Houtte, P., et al. Induction chemotherapy with cisplatin, etoposide and vindesine before radiation therapy for nonsmall-cell lung cancer: a randomized study, in Treatment Modalities in Lung Cancer: Antibiotic Chemotherapy, R. Arriagada, ed. Basel: Karger; 1988:131–137.
376. Schaake-Koning, C., et al. Effects of concomitant cisplatin and radiotherapy on inoperable non-small-cell lung cancer. N Engl J Med 1992. 326:524–530.
377. Ansari, R., et al. A phase III study of thoracic irradiation with or without concomitant cisplatin in locoregional unresectable non small cell lung cancer (NSCLC): a Hoosier Oncology Group (HOG) protocol. Proc ASCO 1991. 10:241.
378. Blanke, C., et al. Phase III trial of thoracic irradiation with or without cisplatin for locally advanced unresectable non-small-cell lung cancer: a Hoosier Oncology Group protocol. J Clin Oncol 1995. 13:1425–1429.
379. Cakir, S., and I. Egehan. A randomised clinical trial of radiotherapy plus cisplatin versus radiotherapy alone in stage III non-small cell lung cancer. Lung Cancer 2004. 43:309–316.
380. Trovo, M.G., et al. Radiotherapy versus radiotherapy enhanced by cisplatin in stage III non-small cell lung cancer. Int J Radiation Oncol Biol Phys 1992. 24:11–15.
381. Groen, H.J.M., et al. Continuously infused carboplatin used as radiosensitizer in locally unresectable non-small-cell lung cancer: a multicenter phase III study 10.1093/annonc/mdh100. Ann Oncol 2004. 15:427–432.
382. Jeremic, B., et al. Randomized trial of hyperfractionated radiation therapy with or without concurrent chemotherapy for stage III non-small-cell lung cancer. J Clin Oncol 1995. 13:452–458.
383. Soresi, E., et al. A randomized clinical trial comparing radiation therapy versus radiation therapy plus cis-dichlorodiammine platinum (II) in the treatment of locally advanced non-small cell lung cancer. Semin Oncol 1988. 15:20–25.
384. Fournel, P., et al. Randomized phase III trial of sequential chemoradiotherapy compared with concurrent chemoradiotherapy in locally advanced non-small-cell lung cancer: Groupe Lyon-Saint-Etienne d'Oncologie Thoracique-Groupe Francais de Pneumo-Cancerologie NPC 95-01 Study 10.1200/JCO.2005.03.070. J Clin Oncol 2005. 23:5910–5917.
385. Belani, C.P., et al. Combined chemoradiotherapy regimens of paclitaxel and carboplatin for locally advanced non-small-cell lung cancer: a randomized phase II locally advanced multimodality protocol 10.1200/JCO.2005.55.405. J Clin Oncol 2005. 23:5883–5891.
386. Zatloukal, P., et al. Concurrent versus sequential chemoradiotherapy with cisplatin and vinorelbine in locally advanced non-small cell lung cancer: a randomized study. 2004. 46:87–98.
387. Thongprasert, S., et al. Relationship between quality of life and clinical outcomes in advanced non-small cell lung cancer: best supportive care (BSC) versus BSC plus chemotherapy. Lung Cancer 1999. 24:17–24.
388. Woods, R.L., et al. A randomised trial of cisplatin and vindesine versus supportive care only in advanced non-small cell lung cancer. Br J Cancer 1990. 61:608–611.

389. Rapp, E., et al. Chemotherapy can prolong survival in patients with advanced non-small-cell lung cancer—report of a Canadian multicenter randomized trial. J Clin Oncol 1988. 6:633–641.
390. Cellerino, R., et al. A randomized trial of alternating chemotherapy versus best supportive care in advanced non-small-cell lung cancer. J Clin Oncol 1991. 9:1453–1461.
391. Cartei, G., et al. Cisplatin-cyclophosphamide-mitomycin combination chemotherapy with supportive care versus supportive care alone for treatment of metastatic non-small-cell lung cancer. J Natl Cancer Inst 1993. 85:794–800.
392. Kaasa, S., et al. Symptomatic treatment versus combination chemotherapy for patients with extensive non-small cell lung cancer. Cancer 1991. 67:2443–2447.
393. Ganz, P.A., et al. Supportive care versus supportive care and combination chemotherapy in metastatic non-small cell lung cancer. Cancer 1989. 63:1271–1278.
394. Helsing, M., et al. Quality of life and survival in patients with advanced non-small cell lung cancer receiving supportive care plus chemotherapy with carboplatin and etoposide or supportive care only. A multicentre randomised phase III trial. Eur J Cancer 1998. 34:1036–1044.
395. Anderson, H., et al. Gemcitabine plus best supportive care (BSC) versus BSC in inoperable non-small cell lung cancer—a randomized trial with quality of life as the primary outcome. U.K. NSCLC Gemcitabine Group. Non-Small Cell Lung Cancer. Br J Cancer 2000. 83:447–453.
396. Roszkowski, K., et al. A multicenter, randomized, phase III study of docetaxel plus best supportive care versus best supportive care in chemotherapy-naive patients with metastatic or non-resectable localized non-small cell lung cancer (NSCLC). Lung Cancer 2000. 27:145–157.
397. Ranson, M., et al. Randomized trial of paclitaxel plus supportive care versus supportive care for patients with advanced non-small-cell lung cancer 10.1093/jnci/92.13.1074. J Natl Cancer Inst 2000. 92:1074–1080.
398. Frasci, G., et al. Gemcitabine plus vinorelbine yields better survival outcome than vinorelbine alone in elderly patients with advanced non-small cell lung cancer. A Southern Italy Cooperative Oncology Group (SICOG) phase III trial. Lung Cancer 2001. 34(suppl. 4):65–69.
399. Cormier, Y., et al. Benefits of polychemotherapy in advanced non-small-cell bronchogenic carcinoma. Cancer 1982. 50:845–849.
400. Kubota, K., et al. Phase III randomized trial of docetaxel plus cisplatin versus vindesine plus cisplatin in patients with stage IV non-small-cell lung cancer: the Japanese Taxotere Lung Cancer Study Group 10.1200/JCO.2004.06.114. J Clin Oncol 2004. 22:254–261.
401. Comella, P., et al. Interim analysis of a phase III trial comparing cisplatin, gemcitabine, and vinorelbine versus either cisplatin and gemcitabine or cisplatin and vinorelbine in advanced non-small-cell lung cancer. A Southern Italy Cooperative Oncology Group Study. Clin Lung Cancer 2000. 1:202–207; discussion 208.
402. Brodin, O., and E. Nou. Patients with non-resectable squamous cell carcinoma of the lung: a prospective, randomized study. Lung Cancer 1991. 75:165.

72

Thoracic and Pulmonary Infections

Frank A. Baciewicz, Jr.

All surgical specialties spend considerable effort to prevent lung infections from occurring and unfortunately even more resources once they have occurred. Due to the often immune-compromised status of surgical patients, the hospital environment, and the infectious nature of many surgical diseases, the surgeon must be vigilant in the diagnosis and treatment of infectious processes of the lung. This chapter outlines the diagnosis, possible preventive measures, and treatment of both common and less-common thoracic infections.

Pneumonia

The most common infectious cause of death and morbidity in the intensive care unit (ICU) is pneumonia. Of admissions in community hospitals, 1% will develop nosocomial pneumonia, and between one-tenth and one-fifth of admissions to the ICU are pneumonia related.[1–3] The mortality of ICU patients who develop pneumonia is as high as 50%, while the overall mortality of ICU patients is only 3.8%.[4] It has been estimated that 6%–20% of ventilated patients will contract pneumonia, and that 50% of these patients will die.[5–10]

Patients with a diagnosis of pneumonia have a large inoculum of an organism that overwhelms the host defenses maintaining the lower respiratory tract. These mechanisms include the cough reflex, mucus in the tracheal bronchial tree, lung macrophages, and physical filtration of air in the upper respiratory tract.

While in the hospital or intensive care unit, other factors contribute to impairment of the host defense mechanisms. Patients with altered mental status secondary to stroke, seizure disorder, or drug overdose are predisposed to develop aspiration pneumonia. Endotracheal intubation or tracheostomy provides access to the lower airway for opportunistic organisms. In addition, the patients themselves are often hypoxic, diabetic, or malnourished; have heart failure; or may be uremic, which contributes to impairment of the normal host mechanisms. There are now a large number of patients who have impaired immunity (i.e., have the human immunodeficiency virus), have had an organ transplant, have malignancies, and have dialysis-dependent renal insufficiency.

The bacteria may gain access to the lung by hematogenous spread, by aspiration either through the oropharynx or indwelling tubes in the airway, or during respiratory therapy.

The most common nosocomial and ICU-acquired pneumonias are secondary to gram-negative bacteria that colonize the upper respiratory tract.[11–14] Factors such as avoiding nasogastric tubes and maintaining the patient in a head-chest elevated position may decrease the incidence of aspiration. Avoiding gastric prophylactic agents, proton pump inhibitors, antacids, and H_2 blockers may decrease the incidence of ICU-acquired pneumonias by lowering the number of gram-negative bacteria in the neutralized gastric fluid, which eventually finds its way to the oropharynx.[15–19] Strict glucose management (80–110 mg/dL) with an insulin drip may also decrease the incidence of ICU pneumonia.[20]

Criteria for the diagnosis of pneumonia have been developed by Andrews et al. and include the presence of a new or progressive infiltrate on chest x-ray, fever, leukocytosis or leukopenia, and purulent tracheal secretions.[21] However, more than 90% of ICU patients met at least three of these criteria, with only 31% actually having pneumonia.[22] A list of noninfectious processes that can be misdiagnosed as pneumonia is given in Table 72.1.[23]

The usual first diagnostic step is an examination of the sputum. A Gram stain can detect bacterial organisms, KOH stain fungal disease, Ziehl-Neelsen stain tuberculosis, and silver methenamine stain *Pneumocystis carinii*. The sputum sample is adequate if it contains 25 polymorphonuclear cells and fewer than 10 epithelial cells per low-power field.[5]

In ventilated patients, bronchoalveolar lavage, which requires a wedged bronchoscope through which 20–60 mm of saline is instilled, or protected-specimen bronchoscopy can be used to diagnose pneumonia. Bronchoalveolar lavage has been shown to have true positive results in up to 80% of patients with known pneumonia.[24–27] The protected-specimen

TABLE 72.1. Noninfectious Processes That Can Mimic Pneumonia.

Congestive heart failure
Chemical aspiration
Pleural effusions
Adult respiratory distress syndrome
Atelectasis
Malignancy
Blood or medication reactions
Oxygen toxicity
Pulmonary embolus
Pulmonary contusion
Hemorrhage

Source: Data from Carlson and Geheb.[23]

bronchoscopy has almost 100% sensitivity and a very low false-negative rate.[28–32] If these diagnostic efforts fail, the patient may be taken to the operating room for a thoracoscopic or open lung biopsy.[33,34]

Since patients in the ICU may be critically ill, delays in treatment cannot be tolerated. The patient's pneumonia will require treatment prior to results of sputum studies, bronchoalveolar lavage, protected specimen bronchoscopy, or lung biopsy. The most common etiologic agents in ICU pneumonia include *Pseudomonas aeruginosa* in 17%–27% of all pneumonias, *Staphylococcus aureus* in 18%–20%, *Acinetobacter* in 6%–8%, and *Enterobacter* in 5%–7%.[35–38] If large numbers of patients with acquired immune deficiency are present, *Pneumoncystis carinii*, fungal, or mycobacterial infection will be noted. In addition, the hospital's unique indigenous flora will reflect antibiotic usage in that hospital and may select antibiotic-resistant bacilli such as vancomycin-resistant entercocous or methacillin-resistant staphylococci. Because of these suspected organisms, when patients must be treated in a declining physical situation without results of the aforementioned tests, the patients usually will receive cefapime, imipenem, or piperacillin tazobactam plus vancomycin, with or without an aminoglycoside. When specific ICU organisms such as methacillin- or vancomycin-resistant staphylococci are present, linezolid may be used initially.[39–41] Prophylactic antibiotics usually are not favored in ICU settings as they may lead to superinfection, and there is a risk of *Clostridium difficile* infection and its associated diarrhea, loss of ability to use enteral feedings, and possibly sepsis. Finally, empiric antibiotics are an inefficient use of financial resources.

Complications of Pneumonia

Parapneumonic Effusion

In the pneumonic inflammatory process, the parietal capillary integrity is disrupted, and fluid leaks into the pleural space. In addition, inflammation can involve the visceral pleura and impair the reabsorption of fluid. Exudative fluid accumulates in the pleural space, resulting in a parapneumonic effusion.

These effusions have been observed to occur in 50% of patients with pneumococcal pneumonia and in 60%–70% of patients with anaerobic pneumonias.[41–43] These are the typical community-acquired organisms. For patients in the ICU, hospital-acquired pneumonias are usually related to *Staphylococcus aureus* or gram-negative rods. In these patients, more than 65% will have a parapneumonic effusion.[42,43]

Initially, the pneumonic process causes an exudative fluid (stage 1) to enter the pleural space. When the pneumonia involves the pleural surface, bacteria can also invade the pleura cavity. With the presence of bacteria in the pleural fluid, the neutrophil concentration increases (stage 2), and the parapneumonic effusion can increase at a rapid rate rather than remain localized. As the neutrophils proliferate, the effusion becomes purulent. If not treated, the parapneumonic effusion may become an empyema. Fibrin deposition (stage 3) then occurs, which may lead to loculated collections of purulent fluid. In the final stage (stage 4), the purulent material is not evacuated; fibroblasts produce a thick peel, which may encase the lung.[44–46] The progression from stage 1 to stage 4 varies from hours to days depending on the organism and the host's underlying resistance to infection.

The chest x-ray is the most straightforward examination for verifying a pleural effusion. Fluid will initially accumulate in the most dependent aspects of the thoracic cavity such that the costophrenic angle will be obliterated when 500mL of fluid are present.[47] In the ICU setting when the patient is not able to have a chest x-ray in an upright position, effusion should be suspected when one hemithorax is more opaque than its contralateral. Ultrasonography and computed axial tomography (CAT) can provide evaluation of much smaller pleural effusions and help differentiate between areas of atelectasis, loculated fluid collections, and parenchymal disease.[48,49]

Thoracentesis

After determining that a significant pleural effusion is present, the pleura needs to be evacuated for both diagnosis and treatment. Thoracentesis is performed in the area where the localized effusion has been noted or in a dependent area with a free-flowing effusion. After prepping the chest and using 1% lidocaine, the needle is introduced over the top of the appropriate rib, usually no lower than the fifth intercostal space to minimize injury to abdominal organs. A representative sample, approximately 20–30mL, is removed if the purpose is diagnostic only. The fluid is grossly inspected and may confirm the clinical diagnosis. If the white cell count is greater than 100,000/mL, the fluid will appear quite cloudy, and an infectious etiology is suspected, either parapneumonic effusion or empyema. Gram stain and cultures should be ordered. The fluid should be analyzed for white cell count, red cell count, glucose, pH, amylase, protein, and lactate dehydrogenase (LDH) and triglyceride and cholesterol if a chylothorax is suspected.[50]

Besides its diagnostic value, thoracentesis can also markedly improve the patient's clinical symptoms. In the event of a parapneumonic effusion, removal of as much of the effusion as possible can be accomplished with thoracentesis, especially if the effusion is relatively small. The recommendation is that no more than 1L be removed initially as greater fluid removal may result in significant reexpansion pulmonary edema and worsen the patient's symptoms.

Pleural effusions, in addition to being related to pneumonic processes, can be a response to subdiaphragmatic infectious processes. About 50% of patients who undergo abdominal surgery will have small pleural effusions within 72h after operation.[51,52] It will often be on the side of the procedure. The exudate may be present in response to peritonitis or a subphrenic abscess. Pancreatitis results in effusions about 20% of the time.[53]

Treatment

If the glucose level is greater than 60mg/dL, the pH greater than 7.3, and the LDH level less than 500IU/L, the effusion will usually resolve with antibiotics and thoracentesis alone.

In the case of a complicated pleural effusion with a pH less than 7.1, glucose less than 40mg/dL, LDH greater than 1000IU, or presence of bacteria on Gram stain, tube thoracostomy drainage should be performed.[54] The placement of a large-bore 32- to 36-French chest tube will prevent the formation of loculated collections that will make it difficult for complete drainage of the pleural space.

Recently, ultrasound or CAT scan has been used to guide placement of a small-caliber catheter directly into the loculated space.[55,56] This technique has the advantage of being more comfortable for the patient. If serial chest x-rays and CAT scan of the chest do not demonstrate that the entire space is adequately drained, a thrombolytic agent such as 250,000IU streptokinase for 3–5 days can be instilled through the chest tube or interventional catheter.[57–61] The strategy is that the streptokinase will cause lysis of the adhesions and result in complete drainage of the pleural space. Streptokinase may result in high-grade fever and if successful will usually result in significantly increased drainage within 24h of placement. This strategy will be successful in over 50% of the patients if the single chest tube is not adequate in draining the pleural space.[62,63] It also has been advocated in patients who are extremely high-risk surgical candidates or who do not qualify as surgical candidates.

Appropriate antibiotics should be administered according to Gram stain or culture of pleural fluid. Parapneumonic effusion is successfully treated with antibiotics and thoracentesis in about 25% of adults.[64] With chest tube placement and lytic agents, at least 50%–60% of patients can avoid operative intervention.[62,63] Surgical drainage will require either thoracoscopic decortication or open decortication via thoracotomy. Thoracoscopic drainage will be successful for stage 2 or stage 3 parapneumonic effusion.

Once the patient reaches stage 4 or the organized fibrotic stage, the lung is trapped under a peel and will require a thoracotomy. The goal in this procedure is to drain the infected area and to eliminate any space with reexpanded lung tissue. If a portion of the lung cannot be reexpanded or is perhaps nonviable and requires resection, then space may become a problem. In this situation, the surgeon has several options. The most successful is to transpose muscle flaps of the latissimus dorsi, serratus anterior, or pectoralis muscle through a limited resection of rib and intercostal space. The greater omentum can also be used.

The chest tubes are typically removed when the drainage becomes serous, less than 50mL a day, and the lung has fully expanded. If the drainage remains high and the lung not completely expanded, the tubes can be converted to open drainage after ensuring that the tubes have no respiratory variation. The tubes converted to open drainage are then slowly withdrawn over the course of several weeks.

Empyema

Parapneumonic effusions can be differentiated from early empyema by the appearance of fluid in the pleural space, the pH, the glucose level, and the presence of bacteria. Empyema patients typically have gross pus in the pleural space on thoracentesis, a pleural pH of 7.0 or less, a glucose level below 40mg/dL, and positive Gram stain for bacteria. Patients with empyema require insertion of a chest tube. At the bedside, a large-bore chest tube, 32- to 36-French, is placed. The chest tube remains in place until the quality of the drainage becomes serous and the volume decreases to less than 50mL per day. The organisms most commonly responsible for empyema include *Staphylococcus aureus*, Gram-negative bacilli, anaerobes, *Streptococcus pneumoniae*, hemolytic streptococcus, and *Haemophilus influenzae*.[65,66]

For patients with chronic empyema or empyema with a bronchopleural fistula, a drainage procedure may be the only option available. In this situation, the most dependent part of the empyema cavity must be localized and a portion of the overlying rib resected. The cavity is opened, pleural space debrided, and lung decorticated. A large-bore chest tube is placed in the cavity, and the tube can be removed out slowly over several weeks. In a particularly ill patient or a patient with a chronic illness, the cavity may be left open permanently (Eloesser flap).[67]

Lung Abscess

If the offending organism is *Staphylococcus aureus*, this may produce a necrotizing pneumonia with cavities and thin-wall abscesses or pneumatoceles. The abscesses may be related to aspirated oral secretions and will often be located in the superior segment of the lower lobes or the posterior segment of the right upper lobe. Anaerobes are typically associated with aspiration-induced abscesses. If the abscess cavity erodes into a bronchus and drains some of its contents, a cavity and an air–fluid level can be seen on an upright chest x-ray. However, the lung abscess may often only be diagnosed with a chest CAT scan.

Lung abscesses are treated with appropriate antibiotics and pulmonary physiotherapy. If the cavity is central, bronchoscopy may result in emptying some of the infected contents of the cavity. Peripheral abscesses may sometimes be treated with CAT scan-guided or ultrasound-guided catheter insertion in an effort to drain the infected fluid and speed recovery. Surgical intervention is required only in patients who have life-threatening hemoptysis, a bronchopleural fistula that does not resolve with conservative management, or a cavity larger than 6.0cm that has failed antibiotic therapy.

Tuberculosis

Mycobacterium tuberculosis, the causative organism for tuberculosis, is acquired by inhalation of the tuberculi bacilli. This involves respiratory contact with a person who has cavitary disease, whose sputum contains the tuberculi bacilli, and who has a cough. The disease is highly contagious.

Currently, there are approximately 10 new cases per 100,000 population in the United States.[68] The rate of infection is higher in males than females, in minority groups, in the elderly, in patients with immunodeficiency syndrome, and in the homeless. It is also prone to develop in immigrants and visitors from underdeveloped countries, intravenous drug abusers, residents of long-term care facilities, and patients with silicosis, gastrectomy, jejunoileal bypass, low body weight, chronic renal failure, diabetes mellitus, on steroids, or with leukemia, lymphoma, or malignancies.[69–73]

Within 6 weeks of infection, the tuberculin skin test will become positive, and infiltrates in the lower two-thirds of the lung may occur. The tuberculi bacteria are contained within the small granulomas in the lung, which heal with fibrosis or undergo central cavitation (caseous necrosis). A Ghon complex is the combination of caseous necrosis or calcification in the periphery of the lung and central lymph nodes. About 5%–10% of adults will have clinical tuberculosis after the initial infection. For those who develop clinical disease, the mortality rate is 30%–40%.[74]

More commonly, secondary or reactivation tuberculosis follows a period of latency that can last up to 60 years. In this case, the infection usually begins as a pneumonitis in the posterior apical segment of the upper lobe or in an apical portion of the lower lobe. The lesions then develop an area of caseous necrosis, granulation tissue, and fibrosis. The caseous material liquefies and then drains into the bronchial tree, at which time the patient becomes contagious.

As the disease progresses, the patient will develop multiple small cavities with irregular walls, or the cavities may fuse to form giant cavities. The blood supply of the tuberculous cavities is the bronchial arterial system, and if erosion occurs into any blood vessel supplying this area, hemoptysis will occur. The tuberculous cavity may also become infected with other bacteria or fungi. Giant bullae may occur as a result of a stenotic bronchus. Life-threatening hemoptysis can occur if the infection erodes into a pulmonary artery (Rasmussen's aneurysm). In the typical clinical course, the patient is asymptomatic early in the disease course. If the disease is not treated, nonspecific symptoms such as weight loss, anorexia, and afternoon fevers will occur. Night sweats are also common later in the disease as well as cough and blood-tinged mucopurulent sputum.

Sputum smears will reveal the acid-fast bacilli in 50%–75% of patients with active pulmonary tuberculosis.[75] Open or closed pleural biopsy may also have a high diagnostic yield (60%–80%) in patients with tuberculous pleural effusions.[76] Culture systems have been developed to increase the speed of verification and susceptibility testing for mycobacterium tuberculosis, but it may still take up to 6 weeks for results. Use of DNA probes that rely on reverse transcriptase polymerase chain reaction can improve the sensitivity of specific DNA sequences and identify mycobacterial isolates from culture and other specimens.[77–84]

Drug Treatment

The current recommendation for treatment of tuberculosis is multiple drugs to which the organism is susceptible. Bactericidal agents are preferred, and first-line drugs include isoniazid (INH), rifampin, ethambutol, and pyrazinamide. These drugs are recommended for a minimum of 6 months.[85] In patients who have evidence of extrapulmonary tuberculosis that may involve the adrenal gland, the vertebral bodies, or pericardium, steroids should be added to the treatment regimen.[86] Patients who have positive skin tests and do not have evidence of active disease are given a 6-month course of INH to prevent the progression to clinical disease.[87]

Surgical Management

Surgical intervention is necessary when patients with pulmonary tuberculosis have persistently positive sputum tests despite appropriate antibiotics. Other surgical indications include tuberculous empyema with or without a bronchopleural fistula, bronchial stenosis with an expanding cavity, cavitating lung parenchyma with persistent infection, or life-threatening hemoptysis.

If a cavity develops in the lung adjacent to the pleura, a bronchopleural fistula may result. In this situation, use of thoracentesis to drain the pleural space and initiation of appropriate antibiotic therapy will hopefully prevent recurrence. If the fluid cavity along with adjacent parenchymal disease remain after several months of antibiotic therapy, decortication and resection of adjacent lung should be considered to prevent the progression of disease. Prior to operation, every effort must be made to convert to a negative sputum culture.

When resection does occur, decortication with resection of underlying lung will usually require at least a lobectomy. When the remaining lung parenchyma does not reexpand to fill the space, the surgeon needs to consider the use of muscle or omental flaps or thoracoplasty to fill the residual space. The granulomatous involvement of peribronchial lymph nodes will make these structures very adherent to the vascular and bronchial structures, which makes any dissection quite hazardous.

If the disease process is extensive and involves all lobes, an extrapleural pneumonectomy may be required. Surgical resection is indicated for a patient who has bled more than 600 mL in 24 h or less. Resection of lung because of bronchial stenosis in an expanding cavity is uncommonly seen with the current early therapy. A large cavity of more than 6.0 cm even with negative sputum may be considered for resection as the incidence of secondary infection, recurrent disease, or hemoptysis is significant. Current mortality rates after extrapleural pneumonectomy are in the 10%–15% range, in the 5% range with lobectomy, and 3%–5% with decortication.[88–91]

Nontuberculous Mycobacterial Infections

The nontuberculous mycobacteria have widespread distribution, with specific species noted in different geographic locations.[92,93] The species have been cultured from water, soil, domestic animals, and birds. They are not considered contagious. The diseases caused by the nontuberculous mycobacteria are more slowly progressive than tuberculosis. Diagnosis is made from sputum samples or transbronchial or open lung biopsy.

Mycobacterium avium and *Mycobacterium intercellulare* are the most common nontuberculosis species isolated in the United States. They usually are seen in patients with autoimmune deficiency disease. A three-drug regimen of clarithromycin, ethambutol, and rifampin for 6 months is recommended.[94]

Mycobacterium kansasii is the second most common nontuberculous bacteria and usually occurs in the Midwest and southern United States. *Mycobacterium fortuitum* is the third most common organism and is resistant to the usual antitubercular drugs. It responds well to conventional antibiotics such as amikacin and cefoxitin. The surgical indications for the atypical mycobacterial infections are the same as for tuberculosis.

Actinomycotic and Nocardial Infections

Actinomyces and *Nocardia* cause bacterial diseases with clinical manifestations similar to the fungal diseases. Both bacteria are also similar to fungi in that they form hyphae with branching and spores.

Actinomycosis

Actinomycosis is caused by the anaerobic actinomycete *Actinomyces israelii*. The common forms of the disease are the cervicofacial form, which is characterized by draining cutaneous sinuses, and the thoracic form, which is due to parenchymal infection of *A. israelii* from the oral cavity, where it is usually not a pathogen. In the lung, there is a focus of infection surrounded by fibrosis and granulomatous inflammatory changes. The disease can extend to the pleura and cause a sinus tract through the chest wall. The disease should be suspected if there is involvement of the rib or vertebral body on chest x-ray.

Diagnosis can be made by culturing the material under anaerobic conditions. Diagnosis can also by made when the classic "sulfur granules" of the gram-positive coccobacillus is seen on stain of the draining material. The drugs of choice are ampicillin or penicillin G for 3 months.[95]

Actinomycoses are usually resected when carcinoma of the lung may be suspected. If no preoperative diagnosis has been made, it is imperative to do an intraoperative biopsy to rule out this benign cause of an infiltrative lesion on radiography.

Nocardiosis

Nocardiosis is caused by the aerobic gram-positive *Nocardia asteroides* bacteria. Nocardia is typically seen in the patient population receiving corticosteroids for immunologic deficiencies such as acquired immunodeficiency syndrome, lymphoma, leukemia, or malignancy. The organism is found in the soil. It is not a common organism in the oropharynx or respiratory tree. The patient usually presents with symptoms of chronic disease, such as cough, fever, weight loss, night sweats, or pleuritic chest pain. Nocardia is often associated with central nervous system involvement, including brain abscess or meningitis. Chest x-rays demonstrate a localized infiltrate, which becomes necrotic and cavitary. It is difficult to isolate the organism from sputum. Typically, bronchoscopy with brush or biopsy or even open lung biopsy is required for diagnosis.

Surgical intervention is usually required if the diagnosis is unknown or if the suspected lung lesion is malignant. The antibiotic of choice at present is trimethoprim-sulfamethoxazole, which is usually continued for 2 to 3 months.[96]

Fungal Infections of the Lung

The major infectious agents for histoplasmosis, coccidiomycosis, and blastomycosis occur in specific geographic areas.[97] In these areas, the infected spores are found in the soil and gain entry to the respiratory tract, where they may cause self-limited infections or progress to more serious pulmonary infections. The cryptococcus and aspergillus are also endemic in the soil. In addition, with the increase in patients receiving immunosuppressive therapy there has been an increase in these opportunistic diseases. The thoracic surgeon may be asked to biopsy lesions in the immunocompromised population, to resect lesions with unknown etiology, or to treat lesions that have not responded to medical therapy.

Histoplasmosis

The most common of the fungal infections is histoplasmosis. It is caused by the fungus *Histoplasma capsulatum*, which is found in soil containing a high concentration of fecal material from chickens, pigeons, or bats. In the United States, the endemic regions are the Mississippi and Ohio River valleys.

Up to 90% of the patients who are infected with *H. capsulatum* spores remain free of symptoms or have minor respiratory illness. Patients who develop clinical disease have cough, shortness of breath, fever, night sweats, myalgias, and arthralgias.[98] Radiologically, areas of bronchopneumonia, nodules, or a solitary pulmonary nodule may be seen on x-ray. The regional lymph nodes are usually involved. With complete healing, calcification may be seen in the peripheral lesion or the involved lymph nodes.

The disseminated form of disease develops in fewer than 1 in 50,000 patients with primary histoplasmosis.[99] The commonly involved organs are those that have reticuloendothelial cells, including the liver, spleen, lymph nodes, bone marrow, and adrenal glands.

Histoplasmosis can also involve the mediastinal lymph nodes and present with a rampant fibrotic reaction or fibrosing mediastinitis. Most of these patients are asymptomatic, but the fibrosis can progress such that there is compression of the esophagus, trachea, or superior vena cava.

A biopsy of the involved tissue and identification of *H. capsulatum* in culture are necessary for the diagnosis of histoplasmosis. The offending organism is usually seen in the caseous material on methenamine silver stain.

The primary treatment for disseminated, cavitary histoplasmosis or fibrosing mediastinitis is an antifungal agent, usually amphotericin B or itraconazole. The surgical indications are the presence of thick-wall cavities that remain after treatment with an antifungal agent or when fibrosing mediastinitis causes symptomatic obstruction of the trachea, esophagus, or superior vena cava.[100–105] Recently, percutaneous stenting has been used to relieve obstructive symptoms.[106]

Coccidiomyocosis

The causative organism of coccidiomycosis, *Coccidiodes immitis*, is ubiquitous to the desert soil of the southwest part of the United States and Mexico. This organism is aerosolized and inhaled. In the endemic region, infection with *C. immitis* is nearly 100%.

Of the patients who inhale the aerosolized spores, 40% develop flu-like symptoms from 1 to 4 weeks later. Fever, cough, pleuritic chest pain, dyspnea, fatigue, and headache are typical complaints. The other 60% remain asymptomatic and develop only positive skin tests as evidence of infection. Patients develop a macular erythematous rash in the inguinal folds and on the hands and feet. When pneumonitis, arthralgias, and erythema nodosum are recognized, the patient is said to have acute Valley fever.[107,108]

With pulmonary involvement due to *C. immitis*, the chest x-ray will demonstrate peripheral cavities and cysts during the first several weeks following the infection. Chronic cavitary lesions are the most frequent long-term result of an acute infection.[109]

Disseminated *C. immitus* usually occurs weeks to months after the initial infection. The central nervous system, the skeletal system, and the genitourinary system (kidney) are the most frequent locations for the disseminated process. Meningitis or involvement of the long bones, vertebrae, and skull can develop.

Diagnosis depends on biopsy of the involved organ or the lung parenchyma or a positive sputum sample. The classic finding is a spherule filled with endospores on potassium hydroxide wet mount. Amphotericin B, itraconazole, and fluconazole are used depending on the severity and extent of disease. Surgical resection is required for chronic cavitary disease.[110]

Blastomycosis

Blastomyces dermatidis is a fungus that causes blastomyocosis in the southeastern and south central parts of the United States. The *B. dermatidis* organism is endemic to the soil and gains access via the respiratory tree.

Some patients will have an acute respiratory infection with pulmonary infiltrates and spread to regional lymph nodes. If there is a hematogenous dissemination with spread to the skin, skeletal system, or genitalia, the chronic disease may manifest. Patients with chronic blastomyocosis can have cutaneous lesions that are raised and crusted with an irregular border. The lesion is usually found on the extremities or on the face.[111]

If there is chronic pulmonary involvement, the upper lobes are usually involved. There are typically cavitary changes, or a nodule may be present. The chronic disease will also involve the skeletal system, with rib involvement suggestive of blastomyocosis. The primary diagnosis is made from the sputum culture, which can take up to 6 weeks to grow. The positive acid-Schiff smear is characterized by spherical cells with a thick-wall contour demonstrating unipolar budding.

The treatment for blastomyocosis is itraconazole or amphotericin B, with a typical duration of 2 to 3 months.[112,113] Surgical therapy is recommended for resection of a large cavity if sputum remains positive following a course of intraconazole or amphotericin B.

Cryptococcosis

Cryptococcus neoformans is found in the soil and dust, particularly contaminated by pigeons. There is no particular geographic area that is favored. In this disease, the organisms gain entry to the host via the respiratory tree. Patients with underlying malignancies or lymphosuppressive diseases are the typical patients who develop disseminated disease.

When the lung is involved, a cavity usually does not develop as this organism does not cause necrosis. Diagnosis can be made from the sputum, by India ink stain, or from tissue with the Mucicarmine stain.

Cryptococcosis has a predilection for the central nervous system. It is a lethal disease and must be treated aggressively with amphotericin B and 5-flucytosine. In fact, if *Cryptococcus* is noted on lung resection, the patient should have a spinal tap performed. Upward of 7%–10% of patients will develop cryptococcal meningeal involvement following a pulmonary resection of the same disease.[114] Only if the cryptococcal lesion in the lung is small without surrounding disease in the infiltrate and it can be completely resected would fluconazole or amphotericin B not be started following resection.

Aspergillosis

Aspergillus fumigatus is a filamentous fungus noted in soil and decaying plants. The airborne spores can produce three distinct clinical entities. The most common is an allergic bronchitis.[115] The second form is the aspergilloma or fungus ball. The organisms are present as branching hyphae in strands or clusters, along with inflammatory cells and fibrin in a necrotic-appearing spherical mass within a previously formed cavity or cyst in the lung. It is usually present in an upper lobe cavity in a patient with preexisting tuberculosis, sarcoidosis, abscess, or cavitating carcinoma.[116] The aspergilloma is resected when an episode of hemoptysis occurs. This occurs in 50% of patients, and in approximately 10% hemoptysis can be severe and recurrent.[117] Dissemination rarely occurs from an aspergilloma. A resection is recommended only in patients with hemoptysis if the patient is a good surgical candidate. Since there is typically significant disease in the area around the aspergilloma, the patient must be able to tolerate a lobectomy as a minimum procedure. The antifungal drugs do not penetrate aspergilloma cavities; consequently, medical therapy is unsatisfactory for aspergilloma.

Patients with simple aspergillomas who have a thin-wall cavity and minimal surrounding parenchymal disease have an operative mortality of less than 5%. However, complex aspergillomas with thick-wall cavities, significant parenchymal disease, and severe adhesions at the apex of the chest have significant operative mortality, up to 30%.[118–122] They also have significant postoperative complications, including air leak, bronchopleural fistula, empyema, and residual space problems.

The third type of aspergillosis is an invasive infection in which there is bronchial pneumonia with necrosis. This disease usually occurs in patients who are in an immunocompromised state. Medical therapy with voriconazole, lipid-based amphotericin B, or a caspofungin and voriconazole has a high failure rate.[123–126] As a result, patients who have invasive aspergillosis localized to one part of the lung without significant involvement of other organs are recommended to have pulmonary resection. The operative mortality is significant, but there are improved outcomes in this patient cohort.[127–130]

References

1. Centers for Disease Control. Nosocomial infection surveillance, 1984. MMWR CDC Surveill Summ 1986;35(ISS):17.
2. Barrett FF, Casey JI, Finland M. Infections and antibiotic use among patients at Boston City Hospital, February 1967. N Engl J Med 1968;278:5.
3. Gross PA, Neu HC, Aswapokee P, et al. Deaths from nosocomial infection: experience in a university and community hospital. Am J Med 1980;68:219.
4. Stevens RM, Teres D, Skillman JJ, et al. Pneumonia in an intensive care unit. A 30 month experience. Arch Intern Med 1974;134:106.
5. Craven DE, Kunches LM, Kilinsky V, et al. Risk factors for pneumonia and fatality in patients receiving continuous mechanical ventilation. Am Rev Respir Dis 1986;133:792.
6. Fagan JY, Chastre J, Domart Y, et al. Nosocomial pneumonia in patients receiving continuous mechanical ventilation. Am Rev Respir Dis 1989;139:877.
7. Lee SC, Hua CC, Yu TJ, et al. Risk factors of mortality for nosocomial pneumonia: importance of initial anti-microbial therapy. Int J Clin Pract 2005;59:39–45.
8. Rello J, Vidaur L, Sandiumenge A, et al. De-escalation therapy in ventilator-associated pneumonia. Crit Care Med 2004;32:2183–2190.
9. Hugonnet S, Eggimann P, Borst F, et al. Impact of ventilator-associated pneumonia on resource utilization and patient outcome. Infect Control Hosp Epidemiol 2004;25:1090–1096.
10. Zapol WM, Snider MT, Hill JD, et al. Extracorporeal membrane oxygenation in severe acute respiratory failure: a randomized prospective study. JAMA 1979;242:2193.
11. Centers for Disease Control. Nosocomial infection surveillance, 1984. MMWR Morb Mortal Wkly Rep 1986;35:17SS.
12. Centers for Disease Control. Nosocomial infections 1980–1982. MMWR Morb Mortal Wkly Rep 1983;32:1SS.
13. Johanson WG, Pierce AK, Sanford JP. Changing pharyngeal bacterial flora of hospitalized patients: emergence of gram-negative bacilli. N Engl J Med 1969;281:1137.
14. Johanson WG, Pierce AK, Sandford JP. Nosocomial respiratory infections with gram-negative bacilli. The significance of colonization of infections of the respiratory tract. Ann Intern Med 1972;77:701.
15. Brennan MT, Bahrani-Mougeot F, Fox PC. The role of oral microbial colonization in ventilator-associated pneumonia. Oral Surg Oral Med Oral Pathol Oral Radiol Endod 2004;98:665–672.
16. Hillman KM, Riordan T, O'Farrell SM, et al. Colonization of the gastric content in critically ill patients. Crit Care Med 1982;10:444.
17. Kahn RJ, Brimioulle S, Vincent JL. Influence of antacid treatment on the tracheal flora in mechanically ventilated patients. Crit Care Med 1982;10:229.
18. Driks MR, Craven DE, Celli BR, et al. Nosocomial pneumonia in intubated patients given sucralfate as compared with antacids or histamine type 2 blockers. N Engl J Med 1987;317:1376.
19. Palmer RH, Gachot B, Jebrak G, et al. Nosocomial pneumonia in intubated patients. N Engl J Med 1988;318:1465.
20. Van den Berghe G, Wouters P, Weekers F, et al. Intensive insulin therapy in critically ill patients. N Engl J Med 2001;345:1359–1367.
21. Andrews CP, Coalson JJ, Smith JD, et al. Diagnosis of nosocomial bacterial pneumonia in acute, diffuse lung injury. Chest 1981;80:254.
22. Fagan JY, Chastre J, Hance AJ, et al. Detection of nosocomial lung infection in ventilated patients: use of a protected specimen brush and quantitative culture techniques in 147 patients. Am Rev Respir Dis 1988;138:110.
23. Carlson RW, Geheb MA. Pneumonia. In: Principles and Practice of Medical Intensive Care. Philadelphia: Saunders; 1993:481.
24. Davis KA, Eckert MJ, Reed RL 2nd, et al. Ventilator-associated pneumonia in injured patients: do you trust your Gram's stain? J Trauma 2005;58:462–467.
25. Cook DJ, Brun-Buisson C, Guyatt GH, et al. Evaluation of new diagnostic technologies: bronchoalveolar lavage and the diagnosis of ventilator-associated pneumonia. Crit Care Med 1994; 22:1314–1322.
26. Rouby JJ, Rossignon MD, Nicolas MH, et al. A prospective study of protected bronchoalveolar lavage in the diagnosis of nosocomial pneumonia. Anesthesiology 1989;7:679.
27. Shorr AF, Sherner JH, Jackson WL. Invasive approaches to the diagnosis of ventilator-associated pneumonia: a meta-analysis. Crit Care Med 2005;33:46–53.
28. Chastre J, Fagon J. Ventilator-associated pneumonia. Am J Respir Crit Care Med 2002;154:867–903.
29. Torres A, Ewig S. Diagnosing ventilator-associated pneumonia. N Engl J Med 2004;35:433–435.
30. Ost DE, Hall CS, Jospeh G, et al. Decision analysis of antibiotic and diagnostic strategies in ventilator-associated pneumonia. Am J Respir Crit Care Med 2003;168:1060–1067.
31. Wood AY, Davit AJ 2nd, Ciraulo DL. A prospective assessment of diagnostic efficacy of blind protective bronchial brushings compared to bronchoscope-assisted lavage, bronchoscope-directed brushings, and blind endotracheal aspirates in ventilator-associated pneumonia. J Trauma 2003;55:825–834.
32. Grossman RF, Fein A. Evidence-based assessment of diagnostic tests for ventilator-associated pneumonia. Chest 2000;117:177S–181S.
33. Dijkman JH, van der Meer JWM, Bakker W, et al. Transpleural lung biopsy by the thoracoscopic route in patients with diffuse interstitial pulmonary disease. Chest 1982;82:76.
34. McCabe RE, Brooks RG, Mark JBD, et al. Open lung biopsy in patients with acute leukemia. Am J Med 1985;78:609.
35. Craven DE, Kunches LM, Lichtenberg DA, et al. Nosocomial infection and fatality in medical and surgical intensive care unit patients. Arch Intern Med 1988;148:1161.
36. Richards MJ, Edwards JR, Culver DH, et al. Nosocomial infections in medical intensive care units in the United States. National Nosocomial Infections Surveillance System. Crit Care Med 1999;27:887–892.
37. El-Solh AA, Aquilina AT, Dhillon RS, et al. Impact of invasive strategy on management of antimicrobial treatment failure in institutionalized older people with severe pneumonia. Am J Respir Crit Care Med 2002;166:1038–1043.
38. Centers for Disease Control: Nosocomial infection surveillance: 1983. MMWR CDC Surveill Summ 1984;33(2SS):9.
39. American Thoracic Society; Infectious Diseases Society of America. Guidelines for the management of adults with hospital-acquired ventilator-assisted, and healthcare-associated pneumonia. Am J Respir Crit Care Med 2005;171:388–416.
40. Thompson DS. Methicillin-resistant *Staphylococcus aureus* in a general intensive care unit. J R Soc Med 2004;97:521–526.
41. Shorr AF, Susla GB, Kollef MH. Quinolones for treatment of nosocomial pneumonia: a meta-analysis. Clin Infect Dis 2005;40:115–122.

42. Taryle DA, Potts DE, Sahn SA. The incidence and clinical correlates of parapneumonic effusions in pneumococcal pneumonia. Chest 1978;74:170.
43. Light RW, Girard WM, Jenkinson SG, et al. Parapneumonic effusions. Am J Med 1980;69:507.
44. Andrews NC, Parker EF, Shaw RR, et al. Management of nontuberculous empyema. Am Rev Respir Dis 1962;85:935.
45. Sahn SA, Reller LB, Taryle DA, et al. The contribution of leukocytes and bacteria to the low pH of empyema fluid. Am Rev Respir Dis 1983.128:811.
46. Light RW, Moller DJ Jr, George RB. Low pleural fluid pH in parapneumonic effusion. Chest 1975;68:273.
47. Collins JD, Burwell D, Furmanski S, et al. Minimal detectable pleural effusions. Radiology 1972;105:51.
48. Roch A, Bojan M, Michelet P, et al. Usefulness of ultrasonography in predicting pleural effusions >500 mL in patients receiving mechanical ventilation. Chest 2005;127:224–232.
49. Stark DD, Federle MP, Goodman PC, et al. Differentiating lung abscess and empyema: radiography and computed tomography. AJR Am J Roentgenol 1983;141:163.
50. Sahn SA. State of the art: the pleural. Am Rev Respir Dis 1988:138:184.
51. Light RW, George RB. Incidence and significance of pleural effusion after abdominal surgery. Chest 1976;69:621.
52. Nielsen PH, Jepsen SB, Olsen AD. Postoperative pleural effusion following upper abdominal surgery. Chest 1989;96:133.
53. McKenna J, Craig RM, Chandraseekhar AJ, et al. The pleuropulmonary complication of pancreatitis. Chest 1977;71:197.
54. Light RW, Girard WM, Jenkinson SG, et al. Parapneumonic effusions. Am J Med 1980;69:507.
55. Klein JS, Schultz S, Heffner JE. Interventional radiology of the chest: image-guided percutaneous drainage of pleural effusions, lung abscess and pneumothorax. AJR Am J Roentgenol 1995; 164:581–588.
56. Ulmer JL, Choplin RH, Reed JC. Image-guided catheter drainage of the infected pleural space. J Thorac Imaging 1991; 6:65–73.
57. Bergh NP, Ekroth R, Larsson S, et al. Intrapleural streptokinase in the treatment of haemothorax and empyema. Scand J Thorac Cardiovasc Surg 1977;11:265.
58. Willsie-Ediger SK, Salzman G, Reisz G, et al. Use of intrapleural streptokinase in the treatment of thoracic empyema. Am J Med 1990;300:296.
59. Park CS, Chung WM, Lim MK, et al. Transcatheter instillation of urokinase into loculated pleural effusion: analysis of treatment effect. AJR Am J Roentgenol 1996;167:649–652.
60. Davies RJ, Traill ZC, Gleeson FV. Randomised controlled trial of intrapleural streptokinase in community acquired pleural infection. Thorax 1997;52:416–421.
61. Basile A, Boullosa-Seoane E, et al. Intrapleural fibrinolysis in the management of empyemas and haemothoraces. Our experience. Radiol Med 2003;105:12–16.
62. Bouros D, Antoniou KM, Chalkiadakis G, et al. The role of video-assisted thoracoscopic surgery in the treatment of parapneumonic empyema after the failure of fibrinolytics. Surg Endosc 2002;Epub 2001.
63. Diacon AH, Theron J, Schuurmans MM, et al. Intrapleural streptokinase for empyema and complicated parapneumonic effusions. Am J Respir Crit Care Med 2004;170:49–53.
64. Renzetti AD. Current treatment of nontuberculous empyema. Pulmonary Perspectives 1986;34:1.
65. Leblan KA, Tucker WY. Empyema of the thorax. Surg Gynecol 1984;158:66.
66. Muskett A, Burton NA, Karwande SV, et al. Management of refractory empyema with early decortication. Am J Surg 1988;156:529.
67. Eloesser L. Of an operation for tuberculosis empyema. Ann Thorac Surg 1969;8:355.
68. Centers for Disease Control. Summary of notifiable diseases, United States, 1989. MMWR Morb Mortal Wkly Rep 1989; 38:43.
69. Bloch AB, Reider HL, Kelly GD, et al. The epidemiology of tuberculosis in the United States. Clin Chest Med 1989; 10:297.
70. Chaisson Re, Schecter GF, Theuer CP, et al. Tuberculosis in patients with acquired immunodeficiency syndrome. Clinical features, response to therapy, and survival. Am Rev Respir Dis 1987;136:570.
71. Rieder HL, Cauthen GM, Kelly GD, et al. Tuberculosis in the United States. JAMA 1989;262:385.
72. Stead WW, Lofgren JP, Warren E, et al. Tuberculosis as an endemic and nosocomial infection among the elderly in nursing homes. N Engl J Med 1985;312:1483.
73. Schieffelbein CW Jr, Snider DE. Tuberculosis control among homeless populations. Arch Intern Med 1988;148:1843.
74. Stead WW. Pathogenesis of a first episode of chronic pulmonary tuberculosis in man: recrudescence of residuals of the primary infection or exogenous reinfection? Am Rev Resp Dis 1967; 95:729.
75. Leonard MK, Osterholt D, Kourbatova EV, et al. How many sputum specimens are necessary to diagnose pulmonary tuberculosis. Am J Infect Control 2005;33:58–61.
76. Willcox PA, Potgieter PD, Bateman ED, et al. Rapid diagnosis of sputum-negative miliary tuberculosis using the flexible fiberoptic bronchoscope. Thorax 1986;41:681.
77. Siddiqi SH, Libonati JP, Middlebrook G. Evaluation of a rapid radiometric method for drug susceptibility testing of *Myobacterium tuberculosis*. J Clin Microbiol 1981;13:908.
78. Daniel TM, Debanne SM. The serodiagnosis of tuberculosis and other mycobacterial diseases by enzyme-linked immunosorbent assay. Am Rev Respir Dis 1987;135:1137.
79. Ellner PD, Kiehn TE, Cammarata R, et al. Rapid detection and identification of pathogenic mycobacteria by combining radiometric and nucleic acid probe methods. J Clin Microbiol 1988;26:1349.
80. Eisenach KD, Cave MD, Bates JH, et al. Polymerase chain reaction amplification of a repetitive DNA sequence specific for *Mycobacterium tuberculosis*. J Infect Dis 1990;161:977.
81. Hermans PW, Schuitema AR, Van Soolinen D, et al. Specific detection of *Mycobacterium tuberculosis* complex strains by polymerase chain reaction. J Clin Microbiol 1990;28:1204.
82. Pao CC, Yen TSB, You JB, et al. Detection and identification of *Mycobacterium tuberculosis* by DNA amplification. J Clin Microbiol 1990;28:1877.
83. Mbulo GM, Kambashi BS, Kinkese J, et al. Comparison of two bacteriophage tests and nucleic acid amplification for the diagnosis of pulmonary tuberculosis in sub Saharan Africa. Int J Tuberc Lung Dis 2004;8:1342–1347.
84. Wang JY, Lee LN, Chou CS, et al. Performance assessment of a nested-PCR assay (the RAPID BA MTB) and the BD ProbeTec ET system for detection of *Mycobacterium tuberculosis* in clinical specimens. J Clin Microbiol 2004;10:4599–4603.
85. American Thoracic Society/Centers for Disease Control. Treatment of tuberculosis and tuberculosis infection in adults and children. Am Rev Respir Dis 1986;134:355.
86. Quale JM, Lipschik GY, Heurich AE. Management of tuberculous pericarditis. Ann Thorac Surg 1987;43:653.
87. Centers for Disease Control: The use of preventive therapy for tuberculous infection in the United States. MMWR Morb Mortal Wkly Rep 1990;39(RR-8):9.
88. Moran JF, Alexander LG, Staub EW, et al. Long-term results of pulmonary resection for atypical mycobacterial disease. Ann Thorac Surg 1983;35:597.
89. Conlan AA, Hurwitz SS, Krige L, et al. Massive hemoptysis. J Thorac Cardiovasc Surg 1983;85:120.

90. Okabayashi K, Yamazaki K, Hamatake D, et al. Pleuropneumonectomy for pulmonary tuberculosis and chronic tuberculous empyema. Kyobu Geka 2004;57:1033–1037.
91. Takeda S, Maeda H, Hayakawa M, et al. Current surgical intervention for pulmonary tuberculosis. Ann Thorac Surg 2005;79:959–963.
92. Timpe A, Runyon EH. The relationship of "atypical" acid-fast bacteria to human disease. J Lab Clin 1954;44:202.
93. Runyon EH. Anonymous mycobacteria in pulmonary disease. Med Clin North Am 1959;43:273.
94. American Thoracic Society. Diagnosis and treatment of disease caused by nontuberculous mycobacteria. Am Rev Respir Dis 1990;142:940.
95. McQuarrie DG, Hall WH. Actinomycosis of the lung and chest wall. Surgery 1968;64:905.
96. Palmer DL, Harvey RL, Wheeler JK. Diagnostic and therapeutic considerations in *Nocardia asteroides* infection. Medicine 1974;53:391.
97. Buechner JA. Management of Fungus Diseases of the Lungs. Springfield, IL: Thomas; 1971.
98. Cole FH, Cole FH Jr, Khandekar A, et al. Management of broncholithiasis: is thoracotomy necessary? Ann Thorac Surg 1986;42:255.
99. Goodwin RA Jr, Owens FT, Snell JD, et al. Chronic pulmonary histoplasmosis. Medicine 1976;55:413–452.
100. Dines DE, Payne WS, Bernatz PE, et al. Mediastinal granuloma and fibrosing mediastinitis. Chest 1979;75:320.
101. Maholtz, MS, Dauber JH, Yousem SA. Case report: fluconazole therapy in histoplasma mediastinal granuloma. Am J Med Sci 1994;307:274–277.
102. Dunn EJ, Ulicny KS Jr, Wright CB, et al. Surgical implications of sclerosing mediastinitis. A report of six cases and review of the literature. Chest 1990;97:338–346.
103. Urschel HC Jr, Razzuk MA, Netto GJ, et al. Sclerosing mediastinitis: improved management with histoplasmosis titer and ketoconazole. Ann Thorac Surg 1990;50:215–221.
104. Garrett HE, Roper CL. Surgical intervention in histoplasmosis. Ann Thorac Surg 1986;42:711–722.
105. Gilliland MD, Scott LD, Walker WE. Esophageal obstruction caused by mediastinal histoplasmosis: beneficial results of operation. Surgery 1984;95:59–62.
106. Doyle TP, Loyd JE, Robbins IM. Percutaneous pulmonary artery and vein stenting: a novel treatment for mediastinal fibrosis. Am J Respir Crit Care 2001;164:657–660.
107. Drutz DJ, Catanzaro A. Coccidioidmycosis. Part I. Am Rev Respir Dis 1978;117:559.
108. Drutz DJ, Catanzaro A. Coccidioidmyocosis. Part II. Am Rev Respir Dis 1978;117:727.
109. Hyde L. Coccidiodal pulmonary cavitations. Dis Chest 1968;54:213.
110. Nelson AR. The surgical treatment of pulmonary coccidioidomycosis. Curr Probl Surg 1974:1–48.
111. Klein BS, Vergeront JM, Weeks RJ, et al. Isolation of *Blastomyces dermatitidis* in soil associated with a large outbreak of blastomycosis in Wisconsin. N Engl J Med 1986;314:529.
112. Chapman SW, Bradsher RW Jr, Campbell GD Jr, et al. Practice guidelines for the management of patients with blastomycosis. Infectious Disease Society of America. Clin Infect Dis 2000;30:679–683.
113. Yamada H, Kotaki H, Takahasi T. Recommendation for the treatment of fungal pneumonias. Expert Opin Pharmacother 2003;8:1241–1258.
114. Hatcher CR Jr, Sehdeva J, Waters WC III, et al. Primary pulmonary cryptococcosis. J Thorac Cardivasc Surg 1971;61:39.
115. Malde B, Greenberger PA. Allergic bronchopulmonary aspergillosis. Allergy Asthma Proc 2004;25:S38–S39.
116. Karas A, Hankins JR, Attar S, et al. Pulmonary aspergillosis: an analysis of 41 patients. Ann Thorac Surg 1976;22:1.
117. Varkey B, Rose HD. Pulmonary aspergilloma: a rational approach to treatment. Am J Med 1976;61:626.
118. Daly RC, Pairolero PC, Piehler JM, et al. Pulmonary aspergilloma: results of surgical treatment. J Thorac Cardiovasc Surg 1986;92:981.
119. Chen JC, Chang YL, Luh SP, et al. Surgical treatment of pulmonary aspergilloma: a 28 year experience. Thorax 1997;52:810–813.
120. el Oakley R, Petrou M, Goldstraw P. Indications and outcome of surgery for pulmonary aspergilloma. Thorax 1997;52:753–754.
121. Babatasi G, Massetti M, Chapelier A, et al. Surgical treatment of pulmonary aspergilloma: current outcome. J Thorac Cardiovasc Surg 200;119:906–912.
122. Kim YT, Kang MC, Sung SW, et al. Good long-term outcomes after surgical treatment of simple and complex pulmonary aspergilloma. Ann Thorac Surg 2005;79:294–298.
123. Boucher HW, Groll AH, Chiou CC, et al. Newer systemic agents: pharmacokinetics, safety and efficacy. Drugs 2004;64:1997–2020.
124. Herbrecht R. Voriconazole: therapeutic review of a new azole antifungal. Expert Rev Anti Infect Ther 2004 2:485–497.
125. Perfect JR. Management of invasive mycoses in hematology patients: current approaches. Oncology 2004 18:5–14.
126. Perfect JR. Use of newer antifungal therapies in clinical practice: what do the data tell us? Oncology 2004 18:15–23.
127. Kontoyiannis DP, Lewis RE. Caspofungin versus liposomal amphotericin B for empirical therapy. N Engl J Med 2005;352:410–414.
128. Temeck BK, Venzon DJ, Moskaluk CA. Thoracotomy for pulmonary mycoses in non-HIV immunosuppressed patients. Ann Thorac Surg 1994;58:333–338.
129. Dunst KM, Mueller LC. Surgical management of bilateral multiple invasive pulmonary aspergillosis. J Thorac Cardiovasc Surg 2004;128:621–622.
130. Matt P, Bernet F, Habicht J, Gambazzi F, et al. Predicting outcome after lung resection for invasive pulmonary aspergillosis in patients with neutropenia. Chest 2004;126:1783–1788.

73

Video-Assisted Thoracic Surgery

Matthew J. Schuchert, James D. Luketich, and Hiran C. Fernando

Minimally invasive techniques have revolutionized the surgical approach to diseases of the lungs and esophagus. Nearly every major thoracic operation has been performed utilizing video-assisted techniques. Although preliminary outcomes data do appear encouraging for some of the more common procedures such as lobectomy, sympathectomy, and thoracic esophagectomy, the majority of such data are derived from individual experiences or institutional series with short- to intermediate-term follow-up. There is a relative paucity of prospective controlled studies that validate long-term efficacy of minimally invasive approaches to diseases of the thoracic cavity. In this chapter, we review the minimally invasive approaches of lobectomy for lung cancer as well as staging and resection for esophageal cancer utilizing an evidence-based analysis. Emphasis is placed on long-term results, complications, and cost-effectiveness.

Video-Assisted Thoracoscopic Surgery Lobectomy

General Considerations

Anatomic resection is generally considered the "gold standard" treatment option for patients with early-stage non-small cell lung cancer (NSCLC). Lobectomy and pneumonectomy, and in certain circumstances segmentectomy, are the preferred operative approaches.[1] Although video-assisted thoracoscopic surgery (VATS) techniques have recently emerged as the method of choice for many thoracic procedures, the use of this modality in the performance of anatomic lung resections remains controversial.[2] One of the first reports on VATS lobectomy was of a procedure performed in Japan in 1993 utilizing a pig model.[3] Later that same year, VATS lobectomy was performed in humans by Kirby and Rice[4] in the United States as well as by Walker et al.[5] in Great Britain. Video-assisted thoracoscopic surgery has the potential advantages of employing small incisions as well as the ability to avoid rib spreading. Although postoperative morbidity and mortality are generally low following lobectomy, postthoracotomy pain, which is directly related to incision size and the spreading of the ribs, has been shown to lengthen hospital stay and prolong recovery.[6] Recent data indicate that a more rapid recovery is attainable when a VATS approach is employed.[7,8]

In theory, a VATS lobectomy should achieve the same result as an open lobectomy in terms of oncologic benefit. Both open and VATS lobectomy can achieve complete removal of the tumor with the ability to perform lymph node dissection or sampling as deemed appropriate. The ideal patients for VATS lobectomy are those with small peripheral tumors. Central hilar tumors may be difficult to manage with the VATS technique. Additional considerations that favor an open approach include plans for a complete mediastinal lymph node dissection, chest wall invasion, prior neoadjuvant therapy, as well as the presence of endobronchial tumor.[9] Although pneumonectomy can be performed via VATS in selected cases, many of the conditions mandating pneumonectomy would potentially complicate the VATS approach.

Techniques

We focus our discussion on three major types of VATS lobectomy described in the literature: video-assisted minithoracotomy,[10,11] video-assisted simultaneously stapled lobectomy,[12,13] and video-assisted non-rib-spreading lobectomy.[4,5] The VATS lobectomy typically includes individual isolation and ligation of the lobar vessel and bronchus and should avoid rib spreading. Lymph node sampling or dissection should be performed in a manner analogous to the open technique.

Video-assisted minithoracotomy remains the technique most commonly used when performing VATS lobectomy.[9] This technique does require a small thoracotomy incision with placement of a rib spreader. Hilar dissection is performed under direct vision through this utility incision, with the added visualization and illumination of the videothoracoscope. The specimen is delivered through the primary incision. The main disadvantage of this technique is that pain remains a significant issue due to the rib spreading. In video-assisted simultaneously stapled lobectomy, a linear stapler is used to create the lobar fissure. The pulmonary artery, vein, and lobar bronchus are then stapled and divided simultaneously. Although Lewis and associates have reported good results with this approach in a series of 250 patients, most surgeons are reluctant to use this technique as this violates the principles of sequential anatomical dissection of the hilar structures.[13] These principles include individual isolation and division of artery, vein, and bronchus as well as hilar and mediastinal lymph node dissection.

The third technique, video-assisted non-rib-spreading lobectomy, represents perhaps the purest form of VATS lobectomy—employing sequential anatomical dissection of the hilar structures while avoiding rib spreading altogether. The specific surgical approach is determined according to the location of the lesion[14] but typically employs two or three port incisions in addition to a small utility incision. The key difference between video-assisted non-rib-spreading lobectomy and video-assisted minithoracotomy is that no rib spreading is involved. A complete description of the VATS lobectomy surgical techniques is detailed elsewhere.[2,6,14] There have been no comparative studies establishing an advantage of one technique over another.

Morbidity and Mortality

Several large, single-institution series have been published that have demonstrated that VATS lobectomy can be performed safely, with acceptable morbidity and mortality (Table 73.1). The two largest series reported on video-assisted non-rib-spreading lobectomy are by McKenna et al.[15] and Yim et al.[16] In the largest series reported to date, in 1998 McKenna and associates reported on 298 consecutive patients undergoing VATS lobectomy.[15] Only 1 patient died in this series, producing a mortality of 0.3%. Morbidity rates were acceptable at 12.4%. Similarly, Yim and colleagues also reported a large series of 214 patients, with similar results (0.5% mortality, 22% morbidity).[16] Landreneau et al. published a prospective, nonrandomized, multicenter study evaluating a mixed group of patients, 44 of whom underwent VAMT.[17] The morbidity rate was 27% (12/44), with no mortalities. Taken together, these results compare quite favorably with the mortality rates seen in the largest and best series (mortality rates ranging from 1.2% to 6.4%) (Table 73.1).

In 1999, Demmy and Curtis[18] reported a case-control series of 22 high-risk surgical patients, indicating both a 13.6% (3/22) morbidity and a 13.6% mortality. Two patients died of pulmonary complications (aspiration, progressive pneumonia), and the third succumbed to perforated diverticulitis, sepsis, and multisystem failure. It should be noted that all three of these deaths occurred in patients with a performance status of 3 and who were at extremely high risk for any surgical intervention. Similarly, McKenna reported his results on VATS lobectomy on very old high-risk patients (age > 80, n = 9). No mortality was observed after video-assisted non-rib-spreading lobectomy, and only 2 patients experienced minor morbidity.[19] In a review by McKenna of the worldwide literature reporting 1120 VATS lobectomies, only 7 (0.6%) deaths were reported.[9]

Only one randomized comparison of VATS and open approaches has been published from Japan.[20] Unfortunately, perioperative morbidity and mortality were not reported for this group of patients as this study focused primarily on long-

TABLE 73.1.
VATS Lobectomy: Morbidity and Mortality.

Reference	*Year*	*Evidence*	*n*	*Follow-up (mo)*	*Morbidity (%)*	*Mortality (%)*
VATS						
Landreneau et al.[17]	1997	Prospective, nonrandomized	44	Median (26)	27.3	0
McKenna et al.[15]	1998	Retrospective	298	Mean (29)	12.4	0.3
Yim et al.[16]	1998	Retrospective	214	Mean (26)	22.0	0.5
Roviaro et al.[10]	1998	Retrospective	171	NR	15	0
Walker[21]	1998	Retrospective	150	Mean (27)	32.0	0.7
Kaseda et al.[22]	1998	Retrospective	128	Median (22)	3.1	0.8
Hermansson et al.[96]	1998	Retrospective	30	NR	3.3	0
Lewis et al.[13]	1999	Retrospective	250	Mean (34)	11.2	0
Demmy and Curtis[18]	1999	Case-control	22	Mean (13)	13.6	13.6
Walker et al.[97]	2003	Retrospective	158	Mean (38)	NR	1.8
Gharagozloo et al.[98]	2003	Prospective	179	Mean (37)	20.7	0.01
Open						
Ginsberg et al. (LCSG)[99]	1983	Retrospective	1,058	NR	NR	2.9
Ginsberg et al. (LCSG)[1]	1995	Prospective, randomized	125	<54	4.8 (Respiratory failure)	1.6
Duque et al.[100]	1997	Retrospective	294	NR	33.3	4.4
Wada et al.[101]	1998	Retrospective	5,609	12	NR	1.2
Thomas et al.[102]	2002	Retrospective	390	35	NR	2.3
Stoelben et al.[103]	2003	Retrospective	699	NR	NR	2.7
Birkmeyer et al.[63]	2003	Retrospective, national database	75,563	NR	NR	4.2 (high volume) 6.4 (low volume)
Deslauriers et al.[104]	2004	Retrospective	184	NR	NR	1.6

NR, not recorded.

term survival and recurrence patterns (these results are described in the next section). Although the vast majority of publications on VATS lobectomy are retrospective in nature, the preponderance of data would suggest that this approach can be performed with acceptable rates of morbidity and mortality when compared with the largest open series. The Cancer and Leukemia Group B (CALGB) (39802) recently completed a prospective multiinstitutional phase II trial assessing the feasibility of VATS lobectomy for solitary, peripheral pulmonary nodules (less than 3 cm). The goal of this trial was to describe a standardized approach to VATS lobectomy and to determine whether this operation was safe in a multicenter setting. In this study, 111 patients were enrolled with peripheral stage I NSCLC. A VATS lobectomy was performed successfully in 97 patients (87%). There were three deaths, producing a 3.1% mortality. Morbidity was documented in 7.2%. One criticism of this study has been that a significant number of the patients enrolled came from a single institution. However, preliminary analysis of the data suggests that VATS lobectomy is safe and effective. These findings will require further validation regarding long-term outcomes as well as cancer recurrence rates and patterns.

Recurrence and Survival

A concern of many surgeons is whether the VATS approach will provide the same oncological control as open operations. Only a few reports with significant numbers of patients have described 5-year survival rates[15,20–23] (Table 73.2). In the only randomized study to date, Sugi et al. (2000) evaluated 100 consecutive patients with clinical stage Ia lung cancer.[20] The group was randomized to VATS lobectomy (n = 48) or standard open lobectomy (n = 52). Radical lymphadenectomy was performed in both groups. Median follow-up was 60 months. The survival was 90% at both 3 and 5 years for the VATS lobectomy group compared with 93% and 85%, respectively, for the conventional open group (P = .91).[20] Locoregional recurrence was equivalent in both groups (3/48 vs. 3/52, respectively).

In 1998, McKenna and his associates reported a retrospective series with 298 patients treated for lung cancer followed over a mean of 29 months.[15] All patients underwent a video-assisted non-rib-spreading lobectomy technique. Three-year survival for patients with stage I disease (n = 233) was 80%, and for those with stage 2 disease (n = 27) it was 66%. Similar results were reported by the retrospective series of Walker,[21] Kaseda et al.,[22] and most recently Iwasaki et al.[23] (Table 73.2). These results are very similar to the expected survival seen after open lobectomy for both stage I and stage II tumors.

When collectively analyzed, the published data would suggest that VATS lobectomy can be performed with recurrence and survival rates comparable to the best open series. It should be emphasized again, however, that the body of published data is almost entirely retrospective, representing individual single-institutional series. Prospective, controlled studies with long-term outcomes will be required to confirm the oncologic efficacy of this approach.

Surgical Outcomes and Quality of Life

Posterolateral thoracotomy has been associated with significant pain and limitation in postoperative function. A VATS lobectomy has been postulated to reduce perioperative pain, allow an earlier return to work, and provide improved quality of life (QOL). Table 73.3 outlines several perioperative variables comparing VATS lobectomy with a conventional open approach. The VATS approach appears to improve perioperative recovery with a trend towards decreased chest tube drainage and decreased length of stay (Table 73.3). Although not presented in the table, mean operative times (133–250 min) from these series were frequently longer in the VATS groups compared with the open groups (110–215 min), though statistical significance is not consistently observed. Interestingly, in the larger series the mean operative times for VATS lobec-

TABLE 73.2.
VATS Lobectomy: Recurrence and Survival.

					Survival (%)				
					Stage 1		*Stage 2*		
Reference	*Year*	*Evidence*	*n*	*Follow-up (mo)*	*3 yr*	*5 yr*	*3 yr*	*5 yr*	*Locoregional recurrence (%)*
VATS									
McKenna et al.[15]	1998	Retrospective	298	Mean (60)	80	60	66	66	NR
Walker[21]	1998	Retrospective	150	Mean (27)	94	75	57	NR	4
Kaseda et al.[22]	1998	Retrospective	103	Median (22)	94	NR	NR	NR	NR
Sugi et al.[20]	2000	Randomized	48	Median (60)	90	90	NR	NR	6
Walker et al.[97]	2003	Retrospective	158	Mean (38)	NRR	NR	78	51	5.7
Gharagozloo et al.[98]	2003	Prospective	179	Mean (37)	86	83	NR	NR	3.9
Iwasaki et al.[23]	2004	Retrospective	140	NR	NR	81	NR	70	NR
Open									
Ginsberg et al. (LCSG)[1]	1995	Prospective, randomized	125	>54	NR	NR	NR	NR	6.4
Mountain[105]	1997	Retrospective	5319	NR	46–71	38–61	31–38	22–34	NR
Thomas et al.[102]	2001	Retrospective	390	35	NR	63	NR	NR	5.8
Deslauriers et al.[104]	2004	Retrospective	185	NR	NR	66	NR	50	22 (sleeve lobectomy)

NR, not recorded.

tomy are quite low (133–135 min) and compare favorably with most open series, suggesting a learning curve effect that is encountered in most minimally-invasive procedures.[11,104] The VATS approach appears to improve perioperative recovery, with a trend toward decreased chest tube drainage and decreased length of stay (Table 73.3). In a series of 895 consecutive VATS patients (including those receiving thoracoscopy, wedge resections, and lobectomies), DeCamp and associates demonstrated that the average hospital stay was 3 days following any simple VATS procedure and 5 days following VATS lung resections.[25]

A significant component of postthoracotomy pain is related to rib spreading. Trauma to the intercostal nerve bundles has been shown to be associated with loss of ipsilateral and contralateral superficial abdominal reflexes within the first week following surgery.[26] There are many studies that have evaluated the intensity of acute pain following VATS lobectomy (Table 73.3). In all of these studies, VATS was associated with reduced postoperative pain within the first weeks after surgery.

Chronic postthoracotomy pain, shoulder function, and return to work are all important issues following thoracic surgery. Most patients are restricted in their function and regular physical activities for the first 6 to 8 weeks following a conventional posterolateral thoracotomy. Stammberger and colleagues assessed the long-term QOL following VATS procedures in 173 patients, of which 16 procedures were lobectomies.[27] Over one-half (53%) of patients said that their pain was insignificant 2 weeks following surgery. Seventy-five percent of patients had no complaints at 6 months following VATS; the remaining 25% had only minimal-to-moderate discomfort. By 2 years, only 4% of patients had any residual discomfort. In this same series, over 89% of patients returned to work within 2 weeks. In another retrospective series of 70 VATS lobectomy patients reported by Walker and associates, there was only mild port site discomfort by 3–6 weeks following surgery, and only 1.2% (1/70) of patients developed chronic pain.[24]

In a retrospective study evaluating acute pain and shoulder dysfunction, Landreneau and coworkers demonstrated that shoulder dysfunction was the same in both the VATS and muscle-sparing thoracotomy groups in the first 3 days after surgery. However, shoulder function was found to return to normal within 3 weeks in the VATS group, whereas it remained significantly impaired in the muscle-sparing thoracotomy group.[7] A follow-up to this study compared pain and shoulder function in 178 patients who had a VATS resection to 165 patients who had a lung resection via thoracotomy.[28] The findings demonstrated that within the first year following surgery, there were quantitatively significant differences in overall pain, pain intensity scores, and shoulder function favoring the VATS approach (shoulder dysfunction 25% in the open group vs. 10% in the VATS group, $P < .001$).[28]

In another retrospective comparison of 22 patients undergoing VATS lobectomy and 22 patients undergoing thoracotomy and lobectomy, Sugiura and associates found that patients who underwent VATS lobectomy had significant decreases in both acute and chronic chest pain as well as in the time to return to preoperative activity. Patients reported overall greater confidence in their wound size as well as the overall impression of their operation.[29]

In a recent prospective, nonrandomized study examining QOL in patients undergoing lobectomy, the European Organization for Research and Treatment of Cancer (EORTC) Quality of Life Questionnaire (QLQ) C30 and EORTC QLQ-LC13 were used to compare VATS (n = 27) and thoracotomy (n = 24) groups. Although there was a trend for the VATS patients to score higher on the QOL and functioning scales as well as to report fewer postoperative symptoms, these differences did not achieve statistical significance.[30]

Several studies have compared pulmonary function following VATS lobectomy and thoracotomy. Nomori and coworkers demonstrated that VATS results in a more rapid recovery of respiratory strength compared with posterolateral thoracotomy.[31] Nagahiro and coworkers also demonstrated significantly improved forced expiratory volume in 1 s (FEV_1) and forced vital capacity (FVC) at postoperative day 14 following VATS lobectomy (n = 13) compared with thoracotomy (n = 9).[8] Kaseda and associates demonstrated a similar improvement in FEV_1 and FVC as long as 3 months following surgery in VATS lobectomy patients compared with standard thoracotomy.[32]

Good preservation of postoperative pulmonary function is of potential great benefit for patients with lung cancer as these patients are often elderly and with poor pulmonary

TABLE 73.3.
VATS Lobectomy: Perioperative Outcomes Data.

			Patient (n)		*Chest tube (days)*		*LOS (days)*		
Reference	*Year*	*Evidence*	*VATS*	*Thor*	*VATS*	*Thor*	*VATS*	*Thor*	*Acute Pain*
Landreneau et al.[7]	1993	Nonrandomized	81	57	NR	NR	5.0	7.5	Less at POD 1, 2[a]
Guidicelli et al.[11]	1994	Nonrandomized	44	23	8	10	12	15	Less at POD 1–4[a]
Kirby et al.[106]	1995	Randomized	30	31	4.6	6.5	7.1	8.3	NR
Tschernko et al.[107]	1996	Randomized	22	25	NR	NR	5.1	9.2	Less at POD 3[a]
Walker et al.[24]	1996	Nonrandomized	70	110	NR	NR	7.0	NR	Less use of pain medications
Ohbuchi et al.[41]	1998	Nonrandomized	35	35	5.3	7.6	15.0	24.0	Less use of pain medications
Demmy and Curtis[18]	1999	Nonrandomized	23	31	4.0	8.3	5.3	12.2	Less use of pain medications
Nagahiro et al.[8]	2001	Nonrandomized	13	9	3.6	3.8	NR	NR	Less pain POD 1, 7, 14[a]

LOS, length of stay; POD, postoperative day; Thor, thoracotomy.
[a]$P < .05$.

reserve. Maintenance of good pulmonary function postoperatively could translate into decreased postoperative complications and promote faster recovery, especially in this group of higher-risk patients. Although the above studies demonstrated an apparent improvement in respiratory dynamics, it should be kept in mind that the data were pooled retrospectively. In addition, other published series have failed to demonstrate any statistical difference in FEV_1 or FVC when comparing VATS lobectomy and open lobectomy.[11,33] Thus, the overall clinical significance of these findings remains uncertain.

Various biologic mediators and cytokines have also been evaluated to investigate differences between VATS and various thoracotomy approaches. A prospective randomized study was performed by Gebhard and associates to evaluate inflammatory cytokine differences between VATS and thoracotomy in the treatment of patients with pneumothorax. Serum levels of C-reactive protein, polymorphonuclear elastase, prostacyclin, and thromboxane A_2 were measurably less in the VATS group compared with the open group.[34] In other studies, postoperative C-reactive protein, interleukin 6 (IL-6), IL-8, and IL-10 levels were all found to be reduced in VATS groups.[35,36] Other studies have demonstrated higher circulating $CD4^+$ T-cell and natural killer cell counts, as well as reduced suppression of lymphocyte oxidation following VATS.[37] When taken together, these data indicate a reduced inflammatory response to surgery following VATS compared with thoracotomy. The overall clinical significance of these findings remains to be established.

Complications

The most common morbidity in all published series was prolonged air leak (Table 73.1). Other complications in these series ranged from major (including empyema, respiratory failure, and bronchopleural fistula) to minor complications, such as subcutaneous emphysema and atrial fibrillation. The causes of mortality included mesenteric venous infarct, massive pulmonary embolism, severe respiratory failure, and unknown causes (Table 73.1). None of the deaths in these series was due to major intraoperative bleeding.

In a review by McKenna of the worldwide literature reporting 1560 VATS lobectomies, only one intraoperative death was reported that was due to bleeding.[9] Conversion rates to thoracotomy were 11.6% in this series. The majority of the conversions were due to oncologic concerns, such as the presence of a T3 tumor or close proximity to the main pulmonary artery. Another 30% of the conversions were due to dense pleural adhesions or poor visualization. The rate of conversions appeared to decrease with increasing experience of the operating surgeon.[38]

VATS Lobectomy Versus Open Lobectomy

The morbidity and mortality following VATS lobectomy compares favorably to open surgery, as discussed above (Table 73.1). In nearly all presented series, the mortality was less than 1%, compared with expected mortality rates of 2%–3% in the open literature. In addition, VATS lobectomy appears to be associated with survival (60%–75% 5-year survival for T1 tumors) and recurrence (4%–6%) rates similar to that published in many open series (Table 73.2). For example, Warren and Faber identified a recurrence rate of 4.9% in patients with stage 1 cancer resected with an open approach.[39] The Lung Cancer Study Group trial comparing open lobectomy with limited resection demonstrated a cancer death rate of 8.5% and a recurrence rate of 9.3% after lobectomy for stage 1A lung cancer.[1]

One concern regarding VATS lobectomy is the adequacy of lymph node dissection. Several studies have addressed this issue and demonstrated that lymph node dissection and sampling are similar between open and VATS approaches (range 10–23 lymph nodes).[40,41] Radical lymphadenectomy can be performed successfully with a VATS approach, if desired.[42] Other authors have raised concerns about the possibility of increased tumor seeding following VATS lobectomy. Large series, however, demonstrated low pleural space or incisional recurrences (0.3%–2%).[43] A VATS lobectomy appears to be associated with less postoperative pain, shorter length of stay, improved pulmonary dynamics, and an overall decreased inflammatory response following surgery, although prospective, controlled studies will be required to delineate the precise benefits.

Cost-Effectiveness

There are no definitive studies establishing cost-effectiveness for VATS lobectomy. In the only study that attempted to address this issue, Sugi and coauthors performed a cost analysis comparing VATS lobectomy (n = 10) and open lobectomy (n = 20). The disposable instrument costs were $3190 higher in the VATS lobectomy group, and the operative time was longer (5.56h for VATS vs. 4.25h for open). In this small series, the length of hospital stay was comparable (25.2 vs. 27.7 days, respectively), thus resulting in a higher total hospital charge in the VATS lobectomy group.[44] These data are difficult to interpret due to the small group size and to the fact that hospital stays were significantly longer than reported in multiple other series in the literature (Table 73.3). A detailed socioeconomic analysis taking into consideration operating room costs, hospital length of stay, total hospital costs, return to work, and productivity will need to be performed to identify any potential societal economic benefit between these procedures.

Summary

Although it would appear that VATS lobectomy is a viable procedure for resection of early (stage 1–2) lung cancers, it should be kept in mind that the preponderance of the data is retrospective, uncontrolled, and single institutional in nature and thereby subject to the traditional biases and potential for error. In an evidence-based review conducted by the American College of Chest Physicians, it was concluded that there were insufficient data to suggest a significant advantage of VATS lobectomy compared to conventional thoracotomy.[45] In addition, there are no adequate prospective, phase III studies to compare VATS versus open lobectomies. There are tremendous obstacles to completing such a randomized study because of market forces as well as physician and patient biases. Experienced surgeons, with good outcomes using either a VATS or open approach, are unwilling to randomize patients to a different approach. Similarly, patients who seek out a surgeon offering a VATS approach are often unwilling to be randomized to a study if there is a 50% chance of requiring a thoracotomy.

The minimally invasive thoracic surgical group who conducted the recent CALBG study is addressing these issues in a follow-up trial that is being developed. The new study will likely be a registry study in which surgeons perform lobectomy using their best approach, with prospective data collection of defined variables and endpoints. For now, VATS lobectomy should be considered feasible. There may be advantages in terms of length of stay, pain severity, recovery of shoulder function, and return to normal activity. Lobectomy utilizing thoracotomy, however, should continue to be considered the gold standard in the surgical management of early-stage lung cancer.

Staging for Esophageal Cancer

General Considerations

Esophageal cancer was estimated to affect 15,560 new patients in the United States in 2007, and over 13,940 patients will die of this disease each year.[46] It is the fastest-growing malignancy in the United States. Most patients will present with advanced disease because dysphagia (the most common symptom), frequently does not develop until a stage III or IV cancer is present. Therefore, the majority of patients will have advanced local, regional, or distant metastases at the time of initial diagnosis. Evidence of extensive locoregional nodal involvement or distant metastases typically precludes curative resection. Therefore, precise preoperative assessment of the extent of disease (staging) will help to identify patients who are unlikely to benefit from radical resection as well as those who may be favorable candidates for aggressive chemotherapy and radiotherapy regimens. In addition, accurate pretreatment staging allows a more rational evaluation and comparison of different treatment modalities.

Currently, several noninvasive modalities are employed in the preoperative assessment of patients with esophageal cancer. The most commonly used are computed tomography (CT) and endoscopic ultrasound (EUS). More recent innovations include the application of positron emission tomography (PET) to esophageal cancer staging. These noninvasive methods frequently overstage or understage esophageal cancer due to the lack of pathologic verification. There is difficulty in discriminating normal lymph nodes from metastatic lymph nodes, inflammatory nodules from metastatic nodules, as well as T3 from T4 invasive lesions.

Video-assisted staging for esophageal cancer utilizing minimally invasive techniques dates back to the report of Murray and colleagues, who described the use of mediastinoscopy and minilaparotomy to evaluate for the presence of pathologic lymph nodes in a retrospective analysis of 30 consecutive patients with esophageal cancer.[47] Whereas mediastinoscopy was positive in 5/18 patients with carcinoma of the mid- to upper esophagus, none of the 12 patients with esophageal cancer of the lower esophagus had abnormal findings at mediastinoscopy. Interestingly, the authors found that celiac lymph node involvement at laparotomy predicted mediastinal extension with an accuracy of 78% (14/18). Of the 7 patients with negative mediastinoscopy and laparotomy findings, 4 were alive and free of disease 14–30 months following resection. The authors therefore concluded that combined mediastinoscopy and laparotomy will help to avoid excessive morbidity in patients with advanced disease and will assist in identifying favorable candidates for aggressive excisional therapy.

Dagnini and coworkers were the first to report the use of laparoscopy for esophageal cancer in 369 patients.[48] They were able to identify intraabdominal metastases in 14% of patients and celiac lymph node metastases in 9.7%, thus preventing unnecessary resection in these patients. In 1993, Krasna and McLaughlin were the first to report the utility of thoracoscopic lymph node staging.[49] Although VATS/laparoscopic staging or laparoscopic staging alone has emerged as the most accurate method of preoperative surgical staging, this is not routinely performed, with most centers preferring noninvasive modalities. However, many surgeons are beginning to employ an initial laparoscopic staging on the table prior to opening for esophagectomy due to adenocarcinoma of the esophagogastric junction.

Noninvasive Staging

Of the noninvasive modalities, EUS is the best clinical instrument for evaluation of the T stage. If T3 or T4 lesions are found, then the patient has locally advanced disease and a high possibility of N1 disease. In patients with a T2 lesion, the prevalence of positive nodes can be as high as 50%. A T3 lesion, whether stricturing or not, is associated with positive lymph nodes in 80% of patients.[50] Although malignant strictures provide a limitation on the use of EUS, the presence of a malignant stricture itself is a reliable predictor of advanced disease, with 90% of such patients exhibiting stage III or IV disease.[51]

The accuracy of EUS for nodal disease is lower. Accuracy rates of 65%–80% have been reported with EUS for nodal status. The identification of N1 disease is extremely important as this finding will frequently influence the management of patients, such as guiding the use of neoadjuvant therapy (Table 73.4).

Positron emission tomography has also been utilized in the pretreatment staging of esophageal cancer. In an evaluation of 35 patents with potentially resectable esophageal cancer, PET detected nine sites of distant metastases missed by conventional scanning (CT plus bone scan), achieving a sensitivity of 88%, specificity of 93%, and accuracy of 91%.[52] Luketich and coauthors also demonstrated that PET can identify distant metastases in 20% of cases if CT scanning and bone scanning were negative, but PET has limited sensitivity (45%) and accuracy (48%) for lymph node metastases smaller than 1 cm.[52] When compared with other noninvasive staging modalities (such as CT), PET appears to afford superior sensitivity and accuracy, especially in the detection of metastatic disease. In a study of 100 consecutive PET scans by Luketich and coworkers, PET scan using ^{18}F-fluorodeoxyglucose was compared with CT scanning in the detection of distant metastases.[53] Minimally invasive staging was used to confirm or refute imaging results, and it identified 70 distant metastases in 39 cases. In this study, PET detected 51 metastases in 27 of the 39 cases (69% sensitivity, 93.4% specificity, and 84% accuracy) compared with CT, which detected 26 metastases in 18 of the 39 cases (46.1% sensitivity, 73.8% specificity,

TABLE 73.4.
Comparison of Staging Modalities.

Reference	*Year*	*Evidence*	*n*	*Modality*	*Sensitivity (%)*	*Specificity (%)*	*Accuracy (%)*	*Comment*
Krasna et al.[56]	1999	Retrospective	47	CT[a]	75 (LN)	76 (LN)	NR	Detection of regional LNs within the chest.
				EUS[a]	0 (LN)	51 (LN)	NR	
				MIS[a]	63 (LN)	100 (LN)	94 (LN)	
			33	CT[a]	0 (LN)	97 (LN)	NR	Detection of regional LNs within the abdomen.
				EUS[a]	22 (LN)	82 (LN)	NR	
				MIS[a]	85 (LN)	100 (LN)	94 (LN)	
Luketich et al.[52]	2000	Retrospective	53	CT[b]	33 (LN)	88 (LN)	59 (LN)	MIS changed the stage originally assigned by CT + EUS in 32% of patients
				EUS[b]	63 (LN)	60 (LN)	NR	
				CT + EUS[b]	86 (LN)	41 (LN)	68 (LN)	
Meltzer et al.[108]	2000	Retrospective	37	PET[b]	41 (LN)	88 (LN)	NR	PET demonstrates higher specificity for the presence of regional tumor and distant metastases.
				CT[b]	87 (LN)	43 (LN)	NR	
				PET[b]	71 (M)	93 (M)	NR	
				CT[b]	57 (M)	97 (M)	NR	
Krasna et al.[58]	2001	Prospective	134	CT[b]	NR	NR	50	CALGB study demonstrated feasibility of MIS. MIS doubled the number of positive LNs identified by conventional staging.
				EUS[b]	NR	NR	70	
Nguyen et al.[109]	2001	Retrospective	33	CT + EUS[a]	NR	91	61	Assessed overall staging accuracy. MIS altered the treatment plan in 36% of patients.
				MIS[a]	NR	100	97	
Parmar et al.[110]	2002	Retrospective	40	CT[a]	30 (M1a)	50 (M1a)	35 (M1a)	EUS/FNA is superior to CT in detecting M1a disease. It directed management in all patients in this study.
				EUS[a]	100 (M1a)	50 (M1a)	90 (M1a)	
				EUS/FNA[a]	100 (M1a)	100 (M1a)	100 (M1a)	

CT, CAT scan; EUS, endoscopic ultrasound; LN, regional lymph nodes; M, metastases; MIS, minimally invasive staging; NR, not recorded.
[a]Modalities compared with final pathology from resected specimens.
[b]Noninvasive modalities compared with and confirmed by minimally invasive staging.

and 63% accuracy) ($P < .01$). Therefore, PET scanning enhances our ability to detect distant metastases in the preoperative staging of esophageal cancer, and is more accurate than CT, but still is only 69% sensitive when compared to minimally invasive staging.

In another retrospective study, Wren and coauthors demonstrated comparable sensitivity and accuracy when comparing CT to PET in the detection of regional nodal involvement or distant metastatic disease.[54] However, PET still demonstrated superior specificity in this study.

It has been suggested that PET may be used to predict biological behavior after neoadjuvant therapy. In a prospective study published by Downy and associates of 39 patients with esophageal cancer, 2-year disease-free and overall survival were 38% and 63%, respectively in patients who had less than a 60% decrease in standardized uptake value (SUV), compared with 67% and 89%, respectively, in patients who had a greater than 60% decrease in SUV following neoadjuvant therapy.[55] The advent of CT-PET combination modalities may further enhance the utility of these tools in the preoperative staging of esophageal cancer.

Minimally Invasive Staging

The most definitive form of staging is one in which precise anatomic and pathologic information can be combined in the assessment of a tumor. As experience with thoracoscopic and laparoscopic techniques has increased, these modalities have been increasingly employed for the staging of esophageal cancer. In addition to providing specific information regarding the primary tumor, such techniques dramatically enhance the detection of regional and distant metastases, simultaneously providing tissue for pathological confirmation. With refinement of technique, success rates have been found to be very high in terms of predicting final pathologic stage.

Results: Minimally Invasive Staging Versus Noninvasive Staging

In 1999, a retrospective comparison study was performed by Krasna and coworkers on 88 patients with esophageal cancer who underwent CT, EUS, or both followed by a thoracoscopic/laparoscopic staging procedure to evaluate the role of the various staging modalities.[56] Of these patients, 82 received both chest and abdominal CT scans, and 62 patients underwent EUS. Thoracoscopic staging was completed in 82 patients, and laparoscopic staging was accomplished in 55 patients; 49 patients underwent both thoracoscopic and laparoscopic staging. Thirty-nine (44%) patients did not undergo resection after staging because of an advanced lesion (T4, 13 patients; M1, 3 patients). Three of 42 patients (6.3%) with N0 disease established by thoracoscopy were found at resection to have paraesophageal lymph node involvement (N1). The overall accuracy of thoracoscopic staging was 93.6%, and for laparoscopic staging it was 93.9%. Based on pathologic evaluation of resected specimens, the sensitivity, specificity, and positive predictive value for staging N1 disease in the chest were 62.5%, 100%, and 100% for thoracoscopy; 75%, 75.6%, and 23.1% with CT; and 0%, 51.4%, and 5.5% by EUS, respectively. For N1 disease in the abdomen, it was 85%, 100%, and 100% by laparoscopy; 0%, 97.1%, and 0% by CT; and 22%, 81.5%, and 28.6% by EUS, respectively. Therefore, thoracoscopic/laparoscopic staging was found to have a higher specificity and accuracy than either CT or EUS, especially for N1 disease in the chest[56] (Table 73.4).

Luketich and associates also found that minimally invasive staging was superior compared to EUS in detecting lymph node metastases in esophageal cancer.[52] In this study, the sensitivity and specificity for EUS in nodal evaluation were found to be 65% and 66%, respectively. Overall accuracy was 65%. The overall incidence of lymph node metastases as detected by laparoscopy/VATS staging was 81%. In the six cases that laparoscopy/VATS detected N1 disease and for which EUS showed N0, the lymph nodes were less than 1 cm in diameter. Although minimally invasive staging never identified a T4 lesion when a T3 lesion was diagnosed by EUS, the sensitivity for nodal metastases smaller than 1 cm was only 44%. Endoscopic ultrasound documented no distant metastases, whereas 4/26 (15%) of patients undergoing minimally invasive staging were found to have liver metastases. An additional limitation of EUS is that in 20%–38% of patients with esophageal cancer a high-grade malignant stricture precludes passage of an echoendoscope. Dilation of such strictures can be performed, but dilation with subsequent EUS carries a significant risk of perforation.[57]

A recent prospective Thoracic Intergroup study (Cancer and Leukemia Group B 9380) evaluated the effectiveness of minimally invasive staging of esophageal cancer in a multi-institutional setting.[58] In this study, 134 patients were evaluated. Thoracoscopic/laparoscopic staging was considered successful if one thoracoscopic lymph node and three laparoscopic lymph nodes were sampled, a confirmed positive node was found, or T4 or M1 disease was documented. If these conditions were met in at least 70% of patients, the method was determined to be feasible. There were no deaths or major complications, the median operative time was 210 min (range 40–865 min), and the postoperative hospital stay was 3 days (range 1–35 days). Seventy-three percent of patients met the definition of feasibility. Positive lymph node disease was found in 43 patients (32%); 10 patients (13%) were found to have T4/M1 disease. Of note, thoracoscopy was not feasible in this study in 30/134 patients. In addition, the number of lymph node stations sampled reliably and the positivity rate of each station were lower in the chest when compared with abdominal lymph node stations. The frequency of positive lymph node by station was 2 (10%), 3 (8%), 4 (10%), 7 (10%), 8 (25%), 9 (10%), 10 (10%), 17 (34%), and 20 (27%). Thirty-two patients (24%) were deemed N0 by thoracoscopic/laparoscopic staging. Of these, 13 went directly to surgery without induction therapy. In final pathologic analysis, only 3 of 13 (23%) were found to have N1 disease, achieving a much higher accuracy of staging compared with the conventional noninvasive modalities. In this study, CT, magnetic resonance imaging (MRI), and EUS incorrectly identified TN staging in 50%, 40%, and 30% of patients, respectively. Thoracoscopic/laparoscopic staging therefore appears to be safe and feasible. It doubles the number of positive lymph nodes detected by conventional noninvasive staging. This helps to establish a more accurate assessment of the patient's stage of disease at the time of presentation and provides optimal information in the assessment of a patient's likelihood of recurrent disease and long-term survival. It now appears clear that the major benefit of staging for adenocarcinoma of the esophagogastric junction is by laparoscopy. We prefer to add thoracoscopy only for a specific indication, such as a pulmonary nodule or midesophageal lesion staging.

Morbidity and Mortality

Laparoscopic (with or without thoracoscopic) staging can be performed with minimal morbidity and mortality. Published series report relatively few major or minor complications. Reported complications following laparoscopic/thoracoscopic staging include pleural effusion, air leak, atelectasis, prolonged ileus, urinary retention, port site infection, and small bowel obstruction. Average hospital stays ranged from 1 to 4 days. Feeding tube and infusaport placement can be performed at the time of surgery. These additional procedures add little in the way of morbidity but enhance the patient's nutritional status and provide access for chemotherapy and blood draws.

A concern that has been raised with the use of minimally invasive staging is the potential for making subsequent resection more difficult due to the obliteration of normal tissue planes and adhesions derived from the staging procedure. Although there have been no formal analyses published in the literature on this topic, many surgeons (including our own group) have suggested that the thoracoscopic staging could be omitted in most cases of gastroesophageal junction adenocarcinoma. In our study, only 3/26 cases were found for which lap staging was negative and thoracoscopic staging was positive.[52] Laparoscopic staging alone permits decreased operative time, decreased length of stay (since there is no need for a chest tube), and a decreased complication rate.

Cost-Effectiveness

In a decision analysis model of cost-effectiveness, Harewood and Wiersema compared the costs of EUS plus fine-needle aspiration (FNA), CT-FNA, and minimally invasive staging.[59] EUS-FNA was the least costly staging strategy ($13,811) when compared to CT-FNA ($14,350) and surgery ($13,992). The statistical and clinical significance of this analysis remains undefined. In a separate analysis, Wallace and colleagues[60] evaluated CT, PET, EUS-FNA, and minimally invasive staging to determine which modality (either alone or in combination) is most cost-effective in the staging of esophageal cancer. The combination of PET and EUS-FNA was found to be the most cost-effective approach and was associated with $60,544 per quality-adjusted life year gained. This marginal cost-effectiveness is in line with other commonly accepted cancer screening methods, such as mammography.[61] The added cost of combining thoracoscopy and laparoscopy appeared offset by the potential increase in accuracy when utilizing this modality in terms of overall cost-efficiency.

Summary

Although minimally invasive staging of esophageal cancer has been shown to be feasible and to provide the most accurate staging information on esophageal cancer, this approach has not been uniformly adopted by many centers. In part, this is due to a lack of familiarity and comfort with these techniques. Other factors include that in many cases management may not be altered, and dissection at the time of resection may be more complex, particularly if an aggressive dissection was performed at the time of staging. At our center, we no longer perform routine VATS staging for the following reasons: (1) Many of the cancers are gastroesophageal junction adenocarcinomas, which are more likely to have abdominal nodal involvement. (2) In our series, there were only 3/26 cases for which laparoscopic staging was negative and thoracoscopic staging was positive. (3) Laparoscopic staging alone would decrease operative times, length of stay, and morbidity. (4) For the reasons alluded to above, resection is technically more difficult after minimally invasive staging with or without neoadjuvant therapy. We continue to use VATS staging to evaluate indeterminate thoracic lesions or to evaluate suspected T4 disease.

As noted above, EUS is the most accurate modality for determining T stage. Since there is an 80% likelihood of nodal disease with T3 disease, we no longer perform as aggressive a lymph node sampling if T3 disease is identified by EUS. All patients with EUS-staged T3 disease are offered neoadjuvant therapy. The purpose of laparoscopy is to rule out unsuspected liver or peritoneal metastases and to evaluate the suitability of the stomach as a conduit at the time of resection. Lymph nodes that are easily accessible are sampled, but an aggressive dissection at the hiatus or in the peritumoral area is not performed.

In conclusion, CT, PET, and EUS are complimentary modalities that are used for clinical staging. Endoscopic ultrasound is most useful for T status, and PET is most useful for assessing distant metastases. Minimally invasive staging combining thoracoscopy and laparoscopy provides the most accurate information on nodal staging but is not routinely performed in most centers for the reasons alluded to above. Laparoscopic staging alone for esophagogastric tumors is a reasonable alternative and can also be done on the table just prior to open esophagectomy to rule out radiologically occult metastatic disease or local resectability.

Minimally Invasive Esophagectomy

General Considerations

Minimally invasive esophagectomy (MIE) is a complex and technically challenging procedure that was initially performed in only a few medical centers worldwide. However, personal communications with our group now indicate well over 50 centers worldwide are performing MIE, and the numbers appear to be growing rapidly. Open esophagectomy remains the standard approach in most medical centers.[62] A number of open approaches are available, with individual centers tending to favor one approach over another. Esophagectomy is associated with significant morbidity and mortality. In centers where there is not a focused approach to esophagectomy, mortality will be higher. In a report documenting statistics from a national database, Birkmeyer and colleagues found that mortality rates from esophagectomy ranged from 8% in high-volume centers to as high as 23% in low-volume centers.[63]

Since the introduction of laparoscopic Nissen fundoplication in 1991, tremendous improvements in instrumentation and optics have fostered the development of minimally invasive approaches to esophageal diseases, including esophagectomy. The earliest descriptions of MIE involved a combination of open surgery with either thoracoscopy or laparoscopy. In 1993, Collard et al. demonstrated that esophageal dissection could be carried out thoracoscopically when combined with laparotomy for gastric mobilization.[64] There have been multiple subsequent reports of esophagectomy for cancer, performed by thoracoscopy and open laparotomy, including those reports by the groups of Liu,[65] Akaishi,[66] Dexter,[67] and Law.[68] These studies demonstrated the feasibility of thoracoscopic-assisted esophagectomy, but the overall benefit was not well established. A concern of all these reports is that all are essentially hybrid operations, with an open approach in one body cavity and a minimally invasive approach in the other.

DePaula and associates from Brazil were the first to describe a completely laparoscopic transhiatal esophagectomy (THE).[69] Swanstrom and Hansen subsequently published their experience using the laparoscopic transhiatal approach. This was the first North American report of esophagectomy using a completely minimally invasive approach. Our group initially adopted this same approach.[70] However, with time the preferred surgical approach has evolved into one combining thoracoscopy and laparoscopy for several reasons. Mobilization of the thoracic esophagus can be tedious and cumbersome via a completely laparoscopic approach. In addition, visualization of paraesophageal structures (such as the inferior pulmonary vein and the mainstem bronchi) and the performance of mediastinal lymph node dissection can be very limited when employing an exclusively transabdominal approach.

In the first 77 patients at the University of Pittsburgh undergoing MIE, Luketich and coworkers utilized a combined thoracoscopic/laparoscopic approach in most patients, achieving a median length of hospital stay of 7 days and a stage-specific survival similar to or better than open surgery results.[71] The authors have now published results on MIE in over 200 patients with high-grade dysplasia or cancer, as detailed by Fernando et al.,[72,73] Nguyen et al.,[74,75] Pierre and Luketich,[76] Litle et al.,[77] and Luketich et al.[78,79]

Techniques

Currently, there remains significant interest in hybrid approaches that combine elements of thoracoscopy or laparoscopy with open techniques. The most widely practiced variant is the thoracoscopic esophagectomy, which utilizes thoracoscopy to achieve esophageal mobilization in combination with standard laparotomy and cervical incisions for the completion of the esophagectomy.[80–83] Other approaches include lap-assisted esophagectomy, in which laparoscopy is utilized for mobilization and preparation of the gastric tube,[84] as well as hand-assisted laparoscopic THE, which introduces a hand port to assist with mediastinal mobilization during THE.[85] Most recently, robotic VATS/laparotomy approaches have been investigated utilizing the da Vinci operating robot.[86]

Totally minimally invasive esophagectomy (total MIE) techniques have been developed utilizing thoracoscopy or laparoscopy exclusively. The initial reports by DePaula et al.[69] and Swanstrom et al.[70] described a laparoscopic THE. Horgan and associates reported their technique of robotic-assisted laparoscopic THE.[87] Ikeda and colleagues have developed a mediastinoscopic esophagectomy technique using carbon dioxide insufflation via a neck approach combined with laparoscopy.[88] Currently, the most popular totally minimally invasive approaches to esophagectomy are the Ivor Lewis[89,90] and three-hole MIE.[79]

Whichever minimally invasive approach is best remains to be determined. Until further randomized data become available, the chosen approach should be based on tumor and patient characteristics as well as the surgeon's personal preference and expertise.

Morbidity and Mortality

To date, there are no prospective, randomized studies involving minimally invasive approaches to esophagectomy. The available data in the literature are composed of single-institution series (Table 73.5). Proponents of MIE contend that a minimally invasive approach will aid in the reduction of morbidity (and potentially mortality) in this patient population. Compared with the largest open series (2.9%–9.8% mortality), minimally invasive approaches to esophagectomy do appear to be associated with lower mortality rates (0%–5.5%). In the largest series (n = 222) by Luketich and coworkers, 1.4% mortality was achieved.[79] The reason for this trend was not established, although lower rates of respiratory and wound-related complications were evident when compared with the open literature, which in turn may account for the lower mortality.[91]

Complications

In the largest series of MIEs published to date, the most frequent minor complication was atrial fibrillation (12%), followed by pleural effusion (6%), which was treated with bedside thoracentesis or pigtail catheter drainage.[79] Major complications occurred in 32% of patients. The most common major complication was anastomotic leak (6%–11%). Most anastomotic leaks were localized to the neck and were managed conservatively. Pneumonia was the second most

TABLE 73.5.
Minimally Invasive Esophagectomy: Surgical Outcomes.

Reference	*Year*	*Evidence*	*n*	*Treatment group*	*Operative time (h)*	*LOS (days)*	*Mortality (%)*
Total MIE							
DePaula et al.[69]	1995	Retrospective	12	Lap THE	4.3	7.6	0
Swanstrom and Hansen[70]	1997	Retrospective	9	Lap THE	6.5	6.4	0
Watson et al.[111]	2000	Retrospective	7	MIE	4.4	12	0
Luketich et al.[79]	2003	Retrospective	222	MIE	NR	7	1.4
Nguyen et al.[109]	2003	Retrospective	46	MIE (41 IL)	5.8	8	4.3
Hybrid							
Gossot et al.[80]	1995	Prospective	29	VATS/laparotomy	2.3[a]	NR	3.8
Jagot et al.[84]	1995	Retrospective	9	Lap-assisted	8.5	10.3	0
Liu et al.[65]	1995	Retrospective	20	VATS/laparotomy	4.6[a]	19	0
Peracchia et al.[81]	1997	Retrospective	18	VATS/laparotomy	5.6	NR	5.5
Law et al.[68]	1997	Retrospective	18	VATS/laparotomy	4	NR	0
Kawahara et al.[112]	1999	Retrospective	23	VATS/laparotomy	1.8[a]	26	0
Smithers et al.[113]	2001	Retrospective	153	VATS/laparotomy	5.0	12	3.3
Osugi et al.[83]	2003	Retrospective	80	VATS/laparotomy	3.7	NR	0
Open							
Mathisen et al. (Duke)[114]	1988	Retrospective	104	TA (64)/IL (40)	NR	NR	2.9
Lerut et al.[115] (Belgium)	1992	Retrospective	198	Open (varied)	NR	18	9.6
Orringer et al.[116] (Mich.)	1999	Retrospective	1085	THE	NR	7[b]	4
Swanson et al.[117]	2001	Retrospective	250	Three hole	NR	13	3.6
Bailey et al. (VA)[118]	2003	Retrospective	1777	Open (varied)	NR	NR	9.8
Rizk et al.[119] (Sloan-Kettering)	2004	Retrospective	510	Open (varied)	NR	23[c] 11[d]	6.1

IL, Ivor Lewis; Lap, laparoscopic; MIE, minimally invasive esophagectomy; TA, left thoracoabdominal; THE, transhiatal esophagectomy; VATS, right thoracoscopic.

[a]VATS portion only.

[b]In last 2 years of series.

[c]Patients with complications.

[d]Patients without complications.

common major complication, occurring in 8% of patients. Vocal cord palsy (4%), chylothorax (3%), and gastric tip necrosis (3%) were uncommon, but serious, complications. These results compare very favorably with both open and minimally invasive series reported to date. Nguyen and coworkers[90] reported a series of 18 combined thoracoscopic and laparoscopic esophagectomies at the University of California, Davis; the most frequent complications included anastomotic leaks (11%), respiratory failure (11%), pulmonary embolism (6%), delayed gastric emptying (6%), and tracheogastric fistula (6%).

Recurrence and Survival

There are scant data on long-term survival and recurrence patterns following minimally invasive approaches to esophagectomy. In the series by Luketich and associates, Kaplan-Meier estimates of survival based on stage were similar to those in the open literature.[79] Although not presented in that original publication, reanalysis of the original data set of 222 patients with esophageal cancer demonstrated 1-, 3-, and 5-year survivals of 69%, 45%, and 36% respectively, which is similar if not better than some open series. In another series of MIE, Nguyen and coworkers documented 87% 1-year and 57% 3-year survival rates in 46 patients[90] (Table 73.6). Locoregional recurrence rates between 16% and 44% have been documented in minimally invasive series (Table 73.6), which is on par with the known natural history of resected esophageal cancer. Prospective, controlled studies will be required to more accurately delineate the survival and recurrence patterns afforded by MIE compared to open techniques.

Operative Outcomes and Comparison to Open Esophagectomy

Minimally invasive esophagectomy techniques require advanced laparoscopic and thoracoscopic skills for optimal outcomes. For this reason, and due to the inherent constraints of visualization and instrumentation, operative times for MIE are longer and encompass a wide range (3.7–7.5 h) (Table 73.5). Most open esophagectomies can be performed within 3 to 6 h. Proponents of MIE endorse the potential benefits of less pain, fewer complications, and shorter length of stay compared to open techniques. To date, however, there are few prospective data to validate any of these potential benefits.

In the only published study comparing minimally invasive (n = 18) and open (n = 16) esophagectomy, Nguyen and coworkers found that the mean operative time (364 min), blood loss (297 mL), and length of intensive care unit stay (6.1 days) were decreased compared with open transthoracic esophagectomy (437 min, 1046 mL, 9.9 days, respectively) and blunt transhiatal esophagectomy (391 min, 1142 mL, 11.1 days, respectively).[92] The incidence of respiratory complications (pneumonia, pulmonary embolism, respiratory failure) was similar between the groups. It should be emphasized that there were significant differences between the groups in this retrospective comparison. The open patients had more advanced cancers. In addition, the open operations were performed by a group of four surgeons with variable experience, whereas the MIE procedures were performed by a single surgeon with expertise in minimally invasive esophageal surgery. The open operations were performed several years before the MIE procedures, so there may have been differences in practice accounting for the longer lengths of stay. In the series by Luketich et al., the median intensive care unit stay was 1 day, time to oral intake was 4 days, and hospital stay was 7 days, which compares favorably with the minimally invasive procedure and is better than most series of open esophagectomy (Table 73.5).[79]

Pain and Quality of Life

Although minimally invasive techniques have been associated with decreased pain in a wide variety of operations, there

TABLE 73.6.
Minimally Invasive Esophagectomy: Recurrence and Survival.

Reference	*Year*	*Evidence*	*n*	*Approach*	*Follow-up (mo)*	*Median*	*Survival (%) 1 yr*	*3 yr*	*5 yr*	*Locoregional recurrence (%)*
Total MIE										
Swanstrom et al.[70]	1997	Retrospective	9	Lap THE	13	NR	NR	NR	NR	22.2
Nguyen et al.[109]	2003	Retrospective	46	MIE (41 IL)	26	NR	87	57	NR	26.1
Luketich et al.[79]	2003	Retrospective	222	MIE	19	26	69	45	36	NR
Hybrid										
Peracchia et al.[81]	1997	Retrospective	18	VATS/laparotomy	17	NR	NR	NR	NR	16.6
Law et al.[68]	1997	Retrospective	18	VATS/laparotomy	13.7	NR	81	NR	NR	44.4
Kawahara et al.[112]	1999	Retrospective	23	VATS/laparotomy	NR	NR	NR	NR	NR	30.4
Smithers et al.[113]	2001	Retrospective	153	VATS/laparotomy	21	29 m	70	NR	40	NR
Open										
Mathisen et al. (Duke)[114]	1988	Retrospective	104	TA (64)/IL (40)	NR	NR	NR	NR	15	5.8
Lerut et al. (Belgium)[115]	1992	Retrospective	198	Open (varied)	>24 months	NR	63	NR	30	NR
Orringer et al. (Michigan)[116]	1999	Retrospective	1085	THE	27	NR	67	34	23	NR
Swanson et al. (B&W)[117]	2001	Retrospective	250	Three hole	24	25	44	NR	NR	5.6
Rizk et al. (Sloan-Kettering)[119]	2004	Retrospective	510	Open (varied)	NR	NR	44	NR	NR	NR

B&W, Brigham and Womens Hospital; IL, Ivor Lewis; MIE, minimally invasive esophagectomy; TA, left thoracoabdominal; THE, transhiatal esophagectomy; VATS, right thoracoscopic.

are no significant analyses of postoperative pain in the MIE literature. Quality of life is a critical factor in the management of patients with esophageal cancer. Headrick and associates have found that, on long-term follow-up, esophagectomy can be performed with little to no impairment to QOL compared with normal patients based on short-form 36 (SF36) scoring.[93] Similarly, Blazeby and coauthors found that QOL initially was diminished in patients undergoing resection for esophageal carcinoma but improved back to baseline in those patients surviving for 2 years following esophagectomy.[94] In our series of 222 patients, the mean postoperative dysphagia score was 1.4 on a scale from 1 (no dysphagia) to 5 (severe dysphagia). Since reflux can be an issue after esophagectomy, heartburn severity was measured using the Health-Related Quality of Life Index (HRQOL). The mean heartburn score was 4.6 (on a scale from 0 to 45), which represents a normal (no reflux) score. The SF36 scores were also measured and were not significantly different compared to age-matched normal values during follow-up.

Cost-Effectiveness

There are no published data regarding the cost-effectiveness of minimally invasive approaches to esophagectomy.

Summary

Minimally invasive esophagectomy is feasible and appeared to be associated with similar, if not better, outcomes than open approaches in several large, single institution experiences. However, it should be reemphasized that esophagectomy, whether performed by an open or minimally invasive approach, is a complex procedure, and outcomes are better in high-volume centers. Another issue with MIE is the steep learning curve required to master these minimally invasive techniques, so it is likely that only a few centers with expertise in both minimally invasive techniques and open esophageal surgery will adopt this approach. Nevertheless, the results are encouraging and may broaden the applicability of this technique to higher-risk patient groups such as the elderly.[95]

Prospective studies will be required to determine whether postoperative pain, recovery time, and cost are improved. A phase II Intergroup Study (E2202) sponsored by ECOG and CALGB has recently opened and will evaluate the feasibility of MIE in a multicenter setting. All MIE procedures in this study will be performed using the same thoracoscopic and laparoscopic approach. If this operation is shown to be feasible in a multicenter setting, further studies, likely registry-oriented series, will be needed to compare open and MIE approaches prospectively.

References

1. Ginsberg R, Rubernstein L. Randomized trial of lobectomy versus limited resection for T1N0 non-small cell lung cancer. Ann Thorac Surg 1995;60:615–623.
2. McKenna RJ Jr, Fischel RJ, Rolf R, et al. Video-assisted thoracic surgery (VATS) lobectomy for bronchogenic carcinoma. Semin Thorac Cardiovasc Surg 1998;10:321–325.
3. Kohno T, Murakami T, Wakabayashi A. Anatomic lobectomy of the lung by means of thoracoscopy: an experimental study. J Thorac Cardiovasc Surg 1993;105:729–731.
4. Kirby TJ, Rice TW. Thoracoscopic lobectomy. Ann Thorac Surg 1993;56:784–786.
5. Walker WS, Carnochan FM, Pugh GC. Thoracoscopic pulmonary lobectomy. Early operative experience and preliminary clinical results. J Thorac Cardiovasc Surg 1993;106:1111–1117.
6. Landreneau RJ, Mack MJ, Dowling RD, et al. The role of thoracoscopy in lung cancer management. Chest 1998;113(1 suppl):6S–12S.
7. Landreneau RJ, Hazelrigg SR, Mack MJ, et al. Postoperative pain-related morbidity: video-assisted thoracic surgery versus thoracotomy. Ann Thorac Surg 1993:56:1285–1289.
8. Nagahiro I, Andou A, Aoe M, et al. Pulmonary function, postoperative pain, and serum cytokine level after lobectomy: a comparison of VATS and conventional procedure. Ann Thorac Surg 2001;72:362–365.
9. McKenna RJ Jr. The current status of video-assisted thoracic surgery lobectomy. Chest Surg Clin N Am 1998;8:775–785.
10. Roviaro G, Varoli F, Vergani C, et al. Video-assisted thoracoscopic surgery (VATS) major pulmonary resections: the Italian experience. Semin Thorac Cardiovasc Surg 1998;10:313–320.
11. Guidicelli R, Thomas P, Lonjon R, et al. Video-assisted minithoracotomy versus muscle-sparing thoracotomy for performing lobectomy. Ann Thorac Surg 1994;58:712–718.
12. Lewis RJ, Caccavale RJ. Video-assisted thoracic surgical non-rib spreading simultaneously stapled lobectomy (VATS(n)SSL). Semin Thorac Cardiovasc Surg 1998;10:332–339.
13. Lewis RJ, Caccavale RJ, Bocage JP, et al. Video-assisted thoracic surgical non-rib spreading simultaneously stapled lobectomy: a more patient friendly oncologic resection. Chest 1999;116:1119–1124.
14. Swanson SJ, Batirel HF. Video-assisted thoracic surgery (VATS) resection for lung cancer. Surg Clin N Am 2002;82:541–559.
15. McKenna RJ Jr, Wolf RK, Brenner M, et al. Is lobectomy by video-assisted thoracic surgery an adequate cancer operation? Ann Thorac Surg 1998;66:1903–1908.
16. Yim AP, Izzat MB, Liu H, et al. Thoracoscopic major lung resections: an Asian perspective. Semin Thorac Cardiovasc Surg 1998;10:326–331.
17. Landreneau RJ, Sugarbaker DJ, Mack MJ, et al. Wedge resection versus lobectomy for stage I (T1N0M0) non-small cell lung cancer. J Thorac Cardiovasc Surg 1997;113:691–700.
18. Demmy TL, Curtis JJ. Minimally-invasive lobectomy directed toward frail and high-risk patients: a case-control study. Ann Thorac Surg 1999;68:194–200.
19. McKenna RJ Jr. Thoracoscopic lobectomy with mediastinal sampling in 80 year old patients. Chest 1994;106:1902–1904.
20. Sugi K, Kaneda Y, Esato K. Video-assisted thoracoscopic lobectomy achieves a satisfactory long-term prognosis in patients with clinical stage IA lung cancer. World J Surg 2000;24:27–31.
21. Walker WS. Video-assisted thoracic surgery (VATS) lobectomy: the Edinburgh experience. Semin Thorac Cardiovasc Surg 1998;10:291–299.
22. Kaseda S, Aoki T, Hangai N. Video-assisted thoracic surgery (VATS) lobectomy: the Japanese experience. Semin Thorac Cardiovasc Surg 1998;10:300–304.
23. Iwasaki A, Shirakusa T, Shiraishi T, et al. Results of video-assisted thoracic surgery for stage I/II non-small cell lung cancer. Eur J Cardiothorac Surg 2004;26:158–164.
24. Walker WS, Pugh GC, Craig SR, et al. Continued experience with thoracoscopic major pulmonary resection. Int Surg 1996;81:235–236.
25. DeCamp MM, Jaklitsch MT, Mentzer SJ, et al. The safety and versatility of videothoracoscopy: a prospective analysis of 895 consecutive cases. J Am Coll Surg 1995;181:113–120.

26. Benedetti F, Amanzio M, Casadio C, et al. Postoperative pain and superficial abdominal reflexes after posterolateral thoracotomy. Ann Thorac Surg 1997;64:207–210.
27. Stammberger U, Steinacher C, Hillinger S, et al. Early and long-term complaints following video-assisted thoracoscopic surgery: evaluation in 173 patients. Eur J Cardiothorac Surg 2000;18:7–11.
28. Landreneau RJ, Mack MJ, Hazelrigg SR, et al. Prevalence of chronic pain after pulmonary resection by thoracotomy or video-assisted thoracic surgery. J Thorac Cardiovasc Surg 1994;107:1079–1086.
29. Sugiura H, Morikawa T, Kaji M, et al. Long-term benefits for the quality of life after video-assisted thoracoscopic lobectomy in patients with lung cancer. Surg Laparosc Endosc Perc Tech 1999;9:403–408.
30. Li WW, Lee TW, Lam SS, et al. Quality of life following lung cancer resection: video-assisted thoracic surgery versus thoracotomy. Chest 2002;122:584–589.
31. Nomori H, Horio H, Fuyuno G, et al. Respiratory muscle strength after lung resection with special reference to age and procedures of thoracotomy. Eur J Cardiothorac Surg 1996;10:352–358.
32. Kaseda S, Aoki T, Hangai N, et al. Better pulmonary function and prognosis with video-assisted thoracic surgery than with thoracotomy. Ann Thorac Surg 2000;70:1644–1646.
33. Nakata M, Saeki H, Yokoyama N, et al. Pulmonary function after lobectomy: video-assisted thoracic surgery versus thoracotomy. Ann Thorac Surg 2000;70:938–941.
34. Gebhard FT, Becker HP, Gerngross H, et al. Reduced inflammatory response in minimal invasive surgery of pneumothorax. Arch Surg 1996;131:1079–1082.
35. Sugi K, Kaneda Y, Esato K. Video-assisted thoracoscopic lobectomy reduces cytokine production more than conventional open lobectomy. Jpn J Thorac Cardiovasc Surg 2000;48:161–165.
36. Yim AP, Wan S, Lee TW, et al. VATS lobectomy reduces cytokine responses compared with conventional surgery. Ann Thorac Surg 2000;70:243–247.
37. Leaver HA, Craig SR, Yap PL, et al. Lymphocyte responses following open and minimally invasive thoracic surgery. Eur J Clin Invest 2000;30:230–238.
38. McKenna RJ Jr, Houck W, Fuller CB. Video-assisted thoracic surgery lobectomy: experience with 1100 cases. Ann Thorac Surg 2006;81:421–425.
39. Warren WH, Faber LP. Segmentectomy versus lobectomy in patients with stage 1 pulmonary carcinoma: 5-year survival and patterns of intrathoracic recurrence. J Thorac Cardiovasc Surg 1994;107:1087–1094.
40. Iwasaki A, Shirakusa T, Kawahara K, et al. Is video-assisted thorascopic surgery suitable for resection of primary lung cancer? J Thorac Cardiovasc Surg 1997;45:13–15.
41. Ohbuchi T, Morikawa T, Takeuchi E, et al. Lobectomy: video-assisted thoracic surgery versus posterolateral thoracotomy. Jpn J Thorac Cardiovasc Surg 1998;46:519–522.
42. Kondo T, Sagawa M, Tanita T, et al. Is complete systematic nodal dissection by thoracoscopic surgery possible? A prospective trial of video-assisted lobectomy for cancer of the right lung. J Thorac Cardiovasc Surg 1998;116:651–652.
43. Swanson SJ, DeCamp MM, Mentzer SJ, et al. Thoracoscopic resection of lung malignancy without port site recurrence: the Brigham and Women's hospital experience. Chest 1997;112:9s.
44. Sugi K, Kaneda Y, Nawata K, et al. Cost analysis for thoracoscopy: thoracoscopic wedge resection and lobectomy. Surg Today 1998;28:41–45.
45. Smythe WR, American College of Chest Physicians. Treatment of stage I non-small cell lung carcinoma. Chest 2003;123(1 suppl):181s–187s.
46. Jemal A, Siegel R, Ward E, et al. Cancer statistics 2007. CA Cancer J Clin 2007;57:43–66.
47. Murray GF, Wilcox BR, Starek PJ. The assessment of operability of esophageal carcinoma. Ann Thorac Surg 1977;23:393–399.
48. Dagnini G, et al. Laparoscopy in abdominal staging of esophageal carcinoma. Gastrointest Endosc 1986;32:400–402.
49. Krasna MJ, McLaughlin JS. Thoracoscopic lymph node staging for esophageal cancer. Ann Thorac Surg 1993;56:671–674.
50. Rice TW, Zuccaro G, Adelstein DJ, et al. Esophageal carcinoma: depth of tumor invasion is predictive of regional lymph node status. Ann Thorac Surg 1998;65:787–792.
51. Vickers J, Alderson D. Influence of luminal obstruction on oesophageal cancer staging using endoscopic ultrasonography. Br J Surg 1998;85:999–1001.
52. Luketich JD, et al. Minimally invasive surgical staging is superior to endoscopic ultrasound in detecting lymph node metastases in esophageal cancer. J Thorac Cardiovasc Surg 1997;114:817–821.
53. Luketich JD, Friedman DM, Weigel TL, et al. Evaluation of distant metastases in esophageal cancer. Ann Thorac Surg 1999;68:1133–1136.
54. Wren SM, Stijns P, Srinivas S. Positron emission tomography in the initial staging of esophageal cancer. Arch Surg 2002;137:1001–1006.
55. Downey RJ, Akhurst T, Ilson D, et al. Whole body ^{18}FDG-PET and the response of esophageal cancer to induction therapy: results of a prospective trial. J Clin Oncol 2003;21:428–432.
56. Krasna MJ, Mao YS, Sonnett J, et al. The role of thoracoscopic staging of esophageal cancer patients. Eur J Cardiothorac Surg 1999;16(suppl 1):S31–S33.
57. Van Dam J, Rice TW, Catalano MF, et al. High-grade malignant stricture is predictive of esophageal tumor stage. Risks of endosonographic evaluation. Cancer 1993;71:2910–2917.
58. Krasna MJ, Reed CE, Nedzwiecki D, et al. CALGB 9380: a prospective trial of the feasibility of thoracoscopy/laparoscopy in staging esophageal cancer. Ann Thorac Surg 2001;71:1073–1079.
59. Harewood GC, Wiersema MJ. A cost analysis of endoscopic ultrasound in the evaluation of esophageal cancer. Am J Gastroenterol 2002;97:452–458.
60. Wallace MB, Nietert PJ, Earle C, et al. An analysis of multiple staging management strategies for carcinoma of the esophagus: computed tomography, endoscopic ultrasound, positron emission tomography, and thoracoscopy/laparoscopy. Ann Thorac Surg 2002;74:1026–1032.
61. Wright TA, Gray MR, Morris AI, et al. Cost-effectiveness of detecting Barrett's cancer. Gut 1996;39:574–579.
62. Kelsen DP, Ginsberg R, Pajak TF, et al. Chemotherapy followed by surgery compared with surgery alone for localized esophageal cancer. N Engl J Med 1998;339:1979–1984.
63. Birkmeyer JD, Siewers AE, Finlayson EVA, et al. Hospital volume and surgical mortality in the United States. N Engl J Med 2002;346:1128–1137.
64. Collard JM, Lengele B, Otte JB, et al. En bloc and standard esophagectomies by thoracoscopy. Ann Thorac Surg 1993;56:675–679.
65. Liu HP, Chang Ch, Lin PJ, et al. Video-assisted endoscopic esophagectomy with stapled intrathoracic esophagogastric anastomosis. World J Surg 1995;19:745–747.
66. Akaishi T, Kaneda I, Higuchi N, et al. Thoracoscopic en bloc total esophagectomy with radical mediastinal lymphadenectomy. J Thorac Cardiovasc Surg 1996;112:1533–1540.
67. Dexter SP, Martin IG, McMahon MJ. Radical thoracoscopic esophagectomy for cancer. Surg Endosc 1996;10:147–151.
68. Law S, Fok M, Chu KM, et al. Thoracoscopic esophagectomy for esophageal cancer. Surgery 1997;122:8–14.
69. DePaula Al, Hashiba K, Ferreira EA, et al. Laparoscopic transhiatal esophagectomy with esophagogastroplasty. Surg Laparosc Endosc 1995;5:1–5.

70. Swanstrom LL, Hansen P. Laparoscopic total esophagectomy. Arch Surg 1997;132:943–949.
71. Luketich JD, Schauer PR, Christie NA, et al. Minimally invasive esophagectomy. Ann Thorac Surg 2000;70:906–912.
72. Fernando HC, Christie NA, Luketich JD. Thoracoscopic and laparoscopic esophagectomy. Semin Thorac Cardiovasc Surg 2000;12:195–200.
73. Fernando HC, Luketich JD, Buenaventura PO, et al. Outcomes of minimally-invasive esophagectomy (MIE) for high-grade dysplasia of the esophagus. Eur J Cardiothorac Surg 2002;22:1–6.
74. Nguyen NT, Schauer PR, Luketich JD. Combined laparoscopic and thoracoscopic approach to esophagectomy. J Am Coll Surg 1999;188:328–332.
75. Nguyen NT, Schauer PR, Luketich JD. Minimally invasive esophagectomy for Barrett's esophagus with high-grade dysplasia. Surgery 2000;127:284–290.
76. Pierre AF, Luketich JD. Technique and role of minimally-invasive esophagectomy for premalignant and malignant diseases of the esophagus. Surg Oncol Clin N Am 2002;11:337–350.
77. Litle VR, Buenaventura PO, Luketich JD. Minimally invasive resection for esophageal cancer. Surg Clin N Am 2002;82:711–728.
78. Luketich JD, Nguyen NT, Weigel T, et al. Minimally invasive approach to esophagectomy. J Soc Laparoendosc Surg 1998;2:243–247.
79. Luketich JD, Alvelo-Rivera M, Buenaventura PO, et al. Minimally invasive esophagectomy: outcomes in 222 patients. Ann Surg 2003;238:486–495.
80. Gossot D, Cattan P, Fritsch S, et al. Can the morbidity of esophagectomy be reduced by the thoracoscopic approach? Surg Endosc 1995;9:1113–1115.
81. Peracchia A, Rosati R, Fumagalli U, et al. Thoracoscopic esophagectomy: are there benefits? Semin Surg Oncol 1997;13:259–262.
82. Smithers BM, Gotley DC, McEwan D, et al. Thoracoscopic mobilization of the esophagus: a 6 year experience. Surg Endosc 2001;15:176–182.
83. Osugi H, Takemura M, Higashino M, et al. Learning curve of video-assisted thoracoscopic esophagectomy and extensive lymphadenectomy for squamous cell cancer of the thoracic esophagus and results. Surg Endosc 2003;17:515–519.
84. Jagot P, Sauvanet A, Berthoux L, et al. Laparoscopic mobilization of the stomach for oesophageal replacement. Br J Surg 1996; 83:540–542.
85. Gerhart CD. Hand-assisted laparoscopic transhiatal esophagectomy using the dexterity pneumo sleeve. J Soc Laparoendosc Surg 1998;2:295–298.
86. Bodner J, Wykypiel H, Wetscher G, et al. First experiences with the daVinci operating robot in thoracic surgery. Eur J Cardiothorac Surg 2004;25:844–851.
87. Horgan S, Berger RA, Elli EF, et al. Robotic-assisted minimally-invasive transhiatal esophagectomy. Am Surg 2003;69:624–626.
88. Ikeda Y, Niimi M, Kan S, et al. Mediastinoscopic esophagectomy using carbon dioxide insufflation via the neck approach. Surgery 2001;129:504–506.
89. Watson DI, Davies N, Jamieson GG. Totally endoscopic Ivor Lewis esophagectomy. Surg Endosc 1999;13:293–297.
90. Nguyen NT, Roberts P, Follette DM, et al. Thoracoscopic and laparoscopic esophagectomy for benign and malignant disease: lessons learned from 46 consecutive procedures. J Am Coll Surg 2003;197:902–913.
91. Schuchert MJ, Luketich JD, Fernando HC. Complications of minimally-invasive esophagectomy. Semin Thorac Cardiovasc Surg 2004;16:133–141.
92. Nguyen NT, Follette DM, Wolfe BM, et al. Comparison of minimally-invasive esophagectomy with transthoracic and transhiatal esophagectomy. Arch Surg 2000;135:920–925.
93. Headrick JR, Nichols FC, Miller DL, et al. High-grade dysplasia: long-term survival and quality of life after esophagectomy. Ann Thorac Surg 2002;73:1697–1702.
94. Blazeby JM, Farndon JR, Donovan J, et al. A prospective longitudinal study examining the quality of life of patients with esophageal carcinoma. Cancer 2000;88:1781–1787.
95. Perry Y, Fernando HC, Buenaventura PO. Minimally-invasive esophagectomy in the elderly. J Soc Laparoendoscop Surg 2002;6:299–304.
96. Hermansson U, Konstantinov IE, Aren C. Video-assisted thoracic surgery (VATS) lobectomy: the initial Swedish experience. Semin Thorac Cardiovasc Surg 1998;10:285–290.
97. Walker WS, Codispoti M, Soon SY, et al. Long-term outcomes following VATS lobectomy for non-small cell bronchogenic carcinoma. Eur J Cardiothorac Surg 2003;23:397–402.
98. Gharagozloo F, Tempesta B, Margolis M, et al. Video-assisted thoracic surgery lobectomy for stage I lung cancer. Ann Thorac Surg 2003;76:1009–1015.
99. Ginsberg RJ, Hill LD, Eagan RT, et al. Modern 30-day operative mortality for surgical resections in lung cancer. J Thorac Cardiovasc Surg 1983;86:654–658.
100. Duque JL, Ramos G, Castrodeza J, et al. Early complications in surgical treatment of lung cancer: a prospective, multicenter study. Ann Thorac Surg 1997;63:944–950.
101. Wada H, Nakamura T, Nakamoto K, et al. Thirty-day operative mortality for thoracotomy in lung cancer. J Thorac Cardiovasc Surg 115:70–73.
102. Thomas P, Cristophe D, Thirion X, et al. Stage I non-small cell lung cancer: a pragmatic approach to prognosis after complete resection. Ann Thorac Surg 2002;73:1065–1070.
103. Stoelben E, Sauerbrei W, Ludwig C, et al. Tumor stage and early mortality for surgical resections in lung cancer. Langenbecks Arch Surg 2003;388:116–121.
104. Deslauriers J, Grégoire J, Jacques LF, et al. Sleeve lobectomy versus pneumonectomy for lung cancer: a comparative analysis of survival and sites of recurrences. Ann Thorac Surg 2004;77:1152–1156.
105. Mountain CF. Revisions in the international system for staging lung cancer. Chest 1997;111:1710–1717.
106. Kirby TJ, Mack MJ, Landreneau RJ, et al. Initial experience with video-assisted thoracoscopic lobectomy. Ann Thorac Surg 1993;56:1248–1252.
107. Tschernko EM, Hofer S, Bieglmeyer C, et al. Early postoperative stress: video-assisted wedge resection/lobectomy versus conventional axillary thoracotomy. Chest 1996;109:1636–1642.
108. Meltzer CC, Luketich JD, Friedman D, et al. Whole-body FDG positron emission tomographic imaging for staging esophageal cancer: comparison with computed tomography. Clin Nucl Med 2000;25:882–887.
109. Nguyen NN, Roberts PF, Follette DM, et al. Evaluation of minimally invasive surgical staging for esophageal cancer. Am J Surg 2001;182:702–706.
110. Parmar KS, Zwischenberger JB, Reeves AL, et al. Clinical impact of endoscopic ultrasound-guided fine needle aspiration of celiac axis lymph nodes (M1a disease) in esophageal cancer. Ann Thorac Surg 2002;73:916–921.
111. Watson DI, Jamieson GG, Devitt PG. Endoscopic cervico-thoracoabdominal esophagectomy. J Am Coll Surg 2000;193:372–378.
112. Kawahara K, Maekawa T, Okabayashi T, et al. Video-assisted thoracoscopic esophagectomy for esophageal cancer. Surg Endosc 1999;13:218–223.
113. Smithers BM, Gotley DC, McEwan D, et al. Thoracoscopic mobilization of the esophagus: a 6 year experience. Surg Endosc 2001;15:176–82.
114. Mathisen DJ, Grillo HC, Wilkins EW, et al. Transthoracic esophagectomy: a safe approach to carcinoma of the esophagus. Ann Thorac Surg 1988;45:137–143.

115. Lerut T, DeLeyn P, Coosemans W, et al. Surgical strategies in esophageal carcinoma with emphasis on radical lymphadenectomy. Ann Surg 1992;216:583–590.
116. Orringer MB, Marshall B, Iannettoni MD. Transhiatal esophagectomy: clinical experience and refinements. Ann Surg 1999;230:392–403.
117. Swanson SJ, Batirel HF, Bueno R, et al. Transthoracic esophagectomy with radical mediastinal and abdominal lymph node dissection and cervical esophagogastrostomy for esophageal carcinoma. Ann Thorac Surg 2001;72:1918–1925.
118. Bailey SH, Bull DA, Harpole DH, et al. Outcomes after esophagectomy: a 10-year prospective cohort. Ann Thorac Surg 2003;75:217–222.
119. Rizk NP, Bach PB, Schrag D, et al. The impact of complications on outcomes after resection for esophageal and gastroesophageal junction carcinoma. J Am Coll Surg 2004;198:42–50.

74

Pleura: Anatomy, Physiology, and Disorders

Joseph S. Friedberg and John C. Kucharczuk

Disorders of the pleura and pleural space reflect some of the oldest diseases encountered in surgical history. Hippocrates described the symptoms of empyema 2400 years ago: "Empyema may be recognized by the following symptoms: In the first place the fever is constant, less during the day and greater at night, and copious sweats supervene. There is a desire to cough and the patient expectorates nothing worth mentioning." He also described an open drainage procedure: "When the fifteenth day after rupture has appeared, prepare a warm bath, set him upon a stool, which is not wobbly, someone should hold his hands, then shake him by the shoulders and listen to see on which side a noise is heard. And right at this place, preferably on the left, make an incision, then it produces death more rarely."[1,2] Beyond providing less-wobbly stools, few advances were made for more than 2000 years that allowed surgeons to routinely enter the pleural cavity, the fear being a potentially fatal pneumothorax. With the advent of positive pressure ventilation in the early 1900s, pneumothorax was no longer a prohibitive risk, and the era of surgical intervention in the pleural cavity had begun.[3]

Empyema represents just one of many disorders of the pleural space that the practicing surgeon may encounter. Disorders of the pleural space may result from a pathological change in the pleura itself or may reflect disease in adjacent or distant organs. The problems span the spectrum from a benign effusion of cardiac origin to mesothelioma, a deadly primary malignancy of the pleura. Despite vastly different etiologies, the presentation and radiographic images of these two conditions may appear very similar. Thus, it is important for the clinician to be familiar with the normal anatomy and physiology of this space as well as the numerous disorders of it. The goal of this chapter is to provide such a background and to give a review of the diagnostic and therapeutic procedures currently employed for pleural diseases.

Anatomy

Embryology and Microscopic Anatomy

Embryologically, the pleural cavity is created during a month, starting in the third week of gestation. Initially, the lateral plate forms two layers, the splanchnopleura and the somatopleura, which subsequently develop into the visceral and parietal pleura, respectively. Eventually, it is the visceral pleura that surrounds the lung and the parietal pleura that lines the remainder of the chest cavity. The different embryological origins of the visceral and parietal pleura are responsible for the separate vascular, lymphatic, and neural supplies of these two structures as seen in the adult. By the end of the seventh week of gestation, the diaphragm has separated the thoracic cavity from the peritoneal cavity, and by the third month of gestation the two pleural cavities have expanded sufficiently to encase the pericardium.[4]

In the adult, both pleural surfaces are approximately 30 to 40 μm thick and are composed of a single layer of mesothelial cells with an underlying layer of connective tissue. Depending on their location, the mesothelial cells may be flat, cuboidal, or columnar. Mesothelial cells characteristically have numerous microvilli that play a role in phagocytosis as well as contributing to the lubricious nature of the pleural surfaces. Surfactant molecules, produced by the mesothelium, line the pleural surfaces and, secondary to similar electrical charge, repulse each other and facilitate sliding, analogous to the lubrication achieved with graphite. It is these apposing layers of mesothelial cells that form the potential space of the pleural cavity and that glide over each other during respiration.

The connective tissue layer contains the neurovascular and lymphatic supply of the pleura. There are certain important differences in this layer between the visceral and parietal pleura. For the visceral pleura, the connective tissue layer is functionally continuous with the fibroelastic network of the lung itself. Functionally, it is this relationship that prevents the visceral pleura from being surgically separated from the surface of a normal lung. Pathological disruption of this connection, however, may result in subpleural air collections known as blebs.[5] The connective tissue layer for the parietal pleura may also be tightly adherent to the underlying structures, as is characteristic of the diaphragmatic pleura. Around the skeletal portion of the thorax, however, the pleura is bound to the underlying tissue by another connective tissue layer called the endothoracic fascia, which forms a natural cleavage plane. It is this plane that the surgeon develops when performing an "extrapleural" dissection.

The blood supply to the visceral pleura in humans is thought to reflect that of the lung itself, with a dual arterial supply from both the pulmonary and bronchial arteries and singular venous drainage into the pulmonary veins. The blood supply to the parietal pleura is from systemic arteries only and drains, predominantly, into peribronchial and intercostal veins, but it may also drain directly into the azygous vein and vena cava.

The visceral pleura is innervated by vagal and sympathetic fibers but has no somatic innervation and is therefore insensate. The parietal pleura is also innervated with sympathetic and parasympathetic fibers, but it is also somatically innervated. Thus, the parietal pleura is capable of sensing and transmitting the sensation of pain. "Pleurisy" from inflammation and pain from chest tubes, during insertion and subsequently as well, are attributable to the somatic intervention of the parietal pleura.

There are also differences in the lymphatic drainage between the two pleural layers. The visceral pleura drains through a lymphatic network into the pulmonary lymphatics, which eventually flow toward the pulmonary hilum. This lymphatic system is richer in the lower lobes than the upper lobes. The parietal pleural lymphatics drain to different locations. The mediastinal pleura drains to the mediastinal and tracheobronchial nodes. The chest wall drains anteriorly to the internal thoracic chain and posteriorly toward the intercostal nodes near the heads of the ribs. The diaphragmatic pleura drains to the parasternal, middle phrenic, and posterior mediastinal lymph nodes. There are also transdiaphragmatic lymphatic communications that allow some degree of lymphatic flow from the peritoneum to the pleural space.

The parietal pleura also differs from the visceral pleura by virtue of the presence of Kampmeier foci and stomata. Kampmeier foci are collections of activated mesothelial and lymphoreticular cells, centered about a lymphatic core, that augment the pleura defensive capabilities. They are concentrated in the lower mediastinal region of the parietal pleura.[6,7] Stomata are 2- to 6-μm pores that communicate directly with the parietal pleural lymphatics. During inspiration, these pores have the capacity to stretch, and their architecture is such that they form functional one-way valves. Thus, they provide for a very effective system for draining both fluid and particles, including both red blood cells and macrophages. It is the presence of these pores on the parietal pleural surface that makes it predominantly, if not exclusively, responsible for clearance of cells and particulate matter from the pleural space. It should be noted that although stomata are well studied and characterized in sheep and other mammals, the definitive presence of stomata in humans is less well established.

Gross Anatomy

In each hemithorax, the visceral pleura is a continuous surface that completely envelops the entire lung, including the fissures. At the pulmonary hilum, it continues on as the parietal pleura to line the mediastinum, chest wall, diaphragm, and cupola of the chest cavity. In humans, the pleural cavities are completely separate, coming into contact with each other for a short distance behind the upper half of the body of the sternum (Fig. 74.1). It is this pleural separation of the right and left chest cavities that prevents bilateral pneumothoraces from occurring as the result of a unilateral chest injury. At the costophrenic and costomediastinal sinuses, the parietal pleural folds back on itself, providing a potential space into which the lungs can expand during inspiration.[8]

Superiorly, the pleura extends above the bony thorax into the base of the neck (Fig. 74.2). This fact explains why pneumothorax may complicate internal jugular central line placement as well as subclavian central line placement. Anteriorly, the pleura extends to the sixth rib, to the ninth rib laterally, and to the twelfth rib posteriorly (Fig. 74.2). In the living patient, the lung can fill the entire posterior recess. In a review of 100 chest radiographs, 80% of patients were found to have lung present at or below the level of the 12th rib, and in 18% it was seen at the level of the first lumbar vertebra.[9] These external landmarks of the pleural space are of practical clinical significance, particularly when evaluating a patient with penetrating trauma.

The pulmonary ligament is a double fold of the mediastinal pleura that tapers down from the root of the lung, where it is in continuity with the visceral pleura, to the caudal mediastinum. This ligament is one of the structures that must be divided to perform a pneumonectomy or lower

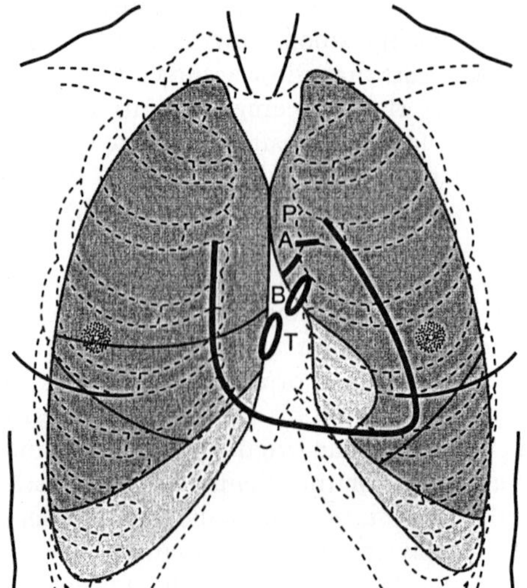

FIGURE 74.1. Relationship of the thoracic skeleton to the heart (line), pleura (light gray), and lungs (dark gray). (Adapted with permission from *Gray's Anatomy*.[76] © 1980 W.B. Saunders Co.)

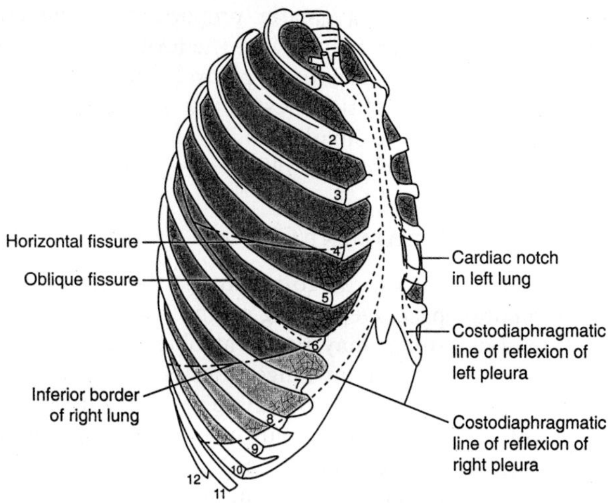

FIGURE 74.2. Relationship of the lung (dark gray) and the parietal pleural envelope, which extends down beyond the edge of the lung (light gray). (Reprinted with permission from *Gray's Anatomy*.[76] © 1980, W.B. Saunders Co.)

lobectomy. It is also routinely divided to its superior border, the inferior pulmonary vein, when attempting to provide mobility to the lower lobe after resecting the upper or middle lobes. The lymph nodes within the pulmonary ligament are the level 9 nodes, which are N2 lymph nodes, and should be routinely harvested when performing a resection for lung cancer.

Physiology

The pleura has both mechanical and physiological functions. It transmits negative pressure from the thorax to the lung, thereby opposing the lung's natural elastic recoil and maintaining pulmonary expansion. During respiration, this function is performed in an environment of very low friction, thereby allowing the lungs to glide smoothly over the internal thoracic surfaces as they expand and contract. The pleura also controls the environment of the chest cavity by maintaining fluid homeostasis, preventing or removing air collections and keeping the space sterile.

Under normal conditions, the pleural cavity is a potential space with a thickness ranging from 10 to 20 µm. The lung is maintained in an expanded state by the maintenance of negative pressure in the pleural space; this allows the expandable chest cavity to overcome the opposing forces exerted by the natural elastic recoil of the lung. The resting pressure in the pleural space, when the lung is at its functional residual capacity, is slightly negative at −2 to −5 cm H_2O. When measured in an upright posture, there is more negative pressure in the apex of the chest than at the diaphragm, likely a gravitational effect. The negative pressure continues to increase through inspiration, with the pressure ranging from −25 to −35 cm H_2O at the vital capacity. Disorders that decrease the compliance of the lung or increase airway resistance further increase the negative pressure in the pleural space with inspiration.[5,9]

Initially, it would seem curious that gas is not drawn out of solution into the pleural space by the negative pressure in the space. It is the lower partial pressure of gases on the venous side of the pleural circulation, as opposed to the arterial side, that prevents spontaneous pneumothorax from occurring under normal conditions. This difference in partial pressures between the two sides of the circulation is mainly a result of oxygen absorption. Unless the pressure in the pleural space decreases to significantly less than −50 cm H_2O, the sum total of the forces under normal conditions favors absorption of gas out of the pleural space.

This diffusion gradient also accounts for reabsorption of gas that is introduced into the pleural space. The clearance rate of gases introduced into the pleural space is dependent on the concentrations of those gases with respect to their partial pressures in the pleural circulation. As the partial pressure of nitrogen is the greatest in the air we breathe, it therefore constitutes the highest partial pressure of the gases that form a pneumothorax. Nitrogen also has the highest partial pressure of the gases in our circulation; this can be decreased by altering the composition of inspired gases. Thus, administration of supplemental oxygen decreases the partial pressure of nitrogen in the bloodstream and thereby increases the nitrogen pressure gradient between the circulation and the pneumothorax, favoring more rapid reabsorption of the trapped gas. This relationship serves as the rationale for placing a patient on supplemental oxygen to facilitate reabsorption of a pneumothorax that is not being externally evacuated.[10]

Under normal conditions, the pleural space contains very little fluid, estimated at approximately 0.3 mL/kg. The fluid is generally hypooncotic, with a protein content of approximately 1 g/dL. The mechanisms of fluid production and reabsorption are complicated and not completely understood. Numerous forces interact from both the parietal and visceral pleura, including their respective hydrostatic and oncotic pressures. Respiratory movement and gravity are both thought to have roles in maintaining the fluid dynamics of the pleural cavity. The predominant factor, however, is thought to be the uptake of fluid into the parietal pleural lymphatics. These lymphatics tend to be concentrated in the dependent portions of the chest cavity. Under normal conditions, this flow rate has been estimated at 0.1 to 0.15 mL/kg/h. The lymphatic flow rate has the capacity to increase and has been estimated to reach as high as 30 mL/h, approximately 700 mL/day in an average-size individual. When the dynamics of this equilibrium are unbalanced beyond the rate at which the lymphatics are able to compensate, pleural effusion accumulates.[7,9,11]

It is interesting to note that the exact purpose of the pleura is still not fully understood. Empirically, it is clear that the pleura maintains fluid and gas homeostasis, mechanically couples the lungs to the bellows mechanism for respiration, and maintains sterility in its described space. To accomplish this, however, it is not clear how important it is to have the configuration of two opposing layers with a small amount of intervening fluid. It has been observed, for instance, that there is little change in pulmonary function tests in patients before and after fusion of the pleural space.[12] It is interesting to note that some mammals do not have a pleural space, similar to patients who have undergone pleurodesis, but that these animals clearly function normally. Thus, the exact necessity for having two pleural membranes defining a potential space remains somewhat of a mystery.

Disorders of the Pleura

There are a large number of pleural disorders. The majority lead to symptoms as a result of mechanical compression of the lung, although many may be asymptomatic or may present with constitutional symptoms or pain. In most cases, the pathology results from the presence of something in the pleural space, which as previously described, is normally a potential space. Therefore, in an effort to organize this large number of disorders, they are grouped according to what abnormal phase of material is occupying the pleural space, that is, gas, liquid, or solid. When gas enters the pleural space, it is referred to as a *pneumothorax*. When liquid enters the pleural space, it may sometimes be broadly referred to as an *exudative* or *transudative effusion* but is frequently classified according to the type of liquid, such as hemothorax, chylothorax, or empyema. Last, solid masses may occupy the pleural space. Most benign masses are pleural plaques, but there are also rare benign tumors of the pleura, some of which may reach enormous size. Malignant masses of the pleura are usually cancers that have metastasized to the pleura, but there are also some rare primary tumors, most commonly mesothelioma. Sometimes, the groups may overlap, with more than one abnormal phase of material filling the pleural space. Such examples include air and blood, a *hemopneumothorax*, after trauma or air and pus, a *hydropneumothorax*, which may be seen with empyemas resulting from a bronchopleural fistula. Frequently, however, there is a predominant, if not sole, etiology for the abnormal accumulation; thus, the following sections review disorders of the pleura according to the state of matter that is abnormally occupying the space—gas, liquid, or solid.

Gas-Phase Disorders of the Pleural Space

Pneumothorax

Pneumothorax is defined as air in the pleural space. It may occur traumatically, iatrogenically, or spontaneously. Spontaneous pneumothorax may be subclassified as primary or secondary, with primary spontaneous pneumothorax arising in an otherwise healthy patient and secondary spontaneous pneumothorax arising as a complication in a patient with known underlying pulmonary disease. Essentially any pneumothorax resulting from pleural disruption can present as a tension pneumothorax. This condition represents a true emergency and is discussed separately.

Pneumothorax Presentation and Diagnosis

Pneumothorax may cause pain or dyspnea, or it may be asymptomatic, depending on its size and the underlying pulmonary function of the patient. Physical findings may range from none to the classic findings seen with a tension pneumothorax: contralateral tracheal deviation, ipsilateral absent breath sounds, and percussive hyperresonance. Electrocardiographic changes may be present, including diminished voltage, right-axis deviation, or T-wave changes that may mimic a subendocardial myocardial infarction.[13]

Except for tension pneumothorax, most cases require an upright chest radiograph to establish the diagnosis. As the pneumothorax occupies a greater proportion of the chest cavity at expiration than inspiration, the former is more sensitive for detecting the diagnostic pleural line. A computed tomographic (CT) scan of the chest is the most sensitive test and may demonstrate a small amount of air in the pleural space that is not visible on the plain radiograph.

Pneumothorax Treatment Options

For all pneumothoraces, the common goal is removal of air from the pleural space. Depending on the etiology, however, prevention of recurrence may also be an objective of the treatment. Options for treatment range from observation to thoracotomy. Selection of the appropriate modality depends on a number of factors, including, but not limited to, presentation, previous history, comorbidities, need for positive pressure ventilation, associated effusion, and even the patient's lifestyle. In addition, the size of the pneumothorax can also play a significant role in determining the appropriate treatment.

The following sections review the basic technique and indications for the different treatment options that are available and give specific recommendations for different pneumothoraces to be described in the following section.

Observation

Observation is generally reserved for patients who are asymptomatic and are diagnosed with a small primary spontaneous pneumothorax or a simple iatrogenic pneumothorax. In such situations, the patient is followed with serial radiographs to ensure that the pneumothorax is decreasing in size. When a patient is breathing room air, gas is absorbed from the pleural cavity at approximately 1.25% of the pleural volume/day, approximately 50 to 70mL/day.[14] Supplemental oxygen, by mechanisms reviewed in the physiology section, can increase this rate up to 4.2%/day.[15] As it is a minimal intervention, it is reasonable to place all hospitalized patients on supplemental oxygen if they are being observed for a pneumothorax.

There are several factors to weigh when considering observation alone for a patient with a pneumothorax. The first is that deaths have been reported in patients with pneumothorax who were being observed. Development of unrecognized tension pneumothorax was believed to have played a role in these cases.[16] This fact highlights the selectivity and judgment required to simply follow these patients, particularly on an outpatient basis. Another consideration is that a lung that has not fully expanded by 2 weeks is at risk for fibrous peel deposition and subsequent entrapment. Correction of this situation commits the patient to a surgical procedure that might have been avoided by initial evacuation of the pneumothorax.

It is recommended that observation be considered only for patients with a simple pneumothorax whose size involves 15% or less of the volume of the chest.[17] If the pneumothorax has not resolved within 1 to 2 weeks, intervention to achieve full expansion should be instituted. Another factor to consider, particularly with primary spontaneous pneumothorax, is that observation alone does nothing to decrease the chance of recurrence. Last, in this age of economic constraints, it may be more cost-effective to definitively treat a pneumothorax on presentation.

SIMPLE ASPIRATION

Simple aspiration can be considered in the case of a simple pneumothorax in which there is no suspicion of an ongoing air leak and the patient is not on positive pressure ventilation. Some authors believe that in select situations aspiration is the treatment of choice.[18] The goal of aspiration is to remove air from the pleural space. It conveys no protection from an ongoing leak or recurrence in the future. The procedure is performed in a manner similar to that used for decompressing a tension pneumothorax. After sterilely preparing the skin and infiltrating with a local anesthetic, a 16- or 18-gauge intravenous catheter is placed into the pleural space in the midclavicular line over the superior surface of the second rib. The needle is then withdrawn, and the catheter is connected to a short length of intravenous tubing capped with a three-way stopcock. A 60-mL syringe is then used to aspirate air from the chest cavity. When air can no longer be aspirated, the catheter is withdrawn, and the first chest x-ray is obtained. If 4 L of air are aspirated and no resistance is met, there is an ongoing air leak, and a chest tube should be placed.

PERCUTANEOUS TUBE THORACOSTOMY

Percutaneous tube thoracostomy is a good option for a simple pneumothorax. Many consider this the procedure of choice for simple pneumothoraces. Cited advantages are therapeutic and cost-effectiveness as well as less trauma compared to standard tube thoracostomy. Depending on the size and etiology of the pneumothorax, success rates for these catheters are reported in the 85% to 90% range.[19] The catheters range in size from 9 to 16 French and are placed using a catheter-over-needle or Seldinger technique. The kits (e.g., Arrow Pneumothorax Kit, Arrow International, Reading, PA) are usually equipped with all the necessary supplies to insert the catheters and an adapter such that the catheter can be connected to a Heimlich valve or a standard suction device such as Pleur-evac (DSP Worldwide, Fall River, MA). These tubes are limited by their size and would be a poor choice for a patient with a large air leak. The principal factor in determining the flow rate through a tube is the diameter of the tube. Thus, a patient with a massive air leak, especially on positive pressure ventilation, should have a standard chest tube placed. As a general guide, it takes at least a 28-French tube to accommodate approximately 15 L/min of flow at −10 cm H_2O suction.[20]

TUBE THORACOSTOMY

A standard chest tube should be placed for failure of a percutaneous tube, a pneumothorax associated with significant fluid collection, or a pneumothorax for which the leak is expected to overwhelm a small-caliber tube, more likely in the setting of positive pressure ventilation. Such tubes are generally placed under local anesthesia and sedation, employing sterile technique. Apical tubes, as employed for drainage of air, are best placed in the mid- or anterior axillary line in the third or fourth intercostal space. It is generally recommended to tunnel the tube subcutaneous up one interspace before entering the pleural cavity. The tunnel serves two purposes. First, it forms a flap valve that helps prevent entrance of air into the chest after the tube is removed. Second, the tunnel allows the surgeon to control the direction of the tube, anteriorly when placed for air or posteriorly when placed to drain fluid. The tube can then be placed for passive or active drainage. Passive drainage may be achieved by connecting the tube to a Heimlich flutter valve or waterseal on a Pleur-evac. For active drainage, most surgeons use a three-bottle system (Fig. 74.3), generally unified as a commercially available unit such as Pleur-evac. Active drainage expedites and facilitates full expansion of the lung. Although also reported with passive drainage, the rare complication of reexpansion pulmonary edema appears to be more common with active suction.[21,22]

Generally viewed as a "floor procedure," chest tube placement should be given all the consideration of a major operation. Although it can be performed with minimal discomfort, utilizing intravenous sedation and strategic local anesthesia, a chest tube placed by an inexperienced operator without expert supervision can be a horrific experience for a patient. In addition to the discomfort, chest tube placement may be accompanied by a number of complications including empyema, lung injury and bleeding, and death.[23] Therefore, coagulation profiles and immunocompetency should be taken into consideration for all patients considered for this procedure. Intravenous analgesia, a short-acting benzodiazepine, or both should be used for an elective chest tube placement.

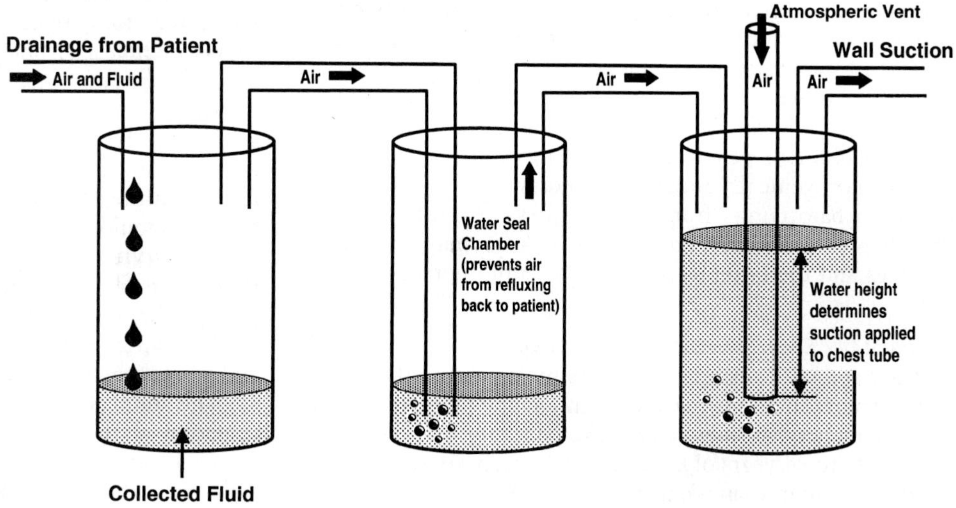

FIGURE 74.3. Three-bottle suction setup for pleural drainage.

Proper use of local anesthesia is critical for patient comfort during the procedure. The amount of local anesthetic that can be administered is limited by toxicity. A small amount of anesthetic is injected for the skin incision, and the remainder is accurately injected along the course of the tunnel that will be created to place the tube. This step allows the surgeon both to locate the superior surface of the rib and, by aspirating, to identify the parietal pleura. A small bolus of anesthesia can be injected at the level of the parietal pleura, and if adequate time is allowed after injection of the pleura, the discomfort of the tube placement can be limited to "pressure" and not sharp pain. As with all procedures under local anesthesia, it is also important to prepare the patient for any anticipated sensations, particularly the entrance into the pleural space as well as the possibility for triggering severe coughing if a collapsed lung is rapidly reexpanded.

Surgery

With the exception of those patients with a large open pneumothorax, essentially all patients considered for surgical treatment for a pneumothorax already have a chest tube in place. With a progressive air leak, tension physiology is imminent once positive pressure ventilation is instituted unless there is a pathway for egress of air from the pleural space or intubation is performed directly with a double-lumen endotracheal tube such that the leaking lung can be immediately isolated. Specific surgical procedures are discussed under the appropriate sections, but it is worth noting that there are two surgical approaches available, video-assisted thoracoscopic surgery (VATS) or standard thoracotomy.

General indications for surgical intervention for a pneumothorax are failure of less-invasive therapy or occurrence of the pneumothorax in the context of additional indications for chest exploration. A VATS approach can be employed, at least initially, for most pneumothoraces. Examples of contraindications to a VATS approach are a pneumothorax secondary to an esophageal perforation, major airway disruption, or a pneumothorax accompanied by significant ongoing bleeding or concomitant trauma to other thoracic organs.

Types of Pneumothorax

Pneumothoraces can be broadly grouped as spontaneous or traumatic. Spontaneous pneumothoraces can be further subclassified as primary or secondary, with primary arising in patients with no known underlying pulmonary disease and secondary spontaneous pneumothoraces arising as a complication of known underlying pulmonary disease. Traumatic pneumothoraces can be subclassified as those that are the result of blunt or penetrating trauma to the chest or those that are iatrogenically induced secondary to an invasive procedure or barotrauma from positive pressure ventilation. In this chapter, the former are referred to as traumatic pneumothoraces and the latter as iatrogenic pneumothoraces.

Primary Spontaneous Pneumothorax

Primary spontaneous pneumothorax most commonly occurs in tall young men but may occur in anyone at any age. The peak incidence has been reported to occur for both men and women 25 to 34 years old. It is approximately six times more common in men than women.

It is thought that the final common pathway for most primary spontaneous pneumothoraces is rupture of subpleural blebs. It is also thought that inflammation of the distal airways plays a significant role in the pathogenesis of this disorder. The lack of communication between these blebs and the distal airways, and hence the inability to rapidly decompress, may explain the increased incidence of primary spontaneous pneumothorax associated with significant drops in atmospheric pressure. The role of inflammation may explain why spontaneous pneumothorax is much more common in smokers. In fact, there appears to be a dose–response relationship, with light smokers (fewer than 13 cigarettes/day) running a risk 7 times that of nonsmokers and those smoking more than 22 cigarettes/day at least 100 times more likely to have a spontaneous pneumothorax than nonsmokers.[24] It is generally accepted that recurrent spontaneous pneumothoraces become increasingly likely with each successive occurrence. The exact statistics vary, but it is estimated that the risk of recurrence in the absence of aggressive preventive measures is in the range of 25% after the first recurrence and 50% after the second recurrence.[25] The chance of recurrence is very much related to the treatment undertaken for the initial spontaneous pneumothorax. Cessation of smoking also decreases the risk of recurrence.

Selection of treatment remains an area of controversy. A consensus statement was released to provide guidance in treatment selection.[26] Observation alone should be selected for treatment on the initial presentation of a small, asymptomatic primary pneumothorax in a patient without any associated comorbidities. It should be reserved for patients who have no barotrauma risks and have ready access to medical help. This treatment may be particularly appropriate for patients who present with heavy cigarette abuse and are willing to stop smoking. Aspiration is another option, but it confers no significant protection from recurrence. Once the decision has been made to violate the pleura for aspiration, it is probably worthwhile leaving a catheter through which air can be continuously aspirated and subsequent pleurodesis can be performed. If a large air leak is anticipated or if there is significant effusion associated with the pneumothorax, then a standard 28-French chest tube should be placed. Neither technique, without pleurodesis, seems to convey significant protection from recurrence.

Surgical treatment remains the gold standard in preventing recurrence of spontaneous pneumothorax. Some of the indications for surgical treatment of a spontaneous pneumothorax include a second pneumothorax (ipsilateral recurrence or a new pneumothorax on the contralateral side); tension physiology; synchronous bilateral pneumothoraces; associated hemothorax (likely secondary to a torn adhesion and complicating approximately 5% of spontaneous pneumothoraces); failure of tube thoracostomy; and lifestyle factors. Surgery should be considered if a leak persists for more than 48h. Lifestyle issues that are accepted indications for surgical therapy at the initial presentation of a primary spontaneous pneumothorax include occupational exposure to barotrauma (scuba diving or flying nonpressurized high-altitude aircraft) and poor accessibility to medical care.

The surgical procedure for spontaneous pneumothorax is resection of the blebs that are usually present, most commonly located in the apex of the upper lobe or the superior segment of the lower lobe. Resection of the blebs is performed

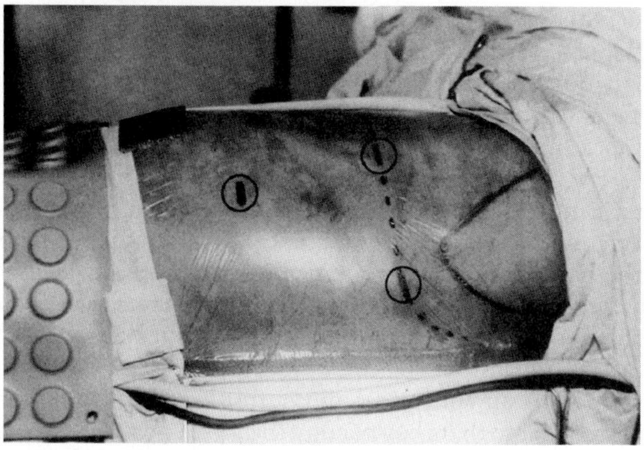

FIGURE 74.4. Typical arrangement of videothoracoscopy ports. The camera, and eventually the chest tube, are introduced through the lowest port (*left*). The remaining two incisions (*right*) are placed along a potential thoracotomy incision. Outline of the scapula is seen on the *right*. (Reprinted with permission from Friedberg and Kniger.[77] © 1998 Greenwich Medical Media Ltd. and by permission of Cambridge University Press.)

with a pulmonary stapling device. Most surgeons also perform a mechanical pleurodesis of the pleura, utilizing an abrasive material such as an electrocautery scratch pad, or perform parietal pleurectomy. Currently, VATS is considered the preferred surgical approach.

A standard triad of video ports can be employed in most cases (Fig. 74.4). Use of a 30° thoracoscope facilitates visualization at the apex of the chest. The thoracoscope is introduced through the inferior port with a grasping device, and the thoracoscopic stapler is introduced through the two superior ports. A sponge stick or folded electrocautery scratch pad can be used for the pleurodesis, with or without a parietal pleurectomy of the bony hemithorax. At the conclusion of the operation, a single 28-French chest tube, with additional ports cut through the radioopaque line, can be placed posteriorly to the apex of the chest. A rongeur is useful for cutting extra holes in chest tubes. If the surgeon is more comfortable placing an anterior and posterior chest tube, two video ports can be created low in the chest at the future chest tube sites, and a single port can be placed in line with a potential thoracotomy incision for grasping and stapling. In skilled hands, the entire lung can be well visualized and mobilized for stapler application, mechanical pleurodesis, and if necessary, pleurectomy (Fig. 74.5). For most of these cases, thoracotomy offers little advantage with respect to visualization or performance of the bleb resections, pleurectomy, and pleurodesis.

Secondary Spontaneous Pneumothorax

Secondary spontaneous pneumothorax is a more serious condition than primary spontaneous pneumothorax because of its occurrence in patients who likely have significantly less pulmonary reserve than the typical patient presenting with a primary spontaneous pneumothorax. As opposed to primary spontaneous pneumothoraces, secondary spontaneous pneumothoraces are associated with a significant mortality.[27] Historically, the most common cause of secondary spontaneous pneumothorax has been chronic obstructive pulmonary disease (COPD). There are many other causes of secondary spontaneous pneumothorax, including, but not limited to, cystic fibrosis, asthma, cancer, many types of infection, sarcoid, collagen vascular diseases, and catamenial pneoumothorax.

The principal factor affecting choice of treatment in these patients is the nature of the underlying pulmonary disease. If the patient is symptomatic, which is far more likely with this patient population, there is no role for observation. Furthermore, an increase in the pneumothorax could possibly place the patient's life in jeopardy. Therefore, observation of a secondary spontaneous pneumothorax is not recommended. Tension physiology is frequently unnecessary to cause clinical decompensation in these patients. Any consideration of employing positive pressure ventilation in a patient with a secondary pneumothorax should serve as an indication for thoracostomy tube placement.

Earnest consideration should be given to sclerosis for prevention in most of these cases. An important exception is the patient who is awaiting lung transplantation because adhesions resulting from sclerosis can significantly complicate explantation of the native lung at the time of transplantation. Another consideration is the nature of the underlying pulmonary disease. If the pneumothorax occurs in the setting of a disease, such as certain malignancies or infections, it may not be possible to staple the lung or to achieve total lung expansion. In these cases, particularly if the patient is terminally ill, consideration should be given to sending the patient home with a chest tube and a Heimlich valve if this provides adequate palliation.

Iatrogenic Pneumothorax

Iatrogenic pneumothorax may be the most common cause of pneumothorax.[28] The most common causes include transthoracic needle biopsy, central line placement, thoracentesis,

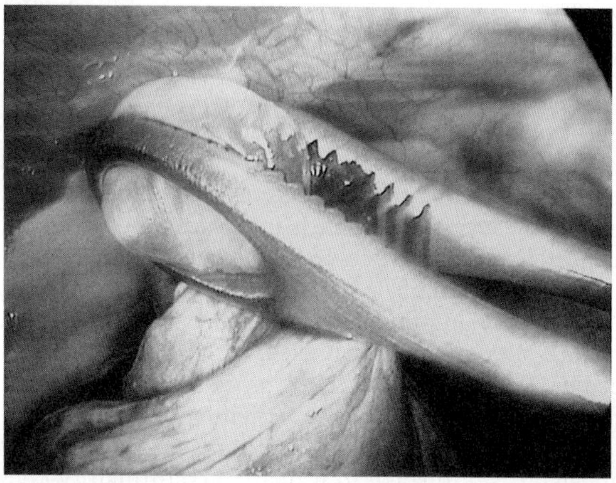

FIGURE 74.5. Intraoperative photograph taken through the videothoracoscope demonstrates an apical bleb (*within the grasping forceps*) in a patient presenting with a recurrent primary spontaneous pneumothorax. The bleb was then resected with a thoracoscopic stapling device, introduced through the third port incision. Subsequently, a parietal pleurectomy of the entire chest wall pleura and a mechanical pleurodesis of the mediastinal and diaphragmatic pleura were performed. A single chest tube was then inserted through the lowest incision, which had been used for the videothoracoscope during the procedure.

transbronchial pulmonary biopsy, and positive pressure ventilation. The management of an iatrogenic pneumothorax must take into account a number of factors, including the etiology, symptoms, and size of the pneumothorax and ventilatory status of the patient. It is logical to consider those patients with pneumothorax secondary to positive pressure ventilation, barotrauma, separately from those who developed pneumothorax secondary to violation of the visceral pleura.

The development of a pneumothorax as a result of barotrauma is an indication for immediate placement of a standard chest tube. This indication is also true for a procedure-induced pneumothorax in a ventilated patient because positive pressure ventilation can rapidly lead to a tension pneumothorax. The clinician should always consider pneumothorax as a cause for instability in a ventilated patient who recently underwent thoracentesis or central line placement.

The majority of iatrogenic pneumothoraces are procedure induced. These pneumothoraces differ from spontaneous pneumothoraces in that the patient is not at an increased risk for recurrence. For small, asymptomatic pneumothoraces, observation is appropriate, and thoracostomy tube placement and sclerosis are not indicated. For larger pneumothoraces or symptomatic pneumothoraces in ambulatory patients, simple aspiration or temporary placement of a small percutaneous catheter is the preferred approach of many clinicians.

Tension Pneumothorax

Any closed pneumothorax arising from visceral pleural disruption has the potential to develop into a tension pneumothorax. Tension pneumothorax occurs when air accumulates in the pleural space in excess of intrapleural pressure and actively compresses the ipsilateral lung. This tension physiology will eventually lead to contralateral mediastinal shift and, in addition to pulmonary embarrassment, can severely limit venous return and compromise cardiac output. Untreated, tension pneumothorax may lead to cardiopulmonary arrest and for this reason is a life-threatening emergency.

Tension pneumothorax is believed to occur when a pleural disruption forms a functional one-way valve allowing air to escape from the lung but not reenter. Such physiology is occasionally well tolerated in a healthy adult and can await chest tube placement under urgent, but controlled, conditions. If, however, the patient is in distress and the diagnosis is suspected, placement of a 16- or 18-gauge intravenous catheter over the second rib, in the midclavicular line, will convert the tension pneumothorax to an open pneumothorax. After decompression has been achieved, a chest tube can then be placed in the usual manner. This procedure should always be performed immediately in any patient who is decompensating and for whom tension pneumothorax is in the differential diagnosis. It is a mistake to wait for a confirmatory chest x-ray in such a situation.

Blebs and Bullae

Although pneumothorax is a disorder of air that has entered into the pleural space, blebs and bullae are also disorders of abnormal air collections, but still contained within the lung. Only blebs can be considered a true pleural disorder. Blebs arise when air escapes from the pulmonary parenchyma and is trapped in the visceral pleura. Simply stated, blebs are subpleural collections of air. They are usually small, less than 2 cm, and tend to occur at the apex of the upper lobe or the apex of the superior segment. The significance of blebs is uncertain. By themselves, it is doubtful that they cause any significant effect on pulmonary function. Their primary clinical significance lies in the fact that they appear to be involved in the pathogenesis of spontaneous pneumothorax. No specific treatment is indicated for the finding of pulmonary blebs in the absence of pneumothorax. Cessation of smoking, as always, is recommended.

Bullae are air collections measuring at least 1 cm, but may become so large that they occupy the greater part of the hemithorax. As opposed to blebs, bullae are formed by destruction and coalescence of alveoli. They may demonstrate trabeculated lumens formed by the residual structural elements from the lung parenchyma they replaced. Blebs may be an incidental finding in patients with otherwise normal lungs, but bullae are likely to be associated with some form of pulmonary disease, most likely emphysema.

Bullous disease is also frequently asymptomatic. In such cases, cessation of smoking and annual chest x-rays are sufficient. In the setting of known underlying lung disease, treatment of that disorder is the priority. Pneumothorax, infection, or hemoptysis can prompt surgical intervention. Surgical intervention can also be indicated for compression of normal lung tissue to improve pulmonary function. Generally, very good results can be anticipated if the bulla is occupying more than 50% of the hemithorax, compressing well-perfused parenchyma.[29]

Liquid-Phase Disorders of the Pleural Space

Pleural effusions are a very common disorder encountered by the clinician. There are many potential causes of effusions (Table 74.1). Occasionally, it is possible to deduce the etiology in the context of the patient's chest radiograph and concurrent morbidities. Frequently, however, the fluid must be sampled to yield a diagnosis. There is a normal composition of pleural fluid (Table 74.2) and a host of tests that can be performed on the fluid in pursuit of a diagnosis (Table 74.3). Once the fluid is sampled, it will fall into one of two categories, transudative or exudative, and 99% of exudative effusions will demonstrate at least one of the following characteristics: pleural fluid protein/serum protein ratio greater than 0.5, pleural fluid lactate dehydrogenase (LDH)/serum LDH greater than 0.6, or pleural fluid LDH more than two-thirds of the upper normal limit for serum LDH.[30]

Transudative effusions result from a perturbation in the hydrostatic or oncotic forces that affect fluid formation and turnover in the pleural space, as described in the physiology section. This imbalance results in fluid accumulation in the pleural space. For transudative effusions, the goal is to drain the effusion for symptomatic relief, if necessary, but to focus on the systemic disease.

Exudative effusions result from diseases that involve the pleura and may be broadly grouped as benign or malignant. The treatment of an exudative effusion is disease specific.

Pleural effusions may be asymptomatic or may cause the patient to present with shortness of breath, secondary to

TABLE 74.1. Differential Diagnoses of Pleural Effusion.

- Transudative pleural effusions
  - Congestive heart failure
  - Cirrhosis
  - Nephrotic syndrome
  - Superior vena cava obstruction
  - Fontan procedure
  - Urinothorax
  - Peritoneal dialysis
  - Glomerulonephritis
  - Myxedema
  - Pulmonary emboli
  - Sarcoidosis
- Exudative pleural effusions
  - Neoplastic disease
    - Metastatic disease
    - Mesothelioma
  - Infectious diseases
    - Bacterial infections
    - Tuberculosis
    - Fungal infections
    - Parasitic infections
    - Viral infections
  - Pulmonary embolization
  - Gastrointestinal disease
    - Pancreatic disease
    - Subphrenic abscess
    - Intrahepatic abscess
    - Intrasplenic abscess
    - Esophageal perforation
    - After abdominal surgery
    - Diaphragmatic hernia
    - Endoscopic variceal sclerosis
    - After liver transplant
  - Collagen vascular diseases
    - Rheumatoid pleuritis
    - Systemic lupus erythematosus
    - Drug-induced lupus
    - Immunoblastic lymphadenopathy
    - Sjögren's syndrome
    - Familial Mediterranean fever
    - Churg-Strauss syndrome
    - Wegener's granulomatosis
  - Drug-induced pleural disease
    - Nitrofurantoin
    - Dantrolene
    - Methysergide
    - Bromocriptine
    - Amiodarone
    - Procarbazine
    - Methotrexate
  - Miscellaneous diseases and conditions
    - Asbestos exposure
    - Postpericardiectomy or postmyocardial infarction syndrome
    - Meigs syndrome
    - Yellow nail syndrome
    - Sarcoidosis
    - Pericardial disease
    - After coronary artery bypass surgery
    - After lung transplant
    - Fetal pleural effusion
    - Uremia
    - Trapped lung
    - Radiation therapy
    - Ovarian hyperstimulation syndrome
    - Postpartum pleural effusion
    - Amyloidosis
    - Electrical burns
    - Iatrogenic injury
  - Hemothorax
  - Chylothorax

Source: Reprinted with permission from Light.[9] © 1995 Lippincott, Williams and Wilkins.

TABLE 74.2. Normal Composition of Pleural Fluid.

Volume	0.1–0.2 mL/kg
Cells/mm³ (%)	1000–5000
Mesothelial cells	3%–70%
Monocytes	30%–75%
Lymphocytes	2%–30%
Granulocytes	10%
Protein (%)	1–2 g/dl
Albumin	50%–70%
Glucose	• plasma level
LDH	<50% plasma level
pH	≥plasma

Data from humans and animals.

Source: Reprinted with permission from Fishman.[29] © 1998 McGraw Hill.

compression of pulmonary parenchyma, as well as other symptoms. A nonspecific sign that is compatible with an effusion is the presence of a nonproductive cough. If the disorder causing the effusion has provoked an inflammatory response in the parietal pleura, the patient may complain of pain with respiration, known as pleuritic chest pain.

Restricted chest wall movement or change in the contour of the hemithorax may be evident, depending on the nature of the effusion and its effect on pleural pressure. If the effusion is unilateral and massive, the trachea may deviate to the contralateral side. Absence of vocal fremitus, dullness to percussion, and decreased breath sounds are all characteristic

TABLE 74.3. Useful Tests in the Evaluation of Pleural Effusion.

Test	*Abnormal value*	*Frequently associated condition*
Red blood cells/mm³	>100,000	Malignancy, trauma, pulmonary embolism
White blood cells/mm³	>10,000	Pyogenic infection
Neutrophils (%)	>50	Acute pleuritis
Lymphocytes (%)	>90	Tuberculosis, malignancy
Eosinophilia (%)	>10	Asbestos effusion, pneumothorax, resolving infection
Mesothelial cells	Absent	Tuberculosis
Protein, PF/S[a]	>0.5	Exudate
LDH, PF/S	>0.6	Exudate
LDH, IU[b]	>200	Exudate
Glucose, mg/dl	<60	Empyema, tuberculosis, malignancy, rheumatoid arthritis
pH	<7.20	Complicated parapneumonic effusion, empyema, esophageal rupture, tuberculosis, malignancy, rheumatoid arthritis
Amylase, PF/S	>1	Pancreatitis
Bacteriological	Positive	Cause of infection
Cytology	Positive	Diagnostic of malignancy

[a]PF/S, pleural fluid-to-serum ratio.

[b]IU, concentration in international units.

findings on physical examination. If the pleura is inflamed, there may be an audible rub. A rub is likely to precede a significant effusion that will separate the roughened pleural surfaces and diminish or resolve the rub. In the case of a hydropneumothorax, there may be an audible "splash," as originally described by Hippocrates.

Plain radiographs of the chest remain the most common test obtained to evaluate a suspected effusion. If the effusion is free flowing, the lateral costophrenic angle may be blunted on an upright posteroanterior radiograph. The lateral radiograph is more sensitive than the posteroanterior view, but neither is as sensitive as the lateral decubitus projection. Additional studies that are commonly used to obtain more information about a suspected effusion include ultrasound and CT scan. Ultrasound is helpful in distinguishing pleural thickening from pleural fluid and determining if an effusion is complex or simple, and it has the advantage of portability. It can be used to help direct the clinician to the best area to perform a thoracentesis at the bedside. CT scans give the most information with respect to exact location of an effusion and may be particularly helpful in distinguishing effusion from pleural disease or parenchymal disease.

If the clinical scenario warrants diagnosis of the effusion, then the next step is to perform a thoracentesis to obtain a specimen for analysis and, possibly, to drain the effusion for relief of symptoms. The decision to perform such a procedure should be taken seriously for the complications can be significant and include pneumothorax, hemothorax, and conversion of a sterile effusion into an empyema. Thus, it is important to make sure the patient is not coagulopathic, and if there is any question regarding the appropriate site to insert the needle, a bedside ultrasound should be performed.

Sterile technique must be observed. The procedure is most easily accomplished with the patient in the sitting position and leaning over a bedside table that has been padded with one or two pillows. For a diagnostic tap, a long 25-gauge needle can be used to infiltrate with lidocaine and can be used as a finder needle. A 22-gauge needle is then used to perform the aspiration.

If a therapeutic tap is indicated, a similar technique is employed, except that a catheter is placed into the chest cavity and connected via tubing to a three-way stopcock, which in turn is connected to a syringe or a vacuum bottle. A number of commercial kits are available for this purpose.

Regardless of the technique, it is generally recommended that not more than 1 L of fluid should be aspirated at one time as this increases the chances of developing reexpansion pulmonary edema. The exact etiology of this syndrome is not fully understood and may be accompanied by 20% mortality.[31] Treatment for reexpansion edema is supportive care.

Transudative Effusions

If the effusion is transudative, then it is most likely secondary to congestive heart failure, hepatic insufficiency, or renal insufficiency. Pleural effusions secondary to congestive failure are the most common transudative effusions.[32] Most of these effusions are bilateral. The presence of a unilateral effusion or bilateral effusions of significantly different sizes does not exclude this diagnosis, but would be unusual. The disorder is thought to result from increased pressure at the pulmonary capillary level secondary to left heart failure. The treatment is the same as for other transudative effusions and is directed at the underlying cause, in this case, congestive failure. If the etiology is unclear or if the effusion remains unchanged after the congestive heart failure has improved, a diagnostic thoracentesis should be performed. Occasionally, it is necessary to perform a therapeutic tap for symptomatic relief.

Approximately 5% of patients with hepatic cirrhosis will develop pleural effusions as a result of their disease.[33] Two-thirds of cirrhotic pleural effusions are right sided. Usually, the patient will have ascites in addition to the pleural effusion. The pleural effusion is thought to result from a one-way communication and fluid flow from the peritoneum, across the diaphragm, to the pleural space. The treatment should be directed at the liver failure and ascites, with diuresis and salt restriction as the initial steps in management. Decompression of the portal circulation, percutaneously or surgically, may be indicated to treat the underlying disease. If the pleural effusion is unresponsive to these measures, or if pulmonary symptoms necessitate intervention, the options include drainage and pleurodesis. Sometimes surgical intervention is indicated, combining closure of a demonstrated peritoneal–pleural communication with pleurodesis; this has been accomplished using VATS techniques as well as thoracotomy.[34,35] Shunting ascites to the venous system is another option; however, these patients are generally poor surgical candidates unless their liver failure is corrected. It is best to avoid placement of a chest tube for drainage of a pleural effusion secondary to cirrhosis as the high drainage rates from decompression of ascites across the diaphragm can make these tubes difficult to remove.

Nephrotic syndrome is another disorder associated with pleural transudates. These effusions tend to be bilateral and result from decreased plasma oncotic pressure. Again, treatment should be aimed at the primary disorder. In severely symptomatic patients, drainage and sclerosis can be considered. Other conditions that may provoke a transudative effusion include, but are not limited to, pulmonary embolism, superior vena cava obstruction, peritoneal dialysis, myxedema, glomerulonephritis, Meigs syndrome, and sarcoidosis.

Exudative Effusions

Exudative effusions can be broadly grouped into benign and malignant effusions. The malignant effusions arise most commonly from metastatic disease but can also herald the presence of a primary malignancy of the pleura. The benign causes of exudative effusion include a long list of conditions, including, but not limited to, infectious diseases, pulmonary embolism, collagen vascular diseases, drug-induced disorders, bleeding, chyle leak, subdiaphragmatic infections, pancreatitis, and esophageal perforation. If the cause is not obvious, then a thoracentesis should be the next step in diagnosing the etiology of the effusion. The following sections discuss the conditions most likely to be encountered by the surgeon.

Malignant Effusions

Malignant effusions represent one of the most common indications for chest tube placement. The tumors most frequently associated with a pleural effusion include lung cancer, breast cancer, ovarian cancer, and lymphoma. Dyspnea from pulmonary compression is the most common symptom produced by a malignant effusion. Malignant effusions are exudative and frequently sanguinous in appearance. The diagnosis can frequently be established by cytological demonstration of cancer cells in the fluid, although up to 40% of effusions yield nondiagnostic cytology.[36] Thus, if malignancy is suspected and the fluid cytology is nondiagnostic, a pleural biopsy should be considered.

The approach of choice is VATS if surgery is required to establish a diagnosis. Depending on their surgical risk, patients may be well served by going to the operating room early in their course for diagnosis and drainage. Under general anesthesia, a single chest tube incision can be created through which the effusion can be drained and the thoracoscope introduced for examination and photodocumentation of the pleural cavity. Pleural biopsies can then be performed through the same incision by sliding the camera port out of the incision onto the proximal scope and sliding a biopsy forceps alongside the scope, through the same incision. A 5-mm 30° thoracoscope is particularly helpful for this procedure as it allows the surgeon to look over the surfaces of the chest cavity and to move the scope off to the side, which facilitates manipulation of the biopsy forceps. If the lung demonstrates the ability to fully expand and a malignant diagnosis is confirmed, intraoperative talc poudrage can be considered. All this can be accomplished through a single 10- to 15-mm incision.

Once the etiology of the malignant effusion is established, a treatment strategy can be formulated.[37] Surgical debulking of metastatic pleural tumor is generally not part of the treatment algorithm outside an experimental protocol. Most patients are relegated to chemotherapy, radiation therapy, or palliative measures directed at preventing further fluid accumulation. Some tumors, such as small cell lung cancer, breast cancer, ovarian cancer, and lymphoma, may respond well to chemotherapy, including resolution of the pleural effusion. Mediastinal radiation therapy may also be indicated in treatment of the patient's tumor, especially if the tumor has involved the thoracic duct and resulted in a chylothorax. If the patient is not receiving treatment for the underlying malignancy or reaccumulates the effusion in spite of treatment, an alternative strategy must be considered if the effusion is causing symptoms. The first choice is pleurodesis, with other options for failure of this technique.

Pleurodesis

If the lung expands completely when fluid has been drained, then pleurodesis is an option. If the lung does not expand, pleural apposition cannot occur, and injection of a sclerosant will not work. In fact, the sclerosant may further hinder the absorptive mechanisms of the pleura, thereby making the effusion worse. The literature does not support the belief that the pleural drainage must be less than 150 mL/day to achieve effective sclerosis. Equal results and greater cost-effectiveness appear to occur if the sclerosis is performed as soon as the lung is fully expanded, regardless of the volume of drainage.[38] There is also no support for the time-honored tradition of "rolling" the patient to achieve even distribution of the sclerosing agent. A prospective, randomized study utilizing instillation of ^{99m}Tc-sestamibi-labeled talc suspension has demonstrated that the dispersion of talc suspension and the overall success rate in patients with malignant effusions is not influenced by the position of the patient.[39]

Choice of Sclerosant

A large number of agents are available for pleural sclerosis. Talc is the most popular chemical sclerosant used. A large metaanalysis reviewing 36 randomized controlled trials including over 1499 patients concluded that: "The currently available evidence supports the need for chemical sclerosants for successful pleurodesis, the use of talc as the sclerosant of choice, and thoracoscopic pleurodesis as the preferred technique for pleurodesis based on efficacy. There was no evidence for an increase in mortality following talc pleurodesis."[40]

Doxycycline is the cheapest of the sclerosing agents. It is also the one that most commonly causes significant discomfort. It is administered dissolved in 50 to 100 mL sterile saline and 200 mg lidocaine via chest tube. Bleomycin generally causes little discomfort but is the most expensive agent. It is administered dissolved in 100 mL of sterile saline via chest tube. Although generally well tolerated, intrapleural bleomycin is absorbed systemically and is therefore not recommended for patients who are receiving chemotherapy, are immunosuppressed, or have renal failure. Support can be found in the literature for using any of these agents in nearly any situation.

A rational approach is to use talc for pleurodesis of malignant effusion and doxycycline for benign indications if the patient can safely tolerate significant sedation with intravenous narcotics and benzodiazepines or if the patient already has an epidural catheter in place. Even with instillation of intrapleural lidocaine, patients will commonly describe doxycycline pleurodesis as one of the most painful experiences of their lives. An argument can be made to avoid the use of talc when there is potential contamination of the pleural space, either primarily or secondarily by some other site of active infection. Talc, as a permanent foreign body, can serve as nidus for infection and result in chronic empyema. In a patient with a malignant effusion, in whom there is concern for possible contamination of the pleural space, bleomycin pleurodesis would be a reasonable option. Table 74.4 summarizes the various agents along with their success and associated complications profile.

Other Options

If the patient's lung does not expand, or if pleurodesis has failed, then chronic drainage becomes the next option. The options include internal or external drainage. For external drainage, the patient may undergo repeat therapeutic thoracenteses or placement of a long-term drainage catheter. Intermittent thoracentesis may be the best for a patient who is minimally symptomatic or has a very short life expectancy. Indwelling catheter placement for intermittent drainage pro-

TABLE 74.4. Commonly Used Sclerosing Agents with Associated Success Rates and Adverse Effects.

Agent	*Success rate*	*Adverse effects*
Talc	93%	Fever 16%
Doxycycline	72%	Pain 40%
Tetracycline	67%	Pain 14%
Bleomycin	54%	Pain 28%, fever 14%

Data from Walker-Renard et al.[78]

vides good palliation.[41] Commercial kits such as the Pleurex catheter (Denver Biomedical, Denver CO) are available. Another option would be placement of a pleuroperitoneal shunt for internal drainage of the pleural space and decompression of the lung. Internal drainage can be accomplished by implanting a shunt, such as the Denver Shunt (Denver Biomaterials), which has a pumping chamber that the patient can press to transfer fluid across the negative pressure gradient from the pleural cavity to the peritoneal cavity. There are a number of downsides to this option. Placement requires an operation, usually under general anesthesia; a small percentage of the shunts will obstruct; and the patient must actively pump the shunt to transfer fluid.

Thoracotomy with decortication, in the presence of a malignant effusion, is rarely indicated. Although highly variable, the average survival of a patient with a malignant effusion from lung cancer is on the order of 4 months, whereas for breast or ovarian cancer it may be more in the range of 7 to 9 months.[42] Thus, recovery from such an operation is likely to result in decreased quality of life for a significant portion of the patient's remaining time.

Benign Effusions

Effusions associated with pneumonia (parapneumonic effusions) are the most common cause of benign exudative effusions. They result from visceral pleural inflammation that alters the normal fluid balance of the pleural space. These effusions may initially be sterile, but if the parenchymal infection spreads to the effusion, an empyema results. There is a continuum that reflects the natural history of untreated parapneumonic effusions, from a thin, clear sterile collection to an infected fibrous peel encasing the lung.

The first stage is the *exudative stage*, characterized by fluid exuding from the lung into the pleural space, likely from the pulmonary interstitial space. This stage should resolve with antibiotic therapy and generally does not require drainage. Normal pH and glucose with a low LDH and white blood cell count are characteristic of the fluid at this stage.

Untreated, the effusion is likely to progress to the *fibropurulent stage*, characterized by increased fluid that is heavily laden with white blood cells, microorganisms, and cellular debris. Fibrin is deposited on the pleural surfaces, and the stage is set for pulmonary entrapment. At this point, the fluid pH and glucose level fall, and the LDH rises. Chest tube drainage is indicated but becomes more difficult as the effusion loculates with fibrinous septae.

The final stage is the *organizational stage*, during which fibroblasts grow into the effusion, laying down a thick fibrous peel that encases the lung and results in entrapment. The remaining effusion is thick and infected and may necessitate through the chest wall or into the lung.

The presentation of a parapneumonic effusion or empyema depends, to a certain extent, on the organism causing the infection. For aerobic organisms, the presence of the effusion has little impact on the clinical picture, which is that of a bacterial pneumonia: fever, chest pain, and a productive cough. An anaerobic infection, frequently as a result of aspiration, is more likely to present in a subacute manner. A patient with an anaerobic empyema may have symptoms for more than a week before seeking medical help, and significant weight loss may be a chief component of their presentation.

Diagnosis

True *empyema thoracis* is simply defined as pus in the pleural space, a clear indication for drainage. For a small simple parapneumonic effusion in a patient being treated with and responding to appropriate antibiotics, there is no indication for drainage. The issue is how to identify the effusion that is not yet frankly purulent but will require drainage to resolve. If the patient with pneumonia continues to have a large or increasing effusion, then a thoracentesis should be performed.

The fluid from the tap should be sent for analysis of glucose, pH, LDH, amylase, protein, complete blood count with differential, Gram stain, aerobic/anaerobic bacterial cultures, and if indicated, special microorganism cultures and stains. If malignancy is suspected, cytology should also be sent. As seen in Table 74.5 from the American College of Chest Physicians Parapneumonic Effusions Panel Evidence-Based Guideline,[43] the risk outcome can be stratified and used to determine whether drainage is warranted. These remain, however, only guidelines, and sound clinical judgment is essential.

Treatment

Once the decision has been made to drain the fluid collection, a number of options are available: aspiration, chest tube drainage, VATS drainage, limited thoracotomy and open drainage, or full thoracotomy with drainage and decortication. For diagnosis and initial treatment of a free-flowing pleural effusion, aspiration is an appropriate initial step. If the clinical situation mandates further drainage, then the clinician has several options. If the effusion is free flowing, then placement of a standard chest tube is a reasonable option. If the effusion is loculated, ultrasound guidance may be helpful either for marking the ideal location for thoracentesis or thoracostomy tube placement or for placement of a percutaneous drainage catheter. The use of intrapleural streptokinase or urokinase has been advocated if drainage fails due to loculations.[44] In several well-constructed studies, however, it has been shown that enzymatic treatment will increase the volume of chest tube output but not affect the clinical course. The role of these agents for treatment of empyema remains undefined.[45]

There are several surgical options for patients with an empyema. The goals of surgical therapy are to establish drainage and, depending on the situation, to eliminate space in the pleural cavity. Space elimination can be accomplished by decortication to allow the lung to expand, collapsing the chest wall with a thoracoplasty, or transposing muscle flaps to fill the space. A critical component is always to establish drainage. The least-invasive option is to explore the chest cavity thoracoscopically, disrupt loculations, debride the visceral pleura, and strategically place chest tubes. Frequently, it is possible to accomplish this procedure utilizing the patient's existing chest tube sites as video ports. This option is most likely to be successful if performed in the exudative or early fibrinopurulent stages.[46]

Once in the organizational stage, the lung is encased in a fibrous peel that most often requires an open thoracotomy to adequately remove. If the patient is able to tolerate such a procedure, then this represents the most effective treatment of the problem. The goal in such a situation is to drain the infection and obliterate any space with reexpanded lung

TABLE 74.5. Categorizing Risk for Poor Outcome in Patients with Parapneumonic Effusions.

Pleural space anatomy		*Pleural fluid bacteriology*		*Pleural fluid chemistry*[a]	*Category*	*Risk of poor outcome*	*Drainage*
A_0 minimal, free-flowing effusion (<10 mm on lateral decubitus)[b]	AND	B_X: culture and Gram stain results unknown	AND	C_X: pH unknown	1	Very low	No[c]
A_1 small-to-moderate free-flowing effusion (>10 mm and < 1/2 hemithorax)	AND	B_0: negative culture and Gram stain[d]	AND	C_0: pH > 7.20	2	Low	No[e]
A_2 large, free-flowing effusion (>1.2 hemithorax,[f] loculated effusion,[g] or effusion with thickened parietal pleura)[h]	OR	B_1: positive culture or Gram stain	OR	C_1: pH < 7.20	3	Moderate	Yes
		B_2: pus			4	High	Yes

[a]pH is the preferred pleural fluid chemistry test, and pH must be determined using a blood gas analyzer. If a blood gas analyzer is not available, pleural fluid glucose should be used (P_0 glucose > 60 mg/dL; P_1 glucose < 60 mg/dL). The panel cautions that the clinical utility and decision thresholds for pH and glucose have not been well established.

[b]Clinical experience indicates that effusions of this size do not require thoracentesis for evaluation but will resolve.

[c]If thoracentesis were performed in a patient with A_0 category pleural anatomy and P_1 and B_1 status found, clinical experience suggests that the P_1 or B_1 findings might be a false-positive result. Repeat thoracentesis should be considered if effusion enlarges or clinical condition deteriorates.

[d]Regardless of prior use of antibiotics.

[e]If clinical condition deteriorates, repeat thoracentesis and drainage should be considered.

[f]Larger effusions are more resistant to effective drainage, possibly because of the increased likelihood that large effusions will also be loculated.

[g]Pleural loculations suggest a worse prognosis.

[h]Thickened parietal pleura on contrast-enhanced CT suggests presence of empyema.

Source: From Colice et al.,[43] with permission from *Chest*.

tissue. If a portion of the lung has already been removed or if the infection has rendered portions nonviable, mandating resection, then space may become an issue. The favored option is to transpose muscle flaps into the chest cavity to obliterate any residual space that exists after the lung has been decorticated and reexpanded. The commonly used muscle flaps are serratus, latissimus, and pectoralis. Omentum is also a good option. A good approach in these cases is to enter the chest through a vertically oriented muscle-sparing thoracotomy such that both serratus and latissimus are spared and can be harvested if necessary.

After a drainage procedure, the clinician is faced with the management of the chest tubes. The classic treatment of a chest tube placed into an empyema is to leave it to closed suction drainage for 2 to 3 weeks. Thereafter, the tubes are taken off suction and converted to open drainage, slowly withdrawing them over the course of several more weeks. Another option is to leave the tubes in place for approximately 1 week on suction. If the lung is fully expanded, drainage is minimal (<50 mL/day), and the patient has no further signs of infection, then the tubes may be removed. The critical point is that the lung must be fully expanded. Cases in which this strategy is safe and effective usually demonstrate full expansion of the lung on the chest x-ray and "walling off" of the chest tube, characterized by essentially no drainage and lack of respiratory variation in the waterseal chamber of the Pleur-evac.

For patients with chronic empyema or empyema with bronchopleural fistula or patients unable to tolerate thoracotomy, an open drainage procedure may represent the best option. These procedures involve localizing the most dependent portion of the empyema cavity and resecting a portion of the overlying rib. The cavity is then entered, the pleural space debrided, and if possible, the lung decorticated. Depending on the size of the cavity, it may close spontaneously or may require reconstruction, usually with a muscle flap. In an elderly or infirm patient, the cavity may be left open. Given enough time, even cavities of substantial size will commonly close.

Benign Effusions, Effusions from Other Causes

Infectious, Nonbacterial

Almost any organism can cause an infection associated with a pleural effusion. Tuberculosis may cause a pleural effusion that tends to be unilateral and of moderate size. They can be difficult to diagnose based on chemical and microbiological evaluation of the pleural fluid but usually demonstrate granulomatous pleuritis on closed pleural biopsy if the diagnosis is in doubt. The effusion usually responds to appropriate antibiotic therapy and, unless symptomatic or part of a mixed empyema, usually does not require drainage or surgery.

Viral effusions usually elude diagnosis and are self-limited. Human immunodeficiency virus (HIV) does not appear to cause pleural effusions, but patients with HIV are more likely to develop pleural complications associated with a bacterial pneumonia.

Effusions may accompany any of a number of fungal pulmonary infections. The primary treatment is appropriate antibiotic therapy and, depending on the infection, drainage. Of note, *Aspergillus* empyemas are almost always associated with a bronchopleural fistula, or a history of previous treatment of tuberculosis with artificial pneumothorax, and almost always require surgical evacuation as part of their treatment.

Although relatively uncommon in the United States, the clinician should be aware that pleural effusions frequently accompany a number of parasitic infections. Again, appropriate drug therapy is essential. Of note, rupture of pleural or hepatic cysts into the pleural space can present with acute symptoms and, as in the case of *Echinococcus*, may represent an indication for urgent thoracotomy to debride and drain the pleural space and to drain the original cyst.

Pulmonary Emboli

Pleural effusions may accompany pulmonary emboli in 30% to 50% of cases. Although the majority of these effusions are exudative, approximately one-quarter may be transudative. This is likely to be determined by the relative contribution to the effusion by the two mechanisms thought to be primarily responsible for the effusion. Transudative effusions are thought to exude from the parietal pleura secondary to right heart failure. Exudative effusions are thought to arise from the visceral pleural secondary to release of local factors from the emboli that increase capillary permeability. The treatment for pulmonary emboli with effusion is the same as for pulmonary emboli without effusion, and as always, the key factor is to consider the diagnosis in a patient with any of the symptoms suggestive of pulmonary embolus.

Subdiaphragmatic Pathology

Inflammation or malignancy below the diaphragm can cause exudative pleural effusions as well as transudative effusions secondary to hepatic or renal dysfunction, as discussed in the transudative effusion section. Acute pancreatitis generally leads to a left-sided effusion, likely as a result of transdiaphragmatic transfer of exudative ascites arising from pancreatic inflammation. The fluid almost always has an elevated amylase, and that amylase is frequently higher than the serum amylase. The fluid generally resolves with resolution of the pancreatic inflammation. Pancreatic abscess can also cause a pleural effusion; again, the treatment is the usual treatment of a pancreatic abscess. A pancreatic pseudocyst can decompress into the pleural space, forming a pancreaticopleural fistula. These effusions tend to be large, usually left sided, very high in amylase, and usually accompanied by chest, not abdominal, symptoms. This finding is thought to be secondary to decompression of the pseudocyst into the thorax. Treatment of this disorder is conservative, the same as the initial treatment of any pancreatic pseudocyst. The role of drainage of the effusion remains controversial, and the clinician should be aware of the risk of infection and the fact that the drainage is likely to be massive and to reaccumulate rapidly until the fistula has closed. Should conservative treatment fail, a percutaneous or surgical drainage procedure should be planned. Subphrenic abscess from any number of intraabdominal sources can lead to an exudative effusion. The effusions rarely are culture positive and tend to have a very high white cell count, yet the pH is usually above 7.20, and the glucose is usually greater than 60 mg/dl. Treatment of the effusion should be symptomatic as the approach is treatment of the abscess and its underlying cause. The effusion usually resolves with these measures.

The clinician is advised always to consider esophageal perforation in the diagnosis of a pleural effusion, particularly after instrumentation of the esophagus or retching. Iatrogenic injury accounts for two-thirds of these injuries, and the patient frequently complains of chest pain. The condition usually presents with a left-sided effusion, but it may be either side or bilateral and accompanied by, or replaced with, a pneumothorax. The fluid is almost always high in amylase from saliva that has leaked into the pleural space. The mortality rate is high, up to 60%, which underscores the imperative of prompt diagnosis. If the diagnosis is being entertained, a contrast swallow study should be obtained. Treatment depends on how early the disruption is diagnosed and ranges from primary repair to esophageal exclusion. Pleural drainage, cessation of ongoing pleural soilage, nutritional support and antibiotics are necessary components of the treatment strategy.

Chylothorax

Chylothorax is an exudative effusion caused by disruption of the lymphatics in the chest, most commonly the thoracic duct, and subsequent drainage of chyle into the pleural space. The initial presentation of a chylothorax is determined by the size of effusion and its mechanical effects within the hemithorax. Once a chest tube is in place, the symptoms are determined by the persistence of the drainage. The longer the drainage continues, the more dangerous it becomes, with the consequences being dehydration, nutritional depletion, and immunocompromise.[47]

More than 50% of chylothoraces are secondary to ductal obstruction and disruption by tumor, with lymphoma accounting for 75% of these cases. Approximately 25% of chyle leaks are traumatic, with iatrogenic trauma the most common. Of the iatrogenic causes, esophageal resection is the leading cause and is more common with transhiatal esophagectomies than transthoracic esophagectomies. The diagnosis is established by analysis of the fluid. Although classically thought of as milky in appearance, chyle may appear serosanguinous, particularly in the fasting state. A triglyceride level in the fluid greater than 110 mg/dL is highly suggestive of chyle, whereas a level below 50 mg/dL essentially excludes the diagnosis of chylothorax. Intermediate values require a lipoprotein analysis to prove the presence of chylomicrons to establish the diagnosis.[48] Some believe that the most reliable test is to give an oral challenge of cream and to observe the tube drainage for gross changes.

The treatment of chylothorax remains controversial; some authors advocate a generous period of conservative treatment, while others recommend early intervention. All agree that a prolonged, high-output leak can be devastating. Conservative therapy involves pleural drainage and total parenteral nutrition. If the leak is secondary to a malignancy, then chemotherapy or radiation therapy may be the treatment of choice.

For other chylothoraces, surgical intervention is indicated when conservative measures have failed. The timing of such intervention is debatable, but most authors agree it is unwise to wait more than 1 week in the setting of an unremitting leak. It is important not to wait until the patient is immunocompromised and nutritionally depleted before deciding to operate as this would unnecessarily increase the risk of the surgery. At the time of surgery, heavy cream is administered via nasogastric tube immediately after intubation; this makes the duct more visible and may also identify the area of leakage. A number of surgical options are available, including parietal pleurectomy, direct ligation of the leak, and mass ligation of the duct. Mass ligation offers at least an 80% chance of resolving the leak.[49] Many advocate performing a ligation of the duct on the right side, just as it emerges from the diaphragm, regardless of the side of the chylothorax. This ligation has traditionally been performed through a small thoracotomy incision in the sixth or seventh interspace. This procedure is

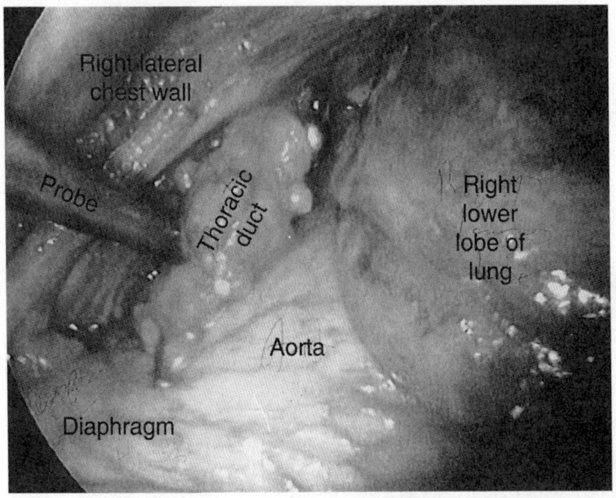

FIGURE 74.6. Intraoperative photograph through a video thoracoscope shows probe under the thoracic duct, which has been dissected free at the level of the diaphragm on the *right side*. Note thoracic duct, aorta, lung, and diaphragm. This duct was clipped and ligated via this VATS (video-assisted thoracoscopic surgery) approach through three 10-mm incisions that resulted in immediate and complete resolution of the patient's chyle leak.

readily accomplished thoracoscopically, utilizing three 1.0- to 1.5-cm port incisions (Fig. 74.6). This procedure seems to offer less morbidity and equal efficacy to the open procedure. If the expertise exists, occlusion of the duct by interventional radiologists may be an option and would be the intermediate step to consider between failure of conservative therapy and surgical ligation of the duct. Should all other measures fail, or if the right chest is hostile, the duct can be approached transabdominally in the aortic hiatus.

HEMOTHORAX

The overwhelming majority of hemothoraces are caused by trauma, including iatrogenic trauma. There are other, significantly less common, causes, including bleeding from metastatic tumors involving the pleura, hemorrhage during anticoagulation therapy for pulmonary emboli, and catamenial hemothorax. The potential consequences of an undrained hemothorax include conversion to an empyema, provocation of a pleural effusion, and conversion to a fibrothorax with lung entrapment. The initial treatment of any hemothorax should be pleural drainage with a large-bore (32- or 36-French) chest tube. If the tube becomes clogged or is inadequate, additional tubes should be strategically placed.

Up to 4% of hemothoraces will become infected. This complication is more common in patients admitted in shock, with gross contamination of the pleura at the time of injury, with prolonged chest tube drainage, and with concomitant abdominal injuries. The pleural effusion associated with hemothoraces may occur after the blood has been evacuated and the chest tubes are removed. If the fluid is infected, it should be treated accordingly. If not, these effusions tend to be self-limited and require no further intervention. Use of VATS is safe and effective in evacuating blood from the chest cavity. In a prospective randomized trial, early VATS drainage of retained hemothorax was found to decrease duration of tube drainage, hospital stay, and cost.[50] The earlier clot evacuation is attempted, the more likely VATS evacuation will be completely successful. In addition, if intervention is instituted early, the entire operation can frequently be performed through the existing chest tube incisions, occasionally requiring one additional videoscopic port incision.

MISCELLANEOUS

Collagen vascular disorders may be associated with pleural effusions. In each case, the treatment of the effusion is symptomatic, with the primary therapy treatment of the underlying disorder. The two most common diseases are rheumatoid arthritis and systemic lupus erythematous. Rheumatoid disease may involve the pulmonary parenchyma as well as the pleura.

There are numerous other causes of exudative effusions. These include but are not limited to cardiac surgery, lung transplantation, asbestos exposure, Dressler's syndrome, Meigs syndrome, yellow nail syndrome, sarcoid, postpartum state, trapped lung, radiation exposure, ovarian hyperstimulation, amyloidosis, acute respiratory distress syndrome (ARDS), electrical burns, and uremia.

Solid Disorders of the Pleural Space

A limited number of benign and malignant solid disorders affect the pleura. The most common benign conditions are fibrothorax, pleural plaques, diffuse pleural thickening, and benign fibrous tumors of the pleura. The most common malignancies are tumors metastatic to the pleura. The primary malignancy of the mesothelium is mesothelioma, and numerous cancers, such as liposarcoma and fibrosarcoma, may arise from any of the elements forming the connective tissue layer of the pleura.

Benign Disorders

Fibrothorax results from deposition of a thick fibrous layer along the pleural surface. This layer may cause entrapment of the lung as well as contraction and immobility of the skeletal hemithorax. The most common causes of fibrothorax are hemothorax, tuberculosis, and bacterial pneumonia.

The treatment of fibrothorax is decortication, which is generally a major operation requiring a full thoracotomy. Patients who are being considered for decortication should be low-risk surgical candidates who are symptomatic from their restriction and have pulmonary parenchyma that is anticipated to expand on release. Generally, the indication is significant pulmonary compromise in a patient whose fibrothorax is stable or has been worsening for at least several months (Fig. 74.7).

The pathogenesis of pleural plaques remains unclear. They are thought to be predominantly caused by asbestos, perhaps secondary to release of local factors in response to the foreign body after macrophage phagocytosis. Pleural plaques are hard, raised, discrete areas involving the parietal pleura, particularly in the lateral, posterior portion of the hemithorax; 80% of pleural plaques that are due to asbestos are bilateral, with the majority of unilateral plaques thought to be secondary to other causes. Pleural plaques do not appear to be predecessors of mesothelioma.[51]

Diffuse pleural thickening, like pleural plaques, appears to be predominantly related to asbestos exposure. Other causes, such as drug reaction, hemothorax, and tuberculosis

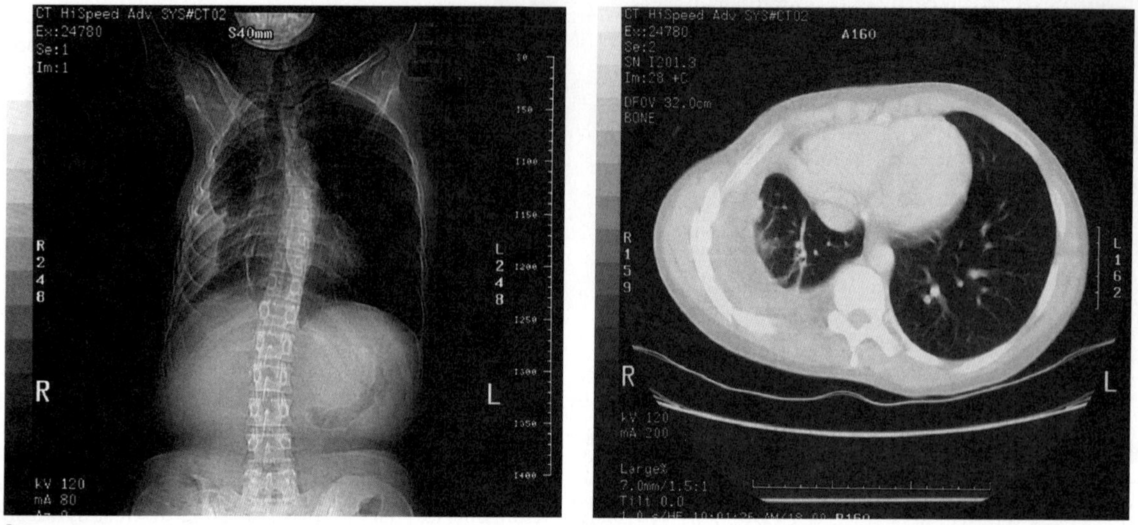

A B

FIGURE 74.7. Anteroposterior radiograph of the chest (**A**) demonstrates scoliosis and volume loss resulting from a fibrothorax caused by a tuberculous empyema. Computed tomographic cross section (**B**) demonstrates the thick parietal pleural peel entrapping healthy lung parenchyma. Notice contraction and overlapping of ribs in both radiographs. The patient underwent a decortication with dramatic improvement of her scoliosis and pulmonary function.

have been reported. Unlike pleural plaques, however, diffuse pleural thickening affects the visceral pleura. Its exact etiology also remains unclear, but it is thought that inflammatory factors are likely to play a major role, particularly in the setting of a resolving asbestos-induced pleural effusion. There appears to be an initial decrease in pulmonary function associated with diffuse pleural thickening that tends to remain stable over time. Again, there is no specific treatment recommended, just routine surveillance.

The benign fibrous tumor of the pleura is rare and primary. These tumors arise from the visceral pleura, are not associated with asbestos, and are frequently discovered incidentally on chest x-ray. These tumors may reach enormous size, thereby causing symptoms by virtue of compression of other structures (Fig. 74.8). Surgery is the treatment of choice and is almost always curative.[52]

Solid Malignancies of the Pleura

The most common malignancies of the pleura are metastatic, predominantly from lung, breast, or colon primaries (Fig. 74.9). There are rare primary sarcomas arising from the connective tissue elements of the pleura, but the most common primary malignancy of the pleura is mesothelioma. Essentially all malignancies of the pleura portend a grim prognosis as a result of either their conferment of metastatic status or the recalcitrance of the vast majority of de novo pleural malignancies to current treatments.

Mesothelioma is a rare tumor, with only 1500 to 3000 cases per year in the United States, but is thought to be on the rise in both the United States and internationally. This is thought to be primarily related to the 20- to 50-year lag between asbestos exposure, with which there is a clear causal link, and the relatively recent or lax restrictions on the use of asbestos.[53–55] Another epidemiological factor of great concern is the link between the simian vacuolating virus 40 (SV40) and mesothelioma. The virus has been demonstrated in human mesotheliomas and is capable of inducing mesothelioma by itself in animal models. It has been identified as a contaminant in millions of vaccines administered in the United States and may be a predisposing factor to mesothelioma formation in humans.[56]

Pleural mesothelioma is almost always unilateral and is diagnosed by pleural biopsy. From the time of diagnosis, the median survival is 4 to 12 months. The tumor usually presents with dyspnea secondary to a pleural effusion but may also present with chest pain or constitutional symptoms. The cancer tends to line the chest cavity as a thick, plaque-like mass, fusing the two pleural layers and invaginating between the lobes of the lung (Fig. 74.10). It progresses inexorably in a locoregional manner, invading lung, diaphragm, pericardium, and chest wall. Contrary to popular belief, the disease also has the capacity to metastasize, but the lethality of the locoregional disease tends to preclude the clinical manifestation of any metastatic disease unless the natural history of the cancer is altered by a successful locoregional treatment.

Although a number of staging systems exist, none has been universally adopted, although most incorporate the usual characteristics of the TNM system. This is likely a reflection of the small number of patients and even smaller number of centers investigating this disease. A staging system should accurately stratify prognosis, and this aspect of a staging system continues to evade researchers. As an example, cell type of mesothelioma (epithelial, sarcomatous, or mixed) is not currently part of any staging system, although some of the best results to date have been reported in patients restricted to the epithelial cell type, with 39% 5-year survival for patients treated with surgery, radiation, and chemotherapy.[57] As a result of this deficiency in macroscopic staging, researchers are looking toward innovative technologies, like genetic profiling, in an effort to better determine prognosis and which patients might benefit from aggressive treatment protocols.[58]

There remains no accepted treatment for mesothelioma. Because of the tumor's diffuse nature, complex anatomic presentation, and inherent recalcitrance to most treatment

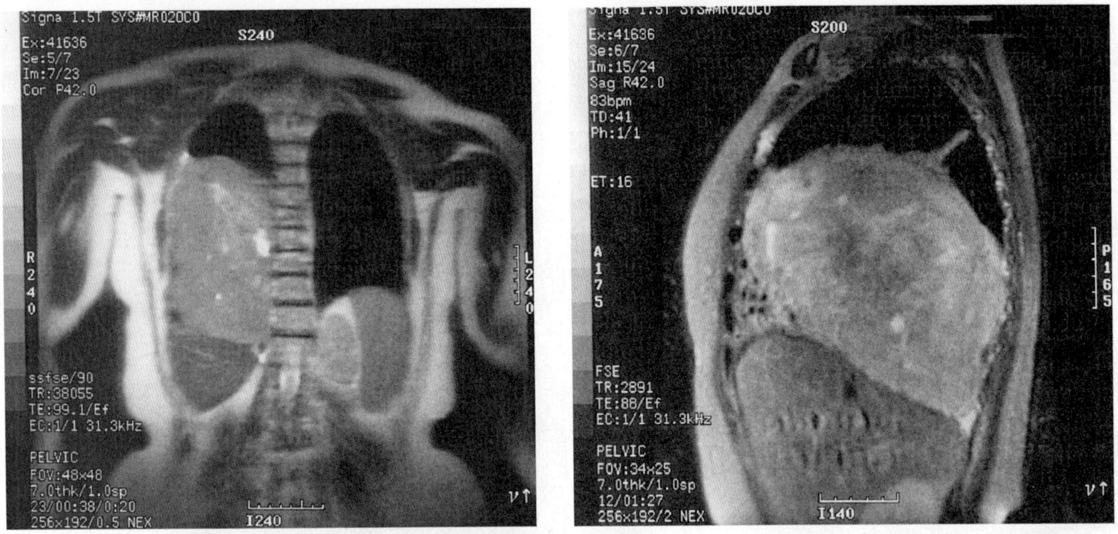

A

B

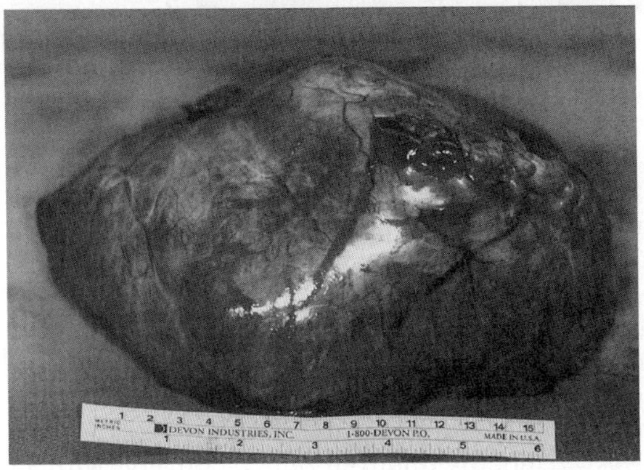

C

FIGURE 74.8. Coronal (**A**) and sagittal (**B**) MRI images demonstrate a large benign fibrous tumor of the pleura occupying the greater part of the right hemithorax. This patient presented with complaints of bilateral lower-extremity swelling that proved secondary to inferior vena cava compression. Photograph (**C**) shows the resected mass that arose from the visceral pleura of the right middle lobe and that was readily separated from the remainder of the lung with a small wedge resection of the affected area.

modalities, it is an extremely difficult cancer to treat. Because of encasement of the lung and potential pulmonary toxicity, there is no role for radiation as single-modality definitive treatment. Radiation can be used with curative intent, as an adjuvant treatment combined with surgery in which the lung has been removed, or in a palliative manner for localized areas of symptomatic invasion. Mesothelioma has proven to be one of the most chemoresistant tumors that oncologists face. Cytotoxic agents have rarely yielded response rates greater than 30%. There have, however, been some encouraging results with newer chemotherapeutic agents, especially antimetabolites, which have shown response rates as high as 45% when used in combination with platinum-based conventional chemotherapy.[59]

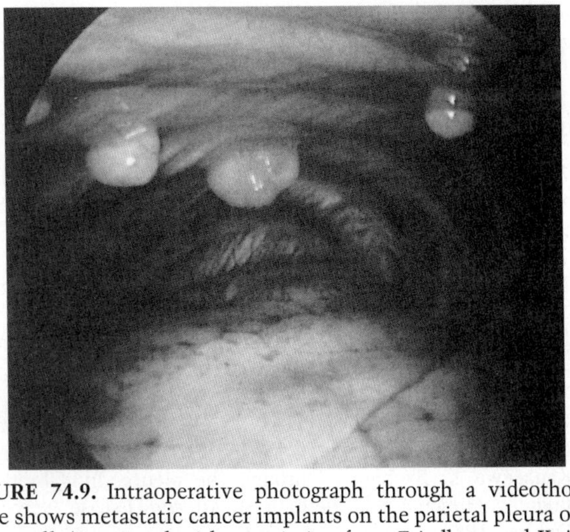

FIGURE 74.9. Intraoperative photograph through a videothoracoscope shows metastatic cancer implants on the parietal pleura on the chest wall. (Reprinted with permission from Friedberg and Kniger.[77] © 1998 Greenwich Medical Media Ltd. and by permission of Cambridge University Press.)

To date, the treatments that have met with the greatest measure of success for pleural mesothelioma are those that combine surgery, for debulking, and other modalities to address the residual disease that almost certainly exists, even after the most "complete" resection. The adjuvant treatments that have been performed, some intraoperatively, include radiation, photodynamic therapy, and hyperthermic chemotherapy intracorporeal lavage. Systemic chemotherapy or immunotherapy have been used in adjuvant and neoadjuvant capacities.[60] Almost all surgery-based multimodality strategies that are performed with curative intent mandate removal of the lung as part of the debulking and preparation for the adjuvant treatments. Some strategies, such as employment of photodynamic therapy for killing residual local disease after surgical debulking, may permit the option of performing lung-sparing procedures.[61]

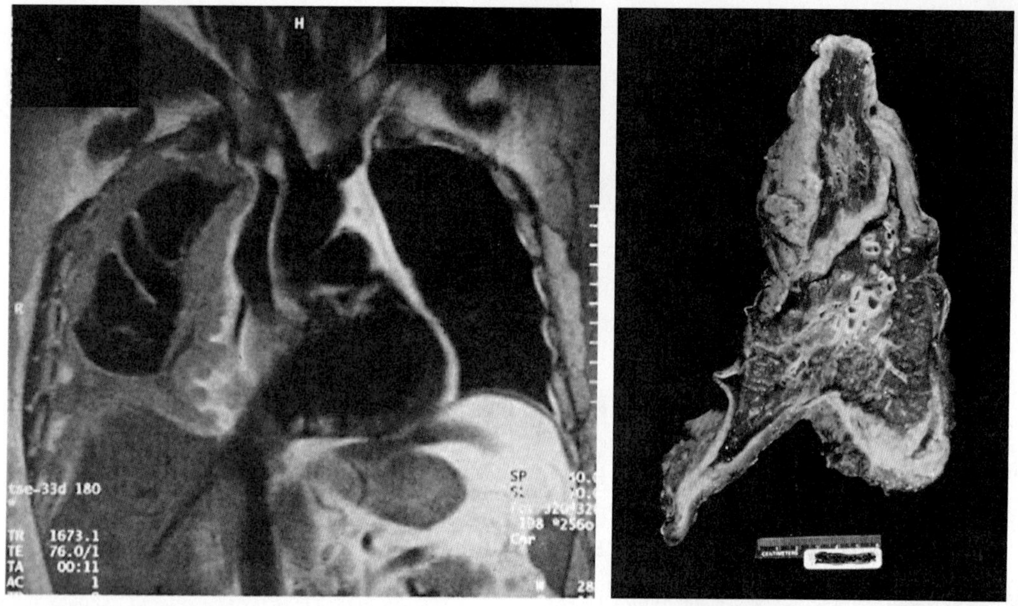

A B

FIGURE 74.10. Coronal MRI image (**A**) demonstrates typical appearance of a mesothelioma. Note the thick rind lining the right hemithorax and invaginating between the lobes of the lung. Photograph (**B**) is a section through an extrapleural pneumonectomy specimen of a resected mesothelioma showing the same pathology as seen on the scan.

Many cancers can metastasize to the pleural space, but one of the most frequently encountered is non-small cell lung cancer (NSCLC), as either bulky disease or a malignancy.[62,63] In the absence of distant metastases, the presence of pleural dissemination confers an International System for Staging Lung Cancer stage of IIIB based on the pleural disease being considered a T4 tumor.[64] The median survival for patients with this subset of stage IIIB NSCLC has been reported from 2 months to greater than 1 year but is generally within the 6- to 9-month range.[64–66] In fact, the survival rate for this subset of stage IIIB patients is so poor that it has been suggested that this disease should be upstaged to stage IV because of the similar survival rates.[67]

The standard of care for patients with NSCLC with pleural dissemination remains palliative chemotherapy, assuming the patient is able to tolerate this treatment, and some intervention to palliate effusion if it is symptomatic. Radiotherapy is rarely administered to these patients because of the pulmonary toxicity from hemithoracic radiotherapy; surgery has been shown to have little impact on survival for these patients and is accompanied by a local failure rate as high as 90%. There are anecdotal reports of long-term survivors after surgery, but it is safe to say that there should be no role for surgery outside of some type of multimodality protocol approach as with mesothelioma.[68–74]

Two recent studies have reported encouraging results for surgery-based multimodality approaches to this disease but require validation in larger studies. In one study, the investigators operated on 22 patients, performing extrapleural pneumonectomies on all 22, but in 11 they also performed intraoperative hyperthermic chemotherapy perfusion. All patients were staged as M0, and the groups were evenly split with respect to nodal status, with the majority being N0 (7/11 and 8/11) and the remainder being N1 (2/11 and 1/11) or N2 (2/11 and 2/11) in the study and control groups, respectively. All patients received adjuvant chemotherapy. The group of evenly matched patients who did not receive intraoperative hyperthermic chemotherapy perfusion had a median survival of 6 months. The group who received intraoperative hyperthermic chemotherapy perfusion had a median survival of 20 months.

Another recent study employed systemic chemotherapy, in a neoadjuvant capacity, and intraoperative photodynamic therapy to address microscopic locoregional disease after surgical debulking. The median survival for all 22 patients enrolled was 22 months from the time of surgery, with 12 of the 20 patients having pneumonectomy; the remainder had parenchymal sparing anatomic resections ranging from bilobectomy to segementectomy. In 18 of the 20 patients having intraoperative photodynamic therapy, N2 disease was present.[75] Both of these studies emphasize the importance of clinical trials that utilize a multimodality approach to cancers involving the pleura and the importance of a component to specifically address the residual microscopic disease that remains after even the most aggressive surgical resection.

References

1. Hippocrates. The Medical Works of Hippocrates. Springfield, IL: Thomas; 1950.
2. Major R. Classic Descriptions of Disease. 2nd ed. Springfield, IL: Thomas; 1939.
3. Eloesser L. Milestones in chest surgery. J Thorac Cardiovasc Surg 1970;60:157–165.
4. Nebut M, Hirsch A, Chretien J. Embryology and anatomy of the pleura. In: Chretien J, Hirsch A, eds. Diseases of the Pleura. New York: Masson; 1982.
5. Pearson F, et al., eds. Thoracic Surgery. New York: Churchill Livingstone; 1995.
6. Kanazawa K. Exchanges through the pleura. In: Chretien J, Bignon J, Hirsch A, eds. Pleura in Health and Disease. New York: Dekker; 1985.
7. Shinohara H. Distribution of lymphatic stomata on the pleural surface of the thoracic cavity and the surface topography of the

pleural mesothelium in the golden hamster. Anat Rec 1997;249:16–23.
8. West J. Respiratory Physiology: The Essentials. 2nd ed. Baltimore: Waverly Press; 1981.
9. Light R. Pleural Diseases. 3rd ed. Baltimore: Lippincott, Williams and Wilkins; 1995.
10. Northfield T. Oxygen therapy for spontaneous pneumothorax. Br Med J 1971;4:86–88.
11. Stewart P. The rate of formation and lymphatic removal of fluid in pleural effusions. J Clin Invest 1963;42:258–262.
12. Ukale V, Bone D, Hillerdal G, Cederlund K, Widstrom O, Larsen F. The impact of pleurodesis in malignant effusion on respiratory function. Respir Med 1999;93:898–902.
13. Walston A, et al. The electrocardiographic manifestations of spontaneous left pneumothorax. Ann Int Med 1974;80:375–379.
14. Kircher LJ, Swartzel R. Spontaneous pneumothorax and its treatment. JAMA 1954;155:24–29.
15. Chadha TS, Cohn MA. Noninvasive treatment of pneumothorax with oxygen inhalation. Respiration 1983;44:147–152.
16. O'Rourke JP, Yee ES. Civilian spontaneous pneumothorax. Treatment options and long-term results. Chest 1989;96:1302–1306.
17. Light RW. Management of spontaneous pneumothorax. Am Rev Resp Dis 1993;148:245–248.
18. Andrivet P, et al. Spontaneous pneumothorax. Comparison of thoracic drainage vs. immediate or delayed needle aspiration. Chest 1995;108:335–339.
19. Conces DJ Jr, et al. Treatment of pneumothoraces utilizing small caliber chest tubes. Chest 1988;94:55–57.
20. Rusch VW, et al. The performance of four pleural drainage systems in an animal model of bronchopleural fistula. Chest 1988;93:859–863.
21. Woodring JH. Focal reexpansion pulmonary edema after drainage of large pleural effusions: clinical evidence suggesting hypoxic injury to the lung as the cause of edema. S Med J 1997;90:1176–1182.
22. Tarver RD, Broderick LS, Conces DJ Jr. Reexpansion pulmonary edema. J Thorac Imag 1996;11:198–209.
23. Waldhausen J, Orringer M. Complications in Cardiothoracic Surgery. St. Louis: Mosby Year Book; 1991.
24. Bense L, Eklund G, Wiman LG. Smoking and the increased risk of contracting spontaneous pneumothorax. Chest 1987;92:1009–1012.
25. Baumann MH, Strange C. Treatment of spontaneous pneumothorax: a more aggressive approach? Chest 1997;112:789–804.
26. Baumann MH, et al. Management of spontaneous pneumothorax. An American College of Chest Physicians Delphi consensus statement. Chest 2001;119:590–602.
27. Tanaka F, et al. Secondary spontaneous pneumothorax. Ann Thorac Surg 1993;55:372–376.
28. Despars JA, Sassoon CS, Light RW. Significance of iatrogenic pneumothoraces. Chest 1994;105:1147–1150.
29. Fishman A, ed. Pulmonary Diseases and Disorders. 3rd ed. New York: McGraw-Hill; 1998.
30. Light RW, et al. Pleural effusions: the diagnostic separation of transudates and exudates. Ann Int Med 1972;77:507–513.
31. Woodring JH. Focal reexpansion pulmonary edema after drainage of large pleural effusions: clinical evidence suggesting hypoxic injury to the lung as the cause of edema. S Med J 1997;90:1176–1182.
32. Kinasewitz GT. Transudative effusions. Eur Resp J 1997;10:714–718.
33. Strauss RM, Boyer TD. Hepatic hydrothorax. Semin Liver Dis 1997;17:227–232.
34. Liu LU, et al. Outcome analysis of cirrhotic patients undergoing chest tube placement. Chest 2004;126:142–148.
35. Assouad et al. Recurrent pleural effusion complication liver cirrhosis. Ann Thorac Surg 2003;75:986–989.
36. Assi Z, et al. Cytologically proved malignant pleural effusions: distribution of transudates and exudates. Chest 1998;113:1302–1304.
37. Marchi E, Teixeira LR, Vargas FS. Management of malignancy-associated pleural effusion: current and future treatment strategies. Am J Respir Med 2003;2:261–273.
38. Villanueva AG, et al. Efficacy of short term versus long term tube thoracostomy drainage before tetracycline pleurodesis in the treatment of malignant pleural effusions [see comments]. Thorax 1994;49:23–25.
39. Mager HJ, et al. Distribution of talc suspension during treatment of malignant pleural effusion with talc pleurodesis. Lung Cancer 2002;36:77–81.
40. Shaw P, Agarwal R. Pleurodesis for malignant pleural effusions (Cochrane Review). In: The Cochrane Library, Issue 4. Chichester, UK: Wiley; 2004.
41. Putnam JB Jr, Walsh GL, Swisher SG, et al. Outpatient management of malignant pleural effusion by a chronic indwelling catheter. Ann Thorac Surg 2000;69:369–375.
42. Sanchez-Armengol A, Rodriguez-Panadero F. Survival and talc pleurodesis in metastatic pleural carcinoma, revisited. Report of 125 cases. Chest 1993;104:1482–1485.
43. Colice et al. Medical and surgical treatment of parapneumonic effusions: an evidence-based guideline for the American College of Chest Physicians Parapneumonic Effusions Panel. Chest 2000;118:1158–1171.
44. Diacon AH, Theron J, Schuurmans MM, Van de Wal BW, Bolliger CT. Intrapleural streptokinase for empyema and complicated parapneumonic effusions. Am J Respir Crit Care Med 2004;170:49–53.
45. Lee YCG. Ongoing search for effective intrapleural therapy for empyema: is streptokinase the answer? Am J Respir Crit Care Med 2004;170:1–2.
46. Striffeler H, et al. Video-assisted thoracoscopic surgery for fibrinopurulent pleural empyema in 67 patients. Ann Thorac Surg 1998;65:319–323.
47. Merrigan BA, Winter DC, O'Sullivan GC. Chylothorax. Br J Surg 1997;84:15–20.
48. Staats BA, et al. The lipoprotein profile of chylous and nonchylous pleural effusions. Mayo Clin Proc 1980;55:700–704.
49. Milsom JW, et al. Chylothorax: an assessment of current surgical management. J Thorac Cardiovasc Surg 1985;89:221–227.
50. Meyer DM, et al. Early evacuation of traumatic retained hemothoraces using thoracoscopy: a prospective, randomized trial. Ann Thorac Surg 1997;64:1396–1400; discussion 1400–1401.
51. Light RW. Pleural Diseases. Baltimore: Lippincott Williams and Wilkins; 2001.
52. Mitchell JD. Solitary fibrous tumor of the pleura. Semin Thorac Cardiovasc Surg 2003;15:305–309.
53. Hanauske AR. The role of Alimta in the treatment of malignant pleural mesothelioma: an overview of preclinical and clinical trials. Lung Cancer 2004;45(suppl 1):S121–S124.
54. O'Brien ME. Malignant mesothelioma—the UK experience. Lung Cancer 2004;45(suppl 1):S133–S135.
55. Pass HI, Vogelzang N, Hahn S, Carbone M. Malignant pleural mesothelioma. Curr Probl Cancer 2004;28:93–174.
56. Carbone M, Pass HI, Miele L, Brochette M. New developments about the association of SV40 with human mesothelioma. Oncogene 2003;22:5173–5180.
57. Sugarbaker DJ, Norberto JJ. Multimodality management of malignant pleural mesothelioma. Chest 1998;113(1 suppl):61S–65S.
58. Pass HI, Liu Z, Wali A, et al. Gene expression profiles predict survival and progression of pleural mesothelioma. Clin Cancer Res 2004;10:849–859.

59. Tomek S, Manegold C. Chemotherapy for malignant pleural mesothelioma: past results and recent developments. Lung Cancer 2004;45(suppl 1):S103–S119.
60. Manegold C. Chemotherapy for malignant pleural mesothelioma: past results and recent developments. Lung Cancer 2004;45(suppl 1):S103–S119.
61. Friedberg JS, Mick R, Stevenson JP, et al. Phase II trial of pleural photodynamic therapy and surgery for patients with non-small-cell lung cancer with pleural spread. J Clin Oncol 2004;22:2192–2201.
62. Werner-Wasik M, Scott C, Cox JD, et al. Recursive partitioning analysis of 1999 Radiation Therapy Oncology Group (RTOG) patients with locally-advanced non-small-cell lung cancer (LA-NSCLC): identification of five groups with different survival. Int J Radiat Oncol Biol Phys 2000;48:1475–1482.
63. Sugiura S, Ando Y, Minami H, et al. Prognostic value of pleural effusion in patients with non-small cell lung cancer. Clin Cancer Res 1997;3:47–50.
64. Mountain CF. Revisions in the International System for Staging Lung Cancer. Chest 1997;111:1710–1711.
65. Martini N, Bains MS, Beattie EJ Jr. Indications for pleurectomy in malignant effusion. Cancer 1975;35:734–738.
66. Reyes L, Parvez Z, Regal AM, et al. Neoadjuvant chemotherapy and operations in the treatment of lung cancer with pleural effusion. J Thorac Cardiovasc Surg 1991;101:946–947.
67. Mott FE, Sharma N, Ashley P. Malignant pleural effusion in non-small cell lung cancer—time for a stage revision? Chest 2001;119:317–318.
68. Mattson K, Holsti LR, Tammilehto L, et al. Multimodality treatment programs for malignant pleural mesothelioma using high-dose hemithorax irradiation. Int J Radiat Oncol Biol Phys 1992;24:643–650.
69. Yokoi K, Matsuguma H, Anraku M. Extrapleural pneumonectomy for lung cancer with carcinomatous pleuritis. J Thorac Cardiovasc Surg 2002;123:184–185.
70. Ichinose Y, Tsuchiya R, Koike T, et al. Prognosis of resected non-small cell lung cancer patients with carcinomatous pleuritis of minimal disease. Lung Cancer 2001;32:55–60.
71. Naruke T, Tsuchiya R, Kondo H, et al. Implications of staging in lung cancer. Chest 1997;112:242S–248S.
72. Ichinose Y, Yano T, Asoh H, et al. Intraoperative intrapleural hypotonic cisplatin treatment for carcinomatous pleuritis. J Surg Oncol 1997;66:196–200.
73. Yokoi K, Miyazawa N. Pleuropneumonectomy and postoperative adjuvant chemotherapy for carcinomatous pleuritis in primary lung cancer: a case report of long-term survival. Eur J Cardiothorac Surg 1996;10:141–143.
74. Shimizu J, Oda M, Morita K, et al. Comparison of pleuropneumonectomy and limited surgery for lung cancer with pleural dissemination. J Surg Oncol 1996;61:1–6.
75. Friedberg JS, Mick R, Stevenson JP, et al. Phase II trial of pleural photodynamic therapy and surgery for patients with non-small-cell lung cancer with pleural spread. J Clin Oncol 2004;22:2192–2201.
76. Geraghty JG, Sackier JM, Young HL, ed. *Gray's Anatomy.* 36th ed. Philadelphia: Saunders; 1980.
77. Friedberg, Kniger. In Minimal Access Surgery in Oncology. Greenwich Medical Media; London; England, 1998.
78. Walker-Renard PB, Vaughan LM, Sahn SA. Chemical pleurodesis for malignant pleural effusion. Ann Intern Med 1994; 120:56.

75

Mediastinum

Mark I. Block

The term *mediastinum* refers to the region of the body located between the two pleural spaces. It is derived from the Latin words *medius* (middle) and *stare* (to stand) and means literally "standing in the middle." Although this definition is anatomically descriptive, it belies the fact that the mediastinum is a complex and tightly knit package of structures immediately vital to the life of the individual—the central airways, the heart, and the great vessels. Also contained within the mediastinum are myriad other tissues, glands, and organs, including the esophagus, thymus, thoracic duct, vagus and phrenic nerves, and lymphatics. The mediastinum extends from the diaphragm to the thoracic inlet and is divided by anatomists into four regions that are defined by their relationship to the pericardium: superior, anterior, middle, and posterior. In this scheme, the middle compartment is equivalent to the pericardial sac and its contents. In contrast, as is discussed in more detail later in this chapter, thoracic surgeons generally divide the mediastinum into just three compartments: anterior, middle, and posterior. In this scheme, the anatomists' superior compartment is divided between the anterior and middle compartments, and the esophagus is included in the middle rather than posterior compartment. This nomenclature is used clinically because it is more helpful for discussions of pathological processes.

Because the mediastinum contains a compact arrangement of vital structures and other tissues, abnormalities such as infection, trauma, and neoplasm can have a profound impact and can present with dramatic symptoms. Sometimes, however, symptoms may be subtle or nonexistent or may manifest as systemic disorders such as myasthenia gravis (MG). Because the mediastinum is relatively inaccessible to physical examination, imaging studies such as computed tomography (CT) play a particularly important role in the evaluation of suspected pathology. Regardless of whether surgical intervention is indicated, successful management of mediastinal pathology requires that the physician is fluent in the embryology, anatomy, and physiology of this complex region. In this chapter, the pathophysiology and management of mediastinal infection (descending necrotizing mediastinitis (DNM), postoperative mediastinitis, and fibrosing mediastinitis); superior vena cava (SVC) syndrome; and the range of primary mediastinal lesions are discussed. Primary cardiac, vascular, and esophageal disorders are not reviewed.

Descending Necrotizing Mediastinitis

Descending necrotizing mediastinitis (DNM) is an uncommon but virulent form of mediastinal infection that arises from infectious sources in the head and neck and descends rapidly through cervical fascial planes to involve the mediastinum. It is distinguished from other forms of mediastinal infection not only by its unique pathophysiology but also by its potential for rapid progression to overwhelming sepsis and death, often within 24 to 48h from the onset of symptoms. Pearse is credited with the first detailed treatment of this syndrome in the literature, describing the clinical presentation and outcome of 110 patients managed before the availability of antibiotics.[1] Surgical therapy was associated with a survival rate of 65%, whereas those treated medically fared far worse, with a survival rate of only 15%. Overall mortality was 60%.

The advent of antibiotics and more aggressive surgical management has improved survival, but DNM remains a potentially lethal condition. Estrera and colleagues[2] reported the first large series following the widespread availability of antibiotics and documented a 42% mortality among 30 cases reviewed. Although more recent large reviews documented mortality rates persistently in excess of 30%,[3,4] a strategy of early and aggressive surgical debridement has been shown to reduce this figure to less than 20%.[4,5]

Epidemiology

More than half of all cases of DNM are odontogenic, arising most commonly from infections of the mandibular molars.[2,3] Less common sources of infection include retropharyngeal abscesses, iatrogenic pharyngeal injuries, cervical lymphadenitis, parotitis, and thyroiditis. The combined effects of gravity and the pressure gradient generated by breathing are thought to facilitate descension of infection into the mediastinum. The mean age of patients is 32 to 36 years, and most are men, with a ratio of men to women as high as 6:1.[3,4,6] Perforation of the cervical esophagus or leakage from a cervical anastomosis following esophagectomy are also potential sources of descending mediastinal infection. However, these circumstances generally require a different management algorithm and therefore should be distinguished from DNM as separate clinical entities.

Anatomy

Infections that arise in the neck can descend into the mediastinum through planes defined by the three layers of deep cervical fascia: superficial, visceral, and prevertebral.[7] These layers divide the neck into three potential spaces. (1) The pretracheal space is bordered by the strap muscles anteriorly and the trachea posteriorly. (2) The retrovisceral space is defined by the prevertebral fascia posteriorly and the esophagus anteriorly and extends from the skull base down to the diaphragm. (3) The perivascular space is surrounded by the carotid sheath and contains the carotid artery, jugular vein, and vagus nerve. The retrovisceral space is the most common avenue for descension of infection into the mediastinum. Infection gains access to this space because the alveolar processes of the second and third mandibular molars extend deep to the posterior origin of the mylohyoid muscle and into the submandibular space. Furthermore, fusion of the anterior visceral fascia with the parietal pericardium and mediastinal pleura at the level of the tracheal carina creates a pathway for development of infected pericardial and pleural effusions. Approximately 20% of cases involve the perivascular space, with the remaining 10% involving the pretracheal space. Because the contents of the carotid sheath are vulnerable to the necrotizing process, infection in the perivascular space can lead to massive hemorrhage and cranial nerve deficits.[2,8]

Microbiology

A variety of organisms have been isolated from patients with DNM, and most patients will harbor a mixed aerobic/anaerobic infection. The most common organisms identified are *Staphylococcus*, *β-hemolytic streptococcus*, *Pseudomonas*, and *Bacteroides*. *Peptostreptococcus* has also been found relatively frequently. Although fungal organisms are uncommon, species of *Aspergillus* and *Candida* are occasionally isolated and should be considered when planning empiric antibiotic therapy.

Diagnosis

Because DNM can progress rapidly, successful management of patients requires early initiation of therapy based on a presumptive diagnosis. Definitive diagnosis is of primarily academic interest and is based on four criteria as described by Estrera and colleagues[2]: (1) clinical manifestations of severe infection; (2) characteristic radiographic features; (3) documentation of necrotizing mediastinal infection at operation or autopsy; and (4) establishment of a relationship between oropharyngeal infection and the development of the necrotizing mediastinal process. It is emphasized, however, that because of the rapid progression and high mortality associated with DNM, appropriate treatment should not await definitive diagnosis. Clinical findings suspicious for DNM include fever, localized cervical or oropharyngeal pain, and respiratory distress. Occasionally, erythema and swelling in the submandibular or cervical region can be identified, while crepitus can be the result of either hollow viscus injury (trachea or esophagus) or advancing anaerobic infection. A recent history of dental work or dental infection combined with signs of infection outside the mouth should prompt immediate initiation of therapy. Respiratory distress is a particularly ominous finding and signals impending airway obstruction from progressive laryngeal edema. Features of DNM appreciable on plain x-rays include widening of the retrovisceral space with or without air–fluid levels, anterior displacement of the tracheal air column, loss of normal cervical spine lordosis, and mediastinal emphysema. However, because these findings may not be apparent until late in the course of the illness, patients in whom the diagnosis is suspected should undergo immediate evaluation by contrast-enhanced CT of the neck and chest. Findings such as soft tissue edema, fluid collections, pleural effusions, and cervical and mediastinal emphysema will establish the diagnosis early and define the extent of infection.[2,4]

Management

Treatment should be initiated as soon as the diagnosis of DNM is suspected and should address three considerations: airway maintenance, antibiotic therapy, and surgical debridement. Cervical infections can lead rapidly to airway obstruction from edema of the larynx and epiglottis. Under these circumstances, if access to the airway is lost, such as by removal of an endotracheal tube, it may be impossible to reestablish. For this reason, some authors advocate routine use of tracheostomy for all patients,[2,3] while others have reported successful results with a more considerate approach, performing tracheostomy only for those patients who have evidence of laryngeal or epiglottic edema.[5,8] Antibiotics should be administered as soon as the diagnosis of DNM is suspected and should not await the results of cultures. High-dose penicillin G (12–20 mU/day) combined with either metronidazole or clindamycin represent front-line therapy, although alternative strategies that include a β-lactam/β-lactamase inhibitor have been recommended.[9,10] Immunosuppressed patients may be appropriate candidates for empiric therapy with cefoxitin, ceftizoxime, or imipenem and antifungal agents. Once antibiotics have been initiated, it is essential to monitor clinical response and results of antibiotic sensitivity testing, making appropriate changes as indicated. In a series of eight patients, Corsten et al.[4] reported that the only death was associated with infection by resistant forms of *Streptococcus pneumoniae* and *Staphylococcus aureus*.

Early and aggressive surgical therapy is critical to successful management of DNM. Exposure and drainage of all three cervical spaces is best accomplished through an incision along the anterior border of the sternocleidomastoid muscle. Routine addition of a thoracotomy to facilitate extensive mediastinal drainage is controversial. Some authors report acceptable results with thoracotomy only when there is evidence by CT of infection extending below the tracheal carina anteriorly or fourth thoracic vertebral body posteriorly.[2,3,8] However, because of the continued high mortality associated with DNM, others recommend routine mediastinal debridement via thoracotomy.[3,4,6] Proponents of this approach report mortality rates consistently less than 20%. In a 1990 review of 43 cases reported in the literature, Wheatley et al.[3] concluded that transcervical drainage alone led to treatment delays and inadequate therapy in 26 of the 33 patients for whom it had been used. In a more recent review of 69 cases from the literature, Corsten et al.[4] reported that mortality was 47% among 30 patients treated with transcervical drainage alone but only 19% among patients for whom thoracotomy for mediastinal debridement was also performed. Freeman and colleagues[5] reported no deaths in a series of 10 patients. They included an oral-maxillofacial surgeon in the operating team and liberally used repeat CT scans and repeat operations. All patients in their series had at least two cervical drainage procedures and two thoracotomies.

Because results are necessarily retrospective, an unbiased analysis of the available data to determine the utility of routine thoracotomy is not possible. However, the relatively low mortality reported by those who advocate routine use of aggressive mediastinal drainage, and the known potential of DNM to progress rapidly to death within 48h of onset, argue strongly for this approach. The decision not to directly debride and drain the mediastinum must be justified by clear and early signs of the patient's clinical improvement. It is likely that the worse the patient's condition, the greater is the extent of debridement required.

Alternatives to a standard thoracotomy for debridement and drainage of the mediastinum have been reported. Median sternotomy offers the advantage of simultaneous bilateral exposure but does not provide good exposure to the posterior mediastinum and can be complicated by wound infection and sternal dehiscence. Bilateral anterior thoracotomies also can be used for wide exposure of the entire chest and mediastinum. Video-assisted techniques have also been applied to facilitate mediastinal drainage. These reports are confined to a few patients with mediastinal infection arising from traumatic esophageal perforation and therefore may not accurately account for the virulent nature of true DNM.[11,12] Regardless of the surgical approach, however, it is important to avoid the use of rigid or stiff drainage devices in close apposition to vascular structures as they can lead to vessel erosion and exsanguinating hemorrhage.[13] Adjuvant use of hyperbaric oxygen therapy has been reported[13] but should not be considered appropriate therapy and should not delay or be used as a substitute for aggressive surgical intervention.

Postoperative Mediastinitis

Milton, an English surgeon working in Cairo, in 1887 introduced the median sternotomy.[14] This approach provided access to mediastinal structures without requiring entry into the pleural space, a potentially lethal complication in the spontaneously breathing anesthetized patient. However, it was not until 1953 when Gibbon introduced cardiopulmonary bypass[15] that the median sternotomy became widely used. The subsequent rapid increase in the number of cardiovascular surgical procedures has made the median sternotomy one of the most commonly used incisions, and as a consequence infection following such procedures, or postoperative mediastinitis, has become an important clinical problem.

Epidemiology

Mediastinitis complicating cardiac surgical procedures has profound implications for the patient as well as the health care system. It is associated with an in-hospital mortality of up to 35%,[16–19] a three- to fourfold increase in long-term mortality,[17,20] and an increase in hospital costs of as much as 4.5 times.[16,21] Worldwide, the incidence of postoperative mediastinitis is between 0.5% and 1.5%. Following heart transplantation, the incidence is 2.5%–2.7%.[22,23] *Staphylococcus* species are the most common causative organisms. *Staphylococcus aureus* and *Staphylococcus epidermidis* are responsible for more than 50% of cases in most reported series. Other important pathogens include *Pseudomonas, Enterobacter, Escherichia coli*, and *Serratia*.

Diagnosis

Establishing the diagnosis of postoperative mediastinitis can be challenging. Suspicious findings include increased incisional pain, sternal instability manifest as a "click" with coughing or palpation, dyspnea, fever, and incisional erythema and drainage. These signs and symptoms usually appear between 5 and 10 days postoperatively but may not become apparent for several months. Diagnosis is made difficult because many patients develop fever and leukocytosis without the finding of sternal instability, and minor sternal instability is not always a consequence of mediastinal infection. Diagnostic evaluation usually includes CT. Although the absence of suspicious findings on CT does not rule out mediastinitis, the presence of soft tissue swelling and fluid and air collections can be important indicators of ongoing infection.[24,25] In the early postoperative period, however, positive findings may not be helpful. Jolles et al.[26] reported a specificity of only 33% when CT was performed within 2 weeks of surgery. As a result, some authors have advocated radiolabeled leukocyte scintigraphy for early diagnosis.[27,28] Prospective comparison of leukocyte scintigraphy with CT found their accuracy to be 95% and 75%, respectively,[27] suggesting that nuclear medicine may be a more helpful tool than CT for early diagnosis.

Risk Factors

Factors contributing to the development of postoperative mediastinitis can be grouped broadly into categories relating to the patient's preexisting conditions, the conduct of the operation, and the postoperative environment of the patient's care. Prospective evaluation of specific postoperative management strategies has shown clearly that excess rates of infection can be eliminated by development of dedicated postoperative care units and strict adherence to principles of infection control.[29,30] A wealth of data from large retrospective studies has identified preexisting conditions such as obesity, chronic obstructive lung disease, prior cardiac surgery, diabetes, and heart failure as significant independent predictors of increased risk.[18–20,31–34] Similarly, these studies identified urgency of the procedure, duration of cardiopulmonary bypass, and overall duration of the procedure as important intraop-

TABLE 75.1.
Comparison of Treatment Options for Postoperative Mediastinitis (Retrospective Studies, Level III Evidence).

Study	*Year*	*Treatment*	*n*	*In-hospital deaths*	*Hospital stay, days (range)*	*Comment*
Song et al.[38]	2003	Twice-daily dressing changes	18	1 (5.6%)	Not given	1.5 ± 0.1 flaps required for closure 0.9 ± 0.07 flaps required for closure, $P < .05$
		Wound VAC	17	3 (17.6%)		
Berg et al.[39]	2000	CI	29	2 (6.9%)	42 ± 22[a,b]	Treatment failure (reexploration of sternal wound within 60 days) = 15 (52%) for CI group, 5 (16%) for VD group; $P = .006$
		VD	31	2 (6.5%)	29 ± 26[a,b]	
El Gamel et al.[40]	1998	Sternal salvage and immediate flap	30	0	22 (13–32)	
		Closed or open drainage (9) or delayed flap (8)	17	8 (47%)	82 (30–110)	
Lopez-Monjardin et al.[41]	1998	Sternectomy followed by flap with				
		Pectoralis major	21	6 (29%)	Not given	Includes only patients with documented osteomyelitis
		Omentum	12	2 (17%)		
Jones et al.[42]	1997	Immediate or delayed muscle or omental flap	171	17 (9.9%)	18.6[a]	For years 1988–1992
					12.4[a]	For years 1992–1996
El Oakley et al.[19]	1997	Debridement and CI	21	3 (14%)	36 (14–69)	
Szerafin et al.[43]	1991	CI ± granulated sugar	15	3 (20%)	92 (76–123)	
Kutsal et al.[44]	1991	CI	50	18 (36%)	Not given	
		Omental transposition	8	1 (13%)	Not given	

CI, continuous irrigation; VD, vacuum drainage.
[a]Hospital stay following procedure for mediastinitis.
[b]Mean ± standard deviation.

erative factors. Bilateral internal mammary artery (BIMA) use is generally accepted as an important risk factor, but the data are inconsistent. Experimentally, dissection of both IMAs has been shown to devascularize the sternum and increase the risk of infection.[35] Clinically, Grover and colleagues[33] found that BIMA grafting was associated with an increased risk of postoperative mediastinitis. However, data from the Cleveland Clinic suggest that a significant increase in risk is seen only in diabetic patients.[16]

There have been two large prospective studies of risk factors and postoperative mediastinitis. Milano and colleagues[17] followed almost 6500 patients and identified only four factors as independent predictors of increased risk: obesity, New York Heart Association heart failure class, previous heart surgery, and duration of cardiopulmonary bypass. In a similar but smaller study, the Parisian Mediastinitis Study Group evaluated 1830 patients from 10 centers over a period of 6 months[36] and found, as did Milano and colleagues, that obesity and previous heart surgery were independent risk factors. In addition, however, they identified BIMA use and requirement for postoperative pressor support as significant risk factors.

Management

Management of patients with postoperative mediastinitis has evolved. Earlier strategies of simple debridement and packing gave way to algorithms that included radical sternal resection with immediate muscle flap reconstruction. Since introduction in 1997 of the wound vacuum-assisted closure (VAC) technique by Morykwas and colleagues,[37] these algorithms have undergone further modification. Following debridement of infected sternum and costal cartilages, the wound can be managed either with immediate muscle flap reconstruction or with open drainage or wound VAC with or without delayed muscle flap closure (Table 75.1). Of these choices, debridement and wound VAC is increasingly the preferred option. Closed drainage with irrigation is of unproven benefit and can lead to systemic absorption and toxicity. Furthermore, Berg and colleagues,[38] in a comparison of 29 patients treated with continuous irrigation and 31 patients treated with wound VAC, found that treatment failure was more than three times as likely in the closed-irrigation group. In general, use of the wound VAC decreases the need for subsequent muscle flap closure. When surgical closure is needed, the wound VAC shortens the time between debridement and muscle flap closure and decreases the likelihood that more complex, large muscle flaps will be needed.[39–45]

Long-Term Sequelae

Aggressive management of postoperative mediastinitis has led to a substantial decrease in mortality. In perhaps the largest published experience on this subject, the group from Emory University described their 20-year experience with debridement and tissue flap closure, reporting an overall mortality of only 8.1%.[42] However, the impact of this management strategy on long-term functional outcome is an important consideration. Closed-irrigation techniques may be associated with higher mortality but are more likely to preserve chest wall stability and function. Although follow-up studies have suggested minimal to no loss of muscle strength and function with tissue flap reconstruction,[46,47] surveyed patients reported a high incidence of persistent pain or discomfort, and half did not return to work. Similar long-term functional results are not yet available for patients treated with wound VAC, but it is likely that this technique marries the functional benefit of closed drainage with the lower mortality risk of immediate flap reconstruction.

Fibrosing Mediastinitis

Fibrosing mediastinitis, also known as sclerosing mediastinitis, is a rare disorder that is characterized by acute and chronic inflammation and progressive fibrosis within the mediastinum. The fibrosis can proceed relentlessly to compromise patency of the SVC, major and minor airways, pulmonary arteries and veins, and the esophagus. It was first described by Oulmont[48] in 1855, and in 1903 Osler reported on several patients who presented with SVC obstruction and mediastinal fibrosis.[49] The association between fibrosing mediastinitis and fungal infection was first suggested by Knox in 1925,[50] and although the precise etiology remains unclear, it is now thought that the most common cause is an abnormal inflammatory response to fungal antigens.

Epidemiology and Clinical Features

Fibrosing mediastinitis usually presents in the second to fourth decade of life, and men are affected slightly more often than are women.[51–53] Although some patients are asymptomatic at the time of diagnosis, more than 60% present with symptoms caused by compression of mediastinal structures.[54] Cough, dyspnea, wheezing, and the sequelae of SVC obstruction are the most common symptoms. Hemoptysis, dysphagia, and chest pain are less-frequent presentations. Some patients develop broncholiths—calcified lymph nodes that erode into the airway and may be expectorated or cause significant hemoptysis.

The fibrosis develops either as a localized hilar or mediastinal mass or as diffuse involvement of the mediastinum. A localized mass is caused by granuloma formation, may or may not be calcified, and causes symptoms by impingement of adjacent structures. Diffuse disease can spread through the entire mediastinum. The SVC, trachea, mainstem bronchi, and right pulmonary artery are most susceptible to compression from diffuse fibrosis. In severe cases, however, the fibrosis may extend to involve the pulmonary hila, leading to segmental perfusion defects and pulmonary venous obstruction. At operation, the mediastinum is often described as appearing as if someone had "poured concrete" into it,[53] with a dense fibrous mass encasing structures and obliterating tissue planes. Biopsies reveal dense hyalinized sclerosis with fibroblasts, infiltration of lymphocytes and plasma cells, collagen bands, and occasional caseating granulomas with calcifications.

Pathophysiology

The progressive fibrosis that characterizes this disorder is a consequence of acute and chronic inflammation and can be triggered by a variety of stimuli. Most commonly, fungal infection is thought to be the inciting event, with more than half the cases reported in the United States linked to *Histoplasma capsulatum*.[52–54] In Britain, where histoplasmosis is far less common, tuberculosis is thought to be the dominant cause.[51] *Aspergillosis*, *Mucormycosis*, *Cryptococcus*, and *Blastomycosis* have also been implicated.[51,55,56] In addition to infectious causes, a variety of noninfectious conditions have been associated with fibrosing mediastinitis; these include autoimmune disease, sarcoidosis, systemic fibrotic disorders such as retroperitoneal fibrosis, sclerosing cholangitis, Riedel's thyroiditis, pseudotumor of the orbit,[51,52] and methysergide therapy (an agent used for the treatment of vascular headaches).[52,57]

Several possibilities have been suggested to explain the relationship between fungal infection and mediastinal fibrosis. Goodwin et al.[58] first proposed that the abnormal fibroproliferative process was the result of a delayed-type hypersensitivity reaction against fungal or mycobacterial antigens. A second hypothesis is that infected granuloma rupture, spreading antigen throughout the mediastinum and initiating a diffuse reaction.[54,55] This theory is supported by observational reports that some patients with localized mediastinal granuloma progress to develop diffuse fibrosis.[54,59] Alternatively, fibrosing mediastinitis may represent an idiosyncratic form of inflammation that can be initiated by exposure to any of a variety of antigens and that is characterized by diffuse collagen deposition and organization.[55]

Diagnosis

Fibrosing mediastinitis is often a diagnosis of exclusion. History and physical examination may reveal exposure to any of the known causative agents as well as signs and symptoms of mediastinal compression. Plain chest x-ray may demonstrate an abnormal mediastinal contour or changes in pulmonary vasculature that indicate pulmonary arterial or venous compromise. Computed tomography is the study of choice for initial evaluation.[60] It readily identifies the extent of fibrosis, the presence of granulomas and calcification, and compression of mediastinal structures. Vascular anatomy is best assessed by combining venography with contrast-enhanced CT. Although magnetic resonance imaging (MRI) is not used routinely to image the mediastinum in this disorder, its superior ability to evaluate vascular structures enables MRI to substitute for the combination of CT and venography in patients for whom contrast administration is contraindicated. Bronchoscopy should be performed to evaluate for the presence of broncholiths and distortion of bronchial anatomy. In general, broncholiths should be left alone as they are often densely adherent to the pulmonary artery, and any attempt to remove them may result in massive hemoptysis.

The decision to pursue additional specific studies such as barium swallow, esophagoscopy, and cardiac catheterization should be guided by clinical signs and symptoms. Although not definitive, serological testing can be suggestive of the diagnosis and may be helpful for planning therapy. Complement fixation titers for fungal antigens are especially valuable because serial measurements of rising titers before the initiation of treatment have been correlated with therapeutic success with antifungal agents. A greater than 1:32 is considered positive.[53] Ultimately, however, because fibrosing mediastinitis is often a diagnosis of exclusion, biopsy may be necessary to rule out other disorders, such as malignancy. Under these circumstances, mediastinoscopy or other attempts at biopsy must be approached with extreme caution. The obliterative nature of the fibrosis eliminates normal tissue planes and pliability and therefore makes any surgical intervention difficult and hazardous.

Therapy

Medical therapy for this disease has met with limited success. Steroids are of no proven benefit,[52,55] but for those patients in whom fungal infection has been implicated, therapy with antifungal agents has been shown effective.[53,61] Ketoconazole is preferred over amphoteracin B because it is better tolerated and easier to take for a prolonged period. Urschel and colleagues[53] reported clinical improvements in six patients treated with ketoconazole at 400mg per day for 1 year and emphasized a strong correlation between ketoconazole therapy, symptoms, erythrocyte sedimentation rate (ESR), and complement fixation titers for histoplasma antigens.

Despite some success with antifungal therapy, many patients require surgical intervention for bypass of the SVC or decompression of central airways and pulmonary vasculature. Airway involvement can lead to distortion and obstruction with chronic postobstructive pneumonia; this is most frequent in the right middle lobe and is known as *middle lobe syndrome*. Treatment may require pulmonary resection. Extensive bronchoplastic procedures, including carinal resection, have been reported but are associated with an operative mortality approaching 45%.[61] The difficulty involved in operating within the mediastinum should not be underestimated, and pulmonary resections may require intrapericardial dissection. Because surgery is likely to be difficult and hazardous, it should only be considered as an appropriate option for patients with progressive disease and severely limiting symptoms. Patients with stable disease and without severe disability may be managed expectantly.

Superior Vena Cava Syndrome

Obstruction of the SVC produces an unmistakable constellation of signs and symptoms known as SVC syndrome. The consequences of impaired venous drainage of the head, arms, and upper torso range from relatively mild to life threatening and in 1757 were first described by Hunter.[62] The severity of symptoms is determined by the adequacy of collateral venous drainage, which is in turn a function of the rapidity with which the SVC obstruction progresses. As a general rule, the more rapid the process, the less time there is for development of collaterals and the more severe the symptoms. Although most patients are symptomatic, in unusual cases when obstruction develops over a prolonged period there may be minimal to no symptoms. Therapy is directed at palliation and, if possible, treatment of the underlying condition.

Epidemiology

Located in the middle mediastinum, the SVC is vulnerable to compression by mediastinal tumors, enlarging paratracheal lymph nodes, and aneurysms of the ascending aorta. Changing disease patterns have led to a change over time in the causes of SVC syndrome. Before the 1950s, almost half of all cases were attributable to benign disorders. Syphilitic aortic aneurysms were responsible for 30% of cases, while mediastinal goiters and tuberculous mediastinitis together accounted for approximately 15%.[63] With the decreasing incidence of tertiary syphilis and the increasing incidence of cancer, SVC syndrome is now rarely caused by aortic aneurysms (<5%) and is instead overwhelmingly the result of malignant disease (90%). Bronchogenic cancer is the most common malignant cause of SVC syndrome (70%–85%), lymphoma is second (5%–15%), and metastases from extrathoracic malignancies, especially breast and testicular cancer, account for most of the rest (5%–10%).[64] Of those patients with primary thoracic malignancies, up to 20% will develop SVC syndrome,[65] including 11% of those with small cell carcinoma.[66]

The most common benign cause of SVC syndrome is thrombosis. Thrombosis is usually iatrogenic and is related to the presence of indwelling central venous catheters or pacemaker leads. The overall risk of SVC thrombosis with pacemaker leads has been estimated[67] at between 0.3 and 4 per 1000 and is higher when leads have been damaged or abandoned.[68] Thrombosis also may compound narrowing of the SVC from other causes, such as encasement by tumor with tumor growth through the vessel wall. In these circumstances, the slowly progressive nature of the primary process may be exacerbated acutely by thrombosis of the residual lumen. A much less common but important benign cause of SVC syndrome is fibrosing mediastinitis.

Venous Collateral Anatomy

There are four routes for collateral venous drainage: (1) the azygous–hemiazygous system, (2) the internal mammary veins (which drain via the inferior epigastric veins to the iliac system), (3) the periesophageal venous plexus (an unusual but important cause of esophageal varices), and (4) subcutaneous collaterals. The relative importance of these various pathways is dependent on the location of the SVC obstruction relative to the cavoazygous junction. In most cases, the cavoazygous junction is obstructed, and blood must drain through multiple visceral and chest wall collaterals, especially the internal mammary and inferior epigastric veins, to reach the inferior vena cava (IVC). However, when the obstruction is below a patent cavoazygous junction, blood flows retrograde from the SVC through the azygous–hemiazygous system to the lumbar and iliac veins and into the IVC. When the obstruction is above a patent cavoazygous junction, blood can drain from prominent collaterals in the neck through the azygous–hemiazygous system, antegrade through the azygous vein, and into the SVC at its junction with the right atrium.

Clinical Presentation and Diagnosis

Clinical findings alone often establish the diagnosis of SVC syndrome. Approximately two-thirds of patients present with facial swelling, dyspnea at rest, orthopnea, and cough. Many patients are sleep deprived because symptoms are worse in the supine position, and they must try to sleep sitting up. Stridor is found in up to one-third of patients and is indicative of laryngeal edema that may progress to complete airway obstruction.[63] In addition to soft tissue edema, the increased

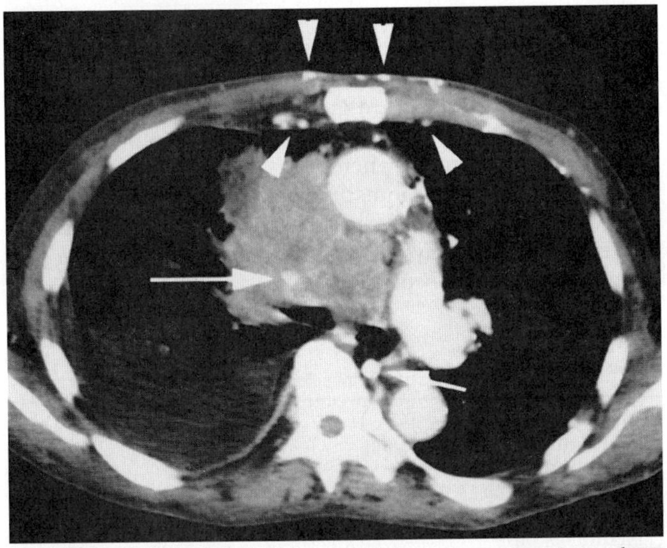

FIGURE 75.1. Superior vena cava syndrome. Contrast-enhanced CT demonstrates near-complete obstruction of the superior vena cava (long arrow) in a patient with small cell lung cancer. Note the large right pleural effusion and prominent collateral venous blood flow through the hemiazygous (short arrow), subcutaneous, and internal mammary (arrowheads) veins.

venous pressures can cause cerebral edema. Headache, vertigo, and stupor are worrisome symptoms of this complication and may presage the development of seizures. Physical examination usually reveals a characteristic plethoric appearance with facial, neck, and arm swelling as well as prominent subcutaneous veins across the neck and upper torso.

Once the diagnosis of SVC syndrome has been made, it is essential to determine the underlying cause and, in some cases, the precise venous anatomy. Computed tomography and MRI are equally valuable for demonstrating the anatomic characteristics of the mediastinum and great vessels and for identifying the existence of synchronous disease elsewhere in the chest. Furthermore, these studies can also assess vessel patency and collateral circulation by demonstrating either opacification with contrast-enhanced CT (Fig. 75.1) or signal loss with MRI. As the majority of cases are caused by malignant disease, tissue diagnosis plays an important role in determining therapy. With improvements in the safety and diagnostic yield of percutaneous biopsy techniques, rarely is there a need for bronchoscopy or mediastinoscopy to obtain adequate tissue specimens. These more invasive procedures should be avoided if possible because they are especially hazardous in the patient with SVC syndrome. Bronchoscopy can worsen laryngeal edema, and mediastinoscopy risks significant hemorrhage from extensive, high-pressure venous collaterals that traverse the mediastinum and chest wall. Although CT and MRI can identify collateral vessels, bilateral upper extremity venography is essential if thrombolysis, surgical bypass, or percutaneous stenting of the SVC is contemplated.

Therapy

Management of patients with SVC syndrome should be designed both to treat the underlying cause of the obstruction and to palliate symptoms. Although definitive therapy may require surgical bypass of the obstructed SVC, medical therapy may be adequate to achieve significant relief of symptoms. Simple measures such as elevation of the head and administration of diuretics should be initiated for all patients regardless of the cause of the obstruction. Diuretics decrease edema generally, decrease the production of cerebrospinal fluid, and decrease cardiac output. Unfortunately, steroids are of no proven benefit for the treatment of laryngeal and cerebral edema in this setting.[63]

Medical Therapy

Additional treatment is guided by the underlying diagnosis. Thrombosis-related SVC syndrome is usually associated with indwelling catheters or pacemaker leads and can produce severe symptoms because of its relatively rapid onset. The foreign body should be removed from the SVC and consideration given to thrombolytic therapy. Although thrombolytics are likely to restore SVC patency, they should be used with caution because they may generate thrombus fragments that can break off and embolize into the pulmonary circulation.[69] Regardless of the decision to use thrombolytics, unless contraindicated, all patients with SVC thrombosis should be treated with long-term anticoagulation.

For most patients, however, SVC obstruction is caused by malignancy and is a consequence of compression from the primary tumor or from lymph node involvement. Once a tissue diagnosis has been made, chemotherapy or radiotherapy can be initiated and in general is associated with an 80% response rate.[63,66,70] Symptoms should improve within 1 to 2 weeks. Superior vena cava syndrome from small cell carcinoma is particularly responsive to medical therapy. For patients presenting with SVC syndrome and a new diagnosis of small cell carcinoma, the response rate to combination therapy can be as high as 94%.[66] Patients with relapsing disease can expect chemotherapy and radiation therapy to produce response rates of 70% and 80%, respectively. Long-term relief of symptoms and a median survival of 6 to 7 months are achieved in the majority of patients, survival results no worse and possibly better than those for patients who present with small cell carcinoma without SVC obstruction.

Surgical Bypass

Definitive palliation is achieved by restoring a functional SVC, which can be accomplished either by surgical bypass using autologous or synthetic materials or by endovascular stenting. Surgical bypass is a major undertaking and is therefore reserved only for those patients with benign disorders and an otherwise good long-term prognosis. In contrast, endovascular stenting has been used most often for patients with malignant disease and limited life expectancy. For surgical bypass, Doty and colleagues[71] have advocated the use of spiral saphenous vein grafts for many years and reported the longest experience with this technique. They documented a patency rate of 88% among 16 patients with follow-up as long as 23 years.

Other options for avoiding synthetic material have been proposed, but none has the proven durability and effectiveness of the spiral vein graft. Large-caliber autologous veins such as the femoral vein provide adequate-size conduits, but their use has been avoided because of significant morbidity from impaired venous drainage distal to the donor site. Pericardial tube grafts, aortic homografts, and extraanatomical bypass with a saphenous vein graft from the jugular vein to the femoral vein have been suggested. The proposed advantage of this last approach is the avoidance of intrathoracic surgery. The experience with these alternatives is limited to isolated case reports with short follow-up,[72–74] and they should not be considered as proven alternatives to the spiral vein graft. In contrast to autologous materials, synthetic grafts are convenient, easy to work with, and readily available in a variety of sizes. However, their patency when used as venous conduits is problematic. Some success has been reported with externally supported polytetrafluoroethylene (PTFE) grafts, but the patency rates remain substantially inferior to vein grafts.[75]

Before construction of a bypass graft, the anatomy and patency of the innominate, jugular, and subclavian veins must be assessed, and a site for the proximal anastomosis should be identified. The operation is conducted through a median sternotomy or partial sternal split. These approaches avoid large chest wall collaterals, provide excellent exposure to the great vessels, and can be extended into the base of the neck for access to the jugular veins in case the intrathoracic veins are not patent. Once exposure is obtained, the graft length is determined based on the distance between the right atrial appendage and the nearest patent central vein.

Doty and colleagues[71] have described in detail the construction and use of a spiral vein graft. Following surgery, the head of the bed should be kept elevated to 30°, and attention should be paid to the airway, which is at risk for obstruction from laryngeal edema. Aspirin therapy is begun, and decompression should be anticipated over the ensuing 24 to 48h. If decompression is not apparent, this suggests early graft failure and thrombosis, necessitating reexploration and thrombectomy.

Endovascular Stents

Endovascular stents are increasingly the preferred method for palliation of SVC obstruction. Initial success rates vary between 70% and 100%, with recurrence of symptoms in 0% to 45% of patients.[76] Frequently, patency is achieved and maintained by a combination of thrombolytics, vessel dilation, and stent placement. Although the procedure requires passage of a guidewire across an obstructed SVC, complete occlusion is not necessarily a contraindication. Reported complications are infrequent but occasionally severe. Kee and colleagues[69] reported a patency rate of 91% in 59 patients with a mean follow-up of 13 months (range 1–27 months). There were two procedure-related deaths. One patient died of multiple pulmonary emboli consequent to the use of thrombolytics, and the other succumbed to cor pulmonale within 24h of the procedure. These results indicate that endovascular stenting is a valuable addition to the therapeutic options available for the treatment of patients with SVC syndrome and can be considered appropriate in a variety of situations.

Mediastinal Lesions

The wide variety and diverse origins of tissues normally found within the mediastinum account for the extraordinary assortment of tumors and cysts that arise from them. These lesions are collectively referred to as *primary mediastinal lesions* (Table 75.2).[77] Secondary lesions of the mediastinum are derived from extramediastinal tissues, such as thyroid, bone, or lung, and either migrate into or metastasize to the mediastinum. Many benign lesions are asymptomatic and are discovered incidentally, whereas malignant lesions are more likely to produce symptoms from compression and invasion of adjacent structures. Mediastinal tumors may also present as a consequence of systemic syndromes caused by the production of bioactive peptides and hormones.

TABLE 75.2. Types of Primary Mediastinal Lesions.

Neurogenic tumors
Neurilemoma (schwannoma)
Neurofibroma
Ganglioneuroma
Ganglioneuroblastoma
Neuroblastoma
Paraganglioma (pheochromocytoma)
Chemodectoma
Cysts
Foregut cysts
Bronchogenic cyst
Duplication (enteric) cyst
Mesothelial cysts
Pleuropericardial cyst
Neurenteric cyst
Unclassified
Thymus
Thymoma
Thymic carcinoma
Thymic cyst
Thymolipoma
Lymphoma
Hodgkin's disease
Non-Hodgkin's lymphoma
Primary mediastinal B-cell lymphoma
Lymphoblastic
Large cell, diffuse
Other
Germ cell tumors
Benign
Epidermoid cyst
Dermoid cyst
Mature teratoma
Malignant
Seminoma
Nonseminomatous germ cell tumor
Mesenchymal tumors
Lipoma/liposarcoma
Fibroma/fibrosarcoma
Leiomyoma/leiomyosarcoma
Myxoma
Mesothelioma
Rhabdomyoma/rhabdomyosarcoma
Hemangioma/hemangiosarcoma
Hemangiopericytoma
Lymphangioma (cystic hygroma)
Lymphangiomyoma
Lymphangiopericytoma
Endocrine
Ectopic parathyroid
Mediastinal thyroid
Carcinoid
Other
Giant lymph node hyperplasia (Castleman's disease)
Granuloma

Source: Adapted from Davis et al.,[77] with permission.

The diagnosis is usually suggested by the patient's age, the location of the lesion within the mediastinum, the presence or absence of symptoms, and its radiographic features. Ultimately, however, definitive diagnosis rests on obtaining tissue through either biopsy or excision. Because appropriate treatment can vary from observation to aggressive multimodality therapy, the surgeon is presented with the challenge of deciding on the extent of preoperative workup and if and when to undertake resection. Although the recent popularization of minimal-access techniques has made the option of surgery more palatable to patients and referring physicians, it should not change the indications for and timing of surgical intervention.

Mediastinal Compartments

Although anatomists divide the mediastinum into four compartments, it is most helpful for discussions of mediastinal lesions to divide the region into only three: anterior, middle, and posterior (Fig. 75.2). The anterior compartment, also known as the anterosuperior or prevascular compartment, extends from the posterior surface of the sternum to the anterior surface of the pericardium and great vessels. It can be readily identified on lateral chest x-ray and contains the thymus and surrounding lymphatic and connective tissues. A line drawn along the border between the esophagus and the anterior longitudinal spinal ligament separates the middle and posterior compartments. This definition can be confusing because, although in this scheme the trachea and esophagus belong to the middle compartment, they are frequently referred to as posterior mediastinal structures. To minimize confusion, Shields[78] suggested replacing *middle* with the more descriptive term *visceral*. This designation emphasizes that the middle compartment contains not only the great vessels and the contents of the pericardium but also the trachea and esophagus. The posterior compartment extends posteriorly from the anterior longitudinal spinal ligament to the costovertebral junction and is equivalent to the bilateral paravertebral sulci.

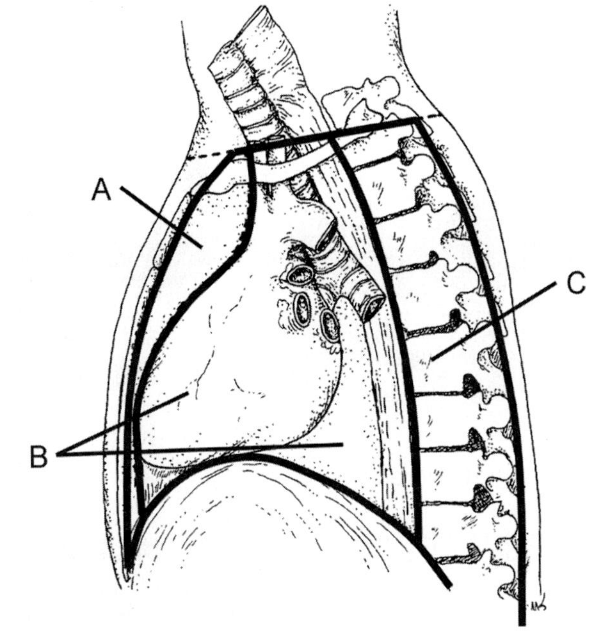

FIGURE 75.2. Mediastinal compartments. **A.** Anterior. **B.** Visceral (middle). **C.** Posterior (paravertebral).

Division of the mediastinum into three compartments facilitates diagnosis because most lesions have a predilection for one of the three (Table 75.3). Thymomas, germ cell tumors, and lymphomas are the predominant primary lesions of the anterior compartment, and tumors of the paravertebral sulcus are typically neurogenic. Primary lesions of the visceral compartment are usually congenital cysts or lymphomas. The most common secondary mediastinal tumor, a substernal thyroid, is found most often in the visceral compartment adjacent to the trachea.

Patient Age

The relative prevalence of specific primary lesions varies with the age of the patient population (Fig. 75.3). In adults, neuro-

TABLE 75.3. Usual Location of Mediastinal Lesions.

	Mediastinal compartment		
Type of lesion	*Anterior*	*Visceral*	*Paravertebral sulci*
Primary			
More common	Thymoma Benign and malignant germ cell tumors Lymphoma	Foregut cyst Pleuropericardial cyst Lymphoma Mediastinal granuloma	Neurilemoma (schwannoma) Neurofibroma Neuroblastoma Malignant schwannoma Ganglioneuroma Ganglioneuroblastoma Foregut cyst Paraganglioma
Less common	Mesenchymal tumors Thymic cyst Parathyroid adenoma	Paraganglioma Neurenteric cyst Thoracic duct cyst	Pheochromocytoma Mesenchymal tumors Lymphoma Extramedullary hematopoiesis
Secondary	Thyroid goiter Bony tumors	Thyroid goiter Metastatic carcinoma Foramen of Morgagni hernia Hiatal hernia Pancreatic pseudocyst	Bony tumors

Source: Adapted from Shields,[78] with permission.

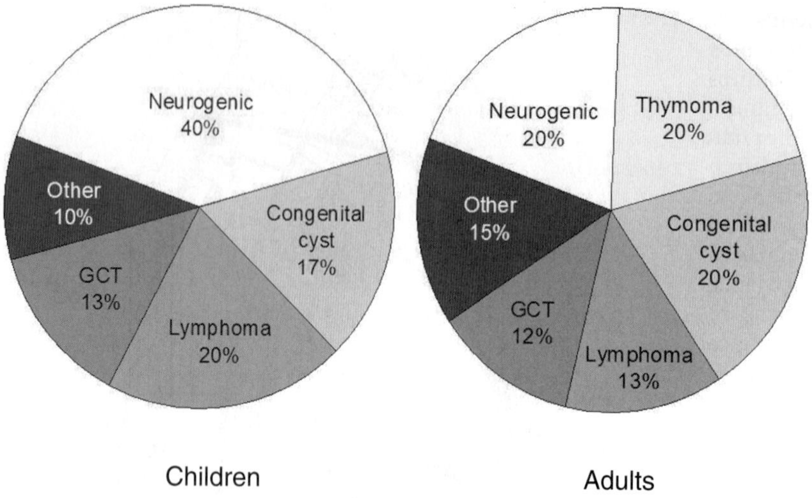

FIGURE 75.3. Common primary mediastinal lesions by patient age. Note that almost half of mediastinal lesions in children are neurogenic tumors, and that thymomas, among the most common in adults, are rare in children. Neurogenic tumors in children under 2 years are most likely neuroblastomas; in children aged 2 to 10 years they are most likely to be ganglioneuromas; and in adults they are most often neurilemomas. GCT, germ cell tumor. (Reprinted from Block,[195] with permission.)

genic tumors and thymomas are equally prevalent and together constitute approximately 40% of all primary lesions.[78,79] In children, neurogenic tumors are the most common by a wide margin, and thymomas are rare, with neurogenic tumors alone accounting for almost 40% of all primary lesions.[78,80] A second important difference is that in children neurogenic tumors are most likely to be neuroblastomas (in children < 2 years of age) and ganglioneuromas (in children 2–10 years),[80,81] while in adults they are most likely to be neurilemomas (schwannomas).[79] Foregut cysts and germ cell tumors each constitute between 10% and 20% of mediastinal lesions in both age groups. Lymphomas also account for approximately 20% in both age groups, with approximately two-thirds of these lesions being non-Hodgkin's lymphoma in both age groups. Thus:

1. An anterior mediastinal mass in an adult is most likely to be a thymoma.
2. An anterior mediastinal mass in a child or young adult is most likely to be a lymphoma or a germ cell tumor.
3. A paravertebral mass in an infant is most likely to be a neuroblastoma (malignant), in a child it is most likely to be a ganglioneuroma (benign), and in an adult it is most likely to be a neurilemoma.

Clinical Presentation

Mediastinal lesions are symptomatic in 50%–75% of patients.[79,80,82] Thus, up to half of all mediastinal lesions are incidental discoveries on chest x-ray or CT scan. Symptoms can be caused by local mass effects, systemic effects of tumor-derived hormones and peptides, or infection. Local effects are dependent on the size and location of the lesion and result from compression of adjacent structures. Examples include cough, stridor, dyspnea, chest pain, and dysphagia. It has been generally accepted that symptoms are more likely to occur in children, although some authors challenged this conclusion.[79,80] Symptoms are also more common with malignant tumors, which, unlike benign lesions, are more likely to fix, encase, and invade adjacent structures. Superior vena cava syndrome, back pain, and neurological deficits such as Horner's syndrome or phrenic nerve palsy are ominous findings. Infection of mediastinal cysts, usually by the hematogenous route, is an important but uncommon presentation. Cysts may also present with rapid enlargement from bleeding into the cavity. Duplication cysts that are lined with gastric mucosa may ulcerate, bleed, and erode into the adjacent airway or esophagus, presenting with hemoptysis or hematemesis.[83]

Many mediastinal tumors are associated with a variety of clinical syndromes (Table 75.4). In some cases, tumor-derived hormones or peptides are directly causative (Table 75.5). Mediastinal carcinoid tumors have not been associated with carcinoid syndrome but can produce corticotropin (ACTH), leading to development of Cushing's syndrome. Neurogenic tumors derived from the ganglion and paraganglion system can produce norepinephrine and, rarely, epinephrine, giving

TABLE 75.4. Mediastinal Tumors and Associated Clinical Syndromes.

Tumor	*Syndrome*
Thymoma	Autoimmune and immune deficiency
	Myasthenia gravis
	Red blood cell aplasia
	White blood cell aplasia
	Aplastic anemia
	Hypogammaglobulinemia
	Polymyositis
	Dermatomyositis
	Progressive systemic sclerosis
	Hemolytic anemia
	Systemic lupus erythematosus
	Rheumatoid arthritis
	Collagen vascular disease
	Endocrine disorders
	Panhypopituitarism
	Addison's disease
	Hyperthyroidism
	Miscellaneous
	Megaesophagus
	Myocarditis
Lymphoma	Anemia
	Myasthenia gravis
Neurofibroma	von Recklinghausen's disease
Thymic carcinoid	Multiple endocrine neoplasia (I and II)
Neurenteric cysts	Vertebral anomalies
Nonseminomatous germ cell tumors	Klinefelter's syndrome

Source: Adapted from Davis et al.,[77] with permission.

TABLE 75.5. Syndromes Caused by Tumor-Derived Products.

Syndrome	*Tumor product*	*Tumor*
Cushing's syndrome	ACTH	Carcinoid
Palpitations/ hypertension	Norepinephrine Epinephrine (rare)	Paraganglioma Pheochromocytoma Chemodectoma Ganglioneuroma Neuroblastoma
Hypoglycemia	Insulin-like hormone	Mesothelioma Teratoma Fibrosarcoma Neurosarcoma
Diarrhea	Vasoactive intestinal polypeptide	Ganglioneuroma Neuroblastoma Neurofibroma
Hypercalcemia	PTH Parathyroid-like hormone	Parathyroid adenoma Hodgkin's disease
Thyrotoxicosis	Thyroid hormone	Substernal thyroid
Gynecomastia	β-HCG	Nonseminomatous germ cell tumor
Precocious puberty	Testosterone	Nonseminomatous germ cell tumor

Source: Adapted from Davis et al.,[77] with permission.

rise to the classic constellation of episodic hypertension, palpitations, and hypermetabolism associated with pheochromocytoma. Nonseminomatous germ cell tumors (NSGCTs) often produce β-human chorionic gonadotropin (β-HCG), which can induce gynecomastia or precocious puberty. Some tumors are associated with specific systemic syndromes. Although the nature of these relationships is not clear, in some cases there is the suggestion of a pathophysiological link, such as the autoimmune and immunodeficient disorders associated with thymoma (e.g., MG, red blood cell aplasia, and hypogammaglobulinemia). In other cases, it is likely that there are common underlying developmental or genetic abnormalities (e.g., Klinefelter's syndrome and NSGCTs; vertebral anomalies and neurenteric cysts; multiple endocrine neoplasia [MEN] and carcinoid tumors).

Evaluation of the Patient with a Mediastinal Lesion

The primary goals of evaluation are to determine the correct diagnosis and to establish anatomical relationships and resectability should surgery be indicated. In some circumstances, a precise tissue diagnosis is not required before proceeding to surgery, but in no case should an extensive resection be undertaken without one.

Radiology

Imaging is essential and is often the only investigation needed before initiating therapy. Typically, CT scanning is the first step. The images obtained clearly demonstrate the precise location of the lesion and its relationships to adjacent structures. Equally valuable is the ability of CT to define important characteristics, such as whether the lesion is solid or cystic, is heterogeneous or homogeneous, or contains fat, fluid, or calcium. Also, CT can demonstrate features that are consistent with either a benign or malignant diagnosis, such as well-defined tissue planes or evidence of local invasion. As an alternative, MRI has several advantages. Because it demonstrates flowing blood and the spinal cord exceptionally well, it is the preferred study for evaluation of suspected vascular lesions and for lesions that may extend into the spinal canal. It is also indicated for those patients who should not receive contrast, either because of a contrast allergy or because they are thought to have a thyroid malignancy and may require radioiodine therapy. Last, the multiplanar imaging features of MRI can be helpful in assessing three-dimensional relationships, particularly when evaluating the potential communication of mediastinal cysts with the pericardium, bronchus, or esophagus. Recent software developments combined with introduction of the multislice CT scanner permit reconstruction of CT images with very high resolution to produce similar three-dimensional perspective.

Ultrasonography has an evolving role in the evaluation of mediastinal lesions. Its once popular use for determination of solid versus cystic features has largely been supplanted by CT and MRI. However, transesophageal echocardiography can be an invaluable tool for assessing the relationship of mediastinal lesions to the heart. A more recent development is esophageal endoscopic ultrasound-guided fine-needle aspiration (EUS-FNA) biopsy.[84] This technique facilitates diagnosis of lesions that may be difficult to reach through more traditional percutaneous approaches. Endoscopic ultrasound nicely demonstrates cystic lesions but cannot distinguish between esophageal duplication and bronchogenic cysts. Fine-needle aspiration should not be done with these lesions because of the risk of introducing infection.

Nuclear medicine offers a variety of functional imaging studies to complement the anatomical imaging of CT, MRI, and ultrasound and can provide definitive diagnostic information in certain circumstances. Fluorodeoxyglucose positron emission tomography (FDG-PET) is now widely used in the evaluation of solid lesions, but sensitivity and specificity for distinguishing benign from malignant primary mediastinal tumors has not been clearly established. The thyroid scan may be helpful for the diagnosis of a substernal goiter, but because many goiters are nonfunctional, a negative study is not helpful; therefore, this study is generally not indicated. Although the thallium-technetium scan can be used to localize a mediastinal parathyroid gland, it is not appropriate for evaluation of a newly discovered mediastinal lesion. In contrast, meta-iodobenzylguanidine (MIBG) scintigraphy should be performed for those rare patients suspected of having a catecholamine-producing tumor, such as paraganglioma. This study is useful both for diagnosis of the primary lesion and for evaluation of metastatic disease. ^{111}In-pentetreotide scintigraphy (octreoscan) can be used to localize neuroendocrine tumors such as neuroblastomas, paragangliomas, and carcinoids. A ^{99}Tc scan can be used to diagnose the rare duplication cyst that is lined with gastric mucosa, but as with EUS in this setting, its use may be superfluous when resection is indicated regardless of the findings.

Serology

Serologic examination for the presence of tumor-specific biochemical markers is not routine for most patients with mediastinal lesions. The most important exception is for males between the ages of 10 and 50 years who present with an anterior mediastinal mass. These patients are likely to have a nonseminomatous germ cell tumor (NSGCT), and therefore their serum α-fetoprotein (AFP) and β-HCG levels should be determined. More than 90% of patients with an NSGCT have elevated levels of one or both, whereas seminomas and benign germ cell tumors (teratomas) characteristically do not produce either.[79] This information is very helpful in planning therapy because NSGCTs typically are aggressive tumors treated primarily with platinum-based chemotherapy. A positive serology is sufficient to proceed with chemotherapy without the need for a tissue diagnosis. Another important exception is when the diagnosis of a catecholamine-producing neurogenic tumor is suspected (e.g., paraganglioma and rare neuroblastomas). These are rare tumors, but in the setting of systemic symptoms suggestive of the diagnosis, measurement of serum catecholamines and urinary vanillylmandelic acid (VMA) and metanephrine is essential. Not only is a positive test diagnostic, but it informs the surgeon that preoperative adrenergic blockade is indicated to prevent intraoperative hypertensive crisis.

Biopsy

Tissue diagnosis is often, but not always, required before proceeding with therapy. As outlined, some imaging and serological information may be diagnostic. Furthermore, resection may be indicated regardless of the results of tissue biopsy. Circumstances in which biopsy is indicated include (1) suspicion of a tumor that is treated primarily with nonoperative therapy (e.g., lymphoma, NSGCT, or seminoma); (2) evidence of local invasion that would require resection and reconstruction of vital structures (e.g., involvement of the SVC by a large anterior mediastinal mass); and (3) evidence of metastatic disease rendering resection inappropriate.

The available techniques for biopsy include FNA cytology, core needle biopsy, cervical and anterior mediastinoscopy, and thoracoscopy. The preference is FNA as it is the least invasive and often simplest approach. Recent series reported an accuracy at cytological diagnosis between 80% and 90% and an accuracy at distinguishing benign from malignant that approaches 100%.[85–87] Most mediastinal lesions can be reached using CT or EUS guidance with minimal risk of complication. Traditional drawbacks to FNA are the inability to subtype lymphomas because of a lack of tissue architecture and difficulty in determining between specific histologies when faced with a poorly differentiated neoplasm. Many of these problems are being overcome by the increasing use of immunohistochemistry for cell-surface markers and cellular products.

If more tissue is required than an FNA can provide, core needle biopsy, open biopsy, or mediastinoscopy is indicated. Cervical mediastinoscopy is appropriate for biopsy of masses within the visceral compartment that are adjacent to the trachea, while anterior mediastinoscopy can be performed on the left (Chamberlain procedure) or right to reach lesions that are anterior and lateral to the aorta or vena cava, respectively. Thoracoscopy is an alternative, but requires one-lung ventilation and is associated with increased morbidity and hospital length of stay compared to mediastinoscopy.[88]

The indication for biopsy of anterior mediastinal masses in adults deserves additional discussion. If the patient is a man under 50 years of age, serum AFP and β-HCG should be determined first. If positive, then a diagnosis of NSGCT is made, and therapy can be initiated without further diagnostic workup. If the patient is a woman or a man older than 50 years or if the serology is negative, then the tumor is most likely to be a thymoma, and the indication for biopsy depends in large part on tumor size. Small (<5-cm) tumors are usually amenable to complete resection with minimal morbidity. Furthermore, thymomas of this size are usually encapsulated and associated with a good prognosis. In this setting, biopsy of an encapsulated thymoma violates the capsule and theoretically risks disseminating disease, possibly worsening prognosis. Resection without preoperative biopsy avoids this possibility, is likely to be uncomplicated, and would not be inappropriate even if the tumor were a lymphoma or a germ cell tumor. In contrast, large tumors can require extensive procedures to achieve complete resection, and thymomas more than 5 cm in diameter are usually invasive and associated with poor prognosis.[89] In this circumstance, biopsy does not risk worsening prognosis and avoids the possibility of undertaking extensive resection for lymphoma. In addition, preoperative chemotherapy may be indicated if a definitive diagnosis of thymoma is made. Consequently, small anterior mediastinal tumors in adults typically are resected without a tissue diagnosis, while larger tumors should first be biopsied.

Operative Considerations

Some mediastinal lesions present unique problems for the surgeon beyond the technical complexities of resection. Large anterior mediastinal masses pose a risk of acute airway obstruction, particularly with induction of general anesthesia and loss of muscle tone. Consequently, rigid bronchoscopy should be immediately available, and consideration should be given to awake intubation with the patient in the semi-Fowler position. For lesions that may require resection and reconstruction of the SVC, lower-extremity venous access is required to ensure that fluids and medications can be administered throughout the procedure.

Secondary Mediastinal Lesions

Substernal Goiter

Substernal goiters are the most common mediastinal lesion of extramediastinal origin, yet fewer than 20% of all resected thyroids have a significant intrathoracic component.[90] Goiters located completely within the mediastinum are rare. Typically, the mass extends down through the thoracic inlet directly into the visceral compartment. It usually lies in continuity with the trachea, either anterior or posterior to it, but in rare cases can be found posterior to the esophagus (Fig. 75.4). Although many substernal goiters may appear to bulge into the superior portion of the anterior compartment, presentation as a truly anterior compartment mass is unusual. Most patients with substernal goiters are in their fourth or fifth decade of life, and women are affected more than twice as often as men.[91,92] Most patients present with an asymptomatic neck mass, but as many as half of patients with a partial or complete substernal goiter have symptoms such as dyspnea, cough, dysphagia, or stridor. Stridor is a particularly worri-

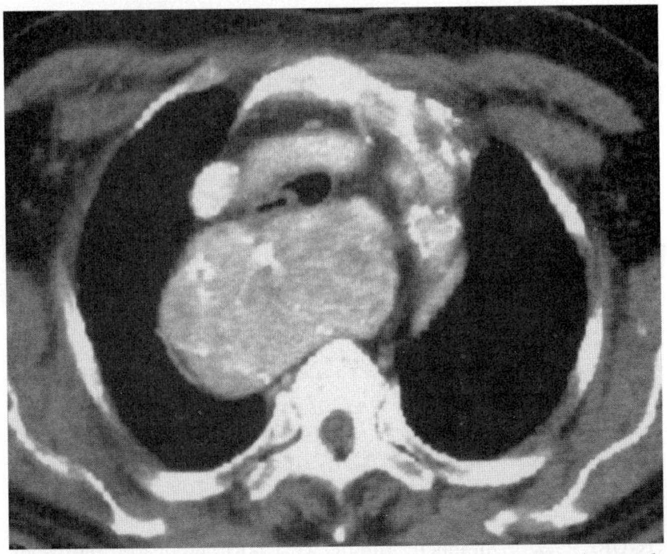

FIGURE 75.4. Mediastinal thyroid. Computed tomography with intravenous contrast of a mediastinal thyroid goiter in an older man with a history of thyroidectomy. Note the characteristic heterogeneity and hypervascularity of the gland as well as scattered punctuate calcifications. The esophagus is displaced anteriorly.

some presentation as it suggests not only impending airway obstruction but also the possibility of tracheomalacia. Thyrotoxicosis is rare, and hoarseness, an uncommon symptom, is highly suggestive of malignancy. Histologically, most lesions are nontoxic multinodular goiters, but as many as 44% may be follicular adenomas.[92] Reports of the prevalence of malignancy vary from 2% to 21%.[92,93]

Both history and physical exam may suggest the diagnosis of substernal goiter as up to 20% of patients have had a thyroidectomy, and almost two-thirds have a palpable low cervical mass.[91–93] Plain films demonstrate a mass in the superior portion of the visceral compartment that may extend anteriorly and appear to be in the anterior compartment. Tracheal or esophageal deviation is often present. Characteristic findings by CT include continuity with the cervical gland, well-defined borders, scattered punctate or coarse calcifications, and a heterogeneous consistency with areas of low density that do not enhance and areas of high attenuation that markedly enhance with contrast. Usually, MRI is redundant but if obtained will demonstrate characteristic flow voids related to the abundant and heterogeneous vascularity of the gland. Further evaluation by thyroid scan (^{131}I scintigraphy) is often unnecessary and usually precluded by the prior administration of intravenous contrast for CT. Although a positive scan is diagnostic, most often the study is negative and unhelpful because most substernal goiters are nonfunctional.[90,93]

Although asymptomatic patients with a definitive diagnosis and a small lesion may be observed in selected circumstances, resection is usually indicated to prevent development of acute airway obstruction and because of the potential for malignancy. Radioactive iodine is contraindicated not only because it is ineffective in treating these large tumors but also because it may initially aggravate airway compression. In the absence of previous thyroidectomy, vascular supply from the inferior thyroid vessels is the rule. Consequently, a cervical incision provides ideal exposure and minimizes the risk of injury to the recurrent laryngeal nerves. Most lesions can be resected without the addition of a partial or complete sternal split. For large lesions posterior to the trachea, simultaneous cervical and thoracic incisions should be considered. An isolated thoracic approach is to be avoided in most circumstances, however, because control of the vascular supply that descends from the neck is difficult, and the risk of recurrent nerve injury is high. Similarly video-assisted thoracic surgery (VATS) is to be used with caution.

Lesions of Skeletal Origin

A variety of lesions that arise in the thoracic skeleton can grow into the mediastinum. Sternal tumors usually are easily distinguished from true mediastinal masses, but lesions that arise from the vertebral bodies may be more difficult to differentiate. These lesions include chordomas, anterior meningoceles, and ectopic extramedullary hematopoietic tissue. Chordomas of the spine are malignant tumors that most often appear in the paravertebral sulcus; they cause erosion of the adjacent vertebral body and therefore are usually symptomatic. Thoracotomy with wide excision and spinal reconstruction is indicated, although the prognosis is poor. Anterior meningocele is a benign lesion that also presents in the paravertebral sulcus and is often confused with neurogenic tumors. It is most often associated with neurofibromatosis and skeletal abnormalities and does not require resection unless symptoms result. Ectopic extramedullary hematopoietic tissue is typically paravertebral and bilateral, is found in patients with hemolytic and hematopoietic disorders such as thalassemia or spherocytosis, and does not require specific therapy.[94] Diagnosis can be confirmed by needle biopsy.

Vascular Lesions

Although they arise from mediastinal structures, vascular abnormalities typically are not included within the spectrum of primary mediastinal lesions. Nevertheless, they should be considered in the differential diagnosis. They may originate from any of the major arteries or veins in the mediastinum and may be either congenital or acquired. Examples include the wide variety of aortic arch and pulmonary arterial anomalies, vascular rings, and aneurysms of the aorta and ductus arteriosus. Angiography is diagnostic, but MRI can be an effective noninvasive substitute.

Lesions of Intraabdominal Origin

Herniation of abdominal viscera through the foramen of Morgagni or the esophageal hiatus can mimic a mediastinal mass on plain chest x-ray. However, careful history and further radiological evaluation should readily differentiate these abnormalities from true mediastinal lesions. Rarely, a pancreatic pseudocyst may present as a mass posteriorly in the visceral compartment, but history and imaging (CT) should discover the true nature of these lesions.[95]

Metastatic Disease

Lymphadenopathy from metastatic lung cancer is the most common mediastinal mass. Mediastinal lymph nodes can also be involved with metastatic disease from a variety of other sources, including colon and rectal cancers, head-and-neck cancer, testicular tumors, and lymphoma. The diagnosis of metastatic cancer is usually straightforward, with a known or suspected primary lesion readily identifiable elsewhere. Furthermore, metastatic disease typically presents as multiple enlarged lymph nodes rather than as a solitary mass that would be more consistent with a primary mediastinal lesion. Evaluation of suspected metastatic disease is usually made with mediastinoscopy, PET, or EUS-FNA.

Primary Mediastinal Lesions

Neurogenic Tumors

In children, neurogenic tumors are the most common mediastinal lesion by a wide margin, whereas in adults neurogenic tumors and thymomas are equally prevalent. Neurogenic tumors can arise from cells of the nerve sheath, the autonomic ganglia, or the paraganglion system and can be either benign or malignant (Table 75.6). Young children are much more likely to have a malignant tumor (neuroblastoma), whereas older children and adults are more likely to have benign lesions (ganglioneuromas and neurilemomas, respectively).[79–81] These tumors arise most often in the paravertebral sulci (posterior compartment), although they can be found in the visceral and anterior compartments. Correspondingly, almost all paravertebral lesions are neurogenic tumors.

Most neurogenic tumors present as incidental findings and are asymptomatic, but symptoms can arise from either local or systemic effects. Local effects are predominantly pain and paresthesias caused by erosion into the vertebral column or chest wall or impingement of nerve roots. Neurological deficits such as Pancoast's or Horner's syndrome may also be present. Systemic effects are uncommon and are a consequence of the rare tumor that produces either catecholamines or vasoactive intestinal polypeptide (VIP) (Table 75.5). Approximately 10% of neurogenic tumors extend through an intervertebral foramen into the spinal canal, producing a characteristic bilobed appearance ("dumbbell tumor") (Fig. 75.5). Evaluation by MRI can be helpful for determination of intraspinal extension and for planning resection.

Tumors of Nerve Sheath Origin

Neurilemomas (schwannomas) and neurofibromas are benign and are the most common neurogenic tumors in adults (Fig. 75.6). The peak incidence is in the second and third decades of life, and although they are associated with von Recklinghausen's disease (neurofibromatosis), they are found mostly in patients without it. Schwannomas are well encapsulated, whereas neurofibromas lack a well-defined capsule. Most dumbbell tumors are schwannomas.

TABLE 75.6. Neurogenic Tumors and Their Origin.

Origin	*Benign*	*Malignant*
Nerve sheath	Neurilemoma (schwannoma)	Malignant schwannoma (neurosarcoma)
	Neurofibroma	
Sympathetic ganglia	Ganglioneuroma	Ganglioneuroblastoma Neuroblastoma
Paraganglion system	Paraganglioma (pheochromocytoma) Chemodectoma	Malignant paraganglioma Malignant chemodectoma

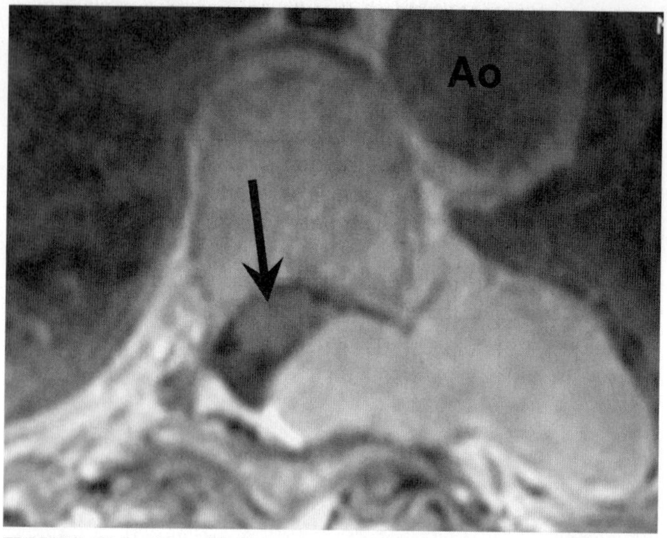

FIGURE 75.5. "Dumbbell" tumor, with MRI demonstrating tumor extending through the vertebral foramen. There is a substantial intraspinal component that abuts the spinal cord (arrow). Ao, descending thoracic aorta. (Reprinted from Block,[195] with permission.)

Complete resection is indicated and curative for both these tumors and may require sacrifice of nerve trunks. Resection of dumbbell tumors should be accomplished in one operation. If the intraspinal component is large, the operation consists of two parts; a laminectomy is performed first, followed by thoracotomy. Akwari and colleagues[96] initially described using separate incisions, whereas Grillo and colleagues advocated a modified approach through a single incision.[97] Most appropriately, however, the size and location of the lesion should determine the choice of exposure. Attempt at removal through a thoracotomy alone (or by VATS) risks disruption of the neck of the lesion, leaving tumor behind and inaccessible in the spinal canal.

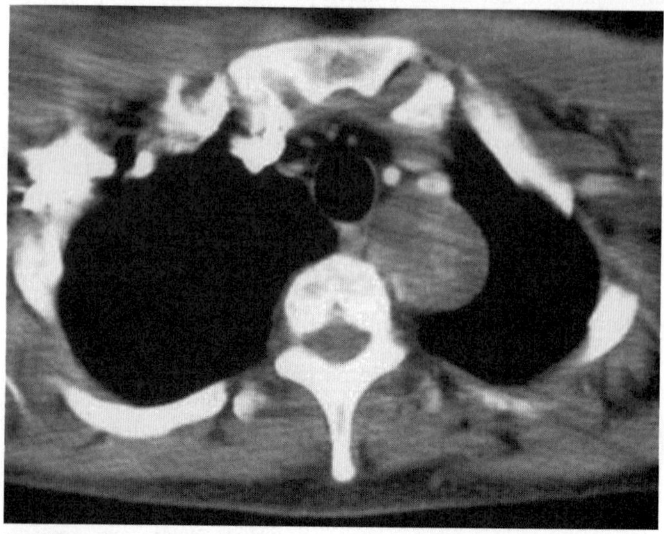

FIGURE 75.6. Mediastinal schwannoma. This was an incidental finding. Note the smooth borders, homogeneous consistency, and the preserved tissue plane between the mass and the esophagus and trachea. The lesion appears to arise from the paravertebral tissues, consistent with a posterior mediastinal mass. (Reprinted from Block,[195] with permission.)

In contrast to these benign lesions, malignant nerve sheath tumors (also called malignant schwannomas or neurosarcomas) are rare aggressive tumors with a poor prognosis. They are locally invasive and typically recur even after wide excision. These tumors have been associated with neurofibromatosis and can produce an insulin-like hormone that precipitates episodic hypoglycemia. They are not responsive to adjuvant therapies, and unless they can be completely resected, the prognosis is poor.

Tumors of Autonomic Ganglia Origin

Ganglioneuromas are derived from cells of the autonomic ganglia and are the most common tumor in older children. They are benign, and complete resection is both indicated and curative. In contrast, neuroblastomas are highly malignant tumors that have frequently metastasized to liver, brain, lung, or lymph nodes by the time of diagnosis. Approximately 20% of all neuroblastomas are found in the mediastinum, and they are the most common mediastinal lesions in children under the age of 2 years.[81] They are less common in older children and unusual in adults.

Histologically, neuroblastomas are distinguished by prominent neurosecretory granules, which may contain catecholamines or VIP. Treatment is stage dependent. Stage I and II tumors (well circumscribed and noninvasive or locally invasive but without extension across the midline, respectively) are treated with resection followed by radiation therapy. Stage III and IV tumors (invasion across the midline or metastatic disease, respectively) require multimodality therapy, with the role of surgery in this setting controversial.[98,99]

As their name implies, ganglioneuroblastomas are intermediate in their differentiation and behavior between benign ganglioneuromas and malignant neuroblastomas. Histologically, ganglioneuroblastomas can be divided into two groups: imperfect or diffuse type, with cellular elements representative of all stages of neural development, and immature or composite type, with focal areas of primitive neuroblasts. Prognosis is highly dependent on histology and is strongly correlated with the presence of neuroblasts. Diffuse-type tumors and composite tumors with individual nests of neuroblasts are associated with a good prognosis (up to 100% survival), whereas composite tumors with aggregates or nodular deposits of neuroblasts have a poor prognosis (67% and 0% survival, respectively).[100] Resection is indicated for early-stage tumors. Adjuvant therapy may be helpful for tumors with high-risk histological features, but its benefit is unproven. Advanced-stage tumors are treated with multimodality therapy.

Tumors of the Paraganglion System

Paragangliomas are catecholamine-producing tumors that arise from sites outside the adrenal gland and are often referred to as extraadrenal pheochromocytomas. Less than 2% of all pheochromocytomas are found in the mediastinum, and not all of these are functional. Although most pheochromocytomas of adrenal gland origin produce both epinephrine and norepinephrine, paragangliomas, including those in the mediastinum, rarely produce epinephrine. Chemodectomas are paragangliomas that are derived from arteries or nerves of branchial arch origin. They are found most often in relation to the carotid body but can also occur in the visceral compartment of the mediastinum. Workup of a suspected paraganglioma should include determination of serum catecholamines, urinary VMA and metanephrine, and MIBG scintigraphy to localize the primary lesion and evaluate for metastases. Metastatic disease from paragangliomas is rare, and primary therapy is complete resection. Radiotherapy with ^{131}I-MIBG has been proposed but should be limited to only those patients whose tumors are demonstrated by MIBG scintigraphy and for whom resection is not feasible.

Thymus

Myasthenia Gravis

Our recognition of the link between the thymus gland and myasthenia gravis (MG) is a consequence of both careful observation and serendipity, and our understanding of the mechanisms underlying this relationship remains incomplete. Myasthenia gravis is an autoimmune disorder of neuromuscular transmission that is characterized by progressive loss of skeletal muscle strength with sustained activity. Antibodies against the acetylcholine receptor (AChR) can be found in 80% of patients with the clinical syndrome and are presumed to mediate the disease by attenuating signal intensity across the neuromuscular junction and hence the strength of muscular contractions. A clinical diagnosis can be made by demonstrating that repetitive exercise produces fatigue of voluntary muscles that resolves with rest. The definitive diagnosis, however, depends on electrophysiological testing and the demonstration of a decremental response of skeletal muscle to repetitive stimuli.

The clinical course is unpredictable, with gradual progression of disease seen in most patients but approximately 10% experiencing spontaneous complete remission.[101,102] Disease severity is usually classified according to the Osserman scale (Table 75.7). Alternatively, disease severity can be graded as ocular, spinal, or bulbar. The prevalence of MG is between 5 and 15 per 100,000, with a female-to-male ratio of almost 2:1.[101,102] Although it can develop at any age, the peak incidence for women is in the third and fourth decades, and for men it is over the age of 50 years. Thymomas are found in approximately 13% of patients presenting with MG (Table 75.8).[103–106]

Primary medical therapy is with acetylcholinesterase inhibitors to increase acetylcholine concentration at the neuromuscular junction and with steroids and cytotoxic drugs to suppress the anti-AChR immune response. Plasmapheresis can be used for severe disease. Although in 1934 Walker first discovered the therapeutic potential of acetylcholinesterase

TABLE 75.7. Osserman Classification for Severity of Myasthenia Gravis.

Class	*Definition*
I	Ocular involvement only (e.g., diplopia, ptosis)
IIA	Generalized muscular involvement without respiratory impairment
IIB	More bulbar manifestations than IIA
III	Rapid onset and progression of bulbar and generalized disease with respiratory muscle weakness
IV	Severe generalized weakness, progressive myasthenic symptoms
V	Muscle atrophy, need for mechanical ventilatory support

Source: From Osserman and Genkins (1971).[103]

TABLE 75.8.
Prevalence of Thymoma in Patients with Myasthenia Gravis (MG).

	All patients			Thymectomy		
Study	*n*	*Number with MG*	*%*	*n*	*Number with MG*	*%*
Papatestas et al. (1987)[104]	2062	226	11	962	174	18
Cosi et al. (1997)[105]	438	92	21	280	92	33
Beekman et al. (1997)[106]	100	12	12	56	12	21
Robertson et al. (1998)[102]	100	12	12	34	12	35
Total	2700	342	13	1332	290	22

inhibitors,[107] the use of these drugs was not popularized until 1954 when Osserman introduced pyridostigmine bromide (Mestinon).[108] The first suggestion of a link between MG and the thymus was made by Hoppe[109] and Weigert[110] at the turn of the century, who independently reported on finding anterior mediastinal masses in patients who died of MG. However, it was not until 1913 that Sauerbruch and Roth performed the first thymectomy on a patient with MG.[111] A 49-g thymoma was removed, and the patient's symptoms improved although did not completely resolve. Although Sauerbruch and Roth's two subsequent patients died of postoperative complications, von Haberer successfully removed a normal thymus from a 27-year-old man with MG and reported 3 years later, in 1917, that the patient's symptoms were better.[112] That same year Bell, from the University of Minnesota, collected a series of 56 patients who died of MG; 27 were found to have a thymoma.[113] Mounting evidence implicating the thymus led Blalock, in 1936, to perform what is generally considered the first thymectomy intended as treatment for MG. Within 1 year, his patient had a near-complete remission, and in 1939 following publication of this result,[114] Blalock undertook a series of thymectomies for MG in 20 patients.[115] His observation that the best results were achieved with total thymectomy early in the course of the disease remains valid today.

The precise mechanisms underlying the role of the thymus gland in the pathophysiology of MG are not completely understood, and a detailed discussion of this subject is beyond the scope of this chapter. The principal role of AChR antibodies has been confirmed in animal models of the disease.[116] Furthermore, the ability to identify these in the serum of most patients and the clinical improvement seen following plasmapheresis provide strong supporting evidence. The possible origin of these antibodies in the thymus can be traced to the presence of thymic myoid cells (TMCs). These cells express AChRs and can be found in the normal thymus. In glands from normal patients, germinal centers rarely contain TMCs. In contrast, TMCs are frequently found in close proximity to antigen-presenting cells in the germinal centers of glands from patients with MG.[117,118]

Although well established as appropriate therapy, the precise role of thymectomy in the management of patients with MG is debated between neurologists and surgeons. This controversy is difficult to resolve because there are no prospective studies comparing medical therapy alone to medical therapy plus thymectomy and because in some patients the disease may stabilize, improve, or even undergo spontaneous complete remission. Buckingham and colleagues[119] from the Mayo Clinic published the first large series addressing the role of thymectomy. They performed a retrospective analysis of 80 patients who had undergone thymectomy compared with 80 patients managed with medical therapy alone. The medically treated patients were matched with the surgically treated patients for age, sex, and severity and duration of disease. Mean follow-up was 20 years. Their results indicated that thymectomy was associated with lower mortality, more complete remissions, and a higher rate of symptom improvement. Advances in medical therapy have substantially reduced mortality overall, but more recent studies have confirmed that patients undergoing thymectomy do better.[102,104–106] Shorter duration of disease, less-severe disease, and no thymoma predict improved prognosis following thymectomy. In a retrospective review of 756 patients, of whom 64% had thymectomy, multivariate analysis found that only age at onset of symptoms (<40 years) and thymectomy were associated with complete stable remission.[120]

Controversy exists regarding the appropriate technique of thymectomy. Because removal of all thymic tissue is a prerequisite to optimal results, Jaretzki et al. advocated a "maximal" approach that combines a cervical incision and dissection with a mediastinal dissection from phrenic nerve to phrenic nerve and diaphragm to innominate vein.[121] Alternatively, Cooper and others[122] described a transcervical approach, facilitated by a specialized retractor to elevate the sternum. They argued that complete thymectomy can be performed through this approach, and that the small, cosmetically acceptable cervical incision is more palatable to the patients with mild disease who stand to benefit the most from thymectomy. Most recently, VATS has been used, and follow-up is now long enough that results can be evaluated.

Comparisons between approaches are difficult for several reasons: (1) all studies are retrospective; (2) few centers report experience with more than one technique; (3) response to thymectomy improves with time, making differences in follow-up intervals confounding; (4) patient groups differ between studies with respect to the important prognostic variables; (5) some studies include poor-prognosis patients with thymoma; and (6) classification schemes for documenting disease severity and response to therapy are not uniform between studies. Nevertheless, overall results from experienced centers are similar for maximal, transcervical, median sternotomy and VATS approaches (Table 75.9).[123–134]

Regardless of approach, however, all agree that complete removal of the entire gland is a prerequisite for good results, and therefore choice of technique should be governed principally by the surgeon's experience and confidence. In a direct, albeit retrospective, comparison between a "basic" and an "extended" thymectomy, both performed through a median sternotomy, Zielinski and colleagues found that the extended approach was associated with a stable 20% absolute improvement in complete remission rates compared to the basic approach. This benefit was seen from 1 through 4 years of follow-up.[135] An extended mediastinal dissection through a median sternotomy with or without a cervical incision is indicated as the procedure of choice, with the transcervical

TABLE 75.9.
Results of Thymectomy for Myasthenia Gravis (Level III Evidence).

Study	Year	n	Median follow-up (years)	Complete response n	Complete response (%)	Partial response n	Partial response (%)	Total benefit n	Total benefit (%)	Comment
Median sternotomy										
Glinjongol et al.[123]	2004	30	3.5	12	(40)	12	(40)	24	(80)	
Roth et al.[124]	2002	26	13	6	(23)	7	(27)	13	(50)	Authors noted late relapses compared to an earlier report on the same patients
Masaoka et al.[125]	1996	194	5	89	(46)	90	(46)	179	(92)	CR = 67% (39/58) at 15-year follow-up
Frist et al.[126]	1994	42	6.3	14	(33)	15	(36)	29	(69)	
Nussbaum et al.[127]	1992	42	4.3	17	(40)	24	(57)	41	(98)	
Mulder et al.[128]	1989	84	3.6	30	(36)	37	(44)	67	(80)	
Maximal										
Jaretzki et al.[120]	1988	72	3.3	33	(46)	36	(50)	69	(96)	CR = 62% at 7.4-year follow-up (n not given; 72 implied)[160]
Transcervical										
Shrager et al.[129]	2002	78	4.6	32	(41)	39	(50)	71	(91)	
Calhoun et al.[130]	1999	52	8.4	23	(44)	24	(46)	47	(90)	
Bril et al.[131]	1998	52	8.4	23	(44)	23	(44)	46	(88)	
DeFillipi et al.[132]	1994	21	>5	9	(43)	8	(38)	17	(81)	
VATS										
Savcenko et al.[133]	2002	36	4.4	5	(14)	25	(69)	30	(83)	
Mineo et al.[134]	2000	31	3.3	8	(26)	22	(71)	30	(97)	

CR, complete response.

and VATS approaches reserved for those with demonstrated expertise in their use. If a thymoma is present, the transcervical approach should not be used. For patients with advanced disease and the potential for respiratory compromise from respiratory muscle weakness, perioperative management should include plasmapheresis both to minimize steroid use and to lower the risk of needing postoperative ventilatory support.

Thymic Epithelial Tumors

The normal thymus gland is composed largely of germinal centers that contain epithelial cells and lymphocytes. Maturing lymphocytes migrate from the medulla to the cortex of the germinal center along the epithelial cell scaffolding. Interaction with epithelial cells is critical for this maturation process. Thymomas and thymic carcinomas are tumors of the thymic epithelial cell. These tumors also contain lymphocytes, but the lymphocytes are benign and do not contribute to the neoplastic behavior of the tumor. In thymomas, the majority of the lymphocytes exhibit an immature phenotype ($CD4^+CD8^+$), suggesting that there is preservation of the epithelial cell biology despite the neoplastic process. In contrast, lymphocytes found in thymic carcinomas are mature "tumor-infiltrating lymphocytes" akin to what is seen with carcinomas of other tissue origin.

The biologic and histologic variability of thymic epithelial cell tumors has led to multiple, confusing classification schemes. Until recently, the histologic subtype of thymomas was based either on the relative abundance of epithelial cells and lymphocytes (epithelial, lymphocytic, mixed, and spindle)[136] or on the morphology of the neoplastic epithelial cell (cortical, medullary, or mixed).[137] Furthermore, neither system included the histologically and biologically distinct thymic carcinoma. However, in 1999 the World Health Organization (WHO) published a new scheme (Table 75.10) that incorporates elements of both preexisting systems and includes a category for thymic carcinoma (type C).[138–144] This scheme is being widely adopted and provides clarity and uniformity to a previously confused field.

Thymoma

Thymoma is the most common neoplasm of the anterior mediastinum and the most common mediastinal lesion in adults (Fig. 75.7). It is rare in children. Most thymomas are found incidentally, but approximately 30% of patients present with MG (Table 75.11). In contrast only 13% of patients with MG are found to have a thymoma (Table 75.8). Other associated autoimmune syndromes include red and white blood cell aplasia, hypogammaglobulinemia, systemic lupus erythematosus, dermatomyositis, and rheumatoid arthritis. Although a TNM staging system is available for thymomas, the Masaoka system is preferred (Table 75.12). Prognosis for patients with thymoma is relatively good. Both Masaoka stage and histologic classification based on the new WHO criteria are independent predictors of survival (Fig. 75.8).[145–148]

Most thymomas are well encapsulated and are clinically benign. These tumors are often called *benign thymomas*. This categorization misrepresents the true nature of these tumors and ignores the potential for continued growth, capsular invasion, and metastasis; more accurately, they should be classified as Masaoka stage I thymomas. Thymomas with evidence of either gross or microscopic capsular invasion

TABLE 75.10. World Health Organization Histologic Classification System for Thymic Epithelial Tumors.

Type	*Definition*
A	A tumor composed of a homogeneous population of neoplastic epithelial cells with spindle/oval shape, lacking nuclear atypia, and accompanied by few or no nonneoplastic lymphocytes.
AB	A tumor in which foci with the features of type A thymoma are admixed with foci rich in lymphocytes; the segregation of two patterns can be sharp or indistinct.
B1	A tumor that resembles the normal functional thymus in that it combines large expanses that have an appearance practically indistinguishable from that of normal thymic cortex with areas resembling thymic medulla.
B2	A tumor in which the neoplastic epithelial component appears as scattered plump cells with vesicular nuclei and distinct nucleoli among a heavy population of lymphocytes; perivascular spaces are common and sometimes very prominent. A perivascular arrangement of tumor cells resulting in a palisading effect may be seen.
B3	A tumor comprised predominantly of epithelial cells with a round or polygonal shape and exhibiting mild atypia admixed with a minor component of lymphocytes; foci of squamous metaplasia and perivascular spaces are common.
C	A thymic tumor exhibiting clear-cut cytologic atypia and a set of cytoarchitectural features no longer specific to the thymus, but rather analogous to those seen in carcinomas of other organs. Type C thymomas lack immature lymphocytes; whatever lymphocytes may be present are mature and usually admixed with plasma cell.

Source: From Rosai and Levine[136] by permission of American Registry of Pathology, Washington, DC 2001.

TABLE 75.11. Prevalence of Myasthenia Gravis (MG) in Patients with Thymoma.

Study	*Year*	*n*	*Number with MG*	*%*
Cowen et al.[139]	1995	149	21	14
Blumberg et al.[89]	1995	118	12	10
Regnard et al.[140]	1996	307	195	64
Venuta et al.[141]	1997	65	24	37
Gripp et al.[142]	1998	70	12	17
Kondo et al.[143]	2005	1089	270	25
Total		1798	534	30

exhibit more malignant behavior and carry a less-favorable prognosis. These tumors are histologically indistinguishable from their benign-behaving counterparts but can be locally aggressive, invading adjacent mediastinal structures and lung. Metastases occur late and predominantly through contiguous spread to pericardium and pleura, although pulmonary metastases are seen occasionally. Hematogenous metastasis is uncommon, and lymphogenous metastasis is rare.

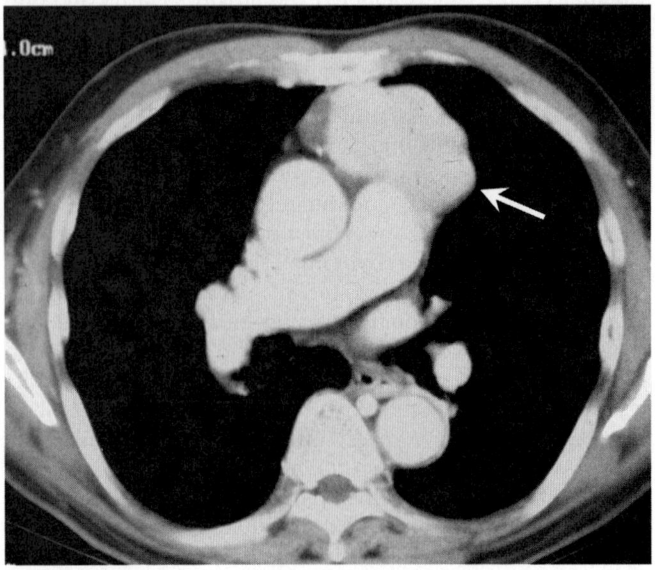

FIGURE 75.7. Thymoma. A 58-year-old man presented with a cough. Chest CT demonstrated a homogeneous anterior mediastinal mass with well-defined borders (arrow). Needle biopsy confirmed a thymoma, and the patient received chemotherapy followed by thymectomy. Final pathology showed evidence of capsular invasion (Masaoka stage II).

Treatment for thymoma is primarily surgical, with complete resection the critical factor in determining long-term survival. Wide resection should be performed, taking all anterior mediastinal tissue from phrenic nerve to phrenic nerve and diaphragm to innominate vein. The pericardium is not routinely removed but should be excised if there is a suggestion of tumor invasion into it. Invasive tumors should be resected en bloc if possible as even in the setting of extensive local invasion requiring reconstruction of major vascular structures such as the SVC and pulmonary artery complete resection remains the strongest predictor of a favorable outcome.[147] One *but not both* phrenic nerves may be sacrificed if complete resection cannot be achieved otherwise. Radiation therapy is not indicated following complete resection of an encapsulated thymoma (Masaoka stage I) but may be considered for patients with stage II disease when tumor approaches or involves the surgical margin.

Recent evidence supports the use of preoperative chemotherapy for patients with stage II or III thymoma (Table 75.13). Venuta and colleagues[141] stratified patients by histology and Masaoka stage. This study pre-dated introduction of the WHO classification, so the authors classified tumors based on the Muller-Hermelink system.[137] Patients with highly invasive tumors that were not considered resectable at initial evaluation received neoadjuvant therapy with cisplatin, epirubicin, and etoposide. All patients underwent surgery, with wide excision of tumor when possible. Adjuvant chemotherapy and radiotherapy were administered to all patients with stage II and above tumors or with stage I cortical thymoma. Results

TABLE 75.12. Masaoka Staging System for Thymoma.

Stage	*Definition*
I	Macroscopically: completely encapsulated Microscopically: no capsular invasion
II	Macroscopic invasion into surrounding fatty tissue or mediastinal pleura Microscopic invasion into capsule
III	Macroscopic invasion into neighboring organ (i.e., pericardium, great vessels, or lung)
IVA	Pleural or pericardial dissemination
IVB	Lymphogenous or hematogenous metastasis

Source: Masaoka et al.[144]

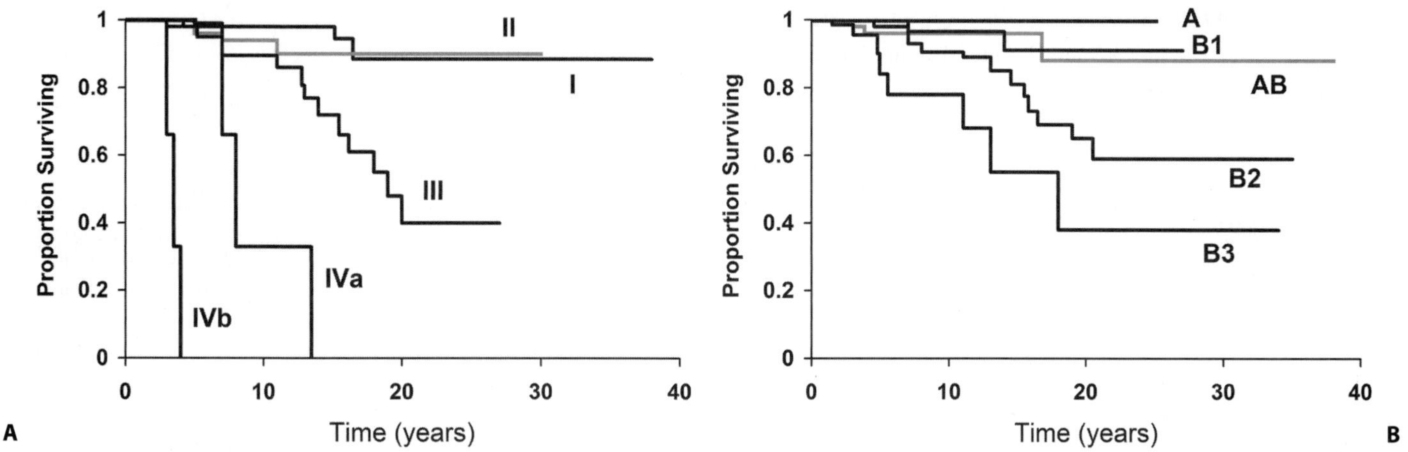

FIGURE 75.8. Survival from tumor death for patients with thymoma. Results from retrospective analysis of 273 patients over a 44-year period at a single institution. All patients underwent thymectomy. Non-tumor-related deaths were censored, so survival is survival from tumor death. **A.** Masaoka stage (number of patients by stage: I = 111; II = 64; III = 56; IVa = 7; IVb = 5). **B.** WHO histologic type (number of patients by type: A = 17; AB = 66; B1 = 49; B2 = 89; B3 = 22). (From Okumura et al.,[145] with permission.)

demonstrated improved resectability rates and improvement in survival at 8-year follow-up for all stages compared to historical controls. Both Shin and colleagues[149] and Kim and colleagues[150] published similar findings from prospective studies of 12 and 22 patients with advanced-stage thymoma, respectively. Induction chemotherapy with cyclophosphamide, cisplatin, doxorubicin, and prednisone produced overall response rates of 92% and 77%, respectively, and improved resectability. All patients received postoperative radiation therapy and consolidation chemotherapy. Five-year survival rates were 100% and 95%, respectively, considerably higher than expected from historical data.

For patients with advanced-stage thymoma (unresectable stage III or stage IV), chemotherapy and radiation therapy is

TABLE 75.13.
Multimodality Treatment for Invasive Thymoma (Phase II Trials, Level II Evidence).

Study	*Year*	*Regimen*	*Median follow-up (years)*	*Stage*[a]	*n*	*Treatment*	*RR (%)*	*Survival (%) 3 yr*	*5 yr*	*8 yr*	*Comments/conclusions*
Kim et al.[149]	2004	PACP	4.2	III	11	CT • resection • CT + RT	77		95	79[b]	Induction CT leads to high resectability rates and long-term survival
				IV	11						
Shin et al.[150]	1998	PACP	3.6	III	4	CT • resection • CT + RT	92	100	100		CT regimen highly effective
				IV	8						Multimodality therapy improves survival for patients with stage III or IV disease
Venuta et al.[141]	1997	PEpE	4.4	II	27	Historical control	100	90	82	77	CT highly effective.
					19	Resection • CT + RT		100	100	100	Adjuvant CT + RT improves survival for patients with stage II disease
				III	27	Historical control		55	48	40	
					12	CT • resection • CT + RT		92	92		
				IV	9	Historical control		55	42	33	Multimodality therapy improves survival for patients with stage III or IV disease
					13	CT • resection • CT + RT		68	68		
Rea et al.[151]	1993	ADRC	2.4	III	13	CT • resection ± RT	100	67	53		CT regimen highly effective
				IV	3			33	33		Induction CT feasible and promising

ADRC, doxorubicin, cisplatin, vincristine, and cyclophosphamide; CT, chemotherapy; PACP, cisplatin, doxorubicin, cyclophosphamide, and prednisone; PEpE, cisplatin, epirubicin, and etoposide; RR, response rate (complete response + partial response) to chemotherapy; RT, radiation therapy.

[a]Masaoka staging system used predominantly.

[b]7-year survival.

TABLE 75.14.
Combination Chemotherapy for Advanced or Recurrent Thymic Tumors (Level II Evidence).

Study	*Year*	*Regimen*	*Median follow-up (years)*	*n*	*RR (%)*	*Median Survival (years)*	*Comments*
Loehrer et al.[152]	2004	Octreotide ± prednisone	Not given	38	32	>3	0/5 PR thymic carcinoma 0/1 PR thymic carcinoid
Palmieri et al.[153]	2002	Octreotide ± prednisone	3.6	16	37	1.3	1/3 PR thymic carcinoma 1/3 PR thymic carcinoid
Loehrer et al.[154]	2001	VIP	3.6	28	32	2.6	2/8 PR thymic carcinoma
Highley et al.[155]	1999	Ifosfamide	Not given	13	46	4.3	Advanced disease
Loehrer et al.[156]	1997	PAC + RT	(1.2–9.2)	23	70	7.8	Limited disease
Giaccone et al.[157]	1996	PE	7	16	56	4.3	Advanced disease
Loehrer et al.[158]	1994	PAC	3	30	50	3.1	Advanced disease

PAC, cisplatin, doxorubicin, and cyclophosphamide; PE, cisplatin and etoposide; PR, partial response; RR, response rate (complete response + partial response) to chemotherapy; RT, radiation therapy; VIP, etoposide, ifosfamide, and cisplatin.

the mainstay of treatment (Table 75.14).[152–158] Recent reports also suggest a potential role for octreotide therapy in appropriately selected patients.[152,153] The role of surgery is controversial. It is only appropriate if complete resection or near-complete debulking can be achieved with acceptable morbidity. Similarly, reresection of recurrent or metastatic disease may be of benefit for highly selected patients. The success of this strategy is dependent on the low propensity for thymoma to metastasize through hematogenous and lymphogenous routes.

Thymic Carcinoma

Thymic carcinomas (Fig. 75.9) are often confused with thymomas, but they are distinct neoplasms that, unlike thymomas, exhibit malignant cytological features and are very aggressive.[159,160] According to the new WHO system, they are now classified as type C thymic epithelial tumors. They often present with extensive local invasion, and imaging reveals areas of necrosis, hemorrhage, calcification, or cyst formation.[161] Their biology is distinct from thymomas and more like other carcinomas in that hematogenous and lymphogenous metastases are common. There is a high incidence of extrathoracic metastases, and the prognosis is very poor. Few patients survive 5 years. Chemotherapy and radiation therapy have limited benefit (Table 75.14), and treatment is wide excision if possible.

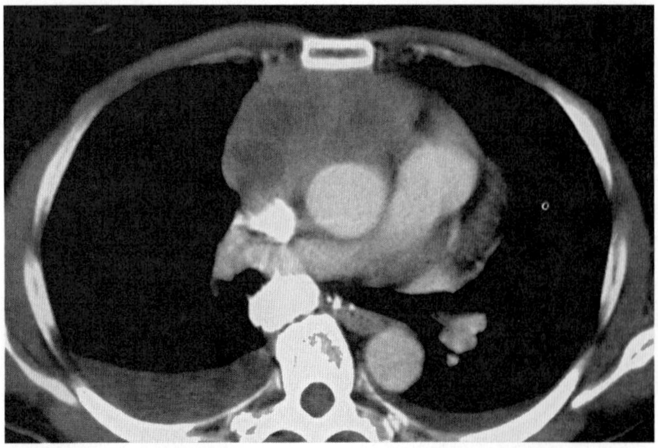

FIGURE 75.9. Thymic carcinoma. Computed tomograph of a patient who presented with chest pain and cough. Note the heterogeneity of the lesion and bilateral pleural effusions. Fine-needle aspiration suggested thymic carcinoma. Induction chemotherapy produced only a minimal response, and at operation the tumor was found to invade lung, pericardium, and myocardium with pericardial metastases.

Other Thymic Tumors

Thymic carcinoid tumors are more common in men than women and are strongly associated with the multiple endocrine neoplasia syndromes.[162,163] Like carcinoids elsewhere, they are derived from Kulchitsky cells of neural crest origin; however, thymic carcinoid tumors have a higher incidence of invasiveness (approximately 50%), and up to 60% will develop regional nodal metastases.[164] Carcinoid syndrome has not been reported with thymic carcinoids, but they can produce ACTH and cause Cushing's syndrome.[163] The octreoscan may be helpful in making the diagnosis.[162] Treatment is by complete resection. Adjuvant radiation therapy has been used to control residual disease, but this is of no proven benefit. Recurrences have been documented late following initial resection,[163] suggesting that regional lymph node dissection should be considered at the time of resection. Octreotide therapy has had disappointing results (Table 75.14).

Thymolipoma is a rare anterior mediastinal mass of mesenchymal origin. It is benign and should be resected to confirm the diagnosis and to prevent complications from growth.[165] *Thymic cyst* is a descriptive term that refers to a variety of lesions of congenital, inflammatory, or neoplastic origin. Occasionally, thymic cysts are seen following therapeutic responses to medical treatment of germ cell tumors or thymoma. Thymic cysts are also seen in patients with human immunodeficiency virus (HIV) infection.

Germ Cell Tumors

Fewer than 5% of all germ cell tumors are found in the mediastinum. They are thought to arise from primordial germ cells that migrate from the urogenital ridge into the mediastinum and thymus gland during embryogenesis, and almost all are found in the anterior compartment. Approximately half of all mediastinal germ cell tumors are benign (teratomas), and although some authors have reported that teratomas are equally prevalent in men and women,[166,167] others have documented either a marked female[168] or male[169] predominance. The peak incidence is during the second through fourth decades of life. Malignant tumors are further classified as either seminomas or nonseminomatous lesions and are much more common in men than women. Until recently, most malignant germ cell tumors were thought to be metastases from occult primary gonadal lesions. It is now believed, however, that solitary metastases to the anterior mediastinum are an exception, and that metastatic disease to the mediastinum typically involves multiple sites, especially lymph nodes in the visceral compartment.[170] As a result, testicular biopsy is not routine and should be performed only if abnormalities are identified on physical examination or ultrasound.

The treatment of malignant germ cell tumors is primarily nonsurgical. Seminomas are very responsive to chemotherapy and radiotherapy and have a good prognosis, but NSGCTs respond less well and carry a less-favorable prognosis. Clinical presentation, radiographic appearance, and serology suggest the diagnosis. Serum AFP and β-HCG levels should be determined for all young male patients with anterior mediastinal masses, and if negative, FNA, open biopsy, or excisional biopsy should be considered.

Benign Germ Cell Tumors

Benign tumors are classified as epidermoid cysts, dermoid cysts (teratodermoids), or mature teratomas. These lesions originate from pluripotent stem cells and characteristically contain multiple tissue elements derived from one or more of the three embryonic germ cell layers. Epidermoid cysts are lined by simple squamous epithelium, while teratodermoids also contain epidermal appendages such as hair follicles and sebaceous glands. Mature teratomas have both soft tissue and cystic components that contain well-differentiated elements from two or more germinal layers. Thus, they may contain a remarkable variety of tissues, such as bone, cartilage, teeth, liver, pancreas, lung, nerve, muscle, and salivary glands. On close examination, most lesions contain tissues derived from more than one germinal layer and therefore are classified as teratomas.

Although most teratomas are benign, as many as 20% may contain elements of undifferentiated primitive embryonic tissue.[168,169] These tumors are considered malignant and are classified as malignant teratomas or teratocarcinomas. Approximately 75% of patients with teratomas present with symptoms such as chest pain, dyspnea, or cough.[166,167,169] Rarely, the cystic components become infected by hematogenous spread and may rupture into the pericardium or pleura, causing tamponade, chest pain, acute respiratory distress, or empyema. Communication with the airway can lead to the dramatic and pathognomonic presentation of trichoptysis, cough productive of hair and sebaceous material.[167]

Rarely, if teeth are present, the diagnosis can be made by chest x-ray. More often, however, CT suggests the diagnosis, demonstrating a heterogeneous anterior mediastinal mass containing soft tissue, fat, and fluid-filled cystic components.[166] Calcification is common and may be seen as globular collections, bone, or teeth. Suspected teratomas should be resected, both as definitive therapy and to ensure that malignant tumors are not missed. Even incomplete resection of a benign lesion is associated with an excellent prognosis, and therefore vital structures should not be sacrificed to achieve complete resection. Adjuvant radiotherapy is not indicated.

Seminoma

From one-third to one-half of malignant mediastinal germ cell tumors are seminomas.[171,172] They are almost exclusively found in men between the ages of 20 and 40 years and are characterized by extensive local invasion. Extrathoracic disease is uncommon, with metastatic spread occurring first through regional lymphatics. Distant metastases are an uncommon and late finding. Up to 70% of patients present with symptoms related to mass effect, local invasion, or both.[173] Constitutional symptoms such as weight loss, lethargy, and fever are also common. Advanced disease can present with SVC syndrome. Chest x-ray and CT typically reveal a large, homogeneous anterior mediastinal mass. If the patient is a young man, the diagnosis of a germ cell tumor should be suspected, and as with all anterior mediastinal masses in young men, serum AFP and β-HCG should be determined. These levels are normal in virtually all patients with pure seminomas but may be elevated if the tumor contains nonseminomatous elements.

Definitive diagnosis is made by FNA or open biopsy. Small, localized tumors may be resected, but because most will have extensive local invasion at the time of diagnosis, resection is usually not feasible. Debulking or attempts at extensive resection are not indicated. Fortunately, seminomas are very sensitive to both radiation therapy and platinum-based chemotherapy (Fig. 75.10), and treatment is associated with a good prognosis. Resection of persistent or residual abnormalities following treatment is not indicated. Recent reports using combination chemoradiotherapy have suggested that long-term survival may approach 100%.[171,172]

Nonseminomatous Germ Cell Tumors

The designation of NSGCT refers to a collection of malignant germ cell tumors that includes embryonal cell carcinomas, teratocarcinomas, choriocarcinomas, and yolk sac (endodermal sinus) tumors. Although most NSGCTs are pure and exhibit histology of only one type, many have elements from more than one type and are classified as mixed. As a group, these lesions may be slightly more common than seminomas and like seminomas are anterior mediastinal masses found almost exclusively in young men.[172,174,175] However, compared to seminomas, they are more aggressive, are more likely to metastasize to extrathoracic sites, and are less sensitive to therapy. Most patients present with constitutional findings of weight loss, fatigue, or fever and symptoms caused by compression or invasion of mediastinal structures. Imaging usually reveals a large tumor with heterogeneous consistency and evidence of local invasion (Fig. 75.11). Furthermore, almost all patients have metastases at the time of diagnosis.[175,176] In contrast to seminomas, most NSGCTs produce β-HCG, AFP, or both, and more than 90% of patients have elevated levels in their serum.[79] This finding is both sensitive and specific and is considered sufficiently diagnostic to initi-

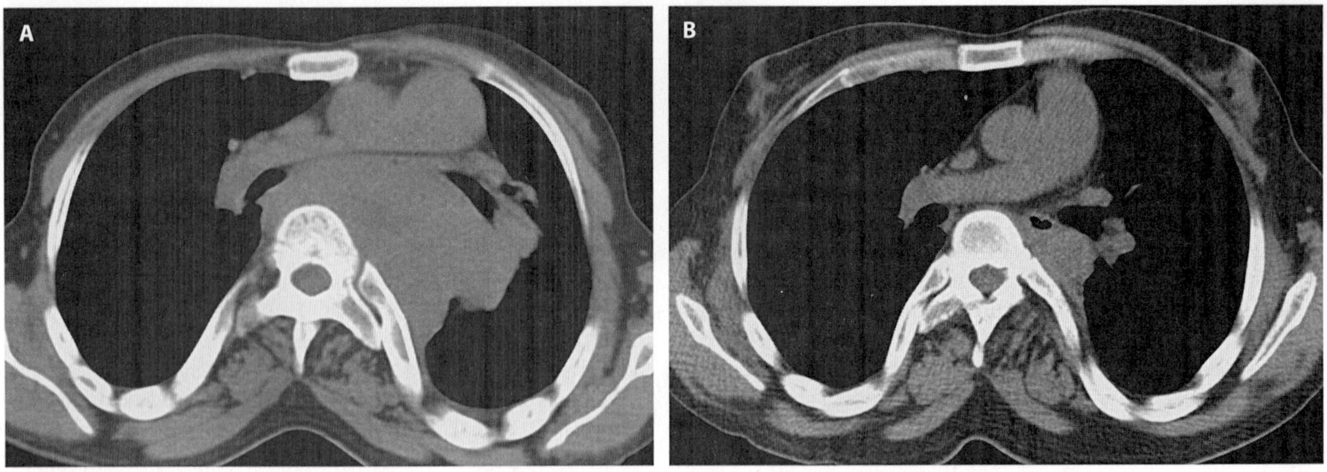

FIGURE 75.10. Mediastinal seminoma. A 47-year-old man presented with chest pain, dyspnea, stridor, dysphagia, and a 30-pound weight loss. A. Chest CT shows a large mediastinal tumor encasing the descending thoracic aorta and displacing the esophagus and mainstem bronchi. Needle biopsy suggested granulomatous inflammation. Serum AFP was 5.3 ng/mL (normal 0–20), and β-HCG was 21 mIU/mL (normal 0–4). Thoracoscopic biopsy confirmed the diagnosis of seminoma. B. Follow-up CT at completion of therapy shows near-complete response. (Reprinted from Block,[195] with permission.)

ate therapy without biopsy confirmation. Increased levels of β-HCG can lead to gynecomastia in men and, presumably through secondary induction of testosterone production by the testes, precocious puberty in boys.[177] NSGCTs have been associated with Klinefelter's syndrome (XXY).[174,177,178]

The NSGCTs are resistant to radiotherapy, and local invasiveness and metastases at the time of diagnosis typically preclude resection. As a consequence, the primary therapeutic modality is platinum-based chemotherapy.[171,174] Response to therapy can be assessed by following AFP and β-HCG levels. If these levels normalize and the tumor has responded completely, no further therapy is indicated. If a residual mass is identified, however, resection is indicated. These residual tumors are often benign teratomas and indicate a good prognosis. Debulking procedures for tumors that are associated with persistently elevated serum markers are of unproven benefit.[171,179] Overall, 5-year survival is between 40% and 70%.[171,172,174]

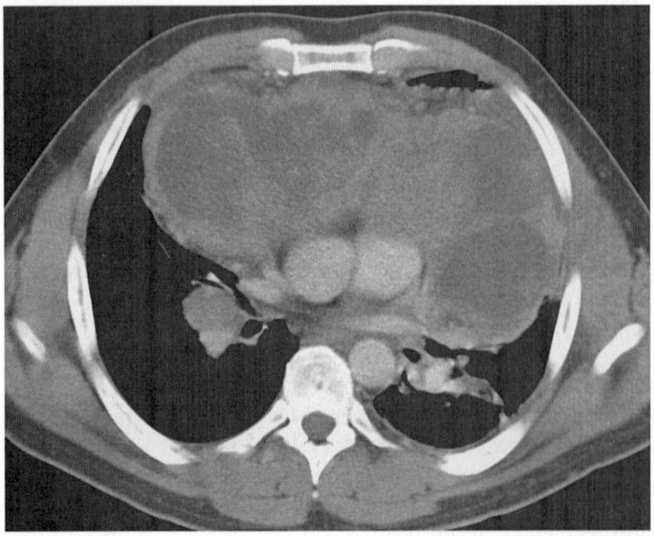

FIGURE 75.11. Nonseminomatous germ cell tumor. Chest CT of a 34-year-old man who presented with cough and chest pain. Serum AFP was 9907 (normal 0–20) and β-HCG was 4654 (normal 0–4). Needle biopsy confirmed the diagnosis of NSGCT. Note the tumor heterogeneity, suggestive of the diagnosis.

Lymphoma

Primary lymphomas of the mediastinum occur predominantly in the anterior compartment and are classified as either Hodgkin's disease or non-Hodgkin's lymphoma. Hodgkin's disease is a malignant tumor of B-cell origin and refers to a single disease, whereas the designation of non-Hodgkin's lymphoma refers to a large collection of lymphoblastic malignancies. Non-Hodgkin's lymphomas are further subdivided into indolent and aggressive forms. The incidence of Hodgkin's disease has a bimodal age distribution, with peak occurrences between 20 and 30 years of age and over 50 years of age. In contrast, the incidence of non-Hodgkin's lymphomas increases with age. Hodgkin's disease is characterized by local or contiguous spread and is more likely to involve the mediastinum. Non-Hodgkin's lymphomas are more diffuse, tend to be disseminated at the time of diagnosis, and less commonly involve the mediastinum. Because non-Hodgkin's lymphomas are approximately six times more common than Hodgkin's disease overall, they account for approximately two-thirds of all primary mediastinal lymphomas despite the greater propensity for Hodgkin's disease to involve the mediastinum.[80–82]

Mediastinal lymphomas usually present with symptoms. Rapidly growing tumors can produce cough, dyspnea, chest pain, stridor, and SVC syndrome. Systemic symptoms are also common. Weight loss, fever, and drenching night sweats are included in the staging criteria and are referred to as B symptoms. (The A classification indicates an absence of well-defined generalized symptoms.) Imaging typically demonstrates a large, heterogeneous, and irregularly shaped anterior mediastinal mass.

The surgeon's role in managing patients with mediastinal lymphoma is primarily to obtain tissue for diagnosis. Traditionally, needle biopsies have not provided adequate material or information about tissue architecture necessary to distinguish among the various types of lymphoma. Because subtyping is critical for planning therapy, more tissue is often required. If extrathoracic nodes are not available for biopsy, anterior mediastinoscopy is typically the procedure of choice (because most of these tumors are in the anterior and not visceral compartment). Cervical mediastinoscopy is performed if paratracheal or subcarinal nodes are involved. The need for surgical biopsies is declining, however, because the use of immunohistochemistry for cell-surface markers is increasingly able to subtype lymphomas from FNA specimens alone.[180] Furthermore, core needle biopsy, rather than FNA, is now more widely performed.

Lymphomas are staged based on the number and location of involved nodal regions and involvement of extralymphatic organs. Stage I disease is defined as disease limited to a single nodal region, and stage II disease involves two or more regions on the same side of the diaphragm. Disease present on both sides of the diaphragm, in the spleen, or in extralymphatic organs is classified as stage III, and disseminated disease is stage IV. Therapy for both Hodgkin's and Non-Hodgkin's lymphoma is guided by the extent of disease and consists of combinations of chemotherapy and radiation therapy. Further discussion of the pathology and therapy of lymphomas is beyond the scope of this chapter.

Congenital Cysts

True cystic lesions of the mediastinum are considered congenital rather than neoplastic abnormalities and can be divided into four major categories based on location and histological features of the cyst lining. *Foregut cysts* are derived from the primitive foregut structures that give rise to the lung and proximal digestive tract. They are lined either by respiratory or digestive tract epithelium and are classified as either bronchogenic or duplication cysts, respectively. Cysts lined by normal mesothelium are termed *pleuropericardial cysts* and are usually found at the cardiophrenic angle. *Neurenteric* cysts are found in the paravertebral sulcus and are derived from the meninges or dura. Some mediastinal cysts do not have a distinctive lining and by default are termed *unclassified*.

Cystic hygromas are congenital cystic masses that present in children and are typically located at the base of the neck and into the chest. These hygromas are more accurately termed lymphangiomas and are classified as mesenchymal tumors rather than as congenital cysts of the mediastinum.

Congenital cysts of the mediastinum are typically benign, although an occasional case report suggests the possibility of malignant degeneration.[181,182] The incidence of symptoms is highly variable, but in general symptoms are recognized as more common in the pediatric population. Local effects from the size of the lesion are the most common cause of symptoms such as cough, stridor, dyspnea, or chest discomfort. Larger cysts may produce dysphagia. Uncommonly, cysts become infected, either by hematogenous spread or as a consequence of communication with the airway. An important iatrogenic cause of infection is EUS-FNA. Duplication cysts that are lined with gastric mucosa may ulcerate and bleed. If the ulcer erodes through the cyst wall, presentation can be with hemoptysis, hematemesis, hemothorax, or pleural abscess.[83] Rapid increase in the size of the cyst from bleeding can lead to acute onset of mass-effect symptoms.

Diagnosis

Definitive diagnosis of mediastinal cysts depends ultimately on histological examination of the cyst lining, but imaging can provide important and sometimes diagnostic clues. The radiographic appearance of the lesion differentiates a true cyst from a cystic mass or other mediastinal lesion, and the location provides clues to a preliminary diagnosis. Although CT is used most often, MRI may be more helpful because its multiplanar imaging capabilities can facilitate identification of subtle communications between the cyst and the airway or pericardium. Endoscopic ultrasound can be used to visualize duplication cysts and may be helpful for planning resection, but FNA should not be performed because of the likelihood of contaminating a sterile cyst. This converts a benign, often asymptomatic, lesion into a source of symptomatic mediastinal infection that requires urgent surgery. Duplication cysts lined with gastric mucosa demonstrate activity with ^{99}Tc scintigraphy.

Foregut Cysts

Bronchogenic cysts are the most common form of congenital mediastinal cyst, constituting as many as 75% of this category in some series.[83] Furthermore, because bronchogenic cysts can occur anywhere along the proximal digestive tract, as many as 75% of presumed duplication cysts may actually be bronchogenic when the histology is examined.[83] The incidence of symptoms is highly variable.[183–186]

Bronchogenic cysts are most commonly found in the visceral compartment of the mediastinum adjacent to the trachea or bronchi or in the lung parenchyma (Fig. 75.12). They are

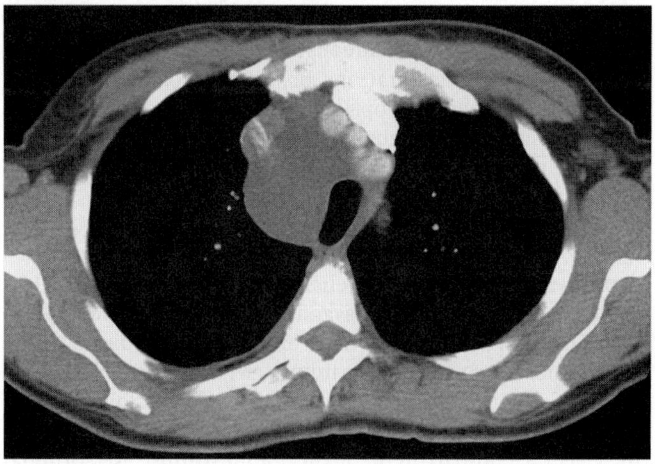

FIGURE 75.12. Bronchogenic Cyst. Chest CT of 72-year-old woman undergoing evaluation for thrombocytopenia. This lesion was discovered incidentally and was asymptomatic. Note that the lesion has smooth borders and is closely associated with the trachea. Hounsfield units were consistent with water density.

known for presenting in the subcarinal space, but in a series of 69 patients of all ages with mediastinal bronchogenic cysts, only 4 (6%) were found in this location.[185]

Bronchial compression by a cyst may produce distal hyperinflation of the lung and appear radiographically as congenital lobar emphysema. It is important to distinguish between this phenomenon and true congenital lobar emphysema so that unnecessary pulmonary resection can be avoided. Bronchogenic cysts can also occur along the esophagus, and may be diagnosed clinically as duplication cysts.

Diagnosis of a bronchogenic cyst rests on finding that the cyst lining is composed of characteristic ciliated respiratory epithelium. Duplication cysts, also known as esophageal duplication cysts or enterogenous cysts, are found alongside the esophagus at the boundary between the visceral and paravertebral compartments of the mediastinum. With enlargement, these cysts will migrate posteriorly and lie in the paravertebral sulcus. Rarely, they can be found in the retroperitoneum. Duplication cysts do not communicate with the esophageal lumen and are lined with esophageal, gastric, or intestinal mucosa. Foregut cysts are benign lesions, but malignant transformation has been reported.[181,182]

Many foregut cysts can be safely observed, but in most circumstances resection is indicated to alleviate symptoms, to prevent complications such as infection or airway compromise, and for definitive diagnosis. Location and size of the lesion determine the surgical approach. Resection is potentially hazardous because of dense adhesions that can make dissection difficult and bloody, and this should be kept in mind if a VATS approach is chosen. The conversion rate to thoracotomy is approximately 10% to 15%.[185–187]

In addition, bronchogenic cysts may be densely adherent to the airway and not amenable to separation from it. One technique for managing this finding is to leave a small portion of the cyst wall on the airway, being careful to ablate completely the mucosal lining to prevent recurrence.[185] Alternatively, a small portion of the airway can be resected and repaired,[188] but this may add unnecessarily to the morbidity of the procedure.

Duplication cysts may be embedded in the esophageal wall, and resection is accomplished by enucleation. Long, tubular cysts may require tedious dissection, and injury to the mucosa should be assiduously avoided.

Given these considerations, observation of an asymptomatic cyst is an acceptable option in appropriate circumstances. Decompression of foregut cysts should be done only as a temporizing measure and should not be considered definitive therapy as the cyst will undoubtedly recur.

Pleuropericardial Cysts

Pleuropericardial or mesothelial cysts are considerably less common than foregut cysts and are caused by incomplete fusion of the fetal lacunae that form the pericardium. Some communicate with the pericardium. Most mesothelial cysts are along the right heart border, one-third are along the left heart border, and the remainder are located centrally within the visceral compartment of the mediastinum. Mesothelial cysts are typically unilocular and contain clear, serous fluid. Radiographically they are round, radiodense, and homogeneous. On CT and MRI, characteristic findings of a simple cyst filled with homogeneous fluid of water density are demonstrated (Fig. 75.13).

Complications from mesothelial cysts such as rupture, cardiac tamponade, right ventricular wall impingement and erosion, bronchial compression, and sudden death have been reported but are rare. Malignant degeneration is exceedingly rare. Because imaging is typically diagnostic, resection is indicated only for symptomatic or enlarging lesions. As these lesions typically are not adherent to adjacent structures and are connected to the mediastinum only by a narrow stalk, VATS is an ideal approach. Often, this stalk originates near the phrenic nerve, so appropriate care should be taken to avoid injury to it.

Neurenteric Cysts

Neurenteric cysts are rare lesions that are thought to arise from the meninges and may communicate with the dural space. They are located in the posterior (paravertebral) compartment and are associated with vertebral column developmental abnormalities such as spina bifida and hemivertebra. Suspected neurenteric cysts should be studied with MRI to evaluate for spinal cord involvement. Resection is indicated.

Mesenchymal Tumors

Because the mediastinum contains a wide variety of tissues of mesenchymal origin, an extraordinary spectrum of mesenchymal tumors has been found there. These tumors occur in men and women with equal incidence, and approximately half are malignant. As with other mediastinal lesions, some are asymptomatic and discovered incidentally, whereas others may cause symptoms by mass effect or local invasion. Rarely, hypoglycemia has been associated with fibrosarcomas that produce an insulin-like hormone.

Lymphangiomas are benign tumors that are more commonly referred to as cystic hygromas. They are characteristically cystic masses derived from abnormal development of lymphatic vessels. More than 90% are diagnosed in children younger than 2 years of age,[189,190] and most arise in the neck. Isolated mediastinal lesions are rare.

The clinical course and management of mesenchymal tumors of the mediastinum are similar to that of mesenchymal tumors elsewhere in the body and are not detailed here.

Castleman's Disease

Also known as giant lymph node hyperplasia, Castleman's disease is a benign disorder of lymphoid proliferation that is often localized to the mediastinum and tends to occur in women in their third and fourth decades.[191,192] It usually presents as a solitary mass, but may be multicentric, and has been associated with HIV infection and Kaposi's sarcoma. Two-thirds are classified histologically as hyaline vascular and one-third as plasma cell types.[191,193] Castleman's disease is usually asymptomatic, but it is characterized by progressive enlargement of nodal tissue and can produce compression of mediastinal structures. Although the lesion is benign, the course of the disease may be fatal. Resection is the primary mode of therapy but can be challenging because of diffuse contiguous nodal involvement and extensive vascularity.[194] Radiation therapy has been recommended for patients with unresectable and multifocal disease.[192]

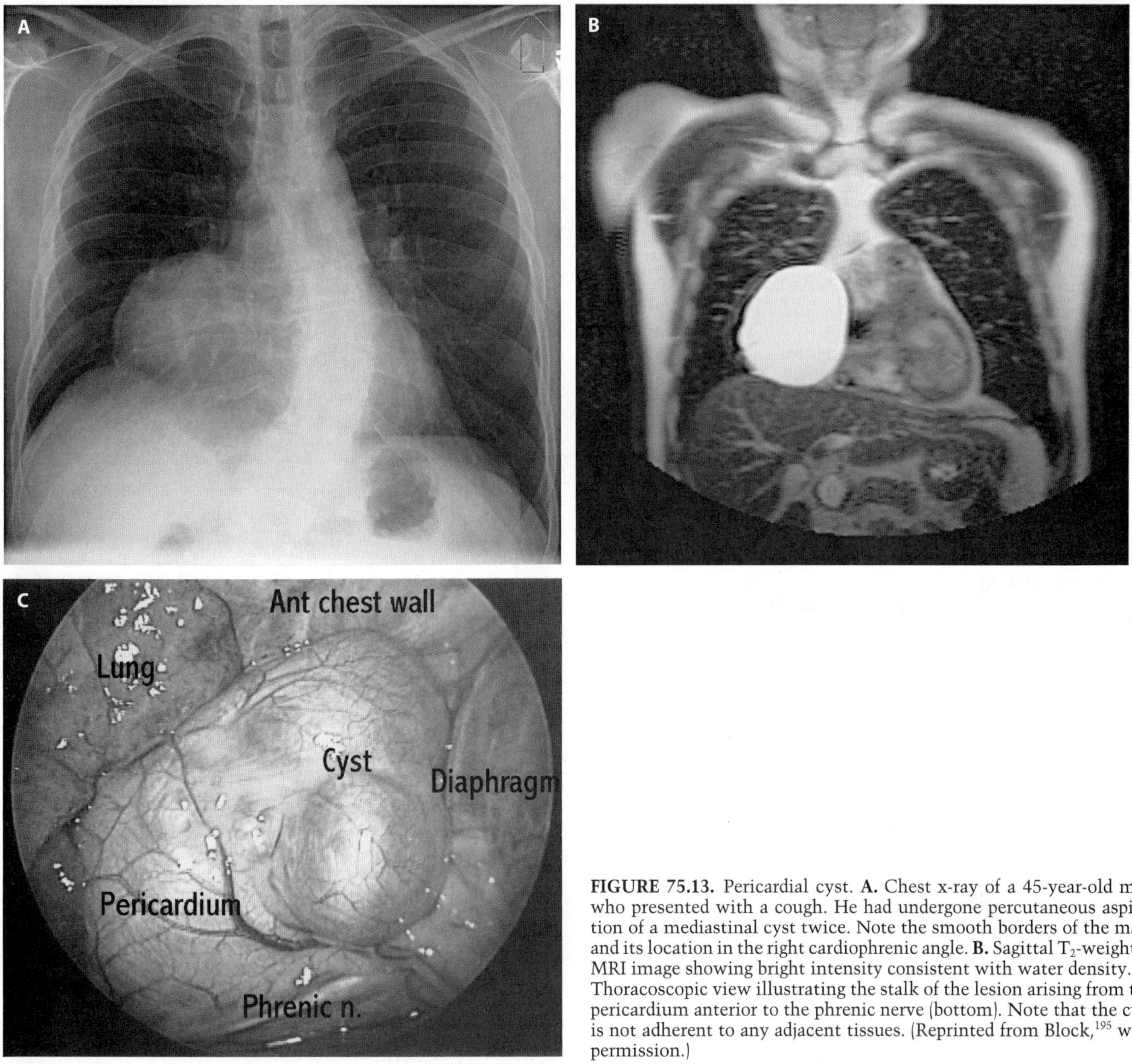

FIGURE 75.13. Pericardial cyst. **A.** Chest x-ray of a 45-year-old man who presented with a cough. He had undergone percutaneous aspiration of a mediastinal cyst twice. Note the smooth borders of the mass and its location in the right cardiophrenic angle. **B.** Sagittal T_2-weighted MRI image showing bright intensity consistent with water density. **C.** Thoracoscopic view illustrating the stalk of the lesion arising from the pericardium anterior to the phrenic nerve (bottom). Note that the cyst is not adherent to any adjacent tissues. (Reprinted from Block,[195] with permission.)

References

1. Pearse HE. Mediastinitis following cervical suppuration. Ann Surg 1938;108:588–611.
2. Estrera AS, Landay MJ, Grisham JM, et al. Descending necrotizing mediastinitis. Surg Gynecol Obstet 1983;157:545–552.
3. Wheatley MJ, Stirling MC, Kirsh MM, et al. Descending necrotizing mediastinitis: transcervical drainage is not enough. Ann Thorac Surg 1990;49:780–784.
4. Corsten MJ, Shamji FM, Odell PF, et al. Optimal treatment of descending necrotising mediastinitis. Thorax 1997;52:702–708.
5. Freeman RK, Vallieres E, Verrier ED, et al. Descending necrotizing mediastinitis: an analysis of the effects of serial surgical debridement on patient mortality. J Thorac Cardiovasc Surg 2000;119:260–267.
6. Marty-Ane CH, Alauzen M, Alric P, et al. Descending necrotizing mediastinitis. Advantage of mediastinal drainage with thoracotomy. J Thorac Cardiovasc Surg 1994;107:55–61.
7. Moncada R, Warpeha R, Pickleman J, et al. Mediastinitis from odontogenic and deep cervical infection. Anatomic pathways of propagation. Chest 1978;73:497–500.
8. Kiernan PD, Hernandez A, Byrne WD, et al. Descending cervical mediastinitis. Ann Thorac Surg 1998;65:1483–1488.
9. Blomquist IK, Bayer AS. Life-threatening deep fascial space infections of the head and neck. Infect Dis Clin North Am 1988;2:237–264.
10. Chow AW. Life-threatening infections of the head and neck. Clin Infect Dis 1992;14:991–1002.
11. Roberts JR, Smythe WR, Weber RW, et al. Thoracoscopic management of descending necrotizing mediastinitis. Chest 1997;112:850–854.
12. Laisaar T. Video-assisted thoracoscopic surgery in the management of acute purulent mediastinitis and pleural empyema. Thorac Cardiovasc Surg 1998;46:51–54.
13. Hang LW, Lien TC, Wang LS, et al. Hyperbaric oxygen as an adjunctive treatment for descending necrotizing mediastinitis: a case report. Chung Hua I Hsueh Tsa Chih 1997;60:52–56.

14. Milton H. Mediastinal surgery. Lancet 1897;1:872–875.
15. Gibbon JH. Application of a mechanical heart and lung apparatus to cardiac surgery. Minn Med 1954;37:171.
16. Loop FD, Lytle BW, Cosgrove DM, et al. J. Maxwell Chamberlain Memorial Paper. Sternal wound complications after isolated coronary artery bypass grafting: early and late mortality, morbidity, and cost of care. Ann Thorac Surg 1990;49:179–186; discussion 186–187.
17. Milano CA, Kesler K, Archibald N, et al. Mediastinitis after coronary artery bypass graft surgery. Risk factors and long-term survival. Circulation 1995;92:2245–2251.
18. Farinas MC, Gald Peralta F, Bernal JM, et al. Suppurative mediastinitis after open-heart surgery: a case-control study covering a 7-year period in Santander, Spain. Clin Infect Dis 1995;20:272–279.
19. El Oakley R, Paul E, Wong PS, et al. Mediastinitis in patients undergoing cardiopulmonary bypass: risk analysis and midterm results. J Cardiovasc Surg 1997;38:595–600.
20. Braxton JH, Marrin CA, McGrath PD, et al. Northern New England Cardiovascular Disease Study Group. Mediastinitis and long-term survival after coronary artery bypass graft surgery. Ann Thorac Surg 2000;70:2004–2007.
21. Taylor GJ, Mikell FL, Moses HW, et al. Determinants of hospital charges for coronary artery bypass surgery: the economic consequences of postoperative complications. Am J Cardiol 1990;65:309–313.
22. Abid Q, Nkere UU, Hasan A, et al. Mediastinitis in heart and lung transplantation: 15 years experience. Ann Thorac Surg 2003;75:1565–1571.
23. Baldwin RT, Radovancevic B, Sweeney MS, et al. Bacterial mediastinitis after heart transplantation. J Heart Lung Transplant 1992;11:545–549.
24. Breatnach E, Nath PH, Delany DJ. The role of computed tomography in acute and subacute mediastinitis. Clin Radiol 1986;37:139–145.
25. Misawa Y, Fuse K, Hasegawa T. Infectious mediastinitis after cardiac operations: computed tomographic findings. Ann Thorac Surg 1998;65:622–624.
26. Jolles H, Henry DA, Roberson JP, et al. Mediastinitis following median sternotomy: CT findings. Radiology 1996;201:463–466.
27. Browdie DA, Bernstein RV, Agnew R, et al. Diagnosis of poststernotomy infection: comparison of three means of assessment. Ann Thorac Surg 1991;51(2):290–292.
28. Bitkover CY, Gardlund B, Larsson SA, et al. Diagnosing sternal wound infections with ^{99m}Tc-labeled monoclonal granulocyte antibody scintigraphy. Ann Thorac Surg 1996;62:1412–1416; discussion 1416–1417.
29. Ferrazzi P, Allen R, Crupi G, et al. Reduction of infection after cardiac surgery: a clinical trial. Ann Thorac Surg 1986;42:321–325.
30. Ehrenkranz NJ, Pfaff SJ. Mediastinitis complicating cardiac operations: evidence of postoperative causation. Rev Infect Dis 1991;13:803–814.
31. Bitkover CY, Gardlund B. Mediastinitis after cardiovascular operations: a case-control study of risk factors. Ann Thorac Surg 1998;65:36–40.
32. Munoz P, Menasalvas A, Bernaldo de Quiros JC, et al. Postsurgical mediastinitis: a case-control study. Clin Infect Dis 1997;25:1060–1064.
33. Grover FL, Johnson RR, Marshall G, et al. Impact of mammary grafts on coronary bypass operative mortality and morbidity. Department of Veterans Affairs Cardiac Surgeons. Ann Thorac Surg 1994;57:559–568; discussion 568–569.
34. Lu JC, Grayson AD, Jha P, et al. Risk factors for sternal wound infection and mid-term survival following coronary artery bypass surgery. Eur J Cardiothorac Surg 2003;23:943–949.
35. Lust RM, Sun YS, Chitwood WR Jr. Internal mammary artery use. Sternal revascularization and experimental infection patterns. Circulation 1991;84:III285–III289.
36. Risk factors for deep sternal wound infection after sternotomy: a prospective, multicenter study [see comments]. J Thorac Cardiovasc Surg 1996;111:1200–1207.
37. Morykwas MJ, Argenta LC, Shelton-Brown EI, et al. Vacuum-assisted closure: a new method for wound control and treatment: animal studies and basic foundation. Ann Plast Surg 1997;38:553–562.
38. Song DH, Wu LC, Lohman RF, et al. Vacuum assisted closure for the treatment of sternal wounds: the bridge between debridement and definitive closure. Plast Reconstr Surg 2003;111:92–97.
39. Berg HF, Brands WG, van Geldorp TR, et al. Comparison between closed drainage techniques for the treatment of postoperative mediastinitis. Ann Thorac Surg 2000;70:924–929.
40. El Gamel A, Yonan NA, Hassan R, et al. Treatment of mediastinitis: early modified Robicsek closure and pectoralis major advancement flaps [see comments]. Ann Thorac Surg 1998;65:41–64; discussion 46–47.
41. Lopez-Monjardin H, de-la-Pena-Salcedo A, Mendoza-Munoz M, et al. Omentum flap versus pectoralis major flap in the treatment of mediastinitis. Plast Reconstr Surg 1998;101:1481–1485.
42. Jones G, Jurkiewicz MJ, Bostwick J, et al. Management of the infected median sternotomy wound with muscle flaps. The Emory 20-year experience. Ann Surg 1997;225:766–776; discussion 776–778.
43. Szerafin T, Vaszily M, Peterffy A. Granulated sugar treatment of severe mediastinitis after open-heart surgery. Scand J Thorac Cardiovasc Surg 1991;25:77–80.
44. Kustal A, Ibrisim E, Catav Z, et al. Mediastinitis after open heart surgery. Analysis of risk factors and management. J Cardiovasc Surg 1991;32:38–41.
45. Domkowski PW, Smith ML, Gonyon DL Jr, et al. Evaluation of vacuum-assisted closure in the treatment of poststernotomy mediastinitis. J Thorac Cardiovasc Surg 2003;126:386–390.
46. Ringelman PR, Vander Kolk CA, Cameron D, et al. Long-term results of flap reconstruction in median sternotomy wound infections. Plast Reconstr Surg 1994;93:1208–1214; discussion 1215–1216.
47. Scully HE, Leclerc Y, Martin RD, et al. Comparison between antibiotic irrigation and mobilization of pectoral muscle flaps in treatment of deep sternal infections. J Thorac Cardiovasc Surg 1985;90:523–531.
48. Oulmont N. Des Obliterations de la Veine Cava Superieure. Paris: Bailliere; 1855.
49. Osler W. On obliteration of the superior vena cava. Bull Johns Hopkins Hosp 1903;14:169–182.
50. Knox LB. Chronic mediastinitis. Am J Med Sci 1925;169:807–820.
51. Mole TM, Glover J, Sheppard MN. Sclerosing mediastinitis: a report on 18 cases. Thorax 1995;50:280–283.
52. Sherrick AD, Brown LR, Harms GF, et al. The radiographic findings of fibrosing mediastinitis. Chest 1994;106:484–489.
53. Urschel HC Jr, Razzuk MA, Netto GJ, et al. Sclerosing mediastinitis: improved management with histoplasmosis titer and ketoconazole. Ann Thorac Surg 1990;50:215–221.
54. Dines DE, Payne WS, Bernatz PE, et al. Mediastinal granuloma and fibrosing mediastinitis. Chest 1979;75:320–324.
55. Dunn EJ, Ulicny KS, Wright CB, et al. Surgical implications of sclerosing mediastinitis: a report of six cases and review of the literature. Chest 1990;97:338–346.
56. Lagerstrom CF, Mitchell HG, Graham BS, et al. Chronic fibrosing mediastinitis and superior vena caval obstruction from blastomycosis. Ann Thorac Surg 1992;54:764–765.

57. Graham JR, Suby HI, LeCompte PR, et al. Fibrotic disorders associated with methysergide therapy for headache. N Engl J Med 1966;274:359–368.
58. Goodwin RA, Nickell JA, Des Prez RM. Mediastinal fibrosis complicating healed primary histoplasmosis and tuberculosis. Medicine (Baltimore) 1972;51:227–246.
59. Rabinowitz JG, Prater W, Silver J, et al. Mediastinal histoplasmosis. Mt Sinai J Med 1980;47:356–363.
60. Rholl KS, Levitt RG, Glazer HS. Magnetic resonance imaging of fibrosing mediastinitis. AJR Am J Roentgenol 1985;145:255–259.
61. Mathisen DJ, Grillo HC. Clinical manifestation of mediastinal fibrosis and histoplasmosis. Ann Thorac Surg 1992;54:1053–1057; discussion 1057–1058.
62. Hunter W. The history of an aneurysm of the aorta with some remarks on aneurysms in general. Med Obs Soc Phys Lond 1757;1:323.
63. Nieto AF, Doty DB. Superior vena cava obstruction: clinical syndrome, etiology, and treatment. Curr Probl Cancer 1986;10:441–484.
64. Ahmann FR. A reassessment of the clinical implications of the superior vena caval syndrome. J Clin Oncol 1984;2:961–969.
65. Escalante CP. Causes and management of superior vena cava syndrome. Oncology 1993;7:61–68; discussion 71–72, 75–77.
66. Wurschmidt F, Bunemann H, Heilmann HP. Small cell lung cancer with and without superior vena cava syndrome: a multivariate analysis of prognostic factors in 408 cases. Int J Radiat Oncol Biol Phys 1995;33:77–82.
67. Goudevenos JA, Reid PG, Adams PC, et al. Pacemaker-induced superior vena cava syndrome: report of four cases and review of the literature. Pacing Clin Electrophysiol 1989;12:1890–1895.
68. Mazzetti H, Dussaut A, Tentori C, et al. Superior vena cava occlusion and/or syndrome related to pacemaker leads. Am Heart J 1993;125:831–837.
69. Kee ST, Kinoshita L, Razavi MK, et al. Superior vena cava syndrome: treatment with catheter-directed thrombolysis and endovascular stent placement. Radiology 1998;206:187–193.
70. Chan RH, Dar AR, Yu E, et al. Superior vena cava obstruction in small-cell lung cancer. Int J Radiat Oncol Biol Phys 1997;38:513–520.
71. Doty JR, Flores JH, Doty DB. Superior vena cava obstruction: bypass using spiral vein graft. Ann Thorac Surg 1999;67:1111–1116.
72. Ohri SK, Lawrence DR, Townsend ER. Homograft as a conduit for superior vena cava syndrome [see comments]. Ann Thorac Surg 1997;64:531–533.
73. Seelig MH, Oldenburg WA, Klingler PJ, et al. Superior vena cava syndrome caused by chronic hemodialysis catheters: autologous reconstruction with a pericardial tube graft. J Vasc Surg 1998;28:556–560.
74. Graham A, Anikin V, Curry R, et al. Subcutaneous jugulofemoral bypass: a simple surgical option for palliation of superior vena cava obstruction. J Cardiovasc Surg 1995;36:615–617.
75. Alimi YS, Gloviczki P, Vrtiska TJ, et al. Reconstruction of the superior vena cava: benefits of postoperative surveillance and secondary endovascular interventions. J Vasc Surg 1998;27:287–299; 300–301.
76. Hochrein J, Bashore TM, O'Laughlin MP, et al. Percutaneous stenting of superior vena cava syndrome: a case report and review of the literature. Am J Med 1998;104:78–84.
77. Davis RW, Oldham HN, Sabiston DC. The mediastinum. In: Sabiston DC, Spencer FC, eds. Surgery of the Chest, Vol. 1. Philadelphia: Saunders; 1995:576–612.
78. Shields TW. Primary lesions of the mediastinum and their investigation and treatment. In: Shields TW, ed. General Thoracic Surgery, Vol. 2. Malvern, PA: Williams and Wilkins; 1994;1724–1769.
79. Davis RD Jr, Oldham HN Jr, Sabiston DC Jr. Primary cysts and neoplasms of the mediastinum: recent changes in clinical presentation, methods of diagnosis, management, and results. Ann Thorac Surg 1987;44:229–237.
80. Azarow KS, Pearl RH, Zurcher R, et al. Primary mediastinal masses. A comparison of adult and pediatric populations. J Thorac Cardiovasc Surg 1993;106:67–72.
81. Massie RJ, Van Asperen PP, Mellis CM. A review of open biopsy for mediastinal masses. J Paediatr Child Health 1997;33:230–233.
82. Whooley BP, Urschel JD, Antkowiak JG, et al. Primary tumors of the mediastinum. J Surg Oncol 1999;70:95–99.
83. Nobuhara KK, Gorski YC, La Quaglia MP, et al. Bronchogenic cysts and esophageal duplications: common origins and treatment. J Pediatr Surg 1997;32:1408–1413.
84. Hunerbein M, Ghadimi BM, Haensch W, et al. Transesophageal biopsy of mediastinal and pulmonary tumors by means of endoscopic ultrasound guidance. J Thorac Cardiovasc Surg 1998;116:554–559.
85. Powers CN, Silverman JF, Geisinger KR, et al. Fine-needle aspiration biopsy of the mediastinum. A multi-institutional analysis. Am J Clin Pathol 1996;105:168–173.
86. Singh HK, Silverman JF, Powers CN, et al. Diagnostic pitfalls in fine-needle aspiration biopsy of the mediastinum. Diagn Cytopathol 1997;17:121–126.
87. Shabb NS, Fahl M, Shabb B, et al. Fine-needle aspiration of the mediastinum: a clinical, radiologic, cytologic, and histologic study of 42 cases. Diagn Cytopathol 1998;19:428–436.
88. Gossot D, Toledo L, Fritsch S, et al. Mediastinoscopy versus thoracoscopy for mediastinal biopsy. Results of a prospective nonrandomized study. Chest 1996;110:1328–1331.
89. Blumberg D, Port JL, Weksler B, et al. Thymoma: a multivariate analysis of factors predicting survival. Ann Thorac Surg 1995;60:908–913; discussion 914.
90. Newman E, Shaha AR. Substernal goiter. J Surg Oncol 1995;60:207–212.
91. Moron JC, Singer JA, Sardi A. Retrosternal goiter: a 6-year institutional review. Am Surg 1998;64:889–893.
92. Katlic MR, Grillo HC, Wang CA. Substernal goiter. Analysis of 80 patients from Massachusetts General Hospital. Am J Surg 1985;149:283–287.
93. Sanders LE, Rossi RL, Shahian DM, et al. Mediastinal goiters. The need for an aggressive approach. Arch Surg 1992;127:609–613.
94. Moran CA, Suster S, Fishback N, et al. Extramedullary hematopoiesis presenting as posterior mediastinal mass: a study of four cases. Mod Pathol 1995;8:249–251.
95. Gentry SE, Harris MA. Posterior mediastinal mass in a patient with chest pain. Chest 1995;107:1757–1759.
96. Akwari OE, Payne WS, Onofrio BM, et al. Dumbbell neurogenic tumors of the mediastinum. Diagnosis and management. Mayo Clin Proc 1978;53:353–358.
97. Grillo HC, Ojemann RG, Scannell JG, et al. Combined approach to "dumbbell" intrathoracic and intraspinal neurogenic tumors. Ann Thorac Surg 1983;36:402–407.
98. Guglielmi M, De Bernardi B, Rizzo A, et al. Resection of primary tumor at diagnosis in stage IV-S neuroblastoma: does it affect the clinical course? J Clin Oncol 1996;14:1537–1544.
99. Martinez DA, King DR, Ginn-Pease ME, et al. Resection of the primary tumor is appropriate for children with stage IV-S neuroblastoma: an analysis of 37 patients. J Pediatr Surg 1992;27:1016–1020; discussion 1020–1021.
100. Aoyama C, Qualman SJ, Reagan M, et al. Histopathologic features of composite ganglioneuroblastoma. Immunohistochemical distinction of the stromal component is related to prognosis. Cancer (St. Louis) 1990;65:255–264.

101. Guidetti D, Sabadini R, Bondavalli M, et al. Epidemiological study of myasthenia gravis in the province of Reggio Emilia, Italy. Eur J Epidemiol 1998;14:381–387.
102. Robertson NP, Deans J, Compston DA. Myasthenia gravis: a population-based epidemiological study in Cambridgeshire, England. J Neurol Neurosurg Psychiatry 1998;65:492–496.
103. Osserman KE, Genkins G. Studies in myasthenia gravis: review of a 20-year experience in over 1200 patients. Mt Sinai J Med 1971;38:497–537.
104. Papatestas AE, Genkins G, Kornfeld P, et al. Effects of thymectomy in myasthenia gravis. Ann Surg 1987;206:79–88.
105. Cosi V, Romani A, Lombardi M, et al. Prognosis of myasthenia gravis: a retrospective study of 380 patients. J Neurol 1997;244:548–555.
106. Beekman R, Kuks JB, Oosterhuis HJ. Myasthenia gravis: diagnosis and follow-up of 100 consecutive patients. J Neurol 1997;244:112–118.
107. Walker MB. Treatment of myasthenia gravis with physostigmine. Lancet 1934;1:1200–1201.
108. Osserman KE, Teng P, Kaplan LI. Studies in myasthenia gravis: preliminary report on therapy with mestinon bromide. JAMA 1954;155:961.
109. Hoppe HH. Ein beitrag zur Kenntnis der bulbärparalyse. Berl Klin Wochenschr 1892;29:332–336.
110. Weigert C. Pathologisch-anatomischer beitrag zur erb'schen krankheit (myasthenia gravis). Neurol Centralbl 1901;13: 597.
111. Sauerbruch DR, Roth D. Thymektomie bei einem Fall von Marbus Basedowi mit Myasthenie. Mitt Grenzgeb Med Chir 1913;25:746–765.
112. von Haberer A. Zur klinischen Bedeutung der Thymus Drüse. Arch Klin Chir 1917;109:193.
113. Bell ET. Tumors of the thymus in myasthenia gravis. J Nerv Ment Dis 1917;45:130–143.
114. Blalock A, Mason MF, Morgan HF, et al. Myasthenia gravis and tumors of the thymic region: report of a case in which the tumor was removed. Ann Surg 1939;110:544–561.
115. Blalock A. Thymectomy in the treatment of mysthenia gravis: report of 20 cases. J Thorac Cardiovasc Surg 1944;13:316.
116. Damjanovic M, Vidic-Dankovic B, Kosec D, et al. Thymus changes in experimentally induced myasthenia gravis. Autoimmunity 1993;15:201–207.
117. Spuler S, Marx A, Kirchner T, et al. Myogenesis in thymic transplants in the severe combined immunodeficient mouse model of myasthenia gravis. Differentiation of thymic myoid cells into striated muscle cells. Am J Pathol 1994;145:766–770.
118. Moran CA, Suster S, Gil J, et al. Morphometric analysis of germinal centers in nonthymomatous patients with mysthenia gravis. Arch Pathol Lab Med 1990;114:689–691.
119. Buckingham JM, Howard FM Jr, Bernatz PE, et al. The value of thymectomy in myasthenia gravis: a computer-assisted matched study. Ann Surg 1976;184:453–458.
120. Mantegazza R, Baggi F, Antozzi C, et al. Myasthenia gravis (MG): epidemiological data and prognostic factors. Ann N Y Acad Sci 2003;998:413–423.
121. Jaretzki AD, Penn AS, Younger DS, et al. "Maximal" thymectomy for myasthenia gravis. Results. J Thorac Cardiovasc Surg 1988;95:747–757.
122. Cooper JD, Al-Jilaihawa AN, Pearson FG, et al. An improved technique to facilitate transcervical thymectomy for myasthenia gravis. Ann Thorac Surg 1988;45:242–247.
123. Glinjongol C, Paiboonpol S. Outcome after transsternal radical thymectomy for myasthenia gravis: 14-year review at Ratchaburi Hospital. J Med Assoc Thai 2004;87:1304–1310.
124. Roth T, Ackermann R, Stein R, et al. Thirteen years follow-up after radical transsternal thymectomy for myasthenia gravis. Do short-term results predict long-term outcome? Eur J Cardiothorac Surg 2002;21:664–670.
125. Masaoka A, Yamakawa Y, Niwa H, et al. Extended thymectomy for myasthenia gravis patients: a 20-year review. Ann Thorac Surg 1996;62:853–859.
126. Frist WH, Thirumalai S, Doehring CB, et al. Thymectomy for the myasthenia gravis patient: factors influencing outcome. Ann Thorac Surg 1994;57:334–338.
127. Nussbaum MS, Rosenthal GJ, Samaha FJ, et al. Management of myasthenia gravis by extended thymectomy with anterior mediastinal dissection. Surgery (St. Louis) 1992;112:681–687; discussion 687–688.
128. Mulder DG, Graves M, Herrmann C. Thymectomy for myasthenia gravis: recent observations and comparisons with past experience. Ann Thorac Surg 1989;48:551–555.
129. Shrager JB, Deeb ME, Mick R, et al. Transcervical thymectomy for myasthenia gravis achieves results comparable to thymectomy by sternotomy. Ann Thorac Surg 2002;74:320–326; discussion 326–327.
130. Calhoun RF, Ritter JH, Guthrie TJ, et al. Results of transcervical thymectomy for myasthenia gravis in 100 consecutive patients. Ann Surg 1999;230:555–559; discussion 559–561.
131. Bril V, Kojic J, Ilse WK, et al. Long-term clinical outcome after transcervical thymectomy for myasthenia gravis. Ann Thorac Surg 1998;65:1520–1522.
132. DeFilippi VJ, Richman DP, Ferguson MK. Transcervical thymectomy for myasthenia gravis. Ann Thorac Surg 1994;57:194–197.
133. Savcenko M, Wendt GK, Prince SL, et al. Video-assisted thymectomy for myasthenia gravis: an update of a single institution experience. Eur J Cardiothorac Surg 2002;22:978–983.
134. Mineo TC, Pompeo E, Lerut TE, et al. Thoracoscopic thymectomy in autoimmune myasthesia: results of left-sided approach. Ann Thorac Surg 2000;69:1537–1541.
135. Zielinski M, Kuzdzal J, Szlubowski A, et al. Comparison of late results of basic transsternal and extended transsternal thymectomies in the treatment of myasthenia gravis. Ann Thorac Surg 2004;78:253–258.
136. Rosai J, Levine GD. Tumors of the thymus. In: Atlas of Tumor Pathology. Second Series, Fascicle 13. Washington, DC: Armed Forces Institute of Pathology; 1976:99.
137. Marino M, Muller-Hermelink HK. Thymoma and thymic carcinoma. Relation of thymoma epithelial cells to the cortical and medullary differentiation of thymus. Virchows Arch A Pathol Anat Histopathol 1985;407:119–149.
138. Rosai J, Sobin LH. Histological typing of tumours of the thymus. In: International Histological Classification of Tumours. 2nd ed. New York: Springer; 1999.
139. Cowen D, Richaud P, Mornex F, et al. Thymoma: results of a multicentric retrospective series of 149 non-metastatic irradiated patients and review of the literature. FNCLCC trialists. Federation Nationale des Centres de Lutte Contre le Cancer. Radiother Oncol 1995;34:9–16.
140. Regnard JF, Magdeleinat P, Dromer C, et al. Prognostic factors and long-term results after thymoma resection: a series of 307 patients. J Thorac Cardiovasc Surg 1996;112:376–384.
141. Venuta F, Rendina EA, Pescarmona EO, et al. Multimodality treatment of thymoma: a prospective study. Ann Thorac Surg 1997;64:1585–1591; discussion 1591–1592.
142. Gripp S, Hilgers K, Wurm R, et al. Thymoma: prognostic factors and treatment outcomes. Cancer (Phila) 1998;83:1495–1503.
143. Kondo K, Monden Y. Thymoma and myasthenia gravis: a clinical study of 1089 patients from Japan. Ann Thorac Surg 2005;79:219–224.
144. Masaoka A, Monden Y, Nakahara K, et al. Follow-up study of thymomas with special reference to their clinical stages. Cancer (Phila) 1981;48:2485–2492.
145. Okumura M, Ohta M, Tateyama H, et al. The World Health Organization histologic classification system reflects the onco-

logic behavior of thymoma: a clinical study of 273 patients. Cancer 2002;94:624–632.
146. Kim DJ, Yang WI, Choi SS, et al. Prognostic and clinical relevance of the World Health Organization schema for the classification of thymic epithelial tumors: a clinicopathologic study of 108 patients and literature review. Chest 2005;127:755–761.
147. Nakagawa K, Asamura H, Matsuno Y, et al. Thymoma: a clinicopathologic study based on the new World Health Organization classification. J Thorac Cardiovasc Surg 2003;126:1134–1140.
148. Yagi K, Hirata T, Fukuse T, et al. Surgical treatment for invasive thymoma, especially when the superior vena cava is invaded. Ann Thorac Surg 1996;61:521–524.
149. Kim ES, Putnam JB, Komaki R, et al. Phase II study of a multidisciplinary approach with induction chemotherapy, followed by surgical resection, radiation therapy, and consolidation chemotherapy for unresectable malignant thymomas: final report. Lung Cancer 2004;44:369–379.
150. Shin DM, Walsh GL, Komaki R, et al. A multidisciplinary approach to therapy for unresectable malignant thymoma. Ann Intern Med 1998;129:100–104.
151. Rea F, Sartori F, Loy M, et al. Chemotherapy and operation for invasive thymoma. J Thorac Cardiovasc Surg 1993;106:543–549.
152. Loehrer PJ Sr, Wang W, Johnson DH, et al. Eastern Cooperative Oncology Group phase II trial. Octreotide alone or with prednisone in patients with advanced thymoma and thymic carcinoma: an Eastern Cooperative Oncology Group phase II trial [erratum in J Clin Oncol 2004;22:2261]. J Clin Oncol 2004;22:293–299.
153. Palmieri G, Montella L, Martignetti A, et al. Somatostatin analogs and prednisone in advanced refractory thymic tumors. Cancer 2002;94:1414–1420.
154. Loehrer PJ Sr, Jiroutek M, Aisner S, et al. Combined etoposide, ifosfamide, and cisplatin in the treatment of patients with advanced thymoma and thymic carcinoma: an intergroup trial. Cancer 2001;91:2010–2015.
155. Highley MS, Underhill CR, Parnis FX, et al. Treatment of invasive thymoma with single-agent ifosfamide. J Clin Oncol 1999;17:2737–2744.
156. Loehrer PJ Sr, Chen M, Kim K, et al. Cisplatin, doxorubicin, and cyclophosphamide plus thoracic radiation therapy for limited-stage unresectable thymoma: an intergroup trial. J Clin Oncol 1997;15:3093–3099.
157. Giaccone G, Ardizzoni A, Kirkpatrick A, et al. Cisplatin and etoposide combination chemotherapy for locally advanced or metastatic thymoma. A phase II study of the European Organization for Research and Treatment of Cancer Lung Cancer Cooperative Group. J Clin Oncol 1996;14:814–820.
158. Loehrer PJ Sr, Kim K, Aisner SC, et al. Cisplatin plus doxorubicin plus cyclophosphamide in metastatic or recurrent thymoma: final results of an intergroup trial. The Eastern Cooperative Oncology Group, Southwest Oncology Group, and Southeastern Cancer Study Group. J Clin Oncol 1994;12:1164–1168.
159. Blumberg D, Burt ME, Bains MS, et al. Thymic carcinoma: current staging does not predict prognosis. J Thorac Cardiovasc Surg 1998;115:303–308; discussion 308–309.
160. Suster S, Moran CA. Thymic carcinoma: spectrum of differentiation and histologic types. Pathology 1998;30:111–122.
161. Quagliano PV. Thymic carcinoma: case reports and review. J Thorac Imaging 1996;11:66–74.
162. Satta J, Ahonen A, Parkkila S, et al. Multiple endocrine neoplastic-associated thymic carcinoid tumour in close relatives: octreotide scan as a new diagnostic and follow-up modality. Two case reports. Scand Cardiovasc J 1999;33:49–53.
163. de Montpreville VT, Macchiarini P, Dulmet E. Thymic neuroendocrine carcinoma (carcinoid): a clinicopathologic study of fourteen cases. J Thorac Cardiovasc Surg 1996;111:134–141.
164. Fukai I, Masaoka A, Fujii Y, et al. Thymic neuroendocrine tumor (thymic carcinoid): a clinicopathologic study in 15 patients. Ann Thorac Surg 1999;67:208–211.
165. Moran CA, Rosado-de-Christenson M, Suster S. Thymolipoma: clinicopathologic review of 33 cases [see comments]. Mod Pathol 1995;8:741–744.
166. Moeller KH, Rosado-de-Christenson ML, Templeton PA. Mediastinal mature teratoma: imaging features. AJR Am J Roentgenol 1997;169:985–990.
167. Lewis BD, Hurt RD, Payne WS, et al. Benign teratomas of the mediastinum. J Thorac Cardiovasc Surg 1983;86:727–731.
168. Dulmet EM, Macchiarini P, Suc B, et al. Germ cell tumors of the mediastinum. A 30-year experience. Cancer (Phila) 1993;72:1894–1901.
169. Moran CA, Suster S. Primary germ cell tumors of the mediastinum: I. Analysis of 322 cases with special emphasis on teratomatous lesions and a proposal for histopathologic classification and clinical staging. Cancer (Phila) 1997;80:681–690.
170. Hejase MJ, Donohue JP, Foster RS, et al. Post-chemotherapy resection of nonseminomatous germ cell testicular tumors metastatic to the mediastinum. J Urol 1996;156:1345–1348.
171. Childs WJ, Goldstraw P, Nicholls JE, et al. Primary malignant mediastinal germ cell tumours: Improved prognosis with platinum-based chemotherapy and surgery. Br J Cancer 1993;67:1098–1101.
172. Jyothirmayi R, Ramadas K, Jacob R, et al. Primary malignant germ cell tumours of the mediastinum—results of multimodality treatment. Acta Oncol 1997;36:317–321.
173. Moran CA, Suster S, Przygodzki RM, et al. Primary germ cell tumors of the mediastinum: II. Mediastinal seminomas—a clinicopathologic and immunohistochemical study of 120 cases. Cancer (Phila) 1997;80:691–698.
174. Hidalgo M, Paz-Ares L, Rivera F, et al. Mediastinal nonseminomatous germ cell tumours (MNSGCT) treated with cisplatin-based combination chemotherapy. Ann Oncol 1997;8:555–559.
175. Moran CA, Suster S, Koss MN. Primary germ cell tumors of the mediastinum: III. Yolk sac tumor, embryonal carcinoma, choriocarcinoma, and combined nonteratomatous germ cell tumors of the mediastinum—a clinicopathologic and immunohistochemical study of 64 cases. Cancer (Phila) 1997;80:699–707.
176. Israel A, Bosl GJ, Golbey RB, et al. The results of chemotherapy for extragonadal germ-cell tumors in the cisplatin era: the Memorial Sloan-Kettering Cancer Center experience (1975 to 1982). J Clin Oncol 1985;3:1073–1078.
177. Bebb GG, Grannis FW Jr, Paz IB, et al. Mediastinal germ cell tumor in a child with precocious puberty and Klinefelter syndrome. Ann Thorac Surg 1998;66:547–548.
178. Logothetis CJ, Samuels ML, Selig DE, et al. Chemotherapy of extragonadal germ cell tumors. J Clin Oncol 1985;3:316–325.
179. Monig SP, Schmidt R, Krug B. Yolk sac tumor of the anterior mediastinum: the role of palliative surgery. Am Surg 1997;63:948–950.
180. Hughes JH, Katz RL, Fonseca GA, et al. Fine-needle aspiration cytology of mediastinal non-Hodgkin's nonlymphoblastic lymphoma. Cancer (Phila) 1998;84:26–35.
181. Okada Y, Mori H, Maeda T, et al. Congenital mediastinal bronchogenic cyst with malignant transformation: an autopsy report. Pathol Int 1996;46:594–600.
182. Bierhoff E, Pfeifer U. Malignant mesothelioma arising from a benign mediastinal mesothelial cyst. Gen Diagn Pathol 1996;142:59–62.
183. Cioffi U, Bonavina L, De Simone M, et al. Presentation and surgical management of bronchogenic and esophageal duplication cysts in adults. Chest 1998;113:1492–1496.
184. Cuypers P, De Leyn P, Cappelle L, et al. Bronchogenic cysts: a review of 20 cases. Eur J Cardiothorac Surg 1996;10:393–396.

185. Ribet ME, Copin MC, Gosselin B. Bronchogenic cysts of the mediastinum. J Thorac Cardiovasc Surg 1995;109:1003–1010.
186. Aktogu S, Yuncu G, Halilcolar H, et al. Bronchogenic cysts: clinicopathological presentation and treatment. Eur Respir J 1996;9:2017–2021.
187. Demmy TL, Krasna MJ, Detterbeck FC, et al. Multicenter VATS experience with mediastinal tumors. Ann Thorac Surg 1998;66:187–192.
188. Tripp HF, Reames MK. Resection of a bronchogenic cyst involving the wall of the mainstem bronchus and repair utilizing a pedicled pericardial flap. Am Surg 1997;63:785–787.
189. Wright CC, Cohen DM, Vegunta RK, et al. Intrathoracic cystic hygroma: a report of three cases. J Pediatr Surg 1996;31:1430–1432.
190. Chong KT, Ong CL. Cystic hygroma in adulthood. Singapore Med J 1997;38:261–262.
191. Kim JH, Jun TG, Sung SW, et al. Giant lymph node hyperplasia (Castleman's disease) in the chest. Ann Thorac Surg 1995;59:1162–1165.
192. Bowne WB, Lewis JJ, Filippa DA, et al. The management of unicentric and multicentric Castleman's disease: a report of 16 cases and a review of the literature. Cancer (Phila) 1999;85:706–717.
193. Shahidi H, Myers JL, Kvale PA. Castleman's disease. Mayo Clin Proc 1995;70:969–977.
194. Pandya A, Baumgartner FJ, Nguyen D, et al. Thoracic Castleman's disease: implications for resection [letter; comment]. Ann Thorac Surg 1998;65:302–303.
195. Block MI. Mediastinal tumors. In: Pass HI, Carbone DP, Johnson DH, Minna JD, Turrisi AT, eds. Lung Cancer: Principles and Practice. 3rd edition. Philadelphia: Lippincott, Williams and Wilkins; 2005:894.

76

Congenital Heart Disease

Carl L. Backer and Constantine Mavroudis

History

The era of surgical correction of congenital heart defects began in 1938 when Robert E. Gross successfully ligated a patent ductus arteriosus (PDA) in a 7-year-old child at Boston Children's Hospital.[1] This historical milestone was followed by several different "closed-heart" operations for children with congenital heart defects, including the Blalock-Taussig shunt,[2] coarctation repair,[3] and pulmonary artery banding.[4] In 1952, the first "open-heart" operation, closure of an atrial septal defect (ASD), was performed by F. John Lewis at the University of Minnesota using hypothermia and inflow occlusion.[5] One year later, John Gibbon performed the first open-heart surgery using cardiopulmonary bypass, also closing an ASD.[6] At the University of Minnesota, C. Walton Lillehei performed the first repair of ventricular septal defect (VSD), tetralogy of Fallot, and atrioventricular canal (AVC) using cross circulation: the parent was the "heart-lung" machine.[7] At the same time, at the Mayo Clinic, Dr. John Kirklin was also pioneering open-heart surgery using a heart-lung machine.[8] The significant historical milestones in congenital heart surgery are summarized in Table 76.1.

Epidemiology/Genetics

Congenital heart defects occur in approximately 6 to 8 of every 1000 live births.[9] The etiology of these defects is multifactorial, with both genetic and environmental influences. There are some clear associations with chromosomal abnormalities, in particular Down syndrome with AVC defects, Turner's syndrome with coarctation of the aorta, Noonan syndrome with pulmonary stenosis and ASD, and Williams syndrome with supravalvar aortic stenosis. If a family has one child with a congenital heart defect, the risk of having a second child with congenital heart disease rises to 2%–6%.[10] The risk of having a child with congenital heart disease to a parent with congenital heart disease is between 2% and 14%, depending on the specific lesion.[11,12]

Clinical Presentation and Diagnosis

In general terms, children with congenital heart defects present in one of two ways: children with left-to-right shunts present with congestive heart failure, and children with right-to-left shunts present with cyanosis (Table 76.2). There are also defects in which the child is clinically asymptomatic but has a cardiac murmur. The diagnosis is based on the history, physical examination, chest x-ray, electrocardiogram, echocardiogram, and cardiac catheterization. There has been a dramatic increase in the use of cardiac magnetic resonance imaging (MRI) and ultrafast computed tomography (CT) scans for diagnosis. Over the past decade, the quality of diagnosis based on the echocardiogram with the use of both two-dimensional and color Doppler flow has greatly improved and has in many cases supplanted cardiac catheterization. Tworetzky and colleagues reported that, in a group of 503 children with major congenital heart defects undergoing repair between 1992 and 1997, 82% underwent surgery after preoperative diagnosis by echocardiography alone.[13]

Cardiac catheterization is now more frequently reserved for difficult diagnostic decisions or for interventional procedures. Echocardiography is used to determine the size, shape, and function of different cardiac chambers. It can also determine the relationship of the great vessels, valve anatomy and function, and anatomic location of specific defects, such as ASD and VSD. Cardiac catheterization is used to evaluate the pressure in the various cardiac chambers along with the oxygen saturation in these chambers and the great vessels; this allows the precise determination of pressure gradients and the magnitude of intracardiac shunting. This information can be used to determine the cardiac output and pulmonary and systemic vascular resistance. Cineangiocardiography permits accurate definition of the anatomy of cardiac chambers and valves as well as the location and particular anatomy of each defect. Much of the anatomic detail previously detected by cardiac catheterization can now be achieved with MRI and CT scan. Also, MRI can be used to calculate intracardiac chamber volume, shunt volume, and regurgitation fractions.

TABLE 76.1. **Congenital Heart Surgery: Historical Milestones.**

Year	*Procedure*	*Surgeon*
Closed heart		
1938	Ligation patent ductus arteriosus	Robert Gross
1944	Blalock-Taussig shunt	Alfred Blalock
1945	Coarctation repair	C. Crafoord
1945	Division of vascular ring	Robert Gross
1952	Pulmonary artery banding	William Muller
Simple open heart		
1952	Closure of atrial septal defect (hypothermia/inflow occlusion)	F. John Lewis
1953	Closure of atrial septal defect (pump oxygenator/ cardiopulmonary bypass)	John Gibbon
1954	Closure of ventricular septal defect ("cross circulation")	C. Walton Lillehei
1955	Repair tetralogy of Fallot	C. Walton Lillehei
1955	Repair atrioventricular canal	C. Walton Lillehei
Complex open heart		
1964	Mustard operation for TGA	William Mustard
1968	Fontan procedure for tricuspid atresia	Francis Fontan
1968	Conduit repair of truncus arteriosus	Dwight McGoon
1976	Arterial switch for TGA	Adib Jatene
1979	Stage I palliation for HLHS	William Norwood
1985	Neonatal cardiac transplantation	Leonard Bailey
1998	Right ventricle to pulmonary artery shunt for HLHS	Shunji Sano

HLHS, hypoplastic left heart syndrome; TGA, transposition of the great arteries.

TABLE 76.2. **Presentation and Classification of Congenital Heart Disease.**

Congestive heart failure	
Left-to-right shunt (increased pulmonary blood flow)	***Obstructive lesions***
Patent ductus arteriosus	Aortic stenosis
Atrial septal defect	Mitral stenosis
Ventricular septal defect	Pulmonic stenosis
Atrioventricular canal	Coarctation of the aorta
Truncus arteriosus	Interrupted aortic arch
Aortopulmonary window	
Cyanosis	
Right-to-left shunt (decreased pulmonary blood flow)	***Complex lesions***
Tetralogy of Fallot With intact ventricular septum With ventricular septal defect	Transposition of the great arteries
Tricuspid atresia	Total anomalous pulmonary venous connection
Pulmonary atresia With intact ventricular septum With ventricular septal defect	Cor triatriatum Hypoplastic left heart syndrome
Miscellaneous	
Anomalous origin of the left coronary artery from the pulmonary artery	
Corrected transposition of the great arteries	
Ebstein's anomaly	
Vascular ring	
Pulmonary artery sling	

Patients with a pure left-to-right shunt have increased pulmonary blood flow and present with symptoms of congestive heart failure. These symptoms are failure to thrive, recurrent upper respiratory tract infections, and sweating with feeding. Signs of heart failure include tachypnea, tachycardia, and hepatomegaly. These patients have pulmonary hypertension, and if left untreated they can develop pulmonary vascular obstructive disease. With progression of this pulmonary vascular disease, the pulmonary vascular resistance steadily increases, and the actual amount of left-to-right shunting decreases. Eventually, a point is reached at which the patient becomes cyanotic and has what is called Eisenmenger's syndrome. At this point, operation to close the intracardiac defect may not help the patient and may actually prove fatal as the child may develop irreversible right ventricular failure. This complication can be prevented by early operative repair.

Patients with intracardiac or extracardiac obstructive lesions may be asymptomatic or present with signs of congestive heart failure. In particular, patients with coarctation of the aorta and interrupted aortic arch may present with severe heart failure and cardiovascular collapse at the time of ductus closure. In fact, there is a group of lesions in which the patient is essentially dependent on a ductus arteriosus for pulmonary blood flow, systemic blood flow, or mixing of blood (Table 76.3). Management of these infants has been greatly enhanced by the use of prostaglandin E_1 (PGE_1) therapy, which was introduced in 1974.[14] The PGE_1 therapy maintains the patency of the ductus arteriosus, and for these critically ill infants can provide the pulmonary blood flow, systemic blood flow, or mixing that they require for survival. By stabilizing these patients with pharmacological management of the ductus, they can undergo complete diagnostic evaluation and elective therapeutic intervention after resolution of hypoxia, acidosis, and ventricular failure.

Patients with a congenital cardiac lesion causing cyanosis can have either a pure right-to-left shunt with decreased pulmonary blood flow or a complex lesion in which there is actually both increased pulmonary blood flow and cyanosis. The most common cause of severe cyanosis in the neonatal period is transposition of the great arteries. These patients have two parallel circulations, and they are usually easily diagnosed because of the intense cyanosis. Another common cause of cyanosis in the newborn is total anomalous pulmonary venous connection, causing both cyanosis and congestive heart failure.

The most common overall cause of cyanotic heart disease is tetralogy of Fallot, but many of these patients do not present until several months of age when they develop progressive hypertrophy of the right ventricular outflow tract. Cyanotic

TABLE 76.3. **Ductal-Dependent Lesions.**

For pulmonary blood flow
Pulmonary atresia
Tricuspid atresia
Severe tetralogy of Fallot
For systemic blood flow
Hypoplastic left heart syndrome
Interrupted aortic arch
Severe coarctation of the aorta
For mixing of blood
Transposition of the great arteries

patients have systemic arterial oxygen desaturation with a resulting stimulus for the bone marrow to produce red blood cells; this results in progressive polycythemia. The right-to-left intracardiac shunt allows the possibility for right-sided thrombi to pass to the systemic circulation, causing cerebral vascular accidents or brain abscess. Another pathophysiological response is the formation of collateral arteries from the systemic circulation to the pulmonary arteries. These collaterals develop as an apparent response to the child's relative hypoxia. These collaterals can become quite large and occasionally erode into the tracheobronchial tree, causing life-threatening hemoptysis. A rather dramatic occurrence in these patients is clubbing at the tips of the fingers, which occurs with prolonged cyanosis. This hypertrophic osteoarthropathy is caused by a proliferation of capillaries and small arteriovenous malformations at the tip of the fingers. Hypercyanotic or "tet" spells are classically seen in patients with tetralogy of Fallot and are caused by muscular spasm of the infundibular muscle in the right ventricular outflow tract.

Surgical Management

Palliation

Historically, many of the first operations for congenital heart disease were palliative in that they were designed to either increase or decrease pulmonary blood flow and temporarily stabilize the patient, allowing for corrective surgery to be performed when the child was older. As surgical and anesthetic techniques improved, along with improvements in cardiopulmonary bypass and myocardial protection, the tendency over the years has been to perform corrective procedures earlier in infancy and to avoid the palliative procedures.

The two most commonly used palliative procedures are the systemic-to-pulmonary artery shunts and pulmonary artery banding. Systemic-to-pulmonary artery shunts provide for increased pulmonary blood flow in patients with a right-to-left shunt and decreased pulmonary blood flow. Pulmonary artery banding is used for patients with increased pulmonary blood flow secondary to a left-to-right shunt.

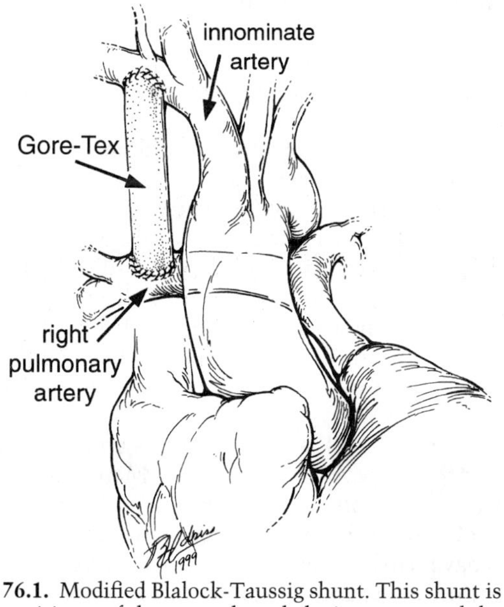

FIGURE 76.1. Modified Blalock-Taussig shunt. This shunt is a Gore-Tex interposition graft between the subclavian artery and the pulmonary artery. The subclavian artery originates from the innominate artery and acts as the regulator of the amount of flow into the shunt. This shunt is best performed through a median sternotomy. The shunt shown is in place in a patient with tetralogy of Fallot.

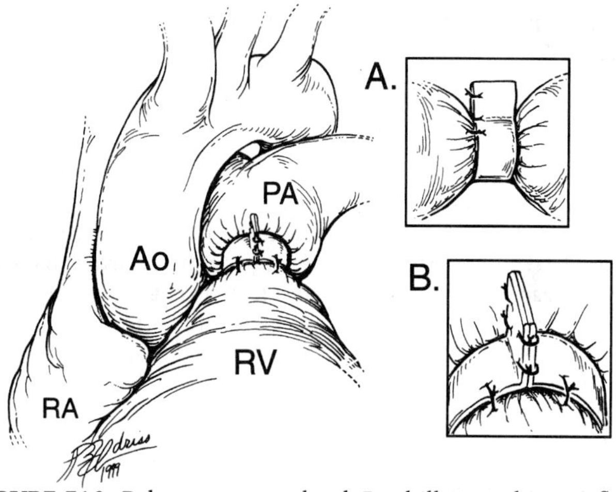

FIGURE 76.2. Pulmonary artery band. Band illustrated is a Teflon-impregnated Dacron band. The band is placed through either a left thoracotomy or a median sternotomy incision. It encircles the pulmonary artery (PA) and is constricted with multiple sutures as illustrated in *inset A* to progressively restrict flow into the pulmonary artery. A pressure-monitoring catheter is usually inserted in the distal pulmonary artery during tightening of the band. The band is fixed to the adventitia of the pulmonary artery (*inset B*) to prevent distal migration of the band. Ao, aorta; RA, right atrium; RV, right ventricle.

Modified Blalock-Taussig Shunt

The most commonly used systemic-to-pulmonary artery shunt is the *modified Blalock-Taussig shunt* (Fig. 76.1). This shunt is a polytetrafluoroethylene (PTFE) interposition graft directed from the subclavian artery to the pulmonary artery and was first reported by de Leval et al.[15] Our center and many others now perform these shunts almost exclusively through a median sternotomy incision instead of through a thoracotomy incision (as originally described). The sternotomy route is technically less challenging and associated with fewer shunt failures than the classic thoracotomy approach.[16] The other advantage of the sternotomy approach is the easy conversion to cardiopulmonary bypass for construction of the shunt should the child have severe cyanosis during the procedure. Other shunts that are now essentially of historical interest only are the Potts, Waterston, and Cooley shunts.

Pulmonary Artery Banding

Pulmonary artery banding was first described for patients with truncus arteriosus by Muller and Dammann.[4] Pulmonary artery banding can be performed through either a left thoracotomy or a median sternotomy. The technique involves encircling the main pulmonary artery with a Dacron or Gore-Tex band that is sequentially tightened while evaluating the pulmonary artery pressure distal to the band (Fig. 76.2). The goal is to reduce the pulmonary artery pressure distal to the band to less than half of the systemic pressure. At the same time, the child's oxygen saturations must be monitored to ensure that they do not drop excessively. If the patient is being prepared for an eventual Fontan procedure, it is preferable to decrease the mean pulmonary artery pressure to less than 20mmHg. The band is then fixed to the wall of the pulmonary artery to ensure that it does not migrate distally and occlude the right pulmonary artery.

Initially, pulmonary artery banding was commonly performed for patients with large left-to-right shunts with the corrective procedure performed later in life. However, the current trend has been to perform pulmonary artery banding for increasingly fewer indications. Current indications for pulmonary artery banding would include multiple VSDs (Swiss cheese VSD) and patients with excessive pulmonary blood flow and single-ventricle physiology without evidence of subaortic stenosis.

Left-to-Right Shunt

Patent Ductus Arteriosus

A *patent ductus arteriosus* is a persistent communication of the normal fetal connection between the pulmonary artery and the descending thoracic aorta (Fig. 76.3). In patients without other congenital heart defects, this creates a left-to-right shunt. In premature infants, it can cause severe congestive heart failure and respiratory distress syndrome. In older children, the patient may be clinically asymptomatic but have a "machinery-type" murmur. In premature infants, the indication for surgical closure is congestive heart failure causing respiratory distress. In older children, simply having a ductus that is audible is an indication for closure. These children are at risk of subacute bacterial endocarditis, aortic aneurysm, pulmonary artery aneurysm, and aortic dissection.

Operative ductus closure is usually performed through a left thoracotomy. The technique (Fig. 76.3) used to close a ductus in premature infants is simple ligation; in older children, we prefer to use the technique of division and oversewing. This technique ensures complete division of the ductus without the potential for recanalization, which can occur in about 3% to 5% of patients who have simple ligation.

Between 1947 and 1993 at the Children's Memorial Hospital, 1108 patients underwent division and oversewing of a

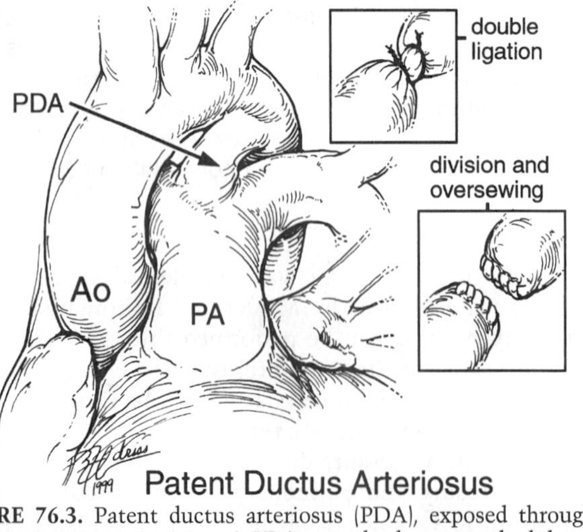

FIGURE 76.3. Patent ductus arteriosus (PDA), exposed through a median sternotomy incision. A PDA may also be approached through a left thoracotomy. The *upper inset* illustrates a double ligation to close the ductus. The *lower inset* shows the ductus divided with the two stumps oversewn. Ao, aorta; PA, pulmonary artery.

PDA.[17] There was no mortality, and there have been no recurrences. Mean hospital stay is now 2 days. Recently, pediatric cardiologists have been using transcatheter techniques to close PDA. Excellent results have been achieved in small PDAs using coil devices that are implanted into the ductus through the descending thoracic aorta.[18] Transcatheter coil occlusion has been shown to be as effective and less costly than surgical closure for small PDAs if silent residual leaks are not considered clinically significant.[19] Our current approach is to recommend coil occlusion for the smaller ductus and surgical division and oversewing for the large ductus. However, there are now PDA occluder devices that are quite effective even for the larger ductus.[20] This device cannot be used in infants because of the potential for protrusion into the descending aorta or pulmonary artery.

Atrial Septal Defect

An *atrial septal defect* is a hole in the intraatrial septum that causes a left-to-right shunt. The degree of shunting is determined by the size of the ASD and the right and left ventricular compliance. Patients with an ASD are often asymptomatic but on physical examination have a fixed split second heart sound and may have a systolic murmur of relative (physiological) pulmonary stenosis. The electrocardiogram will demonstrate right ventricular hypertrophy and the chest x-ray will show cardiomegaly. Any patient who has an audible murmur and documented ASD by echocardiography is a candidate for surgical closure. Patients with an ASD are at risk of atrial arrhythmias, right ventricular dysfunction, pulmonary hypertension, and congestive heart failure. Without surgical intervention, the mean age of death in patients with an ASD is 36 years.[21] Atrial septal defects are classified as ostium secundum (80%), sinus venosus (10%), and ostium primum (10%).

Ostium secundum defects are a simple opening in the atrial septum. Ostium primum and sinus venosus defects are more complex. Ostium primum defects are also called partial AVC defects, and these patients also have a cleft in the mitral valve that must be closed to prevent mitral insufficiency (Fig. 76.4). Sinus venosus defects have partial anomalous pulmonary venous drainage of the right superior pulmonary vein to the superior vena cava.

Between 1990 and 2005 at the Children's Memorial Hospital, 237 patients underwent surgical closure of an ASD.[21a] Mean age at ASD closure was 2.5 years. Approach was through a median sternotomy with the use of cardiopulmonary bypass, aortic cross-clamping, and cold blood cardioplegia to arrest the heart (Fig. 76.5). In 50% of the cases, the defect was closed with a pericardial patch, and in the other 50% direct suture closure was performed. In this series, there have been no deaths and no recurrences of ASD. The mean length of hospital stay was 3.5 days.

"Between 1990 and 2005, 51 patients underwent repair of a sinus venosus type ASD at Children's Memorial Hospital.[21a] Median age was 4.2 years. This defect is high in the atrial septum adjacent to the superior vena cava. Over half of these patients have partial anomalous pulmonary venous return to the superior vena cava. Twenty-one patients had a single pericardial patch repair, 25 patients had a two patch pericardial repair, and 5 patients had a "Warden repair."[21b] There was no mortality and no reoperations."

Several percutaneous transcatheter techniques have been explored for the closure of ASDs. Excellent initial results were

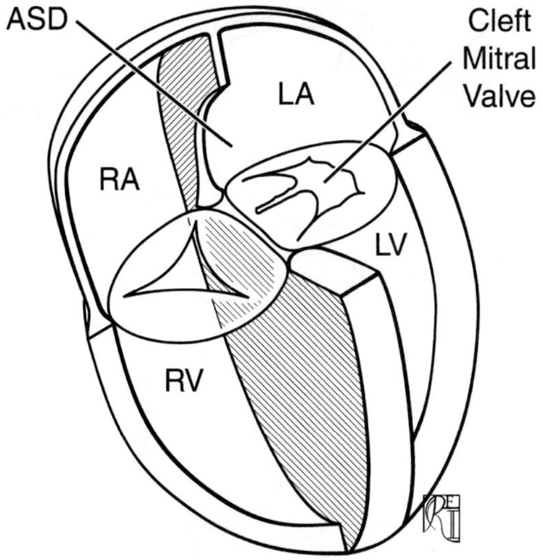

FIGURE 76.4. Partial atrioventricular canal (AVC) defect. There is an ostium primum atrial septal defect (ASD) and a cleft in the mitral valve. LA, RA, left, right atrium, respectively; LV, RV, left, right ventricle, respectively.

described with the clamshell occluder device.[22] On late follow-up, however, the device was taken off the market because of fractures of the struts of the device. More recently, the Amplatzer device, a self-expanding wire mesh, double-mushroom device, has been successfully employed in older patients. Omeish and Hijazi reported 3580 implants of the Amplatzer device. Median patient age was 12 years, median ASD size was 14 mm, and median device size was 18 mm. Closure of the ASD was achieved in 99% of patients; serious complications occurred in fewer than 0.3% of the cases.[23] This device has become the technique of choice for closure of small-to-medium ostium secundum ASDs in older children.

Ventricular Septal Defect

A *ventricular septal defect* is a hole located in the interventricular septum. The degree of left-to-right shunting across the VSD is determined by the size of the defect and the pulmonary vascular resistance. Defects are categorized by their location in the interventricular septum (Fig. 76.6). The anatomical types of VSD are paramembranous (80%), conal (10%), muscular (5%), and inlet (5%). Ventricular septal defects can be further subdivided into two categories, restrictive and nonrestrictive. Nonrestrictive VSDs are the same size as or larger than the aortic valve annulus. These patients have high pulmonary artery pressure and present with severe congestive heart failure. Left untreated, these patients will develop Eisenmenger's syndrome. These patients should undergo elective closure of the VSD at 3 to 6 months of age. In patients with a restrictive VSD, the defect is smaller than the aortic valve annulus. Pulmonary artery pressures are less than systemic. These patients may be managed medically unless they meet the following surgical indications: (1) pulmonary-to-systemic flow ratio greater than 1.5:1; (2) aortic valve prolapse; (3) aortic valve insufficiency; (4) prior episode of endocarditis; (5) conal VSD.

For children with a VSD, the incidence rate of bacterial endocarditis is 14.5 per 10,000 person-years,[24] which is 35 times the normal population-based rate. Surgical closure of the VSD reduces the risk of bacterial endocarditis by more than 50%. Paramembranous and, in particular, conal VSDs may develop aortic valve prolapse as the cusps of the aortic valve sag into the VSD. If the defect is not repaired, these patients may develop aortic valve insufficiency. However, if the VSD is closed, the aortic valve disease does not seem to progress. For this reason, we recommend VSD closure in all patients with conal VSDs.[25]

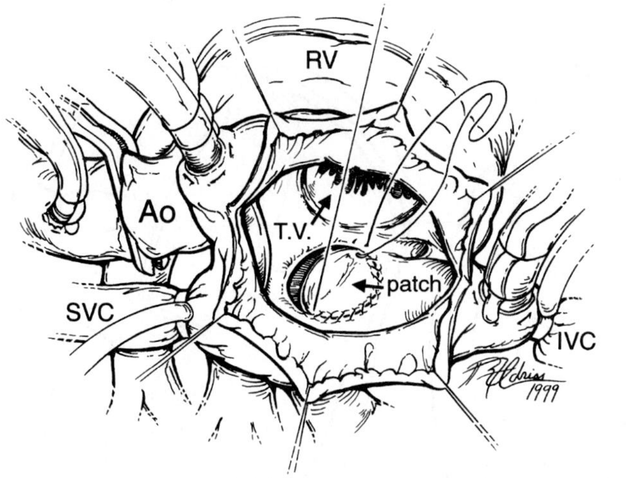

FIGURE 76.5. Atrial septal defect. Surgeon's view of a patient who is on cardiopulmonary bypass with aortic and bicaval venous cannulation. The heart has been arrested with cardioplegic solution injected into the ascending aorta (Ao). The right atrium has been opened, and the atrial septal defect has been partially closed by a patch. This patch is usually autologous pericardium, but Gore-Tex may also be used. The tricuspid valve (T.V.) is immediately above the atrial septal defect. IVC, inferior vena cava; RV, right ventricle; SVC, superior vena cava.

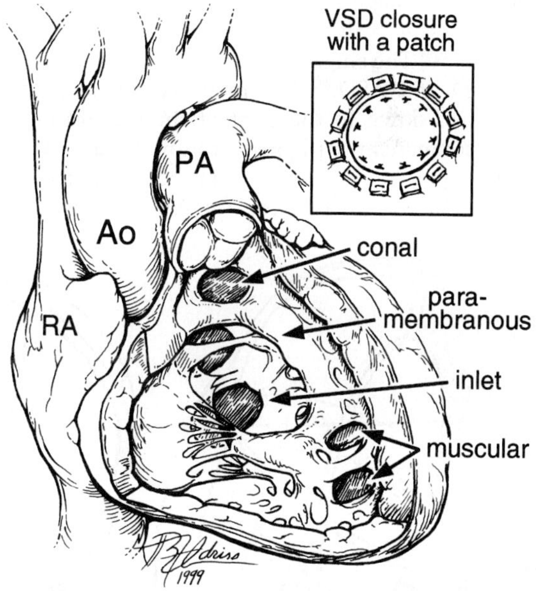

FIGURE 76.6. Ventricular septal defect. A cutaway view of the interventricular septum as it would be seen through a median sternotomy with the anterior right ventricle removed. The four main types of ventricular septal defects are illustrated. Their location within the interventricular septum gives rise to their name. Most ventricular septal defects are closed through the right atrium and through the tricuspid valve (see Fig. 76.5). Conal defects are approached through the pulmonary artery. Most ventricular septal defects are closed with a Dacron or Gore-Tex patch, which can be anchored either with interrupted pledgeted sutures (as shown) or with a running suture technique. In our experience, the interrupted pledgeted suture technique is associated with a lower incidence of residual ventricular septal defects. Ao, aorta; PA, pulmonary artery; RA, right atrium.

At the Children's Memorial Hospital between 1990 and 2004, there were 358 patients who underwent closure of an isolated VSD. All defects were closed with cardiopulmonary bypass, cardioplegia, and a patch (see Fig. 76.6). The median age at VSD closure was 0.7 years. No patients died, 1 of 294 patients without Down syndrome required a permanent pacemaker for atrioventricular (AV) block, and there was 1% incidence of postpericardiotomy syndrome.[26] In a patient population of 141 children over 1 year of age (mean age, 6 years) with a restrictive VSD, there was also no mortality, there were no residual defects, there were no patients with heart block, and mean hospital stay was 3.5 days.[27]

There are currently investigational devices for transcatheter closure of VSD in development.[28] These will be most applicable to muscular VSDs with a rim that does not involve valve or conduction structures and for older children.

Atrioventricular Canal

Atrioventricular canal (AVC) or endocardial cushion defects involve deficiencies of the atrial septum, ventricular septum, and atrioventricular valves (Fig. 76.7). The pathology ranges from partial AVC, to intermediate AVC, to complete AVC. Infants with a complete AVC defect have systemic pulmonary artery pressures and often present in congestive heart failure. More than 80% of patients with AVC defect have trisomy 21 (Down syndrome). We recommend intracardiac repair of AVC defects at the age of 3 to 6 months. The preoperative evaluation is usually adequate with two-dimensional and color flow Doppler echocardiography. Closure may be performed with a single patch, double patch (two patch), or modified single patch (Fig. 76.8A–76.8C). The two-patch technique uses Gore-Tex for the VSD, pericardium for the ASD, and valve reconstruction with mitral valve cleft closure.[29,30] The single-patch technique uses pericardium for the VSD and ASD.[31] The modified single patch pulls the AV valves down to the crest of the septum and closes the atrial component with pericardium.[32] Results with all three techniques are similar: operative mortality 2%–5%, pacemaker 3%–5%, reoperation for AV valve insufficiency 3%–8%.[29–33] However, the modified single patch technique facilitates the operation in smaller, younger patients and can be accomplished with shorter cross-clamp and cardiopulmonary bypass.[33]

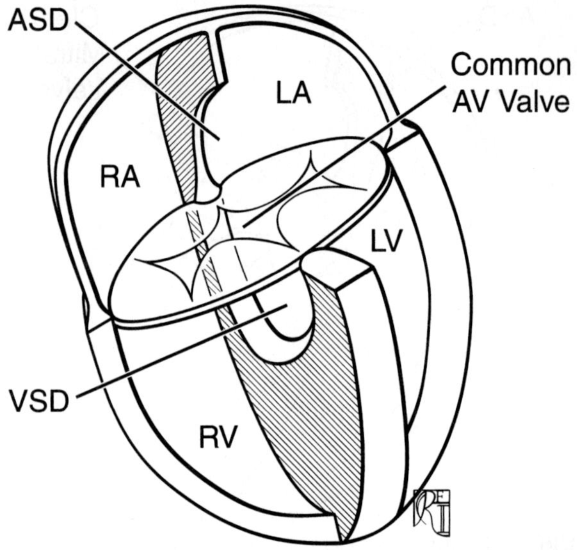

FIGURE 76.7. Complete AV (atrioventricular) canal defect. There is a common AV valve with an ostium primum atrial septal defect (ASD) "above" and a large inlet ventricular septal defect (VSD) "below." LA, RA, left, right atrium, respectively; LV, RV, left, right ventricle, respectively.

Truncus Arteriosus

Truncus arteriosus is a complex lesion in which a single arterial trunk emanates from the ventricular mass of the heart. The systemic, coronary, and pulmonary circulations all arise from this single trunk, and there is a large VSD. Individuals with truncus arteriosus have systemic pulmonary artery pressures and present with severe congestive heart failure in the first several days and weeks of life. Patients with truncus arteriosus have been classified into four groups by Van Praagh;[34] these types are illustrated in Figure 76.9.

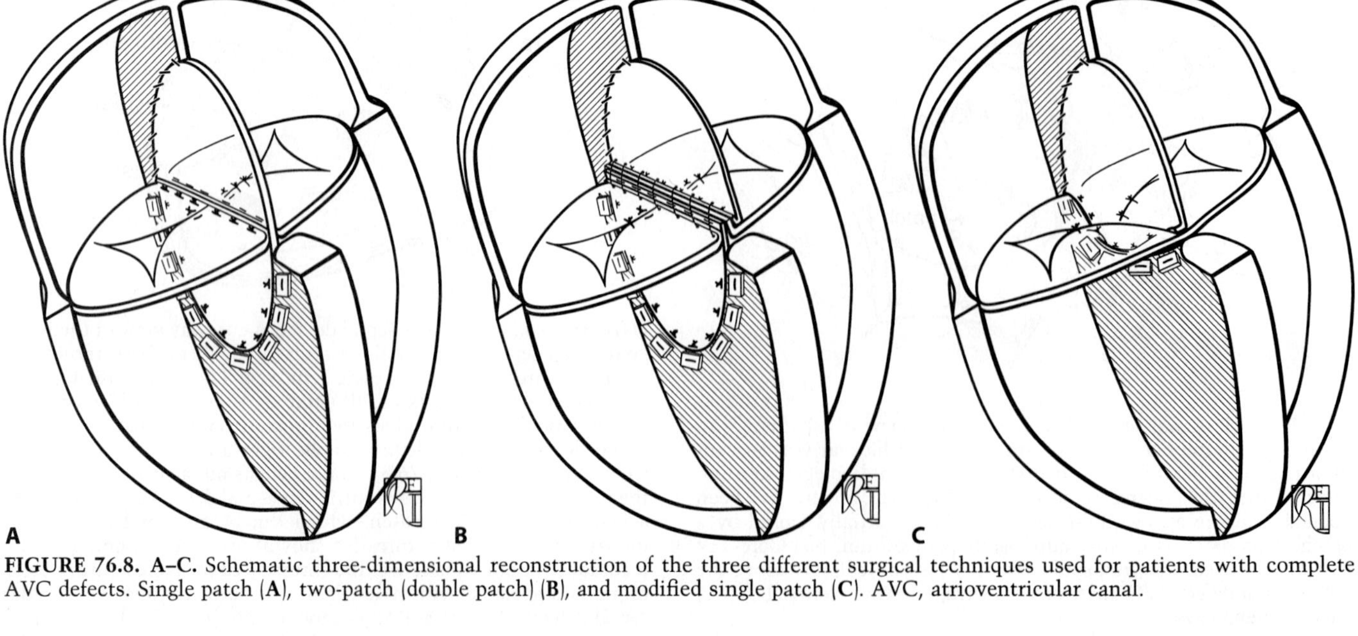

FIGURE 76.8. A–C. Schematic three-dimensional reconstruction of the three different surgical techniques used for patients with complete AVC defects. Single patch (**A**), two-patch (double patch) (**B**), and modified single patch (**C**). AVC, atrioventricular canal.

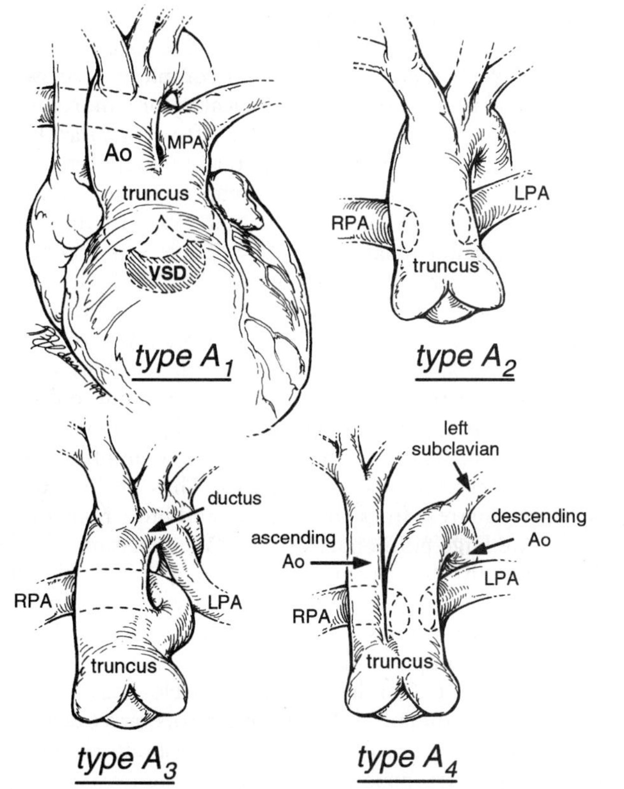

FIGURE 76.9. Truncus arteriosus: the four types as originally described by Van Praagh and Van Praagh. In type A_1, a discrete main pulmonary artery (MPA) originates from the truncus arteriosus. The A_1 illustration also shows the location of the ventricular septal defect beneath the truncal valve. In type A_2, there is separate origin of the right (RPA) and left (LPA) pulmonary arteries from the truncus arteriosus. In type A_3, or "hemitruncus," the LPA originates from the transverse arch from a ductus arteriosus. Type A_4 is both truncus arteriosus and interrupted aortic arch. Note the descending aorta (Ao) originates from the ductus arteriosus, which originates from the truncus arteriosus. There is complete separation of the ascending and descending thoracic aorta (Ao).

These patients were originally palliated with pulmonary artery banding as described in 1952 by Muller and Dammann.[4] The mortality rate of this approach with corrective repair later in life was nearly 50%. Dr. Dwight McGoon from the Mayo Clinic in 1968 described the first physiological correction of truncus arteriosus using a valved conduit from the right ventricle to the main pulmonary artery and VSD closure.[35] In 1984, Dr. Paul Ebert at the University of California, San Francisco (UCSF), reported a series of 100 infants under 6 months of age having repair with VSD closure and placement of a valved conduit with an 11% mortality rate.[36]

Currently, we recommend neonatal repair of truncus arteriosus at the time of diagnosis. The repair involves the use of cardiopulmonary bypass with hypothermia and cardioplegia, detachment of the pulmonary artery from the truncus, VSD closure, and placement of a conduit from the right ventricle to the pulmonary artery (Fig. 76.10); this is commonly called a Rastelli procedure. It should be pointed out that the "Rastelli operation" is one of the more common procedures for complex congenital cardiac lesions. Many patients have the combined problems of a large VSD and pulmonary atresia. The Rastelli procedure addresses this by closing the VSD and placing a conduit from the right ventricle to the pulmonary artery.

Both Bove from Ann Arbor, Michigan, and Hanley at UCSF have reported excellent results with protocols revolving around elective primary repair in the neonatal period.[37,38] Bove reported 46 neonates (mean age, 13 days) repaired between 1986 and 1992 with an 11% mortality.[37] Hanley reported 65 patients operated on between 1992 and 1999. Median age was 10 days; operative mortality was 5%.[38] In that series, truncal valve replacement and weight less than 2.5 kg were important risk factors for perioperative death. Our center has reported excellent results with truncal valve repair for patients with truncal insufficiency using a technique of leaflet excision and reduction annuloplasty.[39]

Aortopulmonary Window

Aortopulmonary window is a very rare congenital lesion in which there is a direct communication between the proximal ascending aorta and the main pulmonary artery. These babies have severe pulmonary hypertension and are at high risk for pulmonary vascular obstructive disease. Commonly associated lesions include interrupted aortic arch (20%) and right pulmonary artery origin from the aorta (20%). We recommend neonatal repair of these patients with a patch placed within the aorta to separate the blood flow in the great arteries. We operated on 22 patients with aortopulmonary window[40] at Children's Memorial Hospital between 1961 and 2001. There has been no mortality in the most recent 7 patients having transaortic patch closure.

Right-to-Left Shunt

Tetralogy of Fallot

Tetralogy of Fallot is the most common cause of cyanotic heart disease. The four components of tetralogy of Fallot are

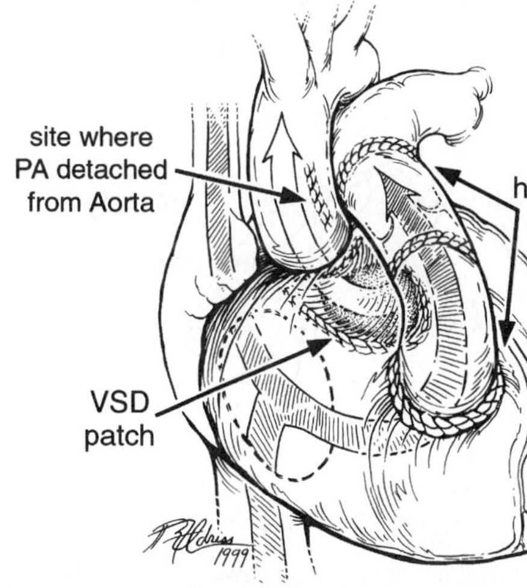

FIGURE 76.10. Rastelli procedure for truncus arteriosus: completed repair of a patient with truncus arteriosus. The pulmonary artery (PA) has been detached from the ascending aorta and the resultant opening closed primarily. A homograft conduit has been inserted from the right ventricle (RV) to the pulmonary artery. Finally, the ventricular septal defect (VSD) has been closed with a patch. Open curved arrows illustrate the flow of blood from the superior and inferior vena cava through the tricuspid valve, into the RV, through the conduit, and into the PA. Blood from the left atrium is deflected by the VSD patch from the LV into the ascending aorta.

VSD, pulmonary stenosis, right ventricular hypertrophy, and an overriding aorta (Fig. 76.11). Tetralogy is caused embryologically by the anterior and superior displacement of the infundibular septum. This displacement of the septum causes the VSD and obstruction of the right ventricular outflow tract. These children usually present with cyanosis within the first several weeks to months of life. Chest x-ray classically shows decreased pulmonary vascularity and a "boot-shaped" heart; 30% of these patients have an aortic arch positioned on the right side. Indications for surgery are hypercyanotic or "tet" spells, progressive polycythemia, or oxygen saturation less than 80% in room air.

In the early years of cardiac surgery, most of these children had an initial modified Blalock-Taussig shunt with complete repair later in life. Currently, an increasing number of centers have changed to performing tetralogy of Fallot repair as soon as the child becomes symptomatic.[41] The operative repair involves closing the VSD (preferably through the right atrium) and relieving the pulmonary stenosis (Fig. 76.11, inset). Relief of pulmonary stenosis may require resection of infundibular muscle, pulmonary valvotomy, and pulmonary artery patching. In patients with a hypoplastic pulmonary valve, a transannular patch may be required.

Although some centers repair all patients with tetralogy of Fallot when symptomatic, we feel that relative contraindications to neonatal (first 30 days of life) repair include hypoplastic pulmonary arteries, multiple VSDs, anomalous origin of the left anterior descending coronary artery from the right coronary artery (7% of patients), and weight below 3 kg. The current results of repair of tetralogy of Fallot are very good. Dr. Roger Mee and associates from Melbourne, Australia, and the Cleveland Clinic reported[42] a cumulative series of 609 patients with tetralogy of Fallot operated on between 1980 and 2000. Median age at the time of complete repair was 15 months, and there were 2 hospital deaths for a mortality rate of 0.3%. The mean right ventricular/left ventricular (RV/LV) pressure ratio postoperatively was 0.46; actuarial survival at 4 years was 97.5%; freedom from reoperation at 5 years was 95%. At Children's Memorial Hospital, 102 patients have had tetralogy of Fallot repair since 1997. There was no operative mortality. Median age was 5.9 months, 24% (25 patients) had a prerepair shunt, 80% (82 patients) had preservation of the pulmonary valve, and reoperation at 5 years was 6%.[43]

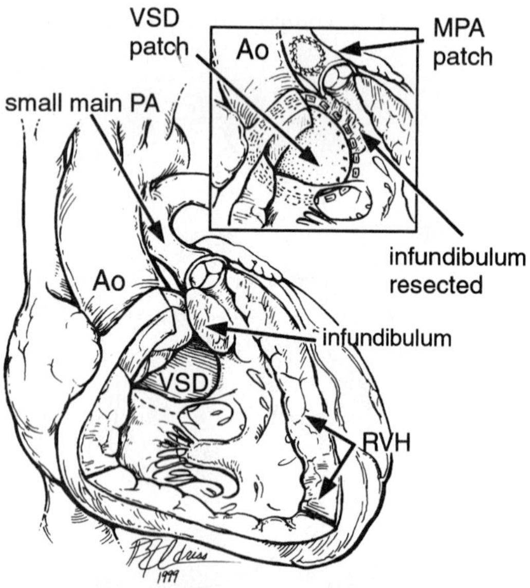

FIGURE 76.11. Tetralogy of Fallot. Cutaway view of the right ventricle illustrates the four components of tetralogy of Fallot: a large ventricular septal defect (VSD); overriding of the ascending aorta (Ao); and anterior and superior displacement of the infundibulum into the right ventricular outflow tract with resultant hypoplasia of the main pulmonary artery (MPA) and right ventricular hypertrophy (RVH). Inset illustrates repair with a Dacron or polytetrafluoroethylene (PTFE) patch closing the VSD. The infundibular muscle has been resected to allow for unobstructed flow of blood to the pulmonary valve, and the area above the pulmonary valve has been opened with a patch.

There is a subgroup of patients with tetralogy of Fallot who have very rudimentary development of the pulmonary valve. These patients develop aneurysmal pulmonary arteries that become quite dilated because of the to-and-fro nature of the pulmonary blood flow in utero. These babies develop respiratory distress from the tracheal and bronchial compression by the large pulmonary arteries. We recommend neonatal repair with VSD closure and a homograft valved conduit from the right ventricle to the pulmonary artery. In addition, the pulmonary arteries are plicated (made smaller) so that they do not compress the tracheobronchial tree. Between 1991 and 1997 at Children's Memorial Hospital, 11 infants underwent this therapy.[44] There were no operative deaths, but there were 2 late deaths secondary to respiratory complications of severe tracheobronchial compression.

Tricuspid Atresia

Patients born with *tricuspid atresia* have no development of the tricuspid valve and as a result no communication between the right atrium and right ventricle. All the blood that returns to the right atrium from the inferior and superior vena cava must traverse an ASD to the left atrium and then pass through the left ventricle and out to the systemic circulation. Some of these patients have a small VSD that gives rise to a small pulmonary artery. If a VSD is not present or if there is associated pulmonary atresia, these patients may be reliant on a PDA for pulmonary blood flow.

The eventual surgical repair of patients with tricuspid atresia is a Fontan type of operation, first performed in 1968 by Francis Fontan of Bordeaux, France.[45] The Fontan operation separates the systemic and pulmonary circulations in a patient with one ventricle. The Fontan procedure, like the Rastelli procedure, is another "signature" congenital heart operation. Because there is no functioning right ventricle, the systemic venous return is connected directly to the pulmonary artery, and the single ventricle becomes the systemic ventricle. Unlike many other pediatric cardiac procedures, the Fontan operation cannot be performed on neonates because of their normally high pulmonary vascular resistance. It is only after about 1.5 to 2 years of age that the pulmonary vascular resistance is low enough to allow the Fontan operation to be performed.

Therefore, the initial palliation of tricuspid atresia is usually with a systemic-to-pulmonary artery shunt, most often a modified Blalock-Taussig shunt as described previously (see Fig. 76.1). Most of these patients then have a second "staging" operation prior to the completion Fontan operation; this staging consists of a bidirectional Glenn (superior cavopulmonary artery anastomosis) at 6 months of age

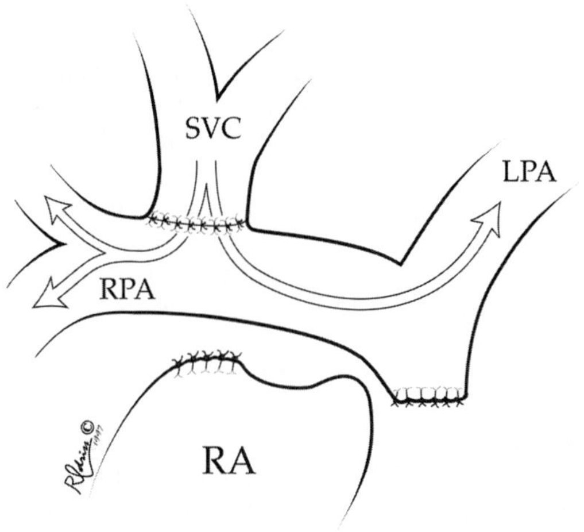

FIGURE 76.12. Bidirectional Glenn: The bidirectional Glenn was first proposed by Hopkins and associates in 1985. The superior vena cava (SVC) is transected, and the cardiac stump on the right atrium (RA) is oversewn as shown. The SVC is then anastomosed to an opening created in the superior aspect of the anatomic right pulmonary artery (RPA). Physiologically, the blood from the SVC can flow into either the RPA or the left pulmonary artery (LPA); hence, the designation *bidirectional Glenn*. The main pulmonary artery has been disconnected from the ventricle so that the only source of pulmonary blood flow is now the SVC. We now call this a *superior caval pulmonary artery anastomosis*.

(Fig. 76.12).[46,47] The Fontan operation is then performed at 2 to 3 years of age. This "three-stage" approach has dramatically improved the outcome of these patients. These patients are evaluated after the bidirectional Glenn with cardiac catheterization to determine whether they satisfy what are now called the "Fontan criteria" for undergoing the Fontan operation (Table 76.4). The Fontan criteria are not rigid but rather are flexible guidelines to indicate the relative risk of the Fontan operation for each patient.

The Fontan operation has evolved considerably since its original description. The original operation was an anastomosis between the superior vena cava and the right pulmonary artery, closure of the ASD, insertion of a homograft valve in the inferior vena cava orifice, and placement of a homograft valved conduit between the right atrium and the left pulmonary artery. The modification described by Kreutzer of Buenos Aires, Argentina, in 1973 omitted the anastomosis from superior vena cava to right pulmonary artery and the inferior vena cava valve.[48]

TABLE 76.4 Original "Criteria" for the Fontan Operation, Now *Relative* Criteria.

Patient age between 2 and 16 years
Normal sinus rhythm
Normal caval anatomy
Normal right atrial volume
Mean pulmonary artery pressure less than 15 mmHg
Pulmonary vascular resistance less than 2 Wood units/m^2
Pulmonary arteries of normal size
Good ventricular function with a normal left ventricular ejection fraction and normal left ventricular end-diastolic pressure
No atrioventricular valve insufficiency
No impairing effects of prior shunts

The two types of Fontan operation that are most commonly used now are the lateral tunnel[49] and extracardiac Fontan.[50] Both are performed after the intermediate procedure, the superior cavopulmonary connection (bidirectional Glenn). The lateral tunnel involves a direct anastomosis of the transected proximal superior vena cava to the inferior aspect of the right pulmonary artery. The inferior vena cava blood is then baffled with a patch through a lateral tunnel in the right atrium to the pulmonary artery (Fig. 76.13).[50] The extracardiac Fontan is a tube graft (usually Gore-Tex) connecting the inferior vena cava and the pulmonary artery (Fig. 76.14).

A modification to this operation is the "fenestrated" Fontan first described by Bridges at Boston Children's Hospital; a small calibrated "ASD" is left in the lateral tunnel at the conclusion of the repair.[51] This allows the left heart to fill with unoxygenated blood and maintain cardiac output at the expense of mild systemic arterial desaturation.[52] This shunt can then be closed later in the cardiac catheterization lab with an ASD closure device or with a surgically placed purse-string suture. At some centers, the small ASD is simply left to close spontaneously over time.

Gentles and associates at the Boston Children's Hospital reported their results with the Fontan operation in 500 consecutive patients.[53] In that series, the incidence of early failure decreased from 27% in the first quartile of the experience to 7% in the last quartile. In a multivariate model, the following variables were associated with early failure: a mean pulmonary artery pressure above 19 mmHg, a right-sided tricuspid

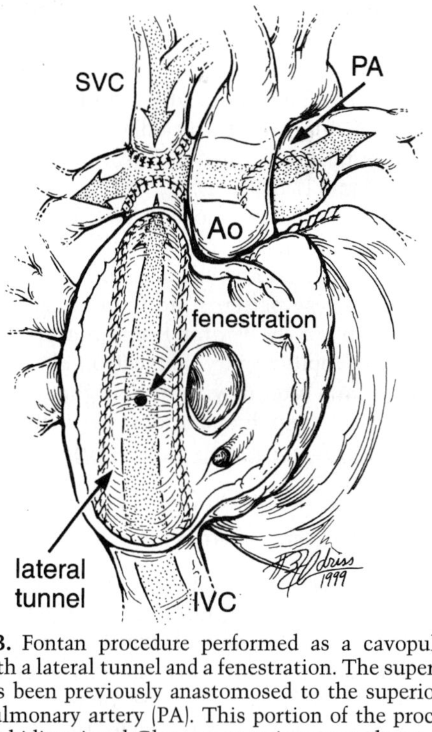

FIGURE 76.13. Fontan procedure performed as a cavopulmonary connection with a lateral tunnel and a fenestration. The superior vena cava (SVC) has been previously anastomosed to the superior aspect of the right pulmonary artery (PA). This portion of the procedure is referred to as a bidirectional Glenn or superior cavopulmonary anastomosis. Flow from the inferior vena cava (IVC) is directed by the lateral tunnel (usually constructed of Gore-Tex), through the cardiac end of the transected SVC, which has been anastomosed to the undersurface of the right PA. A small fenestration, illustrated in the midportion of the Gore-Tex lateral tunnel, allows shunting of blood from right to left to augment the preload in the postoperative period. Ao, aorta.

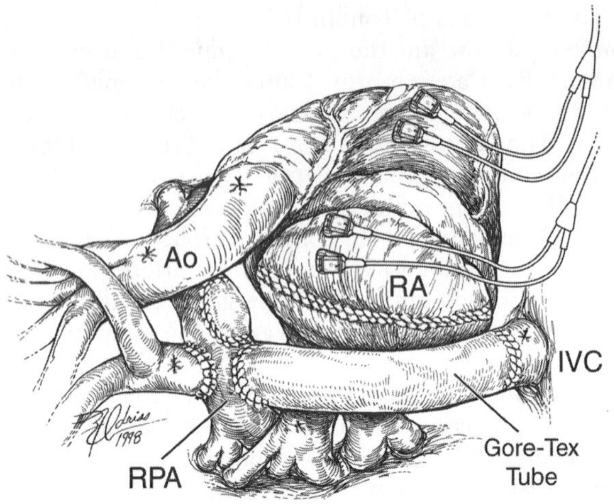

FIGURE 76.14. Extracardiac Fontan: The extracardiac Fontan is typically performed as the third of three stages of palliation for single ventricle. The first stage is some form of modified Blalock-Taussig shunt or Norwood; the second stage is a bidirectional Glenn procedure. The third stage illustrated here is the completion Fontan in which a Gore-Tex tube graft has been anastomosed to the inferior vena cava (IVC) and to the inferior aspect of the anatomic right pulmonary artery (RPA). Now, blood from the IVC may flow into either the right or left pulmonary artery. All desaturated systemic venous blood goes directly to the pulmonary circulation. All of the oxygenated blood returns to the heart and is ejected out of the aorta (Ao). This illustration shows bipolar, steroid-eluting pacing leads on both the atrium and ventricle. It is not uncommon for these patients to have arrhythmias postoperatively. RA, right atrium. (Reprinted from Mavroudis et al.,[113] with permission.)

valve as the only systemic AV valve, atriopulmonary connection instead of a cavopulmonary connection, and absence of a baffle fenestration. Hanley's group from the University of California, San Francisco recently reported their results with 285 patients having an extracardiac Fontan (18 or 20mm gafts).[53a] Early failure defined as death or takedown occurred in only 7 patients (2.5%).

Some older patients who underwent a Fontan with the original atriopulmonary connection have now developed complications of atrial arrhythmias and severe dilation of the right atrium. These patients are increasingly being referred for "conversion" of the Fontan from an atriopulmonary connection to a cavopulmonary connection along with ablation of the arrhythmia circuit within the right atrium.[54] We have now performed 112 such operations (1994–2006) with 1 operative mortality, 6 late deaths, and 6 patients requiring heart transplantation.[54a]

Pulmonary Atresia with Intact Ventricular Septum

Pulmonary atresia means there is no communication between the right ventricle and the pulmonary artery. In many of these patients, the pulmonary valve leaflets are fused. If there is an intact ventricular septum, there is no outlet for the blood within the right ventricle. Because of the small amount of blood flowing into the right ventricle, there is usually hypoplasia of the right ventricle. These patients are dependent on pulmonary blood flow through a PDA. They are broadly divided into three groups based on the size of the right ventricle and whether it contains the inflow, body, and outflow portions of the normal right ventricle. These patients are at risk for coronary sinusoids, which are abnormal communications between the right ventricle and the coronary arteries. These can become quite large and in fact interfere with the coronary circulation. A child with pulmonary atresia with intact ventricular septum presents with cyanosis, which can become severe if the ductus should close. Medical management utilizes intravenous infusion of PGE, which will keep the ductus open and medically stabilize the patient. Diagnosis is usually made by echocardiogram, and the precise surgical decision making is based on a cardiac catheterization, which is used to evaluate the size of the right ventricle and the anatomy of the pulmonary arteries.

We recommend operation through a median sternotomy with pulmonary valvotomy on cardiopulmonary bypass and placement of a modified Blalock-Taussig shunt to provide for adequate pulmonary blood flow. Following the initial procedure, the patient is observed to see how the right ventricle grows. The patients who have a very small right ventricle go on to a bidirectional Glenn and then a Fontan-type procedure. An intermediate group of patients has some growth of the right ventricle but not enough for biventricular repair. In these patients for whom the right ventricle remains between 30% and 60% of predicted normal, the repair involves both ASD closure and placement of a bidirectional Glenn.[55] The bidirectional Glenn decompresses the volume load on the right ventricle. Those patients who have adequate growth of the right ventricle can undergo ASD closure and shunt ligation and division, which is a biventricular repair. Risk factors for surgical intervention are chiefly the extent of the coronary sinusoids. More extensive sinusoids are associated with a higher mortality, and in some of these patients consideration should be given to cardiac transplantation. Roger Mee of Melbourne, Australia, reported[56] on 48 neonates operated on between 1980 and 1992; of these individuals, 31 patients had a valvotomy and a shunt, and 17 patients had a shunt only (small right ventricle). The probability of a biventricular repair was 60%, and the probability of survival at 8 years was 77%.

Pulmonary Atresia with Ventricular Septal Defect

Infants with *pulmonary atresia with VSD* have fusion of the pulmonary valve cusps and a large VSD. This is often considered the most extreme form of tetralogy of Fallot. Although some of these patients have a distinct ductus arteriosus filling the pulmonary arteries, approximately 50% do not have confluent pulmonary arteries but instead have pulmonary blood flow originating from multiple aortopulmonary collateral arteries from the descending thoracic aorta. These babies present with cyanosis, which may or may not improve after prostaglandin infusion because of the small size or absence of a ductus arteriosus. In these patients, cardiac catheterization is necessary to define the pulmonary artery anatomy and the origins of the multiple aortopulmonary collateral arteries.

Initial surgical intervention is usually directed at establishing pulmonary blood flow with a shunt, right ventricular outflow tract patch, or right ventricular-to-pulmonary artery homograft. Because of the VSD, there is adequate development of the right ventricle, and these patients can usually go on to a biventricular repair with a Rastelli-type operation, which includes closing the VSD and placing a valved conduit, often a homograft, between the right ventricle and the pulmonary arteries.

The key to a successful surgical repair in these patients is an adequate pulmonary artery bed. Several approaches may be taken. The most common historical approach is initially to perform right and left unifocalization procedures through thoracotomy incisions; this involves bringing all the pulmonary arteries that originate from the descending thoracic aorta together into a created central pulmonary artery using either a Gore-Tex or pericardial tube connected to a modified Blalock-Taussig shunt.[57] After both the right and left sides have been "unifocalized," a median sternotomy is performed at a later date to close the VSD and anastomose a conduit from the right ventricle to the confluence of these two "created" sets of pulmonary arteries.

Iyer and Mee from Royal Children's Hospital, Australia, reported their results with 58 patients[58]; 121 staging procedures were performed with a 10% mortality, 30 patients underwent hemodynamic repair with an early mortality of 3% and a late mortality of 10%, and 12 patients (21%) failed to achieve minimum requirements for hemodynamic repair. Another technique more recently described by Hanley and associates at UCSF is to operate on the child as an infant and on cardiopulmonary bypass do the unifocalization procedures on the right and the left from the median sternotomy approach. The VSD is then closed, and a conduit of homograft from the right ventricle to the newly reconstructed pulmonary arteries is established. Hanley et al. reported using this technique in 56 patients with a median age of 7 months. Actuarial survival was 80% at 3 years.[59]

Complex Cyanotic Lesions

Transposition of the Great Arteries

Transposition of the great arteries is the most common cause of cyanosis from a cardiac condition in the neonate. Patients with transposition of the great arteries have two parallel circulations. The aorta and coronary arteries originate from the right ventricle, and the pulmonary artery and ductus arteriosus arise from the left ventricle. In one circuit, the oxygenated blood returning from the lungs flows into the left atrium and ventricle, is ejected into the pulmonary artery, and recirculates back to the left atrium. In the other circuit, the unoxygenated blood returning to the right atrium goes into the right ventricle and is ejected out the aorta to recirculate back to the right atrium. With these two parallel circulations, infants with transposition are dependent on mixing of blood at the atrial, ventricular, or ductal levels for initial survival.

Infants with transposition usually present with cyanosis in the first 24h of life. The electrocardiogram shows right ventricular hypertrophy; the chest radiograph shows a narrow superior mediastinum (because of the anteroposterior relationship of the great vessels), increased pulmonary blood flow, and a cardiac silhouette (in relation to the diaphragm) that looks like an egg on its side. The diagnosis is made by two-dimensional echocardiography. Most patients do not go to cardiac catheterization unless there is a question of a coronary artery anomaly, coarctation, or VSD that is not accurately assessed by the echocardiogram.

The initial stabilization of the child with transposition begins with the administration of PGE_1; this maintains patency of the ductus arteriosus and allows mixing of blood at that level. However, some patients will not have enough mixing with PGE_1 infusion and may require an atrial septostomy. This is done percutaneously with a balloon catheter, either at the bedside under echo guidance or in the cardiac catheterization laboratory under fluoroscopy. The catheter is advanced into the left atrium, the balloon is inflated, and when the balloon is pulled back into the right atrium the atrial septum is torn open. This procedure allows for mixing of blood at the atrial level. In the current era, most patients with transposition of the great arteries then undergo a definitive repair, which is an arterial switch operation in the first or second week of life. This technique was first performed successfully by Jatene from Sao Paulo, Brazil, and reported[60] in 1976. Neonatal repair was popularized by Castaneda at Boston Children's Hospital.[61] If the child presents after approximately 4 to 6 weeks of age, primary repair may no longer be possible because the ventricular muscle mass will have "thinned out" and no longer be capable of supporting the systemic circulation after the arterial switch operation. In these patients, the left ventricle must be retrained to prepare for an arterial switch by first banding the pulmonary artery.[62]

The arterial switch operation involves "switching" the great vessels and moving the coronary arteries. This operation is done with cardiopulmonary bypass, hypothermia, and cardioplegic arrest of the heart. The ductus arteriosus is ligated and divided, and the atrial communication created by septostomy is closed. The great vessels are transected and switched, anastomosing the aorta to the left ventricular outflow tract and the main pulmonary artery to the right ventricular outflow tract. The coronary arteries are transferred from the right ventricular outflow tract to the left ventricular outflow tract. This procedure is facilitated by the so-called Le Compte maneuver in which the pulmonary artery is moved anterior to the aorta.[63] When the arterial switch operation is completed, the left ventricle gives rise to the aorta and the coronary arteries, and the right ventricle gives rise to the pulmonary artery.

Wernovsky and colleagues[64] at Boston Children's Hospital reviewed 470 patients who had an arterial switch between 1983 and 1992. Risk of mortality was less than 5%, and risk of reintervention was less than 10%. Long-term follow-up of patients after their arterial switch operation showed that more than 95% were in normal sinus rhythm,[65] and almost all had normal ventricular function.[66] A small percentage (9%) of patients required reoperation for supravalvular pulmonary stenosis, aortic valve insufficiency, or coronary artery stenosis.[67]

This method is a great improvement from the previous operations performed for transposition. The first successful physiological correction was done in 1959 by Ake Senning (Stockholm, Sweden), who performed atrial baffling to direct the superior and inferior caval blood flow to the mitral valve (left ventricle) and the pulmonary venous return to the tricuspid valve (right ventricle). This operation effectively placed the circulation in series with the right ventricle used as the systemic pumping chamber. The Mustard operation (W. Mustard, Toronto, Canada) was also a physiological or "atrial" repair and was first performed in 1964. This technique also redirected the caval flow but used a pericardial patch rather than autologous atrial tissue. This operation was technically easier to perform and became more widely accepted. The difficulty with the atrial baffle procedures were the long-term complications of atrial arrhythmias, AV block, superior vena caval obstruction, baffle leaks, and most seriously, right ventricular dysfunction with tricuspid valve insufficiency. Gelatt and colleagues from the Hospital for Sick Children, Toronto, reviewed the cases of 534 children who had a Mustard operation.[68] Operative mortality was 10%, and survival at 20 years of age was 76%. Sinus rhythm was present in only 40% of patients at 20 years, and 6% of the operative survivors died of sudden death. Some of these patients with severe right ventricular dysfunction are candidates for staged conversion to an arterial switch as described by Cochrane and associates at Royal Children's Hospital, Melbourne.[69] Other patients with severe right ventricular dysfunction will require cardiac transplantation.[70]

Approximately 25% of patients with transposition of the great arteries have an associated VSD. A subset of these patients have the so-called Taussig-Bing heart, which consists of transposition of the great arteries, subpulmonic VSD, double-outlet right ventricle, and subaortic conus. Many of these patients also have a coarctation of the aorta. In the current era, most of these patients are treated with primary repair, either with arterial switch and VSD closure or Kawashima intraventricular repair.[71]

Total Anomalous Pulmonary Venous Connection

In *total anomalous pulmonary venous connection*, there is no direct communication between the pulmonary veins and the left atrium. The common pulmonary vein instead finds a route to the heart via the cardinal, umbilical, or systemic venous channels. These patients require either a large patent foramen ovale or an ASD for survival. Anatomically, there are four types of total anomalous pulmonary venous connection. In the supracardiac type (50%), there is an anomalous vertical vein, usually on the left side of the pericardium, that drains from the common pulmonary vein to the innominate vein. In the cardiac type (30%), the pulmonary veins drain into the coronary sinus, which then drains into the right atrium. In the infracardiac type (15%), the common pulmonary vein drains to a midline vertical vein that can connect to the portal vein, inferior vena cava, or ductus venosus. In the mixed type (5%), there can be any combination of these three types.

These babies have equal oxygen saturations in all four cardiac chambers and the great vessels. They present with cyanosis and congestive heart failure. Chest x-ray reveals a normal heart size with a "ground-glass"-type appearance of the lung fields. Echocardiogram reveals right ventricular diastolic overload and a free space posterior to the left atrium. Color Doppler flow can be used to demonstrate the morphology and flow patterns in the anomalous vein. Most of these babies are referred for cardiac surgical repair without a cardiac catheterization. Babies who have stenosis or obstruction of the venous drainage may present with extreme cyanosis and hypotension and require emergent surgical intervention.

These patients are repaired at the time of diagnosis. Technique of repair is with cardiopulmonary bypass and either low-flow perfusion or circulatory arrest. The repair for supracardiac and infracardiac types is to create an opening in the common pulmonary vein and the left atrium and then suture these two orifices together. The ASD is closed, and the vertical vein draining to the systemic venous system is ligated. The cardiac type of drainage is corrected by widely opening the coronary sinus into the left atrium and then closing the ASD along with the orifice of the coronary sinus. Caldarone and colleagues at the Hospital for Sick Children[72] reported their results in 170 patients treated for total anomalous pulmonary venous connection between 1982 and 1996; median age at repair was 20 days. In the current era, the operative mortality for simple cases was 8% and for complex cases (other cardiac anomalies) was 52%. About 10% of these patients develop pulmonary vein stenosis, and an innovative way of treating them is the "sutureless" repair.[73]

Cor triatriatum is a rare lesion that is part of the spectrum of total anomalous pulmonary venous connection. Although there is a connection between the common pulmonary vein and the left atrium in these patients, this connection is stenotic. Most commonly, this results in a membrane within the atrial chamber that restricts flow to the mitral valve. These patients can present in various ways, depending on the degree of stenosis and whether an ASD is present. Two-dimensional echocardiography provides the diagnosis in most instances. The repair is an excision of the cor triatriatum membrane.

Hypoplastic Left Heart Syndrome

Hypoplastic left heart syndrome is a severe congenital heart defect in which the child does not have a functioning left ventricle. These patients have aortic valve atresia or severe aortic stenosis with mitral valve atresia or severe mitral stenosis. There is hypoplasia of the left ventricle and ascending aorta, and most of these patients have a coarctation. Because the left ventricle is too small to support the systemic circulation, they are candidates for either cardiac transplantation or a series of staged operations leading to an eventual Fontan procedure. These babies present in the first days of life with cyanosis, tachypnea, and when the ductus arteriosus closes, cardiovascular collapse. Electrocardiogram shows severe right ventricular hypertrophy with diminished left ventricular forces. Diagnosis is readily established by two-dimensional and color Doppler echocardiography; most patients do not require cardiac catheterization for the diagnosis.

The medical management of a child with hypoplastic left heart syndrome before operative intervention is quite important. The child is placed on PGE_1 as soon as the diagnosis is made. This medication maintains patency of the ductus arteriosus and thus provides a route for coronary and systemic blood flow. It is important to keep the child on very low or no oxygen support despite low saturation to maintain the systemic cardiac output. In some instances, it is helpful to administer the child supplemental CO_2 to bring oxygen saturations down to the 75% range, which will give the ideal amount of systemic output.

Until the early 1980s, this syndrome was a fatal lesion. The first successful series of palliative operations were reported by Norwood and colleagues[74] on a group of patients operated on between 1979 and 1981. This operation has three components: (1) an atrial septectomy to provide complete mixing of blood at the atrial level, (2) an anastomosis with patch augmentation between the proximal transected main pulmonary artery and the ascending and descending aorta, and (3) a modified Blalock-Taussig shunt to provide for pulmonary blood flow. This operation establishes single-ventricle circulation with pulmonary blood flow maintained through a shunt (Fig. 76.15). The operative mortality of this procedure was initially more than 50%. With refinements in technique, the mortality is now 15% to 20%. These refine-

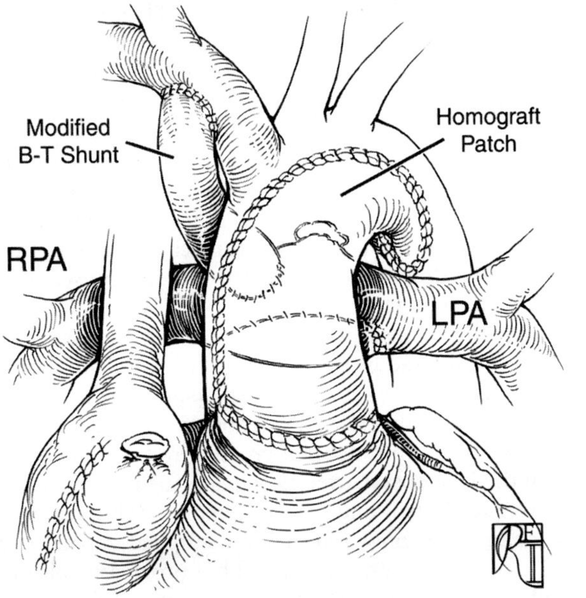

FIGURE 76.15. Norwood procedure: The three primary components of the Norwood procedure are atrial septectomy, a shunt to provide pulmonary blood flow from the systemic circulation, and a connection of the right ventricle to the aorta and coronary arteries along with coarctation repair. The illustration shows a completed Norwood procedure. Atrial septectomy has been performed through the incision in the right atrium. There is a modified Blalock-Taussig shunt that has been constructed from the right innominate artery to the superior aspect of the pulmonary artery. The old pulmonary valve has been converted to a "neoaortic" valve by the anastomosis between the proximal main pulmonary artery and the dimunitive ascending aorta. The large homograft patch is used to augment the ascending aorta and to repair the area of the coarctation distally. LPA, left pulmonary artery; RPA, right pulmonary artery.

ments include use of smaller shunts (3.5–4.0mm), continuous cerebral perfusion, modified ultrafiltration, preoperative steroids, staged chest closure, and more defined postoperative management.

Bove reported[75] on 303 patients undergoing a Norwood operation for hypoplastic left heart syndrome between 1990 and 1998. Overall hospital survival was 76%. Among patients who were considered to be at "standard risk" rather than "high risk," survival was significantly higher at 86%, and actuarial survival at 2 years was 74%.

A recent innovation in the management of these patients that appears to have improved outcomes is the use of a right ventricle-to-pulmonary artery shunt—the Sano modification.[76] After the Norwood (or Sano) operation, these patients undergo a bidirectional Glenn or hemi-Fontan operation (superior cavopulmonary anastomosis) as a second stage at 6 to 9 months of age and a completion Fontan (third stage) at 2 to 3 years of age. Jacobs and Norwood reported on 200 patients (127 with hypoplastic left heart syndrome) who had a completion Fontan after a prior superior cavopulmonary anastomosis.[77] Early mortality was 8%.

An alternative approach to staged palliation is orthotopic cardiac transplantation with extensive aortic arch reconstruction. This was first accomplished successfully in November 1985 by Leonard Bailey.[78] Following this, Mavroudis and others have reported similar success with orthotopic cardiac transplantation and extensive aortic arch reconstruction for infants with hypoplastic left heart syndrome.[79] These patients are maintained on immunosuppression with cyclosporine and CellCept and are weaned from steroids after 6 months of age. Bailey and colleagues from Loma Linda reported 233 infant transplants from 1985 to 1999, with over a 90% operative survival and a 10-year actuarial survival of 70%.[80] At the Children's Memorial Hospital, we also reported a 90% operative survival.[70]

Unfortunately, only 70% to 80% of infants placed on the waiting list for heart transplants will receive a heart.[81] Most centers treating patients with hypoplastic left heart syndrome now recommend staged reconstruction starting with the Norwood procedure and reserve transplant for those who develop ventricular dysfunction.

Obstructive Lesions

Aortic Stenosis

Congenital *aortic stenosis* is an obstruction of flow between the left ventricle and the ascending aorta. There are four congenital types of aortic stenosis: supravalvular, valvular, discrete subvalvular, and hypertrophic muscular subaortic stenosis. Many of these babies have associated lesions, including coarctation of the aorta, supravalvar mitral ring, and parachute mitral valve (Shone's syndrome). The most common type of aortic stenosis is valvular aortic stenosis secondary to a bicuspid aortic valve. If the aortic stenosis is severe, these patients will present in infancy with congestive heart failure and diminished peripheral pulses. Older children present with exercise intolerance, angina, and syncope. Diagnosis is obtained by echocardiography.

Initially, aortic valvotomy was performed with the use of cardiopulmonary bypass. Hawkins and coauthors reported 37 neonates operated on between 1986 and 1996 for critical aortic stenosis.[82] Actuarial survival was 92% at 1 month, 78% at 1 year, and 73% at 10 years. More recently, many centers have advocated balloon dilation of the aortic valve with percutaneous transcatheter techniques in the cardiac catheterization laboratory. McCrindle et al. reported a multiinstitutional study of 110 neonates and infants undergoing either surgical aortic valvotomy (n = 28) or balloon aortic valvuloplasty (n = 82). Survival was 82% at 1 month in both groups.[83] For older children with valvar aortic stenosis, balloon dilation provides good interim palliation. Moore and associates at Boston Children's Hospital reported 148 children over 1 month of age (mean age 7 years) undergoing transcatheter balloon dilation.[84] Procedural mortality was 1%, and dilation was successful in 87%. However, only 50% of patients remained free of repeat intervention at 8 years.

Supravalvular aortic stenosis is relieved by placing a patch in the supravalvar area.[85] Discrete subvalvular aortic stenosis is treated by resecting the fibromuscular ridge. Hypertrophic muscular subaortic stenosis is treated with septal myotomy and myectomy.[86]

Surgeons have become interested in using the Ross operation, not necessarily as the first operation for aortic stenosis, but as the second operation when the aortic stenosis reoccurs after initial aortic valvotomy or balloon valvuloplasty. The Ross operation involves harvesting the pulmonary valve from the patient as an autograft, resecting the aortic valve, and then implanting the pulmonary valve into the aortic annulus.[87] This technique necessitates reimplanting the coronary arteries into the sinuses of the harvested pulmonary autograft. To replace the pulmonary valve, a pulmonary valve homograft is selected and sutured between the right ventricle and the main pulmonary artery. The Ross operation is now performed at many centers and has a very low mortality. Elkins reported[88] on 197 patients (<18 years of age) having the Ross operation between 1986 and 2002. Operative mortality was 3.9%. Actuarial freedom from reoperation for autograft insufficiency was 81% at 16 years and from allograft reoperation was 83% at 16 years. Unlike children with a mechanical valve, these patients do not require anticoagulation. In addition, there is a longer reoperation-free interval when compared to tissue valves, and there is evidence that the neoaortic valve grows in the pediatric population. The hope with these patients is that they will require replacement of only the homograft valve placed in the pulmonic position and that the aortic valve will continue to function throughout their life.

Mitral Stenosis

Congenital *mitral stenosis* patients often have other congenital heart defects, such as coarctation of the aorta or VSD. Mitral stenosis is divided into four anatomical types: (1) typical congenital mitral stenosis, (2) hypoplastic congenital mitral stenosis, (3) supramitral ring, and (4) parachute mitral valve. Surgical options include simple valvotomy, excision of the supravalvular ring, and mitral valve replacement. At the Children's Memorial Hospital, we have reported successful repair of five infants with congenital mitral stenosis.[89]

Pulmonic Stenosis

Pulmonic stenosis is caused by partial fusion of the pulmonary valve cusps. Depending on the degree of valve fusion, these children may present with cyanosis in the newborn period or may be completely asymptomatic and present later in life with a systolic murmur. Isolated pulmonic stenosis is now being treated successfully in the cardiac catheterization laboratory with percutaneous transcatheter balloon dilation in nearly all cases.[90]

Coarctation of the Aorta

Coarctation of the aorta is one of the most common obstructive lesions found in children. The word *coarctation* comes from the Latin "to contract." It is defined as a hemodynamically significant narrowing of the aorta, usually found in the descending thoracic aorta just distal to the left subclavian artery. There are two theories regarding why coarctations form. The first is that ductal tissue from the PDA extends out into the aorta, and at the time of ductus closure this tissue contracts and narrows the aorta. The other theory stems from the observation that many of these patients have an associated intracardiac left-to-right shunt. The left-to-right shunt in utero prevents adequate blood flow through the ascending aorta, and subsequently there is lack of growth of the arch of the aorta distal to the left subclavian artery.

The clinical presentation of the child with coarctation depends on the severity of stenosis and whether the blood flow to the lower extremities is dependent on the ductus arteriosus. Infants with coarctation who have closure of a ductus that is supplying blood to the lower extremities will develop cardiovascular collapse when the ductus closes. These children present with poor perfusion of the lower extremities, acidosis, and renal failure. They also may have severe congestive heart failure because the outflow from the left ventricle is severely obstructed by the coarctation. A chest radiograph in this situation shows cardiomegaly with signs of congestive heart failure.

Older children with a coarctation and even some adults may be asymptomatic. They are usually found to have hypertension in the upper extremities on routine physical examination, often for a school exam. On further evaluation, they are noted to have diminished or absent femoral pulses. A chest radiograph in an older child classically shows the "three sign" in the superior mediastinum. This sign is formed by the combination of a dilated proximal aortic isthmus, the narrowing of the coarctation site itself, and the poststenotic dilation of the descending thoracic aorta. Another radiographic sign in older children is rib notching, created by the collateral flow through the intercostal arteries beneath the ribs. With the use of two-dimensional and color Doppler echocardiography, most infants are now referred for surgical repair without cardiac catheterization. This trend has progressed also to the older child with coarctation, although some of these children will require cardiac catheterization to evaluate other intracardiac anomalies. Cardiac MRI and CT scan are also excellent at showing the anatomy of the coarctation. Older patients are at risk for bacterial endocarditis, rupture of the aorta, hypertension leading to cerebral vascular accidents, and coronary artery disease. For older patients with a coarctation, the mean age at death is 35 years.[91]

Neonates that present with coarctation are resuscitated with a prostaglandin (PGE_1) infusion that opens the ductus arteriosus and the coarctation site itself, restoring blood flow to the lower half of the body. Medical therapy for several days with PGE_1 allows time for resolution of acidosis and renal insufficiency. These children may then be operated on electively when in good physiological condition. Our operative procedure of choice for these infants is currently resection of the coarctation site and ductal tissue with extended end-to-end anastomosis (Fig. 76.16). This approach has resulted in low operative mortality and a very low incidence of recoarctation. We reported on 55 infants operated on from 1991 to 1997 using this technique.[92] Mean age at surgery was 21 days. There was 1 early death, no instances of paraplegia, and a 3.6% recoarctation rate.

Historical operative procedures for infants include a simple resection with end-to-end anastomosis, subclavian flap aortoplasty, and Dacron patch aortoplasty. All these techniques, although popular at one time, have been associated with high recurrence rates and are no longer used at most centers. For older patients with coarctation, we currently recommend Gore-Tex patch aortoplasty. This operation has a very low mortality rate and incidence of recoarctation. We reported[93] on 125 children having PTFE patch aortoplasty between 1979 and 1993. Mean age at repair was 5 years. There was no mortality in patients over 6 months of age, no instances of paraplegia, and a 4% recoarctation rate. One reported complication following this procedure is aneurysm formation in the aortic wall opposite the patch.[94] The incidence of this complication was high in early series if the coarctation ridge was resected, but with current techniques not involving ridge resection, aneurysm formation has become extremely rare.

Following coarctation repair, there is a very low incidence of lower extremity paraplegia related to spinal cord ischemia

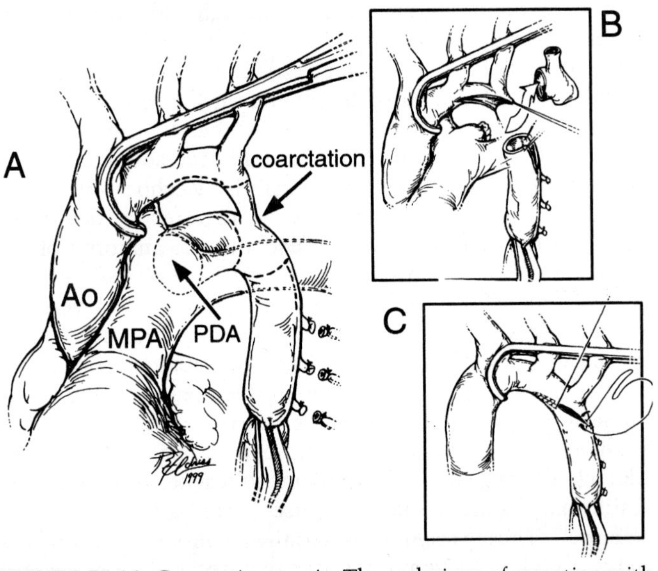

FIGURE 76.16. Coarctation repair. The technique of resection with extended end-to-end anastomosis is illustrated. **A.** Coarctation site is identified along with a large patent ductus arteriosus (PDA) originating from the main pulmonary artery (MPA). A vascular clamp is occluding the left subclavian, left carotid, and a portion of the ascending aorta (Ao). A second vascular clamp is occluding the descending thoracic aorta, and three sets of intercostal collateral arteries have been ligated and divided to allow for mobilization of the descending thoracic aorta. **B.** The ductus arteriosus is ligated proximally, and the ductal tissue and coarctation segment have been excised. Counterincisions have been made on the undersurface of the transverse arch and into the descending thoracic aorta. **C.** The suture line is completed, anastomosing the ascending and descending thoracic aorta with a long oblique anastomosis, which has a very low incidence of recoarctation.

during the time period the aorta is clamped for the repair. Efforts should be made to keep the aortic cross-clamp time under 30 min. The patient should be cooled to 35.5°C and the proximal blood pressure kept artificially high. The incidence of paraplegia[95] after a native coarctation repair is approximately 5 in 1000. We advocate the use of partial cardiopulmonary bypass to prevent this complication.[95] We monitor the femoral artery pressure during the operation (in patients over 1 year of age) and use left atrium to descending aorta bypass if the femoral pressure drops below 45 mmHg. Another unique complication of coarctation repair is paradoxical hypertension postoperatively.[96] These patients have a very elevated blood pressure in the postoperative period despite an adequate anatomical repair of the coarctation. This hypertension is felt to be initially related to the release of the stretch on the high set of the carotid baroreceptors. A second, more prolonged response is thought to be secondary to elevated levels of circulating catecholamines and angiotensin.

Interrupted Aortic Arch

Interrupted aortic arch is physiologically similar to severe coarctation, but in these babies there is complete loss of continuity between the ascending and descending aorta. The blood flow to the descending thoracic aorta is through a PDA (see Fig. 76.9, type A_4). Most of these patients also have a VSD. There are other commonly associated anomalies, including single ventricle (10%); truncus arteriosus (10%); diGeorge syndrome (absent thymus, hypocalcemia, immunological deficiency; 30%); and left ventricular outflow tract obstruction secondary to a malaligned conal septum (25%).[97] Interrupted aortic arch is classified into three types as originally described by Celoria and Patton from Boston Children's Hospital: type A (30%), type B (65%), and type C (5%).[98] Type A involves interruption of the aortic arch just distal to the left subclavian artery; type B, between the left carotid and left subclavian artery; and type C, interruption between the innominate artery and the carotid artery.

These patients present with cardiovascular collapse when the ductus arteriosus closes. They are acidotic, oliguric, and in a low-perfusion state. Similar to a severe coarctation, these patients are medically managed with PGE_1 infusion to open the PDA. The child is intubated, placed on mechanical ventilation, and given inotropic support to improve peripheral perfusion. The diagnosis is made by echocardiography.

There are two approaches to interrupted aortic arch. The two-stage approach is with an initial palliation with repair of the arch and pulmonary artery banding followed by a later procedure to close the VSD and remove the pulmonary artery band.[99] The preferred approach currently is to perform primary repair of the VSD and the aortic arch through a median sternotomy incision under circulatory arrest at the time of diagnosis.

Under deep hypothermia and circulatory arrest, repair is performed by resecting the ductal tissue and anastomosing the ascending and descending aorta together. The VSD is closed with a patch. Serraf et al. reported on 64 patients having a single-stage primary repair between 1985 and 1995. Postoperative mortality since 1990 was 12%.[100] Menahem et al. reported on a series of 50 infants with interrupted aortic arch in which the mortality of neonatal one-stage repair was only 4%.[101] In patients who undergo primary repair, there is a 20% to 30% incidence of recurrent coarctation, which is now often addressed successfully by percutaneous balloon dilation in the cardiac catheterization laboratory.

Miscellaneous Lesions

Anomalous Origin of the Left Coronary Artery from the Pulmonary Artery

An *anomalous origin of the left coronary artery from the pulmonary artery* is a very rare, usually isolated, congenital lesion. The left coronary artery originates from the pulmonary artery, creating left coronary artery insufficiency. In these patients, the blood supply to the left coronary artery distribution is from right coronary artery collaterals. Within the first several weeks of life as the pulmonary vascular resistance drops, the blood flow in the left coronary artery is reversed, and there is a left-to-right shunt into the pulmonary artery. If the collaterals from the right coronary artery are inadequate, these children develop myocardial ischemia followed by myocardial infarction, which leads to left ventricular dysfunction, papillary muscle dysfunction, and mitral valve insufficiency. These patients then present with severe congestive heart failure. A chest radiograph shows cardiomegaly, and the electrocardiogram shows signs of myocardial ischemia or infarction. Echocardiography is diagnostic and reveals an enlarged right coronary artery, a hypokinetic dilated left ventricle, and severe mitral insufficiency. The color Doppler flow may identify the actual entry point of the left coronary artery into the pulmonary artery. The natural history of this lesion is that 80% of untreated infants will die by 1 year of age. All patients diagnosed with anomalous origin of the left coronary artery from the pulmonary artery should receive repair at the time of diagnosis.

The current preferred surgical therapy for anomalous origin of the left coronary artery from the pulmonary artery is to reimplant the anomalous left coronary artery into the ascending aorta.[102] This operation is performed through a median sternotomy with the use of cardiopulmonary bypass. Transfer of the coronary artery is facilitated by transecting the main pulmonary artery completely. A button of pulmonary artery is excised with the coronary artery for the implantation into the ascending aorta. The resulting defect in the pulmonary artery is reconstructed with a patch of pericardium. Between 1989 and 1999, we performed urgent aortic implantation of the anomalous left coronary in 16 consecutive patients with no operative or late deaths. One patient required temporary postoperative support with ECMO. Lambert and colleagues have also reported excellent results with aortic implantation[103]; they reported aortic implantation in 34 patients with 13% mortality. These babies will have, in many cases, nearly complete recovery of what was severe left ventricular dysfunction. Schwartz et al. reported that, of 28 patients having a dual coronary repair with follow-up longer than 1 year, left ventricular function normalized in all patients regardless of preoperative function.[104] Average time to normalization of function was 2 to 7 months.

Corrected Transposition of the Great Arteries

Corrected transposition of the great arteries is a very unusual anomaly in which there are two errors in the connections within the heart. Unlike simple transposition, these patients have the blood flow of the pulmonary and systemic circulations in series. However, the right ventricle is the systemic pumping chamber, and the left ventricle is the pumping chamber of the pulmonary circulation. Blood flow from the right atrium goes into a morphological left ventricle, from which it is directed to the pulmonary artery. The left atrial flow returns to a morphological right ventricle, from which it flows out to the aorta. Many of these patients have an associated VSD and pulmonary stenosis. Many of these patients will develop complete AV heart block spontaneously.

Surgical options for these patients include (1) closure of the VSD and pulmonary valvotomy, (2) a Mustard procedure combined with a Rastelli procedure to make the left ventricle the systemic pumping chamber and the right ventricle the pulmonary pumping chamber,[105] and (3) a double-switch operation combining a Mustard operation with an arterial switch procedure.[106] The last two operations are more complex than the first but make the left ventricle the systemic pumping chamber that is less likely to undergo late deterioration.[106] Another option is a "one and a half" ventricular repair incorporating a bidirectional superior cavopulmonary anastomosis.[106a]

Ebstein's Anomaly

Ebstein's anomaly is an abnormal formation of the tricuspid valve in which the tricuspid valve is displaced downward into the right ventricle. In most of these patients, the anterior leaflet of the tricuspid valve is very large and described as "sail-like." Because of the displacement of the tricuspid valve, there is an abnormal chamber on the right side, which is the so-called atrialized portion of the right ventricle. Most of these patients have an associated ASD and may have pulmonary stenosis. These patients can present with either cyanosis at birth or later in life with congestive heart failure. Approximately 20% of these patients have an accessory connection that can cause tachycardia. Diagnosis is by echocardiography, but cardiac catheterization may be required to determine precisely the right ventricular size and the anatomy of the pulmonary circulation.

The surgical therapy is varied according to the severity of the Ebstein's anomaly. Infants who present with severe cyanosis and cardiomegaly may require neonatal conversion to a single-ventricle-type physiology. In these patients, the initial palliation consists of closure of the tricuspid valve orifice with a pericardial patch, atrial septectomy, and modified Blalock-Taussig shunt. Starnes and colleagues from Stanford, California, reported successful use of this procedure in five infants.[107] These patients will require a Fontan operation later in life. Excellent outcome has been reported with this approach as compared to a nearly 80% mortality with medical management. Older patients who present with congestive heart failure are usually treated by ASD closure and tricuspid valvuloplasty. Danielson et al.[108] at the Mayo Clinic reported 189 patients operated on between 1972 and 1991; 60% had a successful valvuloplasty, 36% required tricuspid valve replacement, and there was a 6% mortality rate.

Vascular Rings

The term *vascular ring* refers to a group of congenital anomalies in which there is a developmental abnormality in the aortic arch system that causes compression of the trachea and esophagus. The two true vascular rings are the double aortic arch and the right aortic arch with left ligamentum and retroesophageal left subclavian artery. These patients have a complete ring of blood vessels around the trachea and esophagus. Other anomalies categorized with vascular rings are pulmonary artery sling and innominate artery compression syndrome.[109] These children typically present with noisy respirations, a brassy cough similar to a seal's bark, cyanosis, apnea, or respiratory distress. In older children, dysphagia for solid foods may be noticed. Diagnosis is suggested by the chest radiograph, which may reveal an abnormal location of the aortic arch. The diagnostic procedure of choice is CT or MRI. These patients should also have an echocardiogram and bronchoscopy.

Operative repair is recommended for all patients with clinical symptoms and evidence of a vascular ring. Dr. Robert Gross from Boston Children's Hospital first reported successful division of a double aortic arch in a 1-year-old boy in 1945. Pulmonary artery sling repair was first reported by Willis J. Potts from Children's Memorial Hospital, Chicago, in 1954.

The true vascular rings (double aortic arch, right aortic arch) are approached through a left thoracotomy. After accurately defining the ring anatomy, the site for ring division is selected. The vascular structures are divided between vascular clamps with oversewing of the stumps similar to the technique described for PDA. Innominate artery compression syndrome is best treated through a right thoracotomy with suspension of the innominate artery to the undersurface of the sternum. For patients with pulmonary artery sling, the

TABLE 76.5. Vascular Ring Surgery at Children's Memorial Hospital, 1947–2003.

Defect	*n*
Double aortic arch	120
Right aortic arch with left ligamentum arteriosum	103
Innominate artery compression syndrome	85
Pulmonary artery sling	36
Complete tracheal rings	40
Total	384

best results are obtained with an approach through a median sternotomy with the use of cardiopulmonary bypass.[110] The left pulmonary artery is transected from its origin at the right pulmonary artery and brought through the space between the trachea and the esophagus. It is then anastomosed to the main pulmonary artery at a site selected to approximate the normal anatomical origin. It should be noted that a high percentage of patients (approximately 50%) with pulmonary artery sling have tracheal stenosis caused by complete cartilaginous rings of the trachea. This defect requires operative attention at the time of the pulmonary artery sling repair with tracheal resection, pericardial tracheoplasty, slide tracheoplasty, or tracheal autograft repair.[111] Since 1947, nearly 400 children have been treated at the Children's Memorial Hospital for vascular rings and slings[112] (Table 76.5). There has been no operative mortality from an isolated vascular ring or pulmonary artery sling since 1959. Over 90% of these infants were free of respiratory symptoms 1 year postoperatively.

There has been enormous progress in the field of congenital heart surgery since the early days of "closed-heart" palliative procedures. The use of cardiopulmonary bypass literally opened the heart to effective complete surgical repairs. Continuous refinements in surgical techniques and in intra- and postoperative care now make possible with outstanding results the repair of newborns who have very complex lesions. Transcatheter techniques have now replaced some of the "simpler" congenital heart operations. Noninvasive imaging techniques have replaced cardiac catheterization for many lesions. Cardiac transplantation for lesions not amenable to repair is now commonplace. Successful outcomes for these patients are dependent on a smooth interaction and team approach of cardiac surgeons, cardiologists, anesthesiologists, intensive care unit attendings, and nursing staff. The future of congenital heart surgery will be based on the steady improvement of current techniques and innovative approaches to complex anomalies.

References

1. Gross RE, Hubbard JP. Surgical ligation of a patent ductus arteriosus. JAMA 1939;112:729–731.
2. Blalock A, Taussig HB. The surgical treatment of malformations of the heart in which there is pulmonary stenosis or atresia. JAMA 1945;128:189–202.
3. Crafoord C, Nylin G. Congenital coarctation of the aorta and its surgical treatment. J Thorac Surg 1945;14:347–361.
4. Muller WH Jr, Dammann JR Jr. The treatment of certain congenital malformations of the heart by the creation of pulmonary stenosis to reduce pulmonary hypertension and excessive pulmonary blood flow. Surg Gynecol Obstet 1952;95:213–219.
5. Lewis FJ, Taufic M. Closure of atrial septal defects with the aid of hypothermia; experimental accomplishments and the report of one successful case. Surgery (St. Louis) 1953;33:52–59.
6. Gibbon JH Jr. Application of a mechanical heart and lung apparatus to cardiac surgery. Minn Med 1954;37:171–180.
7. Lillehei CW, Cohen M, Warden HE, Varco RL. The direct vision intracardiac correction of congenital anomalies by controlled cross circulation. Results in 32 patients with ventricular septal defects, tetralogy of Fallot, and atrioventricularis communis defects. Surgery (St. Louis) 1955;38:11–12.
8. Kirklin JW, DuShane JW, Patrick RT, et al. Intracardiac surgery with the aid of a mechanical pump-oxygenator system (Gibbon type): report of eight cases. Proc Staff Meet Mayo Clin 1955; 30:201–206.
9. Hoffman JI, Kaplan S, The incidence of congenital heart disease. J Am Coll Cardiol 2002;39:1890–1900.
10. Boughman JA, Berg KA, Astemborski JA, et al. Familial risks of congenital heart defect assessed in a population-based study. Am J Med Genet 1987;26:839–849.
11. Hoffman JL. Congenital heart disease: incidence and inheritance. Pediatr Clin North Am 1990;37:25–43.
12. Nora JJ, Nora AH. Recurrence risks in children having one parent with a congenital heart disease. Circulation 1976;53:701–702.
13. Tworetzky W, McElhinney DB, Brock MM, Reddy VM, Hanley FL, Silverman NH. Echocardiographic diagnosis alone for the complete repair of major congenital heart defects. J Am Coll Surg 1999;33:228–233.
14. Heymann MA, Berman W, Rudolph AM, Whitman V. Dilatation of the ductus arteriosus by prostaglandin E_1 in aortic arch abnormalities. Circulation 1979;59:169–173.
15. de Leval MR, McKay R, Jones M, Stark J, Macartney FJ. Modified Blalock-Taussig shunt: use of subclavian artery orifice as flow regulator in prosthetic systemic-pulmonary artery shunts. J Thorac Cardiovasc Surg 1981;81:112–119.
16. Odim J, Portzky M, Zurakowski D, et al. Sternotomy approach for the modified Blalock-Taussig shunt. Circulation 1995;92 (suppl II):II-256–II-261.
17. Mavroudis C, Backer CL, Gevitz M. Forty-six years of patent ductus arteriosus division at Children's Memorial Hospital of Chicago: standards for comparison. Ann Surg 1994;220:402–410.
18. Shim D, Fedderly RT, Beekman RH 3rd, et al. Follow-up of coil occlusion of patent ductus arteriosus. J Am Coll Cardiol 1996; 28:207–211.
19. Prieto LR, DeCamillo DM, Konrad DJ, et al. Comparison of cost and clinical outcome between transcatheter coil occlusion and surgical closure of isolated patent ductus arteriosus. Pediatrics 1998;101:1020–1024.
20. Thanopoulos BD, Hakim FA, Hiari A, et al. Further experience with transcatheter closure of the patent ductus arteriosus using the Amplatzer duct occluder. J Am Coll Cardiol 2000;35:1016–1021.
21. Campbell M. Natural history of atrial septal defect. Br Heart J 1970;32:820–826.

21a. Stewart RD, Bailliard F, Kelle AM, Backer CL, Young L, Mavroudis C. Evolving surgical strategy for sinus venosus atrial septal defect: effect on sinus node function and late venous obstruction. Ann Thorac Surg 2007;84:1651–1655.

21b. Warden HE, Gustafson RA, Tarnay TJ, Neal WA. An alternative method for repair of partial anomalous pulmonary venous connection to the superior vena cava. Ann Thorac Surg 1984;38:601–605.

22. Rome JJ, Keane JF, Perry SB, et al. Double-umbrella closure of atrial defects: initial clinical applications. Circulation 1990;82: 751–758.
23. Omeish A, Hijazi ZM. Transcatheter closure of atrial septal defects in children and adults using the Amplatzer septal occluder. J Interv Cardiol 2001;14:37–44.

24. Gersony WM, Hayes CJ, Driscoll DJ, et al. Bacterial endocarditis in patients with aortic stenosis, pulmonary stenosis, or ventricular septal defect. Circulation 1993;87(suppl 1):121–126.
25. Backer CL, Idriss FS, Zales VR, et al. Surgical management of the conal ventricular septal defect. J Thorac Cardiovasc Surg 1991;102:288–296.
26. Backer CL. American Heart Association Scientific Sessions: Cardiovascular Seminars—Closure of Septal Defects: Catheter or Surgery? American Heart Association, New Orleans, LA, November 8, 2004.
27. Backer CL, Winters RC, Zales VR, et al. The restrictive ventricular septal defect: how small is too small to close? Ann Thorac Surg 1993;56:1014–1019.
28. Holzer R, Balzer D, Cao OL, Lock K, Hijazi ZM, Amplatzer Muscular Ventricular Septal Defect Investigators. Device closure of muscular ventricular septal defects using the Amplatzer muscular ventricular septal defect occluder: immediate and mid-term results of a U.S. registry. J Am Coll Cardiol 2004;43:1257–1263.
29. Backer CL, Zales VR, Alboliras E, Mavroudis C. Repair of complete atrioventricular canal defects: results with the two-patch technique. Ann Thorac Surg 1995;60:530–537.
30. Bando K, Turrentine M, Sun K, et al. Surgical management of complete atrioventricular septal defects: a 20 year experience. J Thorac Cardiovasc Surg 1995;110:1543–1554.
31. Hanley FL, Fenton KN, Jonas RA, et al. Surgical repair of complete atrioventricular canal defects in infancy. J Thorac Cardiovasc Surg 1993;106:387–397.
32. Nicholson IA, Nunn GR, Sholler GF, et al. Simplified single patch technique for the repair of atrioventricular septal defect. J Thorac Cardiovasc Surg 1999;118:642–646.
32a. Wilcox BR, Jones DR, Frantz EG, et al. Anatomically sound, simplified approach to repair of "complete" atrioventricular septal defect. Ann Thorac Surg 1997;64:487–494.
33. Crawford FA Jr, Stroud MR. Surgical repair of complete atrioventricular septal defect. Ann Thorac Surg 2001;72:1621–1629.
34. Van Praagh R, Van Praagh S. The anatomy of common aorticopulmonary trunk (truncus arteriosus communis) and its embryologic implications: a study of 57 necropsy cases. Am J Cardiol 1965;16:406–425.
35. McGoon DC, Rastelli GC, Ongley PA. An operation for the correction of truncus arteriosus. JAMA 1968;205:59–73.
36. Ebert PA, Turley K, Stranger P, et al. Surgical treatment of truncus arteriosus in the first 6 months of life. Ann Surg 1984;200:451–456.
37. Bove EL, Lupinetti FM, Pridjian AK, et al. Results of a policy of primary repair of truncus arteriosus in the neonate. J Thorac Cardiovasc Surg 1993;105:1057–1066.
38. Thompson LD, McElhinney DB, Reddy M, Petrossian E, Silverman NH, Hanley FL. Neonatal repair of truncus arteriosus: continuing improvement in outcomes. Ann Thorac Surg 2001; 72:391–395.
39. Mavroudis C, Backer CL. Surgical management of severe truncal insufficiency: experience with truncal valve remodeling techniques. Ann Thorac Surg 2001;72:396–400.
40. Backer CL, Mavroudis C. Surgical management of aortopulmonary window: a 40-year experience. Eur J Cardiothorac Surg 2002;21:773–779.
41. Van Arsdell GS, Maharaj GS, Tom J, et al. What is the optimal age for repair of tetralogy of Fallot? Circulation 2000;102(19 suppl 3):III123–III129.
42. Mee RB. American Association for Thoracic Surgery 80th Annual Meeting—Symposium on Congenital Heart Disease, Toronto, Ontario, Canada, April 30, 2000.
43. Stewart RD, Backer CL, Young L, Mavroudis C. Tetralogy of Fallot: results of a pulmonary valve-sparing strategy. Ann Thorac Surg 2007;84:1651–1655.
44. Dodge-Khatami A, Backer CL, Holinger LD, et al. Complete repair of tetralogy of Fallot with absent pulmonary valve including the role of airway stenting. J Card Surg 1999;14:82–91.
45. Fontan F, Baudet E. Surgical repair of tricuspid atresia. Thorax 1971;26:240–248.
46. Hopkins RA, Armstrong BE, Serwer GA, Peterson RJ, Oldham HN. Physiological rationale for a bidirectional cavopulmonary shunt. J Thorac Cardiovasc Surg 1985;90:391–398.
47. Chang AC, Hanley FL, Wernovsky G, et al. Early bidirectional cavopulmonary shunt in young infants. Postoperative course and early results. Circulation 1993;88(5 pt 2):II149–II158.
48. Kreutzer G, Galindez E, Bono H, et al. An operation for the correction of tricuspid atresia. J Thorac Cardiovasc Surg 1973; 66:613.
49. de Leval MR, Bull C, Kilner P. Total cavopulmonary connection. A logical alternative to atriopulmonary connection for complex Fontan operations—experimental studies and early clinical experience. J Thorac Cardiovasc Surg 1988;96:682–695.
50. Mavroudis C, Backer CL, Deal BJ: The total cavopulmonary artery Fontan connections using lateral tunnel and extracardiac techniques. Oper Tech Card Thorac Surg 1997;2:180–195.
51. Bridges ND, Lock JE, Castaneda AR. Baffle fenestration with subsequent transcatheter closure. Modification of the Fontan operation for patients at increased risk. Circulation 1990;82:1681–1689.
52. Mavroudis C, Zales VR, Backer CL, Muster AJ, Latson LA. Fenestrated Fontan with delayed catheter closure: effects of volume loading and baffle fenestration on oxygen delivery. Circulation 1992;86(suppl II):II-85–II-92.
53. Gentles TL, Mayer JE, Gauvreau K, et al. Fontan operation in 500 consecutive patients: factors influencing early and late outcome. J Thorac Cardiovasc Surg 1997;114:376–391.
53a. Petrossian E, Reddy VM, Collins KK, et al. The extracardiac conduit Fontan operation using minimal approach extracorporeal circulation: early and midterm outcomes. J Thorac Cardiovasc Surg 2006;132:1054–1063.
54. Mavroudis C, Backer CL, Deal BJ, Johnsrude C, Strasburger J. Total cavopulmonary conversion and maze procedure for patients with failure of the Fontan operation. J Thorac Cardiovasc Surg 2001;122:863–871.
54a. Mavroudis C, Deal BJ, Backer CL, Stewart RD, Franklin WH, Ward K, Tsao S. 111 Fontan Conversions with Arrhythmia Surgery: Surgical Lessons and Outcomes. Ann Thorac Surg 2007;84:1457-1466.
55. Muster AJ, Zales VR, Ilbawi MN, Backer CL, Duffy CE, Mavroudis C. Bidirectional cavopulmonary anastomosis with right ventricle-pulmonary artery continuity (pulsatile bidirectional Glenn) for hypoplastic right ventricle. J Thorac Cardiovasc Surg 1993;105:112–119.
56. Pawade A, Capuani A, Penny DJ, Karl TR, Mee RB. Pulmonary atresia with intact ventricular septum: surgical management based on right ventricular infundibulum. J Card Surg 1993;8:371–383.
57. Puga FJ, Leoni FE, Julsrud PR, Mair DD. Complete repair of pulmonary atresia, ventricular septal defect, and severe peripheral arborization abnormalities of the central pulmonary arteries. Experience with preliminary unifocalization procedures in 38 patients. J Thorac Cardiovasc Surg 1989;98:1018–1029.
58. Iyer KS, Mee RBB. Staged repair of pulmonary atresia with ventricular septal defect and major systemic to pulmonary artery collaterals. Ann Thorac Surg 1991;51:65–72.
59. Reddy VM, McElhinney DB, Amin Z, et al. Early and intermediate outcomes after repair of pulmonary atresia with ventricular septal defect and major aortopulmonary collateral arteries: experience with 85 patients.. Circulation 2000;101:1826–1832.

60. Jatene AD, Fontes VF, Paulista PP, et al. Anatomic correction of transposition of the great vessels. J Thorac Cardiovasc Surg 1976;72:364–370.
61. Castaneda AR, Norwood WI, Jonas RA, et al. Transposition of the great arteries and intact ventricular septum: anatomical repair in the neonate. Ann Thorac Surg 1984;38:438–443.
62. Boutin C, Jonas RA, Sanders SP, Wernovsky G, Mone SM, Colan SD. Rapid two-stage arterial switch operation. Acquisition of left ventricular mass after pulmonary artery banding in infants with transposition of the great arteries. Circulation 1994;90:1304–1309.
63. LeCompte Y, Zannini L, Hazan E, et al. Anatomic correction of transposition of the great arteries. New technique without use of a prosthetic conduit. J Thorac Cardiovasc Surg 1981;82:629–631.
64. Wernovsky G, Mayer JE, Jonas RA, et al. Factors influencing early and late outcome of the arterial switch operation for transposition of the great arteries. J Thorac Cardiovasc Surg 1995;109:289–302.
65. Rhodes LA, Wernovsky G, Keane JF, et al. Arrhythmias and intracardiac conduction after the arterial switch operation. J Thorac Cardiovasc Surg 1995;109:303–310.
66. Colan SD, Boutin C, Castañeda AR, Wernovsky G. Status of the left ventricle after arterial switch operation for transposition of the great arteries. Hemodynamic and echocardiographic evaluation. J Thorac Cardiovasc Surg 1995;109:311–321.
67. Seraf A, Roux D, Lacour-Gayet F, et al. Reoperation after the arterial switch operation for transposition of the great arteries. J Thorac Cardiovasc Surg 1995;110:892–899.
68. Gelatt M, Hamilton RM, McCrindle BW, et al. Arrhythmias and mortality after the Mustard procedure: a 30-year single-center experience. J Am Coll Cardiol 1997;29:194–201.
69. Cochrane AD, Karl TR, Mee RB. Staged conversion to arterial switch for late failure of the systemic right ventricle. Ann Thorac Surg 1993;56:854–862.
70. Backer CL, Zales VR, Idriss FS, Lynch P, Benson DW Jr, Mavroudis C. Heart transplantation in infants and children. J Heart Lung Transplant 1992;11:311–319.
71. Mavroudis C, Backer CL, Muster AJ, Rocchini AP, Rees AH, Gevitz M. Taussig-Bing anomaly: arterial switch versus Kawashima intraventricular repair. Ann Thorac Surg 1996;61: 1330–1338.
72. Caldarone CA, Najm HK, Kadletz M, et al. Surgical management of total anomalous pulmonary venous drainage: impact of coexisting cardiac anomalies. Ann Thorac Surg 1998;66:1521–1526.
73. Yun T-J, Coles JG, Konstantinov IE, et al. Conventional and sutureless techniques for management of the pulmonary veins. J Thorac Cardiovasc Surg 2005:129:167–174.
74. Norwood WI, Lang P, Castaneda AR, Campbell DN. Experience with operations for hypoplastic left heart syndrome. J Thorac Cardiovasc Surg 1981;82:511–519.
75. Bove EL. Surgical treatment for hypoplastic left heart syndrome. Jpn J Thorac Cardiovasc Surg 1999;47:47–56.
76. Sano S, Ishino K, Kado H, et al. Outcome of right ventricle-to-pulmonary artery shunt in first-stage palliation of hypoplastic left heart syndrome: a multi-institutional study. Ann Thorac Surg 2004;78:1951–1958.
77. Jacobs ML, Norwood WI. Fontan operation: influence of modifications on morbidity and mortality. Ann Thorac Surg 1994;58:945–952.
78. Bailey LL, Nehlsen-Cannarella SI, Doroshow RW, et al. Cardiac allotransplantation in newborns as therapy for hypoplastic left heart syndrome. N Engl J Med 1986;315:949–951.
79. Mavroudis C, Harrison H, Klein JB, et al. Infant orthotopic cardiac transplantation. J Thorac Cardiovasc Surg 1988;96:912–924.
80. Fortuna RS, Chinnock RE, Bailey LL. Heart transplantation among 233 infants during the first 6 months of life: the Loma Linda experience. Loma Linda Pediatric Heart Transplant Group. Clin Transpl 1999:263–272.
81. Chiaverelli M, Gundry SR, Razzouk AJ, Bailey LL. Cardiac transplantation for infants with hypoplastic left-heart syndrome. JAMA 1993;270:2944–2947.
82. Hawkins JA, Minich LL, Tani LY, et al. Late results and reintervention after aortic valvotomy for critical aortic stenosis in neonates and infants. Ann Thorac Surg 1998;65:1758–1762.
83. McCrindle BW, Blackstone EH, Williams WG, et al. Are outcomes of surgical versus transcatheter balloon valvotomy equivalent in neonatal critical aortic stenosis? Circulation 2001; 104(12 suppl I):I152–I158.
84. Moore P, Egito E, Mowrey H, et al. Midterm results of balloon dilation of congenital aortic stenosis: predictors of success. J Am Coll Cardiol 1996;27:1257–1263.
85. Brown JW, Ruzmetov M, Vijay P, Turrentine MW. Surgical repair of congenital supravalvular aortic stenosis in children. Eur J Cardiothorac Surg 2002;21:50–56.
86. Deb SJ, Schaff HV, Dearani JA, Nishimura RA, Ommen SR. Septal myectomy results in regression of left ventricular hypertrophy in patients with hypertrophic obstructive cardiomyopathy. Ann Thorac Surg 2004;78:2118–2122.
87. Ross DN. Replacement of aortic and mitral valves with a pulmonary autograft. Lancet 1967;2:956–958.
88. Elkins RC, Elkins CC, Lane MM, Knott-Craig CJ, Trotter TH, Peyton MD. Ross operation—16 year experience. Paper presented at: 85th annual meeting of the American Association for Thoracic Surgery, April 10–13, 2005, San Francisco.
89. Zias EA, Mavroudis C, Backer CL, et al. Surgical repair of the congenitally malformed mitral valve in infants and children. Ann Thorac Surg 1998;66:1551–1559.
90. Caspi J, Coles JG, Benson LN, et al. Management of neonatal critical pulmonic stenosis in the balloon valvotomy era. Ann Thorac Surg 1990;49:273–278.
91. Campbell M. Natural history of coarctation of the aorta. Br Heart J 1970;32:633–640.
92. Backer CL, Mavroudis C, Zias E, Amin Z, Weigel TJ. Repair of coarctation with resection and extended end-to-end anastomosis. Ann Thorac Surg 1998;66:1365–1371.
93. Backer CL, Paape K, Zales VR, Weigel TJ, Mavroudis C. Coarctation of the aorta: repair with polytetrafluoroethylene patch aortoplasty. Circulation 1995;92(suppl II):II-132–II-136.
94. Clarkson PM, Brandt PWT, Barratt-Boyes BG, et al. Prosthetic repair of coarctation of the aorta with particular reference to Dacron onlay patch grafts and late aneurysm formation. Am J Cardiol 1985;56:342–346.
95. Backer CL, Mavroudis C. Coarctation of the aorta and interrupted aortic arch. In: Glenn's Thoracic and Cardiovascular Surgery, Vol. 6. Stamford, CT: Appleton and Lange; 1996:1243–1269.
96. Sealy WC. Paradoxical hypertension after repair of coarctation of the aorta: a review of its causes. Ann Thorac Surg 1990;50:323–329.
97. Freedom RM, Rosen FS, Nada AS. Congenital cardiovascular disease and anomalies of the third and fourth pharyngeal pouch. Circulation 1972;46:165–172.
98. Celoria GC, Patton RP. Congenital absence of the aortic arch. Am Heart J 1959;58:407–413.
99. Mainwaring RD, Lamberti JJ. Mid- to long-term results of the two-stage approach for type B interrupted aortic arch and ventricular septal defect. Ann Thorac Surg 1997;64:1782–1786.
100. Serraf A, Lacour-Gayet F, Robotin M, et al. Repair of interrupted aortic arch: a 10-year experience. J Thorac Cardiovasc Surg 1996;112:1150–1160.
101. Menahem S, Brawn WJ, Mee RBB. Severe subaortic stenosis in interrupted aortic arch in infancy and childhood. J Cardiac Surg 1991;6:373–380.

102. Backer CL, Hillman N, Dodge-Khatami A, Mavroudis C. Anomalous origin of the left coronary artery from the pulmonary artery: successful surgical strategy without assist devices. Semin Thorac Cardiovasc Surg Pediatr Card Surg Annu 2000;3:165–172.
103. Lambert V, Touchot A, Losay J, et al. Midterm results after surgical repair of the anomalous origin of the coronary artery. Circulation 1996;94(suppl II):1138–1143.
104. Schwartz ML, Jonas RA, Colan SD. Anomalous origin of left coronary artery from pulmonary artery: recovery of left ventricular function after dual coronary repair. J Am Coll Cardiol 1997;30:547–553.
105. Ilbawi MN, DeLeon SY, Backer CL, et al. An alternative approach to the surgical management of physiologically corrected transposition with ventricular septal defect and pulmonary stenosis or atresia. J Thorac Cardiovasc Surg 1990;100:410–415.
106. Yagihara T, Kishimoto H, Isobe F, et al. Double switch operation in cardiac anomalies with atrioventricular and ventriculoarterial discordance. J Thorac Cardiovasc Surg 1994;107:351–358.
106a. Backer CL, Stewart RD, Mavroudis C. The classical and the one-and-a-half ventricular options for surgical repair in patients with discordant atrioventricular connections. Cardiol Young 2006;16(Suppl 3):91–96.
107. Starnes VA, Pitlick PT, Bernstein D, et al. Ebstein's anomaly appearing in the neonate. J Thorac Cardiovasc Surg 1991;101:1082–1087.
108. Danielson GK, Driscoll DJ, Mair DD, Warnes CA, Oliver WC. Operative treatment of Ebstein's anomaly. J Thorac Cardiovasc Surg 1992;104:1195–1202.
109. Backer CL, Ilbawi MN, Idriss FS, DeLeon SY. Vascular anomalies causing tracheoesophageal compression: review of experience in children. J Thorac Cardiovasc Surg 1989;97:725–731.
110. Backer CL, Mavroudis C, Dunham ME, Holinger LD. Pulmonary artery sling: results with median sternotomy, cardiopulmonary bypass, and reimplantation. Ann Thorac Surg 1999;67:1738–1745.
111. Backer CL, Mavroudis C, Gerber ME, Holinger LD. Tracheal surgery in children: an 18-year review of four techniques. Eur J Cardiothorac Surg 2001;19:777–784.
112. Backer CL, Mavroudis C, Rigsby CK, Holinger LD. Trends in vascular ring surgery. J Thorac Cardiovasc Surg 2005;129:1339–1347.
113. Mavroudis C, Deal BJ, Backer CL, Johnsrude CL. The favorable impact of arrhythmia surgery on total cavopulmonary artery Fontan conversion. *Semin Thorac Cardiovasc Surg Pediatr Card Surg Annu* 1999;2:143–156.

77

Adult Heart Disease

Todd K. Rosengart, William de Bois, Edgar Chedrawy, and Malica Vukovic

The surgical treatment of acquired cardiac diseases has become increasingly sophisticated in the past two decades—the expected mortality of most cardiac operations in adults has been reduced to extremely low levels—despite the fact that increasingly higher-risk patients are now candidates for surgery.[1–3] In this regard, it is important to recognize that 75% of patients undergoing coronary bypass surgery in the Coronary Artery Surgery Study (CASS) in the late 1970s had an ejection fraction that was greater than 50%, and all patients were younger than 65 years of age, while in the Society of Thoracic Surgery (STS) database for coronary artery bypass in 2002, the *average* patient age was 67 years, and the *average* ejection fraction was 45%. Despite the reality of increasingly higher-risk patients undergoing coronary bypass surgery, the observed operative mortality for coronary bypass surgery in the 2002 STS database was 2.8%. Similarly, morbidity associated with coronary bypass surgery was found to have decreased from 1986 to 1994 in a series of nearly 8000 patients reported from the Cleveland Clinic, despite a significant rise in the patient risk profile in this series.[3] Similar trends can be described for most facets of adult cardiac surgery.

The improvement in outcomes for adult cardiac surgery can be attributed to a number of factors, including (1) the refinement of myocardial preservation technique and the conduct of cardiopulmonary bypass (CPB); (2) advancements in surgical technique; (3) the development of a more sophisticated understanding of the natural history of cardiac diseases, allowing more appropriate timing of interventions; (4) the construction of more accurate predictive models of operative risk, allowing optimized patient selection; (5) the introduction of improved pharmacological agents, such as milrinone, that improve myocardial contractility; and (6) the development of high-performance valve prostheses and cardiac support devices such as the intraaortic balloon pump (IABP). This chapter attempts to delineate the current practice of adult cardiac surgery while focusing on those advancements that have enhanced the outcomes associated with adult cardiac surgery to the present day.

Cardiopulmonary Bypass and Myocardial Preservation

Historical Perspective

The idea of temporarily substituting a mechanical device for a patient's heart and lungs was conceived long before the first successful CPB was first performed. In fact, LeGallois first proposed the idea of artificial circulation in 1812, suggesting that the heart could be replaced by an arterial pump. Although his experiments were inconclusive, this first attempt to perfuse animals initiated the technology that became modern CPB. The subsequent history of the development of CPB includes the first design of a CPB device by von Frey and Gruber in 1885 and the proposal in 1935 by Carrel and Lindbergh of an extracorporeal whole-organ perfusion apparatus that culminated in the seminal developmental work of John Gibbon, from his first published report of experimental animal studies in 1937 to the first clinical application of CPB by Gibbon in 1953. Since that time, although the theoretical function of bypass componentry has actually changed little, dramatic advances have been made in the performance and reliability of CPB owing to improvements in oxygenator function, hemodynamic monitoring, blood conservation, myocardial and neurological protection, and the introduction of disposable circuitry, among other factors.

Principles of Cardiopulmonary Bypass

The primary purpose of CPB is to provide the cardiac surgeon with a bloodless and motion-free operative field. This aim is accomplished by temporarily interrupting the function of the heart and lungs by physiologically substituting a "heart-lung machine" in their place. The "cardiopulmonary bypass" provided by the heart-lung machine (bypass circuit) permits complete cessation of cardiopulmonary activity while allowing the flow of oxygenated blood and preservation of adequate tissue perfusion and organ function systemically. Viewed simplistically, CPB is accomplished by pumping blood

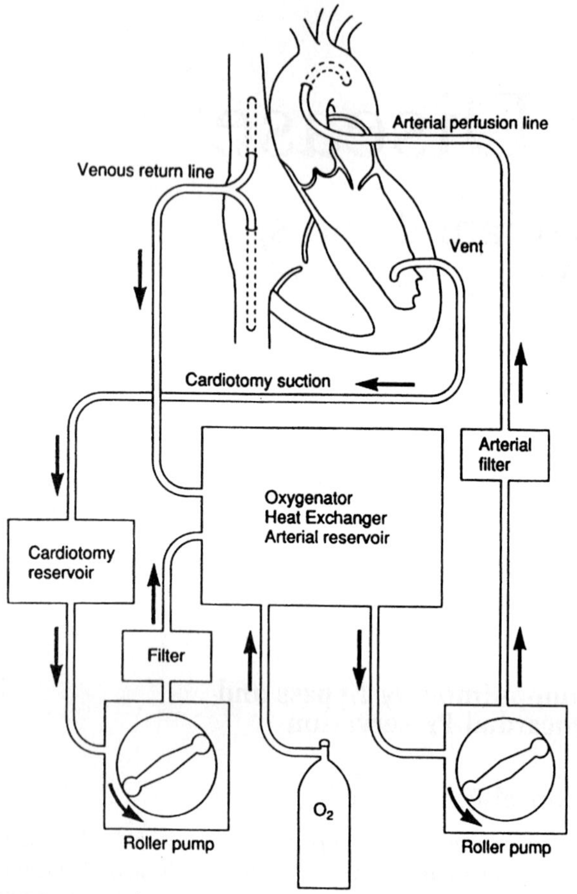

FIGURE 77.1. Schematic representation of the critical components of a cardiopulmonary bypass circuit. (After Callaghan and Wartak,[150] with permission.)

through an extracorporeal circuit, the primary features of which are the allowance of gas and heat exchange.

The circuit by which CPB is provided consists basically of a set of specialized tubing called cannulas, which are inserted into the heart or great vessels to access the circulation; a reservoir, which collects the blood; an arterial pump; and an oxygenator, which provides heat and gas exchange (Fig. 77.1). Commonly added to this system are filters, air emboli safety devices, a myocardial protection system, and a mechanism for hemodynamic monitoring.

Because the performance of CPB necessitates blood flow over a large surface area of artificial materials, a critical feature of this procedure is the administration of heparin, an anticoagulant that prevents the blood from clotting in the CPB circuit. Adequate levels of anticoagulation are monitored throughout CPB, typically utilizing a simple test known as the activated clotting time (ACT). At the completion of CPB, the heparin is reversed by the administration of protamine, a heparin antagonist.

Despite the use of heparin and protamine, the operator's ability to inhibit systemic inflammatory responses to blood exposure to the CPB circuitry is limited, and coagulopathies and other adverse inflammatory responses to CPB are not uncommon (see following). Although the biology of CPB is thus quite complex, the physical parameters that can be manipulated during CPB are quite limited. These variables include flow rate, blood pressure, blood temperature, and blood oxygen and carbon dioxide content.

Strategic Variables in Cardiopulmonary Bypass

Blood Pressure and Flow Rates

Of the several parameters that can be controlled to ensure adequate tissue perfusion during CPB, flow rates and arterial perfusion pressures are among the most important and the most controversial. Because acidosis and lactate production increase in adults when normothermic flow rates are less than 1.6 L/min/m^2 or 50 mL/kg/min, flow rates employed during hypothermia and normothermia commonly range from approximately 1.5 to 2.5 L/min/m^2. Although most centers maintain a minimum arterial pressure of at least 50 mmHg, the optimal arterial perfusion pressure required to maintain nominal tissue perfusion is also largely unknown. In this regard, although autoregulation normally maintains adequacy of blood flow to the vital organs over a wide range of blood pressure, anesthesia and hypothermia associated with CPB are known to affect these mechanisms. The recent literature in fact suggests that maintenance of a mean systemic blood pressure closer to normal levels may help preserve neurological function, especially in patients with evidence of cerebrovascular disease.[4] On the other hand, higher blood pressure during CPB may increase the likelihood of pump circuit problems, increase operative blood loss, and compromise myocardial protection.

Hypothermia

The utilization of systemic and cardiac hypothermia to decrease tissue metabolism and enable lower perfusion rates has been a critical component of the performance of CPB since the work of Bigelow et al.[5] in 1950. In this regard, Woodcock et al., among others, demonstrated that cerebral metabolic requirements were strongly decreased at temperatures below 30°C and thus provided evidence of cerebral protection with hypothermia.[6] It can be further estimated that oxygen consumption decreases about 7% per each 1°C decrease in temperature (Fig. 77.2). Systemic hypothermia thus provides a "margin of error" in providing adequate tissue perfusion during CPB and helps prevent myocardial rewarming by sys-

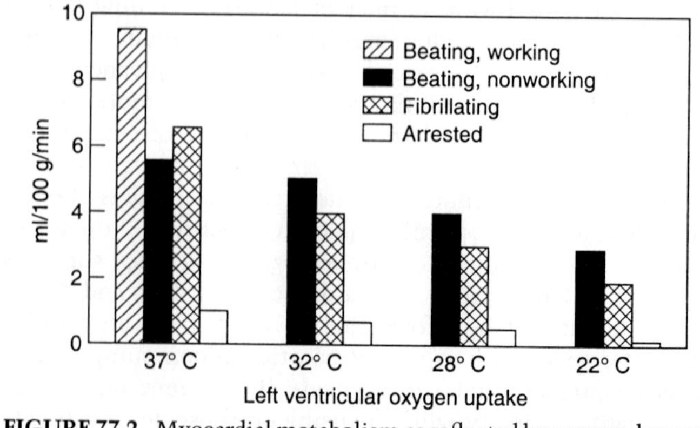

FIGURE 77.2. Myocardial metabolism as reflected by oxygen demand as a function of temperature and working state (beating, nonworking, fibrillating, or arrested). (From Buckberg et al.,[151] with permission.)

temic blood circulating in the thoracic cavity during the period of cold cardioplegic cardiac arrest (see following).

Most CPB procedures employ moderate hypothermia (28°C–32°C) to allow a decrease in CPB flow rates and enhance the safety of CPB. Acceptable cooling rates are approximately 1°C every 1 to 2 min. As opposed to older hypothermia techniques of whole-body immersion in vats of ice water and similar techniques, the modern conduct of CPB provides hypothermia by circulating chilled water around the patient's blood by means of a heat exchanger that is integrated into the CPB circuit oxygenator (Fig. 77.3). Rewarming at the end of CPB to a temperature of 36°C is accomplished in an analogous fashion at a rate of 1°C every 3 to 5 min. Temperature gradients during warming are maintained at no greater than 10°C.

An extension of systemic hypothermia to extremely low levels of less than 20°C allows the performance of deep hypothermic circulatory arrest (DHCA). During DHCA, systemic and cerebral blood flow can be completely halted for safe periods of at least 30 min, and possibly up to 60 min, allowing performance of operations on the heart and aorta without the use of clamps, which may be cumbersome or inappropriate in cases of complex congenital heart disease or aortic disease. Recently, selective arch vessel perfusion or retrograde perfusion of the brain during DHCA via a superior vena cava cannula have been advocated as ways to minimize the risk of neurological injury during circulatory arrest.[7]

In contrast to hypothermic CPB technique, some advocates of normothermic bypass, which can be coupled with continuous warm cardioplegia, note the potential benefits of reduced postoperative bleeding, decreased myocardial ischemia and injury, and shorter intubation times gained by avoiding systemic hypothermia,[8] but substantially increased risk of neurological dysfunction with this technique has been demonstrated by others.[9]

Blood Gas Management

Gas exchange is another variable that can be regulated during CPB. This is accomplished with a "blender" that controls the diffusion of ventilatory gases, oxygen and air, into the blood and carbon dioxide out of the blood as it passes through the oxygenator. Blood levels of respiratory gases are maintained close to normal values, with the exception of Po_2, which is maintained in the range of 150 to 300 mmHg.

Because hypothermia affects blood acid–base balance, two alternative systems may appropriately be utilized to regulate CO_2 levels, Ph-stat and alpha-stat. Briefly, the latter technique aims to keeps the $Paco_2$ close to 40 torr regardless of temperature, while in the Ph-stat strategy, $Paco_2$ is temperature corrected. Debate still exists regarding which of these blood gas management techniques is best based on different interpretations of cerebral blood flow autoregulation as a function of acid–base status. Comparative studies have demonstrated that, in bypass runs longer than 90 min, the relatively greater degree of cerebral vascular dilation associated with pH-stat leads to accumulation of particulate and microgaseous matter that subsequently leads to neural dysfunction.[10]

During DHCA, pH-stat management has, however, been associated with beneficial cerebral effects, including faster recovery of cerebral high-energy phosphates and greater cellular O_2 availability.[11] Alpha-stat management thus appears to be the method of choice for routine CPB when employing moderate-to-normothermic bypass. Alternatively, the method of choice for DHCA may be pH-stat late in the cooling process to ensure adequate cerebral cooling, then returning to alpha-stat during rewarming.

Finally, the hematocrit on bypass is also an important theoretical determinant of oxygen delivery, despite the limitation of oxygen delivery to tissues associated with hypothermia. The current trend is toward lower red blood cell transfusion triggers, but definitive lower limits for safe hematocrits are ambiguous. Our group studied 2738 sequential coronary bypass surgery procedures and determined that the minimum hematocrit on bypass is an independent risk factor for mortality.[12] In high-risk patients, hematocrit levels 17% or less were associated with significantly increased mortality risk in this study. Low-risk patients, however, were able to tolerate hematocrits as low as 15% without any increased risk.

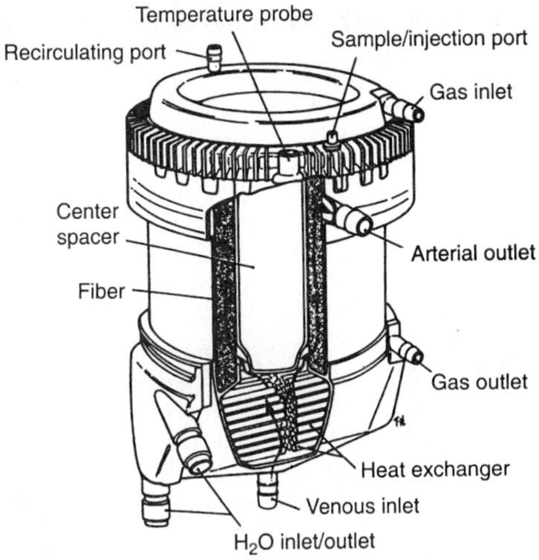

FIGURE 77.3. Example of a modern hollow-fiber oxygenator-heat exchanger. Blood passes around gas-containing capillary tubes. (From Reed and Stafford,[152] with permission.)

The Cardiopulmonary Bypass Circuit

Cannulas

The ascending aorta is the most common site for arterial cannulation and return of blood from the heart-lung machine to the systemic circulation. In previous years and in selected cases today (such as aortic aneurysm surgery), femoral cannulation has been commonly used. The widespread application of femoral cannulation has been limited by its potential complications, including retrograde aortic dissection, which is an often-lethal event. When aortic cannulation may be compromised by atherosclerotic lesions or dissection, axillary artery cannulation has also recently been advocated as an alternative approach to arterial accesss. Access to the ascending aorta is thus typically obtained with a median sternotomy, which is an excellent approach that provides safe and expeditious exposure to the heart and great vessels. Other approaches, including "minimally invasive" partial sternotomies and thoracotomies, may be employed as well.

The arterial cannula, which in the adult patient ranges in size from 20 to 24 French, must be capable of handling nearly the same flow rate as the native aorta despite the fact that the cannula is approximately one-third the size of the native aorta. The potential occurrence of excessively high-pressure gradients and turbulence due to missizing of an aortic cannula can thus lead to complications such as hemolysis, cavitation, dissection, dislodgement of atheromatous plaques, and protein denaturation. The arterial cannula should therefore be appropriately selected such that the pressure gradient across the cannula does not exceed 100 mmHg.

Venous cannulas, typically inserted in the right atrium or cavae, provide venous supply and inflow to the CPB circuit, usually by simple gravity drainage. The most commonly employed venous cannula is the straight two-stage (atrial and inferior vena cava port) device. Common sizes for adult two-stage venous cannulas are 36 to 51 French, while 28 to 42 French can be used in smaller patients (less than 60 kg). Single-stage cannulas are used during procedures in which the right atrium may be opened, for example, tricuspid or mitral valve replacements and repairs or septal defect corrections. These cannulas are inserted via purse-string cannulation into both the superior and inferior vena cavae. Snares placed around the cavae with the cannulas in place allow total diversion of venous return and facilitate intracardiac exposure. Common sizes range from 26 to 36 French, depending on patient blood flow requirements.

Oxygenator

There are three types of oxygenators currently available: the bubble oxygenators, hollow-fiber membrane oxygenators, and sheet or plate membrane devices. Based on cost and performance characteristics, the oxygenator most commonly utilized today is the hollow-fiber membrane device, which incorporates the use of semipermeable tubes separating the blood from the oxygenated gas (see Fig. 77.3). The oxygenator is attached to a gas source via a gas blender, which allows precise titration of both oxygen percentage and gas flow (and thus blood oxygen and carbon dioxide content, respectively). Finally, a heat exchanger is incorporated into the oxygenator and allows warming and cooling of the blood as it passes through this part of the CPB circuit.

Pumps

There are typically four pumps on the heart-lung console: arterial, ventricular vent, cardiotomy suction, and cardioplegia pumps. The arterial pump is commonly of either roller or centrifugal pump-type design (Fig. 77.4). The roller pump consists of two semiocclusive rollers that rotate and compress the tubing within the pump tubing holder ("raceway"). This type of volume-displacement pump provides output in direct relation to the rotation of the rollers and as a result provides accurate blood flow. Unfortunately, roller pumps continue to function even if there is no blood volume available for pumping and therefore can introduce air into the arterial circuit if the venous reservoir empties or if there is an inlet occlusion. Furthermore, because these pumps are not afterload sensitive, line disruption can occur because of overpressurization if there is an occlusion on the outlet side of the pump (pressure transducers on the pump outlet can help mitigate this risk). The more recently introduced centrifugal pump is both preload and afterload sensitive, does not cause the problems associated with roller pumps, and is in many ways a superior device.

Cardioplegia

As it is necessary for the surgeon to operate on a still and bloodless field, the heart is typically arrested and blood flow excluded from the heart during the specific portion of open-heart surgery in which cardiac pathology is corrected surgically, whether that be the performance of a valve replacement or a coronary artery bypass. To thus isolate the heart from the systemic circulation, an aortic cross-clamp is placed across the ascending aorta between the heart and the systemic arterial perfusion cannula (Fig. 77.5). Because myocardial damage caused by an imbalance of energy demands to substrate supply has been shown to follow the ischemic cardiac arrest caused by such a maneuver, techniques of protected cardiac arrest have been developed to protect the heart during the cross-clamp period.

Myocardial protection is typically provided by administration of a cold solution that chemically arrests the heart (cardioplegia); the solution is injected into the coronary circulation following aortic cross-clamping. Ideally, cardioplegia causes an immediate but reversible myocardial arrest that minimizes expenditure of myocardial energy reserves once normal coronary blood flow has been halted by the aortic cross-clamp. After removal of the aortic cross-clamp, the cardioplegic solution is washed out with warm systemic blood, and cardiac rhythm and function return.

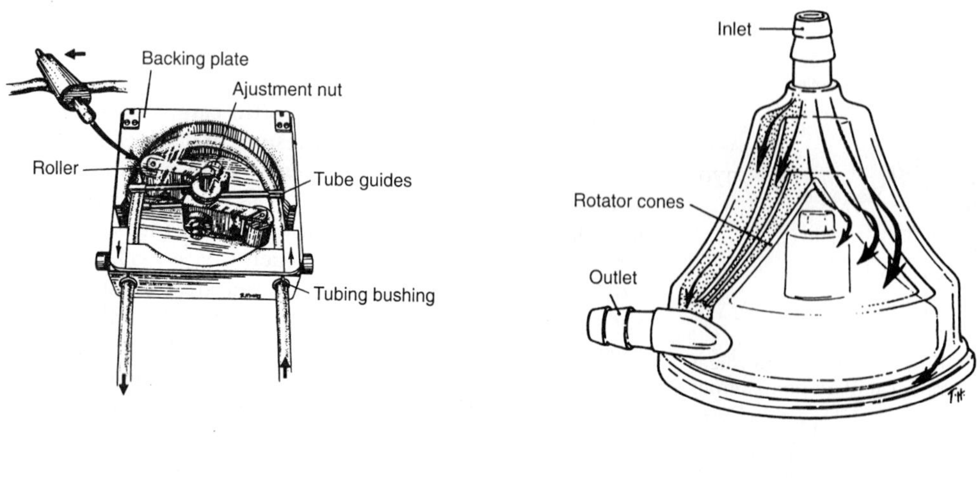

FIGURE 77.4. Debakey-type roller pump (*left*) propels blood through the cardiopulmonary bypass circuit by advancing wave of compression of blood-containing tubing by nonocclusive rollers. Bio-Medicus vortex pump (right) propels blood through tubing by centrifugal force generated by central rotor. (From Reed and Stafford,[152] with permission.)

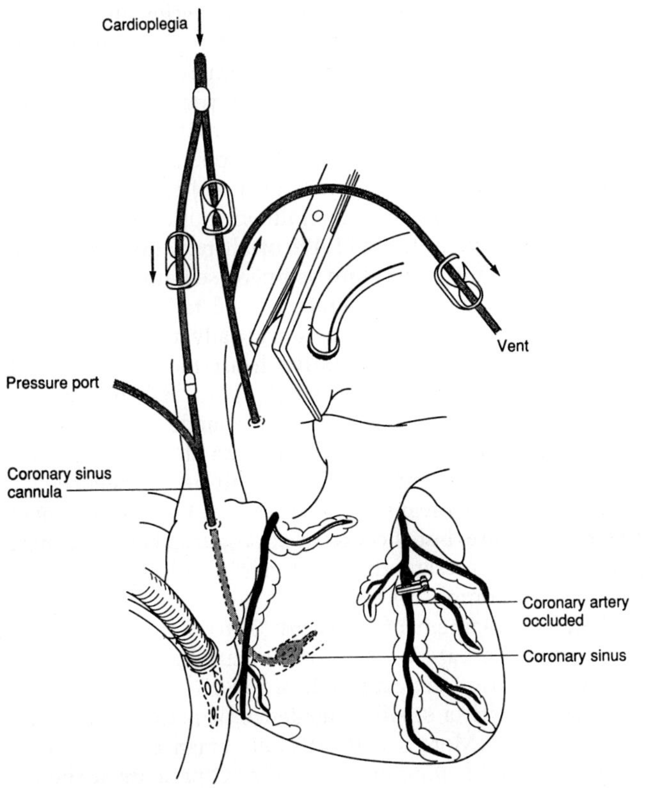

FIGURE 77.5. Typical configuration for antegrade cardioplegia delivery via catheter in aortic root proximal to systemic cannula and aortic cross-clamp and retrograde cardioplegia delivery via a coronary sinus catheter. (From Partington et al.,[153] with permission.)

Cardioplegia may be administered in an antegrade fashion into either the aortic root or directly into the coronary ostia or in a retrograde fashion into the coronary sinus. Retrograde delivery of the cardioplegic solution has been shown to aid in cardioplegia distribution to myocardial territories downstream from arterial obstructions and to improve outcomes in high-risk patients with advanced disease, such as those undergoing reoperation.[13] The retrograde catheter is placed by manual manipulation into the coronary sinus through a stab wound in the right atrium, and isolation of the sinus is accomplished by inflation of a balloon after appropriate catheter positioning.

Although there are many different cardioplegia formulations, potassium is the common ingredient (Table 77.1). By raising the extracellular potassium concentration from approximately 4 to 30 mEq/L, the normal myocyte membrane electrical potential is equalized, leading to myocardial arrest in diastole. Cardiac asystole induced by potassium cardioplegia alone reduces myocardial oxygen utilization by 90%, while hypothermia can be utilized to further decrease myocardial O_2 utilization by 50% for each 10°C decrease in myocardial temperature. Other ingredients added to cardioplegia solution to help improve myocardial protection may include (1) buffers, such as sodium bicarbonate or tromethamine (THAM); (2) respiratory substrates such as oxygen, glucose, and Krebs cycle intermediates such as glutamate or aspartate; (3) coronary vasodilators such as nitroglycerin or L-arginine; and (4) membrane stabilizers such as steroids, magnesium, calcium channel blockers, or O_2 radical scavengers (Table 77.1).[14]

A common configuration for cardioplegia delivery is as a blood crystalloid mixture, in which four parts blood are withdrawn from the oxygenator and one part crystalloid potassium cardioplegia solution is drawn from a premixed bag. This 4:1 ratio results in a solution of approximately 30 mEq KCl. For antegrade delivery, flow rates and pressure are typically 150 to 400 mL/min at 90 mmHg or less, respectively. Adjunctive retrograde cardioplegia is delivered at approximately 150 mL/min with a pressure less than 50 mmHg.

Topical cooling with cold saline or slush further aids in myocardial cooling and helps prevent rewarming of the heart by exposure to the operating room lights, by collateral blood flow, or by the warmer systemic blood circulating in the descending aorta and abdominal viscera. Some data suggest that topical iced slush cooling is associated with a higher incidence of phrenic nerve paralysis, however, and use of iced saline solutions has in many cases been replaced with the use of cold saline alone.

It should be noted that the use of continuous or intermittent warm cardioplegia has been advocated recently as a more effective form of myocardial protection, but problems associated with this technique are loss of hypothermic safety margin, increased hemodilution, higher serum potassium levels, and diminished view of the operative field.[8,9,15]

Conduct of Cardiopulmonary Bypass

After incision has been made and appropriate exposure obtained, sufficient heparin is administered (usually 3–4 mg/kg) to produce an ACT of at least 400 to 450 s. The ascending aorta is cannulated. Venous return is obtained from a two-stage cannula inserted into the right atrium or, for mitral valve or right heart surgery, two single-stage cannulas, each inserted into one of the venae cavae, with total venous bypass provided by caval snares. The venous line is run to the pump oxygenator, and blood is drained. Drainage by gravity from the venous cannulas goes into a venous reservoir chamber. The blood passes through the oxygenator, undergoes gas and heat exchange, as appropriate, and is finally pumped back into the body, usually with a Debakey-type roller pump or Bio-Medicus centrifugal pump (see Figs. 77.1 and 77.4).

Once CPB is established and all other appropriate preparations made as needed for the specific surgical procedures, the heart is arrested by cross-clamping the ascending aorta and

TABLE 77.1. Typical Constituents of Blood Cardioplegia.[a]

Component	*Concentration*	*Purpose*
Blood	Hematocrit 20%–30%	Oxygen delivery/ acid–base buffering
KCl	<20 mEq/L	Maintain cardiac arrest
THAM/$NaHCO_3$[2]	pH 7.5–7.6 (titrated)	Buffer
Glucose	350–400 mOsm	Avoid edema
Heparin	6 U/mL	Anticoagulation
$CaCl_2$	<0.5 mmol/L	Maintain calcium gradients

[a]Other components may include nitroglycerin and Kreb's cycle intermediates.
Source: Modified from Bojar,[148] with permission.

injecting about 10 to 15 mL/kg of a cold potassium cardioplegic solution (30–35 mEq/L potassium concentration) at 4°C to 6°C into the aortic root. Myocardial temperatures are usually maintained at 10°C to 20°C, with reinjections of cold cardioplegic solution about every 20 min as protection during the ischemic cross-clamp period. Injections in the presence of significant aortic valve insufficiency require opening of the aortic root and direct cannulation of the coronary ostia or retrograde cardioplegia delivery via the coronary sinus to prevent reflux of injectate into the left ventricle (LV) and ventricular distension. A topical iced slush or iced saline solution may also be used. After completion of the cardiac intervention, the cross-clamp is removed, the heart is allowed to resume a normal rhythm, and after full rewarming, CPB is discontinued and the cannulas removed.

Complications Associated with Cardiopulmonary Bypass

Catastrophic complications potentially associated with CPB include protamine reactions, oxygenator failures, line disruptions, air embolism, and blood reactions, among other events. Despite the appropriate performance of CPB by current standards, a number of additional delayed events may occur as a result of the physiological trespass imposed by CPB. These complications may be a direct result of the hypothermic nonpulsatile flow characteristic of CPB or may be less directly related to the large number of metabolic and inflammatory response mediator derangements that are also known to occur as a result of CPB. In part, the risk of postoperative systemic dysfunction is also directly related to the level of preoperative organ dysfunction, the length of CPB, and the level of postoperative cardiac dysfunction.

Metabolic derangements associated with CPB affect nearly every aspect of biochemical homeostasis, including perturbations in the coagulation and fibrinolytic cascades, immunosuppression, upregulation of stress hormones such as epinephrine and the adrenocorticoids, and activation of leukocytes and inflammatory mediators such as complement and the interleukins. Anemia, thrombocytopenia, and depletion of clotting factors can lead to immediate or delayed risks of bleeding and cardiac tamponade. Hyperthermia and leukocytosis are also common following CPB and are thus not useful as guides to infection.

Hypothermia and a metabolic acidosis, in part resulting from the washout of regions that were poorly perfused during hypothermia, are commonly seen for the first several hours post-CPB. Sodium and water retention normally seen in surgical patients is exacerbated by the metabolic derangements associated with CPB, and a 5% increase in weight can be expected postbypass. Subsequent physiological diuresis is usually assisted by the administration of exogenous diuretic agents.

One of the most prevalent side effects of CPB is pulmonary dysfunction, which is most severe through the first 3 days after operation but may persist for 7 to 10 days. An increase in total lung and interstitial lung water, increased airway closure rate, and decreased pulmonary compliance may present as tachypnea, an increased alveolar–arterial oxygen gradient, and decreased functional residual capacity. These changes are directly related to preoperative pulmonary function, duration of CPB, and postoperative cardiac function. At a mechanistic level, complement activation and leukocyte aggregation in the pulmonary microcirculation appear to play important roles in pulmonary compromise. Therapy consists of diuresis, pulmonary toilet, and ventilatory support until appropriate extubation parameters are met.

Renal dysfunction (defined as postoperative creatinine of 2 mg/dL or increase of 0.7 mg/dL or more) can be expected to occur in at least 8% of patients following open heart surgery.[16] Eighteen percent of these (1.4% of all patients) will require dialysis. The mortality rate is increased up to 20-fold in patients developing postoperative renal failure. Risk factors for postoperative renal dysfunction are advanced age, a history of moderate-to-severe congestive heart failure (CHF), prior coronary artery bypass grafting (CABG), diabetes mellitus, and preexisting renal disease. Maintenance of a brisk urine output in the perioperative period with the use of diuretics and the early implementation of dialysis, as needed, have been espoused as means of minimizing the risk of postoperative renal failure, but the advent of off-pump coronary bypass surgery may represent the most significant advance in preventing this complication.[17]

The development of transient (3- to 6-month) deterioration in intellectual ability or other neurological dysfunction has been reported to occur in 30% to 80% of patients undergoing CPB, with a smaller incidence of permanent or fixed local defects.[18] More specifically, Newman et al. identified neurocognitive decline in 53% of CABG patients at the time of discharge, 24% of patients 6 months later, but in 42% of patients at 5 years. Gardner et al. reported a persistent decline in cognitive function at 1 year in 10% of patients undergoing coronary bypass, a finding that exceeded changes seen in a noncardiac surgery population.[19] In this study, only 12% of patients demonstrated no decline in cognitive function. In contrast, other prospective studies have shown that neurocognitive performance in patients with CABG does not differ from that of nonsurgical control subjects.[20,20a] The risk of neurological dysfunction has been related to age, preexistent neurological dysfunction, and total CPB time and has been attributed to platelet, thrombin, calcium, cholesterol, and air microemboli or periods of systemic hypotension that appear to result in ischemia in central nervous system watershed zones. Importantly, asymptomatic carotid bruits do not appear to impose an additional risk of neurological events in the absence of hemodynamically significant carotid stenoses. Based on the presumed importance of watershed perfusion, increased systemic pressures during CPB have been advocated as a protective measure. In the absence of identifiable areas of infarct or hemorrhage on head computed tomography (CT), neurological defects can most often be expected to clear in hours to days. Treatment is otherwise supportive. Off-pump bypass surgery may represent the most significant means of mitigating the occurrence of neurologic deficit, especially in high-risk individuals.[21]

Jaundice, acalculous cholecystitis, pancreatitis, gastrointestinal bleeding, peptic ulcer disease, intestinal ischemia, and other acute abdominal complications can also occur with increased frequency following CPB compared to other surgical procedures, occurring in almost 1% of patients after open-heart surgery.[22] The pathophysiology of these complications may in part be related to poor organ perfusion during nonpulsatile CPB or the occurrence of atheromatous embolization. Treatment is specific to the given complication.

Coronary Artery Disease

The surgical treatment of coronary artery disease (CAD) represents one of the greatest and most far-reaching accomplishments in the recent history of medical therapy. The advent of CABG as an operation performed more than 400,000 times annually in the United States has had an immeasurable impact on patient well-being and health care today.

The history of the surgical treatment of CAD represents a decades-long saga that can be traced to the early application of palliative, indirect therapies to ameliorate the symptoms of ischemia, such as sympathectomy, and continues through a period of indirect revascularization techniques, including the use of talc poudrage and the Vineburg procedure (internal mammary artery [IMA] implant into the subepicardium), to the current era of direct coronary artery anastomoses and revascularization.[23] Ironically, the most recent surgical innovations in the treatment of CAD, the use of biological approaches such as angiogenic therapies, in a sense represent a renewal of these treatments of old. Although such "nonbypass" techniques had once been abandoned in favor of the gold standard of direct grafting techniques developed over the past three decades, a number of trials exploring new ways to revascularize the ischemic heart are now underway.

Coronary Anatomy and Physiology

The coronary vasculature typically consists of three major arteries, found on or just below the epicardial surface of the heart, that give rise to several major branches, all of which also typically lie in an epicardial or subepicardial position before dividing into numerous intramyocardial branches (Fig. 77.6). The right coronary artery (RCA) and left (main) coronary artery are the two first branches of the aorta and arise from ostia that are found within the corresponding sinuses of Valsalva, gentle dilations of the aorta just above the aortic valve, the configurations of which are thought to enhance flow into these ostia.

The branching patterns of both the primary coronary arteries are highly variable. The majority of individuals exhibit a right-dominant pattern (Fig. 77.6). In this configuration, the RCA continues beyond the crux of the heart (the juncture of the atrioventricular [AV] and interventricular grooves) in the posterior interventricular groove as the posterior descending artery (PDA). The PDA sends septal perforators into the interventricular septum that anastomose with corresponding branches of the left anterior descending (LAD) branch. Alternatively, a minority of patients exhibit a left-dominant system (Fig. 77.7), in which branches of the circumflex (CX) artery from the left main reach the crux, while the remainder of patients demonstrate a codominant pattern in which both the RCA and left CX supply the crux.

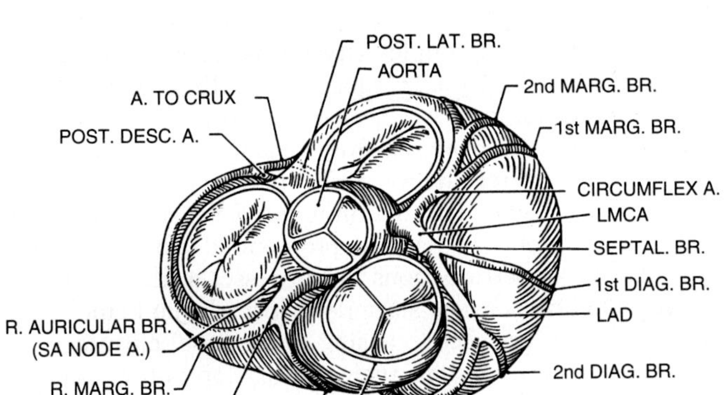

FIGURE 77.6. Overhead view of coronary artery anatomy in the more prevalent right-dominant pattern, with the posterior descending artery derived from the right coronary artery and supplying the posterior interventricular septum. (From Baue et al.,[154] with permission.)

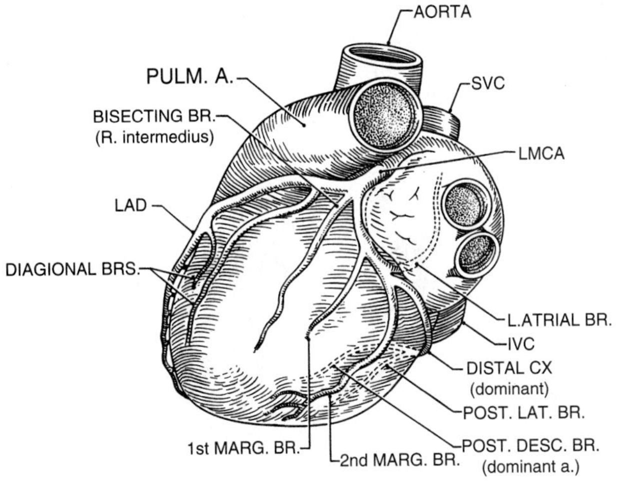

FIGURE 77.7. Lateral view of the left coronary artery system in a left-dominant configuration. Note the major divisions of the left main artery: the left anterior descending (LAD) and the circumflex (CX). In this left-dominant anatomy, the circumflex contributes the posterior descending artery. (Reproduced with permission.[154])

Extending beyond the PDA, additional "posterolateral" branches of the distal RCA extend into the posterior LV free wall. Thus, the RCA typically contributes about 20% to 30% of the cardiac blood supply, including the blood supply to the right ventricle, the posterior third of the septum, the sinus and AV nodes, and the posterior LV. A nondominant RCA, in contrast, may be rudimentary and contribute very little to the cardiac blood supply.

The left coronary artery courses posterior to the pulmonary artery (PA) from its origin in the aorta for approximately 1 cm as the left main coronary artery before it divides into a LAD branch and a CX branch, which travel in the anterior interventricular groove and the left AV groove, respectively. The LAD continues down to the apex of the heart, where it may anastomose with the distal PDA. Diagonal branches from the LAD course obliquely toward the left (obtuse) margin of the heart and supply the anterior LV; obtuse marginal branches correspondingly arise from the CX and supply the posterior LV.

The venous drainage of the heart feeds into a system of epicardial vessels that predominantly run along with the corresponding coronary artery. These coronary veins drain primarily into the great cardiac vein and ultimately into the coronary sinus, which empties into the right atrium (Fig. 77.8). The thebesian veins represent an alternative deep venous drainage system that empties directly into the cardiac chambers, predominantly the right ventricle.

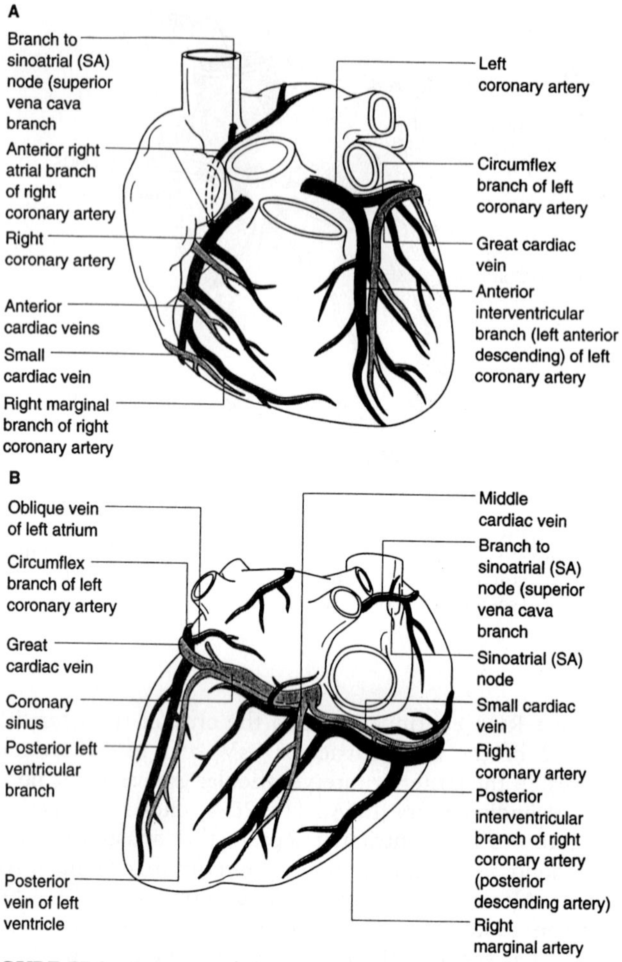

FIGURE 77.8. Anatomy of the coronary venous system, which primarily runs along with the corresponding coronary arteries. The coronary veins contribute to the coronary sinus that empties into the right atrium. (From Greenfield et al.,[155] with permission.)

Physiology of Coronary Blood Flow

Because intramyocardial pressures are greatest during systolic contraction and because the coronary ostia are somewhat obstructed by the opening of the aortic valve leaflets during this interval, pressure gradients favor a unique pattern of intracoronary blood flow that occurs primarily during diastole. Myocardial perfusion is also characterized by a flow gradient during systole such that perfusion of the subendocardium actually ceases during this interval because wall tension is greatest in this area. Conversely, diastolic blood flow is greatest to the subendocardium, thereby equalizing blood flow across the myocardium.

It is not surprising that myocardial oxygen demands are quite high considering the constant energy demands of the contracting myocardium. In this regard, it has been estimated that the heart consumes 4% of total body oxygen consumption while making up only 0.2% of total body weight. Given the extent of myocardial oxygen demand and the normal resting myocardial blood flow to the heart (approximately 20 mL/g/min), the 50% oxygen extraction ratios characteristic of other tissues would be insufficient to adequately supply the myocardium. Myocardial oxygen extraction ratios may therefore typically be as high as 70% at rest and up to 80% with exercise, and coronary sinus (myocardial venous) saturation levels are consequently the lowest of any organ.

Because of the extent of oxygen extraction at rest, it is obvious that little reserve is available during periods of peak increased myocardial oxygen demand to enhance myocardial oxygen delivery by way of increased oxygen extraction. The heart is therefore dependent on increased blood flow to meet this demand. This increased coronary blood flow is provided in part by an overall increase in systemic cardiac output but is also provided dramatically by biochemical regulation of coronary vascular resistance.

Biochemical mediators generated by myocardial hypoxia and ischemia that induce coronary vasodilation include nitric oxide, hydrogen and potassium ions, carbon dioxide, and adenosine. Other locally produced hormonal products that are also involved in coronary vasoregulation include bradykinin, epinephrine, norepinephrine, and prostaglandins, among other substances. In the event that an adequate increase in perfusion is not provided by these mechanisms, the heart can also meet energy demands by adapting into an anaerobic glycolytic metabolic pathway that produces less adenosine triphosphate (ATP) but requires less oxygen than oxidative catabolism. This anaerobic pathway generates lactate, which can be measured in increased quantities in the coronary sinus during ischemic intervals.

Pathogenesis of Coronary Artery Disease

Atherosclerosis remains the leading cause of CAD and the leading cause of death in the Western world. Coronary vasospasm, caused by idiopathic processes or by the intake of vasoreactive substances such as cocaine, is the most common of several other, far less prevalent causes of myocardial ischemia. Congenital anomalies in coronary anatomy, such as origin of the left coronary system from the right ostia or the PA, represent other causes of myocardial ischemia. As opposed to atherosclerosis, these other processes uncommonly lead to myocardial infarction (MI).

The pathophysiology of atherosclerotic CAD is related to the obstruction of the coronary artery lumen by an atheromatous plaque enlarging from within the coronary arterial wall. Atheromatous lesions typically develop gradually over decades, beginning in the early years of life, when they may be represented by a simple fatty streak. A more advanced, subintimal atheromatous plaque is typically comprised of a central lipid core covered by a fibrous cap (Fig. 77.9). The mature lesion is characteristically a complex mass of cholesterol and cholesterol esters, extracellular matrix components and smooth muscle cells, inflammatory cells such as macrophages, and fibroblasts that have proliferated or been recruited by biochemical perturbations in the vessel wall. The nature of the lesion can change abruptly if intraplaque hemorrhage and plaque rupture occur, causing acute vessel closure.

Atherosclerotic lesions typically develop in the proximal one-third to one-half of the epicardial vasculature but may be found more distally at branch points or in the RCA system. Fortuitously, the anatomical localization of CAD to the proximal coronary vasculature typically allows reconstruction by interventional therapies (such as angioplasty and

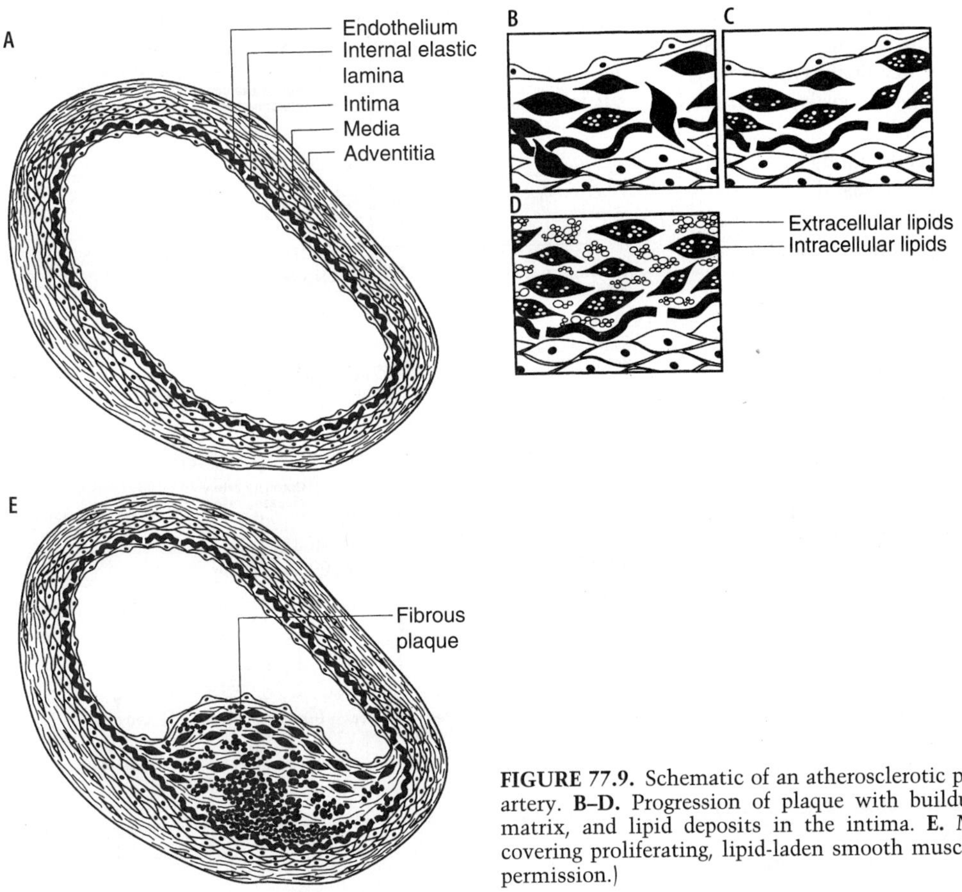

FIGURE 77.9. Schematic of an atherosclerotic plaque. **A.** Depiction of a normal muscular artery. **B–D.** Progression of plaque with buildup of smooth muscle cells, extracellular matrix, and lipid deposits in the intima. **E.** Maturing fibrous plaque with fibroblasts covering proliferating, lipid-laden smooth muscle cells. (After Glomset and Ross,[156] with permission.)

coronary artery bypass) into relatively normal distal vasculature. In contrast, the coronary arteries of diabetic or other patients with advanced disease may be extensively diseased and friable or calcified and inelastic throughout and may not be amenable to conventional therapies. Such patients may be ideal candidates for the "nonbypass" techniques discussed in the following pages.

Risk Factors

The pivotal Framingham study, named after the Massachusetts town whose population was the subject of this study, is one of a number of epidemiological surveys conducted over the past 40 years that have identified a series of risk factors for the development of atherosclerosis. A large number of such risk factors for coronary disease have been identified, the most important of which are hypercholesterolemia, hypertension, smoking, and family history. Reduction of these risk factors, by such measures as diet, weight loss, blood pressure control, cessation of tobacco use, and lifestyle modulation, has most likely contributed significantly to the decreased incidence of fatalities from CAD during the past two decades. Most recently, a series of cholesterol-lowering drugs known collectively as the statins has been introduced; these drugs have directly targeted the major biochemical abnormality associated with hypercholesterolemia. It is expected that the growing use of these and similar agents will substantially lower the incidence of pathological complications associated with atherosclerosis.

Pathophysiology and Clinical Presentation of Coronary Artery Disease

Severe obstructive atherosclerotic disease may compromise adequate coronary blood flow in the resting state, or lesser degrees of obstruction may compromise perfusion only when myocardial oxygen demands increase with exercise and then outstrip blood supply, which is limited by the obstructing coronary lesion. The clinical sequelae of inadequate blood supply, or myocardial ischemia, may present in three major patterns: (1) angina pectoris, which usually develops in the setting of transient mismatches in myocardial oxygen delivery–demand, and that by definition represents a reversible period of myocardial ischemia; (2) myocardial infarction (MI), which occurs in the setting of prolonged periods of ischemia or with cessation of blood flow to a segment of myocardium as the result of complete closure of an atherosclerotic segment; or (3) ischemic cardiomyopathy, which is a state of generalized ventricular dysfunction that may present as fatigue or shortness of breath or heart failure and may occur as the result of repetitive or prolonged episodes of myocardial ischemia or infarction.

Angina Pectoris

Myocardial ischemia typically occurs only with coronary artery obstruction equivalent to at least a 50% reduction of the diameter (equal to 75% reduction of the cross-sectional area) of the arterial lumen. Angina pectoris may present with classical symptoms, crushing substernal pressure that radiates to the left arm, or as "anginal equivalents," such as throat pain, shortness of breath, or other atypical symptoms, and is typically precipitated by events such as exercise, eating, or stress that increase cardiac activity and thus myocardial oxygen demand. Angina can typically be relieved by cessation of the stress event or with nitroglycerin, a vasodilator that increases coronary blood flow and decreases wall stress (see following), although other conditions such as esophageal spasm may also respond favorably to nitroglycerin.

Severe coronary artery stenoses that greatly compromise flow through the coronary lumen may result in unstable angina, which is defined as angina that occurs with a recent (2-month) trend of increasing frequency or severity, or rest (preinfarction) angina, which occurs without provocation. Alternatively, Prinzmetal or atypical angina may also occur at rest but as a result of coronary spasm. Coronary vasospasm typically occurs at or near a site of a fixed atherosclerotic lesion and may occur as a result of plaque ulceration or thrombosis or as a result of smooth muscle cell spasm caused by local production of serotonin, thromboxane, or other vasoactive substances. Rarely, spasm may occur in the absence of atherosclerotic disease, possibly as a result of imbalance in autonomic regulation of coronary tone.

Some patients, typically those with diabetes mellitus, may conversely experience silent ischemia without symptomatology. These patients may be at an increased risk for a catastrophic cardiac event because of the lack of an "early warning system" of angina that allows the halting of provocative stress events and thus the limitation of myocardial ischemia.

Electrocardiographic (ECG) confirmation of myocardial ischemia is essential in confirming that chest pain or related symptomatology in fact represents a myocardial ischemic event. Typical ECG changes consistent with ischemia include ST-segment depression or T-wave inversion. Diagnostic management of the stable patient presenting with angina may include assessment of myocardial flow reserves by one of several provocative tests that induce ischemia by increasing myocardial oxygen demand (Fig. 77.10). An exercise tolerance test that utilizes either a treadmill or bicycle ergonometry to increase cardiac work and incorporates an analysis of provocable symptomatology, ECG, and hemodynamic responses is a commonly performed screening test for myocardial ischemia. Recently, ultrafast CT has been utilized to detect coronary calcifications in the proximal vasculature and was found to be 95% sensitive (although only 44% specific) in screening for significant angiographic disease (at least 50% luminal diameter narrowing of any one vessel).[24]

Studies that are generally considered second-order tests for diagnosing CAD include radionuclide scans that depict myocardial perfusion defects at rest and with pharmacological stresses that vasodilate the coronary bed, such as with the administration of adenosine. Alternatively, echocardiographic assessment of regional wall motion abnormalities at rest and inducibility or reversibility of these abnormalities after administration of the cardiac inotrope dobutamine is another means of documenting myocardial ischemia. Potentially more sensitive tests, including cardiac magnetic resonance imaging (MRI) and positron emission tomographic (PET) scanning, are gaining acceptance when first-order diagnostic exams are not conclusive. Abnormal responses to these

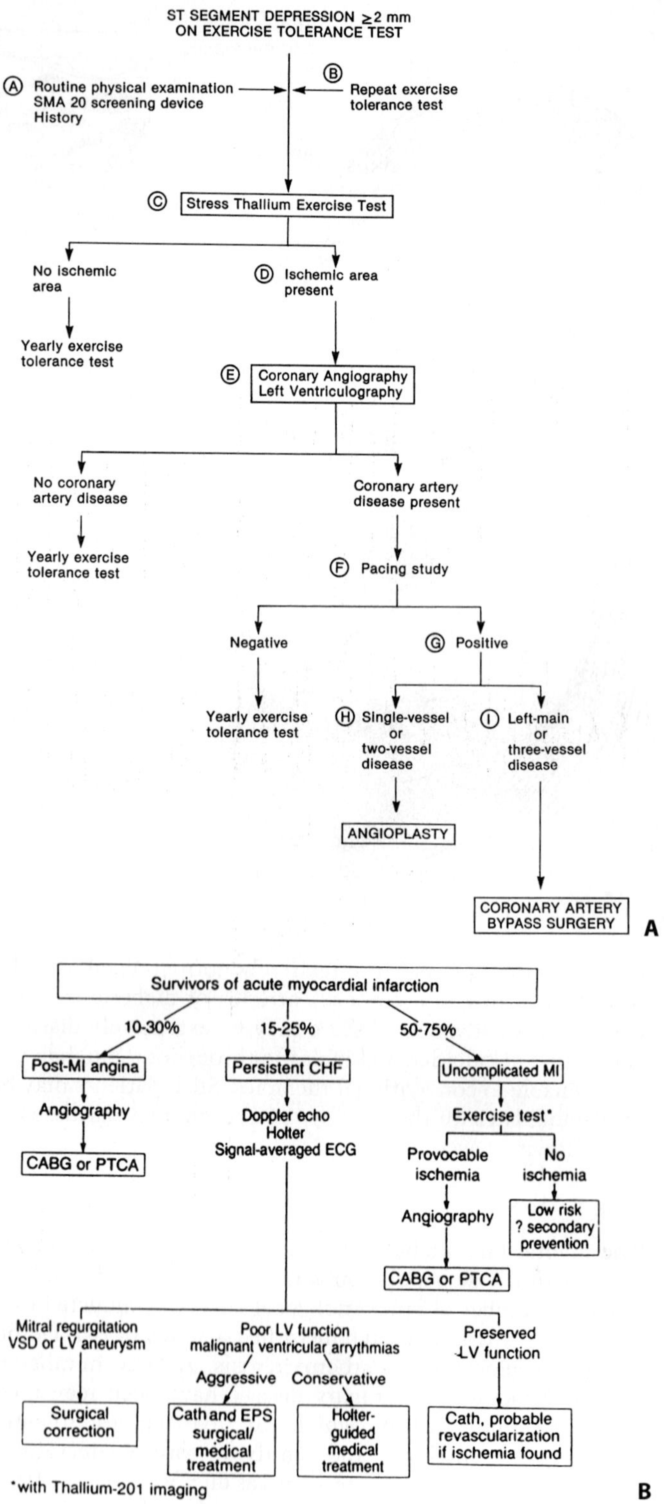

FIGURE 77.10. Typical algorithms for workup of patients with (**A**) stable ischemia pattern or (**B**) following acute myocardial infarction. (From Cohn et al.,[157] with permission.)

screening tests, or a presentation of rest or unstable angina, most likely should result in the performance of coronary angiography that will permit the exact identification of coronary pathology. A presentation of rest or unstable angina will also most likely necessitate interventional therapy, as discussed next. In the near future, however, it is anticipated that highly sophisticated CT scanning technology may allow the performance of noninvasive coronary angiography.

Myocardial Infarction

Although ischemia can usually be viewed as a graded result of gradual lumen encroachment by a progressively enlarging atheromatous plaque, MI typically results from total or near-total occlusion of an epicardial coronary artery by plaque rupture or intraluminal thrombosis. The plaque may rupture as a result of intraplaque hemorrhage, among other causes, and the resultant release into the lumen of vasoactive compounds such as thromboxane A_2 and serotonin results in platelet aggregation and local vasoconstriction at the site of the ruptured plaque. Cholesterol emboli may cause downstream occlusions as well.

Although myocardial contractility is severely diminished within a few minutes of the cessation of blood flow, subsequent myocardial injury is fully reversible for up to 20 min following the onset of ischemia. After about 1 h of profound ischemia, isolated myocyte necrosis progresses to confluent subendocardial necrosis, which then spreads toward the subepicardium. Transmural infarction characteristically ensues after 6 h of coronary occlusion. Healing of the infarct over the ensuing week is characterized by liquefaction necrosis, followed by replacement of the necrotic tissue by fibroblast ingrowth and scar formation. The periinfarct zone around the area of infarction typically remains ischemic and may progress to full infarction if the degree of persistent ischemia overwhelms adaptive responses such as collateral formation and angiogenesis that may revascularize this territory.

An acute coronary occlusion that results in transmural infarction in the region supplied by the occluded vessel is typically diagnosed in the setting of protracted angina or associated symptoms such as nausea, diaphoresis, or shortness of breath and appropriate ECG changes. Development of ST elevation and subsequent ST normalization, T-wave inversion, and, importantly, Q waves, can be anticipated in the ECG leads corresponding to the site of a transmural infarction. In contrast, a subendocardial infarction is typically caused by episodes of perfusion–demand mismatch in a territory supplied by a subtotally occluded or partially collateralized vessel and is characterized by ST depression, T-wave inversion, and the absence of a Q wave.

Laboratory confirmation of MI is made by demonstration of a rise in serum markers of myocardial injury, most notably creatinine phosphokinase (CPK) in association with a prominent myocardial (MB) fraction. CPK-MB fractions typically rise within a few hours after MI and peak 8 to 24 h later. Increases in lactate dehydrogenase (LDH) typically peak over the succeeding 48 to 72 h. Recently, the use of blood troponin assays has been espoused as a more rapid and accurate means of diagnosing MI.

Sudden cardiac death due to ventricular arrhythmias will occur immediately or within the first 24 to 48 h after MI in 20% of patients. This complication can usually be treated or prevented with acute antiarrhythmic medications, and the risk of this complication characteristically resolves within 48 h. Depending on the extent of the infarct, an MI can also be complicated by LV dysfunction, while frank heart failure (cardiogenic shock) will occur in 10% of patients, in association with infarction of at least 40% of the LV (see following). Cardiogenic shock is associated with evidence of poor systemic perfusion (hypotension, tachycardia, renal dysfunction, mental obtundation, and pulmonary edema) and is defined by a cardiac output of less than 2 L/min/m^2.

Mechanical complications of MI caused by transmural necrosis and myocardial rupture involving the free wall, papillary muscle, or septum may occur in 1% to 3% of patients and can lead to cardiac tamponade, acute mitral regurgitation (MR), or acute ventricular septal defect (VSD), respectively (see following). Late mechanical complications of MI include ventricular aneurysm formation, which can be further complicated by the development of life-threatening ventricular arrhythmias.

Ischemic Cardiomyopathy

The combination of a series of small infarcts alone or in combination with one or several larger MIs may lead to progressive loss of viable myocytes and degeneration of ventricular contractility. Alternatively, myocytes that are viable but nonfunctioning or "hibernating" due to inadequate blood supply may also contribute to LV dysfunction. The development of heart failure in this setting has been termed *ischemic cardiomyopathy*. Failure to maintain adequate systolic ejection function leads to an increase in LV end-diastolic volume (LVEDV) and cardiac enlargement, which, according to Laplace's law, results in increases in wall tension and further compromise of subendocardial work/perfusion ratios and further ischemia. Heart failure may be characterized by fatigue or shortness of breath with exertion or even at rest caused by, respectively, diminished cardiac output (forward failure) and increased left ventricular end diastolic pressure (LVEDP), which is transmitted back into the pulmonary circulation and results in pulmonary congestion (backward failure).

Medical Treatment of CAD

The improvement of coronary blood flow and the decrease of myocardial oxygen demands are the cornerstones of medical therapy for CAD. Efficacy of medical therapy can usually be judged on the basis of relief of angina. The three major drug groups used to treat myocardial ischemia have been the nitrates, β-blockers, and calcium channel blockers, as well as the anticholesterol medications used to limit, halt, or reverse the progression of atherosclerotic plaque. More recently, improved survival and preservation of myocardial function have been demonstrated in patients with CAD treated with angiotensin-converting enzyme (ACE) inhibitors.

The nitrates, either long- or short-acting, work by causing vascular smooth muscle cell relaxation and thus vasodilation. By dilating the venous capacitance vessels, nitrates cause pooling of the blood volume in the venous circulation. The primary physiological effect of the nitrates is thus to decrease ventricular filling (myocardial preload) and thereby decrease ventricular wall radius, wall stress, and myocardial oxygen demand. A lesser effect of the nitrates is to directly dilate the coronary bed and improve coronary flow.

The β-blockers work to directly decrease myocardial oxygen demand by decreasing heart rate and contractility. Calcium channel blockers, which are arterial vasodilators, work by decreasing myocardial contractility and blocking

TABLE 77.2.
Coronary Artery Bypass Trials.

Study	*No. of patients*	*Years of enrollment*	*Operative mortality (%)*	*Five-year survival*[a]	
				Medical	*Surgical*
VA Cooperative[37]	686	1972–1974	5.8	64[b]	80[b]
European Cooperative Surgical Study[38]	768	1973–1976	3.3	82	94
Coronary Artery Surgery Study (CASS)[1]	780	1974–1979	1.4	74	92

[a]For patients with LVEF > 50%, triple-vessel disease, class III–IV.
[b]The 30-month survival for patients with left main disease.
Source: Modified from Cohn.[149]

coronary vasospasm and relieve wall stress by decreasing systemic vascular resistance and afterload. Recently, however, the safety of these agents in this setting has been questioned. The ACE inhibitors work through several mechanisms, not all well categorized, including afterload reduction and antiinflammatory mechanisms.

Progression from an ischemic pattern to an infarction event typically signifies acute coronary thrombosis and has been treated by prompt administration of a thrombolytic agent such as urokinase, streptokinase, or tissue plasminogen activator (TPA), with or without heparin. A number of studies have demonstrated that these agents dramatically decrease the mortality associated with acute MI.[25–28] Delivered by intravenous or, occasionally, by direct coronary infusion, these agents can completely reverse the sequelae of acute MI if given within 6h of the onset of symptoms. Contraindications to thrombolytic therapy include anemia, recent surgery or bleeding diatheses, such as peptic ulcer disease, or a recent cerebrovascular accident (CVA).

In the 1980s and 1990s, a surprisingly effective treatment of CAD was found in percutaneous transluminal coronary angioplasty (PTCA), by which the atherosclerotic coronary plaque can be dilated by a balloon catheter placed over a guidewire under fluoroscopic guidance via a peripheral artery. More recently, "simple" PTCA has been nearly completely replaced by ever-more-effective coronary stent technology, by which the dilated coronary segment is kept open by a percutaneously placed intracoronary stent, and most recently, the patency of stenting techniques have been improved by (antihyperplastic) drug-eluting stent technology and sophisticated poststent antiplatelet therapy.[29–36] These current percutaneous coronary interventions (PCIs) today can be expected to be initially successful (6-month patency) in more than 90% of appropriately selected patients, with a 1%–3% complication rate. Late recurrence of stenoses may occur as the result of intimal hyperplasia, arterial recoil, progression of disease, or other factors in 10% to 30% of cases. Most recently, the thrombotic potential of the drug eluting stents have caused a shift back towards "bare metal" stents. These techniques can be used in patients with stable or unstable angina patterns, as described next, or in the setting of an acute MI.

Indications for CABG versus PCI

A number of trials have been conducted over the past three decades comparing CABG to medical therapy for the treatment of CAD and, more recently, comparing CABG to PCI (Tables 77.2 through 77.5). Surprisingly, the cornerstone of the indications for CABG remains the three major trials conducted in the 1970s during the early days of coronary surgery

TABLE 77.3.
CABG Versus Percutaneous Transluminal Coronary Angioplasty (PTCA) Multivessel Disease Trials.

Trial	*CABG (n)*	*PTCA (n)*	*Mean LVEF (%)*	*In-house mortality (%)*		*Follow-up interventions (PTCA or CABG)*[a]		*Angina class ≥CCS II at 3 years (%)*[b]	
				CABG	*PTCA*	*CABG*	*PTCA*	*CABG*	*PTCA*
CABRI (Europe)	513	541	63	0.7	1.3	2.9	2.6	—	—
RITA (United Kingdom)	501	510	—	3.6	3.1	5	41	16	18
EAST (United States)	194	198	61	1.0	1.0	3	50	11	19
GABI (Germany)	177	182	56	2.3	1.0	7	46		
BARI (United States/ Canada)	914	915	57	1.3	1.1	3	47	—	—
Total/average	2299	2346		1.8	1.5	4	44	14	19

[a]Mean number of interventions required subsequent to initial procedure during follow-up period.
[b]Percentage of patients with Canadian Cardiovascular Society angina class II or greater at 3 years postinitial intervention.
Source: Modified from Favaloro (1998).[47]

TABLE 77.4.
CABG Versus Percutaneous Coronary Intervention (PCI) with Stent Trials.[a]

Trial	Extent of CAD	N	Outcome (%) Death	MI[b]	Angina	RR[c] (%) total/PCI/CABG	Follow-up (yr)
SoS	MV	988				6/4/1	1
CABG			2	8	21	21[a]/13/9	
PCI			5[a]	5	34		
ERACI II	MV	450				5/0/0	1.6
CABG			8	6	8	17[a]/0/5	
PCI			3[a]	3	15		
ARTS	MV	1205				4/3/1	1
CABG			3	5	10	21[a]/16/7	
PCI			3	6	21		
AWESOME	MV	454				N/A	3
CABG N/A			N/A	21	N/A		
PCI N/A				20			
SIMA	SV	121				0/0/0	2.4
CABG			4	4	5	24[a]/13/6	
PCI			2	5	9		
Leipzig	SV	220				8/8/0	0.5
CABG			2	5	21	29/25/4	
PCI			0	3	38		

MV, multivessel disease; SV, single vessel.

ARTS, Arterial Revascularization Therapies Study; AWESOME, Angina with Extremely Serious Operative Mortality Evaluation; ERACI II, Coronary Angioplasty with Stenting Versus CABG in Patients with MV Disease; Leipzig, Stenting Versus Minimally Invasive Bypass Surgery; SIMA, Stenting Versus Internal Mammary Artery; SoS, Stent or Surgery Trial.

[a]All trials evidence class I.

[b]Q-wave myocardial infarction.

[c]Repeat revascularization.

Source: From Eagle, Guyton, et al. JACC, 2004; ACC/AHA Practice Guidelines.[61]

and comparing CABG to medical therapy for CAD: the CASS, the Veterans Administration (VA) study, and the European study (Table 77.2).[1,37–39]

This anomaly is particularly significant in that the relevance of these studies has been limited by the subsequent evolutions of surgical techniques *and* medical practices, including the increased use of the internal mammary artery (IMA) as a bypass graft, improved cardioprotection strategies, and on the other hand, the introduction of such drugs such as cholesterol-lowering statins, β-blockers, and ACE inhibi-

TABLE 77.5.
CABG Versus Medical Treatment.

Trial	Number of patients randomized: CABG	Medical treatment	Operative mortality (%)	5-yr mortality (n): CABG	Medical treatment	Odds ratio (95% CI)	10-yr mortality (n): CABG	Medical treatment	Odds ratio (95% CI)
VA (1972–1974)	332	354	5.8	58	79	0.74 (0.5–1.8)	118	141	0.83 (0.61–1.14)
European (1973–1976)	394	373	3.3	30	63	0.4 (0.26–0.64)	91	109	0.72 (0.52–0.99)
CASS (1974–1979)	390	390	1.4	20	32	0.6 (0.34–1.08)	72	83	0.84 (0.59–1.19)
Texas	56	60		10	13	0.79 (0.31–1.97)	23	25	0.97 (0.46–2.04)
Oregon	51	49		4	8	0.44 (0.12–1.56)	23	25	0.94 (0.39–2.26)
New Zealand	51	49		5	7	0.65 (0.19–2.2)	15	16	0.94 (0.38–2.31)
New Zealand	50	50		8	8	1.00 (0.34–2.91)	17	16	1.15 (0.50–2.65)
Total	1324	1325		135 10%	210 16%	0.61 (0.48–0.77) $P < .0001$	350 26%	404 30%	0.83 (0.70–0.98) $P = .03$

Source: From Eagle et al.[61a]

TABLE 77.6. Indications for Coronary Artery Bypass Graft (CABG) Surgery: Class I Recommendations.[a]

Anatomical/physiological indications Subsets of patients
Anatomical/physiological indications
Left main stenosis >50%
Three-vessel disease with impaired LV function
Three-vessed disease with normal LV function but with inducible ischemia on physiological testing
Two-vessel disease including proximal LAD
Cardiogenic shock with appropriate angiographic indications
Positive physiological studies or significant coronary stenosis before major cardiac or noncardiac surgery
Congenital coronary anomalies associated with sudden death
Clinical indications
Unstable or Class III–IV angina refractory to medical therapy (including PTCA/stenting)
Postinfarction angina with appropriate angiographic indications
Failed PTCA with acute ischemia/hemodynamic instability
Acute myocardial infarction <6h with thrombolytic/PTCA therapy contraindicated

[a]Class I recommendations: conditions for which there is evidence or general agreement that a given procedure or treatment is beneficial, useful, and effective.

Source: Eagle, Guyton et al. 2004 ACC/AHA Practice Guidelines.[61]

tors—advancements that have decreased mortalities associated with *both* surgical and medical treatments of CAD. Aside from a number of design and methodologic flaws, further limitations to the application of the results of these landmark studies to current practice include the relatively young age (<65 years) of enrolled subjects, the exclusion of women, and the absence of patients with poor ventricular function and extensive comorbidities—characteristics common to modern cardiac surgery. To a great extent, the relative paucity of subsequent randomized trials nevertheless reflects the important results of these early studies and the ethical challenges to subsequent randomization in the face of their dramatic findings. More recent CABG-versus-angioplasty (Table 77.3) and CABG-versus-stent studies (Table 77.4) have, however, fundamentally confirmed the findings of these initial CABG/medical therapy trials (Table 77.5).

Significant coronary obstruction has generally been defined in these studies as at least a 50% narrowing in luminal diameter on coronary angiography, and *extent of disease* was defined as "single-, double-, or triple-vessel disease" based on the number of major coronary artery territories (LAD, CX, or RCA) involved. Based on long-term survival rates for CABG versus medical therapy in these studies, coronary bypass surgery became indicated for patients with more than 50% narrowing of the left main coronary artery; patients with triple-vessel disease, especially with evidence of LV dysfunction; or patients with refractory angina and double-vessel disease, including the proximal LAD (Table 77.6). Survival benefits are extended in patients with depressed LV function, primarily because of poor longevity if this group is treated medically. In contrast, no survival benefit was conferred by CABG in patients with lesser degrees of single- or double-vessel disease without involvement of the proximal LAD branch, and medical treatment or interventional therapy (PTCA/stent) has become indicated for these cases.

Alternatively, PCI is generally indicated in patients with single- or double-vessel disease or in patients with multiple lesions who are otherwise not appropriate candidates for coronary bypass surgery (Fig. 77.11).[40] Contraindications to PCI generally include left main disease and complex or calcified lesions, especially those that occur at branch points. These considerations are critical in that acute PCI failure due to dissection or thrombosis may infrequently require emergency bypass (currently <1% of cases), which carries an increased operative risk compared with elective cases. The evaluation of sophisticated PCI techniques and the placement of an IABP to improve coronary perfusion and decrease workload are two techniques that have decreased mortality in this setting.

Importantly, on the basis of survival benefits demonstrated in the Bypass Angioplasty Revascularization Investigation (BARI) trial reported in the late 1990s,[41] and confirmed by the Arterial Revascularization Therapies Study (ARTS) trial,[42] CABG also remains indicated for patients with triple-vessel disease and diabetes. The pivotal BARI study randomized 915 patients with clinically severe angina or objective evidence of ischemia to PTCA and 914 patients to CABG. In-house mortality was similar for CABG compared to PTCA (1.3% vs. 1.1%), the MI rate was 4.6% versus 2.1% ($P < .01$), and the stroke rate was 0.8% versus 0.2%, respectively. Respectively, 5-year survival was similar (89% vs. 86%), and the 5-year survival rate free from Q-wave MI was 80% versus 79%. Eight percent of CABG patients versus 54% of PTCA

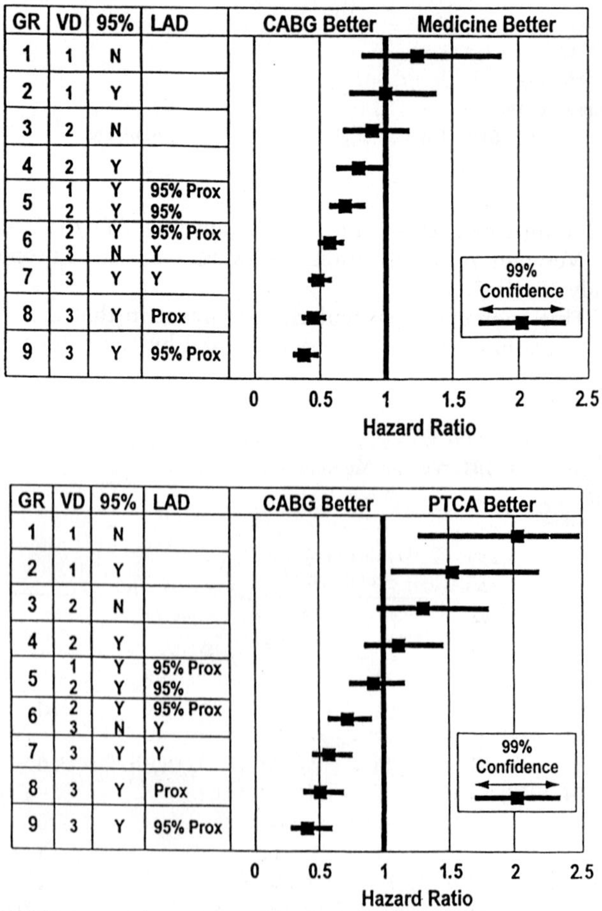

FIGURE 77.11. Adjusted hazard ratios comparing (a) coronary artery bypass grafting (CABG) and medicine and (b) CABG and angioplasty as a function of the extent of coronary artery lesions. VD, number of vessels diseased; 95% ≥ 95% coronary artery stenosis; Prox, proximal; GR, group. (Reproduced with permission from Jones.[46])

patients required subsequent revascularization (multiple in 19%), however, and the number of respective subsequent hospitalizations was 1.9 versus 2.5 ($P < .001$) after 5 years. Importantly, diabetics on insulin or oral hypoglycemics had a 5-year survival of 81% for CABG versus 66% for PTCA ($P = .003$) in the BARI study. The authors concluded that CABG and PTCA yielded similar survival in patients with multivessel disease, although PTCA patients required subsequent interventions significantly more often, and survival at 5 years was significantly better for treated diabetics with multivessel disease undergoing CABG compared with PTCA.

A subsequent analysis of this patient population found significantly more CABG versus PTCA patients to be angina free at early follow-up (95% vs. 73%; $P < .001$) and at 5 years (85% vs. 79%; $P = .007$) compared with PTCA patients. Among angina-free patients at 5 years, 52% of PTCA patients required revascularization after the initial procedure versus 6% of patients who had CABG. Furthermore, another analysis of this study population demonstrated significantly better ($P < .05$) activity status in CABG versus PTCA patients at 3 years, although PTCA patients returned to work 5 weeks earlier than CABG patients ($P < .001$).[43]

As in BARI, in 1 year outcomes for CABG versus ("bare metal") PCI were similar in the ARTS trial, but repeat revascularization rates were higher with stenting at 1 year (17% vs. 4%) versus CABG and at 3 years. Similarly, diabetics required more frequent revascularization (22% vs. 3%) following PCI versus CABG, and event-free survival at 3 years was similarly differentiated (81% vs. 53%). Incomplete revascularization, which was more common in PCI versus CABG patients, resulted in more frequent subsequent interventions (10% vs. 2%) in these studies compared to individuals receiving complete revascularization, supporting the argument for CABG if PCI cannot provide adequate revascularization.

A meta-analysis of recent CABG versus PTCA multivessel disease studies involving a total of 2943 randomized patients demonstrated that the overall risk of death was similar for CABG and PTCA (3.7% vs. 3.9%), whereas CABG patients were more likely to be angina-free (81% vs. 73%; $P < .00001$) and free from subsequent CABG (1% vs. 20%; $P < .00001$) or PTCA (6% vs. 23%; $P < .00001$).[44] A notable exception to these findings was the observation in the single-center Emory (Emory Angioplasty versus Surgery Trial, EAST) trial of a trend toward improved survival with CABG versus PCI in patients with a LAD stenosis (80% vs. 86%) and particularly in those with diabetes (60% vs. 76%).[45]

The Duke study of 10,000 PTCA versus CABG patients summarized the field as follows[46]: (1) Increasing extent of CAD decreases survival whatever the intervention, although to a greater extent with medical therapy compared with CABG; (2) the greatest differences in survival between groups are found in patients with the greatest extent of disease; (3) CABG improves survival compared with medical therapy in patients with at least 95% stenosis of the LAD, and survival increases with increasing severity of CAD; (4) CABG improves survival compared to PTCA in patients with at least double-vessel disease with 95% stenosis of the proximal LAD.

Favaloro has recently contributed an exhaustive review of all the randomized CABG and PTCA trials that elegantly defines the indications for surgery based on risk–benefit ratios in a variety of situations.[47] Finally, an analysis of CABG patients in the BARI study has provided evidence of predictors of improvement in quality-of-life scores following CABG.[48] Of these, patients with heart failure, women, older patients, and diabetics demonstrated significantly less improvement in physical function than other patients at up to 4 years of follow-up. The wealth of outcome data available from these many studies allows an extraordinary opportunity for assigning accurate risk–benefit profiles for CABG versus PTCA and medical therapy to an individual patient with CAD on the basis of patient-specific parameters (Fig. 77.11).

In summary, applying the above-noted indications, CABG and PCI can today generally be expected to yield similar procedural and long-term survival rates as well as MI rates, but with PCI still generally resulting in greater recurrence of angina and revascularization rates.[49] The extent of complete revascularization provided by CABG appears to play an important role in this outcome—a finding that arguably speaks against potentially incomplete revascularization provided by off-pump procedures (see below). On the basis of these outcomes, 65% of all coronary revascularizations performed between 1999 and 2002 were by PCI, with a 7% annual rate of increase in PCI in that interval (majority of these changes occurred between 1999 and 2000). In contrast, CABG volume decreased by 2% per year during this time period. As drug-eluting stent technology improves and revascularization-free outcomes become better with advancements, it can be expected that these indications may further evolve. Importantly, however, the findings of the trials described above employing "bare metal" stents, the basis of current CABG-versus-PCI decision making, will soon be tested in a new set of prospective studies encompassing newer and potentially more effective drug-eluting stent technologies.

Other CABG Indications

Aside from the broad indications for coronary bypass defined in the various CABG and PTCA studies, a series of specific considerations for CABG need also to be considered. First, although a few studies have advocated emergency CABG in the setting of acute MI,[50,51] CABG is generally not indicated in this setting because it is unlikely to achieve revascularization in the 6-h interval immediately following coronary occlusion in which revascularization can prevent myocardial necrosis. For this reason, nonsurgical therapies such as thrombolysis or PCI that can be administered much more expeditiously are generally preferred in this setting. On the other hand, outcome studies suggest that it is not necessary to delay surgery once beyond the 6- to 24-h post-MI interval because further delay beyond this immediate time interval does not significantly alter operative mortality, except possibly in the case of very large infarctions.[52]

Second, patients with postinfarction angina or a positive exercise tolerance test or other positive perfusion–function analysis following MI are usually indicated to undergo coronary angiography and the appropriate intervention, as noted above, because medical treatment of these patients can be expected to result in 1-year mortality of approximately 15% to 50%.[53,54] Finally, most acute complications of MI, such as ventricular rupture, MR, and VSD, require urgent surgical repair and possible revascularization, as discussed below, and CABG is generally indicated for significant CAD in the setting of open-heart surgery for other indications, such as valve replacement.

Operative Procedure

Coronary bypass surgery is usually performed through a median sternotomy utilizing CPB and cardioplegic cardiac arrest. The major morbidities associated with CABG would, however, appear to be the use of CPB and the performance of a median sternotomy. Two alternative schools of thought have emerged in the past 10 years, advocating coronary bypass without the use of CPB or with CPB but via a "minithoracotomy" approach that seek to make CABG a "minimally invasive" procedure by eliminating the need for these respective interventions. While most surgeons rapidly lost enthusiasm for "Heartport" techniques after an initial wave of enthusiasm in the late 1990s, off-pump strategies have evolved from a minithoracotomy approach (MIDCAB, minimally invasive direct coronary artery bypass) to an off-pump strategy via a median sternotomy (OPCAB, off-pump coronary artery bypass). After a gradual, 5-year ramp-up period of adoption by the surgical community, OPCAB is now performed in an apparently plateaued 25% proportion of surgical revascvularization cases.

Preoperative Management

Aside from the preoperative considerations common to any surgical procedure, obligatory preoperative assessments for CABG include an examination of coronary anatomy in terms of the severity of the stenoses and suitability of the distal vessels for bypass, determination of left ventricular ejection fraction (LVEF), and presence or absence of valvular heart disease. This information can be gathered from the cardiac catheterization, with the addition of echocardiography if needed. Additional useful information in terms of the presence of a calcified or extensively atherosclerotic aorta can be obtained from chest x-ray, or transesophageal echo, and may influence operative risk and the approach to cannulation and clamping of the aorta.

The severity of the coronary stenoses alerts the surgical team regarding the risk of hemodynamic instability or arrhythmias during induction; the ejection fraction similarly determines the likelihood of a difficult postbypass course and the potential need for pharmacological or mechanical ventricular support. To help enhance perioperative hemodynamic stability, cardiac medications, usually including any prescribed antiplatelet agents, are usually continued up to the time of surgery.

The nature of the coronary disease, including the extent of distal disease, may suggest the need for additional length of conduit and specify the quality and type of conduit needed; for example, an IMA is more likely than a poor-quality saphenous vein to remain patent when grafted to a small, diffusely diseased LAD. The presence of chronic obstructive pulmonary disease, obesity, or diabetes may contraindicate the use of the IMA as these risk factors all increase the incidence of potential complications, such as sternal wound infection or respiratory compromise with IMA harvest. Inspection of the lower extremities for the presence of saphenous vein varicosities may also determine the need for alternate conduit, including radial artery or, less preferably, the lesser saphenous or cephalic vein.

Determination of the presence of a symptomatic bruit or symptoms of carotid disease is a critical component of the preoperative evaluation. Such findings generally indicate the need for Doppler ultrasound to evaluate the carotid and cerebral vasculature and will possibly warrant carotid surgery in the presence of severe stenoses or symptomatology. With moderate disease, higher on-bypass perfusion pressures may be indicated.

Finally, as with any open-heart procedure, bleeding parameters and potential for coagulopathy should be assessed because of the need for intraoperative heparinization and the coagulopathy sometimes associated with CPB. Patients with significant respiratory compromise should be considered for preoperative pulmonary care, cigarette smoking should be discontinued if possible, and attention should be directed toward improving the nutritional status of the patient. Preoperative enhancement of cardiac function can significantly improve operative mortality; therefore, treatment of congestive failure in the preoperative period and upgrading of functional class, if possible, can have significant effects on the outcome of operation (see later discussion).

Standard Operative Technique

Routine hemodynamic monitoring usually includes the use of an arterial pressure-measuring line, a PA (Swan-Ganz) catheter (a central venous line can be substituted in low-risk patients), and a urinary bladder catheter. (As the safety of bypass surgery has improved, many centers now forgo the use of PA catheter monitoring.) Adequate oxygenation and maintenance of a stable blood pressure, avoiding hypotension or hypertension, are critical to avoiding ischemia during the initial anesthetic induction period. Nitrates or β-blockers may be useful in this setting. Rarely, in the high-risk patient, such as those with a severe left main obstruction or with severely compromised ventricular function, an IABP may be placed preoperatively to provide cardiac support.

With a standard approach, the heart is exposed through a median sternotomy, followed by systemic heparinization and aortic and atrial cannulation, as described previously. Conduit for performing the bypass is harvested simultaneously with the initial stages of accessing the heart and may include preparing one or both internal mammary arteries, saphenous vein, or radial arteries. Alternative, lesser utilized conduits include lesser saphenous vein, cephalic vein, gastroepiploic artery, inferior epigastric artery, or cadaveric vein, although the use of these conduits is usually limited by poor patency or technical difficulties with use. Recently, techniques have been developed for the endoscopic harvest of the saphenous vein, and even the radial artery, an alternative that carries obvious cosmetic and potential wound-healing benefits without apparent compromise in terms of conduit integrity. The arterial conduits are usually prepared by hydrostatic distension with a papaverine solution and the vein conduits with a heparinized saline solution. Avoidance of endothelial trauma during graft harvesting and preparation is thought to be an important principle in terms of preserving long-term graft patency.

The use of the radial artery has been popularized based on the demonstrated benefit of the IMA in comparison to saphenous vein in terms of long-term patency, with advantages perceived to exist with the use of arterial conduit in general. Risks of using the radial artery include that of hand ischemia and tissue loss, which can be minimized with careful testing of collateral flow to the hand, including Doppler testing, Allen test, or other means. The radial artery appears to be prone to a prolonged risk of spasm, and therefore lifelong use of antispasmodic agents such as calcium channel blockers has been suggested with the use of radial artery implants.

Once appropriate conduit is harvested, CPB is initiated. In older or other patients with increased neurological risk due to extensive aortic atherosclerotic disease, systemic perfusion during CPB is maintained at higher pressure, and careful attention to aortic catheter placement, including cannula placement around the arch, is performed under transesophageal or epicardial echo guidance to avoid aortic atheroembolization. In rare cases, hypothermic circulatory arrest and aortic replacement with a "no-clamp" technique may be indicated; alternatively, cannula placement in peripheral arterial branches such as the axillary artery or OPCAB techniques (see later) may be utilized to avoid atheroembolization to the cerebral circulation.

Once bypass has been initiated, the surgeon usually identifies and marks the coronary arteries selected for grafting from preoperative angiographic studies. Occasionally, vessels that are intramyocardial are more easily dissected out once the heart is arrested, and identification of these vessels is deferred to this time.

To institute cardiac arrest, the aorta is cross-clamped proximal to the aortic perfusion cannula and distal to a small cardioplegia delivery cannula placed in the proximal aorta, and approximately 10 to 15 mL/kg of a cardioplegic solution are delivered via the aortic cardioplegia catheter, sometimes with supplemental retrograde cardioplegia delivered via a coronary sinus catheter. This step is usually supplemented by topical cooling and systemic hypothermia to 28°C to 32°C. Iced saline has generally replaced the use of a slush solution to decrease the risk of phrenic nerve injury.

Once the heart is arrested, distal anastomoses are typically performed utilizing ×2.5–3.0 loupe magnification by making a linear arteriotomy approximately 6 mm long in the appropriate coronary artery. The conduit is typically anastomosed utilizing a running 7-0 polypropylene suture, although interrupted anastomoses have been advocated by some to improve graft patency. The pedicled IMA is usually the last of the grafts to be connected to avoid traumatizing this delicate anastomosis and because blood flow throughout this anastomosis will deliver warm systemic blood to the heart and wash out the cardioplegic solution (Fig. 77.12). In critical cases, a vein conduit may therefore be substituted for the IMA for this reason. Occasionally, distal CAD is so diffuse or severe that an endarterectomy is performed, in which the atherosclerotic core of the coronary is excised. Graft occlusion or vessel restenosis appears to be more common with this technique compared with standard grafting, and coronary endarterectomy is therefore not routinely performed.

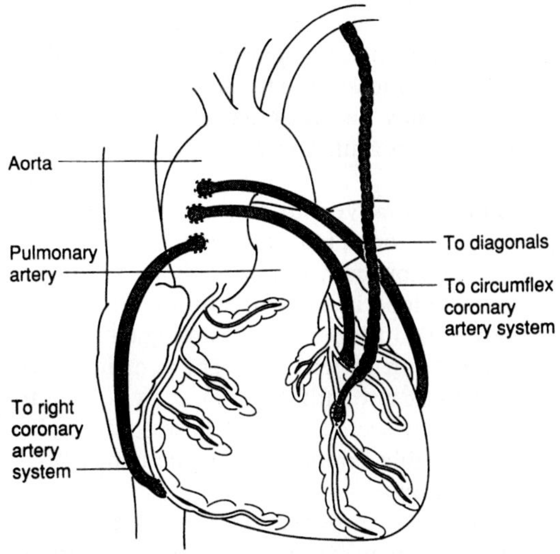

FIGURE 77.12. Depiction of typical arrangement of bypass grafts in patient undergoing coronary artery bypass surgery, including left internal mammary artery to the left anterior descending and saphenous vein grafts. (From Greenfield et al.,[155] with permission.)

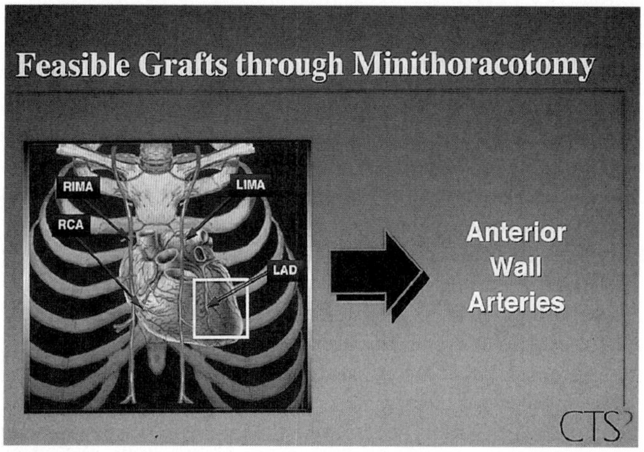

FIGURE 77.13. Depiction of typical configuration of bypasses performed by a "minimally invasive" approach. (Courtesy of CTS.)

The heart is allowed to rewarm with cross-clamp removal once the distal anastomoses are completed. In the normal aorta, a side-biting clamp can be placed and 4.0- or 4.8-cm pledgets punched from the proximal aorta; the proximal ends of the conduits are anastomosed with a 6-0 polypropylene suture. In patients with extensive ascending aortic disease, or routinely in some practices, the proximal anastomoses may be performed with the aortic cross-clamp in place to avoid the potential added risk of embolization associated with placement of a side-biting clamp. Once the proximal anastomoses are completed and hemostasis verified, the patient is then weaned from CPB, heparin is reversed with protamine, and the cannulas are removed. Temporary epicardial atrial and ventricular pacing wires are placed, and the sternum is reapproximated with stainless steel wires.

Off-Pump Coronary Artery Bypass

In performing an OPCAB or "beating heart" procedure, either through a partial or complete median sternotomy or through an anterior third or fourth intercostal (MIDCAB) approach, anastomoses on the coronary arteries are performed utilizing one of several available types of stabilizing devices with occlusive coronary snares or an intracoronary shunt placed to limit blood flow into the area of the anastomosis. The LAD and diagonal coronary arteries are most easily approached with these techniques; all the coronary arteries can now be approached with the introduction of advanced-generation stabilization and cardiac retraction devices (Fig. 77.13). With the use of these stabilizing devices, patency rates have been reported to approach that of formal CABG, although a wide range of results has been reported.[55–57] It is anticipated that the future development of automatic anastomotic devices may improve the technical ease and outcomes of OPCAB.

REOPERATIONS

Compared to first-time cardiac procedures, reoperations pose a number of technical challenges, including avoiding myocardial injury when redividing the sternum and dissecting through scar tissue, provision of adequate myocardial preservation despite the presence of diffuse atherosclerotic disease, and finding appropriate target vessels in the absence of appropriate landmarks and surface features. Other issues relevant to the successful performance of reoperations include the question of regrafting angiographically intact bypasses, appropriate handling of patent IMA grafts, and selection of alternative conduits, when necessary. The use of the oscillating saw to minimize myocardial injury when dividing the sternum and the advent of retrograde cardioplegia to enhance cardioplegia delivery represent two techniques developed to address these issues. The reader is referred elsewhere for focus specifically on the technical challenges of reoperation.[59]

POSTOPERATIVE CARE

One of the primary focuses of the postoperative care of any patient undergoing open-heart surgery must be the maintenance of cardiac output sufficient to provide adequate systemic perfusion. To facilitate this care, the patient's first 12 to 24h following open-heart surgery are usually spent in an intensive care unit with a PA catheter, arterial line, and urinary bladder catheter in place to assist monitoring.

Qualitative assessment of cardiac function can be made by noting the mental status of the patient as well as the color and temperature of the patient's extremities. Urine output is often high immediately after bypass, but it is subsequently a good indicator of organ perfusion. Conversely, systemic blood pressure is often an inaccurate indicator of hemodynamic function. Blood pressure is often elevated in the postoperative period as a result of elevated levels of catecholamines and other endogenous pressor agents and may not appropriately reflect tissue perfusion. The PA thermodilution catheter allows direct quantification of cardiac index, which should be greater than 2 L/min/m^2. Effective treatment of low cardiac output can consist of volume resuscitation to increase preload, the administration of positive inotropic agents, or the use of vasodilators to decrease afterload (Fig. 77.14).

In the usual event of an uncomplicated postoperative course, patients may be extubated within 6–12h of surgery, and with "fast-track" protocols now may be extubated within a few hours of surgery.[60] Care following the first 12 to 24h usually includes pharmacological diuresis to eliminate fluid accumulation that is a by-product of CPB, aggressive pulmonary care, and progressive ambulation. Based on extensive evidence-based and epidemiologic data, most patients are discharged on β-blockers, ACE inhibitors, H_2 blockers to avoid stress gastrointestinal bleeds, digoxin (to help prevent rapid atrial arrythmias, which occur in 25%–30% of patients), and lipid-lowering agents and aspirin to enhance graft patency.[61]

Given the coagulopathy associated with CPB and the need for full systemic heparinization during CPB, excessive bleeding is a unique and critical potential complication following open-heart surgery. High-dose ε-aminocaproic acid (Amikar) and aprotinin are often utilized intraoperatively in patients at

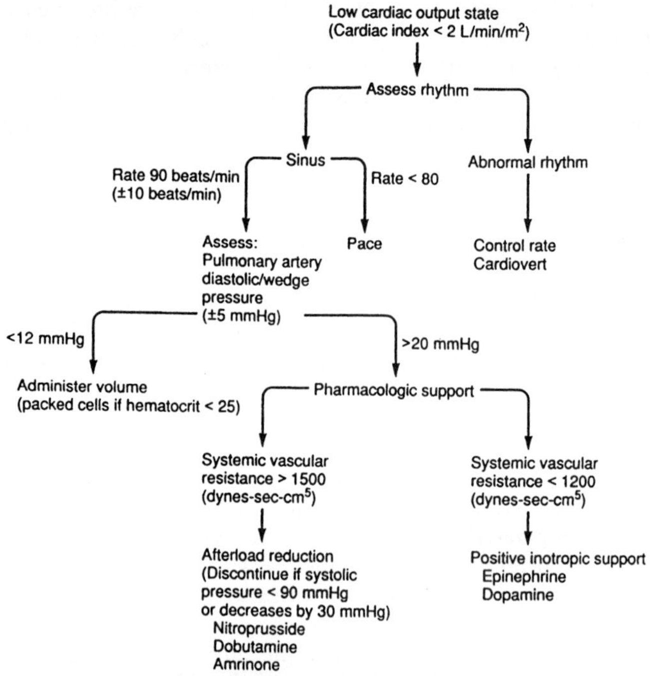

FIGURE 77.14. Algorithm for treatment of low cardiac output syndrome. All hemodynamic parameters and pharmacological agents are suggestions only. (From Greenfield et al.,[155] with permission.)

low and high risk for bleeding, respectively, to minimize the coagulopathy associated with CPB. Despite these measures, approximately 30% of patients require a blood transfusion after CABG, predictably as a function of age, lower weight, low preoperative hemoglobin, and female gender.[62]

Postoperative bleeding is assessed by chest tube output, and algorithms exist to treat with coagulation factors as appropriate. Usually, bleeding in excess of 100 mL/h after the first several hours requires transfusion of platelets, followed by fresh frozen plasma if bleeding persists. Bleeding in excess of 1000 mL in primary operations requires return to the operating room (Fig. 77.15). In the absence of significant bleeding, most surgeons utilize low-dose aspirin starting immediately postoperatively to enhance graft patency rates, and postoperative administration of clopidogrel (Plavix) has recently been advocated as a measure to further enhance graft patency. This precaution may be particularly important in OPCAB patients, in whom coagulation function is not depressed by the effects of CPB.

Elevation of central venous pressure in the setting of low cardiac output syndrome, falling systemic blood pressures, or decreased urine output may indicate cardiac tamponade from accumulation of blood in the pericardium. A central venous pressure above 20 mmHg or echocardiographic evidence of pericardial fluid with or without right ventricular compression are typical but not pathognomonic signs of tamponade, and tamponade can occur without these findings. The diagnosis of postoperative cardiac tamponade invariably requires urgent reexploration.

Occasionally, large pericardial effusions can also be associated with postcardiotomy syndrome, an inflammatory process that presents with unexplained fevers or leukocytosis, chest pain, pericardial friction rub, or diffuse ST/T wave changes. This syndrome can usually be treated with non-

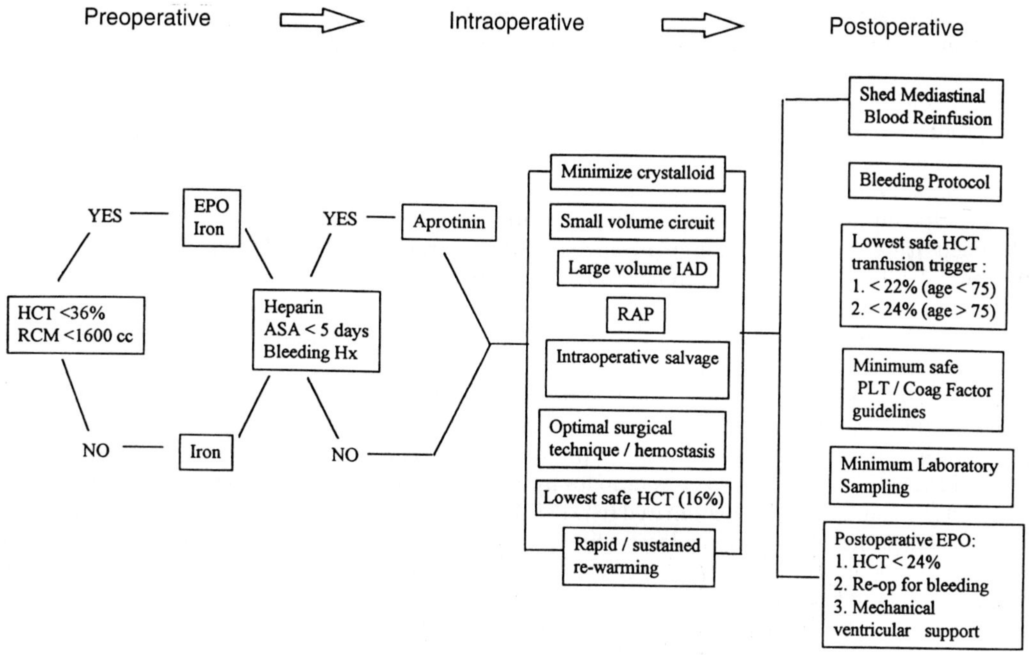

FIGURE 77.15. Algorithm for blood conservation utilizing a multimodality approach. (From Helm et al.,[158] with permission.)

steroidal antiinflammatory agents or steroids but can also necessitate pericardial drainage. Rarely, this can progress to constrictive pericarditis or even result in early graft closures.

Aside from the complications associated with CPB itself, other complications associated with CABG include sternal or leg wound infections, with IMA harvest predisposing to the former. Mediastinitis occurs in approximately 1% to 2% of patients after CABG and carries a mortality rate up to 10%–20% in the absence of other complications. Unexplained fever and leukocytosis, especially in the setting of chest pain, tenderness, or an unstable sternum, should raise the suspicion of mediastinitis. Early-use debridement and placement of a substernal antibiotic irrigation system or the use of muscle flaps based on the pectoralis major or other neighboring muscle groups are each successful in 80% to 90% of cases.

Outcomes

A number of large databases have been established and prospectively applicable computer software now exists, including the STS national database of well over 100,000 cases; these accurately allocate the risk associated with CABG as a function of a large number of patient risk parameters.[63] Analysis of these databases provides several insights into a changing risk factor profile of the patient population undergoing CABG today as opposed to earlier times. First, patients undergoing CABG are increasingly older, sicker (ejection fraction 62% in 1980 and 51% in 1990 in the STS database), and more likely to be women (17% vs. 27%, respectively).[64] They are more likely to be undergoing reoperation (1.9% vs. 9%) or undergoing urgent or emergent surgery (4% vs. 27%) today than in the past. The New England Cardiovascular Disease Study Group similarly reported an increase in age and acuity and a decrease in ejection fraction from 1987 to 1990, with a small increase in mortality during that interval (4.2% vs. 5.2%; $P < .001$).[65] In general, however, the expected operative mortality for CABG is stable or improving, presently about 2.5% to 3% (3.46% in 1994 STS database of 117,000 patients; 2.52% for 19,000 cases in comprehensive 1995 New York State [NYS] database).[66,67]

The LVEF remains one of the most significant of the many risk factors assigned a relative value in predicting the outcome of CABG.[68] The presence of CHF or shock were assigned odds ratios of 2.6 and 7.8, respectively, in the 1995 NYS database and were among the leading predictors of operative mortality in this multivariate logistic regression analysis. Nevertheless, several recent analyses in patients with ejection fractions less than 20% to 30% have showed excellent outcomes in terms of operative mortality and long-term outcomes. One study of 83 consecutive patients with a mean ejection fraction of 24% demonstrated a 36% ($P < .001$) increase in ejection fraction postoperatively.[69] In another study of 74 consecutive patients with similarly depressed mean preoperative ejection fraction, survival at 1 year was 96%, and it was 84% at 7 years, only somewhat less than in patients with greater preoperative ejection fractions.[70] Postoperatively, angina class in this study improved from 2.0 to 1.4 ($P < .0001$), and heart failure class improved from 2.7 to 1.8 ($P < .0001$). One important conclusion of these studies, however, is that patients with extensive areas of salvageable, hibernating tissues, detectable by 24-h rest thallium studies or dobutamine echocardiography, are the most appropriate candidates for CABG in the setting of poor ventricular function.

Other predictors of acute post-CABG mortality include acuity of operations, female gender, the presence of renal failure or previous neurological events, or the need to perform additional procedures such as mitral valve replacement. The presence of female gender as a risk factor may be attributable to physioanatomical considerations, such as smaller coronary vessels or the occurrence of delayed diagnosis and more advanced disease in women as compared with men. Diabetes is not generally associated with increased mortality but is associated with increased infection rates and, in the presence of other risk factors such as female gender and obesity, may represent a contraindication to mammary harvest in this setting.

Reoperation is an important predictor of operative mortality, probably both because of the increased incidence of incomplete revascularization in these cases, itself a short- and long-term survival risk factor, and because of attendant risk factors, including acuity of operation, ejection fraction, advanced patient age, and more advanced atherosclerotic disease.[13,59,71] The risk of inadvertent embolization from diseased grafts and the risk of myocardial injury during dissection through scar tissue are perceived but unproven risks in the reoperative setting as well.

One of the most important predictors of *decreased* early (and late) mortality following CABG, across all major patient and disease groups, is the use of the left internal mammary artery (LIMA).[72–74] The adjusted odds ratio for in-hospital mortality with the use of a LIMA compared to no LIMA is as great as 0.40. Based on these data, at least some have advocated even greater incremental benefits to the use of bilateral, compared to single, IMA bypasses.[75,76]

Although still a highly controversial claim, off-pump surgery may also afford decreased operative mortality compared to conventional CABG, especially in high-risk individuals (e.g., those with neurologic, pulmonary, renal, or hepatic/coagulation system comorbidities or those with diffusely diseased aortas). Puskas et al. randomized 200 patients to OPCAB or conventional CABG and showed that OPCAB achieved similar completeness of revascularization, similar in-hospital and 30-day outcomes, shorter length of stay, reduced transfusion requirement, and less myocardial injury when compared to conventional CABG.[77] Similar results have been obtained in other randomized studies, including those with high-risk patients for whom OPCAB was associated with significantly reduced morbidity and mortality compared to CABG.[78,79] The patency of grafts other than those involving the IMA to the LAD nevertheless still remains uncertain, may be at least 10% lower than that obtained with on-pump procedures,[56] and thus represents a persistent potential limitation of the OPCAB technique.

LONG-TERM OUTCOME

The main benefits of CABG in appropriately selected cases include the relief of angina refractory to medical therapy and increased event-free survival compared to PCI (Table 77.7). It should be noted that although patients with the most severe angina receive the greatest benefit in terms of symptomatic relief and improvement in quality of life, the degree of preoperative angina is generally unrelated to survival benefits. Patients with silent ischemia, for example, can be expected to have survival benefits similar to those with symptoms.

Most CABG trials have demonstrated short-term angina relief in greater than 90% of patients. In contrast, because of graft attrition and progression of native vessel disease, only 50% of patients receiving saphenous vein grafts alone are ischemia-free at 10 years, and only 15% are symptom-free at

TABLE 77.7.
Outcomes of CABG Versus PCI.

			Early outcome (%)			*Late Outcome (%)*						
Trial	*CAD*	*N*	*Death: CABG/ PCI*	*QW-MI: CABG/ PCI*	*Hosp CABG*	*Death CABG/ PCI*	*QW-MI[b] CABG/ PCI*	*Angina*	*RR (%) total/ PCI/CABG CABG PCI*	*Primary end point*	*Primary end point (%) CABG/PCI*	*Follow-up (yr)*
BARI	MV	1829	1.3/1.1	4.6/2.1	na/6.3	15.6/19.1	19.6/21.3	na/na	8/7/1 54/34/31	D	15.6/19.1	8
EAST	MV	392	1.0/1.0	10.3/3.0[a]	na/10.1	17/21	19.6/16.6	12./20[a]	13/13/1 54/41/22	D + MI + T	27.3/28.8	8
GABI	MV	352	2.5/1.1	8/2.3[a]	na/8.5	6.5/2.6	9.4/4.5	26./29	44/27/21	A	26/29	1
Tolouse	MV	152	1.3/1.3	6.6/3.9	na/3.9	10.5/13.2	1.3/5.3	5.3/21.1[a]	9/9/0. 29/15/15	A	5.2/21.1[a]	5
RITA	SV + MV	1011	1.2/0.8	2.4/3.5	na/4.5	3.6/3.1	5.2/6.7	21.5/31.3[a]	4./3/1 31/18/19	D + MI	8.6/9.8	2.5
ERACI	MV	127	4.6/1.5	6.2/6.3	na/1.5	4.7/9.5	7.8/7.8	3.2/4.8	.6/6/3 37/14/22	D + MI + A + RR	23/53[a]	3
MASS	SV(LAD)	142	1.4/1.4	1.4/0	na/11	na/na	na/na	2./18	0/0/0 22/29/14	D + MI + RR	3./24	3
Lausanne	SV(LAD)	134	0/0	0/0	na/2.9	1.5/0	1.5/2.9	5/6.	3/3/0. 25/12/13	D + MI + RR	7.6/36.8	2
CABRI	MV	1054	1.3/1.3	na/na	na/na	2.7/3.9	3.5/4.9	10.1/13.9[a]	9/6/11. 36/21/18	D	2.7/3.9	1

A, angina; D, death; MI, myocardial infarction; RR, repeat revascularization, T, thallium defect.

[a] $p < 0.05$

[b] Q-wave myocardial infarction.

Source: From Eagle et al.,[61] with permission.

15 years.[80] Saphenous vein occlusion rates are 10% to 15% during the first postoperative year, most often the result of technical error, poor runoff, and poor quality of the conduit.[81] Graft attrition rate is then 2% annually for the next 5 years and then doubles to 5% after that because of the development of graft atherosclerotic disease.

The IMA graft has become the conduit of choice because, unlike saphenous vein grafts, the IMA exhibits outstanding short- and long-term patency. Currently used in close to 100% of CABG procedures, LIMA early patency is almost 99% (compared to 94% patency for right IMA anastomoses to major branches of the CX artery).[82,83] Long-term patency of LIMA to an LAD bypass is 95% at 1 year, 94% at 8 years, and 85% at 10 years, and at least 70% of patients receiving a LIMA can be expected to be symptom-free at 10 years.[73,84] Use of IMA has furthermore been shown to significantly decrease the incidence of reoperation, increase the median interval to reoperation from 8 to 12 years, and improve event-free survival. It is therefore anticipated that the long-term benefits of CABG will improve with the greater use in the past decade of the IMA and other arterial conduits in the years to come.

In contrast to the excellent long-term patency and improvements in event-free survival conferred by LIMA bypass to the LAD, evidence of similar benefits with right IMA bypass has been less obvious, although long-term right IMA patency is almost certainly better than that for saphenous vein graft bypasses.[85] A meta-analysis evaluating over 15,000 patients from nine well-designed cohort studies demonstrated increased patient survival with bilateral grafts,[86] but a multivariate analysis prospective study demonstrated that no change in survival, event-free survival, or intervention-free survival was conferred by bilateral IMA use compared with use of unilateral IMA, although the incidence of sternal wound complications was increased (4.8% vs. 1.2%; $P < .02$).[87]

Given the demonstrated benefits of arterial compared to venous bypass conduits, cardiac surgeons have attempted to utilize a variety of different arterial conduits, the most prevalent of these being radial artery. Patency in radial arteries in 141 patients (of 327 study patients) undergoing follow-up angiography demonstrated 92% patency up to 1 year,[88] although more recent data suggest that long-term patency will fall somewhere midway between IMA and vein graft outcomes. Advocates of "total arterial" bypass nevertheless note the lower rates of recurrent angina (2% vs. 13% at 1 year) reported for such procedures compared to standard CABG.[89]

As an alternative to resorting to all-arterial conduit, it finally should also be noted that a number of efforts are underway to inhibit vein graft intimal hyperplasia and improve long-term patency utilizing biopharmacologic strategies. Pretreating vein grafts with rapamycin or paclitaxel or targeting the grafts with ex vivo "gene transfer" or antisense DNA represent some of the most promising of these strategies.[90,91]

Aside from angina relief, enhancement of long-term survival is the primary outcome benefit documented to be conferred by CABG compared to medical therapy in appropriately selected patients (or compared to PCI in diabetics with triple-vessel disease) (Table 77.7). Consistent with the findings of the original VA and European CABG studies, long-term survival following CABG in the CASS study was approximately 25% better (86% vs. 67% at 8 years) than medical therapy in patients with appropriate indications (decreased ejection fraction and triple-vessel disease), but those differences dissipated at longer follow-up, probably because of the attrition of saphenous grafts.

A meta-analysis of 1324 CABG and 1325 medical therapy patients enrolled in seven randomized trials from 1972 to 1984 (including the VA, CASS, and European studies) demonstrated a 41% crossover to CABG at 10 years and lower mortality in the CABG versus medical therapy groups, which was greatest at 5 years but persistent up to 10 years (26.4% vs. 30.5%; $P = .03$).[92] In general, the greatest extension of survival for CABG versus medical therapy was found in patients with the most severe disease, including patients with left main and triple-vessel disease, abnormal LV function, and an abnormal exercise test.

The survival rate for primary CABG patients has more recently been reported to be 90% at 5 years, 80% at 10 years, and 60% at 15 years. In contrast, a recent study of long-term survival of medically treated patients from the CASS study revealed a 12-year survival of only 40% in the presence of triple-vessel disease.[93] Twelve-year survival in this study in patients with at least one-vessel disease and ejection fractions in the range of 35% to 49% was 54% but was only 21% if the ejection fraction was less than 35%. On the other hand, IMA graft utilization has been shown to increase 10-year survival to 90%.

Nonbypass Revascularization

Apart from traditional means of revascularizing the myocardium via direct coronary artery grafting beyond major epicardial obstructions, recent techniques providing "biological revascularization" are under investigation. The first of these techniques, transmyocardial laser revascularization (TMR), which was approved by the Food and Drug Administration in 1998, is thought to provide oxygenated blood from the LV to the ischemic myocardium through formation of transmural channels in subendocardium lased in the area of ischemia (Fig. 77.16).[94] Although it remains controversial whether TMR relieves angina by inducing new blood vessel formation,

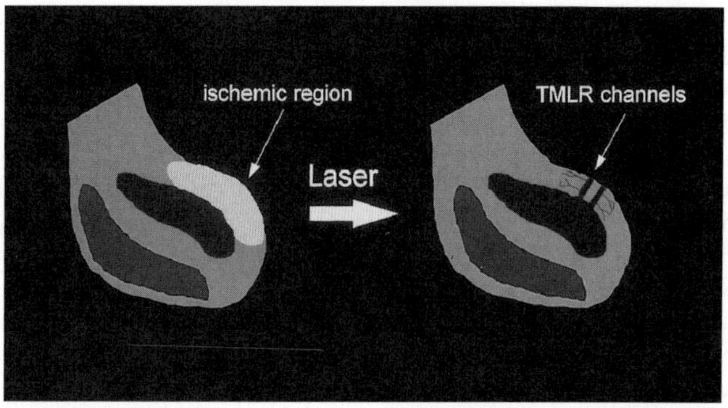

FIGURE 77.16. Schematic of conceptual basis of transmyocardial laser revascularization (TMR) with transmural channels or laser-induced neovasculature contributing to perfusion of ischemic territory.

angiogenesis, or merely creating a denervating injury that masks angina pain, it is notable that the symptomatic improvement seen following TMR has thus far seemed to exceed objective evidence of improved perfusion. Nevertheless, TMR utilizing either of the two approved lasers (CO_2 or holmium:YAG) has been repeatedly demonstrated to relieve angina, although it does not appear to reduce acute or long-term mortality.[95–97]

As an alternative to TMR, a number of investigators are attempting to enhance collateral development by instilling one of several known growth factors, or angiogens, that have been demonstrated to induce angiogenesis.[98–100] Delivery of either the growth factor protein itself or the gene coding for the angiogenic protein (gene therapy) have demonstrated efficacy, especially in terms of improvement of angina and especially when administered via an intramyocardial, as opposed to an intracoronary, approach.

Surgical Treatment of Complications of Coronary Artery Disease

Mechanical complications of MI include free-wall rupture of the ventricle, papillary muscle rupture, VSD, formation of ventricular aneurysm, and mitral valvular regurgitation caused by postinfarction conformational changes in the mitral apparatus. These changes may each occur in the acute period following MI or develop in the chronic remodeling phase of infarct healing. Surgical intervention is usually indicated when clinical manifestations such as tamponade, CHF, or arrhythmias present and lead to further diagnostic evaluation.

Free-Wall Rupture of the Left Ventricle

The free-wall rupture of the LV complication of MI, first described by William Harvey in 1647, is usually a fatal event unless pericardial and fibrous adhesions act to delay tamponade. Ventricular rupture results from transmural infarction and may be preceded by infarct expansion. A contained leak may continue to fill a fibrous sac and thereby form a pseudoaneurysm. The pseudoaneurysms are more likely to be posterior and may present with congestive failure, angina, arrhythmia, or moderate-to-severe MR. Diagnosis may be made by echocardiography showing free intrapericardial fluid. Color flow imaging may show a pseudoaneurysm filling through a small neck that bridges the ventricular cavity and fibrous sac.

Surgical treatment of free rupture involves immediate operation on diagnosis. Methods to repair include infarctectomy and buttressed repair with felt strips or placement of a patch that is then glued to the infarcted area.[101] For pseudoaneurysm repair, patch closure is often performed; however, a chronic pseudoaneurysm may be primarily closed if the neck is fibrotic. Most series of either repair of acute free-wall rupture or repair of pseudoaneurysms have few patients, but patients who have isolated repair of pseudoaneurysms have a low operative mortality (Table 77.8).

Ventricular Aneurysms

The first description of an LV aneurysm was by John Hunter in 1757. In 1931, Sauerbruch resected the sac and ligated the neck of a right ventricular aneurysm that was encountered during exploration for a suspected mediastinal mass. Beck performed an operation to reinforce a ventricular aneurysm using fascia lata in 1944. The first closed resection of an LV aneurysm was performed by Likoff and Bailey in 1955 by application of a clamp to the base of the aneurysm followed by suture and resection. In 1958, Cooley performed the first open resection of an LV aneurysm under CPB. Cooley's technique of linear closure of the aneurysm continues to be a popular method for repair of aneurysms today; however, recently he and several others have developed newer techniques that aim to maintain ventricular geometry following reconstruction.

Ventricular aneurysms are most often the result of transmural MIs, although trauma or congenital cardiac defects may also result in formation of aneurysms. True aneurysms are composed of a wall of thinned myocardial scar with direct communication with the ventricular cavity and a border zone attached to viable myocardial muscle. Ventricular pseudoaneurysms are structures composed of adhesions and pericardium that become contained and develop after acute localized rupture of myocardium from acute infarction, trauma, congenital defect, or endocarditis. The pseudoaneurysm usually has a small neck where it communicates with the ventricular cavity.

The majority of ventricular aneurysms are caused by transmural MI in the distribution of the LAD coronary artery. They appear pathologically as a convex bulging contour of fibrous tissue devoid of functional myocardial cells. Following transmural infarction, there is infarct expansion and replacement of necrotic tissue by fibrous scar. This region is initially akinetic (no contractile wall motion) and with further thinning of the wall and intraventricular pressure loading (Laplace's law) becomes dyskinetic (paradoxical bulging during systole) and may continue to expand. The aneurysm is typically adherent to pericardium and is best identified by contrast ventriculography, which demonstrates dyskinetic or akinetic segments of myocardium. Thrombus may form within the aneurysm, with risk of embolization. The rim and scar may also develop calcification, which may be evident on the ventriculogram or chest radiograph. Intraoperative identification of surgically significant aneurysms is performed by initiation of CPB and total decompression with active venting of the LV followed by inspection of the external surface of the heart for regions totally collapsed because of their lack of structural support by viable trabeculae.

Indications for operation on ventricular aneurysms include mere presence of pseudoaneurysm (because of the high risk of free rupture), symptoms of CHF (dyspnea) because of the loss of effective stroke volume within the aneurysm, angina, ventricular arrhythmias from foci at the border of viable and scarred myocardium, and embolization. Large aneurysms, even if asymptomatic, or those noted intraoperatively at planned cardiac procedures for revascularization should also be repaired.

The repair of ventricular aneurysms is usually through a median sternotomy incision. Strict avoidance of manipulation of the aneurysm (particularly when adherent to pericardium) is maintained as there is risk of dislodging thrombus on the inner surface of the aneurysm. Cardiopulmonary bypass is initiated, and aneurysm borders are identified by the collapsed segment of ventricular wall. Some surgeons prefer LV venting and repair of the aneurysm in the beating heart,

TABLE 77.8.
Selected Series of Surgical Repair of Free Wall Rupture of LV, LV Pseudoaneurysm, and LV Aneurysm.

Author	*No. of patients*	*Mortality (%)*	*Level of evidence*[a]	*Comments*
Free wall rupture of LV				
Lopez-Sendon[159]	33	24	II	Hypotension, tamponade and 0.5 mm pericardial effusion occurred in 70% of patients with rupture.
Schwarz[160]	5	0	III	Two patients in series presented acutely. Three patients had coronary revascularization.
Purcaro[160a]	24	33	II	Diagnosis was usually made by demonstration of hemopericardium and tamponade.
Left ventricular pseudoaneurysm				
Komeda[161]	12	25	III	Deaths occurred in those patients who required mitral valve replacement.
Csapo[162]	5	50	III	Average of 37 days from occurrence of infarction to diagnosis of pseudoaneurysm.
Frances[163]	193	23	III	Data extracted from literature review of articles between 1966 and 1997.
Yeo[164]	42	7	III	Among patients with myocardial infarction as cause of pseudoaneurysm, mortality was 13%.
Ventricular aneurysm				
Cosgrove[165]	1183	5.3	III	Incidence of aneurysm resection shown to be decreasing, and operative risk has maintained fairly constant despite more extensive operations in modern era.
Komeda[166]	336	6.8	III	In patients with poor left ventricular function, the operative mortality was reduced from 12.5% to 6.5% when newer techniques were employed.
Mickleborough[167]	92	3	III	Linear closure method used. Arrhythmia ablation performed in 88% of patients. Objective evidence of clinical improvement shown. Five-year survival was 80%.
Dor[104]	715	7	III	Endoventricular patch method used for repair. Mortality between 15% and 20% when refractory heart failure, VSD, refractory ventricular tachycardia, or emergency procedure.
Cooley[168]	280	11	III	In patients without previous myocardial infarction or cardiac surgery, mortality was 4.7%. Intracavitary repair technique used in all patients.

[a]I, prospective randomized study; II, prospective nonrandomized or case-controlled retrospective study; III, retrospective study.

followed by application of aortic cross-clamping with delivery of cardioplegic solution and subsequent coronary revascularization. Linear resection and closure methods involve aneurysmectomy, removal of embolic material, and repair of the ventriculotomy with layers of felt strips that buttress the free wall of the ventricle. This technique is used most often for small apical, anterior, or posterior aneurysms (Fig. 77.18). For posterior aneurysms, care must be taken to avoid injury to chordal and papillary structures on incision or during repair of the aneurysm. Distortion of these structures may also result in valvular insufficiency.

Methods have also been developed to maintain postrepair ventricular geometry (including septal integrity) by patch and suture remodeling of the ventricular cavity (Fig. 77.17).[102–104] The Jatene repair involves circular reduction of the aneurysmal defect at the endocardial level. The techniques of Cooley and Dor use an endoventricular circular patch repair. These repair methods may incorporate septal or chordal structures to preserve contractile function of remaining myocardium. Several retrospective studies comparing linear repair with the endoaneurysmography method have suggested that the latter results in greater increases in postoperative LVEF and substantially improved long-term functional improvement.[105]

Ventricular arrhythmias are often associated with ventricular aneurysms, and these are believed to arise from border areas between viable myocardium and scar. Electrophysiological studies may confirm foci of inducible arrhythmias. Intraoperative mapping may be used to direct the region of resection or to augment aneurysm repair with cryoablation of the suspected arrhythmia foci, or these lesions may be ignored in favor of implantable defibrillator placement.

Predictors of early mortality following ventricular aneurysm repair, in the range of 3% to 8%, and poor long-term

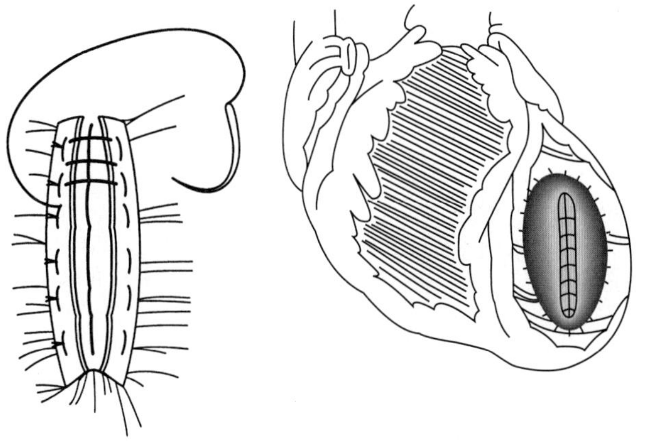

A **B**

FIGURE 77.17. **A.** Linear closure and **(B)** patch reconstruction of left ventricular cavity in the setting of left ventricular aneurysm. (From David,[101] with permission.)

outcomes include acute MI, presence of heart failure, refractory ventricular tachyarrhythmias, advanced age, emergency procedure, left main CAD, and poor ejection fraction. The degree of LV dysfunction and severity of CAD are the most important determinants of long-term outcomes. Actuarial survival after repair of LV aneurysm is 80% at 5 years. Following repair, ejection fraction and New York Heart Association (NYHA) functional class can be expected to improve significantly. In addition, ventricular arrhythmias may be reduced in as many as 90% of patients.

Postinfarction Ventricular Septal Defects

Latham first described rupture of the interventricular septum in 1845, and Cooley reported the first surgical repair of this condition (Table 77.9). Rupture occurs in the anterior portion of the ventricular septum, in the distribution of the LAD coronary artery, slightly more often than posteriorly. Clinical presentation may manifest within hours to weeks following MI. The presence of a new pansystolic murmur following MI and signs of right heart failure may herald this complication. Frank pulmonary edema and cardiogenic shock develop if uncorrected. Mitral regurgitation occurs when the VSD and necrosis involve papillary structures and mitral apparatus. The diagnosis of VSD is obtained by color flow Doppler echocardiography demonstrating a left-to-right intracardiac shunt. This method is also used to evaluate location of the defect, its size, and the degree of mitral and tricuspid valvular dysfunction. The insertion of a PA catheter may also aid in diagnosis as a step up in oxygen saturation is noted between the right atrium and PA. Coronary angiography may be performed to identify correctable ischemic areas, although the significant cardiovascular collapse often associated with postinfarction VSD may preclude this evaluation. The initial clinical management consists of pharmacological and mechanical cardiac support to reduce afterload and avoid further cardiac ischemia and end-organ failure. Intraaortic balloon counterpulsation is used to stabilize patients with VSD; however, *urgent surgical therapy is indicated* despite an initial improvement in the patient's clinical status.

Operative techniques to repair VSDs are usually aimed at resection of grossly infarcted areas surrounding the VSD, reconstruction of the septum, and establishment of the integrity of the mitral apparatus, if involved.[106–108] Appropriate coronary revascularization is also performed to limit the zone of ischemia where possible. Cardiopulmonary bypass is conducted with venting of the LV. Several techniques are used to repair the VSD. Apical septal ruptures may be corrected with amputation of the apex through the infarcted area and reapproximation of septal and ventricular walls with buttressed mattress sutures through felt strips (Fig. 77.18). Anterior septal rupture involves ventriculotomy through the infarct zone and prosthetic patch reconstruction of the interventricular septum. On completion, the ventriculotomy is closed with felt reinforcement. Posterior septal defects represent more difficult closures as they involve patch reconstructions that may require stabilization of the mitral apparatus. The method of Daggett uses infarctectomy with patch closure of the posterior VSD followed by patch reconstruction of the ventriculotomy. Cooley and David have advocated repair of anterior and posterior VSD using infarct exclusion and intracavitary repair with patch reconstruction aimed at pres-

TABLE 77.9.
Selected Series of Surgical Repair of Postinfarction Ventricular Septal Defect (VSD) and Acute Mitral Insufficiency.

Author	*No. of patients*	*Mortality (%)*	*Level of evidence*[a]	*Comments*
Postinfarction VSD				
Skillington[169]	101	20.8	III	Significant factors associated with increase in early death included inferior infarction, cardiogenic shock, and operation more than 7 days after infarction.
Muehrcke[170]	75	24	III	Coronary artery bypass increased long-term survival after VSD repair.
Cooley[107]	126	46.4	III	Mortality was 69% in emergency operations with hemodynamic instability but only 2.9% when patients were stable at operation.
David[171]	52	19	III	Infarct exclusion technique used. Survival at 8 years was 59%.
Dalrymple-Hay[172]	179	26.7	III	Increased cardiopulmonary bypass time was associated with increased mortality.
Acute mitral insufficiency				
Panos[173]	19	10.5	III	Blood cardioplegia used in all cases. All patients had either papillary muscle rupture or dysfunction.
Hendren[174]	11	9.1	III	Five patients were in cardiogenic shock, and three patients had papillary muscle reimplantation. Various repairs performed in all patients.
Horstkotte[175]	8	25	III	Dysfunction of subvalvular apparatus was usually demonstrated by transthoracic echocardiography.
David[176]	20	20	III	All patients were in cardiogenic shock. The 4 deaths occurred among 18 who underwent mitral valve replacement.

Data show subset of acute ischemic mitral regurgitation as defined by each author.

[a]I, prospective randomized study; II, prospective nonrandomized or case-controlled retrospective study; III, retrospective study.

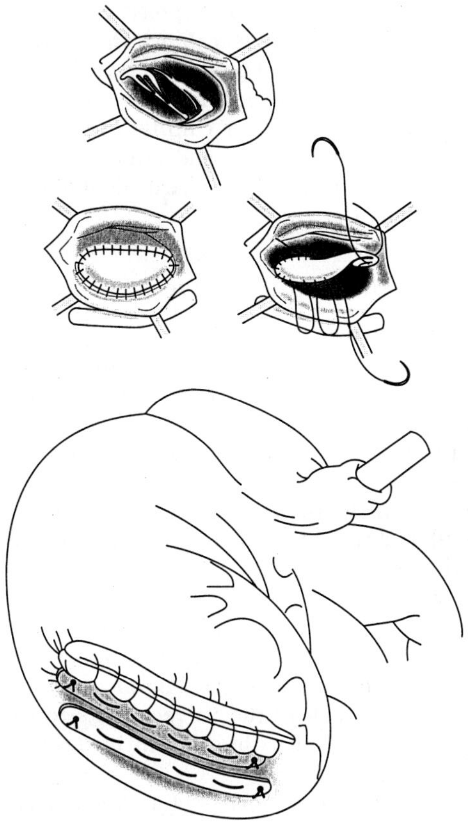

FIGURE 77.18. Repair of posterior ventricular septal defect using infarction exclusion technique. (From David,[101] with permission.)

ervation of ventricular geometry and volume. These methods are adapted in posterior VSD repair to support the mitral apparatus.

The operative mortality for postinfarction VSD ranges from 20% to 40%. The highest mortality rates observed are in patients in cardiogenic shock secondary to posterior VSD. Long-term survival is variable, with 5-year actuarial survival ranging between 40% and 80%. Patients who received coronary revascularization have been shown to have improved long-term survival. A recurrent or residual VSD may occur in 10% to 25% of patients who survive repair.

Mitral Insufficiency

Myocardial infarction may affect the mitral apparatus by several mechanisms. Papillary muscle dysfunction may be the result of localized infarction or fibrosis of the surrounding LV wall. Rupture of chordae tendinae or of the tip of the papillary muscle can lead to acute valvular insufficiency. The posteromedial papillary muscle is more often affected by ischemia, being supplied from the right or CX coronary artery distribution, while the anterolateral muscle typically has a dual blood supply from the LAD and CX coronary arteries. Ischemic MR is also induced by LV dilation that presents in the acute period following infarction. Progressive changes in the LV cavity that elongate papillary muscles and chordae or those that result in dyskinesis of the mitral annular area also result in mitral insufficiency.

Clinical presentation of ischemic mitral insufficiency may be quite variable. Sudden severe insufficiency presents as acute pulmonary edema and cardiogenic shock. Echocardiography may demonstrate ruptured papillary muscle or papillary dysfunction. Chronic mitral insufficiency, however, may present with symptoms of progressive CHF, including dyspnea and pedal edema. Postinfarction angina is often elicited, and three-vessel CAD is often present. Left atrial (LA) dilation from long-standing mitral insufficiency may result in atrial fibrillation (AF), which then amplifies clinical deterioration when cardiac output diminishes without AV synchrony.

Clinical assessment includes cardiac catheterization and echocardiography. Transesophageal echocardiography is particularly useful in defining the mitral valvular anatomy as it may guide operative efforts to repair rather than replace the abnormal valvular structures. Preoperative stabilization consists primarily of afterload reduction and efforts to limit coronary ischemia along with diuresis when pulmonary edema is evident. The IABP may be used to this effect and provides satisfactory hemodynamics with the advantage of delaying operation in the setting of acute MI. When papillary or chordal rupture is not evident by echocardiography, catheter-based reperfusion of the culprit artery is preferred for acute postinfarction MR.

Surgical indications include refractory ischemia and pulmonary edema in the acute setting. For chronic MR, the degree of regurgitation (moderate to severe) along with the associated symptoms and adequacy of ventricular function help define surgical candidates. When CAD is present, coronary artery bypass is combined with a mitral valvular procedure.

Operative approach to the mitral valve may be through either median sternotomy or right thoracotomy. The results of surgical correction of mitral valve regurgitation for ischemic pathology are dependent on the preexisting comorbidities and presentation. Well-compensated moderate-to-severe mitral insufficiency with preserved ventricular function allows elective repair of the mitral valve combined with coronary bypass with mortality under 10%. The operative mortality for patients with acute postinfarction MR and cardiogenic shock, however, is high, ranging from 20% to 90%. In a small series described by David, the actuarial survival at 5 years was approximately 74%.[109] Congestive heart failure, reduced ejection fraction, and advanced age have been associated with poor long-term prognosis following mitral valve surgery for ischemic MR (Table 77.9).

End-Stage Cardiomyopathy

Surgical approaches to end-stage heart failure are rapidly evolving. Current strategies include coronary revascularization in patients with ischemic cardiomyopathy and hibernating myocardium; reconstructive cardiac surgery, particularly the modified Dor procedure (the Batista procedure has been largely abandoned); mitral valve repair in patients with dilated cardiomyopathy; and left ventricular assist devices (LVADs) as a bridge to heart transplantation or as permanent circulatory assistance ("destination therapy"), which are considered elsewhere in this text.

The two principal factors determine the likelihood of improvement in LV function after the revascularization: the extent of myocardial viability and the degree of LV enlargement. Myocardial viability assessment is essential to determine the potential benefit of revascularization and can be done by thallium perfusion imaging, PET scanning, dobutamine echocardiography, or cardiac MRI. A meta-analysis of 24 studies involved 3088 patients with mean LVEF of 32% showed that patients with documented viability had a significant 80% reduction in annual mortality with revascularization compared to medical therapy (3.2% vs. 16%).[110] In contrast, there was no difference in outcome in patients without viability (7.7% vs. 6.2%, respectively). Left ventricular size is also an important determinant of outcome of revascularization in this group. When the LV and diastolic dimension is greater than 7 cm, operative mortality is high, and surgery should be carefully considered.[111]

Left ventricular reconstruction or volume reduction procedures were developed as potential alternatives for cardiac transplantation if revascularization is not likely to restore ventricular performance. These reconstructive procedures seek to restore normal ventricular geometry and thereby enhance ventricular mechanical efficiency. The Dor procedure (also called endoventricular circular patch plasty, EVCPP) utilizes a "purse-string" stitch around the rim of excised, nonviable scarred aneurysm to restore such geometry, covering residual defects with patches made from Dacron, pericardium, or autologous tissue. In a report of the first 661 patients undergoing the Dor procedure, the overall operative mortality was 8%, but there was dramatic improvement in the overall LVEF, the end-diastolic volume index was decreased, symptomatic heart failure status improved, and frequency of ventricular tachycardia decreased at 1-year follow-up.[112]

Valvular Heart Disease

The AV (tricuspid and mitral) and semilunar (pulmonic and aortic) valves allow antegrade flow of blood through the heart and proper functioning of this biological pump. Each valve cycles through more than 30 million cycles of opening and closing in the course of a normal lifetime, a truly amazing bioengineering feat. Given this incredible performance requirement, the occurrence of valve dysfunction is not at all surprising. When dysfunction of the native valves does develop, it may occur as stenosis, improper opening of the valve, which creates a point of fixed obstruction to the antegrade flow of blood, insufficiency, improper closure of the valve that allows upstream reflux (regurgitation) of blood, or a combination of both.

As opposed to coronary artery surgery in which the surgical procedure centers on the epicardial coronary arteries on the surface of the heart, valvular heart surgery within the cardiac chambers truly represents open-heart surgery. The use of CPB, as opposed to off-bypass techniques that can be employed for CABG, will therefore remain a prerequisite for surgical interventions directed toward treating valvular heart disease for the foreseeable future. Indeed, although such pioneers as Cutler, Souttar, Bailey, Harken, and Brok improved the life expectancy of patients with valvular heart disease with "closed" valvotomy techniques, results were usually suboptimal, especially in the setting of valvular insufficiency. It remains to be seen if today's closed percutaneous strategies will prove to be an advance over these efforts.

With the advent of CPB and after many early, unsuccessful iterations of a prosthetic valve, the introduction in 1963 of the Starr-Edwards ball-valve prosthesis ushered in the modern era of valvular surgery. Since then, many modifications and different forms of prosthetic heart valves have been developed, usually with ever-improving outcomes. Partly for these reasons, today well over 1 million valve implants have been successfully performed, and although the ideal prosthetic valve has yet to be designed, excellent long-term results are now to be expected.

Anatomy of the Cardiac Valves

The two AV valves, the right-side tricuspid valve and the left-side bicuspid or mitral valve, so named because of the number of their constituent leaflets, prevent reflux of blood from the ventricle to the atrium during ventricular systole. The tricuspid valve is offset toward the cardiac apex compared with the mitral valve, but the annuli of both are in continuity with the fibrous skeleton of the heart at its base (Fig. 77.19), and these valves are otherwise of analogous anatomical design.

Each valve is made up of a collagenous core lined by endocardium. The leaflets, or cusps, of each valve are continuous with the surrounding annulus fibrosus and meet at attachments called commissures. The chordae tendinae tether the free edges of each of the valve leaflets to the intraventricular papillary muscles, thus preventing reflux during ventricular contraction.

The tricuspid valve consists of a large anterior leaflet, a posterior leaflet at the right margin of the heart, and a smaller, septal leaflet attached to the interventricular septum (Fig. 77.20). A large anterior papillary muscle supports the anterior and posterior leaflets via its chordae, and a variable posterior papillary muscle and a prominent septal, or conus, papillary muscle may each send chordae to the posterior and septal leaflets.

The mitral valve consists of a large anterior (aortic) leaflet, which constitutes about two-thirds of the mitral valve surface area, and a smaller posterior (mural) leaflet, which circumscribes approximately two-thirds of the mitral valve annulus. The anterior and posterior mitral valve leaflets are in continuity with the posterior wall of the aorta and the posterior wall of the heart and the AV groove, respectively. Large anterior and posterior papillary muscles send chordae to each leaflet.

The two anatomically similar semilunar valves, the aortic and pulmonic, bridge the outlets of the two ventricles. *Semilunar* describes the shape of the three valvules, or cusps,

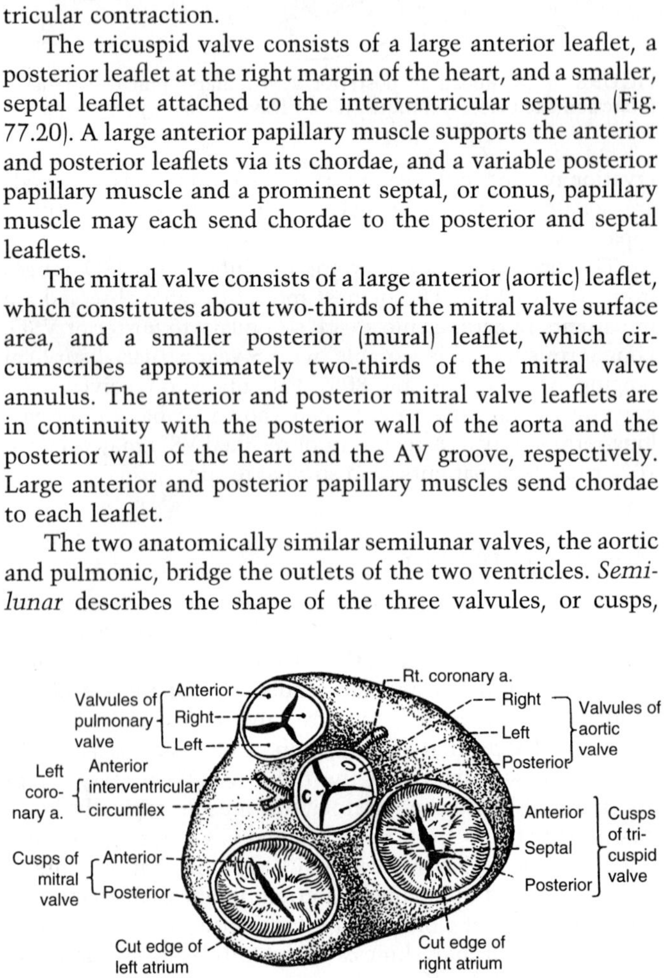

FIGURE 77.19. Anatomy of the cardiac valves, viewed as transverse section at the level of the base of the heart. (From Hollingshead,[177] with permission.)

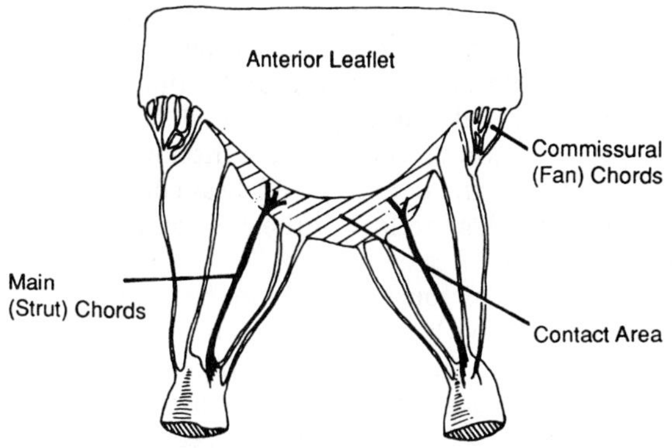

FIGURE 77.20. Schematic of the anatomical makeup of the atrioventricular valves, including the papillary muscles (*bottom*), chordae, and leaflets, as represented by the anterior leaflet of the mitral valve. (From Baue et al.,[154] with permission.)

comprising the valve overlying the valve orifice. The valvules are attached at their base to the valve annulus and are attached to each other at the commissures. As opposed to the complex AV valve apparatus, the aortic and mitral leaflets and their annuli comprise the entire valve structure. The thin, free margins of the valvulae are divided into two lunulae by a thickening at the midpoint, known as the nodulus of Arantius. The three nodules coapt with their opposite members in diastole, thereby sealing the central orifice of the valve.

The sinuses of Valsalva are convexities found in the proximal aortic and pulmonary roots that may play a role in enhancing laminar maximizing blood flow in these great vessels. The left and right coronary sinuses, found above the corresponding valve cusp, give rise to the left and right coronary arteries via ostia in the aortic sinuses, while the third, noncoronary sinus is located posteromedially. Important surgical relationships are the positions of the left and noncoronary cusps of the aortic valve, which are in continuity with the anterior mitral valve leaflet, and the right cusp, which is situated atop the interventricular septum and the conduction system (Fig. 77.21).

Pathology of Valvular Heart Disease

Rheumatic heart disease (RHD) has until recently been the most common cause of heart valve dysfunction and the most common cause of multivalvular disease, but with more pervasive medical therapy of streptococcal infections, the incidence of RHD is undergoing continual decline. Most commonly, RHD affects the mitral valve and is by far the most common cause of mitral stenosis (MS; Table 77.10). Rheumatic aortic valve disease occurs less often than mitral valve involvement but, conversely, is uncommon without mitral valve disease. Tricuspid insufficiency is not uncommon in patients with RHD, but it is almost always a functional complication of left-side disease. Only 5% of RHD patients have significant stenosis of the tricuspid valve, and pulmonic valve disease is unusual.

Rheumatic heart disease produces both stenotic and regurgitant lesions but with a predominantly stenotic hemodynamic profile. Pure MS is seen in 25% of patients with RHD, while 40% of patients exhibit both MS and insufficiency. Rheumatic valvular stenosis appears as a so-called fish-mouth fusion of the valve commissures and cusps but can also produce fusion and shortening of the chordae tendinae. Valvular regurgitation can also result from shortening, fibrosis, and fusion of the valve cusps, chordae tendinae, or papillary muscles.

Nonrheumatic etiologies now supercede RHD as the most common cause of heart valve insufficiency. Myxomatous changes, characteristically becoming clinically prominent in the third or fourth decade of life, most often affect the mitral valve, resulting in mitral valve prolapse or frank insufficiency. As such, degenerative disease was responsible for 63% of MR in patients undergoing mitral valve surgery at the Cleveland Clinic. Less commonly, myxomatous disease can cause insufficiency of the aortic or tricuspid valves.

With the aging population, an increasingly common cause of valve failure are "wear-and-tear" effects that cause valvular calcification and result in immobile leaflets that neither open nor close properly. Such degenerative disease was responsible for aortic stenosis (AS) in 48% of patients more than 70 years of age in a recent report from the Mayo Clinic, while this was the etiology of AS in only 18% of patients less than 70 years old. In younger patients, turbulence caused by preexisting valve deformities, such as a congenitally bicuspid valve, results in AS because of accelerated valve degeneration. In a Mayo Clinic series, 50% of AS in patients less than 70 years of age was secondary to a bicuspid valve. Less frequently, patients with a bicuspid aortic valve present with aortic valve insufficiency, usually at much younger ages. Other causes of AS are far less common (see Table 77.10).

Endocarditis is a somewhat less common cause of valvular failure, usually affecting valves with congenital or acquired deformity. Endocarditis is typically a left-side lesion, reflecting the normal distribution of preexisting valvular disease, but acute endocarditis is increasingly affecting normal valves, including those on the right side. As many as one-third of cases of endocarditis involve normal valves, usually as a result of infection by virulent organisms such as *Staphylococcus aureus* or in immunocompromised patients. Right-side disease is more common with intravenous drug use due to valve seeding with particulate matter from the intravenous injection. Endocarditis associated with central lines also typically involves normal right-side structures.

Endocarditic destruction of the valve or supporting structures can render the valve incompetent and is especially

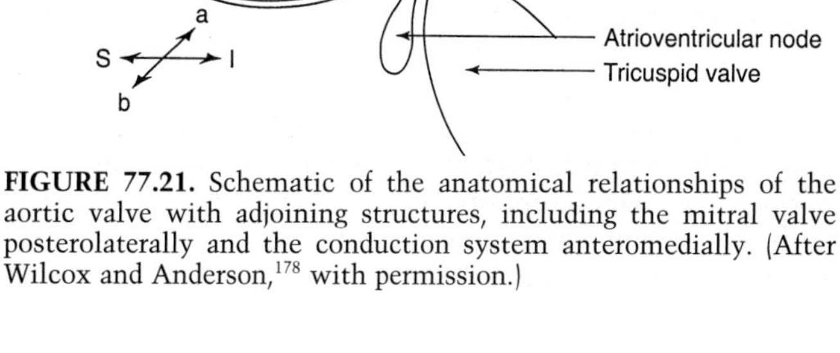

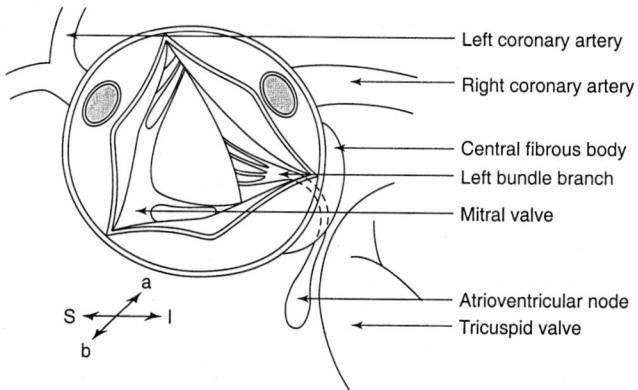

FIGURE 77.21. Schematic of the anatomical relationships of the aortic valve with adjoining structures, including the mitral valve posterolaterally and the conduction system anteromedially. (After Wilcox and Anderson,[178] with permission.)

TABLE 77.10. Prevalent Etiologies of Valvular Heart Disease.

- Mitral stenosis
  - Valvular
    - Rheumatic disease
    - Nonrheumatic disease
      - Infective endocarditis
      - Congenital mitral stenosis
      - Single papillary muscle (parachute valve)
      - Mitral annual calcification
  - Supravalvular
    - Myxoma
    - Left atrial thrombus
- Mitral insufficiency
  - Valvular
    - Rheumatic fever
    - Endocarditis
    - Systemic lupus erythematosis
    - Congenital
      - Cleft leaflet (isolated)
      - Endocardial cushion defect
    - Connective tissue disorders
  - Annular
    - Degeneration
    - Dilation
  - Subvalvular
    - Chordae tendinae
      - Endocarditis
      - Myocardial infarction
      - Connective tissue disorder
      - Rheumatic disease
    - Papillary muscle
      - Dysfunction or rupture
      - Ischemia or infarction
      - Endocarditis
      - Inflammatory disorder
- Malalignment
  - Left ventricular dilation
  - Cardiomyopathy
- Aortic stenosis[a]
  - Acquired
    - Rheumatic disease
    - Degenerative (fibrocalcific) disease
      - Tricuspid valve
      - Congenital bicuspid valve
    - Infective endocarditis
  - Congenital
    - Tricuspid valve with commissural fusion
    - Unicuspid unicommissural valve
    - Hypoplastic annulus
- Aortic insufficiency
  - Valvular
    - Rheumatic disease
    - Congenital
    - Endocarditis
    - Connective tissue disorders (Marfan's)
  - Annular
    - Connective tissue disorders (Marfan's)
    - Aortic dissection
    - Hypertension
    - Inflammatory disease (e.g., ankylosing spondylitis)

[a]Excludes subvalvular and supravalvular processes.

common with acute infections with organisms such as *S. aureus*, as opposed to less-destructive subacute processes, typically caused by *Streptococcus viridans* and other strep species. While endocarditis ranks as the leading etiology of fatal aortic insufficiency (AI) in the adult population, healed endocarditis can also lead to leaflet fibrosis, producing a stenotic lesion. Uncommonly, large vegetations can interfere with normal valvular coaptation and produce insufficiency or functional obstruction.

A number of other disease processes can also induce valvular dysfunction by affecting structures distinct from the valve itself (Table 77.9). Aortic root dilation, whether from dissection, Marfan disease, cystic medial necrosis, or other causes, prevents normal coaptation of the aortic valve leaflets and can produce acute or chronic AI. Less commonly, trauma or dissection can lead to loss of the commissural support for the valve leaflets.

The nonvalvular causes of MR are far greater than those of AI, correlating with the greater complexity of the mitral valve apparatus. For example, chordal rupture caused by endocarditis, myxomatous degeneration, rheumatic heart disease, or acute LV dilation can result in acute, severe MR and rapid cardiac decompensation. Dysfunction of the LV can also produce MR through inadequate contraction of the mitral valve annulus during systole. Papillary muscle ischemia or infarction can cause secondary papillary muscle dysfunction and malalignment of the mitral valve leaflets and MR. The posterior papillary muscle is more commonly implicated in this process, being supplied by branches of the PDA only, whereas the lateral (anterior) papillary muscle receives a dual supply from branches of the LAD and CX marginal arteries. Finally, LV dilation resulting in annulus dilation, or even segmental LV dyskinesis, can create malalignment of the papillary muscles and their respective chordae, also leading to improper leaflet coaptation and MR.

Pathophysiology and Clinical Presentation

Dramatic changes in cardiac structure and function that compensate for the volume and pressure overload stresses imposed on the heart by valvular dysfunction allow individuals with progressing valvular heart disease to persist in an asymptomatic state for many years. The mechanisms that compensate for the hemodynamic derangements associated with valvular heart disease include atrial or ventricular chamber enlargement, shifts along the pressure–function relation (Frank-Starling curve; Fig. 77.22), myocardial hypertrophy, and increased adrenergic stimulation.

More specifically, chamber enlargement allows increased diastolic filling of the ventricle, which increases myocardial sarcomere length, or preload. This change allows optimal overlap between myofilaments, which results in improved ventricular ejection as a function of ventricular filling. These hemodynamic changes are manifested as a shift along the length-active tension relation or Frank-Starling curve (see Fig. 77.23). Increased ventricular wall thickness acts to decrease wall stress according to the Laplace law, by which wall stress is inversely related to wall thickness. Parenthetically, it should be emphasized that cardiac myocytes do not replicate after the neonatal period; increases in myocardial mass and wall thickness are produced by myocyte hypertrophy rather than hyperplasia. Finally, increased adrenergic stimulation enhances myocardial contractility at any given point of ventricular filling.

Eventually, pressure and volume stresses exceed the reserves provided by the cardiac compensatory mechanisms, and CHF ensues. Heart failure may be characterized by fatigue or shortness of breath with exertion or even at rest, caused by, respectively, diminished cardiac output (forward failure) and increased LVEDP, which is transmitted back into the pulmonary circulation and results in pulmonary congestion

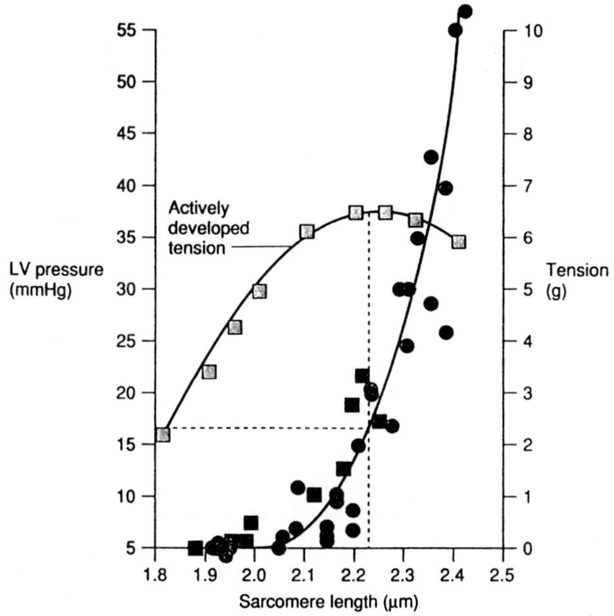

FIGURE 77.22. The Frank-Starling curve. Left ventricular contractility (pressure or tension) increases as a function of volume loading (sarcomere length) at end diastole. *Lower curve* depicts resting ventricular pressures, representing ventricular compliance relationship. (After Spotnitz et al.,[179] with permission.)

(backward failure). Although the different forms of valvular heart disease each share many pathophysiological features, including the ultimate development of CHF, each lesion also presents characteristic pathophysiology, described next.

Mitral Stenosis

Hemodynamic sequelae of MS develop only with reduction of the normal mitral valve orifice area (4–6 cm^2) to an area of 2 cm^2; this is the point at which a transvalvular pressure gradient first appears. Critical MS develops at an orifice area of 1 cm^2, at which point a transvalvular gradient of 20 mmHg is required to maintain a normal resting cardiac output. Calculating back from a low-normal LVEDP of 5 mmHg, this transvalvular gradient results in a LA pressure of 25 mmHg that, when transmitted back through the pulmonary veins to the pulmonary alveolar capillary network, is sufficiently high to cause pulmonary congestion.

The law of Poiseuille dictates that increased flow across a point of fixed resistance results in an increase in the pressure gradient that is equal to the square of the change in flow. Changes in cardiac output therefore result in a disproportionate change in transmitral gradient and LA pressure. Similarly, any increase in heart rate decreases the diastolic filling time available for flow across the stenotic valve, which results in increased flow per unit time and an increase in the transvalvular gradient. The pathophysiology of dyspnea on exertion that is characteristic of MS is related to these mechanisms.

Increased loading of the atrium caused by the pressure gradient imposed by MS eventually results in LA dilation. Atrial fibrillation eventually develops as a consequence of atrial dilation and associated fibrosis and disorganization of atrial fibers, which leads to disparate atrial conduction times and refractory periods. These abnormalities allow the development of ectopic foci and reentrant circuits that ultimately degenerate into supraventricular tachyarrhythmias and AF. In this regard, fewer than 10% of patients with LA diameters of less than 40 mm will develop AF compared with 80% of patients older than 40 years with LA diameters greater than 45 mm who will develop this arrhythmia.

The degeneration of normal sinus rhythm into AF results in a decrease of up to 30% of ventricular diastolic filling that is normally provided by atrial contraction. Atrial pressures must correspondingly increase to adequately load the ventricle, and this compensatory mechanism in turn exacerbates pulmonary congestion in the setting of preexistent increases in LA pressure. The development of AF is often complicated by the occurrence of mural thrombi and thromboembolism, half of which typically enter the cerebral circulation but can also be disseminated to the coronaries, resulting in ischemia or MI; to the kidneys, resulting in hematuria or hypertension; to the splanchnic circulation; or to the periphery. Eighty percent of patients developing thromboembolic complications are in AF, while embolism or stroke is the first symptom of MS in about 10% of cases. Rarely, a large pedunculated thrombus can obstruct the mitral valve orifice, leading to hemodynamic collapse and sudden death.

As opposed to the effects of MS on atrial function, MS does not generally cause LV compromise. When cardiac output is reduced, it is usually caused by decreased preload because of slow filling through the stenotic valve rather than depressed myocardial contractility. In long-standing MS, however, PA pressure can exceed systemic pressure. At PA pressures greater than 70 mmHg, impedance to the right heart outflow frequently results in right-side heart failure, which may be associated with right-ventricular dilation, tricuspid insufficiency, and even pulmonic insufficiency. Further decreases in left heart preload result, and a low cardiac output syndrome can develop.

Aortic Stenosis

The pathophysiological sequelae of aortic valve stenosis develop with a decrease in the normal aortic valve orifice size (2.6–3.5 cm^2) to an area of 1 cm^2. Pressure loading of the ventricle caused by valvular obstruction leads to myocardial sarcomere replication and myocardial hypertrophy. These compensatory mechanisms, which can result in hearts weighing up to 500 to 700 g, allow LV systolic pressures that are 50% to 100% greater than normal and may be as high as 300 mmHg. Adequate systolic ejection and cardiac output and normal systemic pressures are thereby maintained until late in the course of AS. Eventually, however, myocardial hypertrophy leads to significantly decreased ventricular compliance, increased LVEDP, and pulmonary congestion.

Angina pectoris develops in two-thirds of patients with severe AS, although only one-half of these patients also have significant coronary disease. Ischemia caused by AS is multifactorial in origin. First, the absolute increase in LV mass associated with AS acts to outstrip absolute coronary blood supply. Second, the significant increases in systolic ejection pressures and increased LVEDP increase myocardial work and oxygen demand, especially in the subendocardium, thereby lowering the threshold for ischemia. Finally, the prolonged systolic ejection through the stenotic valve decreases the interval available for diastolic coronary blood flow, thus further compromising myocardial perfusion.

Syncope occurs in 25% of symptomatic AS patients. Syncope is probably due to arterial hypotension and decreased cerebral perfusion caused by the presence of a flow-limiting obstruction to cardiac output that limits increases in output during periods of arterial vasodilation or venous pooling, such as with exercise or standing, respectively. Tachycardia can also lead to hypotension in the setting of AS because prolonged ejection times are required to maintain adequate flow through the stenotic valve.

Finally, heart failure develops in patients with AS once maximal LV hypertrophy is achieved. Failure develops as an adequate pressure gradient and systolic ejection across the stenotic aortic orifice can no longer be maintained, which results in a cycle of increases in LVEDP and LVEDV and increasing ventricular systolic dysfunction. Right-side heart failure follows as pulmonary hypertension causes an increase in right-side afterload. Death occurs in 10% to 20% of patients secondary to CHF. Sudden death, possibly secondary to arrhythmia, is responsible for mortality in most of the remainder of cases.

Aortic Insufficiency

As opposed to the pressure-loading strain of AS, AI produces a volume-loading strain on the LV; this is caused by the regurgitant flow returning through the aortic root. The volume-loaded ventricle empties more efficiently and completely than normal, as dictated by the principles of the Frank-Starling curve, compensating somewhat for the net loss of forward cardiac output corresponding to the regurgitant fraction. Increased diastolic loading of the ventricle eventually results in excessive LV chamber enlargement, however, which, according to the law of Laplace, results in increased LV wall tension that is proportional to the increase in LV radius. This increased wall tension represents increased ventricular afterload and translates into increased LV work and myocardial oxygen demand, but increased wall tension also produces a compensatory increase in LV wall thickness, which, also according to Laplace's law, decreases wall stress and consequently decreases myocardial oxygen demands. Maintenance of a normal LV wall thickness-to-volume ratio thus allows a normal amount of noncontractile systolic work to be performed in patients with AI, and the degree of subendocardial ischemia and angina observed with AI is generally far less than that seen in AS patients.

The compensatory mechanisms active with AI can in fact maintain adequate cardiac function through an extensive period of functional derangement. The sum effect of volume enlargement and wall thickening can result in ventricles weighing as much as 1 kg (*cor bovinum*). Increases in LV chamber size and stroke volume in individuals with severe, chronic AI can result in increases in cardiac output to 30 L/min, 20 L of which may return to the heart as regurgitant flow. In this setting, diastolic retrograde flow into the LV results in aortic root decompression and sometimes marked decreases in systemic diastolic pressures.

Compliance of the LV remains relatively high until late in the course of AI, despite the degree of ventricular hypertrophy present, and LVEDP remains low. This effect has been attributed to "slippage" of the myocardial sarcomeres, which replicate in parallel in patients with AI, unlike the sarcomere replication in series associated with AS. Ultimately, however, gradual myocardial decompensation progresses in patients with AI, often before the onset of symptoms. Limitations in cardiac output finally produce symptoms of fatigue and weakness when stroke volume plateaus with end-stage disease. At this point, any additional regurgitant flow cannot be ejected. The LVEDP rises, net forward flow decreases, and cardiac failure ensues.

In comparison with chronic AI, acute AI results in relatively small regurgitant fractions because inadequate time is available for the evolution of chamber enlargement and other compensatory mechanisms. Rapid increases in LVEDP, equalization of systemic and ventricular pressures, and severe pulmonary congestion can result from regurgitation into a small, noncompliant ventricle. Fortunately, high diastolic LV pressures often cause mitral preclosure, thereby providing partial protecting of the pulmonary circuit. Increases in LVEDP and ventricular wall tension can also produce significant myocardial ischemia, and a low cardiac output syndrome or frank cardiovascular collapse can ensue.

Mitral Regurgitation

Because LV chamber pressure exceeds LA pressure well before it reaches aortic root pressure, up to one-half of the ejected LV volume can be ejected through the incompetent mitral valve before the aortic valve has even opened. Thus, as with AI, MR results in the net forward flow of only a portion of the ejected ventricular end-diastolic volume. Diastolic reflow of the regurgitant volume from the atrium volume loads the LV and, as with AI, improves ventricular contractility, as predicted by the Frank-Starling curve. Unlike AI, systolic unloading of the LV into the low-pressure atrium allows enhanced ventricular emptying during systole. "Normal" ejection fractions and fractional shortening ratios in MR patients may thus actually reflect severe LV dysfunction.

Afterload unloading into the low-pressure atrial chamber through the mitral "pop-off" valve yields a net decrease in systolic wall tension, systolic work, and net myocardial oxygen consumption. Left ventricular hypertrophy similarly decreases wall tension, and a constant ratio of LV mass to end-diastolic volume allows maintenance of normal levels of noncontractile work, but diastolic overloading of the LV eventually causes an increase in LV radius and wall tension, as described by the law of Laplace.

With progression of this pathophysiology, dilation of the LA and ventricle causes dilation of the mitral valve orifice, which interferes with proper coaptation of the mitral valve leaflets and worsening MR. Eventually, a point of maximal systolic ejection is reached, and increasing regurgitant diastolic filling of the ventricle in the face of fixed forward ejection results in an increase in end-diastolic volumes. A cycle of deterioration in function and worsening MR eventually ensues, and pulmonary hypertension, pulmonary hypertrophy, and right ventricular dysfunction may develop as well.

Chronic MR characteristically results in a thinned, dilated, high-compliance, low-pressure LA chamber in which sinus rhythm degenerates into AF as a function of LA size. With severe or end-stage MR, the capacitance of the LA is often exceeded, and elevated atrial pressures are transmitted back into the pulmonary system, resulting in the characteristic stigma of pulmonary congestion. In contrast, acute MR is typified by a small, hypertrophied, low-compliance atrium functioning at relatively high pressure but in which sinus rhythm is maintained. Acute MR is thus characterized by the early onset of pulmonary congestion and, possibly, right heart failure because of the lack of atrial capacitance and an associated elevation in LA pressures. "Ventricularization" of the LA in the setting of acute MR is characterized by atrial pressures up to 40 to 70 mmHg. Similarly, LVEDP rises rapidly as the relatively thin-wall but noncompliant, small-capacitance LV is subjected to sudden, severe increases in diastolic filling. Myocardial work is greatly increased, and fulminant cardiac decompensation ensues.

Right-Side and Combined Valvular Dysfunction

Right-side valvular disease is similar to left-side disease in terms of the pathophysiology of these processes, except that elevated right atrial pressure results in systemic venous hypertension rather than pulmonary congestion. Right-side dysfunction may thus be manifested by ascites, jaundice, and other stigmata of cirrhosis, as well as peripheral edema or abdominal swelling.

Tricuspid regurgitation (TR), the predominant form of right-side valve pathology, is primarily caused by the right ventricular dilation secondary to left-side disease and develops in a manner analogous to similar mechanisms causing MR. Tricuspid stenosis, although rarely seen, can produce symptoms of systemic venous hypertension with a tricuspid valve gradient as small as 5 mmHg. Significant hemodynamic sequelae of pulmonary valve dysfunction are rare in the setting of acquired heart disease.

The pathophysiology of multivalvular disease may be quite complex. The downstream lesion is often responsible for producing the more proximal lesion, as, for example, with AS producing MR in the setting of LV dilation and annular enlargement. Alternatively, combined valvular dysfunction can be a part of the same disease process, as in the setting of rheumatic or degenerative valvular heart disease. Complex interactions also mark the effects of combined valvular lesions. The upstream lesion can limit the effects of the downstream. For example, significant MS may retard forward flow to an extent that blocks the development of the pathologic changes of AS or AI. Conversely, multivalvular disease can cause synergistic derangements in hemodynamics. In patients with combined AI and MR, for example, reflux of high-velocity blood flow from the aortic root all the way to the pulmonary circulation can cause severe hemodynamic disorders.

Diagnosis of Valvular Heart Disease

Despite the recent introduction of advanced diagnostic techniques, the initial assessment of patients with valvular heart disease still depends on a careful history and physical examination, which will reveal important information regarding not only the kind of valvular disease present but also the severity, duration, and prognosis of the dysfunction. Data obtained from the chest roentgenogram and 12-lead ECG; M-mode, two-dimensional (2D), and color Doppler echocardiography; the flow-directed PA catheter; and, ultimately, cardiac catheterization provide additional data.

Auscultation is a critical diagnostic tool for detecting and differentiating between the various forms of valvular dysfunction. The midsystolic murmur of AS produced by turbulent, high-velocity flow across the narrowed aortic valve is heard best at the base of the heart and usually radiates to both carotid arteries. Mitral regurgitation is characterized by a constant, blowing holosystolic murmur characteristically heard best at the apex and usually radiating to the axilla. A high-pitched, decrescendo *diastolic* murmur that is best heard in expiration at the left sternal border with the patient leaning forward is found in patients with AI. In contrast, an opening snap, accentuated S1, and a diastolic rumble with presystolic accentuation heard best at the apex is diagnostic of MS (although the auscultory findings of MS may vary widely). Finally, the pansystolic murmur of TR is localized more to the left lower sternal border and tends to increase with inspiration (Carvallo sign) compared with the other systolic murmurs.

Other cardiac and peripheral signs yield additional important diagnostic information. Pulsus parvus et tardus, a late-peaking, low pulse pressure carotid impulse, is usually a late finding of patients with critical AS and indicates severe disease. Similarly, a sustained, forceful, nondisplaced apical impulse (point of maximal impulse [PMI]) is produced by prolonged ventricular ejection through the stenotic aortic valve. High-grade AS lesions can also produce palpable vibrations known as thrills in the aortic auscultation area and a carotid shudder caused by transmission of the turbulent aortic flow. In contrast, the PMI in patients with MR is displaced laterally and is bounding. The hyperdynamic circulation and increased systemic arterial pulse pressure found with AI produce a wide variety of peripheral signs, such as Corrigan water-hammer pulse, Musset sign (head bobbing in time with heartbeat), or Quincke sign (capillary pulsations in fingertips detected with light compression). Finally, TR can be associated with a pulsatile liver, ascites, edema, right ventricular heave, and jugular venous distension with bounding v waves (C-V waves).

Objective ECG data provide further evidence of the extent of valvular heart disease by demonstration, for example, of increased QRS voltage or an LV strain pattern associated with LV hypertrophy, left-axis deviation secondary to ventricular chamber enlargement, or "p" wave changes with or without a hypertrophic pattern indicative of LA enlargement.

The routine posteroanterior and lateral chest roentgenograms may provide nonspecific information about valvular calcification, cardiac chamber enlargement, and pulmonary congestion that may help in assessing the physiological impact of valvular heart disease. Radionuclide scintography yields visual and numeric data regarding cardiac function that can be assessed serially to follow progression of disease. Of all the noninvasive studies now available, however, cardiac echocardiography has revolutionized the diagnosis of valvular heart disease. M-mode and 2D echocardiography allow real-time assessment of chamber size, wall thickness, and valve appearance and motion. Use of 2D echo with color Doppler overlay now provides physiological data at the bedside regarding blood flow across stenotic or regurgitant valves.

Specifically, quantification of mitral orifice size by 2D echo and mitral valve excursion (E-F slope) on M-mode correlate exceptionally well with catheterization data in patients with MS. Evidence of leaflet, chordae, and papillary muscle thickening or fusion, the presence of LA thrombus, as well as accurate LA sizing are additional important diagnostic data provided by echo evaluation for mitral disease. Evidence of ruptured chordae or a flail leaflet can provide an etiology for MR. Aortic valve orifice size and pathological changes such as leaflet thickening and calcification or the presence of a bicuspid valve can also usually be detected by echo. Finally, modification of the Bernoulli principle allows approximation of the pressure gradient across a stenotic valve from Doppler echo as four times the square of blood flow velocity ($P = 4v^2$). Qualitative determination of the severity of regurgitant lesions can be made with pulsed Doppler by measuring how far the high-flow regurgitant jet extends from the incompetent valve and how large is the area of the regurgitant jet.

Cardiac catheterization still remains the only methodology allowing direct and exact measurement of intracardiac pressures and valve gradients. Pressure gradients across stenotic valves are determined by pullback of the catheter from one chamber to the next or, preferably, by simultaneous pressure measurements with catheters placed in each chamber. Valve cross-sectional areas are determined by the Gorlin equations. These equations are derived from a basic hydrodynamic equation, Flow = Pressure/Resistance. A constant that is specific for each valve corrects for resistance to flow caused by blood viscosity and turbulence, predicted by the Poiseuille and Reynold equations, respectively. Because high cardiac output and mixed regurgitant disease are a source of error in these calculations, echocardiographic analyses may be superior to catheter-derived assessments of valvular lesions in these settings.

Regurgitant lesions are graded qualitatively on a scale of 1+ to 4+, based on contrast injections made upstream from the lesion in question. An aortic root injection, for example, is used to assess AI. Regurgitation of scale 1+ corresponds to a regurgitant fraction of about 20%, 21 about 20% to 40%, 3+ between 40% and 60%, and 4+ greater than 60%. Regurgitation that is 2+ or greater is considered hemodynamically significant. Because artifactual TR can be caused by the catheter crossing the tricuspid valve or by ventricular ectopic activity induced by right ventricular injections, TR is best assessed by echocardiography.

Medical Management of Valvular Heart Disease

The medical management of patients with valvular heart disease includes therapies that are specific to the relevant form of valvular dysfunction and other more general strategies that are used to treat CHF, the common end pathway of all forms of valvular heart disease. Also common to the treatment of all patients with valvular heart disease is the required avoidance of negative inotropic agents and the potential need for rate control or cardioversion by electrical or pharmacological means in the event of the onset of AF.

Congestive Heart Failure

Enhancement of cardiac function in patients with congestive failure secondary to valvular dysfunction is directed toward optimizing the three primary determinants of ventricular function: preload, afterload, and myocardial contractility (see Fig. 77.22). Increased preload, or ventricular filling, is an important compensatory mechanism in patients with ventricular failure in that increased volume loading of the ventricle in end diastole shifts ventricular contractility rightward on the Frank-Starling curve. On the other hand, this increase in preload, which is produced by a decrease in water clearance by the kidney, comes at the expense of an increase in total body water and increased total intravascular volume, which in turn may result in edema formation and pulmonary congestion. Venoconstriction caused by adrenergic stimulation and catecholamine release can also increase pulmonary congestion by causing displacement of blood into the intrathoracic vascular compartment. Furthermore, increased ventricular distension represents an unwanted increase in ventricular afterload, with consequent increases in myocardial oxygen consumption and deleterious effects on contractility. Because the ventricle is often operating on the flat portion of the Frank-Starling curve in patients with significant dysfunction, excessive elevation of preload further increases pulmonary congestion and lowers the functional capabilities without significantly improving cardiac output. Excessive preload is therefore lowered with diuretics, such as furosemide, and venodilator agents, such as nitroglycerin, and can effectively improve the symptoms of CHF as well as myocardial performance. Excessive reduction in preload, however, deprives the ventricle of filling volumes needed to maintain effective contraction and thus must be avoided, but that determination usually cannot be discerned a priori. Careful clinical and hemodynamic monitoring of the patient after implementation of therapy is thus mandatory.

Afterload reduction is directed toward lowering the resistance against which the heart must eject and is thus especially effective in patients with decreased cardiac output in the setting of increased systemic vascular resistance. Afterload reduction with vasodilator agents may also be optimally applied to enhance pressure gradients to the periphery in patients with AI or MR, although these patients may already have experienced an intrinsic decrease in vascular tone.

Afterload therapy typically produces a substantial improvement in myocardial performance in patients with LV failure, as demonstrated by an increase in ventricular fiber shortening and stroke volume, as compared with the effects seen in the normal heart. Improved LV emptying results in decreased end-systolic volumes and decreased wall tension. The decrease in systemic vascular resistance induced by vasodilator agents is typically offset by an increase in cardiac output, and blood pressure usually remains stable or decreases only slightly (although excessive use of afterload reducers can also result in significant hypotension).

Afterload reduction can be accomplished with rapidly acting intravenous or oral arterial vasodilators, such as nitroprusside and hydralazine, respectively, or the ACE inhibitors, represented by captopril and enalapril. In the same regard, vasoconstrictor agents such as norepinephrine bitartrate (Levophed) are generally contraindicated because they tend to increase afterload and exacerbate lesions such as AI.

Inotropic agents, which shift the ventricular function curve upward and to the left (see Fig. 77.22), produce more stroke work at any given level of filling and are another important class of drugs for treating heart failure. Because the failing myocardium is working on a decreased length–active tension curve, the relative augmentation of contractility is greater in the failing heart than in the normal heart.

Improvement in cardiac function allows decreased ventricular filling and creates a greater cardiac reserve because the ventricle is able to function at a lower point on the Frank-Starling curve. Decreased levels of LVEDP lead to decreased pulmonary congestion and symptomatic improvement. Increase in cardiac output can result in diuresis and decreased heart rate as sympathetic tone is diminished. A number of inotropic agents are now available that may be useful in enhancing myocardial performance; with all of these, however, a deleterious increase in myocardial oxygen consumption may be produced that must be balanced with the benefits of increased contractility.

Digitalis, the oldest agent available for inotropic effect, can cause improvement in the functional class of the patient, but there is limited evidence that administration of this agent prolongs survival or retards the long-term course of myocardial dysfunction. Dopamine is an endogenous catecholamine that stimulates myocardial contractility by direct action on myocardial β_1-receptors and by indirect release of norepinephrine from sympathetic nerve terminals. At low (1–3 mg/kg/min) doses, dopamine causes vasodilation via dopamine receptors in the coronary, renal, mesenteric, and cerebral vascular beds. Larger doses of dopamine cause vasoconstriction, probably through interaction with serotonin and b_1-receptors.

Dobutamine, a synthetic sympathetamine with b_1 and b_2 activity, usually causes less increase in heart rate and greater decreases in systemic vascular resistance in comparison with dopamine and has been the drug of choice for heart failure in the normotensive or hypertensive patient. A new class of agents, represented by amrinone and milrinone, work through the inhibition of phosphodiesterase F-III, which increases intracellular levels of cyclic adenosine monophosphate (AMP), and produce positive inotropic and vasodilator effects similar to dobutamine. Similarly, nesiritide, which mimics atrial natriuretic factor improves cardiac function as a vasodilator and has potent diuretic effects as well. Because these agents work through a cell pathway entirely separate from that of the sympathetamines, they can be particularly effective when sympathetic mechanisms have already been saturated with other compounds. The long half-life of amrinone and milrinone can, however, be a relative disadvantage to the use of these agents.

Medical Treatment of Specific Valvular Lesions

Despite the broad applicability of the medical therapy of CHF for most patients with valvular heart disease, specific considerations are important in guiding treatment of each specific form. The ventricle of patients with AS, for example, can be significantly noncompliant, leading to large changes in LVEDP with small volume changes. Incremental adjustment of the volume status of these patients may be required in utilizing vasodilator and diuretic therapy to avoid dramatic changes in LVEDP, leading either to pulmonary edema if excessively increased or to vascular collapse with inadequate ventricular filling.

For patients with MR, preload and afterload reduction with vasodilators and improvement of myocardial contractility with inotropes can actually reduce the degree of MR by decreasing the LV–LA gradient and decreasing the mitral valve orifice size. In the setting of acute, severe MR, aggressive afterload reduction with nitroprusside and balloon counterpulsation can also be effective temporizing measures before operation. Peripheral vasodilators are also the keystone to pharmacological treatment of AI, producing a pressure gradient favoring blood flow to the periphery. Importantly, AI is the only lesion for which use of the IABP is strictly contraindicated because balloon inflation during diastole severely exacerbates AI. Valve replacement is often the only effective treatment for cardiac decompensation associated with acute-onset AI.

The primary effects of MS are related to the pulmonary circulation; thus, treatment of pulmonary congestive changes with sodium restriction and diuresis is central to the medical management of MS. As mentioned, excessive dehydration and loss of atrial preload can reduce the needed pressure gradient across the mitral valve, resulting in inadequate LV filling and vascular collapse. Control of ventricular rate with digitalis or negative chronotropes such as the β- and calcium channel blockers is especially important in the medical management of the stenotic valve lesions, especially MS, because of the time dependence of adequate flow across these high-resistance points.

Maintenance of sinus rhythm appears to improve the prognosis of patients with MS, although it is unclear whether this is a reflection of the associated complications of thromboembolism or relates to the underlying status of cardiac function. Antiarrhythmic therapy may therefore be indicated for the frequent premature atrial contractions, often the harbinger of AF. Cardioversion may be indicated for AF, especially if significant hemodynamic compromise develops and if AF is of recent onset (less than 6 months) or if the atrium is less than 55 mm in diameter, in which case the AF is less likely to be recurrent after cardioversion as compared with long-standing AF in a dilated atrium. Finally, percutaneous/catheter-based, open, or even thoracoscopic ablation pathways are now also available to terminate AF, typically in conjunction with, but not as a substitute for, valve repair/replacement procedures.

In cases of right-side valvular dysfunction, correction of the primary left-side disease is of primary importance and should significantly improve the physiological effects of secondary TR. In fact, total excision of the tricuspid valve can (occasionally) be tolerated in the presence of normal right ventricular systolic pressures.

Surgical Treatment of Valvular Disease

Indications for Interventional Therapy

Interventional therapy for patients with valvular heart disease is generally indicated on demonstration of deterioration in ventricular function or development of progressing or refractory symptomatology. An inappropriate delay in definitive therapy can result in an increase in operative mortality and in diminished cardiac and functional improvement postoperatively.

The timing of surgery for AS is well defined and is based on the natural history of this disease. Mean survival after the onset of angina is about 5 years; with syncope, it is 3 years, and with heart failure, 2 years (see Fig. 77.23). Symptomatic patients with significant uncorrected AS have 25% 1-year and 50% 2-year mortality rates.[113] Half these deaths are sudden.

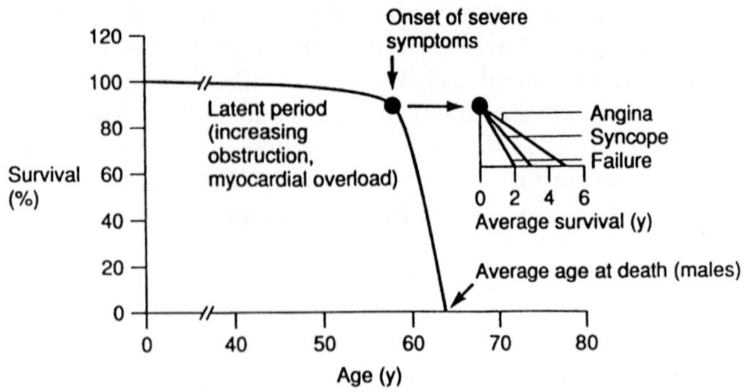

FIGURE 77.23. Life expectancy as a function of symptomatology in patients with aortic stenosis without operation. (After Ross and Braunwald,[180] with permission.)

Operation is thus usually indicated for symptomatic individuals with severe AS, or with evidence of LV systolic dysfunction (EP < 50%), among other ACC/AHA Guidelines.[114]

Intervention in individuals with MS is similarly usually indicated for symptomatic, severe mitral valve stenosis (mitral valve orifice less than 1 cm^2, mean gradient > 10 mmHg, or pulmonary artery systolic pressure > 50 mmHg). Systemic emboli, especially if recurrent, are also an indication for operation. Other mitral valve gradient. The onset of AF has also been suggested as an indication for intervention because prolonged AF seems to worsen the prognosis for patients with MS. On the other hand, early operation does not appear to improve long-term survival in asymptomatic patients. Because the progression of mitral valvular stenosis can stabilize in many individuals and little risk of irreversible myocardial dysfunction is incurred with this disease, some authors therefore advocate deferring interventions in asymptomatic patients with subcritical disease. Conversely, the 5-year survival rate for functional class III patients is only 62%, and it is only 15% for class IV patients.[115]

Symptoms may not develop until after irreversible myocardial dysfunction has occurred in patients with AI or MR, and thus the appropriate timing of intervention in these individuals is significantly more challenging than in patients with stenotic lesions. For example, mean survival after development of symptoms in IA is only 4 years if angina is present and 2 years if congestive failure is present.[116] Thus, operative intervention is most clearly indicated for essentially all symptomatic patients with AI or MR.[114]

Other proposed indications for operation for regurgitant lesions utilize noninvasive technologies such as radionuclide scanning and echo that allow serial assessments of LV function in attempting to guide intervention to the onset of LV dysfunction. For AI, these criteria include progressive LV dilation declining exercise tolerance or an end-systolic LV diameter larger than 55 mm and ejection fraction below 50%, or end-systolic dimension > 75 mmHg, even in the asymptomatic patient.[114,117] Similar criteria established for the timing of operation in MR patients include an ejection fraction less than 30% or fractional shortening less than 30% with an end-systolic diameter of 55 mm.[114]

Analogous to the indications for left-side disease, correction of tricuspid valve stenosis is recommended for a tricuspid valve gradient of at least 5 mmHg or for the rare patient with symptomatic disease. Correction of isolated TR is usually indicated only in the presence of severe, symptomatic disease with clear physical stigmata. Most often, however, TR is functional rather than secondary to primary tricuspid valve pathology and improves on correction of left-side disease. On the other hand, Duran and associates reported a 100% late persistence of uncorrected TR in the presence of significant pulmonary hypertension, compared with a 0% incidence without pulmonary hypertension.[118] Furthermore, TR remained in 47% of patients undergoing mitral valve replacement with associated organic disease of the tricuspid valve compared with no late TR in the absence of organic tricuspid disease.

Options in Interventional Therapy

Percutaneous balloon valvuloplasty is a technique in which a high-pressure balloon catheter introduced via the femoral artery is inflated across a stenotic valve to dilate the obstructing lesion. Initial and intermediate-term results have been favorable for selected cases of MS with limited valvular and subvalvular calcification and fibrosis, as determined by a standardized echocardiographic scoring system.[119] In contrast, percutaneous aortic balloon valvuloplasty suffers from a relatively high complication and recurrence rate and is only occasionally indicated as a bridging technique in critically ill patients.[120] Because results with open repair of either aortic valve stenosis or regurgitation are also generally discouraging, aortic valve replacement remains the primary option in most instances of significant aortic valve disease.

For patients with critical MS in whom balloon valvuloplasty is not indicated, open mitral commissurotomy can be successfully performed if there is limited calcification, leaflet stiffness, chordal fusion, or associated MR. Commissurotomy carries up to a 20% chance of reoperation within 5 years or a 60% chance at 10 years but avoids the potential complications of a valve prosthesis during that time.[121] Repair of MR is now successfully performed in the majority of patients in most reported series. Although excellent long-term results can be expected in appropriately selected patients with degenerative pathology, results are less satisfactory for rheumatic and ischemic etiologies, and repair in these cases must be selected cautiously. Most recently, percutaneous mitral valve techniques have been introduced under investigatory clinical protocols.

Finally, tricuspid valve annuloplasty is the preferred treatment for significant secondary TR, with valve replacement reserved for severe or primary disease. In summary, except for the specific instances just cited, correction of valvular heart disease nearly always requires replacement of the diseased valve with a valve prosthesis or heterograft.

Prosthetic Valves

The ideal prosthetic heart valve should be durable, nonthrombogenic, resistant to infection, and technically easy to insert; it should possess an optimal hemodynamic profile, and it should be subjectively acceptable to the patient. Despite the large number of valves that have been designed and introduced clinically over the past four decades, the ideal valve has not yet been developed. The two major classes of valves—the mechanical and the tissue valves (xenograft [porcine or bovine] or homograft [cadaveric human])—can be viewed as representing strengths in durability versus low thrombogenicity, respectively.

MECHANICAL VALVES

The first generation of mechanical valves, represented by the Starr-Edwards valve, were primarily of the ball-in-cage design. The next generation of mechanical valves consisted of modified versions of the tilting-disk valve, represented by the original Bjork-Shiley valve. Models of the convex–concave Bjork-Shiley valve suffered a 0.17% rate of strut fracture, sometimes associated with catastrophic valve failure, and these valves are not presently available in the United States. Recent modifications of the tilting-disk valve (e.g., the St. Jude valve) use a pivoting bileaflet mechanism made of pyrolite carbon that eliminates the need for retaining struts (Fig. 77.25). The St. Jude valve has enjoyed an excellent long-term performance record but still is subject to a complication rate of approximately 1% to 2%/year, primarily related to the risk of thromboembolism, even with the mandatory use of oral anticoagulant therapy. Although variations of the St. Jude valve have more recently been introduced, one study evaluating hemodymamic and functional outcomes after aortic valve replacement with three different bileaflet mechanical valves (ATS, Carbomedics, or St. Jude Medical) found no clinically relevant differences among these valves.[122]

HETEROGRAFT TISSUE VALVES

Bioprosthetic valves have until recently been primarily represented by the porcine heterografts, generally glutaraldehyde-fixed valves that are harvested from pigs under rigorous specifications (Fig. 77.24). Although these valves enjoy low thromboembolic rates and usually do not require concomitant anticoagulant therapy, the tissue valves are compromised by hemodynamic failure from calcific degeneration at a

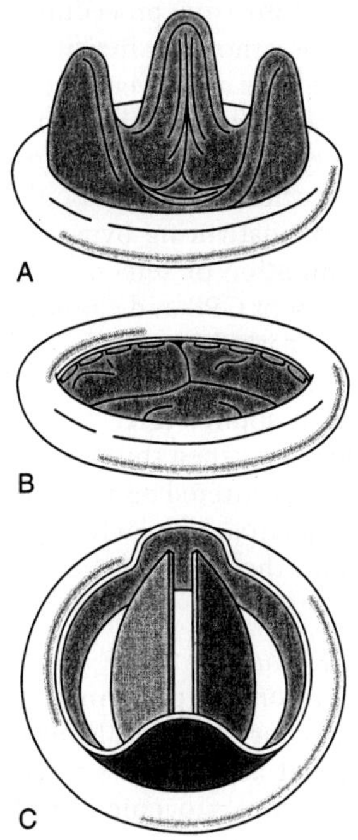

FIGURE 77.24. Representative prosthetic heart valves. **A–B.** Carpentier-Edwards porcine valve. **C.** St. Jude bileaflet mechanical valve. (From Greenfield et al.,[155] with permission.)

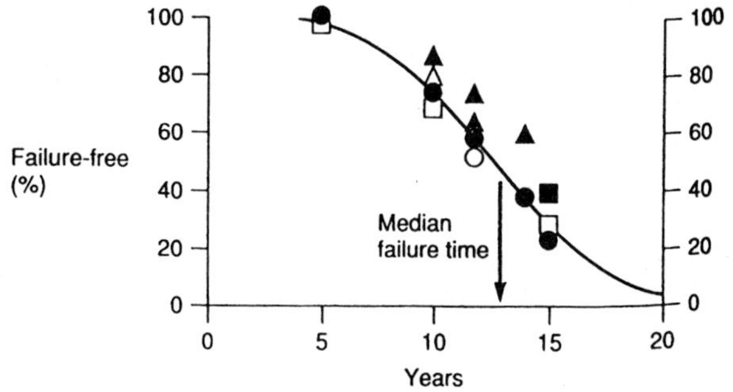

FIGURE 77.25. Failure-free rates for (porcine) tissue heterografts based on published series with more than 10 years follow-up. Median failure time is approximately 13 years. (From Starr and Grunkemeier,[181] with permission.)

median interval of 13 years postimplantation (Fig. 77.25). The specific incidence of structural degeneration for porcine valves in one recent survey was 29% at 10 years and 69% at 15 years.[123] Degeneration of the tissue valves usually involves gradual leaflet calcification and thickening, leading to stenosis or insufficiency, although catastrophic failure due to acute leaflet tears can also occur. Valves implanted in children and young adults (less than 35 years of age), patients with chronic renal failure, and those with high cardiac indices are at the greatest risk for valve failure because of the high mechanical stresses and accelerated calcium metabolism characteristic of these individuals.

The advent of improved preservation technique and advanced antimineralization strategies, including alterations in fixation pressures and use of sodium dodecyl sulfate, as well as the introduction of valves that are manufactured from bovine pericardium provide the possibility of extended durability for tissue valve implants. In this regard, 10–15 years freedom from structural deterioration with "next generation" porcine and bovine pericardial valves have been reported to exceed 90%, especially if implanted in patients older than 65 years.[124]

The new generation of pericardial valves also offers the advantage of improved hemodynamic performance, approaching or equaling that of the mechanical valves, as compared with most porcine valve models, in which design limitations imposed by native valve architecture and constraints imposed by the need for sewing rings result in reductions in effective orifice areas (EOAs) and increased valve gradients (Table 77.11). Improved hemodynamic performances are also characteristic of the recently approved stentless porcine valves. The stentless valves are, however, technically more challenging to implant than the older generation stented valves. Further, while some studies have provided evidence of enhanced regression of LV hypertrophy with stentless compared to stented valves, others have shown that the degree of regression in an LV mass is independent of prosthesis type implanted.[125]

HOMOGRAFT VALVES

Cryopreserved cadaveric human aortic valves have historically been of restricted clinical utility because of limited availability, high cost, and the greater degree of technical expertise required for implantation. The use of homografts has recently been repopularized, however, and these valves remain an important option for aortic valve replacement,

TABLE 77.11. Hemodynamic Performance of Various Valve Prostheses.

Valve	*Peak gradient*	*Effective orifice area (EOA)*
Aortic		
Mechanical		
Starr-Edwards (23 mm)	21	1.2
Bjork-Shiley (21 mm)	24	1.3
St. Jude medical (21 mm)	6	1.7
Biological		
Carpentier-Edwards porcine (21–23 mm)	16	1.5–1.7
Hancock (21 mm)	—	1.3
Carpentier-Edwards pericardial (19 mm)	32	1.08
Mitral		
Mechanical		
Starr-Edwards (27 mm)	5	1.4
Bjork-Shiley (29 mm)	5.5	1.9
St. Jude medical (29 mm)	2.5	2.8
Biological		
Carpentier-Edwards (27–29 mm)	6	2.4
Hancock (modified) (27 mm)	8	1.8

AV, atrioventricular.

Source: Modified from Jamieson.[182]

especially in the young and in patients with endocarditis. The potentially increased durability of homografts due to improved preservation techniques and the adoption of a modified surgical technique in which the homograft valve is implanted as a unit with the aortic root have contributed to this resurgence. This growing acceptance is also related to the increased performance of the Ross procedure, in which the homograft is inserted in the pulmonic position, and the native pulmonic apparatus is transplanted into the aortic position to take advantage of the potentially extended durability of this partial autograft technique. On the other hand, the technical demands of this operation translate into long cross-clamp and CPB times, as well as higher operative mortality rates compared with heterograft implants. The benefits of homograft insertion in terms of excellent hemodynamic performance, low incidences of endocarditis and thromboembolism, and the consequent ability to avoid anticoagulation are potential advantages of this technique, but long-term durability data for these implants are still limited, and recent studies call into question whether any durability advantage at all is provided by homograft compared to heterologous tissue valves.

Based on these relative advantages and disadvantages, mechanical valves are recommended for most patients less than 65 years old. Tissue valves are generally preferred if life expectancy is less than 10 to 15 years; if there is a contraindication to coumadin administration, such as the presence of a known coagulation defect, history of gastrointestinal bleeding, or similar source of potential bleeding; if there is a likelihood of exposure to potential trauma; or if pregnancy is anticipated. Most recently, however, surgeons are increasingly supporting the use of a tissue valve plus reoperation, calculating a lower overall lifetime risk than that associated with life-long anticoagulant therapy (see below). Tissue valves are also considered if there are technical considerations at the time of operation that favor tissue valve implantation, such as a friable or heavily calcified annulus. Finally, tissue valves are usually used for tricuspid valve replacement because of the risk of thrombotic complications associated with the use of mechanical valves in this position.

Operative Procedures for Valvular Disease

Preoperative Care

Careful preoperative preparation of the patient about to undergo heart valve replacement can have important consequences in terms of eventual patient morbidity and mortality. Screening for occult infectious processes such as dental abscesses is critical to prevent contamination of the valvular prosthesis and prosthetic valve endocarditis. As with any open-heart procedure, the potential for coagulopathy should be assessed because of the need for intraoperative heparinization and, specific for valve surgery, postoperative anticoagulation. Intractable or potentially recurrent gastrointestinal tract bleeding in particular will represent a contraindication to mechanical valve implantation.

As with any operative procedure, patients with significant respiratory compromise should be considered for preoperative pulmonary care, cigarette smoking should be discontinued, and attention should be directed toward improving the nutritional status of the patient. Finally, preoperative enhancement of cardiac function can significantly improve operative mortality; therefore, treatment of congestive failure in the preoperative period and upgrading of functional class should be pursued actively (see later discussion).

Surgical Technique

A median sternotomy is the standard approach to the heart for open valve surgery, whether it be for repair or replacement, allowing excellent exposure. Excellent exposure to the mitral valve can also be obtained by way of a standard or small ("mini") thoracotomy incision (aided by femoral vascular access techniques), as has been popularized by the recent interest in minimally invasive procedures. A variety of ministernotomy and parasternotomy incisions for both aortic and mitral valve surgery have also been recently reported.

The aorta is assessed for calcification by palpation and by transesophageal or epiaortic echocardiography before cannulation for CPB. Significant aortic calcification may dictate alternative means of instituting bypass, such as femoral or axillary artery cannulation or selection of other sites on the arch. After institution of CPB and cardioplegic cardiac arrest, the specific valvular pathology is approached. In the case of mitral valve disease, a longitudinal LA incision is made and appropriate retraction applied (Fig. 77.27). Alternatively, the mitral valve can be approached through the right atrium with a transseptal approach centered on the fossa ovalis or through a "superior septal" approach, in which the transseptal incision is extended onto the dome of the LA.

Mitral Valve Repair

A mitral commissurotomy is performed by incising the fused commissures to a point a few millimeters from the valve annulus, ensuring that attachments to the chordae tendinae are left intact to prevent iatrogenic mitral insufficiency (Fig. 77.26). The chordae and even the papillary muscle can similarly be divided to improve valve mobility. Shortened secondary chordae to the mural leaflet can also be divided. Curettage

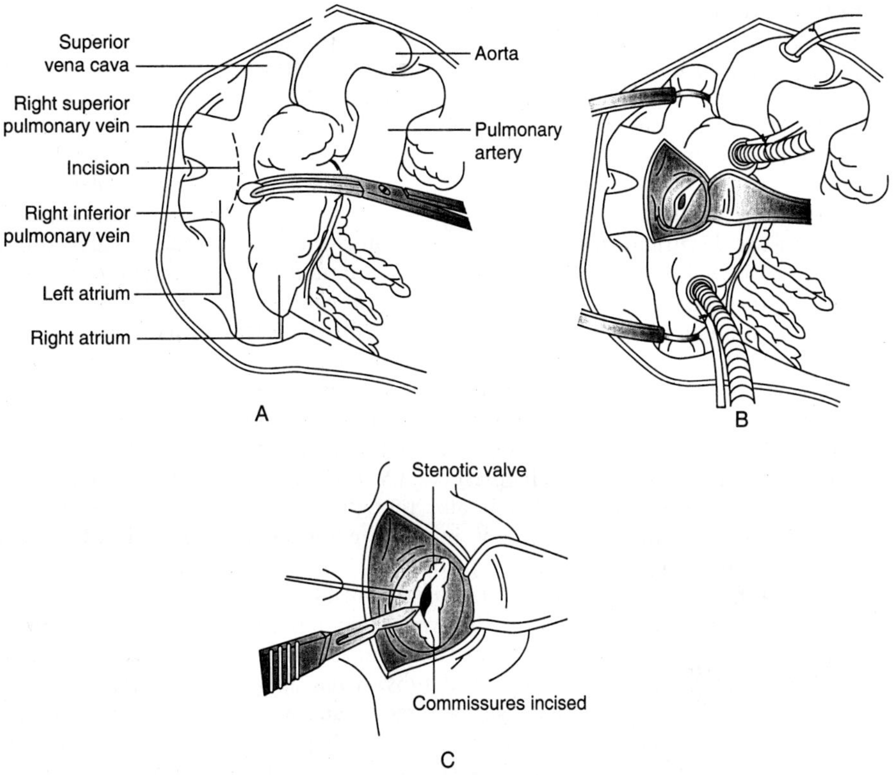

FIGURE 77.26. Mitral commissurotomy for mitral stenosis. **A, B.** Atrial exposure. **C.** Incision of fused leaflets. (From Greenfield et al.,[155] with permission.)

of excessive calcium can be undertaken with care to avoid perforating the ventricle.

Mitral reconstruction for insufficiency most commonly involves mitral annuloplasty, with plication of an enlarged annulus, usually onto a prosthetic ring.[126,127] Recent evidence has suggested that placement of an oversized annuloplasty ring can precipitate systolic anterior motion of the anterior mitral valve leaflet and LV outflow tract obstruction.[128] Placement of a flexible semi-rigid, oval (Carpentier, Duran) ring (Fig. 77.27) or (Cosgrove) semi-ring, avoiding ring placement anteriorly, is thought to alleviate this problem and allows improved LV function as can reduction of posterior leaflet "height".[129]

Mitral reconstruction can be accomplished utilizing a variety of additional techniques, as described by Carpentier and others (see Fig. 77.27). The most commonly performed of the "tailoring" repairs is quadrangular resection of an enlarged posterior (mural) leaflet. Triangular resection of the anterior leaflet, shortening of elongated chordae, transposition of mural leaflet chordae to the aortic (anterior) leaflet, and chordal replacement with polytetrafluorethylene (PTFE) sutures are the most commonly performed of a variety of other techniques. Available for anterior leaflet repair.[127–130]

Exposure of the mitral valve through a right lateral minithoracotomy using video assistance has gained in popularity. This approach allows complex mitral valve repair as well

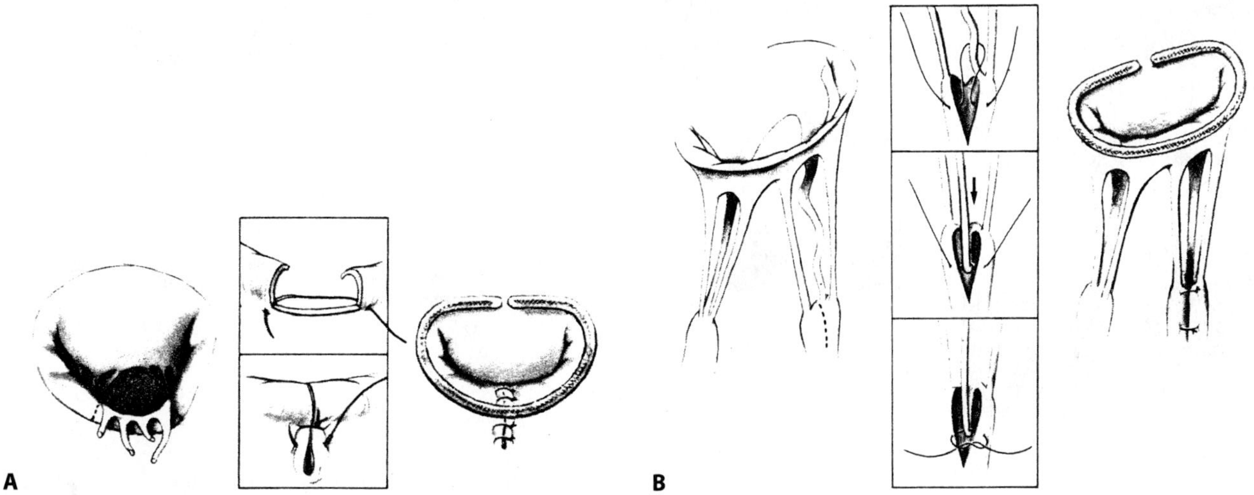

FIGURE 77.27. Mitral valve repair for mitral regurgitation. **A.** Quadrangular resection of posterior leaflet with annuloplasty ring placement. **B.** Chordal shortening via papillary muscle implantation. (From Carpentier,[126] with permission.)

as mitral valve replacement even with biological stentless prostheses with decreased morbidity. The addition of radiofrequency ablation for restoration of sinus rhythm enhances the outcome after mitral valve surgery by alleviating AF with about a 70% success rate and can also be performed through a minithoracotomy approach.

Valve Replacement

Mitral valve replacement has historically consisted of excising the diseased valve some 3 to 4 mm from the annulus and division of the chordae at their junction with the papillary muscles or through the papillary heads (Fig. 77.28). Heavily calcified valves can present difficulties in excision. Many surgeons now preserve the posterior leaflet or at least some of the chordae to the posterior annulus, especially for nonrheumatic MR, due to consideration that maintaining the internal LV architecture will help preserve LV function.[131] Preservation of the posterior leaflet is also thought to help prevent AV groove and posterior LV injuries, potentially lethal complications of mitral valve replacement. The benefits of retaining subvalvular apparatus during mitral valve replacement for chronic MR have been demonstrated in many retrospective investigations. A recent randomized study showed that complete retention of mitral subvalvular apparatus confers a significant early advantage by reducing LV chamber size and systolic afterload compared with partial chordal preservation.[132] Furthermore, LV performance continued to improve over time, probably because of more favorable LV remodeling. In this regard, some surgeons even advocate leaving nearly the entire valve in place, especially if a tissue valve is to be substituted, for which impingement on leaflet motion is less of a concern than with mechanical valve implants.

After valve removal and appropriate debridement of calcium to allow passage of sutures into relatively compliant tissue, the valve orifice is sized with a plastic sizer. While a valve size of at least 25 mm is required to allow adequate transmitral flow, oversizing can lead to outflow tract obstruction, AV groove or posterior wall rupture, or prosthetic dysfunction. Interrupted horizontal mattress sutures of nonabsorbable material, which are buttressed with small Dacron pledgets, are generally utilized to create a hemostatic anastomosis between the valve prosthesis sewing ring and the native valve annulus (see Fig. 77.28). Sutures placed too deep can injure the CX artery in the AV groove posterolaterally, the aortic leaflet mechanism anteriorly, or the AV node medially.

Aortic valve replacement is performed in a similar fashion (Fig. 77.29). After a transverse aortotomy has been made, the aortic valve is completely excised to the level of the valve annulus, making sure that calcium embolization is carefully avoided. The valve orifice is appropriately sized, and the valve prosthesis is sewn into place in a manner analogous to that described for the mitral valve. Orifices that will not accept at least a 19-mm prosthesis may require enlargement, utilizing techniques that extend posteriorly into the anterior mitral valve leaflet (Manoogian procedure) or anteriorly into the interventricular septum and right ventricle (Kono procedure). Homograft techniques, including the Ross procedure, in which a homograft is substituted for the native pulmonic valve, which is then harvested and placed in the aortic position, are considerably more complex, and are described separately.[133]

Closure after valve repair or replacement involves techniques in which the aortotomy or atriotomy incisions are oversewn. These closures are usually not completed until after the critical maneuver of de-airing, in which air is evacuated from the heart to avoid embolization often with the aid of co2 insufflation. Although various other de-airing techniques are used, most involve electrically fibrillating the

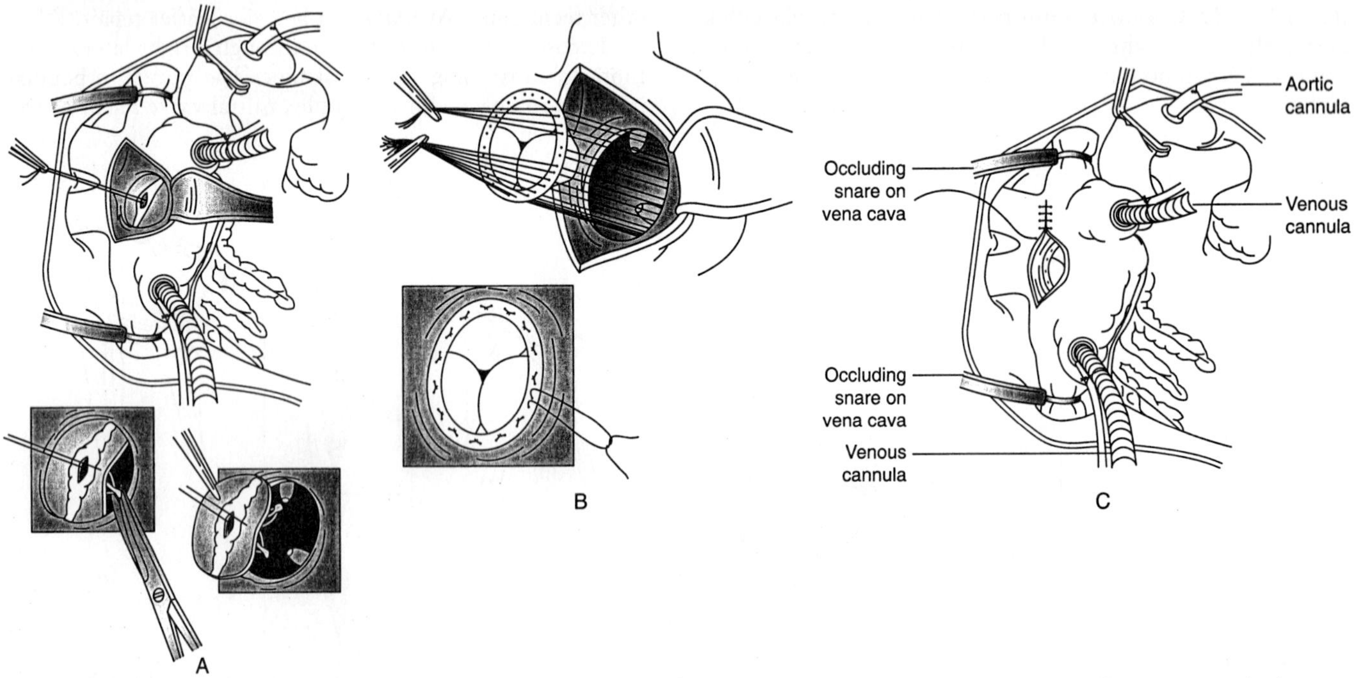

FIGURE 77.28. Mitral valve replacement. **A.** Approach and excision of the diseased valve. **B.** Annular suturing and positioning of a bioprosthetic valve. **C.** Atriotomy closure. (From Greenfield et al.,[155] with permission.)

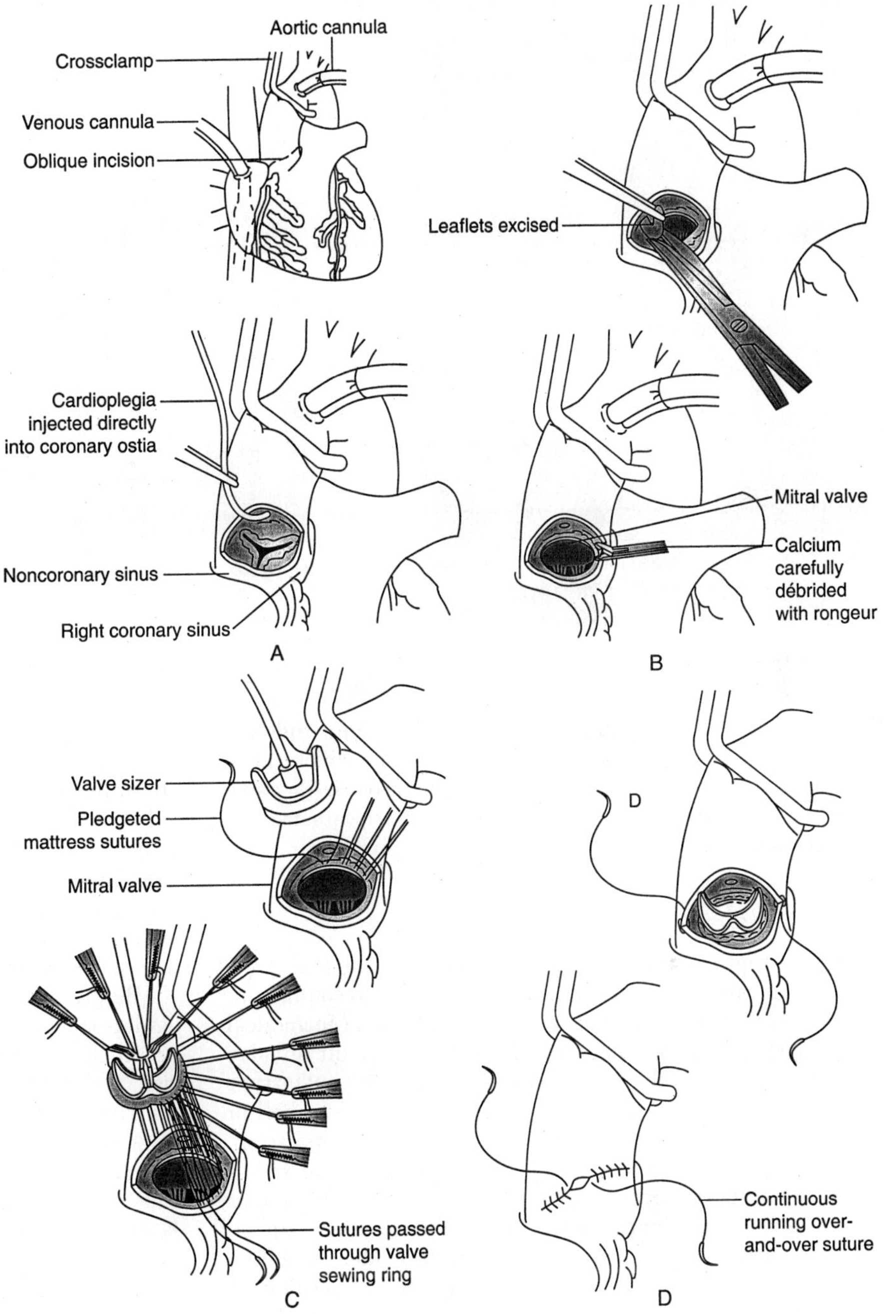

FIGURE 77.29. Aortic valve replacement. **A.** Approach to aortic valve via aorta. **B.** Valve excision. **C.** Suturing of valve prosthesis. **D.** Aortotomy closure. (From Greenfield et al.,[155] with permission.)

heart, ventilating the lungs, filling the left heart chambers by momentarily decreasing the flow through the pump, and allowing air to escape through venting sites placed in superior positions. These maneuvers are assisted by placing the patient in a steep Trendelenburg position, massaging the heart, or partially replacing the aortic cross-clamp.

Surgery is then completed as per other open-heart procedures. The patient is separated from CPB, protamine is given to neutralize the remaining heparin dose, cannulas are removed, atrial and ventricular epicardial pacing wires are placed in the event that they are needed for transient bradycardia or heart block, and appropriate chest tubes are placed.

As noted previously, there is a trend toward implementation of newer minimally invasive techniques in mitral and aortic valve surgery through small mini-thoracotomy incisions or the use of a thoracoscopic or even robotic technique (Fig. 77.30). In addition to percutaneous mitral valve repair techniques, even percutaneous aortic valve replacement is under investigational clinical study.

Postoperative Care

The postoperative course of patients after valve surgery is in many ways similar to that of any patient undergoing operation, with similar neuroendocrine responses to the stress of

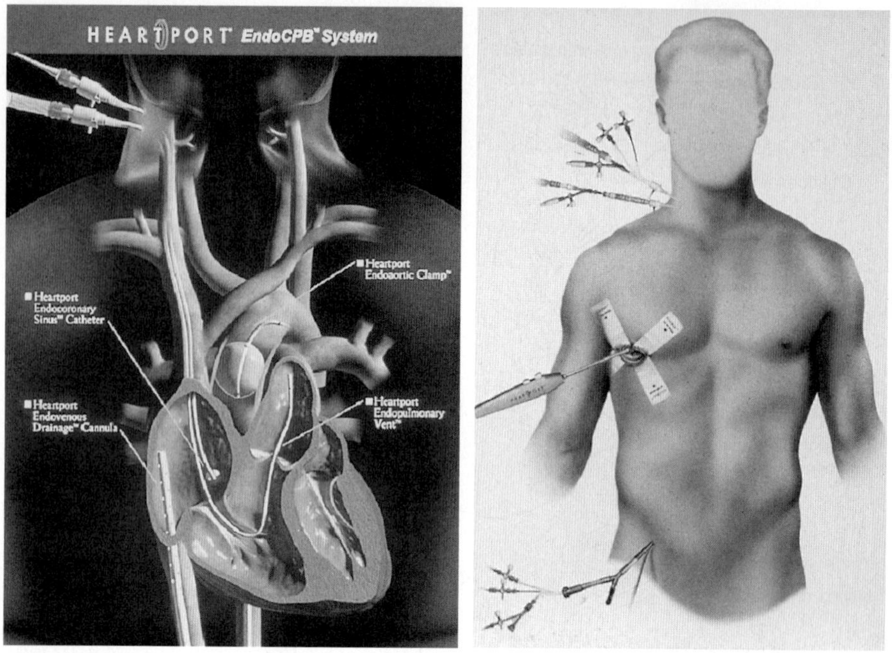

A B

FIGURE 77.30. **A.** Schematic of configuration of catheters employed in minithoracotomy technique, including coronary sinus catheter, venous drainage via femoral venous approach, pulmonary artery vent, and balloon aortic clamp (not shown is arterial cannula in femoral artery). **B.** External appearance of "mini" approach, including small anterior thoracotomy incision and vascular access via internal jugular vein, femoral artery, and femoral vein. (Courtesy of Heartport.)

surgery, and essentially identical to that for patients undergoing coronary artery bypass. Aside from these considerations, complications specifically related to the prosthetic valve implants are the primary and potentially most catastrophic complication associated with valvular heart surgery.

Implant-Related Complications

With appropriate anticoagulant therapy, mechanical prosthetic valves such as the bileaflet valve enjoy freedom from structural failure rates of at least 99% per year. Mechanical valve dysfunction is today predominantly the result of valve thrombosis, although rare causes of failure with older-type valves include strut fracture, ball variance, and even ball or leaflet escape, all of which require emergency reoperation. Although usually more gradual, tissue valve failure manifested by acute leaflet tearing or perforation and development of valvular insufficiency may also necessitate urgent operation and valve re-replacement. The more gradual development of tissue valve fibrosis can usually be managed with elective re-replacement. Auscultation remains one of the most effective means of screening for prosthetic valve dysfunction, and any new or changed murmur or any diminution of prosthetic heart valve sounds should raise the suspicion of valvular dysfunction and be confirmed by Doppler echo studies and cardiac catheterization, if necessary.

The frequency of serious complications such as valve hemorrhage, infection, and structural dysfunction depends on valve type and position and multiple clinical risk factors. The overall incidence of complications is approximately 3% per year. In a meta-analysis of 5837 patients who received aortic valve bioprosthesis, for example, the annual rates of valve thrombosis, thromboembolism, hemorrhage, and nonstructural dysfunction were 0.03%, 0.87%, 0.38%, and 0.38%, respectively.[134] The rate of endocarditis within the first 6 months of implantation was 3.4% but decreased thereafter to an annual rate of 0.68%. Another study evaluated 440 patients receiving a St. Jude mechanical prosthesis in the mitral position who were followed for 19 years; the annualized rates of thromboembolism, thrombosis, and hemorrhage were 0.7%, 0.2%, and 1%, respectively. At 19 years, the freedom from reoperation was 90%.[135] Lifelong anticoagulation therapy is mandated for all mechanical valve implants to avoid an excessive thromboembolic complication rate and carries an additional 1% to 2% per year risk of bleeding complications and a 0.17% mortality rate.[136]

Bioprosthetic implants generally do not require anticoagulation, except for mitral bioprosthetic implants in the presence of AF, which carry an increased thromboembolic risk. It should be noted, however, that approximately 10% of patients with tissue valves in the aortic position and up to 40% to 60% of patients with bioprosthetic valves in the mitral position eventually require anticoagulant therapy, thus partially negating the benefit of a tissue valve implant. Because half of all thromboembolic events for bioprosthetic valves have been reported to occur within the first 12 weeks following surgery, a finding that is probably related to endothelialization of the nonmobile aspects of the prosthesis, anticoagulation is furthermore generally recommended for the first 3 months following bioprosthetic valve implantation, at least in the mitral position, for which an increased risk for thromboembolism exists.

Anticoagulant therapy generally consists of daily dosing of the vitamin K antagonist coumadin, which is regulated by laboratory measurement of prothrombin times or international normalized ratio (INR) on a weekly or monthly basis (home testing is gradually becoming available). In some cases, coumadin therapy may be supplemented by aspirin or Persantine administration in the event of a thromboembolic event with adequate INR levels, under the supposition that an antiplatelet therapy might be beneficial. A wide range of recommendations exists for appropriate anticoagulation levels, depending on the type and location of the valve implant (Table 77.12).

TABLE 77.12. Anticoagulant Recommendations.

Indication	Recommended prothrombin time elevation above control with warfarin administration
Prosthetic heart valves	
Mechanical	1.5–2
Bioprosthetic	1.3–1.5 (3 months postoperatively)
Native valve disease	
Rheumatic mitral valve	
Previous embolism	1.5–2 (1.3–1.5 after 1 year)
Atrial fibrillation	1.3–1.5
Dilated left atrium (0.55 mm in diameter)	1.3–1.5
Aortic valve disease	No treatment[a]
Mitral valve prolapse	No treatment[a]
Mitral annular calcification	No treatment[a]
Infective endocarditis	No treatment[a]
Atrial fibrillation	
Previous embolism	1.5–2 (1.3–1.5 after 1 year)
Mitral valve disease	1.3–1.5
Cardiomyopathy	
Dilated	1.3–1.5
Hypertrophic	1.3–1.5
Thyrotoxicosis	1.3–1.5[b]
Lone atrial fibrillation	No treatment[a]
Cardioversion	1.3–1.5[b+]

[a]Unless other indications exist.

[b]Maintain therapy for 2 to 4 weeks after conversion to sinus rhythm.

Bleeding complications should be treated as appropriate for the specific event, by cessation of coumadin therapy, and by administration of fresh frozen plasma or vitamin K, as appropriate, with continuation of anticoagulant therapy as soon as possible, but preferably within 1 week. It should be noted that vitamin K administration makes subsequent anticoagulation more difficult and should thus be avoided if appropriate. In the event of planned or unanticipated surgical intervention, it should be noted that coumadin therapy can be replaced with intravenous heparin anticoagulation, which can then probably be safely interrupted for 24 to 48 h perioperatively. Finally, a planned or unanticipated pregnancy while on coumadin therapy can adequately be managed by transitioning to subcutaneous heparin, or possibly oral heparin analogues, during the first and third trimesters to avoid coumadin teratogenicity and peripartum hemorrhage during these respective intervals.

Hemolysis is another potential complication of valve implantation, most likely to occur with a prosthesis in the aortic position, with small valve sizes, and in the presence of a periprosthetic leak, especially in the mitral position. Hemolysis is usually mild but can be significant enough to produce clinically apparent jaundice and require transfusion. This usually resolves with time, but valve replacement may be required, especially if a periprosthetic leak exists.

Finally, infection may occur in 1% to 2% of prosthetic valve implants, typically in the aortic position, representing 15% to 30% of all cases of endocarditis. The mortality of prosthetic valve endocarditis is substantial, as high as 80% in patients with infection that is detected in the early postoperative period (less than 60 days after surgery). Endocarditis occurring less than 2 months postoperatively may be related to a break in sterile technique or contamination from skin flora, whereas late endocarditis is usually related to a bacteremic episode. *Staphylococcus epidermidis*, *S. aureus*, or the gram-negative rods are the most common inciting organisms in early cases, while streptococci are more commonly seen in late endocarditis. Patients with prosthetic valves are therefore cautioned to strictly adhere to the recommended guidelines for antibiotic prophylaxis if invasive procedures such as endoscopy or dental procedures are planned.

The onset of fever, chills, or sweats is typical of the clinical presentation for endocarditis and mandates confirmation of the diagnosis by obtaining a set of blood cultures, which will be positive in 90% of cases, before initiating antibiotic therapy. The presence of a new or changed murmur is another important diagnostic sign but may be absent in up to 50% of cases. The classic peripheral stigmata of systemic emboli associated with endocarditis as a function of the more rapid recognition and treatment of this disease are not commonly seen today. Echocardiography has become an increasingly sensitive diagnostic tool, accurate in up to 80% of cases. Healed endocarditis may, however, result in persistent residual vegetations seen on echo, and thus the specificity of echo may be limited.

Antibiotic therapy, typically involving a 6-week course of intravenous antibiotics, is typical therapy for native valve endocarditis, with surgical intervention reserved for treatment failures, recurrent embolization, periprosthetic abscess formation, or hemodynamic compromise caused by valve dysfunction. Prosthetic endocarditis is much less likely to be treatable medically, and thus valve re-replacement is indicated in up to two-thirds of patients who fail antibiotic therapy and possibly all patients with fungal or gram-negative rod endocarditis. Antibiotic cure can be achieved in prosthetic endocarditis when there is evidence of maintained perivalvular integrity. Antibiotic cure can also be achieved without the increased risk of complications in hemodynamically stable patients with nonstaphylococcal endocarditis. The chief cause of death from endocarditis is CHF, and thus evidence of hemodynamic compromise in this setting is an important indication for operation. Operation generally consists of complete excision of the infected valve apparatus, debridement and closure of any abscess, and valve re-replacement. An initially favorable outcome can be expected in 80% to 95% of cases, with a late reinfection rate of 1% to 13%.[137] Late mortality rates of 20% to 60% have been reported.[138]

Surgical Result

Operative Mortality

The overall operative mortality rate for valve repair or replacement ranges from 1% to 12% (Tables 77.13 through 77.15).[139–141] A study from the University of Toronto of almost 2500 patients demonstrated operative mortality rates for aortic and mitral valve replacement of 5.3% and 6.6%, respectively.[138] A retrospective study from the Mayo Clinic of aortic valve replacement for AR demonstrated a 1.2% operative mortality for functional class I/II patients, compared with a mortality of 7.8% for class III/IV patients.[139] Similarly, Blackstone and Kirklin reported nearly a threefold increase in operative mortality for functional class IV compared with functional class I patients.[140] Consistent with these findings, an ejection

TABLE 77.13.
Selected Series of Mitral Valve Replacements.

Valve type	*Years of enrollment*	*n*	*Operative mortality (%)*	*Actuarial survival*	*Freedom from valve-related complications*	*Freedom from reoperation*	*Source*
Mechanical							
St. Jude	1980–1996	514	7.2	8 yr, 89%	—	—	Grossi[142]
St. Jude	1979–1990	397	3.5	10 yr, 73%	3.7% (pt-yr)	—	Jegaden[183]
Carbomedics	1989–1994	330	6.9	5 yr, 77%	10 yr, 69%, 64%	—	Bernal[184]
Bioprosthetic							
Porcine (Carpentier-Edwards)	1975–1995	512	9	10 yr, 52% 15 yr, 24%	—	15 yr. 20%	Jamieson[185]
Porcine (Hancock II)	1982–1994	310	6	15 yr, 30%	15 yr, 87%[b]	15 yr, 69%	David[186]

[a]Freedom from late cardiac death.
[b]Freedom from thromboembolic complications.

TABLE 77.14.
Mitral Valve Repair.

Primary repair technique	*Year of enrollment*	*n*	*Operative mortality (%)*	*15-yr actuarial survival (%)*	*15-yr Freedom from reoperation (%)*	*Comments*	*Study*
Annuloplasty/valvuloplasty	1972–1979	206	5.5	72	87	Freedom from reoperation, 93% for degenerative disease/76% for rheumatic disease ($P < .01$)	Deloche et al.[187]
Annuloplasty	1980–1996	725	5.4	84[a,b]	76[b]	Increased complication/failure rate with rheumatic or multivalve disease	Grossi et al.[142]
Annuloplasty/valvuloplasty	1981–1992	184	0.5	88[a]	95[a]	Failure risk directly related to degree of disease	David et al.[188]
Chordal replacement with e-PTFE[c]	1981–1995	324	0.6	75[d]	96[d]	Chordal replacement for anterior leaflet prolapse	David et al.[130]

[a]Eight-year data.
[b]Freedom from late cardiac death.
[c]Expanded polytetrafluoroethylene.
[d]Ten-year data.

TABLE 77.15. Probability of an Outcome Event at 15 Years After Valve Replacement.

	Aortic valve replacement (%)			*Mitral valve replacement (%)*		
	Mechanical n = 198	*Bioprosthetic n = 196*	**P value**	*Mechanical n = 88*	*Bioprosthetic n = 93*	**P value**
Death from any cause	66 ± 3	79 ± 3	0.02	81 ± 4	79 ± 4	0.3
Any valve-related complication	65 ± 4	66 ± 5	0.26	73 ± 6	81 ± 5	0.56
Systemic embolism	18 ± 4	18 ± 4	0.66	18 ± 5	22 ± 5	0.96
Bleeding	51 ± 4	30 ± 4	0.0001	53 ± 7	31 ± 6	0.01
Endocarditis	7 ± 2	15 ± 5	0.45	11 ± 4	17 ± 5	0.37
Valve thrombosis	2 ± 1	1 ± 1	0.33	1 ± 1	1 ± 1	0.95
Perivalvular regurgitation	8 ± 2	2 ± 1	0.09	17 ± 5	7 ± 4	0.05
Reoperation	10 ± 3	29 ± 5	0.004	25 ± 6	50 ± 8	0.15
Primary valve failure	0 ± 0	23 ± 5	0.0001	5 ± 4	44 ± 8	0.0002

n, number of patients randomised; *P*, significance of difference between mechanical and bioprosthetic valves.
Source: From Hammermeister et al.[189]

fraction less than 30%, emergent surgery, reoperations, concomitant coronary bypass grafting, and MR were independent mortality predictors in a retrospective study[141] of 257 patients with diminished ejection fraction undergoing valve operation at Emory from 1980 to 1993. More specifically, in the Toronto cohort, the presence of significant CAD increased operative mortality to 16% in patients undergoing mitral valve replacement (MVR) for MR, reoperation more than doubled operative risk, as did double-valve replacement and the presence of TR. Although increased age was also noted to be an operative risk factor in the Toronto study, elective valve replacement has been reported in octogenarians with an operative mortality rate as low as 4%.

An increased mortality rate has generally been observed in most studies comparing valve replacement with MR as compared with AI, probably reflecting the pathophysiology of these respective diseases (see following) or technical consideration of the operation. Mitral valve repair has been advocated to result in operative mortality rates less than 5%, significantly lower than that for some reported series of mitral valve replacements, but in a study of 514 mitral valve replacement patients and 725 reconstruction patients, the operative mortalities (7.2% and 5.4%, respectively) were not significantly different.[142]

Hemodynamic and Late Results

Left ventricular chamber size, wall thickness, and LV mass generally tend to decrease as early as 7 to 10 days postoperatively after correction of valvular heart disease. These changes can be related to decreases in afterload and wall stresses related to decreased diastolic filling and improved systolic emptying related to elimination of excessive regurgitant volumes or valvular obstruction in the case of insufficiency and stenotic lesions, respectively. One exception to this is found in patients with significant residual transvalvular gradients following placement of a small aortic valve prosthesis, although the clinical significance of this finding in terms of long-term morbidity and mortality is unknown.

A second exception occurs in patients undergoing correction of MR, in whom ventricular function may only remain stable or may even deteriorate, usually as a function of their underlying baseline LV function. Although it has been suggested that mitral valve repair may help improve long-term outcomes in patients undergoing correction of MR, there was no significance in freedom from late cardiac death, reoperation, and valve-related complications between patients undergoing valve replacement versus valve repair in valve replacement patients (73% versus 65%, respectively) in a study by Grossi et al.[142] Reconstruction did, however, appear to offer benefit in terms of late events in patients with isolated nonrheumatic mitral valve disease in this series.

Excellent functional improvement can also generally be expected for nearly all patients undergoing correction of valvular heart disease, with nearly all patients experiencing functional class I or II symptomatology postoperatively regardless of their preoperative status. Preoperative LV function and the type and durability of surgical correction, with attendant complication rates, are the primary predictors of long-time event-free survival. Significant LV dysfunction in fact can result in up to a 50% decrease in the 5-year survival rates and extent of functional improvement in patients undergoing valve replacement. Five-year survival of hospital survivors in the Emory study of patients with preoperative ejection fractions less than 40% was only 65%.[141] Similarly, 10-year survival in a series of patients undergoing aortic valve replacement (AVR) reported from the Mayo Clinic was significantly decreased for class III/IV patients compared to class I/II patients. In patients undergoing correction of MR, an operation particularly prone to postoperative compromise in ventricular function, predictors of normal postoperative LV function include a preoperative ejection fraction greater than 50%, an end-systolic volume index less than $50\,mL/m^2$, and a mean PA systolic pressure less than 20 mmHg.

Freedom From Reoperation

Aside from operative mortality rates, functional improvement, and thromboembolic and hemorrhagic complication rates, one remaining parameter by which valve surgery must be judged is the freedom from reoperation rate (Table 77.15). In general, this is primarily a consideration for heterograft implants as this rate is less than 1%/year for mechanical implants. In a recent report of 589 patients with a mean age of 67 years undergoing bovine pericardial aortic valve implants, freedom from reoperation at 10 years was 97%, suggesting that previous considerations regarding the limited durability of tissue valve implants may become less significant.[143]

Similarly encouraging results have recently been reported for mitral valve repair (Table 77.14).[144–147] The overall 5-year freedom from reoperation for mitral valve repair has recently been reported at 90%, while 15-year freedom from reoperation has been reported at 87% (93% for degenerative, but only 76% for rheumatic). In the Cleveland Clinic experience, the primary reason for reoperation was technical in 58% of cases, with suture dehiscence and rupture of shortened chordae tendinae a common deficiency.[144] Progression of rheumatic heart valve pathology was also a common cause of reoperation in the Cleveland Clinic series, and RHD (as well as ischemic etiology) must be viewed as a relative contraindication to repair. In support of these findings, David et al., espousing the use of "artificial" (PTFE) chordae, reported freedom from operation and recurrence of severe MR at 10 years of 96% and 93%, respectively, in 324 patients with myxomatous disease.[130] Finally, persistence of MR immediately following repair and failure to use an annuloplasty ring have been demonstrated to represent significant risk factors for reoperation.

In summary, encouraging recent trends have been reported with the use of mitral valve repair, bovine pericardial valves, and, in selected cases, aortic homograft implants in terms of long-term freedom from reoperation and other complications. In other cases for which mechanical implants are required, long-term durability can be expected, although at the expense of a persistent annual risk of thromboembolic and anticoagulant-related complications.

References

1. National Heart, Lung and Blood Institute Coronary Artery Surgery Study. Principal investigators of CASS and their associates. Circulation 1981;63:I1–I81.
2. Edwards FH, Grover FL, Shroyer LW, Schwartz M, Bero J. The society of thoracic surgeons national cardiac surgery database: current risk assessment. Ann Thorac Surg 1997;63:903–908.

3. Estafanous FG, Loop FD, Higgins TL, et al. Increased risk and decreased morbidity of coronary bypass grafting between 1986 and 1994. Ann Thorac Surg 1998;65:383–389.
4. Gold JP, Charlson ME, Williams-Russo P, et al. Improvement of outcomes after coronary artery bypass: a randomized trial comparing intraoperative high versus low mean arterial pressure. J Thorac Cardiovasc Surg 1995;110:1302–1304.
5. Bigelow WG, Callahan JC, Hopps JA. General hypothermia for experimental intracardiac surgery. Ann Thorac Surg 1950;33:52–59.
6. Woodcock TE, Murkin JM, Farrar JK, et al. Pharmacologic EEG suppression during cardiopulmonary bypass: cerebral haemodynamic and metabolic effects of thiopental or isofurane during hypothermia and normothermia. Anesthesiology 1987;67:218–224.
7. Yamashita C, Nakamura H, Nishikawa Y, Yamamoto S, Okada M, Nakamura K. Retrograde cerebral perfusion with circulatory arrest in aortic arch aneurysm. Ann Thorac Surg 1992;54:566–568.
8. Franke UF, et al. Intermittent antegrade warm myocardial protection compared to intermittent cold blood cardioplegia in elective coronary surgery—do we have to change? Eur J Cardiothorac Surg 2003;23:341–346.
9. Martin TC, Craver JM, Gott JP, et al. Prospective randomized trial of retrograde warm blood cardioplegia: myocardial benefit and neurologic threat. Ann Thorac Surg 1994;57:298–304.
10. Stephan H, Weyland A, Kazmaier A, et al. Acid–base management during hypothermic cardiopulmonary bypass does not affect cerebral metabolism but does affect blood flow and neurological outcome. Br J Anaesth 1992;69:51–57.
11. Jonas RA, Bellinger DC, Rappaport LA, et al. Relation of pH strategy and developmental outcome after hypothermic circulatory arrest. J Thorac Cardiovasc Surg 1993;106:362–368.
12. Fang WC, Helm RE, Krieger KH, et al. Impact of minimum hematocrit during cardiopulmonary bypass on mortality in patients undergoing coronary artery surgery. Circulation 1997;96:194–199.
13. Rosengart TK, Krieger K, Lang S, et al. Reoperative coronary artery bypass surgery: improved preservation of myocardial function with retrograde cardioplegia. Circulation 1993;88:330–335.
14. De Paulis R, et al. Troponin I release after CABG surgery using two different strategies of myocardial protection and systemic perfusion. J Cardiovasc Surg 2002;43:153–161.
15. Salerno TA, Christakis GT, Abel J, et al. Technique and pitfalls of retrograde continuous warm blood cardioplegia. Ann Thorac Surg 1991;51:1023–1025.
16. Mangano CM, et al. The multicenter Study of Perioperative Ishemia Research Group: renal disfunction after myocardial revascularization. Ann Intern Med 1998;128:194.
17. Raimondo A, et al. On-pump versus off-pump coronary revascularization: evaluation or renal function. Ann Thorac Surg 1999; 68:493–497.
18. Newman MF, et al. Longitudinal assessment of neurocognitive function after CABG. N Engl J Med 2001;344:395–402.
19. McKhann GM, Goldsborough MA, Borowicz LM, et al. Cognitive outcome after coronary artery bypass: a 1 year prospective study. Ann Thorac Surg 1997;63:510–515.
20. Ola A, et al. Cognitive changes with CAD: a prospective study of CABG and nonsurgical controls. Ann Thorac Surg 2003; 75:1377–1382.
20a. Rosengart T, Sweet J, Finnin E, Wolfe P, Cashy J, Hahn E, Marymont J, Sanborn T. Stable cognition after coronary bypass: comparisons to percutaneous interventions and normal controls. Ann Thorac Surg. 2006;82:597–607
21. Diederik VD, et al. Cognitive outcome after off-pump CABG: a randomized trial. JAMA 2002;287:1405–1411.
22. Lawhorne TW, Davis WL, Smith GW. General surgical complications after cardiac surgery. Am J Surg 1978;136:254–260.
23. Mueller RL, Rosengart TK, Isom OW. The history of surgery for ischemic heart disease. Ann Thorac Surg 1997;63:869–878.
24. Budoff MJ, Georgiou D, Brody A, et al. Ultrafast computed tomography as a diagnostic modality in the detection of coronary artery disease: a multicenter study. Circulation 1996;93:898–904.
25. European Cooperative Study for Streptokinase Treatment in Acute Myocardial Infarction. Streptokinase in acute myocardial infarction. N Engl J Med 1979;301:797–802.
26. The ISAM Study Group. A prospective trial of Intravenous Streptokinase in Acute Myocardial Infarction (ISAM): mortality, morbidity, and infarct size at 21 days. N Engl J Med 1986;314: 1465–1471.
27. Dalen JE, Gore JM, Braunwald E, et al. Six and 12 month follow-up of the phase I Thrombolysis in Myocardial Infarction (TIMI) trial: the TIMI investigators. Am J Cardiol 1988;62:179–185.
28. The European Myocardial Infarction Project. Prehospital thrombolytic therapy in patients with suspected acute myocardial infarction. N Engl J Med 1993;329:383–389.
29. Landau C, Lange RA, Hillis RD. Percutaneous transluminal coronary angioplasty. N Engl J Med 1994;330:981–993.
30. Laham RJ, Ho KKL, Baim DS, Kuntz RE, Cohen DJ, Carozza JP. Multivessel Palmaz-Schatz stenting: early results and 1 year outcome. J Am Coll Cardiol 1997;30:180–185.
31. Fishman DL, Leon MB, Baim DS, et al. A randomized comparison of coronary-stent placement and balloon angioplasty in the treatment of coronary artery disease. N Engl J Med 1994;331:496–501.
32. Grines CL, Browne KE, Marco J, et al. for the Primary Angioplasty in Myocardial Infarction Study Group. A comparison of immediate angioplasty with thrombolytic therapy for acute myocardial infarction. N Engl J Med 1993;328:673–679.
33. Zijlstra F, deBoer MJ, Hoorntje JC, Reiffers S, Reiber JH, Surypantra H. A comparison of immediate angioplasty with intravenous streptokinase in acute myocardial infarction. N Engl J Med 1993;328:680–684.
34. Abizaid at al. CABG vs. PTCA with stent implantation in patients with MVD(the Stent or Surgery Trial): a randomized controlled trial; Lancet 2002;360:956–962.
35. Serruys at al. for the ARTS group. Comparison of CABG and stenting for the MV disease. N Engl J Med 2001;344:1117–1122.
36. Legrand at al. Three year outcome after stenting versus bypass surgery for treatment of CAD. Circulation 2004;109:1114–1121.
37. The Veterans Administration Coronary Artery Bypass Surgery Cooperative Study Group. Eleven year survival in the Veterans Administration randomized trial of coronary bypass surgery for stable angina. N Engl J Med 1984;311:333–339.
38. European Coronary Surgery Study Group. Long-term results of prospective randomised study of coronary artery bypass surgery in stable angina pectoris. Lancet 1982;2:1173–1180.
39. Deter K, Peduzzi P, Murphy M, et al. Effect of bypass surgery on survival in patients in low- and high-risk subgroups delineated by the use of simple clinical variables. Circulation 1981;63:1329–1338.
40. Gibbons RJ, et al. ACC/AHA 2002 guideline update for the management of patients with chronic stable angina-summary article. Circulation 2003;107:149–156.
41. The Writing Group for the Bypass Angioplasty Revascularization Investigation (BARI) Investigators. Five year clinical and functional outcome comparing bypass surgery and angioplasty in patients with multivessel coronary disease. JAMA 1997; 277:715–721.
42. Serruys at al. for the ARTS group. Comparison of CABG and stenting for the MV disease. N Engl J Med 2001;344:1117–1122.

43. Hlatky MA, Rogers WJ, Johnstone I, et al. Medical care costs and quality of life after randomization to coronary angioplasty or coronary bypass surgery. N Engl J Med 1997;336:92–99.
44. Sim I, Gupta M, McDonald K, Bourassa MG, Hlatky MA. A meta-analysis of randomized trials comparing coronary artery bypass grafting with percutaneous transluminal coronary angioplasty in multivessel coronary artery disease. Am J Cardiol 1995;76:1025–1029.
45. King SB, et al. Eight year mortality in the Emory Angioplasty versus Surgery trial (EAST). J Am Coll Cardiol 2000;35:1116–1122.
46. Jones RH, Kesler K, Phillips HR, et al. Long-term survival benefits of coronary artery bypass grafting and percutaneous transluminal angioplasty in patients with coronary artery disease. J Thorac Cardiovasc Surg 1996;111:1013–1025.
47. Favaloro RG. Critical analysis of coronary artery bypass graft surgery: a 30-year journey. J Am Coll Cardiol 1998;31(suppl B):1B–6B.
48. Ryan TJ. Revascularization: reflections of a clinician. J Am Coll Cardiol 1998;31:89B–96B.
49. Mack MJ, et al. Current status and outcomes of coronary revascularization 1999–2002: 148,396 surgical and percutaneous procedures. Ann Thorac Surg 2004;77:761–767.
50. DeWood MA, Notske RN, Berg R, et al. Medical and surgical management of early Q-wave myocardial infarction: effects of surgical reperfusion on survival, recurrent myocardial infarction, sudden death and functional class at 10 or more years of follow-up. J Am Coll Cardiol 1989;14:65–77.
51. Spencer FC. Emergency coronary bypass for acute infarction: an unproved clinical experiment [editorial]. Circulation 1983; 68(suppl II):II17–II19.
52. Cannon CP, McCabe CH, Stone PH, et al. The electrocardiogram predicts 1 year outcome of patients with unstable angina and non-Q wave myocardial infarction: results of the TIMI III registry ECG ancillary study. J Am Coll Cardiol 1997;30:133–140.
53. Gibson RS. Management of acute non-Q-wave myocardial infarction: role of prophylactic pharmacotherapy and indications for predischarge coronary arteriography. Clin Cardiol 1989;12: III26–III32.
54. Bosch X, Theroux P, Waters DD, Pelletier GB, Roy D. Early postinfarction ischemia: clinical, angiographic, and prognostic significance. Circulation 1987;75:988–995.
55. van Dijk RA, Nierich AP, Jansen EW, et al. Early outcome after off-pump versus on-pump coronary bypass surgery. Circulation 2001;104:1761–1766.
56. Khan NE, et al. A randomized comparison of off-pump and on-pump multivessel coronary-artery bypass surgery. N Engl J Med 2004;350:21–28.
57. Straka Z, et al. Off-pump versus on-pump coronary surgery: final results from a prospective randomized study PRAGUE-4. Ann Thorac Surg 2004;73:789–796.
58. Reichenspurner H, Gulielmos V, Wunderlich J, et al. Port-access coronary artery bypass grafting with the use of cardiopulmonary bypass and cardioplegic arrest. Ann Thorac Surg 1998;65:413–419.
59. Machiraju VR. Redo Cardiac Surgery in Adults. CME Network, Southampton, NY; 1997.
60. Engelman RM, Rousou JA, Flack JE III, et al. Fast-track recovery of the coronary bypass patient. Ann Thorac Surg 1994;58:1742–1746.
61. Eagle KA, et al. ACC/AHA 2004 guidelines update for coronary artery bypass graft surgery: summary article. J Am Coll Cardiol 2004;44:1146–1154.
61a. Eagle KA, Guyton RA, et. al. ACC/AHA guidelines for coronary artery bypass graft surgery: executive summary and recommendations. Circulation. 1999;100:1464–1480.
62. Karkouti K, et al. A multivariable model for predicting the need for blood transfusion in patients undergoing first time elective CABG Transfusion 2001;41:1193–1199.
63. Hattler BG, et al. Risk stratification using the Society of Thoracic Surgeons Program. Ann Thorac Surg 1994;58:1348–1355.
64. Edwards FH, Clark RE, Schwartz M. Coronary artery bypass grafting: the Society of Thoracic Surgery national database experience. Ann Thorac Surg 1994;57:12–19.
65. Disch DL, O'Connor GT, Birkmeyer JD, et al. Changes in patients undergoing coronary artery bypass grafting: 1987–1990. Ann Thorac Surg 1994;57:416–423.
66. New York State Department of Health. Coronary Artery Bypass Graft Surgery in New York State. Albany: New York State Department of Health; 1997.
67. Ivanov J, et al. Fifteen year trends in risk severity and operative mortality in elderly patients undergoing CABG. Circulation 1998;97:673–679.
68. Yau TM, et al. Predictors of operative risk for CABG in patients with left ventricular dysfunction. J Thorac Cardiovasc Surg 1999;118:1006–1011.
69. Elefertiades JA, Tolis G, Levi E, Mills LK, Zaret BL. Coronary artery bypass grafting with severe left ventricular dysfunction: excellent survival with improved ejection fraction and functional state. J Am Coll Cardiol 1993;22:1411–1417.
70. Shapira I, Isakov A, Yakirevich VV, Topilsky M. Long-term results of coronary bypass surgery in patients with severely depressed left ventricular dysfunction. Chest 1995;108:1546–1550.
71. Morrison DA, et al. Percutaneous coronary intervention versus repeat CABG for patients with medically refractory myocardial ischemia. AWESOME randomized trial and registry experience with post-CABG patients. J Am Coll Cardiol 2002;40:1951–1956.
72. Leavitt BJ, et al. Use of the internal mammary artery graft and in hospital mortality and other adverse outcomes associated with CABG. Circulation 2001;103:507–512.
73. Loop FD, et al. Influence of the internal mammary artery graft on 10 year survival and other cardiac events. N Engl J Med 1986;314:1–9.
74. Cameron A, et al. CABG surgery with internal-thoracic artery grafts. Effects on survival over a 15 year period. N Engl J Med 1996;334:216–222.
75. Lytle BW, et al. Two internal thoracic arteries are better than one. J Thorac Cardiovasc Surg 1999;117:855–861.
76. Ioannidis JP, et al. Early mortality and morbidity of bilateral versus single internal thoracic artery revascularization: propensity and risk modeling. J Am Coll Cardiol 2001;37:521–527.
77. Puskas JD, et al. Off-pump CABG provides complete revascularisation with reduced myocardial injury, transfusion requirements and length of stay. J Thorac Cardiovasc Surg 2003; 125:797–802.
78. Carrier M, et al. Randomized trial comparing off-pump coronary bypass grafting in high risk patients. Heart Surgery Forum 2003;6:E89–E92.
79. Stamou SC, et al. Operative mortality after conventional versus coronary revascularisation without cardiopulmonary bypass. Eur J Cardiothorac Surg 2004;26:549–555.
80. Bourassa MG, Enjalbert M, Campeau L, Lesperance J. Progression of atherosclerosis in coronary arteries and bypass grafts: 10 years later. Am J Cardiol 1984;53:102C–107C.
81. Grondin CM, Campeau L, Lesperance J, et al. Comparison of late changes in internal mammary artery and saphenous vein grafts in two consecutive series of patients 10 years after operation. Circulation 1984;70(suppl 1):208–212.
82. Berger PB, et al. for the International Multicenter Aprotinin Graft Patency Experience (IMAGE) Investigators. Frequency of

early occlusion and stenosis in a left internal mammary artery to left descending artery bypass graft: benchmark for minimally invasive direct CABG. Circulation 1999;100:2353–2357.
83. Ura M, et al. Analysis by early angiography of right internal thoracic artery graft via the transverse sinus: predictors of graft failure. Circulation 2000;101:640–646.
84. Loop FD, Lytle BW, Cosgrove DM, et al. Influence of the internal mammary artery graft on 10 year survival and other cardiac events. N Engl J Med 1986;314:1–6.
85. Carrel T, Horber P, Turina MI. Operation for two-vessel coronary artery disease: midterm results of bilateral ITA grafting versus unilateral ITA and saphenous vein grafting. Ann Thorac Surg 1996;62:1289–1294.
86. Huddleston CB, Stoney WS, Alford WC, et al. Internal mammary artery crafts: technical factors influencing patency. Ann Thorac Surg 1986;42:5–17.
87. Taggart DP, et al. Effects of arterial revascularisation on survival systematic review of studies comparing bilateral and single internal mammary arteries. Lancet 2001;358:870–877.
88. Acar C, Jebara VA, Portoghese M, et al. Revival of the radial artery for coronary artery bypass grafting. Ann Thorac Surg 1992;54:652–659.
89. Muneretto C, et al. Safety and usefulness of composite grafts for total arterial myocardial revascularization: a prospective randomized evaluation. J Thorac Cardiovasc Surg 2003;125:82.
90. Schachner T, et al. Local application of rapamycin inhibits neointimal hyperplasia in experimental vein grafts. Ann Thorac Surg 2004;77:1580–1588.
91. Mann MJ, et al. Ex-vivo gene therapy of human vascular bypass grafts with E2F decoy: the PREVENT single center randomized, controlled trial. Lancet 1999;354:1493–1499.
92. Yusuf S, Zucker D, Peduzzi P, et al. Effect of coronary artery bypass graft surgery on survival: overview of 10-year results from randomised trials by the Coronary Artery Bypass Graft Surgery Trialists Collaboration. Lancet 1994;344:563–570.
93. Emond M, Mock MB, Davis KB, et al. Long-term survival of medically treated patients in the Coronary Artery Surgery Study (CASS) registry. Circulation 1994;90:2645–2657.
94. Mack CA, Patel SR, Rosengart TK. Myocardial angiogenesis as a possible mechanism for TMLR efficacy. J Clin Laser Med Surg 1997;15:275–279.
95. Schofield PM, et al. Transmyocardial laser revascularisation in patients with refractory angina: a randomized controlled trial. Lancet 1999;252:515–521.
96. Allen KB. Comparison of transmyocardial revascularization with medical therapy in patients with refractory angina. N Engl J Med 1999;341:1029–1035.
97. Frazier OH, et al. Transmyocardial Carbon Dioxide Laser Revascularization Study Group. N Engl J Med 1999;341:1021–1027.
98. Simons M, Banno RO, Chronos N, et al. Clinical trials in coronary angiogenesis: issues, problems, consensus. Circulation 2000;102:E73–E86.
99. Rosengart TK. The era of cardiac biointerventions. Semin Thorac Cardiovasc Surg 2003;15:217–221.
100. Imran IS, Sanborn TA, Rosengart TK. Therapeutic angiogenesis: a biologic bypass. Cardiology 2004;101:131–143.
101. David TE. Surgery for postinfarction rupture of the free wall of the ventricle. In: David TE. Mechanical Complications of Myocardial Infarction, Landes, Austin; 1993.
102. Cooley DA. Ventricular endoaneurysmorrhaphy: a simplified repair for extensive post infarction aneurysm. J Cardiac Surg 1989;4:200–205.
103. Jatene AD. Left ventricular aneurysmectomy: resection or reconstruction. J Thorac Cardiovasc Surg 1985;89:321–331.
104. Dor V. Left ventricular aneurysms: the endoventricular circular path plasty. Semin Thorac Cardiovasc Surg 1997;9:123–130.
105. Menicanti L, et al. The Dor procedure: what has changed after 15 years of clinical practice? J Thorac Cardiovasc Surg 2002;124:886–892.
106. Madsen JC, Daggett WM. Postinfarction ventricular septal defect repair. In: Cox JL, Sundt, TM III, eds. Operative Techniques in Cardiac and Thoracic Surgery, 1997;2:161–169.
107. Cooley DA. Postinfarction ventricular septal rupture. Semin Thorac Cardiovasc Surg 1998;10:100–104.
108. David TE. Repair of postinfarction ventricular septal defect. In: Cox JL, Sundt TM III, eds. Operative Techniques in Cardiac and Thoracic Surgery, 1997;2:170–178.
109. David TE. Techniques and results of mitral valve repair for ischemic mitral regurgitation. J Card Surg 1994;9:274–277.
110. Allman KC, Shaw LJ, Hachamovitch R, et al. Myocardial viability testing and impact of revascularization on prognosis in patients with CAD and LV dysfunction: a meta-analysis. J Am Coll Cardiol 2002;39:1151–1157.
111. Schinkel, et al. Why do patients with ischemic cardiomyopathy and a substantial amount of viable myocardium not always recover in function after revascularisation? J Thorac Cardiovasc Surg 2004;127:385–392.
112. Dor V, Saab M, Coste P, et al. Endoventricular patch plasties with septal exclusion for repair of ischemic left ventricle: technique, results and indications from series of 781 cases. Jpn J Thorac Cardiovasc Surg 1998;46:389–395.
113. Chizner MA, Pearle DL, deLeon AC Jr. The natural history of aortic stenosis in adults. Am Heart J 1980;99:419–425.
114. Bonow RO, et al. ACC/AHA 2006 guidelines for management of patients with valvular heart disease. Circulation 2006;114: e84–e231.
115. Oleson KH. The natural history of 271 patients with mitral stenosis under medical treatment. Br Heart J 1962;24:349–355.
116. Fischl SJ, Gorlin R, Herman MW. Cardiac shape and function in aortic valvular disease: physiologic and clinical implications. Am J Cardiol 1977;39:170–177.
117. Bonow RO, Rosing DR, Kent KM, et al. Timing of operation for chronic aortic regurgitation. Am J Cardiol 1982;50:325–336.
118. Duran CMG, Pomar JI, Colman T, Figueroa A, Revuelta JM, Ubago JI. Is tricuspid valve repair necessary? J Thorac Cardiovasc Surg 1980;80:849–855.
119. Turi ZG, Reyes VP, Raju BS, et al. Percutaneous balloon valvuloplasty versus closed commissurotomy for mitral stenosis: a prospective, randomized trial. Circulation 1991;83:1179–1185.
120. Smerida NG, Ports TA, Merrick SH, Rankin DS. Balloon aortic valvuloplast as a bridge to aortic valve replacement in critically ill patients. Ann Thorac Surg 1993;55:914–918.
121. Hejjer JJ, Wann LS, Weyman AE, Dillon JC, Feigenbaum H. Long term changes in mitral valve area after successful mitral commissurotomy. Circulation 1979;59:443–448.
122. Autschbach R, et al. Prospectively randomized comparison of different mechanical aortic valves. Circulation 2000;102(19 suppl 3):III1–IIII4.
123. Magilligan DJ Jr, Lewis JW Jr, Stein P, Alam M. The porcine bioprosthetic valve: experience at 15 years. Ann Thorac Surg 1989;48:324–329.
124. Auport MR, Sirinelli AL, Diermont FF, et al. The last generation of pericardial valves in the aortic position: ten year follow-up in 589 patients. Ann Thorac Surg 1996;61:615–620.
125. Sensky PR, et al. Does the type of prosthesis influence early left ventricular mass reflection after aortic valve replacement? Assessment with magnetic resonance imaging. Am Heart J 2003;146:E13–E19.
126. Carpentier A. Cardiac valve surgery: the "French correction." J Thorac Cardiovasc Surg 1983;86:323–337.
127. Deloche A, Jebara VA, Relland JYM, et al. Valve repair with Carpentier techniques: the second decade. J Thorac Cardiovasc Surg 1990;99:990–1002.

128. Carpentier AF, Lessana A, Relland JYM, et al. The "Physio-Ring": an advanced concept in mitral valve annuloplasty. Ann Thorac Surg 1993;55:860–863.
129. Cosgrove DM, Arcidi JM, Rodriguez L, Stewart WJ, Powell K, Thomas JD. Initial experience with the Cosgrove-Edwards annuloplasty system. Ann Thorac Surg 1995;60:499–504.
130. David TE, Omran A, Armstrong, et al. Long-term results of mitral valve repair for myxomatous disease with and without chordal replacement with expanded polytetrafluorothylene. J Thorac Cardiovasc Surg 1998;115:1279–1286.
131. Lillehei CW, Levy MJ, Bonnabeau RC. Mitral valve replacement with preservation of papillary muscles and chordae tendinae. J Thorac Cardiovasc Surg 1964;47:532–543.
132. Yun KL, et al. Randomized trail comparing partial versus complete chordal sparing mitral valve replacement: effects on left ventricular volume and function. J Thorac Cardiovasc Surg 2002;123:707–711.
133. Elkins RC. Pulmonary autograft: the optimal substitute for the aortic valve. N Engl J Med 1994;330:59–60.
134. Puvimanasinghe JP, et al. Prognosis after aortic valve replacement with a bioprosthesis: prediction based on meta analysis and microsimulation. Circulation 2001;103:1535–1540.
135. Remadi JP, et al. Isolated mitral valve replacement with St. Jude medical prosthesis: long term results: a follow up of 19 years. Circulation 2001;103:1542–1548.
136. Edmunds LH Jr. Thromboembolic complications of current cardiac valve prostheses. Ann Thorac Surg 1981;34:96.
137. David TE, Bos J, Christakis GT, Brofman PR, Wong D, Feindel CM. Heart valve operations in patients with active endocarditis. Ann Thorac Surg 1990;49:701.
138. Christakis GT, Weisel RD, David TE, et al. Factors of operative survival after valve replacement. Circulation 1988;78(suppl I): I25–I30.
139. Klodas E, Enriquez-Sarano M, Tajik AJ, et al. Optimizing timing of surgical correction in patients with severe aortic regurgitation: role of symptoms. J Am Coll Cardiol 1997;30:746–752.
140. Blackstone EH, Kirklin JW. Death and other time-related events after valve replacement. Circulation 1985;72:753–758.
141. Duarte IG, Murphy CO, Kosinski AS, et al. Late survival after valve operation in patients with left ventricular dysfunction. Ann Thorac Surg 1997;64:1089–1095.
142. Grossi EA, Galloway AC, Miller JS, et al. Valve repair versus replacement for mitral insufficiency: when is a mechanical valve still indicated? J Thorac Cardiovasc Surg 1998;115:389–396.
143. Auport MR, Sirinelli AL, Diermont FF, et al. The last generation of pericardial valves in the aortic position: 10 year follow-up in 589 patients. Ann Thorac Surg 1996;61:615–620.
144. Gillinov MA, Cosgrove DM, Lytle BW, et al. Reoperation for failure of mitral valve repair. J Thorac Cardiovasc Surg 1997;113:467–475.
145. Duran CG. Repair of anterior mitral leaflet chordal rupture or elongation (the flipover technique). J Cardiac Surg 1986;1:161–166.
146. Galloway AC, Colvin SB, Baumann FG, et al. A comparison of mitral valve reconstruction with mitral valve replacement: intermediate term results. Ann Thorac Surg 1989;47:655–661.
147. Spencer FC, Galloway AC, Gross EA, et al. Recent developments and evolving techniques of mitral valve reconstruction. Ann Thorac Surg 1998;65:307–313.
148. Bojar RM. Adult Cardiovascular Surgery. Cambridge, UK: Blackwell Science; 1992.
149. Cohn LH. Coronary artery disease and the indications for coronary revascularization. In: Baue AE, Geha AS, Hammond, et al., eds. Glenn's Thoracic and Cardiovascular Surgery, 5th ed. New York: McGraw-Hill; 1991.
150. Callaghan JC, Wartak J. Open Heart Surgery: Theory and Practice. New York: Praeger; 1986.
151. Buckberg GD, Brazier JR, Nelson RL, Goldstein SM, McConnell DH, Cooper N. Studies of the effects of hypothermia on regional myocardial blood flow and metabolism during cardiopulmonary bypass. I. The adequately perfused beating, fibrillating, and arrested heart. J Thorac Cardiovasc Surg 1977;73:87–94.
152. Reed CC, Stafford TB. Cardiopulmonary Bypass, 2nd ed. Houston: Texas Medical Press; 1985.
153. Partington MT, et al. Studies of retrograde cardioplegia. I. J Thorac Cardiovasc Surg 1989;97:613.
154. Baue AE, Geha AS, et al., eds. Glenn's Thoracic and Cardiovascular Surgery, 5th ed. New York: McGraw-Hill; 1991.
155. Greenfield LO, et al. Surgery, 2nd ed. Philadelphia: Lippincott-Raven; 1977.
156. Glomset JA, Ross R. Atherosclerosis and the arterial smooth muscle cells. Science 1973;180:1332.
157. Cohn LH, et al. Decision Making in Cardiothoracic Surgery. Toronto: Decker; 1987.
158. Helm RE, Rosengart TK, Gomez M, et al. Comprehensive multimodality blood conservation: 100 consecutive CABG operations without transfusion. Ann Thorac Surg 1998;65:125–136.
159. Lopez-Sendon J, Gonzalez A, Lopez de Sa E, et al. Diagnosis of subacute ventricular wall rupture after acute myocardial infarction: sensitivity and specificity of clinical, hemodynamic and echocardiographic criteria. J Am Coll Cardiol 1992;19:1145–1153.
160. Schwarz CD, Punzengruber C, Ng CK, et al. Clinical presentation of rupture of the left ventricular free wall after myocardial infarction: report of five cases with successful surgical repair. Thorac Cardiovasc Surg 1996;44:71–75.
160a. Purcaro A, Costantini C, Ciampani N, et al. Diagnostic criteria and management of subacute ventricular free wall rupture complicating myocardial infarction. Am J Cardiol 1997;80:397–405.
161. Komeda M and David TE. Surgical treatment of postinfarction false aneurysm of the left ventricle. J Thorac Cardiovasc Surg 1993;106:1189–1191.
162. Csapo K, Voith L, Szuk T, et al. Postinfarction left ventricular pseudoaneurysm. Clin Cardiol 1997;20:898–903.
163. Frances C, Romero A and Grady D. Left ventricular pseudoaneurysm. J Am Coll Cardiol 1998;32: 557–561.
164. Yeo TC, Malouf JF, Oh JK, et al. Clinical profile and outcome in 52 patients with cardiac pseudoaneurysm. Ann Intern Med 1998;128:299–305.
165. Cosgrove DM, Lytle BW, Taylor PC, et al. Ventricular aneurysm resection. Trends in surgical risk. Circulation 1989;79(suppl I): I97–I101.
166. Komeda M, David TE, Malik A, et al. Operative risks and long-term results of operation for left ventricular aneurysm. Ann Thorac Surg 1992;53:22–29.
167. Mickleborough LL, Maruyama H, Liu P, et al. Results of left ventricular aneurysmectomy with a tailored scar excision and primary closure technique. J Thorac Cardiovasc Surg 1994;107: 690–698.
168. Cooley DA. Management of left ventricular aneurysm by intracavitary repair. In: Cox JL, Seendt TM III, eds. Operative Techniques in Cardiac and Thoracic Surgery 1997;2:170–178.
169. Skillington PD, Lamb RK, Monro JL, et al. Surgical treatment for infarct related ventricular septal defects: improved early results combined with analysis of late functional status. J Thorac Cardiovasc Surg 1990;99:798–808.
170. Muehrcke DD, Daggett WM Jr., Buckley MJ, et al. Postinfarct ventricular septal defect repair: effect of coronary artery bypass grafting. Ann Thorac Surg 1992;54:876–882.
171. David TE, Armstrong S. Surgical repair of postinfarction ventricular septal defect by infarct exclusion. Semin Thorac Cardiovasc Surg 1998;10:105–110.
172. Dalrymple-Hay MJ, Monro, JL, Livesey SA, et al. Postinfarction ventricular septal rupture: the Wessex experience. Semin Thorac Cardiovasc Surg 1998;10:111–116.

173. Panos A, Christakis GT, Lichtenstein SV, et al. Operation for acute postinfarction mitral insufficiency using continuous oxygenated blood cardioplegia. Ann Thorac Surg 1989;48:816–819.
174. Hendren WG, Nemec JJ, Lytle BW, et al. Mitral valve repair for ischemic mitral insufficiency. Ann Thorac Surg 1999;52:1246–1252.
175. Horstkotte D, Schulte HD, Niehues R, et al. Diagnostic and therapeutic consideration in acute, severe mitral regurgitation: experience in 42 consecutive patients entering the intensive care unit with pulmonary edema. J Heart Valve Disease 1993;2:512–522.
176. David TE. Techniques and results of mitral valve repair for ischemic mitral regurgitation. J Card Surg 1994;9:274–277.
177. Hollingshead WH. The Heart, Abdomen, and Pelvis Anatomy for Surgeons. New York: McGraw-Hill; 1971.
178. Wilcox BR, Anderson RN. Surgical Anatomy of the Heart. New York: Raven Press; 1985.
179. Spotnitz JH, Sonnenblick FH, Spiro D. Relationship of ultrastructure to function in the intact heart: sarcomere structure relative to pressure volume curves of the intact left ventricles of dog and cat. Circ Res 1996;18:57.
180. Ross J Jr, Braunwald E. Aortic stenosis. Circulation 1968;38(suppl 5):61.
181. Starr A, Grunkemeier GL. The expected lifetime of porcine valves. Ann Thorac Surg 1989;48:317–318.
182. Jamieson WR. Bioprostheses are superior to mechanical prostheses. Z Kardiol 1986;75(suppl 2):258–271.
183. Jegaden O, Eker A, Delahaye F, Motagna P, Ossette J, Durand de Gevigney G, Mikaeloff PH. Thromboembolic risk and late survival after mitral valve replacement with the St. Jude Medical valve. Annals of Thoracic Surgery, Vol 58, 1721–1728.
184. Bernal JM, Rambasa JM, Gutierrez-Garcia F, Morales C, Nistal JF, Revuelta JM. The CarboMedics valve: experience with 1,049 implants. Ann Thorac Surg. 1998;65:137–143
185. Jamieson WRE, Munro AI, Miyagishima RT, Allen P, Burr LH, Tyers GFO. Carpentier-Edwards standard porcine bioprosthesis: clinical performance to seventeen years. Ann Thorac Surg. 1995;60:999–006.
186. David TE, Ivanov J, Armstrong S, Feindel CM, Cohen G. Late results of heart valve replacement with the Hancock II bioprosthesis. J Thorac Cardiovasc Surg 2001;121:0268–0278.
187. Deloche A, Jebara VA, Relland JYM, et al. Valve repair with Carpentier techniques: the second decade. J Thorac Cardiovasc Surg 1990;99:990–1002.
188. David TE, Armstrong S, Sun Z, Daniel L. Late results of mitral valve repair for mitral regurgitation due to degenerative disease. Ann Thorac Surg 1993;56:7–12.
189. Hammermeister K, Sethi GK, Henderso WG, Grover FL, Oprian C, Rahimtoola SH. Outcomes 15 years after valvbe replacement with a mechanical versus a bioprosthetic valve: report of the Veterans Affairs randomized trial. J Am Coll Cardiol. 2000;36:1152–1158.

78

Cardiac Replacement Therapy

Benjamin C. Sun

The term *cardiac replacement therapy* until recently was limited only to cardiac transplantation. Indeed, the term only evolved as significant innovations were made in the development and implementation of cardiac assist systems as well as xenotransplantation programs. Long-term implantable left ventricular assist devices (LVADs) are currently in use throughout the world with increasing frequency. In addition, the total artificial heart (TAH) is also making resurgence as a viable therapeutic option. Mechanical circulatory support has evolved from a bridge-to-recovery or bridge-to-transplant therapy to also include destination therapy.

Congestive heart failure (CHF) is a nationwide epidemic, with a prevalence of 4.9 million victims and more than 550,000 new cases per year.[1] Cardiac transplantation as treatment for CHF has been successful with a 5-year survival in these patients approaching 71%,[2] compared to 20%–30% 2-year survival in patients with New York Heart Association class IV heart failure.[1,3,4] However, because of a limited donor organ supply, cardiac transplantation will only treat about 2300 patients in the United States per year.[5]

Cardiac assist devices, TAHs, myoblast transplantation, and other treatments will likely play important complementary roles in the future treatment of CHF. We are only beginning to make an epidemiologic impact on this enormous health care epidemic.

History

The first successful use of an LVAD occurred in 1966 when Michael DeBakey supported a patient with postcardiotomy shock for 4 days using an extrathoracic gas-energized hemispherical pump.[6] The first TAH (the Liotta Heart) was also implanted in 1966 by Denton Cooley and his colleagues as a bridge to cardiac transplantation.[7] The implantation of a TAH as an intent for permanent therapy was first performed by William DeVries et al. in 1981. They used the Jarvik-7-100 (now called the CardioWest) TAH, and the patient survived for 112 days.[8]

There are currently eight ventricular assist systems approved by the Food and Drug Administration (FDA) and one TAH system available for commercial use in the United States. There are over 20 assist devices in development worldwide, with several systems undergoing clinical trials in the United States as well as internationally. This chapter discusses the devices currently in use in the United States (Table 78.1).

Mechanical Circulatory Support

Indications

Mechanical circulatory support devices are currently used for three major indications. All of the commercially available devices are designed to address these specific, although overlapping, indications. They can be further differentiated into ventricular assist devices (VADs) and TAHs.

When a patient is in severe cardiogenic shock from a potentially reversible cardiac insult, a ventricular assist system may be used as a bridge to myocardial recovery. The assist system is implanted to decompress the injured myocardium, allowing it to recover and to provide physiologic support for the patient during this time frame. Specific diagnoses include acute viral cardiomyopathies, postpartum cardiomyopathies, postcardiotomy syndromes, and reperfusion injury from cardiac allografts. As the heart recovers and is able to sustain the circulation, the assist device may be weaned and subsequently explanted.

Cardiac transplant candidates who continue to deteriorate despite aggressive pharmacologic support can become candidates for longer-term assist support or a TAH. The mechanical support system is used as a bridge to cardiac transplantation and is explanted at the time of transplantation.

The third indication for mechanical support systems is as an alternative to cardiac transplantation. This indication is for those patients who remain in class IV heart failure but are not cardiac transplant candidates. The Randomized Evaluation of Mechanical Assistance for the Treatment of

TABLE 78.1. Assist Devices Currently in Use in the United States.

	Device	*Drive mechanism*	*Pump type*	*LVAD only*	*RVAD/ BIVAD*	*Implantable*	*Paracorporeal*	*Anticoagulation*	*Bridge to recovery (short-term)*	*Bridge to transplant (long-term)*	*Permanent/ destination therapy (long-term)*	*Outpatient use*
FDA-approved	Abiomed BVS 5000	Pneumatic/ passive fill	Bladder	No	Yes	No	Yes	Yes	Yes	No	No	No
	Abiomed AB 5000	Pneumatic/ augmented diastole	Bladder	No	Yes	No	Yes	Yes	Yes	?	No	No
	TandemHeart[a]	Electric/ continuous flow	Centrifugal	Yes	No	No	Yes	Yes	Yes	No	No	No
	Thoratec PVAD	Pneumatic/ augmented diastole	Bladder	No	Yes	No	Yes	Yes	Yes	Yes	No	Yes
	Thoratec IVAD	Pneumatic/ augmented diastole	Bladder	No	Yes	Yes	Yes	Yes	Yes	Yes	No	Yes
	Thoratec Heartmate IP	Pneumatic/ passive fill	Pusher plate	Yes	No	Yes	No	No	No	Yes	No	Yes
	Thoratec Heartmate XVE	Electric/passive fill	Pusher plate	Yes	No	Yes	No	No	No	Yes	Yes	Yes
	WorldHeart Novacor	Electric/passive fill	Pusher plate	Yes	No	Yes	No	Yes	No	Yes	?	Yes
FDA investigational	Levotronix	Electric/ continuous flow	Centrifugal	Yes	No	No	Yes	Yes	Yes	No	No	No
	MicroMed DeBakey VAD	Electric/ continuous flow	Axial flow	Yes	No	Yes	No	Yes	No	Yes	?	Yes
	Thoratec Heartmate II	Electric/ continuous flow	Axial flow	Yes	No	Yes	No	Yes	No	Yes	?	Yes

[a]Percutaneous access from the femoral vein, through the interatrial septum, into the left atrium.

Congestive Heart Failure (REMATCH) trial was the first randomized trial to compare optimum medical management (OMM) with placement of a Heartmate® VE LVAD in a group of class IV heart failure patients who were not candidates for cardiac transplantation. The primary endpoint of the study was all-cause mortality. Secondary endpoints included morbidity as well as quality of life. This was a multicenter study supported by the National Institutes of Health (NIH) randomizing 129 patients with a follow-up of 2 years. Kaplan-Meier survival analysis showed a reduction of 48% in the risk of death from any cause in the group that received LVADs as compared with the medical therapy group (relative risk 0.52; 95% 0.34 to 0.78; $P = .001$). The rates of survival at 1 year were 52% in the device group and 25% in the medical therapy group ($P = .002$), and the rates at 2 years were 23% and 8% ($P = .09$), respectively. The frequency of serious adverse events in the device group was 2.35 times that in the medical therapy group (95% confidence interval 1.86 to 2.95), with a predominance of infection, bleeding, and malfunction of the device. The quality of life was significantly improved at 1 year in the device group.[9] This landmark study ushered in the era of long-term mechanical support as a viable alternative for end-stage heart failure patients who are not transplant candidates. The Centers for Medicare & Medicaid Services now has acknowledged this as a reimbursable therapy.

As mechanical support systems become smaller, more reliable, and easier to implant, this indication could eventually become the most frequent utilization of this technology.

Ventricular Assist Devices

Ventricular assist devices can be used for isolated left-side support (LVAD), as a right ventricular assist device (RVAD), or as a biventricular assist device (BIVAD).

These devices are attached to the heart through cannulas that allow the blood to enter the pumping chamber, where it is ejected into the systemic or pulmonary circulation. For left-side or systemic circulatory support, all of the devices can be attached to the left ventricular apex as inflow to the pumping chamber. Indeed, this is the preferential site of LVAD attachment for most of the devices and is the only option for some devices. Some devices can function through cannulation of the left atrium either directly or percutaneously through the interatrial septum. The left atrium is not the ideal cannulation site for long-term support as the left ventricle can form large amounts of thrombi due to blood stasis.[10]

For cardiogenic shock, for which short-term LVAD support is anticipated, left atrial cannulation is a reasonable option. The LVAD outflow graft is anastomosed to the aorta, usually the ascending aorta.

For right-side support, either right atrial or right ventricular cannulation can be used successfully. Substantial thrombus formation in the right ventricle does not appear to occur with right atrial cannulation even in long-term support. The RVAD outflow graft is anastomosed to the pulmonary artery.

The VADs can be implanted without the support of cardiopulmonary bypass (CPB), but CPB is generally used to maintain patient stability.[11]

Current Devices

There are two types of physiologic blood flow-generating mechanisms used: volume displacement pumps and continuous flow pumps. Volume displacement pumps are considered first-generation pumps. Continuous flow pumps can be axial flow devices, centrifugal devices, or magnetic levitation (Mag-Lev) devices. Axial flow pumps are considered second-generation pumps, and Mag-Lev pumps are considered third-generation pumps.

Volume Displacement Pumps

Volume displacement pumps are considered first-generation pumps and are still the most widely used type of circulatory support. They work by ejecting the blood out of a fixed-volume chamber by either a pusher plate mechanism or an air-driven bladder. These pumps can all be run in a fixed-rate pumping mode as well as an automatic mode. In fixed-rate mode, either a pump rate or cardiac output is set; the pump will remain pumping at that set level. In the automatic mode, the pumps are preload responsive and will increase or decrease their outputs depending on the patient's volume status or physiologic demand.

Volume displacement pumps are pulsatile pumps that function independent of the cardiac cycle in either fixed mode or volume (auto) mode. When biventricular assist is used, the RVAD also functions independent of the LVAD.

Abiomed BVS 5000/AB 5000

The Abiomed BVS 5000 is the most widely used system in the United States. The system is easy to implant, requires minimal adjustments to initialize and maintain support, and can be used as univentricular or biventricular support. Its design is only useful as a short-term support system, and it has limited efficacy beyond 1 week of support. There is a large amount of surface area of tubing to which the blood is exposed, and hence the anticoagulation regimen for successful use is quite stringent (Fig. 78.1).

The AB 5000 is the newer design of this pump. It also is a paracorporeal pump and has less surface area for the blood

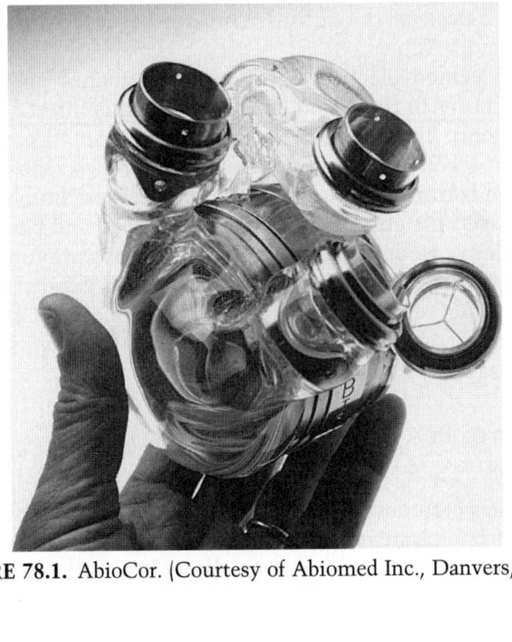

FIGURE 78.1. AbioCor. (Courtesy of Abiomed Inc., Danvers, MA.)

to contact, allowing improved patient mobility. In addition, it adds vacuum assistance for diastolic augmentation of VAD filling.

Thoratec Heartmate

The Thoratec Heartmate is an implantable LVAD that is currently the most widely used system for bridge to transplantation. There is a pneumatically actuated (implantable pneumatic [IP]) as well as an electrically actuated (X vented electric [XVE]) system. The IP is not often implanted anymore as it is not approved for outpatient use. The electrically actuated system is the only system that has received FDA approval for use as destination therapy. The blood contact surfaces for both systems are identical and incorporate a single pusher plate system housed in a titanium shell. A Hall sensor detects the position of the pusher plate at both end systole and end diastole. The pusher plate drives a unique textured polyurethane diaphragm against a sintered titanium shell. The textured surface facilitates the attachment of a neointima along the blood-contacting surface of the diaphragm and effectively prevents thrombus formation. These are currently the only assist systems that do not require anticoagulation.

The pumping chamber is centered between two titanium supported valve housings that hold porcine bioprosthetic inlet and outlet valves. The device can only be attached through the left ventricular apex, and the outlet Dacron graft is attached to the ascending aorta. The chamber is internalized in a preperitoneal pocket or placed intraperitoneally. The driveline is externalized and in the pneumatic version is connected to the drive console through an interconnect cable. The pump has a maximum stroke volume of 85 mL and maximum output of 11 L/min.

The pneumatic drive console actuates the pumping chamber and has a simple efficient display with intuitive adjustment modalities. It displays rate (beats/min), output (L/min), and mode (auto or fixed) as well as an overlapping bar graph that indicates how the pumping chamber is filling and emptying. Alarms chime for flow rates below 2.0 L/min. It is relatively lightweight and moderate size, allowing good patient mobility. An internal battery drives the system for up to 30 min for transport or independent mobility. In the event of a catastrophic console failure, a hand crank is removed from the back of the console and can be used to manually drive the LVAD.

The vented electric (XVE) system attaches an electric torque motor to the pump chamber (which is internalized in the patient). The driveline is attached to a small controller worn on a belt. The system is powered by two rechargeable lead acid batteries that allow 4–6 h of untethered mobility. A powerbase unit charges six batteries at once and can power the device as well. In the event of a catastrophic motor failure, a hand pump that is carried by the patient can be used to manually drive the LVAD. The XVE can be driven by the pneumatic console for diagnostics or during a catastrophic motor failure.

Thoratec Percutaneous/Implantable Ventricular Assist Device

Both the percutaneous VAD (PVAD) and implantable VAD (IVAD) systems are pulsatile pneumatically actuated systems. The PVAD is placed paracorporeally, whereas the IVAD can be placed either paracorporeally or intracorporeally (Fig. 78.2). When placed paracorporeally, the cannulas are internalized but traverse the abdominal wall to the externalized pumping chamber, which rests on the upper abdomen of the patient. They can be configured as an LVAD, RVAD, or BIVAD.

Sandwiched between the cannulas is a single-chamber drive unit separated by two Bjork-Shiley mechanical valves. The blood chamber is a smooth, seamless polyurethane sac housed within a transparent polysulfone shell. A fill switch is used to sense pump chamber filling; however, it is not integrated into the drive system of the console, only the alarm system. In addition, appropriate emptying of the device is performed by manual inspection of the pumping chamber. The device is pneumatically actuated but is one of only two systems that employ suction for preload assistance. An air hose connects the drive console with the pumping chamber as well as the electrical connector to the fill sensor. The system requires manual adjustments of ejection pressure, ejection duration, as well as vacuum levels to optimize output.

The system ejects a relatively constant 65-mL stroke volume and increases output by increasing the rate. The system senses the rate of air displacement (rate of ventricular filling) and responds by either shortening diastole (increasing rate) or lengthening diastole (slowing rate). The maximum output of the device is 7.2 L/min (110 beats/min). It can be used in small patients (<0.8 m^2 body surface area).[12]

The dual-drive console (DDC) display is complex and displays a variety of information, including rate (beats/min), output (L/min), ejection duration (ms), mode (auto or set rate), ejection pressure (mmHg), and vacuum (mmHg). The alarm chimes with console malfunctions or when flows occur below a set threshold. An internal battery drives the system for up to 1 h for transport. In the event of a catastrophic console failure, a suction bulb can be used to manually drive both the RVAD and LVAD individually. A perfusionist is not required for continuous monitoring of this system but is usually required for troubleshooting. The DDC is rather large and limits patient mobility, although it has infinite flexibility in adjustment of the VADs and is most useful early after surgery. A smaller portable drive unit called the TLC II can then be used to facilitate patient mobility and eventual discharge from the hospital. The PVADs/IVADs require anticoagulation

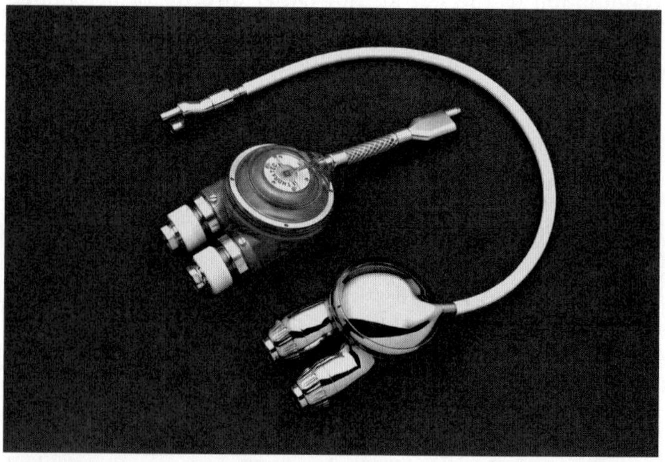

FIGURE 78.2. Thoratec PVAD (left) and IVAD (right). (Reprinted with permission from Thoratec Corporation.)

with heparin or coumadin to maintain an international normalized ratio (INR) of 2.5–3.5 times normal.

WorldHeart Novacor

The Novacor left ventricular assist system (LVAS) is an electromagnetically powered driver attached to two symmetrically opposed pusher plates; it is implanted in the same fashion as the Heartmate. The blood chamber is a smooth, seamless polyurethane sac straddled by two pericardial tissue valves enclosed in a fiberglass-reinforced shell. A percutaneous driveline houses the air vent and wiring that is attached to an external controller and batteries. The pump has a maximum stroke volume of 70mL with a maximum output of 10L/min.

The Novacor system functions in three different modes. Like the Heartmate and Thoratec systems, it can function in fixed mode, but it can also be actuated by an electrocardiogram triggered mode as well as an internal pulse-triggered mode.

The external controller and battery packs are worn similar to the Heartmate XVE, allowing excellent patient mobility and relative independence. The Novacor LVAS requires anticoagulation to maintain an INR above 3.5.[13]

The Novacor system is approved for a bridge to cardiac transplantation and is currently under study as a destination therapy pump.

Limitations

The current ventricular assist systems all require patent outflow valves (aortic or pulmonary) to function appropriately. Even mild preoperative aortic insufficiency (AI) can be problematic since patients in cardiogenic shock will have a low systemic pressure and a high left ventricular end diastolic pressure (LVEDP) and volume (LVEDV). The aortic transvalvular gradient will subsequently be low. With implementation of LVAD support, the LVEDP will be very low, and the mean aortic pressure will be higher; the aortic transvalvular gradient will therefore be much greater. Mild preoperative AI can become severe AI with LVAD support. There are characteristically high device flows as the insufficient valve fills the ventricle and subsequently the VAD. The LVAD may sustain high flow rates and appear to be functioning well; however, this is a circular flow, and the net forward "perfusion" flow will be low. The aortic valve must be addressed in this situation, but the approaches are controversial, and there is insufficient experience to suggest a preferred method.

The presence of an aortic valve prosthesis has been considered a relative contraindication to LVAD support. The aortic valve typically remains closed when on support as the failing heart is usually unable to eject into the higher systemic pressure generated by the LVAD, although there are times when the heart will occasionally eject (i.e., if the heart begins to recover or if the LVAD is being vented). If a prosthetic aortic valve is in place, thrombus can be generated in the outflow tract under the valve. Thromboembolism can then occur if the heart ejects. Methods to address this problem range from oversewing the valve to excising the valve and covering the annulus with a patch.[14] I have personally placed a patch over a mechanical valve (including a Starr-Edwards valve) to keep the valve in the fixed closed position in 12 patients without complication. However, experience with these treatment approaches remains quite limited and anecdotal.

Mitral valve prostheses are generally not considered a contraindication for device support since the valve will continue to open and close provided the apex of the left ventricle is cannulated for device inflow.

Quiescent intracardiac shunts may become clinically apparent and significant with changes in chamber pressures when these devices are initiated. A patent foramen ovale (PFO) is present in up to 20% of the population but is clinically quiescent in the vast majority of these patients. With unloading of the left ventricle and left atrium with LVAD support, right atrial pressure will be higher than left atrial pressure. Even a small PFO in these circumstances can produce a large right-to-left shunt manifested by arterial desaturation and potential air embolism. These shunts should be closed when identified and should be assessed both before and after initiation of device support by transesophageal echo (TEE) flow studies. If identified preoperatively, cannulation techniques for CPB may be altered to facilitate repair.

Physiologic Problems

Thromboembolism was the first great battle that device developers had to face. Common sense would support the idea that creating a blood–surface interface as biologically smooth as possible would minimize blood component activation and thromboembolic events. Indeed, most developers followed this concept with variable success. Flow characteristics of the pumping chamber, valves, and cannula contribute to thromboembolism formation as well, especially if areas of stasis are present. These systems all require stringent anticoagulation to help minimize thromboembolic events, with the notable exception of the Heartmate systems.

The Abiomed, Thoratec, and Novacor systems all employ smooth, seamless blood sacs. The thromboembolic incidence of the Thoratec is about 6% of patients supported.[15] The Novacor LVAS has had a thromboembolic rate of 47% of patients supported.[16] Modifications are under exploration to help decrease this high incidence of events in the Novacor system. The current iteration appears promising.[17]

The Heartmate systems employ a counterintuitive textured surface pumping chamber and cannula. The premise was to create a surface that could facilitate cell adhesion and creation of a stable biologic lining that would prevent thrombus formation. This approach in concert with other unique design features has been quite successful in minimizing thromboembolic events, with incidences around 5%.[18] What makes this low incidence particularly significant is that it is achieved without the use of any anticoagulation. (Some patients do receive anticoagulation for other reasons, such as persistent arrhythmias.)

Infection is currently the major cause of morbidity in the stable supported patient. Device-related infections occur in 20%–70% of patients.[18–23] The vast majority of these infections are driveline-related, and driveline infections appear to predispose patients to LVAD pocket or device "endocarditis," which is infection involving the blood-contacting surface of the device. All of the current systems traverse the skin in some manner. Despite coating the skin exit surfaces with material to facilitate cellular ingrowth and adhesion, true fixation and biologic seal are rarely achieved. In addition, even when fixation is achieved, it can be easily disrupted by torque of any kind at the exit site. Reengineering the drivelines to make them smaller and more flexible have anecdotally improved the infection rate. However, the infection problem will not likely be resolved satisfactorily until totally implantable systems are used, thereby removing any percutaneous component to the systems.

Isolated driveline infections are managed conservatively with suppressive antibiotics until transplantation. Device pocket infections can be treated with suppressive antibiotics alone or in combination with muscle flaps and open drainage with pocket irrigation systems[24] as well as antibiotic-impregnated methylmethacrylate beads.[25]

Device endocarditis can be more problematic. Clinical and laboratory evidence of sepsis combined with embolic events are pathognomonic and can occur in up to half of the patients with the diagnosis. Indeed, the diagnosis can only be confirmed at device explant. However, the diagnosis can be very difficult to make in patients without overt embolism; the associated common symptoms of fatigue, anorexia, and low-grade fevers are nonspecific. Computed tomographic (CT) scanning and ultrasound studies cannot penetrate the device housing and therefore cannot image the device valves for vegetations. Management options for the patient with device endocarditis involve either urgent transplant, including taking a marginal donor, or device replacement.[26]

Increases in panel reactive antibody (PRA) formation have been identified in patients supported by LVADs.[27] This was initially thought to be related to transfusion requirements during device implant despite the routine use of leukodepleted blood products. Three of my own patients developed high PRAs soon after device implant despite not receiving transfusions of any kind. Anecdotal reports were identified at other centers as well.[28] The significance of preformed antibodies with respect to incidence and severity of rejection episodes and long-term survival is controversial. Nevertheless, the idea that the LVAD could stimulate immunologic upregulation is intriguing. Attention has focused on the cells adhered to the surface of the Heartmate LVAD as the potential culprit. Immunopotential cells were identified, including activated macrophages, T-helper cells, B cells, as well as possibly a hematopoietic stem cell (expresses marker for CD34).[29,30]

Despite findings implicating the textured surface pseudoendothelium as the culprit, studies also suggest that the PRA issue is not unique to the Heartmate system but is seen in the Novacor system as well.[31,32] This observation confuses the issue as the Novacor system does not employ a textured blood-contacting surface and therefore does not have a pseudoendothelial layer. This immunologic upregulation may therefore be related to an as-yet-unidentified stimulation related to both these systems, such as an electrical or magnetic field.

Mechanical reliability and durability are issues that only recently have been truly tested. Although these devices have faced stringent in vitro and animal durability trials to satisfy FDA benchmarks, the human experiment is the only way to assess these issues in the manner in which the unpredictable patient will use them. Indeed, these devices were designed to support patients with the assumption that some level of circumspection would be exercised in the level of activity in which the patients would engage. Snowboarding, rock climbing, basketball, and cheerleading were not activities that these devices were expected to tolerate. Nevertheless, these are the types of current and continuing activities of these patients. Therefore, durability and reliability issues are constantly redefined.

Catastrophic device failures have occurred with these systems and have resulted in deaths. Fortunately, it is an uncommon occurrence, only affecting 1%–5% of supported patients.[19] Low-level malfunctions of device controllers requiring bedside change-outs are more common in the Heartmate XVE system, although they are rarely of physiologic significance. Modifications to all these systems to improve durability are constantly implemented as experience grows and issues are identified. Nonetheless, several systems, including the Thoratec PVAD/IVAD and Novacor systems,[32a,32b] have continuously supported patients in excess of 2 years and running. The current successful bridge-to-transplantation rate is 60%–74% for all devices, with the majority of deaths occurring perioperatively (International Society of Heart and Lung Transplantation Mechanical Circulatory Support Data Registry, 2006).

Axial Flow Systems

There are several axial flow systems that are being evaluated as a method for ventricular support. The concept of this approach is the use of an impeller (high-speed rotor) to drive the blood instead of a pusher plate or volume displacement. The potential advantages are many and include primarily a significant reduction in size since a pumping chamber is not required. These pumps are typically the size of a D battery. In addition, inflow and outflow valves are not required, thereby eliminating valve durability issues. A compliance chamber is not required. Anticoagulation is currently required in all of these pumps as well.

There are three systems currently in clinical trials in the United States: the MicroMed Technology Inc. (NASA/DeBakey) assist device,[33,34] the Thoratec Heartmate II,[35,36] and the Jarvik 2000[37,38] (Figs. 78.3 and 78.4). These devices are implanted in much the same way as the current systems, with the inflow attached to the apex of the left ventricle and the outflow graft attached to the ascending or descending thoracic aorta. Their small size permits less-extensive dissec-

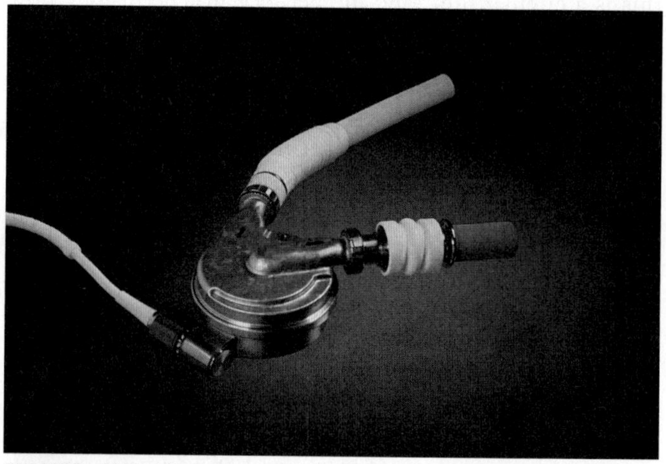

FIGURE 78.3. Heartmate III. (Reprinted with permission from Thoratec Corporation.)

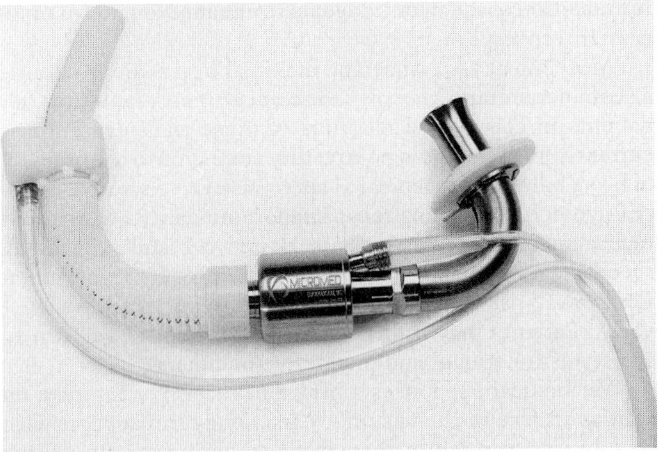

FIGURE 78.4. MicroMed DeBakey VAD. (Courtesy of MicroMed Cardiovascular Inc., Houston, TX.)

tion outside the thoracic cavity. The active issues that are under study include the potential for hemolysis, heat generation from the bearings, device regurgitation if the pump stops (no valves to prevent regurgitant flow), and physiologic tolerance of prolonged low-pulsatile flow. Interestingly, although these pumps have set revolutions per minute, the patient usually will develop a pulsatile blood pressure over time as the heart usually has some level of recovery and begins to eject blood.[39–41]

The maximum pump speeds for all these systems run around 11,000 to 12,500 rpm with power consumptions of 7–12 W.[35,37,42]

The MicroMed and Heartmate II pumps are in trials for bridge to transplantation as well as for destination therapy. There is also a pediatric version of the MicroMed system, the DeBakey VAD *Child*, which is approved under an humanitarian device exemption (HDE) for the pediatric population. The Jarvik 2000 is in a trial for bridge to transplantation.

The Jarvik 2000 system is developing a unique percutaneous carbon pedestal electrical power connector that is mounted in the skull behind the ear. The scalp is highly vascularized and is thought to be more resistant to infection.[42a]

Total Artificial Heart

Indications

The TAH is implanted in the chest after removing the native heart. Early devices had marginal success rates,[43] and enthusiasm for their use waned with the success of the LVAD. Although the LVAD will likely remain the more widely used type of support system, there are certainly patient groups with indications for a TAH.

Patients who have severe biventricular failure requiring long-term biventricular support or patients with severe pulmonary hypertension may benefit from a TAH. Alternatively, they can be treated with the Thoratec systems using biventricular support. Patients who have severe fixed pulmonary vascular resistance currently may require a heart-lung transplant as the donor heart often cannot generate high pressures. The 1-year survival for heart-lung transplantation is 60%, with a survival half-life of 2.6 years.[5] These patients may be better served with a TAH and the donor organs used in patients who would obtain longer survivals from them.

There are also many patients who are poor candidates for LVAD or BIVAD support for anatomical or physiologic reasons. These include patients with large intracardiac shunts, either congenital or acquired (ischemic ventricular septal defect). Patients with prosthetic aortic valves may be better served with a TAH rather than undergoing "creative" surgical interventions to control the thromboembolic risk.

Certain patients would be better served with excision of their native heart, such as heart failure patients with endocarditis or patients with a large ventricular thrombus, a large ventricular aneurysm, or malignant cardiac tumors.

A growing population of heart transplant recipients will develop graft vasculopathy (chronic allograft rejection) over time. This could potentially be the largest population for chronic TAH support as there is presently no good treatment option for this patient population. The actuarial survival rate for retransplantation is 55% at 1 year as compared to a 1-year survival rate of 90% for a first-time heart recipient.[5] Many centers do not perform cardiac retransplantation for chronic allograft rejection because of the limited efficacy derived from this precious commodity. Placement of an LVAD for chronic or permanent support is suboptimal since immunosuppression would still need to be continued to maintain the graft, which could exacerbate infection concerns as well as the other side effects associated with chronic immunosuppression. This rapidly growing patient population could certainly benefit from excision of the graft and chronic support with a TAH.[44,45]

Current Devices

CardioWest

The CardioWest TAH is a pneumatic, implantable system that has recently received FDA approval as a bridge to transplantation. It is the current iteration of the widely publicized Jarvik-7-100 heart used in the patient Barney Clark. It has been utilized worldwide as a bridge to heart transplantation in over 81 patients. Of these patients, 79% were successfully bridged to transplantation. The 1- and 5-year survivals post-transplantation were 86% and 64%, respectively.[46]

Abiomed AbioCor

The AbioCor is the first totally implantable TAH. It is currently in a phase I clinical trial for destination therapy in patients in cardiogenic shock who will not likely survive 30 days without this intervention. It uses a unidirectional, centrifugal hydraulic pump that displaces a fluid (methyl silicon) from one pump chamber to another, which subsequently displaces blood. The system uses a unique hydraulic compliance chamber housed within the right hydraulic chamber, as well as unique proprietary trileaflet polyurethane valves. This system has an implantable controller with internal backup battery capability and employs a transcutaneous energy transfer system (TETS) technology. It is a fairly large pump, and its use will be limited to those who have a fairly large thoracic cavity.[47]

A smaller pump, the AbioCor II, is in development. It is based on a low-friction reversing screw drive motor attached to two pusher plates that alternately compress blood sacs for the right and left circulation. This pump is still a few years away from clinical trial but has the potential for greater application due to its smaller size.

Future Systems

Totally Implantable Systems

Totally implantable systems currently exist in two clinically utilized mechanical support systems, the AbioCor TAH and the Arrow LionHeart. Other device systems are in development with this goal in mind.

To achieve this, the device controller and backup power source (battery) must be implanted. For pusher plate-type systems, a compliance chamber must be introduced. Energy must be transferred through the skin to drive the unit and recharge the battery. Current battery technology is not able to provide batteries that will be sufficient on their own to drive the units for an appropriate length of time with the current power demands of these systems.

The percutaneous driveline will be replaced with TETS. Energy is transmitted through the skin from an external primary TETS coil to a secondary TETS coil that is implanted under the skin. Because no driveline would penetrate the skin, infections should be significantly reduced.

As a pusher plate contracts and displaces the blood from the blood chamber, air is introduced to the opposite chamber to allow the pusher plate to move. This function is facilitated by the driveline as it is the conduit where the air may enter the pump. To internalize the pump, a compliance chamber must be created to allow this movement of air or displacing solution.

Third-Generation Pumps

The third-generation Mag-Lev pumps function on the principle of magnetic bearings. The impeller or rotor would float in this magnetic field and be rotated. The theoretical benefits to this technology include less heat generation as well as improved durability, as there are no traditional bearings to generate friction heat and wear. There is also the possibility of fewer or no anticoagulation requirements in these pumps as well.

Two third-generation pumps, Ventrassist's VentraCor and Impella Cardiosystems AG, are in clinical trials in Australia and Europe.

Enhancing Myocardial Recovery

Mechanical support systems can be used as a tool to support the circulation of a patient and rest the heart. In a small number of patients with chronic heart failure, long-term support has allowed enough recovery of the myocardium to allow explanation of the devices with sustained preservation of myocardial function.[48,49] Therapies are being explored that can be instituted at the time of device implant to help enhance this myocardial recovery. Possibilities include autologous myoblast transplantation,[50] vascular growth factors, and chemotherapy.[51] The VAD can be a tool to facilitate introduction of therapeutic agents to enhance long-term myocardial recovery.

Mechanical assistance and artificial hearts are becoming a complementary therapy to cardiac transplantation for patients in class IV heart failure. Cardiac transplantation is currently an epidemiologic triviality compared to the problem of heart failure. Mechanical support has evolved from a resuscitative tool to a long-term support modality. Outpatient management of these systems is growing and will likely accelerate as patients wait longer and longer for transplantation. Many patients have been supported for greater than 1 year.[52] Patients may return to work or school and return to society as functional and productive members.

Mechanical support as a bridge to recovery may take on a different face in the ensuing years. Long-term support with the ability to institute therapy to "reinvigorate" the ailing heart with gene therapy, cellular transplantation, or chemotherapy is being actively studied.

Our success with mechanical support in patients as bridge to transplantation has set the groundwork for the use of these devices as permanent therapy.[18,19,52–55] Device evolution has been steady and has improved on the shortcomings of the current systems. The limitations of the current systems will be reduced significantly by the systems in development. As device reliability, durability, and patient quality of life continue to improve in the device-supported patient, we may change our criteria for heart transplantation. Patients who are in cardiogenic shock or who are older have historically had poorer survival (International Society of Heart and Lung Transplantation Heart Transplant Data Registry 2006). These patients may receive mechanical support as permanent therapy and reserve cardiac transplantation for those who would get the best/longest survival from the graft (i.e., younger patient without end-organ dysfunction or significant comorbidity).

The use of permanent mechanical support for treatment of end-stage heart failure is in its infancy. Around 200 mechanical support devices have been implanted in the United States for patients as destination therapy. These implants have been limited to about 50 U.S. centers with the multidisciplinary team established to support these patients with intensive needs. The number of device implants will continue to rise modestly over the next few years for all indications. As newer and more durable and reliable pumps become available, the acceptance of this therapy will likely grow more rapidly.

Only when we can achieve this with acceptable morbidity and mortality will we make a significant impact on the treatment of this quiet epidemic.

References

1. American Heart Association. Heart Disease and Stroke Statistics—2005 Update. Dallas, TX: American Heart Association; 2005.
2. Bennett LE, Keck BM, Hertz MI, Trulock EP, Taylor DO. Worldwide thoracic organ transplantation: a report from the UNOS/ISHLT international registry for thoracic organ transplantation. Clin Transpl 2001;25–40.
3. CONSENSUS Trial Study Group. Effects of enalapril on mortality in severe congestive heart failure. N Engl J Med 1987;316:1429–1435.
4. Cowie MR, Mosterd A, Wood DA, et al. The epidemiology of heart failure. Eur Heart J 1997;18:208–225.

5. United Network for Organ Sharing (UNOS) 2003 Annual Report. US Department of Health and Human Resources.
6. DeBakey ME. Left ventricular bypass pump for cardiac assistance. Clinical experience. Am J Cardiol 1971;27:3–11.
7. Cooley DA, Liotta D, Hallman GL, et al. Orthotopic cardiac prosthesis for two staged cardiac replacement. Am J Cardiol 1969;24:723–730.
8. DeVries WC, Anderson JL, Joyce LD, et al. Clinical use of the total artificial heart. N Engl J Med 1984;310:273–278.
9. Rose EA, Gelijns AC, Moskowitz AJ, et al. of the Randomized Evaluation of Mechanical Assistance for the Treatment of Congestive Heart Failure (REMATCH) Study Group. Long-term mechanical left ventricular assistance for end-stage heart failure. N Engl J Med 2001;345:1435–1443.
10. Farrar D. Atrial versus ventricular cannulation for bridge to transplantation with the Thoratec VAD system. Presentation at: Cardiovascular Technology and Science meeting; 1992.
11. Piacentino V 3rd, Jones J, Fisher CA, et al. Off-pump technique for insertion of a HeartMate Vented Electric left ventricular assist device. J Thorac Cardiovasc Surg 2004;127:262–264.
12. Thoratec VAD System Monograph of Clinical Results. Pleasanton: CA, March 1998.
13. Miller PJ, Billich TJ, LaForge DH, et al. Initial clinical experience with a wearable controller for the Novacor left ventricular assist system. ASAIO J 1994;40:M465–M470.
14. Oz MC, Dembitsky W. Personal communication and personal experience.
15. Pennington DG, McBride LR, Miller LW, Swartz MT. Eleven years' experience with the Pierce-Donachy ventricular assist device. J Heart Lung Transplant 1994;13:803–810.
16. Schmid C, Weyand M, Nabavi DG, et al. Cerebral and systemic embolization during left ventricular support with the Novacor N100 device. Ann Thorac Surg 1998;65:1703–1710.
17. Portner PM, Jansen PG, Oyer PE, Wheeldon DR, Ramasamy N. Improved outcomes with an implantable left ventricular assist system: a multicenter study. Ann Thorac Surg 2001;71:205–209.
18. McCarthy PM, Smedira NO, Vargo RL, et al. One hundred patients with the HeartMate left ventricular assist device: evolving concepts and technology. J Thorac Cardiovasc Surg 1998; 115:904–912.
19. Sun B, Catanese K, Spanier T, et al. One hundred long term implantable LVADs: the Columbia Presbyterian interim experience. Ann Thorac Surg 1999;68:688–694.
20. McBride LR, Swartz MT, Reedy JE, Miller LW, Pennington DG. Device related infections in patients supported with mechanical circulatory support devices for greater than 30 days. ASAIO Trans 1991;37:M258–M259.
21. Argenziano M, Catanese KA, Moazami N, et al. The influence of infection on survival and successful transplantation in patients with left ventricular assist devices. J Heart Lung Transplant 1997;16:822–831.
22. Holman WL, Park SJ, Long JW, et al., REMATCH Investigators. Infection in permanent circulatory support: experience from the REMATCH trial. J Heart Lung Transplant 2004;23:1359–1365.
23. Fischer SA, Trenholme GM, Costanzo MR, Piccione W. Infectious complications in left ventricular assist device recipients. Clin Infect Dis 1997;24:18–23.
24. Umaña JP, Ewing D, Sun BC, et al. Use of pedicled muscle flaps successfully manages wound infections in implantable left ventricular assist device (LVAD) patients with a low incidence of device endocarditis [abstract]. J Heart Lung Transplant 1997; 16:93.
25. Holman WL. Personal communication.
26. Prendergast TW, Todd BA, Beyer AJ 3rd, et al. Management of left ventricular assist device infection with heart transplantation. Ann Thorac Surg 1997;64:142–147.
27. Massad MG, Cook DJ, Schmitt SK, et al. Factors influencing HLA sensitization in implantable LVAD recipients. Ann Thorac Surg 1997;64:1120–1125.
28. TCI Investigators and Users Meeting; 1997.
29. Spanier T, Oz M, Levin H, et al. Activation of coagulation and fibrinolytic pathways in patients with left ventricular assist devices. J Thorac Cardiovasc Surg 1996;112:1090–1097.
30. Spanier T, Oz M, Levin H, et al. Activation of coagulation and fibrinolytic-pathways in patients with left ventricular assist devices. Thorac Cardiovasc Surg 1996;112:1090–1097.
31. Ankersmit HJ, Tugulea S, Spanier T, et al. Activation-induced T-cell death and immune dysfunction after implantation of left-ventricular assist device. Lancet 1999;354:550–555.
32. Itescu S, Schuster M, Burke E, et al. Immunobiologic consequences of assist divices. Cardiol Clin 2003;21:119–133, ix–x.
32a. Slaughter MS, Tsui SS, El-Banayosy A, et al. Results of a multicenter clinical trial with the Thoratec Implantable Ventricular Assist Device. J Thorac Cardiovasc Surg 2007;133(6): 1573–1580. Erratum in: J Thorac Cardiovasc Surg 2007;134(3): A34.
32b. Wheeldon DR, LaForge DH, Lee J, Jansen PG, Jassawalla JS, Portner PM. Novacor left ventricular assist system long-term performance: comparison of clinical experience with demonstrated in vitro reliability. ASAIO J 2002;48(5):546–551.
33. Kawahito K, Benkowski R, Ohtsubo S, Noon GP, Nose Y, DeBakey ME. Improved flow straighteners reduce thrombus in the NASA/DeBakey axial flow ventricular assist device. Artif Organs 1997;21:339–343.
34. Mizuguchi K, Damm G, Benkowsky R, et al. Development of an axial flow ventricular assist device: in vitro and in vivo evaluation. Artif Organs 1995;19:653–659.
35. Macha M, Litwak P, Yamazaki K, et al. Survival for up to 6 months in calves supported with an implantable axial flow ventricular assist device. ASAIO 1997;43:311–315.
36. Frazier OH, Delgado RM 3rd, Kar B, Patel V, Gregoric ID, Myers TJ. First clinical use of the redesigned HeartMate II left ventricular assist system in the United States: a case report. Tex Heart Inst J 2004;31:157–159.
37. Westaby S, Katsumata T, Evans R, Pigott D, Taggart DP, Jarvik RK. The Jarvik 2000 Oxford system: increasing the scope of mechanical circulatory support. J Thorac Cardiovasc Surg 1997;114:467–474.
38. Frazier OH, Shah NA, Myers TJ, Robertson KD, Gregoric ID, Delgado R. Use of the Flowmaker (Jarvik 2000) left ventricular assist device for destination therapy and bridging to transplantation. Cardiology 2004;101:111–116.
39. Frazier OH, Shah NA, Myers TJ, Robertson KD, Gregoric ID, Delgado R. Use of the flowmaker (Jarvik 2000) left ventricular assist device for destination therapy and bridging to transplantation. Cardiology 2004;101:111–116.
40. Vitali E, Lanfranconi M, Ribera E, et al. Successful experience in bridging patients to heart transplantation with the MicroMed DeBakey ventricular assist device. Ann Thorac Surg 2003;75: 1200–1204.
41. Myers TJ, Robertson K, Pool T, Shah N, Gregoric I, Frazier OH. Continuous flow pumps and total artificial hearts: management issues. Ann Thorac Surg 2003;75(6 suppl):S79–S85.
42. Kawahito K, Damm G, Benkowski R, et al. Ex vivo phase 1 evaluation of the DeBakey/NASA axial flow ventricular assist device. Artif Organs 1996;20:47–52.
42a. Hohlweg-Majert B, Gutwald R, Siegenthaler MP, Schmelzeisen R. Implantation of the Jarvik 2000 left-ventricular-assist-device: role of the maxillofacial surgeon. Eur J Cardiothorac Surg 2005;28:337–339.
43. Muneretto C, Rabago G Jr, Pavie A, et al. Mechanical circulatory support as a bridge to transplantation: current status of total

artificial heart in 1989 and determinants of survival. J Cardiovasc Surg 1990;31:486–491.
44. Lederman DM, Kung RT, McNair DS. Therapeutic potential of implantable replacement hearts. Am J Cardiovasc Drugs 2002;2:297–301.
45. Frazier OH, Dowling RD, Gray LA Jr, Shah NA, Pool T, Gregoric I. The total artificial heart: where we stand. Cardiology 2004;101:117–121.
46. Copeland JG, Smith RG, Arabia FA, et al., CardioWest Total Artificial Heart Investigators. Cardiac replacement with a total artificial heart as a bridge to transplantation. N Engl J Med 2004;351:859–867.
47. Dowling RD, Gray LA Jr, Etoch SW, et al. Initial experience with the AbioCor implantable replacement heart system. J Thorac Cardiovasc Surg 2004;127:131–141.
48. Helman DN, Maybaum SW, Morales DL, et al. Recurrent remodeling after ventricular assistance: is long-term myocardial recovery attainable? Ann Thorac Surg 2000;70:1255–1258.
49. Farrar DJ, Holman WR, McBride LR, et al. Long-term follow-up of Thoratec ventricular assist device bridge-to-recovery patients successfully removed from support after recovery of ventricular function. J Heart Lung Transplant 2002;21:516–521.
50. Pagani FD, DerSimonian H, Zawadzka A, et al. Autologous skeletal myoblasts transplanted to ischemia-damaged myocardium in humans. Histological analysis of cell survival and differentiation. J Am Coll Cardiol 2003;41:879–888.
51. Hon JK, Yacoub MH. Bridge to recovery with the use of left ventricular assist device and clenbuterol. Ann Thorac Surg 2003;75(6 suppl):S36–S41.
52. Oz MC, Argenziano M, Catanese KA, et al. Bridge experience with long-term implantable left ventricular assist devices. Are they an alternative to transplantation? Circulation 1997;95:1844–1852.
53. DeRose JJ, Argenziano M, Sun BC, Reemtsma K, Oz MC, Rose EA. Implantable left ventricular assist devices: an evolving long-term cardiac replacement therapy. Ann Surg 1997;226:461–468; discussion 468–470.
54. Oz MC, Argenziano M, Catanese KA, et al. Bridge experience with long-term implantable left ventricular assist devices. Are they an alternative to transplantation? Circulation 1997;95:1844–1852.
55. DeRose JJ Jr, Umana JP, Argenziano M, et al. Implantable left ventricular assist devices provide an excellent outpatient bridge to transplantation and recovery. J Am Coll Cardiol 1997;30:1773–1777.

SECTION EIGHT

Transplantation Surgery

79

History of Clinical Transplantation

Thomas E. Starzl

How transplantation came to be a clinical discipline can be pieced together by perusing two volumes of reminiscences collected by Paul I. Terasaki in 1991–1992 from many of the persons who were directly involved. One volume was devoted to the discovery of the major histocompatibility complex (MHC), with particular reference to the human leukocyte antigens (HLAs) that are widely used today for tissue matching.[1] The other focused on milestones in the development of clinical transplantation.[2] All the contributions described in both volumes can be traced back in one way or other to the demonstration in the mid-1940s by Peter Brian Medawar that the rejection of allografts is an immunological phenomenon.[3,4]

Ten years later (1953), Billingham, Brent, and Medawar[5] showed that tolerance to skin allografts could be induced by inoculating fetal or prenatal mice with immunocompetent spleen cells from adult donors. Because of their immunological immaturity, the recipients were incapable of rejecting the spleen cells with progeny that survived indefinitely. Specific nonresponsiveness to donor strain tissues was retained as the recipient animals grew to adult life, while normal reactivity evolved to third-party grafts and other kinds of antigens.

This was not the first demonstration that tolerance could be deliberately produced. Analogous to the neonatal transplant model, Traub[6] showed in 1936 that the lymphocytic choriomeningitis virus (LCMV) persisted after transplacental infection of the embryo from the mother or by injection into newborn mice. However, when the mice were infected as adults, the virus was eliminated immunologically. Similar observations had been made in experimental tumor models. Murphy[7] reported in 1912 on the outgrowth of Rous chicken sarcoma cells on the chorioallantoic membranes of duck or pigeon egg embryos, which could be reversed by inoculation of adult chicken lymphoid cells,[8] whereas sarcoma implantation into adults was not possible.

The observations of Murphy and Traub did not influence the early development of transplantation. Instead, the impetus and rationale for the experiments of Billingham, Brent, and Medawar,[5,9] and similar studies in chickens by Hasek,[10] originated with Owen,[11] who demonstrated that freemartin cattle (the calf equivalent of human fraternal [dizygotic] twins) became permanent hematopoietic chimeras if fusion of their placentas existed in utero, allowing fetal cross-circulation (Fig. 79.1); such animals permanently accept each other's skin.[12] Burnet and Fenner[13] predicted that this natural chimerism and tolerance to other donor tissues and organs could be induced by the kind of experiments successfully performed by Billingham, Brent, and Medawar. However, Billingham and Brent[14,15] soon learned that, in mice, parallel with similar observations by Simonsen[16] in chickens, the penalty for infusion of immunocompetent hematopoietic cells was graft-versus-host disease (GVHD) unless there was a close genetic relationship (i.e., histocompatibility) between the donor and recipient.

This discovery was the beginning of modern transplantation immunology, an extensive history of which has been written by Brent,[17] one of its principal architects. Each cell- and organ-defined branch of transplantation also has had its historians, who have described the stages through which specific kinds of procedures moved to the bedside from experimental laboratories or in some cases directly. The culminating clinical events can be capsulized with a list of the first successful allotransplantation, in humans, of the kidney,[18] liver,[19] heart,[20,21] lung,[22] pancreas,[23] intestine,[24] multiple abdominal viscera,[25] and bone marrow.[26–29]

Although such milestones and dozens of lesser ones are important, the emphasis in this account is on developments that were applicable to all varieties of allografts and responsible for major transitions in transplantation ideology. It will become apparent as the layers of history are peeled away that there were only two seminal turning points in the evolution of clinical transplantation. One was the induction of chimerism-associated neonatal tolerance by Billingham, Brent, and Medawar in 1953. The second was the demonstration in 1962–1963 that organ allografts could self-induce tolerance with the aid of immunosuppression.[30] All subsequent developments in organ transplantation depended on exploitation of this principle, using variations of the drug strategy that had

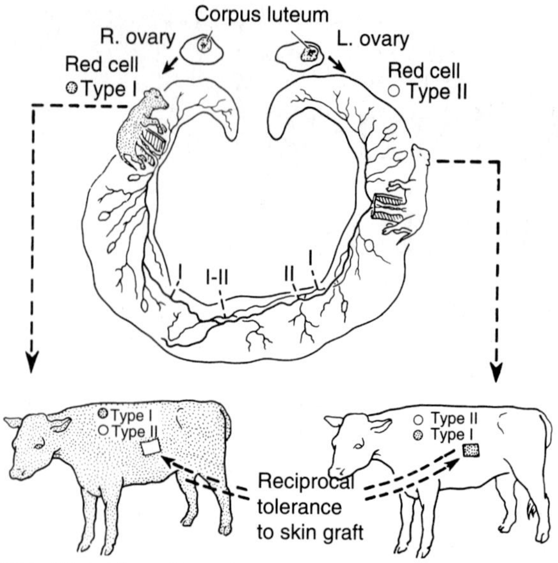

FIGURE 79.1. The chimerism in freemartin (fraternal twins) described by Owen.[11] Cross-tolerance to formed blood elements followed intrauterine circulatory exchange in dizygotic twins. Mutual tolerance to skin grafts was later proved by Anderson with Medawar et al.[12] (From Starzl and Butz,[146] by permission of *Surgical Clinics of North America*.)

made its discovery possible. Ironically, the downside of the resulting revolution in organ transplantation was the early introduction of a conceptual error that distorted the maturation of transplantation immunology and adversely affected the orderly development of general immunology.

The error, which was not corrected until well into the 1990s,[31–33] was the conclusion by consensus that organ allograft acceptance involved different mechanisms compared to the chimerism-dependent ones of neonatal tolerance and its clinical analogue of bone marrow transplantation. Consequently, the vast literature that sprang up in the intervening 30 years admirably documented the progression of improvements in clinical transplantation while failing to explain what was being accomplished.[34] Therefore, the reader may profit by skipping to the last section of this chapter ("Allograft Acceptance Versus Acquired Tolerance") before attempting to understand what went on between 1963 and 1993 and before.

Prehistory: Before Immunosuppression

An indelible mark on the pages of transplantation history was left with the perfection of techniques for organ revascularization by surgical anastomosis in the laboratories of Alexis Carrel at the beginning of the 20th century.[35] Aside from the technical contributions, which also provided the foundation for conventional vascular surgery, Carrel recognized that transplanted organ allografts were not permanently accepted, although he did not know why.

Using vascular surgical techniques, animal research in transplantation was most highly focused on the kidney for most of the next half-century.[36–38] The extrarenal vacuum rapidly was filled between 1958 and 1960 with the development in several laboratories of canine models with which to study all the intra-abdominal[39–43] and thoracic organs.[44–46] Although each organ presented specific technical and physiological issues, the core problems of immunosuppression, tissue matching, and allograft preservation eventually were worked out mainly with the kidney and liver and applied to other organs with minor modifications.

Hetero- (Xeno-)transplantation

The first known attempts at clinical renal transplantation by vascular anastomoses were made between the beginning of the 19th century and 1923 in France,[47] Germany,[48] and elsewhere (summarized by Groth[49]) using pig, sheep, goat, and subhuman primate donors. None of the kidneys functioned for long, if at all, and the human recipients died a few hours to 9 days later. No further animal-to-human transplantations were tried again until 1963, after immunosuppression was available.[50,51]

Homo- (Allo-)transplantation

In 1936, Voronoy of Kiev, Russia, reported the transplantation of a kidney from a cadaver donor of B blood type to a recipient of O blood type,[52] in violation of what have become accepted rules of tissue transfer[53,54] (Table 79.1). In addition, the allograft was jeopardized by the residual risk of acute mercury poisoning (from a suicide attempt) that caused the recipient's renal failure. A final adverse factor was the 6-h lapse between the donor's death and organ procurement. The allograft did not make any urine during the 48 h of the patient's posttransplant survival. Although other attempts may have been made by Voronoy,[55] another 15 years passed before significant kidney transplant activities were resumed in France.

In 1951, Rene Kuss[56] and Charles Dubost[57] in Paris and Marceau Servelle in Creteil[58] carried out a series of renal transplantations with kidneys removed from convict donors immediately after their execution by guillotine. The next year, the French nephrologist Jean Hamburger, in collaboration with the urologist Louis Michon at the Hôpital Necker in Paris, reported the mother-to-son transplantation of a kidney that functioned well for 3 weeks before rejection.[59] The procedure developed by Kuss and the other French sur-

TABLE 79.1. Direction of Acceptable Organ Transfer When the Donor and Recipient Have Different ABO Red Cell Types.

O to non-O	Safe
Rh– to Rh+	Safe
Rh+ to Rh–	Relatively safe
A to non-A	Dangerous
B to non-B	Dangerous
AB to non-AB	Dangerous

For organ transplantation, O is universal donor, and AB is universal recipient. With the transplantation of bone marrow allografts or of lymphoid-rich organ allografts (e.g., intestine or liver), enough antihost isoagglutinins may be produced by the allograft to cause serious or lethal hemolysis in a significant number of cases (humoral GVHD).[54] Consequently, the rules summarized in this table are fully applicable only with leukocyte-poor organs such as the kidney and heart (see the section, "Allograft Acceptance Versus Acquired Tolerance").

Source: From Starzl (1964).[53]

geons and used for this first live donor kidney transplantation has been performed hundreds of thousands of times since then. The operation's relative freedom from chronic morbidity would soon be demonstrated with the identical (monozygotic) twin transplantations of Joseph E. Murray and John Merrill and their associates[60] at the Peter Bent Brigham Hospital in Boston.

The efforts by the French teams were widely known, and visitors flocked to Paris in the early 1950s to learn firsthand from the experience. One of the observers of the extraperitoneal pelvic operation (often called the Kuss procedure in Europe) was John Merrill, as Hume, Merrill, et al.[61] described in their account of the first clinical trials at the Peter Bent Brigham Hospital. In Hume's nine Boston cases, however, all but one of the allografts were placed in the recipient thigh, revascularized from the femoral vessels, and provided with urinary drainage by skin ureterostomies.

The exceptional case in the Boston series[61] was the first one. The donor and recipient operations were performed in Springfield, Massachusetts, on March 30, 1951, by Dr. L.H. Doolittle. The donor kidney was excised because of a carcinoma of the lower ureter and implanted in the vacated renal fossa of the recipient after removal of the native organ. The recipient patient had been under short-term dialysis care at the Brigham, where the first artificial kidney in the United States had been brought from Holland by Wilhelm Kolff and modified by Harvard engineers, as described in detail by Moore.[62]

The next eight operations, in which the allografts were placed in the anterior thigh location, were performed by Hume in Boston between April 23, 1951, and December 3, 1952. The report of the nine cases stands as one of the medical classics of the 20th century, providing an extensive clinical and pathological profile of renal allograft rejection in untreated human recipients. The descriptions complemented the report of Michon and Hamburger of the live donor French case (see earlier[59]) and the pathfinding studies in dogs by the Dane, Morten Simonsen,[37] and W. James Dempster in England.[38] It is noteworthy that Hume treated some of his patients with adrenocortical steroids. It was already known from experimental studies that steroid therapy modestly mitigated primary skin graft rejection[63–65] and even slowed the accelerated rejection of presensitized recipients.[66]

Although compilation of the Boston series postdated the early French efforts (as generously annotated by Hume), the commitment of the Harvard group to transplantation was evident long before the availability of effective immunosuppression. Hume, who moved in 1956 from Boston to the Medical College of Virginia (Richmond), remained a major force in transplantation until his death in the crash of a private plane (of which he was the pilot) near Los Angeles in May 1973. His friend and colleague, John Merrill, who remained in Boston, drowned off the beach of a Caribbean island in 1984.

None of the European and American efforts to this time, or all together, would have had any lasting impact on medical practice were it not for what lay ahead. The principal ingredients of organ transplantation—immunosuppression, tissue matching, and organ procurement (and preservation)—were still unknown or undeveloped. The only unequivocal example of clinically significant allograft function through 1954 was provided by one of the nonimmunosuppressed patients of Hume et al.,[61] whose thigh kidney produced life-supporting urine output for 5 months. Similar claims about function of an allograft transplanted to the orthotopic location[67] (i.e., as in Doolittle's case[61]) or to a nonanatomical site[68] were considered implausible by later critics.

The existence of these cases was public knowledge, but the failure of all the grafts (usually with death of the patients) left very little room for optimism. The perception, if not the reality, of hopelessness was changed at the Peter Bent Brigham Hospital 2 days before Christmas in 1954, when a kidney was removed from a healthy man by the urologist J. Hartwell Harrison and transplanted by Joseph E. Murray to the pelvic location of the donor's uremic identical twin brother.[60,69] Although no effort was made to preserve the isograft, it functioned promptly despite 82 min of warm ischemia. The recipient lived for nearly 25 years before dying of atherosclerotic coronary artery disease.

According to Merrill et al.,[60] exploitation of genetic identity for whole-organ transplantation had been suggested by the recipient's physician, David C. Miller, at the Public Health Service Hospital, Boston. It already was well known that identical twins did not reject each other's skin grafts.[70] To ensure identity, reciprocal skin grafting was performed in the Boston twins. Although the identical twin cases attracted worldwide attention, organ transplantation now had reached a dead end. Further progress in the presence of an immunological barrier would require effective immunosuppression. The possibility of meeting this objective could only be regarded as bleak. To understand why, it is necessary to appreciate not only how barren the landscape of immunology was, but also how slowly the preexisting information had been filled in.

A century had passed between the first vaccination procedure in 1796 (Edward Jenner, smallpox) and the confirmation of the immunization principle by Louis Pasteur (with chicken cholera and rabies). The proof obtained by Robert Koch that microorganisms caused anthrax (1876) and subsequently many other infectious diseases stimulated a search for the host-protective mechanisms. This search yielded components of the immune response: antibodies (Emil Adolf von Behring and Shibasaburo Kitasato, 1890); immune cells (Ilya Metchnikoff, 1884); and complement (Jules Bordet, 1895). In addition, Paul Erlich developed the side-chain theory (1890), according to which each cell has a vital center of protein substance and a series of side chains (later known as receptors) to which toxic substances as well as nutrients were absorbed and then assimilated. In 1910, Erlich introduced the first antimicrobial drug, an arsenical compound effective against syphilis, yaws, and several other infections.

Decades passed between the cluster of great contributions at the turn of the 20th century and the proposal by F. McFarlane Burnet that antibodies were produced in each individual only to those antigens to which he or she was exposed.[13] The lack of major movement between times is evident from a list of Nobel Prizes (Table 79.2). Although 6 of the first 17 Nobel laureates (1901–1919) were honored for work relevant to immunology/transplantation, there was only one further example (Karl Landsteiner, ABO blood groups) among the next 57 (1920–1959). Beginning with Burnet and Medawar, 17 of the 77 laureates since 1960 have been directly responsible for, contributed to, or directly benefited from advances in transplantation (Table 79.2).

TABLE 79.2. Nobel Prizes Related to Immunology/Transplantation.

Year	*Name*	*Accomplishment*
1901	Emil Adolf von Behring	Discovery of antibodies
1905	Heinrich Hermann Robert Koch	Cause and effect of microorganisms and infection
1908	Paul Ehrlich	Side-chain (receptor) concept; champion of humoral immunity; antimicrobial therapy
	Ilya Metchnikoff	Champion of cellular immunity
1912	Alexis Carrel	Vascular surgery and transplantation
1919	Jules Bordet	Discovery of complement
1930	Karl Landsteiner	Discovered ABO blood group antigens
1960	Sir Frank MacFarlane Burnet	Clonal selection hypothesis
	Sir Peter Brian Medawar	Acquired transplantation tolerance
1972	Gerald M. Edelman	Characterized immunoglobulins
	Rodney R. Porter	Clarified structure of antibody molecule
1980	Baruj Benacerraf	Discovered immune response genes and collaborated in discovery of MHC restriction
	Jean Dausset	Discovered first HLA antigen
	George Davis Snell	Discovery of major histocompatibility complex (MHC) gene in mice
1984	Niels Kaj Jerne	Important immunological hypotheses
	Georges J.F. Kohler	Hybridoma technology
	Cesar Milstein	Hybridoma technology
1985	Michael Stuart Brown	Hepatic control of cholesterol metabolism (with Goldstein)[a]
	Joseph Leonard Goldstein	
1987	Susumu Tonegawa	Discovered somatic recombination of immunological receptor genes
1988	Gertrude Belle Elion	Codiscovery (with Hitchings) of 6-mercaptopurine (6-MP) and azathioprine
	George Herbert Hitchings	
1990	Joseph E. Murray	Kidney transplantation
	E. Donnall Thomas	Bone marrow transplantation
1996	Rolf Zinkernagel	Codiscovered (with Doherty) the role of MHC in adaptive immune response to pathogens
	Peter C. Doherty	

[a]Proved with liver transplantation for indication of hypercholesterolemia.[249,250]

In Burnet's original hypothesis of immunity, antibody synthesis was postulated to occur after an antigen locked on to a membrane-bound receptor (a version of the antibody) that was displayed at the surface of an immune cell. After binding the antibody, the cell proliferated, producing a *clone* that secreted identical antibodies (the clonal selection theory). Nossal subsequently proved that the clone rose from a single cell ("one cell/one antibody").[71] Although Burnet's hypothesis was not yet complete, it was to become the cornerstone of modern immunology.

The Concept of Immunosuppression

With Recipient Cytoablation

The transition of tissue and organ transplantation from an exercise in futility to tenuous practicality involved a surprisingly small number of advances that were interspersed with long periods of frustration. After Medawar's demonstration in 1944 that rejection was an immunological event,[3,4] a logical and inevitable question was, why not protect the organ allograft by weakening the immune system? This idea was tested in rabbits in 1950–1951 with cortisone[63,64] and total-body irradiation (TBI).[72] Both prolonged skin graft survival for only a few days.

Neither these results nor those reported with cortisone in 1952 by Cannon and Longmire[65] in a chicken skin graft model, generated much optimism. However, the Cannon-Longmire report contained three observations that, in retrospect, presaged not only the acquired neonatal tolerance produced by Billingham, Brent, and Medawar the following year, but also the most important clinical advances in transplantation of the succeeding decades. First, skin grafts exchanged between 1-day-old chicks of different breeds had a high rate of initial engraftment and a 6% incidence of permanent take. Second, the window of neonatal opportunity was gone by 4 days. Third, and most important, the percentage of permanent engraftment of neonatally transplanted skin was increased to more than 20% by a course of cortisone with no increase of mortality.

The significance of the third observation was recognized by Cannon and Longmire, who wrote:

> Although the cortisone did not entirely prevent a reaction in the homograft, it did decrease the incidence of reaction. Even more important, the increased incidence of reaction [sic] free grafts appeared to maintain itself after the drug was discontinued. This phenomenon is one which up to the present time has not been found in homograft experiments on mammals and humans.

Despite a 1957 confirmatory follow-up study,[73] the neglected Cannon-Longmire article faded quickly from the collective memory of both basic scientists and clinicians. In contrast, the 1953 achievement of acquired neonatal tolerance by Billingham, Brent, and Medawar[5,9] ignited interest in transplantation as never before. Two years later, Main and Prehn[74] attempted to simulate in adult mice the environment that allowed the acquisition of neonatal tolerance. The three steps were first to cripple the immune system with supralethal TBI; next to replace it with allogeneic bone marrow (producing a hematolymphopoietic chimera); and finally to engraft skin from the same inbred strain as the donor of the bone marrow.

The experiments were successful,[74] but as in the neonatal tolerance model, lethal GVHD could be avoided only when there were "weak" histocompatibility barriers.[75] Applying the chimerism strategy for kidney transplantation in beagle dogs in Cooperstown, New York, Mannick et al.[76] reported good renal allograft function in a supralethally irradiated recipient that also was given donor bone marrow and was a hematolymphopoietic chimera; the animal lived for 73 days before dying of pneumonia. Because it was demonstrated later that this kind of outcome depended on the identity of the dog lymphocyte antigens (DLAs),[77,78] an accidental DLA match was suspected in retrospect to have been present in Mannick's experiment. Efforts by Hume et al.[79] and subsequently by Rapaport and coworkers[80] and others to broaden the range of acceptable histoincompatibility inevitably led to lethal GVHD, rejection, or both.

Bone Marrow Transplantation

With the impasse, workers in bone marrow and whole-organ transplantation took separate pathways. Bone marrow transplantation was dependent a priori on the classic chimerism-associated acquired tolerance induction defined at the outset by Billingham, Brent, and Medawar in the neonatal model. In spite of the fact that only highly histocompatible donors could be used, clinical success with bone marrow engraftment was achieved in 1963 by Mathe et al. in Paris,[26] whose patient lived for 2 years with chronic GVHD before committing suicide.

Five years later, Gatti et al. in Minneapolis[28] and Bach et al. at the University of Wisconsin[27] each transplanted bone marrow to recipients who are well today. The lifetime efforts of Thomas,[29] van Bekkum,[81] and others fueled the maturation of bone marrow transplantation into accepted clinical therapy for numerous hematological diseases (including malignancies), acquired immunodeficiency disorders, mesenchymal-based inborn errors of metabolism, and an assortment of other indications.

Bone marrow transplantation was an intellectual triumph. Its development could be traced in a straight line back to the experiments of Main and Prehn[74] and before that to the acquired neonatal tolerance of Billingham, Brent, and Medawar[5,9] and the natural tolerance of Owens' freemartin cattle.[11]

Whole-Organ Transplantation

In contrast, clinical organ transplantation, which preceded bone marrow transplantation by a decade, appeared to be disconnected from a rational base when it was concluded that organ engraftment seemingly was independent of chimerism. An extension of the Main-Prehn strategy (i.e., lethal TBI followed by bone marrow and kidney allografts as in Mannick's dog) was used by Murray et al.[82] in only two cases, both in 1958. The next 10 kidney recipients in Boston were conditioned with sublethal TBI without bone marrow.[18,82,83] Of the 12 irradiated patients, 11 died after 0 to 28 days.

The survivor (who was not given bone marrow) had adequate renal function from the time his fraternal twin brother's kidney was transplanted on January 24, 1959, until he died in July 1979 (Table 79.3). With this historical accomplishment, the genetic barrier to organ transplantation had been definitively breached for the first time in any species.[18] Five months later, Hamburger et al.[84] added a second fraternal twin transplantation using the same treatment (Table 79.3). This second recipient had good renal function until his death 26 years later from carcinoma of the urinary bladder.

In these two dizygotic twin cases, it was conceivable that the donor and recipient placentas had fused during gestation, analogous to Owen's freemartin cattle (see Fig. 79.1). This suspicion was put to rest at the Paris centers of Jean Hamburger[85] and Rene Kuss[86] by four more examples during 1960–1962 of survival of 1 year or more. In Kuss' two cases, the donors were not related (see Table 79.3). During the critical period from January 1959 through the spring of 1962, the cumulative French experience was the principal (and perhaps the only) justification to continue clinical trials in kidney transplantation.

The experience from Boston and Paris summarized in Table 79.3 showed that bone marrow infusion was *not* a necessary condition for prolonged survival of kidney allografts and ostensibly eliminated the requirement of chimerism. The stage was set for drug therapy. In fact, both Hamburger and Kuss mentioned the use of adrenal cortical steroids as an adjunct to TBI (Table 79.3), but neither the dose nor the indication for the steroids was described. In addition, Kuss[86] secondarily administered 6-mercaptopurine (6-MP) to one of his cytoablated patients as early as August 1960 "on the basis of the recent results of the experimental studies conducted by Calne"[87] (see next section). Calne had made an invited visit to the Paris center a few months earlier (Rene Kuss and Roy Calne, personal communication).

TABLE 79.3.
Kidney Transplantation with 6 Months or More Survival as of March 1963.

Case	*City*	*References*	*Date*	*Donor*	*Survival (months)*[b]
1	Boston	18, 82, 83	January 24, 1959	Fraternal twin	>50
2	Paris	84, 85	June 29, 1959	Fraternal twin	>5
3	Paris	86	June 22, 1960	Unrelated[c]	18 (died)
4	Paris	85	December 19, 1960	Mother[c]	12 (died)
5	Paris	86	March 12, 1961	Unrelated[c]	18 (died)
6	Paris	18	February 12, 1962	Cousin[c]	>13
7	Boston	83, 105	April 5, 1962	Unrelated	10

[a]Boston: J.E. Murray (patients 1, 7); Paris: J. Hamburger (patients 2, 4, 6); R. Kuss (patients 3, 5).

[b]The kidneys in patients 1, 2, and 6 functioned for 20.5, 25, and 15 years, respectively. Patient 7 rejected his graft after 17 months and died after return to dialysis.

[c]Adjunct steroid therapy.

Some authorities have considered irradiation-induced and drug-induced graft acceptance to be different phenomena.[49,83,88] More recently, it has become obvious that the variable degree of graft acceptance achieved with sublethal TBI between January 1959 and February 1962 was fundamentally the same as that seen in tens of thousands of drug-treated humans following transplantation of various whole organs (see the section "Allograft Acceptance Versus Acquired Tolerance").

With Drug Immunosuppression

After it was learned that TBI alone could result in prolongation of kidney allografts, it was logical to focus the search for immunosuppressive drugs on myelotoxic agents that mimicked irradiation. In September 1960, Willard Goodwin of Los Angeles produced severe bone marrow depression with methotrexate and cyclophosphamide in a young female recipient of her mother's kidney. The patient subsequently developed several rejections that were associated with bone marrow recovery. They were temporarily reversed with prednisone several times during the 143 days of survival. It was the first example of protracted human kidney allograft function with drug treatment alone.[89] However, the case was not reported until 1963.

Kidney transplant surgeons were quick to realize that bone marrow depression should be avoided, not deliberately imposed, following the demonstration by Schwartz and Dameshek[90] that 6-mercaptopurine (6-MP) in a nontransplant rabbit model was immunosuppressive in submyelotoxic doses. Within a few months after their seminal discovery, Schwartz and Dameshek[91] and Meeker[92] (working with Condie, Weiner, Varco, and Good) showed that 6-MP caused a dose-related delay of skin graft rejection in rabbits. Aware of these results but independent of each other, Calne[93] in London and Zukoski, Lee, and Hume[94] in Richmond, Virginia, demonstrated the same thing in the canine kidney transplant model. In June 1960, Calne moved from the Royal Free Hospital to join Murray at the Peter Bent Brigham Hospital in Boston in further preclinical studies of 6-MP and its analogue, azathioprine.[83,95–97]

The two drugs had been developed originally by Gertrude Elion and George Hitchings as antileukemia agents.[98] Their possible use in transplantation was greeted at first with feverish enthusiasm because it was generally conceded that recipient cytoablation would permit success in only occasional cases of human renal transplantation. Although approximately 95% of the mongrel canine kidney recipients treated with 6-MP or azathioprine died in fewer than 100 days from either rejection or infection, occasional examples were recorded of long-term or seemingly permanent allograft acceptance[99–102] following discontinuance of a 4- to 12-month course of immunosuppression. The number of these animals was discouragingly small, but it was an accomplishment never remotely approached using TBI, with or without adjunct bone marrow. Survival of Mannick's single cytoablated animal for 73 days after combined bone marrow and kidney transplantation had been the previous high-water mark in dogs (see earlier[76]).

The survival of some of Calne's animals beyond 6 months led to the decision at the Brigham to begin clinical trials with chemical immunosuppression. However, the poor therapeutic margin of 6-MP and azathioprine when used alone in dogs was recognized. Calne and Murray also were forewarned by an earlier clinical experience of Hopewell, Calne, and Beswick et al.,[103] which was not published until 1964, in which 6-MP had been used to treat three kidney recipients (including one with a live donor) in 1959–1960; all three recipients had died.

Consequently, the canine studies of 6-MP and azathioprine in Boston were highly focused on finding more effective drug combinations.[83,95,97,104] Although adrenocortical steroids were tested, they did not appear to potentiate the value of azathioprine,[95,97] prompting Murray in his clinical trial to opt for adjunct cytotoxic agents such as azaserine and actinomycin C.[83] Only 1 of the first 10 kidney recipients treated with either 6-MP (n = 2) or azathioprine-based immunosuppression (n = 8) survived for more than 6 months (see the last entry in Table 79.3).[83,105]

At the nadir of the resulting pessimism, two reproducible observations, first in dogs and then in humans, were made at the University of Colorado. Taken together, these events profoundly shaped future developments in transplantation of all organs and eventually of bone marrow. The observations were encapsulated in the title of a report published in October 1963: "The Reversal of Rejection in Human Renal Homografts With the Subsequent Development of Homograft Tolerance."[30]

The reversal was readily accomplished by temporarily adding unprecedented high doses of prednisone (200 mg/day) to baseline immunosuppression with azathioprine. The evidence that the live donor kidneys had self-induced tolerance under an umbrella of immunosuppression was equally clear. Most of the recipients had a subsequent progressively diminishing need for immunosuppression, usually to doses lower than those that initially failed to prevent rejection. The tolerance was complete enough to allow the patients to go home to an unrestricted environment. Nine of the first 10 of these kidney recipients achieved prolonged graft survival,[30] including 2 who bear the longest continuously functioning allografts in the world today (more than 35.5 years) and have been free from immunosuppression for 32 and 4 years, respectively.[106]

The practical as well as theoretical implications of these observations were recognized throughout the report:

> A state of relative immunologic non-reactivity seems to have been produced which has lasted for as long as 6 months. . . . It is not known whether this is due to a change in the antigenic properties of the homograft, or to an alteration in the specific [host] response to the stimulus of the grafted tissues. The apparent host–graft adaptation does, however, provide some hope for prolonged functional survival. . . . It would seem probable that the [therapeutic] principles, as defined with the kidney, can eventually be applied to other organ homografts. . . . The prior knowledge that a rejection crisis is almost a certainty and that it usually can be managed by relatively conservative means should serve as a deterrent to the excessive use of measures that may cause fatal bone marrow depression. . . . It is also conceivable that the avoidance of a primary host–graft reaction by these means [excessive immunosuppression] would prevent the adaptive process.[30]

At the time this bellwether series was compiled between the autumn of 1962 and April 1963, the only other active clinical transplantation programs in the United States were in Richmond (directed by David Hume)[107] and at the Peter Bent Brigham Hospital in Boston (directed by Joseph Murray and John Merrill).[105] The historically important program of Willard Goodwin at the University of California at Los Angeles (UCLA; see earlier[89]) had been closed because all the recipients died in less than 5 months. In Europe, TBI briefly remained the preferred treatment at the long-standing Paris centers of Jean Hamburger and Rene Kuss, while Michael Woodruff of Edinburgh had begun testing azathioprine.[108]

The results in the Colorado series, and more importantly an exact description of the strategy that had been used to induce variable degrees of incomplete tolerance (Table 79.4), created a surge of new activity. Within 12 months, new kidney transplant centers proliferated in North America and Europe. Most of these second-generation programs remain in operation today.

The observations in the original kidney recipients were promptly confirmed. However, the proposed explanation for these successes (i.e., graft alteration plus loss of specific immunological responsiveness)[30] was controversial and remained so for the next three decades (see the section, "Allograft Acceptance Versus Acquired Tolerance"). Except for reports from the University of Colorado, the term *tolerance* was studiously avoided from 1964 onward in referring to the long-surviving dogs and human kidney recipients that were evident by the end of 1963.

The article most often quoted as contravening tolerance was that of Murray et al.,[102] despite the fact that, as the authors took pains to make clear, the evidence in their report was inconclusive and involved only two canine experiments of a potentially crucial nature. The two long-surviving dogs had been given renal homografts 9 and 18 months previously and had been treated for most of these periods with one of the purine analogues. Renal function was deteriorating at the time contralateral kidneys from the original donors were transplanted. The second organs were rejected after 23 and 3 days, respectively, as would be expected.

In commending Murray's 1964 report and conclusions, Medawar wrote[109]:

> There is, however, something special about renal homografts, as [Michael] Woodruff's appraisal in this volume makes very clear. A synoptic survey of more than 1000 renal homografts in dogs carried out by Murray and his colleagues (Murray, Ross Sheil, Moseley, Knight, McGavic & Dammin, 1964)[102] has shown that foreign kidneys do sometimes become acceptable to their hosts for a reason other than acquired tolerance in the technical sense. . . . There has been an adaptation of some kind . . . a possibility Woodruff has long urged us not to overlook[110,111] though there is no reason to believe it an antigenic adaptation.

TABLE 79.4. Empircal Therapeutic Dogma of Immunosuppression.

Ingredients of strategy	*Baseline agents*
Baseline therapy	Azathioprine[a]
Secondary adjustments of prednisone dose, or antilymphoid agents[b]	Cyclosporine
Case-to-case trial (and potential error) of weaning	Tacrolimus

[a]Alone or with prophylactic prednisone. Equivalent results were obtained with cyclophosphamide instead of azathioprine.[173,174]

[b]Initially used for prophylactic "induction."[156]

Medawar continued[109]:

> One possible explanation is the progressive and perhaps very extensive replacement of the vascular endothelium of the graft by endothelium of host origin, a process that might occur insidiously and imperceptibly during a homograft reaction weakened by immunosuppressive drugs. . . . Another possibility, raised by R.Y. Calne (though not mentioned by him in his contribution to this volume) is the laying down of a protective coat of host antibody on the endothelial inner surface of the graft . . . an explanation which would classify the phenomenon under the general heading of "enhancement."

These disclaimers notwithstanding, the commonality of the rejection barrier for different organs was self-evident. So was the likelihood that the means of inducing acceptance of one organ could be used for all the others.[112] There also was evidence from earlier experiments that a liver allograft could protect other donor tissues and organs. It had been noted in 1962 that intestine and pancreas had very little histopathological evidence of rejection in untreated canine recipients if they were components of multivisceral allografts that also included the liver.[113] The observations were confirmed 30 years later in a rat version of the same multivisceral procedures.[114,115]

Most convincingly at an experimental level, it was shown in 1964 that orthotopic canine liver allografts could induce and maintain their own acceptance far more frequently and permanently than renal allografts, even with a treatment course of azathioprine as short as 4 months.[116,117] Soon thereafter, spontaneous engraftment was demonstrated after liver transplantation in untreated outbred pigs,[118–122] many of which passed through self-resolving rejection crises.[121,123,124]

Thus, it already was clear by 1964–1965 that the liver is the most tolerogenic organ. In the late 1960s and early 1970s, Calne, Zimmerman, and Kamada formally proved that the liver tolerization extended to other donor tissues transplanted at the same time or later, first in untreated outbred pigs[125] and then without immunosuppression in selected rat strain combinations.[126–128] Although they were important, the experimental studies with hepatic allografts only affirmed the conclusion reached with the 1962–1963 experience in clinical renal transplantation, suggesting that all organs were capable of inducing tolerance. Just as with liver allografts, the self-induction of donor-specific tolerance by heart and kidney allografts without the aid of immunosuppression was later demonstrated by Corry et al.[129] and Russell and coworkers[130] in selected mouse strain combinations.

The key mechanism of kidney-induced allograft acceptance was suggested as early as 1964 to be clonal exhaustion.[131] This concept was developed[132] more fully for liver allografts in the illustration and caption reproduced in Figure 79.2, published in 1969. Induction of the activated clone by alloantigen was depicted via host macrophages rather than by antigen-presenting dendritic cells, which would not be described[133] until 1973. In the text accompanying the figure, it was pointed out that exhaustion and deletion of an antigen-specific clone had been postulated by Schwartz and Dameshek as early as 1959 to be the mechanism of the tolerance to heterologous protein induced in rabbits with the aid of 6-mercaptopurine.[90] In addition, Simonsen had suggested in 1960 that clonal exhaustion induced by allogeneic

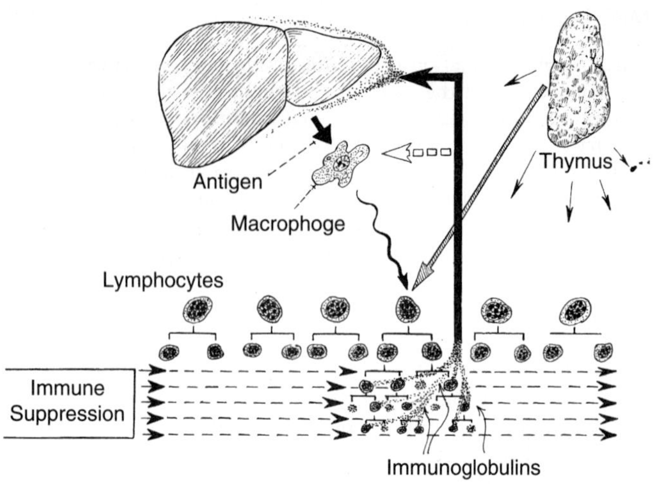

FIGURE 79.2. Hypothesis published in 1969 of allograft acceptance by clonal exhaustion. Antigen presentation was depicted via the macrophages rather than by the dendritic cells (which had not yet been described). A gap in this hypothesis was the failure to stipulate the location of the immune activation. (From Starzl,[132] by permission of W.B. Saunders Co.)

splenocytes could lead to the acquisition of tolerance in adult animals in the absence of immunosuppression.[134]

The error of making a semantic distinction between tolerance and graft acceptance was understandable. The picture that had emerged from the remarkable accomplishments with clinical kidney transplantation between January 1959 and the spring of 1963 was not a product of new insight in immunology. Instead, successful organ transplantation was an intellectually troubling and inexplicable violation of the immunological rules of the time. The revolution in immunology that had already began, and would continue for the next third of a century, did little to change this view.

The Burnet antibody hypothesis of clonal selection (see earlier[13]) was validated and extended to cellular immunity by the late 1950s,[135–137] but this had minimal influence on the clinical development of transplantation; neither did many other key advances in immunology that were either contemporaneous with or came after the rise of organ transplantation. The role of the thymus in the ontology of the immune system and in the postnatal immune function of rodents was discovered in 1961 (by Jacques Miller[138,139]). However, in humans thymectomy did not significantly alter either the early or late course of kidney transplant recipients.[140,141] Lymphocytes were not formally assigned a function until 1963 (by James Gowans[142,143]), although workers in transplantation were aware several years earlier that these mononuclear leukocytes were the cellular agents of allograft rejection[144–146] (Fig. 79.3). By the time the distinction was clearly established between T and B lymphocytes, transplantation was an established specialty of clinical medicine.

Thus, the ascension of organ transplantation came as a surprise to most immunologists. Even as the clinical advances had begun to unfold, Burnet[137] had written in the *New England Journal of Medicine* that, "Much thought has been given to ways by which tissues or organs not genetically and antigenically identical with the patient might be made to survive and function in the alien environment. On the whole, the present outlook is highly unfavorable to success." Pessimism also was deeply ingrained in conventional practitioners of medicine. Well into the 1960s, editorials were published in major clinical journals that questioned both the inherent feasibility and the ethical basis of transplantation procedures.[147] As a consequence, transplantation acquired a renegade image, a burden soon compounded by difficulties in extending its reach to the replacement of vital organs other than the kidney.

One dilemma, as it was perceived at the time, is shown in Figure 79.4.[148] It was feared that chronic drug immunosuppression powerful enough to prevent organ allograft rejection would render the recipient hopelessly vulnerable to indigenous and environmental pathogens. Reports of infectious disease complications in the early Colorado recipients[149] and elsewhere gave warning that dire consequences might, in time, be in store for all recipients. It also was suspected that immune surveillance to tumors would be eroded, a possibility that was verified but by 1958 was shown to be manageable.[150–152]

Autopsy studies in failed clinical cases revealed a typical pattern. Infections for which specific antibiotics were available could be largely controlled. However, opportunistic

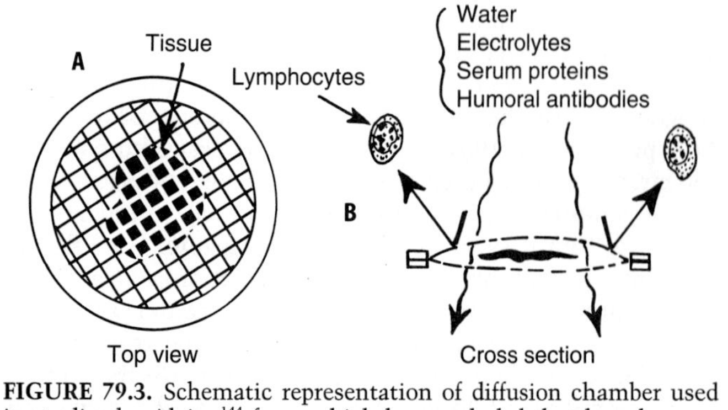

FIGURE 79.3. Schematic representation of diffusion chamber used in studies by Algire,[144] from which he concluded that lymphocytes were the cellular agents of allograft rejection. (From Starzl and Butz,[146] by permission of *Surgical Clinics of North America*.)

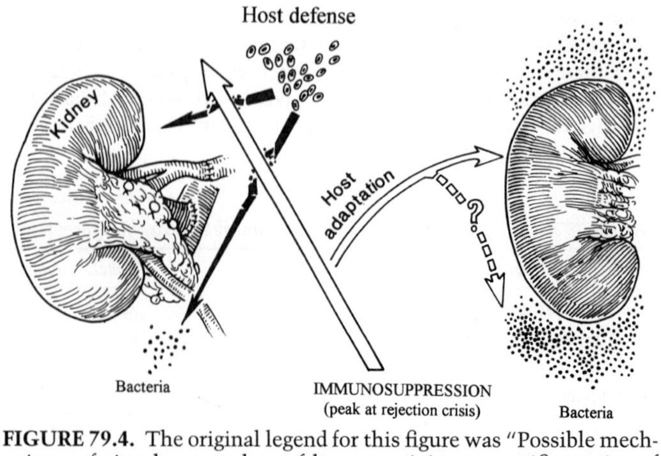

FIGURE 79.4. The original legend for this figure was "Possible mechanisms of simultaneous loss of host reactivity to specific strains of endogenous bacteria, as well as to the alien renal tissue." [From Starzl et al.,[148] by permission of *Surgery (St. Louis)*.]

microorganisms of normally low pathogenicity were overrepresented and appeared at autopsy to be the main cause of death.[153] Of these infections, cytomegalovirus (CMV) was the most common and lethal. The presence of *Pneumocystis carinii* as a coinfection with CMV[154] premonstrated the lethal role of this combination of infectious agents in the acquired immunodeficiency syndrome (AIDS) epidemic in the nontransplant population that lay two decades ahead.

The Maturation of Transplantation

Although it was entirely empirical, the practical framework required for the maturation of clinical transplantation was essentially complete by the end of 1963. Without knowing either the nature of the normal immune response or the way in which it had been subverted, surgeons had learned how to reliably redirect the immune response with the aid of immunosuppression. Surgical (see opening section) and preservation techniques (see later) had been developed for transplantation of all the organs; these are used currently with only minor modifications. Yet, the field of organ transplantation stalled and now entered a phase that was euphemistically termed *consolidation*. The reason was the failure to find improved means of exploiting the principles for control of rejection that had been established with azathioprine and prednisone (see Table 79.4).

Improved Immunosuppression

Antilymphoid Strategies

Between 1963 and 1979, the only significant advance in clinical immunosuppression was the introduction in 1966 of heterologous antilymphocyte globulin (ALG).[155,156] This step was a logical extension of Gowan's demonstration of the immunosuppressive effects of lymphoid depletion with thoracic duct drainage (TDD) in rats.[142,143] In fact, Woodruff and Anderson showed that TDD and antilymphocyte serum (ALS) had additive effects.[157]

Franksson and Blomstrand used TDD clinically in 1963 to treat kidney recipients in Stockholm,[158] an approach that resurfaced periodically during the next two decades (summarized in Ref. 159). Conditioning with TDD before transplantation clearly reduced the frequency and vigor of kidney rejection, but 30 days of pretreatment were required in humans,[159,160] compared to the 5 days in Gowan's rats.[142,143] However, the inconvenience, complexity, and expense of TDD precluded its wide use.[160] For the same reasons, total lymphoid irradiation (TLI),[161] which also was an effective means of lymphoid depletion but with the disadvantage that it was not quickly reversible, did not have a lasting impact on clinical transplantation.[162,163]

In contrast, ALG was a major turning point for two reasons. First, it was a critical factor in the emergence of extrarenal organ transplantation. Second, it was a prototype drug from which numerous variations evolved. The concept of mitigating cellular immunity with heterologous antibodies had been proposed by Ilya Metnikoff at the end of the 19th century[164] and was revitalized by Inderbitzen[165] and Waksman et al.[166] before Woodruff and Anderson,[157] Levey and Medawar,[167] Monaco, Wood, and Russell,[168,169] and other surgeons recognized its potential role in clinical transplantation.

In most of the animal investigations up to 1963, the antilymphocyte antibodies were raised in rabbits, and in all cases the raw ALS was administered. In preparation for clinical trials, horse antidog ALS was prepared, and the active moiety was refined from the gamma globulin.[155] After the product was shown to inhibit or reverse rejection in the canine kidney and liver transplant models,[156] comparable horse antihuman ALG was produced from the serum of horses that had been immunized with leukocytes separated from human lymphoid organs (lymph nodes, spleen, thymus).[155]

The first clinical trial of ALG began in 1966. Daily injections were given to kidney recipients for 1 to 4 postoperative weeks as a short-term adjunct to continuous azathioprine and prednisone.[156] After encouraging results were obtained in the kidney trial, liver transplantation was resumed, with long survival of several patients. The successful liver replacements[19] in the summer of 1967 expanded the horizon of transplantation to the other vital extrarenal organs. Within the succeeding 27 months, heart,[20,21] lung,[22] and pancreas transplantation[23] also were accomplished using variations of the treatment shown in Table 79.4. As had happened with kidney centers in 1963, a wild proliferation of extrarenal (particularly heart) programs followed. However, almost all of them closed within the next 2 years because of an overwhelming failure rate.

Polyclonal ALG was never used in more than about 15% of kidney transplant cases reported to registries up to the early 1980s, in part because it was in no sense a standardized drug like azathioprine and prednisone. Although the use by Najarian and Simmons[170] of known numbers of cultured human lymphoblasts for accurately timed horse immunization improved the predictability of the ALG potency, batch-to-batch variations in potency remained problematic. "Antibody therapy" came of age with production of monoclonal antibodies made feasible by the hybridoma technology of Kohler and Milstein.[171] The first-generation murine monoclonal antibody muromonab CD3 (Orthoclone OKT3) was directed at the CD3 antigen present on all T lymphocytes.[172] Subsequent antibody preparations, which include less-immunogenic humanized "hybrids," have been directed at discrete targets such as T-cell subsets, adhesion molecules, and T-cell or interleukin 2 receptors. However, when these agents are used, the "induction" strategy has been essentially the same as with the original crude ALG.

Cyclophosphamide

Although the experience in this middle era, defined by the first triple-drug regimen, demonstrated the feasibility of transplanting the vital extrarenal organs, it also indicated that further progress would require better baseline immunosuppression. Substitution of the alkylating agent cyclophosphamide for azathioprine was such an effort.[173] The characteristic cycle of immunological confrontation and resolution leading to graft acceptance was no different with this drug than with azathioprine-based therapy. However, when the results with kidney and liver transplantation were almost identical to those using azathioprine but at a higher price of complications, the trials were discontinued.[174] Although cyclophosphamide thereby became a footnote in the history of organ transplantation, it continued to play a role in bone marrow transplantation.

Cyclosporine

Another decade would pass before the greater potency of cyclosporine would make transplantation of the liver and other cadaveric organs (including the kidney) a reliable service. Cyclosporine, an extract from the fungi *Cylindrocarpon lucidum* and *Trichoderma polysporum*, was discovered by Dreyfuss et al.[175] and characterized biochemically by Ruegger et al.[176] and Petcher et al.[177] It was shown to be immunosuppressive by Borel et al.[178–180] with multiple test systems, including skin allotransplantation in mice, rats, and guinea pigs.

The drug depressed humoral and cellular immunity and had a preferential and quickly reversible action against T lymphocytes. Unlike azathioprine and cyclophosphamide, these effects were not accompanied by bone marrow depression or other prohibitive organ toxicity. The ability of cyclosporine to prevent or delay rejection of hearts, kidneys, livers, or pancreases was promptly shown in rats, rabbits, dogs, and pigs by Kostakis,[181] Calne,[182–184] and Green[185] and their associates. There was no hint in these preclinical studies that nephrotoxicity would be the dose-limiting factor in human trials.

The toxicity profile of cyclosporine became evident in Calne's initial evaluation[186,187] of cyclosporine in human recipients of 32 kidneys, 2 pancreases, and 2 livers, reported in 1978–1979. The ability of the drug to prevent rejection, alone or in combination with myelotoxic drugs, exceeded anything previously seen. However, the requisite overdosage caused multiple serious side effects: nephrotoxicity, neurotoxicity, diabetogenicity, a 10% incidence of B-cell lymphoma, and cosmetic changes (gingival hyperplasia, facial brutalization, and hirsutism).

When cyclosporine in lower doses was combined with prednisone in the treatment algorithm shown in Table 79.4, the prognosis of cadaver kidney recipients was improved,[188] and transplantation of the liver,[189] heart,[190,191] and lungs[192] was brought to the level of a practical clinical service. Recapitulating the aborted avalanche of 1967, many new extrarenal programs appeared, joining the five extant liver centers (Denver [from 1963], Cambridge [1968], Hannover [1972], Paris [1974], and Groningen [1977]) and the single remaining heart program (Stanford [from 1968]). This time, most of the programs flourished.

Tacrolimus

Cyclosporine was the unchallenged baseline immunosuppressant for all varieties of transplantation until it was shown in 1989 that intractably rejecting liver allografts could be regularly rescued by replacing cyclosporine with tacrolimus,[193] an extract of *Streptomyces tsukubaensis* discovered by Kino et al.[194] Tacrolimus was tested initially in a rat cardiac transplant model by Ochiai et al.[195] and soon thereafter by Murase et al. in rats[196,197] and by Todo et al. in dogs[198,199] and subhuman primates.[199,200]

TABLE 79.5. Nonimmunological Profile.

	FK 506	*CyA*
Nephrotoxicity	++[a]	++
Neurotoxicity	+	+
Diabetogenicity	+	+
Growth effects		
Hirsutism	0	+++
Gingival hyperplasia	0	++
Facial brutalization	0	+
Hepatotrophic effects	++++	+++
Gynecomastia	0	+
Other metabolic effects		
Cholesterol increase	0[b]	++
Uric acid increase	+?	++

All effects dose-related; ++++, worst.

[a]Less hypertension.

[b]In rats, Van Thiel has shown an increase in cholesterol synthesis and serum concentration.

Source: From Starzl et al.[210]

In addition to numerous confirmatory reports of its ability to rescue about 75% of intractably rejecting human liver allografts,[201] tacrolimus could salvage an equal proportion of rejecting hearts, kidneys, and other organs.[202] In virtually all such cases, a switch back to cyclosporine was never made. Consequently, clinical trials using tacrolimus primarily were begun.[202–204]

By early 1990, more than 150 liver, kidney, heart, and heart-lung recipients had been treated from the time of transplantation with immunosuppression based on tacrolimus (FK 506) rather than cyclosporine (CyA).[205] It was learned from this experience that the three major side effects of the drug (nephrotoxicity, neurotoxicity, and diabetogenicity) were comparable to cyclosporine. Hypertension and hyperlipidemia were less than in historical cyclosporine controls. The cosmetic effects of cyclosporine were not seen (Table 79.5).

The effective use of both cyclosporine and tacrolimus required the same pattern recognition and therapeutic response that have guided organ transplantation since its inception (see Table 79.4). The dose ceilings of the four widely used baseline immunosuppressants were imposed by toxicity: myelotoxicity for azathioprine and cyclophosphamide and the more complex side effects shown in Table 79.5 for cyclosporine and tacrolimus. The dose floors were revealed by the breakthrough of rejection. Because none of the four drugs could be used alone, they had to be incorporated into "cocktails" in which the requisite doses of the individual drug constituents were determined on a case-by-case basis by trial and error. Dose-maneuverable prednisone has remained a constant for 36 years, but steroid dependence declined with the more potent baseline agents.

The lead organ for azathioprine was the kidney. The developmental responsibility for cyclosporine was shared by the kidney and liver, while the liver bore the principal burden for tacrolimus.[193,201,203,205–209] However, progress with one kind of organ allograft inevitably meant progress for all. Thus, survival of each kind of organ graft rose in the same three distinct leaps between 1962 and 1998 (Fig. 79.5). With tacrolimus, the intestine was no longer a "forbidden" organ.[210–212]

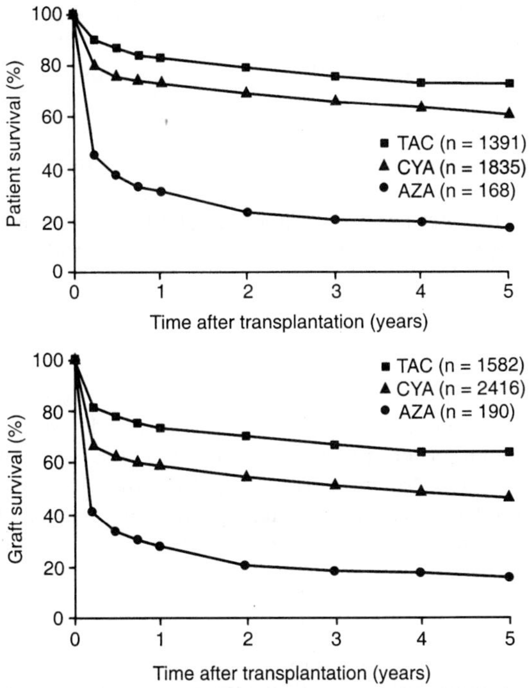

FIGURE 79.5. The three eras of orthotopic liver transplantation at the universities of Colorado (1963–1980) and Pittsburgh (1981–1993), defined by azathioprine (AZA), cyclosporine (CYA), and FK 506 (tacrolimus)-based (TAC) immunosuppression. The same stepwise improvement was seen with all organs. *Top:* Patient survival. *Bottom:* Graft survival. These results were about 10% lower than patient survival in both the cyclosporine (1980–1989) and tacrolimus eras (1989–1993) because of effective retransplantation, an option that did not exist previously.

The Ripple Effect

Organ Procurement and Preservation

The sudden arrival of clinical kidney transplantation in 1962–1963 was so unexpected that little collateral research or other formal preparation had been made to preserve organs. Although kidneys were successfully transplanted in the pioneer identical twin cases despite protracted periods of warm ischemia, the maturation of clinical transplantation could not proceed without effective organ conservation. This was accomplished at first with total body hypothermia of living volunteer kidney donors,[213] using methods developed by cardiac surgeons for open-heart operations.[214] In the experimental laboratory, Lillehei et al.[39] simply immersed the excised intestine in iced saline before its autotransplantation, a method also used by Shumway in developing experimental and clinical heart and heart-lung transplantation.[44–46] Thus, the principle of hypothermia was understood at an early time, although it was not efficiently applied.

The first major innovation in hypothermia was in the laboratory, when canine liver allografts were cooled by infusion of chilled fluids into the vascular bed of hepatic allografts via the portal vein.[42] Before this time, survival of dogs after liver transplantation was almost never obtained, while afterward success became routine. In a logical extension to clinical kidney transplantation, the practice was introduced in 1963 of infusing chilled lactated Ringer's or low molecular weight dextran solutions into the renal artery of kidney grafts immediately after their removal.[215]

Today, intravascular cooling is the first step in the preservation of all whole-organ grafts. For cadaver donors, this is most often done in situ by some variant of the technique described by Marchioro et al.[216] (Fig. 79.6). This method for the continuous hypothermic perfusion of cadaveric livers and kidneys was used clinically long before the acceptance of brain death. Ackerman and Snell[217] and Merkel, Jonasson, and Bergan[218] popularized the simpler core cooling of cadavers with cold electrolyte solutions infused into the distal aorta.

Organ Procurement

Until 1981, transplantation of the extrarenal organs was an unusual event. By late 1981, however, it had become obvious that liver and thoracic organ transplant procedures were going to be widely used. A method of multiple-organ procurement was required by which the kidneys, liver, heart, and lungs or various combinations of these organs could be removed without jeopardizing any of the individual organs. "Flexible techniques" were developed[219,220] that were quickly adopted worldwide. With the methods, all organs to be transplanted are cooled in situ, rapidly removed in a bloodless field, and dissected on a back table. The sharing of organs from a common donor by recipient teams from widely separated centers became routine by the mid-1980s.

Ex Vivo Perfusion

Extension of the safe period after initial cooling has followed one of two prototype strategies, developed either with kidneys

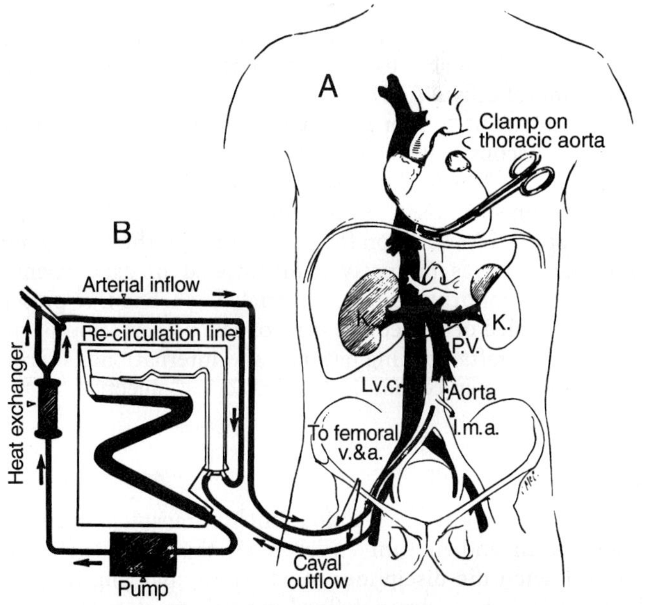

FIGURE 79.6. Technique of extracorporeal perfusion with a heart-lung machine described by Marchioro et al.[216] Catheters are inserted via the femoral vessels into the aorta and vena cava as soon as possible after death. The extracorporeal circuit is primed with a glucose or electrolyte solution to which procaine and heparin are added. The cadaver is thus anticoagulated with the first surge of the pump. Temperature control is provided by the heat exchanger. Cross-clamping the thoracic aorta limits perfusion to the lower part of the body. (From Starzl,[215] by permission of W.B. Saunders Co.)

or livers and applied secondarily to other organs. One approach, which was extensively evaluated by Alexis Carrel and the aviator Charles A. Lindbergh, was to simulate normal physiological conditions with ex vivo perfusion techniques.[221] This concept was modified by Ackerman and Barnard,[222] who provided the isolated organs with a continuous low-flow renal arterial circulation using a perfusate primed with blood and oxygenated within a hyperbaric oxygen chamber. This technique also permitted good preservation of hepatic allografts for as long as a day.[223] However, the complexity of the method precluded its general use.

The elimination of the hemoglobin and hyperbaric chamber components by Belzer et al.[224] resulted in satisfactory kidney preservation for as long as 2 to 3 days. The asanguinous perfusion technique eventually was abandoned in most kidney transplant centers when it was learned that the quality of 2-day preservation was not better than with the simpler "slush" methods (see following). Nevertheless, it is expected that refinement of perfusion technology will someday permit true organ banking.

Slush Preservation

With the so-called static methods, fluids of differing osmotic, oncotic, and electrolyte composition are infused into the allograft before placing it in a refrigerated container.[225,226] The solution described by Collins, Bravo-Shugarman, and Terasaki[225] (which resembles intracellular electrolyte concentrations) or modifications of it were used for almost two decades. Renal allograft preservation was feasible for 1 to 2 days, long enough to allow tissue matching and sharing of organs over a wide geographic area. Experiments with hepatic allografts by Benichou et al.[227] using the Collins-Terasaki solution and by Wall et al.[228] with the plasma-like Schalm solution led directly to liver sharing between cities, but with a time limitation of only 6 to 8 h.

The introduction for liver transplantation of the University of Wisconsin (UW) solution by Belzer, Jamieson, and Kalayoglu,[229,230] was the first major development in static preservation since the Collins-Terasaki solution.[231] The superiority of the UW solution for preservation of the kidney and other organs was promptly demonstrated in experimental models and confirmed in clinical trials.[232–237] The UW preservation doubled or tripled the time of safe preservation of the various allografts, making national and international sharing of most organs an economical and practical objective.

The Life Sciences

While occupying its own unique niche, transplantation has drawn from and in turn enriched all the other basic and clinical scientific disciplines. Aside from changing the philosophy by which organ-defined specialties of surgery and medicine are practiced, transplantation grew parallel with, and contributed in a major way to, advances in immunology, pharmacology, oncology (e.g., the role of tumor immune surveillance[152,238]), infectious disease, intensive care, and anesthesiology. Study of each of the different kinds of allografts has yielded an organ-specific harvest of special information. Examples include a better understanding of diabetes mellitus with pancreas transplantation and of the effects of denervation on cardiopulmonary function with heart and lung transplantation.

The liver became the key organ in unmasking the secrets of acquired tolerance because of its large content of immunocompetent leukocytes (see earlier and the section, "Allograft Acceptance Versus Acquired Tolerance"). In addition, the functional complexity of the liver as well as its metabolic interactions with other abdominal viscera have made hepatic transplantation a "mother lode" for physiological studies.[239]

In the course of determining the optimal revascularization of auxiliary livers transplanted to ectopic sites or to the normal location,[42,240,241] it was found that endogenous insulin is a liver growth factor,[242,243] the first such hepatotrophic factor to be identified. Using transplantation-derived models, a family of other molecules was delineated with insulin-like hepatotrophic properties.[244] Eventually, the gene was discovered that expresses one of these (augmenter of liver regeneration).[245–247] The hepatotrophic factors, most of which are cytokines (e.g., hepatocyte growth factors [HGFs]), regulate liver size, structure, regeneration, and metabolic homeostasis.

Studies of hepatotrophic physiology led directly or indirectly to liver replacement for cure of more than two dozen hepatic-based inborn errors of metabolism,[248] including familial hypercholesterolemia.[249,250] The role of hepatic transplantation in first suggesting, and then proving, that the liver governs cholesterol metabolism has been described elsewhere.[238,249–251] Elucidation of the cellular and molecular mechanisms was rewarded by bestowal of the 1985 Nobel Prize to Brown and Goldstein (see Table 79.2).

Immunological Screening

The importance of the genetically determined major histocompatibility complex (MHC) in determining the immune response to allografts was evident from investigations by George Snell in inbred mice,[252] which in turn derived from the work of Peter Gorer (see "the seminal influence of Gorer and Snell"[253]). However, the information was not clinically applicable. Thus, immunological screening of donors and recipients was not done during the volatile 1959–1963 developmental period.[1] The possibility of tissue matching did not begin to emerge until the discovery in 1958 by Dausset of the first human leukocyte antigen (HLA)[254] and the discovery in the same year by Van Rood et al.[255] of antileukocyte antibodies (soon shown to be HLA directed) in the sera of pregnant women.

The report in 1964 by Terasaki and McClelland[256] of the microcytotoxicity test, with which HLA antigens could be detected serologically in minute quantities of sera, was a critical development in moving forward with the classification of the antigens.

The Crossmatch Principle

As it turned out, the greatest impact of pretransplant tissue matching has been the prevention of hyperacute rejection by observation of ABO compatibility guidelines and the routine use of the cytotoxicity crossmatch.

ABO Compatibility

Hyperacute rejection was first observed more than 30 years ago when ABO-mismatched renal allografts were transplanted into patients who had preformed antigraft ABO isoagglutinins.[53,257] After kidneys were lost on the operating table, arteriograms of the infarcted organs showed nonfilling of the small vessels, correlating histopathologically with widespread thrombotic occlusion of the microvasculature. It was concluded that high-affinity isoagglutinins in the recipient sera had bound to A or B antigens in the graft vessels and parenchymal cells. This finding was consistent with rapid changes in recipient isoagglutinin titers that followed organ revascularization. The guidelines formulated from this experience[53,257] were designed to avoid such antibody confrontations (see Table 79.1).

The ABO rules also apply to heart, liver, and other kinds of organ transplantation. As was originally observed in 1963 with ABO-mismatched kidneys, however,[53,257] not all organs placed in the hostile environment of antigraft isoagglutinins meet the same fate. In fact, the longest continuously functioning renal allograft in the world[106] is a B+ kidney donated to a then-38-year-old A+ male recipient by his younger sister on January 31, 1963. In addition, it was learned at an early time that the liver is more resistant to antibody attack than other organs.[258]

In histocompatibility studies in which human volunteers were sensitized with purified A and B blood group antigens, causing variably increased titers of isoagglutinins, Rapaport et al.[259] showed accelerated or hyperacute (white graft) rejection of ABO-incompatible skin grafts transplanted to recipients with high titers. This result completed the circle of evidence indicating antigraft antibodies as the precipitating cause of hyperacute organ rejection.

With Non-ABO Antibodies

In 1965, hyperacute rejection of a kidney by an ABO-compatible recipient was reported for the first time by Terasaki et al.[260] Terasaki's observation that the serum of the recipient of a live donor kidney contained preformed antigraft lymphocytotoxic antibodies was promptly confirmed in similar cases by Kissmeyer-Nielsen et al.[261] and others.[262,263] The evidence of a cause-and-effect relationship in the single first case was so clear that Terasaki recommended and immediately introduced his now universally applied lymphocytotoxic crossmatch test.[260,264]

It has been shown in presensitized animals and humans that antibodies, clotting factors, and formed blood elements were rapidly cleared by the hyperacutely rejecting grafts.[265,266] Local fibrinolysis from the renal vein also was a consistent finding, and in exceptional cases, there were systemic coagulopathies with disseminated intravascular coagulation (DIC).[267,268] The findings are comparable to those in the Arthus reaction, inverse anaphylaxis, generalized Shwartzman reaction, and other models of innate immunity.[263,267,268]

Non-HLA antibodies such as antivascular endothelial cell antibodies also have been associated with hyperacute or accelerated rejection.[269,270] The vulnerability of extrarenal organs to this kind of rejection was ultimately demonstrated experimentally[271–273] and clinically. Although the liver was the most antibody-resistant,[258] it also was placed at increased risk by the presensitized state.[274] Hyperacute rejection also has been documented in a small number of human organ recipients in the absence of detectable antibodies.[263,275]

Tissue Matching

Historically, it was predicted tissue matching would have to be perfected if long-term engraftment of tissues and organs was to succeed with any degree of reliability and predictability. The prophecy was immediately fulfilled with bone marrow transplantation, in which anything less than a perfect or near-perfect match between the donor and recipient resulted in GVHD or rejection of the graft.[26–29] When similar expectations were not met in studies by Paul Terasaki in kidney transplant recipients, the results initially were treated as a scientific scandal.[276,277] When he later was proved to have been correct, Terasaki emerged as the father of HLA matching and as an enduring symbol of integrity.

Terasaki's investigations began with a retrospective study of the influence of HLA matching on the quality of outcome of patients bearing long-surviving kidney allografts,[278] followed by a prospective trial in live donor kidney recipients treated with azathioprine and prednisone, with or without adjunct ALG.[279] Consistent with the results in the classic skin graft investigations in nonimmunosuppressed healthy volunteers by Rapaport and Dausset,[280–282] HLA-matched allografts had the best survival and function, least dependence on maintenance prednisone, and fewest histopathological abnormalities in routine 2-year postoperative biopsies.[283] Unexpectedly, however, a cumulative adverse effect of mismatching in the kidney recipients could not be identified.

The equally imprecise prognostic discrimination of HLA matching in cadaver kidney transplant cases also was first recognized by Terasaki (with Mickey et al.[284]) and has been evident in analyses up to the present time. With the large sample sizes in United Network for Organ Sharing (UNOS) and European databases, virtually every comparison of the different levels of mismatching showed statistical significance. However, the absence of a large or consistent matching effect unless there is a perfect or near-perfect match has always been the same. In a recent study of more than 30,000 UNOS patients for whom optimal matches had been sought prospectively, approximately 85% of the cases were in the two- to five-HLA-mismatch spectrum in which 1-year survival was clustered within 3%. Subsequent half-life projections thereafter were in the narrow spread of 9 to 11 years.[285]

Terasaki's conclusions nearly three decades ago breathed life into the still-struggling fields of liver, heart, and lung transplantation. It was a relief to know that the selection of donors with random tissue matching would not result in an intolerable penalty. A quarter of a century passed before it could be explained why HLA matching was critical for bone marrow, but not organ, transplantation (see next section).

Allograft Acceptance Versus Acquired Tolerance

During the Festschrift at Harvard honoring Paul Russell's retirement in late November 1990, Norman Shumway told me and Leslie Brent about his text on *Thoracic Transplantation* for which he wanted two chapters: one explaining the

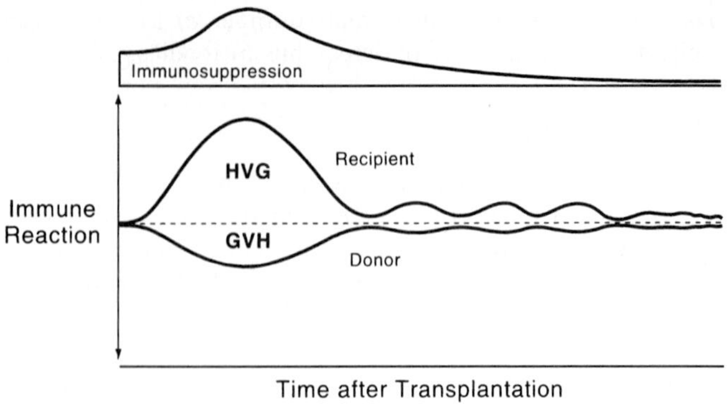

FIGURE 79.7. Contemporaneous host-versus-graft (HVG) and graft-versus-host (GVH) reactions in the two-way paradigm of transplantation immunology. Following the initial interaction, the maintenance of nonreactivity of each leukocyte population to the other is seen as a predominantly low-grade stimulatory state that may wax and wane.

classic immunological tolerance exemplified by bone marrow transplantation and the other defining the presumably different mechanisms of whole-organ allograft acceptance. On learning that I thought the two were the same in principle, Shumway assigned me to the task of defending this opinion.[286]

Evidence was obtained first from investigation of long-surviving human liver, kidney, and other organ recipients[31,32,287–289] and then from detailed confirmatory animal studies.[290–293] The observation that all 30 patients tested had low-level (micro-) chimerism conformed perfectly with the hypothesis being tested that allograft acceptance involved not only chimerism but also a bidirectional immune reaction (Fig. 79.7). The relative strengths of the opposing immune reactions following organ transplantation were simply the reverse of those following bone marrow transplantation to the cytoablated recipient (summarized in Refs. 33 and 106). With this paradigm, it has been possible to view the historical milestones of clinical organ as well as bone marrow transplantation in a coherent way.[34]

Historically, an organ allograft had been envisioned as defenseless and vulnerable to immunological attack in proportion to its histo*in*compatibility (Fig. 79.8, top left). The same dogma in reverse (i.e., the host was the defenseless target) was the conventional view of bone marrow transplantation (Fig. 79.8, top right). Only two pioneer workers raised objections to the definition of transplantation immunology in terms of a unidirectional immune reaction. In 1960–1961, Simonsen[134] and then Michie, Woodruff, and Zeiss[294] postulated that the two populations of immune cells in neonatally tolerant mice managed to coexist in a stable state by becoming mutually nonreactive while retaining the ability to function collaboratively (i.e., in a joint immune response to infection).

Although this heretical suggestion resembled the concept summarized in Figures 79.7 through 79.11, in 1962 the Simonsen-Woodruff hypothesis was recanted,[295] ostensibly because no experimental support could be found for it. More important, however, it had been advanced in a nonreceptive climate in which "group think" had already turned in a different direction. For the next 30 years, transplantation immunity and tolerance were conceived as products of unidirectional immune reactions of the kind that could be studied in vitro by one-way mixed-lymphocyte culture techniques described by Bain, Vas, and Lowenstein[296] and Bach and Hirschhorn.[297]

After chimerism was discovered in 1992–1993 in organ recipients,[31–33] it was recognized that the interaction of the coexisting donor and recipient leukocyte populations was the common factor that underlay both the "acceptance" induced by whole-organ allografts (Fig. 79.8, bottom left) and the

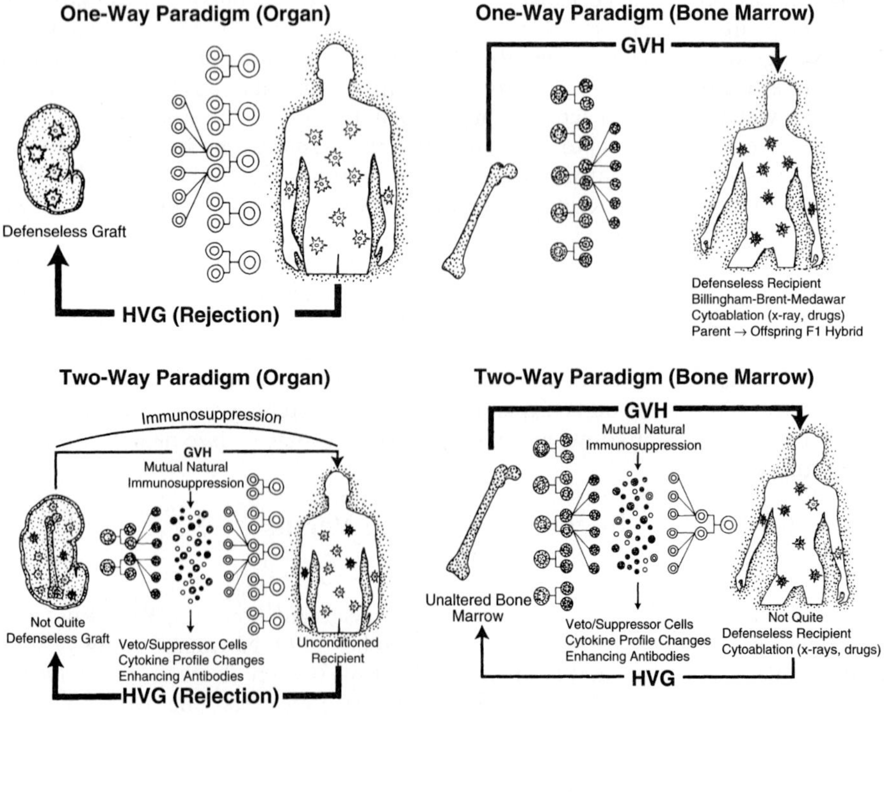

FIGURE 79.8. *Top panels.* One-way paradigm in which transplantation is conceived as involving a unidirectional immune reaction: *left*, host-versus-graft (HVG) with whole organs; *right*, graft-versus-host (GVH) with bone marrow or other lymphopoietic transplants. *Bottom panels.* Two-way paradigm in which transplantation is seen as a bidirectional and mutually canceling immune reaction that is (*left*) predominantly HVG with whole-organ grafts and (*right*) predominantly GVH with bone marrow grafts.

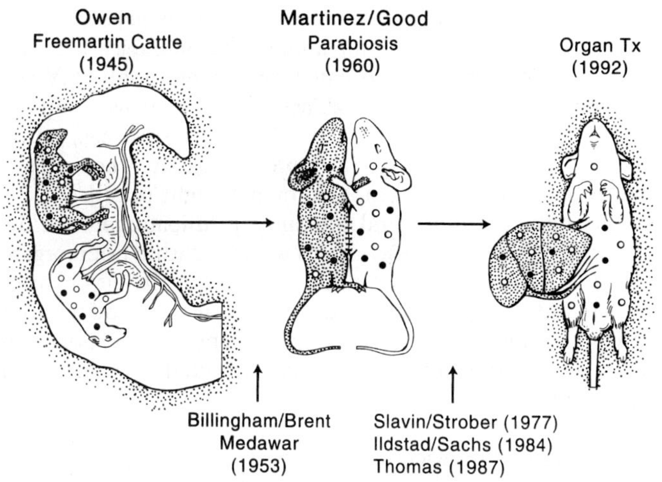

FIGURE 79.9. Continuum of chimerism from observations of Ray Owen in freemartin cattle to the discovery in 1992 of microchimerism in organ recipients.

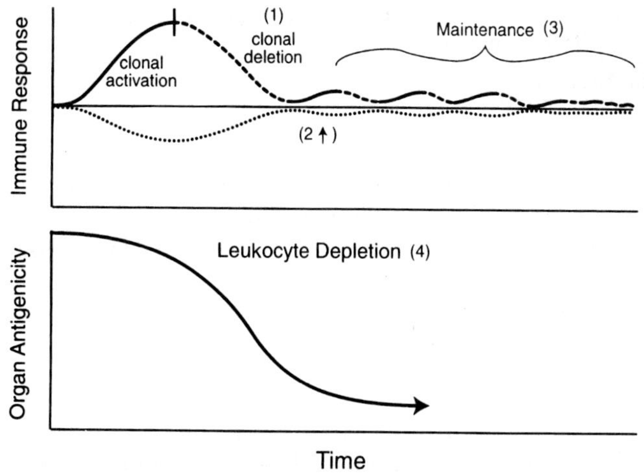

FIGURE 79.10. The four events that occur in close temporal approximation when there is successful organ engraftment. *Top*, double acute clonal exhaustion (*1, 2*) and subsequent maintenance clonal exhaustion (*3*) plus (*bottom*) loss of organ immunogenicity caused by depletion of the graft's passenger leukocytes (*4*).

tolerance induced with bone marrow (Fig. 79.8, bottom right). This context closed the 30-year intellectual gap between the fields of organ and bone marrow transplantation. Organ-associated chimerism then could be identified in a continuum of classic tolerance models,[5,11,161,298–300] beginning with the original observations by Owen in freemartin cattle (Fig. 79.9).

Organ Engraftment

The immunocompetent donor leukocytes in organ transplantation are highly immunogenic multilineage "passenger leukocytes" of bone marrow origin (including stem and dendritic cells) that migrate preferentially to host lymphoid organs and are replaced in the graft by host cells. The result is widespread antigen-specific immune activation of the coexisting donor and recipient cells, each by the other, which proceeds in successful cases to variable reciprocal clonal exhaustion and then deletion (Fig. 79.7).

Engraftment under clinical circumstances requires an umbrella of immunosuppression to prevent one cell population from destroying the other, but in some experimental models it occurs spontaneously (e.g., after pig liver transplantation and in many rodent models). The "nullification" of the two arms explains the poor prognostic value of HLA matching for organ versus bone marrow transplantation (Table 79.6) and the low incidence of GVHD following the engraftment in noncytoablated recipients of immunologically active organs, such as the intestine and liver.

In addition to inducing clonal activation and exhaustion by trafficking to host lymphoid organs, donor leukocytes that survive the initial destructive immune reaction migrate secondarily to nonlymphoid areas, where they do not generate an immune response ("immune indifference"). From here they may "leak" periodically to the host lymphoid organs and maintain clonal exhaustion. With clonal exhaustion/deletion and immune indifference in combination, both of which are regulated by the migration and localization of the antigen,[33] the four interrelated events shown schematically in Figure 79.10 must occur close together to have organ engraftment: double acute clonal exhaustion; maintenance clonal exhaustion, which frequently waxes and wanes; and loss of graft immunogenicity as the organ is depleted of its passenger leukocytes.

Bone Marrow Tolerance

Pretransplant cytoablation renders the recipient susceptible to immune attack by donor immune cells (i.e., GVHD), control of which frequently becomes the principal objective of immunosuppression rather than the prevention of rejection (see Table 79.6). Because complete destruction of host

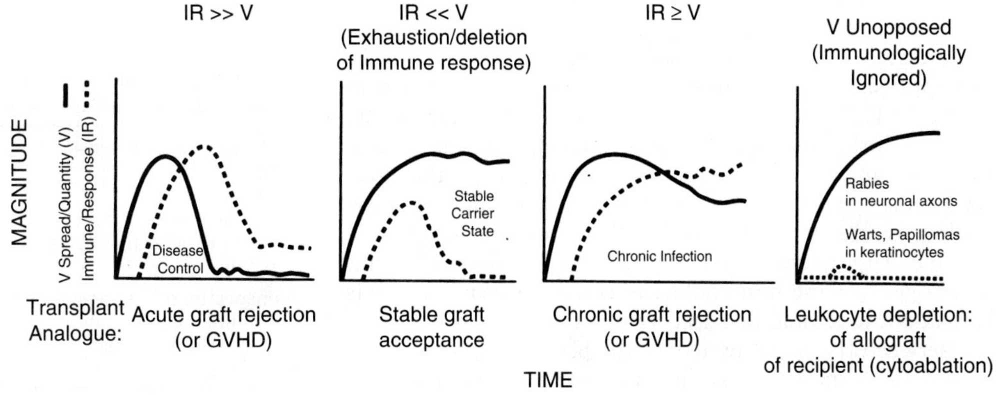

FIGURE 79.11. Variable outcomes after infection with widely disseminated noncytopathic viruses (or other microorganisms) and analogies (in the text below the horizontal axes) to organ and bone marrow transplantation. *Horizontal axis*, time; *vertical axis*, viral load (*v*, *solid line*) and host immune response (*IR*, *dashed line*).

TABLE 79.6. Differences Between Conventional Bone Marrow and Organ Transplantation.

Bone marrow		*Organ*
Yes	•Recipient cytoablation[a]•	No
Critical	•MHC compatibility•	Not critical
GVHD	•Principal complication•	Rejection
Common	•Drug-free state•	Rare
Tolerance	←Term for success→	"Acceptance"[b]

[a]Note: All differences derive from this therapeutic step, which in effect establishes an unopposed GVH reaction in the bone marrow recipient whose countervailing immune reaction is eliminated.

[b]Or "operational tolerance."

leukocytes is not possible with conventional doses of cytoablation,[301] the remaining cells will stimulate an alloresponse by mature or maturing donor T cells. Nevertheless, under immunosuppressive treatment, a weak host-versus-graft reaction mounted by these few recipient cells and a parallel graft-versus-host reaction mounted by the donor bone marrow cells may eventually result in reciprocal tolerance by deletion. These processes represent a mirror image of the events after organ transplantation (see Fig. 79.8, bottom right).

Relation to Infectious Disease

Noncytopathic Microorganisms

Early workers in transplantation[302,303] recognized the resemblance of allograft rejection to the response against infections associated with delayed hypersensitivity, exemplified by tuberculosis. With the demonstration in 1973 of the MHC-restricted mechanisms of adaptive infectious immunity by Doherty and Zinkernagel,[304–307] it became obvious that allograft rejection must be the physiological equivalent of the response to this kind of infection. Microorganisms that generate such an adaptive immune response are generally intracellular and have no or low cytopathic qualities.[308]

Although MHC-restricted host cytolytic T lymphocytes recognize only infected cells, elimination of all the infected cells could disable or even kill the host. Consequently, mechanisms have evolved that can temper or terminate the immune response, allowing both host and pathogen to survive.[308,309] These are the same two mechanisms that allow survival of allografts (i.e., clonal exhaustion/deletion and immune indifference),[33] both of which are governed by antigen migration and localization.[33,308,309] However, unlike the complex dual immune response of transplantation, infectious immunity is essentially a host-versus-pathogen reaction.

The analogies between transplantation and an infection with disseminated noncytopathic microorganisms can be exemplified by the common hepatitis viruses, as shown in Figure 79.11.[33,308,309] The pathogen (antigen) load may rapidly increase during the so-called latent period, but then be dramatically and efficiently controlled by antigen-specific effector T cells, which then subside (left panel). The transplantation analogues are acute irreversible rejection (or intractable GVHD). Alternatively, a continuously high antigen load with an antigen-specific immunological collapse (second panel) is equivalent to unqualified acceptance of an allograft.

Between these two extremes, the persistence of both the infectious agent and a strong immune response result in serious immunopathology (e.g., chronic active hepatitis with a B or C virus infection) comparable to chronic rejection after liver transplantation (third panel) or, uncommonly, GVHD. The conditions in the cytoablated bone marrow recipient mimic those of an infection by microorganisms (e.g., rabies and wart viruses) that avoid immune activation by not migrating through or to host lymphoid organs (right panel).[33]

Because immunity and tolerance to alloantigens follow the same rules as the response to noncytopathic microorganisms,[33] it is not possible with current transplantation practices to induce tolerance to allografts on the one hand without risking unwanted tolerance to pathogens on the other. In this context, the historical anxiety depicted in Figure 79.4 was correct.

Cytopathic Microorganisms

There is no MHC-restricted safety valve for cytopathic microorganisms, which are typically extracellular and generate the full resources of the innate as well as the adaptive immune system.[308,309] An uncontrollable innate immune response involving the effectors shown in Table 79.7 is provoked by discordant xenografts expressing the Gal-α-Gal epitope, an epitope that also is found on numerous cytopathic bacteria, protozoa, and viruses.

The clinical use of such discordant animal donors will require changing the xenogeneic epitope to one that mimics a noncytopathic profile or else elimination of the epitope.[310] Although chimpanzees and baboons do not express the Gal antigen, the clinical xenografts transplanted in 1963 from these subhuman primate donors[50,51] ultimately were damaged by an uncontrollable innate immune reaction, dominated by complement activation. Similar innate immune mechanisms were recognized in the 1960s to be responsible for the hyperacute destruction of ABO-incompatible allografts or allografts transplanted to presensitized recipients (see earlier[263–268]).

Self–Nonself-Discrimination

Survival in a hostile environment requires the ability to mount a protective immune response while avoiding a reaction of the immune system against self. Transplantation has succeeded because it has not lethally eroded this capability, which depends ultimately on the governance of immunological responsiveness or unresponsiveness by migration and localization of antigen.[33] Because the fetus possesses very early T-cell immune function,[311–313] the ontogeny of self–nonself-discrimination during fetal development can be explained by the same mechanisms as acquired tolerance in

TABLE 79.7. Effectors Involved in Response to Cytopathic Parasites and Discordant Xenografts.

The first line of defense
Interferons
Macrophages
Gamma/delta T cells
Natural killer (NK) cells
B cells
Nonspecific or less-specific effectors
Complement
Early interleukins
Phagocytes

later life. Autoimmune diseases then reflect unacceptable postnatal perturbations of the prenatally established localization of self-antigens in nonlymphoid versus lymphoid compartments.[33]

Conclusion

The lesson described in this chapter has been learned many times before: All knowledge can be traced to its roots and ultimately to a seed. For clinical transplantation, the historical beginning was Medawar's recognition that rejection is an immune reaction. Only two primary roots sprang from this seed. One was the demonstration by Billingham, Brent, and Medawar in 1953 that tolerance could be acquired by producing stem cell-driven hematolymphopoietic chimerism[5]; this concept ultimately led to bone marrow transplantation in humans.

The other root was the demonstration during 1962–1963 that kidney allografts could consistently self-induce tolerance with the aid of immunosuppression[30]; all further developments in organ transplantation were derivative from this discovery. The assumption reached by consensus in the early 1960s that the two roots reflected different immune mechanisms led to inadequate explanations of organ allograft acceptance and clouded the meaning of successful bone marrow transplantation.

The false assumption, which promptly became dogma, saddled succeeding generations of scientists and clinicians with a context that precluded the synthesis of a clarifying central principle of immunology that could be applied to all transplant, much less nontransplant, circumstances. After it was discovered in 1992 that organ recipients had persistent microchimerism, it was possible to see the essential commonality of organ and bone marrow transplantation, to relate observations after these procedures to the immune response to infectious diseases and neoplasms, and to explain the genesis of self–nonself-discrimination.

Epilogue

This chapter was originally prepared between August 1997 and August 1998. The immunologic paradigm that had emerged by then[31–34,106,287–293] was finalized in two collaborative reviews with Rolf Zinkernagel (Nobel Laureate, 1996).[314,315] It proved difficult to explain the new concept to persons whose career development (or legacy) during the preceding third of a century depended on not understanding it. The bitter pill that had to be swallowed was the reality that almost all of the clinical and experimental observations in transplantation immunology, and particularly those involved with organ engraftment, had been inserted from 1962 onward into an invalid intellectual framework. The consequence of the error was an epistemologic collapse, that is, a failure to understand.[316] As for the new paradigm, no modifications of the chapter written in 1997–1998 have been necessary. Moreover, the fresh insight into immunoregulation has been systematically exploited for therapeutic purposes under numerous transplant- and nontransplant-related circumstances.[317–319] Thus, both the old and new history of transplantation is a work in progress.

References

1. Terasaki PI, ed. History of HLA: Ten Recollections. Los Angeles: UCLA Tissue Typing Laboratory; 1990:1–269.
2. Terasaki PI, ed. History of Transplantation: Thirty-Five Recollections. Los Angeles: UCLA Tissue Typing Laboratory; 1990:1–704.
3. Gibson T, Medawar PB. The fate of skin homografts in man. J Anat 1943;77:299–310.
4. Medawar PB. The behavior and fate of skin autografts and skin homografts in rabbits. J Anat 1944;78:176–199.
5. Billingham RE, Brent L, Medawar PB. "Actively acquired tolerance" of foreign cells. Nature 1953;172:603–606.
6. Traub E. Persistence of lymphocytic choriomeningitis virus in immune animals and its relation to immunity. J Exp Med 1936;63:847–861.
7. Murphy JB. Transplantability of malignant tumors to the embryos of a foreign species. JAMA 1912;59:874–875.
8. Murphy JB. Factors of resistance to heteroplastic tissue-graftings: studies in tissue specificity. J Exp Med 1914;19:513–522.
9. Billingham R, Brent L, Medawar P. Quantitative studies on tissue transplantation immunity: actively acquired tolerance. Philos Trans R Soc Lond B Biol Sci 1956;239:357–412.
10. Hasek M. Vegetavni hybridisace zivocichu spojenim krevnich obehu v embryonalnim vyvojhi. Cesk Biol 1953;2:265.
11. Owen RD. Immunogenetic consequences of vascular anastomoses between bovine twins. Science 1945;102:400–401.
12. Anderson D, Billingham RE, Lampkin GH, Medawar PB. The use of skin grafting to distinguish between monozygotic and dizygotic twins in cattle. Heredity 1951;5:379–397.
13. Burnet FM, Fenner F. The Production of Antibodies. 2nd ed. Melbourne: Macmillan; 1949:1–142.
14. Billingham R, Brent L. A simple method for inducing tolerance of skin homografts in mice. Trans Bull 1957;4:67–71.
15. Billingham R, Brent L. Quantitative studies on transplantation immunity: induction of tolerance in newborn mice and studies on the phenomenon of runt disease. Philos Trans R Soc Lond B Biol Sci 1959;242:439–477.
16. Simonsen M. The impact on the developing embryo and newborn animal of adult homologous cells. APMIS 1957;40:480–500.
17. Brent L. A History of Transplantation Immunology. London: Academic Press; 1997:1–482.
18. Merrill JP, Murray JE, Harrison JH, Friedman EA, Dealy JB Jr, Dammin GJ. Successful homotransplantation of the kidney between non-identical twins. N Engl J Med 1960;262:1251–1260.
19. Starzl TE, Groth CG, Brettschneider L, et al. Orthotopic homotransplantation of the human liver. Ann Surg 1968;168:392–415.
20. Barnard CN. What we have learned about heart transplants. J Thorac Cardiovasc Surg 1968;56:457–468.
21. Dong E as told by Shumway NE and Lower RR. In: Terasaki PI, ed. History of Transplantation: Thirty-Five Recollections. Los Angeles: UCLA Tissue Typing Laboratory; 1991:435–449.
22. Derom F, Barbier F, Ringoir S, et al. Ten-month survival after lung homotransplantation in man. J Thorac Cardiovasc Surg 1971;61:835–846.
23. Lillehei RC, Simmons RL, Najarian JS, et al. Pancreaticoduodenal allotransplantation: experimental and clinical observations. Ann Surg 1970;172:405–436.
24. Goulet O, Revillon Y, Brousse N, et al. Successful small bowel transplantation in an infant. Transplantation (Baltimore) 1992;53:940–943.
25. Starzl TE, Rowe M, Todo S, et al. Transplantation of multiple abdominal viscera. JAMA 1989;261:1449–1457.
26. Mathe G, Amiel JL, Schwarzenberg L, Cattan A, Schneider M. Haematopoietic chimera in man after allogenic (homologous) bone-marrow transplantation. Br Med J 1963;2:1633–1635.

27. Bach FH. Bone-marrow transplantation in a patient with the Wiskott-Aldrich syndrome. Lancet 1968;2:1364–1366.
28. Gatti RA, Meuwissen HJ, Allen HD, Hong R, Good RA. Immunological reconstitution of sex-linked lymphopenic immunological deficiency. Lancet 1968;2:1366–1369.
29. Thomas ED. Allogeneic marrow grafting: a story of man and dog. In: Terasaki PI, ed. History of Transplantation: Thirty-Five Recollections. Los Angeles: UCLA Tissue Typing Laboratory; 1991:379–393.
30. Starzl TE, Marchioro TL, Waddell WR. The reversal of rejection in human renal homografts with subsequent development of homograft tolerance. Surg Gynecol Obstet 1963;117:385–395.
31. Starzl TE, Demetris AJ, Murase N, Ildstad S, Ricordi C, Trucco M. Cell migration, chimerism, and graft acceptance. Lancet 1992;339:1579–1582.
32. Starzl TE, Demetris AJ, Trucco M, et al. Cell migration and chimerism after whole-organ transplantation: the basis of graft acceptance. Hepatology 1993;17:1127–1152.
33. Starzl TE, Zinkernagel RM. Antigen localization and migration in immunity and tolerance. N Engl J Med 1998;339:1905–1913.
34. Starzl TE, Demetris AJ. Transplantation milestones: viewed with one- and two-way paradigms of tolerance. JAMA 1995;273: 876–879.
35. Carrel A. The operative technique for vascular anastomoses and transplantation of viscera. Lyon Med 1902;98:859.
36. Woodruff MFA. The Transplantation of Tissues and Organs. Springfield, Il: Thomas; 1960:1–777.
37. Simonsen M, Buemann J, Gammeltoft A, et al. Biological incompatibility in kidney transplantation in dogs: experimental and morphological investigations. APMIS 1953;32:36–84.
38. Moore FD, Smith LL, Burnap TK, et al. One-stage homotransplantation of the liver following total hepatectomy in dogs. Transplant Bull 1959;6:103–110.
39. Dempster WJ. Kidney homotransplantation. Br J Surg 1953;40: 447–465.
40. Lillehei RC, Goott B, Miller FB. The physiologic response of the small bowel of the dog to ischemia including prolonged in vitro preservation of the bowel with successful replacement and survival. Ann Surg 1959;150:543–560.
41. Moore FD, Wheeler HB, Demissianos HV, et al. Experimental whole organ transplantation of the liver and of the spleen. Ann Surg 1960;152:374–387.
42. Starzl TE, Kaupp HA Jr, Brock DR, Lazarus RE, Johnson RV. Reconstructive problems in canine liver homotransplantation with special reference to the postoperative role of hepatic venous flow. Surg Gynecol Obstet 1960;111:733–743.
43. Starzl TE, Kaupp HA Jr. Mass homotransplantation of abdominal organs in dogs. Surg Forum 1960;11:28–30.
44. Lower RR, Shumway NE. Studies on orthotopic homotransplantation of the canine heart. Surg Forum 1960;11:18.
45. Lower RR, Stofer RC, Shumway NE. Homovital transplantation of the heart. J Thorac Cardiovasc Surg 1961;41:196–204.
46. Lower RR, Stofer RC, Hurley EJ, Shumway NE. Complete homograft replacement of the heart and both lungs. Surgery 1961;50: 842–845.
47. Jaboulay M. Greffe du reins au pli du coude par soudures arterielles et veineuses [Kidney grafts in the antecubital fossa by arterial and venous anastomosis]. Lyon Med 1906;107:575–577.
48. Unger E. Nierentransplantation [Kidney transplantation]. Wien Klin Wochenschr 1910;47:573–578.
49. Groth CG. Landmarks in clinical renal transplantation. Surg Gynecol Obstet 1972;134:323–328.
50. Reemstsma K, McCracken BH, Schlegel JU, et al. Renal heterotransplantation in man. Ann Surg 1964;160:384–410.
51. Starzl TE, Marchioro TL, Peters GN, et al. Renal heterotransplantation from baboon to man: experience with six cases. Transplantation 1964;2:752–776.
52. Voronoy U. Sobre bloqueo del aparato reticuloendotelial del hombre en algunas formas de intoxicacion por el sublimado y sobre la transplantacion del rinon cadaverico como metodo de tratamiento de la anuria consecutiva a aquella intoxicacion [Blocking the reticuloendothelial system in man in some forms of mercuric chloride intoxication and the transplantation of the cadaver kidney as a method of treatment for the anuria resulting from the intoxication]. Siglo Med 1937;97:296–297.
53. Starzl TE. Patterns of permissible donor-recipient tissue transfer in relation to ABO blood groups. In: Experience in Renal Transplantation. Philadelphia: Saunders; 1964:37–47.
54. Ramsey G, Nusbacher J, Starzl TE, Lindsay GD. Isohemagglutinins of grafts origin after ABO-unmatched liver transplantation. N Engl J Med 1984;311:1167–1170.
55. Hamilton DNH, Reid WA. U Voronoy and the first human kidney allograft. Surg Gynecol Obstet 1984;159:289–294.
56. Kuss R, Teinturier J, Milliez P. Quelques essais de greffe rein chez l'homme. Mem Acad Chir 1951;77:755–764.
57. Dubost C, Oeconomos N, Nenna A, Milliez P. Resultats d'une tentative de greffe renale. Bull Soc Med Hop Paris 1951;67:1372–1382.
58. Servelle M, Soulie P, Rougeulle J. Greffe d'une rein de supplicie a une malade avec rein unique congenital, atteinte de nephrite chronique hypertensive azatemique. Bull Soc Med Hop Paris 1951;67:99–104.
59. Michon L, Hamburger J, Oeconomos N, et al. Une tentative de transplantation renale chez l'homme: aspects medicaux et biologiques. Presse Med 1953;61:1419–1423.
60. Merrill JP, Murray JE, Harrison JH, Guild WR. Successful homotransplantation of the human kidney between identical twins. JAMA 1956;160:277–282.
61. Hume DM, Merrill JP, Miller BF, Thorn GW. Experiences with renal homotransplantation in the human: report of nine cases. J Clin Invest 1955;34:327–382.
62. Moore FD. The development of tissue transplantation. In: Give and Take. Philadelphia: Saunders; 1964:1–182.
63. Billingham RE, Krohn PL, Medawar PB. Effect of cortisone on survival of skin homografts in rabbits. Br Med J 1951;1:1157–1163.
64. Morgan JA. The influence of cortisone on the survival of homografts of skin in the rabbit. Surgery (St. Louis) 1951;30:506–515.
65. Cannon JA, Longmire WP. Studies of successful skin homografts in the chicken. Ann Surg 1952;135:60–68.
66. Krohn PL. Effect of cortisone on second set skin homografts in rabbits. Br J Exp Pathol 1954;35:539.
67. Lawler RH, West JW, McNulty PH, Clancy EJ, Murphy RP. Homotransplantation of the kidney in the human. JAMA 1950;144:844–845.
68. Murray G, Holden R. Transplantation of kidneys, experimentally and in human cases. Am J Surg 1954;87:508–519.
69. Murray JE, Merrill JP, Harrison JH. Renal homotransplantation in identical twins. Surg Forum 1955;6:432–436.
70. Brown JB. Homografting of skin: with report of success in identical twins. Surgery 1937;1:558–563.
71. Nossal GJV. Antibody production of single cells. Nature 1958; 181:1419–1420.
72. Dempster WJ, Lennox B, Boag JW. Prolongation of survival of skin homotransplants in the rabbit by irradiation of the host. Br J Exp Pathol 1950;31:670–679.
73. Cannon JA, Terasaki P, Longmire WP. Studies of factors influencing induced tolerance to skin homografts in the chicken. Ann Surg 1957;146:278–284.
74. Main JM, Prehn RT. Successful skin homografts after the administration of high dosage X radiation and homologous bone marrow. J Natl Cancer Inst 1955;15:1023–1029.

75. Trentin JJ. Mortality and skin transplantibility in X-irradiated mice receiving isologous or heterologous bone marrow. Proc Soc Exp Biol Med 1956;92:688–693.
76. Mannick JA, Lochte HL, Ashley CA, Thomas ED, Ferrebee JW. A functioning kidney homotransplant in the dog. Surgery 1959; 46:821–828.
77. Storb R, Epstein RB, Bryant J, Ragde H, Thomas ED. Marrow grafts by combined marrow and leukocyte infusions in unrelated dogs selected by histocompatibility typing. Transplantation 1968;6:587–593.
78. Epstein RB, Storb R, Ragde H, Thomas ED. Cytotoxic typing antisera for marrow grafting in litter mate dogs. Transplantation 1968;6:45–58.
79. Hume DM, Jackson BT, Zukoski CF, Lee HM, Kauffman HM, Egdahl RH. The homotransplantation of kidneys and of fetal liver and spleen after total body irradiation. Ann Surg 1960; 152:354–373.
80. Rapaport FT, Bachvaroff RJ, Mollen N, Hirasawa H, Asano T, Ferrebee JW. Induction of unresponsiveness to major transplantable organs in adult mammals. Ann Surg 1979;190:461–473.
81. van Bekkum DW. Bone marrow transplantation: a story of stem cells. In: Terasaki PI, ed. History of Transplantation: Thirty-Five Recollections. Los Angeles: UCLA Tissue Typing Laboratory; 1991:395–434.
82. Murray JE, Merrill JP, Dammin GJ, et al. Study of transplantation immunity after total body irradiation: clinical and experimental investigation. Surgery 1960;48:272–284.
83. Murray JE, Merrill JP, Dammin GJ, Dealy JB Jr, Alexandre GW, Harrison JH. Kidney transplantation in modified recipients. Ann Surg 1962;156:337–355.
84. Hamburger J, Vaysse J, Crosnier J, et al. Transplantation of a kidney between nonmonozygotic twins after irradiation of the receiver: good function at the fourth month. Presse Med 1959; 67:1771–1775.
85. Hamburger J, Vaysse J, Crosnier J, Auvert J, Lalanne CL, Hopper J Jr. Renal homotransplantation in man after radiation of the recipient. Am J Med 1962;32:854–871.
86. Kuss R, Legrain M, Mathe G, Nedey R, Camey M. Homologous human kidney transplantation: experience with six patients. Postgrad Med J 1962;38:528–531.
87. Kuss R. Human renal transplantation memories, 1951 to 1981. In: Terasaki PI, ed. History of Transplantation: Thirty-Five Recollections. Los Angeles: UCLA Tissue Typing Laboratory; 1991.
88. Murray JE. Nobel Prize lecture: the first successful organ transplants in man. In: Terasaki PI, ed. History of Transplantation: Thirty-Five Recollections. Los Angeles: UCLA Tissue Typing Laboratory; 1991:121–143.
89. Goodwin WE, Kaufman JJ, Mims MM, et al. Human renal transplantation: clinical experience with six cases of renal homotransplantation. J Urology 1963;89:13–24.
90. Schwartz R, Dameshek W. Drug-induced immunological tolerance. Nature 1959;183:1682–1683.
91. Schwartz R, Dameshek W. The effects of 6-mercaptopurine on homograft reactions. J Clin Invest 1960;39:952–958.
92. Meeker W, Condie R, Weiner D, Varco RL, Good RA. Prolongation of skin homograft survival in rabbits by 6-mercaptopurine. Proc Soc Exp Biol Med 1959;102:459–461.
93. Calne RY. The rejection of renal homografts: inhibition in dogs by 6-mercaptopurine. Lancet 1960;1:417–418.
94. Zukoski CF, Lee HM, Hume DM. The prolongation of functional survival of canine renal homografts by 6-mercaptopurine. Surg Forum 1960;11:470–472.
95. Calne RY. Inhibition of the rejection of renal homografts in dogs by purine analogues. Transplant Bull 1961;28:445–461.
96. Calne RY, Murray JE. Inhibition of the rejection of renal homografts in dogs by Burroughs Wellcome 57-222. Surg Forum 1961;12:118–120.
97. Calne RY, Alexandre GPJ, Murray JE. A study of the effects of drugs in prolonging survival of homologous renal transplants in dogs. Ann N Y Acad Sci 1962;99:743–761.
98. Hitchings GH, Elion GB. The chemistry and biochemistry of purine analogs. Ann N Y Acad Sci 1954;60:195.
99. Pierce JC, Varco RL. Induction of tolerance to a canine renal homotransplant with 6-mercaptopurine. Lancet 1962;I:781–782.
100. Zukoski CF, Callaway JM. Adult tolerance induced by 6-methyl mercaptopurine to canine renal homografts. Nature 1963;198:706–707.
101. Starzl TE. Host-graft adaptation. In: Experience in Renal Transplantation. Philadelphia: Saunders; 1964:164–170.
102. Murray JE, Sheil AGR, Moseley R, Knoght PR, McGavic JD, Dammin GJ. Analysis of mechanism of immunosuppressive drugs in renal homotransplantation. Ann Surg 1964;160:449–473.
103. Hopewell J, Calne RY, Beswick I. Three clinical cases of renal transplantation. Br Med J 1964;I:411–413.
104. Alexandre GPJ, Murray JE. Further studies of renal homotransplantation in dogs treated by combined Imuran therapy. Surg Forum 1962;13:64–66.
105. Murray JE, Merrill JP, Harrison JH, Wilson RE, Dammin GJ. Prolonged survival of human-kidney homografts by immunosuppressive drug therapy. N Engl J Med 1963;268:1315–1323.
106. Starzl TE, Demetris AJ, Murase N, Trucco M, Thomson AW, Rao AS. The lost chord: microchimerism. Immunol Today 1996;17:577–584.
107. Hume DM, Magee JH, Kauffman HM Jr, Rittenbury MS, Prout GR Jr. Renal homotransplantation in man in modified recipients. Ann Surg 1963;158:608–644.
108. Woodruff MFA, Robson JS, Nolan B, Lambie AT, Wilson TI, Clark JG. Homotransplantation of kidney in patients treated by preoperative local radiation and postoperative administration of an antimetabolite (Imuran). Lancet 1963:2:675–682.
109. Medawar PB. Transplantation of tissues and organs: introduction. Br Med Bull 1965;21:97–99.
110. Woodruff MFA, Woodruff HG. The transplantation of normal tissues: with special reference to auto- and homotransplants of thyroid and spleen in the anterior chamber of the eye, and subcutaneously, in guinea pigs. Phil Trans B 1950;234:559–581.
111. Woodruff MFA. Evidence of adaptation in homografts of normal tissue. In: Medawar PB, ed. Biological Problems of Grafting. Oxford: Blackwell Scientific; 1959:83–94.
112. Starzl TE. Precepts of renal homotransplantation applied to homografting of other organs. In: Experience in Renal Transplantation. Philadelphia: Saunders; 1964:360–362.
113. Starzl TE, Kaupp HA Jr, Brock DR, Butz GW Jr, Linman JW. Homotransplantation of multiple visceral organs. Am J Surg 1962;103:219–229.
114. Murase N, Demetris AJ, Kim DG, Todo S, Fung JJ, Starzl TE. Rejection of the multivisceral allografts in rats: a sequential analysis with comparison to isolated orthotopic small bowel and liver grafts. Surgery 1990;108:880–889.
115. Murase N, Demetris AJ, Matsuzaki T, et al. Long survival in rats after multivisceral versus isolated small bowel allotransplantation under FK 506. Surgery 1991;110:87–98.
116. Starzl TE, Marchioro TL, Porter KA, et al. Factors determining short- and long-term survival after orthotopic liver homotransplantation in the dog. Surgery 1965;58:131–155.
117. Starzl TE. Efforts to mitigate or prevent rejection. In: Experience in Hepatic Transplantation. Philadelphia: Saunders; 1969:203–206.
118. Cordier G, Garnier H, Clot JP, et al. La greffe de foie orthotopique chez le porc. Mem Acad Chir (Paris) 1966;92:799–807.
119. Peacock JH, Terblanche J. Orthotopic homotransplantation of the liver in the pig. In: Read AE, ed. The Liver. London: Butterworth; 1967:333.

120. Calne RY, White HJO, Yoffa DE, et al. Observations of orthotopic liver transplantation in the pig. Br Med J 1967;2:478–480.
121. Calne RY, White HJO, Yoffa DE, et al. Prolonged survival of liver transplants in the pig. Br Med J 1967;4:645–648.
122. Starzl TE. Rejection in unmodified animals. In: Experience in Hepatic Transplantation. Philadelphia: Saunders; 1969:184.
123. Hunt AC. Pathology of liver transplantation in the pig. In: Read AE, ed. The Liver. London: Butterworth; 1967:337.
124. Porter KA. Pathology of the orthotopic homograft and heterograft. In: Starzl TE, ed. Experience in Hepatic Transplantation. Philadelphia: Saunders; 1969:427.
125. Calne RY, Sells RA, Pena Jr, et al. Induction of immunological tolerance by porcine liver allografts. Nature 1969;223:472–474.
126. Zimmerman FA, Davies HS, Knoll PP, Gocke JM, Schmidt T. Orthotopic liver allografts in the rat. Transplantation 1984;37: 406–410.
127. Kamada N, Brons G, Davies H. Fully allogeneic liver grafting in rats induces a state of systemic nonreactivity to donor transplantation antigens. Transplantation 1980;29:429–431.
128. Kamada N, Davies HS, Roser B. Reversal of transplantation immunity by liver grafting. Nature 1981;292:840–842.
129. Corry RJ, Winn HJ, Russell PS. Primary vascularized allografts of hearts in mice: the role of H-2D, H-2K, and non-H-2 antigens in rejection. Transplantation 1973;16:343–350.
130. Russell PS, Chase CM, Colvin RB, Plate JMD. Kidney transplants in mice: an analysis of the immune status of mice bearing long-term H-2 incompatible transplants. J Exp Med 1978;147: 1449–1468.
131. Starzl TE. Host graft adaptation. In: Experience in Renal Transplantation. Philadelphia: Saunders; 1964:168–170.
132. Starzl TE. Efforts to mitigate or prevent rejection. In: Experience in Hepatic Transplantation. Philadelphia: Saunders; 1969:228–233.
133. Steinman RM, Cohn ZA. Identification of a novel cell type in peripheral lymphoid organs of mice: morphology, quantitation, tissue distribution. J Exp Med 1973;137:1142–1162.
134. Simonsen M. On the acquisition of tolerance by adult cells. Ann N Y Acad Sci 1960;87:382–390.
135. Burnet FM. The Clonal Selection Theory of Acquired Immunity. Nashville: Vanderbilt University Press; 1959:59.
136. Talmage DW. Immunological specificity. Science 1959;129:1649–1653.
137. Burnet FM. The new approach to immunology. N Engl J Med 1961;264:24–34.
138. Miller JFAP. Immunological function of the thymus. Lancet 1961;2:748–749.
139. Miller JFAP. Effect of neonatal thymectomy on the immunological responsiveness of the mouse. Proc R Soc Lond Biol Sci 1962;156:415.
140. Starzl TE, Marchioro TL, Talmage DW, Waddell WR. Splenectomy and thymectomy in human renal homotransplantation. Proc Soc Exp Biol Med 1963;113:929–932.
141. Starzl TE, Porter KA, Andres G, et al. Thymectomy and renal homotransplantation. Clin Exp Immunol 1970;6:803–814.
142. McGregor DD, Gowans JL. Antibody response of rats depleted of lymphocytes by chronic drainage from the thoracic duct. J Exp Med 1963;117:303–320.
143. McGregor DD, Gowans JL. Survival of homografts of skin in rats depleted of lymphocytes by chronic drainage from the thoracic duct. Lancet 1964;1:629–632.
144. Algire GH, Weaver JM, Prehn RT. Studies on tissue homotransplantation in mice using diffusion chamber methods. Ann N Y Acad Sci 1957;64:1009.
145. Starzl TE, Kaupp HA Jr, Brock DR, Linman JW. Studies on the rejection of the transplanted homologous dog liver. Surg Gynecol Obstet 1961;112:135–144.
146. Starzl TE, Butz GW Jr. Surgical physiology of the transplantation of tissues and organs. Surg Clin North Am 1962;42:55–67.
147. Elkinton JR. Moral problems in the use of borrowed organs, artificial and transplanted. Ann Intern Med 1964;60:309–313.
148. Starzl TE, Marchioro TL, Rifkind D, Holmes JH, Rowlands DT Jr, Waddell WR. Factors in successful renal transplantation. Surgery 1964;56:296–318.
149. Rifkind D. Infectious diseases associated with renal transplantation. In: Starzl TE, ed. Experience in Renal Transplantation. Philadelphia: Saunders; 1964:213–238.
150. Starzl TE. Discussion of Murray JE, Wilson RE, Tilney NL, Merrill JP, Cooper WC, Birtch AG, Carpenter CB, Hager EB, Dammin GJ, Harrison H: 5 years experience in renal transplantation with immunosuppressive drugs. Ann Surg 1968;168:416–435.
151. Penn I, Hammond W, Brettschneider L, Starzl TE. Malignant lymphomas in transplantation patients. Transplant Proc 1969;1:106–112.
152. Starzl TE, Penn I, Putnam CW, Groth CG, Halgrimson CG. Iatrogenic alterations of immunologic surveillance in man and their influence on malignancy. Transplant Rev 1971;7:112–145.
153. Hill RB Jr, Rowlands DT, Rifkind D. Infectious pulmonary disease in patients receiving immunosuppressive therapy for organ transplantation. N Engl J Med 1964;271:1021–1027.
154. Rifkind D, Starzl TE, Marchioro TL, Waddell WR, Rowlands DT Jr, Hill RB Jr. Transplantation pneumonia. JAMA 1964;189:808–812.
155. Iwasaki Y, Porter KA, Amend JR, Marchioro TL, Zuhlke V, Starzl TE. The preparation and testing of horse antidog and antihuman antilymphoid plasma or serum and its protein fractions. Surg Gynecol Obstet 1967;124:1–24.
156. Starzl TE, Marchioro TL, Porter KA, Iwasaki Y, Cerilli GJ. The use of heterologous antilymphoid agents in canine renal and liver homotransplantation and in human renal homotransplantation. Surg Gynecol Obstet 1967;124:301–318.
157. Woodruff MFA, Anderson NF. Effect of lymphocyte depletion by thoracic duct fistula and administration of anti-lymphocytic serum on the survival of skin homografts in rats. Nature 1963;200:702.
158. Franksson C, Blomstrand R. Drainage of the thoracic lymph duct during homologous kidney transplantation in man. Scand J Urol Nephrol 1967;1:123–131.
159. Starzl TE, Weil R III, Koep LJ, Iwaki Y, Terasaki PI, Schroter GPJ. Thoracic duct drainage before and after cadaveric kidney transplantation. Surg Gynecol Obstet 1979;149:815–821.
160. Starzl TE, Klintmalm GBG, Iwatsuki S, Schroter G, Weil R III. Late follow-up after thoracic duct drainage in cadaveric renal transplantation. Surg Gynecol Obstet 1981;153:377–382.
161. Slavin S, Reitz B, Bieber CP, Kaplan HS, Strober S. Transplantation tolerance in adult rats using total lymphoid irradiation (TLI): permanent survival of skin, heart, and marrow allografts. J Exp Med 1978;147:700–707.
162. Najarian JS, Ferguson RM, Sutherland DER, et al. Fractionated total lymphoid irradiation as preparative immunosuppression in high-risk renal transplantation. Ann Surg 1982;196:442–452.
163. Myburgh AJ, Smit AJ, Meyers MA, Botha JR, Browde S, Thomson PD. Total lymphoid irradiation in renal transplantation. World J Surg 1986;10:369–380.
164. Metchnikoff I. Etude sur la resorption des cellules. Ann Inst Pasteur 1899;13:737.
165. Inderbitzen T. Histamine in allergic responses of the skin. In: Shafer JH, LeGrippo GA, Chase MW, eds. Henry Ford Hospital International Symposium on Mechanisms of Hypersensitivity. Boston: Little, Brown and Co.; 1959:493–499.
166. Waksman BY, Arbouys S, Arnason BG. The use of specific "lymphocyte" antisera to inhibit hypersensitive reactions of the "delayed" type. J Exp Med 1961;114:997–1022.

167. Levey RH, Medawar PB. Nature and mode of action of antilymphocytic antiserum. Proc Natl Acad Sci U S A 1966;56:1130–1137.
168. Monaco AP, Wood ML, Russell PS. Adult thymectomy: effect on recovery from immunologic depression in mice. Science 1965;149:432–435.
169. Monaco AP, Wood ML, Russell PS. Studies of heterologous antilymphocyte serum in mice: immunologic tolerance and chimerism produced across the H-2 locus with adult thymectomy and antilymphocyte serum. Ann N Y Acad Sci 1966;129:190–209.
170. Najarian JS, Simmons RL, Gewurz H, Moberg A, Merkel F, Moore GA. Anti-serum to cultured human lymphoblasts: preparation, purification and immunosuppressive properties in man. Ann Surg 1969;170:617–632.
171. Kohler G, Milstein C. Continuous culture of fused cells secreting antibody of predefined specificity. Nature 1975;256:495–497.
172. Cosimi AB, Colvin RB, Burton RC, et al. Use of monoclonal antibodies to T-cell subsets for immunological monitoring and treatment in recipients of renal allografts. N Engl J Med 1981; 305:308–314.
173. Starzl TE, Putnam CW, Halgrimson CG, et al. Cyclophosphamide and whole organ transplantation in human beings. Surg Gynecol Obstet 1971;133:981–991.
174. Starzl TE, Groth CG, Putnam CW, et al. Cyclophosphamide for clinical renal and hepatic transplantation. Transplant Proc 1973;5:511–516.
175. Dreyfuss M, Harri E, Hofmann H, Kobel H, Pache W, Tscherter H. Cyclosporin A and C: new metabolites from *Trichoderma polysporum* (Link ex Pers) Rifai. Eur J Appl Microbiol 1976;3:125–133.
176. Ruegger A, Kuhn M, Lichti H, et al. Cyclosporin A, ein immunosuppressiv wirksamer Peptidmetabolit aus *Trichoderma polysporum* (Link ex Pers) Rifai. Helv Chim Acta 1976;59:1075–1092.
177. Petcher TJ, Weber HP, Ruegger A. Crystal and molecular structure of an iodo-derivative of the cyclic undercepeptide cyclosporin A. Helv Chim Acta 1976;59:1480–1489.
178. Borel JF. Comparative study of in vitro and in vivo drug effects on cell-mediated cytoxicity. Immunology 1976;31:631–641.
179. Borel JF, Feurer C, Gubler HU, Stahelin H. Biological effects of cyclosporin A: a new antilymphocytic agent. Agents Actions 1976;6:468–475.
180. Borel JF, Feurer C, Magnee C, Stahelin H. Effects of the new anti-lymphocytic peptide cyclosporin A in animals. Immunology 1977;32:1017–1025.
181. Kostakis AJ, White DJG, Calne RY. Prolongation of rat heart allograft survival by cyclosporin A. Int Res Commun SystMed Sci 1977;5:280.
182. Calne RY, White DJG. Cyclosporin A: a powerful immunosuppressant in dogs with renal allografts. Int Res Commun Syst Med Sci 1977;5:595.
183. Calne RY, White DJG, Rolles K, Smith DP, Herbertson BM. Prolonged survival of pig orthotopic heart grafts treated with cyclosporin A. Lancet 1978;1:1183–1185.
184. Calne RY, White DJG, Pentlow BD, et al. Cyclosporin A: preliminary observations in dogs with pancreatic duodenal allografts and patients with cadaveric renal transplants. Transplant Proc 1979;11:860–864.
185. Green CJ, Allison AC. Extensive prolongation of rabbit kidney allograft survival after short-term cyclosporin A treatment. Lancet 1978;1:1182–1183.
186. Calne RY, White DJG, Thiru S, et al. Cyclosporin A in patients receiving renal allografts from cadaver donors. Lancet 1978; 2:1323–1327.
187. Calne RY, Rolles K, White DJG, et al. Cyclosporin A initially as the only immunosuppressant in 34 recipients of cadaveric organs: 32 kidneys, 2 pancreases, and 2 livers. Lancet 1979;2:1033–1036.
188. Starzl TE, Weil R III, Iwatsuki S, et al. The use of cyclosporin A and prednisone in cadaver kidney transplantation. Surg Gynecol Obstet 1980;151:17–26.
189. Starzl TE, Klintmalm GBG, Porter KA, Iwatsuki S, Schroter GPJ. Liver transplantation with use of cyclosporin A and prednisone. N Engl J Med 1981;305:266–269.
190. Reitz BA, Wallwork JL, Hunt SA, et al. Heart-lung transplantation: successful therapy for patients with pulmonary vascular disease. N Engl J Med 1982;306:557–564.
191. Griffith BP, Hardesty RL, Deeb GM, Starzl TE, Bahnson HT. Cardiac transplantation with cyclosporin A and prednisone. Ann Surg 1982;196:324–329.
192. Cooper J. The evolution of techniques and indications for lung transplantation. Ann Surg 1990;212:249–256.
193. Starzl TE, Todo S, Fung J, Demetris AJ, Venkataramanan R, Jain A. FK 506 for human liver, kidney and pancreas transplantation. Lancet 1989;2:1000–1004.
194. Kino T, Hatanaka H, Miyata S, et al. FK506, a novel immunosuppressant isolated from *Streptomyces*: immunosuppressive effect of FK-506 in vitro. Jpn J Antibiot 1987;40:1256–1265.
195. Ochiai T, Nakajima K, Nagata M, et al. Effect of a new immunosuppressive agent, FK506, on heterotopic allotransplantation in the rat. Transplant Proc 1987;19:1284–1286.
196. Murase N, Todo S, Lee P-H, et al. Heterotopic heart transplantation in the rat under FK-506 alone or with cyclosporine. Transplant Proc 1987;19:71–75.
197. Lee P, Murase N, Todo S, Makowka L, Starzl TE. The immunosuppressive effects of FR 900506 in rats receiving heterotopic cardiac allografts. Surg Res Commun 1987;1:325–331.
198. Todo S, Podesta L, ChapChap P, et al. Orthotopic liver transplantation in dogs receiving FK-506. Transplant Proc 1987;19:64–67.
199. Todo S, Ueda Y, Demetris JA, et al. Immunosuppression of canine, monkey, and baboon allografts by FK 506 with special reference to synergism with other drugs, and to tolerance induction. Surgery 1988;104:239–249.
200. Todo S, Demetris A, Ueda Y, et al. Renal transplantation in baboons under FK 506. Surgery 1989;106:444–451.
201. Fung JJ, Todo S, Jain A, et al. Conversion of liver allograft recipients with cyclosporine related complications from cyclosporine to FK 506. Transplant Proc 1990;22:6–12.
202. Armitage JM, Kormos RL, Griffith BP, et al. The clinical trial of FK 506 as primary and rescue immunosuppression in cardiac transplantation. Transplant Proc 1991;23:1149–1152.
203. Todo S, Fung JJ, Starzl TE, et al. Liver, kidney, and thoracic organ transplantation under FK 506. Ann Surg 1990;212:295–305.
204. Starzl TE, Fung J, Jordan M, et al. Kidney transplantation under FK 506. JAMA 1990;264:63–67.
205. Starzl TE, Donner A, Eliasziw M, et al. Randomized trialomania? The multicenter liver transplant trials. Lancet 1995;346: 1346–1350.
206. Fung JJ, Todo S, Tzakis A, et al. Conversion of liver allograft recipients from cyclosporine to FK506-based immunosuppression: benefits and pitfalls. Transplant Proc 1991;23:14–21.
207. Fung JJ, Todo S, Jain A, Demetris AJ, McMichael JP, Starzl TE. The Pittsburgh randomized trial of tacrolimus versus cyclosporine for liver transplantation. J Am Coll Surg 1996;183:117–125.
208. The European FK 506 Multicentre Liver Study Group. Randomized trial comparing tacrolimus (FK 506) and cyclosporin in prevention of liver allograft rejection. Lancet 1994;344:423–428.
209. The U.S. Multicenter FK 506 Liver Study Group. A comparison of tacrolimus (FK 506) and cyclosporine for immunosuppression in liver transplantation. N Engl J Med 1994;331:1110–1115.

210. Starzl TE, Abu-Elmagd K, Tzakis A, Fung JJ, Porter KA, Todo S. Selected topics on FK 506: with special references to rescue of extrahepatic whole organ grafts, transplantation of "forbidden organs," side effects, mechanisms, and practical pharmacokinetics. Transplant Proc 1991;23:914–919.
211. Todo S, Tzakis AG, Abu-Elmagd K, et al. Intestinal transplantation in composite visceral grafts or alone. Ann Surg 1992;216:223–234.
212. Todo S, Tzakis AG, Abu-Elmagd K, et al. Cadaveric small bowel and small bowel-liver transplantation in humans. Transplantation (Baltimore) 1992;53:369–376.
213. Starzl TE, Brittain RS, Stonington OG, Coppinger RW, Waddell WR. Renal transplantation in identical twins. Arch Surg 1963; 865:600–607.
214. Owens TC, Prevedel AE, Swan H. Prolonged experimental occlusion of thoracic aorta during hypothermia. Arch Surg 1955;70:95–97.
215. Starzl TE. Experience in Renal Transplantation. Philadelphia: Saunders; 1964:68–71.
216. Marchioro TL, Huntley RT, Waddell WR, Starzl TE. Extracorporeal perfusion for obtaining postmortem homografts. Surgery 1963;54:900–911.
217. Ackerman JR, Snell ME. Cadaveric renal transplantation. Br J Urol 1968;40:515–521.
218. Merkel FK, Jonasson O, Bergan JJ. Procurement of cadaver donor organs: evisceration technique. Transplant Proc 1972;4:585–589.
219. Starzl TE, Hakala TR, Shaw BW Jr, et al. A flexible procedure for multiple cadaveric organ procurement. Surg Gynecol Obstet 1984;158:223–230.
220. Starzl TE, Miller C, Broznick B, Makowka L. An improved technique for multiple organ harvesting. Surg Gynecol Obstet 1987; 165:343–348.
221. Carrel A, Lindbergh CA. The Culture of Organs. New York: Hoeber; 1938.
222. Ackerman JR, Barnard CN. A report on the successful storage of kidneys. Br J Surg 1966;53:525–532.
223. Brettschneider L, Daloze PM, Huguet C, et al. The use of combined preservation techniques for extended storage of orthotopic liver homografts. Surg Gynecol Obstet 1968;126:263–274.
224. Belzer FO, Ashby BS, Dunphy JE. 24-h and 72-h preservation of canine kidneys. Lancet 1967;2:536–538.
225. Collins GM, Bravo-Shugarman T, Terasaki PI. Kidney preservation for transportation: initial perfusion and 30 h ice storage. Lancet 1969;2:1219–1224.
226. Schalm SW. A Simple and Clinically Applicable Method for the Preservation of a Liver Homograft [thesis]. Holland: University of Leyden; 1968.
227. Benichou J, Halgrimson CG, Weil R III, Koep LJ, Starzl TE. Canine and human liver preservation for 6–19 h by cold infusion. Transplantation 1977;24:407–411.
228. Wall WJ, Calne RY, Herbertson BM, et al. Simple hypothermic preservation for transporting human livers long distances for transplantation. Transplantation 1977;23:210–216.
229. Jamieson NV, Sundberg R, Lindell S, et al. Successful 24- to 30-h preservation of the canine liver: a preliminary report. Transplant Proc 1988;29(suppl 1):945–947.
230. Kalayoglu M, Sollinger WH, Stratta RJ, et al. Extended preservation of the liver for clinical transplantation. Lancet 1988;1:617–619.
231. Todo S, Nery J, Yanaga K, Podesta L, Gordon RD, Starzl TE. Extended preservation of human liver grafts with UW solution. JAMA 1989;261:711–714.
232. Hoffman B, Sollinger H, Kalayoglu M, Belzer FO. Use of UW solution for kidney transplantation. Transplantation 1988;46:338–339.
233. Wahlberg JA, Love R, Landegaard L, Southard JH, Belzer FO. 72-h preservation of the canine pancreas. Transplantation 1987;43:5–8.
234. Ploeg RJ, Goossens D, McAnulty JF, Southard JH, Belzer FO. Successful 72-h cold storage of dog kidneys with UW solution. Transplantation 1988;46:191–196.
235. Ueda Y, Todo S, Imventarza O, et al. The UW solution for canine kidney preservation: its specific effect on renal hemodynamics and microvasculature. Transplantation 1989;48:913–918.
236. Belzer FO, Southard JH. Principles of solid-organ preservation by cold storage. Transplantation 1988;45:673–676.
237. Todo S, Podesta L, Ueda Y, et al. A comparison of UW with other solutions for liver preservation in dogs. Clin Transplant 1989;3: 253–259.
238. Starzl TE, Nalesnik MA, Porter KA, et al. Reversibility of lymphomas and lymphoproliferative lesions developing under cyclosporin-steroid therapy. Lancet 1984;1:583–587.
239. Starzl TE. The mother lode of liver transplantation: with particular reference to our new journal. Liver Transplant Surg 1998;4:1–14.
240. Starzl TE, Marchioro TL, Rowlands DT Jr, et al. Immunosuppression after experimental and clinical homotransplantation of the liver. Ann Surg 1964;160:411–439.
241. Marchioro TL, Porter KA, Dickinson TC, Faris TD, Starzl TE. Physiologic requirements for auxiliary liver homotransplantation. Surg Gynecol Obstet 1965;121:17–31.
242. Starzl TE, Francavilla A, Halgrimson CG, et al. The origin, hormonal nature, and action of hepatotrophic substances in portal venous blood. Surg Gynecol Obstet 1973;137:179–199.
243. Starzl TE, Porter KA, Putnam CW. Intraportal insulin protects from the liver injury of portacaval shunt in dogs. Lancet 1975;2: 1241–1246.
244. Francavilla A, Hagiya M, Porter KA, Polimeno L, Ihara I, Starzl TE. Augmenter of liver regeneration (ALR): its place in the universe of hepatic growth factors. Hepatology 1994;20:747–757.
245. Starzl TE, Jones AF, Terblanche J, Usui S, Porter KA, Mazzoni G. Growth-stimulating factor in regenerating canine liver. Lancet 1979;1:127–130.
246. Hagiya M, Francavilla A, Polimeno L, et al. Cloning and sequence analysis of the rat augmenter of liver regeneration (ALR) gene: expression of biology active recombinant ALR and demonstration of tissue distribution. Proc Natl Acad Sci USA 1994;91:8142–8146.
247. Giorda R, Hagiya M, Seki T, et al. Analysis of the structure and expression of the ALR gene. Mol Med 1966;2:97–108.
248. Starzl TE, Demetris AJ, Van Thiel DH. Medical progress: liver transplantation. N Engl J Med 1989;321(pt I):1014–1022.
249. Starzl TE, Bilheimer DW, Bahnson HT, et al. Heart-liver transplantation in a patient with familial hypercholesterolemia. Lancet 1984;1:1382–1383.
250. Bilheimer DW, Goldstein JL, Grundy SC, Starzl TE, Brown MS. Liver transplantation provides low-density-lipoprotein receptors and lowers plasma cholesterol in a child with homozygous familial hypercholesterolemia. N Engl J Med 1984;311:1658–1664.
251. Starzl TE. The little drummer girls. In: The Puzzle People. Pittsburgh: University of Pittsburgh Press; 1992:318–333.
252. Snell GD. Methods for the study of histocompatibility genes. J Genet 1948;49:87–103.
253. Brent L. Immunogenetics: histocompatibility antigens—genetics, structure and function. In: A History of Transplantation Immunology. London: Academic Press; 1997:131–182.
254. Dausset J. Iso-leuco-anticorps. Acta Haematol 1958;20:156.
255. Van Rood JJ, Eernisses JG, van Leeuwen A. Leucocyte antibodies in sera of pregnant women. Nature 1958;181:1735.
256. Terasaki PI, McClelland JD. Microdroplet assay of human serum cytoxins. Nature 1964;204:998–1000.

257. Starzl TE, Marchioro TL, Holmes JH, et al. Renal homografts in patients with major donor-recipient blood group incompatibilities [addendum]. Surgery 1964;55:195–200.
258. Starzl TE, Ishikawa M, Putnam CW, et al. Progress in and deterrents to orthotopic liver transplantation, with special reference to survival, resistance to hyperacute rejection, and biliary duct reconstruction. Transplant Proc 1974;6:129–139.
259. Rapaport FT, Dausset J, Legrand L, Barge A, Lawrence HS, Converse JM. Erythrocytes in human transplantation: effects of pretreatment with ABO group-specific antigens. J Clin Invest 1968;47:2202–2216.
260. Terasaki PI, Marchioro TL, Starzl TE. Sero-typing of human lymphocyte antigens: preliminary trials on long-term kidney homograft survivors. In: Histocompatibility Testing. Washington, DC: National Academy of Science Research Council; 1965:83–96.
261. Kissmeyer-Nielsen F, Olsen S, Peterson VP, Fieldborg O. Hyperacute rejection of kidney allografts associated with preexisting humoral antibodies against donor cells. Lancet 1966;2:662–665.
262. Willimas GM, Hume DM, Hudson RP, Morris PJ, Kano K, Milgrom F. "Hyperacute" renal-homograft rejection in man. N Engl J Med 1968;279:611–618.
263. Starzl TE, Lerner RA, Dixon FJ, Groth CG, Brettschneider L, Terasaki PI. Shwartzman reaction after human renal transplantation. N Engl J Med 1968;278:642–648.
264. Patel R, Terasaki PI. Significance of the positive crossmatch test in kidney transplantation. N Engl J Med 1969;280:735–739.
265. Simpson KM, Bunch DL, Amemiya H, et al. Humoral antibodies and coagulation mechanisms in the accelerated or hyperacute rejection of renal homografts in sensitized canine recipients. Surgery 1970;68:77–85.
266. Boehmig HJ, Giles GR, Amemiya H, et al. Hyperacute rejection of renal homografts: with particular reference to coagulation changes, humoral antibodies, and formed blood elements. Transplant Proc 1971;3:1105–1117.
267. Starzl TE, Boehmig HJ, Amemiya H, et al. Clotting changes, including disseminated intravascular coagulation, during rapid renal-homograft rejection. N Engl J Med 1970;283:383–390.
268. Myburgh JA, Cohen I, Gecelther L, et al. Hyperacute rejection in human-kidney allografts Shwartzman or Arthus reaction? N Engl J Med 1969;281:131–134.
269. Cerilli J, Brasile L, Galouzis T, Lempert N, Clarke J. The vascular endothelial cell antigen system. Transplantation 1985;39:286–289.
270. Brasile L, Zerbe T, Rabin B, Clarke J, Abrahms A, Cerilli J. Identification of the antibody to vascular endothelial cells in patients undergoing cardiac transplantation. Transplantation 1985;40:672–675.
271. Knechtle SJ, Halperin EC, Bollinger RR. Xenograft survival in two species combinations using total-lymphoid irradiation and cyclosporin. Transplantation 1987;43:173–175.
272. Gubernatis G, Lauchart W, Jonker M, et al. Signs of hyperacute rejection of liver grafts of Rhesus monkeys after donor-specific presensitization. Transplant Proc 1987;19:1082–1083.
273. Merion RM, Colletti LM. Demonstration of hyperacute rejection (HAR) in outbred large animal model of liver transplantation (LTX). Transplantation 1990;49:861–868.
274. Takaya S, Bronsther O, Iwaki Y, et al. The adverse impact on liver transplantation of using positive cytotoxic crossmatch donors. Transplantation 1992;53:400–406.
275. Starzl TE, Demetris AJ, Todo S, et al. Evidence for hyperacute rejection of human liver grafts: the case of the canary kidneys. Clin Transplant 1989;3:37–45.
276. Starzl TE. Tissue matching. In: The Puzzle People. Pittsburgh: University of Pittsburgh Press; 1992:118–124.
277. Brent L. Immunogenetics: histocompatibility antigens—structure and function. In: A History of Transplantation Immunology. London: Academic Press; 1997:153–159.
278. Starzl TE, Marchioro TL, Terasaki PI, et al. Chronic survival after human renal homotransplantations: lymphocyte-antigen matching, pathology and influence of thymectomy. Ann Surg 1965;162:749–787.
279. Terasaki PI, Vredevoe DL, Mickey MR, et al. Serotyping for homotransplantation: selection of kidney donors for thirty-two recipients. Ann N Y Acad Sci 1966;129:500–520.
280. Rapaport FT, Lawrence HS, Thomas L, Converse JM, Tillett WS, Mulholland JH. Cross-reactions to skin homografts in man. J Clin Invest 1962;41:2166–2172.
281. Dausset J, Rapaport FT. The Hu-1 system of human histocompatibility. In: Rapaport FT, Dausset J, eds. Human Transplantation. New York: Grune and Stratton; 1968: 369.
282. Rapaport FT, Dausset J. Behavior of HLA-compatible and incompatible skin allografts in human recipients preimmunized with pooled leukocyte extracts obtained from randomly selected donors. Transplantation 1983;36:592–594.
283. Starzl TE, Porter KA, Andres G, et al. Long-term survival after renal transplantation in humans: with special reference to histocompatibility matching, thymectomy, homograft glomerulonephritis, heterologous ALG, and recipient malignancy. Ann Surg 1970;172:437–472.
284. Mickey MR, Kreisler M, Albert ED, Tanaka N, Terasaki PI. Analysis of HL-A incompatibility in human renal transplants. Tissue Antigens 1971;1:57–67.
285. Starzl TE, Eliasziw M, Gjertson M, et al. HLA and cross reactive antigen group (CREG) matching for cadaver kidney allocation. Transplantation 1997;64:983–991.
286. Starzl TE, Demetris AJ, Murase N, Ricordi C, Trucco M. The enigma of graft acceptance. In: Shumway SJ, Shumway NE, eds. Thoracic Transplantation. London: Blackwell Science; 1995:452–470.
287. Starzl TE, Demetris AJ, Trucco M, et al. Systemic chimerism in human female recipients of male livers. Lancet 1992;340:876–877.
288. Starzl TE, Demetris AJ, Trucco M, et al. Chimerism and donor-specific nonreactivity 27 to 29 years after kidney allotransplantation. Transplantation 1993;55:1272–1277.
289. Starzl TE, Demetris AJ, Trucco M, et al. Chimerism after liver transplantation for type IV glycogen storage disease and type I Gaucher's disease. N Engl J Med 1993;328:745–749.
290. Demetris AJ, Murase N, Starzl TE. Donor dendritic cells after liver and heart allotransplantation under short-term immunosuppression. Lancet 1992;339:1610.
291. Demetris AJ, Murase N, Fujisaki S, Fung JJ, Rao AS, Starzl TE. Hematolymphoid cell trafficking, microchimerism, and GVHD reactions after liver, bone marrow, and heart transplantation. Transplant Proc 1993;25:3337–3344.
292. Qian S, Demetris AJ, Murase N, Rao AS, Fung JJ, Starzl TE. Murine liver allograft transplantation: tolerance and donor cell chimerism. Hepatology 1994;19:916–924.
293. Murase N, Starzl TE, Tanabe M, et al. Variable chimerism, graft versus host disease, and tolerance after different kinds of cell and whole organ transplantation from Lewis to Brown-Norway rats. Transplantation 1995;60:158–171.
294. Michie D, Woodruff MFA, Zeiss IM. An investigation of immunological tolerance based on chimera analysis. Immunology 1961;4:413–424.
295. Simonsen M. Graft versus host reactions: their natural history, and applicability as tools of research. Prog Allergy 1962;6:349–467.
296. Bain B, Vas MR, Lowenstein L. The development of large immature mononuclear cells in mixed leukocyte cultures. Blood 1964;23:108–116.

297. Bach F, Hirschhorn K. Lymphocyte interaction: a potential histocompatibility test in vitro. Science 1964;143:813–814.
298. Martinez C, Shapiro F, Good RA. Essential duration of parabiosis and development of tolerance to skin homografts in mice. Proc Soc Exp Biol Med 1960;104:256–259.
299. Ildstad ST, Sachs DH. Reconstitution with syngeneic plus allogeneic or xenogeneic bone marrow leads to specific acceptance of allografts or xenografts. Nature (Lond) 1984;307:168–170.
300. Thomas J, Carver M, Cunningham P, Park K, Gonder J, Thomas F. Promotion of incompatible allograft acceptance in rhesus monkeys given posttransplant antithymocyte globulin and donor bone marrow: in vivo parameters and immunohistologic evidence suggesting microchimerism. Transplantation (Baltimore) 1987;43:332–338.
301. Przepiorka D, Thomas ED, Durham DM, Fisher L. Use of a probe to repeat sequence of the Y chromosome for detection of host cells in peripheral blood of bone marrow transplant recipients. Am J Clin Pathol 1991;95:201–206.
302. Lawrence HS. Homograft sensitivity: an expression of the immunologic origins and consequences of individuality. Physiol Rev 1959;39:811–859.
303. Medawar PB. The immunology of transplantation. In: The Harvey Lectures. Series 52. New York: Academic Press; 1956–1957:144–166.
304. Zinkernagel RM, Doherty PC. Restriction of in vitro T cell-mediated cytotoxicity in lymphocytic choriomeningitis within a syngeneic or semi-allogeneic system. Nature 1974;248:701–702.
305. Zinkernagel RM. Restriction by H-2 gene complex of transfer of cell-mediated immunity to *Listeria monocytogenes*. Nature 1974;251:230–233.
306. Doherty PC, Zinkernagel RM. A biological role for the major histocompatibility antigens. Lancet 1975;1:1406–1409.
307. Zinkernagel RM, Doherty PC. The discovery of MHC restriction. Immunol Today 1997;18:14–17.
308. Zinkernagel RM. Immunology taught by viruses. Science 1996;271:173–178.
309. Zinkernagel RM, Ehl S, Aichele P, Oehen S, Kundig T, Hengartner H. Antigen localization regulates immune responses in a dose- and time-dependent fashion: a geographical view of immune reactivity. Immunol Rev 1997;156:199–209.
310. Starzl TE, Rao AS, Murase N, Fung J, Demetris AJ. Will xenotransplantation ever be feasible? J Am Coll Surg 1998;186:383–387.
311. Sterzl J, Silverstein AM. Development aspects of immunity. Adv Immunol 1967;6:337–459.
312. Matzinger P. Tolerance, danger, and the extended family. Ann Rev Immunol 1994;12:991–1045.
313. Ridge JP, Fuchs EJ, Matzinger P. Neonatal tolerance revisited: turning on newborn T cells with dendritic cells. Science 1996;271:1723–1726.
314. Starzl TE. Zinkernagel R. Antigen localization and migration in immunity and tolerance. N Engl J Med 1998;339:1905–1913.
315. Starzl TE, Zinkernagel R: Transplantation tolerance from a historical perspective. Nat Rev Immunol 2001;1:233–239.
316. Starzl TE. Organ transplantation: a practical triumph and epistemologic collapse. Proc Am Philos Soc 2003;147:226–245.
317. Starzl TE. The saga of liver replacement, with particular reference to the reciprocal influence of liver and kidney transplantation (1955–1967). J Am Coll Surg 2002;195:587–610.
318. Starzl TE, Murase N, Abu-Elmagd K, et al. Tolerogenic immunosuppression for organ transplantation. Lancet 2003;361:1502–1510.
319. Starzl TE, Lakkis FG. The unfinished legacy of liver transplantation: emphasis on immunology. Hepatology 2006;43(2 Suppl 1): S151–163.

80

Immunology of Transplantation

Allan D. Kirk and Eric A. Elster

Tissues transferred between genetically nonidentical individuals are destroyed through a process known broadly as *rejection*. It has been apparent throughout most of medical history that these tissues could provide relief from disease if they were not rejected. Thus, the field of transplantation has grown in tandem with the understanding of the biology of rejection and, to the extent that rejection is an immune-mediated process, of the immune system in general. This close relationship between immunological science and clinical transplantation has fueled remarkable progress in our understanding of immune function and of the fundamental nature of our existence as individuals. The components of the immune system that have been defined in this context are now widely recognized not only for their importance in graft rejection but also for their roles in infection control, shock, tumor growth, autoimmune disease, and the systemic response to trauma. As such, the understanding of immunology that has been born of the study of transplantation has become key to the thorough understanding of the biology of modern medicine and surgery.

It is important to underscore that everything involved in the rejection response evolved under selective pressure to maintain the integrity of the individual, not to prevent the relatively recent and artificial practice of organ sharing. Rejection is a fluke of nature—one that is the result of physiological immunity in a nonphysiological state. The student should remain acutely aware that immune responses to foreign tissues are both similar to and distinct from immune responses to environmental pathogens. Thus, while all maneuvers that interrupt the rejection response are likely to have an impact on natural host defenses, the differences between pathogens and foreign tissues can be exploited to prevent rejection while minimizing the risk of infection.

General Considerations and Terminology

At the most basic level, rejection involves recognition of a tissue that is foreign in a context that is perceived to be appropriate for a defensive response. Put another way, all rejection responses involve something on the graft that is recognized as foreign, some component of the immune system that recognizes it, and something that defines the context of the foreign object as worthy of the immune system's attention. To begin to describe these fundamental aspects of rejection, a rudimentary vocabulary is required. This is followed by a review of physiological immune function and finally a discussion of the biology of transplant rejection.

The word *antigen* is used to describe a molecule or tissue that can be recognized by the immune system. An *epitope* is the portion of the antigen, generally a carbohydrate or peptide moiety, that actually serves as the binding site for a receptor of the immune system. Thus, antigens contain one or many epitopes. Each is bound by one of two types of lymphocyte receptors: the *T-cell receptor* (TCR) of T cells or the *antibody* (or *immunoglobulin*) of B cells. In general, a TCR or antibody binds to one epitope, and each cell expresses a single type of antigen receptor. These receptors allow a given lymphocyte to "see" and respond to one epitope and thus establish the *specificity* of an immune response. The signal from these receptors to the lymphocyte on which they reside defines immune recognition. As discussed below, this general concept of specificity applies well to physiological immunity but is now recognized as imprecise for transplantation immunity. Considerable attention is now directed toward cross-reactive antigen receptors as important mediators of rejection.

The context or appropriateness of an immune response is governed by another set of receptors on lymphocytes broadly referred to as *costimulation* receptors. These receptors bind irrespective of the epitope and allow the lymphocyte to determine whether the specific signal generated by the antigen receptor should evoke a response. By having separate signals for specificity and appropriateness, the immune system can carefully regulate its response to be active when a pathogenic threat is present and inactive as the threat subsides. In general, the ligands for costimulation receptors are expressed most prominently on cells with the job to initiate immune responses, so-called antigen-presenting cells (APCs). Thus, immune responses are typically not initiated unless the antigen is presented to lymphocytes by APCs in a lymphoid organ such as lymph nodes or the spleen. In this way, new immune responses are tightly regulated to avoid autoimmune reactions.

Given the myriad surface receptors involved in lymphocyte function, the descriptive names that are frequently given to a newly discovered molecule are unwieldy. Thus, as new molecules are characterized, they are assigned a cluster of differentiation (CD) number. This nomenclature is vital to any discussion of complex cellular interactions.

Organs transplanted between genetically nonidentical individuals of the same species are termed *allografts*. Antigens from these grafts are thus *alloantigens*, and immunity toward these antigens is known as *alloreactivity*. The word *homograft* was used in earlier literature to describe allografts. The degree to which an allograft shares antigens with the recipient is referred to as the *histocompatibility* of the graft. This term generally refers to the similarity of a cluster of genes on chromosome 6 known as the *major histocompatibility complex* (MHC, also known as human leukocyte antigen [HLA] in humans). Thus, transplant antigens are unique, genetically encoded characteristics of an individual. The structure of the MHC is described in detail in the following section.

Basically, two different classes of MHC gene products are produced, termed *class I* and *class II*. The importance to transplantation of MHC gene products stems from their *polymorphism*. Unlike most genes, which are identical within a given species, polymorphic gene products differ in detail while still conforming to the same basic structure. Thus, polymorphic MHC proteins from one individual are foreign alloantigens to another individual. Allografts that are matched to their recipient at HLA are referred to as *HLA-identical* allografts, and those matched at half of the HLA loci are termed *haplo-identical*.

Note that HLA-identical allografts still differ genetically and are to be distinguished from *isografts*. Isografts are organs transplanted between identical twins, are immunologically inconsequential, and thus do not reject. *Xenografts* are organs transplanted from one species to another and were formerly described as *heterografts*. *Xenografts* are classified based on their genetic similarity to humans. *Concordant* xenografts are closely related species (e.g., Old World monkeys and apes), while *discordant* xenografts are distantly related species (e.g., New World monkeys and pigs).

A Brief History of Transplant Immunology

Many investigators, beginning with Carrel and Guthrie in the early 1900s, recognized that transplanted tissues failed for reasons that were nontechnical in nature.[1,2] Alexis Carrel used organ transplantation as a method for perfecting the technique of vascular anastomosis and was awarded the Nobel Prize in 1912 for his methods.

Murphy was the first to observe that lymphocytes were critical to the process of transplant failure,[3] but it was not until the 1940s that Peter Medawar systematically approached the problem of transplant rejection.[4] His classic studies using skin-grafted rabbits demonstrated that rejection was a genetically controlled, donor-specific event governed by multiple transplant-related antigens, and that it was mediated by lymphocytes and monocytes.[5,6] He went on to show that immunity could be invoked by prior exposure to donor tissues other than the transplanted tissue, that the immunity was remembered by the host immune system, and that active cell division was required for amplification of the host response.[7]

At the time of these studies, Ray Owen demonstrated that freemartin cattle, nonidentical cattle with fused placentas and a shared fetal circulation, could accept skin grafts from their dizygotic twins.[8] Expanding on Owen's studies, Medawar and his colleagues showed that transplant immunity was acquired during ontogeny rather than being an innate property of the host, and thus the barrier to transplantation was not absolute. In other words, he found that *tolerance to self-tissues is an acquired trait* and as such should be able to be developed for nonself-tissues.[9] In 1960, the Nobel Committee recognized Medawar's advances. Mitchison galvanized the importance of lymphocyte-derived immunity in 1954 with his demonstration that leukocyte transfusion could transfer transplant immunity.[10]

It is remarkable to note that, within a period of 10 years, from 1945 to 1955, Medawar and his contemporaries defined the basic barriers to allotransplantation and demonstrated that a biological solution could exist. Their investigations have served as the basis for all subsequent work in the field.

The next two decades were marked by extraordinary progress in the understanding of the genetic basis of immune recognition. This work was guided by a search for the surface alloantigens. Landmark investigations on the immunogenetics of the MHC began with Gorer and Snell's description of the H-2 system in mice, a genetic locus that segregated with transplanted tumor survival.[11–13] This erythrocyte-based system was soon shown by Amos[14] to exist on leukocytes and to elicit an antibody response toward the antigens encoded by H-2. This antibody response became critical for establishing the correlate of H-2 in man. Dausset used this finding together with his observation that antibodies could also be generated by antigen exposure via transfusion or pregnancy to establish the first serologically based typing system for human transplant antigens, the Mac antigens.[15,16] In keeping with the fundamental nature of discoveries in transplant immunobiology, Snell and Dausset shared a Nobel Prize in 1980 for their initial observations.

Class II MHC polymorphism was also defined in this period. Bach demonstrated that lymphocytes would proliferate in response to contact with lymphocytes of a different genetic background.[17] This phenomenon, known as the *mixed lymphocyte culture* (MLC), was found to be based on differences in class II MHC molecules and was defined as HLA-D (eventually shown to be the same molecule as HLA-DR). Thus, both serological and cellular assays had been defined that could determine the degree of similarity between individuals.

These findings set the stage for a series of extraordinary workshops held between 1964 and 1970 to bring the growing number of methods for defining transplant antigens together under one unified system.[4] This effort resulted in the current definition of HLA as six loci on chromosome 6, encoding two related cell surface molecules: class I (HLA-A, -B, and -C) and class II (HLA-DR, -DP, and -DQ) (Fig. 80.1). Stimulated by the increasingly rapid pace in defining HLA polymorphisms, methods for rapid serological definition of HLA were developed and broadly applied to the clinic. The primary methods adopted were the lymphocytotoxicity assay of Terasaki,[18] in which antibodies with known specificities against HLA antigens are reacted with unknown cells to determine the HLA antigens on the unknown sample, and refinements of the MLC of Bach.[17]

In the 1970s, subsequent advancements in molecular biological techniques allowed the genetic basis of HLA polymorphism to be established, eventually leading to the discovery by Bjorkman[19,20] and Brown[21,22] of the three-dimensional structure of HLA antigens. In addition, these methods allowed for the fundamental aspects of antigen recognition to be defined. Particularly important to this effort were the 1987 Nobel Prize-winning contributions of Susumu Tonegawa, which showed that antigen receptors were generated by complex rearrangements of the somatic genes in T and B cells.[23] This principle, described next, offered an explanation of how the immune system could learn not to react toward itself during development and has allowed for further examination of the fundamental nature of neonatal acquired tolerance first described by Medawar. The biological role of HLA as an antigen-presenting molecule was also defined during this period through the work of many investigators, including the 1996 Nobel Prize-winning contributions of Zinkernagel and Doherty.[24,25]

The characterization of HLA also catalyzed numerous fundamental investigations in immunology in the 1980s. With the transplant antigens largely defined, the antigen receptors were quickly characterized. The function and structure of the TCR, the importance of adhesion molecules, and the elucidation of the soluble mediators of cell activation, cytokines, were all products of this period.

The issue of context has been the final major component of the immune response to be elucidated. Bretscher and Cohn were first to propose that antigen recognition was not sufficient to initiate an immune response.[26] Their theory was generalized in the 1970s by Lafferty and Cunningham as the two-signal model for lymphocyte activation, with signal one an antigen-specific signal and signal two a non-

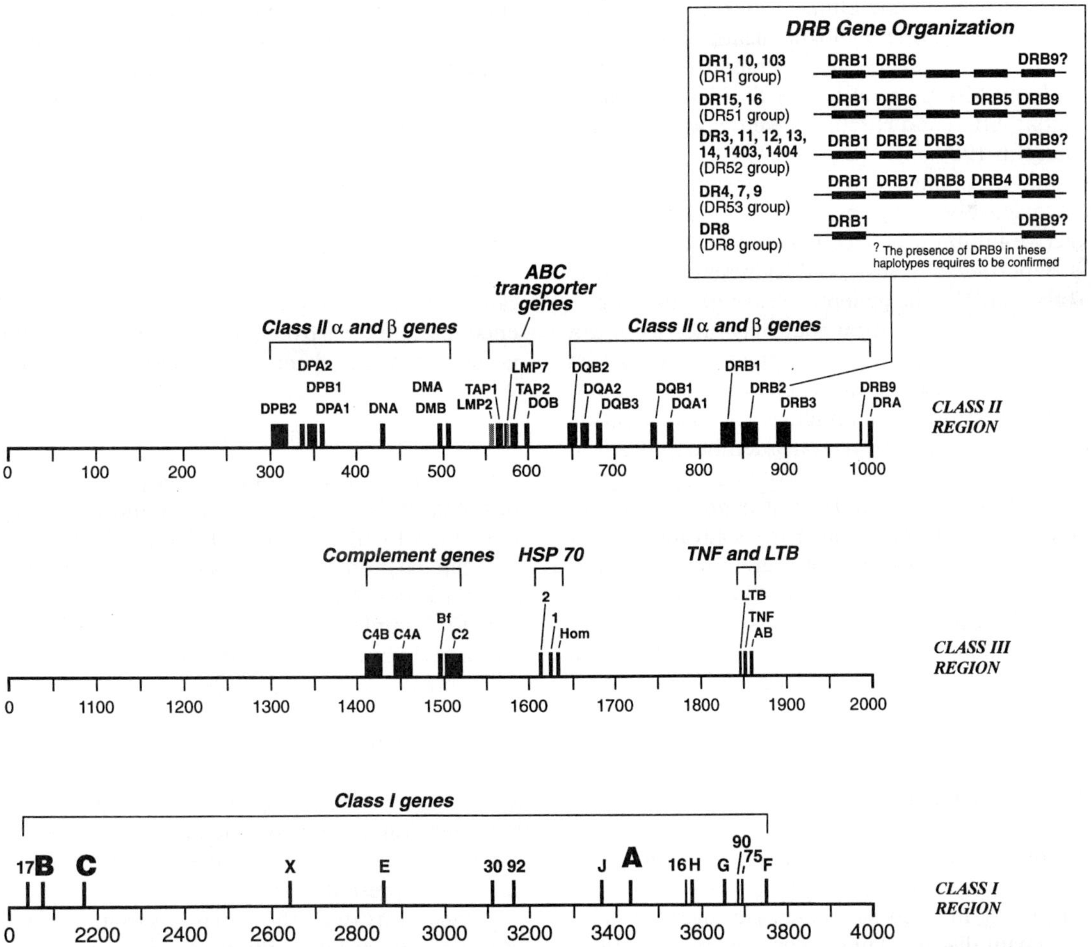

FIGURE 80.1. The human major histocompatibility complex (HLA). An abridged map of the human MHC locus on chromosome 6. One copy of this locus is inherited from each parent, each of which encodes the sequences for the major transplantation antigens HLA-A, -B, -C (class I region), HLA-DR, -DP, and -DQ (class II region). *Inset*: The DR β-chain loci polymorphisms. (From Kirk and Sollinger,[251] with permission.)

specific contextual signal.[27] The components of this second signal, now known as costimulation, have been defined by June, Ledbetter, Linsley, Nadler, and others and are discussed in subsequent sections.[28] The current theory implicating context as a critical element of immune recognition, put forth recently by Matzinger as the "danger" theory of lymphocyte activation, has provided the needed link between an active disease state and antigen recognition. Tissue injury promotes costimulation and makes lymphocyte activation more likely to occur with the appropriate antigen recognition.[29] Together, the studies of the past decade have led to a reasonably comprehensive picture of the mechanism of allograft rejection and of the physiological functions of lymphocytes.

A final historical consideration is particularly germane for students of clinical surgery. The pace of discovery in immunology has been accelerated by a close link between the basic scientific community and surgeons. This in turn has led to the rapid application of new discoveries to the problem of rejection and to clinical observations that have aided greatly in the understanding of basic laboratory studies. There are several particularly notable examples of this symbiosis. Joseph Murray applied the concept that transplant antigens were genetically determined shortly after it was proposed by successfully transplanting a kidney between identical twins.[30] The importance of lymphocyte division was also quickly recognized and exploited. Gertrude Elion and George Hitchings developed a 6-mercaptopurine analogue, azathioprine (Aza), that inhibited lymphocyte nucleic acid metabolism.[31,32] It was applied clinically by Murray to allow for the first successful human allografts.[33] Elion and Hitchings were honored by the Nobel committee in 1988 and Murray in 1990.

The most influential advance in immunosuppression has been the 1976 discovery of cyclosporine by Borel.[34,35] This relatively selective inhibitor of T-cell activation was quickly recognized as important by White and Calne and applied to renal transplantation.[36,37] The general release of this drug in 1983 made clinical transplantation routinely successful not only for kidneys but also for extrarenal organs. The success of cyclosporine has reciprocated a benefit to T-cell biology in general as it has stimulated much of the investigation necessary for understanding overall transmembrane receptor signaling.

As a result of the studies since 1964, it is now rare for an allograft to be lost to acute rejection. Future advances must now focus on the chronic diseases of a growing transplant population, including chronic rejection (CR) and the chronic toxicity associated with lifelong immunosuppression. It is likely that these challenges will be met as were those of the past decades: by cooperation between basic investigators and surgeon scientists.

Physiological Immunity

The mediators of rejection exist not to prevent the well-intended efforts of transplant surgeons, but rather to prevent our bodies from being invaded by foreign pathogens or succumbing to malignant disease. Thus, to understand rejection, and particularly to appreciate the consequences of the pharmacological suppression of rejection, a general understanding of immunity as it functions in a physiological setting is required. This section outlines the constituents of normal immune responses. Subsequent sections discuss these elements of immunity as they relate to transplantation.

Two complementary arms of the immune system have evolved in vertebrates to combat disease: the *innate* and *acquired* immune systems. They differ in their fundamental responsibilities but are now recognized to influence one another to achieve overall homeostasis. Broadly speaking, the innate immune system recognizes *general* motifs that have, through selective evolutionary pressure, come to represent universally pathological states to our species (ischemia, necrosis, trauma, and certain nonhuman cell surfaces).[38] Innate recognition leads to prompt and direct attempts to remove the offending entity. Innate mechanisms of defense are thus direct and are not steeped in regulation. The likelihood that self-reactive innate immunity will occur is low because the molecules that trigger innate processes have been defined by their stark differences from normal tissues. However, the more important role of innate immunity is in recruiting acquired responses to areas where there is clear evidence of a pathological process. Thus, innate responses are frequently precursors of acquired responses rather than protective responses in and of themselves.

In contrast, the acquired immune system recognizes *specific* pathogens through antigen binding. Antigen binding leads to carefully regulated destruction of the antigen-expressing tissue. Obviously, a large number of receptors are required to specifically distinguish the seemingly endless array of pathogens. Highly specific receptors must also respond to very minor differences in antigen structure. With a large and varied assemblage of receptors, the potential for cross-reactivity with self is high. This system must therefore be under constant tight regulation to prevent autoimmunity. Acquired responses are therefore characterized by many regulatory steps designed to prevent autoimmune attack and uncontrolled lymphocyte proliferation. Clearly, an immune system tailor made for one individual will be perturbed when it encounters tissues from another individual. This perturbation is the fundamental cause of allograft rejection.

Physiological Innate Immunity

The innate immune system uses protein receptors encoded in the germ line (passed from one individual to its offspring) to identify foreign or aberrant/damaged tissues.[49] These receptors can exist on cells, such as macrophages, neutrophils, and natural killer (NK) cells, or free in the circulation, as is the case for complement.[38–40] They are limited in specificity but are broadly reactive against common components of pathogenic organisms, for example, lipopolysaccharides on gram-negative organisms or other glycoconjugates. Thus, the receptors of innate immunity are the *same* from one individual to another within a species and, in general, do not play a role in the recognition of a foreign graft per se. They do, however, come into play when an injured tissue (e.g., one that has been made ischemic and moved from one individual to another) is present.

Once activated, the innate system performs two vital functions. It initiates cytolytic pathways for the destruction of the offending organism, primarily through the complement cascade[41] (Fig. 80.2). It also communicates the encounter to the acquired immune system for a more specific response

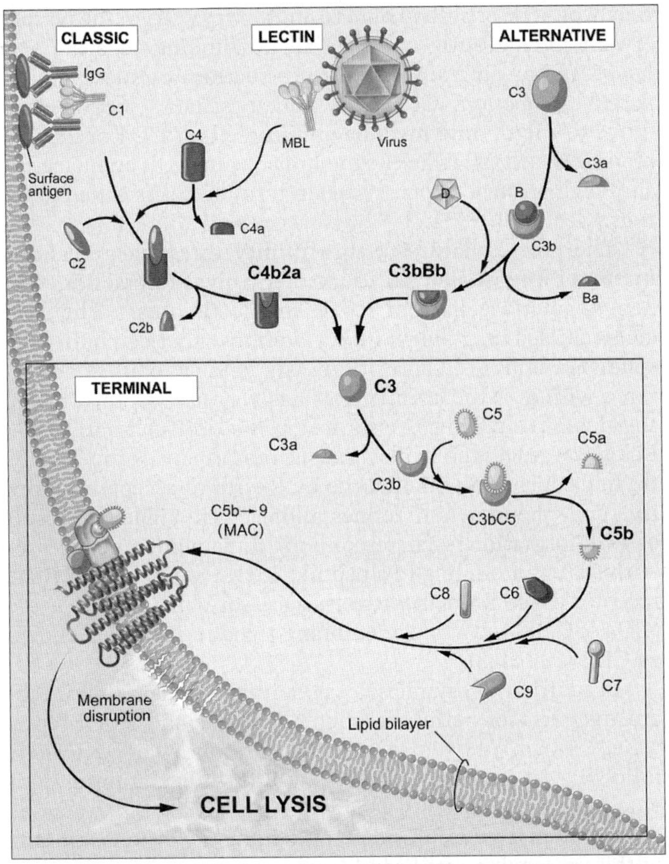

FIGURE 80.2. Complement plays a central role in many innate responses. In a process known as alternative pathway complement activation, C3, the central activating enzyme of the complement cascade, can be activated when carbohydrates lacking sialic acid (a sugar moiety that is not found in most bacteria but is common on human cells) are encountered. One of the cleaved fragments of C3, C3b, is released and binds to the invader, flagging it as foreign, a process known as *opsonization*. C3a, another product of C3 activation, acts to recruit neutrophils to the site, while C3d enhances the immunogenicity of the organism, making it more likely to stimulate a dendritic cell to present the antigen to T cells. C3 activation also leads to formation of the membrane attack complex (MAC). This product is the result of activated C3 catalyzing the activation of C5, which in turn catalyzes the polymerization of C6, C7, C8, and C9, forming the MAC, a pore embedded in the foreign cell that results in disruption of the membrane and lysis.

through by-products of complement activation and through the function of phagocytic cells. Because this system leads to a vigorous and relatively direct response, there can be no room for error; recognition must be based on absolute differences that cannot be present on normal cells.

Macrophages and dendritic cells (DCs) engulf not only foreign cells that have been bound by complement, but also cells identified through receptors for foreign carbohydrates (e.g., mannose receptors).[42] A recently described and highly evolutionarily conserved family of proteins known as Toll-like receptors are now recognized as important activation molecules for innate APCs. They bind to pathogen-associated molecular pattern (PAMP) motifs common to pathogenic organisms.[43] Engulfed cells or tissues are reduced to peptide fragments and presented to the acquired immune system embedded in MHC molecules so that T cells specific for these peptides can be activated. Acquired immunity can also reciprocally activate the innate system. In a pathway known as the classical complement activation cascade, antigen-bound antibody can bind to the complement molecule C1q, which in turn becomes activated and activates C3. The C3 activation products then proceed toward the membrane attack complex (MAC) and serve chemoattractant functions, as described for the alternative pathway. One breakdown product of this pathway (C4d) is now used diagnostically to detect antibody-mediated allograft rejection.[44]

Physiological Acquired Immunity

The hallmark of acquired immunity is *specific* recognition and elimination of cells. Highly specialized antigen receptors (detailed below) for distinguishing infected and transformed cells from normal tissues have evolved to facilitate this goal. The altered cell is recognized as a specific entity, not just as nonself, and a record of that encounter is retained for more rapid response to future encounters, a phenomenon known as *immunological memory*.[45] As discussed previously, the specialized response makes the system more prone to error; thus, the innate response aids the acquired system in determining whether an antigen is worthy of its attention.[46]

The Genetics and Structural Characteristics of Antigen Receptors

Two cell types have evolved with the ability to specifically bind to antigen: T cells and B cells (Fig. 80.3). Their receptors are similar in genetic development but differ in the types of antigens they bind. The T-cell antigen receptors bind peptide antigens that have been processed by cells and combined with MHC molecules, while B-cell antibodies bind antigens in their native conformation on an invading pathogen or free in the extracellular fluid. The TCRs are fixed, while antibodies can be secreted and act at locations remote from the cell.

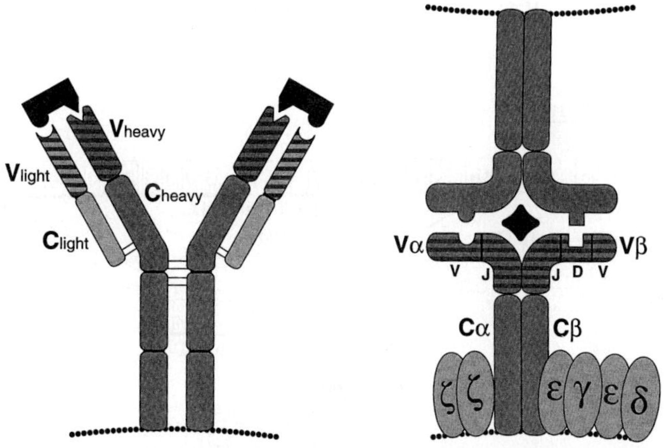

FIGURE 80.3. The general structure of antigen receptors. The two receptor types used by cells of the acquired immune system for specific recognition of antigen. The B-cell antigen receptor (*left*) is an antibody molecule made up of two identical light chains disulfide bonded to two identical heavy chains, thus forming two identical sites for binding soluble antigen. The T-cell antigen receptor (*right*) is associated with a five-chained signal transduction unit called CD3 (shown as the subunits $\zeta_2\varepsilon_2$gd). It has a single antigen-binding site for recognition of a processed peptide antigen bound to an MHC molecule. *Striped areas* represent the regions of most structural variability. (From Kirk and Sollinger,[251] with permission.)

The T-Cell Receptor

The formation of the TCR is fundamental to the understanding of its function.[47,48] The T cells are formed in the fetal liver and bone marrow and migrate to the thymus during the first trimester of fetal development. At this stage, they have no TCR or accessory molecules. On entering the thymus, T cells undergo a remarkable rearrangement of the DNA that encodes the two chains of the TCR (α and β, or γ and δ) (Fig. 80.4).[49] The order of genetic rearrangement recapitulates the evolution of the TCR. The T cells first attempt to recombine the γ and δ TCR genes and then resort to the more diverse α and β TCR genes. The γδ configuration is typically not successful, and thus most T cells are αβ T cells. The T cells expressing the γδ TCR have more primitive functions, including recognition of heat-shock proteins and activity similar to NK cells as well as MHC recognition, while αβ T cells are more typically limited to recognition of MHC-presented peptide.[50] Thus, γδ T cells represent an evolutionary link between the innate and acquired immune systems, possessing the ability to recognize generally injured tissue and specific antigen.

It is important to note that, regardless of the genes used, individual cells recombine to express a TCR with a single specificity. The rearrangements occur randomly, resulting in a population of T cells capable of binding 10^9 different specificities, essentially all combinations of MHC and peptide. These developing T cells also express both CD4 and CD8, accessory molecules that strengthen the TCR binding to MHC (described in more detail following). These accessory molecules further increase the binding repertoire of the population to include either class I or class II MHC molecules.

If these T cells were released unmodified, they would quickly bind to self-cells and destroy the individual. To avoid the release of autoreactive T cells, developing cells undergo a process following recombination known as *thymic selection*[51,52] (Fig. 80.5). Cells initially interact with the MHC-expressing cortical thymic epithelium. If binding does *not* occur to self-MHC, the cells are useless to the individual as they would be unable to bind to and survey cells in the periphery for foreign antigen. Thus, all nonbinding cells undergo *apoptosis*, or programmed self-destruction, a process called *positive selection*. Cells surviving positive selection then move to the thymic medulla and lose either CD4 or CD8. If binding to self-MHC in the medulla occurs with an unacceptably high affinity, apoptosis again results; this is called *negative selection*.

The precise nature of this affinity threshold remains a matter of intense investigation and involves interaction with hematopoietic cells that reside in the thymus.[53] The only cells released into the periphery are those that can both bind self-MHC and avoid activation. Any foreign peptide encountered will alter the affinity that has been preordained in the thymus, resulting in the initial events of T-cell activation. Likewise, MHC molecules that were not part of the T cell's thymic education will bind the TCR with unacceptable affinity. This phenomenon defines alloreactivity. The end result of TCR formation is a heterodimeric transmembrane receptor with a site for binding to a peptide–MHC combination.[54] The receptor is combined with an accessory-binding molecule (CD4 or CD8) and a transmembrane-signaling complex known as CD3 (Fig. 80.3).

In addition to thymic selection, it is now clear that mechanisms exist for peripheral modification of the T-cell repertoire.[53] Much of this is in place for removal of T cells following an immune response and downregulation of activated clones. A molecule known as Fas (CD98) is expressed on activated T cells.[55] Under appropriate conditions, binding of this molecule to its ligand leads to apoptosis. This method is dependent on TCR binding and the activation state of the T cell. In addition to its role in downregulation, the Fas ligand can serve as a molecular barrier to T-cell invasion of certain immunologically privileged sites, for example, testes.[56] Complementing this deletional method to TCR repertoire control are nondeletional mechanisms that selectively anergize (make unreactive) specific T-cell clones. One prominent receptor group mediating this function is the CD28:B7 pair (described in detail later).[28] Binding of the TCR only leads to activation

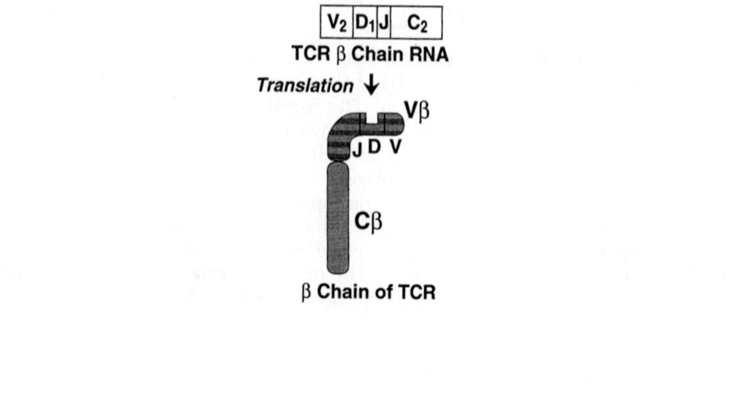

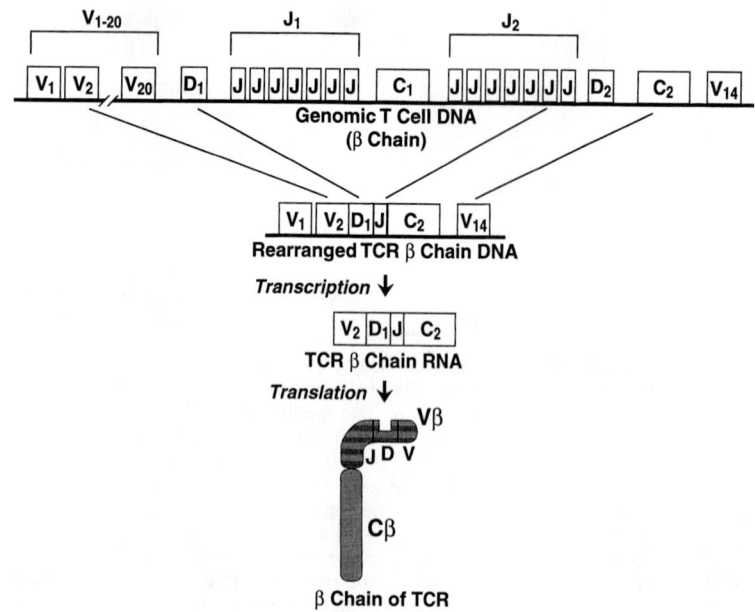

FIGURE 80.4. The genetic rearrangement leading to the formation of a diverse repertoire of T-cell antigen receptors. Genomic DNA is spliced under the direction of specific enzymatic regulation in the T cell during intrathymic T-cell maturation. Random segments from regions termed variable (*V*), joining (*J*), diversity (*D*), and constant (*C*) are brought together to form a unique gene responsible for transcription of a unique TCR chain. The TCR β chain is represented here. Similar rearrangements are required for formation of the α, γ, and δ chains of the TCR, as well as for the heavy and light chains of the B-cell antigen receptor (antibody). Two recombination-activating genes (RAG), RAG-1 and RAG-2, drive this series of genetic deletions and splicing events.[50,51] Four distinct loci (α and δ on chromosome 14 and β and γ on chromosome 7), each made up of a highly polymorphic variable (V), junctional, or diversity (J and D, respectively) region, and a well-conserved constant (C) region, are involved. The recombination event randomly joins C, V, D, and J regions together to form a functional α, β, γ, or δ chain. The γ and δ loci recombine first, and if recombination is successful, a γδ TCR is formed. If this event is not successful, the α and β regions recombine to form an αβ TCR. Approximately 95% of cells progress to express an αβ TCR. (From Kirk and Sollinger,[251] with permission.)

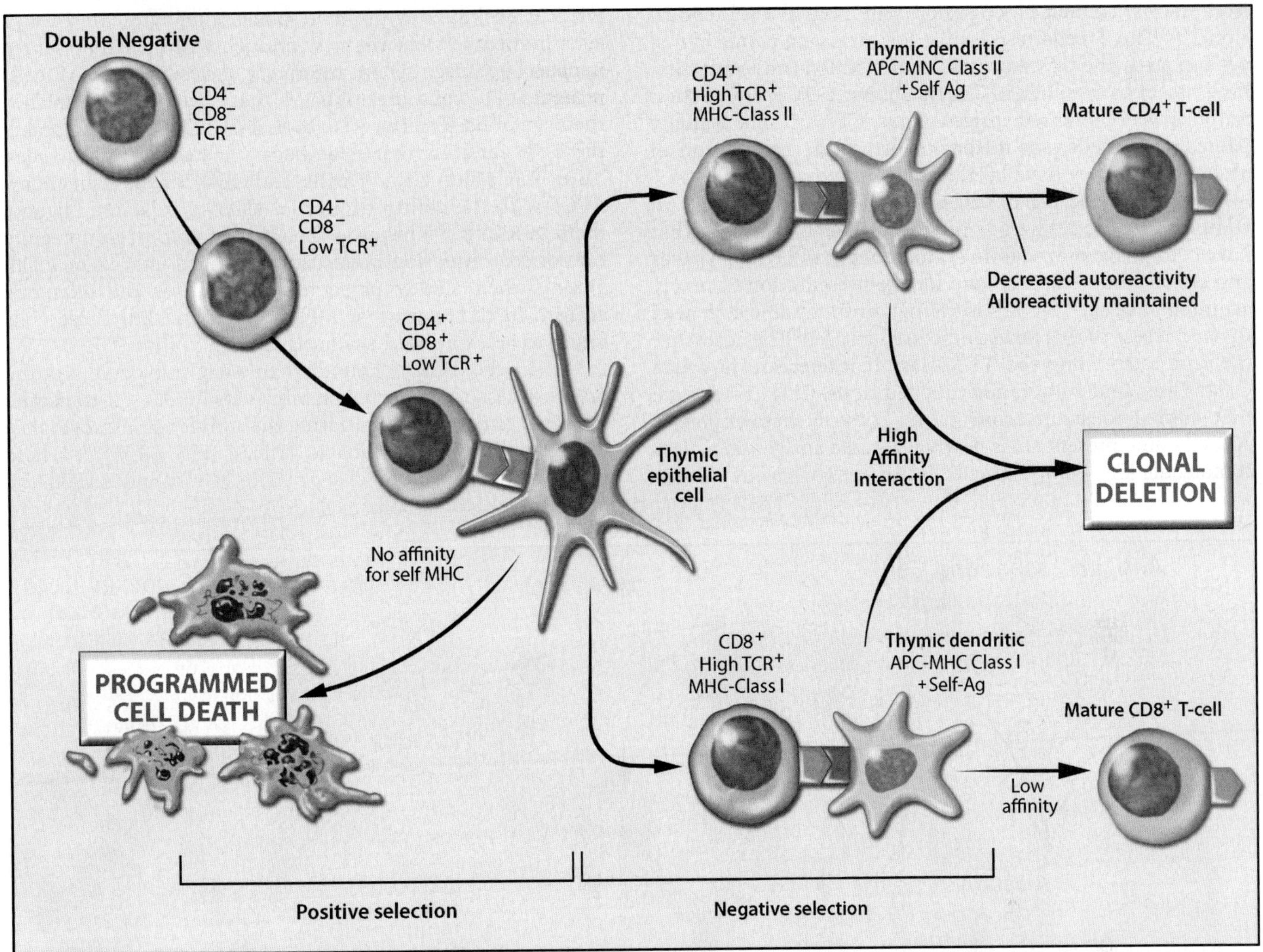

FIGURE 80.5. The T-cell precursors that arrive in the thymus express neither CD4 nor CD8 and are referred to as double-negative cells. This cell population acquires CD4 and CD8, becoming double positive, as well as expression of the αβ TCR and CD3. These double-positive cells initially undergo *positive selection*, in which cells that fail to recognize self-peptide and MHC (class I or II) are deleted via apoptosis. Those remaining cells then undergo *negative selection*, in which T cells with high affinity for self-peptides bound to self-MHC are also deleted via apoptosis. This two-step process ensures that the mature T-cell population retains alloreactivity while decreasing autoreactivity, thereby allowing for a competent immune response.

if the costimulatory molecule B7 is bound to its ligand CD28, generally found on APCs. In the absence of binding, the cell is turned off until exogenous interleukin (IL) 2 is added. Thus, TCR binding that occurs to self in the absence of appropriate antigen presentation or active inflammation fails to lead to self-reactivity. The manipulation of the TCR repertoire by central (thymic) and peripheral mechanisms is responsible for the phenomenon described by Medawar as tolerance. Its understanding will undoubtedly yield the methods required for specific allograft acceptance.

T-Cell Activation

The T cells recognize and destroy cells of the body that make peptide products of mutation or viral infection. They do not recognize these peptide antigens unless they are presented by a self-cell. Molecules of the MHC (described later) perform this presentation. By requiring that T cells only respond to antigen encountered when it is physically embedded in self-cells, the body avoids having its T cells constantly activated by soluble molecules.

Because the number of potential antigens is high, and the likelihood is that self-antigens vary minimally from foreign antigens, the nature of the TCR-binding event has evolved such that a single interaction with an MHC molecule is not sufficient to cause activation. In fact, a T cell must register a signal from approximately 8000 TCR–ligand interactions with the same antigen before a threshold of activation is reached.[57–59] Each event results in the internalization of the TCR. Because resting T cells have low TCR density, sequential binding and internalization over several hours is required. Transient encounters are not sufficient. This threshold is reduced considerably by appropriate costimulation signals (see following).

The binding between the TCR and MHC is governed by *accessory molecules* that improve the TCR-binding affinity and regulate the type of cell that the T cell can "see."[60,61] Parenchymal cells express class I MHC molecules. These class I molecules display peptides from within (e.g., peptides from normal cellular processes or from internal viral replication).[62,63] The T cells responsible for surveying parenchymal cells express the accessory molecule CD8, a molecule that binds to class I, and will only stabilize a TCR interaction with a class I-presented antigen. Thus, $CD8^+$ T cells evaluate parenchymal cells and mediate most of the destruction of altered cells. They have been termed *cytotoxic T cells.*

Hematopoietic cells express class II MHC molecules in addition to class I. Class II molecules display peptides that have been phagocytized from surrounding extracellular spaces and are thus more appropriate for the presentation of newly acquired antigen.[62,63] Cells initiating an immune event need to have access to this newly processed antigen. The accessory molecule stabilizing the TCR–class II interaction is called CD4. Thus, under physiological conditions, $CD4^+$ T cells are first alerted to an invasion of the body by hematopoietic APCs, which present their newly devoured antigen in a class II molecule (Fig. 80.6). These cells are free to present antigen without evoking a cytotoxic response from cytotoxic $CD8^+$ T cells (remember that the new antigen will not be presented in class I because it is not internally derived). The $CD4^+$ cells recognize DCs and macrophages that have an antigen. They then signal back to the APC to activate $CD8^+$ cells to search the body for cells that have been infected by this invader. Thus, APCs alert $CD4^+$ T cells, and $CD4^+$ T cells then endow APCs with the ability to martial $CD8^+$ T cells and "license them to kill."[64,65] This process is mediated through upregulation of *costimulation molecules* (described later). The $CD8^+$ T cells then survey parenchymal cells for the offending antigen in the context of MHC class I and kill those cells found to be expressing the antigen from within.

When the TCR is bound to an MHC molecule and the proper accessory molecule stabilizes its binding, it transmits its signal to the cell by initiating the activity of intracytoplasmic protein tyrosine kinases (PTKs) (Fig. 80.7).[66,67] These PTKs include $p56^{lck}$ (on CD4 or CD8), $p59^{Fyn}$, and ZAP70; the

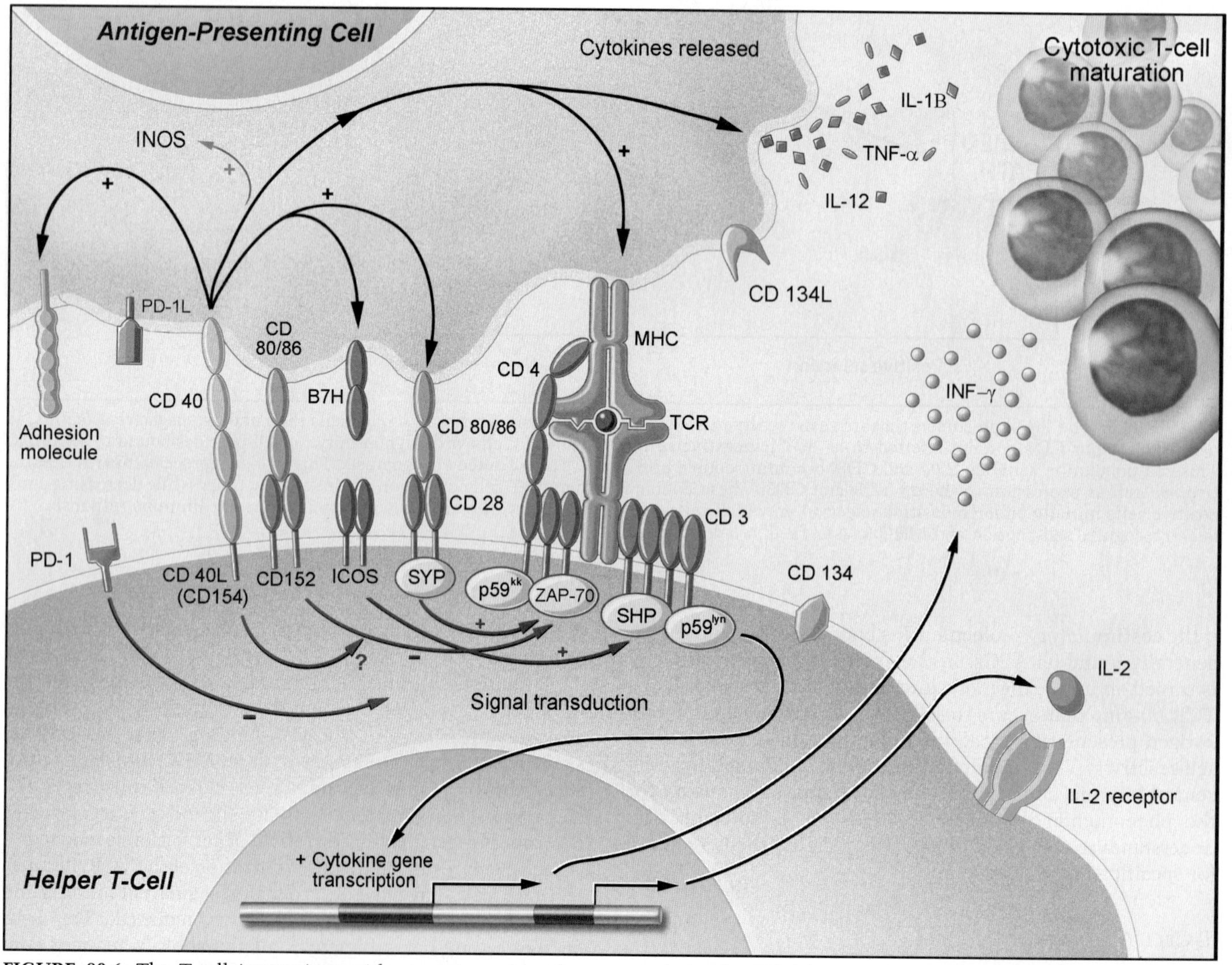

FIGURE 80.6. The T-cell interactions with an antigen-presenting cell (APC). The T-cell receptor (TCR) binds to an MHC molecule (class II is shown). This event is stabilized by an accessory molecule (CD4). The costimulatory molecule CD40 upregulates the expression of the APC costimulation molecules, inducing many critical APC functions. Other costimulatory molecules include PD-1 and ICOS. Costimulatory molecule binding is shifted away from the negative regulation by CTLA4 to positive regulation by CD28. This potentiates signal transduction by the TCR through CD3 and in turn induces IL-2 and interferon-γ synthesis. Interleukin 2 works in an autocrine loop to force the cell into a division cycle. Interferon-γ works in concert with APC-derived cytokines to facilitate cytotoxic T-cell maturation.

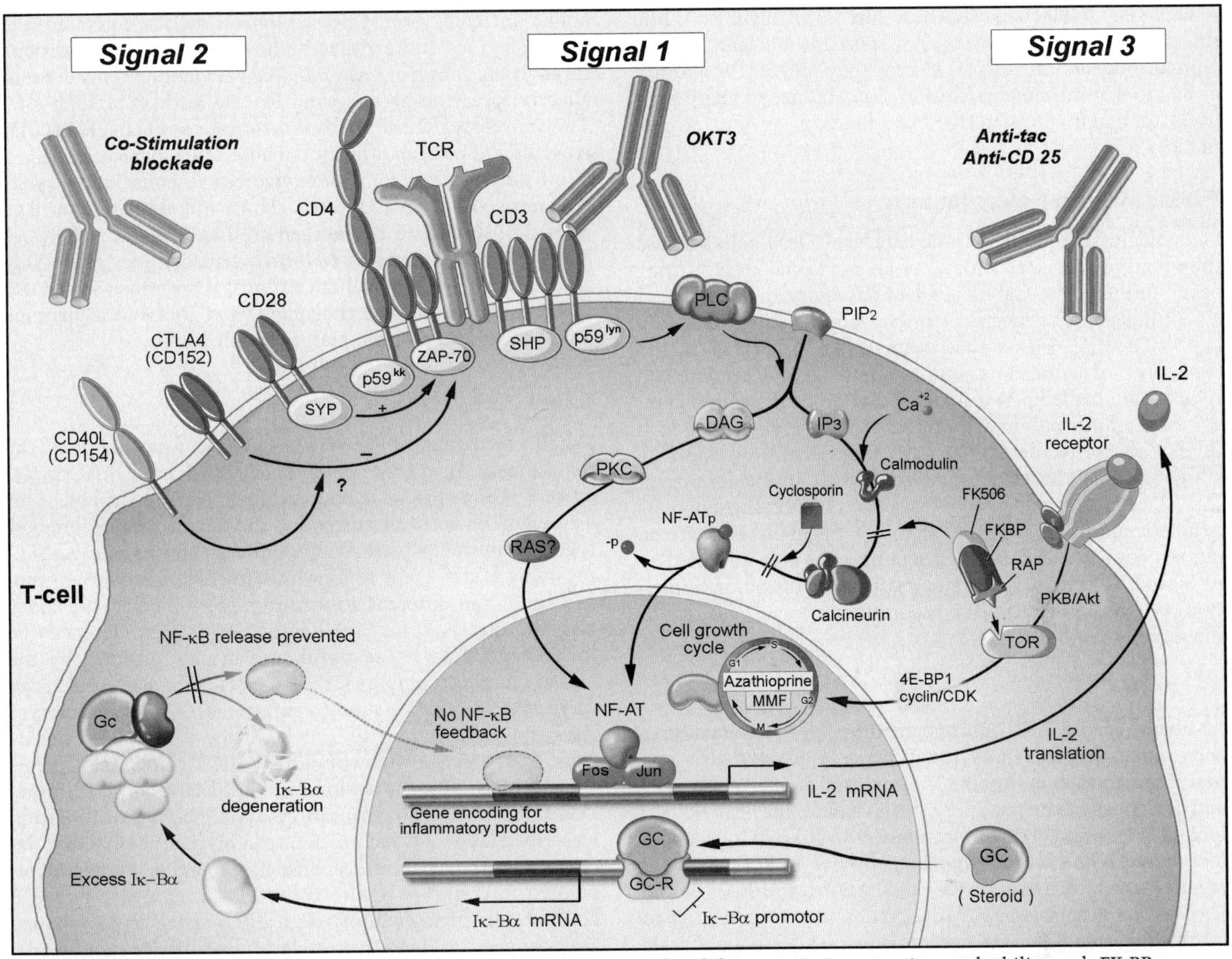

FIGURE 80.7. The T-cell receptor activation signal transduction and the sites of action of various immunosuppressants. The TCR binding facilitates kinase activity by CD3 and CD4 (or CD8). The costimulatory molecules CD28, CD152, and CD154 determine the relative potency of these signals. The TCR signal transduction proceeds via a calcium-dependent dephosphorylation of NF-AT, which enters the nucleus and acts in concert with NF-kB to facilitate cytokine gene expression. Interleukin 2 works in an autocrine loop to force the cell into a division cycle. Cyclosporine A (CyA) and tacrolimus (FK506) both block this signal transduction by blocking the calcineurin/calmodulin-potentiating proteins cyclophilin and FK-BP, respectively. This step limits the access of NF-AT to the nucleus. Rapamycin (RAP) blocks the IL-2 receptor signal transduction by blocking the interaction of RAFT and FKBP. Steroids increase IkBα synthesis and limit the ability of NF-kB to enter the nucleus. Azathioprine (Aza) and mycophenolate mofetil (MMF) interrupt the cell cycle by interfering with nucleic acid metabolism. Monoclonal antibodies (OKT3, anti-IL-2 receptor, and anti-CD40L) interrupt key surface interactions required for T-cell function.

last two are associated with the TCR-associated transmembrane protein complex called CD3. Repetitive binding signals combined with the appropriate costimulation eventually activate phosphokinase-γ (PLC-γ 1), which in turn hydrolyzes the membrane lipid phosphatidyl inositol biphosphate (PIP_2), thereby releasing inositol triphosphate (IP_3) and diacylglycerol (DAG).[68–70] The IP_3 binds to the endoplasmic reticulum, causing a release of calcium that induces calmodulin to bind to and activate calcineurin. Calcineurin dephosphorylates the critical cytokine transcription factor nuclear factor of activated T cells (NF-AT), prompting it, with the transcription factor NF-kB, to initiate transcription of cytokines, including IL-2. Then, IL-2 is released and binds to the T cell in an autocrine loop, potentiating DAG activation of protein kinase C (PKC), which is important in activating many gene regulatory steps critical for cell division.

T-Cell Regulation

The ability of the immune system to act with a "measured" response is thought in part to be due to the activity of regulatory T cells (T_{REG}). A subset of lymphocytes, T_{REG} can down-regulate the immune response by acting on either effector cells or APCs. These cells not only have the ability to suppress cytokines, adhesion molecules, and costimulatory signals, they are also able to focus this response by expression of integrins that allow T_{REG} to home to the location of immune engagement. The most extensively studied[71] population of T_{REG} are those $CD4^+$ T cells that express CD25. These $CD4^+CD25^+$ T cells have been the target of numerous attempts to alter immune function. Other molecules that have been suggested to be unique to regulatory populations include glucocorticoid-induced tumor necrosis factor receptor family-related gene (GITR) and forkhead box P3 (FoxP3).[71,72] While the physiological import of T_{REG} remains unclear, several animal models have suggested that they are vital in control of day-to-day immune activation, and absence of these cells leads to lymphoproliferative syndromes in several animal models.[71,73]

T-Cell-Mediated Cytotoxicity

Physiological cytotoxicity is mediated by $CD8^+$ T cells because they bind to the class I MHC of all nucleated cells. Killing occurs either by a Ca^{2+}-dependent secretory mechanism or a Ca^{2+}-independent mechanism that requires direct cell contact.[74] The Ca^{2+} influx that occurs with activation causes exocytosis of cytolytic granules. These granules contain a lytic protein called perforin and serine proteases called granzymes. Perforin polymerization in the presence of extracellular Ca^{2+} forms defects in the target cell's membrane, allowing granzyme activity to lyse the cell. In the absence of Ca^{2+}, T cells can induce apoptosis of a target cell. Apoptosis is a programmed death that involves fragmentation of the nuclear contents. It occurs when surface *fas* is crosslinked by its ligand. Cytotoxic T cells upregulate *fas* ligand on activation, which can then bind to *fas* on the target cell, leading to the target's death.

Antibody

Antibody, also called immunoglobulin (Ig), is formed in B cells much the same way the TCR is in T cells, although maturation occurs in the bone marrow, and not in the thymus, and continues in the periphery.[23,49] Five different heavy-chain loci (μ, γ, α, ε, and δ) on chromosome 14, and two light-chain loci (κ and λ on chromosome 2, each with V, D or J, and C regions, are brought together randomly by the RAG-1 and RAG-2 recombination-activating genes (RAG) apparatus to form a functional antigen receptor. Antibodies have a basic structure of four chains, two of which are identical heavy chains and two of which are identical light chains (see Fig. 80.3). The heavy-chain usage defines the Ig type as IgM, IgG, IgA, IgE, or IgD. This structure forms two identical antigen-binding sites brought together on a common region known as the Fc portion of the antibody. The Fc portion is critical for opsonization, a process by which Fc receptors on phagocytic cells of the innate immune system bind to antibody, facilitating phagocytic destruction of the antigen to which the antibody is bound and facilitating antigenic peptide processing. The Fc portion of IgM and some classes of IgG also serve to activate complement. The mechanism for regulating B-cell tolerance remains a subject of intense investigation.[75]

Unlike the TCR, the Ig loci undergo continued alteration after B-cell stimulation to improve the affinity and functionality of the secreted antibody. In an alteration known as *isotype switching*, Ig genes change their initial heavy-chain gene usage from the IgM type (used for initial and baseline responses against common carbohydrate antigens) to one of four types, each of which provides heightened specialization for a given purpose.[76] Immunoglobulin G becomes the most significant soluble mediator of opsonization and is clearly the dominant antibody resulting from allostimulation. Immunoglobulin A is formed for mucosal immune responses, IgE for mast cell-mediated immunity, and IgD as a primary cell-bound antibody form. Once a clone of cells is activated, the D and J regions of the utilized gene undergo random additions through the action of terminal deoxynucleotide transferase to slightly alter the gene coding for the antigen-binding site. This process, called *affinity maturation*, results in clones that have altered antigen affinity.[77] Those with increased antigen affinity are retained for a more vigorous response in the event that antigen is reencountered. Thus, individuals who have prior exposure to an alloantigen are likely to have clones of B cells that have mutated to form a gene complex expressing an IgG with extremely high affinity. One must screen for these antibodies before transplantation to avoid a vigorous humoral rejection of the graft (see following).

B-Cell Activation

B cells recognize antigen in its native form without the requirement for processing and presentation on MHC molecules.[78] When antigen is bound by two surface antibodies (or a multimeric form of antibody), the antibodies are brought together on the cell surface in a process known as *crosslinking*. This is the event that stimulates B-cell activation, proliferation, and differentiation into a plasma cell. Like the T cell, the threshold for B-cell activation is high. This can be lowered 100-fold by costimulation signals received by the transmembrane complex CD19–CD21.[79] The B cells also can internalize antigens bound to surface antibodies and process them for presentation to T cells. They can receive signals from T cells via CD40 by binding to the T cell CD154.[80] This signal upregulates expression of B7 molecules on B cells and facilitates antigen presentation and T-cell costimulation (described later). As such, B cells can bind antigen in circulation and initiate a T-cell response to respond to antigen incorporated into tissues of the body. Plasma cells (activated B cells) are distinguished histologically by their hypertrophied Golgi apparatus. They secrete large amounts of monoclonal antibody (antibody with a single specificity). During the activation process, the specificity of the antibody is altered by affinity maturation, as detailed earlier.

In addition to secretion following exposure to an antigen, antibody can be present as part of a natural repertoire in circulation for initial response to common pathogens.[81] Antigen exposure generally leads to B-cell affinity maturation and isotype switching and produces high-affinity IgG antibodies. Naturally occurring antibodies, however, are generally IgM antibodies with low affinity and are generally thought to respond to a broad array of carbohydrate epitopes found on many common bacterial pathogens. Natural antibody is responsible for ABO blood group antigen responses and discordant xenograft rejection (see following).

Antibody-Mediated Cytotoxicity

Antibody facilitates both the destruction and removal of antigenic cells. Once bound to an antigen, antibody serves as an anchoring site for the complement component C1q, as described.[41] Antibody can also serve as an opsonin directly. Most phagocytic cells have receptors for the Fc portion of IgG and actively engulf antibody-coated targets in a process known as *antibody-dependent cellular cytotoxicity* (ADCC).

Cytokines

The entire immune process is dependent on cell-to-cell communication. While receptor interactions can serve this purpose between two cells, soluble mediators of communication are required to facilitate the amplification of the response. *Cytokines* (also known as interleukins [ILs]) (Table 80.1) are polypeptides that are released by many cell types and activate or suppress adjacent cells.[82] They are particularly fundamental to the interactions between CD4+ T cells and APCs.

The prototypical cytokine of T-cell activation is IL-2.[83] The T cells that have bound to their properly presented antigen along with the appropriate costimulation release IL-2 and other cytokines to influence their maturation and that of adjacent cells.[84] They also upregulate a high-affinity chain for the IL-2 receptor (IL-2R), CD25, so that the effects of IL-2 on the activating cell can be amplified without recruiting nonspecific cells into the cycle.[85] The pattern of cytokine expression is thought to influence the type of T-cell response that results.[86,87]

It has been suggested that T cells, once activated, develop into one of two phenotypes based on cytokine expression. The T cells mediating cytotoxic responses, such as delayed-type hypersensitivity, express IL-2, IL-12, IL-15, and interferon (IFN)-γ and have been called Th1 cells. T cells supporting the development of humoral or eosinophilic responses express IL-4, IL-5, IL-10, and IL-13 and have been called Th2 cells. This dichotomy is supported by the fact that many Th1 cytokines have a common receptor chain called γ that is not used by Th2-type cytokines.[88] Cytokine receptors are now known to function through the Janus Kinase (Jak) signal transduction proteins. They convey signals to the signal transducers and activators of transcriptions (STATs), DNA-binding proteins that translocate to the nucleus to influence gene transcription. Resulting transcripts known as suppressors of cytokine signaling (SOCS) proteins feed back onto Jak proteins to control their response to cytokines. The pattern of Jak/STAT/SOCS activity is known to influence the Th1/Th2 phenotype of activated cells. The Th1 cytokines tend to encourage cytotoxic CD8+ T-cell activity.[89] Although these groupings seem to apply to the responses to many environmental pathogens, the response to alloantigens is more typically heterogeneous.[90–92] In addition to cytokines, many other soluble chemicals released during an immune response or other types of inflammation increase blood flow to the area and improve the exposure of the area to lymphocytes and the innate immune system.

Costimulation

As mentioned, TCR binding is not usually sufficient to cause a new T-cell response. Rather, receptor–ligand pairs known as costimulation molecules determine how the T cell will respond[93,94] (Fig. 80.8). Depending on the type of costimulation that is given to the T cell, TCR signal transduction can lead to activation or a state in which the T cell becomes dormant. Costimulatory molecules include the T-cell-based molecules CD28 and CD152 (CTLA4) (Fig. 80.6). In general terms, CD28 binding permits the TCR signal to lead to activation, while CTLA4 binding directs the TCR signal to induce anergy. The ligands for CD28 and CTLA4 are the B7 molecules (CD80, CD86). Both B7 molecules can bind to either CD28 or CD152, but their affinity is much greater for CD152. Generally, B7 is not found on resting parenchymal cells. Rather, it is expressed on cells with potent APC function (so-called professional APCs, such as DCs and macrophages). In this way, T-cell interactions with self-MHC class I on normal tissues do not induce a response but rather reinforce the quiescence of autoreactive T cells that have escaped thymic selection. When B7 is limiting, CD152 has the dominant effect by virtue of its higher affinity. Thus, in the absence of APC activity actively driving an immune response, the default is for T-cell activity to wane.

An additional costimulation molecule pair is CD40, a molecule found on endothelium, DCs, and other APCs, and its T-cell-based ligand CD154 (CD40L)[95,96] (Fig. 80.6). Binding of CD40 is required for APCs to stimulate a cytotoxic T-cell response. It leads to the release of activating cytokines, particularly IL-12, and the upregulation of B7 molecules.[97,98] It also stimulates innate functions of APCs, including nitric oxide synthesis and phagocytosis. Its ligand CD40L is upregulated on T cells after the TCR binds antigen and provides positive feedback for the APC during its interaction with the T cell. Also, CD40L may directly influence the T cell. Interestingly, CD40L is also found in and released in soluble form by activated platelets.[99] Thus, sites of trauma that recruit activated platelets simultaneously recruit the ligand required to activate tissue-based APCs, providing a link between innate and acquired immunity.[100]

The mechanism of costimulation remains an area of active investigation. Binding of CD28 directly potentiates the TCR-initiated tyrosine phosphorylation,[67] allowing more efficient signal transduction and lowering the number of binding events required for T-cell activation from 8000 to about 1500.[57,58] In contrast, when CTLA4 is bound to B7, the T cell becomes unable to make IL-2 during the encounter and, remarkably, when it encounters antigen at a later time.[101] Clearly, CD28 signaling is a fundamental part of T-cell responses to antigen, and CTLA4 function is critical to the downregulation of T cells after the antigen has been eliminated.[102,103] Also, CTLA4 is likely to play a role in preventing autoimmunity. Temporal changes in expression and differences in binding kinetics control the function of costimulation molecules.[104]

Evidence from small animal models also suggests that activation is dependent on the presence of a "danger" signal.[31,101] Spontaneous T-cell activation is prevented by requiring that there is some indication that the antigen-binding event is occurring in a location undergoing injury. Dendritic cells activated by injured or opsonized material or by complement may give this signal. While thought to play a key role in immune activation, allograft rejection has been demonstrated in the absence of "danger," reinforcing the fact that multiple mechanisms are involved in the immune response.[105,106]

Several other molecules have been characterized that demonstrate costimulatory activity. Inducible costimulator (ICOS), expressed on T cells, and its ligand (ICOSL or B7-H2), expressed on APCs, interact with one another on activated T cells.[107] While CD154 and ICOS are positive regulators of the immune response, the cell surface receptor PD-1 (programmed cell death) works in a similar fashion to CTLA4 in providing negative regulation of immune interaction.[107] In addition,

TABLE 80.1. Properties of Some Human Cytokines.

Cytokine	*Alternative name*	*Source(s)*	*Target cell types*	*Actions*
IFN-α and IFN-β	—	Activated T cells, endothelial cells, macrophages, fibroblasts	Activated T and B cells, NK and LAK cells	Induces antiviral state, antitumor activity, fever; increases class I and II MHC expression; stimulates activated B-cell differentiation and proliferation and NK activity; inhibits T and LAK cell activity
IFN-γ	—	Activated T cells, LAK cells	Activated and resting B and plasma cells; NK, endothelial, and LAK cells; macrophages	Induces antiviral state, antitumor activity, fever; increases class I and II MHC expression; stimulates activated B-cell differentiation and proliferation and NK and LAK activity; activates macrophages and endothelial cells, stimulates IgG2a isotype switch
TGF-γ	—	T cells, macrophages, NK cells	Monocytes, fibroblasts	Chemotactic for fibroblasts and monocytes; induces extracellular matrix remodeling, repair, and fibrosis; induces B-cell differentiation and isotype switching, T-cell proliferation, and angiogenesis
TNF	—	Activated T cells, LAK cells, macrophages	Resting T, activated T and B cells; plasma, stem, and endothelial cells; eosinophils, fibroblasts, macrophages	Induces antiviral state, antitumor activity, fever; increases class I MHC expression; activates macrophages, granulocytes, eosinophils, and endothelial cells, chemotactic and angiogenic activity
IL-l	Endogenous pyrogen	Activated T and B cells, LAK cells, endothelial cells, macrophages, fibroblasts	Resting T and B cells; activated T and B cells; plasma, stem, and endothelial cells; eosinophils, fibroblasts, macrophages	Induces antiviral state, antitumor activity, fever; stimulates activated B-cell differentiation and proliferation; activates and stimulates proliferation of T cells; activates granulocytcs and endothelial cells; stimulates hematopoiesis
IL-2	T-cell growth factor	Activated T cells, LAK cells	Activated T cells; activated and resting B cells; NK and LAK cells, macrophages	Activates macrophages, T, NK, and LAK cells; stimulates differentiation of activated B cells; stimulates proliferation of activated B and T cells; induces fever
IL-3	Multi-CSF	Activated T cells	Stem cells, activated B cells, eosinophils	Stimulates hematopoiesis; activates B-cell proliferation and eosinophil activity
IL-4	B-cell-stimulating factor-l	Activated T cells	Activated T cells; activated and resting B cells; plasma LAK cells; macrophages	Activates macrophages, T and B cells; stimulates differentiation of activated B cells; stimulates proliferation of activated B and T cells; induces IgE receptors on B cells; stimulates IgE and IgGI isotype switch
IL-5	B-cell growth factor-2	Activated T cells	Activated and resting B cells, plasma cells, eosinophils	Stimulates IgA isotype switch and eosinophil activity
IL-6	B-cell-stimulating factor-2, B-cell-differentiating factor, interferon-β2	Activated T cells, endothelial cells, fibroblasts, macrophages	Activated T, resting B, and stem cells	Activates T cells; stimulates activated B-cell differentiation and activated T- and B-cell proliferation
IL-7	—	Activated T cells	Activated T and resting B cells	Stimulates activated T-cell and resting B-cell proliferation
IL-8	—	Activated T cells	Granulocytes	Stimulates granulocyte activity, chemotactic activity
IL-9	—	Activated T cells	T cells	Stimulates T-cell proliferation
IL-10	—	Macrophages, B and T cells	Macrophages, B and T cells	Inhibits macrophage cytokine release; induces B-cell differentiation and isotype switching; induces class II expression, T-cell stimulation
IL-11	—	Bone marrow stromal cells	Hematopoietic stem cells	Stimulates megakaryocyte and B lineage stem cell maturation
IL-12	—	NK cells and macrophages	T cells	Induces T-cell maturation and cytotoxic activity
G-CSF	—	Endothelial cells, fibroblasts, macrophages	Granulocytes	Stimulates granulocyte activity and hematopoiesis
M-CSF	—	Macrophages	Macrophages	Activates macrophages
GM-CSF	—	Endothelial cells, fibroblasts, activated T cells	Stem cells, granulocytes, macrophages, eosinophils	Activates macrophages; stimulates granulocyte and eosinophil activity and hematopoiesis

CSF, colony-stimulating factor; IL, interleukin; INF, interferon; LAK, lymphokine-activated killer; NK, natural killer; TGF, transforming growth factor; TNF, tumor necrosis factor.

Cytokines are secreted polypeptides that mediate autocrine and paracrine cellular communication but do not bind antigen. They include those compounds previously termed interleukins and lymphokines.

Source: Based on the consensus cytokine chart of the British Cytokine Group.[250]

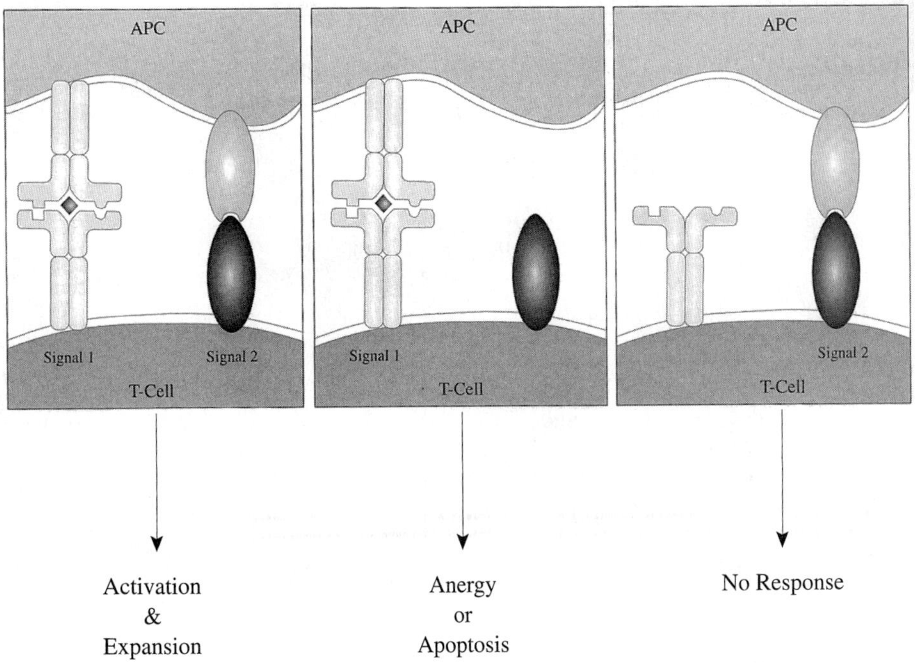

FIGURE 80.8. Costimulation of T-cells. The T-cell responses depend on two signals; signal one is given by antigen through the TCR, and signal two is given by costimulatory receptors. Both are required for activation. Signal one alone leads to T-cell anergy or death. Signal two has no independent effect.

many other adhesion molecules (intercellular adhesion molecule [ICAMs], selectins, integrins, etc.) control the movement of immune cells through the body, monitor their trafficking to specific areas of inflammation, and nonspecifically strengthen the TCR–MHC binding interaction.[102,103] They differ from costimulation molecules in that they enhance the interaction of the T cell with its antigen without influencing the quality of the TCR response. Almost all are upregulated by cytokines released during T cell and endothelial activation.

Transplant Immunity

The Genetics and Structural Characteristics of Transplant Antigens

The antigens primarily responsible for human allograft rejection are those encoded by the HLA region of chromosome 6 (see Fig. 80.1).[108] The polymorphic proteins encoded by this locus include class I molecules (HLA-A, -B, and -C) and class II molecules (HLA-DR, -DP, and -DQ). Class I genes with limited polymorphism (E, F, G, H, and J) are not currently typed and are not considered here. Other genes encoded by HLA are the tumor necrosis factors α and β, components of the complement cascade (class III molecules), the heat-shock protein HSP 70 (which may be involved in danger signaling), and genes necessary for class I and class II presentation of peptides to the body's T cells (peptide transporter proteins TAP-1 and TAP-2 and proteosome proteases LMP-2 and LMP-7). Although other polymorphic genes, referred to as minor histocompatibility antigens, exist in the genome, they are not covered in this section. It is, however, important to point out that even HLA-identical individuals are subject to rejection on the basis of these minor differences. The blood group antigens of the ABO system must also be considered polymorphic transplant antigens, and their biology is critical to humoral rejection.

Each class I molecule is encoded by a single polymorphic gene that is combined with the nonpolymorphic protein β_2-microglobulin (β_2M, from chromosome 15) for expression[19,20] (Fig. 80.9). The polymorphism of each class I molecule is extreme, with 30 to 50 alleles per locus. Class II molecules are made up of two chains, α and β, and individuals differ not only in the alleles represented at each locus, but also in the number of loci present in the HLA class II region.[22] The polymorphism of class II is thus increased by combinations of α and β chains as well as of hybrid assembly of chains from one class II locus to another.[109] As the HLA sequence varies, the ability of various peptides to bind to the molecule and be presented for T-cell recognition changes. Teleologically, this extreme diversity is thought to improve the likelihood that a given pathogenic peptide will fit into the binding site of these antigen-presenting molecules, thus preventing a single viral agent from evading detection by T cells of an entire population.[110,111] The importance of class I and class II structure is also underscored by the relationship of HLA allotypes to many viral and autoimmune diseases.

While the structure of HLA is complex, the clinical importance of the region with respect to transplantation is easily understood by simple Mendelian genetics. Recombination within the locus is uncommon, occurring in approximately 1% of molecules. The HLA type of the offspring is therefore predictable. The unit of inheritance is the haplotype, which consists of one chromosome 6 and therefore one copy of each class I and class II locus (HLA-A, -B, -C, -DR, -DP, and -DQ). The genetics of HLA is particularly important in understanding clinical living-related donor (LRD) transplantation. Each child inherits one haplotype from each parent; therefore, the chance of siblings being HLA-identical is 25%. Haploidentical siblings occur 50% of the time and completely nonidentical or HLA-distinct siblings occur 25% of the time. Biological parents are haploidentical with their children unless there has been a rare recombination event. The degree of HLA match can also improve if the parents are homozygous for a given allele, thus giving the same allele to all children. Likewise, if

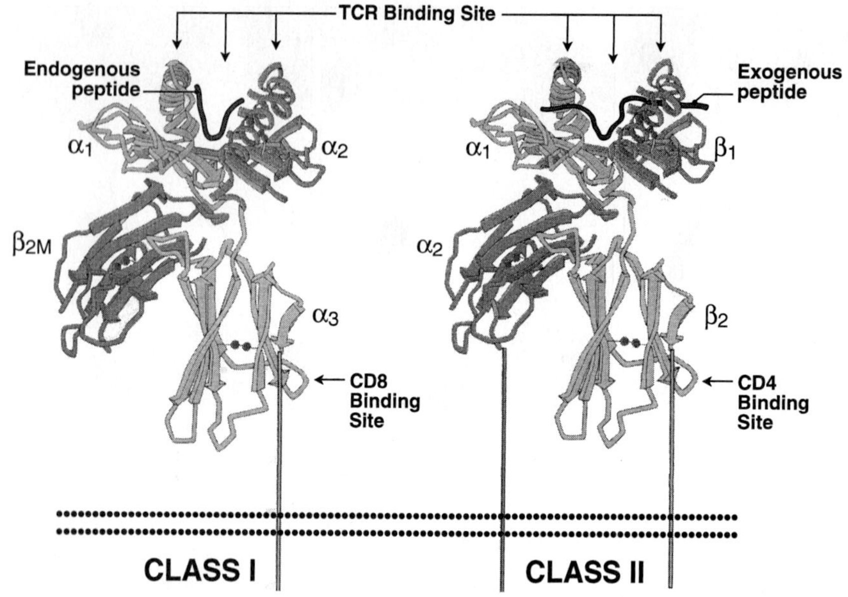

FIGURE 80.9. The three-dimensional structure of MHC class I and class II molecules. The structure of the two major classes of transplantation antigens is shown. Note that while class I molecules are made of a single chain combined with β_2-microglobulin (β_2M) and class II molecules are two separate chains, the general structure is very similar. Two α helices form a groove on top of a β-pleated sheet to present peptide antigens for TCR binding. The peptide presented by class I is short (9 amino acids) and derived from endogenous proteins. The peptide presented by class II varies in length (up to 22 amino acids) and is derived from exogenous proteins engulfed by the cell and is substantially larger (up to 23 amino acids long) than the peptide found in class I. Like class I, the sequence polymorphism of class II is located at this TCR interface region. The binding sites for the T-cell accessory molecules $CD4^+$ and $CD8^+$ are also shown. They regulate the type of T cell that can bind to each MHC molecule. (From Kirk and Sollinger,[251] with permission.)

the parents share the same allele, the likelihood of that allele being inherited improves to 50%. The inheritance of HLA is also affected by linkage disequilibrium, or a propensity of certain class I and class II genes to be located on the same chromosome.

The three-dimensional structure of class I molecules (HLA-A, -B, and -C) was first elucidated in 1987 and is shown in Figure 80.9.[19,20] Class I is expressed as a single MHC-encoded, transmembrane α chain, in combination with β_2M. The α chain has three domains, α_1, α_2, and α_3. The critical structural feature of class I molecules is the presence of a groove formed by two α helices mounted on a β-pleated sheet in the α_1 and α_2 domains. Within this groove, a nine-amino-acid peptide, formed from fragments of proteins being synthesized in the cell's endoplasmic reticulum, is mounted for presentation to the body's T cells. Almost all the significant sequence polymorphism of class I is located in the region of the peptide-binding groove and in areas that directly contact T cells. It is this variation in sequence at the HLA–TCR interface that is the essence of alloreactivity. The TCR repertoire formed in the thymus is formed on the basis of its ability to bind to these α helices without becoming activated. When the amino acid structure of the α helices on MHC molecules is different from that presented in the thymus, the TCR is likely to interpret this interaction as one with a foreign antigen. Organs reject because recipient T cells were not educated with donor MHC in the thymus.

The three-dimensional structure of class II molecules (HLA-DR, -DP, and -DQ) was inferred in 1988 by sequence homology to class I[21] and eventually proven in 1993 by x-ray crystallography.[22] The structural features of class II molecules are strikingly similar to those of class I molecules (see Fig. 80.9). Class II molecules are found primarily on cells of the innate immune system, particularly phagocytes, such as DCs, macrophages, and monocytes, but can be upregulated to appear on other parenchymal cells by cytokines released during an immune response or injury.

Another important sequence-related difference between class I and class II molecules is located on the supporting subunits (α_3 domain for class I and the β_2 domain for class II). A loop extends outward and serves as a binding site for accessory molecules associated with the TCR. The TCR accessory molecule CD8 selectively binds the loop of class I,[112] while the accessory molecule CD4 binds the loop of class II.[113] In this way, T cells geared toward the initial recognition of intruders and subsequent amplification of the immune response ($CD4^+$ helper T cells) are targeted to bind the cells with the ability to capture and present these antigens. Similarly, T cells that survey the body's parenchyma for signs of entrenched intracellular pathogens and destroy infected cells ($CD8^+$ cytotoxic T cells) are outfitted to perform this duty.

The Biology of Transplant Antigens

The physiological role of MHC molecules is twofold: to provide a mechanism for T-cell inspection of parenchymal cells and to provide an interface between APCs and T cells. For the structural reasons just detailed, class I molecules serve the first role, while class II molecules serve the second. It is important to reiterate, however, that organ transplantation is not a physiological process, but rather an artificial situation. Thus, T-cell responses to either class of MHC molecule can generate a rejection episode.

The assembly of class I is dependent on association of the α chain with β_2M and occupation of the peptide groove with a native peptide. Incomplete molecules are not expressed.[114] In general, all peptides made by a cell are candidates for presentation, although sequence alterations in this region favor certain sequences over others. Human class I presentation occurs on all nucleated cells in contact with blood, thus allowing the acquired immune system to inspect and approve ongoing protein synthesis. Deviation of the peptide content from that present during thymic maturation can induce T-cell activation if it is presented in the proper context. In the case of transplantation, this alteration is possible not only with the peptide but also with the presenting molecule itself or with the allo-MHC engulfed by APCs and presented remote from the allograft.

Class II molecule assembly requires association of an α chain and a β chain in combination with a temporary protein called the invariant chain.[115] This third protein covers the peptide-binding groove until the class II molecule is out of the endoplasmic reticulum and is sequestered in an endosome. Proteins that are engulfed by a phagocytic cell are degraded at the same time as the invariant chain is removed, allowing peptides of external sources to be associated with and presented by class II. In this way, the acquired immune system can inspect and approve of proteins that are present free in circulation. The T cells that bind class II molecules are $CD4^+$ and have enhanced abilities for directing the APC-mediated activation of $CD8^+$ T cells and antibody-producing B cells.

When an inappropriate peptide is detected in the appropriate setting, an alloreactive response is generated in which $CD4^+$ T cells release cytokines to activate APCs to recruit $CD8^+$ cells into the area to inspect nearby cells for intracytoplasmic presence of the offending peptide. As alloreactive T cells have a much higher precursor frequency than naive cells, the stage is set for clonal expansion of this population and an aggressive response. This is in contrast to a physiologic response to antigens (such as viral peptides), by which naive cells have a much lower precursor frequency and expansion proceeds in a more leisurely fashion. The high frequency of alloreactive thymic precursors is thought to be a consequence of the collective immunologic memory of viral (and other antigen) peptides and resulting cross-reactivity, a phenomenon entitled *heterologous immunity*.[116]

Once the immune response has been engaged, B cells are also stimulated to release antibody to bind the offending peptide (in its native form) and aid in its clearance by the innate immune system. The cytokines released by $CD4^+$ cells, particularly IFN-γ, also induce expression of class II molecules on local cells and increase expression of class I molecules locally.[117] This reaction increases the chance that infected cells will be detected. In the case of transplanted organs, ischemic injury at the time of transplantation accentuates the potential for T-cell activation by upregulation of both class I and class II molecules.[118] Surgical trauma and ischemia also upregulate class II (as well as B7 and adhesion molecules) on all cells of an allograft, making antigen more abundant.

If rejection can be prevented until the cells of the graft can return to their baseline state of antigen expression, the chance of a T cell encountering foreign antigen in sufficient density to become activated is greatly reduced. This alteration is the primary reason that immunosuppression is heavily administered in the immediate postoperative period and tapered to lower, less-toxic levels over time.

Clinical Definition of Transplant Antigens

For the reasons already discussed, closely matched transplants are less likely to be recognized and rejected than are similar grafts differing at the MHC. Historically, an MHC match has been defined using two assays: the lymphocytotoxicity assay and the MLC.[17,18] Both assays define MHC epitopes but do not comprehensively define the entire antigen or the exact genetic disparity involved. Techniques now exist for precise genotyping that distinguishes the nucleotide sequence of an individual's MHC.

The lymphocytotoxicity assay is performed by taking serum from individuals with anti-MHC antibodies of known specificity and mixing it with lymphocytes from the individual in question. Rabbit complement is added, as is a vital dye such as trypan blue, which is not taken up by intact cells. If the antibody binds to MHC, it activates the complement, leads to cell membrane disruption, and stains the cell. Microscopic examination of the cells can then determine if the MHC antigen exists on the cells. Although this assay has been extremely valuable, it is limited by the nature of the reagents. Antibodies bind to epitopes. The presence of one epitope does not preclude the presence of other epitopes that may differ from the desired MHC type. Thus, many antibodies cross-react with MHC antigens other than the one to which they were raised. Fortunately, the pattern of these cross-reactivities is reasonably well established such that use of a large panel of antibodies allows for reasonable definition of the genetic locus in question.

The MLC is performed by incubating recipient T cells with irradiated donor cells in the presence of ^{3}H-thymidine. If the cells differ at the class II MHC locus, the recipient cells proliferate and incorporate the radionucleotide into the new cells. This incorporation can be detected and quantified. While class II polymorphism is detected by this assay, it takes several days to complete one assay (unlike the lymphocytotoxicity assay, which takes 4–6h). Thus, use of MLC as a prospective typing assay is limited to LRDs. Again, the antigen receptor is the biological reagent of this assay, and the genetic basis for the reaction can only be inferred from a series of reactions.

The sequencing of the class I and class II HLA loci has allowed several genetic-based techniques to be used for histocompatibility testing.[119,120] These methods include restriction fragment length polymorphism (RFLP),[121] oligonucleotide hybridization,[122] and polymorphism-specific amplification using the polymerase chain reaction and sequence-specific primers (PCR-SSPs).[123,124] Of these methods, the PCR-SSP technique is most commonly employed for class II typing. Serological techniques are still the predominant method for class I typing because of the complexity of class I sequence polymorphism. It is important to point out that sequence polymorphisms that do not alter the TCR–MHC interface are unlikely to affect allograft survival; thus, the enhanced precision of molecular typing may provide more information than is clinically relevant.

While HLA matching donors and recipients has clearly been shown to improve outcome following kidney, heart, and pancreas transplantation, no such correlation exists with liver transplantation. Indeed, matching may in fact reduce overall survival.[124,125] The reasons for this lie in the dualistic nature of HLA in the pathophysiology of liver disease. The T-cell-mediated rejection of the liver is mechanistically the same as with other organs; therefore, rejection is reduced with improved HLA compatibility. However, the physiological role of HLA is the presentation of viral peptides to T cells to initiate destruction of virally infected cells. Thus, HLA compatibility potentiates the inflammation during viral reinfection following transplantation for viral hepatitis and increases the chance for clinical recurrence of the original disease. Similarly, T-cell-mediated autoimmune diseases, such as primary biliary cirrhosis, are etiologically based on T-cell recognition of HLA-presented peptides. As such, recurrence

TABLE 80.2. Degree of Mismatch Critically Influences Graft Survival.

Degree of match (mismatch for CAD)	*Graft half-life (years)*
HLA identical (siblings)	23.1
LRD (siblings)	14
LURD (spousal)	14.5
0 antigen mismatch CAD	13
1 antigen mismatch CAD	11
2 antigen mismatch CAD	9.3
3 antigen mismatch CAD	9.5
4 antigen mismatch CAD	8.6
5 antigen mismatch CAD	8.4
6 antigen mismatch CAD	8.2

Source: Data from Refs. 127 and 128.

of autoimmune diseases may be potentiated as well. Further knowledge regarding specific disease states worsened by certain HLA matches may be useful for selective typing in the future.

Matching is only temporally feasible before cadaveric renal transplantation and living-related allografts. While of paramount importance in predicting long-term success of cadaveric grafts, the degree of HLA matching plays a limited role in living kidney donation[126–128] (Table 80.2). It seems apparent that the quality of the allograft (from healthy donors) and the amount of associated ischemic injury are key factors that dictate long-term renal allograft survival.[127] For nonrenal transplants, some centers now use HLA typing to dictate pancreas allocation as well. Other organs are MHC typed retrospectively. As would be predicted, the incidence of acute rejection declines with decreasing MHC disparity.[127,128] However, any mismatch puts the patient at risk for antibody or T-cell-mediated graft destruction and mandates T-cell-specific immunosuppression. As immunosuppression has improved, the relative importance of MHC matching, even for renal allotransplantation, has decreased, even allowing for transplantation in the face of a positive crossmatch or ABO incompatability.[129,130] Now, when determining the destination of an organ, significant emphasis is also placed on the recipient's physical condition and time on the waiting list.

Mechanisms of Allograft Rejection

T-Cell-Mediated Rejection

The T cells are the primary mediators of acute allograft rejection.[131–132] They can respond to transplant antigens either directly, through TCR binding to foreign MHC molecules expressed on transplanted tissues in the presence of donor costimulation, or indirectly, by encountering self-APCs that have phagocytosed alloantigens and processed them for presentation on self-MHC. It is also probable that recipient T cells can bind to donor APCs, particularly DCs, activating them and allowing them to direct recipient cytotoxic T-cell maturation. Regardless of the source of the activating MHC, however, the ensuing internal T-cell events proceed as described for physiological T-cell function. Knowledge of this process has been exploited at almost every critical step along the T-cell activation pathway to prevent acute rejection, and its understanding is key to the rational use of immunopharmaceuticals (see Fig. 80.7).

Initial T-cell binding to a donor APC or endothelial cell is nonspecific and mediated by adhesion molecules.[133] These molecules, including ICAM-1, VCAM-1, LFA-1, and other integrin family molecules, are all upregulated on donor cell activation. This reaction is most critical on donor endothelium and APCs and is mediated at least in part by activation through the CD40 surface molecule.[134] CD40 is activated when bound by CD154, a molecule expressed by platelets and T cells. Thus, both activated T cells and activated platelets likely have the ability to drive allograft rejection.

Once nonspecific adhesion has formed, MHC recognition can occur. The costimulatory environment of the donor tissue is affected by many factors, most of which are related to the mechanics of transplantation. Ischemia and surgical trauma induce B7 expression on the endothelium.[135] Platelet interactions and C3d deposition greatly improve the antigen-presenting ability of the donor tissues[42]; MHC class II is upregulated, as are many nonspecific adhesion molecules.[118]

Once T-cell activation occurs, cytokines, particularly IL-2 and IFN-γ from T cells and IL-12 from APCs, create a potent milieu recruiting other T cells into the response and potentiating clonal expansion.[82,91,92,136] Interleukin 2 works on the cell that is secreting it, so-called autocrine secretion, and leads to upregulation of CD25, the high-affinity receptor for IL-2. To amplify the effect of local IL-2, CD25 combines with two additional constitutively expressed IL-2R chains.[85] The central roles of IL-2 and the IL-2R have been exploited to prevent allospecific T-cell activation by drugs such as cyclosporine, tacrolimus, and anti-CD25 monoclonal antibodies (see following). Also, IFN-γ induces nonlymphoid graft tissues to express class II molecules and to upregulate expression of class I molecules, making alloantigen more prevalent.[117] It also fosters cytotoxic T-cell maturation. Mediation of B-cell activation also occurs through cytokine secretion. Cytokines are responsible for many of the systemic symptoms of fever and malaise that can be associated with severe graft rejection.

As discussed, many physiological responses lead to predictable differential cytokine expression that clearly alters the character of the effector response. More recent study has shown that the response to alloantigen is not easily categorized into Th1 versus Th2 responses.[82,90–92,136,137] Rather, responses during transplant rejection are characterized by both Th1 and Th2 cytokines, including IFN-γ, TNF-α, IL-2, IL-5, IL-6, IL-10, IL-12, and IL-15. Immunosuppression also produces artificial patterns of gene expression. Responses also vary based on the organ targeted for rejection. Kidneys are infiltrated by T cells, leading to a Th1-type milieu plus IL-10, but livers have a significant eosinophil infiltration and a striking presence of IL-5. Thus, the patterns of inflammation seen during allograft rejection result from cytokine-mediated amplification but vary considerably based on many other factors.

In the late phases of rejection, the inflammatory response recruits cells with nonspecific cytotoxic activity to the organ. The T cells expressing the γδ TCR as well as other T-lineage cells, such as lymphokine-activated killer cells, are activated to destroy surrounding tissue in an MHC-unrestricted fashion.[50] Interleukin 8, released by activated macrophages and T cells, also recruits neutrophils to remove necrotic tissue.[92]

Although cytotoxicity is best mediated by $CD8^+$ cells, in the artificial situation presented by allotransplantation, both $CD4^+$ and $CD8^+$ cells have been shown to mediate cytotoxicity.[132] Both perforin/granzyme-dependent mechanisms and *fas*-dependent mechanisms for graft destruction are involved.[137] It is now clear that, following activation, non-MHC-restricted, T-cell-mediated cytotoxicity occurs in addition to MHC-directed killing.[88] This reaction allows the utilization of T cells activated in the area of inflammation but without a TCR specific to the antigen to take part in protective or, in the case of transplant rejection, detrimental immunity. It is likely that this additional promiscuous killing is spurred forward by a failure to eliminate the antigen. The mechanisms of direct T-cell-mediated destruction of microorganisms or non-MHC-expressing tissue remain poorly defined.[138] It is, however, clear that T cells expressing the γδ TCR are prominent effectors of non-MHC-restricted cytotoxicity. This type of activity is induced by high concentrations of IL-2, which may be relevant in the local milieu of a rejecting allograft.

Antibody-Mediated Rejection

Although acute rejection is always the result of T-cell recognition and activation, most acute rejections are accompanied by an antibody response.[139] In addition, antibody can be the primary mediator of two types of rejection: hyperacute rejection (HAR) and acute vascular rejection. Furthermore, antibody formed during the course of an allograft rejection remains in the circulation even after the acute event has been successfully controlled. Many investigators believe that chronic exposure to donor-specific antibody can have progressively damaging effects on the graft and contribute significantly to CR.

Donor-specific antibody has multiple effects on the graft. Direct cell lysis occurs as a result of classical pathway complement activation. Antibody opsonization increases the phagocytic uptake of donor antigen and as such increases the antigen presentation to the recipient immune system. Antibody also directly alters the activation status of the endothelial cell. This change leads to cellular retraction and exposure of the underlying matrix, which in turn potentiates platelet activation and aggregation. Endothelial activation also alters its usually anticoagulant environment in favor of a procoagulant one.[140,141] Heparan sulfate is shed, as is thrombomodulin; this prevents thrombomodulin-mediated activation of protein C and the interaction of activated protein C with protein S. The result is microvascular thrombosis, a hallmark for antibody-mediated graft rejections.

Clinical Rejection Syndromes

There are three major types of rejection: hyperacute, acute, and chronic. They differ in their general pathophysiology and in the effector arm of the immune system involved with current immunosuppression. Of these, only acute rejection can be successfully reversed once it is established. As the transplant community has become more sophisticated in its use of immunopharmaceuticals, graft loss from acute rejection has become increasingly rare. Although untreatable, HAR can be prevented more than 99% of the time with proper use of the lymphocytotoxic crossmatch before transplantation. Thus, most graft loss is now the result of CR, a disease that is only now being defined.

Hyperacute Rejection

Hyperacute rejection (HAR) is caused by donor-specific antibody present in the recipient's serum at the time of transplantation.[139] The antibody is not a result of the transplant but rather is a result of prior sensitization to donor antigens or to antigens that are sufficiently similar to those of the donor to elicit cross-reactivity. Presensitization is usually the result of prior transplant, transfusion, or pregnancy. Hyperacute rejection develops in the first minutes to hours following graft reperfusion. Antibodies bind to the donor tissue, initiating complement-mediated lysis, endothelial cell activation, a procoagulant state, and immediate graft thrombosis.

Although there is no proven treatment for HAR, a thorough understanding of its cause has resulted in its avoidance through the use of two preoperative screening tests, namely, the lymphocytotoxic crossmatch (described earlier) and ABO blood group typing. These two tests identify donor-to-recipient combinations in which HAR would likely occur.

The crossmatch is performed by mixing cells (generally nonactivated T cells that express class I but not class II MHC antigens on their surface) from the donor with serum from the recipient. Lysis of the donor cells indicates that antibodies directed against the donor are present in the recipient serum; this is called a *positive* test result. A positive test can result from IgG or IgM antibodies. The IgM antibodies are frequently not directed at HLA antigens and are considered false-positive results. By adding dithiothreitol, IgM molecules can be broken down. If the lysis is due to IgM, it will not occur in the presence of dithiothreitol. In general, only detection of IgG antibodies directed against class I MHC molecules represents a positive test and an absolute contraindication to transplantation. Preoperative verification of proper ABO matching and a negative crossmatch effectively prevent HAR in 99.5% of transplants.

The overall purpose of the crossmatch is to detect clinically relevant antibodies and to prevent antibody mediated-rejection. As such, many variations of the crossmatch exist[142,143]; these include crossmatch studies performed with class II-expressing B cells. As graft cells can express class II molecules, particularly during rejection or following an ischemic insult, antidonor class II antibodies can initiate graft injury. Noncytotoxic assays can also be performed. These studies involve flow cytometry, a technique in which antibodies that bind to a target can be stained using fluorescent dyes and detected using specialized equipment. Although this assay is very sensitive at detecting and characterizing antidonor antibodies, some of the antibodies that are detected represent autoantibodies or IgM HLA antibodies and have little functional consequence (77% of positive B-cell crossmatches are not from HLA antibodies).[144] Other techniques involve bead-based screening assays, which increase the specificity of flow cytometry by removing interference from non-HLA antibodies. When relevant antibodies are detected and the flow crossmatch is positive, graft survival is significantly decreased.[145] Thus, a positive flow cytometric crossmatch for donor T- or B-cell reactive IgG antibodies represents a high risk of humoral rejection and a relative contraindication to transplantation.

As one might expect, the sensitization status of a patient can change over time. New exposures through transfusions can lead to new antibody formation. Existing sensitivities can wane with prolonged time on the waiting list. Thus, serum from patients awaiting transplantation is frequently screened against a battery of random donor cells to assess their level of sensitization. The screening assay is known as the *panel reactive antibody* assay, or PRA. A nonsensitized patient has a PRA of 0%; in other words, that patient's serum lyses 0% of randomly selected cells. The chance of that patient having a positive crossmatch is very low. Patients who have had multiple exposures to other human tissues have higher reactivity to random cells. As their PRA rises, the likelihood of their receiving an organ that elicits a negative crossmatch diminishes. Clinical desensitization protocols exist that use plasmapheresis or intravenous immune globulin (IVIG) to reduce circulating antibody (see following sections).

A delayed variant of HAR known as vascular rejection is also mediated by humoral factors.[146] Vascular rejection occurs when offending alloantibodies exist in circulation at levels undetectable by the crossmatch assay, even though presensitization has taken place. Frequently, this is seen in a patient with a high PRA that decreases with time. Serum tested at the time of the transplant is negative, but serum from an archived sample is positive. Reexposure leads to restimulation of the memory B cells responsible for the donor-specific antibodies. The result is initial graft function, followed by rapid deterioration on or about postoperative day 3. Enhanced immunosuppression with steroids, combined with nonspecific antibody depletion with plasmapheresis, or administration of nonspecific Ig (see following sections) is occasionally successful in reversing vascular rejection.

Because of these preoperative screening techniques, HAR is rarely seen clinically. As a result of our inability to treat this disease and the resulting extended waiting times for transplantation, several protocols have been developed for transplanting across ABO barriers or a positive crossmatch. Using a combination of plasmapheresis, IVIG, rituximab (see below), or splenectomy, several groups have gained significant experience and good outcomes in this difficult patient population.[129,130] As a result of these efforts, this group of patients who otherwise would likely never receive a suitable organ and would die without being transplanted now have a potential option.

Acute Rejection

The T cells cause acute rejection.[131,132] Acute rejection can occur at any time after the first 4 days postoperatively but is most common in the first 6 months posttransplant. It evolves over a period of days to weeks and is the inevitable result of an allotransplant unless immunosuppression directed against T cells is employed. To initiate acute rejection, T cells bind alloantigen via their TCR directly or following phagocytosis of donor tissue and representation of MHC peptides by self-APC. This then leads to cell activation, as described. The result is a massive infiltration of the graft of T cells (Fig. 80.10), with destruction of the organ through direct cytolysis and endothelial perturbation leading to thrombosis.

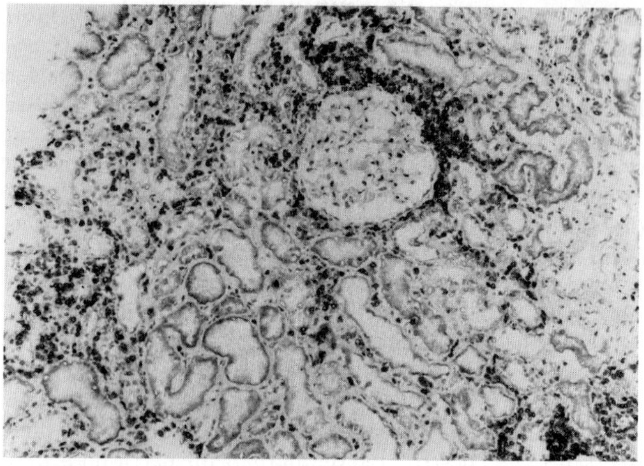

FIGURE 80.10. The histology of acute rejection. A photomicrograph of a renal biopsy with T cells stained dark (immunoperoxidase technique) shows infiltration of the kidney with activated T cells and renal tubular damage. (From Kirk and Sollinger,[251] with permission.)

Knowledge regarding the pathophysiology of acute rejection and the normal physiology of T cells has grown substantially in the past 20 years. This understanding has led to the development of relatively specific treatments, described next, that are capable of counteracting this disease. In approximately 70% of allotransplants, T-cell-specific treatment leads to prevention of acute rejection. When it does occur, it can be reversed in most cases.

Prompt recognition of acute rejection is imperative because prolonged rejection leads to recruitment of multiple arms of the immune system that do not respond to T-cell-specific therapies. In addition, graft damage, particularly for kidney, pancreas, and heart, is generally accompanied by a permanent loss of function that is proportional to the magnitude of involvement. Most acute rejection episodes for patients on modern immunosuppression are asymptomatic until the secondary effects of organ dysfunction occur. By this time, the rejection is well entrenched and difficult to reverse. For this reason, monitoring for acute rejection must be intense, particularly during the first year following transplantation. Generally, unexplained graft dysfunction should prompt biopsy and evaluation for the lymphocytic infiltration and graft parenchymal necrosis characteristic of acute rejection.

Like HAR resulting from humoral presensitization, T-cell presensitization will result in an accelerated form of cellular rejection mediated by memory T cells. It occurs within 3 days of transplant and is usually accompanied by a significant humoral response.

Chronic Rejection

Unlike acute rejection and HAR, chronic rejection (CR) remains poorly understood.[147,148] In many instances, it is likely a combination of immune and nonimmune factors and represents the aggregate effect of many offending pathways. Thus, the term chronic *rejection* is falling out of favor in lieu of terms acknowledging the multifactorial etiology[149]: chronic allograft nephropathy for kidneys, chronic coronary vasculopathy for hearts, vanishing bile duct syndrome for livers, and bronchiolitis obliterans for lungs. Chronic graft disease is insidious, occurring over a period of months to years, and because the pathophysiology is not well defined, it remains untreatable. Heightened immunosuppression is not effective in reversing or retarding its progression. Thus, its distinction from acute rejection by biopsy is important.

Chronic rejection tends to be poorly defined even by histological criteria. Regardless of the organ involved, it is characterized by parenchymal replacement by fibrous tissue and a relatively sparse lymphocytic infiltrate. Infiltrates may contain macrophages and DCs. Those organs with epithelium show a dropout of the epithelial cells as well as endothelial destruction. Chronic rejection is clearly related to the events associated with transplantation, including allorecognition and ischemic injury, which set the stage for tissue remodeling. These effects set the stage for expression of various soluble factors, including TGF-β and the remodeling of the organ's parenchyma and its replacement by fibrous scar.

Immunosuppression

The redundancy and plasticity of the immune system has to date prevented any single agent from specifically preventing graft destruction. In addition, as allograft recognition is mediated by an immune system formed for the detection and elimination of pathogens, manipulations altering this system do so at the expense of a vital defense network. Thus, no immunosuppressive intervention is allograft-specific, or put another way, all drugs preventing allograft loss put the recipient at increased risk for infection and malignancy. Rational, selective use of several immunosuppressive agents acting through different synergistic mechanisms is required to successfully prevent rejection without completely removing the body's defense.

For all organs, it is clear that the events occurring at the time of the initial antigen exposure are the most critical in establishing a lasting state of immune unresponsiveness. For this reason, immunosuppression is extremely intense in the early postoperative period and tapered thereafter. This initial conditioning of the recipient's immune system is known as *induction* immunosuppression. It usually involves deletion of the T-cell response completely and as such cannot be maintained indefinitely without lethal consequences. Medications used to prevent acute rejection for the life of the patient are called *maintenance* immunosuppressants. These agents tend to be well tolerated acutely if dosed appropriately, but all have chronic side effects. Immunosuppressants used to reverse an acute rejection episode are called *rescue* agents. They are generally the same as those agents used for induction therapy. The mechanisms of immunosuppressants are described next, and the pivotal clinical trials demonstrating their efficacy and mechanism are outlined in Table 80.3; the clinical use of these agents is detailed in the chapter on rejection (see chapter 81).[150–156]

Corticosteroids

Corticosteroids, particularly glucocorticosteroids, remain a central tool in the prevention and treatment of allograft rejection. Used alone at maintenance doses, they are ineffective in preventing allograft rejection, but used in combination with other agents, they significantly improve graft survival. When used in higher doses, they effectively rescue acute cellular rejection. Although steroids have a desirable immuno-

TABLE 80.3.
Immunosuppression Approaches.

Reference	*Year*	*Approach*	*Optimized regimen*	*Organ*	*Patients*	*Results*	*Comment*
150	2001	Calcineurin inhibition	Tacrolimus + MMF	Kidney	223	23% increase in allograft survival in DGF	2-year follow-up; compared with CsA + MMF and TAC + AZA (all with steroids)
151	1998	Calcineurin inhibition	Tacrolimus + AZA	Kidney	412	Reduction in AR versus CyA (30.7% vs. 46.6%) and need for antibody therapy	All patients with induction therapy; high percentage of African Americans
152	1998	Antiproliferative	CyA + MMF	Kidney	503	50% reduction in AR when compared with AZA	No difference at 3 years
153	1998	T-cell depletion for AR	rATG	Kidney	163	88% AR reversal and 17% recurrent AR (vs. ATGAM at 76% and 36%)	Increased and prolonged depletion with rATG without increase in side effects
154	2000	TOR inhibition	CyA + prednisone + sirolimus	Kidney	719	Decreased rate of AR (12%) versus AZA (32.3%)	Similar 12-month patient and graft survival
155	1998	Anti-IL2	Daclizimab	Kidney	260	Decreased rate of AR (22%) versus placebo (35%)	Induction with triple therapy (CyA, AZA, prednisone)
156	2004	T-cell depletion for induction	rATG	Kidney	72	Increased graft survival (77%) and freedom from rejection (92%) versus ATGAM (55 and 66%)	5-year follow-up

suppressive effect, they can contribute significantly to the morbidity of transplantation.

The mechanism of the immunosuppressive effect of glucocorticosteroids has only recently been elucidated.[157,158] Glucocorticosteroids bind to an intracellular receptor after nonspecific uptake into the cytoplasm (see Fig. 80.7). The receptor–ligand complex then enters the nucleus, where it acts as a DNA-binding protein and increases the transcription of several genes. The most important gene affected is probably the gene for IkBα. This protein binds to and prevents the function of NF-kB, a key activator of proinflammatory cytokines and an important transcription factor used in T-cell activation. By increasing IkBα in the cell, steroids prevent the primary mechanism by which lymphocytes amplify their responsiveness. The resulting effects are predictably diverse. Steroids block transcription of IL-1 and TNF-α by APCs. They also block IFN-γ production by T cells and migration and lysosomal enzyme release by neutrophils. Phospholipase A_2, and consequently the entire arachidonic acid cascade, is inhibited. Steroids also mute the upregulation of MHC. By blocking the response of leukocytes to chemotactins and by inhibiting vasodilators such as histamine and prostacyclin, steroids dampen the inflammatory response and decrease the costimulation environment. Steroids do not have a significant influence on antibody production. The most commonly used form of steroid is prednisone or its intravenous substitute, methylprednisolone.

Antiproliferative Agents

Azathioprine

The antimetabolite azathioprine (Aza) was the first immunosuppressive pharmaceutical used in organ transplantation and remains a part of many maintenance protocols.[31–33] Azathioprine undergoes hepatic conversion first to 6-mercaptopurine (6-MP) and then to 6-thio-inosine monophosphate (6-tIMP). These derivatives in turn inhibit DNA synthesis by alkylating DNA precursors and inducing chromosomal breaks through interference with DNA repair mechanisms. In addition, they inhibit the enzymatic conversion of IMP to adenosine monophosphate (AMP) and guanosine monophosphate (GMP). The primary effect is to deplete the cell of adenosine. The effects of Aza are relatively nonspecific. It acts not only on proliferating lymphocytes and polymorphonuclear cells (PMNs), but also on all rapidly dividing cells. As such, its primary toxicity is directed at the bone marrow, gut mucosa, and liver. Azathioprine is relatively ineffective alone and has no efficacy as a rescue agent. It does effectively inhibit rejection when given as a maintenance agent in combination with steroids and a calcineurin inhibitor.

Mycophenolate Mofetil

Mycophenolate mofetil (MMF) is an immunosuppressive agent approved in 1995 for use in adults.[159] It is a morpholinoethyl ester of mycophenolic acid (MPA), an established noncompetitive, reversible inhibitor of IMP dehydrogenase. This modification improves the bioavailability of MPA.

Physiological purine metabolism requires that GMP be synthesized for subsequent synthesis of guanosine triphosphate (GTP) and deoxyguanosine monophosphate (dGTP). For RNA synthesis, GTP is required, and dGTP is required for DNA synthesis. Guanosine monophosphate is formed from IMP by IMP dehydrogenase. Therefore, MMF prevents a critical step in RNA and DNA synthesis. Of major importance, however, is the presence of a "salvage pathway" for GMP production in most cells *except* lymphocytes (hypoxanthine-guanine phosphoribosyl transferase-catalyzed GMP production directly from guanosine). Thus, MMF exploits a critical difference between lymphocytes and other body tissues, including PMNs, to produce relatively lymphocyte-specific immunosuppressive effects. Mycophenolate mofetil blocks the proliferative response of both T and B cells, inhibits antibody formation, and prevents the clonal expansion of cytotoxic T cells.

Mycophenolate mofetil decreases the rate of biopsy-proven rejection and the need for antilymphocyte agents in rescue therapy compared to Aza.[160,161] As such, MMF has replaced Aza in most patients and is used in combination with either a calcineurin inhibitor or sirolimus by many centers in steroid-sparing protocols. Subsequent study has shown that MMF also has some effect as a rescue agent when used with steroids. In addition, treatment with MMF has been suggested to slow the progression of chronic allograft nephropathy. Despite these improvements, MMF is not effective enough to use without either steroids or calcineurin inhibitors. Tacrolimus may interact with MMF, potentiating the effect and toxicity of both drugs.

Calcineurin Inhibitors

Cyclosporine

The T-cell-specific immunosuppressive drug cyclosporine A (CyA) is a cyclic endecapeptide isolated from the fungus *Tolypocladium inflatum gams*.[34,162] Its mechanism of action is mediated primarily through its ability to bind to cytoplasmic protein cyclophilin (Cn)[154] (see Fig. 80.7). The CyA–Cn complex binds with high affinity to the calcineurin–calmodulin complex and, in doing so, blocks its role in the calcium-dependent phosphorylation and activation of the transcription-regulating factor NF-AT. This prevents the transcription of the IL-2 gene. Cellular cytotoxicity is also probably interrupted through calcineurin inhibition. The transcription of other genes critical for T-cell activation is also altered. Cyclosporine A increases TGF-β transcription.[163,164] This cytokine is part of the natural downregulatory milieu present after injury. It effectively inhibits T-cell activation, reduces regional blood flow, and activates many pathways critical in tissue remodeling and wound repair. The toxicity of CyA may be related to the last two of these three TGF-β-mediated effects. Also, CyA blocks Cn function as a *cis-trans* peptidyl-prolyl isomerase, which is critical for the proper folding of proteins. This function is not critical to the immunosuppressive effects of CyA but may relate to the toxic side effects of the drug.

Cyclosporine A blocks TCR signal transduction but does not inhibit costimulation signals.[165] As such, on withdrawal of CyA, the T cell is not rendered anergic but rather is capable of mounting an attack on its intended antigen. The effects of CyA can be overcome with exogenous (or in the case of an ongoing rejection episode, ambient) IL-2. For this reason, once IL-2 is present in the graft cytokine milieu, CyA is ineffective.

Cyclosporine therefore works solely as a maintenance agent and is ineffective as a rescue agent.

Cyclosporine is insoluble in aqueous solutions but soluble in lipids and organic solvents. Because of this, the gastrointestinal absorption of CyA is dependent on bile flow (a significant concern in liver transplantation). A newer microemulsion form is less bile-dependent. Cyclosporine is metabolized by the hepatic cytochrome P-450 enzymes, and blood levels are therefore increased by inhibitors of cytochrome P-450 (ketoconazole, erythromycin, calcium channel blockers) and decreased by cytochrome P-450 inducers (rifampin, phenobarbital, phenytoin). Liver failure slows the clearance of CyA because 90% of its metabolites are cleared in the bile. Renal failure only minimally alters the clearance of CyA.

Cyclosporine has much toxicity that governs its use. It has a significant vasoconstrictor effect on proximal renal arterioles that decreases the renal blood flow by approximately 30%. This action is most likely mediated through the induction of TGF-β, which in addition to suppressing T-cell activation, increases the transcription of endothelin.[163,164] Endothelin-mediated vasoconstriction activates the renin–angiotensin pathway, promoting hypertension. The remodeling effects of TGF-β also induce fibrin deposition, which may promote the fibrosis typically seen during CR. The vascular effects of CyA tend to increase vascular resistance in the kidney and delay the resolution of acute tubular necrosis (ATN) or hepatorenal insufficiency. An additional renal effect is an idiosyncratic reaction producing hemolytic uremic syndrome. Hyperkalemia may also result from its effects on both the proximal and distal renal tubules.

Discontinuing the drug can reverse most of the toxic effects of CyA. Cyclosporine frequently causes neurological side effects consisting of tremors, paresthesias, headache, depression, confusion, somnolence, and, rarely, seizures. Hypertrichosis of the face, arms, and back is seen in about 50% of patients. Gingival hyperplasia may also occur. CyA also may promote malignant transformation of some cell types.[166]

Tacrolimus

Tacrolimus, previously described investigationally as FK506, is a macrolide produced by *Streptomyces tsukubaensis* that was discovered in 1984 in Japan during a search for new immunosuppressive agents. In 1987, Kino and coworkers first demonstrated its in vitro immunosuppressive properties.[167] Tacrolimus, like CyA, blocks the effects of NF-AT, prevents cytokine transcription, and arrests T-cell activation[168] (Fig. 80.7). The intracellular target is an immunophilin protein distinct from cyclophilin known as FK-binding protein (FKBP); thus, the effect is additive to that of CyA. As such, the use of tacrolimus with CyA produces prohibitive toxicity. Tacrolimus increases TGF-β transcription, leading to both the beneficial and toxic effects of this cytokine.[163,164] It is 100 times more potent in blocking IL-2 and IFN-γ production than CyA, but its toxicity limits its dose to approximately 1% of CyA. Like CyA, the effects of tacrolimus are relatively T-cell-specific, but in addition to its role as a maintenance agent, tacrolimus has also shown promise as a rescue agent.[169]

The side-effect profile for tacrolimus is similar to that of CyA with regard to renal toxicity. As compared with CyA, neurotoxicity, in the form of tremors and mental status changes, is somewhat more pronounced, as is its diabetogenic effect. In addition, as tacrolimus and CyA are both metabolized by cytochrome P-450 enzymes, they share similar drug interactions. Cosmetic side effects are substantially reduced. Tacrolimus has been shown to be extremely effective for liver transplantation and has become the drug of choice for most centers.

Antilymphocyte Preparations

Antithymocyte Globulin

Antilymphocyte globulin (ALG) is produced by inoculating heterologous species with human lymphocytes, collecting the plasma, and purifying the IgG fraction. The resulting preparation, known as a *polyclonal antibody preparation*, contains antibodies directed against many antigens on lymphocytes. Thymocytes rather than lymphocytes are sometimes used as the immunogen, and antibodies formed from this process are known as antithymocyte globulin (ATG). The most commonly used preparation in the United States is a rabbit ATG (Thymoglubulin, Sangstat).

Antibodies in ATG coat multiple epitopes on the T cell.[170,171] This has many effects, including promoting T-cell clearance through complement-mediated lysis and opsonin-induced phagocytosis, as well as limiting the ability of the T cell to generate an effective TCR signal by internalization of key surface receptors. In addition, the antibodies crosslink several key molecules, including adhesion and costimulation molecules[171]; crosslinking has the effect of impairing or altering signals generated by these receptors and either preventing activation or possibly leading to an anergic phenotype. The overall result is to reduce the precursor frequency of the primary effector cells below that required for acute rejection and allow for slow repopulation during the critical time posttransplantation.

When used as an induction agent, the profound and long-term T-cell depletion reduces the possibility that T-cell-mediated antigen recognition will occur when the graft is in its most vulnerable state. Cell surface crosslinking prevents appropriate costimulation for those cells that do encounter antigen. The costimulatory milieu produced by organ preservation and postischemic reperfusion can subside before the introduction of T cells, which lessens the possibility that T cells will encounter alloantigen in an environment that will foster a positive TCR signal. When ATG is used as a rescue agent, antigen recognition has already occurred, and the beneficial effects of ATG are likely related solely to its ability to destroy cytotoxic T cells.

Antithymocyte globulin is most commonly used as part of a multidrug induction immunosuppression protocol with CyA, Aza or MMF, and prednisone and more recently as a key depletional agent in minimization protocols.[172–174] Often, ATG is used sequentially with CyA or tacrolimus in the early postoperative period following renal transplantation to avoid the nephrotoxicity of these drugs early in the transplant course. In addition, ATG is an effective rescue agent in cases of steroid-resistant acute rejection.

Most of the side effects of ATG stem from its heterologous origin and heterogeneous composition. Because ATG is polyclonal, antibodies specific for antigens on both T- and B cells, as well as to other cells, are present. In fact, only a small fraction of the serum is estimated to be biologically active against T cells. One prominent side effect related to this promiscuous specificity is thrombocytopenia resulting from cross-reactivity with platelets. In addition, leukopenia and anemia may also occur. Despite this, major side effects are rare, and the drug is well tolerated by most transplant recipients. The most common symptoms are the result of transient cytokine release following antibody binding. Chills and fevers occur in up to 20% of patients and are easily treated with antipyretics and antihistamines. The use of ATG has been associated with an increase in the reactivation and development of primary viral disease caused by cytomegalovirus (CMV), herpes simplex virus (HSV), Epstein-Barr virus (EBV), and varicella.

Muromonab (OKT3)

Although polyclonal antibody preparations have many binding specificities, monoclonal antibodies have a single specific target antigen. The first, and for years only, commercially available monoclonal antibody preparation for use in organ transplantation was muromonab (OKT3, Orthoclone; Ortho Pharmaceuticals, Raritan, NJ). This murine monoclonal antibody is directed at the signal transduction subunit on human T cells (CD3)[175] (see Fig. 80.7).

There are several ways in which OKT3 is thought to have its effect.[175,176] The CD3 determinant, as described earlier, is a cluster of transmembrane proteins found on the surface of all mature T lymphocytes. When OKT3 binds to CD3, it leads to internalization of the TCR complex, thus preventing antigen recognition and TCR signal transduction. In addition, T-cell opsonization and clearance by the reticuloendothelial system occur. Following the administration of OKT3, there is a rapid decrease in the number of circulating $CD3^+$ lymphocytes. Effect is minimal on T cells residing in the thymus, lymph nodes, or spleen. Following several days of administration, there is a return of T cells expressing the accessory binding molecules $CD4^+$ and $CD8^+$ but lacking the TCR. These "blind" T cells remain incapable of binding to antigen. In addition to interfering with the generation of cytotoxic T cells and the modulation of cell surface proteins, OKT3 blocks the cytotoxic activity of already activated T cells; this is the result of inappropriate activation and degranulation that results when the CD3 is bound by OKT3. This reaction is perhaps its most important function but leads to its substantial side-effect profile.

The T-cell-derived cytokines have evolved as activators of adjacent cells.[177] Their release is strongly polarized to the side of the cell actively engaged in cell-to-cell contact. Indeed, the most potent T-cell activator, IL-2, exerts most of its effect in an autocrine loop. Pan-activation of the body's T cells leads to transient activation and systemic cytokine release, similar to the effect of the superantigen staphylococcal exotoxin, the etiological agent for toxic shock syndrome. As such, administration of OKT3 leads to profound, systemic cytokine release syndrome that can result in hypotension, pulmonary edema, and fatal cardiac myodepression. In approximately 2% of patients, the inflammatory response manifests itself as aseptic meningeal inflammation. Administration of high-dose methylprednisolone before OKT3 administration is required to blunt this adverse response, but it is rarely avoided altogether. The syndrome abates with subsequent dosages as the target cells available for degranulation become consumed or exhausted.

Measurement of serum levels of OKT3 is possible but is not done routinely.[178] More commonly, the percentage of $CD3^+$ cells is determined by flow cytometry. The presence of less than 10% $CD3^+$ cells is usually associated with therapeutic efficacy. Greater than 10% $CD3^+$ cells usually indicates the presence of anti-OKT3 antibodies, which may limit the desired therapeutic effect. Because OKT3 is a foreign protein, it is itself an antigen that will elicit an immune response. Antimurine antibodies may be directed against structural regions of the antibody (constant or variable regions) or the actual binding site (idiotypic) of the OKT3 antibody; they usually arise after a prolonged course of OKT3 or following the cessation of therapy. As would be expected, the use of MMF or other immunosuppressants with anti-B-cell activity during treatment with OKT3 may reduce the formation of anti-OKT3 antibodies.

Much like ATG, OKT3 was first used as a rescue agent to treat acute renal allograft rejection.[179,180] It is greatly superior to conventional steroid therapy in reversing rejection and, consequently, in improving allograft survival. However, its side effects and the limiting nature of the antimurine antibody response have limited its use to steroid-resistant rejection, during which maintenance immunosuppression is reduced. Use of OKT3 in induction immunosuppressive protocols for kidney transplants is now less frequent due to the availability of both ATG and alemtuzumab. As with other antilymphocyte preparations, OKT3 has been shown to cause a very high reactivation rate of CMV and other viruses.

Anti-IL-2 Strategies

Two other monoclonal antibodies are currently approved for use in transplantation induction protocols: daclizumab (Zenapax; Roche Pharmaceuticals, Nutley, NJ) and basiliximab (Simulect; Novartis Pharmaceuticals, Basel, Switzerland).[155,181,182] They are either humanized (daclizumab) or chimeric (basiliximab), and both are directed against CD25, the high-affinity chain of the IL-2R (Fig. 80.7). As discussed in previous sections, a high-affinity form of the IL-2R is required for T-cell clonal expansion. This form of the receptor is dependent on the upregulation of CD25, a 55-kDa α chain that combines with a β and γ chain to form a heterotrimer. Targeting this receptor has many potential advantages. It is only present on activated T cells, and thus the effects are limited to those T cells that have become activated in the face of an allotransplant. Theoretically, only allograft-specific cells are affected, leaving T cells with physiological specificity undisturbed. It should be pointed out, however, that because alloreactivity is the result of cross-reactivity, even removal of alloreactive cells might remove cells with important specificity against pathogenic antigens. An additional benefit of anti-CD25 therapy is that it is monoclonal, and the binding of its target does not precipitate a T-cell signal that induces cytokine release. Thus, no acute side effects occur. Finally, both these antibodies are the products of genetic engineering. While the antigen-binding regions of their parent murine antibodies have been retained, the structural components have been replaced with human IgG. Thus, they are mostly human proteins, and their propensity to generate a neutralizing immune response is greatly reduced.

Both anti-CD25 antibodies function as induction agents only. The prevention of IL-2R function efficiently prevents the activation of nonactivated T cells. However, IL-2 is only required very early in the activation process. Once a rejection episode has been initiated, cytotoxic T cells can function without high-affinity IL-2R signaling. As such, these agents do not readily reverse rejection.

Experience in the form of several experimental and clinical trials with anti-CD25 monoclonal antibodies has been encouraging.[155,181,182] Induction with anti-CD25 has been shown to prevent or reduce the frequency of early rejection episodes when used in combination with a calcineurin inhibitor, an antiproliferative agent, and steroids. In addition, several trials have shown success with the incorporation of anti-IL-2 agents in steroid or calcineurin avoidance protocols with the added benefit of reduced toxicity as compared with other induction regimens.[183]

New Immunosuppressive Agents

Sirolimus/Everolimus

Sirolimus and everolimus are macrolide antibiotics derived from *Streptomyces hygroscopicus*.[184–186] The effects of these agents depend on binding to the immunophyllin FKBP12, which is also the intracellular target for tacrolimus. However, these agents do not affect calcineurin activity.[187–189] As a result, sirolimus and everolimus do not inhibit the expression of NF-AT or IL-2 expression. Rather, they impair signal transduction by the IL-2R through interaction of the rapamycin–FKBP (FRAP) complex with the cytoplasmic protein RAFT-1, a critical kinase in IL-2R-associated activation (Fig. 80.7). In doing so, the p70 S6 kinase cascade is arrested, and T cells are prevented from progressing from G1 to the S phase of cell replication[190]; this has the advantage of interrupting the T-cell activation pathway even if IL-2 is present from an exogenous source or ongoing rejection. Other receptors are also affected, including those for IL-4, IL-6, and platelet-derived growth factor (PDGF). An additional benefit may lie in the ability of sirolimus to antagonize B-cell lymphomas and the ability of everolimus to prevent the growth of EBV.[191,192] As such, their use may potentially prevent the development of posttransplant lymphoproliferative disease.

Both agents have been shown to dramatically prolong allograft survival in multiple animal models. This effect has been carried to the clinic, where sirolimus has become an alternative to calcineurin inhibition in selected patients. In addition, both have demonstrated synergy with cyclosporine,[154] tacrolimus,[193] and steroids, thus allowing reduction in their dose.[194]

As with calcineurin inhibition, the use of both of these agents has been limited by their side effects. The increased incidence of hypercholesterolemia and hypertriglyceridemia seen with both agents often mandates treatment with a cholesterol-lowering agent or changing to a calcineurin inhibitor. In addition, thrombcytopenia is a common side effect of both agents, and impaired wound healing and oral ulcers remain a frequent problem with sirolimus. Overall, both agents offer an adjunct or alternative to calcineurin inhibition, albeit with a different side-effect profile that is generally manageable with dose adjustment.

Alemtuzumab

While lymphocyte depletion with ATG utilizes a polyclonal preparation, other depletion strategies focus on monoclonal antibodies directed against specific cell populations. Alemtuzumab (Campath, Berlex Laboratories, Seattle, WA) is a humanized monoclonal antibody directed against CD52, which is present on lymphocytes and monocytes but not on leukocyte precursors in the bone marrow. As with ATG, treatment with alemtuzumab results in a profound reduction in the number of central and peripheral T lymphocytes at the time of transplantation, therefore decreasing the frequency of alloreactive cells at a time of increased immune susceptibility. Alemtuzumab also depletes B cells and monocytes to a lesser degree. Alemtuzumab is approved for use in the treatment of hematogenous malignancies.

Initial groundbreaking work by Calne[195] using alemtuzumab and subsequent drug minimization[196,197] with cyclosporine has set the stage for several studies demonstrating the efficacy of this drug as an induction agent in both minimization strategies and attempts at tolerance (Table 80.4). Both of these approaches (depletion with either ATG or alemtuzumab) should be considered complementary and usage should be directed by patient considerations.

Deoxyspergualin

The antitumor antibiotic spergualin was isolated from *Bacillus laterosporus* in 1981. Its derivative deoxyspergualin (DSG) was shown to have strong antiproliferative and immunosuppressant properties.[198] Although the mechanism of DSG is not completely understood, there is evidence that it is immunosuppressive via a predominantly anti-APC effect.[199] It does prevent the nuclear translocation of NF-kB, perhaps through its association with the heat-shock proteins HSP 70 and HSP 90. This interaction inhibits the release of IkB, perhaps mimicking a critical part of the steroid mechanism of action. The close relationship with HSPs, combined with evidence that the inhibitory effect of DSG on cytotoxic T cells can be abolished by the MHC-upregulating cytokine IFN-γ, suggests that the primary effect of DSG is to inhibit antigen presentation or the costimulatory function of APCs. Deoxyspergualin has been shown to effectively prolong allograft survival in many animal models.[198] Early clinical studies have not been as promising, and it is thought that DSG will have a minor role in the transplantation armamentarium.[200]

FTY720

FTY720 (2-amino-2-(2-[4-octylphenyl]ethyl)-1,3-propanediol) is a chemical derivative of the fungus *Isaria sinclairii* and functions to produce a profound, yet reversible, state of lymphopenia by sequestering lymphocytes in lymphatic tissues.[201] This agent traps lymphocytes (T and B cells) in lymphoid organs by rendering them unresponsive to the egress signal provided by the lysophospholipid sphingosine 1-phosphate (S1P). In addition, FTY720 decreases vascular permeability associated with ischemic injury via a similar mechanism, thereby enhancing its effect. The major reported side effect of

TABLE 80.4.
Results of Recent Tolerance and Minimization Trials.

Reference	*Year*	*Approach*	*Optimized regimen*	*Organ*	*Patients*	*Results*	*Comment*
207	2001	Costimulation blockade	Anti-CD154	Kidney	7	7 AR	3 thromboembolic events; all grafts rescued
195	1998	T-cell depletion	Alemtuzumab and low-dose CYA	Kidney	13	2 AR	Prope tolerance; low-dose CYA as maintenance
208	1999	T-cell depletion	Alemtuzumab and low-dose CYA	Kidney	31	6 AR (steroid-responsive)	Follow-up of above study; 29 functioning grafts (21 months)
196	2003	T-cell depletion	Alemtuzumab	Kidney	7	7 AR	Placed on monotherapy sirolimus after AR
209	2003	T-cell depletion	Alemtuzumab and DSG	Kidney	5	5 AR	Placed on monotherapy sirolimus after AR
211	2000	Chimerism	TLI, RATG, steroid withdrawal	Kidney	25	3 patients off immunosuppression	>10 years after transplantation
212	2002	Chimerism	TLI, RATG, stem cells	Kidney	4	2 patients weaned off immunosuppression, both with AR	HLA nonidentical
210	1999	Chimerism	Cyclophosphamide, ATGAM, TLI, BM	Kidney (Multiple Myeloma)	2	No AR (2 to 4 years) off immunosuppression	HLA identical patients with multiple myeloma; no GVHD and minimal disease recurrence

ATGAM, antithymocyte globulin; AR, acute rejecton; BM, bone marrow; CYA, cyclosporine A; DSG, deoxyspergualin; RATG, rabbit antithymocyte globulin; TLI, total lymphoid irradiation.

FTY720 administration has been bradycardia. Currently, these two properties of reversible lymphopenia and reduction of ischemia reperfusion injury are being evaluated in renal transplantation clinical trials.

Other Agents

Rituximab

Rituximab is a murine antihuman anti-CD20 chimeric antibody that has been used successfully in the treatment of non-Hodgkin's lymphoma and posttransplant lymphoproliferative disorder (PTLD). In addition, this agent has been used in lieu of splenectomy in renal transplantation across ABO and HLA boundaries (see hyperacute rejection section). Rituximab inhibits B-cell proliferation by apoptosis, Fc receptor-mediated ADCC, and complement-dependent cytotoxicity (CDC) and therefore limits antibody production. Recent reports have highlighted the use of rituximab in highly sensitized patients in whom humoral-mediated rejection ensues.[202] The success of this approach in certain circumstances helps illustrate the importance of B-cell responses in the immune response.

Intravenous Immune Globulin

Intravenous immune globulin (IVIG) is a clinically available blood product and is currently used for the treatment of various diseases, such as immune thrombocytopenia, humoral-mediated rejection, Guillian-Barré syndrome, uveitis, and myasthenia gravis. It is prepared from the pooled plasma of 50,000 to 100,000 human plasma donors and is comprised of more than 90% IgG antibodies directed against the multitude of antigens present in such a large population.

The roles of IVIG in transplantation have focused mainly on pretreatment of the highly sensitized patient and on the treatment of humoral-mediated rejection and hemolytic uremic syndrome associated with calcineurin use. The mechanisms behind IVIG's actions are varied but focus on inhibition of antibody formation via Fc-mediated effects, direct antiidiotypic antibodies present in IVIG, and antiinflammatory activities mediated by complement. Of these, the saturation of the neonatal Fc receptor (FcRn) on IVIG administration and the subsequent catabolism of IgG, including alloantibodies, seems the most compelling regarding the elimination of alloantibody.[203,204] Currently, treatment with high-dose IVIG (1–2 g/kg) is the cornerstone of attempts at antibody removal either before transplantation in highly sensitized individuals to reduce the PRA and potential positive crossmatch or after transplantation in the treatment of antibody-mediated rejection.[205] In addition, IVIG is also used in ABO-incompatible renal transplants with reasonable success.[129]

Tolerance

Physicians have long dreamed of a method that would allow for organs to be transplanted and specifically accepted as self-organs. Since the middle of the twentieth century, it has been clear that one *acquires* the ability to respond to certain antigens and not respond to others. More recently, it has become apparent that tolerance to self-tissues is rarely absolute, is closely regulated, and is probably *maintained* by repetitive exposure to self-antigen in a context that fosters T-cell anergy rather than T-cell activation. Several investigators are now aggressively pursuing means to apply the body's natural ability to acquire and maintain tolerance to transplanted organs rather than relying on toxic immunosuppression for graft survival. Extraordinary success has been achieved in animals

TABLE 80.5.
Preclinical Tolerance.

Reference	Year	Approach	Optimized regimen	Animal	Organ	MST (days)	MaxST	Comment
213	1997	Costimulation blockade	Anti-CD154 and CTLAIg	Rhesus	Kidney	20–30	>6 months	
214	1999	Costimulation blockade	Anti-CD154	Rhesus	Kidney	750	>5 years	20mg/kg dose, 6-month treatment, conventional agents decreased survival
215	2001	Costimulation blockade	Anti-CD154 and DST	Rhesus	Skin	236	>365 days	No difference with DST
218	2001	Costimulation blockade	Anti-CD80/86	Rhesus	Kidney	191		
217	2002	Costimulation blockade	Anti-CD80/86 and anti-CD154	Rhesus	Kidney	565		Delayed antidonor Ab; no difference versus anti-CD154 alone
216	2002	Costimulation blockade	Anti-CD40	Rhesus	Kidney	49		
219	1998	T-cell depletion	FN18-CRM9 immunotoxin	Rhesus	Kidney	>100 (8 of 14 animals)		5 of 6 animals maintained repeat challenge skin grafts
220	2003	T-cell depletion	Immunotoxin and DSG	Rhesus	Kidney	1495		Tolerant group with high IL-10/IFN-γ ratio
221, 222	1999, 2001	Chimerism	TBI, thymic XRT, ALG, BM, CYA ± splenectomy or anti-CD154	Cynomolgus	Kidney	>200		Transient macrochimerism (less than 2 months)

ALG, antilymphocyte globulin; BM, bone marrow; CYA, cyclosporine A; DSG, deoxyspergualin; XRT, X irradiation.

using several techniques.[206] Indeed, transplantation of kidneys and hearts without any chronic immunosuppression is now routinely successful in nonhuman primates, and early human trials have been initiated (although none with definitive success as yet). Several of the more promising approaches are briefly outlined next, and both preclinical and clinical trials are highlighted in Tables 80.4 and 80.5.[195,196,207–222]

T-Cell Ablation

It is becoming increasingly clear that postischemic reperfusion and surgical trauma significantly increase immune recognition following transplantation.[118,135] This concept has been the rationale for the use of induction therapy. Current antilymphocyte preparations successfully remove T cells from the circulation for several days and render those that are present inert, but they do not have a significant impact on a subset of memory T cells, which appear to be sensitive to calcineurin inhibition with tacrolimus.[223] It has been demonstrated that tolerance can be achieved by complete ablation of all mature T cells at the time of engraftment.[224] In nonhuman primates, a T-cell-specific immunotoxin has been used to deplete all T cells from the body. Reconstitution does not occur for approximately 1 month. When the cells return, cells reactive to the graft are not found in the circulation, and acute rejection does not occur. The animal is, however, capable of rejecting a subsequent graft or fighting infection. Because the T-cell ablation is nonspecific, the specific effect must be the result of regulation occurring in the repopulated thymus or in the peripheral lymphoid tissues.

Based on these preclinical data, depletion has been studied with both globulin and alemtuzumab in an attempt to institute tolerance or minimize immunosuppression. As demonstrated in Table 80.4, although depletion alone has not been able to establish tolerance, the minimization of immunosuppression to single-agent therapy has been a tremendous step toward achieving tolerance. The success of lymphocyte depletion suggests the reduction in the number of alloreactive cells available to institute graft rejection allows for a decreased level of maintenance immunosuppression.

Mixed Chimerism

Donor antigen is clearly required for any specific immune event to occur, be it rejection or tolerance. It has become increasingly clear that the character of that antigen and the means by which it is administered are important factors in determining the direction the immune system will take. Several investigators have had success achieving tolerance by supplementing the transplanted organ antigen with additional antigen in the form of bone marrow.[225–227] Using a variety of conditioning regimens, donor bone marrow is transplanted and engrafts throughout the body. This situation is known as *mixed chimerism* because donor and recipient hematopoietic elements coexist. The mechanism by which this promotes graft acceptance remains unclear. Thymic reeducation in the face of the new "self"-antigen has been proposed, and some investigators have improved their experimental success by directly injecting donor antigen into the recipient thymus.[228] There is also evidence that the marrow cells establish a self-regulating network that maintains a state of unresponsiveness to the graft.[229] There is growing speculation that the identification of mixed chimerism in a patient may in fact denote a state of potential tolerance.[230]

Despite promising results in preclinical models, the only successful deliberate attempts at tolerance induction with this strategy have been in human renal transplant recipients with multiple myeloma and end-stage renal failure (Tables 80.4 and 80.5). In these patients, mixed chimerism was transiently established after either total lymphoid irradiation (TLI) or nonmyeloablative conditioning, and immunosuppression was withdrawn without graft loss.[211,212] The applicability of this approach to the broader transplant population is currently under investigation.

Costimulation Blockade

Current immunosuppressive regimens have relied on agents that dramatically curtail normal T-cell functions, including TCR signal transduction. As specificity is mediated through the TCR, blocking this signal ensures that a nonspecific effect is elicited. With a growing awareness that T cells can be important mediators of tolerance, there has been growing interest in using the T-cell response in the absence of activating costimulation to foster persistent T-cell tolerance.

As has been discussed, once the TCR is engaged, the T cell can follow one of two paths: activation, through CD28 binding to B7, or anergy, in the absence of CD28 binding or in the presence of CTLA4 binding (see Fig. 80.7). A toleragenic phenotype will also result if the APCs cannot be appropriately activated to foster helper T-cell function and induce cytotoxic T-cell maturation. Interruption of the CD28 or CD40 pathways at the time of transplantation should thus selectively anergize only those cells undergoing binding to the allograft, leaving nonreactive cells unaffected. Preexisting immunity and innate immunity should be unaffected by this approach. There are an increasing number of reports in the literature that verify this approach using specific biological blockade of the CD28 or CD40 pathways.[96,213,231] Most encouraging are data showing, in rodents and primates, that simultaneous blockade of CD28 and CD40 at the time of transplantation can allow for prolonged survival of cardiac and renal allografts without the need for any subsequent immunosuppression and without any infectious or malignant side effects.

The extrapolation of these results to clinical practice has been disappointing thus far. In the only human tolerance trial of costimulation blockade, hu5C8, a humanized anti-CD154 monoclonal antibody, demonstrated limited efficacy and was associated with potential thromboembolic toxicity[207] (see Table 80.4). Currently, these agents are being reevaluated in preclinical models and will most likely be added to the armamentarium of transplant therapeutics.

Xenotransplantation

Transplantation has now become the treatment of choice for most end-stage diseases of most solid organs. Unfortunately, the indications for organ replacement have expanded at a rate far exceeding the available donor supply. As such, most people who could benefit from a transplanted organ are unable to receive one. Those who do receive one generally must wait a significant amount of time, during which they undergo deterioration in their fitness for surgery. Many investigators are now examining the feasibility of xenotransplantation to improve the availability of organs.[232] In addition to increasing the supply of transplantable organs, xenotransplantation also offers some of the same benefits achieved with living donors, including decreased ischemic injury to the organ and optimization of recipient health status, albeit at the cost of potential zoonotic viral transmission. In general, there are two types of xenografts, discordant and concordant. The immunology of these two types of xenografts differs markedly.

Concordant Xenografts

Concordant grafts are derived from closely related species. For humans, these include Old World monkeys and apes. The critical element defining an animal as concordant is the assembly of carbohydrate antigens on the surface of their cells. In particular, the enzyme galactosyl transferase is absent in these animals, and as a result their carbohydrates are the typical blood group antigens of the ABH system and lack the N-linked disaccharide galactose α (1–3) galactose [GALα(1–3)GAL].[233,234] Thus, the antibodies present in circulation of potential human recipients can be predicted by straightforward ABH typing, thereby avoiding the problem of HAR. With HAR removed as a threat, the typical mechanisms of graft rejection are left, including acute cellular rejection, acute vascular rejection, and, presumably, CR.

It is now clear that most of the critical molecular elements responsible for antigen presentation and T-cell-mediated rejection are evolutionarily conserved in mammals. Xenogeneic MHC polymorphism is, for the most part, restricted to the antigen-binding region.[235] The areas responsible for accessory molecule binding are also conserved. In addition, costimulatory and adhesion molecules required for adequate T-cell interaction function well across the species barrier.[236,237] For these reasons, cellular rejection and T-cell-dependent humoral rejection proceed as they do for an allograft completely mismatched at the HLA locus.

Several experimental models of concordant xenograft rejection, as well as occasional ventures into the clinical arena, have clearly demonstrated that concordant xenotransplantation is feasible given currently available immunosuppressive pharmaceuticals.[238–240] Prevention of concordant xenograft rejection would require induction with a T-cell-specific biological agent and chronic cellular suppression, including calcineurin inhibition, an antiproliferative agent such as MMF, and steroids. Results matching those seen for poorly matched allografts could be expected, including the complications from the immunosuppression required for engraftment.

With the possible exception of neonatal cardiac transplantation, however, the use of endangered, intelligent species with little ability to be bred or genetically altered could not meet the need for readily available, size-matched organs. Widespread application of concordant xenografts would quickly deplete the supply of nonhuman primates, particularly when a loss rate extrapolated from poorly matched allografts is taken into consideration. In addition, there is significant concern that zoonotic transfer of disease, in particular retroviral illness, will put the patient and the public at undue risk. It is therefore anticipated that concordant xenotransplantation will not remedy the organ shortage.

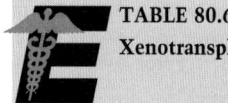

TABLE 80.6.
Xenotransplantation.

Reference	*Year*	*Approach*	*Optimized regimen*	*Animal*	*Organ*	*No. of Animals*	*MST (days)*	*Max ST*	*Comment*
247	2000	Transgenic	hDAF porcine	Cynomolgus	Kidney	14	>50 days (4/9 animals)	78 days	Splenectomy and triple therapy
248	1999	Transgenic	hDAF porcine	Baboon	Heart	9	26	99 days	Heterotopic heart; triple therapy
249	2000	Transgenic	hDAF porcine	Baboon	Heart	1	N/A	39 days	Orthotopic; triple therapy

hDAF, human decay-accelerating factor.

Discordant Xenografts

Discordant grafts are derived from distantly related species that express galactosyl transferase. For the purposes of human application, these include New World monkeys and nonprimates such as pigs. When transplanted into humans, these organs rapidly undergo HAR.[241] The primary cause of the rejection varies from species to species, but generally involves preformed IgM antibodies directed against atypical carbohydrate residues, such as GALα(1–3)GAL, acting in concert with complement.[233,234] These preformed antibodies serve an innate protective role by binding to GAL residues on bacteria. Vigorous T-cell-mediated rejection can also occur as human T cells can still be bound and activated by discordant MHC and costimulated by discordant B7.[236,237] Induced antibody responses similar to a vigorous vascular rejection are seen. In addition to the typical patterns of cellular rejection, there may also be a substantial detrimental effect of NK cells and other innate cellular elements.[236,242]

Given the spectrum of effectors involved in discordant rejection, intervention at all levels of both innate and acquired immunity will be required for successful engraftment. As such, a multimodal approach will be required. Despite this formidable challenge, significant headway has been made, particularly in the pig, toward establishing a xenogeneic source of donor organs.[242–244] Several groups have now transgenically altered pigs to express human complement regulator proteins such as CD59, decay-accelerating factor (DAF), and membrane cofactor protein (MCP). Others have altered the balance of carbohydrate processing to produce α(1–3) galactosylantransferase knockout animals, which would eliminate the expression of GALα(1–3)GAL in homozygotes, removing the major target of complement activation.[245,246] Using such an approach with transgenic swine that express human DAF, prolonged cardiac allograft survival has been demonstrated[247–249] (Table 80.6). Added to conventional immunosuppression, these interventions, as well as several inhibitors of complement, including anti-C5 monoclonal antibodies, cobra venom factor, and soluble complement receptor type 1, have been successful in abrogating HAR and extending survival in primates from minutes to weeks. While clinical application remains several years away, it is clear that the flexibility afforded by genetic engineering will one day allow for custom organs available as necessary to combat end-organ failure.

References

1. Carrel A. La technique operatoire des anastomoses vasculaires et la transplantation des visceres. Lyon Med 1902;98:859.
2. Carrel A. Results of the transplantation of blood vessels, organs and limbs. JAMA 1908;51:1662.
3. Converse JM, Casson PR. The historical background of transplantation. In: Rapaport F, Dausset J, eds. Human Transplantation. New York: Grune and Stratton; 1968.
4. Terasaki PI, ed. History of Transplantation: Thirty-Five Recollections. Los Angeles: UCLA Tissue Typing Laboratory; 1991.
5. Medawar PB. The behaviour and fate of skin autografts and skin homografts in rabbits. J Anat 1944;78:176–199.
6. Medawar PB. A second study of the behaviour and fate of skin homografts in rabbits. J Anat 1945;79:157–176.
7. Medawar PB. Immunity to homologous graft skin, I: the suppression of cell division in grafts transplanted to immunized animals. Br J Exp Pathol 1946;27:9.
8. Owen RD. Immunogenetic consequences of vascular anastomoses between bovine twins. Science 1945;102:400–401.
9. Billingham RE, Brent L, Medawar PB. Actively acquired tolerance of foreign cells. Nature 1953;172:603–606.
10. Mitchison NA. Passive transfer of transplantation immunity. Proc R Soc Lond B Biol Sci 1954;142:72.
11. Gorer PA. The antigenic basis of tumour transplantation. J Pathol Bacteriol 1938;47:231–252.
12. Gorer PA, Lyman S, Snell GD. Studies on the genetic and antigenic basis of tumour transplantation: linkage between a histocompatibility gene and "fused" in mice. Proc Soc Lond B Biol Sci 1948;135:499.
13. Snell GD. Methods for the study of histocompatibility genes. J Genet 1948–1949;49:87–108.
14. Amos DB, Gorer PA, Mikulska ZB. The antigenic structure and genetic behavior of a transplanted leukosis. Br J Cancer 1955;9:209.
15. Dausset J, Nenna A, Présence d'une leuco-agglutinine dans le sérum d'un cas d'agranulocytose chronique [Presence of leukoagglutinin in the serum of a case of chronic agranulocytosis]. Compt Rendus Soc Biol (Paris) 1952;146:1539.
16. Dausset J. Iso-leuco-anticorps. Acta Haematol 1958;20:156–166.
17. Bach F, Hirschhorn K. Lymphocyte interaction: a potential histocompatibility test in vitro. Science 1964;143:813–814.
18. Terasaki PI, McClelland JD. Microdroplet assay of human serum cytotoxins. Nature 1964;204:998–1000.
19. Bjorkman PJ, Saper MA, Samraoui B, et al. Structure of the human class I histocompatibility antigen, HLA-A2. Nature 1987;329:506–511.

20. Bjorkman PJ, Saper MA, Samraoui B, et al. The foreign antigen binding site and T cell recognition regions of class I histocompatibility antigen. Nature 1987;329:512–518.
21. Brown JH, Jardetzky T, Saper MA, et al. A hypothetical model of the foreign antigen binding site of class II histocompatibility molecules. Nature 1988;332:845–850.
22. Brown JH, Jardetzky T, Gorga JC, et al. Three-dimensional structure of the human class II histocompatibility antigen HLA-DR1. Nature 1993;364:33–39.
23. Hozumi N, Tonegawa S. Evidence for somatic rearrangement of immunoglobulin genes coding for variable and constant regions. Proc Natl Acad Sci U S A 1976;73:3628–3632.
24. Zinkernagel RM, Doherty PC. Restriction of in vitro T cell-mediated cytotoxicity in lymphocytic choriomeningitis within a syngeneic or semiallogeneic system. Nature 1974;248:701–702.
25. Doherty PC, Zinkernagel RM. T cell-mediated immunopathology in viral infections. Transplant Rev 1974;19:89–120.
26. Bretscher P, Cohn M. A theory of self-non-self discrimination. Science 1970;169:1042–1049.
27. Lafferty KJ, Cunningham AJ. A new analysis of allogeneic interactions. Aust J Exp Biol Med Sci 1975;53:27–42.
28. June CH, Bluestone JA, Nadler LM, Thompson CB. The B7 and CD28 receptor families. Immunol Today 1994;15:321–331.
29. Ridge JP, Fuchs EJ, Matzinger P. Neonatal tolerance revisited: turning on newborn T cells with dendritic cells. Science 1996; 271:1723–1726.
30. Murray JE, Merrill JP, Harrison JH. Renal homotransplantation in identical twins. Surg Forum 1955;6:432.
31. Hitchings GH, Elion GB, Falco EA, et al. Antagonists of nucleic acid derivatives, I: the *Lactobacillus casei* model. J Biol Chem 1950;183:1.
32. Hitchings GH, Elion GB. Chemical suppression of the immune response. Pharmacol Rev 1963;15:365.
33. Calne RY, Murray JE. Inhibition of rejection of renal homografts in dogs by Burroughs-Wellcome 57-322. Surg Forum 1961;12: 118–120.
34. Borel JF, Feurer C, Gubler HU. Biological effects of cyclosporine A: a new antilymphatic agent. Actions Agents 1976;6:468–475.
35. Borel JF. Comparative study of in vitro and in vivo drug effects on cell-mediated cytotoxicity. Immunology 1976;31:631–641.
36. Calne RY, White DJ, Rolles K, et al. Prolonged survival of pig orthotopic heart grafts treated with cyclosporin A. Lancet 1978; 1:1183–1185.
37. Calne RY, White DJ, Thiru S, et al. Cyclosporin A in patients receiving renal allografts from cadaver donors. Lancet 1978;2: 1323–1387.
38. Dempsey PW, Allison MED, Akkaraju S, et al. C3d of complement as a molecular adjuvant: bridging innate and acquired immunity. Science 1996;271:348–350.
39. Fearon DT, Locksley RM. The instructive role of innate immunity in the acquired immune response. Science 1996;272:50–53.
40. Wright SD, Ramos RA, Tobias PS, et al. CD14, a receptor for complexes of lipopolysaccharide (LPS) and LPS binding protein. Science 1990;249:1431–1433.
41. Baldwon WM, Pruitt SK, Brauer RB, et al. Complement in organ transplantation. Transplantation 1995;59:797–808.
42. Hart DNJ. Dendritic cells: unique leukocyte populations which control the primary immune response. Blood 1997;90:3245–3287.
43. Akira S, Takeda K. Toll-like receptor signaling. Nat Rev Immunol 2004;4:499–511.
44. Koo, DDH, Roberts, ISD, et al. C4d deposition in early renal allograft protocol biopsies. Transplantation 2004;78:398–403.
45. Ahmed R, Gray D. Immunological memory and protective immunity: understanding their relation. Science 1996;272:54–60.
46. Fearon DT. Seeking wisdom in innate immunity. Nature 1997;388:323–324.
47. Davis MM, Bjorkman PJ. T cell antigen receptor genes and T cell recognition. Nature 1988;334:395–402.
48. Cooper MD. B lymphocytes: normal development and function. N Engl J Med 1987;317:1452–1457.
49. Gill JI, Gulley ML. Immunoglobulin and T cell receptor gene rearrangement. Hematol Oncol Clin North Am 1994;8:751–770.
50. Kirk AD, Ibrahim S, Dawson DV, et al. Characterization of T cells expressing the γ/δ antigen receptor in human renal allografts. Hum Immunol 1993;36:11–19.
51. Kappler JW, Marrack P. T cell tolerance by clonal elimination in the thymus. Cell 1987;49:273–280.
52. Bevan MJ. In thymic selection, peptide diversity gives and takes away. Immunity 1997;7:175–178.
53. Fowlkes BJ, Ramsdell F. T cell tolerance. Curr Opin Immunol 1993;5:873–879.
54. Itoh N, Yonehara S, Ishii A, et al. The polypeptide encoded by the cDNA for human cell surface antigen Fas can mediate apoptosis. Cell 1991;66:233–243.
55. Griffith TS, Brunner T, Fletcher SM, et al. Fas ligand-induced apoptosis as a mechanism of immune privilege. Science 1995; 270:1189–1192.
56. Wilson IA, Garcia KC. T cell receptor structure and TCR complexes. Curr Opin Struct Biol 1997;7:839–848.
57. Rothenberg EV. How T cells count. Science 1996;273:78–79.
58. Viola A, Lanzavecchia A. T cell activation determined by T cell receptor number and tunable thresholds. Science 1996;273:104–106.
59. Kumagai N, Benedict SH, Mills GB, et al. Requirements for the simultaneous presence of phorbol esters and calcium ionophores in the expression of human T lymphocyte proliferation-related genes. J Immunol 1987;139:1393–1399.
60. Saizawa K, Rojo J, Janeway CA Jr. Evidence for a physical association of CD4 and the CD3: alpha:beta T cell receptor. Nature 1987;328:260–263.
61. Leahy DJ, Axel R, Hendrickson WA. Crystal structure of a soluble form of the human T cell coreceptor CD8 at 2.6 Å resolution. Cell 1992;68:1145–1162.
62. Germain RN. MHC-dependent antigen processing and peptide presentation: providing ligands for T lymphocyte activation. Cell 1994;76:287–299.
63. Monaco JJ. Structure and function of genes in the MHC class II region. Curr Opin Immunol 1993;5:17–20.
64. Ridge JP, Di Rosa F, Matzinger P. A conditioned dendritic cell can be a temporal bridge between a $CD4^+$ T-helper and a T-killer cell. Nature 1998;393:474–478.
65. Lanzavecchia A. License to kill. Nature 1998;393:413–414.
66. Plas DR. Johnson R, Pingel JT, et al. Direct regulation of ZAP-70 by SHP-1 in T cell antigen receptor signaling. Science 1996; 272:1173–1176.
67. Marengere LEM, Waterhouse P, Duncan GS, et al. Regulation of T cell receptor signaling by tyrosine phosphatase SYP associated with CTLA-4. Science 1996;272:1170–1173.
68. Crabtree GR. Contingent genetic regulatory events in T lymphocyte activation. Science 1989;243:355–361.
69. Ullman KS, Northrop JP, Verweij CJ, Crabtree GR. Transmission of signals from the T lymphocyte antigen receptor to the genes responsible for cell proliferation and immune function: the missing link. Annu Rev Immunol 1990;8:421–452.
70. Siegel JN, June CH. Signal transduction in T cell activation and tolerance. In: Gupta S, Griscelli C, eds. New Concepts in Immunodeficiency Diseases. New York: Wiley; 1993;85–129.
71. Karthryn Wood and Shimon Sakaguchi. Regulatory T cells in transplant tolerance. Nat Rev Immunol 2003;3:199–210.
72. Shimizu J, Yamazaki S, Takahashi T, Ishida Y, Sakaguchi S. Stimulation of CD25(+)CD4(+) regulatory T cells through GITR

breaks immunological self-tolerance. Nat Immunol 2002;3:135–142.

73. Baecher-Allan at al. CD4+CD25+ highly regulatory cells in human peripheral blood. J Immunol 2001;167:1245–1253.
74. Berke G. The CTL's kiss of death. Cell 1995;81:9–12.
75. Zouali M. B cell superantigens: implications for selection of the human antibody repertoire. Immunol Today 1995;16:399–405.
76. Jung S, Rajewsky K, Radbruch A. Shutdown of class switch recombination by deletion of a switch region control element. Science 1993;259:984–987.
77. Griffiths GM, Berek C, Kaartinen M, Milstein C. Somatic mutation and the maturation of immune response to 2-phenyloxazolone. Nature 1984;312:271–275.
78. Cambier JC, Pleiman CM, Clark MR. Signal transduction by the B cell antigen receptor and its coreceptors. Annu Rev Immunol 1994;12:457–486.
79. Tedder TF, Zhou LJ, Engel P. The CD19/CD21 signal transduction complex of B lymphocytes. Immunol Today 1994;15:437–442.
80. Lederman S, Yellin MJ, Inghirami G, et al. Molecular interactions mediating T-B lymphocyte collaboration in human lymphoid follicles: roles of the T cell-B cell activating molecule (5c8 antigen) and CD40 in contact dependent help. J Immunol 1992; 149:3817–3826.
81. Takeuchi Y, Porter CD, Strahan KM, et al. Sensitization of cells and retroviruses to human serum by (a1–3) galactosyltransferase. Nature 1996;379:85–88.
82. Arai KI, Lee F, Miyajima A, et al. Cytokines: coordinators of immune and inflammatory responses. Annu Rev Biochem 1990; 59:783–836.
83. Waldmann T, Tagaya Y, Bamford R. Interleukin-2, interleukin-15, and their receptors. Int Rev Immunol 1998;16:205–226.
84. Feldman M, Londei M, Haworth C. T cells and lymphokines. Br Med Bull 1989;45:361–370.
85. Leonard WJ, Depper JM, Robb RJ, et al. Characterization of the human receptor for T cell growth factor. Proc Natl Acad Sci U S A 1983;8:6957–6961.
86. Mosmann TR, Cherwinski H, Bond MW, et al. Two types of murine helper T cell clone, I: definition according to profiles of lymphokine activities and secreted proteins. J Immunol 1986;136:2348–2357.
87. Mosmann TR. Cytokines: is there biological meaning? Curr Opin Immunol 1991;3:311–314.
88. Sugamura K, Asao H, Kondo M, et al. The common gamma-chain for multiple cytokine receptors. Adv Immunol 1995;59:225–277.
89. Aaronson DS, Horvath CM. A road map for those who don't know JAK-STAT. Science 2002;296:1653–1655.
90. Kelso A. Th1 and Th2 subsets: paradigms lost? Immunol Today 1995;16:374–380.
91. Krams SM, Falco DA, Villaneuva JC, et al. Cytokine and T cell receptor gene expression at the site of allograft rejection. Transplantation 1992;53:151–156.
92. Kirk AD, Bollinger RR, Finn OJ. Rapid, comprehensive analysis of human cytokine mRNA and its application to the study of acute renal allograft rejection. Hum Immunol 1995;43:113–128.
93. Allison JP, Krummel MF. The yin and yang of T cell costimulation. Science 1995;270:932–933.
94. Chambers CA, Allison JP. Co-stimulation in T cell responses. Curr Opin Immunol 1997;9:396–404.
95. Larsen CP, Pearson TC. The CD40 pathway in allograft rejection, acceptance, and tolerance. Curr Opin Immunol 1997;9:641–647.
96. Harlan DM, Kirk AD. Anti-CD154 therapy to prevent graft rejection. Graft 1998;1:63–70.
97. Bennett SRM, Carbone FR, Karamalis F, et al. Help for cytotoxic T cell responses is mediated by CD40 signalling. Nature 1998; 393:478–480.
98. Schoenberger SP, Toes REM, van der Voort EIH, et al. T cell help for cytotoxic T lymphocytes is mediated by CD40-CD40L interactions. Nature 1998;393:480–483.
99. Henn V, Slupsky JR, et al. CD40 ligand on activated platelets triggers an inflammatory reaction of endothelial cells. Nature 1998;391:591–594.
100. Czapiga M, Kirk AD, Lekstrom-Himes J. Platelets deliver costimulatory signals to antigen-presenting cells: a potential bridge between injury and immune activation. Exp Hematol 2004;32:135–139.
101. Blair PJ, Riley JL, Levine BL, et al. CTLA-4 ligation delivers a unique signal to resting human CD4 T cells that inhibits interleukin-2 secretion but allows Bcl-X_L induction. J Immunol 1998; 160:12–15.
102. Waterhouse P, Penninger JM, Timms E, et al. Lymphoproliferative disorders with early lethality in mice deficient in CTLA-4. Science 1995;270:985–988.
103. Walunas TL, Lenschow DJ, Bakker CY, et al. CTLA-4 can function as a negative regulator of T cell activation. Immunity 1994;1:405–413.
104. Linsley PS, Greene JL, Brady W, et al. Human B7-1 (CD80) and B7-2 (CD86) bind with similar avidities but distinct kinetics to CD28 and CTLA-4 receptors. Immunity 1994;1:793–801.
105. Pennisi E. Teetering on the brink of danger. Science 1996;271: 1665–1667.
106. Bingaman AW, Ha J, et al. Vigorous allograft rejection in the absence of danger. J Immunol 2000;164:3065–3071.
107. Okazaki T, Iwai Y, Honjo T. New regulatory co-receptors: inducible co-stimulator and PD-1. Curr Opin Immunol 2002;14:779–82.
108. Campbell RD, Trowsdale J. Map of the major histocompatibility complex. Immunol Today 1993;14:349–352.
109. Lotteau V, Teyton L, Borroghs D, Charron D. A novel HLA class II molecule (DRalpha-DQbeta) created by mismatched isotype pairing. Nature 1987;329:339–341.
110. Parham P, Ohta T. Population biology of antigen presentation by MHC class I molecules. Science 1996;272:67–74.
111. Nowak MA, Bangham CRM. Population dynamics of immune responses to persistent viruses. Science 1996;272:74–79.
112. Salter RD, Benjamin RJ, Wesley PK, et al. A binding site for the T cell co-receptor CD8 on the a3 domain of HLA-A2. Nature 1990;345:41–46.
113. Doyle C, Strominger JL. Interaction between CD4 and class II MHC molecules mediates cell adhesion. Nature 1987;330:256–259.
114. Williams DB, Barber BH, Flavell RA, et al. Role of b_2-microglobin in the intracellular transport and surface expression of murine class I histocompatibility molecules. J Immunol 1989; 142:2796–2806.
115. Teyton L, O'Sullivan D, Dickson PW, et al. Invariant chain distinguishes between the exogenous and endogenous antigen presenting pathways. Nature 1988;348:39–44.
116. Adams AB, Pearson TC, Larsen CP. Heterologous immunity: an overlooked barrier to tolerance. Immunol Rev 2003;196: 147.
117. Halloran PF, Madrenas J. Regulation of MHC transcription. Transplantation 1990;50:725–738.
118. Gerritsen ME, Bloor CM. Endothelial cell gene expression in response to injury. FASEB 1993;7:523–533.
119. Marsh SGE, Bodmer JG. HLA class II nucleotide sequences, 1992. Immunogenetics 1993;37:79–94.
120. Zemmour J, Parham P. HLA class I nucleotide sequences, 1992. Immunogenetics 1993;37:239–250.
121. Bidwell J. DNA-RFLP analysis and genotyping of HLA-DR and DQ antigens. Immunol Today 1998;9:18–23.

122. Nevinny-Stickel C, Bettinotti MP, Andreas A, et al. Nonradioactive HLA class II typing using polymerase chain reaction and digoxigenin-11-29-39-didesoxy-uridinetriphosphate labeled oligonucleotide probes. Hum Immunol 1991;31:7–13.
123. Nevinny-Stickel C, Hinzpter M, Andreas A, et al. Nonradioactive oligotyping for HLA-DR1-DRw10 using polymerase chain reaction, digoxigenin-labeled oligonucleotides and chemiluminescence detection. Eur J Immunogenet 1991;18:323–332.
124. Olerup O, Zetterquist H. HLA DR typing by PCR amplification with sequence-specific primers (PCR-SSP) in 2 hours: an alternative to serological typing in clinical practice including donor-recipient matching in cadaveric transplantations. Tissue Antigens 1992;39:225–235.
125. Markus BH, Duquesnoy RJ, Gordon RD, et al. Histocompatibility and liver transplantation. Does HLA exert a dualistic effect? Transplantation (Baltimore) 1988;46:372–377.
126. Steinhoff G. HLA/ABO matching. In Neuberger J, Adams D, eds. Immunology of Liver Transplantation. London: Edward Arnold; 1993:261–266.
127. Terasaki PI, Cecka JM, Gjertson DW, Takemoto S. High survival rates of kidney transplants from spousal and living unrelated donors. N Engl J Med 1995;333:333–336.
128. Terasaki PI, Cecka JM, Gjertson DW, Cho YW. Spousal and Other Living Renal Donor Transplants. Los Angeles: UCLA Tissue Typing Laboratory, Clinical Transplants; 1997.
129. Gloor JM, DeGoey SR, et al. Overcoming a positive crossmatch in living-donor kidney transplantation. AJT 3:1017, 2003:1017–1023.
130. Takahashi K, Saito K, et al. Excellent long-term outcome of ABO-incompatible living donor kidney transplantation in Japan. Am J Transplant 2004;4:1089–1096.
131. Burdick JF. An anatomy of rejection. Transplant Rev 1991;5:81–90.
132. Kirk AD, Ibrahim MA, Bollinger RR, et al. Renal allograft infiltrating lymphocytes: a prospective analysis of in vitro growth characteristics and clinical relevance. Transplantation 1992; 53:329–338.
133. Fuggle SV, Koo DDH. Cell adhesion molecules in clinical renal transplantation. Transplantation 1998;65:763–769.
134. Henn V, Slupsky JR, Grafe M, et al. CD40 ligand on activated platelets triggers an inflammatory reaction of endothelial cells. Nature 1998;391:591–594.
135. Takada M, Chandraker A, Nadeau KC, et al. The role of the B7 costimulatory pathway in experimental cold ischemia/reperfusion injury. J Clin Invest 1997;100:1199–1203.
136. Dallman MJ, Clark GJ. Cytokines and their receptors in transplantation. Curr Opin Immunol 1991;3:729–734.
137. Strehlau J, Pavlakis M, Lipman M, et al. Quantitative detection of immune activation transcripts as a diagnostic tool in kidney transplantation. Proc Natl Acad Sci U S A 1997;94:695–700.
138. Levitz SM, Mathews HL, Murphy JW. Direct antimicrobial activity of T cells. Immunol Today 1995;16:387–391.
139. Baldwin WM III, Pruitt SK, Sanfilippo F, et al. Alloantibodies: basic and clinical concepts. Transplant Rev 1991;5:100–119.
140. Saadi S, Platt JL. Transient perturbation of endothelial integrity induced by natural antibodies and complement. J Exp Med 1995;181:21–31.
141. Bach FH, Winkler H, Ferran C, et al. Delayed xenograft rejection. Immunol Today 1996;17:379–384.
142. Gebel HM, Lebeck LK. Crossmatch procedures used in organ transplantation. Clin Lab Med 1991;11:603–620.
143. Talbot D. The flow cytometric crossmatch in perspective. Transplant Immunol 1993;1:155–162.
144. Le Bas-Bernardet S, Hourmant M. Identification of the antibodies involved in B-cell crossmatch positivity in renal transplantation. Transplantation 2003;75:477–482.
145. Noreen HJ, McKinley DM, et al. Positive remote crossmatch: impact on short-term and long-term outcome in cadaver renal transplantation. Transplantation 2003;75:501–505.
146. Colvin RB. The pathogenesis of vascular rejection. Transplant Proc 1991;23:2052–2055.
147. Paul LC. Chronic renal transplant loss. Kidney Int 1995;47:1491–1499.
148. Almond PS, Matas A, Gillingham KJ, et al. Risk factors for chronic rejection in renal allograft recipients. Transplantation 1993;55:752–757.
149. Gourishankar S, Halloran PF. Late deterioration of organ transplants: a problem in injury and homeostasis. Curr Opin Immunol 2002;14:576–583.
150. Ahsan N, Johnson C, et al. Randomized trial of tacrolimus plus mycophenolate mofetil or azathioprine versus cyclosporine oral solution (modified) plus mycophenolate mofetil after cadaveric kidney transplantation: results at 2 years. Transplantation. 2001; 72:245–250.
151. Jensick SC. Tacrolimus in kidney transplantation: 3-year survival results of the US multicenter, randomized, comparative trial. FK506 Kidney Transplant Study Group. Transplant Proc 1998;30:1216–1218.
152. Mathew TH. A blinded, long-term, randomized multicenter study of mycophenolate mofetil in cadaveric renal transplantation: results at 3 years. Tricontinental Mycophenolate Mofetil Renal Transplantation Study Group. Transplantation 1998;65: 1450–1454.
153. Gaber A. Results of the double-blind, randomized, multicenter, phase III clinical trial of thymoglobulin versus ATGAM in the treatment of acute graft rejection episodes after renal transplantation. Clin Transplant 1998;66:29–37.
154. Kahan BD. Efficacy of sirolimus compared with azathioprine for reduction of acute renal allograft rejection: a randomized multicentre study. Lancet 2000;356:194–202.
155. Vincenti F. Interleukin-2-receptor blockade with daclizimab to prevent acute rejection in renal transplantation. N Engl J Med 1998;338:161–165.
156. Hardinger KL, Schnitzler MA, et al. Five-year follow up of thymoglobulin versus ATGAM induction in adult renal transplantation. Transplantation 2004;78:136–141.
157. Auphan N, DiDonato JA, Rosette C, et al. Immunosuppression by glucocorticoids: inhibition of NF-kB activity through induction of IkB synthesis. Science 1995;270:286–290.
158. Scheinman RI, Cogswell PC, Lofquist AK, et al. Role of transcriptional activation of IkBα in mediation of immunosuppression by glucocorticoids. Science 1995;283:283–286.
159. Plaz KP, Sollinger HW, Hullet DA, et al. RS-61443, a new, potent immunosuppressive agent. Transplantation 1991;51:27–31.
160. Sollinger HW, Deierhoi MH, Belzer FO, et al. RS-61443: a phase I clinical trial and pilot rescue study. Transplantation 1992;53: 428–432.
161. Sollinger HW. US Renal Transplant Mycophenolate Mofetil Study Group. Mycophenolate mofetil for the prevention of acute rejection in primary cadaveric renal allograft recipients. Transplantation 1995;60:225–232.
162. Kahan BD. Role of cyclosporine: present and future. Transplant Proc 1994;26:3082–3087.
163. Khanna A, Sharma VK, Suthanthiran M. Immunoregulatory and fibrogenic activities of cyclosporine: a unifying hypothesis based on transforming growth factor-b expression. Transplant Proc 1996;28:2015–2019.
164. Kirk AD, Jacobson LM, Heisey DM, et al. Post-transplant diastolic hypertension: associations with intragraft TGF-β, endothelin and renin transcription. Transplantation 1997;64: 1716–1720.
165. June CH, Ledbetter JA, Gillespie MM, et al. T cell proliferation involving the CD28 pathway is associated with cyclosporine-

resistant interleukin-2 gene expression. Mol Cell Biol 1987;7:4472–4481.
166. Hojo M, Morimoto T, Maluccio M, et al. Cyclosporine induces cancer progression by a cell-autonomous mechanism. Nature 1999;397:530–534.
167. Kino T, Hatanaka H, Miyata S, et al. FK-506, a novel immunosuppressant isolated from streptomyces, II: immunosuppressive effect of FK-506 in vitro. J Antibiot 1987;40:1256–1265.
168. Fruman DA, Klee CB, Bierer BE, Burakoff SJ. Calcineurin phosphatase activity in T lymphocytes is inhibited by FK506 and cyclosporin A. Proc Natl Acad Sci U S A 1992;89:3686–3690.
169. Starzl TE, Fung JJ, Venkataramanan, et al. FK-506 for liver, kidney, and pancreas transplantation. Lancet 1989;334:1000–1004.
170. Gaber AO, First MR, Tesi RJ, et al. Results of the double-blind, randomized, multicenter, phase III clinical trial of thymoglobulin versus ATGAM in the treatment of acute graft rejection episodes after renal transplantation. Transplantation 1998;66:29–37.
171. Merion RM, Howell T, Bromberg JS. Partial T cell activation and energy induction by polyclonal antithymocyte globulin. Transplantation 1998;65:1481–1489.
172. Swanson SJ, Hale DA, Mannon RB, et al. Kidney transplantation with rabbit antithymocyte globulin induction and sirolimus monotherapy. Lancet 2002;360:1662.
173. Starzl TE, Murase N, et al. Tolerogenic immunosuppression for organ transplantation. Lancet 2003;361:1502–1510.
174. Brennan DC, Flavin K, Lowell JA, et al. A randomized, double-blinded comparison of Thymoglobulin versus Atgam for induction immunosuppressive therapy in adult renal transplant recipients. Transplantation 1999;67:1011–1018.
175. Wilde MI, Goa KL. Muromonab CD3: a reappraisal of its pharmacology and use as prophylaxis of solid organ transplant rejection. Drugs 1996;51:865–894.
176. Delmonico FL, Cosimi AB. Monoclonal antibody treatment of human allograft recipients. Surg Obst Gynecol 1988;166:89–98.
177. Kupfer A, Mosmann TR, Kupfer H, et al. Polarized expression of cytokines in cell conjugates of helper T cells and splenic B cells. Proc Natl Acad Sci U S A 1991;88:775–779.
178. Shield CF III, Norman DJ. Immunological monitoring during and after OKT3 therapy. Am J Kidney Dis 1988;11:120–124.
179. Ortho Multicenter Transplant Study Group. A randomized clinical trial of OKT3 monoclonal antibody for acute rejection of cadaveric renal transplants. N Engl J Med 1985;313:337–342.
180. Light JA, Khawand N, Aquino A, et al. Quadruple immunosuppression: comparison of OKT3 and Minnesota antilymphocyte globulin. Am J Kidney Dis 1989;14:10–13.
181. Soulillou JP, Le Mauff B, Olive D, et al. Prevention of rejection of kidney transplants by a monoclonal antibody directed against interleukin 2. Lancet 1987;1:1339–1342.
182. Nashan B, Moore B, Amlot P, et al. Randomised trial of basiliximab versus placebo for control of acute cellular rejection in renal allograft recipients. Lancet 1997;350:1193–1198.
183. Flechner M, Goldfarb D, Modlin C, et al. Kidney transplantation without calcineurin inhibitor drugs: A prospective, randomized trial of sirolimus versus cyclosporine. Transplantation 2002;74:1070–1076.
184. Segal SN, Baker H, Vezina C, et al. Rapamycin (AY-22,989), a new antifungal antibiotic, II: fermentation, isolation and characterization. J Antibiot (Tokyo) 1975;28:727–732.
185. Martel RR, Klicius J, Galet S. Inhibition of the immune response by rapamycin, a new antifungal antibiotic. Can J Physiol Pharmacol 1977;55:48–51.
186. Baker H, Sidorowicz A, Sehgal SN, Vezina C. Rapamycin (AY-22,989), a new antifungal antibiotic, III: In vitro and in vivo evaluation. J Antibiot 1978;31:539–545.
187. Molnar-Kimber KL. Mechanism of action of rapamycin (sirolimus, rapamune). Transplant Proc 1996;26:964–969.
188. Dumont FJ, Melino MR, Staruch MJ, et al. The immunosuppressive macrolides FK-506 and rapamycin act as reciprocal antagonists in murine T cells. J Immunol 1990;144:1418–1424.
189. Dumont FJ, Staruch MJ, Koprak SL, et al. Distinct mechanisms of suppression of murine T cell activation by the related macrolides FK-506 and rapamycin. J Immunol 1990;144:251–258.
190. Kuo CJ, Chung J, Fiorentino DF, et al. Rapamycin selectively inhibits interleukin 2 activation of p70 S6 kinase. Nature 1992;358:70–73.
191. Muthukkumar S, Ramesh TM, Bondada S. Rapamycin, a potent immunosuppressive drug, causes programmed cell death in B lymphoma cells. Transplantation 1995;60:264–270.
192. Bjorn Nashan. Review of the proliferation inhibitor everolimus. Exper Opin Invest Drug 2002;11:1845–1857.
193. McAlister VC, Gao Z, et al. Sirolimus-tacrolimus combination immunosuppression. Lancet 2000;355:376–377.
194. Morris RE. Rapamycins: antifungal, antitumor, antiproliferative and immunosuppressive macrolides. Transplant Rev 1992;6:39–87.
195. Calne RY, Friend P, Moffatt S, et al. Prope tolerance, perioperative campath 1H, and low-dose cyclosporin monotherapy in renal allograft recipients. Lancet 1998;351:1701.
196. Kirk AD, Hale DA, Mannon RB, et al. Results from a human renal allograft tolerance trial evaluating the humanized CD52-specific monoclonal antibody alemtuzumab (CAMPATH-1H). Transplantation 2003;76:120.
197. Knechtle SJ, Pirsch JD, Fechner H, et al. Campath-1H induction plus rapamycin monotherapy for renal transplantation: results of a pilot study. Am J Transplant 2003;3:722.
198. Kaufman DB. 15-Deoxyspergualin in experimental transplant models: a review. Transplant Proc 1996;28:868–870.
199. Ramos EL, Nadler SG, Grasela DM, Kelly SL. Deoxyspergualin: mechanism of action and pharmacokinetics. Transplant Proc 1996;28:873–875.
200. Kirk A. Results from a human tolerance trial using alemtuzumab (campath-1H) with deoxyspergualin (DSG). Am J Transplant 2003;3(S5):S310.
201. Brinkmann V, Cyster JG, Hla T. FTY720: sphingosine 1-phosphate receptor-1 in the control of lymphocyte egress and endothelial barrier function. Am J Transplant 2004;4:1019.
202. Becker YT, Becker BN, et al. Rituximab as treatment for refractory kidney transplant rejection. Am J Transplant 2004;4:996.
203. Samuelsson A, Towers TL, Ravetch JV. Anti-inflammatory activity of IVIG mediated through the inhibitory Fc receptor. Science 2001;291:484.
204. Bleeker WK, Teeling JL, Hack CE. Accelerated autoantibody clearance by intravenous immunoglobulin therapy: studies in experimental models to determine the magnitude and time course of the effect. Blood 2001;98:3136–3142.
205. Takemoto SK, Zeevi A, et al. National Conference to Assess Antibody-Mediated Rejection in Solid Organ Transplantation. Am J Transplant 2004;4:1033–1041.
206. Kirk AD. Transplant tolerance: a look at the non-human primate literature in the view of modern tolerance theories. Crit Rev Immunol 1999;19:349–388.
207. Kirk AD, Knechtle SJ, Sollinger H, Vincenti FG, Stecher S, Nadeau K. Preliminary results of the use of humanized anti-CD154 in human renal allotransplantation. Am J Transplant 2001;1:S191.
208. Calne R, Moffatt SD, Friend PJ, et al. Campath IH allows low-dose cyclosporine monotherapy in 31 cadaveric renal allograft recipients. Transplantation 1999;68:1613–1616.
209. Kirk A. Results from a human tolerance trial using alemtuzumab (campath-1H) with deoxyspergualin (DSG). Am J Transplant 2003;3(S5):S310.
210. Spitzer TR, Delmonico F, Tolkoff-Rubin N, et al. Combined histocompatibility leukocyte antigen-matched donor bone marrow and renal transplantation for multiple myeloma with

end stage renal disease: the induction of allograft tolerance through mixed lymphohematopoietic chimerism. Transplantation 1999;68:480.
211. Strober S, Benike C, Krishnaswamy S, Engleman EG, Grumet FC. Clinical transplantation tolerance 12 years after prospective withdrawal of immunosuppressive drugs: studies of chimerism and anti-donor reactivity. Transplantation 2000;69:1549.
212. Millan MT, Shizuru JA, Hoffmann P, et al. Mixed chimerism and immunosuppressive drug withdrawal after HLA-mismatched kidney and hematopoietic progenitor transplantation. Transplantation 2002;73:1386.
213. Kirk AD, Harlan DM, Armstrong NN, et al. CTLA4-Ig and anti-CD40 ligand prevent renal allograft rejection in primates. Proc Natl Acad Sci U S A 1997;94:8789.
214. Kirk AD, Burkly LC, Batty DS, et al. Treatment with humanized monoclonal antibody against CD154 prevents acute renal allograft rejection in nonhuman primates. Nat Med 1999; 5:686.
215. Elster EA, Xu H, Tadaki DK, et al. Treatment with the humanized CD154-specific monoclonal antibody, hu5C8, prevents acute rejection of primary skin allografts in nonhuman primates. Transplantation 2001;72:1473.
216. Pearson TC, Trambley J, Odom K, et al. Anti-CD40 therapy extends renal allograft survival in rhesus macaques. Transplantation 2002;74:933.
217. Montgomery SP, Xu H, Tadaki DK, et al. Combination induction therapy with monoclonal antibodies specific for CD80, CD86, and CD154 in nonhuman primate renal transplantation. Transplantation 2002;74:1365.
218. Kirk AD, Tadaki DK, Celniker A, et al. Induction therapy with monoclonal antibodies specific for CD80 and CD86 delays the onset of acute renal allograft rejection in non-human primates. Transplantation 2001;72:377–384.
219. Knechtle SJ, Fechner JH Jr, Dong Y, et al. Primate renal transplants using immunotoxin. Surgery 1998;124:438.
220. Hutchings A, Wu J, Asiedu C, et al. The immune decision toward allograft tolerance in non-human primates requires early inhibition of innate immunity and induction of immune regulation. Transpl Immunol 2003;11:335.
221. Kawai T, Poncelet A, Sachs DH, et al. Long-term outcome and alloantibody production in a non-myeloablative regimen for induction of renal allograft tolerance. Transplantation 1999; 68:1767.
222. Kawai T, Abrahamian G, Sogawa H, et al. Costimulatory blockade for induction of mixed chimerism and renal allograft tolerance in nonhuman primates. Transplant Proc 2001;33: 221.
223. Pearl JP, Parris J, Hale DA, et al. Immunocompetent T-cells with a memory-like phenotype are the dominant cell type following antibody-mediated T-cell depletion. Am J Transplant 2005;5:465–474.
224. Knechtle SJ, Vargo D, Fechner J, et al. FN18-CRM9 immunotoxin promotes tolerance in primate renal allografts. Transplantation 1997;63:1–6.
225. Sykes M, Sachs DH. Mixed allogeneic chimerism as an approach to transplant tolerance. Immunol Today 1998;9:23–27.
226. Sharabi Y, Sachs DH. Mixed chimerism and permanent specific transplantation tolerance induced by a nonlethal preparative regimen. J Exp Med 1989;169:493–502.
227. Kaufman CL, Ildstad ST. Induction of donor-specific tolerance by transplantation of bone marrow. Ther Immunol 1994;1:101–111.
228. Odorico JS, O'Connor T, Campos L, et al. Examination of the mechanisms responsible for tolerance induction after intrathymic inoculation of allogeneic bone marrow. Ann Surg 1993; 218:525–531.
229. Qin S, Cobbold SP, Pope H, et al. Infectious transplant tolerance. Science 1993;259:974–977.
230. Starzl TE, Demetris AJ, Murase N, et al. Cell migration, chimerism and graft acceptance. Lancet 1992;339:1579–1582.
231. Larsen CP, Elwood ET, Alexander DZ, et al. Long-term acceptance of skin and cardiac allografts after blocking CD40 and CD28 pathways. Nature 1996;381:434–438.
232. Kirk AD, Harlan DM, Armstrong NN, et al. CTLA4-Ig and anti-CD40 ligand prevent renal allograft rejection in primates. Proc Natl Acad Sci U S A 1997;94:8789–8794.
233. Auchincloss H Jr, Sachs DH. Xenogeneic transplantation. Annu Rev Immunol 1998;16:433–470.
234. Sandrin MS, Vaughan HA, et al. Anti-pig IgM antibodies in human serum react predominantly with gal(a1–3)gal epitopes. Proc Natl Acad Sci U S A 1993;90:11391–11395.
235. Cooper DKC, Good AH, et al. Identification of alpha-galactosyl and other carbohydrate epitopes that are bound by human anti-pig antibodies: relevance to discordant xenografting in man. Transpl Immunol 1993;1:198–205.
236. Prilliman K, Lawlor D, Ellexson M. Characterization of baboon class I major histocompatibility molecules. Transplantation 1996;61:989–996.
237. Kirk AD, Li RA, Kinch MS, et al. The human antiporcine cellular repertoire. In vitro studies of acquired and innate cellular responsiveness. Transplantation 1993;55:924–931.
238. Tadaki D, Saini A, Craighead N, et al. Costimulatory pathways are active in xenogeneic immune responses [abstract]. Transplantation 1998;65:87.
239. Reemtsma K, McCracken BH, et al. Renal heterotransplantation in man. Ann Surg 1964;160:384.
240. Starzl TE, Marchioro TL, et al. Renal heterotransplantation from baboon to man: experience with six cases. Transplantation 1964;2:752–759.
241. Bailey LL, Nehlsen-Cannarella SL, et al. Baboon-to-human cardiac xenotransplantation in a neonate. JAMA 1985;254:3321–3329.
242. Platt JL, Fischel RJ, et al. Immunopathology of hyperacute xenograft rejection in a swine-to-primate model. Transplantation 1991;52:214–220.
243. Goodman DJ, von Albertini M, et al. Direct activation of porcine endothelial cells by human natural killer cells. Transplantation 1996;61:763–771.
244. McCurry KR, Kooyman DL, et al. Human complement regulatory proteins protect swine-to-primate cardiac xenografts from humoral injury. Nat Med 1995;1:423–427.
245. Sandrin MS, Fodor WL, et al. Enzymatic remodeling of the carbohydrate surface of a xenogeneic cell substantially reduces human antibody binding and complement-mediated cytolysis. Nat Med 1996;1:1261–1267.
246. Lai L, Kolber-Simonds D, et al. Production of α-1,3-galactosyltransferase knockout pigs by nuclear transfer cloning. Science 2002:295:1089–1092.
247. Cozzi E, Bhatti FNK, Schmoeckel M, et al. Long-term survival of nonhuman primates receiving life-supporting transgenic porcine kidney xenografts. Transplantation 2000;70:12–21.
248. Bhatti FNK, Schmoeckel M, Zaidi A, et al. Three-month survival of HDAFF transgenic pig hearts transplanted into primates. Transplant Proc 1999;31:958.
249. Vial CM, Ostlie DJ, Bhatti FNK, et al. Life supporting function for over one month of a transgenic porcine heart in a baboon. J Heart Lung Transplant 2000;19:224–229.
250. Burke F, Naylor MS, et al. The cytokine wall chart. Immunol Today 1993;14:165.
251. Kirk AD, Sollinger HW. Transplant immunology and immunosuppression. In: Schwartz S, ed. Principles of Surgery, 7th Ed. New York; McGraw-Hill, 1998.

81

Rejection

J. Richard Thistlethwaite and David Bruce

The mammalian immune system is specialized for the discrimination between self and nonself. The appearance of new macromolecules (or *antigens*) normally signifies a threat, such as an infection or malignant tumor. In these settings, the prompt destruction of antigen-bearing cells is a valuable adaptation. Unfortunately, the same defense mechanisms are also efficiently invoked by the clinical transplantation of potentially lifesaving organs.

The term *rejection* refers to any immune response to foreign tissue that can cause graft destruction. Three immunopathological types of rejection have been defined: hyperacute, acute, and chronic. Although some authors have defined *accelerated acute rejection* as a separate category, this term essentially refers to acute rejection that proceeds at a rapid pace as the result of prior antigenic exposure resulting in immunological memory. While this categorization is conceptually useful, it should be noted that these types of rejection are not mutually exclusive. For example, early acute rejection episodes are occasionally accompanied by a component of humoral ("delayed hyperacute") rejection. Similarly, an allograft with advanced chronic rejection may develop severe acute rejection following cessation of immunosuppression. This chapter focuses on the clinical manifestations of the various forms of rejection as well as their prevention, diagnosis, and management. Basic mechanisms of rejection and immunosuppressive drug action are discussed elsewhere in this text (see Mechanisms of Allograft Regection and Immunosuppression in Chapter 80, "Immunology of Transplantation").

Acute (Cellular) Rejection

Clinical Manifestations of Acute Rejection

Acute cellular rejection is the form of early rejection most commonly encountered in transplantation, and most clinical immunosuppression is directed toward its prevention or treatment. Acute rejection most commonly occurs between 1 and 6 weeks after transplantation but may occur at any time, particularly if immunosuppression is reduced or discontinued.

As acute rejection develops, activated T lymphocytes infiltrate the allograft and begin to destroy their target cells. The clinical presentation of acute rejection obviously varies according to the organ transplanted. With current immunosuppression, most patients with rejection are asymptomatic, although severe rejection of any organ can cause fever and allograft tenderness. The diagnosis is usually suspected when patients develop laboratory evidence of allograft inflammation or dysfunction. For example, liver transplant recipients experiencing rejection often have elevations in serum activities of transaminases, alkaline phosphatase, or serum bilirubin, whereas kidney transplant recipients usually develop a rise in serum creatinine concentration. Percutaneous allograft biopsy is generally used to establish the diagnosis as the differential diagnosis for allograft dysfunction is extensive. Heart transplant recipients may have rejection with no clinical abnormalities whatsoever. These patients periodically undergo transvenous endomyocardial biopsy in the early posttransplant period for surveillance for rejection.

Prevention of Acute Rejection

The present field of transplantation was made possible by the significant advances in the prevention and treatment of rejection during the past four decades. While it is not the purpose of this chapter to provide a detailed review of immunosuppressive drugs, an overview of general strategies of immunosuppression is indicated. Table 81.1 lists the immunosuppressive agents that are currently in clinical use. It is conceptually useful to subdivide clinical transplant immunosuppression into prevention of rejection and treatment of rejection.

For prevention of rejection, two or three drugs are usually begun at or soon after the time of transplantation and continued chronically. These combinations generally consist of a calcineurin inhibitor and corticosteroids, with the frequent addition of either mycophenolate mofetil (MMF) or sirolimus (Table 81.2). Azathioprine is occasionally used but has largely been supplanted by mycophenolate and sirolimus. The calcineurin inhibitors cyclosporine and tacrolimus are generally considered the mainstays of current immunosuppression.[1,2]

TABLE 81.1. Immunosuppressive Drugs in Clinical Use.

Lymphocyte activation inhibitors
Cyclosporine
Tacrolimus
Sirolimus
Everolimus
Antiproliferative agents
Azathioprine
Mycophenolate mofetil
Mycophenolate sodium
Corticosteroids
Prednisone
Methylprednisolone
Antilymphocyte antibodies
Antithymocyte globulin
Muromonab-CD3
Daclizumab
Basiliximab
Alemtuzumab (not approved for this indication by regulatory agencies)
Rituxumab (not approved for this indication by regulatory agencies)

Cyclosporine is a cyclic peptide, whereas tacrolimus is a macrolide structurally related to erythromycin. These drugs share a very similar mechanism of action. Their major effect is suppression of interleukin (IL)-2 production, thereby preventing T-cell proliferation and expansion of antigen-reactive clones. Nearly all immunosuppressive regimens for solid organ transplantation utilize one of these agents.

The efficacy and adverse-event profile of cyclosporine and tacrolimus are grossly comparable. Cyclosporine, the older of the two agents, led to dramatically improved outcomes in transplantation when it was introduced in the early 1980s.[3] Although some controversy persists, the bulk of available data indicate that tacrolimus tends to be somewhat more effective than cyclosporine for prevention of acute rejection.[4–7] Both agents are nephrotoxic and may cause tremor, paresthesias, and even seizures and coma; the more serious neurological sequelae fortunately are infrequent. An important difference is that cyclosporine causes hirsutism and gingival hyperplasia, while tacrolimus lacks these side effects. Although these cosmetic issues might seem less important, they are an important cause of noncompliance with prescribed immunosuppression, which can lead to severe rejection and graft loss. One disadvantage of tacrolimus is that it is significantly more diabetogenic than is cyclosporine. Approximately 10% of kidney transplant recipients receiving tacrolimus develop posttransplant diabetes, compared to fewer than 5% of patients treated with cyclosporine.[7] An important advance in the clinical use of cyclosporine has been the realization that blood levels obtained 2h after a dose (C2 monitoring) correlate better with drug exposure than do 12-h trough levels.[4] With C2 monitoring, the efficacy of cyclosporine and tacrolimus appear to be virtually equivalent.[8–11]

Sirolimus (rapamycin) is a macrolide compound structurally related to tacrolimus.[12] Although sirolimus binds to the same intracellular protein as tacrolimus, subsequent cellular effects are quite different. Tacrolimus and cyclosporine act predominantly by suppressing IL-2 production, but sirolimus interferes with signaling through the IL-2 receptor. Sirolimus was initially tested clinically in combination with cyclosporine and corticosteroids in kidney transplantation and was approved for that indication.[13–15] As both sirolimus and tacrolimus bind to the same protein, it was initially believed that they could not be used together, but subsequent clinical experience has shown that this is not the case. The side-effect profile of sirolimus is quite different from that of the calcineurin inhibitors. It has no nephrotoxicity or neurotoxicity but can lead to hyperlipidemia, thrombocytopenia, and leukopenia. It also interferes with wound healing and has been associated with a greater incidence of wound complications in liver transplantation[16] and lymphoceles in kidney transplantation.[17] Due to the lack of nephrotoxicity, there is great current interest in using sirolimus as a replacement for calcineurin inhibitors to avoid chronic calcineurin inhibitor toxicity (Table 81.2). Sirolimus is currently approved for kidney and heart transplantation but not for liver or lung transplantation. Everolimus is an agent closely related to sirolimus that has recently been approved for use in kidney transplantation.[18] It has a shorter half-life, which may make it easier to achieve target levels more quickly. It is unclear whether it will offer significant advantages over sirolimus. These two drugs are often called TOR (target of rapamycin) inhibitors.

Azathioprine and MMF are both antagonists of purine metabolism. Azathioprine is a purine analogue that is converted by the liver to 6-mercaptopurine (6-MP). Because 6-MP competitively inhibits DNA synthesis nonselectively, it has

TABLE 81.2.
Studies of Calcineurin Inhibitor Withdrawal or Avoidance.

Author	*Year*	*Study type*	*Allograft*	*Design*	*Conclusions*
Grimbert[66]	2002	Single-center randomized trial (n = 167)	Kidney	ALG/Aza/prednisone ± CsA in low-risk renal transplants	Similar graft survival with poorer renal function in CsA group at 12 years
Tran[67]	2001	Single-center pilot study (n = 45)	Kidney	Daclizumab/MMF/prednisone in 45 renal transplants	ACR 31%, all controlled; 1-year graft survival 95%
Stegall[68]	2003	Single-center randomized trial	Kidney	Sirolimus or tacrolimus + MMF/prednisone/thymo	Very little rejection (<10%) either way
Schrama[69]	2003	Single-center pilot study (n = 15)	Kidney	15 stable renal transplants switched to MMF/prednisone	1/15 rejection; hypertension improved

ACR, acute rejection; ALG, antilymphocyte globulin; Aza, azathioprine; CsA, cyclosporine; MMF, mycophenolate mofetil; thymo, thymoglobulin.

TABLE 81.3.
Studies of Alemtuzumab (Campath) for Induction.

Author	*Year*	*Study type*	*Allograft*	*Design*	*Conclusions*
Tzakis[105]	2004	Single-center comparative trial	Liver	Campath + FK vs. steroid + FK in 40 liver transplants	Less early rejection with Campath; similar overall rejection; well tolerated
Kirk[106]	2003	Single-center pilot study	Kidney	Campath alone in 7 renal transplants	All had ACR within 1 month; successfully treated
Friend[37]	1989	Single-center randomized trial	Kidney	High-dose CsA ± 10 days Campath in renal transplants	Campath had less rejection but more infections; overall outcome similar

ACR, acute rejection; CsA, cyclosporine; FK, tacrolimus.

the greatest effect on rapidly dividing cells, such as the lymphocytes participating in an immune response. As might be expected, the chief side effect of azathioprine is bone marrow depression, with leukopenia and occasionally anemia or thrombocytopenia. Mycophenolate mofetil is an orally absorbable ester of the active drug mycophenolic acid (MPA).[19] MPA is a reversible inhibitor of inosine monophosphate dehydrogenase, an important enzyme in the de novo pathway of purine synthesis. Lymphocytes are unusual in that they lack an effective salvage pathway for purine synthesis and are thus highly dependent on de novo purine synthesis. As such, MMF is a relatively lymphocyte-selective inhibitor of purine metabolism. In combination with cyclosporine and corticosteroids, MMF has been shown to be significantly more effective than either azathioprine or placebo for preventing acute renal allograft rejection.[20–22] An enteric-coated formulation of mycophenolate sodium has been developed in an attempt to reduce gastrointestinal side effects. In practice, this drug appears to be therapeutically equivalent to MMF.[23,24]

Corticosteroids are also a component of nearly all immunosuppressive regimens. The adverse effects of these drugs are well known and account for much of the long-term morbidity of chronic immunosuppression. Thus, there is great interest in either eliminating or reducing the duration of steroid use in transplant recipients. In the era of cyclosporine/azathioprine-based immunosuppression, data were equivocal on whether steroid withdrawal was advisable.[25] With newer immunosuppressive agents, it appears quite clear that steroids can be avoided or withdrawn very early after transplant (7 days or less) with excellent short-term graft survival and an acceptable incidence of acute rejection, particularly if induction therapy is used (see below).[26–31] Although the effects of steroid withdrawal on long-term graft and patient survival remain a topic of controversy, there has been a clear trend toward reducing corticosteroid use in transplant recipients in recent years.

An additional strategy for prevention of rejection is the perioperative use of antilymphocyte antibody preparations. Unlike the baseline immunosuppressant drugs mentioned above, antilymphocyte antibodies are only used for a limited duration (*induction therapy*). Several agents are available that target all T cells for depletion. The currently available rabbit-derived antithymocyte globulin (ATG) (Thymoglobulin) is the agent most commonly used in the United States for this indication.[32,33] Muromonab-CD3 (OKT3) is a monoclonal antibody that binds to all T cells and causes receptor modulation and coating as well as T-cell activation and cytokine release.[34] Alemtuzumab (Campath-1H) is a monoclonal antibody against CD52 that is exceptionally potent at depleting both T and B cells.[35–37] It is currently approved only for treatment of leukemia, but ongoing trials suggest it may be of significant value in transplantation (Table 81.3). With perioperative use of any of these agents, early acute rejection is effectively prevented. However, rejection may occur following cessation of antibody therapy. The overall incidence of rejection does not appear to be reduced by perioperative use of OKT3. Antithymocyte globulin has largely replaced OKT3 for both induction and rejection therapy, and data suggest that it may help to reduce the overall incidence of rejection.[32,38–43]

The monoclonal antibodies daclizumab and basiliximab represent an attempt to target alloreactive T cells more specifically.[44,45] Both of these antibodies are directed toward the α chain of the IL-2 receptor (CD25). By interfering with the binding of IL-2 to its receptor, basiliximab and daclizumab block proliferation of alloreactive T cells. Basiliximab is a chimeric antibody, meaning that it consists of the variable region of a murine antibody grafted onto the constant region of a human antibody. Daclizumab is a so-called humanized antibody, meaning that it is a human antibody with hypervariable regions that have been altered by site-directed mutagenesis to recreate the antigen-binding specificity of the original murine monoclonal antibody. Humanized and chimeric antibodies, because they are largely human immunoglobulins, have much longer half-lives in the human circulation than murine antibodies. Also, the problem of antimurine antibody formation is largely avoided. Basiliximab and daclizumab were first shown to reduce the incidence of acute rejection by approximately one-third in kidney transplant recipients receiving cyclosporine and corticosteroids. This effect has subsequently been confirmed in numerous studies, as shown in Table 81.4. These agents are extremely well tolerated, with essentially no adverse effects attributed to them.

Treatment of Acute Rejection

Acute rejection is becoming a less-frequent occurrence in clinical transplantation due to the above-mentioned advances. Nonetheless, some transplant recipients experience acute

TABLE 81.4.
Studies of Anti-IL2R (Anti-CD25) Antibodies.

Author	*Year*	*Study type*	*Allograft*	*Design*	*Conclusions*
Chow[78]	2003	Single-center comparative trial with historical control	Kidney-pancreas	Basiliximab or OKT3 + CsA/MMF/ prednisone in SPK (n = 28)	Similar survival and rejection; OKT3 had more infections and side effects
Mocarquer[79]	2003	Multicenter uncontrolled pilot	Kidney	Basiliximab/CsA/Aza/prednisone in renal transplants (n = 23)	ACR 17%; well tolerated
Martin Garcia[80]	2003	Multicenter randomized trial	Kidney	CsA/prednisone vs. CsA/basiliximab vs. FK/basiliximab in 95 renal transplants	Less rejection in basiliximab groups (26% vs. 0% vs. 4%); well tolerated
Kode[81]	2003	Single-center comparative trial with historical control	Kidney	Basiliximab/CsA/MMF/prednisone vs. OKT3/CsA/MMF/prednisone in renal transplants	Less rejection in basiliximab group (14% vs. 35%); well tolerated
Sheashaa[82]	2003	Single-center randomized trial	Kidney	CsA/Aza/prednisone ± basiliximab (50 each) in LDRT	Less rejection in basiliximab group (36% vs. 62%); well tolerated
Lawen[83]	2003	Multicenter randomized trial	Kidney	CsA/MMF/prednisone ± basiliximab in 123 renal transplants	Trend toward less rejection in basiliximab group (15% vs. 26%)
Offner[84]	2002	Multicenter uncontrolled pilot	Kidney	Basiliximab/CsA/prednisone in pediatric renal transplants	ACR 22%; few adverse events
Lebranchu[85]	2002	Multicenter randomized trial	Kidney	Basiliximab or ALG + CsA/MMF/ prednisone in renal transplants	Same survival and rejection, more CMV in thymo group
Neuhaus[86]	2002	Multicenter randomized trial	Liver	CsA/prednisone ± basiliximab in liver transplants	Less rejection/death/graft loss/HCV recurrence in basiliximab group
Calmus[87]	2002	Single-center pilot study	Liver	CsA/Aza/prednisone/basiliximab in liver transplants	Well tolerated; satisfactory outcomes
Sollinger[88]	2001	Multicenter randomized trial	Kidney	CsA/MMF/prednisone + basiliximab vs. ATGAM in kidney transplants	Similar rejection; fewer side effects with basiliximab
Ponticelli[89]	2001	Multicenter randomized trial	Kidney	CsA/Aza/prednisone ± basiliximab in 340 renal transplants	Less rejection (35% vs. 21%) with basiliximab
Kahan[90]	1999	Multicenter randomized trial	Kidney	CsA/prednisone ± basiliximab in 348 renal transplants	Less rejection (49% vs. 35%) with basiliximab
Nashan[91]	1997	Multicenter randomized trial	Kidney	CsA/prednisone ± basiliximab in 376 renal transplants	Less rejection (44% vs. 30%) with basiliximab
Pescovitz[92]	2003	Multicenter randomized trial	Kidney	CsA/MMF/prednisone ± daclizumab in 75 renal transplants	Less rejection (20% vs. 14%) with daclizumab
Abou-Jaoude[93]	2003	Single-center randomized trial	Kidney	Daclizumab vs. ATG in 45 renal transplants	Similar outcomes; less toxicity with daclizumab
Heffron[94]	2003	Single-center pilot study	Liver	FK/MMF/prednisone ± daclizumab in pediatric liver transplantation	Less rejection with daclizumab
Kuypers[95]	2003	Single-center randomized trial	Kidney	FK/MMF/prednisone ± daclizumab in kidney transplantation	Less rejection (17% vs. 41%) with daclizumab
Stratta[96]	2003	Multicenter randomized trial	Kidney-pancreas	FK/MMF/prednisone ± 2- or 5-dose daclizumab in SPK	2- and 5-dose daclizumab both effective
Ahsan[97]	2002	Single center randomized trial	Kidney	FK/MMF/prednisone ± single-dose daclizumab in kidney transplantation	Less rejection (6% vs. 16%) with daclizumab
Stratta[98]	2002	Multicenter randomized trial	Kidney-pancreas	FK/MMF/prednisone ± 2- or 5-dose daclizumab in SPK	2- and 5-dose daclizumab both effective
Brock[99]	2001	Single-center "controlled" trial	Lung	OKT3 vs. ATG vs. daclizumab in 87 lung transplants	OKT3 had most infections, daclizumab had fewest
Bumgardner[100]	2001	Multicenter randomized trial	Kidney	CsA/Aza/prednisone or CsA/prednisone with or without daclizumab in renal transplants	Less rejection with daclizumab for both double and triple therapy
Ekberg[101]	2000	Multicenter randomized trial	Kidney	CsA/Aza/prednisone with or without daclizumab in 535 renal transplants	Less rejection (15% vs. 43%) with daclizumab
Beniaminovitz[102]	2000	Single-center randomized trial	Heart	CsA/MMF/prednisone with or without daclizumab in 55 heart transplants	Less rejection (18% vs. 63%) with daclizumab
Nashan[103]	1999	Multicenter randomized trial	Kidney	CsA/prednisone ± daclizumab in 275 renal transplants	Less rejection (28% vs. 47%) with daclizumab
Vincenti[104]	1998	Multicenter randomized trial	Kidney	CsA/Aza/prednisone ± daclizumab in 260 renal transplants	Less rejection (22% vs. 35%) with daclizumab

ACR, acute rejection; ALG, antilymphocyte globulin; ATGAM, antithymocyte globulin; Aza, azathioprine. CsA, cyclosporine; FK, tacrolimus; LDRT, living donor renal transplantation, MMF, mycophenolate mofetil; SPK, simultaneous pancreas and kidney; thymo, thymoglobulin.

rejection, usually within the first several weeks. The incidence depends on the transplanted organ, the baseline immunosuppressive drugs used, and whether antibody induction is used. Most series report rejection in 10%–20% of recipients, except in highly immunogenic organs such as small bowel and lung. Late rejection episodes are often a manifestation of noncompliance. With currently available agents, acute rejection can be arrested in virtually all cases. Depending on the amount of damage done as well as the reparative capacity of the organ involved, the lasting effects on allograft function range from negligible to catastrophic. Timeliness of diagnosis is paramount, particularly in allografts that have less reparative capacity, such as the kidney, heart, and pancreas. Clinicians should have a low threshold for performing an allograft biopsy when the clinical picture is compatible with the diagnosis of rejection. The effects of treated rejection episodes on long-term graft survival are considered later in this chapter.

High-dose corticosteroids are the most widely used initial therapy for acute rejection. The doses employed in this situation (typically methylprednisolone, 500–1000 mg daily for 3 days) greatly exceed those used for chronic maintenance (typically prednisone, 5–10 mg daily). Approximately 75% of acute rejection episodes will resolve with "pulse" corticosteroid therapy.[34] In most settings, a single course of high-dose steroid therapy carries little risk, an exception being liver transplant recipients with hepatitis C. Repeated courses of high-dose steroids carry significant morbidity and are rarely used now that many other therapeutic options are available.

Antilymphocyte antibodies have traditionally been the "gold standard" for rejection therapy. Antithymocyte globulin is most frequently used for steroid-resistant rejection. The currently available ATG preparation is extremely effective at reversing acute rejection and seems to be associated with a low incidence of "rebound" rejection following cessation of antibody therapy. It may cause fever, tachycardia, and hemodynamic instability that appears to be due to cytokine release. These side effects can be minimized by infusing the dose over several hours. Also, OKT3 can be used for this indication. It is also nearly universally effective at halting rejection, but the acute side effects may be more severe than those of ATG.[34] Rare but serious effects include seizures, cardiovascular collapse, and death. Although OKT3 arrests nearly 100% of cellular rejection episodes, recovery of function may not be complete if the allograft has been significantly injured. Furthermore, rejection frequently returns in the weeks following OKT3 treatment. Both OKT3 and ATG predispose to cytomegalovirus (CMV) and other viral infections as well as the posttransplant lymphoproliferative disorder.

A conceptual limitation of short-term rejection therapy is that rejection may recur following the brief treatment period. It is generally considered advisable to augment baseline immunosuppression for several weeks after rejection therapy by either increasing medication doses or adding additional agents. Sometimes, rejection therapy may consist solely of increasing baseline immunosuppression without giving either antibody treatment or large steroid boluses. This is often done in settings where intense immunosuppression may have serious adverse consequences, as in liver transplant recipients with hepatitis C. There is significant evidence indicating that rejection occurring in patients receiving cyclosporine can usually be reversed by switching to tacrolimus, so-called tacrolimus/FK506 rescue therapy.[46–48]

Hyperacute (Humoral) Rejection

Mechanism of Humoral Rejection

Humans ordinarily do not have circulating antibodies against allogeneic human leukocyte antigen (HLA). Such antibodies reflect previous exposure to allogeneic tissue, which may occur as a result of a blood transfusion, a previous organ transplant, or maternal exposure to fetal-derived cells at the time of delivery. The term *hyperacute rejection* refers to rapid allograft damage or destruction caused by preformed antibodies against donor cell surface antigens, particularly class I HLA. Binding of antibodies leads to complement activation and endothelial cell death. Subsequent events include activation of the coagulation cascade, small-vessel thrombosis, and infarction. As the process is caused by preformed antibodies, hyperacute rejection becomes evident within a few minutes of allograft reperfusion. The process may be considered analogous to a hemolytic transfusion reaction.

Antibody-mediated rejection may also develop following transplantation as a result of formation of new antidonor antibodies. The pathophysiology is similar to that of hyperacute rejection, but the pace is slower, and there is more potential for therapeutic intervention. This process is sometimes given the confusing name *delayed hyperacute rejection*. For the purposes of this discussion, *humoral rejection* refers to any rejection process mediated by antidonor antibodies. The term *hyperacute rejection* is reserved for humoral rejection occurring immediately as a result of preformed antibodies.

Prevention of Humoral Rejection

In general, hyperacute rejection can be prevented by testing the recipient's serum for antibodies against cells from the potential donor. Such testing is termed a *crossmatch*. Several types of crossmatch procedures are in clinical use. A so-called standard (or "NIH," National Institutes of Health) crossmatch tests the ability of recipient serum to lyse donor cells in the presence of complement. The sensitivity of the assay may be increased by an additional step in which antihuman immunoglobulin is added to further crosslink bound antibody molecules (antiglobulin crossmatch test).

Flow cytometry is an even more sensitive method to detect antidonor antibodies. After incubating donor cells with recipient serum, bound antibodies can be detected using fluorochrome-labeled antihuman immunoglobulin (IgG). Although flow cytometry is more sensitive than a conventional cytotoxic crossmatch, the specificity is accordingly decreased. A positive flow crossmatch does not necessarily preclude successful transplantation, but there is increasing agreement that HLA-specific antidonor antibodies generally tend to have detrimental effects on renal allograft survival (Table 81.5).

With either crossmatch technique, recipient sera can be tested against either donor T lymphocytes or B lymphocytes. Resting T lymphocytes express class I HLA but not class II HLA, whereas B lymphocytes express both class I and class II

TABLE 81.5.
Effects of Positive Flow or B-Cell Crossmatch on Transplant Outcome.

Author	*Year*	*Study type*	*Allograft*	*Design*	*Conclusions*
Kotb[70]	1999	Single-center retrospective analysis (n = 106)	Kidney	Compared acute rejection incidence based on B-cell flow crossmatch (cytotoxic crossmatch negative)	Positive B-cell flow crossmatch is a risk factor for acute rejection
Pelletier[71]	1997	Single-center retrospective analysis (n = 168)	Kidney and kidney-pancreas	Compared acute rejection incidence based on flow crossmatch (cytotoxic crossmatch negative)	No effect of positive flow crossmatch on rejection, function, or survival
Christiaans[72]	1996	Single-center retrospective analysis (n = 180)	Kidney	Compared acute rejection incidence based on flow crossmatch (cytotoxic crossmatch negative)	No effect of positive flow crossmatch on rejection, function, or survival
Mahoney[73]	1996	Multicenter retrospective analysis (n = 103)	Kidney	Compared immunologic graft loss in second transplants based on flow crossmatch and duration of function of first graft	Positive flow crossmatch in second transplants does not predict poor outcome unless first graft failed within 3 months
Scornik[74]	1994	Single-center retrospective analysis (n = 230)	Kidney	Compared acute rejection incidence based on flow crossmatch (cytotoxic crossmatch negative); nonsensitized primary recipients only	No effect of positive flow crossmatch on rejection, function, or survival
Ogura[75]	1993	Single-center retrospective analysis (n = 841)	Kidney	Compared graft survival based on flow crossmatch (cytotoxic crossmatch negative); primary recipients only	1-year graft survival worse (75% vs. 82%) if flow crossmatch positive; allocate kidneys to flow-negative recipients if possible
Ogura[76]	1994	Single-center retrospective analysis (n = 82)	Liver	Compared graft survival based on flow and cytotoxic crossmatch	Worse outcome if either crossmatch positive, flow more predictive than cytotoxic
Bishay[77]	2000	Single-center retrospective analysis (n = 357)	Heart	Compared patient survival and rejection based on flow crossmatch	Worse outcome if T-cell flow crossmatch positive; B cell has no effect

HLA. Thus, a positive T-lymphocyte crossmatch implies the presence of alloantibodies against donor class I HLA and represents a stronger contraindication to proceeding with transplantation. Nonetheless, class II alloantibodies can also be clinically significant, and the inclusion of a B-lymphocyte crossmatch allows the clinician to avoid transplantation in the presence of these antibodies.

Clinical utilization of crossmatch data varies according to the organ to be transplanted. Due to time considerations, crossmatching was historically not utilized in heart transplantation. With the current option of obtaining inguinal lymph nodes or peripheral blood lymphocytes before the organ recovery operation, crossmatching for heart transplantation is now feasible. Crossmatching is employed selectively in heart transplantation, generally for patients with an elevated panel reactive antibody (PRA) or others deemed to be at increased immunological risk. Crossmatches are obtained routinely before kidney and pancreas transplants. These transplants are not performed in the presence of a positive cytotoxic T-cell crossmatch, and even a positive flow or B-cell crossmatch is a significant relative contraindication. Interestingly, the liver is quite resistant to antibody-mediated damage. Even in the presence of preformed antibodies, the liver usually suffers no clinically evident injury. The reasons for this resistance to humoral injury are uncertain. Possible explanations include the sinusoidal hepatic microcirculation as well as the greater size of the liver allograft as the quantity of preformed antibody in circulation may be insufficient to cause significant hepatic injury. Thus, crossmatching does not play a role in organ allocation in clinical liver transplantation.

It should be noted that crossmatching detects antibodies currently in circulation but provides little information about previous sensitization as immunological memory may be present even though antibody titers have declined to undetectable levels. With the antigenic challenge of the new transplant, a vigorous humoral response may arise within the first several days. To reduce this possibility, crossmatches for renal transplants are performed on both a current serum specimen and on a sample obtained 1 to 2 months previously. For second kidney transplants, donors with mismatched HLA antigens in common with those of a previously rejected kidney are usually excluded.

The literature contains a variety of recommendations in cases in which the T-cell cytotoxic crossmatch is negative but other assays (B-cell cytotoxic or flow cytometry crossmatch) are positive. Most available data concern kidney transplantation, as summarized in Table 81.5. In this setting, transplantation can be performed successfully in most cases, although some studies show an increased incidence of rejection and immunological graft loss. Many clinicians attach greater significance to positive flow crossmatches if the patient has had a previous transplant as the low titers of antibodies detectable by these assays may be a marker of sensitization from prior antigenic exposure.

In view of the increasing disparity between organ supply and demand, a great deal of effort has focused on allowing kidney transplant candidates to receive organs from donors against whom they have demonstrable antibody. For logistic reasons, most of this experience has been in living donor kidney transplantation. The prospective recipient is treated with intravenous human immunoglobulin (IVIG), plasmapheresis, and sometimes other immunosuppression in an attempt to clear antidonor antibodies. If the crossmatch becomes negative, living-donor transplantation is carried out. Short-term graft survival has been acceptable, although a substantial fraction of patients experience early humoral rejection.

Clinical Presentation and Treatment of Humoral Rejection

In the case of kidney transplantation, a fully developed hyperacute rejection response rapidly causes irreversible allograft destruction. Treatment consists of allograft nephrectomy and continuation of chronic dialysis. Comparable episodes in heart transplant recipients are generally fatal. Humoral rejection of lesser severity (delayed hyperacute rejection) may present several days after transplantation, particularly in recipients who have received previous transplants.

Humoral rejection should be suspected in any renal transplant whose function abruptly deteriorates within the first several days, particularly if the recipient has had a previous transplant or is otherwise sensitized. The diagnosis is made by renal allograft biopsy. Conventional histology typically shows vascular injury and neutrophilic infiltration in glomeruli and peritubular capillaries. A valuable recent advance has been the clinical availability of immunostaining for the complement product C4d, which is sensitive and specific for humoral rejection.[49,50] Demonstration of donor-specific antibody (DSA), if possible, may provide further confirmation of the diagnosis.

The therapy of humoral rejection is not well standardized. Most commonly, plasma exchange or plasmapheresis is used in combination with ATG and IVIG.[51,52] Rituximab is an anti-CD20 monoclonal antibody that depletes B cells and has sometimes been used in regimens to prevent or treat humoral rejection.[53–56] It should be noted that antibodies are actually produced by differentiated plasma cells that do not express CD20, making the role of rituximab in acute humoral rejection theoretically debatable. Although many allografts with humoral rejection can be salvaged with aggressive therapy, the prognosis is worse than that of cellular rejection.

Chronic Rejection

Mechanisms of Chronic Rejection

Chronic rejection is the least well understood of the three forms of rejection. This term refers to a gradual loss of allograft function that typically occurs months to years after transplantation. The mechanism by which this occurs remains largely unknown. Indeed, the extent to which this is an immune process is open to question. The term *chronic allograft nephropathy* is now preferred to reflect the possible contribution of nonimmunological factors to progressive allograft dysfunction.[57] Such factors may include hyperfiltration and chronic exposure to nephrotoxic drugs, as well as hypertension and other conditions leading to renal damage in the nontransplant setting.

In most organs, small vessels appear to be a major target of chronic rejection. Biopsies of renal allografts with chronic rejection reveal varying degrees of tubular loss with interstitial fibrosis. In the liver, chronic rejection causes destruction of small bile ducts, leading to progressive cholestasis, hence the term *ductopenic rejection* or vanishing bile duct syndrome. Hepatocytes are comparatively unaffected in most cases. Cardiac allografts develop disease of small coronary arteries that may lead to myocardial ischemia and infarction. In the transplanted lung, small airways are destroyed. This process is termed *bronchiolitis obliterans.*

The relationship of acute and chronic rejection remains incompletely defined. In kidney transplantation, acute rejection is clearly a risk factor for late allograft loss.[58] Patients experiencing no acute rejection episodes have superior long-term graft survival compared to patients with even a single rejection episode. There is evidence indicating that the impact of acute rejection on long-term graft survival is mitigated by prompt and effective treatment of acute rejection when it occurs.[59,60] In liver allograft recipients, single episodes of acute rejection appear to have no effect on late allograft failure.[61–63] However, patients experiencing recurrent or refractory liver allograft rejection are at increased risk of late graft failure.[64]

Clinical Manifestations and Management of Chronic Rejection

In all transplanted organs, chronic rejection leads to a progressive loss of allograft function. At present, the treatment of chronic rejection is unsatisfactory, and most cases eventually lead to graft failure. In liver transplantation, there is some evidence that conversion from cyclosporine to tacrolimus in the early stage of chronic rejection may reduce graft loss.[65] Kidney transplant recipients with chronic allograft nephropathy may benefit from the withdrawal of the nephrotoxic calcineurin inhibitors and substitution of sirolimus. In other organs, there is little evidence that the course of established chronic rejection can be altered. Management consists of avoiding additional insults to the graft, monitoring graft function carefully, and offering retransplantation at the appropriate time if the patient remains a suitable candidate.

References

1. Calne RY WD, Thiru S, et al. Cyclosporin A in patients receiving renal allografts from cadaver donors. Lancet 1978;2:1323–1327.
2. Fung JJ, Starzl TE. FK506 in solid organ transplantation. Ther Drug Monit 1995;17:592–595.
3. A randomized clinical trial of cyclosporine in cadaveric renal transplantation. N Engl J Med 1983;309:809–815.

4. Randomised trial comparing tacrolimus (FK506) and cyclosporin in prevention of liver allograft rejection. European FK506 Multicentre Liver Study Group. Lancet 1994;344:423–428.
5. A comparison of tacrolimus (FK 506) and cyclosporine for immunosuppression in liver transplantation. The U.S. Multicenter FK506 Liver Study Group. N Engl J Med 1994;331:1110–1115.
6. Two-year follow-up study of the efficacy and safety of FK 506 in kidney transplant patients. Japanese FK 506 Study Group. Transpl Int 1994;7(suppl 1):S247–S251.
7. Laskow DA, Vincenti F, Neylan JF, Mendez R, Matas AJ. An open-label, concentration-ranging trial of FK506 in primary kidney transplantation: a report of the United States Multicenter FK506 Kidney Transplant Group. Transplantation 1996;62:900–905.
8. Randomized, international study of cyclosporine microemulsion absorption profiling in renal transplantation with basiliximab immunoprophylaxis. Am J Transplant 2002;2:157–166.
9. Villamil F, Pollard S. C2 monitoring of cyclosporine in de novo liver transplant recipients: the clinician's perspective. Liver Transpl 2004;10:577–583.
10. Pape L, Ehrich JH, Offner G. Advantages of cyclosporin A using 2-h levels in pediatric kidney transplantation. Pediatr Nephrol 2004;19:1035–1038.
11. Morton JM, Aboyoun CL, Malouf MA, Plit ML, Glanville AR. Enhanced clinical utility of de novo cyclosporine C2 monitoring after lung transplantation. J Heart Lung Transplant 2004;23: 1035–1039.
12. Thomson AW. The immunosuppressive macrolides FK-506 and rapamycin. Immunol Lett 1991;29:105–111.
13. Kahan BD, Podbielski J, Napoli KL, Katz SM, Meier-Kriesche HU, Van Buren CT. Immunosuppressive effects and safety of a sirolimus/cyclosporine combination regimen for renal transplantation. Transplantation 1998;66:1040–1046.
14. Groth CG, Backman L, Morales JM, et al. Sirolimus (rapamycin)-based therapy in human renal transplantation: similar efficacy and different toxicity compared with cyclosporine. Sirolimus European Renal Transplant Study Group. Transplantation 1999; 67:1036–1042.
15. Kahan BD. Efficacy of sirolimus compared with azathioprine for reduction of acute renal allograft rejection: a randomised multicentre study. The Rapamune US Study Group. Lancet 2000;356: 194–202.
16. Guilbeau JM. Delayed wound healing with sirolimus after liver transplant. Ann Pharmacother 2002;36:1391–1395.
17. Langer RM, Kahan BD. Incidence, therapy, and consequences of lymphocele after sirolimus-cyclosporine-prednisone immunosuppression in renal transplant recipients. Transplantation 2002;74:804–808.
18. Nashan B, Curtis J, Ponticelli C, Mourad G, Jaffe J, Haas T. Everolimus and reduced-exposure cyclosporine in de novo renal-transplant recipients: a 3-year phase II, randomized, multicenter, open-label study. Transplantation 2004;78:1332–1340.
19. Sollinger HW, Belzer FO, Deierhoi MH, et al. RS-61443 (mycophenolate mofetil). A multicenter study for refractory kidney transplant rejection. Ann Surg 1992;216:513–518; discussion 8–9.
20. Placebo-controlled study of mycophenolate mofetil combined with cyclosporin and corticosteroids for prevention of acute rejection. European Mycophenolate Mofetil Cooperative Study Group. Lancet 1995;345:1321–1325.
21. Sollinger HW. Mycophenolate mofetil for the prevention of acute rejection in primary cadaveric renal allograft recipients. US Renal Transplant Mycophenolate Mofetil Study Group. Transplantation 1995;60:225–232.
22. A blinded, randomized clinical trial of mycophenolate mofetil for the prevention of acute rejection in cadaveric renal transplantation. The Tricontinental Mycophenolate Mofetil Renal Transplantation Study Group. Transplantation 1996;61:1029–1037.
23. Sollinger HW. Mycophenolates in transplantation. Clin Transplant 2004;18:485–492.
24. Salvadori M, Holzer H, de Mattos A, et al. Enteric-coated mycophenolate sodium is therapeutically equivalent to mycophenolate mofetil in de novo renal transplant patients. Am J Transplant 2004;4:231–236.
25. Ratcliffe PJ, Dudley CR, Higgins RM, Firth JD, Smith B, Morris PJ. Randomised controlled trial of steroid withdrawal in renal transplant recipients receiving triple immunosuppression. Lancet 1996;348:643–648.
26. Grewal HP, Thistlethwaite JR Jr, Loss GE, et al. Corticosteroid cessation 1 week following renal transplantation using tacrolimus/mycophenolate mofetil based immunosuppression. Transplant Proc 1998;30:1378–1379.
27. Wiland AM, Fink JC, Weir MR, et al. Should living-unrelated renal transplant recipients receive antibody induction? Results of a clinical experience trial. Transplantation 2004;77:422–425.
28. ter Meulen CG, van Riemsdijk I, Hene RJ, et al. Steroid-withdrawal at 3 days after renal transplantation with anti-IL-2 receptor alpha therapy: a prospective, randomized, multicenter study. Am J Transplant 2004;4:803–810.
29. Pageaux GP, Calmus Y, Boillot O, et al. Steroid withdrawal at day 14 after liver transplantation: a double-blind, placebo-controlled study. Liver Transpl 2004;10:1454–1460.
30. Hocker B, John U, Plank C, et al. Successful withdrawal of steroids in pediatric renal transplant recipients receiving cyclosporine A and mycophenolate mofetil treatment: results after 4 years. Transplantation 2004;78:228–234.
31. Kaufman DB, Iii GW, Bruce DS, et al. Prospective, randomized, multi-center trial of antibody induction therapy in simultaneous pancreas-kidney transplantation. Am J Transplant 2003;3:855–864.
32. Lebranchu Y, Bridoux F, Buchler M, et al. Immunoprophylaxis with basiliximab compared with antithymocyte globulin in renal transplant patients receiving MMF-containing triple therapy. Am J Transplant 2002;2:48–56.
33. Zuckermann AO, Grimm M, Czerny M, et al. Improved long-term results with thymoglobuline induction therapy after cardiac transplantation: a comparison of two different rabbit-antithymocyte globulines. Transplantation 2000;69:1890–1898.
34. A randomized clinical trial of OKT3 monoclonal antibody for acute rejection of cadaveric renal transplants. Ortho Multicenter Transplant Study Group. N Engl J Med 1985;313:337–342.
35. Tzakis AG, Kato T, Nishida S, et al. Alemtuzumab (Campath-1H) combined with tacrolimus in intestinal and multivisceral transplantation. Transplantation 2003;75:1512–1517.
36. Calne R, Moffatt SD, Friend PJ, et al. Campath IH allows low-dose cyclosporine monotherapy in 31 cadaveric renal allograft recipients. Transplantation 1999;68:1613–1616.
37. Friend PJ, Hale G, Waldmann H, et al. Campath-1M—prophylactic use after kidney transplantation. A randomized controlled clinical trial. Transplantation 1989;48:248–253.
38. Abou-Jaoude MM, Ghantous I, Almawi WY. Comparison of daclizumab, an interleukin 2 receptor antibody, to anti-thymocyte globulin-Fresenius induction therapy in kidney transplantation. Mol Immunol 2003;39:1083–1088.
39. Ault BH, Honaker MR, Osama Gaber A, et al. Short-term outcomes of Thymoglobulin induction in pediatric renal transplant recipients. Pediatr Nephrol 2002;17:815–818.
40. Mourad G, Garrigue V, Squifflet JP, et al. Induction versus non-induction in renal transplant recipients with tacrolimus-based immunosuppression. Transplantation 2001;72:1050–1055.
41. Hesse UJ, Troisi R, Jacobs B, et al. A single center's clinical experience with quadruple immunosuppression including ATG or IL2 antibodies and mycophenolate mofetil in simultaneous pancreas-kidney transplants. Clin Transplant 2000;14(4 pt 1):340–344.

42. Palmer SM, Miralles AP, Lawrence CM, Gaynor JW, Davis RD, Tapson VF. Rabbit antithymocyte globulin decreases acute rejection after lung transplantation: results of a randomized, prospective study. Chest 1999;116:127–133.
43. Thibaudin D, Alamartine E, de Filippis JP, Diab N, Laurent B, Berthoux F. Advantage of antithymocyte globulin induction in sensitized kidney recipients: a randomized prospective study comparing induction with and without antithymocyte globulin. Nephrol Dial Transplant 1998;13:711–715.
44. Kovarik J, Wolf P, Cisterne JM, et al. Disposition of basiliximab, an interleukin-2 receptor monoclonal antibody, in recipients of mismatched cadaver renal allografts. Transplantation 1997;64: 1701–1705.
45. Waldmann TA, O'Shea J. The use of antibodies against the IL-2 receptor in transplantation. Curr Opin Immunol 1998;10:507–512.
46. Millis JM, Cronin DC, Newell KA, et al. Tacrolimus treatment of steroid-resistant rejection provides economic advantages compared with OKT3 therapy. Transplant Proc 1997;29:1549.
47. Woodle ES, Thistlethwaite JR, Gordon JH, et al. A multicenter trial of FK506 (tacrolimus) therapy in refractory acute renal allograft rejection. A report of the Tacrolimus Kidney Transplantation Rescue Study Group. Transplantation 1996;62:594–599.
48. Woodle ES, Cronin D, Newell KA, et al. Tacrolimus therapy for refractory acute renal allograft rejection: definition of the histologic response by protocol biopsies. Transplantation 1996;62:906–910.
49. Shimizu T, Tokiwa M, Yamaguchi Y. A case of acute antidonor antibody-mediated humoral rejection after renal transplantation with specific consideration of serial graft biopsy histology. Clin Transplant 2002;16(suppl 8):62–67.
50. Crespo M, Pascual M, Tolkoff-Rubin N, et al. Acute humoral rejection in renal allograft recipients: I. Incidence, serology and clinical characteristics. Transplantation 2001;71:652–658.
51. Aichberger C, Nussbaumer W, Rosmanith P, et al. Plasmapheresis for the treatment of acute vascular rejection in renal transplantation. Transplant Proc 1997;29:169–170.
52. Berglin E, Kjellstrom C, Mantovani V, Stelin G, Svalander C, Wiklund L. Plasmapheresis as a rescue therapy to resolve cardiac rejection with vasculitis and severe heart failure. A report of five cases. Transpl Int 1995;8:382–387.
53. Faye A, Van Den Abeele T, Peuchmaur M, Mathieu-Boue A, Vilmer E. Anti-CD20 monoclonal antibody for post-transplant lymphoproliferative disorders. Lancet 1998;352:1285.
54. Aranda JM Jr, Scornik JC, Normann SJ, et al. Anti-CD20 monoclonal antibody (rituximab) therapy for acute cardiac humoral rejection: a case report. Transplantation 2002;73:907–910.
55. Garrett HE Jr, Groshart K, Duvall-Seaman D, Combs D, Suggs R. Treatment of humoral rejection with rituximab. Ann Thorac Surg 2002;74:1240–1242.
56. Becker YT, Becker BN, Pirsch JD, Sollinger HW. Rituximab as treatment for refractory kidney transplant rejection. Am J Transplant 2004;4:996–1001.
57. Solez K. International standardization of criteria for histologic diagnosis of chronic rejection in renal allografts. Clin Transplant 1994;8(3 pt 2):345–350.
58. Matas AJ, Burke JF Jr, DeVault GA Jr, Monaco A, Pirsch JD. Chronic rejection. J Am Soc Nephrol 1994;4(8 suppl):S23–S29.
59. Tesi RJ, Elkhammas EA, Henry ML, Ferguson RM. OKT3 for primary therapy of the first rejection episode in kidney transplants. Transplantation 1993;55:1023–1029.
60. Ashraf S, Parrott NR, Dyer P, Roberts I, Johnson RW. Clinical response and temporal patterns of acute cellular rejection: relationship to chronic transplant nephropathy. Transpl Int 1998; 11(suppl 1):S5–S9.
61. Klintmalm GB, Nery JR, Husberg BS, Gonwa TA, Tillery GW. Rejection in liver transplantation. Hepatology 1989;10:978–985.
62. Mor E, Gonwa TA, Husberg BS, Goldstein RM, Klintmalm GB. Late-onset acute rejection in orthotopic liver transplantation—associated risk factors and outcome. Transplantation 1992;54: 821–824.
63. Dousset B, Conti F, Cherruau B, et al. Is acute rejection deleterious to long-term liver allograft function? J Hepatol 1998;29:660–668.
64. Snover DC, Freese DK, Sharp HL, Bloomer JR, Najarian JS, Ascher NL. Liver allograft rejection. An analysis of the use of biopsy in determining outcome of rejection. Am J Surg Pathol 1987;11:1–10.
65. McDiarmid SV, Klintmalm GB, Busuttil RW. FK506 conversion for intractable rejection of the liver allograft. Transpl Int 1993; 6:305–312.
66. Grimbert P, Baron C, Fruchaud G, et al. Long-term results of a prospective randomized study comparing two immunosuppressive regimens, one with and one without CsA, in low-risk renal transplant recipients. Transpl Int 2002;15:550–555.
67. Tran HT, Acharya MK, McKay DB, et al. Avoidance of cyclosporine in renal transplantation: effects of daclizumab, mycophenolate mofetil, and steroids. J Am Soc Nephrol 2000;11: 1903–1909.
68. Stegall MD, Larson TS, Prieto M, et al. Kidney transplantation without calcineurin inhibitors using sirolimus. Transplant Proc 2003;35(3 suppl):125S–127S.
69. Schrama YC, Joles JA, van Tol A, Boer P, Koomans HA, Hene RJ. Conversion to mycophenolate mofetil in conjunction with stepwise withdrawal of cyclosporine in stable renal transplant recipients. Transplantation 2000;69:376–383.
70. Kotb M, Russell WC, Hathaway DK, Gaber LW, Gaber AO. The use of positive B cell flow cytometry crossmatch in predicting rejection among renal transplant recipients. Clin Transplant 1999;13(1 pt 2):83–89.
71. Pelletier RP, Orosz CG, Adams PW, et al. Clinical and economic impact of flow cytometry crossmatching in primary cadaveric kidney and simultaneous pancreas-kidney transplant recipients. Transplantation 1997;63:1639–1645.
72. Christiaans MH, Overhof R, ten Haaft A, Nieman F, van Hooff JP, van den Berg-Loonen EM. No advantage of flow cytometry crossmatch over complement-dependent cytotoxicity in immunologically well-documented renal allograft recipients. Transplantation 1996;62:1341–1347.
73. Mahoney RJ, Norman DJ, Colombe BW, Garovoy MR, Leeber DA. Identification of high- and low-risk second kidney grafts. Transplantation 1996;61:1349–1355.
74. Scornik JC, Brunson ME, Schaub B, Howard RJ, Pfaff WW. The crossmatch in renal transplantation. Evaluation of flow cytometry as a replacement for standard cytotoxicity. Transplantation 1994;57:621–625.
75. Ogura K, Terasaki PI, Johnson C, et al. The significance of a positive flow cytometry crossmatch test in primary kidney transplantation. Transplantation 1993;56:294–298.
76. Ogura K, Terasaki PI, Koyama H, Chia J, Imagawa DK, Busuttil RW. High 1-month liver graft failure rates in flow cytometry crossmatch-positive recipients. Clin Transplant 1994;8(2 pt 1): 111–115.
77. Bishay ES, Cook DJ, Starling RC, et al. The clinical significance of flow cytometry crossmatching in heart transplantation. Eur J Cardiothorac Surg 2000;17:362–369.
78. Chow FY, Polkinghorne K, Saunder A, Kerr PG, Atkins RC, Chadban SJ. Historical controlled trial of OKT3 versus basiliximab induction therapy in simultaneous pancreas-renal transplantation. Nephrology (Carlton) 2003;8:212–216.
79. Mocarquer A, Pinto V, Buckel E, et al. of the Simulect Multicenter Study Group of Chile. Basiliximab: efficacy and tolerability in adults and children. Transplant Proc 2003;35:2518–2519.
80. Martin Garcia D, Martin Gago J, Mendiluce A, et al. Tacrolimus-basiliximab versus cyclosporine-basiliximab in renal transplan-

tation "de novo": acute rejection and complications. Transplant Proc 2003;35:1694–1696.
81. Kode R, Fa K, Chowdhury S, et al. Basiliximab plus low-dose cyclosporin versus OKT3 for induction immunosuppression following renal transplantation. Clin Transplant 2003;17:369–376.
82. Sheashaa HA, Bakr MA, Ismail AM, Sobh MA, Ghoneim MA. Basiliximab reduces the incidence of acute cellular rejection in live-related-donor kidney transplantation: a three-year prospective randomized trial. J Nephrol 2003;16:393–398.
83. Lawen JG, Davies EA, Mourad G, et al. of the Simulect International Study Group. Randomized double-blind study of immunoprophylaxis with basiliximab, a chimeric anti-interleukin-2 receptor monoclonal antibody, in combination with mycophenolate mofetil-containing triple therapy in renal transplantation. Transplantation 2003;75:37–43.
84. Offner G, Broyer M, Niaudet P, et al. A multicenter, open-label, pharmacokinetic/pharmacodynamic safety, and tolerability study of basiliximab (Simulect) in pediatric de novo renal transplant recipients. Transplantation 2002;74:961–966.
85. Lebranchu Y, Bridoux F, Buchler M, et al. Immunoprophylaxis with basiliximab compared with antithymocyte globulin in renal transplant patients receiving MMF-containing triple therapy. Am J Transplant 2002;2:48–56.
86. Neuhaus P, Clavien PA, Kittur D, et al. of the CHIC 304 International Liver Study Group. Improved treatment response with basiliximab immunoprophylaxis after liver transplantation: results from a double-blind randomized placebo-controlled trial. Liver Transpl 2002;8:132–142.
87. Calmus Y, Scheele JR, Gonzalez-Pinto I, et al. Immunoprophylaxis with basiliximab, a chimeric anti-interleukin-2 receptor monoclonal antibody, in combination with azathioprine-containing triple therapy in liver transplant recipients. Liver Transpl 2002;8:123–131.
88. Sollinger H, Kaplan B, Pescovitz MD, et al. Basiliximab versus antithymocyte globulin for prevention of acute renal allograft rejection. Transplantation 2001;72:1915–1919.
89. Ponticelli C, Yussim A, Cambi V, et al. of the Simulect Phase IV Study Group. A randomized, double-blind trial of basiliximab immunoprophylaxis plus triple therapy in kidney transplant recipients. Transplantation 2001;72:1261–1267.
90. Kahan BD, Rajagopalan PR, Hall M. Reduction of the occurrence of acute cellular rejection among renal allograft recipients treated with basiliximab, a chimeric anti-interleukin-2-receptor monoclonal antibody. United States Simulect Renal Study Group. Transplantation 1999;67:276–284.
91. Nashan B, Moore R, Amlot P, Schmidt AG, Abeywickrama K, Soulillou JP. Randomised trial of basiliximab versus placebo for control of acute cellular rejection in renal allograft recipients. CHIB 201 International Study Group. Lancet 1997;350:1193–1198.
92. Pescovitz MD, Bumgardner G, Gaston RS, et al. Pharmacokinetics of daclizumab and mycophenolate mofetil with cyclosporine and steroids in renal transplantation. Clin Transplant 2003;17:511–517.
93. Abou-Jaoude MM, Ghantous I, Najm R, Afif C, Almawi WY. Daclizumab versus anti-thymocyte globulin-fresenius as induction therapy for low-risk kidney transplant recipients. Transplant Proc 2003;35:2731–2732.
94. Heffron TG, Pillen T, Smallwood GA, Welch D, Oakley B, Romero R. Pediatric liver transplantation with daclizumab induction. Transplantation 2003;75:2040–2043.
95. Kuypers DR, Vanrenterghem YF. Monoclonal antibodies in renal transplantation: old and new. Nephrol Dial Transplant 2004;19:297–300.
96. Stratta RJ, Alloway RR, Lo A, Hodge E. Two-dose daclizumab regimen in simultaneous kidney-pancreas transplant recipients: primary endpoint analysis of a multicenter, randomized study. Transplantation 2003;75:1260–1266.
97. Ahsan N, Holman MJ, Jarowenko MV, Razzaque MS, Yang HC. Limited dose monoclonal IL-2R antibody induction protocol after primary kidney transplantation. Am J Transplant 2002;2:568–573.
98. Stratta RJ, Alloway RR, Hodge E, Lo A; Pancreas Investigators Vital Outcomes Trial (PIVOT) Study Group. A multicenter, open-label, comparative trial of two daclizumab dosing strategies versus no antibody induction in simultaneous kidney-pancreas transplantation: 6-month interim analysis. Transplant Proc 2002;34:1903–1905.
99. Brock MV, Borja MC, Ferber L, et al. Induction therapy in lung transplantation: a prospective, controlled clinical trial comparing OKT3, anti-thymocyte globulin, and daclizumab. J Heart Lung Transplant 2001;20:1282–1290.
100. Bumgardner GL, Hardie I, Johnson RW, et al. of the Phase III Daclizumab Study Group. Results of 3-year phase III clinical trials with daclizumab prophylaxis for prevention of acute rejection after renal transplantation. Transplantation 2001;72:839–845.
101. Ekberg H, Backman L, Tufveson G, Tyden G, Nashan B, Vincenti F. Daclizumab prevents acute rejection and improves patient survival post transplantation: 1 year pooled analysis. Transpl Int 2000;13:151–159.
102. Beniaminovitz A, Itescu S, Lietz K, et al. Prevention of rejection in cardiac transplantation by blockade of the interleukin-2 receptor with a monoclonal antibody. N Engl J Med 2000;342:613–619.
103. Nashan B, Light S, Hardie IR, Lin A, Johnson JR. Reduction of acute renal allograft rejection by daclizumab. Daclizumab Double Therapy Study Group. Transplantation 1999;67:110–115.
104. Vincenti F, Nashan B, Light S. Daclizumab: outcome of phase III trials and mechanism of action. Double Therapy and the Triple Therapy Study Groups. Transplant Proc 1998;30:2155–2158.
105. Tzakis AG, Tryphonopoulos P, Kato T, et al. Preliminary experience with alemtuzumab (Campath-1H) and low-dose tacrolimus immunosuppression in adult liver transplantation [erratum in Transplantation 2004;78:489]. Transplantation 2004;77:1209–1214.
106. Kirk AD, Hale DA, Mannon RB, et al. Results from a human renal allograft tolerance trial evaluating the humanized CD52-specific monoclonal antibody alemtuzumab (CAMPATH-1H). Transplantation 2003;76:120–129.

82 Principles of Organ Preservation

Brian Lima and J.E. Tuttle-Newhall

Organ preservation refers to the maintenance of ex vivo organ viability and restoration of normal organ function when physiologic blood flow is reestablished.[1] This paradigm defines the basis for current clinical and research models of organ transplantation. If an organ does not regain normal function rapidly after clinical implantation surgery and reperfusion, either delayed graft function (DGF) or primary nonfunction (PNF) has occurred. *Delayed graft function* is defined as impaired function that eventually returns to normal. *Primary nonfunction* indicates complete failure of the organ to restore function or the inability of the transplanted organ to sustain life.

Clinically, DGF occurs in 10%–15% of all liver grafts and 30%–50% of cadaveric kidneys transplanted within 24h of cold preservation.[2] In heart, lung, or liver transplants, DGF can have devastating results in the individual patient, with prolonged intensive care unit and hospital stays due to compromised organ function. Primary nonfunction of a vital organ is a fatal event unless a retransplant is rapidly performed. In the initial postoperative setting, the clinical distinction between DGF and PNF is often difficult to discern, and the decision to relist a patient for retransplantation may be particularly challenging. Attempts to predict graft function in individuals and large cohorts of patients has revealed numerous factors that have an impact on the extent to which a transplanted organ regains normal function. These factors include preexisting donor organ diseases, events occurring during the process of death of the donor and organ harvest, the duration of cold preservation, events during implantation surgery, and the medical conditions of the recipients. Acceptance or refusal of an organ for transplantation requires careful consideration of all these factors to optimize the clinical outcome in each individual case.

In the laboratory, organs can be preserved in the University of Wisconsin (UW) preservation solution for up to 72h with 100% immediate graft function in some animal models.[3] Despite these findings, DGF is often attributed to hypothermic preservation techniques that are currently utilized in clinical organ transplants; however, it is clear that other variables are critical, such as donor and recipient characteristics as well as immunologic issues. Specifically, conditions during preprocurement, cold storage, and cellular ischemia lead to a cascade of events that cause further graft injury with reperfusion. With hypothermia and ischemia, there is a slowing of cellular metabolism, a loss of homeostatic processes, and a time-dependent loss of cellular energy that accentuate the injuries detected after reperfusion.[1,4] To reduce the incidence of DGF and PNF, it is paramount to understand the mechanisms of graft injury during preprocurement, ex vivo transport, and subsequent reperfusion. Notable recent advances have been made in furthering our understanding of the mechanisms underlying preservation and reperfusion injury. This progress has led to the development of innovative therapies for improvements of graft and patient outcomes. In this chapter, we discuss the physiologic principles that underlie current preservation techniques and inherent injuries, the specific components of flush solutions, the current state-of-the-art in organ preservation methods, research, and future trends.

Mechanisms of Preservation Injury

To reduce the incidence of DGF and PNF, it is important to understand the types of injuries that occur at the cellular level. Discussion of preservation and reperfusion injury requires analysis of four different time periods: prepreservation, cold preservation, rewarming, and reperfusion.[1] Although the prepreservation time period is distinct, the other three time periods are interrelated and codependent, comprising the classic ischemia–reperfusion interval. Our discussion emphasizes injuries sustained by the liver as an illustrative example; however, other solid organs are discussed as well.

Prepreservation

Injury to solid organs can occur prior to the procurement process. Nonimmune-mediated processes may be critical to both short- and long-term patient and graft outcomes. On reviewing the current United Network of Organ Sharing (UNOS) database, immediate function and long-term graft survival are superior in grafts from living donors compared to those procured from cadaveric sources. Survival rates of kidneys from living unrelated donors and one haplotype-matched living related donors are identical despite clearly defined differences in genetics. Both types of living donor kidneys have decreased incidence of DGF and increased 2- to 5-year graft survival compared to similarly matched cadaveric kidneys.[5] These findings suggest that nonimmunological factors may be responsible for early graft injury leading to delayed or limited function.

Donor organ disease may be incompatible with graft survival after transplantation (e.g., severe hepatic steatosis) or may result in transmissible diseases such as hepatitis C or B. Brain death triggers specific injuries in the cadaveric donor. Until recently, brain death itself had not been considered a significant risk factor in the prepreservation period;[6] however, brain death causes severe and profound derangement of the hemodynamic and endocrine systems as well as striking structural changes in the organs themselves. These effects may activate various cellular pathways, leading to increased immunogenicity and exacerbation of preservation and reperfusion injuries.

Cardiovascular Effects of Brain Death

The effects of brain death on the cardiovascular system can be divided into two phases: an early hypertensive phase followed by a later normotensive or hypotensive phase. Immediately prior to brain herniation, there is increased parasympathetic tone with bradycardia in response to increased intracranial pressure. As brain death occurs, there is a pronounced increase in sympathetic outflow. This process produces marked alterations in blood pressure and heart rates as well as variable perfusion of the potential donor organs. Prolonged episodes of hypoperfusion severely damage potential allografts, as evidenced by significantly increased rates of DGF or acute tubular necrosis (ATN) in renal transplants from unstable cadaveric donors. Elevated expression of class II major histocompatibility complex (MHC) antigens and consequent increased immunogenicity have been noted in response to the ischemic insult.[7]

Donor organs are often subjected to varying levels of systemic vascular resistance secondary to release of endogenous catecholamines. Severe vasoconstriction can lead to organ hypoperfusion even in the setting of increased blood pressure.[8] Increased catecholamine production may cause ischemic damage to donor organs.[9] Some authors have suggested that there is a global energetic failure secondary to a cellular oxygen deficit despite measurements of blood pressure within the normal range. This "energetic failure" may be associated with normal-to-high levels of oxygen delivery. The finding of high mixed venous oxygen saturation in the pulmonary venous circulation suggests a defect at the cellular level in peripheral oxygen extraction leading to a cellular oxygen debt.[10] The rapid rise in systemic catecholamines and the resulting decrease in cellular energy (adenosine triphosphate, ATP) lead to an increase in cytosolic calcium, thereby activating intracellular enzyme systems, which can disrupt normal cellular structure and physiology. Activation of nitric oxide synthases may lead to production of free-oxygen radicals, lipid peroxidation, and subsequent loss of membrane channel integrity. Adenosine is a byproduct of ATP catabolism, and its production parallels ATP breakdown. Adenosine deaminase and xanthine oxidase participate in adenosine breakdown and the generation of cytotoxic oxygen free radicals. Oxygen free radicals also participate in membrane lipid peroxidation, which impairs cell membrane integrity and can lead to injury of vascular endothelium.[9]

Endocrine Effects of Brain Death

In addition to the cardiovascular and subsequent cellular effects of brain death, deleterious effects on the endocrine system also occur with substantial impairment of normal energy homeostasis. The endocrine changes associated with brain death can be divided into two phases: the autonomic sympathetic storm and the failure of the hypothalamic–pituitary axis. In animal models of brain death, there is documented reduction in serum levels of free triiodothyronine (free T_3) and thyroxine (T_4) in the presence of normal thyroid-stimulating hormone (TSH) levels. There is also a decrease in serum cortisol, insulin, and antidiuretic hormone.[11]

Despite apparent clinical responses to hormone replacement therapy, the actual changes in hormone levels during the process of brain death in human donors remain somewhat controversial. One group studied 32 potential organ donors prospectively to determine serum and plasma concentrations of hypothalamic–pituitary hormones, thyroid hormones, and cortisol over a period of up to 80h. While 78% of the organ donors developed diabetes insipidus, none of the circulating hormones of the anterior pituitary gland showed a progressive decline in concentration according to their plasma half-lives. With the exception of arginine vasopressin, no hormone concentration was found to be subnormal due to the onset of brain death. The low free T_3 values and cortisol levels in 62% of cases were similar to the control group of patients with severe head injuries. While the corticotropin concentrations remained constant during the study period, TSH and human growth hormone concentrations showed a 12- and 35-fold increase from baseline values, respectively, after 30–40min.[12]

Patients who suffer brain death may have various degrees of pituitary injury, perfusion, and viability. In laboratory models, alterations in endocrine function are implicated in diffuse mitochondrial injury, leading to impaired aerobic metabolism and decreased cellular energy stores.[11] These findings were noted in animal models using the principle of single-bolus kinetics with labeled carbon compounds, with measurement of both plasma activity and of exhaled O_2 to study glucose, pyruvate, and palmitate utilization under conditions of brain death. Using the labeled substrate and oxygen compounds, the rate of glucose, pyruvate, and palmitate utilization was found to be markedly reduced after brain death. In this model, there was an accumulation of lactate and free fatty acids in the plasma as well, indicating a general shift from aerobic to anaerobic metabolism. The administration of T_3 resulted in a dramatic increase in the rate of metabolite utilization and a reduction in the plasma concentrations of lactate and free fatty acids, indicating an apparent reversal from anaerobic to aerobic metabolism within the tissues.[13]

TABLE 82.1. The Impact of T_3 Therapy on Dopamine Requirements.

Group	*Dopamine range*	*n*	*Pre-T3*	*Post-T_3*	P
1	0–5	46	1.52 (0.3)	1.24 (0.28)	—
2	6–10	53	8.92 (0.19)	5.71 (0.40)	<.02
3	11–15	12	13.5 (0.48)	6.75 (1.52)	<.0001
4	16–20	28	18.69 (0.34)	7.5 (0.69)	<.0001
5	>20	15	34 (1.48)	7.81 (0.95)	<.0001

Source: Modified from Novitzky.[84]

In addition to T_3, cortisol and insulin have been added to the brain-dead donor as part of preprocurement management to limit the need for exogenous inotropic and pressor support. This strategy may limit the hypoperfusion injury mediated by catecholamines. Using prospective donors in his institution, Novitsky modified T_3 infusion based on the required doses of dopamine needed to maintain an acceptable blood pressure. Donors supported with dopamine doses greater than 21 µg/kg/min required several boluses of intravenous T_3 before their pressor support was weaned to doses less than 10 µg/kg/min (Table 82.1). Donors requiring large doses of dopamine required higher doses of T_3 to achieve hemodynamic stability. Despite differing requirements of pressor support, all donors responded to varying doses of T_3 therapy by decreasing their requirement for dopamine support.[9]

Data from living related kidney transplantation is suggestive of increased immunogenicity associated with the use of cadaveric organs, regardless of the degree of antigen matching. To further characterize the nature of this effect, researchers have investigated the release of soluble immunologic mediators at the time of brain death and cellular activation. In one animal model of rapid onset brain death, investigators found elevated levels of macrophage and T-cell products, including interleukin (IL)-6 and IL-1 and tumor necrosis factor (TNF)-α.[14] Similarly, others have suggested a role for increased levels of interferon-γ (IFN-γ).[6] Immunohistochemical staining of peripheral organs in this rat model revealed augmented expression of MHC class I and II antigens as well as other costimulatory molecules. This increased antigen expression is often thought to be induced by cytokine production and can lead to increased T-cell recognition in the recipient, thereby contributing to increased incidence and severity of acute rejection.

Several studies in renal transplantation have suggested that the number and severity of acute rejection episodes in combination with other factors, such as incidence of DGF and high donor age, raise the risk of donor graft loss from chronic rejection within 5 years of transplantation.[7,15] One can infer from these data that brain death upregulates production of proinflammatory cytokines and adhesion molecules, with resultant increased expression of certain classes of MHC. These events may be causative for the injuries sustained during the periods of cold ischemia and reperfusion.

Ischemic Injury

The current clinical methods used to preserve organs for ex vivo transport and later implantation in a suitable recipient are based on the suppression of metabolism by hypothermia at the time of explantation. Organs are prepared for hypothermia by removing blood and replacing it with solutions designed to limit the physiologic consequences of hypothermic preservation. In addition to cellular injury sustained during hypothermia, there are also organ-specific homeostatic mechanisms that are perturbed in ways that prime them for augmentation of injury during reperfusion.

Hypothermia decreases the cellular metabolic rate and the rate at which cellular enzyme systems function. Southard reported that, in most animal enzyme systems, there is a substantial enzyme activity decrease over a range of temperature decline. When the temperature is decreased from normothermia, 37°C, to 0°C–4°C, there is 12- to 13-fold decrease in metabolism[16]; however, cellular metabolism during this hypothermic state does not cease completely. While hypothermia is essential to organ preservation, residual cellular energy requirements exceed the capacity of the cell to generate energy from anaerobic metabolism. This in turn leads to diminished intracellular energy, ATP and adenosine diphosphate (ADP) levels, as demonstrated in several laboratory models.[17] A direct correlation between energy content of transplanted livers in patients and clinical outcome has been reported but not substantiated by laboratory models.[1,18]

In clinical transplantation, the period of warm ischemia during implantation may cause further reduction in intragraft ATP. In 30 liver transplantations, ATP levels were assessed as well as clinical markers of bile production and transaminase levels postimplantation. The level of recovery of ATP was inversely related to the period of warm ischemia during implantation. Bile production, used as a parameter of initial function, was observed shortly after implantation in 17 of 24 grafts that functioned satisfactorily but in only 1 of 6 poorly functioning grafts. The authors concluded that loss of adenine nucleotides and lack of bile production during transplantation were markers of graft viability in the clinical setting.[18]

One mechanism of cellular injury during ischemic hypothermia is the loss of mitochondrial respiration and resultant ATP depletion.[19] The energy debt created during hypothermic conditions leads to several other intracellular events. One key event is the shift toward anaerobic metabolism and ensuing intracellular lactic acidosis. There are data to suggest that intracellular acidosis may actually be protective[20,21]; however, following a critical period of ischemia, reperfusion results in irreversible injury. Reperfusion injury to several cell lines and experimental models was accompanied by a rapid return to physiological pH, the phenomenon known as a *pH paradox*. In this paradox, cellular injury and death are not secondary to the acidosis caused by anaerobic metabolism but instead the rapid return to normal pH during reperfusion.[20] In reperfusion models, protection from the pH paradox was associated with maintenance of an acidotic pH. Free intracellular Ca^{2+} progressively increased during experimental ischemia. After reperfusion without pH protection, free Ca^{2+} increased further, suggesting a Ca^{2+}-mediated form of cell injury.[21]

Another well-described mechanism of hypothermic cell injury is cellular swelling. Across cell membranes, K^+ and Cl^- are in equilibrium, and their distribution is affected by the presence of negatively charged intracellular ions such as proteins and nucleotides. In normothermic conditions, Na^+/K^+ adenosine triphosphatase (ATPase) is a principal membrane-bound enzyme system that prevents cell swelling by the active extrusion of intracellular Na^+, decreasing the osmotic pressure of the cytoplasm.[22] This enzyme is inhibited in hypothermic conditions, resulting in intracellular accumulation of Na^+ accompanied by influx of water and eventual cell swelling.[23]

Initial studies suggested that reactive oxygen species played a large role in the initial cellular injury that occurred at the time of reperfusion.[19] Briefly, ATP degradation during hypothermia results in the accumulation of hypoxanthine with conversion of xanthine dehydrogenase and xanthine oxidase to an activated state. This conversion may also be associated with increasing levels of cytosolic calcium and protease activity. On reperfusion, xanthine oxidase further catalyzes hypoxanthine to xanthine and uric acid, which is responsible for producing reactive oxygen intermediates. While some reactive oxygen species are produced during cold ischemia, the majority occur at reperfusion.[24] Nonetheless, further investigations have failed to prove that reactive oxygen intermediates play a large role in cellular injury.[25,26] The activation of xanthine dehydrogenase and xanthine oxidase occurs very slowly and does not correlate with injury. Second, hepatocytes tolerate a large degree of intracellular oxidative stress even after ischemia.[26] Finally, the destruction of damaged cells occurs primarily via cell-mediated immune responses, with a limited significance attributed to the effects of intracellular reactive oxygen species.[27]

Preservation Solutions

Successful ex vivo transport and reimplantation of graft organs depends on the ability of the graft to survive hypothermic preservation. In the late 1960s, Belzer and Collins made landmark developments in preservation solutions. Belzer and colleagues demonstrated that a kidney could be maintained 3 days by continuous perfusion at 6°C with a preservation solution made from plasma. Unfortunately, plasma was found to contain lipid moieties that occluded renal microvasculature in the cold. Once the lipids were removed, they demonstrated that canine kidneys could be kept viable with continuous perfusion for eventual transplantation with 100% immediate function. Due to the human origin of this preservation solution, its main disadvantage was the implicit risk of spreading transmissible human diseases.[2]

Collins eventually developed a simpler method of organ preservation via cold storage after removal of the blood of the organ and perfusing it with a cold preservation solution known as Collins solution (Table 82.2) at the time of procurement. The concept in the composition of the fluid was that it would resemble the intracellular compartment because of the high K^+ and low Na^+ content. To make the solution hyperosmotic, glucose was added in a large amount. Cold storage with Collins solution replaced machine perfusion as the method of choice for preservation of kidneys by the early 1970s. It was simple, less cumbersome, and cheaper with equivalent clinical results in kidney transplants.[28,29]

TABLE 82.2. Components of the Original Collins Solution.

Component	*Amount (mmol/L)*
Potassium	115
Sodium	10
Phosphate	57.5
Magnesium	30
Sulfate	30
Glucose	140

Osmolality (mOsm/L) = 350, pH = 7.1.

Modifications of the Collins solution were numerous. With 30 m*M* phosphate and 57.5 m*M* magnesium, the solubility product of the solution was exceeded, and often magnesium phosphate crystals were found in the preservative. Consequently, magnesium was removed from the solution, and it became known as Euro-Collins solution. While Euro-Collins was highly effective in preserving kidneys for transplants, this solution was less effective for the preservation of heart, lung, liver, or pancreas grafts.

Given the increasing need for prolonged preservation periods for all solid organs during the 1980s, several groups aggressively pursued new preservation strategies. Applying basic knowledge about hypothermic cellular injury, Belzer and Southard described the characteristics of the ideal preservation solution: (1) It must contain substrates to regenerate high-energy phosphate compounds; (2) it must have an alkaline pH to counteract acidosis; (3) it must contain materials to prevent injury from reactive oxygen intermediates; and (4) it must minimize cell swelling in hypothermic conditions.[16]

From these principles emerged the UW solution, which contains several agents not found in Euro-Collins thought to facilitate storage of the liver, pancreas, and other organs, such as heart and lung (Table 82.3). Adenosine and phosphate were added to provide substrate for ATP to facilitate energy preservation and support energy requiring cellular mechanisms. Acidosis was limited by using a phosphate buffer. Less magnesium was added to facilitate cation-dependent events. Allopurinol and glutathione were added to minimize damage by reactive oxygen intermediates. To prevent cell swelling, several large molecular weight anions, lactobionate (a disaccharide, 4-0-β-D-galactopyranosyl-D-gluconic acid) and raffinose (a trisaccharide), were added as the major impermeant molecular species in the solution. The solution also contains a colloid, hydroxyethyl starch, to prevent the expansion of the extracellular space.[2,30] A precise explanation of the role of each component in UW solution is difficult as each compo-

TABLE 82.3. Components of University of Wisconsin Solution.

Component	*Amount (mmol/L)*
KH_2PO_4	25
$MgSO_4$	5
Raffinose	30
Pentafraction (HES)	50 (g/L)
Penicillin	200,000 U/L
Insulin	40 U/L
Dexamethasone	16 (mg/dl)
K Lactobionate	100
GSH	3
Adenosine	5
Allopurinol	1
Na	25
K	125

GSH, glutathione; HES, hydroxyethyl starch.

nent appears to act in concert with the others to prevent the untoward summation of events that occur in hypothermic preservation.

Although Euro-Collins and UW can be utilized relatively interchangeably for the preservation of kidneys, UW enables the longest period of safe preservation of liver, pancreas, bowel, and lungs. It is also the only solution that is effective for prolonged preservation of isolated transplantable cells, such as pancreatic islet cells.[31–33]

Even though it is clear that UW is the preferred storage solution for organs other than kidneys, the effectiveness of some of the additives has been questioned, as has its efficacy compared to other preservation solutions. For example, recent prospective trials comparing UW to Celsior solution for kidney and liver preservation provide convincing evidence that these solutions have equivalent efficacy.[34,35] Celsior, a new extracellular-type, low-K^+, low-viscosity perfusate originally applied for heart and lung preservation, is deemed theoretically advantageous compared to UW given its low cost, more rapid organ flushing capacity due to its low viscosity, and its higher buffering capacity.

One important additive in UW, lactobionate, chelates Ca^{2+} and iron in hypothermic conditions, potentially limiting certain oxidative reactions that depend on divalent ions. Substituting other large anion molecules (i.e., gluconate) for lactobionate does not produce the same effect.[2] The presence of colloid in the solution has also been studied. Colloid was originally added to maintain hydrostatic pressure during continuous pulsatile perfusion. Several studies have shown that effective osmotic ingredients are essential for heart and pancreas preservation,[31,36] although these ingredients might be less important for lung preservation.[37] Phosphate was originally added to promote energy stability, but it also functions as a hydrogen ion acceptor. Dexamethasone was added due to the theoretical ability of steroids to stabilize membranes, but outcomes of organ preservation have been similar with and without this agent.[30] Allopurinol has been studied as well and has been shown to improve the quality of kidney preservation but not to change the eventual outcome of the graft.[38]

While hypothermic preservation with UW solution prevents most global tissue injury by a variety of mechanisms, it also ameliorates certain organ-specific injuries. The solution is superior to other solutions in the preservation of hepatic grafts due to its ability to protect the sinusoidal endothelial cell (SEC) from hypothermic injury. Preservation of the SEC has been shown to be directly related to graft viability.[1] During cold preservation, the SEC detaches from the perisinusoidal matrix and rapidly dies on reperfusion. There is growing evidence that the injury and eventual death of the detached SEC is a major component of hepatic injury during ischemia and reperfusion. Changes in the SEC/perisinusoidal matrix attachment involve a protease-mediated alteration in the cellular cytoskeleton and extracellular matrix.[39] As in the process of angiogenesis, SEC injury is accompanied by Kupffer cell activation and production of angiogenic mediators during hypoxic conditions.[37,40,41] These angiogenic mediators are suspected to induce the release of proteases, resulting in disruption of the cellular cytoskeleton and extracellular matrix and subsequent SEC detachment.

Several groups have demonstrated increased proteolytic activity in clinical transplantation. Calmus et al. showed that increased free amino acids in the preservation fluid of cold-stored hepatic allografts were related to graft function and patient outcome.[42] In their study, 30 recipients of 32 liver allografts were studied prospectively. The amino acid content of the preservation fluid was analyzed at the end of cold storage as an indicator of proteolysis. Concentrations of amino acids and transaminases in the preservation fluid correlated with the duration of cold ischemia as well as indices of graft dysfunction.[42]

Likewise, others have demonstrated an important role for matrix metalloproteinases (MMPs), namely gelatinases, in preservation injury.[43] Lactobionate interestingly has strong inhibitory effects on these specific proteases, most likely via chelation of calcium and zinc. This suggests that the protective effect of UW solution may be related to its ability to limit the action of these proteases.[39]

The utilization of perfluorocarbons (PFCs) in organ preservation has been extensively explored in experimental animal models.[44,45] Perfluorocarbons comprise a hydrocarbon solution in which a large proportion of the hydrogen atoms have been replaced by fluorine. This atomic substitution enables an efficient oxygen delivery system given the 20- to 25-fold increased oxygen solubility in PFC versus plasma and its negligible oxygen-binding capacity.

Several groups have investigated the so-called two-layer method (TLM), in which the organ is submerged in a chamber containing fully preoxygenated PFC with UW preservation solution (Fig. 82.1).[44,45] The two fluids separate given that PFC is lipophilic and has a higher density. The explanted organ floats at the interface of these two fluids, with adequate oxygen available via simple diffusion from the PFC to support ATP synthesis without the need for continuous perfusion equipment. Experimentally, the TLM has allowed significant prolongation of organ preservation and improved outcomes in limited clinical evaluations[45]; however, before widespread clinical application of the TLM, further studies and randomized prospective clinical trials comparing TLM to UW alone are necessary.

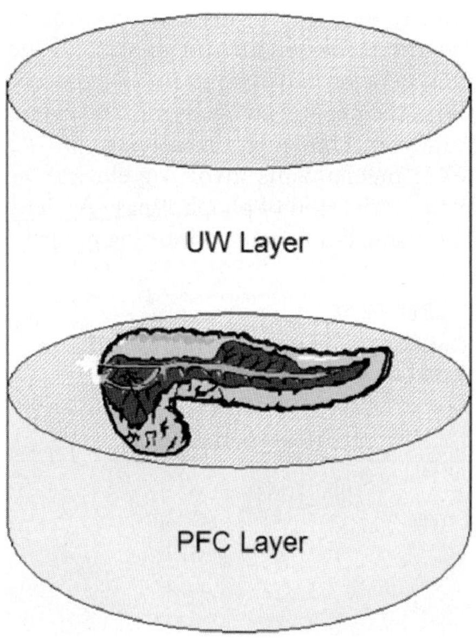

FIGURE 82.1. Two-layer method of organ preservation using preoxygenated PFC and UW solution. The pancreas floats at the interface of this mixture with oxygenation provided by PFC.

Reperfusion Injury

During the ischemic phase of injury, particularly in the liver, the extent of injury is not uniformly distributed. The SECs are highly sensitive to hypothermia and reperfusion, while hepatocytes appear quite resistant. Periods of normothermic ischemia, in contrast, exacerbate injury in hepatocytes at the time of reperfusion.[46] The key to limiting the degree of cellular preservation injury is to restore normal physiologic blood flow as soon as possible, that is, to limit the duration of hypothermic and normothermic ischemia. (See Table 82.4 for optimal cold ischemia times for specific organs.) While the mechanism of reperfusion injury is multifactorial and not completely mechanistically defined, it primarily involves activation of specific cell types, expression of certain cell markers, increased production of immunomodulators, microvascular perfusion failure, and programmed cell death.

Although generation of intracellular reactive oxygen species may not have a significant impact on cell injury during hypothermic ischemia, free oxygen radicals may have a prominent role in reperfusion of ischemic grafts. When rat livers were subjected to varying periods of cold preservation in standard preservation solutions and subsequently reperfused, Kupffer cells exhibited progressive rounding, ruffling of the cell surface, polarization, appearance of wormlike densities, vacuolization, and degranulation as demonstrated by electron microscopy.[47] These activated cells from reperfused livers also revealed increased production of reactive oxygen intermediates. If production of these oxygen species were blocked using cell-specific interventions such as methyl palmitate, injury during reperfusion and reoxygenation was attenuated.[48] In vitro studies utilizing an isolated rat liver perfusion model revealed that neither the presence nor the absence of Kupffer cells had a significant impact on the extent of reperfusion injury.[49] This is in contrast to in vivo data, for which downregulation of Kupffer cells with calcium blockers or pentoxifylline improved graft survival.[50]

The early reperfusion time period is also characterized by infiltration of neutrophils into hepatic vasculature with detectable injury by 3–5h.[51] This delay may be theoretically related to the time required for upregulation of adhesion molecules, attachment of neutrophils to SECs, extravasation of those cells into the hepatic parenchyma, and eventual damage to the hepatocytes. Upregulation of neutrophils occurs by a complex set of mechanisms involving elevated intracellular calcium levels, activation of phopholipase A_2, leukotriene B_4, hydrolysis of arachadonic acid-containing phopsholipids, and production of platelet-activating factor (PAF) and bioactive eicosanoids thromboxane A_2 and prostacyclin.[52] Platelet-activating factor may contribute significantly to the activation of neutrophils because it is presented by the activated SEC and remains anchored on the cell surface as it interacts with the specific receptor on the activated cell.[53]

TABLE 82.4.
Optimal Cold Ischemia Time for Different Organs Based on Class of Evidence.

Organ	*Cold ischemia time (UW)*	*Evidence*
Kidney	<24h	II[85]
Kidney/pancreas	<21h	II[86]
Liver	<12h	II[87]
Lungs	4–6h	I[88,89]
Heart	4h	I[90]
Small intestine	6–10h	II[91,92]

Source: Data from References 85–92.

There is also upregulation of certain adhesion molecules on the cell surfaces of the SECs, neutrophils, and hepatocytes. Neutrophils express β_2 integrin, adhesion molecule Mac-1 (CD11b/CD18), which in turn reacts with its counterreceptor intercellular adhesion molecule 1 (ICAM-1), expressed by SECs and hepatocytes.[54] The counterreceptor ICAM-1 is important for transendothelial migration of activated neutrophils and adherence to parenchymal cells. Oxygen free radicals produced by activated Kupffer cells also cause prolonged expression of P-selectin on the surface of the endothelial cell. The coexpression of PAF and P-selectin also augment the tethering to the SECs and activation of neutrophils.[52] Ischemia and reperfusion induce the expression of ICAM-1 protein via activation of the transcription factor, nuclear factor kappa B (NF-κB).[55] Monoclonal antibodies against both MAC-1 and ICAM-1 in the experimental setting are beneficial against reperfusion injury. These antibodies are effective when given early in the course of reperfusion, suggesting that Kupffer cell injury can be diminished if neutrophil infiltration can be limited.[19]

This early reperfusion time period is also marked by increased production of many nonspecific inflammatory mediators, such as TNF-α, IL-1, and IFN-γ. These cytokines are critically important in initial leukocyte adherence in models of nonspecific inflammation and mediate multiple effects on endothelial cells, neutrophils, and hepatocytes.[1] Also, TNF-α and IL-1 can induce transcription expression of ICAM-1 in endothelial cells and hepatocytes. These inflammatory mediators also elicit chemotactic factors such as IL-8, which may be important for hepatic neutrophil extravasation and sequestration.[54]

Other cytokines, however, have been found to engage in a protective role against injury and in the liver promote recovery via regeneration. Interleukin-6 has been found to prevent injury in a rodent model of acute hepatitis through downregulation of TNF-α.[56] Using a model of warm ischemia and reperfusion in rats, IL-6 was shown to be protective against hepatic necrosis and elevated transaminases as a marker of injury. It was also found to promote hepatic regeneration. Interleukin 6 may therefore limit hepatic ischemia/reperfusion injury by way of its antiinflammatory properties and modulation of TNF-α.[56]

Complement activation has also been described during reperfusion. Complement activation increases MAC-1 expression on neutrophils, induces neutrophil sequestration in the liver, and causes increased superoxide formation in neutrophils and Kupffer cells.[57]

Based on these numerous experimental findings, it is evident that nonspecific inflammation and soluble mediators are critical components of reperfusion injury through upregulation of adhesion molecules, cell adherence and sequestration, and priming of neutrophils and Kupffer cells for increased cytotoxicity. Clinically, the release of these mediators may reflect the degree of ischemia reperfusion injury and may stimulate a specific immune response that leads to an increased risk of acute allograft rejection.

Mueller et al. studied 85 patients undergoing liver transplantation.[58] Using hepatic and peripheral venous samples at the time of reperfusion and the following 48 h, they measured various soluble mediators such as TNF-α, Il-8, Il-10, L-selectin, ICAM-1, and molecules involved in the production of extracellular matrix such as hyaluronic acid and laminin. The levels of these mediators correlated significantly with the extent of preservation and reperfusion injury (Fig. 82.2). In patients with elevated levels of TNF-α, E-selectin, and laminin, there was a statistically significant increased risk of acute allograft rejection.[58] An understanding of the potential mechanisms underlying these events may allow for strategic intervention at key points in this inflammatory cascade in the future.

Another confounding variable in the early phase of reperfusion is the failure of microvascular perfusion. Although there is ample evidence suggesting that the integrity of the microcirculation is an important determinant of tissue viability during reperfusion after ischemia in the liver, kidney, and other tissues, the mechanisms responsible for microvascular failure have not been fully elucidated. It is known that the microvascular response to reperfusion, as in the response to shock, can consist of either a rapid exacerbation of injury after a severe ischemic episode or more of a slowly developing alteration in responsiveness that occurs after a less-severe insult.[59]

Poor sinusoidal perfusion was once thought to result exclusively from cellular debris accumulating in the sinusoids leading to impaired blood flow. Neutrophils are found in the sinusoids but do not cause cellular or microvascular injury in spite of microvascular accumulation unless they are in an activated state. Activated neutrophils damage microcirculation or hepatocytes depending on the nature of the activation.[60] Platelets are also found at sites of activated endothelial cells and exposed matrix components, forming activated "plugs" that restrict microcirculatory flow and may further graft injury.[61]

Mediators that regulate sinusoidal blood flow are also affected during reperfusion. In the more slowly developing response to reperfusion, upregulation of stress-induced vascular mediators such as endothelin, nitric oxide synthase, and heme oxygenase can alter the status of the microvasculature.[59] Of note, supplying excess nitric oxide does reverse the ischemic component of reperfusion but does not change the Kupffer cell or neutrophil mediated injury.[62]

Others have shown that poor sinusoidal perfusion may occur as a combination of physical impairment of blood flow due to leukocyte adhesion and clot formation involving other soluble mediators, such as L-selectin and ICAM-1 receptors.[52] Sinusoidal blood flow during reperfusion is impaired mainly by excess formation of vasoconstrictors, resulting in focal ischemia and propagation of injury.[59,63] Superoxide produced by Kupffer cells can contribute to an imbalance favoring vasoconstriction.[64]

Finally, recent attention has focused on programmed cell death at the time of reperfusion as a mechanism of graft injury.[39] Within the realm of liver transplantation, preservation strategies dealing with ischemia/reperfusion injury have concentrated on minimizing the biochemical and histologic correlates associated with classic cellular and tissue necrosis.[64] Apoptosis, or programmed cell death, is a tightly regulated process that requires the involved cell to activate intrinsic proteases via multiple intracellular signaling pathways to commit cellular "suicide." Apoptotic cells are characterized by cytoplasmic blebbing and nuclear and cytoplasmic condensation, followed by the disintegration of the nuclear membrane and formation of condensed nuclear material in the cytoplasm, so-called apoptotic bodies. During this process, however, mitochondria appear well preserved. Apoptotic cells are then removed by phagocytosis (Fig. 82.3) without accompanying inflammation.[65] Conversely, necrosis is a passive cell process that requires no intrinsic activation of cell processes. Morphologically, necrosis is characterized by nuclear and cytoplasmic destruction.[66]

Several studies have implicated apoptosis as a major mechanism of graft injury at the time of reperfusion[64,67,68] not only in liver but also in pancreas and heart allografts as well.[69,70] In a rat model of liver transplantation, apoptosis of endothelial cells occurred rapidly on reperfusion, with the number of apoptotic SECs correlating with the duration of cold ischemia and graft survival following implantation.[67] These data and that of others[71,72] favor apoptosis, not coagulative necrosis, as the more prominent cause of graft failure in transplantation.

The pathogenesis of cellular "self-destruction" has yet to be identified, but hypoxia has been implicated in apoptosis in renal and heart allografts.[73] Other authors have suggested that it is a combination of hypoxia and hypothermia that triggers rapid apoptosis following reperfusion (Fig. 82.4). Hypothermia leads to low oxygen tension, which in turn can trigger the release of angiogenic factors. These angiogenic

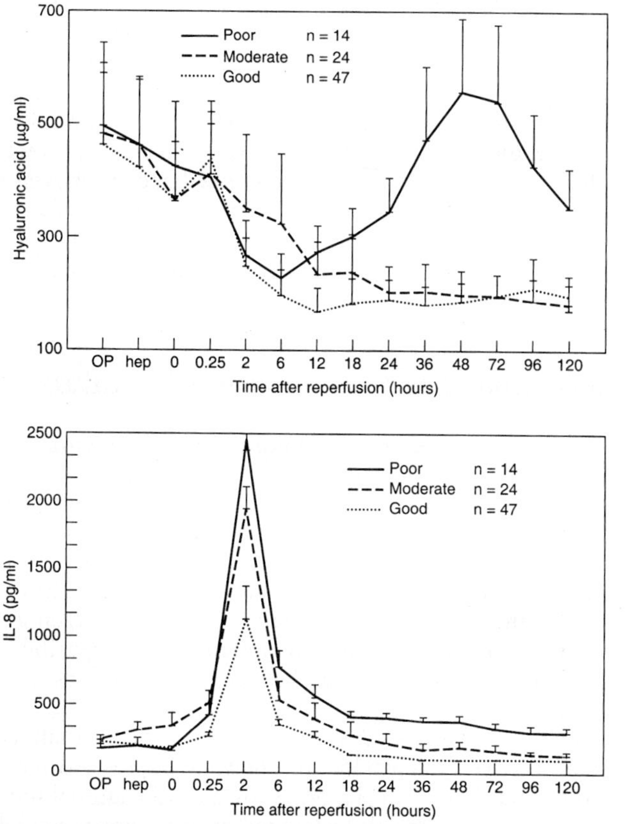

FIGURE 82.2. Levels of hyaluronic acid and IL-8 in patients with good, moderate, and poor initial graft function. (From Mueller et al.,[58] by permission of *Transplantation*.)

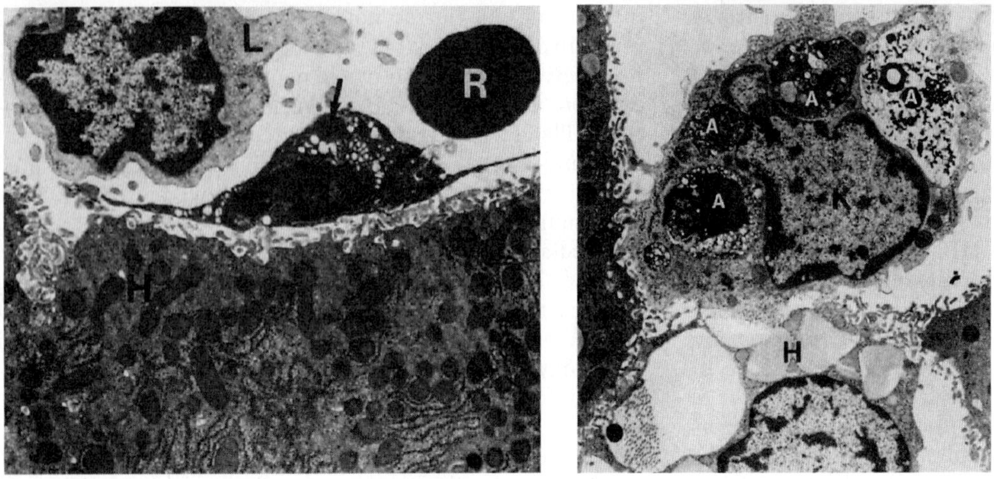

A B

FIGURE 82.3. (A) and (B) Activated Kupffer cell (K) and apoptotic sinusoidal epithelial cell (SEC). (From Gao et al.,[67] by permission of *Hepatology*.)

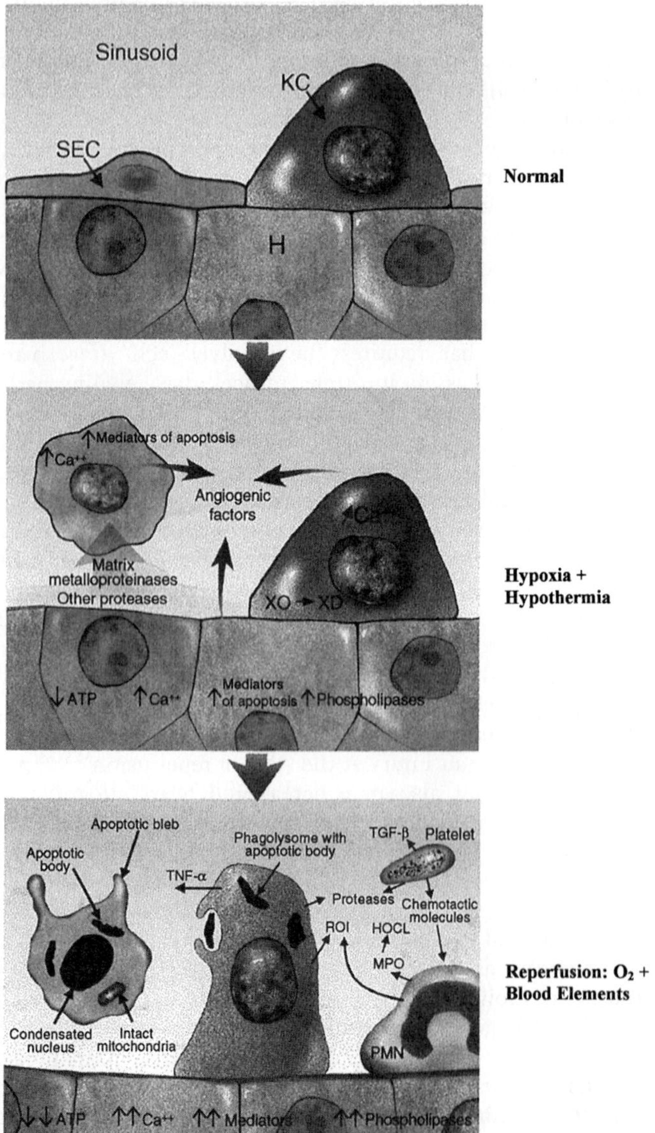

FIGURE 82.4. Potential mechanisms of injury during cold preservation and reperfusion.

mediators may generate proteases such as MMPs, specifically gelatinases, which destroy the SEC cytoskeleton and extracellular matrix.[43] These proteases have been implicated in SEC injury during cold preservation.[1,39,43,67] After exiting the basement membrane, the SEC becomes rounded and loses its cytoplasmic processes. Intracellular ATP is also reduced, with a concomitant rise in intracellular calcium. Increases in intracellular calcium may play an important role in apoptosis by activation of calcium-sensitive proteases such as calpain.[74]

Another component of this process is the increased production of reactive oxygen intermediates by activated Kupffer cells and neutrophils. Apoptosis of the SEC shortly follows reperfusion probably secondary to reactive oxygen intermediates, the release of extracellular proteases, as well as proapoptotic mediators such as TNF-α and transforming growth factor-β (TGF-β).[39,75] Recently, IL-6 has been shown to prevent apoptosis in a leukemia model, which may explain in some part the mechanism of its protective effect in preventing ischemia reperfusion injury as discussed above.[56] Given the distinct nature of apoptosis and the highly regulated pathway for its initiation, inhibition of apoptosis with specific molecular targets may serve to decrease allograft reperfusion injury.

Prevention of Ischemia Reperfusion Injury

To recapitulate, preservation injury results from cumulative effects of brain death, cold and warm ischemia, as well as reperfusion. The relative contributions of these separate events to the extent of preservation injury have yet to be clearly defined. Empirically, preservation injury can be obviated or significantly limited by using living donors or limiting storage times. Specific donor qualities, reactive oxygen intermediates, soluble mediators of inflammation, specific cell types, or preconditioning may be manipulated to hinder preservation injury.

Some have suggested that the quality of the liver allograft is not necessarily dependent on the time of preservation but on the condition of the donor. Using a fasting animal model, increased hepatic injury was noted at 48h after reperfusion and attributed to the loss of glycogen that may be an essential source of energy in the initial posttransplant period.[17] Conversely, there are data that fasting donor livers tolerate hypothermic preservation better than nonfasted donors.

In attempt to clarify this controversy, Southard et al. used a rat transplant model to compare markers of liver viability in prolonged fasted and fed donors. They theorized that the enhanced survival of fasted donors may be due to inactivation of Kupffer cells from nutritional depletion of the liver. Although livers from fasted donors showed improved survival, there was extensive hepatocellular injury. Feeding rats glucose elevated liver glycogen and significantly reduced hepatocellular injury. These results showed that both extensive donor fasting and glucose feeding enhanced outcome in orthotopic liver transplantation.[76]

Donor infection and presence of endotoxin can also affect graft function and recipient outcomes. Prolonged exposure of the liver to high levels of endotoxin can increase the incidence of PNF.[77] Due to the activated state of Kupffer cells in the reperfused allograft, exposure to additional stimulation from infection or endotoxin can potentiate the production of reactive oxygen intermediates and increase the degree of cellular damage.[78] This phenomenon is not isolated to the liver and occurs in transplanted lung grafts as well.[79] Using organs from donors without significant hemodynamic instability or sepsis can improve the chances for clinical success. Nutritional issues in donors are more difficult to control, and it is unclear in the clinical arena how to optimize donor nutritional status and intraorgan energy levels.

Another strategy to limit injury may involve the technique of preconditioning. Single or repeated periods of ischemia can provide a protective effect against subsequent prolonged episodes of ischemia. The proposed mechanism for this phenomenon may be the induction of endogenous antioxidant systems prior to longer periods of ischemia.[80] A short time of warm ischemia before reperfusion has been shown to improve the tolerance of the heart and the liver to a prolonged warm ischemia; however, in cold ischemia reperfusion models, preliminary results would suggest that preservation injury is increased in preconditioned groups. Preconditioning may also have a deleterious effect on hepatic tolerance to the extended cold ischemia time required for transplantation.[81]

Recent advances in the mechanistic description of programmed cell death based on angiogenic mediators and proteases have and will lead to new avenues of prevention of ischemia reperfusion injury. Adding specific inhibitors of MMPs or calpain to preservation solutions may limit SEC detachment and graft injury. Administration of antiangiogenic agents such as IFN-α to donors may prolong graft tolerance to hypothermic preservation.[82] Modulation of transcription factors such as NF-κB may limit the expression of specific adhesion molecules and the production of TNF-α, an inducer of apoptosis.[82] While it is clear that a better understanding of the mechanisms of apoptosis will guide preventive interventions, it is likely that multiple interventions will be required for the best chance at preventing SEC injury.[39]

Genetic modification of organs during preservation may potentially offer an additional therapeutic strategy to minimize the extent of ischemia–reperfusion injury and inhibit or delay allograft rejection. Gene transfer of numerous cytoprotective and immunodulatory molecules has yielded very promising experimental results.[44,83] Some of the cytoprotective molecules genetically transferred to explanted organs include heme oxygenase 1, endothelial nitric oxide synthase, superoxide dismutase, and antisense (decoy) oligodeoxynucleotides specific for transcription factor NF-κB or ICAM-1.[83] Other gene therapy approaches have included transfer of immunomodulatory cytokines IL-4, IL-10, and TGF-β. The majority of these gene therapies have relied on a replication-deficient, recombinant adenoviral vector as the mode of gene delivery. However, this approach is limited given that adenovirus elicits a significant inflammatory response and provides only transient transgene expression, up to only 2–4 weeks. A more prolonged period of transgene expression has been observed in alternative viral vectors, such as adeno-associated virus (AAV) and retroviruses.[83] Further investigation of therapeutic gene transfer, both experimentally and clinically, is warranted and may truly ameliorate current organ preservation practices.

Conclusion

The series of events that lead to ischemia reperfusion injury are complex. While the understanding of specific organ injuries during preservation is just emerging, a significant breakthrough has yet to come. Preservation injury depends on the condition of the donor organ and the length of cold and warm ischemia. Although injury to the graft cannot be completely avoided during reperfusion, the goal is to limit the degree of injury and minimize the risk of DGF and PNF. As our understanding of the mechanisms of injury continues to increase, broader application of innovative therapies may be possible.

References

1. Clavien PA, Harvey RC, Strasberg SM. Preservation and reperfusion injuries in liver allografts. Transplantation 1992;53:957–978.
2. Southard J, Belzer F. Organ preservation. Annu Rev Med 1995; 46:235–247.
3. Wahlberg JA, Lover R, Landegaard L, Southard JH, Belzer FO. 72-hour preservation of the canine pancreas. Transplant Proc 1987;43:5–8.
4. Southard J. Improving early graft function. Transplant Proc 1997;29:3510–3511.
5. United Network of Organ Sharing. UNOS 1996 Annual Report. Washington, DC: Department of Health and Human Services; 1996.
6. Pratschke J, Wilhelm MJ, Kuska M, et al. Brain death and its influence on donor organ quality and outcome after transplantation. Transplantation 1999;67:343–348.
7. Nagano H, Tilney N. Chronic allograft failure: the clinical problem. Am J Med Sci 1997;313:305–309.
8. Herijgers P, Leunens V, Tjandra-Maga TB, Mubagwa K, Flameng W. Changes in organ perfusion after brain death in the rat and its relation to circulating catecholamines. Transplantation 1996;62:330–335.
9. Novitzky D. Donor management: state of the art. Transplant Proc 1997;29:3773–3775.
10. Depret J, Teboul JL, Benoit G, Mercat A, Richard C. Global energetic failure in brain-dead patients. Transplantation 1995; 60:966–971.
11. Novitzky D. Detrimental effects of brain death on the potential organ donor. Transplant Proc 1997;29:3770–3772.
12. Gramm HJ, Meinhold H, Bickel U, et al. Acute endocrine failure after brain death? Transplantation 1992;54:851–857.
13. Novitzky D, Cooper DK, Morrell D, Isaacs S. Change from aerobic to anaerobic metabolism after brain death, and reversal

following triiodothyronine therapy. Transplantation 1988;45:32–36.
14. Takada M, Nadeau KC, Hancock WW, et al. Effects of explosive brain death on cytokine activation of peripheral organs in the rat. Transplantation 1998;65:1533–1542.
15. Schneeberger H, Aydemir S, Illner WD, Land W. Nonspecific primary ischemia/reperfusion mediated injury in combination with secondary specific acute rejection-mediated injury of human kidney allografts contributes mainly to development of chronic transplant failure. Transplant Proc 1997;29:948–949.
16. Belzer FO, Southard JH. Principles of solid-organ preservation by cold storage. Transplantation 1988;45:673–676.
17. Boudjema K, Lindell SL, Southard JH, Belzer FO. The effects of fasting on the quality of liver preservation by simple cold storage. Transplantation 1990;50:943–948.
18. Kamiike W, Burdelski M, Steinhoff G, Ringe B, Lauchart W, Pichlmayr R. Adenine nucleotide metabolism and its relation to organ viability in human liver transplantation. Transplantation 1988;45:138–143.
19. Jaeschke H. Preservation injury: mechanisms, prevention and consequences. J Hepatol 1996;25:774–780.
20. Bond JM, Herman B, Lemasters JJ. Protection by acidotic pH against anoxia/reoxygenation injury to rat neonatal cardiac myocytes. Biochem Biophysiol Res Commun 1991;179:798–803.
21. Bond JM, Chacon E, Herman B, Lemasters JJ. Intracellular pH and Ca^{2+} homeostasis in the pH paradox of reperfusion injury to neonatal rat cardiac myocytes. Am J Physiol 1993;265:C129–C137.
22. Levy MN, Berne RM. Physiology. St. Louis, MO: Mosby; 1988;26–27.
23. Raison J. The influence of temperature-induced phase changes on the kinetics of respiratory and other membrane associated enzyme systems. Bioenergetics 1973;4:285–290.
24. Adkinson D, Hoellwarth ME, Benoit JN, Parks DA, McCord JM, Granger DN. Role of free radicals in ischemia reperfusion injury to the liver. Acta Physiol Scan Suppl 1986;548:101–107.
25. Engerson TD, McKelvey TG, Rhyne DB, Boggio EB, Synder SJ, Jones HP. Conversion of xanthine dehydrogenase to oxidase in ischemic rat tissue. J Clin Invest 1987;79:1564–1570.
26. de Groot H, Littaurer A. Reoxygenation injury in isolated hepatocytes: cell death precedes conversion of xanthine dehydrogenase to xanthine oxidase. Biochem Biophysiol Res Commun 1988;155:278–282.
27. Jaeschke H. Reactive oxygen and ischemia/reperfusion injury of the liver. Chem Biol Interact 1991;79:115–136.
28. Collins GM, Bravo-Shugarman MB, Terasaki PI. Kidney preservation for transplantation: initial perfusion and 30h ice storage. Lancet 1969;2:1219–1225.
29. Opelz G, Teraski PI. Advantage of cold storage over machine perfusion for preservation of cadaver kidneys. Transplantation 1982;33:64–68.
30. Southard JH, van Gulik TM, Ametani MS, et al. Important components of the UW solution. Transplantation 1990;49:251–257.
31. Jeevanandam V, Auteri JS, Marboe CC, et al. Extending the limits of donor heart preservation: a trial with UW Solution. Transplant Proc 1991;23:697–698.
32. Kawahara K, Ikari H, Hisano H, et al. Twenty four hour canine lung preservation using UW solution. Transplantation 1991;51: 584–587.
33. Zucker PF, Bloom AD, Strasser S, et al. Successful cold storage preservation of canine pancreas with UW-1 solution prior to islet isolation. Transplantation 1988;168–170.
34. Montalti R, Nardo B, Capocasale E, et al. Kidney transplantation from elderly donors: a prospective randomized study comparing Celsior and UW solutions. Transplant Proc 2005;37:2454–2455.
35. Pedotti P, Cardillo M, Rigotti P, et al. A comparative prospective study of two available solutions for kidney and liver preservation [erratum in Transplantation 2004;78:489]. Transplantation 2004; 77:1540–1545.
36. Ploeg RJ, Boudjema K, Marsh D, et al. The importance of a colloid in canine pancreas preservation. Transplantation 1992; 53:735–741.
37. Moriyasu K, McKeown PP, Novitzky D, Snow TR. Preservation of competent rabbit lung function after 30h of storage with a low-potassium dextran solution. J Heart Lung Transplant 1995;14:75–79.
38. Marshall VC, Biguzas M, Jablonski P, et al. Rat kidney preservation with UW solution. Transplant Proc 1988;21:3783–3788.
39. Clavien PA. Sinusoidal endothelial cell injury during hepatic preservation and reperfusion. Hepatology 1998;28:281–285.
40. Gao W, Washington MK, Bentley RC, Clavien PA. Antiangiogenic agents protect liver sinusoidal lining cells from cold preservation injury in rat liver transplantation. Gastroenterology 1997;113:1692–1700.
41. Folkman M. Clinical application of research on angiogenesis. N Engl J Med 1995;333:1757–1763.
42. Calmus Y, Cynober L, Dousset B, et al. Evidence for the detrimental role of proteolysis during liver preservation in humans. Gastroenterology 1995;108:1510–1516.
43. Upadhya GA, Harvey PRC, Howard TK, et al. Evidence for a role for matrix metalloproteinases in preservation injury of the liver in humans and in rats. Hepatology 1997;26:922–928.
44. McKeown CMB, Edwards V, Phillips MJ, et al. Sinusoidal cell lining damage: the critical injury in cold preservation of liver allografts in the rat. Transplantation 1988;46:178–191.
45. Matsumoto S, Kuroda Y. Perfluorocarbon for organ preservation before transplantation. Transplantation 2002;74:1804–1809.
46. McLaren AJ, Friend PJ. Trends in organ preservation. Transplant Int 2003;16:701–708.
47. Caldwell-Kenkel JC, Currin RT, Tanaka Y, Thurman RG, Lemasters JJ. Kupffer cell activation and endothelial cell damage after storage of rat livers: effects of reperfusion. Hepatology 1991;13:83–95.
48. Lindert KA, Caldwell-Kenkel JC, Nukina S, Lemasters JJ, Thurman RG. Activation of Kupffer cells on reperfusion following hypoxia: particle phagocytosis in a low-flow, reflow model. Am J Physiol 1992;262:G345–G350.
49. Imamura H, Sutto F, Brault A, Huet PM. Role of Kupffer cells in cold ischemia/reperfusion injury of rat liver. Gastroenterology 1995;109:189–197.
50. Lemasters JJ, Thurman RG. Reperfusion injury after liver preservation for transplantation. Annu Rev Pharmacol Toxicol 1997;37:327–338.
51. Yadav SS, Howell DN, Gao W, Steeber DA, Harland RC, Clavien PA. L-Selectin and ICAM-1 mediate reperfusion injury and neutrophil adhesion in the warm ischemic mouse liver. Am J Physiol 1998;275:G1341–G1352.
52. Grinyo J. Reperfusion injury. Transplant Proc 1997;29:59–62.
53. Zimmerman GA, Prescott SM, McIntyre TM. Endothelial cell interactions with granulocytes: tethering and signaling molecules. Immunol Today 1992;13:93–100.
54. Essani NA, Fisher MA, Farhood A, Manning AM, Smith CW, Jaeschke H. Cytokine-induced upregulation of hepatic intercellular adhesion molecule-1 (ICAM-1) mRNA expression and its role in the pathophysiology of murine endotoxin shock and acute liver failure. Hepatology 1995;21:1632–1639.
55. Bell FP, Manning AM, Jaeschke H. Activation of nuclear factor-kB and expression of intra-cellular molecule-1 mRNA during hepatic ischemia and reperfusion. Hepatology 1995;22:381A.
56. Camargo CA Jr, Madden JF, Gao W, Selvan RS, Clavien PA. Interleukin-6 protects liver against warm ischemia/reperfusion injury and promotes hepatocyte proliferation in the rodent. Hepatology 1997;26:1513–1520.

57. Jaeschke H, Farhood A, Bautista AP, Spolarics Z, Spitzer JJ. Complement activates Kupffer cells and neutrophils during reperfusion after hepatic ischemia. Am J Physiol 1993;264:801–809.
58. Mueller A, Platz KP, Haak M, et al. The release of cytokines, adhesion molecules, and extra-cellular matrix parameters during and after reperfusion in human liver transplant. Transplantation 1997;62:1118–1126.
59. Clemens MG, Bauer M, Pannen BH, Bauer I, Zhang JX. Remodeling of hepatic microvascular responsiveness after ischemia/reperfusion. Shock 1997;8:80–85.
60. Zhang JX, Jones DV, Clemens MG. Effect of activation on neutrophil-induced hepatic microvascular injury in isolated rat liver. Shock 1994;1:273–278.
61. Cywes R, Packham MA, Tietze L, et al. Role of platelets in hepatic allograft preservation injury in the rat. Hepatology 1993;18:635–647.
62. Wang CY, Mathews WR, Guido DM, et al. Inhibition of nitric oxide synthesis aggravates reperfusion injury after hepatic ischemia and endotoxemia. Shock 1995;4:282–288.
63. Bauer M, Zhang JX, Bauer I, Clemens MG. Endothelin-1 as a regulator of hepatic microcirculation: sublobular distribution of effects and impact on hepatocellular secretory function. Shock 1994;1:457–465.
64. Kuo PC, Drachenberg CI, de la Torre A, et al. Apoptosis and hepatic allograft reperfusion injury. Clinical Transplantation 1998;12:219–223.
65. Krams SM, Martinez OM. Apoptosis as a mechanism of tissue injury in liver allograft rejection. Semin Liver Dis 1998;18:153–167.
66. Manjo GIJ. Apoptosis, oncosis, and necrosis. Am J Pathol 1995;146:3–15.
67. Gao W, Bentley RC, Madden JF, Clavien PA. Apoptosis of sinusoidal endothelial cells is a critical mechanism of preservation injury in rat liver transplantation. Hepatology 1998;27:1652–1660.
68. Sedivy R, Gollackner B, Casati B, et al. Apoptotic hepatocytes in rejection and vascular occlusion in liver allograft specimens. Histopathology 1998;32:503–507.
69. Boonstra JG, Wever PC, Laterveer JC, et al. Apoptosis of acinar cells in pancreas allograft rejection. Transplantation 1997;64: 1211–1213.
70. Shaddy RE. Apoptosis in heart transplantation. Coronary Artery Dis 1997;8:617–621.
71. Natori S, Selzner M, Valentino K, et al. Apoptosis of sinusoidal endothelial cells occurs during liver preservation injury by a capase dependent mechanism. Transplantation 1999;68:89–96.
72. Sindram D, Kohli V, Madden JF, Clavien PA. Calpain inhibition prevents sinusoidal endothelial cell apoptosis in the cold ischemic rat liver. Transplantation 1999;68:136–140.
73. Schumer M, Colombel MC, Swaczuk IS, et al. Morphological, biochemical, and molecular evidence of apoptosis during the reperfusion phase after brief periods of ischemia. Am J Pathol 1992;140:831–838.
74. Kohli V, Madden JF, Bentley RC, Clavien PA. Calpain mediates ischemic injury of the liver through modulation of apoptosis and necrosis. Gastroenterology 1999;116:168–178.
75. Clavien PA, Camargo CA Jr, Gorczynski R, et al. Acute reactant cytokines and neutrophil adhesion after warm ischemia in cirrhotic and noncirrhotic human livers. Hepatology 1996;23:1456–1463.
76. Lindell SL, Hansen T, Rankin M, Danielewicz R, Belzer FO, Southard JH. Donor nutritional status—a determinant of liver preservation injury. Transplantation 1996;61:239–247.
77. Yokoyama I, Todo S, Miyata T, Selby R, Tzakis AG, Starzl TE. Endotoxemia and human liver transplantation. Transplant Proc 1989;21:3833–3841.
78. Liu P, Vonderfecht SL, Fisher MA, McGuire GM, Jaeschke H. Priming of phagocytes for reactive oxygen production during hepatic ischemia and reperfusion increases the susceptibility for endotoxin induced liver injury. Circulatory Shock 1994;43: 9–17.
79. McGuire GM, Liu P, Jaeschke H. Neutrophil induced lung damage after hepatic ischemia and endotoxemia. Free Radical Biol Med 1996;20:189–197.
80. Yamashita N, Nishida M, Hoshida S, et al. Induction of manganese superoxide dismutase in rat cardiac myocytes increases tolerance to hypoxia 24h after pre-conditioning. J Clin Invest 1994;94:2193–2196.
81. Adam R, Arnault I, Bao YM, Salvucci M, Sebagh M, Bismuth H. Effect of ischemic preconditioning on hepatic tolerance to cold ischemia in the rat. Transplant Int 1998;11:S168–S170.
82. Liu Z, Hsu H, Goeddel D, Karin M. Dissection of TNF receptor 1 effector functions: JNK activation is not linked to apoptosis while NFKB activation prevents apoptosis. Cell 1996;87:565–576.
83. Vassalli G, Fleury S, Li J, et al. Gene transfer of cytoprotective and immunomodulatory molecules for prevention of cardiac allograft rejection. Eur J Cardiothorac Surg 2003;24:794–806.
84. Novitzky D. Donor management: state of the art. Transplant Proc 1997;29:3774.
85. Pita S, Valdez F, Alonzo A, et al. The role of cold ischemia on graft survival in recipients of renal transplants. Transplant Proc 1997;29:3596–3697.
86. Stratta R. Donor age, organ import, and cold ischemia: effect on early outcomes after simultaneous kidney pancreas transplantation. Transplant Proc 1997;29:3291–3292.
87. Klar E, Angelescu M, Zapletal C, et al. Definition of cold ischemia time without reduction of graft quality in clinical liver transplantation. Transplant Proc 1998;30:3683–3685.
88. Serrick C, Giaid A, Reis A, Shennib H. Prolonged ischemia is associated with more pronounced rejection in the lung allograft. Ann Thorac Surg 1997;63:202–208.
89. Binns ORA, Delima N, Buchanan S, et al. Both blood and crystalloid-based extracellular solutions are superior to intracellular solutions for lung preservation. J Thorac Cardiovasc Surg 1996;112:1515–1526.
90. Schmid C, Heemann U, Tilney NL. Factors contributing to the development of chronic rejection in heterotopic rat heart transplantation. Transplantation 1997;64:222–228.
91. Balaz P, Matia I, Jackanin S, et al. Preservation injury of jejunal grafts and its modulation by custodiol and university of wisconsin perfusion solutions in wistar rats. Eur Surg Res 2004;36:192–197.
92. Cicalese L, Sileri P, Green M, Abu-Elmagd K, Kocoshis S, Reyes J. Bacterial translocation in clinical intestinal transplantation. Transplantation 2001;71:1414–1417.

83

Kidney Transplantation

Stuart J. Knechtle

In 2002 in the United States, 431,281 patients received treatment for end-stage renal disease (ESRD), including 308,910 on dialysis and 122,374 with a functioning renal transplant.[1] The prevalence of ESRD is increasing at an annual rate of 4%, down from 9% a decade ago. In 2004, there were 15,977 renal transplants performed in the United States, and two-thirds of renal transplant patients are now alive 5 years after transplantation, compared to one-third on either hemodialysis or peritoneal dialysis. The 1-year mortality of renal transplant patients is 6% for deceased donor recipients and 3% for living donor kidney recipients compared to 25% for patients treated with dialysis, reflecting the fact that transplant recipients represent a relatively healthier subset of patients with ESRD compared to dialysis patients.[2] Nevertheless, the death rate on dialysis is higher than after transplantation even after adjusting for patient characteristics.[3]

With both dialysis and transplantation, deaths are primarily caused by cardiovascular disease (50%), infection (15%), and malignancy (10%).[4,5] Figure 83.1 shows the impact of length of time on dialysis prior to transplantation as it influences cardiovascular mortality.[6] Clearly, there is a benefit to minimizing time on dialysis. With the increasing application of renal transplantation, a failed kidney transplant has become a major reason for initiation of dialysis, recently moving up from the fourth to the third leading cause of ESRD.

Should Patients Be Dialyzed or Transplanted?

In patients with known renal disease in whom end-stage renal failure gradually approaches, there is time to anticipate and plan renal replacement therapy. If such a patient is fortunate to have a living donor, a renal transplant can be planned to occur when the recipient's renal failure reaches the critical point at which replacement therapy is necessary to control fluid volume or potassium. Such is the ideal setting, in which transplantation occurs as primary treatment without the need for dialysis and the availability of a living donor removes the indefinite waiting period for a deceased donor. A recent study showed that, for HLA-identical living related renal transplants, the major risk factor for shorter graft survival is time on dialysis pretransplant.[6] This finding highlights the advantage of preemptive renal transplantation and the benefit of avoiding dialysis. However, it is advisable to wait until the serum creatinine is at least 3 mg/dL prior to transplantation to be able to subsequently monitor kidney transplant function.

The relative proportion of patients with renal failure proceeding directly to renal transplantation without dialysis has varied over time at the University of Wisconsin but averages 39% for recipients of living donor kidneys and 12% for deceased donor recipients. Early referral for transplantation is largely responsible for this shift and is to be encouraged. Increasing reliance on living donation is also responsible and to be encouraged. Factors influencing waiting time for deceased donor renal transplantation include the patient's blood type (with B blood type waiting the longest), panel reactive antibody (PRA), the rate of deceased donor organ donation, and the size of the waiting list. The PRA measures recipient sensitization; the higher the PRA is, the more difficult it is to locate immunologically compatible donors. A previous transplant, blood transfusion, or pregnancy may lead to allosensitization, raising the PRA.

Often, patients initially present in end-stage renal failure and must begin renal replacement therapy immediately. Hemodialysis or peritoneal dialysis can be started immediately and can be used as either definitive therapy when appropriate or as a bridge to deceased donor or living donor renal transplantation. Patients with contraindications to renal transplantation (Table 83.1) are treated with dialysis.

Prospective studies comparing the costs, quality of life, and the expected length of life of patients on hemodialysis, peritoneal dialysis, and with renal transplants have been done[7–10] and serve as the basis of the following conclusions: Quality of life with a renal transplant is superior to quality of life on peritoneal dialysis, which in turn is superior to quality of life on hemodialysis. This conclusion is true because of the greater level of independence as well as greater sense of well-being physically and psychologically. Nevertheless, transplant patients do not rate their quality of life as normal.[7] Despite the greater initial cost of renal transplantation compared to dialysis, cost-effectiveness studies have shown that if the renal transplant functions for at least 2.5 years, the transplant becomes less expensive than dialysis, and quality of life is superior.[10]

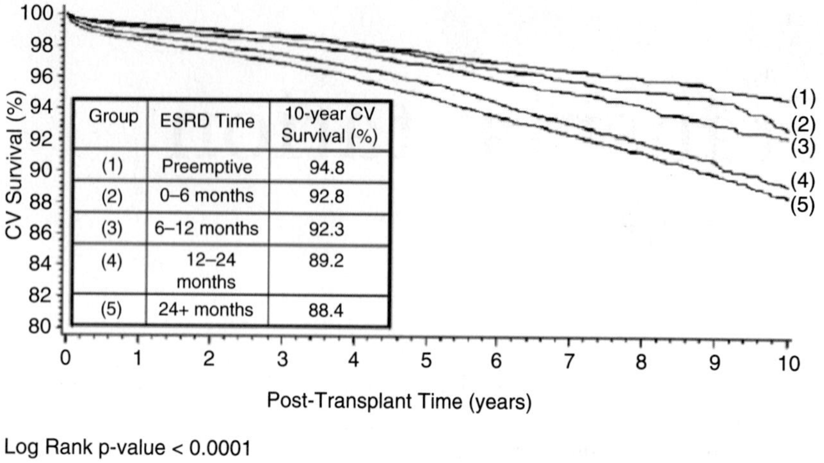

FIGURE 83.1. Kaplan-Meier plot of cardiovascular death by pretransplant dialysis time (transplants 1990–2000). (From Meier-Kriesche et al.,[6] by permission of *American Journal of Transplantation*.)

Patient survival rates can be compared among hemodialysis, peritoneal dialysis, and renal transplantation overall as well as by specific disease etiology. Hospital admissions and mortality are significantly lower for patients who have received a transplant compared to those on peritoneal dialysis or hemodialysis (Figs. 83.2 and 83.3). On average, the annual mortality among patients being treated with dialysis is nearly 25%[1] but depends on disease etiology. Diabetics with renal failure who are treated with dialysis have a 2-year survival of 30%, while those treated with renal transplantation have a 2-year survival of 70%. Patients with ESRD who are waiting for a suitable living donor or deceased donor kidney or who have a contraindication to transplantation are maintained with dialysis. Table 83.2 shows the impact of disease etiology on outcomes of renal transplantation stratified according to donor source with living donor, standard criteria deceased donor, or extended criteria deceased donor. Extended criteria deceased donor is defined as a deceased donor older than 60 years or 51–59 years with any two risk factors that include (1) history of hypertension, (2) death from cerebral hemorrhage, or (3) creatinine above 1.5 mg/dL.

Renal Transplantation

Patient Selection

Because of increasingly successful outcomes in renal transplantation, indications have expanded continually, and the average age of renal transplant recipients has risen progressively. For instance, the average age of renal transplant recipients has risen from 38 to 46 years during the cyclosporine era at the University of Wisconsin.[5] Guidelines for patient selection and evaluation have been developed by the American Society of Transplantation and have been reviewed in detail.[11] Patients interested in pursuing renal transplantation should be screened appropriately for coronary artery disease because renal failure itself, as well as hypertension, hyperlipidemia, smoking, and family history of heart disease, is a risk factor for accelerated coronary atherosclerosis. A high proportion of patients in renal failure have multiple risk factors. Noninvasive screenings using thallium stress tests are generally satisfactory, reserving cardiac catheterization for patients with positive findings by radionuclide imaging. Careful attention should be paid to addressing cardiac risk factors because cardiovascular disease accounts for the vast majority of deaths following renal transplantation. Coronary angioplasty or revascularization may be appropriate before renal transplantation.

TABLE 83.1. Contraindications to Renal Transplantation.

Cancer present
Active infection
Severe liver disease
Severe lung disease
Severe heart disease
Noncompliance with medical therapy
Active alcohol or substance abuse
Advanced systemic disease (amyloidosis, hemochromatosis)
Advanced age (relative)
Severe obesity (relative)

Frequently, patients are referred with renal failure of unknown etiology. While a biopsy is in some instances performed, it is only helpful if the patient's underlying disease carries a significant risk of recurrence in the transplanted kidney. This risk should be explained to the patient as well as their potential living donor. Table 83.3 lists the diseases that recur most commonly following renal transplantation.[12,13] Some diseases, such as immunoglobulin A (IgA) nephropathy, have a high likelihood of recurring posttransplant (50%–70%) but a low likelihood of leading to graft loss (10%). Similarly, diabetic nephropathy is likely to recur if the graft survives long enough. In most cases of type 2 diabetes, neither the patient nor the graft survives long enough for recurrence of diabetic nephropathy to be the principal cause of graft failure. In young patients with type 1 diabetes, combined pancreas-kidney transplantation prevents recurrence of diabetic nephropathy, and long-term survival is excellent.

Bilateral native nephrectomy is not indicated in most patients undergoing renal transplantation and is not helpful from an immunological standpoint.[14] Appropriate indications for bilateral native nephrectomy include recurrent pyelonephritis with significant risk of infection posttransplantation or polycystic kidney disease with significant hematuria, pain, or infected cysts. Unilateral nephrectomy would be indicated for a mass in a kidney suspicious of malignancy.

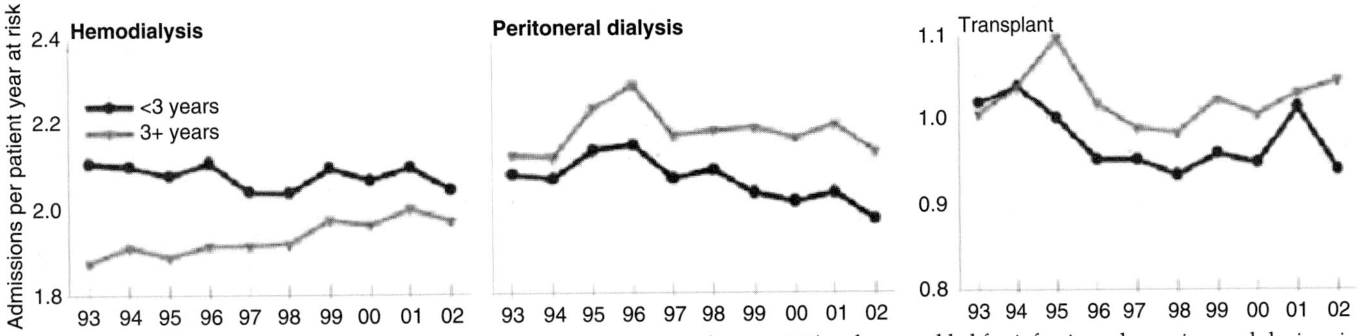

FIGURE 83.2. Adjusted hospital admissions by modality and patient vintage: prevalent patients. Period-prevalent ESRD patients; adjusted for age, gender, race, and primary diagnosis. All ESRD patients, 2002, used as reference cohort. At the end of 1998, a new *International Classification of Diseases, Ninth Revision, Clinical Modification* (*ICD-9-CM*) code was added for infections due to internal devices in peritoneal dialysis patients; data prior to this date are omitted. Note the differences in the scales of the ordinate axis. (From U.S. Renal Data System 2004 Annual Data Report.[1])

Patients with Malignancy

Because immunosuppression favors the development and recurrence of malignancies, patients with solid tumors are generally not transplanted unless they are free of disease at least 2 years following curative surgical excision. Depending on the type of tumor, a workup may be appropriate to exclude persistent or recurrent tumor. Especially for hematological malignancies, it is important to be sure that the underlying disease is indeed cured. Involvement of an oncologist experienced in management of patients with malignancy and immunosuppression is helpful. Patients with premalignant conditions, such as myeloproliferative disorders, should be carefully evaluated by oncologists experienced with hematological diseases before being considered for renal transplantation.

Infection

Patients with infections of any kind should have the infection treated completely before undergoing renal transplantation. Patients with recurrent antibiotic-resistant urinary tract infections and reflux with or without chronic pyelonephritis should be considered for pretransplant bilateral native nephrectomy. Patients with tuberculosis should be treated for 1 year with antitubercular agents and then reassessed for cure before proceeding to renal transplantation.

Compliance

Noncompliance with drug therapy, blood draws for lab testing, or follow-up visits is likely to lead to failure of a renal transplant whether the noncompliance is due to financial or nonfinancial reasons. Therefore, pretransplant assessment of compliance is crucial, although admittedly difficult. Patients who have lost a renal transplant as a result of noncompliance and who request retransplantation must be carefully screened. Often, a period of several months of hemodialysis increases compliance following retransplantation.

Immunological Considerations

Tissue Typing

All patients considered for renal transplantation undergo tissue typing to determine their HLA class I and class II types. Because acute rejection is mediated predominantly by lymphocytes, which recognize major histocompatibility complex (MHC) classes I and II, it is logical and compelling to optimize the matching of MHC antigens between donor and recipient.[15] Because of the substantial polymorphism of HLA (the human MHC) and because of the significant impact of HLA matching on renal transplant outcome, HLA typing is one criterion for donor–recipient selection[16] (see "Transplant Immunity" in "Immunology of Transplantation," chapter 80). In many tissue-typing laboratories, DNA typing of MHC is used.

Antidonor Antibody

Before performing a renal transplant, recipient serum is tested against donor lymphocytes to assess the presence of preformed antidonor antibody. Termed a *crossmatch test*, this

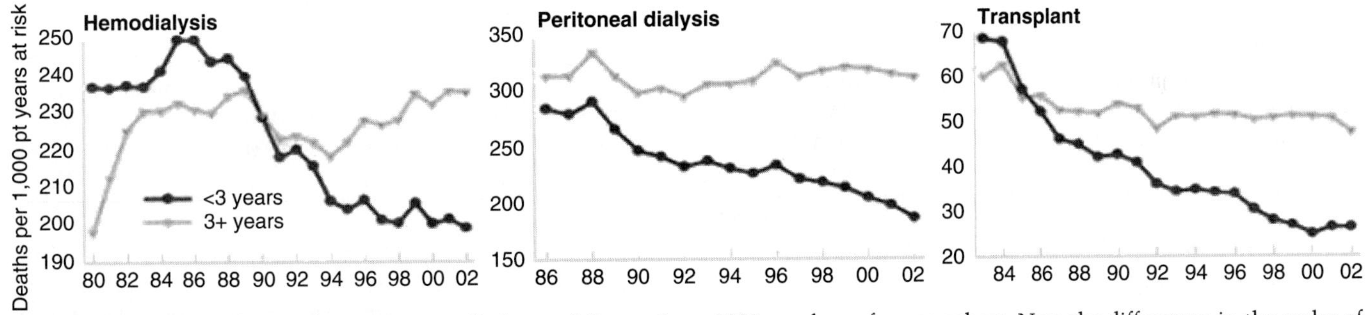

FIGURE 83.3. Adjusted mortality rates, overall, by modality and patient vintage: prevalent patients. Period-prevalent ESRD patients; adjusted for age, gender, race, and primary diagnosis. ESRD patients, 2001, used as reference cohort. Note the differences in the scales of the ordinate axis. (From U.S. Renal Data System 2004 Annual Data Report.[1])

TABLE 83.2. Distribution of Diseases Leading to First Transplant According to Donor Source.

	LD			SCD			ECD		
Disease	*N*	*1 yr (%)*	*3 yr (%)*	*N*	*1 yr (%)*	*3 yr (%)*	*N*	*1 yr (%)*	*3 yr (%)*
Diabetes									
Kidney alone	1918	95.8	88.6	1772	90.3	79.0	316	85.4	70.1
Simultaneous kidney-pancreas	19	100.0	80.0	4319	92.4	83.7	50	89.2	81.3
Hypertensive nephrosclerosis	2478	94.4	85.9	4948	89.4	76.9	1066	79.4	65.2
Unknown	3838	94.1	87.5	4173	90.0	80.8	784	79.7	63.3
Polycystic kidneys	2151	96.4	93.0	2756	93.3	87.6	526	86.6	76.8
Non-insulin-dependent diabetes mellitus (adult)	1400	93.1	86.2	2378	90.0	79.6	656	79.8	63.0
Adult diabetes	1266	92.1	83.2	1933	88.8	78.1	468	82.2	63.3
Chronic glomerulonephritis	1203	95.9	89.6	1663	91.4	81.3	261	82.7	70.8
Malignant hypertension	837	95.6	86.9	1454	90.0	77.1	270	82.3	63.1
Focal sclerosis	1188	94.6	89.7	1325	91.3	80.2	165	80.6	72.6
IgA nephropathy	1461	96.9	93.6	995	94.2	86.8	144	88.0	79.0
Systemic lupus	813	94.7	89.0	933	90.4	79.3	116	90.0	67.2
Membranous glomerulonephritis	606	95.2	86.2	647	92.9	85.3	112	86.1	77.4
Pyelonephritis	612	94.0	88.0	499	91.9	87.7	57	89.2	72.4
Focal segmental glomerulosclerosis	404	93.0	86.6	369	90.9	81.5	31	96.7	87.0
Nephritis	321	93.9	84.4	333	91.2	80.7	57	69.9	55.7
Alport syndrome	276	96.3	93.0	274	94.4	88.6	24	83.1	63.3
Congenital obstructive uropathy	376	96.5	92.1	274	90.9	83.7	29	85.3	63.6
Glomerular sclerosis	173	94.5	88.7	227	89.3	76.1	46	80.0	67.7
Hypoplasia/dysplasia	272	95.5	89.9	197	93.7		11	81.8	54.5
Postinfectious glomerulonephritis	166	94.8	86.6	174	90.7	84.3	25	87.6	70.1
Obstructive uropathy	135	94.8	90.8	142	90.6	78.2	25	72.0	55.4
Wegener glomerulomatosis	175	95.9	93.6	135	93.2	80.4	33	90.9	79.7
Membranoproliferative glomerulonephritis	90	98.8	76.8	100	93.7	86.0	15	86.7	66.0
Non-insulin-dependent diabetes mellitus (juvenile)	79	91.8	89.4	95	91.3	83.2	9	100.0	32.1
Analgesic nephropathy	76	90.6	78.5	93	91.3	81.2	20	95.0	78.4
Hemolytic uremia	112	88.7	77.8	86	87.9		7	71.4	
Nephrosclerosis	58	91.1	91.1	76	93.3	82.0	17	88.2	71.3
Membranous nephropathy	81	92.5	84.3	71	91.0	86.5	16	86.7	78.8
Familial nephropathy	57	100.0	90.9	70	91.2	84.5	9	64.8	
Goodpasture's syndrome	91	96.5	87.7	67	84.4	79.0	4		
Medullary cystic disease	60	100.0	88.2	57	94.7		2		
Renal cell carcinoma	54	92.5	82.4	54	86.5	66.9	10	77.1	61.7
Nephrolithiasis	38	97.4	92.7	50	93.9	93.9	8	87.5	
Henoch-Schönlein purpura	45	100.0	93.8	48	100.0	89.3	3		
Scleroderma	35	85.7	68.9	40	69.5	50.6	5	100.0	66.7
Sickle cell anemia	22	95.5	80.9	39	83.8		1		
Amyloidosis	45	91.9	69.4	34	85.2	76.4	12	82.5	70.7
Nephronophthisis	37	94.4	69.7	33	90.5	83.0	5	100.0	
Prune-belly syndrome	66	98.5	96.0	33	97.0	97.0	3		
Drug interstitial nephritis	37	86.4	57.6	31	90.3	90.3	8	70.0	
Type 2 glomerulonephritis	12	100.0	90.0	23	95.5	73.6	5	80.0	
Dysplasia	55	94.5	94.5	23	95.7	95.7	2		
Fabry's disease	20	95.0	86.4	22	95.2	89.3	0		
Oxalosis	22	86.4	69.4	20	89.7	89.7	1		

ECD, extended criteria deceased donor; LD, living donor; SCD, standard criteria deceased donor.

Source: From Cecka,[16] OPTN/UNOS Renal Transplant Registry, 2003.

TABLE 83.3. Recurrent Diseases in the Kidney Transplant.

Systemic diseases	*Primary renal diseases*
Systemic lupus erythematosus	Focal and segmental glomerulosclerosis
Hemolytic uremic syndrome	IgA nephropathy
Schönlein-Henoch purpura	Membranoproliferative glomerulonephritis type I
Diabetes mellitus	Membranoproliferative glomerulonephritis type II
Monoclonal gammopathies and mixed cryoglobulinemia	Membranous glomerulonephritis
Essential mixed cryoglobulinemia	Anti-GBM disease
Multiple myeloma	
Waldenström macroglobulinemia	
Light-chain deposition disease	
Fibrillary glomerulonephritis	
Wegener's granulomatosis	
Primary hyperoxaluria type I	
Cystinosis	
Fabry's disease	
Sickle cell disease	
Systemic sclerosis (scleroderma)	
Alport's syndrome	

Source: Data from Ramos and Tisher[12] and Hariharan et al.[13]

can be done either by using a standard National Institutes of Health (NIH) method or by flow cytometry. Patients awaiting a deceased donor renal transplant have serum samples tested monthly to assess for panel reactive antibody (PRA). The PRA test measures the patient's serum against a standard panel of cells from different donors who are theoretically representative of the regional donor population. Patients who have a positive crossmatch with a high proportion of the panel are highly sensitized, and it is more difficult to identify a crossmatch-negative donor for them. Such patients typically wait for a renal transplant for a prolonged period. They in particular benefit from national sharing of zero-mismatched kidneys. Renal transplantation in the setting of a positive crossmatch test is contraindicated because the risk of hyperacute rejection is greater than 85%.[17,18] The risk of hyperacute rejection in the setting of a negative T-cell crossmatch is close to 0%. Recently, some centers treat patients who have antidonor antibody with plasmapheresis or intravenous immune globulin to remove alloantibody, converting the crossmatch test to negative (or positive at low titer only) and render transplantation in such patients successful.[19] Similarly, donor–recipient pairs incompatible in ABO blood type may with treatment undergo successful transplantation.[20]

TABLE 83.4. Criteria for Brain Death.

Prerequisite

All appropriate diagnostic and therapeutic procedures have been performed, and the patient's condition is irreversible. The patient is free of sedative drugs or hypothermia.

Criteria (to be present for 30 min at least 6 h after the onset of coma and apnea)

1. Coma
2. Apnea (no spontaneous respirations)
3. Absent cephalic reflexes (pupillary, corneal, oculoauditory, oculovestibular, oculocephalic, cough, pharyngeal, and swallowing)

Confirmatory tests

Absence of cerebral blood flow by radionuclide brain scan

Absence of electrical activity by electroencephalogram

Source: From Van der Werf et al.,[21] by permission of *Surgical Clinics of North America*.

TABLE 83.5. Absolute and Relative Contraindications to Deceased Donor Kidney Donation.

Absolute	*Relative*
Malignancy outside central nervous system	Age >70 years
Prolonged warm ischemia	Age <3 years
Sepsis/active infection	Hypertension
Human immunodeficiency virus	Hepatitis B, C virus
	Intravenous drug abuse
	Prolonged cold ischemia
	Acute tubular necrosis in older donors
	Donor diabetes of long duration
	Biopsy showing >20% glomerulosclerosis

ABO Matching

A donor–recipient pair must generally be ABO compatible. Otherwise, hyperacute rejection mediated by complement-fixing preformed natural antibody is very likely. Some groups are performing renal transplantation in ABO-incompatible donor–recipient combinations using living donors, but this is a high-risk proposition.[20]

Procurement and Preservation of Deceased Donor Kidneys

Any patient who has been declared brain dead or is to be withdrawn from life support is a potential multiorgan (including kidney) donor. *Brain death* is defined as complete and irreversible loss of all brain and brainstem function and presents clinically as apnea, brainstem areflexia, and cerebral unresponsiveness. Table 83.4 lists criteria for brain death.[21]

Evaluation of a potential kidney donor includes obtaining history on the mechanism of death, length of time during cardiac or pulmonary arrest, duration of hypotension, vasopressor use, and donor social and medical history. Laboratory evaluation includes measurement of serum creatinine, serum urea nitrogen (BUN), electrolytes, hemoglobin, white blood cells (WBCs), arterial blood gas, urinalysis, prothrombin time/partial thromboplastin time, ABO typing, and viral screening, including evaluation for hepatitis B, hepatitis C, human immunodeficiency virus (HIV), human T-lymphotrophic virus (HTLV) 1, and cytomegalovirus (CMV). Table 83.5 lists contraindications to deceased donor kidney donation.

Use of the Marginal Donor

Table 83.6 summarizes the number of patients in 2002 awaiting deceased donor renal transplantation, the number of deceased donors, the number of kidneys recovered from these donors, and the number of kidneys transplanted in the United States.[2] The distribution of waiting times for deceased donor renal transplants is shown in Figure 83.4.[1] Because only about

TABLE 83.6. Kidneys Transplanted in the United States, 2002.

Number of kidneys transplanted	14,523
Number of deceased donor kidneys transplanted	8,287
Number of living donor transplants	6,236
Number of patients awaiting kidney	50,855

Source: From OPTN/SRTR 2003 Annual Report.[2]

one-fourth of patients on the waiting list are transplanted each year, there continues to be an interest in expanding the donor pool to make kidney transplantation available to more needy recipients.

Increasing experience with marginal donors who do not meet one of the relative contraindications listed in Table 83.5 suggests that these kidneys ultimately function well. Terasaki et al. have shown the usefulness of matching older donor kidneys with older recipients because the older recipients have lower muscle mass and shorter potential longevity.[22] A donor kidney biopsy demonstrating less than 15% glomerulosclerosis may be used as a criterion to transplant kidneys from older donors. Use of donors after cardiac death (DCD) is another potential way to expand the donor pool by as much as 20%. Before the acceptance of brain death criteria, DCD donors were the sole type of kidney retrieved for transplantation, and this practice is now returning. Although a period of warm ischemia associated with the DCD donor may lead to a higher acute tubular necrosis (ATN) rate and higher discharge creatinine, the 10-year graft survival of 52% reported for DCD donors was similar to the graft survival of 45% for brain dead donors.[23]

Donors with a serum creatinine above 2.5 mg/dL may be considered as kidney donors. Despite ATN from hypotension, kidneys from a young donor will usually recover after transplantation, especially if rehydration prior to donation results in a fall in creatinine and continued diuresis.

Deceased donors with a history of hypertension, diabetes, or age greater than 55 years are considered extended criteria donors and have been shown to be associated with slightly poorer outcomes. Therefore, it is recommended that this reality be discussed with kidney transplant recipients in advance of the transplant so that informed consent is obtained to use these kidneys.

Donor Management

Following declaration of brain death, it is crucial for the donor to receive appropriate medical management to optimize successful organ recovery. Increased intracranial pressure following head injury or cerebrovascular accident results in a massive catecholamine release in an effort to compensate for cerebral ischemia by increasing systemic pressure.[24] However, after the brain becomes necrotic, catecholamine levels drop to less than 10% of baseline within hours.[25] Such patients have often been managed by a strategy of dehydration to minimize brain edema. These factors in combination often result in a hemodynamically unstable donor who is vasodilated. Most brain dead donors also develop diabetes insipidus, which exacerbates hypovolemia. Diabetes insipidus is managed by replacing urine output (mL/mL) with hypotonic crystalloid solution. When urine output exceeds 200 mL/h, vasopressin (Pitressin) is administered at a dose of 40 U/L at 120 mL/h for 15 min and repeated every 4 h. Alternatively, desmopressin (DDAVP) can be given at a dose of 1 to 2 mg every 8 h.

Hypothalamic regulation of body temperature is lost in up to 86% of donors.[26] Hypothermia shifts the oxygen dissociation curve to the left and results in more diuresis from renal tubules. It is important to maintain the donor's body temperature. Systolic blood pressures are maintained above 100 mmHg using blood or crystalloid resuscitation as appropriate to maintain a hematocrit of 25% to 30%. Dopamine, norepinephrine, phenylephrine, and epinephrine infusions may be necessary. In summary, the goal of preoperative and intraoperative donor management is to maintain adequate intravascular volume, tissue oxygenation, and normothermia.

Donor Nephrectomy

Isolated Renal Procurement

If only the kidneys are to be procured from the donor abdomen, a midline abdominal incision is used for exposure. Supraceliac aortic control is attained. The right colon and distal small bowel are mobilized from their retroperitoneal attachments. The duodenum is mobilized to expose the inferior vena cava

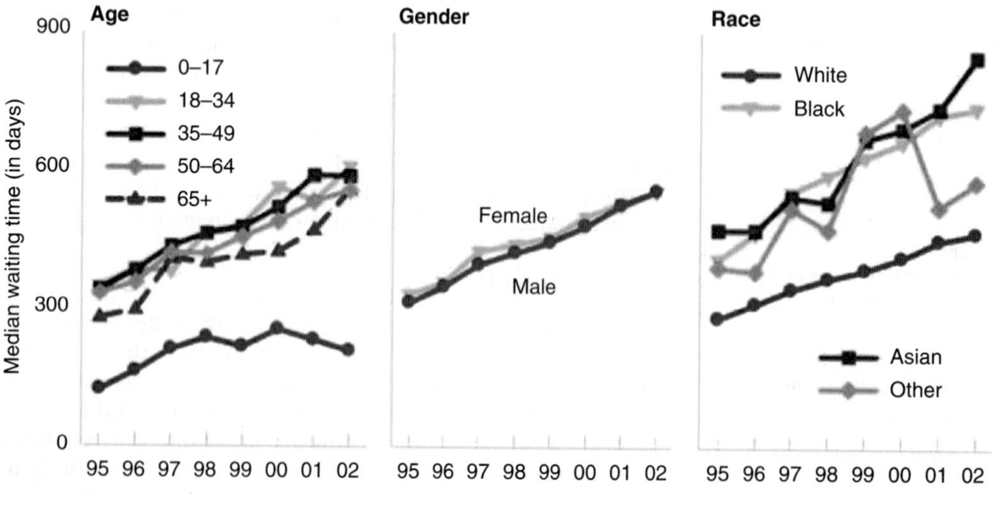

FIGURE 83.4. Waiting times, by age, gender, and race. Patients receiving deceased donor, kidney-only first transplants; unadjusted. Year is the year of transplant, not the year the patient was first listed. (From U.S. Renal Data System 2004 Annual Data Report.[1])

and left renal vein. The adrenal and gonadal branches of the left renal vein are ligated. The distal aorta is cannulated, and the donor is administered 20,000U heparin and 10mg phentolamine (Regitine). The supraceliac aorta is cross-clamped, the vena cava is divided, and 1L of ice-cold University of Wisconsin (UW) solution is infused through the aorta cannula. The kidneys are bathed in iced saline. When the aortic flush is complete, the renal veins are divided at the level of the vena cava to leave a patch of vena cava attached to the left renal vein and the remainder of the vena cava attached to the shorter right renal vein. The aorta is opened anteriorly, and all renal arteries are identified and preserved with a Carrel patch of aorta. The ureters are divided distal to where they cross the iliac vessels, and care is taken to avoid skeletonizing or devascularizing the ureters. The retroperitoneal attachments to the kidney are divided, and the kidneys are excised and transferred to a back table, where they are flushed with 250 to 500mL of cold UW solution or until the effluent is clear.

If the donor nephrectomy is part of a multivisceral procurement, the foregoing procedure should be incorporated into the liver and pancreas procurement as the last step. Dissection of the kidneys from the retroperitoneum should be delayed until final nephrectomy because dissection generally induces vasospasm.

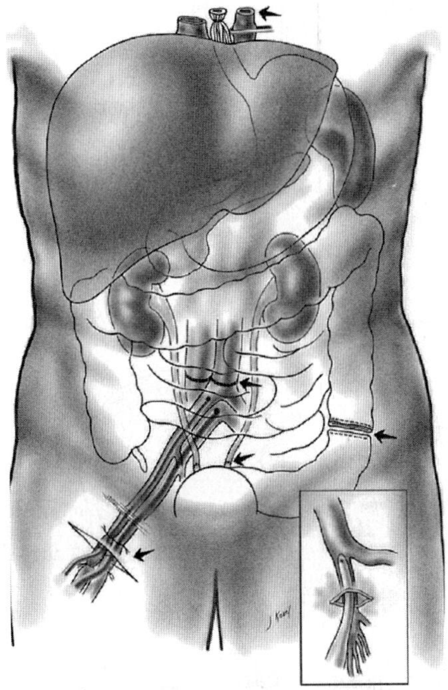

FIGURE 83.5. Technique of combined hepatic, pancreatic, and renal retrieval. *Arrows* indicate major steps in en bloc removal of intra-abdominal organs. *Insert* depicts flush-out of portal circulation through a branch of the superior mesenteric vein. (From D'Alessandro et al.,[27] by permission of *Transplantation*.)

Nephrectomy After Donor Cardiac Death

In nephrectomy after donor cardiac death, ventilatory support is withdrawn in the intensive care unit or in the operating room according to the family's wishes. Heparin and phentolamine are administered as above, and the donor is extubated. Once cardiopulmonary arrest and death are declared by a physician not associated with the transplant team, a midline incision is made, and the kidneys are removed quickly and flushed with cold UW solution on the back table.

If procurement is to include the liver and pancreas, the procedure is as follows (Fig. 83.5). The femoral artery and vein are cannulated before withdrawing support if the family has consented to this. Support is then withdrawn. The femoral artery catheter is used to flush the patient with iced UW solution as soon as death is declared. A midline incision is made from the manubrium to the pubis to open chest and abdomen. The aorta is clamped above the diaphragm. All abdominal viscera are removed en bloc during the cooling process after stapling and dividing the esophagus and rectum. The ureters are divided at the bladder, and the entire abdominal viscera are excised. Organs are individually flushed on ice on the back table. Excellent results have been obtained transplanting kidneys from non-heart-beating donors using this method.[27]

Recipient Operation

Regardless of the source of the donor kidney, the preferred site for implantation of the kidney in the recipient is the right pelvis, heterotopically implanting the kidney on the right-sided iliac vessels. The operation is performed through a right lower quadrant oblique incision. The right is preferable to the left because the iliac vein is more superficial, but some surgeons place a right kidney on the left and a left kidney on the right to keep the renal pelvis anterior to the renal vessels should the pelvis need to be accessed. The peritoneum is reflected medially, and the common, external, and internal iliac artery and vein are exposed. The donor renal vein is anastomosed end-to-side to either the right external iliac vein, common iliac vein, or inferior vena cava. The donor renal artery is anastomosed end-to-side to the right common or external iliac artery. An alternative is to anastomose the renal artery end-to-end to the divided internal iliac artery. Following completion of the vascular anastomoses, the kidney is reperfused.

The ureter is then anastomosed to the bladder using one of several acceptable techniques. The Leadbetter-Politano approach is an open technique performed through an anterior cystostomy and tunneling the ureter through the posterior wall of the bladder.[28] The Lich-Gregoire technique is an extravesical approach that is technically less challenging.[29] Modifications of these techniques have been described,[30] including right native nephrectomy and ureteropyelostomy using the native right ureter to anastomose to the pelvis of the transplanted kidney. The abdominal wall incision is then closed. Figure 83.6 shows the completed kidney transplant procedure.

The patient may be administered furosemide (100mg) and mannitol (12.5g) to encourage diuresis. However, if no diuresis ensues, intraoperative and postoperative management is aimed at maintaining euvolemia, an adequate hemoglobin concentration, normal blood pressure, and good oxygen delivery. Primary nonfunction resulting from donor factors, preservation injury, or recipient immune response will not respond to diuretics. Patients with initial good function following renal transplantation have a better outcome than patients who experience ATN and require dialysis posttransplant.[31] A native nephrectomy is generally not performed at the time of renal transplantation.

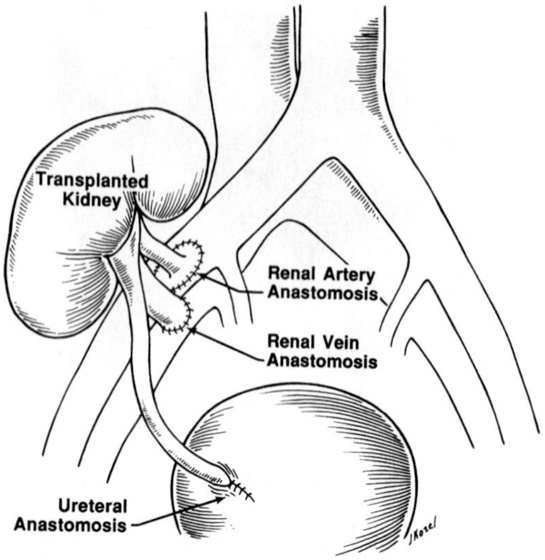

FIGURE 83.6. Completed kidney transplant procedure showing vascular anastomoses to iliac vessels and ureteroneocystostomy.

Postoperative Complications and Their Management

Thrombosis

Renal artery or renal vein thromboses are rare (<1% incidence) but are devastating because they almost always result in loss of the renal allograft as their recognition and treatment with thrombectomy are generally not performed rapidly enough (within an hour of occurrence) to salvage the graft. The diagnosis is made by sudden drop in urine output and an ultrasound showing no flow through the renal artery or vein. Renal vein thrombosis may be heralded by gross hematuria. The patient should return to the operating room for exploration and possible transplant nephrectomy because the acutely thrombosed kidney will ultimately cause fever and systemic illness unless removed. Thrombosis occurring years after kidney transplantation as a result of gradual rejection is not clinically apparent in most cases and does not require transplant nephrectomy.

Urine Leak/Obstruction

A urine leak following renal transplantation presents with local pain and tenderness over the kidney, falling urine output, rise in creatinine, and an ultrasound showing fluid collection around the kidney. Alternatively, a radionuclide scan demonstrates extravasation of urine into the retroperitoneum. This complication should be managed surgically in an urgent manner by opening the transplant incision and repairing the leak.

The diagnosis of urinary obstruction is made most directly by ultrasound showing hydronephrosis. If the cause of obstruction is bladder outlet obstruction or neurogenic bladder dysfunction, this should resolve with Foley catheter placement and repetition of the renal transplant ultrasound 24h later. If hydronephrosis persists despite decompression of the bladder with a Foley catheter, a percutaneous nephrostomy tube can be placed in the renal pelvis by an invasive radiologist. A Whitaker test may be performed by infusing saline through the nephrostomy tube and measuring pressures. Pressures should be less than 12cm H_2O. A ureterogram can be performed by injecting dye through the nephrostomy tube to identify the site of obstruction.

Short strictures, most commonly at the site of the ureteroneocystostomy, can be balloon dilated and stented using the percutaneous nephrostomy as access. However, longer strictures are generally caused by ischemic injury of the transplant ureter and consequent fibrosis and require surgical repair. Short strictures not responding to balloon dilation and stenting also require surgical repair. Typically, pyeloureterostomy or ureteroureterostomy using the ipsilateral native ureter is the operation of choice. The proximal native ureter can be ligated with impunity in at least 90% of cases and the distal ureter anastomosed to the transplant renal pelvis or ureter. The spatulated ends of the two ureters are anastomosed over a double-J stent. The stent is removed cystoscopically 4 to 6 weeks later.

Lymphocele

Because of the retroperitoneal dissection involved in the renal transplant procedure, lymphatics in this area may be disrupted and leak a significant amount of lymph into the potential space surrounding the renal transplant. If such a fluid collection becomes substantial, it may compress the adjacent iliac vein, causing leg edema, and ultimately compress the transplant ureter, causing urinary obstruction. The diagnosis is made clinically by a swollen leg on the side of the kidney transplant and a rise in the serum creatinine. The diagnosis is confirmed by ultrasound demonstrating a substantial (i.e., >4cm in diameter) fluid collection adjacent to the kidney with hydronephrosis.

Although percutaneous drainage and injection of sclerosing agents have been attempted, these methods are generally unsuccessful, and surgical repair is indicated. While open surgical drainage by creation of a peritoneal window is effective, laparoscopic lymphocele drainage has proven to be an effective remedy for the peritransplant lymphocele.[32] By inserting the laparoscopic camera through a periumbilical incision, the lymphocele can generally be visualized as a bulge in the retroperitoneum with a bluish tint. This collection may be aspirated to confirm the presence of straw-colored fluid before using electrocautery to create a peritoneal window between the lymphocele and the peritoneal cavity. The peritoneal surfaces are usually able to reabsorb this lymphatic fluid.

Acute Rejection/Ruptured Kidney

Severe acute rejection may result in graft loss if it is unresponsive to antirejection therapy. Severe acute rejection may be manifested by a swollen tender kidney with marked enlargement of the kidney by ultrasound. A severely swollen kidney is at high risk for rupture, especially if percutaneously biopsied. Therefore, ultrasound should be performed before attempting to biopsy the kidney, and if it is markedly enlarged, the biopsy should be aborted. A ruptured kidney is diagnosed clinically by a fall in the hematocrit and a tender enlarged kidney. This is a surgical emergency and should be managed by opening the transplant incision, evacuating hematoma, and obtaining hemostasis by wrapping the kidney in a material such as Surgicell. Remarkably, most of the kidneys do not need to be removed and can be salvaged by this technique combined with antirejection therapy.

A severe acute rejection episode unresponsive to antirejection therapy may also progress to thrombosis of the kidney; this can be diagnosed by radionuclide imaging study showing absent blood flow to the kidney. Kidneys undergoing severe acute rejection with graft loss in this manner should be removed because the necrotic kidney will cause systemic illness and fever.

Renal Artery Stenosis/Pseudostenosis

Transplant renal artery stenosis can be diagnosed clinically by extreme sensitivity to cyclosporine or tacrolimus (calcineurin inhibitor, CNI) therapy. Because these drugs cause constriction of the renal afferent arteriole, when this occurs in series with a proximal renal artery stenosis the patient's creatinine may rise precipitously following CNI administration. Such patients also commonly present with fluid retention, a rise in serum creatinine, and worsening hypertension. The diagnosis requires either a renal transplant arteriogram or gadolinium magnetic resonance imaging (MRI). If the patient's serum creatinine has not been chronically elevated (>3.0 mg/dL), this lesion is worth repairing quickly to restore normal renal function. A variety of surgical techniques can be used. Bypass of the stenosis using a segment of donor (third-party) iliac artery of a compatible blood type is an attractive option. Alternatively, balloon angioplasty, if feasible, may be effective and spare the patient another operation.[33]

As older patients and patients with advanced vascular disease are more commonly undergoing renal transplantation, *pseudorenal artery stenosis* is becoming more common. This term refers to a clinical syndrome mimicking renal artery stenosis but actually caused by atherosclerotic plaque in the iliac artery proximal to the transplant renal artery. This can be addressed either by balloon angioplasty (which risks distal embolization to the kidney), aortofemoral bypass, or endarterectomy.

Living Donor

Living donors are screened for overall health to ensure that they are at low risk for a general anesthetic and a major surgical procedure. Second, they must have no evidence of risk factors for renal failure, such as hypertension, diabetes, or underlying kidney disease. Serum urea nitrogen and creatinine are measured, although a glomerular filtration rate (GFR) test is not routinely done. Urinalysis is checked to rule out proteinuria or hematuria. Blood type compatibility, tissue typing, and crossmatching are assessed. Finally, an arteriogram or a spiral computed tomographic (CT) scan is performed to identify the vascular anatomy of the kidneys and to assess for presence of multiple renal arteries. The kidney with the fewest arteries is generally chosen for removal. The advantage of the spiral CT is that it also screens for a renal parenchymal mass. Alternatively, an intravenous pyelogram (IVP) and arteriogram can be done to accurately delineate the vascular anatomy and collecting system of the donor.

Donors are usually adults between the ages of 18 and 60 years, although older donors have been used successfully, and minors may be used as well. Although most donors have traditionally been blood relatives of the recipient, a substantial number of living-unrelated renal transplants have been done, primarily between spouses, but sometimes between individuals with no emotional or personal relationship.[34] Criteria for living donors are under continual review by the United Network for Organ Sharing (UNOS) and by local institutional review boards (IRBs). It is illegal to sell organs for transplantation in the United States. Programs are in place to pair recipients of different families who may have blood type incompatibility with their own family donor but share blood type with the other family's donor.[35]

Living Donor Nephrectomy: Open Technique

The open donor nephrectomy technique has been traditionally used for living-related transplantation, although the laparoscopic donor nephrectomy has received recent attention and is described below. Using the open technique, the patient under general anesthesia is placed in the lateral decubitus position. A flank incision is made below the costal margin and dissection carried down through Gerota's fascia to the kidney. To obtain exposure, the tip of the 12th rib may be resected, although this is typically not necessary. Care must also be taken to avoid entering the pleural space, but if this occurs, a chest tube is placed. The ureter is identified and is ligated distally to allow procurement of at least 15 cm of ureter. The donor renal artery and vein are dissected free, with care taken to preserve all renal artery branches. The renal artery and vein are ligated as close to the aorta and inferior vena cava as possible to preserve vessel length on the donor kidney. The kidney is excised and immediately flushed with iced preservation solution. The vessels are prepared for implantation, and if there are multiple renal arteries, these are reconstructed on the back table. Heparin typically does not need to be administered before removal of the kidneys, although this may be advantageous, particularly if there are multiple vessels.

Laparoscopic Donor Nephrectomy

Laparoscopic donor nephrectomy has been advanced as a means of reducing the morbidity associated with donor nephrectomy and has become the predominant surgical method at most large U.S. transplant centers. Advantages include shorter hospital stay, less postoperative pain, and more rapid return to normal activity. The disadvantage is that advanced laparoscopic surgical experience is required.[36,37]

From a laparoscopic perspective, the left kidney is preferable to the right for laparoscopic nephrectomy because its renal vein is longer and has a thicker wall. Laparoscopic left donor nephrectomy is performed with the donor in the right lateral decubitus position. The patient is draped to allow for a standard left flank incision as well as the midline, permitting conversion to an urgent laparotomy if necessary. Following creation of a 15-mmHg carbon dioxide pneumoperitoneum, three 12-mm operating ports and one 5-mm port are placed in the left subcostal and flank regions. A 15-mm operating port is placed later during the operation through a 6- to 7-cm midline incision used for kidney extraction.

The splenic flexure of the colon is taken down from its retroperitoneal attachments. The renal vein and artery and ureter are dissected free. To avoid early graft dysfunction, the donor is vigorously hydrated during the procedure. The kidney is mobilized from its fatty attachments after opening Gerota's fascia. The patient is systemically anticoagulated before division of the renal artery and vein. A laparoscopic stapler is used to divide the renal vessels. An extraction incision is made in a Pfannenstiel manner (lower transverse abdominal), and the kidney is excised and removed using an extraction bag.

Centers experienced in laparoscopic nephrectomy have achieved excellent results, as measured by graft function and survival and perioperative morbidity to the donor.[36] An alternative to the method described above is a hand-assisted laparoscopic approach that is a hybrid of open and laparoscopic approaches. Robotic assistance for laparoscopic donor nephrectomy is also being performed at an increasing number of centers.[38]

Medical Complications and Their Management

Diagnosis of Renal Dysfunction

Table 83.7 lists the differential diagnosis of renal transplant dysfunction, dividing causes into early and late and subdividing early complications into surgical (covered earlier) and medical. Acute rejection is the most common cause of early graft dysfunction. Its diagnosis can be accurately based on histological evaluation of a needle biopsy. A biopsy can be safely performed under ultrasound guidance with the additional benefit of the ultrasound, excluding other complications such as hemorrhage, hydronephrosis, thrombosis, and lymphocele. The histology of renal transplant biopsies is classified according to the Banff criteria.[39] Treatment of acute, hyperacute and chronic rejection are discussed in the preceding chapter (see "Rejection" chapter 81). Additional information obtainable from a biopsy includes ischemic injury, ATN, recurrence of original disease, CNI toxicity, vascular rejection, or chronic rejection. With the exception of the swollen tender kidney, which is susceptible to rupture at the time of biopsy, a renal transplant biopsy can be performed safely in the setting of graft dysfunction. Of acute rejection episodes, 85% occur during the first year posttransplant.[40]

Although a successfully treated rejection episode may result in a return of the serum creatinine to baseline levels, patients who have one or more rejection episodes are at increased risk of graft loss compared to patients without rejection.[31] Repeated episodes of acute rejection appear to increase the risk of chronic rejection. Initial good function of a kidney transplant also favors a successful long-term outcome.[31] Patients who require dialysis posttransplant have poorer graft survival compared to patients not dialyzed posttransplant.[31]

TABLE 83.7. Differential Diagnosis of Renal Transplant Dysfunction.

Surgical/mechanical	*Medical*
Early	Early
Lymphocele	Acute rejection
Urine leak	Ureteral obstruction
Renal artery stenosis	Delayed graft function
Vascular thrombosis	Acute CNI nephrotoxicity
	Prerenal/volume contraction
	Drug toxicity
	Infection
	Recurrent disease
Late	Late
Ureteral obstruction	Acute or chronic rejection
Renal artery stenosis	CNI nephrotoxicity, drug toxicity
	Volume contraction
	Infection
	De novo/recurrent disease

Urinary tract infection is the most common infection occurring following renal transplantation and occasionally is accompanied by transplant pyelonephritis causing a rise in serum creatinine. Hypovolemia may cause a rise in creatinine and can be related to dehydration from vomiting, diarrhea, or glucosuria in poorly controlled diabetics. Excessive use of diuretics may also be responsible.

Nephrotoxicity related to CNIs results from vasoconstriction of afferent arterioles of the kidney, which in turn leads to hypertension. Acute CNI toxicity is reversible with a reduction in CNI dose. The CNIs can also cause structural damage characterized by endothelial proliferation of arterioles, causing obliterative arteriopathy.[41–43] This then results in ischemic injury to tubules and a striped pattern of interstitial fibrosis. These ultrastructural changes in the kidney are irreversible. Although long-term injury from CNI has raised concern about long-term therapy, the safety and efficacy of long-term CNI therapy is well documented in renal transplant recipients, and the danger of CNI withdrawal is late rejection in 20% to 40% of patients.[44,45]

Chronic rejection remains one of the unsolved problems in renal transplantation. It is defined histologically by interstitial fibrosis, neointimal hyperplasia with narrowing of the arteriolar lumen, and a characteristic glomerulopathy with reduplication of the glomerular basement membrane seen on silver stain. There is no effective treatment for chronic rejection, and it generally leads to inexorable deterioration of graft function. Its cause remains poorly defined but probably includes specific and nonspecific immunological injury as well as nonimmunological causes. Despite improvements in immunosuppressive therapy over the past 25 years with a marked reduction in graft loss due to acute rejection, there has not been a coincident decline in the rate of chronic rejection of long-surviving renal allografts.[3,31]

Cardiovascular Disease

Fifty percent of deaths in renal transplant patients are caused by cardiovascular disease, making it the most common cause of death following transplantation.[5] Transplant patients commonly have multiple risk factors for cardiovascular disease, including hypertension, hyperlipidemia, and diabetes. Many patients also have a smoking history and family history of cardiovascular disease. Improving long-term patient survival requires intensive management of cardiovascular factors. Table 83.8 lists the advantages and disadvantages of antihypertensive drugs in transplant recipients. Patients with difficult-to-control hypertension who are on three or more antihypertensive drugs may benefit from native nephrectomy.

Hyperlipidemia

Posttransplant hyperlipidemia is manifested by increased or unchanged triglyceride and high-density lipoprotein (HDL) levels and by increased low-density lipoprotein (LDL) and total cholesterol levels.[46] Patients treated with tacrolimus have lower LDL and total cholesterol levels than patients treated with cyclosporine. Pharmacological therapy of hyperlipidemia is problematic in renal transplant patients because of potential side effects. Table 83.9 lists agents useful in managing hyperlipidemia in renal transplant patients. Close monitoring of side effects is necessary with these agents.

Infection

During the first month posttransplant, infections are most commonly of bacterial origin and related to urinary tract infection, line sepsis, pneumonia, or wound infection. Between 30 and 90 days, fever not caused by bacterial infection is most often due to CMV infection. The risk of CMV infection is increased when the donor or recipient is seropositive for CMV infection before transplant. Prophylaxis with acyclovir or ganciclovir significantly reduces the incidence of posttransplant CMV infection, and these drugs are used to effectively treat infection as well.

Routine prophylaxis with trimethoprim-sulfamethoxazole (TMP-SMX) has made *Pneumocystis carinii* infection rare in transplant patients. Prophylaxis is continued for 1 year after transplantation. After the first 6 months following successful renal transplantation, opportunistic infections become less likely.

TABLE 83.9. Pharmacological Agents Useful in Posttransplant Hyperlipidemia.

Drug	*Side effects*	*Recommendations*
Cholestyramine/ colestipol	Poor compliance	Schedule doses 1–2 h after immunosuppressive therapy
	May interfere with drug absorption	
Niacin	Hepatotoxicity	Monitor closely
	Hyperuricemia	Aspirin to prevent flushing
	Hyperglycemia	
	Flushing	
Gemfibrozil inhibitors	Hepatotoxicity	Do not use with HMG-CoA inhibitors
	Myositis	Monitor hepatic enzymes
HMG-CoA inhibitors	Hepatotoxicity	Do not use with gemfibrozil
	Myositis	Low dose preferred

Malignancy

Skin cancers occur 100 times more commonly in renal transplant patients compared to the general population because of immunosuppressive therapy. Infection with papillomavirus may be related, as is significant sun exposure. Infection with Epstein-Barr virus (EBV) may lead to posttransplant lymphoproliferative disease (PTLD), particularly in patients on high doses of immunosuppressive drugs. Posttransplant lymphoproliferative disease presents with fever and adenopathy with or without graft dysfunction. Successful treatment requires early diagnosis based on EBV serologies and histological evaluation of lymphoid tissue and, most recently, DNA analysis based on polymerase chain reaction (PCR). Withdrawal of immunosuppressive drugs is the most important step in therapy. Kidney transplant patients do not appear to be at increased risk for carcinomas of solid tissue.[47]

TABLE 83.8. Advantages and Disadvantages of Antihypertensive Drugs in Transplant Recipients.

Class	*Advantages and indications*	*Potential side effects*
Diuretics	Salt-sensitive hypertension	Hyperuricemia
		Adverse impact on lipids
β-Blockers	Large selection	Adverse impact on lipids (some)
	Selective agents preferred	Relative contraindication in diabetes and vascular disease
α-Blockers	Young patients	Postural hypotension (first dose)
	Clonidine useful in diabetic patients	Rebound hypertension with clonidine
Calcium channel blockers	Improve renal blood flow	Verapamil and diltiazem increase CNI levels
	May ameliorate CNI nephrotoxicity	
	Nifedipine/isradipine preferred	
ACE inhibitors	Native kidney hypertension	May precipitate renal failure
		Anemia with enalapril

Outcomes

The UNOS compiles the national data on transplant statistics from U.S. centers. The oversight of the data is managed by the U.S. Organ Procurement and Transplantation Network and the Scientific Registry of Transplant Recipients.[2] The United States Renal Data System also publishes the data with respect to renal disease annually.[1] The following results summarize U.S. national data for renal transplantation.

Figures 83.7 and 83.8 show graft and patient survival associated with deceased donor kidney transplants and living donor kidney transplants, respectively.[1] Apparent from these results is the substantial benefit of living donor kidney transplants compared to deceased donor transplants and the gradually improving outcomes in more recent years related to improvements in patient management.

Recipients who required dialysis within the first week posttransplant had lower graft and patient survival rates at all time points than those who did not require dialysis. Graft survival rates for the dialysis group were 80% at 1 year and 53% at 5 years posttransplant, compared with 91% at 1 year and 67% at 5 years posttransplant for the nondialysis group.

Since 1995, the 1-year graft survival rate has steadily improved but without a change in late graft failure (Figs. 83.7 and 83.8).[1] For deceased donor kidney transplants, the 1-year graft survival rate was 87%; the 1-year patient survival rate

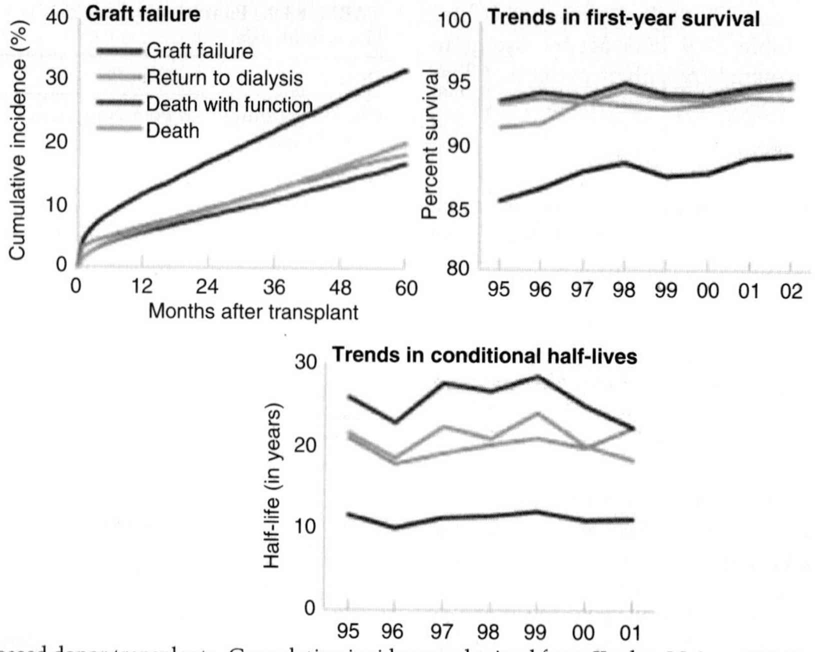

FIGURE 83.7. Survival: deceased donor transplants. Cumulative incidences obtained from Kaplan-Meier estimate, 1998–2002 combined. Half-life estimates are conditional on first-year graft survival. (From U.S. Renal Data System 2004 Annual Data Report.[1])

was 95%. Patient survival rates for recipients with diabetes were lower at all time points than for recipients with any other diagnosis. Deceased donor kidney transplants with a zero HLA mismatch had the highest graft survival rates at all time points.

The influence of race on renal transplant outcomes is demonstrated by the relatively poorer graft survival among black recipients. Conversely, Asian recipients had better graft survival rates than any other race.

The substantial improvement during the past 20 years in patient and graft survival following kidney transplantation is the result of multiple factors, including improved diagnostic methods, more effective immunosuppressive agents, and better infection prophylaxis. As the success rate for renal transplantation has improved over the past 20 years, so has the demand for its application to patients with renal failure. There must be a significant increase in organ donation if this demand is to be met successfully.

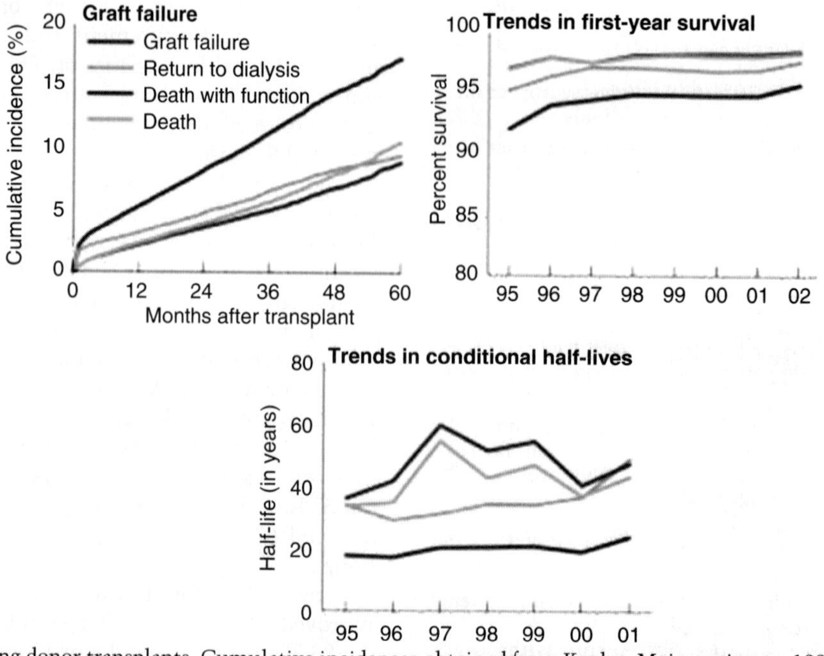

FIGURE 83.8. Survival: living donor transplants. Cumulative incidences obtained from Kaplan-Meier estimate, 1998–2002 combined. Half-life estimates are conditional on first-year graft survival. (From U.S. Renal Data System 2004 Annual Data Report.[1])

References

1. U.S. Renal Data System. USRDS 2004 Annual Data Report: Atlas of End-Stage Renal Disease in the United States, National Institutes of Health, National Institute of Diabetes and Digestive and Kidney Diseases, Bethesda, MD. Available at: www.usrds.org.
2. HHS/HRSA/SPB/DOT, UNOS, URREA. 2003 OPTN/SRTR Annual Report: Transplant Data 1993–2002. Available at: www.ustransplant.org.
3. Meier-Kriesche HU, Ojo AO, Port FK, et al. Survival improvement among patients with end-stage renal disease: trends over time for transplant recipients and wait-listed patients. J Am Soc Nephrol 2001;12:1293–1296.
4. Pastan S, Bailey J. Dialysis therapy. N Engl J Med 1998;338:1428–1437.
5. Knechtle SJ, Pirsch JD, D'Alessandro AM, et al. Renal transplantation at the University of Wisconsin in the cyclosporine era. In Terasaki PI, Cecka JM, eds. Clinical Transplants 1993. Los Angeles: UCLA Tissue Typing Laboratory; 1994;211–218.
6. Meier-Kriesche HU, Schold JD, Srinivas TR, et al. Kidney transplantation halts cardiovascular disease progression in patients with end-stage renal disease. Am J Transplant 2004;4:1662–1668.
7. Laupacis A, Keown P, Pus N, et al. A study of the quality of life and cost-utility of renal transplantation. Kidney Int 1996;50:235–242.
8. Krmar RT, Eymann A, Ramirez JA, Ferraris JR. Quality of life after kidney transplantation in children. Transplantation 1997;64:540–541.
9. Joseph JT, Baines LS, Morris MC, Jindal RM. Quality of life after kidney and pancreas transplantation: a review. Am J Kidney Dis 2003;42:431–445.
10. Karam VH, Gasquet I, Delvart V, et al. Quality of life in adult survivors beyond 10 years after liver, kidney, and heart transplantation. Transplantation 2003;76:1699–1704.
11. Danovitch GM, Hariharan S, Pirsch JD, et al. for the Clinical Practice Guidelines Committee of the American Society of Transplantation. Management of the waiting list for cadaveric kidney transplants: report of a survey and recommendations by the Clinical Practice Guidelines Committee of the American Society of Transplantation. J Am Soc Nephrol 2002;13:528–535.
12. Ramos EL, Tisher CC. Recurrent diseases in the kidney transplant. Am J Kidney Dis 1994;24:142–154.
13. Hariharan S, Adams MB, Brennan DC, et al. Recurrent and de novo glomerular disease after renal transplantation: a report from Renal Allograft Disease Registry (RADR). Transplantation 1999;68:635–641.
14. Odorico JS, Knechtle SJ, Rayhill SC, et al. The influence of native nephrectomy on the incidence of recurrent disease following renal transplantation for primary glomerulonephritis. Transplantation 1996;61:228–234.
15. Sayegh MH, Turka LA. The role of T-cell costimulatory activation pathways in transplant rejection. N Engl J Med 1998; 338:1813–1821.
16. Cecka JM. The OPTN/UNOS Renal Transplant Registry 2003. In Cecka JM, Terasaki PI, eds. Clinical Transplants 2003. Los Angeles: UCLA Immunogenetics Center; 2004;1–12.
17. Kissmeyer-Nielsen F, Olsen S, Petersen VP, Fjeldborg O. Hyperacute rejection of kidney allografts, associated with pre-existing humoral antibodies against donor cells. Lancet 1966;2:662–665.
18. Patel R, Terasaki PI. Significance of the positive crossmatch test in kidney transplantation. N Engl J Med 1969;280:735–739.
19. Gloor JM, DeGoey S, Ploeger N, et al. Persistence of low levels of alloantibody after desensitization in crossmatch-positive living-donor kidney transplantation. Transplantation 2004; 78:221–227.
20. Stegall MD, Dean PG, Gloor JM. ABO-incompatible kidney transplantation. Transplantation 2004;78:635–640.
21. Van der Werf WJ, D'Alessandro AM, Hoffmann RM, Knechtle SJ. Procurement, preservation, and transport of cadaver kidneys. Surg Clin North Am 1998;78:41–54.
22. Terasaki PI, Cho YW, Cecka JM. Strategy for eliminating the kidney shortage. In Cecka JM, Terasaki PI, eds. Clinical Transplants 1997. Los Angeles: UCLA Tissue Typing Laboratory; 1998;265–267.
23. D'Alessandro AM, Hoffmann RM, Belzer FO. Non-heart-beating donors: one response to the organ shortage. Transplant Rev 1995;9:168–176.
24. Chen EP, Bittner HB, Kendall SW, Van Trigt P. Hormonal and hemodynamic changes in a validated animal model of brain death. Crit Care Med 1996;24:1352–1359.
25. Novitzky D, Wicomb WN, Cooper DKC, et al. Electrocardiographic, hemodynamic and endocrine changes occurring during experimental brain death in the chacma and baboon. J Heart Transplant 1984;4:63–69.
26. Griepp RB, Stinson EB, Clark DA, et al. The cardiac donor. Surg Gynecol Obstet 1971;133:792–798.
27. D'Alessandro AM, Hoffmann RM, Knechtle SJ, et al. Successful extrarenal transplantation from non-heart-beating donors. Transplantation 1995;59:977–982.
28. Politano VA, Leadbetter WF. An operative technique for the correction of vesicoureteral reflux. J Urol 1958;79:932–941.
29. Mangus RS, Haag BW, Carter CB. Stented Lich-Gregoir ureteroneocystostomy: case series report and cost-effectiveness analysis. Transplant Proc 2004;36:2959–2961.
30. Knechtle SJ. Ureteroneocystostomy for renal transplantation. J Am Coll Surg 1999;188:707–709.
31. Cecka JM. The UNOS Scientific Renal Transplant Registry—10 years of kidney transplants. In Cecka JM, Terasaki PI, eds. Clinical Transplants 1997. Los Angeles: UCLA Tissue Typing Laboratory; 1998;1–14.
32. Gruessner RW, Fasola C, Benedetti E, et al. Laparoscopic drainage of lymphoceles after kidney transplantation: indications and limitations. Surgery 1995;117:288–295.
33. Sankari BR, Geisinger M, Zelch M, et al. Post-transplant renal artery stenosis: impact of therapy on long-term kidney function and blood pressure control. J Urol 1996;155:1860–1864.
34. D'Alessandro AM, Pirsch JD, Knechtle SJ, et al. Living unrelated renal donation: the University of Wisconsin experience. Surgery 1998;124:604–611.
35. Ross LF, Rubin DT, Siegler M, et al. Ethics of a paired-kidney-exchange program. N Engl J Med 1997;336:1752–1755.
36. Flowers JL, Jacobs S, Cho E, et al. Comparison of open and laparoscopic live donor nephrectomy. Ann Surg 1997;226:483–490.
37. Ratner LE, Kavoussi LR, Sroka M, et al. Laparoscopic assisted live donor nephrectomy—a comparison with the open approach. Transplantation 1997;63:229–233.
38. Horgan S, Benedetti E, Moser F. Robotically assisted donor nephrectomy for kidney transplantation. Am J Surg 2004;188:45S–51S.
39. Racusen LC, Halloran PF, Solez K. Banff 2003 meeting report: new diagnostic insights and standards. Am J Transplant 2004;4:1562–1566.
40. Pirsch JD, Friedman R. Primary care of the renal transplant patient. J Gen Intern Med 1994;9:29–37.
41. Mihatsch MJ, Thiel G, Spichtin HP, et al. Morphological findings in kidney transplants after treatment with cyclosporine. Transplant Proc 1983;15:2821.
42. Nankivell BJ, Borrows RJ, Fung CL, et al. Calcineurin inhibitor nephrotoxicity: longitudinal assessment by protocol histology. Transplantation 2004;78:557–565.

43. Nankivell BJ, Borrows RJ, Fung CL, et al. The natural history of chronic allograft nephropathy. N Engl J Med 2003;349:2326–2333.
44. Stoves J, Newstead CG, Baczkowski AJ, et al. A randomized controlled trial of immunosuppression conversion for the treatment of chronic allograft nephropathy. Nephrol Dial Transplant 2004;19:2113–2120.
45. Bakker RC, Hollander AA, Mallat MJ, et al. Conversion from cyclosporine to azathioprine at three months reduces the incidence of chronic allograft nephropathy. Kidney Int 2003;64:1027–1034.
46. Miller LW. Cardiovascular toxicities of immunosuppressive agents. Am J Transplant 2002;2:807–818.
47. Morath C, Mueller M, Goldschmidt H, et al. Malignancy in renal transplantation. J Am Soc Nephrol 2004;15:1582–1588.

84

Pancreas and Islet Transplantation

Robert C. Harland and Marc R. Garfinkel

Diabetes mellitus is a systemic disease that currently affects 6% of the population and ranks as the third most common disease.[1] In the United States, 1 to 2 million of these people have type 1 diabetes mellitus, previously referred to as juvenile-onset diabetes.[2] Type 1 diabetes is characterized by deficient insulin production due to destruction of insulin-producing beta cells in the pancreas. The etiology of this cell destruction has not been fully elucidated, but autoimmune attack, genetic factors, and environmental influences, including infectious agents, have all been implicated. Some insulin-deficient patients have glucose intolerance from loss of pancreas function following pancreatitis, with or without surgical pancreatic resection. Such patients are also insulin deficient and have many of the characteristics and complications seen in patients with autoimmune type 1 diabetes.

Insulin-deficient diabetics require exogenous insulin administration to avoid hyperglycemia and ketoacidosis. While the discovery of insulin provided a method to prolong the life of the diabetic, it also led to the discovery of the many long-term complications of diabetes. Diabetes is currently the leading cause of end-stage renal disease. Approximately 100,000 people with diabetes undergo dialysis or kidney transplantation each year.[3] Diabetes is also the leading cause of new cases of blindness in adults. Diabetic retinopathy causes from 12,000 to 24,000 new cases of blindness each year.

Diabetes is also the leading disease cause of amputations and impotence. Abnormal glucose control is associated with accelerated atherosclerosis and abnormalities in lipid metabolism, making it a leading contributor to cardiovascular deaths.[4] The disruption of daily life by the need for glucose monitoring and insulin administration in otherwise young active patients, combined with the chronic complications described above, leads to diabetes as a significant contributor to health care costs.[5,6] It is estimated that the total direct and indirect medical costs of diabetes, including disability, work loss, and premature mortality, exceeds $100 billion per year in the United States.

The progression of some of the complications of diabetes can be slowed by intensive control of hyperglycemia. This was demonstrated convincingly by the Diabetes Control and Complication Trial, although tight glucose control was complicated by a significant increase in the incidence of hypoglycemic events.[7] Transplantation of a vascularized pancreas allograft (and, possibly, isolated islet transplantation) is currently the only therapy that reliably establishes a euglycemic state without the need for exogenous insulin therapy, normalizing the glycosylated hemoglobin level in previously hyperglycemic type 1 diabetics.

The rate of pancreas transplantation has increased dramatically since 1980, but it still remains a relatively uncommon procedure. Figure 84.1 demonstrates that slightly more than 1300 pancreas transplants were performed in the United States in 2003, a rate that lags behind most other solid-organ transplants and appears to have leveled off since 2000. A number of factors might be responsible for this, including a practice of only transplanting those pancreata procured from "ideal" donors and the existence of fewer appropriate recipient candidates on the waiting list compared to other organs. In recent years, funding for simultaneous pancreas and kidney (SPK) transplantation, pancreas-after-kidney (PAK) transplant, and even pancreas transplant alone (PTA) has become standard for many insurance providers, including Medicare.

Anatomy and Physiology

The pancreas is a mixed exocrine and endocrine organ with the majority of its mass composed of acinar cells that secrete bicarbonate and digestive enzymes. Scattered throughout the gland are 1 to 2 million endocrine cells in clusters called the islets of Langerhans. These cells arise as part of the APUD (amine precursor uptake and decarboxylation) system. Within these clusters, beta cells provide insulin, alpha cells secrete glucagon, and delta cells are a source of somatostatin.

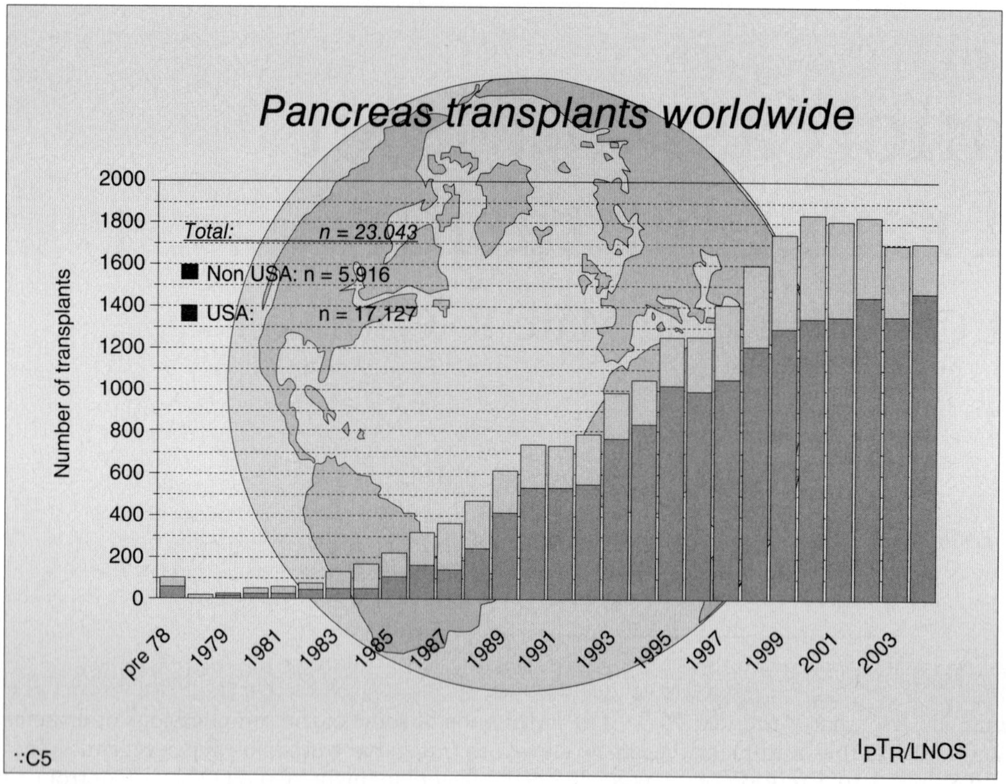

FIGURE 84.1. Annual number of pancreas transplants reported to the International Pancreas Transplant Registry (IPTR). Reporting is obligatory in the United States but not elsewhere. Non-U.S. transplants are likely underrepresented. (From International Pancreas Transplant Registry, Department of Surgery, University of Minnesota, Minneapolis.)

Additional cells located in islets secrete other hormones, including pancreatic polypeptide, gastrin, and vasoactive intestinal peptide.[8] The ability to provide only the endocrine tissue for a diabetic patient without the surrounding exocrine tissue is attractive and increasingly successful and is discussed at the end of this chapter. Nonetheless, transplantation of the entire vascularized exocrine and endocrine pancreas, including a portion of the donor duodenum, has been to date the most reliably successful method of treating diabetes through transplantation.

Recipient Selection

The initial challenge of clinical pancreas transplantation is the selection of appropriate recipients. The rate of development of diabetic complications is variable, as is their severity, making it difficult to discern which patients might benefit from pancreas transplantation. At this point in time, the risks of the surgical procedure combined with the long-term risks and cost of immunosuppressive medications has largely limited the application of pancreas transplantation to those patients with established secondary diabetic complications. The most common of these is diabetic nephropathy, which occurs in 40% to 50% of type 1 diabetics. The ability to treat end-stage diabetic nephropathy with renal transplantation, either before or simultaneously with pancreas transplantation (SPK), has resulted in most pancreas transplants (90%) being performed in diabetics who have significant renal involvement.[9]

The majority of these patients undergo SPK transplantation. Simultaneous transplantation confers the economic benefits of only one transplant procedure and the associated hospitalization. Furthermore, the ability to detect (by monitoring the serum creatinine) and diagnose (by renal biopsy) rejection allows early detection and treatment of rejection, thereby reducing immunologic pancreas graft loss. Finally, the observation that pancreas graft survival is consistently better in SPK recipients compared to recipients of pancreas transplants alone may be due to the relatively immunosuppressed state induced by uremia.[10]

An increasing number of type 1 diabetics with nephropathy undergo pancreas transplantation at some time after successful kidney transplantation (PAK).[9] As more patients are listed for SPK transplantation and waiting times increase, many patients with a suitable living donor may opt for immediate renal transplantation with a subsequent PAK transplant. This strategy allows elective transplantation utilizing a living donor kidney, with the known benefits of better immediate and long-term renal function. This strategy essentially "adds a kidney" to the pool of available organs for transplantation into patients with end-stage renal disease. After recovery from kidney transplantation, deceased donor pancreas transplant alone (PTA) can then be performed. Monitoring for pancreas transplant rejection can be more challenging in PAK transplants, but improved immunosuppression and alternative monitoring methods have led to graft survival that is close to or equal to that seen in SPK transplant recipients.[9]

Currently, fewer than 10% of pancreas transplants are performed in patients who have only mild renal impairment or normal renal function. These PTA procedures are most often performed in patients with demonstrated progressive secondary complications such as neuropathy (autonomic or peripheral), proliferative retinopathy, or early nephropathy (proteinuria with a serum creatinine of 2.0). The presence of hyperlabile diabetes, especially the occurrence of frequent hypoglycemic episodes, is a further indication to pursue PTA.[11]

The challenge for those contemplating PTA transplantation is the achievement of benefits that outweigh the risks of a surgical procedure and the need for chronic immunosuppression. The appropriateness of PTA has been challenged by Venström et al.,[12] who analyzed United Network of Organ Sharing (UNOS) data to demonstrate an increased mortality (relative risk of death) for PTA compared to patients on the waiting list. This conclusion was challenged by Gruessner et al.,[13] who observed no increase in mortality after PTA versus remaining on the waiting list and suggested that unaccounted multiple listings and PTA wait list removal for deteriorating kidney function and renal transplantation as confounding factors in the Venström study. Nonetheless, this debate supports the contention that PTA be reserved for selected patients with brittle diabetes, hypoglycemic unawareness, or progressive neuropathy.

Pretransplant Evaluation

The presence of a chronic systemic disease mandates a thorough, multidisciplinary pretransplant evaluation of all potential pancreas transplant recipients. This workup should include a determination of the patient's ability to withstand a major operation and an assessment of the social and psychological state of the patient with attention to the potential for noncompliance. Specific attention should be given to the cardiovascular evaluation, which should include routine noninvasive rest and stress cardiac testing. Coronary angiography was often performed routinely in all potential candidates in the past but is less necessary with improved noninvasive testing.[14] Smoking constitutes a contraindication to pancreas transplantation at our institution. The presence of coronary disease is not an absolute contraindication to transplantation, although revascularization with angioplasty or coronary artery bypass grafting may first be required to safely undergo the transplant procedure.[15]

Cadaver Donor Selection, Preservation, and Preparation

Cadaver donors in the age range of 8 to 55 years without a history of diabetes or pancreatic trauma have generally been utilized for pancreas transplantation. Donors less than 20 to 25 kg may present a technical challenge due to the small size of the vasculature and corresponding low graft perfusion rates. Age-related loss of islet mass occurs and may limit the success rate of pancreas transplants from older cadaver donors. Indeed, in one study, the use of donors older than 45 years was associated with an elevated glycosylated hemoglobin in recipients, an increased need for oral hypoglycemic use, and a lower graft survival rate.[16] An extended period of time (15 h) between the occurrence of brain death and organ procurement has been shown to be an independent risk factor for pancreas graft failure in a single-center study.[17] Donor hyperglycemia has been shown to have a deleterious effect on allograft function in some, but not all, series. In general, hyperglycemia or hyperamylasemia is not an absolute contraindication to successful pancreas procurement and transplantation.[18,19]

The observation has been made that the presence of significant fatty infiltration of the pancreas as well as significant pancreatic edema are associated with poor pancreas graft outcome. This has placed a great deal of importance on subjective assessment by an experienced transplant surgeon in the operating room to determine whether a pancreas is acceptable for transplantation.[18]

Simultaneous procurement of the liver, kidneys, and other organs can occur in essentially all donors despite vascular anomalies.[20,21] The splenic artery is divided just distal to its origin from the celiac axis, and the superior mesenteric artery is preserved as the blood supply for the head of the pancreas. An aberrant right hepatic artery arising from the superior mesenteric artery is a frequent anomaly but can almost always be separated from the posterior aspect of the pancreas, allowing successful transplantation of both liver and pancreas. Especially in the presence of arterial anomalies, en bloc procurement of liver and pancreas with back-table dissection can avoid in situ manipulation and assist in the identification of aberrant anatomy to preserve the arterial blood supply of all transplanted organs. Preservation with an intraarterial infusion of University of Wisconsin (UW) solution (Viaspan, Dupont) is universally used in North America; this allows safe cold storage for at least 24 h without compromise of graft function,[22] although more recently organ preservation with histidine-tryptophan-ketoglutarate preservation solution has also gained acceptance.[23]

Living Donor Versus Deceased Donor Pancreas Transplantation

Experience with living donor, segmental pancreas transplantation is largely limited to the University of Minnesota. This institution has reported a series with more than 100 such transplants.[24] While the risk of immunological graft loss is less than that seen with cadaver pancreas transplants, the incidence of graft loss to thrombosis was much greater (18.5%) in living donors, most likely due to the segmental nature of the living donor transplant with a relatively low blood flow. This, combined with the potential morbidity for the donor (including a risk of glucose intolerance), has decreased the enthusiasm for living donor transplantation.[25] Still, some living donor transplants are reported each year, including those performed with simultaneous living donor renal transplantation.[26,27] One suggested indication for such transplants is the recipient who is highly sensitized and thus unlikely to locate a crossmatch-negative deceased donor.

Operative Procedure

Back-Table Preparation

Topical hypothermia is maintained in a bath of preservation solution while the arterial supply of the pancreas is reconstructed. Usually, a Y-graft of donor iliac artery is utilized to join the superior mesenteric artery and the splenic artery of the pancreas graft (Fig. 84.2). The portal vein is generally left quite short (1–2 cm) to avoid kinking and subsequent thrombosis. The staple lines on the duodenum are oversewn, as are the mesenteric vascular branches on the anterior surface of the pancreas.

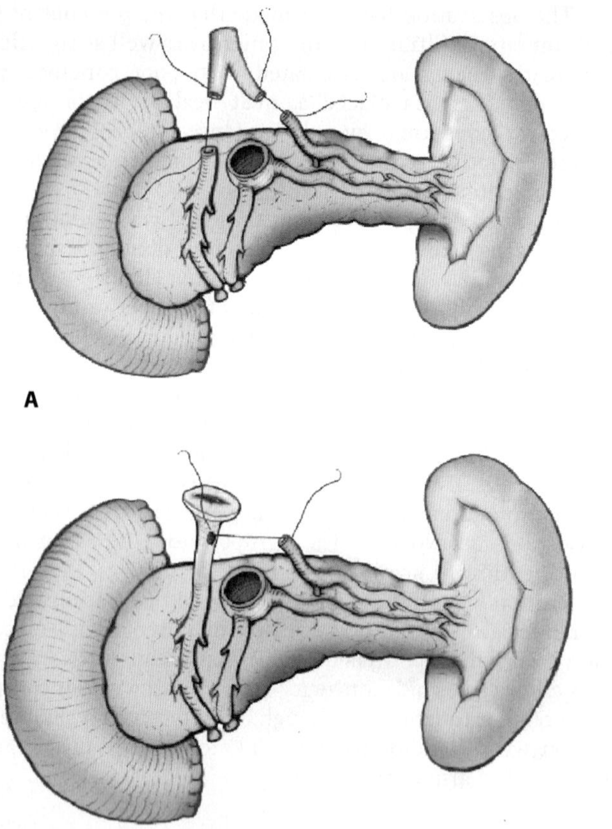
A

B

FIGURE 84.2. A. Donor iliac artery conduit is anastomosed to the splenic artery and the superior mesenteric artery of the pancreas on the back table. **B.** Alternatively, the blood supply to the donor pancreas can be reconstituted by direct anastomosis of the splenic artery to the superior mesenteric artery.

Systemic Venous Drainage Versus Portal Venous Drainage

The pancreas is usually transplanted in the right iliac fossa to the mobilized iliac vein or inferior vena cava. The Y-graft of donor iliac artery is anastomosed to the iliac artery (Fig. 84.3). In this position, the donor duodenum can easily be attached to the bladder to drain the exocrine output of the pancreas.

More physiological insulin secretion might be observed with venous outflow from the pancreas to the portal system. To accomplish this, the portal vein of the transplanted pancreas is anastomosed to a branch of the superior mesenteric vein (SMV) inferior to the transverse mesocolon. Arterial inflow is accomplished via the donor iliac artery graft attached to the iliac artery or to the aorta and tunneling this conduit through a defect created in the small bowel mesentery (Fig. 84.4). This allows more physiological glucose control, avoiding the hyperinsulinemia observed in systemically drained transplants. Hyperinsulinemia has been associated with elevated serum lipid levels and atherosclerosis.[26] The attachment of the venous outflow of the pancreas to the portal system may also confer an immunological advantage. The Memphis group, in a single-center series, observed nearly a 50% decrease in rejection episodes occurring in the kidney and in the pancreas in SPK recipients who had portal venous drainage versus systemic venous drainage of their pancreas transplants. There was a similar decrease in the number of pancreas grafts lost to rejection.[28] A subsequent report from the same group[29] demonstrated the safety of this technique in a series of 126 patients. Although bladder drainage of exocrine secretions is usually not possible with portal venous drainage, enteric anastomosis to the proximal recipient jejunum is easily accomplished.

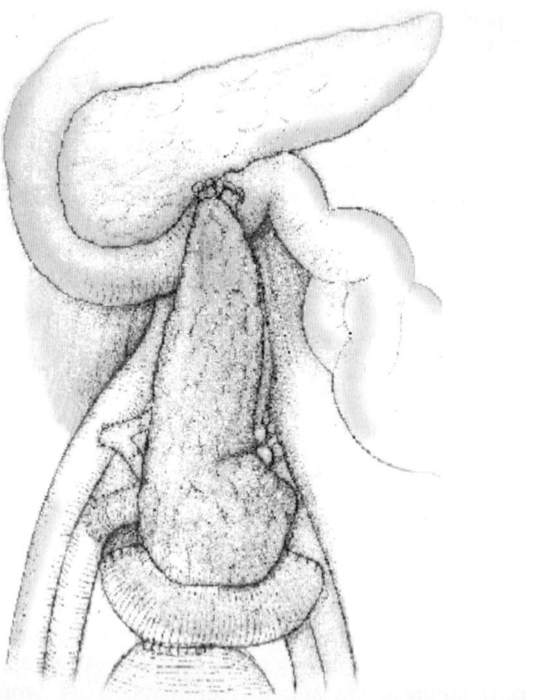

FIGURE 84.3. Pancreas transplant in the right lower quadrant with systemic venous drainage to the iliac vein and exocrine drainage via duodenocystostomy.

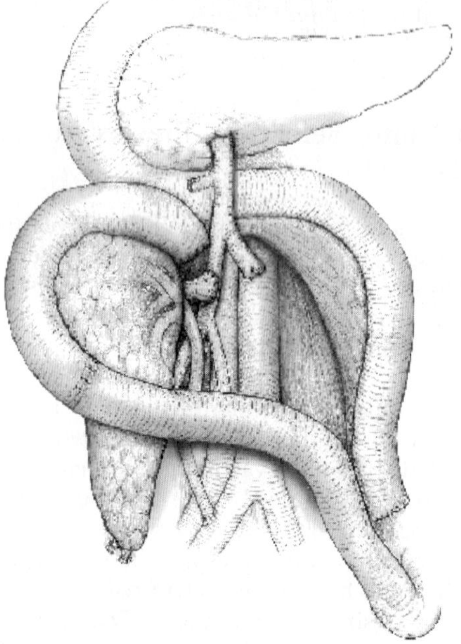

FIGURE 84.4. Pancreas transplant with venous drainage to the portal system via the superior mesenteric vein and enteric drainage of exocrine secretions to a Roux-en-Y limb of jejunum.

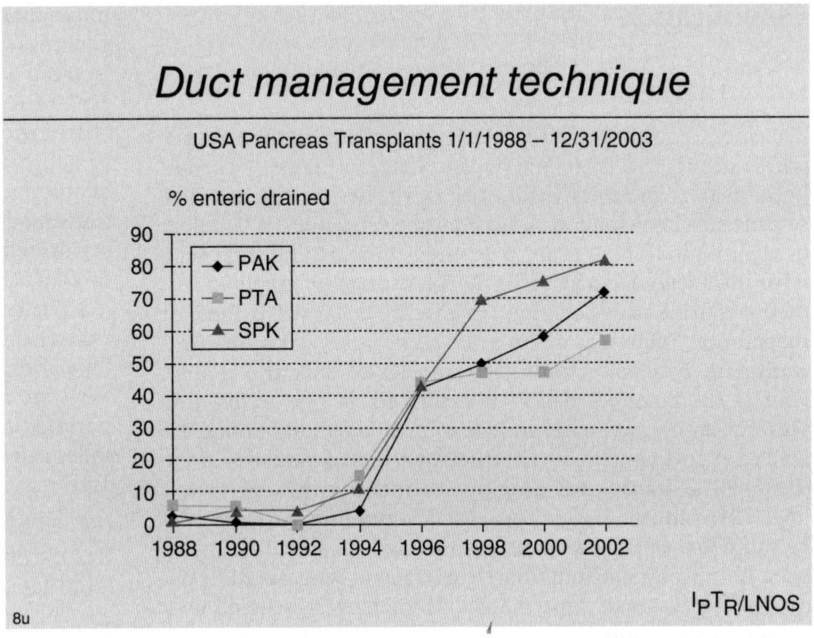

FIGURE 84.5. Duct management technique as percentage of transplants performed by category with enteric drainage (vs. bladder drainage). Note that today most are done with enteric drainage, a change from the 1980s and early 1990s. (From International Pancreas Transplant Registry 2004 annual report.)

Bladder Drainage Versus Enteric Drainage of Exocrine Secretions

Throughout the 1980s and early 1990s bladder drainage of the exocrine output of the pancreas was preferred as it had been demonstrated to be superior to enteric drainage.[30] This finding was attributed to a decreased risk of intraabdominal infection and the ability to monitor the pancreas transplant with urinary amylase secretion. Bladder-related and metabolic complications, including cystitis, dehydration, and metabolic acidosis (from the loss of bicarbonate-rich pancreatic exocrine secretion into the bladder), however, plagued many pancreas recipients managed by bladder drainage.

In recent years, there has been increased interest in and performance of enteric drainage of pancreas transplants. Currently, more than half of pancreas transplants performed in the United States utilize the enteric drainage technique (see Fig. 84.5).[31] Not only does this avoid many of the urological and metabolic complications seen in bladder-drained transplants, it also allows the option of portal venous drainage of the transplant with improved glucose control while avoiding hyperinsulinemia, as described above. Enteric drainage can be performed with either a Roux limb or a side-to-side anastomosis between the transplant duodenum and the small intestine.

More recently, enteric drainage via an "omega" reconstruction, in which a direct side-to-side anastomosis between transplant duodenum and recipient jejunum is combined with a jejunojejunostomy between segments proximal and distal to the site of anastomosis to the pancreas, has been described.[32] This technique, currently routinely employed at the University of Chicago, allows the advantages of the Roux-en-Y reconstruction without the need for dividing the bowel or its mesentery.

Demartinesa et al.[33] conducted an evidence-based analysis of pancreas transplantation outcomes, including bladder versus enteric drainage, and concluded that there is no difference in graft survival rate between the two techniques. However, from their analysis of six studies, the authors concluded that the use of enteric drainage reduced the incidence of urological complications, anastomotic leaks, and opportunistic infections, thus favoring enteric drainage overall as the technique of choice.

Immunosuppression

When comparing SPK transplant recipients to recipients of kidney transplants alone, several series demonstrated a 50% to 100% increase in the incidence of acute rejection episodes,[34,35] suggesting that pancreas transplant recipients require a greater degree of immunosuppression than recipients of kidney-alone transplants. The use of either a polyclonal or monoclonal anti-T-cell induction agent was shown to be effective in improving the outcome of both the kidney and the pancreas in such transplants, despite the increased rate of acute rejection.[36] Incremental improvements in graft survival have been observed with the introduction of newer, more potent agents. This is especially true with the addition of mycophenolate mofetil to the immunosuppressive armamentarium. Many centers now base therapy on the more potent calcineurin inhibitor tacrolimus. Clinical observations suggest that even better results will be observed with the use of interleukin (IL)-2 receptor-blocking agents. Both daclizumab and basiliximab have been effective in reducing the incidence of acute rejection episodes in renal allotransplantation, and more recently, the benefits of induction therapy have been demonstrated in an evidence-based analysis of five trials using these agents in pancreas transplant recipients as well.[33]

Complications

Graft Thrombosis

The most common cause of early graft loss is thrombosis, which occurs in 5% to 19% of pancreas transplants.[37] Thrombosis usually presents with a rise in the serum glucose. The serum amylase may or may not be elevated. A nuclear medicine blood flow scan, computed tomographic (CT) scan with intravenous contrast, or Doppler ultrasonography documents a lack of blood flow to the transplanted organ. At reoperation, infarction of the pancreas is observed and requires transplant pancreatectomy. Thrombosis of only the splenic vein of the pancreas has been described. In one series, this was not associated with graft loss in SPK recipients but did lead to eventual graft loss in three-quarters of pancreas-alone (PAK, PTA) transplants despite treatment with heparin followed by warfarin for 6 to 8 weeks.[38] Nonuremic patients may be more susceptible to pancreas thrombosis since they may have better platelet function than patients who are dialysis-dependent. In most centers, aspirin therapy is utilized as a preventive measure. Hemorrhagic complications have been seen with routine use of more aggressive anticoagulation.

Pancreatitis and Exocrine Leaks

Graft pancreatitis is observed in as many as one-third of recipients and may be associated with prolonged preservation times or an elevated serum amylase in the donor. The etiology of pancreatitis may be related to preservation injury or reflux of bladder contents. In severe cases, a picture very similar to that seen in native pancreatitis can be seen, including fever, hypovolemia, and renal dysfunction. Intraabdominal fluid collections may develop and can lead to intraabdominal abscesses.

Similarly, a leak of exocrine secretions from the transplanted duodenum or its anastomosis to either the bladder or recipient intestine can lead to intraabdominal fluid collections that contain digestive enzymes. One or more abdominal explorations may be required if percutaneous drainage does not result in rapid improvement.[39] At exploration, attempted repair of the leak and drainage of the area may be attempted, but graft pancreatectomy is the most reliable way of improving the patient's health and should be applied early in unstable patients or in those with significant intraabdominal infection.

Rejection

Symptoms of pancreas transplant rejection can include fever and graft tenderness. The serum amylase and lipase may be elevated, and in bladder-drained transplants, urinary amylase excretion will decrease. These findings are relatively sensitive but are not very specific for rejection. Other tests, such as measurement of soluble HLA and serum anodal trypsinogen, have demonstrated some correlation with rejection but have not had widespread application.[40] The glucose disappearance curve obtained by a brief (1-h) glucose tolerance test has proven useful as an indicator of graft dysfunction.[41]

For those patients undergoing SPK transplantation, the best indicator of rejection is evidence of renal dysfunction. In more than 75% of cases, rejection is observed in both the pancreas and kidney transplanted from the same donor. Isolated pancreas rejection can occur, however, in as many as 20% of SPK transplant patients who have a rejection episode. Histological confirmation of pancreas transplant rejection can be achieved by biopsy of the transplanted pancreas. Percutaneous core biopsies and fine-needle aspiration, as well as transduodenal biopsies via the cystoscope, have all been performed and provide adequate tissue on which to make therapeutic decisions.[42]

Treatment of acute rejection episodes consists of an initial trial of methylprednisolone boluses given for 3 to 5 days. If the patient fails to have an adequate response, then treatment with an antilymphocyte agent, usually Thymoglobulin, is initiated and continued for 7 to 14 days. Most rejection episodes can now be reversed without significant long-term graft dysfunction.

Recurrence of Autoimmune Islet Destruction

The hypothesis that transplanted islets are also susceptible to autoimmune attack has been tested by the performance of at least nine living donor pancreas transplants between identical twin siblings. The initial three transplants were performed without immunosuppression, and isletitis and recurrent diabetes developed within 3 months.[43] The next identical twin recipient was treated with azathioprine and required 4 years before recurrence of diabetes was observed.[44] The last four cases that have been reported were treated with cyclosporine and azathioprine, but at doses lower than that usually utilized in nontwin allografts. These patients have all demonstrated freedom from recurrent diabetes with normal histology of their transplanted pancreas from 1 to more than 7 years posttransplant.[45,46] This is in concordance with the observation that immunosuppressive agents can modify the autoimmune islet destruction seen in early type 1 diabetes.[47] The universal use of immunosuppression for allografts explains why recurrence of diabetes has not been observed in patients receiving pancreatic allografts.

Urological Complications

Urological complications, including hematuria, urinary tract infections, leak from the duodenocystostomy, urethritis, and urethral strictures, have been observed following bladder-drained pancreas transplantation. Hematuria may be caused by mucosal damage from digestive enzymes. Urinary tract infections can be related to foreign bodies, such as sutures, in the bladder as well as the high urine pH caused by bicarbonate excretion by the pancreas. Duodenocystostomy leaks can present with graft pancreatitis, urgency, and urinary frequency.[48]

Some of these complications can be treated conservatively with bladder catheter drainage and appropriate medical care. Persistent or recurrent symptoms should be treated with operation, usually conversion from bladder drainage to enteric drainage (Fig. 84.5). Overall, 10% to 30% of patients with a bladder-drained pancreas transplant require conversion to enteric drainage at some point following transplantation, which is one of the main factors leading to the increase in enteric-drained transplants.[9]

TABLE 84.1. Outcome of U.S. Cadaveric Pancreas Transplants by Era of Transplant (Level II Evidence).

Type of transplant	*Era*	*1-year pancreas graft survival (%)*
Simultaneous pancreas-kidney	1987–1992	77
	1993–1995	80
	1996–1998	84
	1999–2000	84
	2001-2003	85
Pancreas after kidney	1987–1992	57
	1993–1995	64
	1996–1998	71
	1999–2000	78
	2001–2003	80
Pancreas transplant alone	1987–1992	55
	1993–1995	54
	1996–1998	77
	1999–2000	80
	2001–2003	77

Source: Data from 2003 Annual Report, International Pancreas Transplant Registry (IPTR), Department of Surgery, University of Minnesota, Minneapolis, MN.

Outcome

Patient and Pancreas Graft Survival

The International Pancreas Transplant Registry (IPTR) has collected results of clinical pancreas transplantation. Reporting has been obligatory in the United States since 1987. The outcome data are prospective but not randomized (level II). As expected, results have improved over time, presumably because of improved graft preservation, more potent immunosuppression, and better surgical techniques. Table 84.1 demonstrates the improved graft survival seen over the past decade in U.S. transplants reported to the IPTR. Single-center series have demonstrated even better patient and graft outcomes,[49] but registry data provide data based on large numbers, with less possibility of significant "center effect."

TABLE 84.2. Outcomes According to Method of Exocrine Drainage. U.S. Pancreas Transplants Performed Between January 1, 2000, and June 6, 2004.

	Pancreas graft function at 1 year (%)		
Type of exocrine drainage	*SPK*	*PAK*	*PTA*
Bladder	87	80	79
Enteric	85	77	72

Source: Data from 2004 Annual Report, International Pancreas Transplant Registry (IPTR), Department of Surgery, University of Minnesota, Minneapolis, MN.

The ability to promptly detect rejection in the transplanted kidney and the additional immunosuppression of the uremic state have both been utilized as explanations why SPK recipients enjoy better graft survival than PAK or PTA recipients (Fig. 84.6). Bladder drainage of exocrine secretions from the pancreatic allograft was associated with better graft survival in all categories of pancreas transplants in the past.[50] The most recent era, however, demonstrates no significant difference in graft survival whether bladder drainage or enteric drainage is initially performed (Table 84.2), except in the PTA category, for which there was an increased risk of technical failure due to anastomotic leakage (Table 84.3).

The type of maintenance immunosuppression also influences graft outcome, with improved graft survival seen with the use of one or both of the newer immunosuppressive agents (mycophenolate mofetil, tacrolimus). This is observed in all categories of pancreas transplants (Table 84.4). Recipient age has an effect on patient, pancreas, and kidney graft survival in SPK recipients, with older (≥45 years) patients experiencing lower survival rates at 1 year. This effect is not observed in PAK or PTA recipients, perhaps because of the restriction of these more "elective" transplants to healthier diabetics with fewer comorbidities (Table 84.4).

The beneficial effect of a very well matched donor–recipient combination has been demonstrated in pancreas transplantation as in kidney transplantation. Registry data

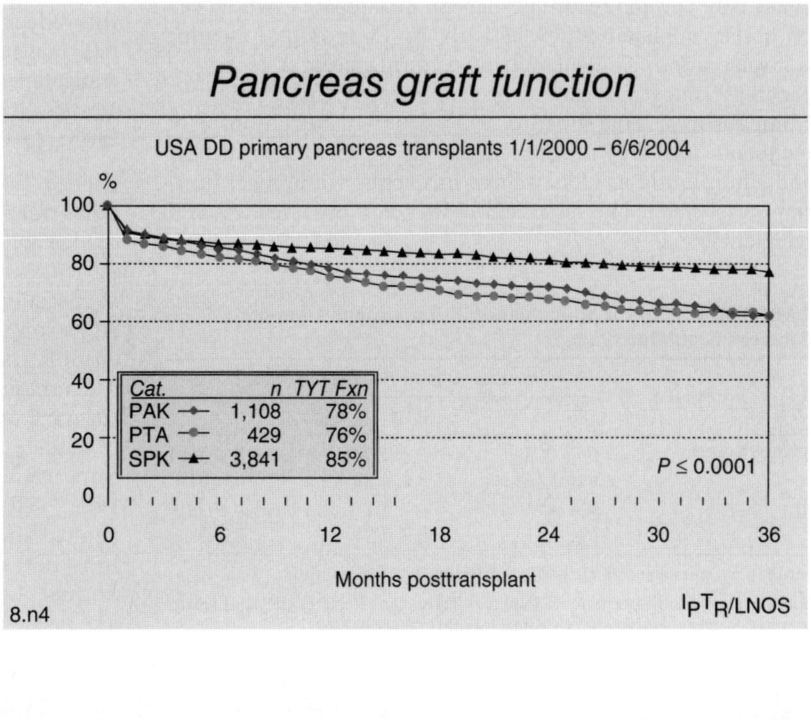

FIGURE 84.6. Pancreas graft function from 2000 to 2004. (From International Pancreas Transplant Registry, Department of Surgery, University of Minnesota, Minneapolis.)

TABLE 84.3. Reasons for Early Technical Pancreas Graft Loss by Duct Management Technique (U.S. DD Primary Pancreas Transplants January 1, 2000–June 2004).

	SPK			PAK			PTA		
Variables	*BD (%)*	*ED (%)*	P	*BD (%)*	*ED (%)*	P	*BD (%)*	*ED (%)*	P
Graft thrombosis	2.7	5.4	.003	3.6	6.1	.06	6.5	8.0	.57
Infection	1.0	1.3	.53	1.4	1.4	.99	1.6	1.75	.96
Pancreatitis	0.4	0.3	.60	0.3	0.1	.60	1.6	0.0	.04
Anastomosis leak	0.6	1.3	.09	0.8	1.5	.35	0.0	2.1	.05
Bleed	0.1	0.5	.20	0.0	0.5	.15	1.1	1.7	.60

BD, bladder drainage; ED, enteric drainage; DD, deceased donors.

reveal that a high degree of HLA match confers a high probability of freedom from acute rejection and excellent graft survival. These data led to UNOS policies that mandate a cadaveric pancreas first be offered to potential recipients who are a zero antigen mismatch (six-antigen match) with the donor. The beneficial effect of lesser degrees of HLA mismatching is especially evident in PAK and PTA recipients, leading most programs to specify a maximum of three HLA mismatches (three-antigen match).

Benefits of Pancreas Transplantation

Many of the goals of normalization of glucose control are related to the long-term avoidance of the end-organ complications from diabetes mellitus. As discussed earlier, most recipients of pancreas transplants already suffer from some of the complications of the disease. Therefore, the expectation that these end-organ changes will completely and rapidly reverse is unrealistic. The ultimate test of the beneficial effect of achieving normal glucose homeostasis via transplantation awaits long-term follow-up of transplanted patients as well as the application of pancreas transplantation to those at an earlier stage of diabetes. Some beneficial effects, however, have been observed, as are outlined next.

Protection from Nephropathy

Diabetics who are recipients of a functioning renal allograft eventually develop recurrent diabetic nephropathy, which can be observed histologically as early as 18 months following transplantation. The subsequent performance of a successful pancreas transplant can reverse or prevent this finding.[51,52] Comparison of renal function at 2 years in diabetic transplant recipients has shown deterioration in the serum creatinine and albuminuria in kidney-alone recipients, while renal function was stable and proteinuria was not observed in SPK recipients.[53]

TABLE 84.4. Type of Maintenance Immunosuppression on Pancreas Graft Outcome.

	Pancreas graft function at 1 year		
	SPK	*PAK*	*PTA*
TAC&MMF	*P* = .008 RR 0.74	*P* = .0001 RR 0.51	*P* = .014 RR 0.46
SIR	*P* = .17 RR 0.81	*P* = .01 RR 0.54	*P* = .001 RR 0.16

MMF, mycophenolate mofetil; SIR, sirolimus; TAC, tacrolimus.

Source: Data from International Pancreas Transplant Registry (IPTR), Department of Surgery, University of Minnesota, Minneapolis, MN.

Diabetic Neuropathy

Both peripheral and autonomic neuropathy have consistently shown improvement following pancreas transplantation, as has been documented by nerve conduction studies,[54] cardiorespiratory reflexes, and studies of gastric emptying. One long-term study suggested that continued improvement in nerve conduction is observed even 5 years following pancreas transplantation, suggesting the improvement of a long-standing condition may require many years. Severe autonomic neuropathy is a risk factor for sudden cardiac death. Recipients of a successful pancreas transplant have a significantly higher probability of survival than those who are not transplanted or who have unsuccessful transplants, presumably in part due to improvement in autonomic neuropathy.[55]

Retinopathy

Many of the diabetics who undergo pancreas transplantation have severe visual impairments, making it difficult to assess the beneficial effect of transplantation. Short-term studies have shown no significant improvement in diabetic retinopathy in patients who undergo transplantation.[56] In the presence of a long-term functioning pancreas allograft, however, retinopathy tended to stabilize, while continued deterioration in vision was observed in patients whose grafts had failed.[57] A rapid improvement in the degree of glycemic control has been shown to acutely worsen diabetic retinopathy. Fortunately, this effect was not observed in studies in which patients had rapid normalization of glucose control by way of SPK transplantation.

Quality of Life

Kidney transplantation alone or in combination with pancreas transplantation has been shown to provide an improved quality of life for recipients as measured by the patients.[58] Patients who underwent SPK transplantation scored higher in measures of general satisfaction and diabetes-specific measures compared to patients with a kidney transplant alone or an SPK transplantation with subsequent failure of the pancreas transplant. Freedom from the need for glucose monitoring, lack of hypoglycemic episodes, and overall improvement in subjective well-being were the most commonly cited improvements following successful pancreas transplantation.[59] Given that pancreas transplantation is generally applied after significant end-organ complications are present, it is not surprising that quality of life does not revert to normal. Long-term studies with appropriate control groups are needed to ascertain what economic impact successful pancreas transplantation has on changes in quality of life and employment.

Islet Cell Transplantation

Only a small percentage of the cells comprising the pancreas (the islets of Langerhans) is necessary for glucose homeostasis. The remainder of the tissue is composed of exocrine tissue that not only provides little useful function in the diabetic recipient but also is responsible for many of the serious complications of pancreas transplantation. The ability to transplant only the cellular elements providing endocrine function is therefore attractive and has been the focus of intense research efforts for more than 40 years.

The technical feasibility of isolating islet cells from human pancreata and transplanting them has been demonstrated in a series of 48 patients undergoing pancreatectomy for chronic pancreatitis with subsequent autologous transplantation of the digested pancreatic tissue. Intraportal transplantation of an adequate number of islets (300,000) was associated with a 74% probability of freedom from insulin therapy for more than 2 years following transplantation.[60]

Until recently, the application of this technology to allotransplantation, which presents the additional barriers of rejection and potential toxicity of immunosuppressive agents, had resulted in limited success. A review of all islet transplants performed and reported between 1990 and 1998 to the International Islet Transplant Registry[61] revealed 1-week and 1-year insulin independence rates of 12% and 8%, respectively. Transplants in which only one pancreas was used per recipient had even poorer results, with insulin independence rates at the same time points of 10% and 7%, respectively.

In July 2000, the publication of a clinical report[62] from the University of Alberta in Edmonton, Canada, described seven patients with type 1 diabetes with histories of severe hypoglycemia and metabolic instability who underwent islet transplantation with islets derived from two or three donor pancreata. All seven of these patients remained insulin-independent at a mean follow-up of 11.9 months. A follow-up article from the same group[63] provided further data after a total enrollment of 12 patients, with 9 of the 12 insulin independent at a mean follow-up of 10.2 months. This relative success was attributed to transplantation of sufficient numbers of islets and a new immunosuppressive regimen that minimized tacrolimus and completely eliminated prednisone. The immunosuppressive and isolation schemes used for this trial became known as the Edmonton protocol, and these initial results renewed worldwide enthusiasm and optimism for the future of islet allograft transplantation.

Since the publication of the initial report from Edmonton, at least three major multicenter initiatives have been undertaken to reproduce and expand on the University of Alberta's initial success. First, the Immune Tolerance Network (ITN) identified and funded 10 centers around the world, 7 of which are in North America, to participate in a multicenter trial of the Edmonton protocol. Second, a request for applications (RFA) released by the National Institutes of Health (NIH) January 3, 2001, "Human Pancreatic Islet Cell Resources (ICRs)," the NIH proposed six (and has since funded nine[64]) U.S. centers to become "Islet Cell Resources (ICRs) for the isolation, purification, and characterization of human pancreatic islet cells for transplantation into diabetic patients." Third is the Clinical Islet Transplant Consortium, also funded by the NIH, which has allocated $75 million to five centers to conduct a large-scale clinical trial of islet transplantation and to translate the practice of islet transplantation from clinical research to standard of care. These and other funding initiatives at the international level illustrate the optimism associated with a new era of islet transplantation immediately following the release of the Edmonton data.

Recipient Selection

Islet transplantation continues to be an experimental procedure worldwide. Therefore, recipient selection has generally been matched to a particular clinical protocol. Candidates for islet transplantation tend to fall into one of two broad groups: (1) persons with type 1 diabetes already receiving immunosuppression after another solid organ transplant (most often a kidney; this group is referred to as islet after kidney or IAK) and (2) persons with type 1 diabetes and without another transplant (islet transplant alone or ITA) who, despite intensive medical management, including frequent blood sugar assessments and more than three insulin injections/day or an insulin pump, suffer from extreme metabolic lability characterized by wide swings in blood glucose, hypoglycemic unawareness, or progressive secondary complications of the disease.[65] As is the case for PTA recipients discussed above, the major challenge for those considering ITA is weighing the relative benefit of insulin independence with the risks of chronic immunosuppression. Pre-transplant assessment is otherwise similar to that for pancreas transplant candidates.

Donor Selection and Organ Preservation

Successful islet transplantation depends on the infusion of an adequate amount of islet tissue. Many centers classify islet yield as adequate if at least 5000 islet equivalents (IEq; defined as a standardized islet volume assuming an "ideal" islet of 150-μm diameter) per kilogram recipient body weight are obtained from a single processed pancreas. Islet yield is enhanced by the use of older donors,[66] which is convenient given the greater success of younger donors in whole-organ pancreas transplantation. Other donor variables correlated with a successful outcome (sufficient yield) include a value above 25 for body mass index[67] and a local procurement team, whereas those correlated with an unsuccessful outcome are rising serum glucose, duration of cardiac arrest, and duration of cold ischemic time.[7] The observed positive effect of a local procurement team may result from special attention given to maintaining low core pancreatic temperature during procurement by careful packing of iced saline slush around the pancreas and in the lesser sac.[68]

Organ preservation has traditionally been carried out in cold (4°C) UW solution as for solid organs, but recently the two-layer method (TLM) of cold storage, which employs UW and perfluorocarbon (PFC) with preoxygenation, has come into use for whole pancreas[69–71] and, later, islet transplantation.[72–75] The PFC, one of the two components in TLM, is a hydrocarbon in which most or all the hydrogen atoms have been replaced with fluorine.[76] Because PFC is hydrophobic and has a high density, PFC and UW solutions are immiscible and thus form two layers when placed together in a container. One of the unique features of PFC is that it can dissolve large amounts of respiratory gases, such as carbon dioxide, oxygen, and nitrogen. Once oxygenated, PFC can be used as an oxygen source for applications such as surrogate blood[77] and cell culture.[76] The other key component in TLM, UW contains glutathione, adenosine, and different electrolytes.[78–80] By combining these two liquids and proper oxygenation, TLM provides sufficient metabolic substrates (O_2 and adenosine) for adenosine triphosphate (ATP) generation during preservation.[70,81] Studies have shown the superiority of TLM to traditional cold UW pancreas preservation in areas such as extended preservation of ischemically damaged pancreas,[82] increased islet yield,[17] improved ATP metabolism,[81] and maintenance of the integrity of intracellular and cellular membranes of the preserved pancreas.[83]

Isolation Procedure

Islet isolation is performed by a semiautomated technique described by Ricordi.[84] After procurement and storage, the pancreas is dissected from the duodenum, spleen, external vessels, and extraneous fat while leaving the thin capsule intact. The neck of the pancreas is partially divided, and the main pancreatic duct is identified and cannulated in an antegrade and retrograde fashion. Both the head and the tail of the organ are then distended with a collagenase- and neutral protease-containing solution while maintaining topical hypothermia. Once distended, the pancreas is minced into variable size pieces and placed in a specialized chamber containing marbles and a screen filtering the outlet to allow for mechanical and enzymatic digestion to occur. A continuous digestion circuit is established, with collagenase solution passing through a heating element[85] to sustain 37°C to activate the digestive enzymes. The digestion is monitored by taking sample aliquots from the continuously circulating enzyme solution and examining microscopically. When islets are free of acinar tissue but still intact, the digestion is stopped by cooling (thus inactivating) the solution. The slurry of digested pancreas is washed several times and recombined prior to purification via density gradient centrifugation in a Ficoll gradient.

Final islet preparations are then assessed prior to release for transplant to ensure adequacy of islet yield, sterility, viability, and sometimes function. At the University of Chicago, prerelease criteria are typical of most programs and include a minimum yield of 5000 IEq/kg recipient body weight, a negative Gram stain, maximum endotoxin level of 5 endotoxin units per kilogram/recipient, 70% viability, and 10 mL maximum tissue volume. Because islets are transplanted as soon as practical after the completion of isolation and testing, in vitro and in vivo functional assays are performed postinfusion. Some programs have elected to culture islets, usually for 48 h, prior to infusion, thus allowing for in vitro functional testing prior to infusion,[86] as well as the logistical considerations of recipient travel and pretransplant immunosuppression.

Islet Infusion Procedure

Despite multiple potential sites for islet implantation, including immunologically privileged sites such as the testis, cornea, and thymus, most programs use intraportal infusion into the liver.[87] The portal vein can be accessed with limited laparotomy and mesenteric vein cannulation or through sonographically and fluoroscopically guided percutaneous transhepatic portal vein puncture. The latter approach has the appeal of minimal invasiveness and accommodation to local anesthesia and mild intravenous sedation.[88] Heparin is administered along with the suspended islets to prevent portal vein thrombosis. Portal vein pressures are measured periodically throughout the procedure with stopping parameters that, at the University of Chicago, include opening portal pressure above 20 mmHg, sustained portal pressure at any time above 22 mmHg, doubling of portal pressure to above 18 mmHg, or subject inability to tolerate the procedure due to symptoms. After infusion, the hepatic parenchymal tract is embolized with coils or gelatin sponge (Gelfoam) plugs during catheter withdrawal.[89]

Uncommon but observed complications from this procedure include inability to achieve access, portal venous hypertension[90]; intraabdominal bleeding (requiring or not requiring transfusion or corrective laparatomy); adjacent organ (e.g., gallbladder) puncture[91]; portal vein thrombosis[92]; abdominal pain; and nausea. Transient elevations in transaminase levels are nearly universal.[89]

Immunosuppression

In addition to enhanced isolation techniques, much of the success of the initial report from Edmonton[62] is attributed to a novel immunosuppressive regimen involving a complete avoidance of steroid and minimal doses of tacrolimus (trough levels 3–6 ng/mL), both of which are diabetogenic. The lower doses of these drugs were thought possible by the availability of two relatively more recent drugs: the mTOR (mammalian target of rapamycin) inhibitor of rapamycin and the IL-2 receptor blocker daclizimab.

Additional reports detail small islet transplant series with immunosuppressive regimens including the monoclonal anti-CD3 antibody hOKT3γ1 (Ala-Ala),[93] and antithymocyte globulin with the tumor necrosis factor (TNF)-α receptor etanercept,[86] but due to small sample size and other variables, none has been demonstrated to be clearly superior.

Outcomes

To date, no large multicenter trial of islet transplantation has been reported, and most clinical reports contain data from single-institution experiences. Variable reporting styles inhibit meta-analysis. The ITN trial mentioned at the beginning of this section enrolled 36 patients, and a preliminary report published in 2003 suggested an initial insulin independence rate of 52%, with 2 voluntary withdrawals due to immunosuppressive side effects, 6 graft losses, and intercenter variability in transplant success.[94] The final results of this trial were subsequently reported.[95] Similar to the preliminary report, 44% of subjects met the primary endpoint of insulin independence 1 year after the final infusion of islets, and only 31% of those remained insulin-independent at 2 years.

The group from Edmonton continues to have the largest single-center experience in the world. The most recent published report of this series[96] describes the Edmonton group's experience with the first 65 islet recipients in their series, transplanted by November 1, 2004. The actual number of recipients in that series now approaches 100. Of the 65 reported patients, 44 achieved insulin independence at some time after islet transplant, but only 10% retained insulin independence at 5 years. Median duration of insulin independence was reported to be 15 months, with an interquartile range of 6.2 to 25.5 months. Despite this, evidence of ongoing islet function as determined by positive C-peptide measurements was 80% at 5 years. Those recipients with continued islet function (insulin independence *or* positive C-peptide) had markedly improved HbA_{1c} compared with recipients who lost all detectable islet function (insulin-independent 6.4%, C-peptide-positive but not insulin-independent 6.7%, C-peptide-negative 9%). Regardless of insulin independence, recipients with functioning islet allografts experienced less hypoglycemia as measured by a validated self-reported survey instrument[97] and less glycemic lability. These results suggest clinical benefit in terms of diabetes management in the majority of islet recipients despite a high rate of return to some degree of insulin independence and the need to further study and enhance means of engraftment and allograft protection of transplanted islets.

Many of the Edmonton-transplanted patients have received more than one infusion of islets, thus requiring multiple cadaveric pancreata to achieve these results. Some centers now report experience with single-donor islet transplantation. The University of Minnesota recently reported eight subjects who underwent single-donor transplantation.[86] In this series, all eight achieved insulin independence, while five sustained this independence for greater than 1 year. Similarly, the University of Pennsylvania recently reported[98] a series of nine patients; seven had completed therapy at the time of publication. All seven had achieved insulin independence, and five of the seven achieved this independence with only one infusion. Common to both reports is the observation that achievement of insulin independence with single-donor infusions requires adequate numbers and quality of islet mass, but the centers differ in many aspects, including the use of TLM for organ preservation, immediate infusion versus preinfusion culture, and immunosuppressive regimen.

Future Directions

Despite these relatively recent successes, islet transplantation remains severely limited in its widespread applicability because of two major problems: a significant shortage of donor tissue and the ongoing need for immunosuppression. Regarding donor supply, enhanced utilization of available organs through improved immunosuppressives, better engraftment, and single-donor success are important measures. The recent report of a successful living donor islet allotransplantation[99] highlights the importance of this potential donor source and presents the possibility of enhanced islet quality from living donors. Stem cell-based approaches to this problem have been thoroughly reviewed by Street et al.[100] According to these authors, embryonic stem cells are conceptually attractive due to expandability, multipotentiality, and potential nonimmunogenicity but have been limited by technical difficulties in obtaining homogeneous differentiation toward islet tissue. Although adult pancreatic ductal cells have received much attention as potentially harboring islet precursor cells, no specific cellular phenotype demonstrating endocrine capabilities has been defined.

The concept of immunoisolation, in which transplanted tissue is separated by a semipermeable membrane from the recipient, has been evaluated as a potential remedy to problems of both donor tissue source and immunosuppression.[101] Theoretically, this membrane serves as a mechanical barrier isolating the graft from recipient complement, leukocytes, and antibodies while continuing to allow the diffusion of glucose, water, insulin, oxygen, nutrients, and cellular waste. Therefore, in addition to potentially eliminating the need for immunosuppression in the allograft setting, immunoisolation has the potential to expand donor tissue availability by enabling xenotransplantation without exposing islets to mediators of hyperacute rejection.[102]

Immunoisolation devices have taken a number of forms, including intravascular hollow tubes,[103] extravascular macrocapsules in shapes ranging from spheres to planes to hollow fibers,[101,104] micromachined interfaces,[105] and microencapsulation.[106] Of these, microencapsulation avoids many of the limitations of the other techniques, including vascular thrombosis, larger diffusion distances,[101] and mechanical complexity.

References

1. Harris M, Hadden WC, Knowles WC, Bennett PH. Prevalence of diabetes and impaired glucose tolerance and plasma glucose levels in the U.S. population aged 20–74 years. Diabetes 1987;36:523–534.
2. Libman I, Songer T, Lapote R. How many people in the U.S. have IDDM? Diabetes Care 1993;16:841–842.
3. National Diabetes Data Group, National Institutes of Health. Diabetes in America, 2nd ed. Bethesda, MD: National Institutes of Health; 1995.
4. Nathan DM. Long-term complications of diabetes mellitus. N Engl J Med 1993;328:1676–1684.
5. Selby JV, Fitzsimmons SC, Newman JM, et al. The natural history and epidemiology of diabetic nephropathy: implications for prevention and control. JAMA 1990;263:1954–1960.
6. American Diabetes Association. Economic consequences of diabetes mellitus in the U.S. in 1997. Diabetes Care 1998;21: 296–309.
7. The Diabetes and Control and Complications Trial Research Group. The effect of intensive treatment of diabetes on the development and progression of long-term complications in insulin-dependent diabetes mellitus. N Engl J Med 1993;329:977–986.
8. Munger B. Morphologic characterization of islet cell diversity. In: Cooperstein S, Watkins D, eds. The Islets of Langerhans: Biochemistry, Physiology, and Pathology. New York: Academic Press; 1981:3–34.
9. Gruessner AC, Sutherland DER. Analysis of United States and non-U.S. pancreas transplants as reported to the International Pancreas Transplant Registry (IPTR) and to the United Network for Organ Sharing (UNOS). Clinical Transplants 1998. Los Angeles: UCLA Tissue Typing Laboratory; 1999:1–19.
10. Sollinger HW, Ploeg RJ, Eckhoff DE, et al. Two hundred consecutive simultaneous pancreas-kidney transplants with bladder drainage. Surgery 1993;114:736–744.
11. Kuo PC, Johnson LB, Schweitzer EJ, et al. Solitary pancreas allografts. Arch Surg 1997;132:52–57.
12. Venström JM, McBride MA, Rother KI, et al. Survival after pancreas transplantation in patients with diabetes and preserved kidney function. JAMA 2003;290:2817–2833.

13. Gruessner RWG, Sutherland DER, Gruessner AC. Mortality assessment for pancreas transplants. Am J Transplant 2005; 4:2018–2026.
14. Stratta RJ, Taylor RJ, Larsen JL, Cushing K. Pancreas transplantation. Int J Pancreatol 1995;17:1–13.
15. Schweitzer EJ, Anderson L, Kuo PC, et al. Safe pancreas transplantation in patients with coronary artery disease. Transplantation 1997;63:1294–1299.
16. Odorico JS, Heisey DM, Voss BJ, et al. Donor factors affecting outcome after pancreas transplantation. Transplant Proc 1998;30: 276–277.
17. Doudzdjian V, Gugliuzza KG, Fish JC. Multivariate analysis of donor risk factors for pancreas allograft failure after simultaneous pancreas-kidney transplantation. Surgery 1995;118:73–81.
18. Gores PF, Gillingham KJ, Dunn DL, Moudry-Munns KC, Najarian JS, Sutherland DER. Donor hyperglycemia as a minor risk factor and immunologic variables as major risk factors for pancreas allograft loss in multivariate analysis of a single institution's experience. Ann Surg 1992;215:217–230.
19. Hesse UJ, Sutherland DER. Influence of serum amylase and plasma glucose levels in pancreas cadaver donors on graft function in recipients. Diabetes 1989;38(suppl 1):1–3.
20. Bunzendahl H, Ringe B, Meyer HJ, Gubernatis G, Pichlmayr R. Combination harvesting procedure for liver and whole pancreas. Transpl Int 1988;1:99–102.
21. Dunn DL, Morel P, Schlumpf R, et al. Evidence that combined procurement of pancreas and liver grafts does not affect transplant outcome. Transplantation 1991;51:150–157.
22. Belzer FO, D'Alessandro AM, Hoffman RM, et al. The use of UW solution in clinical transplantation. Ann Surg 1992;215:579–585.
23. Englesbe MJ, et al. Early pancreas outcomes with histidine-tryptophan-ketoglutarate preservation: a multicenter study. Transplantation 2006;82:136–139.
24. Humar A, Gruessner RWG, Sutherland DER. Living related donor pancreas and pancreas-kidney transplantation. Br Med Bull 1997;53:879–891.
25. Seaquist ER, Robertson RP. Effects of hemipancreatectomy on pancreatic alpha and beta cell function in healthy human donors. J Clin Invest 1992;89:1761–1766.
26. Gruessner RW, Kendall DM, Drangstveit MB, Gruessner AC, Sutherland DE. Simultaneous pancreas-kidney transplantation from live donors. Ann Surg 1997;226:471–480.
27. Zieliski A, et al. Simultaneous pancreas-kidney transplant from living related donor: a single-center experience. Transplantation 2003;76:547–552.
28. Nymann T, Hathaway DK, Shokouh-Amiri MH, et al. Patterns of acute rejection in portal-enteric versus systemic-bladder pancreas-kidney transplantation. Clin Transplant 1998;12:175–183.
29. Stratta RJ, Gaber AO, Shokouh-Amiri MH, et al. A 9-year experience with 126 pancreas transplants with portal enteric drainage. Arch Surg 2001;136:1141–1149.
30. Gruessner AC, Sutherland DER. Pancreas transplants for United States and non-U.S. cases as reported to the International Pancreas Transplant Registry (IPTR) and to the United Network for Organ Sharing (UNOS). Clinical Transplants 1997. Los Angeles: UCLA Tissue Typing Laboratory; 1998:40–45.
31. Gaber AO, Shokouh-Amiri MH, Hathaway D, et al. Results of pancreas transplantation with portal venous and enteric drainage. Ann Surg 1995;221:613–624.
32. Losanoff JE, Harland RC, Thistlethwaite JR, et al. Omega jejunoduodenal anastomosis for pancreas transplant. J Am Coll Surg 2005;202:1021–1024.
33. Demartinesa N, Schiessera M, Claviena PA. An evidence-based analysis of simultaneous pancreas-kidney and pancreas transplantation alone. Am J Transplant 2005;5:2688–2697.
34. Sollinger HW, Stratta RJ, D'Alessandro AM, Kalayoglu M, Pirsch JD, Belzer FO. Experience with simultaneous pancreas-kidney transplantation. Ann Surg 1988;208:475–483.
35. Rosen B, Frohnert PP, Velosa JA, et al. Morbidity of pancreas transplant during cadaveric renal transplantation. Transplantation 1991;51:123–127.
36. Stratta RJ, Taylor RJ, Lowell JA, et al. OKT3 induction in 100 consecutive pancreas transplants. Transplant Proc 1994;55:509–516.
37. Sutherland DER, Gruessner A. Pancreas transplantation as reported to the United Network for Organ Sharing and analyzed by the International Pancreas Transplant Registry. Clinical Transplants 1995. Los Angeles: UCLA Tissue Typing Laboratory; 1996:49.
38. Kuo PC, Wong J, Schweitzer EJ, Johnson LB, Lim JW, Bartlett ST. Outcome after splenic vein thrombosis in the pancreas allograft. Transplantation 1997;64:933–935.
39. Troppman C, Gruessner MS, Dunn DL, Sutherland DER, Gruessner RWG. Surgical complications requiring early relaparotomy after pancreas transplantation. Ann Surg 1998;227:255–268.
40. DeVito-Haynes LD, Jankowska-Gan E, Sollinger HW, Knechtle SJ, Burlingham WJ. Monitoring of kidney and simultaneous pancreas-kidney transplantation rejection by release of donor-specific, soluble HLA class I. Hum Immunol 1994;40:191–201.
41. Elmer DS, Hathaway DK, Bashar Abdulkarim A, et al. Use of glucose disappearance rates (kG) to monitor endocrine function of pancreas allografts. Clin Transplant 1998;12:56–64.
42. Drachenberg CB, Papadimitriou JC, Klassen DK, et al. Evaluation of pancreas transplant needle biopsy. Transplantation 1997;63:1579–1586.
43. Sutherland DER, Sibley RK, Xu XZ, et al. Twin-to-twin pancreas transplantation: reversal and reenactment of the pathogenesis of type 1 diabetes. Trans Assoc Am Phys 1984;97:80–87.
44. Sutherland DER, Goetz FC, Sibley RK. Recurrence of disease in pancreas transplants. Diabetes 1989;38:85–87.
45. Sutherland DER, Gruessner RWG, Dunn DL, Moudry-Munns KC, Gruessner AC, Najarian JS. Pancreas transplants from living related donors. Transplant Proc 1994;26:443–445.
46. Benedetti E, Dunn T, Massad MG, et al. Successful living related simultaneous pancreas-kidney transplant between identical twins. Transplantation 1999;67:915–934.
47. Voltarelli JC, et al. Autologous nonmyeloablative hematopoietic stem cell transplantation in newly diagnosed type 1 diabetes mellitus. JAMA 2007;297:1568–1576.
48. D'Alessandro AM, Kalayoglu M, Hammes R, et al. Diagnosis of intestinal transplant rejection using technetium-99m-DTPA. Transplantation 1994;58:112–113.
49. Sollinger HW, Odorico JS, Knechtle SJ, D'Alessandro AM, Kalayoglu M, Pirsch JD. Experience with 500 simultaneous pancreas-kidney transplants. Ann Surg 1998;228:284–296.
50. Gruessner AC, Sutherland DER. Pancreas transplants for United States and non-U.S. cases as reported to the International Pancreas Transplant Registry (IPTR) and to the United Network for Organ Sharing (UNOS). Clinical Transplants 1997. Los Angeles: UCLA Tissue Typing Laboratory; 1998:40–45.
51. Bohman S-O, Wilsczek H, Tyden G, Jaremko G, Lundgren G, Groth CG. Recurrent diabetic nephropathy in renal allografts placed in diabetic patients and protective effect of simultaneous pancreatic transplantation. Transplant Proc 1987;19:2290–2293.
52. Wilczek HE, Jaremko G, Tyden G, Groth CG. Evolution of diabetic nephropathy in kidney grafts: evidence that a simultaneously transplanted pancreas exerts a protective effect. Transplantation 1995;59:51–57.
53. el-Gebely S, Hathaway DK, Elmer DS, Gaber LW, Acchiardo S, Gaber AO. An analysis of renal function in pancreas-kidney and diabetic kidney-alone recipients at 2 years following transplantation. Transplantation 1995;59:1410–1415.

54. Muller-Felber W, Landgraf R, Scheuer R, et al. Diabetic neuropathy 3 years after successful pancreas and kidney transplantation. Diabetes 1993;42:1482–1486.
55. Navarro X, Kennedy WR, Loewensen RB, Sutherland DER. Influence of pancreas transplantation on cardiorespiratory reflexes, nerve conduction, and mortality in diabetes mellitus. Diabetes 1990;39:802–806.
56. Wang Q, Klein R, Moss SE, et al. The influence of combined kidney-pancreas transplantation on the progression of diabetic retinopathy: a case series. Ophthalmology 1994;101:1071–1076.
57. Sutherland DER, Kendall DM, Moudry KC, et al. Pancreas transplantation in nonuremic, type 1 diabetic recipients. Surgery 1988;104:453–464.
58. Gross CR, Limwattananon C, Matthees BJ. Quality of life after pancreas transplantation: a review. Clin Transplant 1998;12:351–361.
59. Milde FK, Hart LK, Zehr PS. Pancreatic transplantation: impact on the quality of life of diabetic renal transplant recipients. Diabetes Care 1995;18:93–95.
60. Wahoff DC, Papalois BE, Najarian JS, et al. Autologous islet transplantation to prevent diabetes after pancreatic resection. Ann Surg 1995;222:562–579.
61. Brendel M, et al. International Islet Transplant Registry Report. Giessen, Germany: University of Giessen; 1999.
62. Shapiro AM, Lakey JR, Ryan EA, et al. Islet transplantation in seven patients with type 1 diabetes mellitus using a glucocorticoid-free immunosuppressive regimen. N Engl J Med 2000; 343:230–238.
63. Ryan EA, Lakey JR, Rajotte RV, et al. Clinical outcomes and insulin secretion after islet transplantation with the Edmonton protocol. Diabetes 2001;50:710–719.
64. NCRR launches $10.4 million initiative to create islet cell resource centers. Transplant News 2001;11(20):4.
65. Bertuzzi F, Secchi A, DiCarlo V. Islet transplantation in type 1 diabetics. Transplant Proc 2004;36:603–604.
66. Lakey JR, Warnock GL, Rajotte RV, et al. Variables in organ donors that affect the recovery of human islet of Langerhans. Transplantation 1996;61:1047–1053.
67. Toso C, Oberholzer J, Ris F, et al. Factors affecting human islet of Langerhans isolation yields. Transplant Proc 2002;34:826–827.
68. Lakey JR, Kneteman NM, Rajotte RV, Wu DC, Bigam D, Shapiro AMJ. Effect of core pancreas temperature during cadaveric procurement on human islet isolation and functional viability. Transplantation 2002;73:1106–1110.
69. Kawamura T, Kuroda Y, Suzuki Y, Fujiwara H, Yamamoto K, Saitoh Y. A new simple two layer (Euro-Collins' solution/perfluorochemical) cold storage method for pancreas preservation. Transplant Proc 1989;21(1 pt 2):1376–1377.
70. Fujino Y, Kuroda Y, Suzuki Y, et al. Preservation of canine pancreas for 96 hours by a modified two-layer (UW solution/perfluorochemical) cold storage method. Transplantation 1991; 51:1133–1135.
71. Kuroda Y, Kawamura T, Suzuki Y, Fujiwara H, Yamamoto K, Saitoh Y. A new, simple method for cold storage of the pancreas using perfluorochemical. Transplantation 1988;46:457–460.
72. Matsumoto S, Rigley TH, Reems JA, Kuroda Y, Stevens RB. Improved islet yields from macaca nemestrina and marginal human pancreata after two-layer method preservation and endogenous trypsin inhibition. Am J Transplant 2003;3:53–63.
73. Matsumoto S, Kuroda Y. Perfluorocarbon for organ preservation before transplantation. Transplantation 2002;74:1804–1809.
74. Lakey JR, Tsujimura T, Shapiro AM, Kuroda Y. Preservation of the human pancreas before islet isolation using a two-layer (UW solution-perfluorochemical) cold storage method. Transplantation 2002;74:1809–1811.
75. Ricordi C, Fraker C, Szust J, et al. Improved human islet isolation outcome from marginal donors following addition of oxygenated perfluorocarbon to the cold-storage solution. Transplantation 2003;75:1524–1527.
76. Lowe KC DM, Power JB. Perfluorochemicals: Their applications and benefits to cell culture. Trends Biotechnol 1998;16:272.
77. Lowe KC. Perfluorinated blood substitutes and artificial oxygen carriers. Blood Rev 1999;13:171–184.
78. D'Alessandro AM, Kalayoglu M, Sollinger HW, Pirsch JD, Southard JH, Belzer FO. Current status of organ preservation with University of Wisconsin solution. Arch Pathol Lab Med 1991;115:306–310.
79. Palombo JD, Pomposelli JJ, Hirschberg Y, Blackburn GL, Bistrian BR. Glycolytic support of adenine nucleotides in rat liver flush-preserved with UW or Collins' II. Importance of donor nutritional status. Transplantation 1989;48:901–905.
80. Southard JH, van Gulik TM, Ametani MS, et al. Important components of the UW solution. Transplantation 1990;49:251–257.
81. Kuroda Y, Fujino Y, Kawamura T, et al. Mechanism of oxygenation of pancreas during preservation by a two-layer (Euro-Collins' solution/perfluorochemical) cold-storage method. Transplantation 1990;49:694–696.
82. Kuroda Y, Fujino Y, Morita A, et al. Successful 96-hour preservation of the canine pancreas. Transpl Int 1992;5(suppl 1):S388–S390.
83. Iwanaga Y, Suzuki Y, Okada Y, et al. Ultrastructural analyses of pancreatic grafts preserved by the two-layer cold-storage method and by simple cold storage in University of Wisconsin solution. Transpl Int 2002;15:425–430.
84. Ricordi C, Lacy PE, Finke EH, Olack BJ, Scharp DW. Automated method for isolation of human pancreatic islets. Diabetes 1988;37:413–420.
85. Garfinkel MR, Connors M, Ostrega D, Jarosz J, Philipson L, Millis JM. Islet isolation under cGMP conditions: replacing the coil. Transplant Proc 2004;36:1031–1033.
86. Hering BJ, Kandaswamy R, Ansite JD, et al. Single-donor, marginal-dose islet transplantation in patients with type 1 diabetes. JAMA 2005;293:830–836.
87. Brunicardi FC, Mullen Y. Issues in clinical islet transplantation. Pancreas 1994;9:281–290.
88. Larson-Wadd K, Belani KG. Pancreas and islet cell transplantation. Anesthesiol Clin North Am 2004;22:633–674.
89. Goss JA, Soltes G, Goodpator SE, et al. Pancreatic islet transplantation: the radiologic approach. Transplantation 2003;76:199–203.
90. Casey JJ, Lakey JRT, Ryan EA, et al. Portal venous pressure changes after sequential clinical islet transplantation. Transplantation 2002;74:913–915.
91. Ryan EA, Lakey JRT, Paty BW, et al. Successful islet transplantation: continued insulin reserve provides long-term glycemic control. Diabetes 2002;21:2148–2157.
92. Shapiro AMJ, Lakey JRT, Rajotte RV, et al. Portal vein thrombosis after transplantation of partially purified pancreatic islets in a combined human liver/islet transplant. Transplantation 1995;59:1060–1063.
93. Hering BJ, Kandaswamy R, Harmon JV, et al. Transplantation of cultured islets from two-layer preserved pancreases in type 1 diabetes with anti-CD3 antibody. Am J Transplant 2004;4:390–401.
94. Immune Tolerance Network. Preliminary Results of ITN Multicenter Islet Transplant Trial Confirm Potential Patient Benefits, Underscore Steep Learning Curve. In: ITN News and Announcements; 2003.
95. Shapiro AMJ, et al. International trial of the Edmonton protocol for islet transplantation. N Engl J Med 2006;355:1318–1330.
96. Ryan EA, Paty BW, Senior PA, et al. Five-year follow-up after clinical islet transplantation. Diabetes 2005;54:2060–2069.

97. Ryan EA, Shandro T, Green K, et al. Assessment of the severity of hypoglycemia and glycemic lability in type 1 diabetic subjects undergoing islet transplantation. Diabetes 2004;53:955–962.
98. Markmann JF, Deng S, Huang X, et al. Insulin independence following isolated islet transplantation and single islet infusions. Ann Surg 2003;237:741–750.
99. Matsumoto S, Okitsu T, Iwanaga Y, et al. Insulin independence after living-donor distal pancreatectomy and islet allotransplantation. Lancet 2005;365:1642–1644.
100. Street CN, Sipione S, Helms L, et al. Stem cell-based approaches to solving the problem of tissue supply for islet transplantation in type 1 diabetes. Int J Biochem Cell Biol 2004;36:667–683.
101. deVos P, Hamel AF, Tatarkiewicz K. Considerations for successful transplantation of encapsulated pancreatic islets. Diabetologia 2002;45:159–173.
102. Sun Y, Ma X, Zhao D, Vacek I, Sun AM. Normalization of diabetes in spontaneously diabetic cynomologus monkeys by xenografts of microencapsulated porcine islets without immunosuppression. J Clin Invest 1996;98:1417–1422.
103. Chick WL, et al. A hybrid artificial pancreas. Transam Soc Artif Internal Organs 1975;21:8–15.
104. Scharp DW, Mason NS, Sparks RE. Islet immunoisolation: the use of hybrid artificial organs to prevent islet tissue rejection. World J Surg 1984;8:221–229.
105. Desai TA, Hansford DJ, Ferrari M. Micromachined interfaces: new approaches in cell immunoisolation and biomolecular separation. Biomol Eng 2000;17:23–36.
106. Lim F, Sun AM. Microencapsulated islets as bioartificial endocrine pancreas. Science 1980;210:908–910.

85

Liver Transplantation

Douglas W. Hanto, Scott R. Johnson, Seth J. Karp, and Khalid Khwaja

Chronic liver disease (CLD) is a major health problem in the United States, affecting millions of Americans and resulting in large health care expenditures and economic losses. The incidence of newly diagnosed CLD in the United States is 72.3 per 100,000 population.[1] The most common etiologies of CLD include hepatitis C virus (HCV) (57%), alcohol (24%), nonalcoholic fatty liver disease (NAFLD) (9.1%), and hepatitis B virus (HBV) (4.4%). Approximately 3.9 million Americans (1.8% of the population) have been infected with HCV, and 70% or 2.7 million have evidence of chronic infection based on detection of serum HCV RNA.[2] Fortunately, the incidence of new infections is decreasing from a peak of 100 cases per 100,000 in the 1980s to 20 cases per 100,000 or 40,000 new infections annually currently. Because HCV is a chronic infection, however, the projections are for a fourfold increase between 1990 and 2015 in the number of individuals with a 20-year history of HCV infection[1,3] (Fig. 85.1). This is important because of the increased risk in this population of life-threatening complications of CLD and the development of hepatocellular carcinoma (HCC). Estimates are that 14 million Americans (7.4% of the population) 18 years and older meet established criteria for alcohol abuse or dependence,[1] and alcohol accounts for 28% of the deaths from CLD. Nonalcoholic fatty liver disease is probably the most common cause of asymptomatic elevation of liver function tests occurring in 10% to 40% of the population. It is estimated that 1.25 million people have chronic HBV infection, and there are over 78,000 new cases of HBV each year.

Chronic liver disease is estimated to be the eighth leading cause of death (44,677 deaths) in the United States, between diabetes and suicide and higher than deaths from kidney disease.[1] Although the age-adjusted death rate from CLD declined from 1990 to 1994, it remained unchanged from 1995 to 1998.[4] The death rate for alcohol declined from 1990 to 1998, and the death rate for HBV remained unchanged, but the death rate for HCV increased 220% from 1993 to 1998 at the same time that there was a 45% decrease in deaths from unspecified viral hepatitis[4]. Although it is difficult to estimate all the costs associated with CLD, current estimates place the direct and indirect health care costs at approximately \$3 billion per year.[1] It is estimated that from 2010 to 2019 there will be 165,900 deaths from CLD, 27,200 deaths from HCC, and \$10.7 billion in direct expenditures.[5]

Liver transplantation is the only treatment left for many patients with end-stage liver disease. The number of patients waiting for a liver transplant increased from 3,955 in 1994 to 17,171 in 2003 (Fig. 85.2), and 10,856 new patients were added to the waiting list in 2004 according to recent summary data.[6] The number of patients undergoing liver transplantation only increased from 3574 to 5344 in 2003, illustrating the continued gap between demand and supply[7] (Fig. 85.3). The death rate on the waiting list, however, has declined from 225 deaths per 1000 patient-years in 1994 to 124 per 1000 in 2003 due to improvements in the care of patients with end-stage liver disease and allocation policies that favor transplanting the sickest patients. Patient survival after liver transplantation is now 88%, 80%, and 74% at 1, 3, and 5 years, respectively. There are currently 35,000 patients alive with a functioning liver transplant and a markedly improved quality of life (QOL).

Indications

Liver transplantation should be considered for patients with (1) debilitating or life-threatening complications of liver disease or (2) early-stage hepatocellular cancer when resection is not possible due to concomitant liver disease or tumor location. Disease states that may lead to the need for liver transplantation may be divided into seven categories: noncho-

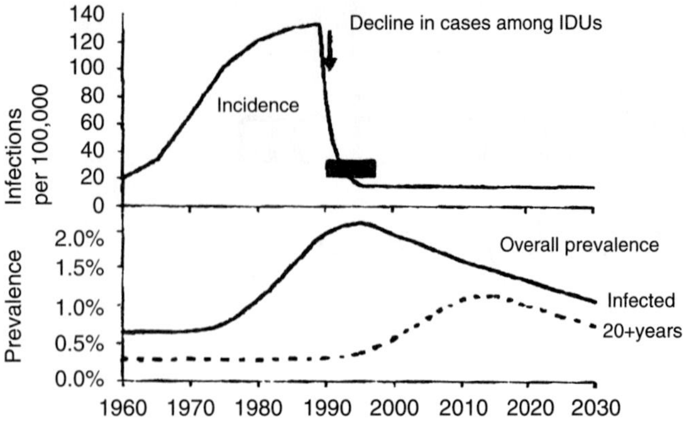

FIGURE 85.1. The incidence and prevalence of HCV infection in the United States. IDU, injecting drug user. (From Kim et al.,[1] by permission of *Hepatology*.)

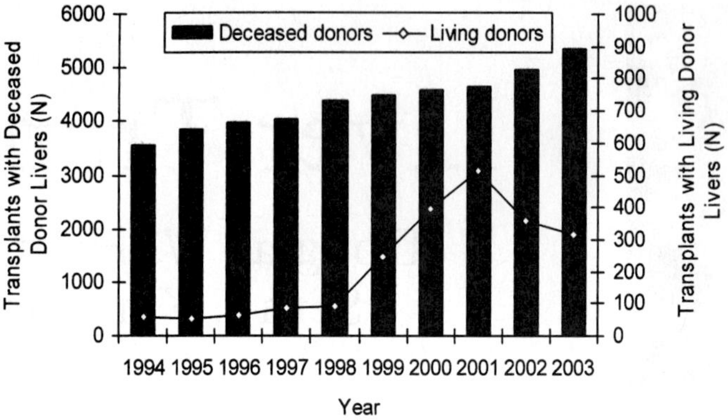

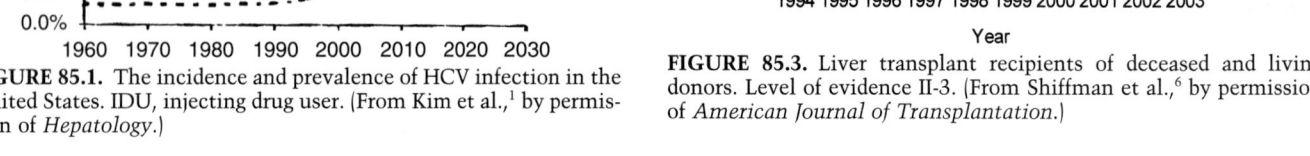

FIGURE 85.3. Liver transplant recipients of deceased and living donors. Level of evidence II-3. (From Shiffman et al.,[6] by permission of *American Journal of Transplantation*.)

lestatic cirrhosis, cholestatic cirrhosis, fulminant liver failure, metabolic diseases, cancer, biliary atresia, and a miscellaneous group (Table 85.1).

Noncholestatic Cirrhosis

Ongoing hepatocyte injury is the defining aspect of this diverse group of diseases. Cirrhosis is the ultimate result, with the subsequent development of portal hypertension (Table 85.2). Gastric and esophageal varices, ascites, and hydrothorax frequently develop as a consequence of portal hypertension as blood flow through the liver meets increasing resistance. In later stages, synthetic dysfunction can result in coagulopathy and failure of bilirubin metabolism and excretion, leading to jaundice and pruritus. Malnutrition results in impaired energy production, muscle wasting, and fatigue. Inadequate detoxification of portal blood causes hepatic encephalopathy. Other complications of advanced disease that are not well understood but can be devastating are hepatorenal syndrome and hepatopulmonary syndrome.

Hepatitis C

Infection with hepatitis C is the most common reason for liver transplantation, accounting for up to 50% of adult transplants at some centers.[5] Approximately 4 million people in the United States have chronic hepatitis C infection.[8] Viral infection occurs primarily via exposure to infected blood. Common mechanisms include blood transfusions given prior to 1992 when accurate tests for the virus became available; tattoos, especially if not done using sterile technique; or intravenous drug abuse when using shared needles. Acute symptoms include jaundice, malaise, nausea, and right upper quadrant pain but only occur in 25% of patients.

Approximately 70% of infections will result in chronic hepatitis manifested by persistently elevated liver enzymes, and 10%–15% of these patients will go on to develop cirrhosis.[9] Concurrent alcohol use or coinfection with hepatitis B greatly increases the risk of progression to cirrhosis.[10] Patients coinfected with HIV (human immunodeficiency virus) who are well controlled on HAART (highly active antiretroviral therapy) and have CD4 counts above 100 are currently being transplanted in a prospective multicenter study sponsored by the National Institutes of Health (NIH) to evaluate the safety and efficacy of kidney and liver transplantation in HIV-infected patients. Results from single-center studies have been mixed.

One particularly troubling aspect of hepatitis C is that it is responsible for approximately one-third of hepatocellular cancers in the United States; approximately 25% to 30% of HCV-positive patients will develop HCC.[11,12] Once cirrhosis is established, the risk of HCC is as high as 4% per year.[9] Patients with HCV should be screened every 3 to 6 months by α-fetoprotein (AFP) measurements and ultrasonography or computed tomographic (CT) scan.[11–13]

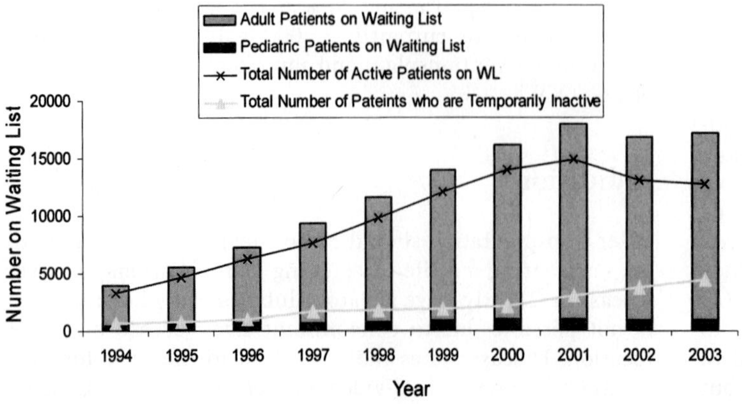

FIGURE 85.2. Pediatric and adult liver waiting list (WL) candidates. Level of evidence II-3. (From Shiffman et al.,[6] by permission of *American Journal of Transplantation*.)

TABLE 85.1. Indications for Liver Transplantation.

Noncholestatic cirrhosis	<68.0%
Hepatitis C virus (HCV)	28.1%
Alcohol	15.0%
Alcohol + HCV	6.0%
Cryptogenic	8.6%
Autoimmune	4.1%
Hepatitis B virus (HBV)	3.6%
Nonalcoholic steatohepatitis (NASH)	1.8%
Other	0.8%
Cholestatic cirrhosis	12.0%
Primary biliary cirrhosis (PBC)	4.2%
Primary sclerosing cholangitis (PSC)	4.9%
Caroli's disease	0.1%
Other	1.1%
Fulminant liver failure	4.3%
Metabolic diseases	1.8%
Malignant neoplasms	1.0%
Hepatoblastoma	<0.1%
Hemangioendothelioma	<0.1%
Hemangiosarcoma	<0.1%
Hepatocellular carcinoma (HCC)	0.8%
Cholangiocarcinoma	<0.1%
Metastatic	<0.1%
Biliary atresia	1.7%
Other	1.3%
Budd-Chiari syndrome	0.6%
Polycystic liver disease	0.2%
Total parenteral nutrition (TPN)	0.4%
Benign hepatic tumors	0.1%
Miscellaneous	
Other not classified	5.9%
Not reported	5.7%

Candidates waiting for liver transplantation on the United Network for Organ Sharing (UNOS) list as of April 7, 2005 (http://www.optn.org/latestdata/rptdata.asp).

Alcohol

Chronic alcohol ingestion is the second most common indication for liver transplantation, accounting for approximately 25% of adult transplants. Acute alcohol ingestion can produce fatty changes in the liver that occur predominantly around the central vein. Chronic exposure leads to pericentral fibrosis and ultimately to panlobular fibrosis and liver failure. Laboratory examination typically reveals an aspartate aminotransferase/alanine aminotransferase (AST/ALT) ratio of greater than 2, a level uncommon in other forms of liver disease, and a relatively mild elevation in the transaminases (<500). Common clinical complications include spontaneous bacterial peritonitis, upper gastrointestinal hemorrhage from ulcers or varices, encephalopathy, and synthetic failure.

Recidivism after liver transplantation places the graft at high risk. Sobriety of greater than 6 months prior to transplantation is associated with higher success rates for alcohol abstinence, and most centers and insurance companies require this period before considering a patient for transplantation. Other reasonable requirements include that the patient be involved in a chemical dependency recovery program, have adequate social support, and agree to random blood and urine toxin screens. An interesting issue involves patients who have rapid decompensation and require liver transplantation prior to a 6-month period of sobriety. Consideration of the individual circumstances is recommended in these cases, consistent with a Michigan court decision that stated a period of abstinence greater than the patient's expected survival should not be a requirement before listing a patient for transplantation.[14]

Cryptogenic

Although much of what was termed cryptogenic cirrhosis in the past is now identified as nonalcoholic steatohepatitis (NASH), approximately 3% percent of patients still undergo liver transplantation when the cause is not known.[15] Diagnosis necessitates a negative history of alcohol abuse, lack of exposure to hepatotoxins, no serologic evidence of viral hepatitis, no family history of liver disease, and no autoimmune disease.[16] Possible causes include occult alcohol use, ingestions, and viral hepatitis. There may be an autoimmune component in some patients as posttransplant liver inflammation is common in these patients.[17,18]

Autoimmune

The diagnosis of autoimmune hepatitis (AIH) relies on a constellation of signs and symptoms and the exclusion of all other causes. Patients generally present with features of CLD, including fatigue, weight loss, and abdominal pain. Skin rash and musculoskeletal complaints are common. Liver function tests typically demonstrate elevated ALT, AST, and bilirubin but relatively normal alkaline phosphatase. Patients are more commonly female. Biopsy generally reveals a predominantly periportal inflammation. Serological examination reveals an elevated immunoglobulin (Ig) G; and antinuclear antibody (ANA), smooth muscle antibodies (SMA), anti liver/kidney microsome (anti-LKM1), perinuclear antineutrophil cytoplasmic antibodies (p-ANCA) and anti soluble liver antigens and liver-pancreas antigens (anti-SLA/LP) (the only autoantibodies specific for AIH) are positive, while AMA (antimitochondrial antibodies) are negative. Antibody titers and disease severity may fluctuate. Response to corticosteroid therapy supports the diagnosis.

Hepatitis B

Despite the availability of effective vaccines against hepatitis B, it remains an important reason for liver failure in the United States and worldwide. Approximately 300 million people in the world are infected with the virus, and 250,000 die each year as a consequence. The majority of acute infec-

TABLE 85.2. Complications of Chronic Liver Disease Leading to Liver Transplantation.

Portal hypertension
Intractable ascites
Spontaneous bacterial peritonitis
Bleeding esophageal/gastric varices
Hydrothorax
Hepatorenal syndrome
Hepatic encephalopathy
Reduced hepatic synthetic function
Malnutrition and muscle wasting
Fatigue
Pruritus
Hepatopulmonary syndrome
Recurrent cholangitis in patients with primary sclerosing cholangitis
Malignancy

tions in adults result in clearance of the virus and no sequelae. In up to 5% of patients, however, chronic infection will occur. Cirrhosis will occur in 15% of these patients, and a further 20% of these patients will progress to decompensated cirrhosis requiring liver transplantation. Similar to hepatitis C, hepatitis B is a risk factor for the development of HCC, and 10% of patients with hepatitis B cirrhosis will develop hepatocellular cancer.

Adjunctive therapy with hepatitis B immune globulin (HBIG) and lamivudine has revolutionized the treatment of hepatitis B-induced liver failure. Transplantation produced poor results initially, with only 50% 3-year actuarial survival due to recurrent hepatitis B causing fulminant failure.[19–21] In the 1990s, passive immunization with HBIG reduced the risk of recurrent HBV and improved survival.[22] Pilot studies in 1999 demonstrated efficacy of lamivudine against HBV in liver transplant patients.[23] These studies were extended over the next few years, including one study that demonstrated no recurrences in 17 patients who were HBsAg (hepatitis B surface antigen)-positive but HBV DNA-negative with a combination of lamivudine and HBIG.[24–26] The combination of the antiviral lamivudine and HBIG demonstrates recurrence rates of less than 5% in most studies, even when patients with HBV DNA are included.[26–33]

Hepatitis B is now considered a manageable disease in the setting of liver transplantation. Selected patients coinfected with HIV (CD4 count >100, viral load undetectable) can also be successfully transplanted and generally have better outcomes than HIV/HCV coinfected patients.[34]

Nonalcoholic Steatohepatitis

Recognized in 1999 as a cause of end-stage liver disease, NASH is responsible for about half of the cases of what was formerly termed cryptogenic cirrhosis, approximately 3% of all transplants. Obesity is a strong risk factor, and although many patients with NASH have a normal body mass index, there is suggestion of insulin resistance in many of these patients.[35,36] Up to 20% of the obese population will have NASH, and progression to cirrhosis will occur in 3%–15%.[37–41]

Pathological examination reveals predominantly macrosteatosis and lobular inflammation consisting of polymorphonuclear leukocytes and mononuclear cells. This disease is part of a continuum between NAFLD and cirrhosis. Although not all obese patients have NAFLD, and not all patients with NAFLD are obese, there is a strong association between the two groups. Nearly 70% of obese patients will have NAFLD, compared with 35% of nonobese patients, and NASH will occur in 18.5% of obese patients and fewer than 3% of nonobese patients.[42] Disease severity seems to be influenced by advanced age, hyperlipidemia, diabetes, and female gender.[40,41,43–46] The disease may be part of the metabolic syndrome.

Cholestatic Liver Disease/Cirrhosis

Chronic biliary damage characterizes the cholestatic liver disease/cirrhosis group of diseases. Progressive impairment of bile flow leads to a cycle of obstruction and infection, which in turn exacerbates the biliary damage. Obstruction initially most often causes pruritis, which can be severe and debilitating, and later jaundice. Cholangitis may also result, producing fever and right upper quadrant pain and even biliary sepsis. In general, the ongoing biliary damage predisposes the patient to the development of cholangiocarcinoma, an aggressive malignancy that is generally a contraindication to transplantation.

Primary Biliary Cirrhosis

Primary biliary cirrhosis (PBC) is a progressive autoimmune disorder for which there is no currently effective medical therapy; it is the fourth most common indication for liver transplantation. The disease is characterized by granulomatous destruction of the intralobar bile ducts, leading to obstruction, jaundice, and biliary sepsis. Middle-aged women are most commonly affected. Diagnosis is often made in asymptomatic patients on the basis of elevated alkaline phosphatase on routine examination, although common symptoms include fatigue, pruritis, and xanthomata. Osteoporosis commonly develops. Positive AMA is the hallmark of the disease. Although PBC can recur in the transplanted liver, this is a rare event and does not affect suitability for transplantation.

Primary Sclerosing Cholangitis

Primary sclerosing cholangitis (PSC) is a chronic cholestatic liver disease of unknown etiology and is characterized by inflammatory fibrosis of the intrahepatic or extrahepatic biliary tree, leading to diffuse stricturing.[47] Pretransplant management of strictures includes medical, radiologic, endoscopic, or surgical interventions and can delay the development of liver failure. When cirrhosis and portal hypertension develop, patients usually require transplantation.[48] Approximately 60% of PSC patients have concomitant inflammatory bowel disease that is progressive in 30% posttransplant. Careful monitoring for dysplasia and carcinoma of the colon must continue posttransplant, and some patients may require colectomy.[49]

A particularly dangerous aspect of the disease is the development of cholangiocarcinoma in up to 30% of patients with long follow-up.[49–51] Primary sclerosing cholangitis should be viewed as a premalignant condition and managed with careful screening. Brushings of the biliary tree for cytology should be obtained at the time of endoscopic retrograde cholangiopancreatography (ERCP) or percutaneous transhepatic cholangiography (PTC). The tumor marker CA19-9 should be followed serially and can aid in the differentiation of cholangiocarcinoma from benign strictures of PSC.[52] Diagnosis of cholangiocarcinoma is considered a contraindication to transplantation, although there is one current trial examining the feasibility of transplanting patients with early-stage cholangiocarcinoma.[53]

Caroli's Disease

Caroli's disease is a rare indication for liver transplantation caused by a genetic defect in a protein named PKHD1, the polycystic kidney and hepatic disease 1 gene, that may be involved in hepatocyte growth.[54] Segmental dilations of large intrahepatic bile ducts lead to chronic biliary stasis. Intraductal lithiasis is common and can be difficult to treat. Recurrent biliary obstruction may produce sepsis and intrahepatic abscesses. Commonly, Caroli's disease is associated with congenital hepatic fibrosis and is then termed Caroli's syndrome.[55]

Biliary Atresia

The most common indication for liver transplantation in children is biliary atresia (53.3%). Most infants with biliary atresia undergo a portoenterostomy (Kasai procedure), which reestablishes bile flow in 60% if done prior to the third month of life. Recurrent cholestasis, cholangitis, cirrhosis, and portal hypertension develop in most patients, and the 5-year survival after a portoenterostomy is 40% to 60%. Indications for liver transplantation after a failed portoenterostomy include poor nutrition, growth, and development; recurrent cholangitis; and variceal hemorrhage. Approximately 60% to 70% of patients with biliary atresia require liver transplantation. Results have continued to improve, with 1-, 2-, and 5-year actuarial patient survival rates of 83%, 80%, and 78%, respectively.[56]

Fulminant Liver Failure

Liver failure within 8 weeks of the onset of symptoms in patients without preexisting liver disease (except in the case of Wilson's disease) is defined as fulminant hepatic failure by UNOS for listing purposes. Encephalopathy is the sine qua non of this disease. Prognosis seems to be better in patients in whom the time between the development of jaundice and encephalopathy is short, although attempts to classify fulminant hepatic failure into groups based on duration of disease are not clinically useful.

Fulminant hepatic failure is most commonly caused by acetaminophen overdose (20%), followed by cryptogenic liver failure (15%), idiosyncratic drug reactions (12%), hepatitis B (10%), and hepatitis A (10%).[57] Other important causes include Budd-Chiari syndrome, herpes simplex infection, Epstein-Barr infection, paramyxovirus infection, *Amanita* poisoning, acute fatty liver disease of pregnancy, autoimmune hepatitis, and neonatal hemochromatosis. Wilson's disease is unique in that fulminant hepatic failure can occur in these patients regardless of preexisting disease. The diagnosis of fulminant hepatic failure from hepatitis C is so rare that it should prompt careful reevaluation of possible causes.

Deciding which patients with fulminant liver failure should undergo transplantation is one of the most difficult decisions in all of transplantation. Transplantation of the liver in the setting of acute failure has a 1-year survival rate of 71%[57,58] and carries the additional morbidity of immunosuppression, operative complications, and chronic rejection. Conversely, in patients who do recover without a transplant, most will have no long-term morbidity.

Seminal work determining which patients with acute liver failure should undergo transplantation comes from King's College in London.[59] Statistical analysis of almost 600 patients between 1973 and 1985 identified prognostic factors for poor prognosis, which were then analyzed prospectively for accuracy. Validation of these criteria was performed both in the original paper and in numerous subsequent studies.[60] Prognostic indices segregate fulminant failure by cause. Poor survival after Tylenol overdose is best predicted by either an arterial pH less than 7.3 after volume resuscitation or the combination of a prothrombin time (PT) greater than 100, creatinine greater than 3.3 mg/dL, and grade III or IV encephalopathy (arousable but unable to perform mental tasks or worse). Poor survival after the development of fulminant liver failure after all other causes is best predicted by either a PT greater than 100 s or any three of the following: age less than 10 or greater than 40, interval between jaundice and encephalopathy greater than 7 days, bilirubin greater than 300 μmol/L, PT greater than 50 s, and a cause of either drug-induced, nonA/nonB-, or halothane-induced hepatitis.

Evaluation of the criteria is extremely difficult. Most clinicians are reluctant to overrule their clinical judgment, and it is hard to envision how an ethical prospective randomized trial could be performed. Retrospective studies are inherently biased. Patients who did not receive a transplant were probably less ill to begin. Furthermore, the relatively small number of patients transplanted for acute failure limits the robustness of the statistical analysis.

Survival after acetaminophen overdose has been assessed[60] in two prospective and eight retrospective studies reviewed in 2003. These demonstrated the sensitivity of the King's College criteria to be 69% and the specificity to be 92%. Assessment of these numbers justifies transplantation in all patients who meet the criteria. Unfortunately, many patients who do not meet criteria may still die without a transplant.

For patients with nonacetaminophen-induced liver injury, the positive predictive value, negative predictive value, and predictive accuracy were 79%, 50% and 68%, respectively,[61] again suggesting the criteria are best for identifying patients with poor prognosis who require transplantation.

Metabolic Diseases

In many pediatric transplant centers, metabolic diseases caused by inherited genetic defects constitute the second most common indication for liver transplantation after biliary atresia. These diseases can be categorized as metabolic diseases that cause structural liver damage leading to liver failure (e.g., α-1-antitrypsin deficiency, Wilson's disease, tyrosinemia, urea cycle defects such as ornithine carbamoyltransferase [OTC] deficiency, galactosemia, glycogen storage disease IA and IV) or metabolic diseases that do not cause structural damage (e.g., familial hypercholesterolemia, primary oxalosis, protein C deficiency, hemophilia A or B). Liver transplantation can replace the missing enzyme and be curative of the metabolic disease as well as the liver failure.

Malignant Neoplasms

Hepatoblastoma

Hepatoblastoma accounts for approximately 75% of primary liver tumors in children.[62] Cisplatin-based chemotherapy in conjunction with complete resection provides 60%–80% long-term survival. Transplantation is an option for patients with unresectable disease and has good survival as both an initial therapy and for patients with recurrence after resection who are found to be unresectable at laparotomy.[62]

Hemangioendothelioma, Angiosarcoma

Hemangioendothelioma is a rare malignancy that is generally slow growing. Radical resection is the treatment of choice;

however, this is often precluded by the multifocal nature of the lesion.[63] Good outcomes with transplantation have been reported even in the presence of extrahepatic lymph node involvement.[64] Care must be taken not to confuse this lesion with angiosarcoma, a much more aggressive malignancy in which results after transplantation are very poor.[65,66]

Hepatocellular Carcinoma

Hepatocellular carcinoma is one of the most common malignancies worldwide. In the United States, the incidence has doubled since 1990 to approximately 3 per 100,000. Risk factors include most CLDs. Worldwide, this is most commonly from chronic infection with hepatitis B, while in the United States this is most commonly due to infection with hepatitis C. Diagnosis can be made on the basis of elevated AFP (>500 µg/L) in patients with a suggestive history and characteristic lesions on CT, although as many as 25% of patients with HCC will have normal AFP.

Treatment of hepatocellular cancer is best administered via a multimodality approach combining chemotherapy, interventional radiology, and surgery. Chemoembolization and radio-frequency ablation are relatively new modalities that hold promise. Resection is the mainstay of treatment.

Resection is not possible in all patients. Tumor location, size, or multifocality may preclude primary resection. Concomitant liver disease may make a major hepatic resection too dangerous. In these cases, liver transplantation should be considered.

Early experience with transplantation for hepatocellular cancer demonstrated high recurrence rates and only 10% to 20% 5-year survival.[67] Review of the data demonstrated poor outcomes primarily in patients with stage III or IV disease by TNM classification.[68] This led to a stratification of patients with early-stage tumors that could be cured by liver transplantation and patients with later-stage tumors that would not benefit from transplantation. Two studies, the first demonstrating an 83% disease-free survival for patients undergoing liver transplantation with up to three tumors all less than 3 cm, as compared with an 18% disease-free survival following liver resection,[69] and a second demonstrating patients with a solitary lesion less than 5 cm or up to three tumors all less than 3 cm and with patients having a 4-year recurrence-free survival of 92%,[70] form the basis for the current UNOS policies regarding the transplantation of these patients. Under this system, patients with early-stage cancers that cannot be resected due to location or concomitant disease receive extra MELD (model for end-stage liver disease) points that move them higher on the waiting list. A subsequent review of patients with HCC, some of whom had larger tumors, concluded that equivalent survival rates could be obtained in patients with a solitary tumor smaller than 6.5 cm or fewer than three nodules, with the largest lesion smaller than 4.5 cm and total tumor diameter less than 8 cm (90% and 75.2% survival at 1 and 5 years, respectively) compared to 50% 1-year survival for patients who exceeded these limits.[71]

Cholangiocarcinoma

Patients with known cholangiocarcinoma have very poor survival with or without transplant, and resection is the preferred treatment. The 3-year survival in almost all series is less than 40%, and in some it is 0%.[72] Liver transplantation for these patients should only be considered as part of a research protocol. Currently, data from the Mayo Clinic suggest 50% 5-year survival for selected patients with stage 1 or 2 disease with perihilar cancer who underwent external beam irradiation, brachytherapy, and chemotherapy.[53]

Other

Budd-Chiari Syndrome

Budd-Chiari syndrome is characterized by occlusion of the main hepatic veins (HV) and presents acutely with right upper quadrant abdominal pain, hepatomegaly, and massive ascites. These patients should be evaluated for underlying hypercoagulable states such as polycythemia vera, protein C deficiency, protein S deficiency, or antithrombin III deficiency. Before the development of cirrhosis, the treatment of choice is a side-to-side portacaval shunt that decompresses the liver, prevents continued hepatic necrosis and cirrhosis, and is associated with excellent long-term survival.[73] Even in patients with early cirrhosis, caudate hypertrophy, and vena caval obstruction, a side-to-side portacaval shunt can be efficacious.[74] Once patients have cirrhosis and secondary complications related to their liver failure, portal vein (PV) or inferior vena caval thrombosis, or a failed portacaval shunt, liver transplantation is indicated. Five-year survival rates are approximately 70%.[75,76]

Additional Indications for Liver Transplantation

A number of indications do not fit into the above categories. Total parenteral nutrition (TPN)/hyperalimentation-induced liver disease typically requires combined liver/intestinal transplant. Patients with massive liver enlargement due to polycystic liver disease may be candidates for liver transplantation. Most hepatic adenomas can be treated with resection, but large, unresectable hepatic adenomas may be indications for transplant due to concern for malignancy, bleeding, or pain.

Treatment of Patients with Liver Failure

Acute Liver Failure

Patients with acute fulminant liver failure require urgent evaluation and consideration of listing for liver transplantation. Admission to the intensive care unit is mandatory with aggressive multisystem support. The proximate cause of death in most patients is sepsis or cerebral ischemia, and care is directed toward preventing these complications. Prophylactic antibiotics are generally started. Prevention of cerebral ischemia is critical and consists of maintaining the cerebral perfusion pressure (CPP) (mean arterial blood pressure minus intracranial pressure) above 60 mmHg. This is accomplished by minimizing cerebral edema with hypoventilation, fluid restriction, and mannitol as needed. Serum osmolality is maintained at approximately 325 mOsm/dL. Placement of an intracranial pressure monitor is controversial. No studies demonstrated improved outcomes with these devices, but they allow precise management of CPP and may be a useful guide to prognosis if the CPP is less than 60 mmHg for extended periods of time. Often, these patients develop high-output cardiac failure with low systemic vascular resistance requiring vasopressor support. When renal failure occurs, continuous venovenous hemodialysis is recommended as it produces less circulatory stress than conventional hemodialysis. Patients in stage III or IV coma are intubated when there is concern regarding respiratory insufficiency or a risk of aspiration. Lactulose may be given by nasogastric tube to improve encephalopathy. Risk of bleeding is minimized with fresh frozen plasma and cryoprecipitate to decrease the international normalized ratio (INR) below 1.5 and platelet infusions to keep the platelet count above 100.

Other options for treatment in these patients or as bridges to transplantation have included auxiliary heterotopic or orthotopic cadaver liver transplantation, the use of bioartificial liver support devices, hepatocyte transplantation, and ex vivo liver perfusion.[77–79] Artificial and bioartificial support systems reduce mortality in acute liver failure superimposed on chronic liver failure, but not acute liver failure alone.[80] Management of patients with Tylenol overdose involves the above considerations as well as the administration of n-acetylcysteine and activated charcoal.

Chronic Liver Failure

Principles of managing patients with chronic liver failure include treating the manifestations of portal hypertension, including controlling ascites, prevention of infection and bleeding, treating hepatic encephalopathy, maintaining adequate nutrition, and symptomatic relief (Table 85.2). Feeding tubes can be placed for nutritional support. Infection prevention occurs through careful surveillance and rapid treatment. Prevention of bleeding involves monitoring for the development of varicies and banding. Transjugular intrahepatic portosystemic shunts (TIPS) are sometimes necessary to prevent bleeding. They complicate but are not a contraindication to transplant. Symptomatic relief may involve interval paracentesis or thoracocentesis and lactulose for encephalopathy.

Listing and Liver Allocation

Each patient listed for liver transplantation is assigned a MELD score based on three laboratory values: creatinine, INR, and bilirubin. The MELD score calculated by the formula MELD = (0.957 × log(serum creatinine) + 0.378 × log(serum bilirubin) + 1.12 × log(INR) + 0.643) × 10. The MELD score has been shown to predict short- and medium-term mortality of patients with cirrhosis, with mortality increasing with increasing MELD scores (Table 85.3). Livers are allocated to patients with the highest MELD score (i.e., to the sickest, most needy patients).

TABLE 85.4. Unadjusted Waiting List and Transplant Mortality Rates by MELD Category.

	Waiting list deaths	*Transplant deaths (1-year follow-up)*		
MELD	*Rate per 1000 patient-years*	*Rate per 1000 patient-years*	*Hazard ratio*[a]	*P values*
6–11	44.8	163.3	3.64	<.001
12–14	52.5	127.4	2.35	<.001
15–17	146.4	164.7	1.21	.41
18–20	271.9	174.1	0.62	<.01
21–23	514.9	178.4	0.38	<.001
24–26	840.7	176.9	0.22	<.001
27–29	1,663.8	195.9	0.18	<.001
30–39	4,634.1	245.5	0.07	<.001
40[b]	13,152.7	254.6	0.04	<.001
Total	217.3	183.5	—	—

MELD, model for end-stage liver disease.

Level of evidence II-2.

[a]Comparison of mortality risk expressed as hazard ratio by MELD score for recipients of liver transplants compared to candidates on the liver transplant waiting list.

[b]Includes patients whose MELD score was capped at 40.

Source: From Merion et al.,[81] by permission of *American Journal of Transplantation.*

A number of features of this system are worth comment. Indices that determine the MELD score are all objective and quantifiable, eliminating the potential interphysician variability and minimizing the effect of subjective indices. Statistical analysis is facilitated because of the high degree of standardization. Refinements can be made to the system as more data become available. Principles of justice derive from the prioritization based on expected mortality. Recent data suggest that at MELD scores 18 and higher, there is a significant survival benefit from a transplant that increases with increasing MELD score without an upper limit, and at MELD score less than 15, patients have a survival benefit on the waiting list compared to transplantation.[81] Patients with MELD scores 15–17 have roughly equivalent mortality rates with or without transplant (Table 85.4). It is unclear, however, if allocation in this manner provides the highest aggregate utility.

Flexibility in the MELD system allows diseases that portend high mortality but that do not result in a high MELD score to be incorporated into the current system by assigning these patients a higher MELD score. Currently recognized

TABLE 85.3. Three-Month Death Rates by MELD Score.

MELD	*≤9*	*10–19*	*20–29*	*30–39*	*≥40*
Hospitalized	4% (6/148)	27% (28/103)	76% (16/21)	83% (5/6)	100% (4/4)
Ambulatory noncholestatic	2% (5/213)	5.6% (14/248)	50% (15/30)	—	—
Ambulatory PBC	1% (3/308)	13% (2/16)	0% (0/2)	—	—
Historical	8% (55/711)	26% (90/344)	56% (47/84)	66% (23/35)	100% (5/5)

MELD, model for end-stage liver disease; PBC, primary biliary cirrhosis.

Level of evidence II-2.

Source: From Kamath et al.,[225] with permission.

diseases outside the MELD platform include hepatocellular cancer, hepatopulmonary syndrome, familial amyloidosis, primary oxaluria, and metabolic syndromes. The ease with which these diseases can be incorporated based on the probability of death is one of the strongest parts of the MELD system.

Patients with stage II hepatocellular cancer (2- to 5-cm lesion or no more than three lesions, the largest less than 3 cm) receive MELD points equal to the probability of death on the waiting list of 15% within 3 months. This results in a significant number of transplants for HCC. The decision not to grant points for small lesions reflects the low rate of metastases of these lesions. Larger lesions do not receive points due to the poor outcomes observed when transplanting patients with advanced disease.

Timing

Introduction of the MELD system resulted in sicker patients being transplanted and fewer deaths on the waiting list.[82] In the past, the question of when to transplant patients, especially those with PBC and PSC, was a difficult one. Introduction of the MELD system directly linked expected mortality with rank on the waiting list so that, in the current system, when a liver becomes available for a patient it should generally be used.

There are, however, instances when liver transplantation should not be performed. Considering that liver transplantation has a 2% perioperative mortality, a 10%–15% 1-year mortality, and significant morbidity, transplantation may not improve outcomes in healthier patients whose morbidity and mortality from liver disease is low. Fortunately, the MELD system is designed to compare mortality between groups. Analysis of the data is ongoing, but it seems likely that patients with very low scores should not be transplanted unless there are extenuating circumstances.[81] Similar issues arise when discussing live donation. Data are accumulating that mortality after live donation increases as MELD score increases. It is imperative therefore that patients be identified and evaluated quickly so they can be transplanted at the optimum time.

Contraindications

Absolute and relative contraindications to liver transplantation have decreased over the past several years as our ability to successfully transplant sicker and more complex patients has improved. Absolute contraindications include advanced uncorrectable cardiac or pulmonary disease, severe irreversible pulmonary hypertension, irreversible neurological impairment, uncontrolled sepsis, and most instances of extrahepatic cancer (Table 85.5). Protocols exist for a number of diseases that were previously thought to be absolute contraindications for transplantation. These include HIV infection, advanced hepatocellular cancer, and cholangiocarcinoma. Interestingly, some of the most difficult problems to overcome do not relate to the operation but rather to the patient's ability to follow the prescribed immunosuppressive regimens and take care of the liver. Included in this group is lack of social and economic support, patients who are actively using alcohol, and those with a history of noncompliance with medical care. Liver transplant programs generally include specialists in social, psychiatric, and financial issues so that full evaluation and maximization of resources is possible.

TABLE 85.5. Contraindications to Liver Transplantation.

Absolute
Advanced, uncorrectable cardiac or pulmonary disease
Severe, irreversible pulmonary hypertension (>50 mmHg)
Hypotension requiring vasopressor support
Cerebral perfusion pressure below 60 mmHg in acute liver failure
Recent intracranial hemorrhage
Irreversible neurological impairment
Uncontrolled sepsis
Extrahepatic malignancy[a]
Inability to comply with the posttransplant regimen
Active substance abuse
Relative
Stage III or IV HCC
HBV-DNA+ and HBeAg+ hepatitis B
Cholangiocarcinoma
HIV infection
Advanced age (>75 years)
Severe obesity (BMI > 40)

[a]With the exception of skin cancer and some neuroendocrine tumors and sarcomas.

Preoperative Evaluation and Management

Patients undergoing evaluation as potential liver transplant candidates may do so as an outpatient or inpatient depending on the disease and its severity. This is a multidisciplinary evaluation that begins with a complete history, physical examination, routine laboratory studies, chest x-ray, and electrocardiogram. All patients need current hepatitis (A, B, C) serological results; viral serology (herpes simplex virus [HSV], cytomegalovirus [CMV], Epstein-Barr virus [EBV], HIV, and varicella zoster virus [VZV]; infectious serology (rapid plasma reagin [RPR], toxoplasmosis, rubella); AFP, CA19-9 (in patients with suspected cholangiocarcinoma or PSC), and ABO typing. Visualization of the liver by CAT (computerized axial tomography), MRI (magnetic resonance imaging), or MRA (magnetic resonance angiography) is performed for vessel patency and liver volume and to rule out liver tumors. A dental evaluation, Papanicolaou test, mammogram in women more than 40 years of age, and prostate-specific antigen (PSA) in men more than 40 years of age are required.

Other studies that are obtained less frequently, depending on the patient's history and disease, include upper gastrointestinal endoscopy, pulmonary function tests with arterial blood gases, colonoscopy in patients over 40 years, echocardiogram, dipyridamole stress thallium study, cardiac catheterization with coronary angiography, and psychiatric evaluation for all patients with a history of substance abuse, alcohol abuse, or psychiatric illness. If portal vein (PV) occlusion is suspected, imaging to clearly define the patency of the superior mesenteric vein (SMV), splenic vein, and PV is necessary. Appropriate consultations from physicians in cardiology, pulmonary disease, neurology, and infectious disease are obtained as needed.

TABLE 85.6. Unadjusted Patient and Graft Survival Rates After Liver Transplantation.

	N	*3 months (%)*	*1 year (%)*	*3 years (%)*	*5 years (%)*
Deceased donor					
Patient	8275	92.3	86.5	78.5	72.7
Graft	9131	88.2	81.4	72.2	65.9
Live donor					
Patient	852	92.7	86.6	77.5	77.8
Graft	285	94.0	90.9	88.1	85.6

Level of evidence III.

Source: Data from 2004 OPTN/SRTR Annual Report, Tables 9.12a, 9.12b, 9.9a, 9.9b.

Outcomes

The overall death rate while on the liver transplant waiting list has decreased from 225 deaths per 1000 patient-years in 1994 to 124 in 2003. The posttransplant death rates have also decreased. The death rate in the first year following deceased donor liver transplant was 156 deaths per 1000 patient-years in 2002 compared to 197 in 1994.

Patient survival rates following deceased donor liver transplantation are 93% at 3 months, 88% at 1 year, 80% at 3 years, and 74% at 5 years. Graft survival rates are 88% at 3 months, 81% at 1 year, 72% at 3 years, and 66% at 5 years[6] (Table 85.6). Overall survival for living donor recipients is nearly identical at the same time points.[83]

The etiology of liver disease affects patient survival of deceased donor livers. The highest 1-year survival rates are seen in patients with metabolic diseases (91%), biliary atresia (91%), and cholestatic liver disease (90%) (Table 85.7). This trend continues at 3 and 5 years. In contrast, patients with acute hepatic necrosis had the lowest 1-year patient survival rate (81%). Although 1-year survival among patients with malignancy was 86%, this number dropped to 60% at 5 years, presumably due to recurrent malignancy. Patients with MELD scores greater than 30 have an 86% survival at 3 months and a 76% 1-year survival, compared to 93% and 88%, respectively, for MELD scores of 21–30, significantly worse than other groups based on MELD.[6] Graft survival rates at 3 months and 1 year were 83% and 73%, respectively, compared to 91% and 85%, respectively, for MELD scores of 21–30. A recent analysis of risk factors for death after liver transplantation cited hemodialysis pretransplantation, age at the time of transplantation, and the etiology of underlying liver disease as independent predictors of survival after liver transplantation, whereas MELD score, Child-Pugh class, and the presence of diabetes mellitus or heart disease were not[84] (Table 85.8).

TABLE 85.8. Risk Factors for Death After Liver Transplantation.

Demographic	P *value*	*Risk ratio (95% CI)*
Pretransplant hemodialysis	<.001	5.1 (2.6–10.2)
Age > 42 years	<.001	3.4 (1.7–7.0)
Etiology of liver disease[a]		
PBC		1.0
Alcohol	.002	4.4 (1.7–11.3)
α-1-Antitrypsin deficiency	.005	4.9 (1.6–4.6)
Autoimmune hepatitis	.002	6.3 (2.0–20.2)
Malignancies	.028	4.8 (1.2–19.4)
PSC	.291	1.7 (0.6–4.5)
Viral hepatitis	.004	3.8 (1.5–9.4)
Other	<.001	5.5 (2.1–14.4)

Level of evidence III. Retrospective univariate logistic regression analysis and multiple variate analysis of 499 consecutive liver transplant patients at the Mayo Clinic between June 1990 and February 1998.

[a]Relative to a diagnosis of PBC.

Source: From Merion et al.[81]

Patients with HCV at a single center had overall 1-, 5-, and 10-year patient and graft survival rates of 84%, 68%, and 60% and 73%, 56%, and 49%, respectively.[85] In patients with HCV viremia, recurrent HCV infection is universal after transplant, and patient and graft survival rates are decreased in these patients.[86,87] In addition, the natural history of chronic HCV after liver transplantation is accelerated compared with nontransplant patients, with 20% to 40% of recipients progressing to cirrhosis within 5 years compared with 5% in the general population.[86] The rate of progression from cirrhosis to decompensation is more rapid for transplant recipients with recurrent chronic HCV infection compared with nontransplant patients, and time from decompensation to death is also decreased. Nonviral factors such as advanced donor age, prolonged donor hospitalization, increasing recipient age, and elevated recipient MELD score have been shown to increase the risk of HCV disease progression.[88] Donor age in particular has been shown in several studies to have an impact on patient and graft survival rates and fibrosis progression.[89] Treatment of HCV posttransplant with pegylated interferons

TABLE 85.7. Unadjusted Patient and Graft Survival of Deceased Donor Liver Recipients by Primary Diagnosis.

	3 months (%)		*1 year (%)*		*3 years (%)*		*5 years (%)*	
	Patient	*Graft*	*Patient*	*Graft*	*Patient*	*Graft*	*Patient*	*Graft*
Noncholestatic cirrhosis, N (P/G*) = 5453/5790	92.6	89.4	86.3	82.3	77.6	71.9	71.0	65.5
Cholestatic cirrhosis, N (P/G) = 824/923	93.8	90.0	90.2	84.5	88.3	78.0z5	80.0	72.1
Acute hepatic necrosis, N (P/G) = 646/765	88.1	82.6	80.8	74.5	75.4	68.3	71.0	62.4
Biliary atresia, N (P/G) = 282/328	92.9	83.8	90.8	80.8	88.7	79.5	80.0	67.0
Metabolic diseases, N (P/G) = 288/302	93.8	90.7	91.0	87.1	83.7	76.6	81.8	73.7
Malignant neoplasm, N (P/G) = 397/418	93.7	88.8	86.1	80.1	63.4	59.4	60.2	53.3
Other, N (P/G) = 385/609	89.6	82.3	84.7	75.5	75.6	67.4	69.1	56.5

G, graft; P, patient.

Level of evidence II-2.

Source: Data from 2004 OPTN/SRTR Annual Report, Tables 9.9a and 9.12a.

(IFNs) and ribavirin has largely been ineffective because of low response rates and tolerability, although recent studies provide some hope.[5]

Quality of life after transplant is an important measure of the success of liver transplantation. Short-term prospective studies have shown improved QOL at 9 and 18 months after liver transplant as compared with control groups. In addition, there was cognitive improvement in patients after liver transplantation.[90] These improvements persist to 5 years after transplantation.[91]

Analysis of outcomes for each MELD category revealed that the survival benefit of a transplant for an individual patient increases with increasing MELD score above 18. At the bottom MELD group (<11), 1-year mortality was much higher with a transplant, while at the other extreme, patients with a MELD of greater than 40 had a 96% reduction in mortality with a transplant.[81]

Donor Selection and Evaluation

The Deceased Donor

Donor selection and liver procurement are critical to prevent primary nonfunction (PNF) or delayed primary function of the transplanted liver and to prevent disease transmission. When a donor liver is offered for a listed recipient, ABO and size compatibility are the first two criteria that need to be met. Additional donor factors that must be considered include age; cause of death; hemodynamic stability and the need for vasopressors; other medical conditions (e.g., history of atherosclerotic cardiovascular disease, diabetes mellitus, HIV, hepatitis B or C, malignancy, cancer, infection); social history (e.g., alcoholism, intravenous drug use, sexual promiscuity); and laboratory values, including complete blood count (CBC), renal and liver function tests, arterial blood gases, chest x-ray, coagulation studies, and viral serology (hepatitis B, C, HIV, RPR, CMV).

Primary nonfunction of liver allografts occurs in 5% to 15% of cases, requires urgent retransplantation, and is a significant cause of morbidity and mortality after liver transplantation.[92,93] Donor risk factors for PNF include prolonged cold and warm ischemia, severe macrovesicular steatosis, ABO incompatibility, donor age over 50 years, elevated donor transaminase levels, prolonged intensive care unit stay, increased bilirubin, and the need for vasopressors in the donor[92–96] (Table 85.9).

Because there continues to be a critical shortage of deceased donor livers and patients continue to die on the waiting list, many centers are now using livers that previously were discarded and have thereby expanded the donor pool. For example, livers from donors older than 80 years of age have been successfully transplanted with success in HCV-negative recipients.[97] Older donor livers, however, do not tolerate long cold ischemia times and ideally should be transplanted within 6h.[98,99] Moreover, donor age older than 60 years is a strong predictor of graft loss and death.[100] Transplants of ABO-incompatible livers have been performed with a 1-year survival rate of 87% when a combination of pre- and posttransplant plasmapheresis, splenectomy, OKT3 induction, and Cytoxan, prednisone, and cyclosporine are used.[101]

TABLE 85.9. Deceased Donor Risk Factors for Primary Nonfunction.

Prolonged cold and warm ischemia
Severe macrovesicular steatosis
ABO incompatibility
Donor age > 50 years
Elevated donor transaminase levels
Prolonged intensive care unit stay
Increased bilirubin
Need for vasopressors in the donors

Severe steatosis has been considered a major risk factor for the development of PNF, and donor livers with moderate-to-severe steatosis are frequently discarded or used in high-risk recipients with an urgent need for transplantation. Most studies, however, have not distinguished between microvesicular and macrovesicular steatosis (Fig. 85.4). A Sudan black or oil red O stain can facilitate the quantitation of fat in the liver biopsy. A recent study of 120 donor livers with mild (<30%), moderate (30% to 60%), to severe (>60%) macrovesicular steatosis that underwent transplantation demonstrated no increase of PNF, although the incidence of initial poor graft function was higher with moderate and severe steatosis, and 1-year graft survival was significantly lower.[102] The risks associated with use of fatty livers are compounded by increasing donor age, prolonged ischemic times, and recipient HCV positivity.[102,103]

A recent analysis of PNF in the MELD era identified donor age, serum creatinine above 1.5mg/dL, hypertension, and cerebrovascular accident (CVA) as risk factors for PNF, and recipient factors included life support, mechanical ventilation, use of inotropes, hemodialysis, initial status 1, and use of a shared transplant.[104] Of interest is that the incidence of PNF has not increased in the MELD era even with sicker recipients and more liberal donor acceptance criteria.

Recently, the concept of a donor risk index has been introduced to identify and quantify donor characteristics that predict the risk of graft failure.[105] Donor age over 40 years and especially over 60 years, donation after cardiac death (DCD), and split/partial grafts were the greatest risk factors for graft failure. African American race, shorter height, CVA, and other causes of brain death were also associated with an increased risk but much less than the other factors noted (Table 85.10). These data can be used to select appropriate recipients and to inform the recipient of the risks associated with particular donors.

Another goal of proper donor selection is to prevent transmission of disease, particularly hepatitis B, C, HIV, and malignancy; therefore, careful screening and serological testing of donors is performed. The donor pool can be expanded further, however, by the use of HBsAg–, HBcAb+, HBIgM– donors, who have a low risk of transmitting HBV to kidney recipients[106] but a 30% to 50% chance of transmitting HBV to an unmodified liver recipient.[107] Livers from these donors are currently being transplanted into HBsAb+ and HBsAb– recipients along with HBIG or lamivudine prophylaxis with minimal risk of the recipient becoming HBsAg+. Livers from HCV-positive donors with normal liver histology have been used for HCV-positive recipients.[108]

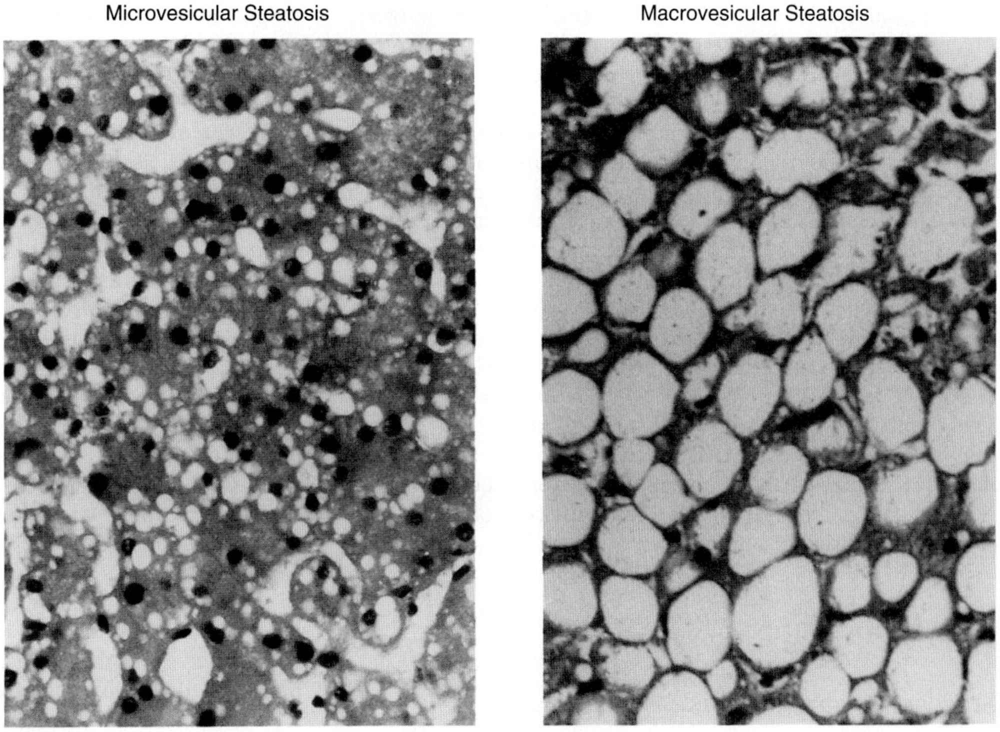

FIGURE 85.4. Deceased donor liver biopsies demonstrating severe microvesicular steatosis (*left panel*) and macrovesicular steatosis (*right panel*). (Hematoxylin-eosin, ×66.)

Splitting of livers from deceased donors is a novel way of expanding the donor pool. Candidate donors are very carefully selected. In general, these donors should be young, hemodynamically stable with short hospitalization, and have normal liver function tests and no period of arrest.[109] Also, the liver should be of a size adequate enough to sustain two recipients.

The Living Donor

The medical and psychological assessment of the living donor is a rigorous process, even more so since a well-publicized death in New York that led to state guidelines for donor evaluation, surgery, and postoperative treatment.[110] Briefly, donors should be between 18 and 55 years of age; related to the recipient or have established emotional ties; ABO-compatible with the recipient; and without medical problems that would increase the surgical risk. The donor must be competent, willing to donate, and free from coercion. The family psychosocial support systems must be adequate as determined by a psychiatric and social work evaluation. The donor should have a normal history, physical examination, hematological and serum chemistry profile, along with normal kidney and liver function tests. An electrocardiogram (EKG) and chest x-ray are obtained and should be normal. The donor must have negative hepatitis B and C and HIV serological tests. An independent donor advocacy group should confirm candidate suitability. The donor must be fully informed of risks and benefits to donation and the alternate treatments available to the recipient (Table 85.11).

The anatomical suitability of the liver for living donation must then be determined. Noninvasive imaging techniques have all but replaced arteriography and endoscopic retrograde cholangiopancreatography (ERCP). Imaging modalities based on CT or MR can accurately define liver volumes and arterial, venous, and biliary anatomy.[111,112] Precise three-dimensional (3D) rendering of these images allows calculation of individ-

TABLE 85.10. Donor Factors Significantly Associated with Liver Allograft Failure (1998–2002).

Donor parameter	*RR*	*95% CI*	P *value*
Age			
<40	1.00		
40–49	1.17	1.08–1.26	.0002
50–59	1.32	1.21–1.43	<.0001
60–69	1.53	1.39–1.68	<.0001
>70	1.65	1.46–1.87	<.0001
African American race (vs. white)	1.19	1.10–1.29	<.0001
Donor height (per 10 cm decrease)	1.07	1.04–1.09	<.0001
COD = CVA	1.16	1.08–1.24	<.0001
COD = Other	1.20	1.03–1.40	.018
DCD	1.51	1.19–1.91	.0006
Partial/split	1.52	1.27–1.83	<0.0001

COD, cause of death; DCD, donation after cardiac death.
Source: From Feng et al.[105]

TABLE 85.11. Informed Choice in Living Donation.

Potential donors should be
- Competent
- Willing to donate
- Free from coercion
- Medically and psychologically suitable
- Fully informed of risks and benefits of donation
- Fully informed of alternate treatments available to recipient
- Likely to benefit in a nonmonetary way

Source: From Barr ML, et al.[110] and New York State Committee on Quality Improvements in Living Liver Donation.[227]

ual vascular territories and is an invaluable aid to surgery. Liver steatosis can be assessed by analysis of liver/spleen attenuation ratios.[113] A percutaneous liver biopsy may be required in some cases.[114]

Size matching is critically important. The healthy native liver is 2% to 3% of body weight, but the minimum amount of transplanted liver needed to survive is estimated to be approximately 25% of the recipient's ideal liver mass.[115,116] The risk of delayed and poor function increases, however, when grafts with less than 50% of the recipient's ideal liver mass are used.[117] The donor segmental volume can be accurately determined within 3% by cross-sectional imaging,[118] as can the available space in the recipient. The ideal liver volume of both donor and recipient can be calculated based on body surface area (BSA) [LV (mL) = $706.2 \times \text{BSA (m}^2) + 2.4$] to match the volume of the potential donor segmental graft with the recipient requirements.[119] Liver regeneration occurs throughout the first postoperative year, with livers regaining about 80% of their original volume.[120]

Donor Procedures

Standard Technique: Deceased Donor

A midline incision is made from the suprasternal notch to the symphysis pubis. This includes a sternotomy. In obese donors, a cruciate incision made at the level of the umbilicus may improve exposure (Fig. 85.5). The abdomen is thoroughly inspected to exclude malignancies or other disease processes that would preclude organ retrieval.

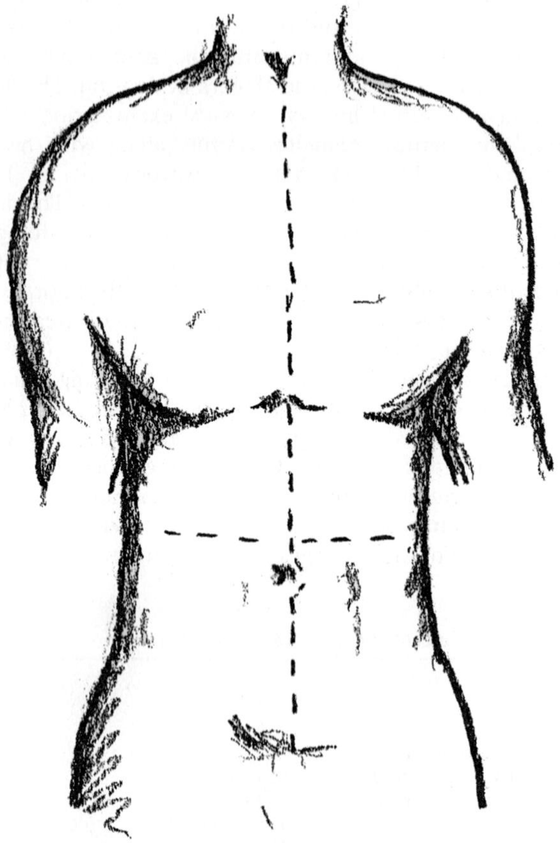

FIGURE 85.5. Incision(s) for deceased donor operation. The incision is made from the suprasternal notch to the pubic bone and may be "cruciated" if necessary. (Courtesy of Khalid Khwaja, MD.)

The liver is then carefully examined, including palpation of both the lobes. This is facilitated by division of the right and left coronary and triangular ligaments. It is particularly important to assess for steatosis: Fatty livers have a characteristic yellowish hue and rounded edges and tend to be large. A tru-cut or wedge biopsy is taken for frozen section if an abnormality is suspected.

The dissection can now proceed in one of several ways depending on the surgeon's preference. In the standard technique, most of the dissection is performed in the "warm," while the heart is still beating. It is prudent to gain early control of both the supraceliac and infrarenal aorta in case the donor becomes unstable; this allows for rapid cannulation and aortic cross-clamping should the need arise. The right-sided peritoneal reflection is incised and the cecum, ascending colon, and small bowel mesentery mobilized toward the left. This provides excellent exposure of the retroperitoneal structures. Care must be taken to avoid injury to the right ureter during this maneuver. The aorta can now be dissected and looped just proximal to its bifurcation. Next, the supraceliac aortic is controlled; the left coronary and triangular ligaments are incised and the left lobe of the liver gently retracted toward the right. The peritoneum overlying the gastroesophageal junction is divided and the esophagus retracted toward the left. The diaphragmatic crura can then be divided to expose the supraceliac aorta, which is looped.

The dissection then continues in the gastrohepatic ligament. The clear portion of this ligament is incised to expose the caudate lobe. A search is now made for a replaced left hepatic artery (HA) arising from the left gastric artery, which occurs in approximately 17% of donors. If a replaced left HA is present, it is carefully preserved and dissected to its junction with the left gastric artery. The left gastric artery is then traced to its origin at the celiac trunk, identifying and ligating any arterial branches to the stomach. Next, the dissection proceeds to the hepatoduodenal ligament. This ligament is opened layer by layer to expose the underlying structures. The proper HA is isolated and followed proximally along the superior border of the pancreas. As one proceeds toward the celiac artery, the gastroduodenal artery (GDA) and right gastric arteries are identified and ligated. The splenic artery is identified and preserved if the pancreas is being retrieved. The common HA is then freed to the level of the celiac artery. Next, the tissue between the proper HA and common bile duct (CBD) overlying the PV is incised and the anterior surface of the PV exposed. The PV is mobilized and isolated. This dissection should not proceed caudad to the upper border of the pancreas if it is being retrieved for transplant.

A replaced right HA, arising from the superior mesenteric artery (SMA), occurs in approximately 19% of donors. It is usually present lateral and slightly deep to the CBD and is readily felt by passing an index finger into the foramen of Winslow. If such a vessel is identified, it is traced to its origin from the SMA. This is accomplished by "Kocherizing" the duodenum and head of the pancreas. In the majority of cases, the replaced right HA can be separated from the head of the pancreas, allowing preservation of the pancreas for transplant if necessary. The proximal part of the SMA trunk is kept with the replaced right HA, and the distal part of the SMA is preserved with the pancreas.

The portal dissection is completed by identifying the CBD and then encircling it distal to the entry of the cystic duct. As much tissue as possible is preserved around the CBD to avoid subsequent devascularization. The CBD is then divided close to the head of the pancreas. The gallbladder is irrigated through an opening made in its fundus. This prevents necrosis of the biliary tract mucosa caused by bile remaining in contact with the mucosa during cold storage. Next, a site is selected for placement of the portal infusion catheter. This can be placed directly into the PV itself, into the SMV, or into the inferior mesenteric vein (IMV). The SMV can be easily isolated at the root of the small bowel mesentery. The IMV can be found just toward the left of the ligament of Trietz.

If the kidneys and pancreas are being retrieved, further dissection of these structures can be performed at this point or after cross-clamp. In coordination with the other teams, the patient is systemically heparinized. Usually, a dose in the range of 300 U/kg is administered. A perfusion catheter is then inserted and secured in the distal aorta. A 10- to 14-French catheter is inserted into the portal system, either through the IMV or SMV or directly into the portal vein (PV). In coordination with the cardiac retrieval team, the supraceliac aorta is cross-clamped, and the vena cava is vented in the right chest by incising the inferior vena cava–right atrium junction (Fig. 85.6). Alternatively, the venting may take place through a cannula placed in the distal vena cava. Surface cooling of the liver, pancreas, and kidneys is achieved by placing cold slush solution in the abdomen. Usually, 3 L of University of Wisconsin (UW) solution is infused into the aorta (500 to 2000 mL in children) and 2 L into the portal system (100 to 250 mL in children) over approximately 10–15 min. The liver edge should be carefully observed for signs of overperfusion, manifest by a liver tense to palpation with rounding of the edges. The heart and lungs are usually removed while the abdominal organs are being flushed.

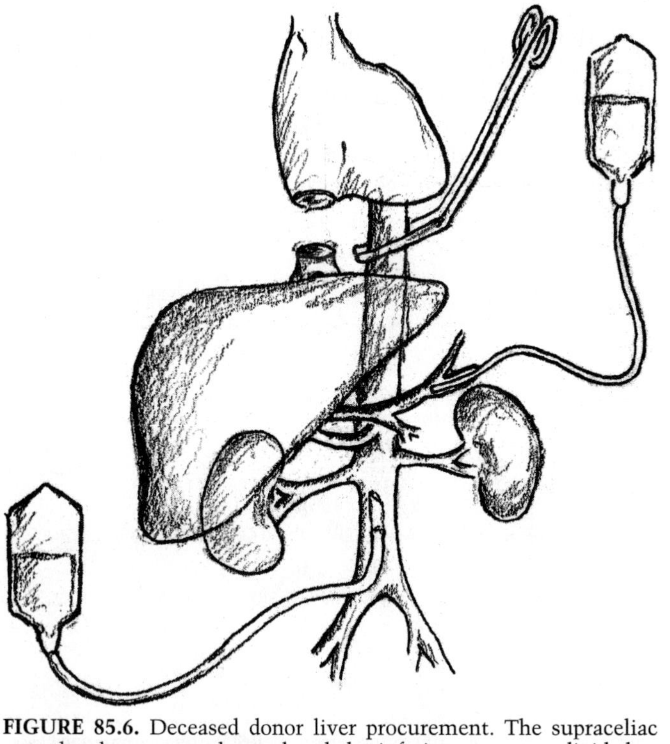

FIGURE 85.6. Deceased donor liver procurement. The supraceliac aorta has been cross-clamped and the inferior vena cava divided at the atriocaval junction. Preservative solution is flushed into both systemic and portal circulations. (Courtesy of Khalid Khwaja, MD.)

When flushing is complete, the liver can be removed. The remaining dissection around the celiac axis is completed. The splenic artery can be divided, leaving a small stump on the "liver side." The left gastric artery can also be ligated or preserved if there is a replaced left HA present. The thick, ganglionic tissue around the celiac trunk is dissected free and the anterior surface of the aorta preserved. The celiac trunk is then separated from the aorta, preserving a generous cuff of aortic tissue around it for subsequent reconstruction. In the presence of a replaced right HA, the aortic patch should include the origin of the SMA. Next, the PV is divided, maintaining adequate length for both the liver and pancreas grafts. The hilar structures are then retracted upward and protected. The infrahepatic vena cava can now be readily exposed, circumferentially dissected, and divided just above the left and right renal veins. The remaining attachments of the liver are sharply freed. The diaphragm is divided around the suprahepatic vena cava, allowing removal of the liver.

The liver is then taken to the back table and placed in cold UW solution. Additional UW is infused into the HA, PV, and a small amount into the CBD. The liver is then packaged in UW solution for transport. The iliac veins and arteries are excised and stored in cold UW in the event that vascular reconstruction is required in the recipient.

Before transplantation into the recipient, the deceased donor liver must be prepared on the back table. The remaining diaphragm is removed, the suprahepatic vena cava isolated, and phrenic veins are identified and suture ligated. The infrahepatic vena cava is identified and ligated or oversewn if a piggyback liver transplant is to be performed. The divided adrenal vein is ligated along with any other small branches divided during retrieval. The PV and HA are isolated, and if desired the gallbladder is removed after ligation of the cystic artery and duct. Alternatively, the gallbladder may be removed in situ after reperfusion of the liver. Then, UW solution is infused into the HA, PV, and vena cava to check for leaks.

If there is a replaced right HA, it can be reconstructed in one of several ways. The simplest and most common technique is the anastomosis of the proximal end of the SMA to the celiac axis and an anastomosis of the distal SMA to the recipient's HA. The replaced right HA can also be sewn to the stump of the splenic artery or GDA.

Rapid Flush Technique

The technique just described is the traditional method for liver procurement. The rapid flush technique minimizes the amount of dissection before aortic cross-clamping.[121] Although some surgeons use this technique or a variant routinely, it is most applicable in an unstable donor from whom the expeditious removal of the liver is necessary or in non-heart-beating donors, thereby minimizing warm ischemia time.

The key steps involve placement of an aortic perfusion cannula in the distal aorta; placement of a portal perfusion cannula in the IMV or SMV; and isolation of the supraceliac aorta for cross-clamping. The proximal aorta is clamped and infusion of cold UW to the portal cannula and aortic catheters begun. The inferior vena cava can be vented either in the abdomen distally or in the chest at the junction of the right atrium. Cold slush solution is placed on all the abdominal organs. Once the organs have been cooled and flushed, the dissection can proceed in a more controlled manner, similar to that described for the traditional technique, except that the operative field is now bloodless. Again, particular care must be taken to identify replaced left or right HAs.

En Bloc Procurement

En bloc procurement of multiple abdominal organs is preferred by some surgeons. The ascending colon and small bowel are mobilized toward the right, and control is obtained of the distal aorta and vena cava just above the bifurcation. The liver is mobilized by dividing the triangular and coronary ligaments, and control of the supraceliac aorta is obtained. If the small bowel is being procured for transplant, then the SMA and superior mesenteric vein are isolated close to the uncinate process and looped. The small intestine is divided just proximal to the ileal cecal valve.

In coordination with the cardiac team, aortic cross-clamping and perfusion is then started. The aorta is perfused with 3 to 4L UW solution via a large cannula placed in the distal aorta. Venting takes place by division of the suprahepatic vena cava in the chest. Slush solution is packed in all four quadrants of the abdomen.

The dissection proceeds once the flushing is complete. The small bowel is removed by division of the superior mesenteric vessels. Care must be taken not to injure the inferior pancreaticoduodenal artery during this maneuver as it supplies the head of the pancreas. The gastrocolic ligament is incised and the duodenum divided with a stapler just distal to the pylorus. Dissection then continues sharply up the lesser curve of the stomach, allowing it to be retracted upward and out of the operative field. The entire colon is then mobilized. It is best to divide the mesentery just under the colon to avoid injury to underlying structures. Mobilization is continued down to the rectum, and the colon is retracted away from the operative field. Both ureters are then identified and transected as far distal as possible and mobilized off the retroperitoneum, leaving a generous amount of surrounding tissue. The distal aorta and vena cava are then divided just above the bifurcation. Next, the supraceliac aorta and suprahepatic vena cava are divided. The whole block containing the liver, pancreas, and kidneys is then mobilized in a cephalad-to-caudad direction. Injury to the underlying aorta, cava, and pancreas is avoided by maintaining a lateral plane. Dissection proceeds sequentially on the left and right sides, incorporating the kidneys in the block.

The multiorgan block is then removed from the abdominal cavity and placed in cold UW solution. The organs are carefully separated on the back table. Any anatomical variants can be readily identified. Portal venous flushing of the liver is accomplished on the back table. The gallbladder is also incised and flushed. Several variations of this technique have been described but the principle remains the same.[122,123]

Donor After Cardiac Death

Organs from donors after cardiac death (DCD) or non-heart-beating donors are increasingly being used to expand the donor pool.[124–127] In a recent analysis of UNOS data, 144 DCD liver transplants were reported with a 1-year graft survival of 70%.[124] However, the rate of PNF was significantly higher than grafts from heart-beating donors (11.8% vs. 6.4%), as was the retransplant rate (13.9% vs. 8.3%) (Table 85.12).

Other factors that influenced DCD graft failure included life support at the time of transplantation, dialysis at the time of transplantation, preoperative PT, and cold ischemia time (Table 85.13). Other series have also noted higher rates of PNF, requirement for retransplantation, and biliary complications leading to a significant decrease in graft survival rates (Table 85.12).

Although the surgical technique is similar to those already described, the key to successful procurement is minimization of warm ischemia. Once the decision to withdraw support has been made and consent obtained, the sequence of events is planned. Individual centers have specific protocols that require careful adherence. Withdrawal of support usually

TABLE 85.12.
Liver Transplantation from Donors After Cardiac Death.

Reference	*Year*	*Level of evidence*	*Donor*	*N*	*Patient survival, 1 yr*	*Patient survival, 3 yr*	*Graft survival, 1 yr*	*Graft survival, 3 yr*	*PNF*	*ReTx*	*Ischemic bile duct strictures*
Abt[124]	2004	II-3	DCD	144	79.7%	72.1%	70.2%	63.3%	11.8%	13.9%	
			HBD	26,856	85%	77.4%	80.4%	72.1%	6.4%	8.3%	
					$P = .082$	$P = .146$	$P = .003$	$P = .012$	$P = .008$	$P = .04$	
Reich[125]	2000	III	DCD	8	100%			100%	0	0	0
D'Alessandro[126]	2000	II-3	DCD	19		72.6%		53.8%	10.5%	21.1%	5.3%
			HBD	364		84.8%		80.9%	1.3%	—	4.6%
						$P = .36$		$P = .007$	$P = .04$		$P =$ NS
Casavilla[127]	1995	II-3	DCD-UC	6	67%		17%		50%	83.3%	
			DCD-C	6	50%		50%		0%	33.3%	

C, controlled; DCD, donors after cardiac death; HBD, heart-beating donors; NS, not significant; PNF, primary nonfunction; ReTx, retransplantation; UC, uncontrolled.

TABLE 85.13. Risk Factors for Early Graft Failure After Liver Transplantation Using Donors After Cardiac Death.

Variable	*Hazard ratio*	*95% CI*	*P value*
Life support at the time of transplant	5.13	2.2–12.2	<.001
Dialysis at the time of transplant	5.25	1.2–22.6	.026
Preoperative prothrombin time (per second change)	1.08	1.01–1.2	.024
Cold ischemic time	1.17	1.05–1.33	.007

Level of evidence II-3.
Source: From Abt et al.[124]

takes place in an intensive care unit setting[128] or in the operating room if consent has been obtained. Cannulation of the femoral artery and vein may be performed prior to extubation. Also, the donor may be systemically heparinized after extubation. After withdrawal of life support, if the potential donor does not proceed to asystole within 2h, the procedure is usually abandoned. Incision is only made after 5min of confirmed asystole. If life support has been withdrawn in the intensive care unit, the patient is rapidly transported to the operating room.

A standard midline incision is fashioned, and the abdominal cavity is immediately packed with cold slush solution. The distal aorta is quickly cannulated with a large-bore catheter and perfusion begun with UW solution. Alternatively, the perfusion can be through the femoral arterial cannula. It is usually easiest to vent through the distal vena cava or alternatively through the femoral venous line if in place. The supraceliac aorta is then cross-clamped. The organs and abdominal contents are carefully inspected during the flushing procedure. On completion of flushing, the procurement can then proceed using one of the techniques already described. Minimization of both cold and warm ischemia times is important.

Split Liver Procurement: Deceased Donor

A deceased donor liver may be split along anatomical planes, allowing transplantation into two separate recipients. In the early 1980s, investigators reported reducing donor livers so that they could be accommodated into pediatric recipients.[129,130] Usually, the right side of the liver was discarded and the viable left hemigraft transplanted into the recipient. However, with increasing need for donor livers, several groups started using the right hemigraft for implantation into smaller adults. This gradually evolved into a true splitting of the liver by which the liver was divided into left and right lobes and the resultant halves grafted into two adults.

Adult/Pediatric Split

In the adult/pediatric split technique, a left lateral segment graft is split from the main liver for use in a pediatric recipient. The operation follows the principles of segmental liver anatomy as described by Couinaud.[131] The split may be performed in situ or ex situ. Although in situ splitting is more time-consuming and requires careful coordination with the other procurement teams, it results in fewer biliary complications, less bleeding from the cut surface of the liver, and less risk of warm ischemic injury to the liver as it avoids back-table manipulation of the allograft.

Standard principles of liver procurement are initially followed. The suprahepatic vena cava is exposed, and the left HV is identified. The left HV is isolated separately from the middle HV. If there is a long common trunk, the left HV may be isolated during subsequent hepatic parenchymal transection. Dissection is then continued in the left hepatic hilum. This is best identified by following the umbilical ligament into the umbilical fissure. The left PV is isolated for its entire length. Small venous branches to segment 4 of the liver may be transected and ligated at this point. The left HA is also dissected. The segment 4 arterial branch is identified and preserved. Transection of the HA must be at a point distal to the origin of the segment 4 branch. Anatomical variations may be encountered and are dealt with accordingly. For example, a replaced left HA may be present, and this is kept with the lateral segment graft.

Hepatic transection then begins in a plane just toward the right of the falciform ligament. Once parenchymal transection is complete, the vascular structures are left intact for the time being. The aorta is cross-clamped, and flushing is performed per standard protocol. The liver graft can then be removed and the remaining transection completed ex situ. In this manner, a left lateral segment consisting of segments 2 and 3 is isolated. A larger, right-sided segment consisting of segments 4, 5, 6, 7, and 8 with the caudate lobe (segment 1) is also preserved for transplantation.

Adult/Adult Split

The adult/adult split is a true left-right split by which both hemilivers are transplanted into two small adults (Figs. 85.7 and 85.8). Procurement begins in standard fashion. Again, the split is best accomplished in situ. All hilar structures are carefully identified. Bifurcations of the HA, PV, and CBD are identified. The left hepatic vasculature can be temporarily clamped to identify a plane of transection. This is usually just toward the right of the middle HV. The liver parenchyma is carefully transected along this plane using standard methods. Once parenchymal transection is complete, the aorta is cross-clamped, and flushing proceeds in the standard fashion. The liver is then removed and the final separation takes place on the back table.

There are several variations in the splitting of the vasculature. Typically, the main PV is kept with the right-sided graft because of the longer left PV (Figs. 85.7A and 85.8A). The celiac trunk, proper HA, and left HA are kept with the left-sided graft. This allows preservation of the segment 4 artery with the left-sided graft. The CBD is usually kept with the right-sided graft, with the division taking place at the left hepatic duct just beyond the bifurcation. The vena cava can be kept with either side (Figs. 85.7A and 85.8A). Maintaining the cava with the right graft allows small and large HVs draining the right to be kept intact (Fig. 85.8A).[132] The final result is a right-sided graft consisting of segments 5, 6, 7, and 8 and a left-sided graft consisting of segments 4, 3, and 2. Part of the caudate lobe may go to each side depending on where the cava is preserved. Vascular structures may require reconstruction on the back table prior to implantation.

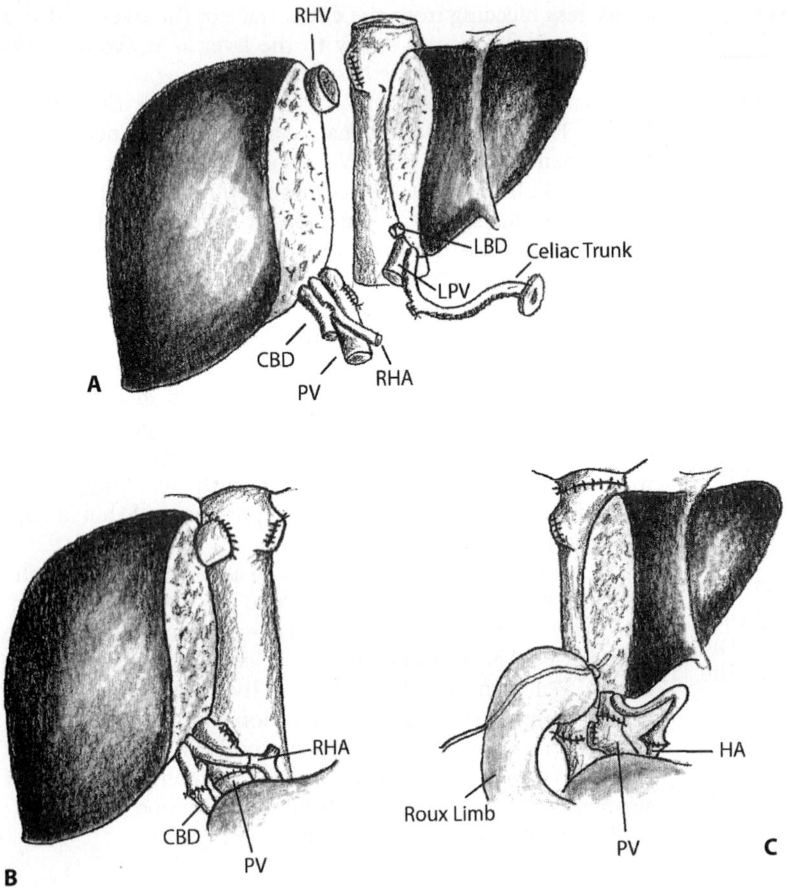

FIGURE 85.7. Deceased donor liver split. **A.** The liver is split in a plane just to the right of the middle hepatic vein, resulting in two hemigrafts. In this instance, the cava is preserved with the left lobe. CBD, common bile duct; LBD, left bile duct; LPV, left portal vein; PV, portal vein; RHA, right hepatic artery; RHV, right hepatic vein. **B.** Right lobe recipient operation. The donor RHV is anastomosed to the widened orifice of the recipient RHV. **C.** Left lobe recipient operation. The cava can be sewn orthotopically (depicted) or in a piggyback fashion. The left bile duct is anastomosed to a Roux-en-Y limb over a stent (depicted) or may be directly anastomosed to the recipient duct. HA, hepatic artery. (Courtesy of Khalid Khwaja, MD.)

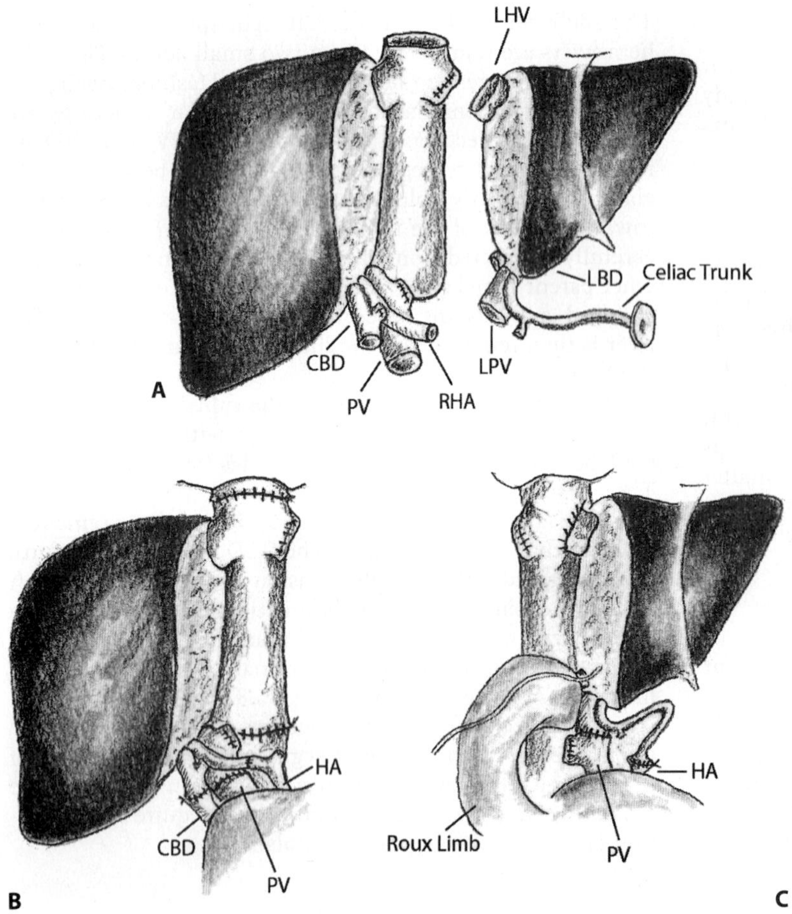

FIGURE 85.8. Deceased donor split. **A.** The liver is split in a plane just to the right of the middle hepatic vein, resulting in two hemigrafts. In this instance, the cava is preserved with the right lobe. CBD, common bile duct; LBD, left bile duct; LPV, left portal vein; PV, portal vein; RHA, right hepatic artery; RHV, right hepatic vein. **B.** Right lobe recipient operation. The cava can be sewn orthotopically (depicted) or in a piggyback fashion. **C.** Left lobe recipient operation. The donor LHV is anastomosed to the widened orifice of the recipient LHV. The left bile duct is anastomosed to a Roux-en-Y limb over a stent (depicted) or may be directly anastomosed to the recipient duct. HA, hepatic artery. (Courtesy of Khalid Khwaja, MD.)

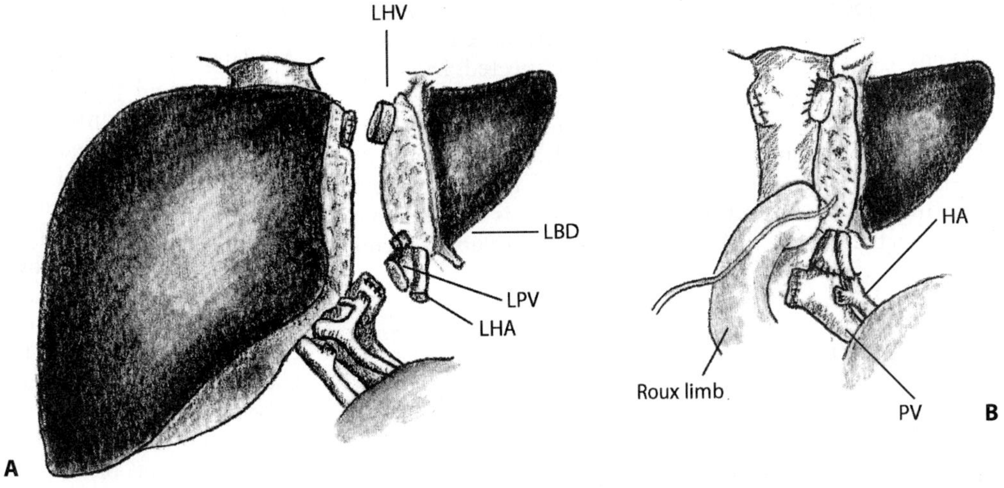

FIGURE 85.9. **A.** Living donor left lateral segmentectomy. The liver is transected at the falciform ligament. Portal and arterial branches to the medial segment are preserved on the recipient side. LBD, left bile duct; LHA, left hepatic artery; LHV, left hepatic vein; LPV, left portal vein. **B.** The recipient operation. The bile duct is anastomosed to a Roux-en-Y limb over a stent. Extension grafts may be used for vascular reconstruction. HA, hepatic artery; PV, portal vein. (Courtesy of Khalid Khwaja, MD.)

Living Donor Hepatectomy

Left Lateral Segmentectomy

The surgical technique of removing the left lobe or left lateral segment in the living donor has been well described.[133] The left HA, left PV, and left hepatic duct are isolated far to the left of the porta hepatis at the base of the falciform ligament (Fig. 85.9A). A segment 4 branch arising from the left HA is identified and preserved on the donor side. Similarly, any obvious portal venous branches supplying segment 4 should also be preserved. The left lateral segment HV is also identified and looped. Parenchymal transection takes place in a plane just to the right of the falciform ligament. The vessels are divided after systemic heparinization, and the liver is flushed on the back table with cold UW solution. If necessary, a segment of recipient saphenous vein may be used to lengthen the HA. Portal vein grafts are avoided if possible.

Right Donor Hepatectomy

The technique for a right donor hepatectomy has been well described[134,135] (Fig. 85.10A). Dissection begins in the hepatoduodenal ligament. The proper HA and its left and right bifurcation are identified. Occasionally, a segment 4 HA may arise from the right HA, and this should be identified and preserved on the donor side. The gallbladder is excised, and an intraoperative cholangiogram is obtained through the stump of the cystic duct. It is of paramount importance to carefully delineate biliary anatomy as anatomical variations are common. If there is an early division of the right hepatic duct into anterior and posterior sectoral branches, it may not be possible to obtain a single duct, and two separate biliary anastomoses will have to be performed in the recipient.

After cholangiography, the CBD is circumferentially dissected and the left and right hepatic ducts exposed. This usually involves taking down the hilar plate. The PV and its left and right divisions can be exposed by retracting the freed HA toward the left side. Next, the right HV is identified and controlled. The right lobe of the liver is completely mobilized. The hepatocaval ligament is divided, and small venous branches from the caudate lobe are ligated. Intraoperative ultrasound is particularly helpful in identifying the course of the middle HV, which guides parenchymal transection. Parenchymal transection is usually performed in a plane just toward the right of the middle HV. However, others prefer to transect the liver just to the left of the middle HV, keeping that structure with the graft.[136]

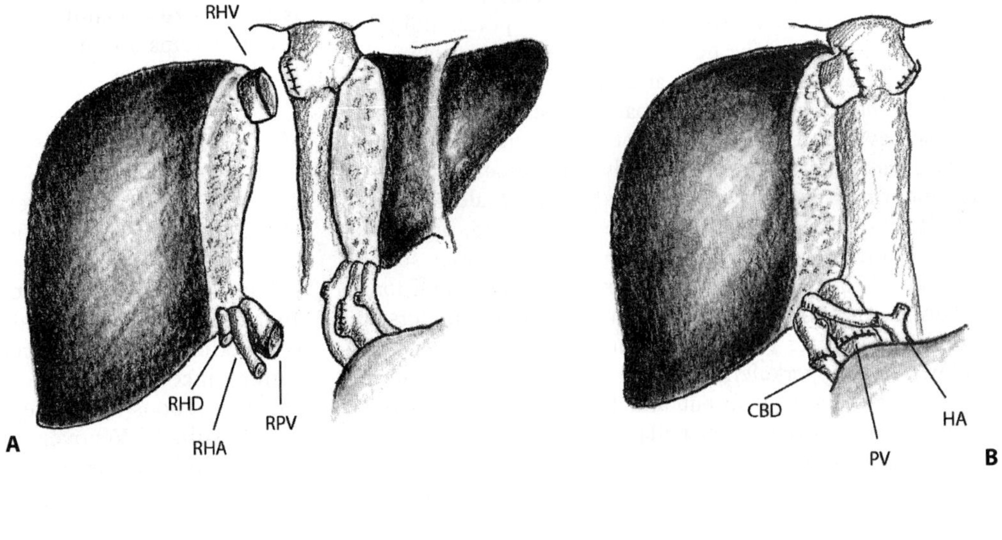

FIGURE 85.10. **A.** Living donor right hepatectomy. The liver is transected in a plane to the right of the middle hepatic vein. RHA, right hepatic artery; RHD, right hepatic duct; RHV, right hepatic vein; RPV, right portal vein. **B.** The recipient operation. Donor RHV is anastomosed to the widened orifice of the recipient RHV. (Courtesy of Khalid Khwaja, MD.)

On completion of parenchymal transection, the vessels are divided, and the liver is flushed on the back table with cold UW solution. The liver is carefully inspected. Large segmental veins (draining segment 5 or 8) may require separate implantation, either directly into the recipient's vena cava or via a saphenous vein graft. Early bifurcation of the right PV may result in two separate portal venous branches. These can sometimes be spatulated together or, if this is not possible, reconstructed using a "Y" graft taken from explanted recipient PV.

Recipient Procedures

Intraoperative Management

The recipient is taken to the operating room, often with a full stomach, where he or she undergoes induction of general anesthesia. A rapid sequence induction with cricoid pressure is used for intubation. General anesthesia is maintained with an inhalation agent, a neuromuscular blocking agent, and intravenous narcotics. Monitoring and infusion lines are placed, including two radial arterial lines (one for continuous measurement of arterial pressure and one for intermittent blood drawing), a right internal jugular vein Swan-Ganz catheter for hemodynamic monitoring, a 9-French trauma catheter for use with the rapid infuser placed in an internal jugular or a subclavian vein, and two 14-gauge peripheral intravenous lines. As is standard for any general anesthetic, continuous EKG, pulse oximetry, capnography, and core temperature monitoring are performed. A Foley catheter and nasogastric tube are placed, and a forced air warmer is used to maintain the body temperature. Intraoperatively, arterial blood pressure, central venous and pulmonary artery pressures, cardiac output, systemic vascular resistance, stroke volume, and urine output are monitored. Laboratory studies are measured at least hourly, including platelet count, electrolytes, ionized calcium, PT, partial thromboplastin time (PTT), factor and fibrinogen levels, fibrin degradation products, and arterial blood gases.

Several major events occur during a liver transplant that require attention. During the recipient hepatectomy, it is critical to carefully replace ongoing blood loss and to maintain normal fluid, electrolyte, and coagulation studies. After initiation of venovenous bypass and just before removing the liver, additional replacement is usually necessary because of a decrease in venous return that occurs when portal and vena caval blood return to the heart is interrupted. Increasing the venovenous bypass flow rate after the liver is removed is usually helpful. During the anhepatic phase, while hemostasis is achieved in the retroperitoneum and the liver is sewn in place, careful attention to hemodynamic changes, electrolyte abnormalities (hypocalcemia and hyperkalemia), and coagulation abnormalities (decreased fibrinogen, increased PT) is important, and correction of any abnormalities should be accomplished. Before unclamping the liver, additional calcium, sodium bicarbonate, and fluid or blood products are administered. After the liver is unclamped, there can be a brief period of hyperkalemia, hypocalcemia, metabolic acidosis, depressed cardiac output and hypotension, pulmonary hypertension and right ventricular dysfunction, and fibrinolysis that require correction.

Recipient Hepatectomy

A bilateral subcostal skin incision with a midline extension to the xiphoid process is used. The falciform ligament is divided cephalad until the anterior surface of the suprahepatic vena cava is identified. The left lobe is mobilized by dividing the left triangular and coronary ligaments and the gastrohepatic ligament. The hilar dissection begins with division of the cystic duct and artery. The left and right HAs are divided close to the liver to provide adequate length for a branch-patch anastomosis to the donor HA. The HAs are then dissected free proximal to the bifurcation, and a length of the common HA is isolated for subsequent clamping. If the HA is unsuitable for anastomosis at this point, further dissection to or beyond the takeoff of the GDA may be necessary.

The tissue posterior to the HA is divided, exposing the anterior aspect of the PV, which is mobilized distal to the bifurcation and proximal to the head of the pancreas. The lymph node tissue inferolateral and posterior to the CBD is divided, and the posterior aspect of the PV is identified. An opening anterior to the PV and posterior to the CBD is then made, leaving much of the surrounding tissue adjacent to the bile duct intact to avoid its devascularization. The CBD is ligated adjacent to the liver and divided.

The infrahepatic vena cava is then isolated. Mobilization of the right lobe of the liver is performed by dividing the right triangular and coronary ligaments. At this point, there are three options for completing the hepatectomy, depending on the procedure to be performed. In the traditional procedure in which the recipient vena cava is removed as part of the liver with the patient on venovenous bypass, the infrahepatic vena cava is completely mobilized from the level of the renal veins to the suprahepatic vena cava. The danger is bleeding from retroperitoneal collaterals. Alternatively, the infrahepatic and suprahepatic vena cavae can simply be isolated enough to allow clamping and the back wall of the vena cava left in place when the liver is excised. A third option is to divide the HVs entering the liver posteriorly from the anterior surface of the inferior vena cava and the liver dissected off the vena cava. The inferior vena cava is left in situ, which eliminates the need for venovenous bypass. The donor suprahepatic vena cava is then sewn into the confluence of the HV ("piggyback").

To remove the liver with the patient on venovenous bypass, the infrahepatic and suprahepatic vena cavae are clamped and divided and the liver removed. If the vena cava is left in situ, a clamp is placed across the confluence of the HV, the veins are divided within the liver parenchyma, and the liver is removed.

Venovenous Bypass

The advantages of venovenous bypass include maintenance of venous return and splanchnic venous drainage during the anhepatic phase with improved hemodynamic stability and reduction in mesenteric edema, improved renal perfusion, and provision of additional time to obtain hemostasis in the retroperitoneum, for placement of vascular grafts, and for performance of vascular anastomoses.[137,138] Many surgeons use venovenous bypass selectively or not at all with comparable results.[139] Venovenous bypass can be performed as an open technique with left saphenous vein and axillary vein

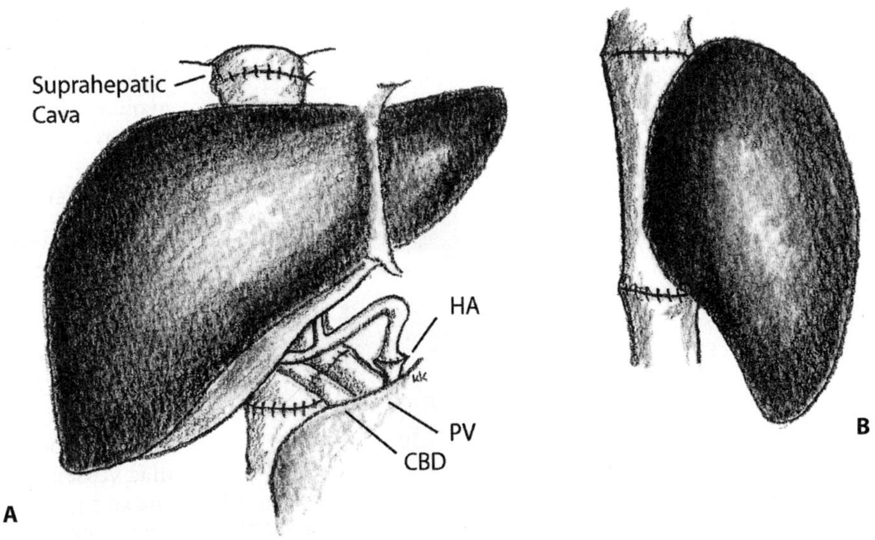

FIGURE 85.11. **A.** Orthotopic deceased donor liver transplant. Supra- and infrahepatic cavae are separately anastomosed. Corresponding donor and recipient hepatic arteries (HA), portal veins (PV), and bile ducts are anastomosed end to end. CBD, common bile duct. **B.** "Profile" view depicting donor inferior vena cava (IVC) interposed into recipient IVC. (Courtesy of Khalid Khwaja, MD.)

cutdowns. Alternatively, a percutaneous technique has been used, which is as effective and has an advantage of a significant reduction in wound complications.[140]

Deceased Donor Transplant

In deceased donor transplant, the suprahepatic vena caval anastomosis is performed first as an end-to-end anastomosis (Fig. 85.11A and 85.11B). The donor infrahepatic vena caval anastomosis is then performed while infusing 1 L cold lactated Ringer's solution through the PV cannula. This flushes the liver of UW solution, which is high in potassium and contains heparin. It also flushes air from the liver and reduces the risk of air emboli. The portal venovenous bypass cannula is clamped and removed from the recipient PV that is clamped. The PV anastomosis is completed end to end with a loosely tied corner ("growth stitch") to allow expansion of the PV after unclamping. If the PV is thrombosed, a long donor iliac vein graft can be sewn end to side to the SMV, which is isolated in the mesentery of the transverse colon. It is tunneled retrocolic, posterior to the antrum and anterior to the pancreas for anastomosis to the PV.

There are several techniques for performing the arterial anastomosis, depending on the size of the vessels and the arterial anatomy. It can be performed as an end-to-end anastomosis between the recipient proper HA and the donor common HA. Our preferred technique is to longitudinally open the recipient right and left HA branches to create a "branch patch" (Fig. 85.12). An end-to-end anastomosis of the branch patch to the donor celiac axis with a Carrel patch is completed. Alternatively, the donor common HA can be sewn end to side to the junction of the common HA and the GDA. If there is inadequate inflow via the recipient HA or celiac axis, a donor iliac arterial graft can be placed to the supraceliac or infrarenal aorta. After completion of the vascular anastomoses, the clamps are removed sequentially. First, the PV clamp is removed and the liver perfused, followed by the suprahepatic vena cava clamp, HA clamp, and inferior vena cava clamp. Hemostasis is obtained, and the patient is taken off venovenous bypass.

The bile duct is usually reconstructed as an end-to-end choledochostomy using interrupted absorbable sutures. Traditionally, this has been performed over a T tube brought out through a separate choledochotomy. However, because 10% to 15% of patients develop a bile duct leak after T-tube removal, necessitating an ERCP and nasobiliary drain or stent placement, some centers have eliminated the use of T tubes

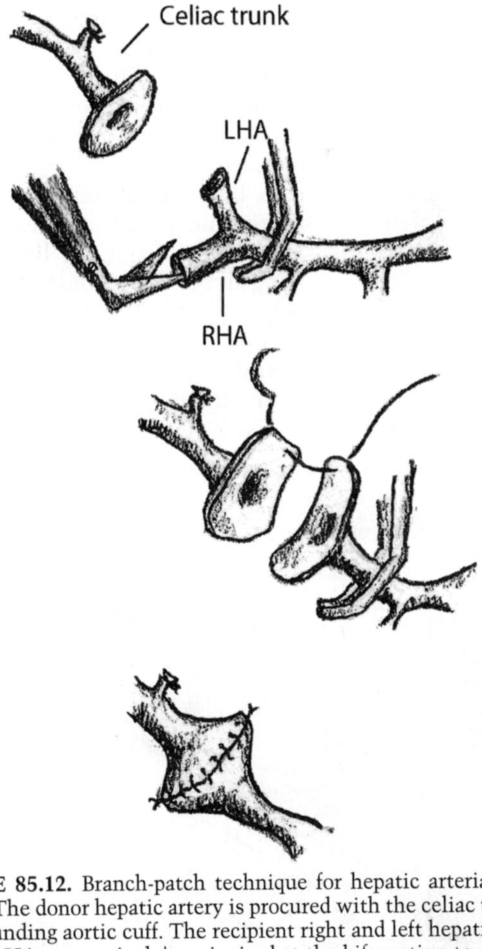

FIGURE 85.12. Branch-patch technique for hepatic arterial anastomosis. The donor hepatic artery is procured with the celiac trunk and a surrounding aortic cuff. The recipient right and left hepatic arteries (RHA, LHA, respectively) are incised at the bifurcation to create the branch patch; this is anastomosed to the aortic cuff. (Courtesy of Khalid Khwaja, MD.)

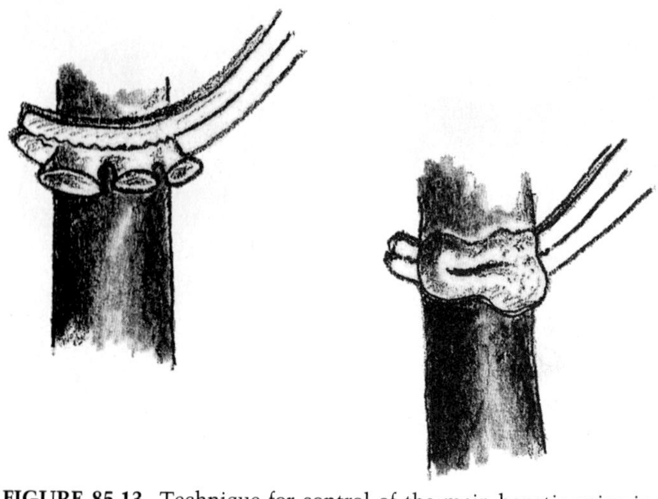

FIGURE 85.13. Technique for control of the main hepatic veins in preparation for piggyback liver transplantation. (Courtesy of Khalid Khwaja, MD.)

with comparable results.[141,142] If the recipient bile duct is not usable secondary to disease (e.g., PSC or large periductal varices) or there is a marked size discrepancy with the donor duct, an end-to-side Roux-en-Y choledochojejunostomy should be performed. A small 5-French feeding tube is placed through the anastomosis and brought out through a tunnel in the Roux loop. The anastomosis is done as a single-layer anastomosis using absorbable sutures. Careful hemostasis is obtained, all anastomoses are reinspected, the abdomen is irrigated with antibiotic-containing saline solution, and drains are placed. The abdomen is closed.

An alternative method for liver transplantation is the piggyback technique.[143] This technique involves leaving the recipient vena cava in situ and mobilizing the liver off the interior vena cava by dividing all the HVs entering the posterior aspect of the liver. Only the left, middle, and right HVs are left in place. A clamp is placed across the HVs and the confluence of the veins opened (Fig. 85.13). The donor infrahepatic vena cava is oversewn on the back table, eliminating one anastomosis, and the donor suprahepatic vena cava is sewn end to end to the confluence of the recipient HVs (Fig. 85.14A and 85.14B). Venovenous bypass is not required. In addition, there is significantly less blood loss as a result of avoiding dissection posterior to the vena cava where bleeding from retroperitoneal collaterals can be encountered.

Split Liver Transplants

The surgical techniques for split liver implantation are similar to those described for living donor transplants. Generally, left lateral segments are transplanted into pediatric recipients (see Fig. 85.9B). The right lobe can be transplanted into an adult recipient via orthotopic (Fig. 85.8B) or piggyback placement (see Fig. 85.7B). The left lobe can be transplanted into small adults orthotopically (see Fig. 85.7C) or piggyback (see Fig. 85.8C), depending on how the split was performed. Donor iliac vessels are used as extension grafts if necessary. Recipient and graft survival rates are similar to those reported for whole-organ transplants, but biliary complications are in the 20%–30% range[144,145] (Table 85.14).

Living Donor Transplants

Left Lateral Segment Grafts

The left lateral segment graft is procured and prepared as previously described (Fig. 85.9A). The recipient hepatectomy is similar to that described for the piggyback technique, with preservation of the entire vena cava, and as much length as possible on the left PV and HA. The donor left HV is sewn to the confluence of the left and middle HVs in the recipient (Fig. 85.9B). Attention to graft orientation within the abdomen and construction of a widely patent venous outflow is important to avoid postoperative congestion.[146,147] The donor HA is anastomosed to the recipient HA if length allows. A saphenous vein graft may be used to anastomose the HA directly to the aorta,[133] and the use of a surgical microscope has led to a significant reduction in arterial complications.[148] Not all arterial branches need to be revascularized as long as pulsatile backbleeding is noted following anastomosis of the largest trunk.[149] The graft PV can generally be sewn to the recipient left (or main) PV. Roux-en-Y biliary reconstruction, in some cases to separate segment 2 and 3 ducts, is performed.

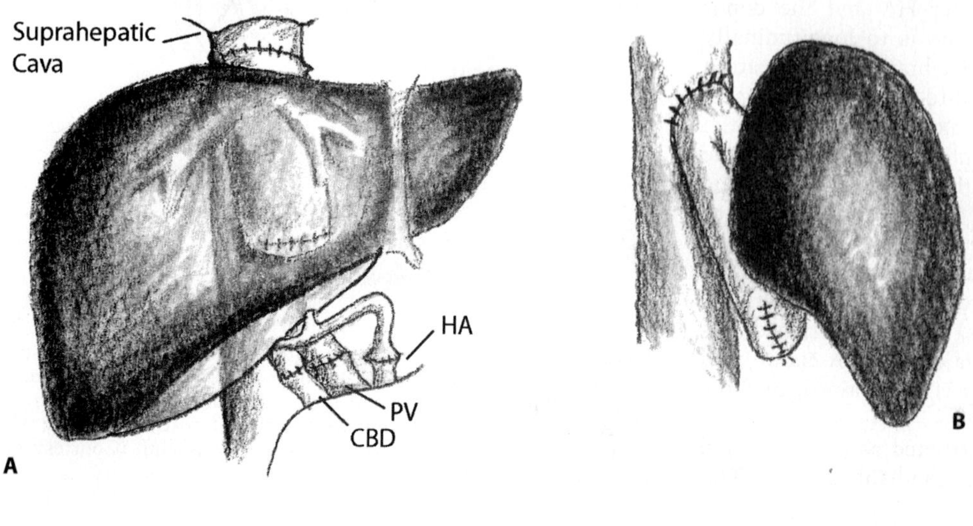

FIGURE 85.14. A. Piggyback deceased donor liver transplant. The distal donor inferior vena cava (IVC) is oversewn and the suprahepatic end piggybacked onto the recipient IVC, usually at the orifices of the hepatic veins. Donor and recipient hepatic arteries (HAs), portal veins (PVs), and bile ducts are anastomosed end to end. CBD, common bile duct. B. "Profile" view depicting donor IVC piggybacked onto recipient IVC. (Courtesy of Khalid Khwaja, MD.)

TABLE 85.14.
Adult/Adult Split Liver Transplantation.

Reference	Year	Level of evidence	N	Patient survival (%)	Graft survival	Follow-up (mo)	PNF (%)	Biliary complications (%)	HA thrombosis (%)	Comments
Humar[226]	2004	III	28	79	79%	28	3	21	7	Splits all performed in situ
Azoulay[145]	2001	III	34	84	75%	24	9	21	6	30 splits were ex situ
Adorno[144]	2001	III	8	88	72%	10–18	12	Not reported	12	All in situ

HA, hepatic artery; PNF, primary nonfunction.

Right Lobe Grafts

For right lobe grafts, the recipient hepatectomy is performed in a similar manner. The right and left hepatic ducts are individually ligated beyond the common duct bifurcation. As much length as possible is maintained on the right HA. The right lobe graft is procured and prepared as previously described (Fig. 85.10A). The donor right HV is anastomosed to the orifice of the recipient right HV (Fig. 85.10B). Accessory HVs draining segments 5 or 8 that are larger than 5 mm should be reimplanted, either directly into the cava or through saphenous vein grafts[150,151] (Fig. 85.15). The donor PV is sewn to the recipient right (or main) PV (Fig. 85.10B). The donor and recipient right HAs are anastomosed end to end. Several innovative variations in arterial reconstruction have been described, including Y grafts from the recipient HA bifurcation if there are two donor arteries (ex situ reconstruction).[152] Biliary reconstruction can be performed as an end-to-end anastomosis. Often, two separate anastomoses to anterior and posterior sectoral ducts have to be performed, and in this situation, the donor right and left ducts may be used separately. Alternatively, Roux-en-Y biliary reconstruction may be employed.

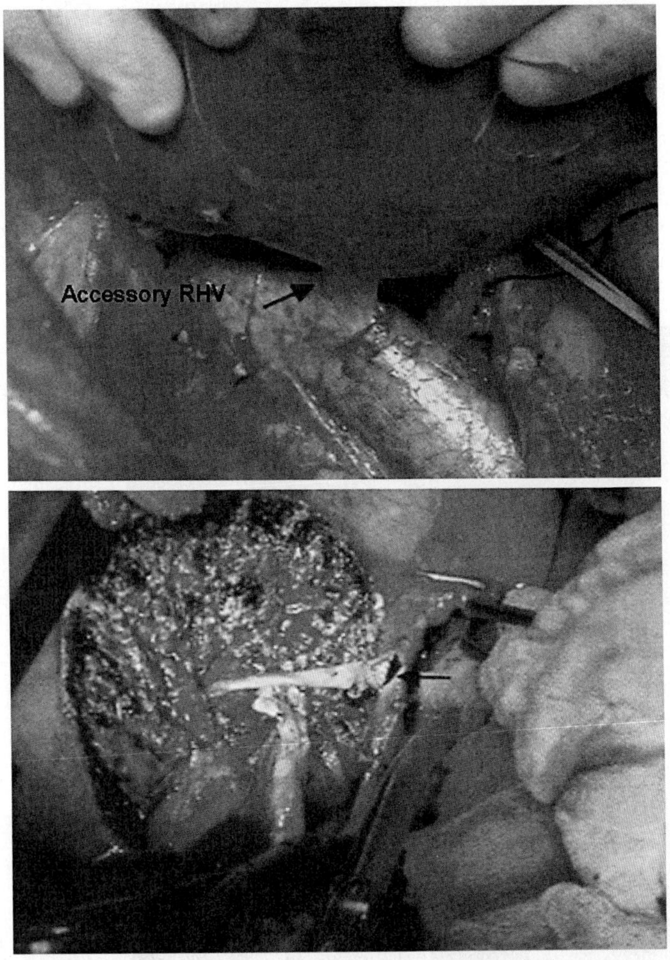

FIGURE 85.15. In the *top panel*, a large accessory right hepatic vein enters the posterior right lobe of the liver. In the *lower panel*, a saphenous vein extension graft is used to reimplant the hepatic vein into the recipient vena cava (*arrow*). (From Humar et al.,[151] by permission of *Liver Transplantation*.)

Postoperative Surgical Complications

Vascular Complications

Hepatic Artery

Compromise of the arterial flow to the graft can be caused by HA thrombosis (HAT), stenosis, pseudoaneurysm, mycotic aneurysm, rupture, or compression by the arcuate ligament. All are serious complications that require urgent diagnosis and treatment.

Hepatic artery thrombosis occurs in between 3% and 12% of patients.[153] Review of published data from large centers reveals a mortality rate of 31% and a retransplantation rate of 53%.[153] Usually, HAT occurs within the first 2 months posttransplant and can be associated with one of three syndromes: (1) acute, massive hepatic necrosis leading to fulminant hepatic failure; (2) biliary tract ischemia leading to bile duct necrosis and leak; or (3) relapsing bacteremia with recurrent febrile illnesses due to cholangitis from biliary strictures and bilomas.[154] Nearly 75% of patients with HAT require retransplantation, although some grafts can be salvaged if HAT is recognized early and revascularization of the HA is urgently accomplished.[155–157]

Early diagnosis correlates with improved outcomes, so screening Doppler ultrasound is recommended.[158] Presentation, diagnosis, and management differ depending on whether the thrombosis occurs less than or greater than 1 month after transplant. Early thrombosis raises concern for graft failure. Indeed, UNOS elevates patients with HAT within 1 week after transplantation to status I in recognition of the poor prognosis of this lesion. Almost all will present with increases in transaminase levels; cholestasis is also very common.[153] Risk factors include donor age greater than 60 and reconstruction of variant arterial anatomy.[159]

Treatment options include operative revision of the artery; interventional radiologic approaches, including fibrinolysis, angioplasty, and stenting (Fig. 85.16); retransplantation; or if the symptoms are mild, expectant management. It is possible to reopen arteries percutaneously with good long-term results.[160]

Risk factors for late HAT include interposition grafts and donors dying of a CVA.[159] Although generally considered to have a more benign course than early HAT, this is not born out in the literature. Complications include biliary ischemia, recurring cholangitis, and intrahepatic abscesses. These complications require retransplantation in as many as 75% of patients.[161] Small sample size and lack of randomized data make it difficult to base specific clinical decisions on the data. For example, it would be incorrect to conclude native arterial supply should be used preferentially to a conduit as the data are biased toward using conduits when the arterial supply is poor.

Hepatic artery stenosis occurs in approximately 4.8%–11% of patients,[162] and these patients are at markedly increased risk of biliary complications compared to control groups (67% vs. 28%).[162] Patient survival of 65% at 4 years following arterial revision has been achieved using either operative or percutaneous approaches.[156,160]

Hepatic artery pseudoaneurysms are rare (0.2%–0.9%), usually occur at the anastomosis, are often infected, and may rupture and cause fatal hemorrhage, making early diagnosis and treatment imperative. They may occur after percutaneous attempts at arterial revascularization.[163] Scanning by CT is accurate in two-thirds of patients, ultrasound in one-third, and angiography in all cases. Resection and primary anastomosis or reconstruction with an interposition graft can be performed in the absence of infection. In the presence of infection, excision and ligation of the HA is advisable even though retransplantation may be required.

Arcuate ligament syndrome occurs when the muscular and fibrous bands overlying the celiac axis compromise HA supply.[164,165] This problem can be treated by division of the arcuate ligament or by reconstruction of the HA with an iliac artery conduit from the supraceliac or infrarenal aorta.

Portal Vein

Rates of PV thrombosis (PVT) after liver transplantation vary from 1% in uncomplicated adult transplants to as high as 13% in the presence of PVT prior to transplantation, use of split livers, use of PV conduits, and pediatric transplantation. The diagnosis is usually made by ultrasound, CT angiography, MR, or angiography. Treatment options include operative thrombectomy, construction of a donor iliac vein conduit from the SMV to PV, or percutaneous transhepatic thrombolytic therapy and possible stent placement. Portal vein thrombosis may lead to liver failure, requiring retransplantation, or to recurrent portal hypertension.

Biliary Tract Complications

Approximately 10%–15% of patients will develop biliary complications after standard adult-to-adult deceased donor liver transplant.[166,167] Split liver and live donor grafts have a

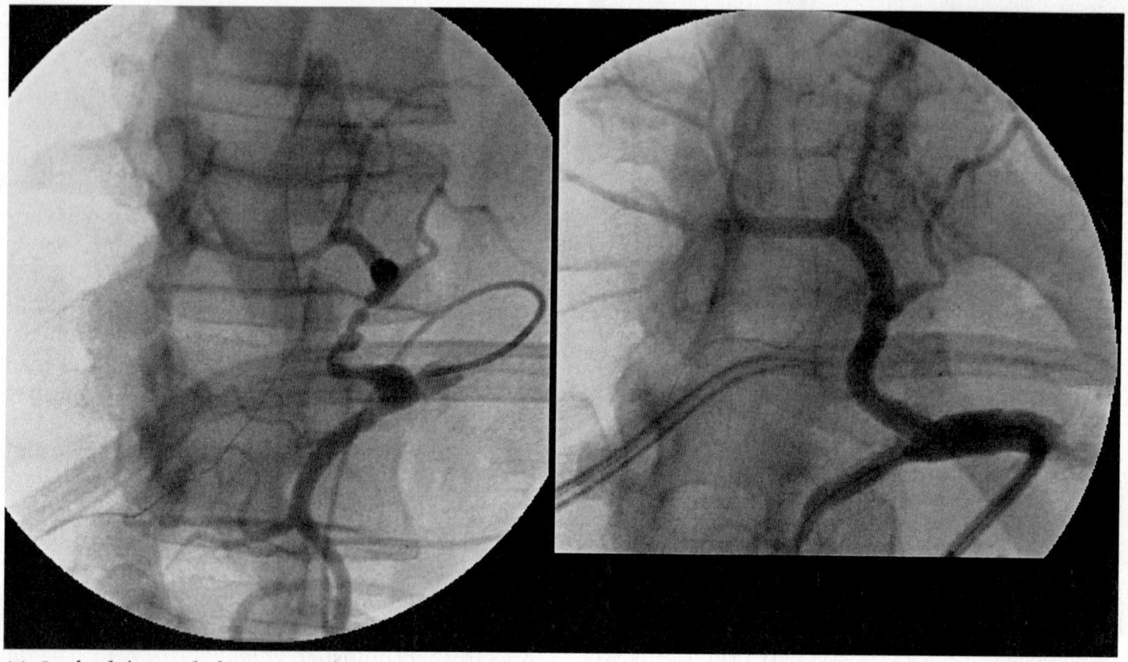

FIGURE 85.16. In the *left panel*, three areas of stenosis are demonstrated in the donor proper hepatic artery distal to the donor–recipient anastomosis and just proximal to the bifurcation of the hepatic artery into left and right branches. In the *right panel*, the artery is visualized after successful balloon dilation and stenting with a normal lumen. (Courtesy of Duane Pinto, MD, Beth Israel Deaconess Medical Center, Boston, MA.)

higher incidence of biliary complications, as do grafts from donors after cardiac death.[168,169] Complications include leaks from anastomotic sites or T-tube entry or exit sites; strictures at the anastomosis or of the biliary tree; obstruction from sludge, stones, or stents; and biliary fistula from stent migration. Approximately two-thirds of biliary tract complications occur in the first 4 weeks posttransplant. These are usually anastomotic bile duct leaks related to technical errors or ischemia of the distal bile duct. Late complications are primarily anastomotic and intrahepatic strictures. These complications are potentially serious and result in graft loss in about 2% of patients.

Anastomotic leaks usually present with bilious drainage from surgically placed drains or from the wound or with signs of intraabdominal infection. Cholangiography through the T tube or biliary stent can determine the site and severity of the leak. Patency of the HA should be confirmed by ultrasonography or angiography. A CAT scan should be obtained to rule out a subhepatic biloma. Anastomotic strictures may present with elevated liver function tests, cholangitis, or signs of obstruction on liver biopsy. The diagnosis is made by T-tube cholangiography, if still in place, by ERCP, or by PTC in patients with a Roux-en-Y hepaticojejunostomy.

Routine use of T tubes is controversial (Table 85.15). Placement involves inserting the top of the T into the donor bile duct so that one limb passes through the anastomosis and the other is directed up into the liver. The body of the tube is passed out through the skin. The advantage of the tube is easy access to the biliary tree. The disadvantages include leaks, tube dislodgement, and obstruction. Two randomized controlled studies failed to show any benefit of routine use of T tubes. One study demonstrated increased rates of cholangitis and biliary fistula with T-tube use.[170] In another, smaller study, Vougas et al.[142] found similar complication rates in 60 patients randomized to T tube or no T tube. Other retrospective studies also failed to demonstrate the superiority of routine T-tube placement, including the University of California at Los Angeles experience, which centered on cost-effectiveness and demonstrated longer hospital stay, higher rates of complications, and greater cost associated with T-tube use.[171]

Recent evidence demonstrates good outcomes with nonoperative management of most of these complications. A combination of ERCP, transhepatic catheter placement, balloon dilation, and stenting will be definitive management in the majority of patients.[172] In addition, endoscopic management can be useful not only as definitive therapy but also as a temporizing measure prior to operative management.[173]

Live Donor Complications

Complications in the right lobe of adult live donors are an important issue because of medical and ethical concerns over donor morbidity and mortality in otherwise healthy individuals. It is generally believed that donor complications are underreported and therefore underestimated. The overall morbidity is estimated to be between 20% and 50%,[174] including biliary tract complications (injury to the common or right hepatic bile duct, bile duct leak from the cut surface of the liver, bile duct stricture) in 3% to 8%, PVT, small bowel obstruction, wound infection, incisional hernia, splenic rupture, pneumonia, pleural effusion, neuropraxia, thrombophlebitis and pulmonary emboli, and duodenal ulcer. Fatal postoperative pulmonary emboli have been reported in both the United States and Europe. A recent review of documented deaths places the estimated rate of donor death between 0.15% and 0.20%.[175]

TABLE 85.15.
Routine Use of T Tubes.

Author	*Year*	*Type of evidence*	*Randomization*	*Study type*		*Length of stay*	*Biliary complications*	*Cost*	*Retransplantations*	*Patient survival*	*Comments*
Vougas[142]	1996	I	Yes	Randomized, controlled	T tube No T tube	—	16.6% 20% (NS)	—	—	—	60 patients; no evidence that T tubes improve outcomes
Scatton[170]	2001	I	Yes	Randomized, controlled	T tube No T tube	—	33.3% 15.5% (P < .005)	—	4.4% 3.3% (NS)	72.8% 80.15% (NS)	180 patients; higher incidence of biliary complications due primarily to increased cholangitis and biliary fistula
Shimoda[171]	2001	II-2	No	Retrospective	T tube No T tube	31.1 days 18.8 days ($P < .001$)	32.9% 15.5% (P < .01)	Higher Lower (NS)	80% graft survival 89.5% graft survival (NS)	83% 89.5% (NS)	147 patients; not randomized
Randall[222]	1996	II-2	No	Retrospective	T tube No T tube	—	22% 13.7% (NS)	—	—	84.7% 90.6% (NS)	110 patients; no benefit with T tubes

NS, not significant.

Immunosuppression

The optimal immunosuppressive regimen after liver transplantation has yet to be established. There are several immunosuppressive drugs, polyclonal antibodies, and monoclonal antibodies currently available that are used in various combinations to optimize the degree of immunosuppression, thereby minimizing the incidence of acute and chronic rejection, while attempting to decrease the adverse side effects, including drug toxicity, infections, and malignancy. They have different sites of action in the cascade of immunological events that lead to allograft rejection (Fig. 85.17).

Immunosuppressive Drugs (Table 85.16)

Antimetabolites

Mycophenolate mofetil (MMF) is the morpholinoethylester of mycophenolic acid (MPA) and is rapidly converted to MPA after oral administration or intravenous administration. Mycophenolic acid inhibits inosine monophosphate dehydrogenases, thereby blocking proliferation of T and B lymphocytes and inhibits antibody formation and the generation of cytotoxic T cells. Also, MPA downregulates the expression of adhesion molecules on lymphocytes. It is glucuronidated in the liver and excreted primarily by the kidneys. Mycophenolic acid can be administered orally or intravenously in doses from 250 to 1000mg two to three times per day (total dose 1–3g/day). It has been used to rescue patients with resistant rejection and as part of triple or quadruple immunosuppressive protocols. The primary side effects, which in general are dose-dependent, include nausea, diarrhea, gastritis, leukopenia, anemia, and viral infections.

Azathioprine (AZA), a purine synthesis inhibitor, and cytoxan, an alkylating agent, were commonly used in the past, but their use has largely been replaced by MMF.

TABLE 85.16. Immunosuppressive Agents.

Generic names	*Brand names*
Antimetabolites	
Azathioprine	Imuran
Cyclophosphamide	Cytoxan, Neosar
Mycophenolate mofetil	CellCept
Mycophenolate sodium	Myfortic
Corticosteroids	
Prednisone	
Methylprednisolone	
Calcineurin inhibitors	
Cyclosporine (cyclosporine A)	Sandimmune, Neoral, Gengraf, Eon, SangCya, generic cyclosporine
Tacrolimus (FK506)	Prograf
Target of rapamycin (TOR) inhibitors	
Sirolimus	Rapamune
Everolimus	Certican
Polyclonal antibodies	
Antithymocyte globulin (rabbit)	Thymoglobulin
Antithymocyte globulin (equine)	ATGAM
Monoclonal antibodies	
Anti-CD3	
Muromonab-CD3	Orthoclone OKT3
Anti-CD25 (IL-2 receptor)	
Basiliximab	Simulect
Daclizumab	Zenapax
Anti-CD52	
Alemtuzumab	Campath 1-H

Corticosteroids

Corticosteroids have been the mainstay of immunosuppression since first introduced in 1960 to treat acute allograft rejection. The actions of corticosteroids are complex, but they have been shown to alter the transcription and translation of several genes responsible for cytokine synthesis. They inhibit T-cell activation by blocking interleukins 1, 2, and 6 and

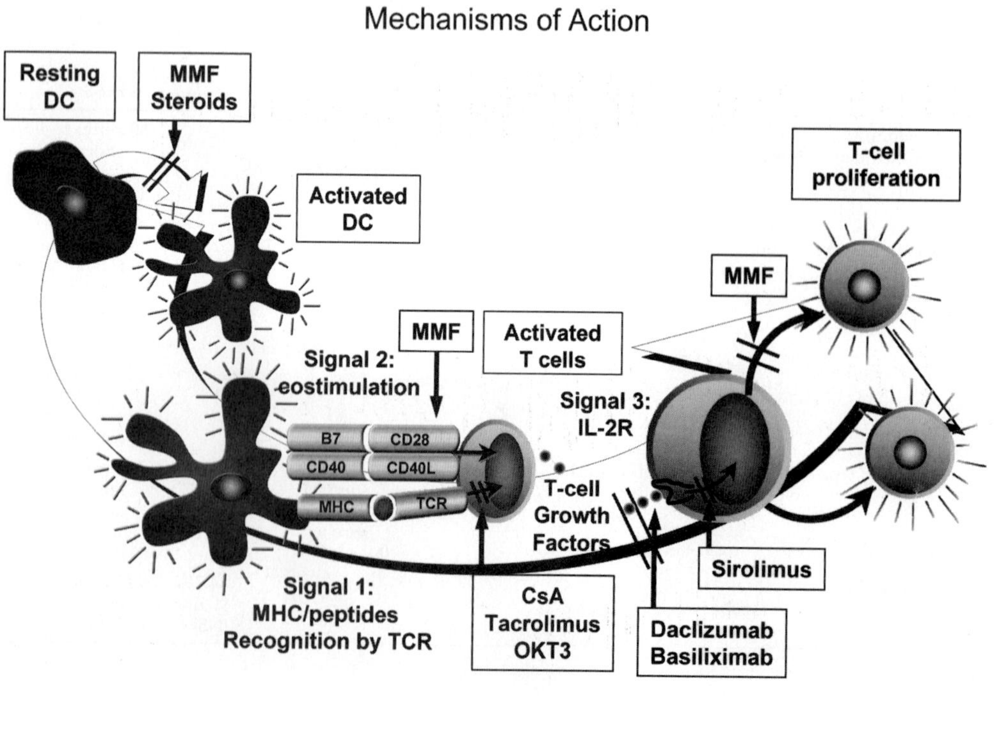

FIGURE 85.17. Sites of action of commonly used immunosuppressive drugs in the cascade of events leading to allograft rejection. MHC, major histocompatibility complex.

IFN-γ synthesis. They also have local antiinflammatory effects. Corticosteroids are used as part of many induction and maintenance immunosuppressive regimens and are usually the first-line treatment for allograft rejection.

Many protocols now incorporate early corticosteroid withdrawal to avoid their long-term side effects. These side effects include Cushingoid features (moon facies, acne, centripetal obesity, striae), hypertension, increased appetite and weight gain, hyperglycemia, osteoporosis, avascular necrosis, posterior lenticular cataracts, growth retardation in children, poor wound healing, thinning of the skin with increased fragility and ecchymoses, pancreatitis, peptic ulceration, colonic perforation, steroid-induced hyperactivity or psychosis, and predisposition to infectious and malignant complications.

Calcineurin Inhibitors

Cyclosporine A (CsA) and tacrolimus (TAC) are calcineurin inhibitors (CNIs) due to their similar mechanism of action of binding to their specific immunophilins, which inhibits calcineurin activity and blocks signal transduction necessary for the transcription of several early T-cell activation genes, including IL-2, IL-3, IL-4, and IFN-γ. This action blocks the development of sensitized cytotoxic and helper T cells. The introduction of CNIs for use in liver transplant recipients dramatically improved patient and graft survival rates and reduced the incidence of rejection.

Cyclosporine A can be administered orally or intravenously and trough (C_0) or 2-h postdose (C_2) blood levels monitored. Neoral (Novartis) is a microemulsion formulation that has better bioavailability than earlier formulations and is not dependent on bile for its absorption. Neoral is usually started posttransplant orally in two divided doses with a target C_0 level of 350 to 450 ng/mL or C_2 level of 0.8 to 1.2 µg/mL for the first month posttransplant. Monitoring with C_2 levels has been associated with a reduction in the incidence and severity of acute rejection without an increase in toxicity.[176] Tacrolimus can be administered orally or intravenously and trough (C_0) levels monitored. TAC is usually started at 0.1 to 0.15 mg/kg/day for the first month, with target levels of 5 to 15 ng/mL. Typically, CsA and TAC are used clinically in various combinations with MMF, corticosteroids, rapamycin (RAPA), and polyclonal or monoclonal antibodies.

Side effects of CsA include nephrotoxicity; hypertension; hyperkalemia; hyperuricemia and gout; gingival hypertrophy; hirsutism; neurological abnormalities (tremors, seizures, hyperactivity, insomnia, confusion, depression, somnolence); hyperglycemia; hypomagnesemia; hypercholesterolemia; hypertriglyceridemia; hepatotoxicity; and the development of de novo hemolytic uremic syndrome. The adverse effects of TAC are similar to CsA and include nephrotoxicity; neurological complications (headaches, tremors, paresthesias); and hyperglycemia. Hypertension and hirsutism are more commonly associated with CsA and neurological side effects and hyperglycemia are usually associated with TAC.

Polyclonal Antibodies

Polyclonal antibodies are heterologous antisera made most commonly in horses, goats, or rabbits against human lymphocytes or thymocytes. They cause a rapid decline in circulating T and B lymphocytes as a result of apoptosis, complement-dependent lysis, and opsonization of lymphocytes with subsequent removal in the reticuloendothelial system. Horse antithymocyte globulin (ATGAM, Pfizer) and rabbit antithymocyte globulin (Thymoglobulin, Genzyme) are currently the only polyclonal antibodies approved for use by the U.S. Food and Drug Administration. ATGAM is administered intravenously in a dose of 10 to 30 mg/kg/day for 3 to 14 days posttransplant, and Thymoglobulin is dosed 1.5 mg/kg/day for 3 to 14 days for rejection prophylaxis and to reduce CNI exposure. ATGAM and Thymoglobulin are also used for the treatment of steroid-resistant rejection. The most frequent side effects include fever, chills, nausea, vomiting, diarrhea, athralgias, headache, myalgias, rash, pruritus, urticaria, phlebitis, leukopenia, thrombocytopenia, and predisposition to viral infections.

Monoclonal Antibodies

Muromonab-CD3 (OKT3) is a murine IgG_{2a} monoclonal antibody that reacts with the T3 recognition complex on the surface of mature T lymphocytes and blocks the recognition of class I and class II antigens, resulting in the inhibition of the generation and function of effector T cells. Its primary mechanism of action in vivo involves the binding of OKT3 to circulating T cells with increase in the opsonization and destruction of these cells by the reticuloendothelial system. Also, OKT3 acts by modulation of the T3 antigen recognition complex of circulating T cells and by inhibiting the function of sessile T cells. It is administered intravenously at a dose of 2.5 to 5 mg/day for 3 to 14 days posttransplant for rejection prophylaxis, to reduce CNI exposure, and for the treatment of steroid-resistant rejection. Levels of CD3 and antimurine antibody titers are monitored. Side effects are most commonly seen with the first two doses and include fever, chills, diarrhea, headache, nausea, vomiting, dyspnea, wheezing, pulmonary edema, tachycardia, hypotension, aseptic meningitis, seizures, and coma. These side effects result from the release of tumor necrosis factor (TNF), IFN-γ, and IL-1. This symptom complex can be reduced by pretreatment of the patient with high-dose steroids, acetaminophen, diphenhydramine hydrochloride, and indomethacin. Between 15% and 40% of patients develop antimurine antibodies.

Basiliximab (Simulect, Novartis) is a chimeric anti-CD25 monoclonal antibody bearing the murine variable IgG_{2a} antigen-combining site and IgG_1 human constant regions. The advantage over murine antibodies is that it does not have the xenogeneic murine Fc region structures but retains the variable region-combining site of the murine antibody and therefore does not stimulate a host antimurine immune response. The chimeric antibody binds to the high-affinity IL-2 receptor (IL-2R) and prevents binding of IL-2 to the receptor and blocks IL-2-driven proliferative responses, the duration of which is dose-dependent. It has a mean half-life of 1 to 2 weeks. Basiliximab is administered intravenously at a dose of 20 mg at the time of transplant and 4 days later. This regimen produces a 30- to 45-day blockade of IL-2R expression in adult patients. Basiliximab is used primarily for rejection prophylaxis. No adverse side effects compared to placebo have been reported.

Daclizumab (Zenapax, Hoffman-LaRoche) is a humanized monoclonal antibody that is a human IgG_1 containing the antigen-binding regions of a murine anti-CD25 monoclonal antibody that binds to the high-affinity IL-2R in a similar fashion to basiliximab. Daclizumab is administered intravenously in a dose of 1 mg/kg before transplantation and then every 2 weeks for a total of five doses. Its effects on IL-2R suppression last up to 10 weeks, and it is used primarily for rejection prophylaxis. No adverse side effects have been reported.

Alemtuzumab (Campath-1H) (C-1H) is a humanized, recombinant anti-CD52 monoclonal antibody that results in profound depletion of mature T cells and to a lesser degree B cells and monocytes for over a month. It is administered intravenously at the time of transplant and posttransplant at a dose of 0.3 mg/kg for one to three doses for rejection prophylaxis and CNI sparing.[177] It has also been given for long-term therapy by redosing based on recovery of the lymphocyte count.

Mammalian Targets of Rapamycin Inhibitors

Sirolimus or rapamycin (RAPA) (Rapamune, Wyeth-Ayerst) is a macrolide antibiotic that binds to the same intracellular receptors as TAC, termed FKBPs and specifically to the isoform FKBP12.[178,179] The sirolimus–FKBP12 complex inhibits targets of rapamycin (TOR) and the signal III pathway blocking T-cell activation and proliferation after cytokine stimulation and costimulation interactions. It blocks G_1-to-S transition, translation, and cytokine-induced T-cell proliferation. Also, RAPA inhibits fibroblast activity that interferes with wound healing. It is administered orally at a dose of 1 to 5 mg per day posttransplant and is rapidly absorbed but has a long half-life of 62 h and reaches steady state in 7–14 days. Drug levels are monitored with target trough levels between 5 and 15 ng/mL depending on the time posttransplant. Side effects include anemia, leukopenia, thrombocytopenia, elevated serum cholesterol and triglycerides, gastrointestinal side effects, poor wound healing and lymphoceles, pneumonitis, and oral ulcerations. A significant advantage of RAPA is less nephrotoxicity than CNIs and the protection against posttransplant malignancies.[180]

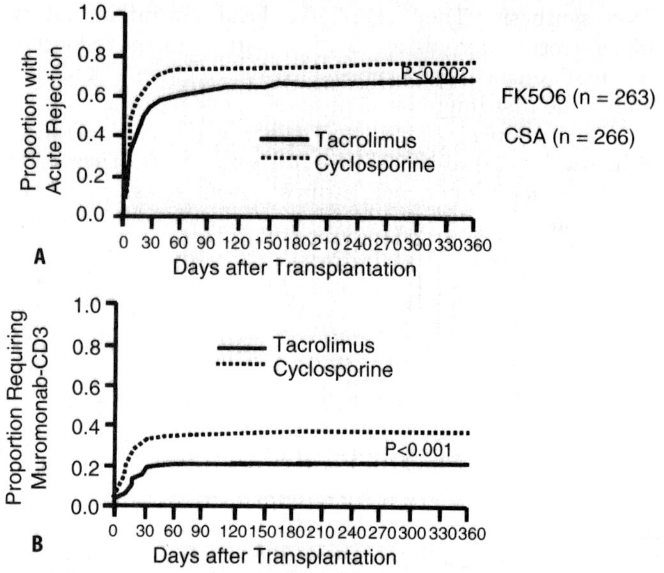

FIGURE 85.19. **A** and **B.** Data from the U.S. multicenter FK506 liver study group showing a lower incidence of rejection and rejection requiring monoclonal anti-CD3 antibody treatment. Level of evidence I. (Adapted from The U.S. Multicenter FK506 Liver Study Group,[185] by permission of *New England Journal of Medicine.*)

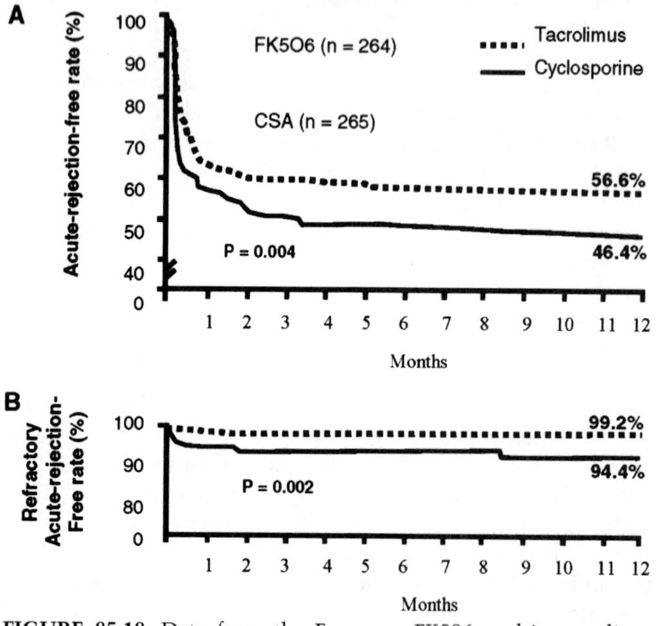

FIGURE 85.18. Data from the European FK506 multicenter liver study group showing a lower incidence of rejection and refractory rejection with FK506 compared to cyclosporine. Level of evidence I. (Adapted from European FK506 Multicentre Liver Study Group,[186] by permission of *Lancet.*)

Immunosuppressive Protocols

Most liver transplant recipients are treated with a combination of immunosuppressive drugs, most commonly MMF (54%), corticosteroids (82%), and TAC (89%) or cyclosporine (10%).[181] The percentage of patients receiving corticosteroids has been decreasing because of their side effects and apparent negative impact on HCV infection posttransplant. Furthermore, several studies have demonstrated that liver transplantation can be performed with complete avoidance or early withdrawal of corticosteroids.[182–184]

Tacrolimus is by far the most common CNI administered posttransplant based on a lower incidence of rejection in two early multicenter trials, one in the United States and one in Europe, comparing TAC to cyclosporine (Figs. 85.18–85.20).[185,186] Data with Neoral and C_2 monitoring show com-

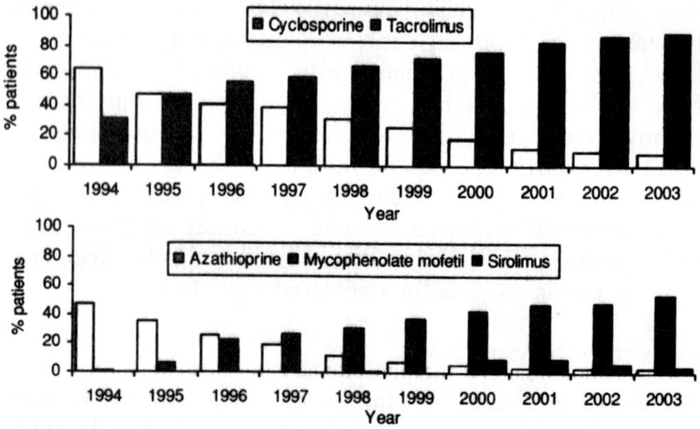

FIGURE 85.20. Trends in maintenance immunosuppression prior to discharge for liver transplantation 1994–2003. Level of evidence II-3. (From 2004 OPTN/SRTR Annual Report, Table 9.6b; from Shapiro et al.,[181] by permission of *American Journal of Transplantation.*)

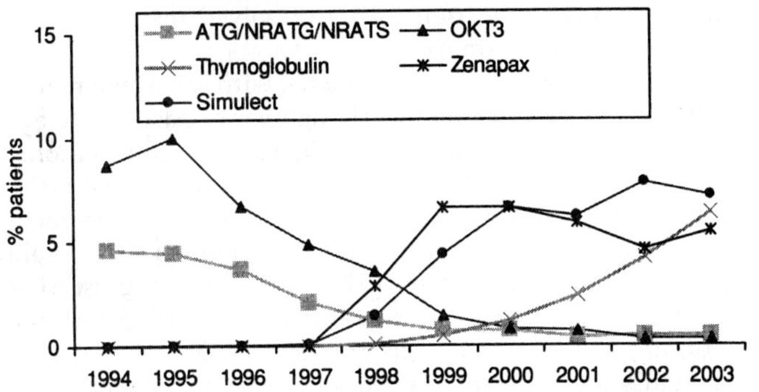

FIGURE 85.21. Trends in induction immunosuppression for liver transplantation 1994–2003. Level of evidence II-3. (From 2004 OPTN/SRTR Annual Report, Table 9.6a; from Shapiro et al.,[181] by permission of *American Journal of Transplantation*.)

parable rates of rejection,[176] but it is unlikely that centers will alter their established practices.

The most commonly prescribed antimetabolite is MMF, and it has largely replaced azathioprine based on a randomized double-blind comparative study of MMF and azathioprine showing a lower incidence of rejection (47.7% in the azathioprine patients compared to 38.5% in the MMF patients; $P < 03$).[187] Only 4% of patients receive sirolimus in the early posttransplant period because of concerns about an increased risk of HAT and poor wound healing. As many as 14% of patients receive sirolimus after discharge, however.

Induction therapy with polyclonal or monoclonal antibodies is unusual in the current era except in patients with renal insufficiency to avoid the nephrotoxicity of cyclosporine and TAC (Fig. 85.21). Because of the increasing prevalence of renal disease in liver transplant recipients, the use of induction therapy increased from 7% in 1997 to 20% in 2003. Basiliximab (7%) is the most commonly administered, followed by rabbit antithymocyte globulin (ATG) (6%) and daclizumab (6%).

Liver Allograft Rejection

Classification

Allograft rejection can be broadly classified as antibody-(humoral-) mediated rejection or cellular rejection. Antibody-mediated rejection can be further characterized as hyperacute or chronic rejection and cellular rejection as acute or chronic rejection.

Diagnosis

The presumptive diagnosis of rejection can often be made on the basis of clinical and laboratory studies. Studies such as liver function tests, immunological monitoring parameters, radiologic studies, drug levels, and fine-needle aspirates may provide useful information, but the standard against which all studies are compared is the biopsy. Biopsy can confirm the diagnosis and determine the severity of rejection, therefore providing important information for therapy and prognosis. Biopsy also can detect the presence of other diseases responsible for organ dysfunction (preservation injury, ischemia, infection, bile duct obstruction, recurrent disease, etc.) and can be used to follow the effectiveness of therapeutic interventions.

Hyperacute Rejection

Hyperacute rejection, first described in renal allograft recipients, is mediated by anti-HLA (donor-specific lymphocytotoxic) antibodies or by isohemagglutinins directed against donor AB blood group antigens. Within minutes to hours of revascularization, complement activation by alloantibody causes microvascular occlusion by platelet and fibrin aggregates, infiltration of neutrophils and mononuclear cells, and endothelial destruction. Vascular thrombosis rapidly ensues. Immunofluorescence studies demonstrate the deposition of immunoglobulin and complement in the blood vessel walls. The heart, kidney, and pancreas are particularly susceptible to hyperacute rejection mediated by anti-HLA antibodies and by anti-A or anti-B isoagglutinins. As a result, for these organs a negative T-cell crossmatch and ABO compatibility are prerequisites for transplantation.

In contrast, the liver is less susceptible to antibody-mediated rejection both in experimental animals and in humans. Experimentally, it has been shown that hyperacute rejection of the liver can occur in sensitized animals.[188] Previously, it was thought that hyperacute rejection did not occur in humans because liver transplants were routinely performed in the face of a positive crossmatch and frequently from ABO-incompatible donors without apparent hyperacute rejection. It is now clear that anti-HLA antibody-mediated rejection, although rare, can occur in humans.[189–191] The time course of hyperacute rejection of the liver is longer (3–7 days), perhaps related to the liver's large capacity to absorb antibodies. Histologically, hyperacute rejection in the liver is characterized by a predominantly centrilobular infiltrate of polymorphonuclear leukocytes and by aggregates of fibrin within and around the walls and lumina of the central veins and, subsequently, small arteries, leading to hemorrhagic necrosis and infarction. More than one-third of patients undergoing ABO-incompatible transplants may develop antibody-mediated rejection leading to graft failure, but the risk may be reduced by plasmapheresis, splenectomy, and intensive immunosuppression.[192]

The liver's capacity to absorb anti-HLA antibodies is also illustrated in patients who have a positive antidonor T-cell crossmatch before transplant that becomes negative several hours after the liver transplant is completed. This change has been used to advantage in patients requiring combined kidney and liver transplants. The kidney has been successfully transplanted after the liver and after the crossmatch has become negative without the development of hyperacute rejection,[193] although this is not universally true.[194]

Acute Rejection

Acute hepatic allograft occurs in 30% to 75% of recipients, depending on the type of induction immunosuppression used.[195] The proportion of patients treated for rejection has been steadily decreasing according to national data from the SRTR (Scientific Registry of Transplant Recipients),[181,196] from 47% in 1992 to 28% in 2001 and 24% in 2002 (Fig. 85.22).

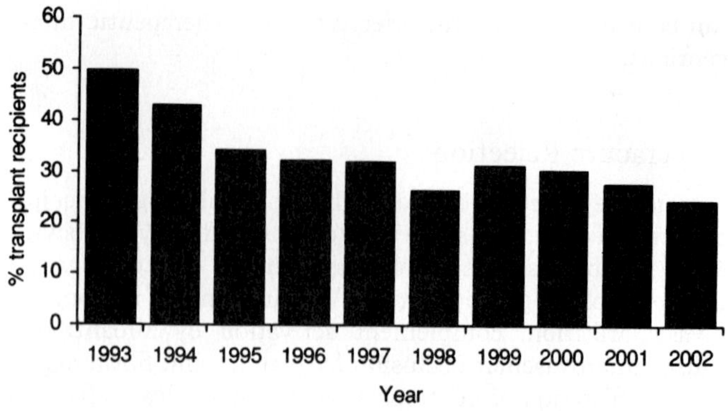

FIGURE 85.22. Incidence of rejection during the first year among liver transplant recipients, 1993–2002. Level of evidence II-3. (From 2004 OPTN/SRTR Annual Report, Table 9.6d; From Shapiro et al.,[181] by permission of *American Journal of Transplantation*.)

Clinical features include a decrease in bile output and change in color and consistency from a thin, clear, golden yellow to a thicker, dark green. Elevated liver function tests may include elevated transaminases, alkaline phosphatase, or bilirubin, alone or in combination. Rejection can be difficult to diagnose clinically, however, because the differential diagnosis of abnormal liver function tests is broad, including preservation injury, ischemia, viral infection, bacterial cholangitis, bile duct obstruction, and recurrent disease. Therefore, a biopsy is usually obtained when acute rejection is suspected or any time the etiology of elevated hepatic function tests is in question. Other studies useful in determining the etiology of elevated liver function tests include cholangiography, duplex ultrasonography of the hepatic vasculature, and if necessary, CT angiography with computerized reconstructions or hepatic arteriography.

Acute rejection is histologically characterized by three features: (1) a portal mononuclear infiltrate (primarily small lymphocytes, but also variable numbers of eosinophils and polymorphonuclear leukocytes); (2) bile duct epithelial damage and infiltration by small lymphocytes; and (3) subendothelial inflammation of portal or terminal HVs (endothelialitis)[195,197] (Figs. 85.23 and 85.24). The international consensus conference on the Banff schema for grading liver allograft rejection agreed that the diagnosis of rejection requires at least two of these histopathological findings (mixed portal infiltrate and bile duct damage) and biochemical evidence of liver damage (Table 85.17). The diagnosis is even more ensured if more than 50% of the bile ducts are damaged or if unequivocal endothelialitis is demonstrated. After a global assessment of severity, the Banff schema proposed a semiquantitative grading (0–3, mild, moderate, severe) be performed on the basis of scoring of portal inflammation, bile duct damage, and venular inflammation to arrive at a rejection activity index (RAI) (Table 85.17).

Most rejection episodes are classified as mild (60%–70%), with fewer classified as moderate (25%–30%) and severe (5%–10%).[195] The histological severity of rejection correlates with outcome. By the time the additional immunosuppression used to treat acute rejection is stopped, 97% of mild acute rejection episodes have resolved, whereas 18% of recipients with severe rejection have unresolved rejection, have died, or have been retransplanted.

Risk factors shown to be associated with the development of acute rejection include underlying liver disease (acute fulminant hepatic failure, hepatitis B, and autoimmune chronic active hepatitis), younger age of recipient, lower Karnofsky score, serum creatinine below 2.0 mg/dL, lack of edema, renal failure, ascites, fewer HLA-DR matches, donor age, and cold ischemia time greater than 15 h. These data suggest that healthier recipients, recipients poorly HLA matched with the donor, and recipients of livers that are more predisposed to liver injury are at greater risk for developing acute rejection. When the impact of acute rejection on patient and graft survival is analyzed, it has been shown that patient and graft survival rates are better in patients with acute rejection because the highest incidence of rejection is in the healthiest recipients. Adjusting for these risk factors, acute rejection was not shown to have a significant effect on patient or graft survival rates. This finding is in direct contrast to kidney transplantation, for which acute rejection episodes have been shown to correlate with poorer patient and graft survival rates.

Chronic Rejection

Chronic rejection is a slowly progressive immunological process characterized by increasing cholestasis with an elevation in alkaline phosphatase, g-glutamyl transpeptidase, or 5′-nucleotidase and eventually bilirubin that occurs uncommonly in the current era of potent immunosuppressive drugs. Histologically, it is characterized by obliterative vasculopathy and loss of bile ducts (vanishing duct syndrome or paucity of bile ducts) involving more than 50% of the portal triads (Table 85.18; Fig. 85.25).[198] Early signs of chronic rejection can include the subendothelial accumulation of foamy histiocytes with subsequent subintimal fibrosis and occlusion (Fig. 85.26).

Chronic rejection is often difficult to diagnose because arteries of the size involved with chronic rejection are not usually present on needle biopsies. Therefore, it has been shown that centrilobular ballooning degeneration and necro-

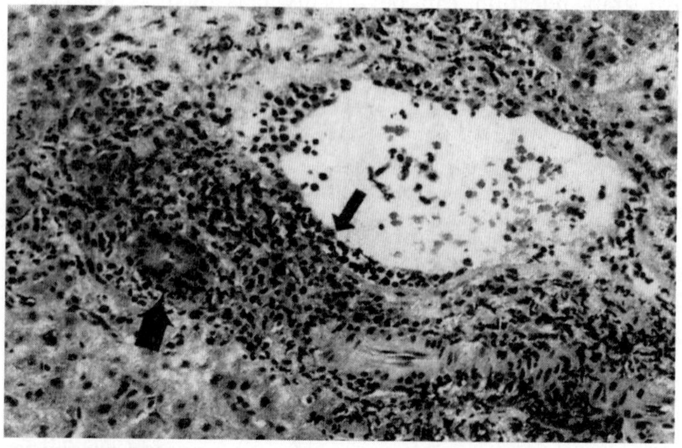

FIGURE 85.23. Acute liver allograft rejection. Portal inflammation, endothelialitis, and damage of bile ducts. (From Demetris et al.,[197] by permission of *Hepatology*.)

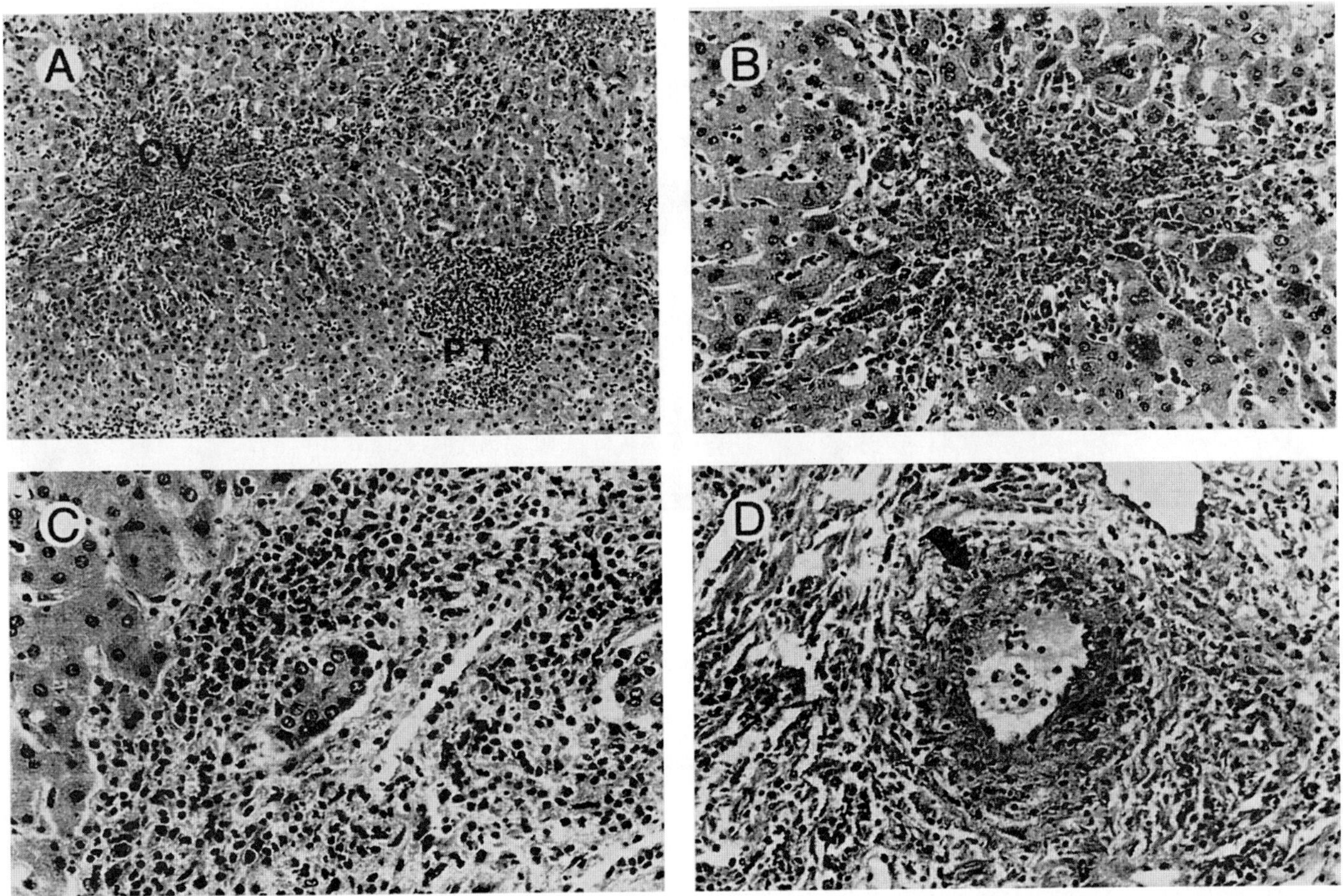

FIGURE 85.24. Failed liver allograft with severe acute rejection. **A.** Portal triad (PT) and central vein (CV) inflammation. **B.** Confluent perivenular necrosis. **C.** Bile duct inflammation. **D.** Necrotizing arteritis. (From Demetris et al.,[197] by permission of *Hepatology*.)

TABLE 85.17. Banff Schema for Grading Acute Liver Allograft Rejection.

Major criteria[a]
1. Mixed, but predominantly mononuclear portal inflammation, containing activated lymphocytes, neutrophils, and frequently eosinophils
2. Bile duct inflammation/damage
3. Subendothelial inflammation or portal veins or terminal hepatic venules

Global assessment
1. Indeterminate: portal inflammatory infiltrate that fails to meet the criteria for the diagnosis of rejection
2. Mild: rejection infiltrate in a minority of the triads, which is generally mild, and confined within the portal spaces
3. Moderate: rejection infiltrate expanding most or all of the triads
4. Severe: as above for moderate, with spillover into the periportal areas and moderate-to-severe perivenular inflammation that extends into the hepatic parenchyma and is associated with perivenular hepatocyte necrosis

Rejection activity index (score 1–3)
1. Portal inflammation
2. Bile duct inflammation damage
3. Venous endothelial inflammation

[a]Two of these three features are required; diagnosis strengthened if more than 50% of the ducts are damaged or if unequivocal endothelialitis is present.

Source: From Demetris et al.,[197] by permission of *Hepatology*.

sis in the setting of previous acute rejection episodes and loss of bile ducts suggest chronic rejection. Chronic rejection usually develops following an unresolved acute rejection episode, after multiple acute rejection episodes, or slowly over many years in patients with a history of remote acute rejection episodes or no apparent episodes of acute rejection. Chronic rejection is not always irreversible, and bile duct regeneration can occur.

Treatment

The rate of treatment of acute rejection has decreased from 50% in 1993 to 24% in 2002.[181] This is most likely due to

TABLE 85.18. International Banff Schema for Histopathologic Staging and Reporting of Chronic Rejection.

1. Appropriate clinical, radiological, laboratory, and histopathologic findings
2. Bile duct atrophy/pyknosis, affecting a majority of the bile ducts, with or without bile duct loss
3. Convincing foam cell obliterative arteriopathy
4. Bile duct loss affecting greater than 50% of the portal tracts

Source: From Demetris et al.,[198] by permission of *Hepatology*.

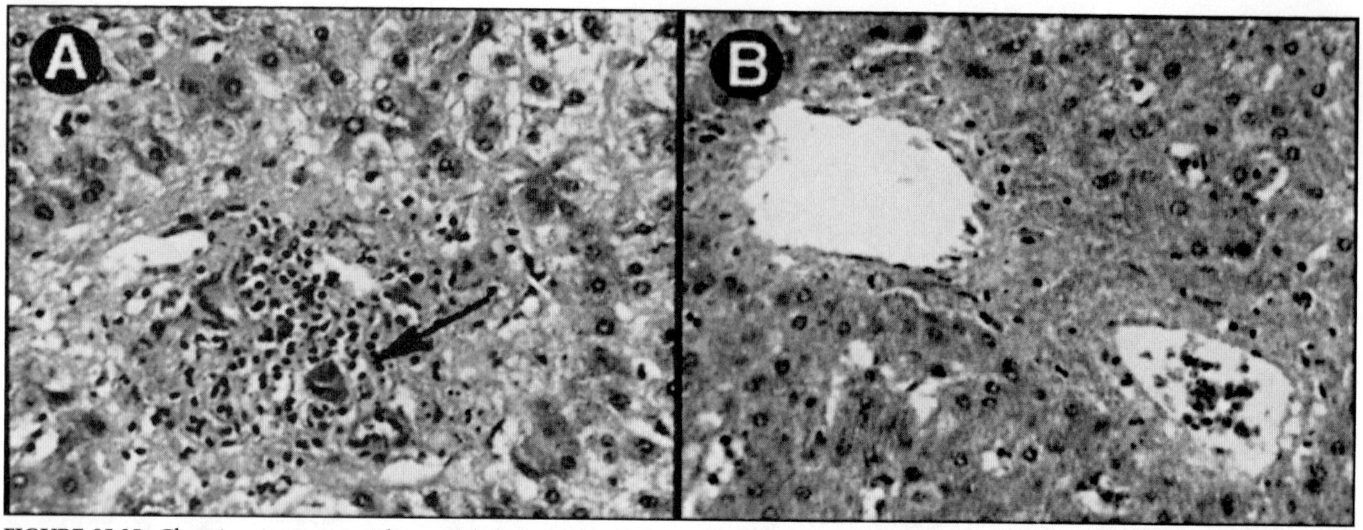

FIGURE 85.25. Chronic rejection. A. Biliary epithelial atrophy. B. Loss of bile duct and hepatic artery branches. (From Demetris et al.,[198] by permission of *Hepatology*.)

improved immunosuppressive drugs, a lower incidence of rejection, and a reluctance to treat mild rejection in patients with HCV because of its negative impact on progression of the disease. Treatment of rejection with corticosteroids is used in 90% and can be accomplished by a short course of intravenous methylprednisolone boluses (e.g., 250–1000 mg/day for 3–5 days) or by an increase in the oral prednisolone dose (e.g., 2 mg/kg/day) with a tapering schedule over 2 to 4 weeks. The only controlled study in liver transplant recipients showed that the administration of 1000 mg methylprednisolone followed by a 6-day taper from 200 to 20 mg/day is more effective and safer than 1000 mg of methylprednisolone for 3 days consecutively in the treatment of acute cellular rejection.[199] Antibody therapy is given to approximately 18% of patients, muromonab-CD3 (6%), rabbit ATG (6%), and basiliximab (4%). Both MMF and TAC have been used to rescue patients with steroid-resistant rejection.[181]

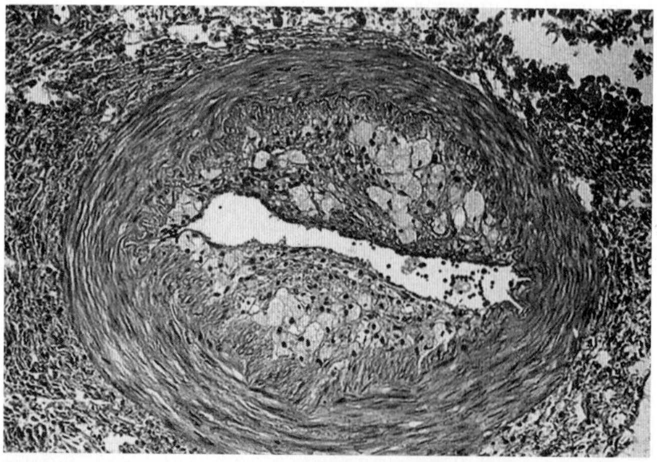

FIGURE 85.26. Chronic rejection. Subendothelial accumulation of foamy histiocytes, subintimal fibrosis and thickening.

Infections

The incidence and severity of infections after liver transplantation are influenced by the type, intensity, and duration of immunosuppression, by the incidence of technical complications, and by the infectious diseases that the patient encounters in the hospital and community.[200] More than 60% to 80% of liver transplant recipients will have at least one infection after transplant, with an overall incidence of 1.5 to 1.7 infections per patient, an incidence that is similar in induction and noninduction series.[185,186,201] In the current era of antibiotic, antiviral, and antifungal prophylaxis, 70% of posttransplant infections are bacterial, 20% are viral, and 10% are fungal. Although early series reported an infection-related mortality rate of 40%, current series report a mortality rate of less than 10%.[201,202]

Posttransplant infections can be classified by the time period after transplantation in which they are most likely to occur; whether they are bacterial, viral, fungal, or protozoal; and by the clinical disease they cause. Most infections occurring in the first month are bacterial or fungal and are related to the surgical procedure, including intraabdominal infections, cholangitis, pneumonitis, urinary tract infections, wound infections, and central venous catheter infections. From 1 to 6 months after transplant, viral infections, including CMV, HSV, and EBV, are most common, although late fungal infections may occur. After 6 months, the risk of infection is low.

Bacterial Infections

Bacterial infections account for 50% to 70% of infections after liver transplantation and are most common in the first month posttransplant. Risk factors for the development of bacterial infections include length of operation (>12 h), multiple abdominal operations, retransplantation, pretransplant bilirubin 12 mg/dL or more, length of antibiotic therapy posttransplant (5 days), and intraoperative transfusions (25 units of packed red cells and 30 units of fresh frozen plasma). The most common diagnoses include wound infections; intraabdominal infections (peritonitis, hepatic and extrahepatic abscesses, and cholangitis); pneumonias; urinary tract infections; central venous catheter infections; and bacteremias.

Gram-positive infections make up 60% to 70% of the bacterial infections and gram-negative infections make up 30% to 40%. The most frequent organisms isolated include *Enterococcus* species, *Staphylococcus epidermidis*, *Staphylococcus aureus*, *Pseudomonas aeruginosa*, *Enterobacter* species, *Clostridia difficile*, *Klebsiella* species, *Citrobacter* species, and *Escherichia coli*.[201]

The diagnosis of bacterial infections depends on their site but involves cultures (blood, urine, sputum, wounds, drains, bile); ultrasonography; CAT scan; cholangiography; angiography; liver biopsy; chest x-ray; bronchoscopy and bronchoalveolar lavage; and open lung biopsy. Antibiotic therapy is dictated by the organism and its antibiotic sensitivities. In many intraabdominal infections, fungal organisms will also be cultured and require appropriate antifungal therapy.

Similarly, directed therapy of the infection will depend on its etiology and location. Superficial wound infections require drainage and local wound care. Subhepatic or subphrenic fluid collections, hematomas, and abscesses, as well as intrahepatic abscesses, usually can be effectively drained percutaneously but may require operative drainage. Associated bile duct leaks should be excluded by cholangiography and, if present, HAT should be ruled out. Bacterial pneumonias and urinary tract infections usually respond to antibiotic therapy. Infected central venous catheters should be removed and antibiotics administered.

Prophylaxis of bacterial infections usually involves perioperative administration of a third-generation cephalosporin along with ampicillin or vancomycin or ampicillin–sulbactam as a single agent for gram-positive and gram-negative coverage. Some centers use selective bowel decontamination protocols involving the administration of oral nystatin, gentamicin, and polymyxin. Fibers (prebiotics) and living lactic acid bacteria (LAB, probiotics) were recently shown in a prospective randomized trial to decrease the incidence of bacterial infections from 48% to 13% compared to selective bowel decontamination.[203]

Viral Infections

The most important viral infections after liver transplantation include CMV, EBV, HSV, and VZV. These viruses exhibit latency, which refers to their ability to persist indefinitely in a dormant state and to be reactivated at any time by a variety of factors, including immunosuppression. These viruses are also potentially oncogenic. Other viral infections that can occur posttransplant include human herpes viruses (HHV) 6, 7, and 8; papovavirus; and adenovirus.

Herpes Simplex Virus

Herpes simplex virus infections are uncommon posttransplant because of the widespread use of valganciclovir and ganciclovir prophylaxis. Usually, HSV infections occur during the first 6 weeks after transplantation and can be primary or reactivation infections due to HSV-1 or HSV-2. The HSV-1 infections are usually mucocutaneous infections in and around the oral cavity, but esophagitis, hepatitis, encephalitis, pneumonitis, and ocular HSV infections can occur. Herpes simplex virus 2 can cause penile vesicular lesions, cervicovaginitis, and proctitis. The diagnosis can be made by physical examination, endoscopy and biopsy, liver biopsy, bronchoscopy, and culture of vesicular lesions. Serology is rarely helpful. Intravenous or oral acyclovir is effective therapy in most patients.

Cytomegalovirus

Cytomegalovirus infection is still the most important opportunistic infection occurring in liver transplant recipients. Primary or reactivation CMV infection occurs in 25%–75% of liver transplant recipients, and about 50% of these patients will develop CMV disease. The incidence of CMV appears to be decreasing with the widespread use of antiviral prophylaxis and new immunosuppressive regimens.[204,205] Most commonly, CMV occurs in the first 3 to 6 months after transplant, with a peak incidence at 4 to 6 weeks. The classic clinical signs and symptoms include fever, malaise, myalgias, athralgias, and leukopenia. It may involve several organ systems, resulting in pneumonitis; ulceration and hemorrhage in the stomach, duodenum, or colon; hepatitis; esophagitis; mononucleosis; retinitis; encephalitis; glomerulopathy; and pancreatitis.

The diagnosis is now most often made by pp65 antigenemia assay or plasma or cell-free quantitative polymerase chain reaction (PCR) or other viral DNA capture method, but biopsy (presence of viral inclusions, immunohistochemical stains for CMV antigens, or in situ hybridization) is often useful. The risk of developing CMV depends on the donor–recipient serology, with the greatest risk (60%) present in seronegative recipients of organs from seropositive donors (D+R–). Seronegative recipients of organs from seronegative donors (D–R–) who only receive seronegative blood products virtually never develop clinical CMV disease.

The incidence of CMV infection can be reduced by prophylactic antiviral therapy with intravenous ganciclovir or oral valganciclovir for 3 months, except in D+/R–, for which 6 months of valganciclovir is recommended, and by using less immunosuppression[204–207] (Table 85.19). Ganciclovir or valganciclovir are effective therapies with some of the lowest described incidences of CMV with 14 days of intravenous ganciclovir followed by 12 weeks of oral ganciclovir (Table 85.19). Foscarnet is an effective alternative in ganciclovir-resistant disease, but CMV still negatively affects outcomes in terms of patient and graft survival, other infections, severity of recurrent hepatitis C, and cost.

Epstein-Barr Virus

Infection with EBV occurs in 5% to 10% of liver transplant recipients as a primary or reactivation infection and causes a spectrum of posttransplant lymphoproliferative diseases (PTLDs). There are four primary types of disease, the classification of which have important therapeutic and prognostic implications: uncomplicated infectious mononucleosis; benign polyclonal B-cell hyperplasia without evidence of malignant transformation as shown by the absence of cytogenetic abnormalities or immunoglobulin gene rearrangements; the intermediate polymorphic B-cell lymphoma, which is predominantly a polyclonal B-cell proliferation but contains a subpopulation of malignantly transformed cells with clonal

TABLE 85.19.
Prevention of CMV Disease in Liver Transplant Recipients.

Author	*Year*	*Level of evidence*	*Type of trial*	*Subjects*	*Study groups*	*CMV disease*	*CMV viremia*	*Death from CMV*	*Neutropenia*	*Conclusions*
Paya[223]	2004	I	Prospective, randomized, double-blind, double-dummy	Liver (177), kidney (120), H (50), P (11) recipients; D/R ±	VGCV 900 mg daily (100 days)	12.1%	2.9%	0	9.2%	Once daily VGCV was as clinically effective as oral GCV for CMV disease prevention in SOT
					GCV 1000 mg three times daily (100 days)	15.2%, P = NS	10.4%, $P < .001$	0	3.2%, $P < .0631$	
Winston[207]	2004	I	Prospective, randomized	CMV D/R ± liver recipients	Intravenous GCV[a] (1–14 d) + oral GCV (15–100 d)	3/32 (9.3%)		0		After 14 days of intravenous GCV, oral GCV is as effective as intravenous GCV in high-risk D+/R– patients
					Intravenous GCV (100 d)	4/32 (12.5%), $P > .2$		0		
Winston[224]	2003	I	Prospective, randomized	CMV-seropositive liver recipients	Intravenous GCV (1–14 d) + oral GCV (15–100 d)	1/110 (0.9%)		0	38/110 (35%)	14 days of intravenous GCV followed by 12 weeks of oral GCV superior to intravenous GCV plus oral ACV and almost completely eliminates CMV disease after liver transplantation
					Intravenous GCV (1–14 d) + oral ACV (15–100 d)	8/109 (7.3%), $P = .019$		1	20/109 (18%), $P = .009$	

ACV, acyclovir; CMV, cytomegalovirus; D, donor; GCV, ganciclovir; H, heart; P, pancreas; R, recipient; VGCV, valganciclovir.
[a]Intravenous GCV dose = 6 mg/kg once daily; oral GCV 1000 mg three times daily; and oral ACV 800 mg three times daily.

cytogenetic abnormalities and immunoglobulin gene rearrangements; and malignant monoclonal or oligoclonal B-cell lymphoma with clonal cytogenetic abnormalities and immunoglobulin gene rearrangements in a majority of cells.[208,209]

The incidence of PTLD ranges from 0.85% to 20% depending on age, type of transplant, degree and type of immunosuppression, and EBV serology and may be localized or disseminated with mortality rates of 50% or greater.[210,211] Treatment usually involves reduction or withdrawal of immunosuppression as first-line therapy along with ganciclovir antiviral therapy. Other treatment modalities include IFN-α, cytotoxic chemotherapy, anti-B-lymphocyte antibodies, and humanized anti-CD20 monoclonal antibody (Rituximab).[212] Mortality ranges from 25% to 75%. Prolonged antiviral prophylaxis and serial measurements of EBV viral load may be helpful in reducing the risk of PTLD.

Varicella Zoster Virus

Varicella zoster virus infections occur as primary or reactivation infections. Primary VZV infections in immunosuppressed patients can be severe, leading to rapid dissemination and death. They are often characterized by severe pneumonia; gastrointestinal tract ulceration and hemorrhage; and severe central nervous system, skin, and eye involvement. Reactivation VZV infections occur in about 7% to 10% of patients months to years after transplantation and present as typical vesicular lesions in a dermatomic distribution (zoster).[213] Visceral dissemination in these patients is rare.

The diagnosis of VZV is made on the basis of physical examination of the classic cutaneous vesicular lesions, by direct fluorescent antibody or PCR. Intravenous acyclovir is used for treatment of disseminated VZV along with a reduction in immunosuppression. Intravenous or oral acyclovir may be used for herpes zoster infections, depending on the severity of the disease. In patients who have never had chicken pox, a history of recent exposure should be treated immediately with varicella zoster immune globulin, and acyclovir should be started at the earliest sign of disease.

Human Herpes Virus

Human herpes viruses 6 and 7 infection have been noted to be associated with encephalitis, rejection, CMV infection, and bone marrow suppression. Infection with HHV-8 has been causally associated with Kaposi's sarcoma. Treatment with standard antiherpes viral therapies is not well established, although successes in HHV-6 treatment have been reported with foscarnet and, in some cases, ganciclovir. The specific agent of choice depends on the HHV-6 subtype. Human herpes virus 8 disease with Kaposi's sarcoma may be treated locally with intralesional injections of IFN or doxorubicin or systemically if disseminated or visceral disease has developed. Like the treatment for EBV disease, these are adjunctive therapies, and the mainstay is reduction in immunosuppression to balance graft survival. Sirolimus has recently been shown to inhibit the progression of dermal KS in kidney transplant recipients while preventing rejection.[214]

Fungal Infections

Invasive fungal infections have been reported to occur in 5% to 42% of liver transplant recipients, with the most frequent organisms being *Candida* species, followed by *Aspergillus* species.[201,215–217] Seventy percent occur in the first month posttransplant. The mortality rate from fungal infections has varied from 25% to 71%. The risk factors have changed over time, with variables related to operative time and transfusions less important now than in the 1980s and 1990s. Instead, preoperative antibiotic prophylaxis for spontaneous bacterial peritonitis and postoperative complications including retransplantation, posttransplant dialysis, and CMV viremia are associated with invasive candidiasis.[205] *Candida* species account for 80% of posttransplant fungal infections. *Candida albicans* accounts for 65% of candidiasis cases, followed by *Candida glabrata* in 21%, *Candida tropicalis* in 9%, and *Candida parapsilosis*, *Candida lusitaniae*, and *Candida krusei* account for the rest. *Aspergillus* accounts for 20% of fungal infections. *Mucormycosis* and *Cryptococcus* can also occur posttransplant.

Candida infections include candidemia in 40%, peritonitis in 40%, and intraabdominal abscesses in 11% with empyema, pneumonitis, endophthalmitis, esophagitis, stomatitis, urinary tract infections, and wound infections also occurring. Treatment of invasive *Candida albicans* may include high-dose fluconazole if the patient is fluconazole-naïve, or amphotericin B, liposomal amphotericin, or caspofungin[218] along with removal of the inciting cause (e.g., intraabdominal abscess). Treatment of the non-albicans *Candida* species includes amphotericin B, liposomal amphotericin B, caspofungin, or newer triazole antifungal agents such as voriconazole.

Aspergillus fumigatus and *Aspergillus flavus* are hyphal saprophytic fungi that are contracted by the inhalation of spores. The lungs are the primary site of infection. *Aspergillus* infections usually begin as upper lobe pulmonary infiltrates that undergo cavitation. Central nervous system infection, including brain abscesses, and dissemination are not uncommon. The diagnosis is usually made by bronchoscopy and transbronchial biopsy, open-lung biopsy, or brain biopsy. In cases of angioinvasive aspergillosis, antigen assays such as galactomannan or 1,3-β-glucan can also be useful. Treatment is evolving, with options including high-dose liposomal amphotericin (up to 12 mg/kg/day), caspofungin, or voriconazole. The mortality is extremely high in spite of antifungal treatment.

Prophylaxis with nystatin or clotrimazole is effective in preventing oral candidiasis (thrush) and esophagitis posttransplant but is less effective in preventing invasive fungal infections. Prophylaxis with low-dose systemic amphotericin has been effective in decreasing the risk of invasive fungal infections, but nephrotoxicity limits its use. Liposomal amphotericin can reduce the risk of fungal infection without nephrotoxicity. Oral fluconazole has been shown in a randomized, double-blind, placebo-controlled trial to reduce fungal infections in liver transplant recipients[219] and to be superior to nystatin in decreasing posttransplant fungal infections.[220] Fluconazole is now used in many centers, but a randomized placebo-controlled trial showed the broad-spectrum triazole–itraconazole oral solution safely reduces the risk of fungal infections and may be superior because of its greater activity against *Aspergillus* species.[221]

Protozoal Infections

Pneumocystis carinii causes dyspnea, fever, and cough associated with diffuse bilateral interstitial pulmonary infiltrates.

The diagnosis is usually made by the identification of the organism using the methenamine silver stain on bronchoalveolar lavage fluid or by transbronchial or open-lung biopsy. Treatment with trimethoprim–sulfamethoxazole or pentamidine is usually effective. Trimethoprim–sulfamethoxazole prophylaxis has essentially eliminated pneumocystis infections in transplant recipients.

References

1. Kim WR, Brown RS Jr, Terrault NA, El-Serag H. Burden of liver disease in the United States: summary of a workshop. Hepatology 2002;36:227–242.
2. Alter MJ, Kruszon-Moran D, Nainan OV, et al. The prevalence of hepatitis C virus infection in the United States, 1988 through 1994. N Engl J Med 1999;341:556–562.
3. Armstrong GL, Alter MJ, McQuillan GM, Margolis HS. The past incidence of hepatitis C virus infection: implications for the future burden of chronic liver disease in the United States. Hepatology 2000;31:777–782.
4. Vong S, Bell BP. Chronic liver disease mortality in the United States, 1990–1998. Hepatology 2004;39:476–483.
5. Curry MP. Hepatitis B and hepatitis C viruses in liver transplantation. Transplantation 2004;78:955–963.
6. Shiffman ML, Saab S, Feng S, et al. Liver and intestine transplantation in the United States, 1995–2004. Am J Transplant 2006;6(part 2):1170–1187.
7. Hanto DW, Fishbein TM, Pinson CW, et al. Liver and intestine transplantation: summary analysis, 1994–2003. Am J Transplant 2005;5(4 pt 2):916–933.
8. Alter MJ. The epidemiology of acute and chronic hepatitis C. Clin Liver Dis 1997;1:559–568, vi–vii.
9. Lauer GM, Walker BD. Hepatitis C virus infection. N Engl J Med 2001;345:41–52.
10. Zarski JP, Bohn B, Bastie A, et al. Characteristics of patients with dual infection by hepatitis B and C viruses. J Hepatol 1998;28:27–33.
11. Tanaka H, Hiyama T, Tsukuma H, et al. Cumulative risk of hepatocellular carcinoma in hepatitis C virus carriers: statistical estimations from cross-sectional data. Jpn J Cancer Res 1994;85: 485–490.
12. Curley SA, Izzo F, Gallipoli A, de Bellis M, Cremona F, Parisi V. Identification and screening of 416 patients with chronic hepatitis at high risk to develop hepatocellular cancer. Ann Surg 1995;222:375–380; discussion 380–383.
13. Ikeda K, Saitoh S, Koida I, et al. A multivariate analysis of risk factors for hepatocellular carcinogenesis: a prospective observation of 795 patients with viral and alcoholic cirrhosis. Hepatology 1993;18:47–53.
14. Beresford TP, Turcotte JG, Merion R, et al. A rational approach to liver transplantation for the alcoholic patient. Psychosomatics 1990;31:241–254.
15. Charlton M, Kasparova P, Weston S, et al. Frequency of nonalcoholic steatohepatitis as a cause of advanced liver disease. Liver Transpl 2001;7:608–614.
16. Heneghan MA, Sylvestre PB. Cholestatic diseases of liver transplantation. Semin Gastrointest Dis 2001;12:133–147.
17. Maor-Kendler Y, Batts KP, Burgart LJ, et al. Comparative allograft histology after liver transplantation for cryptogenic cirrhosis, alcohol, hepatitis C, and cholestatic liver diseases. Transplantation 2000;70:292–297.
18. Ong J, Younossi ZM, Reddy V, et al. Cryptogenic cirrhosis and posttransplantation nonalcoholic fatty liver disease. Liver Transpl 2001;7:797–801.
19. Freeman RB, Sanchez H, Lewis WD, et al. Serologic and DNA follow-up data from HBsAg-positive patients treated with orthotopic liver transplantation. Transplantation 1991;51:793–797.
20. Rizzetto M, Recchia S, Salizzoni M. Liver transplantation in carriers of the HBsAg. J Hepatol 1991;13:5–7.
21. O'Grady JG, Smith HM, Davies SE, et al. Hepatitis B virus reinfection after orthotopic liver transplantation. Serological and clinical implications. J Hepatol 1992;14:104–111.
22. Sawyer RG, McGory RW, Gaffey MJ, et al. Improved clinical outcomes with liver transplantation for hepatitis B-induced chronic liver failure using passive immunization. Ann Surg 1998;227:841–850.
23. Yao F, Gish RG. Treatment of chronic hepatitis B: new antiviral therapies. Curr Gastroenterol Rep 1999;1:20–26.
24. Dumortier J, Chevallier P, Scoazec JY, Berger F, Boillot O. Combined lamivudine and hepatitis B immunoglobulin for the prevention of hepatitis B recurrence after liver transplantation: long-term results. Am J Transplant 2003;3:999–1002.
25. Yao FY, Osorio RW, Roberts JP, et al. Intramuscular hepatitis B immune globulin combined with lamivudine for prophylaxis against hepatitis B recurrence after liver transplantation. Liver Transpl Surg 1999;5:491–496.
26. Lo CM, Fan ST, Liu CL, Lai CL, Wong J. Prophylaxis and treatment of recurrent hepatitis B after liver transplantation. Transplantation 2003;75(3 suppl):S41–S44.
27. Markowitz JS, Martin P, Conrad AJ, et al. Prophylaxis against hepatitis B recurrence following liver transplantation using combination lamivudine and hepatitis B immune globulin. Hepatology 1998;28:585–589.
28. Angus PW, McCaughan GW, Gane EJ, Crawford DH, Harley H. Combination low-dose hepatitis B immune globulin and lamivudine therapy provides effective prophylaxis against posttransplantation hepatitis B. Liver Transpl 2000;6:429–433.
29. Marzano A, Salizzoni M, Debernardi-Venon W, et al. Prevention of hepatitis B virus recurrence after liver transplantation in cirrhotic patients treated with lamivudine and passive immunoprophylaxis. J Hepatol 2001;34:903–910.
30. Rosenau J, Tillmann HL, Bahr MJ, et al. Successful hepatitis B reinfection prophylaxis with lamivudine and hepatitis B immune globulin in patients with positive HBV-DNA at time of liver transplantation. Transplant Proc 2001;33:3637–3638.
31. Roche B, Samuel D. Treatment of hepatitis B and C after liver transplantation. Part 1, hepatitis B. Transpl Int 2005;17:746–758.
32. Han SH, Ofman J, Holt C, et al. An efficacy and cost-effectiveness analysis of combination hepatitis B immune globulin and lamivudine to prevent recurrent hepatitis B after orthotopic liver transplantation compared with hepatitis B immune globulin monotherapy. Liver Transpl 2000;6:741–748.
33. Steinmuller T, Seehofer D, Rayes N, et al. Increasing applicability of liver transplantation for patients with hepatitis B-related liver disease. Hepatology 2002;35:1528–1535.
34. Terrault NA, Carter JT, Carlson L, Roland ME, Stock PG. Outcome of patients with hepatitis B virus and human immunodeficiency virus infections referred for liver transplantation. Liver Transpl 2006;12:801–807.
35. Lee RG. Nonalcoholic steatohepatitis: a study of 49 patients. Hum Pathol 1989;20:594–598.
36. Pagano G, Pacini G, Musso G, et al. Nonalcoholic steatohepatitis, insulin resistance, and metabolic syndrome: further evidence for an etiologic association. Hepatology 2002;35:367–372.
37. Burke A, Lucey MR. Non-alcoholic fatty liver disease, non-alcoholic steatohepatitis and orthotopic liver transplantation. Am J Transplant 2004;4:686–693.
38. Powell EE, Cooksley WG, Hanson R, Searle J, Halliday JW, Powell LW. The natural history of nonalcoholic steatohepatitis: a follow-up study of 42 patients for up to 21 years. Hepatology 1990;11:74–80.
39. Evans CD, Oien KA, MacSween RN, Mills PR. Non-alcoholic steatohepatitis: a common cause of progressive chronic liver injury? J Clin Pathol 2002;55:689–692.

40. Angulo P, Lindor KD. Non-alcoholic fatty liver disease. J Gastroenterol Hepatol 2002;17(suppl):S186–S190.
41. Angulo P, Lindor KD. Insulin resistance and mitochondrial abnormalities in NASH: a cool look into a burning issue. Gastroenterology 2001;120:1281–1285.
42. Wanless IR, Shiota K. The pathogenesis of nonalcoholic steatohepatitis and other fatty liver diseases: a four-step model including the role of lipid release and hepatic venular obstruction in the progression to cirrhosis. Semin Liver Dis 2004;24:99–106.
43. Dixon JB, Bhathal PS, Hughes NR, O'Brien PE. Nonalcoholic fatty liver disease: improvement in liver histological analysis with weight loss. Hepatology 2004;39:1647–1654.
44. Marchesini G, Bugianesi E, Forlani G, et al. Nonalcoholic fatty liver, steatohepatitis, and the metabolic syndrome. Hepatology 2003;37:917–923.
45. Dixon JB, Bhathal PS, O'Brien PE. Nonalcoholic fatty liver disease: predictors of nonalcoholic steatohepatitis and liver fibrosis in the severely obese. Gastroenterology 2001;121:91–100.
46. Poonawala A, Nair SP, Thuluvath PJ. Prevalence of obesity and diabetes in patients with cryptogenic cirrhosis: a case-control study. Hepatology 2000;32(4 pt 1):689–692.
47. Lee YM, Kaplan MM. Primary sclerosing cholangitis. N Engl J Med 1995;332:924–933.
48. Ahrendt SA, Pitt HA, Kalloo AN, et al. Primary sclerosing cholangitis: resect, dilate, or transplant? Ann Surg 1998;227:412–423.
49. Narumi S, Roberts JP, Emond JC, Lake J, Ascher NL. Liver transplantation for sclerosing cholangitis. Hepatology 1995;22:451–457.
50. Farges O, Malassagne B, Sebagh M, Bismuth H. Primary sclerosing cholangitis: liver transplantation or biliary surgery. Surgery 1995;117:146–155.
51. Ismail T, Angrisani L, Powell JE, et al. Primary sclerosing cholangitis: surgical options, prognostic variables and outcome. Br J Surg 1991;78:564–567.
52. Nichols JC, Gores GJ, LaRusso NF, Wiesner RH, Nagorney DM, Ritts RE Jr. Diagnostic role of serum CA 19–9 for cholangiocarcinoma in patients with primary sclerosing cholangitis. Mayo Clin Proc 1993;68:874–879.
53. Heimbach JK, Gores GJ, Haddock MG, et al. Liver transplantation for unresectable perihilar cholangiocarcinoma. Semin Liver Dis 2004;24:201–207.
54. Onuchic LF, Furu L, Nagasawa Y, et al. PKHD1, the polycystic kidney and hepatic disease 1 gene, encodes a novel large protein containing multiple immunoglobulin-like plexin-transcription-factor domains and parallel beta-helix 1 repeats. Am J Hum Genet 2002;70:1305–1317.
55. Desmet VJ. Ludwig symposium on biliary disorders—part I. Pathogenesis of ductal plate abnormalities. Mayo Clin Proc 1998;73:80–89.
56. Goss JA, Shackleton CR, Swenson K, et al. Orthotopic liver transplantation for congenital biliary atresia. An 11-year, single-center experience. Ann Surg 1996;224:276–284; discussion 284–287.
57. Schiodt FV, Atillasoy E, Shakil AO, et al. Etiology and outcome for 295 patients with acute liver failure in the United States. Liver Transpl Surg 1999;5:29–34.
58. Wall WJ, Adams PC. Liver transplantation for fulminant hepatic failure: North American experience. Liver Transpl Surg 1995;1:178–182.
59. O'Grady JG, Alexander GJ, Hayllar KM, Williams R. Early indicators of prognosis in fulminant hepatic failure. Gastroenterology 1989;97:439–445.
60. Bailey B, Amre DK, Gaudreault P. Fulminant hepatic failure secondary to acetaminophen poisoning: a systematic review and meta-analysis of prognostic criteria determining the need for liver transplantation. Crit Care Med 2003;31:299–305.
61. Anand AC, Nightingale P, Neuberger JM. Early indicators of prognosis in fulminant hepatic failure: an assessment of the King's criteria. J Hepatol 1997;26:62–68.
62. Otte JB, Pritchard J, Aronson DC, et al. Liver transplantation for hepatoblastoma: results from the International Society of Pediatric Oncology (SIOP) study SIOPEL-1 and review of the world experience. Pediatr Blood Cancer 2004;42:74–83.
63. d'Annibale M, Piovanello P, Carlini P, et al. Epithelioid hemangioendothelioma of the liver: case report and review of the literature. Transplant Proc 2002;34:1248–1251.
64. Madariaga JR, Marino IR, Karavias DD, et al. Long-term results after liver transplantation for primary hepatic epithelioid hemangioendothelioma. Ann Surg Oncol 1995;2:483–487.
65. O'Grady JG, Polson RJ, Rolles K, Calne RY, Williams R. Liver transplantation for malignant disease. Results in 93 consecutive patients. Ann Surg 1988;207:373–379.
66. O'Grady JG. Treatment options for other hepatic malignancies. Liver Transpl 2000;6(6 suppl 2):S23–S29.
67. Pichlmayr R, Weimann A, Ringe B. Indications for liver transplantation in hepatobiliary malignancy. Hepatology 1994;20(1 pt 2):33S–40S.
68. Ismail T, Angrisani L, Gunson BK, et al. Primary hepatic malignancy: the role of liver transplantation. Br J Surg 1990;77:983–987.
69. Bismuth H, Chiche L, Adam R, Castaing D, Diamond T, Dennison A. Liver resection versus transplantation for hepatocellular carcinoma in cirrhotic patients. Ann Surg 1993;218:145–151.
70. Mazzaferro V, Regalia E, Doci R, et al. Liver transplantation for the treatment of small hepatocellular carcinomas in patients with cirrhosis. N Engl J Med 1996;334:693–699.
71. Yao FY, Ferrell L, Bass NM, et al. Liver transplantation for hepatocellular carcinoma: expansion of the tumor size limits does not adversely impact survival. Hepatology 2001;33:1394–1403.
72. Shimoda M, Farmer DG, Colquhoun SD, et al. Liver transplantation for cholangiocellular carcinoma: analysis of a single-center experience and review of the literature. Liver Transpl 2001;7:1023–1033.
73. Orloff MJ, Daily PO, Orloff SL, Girard B, Orloff MS. A 27-year experience with surgical treatment of Budd-Chiari syndrome. Ann Surg 2000;232:340–352.
74. Vons C, Smadja C, Bourstyn E, Szekely AM, Bonnet P, Franco D. Results of portal systemic shunts in Budd-Chiari syndrome. Ann Surg 1986;203:366–370.
75. Hemming AW, Langer B, Greig P, Taylor BR, Adams R, Heathcote EJ. Treatment of Budd-Chiari syndrome with portosystemic shunt or liver transplantation. Am J Surg 1996;171:176–180; discussion 180–181.
76. Ringe B, Lang H, Oldhafer KJ, et al. Which is the best surgery for Budd-Chiari syndrome: venous decompression or liver transplantation? A single-center experience with 50 patients. Hepatology 1995;21:1337–1344.
77. Moritz MJ, Jarrell BE, Munoz SJ, Maddrey WC. Regeneration of the native liver after heterotopic liver transplantation for fulminant hepatic failure. Transplantation 1993;55:952–954.
78. Chari RS, Collins BH, Magee JC, et al. Brief report: treatment of hepatic failure with ex vivo pig-liver perfusion followed by liver transplantation. N Engl J Med 1994;331:234–237.
79. Watanabe FD, Mullon CJ, Hewitt WR, et al. Clinical experience with a bioartificial liver in the treatment of severe liver failure. A phase I clinical trial. Ann Surg 1997;225:484–491; discussion 491–494.
80. Kjaergard LL, Liu J, Als-Nielsen B, Gluud C. Artificial and bioartificial support systems for acute and acute-on-chronic liver failure: a systematic review. JAMA 2003;289:217–222.
81. Merion RM, Schaubel DE, Dykstra DM, Freeman RB, Port FK, Wolfe RA. The survival benefit of liver transplantation. Am J Transplant 2005;5:307–313.

82. Wiesner RH, Freeman RB, Mulligan DC. Liver transplantation for hepatocellular cancer: the impact of the MELD allocation policy. Gastroenterology 2004;127(5 suppl 1):S261–S267.
83. Olthoff KM, Merion RM, Ghobrial RM, et al. Outcomes of 385 adult-to-adult living donor liver transplant recipients. A report from the A2LL consortium. Ann Surg 2005;242:314–325.
84. Menon KV, Nyberg SL, Harmsen WS, et al. MELD and other factors associated with survival after liver transplantation. Am J Transplant 2004;4:819–825.
85. Ghobrial RM, Steadman R, Gornbein J, et al. A 10-year experience of liver transplantation for hepatitis C: analysis of factors determining outcome in over 500 patients. Ann Surg 2001;234: 384–393; discussion 393–394.
86. Forman LM, Lewis JD, Berlin JA, Feldman HI, Lucey MR. The association between hepatitis C infection and survival after orthotopic liver transplantation. Gastroenterology 2002;122:889–896.
87. Gane E. The natural history and outcome of liver transplantation in hepatitis C virus-infected recipients. Liver Transpl 2003;9:S28–S34.
88. Cameron AM, Ghobrial RM, Hiatt JR, et al. Effect of nonviral factors on hepatitis C recurrence after liver transplantation. Ann Surg 2006;244:563–571.
89. Khapra AP, Agarwal K, Fiel MI, et al. Impact of donor age on survival and fibrosis progression ini patients with hepatitis C undergoing liver transplantation using HCV+ allografts. Liver Transpl 2006;12:1496–1503.
90. Moore KA, Jones RM, Burrows GD. Quality of life and cognitive function of liver transplant patients: a prospective study. Liver Transpl 2000;6:633–642.
91. Levy MF, Jennings L, Abouljoud MS, et al. Quality of life improvements at 1, 2, and 5 years after liver transplantation. Transplantation 1995;59:515–518.
92. Ploeg RJ, D'Alessandro AM, Knechtle SJ, et al. Risk factors for primary dysfunction after liver transplantation—a multivariate analysis. Transplantation 1993;55:807–813.
93. Mor E, Klintmalm GB, Gonwa TA, et al. The use of marginal donors for liver transplantation: a retrospective study of 365 liver donors. Transplantation 1992;53:383–386.
94. Strasberg SM, Howard TK, Molmenti EP, Hertl M. Selecting the donor liver: risk factors for poor function after orthotopic liver transplantation. Hepatology 1994;20:829–838.
95. Gaffey MJ, Boyd JC, Traweek ST, et al. Predictive value of intraoperative biopsies and liver function tests for preservation injury in orthotopic liver transplantation. Hepatology 1997;25:184–189.
96. D'Alessandro AM, Kalayoglu M, Sollinger HW, et al. The predictive value of donor liver biopsies for the development of primary nonfunction after orthotopic liver transplantation. Transplantation 1991;51:157–163.
97. Cescon M, Grazi GL, Ercolani G, et al. Long-term survival of recipients of liver grafts from donors older than 80 years: is it achievable? Liver Transpl 2003;9:1174–1180.
98. Wall WJ, Mimeault R, Grant DR, Bloch M. The use of older donor livers for hepatic transplantation. Transplantation 1998;49:377–381.
99. Hoofnagle JH, Lombardero M, Zetterman RK, et al. Donor age and outcome of liver transplantation. Hepatology 1996;24:89–96.
100. Lake JR, Shorr JS, Steffen BJ, et al. Differential effects of donor age in liver transplant recipients infected with hepatitis B, hepatitis C and without viral hepatitis. Am J Transplant 2005;5:549–557.
101. Hanto DW, Fecteau AH, Alonso MH, Valente JF, Whiting JF. ABO-incompatible liver transplantation with no immunological graft losses using total plasma exchange, splenectomy, and quadruple immunosuppression: evidence for accommodation. Liver Transpl 2003;9:22–30.
102. Verran D, Kusyk T, Painter D, et al. Clinical experience gained from use of 120 steatotic donor livers for orthotopic liver transplantation. Liver Transpl 2003;9:500–505.
103. Salizzoni M, Franchello A, Zamboni F, et al. Marginal grafts: finding the correct treatment for fatty livers. Transpl Int 2003;16:486–493.
104. Johnson SR, Alexopoulos S, Curry M, Hanto DW. Primary nonfunction (PNF) in the MELD era: an SRTR database analysis. Am J Transplant 2007;7:1003–1009.
105. Feng S, Goodrich NP, Bragg-Gresham JL, et al. Characteristics associated with liver graft failure: the concept of a donor risk index. Am J Transplant 2006;6:783–790.
106. Satterthwaite R, Ozgu I, Shidban H, et al. Risks of transplanting kidneys from hepatitis B surface antigen-negative, hepatitis B core antibody-positive donors. Transplantation 1997;64:432–435.
107. Wachs M, Amend WJ, Ascher NL, et al. The risk of transmission of hepatitis B from HBsAG2, HBcAB1, HBIgM2 organ donors. Transplantation 1995;59:230–234.
108. Arenas JI, Vargas HE, Rakela J. The use of hepatitis C-infected grafts in liver transplantation. Liver Transpl 2003;9:S48–S51.
109. Renz JF, Yersiz H, Reichert PR, et al. Split-liver transplantation: a review. Am J Transplant 2003;3:1323–1335.
110. Barr ML, Belghiti J, Villamil FG, et al. A report of the Vancouver Forum on the care of the live organ donor: lung, liver, pancreas, and intestine data and medical guidelines. Transplantation 2006;81:1373–1387.
111. Harms J, Bourquain H, Bartels M, et al. Surgical impact of computerized 3D Ct-based visualization in living donor liver transplantation. Surg Technol Int 2004;13:191–195.
112. Sahani D, D'souza R, Kadavigere R, et al. Evaluation of living liver transplant donors: method for precise anatomic definition by using a dedicated contrast-enhanced MR imaging protocol. Radiographics 2004;24:957–967.
113. Iwasaki M, Takada Y, Hayashi M, et al. Noninvasive evaluation of graft steatosis in living donor liver transplantation. Transplantation 2004;78:1501–1505.
114. Trotter JF, Campsen J, Bak T, Wachs M, Forman L, Everson G, Kam I. Outcomes of donor evaluations for adult-to-adult right hepatic lobe living donor liver transplantation. Am J Transplant 2006;6:1882–1889.
115. Lo CM, Chan KL, Fan ST, et al. Living donor liver transplantation: the Hong Kong experience. Tranplant Proc 1996;28:2390–2392.
116. Lo CM, Fan ST, Chan JKF, Wei W, Lo RJW, Lai CL. Minimum graft volume for successful adult-to-adult living donor liver transplantation for fulminant hepatic failure. Transplantation 1996;62:696–698.
117. Emond JC, Renz JF, Ferrell LD, et al. Functional analysis of grafts from living donors. Implications for the treatment of older recipients. Ann Surg 1996;224:544–552; discussion 552–554.
118. Gonzalez Chamorro A, Loinaz Segurola C, Moreno Gonzalez E, et al. Graft mass and volume calculation in living related donors for liver transplantation. Hepatogastroenterology 1998;45:510–513.
119. Urata K, Kawasaki S, Matsunami H, et al. Calculation of child and adult standard liver volume for liver transplantation. Hepatology 1995;21:1317–1321.
120. Pomfret EA, Pomposelli JJ, Gordon FD, et al. Liver regeneraton and surgical outcome in donors of right-lobe liver grafts. Transplantation 2003;76:5–10.
121. Emre S, Schwartz ME, Miller CM. The donor operation. In: Busuttil RW, Klintmalm GB, eds. Transplantation of the Liver. Philadelphia: Saunders; 1996:392–404.
122. Nakazato PZ, Concepcion W, Bry W, et al. Total abdominal evisceration: an en bloc technique for abdominal organ harvesting. Surgery 1992;111:37–47.

123. Boggi U, Vistoli F, Del Chiaro M, et al. A simplified technique for the en bloc procurement of abdominal organs that is suitable for pancreas and small-bowel transplantation. Surgery 2004; 135:629–641.
124. Abt PL, Desai NM, Crawford MD, et al. Survival following liver transplantation from non-heart-beating donors. Ann Surg 2004; 239:87–92.
125. Reich DJ, Munoz SJ, Rothstein KD, et al. Controlled non-heart-beating donor liver transplantation. Transplantation 2000; 70:1159–1166.
126. D'Alessandro AM, Hoffmann RM, Knechtle SJ, et al. Liver transplantation from controlled non-heart-beating donors. Surgery 2000;128:579–588.
127. Casavilla A, Ramirez C, Shapiro R, et al. Experience with liver and kidney allografts from non-heart-beating donors. Transplantation 1995;59:197–203.
128. Johnson SR, Pavlakis M, Khwaja K, et al. Intensive care unit extubation does not preclude extrarenal organ recovery from donors after cardiac death. Transplantation 2005;80:1244–1250.
129. Bismuth H, Houssin D. Reduced-size orthotopic liver graft in hepatic transplantation in children. Surgery 1984;95:367–370.
130. Broelsch CE, Emond JC, Thistlethwaite JR, Rouch DA, Whitington PF, Lichtor JL. Liver transplantation with reduced-size donor organs. Transplantation 1988;45:519–524.
131. Couinaud C. Le Foie. Etudes Anatomiques et Cirurgicales. Paris: Masson; 1957.
132. Humar A, Khwaja K, Sielaff TD, Lake JR, Payne WD. Split-liver transplants for two adult recipients: technique of preservation of the vena cava with the right lobe graft. Liver Transpl 2004;10:153–155.
133. Broelsch CE, Whitington PF, Emond JC, et al. Liver transplantation in children from living related donors. Surgical techniques and results. Ann Surg 1991;214:428–437; discussion 437–439.
134. Bak T, Wachs M, Trotter J, et al. Adult-to-adult living donor liver transplantation using right-lobe grafts: results and lessons learned from a single-center experience. Liver Transpl 2001;7: 680–686.
135. Wachs ME, Bak TE, Karrer FM, et al. Adult living donor liver transplantation using a right hepatic lobe. Transplantation 1998;66:1313–1316.
136. Lo CM, Fan ST, Liu CL, et al. Lessons learned from one hundred right lobe living donor liver transplants. Ann Surg 2004;240:151–158.
137. Shaw BWJ, Martin DJ, Marquez JM, et al. Venous bypass in clinical liver transplantation. Ann Surg 1984;200:524–534.
138. Grande L, Rimola A, Cugat E, et al. Effect of venovenous bypass on perioperative renal function in liver transplantation: results of a randomized, controlled trial. Hepatology 1996;23:1418–1428.
139. Wall WJ, Grant DR, Duff JH, Kutt JL, Ghent CN, Block MS. Liver transplantation without venous bypass. Transplantation 1987;43:56–61.
140. Johnson SR, Marterre WF, Alonso MH, Hanto DW. A percutaneous technique for venovenous bypass in orthotopic cadaver liver transplantation and comparison with the open technique. Liver Transplant Surg 1996;2:354–361.
141. Rouch DA, Emond JC, Thistlewaite JRJ, Mayes JT, Broelsch CE. Choledochostomy without a T tube or internal stent in transplantation of the liver. Surg Gynecol Obstet 1990;170:239–244.
142. Vougas V, Rela M, Gane E, et al. A prospective randomised trial of bile duct reconstruction at liver transplantation: T tube or no T tube? Transpl Int 1996;9:392–395.
143. Busque S, Esquivel CO, Concepcion W, So SKS. Experience with the piggyback technique without caval occlusion in adult orthotopic liver transplantation. Transplantation 1998;65:77–82.
144. Andorno E, Genzone A, Morelli N, et al. One liver for two adults: in situ split liver transplantation for two adult recipients. Transplant Proc 2001;33:1420–1422.
145. Azoulay D, Castaing D, Adam R, et al. Split-liver transplantation for two adult recipients: feasibility and long-term outcomes. Ann Surg 2001;233:565–574.
146. Egawa H, Inomata Y, Uemoto S, et al. Hepatic vein reconstruction in 152 living-related donor liver transplantation patients. Surgery 1997;121:250–257.
147. Emond JC. Clinical application of living-related liver transplantation. Gastroenterol Clin North Am 1993;22:301–315.
148. Inomoto T, Nishizawa F, Sasaki H, et al. Experiences of 120 microsurgical reconstructions of hepatic artery in living related liver transplantation. Surgery 1996;119:20–26.
149. Ikegami T, Kawasaki S, Matsunami H, et al. Should all hepatic arterial branches be reconstructed in living-related liver transplantation? Surgery 1996;119:431–436.
150. Kubota T, Togo S, Sekido H, et al. Indications for hepatic vein reconstruction in living donor liver transplantation of right liver grafts. Tranplant Proc 2004;36:2263–2266.
151. Humar A, Khwaja K, Sielaff TD, Lake JR, Payne WD. Technique of split-liver transplant for two adult recipients. Liver Transpl 2002;8:725–729.
152. Marcos A, Killackey M, Orloff MS, Mieles L, Bozorgzadeh A, Tan HP. Hepatic arterial reconstruction in 95 adult right lobe living donor liver transplants: evolution of anastomotic technique. Liver Transpl 2003;9:570–574.
153. Stange BJ, Glanemann M, Nuessler NC, Settmacher U, Steinmuller T, Neuhaus P. Hepatic artery thrombosis after adult liver transplantation. Liver Transpl 2003;9:612–620.
154. Tzakis AG, Gordon RD, Shaw BW Jr, Iwatsuki S, Starzl TE. Clinical presentation of hepatic artery thrombosis after liver transplantation in the cyclosporine era. Transplantation 1985;40: 667–671.
155. Langnas AN, Marujo W, Stratta RJ, Wood RP, Li SJ, Shaw BW. Hepatic allograft rescue following arterial thrombosis. Role of urgent revascularization. Transplantation 1991;51:86–90.
156. Abbasoglu O, Levy MF, Vodapally MS, et al. Hepatic artery stenosis after liver transplantation—incidence, presentation, treatment, and long term outcome. Transplantation 1997;63:250–255.
157. Sheiner PA, Varma CV, Guarrera JV, et al. Selective revascularization of hepatic artery thromboses after liver transplantation improves patient and graft survival. Transplantation 1997;64: 1295–1299.
158. Cavallari A, Vivarelli M, Bellusci R, Jovine E, Mazziotti A, Rossi C. Treatment of vascular complications following liver transplantation: multidisciplinary approach. Hepatogastroenterology 2001;48:179–183.
159. Vivarelli M, Cucchetti A, La Barba G, et al. Ischemic arterial complications after liver transplantation in the adult: multivariate analysis of risk factors. Arch Surg 2004;139:1069–1074.
160. Cotroneo AR, Di Stasi C, Cina A, et al. Stent placement in four patients with hepatic artery stenosis or thrombosis after liver transplantation. J Vasc Interv Radiol 2002;13:619–623.
161. Valente JF, Alonso MH, Weber FL, Hanto DW. Late hepatic artery thrombosis in liver allograft recipients is associated with intrahepatic biliary necrosis. Transplantation 1996;61: 61–65.
162. Orons PD, Sheng R, Zajko AB. Hepatic artery stenosis in liver transplant recipients: prevalence and cholangiographic appearance of associated biliary complications. AJR Am J Roentgenol 1995;165:1145–1149.
163. Narumi S, Osorio RW, Freise CE, Stock PG, Roberts JP, Ascher NL. Hepatic artery pseudoaneurysm with hemobilia following angioplasty after liver transplantation. Clin Transplant 1998; 12:508–510.
164. Fukuzawa K, Schwartz ME, Katz E, et al. The arcuate ligament syndrome in liver transplantation. Transplantation 1993;56:223–224.

165. Jurim O, Shaked A, Kiai K, Millis JM, Colquhoun SD, Busuttil RW. Celiac compression syndrome and liver transplantation. Ann Surg 1993;218:10–12.
166. Moser MA, Wall WJ. Management of biliary problems after liver transplantation. Liver Transpl 2001;7(11 suppl 1):S46–S52.
167. Thethy S, Thomson B, Pleass H, et al. Management of biliary tract complications after orthotopic liver transplantation. Clin Transplant 2004;18:647–653.
168. Busuttil RW, Tanaka K. The utility of marginal donors in liver transplantation. Liver Transpl 2003;9:651–663.
169. Abt P, Crawford M, Desai N, Markmann J, Olthoff K, Shaked A. Liver transplantation from controlled non-heart-beating donors: an increased incidence of biliary complications. Transplantation 2003;75:1659–1663.
170. Scatton O, Meunier B, Cherqui D, et al. Randomized trial of choledochocholedochostomy with or without a T tube in orthotopic liver transplantation. Ann Surg 2001;233:432–437.
171. Shimoda M, Saab S, Morrisey M, et al. A cost-effectiveness analysis of biliary anastomosis with or without T-tube after orthotopic liver transplantation. Am J Transplant 2001;1:157–161.
172. Thuluvath PJ, Atassi T, Lee J. An endoscopic approach to biliary complications following orthotopic liver transplantation. Liver Int 2003;23:156–162.
173. Pfau PR, Kochman ML, Lewis JD, et al. Endoscopic management of postoperative biliary complications in orthotopic liver transplantation. Gastrointest Endosc 2000;52:55–63.
174. Pomfret EA. Early and late complications in the right-lobe adult living donor. Liver Transpl 2003;9(10 suppl 2):S45–S49.
175. Trotter JF, Adam R, Lo CM, Kenison J. Documented deaths of hepatic lobe donors for living donor transplantation. Liver Transpl 2006;12:1485–1488.
176. Levy G, Burra P, Cavallari A, et al. Improved clinical outcomes for liver transplant recipients using cyclosporine monitoring based on 2-h post dose levels (C_2). Transplantation 2002;73:953–969.
177. Tzakis AG, Tryphonopoulos P, Kato T, et al. Preliminary experience with alemtuzumab (Campath-1H) and low-dose tacrolimus immunosuppression in adult liver transplantation. Transplantation 2004;77:1209–1214.
178. Neuhaus P, Klupp J, Langrehr JM. mTOR inhibitors: an overview. Liver Transpl 2001;6:473–484.
179. Fung J, Kelly D, Kadry Z, Patel-Tom K, Eghtesad B. Immunosuppression in liver transplantation. Beyond calcineurin inhibitors. Liver Transpl 2005;11:267–280.
180. Kauffman HM, Cherikh WS, Cheng Y, Hanto DW, Kahan BD. Maintenance immunosuppression with target-of-rapamycin inhibitors is associated with a reduced incidence of de novo malignancies. Transplantation 2005;80:883–889.
181. Shapiro R, Young JB, Milford EL, Trotter JF, Bustami RT, Leichtman AB. Immunosuppression: evolution in practice and trends, 1993–2003. Am J Transplant 2005;5(4 pt 2):874–886.
182. Eason JD, Nair S, Cohen AJ, Blazek JL, Loss GE Jr. Steroid-free liver transplantation using rabbit antithymocyte globulin and early tacrolimus monotherapy. Transplantation 2003;75:1396–1399.
183. Greig P, Lilly L, Scudamore C, et al. Early steroid withdrawal after liver transplantation: the Canadian tacrolimus versus microemulsion cyclosporin A trial: 1-year follow-up. Liver Transpl 2003;9:587–595.
184. Trotter JF, Wachs M, Bak T, et al. Liver transplantation using sirolimus and minimal corticosteroids (3-day taper). Liver Transpl 2001;7:343–351.
185. The U.S. Multicenter FK506 Liver Study Group. A comparison of tacrolimus (FK506) and cyclosporine for immunosuppression in liver transplantation. N Engl J Med 1994;331:1110–1115.
186. European FK506 Multicentre Liver Study Group. Randomised trial comparing tacrolimus (FK506) and cyclosporin in prevention of liver allograft rejection. Lancet 1994;344:423–428.
187. Wiesner RH, Rabkin J, Klintmalm G, et al. A randomized double-blind comparative study of mycophenolate mofetil and azathioprine in combination with cyclosporine and corticosteroids in primary liver transplant recipients. Liver Transpl 2001;7:442–450.
188. Knechtle SJ, Kolbeck PC, Tsuchimoto S, Coundouriotis A, Sanfilippo AP, Bollinger RR. Hepatic transplantation into sensitized recipients: demonstration of hyperacute rejection. Transplantation 1987;43:8–12.
189. Hanto DW, Snover DC, Noreen HJ, et al. Hyperacute rejection of a human orthotopic liver allograft in a presensitized recipient. Clin Transplant 1987;1:304–310.
190. Demetris AJ, Jaffe R, Tzakis A, et al. Antibody-mediated rejection of human orthotopic liver allografts. A study of liver transplantation across ABO blood group barriers. Am J Pathol 1988;132:489–502.
191. Ratner L, Phelan D, Brunt EM, Mohanakumar T, Hanto DW. Probable antibody-mediated failure of two sequential ABO-compatible hepatic allografts in a single recipient. 1993;55:814–819.
192. Hanto DW. A 50-year-old man with hepatitis C and cirrhosis needing liver transplantation. JAMA 2003;290:3238–3246.
193. Neumann UP, Lang M, Moldenhauer A, et al. Significance of a T-lymphocytotoxic crossmatch in liver and combined liver-kidney transplantation. Transplantation 2001;71:1163–1168.
194. Eid A, Moore SB, Wiesner RH, DeGoey SR, Nielson A, Krom RAF. Evidence that the liver does not always protect the kidney from hyperacute rejection in combined liver-kidney transplantation across a positive lymphocyte crossmatch. Transplantation 1990;50:331–334.
195. Wiesner RH, Demetris AJ, Belle SH, et al. Acute hepatic allograft rejection: incidence, risk factors, and impact on outcome. Hepatology 1998;28:638–645.
196. Kaufman DB, Shapiro R, Lucey MR, Cherikh WS, Bustami RT, Dyke DB. Immunosuppression: practice and trends. American Journal of Transplantation 2004;4(suppl 9):38–53.
197. Demetris AJ, Batts KP, Dhillon AP, et al. Banff schema for grading liver allograft rejection: an international consensus document. Hepatology 1997;25:658–663.
198. Demetris A, Adams D, Bellamy C, et al. Update of the International Banff Schema for Liver Allograft Rejection: working recommendations for the histopathologic staging and reporting of chronic rejection. An international panel. Hepatology 2000;31:792–799.
199. Volpin R, Angeli P, Galioto A, et al. Comparison between two high-dose methylprednisolone schedules in the treatment of acute hepatic cellular rejection in liver transplant recipients: a controlled clinical trial. Liver Transpl 2002;8:527–534.
200. Fishman JA, Rubin RH. Infection in organ transplant recipients. N Engl J Med 1998;338:1741–1751.
201. Whiting JF, Rossi SJ, Hanto DW. Infectious complications after OKT3 induction in liver transplantation. Liver Transplant Surg 1997;3:563–570.
202. Wade JJ, Rolando N, Hayllar K, Philpott-Howard J, Casewell MW, Williams R. Bacterial and fungal infections after liver transplantation: an analysis of 284 patients. Hepatology 1995;21:1328–1336.
203. Rayes N, Seehofer D, Theruvath T, et al. Supply of pre- and probiotics reduces bacterial infection rates after liver transplantation—a randomized, double-blind trial. Am J Transplant 2005;5:125–130.
204. Trotter JF, Wallack A, Steinberg T. Low incidence of cytomegalovirus disease in liver transplant recipients receiving sirolimus primary immunosuppression with 3-day corticosteroid taper. Transplant Infect Dis 2003;5:174–180.

205. Gane E, Saliba F, Valdecasas FJC, O'Grady J, Pescovitz MD, Lyman S. Randomised trial of efficacy and safety of oral ganciclovir in the prevention of cytomegalovirus disease in liver-transplant recipients. Lancet 1997;350:1729–1733.
206. Couchoud C, Chucherat M, Haugh M, Pouteil-Noble C. Cytomegalovirus prophylaxis with antiviral agents in solid organ transplantation: a meta-analysis. Transplantation 1998;65:641–647.
207. Winston DJ, Busuttil RW. Randomized controlled trial of sequential intravenous and oral ganciclovir versus prolonged intravenous ganciclovir for long-term prophylaxis of cytomegalovirus disease in high-risk cytomegalovirus-seronegative liver transplant recipients with cytomegalovirus-seropositive donors. Transplantation 2004;77:305–308.
208. Hanto DW. Classification of Epstein-Barr virus-associated post-transplant lymphoproliferative diseases: implications for understanding their pathogenesis and developing rational treatment strategies. Annu Rev Med 1995;46:381–394.
209. Nalesnik MA. The diverse pathology of post-transplant lymphoproliferative disorders: the importance of a standardized approach. Transpl Infect Dis 2001;3:88–96.
210. Paya CV, Fung JJ, Nalesnik MA, et al. Epstein-Barr virus-induced posttransplant lymphoproliferative disorders. ASTS/ASTP EBV-PTLD Task Force and the Mayo Clinic Organized International Consensus Development Meeting. Transplantation 1999;68: 1517–1525.
211. Cherikh WS, Kauffman HM, McBride MA, et al. Association of the type of induction immunosuppression with posttransplant lymphoproliferative disorder, graft survival, and patient survival after primary kidney transplantation. Transplantation 2003; 76:1289–1293.
212. Savoldo B, Rooney CM, Quiros-Tejeira E, et al. Cellular immunity to Epstein-Barr virus in liver transplant recipients treated with rituximab for post-transplant lymphoproliferative disease. Am J Transplant 2005;5:566–572.
213. Levitsky J, Kalil A, Meza JL, Hurst GE, Freifeld A. Herpes zoster infection after liver transplantation: a case-control study. Liver Transpl 2005;11:320–325.
214. Stallone G, Schena A, Infante B, et al. Sirolimus for Kaposi's sarcoma in renal-transplant recipients. N Engl J Med 2005;352: 1317–1323.
215. Rabkin JM, Orloff SL, Corless CL, et al. Association of fungal infection and increased mortality in liver transplant recipients. Am J Surg 2000;2000:426–430.
216. Paya CV. Prevention of fungal and hepatitis virus infections in liver transplantation. Clin Infect Dis 2001;33(suppl 1):S47–S52.
217. Husain S, Tollemar J, Dominguez EA, et al. Changes in the spectrum and risk factors for invasive candidiasis in liver transplant recipients: prospective, multicenter, case-controlled study. Transplantation 2003;75:2023–2029.
218. Walsh TJ, Teppler H, Donowitz GR, et al. Caspofungin versus liposomal amphotericin B for empirical antifungal therapy in patients with persistent fever and neutropenia. N Engl J Med 2004;351:1391–1402.
219. Winston DJ, Pakrasi A, Busuttil RW. Prophylactic fluconazole in liver transplant recipients. Ann Internal Med 1999;131:729–737.
220. Lumbreras C, Cuervas-Mons V, Jara P, del Palacio A, Turrion S, Barrios C. Randomized trial of fluconazole versus nystatin for the prophylaxis of Candida infection following liver transplantation. J Infect Dis 1996;174:583–688.
221. Sharpe MD, Ghent C, Grant D, et al. Efficacy and safety of itraconazole prophylaxis for fungal infections after orthotopic liver transplantation: a prospective, randomized, double-blind study. Transplantation 2003;76:977–983.
222. Randall HB, Wachs ME, Somberg KA, et al. The use of the T tube after orthotopic liver transplantation. Transplantation 1996;61:258–261.
223. Paya C, Humar A, Dominguez E, et al. Efficacy and safety of valganciclovir versus oral ganciclovir for prevention of cytomegalovirus disease in solid organ transplant recipients. Am J Transplant 2004;4:611–620.
224. Winston DJ, Busuttil RW. Randomized controlled trial of oral ganciclovir versus oral acyclovir after induction with intravenous ganciclovir for long-term prophylaxis of cytomegalovirus disease in cytomegalovirus-seropositive liver transplant recipients. Transplantation 2003;75:229–233.
225. Kamath PS, Wiesner RH, Malinchoc M, et al. A model to predict survival in patients with end-stage liver disease. Hepatology 2001;33:464–470.
226. Humar A, Sielaff RT, Lake JR, Payne WD. Split liver transplant for two adult recipients—evolution of the surgical procedure. Paper presented at: American Transplant Congress 2004; Boston; May 15–19, 2004.
227. New York State Committee on Quality Improvements in Living Liver Donation. A report to the New York State Transplant Council and New York State Department of Health. New York State Department of Health, Albany, NY; December 2002.`

86

Transplantation of the Intestine

Fady M. Kaldas and Douglas G. Farmer

The intestine was one of the last solid organs to be successfully transplanted. The reasons behind the barriers to successful intestinal transplantation (ITx) in humans are multifactorial. No doubt, the fact that the bowel is one of the largest and most active immune "organs" in the human body and the fact that bacteria and fungi reside in symbiosis within the lumen of the gut play a significant role. In fact, the immunogenicity of the intestine is so strong that successful transplantation was not possible without the advent of powerful immunosuppressive medications. This chapter outlines the development of this field, the surgical techniques used, the outcomes, as well as the major problems commonly seen after ITx.

Historical Perspective

The foundation for the early human ITx attempts came from two arenas in the 1950s and 1960s. The first was the successful renal transplants performed under the immunosuppressive cocktails of that time period. The second was the canine intestinal models developed in 1959 by Lillehei[1] and in 1960 by Starzl[2] that outlined the technical and immunologic parameters for ITx. Coupled with the fact that no suitable medical therapy existed at that time for patients who acutely developed short gut syndrome (SGS), these events formed the basis that resulted in the 10 unsuccessful human intestinal transplants performed between 1964 and 1972.[3] All recipients died as a result of sepsis, rejection, or technical complications.[4] Despite the relative efficacy of steroids, azathioprine, and antilymphocyte globulin immunosuppressive regimens in other organ transplants, these regimens proved inadequate for controlling intestinal graft rejection. With the development of total parenteral nutrition (TPN) by Dudrick et al.[5] in 1968 and long-term central venous access catheters (CVCs) in 1972 by Broviac and Scribner,[6] an effective means of long-term nutritional support was established and enabled the survival of patients with SGS, thus relegating ITx to an entity of academic interest rather than clinical applicability.

Despite the utility of TPN in most patients with SGS/intestinal failure (IF), it became evident subsequently[4] that there was a cohort of patients with high mortality rates and a poor prognosis due to TPN dependence, prompting renewed interest in ITx. This interest was fueled by the clinical introduction of cyclosporine in the early 1980s, which showed promising results in other solid organ transplants.[7] Reports from several centers[8–11] demonstrated that ITx was possible, albeit on a case-by-case basis. During this era, the first successful human mutivisceral transplant was performed in 1987 by Starzl et al.,[9] the first successful combined liver-intestinal transplant was reported in 1988 by Grant et al.,[8] and the first successful isolated intestinal transplant was performed in 1988 by Deltz et al.[12]

It was not until the introduction of FK506 (tacrolimus; Prograf, Fujisawa, Deerfield, IL) that reports with larger series of intestinal recipients became a clinical reality. Today, almost all intestinal transplant recipients are treated with tacrolimus-based immunosuppression. This immunosuppressive regimen has been pivotal in establishing ITx as a standard treatment for IF and life-threatening TPN-related complications.

Intestinal Failure

Intestinal failure is defined as loss or nonfunction of the gut that results in the need for life-saving supplemental TPN.[4] The diagnosis of IF and the documentation of its irreversibil-

TABLE 86.1. Causes of Intestinal Failure.

Pediatric	*Cases (%)*	*Adults*	*Cases (%)*
Gastroschisis	21	Ischemia	23
Volvulus	17	Crohn's disease	14
Necrotizing enterocolitis	12	Trauma	10
Pseudoobstruction	9	Desmoid	9
Atresia	8	Short gut, other	9
Retransplant	8	Motility	8
Hirshsprung's	7	Volvulus	7
Microvillus occlusion disease	6	Retransplant	6
Short gut, other	5	Other tumor	5
Malabsorption	3	Gardner's familial polyposis	3
Tumor	1	Miscellaneous	5
Motility	1		
Other	2		

Source: Adapted from Grant et al.,[14] by permission of *Annals of Surgery*.

ity are essential prerequisites for ITx.[13] The most common causes of chronic IF are listed in Table 86.1[14] and include functional disorders of intestinal motility and absorption in addition to surgical disorders. In the pediatric population, gastroschisis, volvulus, and necrotizing enterocolitis are the most common causes of SGS/IF leading to ITx, whereas ischemia, Crohn's disease, and trauma are the most common diagnoses in adults.

Indications for Intestinal Transplantation

In general, ITx is indicated for patients with IF and TPN dependence who have developed one or more major complications related to chronic TPN therapy. This approach relies on the premise that outcomes after ITx, although improving, have not yet surpassed those for patients on chronic TPN who do not have any major TPN-related complications. The most common complications leading to consideration for ITx include parenteral nutrition-associated liver disease (PNALD), limited central venous access due to deep venous thrombosis, and recurrent CVC sepsis.[15]

Perhaps PNALD is the most devastating complication associated with IF[16] and is a clear indication for ITx. Its prevalence and clinical presentation seem to vary based on several clinical characteristics, including patient age, time on TPN, length of remnant bowel, and amount of enteral nutritional support. The complication is not well understood and probably represents a spectrum of liver diseases that arise in this patient population. Patients at highest risk for PNALD appear to be young children as well as those with total loss of midgut or gastrocolonic discontinuity. The degree of liver disease present tends to dictate the need for combined liver-intestinal grafts. In general, PNALD characterized by advanced fibrosis (or cirrhosis) along with portal hypertension necessitates combined grafts. However, early PNALD with lesser degrees of fibrosis in the absence of portal hypertension can be rescued/reversed with isolated intestinal grafts.[17] It is therefore imperative that patients with IF and progressive liver disease be referred to a transplant center at the first sign of liver disease.

Scarce central venous access is a common problem that occurs in both the pediatric and adult patient population. The generally accepted consensus is that loss of half of the standard central venous access sites, bilateral subclavian, internal jugular, and iliac veins (older children and adults), constitutes an indication to refer the patient for transplant evaluation. Given the need for peri- and postoperative central venous access in ITx recipients, referral should not be delayed until difficult, more invasive approaches such as intrahepatic, intrathoracic, or intracardiac access lines are necessary.

Recurrent and problematic CVC infections represent a third common indication for ITx consideration. Chronic home TPN patients are generally reported in large series to average approximately one CVC infection every 1–2 years on TPN. Messing et al.[18] demonstrated that 15% of all deaths of patients receiving home TPN was a result of central line-related sepsis. When patients experience frequent CVC infections, infections involving multidrug-resistant microbial organisms or yeast; septic foci such as abscesses, endocarditis, or arthritis; or any septic episode associated with multisystem organ failure, referral for consideration for ITx is warranted.

Several groups of patients with poor prognosis on TPN should be referred early for ITx evaluation. Patients with very short lengths of remnant intestine (<10 cm of intestine) constitute such a group. Although there have been case reports of patients with remnant bowel as short as 11 cm being completely weaned to enteral nutrition,[19] the majority of these patients face a dismal chance of long-term survival without transplant. Congenital epithelial disorders, including microvillus inclusion disease, tufting enteropathy, and untreatable villous atrophies, carrying no realistic hope for bowel adaptation also warrant prompt referral for transplantation.

The second group of patients consists of those patients suffering from significant impairment in their quality of life (QOL) caused by severe pain in the cases of chronic motility disorders or a persistent need for hospitalization to manage erratic metabolic parameters resulting from lack of enteral nutrition. These groups warrant consideration for ITx on a case-by-case basis.

Contraindications for Intestinal Transplantation

In general, the contraindications for ITx are similar to those for other solid organ transplants. Patients with uncontrolled sepsis, major cardiopulmonary diseases, or malignancy not resectable by transplantation should not be considered candidates for transplantation. Other commonly cited contraindications as outlined by Kaufman et al.[15] include the presence of profound neurological disabilities, severe immunodeficiencies, multisystem autoimmune diseases, life-threatening illnesses not related to the gastrointestinal tract, and insufficient vascular access to allow peritransplant monitoring/management.

Wait-List Mortality

One of the most reliable predictive factors of posttransplant graft and patient outcome has been pretransplant patient status. Therefore, optimizing transplant candidates' clinical status is imperative for improving outcomes. Unfortunately, ITx candidates have tended to fare poorly while waiting for transplantation. In an extensive analysis of United Network of Organ Sharing (UNOS) data, Fryer et al. demonstrated that patients awaiting any type of intestinal graft (combined with liver or intestine alone) had a mortality rate three times higher than patients awaiting liver grafts.[20] Langnas also reported that the mortality rate for patients awaiting ITx was far greater than that of candidates awaiting other organ transplants.[4] This was of particular prominence in the pediatric population. Candidates awaiting combined liver-intestine transplants had a mortality rate 3.6 times higher than patients with comparable pediatric end-stage liver disease (PELD) scores awaiting liver transplantation alone.[21]

These data in retrospect are not surprising for a number of reasons. First, the PELD scoring system was designed to predict the mortality of pediatric patients awaiting isolated liver transplantation with the most common causes of pediatric liver diseases such as biliary atresia.[22] In fact, the PELD score was tested to the exclusion of patients with PNALD. In addition, ITx candidates represent unique wait-list challenges. Their histories of multiple prior abdominal surgeries and loss of abdominal cavity domain have traditionally limited the donor options for these candidates to pediatric donors of smaller size. This has compounded the wait-list mortality issues.

The wait-list mortality data have resulted in several changes in the UNOS listing system designed to alter these findings. First, modifications in the PELD scoring system by which patients awaiting a combined liver-intestine graft are allotted 12 additional points and regular increases in PELD points to help reduce wait-list mortality for those patients have been instituted. Policies by which pediatric donors are offered to pediatric recipients and multiorgan recipients are offered donors ahead of single-organ recipients have been put into place. The efficacy of these changes remains to be determined. Other center-specific modifications have included the use of reduced or split-donor organs, allowing the retrieval of larger donor grafts.[23] Other more simple mechanisms are earlier referral and listing for transplantation, allowing more time to allocate suitable donor organs. As the wait for liver donors is most competitive, transplanting appropriate candidates with isolated intestinal grafts prior to the development of advanced PNALD is most logical. As the wait-list mortality continues to be an issue, further study and follow-up are mandatory.

Graft Options

There are several graft options available to candidates for ITx depending on the underlying cause of the SGS/IF, the visceral organs affected by the underlying disease state, and the degree of liver disease. The graft options, outlined below, include an isolated intestinal graft, a combined liver-intestinal graft, a multivisceral graft, a modified multivisceral graft, and an isolated liver graft. The most common graft type used in this patient population is the combined liver-intestinal graft.[24]

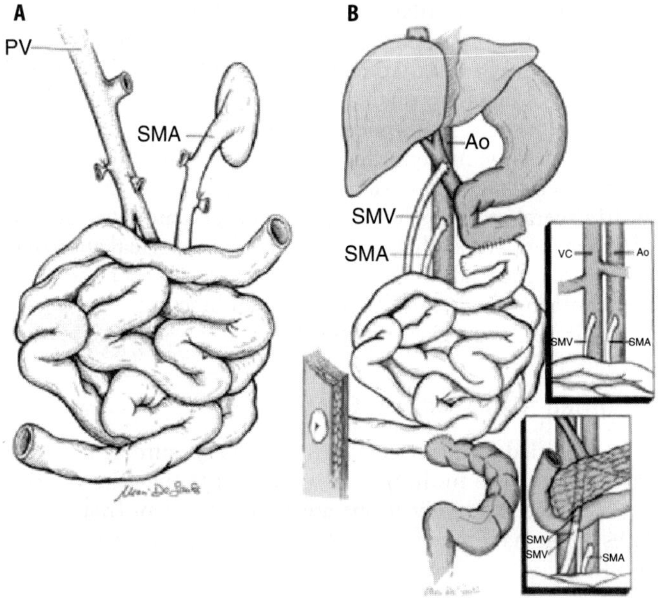

FIGURE 86.1. (A) Isolated intestinal allograft (B) Isolated intestinal transplant. Intestinal piggyback method, superior mesenteric vein (SMV) drainage (*inset, below*), mesocaval drainage (*inset, above*). Ao, aorta; PV, portal vein; SMA, superior mesenteric artery; VC, vena cava. (From Kato et al.,[25] by permission of *World Journal of Surgery*.)

Isolated Intestinal Graft

The isolated intestinal graft, usually comprising the entire jejunoileum with a vascular pedicle including the superior mesenteric artery (SMA) and superior mesenteric vein, is the procedure of choice in patients with disease confined to the intestine and reversible/early in other abdominal viscera (Fig. 86.1A).[25] This is particularly important and difficult for patients with liver disease. In general, as outlined above, if the liver disease is reversible and no evidence of portal hypertension exists, then isolated intestinal grafts are indicated.

Combined Liver-Intestinal Graft

The liver-intestinal graft is most frequently procured en bloc with or without the duodenum/head of the pancreas.[26] The arterial inflow usually is derived from the aorta and includes both the SMA and celiac trunk, and the venous outflow remains intact via the suprahepatic vena cava (Fig. 86.2A).[25] This graft type is indicated for patients with irreversible liver disease of any cause combined with SGS/IF. Technical and therapeutic indications make it necessary to offer combined grafts to IF patients with portomesenteric thrombosis or patients with metabolic or enzymatic defects of the liver.[27]

Multivisceral Graft

The true multivisceral graft constitutes an en bloc set of organs that include the liver, pancreas, duodenum, and jejunoileum with or without the stomach. The vascular inflow and outflow are similar to that described above for liver-intestine grafts (Fig. 86.3A).[25] This graft option is reserved for patients with advanced, irreversible liver disease plus pangastrointestinal disorders such as motility disorders or gastrointestinal polyposis syndromes. Other indications include the presence of large mesenteric desmoid tumors or diffuse mesenteric venous thrombosis. More recently, the use of the multivisceral graft has been reported for patients with severe adhesions or fistulas that prevent a standard surgical approach to the abdomen and require removing other viscera such as the stomach, duodenum, or pancreas en bloc with the bowel to facilitate the surgical technique.[3,25]

Modified Multivisceral Graft

The modified multivisceral graft is very similar to that described for the multivisceral graft except that the liver is not included. The indications are as above except that candidates must have reversible liver disease or no liver disease at all.

Isolated Liver Graft

Rarely, isolated liver grafts are appropriate options for patients with advanced liver disease and SGS. In these cases, candidates for this procedure must be deemed to have adequate intestinal length and function to facilitate adaptation from TPN after transplantation. The determination/prediction of adaptation can be quite difficult and should really only be undertaken at specialized transplant centers. Outcomes can be quite good[28] in select candidates. However, the inappropriate selection of such candidates can be disastrous if SGS/IF persists, leading in most instances to posttransplant liver failure with the need for retransplantation.

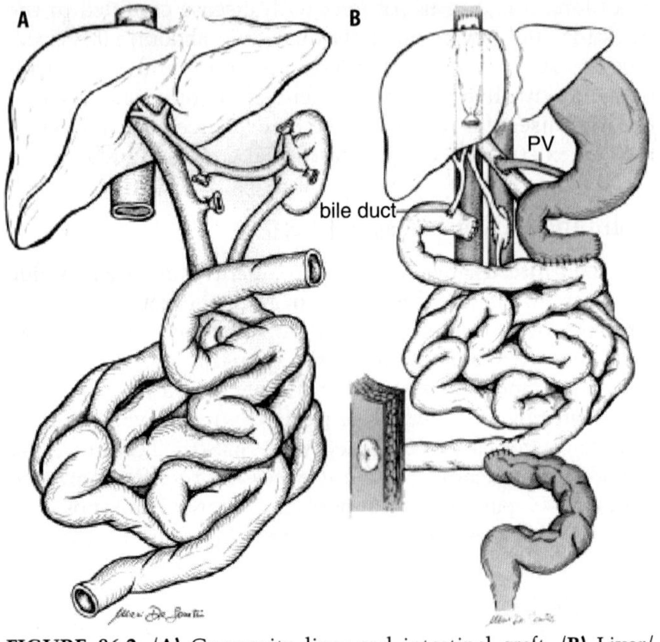

FIGURE 86.2. (A) Composite liver and intestinal graft. (B) Liver/intestinal transplant. An anastomosis from native portal vein to donor portal vein and a donor biliary reconstruction with choledocojejunostomy. (From Kato et al.,[25] by permission of *World Journal of Surgery*.)

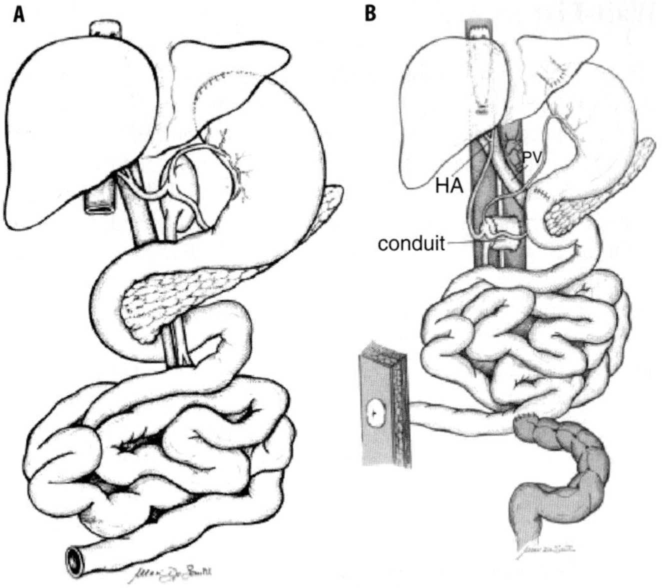

FIGURE 86.3. (A) Multivisceral graft. (B) Multivisceral transplant. An arterial anastomosis with a conduit. HA, hepatic artery. (From Kato et al., [25] by permission of *World Journal of Surgery*.)

Donor Operation/Selection

Donor selection criteria are quite strict in general. First, the recipient characteristics, which include loss of abdominal cavity domain coupled with the small stature of most candidates, dictate that the potential donor is no more than equal in size to the recipient. In fact, most centers prefer donors who are smaller than the recipient to ensure adequate abdominal cavity for allograft placement. Therefore, most intestinal donors are children or young adults, representing 68% of the donors used to date.[29] Furthermore, donors should not have a history of intestinal or liver disorders and should not have had intestinal resections. Donors should be hemodynamically stable with minimal pressor requirements. Donors with extensive downtime or recent cardiopulmonary resuscitation are generally avoided. Donors with hepatitis virus or HIV-positive donors have never been used for ITx.

Recipient Operative Procedure

The conduct of the operation is divided into several phases. Vascular access is the first phase. This may be quite challenging in patients with limited vascular access. As a result, pretransplant evaluation testing should be targeted to identify potential access sites to avoid operative delays required for difficult venous access cases. Multiple central venous lumens are generally required for intra- and postoperative management and monitoring.

The second operative phase is the abdominal operation. The incision is crucial for later successful closure. Prior operative scars, tube sites, and ostomy sites will have an impact on this decision. Generally, for patients requiring liver inclusive grafts, a bilateral subcostal incision is used. For recipients of modified multivisceral grafts or isolated intestinal grafts, a midline incision is used. The abdominal portion of the surgery is then further subdivided into liver hepatectomy (for liver recipients), establishing vascular inflow/outflow targets/conduits, graft implantation and reperfusion, removal of diseased/dysfunctional gastrointestinal organs, restoration of gastrointestinal continuity, placement of enteral feeding tubes, and abdominal wall closure.

Hepatectomy is generally performed in a fashion similar to that done for isolated liver transplantation with mobilization of the ligament attachments, dissection of the porta hepatis, and control of the vena cava. The piggyback technique is frequently used. Many centers today perform a native end-side portocaval shunt during the anhepatic phase. An alternative technique for draining the native portal circulation is an anastomosis onto the transplanted portal vein. In this case, this anastomosis is delayed until the allograft organs are in situ. It is also noteworthy that recipients of multivisceral grafts usually require a more extensive resection than that described above. In general, the entire foregut and midgut are removed by mobilizing the liver, stomach, duodenum, pancreas, spleen, and small bowel en bloc. The celiac trunk and SMA are controlled at their origins and the liver is taken off the retrohepatic inferior vena cava (IVC). Obviously, there is no native portomesenteric circulation for anastomosis in this case. In some ways, this approach simplifies the later operative plan as outlined below.

Establishing optimal vascular inflow and outflow are the next steps. For the inflow, the aorta is usually the vessel of choice, with the infrarenal aorta used for some modified multivisceral and isolated intestinal grafts (Fig. 86.1B)[25] and supraceliac aortic conduits used for liver-intestinal (Fig. 86.2B)[25] and multivisceral grafts (Fig. 86.3B).[25] The liberal use of conduits is recommended. In some cases of isolated intestinal grafts, the SMA of the recipient provides excellent arterial inflow. Venous outflow is also important. The outflow vessel must be large enough to avoid congestion of the viscera. Again, the liberal use of short conduits is recommended. For liver-inclusive grafts, the outflow is via the suprahepatic IVC (Fig. 86.2B).[25] For cases of isolated ITx (Fig. 86.1B)[25] and modified multivisceral grafts, the outflow can be via the IVC, portal vein, splenic vein, or SMV depending on recipient anatomy. There are no human data to support the superiority of one target outflow vessel over the other.

Implantation of the allograft follows. The venous outflow is sutured first using fine monofilament suture. For liver-inclusive grafts, the suprahepatic vena cava anastomosis is similar to that commonly performed in liver transplantation. With use of the piggyback technique, the donor infrahepatic IVC is simply oversewn. The recipient portal vein, if not already shunted into the recipient vena cava, can then be addressed. The arterial anastomosis involves suturing the aortic conduits onto the supraceliac aorta of the donor. For other visceral grafts, the SMV is sutured to the target outflow venous graft using fine monofilament suture. This is followed by anastomosis between the donor SMA and the aortic conduit. Once all vascular anastomoses are completed, reperfusion is undertaken by releasing the venous outflow, followed by the arterial inflow. Adequate vascular flow is then ensured.

The next phase of the transplant procedure is gastrointestinal surgery. First, target gastrointestinal sites are chosen for the proximal and distal anastomoses. The proximal jejunum is usually the proximal target, but the recipient duodenum or stomach is also possible. The latter is used for patients with poor gastric emptying or recipients of multivisceral grafts that include the stomach. Sparing as much distal colon as possible is also important, depending on the recipient length of remnant bowel. Then, once these targets are established, the remnant native gut should be resected. Anastomosis between the native bowel and the transplanted bowel is then performed. Our standard is a double-layer hand-sewn anastomosis. We also perform the distal ileocolostomy at the initial transplant surgery as well as a terminal ileostomy. This facilitates later ileostomy takedown for eligible patients.

A crucial portion of the transplant procedure is the placement of enteral access. Proper placement facilitates medication administration and postoperative enteral feeding. Both a gastrostomy and jejunostomy are required in most cases due to the high prevalence of posttransplant gastroparesis. We prefer a combined gastrojejunostomy tube rather than separate gastric and jejunal feeding tubes.

Abdominal wall closure is the last and many times most complex portion of the procedure. For a detailed discussion of this topic, the reader is referred to a publication by Carlsen et al.[30] Prior laparotomies, surgical scars, enteral feeding tubes, loss of abdominal wall domain, donor organ size mismatch, postreperfusion graft edema, as well as recipient abdominal wall edema create the surgical challenge. The foremost principle is never to close under tension. We prefer to use a polytetrafluoroethylene (PTFE) patch closure for all abdominal walls that do not easily come together. This allows for diuresis and reduction in swelling to occur over the first several postoperative days, followed by a return to the operating room for definitive closure.

As always, the primary goal is to reapproximate the fascia. To accomplish this goal, creation of an intraabdominal domain is sometimes necessary. Options available to do so include lysis of all intraabdominal adhesions, splenectomy, partial enterectomy, and partial hepatectomy. In general, if size-matched organs are obtained, these measures are not needed. Furthermore, alternative abdominal wall closure options are available. Serial PTFE patches can allow reapproximation of the fascia. A skin-only closure is an option. Particularly large defects can be managed with PTFE grafts until a granulation bed is established on the allograft. The coverage with a split-thickness skin graft may be used. Usually, rotational or free flaps are not optimal in this patient population due to concurrent illness, debilitation, and immunosuppression. Abdominal wall transplantation has been used successfully in a small number of patients.[31]

Immunosuppression

One of the most critical factors influencing the advancement of clinical ITx has certainly been the development and refinement of immunosuppressive regimens over time. Although immunosuppression plays an important role in the field of transplantation as a whole, several aspects pertaining to anatomy and physiology of the intestine illustrate why intestinal grafts in particular have proven difficult to manage, requiring delicate immunosuppressive protocols.

First, the intestine is a lymphoid-rich organ with large aggregates of leukocytes rendering it particularly immunogenic. Second, the intestine naturally contains luminal bacteria, fungi, and toxins that are potentially capable of translocating into the bloodstream, thus requiring constant immunologic surveillance by the host. This issue is of particular relevance in the setting of transplantation since injuries incurred from ischemia or rejection serve to facilitate bacterial translocation, making recipients of intestinal grafts vulnerable to infections.

Tacrolimus-based immunosuppression became the mainstay for ITx throughout the 1990s. Steroids alone or steroids with azathioprine, cyclophosphamide, or mycophenolate mofetil are often employed in various combinations with tacrolimus.[32,33] Recent data from the International Transplant Registry (ITR)[34] represent an analysis of nearly 1000 transplants performed in 61 centers worldwide. Overall 5-year graft survival rates ranged between 35% and 45% depending on the type of intestinal allograft, with rejection rates ranging between 39% and 57%.

Despite improved outcomes with tacrolimus, persistently high rejection rates and immunosuppression-related complications of neuro- and nephrotoxicity left a lot to be desired in the way of more potent, specific, and less-toxic immunosuppressive regimens.

Several new therapies have had varying degrees of success in the clinical arena when combined with tacrolimus.[35] The first of these is bone marrow augmentation, a therapy based on the rationale that infusion of large numbers of donor lymphoid cells simultaneously with transplantation of solid organs would induce peripheral immune tolerance and an anergic state. Initially pioneered at the Universities of Miami and Pittsburgh,[32,36] this modality has not reduced rejection or eliminated the need for immunosuppression, showing only minimal benefit in nonvisceral organs.[32,36,37] Donor-derived bone marrow augmentation has thus lost momentum in favor of other therapies.

The second significant modification emerged with the introduction of interleukin-2 receptor antagonists (IL-2RAs) such as basiliximab (Simulect, Novartis Pharmaceutical Corporation, East Hanover, NJ) or daclizumab (Zenapax, Roche Pharmaceuticals, Nutley, NJ). Protocols using these agents have been used at the Universities of Pittsburgh, Miami, and Nebraska and the University of California at Los Angeles (UCLA).[38–41] The use of IL-2RA reduced the incidence of rejection significantly without increasing the incidence of infection. Furthermore, survival and renal function were improved by allowing the administration of reduced doses of nephrotoxic agents such as tacrolimus.

Rabbit antithymocyte thymoglobulin (ATG; Thymoglobulin, Sangstat Medical Corporation, Freemont, CA) has been introduced as an induction agent after ITx and was used initially at the University of Pittsburgh.[42,43] Protocols entail the use of high-dose Thymoglobulin and tacrolimus monotherapy with or without ex vivo allograft irradiation combined with posttransplant infusion of donor-specific bone marrow. Early results in a cohort of about 90 ITx recipients had patient and graft survival of 92% and 89%, respectively.[43] These findings are supported by data generated from the ITR (Fig. 86.4).[24]

Other agents such as sirolimus (Rapamune, Wyeth-Ayerst, Philadelphia, PA), an agent that impairs lymphocyte activation,[44] and alemtuzumab (Campath-1H, Berlex Laboratories, Montville, NJ), a monoclonal antibody against panlymphocyte marker CD52,[45] have also been introduced to the clinical arena, with mixed results. Longer follow-up times and adequate assessment of drug-related complications are needed to

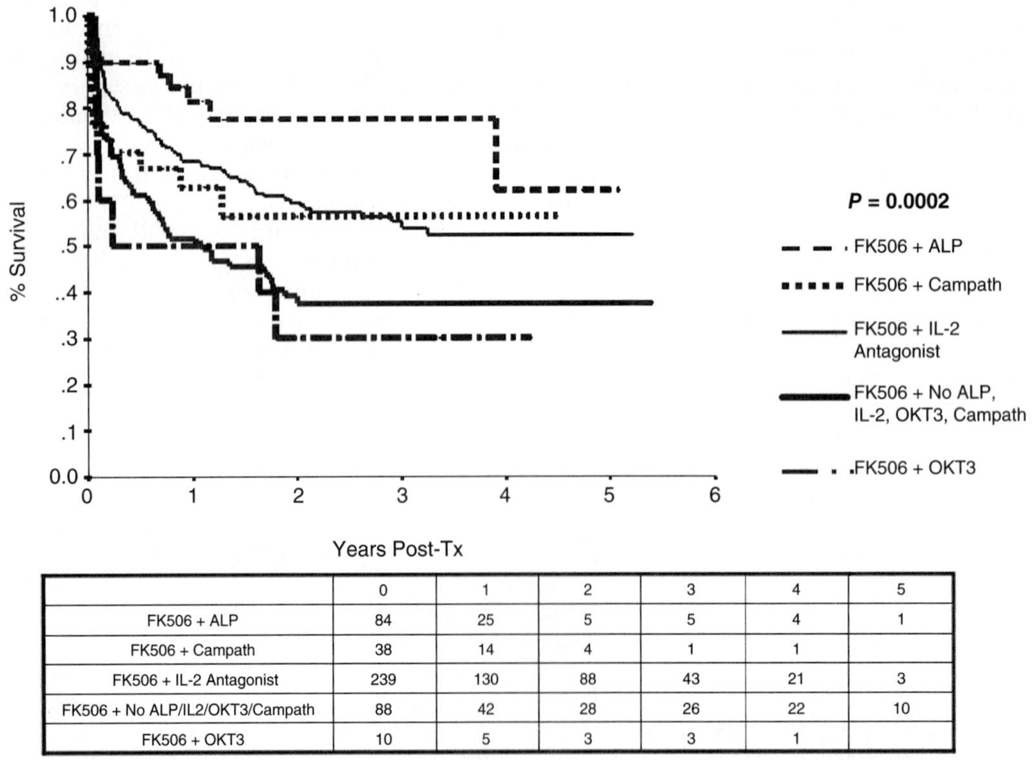

	0	1	2	3	4	5
FK506 + ALP	84	25	5	5	4	1
FK506 + Campath	38	14	4	1	1	
FK506 + IL-2 Antagonist	239	130	88	43	21	3
FK506 + No ALP/IL2/OKT3/Campath	88	42	28	26	22	10
FK506 + OKT3	10	5	3	3	1	

ALP, anti-lymphocyte product; campath, alemtuzumab; FK506, tacrolimus; OKT3, muromonab-CD3.

FIGURE 86.4. Graft survival after intestinal transplantation for transplants performed between 1998 and 2003 based on type of maintenance immunosuppression used. Survival curve is shown as (%) survival on *y*-axis and year after intestinal transplant on *x*-axis. (From ITR.[24])

assess the true clinical applicability of these agents. It is clear, however, that newer, more refined immunosuppressive agents are already having a positive impact on ITx.

Outcomes

There is clear evidence indicating that significant progress has been made in the way of improving the survival of ITx recipients, especially in recent years. Table 86.2[16,29,32,46–54] represents an analysis of patient survival data sets from most major available data sources. Overall 1- and 5-year survival rates range between 40% and 88% and between 38% and 60%, respectively, with the most recent reports demonstrating the highest rates of patient survival. Furthermore, isolated intestinal grafts are reported to have the highest early survival rates.

Similarly, Table 86.3[16,29,32,46–54] represents single-center and worldwide 1- and 5-year overall graft survival ranging between 37% and 78% and between 34% and 54%, respectively. Highest rates of graft survival were more likely to be reported in more recent series. However, follow-up is short in most series.

Several factors have had an impact on the improvement in both patient and graft outcomes. The standardization of surgical techniques and postoperative care go hand in hand with the experience of the transplant team/center. The ITR data have shown that statistically significant improved outcomes are seen in transplant centers that have performed more than 10 intestinal-type transplants. Earlier referral for transplantation has clearly had a significant impact on improving outcomes. This pattern is probably reflected in the pretransplant location of a recipient. In examining ITR data, the number of patients home at time of transplant was 73% among patients transplanted since 2001, compared to 55% across all registered transplants. In this same data set, statistical analysis of outcomes indicated that survival was significantly better in nonhospitalized patients (Fig. 86.5).[24] The correlation of these data with improved outcomes should come as no surprise since patients who are in better medical condition have tended to fare better postoperatively in other solid organ transplants as well. Other factors con-

TABLE 86.2.
Patient Survival.

Reference	*Center*	*Year*	*N*	*1 yr (%)*	*3 yr (%)*	*5 yr (%)*	*Comment*
46	ITR	1996	69	83	40	—	SBT
46	ITR	1996	83	66	40	—	LSBT
46	ITR	1996	28	59	43	—	MVT
47	ITR	1999	113	68	48	43	SBT
47	ITR	1999	130	61	40	40	LSBT
47	ITR	1999	30	43	40	38	MVT
47	ITR	1999	—	64	—	—	SBT 1995–1997
47	ITR	1999	—	64	—	—	LSBT 1995–1997
47	ITR	1999	—	64	—	—	MVT 1995–1997
29	USA	2004	77	62–83	33–80	51–60	Pediatric
48	Paris	2002	39 GFT/36 PT	77	77	—	Pediatric
49	Mt Sinai	2002	37 GFT/34 PT	74	—	—	Total
49	Mt Sinai	2002	14	87	—	—	SBT
49	Mt Sinai	2002	20	63	—	—	MVT
50	Mt Sinai	2003	28 GFT/26 PT	88	88	—	SBT
51	UCLA	2001	21 GFT/17 PT	63	55	—	Total
52	UCLA	2004	37 GFT/33 PT	77	—	52	Total
53	Miami	2002	16	84	—	—	SBT 1997–2002
53	Miami	2002	28	40	—	—	LSBT all
53	Miami	2002	40	48	—	—	MVT all
53	Miami	2005	124 GFT/108 PT	59	—	41	Pediatric
32	Pittsburgh	1998	104 GFT/98 PT	72	—	48	Total
54	Pittsburgh	2001	165 GFT/155 PT	75	—	54	Total
54	Pittsburgh	2001	93	78	—	63	>1994
16	Pittsburgh	2002	89 GFT/84 PT	74	59	56	Pediatric
16	Pittsburgh	2002	50	77	68	64	Pediatric >1994

The patient survival reported in the data sources analyzed is shown.

GFT, intestinal transplant graft; ITR, Intestinal Transplant Registry; LSBT, combined liver-small bowel transplants; MVT, multivisceral transplants; N, patient number; PT, patient; REF, reference number; SBT, isolated small bowel transplants.

TABLE 86.3.
Graft Survival.

Reference	*Center*	*Year*	*N*	*1 yr (%)*	*3 yr (%)*	*5 yr (%)*	*Comment*
46	ITR	1996	69	60	30	—	SBT
46	ITR	1996	83	60	40	—	LSBT
46	ITR	1996	28	52	40	—	MVT
47	ITR	1999	—	50	—	—	SBT 1995–1997
47	ITR	1999	—	62	—	—	LSBT 1995–1997
47	ITR	1999	—	62	—	—	MVT 1995–1997
29	USA	2004	77	56.5–77	31–73	41–54	Pediatric
48	Paris	2002	39 GFT/36 PT	46	31	—	Pediatric
49	Mt Sinai	2002	37 GFT/34 PT	64	—	—	Total
49	Mt Sinai	2002	16	73	—	—	SBT
49	Mt Sinai	2002	21	58	—	—	MVT
50	Mt Sinai	2003	28 GFT/26 PT	78	71	—	SBT
51	UCLA	2001	21 GFT/17 PT	73	55	—	Total
52	UCLA	2004	37 GFT/33 PT	64	—	34	Total
53	Miami	2002	16	72	—	—	SBT 1997–2002
53	Miami	2002	28	37	—	—	LSBT
53	Miami	2002	40	40	—	—	MVT
32	Pittsburgh	1998	104 GFT/98 PT	64	—	40	Total
54	Pittsburgh	2001	165 GFT/155 PT	65	—	45	Total
16	Pittsburgh	2002	89 GFT/84 PT	67	53	47	Pediatric

The graft survival reported in the data sources analyzed is shown.

GFT, intestinal transplant graft; ITR, Intestinal Transplant Registry; LSBT, combined liver-small bowel transplants; MVT, multivisceral transplants; N, patient number; PT, patient; SBT, isolated small bowel transplants.

tributing to improved outcomes include a reduction in rejection rates and infection rates, both related to refined immunotherapy as discussed below. Finally, adjustments in MELD (model for end-stage liver disease) and pediatric end-stage liver disease (PELD) scores for candidates awaiting combined liver-small bowel grafts are yet to be adequately evaluated but may also further improve outcomes.

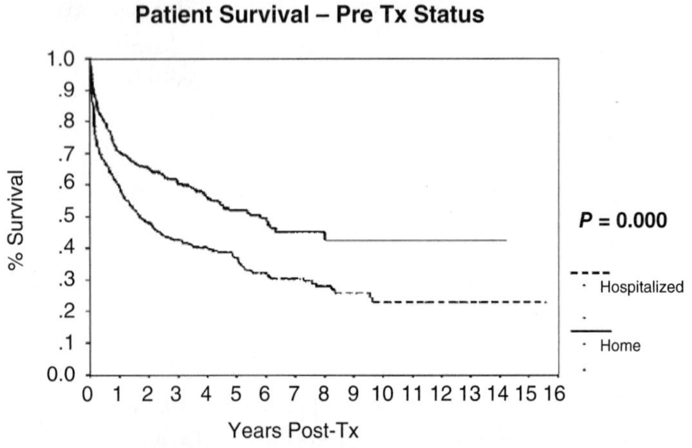

	0	1	2	3	4	5	6	7	8	9	10	11	12
Hospitalized	437	230	173	129	110	81	56	39	29	20	15	9	5
Home	541	302	209	152	108	76	48	23	17	9	4	1	1

FIGURE 86.5. Patient survival based on pre-SBTx (pre-small bowel transplant) status. Patients hospitalized prior to transplantation are denoted by the *dotted line*, while the *solid line* represents patients who came from home at time of transplantation. There is a marked improvement in survival seen in the patient population whose health allowed them to wait at home until the time of transplantation. (From Intestinal Transplant Registry, www.intestinaltransplant.org.)

Risk Factors

The most common causes of patient death posttransplantation are listed in Table 86.4.[24] Sepsis is the most common cause of post-ITx patient mortality, while rejection remains the most common cause of graft loss.

TABLE 86.4. Causes of Death.

Lymphoma	27
Rejection	49
Sepsis	202
Multisystemic organ failure	11
Other	27
Renal failure	5
Technical	27
Respiratory causes	29
Cardiac	14
Cerebral	15
Thrombosis/ischemia/bleeding	14
Hepatitis C	2
Liver failure	10
Pancreatitis	3
Total	435

Source: From Intestinal Transplant Registry, www.intestinaltransplant.org.

Rejection

Although the arrival of newer immunosuppressive therapies to the clinical arena has decreased the severity and overall incidence of rejection, it remains the primary cause of graft failure, resulting in removal of 56% of all transplanted grafts.[24] Of ITx patient mortality, 11% is also attributed to rejection.[24] The ITR results from 1997 revealed that rejection occurred in 73% of patients, with some data sources reporting acute rejection rates as high as 93%. Overall, rejection rates continue to improve with the introduction of novel immunosuppressive regimens such as ATGs,[35] induction interleukin-2 receptor antagonists,[41] and alemtuzumab,[55] reducing rejection rates to levels between 19% and 44%.

Detection of ITx rejection is complicated by the lack of specific symptoms or serum markers. Instead, vague constitutional symptoms such as fevers, changes in gastrointestinal outputs, nausea, vomiting, or abdominal pain are relied on to help diagnose acute rejection. Serum markers such as intestinal fatty acid-binding protein,[56] citruline,[57,58] and granzyme b[59] have shown little clinical utility in reliably diagnosing rejection mainly due to the lack of specificity for intestinal rejection.

Endoscopy with biopsy is the gold standard for diagnosis of rejection in ITx patients, and biopsies at intervals according to protocol are the norm in most centers to enable rejection detection. Newer modalities such as the zoom videoendoscopy and capsule endoscopy showed promise in small groups of nonrandomized patients to help diagnose rejection. Acute rejection is classified by standards set forth at the Eighth International Small Bowel Transplant Symposium.[60]

Chronic rejection is an entity reported more often now that patients are surviving longer after ITx. The most common presenting symptoms are again vague constitutional symptoms—fatigue, weight loss, and diarrhea. Not surprisingly, ITx recipients are probably at higher risk for chronic rejection due to the susceptibility of the intestine to ischemia and reperfusion injury, the common occurrence of acute rejection episodes, and the common occurrence of cytomegalovirus (CMV) infections. Accurate diagnosis of chronic rejection remains elusive, however, resulting in its underdiagnosis in ITx recipients and making it difficult to assess its prevalence in the ITx patient population. Likewise, antibody-mediated vascular rejection is probably underdiagnosed and reported in the literature.

Treatment of both acute and chronic rejection depends on the severity of the episode and the condition of the patient. Most episodes are addressed with increases in immunosuppression. The most common first-line treatment is pulse steroids. More severe episodes or steroid-refractory episodes are generally treated with antibody therapy, such as OKT3 or ATG. Enterectomy may be required for severe cases or cases that do not respond to conventional immunotherapy.

Infectious Complications

Sepsis continues to be the primary cause of patient mortality among ITx recipients, accounting for approximately 50% of overall mortality.[24] Sepsis is also the culprit, resulting in 6.6% of total graft loss.[24] The spectrum of infection includes line sepsis, wound infection, intraabdominal abscesses, pneumonia, urinary tract infection, and sepsis during rejection.[61] Although present in most other solid organ transplants, infection is a particularly formidable cause of morbidity and mortality in ITx for several reasons. Rejection increases the risk of infection by facilitating microbial translocation. The transplant operation is lengthy, involving gastrointestinal procedures, thus increasing the likelihood of infection. Furthermore, most intestinal transplant recipients have suffered multiple episodes of infection prior to their transplant and therefore are more likely to harbor resistant organisms that are difficult to treat. Finally, ITx recipients receive heavy doses of immunosuppression, rendering them more susceptible to infection.

More than 90% of recipients suffer an episode of bacterial infection,[62–64] with most of these episodes occurring within the first postoperative month.[64] In 50% of bacterial infections, more than one type of bacterium is isolated.[62] Aggressive measures must be pursued to investigate and treat infections as early as possible to avoid the deleterious sequelae of sepsis and rejection that often ensue. In a study by Sigurdsson et al., 74 of 107 episodes of bacteremia correlated with ongoing rejection identified by histology.[65] Bacteremia should therefore prompt biopsy surveillance of the intestinal allograft to ensure that rejection is not present as both are associated entities.

Infectious enteritis is an entity unique to ITx recipients and frequently implicated as a cause of graft loss. These infections may mimic rejection in their presentation and may be mistreated as rejection. Furthermore, infectious enteritis may precipitate rejection and subsequent graft loss. Adenovirus, CMV, cryptosporidium, *Giardia lamblia*, and *Clostridium difficile* have been seen in cases of infectious enteritis.[66]

Cytomegalovirus/Epstein-Barr Virus

Cytomegalovirus and Epstein-Barr virus (EBV) infections/disease are a major problem after ITx. As common pathogens of both the liver and intestine, CMV and EBV can cause significant morbidity and mortality in the immunosuppressed patient, manifesting as tissue-invasive disease in the case of CMV or causing subsequent posttransplant lymphoproliferative disease (PTLD)[67] in the case of EBV. Infection rates have been reported as high as 36% in some reports.[68,69]

This has prompted the development of an aggressive prophylactic regimen aimed at reducing the incidence of CMV and EBV disease and their sequelae. At UCLA, intravenous ganciclovir (Cytovene, Roche Pharmaceuticals) prophylaxis is administered for 100 days after ITx, followed by conversion to oral acyclovir.[70] Vigilant surveillance of blood for viral DNA or early antigens is employed. Patients who test positive for viral DNA receive preemptive treatment with intravenous ganciclovir or CMV immune globulin (Cytogam, Medimmune Pharmaceuticals, Gaithersburg, MD). This protocol has been instrumental in significantly reducing the incidence of tissue-invasive CMV infection and PTLD in our cohort of ITx recipients.

Nutritional Autonomy

Perhaps one of the most important measures of the success of ITx is nutritional autonomy. Unfortunately, there has been little consistency between centers in the methodology used to assess the degree of nutritional autonomy and patient growth. Furthermore, TPN independence has not been consistently reported, making it difficult to draw reliable conclusions in this regard. Most data sources report rates of nutritional autonomy ranging from 77% to 95% (Table 86.5).[16,24,32,46–48,50,51,54] That is, this percentage of patients comes off TPN after ITx. Unanswered questions remain regarding length of time off TPN and patient growth and nutritional status off TPN.

The UCLA nutritional experience after ITx has been similarly successful. Enteral tube feeds have been initiated an average of 9.6 ± 4.3 days after ITx. Independence from TPN occurred an average of 34 days after ITx and was achieved in 81.3% of patients surviving more than 30 days after ITx.[51,52]

Few studies examined other nutritional parameters after ITx, and most have focused on small series in the pediatric population. At the University of Pittsburgh, reports addressing post-ITx nutrition in children showed improved serum and anthropometric indices.[71] Insulin-like growth factor 1 and insulin-like growth factor-binding protein 3 have also been noted to normalize in ITx recipients.[72] In a questionnaire administered by Sudan et al.[73] surveying nutritional outcome 1 year after ITx, 35% required a period of supplemental parenteral nutrition after achieving nutritional autonomy. Examination of Z scores for growth and weight by Iyer et al.[74] showed continued linear growth retardation up to 2 years after ITx, without evidence of catch-up growth. As ITx recipients suffer from severe pre-ITx growth failure and postoperative complications and receive postoperative immunosuppression, it is therefore not surprising that they do not exhibit impressive adequate catch-up growth, particularly in these early, limited studies. As efforts continue to minimize wait-list times and postoperative complications, the degree of nutritional autonomy is likely to improve as well. Clearly, nutritional outcomes need to be evaluated further in larger series using standardized parameters.

TABLE 86.5.
Nutritional Autonomy.

Reference	*Center*	*Year*	*N*	*Total (%)*
46	ITR	1996	180 GFT/170 PT	78
47	ITR	1999	273 GFT/260 PT	77
24	ITR	2003	989 GFT/923 PT	80
48	Paris	2002	39 GFT/36 PT	95
51	UCLA	2001	16	81
50	Mt Sinai	2003	28 GFT/26 PT	81
32	Pittsburgh	1998	104 GFT/98 PT	91
54	Pittsburgh	2001	76 PT	93
16	Pittsburgh	2002	89 GFT/84 PT	87

The rates of parenteral nutrition independence after intestinal transplantation as defined by cessation of parenteral nutrition in the data sources analyzed are shown.

GFT, intestinal transplant graft; ITR, Intestinal Transplant Registry; N, patient number; PT, patient.

Quality of Life

The severity of underlying illness in patients undergoing ITx is a major confounding factor[75] when determining their QOL. This has made it difficult to assess the QOL of ITx recipients compared to patients who are maintained on TPN. As a result, reports on the QOL of ITx recipients have been scarce, with few patients reported in each series. Perhaps one of the more reliable and direct measures of QOL is hospital length of stay. Although length of stay decreased slightly in the era from 1998 to 2001, it remains long, ranging from 39.9 ± 32.9 to 84.4 ± 60.9 days.[54] The type of graft appears to play a role in the length of stay; according to ITR data, isolated intestinal transplants have the shortest length of stay, while multivisceral graft recipients have the longest.[24]

These reports give a fragmented picture of the QOL after ITx, however. More comprehensive studies are needed that would correct for confounders such as rehospitalizations, clinic visits, ostomy care, and other factors to adequately ascertain the QOL of ITx recipients compared to those with other solid organ transplants and patients maintained on TPN.

Conclusion

Clearly, ITx has evolved from an experimental entity to an efficacious life-saving clinical procedure. With the refinement of immunosuppressive therapies, aggressive treatment of infections such as CMV and EBV, and standardization of surgical approaches, patient and graft outcomes continue to improve. As perioperative morbidity and mortality are reduced, increasing numbers of ITx will be performed. Finally, larger cohorts of ITx recipients will allow for more accurate determination of important parameters such as nutritional independence and QOL.

References

1. Lillehei RC, Goott B, Miller FA. The physiological response of the small bowel of the dog to ischemia including prolonged in vitro preservation of the bowel with successful replacement and survival. Ann Surg 1959;150:543–560.
2. Starzl TE, Kaupp HA Jr, Brock DR, et al. Homotransplantation of multiple visceral organs. Am J Surg 1962;103:219–229.
3. Fishbein TM, Gondolesi GE, Kaufman SS. Intestinal transplantation for gut failure. Gastroenterology 2003;124:1615–1628.
4. Langnas AN. Advances in small-intestine transplantation. Transplantation 2004;77(9 suppl):S75–S78.
5. Dudrick SJ, Wilmore DW, Vars HM, Rhoads JE. Long-term total parenteral nutrition with growth, development, and positive nitrogen balance. Surgery 1968;64:134–142.
6. Broviac JW, Scribner BH. Prolonged parenteral nutrition in the home. Surg Gynecol Obstet 1974;139:24–28.
7. Calne RY, Rolles K, White DJ, et al. Cyclosporin A initially as the only immunosuppressant in 34 recipients of cadaveric organs: 32 kidneys, 2 pancreases, and 2 livers. Lancet 1979;2:1033–1036.
8. Grant D, Wall W, Mimeault R, et al. Successful small-bowel/liver transplantation. Lancet 1990;335:181–184.
9. Starzl TE, Rowe MI, Todo S, et al. Transplantation of multiple abdominal viscera. JAMA 1989;261:1449–1457.

10. Williams JW, Sankary HN, Foster PF, et al. Splanchnic transplantation. An approach to the infant dependent on parenteral nutrition who develops irreversible liver disease. JAMA 1989;261:1458–1462.
11. Goulet O, Jan D, Sarnacki S, et al. Isolated and combined liver-small bowel transplantation in Paris: 1987–1995. Transplant Proc 1996;28:2750.
12. Deltz E, Schroeder P, Gundlach M, et al. Successful clinical small-bowel transplantation. Transplant Proc 1990;22:2501.
13. Abu-Elmagd K, Bond G, Reyes J, Fung J. Intestinal transplantation: a coming of age. Adv Surg 2002;36:65–101.
14. Grant D, Abu-Elmagd K, Reyes J, et al. 2003 report of the intestine transplant registry: a new era has dawned. Ann Surg 2005;241:607–613.
15. Kaufman SS, Atkinson JB, Bianchi A, et al. Indications for pediatric intestinal transplantation: a position paper of the American Society of Transplantation. Pediatr Transplant 2001;5:80–87.
16. Reyes J, Mazariegos GV, Bond GM, et al. Pediatric intestinal transplantation: historical notes, principles and controversies. Pediatr Transplant 2002;6:193–207.
17. Sudan DL, Kaufman SS, Shaw BW Jr, et al. Isolated intestinal transplantation for intestinal failure. Am J Gastroenterol 2000;95:1506–1515.
18. Messing B, Crenn P, Beau P, et al. Long-term survival and parenteral nutrition dependence in adult patients with the short bowel syndrome. Gastroenterology 1999;117:1043–1050.
19. Dorney SF, Ament ME, Berquist WE, et al. Improved survival in very short small bowel of infancy with use of long-term parenteral nutrition. J Pediatr 1985;107:521–525.
20. Fryer J, Pellar S, Ormond D, et al. Mortality in candidates waiting for combined liver-intestine transplants exceeds that for other candidates waiting for liver transplants. Liver Transpl 2003;9:748–753.
21. Horslen S. Organ allocation for liver-intestine candidates. Liver Transpl 2004;10(10 suppl 2):S86–S89.
22. McDiarmid SV, Anand R, Lindblad AS. Development of a pediatric end-stage liver disease score to predict poor outcome in children awaiting liver transplantation. Transplantation 2002;74:173–181.
23. de Ville de Goyet J, Mitchell A, Mayer AD, et al. En block combined reduced-liver and small bowel transplants: from large donors to small children. Transplantation 2000;69:555–559.
24. The Intestinal Transplant Registry, http://www.intestinal transplant.org/, Current Results, Intestinal Transplant Registry Final Summary 2003. Accessed 2006.
25. Kato T, Ruiz P, Thompson JF, et al. Intestinal and multivisceral transplantation. World J Surg 2002;26:226–237.
26. Sudan DL, Iyer KR, Deroover A, et al. A new technique for combined liver/small intestinal transplantation. Transplantation 2001;72:1846–1848.
27. Abu-Elmagd K, Bond G, Reyes J, Fung J. Intestinal Transplantation: Coming of Age, Vol. 36. Mosby; 2002.
28. Horslen SP, Sudan DL, Iyer KR, et al. Isolated liver transplantation in infants with end-stage liver disease associated with short bowel syndrome. Ann Surg 2002;235:435–439.
29. U.S. Department of Human Services, Health Resources and Services Administration's Division of Transplantation 2006 OPTN/SRTR Annual Report: Transplant Data 1996–2005, http://www.optn.org/AR2006/survival_rates.htm Survival Rate Data Tables. Accessed 2006.
30. Carlsen BT, Farmer DG, Busuttil RW, Miller TA, Rudkin GH. Incidence and management of abdominal wall defects after intestinal and multivisceral transplantation. Plast Reconstr Surg 2007;119:1247–1255; discussion 1256–1258.
31. Tzakis AG, Tryphonopoulos P, Kato T, et al. Intestinal transplantation: advances in immunosuppression and surgical techniques. Transplant Proc 2003;35:1925–1926.
32. Abu-Elmagd K, Reyes J, Todo S, et al. Clinical intestinal transplantation: new perspectives and immunologic considerations. J Am Coll Surg 1998;186:512–525; discussion 525–527.
33. Tzakis AG, Nery JR, Thompson J, et al. New immunosuppressive regimens in clinical intestinal transplantation. Transplant Proc 1997;29:683–685.
34. Grant D. Oral presentation, Eighth International Small Bowel Transplant Symposium; September 23, 2003; Miami, FL.
35. Farmer DG. Clinical immunosuppression for intestinal transplantation. Curr Opin Organ Transplant 2004;9:214–219.
36. Ricordi C, Karatzas T, Nery J, et al. High-dose donor bone marrow infusions to enhance allograft survival: the effect of timing. Transplantation 1997;63:7–11.
37. Salgar SK, Shapiro R, Dodson F, et al. Infusion of donor leukocytes to induce tolerance in organ allograft recipients. J Leukoc Biol 1999;66:310–314.
38. Abu-Elmagd K, Fung J, McGhee W, et al. The efficacy of daclizumab for intestinal transplantation: preliminary report. Transplant Proc 2000;32:1195–1196.
39. Carreno MR, Kato T, Weppler D, et al. Induction therapy with daclizumab as part of the immunosuppressive regimen in human small bowel and multiorgan transplants. Transplant Proc 2001;33:1015–1017.
40. Sudan DL, Chinnakotla S, Horslen S, et al. Basiliximab decreases the incidence of acute rejection after intestinal transplantation. Transplant Proc 2002;34:940–941.
41. Farmer DG, McDiarmid SV, Edelstein S, et al. Induction therapy with interleukin-2 receptor antagonist after intestinal transplantation is associated with reduced acute cellular rejection and improved renal function. Transplant Proc 2004;36:331–332.
42. Gaber AO, First MR, Tesi RJ, et al. Results of the double-blind, randomized, multicenter, phase III clinical trial of Thymoglobulin versus Atgam in the treatment of acute graft rejection episodes after renal transplantation. Transplantation 1998;66:29–37.
43. Starzl TE, Murase N, Abu-Elmagd K, et al. Tolerogenic immunosuppression for organ transplantation. Lancet 2003;361:1502–1510.
44. Fung J, Marcos A. Rapamycin: friend, foe, or misunderstood? Liver Transpl 2003;9:469–472.
45. Calne R, Friend P, Moffatt S, et al. Prope tolerance, perioperative campath 1H, and low-dose cyclosporin monotherapy in renal allograft recipients. Lancet 1998;351:1701–1702.
46. Grant D. Current results of intestinal transplantation. The International Intestinal Transplant Registry. Lancet 1996;347:1801–1803.
47. Grant D. Intestinal transplantation: 1997 report of the international registry. Intestinal Transplant Registry. Transplantation 1999;67:1061–1064.
48. Goulet O, Lacaille F, Colomb V, et al. Intestinal transplantation in children: Paris experience. Transplant Proc 2002;34:1887–1888.
49. Fishbein T, Kaufman S, Schiano T, et al. Intestinal and multiorgan transplantation: the Mount Sinai experience. Transplant Proc 2002;34:891–892.
50. Fishbein TM, Kaufman SS, Florman SS, et al. Isolated intestinal transplantation: proof of clinical efficacy. Transplantation 2003;76:636–640.
51. Farmer DG, McDiarmid SV, Yersiz H, et al. Outcome after intestinal transplantation: results from one center's 9-year experience. Arch Surg 2001;136:1027–1031; discussion 1031–1032.
52. Farmer DG, McDiarmid SV, Edelstein S, et al. Improved outcome after intestinal transplantation at a single institution over 12 years. Transplant Proc 2004;36:303–304.
53. Kato T, Gaynor JJ, Selvaggi G, et al. Intestinal transplantation in children: a summary of clinical outcomes and prognostic

factors in 108 patients from a single center. J Gastrointest Surg 2005;9:75–89; discussion 89.
54. Abu-Elmagd K, Reyes J, Bond G, et al. Clinical intestinal transplantation: a decade of experience at a single center. Ann Surg 2001;234:404–416; discussion 416–417.
55. Garcia M, Weppler D, Mittal N, et al. Campath-1H immunosuppressive therapy reduces incidence and intensity of acute rejection in intestinal and multivisceral transplantation. Transplant Proc 2004;36:323–324.
56. Kaufman SS, Lyden ER, Marks WH, et al. Lack of utility of intestinal fatty acid binding protein levels in predicting intestinal allograft rejection. Transplantation 2001;71:1058–1060.
57. Gondolesi G, Fishbein T, Chehade M, et al. Serum citrulline is a potential marker for rejection of intestinal allografts. Transplant Proc 2002;34:918–920.
58. Pappas PA, Saudubray JM, Tzakis AG, et al. Serum citrulline as a marker of acute cellular rejection for intestinal transplantation. Transplant Proc 2002;34:915–917.
59. McDiarmid SV, Farmer DG, Kuniyoshi JS, et al. Perforin and granzyme B. Cytolytic proteins up-regulated during rejection of rat small intestine allografts. Transplantation 1995;59:762–766.
60. Ruiz P, Bagni A, Brown R, et al. Histological criteria for the identification of acute cellular rejection in human small bowel allografts: results of the pathology workshop at the Eighth International Small Bowel Transplant Symposium. Transplant Proc 2004;36:335–337.
61. Nishida S, Levi D, Kato T, et al. Ninety-five cases of intestinal transplantation at the University of Miami. J Gastrointest Surg 2002;6:233–239.
62. Loinaz C, Kato T, Nishida S, et al. Bacterial infections after intestine and multivisceral transplantation. Transplant Proc 2003;35:1929–1930.
63. Langnas A, Chinnakotla S, Sudan D, et al. Intestinal transplantation at the University of Nebraska Medical Center: 1990 to 2001. Transplant Proc 2002;34:958–960.
64. Guaraldi G, Cocchi S, De Ruvo N, et al. Outcome, incidence, and timing of infections in small bowel/multivisceral transplantation. Transplant Proc 2004;36:383–385.
65. Sigurdsson L, Reyes J, Kocoshis SA, et al. Bacteremia after intestinal transplantation in children correlates temporally with rejection or gastrointestinal lymphoproliferative disease. Transplantation 2000;70:302–305.
66. Ziring D, Tran R, Edelstein S, et al. Infectious enteritis after intestinal transplantation: incidence, timing, and outcome. Transplantation 2005;79:702–709.
67. Kocoshis SA. Small bowel transplantation in infants and children. Gastroenterol Clin North Am 1994;23:727–742.
68. Bueno J, Green M, Kocoshis S, et al. Cytomegalovirus infection after intestinal transplantation in children. Clin Infect Dis 1997;25:1078–1083.
69. Manez R, Kusne S, Green M, et al. Incidence and risk factors associated with the development of cytomegalovirus disease after intestinal transplantation. Transplantation 1995;59:1010–1014.
70. Farmer DG, McDiarmid SV, Winston D, et al. Effectiveness of aggressive prophylactic and preemptive therapies targeted against cytomegaloviral and Epstein-Barr viral disease after human intestinal transplantation. Transplant Proc 2002;34:948–949.
71. Rovera GM, Strohm S, Bueno J, et al. Nutritional monitoring of pediatric intestinal transplant recipients. Transplant Proc 1998;30:2519–2520.
72. Nucci AM, Reyes J, Yaworski JA, et al. Serum growth factors and growth indices pre- and post-pediatric intestinal transplantation. J Pediatr Surg 2003;38:1043–1047.
73. Sudan DL, Iverson A, Weseman RA, et al. Assessment of function, growth and development, and long-term quality of life after small bowel transplantation. Transplant Proc 2000;32:1211–1212.
74. Iyer K, Horslen S, Iverson A, et al. Nutritional outcome and growth of children after intestinal transplantation. J Pediatr Surg 2002;37:464–466.
75. Cameron EA, Binnie JA, Jamieson NV, et al. Quality of life in adults following small bowel transplantation. Transplant Proc 2002;34:965–966.

87

Lung Transplantation

Christine L. Lau, G. Alexander Patterson, and R. Duane Davis

The first successful human lung transplant was performed in 1983 by the Toronto Lung Transplant Group.[1] More than two decades have passed since this landmark procedure, and in the interim over 17,000 lung transplants have been performed.[2] Lung transplantation currently is the preferred treatment option for a variety of end-stage pulmonary diseases. Remarkable progress has occurred through refinement in technique and improved understanding of transplant immunology and microbiology. The 1-, 3-, 5-, and 10-year actuarial survival rates for all lung transplants are 74%, 58%, 47%, and 24%, respectively.[2] Despite these improvements, donor shortages and chronic lung allograft rejection continue to plague the field and prevent it from reaching its full potential. Chronic rejection of the lung allograft is currently the major hurdle limiting long-term survival. To date, prevention of known risk factors and treatment strategies have not lessened the devastating toll this process has on lung transplant survival.

Historical Aspects

Dr. James D. Hardy performed the first human lung transplantation more than four decades ago.[3] The patient was a 58-year-old male prisoner with lung cancer, and the donor was a male who had died from a massive myocardial infarction. Notably, the recipient was blood group A, yet the donor was blood group B. Succumbing to renal failure, the recipient survived 18 days. Over the next 20 years, approximately 40 lung transplants were attempted, with none achieving long-term success.[4]

The Toronto Lung Transplant Group's initial attempt at lung transplantation was in 1978, ending with the patient dying following bronchial dehiscence.[5] Based on this patient and the poor results of other lung transplants reported, this group began experimental studies into the causes of lung transplant failure. Through these investigations, they discovered that perioperative steroid usage contributed significantly to poor bronchial anastomotic healing.[6] Wrapping an omental pedicle around the bronchus resulted in restoration of blood supply and protection from dehiscence.[7] In addition, recognizing that most of the early attempts had been in acutely ill, often ventilator-dependent, patients, recipient selection issues were addressed. On November 7, 1983, the first successful isolated lung transplant was performed in a 58-year-old man with pulmonary fibrosis.[1] This patient eventually returned to work. In subsequent analysis, it appears to be the use of cyclosporine and the attention to detail that this group practiced that led to long-term transplant success. The use of the omental flap and the concept of withholding steroids perioperatively have now been largely abandoned.

Following this success, Patterson and colleagues expanded the use of lung transplantation with the en bloc double-lung transplant technique.[8] As for the single-lung technique, this procedure was initially perfected in the laboratory prior to attempts in humans.[9] The en bloc double-lung transplant, however, had several drawbacks: It was technically difficult, requiring cardiopulmonary bypass; tracheal anastomotic ischemic complications occurred frequently; cardiac denervation occurred; and bleeding into the posterior mediastinum was common because of poor operative exposure. In an effort to avoid these problems, Pasque and colleagues[10] devised the technique of bilateral sequential pulmonary transplantation, which is still in use.

Recipient Selection

International guidelines for selection of lung transplant candidates have been proposed.[11] As these are general guidelines (Table 87.1), they may be relaxed at times, depending on the specifics of individual cases. The presence of declining end-stage lung disease with a life expectancy of less than 24–48 months despite optimal medical therapy and the potential for improvement in survival or quality of life with transplantation are absolute criteria. Abstinence from smoking for at least 6 months is an another absolute requirement. Recipient age has been shown to be a significant predictor of adverse outcome.[12] In general, we do not transplant patients older than 65. Medical management of the patient's pulmonary disease needs to be maximized and other possible options considered (e.g., lung volume reduction surgery for patients with chronic obstructive pulmonary disease [COPD]; epoprostenol for primary pulmonary hypertension [PPH]) prior to lung transplant listing.

Potential transplant recipients should be without significant comorbid diseases. Clinically relevant coronary artery disease that cannot be revascularized, systemic vascular diseases, poorly controlled insulin-dependent diabetes mellitus, symptomatic osteoporosis, or end-stage hepatic or renal failure usually contraindicate isolated lung transplantation. The steroid requirements after transplantation can exacerbate osteoporosis[13] and insulin-dependent diabetes. In addition, attempts are made to wean steroids preoperatively in patients who require them to doses below 20 mg/day of prednisone to minimize the complications related to their use. On occasion, combined lung and liver or kidney transplants have been performed. Treatable coronary disease can be addressed and if resolved does not prevent listing for lung transplantation.

TABLE 87.1. Absolute or Relative Criteria for Recipient Selection.

End-stage pulmonary disease
Maximization of medical therapy
Functional limitations (NYHA class III or IV)
Life expectancy anticipated less than 2 years
Life expectancy and quality of life anticipated to be improved following pulmonary transplantation
Without significant comorbid diseases Symptomatic osteoporosis Severe musculoskeletal disease Other major organ dysfunction Creatinine clearance <50 mg/mL/min Coronary artery disease or left ventricular dysfunction
HIV negative/no active hepatitis B or C
Proven smoking cessation for 6 months
Without alcohol or drug addiction
Medically compliant
Single lung transplants 65 years of age or younger
Bilateral lung transplants 60 years of age or younger
Without active or recent malignancy (within 5 years) except basal/squamous skin cancers and some cases of bronchioloalveolar lung cancer
Inadequate nutrition, <70% ideal body weight
Morbid obesity >130%
Ambulatory with oxygen if required
Systemic steroids <20 mg prednisone/day
Psychosocial stability
Completion of pulmonary rehabilitation
Adequate support

Source: Data from Davis et al.[196]; McCurry et al.[197]; and Lau et al.[198]

TABLE 87.2. Studies Obtained During Lung Transplant Evaluation.

Full lung function tests
Exercise performance measured by a standardized test, such as a 6-min walk
Electrocardiogram
Echocardiogram
High-resolution computed tomography (CT) of the thorax in patients with parenchymal disease, pleural disease, or previous thoracic surgical procedures
Stress echocardiogram—such as dobutamine, dobutamine positron emission tomography, and sestamibi—or coronary angiograms in patients at high risk for coronary artery disease
A 24-h creatinine clearance
Liver function studies

Source: From Maurer et al.,[11] reprinted with permission.

Adequate nutrition is particularly important to address. Patients with an ideal body weight less than 70% or more than 130% predicted are not considered for transplantation. Patients with cystic fibrosis (CF) and COPD are particularly prone to cachexia.[14] Dietary consultation and oral supplements may suffice, but the placement of a percutaneous endoscopic gastrostomy tube for tube feedings prior to transplantation may also prove useful. Morbid obesity is most commonly seen in patients with idiopathic pulmonary fibrosis (IPF), pulmonary hypertension, and sarcoidosis. Weight reduction via a supervised diet and routine exercise to the degree possible given physiologic constraints of the disease (particularly pulmonary hypertension) are undertaken by these patients prior to transplant listing.

Noncutaneous malignancy unless longer than 5 years from diagnosis and curative treatment remains a contraindication. Prior thoracic surgery may increase the technical difficulty, with greater risk of hemorrhage and nerve injury, but is not a contraindication to lung transplantation. Active infection outside the thorax is a contraindication to transplantation.

After initial evaluation, patients with end-stage lung disease who are being considered for lung transplantation undergo extensive preoperative testing to assess their overall medical condition as well as the severity of their lung disease. The transplant evaluation consists of the tests shown in Table 87.2. Laboratory tests consisting of general blood work, blood typing, and immunologic determination of preformed antibodies against HLA antigens are done. Excluding patients with pulmonary vascular diseases, potential recipients are required to complete pulmonary rehabilitation to improve cardiac conditioning prior to transplantation. Consults with nutrition and social work are obtained, and financial issues are addressed.

Disease-Specific Guidelines

Prior to consideration for pulmonary transplantation, patients with COPD should have maximization of medical therapy, consisting of bronchodilator therapies and oxygen therapy. Consideration should be given to lung volume reduction surgery (LVRS) in ideal patients (hyperinflation, heterogeneous distribution of disease with upper lobe predominant disease, FEV_1 (forced expiratory volume in 1 s) of more than 20%, and normal Pco_2).[15] We have not found LVRS to be an ideal option in patients with α_1-antitrypsin deficiency as in general these patients have diffuse disease.[15] Preliminary LVRS does not jeopardize subsequent successful lung transplantation.[16] Generally, in patients with COPD, the FEV_1 should be significantly less than 25% predicted and not reversible, with most patients actually having an FEV_1 of less than 20% predicted at the time of transplantation. Progressive deterioration as evidence by hypercarbia ($Paco_2 \geq$ 55 mmHg), increasing oxygen requirement (resting $Pao_2 <$ 55 mmHg), the development of secondary pulmonary hypertension, rapid decline of FEV_1, or frequent life-threatening infections indicates decreased survival, suggesting the need for transplantation.[11]

Recent debate has centered on whether bilateral lung transplants are preferred to single-lung transplants in this population of patients.[17–19] According to the International Society for Heart and Lung Transplantation (ISHLT) registry, a survival advantage is seen in COPD recipients who receive bilateral versus single-lung transplants.[12] This survival benefit, however, may not extend to older, less-healthy recipients.[19] Our results have been consistent with the ISHLT data, and we have also reported improved lung function and exercise tolerance in the bilateral lung transplant patients.[17] For these reasons, when possible we prefer to perform bilateral lung transplantation of patients with COPD, particularly in patients with recurrent infections and especially patients with atypical mycobacterial organisms.

Patients with septic lung diseases (CF, bronchiectasis) presenting with $FEV_1 \leq 30\%$ predicted or rapidly progressive disease despite optimal medical management should be evaluated for potential lung transplantation. Progressive disease is indicated by an increasing number of hospitalizations, rapid decline in FEV_1, massive hemoptysis, or increasing weight loss.[11] Young female patients with CF have a tendency to do poorly, and early consideration is appropriate.[20] Evidence of hypercarbia ($Pco_2 > 50$) or hypoxemia ($Pao_2 < 55$ mmHg) indicates the need for transplant evaluation.[11] Liou and colleagues[21] have suggested that the use of a nine-parameter model to stratify pretransplant CF patients into five categories based on predicted survival (ranging from 30% to approaching 100%) would more accurately predict the group who would most benefit from lung transplantation. Bilateral transplantation is required for patients with septic lung diseases.

Patients with septic lung disease or those with significant sputum production are evaluated with frequent sputum cultures to assess bacterial sensitivities. Inhaled high-dose aminoglycosides or colistin are frequently used in this population. Patients with multidrug-resistant organisms, especially panresistant *Burkholderia cepacia*, are considered high-risk, and many centers consider this a contraindication to transplantation. Early mortality in patients with CF infected with *B. cepacia* is significantly increased.[22,23] However, the increased risk appears to be limited to primarily the genovariant III strain of *B. cepacia*, now named *B. cenocepacia*.[23] Transplant results for recipients colonized with the other genovariant strains of *B. cepacia* have results comparable to other CF recipients not infected with the organism. Successful transplantation in these patients often requires the use of multiple combinations of intravenous antibiotics using in vitro synergy testing to guide antibiotic selection. Although some centers consider the absence of a susceptible antibiotic regimen determined by synergy testing a contraindication, other centers utilize an empiric multidrug (more than five) antibiotic regimen at the time of transplantation.

Patients with IPF should be evaluated for transplantation when they become symptomatic. This disease is associated with the highest mortality while waiting for transplantation.[24] For this reason, potential recipients with pulmonary fibrosis in the United States are credited with 90 days waiting time at transplant listing.[25] Although initially helpful, this added time no longer appears to be substantial enough to significantly alter wait-list mortality. Review of histologic diagnosis is important because a minority of patients with IPF may have disease processes such as desquamative interstitial pneumonitis (DIP), which may be responsive to steroids, preventing the need for transplantation.[26] In addition to symptomatic presentation, physiologic parameters may be utilized, including a fall in vital capacity to below 60%–70% predicted or a fall in diffusion capacity to below 50%–60% predicted, as requirements for transplant evaluation. If the pulmonary fibrosis is part of a systemic disease process, the systemic symptoms should be under control and preferably in remission.[11] We prefer bilateral lung transplantation in this group, although a survival benefit has not been seen in bilateral versus single-lung transplant patients with IPF.[12,27]

Patients with pulmonary hypertension were previously considered for lung transplantation early in the course of their disease because of the poor outcome of this disease process. Recently, with the use of intravenous prostacyclin (Flolan) and other vasodilator therapies, an improvement in pulmonary artery (PA) pressures and relief of symptoms is seen in the majority of patients with PPH.[28] Transplantation may be delayed as long as patients remain clinically stable on vasodilatory therapy. For patients with pulmonary hypertension secondary to congenital heart defects or thromboembolic diseases, consideration for surgical intervention for the primary diagnosis (atrial septostomy or thromboendarterectomy) should be given. Current indication for transplantation is progressive deterioration despite optimal therapy (i.e., New York Heart Association [NYHA] class III or IV, mean PA pressure above 50, right atrial pressure above10 mmHg, cardiac index below 2.5 L/min/m^2, syncopal episodes).[11] With the widespread use of Flolan, patients with pulmonary hypertension often are in much worse medical condition with very shortened life spans by the time they require transplantation. We prefer bilateral lung transplantation in this group; however, a survival advantage with bilateral lung transplantation has not been appreciated.[12] If the patient is to undergo single-lung transplantation, we do not use a marginal donor lung as the through of the cardiac output will be through the transplanted lung. Patients with Eisenmenger's syndrome and secondary pulmonary hypertension have not shown an improvement in survival following lung transplantation.[29,30] It has been suggested that heart-lung transplantation may be preferable to isolated lung transplant in this group.[31]

Donor Selection

Despite aggressive measures, including the use of marginal donors, efforts to boost organ donations, and the use of lobar and non-heart-beating donors, there remains a critical shortage of donor lungs. Further contributing to this shortage is the estimate that only 10%–15% of multiorgan donors have lungs suitable for procurement.[32,33]

Careful donor selection is required (Table 87.3). The donor's medical history is obtained, with particular emphasis and attention paid to the donor's age, cause of death, timing of death, smoking history, and prior thoracic procedures. Older donor age (older than 60) is considered a significant risk factor for adverse outcome after pulmonary transplantation, and in general donors younger than 55 are preferred.[12] Although a significant smoking history (≥30 pack-years) in the donor is concerning, it is not an absolute contraindication to the use of otherwise suitable donor lungs. Absolute contraindications to donor lung procurement are ABO incompatibility between donor and recipient, human immunodeficiency virus (HIV) positivity, active malignancies (outside the central nervous system), and active hepatitis infections. Histocompatibility antigen (HLA) matching currently is not usually performed between donor and recipient prior to transplantation unless the patient has an elevated panel reactive antibody (PRA) or known HLA antibodies from prior sensitization.

Ideally, the donor chest radiograph should be clear. Preferably both lung fields should be free of pulmonary contusions, pneumonia, or atelectasis. The presence of a radiologic abnormality does not preclude further assessment by the harvest team, but it needs to be correlated with manual evaluation.[34] Size matching is primarily based on comparison of donor and recipient heights and sex. Donor lungs that are substantially larger than the recipient's chest cavity but are otherwise usable should not preclude transplantation. Anatomic donor upper lobectomy is easily performed on the back table. In our experience, this downsizing of donor lungs for smaller recipients can be done safely with minimal morbidity. We prefer this option to multiple wedge resections after implantation.[35]

TABLE 87.3. Criteria for Donor Lung Suitability.

Preliminary
Age <60 years
ABO compatibility
Chest roentgenogram
Clear
Allows estimate of size match
History
≤20 pack-years
No significant trauma (blunt, penetrating)
No aspiration/sepsis
Gram stain and culture data if prolonged intubation
No prior cardiac/pulmonary operation
Oxygenation
Arterial oxygen tension ≥300 mmHg on inspired oxygen fraction of 1.0, 5 cm H_2O positive end-expiratory pressure
Adequate size match
Final assessment
Chest roentgenogram shows no unfavorable changes
Oxygenation has not deteriorated
Bronchoscopy shows no aspiration or mass
Visual/manual assessment
Parenchyma satisfactory
No adhesions or masses
Further evaluation of trauma

Source: Adapted from Sundaresan et al.,[32] with permission from the Society of Thoracic Surgeons. *Ann Thorac Surg.*

Confirmation of satisfactory gas exchange, utilizing the standard gas exchange parameters of Pa_{O_2} above 300 mmHg on F_{IO_2} (fraction of inspired oxygen) of 100%, and positive end-expiratory pressure (PEEP) of 5 cm H_2O is obtained on the donor lungs. In addition, lung parameters, including mean airway pressures and compliance, are evaluated. Mean airway pressures above 30–32 mmHg with standard volume ventilation are considered a relative contraindication for lung donation unless a nonparenchymal explanation (i.e., a small endotracheal tube or morbid obesity) is evident.

Bronchoscopy is performed to assess the airways. The presence of mucopurulent secretions that are easily cleared is acceptable, but the presence of frank pus, significant airway erythema, or evidence of aspiration contraindicates the use of the lung from which these findings arise (but not necessarily the contralateral lung). Median sternotomy provides adequate exposure for thorough gross inspection of both lungs. The presence of a mass, consolidation, or significant pulmonary contusions contraindicates the use of the lungs. Recipients without pulmonary hypertension receiving bilateral sequential lung transplants may tolerate one lung that has a small contusion when the other lung is free from injury. The noninjured lung is transplanted first if possible, followed by the slightly injured lung with a low threshold for utilizing cardiopulmonary bypass.

The primary reasons that lungs from a multiorgan donor are not suitable for transplantation are pulmonary contusions, pulmonary sepsis, and pulmonary edema.[36] Various techniques have been suggested to increase the recoverability of donor lungs, including use of high-dose steroids early during the management of brain dead patients, maximization of pulmonary toilet, and strict monitoring of ventilator support and fluid administration.[33,36,37]

Living lobar transplantation using a lobe from two separate donors has been successfully employed in CF patients and other recipients.[38,39] This strategy was pioneered by the University of Southern California (USC) program.[40] They have reported impressive results in adults and children.[41] In the USC experience, pediatric patients receiving living lobar transplants had less bronchiolitis obliterans syndrome (BOS) and better pulmonary function than pediatric recipients receiving cadaveric donor lungs; this group believes living lobar transplantation is the preferred method for children.[41] Living lobar transplant has been conducted in other centers with reasonable results. Thus far, there have been no reports of donor fatality, but a significant number of complications have been encountered.[42]

Two novel techniques to optimize donor usage have recently been introduced. The first is a split-lung technique that bipartitions the left lung of a large cadaveric donor and uses the two lobes to perform a bilateral lobar transplant in the smaller recipient.[43] It requires significant expertise in lung transplantation but has been performed successfully with good outcomes at certain institutions.[43,44] The second technique is the use of non-heart-beating donors.[45] Although non-heart-beating donors have not provided many lungs, with further modifications this technique may significantly increase the donor supply.

Xenotransplantation is one solution to overcoming the donor shortage and offers the potential of an unlimited supply. Unfortunately, advances in this area have been hindered not only by the severe immune response of the recipient but also by apparent incompatibilities between the coagulation systems of different species.[46] It has therefore remained relegated to the research realm.

Operative Procedure

Donor Harvest

The donor harvest technique has been described by Sundaresan and colleagues[32] and allows en bloc removal of the lungs and preservation of the heart, with the potential therefore of performing three separate transplants. A median sternotomy provides excellent exposure to both lungs. The pericardium is opened, and stay sutures are placed to allow exposure of the great vessels. The superior vena cava (SVC) is encircled caudal to the azygous vein with silk sutures. The inferior vena cava (IVC) is also encircled unless hemodynamic instability occurs on attempt to do so. The periadventitial tissue overlying the right PA is dissected, cleaning the plane between the artery and the SVC. The same is done to separate the right PA from the back of the ascending aorta.

The aorto-pulmonary artery window is dissected in preparation for placement of the aortic cross-clamp. The SVC and the aorta are gently retracted laterally, and the posterior pericardium is incised above the right PA, allowing access to the trachea. The plane of the trachea is manually developed, and the trachea can be encircled with an umbilical tape. Following completion of the thoracic dissection, the donor is heparinized (250–300 U/kg). The ascending aorta and main PA are then cannulated for cardioplegia and pulmonary flush. Following this, a bolus dose of prostaglandin E_1 (PGE_1) is given directly into the PA. Immediately after the PGE_1, the SVC is ligated, and the IVC is divided, allowing the right heart to decompress. The aorta is cross-clamped, and cardioplegia is initiated. The left atrial appendage is incised, decompressing the left side of the heart (Fig. 87.1). The pulmonary flush is initiated and consists of several liters (50–75 mL/kg) of Perfadex solution at 4°C. While the heart and lung preservation fluids are running, the chest cavity is cooled with ice-slush normal saline. Ventilation is continued throughout.[32]

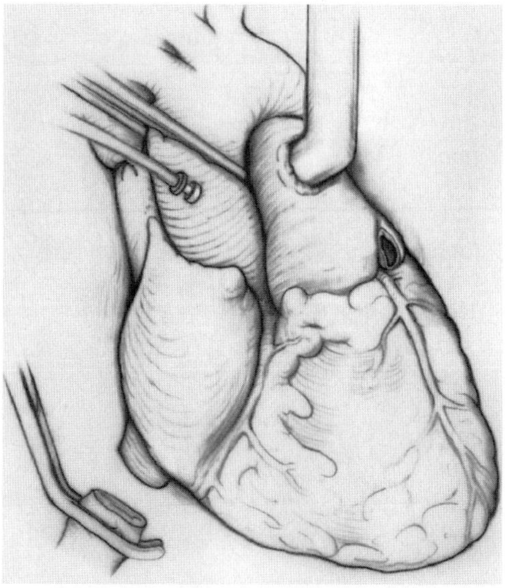

FIGURE 87.1. Drawing at time of cross-clamping showing placement of cannulas and venting of right and left side of the heart. (Reprinted from Sundaresan et al.,[32] with permission from the Society of Thoracic Surgeons.)

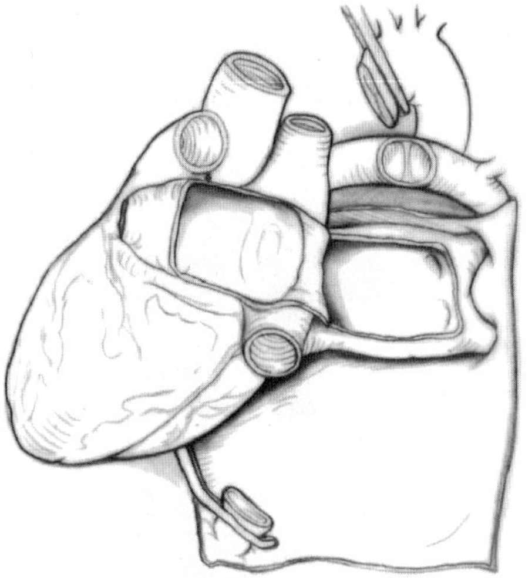

FIGURE 87.2. The heart is removed, leaving a cuff of left atrium. (Reprinted from Sundaresan et al.,[32] with permission from the Society of Thoracic Surgeons.)

After completion of the pulmonary flush and the cardioplegia, the cardiac team extracts the heart (Fig. 87.2). This step is best performed as described by Sundaresan and colleagues.[32] The SVC is transected between ties, the aorta is divided proximal to the cross-clamp, and the PA is divided at the bifurcation of the main PA. The left atrium is carefully divided midway between the coronary sinus and the left pulmonary veins. The remaining cusp of left atrium can be transected while internally visualizing orifices of the right pulmonary veins. The heart is carefully removed from the table, and the pulmonary team proceeds with the en bloc lung removal.[32]

Complete encirclement of the trachea is substantially easier now that the great vessels have been divided. While ventilation is continued, the TA-30 stapler is used twice, and the trachea is transected between the staple lines. This division should be performed two to three rings above the carina, and the lungs should remain in moderate inflation for transport. It is important to avoid overinflation (Fig. 87.3). The contents of the thoracic cavity are removed en bloc to prevent injury to the membranous trachea, pulmonary arteries, and pulmonary veins. This removal proceeds by division of the esophagus using a GIA stapler at approximately the level of the transected trachea. The tissue back along the thoracic spine is sharply dissected. The pericardium near the diaphragm is transected, and the inferior pulmonary ligaments are divided. Completion esophagectomy is performed with a GIA stapler, the thoracic aorta is transected, and the lungs are removed en bloc. If the lungs are returning to the same institution, they are triple bagged together with cold preservation solution and transported on ice. Alternatively, if the lungs are to be used at separate institutions, they are divided on the back table by division of the posterior pericardium, left atrium between the pulmonary veins, division of the main PA at the bifurcation, and division of the left bronchus above the takeoff of the upper lobe bronchus. The left bronchus is

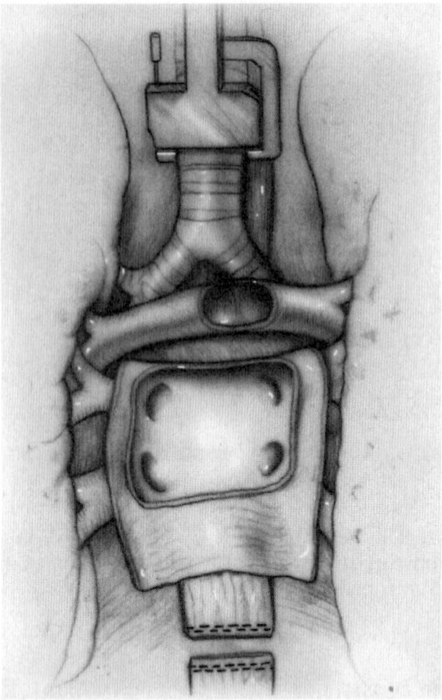

FIGURE 87.3. Drawing after removal of the heart, esophagectomy, and division of trachea prior to double-lung bloc extraction. (Reprinted from Sundaresan et al.,[32] with permission from the Society of Thoracic Surgeons.)

divided between staples to maintain the inflation of each lung.[32]

Recipient Implantation

All recipients should have complete hemodynamic monitoring, including a Swan-Ganz catheter. Transesophageal echocardiography is routinely performed and should be available. Double-lumen endotracheal intubation is performed for adults, followed by replacement with a single-lumen tube at the completion of the procedure. In children and small adults in which a suitable-size double-lumen endotracheal tube cannot be inserted, single-lumen intubation is performed with the routine use of cardiopulmonary bypass.

For single-lung transplantation, the choice of side of transplant is based on several factors, but when possible, the side with the poorest function determined by preoperative ventilation perfusion scanning is transplanted, providing the presence of a normal thoracic cavity. The standard incision is the posterolateral thoracotomy. For sequential double-lung transplantation, bilateral anterior thoracotomies and transverse sternotomy (clamshell incision) are performed, which provides excellent exposure to both pleural spaces. Alternatively, bilateral anterior thoracotomies without sternal division can be performed with the benefit of avoiding sternal wound problems.[47] The lung with the worst function is gently explanted first. The decision to place the patient on cardiopulmonary bypass is made based on the patient's status (right ventricular failure, hypoxia) or, once the first allograft is in, with the development of pulmonary hypertension or pulmonary edema.

A pneumonectomy is performed via standard technique. The PA, left atrium, and bronchus are mobilized and dissected back toward the mediastinum to prepare for implantation of the donor lung.

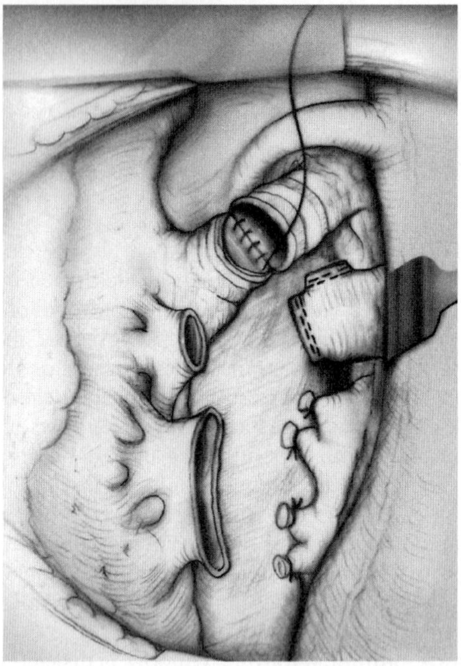

FIGURE 87.4. Single right lung transplant procedure showing bronchial anastomosis as continuous 4.0 PDS suture. (Adapted with permission from Patterson GA, Cooper JD. Lung transplantation. In: Shields TW, ed. General Thoracic Surgery, Vol. 1. Baltimore: Williams & Wilkins, 1994:1074.)

The donor lung is placed within the recipient's chest cavity covered by a cold lap pad. The bronchial anastomosis is usually performed first (Fig. 87.4). A continuous 4.0 PDS synthetic absorbable suture is used for the anastomosis, beginning with the posterior membranous trachea and proceeding anteriorly. On completion of the anastomosis, the anterior portion is covered with peribronchial tissue for protection (Fig. 87.5). Following this, the PA of the donor and

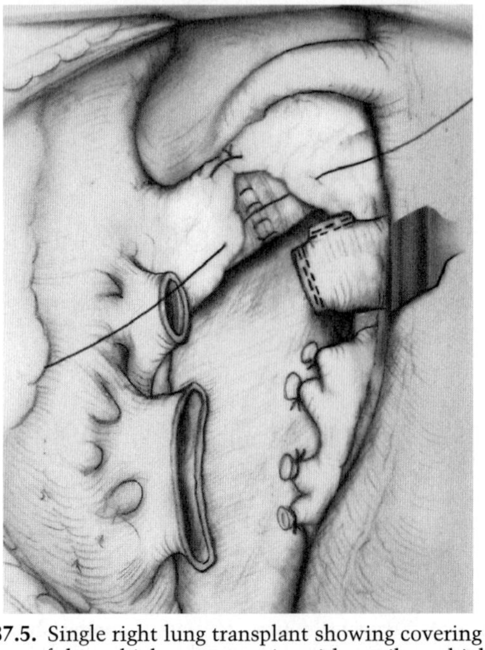

FIGURE 87.5. Single right lung transplant showing covering of anterior portion of bronchial anastomosis with peribronchial tissue. (Adapted with permission from Patterson GA, Cooper JD. Lung transplantation. In: Shields TW, ed. General Thoracic Surgery, Vol. 1. Baltimore: Williams & Wilkins, 1994:1074.)

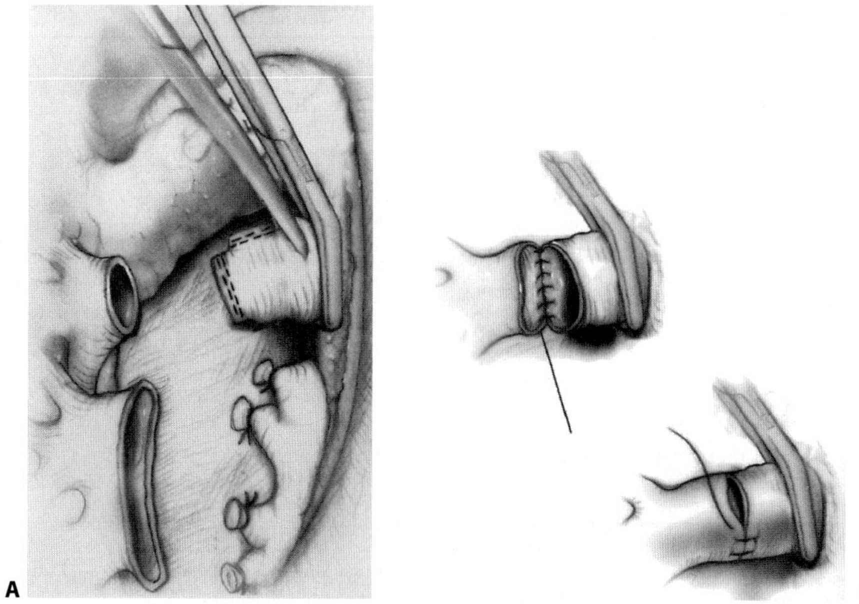

FIGURE 87.6. A. Single right lung transplant showing preparation of pulmonary artery for anastomosis. B. Continuous end-to-end anastomosis of pulmonary artery using a 5.0 or 6.0 polypropylene suture. (Adapted from Patterson and Cooper,[195] with permission.)

recipient are aligned in proper orientation and trimmed to prevent excessive length and possible kinking of the PA postoperatively. The anastomosis is performed end to end using 5.0 or 6.0 polypropylene suture in a continuous stitch (Fig. 87.6). Finally, the left atrial cuff of the donor containing the superior and inferior pulmonary veins is anastomosed to the recipient's left atrium (Fig. 87.7). Controlled reperfusion of the lung allografts with low pressure and high flow using minimal inspired oxygen to maintain adequate systemic oxygenation has been associated with a marked decrease in reperfusion injury. Following completion of the transplantation and closure of the incision, bronchoscopy is performed before leaving the operating room to check for adequacy of the bronchial anastomosis.

Postoperative Care

Immediately postoperatively, patients are transported intubated to the intensive care unit for constant monitoring. Once stabilized, a standard ventilator pressure support weaning protocol is initiated. All attempts are made to limit mean airway pressures to prevent barotrauma to the new anastomosis. Postoperatively, a quantitative lung perfusion scan to assess for adequate patency and graft flow is usually performed. If a lobar or greater perfusion defect is appreciated, further interrogation for the cause should be undertaken either by catheterization or operative exploration. Recently, we have used three-dimensional computed tomographic (CT) scanning as a method of evaluating the anastomosis.

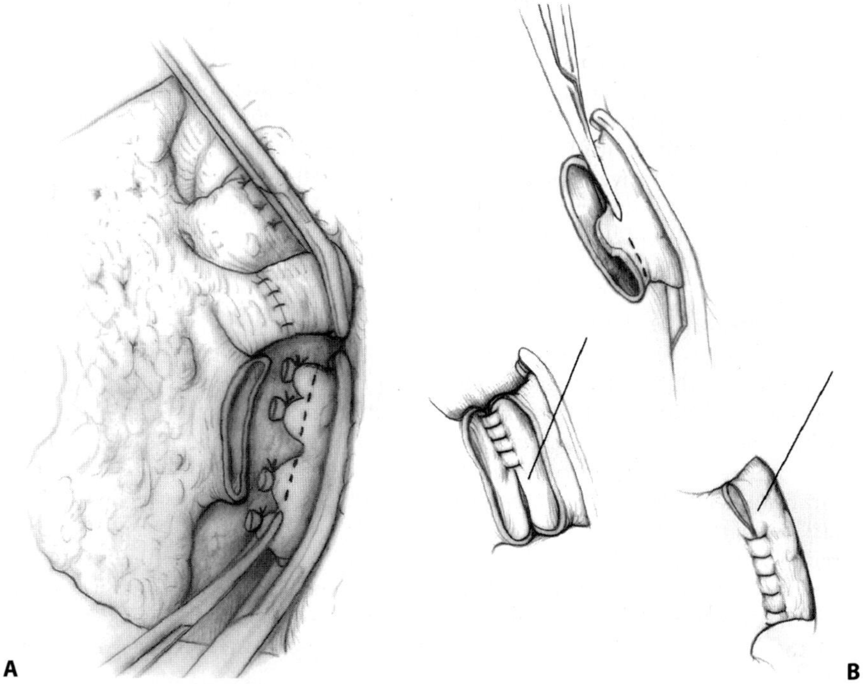

FIGURE 87.7. A. Single right lung transplant showing preparation of left atrial cuff. B. Continuous suture anastomosis of left atrial cuffs. (Adapted from Patterson and Cooper,[195] with permission.)

TABLE 87.4. Immunosuppressive Regimen at Barnes-Jewish Hospital.

	Induction of anesthesia	*Time of reperfusion*	*Postoperative*
Cyclosporine A (Neoral, Novartis)			Usually start 50–75 mg IV/PO POD 1 and increase for target trough 250–350 for first 6 months, then after 6 months 200–300
Azathioprine	2 mg/kg IV one time		2 mg/kg IV/PO daily (round to nearest 25, maximum dose 150 mg daily)
Corticosteroids		500 mg IV methylprednisolone	Methylprednisolone or prednisone 0.5 mg/kg twice daily for six doses, then 0.5 mg/kg PO daily for first 3 months, taper to 15 mg daily between 3 and 6 months, then after 6 months decrease to 7.5 mg daily for diabetic patients or 15 mg every other day for nondiabetic patients
Induction therapy (IL-2 receptor antagonist)	20 mg IV basiliximab (Simulect®, Novartis) one time		20 mg IV basiliximab POD 4

POD, postoperative day.
If switched to tacrolimus, adjust for target trough 10–14 first 6 months, then decrease to 8–12 after 6 months.
If switched to mycophenolate mofetil (CellCept), dose is 1–2 g/day given twice daily.

Careful fluid management is necessary to avoid substantial transplant lung edema, and usually negative fluid balance is attempted within the first 48 h. Prior to extubation, patients undergo bronchoscopy to ensure adequate clearance of secretions. Following extubation, the apical chest tubes are removed in the absence of an air leak, commonly within 48 h postoperatively. Because of the frequent occurrence and reoccurrence of pleural effusions postoperatively, especially in bilateral lung transplant candidates, the basal chest tubes remain for several days, usually being removed on postoperative day 5–7 (chest tube drainage <150 mL/24 h).

Vigorous chest physiotherapy, postural drainage, inhaled bronchodilators, and frequent clearance of pulmonary secretions are required in the postoperative care of these patients. Early and constant involvement of the physical therapy team ensures that transplant recipients are out of bed to chair, ambulatory with assistance, and utilizing the treadmill or exercise bikes as soon as possible even if they remain intubated. In patients with early allograft dysfunction requiring prolonged intubation, early tracheostomy allows easier mobility and better patient comfort, oral hygiene, and clearance of pulmonary secretions.

Adequate pain control is a necessity to prevent atelectasis from poor chest movement and inadequate coughing effort secondary to postthoracotomy incisional pain. An epidural catheter typically is used to provide this relief.

Immunosuppression

According to the ISHLT registry, most lung transplant recipients are maintained on steroids plus a calcineurin inhibitor (CNI; cyclosporine vs. tacrolimus) and a purine synthesis antagonist (azathioprine vs. mycophenolate mofetil [MMF]). Sirolimus (rapamycin; Rapamune, Wyeth; and RAD rapamycin derivative, Novartis) is a component in maintenance regimens in approximately 9% of recipients at both 1 and 5 years. Sirolimus has been associated with anastomotic dehiscence when used early following transplantation.[48] According to the ISHLT registry, fewer than 50% of recipients have received induction therapy over recent years. The most noticeable recent trend has been the shift away from polyclonal antilymphocyte/antithymocyte preparations toward interleukin-2 receptor (IL-2R) antagonists.

Our standard immunosuppression regimen is shown in Table 87.4. Preoperatively, we give azathioprine, and at the time of graft reperfusion we give 500 mg IV methylprednisolone. Our postoperative regimen consists of triple therapy with cyclosporine A (Neoral, Novartis), azathioprine, and corticosteroids and perioperative use of an induction agent. We have chosen to use induction agents in our program because they have been shown to decrease the incidence of acute rejection.[49,50] Recently, freedom from acute rejection has been shown to be the same whether using a cytolytic agent or IL-2R antagonists as induction strategy.[51] We have switched to using IL-2R antagonists because of their ease of administration (no premedication, central venous access not needed), fewer side effects, and potentially fewer secondary infections.

Infection Prophylaxis

Our standard infectious prophylaxis regimen consists of intravenous cefepime and vancomycin. In patients with septic lung disease, antibiotic coverage is based on previously isolated bacterial organisms and their antibiotic sensitivities. Modifications are made based on intraoperative cultures. If *Candida albicans* is detected from airway cultures, we treat with fluconazole, and if in the past the recipient was known to be colonized with *Aspergillus* species, we use voriconazole.

In general, we treat positive cultures for a total of 10–14 days, but if cultures are negative we discontinue antibiotics after 7 days. For the first year after transplantation, we routinely give acyclovir (unless on ganciclovir or valcyte) for herpes simplex prophylaxis. To prevent *Candida albicans*, we use nystatin (unless on fluconazole). In patients at high risk for cytomegalovirus (CMV) (donor-positive/recipient-negative mismatch), our standard prophylaxis is 12 weeks of intravenous ganciclovir (5 mg/kg daily), usually starting 7–14 days posttransplantation. For patients at high risk for CMV infections such as donor-seropositive and recipient-seronegative (highest risk) or recipient-seropositive, prolonged prophylaxis with valganciclovir may provide improved results.[52] For transplants, we use CMV-negative or leukocyte-reduced blood products.[53] We give lifelong prophylaxis for pneumocystis with Bactrim DS or pentamidine starting approximately 3 weeks after transplantation.

General Follow-up

We perform scheduled surveillance bronchoscopies with bronchoalveolar lavage (BAL) and transbronchial biopsies (TBBxs) at 3 weeks, 6 weeks, 12 weeks, 6 months, and 12 months postoperatively. In 25% of patients undergoing surveillance bronchoscopy with TBBx and BAL, unsuspected infection or rejection requiring treatment is detected.[54] Considering that some of these bronchoscopies are done as follow-up after treatment, this number may actually be even higher. Our routine is to obtain at least 8–10 adequate-size biopsy specimens.

Debate continues about the necessity of surveillance bronchoscopy,[54–60] and a few centers have elected to perform only diagnostic bronchoscopies based on clinical indications.[61] The time period that surveillance biopsies should be performed is also debated. Kesten and colleagues reported the yield of surveillance TBBxs beyond 4 years was very low.[62] Baz and colleagues reported that patients free of acute rejection during the first 4 months following transplantation remained free, and therefore surveillance bronchoscopy could be discontinued in this group after 4 months.[59]

Since 10% of our patients who are free of acute rejection during the first 100 days still develop acute rejection during the remainder of the year, we perform surveillance bronchoscopy in all our recipients for the first year. After 1 year, we perform bronchoscopy based on clinical or functional decline in the recipient lung function. Samples from the BAL are routinely sent for cytology, Gram, KOH, and acid-fast bacillus (AFB) stains and immunostain for respiratory viruses, herpes simplex virus, and CMV. In addition, bacterial, mycobacterial, fungal, and viral cultures are performed. Open lung biopsies are performed on occasion when necessary and may be particularly useful at later time points.[63]

Postoperative Complications

It is important to have a working knowledge of the common complications that arise after lung transplantation. Space precludes a more through review of potential complications, but the reader is referred to recent articles.[64]

Ischemia–Reperfusion Injury

Ischemia–reperfusion is characterized by noncardiogenic pulmonary edema and progressive lung injury over the first few hours following implantation (Fig. 87.8A and 87.8B). In its most severe form, ischemia–reperfusion injury is described as primary graft failure that pathologically appears as diffuse alveolar damage (Fig. 87.8C). A variety of factors such as poor preservation techniques, prolonged ischemic time, or unsuspected donor lung pathology (e.g., contusion, pulmonary thromboembolism, or aspiration) all play a role in the development of primary graft dysfunction. Secondary causes of early allograft dysfunction, such as a technically inadequate vascular anastomosis, must be ruled out. Hyperacute rejection is exceedingly rare, but it must be a consideration in cases of early severe lung dysfunction. The condition is characterized by noncardiogenic pulmonary edema and progressive lung injury over the first few hours following implantation.

Irrespective of its cause, it is important to establish a diagnosis of early graft dysfunction and rule out other treatable conditions. We perform open lung biopsy at the time of implantation if graft dysfunction is immediately apparent in the operating room. In addition, serological evaluation for anti-HLA antibodies may reveal evidence for hyperacute rejection in some of these patients.

Fortunately, severe reperfusion injury has not been so commonly encountered in recent years. Superior strategies of lung preservation have evolved.[65] It is clear from experimental[66,67] and clinical work[68] that low-potassium dextran solution provides superior preservation over high-potassium preservation solutions previously in use. In addition, experimental work suggests that nitric oxide added to the flush

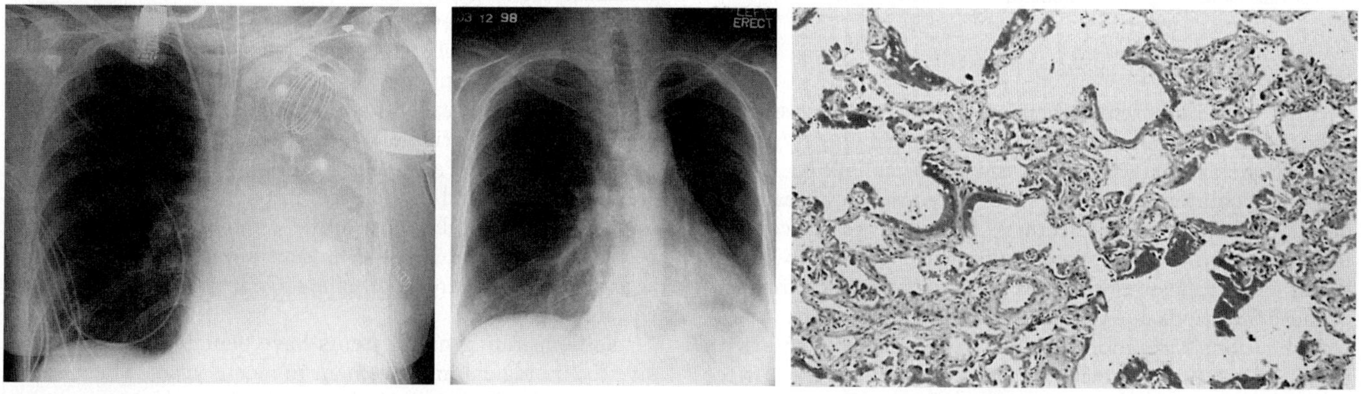

A B C

FIGURE 87.8. **A.** Chest radiograph showing diffuse consolidation typical of primary graft failure. **B.** Radiograph of same patient after complete recovery. **C.** Transbronchial biopsy showing diffuse alveolar damage characteristic of ischemia–reperfusion injury.

solution or inhaled at the time of harvest provides a preservation advantage.[69,70] Lung hyperinflation is an excellent model of pulmonary edema. Therefore, we are particularly careful to avoid lung hyperinflation during harvest and storage of the donor lungs. Each of these factors has contributed to a reduction in the frequency of ischemia–reperfusion injury.

The use of controlled reperfusion in combination with leukocyte depletion[71–77] has shown promise as a preventive strategy for ischemia–reperfusion injury. Lick and colleagues[78] reported a nonrandomized small series in humans utilizing this technique and reported no reperfusion injury in the treated cohort of patients. At the time of reperfusion, leukocyte-filtered, pharmacologically modified perfusate is pumped into the newly implanted PA at a controlled rate (200 mL/min) and pressure (less than 20 mmHg) for 10 min. The lung is ventilated with 50% inspired oxygen concentration during the period to further reduce the opportunity for oxygen radical-mediated reperfusion injury.

In cases of established ischemia–reperfusion injury, proper treatment includes diuresis and maximal ventilatory support with simultaneous avoidance of additional ventilator-induced injury. In most cases, the reperfusion injury will resolve over 24–48 h. We have previously demonstrated that inhaled nitric oxide is of benefit in severe reperfusion injury as it decreases PA pressure and improves Pa_{O_2}/Fi_{O_2} ratio.[79] Recently, inhaled prostacyclin has been investigated and has shown promise as an economical alternative to nitric oxide.[80] Paralytics and sedatives are used to minimize oxygen consumption. In severe cases, extracorporeal membrane oxygenation (ECMO) is a suitable treatment option if employed early.[81] Improved results have been obtained using venovenous ECMO preferentially.

Anastomotic Complications

The bronchial circulation to the donor lung is severed during extraction, and after implantation, the donor bronchus depends on retrograde flow from the pulmonary circulation until systemic collaterals develop. Anastomotic complications resulting from airway ischemia include infection, dehiscence, stenosis, and malacia. The reported incidence of these complications is 7% to 14%[82–85] of patients, although improvement in anastomotic techniques, pulmonary preservation, and care in preserving collateral circulation during harvesting have lessened their occurrence. In our recent experience, the incidence of airway complications was only 4%.[86]

Anastomotic Infections

Because of the inherent ischemia occurring at the bronchial anastomosis after lung transplantation, fungal infections may develop at this site. *Aspergillus* and *Candida* have been identified as potential pathogens that can cause life-threatening bronchial anastomotic infection.[87] Nunley and colleagues[88] identified 15 (24.6%) saprophytic fungal infections involving the bronchial anastomoses in 61 recipients, with the majority of these infections due to *Aspergillus* species. Stenotic airway complications were more frequently seen in recipients with these anastomotic infections (46.7%) compared to those without fungal infections (8.7%). Specific complications from fungal infections arising at the bronchial anastomoses included bronchial stenosis, bronchomalacia, and fatal hemorrhage. A variety of interventions, including bronchial stenting, balloon dilation, electrocauterization, laser debridement, and radiation brachytherapy, were utilized to treat these complications. In addition, in this series, three fatalities were associated (4.9%) with saprophytic bronchial anastomotic infections.

If bronchoscopic inspection reveals extensive anastomotic pseudomembranes, a biopsy of the site should be performed to rule out an invasive fungal infection. The optimal treatment of bronchial anastomotic fungal infection is unknown. Success has been reported with a combination of systemic and inhaled antifungal agents. The addition of the inhaled antifungal therapy seems appropriate because aerosolization allows direct drug delivery to the poorly vascularized anastomosis. Debridement of the site may also be necessary.[89,90]

Dehiscence

Anastomotic dehiscences are often initially detected by bronchoscopy. Membranous wall defects generally heal without any airway compromise, whereas cartilaginous defects usually result in some degree of late stricture. Significant dehiscence (greater than 50% of the bronchial circumference) may result in compromise of the airway. This problem should be managed expectantly by mechanical debridement of the area to maintain satisfactory airway patency. A stent can only be placed if the distal main airway remains intact.

Occasionally, a significant dehiscence results in direct communication with the pleural space, resulting in pneumothorax and a significant air leak following chest tube insertion. If the lung remains completely expanded and the pleural space is evacuated, the leak will ultimately seal, and the airway may heal without significant stenosis. Similarly, a dehiscence may communicate directly with the mediastinum, resulting in significant mediastinal emphysema. If the lung remains completely expanded and the pleural space is filled, adequate drainage of the mediastinum can be achieved by placing a drain close to the anastomotic line by way of mediastinoscopy. This step will also result in satisfactory healing of the anastomosis, often without stricture.

Anastomotic Stenosis/Malacia

Late complications from airway ischemia, infection, and dehiscence include bronchial stricture or malacia and may present as stridor and wheezing. Bronchoscopic assessment confirms the diagnosis. Bronchial stenosis and bronchomalacia can be successfully treated with serial balloon dilation in the case of bronchial stenosis and stent placement in cases of refractory bronchial stenosis and bronchomalacia. Silastic stents are tolerated exceptionally well. Patients may, however, require daily inhalation of *N*-acetylcysteine to keep the stents patent. DeHoyos, Patterson, and Maurer[91] reported that the stents have resulted in dramatic improvement in pulmonary function. Fortunately, most of these stents have proven to be required only temporarily. After several months, most stented anastomotic strictures maintain satisfactory patency without the stent in place.

Self-expanding metal stents have benefited from impressive technological improvement in recent years. These stents come in a wide variety of lengths and diameters, and they have been exceptionally easy to insert. In rare situations in which the airways distal to an anastomotic stricture are too small to accept a Silastic stent or when a Silastic stent will obstruct one bronchus while stenting another, the use of a self-expanding metal stent may suit the purpose perfectly. The only caveat is that granulation tissue will rapidly overgrow an uncovered metal mesh stent, sometimes making it impossible to remove.

Finally, a recent addition to the armamentarium is a self-expanding plastic stent without interstices that allow granulation tissue ingrowth. This stent (Polyflex, Rüsch, http://www.ruesch.de) appears to incorporate the best aspects of the two predecessor stents and combine them in a useful device. Long-term data concerning stability and function of these stents are lacking.

TABLE 87.5. Grading of Acute Pulmonary Allograft Rejection.

A. Acute rejection	
Grade 0	None
Grade 1	Minimal
Grade 2	Mild
Grade 3	Moderate
Grade 4	Severe
B. Airway inflammation	
With or without lymphocytic bronchitis/bronchiolitis may grade	
Grade 0	None
Grade 1	Minimal
Grade 2	Mild
Grade 3	Moderate
Grade 4	Severe
Grade X	Ungradable

Source: Adapted from Yousem et al.[103] J Heart Lung Transplant.

Rejection

Both acute and chronic lung allograft rejection contribute substantially to morbidity seen in lung transplant recipients. Chronic lung rejection remains the major limitation to long-term success in lung transplantation. Hyperacute rejection has only anecdotally been reported in the literature.[92–94] Saint Martin and colleagues[95] performed immunofluorescence with C3, immunoglobin M, and immunoglobin G and found no evidence of humoral rejection in 106 biopsies. In this particular report, only one patient had a high reactivity pretransplant PRA, suggesting a low risk for hyperacute rejection. Conversely, we have reported immunohistochemical findings of humoral injury in some recipients with high PRA.[96] Interestingly, Magro and colleagues[97] have reported evidence suggesting that a frequently occurring septal capillary injury syndrome may represent humoral injury in lung allografts.

Acute Rejection

Acute rejection remains the "thorn in the side" of lung transplantation, more prevalent in the lung than in any other solid organ transplant.[98,99] While it is an uncommon cause of mortality, it is strongly linked with the development of chronic rejection. The majority of episodes of acute rejection occur early in the postoperative period, and the incidence steadily declines after the first 3 months.[55,56,100] The clinical diagnosis of acute rejection remains imprecise. Normally, symptomatic episodes present with dyspnea, hypoxemia, low-grade fever, and moderate leukocytosis, which can be difficult to differentiate from early infection. The chest radiograph findings of diffuse-perihilar interstitial infiltrates along with these clinical findings are consistent with rejection. Trulock[101] reported the frequent occurrence of radiographic abnormalities with early episodes of rejection, while episodes occurring after the first month frequently had a normal-appearing chest radiograph. Monitoring of the allograft by spirometry is useful, and a 10% or greater decline in baseline FEV_1 or FVC (forced vital capacity) indicates the need for further evaluation.

Suspicion of acute rejection should be evaluated by bronchoscopy with TBBx to confirm the diagnosis and rule out infection. A uniform grading system for classification of pulmonary transplant rejection (acute and chronic) was initially proposed in 1990[102] and subsequently was revised in 1995 by the Lung Rejection Study Group (LRSG).[103] For acute rejection, this grading system is based on histologic criteria found on biopsy, with emphasis on perivascular and interstitial infiltration of mononuclear cells (Table 87.5; Fig. 87.9A and 87.9B). Each grade should also note the coexistence of airway

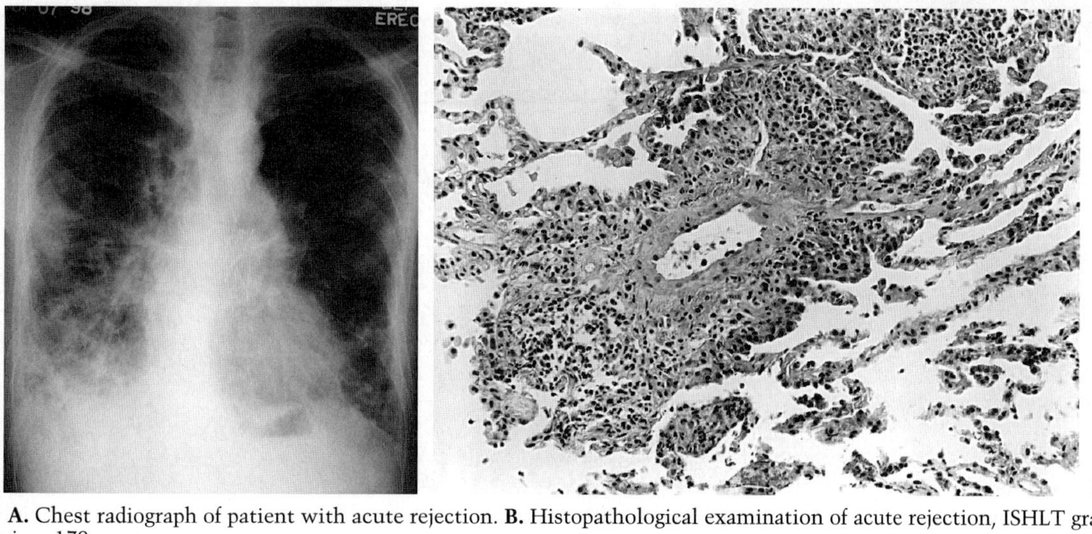

A B

FIGURE 87.9. A. Chest radiograph of patient with acute rejection. **B.** Histopathological examination of acute rejection, ISHLT grade 3. Hematoxylin and eosin, ×170.

inflammation. The degree of perivascular inflammation is graded in the A category from 0 (no rejection) to 4 (severe rejection). The presence of small and large airway inflammation is listed as a B category and divided into five grades of increasing intensity or, based on institutional preference, simply noted as present or absent. While perivascular infiltrates are the primary focus in this classification scheme, it was felt that the correlation of airway inflammation with the development of chronic rejection could not be ignored.[103]

Acute rejection is usually treated with intravenous methylprednisolone, 10–15 mg/kg/day for 3–5 days. Usually, there is improvement in symptoms and radiographic findings within 8–12 h. Often, this is followed with a steroid taper over 2–3 weeks. Another goal with therapy is to prevent future episodes; with this in mind, the patient's maintenance therapy should be evaluated. New medications should be considered as they can decrease drug levels of CNIs by activating the cytochrome P450 enzyme pathway and increasing their metabolism.

The optimal initial maintenance immunosuppression regimen has not been clearly delineated. Two studies have shown a decrease in acute rejection episodes when tacrolimus (FK506; Prograf, Fujisawa) is chosen as the initial CNI.[104,105] Other studies have shown decreased recurrence in acute rejection after switching from cyclosporine to tacrolimus.[106,107] Based on these studies, we often discontinue cyclosporine and start tacrolimus in patients with severe or recurrent acute rejection episodes. Mycophenolate mofetil (Cellcept, Hoffman LaRoche) has not been shown to decrease acute rejection episodes compared to azathioprine in lung transplantation,[108,109] but based on its success in other organ transplants, we often switch to this cell cycle inhibitor when patients have recurrent acute rejection episodes.[110] Novel immunosuppressive agents such as sirolimus (rapamycin, Rapamune, Wyeth; and RAD rapamycin derivative, Novartis), a newer immunosuppressive agent that acts synergistically with CNIs plus has antiproliferative properties, and Leflunomide (Arava), a de novo pyrimidine nucleotide synthesis inhibitor, have shown promise in other organ transplants.[111–113] Their role in acute rejection in lung transplantation is being evaluated.[114]

After treatment of acute rejection, we repeat bronchoscopy in 3–6 weeks to confirm an appropriate response to therapy. In approximately one-third of cases, persistence of acute rejection is detected on follow-up.[54,56,57,115]

Treatment of acute rejection refractory to the above acute (steroids) and maintenance interventions is not uniform. A trial of cytolytic therapy is often initiated.[49,116–118] Other regimens have been attempted, including aerosolized cyclosporine,[119] alemtuzumab (Campath),[120] methotrexate,[121] extracorporeal photopheresis,[122,123] and total lymphoid irradiation.[124] No controlled trials have been performed comparing these therapies, and reported studies are small with varying degrees of success reported.

Chronic Rejection

Chronic rejection of the lung allograft is the major limitation to long-term recipient survival. Five years after transplantation, approximately 50% of recipients have developed chronic rejection.[12] Bronchiolitis obliterans (BO) is the histologic finding of chronic rejection in the lung allograft (Fig. 87.10A and 87.10B). This entity, characterized by scarring and fibrosis of the small airways with or without an inflammatory component, was first described at Stanford in heart-lung recipients.[125] In the revised classification of pulmonary allograft rejection by the LRSG,[103] chronic rejection was categorized as C grade for chronic airway rejection (BO) and D grade for chronic vascular rejection. In the C grade subcategories, a and b were used to note the presence or absence of active airway inflammation (mononuclear cell infiltrates), respectively.

Bronchiolitis obliterans is a patchy heterogeneous process. While TBBx is useful for the diagnosis of infection and acute rejection, it is insensitive in the diagnosis of chronic rejection. Chamberlain and colleagues, in a review of over 1000 TBBxs, estimated the sensitivity to be only 17%.[126]

Because of the difficulties documenting BO histologically, a classification system based on clinical parameters was proposed by the ISHLT, termed bronchiolitis obliterans syndrome (BOS).[127] In this classification scheme, posttransplant

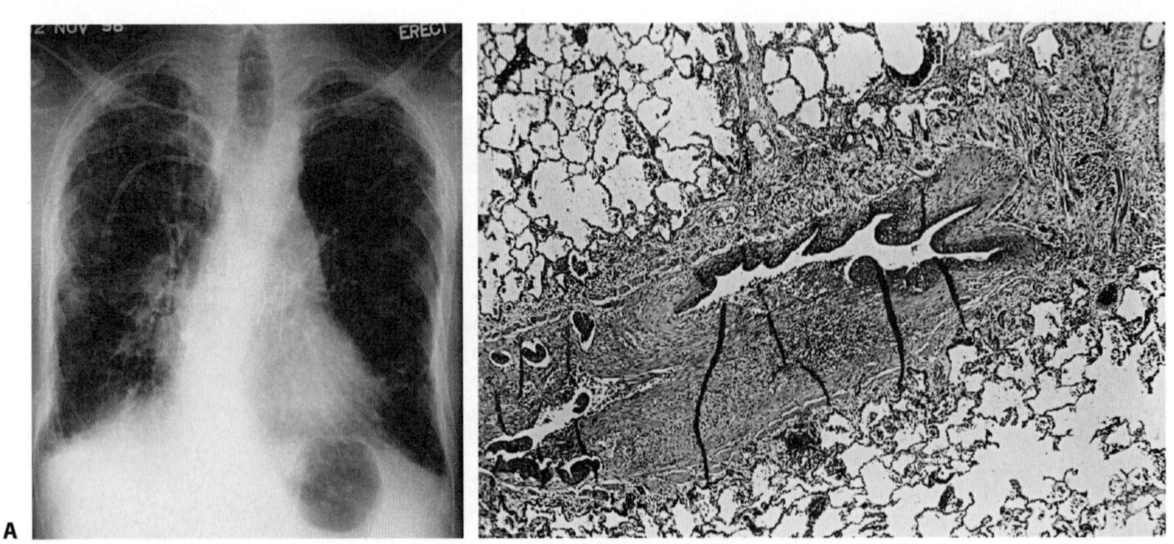

FIGURE 87.10. A. Chest radiograph of patient with bronchiolitis obliterans. **B.** Histopathological examination of bronchiolitis obliterans. Hematoxylin and eosin, ×40.

TABLE 87.6. **Criteria for Bronchiolitis Obliterans Syndrome.**

BOS score	*Degree*	*Baseline FEV_1*
0	None	>90% and FEF_{25-75} >75%
0-p	Potential	81%–90% and/or FEF_{25-75} ≤75%
1	Mild	66%–80%
2	Moderate	51%–65%
3	Severe	≤50%

Each BOS score or grade has a subcategory noting absence or presence of documented bronchiolitis obliterans histologically: (a) without pathologic evidence of bronchiolitis obliterans; (b) with pathologic evidence of bronchiolitis obliterans.

Data from ISHLT et al.[127] and J Heart Lung Transplant; Estenne et al.,[128] J Heart Lung Transplant.

FEV_1 is used to assess graft function. The best posttransplant FEV_1 is determined and defined as BOS 0. A decline from this baseline determines the stage of BOS, with stages 1–3 representing progressively worse pulmonary function. Importantly, other causes for a decrease in FEV_1 (i.e., infection, acute rejection) must be excluded. Patients cannot receive a diagnosis of BOS until at least 3 months after transplantation. Bronchiolitis obliterans syndrome is a surrogate marker for chronic allograft rejection and does not require the presence of histologically documented BO. The absence or presence of BO, however, is noted by subcategories a and b, respectively.

Revision, with the addition of a potential BOS stage (BOS 0-p), has recently been proposed based on limitations in the original staging system (Table 87.6).[128] Stage BOS 0-p is defined by a drop in FEV_1 of 10%–19% or a 25% or greater decline in baseline midexpiratory flow rate (FEF_{25-75}). The FEF_{25-75} has been shown in several studies to be more sensitive than the FEV_1 in detection of early airflow obstruction in bilateral lung transplant recipients, but it has a wide variability with single-lung transplants. The goal of introducing this potential stage of BOS is to raise clinical concern and increase surveillance.[128]

Numerous publications attempting to identify risk factors for BOS have been reported. Sharples and colleagues[129] reviewed these studies and defined the reported risk factors as accepted, potential, or hypothetical based on the available evidence (Table 87.7).

Treatment of patients with BOS/BO rarely reverses the lung dysfunction. Several therapies have been reported, but in general the studies have been nonrandomized, small, and with short follow-up. Further complicating assessment of therapeutic benefit of a particular treatment has been the uncertain natural history of BOS. Although almost certain decline in pulmonary function is seen after the onset of BOS, the rate of this decline can vary dramatically between individuals. The acute and chronic onset of BOS have been suggested to represent different entities.[130]

In general, therapy consists of augmenting standard immunosuppression regimens, addition of new immunosuppressive medicines, and immune-modulating therapies.[131–146] Our standard therapy usually consists of modification of standard immunosuppression with a switch from cyclosporine to tacrolimus and possibly azathioprine to MMF. More recently, we have added Rapamune, which has unique properties (antiproliferative, tolerogenic) that may make it particularly useful for treatment of BO/BOS. We have tried leflunomide on one occasion without success.

Cytolytic therapy is utilized if continued decline in pulmonary function is seen despite these changes. On occasion, we have used total lymphoid irradiation. Other treatment options that have been tried include inhaled steroids,[142] aerosolized cyclosporine,[143] methotrexate,[141] cyclophosphamide,[137] and extracorporeal photopheresis;[145,146] a few have resulted in stabilization of the patients' pulmonary status, but generally treatment was disappointing.

A surgical treatment for BOS has been proposed by the Duke Lung Transplant Group[147–149] for use in patients with BOS found to have gastroesophageal reflux disease (GERD). Gastroesophageal reflux with resultant aspiration may contribute to BOS. It is prevalent in lung transplant recipients, and for multiple reasons this group may be more likely to be affected, even by silent aspiration of acid contents. Host defense mechanisms such as cough and mucociliary clearance of foreign bodies are markedly impaired after lung transplantation. Furthermore, vagal nerve injury during the transplant and the use of immunosuppressive agents after transplantation may result in delayed gastric emptying and decreased gastrointestinal motility. The Duke University Lung Transplant Group has reported improvement in pulmonary function following a laparoscopic Nissen fundoplication for treatment of GERD.[149] Patients treated before they progressed to the later stages of BOS showed the most benefit. A survival advantage was also seen in the lung transplant group surgically treated for their GERD. Currently, a prospective, randomized, multiinstitutional trial is planned to further evaluate the role played by GERD in BOS.

Prevention of BOS through the promotion of immune tolerance of transplanted organs is under investigation. Long-term surviving transplant recipients have been found to have donor cells present in their tissues and blood (chimerism).[150,151] Based on these findings, the Pittsburgh Lung Transplant Group[151] attempted to increase chimerism in lung transplant recipients with concurrent infusion of donor bone marrow (BM) cells at the time of transplantation. Overall, these results were unimpressive but not surprising. Preconditioning (±BM infusion) of the host using different regimens may be required to achieve tolerance and chimerism in adults. Much ongoing research is now directed toward achieving the state of tolerance in clinical transplantation.

Retransplantation may be an option in carefully selected patients with BOS. Bronchiolitis obliterans syndrome does not appear to occur in an accelerated manner after retransplantation. In the pulmonary retransplant registry, 81% and 56% were free of BOS at 1 and 4 years after retransplantation, respectively.[152]

TABLE 87.7. **Risk Factors for BOS/OB.**

Definitive role (accepted risk factors)
Acute rejection
Late rejection
Lymphocytic bronchitis/bronchiolitis
Late onset
Less clear role (potential risk factors)
CMV
Other infectious organisms
HLA matching
Little or no role (hypothetic risk factors)
Recipient and donor characteristics

Source: Adapted from Sharples et al.[129]

Infectious Complications

Lung transplant recipients are at increased risk for a variety of infectious complications due to the chronic immunosuppression and abnormal physiology of the posttransplant lung. Infections with typical bacterial pathogens as well as opportunistic infections like CMV are common. Collectively, infections represent the leading cause of death in the early postoperative period and remain an important cause of morbidity and mortality throughout the posttransplant period. Furthermore, evidence suggests that many infections may induce immune and inflammatory responses that predispose to either acute or chronic allograft rejection or both.

Bacterial Infections

Bacterial infections are most common in the early posttransplant period and remain the primary cause of mortality in this period.[153] The most common organisms involved are those colonizing the donor, the recipient, or iatrogenic bacteria that populate individual institutions' intensive care units. Gram-negative pathogens such as *Pseudomonas* species, *Klebsiella*, and *Haemophilus influenzae* are responsible for most early posttransplant bacterial pneumonias, but gram-positive organisms such as *Staphylococcus aureus* are also causes. Less commonly, *Actinomyces, Mycobacterium tuberculosis*, and atypical mycobacterium have been seen in lung transplant recipients.[153,154] Analysis of trends in individual hospital bacterial susceptibilities should guide selection of empiric therapy, with adjustments as necessary when sensitivities are available. At our institution, all lung transplant patients receive a 7- to 10-day course of postoperative broad-spectrum antimicrobial prophylaxis (e.g., vancomycin and cefipime). This antibiotic regimen is modified depending on results of the cultures obtained from the donor and recipient prior to transplantation (especially in patients with CF who have preoperative pathogens with known sensitivities). Antibiotics may be continued longer depending on the recipient's bronchial cultures after transplantation.

Bloodstream infections (BSIs) have been identified as an important cause of early postoperative morbidity and mortality. In one report, BSI was documented in 25% of lung transplant recipients, with *Staphylococcus aureus* and *Pseudomonas aeruginosa* singled out as the most common pathogens. Pneumonia and catheter-related infection represented the most common etiology for posttransplant BSI, and infection was associated with a significantly increased risk for postoperative death. These results highlight the importance of appropriate antibiotic selection and the need to minimize the duration of central lines.[155]

Viral Infections

Cytomegalovirus

Cytomegalovirus (CMV) disease is the most common infectious postoperative complication after lung transplantation. This virus causes infection in 13%–75% of transplant patients depending on the specific definitions of infection and on the type and duration of pharmacologic CMV prophylaxis.[53,156] Lung transplant recipients who are serologically CMV negative preoperatively and receive serologically CMV-positive donor lungs are at the highest risk of developing severe, life-threatening disease from primary infection. On the contrary, such infection is not usually seen in donor-negative/recipient-negative transplants.[53]

The optimal approach to the prevention of posttransplant CMV infection remains controversial. Most centers, including our own, will employ a regimen of 12 weeks of intravenous ganciclovir (5 mg/kg daily) posttransplantation in the high-risk (donor-positive/recipient-negative) mismatch patients. Some centers employ a shorter course of intravenous ganciclovir (e.g., 4 weeks) in all "at-risk" lung recipients. In a randomized prospective trial, Kruger and colleagues demonstrated that hyperimmune globulin against CMV (e.g., Cytogam) alone is ineffective in the prevention of CMV viremia or pneumonitis after lung transplant.[157] As an additional preventive measure, we use CMV-negative or leukocyte-reduced blood products in all instances except major bleeding requiring large-volume rapid transfusion.[53]

Cytomegalovirus infection refers to detection of the virus in the serum or BAL using conventional culture, shell vial assay, or qualitative serum assay (e.g., polymerase chain reaction or CMV DNA by hybrid capture). *Cytomegalovirus disease*, on the other hand, is defined by the presence of "cytomegalic"cells (CMV inclusion bodies or cells positive on immunoperoxidase stain) on tissue biopsies (Fig. 87.11A

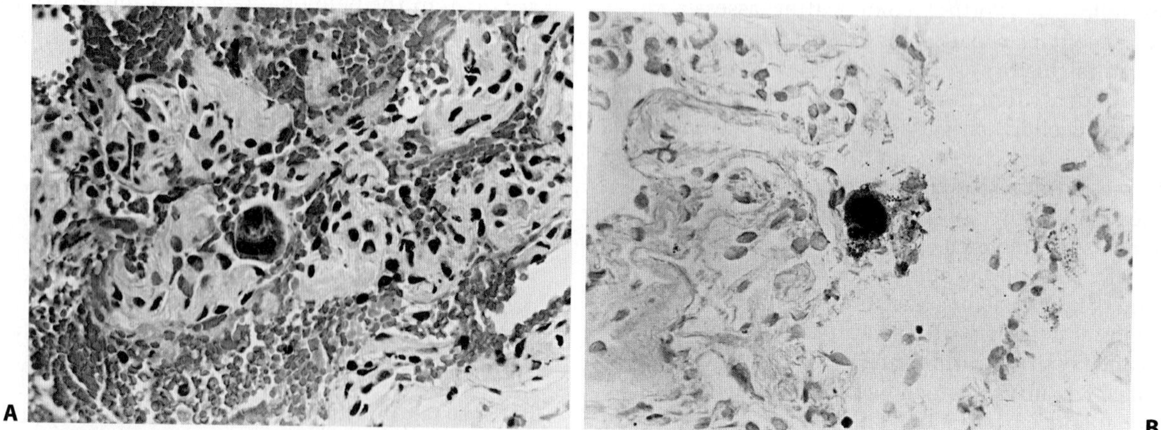

FIGURE 87.11. A. Demonstration of CMV inclusion bodies in lung biopsy. Hematoxylin and eosin, ×400. **B.** Demonstration of CMV inclusion bodies by immunoperoxidase.

and 87.11B) or the isolation of CMV from a tissue specimen in the presence of clinical findings consistent with CMV infection.

Most CMV infections respond to 14–21 days of intravenous ganciclovir (5 mg/kg twice daily). The dose should be adjusted for leukopenia and renal dysfunction. When patients fail to respond to intravenous ganciclovir therapy, drug resistance should be considered, and the addition of Foscarnet or Cidofovir therapy may be instituted.[52] However, because of the significant nephrotoxicity of these second-line agents, formal testing for ganciclovir resistance should be performed when suspected. Acute renal failure has been reported in a lung transplant recipient treated with Cidofovir.[158] Valganciclovir (Roche, Palo Alto, CA), an oral ganciclovir derivative with bioavailability comparable to intravenous formulations of ganciclovir, has recently been introduced for use in transplantation. Ongoing prospective studies will define the indications, efficacy, and cost-effectiveness of oral valganciclovir in the lung transplant population.

Community-Acquired Respiratory Viral Infections

Community-acquired respiratory viral infections, including respiratory syncytial virus (RSV) adenovirus, parainfluenza, and influenza, cause significant morbidity and mortality in lung transplant recipients.[159–163] These viral respiratory infections occur over a broad time range after transplantation, and different mechanisms may account for early and late posttransplant infection. Early viral infection may result from nosocomial transmission or reactivation of latent virus. In contrast, late posttransplant respiratory viral infection is more likely to be community acquired. A seasonal variation is seen with RSV (January to April), while infection with adenovirus and parainfluenza occur throughout the year.

The majority of viral infections produce acute symptoms, including cough, wheeze, dyspnea, and fever. Presentation of influenza may be atypical, with gastrointestinal symptoms predominating. New radiographic findings in lung transplant recipients with viral respiratory infections indicate severe infection and are a marker for poor prognosis.[161] Symptomatic adenoviral infection in particular is typically associated with new radiologic abnormalities and is frequently fatal.[161]

Treatment options for respiratory viral infections are limited. Aerosolized ribavirin has shown benefit in the treatment of RSV and parainfluenza infection in children.[164] Intravenous immunoglobulin to RSV has been used in prevention and treatment of RSV infections in infants.[165] While the efficacy of these agents in lung transplant recipients remains unclear, it has been recommended that all patients with severe symptomatic RSV or parainfluenza infection receive aerosolized ribavirin. Ribavirin is also recommended in patients with radiographic abnormalities in the setting of RSV or parainfluenza infection given the increased potential to progress to respiratory failure.

Care for adenovirus is currently supportive as there are no definitive therapies available. A trial of reduced immunosuppression appears worthwhile, although the risk for rejection must be considered. Reports of the use of intravenous ribavirin or immunoglobulin have suggested potential value in adenoviral infections in pediatric, BM recipients, and patients with acquired immunodeficiency syndrome (AIDS).[166–169] Intravenous ribavirin has also been used with some success in a pediatric patient with adenoviral infection after liver transplantation.[170]

Treatment for influenza in nonimmunocompromised patients consists of several potential drugs, including amantadine, rimantadine, and the newer neuraminidase inhibitors such as zanamivir and oseltamivir.[171,172] The use of these agents in lung transplant recipients requires further study.

Because treatment options for community-acquired viral infections in lung transplant recipients are limited, the main goal in this population is prevention. It is routine for all our lung transplant recipients to receive yearly influenza vaccines. Unfortunately, the response to influenza vaccine in solid organ transplant recipients has been noted to be impaired, and revaccination does not seem to improve the vaccine response.[164] In a series of heart transplant patients, the efficacy of the influenza vaccine was significant impaired. Although vaccination was less effective compared to nonimmunosuppressed individuals, 50% of patients still reached protective serum antibody titers against two of three virus strains.[173] Therefore, routine influenza immunization is still recommended, but serologic testing may be indicated.[162]

Importantly, all close contacts should receive influenza vaccination with the intended goal of decreasing the risk of infection to the transplant patient. Lung transplant recipients should avoid contact with family and friends with respiratory symptoms, especially children, to minimize risks of acquiring community viral infections. Frequent hand washing should be encouraged after contact with infected patients.

Fungal Infections

Fungal infections are a major problem after lung transplantation and occur early and late after transplant. *Aspergillus* and *Candida* account for the majority of these fungal infections[174] (Fig. 87.12). *Candida albicans* is commonly isolated from bronchial washings after transplant, and its presence usually represents colonization,[153] but it may also be invasive.[175] Presence of *Aspergillus* can also represent colonization, but because of the potential for invasive life-threatening infections, strong consideration needs to be given to treatment. Greater than 50% of cases of *Aspergillus* colonization and infection occur within 6 months after transplantation. Mortality rates associated with invasive *Aspergillus* pneumonia or disseminated infection approached 60% in one series of lung transplant recipients.[176]

Although risk factors for posttransplant fungal infection are not well defined, pretransplant colonization or prior treated infection may identify patients at higher risk for posttransplant infection. In patients with a single-lung transplant, one obvious potential reservoir of persistent *Aspergillus* is the native lung.[153,177] Aspergilloma lesions found in the recipient explanted lungs have been associated with reduced posttransplant survival.[178] Patients with CF and positive preoperative sputum cultures for *Aspergillus* are at higher risk for postoperative infections.[179]

Nocardia infections are increasingly recognized as complications of lung transplantation.[180] While *Nocardia asteroides* accounts for the most transplant-related nocardiosis, a case of disseminated infection with *Nocardia brasiliensis*[181] in a single-lung transplant recipient has been reported. While the mortality is high for immunocompromised patients with

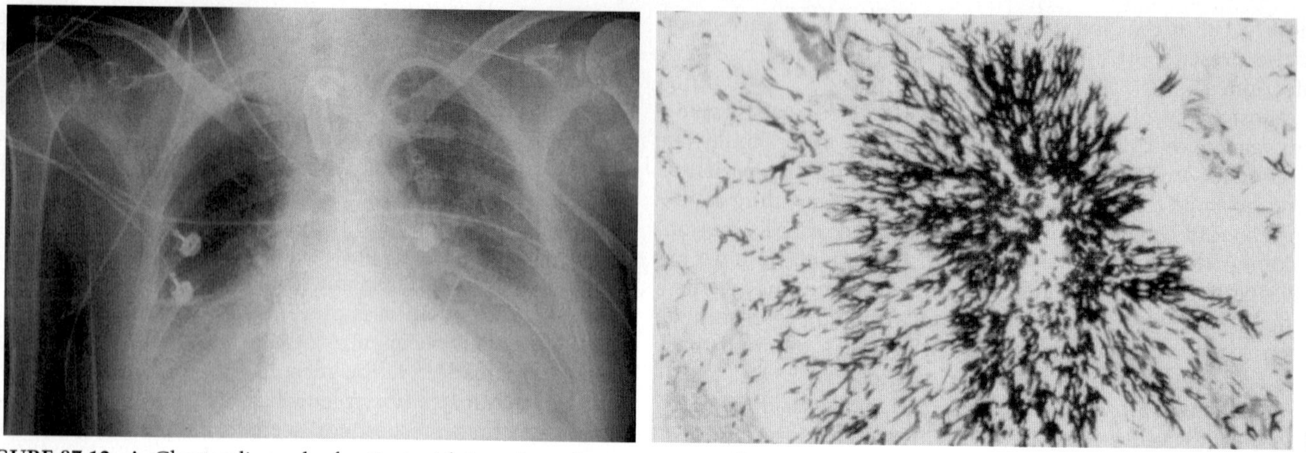

A B

FIGURE 87.12. A. Chest radiograph of patient with invasive pulmonary *Aspergillus*. **B.** Histopathologic examination of patient with *Aspergillus* (hematoxylin and eosin, ×20).

N. brasiliensis, prompt diagnosis and early initiation of appropriate therapy may improve outcome.

Reports of other fungal infections, such *as Histoplasma, Coccidiomycosis, Mucormycosis, Zygomycetes*, and *Cryptococcus*, are also documented.[153] *Scedosporium apiospermum* is an uncommon cause of disseminated infection, but importantly it is resistant to amphotericin B.[182] *Pneumocystis carinii*, now classified as a fungus, remains a rare cause of infection because of the routine use of effective prophylaxis in all lung transplant recipients. Dematiaceous fungi, such as *Mucormycosis*, are also infrequent causes of postoperative infection.

Treatment for fungal infection is based on the specific organism causing the infection; amphotericin B has been the drug of choice for *Aspergillus* and *Fusarium*. Newer options that may be as effective with less toxicity include liposomal formulations of amphotericin, voriconazole, and caspofungin. Voriconazole in particular must be used with caution in lung transplant recipients because of its extensive list of known drug interactions. High-dose azole therapy (itraconazole, voriconazole) may be used for *Scedosporium*. Nocardia infections are treated with trimethoprim-sulfamethoxazole. Most candidal infections can be treated with fluconazole. Non-albicans *Candida* species, however, are increasingly resistant to Diflucan but can be effectively treated by new drugs such as voriconazole. Single-lung transplant should probably not be performed in patients with mycetomas as adequate removal of fungal organisms cannot be achieved, and the newly transplanted lung will be at increased risk of colonization and infection.[178] Prolonged therapy is required for all fungal infections.

Because of the potential morbidity and mortality associated with fungal infections, several antifungal prophylactic strategies have been used in lung transplant recipients, often employing systemic or inhaled antifungal agents or both.[183] However, enthusiasm for the use of systemic antifungal therapies is limited by the lack of in vitro activity against some infections, drug interactions, and significant treatment-limiting toxicities. Furthermore, the use of inhaled amphotericin B has been associated with significant subjective intolerance, leading to treatment discontinuation in up to 50% of patients.[184]

The Duke lung transplant group has recently demonstrated the safety and tolerability of inhaled amphotericin B lipid complex, or ABLC (Abelcet®, Elan Pharmaceuticals), in over 50 lung transplant recipients. Because of the lipid properties, it was hypothesized that ABLC would be more effectively nebulized with greater pulmonary deposition than conventional amphotericin B. Consistent with this hypothesis, very low rates of intolerance and very low rates of fungal infection were seen in patients who received nebulized ABLC.[185] Although further study is needed, nebulized ABLC seems a promising approach to prevent fungal infections without systemic toxicities after lung transplantation.

Results

Since 1990, over 16,000 lung transplants, including almost 9000 single-lung and over 7000 double-lung transplants, have been performed.[2] The major recipient indications for transplantation in the ISHLT registry include COPD (39%), IPF (17%), CF (16%), α_1-antitrypsin deficiency emphysema (9%), and PPH (4%). The 1-, 3-, 5-, and 10-year survival rates reported in this registry were 74%, 58%, 47%, and 24% respectively. The mortality rate was highest in the first year. Bilateral lung transplant recipients after the first year had higher survival rates compared to single-lung transplant recipients. However, bilateral and single-lung transplant recipients vary in their comorbidities and indication for transplantation, so a direct comparison without consideration of influential variables is difficult to interpret. The most common causes of early deaths are graft failure and non-CMV infections, with BOS the primary cause of late death.[2]

Our combined centers have performed over 1300 lung transplants. As in the ISHLT database, COPD leads as the cause of transplantation, followed by CF, IPF, and PPH.

Hosenpud and colleagues,[24] based on data from the joint United Network for Organ Sharing/International Society of Heart and Lung Transplantation Thoracic registry, reported a survival benefit for patients undergoing lung transplantation for CF and IPF but not for patients transplanted for end-stage emphysema. Other studies have shown a survival benefit for emphysema in addition to IPF, CF, and pulmonary hypertension.[30]

Multiple studies have addressed quality of life in lung transplant recipients.[186–190] Improvement in quality of life is seen posttransplant and usually becomes evident after 3–6 months. Mobility, energy, sleep, activities of daily living, dependency level, and dyspnea were reported to be improved following lung transplantation.[190] Pretransplant psychological status appears to affect posttransplant quality of life and adjustment.[187] Paris and colleagues evaluated return to work after lung transplantation and reported 22% were employed, 38% were unemployed but medically able to work, 29% were disabled, and 10% had retired.[191]

The economic impact of lung transplantation has been assessed in the United Kingdom. Anwanyu and colleagues[192] compared the costs of lung transplantation to the cost of remaining on the waiting list. They concluded that, although lung transplantation is an expensive treatment, benefits in survival and quality-of-life gains are seen, and bilateral lung transplantation appears to be more cost-effective than single-lung transplantation.

Pediatric Lung Transplantation

According to the ISHLT registry, approximately 60 pediatric lung transplants are performed each year, with approximately 800 total having been reported.[193] While most pediatric lung transplants are performed after the age 10, because of congenital anomalies there are a number performed in the first year of life. Many donor lungs come from adults. In infants, congenital heart disease, PPH, and pulmonary vascular disease are the main indications for lung transplantation. During childhood and adolescence, CF accounts for the majority of lung transplants. Approximately 40% of pediatric lung transplant recipients survive 5 years. Most mortality occurs early following transplantation. If only recipients surviving the first year of transplantation are included, 50% are alive at 6.7 years. Bilateral lung transplant recipients show an improved survival compared to single-lung transplant recipients, but this may be an effect of underlying disease and other recipient factors. The vast majority of pediatric lung transplants are bilateral (89%). As in adults, early mortality after pediatric lung transplantation is secondary to infections and graft failure, and late mortality is attributed mostly to BO.[193] Functional status in pediatric lung transplants is excellent, with more than 80% reporting no activity limitations at 5 years.

Living lobar transplantation has been used most commonly in pediatric lung transplantation. The procedure involves harvest of a left lower lobe from one healthy donor and a right lower lobe from another donor. Both lobes are implanted as bilateral grafts into a single recipient. This strategy was pioneered by the University of Southern California program.[40] They have reported that pediatric patients receiving living lobar transplants have less BOS and better pulmonary function than pediatric recipients receiving cadaveric donor lungs.[41] Living lobar transplant has been conducted in other centers as well; however, the success of the USC program has been difficult to duplicate. Thus far, there have been no reports of donor fatality, but a significant number of complications have been encountered.[42] In the recipients undergoing lobar transplants for CF, the 1-year survival is 73.8%, and in the recipients with other lung diseases, the 1-year survival is 75%.[39]

Only 20–30 centers are currently performing pediatric lung transplants. One of our centers began its pediatric lung transplant program in July 1990 and performed its first infant lung transplant in 1993. Currently, the largest pediatric lung transplant program worldwide, our center has performed 262 pediatric lung transplants (and 16 heart-lung transplants) since its inception. Of these, the vast majority (>75%) have been bilateral, but over 40 have been bilateral lobar (living donor) (St. Louis Children's Hospital Lung Transplant Registry; Huddleston, personal communication). The indications for lung transplantation were, in decreasing order, CF (42%), pulmonary vascular disease (21%), BO (10%), pulmonary alveolar proteinosis (6%), pulmonary fibrosis (7%), and other (12%). The average age of recipients at the time of transplantation was 9.5 ± 5.9 years.[194] Actuarial survival at our center was 77% at 1 year, 62% at 3 years, and 55% at 5 years. The most common cause of early mortality was graft failure. Late mortality was most commonly secondary to BO (57%), infection (21%), and posttransplant malignancies (18%).[194]

Conclusion

Lung transplantation currently is the preferred treatment option for a variety of end-stage pulmonary diseases. Improvements in organ preservation, surgical techniques, infection prophylaxis, and immunosuppression medications have resulted in durable and steady improvements in transplant outcomes and have allowed for expanded uses of lung transplantation.

As we now advance through the third decade of successful clinical lung transplantation, the major obstacle to long-term survival in recipients remains chronic rejection. While our understanding of chronic rejection is continuing to evolve, it has proven to be a challenging adversary. Despite identification of risk factors and development of treatment strategies, chronic rejection remains a major source of morbidity and mortality. Hope may lie with the promotion of immune tolerance.

References

1. Toronto Lung Transplantation Group. Unilateral lung transplantation for pulmonary fibrosis. N Engl J Med 1986;314:1140–1145.
2. Trulock EP, Edwards LB, Taylor DO, et al. The Registry of the International Society for Heart and Lung Transplantation: 21 official adult lung and heart-lung transplant report—2004. J Heart Lung Transplant 2004;23:804–815.
3. Hardy JD, Webb WR, Dalton ML, Walker GR. Lung homotransplantation in man. JAMA 1963;186:1065–1074.
4. Wildevuur CRH, Benfield JR. A review of 23 human lung transplantations by 20 surgeons. Ann Thorac Surg 1970;9:489–515.
5. Nelems W. Human lung transplantation. Chest 1980;78:569.
6. Lima O, Cooper JD, Peters WJ, et al. Effects of methylprednisolone and azathioprine on bronchial healing following lung autotransplantation. J Thorac Cardiovasc Surg 1981;82:211.

7. Lima O, Goldberg M, Peters WJ, et al. Bronchial omentopexy in canine lung transplantation. J Thorac Cardiovasc Surg 1982;83:418–421.
8. Patterson GA, Cooper JD, Goldman B, et al. Technique of successful clinical double-lung transplantation. Ann Thorac Surg 1988;45:626–632.
9. Dark JH, Patterson GA, Al-Jilaihawi AN, et al. Experimental en bloc double-lung transplantation. Ann Thorac Surg 1986;42:394–398.
10. Pasque MK, Cooper JD, Kaiser LR, et al. An improved technique for bilateral lung transplantation: rationale and initial clinical experience. Ann Thorac Surg 1990;49:785–791.
11. Maurer JR, Frost AE, Estenne M, et al. International guidelines for selection of lung transplant candidates. J Heart Lung Transplant 1998;17:703–709.
12. Hertz MI, Taylor DO, Trulock EP, et al. The Registry of the International Society for Heart and Lung Transplantation: 19th official report—2002. J Heart Lung Transplant 2002;21:950–970.
13. Aris RM, Neuringer IP, Weiner MA, et al. Severe osteoporosis before and after lung transplantation. Chest 1996;109:1176–1183.
14. Gray-Donald K, Gibbons L, Shapiro SH, et al. Nutritional status and mortality in chronic obstructive pulmonary disease. Am J Respir Crit Care Med 1996;153:961–966.
15. Meyers BF, Patterson GA. Lung transplantation versus lung volume reduction as surgical therapy for emphysema. World J Surg 2001;25:238–243.
16. Meyers BF, Yusen RD, Guthrie TJ, et al. Outcome of bilateral lung volume reduction in patients with emphysema potentially eligible for lung transplantation. J Thorac Cardiovasc Surg. 2001;122:10–17.
17. Sundaresan S, Shiraishi Y, Trulock EP, et al. Single or bilateral lung transplantation for emphysema? J Thorac Cardiovasc Surg 1996;112:1485–1495.
18. Weill D, Keshavjee S. Lung transplantation for emphysema: two lungs or one. J Heart Lung Transplant 2001;20:739–742.
19. Meyer DM, Bennett LE, Novick RJ, Hosenpud JD. Single versus bilateral, sequential lung transplantation for end-stage emphysema: influence of recipient age on survival and secondary endpoints. J Heart Lung Transplant 2001;20:935–941.
20. Dodge JA, Morison S, Lewis PA, et al. Cystic fibrosis in the United Kingdom, 1968–1988: incidence, population, and survival. Paediatric Perinatal Epidemiol 1993;7:157–166.
21. Liou TG, Adler FR, Cahill B, et al. Survival effect of lung transplantation among patients with cystic fibrosis. JAMA 2001;286:2683–2689.
22. Chaparro C, Maurer J, Gutierrez C, et al. Infection with *Burkholderia cepacia* in cystic fibrosis: outcome following lung transplantation. Am J Respir Crit Care Med 2001;163:43–48.
23. Aris RM, Routh JC, LiPuma JJ, et al. Lung transplantation for cystic fibrosis patients with *Burkholderia cepacia* complex. Survival linked to genomovar type. Am J Respir Crit Care Med 2001;164:2102–2106.
24. Hosenpud JD, Bennett LE, Keck BM, et al. Effect of diagnosis on survival benefit of lung transplantation for end-stage lung disease. Lancet 1998;351:24–27.
25. United Network of Organ Sharing. UNOS Policy 3.7.5.1. Allocation of Thoracic Organs, Waiting Time Accrual for Lung Candidates With Idiopathic Pulmonary Fibrosis (IPF). Richmond, VA: UNOS; 1997.
26. Trulock EP. Recipient selection. Chest Surg Clin North Am 1993;3:1–18.
27. Meyers BF, Lynch JP, Trulock EP, et al. Single versus bilateral lung transplantation for idiopathic pulmonary fibrosis: a 10-year institutional experience. J Thorac Cardiovasc Surg 2000;120:99–107.
28. McLaughlin VV, Genthner DE, Panella MM, Rich S. Reduction in pulmonary vascular resistance with long-term epoprostenol (prostacyclin) therapy in primary pulmonary hypertension. N Engl J Med 1998;338:273–277.
29. De Meester J, Smits JM, Persijn GG, Haverich A. Listing for lung transplantation: life expectancy and transplant effect, stratified by type of end-stage lung disease, the Eurotransplant experience. J Heart Lung Transplant 2001;20:518–524.
30. Charman SC, Sharples LD, McNeil KD, Wallwork J. Assessment of survival benefit after lung transplantation by patient diagnosis. J Heart Lung Transplant 2002;21:226–232.
31. Waddell TK, Bennett L, Kennedy R, et al. Heart-lung or lung transplantation for Eisenmenger syndrome. J Heart Lung Transplant 2002;21:731–737.
32. Sundaresan S, Trachiotis GD, Aoe M, et al. Donor lung procurement: assessment and operative technique. Ann Thorac Surg 1993;56:1409–1413.
33. Straznicka M, Follette DM, Eisner MD, et al. Aggressive management of lung donors classified as unacceptable: excellent recipient survival 1 year after transplantation. J Thorac Cardiovasc Surg 2002;124:250–258.
34. Sundaresan S, Semenkovich J, Ochoa L, et al. Successful outcome of lung transplantation is not compromised by the use of marginal donor lungs. J Thorac Cardiovasc Surg 1995;109:1075–1080.
35. Lau CL, Guthrie TJ, Scavuzzo M, et al. Lobectomy to downsize donor lungs for use in small recipients. J Heart Lung Transplant 2003;22:S116–S117.
36. Follette DM, Rudich SM, Babcock WD. Improved oxygenation and increased lung donor recovery with high-dose steroid administration after brain death. J Heart Lung Transplant 1998;17:423–429.
37. Cummings J, Houck J, Lichtenfeld D. Positive effect of aggressive resuscitative efforts on cadaver lung procurement. J Transplant Coord 1995;5:103–106.
38. Barbers RG. Cystic fibrosis: bilateral living lobar versus cadaveric lung transplantation. Am J Med Sci 1998;315:155–160.
39. Starnes VA, Barr ML, Schenkel FA, et al. Experience with living-donor lobar transplantation for indications other than cystic fibrosis. The J Thorac Cardiovasc Surg 1997;114:917–922.
40. Cohen RG, Barr ML, Schenkel FA, et al. Living-related donor lobectomy for bilateral lobar transplantation in patients with cystic fibrosis. Ann Thorac Surg 1994;57:1423–1428.
41. Starnes VA, Woo MS, MacLaughlin EF, et al. Comparison of outcomes between living donor and cadaveric lung transplantation in children. Ann Thorac Surg 1999;68:2279–2283; discussion 2283–2284.
42. Battafarano RJ, Anderson RC, Meyers BF, et al. Perioperative complications after living donor lobectomy. J Thorac Cardiovasc Surg 2000;120:909–915.
43. Couetil JA, Tolan MJ, Loulmet DF, et al. Pulmonary bipartitioning and lobar transplantation: a new approach to donor organ shortage. J Thorac Cardiovasc Surg 1997;113:529–537.
44. Artemiou O, Birsan T, Taghavi S, et al. Bilateral lobar transplantation with the split lung technique. J Thorac Cardiovasc Surg 1999;118:369–370.
45. Steen S, Sjoberg T, Pierre L, et al. Transplantation of lungs from a non-heart-beating donor [comment]. Lancet 2001;357:825–829.
46. Gaca JG, Lesher A, Aksoy O, et al. Disseminated intravascular coagulation in association with pig-to-primate pulmonary xenotransplantation. Transplantation 2002;73:1717–1723.
47. Meyers BF, Sundaresan RS, Guthrie T, et al. Bilateral sequential lung transplantation without sternal division eliminates posttransplantation sternal complications. J Thorac Cardiovasc Surg 1998;117:358–364.

48. King-Biggs MB, Dunitz JM, Park SJ, et al. Airway anastomotic dehiscence associated with use of sirolimus immediately after lung transplantation. Transplantation 2003;75:1437–1443.
49. Palmer SM, Miralles AP, Lawrence CM, et al. Rabbit antithymocyte globulin decreases acute rejection after lung transplantation: results of a randomized, prospective study. Chest 1999;116: 127–133.
50. Garrity ER Jr, Villanueva J, Bhorade SM, et al. Low rate of acute lung allograft rejection after the use of daclizumab, an interleukin 2 receptor antibody. Transplantation 2001;71:773–777.
51. Brock MV, Borja MC, Ferber L, et al. Induction therapy in lung transplantation: a prospective, controlled clinical trial comparing OKT3, anti-thymocyte globulin, and daclizumab. J Heart Lung Transplant 2001;20:1282–1290.
52. Zamora MR. Controversies in lung transplantation: management of cytomegalovirus infections. J Heart Lung Transplant 2002;21:841–849.
53. Ettinger NA, Bailey TC, Trulock EP, et al. Cytomegalovirus infection and pneumonitis. Impact after isolation lung transplantation. Am Rev Respir Dis 1993;147:1017–1023.
54. Guilinger RA, Paradis IL, Dauber JH, et al. The importance of bronchoscopy with transbronchial biopsy and bronchoalveolar lavage in the management of lung transplant recipients. Am J Respir Crit Care Med 1995;152:2037–2043.
55. Hopkins PM, Aboyoun CL, Chhajed PN, et al. Prospective analysis of 1235 transbronchial lung biopsies in lung transplant recipients. J Heart Lung Transplant 2002;21:1062–1067.
56. Trulock EP, Ettinger NA, Brunt EM, et al. The role of transbronchial lung biopsy in the treatment of lung transplant recipients: an analysis of 200 consecutive procedures. Chest 1992;102:1049–1054.
57. Sibley RK. The role of transbronchial biopsies in the management of lung transplant recipients. J Heart Lung Transplant 1993;12:308–324.
58. Boehler A, Vogt P, Zollinger A, et al. Prospective study of the value of transbronchial lung biopsy after lung transplantation. Eur Respir J 1996;9:658–662.
59. Baz MA, Layish DT, Govert JA, et al. Diagnostic yield of bronchoscopies after isolated lung transplantation [comment]. Chest 1996;110:84–88.
60. Yousem SA. Significance of clinically silent untreated mild acute cellular rejection in lung allograft recipients. Hum Pathol 1996;27:269–273.
61. Valentine VG, Taylor DE, Dhillon GS, et al. Success of lung transplantation without surveillance bronchoscopy. J Heart Lung Transplant 2002;21:319–326.
62. Kesten S, Chamberlain D, Maurer J. Yield of surveillance transbronchial biopsies performed beyond two years after lung transplantation. J Heart Lung Transplant 1996;15:384–388.
63. Chaparro C, Maurer JR, Chamberlain DW, Todd TR. Role of open lung biopsy for diagnosis in lung transplant recipients: 10-year experience. Ann Thorac Surg 1995;59:928–932.
64. Lau CL, Patterson GA, Scott M. Palmer J. Critical care aspects of lung transplantation. J Intensive Care Med 2004;19:83–104.
65. Matsuzaki Y, Waddell TK, Puskas JD, et al. Amelioration of post-ischemic lung reperfusion injury by PGE1. Am Rev Respir Dis 1993;148:882–889.
66. Keshavjee S, Yamazaki F, Cardoso PF, et al. A method for safe 12-hour pulmonary preservation. J Thorac Cardiovasc Surg 1989;98:529–534.
67. Maccherini M, Keshavjee SH, Slutsky AS, et al. The effect of low-potassium-dextran versus Euro-Collins solution for preservation of isolated type II pneumocytes. Transplantation 1991; 52:621–626.
68. Fischer S, Matte-Martyn A, De Perrot M, et al. Low-potassium dextran preservation solution improves lung function after human lung transplantation. J Thorac Cardiovasc Surg. 2001;121: 594–596.
69. Yamashita M, Schmid RA, Ando K, et al. Nitroprusside ameliorates lung allograft reperfusion injury. Ann Thorac Surg 1996;62: 791–797.
70. Fujino S, Nagahiro I, Triantafillou AN, et al. Inhaled nitric oxide at the time of harvest improves early lung allograft function. Ann Thorac Surg 1997;63:1383–1390.
71. Halldorsson A, Kronon M, Allen BS, et al. Controlled reperfusion prevents pulmonary injury after 24-hours of lung preservation. Ann Thorac Surg 1998;66.
72. Halldorsson A, Kronon M, Allen BS, et al. Controlled reperfusion after lung ischemia: implications for improved function after lung transplantation. J Thorac Cardiovasc Surg 1998;115: 415–425.
73. Clark SC, Sudarshan C, Khanna R, et al. Controlled reperfusion and pentoxifylline modulates reperfusion injury after single lung transplantation. J Thorac Cardiovasc Surg 1998;115:1335–1341.
74. Bhabra MS, Hopkinson DN, Shaw TE, et al. Controlled reperfusion protects lung grafts during a transient early increase in permeability. Ann Thorac Surg 1998;65:187–192.
75. Halldorsson AO, Kronon MT, Allen BS, et al. Lowering reperfusion pressure reduces the injury after pulmonary ischemia. Ann Thorac Surg 2000;69:198–203.
76. Clark SC, Sudarshan CD, Dark JH. Controlled perfusion of the transplanted lung [comment]. Ann Thorac Surg 2001;71:1755–1756.
77. Fiser SM, Kron IL, Long SM, et al. Controlled perfusion decreases reperfusion injury after high-flow reperfusion. J Heart Lung Transplant 2002;21:687–691.
78. Lick SD, Brown PS, Jr., Kurusz M, et al. Technique of controlled reperfusion of the transplanted lung in humans [comment]. Ann Thorac Surg 2000;69:910–912.
79. Date H, Triantafillou A, Trulock E, et al. Inhaled nitric oxide reduces human lung allograft dysfunction. J Thorac Cardiovasc Surg 1996;111:913–919.
80. Fiser SM, Cope JT, Kron IL, et al. Aerosolized prostacyclin (epoprostenol) as an alternative to inhaled nitric oxide for patients with reperfusion injury after lung transplantation [erratum appears in J Thorac Cardiovasc Surg 2001;121:1136]. J Thorac Cardiovasc Surg 2001;121:981–982.
81. Meyers BF, Sundt TM 3rd, Henry S, et al. Selective use of extracorporeal membrane oxygenation is warranted after lung transplantation. J Thorac Cardiovasc Surg 2000;120:20–26.
82. Chhajed PJ, Malouf MM, Tamm M, et al. Interventional bronchoscopy for the management of airway complications following lung transplantation. Chest 2001;120:1894–1899.
83. Griffith BP, Hardesty RL, Armitage JM, et al. A decade of lung transplantation. Ann Surg 1993;218:310–320.
84. Schafers HJ, Haydock DA, Cooper JD. The prevalence and management of bronchial anastomotic complications in lung transplantation. J Thorac Cardiovasc Surg 1991;101:1044–1052.
85. Shennib H, Massard G. Airway complications in lung transplantation. Ann Thorac Surg 1994;57:506–511.
86. Date H, Trulock EP, Arcidi JM, et al. Improved airway healing after lung transplantation. An analysis of 348 bronchial anastomoses. J Thorac Cardiovasc Surg 1995;110:1424–1432; discussion 1432–1433.
87. Kramer MR, Denning DW, Marshall SE, et al. Ulcerative tracheobronchitis after lung transplantation. A new form of invasive aspergillosis. Am Rev Respir Dis 1991;144:552–556.
88. Nunley DR, Gal AA, Vega JD, et al. Saprophytic fungal infections and complications involving the bronchial anastomosis following human lung transplantation. Chest 2002;122:1185–1191.
89. Palmer SM, Perfect JR, Howell DN, et al. Candidal anastomotic infection in lung transplant recipients: successful treatment with a combination of systemic and inhaled antifungal agents. J Heart Lung Transplant 1998;17:1029–1033.

90. Hadjiliadis D, Howell DN, Davis RD, et al. Anastomotic infections in lung transplant recipients. Ann Transplant 2000;5:13–19.
91. de Hoyos A, Patterson GA, Maurer J. Pulmonary transplantation: early and late results. J Thorac Cardiovasc Surg 1992;103:295–306.
92. Frost AE, Jammal CT, Cagle PT. Hyperacute rejection following lung transplantation. Chest 1996;110:559–562.
93. Bittner HB, Dunitz J, Hertz M, et al. Hyperacute rejection in single lung transplantation—case report of successful management by means of plasmapheresis and antithymocyte globulin treatment. Transplantation 2001;71:649–651.
94. Choi JK, Kearns J, Palevsky HI, et al. Hyperacute rejection of a pulmonary allograft. Immediate clinical and pathologic findings. Am J Respir Crit Care Med 1999;160:1015–1018.
95. Saint Martin GA, Reddy VB, Garrity DR, et al. Humoral (antibody-mediated) rejection in lung transplantation. J Heart Lung Transplant 1996;15:1217–1222.
96. Lau CL, Palmer SM, Posther KE, et al. Influence of panel-reactive antibodies on posttransplant outcomes in lung transplant recipients. Ann Thorac Surg 2000;69:1520–1524.
97. Magro CM, Deng A, Pope-Harman A, et al. Humorally mediated posttransplantation septal capillary injury syndrome as a common form of pulmonary allograft rejection: a hypothesis. Transplantation 2002;74:1273–1280.
98. Levine SM, Bryan CL. Bronchiolitis obliterans in lung transplant recipients. The "thorn in the side" of lung transplantation [comment]. Chest 1995;107:894–897.
99. Trulock EP. Lung transplantation. Am J Respir Crit Care Med 1997;155:789–818.
100. De Hoyos A, Chamberlain D, Schvartzman R, et al. Prospective assessment of a standardized pathologic grading system for acute rejection in lung transplantation. Chest 1993;103:1813–1818.
101. Trulock EP. Management of lung transplant rejection. Chest 1993;13:1566–1576.
102. Yousem SA, Berry GJ, Brunt EM, et al. A working formulation for the standardization of nomenclature in the diagnosis of heart and lung rejection: lung rejection study group. J Heart Lung Transplant 1990;9:593–601.
103. Yousem SA, Berry GJ, Cagle PT, et al. Revision of the 1990 working formulation for the classification of pulmonary allograft rejection: lung rejection study group. J Heart Lung Transplant 1996;15:1–15.
104. Keenan RJ, Konishi H, Kawai A, et al. Clinical trial of tacrolimus versus cyclosporine in lung transplantation. Ann Thorac Surg 1995;60:580–585.
105. Treede H, Klepetko W, Reichenspurner H, et al. Tacrolimus versus cyclosporine after lung transplantation: a prospective, open, randomized two-center trial comparing two different immunosuppressive protocols. J Heart Lung Transplant 2001; 20:511–517.
106. Vitulo P, Oggionni T, Cascina A, et al. Efficacy of tacrolimus rescue therapy in refractory acute rejection after lung transplantation. J Heart Lung Transplant 2002;21:435–439.
107. Horning NR, Lynch JP, Sundaresan SR, et al. Tacrolimus therapy for persistent or recurrent acute rejection after lung transplantation. J Heart Lung Transplant 1998;17:761–767.
108. Palmer SM, Baz MA, Sanders L, et al. Results of a randomized, prospective, multicenter trial of mycophenolate mofetil versus azathioprine in the prevention of acute lung allograft rejection. Transplantation 2001;71:1772–1776.
109. Corris PA, Glanville A, McNeil K, et al. One year analysis of an ongoing international randomized study of mycophenolate mofetil (MMF) versus azathioprine (AZA) in lung transplantation [abstract]. J Heart Lung Transplant 2001;20:149–150.
110. Sollinger HW, Group USRTMMS. Mycophenolate mofetil for the prevention of acute rejection in primary cadaveric renal allograft recipients. Transplantation 1995;60:225–232.
111. Kahan BD. Efficacy of sirolimus compared with azathioprine for reduction of acute renal allograft rejection: a randomised multicentre study. The Rapamune U.S. Study Group [comment]. Lancet 2000;356:194–202.
112. Hong JC, Kahan BD. Sirolimus rescue therapy for refractory rejection in renal transplantation. Transplantation 2001;71:1579–1584.
113. Williams JW, Mital D, Chong A, et al. Experiences with leflunomide in solid organ transplantation. Transplantation 2002;73:358–366.
114. Snell GI, Levvey BJ, Chin W, et al. Rescue therapy: a role for sirolimus in lung and heart transplant recipients. Transpl Proc 2001;33:1084–1085.
115. Aboyoun CL, Tamm M, Chhajed PN, et al. Diagnostic value of follow-up transbronchial lung biopsy after lung rejection. Am J Respir Crit Care Med 2001;164:460–463.
116. Sheenib H, Massard G, Reynaud M, Noirclerc MJ. Efficacy of OKT3 therapy for acute rejection in isolated lung transplantation. J Heart Lung Transplant 1994;13:514–519.
117. Griffith BP, Hardesty RL, Armitage JM, et al. Acute rejection of lung allografts with various immunosuppressive protocols. Ann Thorac Surg 1992;54:846–851.
118. Barlow CW, Moon MR, Green GR, et al. Rabbit antithymocyte globulin versus OKT3 induction therapy after heart-lung and lung transplantation: effect on survival, rejection, infection, and obliterative bronchiolitis. Transplant Int 2001;14:234–239.
119. Iacono AT, Smaldone GC, Keenan RJ, et al. Dose-related reversal of acute lung rejection by aerosolized cyclosporine. Am J Respir Crit Care Med 1997;155:1690–1698.
120. Reams BD, Davis RD, Curl J, Palmer SM. Treatment of refractory acute rejection in a lung transplant recipient with campath 1H. Transplantation 2002;74:903–904.
121. Cahill BC, O'Rourke MK, Strasburg KA, et al. Methotrexate for lung transplant recipients with steroid-resistant acute rejection. J Heart Lung Transplant 1996;15:1130–1137.
122. Andreu G, Achkar A, Couetil JP, et al. Extracorporeal photochemotherapy treatment for acute lung rejection episode. J Heart Lung Transplant 1995;14:793.
123. Villanueva J, Bhorade SM, Robinson JA, et al. Extracorporeal photopheresis for the treatment of lung allograft rejection. Ann Transplant 2000;5:44–47.
124. Valentine VG, Robbins RC, Wehner JH, et al. Total lymphoid irradiation for refractory acute rejection in heart-lung and lung allografts. Chest 1996;109:1184.
125. Burke CM, Theodore J, Dawkins KD, et al. Post-transplant obliterative bronchiolitis and other late lung sequelae in human heart lung transplantation. Chest 1984;86:824–829.
126. Chamberlain D, Maurer J, Chaparro C, Idolor L. Evaluation of transbronchial lung biopsy specimens in the diagnosis of bronchiolitis obliterans after lung transplantation. J Heart Lung Transplant 1994;13:963–971.
127. ISHLT, Cooper JD, Billingham M, et al. A working formulation for the standardization of nomenclature and for clinical staging of chronic dysfunction in lung allografts. J Heart Lung Transplant 1993;12:713–716.
128. Estenne M, Maurer JR, Boehler A, et al. Bronchiolitis obliterans syndrome 2001: an update of the diagnostic criteria. J Heart Lung Transplant 2002;21:297–310.
129. Sharples LD, McNeil K, Stewart S, Wallwork J. Risk factors for bronchiolitis obliterans: a systematic review of recent publications. J Heart Lung Transplant 2002;21:271–281.
130. Jackson CH, Sharples LD, McNeil K, et al. Acute and chronic onset of bronchiolitis obliterans syndrome (BOS): are they different entities? J Heart Lung Transplant 2002;21:658–666.
131. Ross DJ, Lweis MI, Kramer M, et al. FK 506 "rescue" immunosuppression for obliterative bronchiolitis after lung transplantation. Chest 1997;112:1175–1179.

132. Kesten S, Chaparro C, Scavuzzo M, et al. Tacrolimus as rescue therapy for bronchiolitis obliterans syndrome. J Heart Lung Transplant 1997;16:905–912.
133. Revell MP, Lewis ME, Llewellyn-Jones CG, et al. Conservation of small-airway function by tacrolimus/cyclosporine conversion in the management of bronchiolitis obliterans following lung transplantation. J Heart Lung Transplant 2000;19:1219–1223.
134. Sarahrudi K, Carretta A, Wisser W, et al. The value of switching from cyclosporine to tacrolimus in the treatment of refractory acute rejection and obliterative bronchiolitis after lung transplantation. Transplant Int 2002;15:24–28.
135. Whyte RI, Rossi SJ, Mulligan MS, et al. Mycophenolate mofetil for obliterative bronchiolitis syndrome after lung transplantation. Ann Thorac Surg 1997;64:945–949.
136. Speich R, Boehler A, Thurnheer R, Weder W. Salvage therapy with mycophenolate mofetil for lung transplantation bronchiolitis obliterans: importance of dosage. Transplantation 1997;64:533–535.
137. Verleden GM, Buyse B, Delcroix M, et al. Cyclophosphamide rescue therapy for chronic rejection after lung transplantation. J Heart Lung Transplant 1999;18:1139–1142.
138. Date H, Lynch JP, Sundaresan S, et al. The impact of cytolytic therapy on bronchiolitis obliterans syndrome. J Heart Lung Transplant 1998;17:869–875.
139. Snell GI, Esmore DS, Williams TJ. Cytolytic therapy for the bronchiolitis obliterans syndrome complicating lung transplantation. Chest 1996;109:874–878.
140. Kesten S, Rajagopalan N, Maurer J. Cytolytic therapy for the treatment of bronchiolitis obliterans syndrome following lung transplantation. Transplantation 1996;61:427–430.
141. Dusmet M, Maurer J, Winston T, Kesten S. Methotrexate can halt the progression of bronchiolitis obliterans syndrome in lung transplant recipients. J Heart Lung Transplant 1996;15:948–954.
142. Speich R, Boehler A, Russi EW, et al. A case report of a double-blind, randomized trial of inhaled steroids in a patient with lung transplant bronchiolitis obliterans. Respiration 1997;64:375–380.
143. Iacono AT, Keenan R, Duncan SR, et al. Aerosolized cyclosporine in lung recipients with refractory chronic rejection. Am J Respir Crit Care Med 1996;153:1451–1455.
144. Diamond DA, Michalski JM, Lynch JP, Trulock EP. Efficacy of total lymphoid irradiation for chronic allograft rejection following bilateral lung transplantation. Int J Radiat Oncol 1998;41:795–800.
145. Slovis BS, Loyd JE, L.E. King J. Photopheresis for chronic rejection of lung allografts. N Engl J Med 1995;332:962.
146. O'Hagan AR, Stillwell PC, Arroliga A, Koo A. Photopheresis in the treatment of refractory bronchiolitis obliterans complicating lung transplantation. Chest 1999;115:1459–1462.
147. Palmer SM, Miralles AP, Howell DN, et al. Gastroesophageal reflux as a reversible cause of allograft dysfunction after lung transplantation. Chest 2000;118:1214–1217.
148. Lau CL, Palmer SM, Howell DN, et al. Laparoscopic anti-reflux surgery in the lung transplant population. Surg Endosc 2002;16:1674–1678.
149. Davis RD, Lau CL, Eubanks S, et al. Improved lung allograft function following fundoplication in lung transplant patients with GERD. J Thorac Cardiovasc Surg 2003;125:533–542.
150. Starzl TE, Demetris AJ, M. T, et al. Systemic chimerism in human female recipients of male livers. Lancet 1992;340:876–877.
151. Pham SM, Rao AS, Zeevi A, et al. Effects of donor bone marrow infusion in clinical lung transplantation. Ann Thorac Surg 2000;69:345–350.
152. Novick RJ, Stitt LW, Al-Kattan K, et al. Pulmonary retransplantation: predictors of graft function and survival in 230 patients. Ann Thorac Surg 1998;65:227–234.
153. Chaparro C, Kesten S. Infections in lung transplant recipients. Clin Chest Med 1997;18:339–351.
154. Bassiri AG, Girgis RE, Theodore S. Actinomyces odontolyticus thoracopulmonary infections. Two cases in lung and heart-lung transplant recipients and review of the literature. Am J Respir Crit Care Med 1995;152:374–376.
155. Palmer SM, Alexander BD, Sanders LL, et al. Significance of blood stream infection after lung transplantation: analysis in 176 consecutive patients. Transplantation 2000;69:2360–2366.
156. Gutierrez CA, Chaparro C, Drajden M, et al. Cytomegalovirus viremia in lung transplant recipients receiving ganciclovir and immune globulin. Chest 1998;113:924–932.
157. Kruger RM, Paranjothi S, MD GAS, et al. Impact of prophylaxis with cytogam alone on the incidence of CMV viremia in CMV-seropositive lung transplant recipients. J Heart Lung Transplant 2003;22:754–763.
158. Zedtwitz-Liebenstein K, Presterl E, Deviatko E, Graninger W. Acute renal failure in a lung transplant patient after therapy with cidofovir. Transplant Int 2001;14:445–446.
159. Palmer SM Jr, Henshaw NG, Howell DN, et al. Community respiratory viral infection in adult lung transplant recipients [comment]. Chest 1998;113:944–950.
160. Holt ND, Gould FK, Taylor CE, et al. Incidence and significance of noncytomegalovirus viral respiratory infection after adult lung transplantation. J Heart Lung Transplant 1997;16:416–419.
161. Matar LD, McAdams HP, Palmer SM, et al. Respiratory viral infections in lung transplant recipients: radiologic findings with clinical correlation. Radiology 1999;213:735–742.
162. Garantziotis S, Howell DN, McAdams HP, et al. Influenza pneumonia in lung transplant recipients: clinical features and association with bronchiolitis obliterans syndrome [comment]. Chest 2001;119:1277–1280.
163. McCurdy LH, Milstone A, Dummer S. Clinical features and outcomes of paramyxoviral infection in lung transplant recipients treated with ribavirin. J Heart Lung Transplant 2003;22:745–753.
164. Blumberg EA, Albano C, Pruett T, et al. The immunogenicity of influenza virus vaccine in solid organ transplant recipients. Clin Infect Dis 1996;22:295–302.
165. Wandstrat TL. Respiratory syncytial virus immune globulin intravenous. Ann Pharmacother 1997;31:83–88.
166. Zahradnik JM. Adenovirus pneumonia. Semin Respir Infect 1987;2:104–111.
167. Jurado M, Navarro JM, Hernandez J, et al. Adenovirus-associated haemorrhagic cystitis after bone marrow transplantation successfully treated with intravenous ribavirin. Bone Marrow Transplant 1995;15:651–652.
168. McCarthy AJ, Bergin M, De Silva LM, Stevens M. Intravenous ribavirin therapy for disseminated adenovirus infection. Pediatr Infect Dis J 1995;14:1003–1004.
169. Maslo C, Girard PM, Urban T, et al. Ribavirin therapy for adenovirus pneumonia in an AIDS patient. Am J Respir Crit Care Med 1997;156:1263–1264.
170. Shetty AK, Gans HA, So S, et al. Intravenous ribavirin therapy for adenovirus pneumonia. Pediatr Pulmonol 2000;29:69–73.
171. Cox NJ, Subbarao K. Influenza. Lancet 1999;354:1277–1282.
172. Anonymous. Randomised trial of efficacy and safety of inhaled zanamivir in treatment of influenza A and B virus infections. The MIST (Management of Influenza in the Southern Hemisphere Trialists) Study Group [comment] [erratum appears in Lancet 1999;353:504]. Lancet 1998;352:1877–1881.
173. Dengler TJ, Strnad N, Buhring I, et al. Differential immune response to influenza and pneumococcal vaccination in immunosuppressed patients after heart transplantation. Transplantation 1998;66:1340–1347.
174. Grossi P, Farina C, Fiocchi R, Dalla Gasperina D. Prevalence and outcome of invasive fungal infections in 1963 thoracic organ

transplant recipients: a multicenter retrospective study. Italian Study Group of Fungal Infections in Thoracic Organ Transplant Recipients. Transplantation 2000;70:112–116.
175. Kanj SS, Welty-Wolf K, Madden J, et al. Fungal infections in lung and heart-lung transplant recipients. Report of nine cases and review of the literature. Medicine 1996;75:142–156.
176. Mehrad B, Paciocco G, Martinez FJ, et al. Spectrum of *Aspergillus* infection in lung transplant recipients: case series and review of the literature. Chest 2001;119:169–175.
177. Westney GE, Kesten S, DeHoyos A, et al. *Aspergillus* infection in single and double lung transplant recipients. Transplantation 1996;61:915–919.
178. Hadjiliadis D, Sporn TA, Perfect JR, et al. Outcome of lung transplantation in patients with mycetomas [comment]. Chest. 2002;121:128–134.
179. Nunley DR, Ohori P, Grgurich WF, et al. Pulmonary aspergillosis in cystic fibrosis lung transplant recipients. Chest 1998;114:1321–1329.
180. Husain S, McCurry K, Dauber J, et al. *Nocardia* infection in lung transplant recipients. J Heart Lung Transplant 2002;21:354–359.
181. Palmer SM, Kanj SS, Davis RD, Tapson VF. A case of disseminated infection with *Nocardia brasiliensis* in a lung transplant recipient. Transplantation 1997;63:1189–1190.
182. Raj R, Frost AE. *Scedosporium apiospermum* fungemia in a lung transplant recipient. Chest 2002;121:1714–1716.
183. Calvo V, Borro JM, Morales P, et al. Antifungal prophylaxis during the early postoperative period of lung transplantation. Valencia Lung Transplant Group. Chest 1999;115:1301–1304.
184. Erjavec Z, Woolthuis GM, de Vries-Hospers HG, et al. Tolerance and efficacy of amphotericin B inhalations for prevention of invasive pulmonary aspergillosis in haematological patients. Eur J Clin Microbiol Infect Dis 1997;16:364–368.
185. Palmer SM, Drew RH, Whitehouse JD, et al. Safety of aerosolized amphotericin B lipid complex in lung transplant recipients. Transplantation 2001;72:545–548.
186. Ramsey SD, Patrick DL, Lewis S, et al. Improvement in quality of life after lung transplantation: a preliminary study. J Heart Lung Transplant 1995;14:870–877.
187. Cohen L, Littlefield C, Kelly P, et al. Predictors of quality of life and adjustment after lung transplantation. Chest 1998;113:633–644.
188. Limbos MM, Chan CK, Kesten S. Quality of life in female lung transplant candidates and recipients. Chest 1997;112:1165–1174.
189. Gross CR, Raghu G. The cost of lung transplantation and the quality of life post-transplant. Clin Chest Med 1997;18:391–403.
190. TenVergert EM, Essink-Bot M-L, Geertsma A, et al. The effect of lung transplantation on health-related quality of life. Chest 1998;113:358–364.
191. Paris W, Diercks M, Bright J, et al. Return to work after lung transplantation. J Heart Lung Transplant 1998;17:430–436.
192. Anyanwu AC, McGuire A, Rogers CA, Murday AJ. An economic evaluation of lung transplantation [comment]. J Thorac Cardiovasc Surg 2002;123:411–418; discussion 418–420.
193. Boucek MM, Edwards LB, Keck BM, et al. Registry for the International Society for Heart and Lung Transplantation: seventh official pediatric report—2004. J Heart Lung Transplant 2004;23:933–947.
194. Huddleston CB, Bloch JB, Sweet SC, et al. Lung transplantation in children. Ann Surg 2002;236:270–276.
195. Patterson GA, Cooper JD. Lung transplantation. In: Shields TW, ed. General Thoracic Surgery, Vol. 1. Baltimore: Williams and Wilkins; 1994:1074.
196. Davis RD, Pasque MK. Pulmonary transplantation. Ann Surg 1995;221:14–28.
197. McCurry KR, Iacono AT, Dauber JH, et al. Lung and heart-lung transplantation at the University of Pittsburgh. Clin Transpl 1997;11:209–218.
198. Lau CL, Palmer SM, D'Amico TA, et al. Lung transplantation at Duke University Medical Center. Clin Transpl 1998;12:327–340.

88

Heart Transplantation

Catherine Sudarshan, Daniel Kreisel, and Bruce R. Rosengard

Donor Issues

The clinical success of cardiac transplantation for patients suffering from end-stage heart failure has led to an increased demand for heart donors. Currently, 1.7% of all patients and 45% of the status 1 patients listed for transplantation die while awaiting a suitable donor organ.[1] The availability of donor organs is presently the primary limiting factor to cardiac transplantation. As in the case of abdominal organs, a common approach has been to extend the acceptance criteria for hearts. Donor parameters such as advanced age, high-dose inotropic support, seropositivity for hepatitis C, size mismatch, echocardiographic abnormality, and prolonged cold ischemic time have been reconsidered as relative contraindications to organ usage. Certain criteria such as donor seropositivity for human immunodeficiency virus (HIV), intractable ventricular dysrhythmias, extracranial malignancy, documented prior myocardial infarction, severe coronary artery or valvular disease, and death from carbon monoxide poisoning with a blood carboxyhemoglobin level greater than 20% remain absolute contraindications. Patients are listed according to priority. A large proportion—more than 90% of recipients—are inpatients at the time of transplantation.[2]

Donor Age

There exist conflicting reports with respect to impact of donor age on clinical outcome. The registry of the International Society for Heart and Lung Transplantation considered donor age over 40 years to represent an adverse prognostic feature.[3] Similarly, the United Network for Organ Sharing (UNOS) data on more than 9000 cardiac allograft recipients suggested that donor age was second only to retransplantation as a predictor of early postoperative mortality.[4]

In an attempt to expand the donor pool, cardiac transplant centers have increasingly liberalized age criteria for donor acceptability, and utilization of donors up to the age of 60 years has been reported by several centers. Grafts from old donors are often reserved for older recipients or for emergent situations. Livi et al. compared results of heart transplantation with donors over the age of 40 years with younger donors and found equivalent survival rates and graft performance assessed by echocardiography at 5-year follow-up.[5] Patients who had received grafts from older donors experienced a higher rate of major conduction disturbances, which were mainly observed in the early postoperative period; this can be explained by higher susceptibility of older grafts to ischemia of the conduction tissue.

Similarly, Chau et al. reported an increased incidence of conduction abnormalities in patients who received hearts from a donor over the age of 40 years.[6] The majority of these patients required implantation of permanent pacemakers. Survival rates were comparable with young and old donor hearts, and the authors concluded that older donor hearts may be used successfully with careful selection of the recipients.

A study from Papworth Hospital found a significant increase in incidence of cardiac allograft vasculopathy as assessed by coronary angiography 2 years after transplantation in hearts from donors above the age of 49 years.[7] Despite the increased evidence of vasculopathy, there was no significant difference in patient survival.

Gao et al. analyzed the influence of donor age and preexisting donor coronary artery disease on the later development of cardiac allograft vasculopathy and survival.[8] While patients who had received hearts from donors over the age of 40 years had a higher incidence of cardiac allograft vasculopathy at 3 years posttransplantation, no significant differences were observed at the 6-year mark.

There is little question that hearts recovered from older donors have higher rates of both early and late graft failure. The early failure rate can be minimized by careful screening comprising coronary angiography, invasive hemodynamic monitoring with a pulmonary artery catheter, and echocardiography. Unfortunately, there are no effective strategies to retard the development of cardiac allograft vasculopathy, which has a high incidence in grafts from older donors as a result of preexisting, hemodynamically insignificant coronary artery lesions. Such lesions are frequently not seen on angiograms but are readily apparent when intracoronary ultrasound (ICUS) is used. However, it is not practical to screen donors with ICUS.

Thus, judicious use of older donor hearts is necessary. The authors would favor the use of such hearts in older recipients, highly presensitized recipients with a negative prospective crossmatch, or in desperately ill recipients, particularly those patients in whom ventricular-assist systems are problematic or contraindicated. Thus, the use of older donor hearts in younger, lower-risk recipients should be avoided.

Hepatitis B

Evidence of previous hepatitis B infection is not a contraindication for heart donation. The presence of antibody against the core of hepatitis B with the absence of surface antigen is considered to be safe.[9] However, Ko and colleagues claimed that active infection should not be a contraindication for either receiving or donating a heart. They reported that hepatitis B reactivation after the heart transplantation was common but usually well controlled with lamivudine treatment, and therefore hepatitis B carrier status should not be a contraindication for heart transplantation.[10]

Informed consent should be obtained from the recipient. In suspicious cases of active infection, administration of anti-hepatitis B immunoglobulin and lamivudine should be considered. All recipients who have not been exposed to the virus should be vaccinated once listed.

Hepatitis C

The utilization of organs from hepatitis C virus-positive donors is highly controversial. Seropositivity for hepatitis C among potential organ donors has been reported to be as high as 13% in some geographic regions. It has been clearly established that hepatitis C virus is transmitted through organ transplantation. Transmission rates based on seroconversion have been reported to be between 6% and 100%. This variation in the incidence of transplantation-related transmission reflects differences in the sensitivity of assays used, the variable time to seroconversion, and the differential ability among immunosuppressed patients to mount a detectable antibody response. More recent studies utilizing reverse transcriptase polymerase chain reaction (RT-PCR) to probe for viral antigen reported transmission rates approaching 100%.

There are several case reports of adverse and even fatal outcomes among heart transplant recipients of hepatitis C virus-infected organs.[11] It is generally accepted that the virus replicates more quickly in the setting of immunosuppression and can lead to liver failure over a shorter period of time. Nevertheless, proponents of acceptance of these grafts into the donor pool argue that, in light of the donor organ shortage, the risk of acquiring hepatitis C seropositivity associated with adverse effects in an immunosuppressed state is preferable to death from end-stage heart failure on the waiting list.

Policies regarding acceptance of these organs vary among transplant centers. A study conducted by Lake et al. in 1994 showed that hepatitis C-positive donor organs were utilized by 71% of 72 transplant centers surveyed.[12] The vast majority of centers restricted the use of these grafts and selectively allocated them to hepatitis C-positive candidates and patients who were listed as UNOS status 1. However, transplanting a hepatitis C-positive organ into a hepatitis C-positive recipient carries the risk of superinfection with a more virulent strain, which could lead to rapid progression of preexisting hepatic pathology.[13] Reactivation of the virus should be treated with a combination of once-weekly subcutaneous pegylated α-interferon plus daily oral ribavirin for prolonged periods.[14]

The increasing incidence of hepatitis C in the general population has led to an increasing number of anatomically and physiologically suitable hearts that are not utilized because of positive donor serologies. This loss is particularly true for inner-city trauma victims, with certain organ procurement organizations (OPOs) reporting a 20% discard rate. Although a small percentage of patients receiving a heart from a hepatitis C-positive donor will develop early, fulminant hepatitis, most patients will follow the usual indolent clinical course, perhaps with a slightly accelerated development of cirrhosis. Given the fact that the 10-year survival following heart transplantation is 45%, it is clear that most patients will succumb to cardiac causes long before hepatitis C-related cirrhosis becomes manifest. The authors would, therefore, favor aggressive utilization of hearts from hepatitis C-positive donors, particularly in higher-risk, older, and unstable (status 1A) recipients.

Size Mismatching

Traditionally, careful matching of donor and recipient body weight has been performed in an attempt to avert acute graft failure from utilization of an undersize organ. In general, body weights were matched within 10% of recipient weight. Problems associated with undersize cardiac allografts are primarily failure of the right ventricle in the immediate post-transplant period and reduced left ventricular stroke volume with inability to maintain circulatory support. However, in an attempt to expand the donor heart pool, acceptable weight ranges have been extended, particularly because the correlation between body weight and heart size has been shown to be quite inaccurate.[15] A study by Hosenpud et al. suggested that undersizing by 35% is acceptable for orthotopic heart transplantation.[16]

An intriguing approach to expand the donor pool by downsizing was outlined by Jeevanandam et al.[17] Of currently available donor hearts, 10% come from brain-dead patients between 6 and 14 years of age, a population who make up less than 2% of candidates on the waiting list. Therefore, many donor organs from this age group are not utilized for transplantation. These hearts represent an underused resource, and Jeevanandam et al. showed that these small hearts were able to salvage six adult patients, who had deteriorated rapidly and were in emergent need of a donor organ. Similarly, grossly undersize hearts have been used successfully as heterotopic auxiliary hearts.[18]

In contrast, in the setting of an elevated pulmonary vascular resistance, caution must be exercised in the use of undersize grafts for orthotopic transplants. Tamisier et al. observed an increased rate of early heart failure associated with a higher mortality rate when undersize hearts were used.[19] Reversible pulmonary hypertension, however, is not a contraindication to utilization of undersize hearts.[20]

In general, the best method for size matching donor and recipient is to use height rather than body weight. In most situations, it is safe to use a heart from a donor who is as much as 6 inches (15 cm) shorter than the recipient. This factor is particularly true when the donor is young (≤40), the projected ischemic time is short (≤2.5 h), the donor is hemodynamically stable on minimal doses of inotropes, and the recipient has normal pulmonary vascular resistance. In cases not fitting the aforementioned criteria, caution must be exercised, especially when the donor is female and the recipient is male. The time-honored warning to beware the heart of a middle-aged woman donor dying of a cerebrovascular accident should be strictly observed in size-mismatch situations.

A new twist to the problem in size matching is the shrinkage of the pericardial space consequent to chronic ventricular-assist device (VAD) placement. The combination of complete decompression of the ventricle and pericardial fibrosis induced by the conduits often leads to a small pericardial space. If too large a heart is implanted, tamponade physiology can develop and create difficulties perioperatively.

Gender Mismatching

Several factors, including pregnancy-related exposure to alloantigens, higher baseline levels of circulating antibody, and the immunomodulatory influences of estrogen, are thought to contribute to a more vigorous host-versus-graft response in female organ recipients. The impact of gender mismatching on graft performance and outcome has not been conclusively elucidated. There are several reports that suggested higher susceptibility of female allografts to development of cardiac allograft vasculopathy. Cardiac allograft vasculopathy is thought to be an immunological phenomenon that is associated with upregulation of class I and II major histocompatibility antigens on vascular endothelium.

A study from Papworth Hospital demonstrated that transplanting a female heart into a male recipient was associated with a higher incidence of cardiac allograft vasculopathy, as demonstrated by coronary angiography, as compared to transplants of male hearts into female recipients or gender-matched transplants.[21] Similarly, Mehra et al. reported a higher degree of vascular intimal thickening detected at 1 year posttransplant by intravascular ultrasound in male recipients of female allografts as compared to male recipients of male allografts or female recipients of male allografts.[22] However, recent reports from Creteil, France,[23] and Temple University[24] reached an opposite conclusion. In these studies, female recipients of male hearts had the least-favorable long-term outcome.

Although the question of the impact of gender mismatching on the alloimmune response is interesting biologically, the differences in outcomes are not sufficiently different to alter organ allocation schemes. The data are more convincing that a male-to-female transplant poses a more substantial immunological barrier. Whether it is the presence of the H-Y antigen, coded by the Y chromosome on male grafts; the effect of alloantigen exposure during pregnancy; or differences in the hormonal milieu, there is little doubt that rejection is more problematic in male-to-female transplants. In contrast, female-to-male transplantation has an increased risk of early graft dysfunction on physiological grounds. There is no doubt that gender matching would be desirable. However, the current system of organ allocation has established time on the waiting list and severity of illness as the criteria to ensure fairness in organ distribution. Nevertheless, in selected cases it may be appropriate to require a gender match.

Hormonal Resuscitation

Brain death leads to a variety of well-characterized pathophysiological changes in the donor. Hemodynamic instability consequent to these derangements is best avoided by invasive monitoring in an intensive care unit (ICU). The catecholamine surge associated with herniation leads to severe systemic hypertension and coronary vasoconstriction, which results in subendocardial ischemia. After the initial catecholamine storm, there is a loss of vasomotor tone, which results in systemic hypotension. Transient dysrhythmias are usually secondary to electrolyte or acid–base imbalances and can be managed accordingly. Central diabetes insipidus is commonly observed with brain death because of the markedly decreased levels of antidiuretic hormone. Pituitary damage associated with brain death can lead to decreased triiodothyronine (T_3) and thyroxine levels, leading to a bodywide shift toward anaerobic metabolism with depletion of high-energy phosphate stores and accumulation of lactate, which is most pronounced in the heart and kidney. Myocardial dysfunction in these cases is characterized by global hypokinesis or elevated filling pressures in the absence of significant coronary artery disease.

Jeevanandam and colleagues studied the effects of exogenously administered triiodothyronine on myocardial function in predominantly young donor hearts that would not have been used as transplants because of high inotrope requirements, decreased global myocardial function, and elevated left atrial pressures.[25] Bolus administration of triiodothyronine led to a decreased requirement for inotropic support and significantly lowered central venous and left atrial pressures. Postoperative ejection fractions were satisfactory, and all recipients of these "marginal" hearts were successfully discharged to home. Although a prospective, randomized study failed to confirm these findings,[26] problems in the design of the study limited its ability to demonstrate the efficacy of T_3.

Using a comprehensive system of invasive hemodynamic monitoring, normalization of preload and afterload, and aggressive hormonal resuscitation, the Transplant Unit at Papworth Hospital reported that 30% of hearts considered functionally unsuitable on initial evaluation could be resuscitated and successfully implanted.[27] Each component of the "Papworth cocktail" (Table 88.1) is designed to reverse a well-described hormonal deficiency in brain-dead patients. Arginine vasopressin reverses peripheral vasodilation without increasing myocardial oxygen demand and effectively treats diabetes insipidus. Triiodothyronine promotes aerobic metabolism in the myocardium and improves myocyte function directly through a calcium-dependent mechanism. Insulin maintains normal serum electrolytes and directly enhances

TABLE 88.1. Papworth Hormonal Resuscitation Cocktail.

Triiodothyronine (T_3): 4-μg bolus, 3-mg/h IV infusion
Arginine vasopressin: 1-U bolus, 1–8 U/h IV infusion (titrate SVR 800–1200)
Methylprednisolone: 15 mg/kg/day IV
Insulin: Intravenous infusion (minimum rate 1 U/h, titrate blood sugar 0–150 mg/dL)

SVR, systemic vascular resistance.

the functional recovery of ischemic myocardium. Last, methylprednisolone corrects the disruption of the hypothalamic–adrenal axis.

There is a wealth of experimental and clinical evidence in support of hormonal resuscitation for brain-dead donors. A retrospective analysis of more than 4500 donors from the UNOS database revealed that hormonal resuscitation with methylprednisolone, triiodothyronine, and vasopressin resulted in an increased number of transplanted hearts with better shorter term graft function.[28] The issue, however, remains controversial because a well-controlled prospective, randomized study has not been conducted. The multicenter T_3 study failed to convincingly demonstrate efficacy, but the bulk of the retrospective evidence in support of hormonal therapy involves "complete" hormonal resuscitation along with aggressive management of hemodynamics based on invasive monitoring of all donors.

To resolve this controversy, a multicenter, prospective, randomized trial of aggressive donor management, including complete hormonal resuscitation, is underway in the United States. An algorhithm has been recommended following the conference "Maximizing Use of Organs Recovered from the Cadaver Donor" until the data from the trial are available.[29]

Recipient Issues

Pulmonary Hypertension

Pulmonary hypertension in heart transplant recipients most commonly arises as a consequence of long-standing left ventricular dysfunction. An elevated pulmonary vascular resistance is the primary risk factor for right heart failure in the perioperative period. Right heart failure is thought to occur as a result of the sudden increase in right ventricular afterload when a heart is implanted into a patient with pulmonary hypertension. Hence, evaluation of the severity and the reversibility of pulmonary hypertension with serial right heart catheterization is a critical component of heart transplant candidate selection.[30] Reversibility can be assessed by administration of several vasodilators, sodium nitroprusside, or inhaled nitric oxide. It is generally held that the selective action of nitric oxide on the pulmonary vasculature makes it a better agent for preoperative assessment of pulmonary hypertension.[31] It is particularly useful for discriminating between candidates for cardiac and combined cardiopulmonary transplantation.

Patients with reversible pulmonary hypertension can safely undergo heart transplantation because pulmonary artery pressures normalize after implantation of a graft with normal left ventricular function. However, a study by Chen and colleagues suggested that reversibility of preoperative pulmonary hypertension improves but does not eliminate the increased risk of perioperative mortality.[32] Fixed pulmonary hypertension occurs most commonly in the setting of chronic pulmonary emboli and congenital heart disorders (Eisenmenger's syndrome) but can be seen in patients with primary cardiomyopathy. In addition, great attention must be given to donor selection because size mismatch, prolonged ischemic time, and a high donor inotrope requirement can aid and abet postoperative right heart failure.

Controversy exists regarding which of the three major calculated indices—pulmonary vascular resistance, pulmonary vascular resistance index, or transpulmonary gradient—predicts postoperative mortality most accurately. While some centers argue that the determination of indexed and nonindexed pulmonary vascular resistances is inaccurate at low cardiac outputs, others stress that pulmonary vascular resistance indices are required to account for variations in body size. The majority of centers consider severe pulmonary hypertension with a fixed pulmonary vascular resistance index greater than 6 Wood units/m^2 or a transpulmonary gradient greater than 20 mmHg to represent an absolute contraindication to cardiac transplantation.

Based on the cardiac transplantation experience at Columbia-Presbyterian Medical Center, Michler et al. stratified heart transplant recipients into three categories based on severity and reversibility of pulmonary hypertension and correlated these data with 30-day mortality.[33] Patients with fixed pulmonary hypertension had a fourfold increase in the risk of 30-day mortality when compared to patients with normal pulmonary artery pressures. Patients with reversible pulmonary hypertension were in an intermediate risk category. Kirsch et al. reported that preoperative pulmonary vascular resistance exceeding 3 Wood units was associated with a significantly higher incidence of death in the postoperative period.[34] McCarthy et al. reported an early mortality rate of almost 30% in patients with pulmonary vascular resistance exceeding 5 Wood units.[35]

On the other hand, a recently published single-center study by Tenderich and colleagues failed to demonstrate an increase in early and late postoperative mortality in a population of 83 patients who had preoperative pulmonary hypertension as defined by a transpulmonary gradient greater than 15 mmHg or pulmonary vascular resistance exceeding 5 Wood units. They attributed this outcome to use of vasodilators in the preoperative phase and administration of inhaled nitric oxide postoperatively.[36] Inhaled iloprost, a potent acute pulmonary vasodilator, has been used in some centers and is preferred therapy over inhaled nitric oxide due to the ease of administration in extubated patients. Its action lasts for approximately an hour, and it is usually administered every 3 h. The frequency of dosing is weaned gradually according to clinical response.

Pulmonary hypertension remains a major risk factor for acute cardiac allograft failure. There is no doubt that patients with a fixed pulmonary resistance in excess of 6 Wood units should not be considered for orthotopic cardiac transplantation. These patients are better served with heterotopic cardiac transplantation or combined heart-lung transplantation. Fortunately, there have been significant advances in the diagnosis and treatment of pulmonary hypertension over the last decade.

The introduction of inhaled nitric oxide into clinical practice has made an enormous impact on the perioperative management of patients with elevated pulmonary vascular resistance as a result of long-standing left heart failure. The authors routinely place all patients with a mean pulmonary artery pressure in excess of 25 mmHg on nitric oxide at 40 ppm during the perioperative period. In general, we have been able to wean nitric oxide and extubate patients within 24 h of transplant. In a subgroup of patients having more significant elevations in pulmonary vascular resistance or those receiving small grafts or grafts with prolonged ischemic time, we have prolonged nitric oxide therapy for up to 72 h with excellent success.

One question that remains unanswered is whether nitric oxide would allow programs to transplant patients with higher degrees of pulmonary vascular resistance, particularly those patients who have a poor initial response at right heart catheterization. Careful study is required before routine recommendations for a pulmonary vascular resistance cutoff can be liberalized.

Diabetes Mellitus

Diabetic patients are often excluded from transplantation because of the systemic consequences of long-standing disease and an increased baseline susceptibility to infections, which is exacerbated by immunosuppressive therapy. It is well known that hyperglycemia can lead to impairment of the immune system. Because high-dose corticosteroids make blood sugar control in diabetics extremely difficult, this increases the infectious risk in the perioperative period. The high prevalence of atherosclerosis in the diabetic population increases the risk of peripheral vascular complications. Last, the nephrotoxicity of cyclosporine and tacrolimus in the setting of diabetic nephropathy can lead to frank renal failure. At the same time, the increased incidence of coronary artery disease and cardiomyopathy in diabetics results in a significant number of potential heart transplant recipients in this patient population.

Improvements in immunosuppression, leading to reduced doses of corticosteroids, as well as refinements in operative and perioperative management have led an increasing number of centers to consider selected diabetic patients for cardiac transplantation. The policies on listing of diabetics with significant end-organ damage, including nephropathy, retinopathy, and peripheral vascular disease, vary among transplant centers.

Ladowski et al. reviewed the experience with heart transplantation in 19 adult-onset diabetic patients at the University of Pittsburgh; 6 of these patients were insulin-dependent before surgery.[37] Diabetic patients received immunosuppressive regimens with lower glucocorticoid doses. Approximately 40% of patients who were not insulin-dependent before transplant required insulin after the transplant. At a mean follow-up of 17 months, a greater incidence of rejection, coronary artery disease, or lethal infections was not observed in diabetic recipients as compared to matched nondiabetic controls. They concluded that midterm outcomes in selected diabetic patients were comparable to nondiabetics.

A similar report from the Texas Heart Institute examined outcomes of 37 diabetic patients after heart transplantation.[38] Unlike the Pittsburgh study, a small number of diabetics with evidence of end-organ damage were also included in this series, which had a mean follow-up period of almost 3 years. Similar to Ladowski et al.'s study, there was an increase in insulin dependence among diabetics after the operation. However, because corticosteroid doses were not minimized in the early posttransplant period, the incidence of developing insulin dependence approached 80%. The authors tolerated this high incidence of insulin dependence because they believed that rapid tapering of steroids leads to an unacceptably high rate of rejection. There was no significant difference with respect to the frequency of infectious complications, rejection episodes, cardiac allograft vasculopathy, or actuarial survival between diabetics and nondiabetics. Furthermore, although the creatinine levels increased in both patient cohorts over time, presumably as a result of cyclosporine toxicity, there were no differences between the two groups.

Although several groups have reported successful transplantation in the diabetic population, the authors remain somewhat skeptical that this is an optimal use of a scarce resource. We believe that long-standing insulin-dependent diabetes remains a contraindication to transplantation, even if end-organ damage cannot be clearly identified. Furthermore, a combination of advanced age (>60 years) and diabetes mellitus is a certain recipe for a poor long-term outcome. We believe that diabetes mellitus represents a high-risk category for transplantation, which should be considered in the context of dual listing.

Dual Listing

In 1991, cardiologists and cardiothoracic surgeons from the University of California at Los Angeles (UCLA) proposed an "alternate" recipient list as an approach to maximize the utilization of marginal donor hearts and thereby expand the number of organ recipients.[39] The guiding principle behind their method was matching the higher-risk patients with the higher-risk donors. High-risk candidates constituted patients over the age of 65 years and those who were being considered for a third heart transplant. Criteria that defined marginal donors included ventricular dysfunction requiring high-dose inotropic support, wall motion abnormalities on echocardiography, coronary artery disease, donor age greater than 55 years, a history of cardiac risk factors (e.g., smoking), and prolonged ischemia time.

Laks and colleagues reported their experience with cardiac transplantation in 17 patients from the "alternate" waiting list.[40] There were 2 early deaths (1 hyperacute rejection and 1 ventricular failure) and 2 late deaths at a median follow-up period of 8.5 months. There was no significant difference between this patient population and "standard" heart transplant recipients with respect to length of stay in the ICU, duration of hospitalization, postoperative cardiac function, frequency of acute rejection, incidence of infectious complications, or actuarial survival at 1 year. The early outcomes of the UCLA group justified the "alternate" list as a potential approach to expand the recipient population to include patients who would otherwise not be considered for this lifesaving procedure.

Dual listing is an extremely logical and reasonable approach given the ethical conundrum produced by the scarcity of donor organs. However, the criteria for discarding hearts vary widely across the United States. In a recent survey conducted by the American Society of Transplant Surgeons, it was found that the discard rate for hearts ranged between 20% and 55%. Clearly, hearts considered "too marginal" in certain regions are thought to be suitable in others. Development of universal criteria for organ utilization will help address this problem. In addition, certain disease states, such as hepatitis C, will always place a donor organ in the marginal category, despite excellent physiological function. The authors believe strongly that all such hearts should be utilized. The authors is likely that dual listing will continue to expand at several high-volume programs across the United States. Careful, multicenter studies should be undertaken to determine the limits of this approach.

Elderly

Age greater than 60 years has traditionally been considered to be an exclusion criterion for heart transplantation, based on several studies that found advanced age adversely influences outcome.[41,42] In view of the shortage of donor organs, it was thought that hearts should be allocated to patients with the best prognosis. The question of heart transplantation in the elderly is marked by both ethical and economic considerations. Opponents of heart transplantation in the elderly population argue that postoperative care is substantially more expensive, and that long-term outcomes are less favorable. One solution is to allocate older donor hearts to elderly patients on an alternate waiting list to avoid using "good hearts" for high-risk patients with naturally shorter life expectancies.

However, these concepts have recently been challenged by several transplant centers. Age limits have been increasingly relaxed, and it is not unusual to encounter reports of successful heart transplantations in septuagenarians.[43] The experience from Cedars-Sinai Medical Center reflects the growing percentage of elderly among heart transplant recipients; 36% of their heart transplant recipients between 1988 and 1993 were over the age of 60 years. This patient group has similar operative mortalities, 1-year survival rates, and quality-of-life indices when compared to the younger cohort. Frazier et al.'s series of heart transplantation in elderly individuals included 95 patients over the age of 60 years, one-quarter of whom were older than 65 years. Their survival rates at a mean follow-up period of 3.2 years were comparable to a cohort of younger heart transplant recipients.[44] In addition, the quality-of-life indices of the elderly patient group were quite satisfactory.

There is no doubt that excellent early results after heart transplantation can be achieved in highly selected patients above the age of 60. However, there is also no question that the long-term outcomes are somewhat less satisfactory consequent to comorbidities associated with aging. Given the scarcity of donor hearts, the authors believe that the elderly should not be disenfranchised from transplantation, but rather that elderly patients are ideal for dual listing. Furthermore, we believe that donor age restrictions should be relaxed as long as there is adequate documentation of suitable physiology in the absence of significant coronary or valvular disease. We consider it quite reasonable to transplant a 69-year-old recipient with end-stage heart failure with a donor heart from a 64-year-old brain-dead patient.

Ventricular Assist

Temporary circulatory support with VADs has become a well-established treatment option for patients awaiting cardiac transplantation. Recent studies demonstrated that transplantation after mechanical support offers satisfactory outcomes to a population of patients who otherwise would have faced certain death.[45] However, bridge-to-transplant patients, who have usually suffered hemodynamic deterioration with consequent end-organ dysfunction, have a lower overall survival rate after heart transplantation than non-bridged controls, and this is shown to be an independent risk factor following transplantation.[46] However, the opposite had been reported by Rajasinghe et al. from their series of more than 500 consecutive heart transplants.[47]

Despite continuous advances in this field, mechanical ventricular assistance is associated with the potential for several sometimes-fatal complications that can preclude transplantation. These disadvantages include bleeding, infection, thromboembolic events, immune sensitization, and end-organ dysfunction. Approximately one-third of VAD patients suffer from significant infectious complications, and many of these patients are excluded from transplantation. Cases in which the device itself is infected can be especially devastating. In a recent comprehensive review of infections in VAD patients, the authors reported that even "low-grade" driveline infections were associated with prolonged pretransplant waiting times.[48] Moreover, left VAD endocarditis, which can arise from a driveline infection, carries a mortality rate of approximately 50%. However, the study also demonstrated that infections treated early and aggressively are not a negative predictor for success after transplantation if the infection is cleared successfully. Almost 60% of patients who had infections during left VAD therapy eventually underwent successful transplantation. Furthermore, pretransplant infections did not seem to predict higher rates of postoperative infectious complications.

In addition to the infectious risks associated with VADs, their prolonged use can be associated with mechanical failure. Furthermore, patients who are on mechanical support before transplantation are at an increased risk for the development of anti-HLA lymphocytotoxic antibodies. Such patients are at a higher risk for both hyperacute rejection with immediate graft failure and resistant, persistent, or recurrent acute rejection. Because the presence of lymphocytotoxic antibodies has also been implicated in the development of cardiac allograft vasculopathy, patients who were bridged with mechanical assist devices may be at risk for late complications as well.

Itescu et al. confirmed a higher frequency of immunoglobulin (Ig) G antibodies directed against class I and class II major histocompatibility complex (MHC) antigens among patients with left VADs.[49] The presence of anti-MHC class I antibodies led to increased waiting times because of the need for prospective crossmatching to eliminate the risk of hyperacute rejection. Moreover, the authors showed that the presence of IgG directed against class II MHC antigens in the serum of recipients before transplantation led to an increased incidence of early high-grade cellular rejection and an increased cumulative rate of annual rejection.

Although the clinical use of implantable left VADs and paracorporeal right VADs has increased dramatically over the

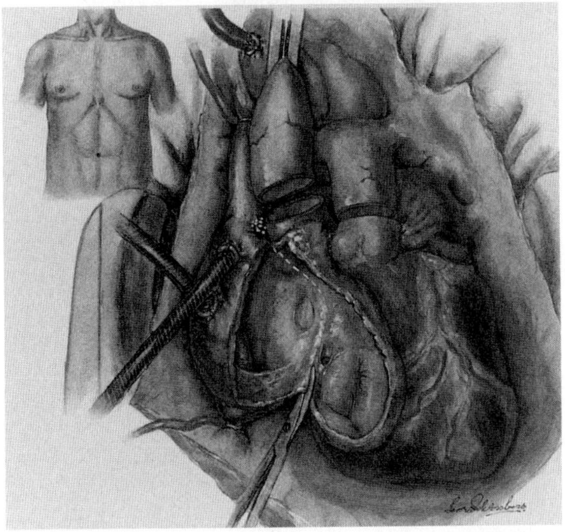

FIGURE 88.1. Recipient cardiectomy for standard heart transplantation.

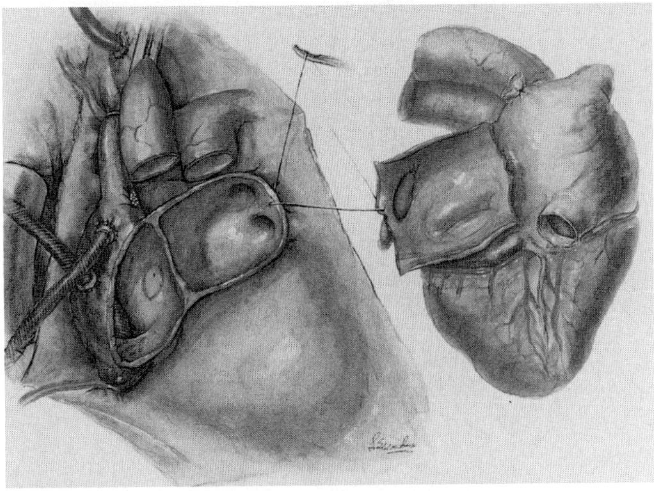

FIGURE 88.2. Left atrial anastomosis at the initiation of the graft implantation.

last 10 years, VADs still remain primarily as a bridge to transplantation. Until VADs can be routinely used as destination therapy, it is imperative that the long-term outcome of patients bridged to transplantation with a VAD are similar to patients not requiring bridging, given the scarcity of donor organs. Unfortunately, even in the best series short-term and midterm outcomes on bridged patients are somewhat less satisfactory. What is most concerning is the degree of presensitization consequent to VAD bridging. As more data become available, it is likely that VAD patients may need to be considered for dual listing because they represent a "high-risk" group. As destination therapy devices become better defined, easier to implant, and therefore more popular, bridge to transplantation and even scarcity of donor organs would become less of an issue.

Surgical Issues

Bicaval Versus Biatrial

Orthotopic heart transplantation is usually performed using one of two different techniques. The biatrial technique developed by Shumway and Lower, which is considered to be the standard method, has been in clinical use since the introduction of cardiac transplantation in the 1960s. The recipient cardiectomy is performed by removing the ventricles at the AV groove and then trimming the atria, leaving a cuff of atrial wall behind. The recipient heart is implanted using four anastomoses: the left and right atria, the pulmonary artery, and the aorta.

The alternative method is termed *bicaval orthotopic heart transplantation*. The first use of bicaval anastomoses came with the domino procedure in 1990, in which the native heart of a combined heart-lung recipient was used as a donor allograft.[50] In most cases, bicaval implantation is performed with a left atrial anastomosis, identical to that performed using the standard biatrial technique. Thus, the procedure requires five anastomoses. Total orthotopic heart transplantation involves complete excision of the recipient heart except for two pulmonary venous cuffs and two caval cuffs. Bilateral pulmonary venous anastomoses and individual anastomoses of the cavae are performed during implantation, for a total of six anastomoses. For this reason, total orthotopic transplantation has not gained widespread application.

Several nonrandomized studies have demonstrated improved atrial function,[51,52] a reduction in atrial arrhythmias,[53,54] fewer left atrial thrombi,[55] and improved tricuspid and mitral valve function.[56] There have been three prospective randomized trials.[57–59] These studies all showed fewer atrial arrhythmias and smaller atrial dimensions. What remains entirely unclear is whether these improvements translate into a long-term survival advantage or improved exercise capacity in the long term. For these techniques, see Figures 88.1 through 88.20.

Recent interest has been shown in prophylactic annuloplasty of the tricuspid valve to prevent postoperative tricuspid regurgitation. Jeevanandam and colleagues have demonstrated that simple De Vega annuloplasty prior to bicaval anastomosis of the heart improves right ventricular function and reduces mortality.[60] Similar findings have been reported by Brown et al.[149]

Prospective, randomized studies of biatrial versus bicaval implantation have demonstrated a clear reduction in atrial arrhythmias. In addition, these studies have suggested that atrial transport and valvular function may be improved. However, these echocardiographic findings have yet to be correlated to clinical endpoints. Therefore, most surgeons believe that the bicaval operation has a marginal benefit in terms of arrhythmia and right atrial function. This small advantage, however, must be balanced against the longer ischemic times consequent to bicaval implantation and the risk for anastomotic complications, particularly at the level of the superior vena cava anastomosis. Currently, all organs that arrive at the operating room with 2 h or less of cold ischemia are implanted bicavally, assuming that there are no technical contraindications. The authors continue to use biatrial implantation for hearts with longer ischemic times or when there is gross disparity between the size of donor and recipient cavae. We remain unconvinced that there is any benefit to total orthotopic cardiac transplantation. Although elegant,

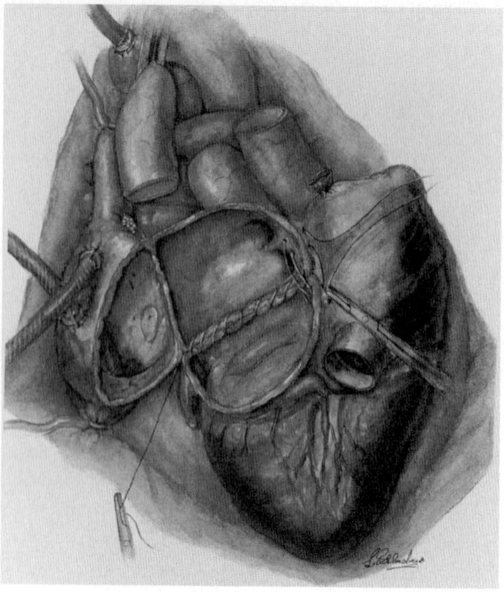

FIGURE 88.3. Completion of left atrial anastomosis.

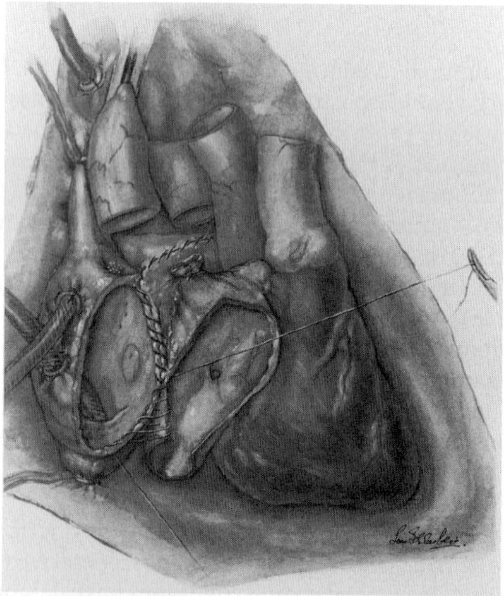

FIGURE 88.4. Initiation of right atrial anastomosis.

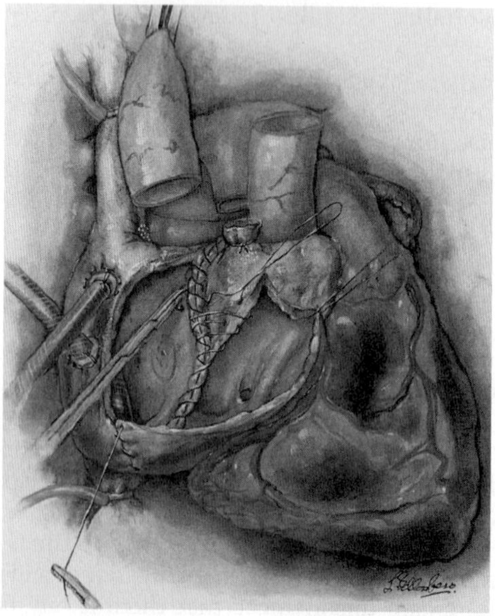

FIGURE 88.5. Completion of right atrial anastomosis.

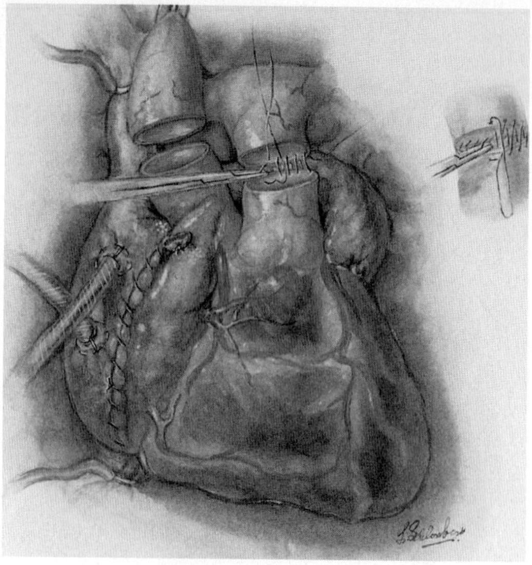

FIGURE 88.6. Anastomosis of the pulmonary artery.

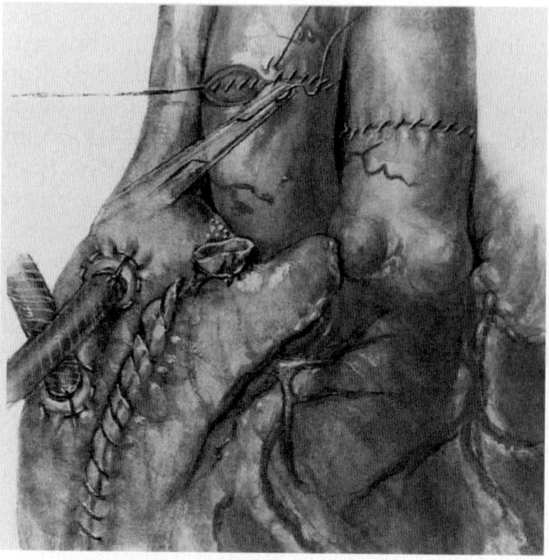

FIGURE 88.7. Anastomosis of the aorta.

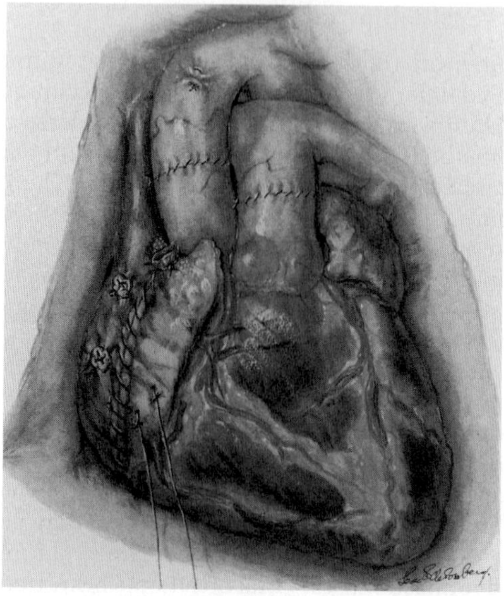

FIGURE 88.8. Graft after completed implantation.

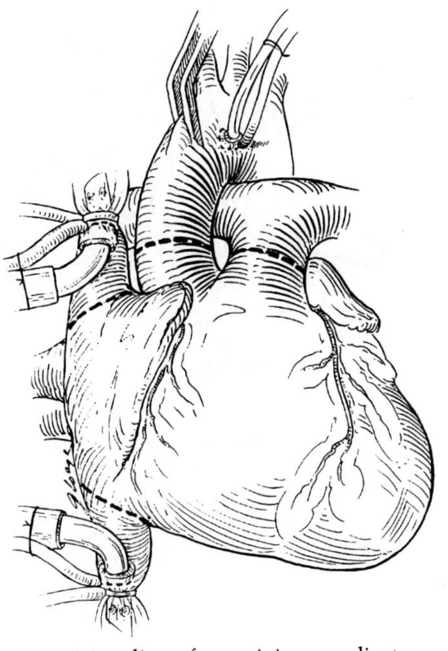

FIGURE 88.9. Incision lines for recipient cardiectomy in bicaval heart transplantation.

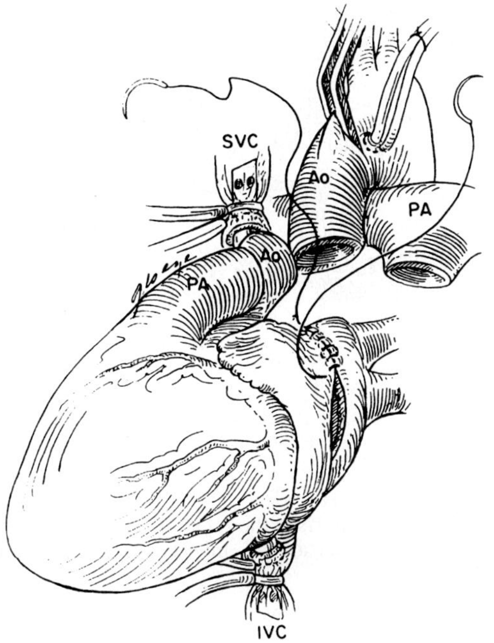

FIGURE 88.11. Initiation of left atrial anastomosis.

this procedure is more time-consuming and increases the risk of anastomotic complications.

Cardioplegia

The need to expand the donor pool has led to a renewed interest in improving techniques for myocardial protection. Remote procurement of cardiac allografts is greatly limited by the lack of methods for prolonged myocardial preservation. The incidence of primary graft failure that occurs as a result of suboptimal preservation techniques is still unacceptably high. Although primary nonfunction of the graft may not be life-threatening in kidney transplantation, the heart transplant recipient depends on immediate function of the allograft. Unlike the case with kidneys and livers, there is great variability among heart transplant centers with respect to preservation methods. Research has focused on methods of cardioplegic induction, efficacy of different cardioplegic solutions, choice of the transport medium and storage modalities, and reperfusion strategies.

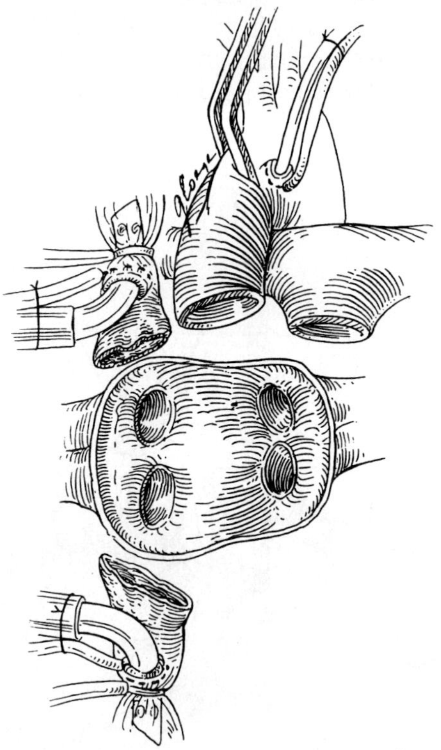

FIGURE 88.10. Completion of recipient cardiectomy.

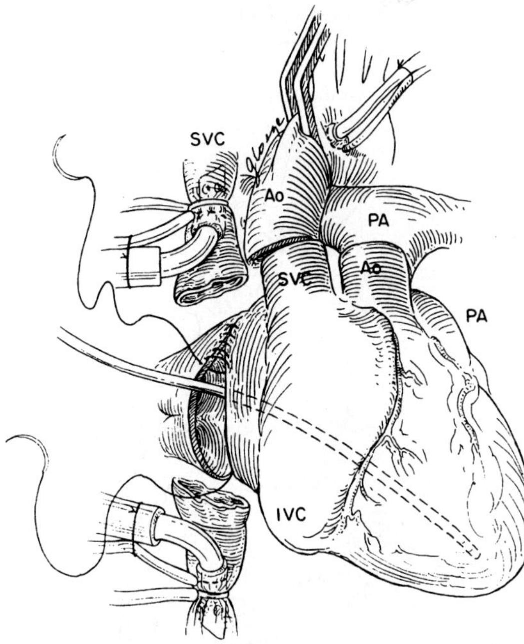

FIGURE 88.12. Completion of left atrial anastomosis. Left ventricular vent placed across mitral valve.

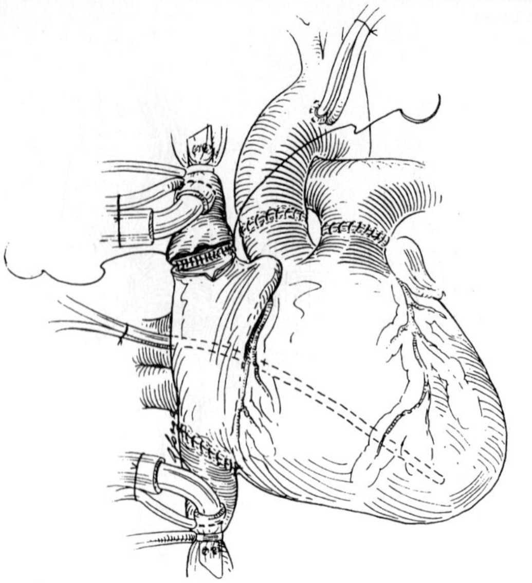

FIGURE 88.13. Anastomosis of the superior vena cava. Anastomoses of pulmonary artery, aorta, and inferior vena cava have been completed.

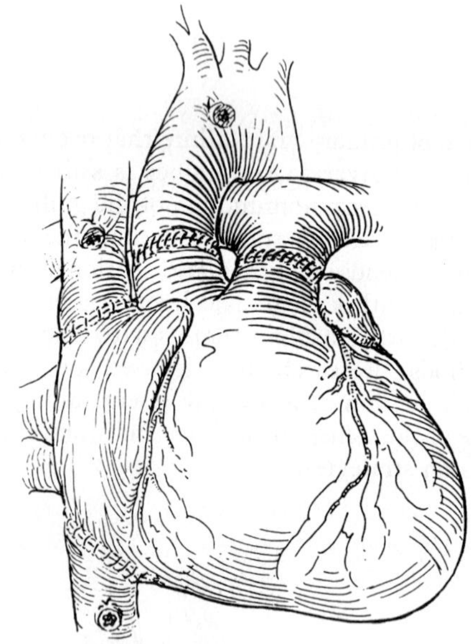

FIGURE 88.14. Graft after completed implantation.

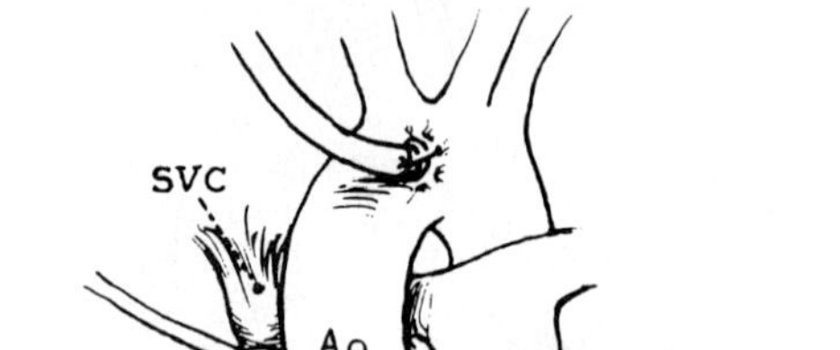

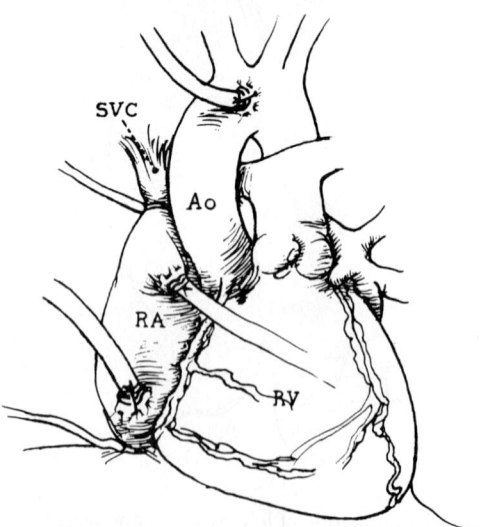

FIGURE 88.15. Cannulation of the recipient heart for heterotopic heart transplantation.

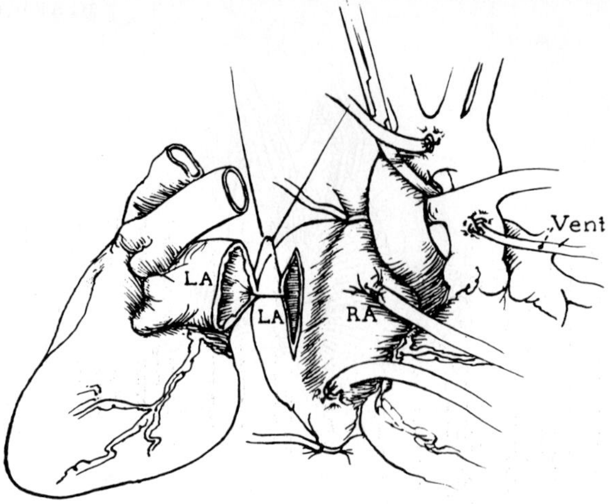

FIGURE 88.16. Initiation of left atrial anastomosis.

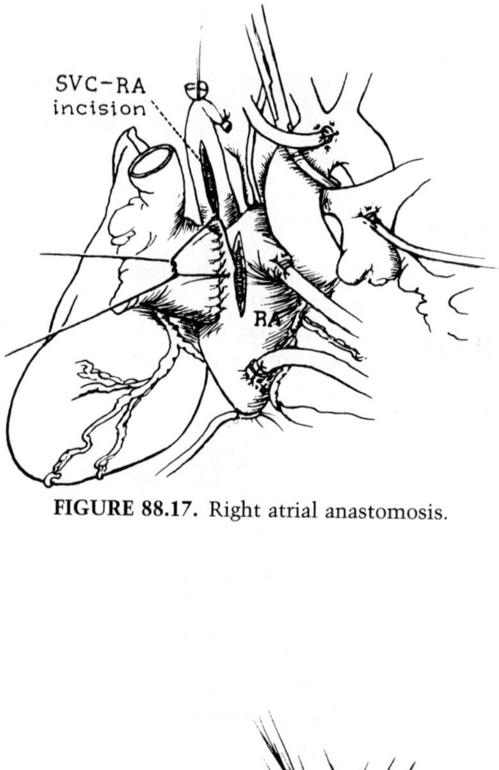

FIGURE 88.17. Right atrial anastomosis.

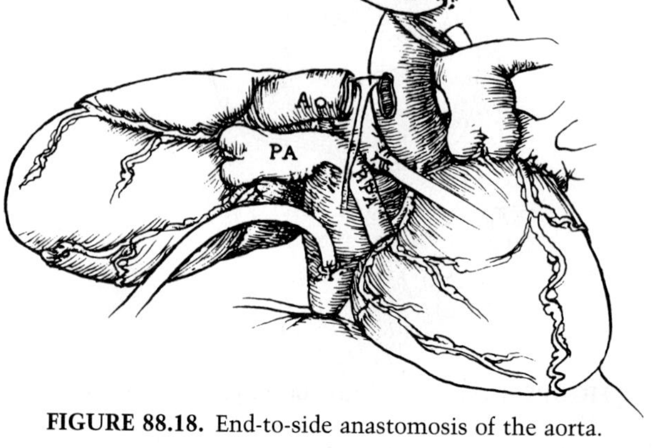

FIGURE 88.18. End-to-side anastomosis of the aorta.

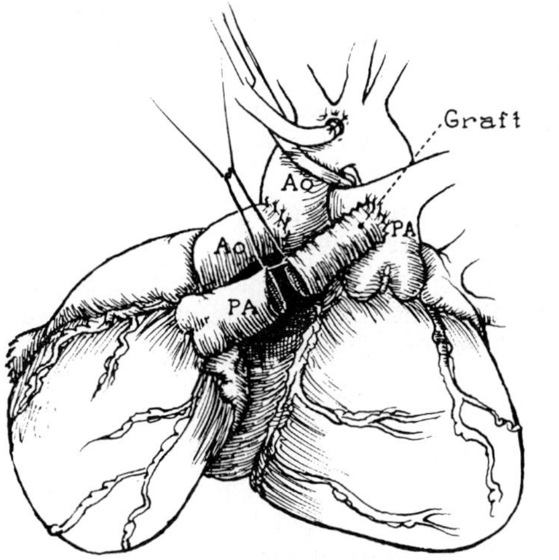

FIGURE 88.19. Anastomosis of the pulmonary arteries with synthetic interposition graft.

In most cases, antegrade cardioplegia is administered through the aortic root during the procurement. Traditionally, cardioplegia has consisted of cold, high-potassium crystalloid solutions, which led to a quick diastolic arrest of the heart. There are numerous cardioplegic solutions in clinical use,[61] and they are commonly subdivided into those with electrolyte compositions resembling the intra- or extracellular milieu. A variety of agents have been added to cardioplegic solutions to improve the heart's tolerance of ischemic storage; these include free-radical scavengers, calcium channel antagonists, osmotic agents, buffer systems, energy substrates, and oxygen.

In the routine practice of cardiac surgery, investigators have described improved myocardial protection by using blood-based cardioplegia. Several theoretical advantages exist for using blood-based cardioplegia for donor hearts. Brain-dead donors have a variety of physiological derangements, which lead to significant metabolic changes in the myocardium. Increased lactate levels reflect ongoing anaerobic metabolism, and high-energy phosphates, glycogen, and amino acids are depleted. As compared to crystalloid solutions, blood cardioplegia provides osmotic support that reduces myocardial edema, excellent buffering capacity that minimizes intracellular acidosis, free-radical scavengers, and improved rheological properties. In addition, blood cardioplegia can provide oxygen for aerobic metabolism, although this effect is minimized when the solution is delivered at low temperatures.

Luciani and associates reported favorable results with induction of cardiac arrest in the donor with cold blood cardioplegia as compared to a cold crystalloid solution.[62] They observed lower incidences of both graft failure and atrioventricular conduction disturbances. The optimal temperature of blood cardioplegia is a topic of debate.[63] The goal of hypothermia (4°C) is rapid reduction in myocardial oxygen demand and metabolic rate. This concept, however, is less relevant when oxygenated cardioplegia solutions are used. The advantages of hypothermia with blood cardioplegia must be balanced against its disadvantages: Oxygen release from hemoglobin is impaired at lower temperatures, and the function of membrane pumps is retarded.

Controlled reperfusion with normothermic cardioplegia (37°C) has been shown to reduce reperfusion injury by enhancing metabolic repair.[64] Similarly, in a large-animal model, functional recovery following orthotopic heart transplantation was improved after perfusion of the donor graft with donor blood during prolonged storage.[65]

Despite the metabolic advantage of normothermic blood cardioplegia, this would require continuous perfusion, which would increase the complexity of recovery efforts. As a result, this approach has not achieved widespread application. Wheeldon et al. found that most cardiac transplant surgeons use single-flush, cold, crystalloid cardioplegic induction.[61] Induction of cardioplegia with blood-based solutions was used in only 1.4% of all patients. Interestingly, only 12% of the centers surveyed used the same crystalloid solution for induction and storage.

Reperfusion is the final component of preservation of the cardiac allograft. Controversial areas include the composition, temperature, and infusion pressure of reperfusion solutions. Wheeldon et al.[61] reported that 55% of transplant centers used some form of reperfusion modification. Common regimens include intermittent doses of cold blood or cold oxygenated crystalloid cardioplegia during graft implantation and delivery of a warm, blood-based solution before release of the aortic cross-clamp.

Important characteristics of the ideal reperfusion solution are the capacity for oxygen delivery, the provision of substrate, the maintenance of asystole with high concentrations of potassium, and normothermic conditions to enhance anabolism and cellular repair. The goal is to facilitate metabolic recovery and thus improve early graft function. It was recommended by Kirklin and coworkers to perform the reperfusion at low pressures and flows.[66] Pradas and associates reported their results with continuous warm reperfusion with blood during cardiac transplantation.[67] Reperfusion was started at the time when the organ was removed from cold storage, thereby reducing ischemic time. Continuous normothermic reperfusion was associated with lower rates of postoperative dysrhythmias and decreased duration of catecholamine administration. In practice, most surgeons are reluctant to use continuous warm perfusion, particularly via the coronary sinus, because of concerns about the adequacy of right ventricular perfusion.

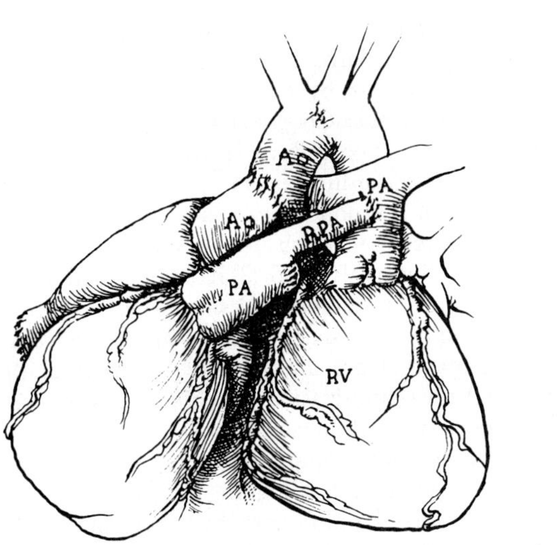

FIGURE 88.20. Anastomosis of the pulmonary arteries using donor right pulmonary artery.

Single-dose, antegrade, crystalloid cardioplegia remains the standard in clinical practice and is very unlikely to change due to the simplicity of the approach. In the early days of transplantation, there was far greater focus on recovery of hearts from geographically distant sites. With the proliferation of transplant programs across the United States, the need to develop strategies for 6- to 8-h preservation has been virtually eliminated. In fact, the authors consider such efforts to be misdirected. Rather, the focus should be on optimizing logistics to minimize ischemic time and to improve short-term myocardial preservation. Although it is likely that some incremental improvement can be made in preservation solutions, we suspect that novel reperfusion strategies will be the most effective avenue in the future.

Excellent preservation can be achieved during implantation using a variety of techniques. The simplest method is topical hypothermia, which can be achieved with a continuous cold saline drip or a cooling jacket placed within the pericardium. The use of slush should be avoided due to myocardial injury at temperatures below 4°C. The authors continue to use topical hypothermia as the sole method of preservation for routine transplants. In higher-risk situations such as prolonged graft cold ischemic time, recipient pulmonary hypertension, an undersize graft, or a donor managed with high-dose catecholamines, we combine topical hypothermia with continuous, high-potassium, blood cardioplegia delivered via the coronary sinus. We do not use a brief retrograde "hot shot" before removing the aortic cross-clamp because we are unconvinced that any significant anabolism is achieved with such a maneuver. Rather, we allow the serum potassium to rise during graft implantation by using high-potassium blood cardioplegia. This technique maintains asystole for several minutes after removal of the aortic cross-clamp. We consider this period of time to be a prolonged antegrade hot shot. Moreover, we rest the heart on cardiopulmonary bypass for 15 min for each hour of ischemia before attempting to wean. Using this approach, we have successfully avoided acute graft failure and have utilized hearts with as much as 6 h of cold ischemia.

Heterotopic Auxiliary Heart Transplantation

The first human heterotopic heart transplantation was performed in 1974 by Barnard and Losman.[68] The donor heart is implanted in parallel by anastomosing donor and recipient atria and great vessels. Cooper et al.[69] summarized the limited indications for this procedure: (1) patients in whom recovery of the native myocardium is possible; (2) situations in which the function of the donor heart is considered inadequate to maintain the recipient's circulation alone (undersize donors, long ischemic intervals, etc.); (3) recipients with elevated pulmonary vascular resistance; (4) situations requiring a bridge to orthotopic heart transplantation; and (5) certain cases of severe angina that are unresponsive to medical therapy or myocardial revascularization in which left ventricular function is preserved. Because several reports suggested that undersize donor hearts implanted heterotopically are not detrimental to long-term allograft function, it is generally thought that fixed pulmonary hypertension in the recipient is the only absolute indication for heterotopic heart transplantation.[70]

Heterotopic heart transplantation brings with it a unique set of complications, which may contribute to slightly worse outcomes as compared to orthotopic heart transplantation. Since 2000, heterotopic auxiliary heart transplants have been performed worldwide with a 1-year survival of 71% as compared to a 1-year survival rate of 91% for orthotopic transplants. However, as heterotopic auxiliary heart transplantation is reserved for selected high-risk situations, it is not clear that the procedure is, in fact, any less successful or any more morbid. Complications of the heterotopic procedure include an increased risk of pulmonary infections due to obstructive atelectasis of the right lower lobe, an increased high risk of thromboembolic events from thrombus formation in the native heart, and mitral regurgitation in donor and native hearts.

Kawaguchi et al. compared the results of orthotopic versus heterotopic heart transplantation in situations of a significantly undersize donor.[71] They compared a nonrandomized population of patients who received undersize hearts in an orthotopic position with a group of patients who underwent a heterotopic heart transplant exclusively for reasons of size mismatch. Although postoperative allograft function in orthotopic heart transplant recipients from undersize donors was worse than in size-matched (±10% body weight) controls, the overall risk of graft failure was higher in recipients in whom similarly undersize hearts were implanted in a heterotopic position. The authors believed that their findings in combination with the high degree of postoperative complications in heterotopic heart transplant recipients did not justify this procedure when the indication was limited to size mismatch.

This belief was challenged by Sekela and colleagues, who utilized small donor hearts, the majority of which had been previously rejected by other centers, to perform heterotopic heart transplants in large recipients who were not at high risk at the time of the operation.[18] Utilizing this policy, they were able to significantly reduce waiting times and overall mortality (waiting time plus perioperative time) for large patients.

The reluctance of most centers to accept small hearts for large recipients has created prolonged waiting times. Sekela et al.[18] argued that the relatively poor outcomes after heterotopic heart transplants are usually related to the fact that recipients of heterotopic grafts are often in extremis before transplant. Moreover, outcomes equivalent to those of orthotopic heart transplants could be obtained if the indications were comparable and the procedure was performed in expert hands.

Supporting this notion, Khaghani and associates reported their experience with using heterotopic heart transplants as auxiliary pumps in infants and children, a patient population particularly affected by the shortage of suitable donor organs.[72] Twelve children between the ages of 11 months and 15 years, 8 of whom suffered from pulmonary hypertension, were the recipients of heterotopic hearts. The authors achieved a 1-year survival rate greater than 80%. Furthermore, mean pulmonary pressures were markedly reduced in patients who had pulmonary hypertension preoperatively. Although longer follow-up is necessary, Khaghani's results are encouraging and demonstrate that heterotopic heart transplantation should be considered in selected pediatric patients. The same group reported favorable results with heterotopic heart transplants that were performed in conjunction with operations on the native heart in patients who suffered from end-stage ischemic heart disease.[73] Survival rates for 1 year and 5 years were 79% and 63%, respectively. The majority of survivors experienced marked improvements in their functional status. In the majority of survivors, the donor allograft made the major contribution to cardiac output.

Auxiliary heart transplantation remains an acceptable option in certain, selected clinical situations. The authors believe that it is no longer reasonable to use heterotopic heart transplants when recovery of the native myocardium is possible or in situations requiring a bridge to orthotopic transplant, given the improvement in VAD technology. Furthermore, transmyocardial laser revascularization and novel gene therapy approaches to achieve myocardial angiogenesis make heterotopic transplantation a poor option for patients with intractable angina and preserved left ventricular function. However, heterotopic transplants are still reasonable in the setting of a grossly undersize donor heart or in the setting of a recipient with fixed pulmonary vascular resistance. However, expansion of pediatric and adolescent transplant programs make it more reasonable to use smaller donor hearts for smaller recipients rather than perform a suboptimal procedure. Last, heterotopic transplantation will have to compete against combined heart-lung transplantation in patients with severe fixed pulmonary hypertension. Perhaps the most important use of heterotopic, auxiliary heart transplantation will come in the development of xenotransplantation technology. Given that the clinical development of cardiac xenotransplantation will undoubtedly be an iterative process, many investigators believe it is reasonable to first use xenotransplants as biological biventricular-assist devices.

Postoperative Management: Intensive Care Unit Phase

Inotropic Support

Right ventricular dysfunction is a common occurrence in the early posttransplant period that requires the administration of pulmonary vasodilators and inotropes. Isoproterenol, a pure β-agonist, is a positive inotrope and chronotrope that also reduces right ventricular afterload by dilating the pulmonary arterial tree. It is a first-line agent and is used prophylactically by virtually all surgeons and intensivists for the transplant recipient. The dose is titrated to a heart rate of 90 to 120 beats per minute. Low-dose dopamine is also frequently administered routinely to increase heart rate and splanchnic and renal perfusion in the hope of mitigating the toxicity of cyclosporine or tacrolimus. Other inotropes or vasoconstrictors are often added, depending on the clinical situation. Pulmonary hypertension often necessitates the use of milrinone, amrinone, or enoximone. However, the peripheral vasodilating effects of these agents often limits their utility, particularly in patients who have been managed for long periods of time on angiotensin-converting enzyme (ACE) inhibitors.

Inhaled nitric oxide, which is selective for the pulmonary vasculature by dint of its route of administration, has become an essential component in postoperative management.[74] Although there are no prospective randomized studies confirming the efficacy of inhaled nitric oxide, it has made a significant impact on clinical practice and has led many groups to rethink exclusion criteria for patients with a high pulmonary vascular resistance.[29]

In addition to perioperative right heart dysfunction, the other common hemodynamic derangement in the postoperative period is a low systemic vascular resistance due to a combination of the effects of cardiopulmonary bypass and chronic therapy with ACE inhibitors. The α-agonists such as phenylephrine and norepinephrine have traditionally been used as vasoconstrictors. Recently, the use of vasopressin has been popularized by several groups.[75] The primary advantage of vasopressin is that it increases systemic vascular resistance without altering myocardial oxygen demand.

Although issues regarding inotropic support after transplantation are not highly controversial, it is a field in which there have been several recent advances. Moreover, a number of novel, intravenous, inotropic agents such as levosimendan, a calcium-sensitizing agent that has been shown to be of prognostic benefit in patients with severe low-output heart failure in a multicenter randomised double-blind trial[76] may have significant impact in the management of freshly transplanted hearts. The authors believe that the two most significant advances in the field are the widespread use of inhaled nitric oxide and intravenous arginine vasopressin. Both drugs have become a standard part of our armamentarium in addition to the routine use of isoproterenol and renal-dose dopamine.

Pacing

The transplanted heart is devoid of autonomic innervation and has a resting heart rate of approximately 100 beats per minute. Although bradyarrhythmias are common in the early postoperative period, tachyarrhythmias are far less common and are often associated with acute allograft rejection. Dysfunction of the donor sinus node is the most common cause for bradyarrhythmias, followed by atrioventricular block. The increasing use of amiodarone, an antiarrhythmic with an extraordinarily long half-life, in patients awaiting transplantation has led to a substantial increase in bradyarrhythmias in some centers. Most surgeons believe that sinoatrial and atrioventricular nodal dysfunction is primarily related to alteration of blood supply consequent to surgical trauma, but other factors such as the ischemic interval, the composition of cardioplegia, and the duration of cardiopulmonary bypass have been implicated as well. Moreover, a clear correlation exists between low preimplantation donor heart myocardial temperature (topical slush during implantation) and development of early bradyarrhythmias.[77] As the sinus node usually resumes normal function within 3 weeks, the majority of these cases respond well to pharmacological agents or temporary pacing via epicardial wires. In most series, the incidence of perioperative nodal dysfunction requiring permanent pacing is approximately 5%.

Advantages of early implantation of a permanent pacemaker include increased mobility and shortened hospital stay. However, the potential for long-term complications such as endocarditis or thrombosis and the interference with endomyocardial biopsies requires the decision to place a permanent pacemaker to be made carefully. In addition, there is controversy surrounding the choice of pacing mode. Scott et al. studied the need for long-term pacing and the optimum mode of pacing in a cohort of 191 orthotopic heart transplant recipients who survived at least 1 month.[78] Eleven percent of their patients received permanent pacers for either sinus node dysfunction or atrioventricular node block. Roughly three-quarters of their patients received ventricular pacers, and the selection between rate-responsive and rate-adaptive systems was made on an individual basis. The frequency of pacing as assessed by electrocardiogram declined from 40% at 3 months to 10% at 3 years. After reprogramming, they observed that continued pacing was more common in a subgroup of patients who had sinus node dysfunction persistent beyond the second postoperative week. Therefore, premature implantation of permanent pacers was discouraged, and it was recommended to delay the decision for pacemaker placement until 3 weeks after the transplantation.

Although a certain percentage of patients ultimately require pacing, the authors do not advocate early implantation of pacemaker systems. As long as patients are without hemodynamic embarrassment, we rarely implant pacemakers before the 1-month posttransplant mark. Oral theophylline is often helpful in patients with perioperative bradyarrhythmias, but it has been our experience that many patients have spontaneous resolution of rhythm disturbances. We favor implantation of dual-chamber pacemakers when pacing becomes necessary.

Pulmonary Hypertension

As mentioned previously, failure of the right ventricle in the immediate and the early postoperative period accounts for nearly half of all cardiac complications following heart transplantation. It can be associated with inability to separate the patient from cardiopulmonary bypass and represents one of the major risk factors for death. In recipients with elevated pulmonary vascular resistance, the etiology of right ventricular dysfunction is the abrupt increase in afterload at the time of the operation, aided and abetted by ischemia–reperfusion injury. To avert acute graft failure, it is imperative to effectively control the recipient's hemodynamics immediately after discontinuation of cardiopulmonary bypass. There are several agents in clinical use that dilate the pulmonary vasculature and thus lower the pulmonary vascular resistance and hence reduce right ventricular afterload. The pulmonary vasodilators differ in their selectivity of action and therefore in their systemic side effects.

Kieler-Jensen et al. compared the effects of intravenous sodium nitroprusside, prostacyclin, prostaglandin E_1, and inhaled nitric oxide on hemodynamics within 48h after orthotopic heart transplantation.[79] Prostaglandin E_1 has a pronounced first-pass elimination in the pulmonary vasculature, and inhaled nitric oxide selectively dilates vessels of ventilated areas of the lung. The authors found that inhaled nitric oxide at 20ppm decreased pulmonary artery pressure, pulmonary vascular resistance, transpulmonary gradient, and central venous pressure. It had no significant effect on mean arterial pressure, pulmonary capillary wedge pressure, heart rate, or systemic vascular resistance and led to an increase in cardiac output.

The three intravenous vasodilators were compared[79] at a predetermined desired level of mean arterial pressure. They all led to a decrease in both pulmonary vascular and systemic vascular resistance. Unlike sodium nitroprusside and prostaglandin E_1, prostacyclin led to a mild increase in cardiac output and stroke volume. The authors concluded that while prostacyclin appeared to be the ideal intravenous vasodilator, the high degree of pulmonary selectivity makes inhaled nitric oxide the preferred treatment for pulmonary hypertension in the postoperative phase.

A study by Auler et al. confirmed Kieler-Jensen et al.'s findings. The trial evaluated the effects of a brief course of inhaled nitric oxide at 20ppm in the immediate postoperative period, within 2h after the surgical procedure.[80] Inhaled nitric oxide selectively dilated the pulmonary vasculature without having deleterious effects on systemic hemodynamics. The authors also observed transient increases in cardiac indices. The maximal effects were reached at 30min of drug action, and the examined parameters returned to baseline after discontinuation of therapy.

The authors are extremely aggressive in our postoperative therapy for pulmonary hypertension secondary to left ventricular failure. We continue to use reversibility of pulmonary vascular resistance elevations as a criterion for listing for orthotopic cardiac transplantation. In the perioperative period, patients with pulmonary hypertension are treated with inhaled nitric oxide or inhaled iloprost. We are also aggressive in our use of intravenous milrinone so long as the patient's systemic blood pressure can tolerate the drug. Other strategies employed include hyperventilation and aggressive diuresis in patients with demonstrated volume overload. We are particularly careful with renal function in patients with pulmonary hypertension as they appear to be more sensitive to drug-related nephrotoxicity. We tend to favor cytolytic therapy in the early postoperative period to avoid cyclosporine-related nephrotoxicity.

Immunosuppression

The dramatic improvement in long-term survival after orthotopic heart transplantation over the past two decades is mainly the result of advances and refinements in immunosuppression. In the early years of cardiac transplantation, polyclonal antilymphocyte sera, azathioprine, and corticosteroids were the only available immunosuppression. Despite their ability to suppress immune responses leading to acute rejection, the nonspecific mode of action of these agents posed significant risks to recipients, particularly susceptibility to infection and bone marrow suppression. The introduction of cyclosporine to clinical cardiac transplantation in 1980 revolutionized the field. This drug inhibits the production of interleukin (IL)-2 and thus suppresses the proliferation of helper T lymphocytes. Through its selective action, cyclosporine spares the remainder of the immune system and does not lead to suppression of the bone marrow. The drug has a broader therapeutic index; it is a more effective immunosuppressant and at the same time is associated with a lower risk of opportunistic infections.

Tacrolimus (FK506), which has similar mechanisms of action to cyclosporine has now become recognized therapy in patients who cannot tolerate cyclosporine or experience rejection despite therapeutic serum levels. In a similar manner, mycophenate mofetil (MMF) has replaced azathioprine as part of the standard triple maintenance therapy in most cardiac transplant centers. Newer, small-molecule immunosuppressants with different mechanisms of action have been developed over the last few years; these include rapamycin, everolimus, and leflunomide. In addition, a variety of new antilymphocyte preparations have entered the clinic; OKT3, a murine monoclonal directed at the CD3 molecule, is the most effective rescue agent available. Polyclonal cytolytic agents such as horse or rabbit antithymocyte globulin are primarily used as induction therapy. Moreover, humanized and chimeric monoclonal antibodies against IL-2 receptors have been used effectively as induction agents in renal and cardiac transplant recipients.[81] Last, costimulation blockers are now in clinical trials. Nonpharmacological immunosuppressive strategies such as total lymphoid irradiation, plasmapheresis, and particularly photopheresis[82] have received increased attention, especially in the setting of presensitized recipients or those with persistent, recurrent, or resistant rejection.

Until the successful induction of transplantation tolerance in humans, immunosuppression will remain as a necessary evil. All immunosuppressive regimens in clinical use are associated with significant side effects and toxicities. In fact, immunosuppression is the most common cause of major complications after a transplant. In addition to increasing susceptibility to infection, immunosuppressants have toxic effects on the kidneys, brain, and bone marrow. In addition, they have adverse effects on lipid metabolism and glucose regulation. These considerations are the main motivation to investigate means to induce tolerance and to develop new drugs with increased specificities and fewer side effects. Current practice is based on observational data rather than on randomized clinical trials.[83] At most transplant centers, immunosuppressive regimens are guided mainly by two principles: high levels of immunosuppression in the immediate postoperative period to prevent acute rejection and the administration of multiple drugs having different mechanisms of action to lower the dose of each drug, thereby reducing toxicity. Traditionally, most centers have tried to use a single immunosuppression regimen, although the advent of new agents has shifted the focus toward individualizing immunosuppression.

The lack of generally accepted guidelines and newly emerging regimens led to divergent policies at different heart transplant centers. Controversies are not just limited to maintenance immunosuppression but extend to monitoring for rejection and treatment of rejection episodes.

Induction Therapy

There is great controversy in the literature with respect to the necessity for induction therapy with cytolytic agents in heart transplantation. Clinical practice often relies on personal preference rather than on scientifically proven fact. This issue is further complicated by the variety of cytolytic agents available as well as by differences in dosing schedules and maintenance immunosuppressive agents.

Induction therapy refers to the administration of cytolytic agents for 7 to 14 days in the immediate postoperative period. The principal cytolytics in clinical use include the polyclonal agents horse antithymocyte globulin (ATGAM), rabbit antithymocyte globulin (Thymoglobulin), and the murine monoclonal antibody OKT3. Waid and colleagues reported favorable preliminary results after induction therapy with the monoclonal agent T10B9.[84] This agent, which is directed against the T-cell receptor, does not lead to the massive cytokine release that can be observed with OKT3 and hence has been shown not to display the same spectrum of untoward effects. Last, monoclonals directed against the IL-2 receptor have been approved for use in renal transplantation. In one small trial comparing OKT3 with an anti-IL-2 receptor monoclonal antibody, similar efficacy was demonstrated, and no side effects were noted.[85]

The use of cytolytic induction therapy with antithymocyte globulin (ATG) is most advantageous in patients who have preexisting renal dysfunction. The first dose of ATG is given at 1 mg/kg body weight according to the weight of the patient. Calculation of the next dose is dependent on CD3 cell count measured on the morning after the completion of the infusion. This avoids complete suppression of the T-cell population and has therefore significantly reduced the incidence of posttransplant sepsis. Early postoperative administration of cyclosporine in such patients with preexisting renal dysfunction can lead to oliguria or anuria and, consequently, poor outcome.[86] Cytolytics postpone the need to begin cyclosporine until hemodynamic parameters improve and the effects of cardiopulmonary bypass resolve, thus reducing the toxic effects of the drug. Induction therapy is also beneficial in heart recipients who are at a higher risk for acute rejection (e.g., retransplantation candidates or presensitized patients). Several investigators have suggested that the use of induction therapy may permit subsequent discontinuation of steroids.[87] Finally, there is controversy as to whether induction therapy has any impact on later episodes of rejection. While a European multicenter trial reported increased rejection-free rates at 1 year with the use of induction therapy with antithymocyte globulin, a U.S. trial failed to show significant differences in rejection frequencies between heart transplant recipients who received induction therapy with OKT3 and a control group who were treated with triple-drug therapy.[88]

The risk of infection and the question of an association with lymphoproliferative disorders are the main arguments against the use of cytolytic induction therapy. However, the available data are rather inconclusive. A study by Alonso-Pulpon et al. showed that lowering the dose of OKT3 from 5 to 2.5 mg/day for 7 consecutive days led to a decrease in bacterial, fungal, and viral infections, but the infection rate still exceeded that in a control population who did not receive induction.[89] Others have found an association between the use of OKT3 and the development of cytomegalovirus (CMV) infections.[90] An increased cumulative dose of OKT3 has been shown to correlate with an increase in the incidence of lymphoproliferative disorders.[91] Epstein-Barr virus (EBV) is thought to play a role in the development of posttransplantation lymphoproliferative disorders by inducing uncontrolled proliferation of B lymphocytes. Although the aforementioned study was not definitive, the EBV seroconversion rate was suggestive of a pathogenic link.

Interleukin 2 Blockers

Recently, human IgG_1 monoclonal antibody daclizumab, which blocks the high-affinity IL-2 receptors present on the surface of activated T cells, has been shown to reduce the frequency and severity of allograft rejection in the induction period in cardiac transplant recipients.[81]

In general, the authors favor selective use of induction cytolytic therapy. We believe that the risks of CMV and lymphoproliferative disorders make routine use of induction therapy undesirable. However, patients with renal dysfunction, particularly elderly patients or those with diabetes, and presensitized patients clearly benefit from judicious use of cytolytic therapy. We favor the use of polyclonal agents for induction and carefully titrate the dose of antilymphocyte globulin to the patient's peripheral CD3 count. Using this approach, we have been able to demonstrate dramatic reductions in dosing of antilymphocyte globulin and have not seen any increased incidence in rejection. We suspect that the 5- to 10-fold reduction in total exposure to antilymphocyte globulin will reduce the incidence of long-term complications of CMV infection and lymphoproliferative disorders. Most clinical experience with induction therapy has been without peripheral T-cell monitoring. Therefore, conclusions about the downside effects of cytolytic therapy may not be warranted in the setting of careful monitoring. Moreover, newer agents such as IL-2 receptor blockers and costimulation blockers may dramatically enhance the therapeutic index of induction therapy.

Mycophenolate Mofetil Versus Azathioprine

Mycophenolate mofetil (MMF) inhibits de novo purine synthesis. Mycophenolate mofetil was designed to exert preferential effects on both B and T lymphocytes because lymphocytes lack the salvage pathway for purine synthesis. This selective action may represent an advantage of MMF over azathioprine, which inhibits both the de novo and the salvage pathways of purine biosynthesis and thereby suppresses erythropoiesis and neutrophil production in addition to blocking lymphopoiesis.

The first clinical trials with MMF were conducted in cadaveric renal transplantation, where it has shown promise both in prophylaxis of rejection and in the treatment of refractory rejection.[92] While there was no suggestion of bone marrow suppression, the main adverse side effects were related to gastrointestinal disturbances that led to discontinuation of the drug in several cases. It was suggested that mycophenolate mofetil could eventually replace azathioprine in the immunosuppressive regimen for renal transplantation. Favorable results of an uncontrolled, nonrandomized phase I trial of the efficacy and safety of MMF in heart transplant recipients were published in 1993 by the Utah group.[93]

More recently, a randomized multicenter double-blind trial comparing the efficacies of MMF and azathioprine in 650 heart transplant recipients also receiving cyclosporine and corticosteroids as maintenance immunosuppressants has been reported.[94] Patients who were treated with MMF had higher 1-year survival rates as well as higher rates of freedom from allograft rejection at 6 months. Although angiography did not detect significant differences with respect to development of cardiac allograft vasculopathy, there were indications on ICUS that MMF may have beneficial effects on remodeling of the coronary arteries. This finding is in agreement with animal experiments that described decreases in intimal proliferation in a rat aortic allograft model after administration of MMF. Gastrointestinal toxicity, which has been shown to be associated with administration of MMF in previous renal trials, was also noted in the heart trial. In addition, the MMF-treated patient group had a higher incidence of infectious complications, approximately 60% of which were caused by herpes simplex or herpes zoster. Overall, substitution of MMF for azathioprine in maintenance immunosuppression appeared beneficial.

The authors believe that MMF is slightly superior to azathioprine as a maintenance immunosuppressant. Although the results of the multicenter trial in cardiac transplantation are equivocal, our experience with the drug suggests that it does help to reduce the incidence of acute rejection. However, the differences are not dramatic, and a substantial number of patients are unable to tolerate the drug because of gastrointestinal toxicity. Obviously, the hope is that MMF will reduce the incidence of cardiac allograft vasculopathy. Thus far, there are insufficient data to make any conclusions on this issue.

Cyclosporine Versus Tacrolimus

Cyclosporine represented a major advance in immunosuppression due to its selective action on T lymphocytes. Introduced into the clinical arena in 1983, cyclosporine has fundamentally changed the field of organ transplantation. However, administration of cyclosporine is associated with significant toxicities. The spectrum of renal side effects—reversible acute dysfunction, chronic progressive insufficiency, and arterial hypertension—are well known to all transplant clinicians. In addition, cyclosporine is associated with neurotoxicity, gingival hyperplasia, hirsutism, hyperlipidemia, and osteoporosis. More recently, animal experiments have suggested an association between the chronic use of cyclosporine and the development of cardiac allograft vasculopathy.[95] Despite the obvious efficacy of cyclosporine, the adverse effects of the drug led to a search for other immunosuppressive drugs.

Tacrolimus is a naturally occurring macrolide antibiotic that shares many pharmacological characteristics with cyclosporine. However, it has been shown to be 10- to 100-fold more potent than cyclosporine at inhibiting the activation of alloreactive T lymphocytes when compared on a molar basis. The spectrum of adverse effects resembles that of cyclosporine, including nephrotoxicity, central nervous system toxicity, hypertension, and gastrointestinal disturbances. Last, there is an association between the use of tacrolimus and a reduction in bone mineral density in a subgroup of heart transplant recipients, which may be related to an impairment of testosterone biosynthesis.[96]

Three recent randomized trials have compared the efficacy of cyclosporine and tacrolimus in preventing acute rejection in heart transplant recipients.[97–99] The studies demonstrated equivalent survival rates and incidences of acute rejection. The primary differences noted were the distribution of drug-related complications. Nephrotoxicity was slightly more frequent in patients treated with tacrolimus. Moreover, tacrolimus was frequently associated with hyperglycemia. In contrast, cyclosporine was associated with higher incidences of hirsutism, hypertension, and hypercholesterolemia. Neurotoxocity was equivalent.

The authors believe that cyclosporine and tacrolimus are essentially equivalent as first-line maintenance immunosuppressants. Although it is clear that switching from cyclosporine to tacrolimus is efficacious in circumstances of recurrent rejection, the same cannot be said for switching from tacrolimus to cyclosporine. As a result, we continue to use cyclosporine as our primary immunosuppressant in conjunction with MMF and steroids and then escalate therapy to tacrolimus in patients with recurrent, steroid-resistant, or persistent rejection. Given that the drugs have a different spectrum of side effects, we also use tacrolimus selectively as primary immunosuppression in certain patients. Finally, it is questionable whether tacrolimus will be useful in combination with rapamycin or rapamycin derivative (RAD) as these drugs compete for the same binding protein.

Steroids

Triple-drug immunosuppression with cyclosporine, azathioprine, and corticosteroids after heart transplantation has been shown to be associated with improvements in short- and long-term survival.[100] The ability of this combination to significantly reduce the incidence of acute rejection has made it the most commonly used regimen in both adult and pediatric populations. Concerns about side effects, including hyperlipidemia, arterial hypertension, and weight gain, which may predispose to the development of cardiac allograft vasculopathy, have stimulated efforts to modify this regimen. While the antiinflammatory and immunosuppressive effects of corticosteroids are clearly beneficial in preventing early rejection and in reversing acute rejection, steroids have multiple adverse effects. Steroid-induced diabetes mellitus, hypertension, gastrointestinal disturbances, truncal obesity, fluid retention, and osteoporosis are poorly tolerated by transplant recipients. Moreover, growth retardation consequent to steroid use is a major concern in the pediatric population.

Approaches to decrease morbidity from steroid use have varied from late weaning many months posttransplant[101] to protocols that exclude steroids entirely from maintenance immunosuppression. Olivari[100] reported the results of a corticosteroid-tapering protocol that was initiated a few days postoperatively and resulted in complete cessation of steroids by 6 months after heart transplantation.[100] At 1-year follow-up, steroid withdrawal had no adverse effect on survival or on allograft function as assessed by hemodynamic data. Moreover, there was no difference in vasculopathy as assessed by angiography. Patients who were withdrawn from steroids not only had a higher incidence of allograft rejection but also a decrease in infectious complications and a reduction in bone loss. The authors concluded that even in the absence of induction therapy, early withdrawal from steroids was safe for the majority of patients. They found that the higher incidence of acute rejection did not compromise overall survival because of the lower incidence of infectious complications. Potential benefits of withdrawing steroids early in female heart recipients to avoid osteoporosis need to be weighed against the higher risk of acute rejection in this patient population. There is also a controversy in the literature with respect to the predictive power of donor-recipient HLA-DR class II histocompatibility antigen matching on successful steroid withdrawal.[102]

Last, steroid withdrawal is recommended in patients with a history of multiple previous rejection episodes. A prospective study addressed the issue of steroid discontinuation among the pediatric heart transplant population.[103] Initial immunosuppression was a triple-drug regimen without induction therapy. Steroids were weaned 6 to 12 months after transplantation. Twenty-four percent of their patients showed evidence of rejection on endomyocardial biopsy between 2 weeks and 6 months after discontinuation of steroids. The study was unable to correlate the likelihood of rejection after discontinuation of steroids with the child's chronological age at transplantation, the time point of steroid withdrawal, number of rejection episodes before steroid withdrawal, or the degree of HLA matching. Although the study demonstrated that it was feasible to withdraw steroids successfully in the majority of their patients, the potentially devastating consequences of rejection in children necessitates frequent surveillance endomyocardial biopsies after complete steroid discontinuation.

There is little question that the side effects of steroids are the most disabling and difficult for patients and for transplant physicians. Therefore, the authors believe that efforts to aggressively wean steroids are warranted. Furthermore, with the advent of a variety of new small-molecule and biological immunosuppressants, it may be reasonable to reconsider the universal practice of steroid pulsing as primary therapy for acute rejection. Although the initial clinical trials of RAD in cardiac transplant patients will compare this drug to azathioprine, we suspect that future multicenter, prospective randomized trials will use novel drug combinations to eliminate steroids completely for maintenance immunosuppression.

New Immunosuppressants

The target of rapamycin (TOR) inhibitors sirolimus and its derivative everolimus act on specific intracellular receptors within lymphocytes. They are being used more widely in renal transplant recipients and seem to be making their way into the cardiac population.

Sirolimus

Sirolimus is a highly potent immunosuppressant that has recently undergone phase one/two trials in renal transplantation.[104] It is a macrocyclic antibiotic and is structurally related to tacrolimus. It therefore forms a complex with FK-binding proteins but differs in its mechanism of suppression. Unlike the calcineurin inhibitors (CNIs), sirolimus prevents progression of the T-cell cycle from G1 to S phase by blocking signaling downstream of the IL-2 receptors. It also inhibits T-cell responses to cytokines. On the other hand, it blocks lymphocytic proliferation at a point that is upstream from the CNIs. It therefore should have a synergistic action with antiproliferatives and CNIs. It could cause hyperlipidemia, thrombocytopenia, and leucopenia.[105] Pneumonitis as a result of sirolimus therapy has been a well-recognized complication in renal transplant recipients and has been persistent despite cessation of treatment in some.[106] Heart transplant recipients are no exception.

Everolimus is one of the new immunosuppressants being developed for prevention of rejection. It is a novel proliferation signal inhibitor, blocking growth factor-driven proliferation of both hematopoietic and nonhematopoietic cells. It synergizes with cyclosporine to prevent and reverse acute rejection in preclinical models of kidney, heart, or lung transplantation.[107] It blocks growth factor-driven transduction signals in the T-cell response to alloantigen. After stimulation of the IL-2 receptor on the activated T cell, everolimus inhibits p70S6 kinase, acting at a later stage in the T-cell-mediated response than cyclosporine and other CNIs. These activities are complementary to those of cyclosporine and provide a rationale for the addition of this drug to cyclosporine-based immunosuppression, with the potential for minimizing nephrotoxicity, reducing the incidence of acute rejection, and favoring long-term graft survival. The manifestations of chronic rejection that may contribute to graft loss are also inhibited by everolimus in preclinical models.

Although everolimus is metabolized by the cytochrome P450 CYP3A isoenzyme, coadministration with cyclosporine does not alter the pharmacokinetics of cyclosporine, but cyclosporine coadministration increases exposure to everolimus. Everolimus interacts with inhibitors and inducers of this system; its clearance is reduced in patients with hepatic impairment. In an immunosuppressive regimen with cyclosporine microemulsion formulation and corticosteroids, transplant recipients treated with everolimus show low rates of acute rejection and, in one heart and one renal trial, lower rates of CMV infection. Acute rejection rates are lower than those seen with azathioprine in cardiac transplant recipients[108] and similar to those seen with MMF in renal transplant recipients.

Low rates of acute rejection are maintained when everolimus is given as part of a quadruple immunosuppressive regimen with low-dose cyclosporine in renal transplant recipients, with the added benefit of better renal function compared with full-dose cyclosporine. Use of C(2) monitoring to optimize cyclosporine exposure and enhance efficacy and safety of everolimus is planned in future studies. Hypertriglyceridemia and hypercholesterolemia have been associated with everolimus, but these effects are not dose-limiting.

There is no clear upper therapeutic limit of everolimus. However, thrombocytopenia occurs at a rate of 17% at everolimus trough serum concentrations above 7.8 ng/mL in renal transplant recipients. There are limited safety data available in patients with trough concentrations above 12 ng/mL. Studies suggest everolimus targets primary causes of chronic rejection by reducing acute rejection, allowing for cyclosporine dose reduction (which may lead to improved renal function relative to full-dose cyclosporine) and by reducing CMV infection and inhibiting vascular remodeling. Everolimus has also been shown to inhibit the early phase of cardiac allograft vasculopathy.

Anti-CD25 Monoclonal Antibodies

Basiliximab, a new monoclonal antibody against CD25, has been used in patients with acute renal dysfunction due to CNI therapy. Patients are given a break from CNIs (a CNI holiday) after being administered a single dose of the monoclonal antibody. This provides a rejection-free period and enables renal function to return to normal.[109,110]

As more information is revealed about immunosuppression alongside the increasing number of products that are available for current practice, the "one-size-fits-all" institutional policies should be abolished in favor of individualized regimes.

Endomyocardial Biopsy

The routine use of postoperative surveillance endomyocardial biopsies has contributed to an overall increase in survival after cardiac transplantation. Biopsy allows allograft rejection to be detected and therefore treated before the onset of hemodynamically significant dysfunction. Because allograft rejection is most common early after transplantation, endomyocardial biopsies have been traditionally performed weekly for the first month and progressively less frequently thereafter. Despite ongoing attempts to develop noninvasive techniques to monitor allograft rejection, transvenous endomyocardial biopsy has remained the gold standard for diagnosis of rejection.

Endomyocardial biopsy is not without limitations. It is an invasive procedure that is uncomfortable and is occasionally associated with injury to the tricuspid valve or with right atrial or ventricular perforation. Moreover, the diagnostic accuracy of the procedure can be limited by sampling error. Furthermore, the specificity of certain histological findings is controversial. For example, the Quilty effect, a focal endocardial or myocardial lymphocytic aggregation, is observed in up to one-third of all biopsies. It is often difficult to distinguish the Quilty effect from actual rejection. While some believe that the Quilty effect is a predictor of rejection, others think that it is a benign phenomenon. Last, a single endomyocardial biopsy generates more than $1000 in health care costs.

These considerations have led several investigators to challenge the long-accepted practice of indefinite endomyocardial biopsies. As the incidence of allograft rejection decreases with time, the necessity of biopsies late after transplantation has become a focus of interest. White et al. addressed this issue in a study of more than 1100 routine endomyocardial biopsies that were performed in 235 heart recipients at least 1 year after the transplantation.[111] Less than 1% of all biopsies showed evidence of significant rejection that necessitated adjustment in the immunosuppressive regimen. The authors concluded that routine endomyocardial biopsies beyond 1 year are unnecessary and recommended their use only if clinically indicated. Sethi et al. reached a similar conclusion after reviewing routine surveillance endomyocardial biopsies that were performed at least 6 months after the transplantation.[112] Compared to a group of historical control patients who had undergone routine biopsies indefinitely, recipients in whom routine biopsies were curtailed 6 months after transplant had no difference.

A study conducted by Brunner-La Rocca and Kiowski at the University of Zurich attempted to identify patient characteristics associated with higher risk for late rejection that would justify long-term follow-up with routine endomyocardial biopsy.[113] They found several predictors that correlated with higher incidences of late graft rejection, including a history of previous graft rejection, young recipient age, low cyclosporine blood levels during the first 2 years after transplantation, and reduction or withdrawal of steroids. They recommended routine long-term endomyocardial biopsies for patients who fall into these high-risk categories for late rejection.

Endomyocardial biopsy remains the gold standard for the diagnosis of acute rejection, and the authors believe that an aggressive surveillance biopsy program is particularly important in the first year after transplantation. In general, we do not believe annual biopsies are particularly intrusive or risky, although we recognize that maintenance immunosuppression is rarely changed as a result of such long-term surveillance biopsies in asymptomatic patients. In general, we have stopped doing surveillance biopsies 2 years after transplantation.

Rejection Therapy

Cardiac allograft rejection accounts for approximately one-third of all deaths related to the procedure. Treatment of rejection episodes depends on histological grade and on clinical symptoms. The rationale to treat even mild acute cardiac rejection without hemodynamic compromise early and aggressively stems from the beliefs that low-grade rejection is a precursor to high-grade rejection and that repetitive episodes of untreated low-grade rejection can compromise long-term cardiac function and may predispose to cardiac allograft vasculopathy. This notion that low-grade rejection portends high-grade rejection is supported by the observation that increasing immunosuppression in patients with low-grade rejection prevents progression to moderate rejection on subsequent biopsies.[114]

A variety of both pharmacological and nonpharmacological strategies can be employed for the treatment of allograft rejection. Corticosteroids have been used most commonly to treat episodes of cellular rejection with or without hemodynamic compromise. Policies differ with respect to dose, route of administration, and tapering after the bolus therapy. Traditionally, the treatment consists of intravenous administration of 1 g methylprednisolone per day for 3 consecutive days. However, comparable results in the treatment of asymptomatic moderate rejection have been achieved by administering an oral prednisone pulse therapy of 100 mg per day for 3 consecutive days followed by a taper over 2 weeks.[115] Moreover, health care costs with the oral regimen were substantially lower.

Other small-molecule immunosuppressants can reverse acute rejection. Tacrolimus has been shown to reverse steroid-resistant acute rejection. Moreover, if substituted for cyclosporine in the maintenance regimen, it will also prevent recurrent acute rejection. Methotrexate, a folic acid analogue that inhibits the biosynthesis of purine, has been utilized successfully in the treatment of recurrent cellular rejection in heart transplant recipients receiving triple-drug immunosuppression.[116] However, unlike tacrolimus, methotrexate does not decrease the risk of subsequent rejection episodes. Despite a persistent risk of acute rejection, methotrexate-treated patients did not show an increased incidence of allograft vasculopathy. This finding challenges the notion that a relationship exists between acute rejection rates and later development of cardiac allograft vasculopathy. Moreover, it suggests that methotrexate may have a protective effect against the development of this morbid complication.[117] It has been suggested that antimetabolites, particularly methotrexate and MMF, inhibit the activation of the endothelium and the proliferation of vascular smooth muscle.[118]

Cytolytic therapy has been the preferred treatment for steroid-resistant, hemodynamically significant, and acute vascular rejection for many years. Haverty et al. treated acute heart rejection with OKT3 in more than 100 patients who had failed "conventional" strategies like high-dose intravenous steroids or in whom conventional therapy was medically contraindicated.[119] Primary and recurrent episodes of acute rejection could be reversed in approximately 90% of their patients after 10- to 14-day courses of OKT3. The authors reported 12-month graft and patient survivals of approximately 70% after OKT3 treatment for both primary and recurrent rejection. In contrast, a study conducted by Wagner et al. at the University of Munich was far less encouraging.[120] Complete resolution of steroid-resistant acute rejection was achieved in only 17% of patients with 10-day courses of OKT3. The remainder of the OKT3-treated patients did not show any improvement in rejection as assessed by biopsy or experienced a recurrent rejection within 3 weeks of the initial resolution. These patients, who failed OKT3 therapy, were treated successfully with methotrexate.

The main nonpharmacological modalities for the treatment of allograft rejection are photopheresis and total lymphoid irradiation. Photopheresis is an immunomodulatory therapy in which the patient's mononuclear cells are treated with 6-methylpsoralen, a photosensitizing agent, and subsequently exposed to ultraviolet A ex vivo. After photoexposure, these cells are then returned to the patient. It is postulated that these cells stimulate a suppressor response by altering antigen presentation. Initially used in the treatment of cutaneous T-cell lymphoma, the indications for photopheresis were expanded to several autoimmune diseases and more recently to bone marrow and solid-organ transplantation.

Although its specific mechanisms of action have not been clearly elucidated, preliminary results from animal experiments and small clinical series are encouraging. Several authors have demonstrated that photopheresis can reverse steroid-resistant, cytolytic-resistant, or recurrent acute rejection.[121–123] Photochemotherapy also can reduce panel reactive antibodies in multiparous women or candidates for retransplantation.[124] Last, prophylactic photopheresis clearly reduces the incidence of acute rejection and may help prevent allograft vasculopathy.[125,126]

The authors continue to use pulse steroids as our primary therapy for acute allograft rejection, although the advent of several new immunosuppressive agents may challenge this time-honored clinical approach. We continue to use cytolytic therapy in all circumstances in which allograft rejection leads to hemodynamic compromise. In addition to reversing the rejection episodes, we believe strongly that any rejection episode that is grade IIIA or higher warrants alteration of maintenance immunosuppression in addition to rescue therapy. We have also been aggressive about the use of photopheresis therapy and have had excellent results using this approach. Although somewhat cumbersome, logistically difficult, and expensive, photopheresis is without significant side effects. Therefore, a long-term cost–benefit analysis would likely favor photopheresis therapy. We believe that photopheresis in addition to other biological strategies for mitigating allograft rejection will play an increasingly important role in the future.

Complications

Infections

The drug-induced immunosuppressive state in solid-organ recipients places this population at risk for life-threatening infections. Infectious complications following heart transplantation are one of the leading causes of morbidity and mortality, as is clearly illustrated by the fact that more than two-thirds of all heart transplant recipients develop at least one infectious episode within the first year after the operation. Among heart transplant recipients, infections are responsible for 18% of early and 38% of late mortality. The type of infection depends on several factors, including the patient's environment, the time period that has elapsed since the operation, and the net state of immunosuppression.

Grossi and colleagues examined the relationship between immunosuppressive regimens and infectious complications in a population of more than 600 heart transplant recipients.[127] They observed a peak incidence of infections within the first 6 months postoperatively. A clear correlation between the use of pulsed steroids or cytolytics and the incidence of infectious complications was demonstrated.

Bacterial infections are common in the perioperative period (0–6 months posttransplant) and warrant aggressive workup and expeditious treatment. Opportunistic infections (fungal, parasitic, viral) tend to occur later in the postoperative course.

The most common fungal pathogens encountered after transplant are *Candida*, *Aspergillus*, and *Cryptococcus*. Disseminated infections with *Candida* or *Aspergillus* can often be fatal complications and must be treated with an extended course of amphotericin B, followed by lifelong azole therapy. Mayer et al. reported a case of a heart transplant recipient who suffered from an isolated pulmonary *Aspergillus* infection that was diagnosed approximately 2 weeks after treatment of acute rejection with intravenous corticosteroids.[128] Despite a prolonged course of antifungal therapy, the pulmonary lesion persisted and eventually necessitated surgical resection. This case illustrates the difficulty in eradicating fungal infections in immunosuppressed patients.

Infections with intracellular parasites are also increased in immunosuppressed patients. A review by Munoz et al. documented an increased incidence of tuberculosis and atypical mycobacterial infections among heart transplant recipients.[129] *Toxoplasma gondii* and *Pneumocystis carinii* are also common opportunistic pathogens in immunosuppressed heart transplant recipients. In the case of toxoplasmosis, the importance of prophylactic treatment for seronegative recipients of hearts from seropositive donors has been demonstrated by Holliman et al.[130] Moreover, all heart transplant recipients should receive prophylaxis against *Pneumocystis*.

Heart transplant recipients are particularly susceptible to infections with the herpesviruses, namely CMV, EBV, varicella zoster virus (VZV), and herpes simplex virus types 1, 2, and 6. Because CMV is a major cause of morbidity and mortality, a large body of work on prophylaxis and treatment of CMV infections exists. Infections with CMV are usually asymptomatic in an immunocompetent host; they are often severe and potentially fatal in immunosuppressed patients. The disease process affects several target organs, particularly the lungs, liver, intestines, and bone marrow. Also, CMV has been implicated as a predisposing factor for the development of cardiac allograft vasculopathy. Infection can result from reactivation of latent virus in a seropositive recipient, or de novo infection can occur in seronegative recipients of organs from seropositive donors. To avoid mortality and morbidity of de novo infection, several groups favor donor-recipient CMV matching; this is particularly true in the setting of heart-lung transplantation because of the risk of CMV pneumonitis in the transplanted lung.[131] Because treatment of established disease is difficult and there is not a single placebo-controlled, double-blind, randomized trial that showed clinical benefit against established CMV disease for any drug with anti-CMV activity, the development of prophylactic strategies to prevent disease has become a main focus of investigation.[132]

The Stanford group led the first multicenter, placebo-controlled, double-blind study with ganciclovir prophylaxis in a population of heart transplant recipients who were at high risk for development of CMV disease.[133] The trial showed that a prophylactic 28-day course of intravenous ganciclovir starting 1 day after transplantation was able to significantly reduce the incidence of CMV disease in heart transplant recipients who were seropositive before transplantation. On the other hand, the incidence of illness was not reduced in seronegative recipients of organs from seropositive donors. Numerous studies in other organ transplants have not confirmed this observation.

In general, prophylaxis appears to be most important in mitigating the clinical sequelae of de novo infections. Most current prophylactic regimens employ ganciclovir, valacyclovir, or foscarnet alone or in combination with anti-CMV hyperimmune globulin in high-risk patients. However, although the incidence of life-threatening infections can be reduced or delayed with these strategies, these infections cannot be prevented completely.

The primary controversy that exists regarding management of infectious complications after heart transplantation involves the choice between expectant and prophylactic management for CMV. In all circumstances of donor or recipient seropositivity, the authors support aggressive prophylaxis with intravenous ganciclovir during the hospitalization, followed by oral ganciclovir on discharge. We extend therapy with intravenous ganciclovir to 6 weeks for seronegative recipients of seropositive organs. Currently, we use hyperimmune globulin only for those patients with severe symptomatic CMV.

Cardiac Allograft Vasculopathy

Improvements in immunosuppression and perioperative management have led to increased survival rates after heart transplantation, with 1-year survival rates of 91%. Despite these advances in short-term survival, long-term morbidity and mortality still remain a serious problem in this patient population. The major cause for late morbidity and mortality is cardiac allograft vasculopathy, which is a pathological process distinct from atherosclerotic coronary artery disease. The disease process is not only limited to the epicardial coronary arteries but also involves intramyocardial arterioles, venous structures, and the great vessels of the allograft.

Cardiac allograft vasculopathy is diffuse in nature, begins distally and progresses proximally, and is characterized by concentric proliferation of the intima. The pathological anatomy is associated with abnormalities in the vasodilatory response of the coronary circulation.[134] Most investigators believe that chronic, sublethal injury to the endothelium leads to alterations in cytokine production that induce the proliferative process.[135] It is interesting to note that these obliterative changes in the coronary circulation were first described in the autopsy specimen of Barnard's second heart transplant recipient, who survived for nearly 2 years.[136]

Immune-mediated mechanisms are thought to be primarily responsible for the development of cardiac allograft vasculopathy. In addition, a variety of nonimmunological mechanisms have been implicated as etiologic factors. Mismatches of HLA at the DR locus are closely associated with a higher incidence of cardiac allograft vasculopathy.[137] Controversy exists regarding the pathogenetic link between acute rejection and cardiac allograft vasculopathy. Although early studies suggested that the frequency of acute rejection portends vasculopathy,[138] subsequent studies employing triple-drug therapy were equivocal.[139] Controversy also exists regarding the dominant mechanism responsible for the problem. Experimental studies using B-cell knockout mice suggested that humoral immunity plays a dominant role in cardiac allograft vasculopathy.[140] However, analysis of humoral and cellular responses of human recipients to purified donor-specific endothelial cells suggested that cell-mediated immunity is more important.[141]

Multiple nonimmunological risk factors that have been discussed in the literature include donor ischemia–reperfusion injury and side effects of immunosuppressants, as well as recipient factors such as obesity, hyperlipidemia, hypercholesterolemia, and hypertension. Escobar et al. conducted a study examining the predictive power of several nonimmunological risk factors for the development of cardiac allograft vasculopathy.[142] Unlike other studies, the presence and severity of cardiac allograft vasculopathy was assessed by intravascular ultrasonography rather than coronary angiography. This modality is more sensitive than coronary angiography and is able to detect coronary lesions during earlier stages of development. The authors found that hyperlipidemia, specifically high levels of low-density lipoprotein cholesterol; weight gain; donor age above 25 years; and time elapsed since cardiac transplantation were independent predictors of severity of this multifactorial disease.

There is increasing evidence that the ischemic injury to the graft sustained during the perioperative time period plays a major role in the development of cardiac allograft vasculopathy.[143] Ischemia leads to complement-mediated endothelial injury, upregulation of MHC antigens, and upregulation of adhesion molecules, which increase graft immunogenicity and antigenicity. A clinical trial of superoxide dismutase, which reduces ischemia–reperfusion injury, demonstrated a reduction in acute and chronic rejection rates of cadaveric kidney grafts.[144] Preliminary studies with the potent complement inhibitor soluble complement receptor type 1 (sCR1) are yielding similar results.

It is imperative to continue research efforts to further elucidate the underlying mechanisms responsible for the development of cardiac allograft vasculopathy and to direct efforts toward preventive strategies. To date, the only definitive therapy for this potentially fatal late complication of cardiac transplantation remains retransplantation.

There is little doubt that the pathological process of cardiac allograft vasculopathy is driven primarily by histoincompatibility. Although nonimmunological factors are important and demand further investigation with development of novel therapies, efforts to eradicate cardiac allograft vasculopathy will undoubtedly depend on better immunosuppression or the induction of donor-specific tolerance. The authors believe that early episodes of acute rejection increase the incidence of late vasculopathy by upregulating HLA antigens, adhesion molecules, and costimulatory molecules on the surface of vascular endothelium. Therefore, we advocate intense maintenance immunosuppression for the first 3 to 6 months after transplantation. After 6 months, highly immunostimulatory donor-type bone marrow-derived antigen-presenting cells have disappeared, thus largely eliminating direct allorecognition.

Reduction in immunosuppression at this point is theoretically appealing. Reduction in acute rejection is likely to reduce the long-term incidence of cardiac allograft vasculopathy. In addition, a variety of new pharmacological agents, particularly rapamycin and RAD, may act directly to prevent this feared complication as a result of the direct antiproliferative effects of these agents. Last, clinical trials of tolerance induction employing several strategies are likely to be undertaken in the next several years. Experimental work has consistently shown that the induction of antigen-specific tolerance will eliminate both acute allograft rejection and cardiac allograft vasculopathy.

Retransplantation

The question of cardiac retransplantation involves both ethical and scientific issues. Although it is the only possible lifesaving intervention for an individual patient, society is faced with a scarcity of donor organs. There are no universal guidelines, and health care professionals must make this difficult decision on a case-by-case basis because a decision for retransplantation will deny a potential recipient access to a transplant. The outcome after retransplantation is generally worse than after a primary transplant. The Stanford group reported a 1-year survival rate of 49% and a 5-year survival rate of 24% for retransplanted patients, while in the case of primary transplants these figures were 82% and 62%, respectively.[145]

Indications for retransplantation in the early postoperative period are usually allograft failure on the basis of nonimmunological factors (ischemia, high pulmonary vascular resistance, etc.) or immune-mediated injury. There are several isolated reports in the literature of favorable outcomes when patients were bridged for several hours with assist devices for nonimmunological primary graft failure before a second heart became available. Because patients with immediate or early primary cardiac allograft failure are generally hemodynamically unstable, the urgency of the situation often leads to acceptance of marginal hearts for this already high-risk group. As a result, a recent study found that three of four patients who underwent retransplantation for primary graft failure died within 2 weeks of the operation.[146] The aforementioned retransplantation from Stanford had equally disappointing results, with five of nine patients dying in the perioperative period. It is not surprising that strong criticism against utilizing donor hearts under these circumstances has been voiced.[147]

Equally disappointing are results from patients who undergo retransplantation for intractable rejection due to the high incidence of postoperative rejection.[148] Of all patients who underwent retransplantation for intractable rejection at Stanford, nearly one-quarter died during the first 6 months of acute allograft rejection.

Thus, the main indication for cardiac retransplantation is for cardiac allograft vasculopathy in the late postoperative period as this patient population has more favorable outcomes after retransplantation. In the Stanford series, the 1-year and 5-year survival rates for patients who underwent retransplantation for graft atherosclerosis were 69% and 34%, respectively. Although these results are clearly inferior to primary transplants, they are not poor enough to clearly contraindicate retransplantation in this subgroup of patients.

The population of long-term heart transplant survivors who are at risk for developing graft atherosclerosis is increasing. Thus, the issue of retransplantation will become more important in the future. Some health care professionals call for the implementation of universal policies to absolve physicians of the burden of making the ultimate decision about allocation of a limited supply of organs. Several authors believe that these rationing decisions need to be made at the level of organizations such as UNOS. Many ethicists contend, on the basis of survival statistics and the principle of justice, each individual should receive only one chance at an organ. However, the advent of long-term assist devices and xenotransplants may help to defuse this ethical conundrum.

Retransplantation is only reasonable for young people with late-occurring cardiac allograft vasculopathy. The outcome of retransplantation in all other subgroups of patients does not warrant the use of a scarce resource of donor hearts. In general, the authors believe that patients undergoing retransplantation should only be given organs from high-risk donors.

Summary

Heart transplantation is currently the best therapy for end-stage heart failure. Nevertheless, it remains an imperfect science. Unfortunately, the proliferation of heart transplant programs with consequent dilution of experience has hampered progress in the field. Until recently, very few prospective, randomized studies of sufficient statistical power have been undertaken in the field of heart transplantation. In fact, many of the controversies discussed in this chapter cannot be settled because of the lack of sufficient data. Given that heart transplantation is an "orphan" procedure (2500 cases per annum) due to the lack of suitable donor organs, it would make sense to restrict the number of centers performing the procedure in an effort to concentrate experience, improve patient care through careful clinical research, and reduce the financial burden to society via enhanced efficiency.

References

1. 1999 Annual Report of the U.S. Scientific Registry of Transplant Recipients and the Organ Procurement and Transplantation Network: Transplant Data 1989–1998. Richmond, VA: HHS/GRSA/OSP/DOT and United Network for Organ Sharing; 1999.
2. Hoercher KJ, Gonzalez-Stawinski GV, Taylor DO, McCarthy PM, Young JB, Starling RC. Cardiac transplantation at the Cleveland Clinic. Clin Transpl 2003;267–274.
3. Hosenpud JD, Novick RJ, Breen TJ, et al. The registry of the International Society for Heart and Lung Transplantation: 11th official report-1994. J Heart Lung Transplant 1994;13:561–570.
4. Breen TJ, Keck B, Daily OP, et al. The use of older donors results in a major increase in early mortality following orthotopic cardiac transplantation. J Heart Lung Transplant 1994;13:S51.
5. Livi U, Bortolotti U, Luciani GB, et al. Donor shortage in heart transplantation: is extension of donor age limits justified? J Thorac Cardiovasc Surg 1994;107:1346–1355.
6. Chau EMC, McGregor CGA, Rodeheffer JR, et al. Increased incidence of chronotropic incompetence in older donor hearts. J Heart Lung Transplant 1995;14:743–748.
7. Mercer P, Sharpies L, Edmunds J, et al. Evaluating the donor pool: impact of using hearts from donors over the age of 49 years. Transplant Proc 1997;29:3293–3296.
8. Gao, S-Z, Hunt SA, Alderman EL, et al. Relation of donor age and preexisting coronary artery disease on angiography and intracoronary ultrasound to later development of accelerated allograft coronary artery disease. J Am Coll Cardiol 1997;29:623–629.
9. Blanes M, Gomez D, Cordoba J, et al. Is there any risk of transmission of hepatitis B from heart donors hepatitis B core antibody positive? Transplant Proc 2002;34:61–62.
10. Ko WJ, Chou NK, Hsu RB, et al. Hepatitis B virus infection in heart transplant recipients in a hepatitis B endemic area. J Heart Lung Transplant 2001;20:865–875.
11. Lim HL, Lau GK, Davis GL, et al. Cholestatic hepatitis leading to hepatic failure in a patient with organ-transmitted hepatitic C virus infection. Gastroenterology 1994;106:248–251.
12. Lake KD, Smith CI, Laforest SKM, et al. Policies regarding the transplantation of hepatitis C-positive candidates and donor organs. J Heart Lung Transplant 1997;16:917–921.
13. Widell A, Mansson S, Persson NH, et al. Hepatitis C superinfection in hepatitis C virus (HCV)-infected patients transplanted with an HCV-infected kidney. Transplantation (Baltimore) 1995;60:642–647.
14. Ferenci P. Current treatment for chronic hepatitis C. Curr Treat Options Gastroenterol 2004;7:491–499.
15. Chan BB, Fleischer KJ, Bergin JD, et al. Weight is not an accurate criterion for adult cardiac transplant size. Ann Thorac Surg 1991;52:1230–1235.
16. Hosenpud JD, Pantely GA, Morton MJ, et al. Relation between recipient: donor body size match and hemodynamics 3 months after heart transplantation. J Heart Transplant 1989;8:241–243.
17. Jeevanandam V, Mather P, Furukawa S, et al. Adult orthotopic heart transplantation using undersized pediatric donor hearts. Circulation 1994;90(pt 2):1174–1177.
18. Sekela ME, Smart FW, Noon GP, et al. Attenuation of waiting time mortality with heterotopic heart transplantation. Ann Thorac Surg 1992;54:547–551.
19. Tamisier D, Vouhe P, Le Bidois J, et al. Donor-recipient size matching in pediatric heart transplantation: a word of caution about small grafts. J Heart Lung Transplant 1996;15:190–195.
20. Iberer F, Wasler A, Tscheliessnigg K, et al. Prostaglandin E1-induced moderation of elevated pulmonary vascular resistance: survival on waiting list and results of orthotopic heart transplantation. J Heart Lung Transplant 1993;12:173–178.
21. Sharples LD, Caine N, Mullins P, et al. Risk factor analysis for the major hazards following heart transplantation—rejection, infection, and coronary occlusive disease. Transplantation 1991; 52:244–252.
22. Mehra MR, Stapleton DD, Ventura HO, et al. Influence of donor and recipient gender on cardiac allograft vasculopathy: an intravascular ultrasound study. Circulation 1994;90(pt 2):1178–1182.

23. Kirsh M, Baufreton C, Naftel DC, et al. Pretransplantation risk factors for death after heart transplantation: the Henri Mondor experience. J Heart Lung Transplant 1998;17:268–277.
24. Prendergast TW, Furukawa S, Beyer AJ III, et al. The role of gender in heart transplantation. Ann Thorac Surg 1998;65:88–94.
25. Jeevanandam V, Todd B, Regillo T, et al. Reversal of donor myocardial dysfunction by triiodothyronine replacement therapy. J Heart Lung Transplant 1994;13:681–687.
26. Jeevanandam V. Triiodothyronine: spectrum of use in heart transplantation. Thyroid 1997;7:139–145.
27. Wheeldon DR, Potter CD, Jonas M, et al. Transplantation of "unsuitable" organs? Transplant Proc 1993;25:3104–3105.
28. Rosendale JD, Kauffman HM, McBride MA, et al. Hormonal resuscitation yields more transplanted hearts, with improved early function. Transplantation 2003;75:1336–1341.
29. Zaroff JG, Rosengard BR, Armstrong WF, et al. Consensus conference report: maximizing use of organs recovered from the cadaver donor: cardiac recommendations, March 28–29, 2001, Crystal City, VA. Circulation 2002;106:836–841.
30. Stein JH, Neumann A, Preston LM, et al. Echocardiography for hemodynamic assessment of patients with advanced heart failure and potential heart transplant recipients. J Am Coll Cardiol 1997;30:1765–1772.
31. Adatia I, Perry S, Landzberg M, et al. Inhaled nitric oxide and hemodynamic evaluations of patients with pulmonary hypertension before transplantation. J Am Coll Cardiol 1995;25:1565–1564.
32. Chen JM, Levin HR, Michler RE, et al. Reevaluating the significance of pulmonary hypertension before cardiac transplantation: determination of optimal thresholds and quantification of the effect of reversibility on perioperative mortality. J Thorac Cardiovasc Surg 1997;114:627–634.
33. Michler RE, Chen JM, Itescu S, et al. Two decades of cardiac transplantation at the Columbia-Presbyterian Medical Center: 1977–1997. Clin Transpl 1996;153–165.
34. Kirsch M, Baufreton C, Naftel D, et al. Pretransplantation risk factors for death after heart transplantation: the Henri Mondor experience. J Heart Lung Transplant 1998;17:268–277.
35. McCarthy JF, McCarthy PM, Massad MG, et al. Risk factors for death after heart transplantation: does a single-center experience correlate with multicenter registries? Ann Thorac Surg 1998;65:1574–1579.
36. Tenderich G, Koerner MM, Stuettgen L, et al. Does preexisting elevated pulmonary vascular resistance (transpulmonary gradient >15 mmHg or >5 Wood) predict early and long-term results after orthotopic heart transplantation? Transplant Proc 1998;30:1130–1131.
37. Ladowski JS, Kormos RL, Uretsky BF, et al. Heart transplantation in diabetic recipients. Transplantation 1990;49:303–305.
38. Munoz E, Lonquist JL, Radovancevic B, et al. Long-term results in diabetic patients undergoing heart transplantation. J Heart Lung Transplant 1992;11:943–949.
39. Stevenson LW, Warner SL, Steimle AE, et al. The impending crisis awaiting cardiac transplantation: modeling a solution based on selection. Circulation 1994;89:450–457.
40. Laks H, Scholl GF, Drinkwater DC, et al. The alternate recipient list for heart transplantation: does it work? J Heart Lung Transplant 1997;16:735–742.
41. Anguita M, Arizon JM, Valles F, et al. Influence on survival after heart transplantation of contraindications seen in transplant recipients. J Heart Lung Transplant 1992;11:708–715.
42. Miller LW, Kubo SH, Young JB, et al. Report of the consensus conference on candidate selection for heart transplantation—1993. J Heart Lung Transplant 1995;14:562–571.
43. Blanche C, Matloff JM, Denton TA, et al. Heart transplantation in patients 70 years of age and older: initial experience. Ann Thorac Surg 1996;62:1731–1736.
44. Frazier OH, Macris MP, Duncan JM, et al. Cardiac transplantation in patients over 60 years of age. Ann Thorac Surg 1997;64:1866–1867.
45. Masters RG, Hendry PJ, Davies RA, et al. Cardiac transplantation after mechanical circulatory support: a Canadian perspective. Ann Thorac Surg 1996;61:1734–1739.
46. Bonet LA. Predictors of mortality following heart transplantation: Spanish Registry of Heart Transplantation 1984–2001. Transplant Proc 2003;35:1946–1950.
47. John R, Rajasinghe H, Chen JM, et al. Impact of current management practices on early and late death in more than 500 consecutive cardiac transplant recipients. Ann Surg 2000;232:302–311.
48. Arzenziano M, Catanese KA, Moazami N, et al. The influence of infection on survival and successful transplantation in patients with left ventricular assist devices. J Heart Lung Transplant 1997;16:822–831.
49. Itescu S, Tung TC, Burke EM, et al. Preformed IgG antibodies against major histocompatibility complex class II antigens are major risk factors for high-grade cellular rejection in recipients of heart transplantation. Circulation 1998;98:786–793.
50. Cavarocchi NC, Badellino M. Heart/heart-lung transplantation: the domino procedure. Ann Thorac Surg 1989;48:130–133.
51. Traversi E, Pozzoli M, Grande A. The bicaval anastomosis technique for orthotopic heart transplantation yields better atrial function than the standard technique: an echocardiographic automatic boundary detection study. J Heart Lung Transplant 1998;17:1065–1074.
52. Blanche C, Nessim S, Quartel A, et al. Heart transplantation with bicaval and pulmonary venous anastomoses. A hemodynamic analysis of the first 117 patients. J Cardiovasc Surg 1997;38:561–566.
53. Brandt M, Harringer W, Hirt SW, et al. Influence of bicaval anastomoses on late occurrence of atrial arrhythmia after heart transplantation. Ann Thorac Surg 1997;64:70–72.
54. Rothman SA, Jeevanandam V, Combs WG, et al. Eliminating bradyarrhythmias after orthotopic heart transplantation. Circulation 1996;suppl 9:II178–II182.
55. Bouchart F, Derumeaux G, Mouton-Schleifer D, et al. Conventional and total orthotopic cardiac transplantation: a comparative clinical and echocardiographical study. Eur J Cardiothorac Surg 1997;12:555–559.
56. Aleksic I, Freimark D, Blanche C, et al. Resting hemodynamics after total versus standard orthotopic heart transplantation in patients with high preoperative pulmonary vascular resistance. Eur J Cardiothorac Surg 1997;11:1037–1044.
57. Deleuze PH, Benvenuti C, Mazzucotelli JP, et al. Orthotopic cardiac transplantation with direct caval anastomosis: is it the optimal procedure? J Thorac Cardiovasc Surg 1995;109:731–737.
58. elGamel A, Yonan NA, Grant S, et al. Orthotopic cardiac transplantation: a comparison of standard and bicaval Wythenshawe techniques. J Thorac Cardiovasc Surg 1995;109:721–730.
59. Sievers HH, Leyh R, Jahnke A, et al. Bicaval versus atrial anastomoses in cardiac transplantation: right atrial dimension and tricuspid valve function at rest and during exercise up to 36 months after transplantation. J Thorac Cardiovasc Surg 1995;109:1257–1259.
60. Jeevanandam V, Russell H, Mather P, et al. A 1-year comparison of prophylactic donor tricuspid annuloplasty in heart transplantation. Ann Thorac Surg 2004;78:759–766.
61. Wheeldon D, Sharples L, Wallwork J, et al. Donor heart preservation survey. J Heart Lung Transplant 1992;11:986–993.
62. Luciani GB, Faggian G, Forni A, et al. Myocardial protection during heart transplantation using blood cardioplegia. Transplant Proc 1997;29:3386–3388.

63. Engelman RM, Pleet AB, Rousou JA, et al. What is the best perfusion temperature for coronary revascularization? J Thorac Cardiovasc Surg 1996;112:1622–1633.
64. Tixier D, Matheis G, Buckberg GD, et al. Donor hearts with impaired hemodynamics. J Thorac Cardiovasc Surg 1991;102: 207–214.
65. Rao V, Feindel CM, Weisel RD, et al. Donor blood perfusion improves myocardial recovery after heart transplantation. J Heart Lung Transplant 1997;16:667–673.
66. Kirklin JK, Neves J, Naftel DC, et al. Controlled initial hyperkalemic reperfusion after cardiac transplantation: coronary vascular resistance and blood flow. Ann Thorac Surg 1990;49: 625–631.
67. Pradas G, Cuenca J, Juffe A. Continuous warm reperfusion during heart transplantation. J Thorac Cardiovasc Surg 1996; 111:784–790.
68. Barnard CN, Losman JG. Left ventricular bypass. South African Med J 1975;49:303–312.
69. Cooper DK, Novitzky D, Becerra E, et al. Are there indications for heterotopic heart transplantation in 1986? A 2- to 11-year follow-up of 49 consecutive patients undergoing heterotopic heart transplantation. Thorac Cardiovasc Surgeon 1986;34:300–304.
70. Baumgartner WA. Heterotopic transplantation: is it a viable alternative? Ann Thorac Surg 1992;54:401–402.
71. Kawaguchi AT, Gandjbakhch I, Desruennes M, et al. Orthotopic versus heterotopic heart transplantation in donor/recipient size mismatch. Transplant Proc 1995;27:1227–1281.
72. Khaghani A, Santini F, Dyke CM, et al. Heterotopic cardiac transplantation in infants and children. J Thorac Cardiovasc Surg 1997;113:1042–1049.
73. Ridley PD, Khaghani A, Musumeci F, et al. Heterotopic heart transplantation and recipient heart operation in ischemic heart disease. Ann Thorac Surg 1992;54:333–337.
74. Chester AH, Birks EJ, Yacoub MH. Role of nitric oxide following cardiac transplantation. J Hum Hypertens 1998;12:883–887.
75. Argenziano M, Chen JM, Choudri AF, et al. Management of vasodilatory shock after cardiac surgery: identification of predisposing factors and use of a novel pressor agent. J Thorac Cardiovasc Surg 1998;116:973–980.
76. Follath F, Cleland JG, Just H, et al. Efficacy and safety of intravenous levosimendan compared with dobutamine in severe low-output heart failure (the LIDO study): a randomised double-blind trial. Lancet 2002;360:196–202.
77. Montero JA, Anguita M, Concha M, et al. Pacing requirements after orthotopic heart transplantation: incidence and related factors. J Heart Lung Transplant 1992;11:799–802.
78. Scott CD, McComb JM, Dark JH, et al. Permanent pacing after cardiac transplantation. Br Heart J 1993;69:399–403.
79. Kieler-Jensen N, Lundin S, Ricksten SE. Vasodilator therapy after heart transplantation: effects of inhaled nitric oxide and intravenous prostacyclin E_l, and sodium nitroprusside. J Heart Lung Transplant 1995;14:436–443.
80. Auler JOC, Carmona MJC, Bocchi EA, et al. Low doses of inhaled nitric oxide in heart transplant recipients. J Heart Lung Transplant 1996;15:443–450.
81. Beniaminovitz A, Itescu S, Lietz K, et al. Prevention of rejection in cardiac transplantation by blockade of the interleukin-2 receptor with a monoclonal antibody. N Engl J Med 2000;342:613–619.
82. Dall'Amico R, Montini G, Murer L, et al. Extracorporeal photochemotherapy after cardiac transplantation: a new therapeutic approach to allograft rejection. Int J Artif Organs 2000;23:49–54.
83. Valantine HA. Individualizing immunosuppression for heart transplantation: strategies for the next decade. Transplant Proc 1999;29(suppl 8A):5S–8S.
84. Waid TH, Johnson JS, McKeown JW, et al. Induction immunotherapy in heart transplantation with T10B3. 1A-31: a phase I study. J Heart Lung Transplant 1997;16:913–916.
85. vanGelder T, Balk AH, Jonkman FA, et al. A randomized trial comparing safety and efficacy of OKT3 and a monoclonal anti-interleukin-2 receptor antibody (BT563) in the prevention of acute rejection after heart transplantation. Transplantation 1996;62:51–55.
86. Wahlers T. Cytolytic induction therapy in heart and lung transplantation: the protagonist opinion. Transplant Proc 1998; 30:1100–1103.
87. Keogh A, Macdonald PO, Harvison A, et al. Initial steroid-free versus steroid-based maintenance therapy and steroid withdrawal after heart transplantation: two views of the steroid question. J Heart Lung Transplant 1992;11:421–427.
88. Barr ML, Sanchez JA, Seche LA, et al. Anti-CD3 monoclonal antibody induction therapy: immunological equivalency with triple-drug therapy in heart transplantation. Circulation 1990; 82(suppl 5):IV291–IV294.
89. Alonso-Pulpon L, Serrano-Fiz S, Rubio JA, et al. Efficacy of low-dose OKT3 as cytolytic induction therapy in heart transplantation. J Heart Lung Transplant 1995;14:136–142.
90. Costanzo-Nordin MR, Sinnen LJ, Fisher SG, et al. Cytomegalovirus infections in heart transplant recipients: relationship to immunosuppression. J Heart Lung Transplant 1992;11:837–846.
91. Swinnen LJ, Costanzo-Nordin MR, Fisher SG, et al. Increased incidence of lymphoproliferative disorder after immunosuppression with the monoclonal antibody OKT3 in cardiac transplant recipients. N Engl J Med 1990;323:1723–1728.
92. Sollinger HW, U.S. Renal Transplant Mycophenolate Mofetil Study Group. Mycophenolate mofetil for the prevention of acute rejection in primary cadaveric renal allograft recipients. Transplantation 1995;60:225–232.
93. Ensley RD, Bristow MR, Olsen SL, et al. The use of mycophenolate mofetil (RS-61443) in human heart transplant. Transplantation 1993;56:75–82.
94. Kobashigawa J, Miller L, Renlund D, et al. A randomized active-controlled trial of mycophenolate mofetil in heart transplant recipients. Transplantation 1998;66:507–515.
95. Haverich A, Costard-Jackle A, Cremer J, et al. Cyclosporin A and transplant coronary disease after heart transplantation. Transplant Proc 1994;26:2713–2715.
96. Stempfle HU, Werner C, Echtler S, et al. Rapid trabecular bone loss after cardiac transplantation using FK506 (tacrolimus)-based immunosuppression. Transplant Proc 1998;30:1132–1133.
97. Meiser BM, Uberfuhr P, Fuchs A, et al. Single-center randomized trial comparing tacrolimus and cyclosporine in the prevention of acute myocardial rejection. J Heart Lung Transplant 1998; 17:782–788.
98. Reichart 13, Meisr B, Vigano M, et al. European multicenter tacrolimus (FK506) heart pilot study: 1-year-results—European tacrolimus multicenter heart study group. J Heart Lung Transplant 1998;17:775–781.
99. Pham SM, Kormos RL, Hattler BG, et al. A prospective trial of tacrolimus (FK506) in clinical heart transplantation: intermediate-term results. J Thorac Cardiovasc Surg 1996;111:764–772.
100. Olivari MT, Jesse ME, Baldwin BJ, et al. Triple-drug immunosuppression with steroid discontinuation by 6 months after heart transplantation. J Heart Lung Transplant 1995;14:127–135.
101. Kobashigawa JA, Stevenson LW, Brownfield ED, et al. Initial success of steroid weaning late after heart transplantation. J Heart Lung Transplant 1992;11:428–430.
102. Miller LW, McBride WT, Peigh P, et al. Successful withdrawal of corticosteroids in heart transplantation. J Heart Lung Transplant 1992;11:431–434.
103. Canter CEW, Moorhead S, Saffitz JE, et al. Steroid withdrawal in the pediatric heart transplant recipient initially treated with

triple immunosuppression. J Heart Lung Transplant 1994;13:74–80.
104. Kahan BD. Efficacy of sirolimus compared with azathioprine for reduction of acute renal allograft rejection: a randomised multicentre study. The Rapamune U.S. Study Group. Lancet 2000; 356:194–202.
105. Groth CG, Backman L, Morales JM, et al. Sirolimus (rapamycin)-based therapy in human renal transplantation: similar efficacy and different toxicity compared with cyclosporine. Sirolimus European Renal Transplant Study Group. Transplantation 1999; 67:1036–1042.
106. Shefet D, Ben-dor I, Lustig S. Sirolimus-induced interstitial pneumonitis after renal transplantation. Transplantation 2004; 78:950.
107. Schuler PB, Lloyd LK, Leblanc PA, Clapp TA, Abadie BR, Collins RK. The effect of physical activity and fitness on specific antibody production in college students. J Sports Med Phys Fitness 1999;39:233–239.
108. Eisen HJ, Tuzcu EM, Dorent R, et al. of the RAD B253 Study Group. Everolimus for the prevention of allograft rejection and vasculopathy in cardiac-transplant recipients. N Engl J Med 2003;349:847–858.
109. Doggrell SA. Is everolimus useful in preventing allograft rejection and vasculopathy after heart transplant? Expert Opin Investig Drugs 2004;13:161–163.
110. Cantarovich M, Metrakos P, Giannetti N, Cecere R, Barkun J, Tchervenkov J. Anti-CD25 monoclonal antibody coverage allows for calcineurin inhibitor "holiday" in solid organ transplant patients with acute renal dysfunction. Transplantation 2002;73:1169–1172.
111. White JA, Guiraudon C, Pflugfelder PW, et al. Routine surveillance myocardial biopsies are unnecessary beyond 1 year after heart transplantation. J Heart Lung Transplant 1995;14:1052–1056.
112. Sethi GK, Kosaraju S, Arabia FA, et al. Is it necessary to perform surveillance endomyocardial biopsies in heart transplant recipients? J Heart Lung Transplant 1995;14:1047–1051.
113. Brunner-La Rocca HP, Kiowski W. Identification of patients not requiring endomyocardial biopsies late after cardiac transplantation. Transplantation 1998;65:533–538.
114. Kobashigawa JA, Stevenson LW, Moriguchi J, et al. Randomized study of high dose oral cyclosporine therapy for mild acute cardiac rejection. J Heart Lung Transplant 1989;8:53–58.
115. Kobashigawa JA, Stevenson LW, Moriguchi JD, et al. Is intravenous glucocorticoid therapy better than an oral regimen for asymptomatic cardiac rejection? A randomized trial. J Am Coll Cardiol 1993;21:1142–1144.
116. Bourge RC, Kirklin JK, White-Williams C, et al. Methotrexate pulse therapy in the treatment of recurrent acute heart rejection. J Heart Lung Transplant 1992;11:1116–1124.
117. Costanzo MR, Koch DM, Fisher SG, et al. Effects of methotrexate on acute rejection and cardiac allograft vasculopathy in heart transplant recipients. J Heart Lung Transplant 1997;16:169–178.
118. Kirklin JK, Bourge RC, Naftel DC, et al. Treatment of recurrent heart rejection with mycophenolate mofetil (RS-61443): initial clinical experience. J Heart Lung Transplant 1994;13:444–450.
119. Haverty TP, Sanders M, Sheahan M. OKT3 treatment of cardiac allograft rejection. J Heart Lung Transplant 1993;12:591–598.
120. Wagner FM, Reichenspurner H, Uberfuhr P, et al. How successful is OKT3 rescue therapy for steroid-resistant acute rejection episodes after heart transplantation? J Heart Lung Transplant 1994;13:438–443.
121. Dall'Amico R, Livi U, Milano A, et al. Extracorporeal photochemotherapy as adjuvant treatment of heart transplant recipients with recurrent rejection. Transplantation 1995;60:45–49.
122. Costanzo-Nordin MR, Hubbell EA, O'Sullivan EJ, et al. Photophoresis versus corticosteroids in the therapy of heart transplant rejection: preliminary clinical report. Circulation 1992;86(suppl 5):11242–11250.
123. Costanzo-Nordin MR, Hubbell EA, O'Sullivan EJ, et al. Successful treatment of heart transplant rejection with photophoresis. Transplantation 1992;53:808–815.
124. Rose EA, Barr ML, Xu H, et al. Photochemotherapy in human heart transplant recipients at high risk for fatal rejection. J Heart Lung Transplant 1992;11:746–759.
125. Barr ML, Meisser BM, Eisen HJ, et al. Photophoresis for the prevention of rejection in cardiac transplantation: photophoresis transplantation study group. N Engl J Med 1998;339:1744–1751.
126. Ross HJ, Gullestad L, Pak J, et al. Methotrexate of total lymphoid radiation for treatment of persistent or recurrent allograft cellular rejection: a comparative study. J Heart Lung Transplant 1997;16:179–189.
127. Grossi P, De Maria R, Caroli A, et al. Infections on heart transplant recipients: the experience of the Italian heart transplantation program. J Heart Lung Transplant 1992;11:847–866.
128. Mayer JM, Nimer L, Carroll K. Isolated pulmonary *Aspergillus* infection in cardiac transplant recipients: case report and review. Clin Infect Dis 1992;15:698–700.
129. Munoz P, Palomo J, Munoz R, et al. Tuberculosis in heart transplant recipients. Clin Infect Dis 1995;21:398–402.
130. Holliman RE, Johnson JD, Adams S, et al. Toxoplasmosis and heart transplantation. J Heart Transplant 1991;10:608–610.
131. Huffer JA, Scott J, Wreghitt T, et al. The importance of cytomegalovirus in heart-lung transplant recipients. Chest 1989; 95:627–631.
132. Griffiths PD. Prophylaxis against CMV infection in transplant patients. J Antimicrob Chemother 1997;39:299–301.
133. Merigan TC, Renlund DG, Keay S, et al. A controlled trial of ganciclovir to prevent cytomegalovirus disease after heart transplantation. N Engl J Med 1992;326:1182–1186.
134. Kofoed KF, Czernin J, Johnson J, et al. Effects of cardiac allograft vasculopathy on myocardial blood flow, vasodilatory capacity, and coronary vasomotion. Circulation 1997;95:600–606.
135. Libby P, Tanaka H. The pathogenesis of coronary arteriosclerosis ("chronic rejection") in transplanted hearts. Clin Transplant 1994;8:313–318.
136. Thomson JG. Production of severe athero in a transplanted human heart. Lancet 1969;2:1088–1092.
137. Costanzo-Nordin MR. Cardiac allograft vasculopathy: relationship with acute cellular rejection and histocompatibility. J Heart Lung Transplant 1992;11:S90–S103.
138. Uretsky BF, Murali S, Reddy S, et al. Development of coronary artery disease in cardiac transplant patients receiving immunosuppressive therapy with cyclosporine and prednisone. Circulation 1987;76:827–834.
139. Olivari MT, Homans DC, Wilson RF, et al. Coronary artery disease in cardiac transplant patients receiving triple drug immunosuppressive therapy. Circulation 1989;80:III111–III115.
140. Russell PS, Chase CM, Winn HF, et al. Coronary atherosclerosis in transplanted mouse hearts, II: importance of humoral immunity. J Immunol 1994;152:5135–5141.
141. Hosenpud JD, Everett JP, Morris TE, et al. Cellular and humoral immunity to vascular endothelium and the development of cardiac allograft vasculopathy. J Heart Lung Transplant 1995;14: S185–S187.
142. Escobar A, Ventura HO, Stapleton DD, et al. Cardiac allograft vasculopathy assessed by intravascular ultrasonography and nonimmunologic risk factors. Am J Cardiol 1994;74:1042–1046.
143. Day JD, Rayburn BK, Gaudin PB, et al. Cardiac allograft vasculopathy: the central pathogenetic role of ischemia-induced endothelial cell injury. J Heart Lung Transplant 1995;14:S142–S149.
144. Land W, Schneeberger H, Schleibner S, et al. The beneficial effect of human recombinant superoxide dismutase on acute and

chronic rejection events in recipients of cadaveric renal transplants. Transplantation 1994;57:211–217.

145. Smith JA, Ribakove GH, Hunt SA, et al. Heart retransplantation: the 25-year experience at a single institution. J Heart Lung Transplant 1995;14:832–839.

146. Schnetzler B, Pavie A, Dorent R, et al. Heart retransplantation: a 23-year single-center clinical experience. Ann Thorac Surg 1998;65:978–983.

147. Mullins P, Scott J, Chauhan A, et al. Acute heart retransplantation. Lancet 1991;337:1158.

148. Collins EG, Mozdzierz G. Cardiac retransplantation: determining limits. Heart Lung 1993;22:206–212.

149. Brown NE, Muehlebach GF, Jones P, et al. Tricuspid annuloplasty significantly reduces early tricuspid regurgitation after biatrial heart transplantation. J Heart Lung Transplant 2004;23:1160–1162.

SECTION NINE

Cancer Surgery

89

History of Surgical Oncology

Walter Lawrence, Jr.

The history of the special interest area within general surgery that is now called surgical oncology began long before this nomenclature was conceived. It seems fair to say that the therapeutic approach to cancer, or "oncology," has been intimately linked to the field of surgery since ancient times. Certainly, it is only in the past 100 years that there has been any useful treatment to offer the cancer patient other than an operation. Even though the effect of radiation was discovered just before the turn of the last century, this modality was only of limited clinical value until about 50 years ago. As the anticancer drugs and various hormonal alterations appeared on the scene as therapy at about the same time, we must consider all but the most recent history of oncology to be a purely surgical story.

Early History of Surgery for Cancer

Most recorders of the history of oncology refer to statements about cancer appearing in the Edwin Smith and Ebers Papyri (1600–1700 BC). In addition to a description in these ancient documents of the clinical manifestations of breast cancer by these Egyptian "authors," there is a brief description of cautery destruction of the cancer as a potential surgical approach[1] (Fig. 89.1). It seems safe to assume that the less visible, visceral cancers were not really known as disease entities to people of those times. Much later, in the fifth century BC the famous Greek physician, Hippocrates (Fig. 89.2), made some observations about breast cancer, but he had a negative view on local surgical management. He cautioned against it with the admonition that it would shorten survival, and he seemed to apply this philosophy to the treatment of all cancers.[2]

Celsus and Galen, Roman physicians of the first and second centuries AD, wrote extensively about both operations and dietary treatment for cancer of the breast. Lenoidas, a Greek physician in the fifth century AD, was actually the first to describe a mastectomy for cancer, an operative procedure that utilized cautery to achieve hemostasis. Surgical treatment methods for all cancers were clearly crude at that time and were applicable only to superficial tumors, such as those arising in the skin or in the breast. Cancer of the uterine cervix, although relatively superficial, was described clinically by Archigenes, another Greek physician of that era, but he considered this an incurable disease despite the use of various topical medications that he recommended. Oncological therapy and surgical therapy, in general, appeared to be at a standstill throughout the dark ages of medicine, which lasted from this time until the seventeenth century. It was about that time that the humoral theories of disease (blood, phlegm, white bile, and black bile) began to be replaced by scientific hypotheses and experimentation, of a sort. John Hunter (1728–1793) (Fig. 89.3), who is considered the father of surgery, added many new and useful concepts in a number of fields, including oncology. He believed that cancer was a localized process and amenable, in some instances, to surgical removal, but he was worried about the "constitutional effects" of the disease. He had some surprisingly modern concepts in terms of cancer biology, and he stressed the need for total removal of cancers when feasible as well as their potential areas of lymphatic spread. Many of his thoughts on breast cancer were similar to the concepts expressed much later by Dr. William Stewart Halsted,[3,4] a surgical leader in the late 1800s (Fig. 89.4).

Anatomic studies, a more thorough understanding of gross pathology, and the use of autopsies added to a much better understanding of disease, in general, and cancer, in particular. However, major advances in the surgical treatment of cancer in the United States had to await the first use of general anesthesia by Crawford Long in 1842 and the demon-

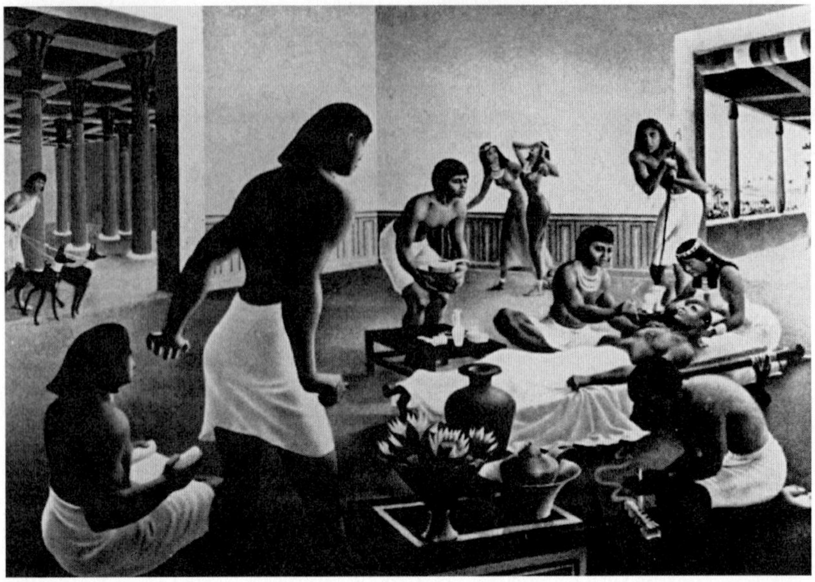

FIGURE 89.1. Artist's conception of treatment of breast disease by cauterization with the fire drill. (From Lewison.[1])

stration of its effectiveness for major surgery by Morton in 1846 at the Massachusetts General Hospital. The development of the principles of antisepsis was advanced by Lister in 1867, and this was the other major development that allowed major surgical procedures for cancer. It is true that Ephraim McDowell of Kentucky[5] had removed a massive ovarian tumor in a patient's home as early as 1809, but it was not until the middle of the nineteenth century, when anesthesia and antisepsis were introduced, that effective intraabdominal surgery for cancer was considered either practical or feasible.

The latter half of the nineteenth century saw the development of a number of extensive surgical resections for cancer, with breast cancer continuing to be a major focus. Valpeau of France, Moore of London, and Gross and Pancoast of Philadelphia all wrote extensively regarding the principles and techniques of mastectomy for cancer. However, it remained for William Stewart Halsted, of Johns Hopkins Hospital in Baltimore, to first define the optimal technique of operation for breast cancer in 1891.[3] His operation, the radical mastectomy, survived as the classical surgical approach to breast cancer in the United States until only a little more than a decade ago, despite the progressive addition of various nonoperative treatments earlier in the twentieth century. The long-term survival of breast cancer patients quoted by Valpeau was only in the 5% to 10% range, but the Halsted surgical method increased the cure rate to more than 40%, a fantastic improvement in end results.[4]

In the same era, the latter half of the nineteenth century, major operations for cancer were developed for the gastrointestinal tract, the head and neck area, the genitourinary system, and in gynecology. There were no useful alternative therapies, so operation was the only available and practical approach to cancer treatment.

Stomach

Theodor Billroth (Fig. 89.5) of Vienna conducted the first successful partial gastrectomy for cancer in 1881 and published

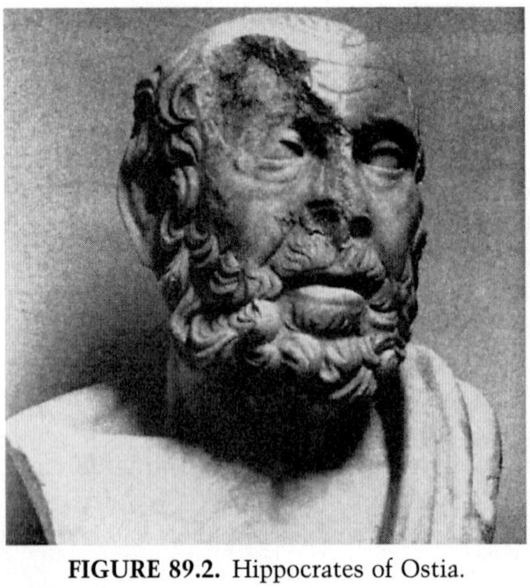

FIGURE 89.2. Hippocrates of Ostia.

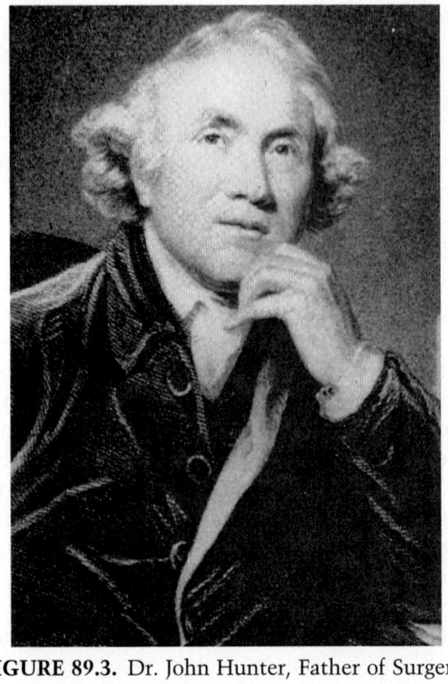

FIGURE 89.3. Dr. John Hunter, Father of Surgery.

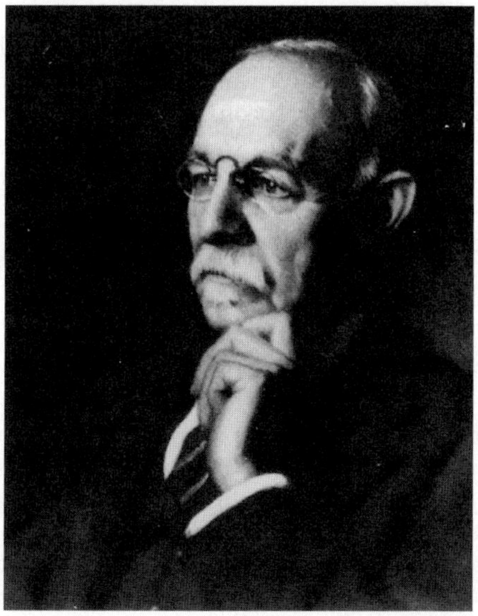

FIGURE 89.4. William Stewart Halsted of Johns Hopkins Hospital.

his accomplishment 7 days later. His patient, Ms. Teresa Heller, survived the postoperative period and succumbed months later of recurrent cancer. According to Rutledge,[6] Billroth made more contributions to cancer surgery than anyone else of his time. He made a number of valuable additions to the pathology of cancer, as well as being the first in performing a number of extensive operations for cancers other than gastric cancer: these included the first successful total laryngectomy (in 1873), the first hemipelvectomy (albeit unsuccessful) in 1891, the first perineal prostatectomy for cancer, and the first suprapubic removal of a bladder tumor.[7] He would certainly have been considered the "compleat" surgical oncologist, if that term had existed at that time. The first total gastrectomy with patient survival was performed in Zurich by Carl Schlatter in 1897.[8] This procedure was only rarely performed until the middle of the twentieth century because the operative mortality was almost prohibitive. In a collective review by Pack and McNeer[9] as late as 1943, the operative mortality was 37%.

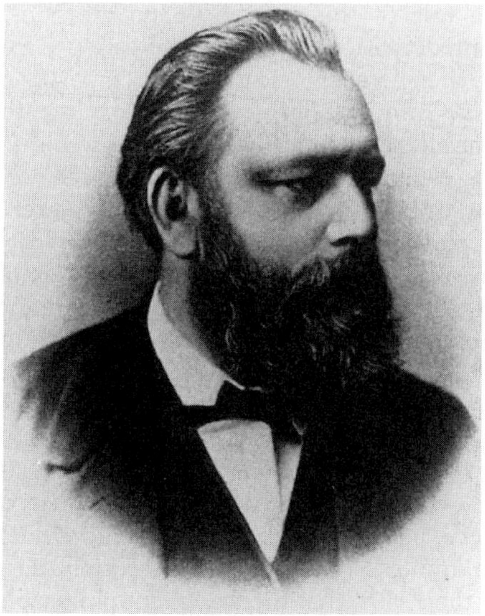

FIGURE 89.5. Theodor Billroth of Vienna (1867).

Colon and Rectum

Soon after Billroth described gastrectomy, Robert Weir reported resection of colon cancer in 1885, the proximal bowel being brought out as a permanent colostomy.[10] In 1895, von Mikulicz described a two-stage colon resection for cancer with colostomy closure,[11] and Charles Mayo described 14 cases of colon resection with anastomosis for cancer that same year.[12] Shortly thereafter, in 1908, Ernest Miles[13] described combined abdominoperineal resection of cancer of the rectum, an approach still very much in use today for lesions not suitable for sphincter-saving procedures. Many of these colorectal cancer operations have continued, with some refinements, until the present day.

Head and Neck Cancer

Although J. Marion Sims actually attained international prominence as the gynecologist who first successfully treated vesicovaginal fistula, the second paper of his career in 1847 described removal of the superior maxilla for a tumor of the maxillary antrum.[14] A short time later, again in 1847, he reported successful intraoral resection of the mandible for osteosarcoma. Professor Billroth's first successful total laryngectomy for cancer in 1873 warrants mention again in this listing of historical accomplishments in head and neck surgery. Theodor Kocher of Berne pioneered thyroid resection for both benign and malignant disease, with a report of 100 such operations in 1883,[15] while Charles Mayo and George Crile were the U.S. surgeons who were the leaders in this anatomic area over the next couple of decades. Nicholas Senn, Professor of Surgery at Rush Medical College in Chicago, had a wide range of surgical interests as shown by his book on the pathology and treatment of tumors published in 1900,[16] but he was well known also for developing a wide range of new operations for cancers arising in the oral cavity and pharynx. It remained for George Crile to describe radical neck dissection in a beautifully illustrated article in 1906,[17] and to establish the importance of this technique in the management of various cancers of the head and neck (Fig. 89.6). Much of the

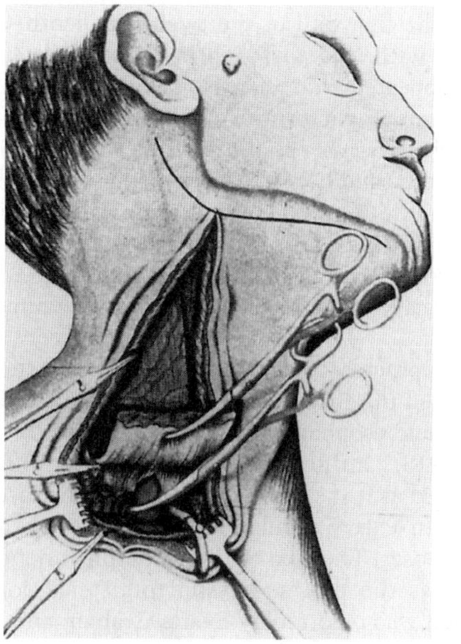

FIGURE 89.6. Drawing from Dr. Crile's paper on radical neck dissection.[17]

history of head and neck surgery would be later altered by the introduction of radiation techniques, but operation was the only available treatment for head and neck cancer until this century.

Uterine Cancer

John G. Clark of the Johns Hopkins Hospital in Baltimore, Maryland, a resident of the famous gynecologist, Howard Kelly, was the first to perform radical hysterectomy for cancer, in 1895.[18] As with head and neck cancer, the introduction of radium and its use by Kelly led to a change in treatment approach in the United States for this disease, but the surgical approach to uterine cancer remained paramount in both Germany and Austria. Ernst Wertheim of Vienna had perfected the operation described first by Clark and, in later years, Victor Bonney in England continued the tradition. It was many years later, in 1933, when Joe Meigs of Boston brought a surgical approach for cancers of the cervix back to the United States after observing Bonney in England.[19]

Surgical Oncology in the Early Twentieth Century

Probably the most important new development in oncology at the turn of the century was the discovery of the effect of radiation. Roentgen's discovery of what we now call X-rays in 1896, and the discovery of radium by Madame Curie in 1898, added the potential for a new treatment modality. Cancer treatment by extensive operations with high morbidity and mortality created a grim situation, and there was much hope for this new treatment method. Those cancers applicable to surface treatments with various forms of applicators or needle insertions, such as cancer of the cervix, head and neck cancer, and breast cancer, were those first subjected to this approach. Equipment for producing low-voltage therapeutic X-rays was available also and this was employed as well. Although modern techniques in radiation therapy have revolutionized the role of these treatments, the local side effects, toxicities, and limitations associated with radiation therapy in the first half of the twentieth century led to dissatisfaction with this approach in clinical situations where operation appeared to be a reasonable alternative. The subsequent development of a capability for plasma and whole blood transfusions, as a result of studies by John Scudder and Charles Drew, and the discovery of antimicrobial agents made more extensive operations even more feasible. Radiation technology in the first half of this century seemed a poor substitute for the surgical treatment of cancer, and the more radical operative procedures became the new hope for cancer treatment.

Surgical progress during the first half of the twentieth century added the thorax to the theater of operation. Cancer of the thoracic esophagus was first successfully resected by Torek in 1913,[20] although restoration of continuity was not accomplished as it is today. The cervical esophagus was connected by an external rubber tube to the gastrostomy for feeding purposes. The next major accomplishment in thoracic oncology was the first successful total pneumonectomy in 1933, which was reported by Evarts Graham and J.J. Singer,[21] Dr. Graham's pulmonologist. William Adams and Dallas Phemister were the first to describe distal thoracic esophagectomy with esophagogastric anastomosis in the United States in 1938.[22] This writer was privileged to continue laboratory studies on this approach in their laboratories in the following decade. Long-term results from the surgical approach to thoracic cavity cancers were not very good at that time, but there had been no alternative therapy for these lesions before these new surgical initiatives.

Cancer Treatment at the Mid-Twentieth Century

Although there were radiation treatment techniques available as a result of earlier discoveries of the effects of these energies on tumors, the newfound capabilities for extending the operative attack and the less than ideal results of radiation treatment led to surgical domination of cancer care—for a while. Dr. Allen O. Whipple first performed a two-stage pancreatoduodenectomy for cancer in 1935,[23] and Pack and McNeer,[24] Longmire,[25] and Lahey and Marshal[26] extended the scope of operations for gastric cancer in the 1940s. Major liver resection for primary and limited metastatic cancer was next added to the cancer surgery armamentarium by Pickrell and Clay,[27] Lortat-Jacob in France,[28] and Pack and Baker.[29] Most of these extensive operations continue to be the standard of care for a number of these cancers, with the major difference occurring in recent years being that of a markedly reduced morbidity and mortality.

Grant Ward of Johns Hopkins Hospital in Baltimore and Hayes Martin of Memorial Hospital in New York, both well experienced in radiation techniques, reverted to a more radical surgical approach to head and neck cancer in the 1940s and 1950s as dissatisfaction with radiation results developed. Aspiration biopsy for diagnosis was introduced by Martin and Ellis[30] in that same era. Alexander Brunschwig of Chicago[31] had been an exponent of extended and radical operations for advanced abdominal cancers while a professor of surgery at the University of Chicago in the 1930s and 1940s, and he then developed an interest in applying these more radical surgical principles to uterine cancer. He performed his first total pelvic exenteration for recurrent carcinoma of the cervix or its radiation complications in 1946 (Fig. 89.7) and went on to explore the role of this extensive and disabling operation when recruited to Memorial Sloan-Kettering Cancer Center as chief of their gynecological service in 1948.[32] This new position gave him the opportunity to explore the surgical approach for all stages of cancer of the cervix instead of the then more established treatment approach of radiation therapy. Dr. Meigs of Boston, long a supporter of radical surgery for cancer of the cervix,[19] Howard Ulfelder of Boston, and Eugene Bricker of St. Louis, the initiator of the ileal conduit for urinary diversion,[33,34] all participated in this new emphasis on radical surgery for pelvic cancer.

The other major cancer in females, cancer of the breast, had been treated by a radical surgical approach since the turn of the century when Dr. Halsted popularized radical mastectomy. However, Jerome Urban[35] of Memorial Hospital, Everett Sugarbaker[36] of Columbia, Missouri, and Eduardo Caceres[37] of Lima, Peru, extended this operation to include ipsilateral internal mammary lymph node dissection (Fig. 89.8). It seemed, in the 1950s, that the treatment philosophy for most

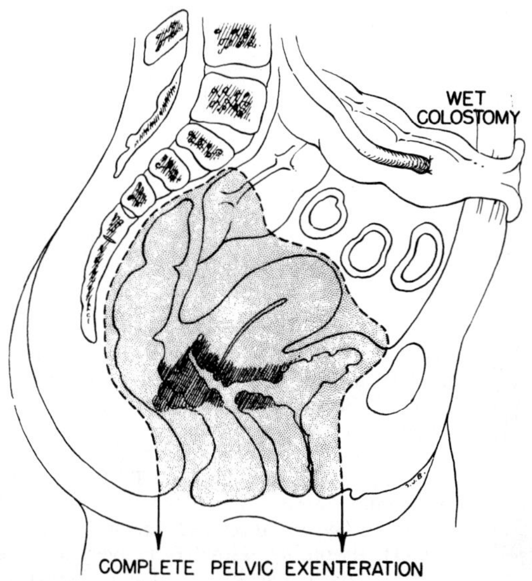

FIGURE 89.7. Diagram of technique of Alexander Brunschwig for total pelvic exenteration. (Reprinted with permission from Meigs JV. Surgical Treatment of Cancer of the Cervix. ©1954 WB Saunders Co.)

human cancers was primarily surgical and the larger the operation, the greater the hope for cure. All these extensions of operation just described were then considered the truly major advances in cancer care, and "cancer surgeons" were the clinical leaders in the dedicated cancer centers that existed in this country at that time. The term *surgical oncology* had not yet been heard here in the United States, but cancer surgeons were in abundance at the major medical centers and cancer centers.

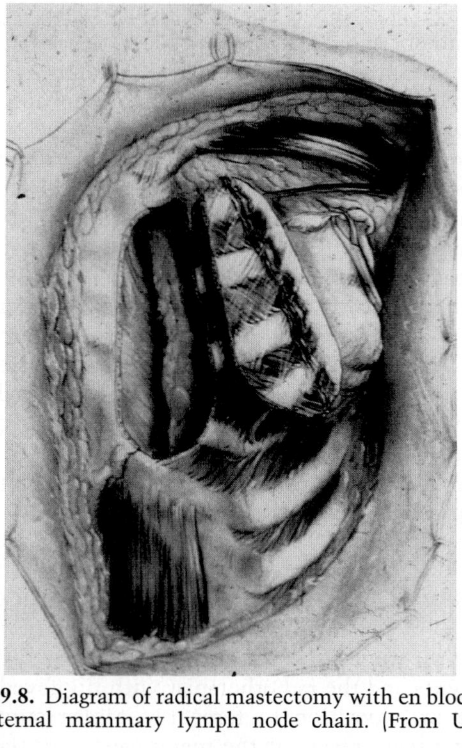

FIGURE 89.8. Diagram of radical mastectomy with en bloc resection of the internal mammary lymph node chain. (From Urban and Baker.[35])

Winds of Change

Major shifts in the focus of cancer management began to occur following World War II (WW II), and this began to impact on the surgical situation just described. The science of radiation oncology became better developed, and this treatment approach was improved both by the identification of physicians specifically trained in radiation oncology and by major technological advances. The famous pathologist and oncologist, Dr. James Ewing (Fig. 89.9), was convinced that radiation treatment was superior to the surgical approach to cancer, and he imposed his beliefs in this regard on the cancer surgeons at Memorial Hospital in New York in the 1920s and 1930s (Fig. 89.10). His confidence regarding this radiation approach was augmented by a gift to the Memorial Hospital of a generous supply of radium and by the presence on his staff of two outstanding physicists, G.P. Fialla and Edith Quimby. However, the rapid growth of the field of surgery, as just described, and the death of Dr. Ewing in 1943 led to the pendulum swing from radiation to the surgical treatment emphasis described. The radiation oncologists had maintained a stronger foothold in some cancer centers in Europe, but resurgence of radiation therapy as a treatment tool did not occur in the United States until major advances had occurred in technology in the post-WW II era and when the medical oncologists appeared on the scene as teammates in the nonoperative approach.

The potential benefits of the first effective anticancer agent, the alkylating agent nitrogen mustard, were first revealed by scientists working in a chemical warfare facility (Edgewood Arsenal in Maryland) near the end of WW II.[38] The major impact of nitrogen mustard was appreciated after the WWII bombing of a U.S. cargo ship in an Italian port that was carrying this compound as a possible deterrent to the use of poison gas by enemy forces. C.P. Rhoads, David Karnofsky, and Joseph Burchenal explored the clinical usefulness of this alkylating agent at the Memorial Hospital after the war, and others (Gilman, Phillips, and Goodman) made similar observations. The radiomimetic effect of alkylating agents proved useful, particularly in the management of hematopoietic neoplasms, but benefits were limited for the more common solid tumors. The folic acid antagonists first reported by Farber in

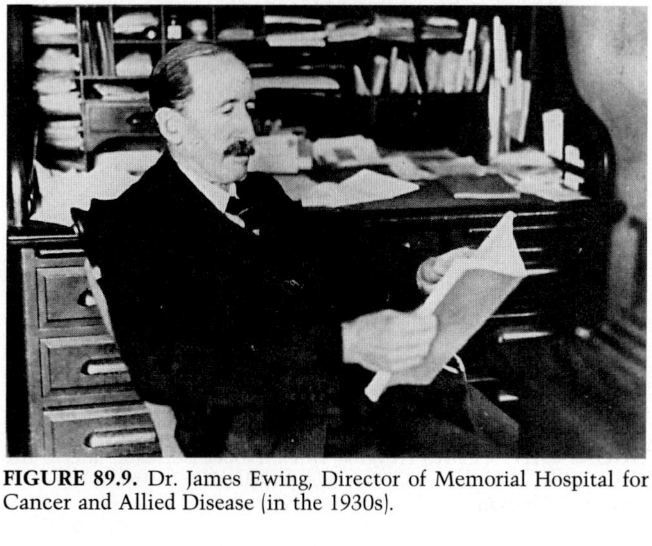

FIGURE 89.9. Dr. James Ewing, Director of Memorial Hospital for Cancer and Allied Disease (in the 1930s).

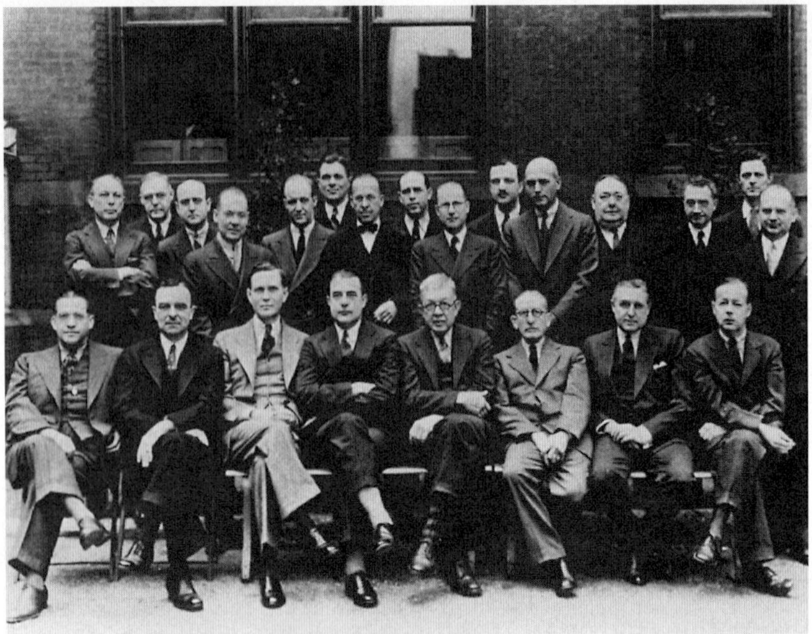

FIGURE 89.10. Attending staff of Memorial Hospital in 1938 included (seated) Drs. Norman E. Treves, George E. Binkley, Hayes E. Martin, Bradley L. Coley, Benjamin S. Barringer, James Ewing, Frank E. Adair, and Fred W. Stewart; (standing) Drs. Ralph E. Heredeen, Edward King, George T. Pack, William S. MacComb, Gordon P. McNeer, Alfred E. Hocker, George H. Hyslop, Joseph H. Farrow, Archie L. Dean, Gray H. Twombly, Lloyd F. Craver, Mr. George F. Holmes, Drs. Gioacchino Failla, E. Leonard Frazell, and Frank R. Smith. (Reprinted from A Century of Commitment. Produced by the Archives Committee of Memorial Sloan Kettering Cancer Center, 1984.)

1948,[39] and the description of mercaptopurine and its effects by Hitchings and Elion in 1951,[40] expanded the anticancer drug armamentarium. Karnofsky, Burchenal, Holland, Gellhorn, Haddow, Freireich, Frei, and others began extensive studies of this limited number of new agents with an emphasis on leukemia and related neoplasms. They began to train scientific progeny of their own and these new players in the cancer game, the forerunners of today's hematologists/oncologists, had successes in the treatment of both leukemias and lymphomas. A bit later, these drugs and other agents demonstrated effects on the more common, traditionally surgical, cancers. The clinical chemotherapist quickly became known as the oncologist, and this seriously threatened the roles of both the "cancer surgeon" and the radiotherapist. As we entered the latter half of the twentieth century, the surgeon who formally dominated cancer care began to see competition in his or her role as the primary specialty representative in this area. By the mid-1960s general surgeons who had been focusing on the field of cancer surgery began to use the term "surgical oncology," mainly as a defense against the rapidly developing concept of the nonsurgical oncologists being considered the experts on all aspects of cancer care.

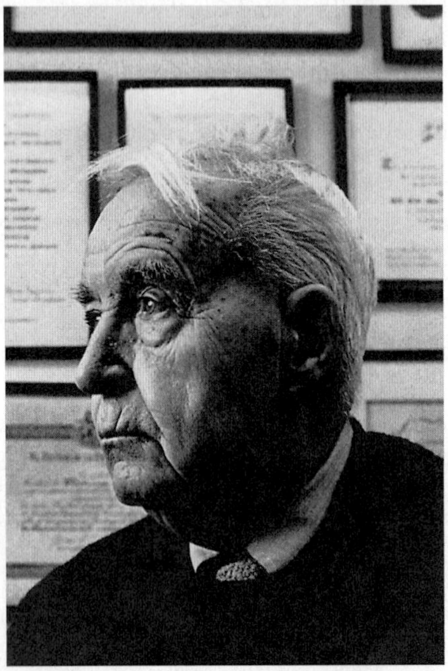

FIGURE 89.11. Charles Huggins, M.D., Nobel Laureate, late in life after almost 70 illustrious years as a physician scientist at the University of Chicago.

A comment should be made about hormonal approaches to cancer, as these approaches had a long-term association with surgeons. The benefits of various hormonal alterations on cancer growth had been demonstrated in animal systems years before and in women with advanced breast cancer by Beatson as early as 1896.[41] However, the first real exploitation of the concept of hormonal alteration was that of Nobel laureate Charles Huggins in 1941[42] when he demonstrated the effect of male castration on prostate cancer (Fig. 89.11). Subsequent treatment of human cancer by oophorectomy, adrenalectomy, and hormonal administration was primarily the domain of the surgeon at medical centers, but later nonoperative hormonal manipulations further diminished the role of operation in cancer care. By this time, it was clear that cancer treatment using more than one modality was emerging, but coordinated cooperative ventures, or the multidisciplinary approach, were still quite far off.

The Changing Role of the Cancer Surgeon

Almost at the same time, the chemotherapist with new anticancer agents and the radiotherapist with improved technology were in a position to force the cancer surgeon into becoming a team player at the major cancer centers. Often, these early multidisciplinary cancer care efforts were investigational, and it was then that the era of clinical trials actually began.

The chemotherapists were active at categorical cancer centers but by the middle of the 1950s had not made many inroads in university centers or in the community centers. Most of the care for patients with solid tumors at these geographic sites was still the primary responsibility of the surgeon. With increasing use of chemotherapeutic agents for advanced disease, many surgeons outside the cancer centers, both in university departments and the community, began to add the use of these agents to their own portfolio of treatments. Anthony Curreri at the University of Wisconsin and his scientific successor, Robert Johnson, were two such examples of this trend, but many other surgeons focusing on cancer considered that the administration of chemotherapy, particularly as an adjuvant measure, was the responsibility of the surgeon. Part of the reason for this was the limited number of nonsurgeons in the community who had an interest in chemotherapy for "solid" tumors, particularly those cancers arising in the gastrointestinal tract. Other surgeons acquiesced to the expanding population of chemotherapists at medical centers, now termed medical oncologists, and they developed more of a teamwork approach. The science of anticancer drugs and the toxicity problems associated with the newer and more effective drugs then began to convince most surgeons that a team approach to cancer, rather than a purely surgical approach, was preferable.

It became clear that, to maintain their role and prominence on the team and to be equal partners with the nonsurgical oncologists, surgeons needed the concept of surgical oncology to become better established. Oncologists within medicine were a specialty—medical oncology and, later, hematology/oncology; oncologists within radiology were radiation therapists and later radiation oncologists; but general surgeons remained surgeons. The age of specialization had arrived in many areas within medicine (rheumatology, allergy, nephrology, cardiology, etc.), and it was time for surgical oncology to evolve as an area of special interest in general surgery.

Although those general surgeons with a particular focus, interest, or expertise in cancer management were pleased to adopt the concept of being surgical oncologists, there remained a number of problems with the identification of the field of surgical oncology by others, both in and out of the field of surgery. Medical oncology, pediatric oncology, and radiation oncology were all quickly embraced by their colleagues as legitimate subspecialties within these broad disciplines as each of these oncology fields filled large voids, both clinical and investigational. For general surgery, however, it was (and still is) a very different situation. The general surgeon had been performing surgical procedures for cancer from the beginning of history. In contrast to these other disciplines, there was really no void to fill.

Although the concept of surgical oncology might well apply to surgeons within the various established surgical specialties who focus on cancer in their specialty area, the term surgical oncologist generally began to refer to the surgeon who, through both training and practice, focused his or her clinical efforts on the surgery of our more common cancers. Because most well-trained general surgeons were technically capable of this type of surgical care under most circumstances, this new breed of general surgical oncologist usually, but not always, was affiliated with medical centers or university hospitals where the administrative structure had allowed such a focus on surgical subspecialization. By the mid-1960s, the first formal division of surgical oncology in a university department of surgery was established at The Medical College of Virginia in Richmond, and many other departments of surgery soon followed suit. A later study of surgical oncology in university departments of surgery in 1986[43] showed that 47 of 126 departments (38%) had established formal divisions of surgical oncology. Adding this to the number of departments that had a separate general surgical service with a cancer focus yielded 70% of surgical departments with a surgical oncology emphasis. By the early twenty-first century, this trend has become even more prominent. Most academic departments of surgery have now developed a clear-cut surgical oncology "presence" of some type (division, section, or service). Academic medicine has recognized the importance of surgical oncology as a field of special importance within general surgery.

Profile of the New Surgical Oncologist

The evolution of the surgical oncologist during the 1960s and 1970s led to many changes in the classic practice of the cancer surgeon of earlier decades. Two major attributes of surgical trainees from cancer centers in the earlier years were the capability for radical head and neck cancer surgery and the ability to conduct extensive operations for gynecological cancer, particularly the more advanced lesions. As this trend toward specialization in oncology developed within general surgery and in medicine in general, both these anatomic areas traditionally served by "cancer surgeons" became a focus of other specialty groups rather than the sole domain of the general surgical oncologist. Head and neck cancer operations, except thyroid and parotid surgery, had long been a weakness of most practicing general surgeons, and most otolaryngology training programs did not include major head and neck surgery. General surgeons had included the standard but not the radical gynecological surgical procedures in their practices for many years, and gynecological surgery training in earlier years had never encompassed operations of the magnitude required for advanced gynecological cancer. However, both these fields (otolaryngology and gynecology) then began to develop special advanced training in oncology surgery for these anatomic areas in the 1960s, at the same time that surgical oncology was evolving within general surgery. In both these specialties (head and neck oncology and gynecological oncology), oncologists with additional training were able to focus efforts entirely on the specific anatomic sites associated with their specialty. In gynecological oncology, this focus allowed the development of expertise in administration of chemotherapy as well as in the specialized operative procedures required. In head and neck oncology, the total focus of specialized otolaryngological surgeons on the performance of extensive resections in the head and neck area led to developing the increased technical skills in the reconstructive surgery required after these radical resections. Despite both the complaints and the territorial claims of the general surgical establishment, these two surgical oncology areas of great interest were slowly removed as major activities from the purview of both the practicing general surgeon and the emerging surgical oncologist. It is truly of interest that these were the two areas of surgical activity that had specifically identified the cancer surgeon a couple of decades earlier, and now each had their own special brand of oncologist fulfilling cancer patient care needs. It is clear that the surgical oncologist in general surgery had become a different commodity than the old-time "cancer surgeon" as a result of the growth of both nonsurgical and other surgical oncology disciplines.

In view of these "invasions" of the areas of interest of the surgical oncologist, there was some interest in making this practice area more of a specialty, thereby excluding other less focused general surgeons from the territory. This notion was not widely accepted by general surgeons. As the large proportion of the operative effort of the active general surgeon has been and continues to be related to cancer, the general surgeon has seen little reason for rearranging operative responsibilities in such a way as to reduce or eliminate cancer surgery from his armamentarium. In spite of the fact that there was an increasing need for vigorous and expert surgical oncology involvement on our newly developed multidisciplinary oncology teams, it is clear that many general surgeons thought that they were still quite capable of playing this specialized role. The general surgeon who had been so intimately involved with cancer thus far seriously questioned the development of this upstart subspecialty in surgical oncology that threatened to diminish the clinical roles they had played for so long. The concept of a specially trained general surgeon who is focused on the cancer problem as a full-time oncologist has finally now emerged in spite of these concerns, primarily because of the increasing complexity of the process of cancer management. It has become increasingly apparent that the quality of cancer patient care is improved by the development of a few surgical oncologists to provide leadership in the area of cancer management to the overall community of general surgeons. To put the role of this new oncology specialist in perspective, however, a specific definition of this emerging field is needed.

A useful definition of the field of surgical oncology began to evolve in the 1960s, but it is not fully agreed upon, even at the present time, by those who consider themselves surgical oncologists. A few surgeons continue to propose that all operative procedures for cancer be performed by surgical oncologists. Having the surgical oncologist monopolize the operations for cancer within the field of general surgery might be both satisfying and convenient for many of our nonsurgical colleagues who themselves work full time in oncology, but the practical problems associated with this minority view are many. Instead, what has become both a simple and more workable definition of the surgical oncologist is that he or she is an individual who is a fully qualified general surgeon who has had additional training and experience in all aspects of oncology, is capable of collaborating well with other oncology disciplines, has a full-time commitment to oncology, and serves the important role of leader (rather than competitor) of his fellow general surgeons in the care of the cancer patient. This description is the product of thoughtful conferences that were sponsored by the Society of Surgical Oncology (SSO) and the National Cancer Institute (NCI) in the late 1970s.[44]

The foregoing concept of the leadership role of a surgical oncologist now seems reasonably well accepted by the majority of general surgeons and surgical oncologists, but the borders of the definition are a bit "fuzzy." Most surgical oncologists have developed the capability and the experience of performing some less frequently utilized operative procedures for neoplastic disease that are not usually employed by the general surgeon. However, this additional specialized experience of the surgical oncologist, by virtue of the background described, more often relates to the proper selection of operation, as opposed to other treatment options, than to the actual performance of the operation itself. The surgical oncologist is able to review and evaluate all operative procedures for cancer with the perspective of the total care of the patient being provided by other oncology disciplines rather than viewing the operation as an isolated treatment method. Another major contribution to patient care that the surgical oncologist has been able to make is an in-depth understanding of the natural history of the wide range of diseases we know as cancer. This understanding gives the surgical oncologist the ability to provide expert consultation and leadership to both surgical and nonsurgical colleagues in a large variety of circumstances, and is accomplished in a fashion similar to that of other general surgeons who have focused their professional activities on a special area in general surgery, such as trauma, burns, endocrine surgery, peripheral vascular disease, or inflammatory bowel disease.

Role of the Surgical Oncologist in Clinical Trials

Clinical trials and randomized clinical trials began in earnest in the mid-1970s when the U.S. Congress responded to the pleas of the national leaders, Jonathan Rhoads and Sidney Farber, to establish a national chemotherapy center at the National Cancer Institute (NCI). The early trials initiated with NCI support focused on leukemia, a nonsurgical cancer, but metastatic forms of breast and lung cancer, melanoma, and Hodgkin's disease were the next treatment targets using several of the available alkylating agents. Surgeons were not really involved in these early trials of metastatic and advanced disease but were first involved in a major way in 1957 with the initiation of the National Surgical Adjuvant Breast Project (NSABP) under the direction of Rudolph Noer.[45] Subsequently, this multiinstitutional cooperative project was headed by Bernard Fisher and his colleagues, who embarked on truly landmark studies of breast and colon cancer. William Longmire, William Holden, and George Higgins were pioneer surgical leaders in additional randomized clinical trials of breast, gastric, and colorectal cancer of that era and established this key role for all surgical oncologists in the surgical community, that of being the local leader in clinical trial research. Currently, surgical oncologists in both university departments and nonuniversity medical centers are serving as both leaders and participants in multidisciplinary cooperative group trials of cancer prevention, early detection, and treatment. Also, they are serving as facilitators, in terms of encouraging participation of the general surgical community in these trials.

The American College of Surgeons, under the leadership of Dr. Samual A. Wells, Jr., formed a cooperative clinical trial group for studies designed specifically to evaluate the surgical aspects of cancer management. This organization known as The American College of Surgeons Oncology Group

(ACOSOG) was planned in the late 1990s and by 2003 had 2644 physician members (1878 of these being surgeons) and more than 8500 patients already accrued in sixteen clinical trials. The ACOSOG office is located at the Duke University Medical Center, has ten organ site committees for planning these trials, and includes a broad participation of surgical oncologists from both academic medical centers and private practice. It has accomplished all of this by developing a strong commitment from members of the SSO and many other surgical speciality societies concerned with cancer management.

The Society of Surgical Oncology

The SSO was established in 1975, at a time the concept of surgical oncology was being formulated. It was an outgrowth of the James Ewing Society, which was founded in 1940 both to "further our knowledge of cancer" and to honor Dr. James Ewing, the famous pathologist/oncologist, who was the director of the Memorial Hospital in New York from its inception in 1913 until his retirement in 1939.[45] It was not a purely surgical or surgical oncological society, but surgeons dominated this multidisciplinary oncology society as they had dominated the oncology field during those years before and immediately after World War II. At a time when some academic surgeons (primarily Donald Morton and Tapas Das-Gupta) were suggesting the formation of an academic surgical oncology society, it appeared that the transformation of this well-established oncology society, with strong surgical oncology input, would be a better solution to this need for a national subspecialty organization. The field of surgical oncology, poorly defined as it was at that time, could hardly undergo the further confusion of having two separate organizations representing it. There was considerable controversy in the James Ewing Society over this name change; however, the major argument against it was the potentially negative impact on the memory of the beloved Dr. James Ewing, a true hero of all the membership as well as the oncology community of the day. Many of us believed that the creation of an entirely new and separate national surgical oncology society, rather than merely changing the name of this society, would seriously threaten the future of the James Ewing Society by leading to the loss of valuable surgical members whereas a name change would give this society an expanded role and purpose. The impasse at a rather emotional meeting on this topic, under the chairmanship of President Edward Scanlon in 1975, was broken by the strong supportive comments of Harvey Baker and those of the pioneer surgical oncologist Murray Copeland.[46] Dr. Copeland committed all to the promise that surgical oncologists would continue to be true to the memory and the inspiration of Dr. Ewing, despite the name change, and most of us believe that this has been the case. In addition, the major foundation associated with the SSO, the James Ewing Foundation, proudly maintains his name.

Since its formation, the SSO has developed guidelines for training and a review and approvals process for training programs, and has continued and expanded scientific interchange at an annual scientific meeting. An early attempt at initiating clinical trials through the aegis of the SSO was not very successful, but the national organization has continued to grow both in size and stature. By 2004 the total membership was roughly 1900 members in 48 states and 43 foreign countries, more than double the number of members at the time of the formation of this society in 1975. This growth represents not only an increasing interest in surgical oncology, but an appreciation of its importance in the multidisciplinary approach to cancer management.

The American College of Surgeons and the American Cancer Society

Most surgeons concerned with cancer have been active participants in these two organizations for several generations, both societies having their origin in 1913. The American Association for the Advancement of Cancer began then, but later became the American Cancer Society (ACS) in 1946 with a well-known New York breast cancer surgeon, Frank Adair (Fig. 89.12), serving as its first president. Many leaders in surgical oncology and the SSO have served in leadership positions in the ACS since that time, and this has maintained the ties of surgical oncology to public cancer education and cancer control programs.[47] The surgical oncology connection with the American College of Surgeons has been strengthened through its highly effective cancer program, which began in 1913, at the time of the formation of the College with its focus first on cancer clinics and later on cancer registries. The cancer program expanded in 1965 with the formation of the multidisciplinary Commission on Cancer. At the same time as the formulation of guidelines for postresidency surgical oncology training by the SSO in the early 1980s, the Commission on Cancer began CME courses on cancer care for all general surgeons as well as developing special surgical oncology educational presentations at both the spring and the

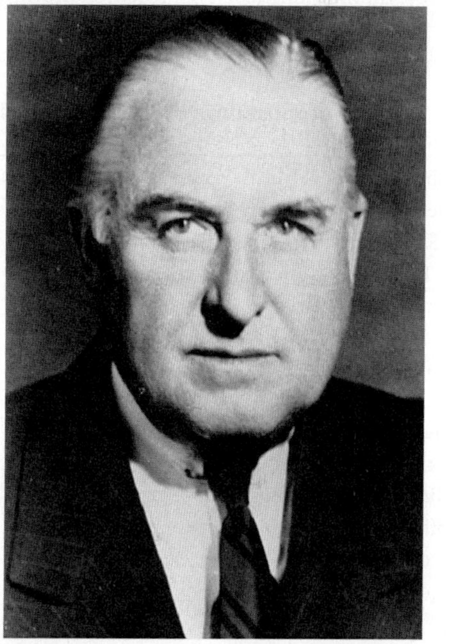

FIGURE 89.12. Dr. Frank Adair, chairman of the Committee on Cancer of the American College of Surgeons 1940–1946 and first president of the American Cancer Society (1946), the year of the name change from American Society for the Control of Cancer.

annual congresses of the American College of Surgeons. At this time, these programs are extensive and well attended.

The continued contributions of these two national organizations to the surgical oncology effort in the United States was well demonstrated in 1997 by the initiation of the TRIAD program by the Commission on Cancer. This is a regional cooperative program with representatives from the Field Liaison program (primarily surgical oncologists), the volunteers and the staff of the ACS, and the regional representatives of the American Association of Cancer Registries. This cooperative effort allows surgical oncologists to better accomplish their mission at the regional level.

Training in Surgical Oncology

Any history of surgical oncology must include comments regarding the development of the training process for surgical oncologists. As with any specialty in medicine, this training must be related to the ultimate roles and responsibilities of such a "specialist." Since the relatively newly hatched specialty of surgical oncology has thus far primarily been a clinical research field as well as a field committed to the coordination of others, both surgical and nonsurgical, most surgical oncologists have continued to serve in either university or other tertiary care centers. For this reason the training centers for these surgical oncologists have been located either in the categorical cancer centers or the university departments of surgery that have developed formal free-standing divisions of surgical oncology. Training programs at cancer centers have existed for many years, but the university-based training programs in surgical oncology have slowly developed over the past three decades.

A review of the training programs that now exist (2004) demonstrates the fact that there is no one prescribed training pathway. However, most postresidency fellowships in surgical oncology include clinical and research training because most products of these programs have both clinical and research roles to play. General guidelines for such training have been developed by the SSO and by the NCI, with the SSO assuming responsibility for voluntary review of all such training programs. Currently, there are 16 institutions with surgical oncology training programs approved by the training committee of the SSO, and the output from this group of training programs approaches 40 trainees per year (Table 89.1). There are some additional institutions that have specialized training programs, often with surgical oncology research fellowship support (T32) from the NCI, but many of these have not fulfilled all the clinical training requirements of the SSO. However, the academic output of these research training programs contributes also to the manpower in surgical oncology. By 2003 there were 15 funded T32 programs supporting 62 trainees, with many of such programs not being represented in the SSO group of approved clinical programs (Cancer Training Branch, NCI, personal communication, 2004) (Table 89.2).

TABLE 89.1. Society of Surgical Oncology: 18 Approved Training Programs, 2007.

City of Hope National Medical Center
M. D. Anderson Cancer Center
Memorial Sloan-Kettering Cancer Center
Ohio State University College of Medicine
Roswell Park Cancer Institute
University of Miami School of Medicine
University of Chicago
Fox Chase Cancer Center
John Wayne Cancer Institute
Johns Hopkins Hospital
Roger Williams Hospital—Boston University
H. Lee Moffit Cancer Center & Research Institute
University of Pittsburgh
University of Toronto
University of Calgary
Virginia Commonwealth University (Massey Cancer Center)
University of Louisville
University of Miami School of Medicine

TABLE 89.2. National Research Awards in Surgical Oncology (FY 2003).

Institutions	*Positions*
Duke University (2 awards)	11
University of Alabama, Birmingham	6
University of Wisconsin	3
Weill Medical College of Cornell	6
University of Texas MD Anderson (2 awards)	8
Memorial Sloan Kettering Cancer Center (2 awards)	8
University of North Carolina Chapel Hill	2
University of Michigan	4
Washington University	4
Fred Hutchinson Cancer Center Seattle	6
Brigham and Womens' Hospital	2
University of Pittsburgh	2
Total positions:	62

At this time, the SSO guidelines for approval of a training program in surgical oncology specify a minimum of 2 years of postresidency training, at least 18 months of this being clinical. The goals of the program include developing clinical and technical skills in the management of the cancer patient, developing a broad knowledge of cancer management modalities other than surgery, and acquiring the scientific background needed for leadership in the multidisciplinary approach to the cancer patient, leadership in clinical trials research, and leadership in institutional and educational programs. Interaction with other surgical oncological specialities on specific rotations is considered important, and experience with the management of complicated cancer cases is assured by the establishment of minimum numbers of operative cases of various kinds. The research experience appears to vary widely in both type and duration; the programs receiving NCI grant support require at least 2 years of research training.

Evaluation of the trainees by examination has been encouraged for self-assessment purposes and for the individual program director's evaluation, but as yet there is no official certifying examination. Each program is evaluated by the Training Committee of the SSO and by periodic site visit review teams, rather than evaluation of the individual trainees; these include representatives of nonsurgical oncological disciplines, surgical oncologists from the SSO, and nonmember general surgeons who are familiar with the standards of postgraduate education.

The current annual output of "new" surgical oncologists from all these programs is probably appropriate for fulfilling the national manpower needs in surgical oncology if the role of the surgical oncologist is to remain limited to the leadership activity outlined earlier in this chapter. The distribution of surgical oncologists at present is clearly not totally limited to faculty positions in university divisions of surgical oncology and cancer centers, as evidenced by the current membership number in the SSO. However, it is probably fair to say that most surgical oncologists serve as leaders of fellow general surgeons in their communities rather than assuming a monopoly position in surgical cancer care.

Credentialing Surgical Oncologists

Any discussion of a new clinical field, or subspeciality, always raises the question of a certification process for assuring quality performance; this has been the basis for the establishment of new boards and/or certificates within major clinical disciplines. Certification in vascular surgery, cardiothoracic surgery, or other technically highly demanding areas, from the standpoint of technical expertise, provides examples of this trend. Ever since surgical oncology appeared as a "player" on the scene in the mid-1960s, there has been pressure from a number of surgical oncologists to develop a certification process for the specific identification of this expertise. Some surgeons who have focused their professional efforts on surgical oncology believed this certification was essential to progress, while others thought identification of this special interest and skill could be better demonstrated by active membership and participation in the national society devoted to this field, the SSO. Those who were against formal certification feared that this certification would become a franchise, to be used at the local level, and designed to give an outright monopoly to surgical oncologists for all general surgical cancer problems; this would clearly obviate the role of the surgical oncologist as the leader for fellow general surgeons. The other uneasiness about board certification or official designation of special expertise was that surgical oncology seems to be more of a conceptual than a technical specialty. The advantages provided to cancer care by the surgical oncologist are increased knowledge of the natural history of the disease, increased knowledge of the role of other oncological specialities, and increased ability in clinical trials research. None of these special skills appeared to have a specific reason for board certification in the view of many, and in the view of the American Board of Surgery. However, in 1998, the American Board of Surgery did establish a Surgical Oncology Advisory Council, a move suggesting a stronger acknowledgment of this special area of surgical interest in the future. The leadership role of this council is evidenced by the fact that one of its primary functions is to review the oncology content of the Board's written and oral examinations to assure that it is consonant with current knowledge and standards of care. As the pattern of medicine changes in future decades, more specific identification of surgical oncologists by formation of a "subboard" may take place, as happened with vascular surgery and with pediatric surgery (R.S. Rhodes, American Board of Surgery, personal communication, 2004). However, it does seem probable that the current status of a surgical oncologist as a regional leadership individual for fellow general surgeons will remain relatively constant for some time to come.

Comment

During the past 30 years the status and, hopefully, the appropriate status of the general surgical oncologist has evolved on the basis of the needs of the cancer patient. The sophistication required in the use of some of the newer diagnostic and therapeutic techniques, the refinement of technology now available in radiation therapy, and the development of improved drug management approaches for both adjuvant benefit and palliation made it mandatory for a few general surgeons to have the needed additional experience and commitment to the cancer field to put these new approaches in proper perspective. The general surgeon needed colleagues from his own specialty to provide leardership in multidisciplinary cancer programs and to ensure complementary support and consultation in the management of difficult patient management problems, as well as facilitating the collaboration of each and every general surgeon in vital clinical research activity. Clinical trials of adjuvant chemotherapy after operations, immunotherapy, and the choice of the optimal operative procedures have required and will continue to require the presence of surgical oncologists who are frequently the leaders in these activities. The need for, and the appreciation of, the role of surgical oncologists here in the United States is well demonstrated by the gradual increase in the membership of the SSO during the past two decades, acknowledgment of this field of endeavor by the leading national surgical organizations, and recognition by the nonsurgical oncological disciplines.

References

1. Lewison EF. Breast Cancer and its Diagnosis and Treatment. Baltimore: Williams & Wilkins, 1955.
2. Hippocrates. Works. Jones WHS, Withington ET, eds, 4 vols. New York: Putnam, 1923–1931.
3. Halsted WS. The treatment of wounds with special reference to the value of the blood clot in the management of dead spaces. Johns Hopkins Hosp Rep 1890–1891;2:255–314.
4. Halsted WS. The results of radical operations for the cure of cancer of the breast. Ann Surg 1907;46:1–19.
5. McDowell E. Three cases of extirpation of diseased ovaries. Eclectic Repertory and Analytic Review 1817;7:242.
6. Rutledge RH. Theodore Billroth: a century later. Surgery (St. Louis) 1995;118:36–43.
7. Caldamone AA. Theodore Billroth: the urologist. Urology 1981;18:316–324.
8. Schlatter C. Beitr Klin Chir 1897;19:757–776.
9. Pack GT, McNeer GP. Total gastrectomy for cancer: a collective review of the literature and an original report of 20 cases. Int Abstr Surg 1943;77:265–299.
10. Weir R. Resection of the large intestine for carcinoma. Ann Surg 1886;3:469–489.
11. Von Mikulicz-Radciki J. Small contributions to the surgery of the intestinal tract. Bost Med Surg J 1903;148:608–611.

12. Mayo CH. Gastroenterostomy by means of Murphy button with table of late cases of anastomosis by this method. Ann Surg 1895;21:41–44.
13. Miles WE. A method for performing abdominoperineal excision for carcinoma of the rectum and terminal portion of the pelvic colon. Lancet 1908;2:1812–1813.
14. Sims JM. Removal of the superior maxilla for a tumor of the antrum; apparent cure; return of the disease [Sequel]. Am J Med Sci 1847;13:310–314.
15. Meade RH. Surgery of the thyroid and parathyroid: In: An Introduction to the History of General Surgery. Philadelphia: Saunders, 1968.
16. Senn N. Pathology and Treatment of Tumors. Philadelphia: Saunders, 1900.
17. Crile GW. Excision of cancer of the head and neck. JAMA 1906;XLVII:1780.
18. Clark JG. A more radical method for performing hysterectomy for cancer of the cervix. Johns Hopkins Bull 1895;6:121.
19. Meigs JV. Carcinoma of the cervix: the Wertheim operation. Surg Gynecol Obstet 1944;78:195.
20. Torek F. The first successful case of resection of the thoracic portion of the esophagus for carcinoma. Surg Gynecol Obstet 1913;16:614–617.
21. Graham EA, Singer JJ. Successful removal of an entire lung for carcinoma of the bronchus. JAMA 1933;101:371–374.
22. Adams WE, Phemister DB. Carcinoma of the lower esophagus. Report of a successful resection and esophagogastrostomy. J Thorac Surg 1938;7:621–632.
23. Whipple AD, Parsons WB, Mullins CR. Treatment of carcinoma of the ampulla of vater. Ann Surg 1935;102:763–779.
24. Pack GT, McNeer GP, Booher RJ. Principles governing total gastrectomy. Arch Surg 1947;55:457–485.
25. Longmire WP Jr. Total gastrectomy for carcinoma of the stomach. Surg Gynecol Obstet 1947;84:21–30.
26. Lahey FH, Marshal SF. Should total gastrectomy be employed in early carcinoma of the stomach? Experience with 139 total gastrectomies. Ann Surg 1950;132:54–56.
27. Pickrell KL, Clay RC. Lobectomy of the liver: report of three cases. Arch Surg 1944;48:267–277.
28. Lortat-Jacob JL, Robert HG. Hepatectomie droite reglée. Presse Med 1952;60:549–551.
29. Pack GT, Baker HW. Total right hepatic lobectomy. Ann Surg 1953;138:253–258.
30. Martin HE, Ellis EB. Biopsy by needle puncture and aspiration. Ann Surg 1930;92:169–181.
31. Brunschwig A. Radical Surgery in Advanced Abdominal Cancer. Chicago: University of Chicago Press, 1947.
32. Brunschwig A. Complete excision of the pelvic viscera for advanced carcinoma. Cancer (Phila) 1948;1:177–183.
33. Bricker EM. Bladder substitutions after pelvic evisceration. Surg Clin N Am 1950;30:1511.
34. Bricker EM, Butcher HR Jr, Lawler WH Jr, McAfee CA. Surgical treatment of advanced and recurrent cancer of the pelvic viscera: an evaluation of 10 years experience. Ann Surg 1960;152:388–402.
35. Urban JA, Baker HW. Radical mastectomy with en bloc resection of the internal mammary lymph node chain. Cancer (Phila) 1952;5:992–1008.
36. Sugarbaker ED. Extended radical mastectomy: its superiority in the treatment of breast cancer. JAMA 1964;186:999.
37. Caceres E. An evaluation of radical mastectomy and extended radical mastectomy for cancer of the breast. Surg Gynecol Obstet 1967;125:337–341.
38. Krakoff IH. Progress and prospects in cancer treatment: the Karnofsky legacy. J Clin Oncol 1994;12:432–438.
39. Farber S, Diamond LK, Mercer RD, et al. Temporary remissions in acute leukemia in children produced by folic acid antagonist, aminopteroyl-glutamic acid. N Engl J Med 1948;238:693.
40. Hitchings GH, Elion GB, Falco EA, et al. J Biol Chem 1950; 183:1.
41. Beatson GT. On the treatment of inoperable carcinoma of the mama: suggestions for a new method of treatment with illustrated cases. Lancet 1896;2:104–107.
42. Huggins CB, Hodges CV. Studies on prostatic cancer: the effect of castration, of estrogen and of androgen injection on serum phosphatases in metastatic carcinoma of the prostate. Cancer Res 1941;1:293–297.
43. Lawrence W Jr, Wilson RE, Shingleton WW, et al. Surgical oncology in university departments of surgery in the United States. Arch Surg 1986;121:1088–1093.
44. Schweitzer RJ, Edwards MH, Lawrence W Jr, et al. Training guidelines for surgical oncology. Cancer (Phila) 1981;48:2336–2340.
45. Fleming ID. Society of Surgical Oncology, oral presentation, March 1997.
46. Lawrence W Jr. Some problems with clinical trials (James Ewing lecture). Arch Surg 1991;126:370–378.
47. Lawrence W Jr. The Commission on Cancer and the American Cancer Society: partners in cancer control. Bull Am Coll Surg 1993;78:19–24.

90

Genetics of Cancer

John E. Phay and Jeffrey F. Moley

Numerous discoveries of genetic abnormalities in cancer cells have pointed to the paramount importance of genetic defects in the origin and development of cancer. Although other factors certainly play a role in the growth and maintenance of the transformed state (such as hormones, growth factors, and cytokines), defects in critical genes in cancer cells are undoubtedly at the heart of most malignant states.

Chromosome Number and Nomenclature

Each human somatic cell contains 46 chromosomes organized as 23 pairs. Chromosomes 1 through 22 are referred to as autosomes. The 23rd pair is the sex chromosomes, XX in females and XY in males. The autosomes are numbered based on their relative size as seen on karyotype analysis. Chromosome 1 is the longest chromosome, and chromosome 22, the smallest. One chromosome of each pair is inherited from the mother, the other from the father. During meiosis, the process in which the cells with only 23 chromosomes are formed (sperm cells and oocytes), recombination events occur in which hybrid chromosomes are formed containing part of each parental chromosome, contributing to variation in individuals in a population. This phenomenon of reassortment of parental chromosome makeup is fundamental to maintaining variation within the population and is the basis of gene mapping studies by linkage analysis.

Chromosome preparations from individual cells can be studied by staining techniques that give the chromosomes characteristic banding patterns, making their identification and arrangement into a karyotype possible. Each chromosome is divided into two major regions or arms, separated by the centromere, generally but not always near the middle of the chromosome. The shorter arm is pictorially represented on top and is designated the p-arm. The longer arm is pictorially represented on the bottom and is called the q-arm. The ends of each chromosome are called telomeres. Within each chromosomal arm, regions are designated numerically based on their banding pattern, and these are subdivided into smaller regions. Therefore, as noted in Figure 90.1, chromosome 1p has three major subregions, designated 1p1, 1p2, and 1p3. These regions are subdivided (e.g., 1p32), and further subdivided (1p32.2), based on their banding pattern. A gene or DNA sequence can be localized, or "mapped," to the chromosome and chromosomal subregion at which it resides by genetic linkage or chromosomal in situ hybridization.

Cancer cells very frequently have multiple chromosomal abnormalities that are apparent cytogenetically. These aberrations include gains or losses of chromosomes, deletions, inversions, and translocations. Gain of a chromosome is described as a trisomy for that chromosome, and loss of a copy of a chromosome is designated a monosomy. If a cell has more than 46 chromosomes, it is said to be hyperdiploid, and if its chromosome complement is less than 46, it is called hypodiploid. In a deletion, a band, subband, or even an entire arm of a chromosome is missing. Inversions and translocations involve rearrangements of parts of chromosomes to either the same or other chromosomes. Tumors may contain multiple clonal populations of cells that contain different karyotypic abnormalities.

Historical Aspects

Cancer is a genetic disease. That is not to say that that cancer is always a hereditary disease, but that the cause of the malignant transformation of a cell resides in its genetic material (DNA), which has been altered to produce a phenotype with malignant characteristics. Historically, several lines of evidence supported this hypothesis. First, malignant tumors are generally clonal, which means that tumors are composed of

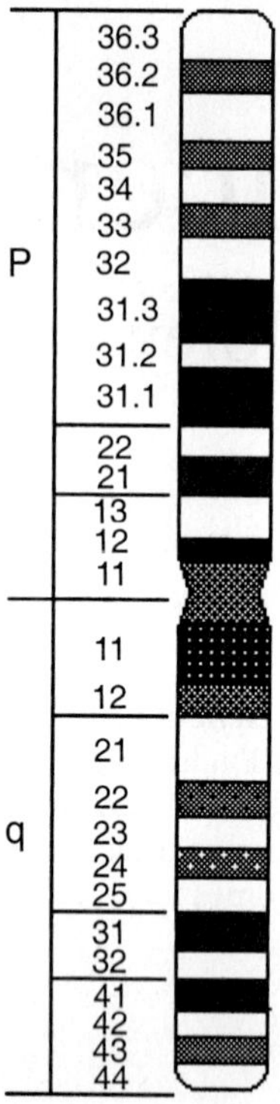

FIGURE 90.1. Diagrammatic representation of chromosome 1, showing subregions based on banding patterns. The chromosome consists of a p-arm and a q-arm joined by the centromere. (See text for discussion.) (Reprinted with permission from Moley JF, Kim SH. Molecular Genetics in Surgical Oncology. Austin: Landes, 1994.)

groups of cells that are derived from a single malignant cell.[1] Second, most carcinogens are mutagens for DNA. Third, there are several hereditary types of cancer in which individuals in a family are predisposed to develop cancer. In most of these genetic cancer syndromes, the cancer predisposition is inherited as an autosomal dominant trait, as is discussed later in this chapter. Fourth, individuals who have acquired specific chromosomal defects are often noted to develop certain types of cancer (e.g., patients with Down syndrome often develop acute lymphocytic leukemia). Last, certain types of cancer are known to be associated with specific chromosomal anomalies that occur in the cancer cells themselves (e.g., the Philadelphia chromosome in chronic myelogenous leukemia). These associations suggested that cancer was caused by defects in genes and/or chromosomes.

Viruses and Cancer

A viral etiology for cancer was suggested by the fact that a number of viruses can cause cancer in animals and can transform cells in culture. In 1907, Peyton Rous discovered a virus that causes sarcomas in chickens (RSV, or Rous sarcoma virus).[2] Subsequently, a number of viruses that cause cancer in animals were discovered, and the association of viral infection with several types of human cancer (e.g., hepatitis B and hepatocellular carcinoma) was documented (Table 90.1).

There are two main types of tumor viruses, DNA tumor viruses and RNA tumor viruses. After incorporating their viral DNA into the host cell DNA, DNA tumor viruses (including SV40, polyoma, and adenoviruses) make viral oncoprotein products, some of which have transforming properties. RNA tumor viruses (retroviruses) infect susceptible cells, copy their RNA genome into double-stranded DNA using the enzyme reverse transcriptase, and then integrate their viral DNA into the host cell genome. Many of these viruses carry oncogenes, which enable the virus to transform cells. In 1976, the Rous sarcoma virus oncogene was identified and called *SRC* (or v-*SRC* for viral SRC).[3] *SRC* encodes a 60-kDa protein that is a membrane tyrosine kinase. Shortly thereafter, it was discovered that a gene very similar to v-*SRC* was present in the genome of normal chicken cells (c-*SRC*). This spectacular finding indicated that the viral *SRC* gene was not a viral gene at all but was a normal vertebrate gene that had been captured and incorporated into the viral genome at some time in the past. The viral *SRC* gene had been mutated in a way that modified tyrosine kinase activity, and, under control of viral promoters, the gene is overexpressed in infected cells, leading to cell proliferation and tumor formation. The virus is perpetuated by horizontal transmission between animals of the affected species. Ultimately, this highly conserved *SRC* gene was identified in normal human cells.

A number of RNA tumor virus oncogenes have been described (Table 90.2), and screening of the vertebrate genome has indicated that many of the viral oncogenes are modified vertebrate genes (called proto-oncogenes). Normal genes have been incorporated into viral genomes and can cause transformation in a retroviral infection. It was then found that human tumors often contained activated oncogenes derived from normal genes, called proto-oncogenes, which were homologous to viral oncogenes. To summarize, RNA tumor viruses

TABLE 90.1. Human Malignancies Associated with Viral Infection.

Virus	*Tumor*
Human papilloma virus (HPV)	Cervical cancer Vulvar cancer Penile cancer Anal cancer
Epstein–Barr virus (EBV)	Burkitt's lymphoma Nasopharyngeal cancer B-cell lymphoma
Hepatitis B virus (HBV)	Hepatocellular cancer
Human T-cell leukemia virus type 1 (HTLV-1)	T-cell leukemia
Human immunodeficiency virus (HIV)	Kaposi's sarcoma

TABLE 90.2. Viral Oncogenes and Human Homologues.

Virus	*Viral oncogene*	*Human oncogene*
Rous sarcoma virus	v-*src*	*src*
Maloney murine sarcoma virus	v-*mos*	*mos*
Harvey murine sarcoma virus	v-Ha-*ras*	H-*ras*
Simian sarcoma virus	v-*sis*	PDGFB (platelet-derived growth factor)
Avian erythroblastosis virus	v-*erbB*	EGFR (epidermal growth factor receptor)

carry oncogenes (v-*ONC*) that are homologous to normal human genes (proto-oncogenes). In the absence of viral infection (which is a rare cause of human cancer), human proto-oncogenes can be activated in a number of ways to form oncogenes that can cause tumors.

Human Oncogenes

The discovery of the human *RAS* oncogenes illustrates the link between tumor viruses and human cancer and the difference between oncogenes and proto-oncogenes. In 1982, researchers used the DNA transfection assay, in which human tumor DNA (without any viral exposure) is passed into rodent cells and later isolated, to identify an oncogene from a human bladder cancer.[4,5] A DNA probe was made from the oncogene and used to analyze normal (nontumor) human DNA. This finding revealed that all normal human cells had copies of this gene. Characterization of the normal human cellular gene revealed that it was the H-*RAS* (Harvey ras) gene, which had already been characterized. The H-*RAS* gene (see Table 90.2) was known to be the human homologue of the viral oncogene of the Harvey sarcoma virus! Analysis of the sequence of the H-*RAS* oncogene from the bladder tumor revealed a minor sequence difference (mutation) from the normal cellular H-*ras* proto-oncogene. This mutation caused a different amino acid to be present at position 61. This single amino acid change results in an abnormal H-*RAS* protein that has transforming properties. Mutated *RAS* oncogenes have now been described in a number of human cancers.

In the case just described, a single point mutation in a normal cellular gene results in an oncogene with transforming properties. Normal cellular genes can become oncogenic in a number of other ways, some of which can be detected cytogenetically by examining tumor cell karyotypes.[6] Examination of karyotypes of cells derived from human neuroblastomas revealed the presence of small bits of extra chromosomal material (double minute bodies) that, on analysis, were found to be extrachromosomal pieces of chromosome 8 carrying the N-*MYC* gene.[7] By breaking off and replicating independently, the small bits of DNA result in amplification of the N-*MYC* oncogene, whose resultant overexpression contributes to the malignant phenotype. N-*MYC* amplification in tumor DNA can be detected at the molecular level by Southern blotting with a radioactive N-*MYC* probe. Tumors with N-*MYC* amplification demonstrate an increase in intensity of the corresponding band on the autoradiogram, and tumors with N-*MYC* amplification have been found to have a poorer prognosis than tumors without.[8] Other tumors with oncogene amplification are listed in Table 90.3.

Another chromosomal abnormality, detected initially by examination of tumor cell karyotypes, led to the discovery of a different mechanism of oncogene activation. The Philadelphia chromosome is the result of reciprocal translocation between chromosomes 9 and 22.[9] This alteration occurs in 90% of patients with chronic myelogenous leukemia and in some patients with acute lymphocytic leukemia. Molecular analysis has revealed that this translocation results in the juxtaposition of the 59-coding sequence of the *BCR* (breakpoint cluster region) gene with the *ABL* oncogene.[10–12] This then results in the production of hybrid *BCR-ABL* fusion proteins that have increased tyrosine kinase activity, compared to the normal, smaller C-*ABL* protein which is normally found in both the cellular cytoplasm and nucleus. Expression of the BCR-ABL protein in mice produces an illness similar to myelogenous leukemia. Other examples of translocations resulting in fusion oncogenes include papillary thyroid carcinoma [inv10(q11.2;q21)], Ewing's sarcoma [t(11;22)(q24;q12)], and liposarcoma [t(12;16)(q13;p11)].[13]

TABLE 90.3. Oncogene Amplification in Human Tumors.

Tumor	*Amplified gene*
Neuroblastoma	N-*myc*
Retinoblastoma	N-*myc*
Glial brain tumors	Epidermal growth factor (c-*erb*-B)
Breast cancer	Her 2-*neu* (*erb*-B2)
Ovarian cancer	Her 2-*Neu* (*erb*-B2)

Proto-oncogenes are normal cellular genes that become oncogenes when mutated, amplified, or overexpressed in a way that causes malignant transformation. Oncogenes produce an overexpressed or abnormally activated gene product. This protein typically has an important function in cellular proliferation or differentiation. Therefore, an abnormal *gain of function* of a proto-oncogene has occurred. An often-used analogy is that of the cell as an automobile. The proto-oncogene is the accelerator, resulting in movement of the car or growth of the cell. When the accelerator is fixed in the engaged position, the car travels uncontrollably fast, similar to the actions of an oncogene.

Tumor Suppressor Genes

In apposition to dominant-acting oncogenes is another class of genes known as tumor suppressor genes. Although oncogenes achieve their effect on cell proliferation by producing abnormal stimulatory effects, tumor suppressor genes normally inhibit abnormal cell growth and differentiation. Tumor suppressor genes contribute to tumorigenesis when they are mutated or otherwise inactivated so as to cause a *loss of function*. Using the automobile analogy, the normal tumor suppressor gene is the car's brakes. When mutated, failure or inactivation of the brakes occurs, resulting in uncontrolled cell proliferation.

The first evidence for the existence of tumor suppressor genes came from hybrid cell experiments.[14] Hybrid cells generated by fusion of malignant and normal cells lost the characteristics of the transformed cell and were unable to form tumors in nude mice. Loss of chromosomal material from these unstable hybrids, however, occasionally resulted in restoration of the malignant phenotype. This result suggested that the malignant phenotype was the result of a recessive genetic effect, and that complementation of that effect with the normal gene abolished the cancerous phenotype.

More direct evidence of the existence of tumor suppressor genes came with the observation that malignant cells often have loss of chromosomal material. Tumor cell karyotypes often show deletions of small or large regions on individual chromosomes, and sometimes even have loss of entire chromosomes or chromosomal arms. Several tumor suppressor genes have been cloned from these deleted regions. Loss of one tumor suppressor allele can result in failure to suppress abnormal growth if the other allele is inactivated by a mutation or deletion. Generally both alleles of a tumor suppressor gene need to be inactivated to result in a cancer phenotype. In some cases it may also be possible that loss of one allele results in a decrease in the normal amount of gene product required to maintain normal growth, a situation called gene dosage effect.

The classic case of a tumor suppressor gene is the retinoblastoma gene. Knudson initially postulated that the development of hereditary and sporadic types of retinoblastomas could be explained by a two-mutation model of tumorigenesis.[15] In hereditary neoplasms, the first mutation is at a germline mutation and predisposes certain cell populations to the development of neoplasia. The second mutation is a somatic mutation that transforms the predisposed cell into a tumor cell. In the sporadic form of these tumors, both mutations occur at a somatic level (Fig. 90.2). Support for this theory came with the observation that individuals with hereditary retinoblastoma often had constitutional deletions of chromosome 13q14.[16] It was then found that retinoblastoma tumors in these individuals often had deletions of the normal chromosome 13. In nonhereditary (sporadic) retinoblastomas, it was then noted that tumors often demonstrated deletions at this locus also. These observations eventually led to the cloning and characterization of the retinoblastoma gene in 1987.[17,18] This gene encodes a protein that negatively regulates entry into the cell cycle. Knockout or mutation of this gene in retinoblastomas and other tumors results in failure of the cell to arrest mitosis at appropriate times and thus contributes to uncontrolled growth.

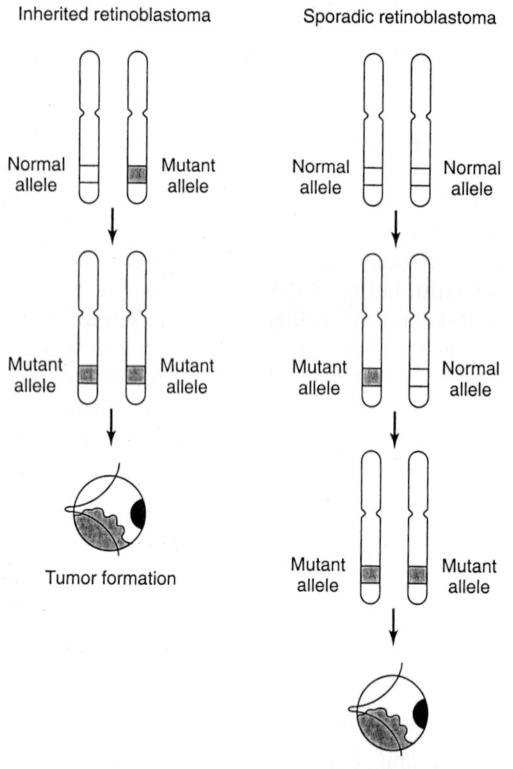

FIGURE 90.2. Proposed sequence of genetic events in formation of sporadic and hereditary retinoblastomas. *Left*: In hereditary cases, the mutant allele is inherited and is present in all cells of the body. When the normal allele becomes mutated, deleted, or rearranged, this results in the absence of functional protein product, and tumor formation ensues. *Right*: In sporadic cases, both mutations develop as separate events. This mechanism accounts for the fact that hereditary tumors have an earlier age of onset. (Reprinted with permission from Moley JF, Kim SH. Molecular Genetics in Surgical Oncology. Austin: Landes, 1994.)

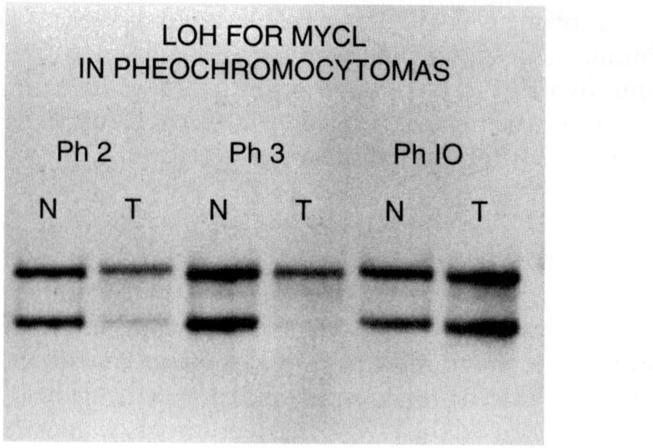

FIGURE 90.3. Loss of heterozygosity (*LOH*) in human pheochromocytomas. Autoradiogram of a Southern hybridization shows *Eco*RI-digested pheochromocytoma and normal DNA probed with a chromosome 1p gene product (MYCL). Three normal tumor pairs are shown. *N*, normal DNA obtained from patient's blood; *T*, tumor DNA. In Ph2 and Ph3, the tumor DNA lacks the lower band, which represents the smaller allele detected by the MYCL probe in the normal DNA. In Ph10 both alleles are present in the tumor. (Reprinted with permission from Moley JF, Kim SH. Molecular Genetics in Surgical Oncology. Austin: Landes, 1994.)

On a molecular level, normal cells generally exhibit a heterozygosity at different genetic markers reflecting the two different chromosomes. In tumors, deletions of chromosomal material are detected as absence of the expected pattern of bands in Southern hybridization or polymerase chain reaction (PCR) experiments (Fig. 90.3). This phenomenon, generally referred to as *loss of heterozygosity* (or LOH), is seen in many types of cancer at many chromosomal locations. LOH frequently reflects deletion of tumor suppressor gene alleles. The phenomenon of genomic instability is so widespread in human cancer cells that much of LOH is probably random and may reflect a loss of regulatory and repair mechanisms that occur as a result of the genetic abnormalities accumulated by cancer cells.

DNA Repair Systems and Cancer

A third category of molecular genetic defects that characterizes tumors is abnormal DNA repair associated with mutations in DNA repair genes. All cells have complex enzyme systems that identify and repair mistakes which occur in DNA replication. Many colorectal tumors, both hereditary and sporadic forms, have been found to have mutations in genes that encode proteins responsible for repair of short stretches of repetitive DNA. A failure in the normal DNA repair systems results in the accumulation of genetic defects in the cells. The genes responsible for the hereditary nonpolyposis coli (HNPCC) syndromes are examples of such genes.[18–21] The TP53 and ataxia telangiectasia (ATM) genes are involved in surveillance and repair of DNA damage as well. These genes are frequently mutated in human cancers, and are discussed later in this chapter.

Multistep Nature of Carcinogenesis

In the case of retinoblastoma, abnormalities of a single gene appear to result in the development of a tumor. In the more common types of cancer, such as colon, breast, lung, and head and neck, multiple genetic abnormalities are found in tumor cells, and it is likely that these cancers arise after multiple defects in different genes have occurred. Dr. Bert Vogelstein at Johns Hopkins has most elegantly described this idea in colorectal neoplasia.[22–25] He and his colleagues have described the occurrence of *RAS* gene mutations, DNA hypomethylation, and deletion of multiple tumor suppressor loci (*DCC, APC, TP53, MCC*) in colonic adenomas and carcinomas. He has postulated that these genetic insults may occur in a cumulative fashion, and that adenomas progress to carcinomas after accumulating several critical mutations or deletions. There are certainly many more defects that contribute to the development of these cancers; this applies even to the best characterized tumors. In time, it may be possible to obtain a genetic profile of tumors that will entail the testing of multiple oncogenes, tumor suppressor genes, and growth factor-receptor genes, which may enable directing therapy or determining prognosis.

Cancer Susceptibility Genetics

Because some of the tumor-causing genetic alterations can be inherited, there are a variety of syndromes that predispose individuals to develop certain types of cancer. Much of our knowledge of the genetic basis of cancer has been derived from the study of these inherited cancer syndromes, because inherited cancer syndromes are typically the result of a single mutated gene that is passed from generation to generation whereas individual tumors have acquired multiple genetic changes. Genetic mutations that are inherited from one's parents and are present in all cells of the body are germline or constitutional mutations; mutations which are acquired during an individual's lifetime and cannot be passed on to one's children are somatic mutations. Somatic mutations may be caused by radiation, chemicals, or chronic inflammation, or they may occur without any obvious triggering event. In some hereditary cancer syndromes, including Li–Fraumeni, ataxia-telangiectasia, and hereditary nonpolyposis colon cancer, the germline mutation causes a tendency for the cell to accumulate somatic mutations and DNA damage that cause malignant transformation in some cells.

A tumor that arises in an individual may be classified as either hereditary or sporadic. In hereditary cases, an inherited germline mutation is responsible for the predisposition to neoplasia, and multiple somatic alterations need also to occur to lead to tumor development. If the patient with a tumor does not have an inherited predisposition, presumably the mutations in the tumor DNA are all somatic, and then the tumor is classified as sporadic. The index case or *proband* is the individual who is first diagnosed as having the syndrome, even if earlier generations are later recognized as also having the syndrome. De novo cases of familial cancer arise when a mutation occurs in a germ cell that may be passed on to offspring.

The specific mutations responsible for hereditary and sporadic cancer often overlap. For example, familial adenomatous polyposis (FAP) is caused by a germline mutation in the adenomatous polyposis coli gene (*APC*). More than 80% of *sporadic* colorectal cancers also have a somatic mutation of this same gene; the same is true for medullary thyroid carcinoma (MTC). Germline mutations of the *RET* proto-oncogene are responsible for the predisposition to development of MTC in patients with multiple endocrine neoplasia type 2 (MEN 2). Somatic mutations of *RET* are found in approximately 50% of sporadic MTCs. Understanding inherited cancer genetic defects has provided significant insight into the mechanisms of sporadic cancers as well.

In families affected by an inherited cancer syndrome, predisposition to neoplasia is usually transmitted in an autosomal dominant manner to the next generation. When this is the case, each child has a 50% risk of inheriting the mutated gene. Any individual who inherits one of these cancer susceptibility genes from a parent has an increased risk of developing the syndrome. Not all these individuals will develop the disorder because not all these genes have complete penetrance. The penetrance of a genetic mutation is the likelihood that an individual will develop a phenotype (such as cancer) from a specific genotype. Penetrance can vary widely, ranging from close to 100% (e.g., colon cancer in FAP, and MTC in MEN 2) to less than 1% (e.g., pheochromocytomas in neurofibromatosis). Penetrance can also vary considerably for different characteristics of the same syndrome. The factors determining penetrance remain largely unknown. A few exceptions to the autosomal dominant pattern of inheritance exist. Specifically, ataxia-telangiectasia and xeroderma pigmentosum are transmitted in an autosomal recessive manner. An individual must inherit a defective gene from each parent to develop these syndromes. In these kindreds, each parent may only have one affected gene and not exhibit the syndrome, conferring to their children a 25% risk of inheriting both genes, resulting in the syndrome. Therefore, the syndrome may skip generations.

Most familial cancer syndromes are the result of a germline mutation in a tumor suppressor gene or are involved in DNA repair. Because these mutations make the gene product nonfunctional, the abnormality may be a mutation, deletion, or rearrangement anywhere in the gene. Some of these genes are quite large (e.g., BRCA2), which makes identification of a mutation in an individual or family difficult. Some mutations have even been found in noncoding regions of DNA, causing an error in splicing the final gene, and this can make identifying the specific mutation in a family more difficult. Because oncogenes develop a gain of function, generally there are only several specific areas in the gene where the mutation occurs, which typically makes finding the mutation in a family easier. Currently, there are only two known oncogenes resulting in a familial cancer syndrome, the RET gene causing MEN2 and the similar MET gene causing kidney cancer.

Basic Principles When Evaluating a Patient with a Suspected Familial Cancer Syndrome

There are several features of familial cancer syndromes that should be kept in mind when evaluating a patient with cancer. First, familial cancers tend to occur at an earlier age than sporadic cases, because one of the mutations needed for

TABLE 90.4. Characteristics of Familial Cancer Syndromes.

Early age of cancer (under 50)
Similar cancers occur in several family members
Multifocal or bilateral cancers
Multiple cancers (especially rare) diagnosed in multiple family members
More than one cancer occurs in an individual

neoplastic transformation is already present as a germline mutation. Second, close relatives are usually affected by the same type of cancer, often in several generations. Third, inherited cancers are often multifocal or bilateral. Last, familial cancer syndromes may not be limited to a specific type of cancer, but can involve a variety of cancers. The Li–Fraumeni syndrome can give rise to breast cancer, sarcomas, brain tumors, adrenocortical carcinomas, and others. If one finds any of these trends in a patient and their family, one should suspect a familial cancer syndrome (Table 90.4).

All patients with cancer should be questioned about family history of malignancy and other medical conditions. If an inherited cancer is suspected, then a family pedigree should be created (Fig. 90.4). Circles are drawn for all females and boxes for all males in rows by generation. All married couples are joined by a horizontal line. Their offspring are all connected to this line. Affected individuals are represented by a completely or partially filled circle or box, often with the type of cancer and their age of diagnosis written next to them. All deceased individuals are represented by a diagonal slash through their symbol. Once a pedigree is established, at-risk individuals can be identified and appropriate counseling and testing can be done.

Chromosomal alterations, which can give rise to associated conditions such as physical deformities and mental retardation, may be associated with cancer. The loss or addition of specific chromosomes can provide important clues to the location of the gene responsible for a syndrome. A karyotype of the individual may be helpful in locating the defective gene. The initial clue that the *APC* gene resides on chromosome 5 was the karyotype of an institutionalized patient with polyposis, mental retardation, and congenital abnormalities. The karyotype revealed an interstitial deletion on the long arm of chromosome 5,[26] which led to the positional cloning of the *APC* gene.

Genetic Testing and Counseling

Genetic testing should be considered when a patient presents with a suspected familial malignancy. The American Society of Clinical Oncology (ASCO) recommends that a genetic test be offered when a family history is suggestive of an inherited cancer syndrome, if the test can be adequately interpreted, and if the results will aid future management of the individual or their family.[27] If a germline mutation is found, this patient will need close surveillance and possible prophylactic surgery or chemotherapy. Testing and surveillance of family members and especially children of affected individuals should be recommended. In those found not to have inherited a mutation in the setting of a known kindred mutation, the emotional stress and financial costs of surveillance can be lessened. Conversely, a positive result will necessitate the need for lifelong testing and intervention; therefore, all outcomes must be thoroughly discussed beforehand. Comprehensive pre- and posttest counseling should be provided.

The involvement of trained genetic health professionals is an important complement to the nurses and surgeons who discuss therapeutic options with family members. More than 30% of physicians misinterpreted the test results of a commercial APC gene test in a study evaluating its use.[26] Genetic health professionals include medical geneticists (M.D.s or Ph.D.s who are board certified by the American Board of Medical Genetics), genetic counselors (masters degree trained who are board certified by the American Board of Genetic Counselors), and oncology nurses specializing in genetics. A cancer genetic services directory can be found on the NCI website (www.cancer.gov/search/genetics_services/). Genetic professionals are trained in the communication skills necessary for transmitting complicated information to family members. They are primarily involved in explaining test results and therapeutic options available in a nonbiased way. Patients consider them a valuable resource for obtaining information and understanding these complex issues. Proper pretesting counseling cannot be overemphasized.

A comprehensive searchable database of genetic tests and which laboratories perform them can be found at the Gene Tests website (www.genetests.org). Gene Tests is a free, National Institutes of Health (NIH)-funded resource containing detailed information on more than 1000 inherited diseases that is easily searchable by cancer type. Also provided is a genetics clinic directory. Another valuable resource is the Online Mendelian Inheritance in Man (OMIM) website (www.ncbi.nlm.nih.gov/entrez/query.fcgi?db=OMIM) within the National Center for Biotechnology Information. Searching

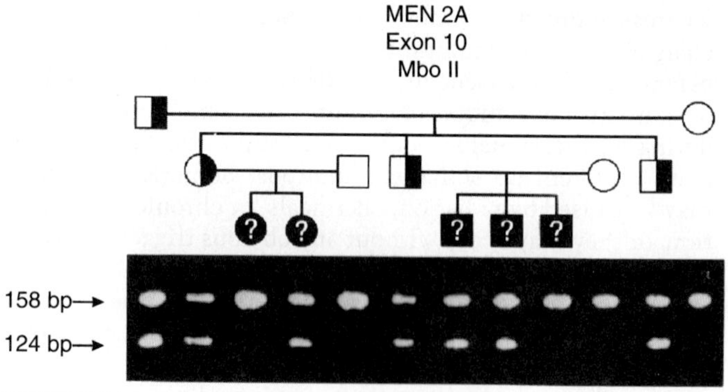

FIGURE 90.4. *Top*: Pedigree of kindred affected by MEN-2A (*circles*, females; *squares*, males; *shaded right hemicircle*, affected by medullary thyroid carcinoma). *Bottom*: Restriction digest patterns for the 12 family members shown in pedigree. The portion of the RET gene that is mutated in this family was amplified by polymerase chain reaction and then cut with a restriction enzyme that gives a different cleavage pattern for normal and mutant alleles. The normal allele contains one restriction site producing a fragment of 158 bp, whereas the mutant 158-bp fragment is cleaved into fragments of 124 and 61 bp (only the 158- and 124-bp fragments are resolved in the picture). bp, fragment size in base pairs; DNA size standard (1-kb ladder). Four individuals with clinical signs of MEN-2A demonstrate the mutant RET digestion pattern. Three of the third-generation presymptomatic at-risk individuals have inherited the mutant allele (female with question mark on right, and left and middle males with question marks). (Reprinted with permission from Chi D, Toshima K, Donis-Keller H, Wells SA Jr. Predictive testing for multiple endocrine neoplasia type 2A: based on the detection of mutations in the RET proto-oncogene. Surgery (St. Louis) 1994;116:128.)

their database with different terms describing a possible syndrome, such as breast cancer and trichilemmomas, produces possible responsible syndromes and genes, such as Cowden syndrome caused by PTEN mutations. Because inherited cancer syndromes are a rapidly changing field, these websites provides an essential up-to-date reference on the topic.

Specific Cancer Syndromes

For a list of cloned genes for familial cancer syndromes, see Table 90.5. For a table of the syndromes with their associated cancers, see Table 90.6.

TABLE 90.5. Cloned Genes of Familial Cancer Syndromes.

Syndrome	*Tumor*	*Associated tumors and traits*	*Gene*	*Chromosome*
Familial adenomatous polyposis	Colorectal cancer	Colonic polyposis, CHRPE, desmoids, osteomas, upper GI cancer	APC MYH	5q21 1p31.1–34.3
Hereditary nonpolyposis colon cancer	Colorectal cancer	Endometrial and ovarian cancer	MLH1, MSH2, MSH6, PMS2	3p21, 2p22, 2q16, 7p22
Muir–Torre	Colorectal cancer	Sebaceous gland tumor	MSH2, MLH1	3p21. 2p22
Puetz–Jeghers	Colorectal cancer	Polyposis, GI, lung, breast, ovary, endometrial, pancreatic cancer	STK11 (LKB1)	19p13.3
Juvenile polyposis	Colorectal cancer	Hamartomatous and adenomatous polyps, vascular anomalies	MADH4 BMPR1A	18q21 10q22.3
Hereditary early-onset breast cancer	Breast cancer	Ovarian cancer	BRCA1, BRCA2	17q21.1, 13q12–13
Li–Fraumeni syndrome	Sarcoma, breast	Pediatric malignancies	p53	17p13
Cowden's disease	Breast cancer	Facial lesions	PTEN	10q23
Ataxia-telangiectasia	Leukemia, lymphoma, breast cancer	Cerebellar ataxia, telangiectasias	ATM	11q22–23
MEN 1	Pancreatic islet cell	Parathyroid hyperplasia, pituitary adenoma	MENIN	11q13
MEN 2A	Medullary thyroid cancer	Pheochromocytoma, parathyroid hyperplasia	RET	10q11.2
MEN 2B	Medullary thyroid cancer	Pheochromocytoma, ganglioneuromatosis, marfanoid habitus	RET	10q11.2
Familial medullary thyroid cancer	Medullary thyroid cancer		RET	10q11.2
Paraganglioma	Pheochromocytoma	Paraganglioma	SDHB, SDHC SDHD	1p36.1, 1q21, 11q23
Hyperparathyroidism-Jaw tumor	Parathyroid cancer	Hyperparathyroidism, jaw tumors	HRPT2	1q25
Carney complex	Endocrine tumors	Lentiginoses, myxomas	PRKAR1A	17q23
Diffuse gastric cancer	Gastric cancer	Breast cancer	E-cadherin	16q22.1
Werner	Sarcoma	Premature aging, DM, MI	WRN	8p12
Neurofibromatosis type I	Neurofibrosarcomas	Neurofibromas, cafe au lait spots, Lisch nodules	NF1	17q11.2
Neurofibromatosis type II	Neurofibrosarcomas	Neurofibromas, bilateral vestibular schwannomas	Merlin	22q12
Familial retinoblastoma	Retinoblastoma	Development retardation, osteosarcomas	Rb	13q14
Familial atypical multiple-mole syndrome	Melanoma	Atypical melanocytic nevi, pancreatic cancer	CDKN2, CDK4	9p21 12q14
Wilms' tumor syndrome	Wilms' tumor	WAGR, Denys–Drash syndrome	WT1	11p13
Von Hippel–Lindau	Hemangioblastoma, renal cancer	Multiple cysts, pheochromocytomas	VHL	3p25
Birt-Hogg-Dubé	Renal cancer	Cutaneous nodules, pulmonary cysts	BHD	17p11.2
Leiomyomatosis renal cell	Papillary renal cancer	Leiomyomatosis	Fumarate hydratase	1q42.1
Hereditary papillary renal carcinoma	Papillary renal cancer		MET	7q31–34
Hereditary pancreatitis	Pancreatic cancer	Pancreatitis	PRSS1 SPINK1	7q34 5q32

TABLE 90.6. Familial Cancer Syndromes and Associated Cancers and Traits.

	Cancer or characteristic																																						
Syndrome	Adrenal tumors	Biliary tumors	Breast (female)	Breast (male)	Carcinoid	Cervix	CNS tumors	Colon/rectum	Endolymphatic sac tumor	Endometrium	Esophogus	Hepatocellular	Gastric	Genitourinary	Leukemia	Lentiginoses	Lung	Lymphoma	Melanoma	Neuroblastoma	Osteosarcoma	Ovarian	Pancreas (endocrine)	Pancreas (exocrine)	Parathyroid	Peripheral Nerve Sheath	Pheochromocytoma	Pituitary	Prostate	Renal cell (clear)	Renal cell (papillary)	Retinoblastoma	Schwannoma	Small bowel/duodenal	Soft tissue sarcoma	Testicular	Thyroid (non-medullary)	Thyroid (medullary)	Wilms' tumor
Ataxia-telangiectasia			X				X			X			X	X	X			X				X		X						X									
Birt-Hogg-Dubé																																							
Breast-ovarian (BRCA1)			X					X					X						X			X							X										
Breast-ovarian (BRCA2)			X	X				X					X						X			X		X					X										
Carney complex	X															X												X					X			X	X		
Colon (FAP)									X				X																					X			X		
Colon (HNPCC)		X	X				X	X		X		X	X	X								X		X						X				X			X		
Cowden syndrome			X							X																													
Diffuse gastric cancer			X										X																										
Juvenile polyposis								X																															
Li–Fraumeni	X		X				X						X		X		X	X	X		X	X		X					X						X	X			X
Leiomyomatosis renal																															X				X				
Melanoma (FAMMM)																X			X					X															
MEN 1	X				X																		X		X		X	X											
MEN 2A																									X		X											X	
MEN 2B																											X											X	
Muir–Torre								X						X																									
NF1					X		X								X					X						X	X						X						X
NF2							X																			X							X						
Pancreatitis syndrome																								X															
Paraganglioma																												X											
Parathyroid (HPJT)																										X													X
Peutz–Jeghers			X			X		X		X	X		X			X	X					X		X										X		X			
Renal cancer (papillary)																															X								
Retinoblastoma															X			X	X		X											X			X				
von Hippel–Lindau					X		X		X														X				X			X									
Werner																			X		X														X		X		
Wilms' tumor	X																			X															X				X

Colorectal Cancer

About 150,000 new cases of colorectal cancer are diagnosed annually in the United States. Familial cancers may account for as many as 15% of these cases.[28] Although there are several rare hereditary syndromes associated with colorectal cancer, most known hereditary colorectal cancer can be divided into two main categories, familial adenomatous polyposis (FAP) and hereditary nonpolyposis colorectal cancer (HNPCC). Historically, FAP has received the greatest amount of attention, as it is characterized by an obvious phenotype, florid colonic polyposis, and its inherited nature was appreciated by 1900. During the explosion of molecular genetics, the research community has used this disease as a paradigm for familial cancer, leading to the identification of the responsible gene, adenomatous polyposis coli gene (*APC*). More recently, HNPCC, lacking a striking precancerous phenotype, has gained recognition as the more prevalent form.

Although 5% of colorectal cancer has been ascribed to defined inherited syndromes, another 10% of colorectal cancer appears to have a hereditary component. The genes or factors responsible for these cases are unknown. One explanation is that certain mutations in cancer-related genes which initially appear harmless actually make the region more likely to be mutated. The inherited mutation does not alter the function of the gene but makes further mutations more common during DNA replication. Volgelstein et al. reported one such mutation in the APC gene in Ashkenazi Jews that doubled an individual's risk for colorectal cancer.[29]

Familial Polyposis Syndrome

Familial adenomatous polyposis (FAP) is typically an autosomal dominant inherited disease caused by mutations in the tumor suppressor gene, APC. The penetrance is extremely high, with more than 90% of affected individuals developing colorectal cancer if not treated. Carriers typically develop adenomatous polyps that progress to carpet the large intestine during the second or third decades of life. The polyps are histologically indistinguishable from sporadic polyps, and individually these polyps do not have a greater propensity to undergo malignant transformation than sporadic polyps. Because of the enormous number of polyps (typically hundreds to thousands) and the early age at which the polyps develop, the risk that one of these will undergo further genetic changes to progress to malignancy is close to 100%. The median age of cancer diagnosis for untreated individuals is 39 years, almost 30 years earlier than the median age for sporadic colorectal cancer. Affected individuals are also prone to develop duodenal, gastric, and ileal polyps, and are at risk for developing duodenal, stomach, periampullary, thyroid, and other cancers.

The *APC* gene was positionally cloned in 1991[30,31] after cytogenetic analysis of a patient with congenital abnormalities and intestinal polyposis suggested that the gene was on the long arm of chromosome 5 (5q).[26] The gene encodes a 300-kDa protein expressed in a variety of cell types and appears to have a variety of functions. The protein interacts with β-catenin, likely playing a role in WNT signaling pathway and possibly cell adhesion. A mouse model has been developed in which the mice carry a germline mutation in the mouse homologue of the *APC* gene and develop multiple intestinal neoplasia (*MIN*).

Germline mutations of the *APC* gene have been found in many FAP kindreds. Somatic mutations in the APC gene also occur in more than 80% of sporadic cases of colorectal cancer as well as sporadic adenomas. These mutations have been found in early adenomas, suggesting these mutations are one of the early genetic events in the development of colonic malignancy.

The complex relationship between genotype and phenotype is becoming more clear.[32] The location of a mutation within the gene can produce different phenotypes. Congenital hypertrophy of the retinal pigment epithelium (CHRPE), which was once thought to be a signature of the disease, is associated with mutations between codons 463 and 1387. There are several phenotypic variations of FAP that were once thought to be distinct syndromes but are probably a family of disorders related to the *APC* gene. Gardner syndrome, associated with mutations in codons 1403 to 1578, is characterized by desmoid tumors (especially of the abdominal wall and mesentery), osteomas of the mandible or skull, and sebaceous cysts. Turcot's syndrome is associated with malignant central nervous system tumors, gastrointestinal polyposis, and colorectal cancer.

Attenuated FAP occurs in patients who have a relatively sparse number of polyps, 5 to 300. These patients generally develop polyps and cancer at a later age but still are at increased risk of colorectal cancer. Polyps tend to be more proximal in the colon than in classic FAP, necessitating surveillance via colonoscopy rather than sigmoidoscopy. Mutations in both ends of the APC gene have been identified in these individuals. Other genes that modify or regulate the *APC* gene may also cause similar phenotypes. Two *MIN* mice can have a significant variation in the number of gastrointestinal polyps, even though they possess the same mutation in the mouse *APC* homologue gene. Apparently this variation of polyp number is caused by a gene on a different chromosome, *MOM*1 (modifier of *MIN*), which affects the mouse *APC* homologue.

Recently another gene, MYH, has been found to cause an autosomal recessive form of FAP. Germline mutations were found in both alleles of the MYH gene in affected individuals.[33] When there is not a clear generational, vertical transmission of FAP, MYH mutations should be considered. Individuals must inherit a mutated gene from each parent, who themselves may not exhibit the syndrome. Although the MYH phenotype has not clearly been defined, these patients tend to have fewer polyps and develop cancer at a later age. MYH gene function is involved in DNA base excision repair.

Screening and Diagnosis

Because of the high penetrance and the early age at which tumors develop, close surveillance is essential. For children of an affected individual, the colon should be examined via flexible sigmoidoscopy beginning in their preteenage years. After a baseline procedure, sigmoidoscopy should be done annually.

Currently there are about 10 centers in North America that perform analysis for the *APC* gene, via direct sequencing, linkage analysis, or protein truncation. In addition to the at-risk individual, linkage testing requires other affected and unaffected individuals within the kindred. More than 80% of the mutations result in a truncated protein product. A protein truncation assay has been developed that is quicker and cheaper, but should only be used on family members, once a truncation mutation is confirmed in the proband.

Genetic testing may eliminate some of the emotional stress and financial cost of surveillance, if the patient or at-risk family member is found not to have inherited a mutation in the setting of a known mutation in the family. Two to three sigmoidoscopies should still be done to guard against a false-negative result. Genetic testing is also appropriate when a patient presents with a large number of intestinal polyps, with or without the presence of colorectal cancer. If a mutation in the *APC* gene is found, they will need lifelong surveillance of their upper gastrointestinal tract for a second malignancy and genetic counseling of family members.

Surgical Management

The primary treatment for FAP is surgical. Surgery should be done when florid polyposis is detected, usually in the late teen years or early twenties. There are three main surgical options: a total proctocolectomy with an ileal pouch–anal anastomosis, a colectomy with an ileorectal anastomosis, or a proctocolectomy with ileostomy. Proctocolectomy with ileostomy is almost never done as a first operation. By leaving rectal mucosa after an ileorectal anastomosis, there is still a significant risk for developing rectal cancer. Close surveillance of this mucosa is necessary. Iwama and Mishima found the risk for rectal carcinoma after ileorectal anastomosis to be 24% at 15 years for 322 patients who underwent rectum-preserving surgery.[34] Two factors were found to correlate with an increased risk of rectal cancer: length of the rectal stump greater than 7cm and a high rectal polyp density. Ambroze et al. reported the rates to be 13% at 25 years from St. Marks Hospital, 12% at 20 years from the Cleveland Clinic, and 20% at 20 years from the Mayo Clinic.[35] Generally, rectal screening should be done every 6 months and possibly more frequently, especially after the age of 45.

Total proctocolectomy with ileal pouch–anal anastomosis also has disadvantages: sphincter dysfunction, greater morbidity, including loss of sexual function in men, and more technically challenging surgery. Because many FAP patients are asymptomatic at the time of surgery, these patients may not tolerate the functional problems of an ileal pouch as well as patients who undergo this surgery for ulcerative colitis. Endoscopic evaluation of the pouch is recommended every 2 years. Multiple factors should be considered when deciding the appropriate surgical procedure, including extent of rectal disease, location of any cancer, sphincter function, extracolonic disease, surgeon experience, and patient follow-up.

After the colorectal cancer risk, the greatest risk of mortality is from upper gastrointestinal cancer, primarily periampullary, duodenal, and stomach tumors. Jejunal and ileal cancers are rare. Upper endoscopic surveillance is strongly recommended for these individuals. Generally duodenal polyposis progresses slowly, but the natural history is not well understood.[36,37] Upper endoscopy is recommended every 3 years beginning at age 25. Polypectomy, if possible, is thought to be adequate treatment for most polyps, followed by annual screening. Currently, prophylactic resection is not recommended.

Desmoids appear as a phenotypic characteristic in 10% to 20% of FAP patients. Although not malignant, they can be locally aggressive and a significant cause of morbidity. Desmoids often arise in surgical scars or in the small bowel mesentery after abdominal surgery. Diffuse fibrosis may lead to ureteral, vascular, or gastrointestinal obstruction. Further surgical resection may not be possible, and after initial success, desmoids often recur. Rodriguez-Bigas et al. found only 9 of 21 patients who underwent surgery for desmoids were potentially cured, and 7 of these 9 had a recurrence at a median of 61 months postoperatively.[38] Overall, only 2 of 21 were thought to have a long-term cure. Desmoids may also prevent an ileorectal anastomosis from being converted to a restorative proctectomy. Radiation, sulindac, tamoxifen, and cytotoxic chemotherapy have been used to treat desmoids with varying success. According to the American Society of Colon and Rectal Surgeons guidelines, desmoids in the small bowel mesentery should be treated based on their growth rate and clinical presentation. Aggressive therapy with high-dose tamoxifen or chemotherapy is reserved for rapidly growing tumors.[39]

Hereditary Nonpolyposis Colorectal Cancer Syndrome

Hereditary nonpolyposis colorectal cancer syndrome (HNPCC), also known as Lynch syndrome I and II, is an autosomal dominant disease caused by mutations in one of at least four DNA mismatch repair genes. When Lynch initially described this syndrome, he divided kindreds into those having only colorectal cancer (Lynch syndrome I) and those who also had extracolonic cancers (Lynch syndrome II), which is the more common form. The colorectal cancer penetrance is around 80%, with a mean age at diagnosis of about 45 years. As in sporadic and FAP colorectal cancer cases, these patients still develop cancer through the progression of adenomatous polyps to frank malignancy, but lack the diffuse colonic polyposis seen in FAP. The incidence of polyps is believed to be equal to that seen in individuals who develop sporadic colorectal cancer, but once a polyp develops there appears to be an increased rate of tumor progression. In contrast to sporadic tumors, about 10% of HNPCC patients develop a colorectal cancer within 5 years after colonoscopy or colon resection, with the median age of cancer development being 44 years.[40]

HNPCC was initially defined based on its clinical manifestations, termed the Amsterdam criteria. These criteria consist of (1) a family with at least three relatives having proven colorectal cancer and one individual being a primary relative of the other two, (2) at least two generations being affected, and (3) one individual being diagnosed before age 50. Broader sets of criteria include the Bethesda and Modified Bethesda criteria, which may more accurately define the syndrome. There are several other clinical characteristics of these cancers. The lesions have a right-sided colon predominance (70% proximal to the splenic flexure). There is an excess of synchronous and metachronous colorectal cancers. Anecdotal reports suggest that these patients do better, stage for stage, than their sporadic counterparts. Extracolonic malignancies are also seen, especially endometrial and ovarian cancer. The lifetime risk of endometrial cancer is 30% to 60% and that of ovarian cancer 10% to 13%. Other associated cancers include stomach, small bowel, pancreas, urological tract, bladder, biliary tract, and possibly larynx and breast cancer.

The process that led to the discovery of the responsible genes was aided both by linkage analysis in affected families and by microbiologists studying mutations in bacteria and yeast. Tumor DNA of affected patients were found to have widespread instability in short repeat sequences, termed microsatellite instability, detected as extra bands on PCR-amplified short repetitive segments of DNA. Similar DNA instability is seen in bacteria and yeast that have induced mutations in their DNA mismatch repair genes: this led to the identification of mutations in the human versions of the same genes, *MSH2*, *MLH1*, *MSH6*, and *PMS2* in families with hereditary colorectal cancer.[41] Currently, *MSH2* and *MLH1* are estimated to account for greater than 80% of HNPCC, and *MSH6* and *PMS2* cause less than 15% of cases. When the normal corresponding allele to one of these mismatch repair genes is mutated, the cell cannot repair mistakes made by DNA polymerase during DNA replication, leading to genome-wide mutations. The mutation rate in tumors of these patients has been shown to be two to three times higher than in normal cells.[32] Consequently, mutations in proto-oncogenes and tumor suppressor genes occur much more frequently, leading to cancer.

HNPCC accounts for about 5% of all colorectal cancers. Microsatellite instability is seen in 10% to 15% of sporadic tumors. These sporadic tumors also occur predominantly in the proximal colon.[42] Some, but not all, have somatic mutations in the genes that cause HNPCC. There is an inverse relationship between microsatellite instability and aneuploidy, suggesting that one of these two forms of instability is found in all colorectal cancer.[43]

Screening and Treatment

Currently, genetic testing for *MSH2* and *MLH1* is only done at several centers. Microsatellite instability is sometimes used as the initial screening test on a tumor suspected to be a hereditary tumor. Microsatellite instability testing is generally simpler to perform than sequencing the entire mismatch repair genes. For individuals known to carry a germline mutation or strongly suspected to have one, the Cancer Genetics Study Consortium suggests screening with colonoscopy every 1 to 3 years beginning between the ages of 20 and 25 years.[44] Women carriers should undergo endometrial aspiration curettage annually beginning at age 30. Surveillance for ovarian cancer is limited, but transvaginal ultrasound and CA-125 should be considered.

Treatment for HNPCC kindreds has not been well defined. If a germline mutation is found in an individual, then prophylactic surgery should be considered. The same general surgical principles of treatment exist as for FAP, but a colectomy with an ileorectal anastomosis may be a more reasonable alternative because these tumors have a proximal predilection. Alternatively, nonoperative management with screening colonoscopy every 1 to 2 years in known gene carriers is a reasonable option. At this point there have been no significant clinical trials examining the various treatment options. Prophylactic total abdominal hysterectomy and bilateral salpingo-oophorectomy could be considered for women who have completed their families. Carriers need to be forewarned that removal of both ovaries, even if they appear histologically normal, does not completely eliminate the risk of ovarian cancer.

Muir–Torre Syndrome

Muir–Torre syndrome (MTS) is a rare autosomal dominant disorder characterized by the presence of at least one sebaceous gland tumor and a visceral cancer and is sometimes considered a variant of HNPCC. The sebaceous gland tumors often appear as yellow facial papules and are considered a hallmark of this syndrome. The most common internal malignancy is colorectal cancer, but other tumors occur, especially genitourinary. The clinical similarities with HNPCC include an inherited susceptibility to colorectal cancer at an early age. Both have a tendency to form proximal colon cancers, and patients tend to have better survival than with sporadic cancers. Recently, genetic similarities have strengthened this association. Microsatellite instability is found in the sebaceous tumors and other malignancies in about half the affected individuals.[45] Germline mutations have been found in both the *MSH2* and *MLH1* genes in different kindreds.[46]

Peutz–Jeghers Syndrome

Peutz–Jeghers syndrome is a rare autosomal dominant disease, characterized by gastrointestinal polyposis and mucocutaneous pigmentations. The pigmentations are melanin deposits that can occur on and around the lips, oral mucosa, hands, feet, perianal region, and umbilical area, usually appearing in childhood. Those on the skin may fade, but generally not those of the mucous membranes. The gastrointestinal polyps are hamartomas with a prominent smooth muscle component derived from the muscularis mucosa. These polyps are distinctly different from those seen in FAP and HNPCC. Their malignant potential is uncertain, but it is likely that carcinomas arise from coexisting adenomatous polyps. Hamartomas can be found anywhere along the gastrointestinal tract, but are more frequent in the small bowel and are usually multiple. Obstruction, intussusception, and bleeding are the most common manifestations.

Individuals have an overall increased lifetime relative risk of cancer between 9 and 15. Malignancies of the gastrointestinal tract occur with increased frequency, including colon, stomach, esophageal, pancreatic, and small bowel cancer. There also is an increased risk of extragastrointestinal malignancies including lung, breast, ovary, and endometrial.[47] Spigelman et al. found the mortality from any cancer by age 57 was 50%.[48]

Mutations in the serine/threonine-kinase 11 gene (STK11; also called LKB1) have been identified in many kindreds. The protein is involved in cell polarity and inhibition of mTOR, which controls vascular endothelial growth factor (VEGF) and hypoxia-inducible factor (HIF).[49] Genetic testing is available in a few centers through sequencing the gene. Individuals should have a baseline upper endoscopy and colonoscopy around age 20 with frequent surveillance thereafter. Some authors have advocated a subtotal colectomy if the polyps are too numerous to follow.

Juvenile Polyposis

Juvenile polyposis is another rare autosomal dominant disease characterized not by adenomatous polyps but by juvenile polyps. Typically, juvenile polyps are found as solitary lesions in children with no known malignant potential and not associated with a familial syndrome. Histologically, juvenile polyps consists of stromal elements overlaid with normal epithelium. In the polyposis syndrome, the polyps usually number 50 to 200, and primarily occur in the colon and rectum, but can be found in the stomach and duodenum. The polyps may be "atypical," containing epithelial dysplasia, or "mixed," containing regions that resemble an adenoma. Individuals usually present with diarrhea during childhood or rectal bleeding during the second decade. Associated congenital abnormalities include cerebral and pulmonary arteriovenous malformations, cardiac anomalies, polydactyly, malrotation, and cranial malformations. Germline mutations in the MADH4 (formerly called *SMAD* 4) gene have been reported in about 20% of juvenile polyposis families.[50] Mutations in BMPR1A have also been identified in about 20% of kindreds. The gene product of both genes is involved in the transforming growth factor-beta (TGF-β) signaling pathway. Sequence analysis of both genes is available at a few centers.

The lifetime risk for developing colorectal cancer is estimated to be 10% to 50%, usually at an early age. Patients need frequent colonoscopies to remove polyps. If not all the polyps can be removed, then a colectomy should be performed, either a subtotal colectomy with ileorectal anastomosis or a total proctocolectomy with an ileal pouch–anal anastomosis. Periodic surveillance of the ileal pouch is necessary because polyps may arise in the ileal pouch.

Breast Cancer

Breast cancer is one of the most common cancers treated by the general surgeon. For more than 100 years, it has been recognized that certain families have a very high incidence of breast and ovarian cancer. About 5% to 10% of breast cancers demonstrate an autosomal dominant inheritance pattern, accounting for 9,000 to 18,000 cases per year in the United States.[51] For all inherited forms of breast cancer, family histories need to include the paternal as well as the maternal side, as defective genes can be passed on from either parent.

BRCA1 and BRCA2

The cloning of the *BRCA*1 and *BRCA*2 genes has provided a great deal of insight into these familial cancer syndromes but has also raised difficult screening, treatment, and ethical issues. Hereditary early-onset breast cancer was initially linked to the long arm of chromosome 17 (17q 12–21) by King in 1990. Four years later, after an intense international search, the *BRCA*1 gene was positionally cloned by Skolnick using the family pedigrees of the Mormon community.[52] Just over a year later, a second hereditary early-onset breast cancer gene was identified on chromosome 13, *BRCA*2.[53] The highly publicized discovery of these genes has created great expectations from the general public and the medical community of being able to control these relatively prevalent diseases, but certain characteristics of these genes have made this difficult. *BRCA*1 is a large gene spanning about 100,000 nucleic acids, and BRCA2 is even larger. More than 1,500 different site mutations have been found spread across both genes, which makes identifying a mutation, as well as determining the significance of a mutation, an arduous task. To detect a new mutation in an individual whose family has not been studied, the entire gene needs to be examined, not just a specific region of a gene. Finally, there is no functional assay of the *BRCA* gene products, which could provide the quickest method to screen for abnormalities. The gene products are involved with maintaining chromosomal stability and the transcriptional regulation of other genes important in DNA repair, cell cycle, and apoptosis.[54] For a physician and patient to make an informed decision regarding management of *BRCA* mutations, the lifetime risk of developing cancer needs to be known. Current estimates have been largely based on genetic linkage analysis of large families with multiple members with breast or ovarian cancer or both. Assessment of risk based on these families may overestimate the risk for other families. Penetrance may depend on the specific *BRCA* mutation, other related genes, or environmental factors. Initial estimates reported that a *BRCA*1 mutation confers an 87% lifetime risk of developing breast cancer, as opposed to a 12% risk for the general public.[55] The lifetime risk for carriers of *BRCA*2 mutations has been estimated to be 80%. On the other hand, a study from the National Cancer Institute of specific *BRCA*1 and *BRCA*2 mutations in the Ashkenazi Jewish population found the risk at age 70 to be only 56%.[56] These differences may influence physician and patient decisions about prevention. Clearly, more broad-based studies need to be done to determine the actual risks for specific mutations.

Carriers of *BRCA* mutations are also at higher risk for other cancers, especially ovarian cancer. The estimates of the lifetime risk of ovarian cancer in a patient with a *BRCA*1 mutation have ranged from 16% to 84% with a generally accepted rate of 40% to 60%.[53] About 5% of all ovarian cancers are believed to arise from *BRCA*1 germline mutations. For *BRCA*2 mutation carriers, the risk of ovarian cancer is believed to be much lower than for *BRCA*1, closer to 15% to 20%. Prostate and pancreatic cancer appears to be more common in these kindreds, and a few studies have found colon and stomach cancer to be more prevalent. BRCA2 mutation carriers have an increased risk of melanoma (skin and ocular). Men who are carriers for *BRCA*2 mutations have a significantly higher risk themselves of breast cancer (about 7%), whereas for male BCRA1 carriers there is a slight increased risk.[57]

Mutations in the *BRCA*1 gene are generally believed to account for 45% of hereditary early-onset breast cancer and 5% of all breast cancers. These estimates again are based on large families with multiple members. A study based on all women (not only early-onset) with a family history of breast cancer found the rate of *BRCA*1 mutations to be only 16% for patients who had breast cancer with a positive family history.[58] BRCA2 mutations are estimated to be responsible for 70% of the remaining cases of familial breast cancers. The accuracy of these numbers is important for counseling a family who has a negative genetic analysis for the *BRCA* genes.

Diagnosis and Screening

BRCA1 and -2 mutations should be suspected when an individual has one or more of the following: breast cancer before age 40, bilateral breast cancer, breast and ovarian cancer, a family history of at least two family members with breast cancer before age 50, a family history of breast and ovarian cancer, and a family history of male breast cancer. There are

TABLE 90.7. Consensus Statement for Screening Recommendations for BRCA Mutation Carriers.

Screening Test	*Beginning age*	*Interval*
Self breast exam	18–21 years	Monthly
Clinical breast exam	25–35 years	6–12 months
Mammogram	25–35 years	6–12 months
Transvaginal ultrasound	25–35 years	6–12 months
CA-125	25–35 years	6–12 months

Source: From Burke W, Petersen G, Lunch P, et al.,[44] by permission of JAMA.

several models used to predict the likelihood of a BRCA1 or -2 mutation. Each model has strengths and limitation, with the Frank and BRCAPRO models most widely used. Genetic analysis for mutations in the *BRCA1* and *BRCA2* genes is commercially available. Unless a mutation is already known in a patient's family, a method that sequences the entire gene is preferable. These tests should only be used for patients at risk for having a mutation, and not as a screening test for the general population. Genetic counseling is essential before any test is administered and should also be given with the test results. Because of the nature of these genes, genetic testing may identify a mutation of unknown significance, which the physician needs to be prepared to explain to the patient.

Treatment for carriers of BRCA mutations has not been well studied or defined. The NIH consensus panel screening recommendations are given in Table 90.7. The panel also recommended that prophylactic bilateral mastectomies and oopherctomies be offered and decided on an individual basis. A decision analysis study based on a lifetime risk of breast cancer ranging from 40% to 85% found prophylactic bilateral mastectomies increased life expectancy 2.9 to 5.3 years for a 30-year-old woman but only 0.2 to 0.5 years for a 60-year-old woman.[59] A study of more than 600 women with a family history of breast cancer found a reduction of breast cancer by 90% after bilateral prophylatic mastectomies.[60] After mastectomy, the subsequent risk of cancer is not zero, because a small amount of breast tissue is invariably left behind. If mastectomies are performed, it is critical that the patient continues to have close follow-up of her remaining breast tissue.

Although *BRCA1* and *BRCA2* comprise most of the inherited breast cancer cases, there are some other important syndromes that the clinician should consider when treating a patient with familial breast cancer.

Li–Fraumeni Syndrome

Li–Fraumeni syndrome (LFS) is a rare autosomal dominant disease, also known as SBLA syndrome (sarcoma, breast cancer, leukemia, and adrenocortical cancer). It is characterized by an inherited predisposition to at least five childhood cancers—soft tissue sarcomas, osteosarcomas, leukemias, brain tumors, and adrenocortical carcinomas—and breast cancer. Other tumors have been reported in these patients, including germ cell tumors, neuroblastoma, melanoma, Wilms' tumor, and carcinoma of the lung, prostate, stomach, and pancreas. Breast cancer is the most common cancer seen in LFS, and almost 90% of carriers develop it by age 50 in classic kindreds.[51] Because the syndrome is rare, LFS accounts for less than 1% of all breast cancers. The penetrance for any invasive cancer is approximately 50% by age 30. Patients appear to have an increased sensitivity to radiation as second primaries are prone to develop in the bed of an irradiated field.

Germline mutations in the TP53 tumor suppressor gene were identified in five LFS kindreds in 1990, and since then about 50% of LFS families have been found to have germline mutations in this gene.[61] There are also a significant number of LFS kindreds who do not have TP53 germline mutation, suggesting genetic heterogeneity. One possibility is that genes involved in regulation of TP53 may be mutated. Another study found germline TP53 mutations in a family without classic LFS characteristics, having a high rate of gastric cancer instead. Nonetheless, when a germline TP53 mutation is discovered in a kindred, genetic testing can identify carriers.

The TP53 gene is considered to be the most commonly mutated gene in all cancer. The protein product of the TP53 gene, p53, appears to function as a transcription factor. The product likely has a role in preventing DNA synthesis when damage has occurred to the cell's DNA. The types of germline mutations in LFS are similar to those TP53 mutations found in sporadic tumors, mostly occurring in exons 5 to 9.

Cowden Syndrome

Cowden syndrome is one of several syndromes that fall within the PTEN hamartoma tumor syndrome family, along with Bannayan–Riley–Ruvalcaba syndrome, Proteus syndrome, and a Proteus-like syndrome. Cowden syndrome, named after the patient Rachel Cowden, is an autosomal dominant syndrome best characterized by cutaneous facial lesions, seen in 96% of patients. The spectrum of disease includes multiple facial trichilemmomas, oral papillomas, lingua plicata ("cobblestoning" of the tongue), acral keratoses, macrocephaly, bilateral breast cancer, gastrointestinal hamartomas, and thyroid and endometerial tumors. Lipomas, hemangiomas, skin, renal, and brain tumors have also been reported. Breast cancer develops in 25% to 50% of patients by age 50. The risk of thyroid cancer is about 10%. Germline mutations in the gene *PTEN* (also known as *MMAC1*) were initially described in affected individuals in four of five kindreds.[62] The protein is a tumor suppressor with tyrosine phosphatase activity that suppresses growth. Testing via sequence analysis is available in a few centers.

Ataxia-Telangiectasia

Ataxia-telangiectasia (AT) is an autosomal recessive disease with a varied phenotype including progressive cerebellar ataxia, oculocutaneous telangiectasias, progeric skin changes, immune dysfunction, and increased cancer susceptibility. The hallmark of AT is cerebellar ataxia, often seen at a very young age. Most are unable to walk by age 10. These individuals are extremely sensitive to ionizing radiation. Cells from individuals display characteristics suggesting that the AT gene plays a role in DNA repair. *ATM* (AT mutated) gene has been identified on the long arm of chromosome 11. *ATM* appears to be required for the transcription of TP53 in response to radiation damage. Most of the mutations in the gene lead to a truncation of the protein; therefore, a protein truncation assay may be useful for detection in the future. Currently, genetic testing is done only at a few centers through sequencing.

Individuals are prone to a variety of cancers, particularly leukemia and lymphoma, but also breast cancer, as well as pancreatic, stomach, bladder, and ovarian cancer. Heterozygous carriers also are reported to have an increased risk of breast cancer, as much as a five- to eightfold increase over the normal population, and an earlier incidence of cancer. As about 1% of the population are heterozygous carriers of AT, these individuals may account for up to 7% of all breast cancers.[63] A study of 401 women with early-onset breast cancer found only 0.5% of them to be AT carriers, suggesting that the gene may not be involved in as large a number of cases as originally believed.[64]

Endocrine Cancers

The multiple endocrine neoplasia (MEN) syndromes are a group of familial endocrinopathies that include MEN 1, MEN 2A, and MEN 2B. In 1993, the RET proto-oncogene was found to be the predisposition gene for MEN 2A, MEN 2B, and familial medullary thyroid cancer (FMTC).[65–67] This finding made possible the institution of presymptomatic genetic testing for at-risk members of affected kindreds and led the way to early, preventative treatment of gene carriers. The predisposition gene for MEN-1 was cloned and characterized more recently[68] and presymptomatic genetic screening is only recently available. These recent discoveries and their influence upon patient management reflect the rapid changes in clinical medicine that are occurring as a result of advances in basic science research. Now it is possible to recommend an operation based solely on the results of a genetic test. Surgeons must exercise particular diligence and attention to detail when performing preventative operations and when recommending treatment and follow-up of patients and their relatives.

Multiple Endocrine Neoplasia Type 1

In MEN 1, patients develop tumors of the parathyroid glands, the pancreatic islet cells, and the pituitary gland. Lipomas, carcinoids, and benign tumors of the thyroid and adrenal cortex may also develop. Hyperparathyroidism occurs in virtually all patients with MEN 1. Clinical symptoms of pituitary and pancreatic islet cell tumors develop in 25% and 50% of patients, respectively. MEN 1 patients who do not manifest clinical evidence of hyperfunction of either the pituitary gland or the pancreatic islets have neoplastic changes noted at autopsy. The diagnosis of MEN 1 is confirmed clinically by the presence of at least three of these four criteria: primary hyperparathyroidism, pancreatic islet cell tumor (Zollinger–Ellison syndrome, insulinoma, VIPoma), a pituitary tumor, or a positive family history. The gene responsible for MEN 1 is the tumor suppressor gene, *Menin*, located on chromosome 11q13.[69] Menin has been shown to regulate cyclin-dependent kinase inhibitors, p27(Kip1) and p18(Ink4c).[69] Presymptomatic diagnostic testing is available at a few locations. Relatives of patients with MEN 1 should be screened for this disorder, starting in their early teens. Because hyperparathyroidism is almost always the first detectable abnormality in patients with MEN 1, serum calcium measurements should be performed yearly on asymptomatic kindred members at risk for the disease. If the history or physical examination suggests pituitary or pancreatic tumors, an appropriate diagnostic evaluation, including biochemical testing and radiologic imaging studies, should be initiated. A few patients present with renal stones or bone disease. Patients with MEN 1 have generalized (four-gland) parathyroid enlargement. Occasionally there is a marked discrepancy in the size of the parathyroid glands, but patients should be treated as if they have four-gland disease. Surgery is the appropriate treatment for these patients. Three-and-one-half gland parathyroidectomy is the procedure of choice of many surgeons. However, there are reported rates of persistent or recurrent hypercalcemia up to 50%. Therefore, we perform total parathyroidectomy with autotransplantation of parathyroid tissue to the forearm. This method achieves an immediate cure rate of more than 90% with an incidence of hypoparathyroidism of less than 5%. Approximately 50% of patients having total parathyroidectomy and autotransplantation develop graft-dependent hyperparathyroidism, but this can be effectively managed by resecting a portion of the autografted tissue under local anesthesia.[70]

Pituitary tumors occur in 40% of patients with MEN 1. The most common type of tumor is a benign prolactin-producing adenoma, although a few patients have tumors that produce growth hormone or adrenocorticotrophic hormone (ACTH). Patients present with headache, diplopia, and symptoms referable to hormone overproduction. Prolactinomas cause amenorrhea-galactorrhea in females and impotence in men. Hypopituitarism may also be present. Patients with growth hormone-producing tumors present with symptoms of acromegaly, and ACTH-producing tumors result in Cushing's disease. Most patients achieve effective inhibition of prolactin production by administration of bromocriptine, an ergot derivative with dopaminergic activity. Use of this drug may also reduce tumor bulk and obviate the need for surgical intervention, although transsphenoidal hypophysectomy may be necessary in patients who fail bromocriptine treatment and in patients with growth hormone-producing tumors. Patients with MEN 1 who do not have known pituitary disease should be screened by monitoring serum prolactin and growth hormone levels.

Pancreatic islet cell tumors occur in 60% of patients with MEN 1. Although these tumors often secrete more than one type of polypeptide hormone, they rarely produce a mixed clinical picture. The most common islet cell tumor in patients with MEN 1 is gastrinoma, producing the clinical picture of Zollinger–Ellison syndrome. Vasoactive intestinal polypeptide-secreting tumors (VIPomas), insulinomas, glucagonomas, and somatostatinomas are also encountered. As opposed to the management of sporadic islet cell tumors, the management of pancreatic tumors in patients with the MEN 1 syndrome is complicated by the fact that the pancreas is usually diffusely involved with islet cell hyperplasia and multifocal tumors. Islet cell tumors (particularly gastrinomas) may also be found in the proximal duodenum and peripancreatic areas (gastrinoma triangle), and the tumors are often malignant. Therefore, the treatment of these tumors must be focused on two goals: relief of symptoms related to excessive hormone production, and cure or palliation of the malignant process. Patients with islet cell tumors almost always suffer from the systemic effects of overproduction of a specific hormone rather than the effects of a space-occupying mass. Before surgical exploration for an islet cell tumor, the patient should be evaluated for the presence of an adrenal tumor by measuring urinary excretion rates of glucocorticoids, mineralocorticoids, and sex hormones.

Follow-Up of Patients with MEN 1

Patients with known MEN 1 and their children should be closely followed for development of new abnormalities and recrudescence of endocrinopathies already treated. This follow-up should include yearly determinations of plasma calcium, glucose, gastrin, fasting insulin, VIP, prolactin, growth hormone, and beta-human gonadotropin hormone. In addition, a detailed history and physical examination should be directed toward detecting abnormalities in the parathyroid, pituitary, or pancreatic islet cell systems. Because the gene responsible for MEN 1 has been identified, routine genetic testing allows identification of MEN 1 gene carriers in most affected families, and this will obviate the need to continue following individuals found not to have inherited the mutation.[71]

Multiple Endocrine Neoplasia Type 2

MEN 2 comprises three syndromes: MEN 2A, MEN 2B, and familial medullary thyroid cancer (FMTC) which are all characterized by a very high penetrance (nearly 100%) of medullary thyroid cancer (MTC). These syndromes are all autosomal dominant caused by germline mutations in the RET proto-oncogene. Besides MTC, MEN 2A is characterized by the development of pheochromocytoma in approximately 50% and hyperplasia of the parathyroid glands in approximately 25%. MEN 2B individuals develop MTC and pheochromocytomas, as well as megacolon, ganglioneuromatosis, and a characteristic physical appearance, with hypergnathism of the midface, marfanoid body habitus, and multiple musocal neuromas; they do not develop hyperparathyroidism (Fig. 90.5). Familial MTC (FMTC) patients develop MTC only. In all these disorders, MTC develops on a background of C-cell hyperplasia, and pheochromocytomas arise in the setting of hyperplastic adrenal chromaffin cells. MTC shows a spectrum of histological and clinical malignancy that ranges from C-cell hyperplasia to minimally aggressive disease in patients with FMTC, intermediate-grade behavior in patients with MEN 2A, and aggressive growth in patients with MEN 2B. Predicting the clinical behavior of these tumors based on the histological appearance alone is frequently difficult. Most pheochromocytomas in these patients are not invasive and have a low metastatic potential.

Diagnosis, Screening, and Biochemical Testing

Because the MEN 2 disorders are inherited in an autosomal dominant fashion, first-degree relatives and children of patients with the disorder have a 50% chance of inheriting the mutated gene for the disease. RET encodes a transmembrane tyrosine kinase receptor, whose ligand is glial cell line-derived neurotrophic factor (GDNF). The mutations found in MEN 2A, -2B, and FMTC cause constitutive activation (tyrosine phosphorylation) of the *RET* protein, which drives tumorigenesis through mechanisms that are currently being elucidated.[72] These mutations are gain-of-function mutations with a dominant oncogenic affect. There is a close phenotype–genotype correlation. Activating mutations of *RET* that have been described in MEN 2A and FMTC affect exon 10 (codons 609, 611, 618, or 620), exon 11 (codons 630 or 634), exon 13 (codon 768), or exon 14 (codon 804). Patients with MEN 2B almost all have a mutation in codon 918.[73] Testing for the presence of a *RET* gene mutation is done by polymerase chain-based methods that involve restriction digestion, band migration on acrylamide gels, or direct sequencing and is available in a variety of centers.

C-cells and MTC cells produce calcitonin, which can be measured in blood samples, and has been invaluable in screening patients for recurrent or residual disease after treatment for MTC. The sequential infusion of calcium gluconate and pentagastrin is a very potent calcitonin secretagogue and provides more reliable results than basal, or unstimulated

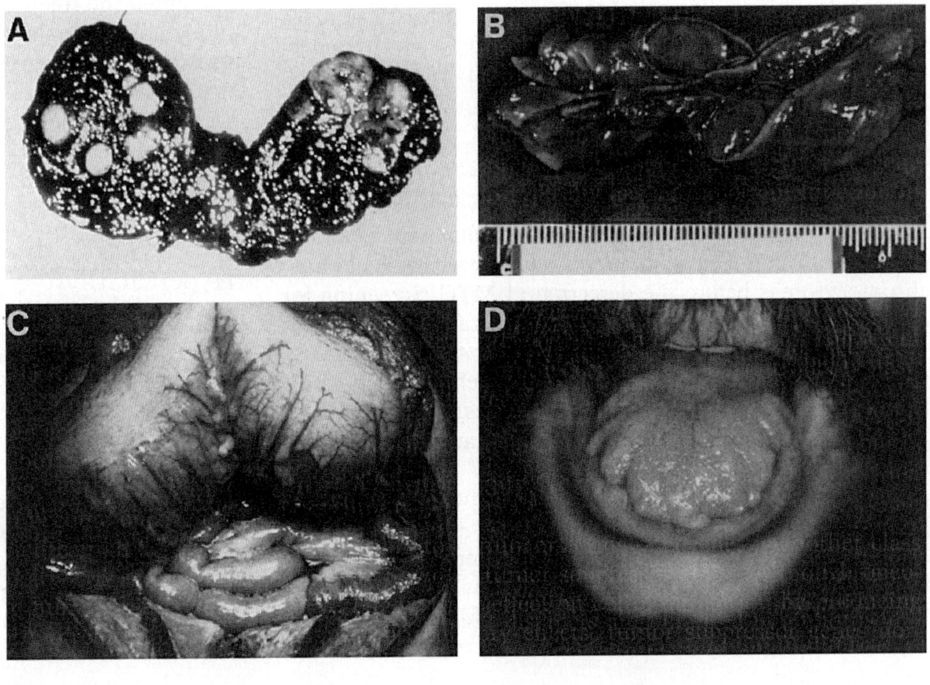

FIGURE 90.5. Features of patients with hereditary medullary thyroid carcinoma (MTC). **A.** Bisected thyroid gland from a patient with MEN 2A showing multicentric, bilateral foci of MTC. **B.** Adrenalectomy specimen from patient with MEN 2B demonstrating pheochromocytoma. **C.** Megacolon in patient with MEN 2B. **D.** Midface and tongue of patient with MEN-2B showing characteristic tongue notching secondary to plexiform neuromas. (Photograph **A** courtesy of Dr. S.A. Wells; photographs **B, C, D** courtesy of Dr. R. Thompson.) (Reprinted with permission from Moley, JF. Medullary thyroid cancer. In: Clark OH, Duh Q-Y, eds. Textbook of Endocrine Surgery. Philadelphia: WB Saunders Co. 1997.)

calcitonin levels. Blood is collected before and at 1, 2, 3, and 5 min following injection, and calcitonin levels are measured by radioimmunoassay.[74]

Surgical Management of Medullary Thyroid Carcinoma

Because MTC in patients with MEN 2 is virtually always present in both thyroid lobes, the preferred treatment is total thyroidectomy with resection of lymph nodes in the central region of the neck.[75] Central node dissection entails removal of all nodes and fatty tissue between the carotid sheaths from the level of the hyoid to the innominate artery. We also perform parathyroidectomy with autotransplantation of parathyroid tissue into the forearm (MEN 2A) or sternocleidomastoid (MEN 2B, FMTC, sporadic disease). Other experts attempt to leave the parathyroids in situ.

Patients who are at risk for development of MTC because they are in known MEN 2A, MEN 2B, or FMTC kindreds should undergo genetic testing for the presence of a mutation in the *RET* proto-oncogene and stimulated calcitonin testing. If an individual is found to have a mutation, they should undergo screening for a pheochromocytoma and, if there is no evidence of pheochromocytoma, thyroidectomy should be performed. Over the past 10 years at Washington University, we have studied more than 132 kindred members at direct risk for inheriting MEN 2A, FMTC, or MEN 2B.[76,77] More than 50 "preventative" thyroidectomies in patients found to be *RET* gene mutation carriers have been performed; 32 of these patients were under 15 years of age. The operative treatment was total thyroidectomy, regional lymph node dissection, and autotransplantation of the parathyroid to the forearm (MEN-2A) or sternocleidomastoid muscle (MEN-2B). In all except 2 patients (5 years old and 13 years old), a C-cell disorder was identified in the resected specimen. Three patients were found to have lymph node metastases (two 10-year-olds with MEN-2A and one 6-year-old with MEN-2B). This series and others indicate that genetic testing allows earlier intervention in these patients, which will result in more long-term cures. Generally, it is recommended that children with MEN2B have a thyroidectomy by age 6 months, those with mutations in codons 611, 618, 620, and 634 have thyroidectomies by age 5 years, and others have thyroidectomies by age 5 to 10 years.

Pheochromocytomas

Most patients with MEN-2A and MEN-2B who develop pheochromocytomas do so subsequent to development of MTC. Only about 10% of patients present with symptoms of pheochromocytomas before the detection of MTC. Screening for pheochromocytomas should be done at the same time as screening for MTC; this traditionally consists of measurement of 24-h urinary excretion rates of catecholamines, vanillylmandelic acid (VMA), and metanephrines. Eisenhofer et al. found measuring plasma normetanephrine and metanephrine a more sensitive test in familial diseases.[78] In another comparison of the two tests, Sawka et al. found the sensitivity of plasma metanephrines greater, making it more suitable for high-risk individuals (inherited forms), whereas 24-h urinary metanephrines and catecholamines yielded fewer false-positive results, making it more suitable for low-risk patients.[79] If urinary or plasma values are positive, computed tomography or magnetic resonance imaging of the adrenals is obtained. It is critical to identify pheochromocytomas in these patients before performing other surgeries because of the high mortality rate in patients undergoing operations who have an undetected pheochromocytoma.

Pheochromocytoma and Paraganglioma Syndromes

Pheochromocytomas and paragangliomas are tumors of the paraganglionic nervous system extending from the skull base to the pelvic floor and derived from the neuroectoderm. The most common of these tumors arise from the adrenal medulla (pheochromocytoma) and typically are functional, followed by nonfunctional head and neck tumors (paragangliomas, which include glomus and carotid body tumors), and then intraabdominal extraadrenal pheochromocytomas (which are also sometimes called paragangliomas). Pheochromocytomas occur in several familial syndromes, most commonly in MEN 2 (previously described) and von Hippel–Lindau (described later) and less commonly in neurofibromatosis type 1 (described later). Recently, three related genes have been identified that cause susceptibility to paragangliomas and/or pheochromocytomas. Familial paraganglioma type 1 (PGL-1) results from germline mutations in succinate dehydrogenase subunit type D (SDHD), PGL-type 3 from mutations in succinate dehydrogenase subunit type C (SDHC), and PGL-type 4 from mutations in succinate dehydrogenase subunit type B (SDHB). Together these subunits, along with a fourth, form the enzyme succinate dehydrogenase, which oxidizes succinate to fumarate as part of the Krebs cycle on the inner mitochondrial membrane. Succinate dehydrogenase is also directly linked to electron transfer in oxidative phosphorylation. In a comparison of SDHD and SDHB mutation carriers, individuals with SDHD mutations were more likely to have head and neck paragangliomas and multifocal disease, but individuals with SDHB mutations were much more likely to have metastatic disease.[80] These findings clearly have screening and treatment implications. Neumann et al. also examined the frequency of germline mutations in pheochromocytoma patients who presented with an apparent sporadic tumor, not in the context of one of these syndromes and with no family history of the disease.[81] One-fourth of these patients were found to have germline mutations in either von Hippel–Lindau, RET, SDHD, or SDHB genes, which dispels the previously held idiom that 10% of pheochromocytomas are inherited.

Hyperparathyroidism-Jaw Tumor Syndrome

A hereditary predisposition to parathyroid hyperplasia with hyperparathyroidism is seen in multiple endocrine neoplasia MEN 1, MEN 2A, (not MEN 2B), hyperparathyroidism–jaw tumor syndrome(HPT-JT), and familial isolated hyperparathyroidism (FIHP). HPT-JT is characterized by hyperparathyroidism with a high frequency of parathyroid carcinomas, up to 25% of these in kindreds. These patients may also have fibro-osseous tumors of the mandible or maxilla, and renal cysts and tumors, including Wilms' tumor, and possibly uterine tumors. Germline, inactivating mutations in the gene *HRPT2* have been identified in about one-half of kindreds.[82] HRPT2 produces the protein parafibromin, which has been shown to block cyclin D1/PRAD1 expression and can associate with a histone methyltransferase complex important in transcription.[83] Germline mutations have also been detected in a few FIHP kindreds as well as in parathyroid carcinomas thought to be sporadic.

Carney Complex

The Carney complex is an autosomal dominant syndrome characterized by lentiginoses, myxomas, and endocrine tumors. Lentigines are pigmented, brown-to-black skin macules, very similar histologically to freckles except they contain melanocyte hyperplasia. Lentigines can also be more deeply pigmented and found in certain anatomic areas making a lentiginoses suspected, namely the mucosa of the lips, vulva, and the inner and outer canthi of the conjunctivae.[84] Skin lesions also include blue nevi and other pigmented lesions. Individuals are predisposed to myxomas (cardiac, skin, breast, and others) and endocrine tumors (adrenal, thyroid, pituitary, and testis). The adrenal disease is primary pigmented nodular adrenal disease (PPNAD), which is bilateral and can lead to Cushing syndrome, seen in one third of patients. These patients often have atypical Cushing syndrome, characterized by a thin body habitus from muscle wasting and osteoporosis and normal or near-normal 24-h urinary free cortisol levels with a loss of the normal circadian rhythm. Cushing syndrome is usually managed with bilateral adrenalectomies. Pituitary adenomas are common and can secrete growth hormone or prolactin. More than three-fourths of men develop testicular tumors. Thyroid cancer has also been reported in several kindreds. Some kindreds have been found to have germline mutations in the PRKARIA gene, which encodes the type Iα regulatory subunit of protein kinase A (PKA).[85] Other families localize to the short arm of chromosome 2, without the identification of a specific gene as yet.

Gastric Cancer

Gastric cancer is divided histologically into two major histopathological types (diffuse and intestinal), both with their own familial syndromes. Hereditary diffuse gastric cancer syndrome is an autosomal dominant disease caused in part by mutations in the E-cadherin (CHD1) gene with a penetrance up to 70%. Although initially described in Maori (New Zealand) kindreds, germline mutations have also been found in European, African-American, Pakastani, and Asian kindreds. E-cadherin is a transmembrane glycoprotein important in cell–cell adhesion and signal transduction. Mutations cause a loss of function of the protein.[86] The consensus statement from the International Gastric Cancer Linkage Consortium recommended genetic testing for families that have two or more diffuse gastric cancers in close relatives with one before age 50 or three or more cancers at any age.[87] Prophylactic total gastrectomy carries a high morbidity, but should be strongly considered because mucosal abnormalities may not be detected endoscopically until late in the disease. Lobular breast carcinoma has been described in some of these kindreds. Hereditary intestinal gastric cancer has not been as well defined.

Sarcoma

Soft tissue carcinomas, including Ewing's sarcoma and liposarcoma, frequently have characteristic cytogenetic abnormalities.[13] A predisposition to soft tissue sarcomas has been identified in several familial cancer syndromes, including Li–Fraumeni (described in the breast section), Werner syndrome, familial retinoblastoma, and neurofibromatosis.

Werner Syndrome

Werner syndrome is an autosomal recessive syndrome characterized by the premature development of many features of aging including graying of hair, cataracts, scleroderma skin changes, osteoporosis, diabetes mellitus, wizened facies, and early death by either myocardial infarction or cancer. There is an increased risk of cancer, primarily soft tissue sarcomas, osteosarcomas, thyroid cancers (primarily follicular), and melanomas. Germline mutations in the WRN gene are responsible for the syndrome and encodes a DNA helicase.[88]

Familial Retinoblastoma

Familial retinoblastoma is characterized by bilateral retinoblastomas in infants and young children, but also by an increased risk of pinealomas (tumors of the pineal gland) and sarcomas (primarily osteosarcomas), especially in irradiated beds. The syndrome is an autosomal dominantly inherited disorder with 90% penetrance. The retinoblastoma gene, *RB*, is located on chromosome 13q14. Most familial cases have no prior family history, indicating that they are de novo cases. Early screening includes ophthalmological exams every 3 months to age 2, then every 4 months to age 4, and then every 6 months to age 10, and can reduce mortality by 55%. Treatment includes cryocoagulation, photocoagulation, radiation, or enucleation for advanced cases.

Neurofibromatosis

Neurofibromatoses are a group of inherited neurocutaneous syndromes that confer a much greater risk for developing malignant peripheral nerve sheath tumors (MPNST), also called neurofibrosarcoma. These syndromes primarily affect neural crest-derived tissues and have a wide clinical heterogeneity. Predisposition genes for two distinct forms have been cloned: neurofibromatosis type I and neurofibromatosis type II. Neurofibromatosis type 1 (NF-1), also called von Recklinghausen disease, is a common autosomal dominant disorder, affecting more than 80,000 people in the United States. The three hallmarks of the disease are multiple neurofibromas, café-au-lait spots, and Lisch nodules (benign iris hamartomas). Neurofibromas are benign tumors arising from Schwann cells. Surgical excision may be required for pain, functional impairment, or cosmetic reasons. Complete surgical resection is often needed because of the aggressive nature of the tumors. Neurofibromas can also occur along the gastrointestinal tract, resulting in bleeding, obstruction, or intussusception. Although more than 90% of NF1 patients demonstrate each of the three characteristic features, the number of lesions can be extremely variable. Other characteristics of NF-1 include learning disabilities, macrocephaly, scoliosis, short stature, seizures, pseudoarthrosis, and malignancies.[89] NF-1 tends to be a progressive disease, with many of these features appearing in childhood.

Neurofibromatosis type 1 patients have a much greater likelihood to develop MPNST and are also at risk for pheochromocytomas, astrocytomas, and leukemias. The increased risk for developing a MPNST is estimated to be 10,000 to 100,000 times greater than for the normal population.[90] Thus, 3% to 13% of all patients with NF-1 develop MPNST.[91] These tumors are believed to arise from neurofibromas, especially the plexiform type, and can be aggressive and invasive (Fig. 90.6). An enlarging mass, localized pain, or neuropathy should be considered a MPNST until proven otherwise. After a tissue diagnosis is made, complete surgical removal should be performed as early as possible. These tumors are generally resistant to radiation and chemotherapy.

The tumor suppressor gene responsible for NF1 was positionally cloned in 1990 to the long arm of chromosome 17 at q11.2 and is termed the *NF*1 gene.[92,93] The gene is extremely large, spanning more than 350 kb DNA with at least 59 exons. Within one of its introns are three other genes that are read in the opposite orientation. The gene product, neurofibromin, has a GTPase-activating protein domain, which has been shown to downregulate the proto-oncogene Ras. Occasionally this locus is deleted in other sporadic tumors, especially colon cancer. Presently there are several centers that provide genetic testing for the *NF*1 gene.

A

B

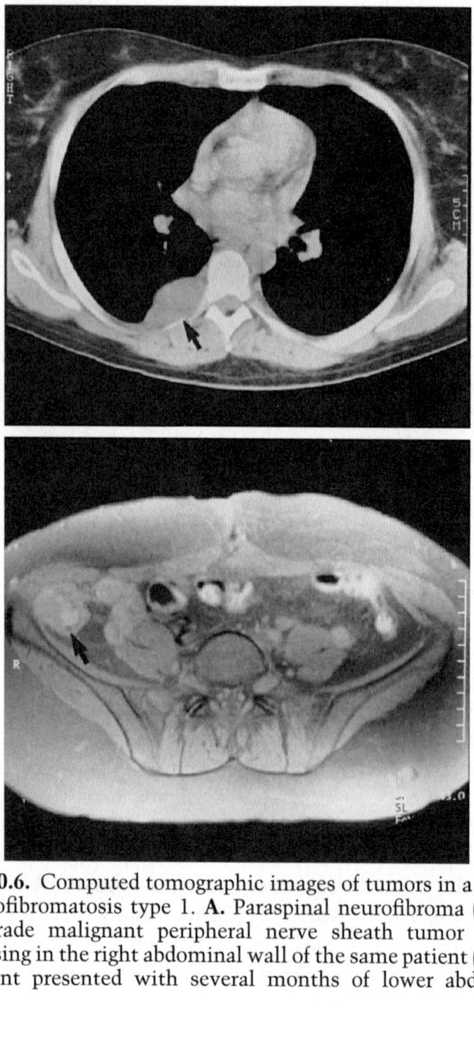

FIGURE 90.6. Computed tomographic images of tumors in a patient with neurofibromatosis type 1. **A.** Paraspinal neurofibroma (*arrow*). **B.** High-grade malignant peripheral nerve sheath tumor (Triton tumor) arising in the right abdominal wall of the same patient (*arrow*). This patient presented with several months of lower abdominal pain.

Neurofibromatosis type 2 (*NF*2) is a much more rare disorder, characterized by the defining feature of bilateral vestibular schwannomas (previously referred to as acoustic neuromas). The syndrome shares similarities with *NF*1, namely skin neurofibromas and café-au-lait spots. The syndrome also is characterized by cataracts and other CNS tumors, including gliomas, meningiomas, schwannomas, and neurofibromas.

NF2 is inherited in an autosomal dominant manner with a high degree of penetrance. In 1993 the gene, called Merlin or Schwannomin, was cloned and localized to chromosome 22 q11.1–13.1.[94,95] Its predicted protein product has sequence similarity to the exrin family of proteins, which play a role in attaching the cell cytoskeleton to the cell membrane. Studies of neurofibrosarcomas and meningiomas have found somatic mutations in this gene, suggesting that it is a tumor suppressor gene.

Melanoma

The incidence of cutaneous malignant melanoma has been rising faster than any other cancer. Approximately 10% of melanoma cases are familial, often associated with multiple atypical moles. These moles have been suggested as precursor lesions for melanoma. In 1820 Norris probably described the first family with familial atypical multiple-mole melanoma syndrome (FAMMM). The syndrome has been called several names, including dysplastic nevus syndrome, B-K syndrome, and large atypical nevus syndrome. Because these syndromes have not been defined uniformly either clinically or histopathologically, controversy has surrounded their description, inheritance, and predisposition toward melanoma. The number and size of the moles can vary considerably, as well as their associated risk of developing melanoma. The NIH Consensus Conference defined FAMMM as having (1) the occurrence of malignant melanoma in one or more first- or second-degree relatives, (2) a large number of melanocytic nevi, usually more that 50, some of which are atypical and variable in size, and (3) melanocytic nevi that have certain histopathological features, including asymmetrical architecture disorders, subepidermal fibroplasia, and lentiginous melanocytic hyperplasia with spindle or epithelial melanocyte nests.[96] The lesions predominantly occur on the trunk, but are also found on the buttocks, scalp, and lower extremities. Previously, the syndrome was believed to have an autosomal dominant inheritance, but a Genetics Analysis Workshop Study Group focusing on melanoma concluded this was not necessarily the case.[97] They also found that the most difficult issue in the analysis of this syndrome was the definition of affected individuals. The increased risk for developing melanoma in the presence of FAMMM is significant but has not been well established. The relative risk based on nine studies of patients with atypical moles ranged from 1.6 to 70, but most studies found the range to be from 5 to 11 when multiple atypical moles were present.[98]

The diverse clinical and histopathological definitions of FAMMM have also made cloning the genes by linkage analysis difficult. Initial studies pointed to a gene on the short arm of chromosome 1. Four other independent studies since did not show linkage to this area, suggesting multiple genes are responsible for the syndrome, possibly each with their own characteristics. Overwhelming evidence based on linkage, cytogenetic studies, and LOH has implicated the region 9p21 as having at least one tumor suppressor gene related to melanoma. Germline mutations in 13 of 18 kindreds were found in a cell cycle gene, *CDKN2*, also called p16.[99] *CDNK2* encodes a 16-kDa protein (p16INK4) that inhibits cyclin-dependent kinase 4 (CDK-4). Normally, CDK-4 combines with cyclin and phosphorylates the retinoblastoma (*RB*) protein; this releases RB-bound transcription factors necessary for the transition from the G_1 to the S phase in the cell cycle. When p16INK4 binds to CDK4, Rb does not become phosphorylated, therefore arresting the cell in G_1. Knocking out CDKN2 removes a break on the cell cycle, leading to uncontrolled cell growth. Another candidate for a 9p tumor suppressor gene is p15 *INK*4B, which is located close to the *CDKN2* gene and has structural and functional homology. Abnormalities in 9p have been found in a high number of dysplastic nevi as well as melanomas, suggesting it plays an early role in tumor development. The penetrance of melanomas in three 9p kindreds was calculated to be 53% by age 80.[100] Gene carriers that developed melanoma were found to have more sun exposure than those that did not develop melanoma, suggesting environmental and other genetic factors may be involved. More recently, other implicated genes include CDK4 on chromosome 12q14 and genes located on 1p36 and 1p22.[101,102]

Screening

Testing for *CDKN2* is available at several locations. There are several actions that should be taken for members of FAMMM kindreds and others with a strong family history of malignant melanoma.[98] These patients should have physical exams yearly, which should include a total cutaneous exam in which they are completely undressed. In a prospective study of patients with atypical moles, the only melanomas found greater than 0.76mm thick were those in patients who did not have routine skin examinations.[103] Screening should begin around puberty. A recent study found the median age for melanoma diagnosis was 34 years for 9p kindreds. For patients who have a large number of moles, baseline photographs may be helpful. Patients should examine their own skin regularly. Suspicious lesions should undergo biopsy. Regular ophthalmological exams should also be a part of their care as there is an increased risk of ocular nevi and ocular melanoma. Sun exposure should be avoided. Other malignancies have been related to mutations in the *CDKN2* gene, especially pancreatic cancer.[103–106]

Kidney Cancer

The kidney is host to several forms of hereditary cancer, including renal cell carcinoma associated with von Hippel–Lindau (VHL) disease, Birt-Hogg-Dubé, hereditary papillary renal carcinoma (HPRC), hereditary leiomyomatosis renal cell carcinoma (HLRCC), and Wilms' tumor, an embryonic malignancy arising from immature kidney remnants in children. Estimates are that up to 4% of adult renal carcinomas are familial. Histologically, the most common type of renal carcinoma is clear cell, whereas the papillary variant represents a small subset (5%–15%). VHL patients develop exclusively clear cell renal carcinoma.

The first clues to a gene responsible for renal carcinoma came from a kindred with multifocal clear cell carcinoma who had a translocation from the short arm of chromosome 3 (3p) to chromosome 8. Translocations of 3p have been shown to be a common trait of these kindreds. LOH of 3p has been found in 90% of all sporadic renal carcinomas, but not in papillary renal carcinomas, strongly suggesting the presence of a tumor suppressor gene for nonpapillary cancer in this area. The von Hippel–Lindau gene was subsequently localized on 3p25–p26, cloned,[107] and found to be mutated frequently (50%) in sporadic clear cell renal carcinomas.[108] No mutations in the *VHL* gene have been found in papillary renal cell carcinomas. Despite frequent 3p deletions in other types of cancers, *VHL* mutations have not been found in other sporadic tumors including pheochromocytomas, lung, ovarian, colon, or bladder cancers.

Von Hippel–Lindau

Von Hippel–Lindau disease is an autosomal dominant familial cancer syndrome in which benign and malignant tumors develop in a variety of organs. Organs involved include the kidneys, brain, spine, eyes, adrenal glands, pancreas, inner ear, and epididymis. The penetrance of the *VHL* gene is about 90% by age 65, with the mean age at diagnosis being 26 years. Maher found the frequency of the different tumors to be 59% for retinal hemangioblastomas, 59% for cerebellar hemangioblastomas, 28% for renal cell carcinomas, 13% for spinal hemangioblastomas, and 7% for pheochromocytomas.[109] The median age for diagnosis of retinal hemangioblastomas (25.4 years) and of cerebellar hemangioblastomas (29 years) was significantly less than that for renal cell carcinomas (44 years). Multiple, bilateral renal cysts are also common, with up to 75% of VHL patients developing cysts, tumors, or both. Pancreatic and epididymal cysts can also occur and are usually asymptomatic. The number of renal cysts can be greater than 100 with up to 600 clear cell carcinomas. Tumors can even be found growing inside renal cysts. The cancers have been found to metastasize in up to 40% of untreated patients. Renal cell carcinoma and cerebellar hemangioblastomas are the most common cause of death.

The function of the *VHL* protein appears to be regulating the transcription of DNA to mRNA by RNA polymerase II. Normally the VHL product binds to at least four subunits (elongin B and C, Cul2, and Rbx 1), which helps degrade the transcriptional activator hypoxia-inducible factor (HIF) in the presence of oxygen. Normally, only when oxygen levels are low, is HIF abundant, resulting in upregulation of angiogenic genes such as VEGF (vascular endothelial growth factor) and PDGF-β (platelet-derived growth factor-β chain). By mutating VHL, transcription of these genes proceeds even in the presence of oxygen. The protein also appears to help control extracellular matrix formation and the cell cycle.

There is extensive clinical variation of the disease, and several investigations have examined the correlation between genotype and phenotype. Crossey et al. found that more than 80% of kindreds with pheochromocytomas had missense mutations, compared to 25% of families without pheochromocytomas.[110] Mutations causing a truncation of the protein were much more common in kindreds without pheochromocytomas than those with them. Other studies have found a specific mutation to be correlated with a phenotype having pheochromocytomas, but not renal cell carcinomas. This finding has led to classifying VHL into different types based on phenotypes. In type I, pheochromocytomas do not occur: in type 2A, pheochromocytomas are present, but have a low risk of renal cell carcinomas; in type 2B, both pheochromocytomas and renal cell carcinomas are in the kindred; and in type 2C, only pheochromocytomas occur and hemangiomas or renal cell carcinomas do not.[111] This classification may prove to be helpful in presymptomatic counseling and screening.

Screening and Management

The management of VHL patients requires a multidisciplinary approach. Direct testing of the gene as well as prenatal testing are possible in a handful of centers; this testing enables physicians to tailor presymptomatic screening. Renal cysts should be regarded as potentially malignant, particularly any solid or rapidly growing areas, because their epithelial lining can undergo malignant transformation. Because renal cell carcinomas in VHL are usually bilateral and multiple, nephron-sparing surgery is the treatment of choice to preserve as much renal function as possible.[112] The rate of recurrence is 40% to 50%, necessitating close follow-up. Renal transplantation has also been used successfully for extensive disease. Retinal hemangioblastomas frequently are symptomatic and are usually controlled with laser treatment. Therefore, regular examinations by an ophthalmologist can lower the risk of blindness. Spinal and cerebellar hemangioblastomas should be removed so that functional damage does not occur. Pheochromocytomas should be removed when found.

Birt-Hogg-Dubé

Birt-Hogg-Dubé (BHD) syndrome is characterized by the development of cutaneous nodules, pulmonary cysts, and a variety of renal tumors. These individuals may develop chromophobe renal carcinoma, chromophobe/oncocytic hybrid, oncocytoma, or clear cell renal carcinoma with a penetrance of 15% to 30%.[113] The BHD gene has recently been identified and appears to be a tumor suppressor gene.[114]

Hereditary Papillary Renal Carcinoma

Hereditary papillary renal carcinoma (HPRC) was only recognized as a distinct form of familial renal carcinoma in 1994. HPRC is characterized by the development of multiple, bilateral type I papillary renal cell carcinomas. Based on an investigation of 10 kindreds, the median age of survival is 52 years.[115] The carcinomas were often detected incidentally in asymptomatic patients or during screening of asymptomatic patients. None of the kindreds have VHL or other 3p mutations. The *MET* proto-oncogene on chromosome 7q31–34 was found to be the predisposition gene.[116] The MET proto-oncogene encodes a transmembrane tyrosine kinase receptor, which is activated by hepatocyte growth factor and induces cellular proliferation, motility, and invasiveness. This receptor has been found to be overexpressed in a variety of cancers.[117,118] The gene is similar to the *RET* proto-oncogene, and its mutations are homologous to those seen in *RET*, suggesting that they cause constitutive activation of the protein. The *RET* and *MET* genes are the only known proto-oncogenes to cause a human inherited cancer syndrome.

Hereditary Leiomyomatosis Renal Cell Carinoma

Hereditary leiomyomatosis renal cell carinoma (HLRCC) is characterized by cutaneous and uterine leiomyoma, uterine leiomyosarcoma, and an aggressive form of type 2 papillary renal carcinoma. In 2003, germline mutations in the fumarate hydratase gene were found to be predisposing to the syndrome.[119] Fumarate hydratase cataylzes the hydration of fumarate to malate as a part of the Krebs cycle. The enzyme appears to be a tumor suppressor, because loss of the second allele is found in the kidney cancers in these kindreds.

Wilms' Tumor

Wilms' tumor, or nephroblastoma, is the most common intraabdominal solid tumor in children. The peak incidence occurs at age 3 to 4 years. Bilateral tumors occur in 5% to 10% of cases, with the peak incidence between ages 2 and 3. Most tumors are sporadic, with 1% to 2% being inherited. Three distinct syndromes have a genetic predisposition to Wilms' tumor: WAGR syndrome (Wilms' tumors, aniridia, genitourinary malformations, and mental retardation), Denys–Drash syndrome, and Beckwith–Wiedemann syndrome. There is also a familial form that lacks any other associated conditions. The first gene linked to Wilms' tumor was discovered through the investigations of the WAGR syndrome. Within this syndrome there is a greater than 30% chance of developing a Wilms' tumor. Karyotypic analysis of patients with WAGR found deletions in chromosome 11q13. This deletion has been found to encompass several genes, including PAX6, which causes aniridia, and WT1, which is a Wilms' tumor suppressor gene. Although loss of only one allele of the PAX6 gene causes aniridia, both alleles of WT1 must be mutated for a Wilms' tumor to develop. The product of WT1 is a zinc-finger transcription factor that plays a role in embyogenesis and organ formation. The tissue distribution of WT1 expression is limited, in contrast to some other tumor suppressor genes, such as p53 and Rb, which are found throughout the body. Renal expression is limited to blastemal cells, renal vesicles, and glomerular epithelium, and peaks at birth only to fall rapidly with age. WT1 expression is also found in mesothelial cells, Sertoli cells of the testis, and granulosa cells of the ovary. WT1 mutations are also found in 10% of sporadic cases of Wilms' tumors. Another gene has already been named WT2 and lies in the 11p15 area.

Denys–Drash syndrome (DDS) is characterized by Wilms' tumors, mesangial sclerosis leading to progressive renal failure, and ambiguous genitalia. The severity of the genital anomalies is highly variable, and there can be phenotypic overlap with WAGR. Germline point mutations in the *WT1* gene can be found in most DDS patients.[120]

Beckwith–Wiedemann syndrome (BWS) is characterized by overgrowth, congenital malformations (especially omphalocele), and a predisposition to embryonic malignancies, the most common of which is Wilms' tumor. The overgrowth can involve half the body in the form of hemihyperplasia, or it can be regional, as of an extremity or certain organs such as the tongue, kidneys, pancreas, adrenal cortex, and liver. Patients with hemihyperplasia appear to have a greater risk for malignancy (12.5%). Besides Wilms' tumors, other cancers include hepatoblastoma, neuroblastoma, rhabdomyosarcoma, and adrenocortical carcinoma. BWS is usually sporadic, but when inherited it follows an autosomal dominant pattern with variable penetrance. The genetic locus for BWS has been narrowed to chromosome 11p15, with a subset of these patients having chromosomal duplication. Presently it is unclear whether the gene causing BWS is WT2. BWS is a genetically heterogeneous disorder, probably affected by imprinting from different methylation patterns from the paternal and maternal allele.[121]

Finally, Wilms' tumor can be familial without any of the associated syndromes. Two familial Wilms' tumor genes have been mapped but not identified: FWT1 at 17q12–q21 and FWT2 at 19q13.4.[122] Isolated cases have also been reported in several other inherited cancer syndromes including Li–Fraumeni, Bloom, neurofibromatosis type 1, and hyperparathyroidism-jaw tumor syndromes.

SCREENING AND MANAGEMENT

The best method for surveillance for patients with a predisposition to Wilms' tumor is with abdominal ultrasound. Generally it is agreed that the exams should occur every 3 months until age 5 to 7.[123] A baseline abdominal CT should be performed in those patients at risk for other malignancies. Genetic testing is only available at a few centers, and is done largely on a research basis, but can be helpful in identifying a high-risk individual. In the presence of aniridia, genetic evaluation can distinguish whether only the *PAX6* gene has a mutation, or if the WT1 gene is also affected. The treatment of Wilms' tumor consists of resection for local control and chemotherapy for most patients, and radiation therapy for advanced disease. Generally patients with Wilms' tumors have a survival rate of greater than 90%.

Pancreatic Cancer

Because of the fairly high incidence of pancreatic cancer and its extremely high mortality rate, discovering genes that predispose to pancreatic cancer could provide a significant improvement in healthcare. Genetic factors are thought to play a role in 3% to 5% of all pancreatic cancers.[124] Several inherited syndromes have pancreatic cancer as a component of their disorder, including hereditary pancreatitis, familial atypical multiple mole melanoma syndrome (FAMMM), hereditary nonpolyposis colorectal cancer syndrome (HNPCC), Peutz–Jeghers syndrome, hereditary breast and ovarian cancer (BRCA2), and possibly ataxia-telangiectasia.[125] Endocrine pancreatic tumors are seen in multiple endocrine neoplasia type 1 and have been reviewed earlier. There have also been reports of familial pancreatic cancer, which is not related to any other syndrome.

Hereditary pancreatitis usually affects individuals at an early age (frequently in childhood) with recurrent episodes of pancreatitis. Affected patients often develop the sequelae of chronic pancreatitis, namely diabetes, pancreatic insufficiency, and pseudocysts, and can also develop portal and splenic vein thrombosis. The syndrome is transmitted in an autosomal dominant fashion by the cationic trypsin gene (PRSS1) gene in 70% of kindreds. Mutations prevent the normal inhibition of trypsin, allowing autodigestion of the pancreas.[126] The serine protease inhibitor, Kazal type 1 (SPINK1) gene has also been found to be mutated in children with idiopathic or hereditary chronic pancreatitis.[127] The prevalence of pancreatic cancer was found to be 20% in 21 kindreds and may be as high as 40% by age 70.[128] This is a higher rate of pancreatic cancer than found in individuals with pancreatitis for other reasons. The longer period of time for which the patients with the inherited form of pancreatitis are exposed to this insult may account for this difference. Presently, it is unknown whether the increased risk of pancreatic cancer is the result of a genetic susceptibility or if it is caused by the pancreatitis itself.

Kindreds with FAMMM (previously described) with a germline mutation in CDKN2 have an increased risk of pancreatic cancer.[105] In sporadic pancreatic tumors, this genetic region was found to be lost in 85% of the cases, suggesting that this gene plays an important role in all pancreatic cancers.[129]

Conclusion

Inherited cancer syndromes have provided tremendous insight into the genetics of cancer. This understanding has translated into elucidating the mechanisms of sporadic cancer as well as improved treatment for those with familial cancer. A new paradigm in surgery has emerged: the recommendation that an operation be performed based on the results of a genetic test. Surgeons must now face a number of related, and sometimes unfamiliar, issues related to genetic testing: ethics, confidentiality, liability, and insurance coverage. It is an exciting and challenging time for clinicians involved in care of these patients. The field of inherited cancer susceptibility is growing so rapidly that it is impossible for a book to provide the most current information. The past several years has seen the discovery of a different type of gene contributing to these syndromes, namely metabolic genes, such as succinate dehydrogenase and fumarate hydratase. New predisposition genes are constantly being isolated and characterized; therefore, enlistment of a genetic counselor can help keep one abreast of the changing field.

References

1. Fialkow P. The origin and development of human tumors studied with cell markers. N Engl J Med 1974;291:26–35.
2. Rous P. A Sarcoma of fowl transmissable by an agent separable from the tumor cells. J Exp Med 1911;13:397.
3. Wang L, Galehouse D, Mellon P, Duesberg P, Mason WS, Vogt PK. Mapping oligonucleotides of the Rous sarcoma virus that segregate with polymerase group-specific antigen markers in recombinants. Proc Natl Acad Sci U S A 1976;73:3952–3956.
4. Shih C, Weinberg R. Isolation of transforming sequence from a human bladder carcinoma cell line. Cell 1982;29:161–169.
5. Perucho M, Goldfarb M, Shimizu K, Lama C, Fogh J, Wigler M. Humor tumor-derived cell lines contain common and different transforming genes. Cell 1981;27:467–476.
6. Schimke R. Gene Amplification. Cold Spring Harbor, NY: Cold Spring Harbor Laboratory, 1982.
7. Shwab M, Alitalo K, Klemphauer K, et al. Amplified DNA with limited homology to myc cellular oncogene is shared by human neuroblastoma tumor. Nature (Lond) 1983;305:245–248.
8. Brodeur G, Seeger R, Schwab M, et al. Amplification of N-myc in untreated human neuroblastomas correlates with advanced disease stage. Science 1984;224:1121–1124.
9. Rowley J. A new consistent chromosomal abnormality in chronic myelogenous leukemia identified by quinacrine fluorescence and giemsa staining. Nature (Lond) 1973;243:290–293.

10. deKlein A, Van Kessel A, Grosveld G, et al. A cellular oncogene is translocated to the Philadelphia chromosome in chronic myelocytic leukaemia. Nature (Lond) 1982;300:765–767.
11. Heisterkamp N, Stam K, Groffen J, et al. Structural organization of the bcr gene and its role in the Ph9 translocation. Nature (Lond) 1985;315:758–761.
12. Kurzrock R, Gutterman J, Talpaz M. The molecular genetics of Philadelphia chromosome-positive leukemias. N Engl J Med 1988;319:990–998.
13. Rabbitts T. Chromosomal translocations in human cancer. Nature (Lond) 1994;372:143–149.
14. Pereira-Smith O, Smith J. Evidence for the recessive nature of cellular immortality. Science 1983;221:964–966.
15. Knudson AG. Mutation and cancer: statistical study of retinoblastoma. Proc Natl Acad Sci U S A 1971;68:820–823.
16. Cavanee W, Dryja T, Phillips R, et al. Expression of recessive alleles by chromosomal mechanisms in retinoblastoma. Nature (Lond) 1983;305:779–784.
17. Friend S, Bernards R, Rogelj S, et al. A human DNA segment with properties of the gene that predisposes to retinoblastoma and osteosarcoma. Nature (Lond) 1986;323:643–646.
18. Leach FS, Nicolaides NC, Papadopoulos N, et al. Mutations of a mutS homolog in hereditary nonpolyposis colorectal cancer. Cell 1993;75:1215–1225.
19. Bronner CE, Baker SM, Morrison PT, et al. Mutation in the DNA mismatch repair gene homologue hMLH1 is associated with hereditary non-polyposis colon cancer. Nature (Lond) 1994;368: 258–261.
20. Papadopoulos N, Nicolaides NC, Wei YF, et al. Mutation of a mutL homolog in hereditary colon cancer. Science 1994;263:1625–1629.
21. Fishel R, Lescoe MK, Rao MRS, et al. The human mutator gene homolog MSH2 and its association with hereditary nonpolyposis colon cancer. Cell 1993;75:1027–1038.
22. Vogelstein B, Fearon E, Hamilton S. Genetic alterations during colorectal tumor development. N Engl J Med 1988;319:525–532.
23. Vogelstein B, Fearon ER, Kern SE, et al. Allelotype of colorectal carcinomas. Science 1989;244:207–211.
24. Powell SM, Zilz N, Beazer-Barclay Y, et al. APC mutations occur early during colorectal tumorigenesis. Nature (Lond) 1992;359: 235–237.
25. Herrera L, Kakati S, Gibas L, Pietrzak E, Sandberg AA. Gardner syndrome in a man with an interstitial deletion of 5q. Am J Med Genet 1986;25:473–476.
26. Giardiello FM, Brensinger JD, Petersen GM, et al. The use and interpretation of commercial APC gene testing for familial adenomatous polyposis [see comments]. N Engl J Med 1997;336:823–827.
27. American Society of Clinical Oncology. American Society of Clinical Oncology policy statement update: genetic testing for cancer susceptibility. J Clin Oncol 2003;21:2397–2406.
28. Houlston RS, Collins A, Slack J, Morton NE. Dominant genes for colorectal cancer are not rare. Ann Hum Genet 1992;56:99–103.
29. Laken SJ, Petersen GM, Gruber SB, et al. Familial colorectal cancer in Ashkenazim due to a hypermutable tract in APC. Nat Genet 1997;17:79–83.
30. Kinzler KW, Nilbert MC, Su LK, et al. Identification of FAP locus genes from chromosome 5q21. Science 1991;253:661–665.
31. Groden J, Thliveris A, Samowitz W, et al. Identification and characterization of the familial adenomatous polyposis coli gene. Cell 1991;66:589–600.
32. Kinzler KW, Vogelstein B. Lessons from hereditary colorectal cancer. Cell 1996;87:159–170.
33. Jones S, Emmerson P, Maynard J, et al. Biallelic germline mutations in MYH predispose to multiple colorectal adenoma and somatic G:C to T:A muatations. Hum Mol Genet 2002;11:2961–2967.
34. Iwama T, Mishima Y. Factors affecting the risk of rectal cancer following rectum-preserving surgery in patients with familial adenomatous polyposis. Dis Colon Rectum 1994;37:1024–1026.
35. Ambroze WL Jr, Orangio GR, Lucas G. Surgical options for familial adenomatous polyposis. Sem Surg Oncol 1995;11:423–427.
36. Debinski HS, Spigelman AD, Hatfield A, Williams CB, Phillips RK. Upper intestinal surveillance in familial adenomatous polyposis. Eur J Cancer 1995;31A:1149–1153.
37. Lynch HT, Smyrk T, Watson P, et al. Hereditary colorectal cancer. Semin Oncol 1991;18:337–366.
38. Rodriguez-Bigas MA, Mahoney MC, Karakousis CP, Petrelli NJ. Desmoid tumors in patients with familial adenomatous polyposis. Cancer (Phila) 1994;74:1270–1274.
39. Church J, Simmang C. Practice parameters for the treatment of patients with dominantly inherited colorectal cancer. Dis Colon Rect 2003;46:1001.
40. Lynch HT, Smyrk T, Lanspa S, Lynch J. Colonoscopy in relation to the evolving genetics of familial colorectal cancer. Endoscopy 1995;27:43–49; discussion 61–62.
41. Nystrom-Lahti M, Parsons R, Sistonen P, et al. Mismatch repair genes on chromosomes 2p and 3p account for a major share of hereditary nonpolyposis colorectal cancer families evaluable by linkage. Am J Hum Genet 1994;55:659–665.
42. Lynch HT, Smyrk T, Lynch J, Fitzgibbons R Jr, Lanspa S, McGinn T. Update on the differential diagnosis, surveillance and management of hereditary non-polyposis colorectal cancer. Eur J Cancer 1995;31A:1039–1046.
43. Lengauer C, Kinzler KW, Vogelstein B. Genetic instability in colorectal cancers. Nature (Lond) 1997;386:623–627.
44. Burke W, Petersen G, Lunch P, et al. Recommendations for follow-up care of individuals with an inherited predisposition to cancer. I. Hereditary nonpolyposis colon cancer. Cancer genetics studies consortium. JAMA 1997;277:915–919.
45. Honchel R, Halling KC, Schaid DJ, Pittelkow M, Thibodeau SN. Microsatellite instability in Muir–Torre syndrome. Cancer Res 1994;54:1159–1163.
46. Bapat B, Xia L, Madlensky L, et al. The genetic basis of Muir–Torre syndrome includes the hMLH1 locus [letter]. Am J Hum Genet 1996;59:736–739.
47. Giardello FM, Brensinger JD, Termette AC, et al. Very high risk of cancer in familial Peutz–Jeghers syndrome. Gastroenterology 2000;119:1447–1453.
48. Spigelman AD, Arese P, Phillips RK. Polyposis: the Peutz–Jeghers syndrome. Br J Surg 1995;82:1311–1314.
49. Brugarolas J, Kaelin WG. Dysregulation of HIF and VEGF is a unifying feature of the familial hamartoma syndromes. Cancer Cell 2004;6:7–10.
50. Howe JR, Roth S, Ringold JC, et al. Mutations in the SMAD4/DPC4 gene in juvenile polyposis. Science 1998;280:1086–1088.
51. Radford DM, Zehnbauer BA. Inherited breast cancer. Surg Clin N Am 1996;76:205–220.
52. Miki Y, Swensen J, Shattuck-Eidens D, et al. A strong candidate for the breast and ovarian cancer susceptibility gene BRCA1. Science 1994;266:66–71.
53. Wooster R, Bignell G, Lancaster J, et al. Identification of the breast cancer susceptibility gene BRCA2 [see comments]. Nature (Lond) 1995;378:789–792.
54. Yoshida K, Miki Y. Role of BRCA1 and BRCA2 as regulators of DNA repair, transcription, and cell cycle in response to DNA damage. Cancer Sci 204;95:866–871.
55. Easton DF, Ford D, Bishop DT. Breast and ovarian cancer incidence in BRCA1-mutation carriers: Breast Cancer Linkage Consortium. Am J Hum Genet 1995;56:265–271.

56. Struewing JP, Hartge P, Wacholder S, et al. The risk of cancer associated with specific mutations of BRCA1 and BRCA2 among Ashkenazi Jews [see comments]. N Engl J Med 1997;336:1401–1408.
57. Liede A, Karlan BY, Narod SA. Cancer risks for male carriers of germline mutations in BRCA1 or BRCA2: a review of the literature. J Clin Oncol 2004;22:735–742.
58. Couch FJ, DeShano ML, Blackwood MA, et al. BRCA1 mutations in women attending clinics that evaluate the risk of breast cancer [see comments]. N Engl J Med 1997;336:1409–1415.
59. Schrag D, Kuntz KM, Garber JE, Weeks JC. Decision analysis—effects of prophylactic mastectomy and oophorectomy on life expectancy among women with BRCA1 or BRCA2 mutations [see comments]. N Engl J Med 1997;336:1465–1471.
60. Hartmann LC, Schaid DJ, Woods JE, et al. Efficacy of bilateral prophylactic mastectomy in women with a family history of breast cancer. N Engl J Med 1999;340:77–84.
61. Frebourg T, Barbier N, Yan YX, et al. Germ-line p53 mutations in 15 families with Li–Fraumeni syndrome. Am J Hum Genet 1995;56:608–615.
62. Liaw D, Marsh DJ, Li J, et al. Germline mutations of the PTEN gene in Cowden disease, an inherited breast and thyroid cancer syndrome. Nat Genet 1997;16:64–67.
63. Athma P, Rappaport R, Swift M. Molecular genotyping shows that ataxia-telangiectasia heterozygotes are predisposed to breast cancer. Cancer Genet Cytogenet 1996;92:130–134.
64. FitzGerald MG, Bean JM, Hegde SR, et al. Heterozygous ATM mutations do not contribute to early onset of breast cancer [see comments]. Nat Genet 1997;15:307–310.
65. Mulligan L, Kwok J, Healy C. Germ-line mutations of the RET proto-oncogene in multiple endocrine neoplasia type 2A (MEN 2A). Nature (Lond) 1993;363:458–460.
66. Donis-Keller H, Dou S, Chi D, et al. Mutations in the RET proto-oncogene are associated with MEN 2A and FMTC. Hum Mol Genet 1993;2:851–856.
67. Hofstra RM, Landsvater RM, Ceccherini I, et al. A mutation in the RET proto-oncogene associated with multiple endocrine neoplasia type 2B and sporadic medullary thyroid carcinoma [see comments]. Nature (Lond) 1994;367:375–376.
68. Chandrasekharappa SC, Guru SC, Manickam P, et al. Positional cloning of the gene for multiple endocrine neoplasia-type 1. Science 1997;276:404–407.
69. Milne TA, Hughes CM, Lloyd R, et al. Menin and MLL cooperatively regulate expression of cyclin-dependent kinase inhibitors. Proc Natl Acad Sci U S A 2005;102(3):749–754.
70. Wells SA Jr, Farndon JR, Dale JK, Leight DS, Dilley WG. Long-term evaluation of patients with primary parathyroid hyperplasia managed by total parathyroidectomy and heterotopic autotransplantation. Ann Surg 1980;192:451–458.
71. Moley JF, Wells SA. Multiple endocrine neoplasia. In: Niederhuber JE, ed. Current Therapy in Oncology. St. Louis: Mosby Year Book, 1993:282–292.
72. Santoro M, Carlomango F, Romano A, et al. Activation of *RET* as a dominant transforming gene by germline mutations of MEN2A and MEN2B. Science 1995;267:381–383.
73. Goodfellow PJ, Wells SA Jr. RET gene and its implications for cancer. J Natl Cancer Inst 1995;87:1515–1523.
74. Wells S, Baylin S, Linehan W, Farrel R, Cox E, Cooper C. Provocative agents and the diagnosis of medullary carcinoma of the thyroid gland. Ann Surg 1978;188:139–141.
75. Moley JF. Medullary thyroid cancer. Surg Clin N Am 1995; 75:405–420.
76. Wells SA, Chi DD, Toshima K, et al. Predictive DNA testing and prophylactic thyroidectomy in patients at risk for multiple endocrine neoplasia type 2A. Ann Surg 1994;220:237–250.
77. Wells SAJ, Moley JF, DeBenedetti MK, Skinner MA. Prophylactic thyroidectomy in patients with MEN2A and familial medullary thyroid carcinoma. Sixth International Workshop on Multiple Endocrine Neoplasia and Von Hippel–Lindau Disease. Noordwijkerhout, The Netherlands: Leeuwenhorst Congress Center, 1997.
78. Eisenhofer G, Lenders JWM, Linehan WM, et al. Plasma normetanephrine and metanephrine for detecting pheochromocytoma in von Hippel–Lindau disease and multiple endocrine neoplasia type 2. N Engl J Med 1999;340:1872–1879.
79. Sawka AM, Jaeschke R, Singh RJ, Young WF. A comparison of biochemical tests for pheochromocytoma: measurement of fractionated plasma metanephrines compared with the combination of 24-hour urinary metanephrines and catecholamines. J Clin Endocrinol Metab 2003;88:553–558.
80. Neumann HPH, Pawlu C, Peczkowska M, et al. Distant clinical features of paraganglioma syndromes associated with SDHB and SDHD gene mutations. JAMA 2004;292:943–951.
81. Neumann HPH, Bausch B, McWinney SR, et al. Germ-line mutations in nonsyndromic pheochromocytoma. N Engl J Med 2002;346:1459–1466.
82. Carpten JD, Robbins CM, Villablanca A, et al. HRPT2, encoding parafibromin, is mutated in hyperparathyroidism-jaw tumor syndrome. Nat Genet 2002;32:584–588.
83. Rozenblatt-Rosen O, Hughes CM, Nannepaga SJ, et al. The parafibromin tumor suppressor protein is part of a human Paf1 complex. Mol Cell Biol 2005;25:612–620.
84. Stratakis CA. Genetics of Peutz–Jeghers syndrome, Carney complex and other familial lentiginoses. Horm Res 2000;54:334–343.
85. Kirschner LS, Carney JA, Pack S, et al. Mutations in the gene encoding the type Ia regulatory subunit of the protein kinase A (PRKARIA) in patients with Carney complex. Nat Genet 2000;26:89–92.
86. Brooks-Wilson AR, Kaurah P, Suriano G, et al. Germline E-adherin mutations in hereditary diffuse gastric cancer: assessment of 42 new families and review of genetic screening criteria. J Med Genet 2004;41:508–517.
87. Caldas C, Carneiro F, Lynch HT, et al. Familial gastric cancer: overview and guidelines for management. J Med Genet 1999;36:873–880.
88. Yu CE, Oshima J, Fu YH, et al. Positional cloning of the Werner's syndrome gene. Science 1996;272:258–262.
89. Goldberg Y, Dibbern K, Klein J, Riccardi VM, Graham JM Jr. Neurofibromatosis type 1: an update and review for the primary pediatrician. Clin Pediatr 1996;35:545–561.
90. Riccardi VM, Powell PP. Neurofibrosarcoma as a complication of von Recklinghausen neurofibromatosis. Neurofibromatosis 1989;2:152–165.
91. Arun D, Gutmann DH. Recent advances in neurofibromatosis type 1. Curr Opin Neurol 2004;17:101–105.
92. Wallace MR, Marchuk DA, Andersen LB, et al. Type 1 neurofibromatosis gene: identification of a large transcript disrupted in three NF1 patients [published correction appears in Science 1990;250:1749]. Science 1990;249:181–186.
93. Cawthon RM, Weiss R, Xu GF, et al. A major segment of the neurofibromatosis type 1 gene: cDNA sequence, genomic structure, and point mutations [published correction appears in Cell 1990;62: following 608]. Cell 1990;62:193–201.
94. Rouleau GA, Merel P, Lutchman M, et al. Alteration in a new gene encoding a putative membrane-organizing protein causes neuro-fibromatosis type 2 [see comments]. Nature (Lond) 1993; 363:515–521.
95. Trofatter JA, MacCollin MM, Rutter JL, et al. A novel moesin-, ezrin-, radixin-like gene is a candidate for the neurofibromatosis 2 tumor suppressor. Cell 1993;75:826.
96. Anonymous, NIH Consensus Conference. Diagnosis and treatment of early melanoma [see comments]. JAMA 1992;268:1314–1319.

97. Risch N, Sherman S. Genetic Analysis Workshop 7: summary of the melanoma workshop. Cytogenet Cell Genet 1992;59:148–158.
98. Slade J, Marghoob AA, Salopek TG, Rigel DS, Kopf AW, Bart RS. Atypical mole syndrome: risk factor for cutaneous malignant melanoma and implications for management. J Am Acad Dermatol 1995;32:479–494.
99. Hussussian CJ, Struewing JP, Goldstein AM, et al. Germline p16 mutations in familial melanoma [see comments]. Nat Genet 1994;8:15–21.
100. Cannon-Albright LA, Kamb A, Skolnick M. A review of inherited predisposition to melanoma. Semin Oncol 1996;23:667–672.
101. Gillanders E, Juo SHH, Holland EA, et al. Localization of a novel melanoma susceptibility locus to 1p22. Am J Hum Genet 2003;73:301–313.
102. Soufir N, Avril MF, Chompret A, et al. Prevalence of p16 and CDK4 germline mutations in 48 melanoma-prone families in France: the French Familial Melanoma Study Group. Hum Mol Genet 1998;7:209–216.
103. Tucker MA, Fraser MC, Golstein AM, Elder DE, Guerry DT, Organic SM. Risk of melanoma and other cancers in melanoma-prone families. J Invest Dermatol 1993;100:350S–355S.
104. Goldstein AM, Fraser MC, Struewing JP, et al. Increased risk of pancreatic cancer in melanoma-prone kindreds with p16INK4 mutations [see comments]. N Engl J Med 1995;333:970–974.
105. Whelan AJ, Bartsch D, Goodfellow PJ. Brief report: a familial syndrome of pancreatic cancer and melanoma with a mutation in the CDKN2 tumor- suppressor gene [see comments]. N Engl J Med 1995;333:975–977.
106. Goldstein AM, Struewing JP, Fraser MC, Smith MW, Tucker MA. Prospective risk of cancer in CDKN2A germline mutation carriers. J Med Genet 2004;41:421–424.
107. Latif F, Tory K, Gnarra J, et al. Identification of the von Hippel–Lindau disease tumor suppressor gene [see comments]. Science 1993;260:1317–1320.
108. Gnarra JR, Tory K, Weng Y, et al. Mutations of the VHL tumour suppressor gene in renal carcinoma. Nat Genet 1994;7:85–90.
109. Maher ER, Yates JR, Harries R, et al. Clinical features and natural history of von Hippel–Lindau disease [see comments]. Q J Med 1990;77:1151–1163.
110. Crossey PA, Richards FM, Foster K, et al. Identification of intragenic mutations in the von Hippel–Lindau disease tumour suppressor gene and correlation with disease phenotype. Hum Mol Genet 1994;3:1303–1308.
111. Hoffman MA, Ohh M, Yang H, et al. von Hippel–Lindau protein mutants linked to type 2C VHL disease preserve the ability to downregulate HIF. Hum Mol Genet 2001;10:1019–1027.
112. Steinbach F, Novick AC, Zincke H, et al. Treatment of renal cell carcinoma in von Hippel–Lindau disease: a multicenter study. J Urol 1995;153:1812–1816.
113. Pavlovich CP, Walther MM, Eyler Ra, et al. Renal tumors in the Birt–Hogg–Dube syndrome. Am J Surg Pathol 2002;26:1542–1552.
114. Nickerson ML, Warren MB, Toro JR, et al. Mutations in a novel gene lead to kidney tumors, lung wall defects, and benign tumors of the hair follicle in patients with the Birt–Hogg–Dube syndrome. Cancer Cell 2002;2:157–164.
115. Zbar B, Glenn G, Lubensky I, et al. Hereditary papillary renal cell carcinoma: clinical studies in 10 families [see comments]. J Urol 1995;153:907–912.
116. Schmidt L, Duh FM, Chen F, et al. Germline and somatic mutations in the tyrosine kinase domain of the MET proto-oncogene in papillary renal carcinomas. Nat Genet 1997;16:68–73.
117. Di Renzo MF, Olivero M, Katsaros D, et al. Overexpression of the Met/HGF receptor in ovarian cancer. Int J Cancer 1994; 58:658–662.
118. Ferracini R, Di Renzo MF, Scotlandi K, et al. The Met/HGF receptor is overexpressed in human osteosarcomas and is activated by either a paracrine or an autocrine circuit. Oncogene 1995;10:739–749.
119. Toro JR, Nickerson ML, Wei MH, et al. Mutations in the fumarate hydrratase gene cause hereditary leiomyomatosis and renal cell carncer in families in North America. Am J Hum Genet 2003;73:95–106.
120. Coppes MJ, Haber DA, Grundy PE. Genetic events in the development of Wilms' tumor. N Engl J Med 1994;331:586–590.
121. Weksberg R, Squire JA. Molecular biology of Beckwith–Wiedemann syndrome. Med Pediatr Oncol 1996;27:462–469.
122. Ruteshouser EC, Huff V. Familial Wilms' tumor. Am J Med Genet 2004;129C:29–34.
123. Clericuzio CL, Johnson C. Screening for Wilms' tumor. Am J Med Genet 2004;129C:29–34.
124. Lynch HT, Smyrk T, Kern SE, et al. Familial pancreatic cancer: a review. Semin Oncol 1996;23:251–275.
125. Rieder H, Bartsch DK. Familial pancreatic cancer. Fam Cancer 2004;3:69–74.
126. Whitcomb DC, Gorry MC, Preston RA, et al. Hereditary pancreatitis is caused by a mutation in the cationic trypsinogen gene. Nat Genet 1996;14:141–145.
127. Witt H, Luck W, Hennies HE, et al. Mutations in the gene encoding the serine protease inhibitor, Kazal type 1 are associated with chronic pancreatitis. Nat Genet 2000;25:213–216.
128. Kattwinkel J, Lapey A, Di Sant'Agnese PA, Edwards WA. Hereditary pancreatitis: three new kindreds and a critical review of the literature. Pediatrics 1973;51:55–69.
129. Caldas C, Hahn SA, da Costa LT, et al. Frequent somatic mutations and homozygous deletions of the p16 (MTS1) gene in pancreatic adenocarcinoma. Nat Genet 1994;8:27–32.

91

Fundamentals of Cancer Genomics and Proteomics

Jimmy C. Sung, Alice Y. Lee, and Timothy J. Yeatman

The foundation of modern surgery has long been based on a clear understanding of anatomy and physiology. This structural and functional paradigm has produced tremendous progress in the comprehension and treatment of human disease. The advent of molecular biology and the completion of the Human Genome Project, however, have brought forth a new scientific basis for surgical investigation and practice. In the era of genomic medicine, molecular structures and gene functions are the foundation for the conceptualization of surgical diseases. Because genetic mutation is the basis for the abnormal phenotypic presentation in tumors, surgical oncology is an excellent field in which to translate the discoveries of genomic research into novel therapeutic approaches. The aim of this chapter is to provide a primer for oncologists and surgeons to understand the relevance and applications of genomics and proteomics in surgical oncology.

Translating the Genome, Transcriptome, and Proteome

In the genomic era, the "structure and function" paradigm of modern medicine has remained, but the focus has shifted toward identifying the sequence structure of the genome (genomics), interrogating the expression of critical messenger RNA transcripts (transcriptomics), and understanding the expression and function of the final protein product (proteomics).

The human genome is composed of 2.9 billion nucleotides. This large sequence of genetic code is made up of introns, which are the noncoding regions, and exons, the coding regions. It is these coding regions—comprising only 1% of all human DNA—that define nearly 55,000 genes, which serve as the template for all biological functions.

The central dogma of molecular biology summarizes the relationship between DNA, RNA, and protein. DNA codes for the production of messenger RNA (mRNA), which in turn codes for protein production. By translating these individual mRNAs, distinct polypeptide chains can be made using 20 amino acids as building blocks. Once assembled, these chains of amino acids can be further modified by posttranslational processes such as glycosylation and phosphorylation and folded into three-dimensional structures known as proteins. It is estimated that there are 1000 to 5000 distinct protein structures involved in the wide spectrum of human biological activity. Thus hidden within the genetic code is a description of the precise mechanism of human disease.[1]

High-Throughput Technology: DNA Microarray, Proteomics, and Tissue Array

In 1953, James Watson and Francis Crick discovered the structure of deoxyribonucleic acid, DNA, the "blueprint of life"; however, it was not until a half a century later that the first draft of the human genome was published. In 2001, both the International Consortium and Celera Genomics, using two different technological approaches, separately completed the first draft of the entire human genome.[2,3] This gap of almost 50 years was not caused by lack of vision or ambition but rather resulted from the need for the development of many technological advances required for large-scale sequencing and genomic analysis. The sequence of the human genome was deciphered only after significant advancements were made in both molecular biology and computer science permitting high-throughput sequencing and sequence alignment. Defining the structure of the genome was just the first step in understanding the molecular basis of human diseases. The challenge lies in determining the function of each gene and its relationship to other genes (gene and protein interactions, protein and protein interactions) under various biological circumstances.

Gene Expression Profiling Using Microarray

In 1995, Schena et al.[4] developed a new technology known as the DNA microarray capable of monitoring the expression of multiple genes simultaneously. A microarray is an ordered array of microscopic elements on a planar substrate that allows the specific binding of genes or gene products. Currently, gene expression profiling is accomplished by two principal microarray platforms by using either oligonucleotides or complementary DNAs (cDNAs) to interrogate RNA-derived biological samples (Fig. 91.1). These arrays are all based on DNA sequences from the Human Genome Project database. Oligonucleotide arrays generally use small DNA sequences, 21- to 70-mer, to recognize and distinguish individual genes. Spotted cDNA arrays are constructed by spotting down thousands of longer portions of DNA, each representing an individual gene. The oligonucleotide arrays have the potential benefit of identifying splice products, whereas the cDNA arrays generally cannot.[1]

The process of hybridization underlies all chip-based microarray technology. Hybridization is the chemical process by which two complementary DNA or RNA strands combine to form a double-stranded molecule. In a microarray assay, a copy of the mRNA (either cDNA or cRNA) is labeled with fluorescent dye and hybridized to a known DNA sample tethered onto the microarray chip. Larger quantities of mRNA for any particular gene result in higher degrees of hybridization and stronger fluorescent intensity. One of the potential shortcomings of this technology is the faulty assumption that all probes work equally well under the same hybridization condition used to process the GeneChip or microarray. For this very reason, normalization processes such as robust multiarray average (RMA) attempt to control this sort of inherent variability. By analyzing a digital image of the fluorescent intensity across the microarray, one can determine the degree of expression of all the genes on the chip. Currently, a typical high-intensity microarray chip contains 12,000 to 60,000 genes, thus allowing the generation of global gene expression patterns that are unique to various biological processes. Using microarray technology, diseases can now be identified, classified, and treated based on global analysis of gene expression.[1]

Proteomics

Although the ability to monitor genome-wide activity is a significant advancement in the understanding of disease, the final molecular interactions of biological processes occur at the protein level. However, in large part because of posttranslational modification and limitations of current protein annotations, gene expression levels do not always correlate with protein activity. The field of proteomics involves the development of high-throughput methods that facilitate the comprehensive analyses of the protein activity in various biological states.

Two-dimensional gel electrophoresis (2-D gel) and mass spectrometry are most representative of the current state of the art in proteomics. The three crucial aspects of proteomic analysis are (1) isolation of individual proteins from a biological specimen; (2) generation of a unique fingerprint based on molecular mass; and (3) identification of the protein using computational analysis.[5] The analysis may begin with the physical separation of proteins by mass and charge using 2-D gels, a technique that exploits the differences in isoelectric points (the first dimension) and molecular mass (the second dimension) of various proteins, separating them into spots on a gel. Each protein spot is cut out and digested with trypsin, producing a set of peptide fragments that may then be further

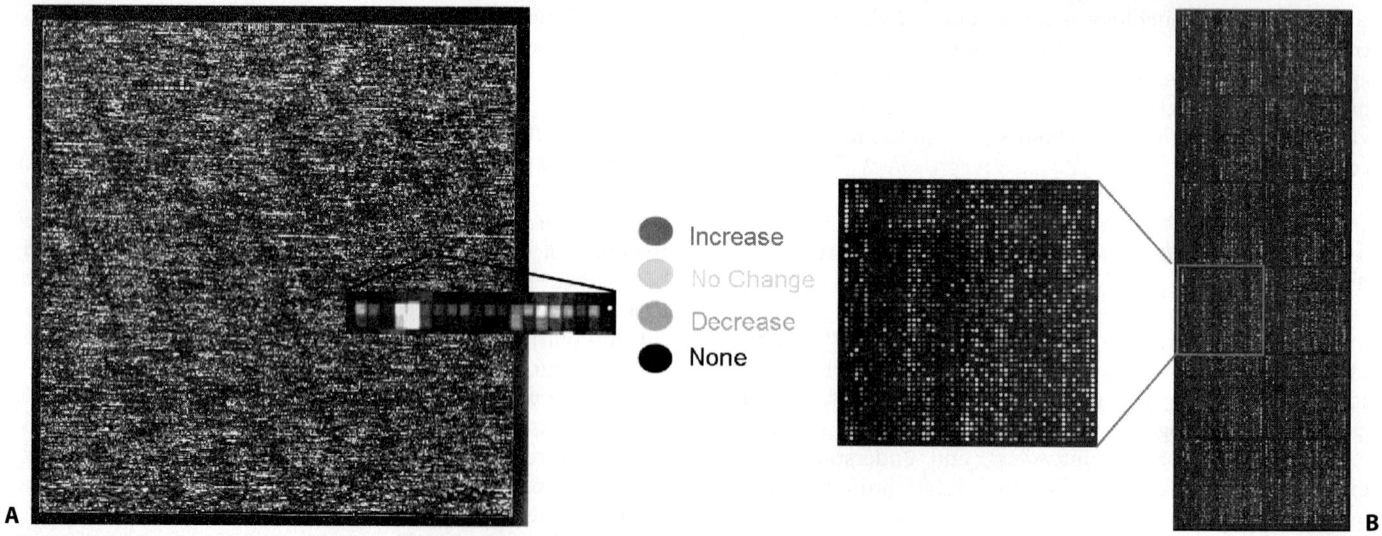

FIGURE 91.1. Two available platforms for gene expression profiling. **A.** Affymetrix GeneChip utilizes a large number of short oligonucleotide probes (21 bp in length) (see *inset*) and probe sets to discriminate the expression of one gene versus another. Each gene may be interrogated by one or more probe sets. cRNA produced from RNA is hybridized to the GeneChip and the degree of hybridization (or measured fluorescence) is a measure of relative gene expression. Numerous probes and probesets are used to measure the expression of each individual gene. **B.** Custom cDNA microarray utilizes a large number of long cDNA probes (averaging 1.4 kb in length) to measure each gene's expression. These microarrays require two experiments to be performed on each sample, one test and one control sample, such that a ratio of gene expression of test to control is constructed.

separated by a microscale capillary high performance liquid chromatography (HPLC) column based on the hydrophobicity of each fragment. Once separated, these peptides are ionized by either electrospray ionization or matrix-assisted laser desorption/ionization (MALDI) before introduction into the vacuum of a mass spectrometer (Fig. 91.2).

All mass spectrometers consist of three distinct components: an ionizer, ion analyzer, and detector. The types of mass spectrometers most commonly used in proteomics are the quadrupole mass spectrometer, the time of flight (TOF) mass spectrometer, and the "ion trap." A quadrupole mass analyzer consists of four parallel rods that generate an electric field. As peptide ions pass through the quadrupoles, their motion depends on their mass-to-charge ratio (m/z). Ions with a large m/z ratio follow a path with a larger radius than ions with a small m/z ratio. The quadrupole mass spectrometer adjustable four-sided electronic array allows only ions with specific m/z ratios to pass through. Whenever an ion reaches a detector, an electronic signal is generated. The signals produced during the course of the scan produce a mass spectrum illustrating at which point the m/z ions are present (Fig. 91.3).

Time-of-flight mass spectrometers measure the time it takes for each ion to reach the detector, as the speed an ion travels is directly related to its mass. After charging all the ions to the same kinetic energy by passage through an electric field, the spectrometer measures the time each ion takes to travel the field. On the other hand, the ion trap mass analyzer consists of three hyperbolic electrodes. These electrodes form a cavity that traps and analyzes ions. Ions produced from the source enter the trap, and various voltages are applied to the electrodes to trap and eject ions according to their mass-to-charge ratios. The ions are ejected in order of increasing mass-to-charge ratio and detected by the ion detector system.

Once the molecular fingerprint of a specific set of peptide fragments is generated by mass spectrometry, the identity of the protein can be determined by searching against a known protein database. Search engines such as Sequest and Mascot use mass spectrometry data to identify proteins from primary sequence databases.[6] Therefore, as in genomic profiling, differential protein expression between various biological processes or pathological states also holds promise to identify, classify, and treat human disease.

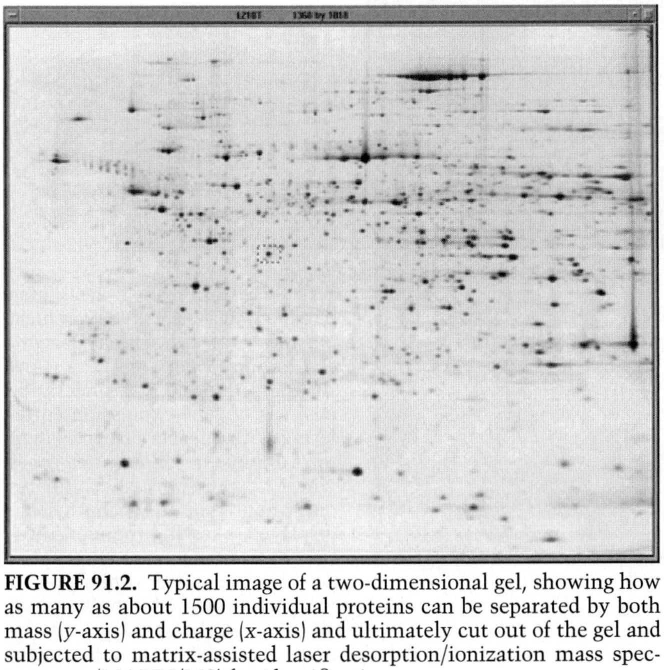

FIGURE 91.2. Typical image of a two-dimensional gel, showing how as many as about 1500 individual proteins can be separated by both mass (y-axis) and charge (x-axis) and ultimately cut out of the gel and subjected to matrix-assisted laser desorption/ionization mass spectrometry (MALDI/MS) for identification.

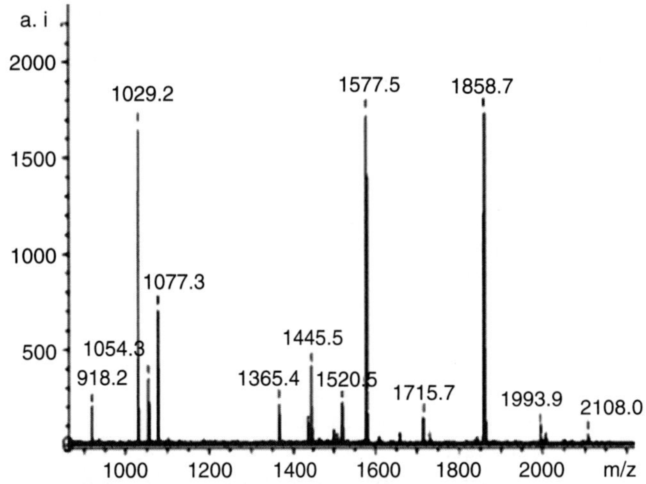

FIGURE 91.3. Spectra derived from a mass spectrometer delineate multiple peaks with potentially distinctive mass/charge ratios.

Tissue Arrays

Novel candidate tumor markers identified using genomics or proteomics technology can be validated with another high-throughout method known as tissue microarray (TMA). The making of the tumor tissue microarray begins with taking a sample from the paraffin-embedded tumor specimen. A collection of these tumor samples is then spotted on to a glass slide in the format of an array. Each individual tumor array contains tissues samples of hundreds of different patients.[7] A good example of the applications of this technology can be seen in the set of breast cancer tissue arrays developed by Torhorst et al.[8] On each breast cancer TMA chip are tissue samples from 553 patients linked with detailed clinical data. Using this technology in conjunction with standard immunohistochemical techniques, the investigators studied the prognostic significance of estrogen receptors (ERs), progesterone receptors (PRs), and p53 in a single experiment under identical hybridization conditions. This study demonstrated that minute tissue samples (0.6-mm biopsies) in an array format are sufficient for the analysis of the association between genomics alterations and clinical outcomes. As the use of proteomics and genomics technologies continue to identify a large number of potential molecular markers, TMA provides a very efficient and statistically robust method to validate novel tumor markers and translate the information into clinical applications.

Computational Analysis of Genomic Data

The analysis of complex data generated by high-throughput approaches has required multidisciplinary interaction between molecular biologists, computational biologists, mathematicians, and statisticians. The two mortal sins of genomics and proteomics are poor specimen collection and faulty analyses. As the quality and success of molecular analysis depends on clear communication among members of an interdisciplinary team, some minimal understanding of computational analysis is essential for the surgical oncologist.

The major goal of computational techniques for the analysis of microarray data is to group together genes or samples (representing, for example, different experimental conditions or individual patients) that share similar patterns of gene expression. These data analysis techniques are generally divided into two groups: *unsupervised* methods, which can be used to discover previously unknown groupings or classes, and *supervised* methods, which are used to learn discriminating features of already established classifications to classify uncategorized objects.[9]

Hierarchical clustering is the most widely used of the unsupervised techniques. It is an agglomerative process that groups together closely related genes (or samples) using a distance metric that defines objects with similar patterns of gene expression as close to one another. The process begins with each individual object as its own cluster. Subsequently, the two clusters with the smallest distance between one another are merged, with the process repeating itself until all clusters are joined into one. This gradual fusing of the groups results in a visual representation of patterns hidden in the data, typically in the format of a heat map and dendrogram. A heat map consists of many small colored boxes, each illustrating the level of gene expression by degree of light intensity. Customarily, red spots indicate high expression; green spots indicate low expression. The dendrogram is a hierarchical tree with branches representing the degrees of similarity among the clusters, showing relationships among genes or samples that might have previously been unknown (Fig. 91.4).

If there is some previous knowledge about which samples should group together, such as cancer stage or length of survival, supervised methods that classify gene expression data represent a powerful alternative to unsupervised methods. The general process of classification is to train a classifier to recognize patterns from training data (a set of samples whose classification is already known) so that independent test data (new samples) can be accurately classified.

Machine learning classification techniques that have been used to analyze microarray data include approaches such as neural networks (ANN) and support vector machines (SVM). The ANN is a nonlinear machine learning paradigm modeled on how biological neural networks, such as the brain, learn and process information. An ANN is composed of large number of interconnected "neurons," each of which consists of a set of inputs, a processing element that evaluates these inputs, and a set of outputs. Each neural connection, or

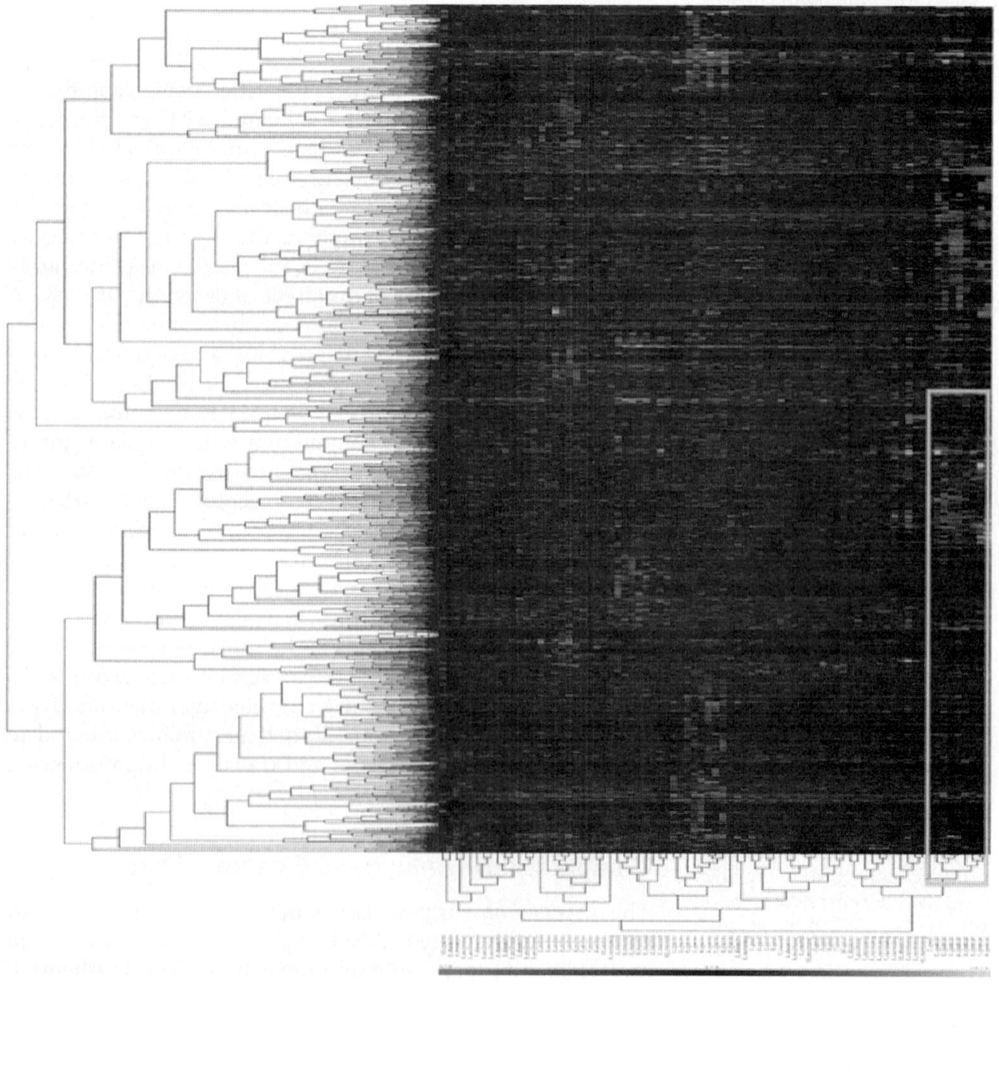

FIGURE 91.4. Typical heat map demonstrates the hierarchical clustering of genes (*left margin*) and tumors (*top margin*) can allow the discrimination of underlying patterns of gene expression correlating with subsets of experimental samples. In this figure, genes whose expression discriminates one tumor type from another are displayed, allowing the identification of multiple tumor types that actually are quite similar histologically. (Modified from Bloom G, Yang IV, Boulware D, et al.,[23] by permission of American Journal of Pathology.)

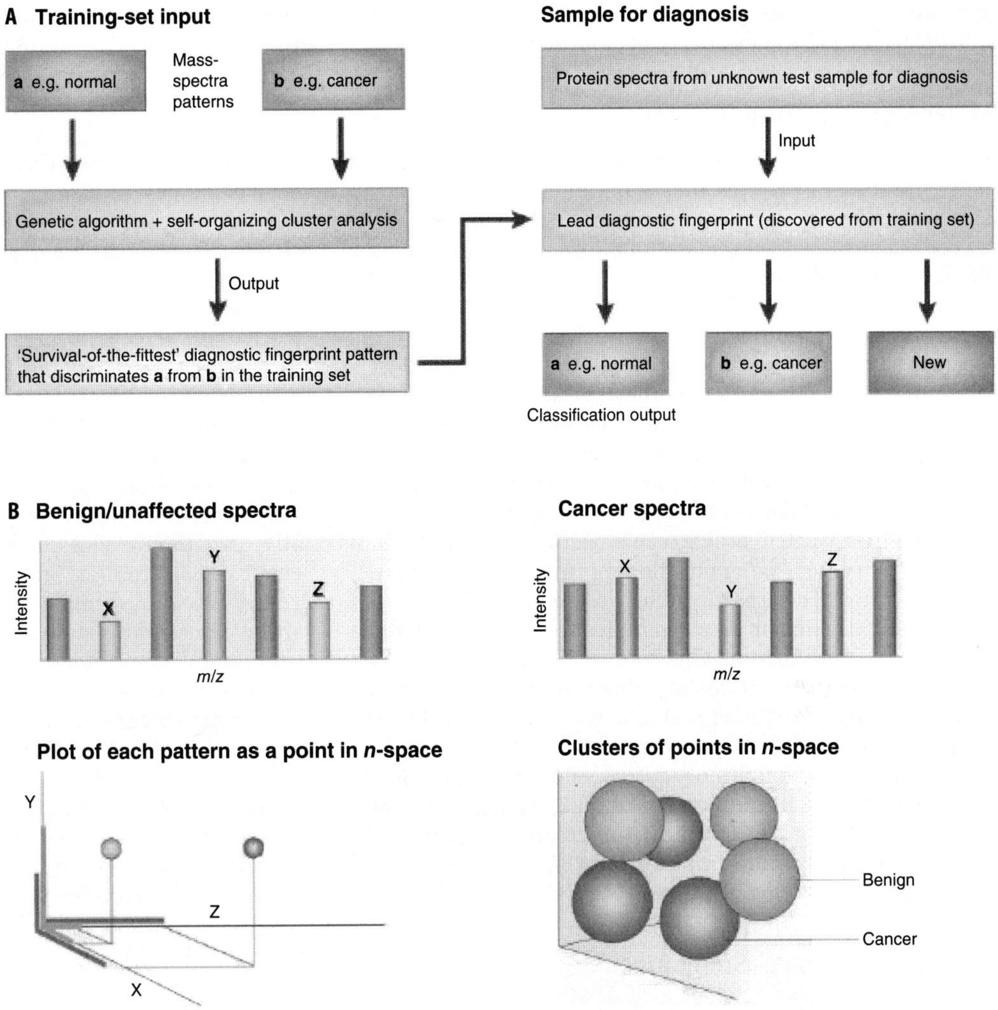

FIGURE 91.5. Analysis of training and test sets is a common and effective means to identify gene- and protein-based prognostic signatures. (From Petricoin EF, Zoon KC, Kohn EC, Barrett JC, Liotta LA. Clinical proteomics: translating benchside promise into bedside reality. By permission of Nature Reviews Drug Discovery 2002;1(9):683–695.)

"synapse," has a weight assigned to it, indicating the strength of the incoming signal to the receiving neuron. A set of training data, such as the gene expression profiles of samples with known cancer types, is initially fed to a small group of neurons within the network. When a neuron receives information from all its inputs, it calculates a weighted sum of these values and determines whether this sum meets a certain threshold value. If the threshold is met, the neuron "fires" to all other neurons to which it is connected, with each of these neurons calculating the sum of their inputs and "firing" in a similar fashion. Eventually, the information is transformed and propagated throughout the entire network until a set of neurons outputs the results, which are used to adjust the weights of the synapses in the network. In this way the ANN is trained to recognize complex patterns and characteristic features of the classes so that it can be used to classify new data into their appropriate categories.[10]

Another supervised learning technique that has been gaining popularity recently is the support vector machine (SVM). The SVM is a binary linear classifier that attempts to divide genes or samples into two classes by defining a mathematical plane separating members of a class from nonmembers. The mathematical plane is known as a "decision surface" that the SVM defines by learning. SVMs and other machine-learning techniques that analyze microarray data could prove extremely useful in the predictive analysis of cancer.[11]

The use of these sophisticated techniques of computational analysis has allowed researchers to analyze large and complex sets of genetic data in many areas of medical research. With adequately powered training and test sets, mathematical models can be formulated to predict clinical outcomes that are not otherwise possible with current pathological or other approaches. These approaches utilizing training and test sets to discern prognostic gene expression patterns are germane to both RNA-based microarrays as well as to mass spectrometry-based proteomics (Fig. 91.5).

Application of Genomics and Proteomics in Surgical Oncology

It is not surprising that oncology researchers have been taking advantage of these technologies and leading the development of genomic medicine. After all, cancer is a disease that is defined by a series of hereditary and somatic genetic alterations. Although the application of proteomics in oncology is still in its infancy as a consequence of complex technical challenges, genomics has become a widely used tool in the study of cancer. Using gene-profiling technologies, new diagnostic, prognostic, and therapeutic methods are being discovered and developed. These new technologies overcome the limitations of traditional cancer diagnosis with the promise of more accurate cancer classification, improved treatment stratification, and the discovery of new therapeutic targets.

Molecular Signature of Cancer

The advancement in molecular profiling represents a paradigm shift in the classification and diagnosis of cancer. Traditionally, histomorphology has been the cornerstone of cancer diagnosis. However, the quality and accuracy of the diagnosis depends on the subjective interpretations of the examiner and the morphological appearance of the tumor. Gene expression profiling offers an objective adjunct to the process. Furthermore, it also provides the sensitivity necessary to identify the genomic profile of each specimen, that is, a unique molecular signature that is particular to a particular pathological state and individual patient.

Analyzing biological specimens with microarrays creates a gene expression signature—a cluster of genes coordinately expressed by a particular cell type or during a particular biological activity. Molecular profiling using microarray technology has great potential as a systematic and unbiased approach for assigning particular tumor samples to previously defined pathological classification. Golub et al.[12] were among the first to demonstrate that patterns in gene expression data could be used to distinguish among different types of cancer. On the basis of gene expression profiling alone, it was possible to distinguish tumor samples of acute myeloid leukemia (AML) from acute lymphoblastic leukemia (ALL). Using a gene predictor derived from an analysis of microarray data from 38 known acute leukemia samples, 29 of 34 new independent leukemia samples were accurately classified.

Discovery of Novel Subgroups

As researchers begin to characterize the molecular fingerprints of various cancers, gene expression profiling has proven a valuable tool for pattern-based class discovery. An important advancement in the use of gene profiling in cancer classification is the ability to detect clinically distinct subgroups of a pathological condition within a previously defined disease. Often, surgeons encounter patients whose clinical course differs from their pathological or clinical staging. This diagnostic confusion may, on the whole, adversely affect the quality of patient care while unnecessarily increasing healthcare expenditure. Recent research suggests that such errors in prognostication are in part caused by the distinct subgroups that traditional classification methods have failed to identify.

The correlation between gene expression patterns and clinical outcomes was first demonstrated by Alizadeh et al.[13] in a cDNA microarray-based study of diffuse large B-cell lymphoma (DLBCL), the most common subtype of non-Hodgkin's lymphoma. DLBCL is also well known to be clinically heterogeneous: 40% of patients respond favorably to standard therapy, achieving a durable remission, whereas the remainder succumbs to the disease. This variability in clinical outcome was shown to reflect molecular heterogeneity within the tumors. Hierarchical clustering identified two molecularly distinct types of DLBCL with gene expression patterns indicative of different stages of B-cell differentiation. The investigators found one type had a gene expression pattern characteristic of germinal center B cells whereas the second type expressed genes normally induced during in vitro activation of peripheral blood B cells. Patients with the germinal center B cell-like DLBCL showed a significantly higher post-treatment survival rate (76% versus 16%) than patients with the peripheral blood B type, demonstrating that gene expression-based tumor classification can identify clinically significant subtypes of cancer. In fact, the clinical divergence between the two types was so remarkable that the researchers suggested that the two subtypes be regarded as distinct diseases.

Alizadeh et al.[13] also anticipated that such large-scale microarray data analyses would identify a small group of marker genes that could be used to stratify patients into molecularly distinct categories, thus improving the power and precision of clinical therapies. For example, by determining which patients are unlikely to respond to standard chemotherapy, more aggressive therapies, such as bone marrow transplantation, could be recommended early on. Additionally, as the two classes of DLBCL differentially expressed entire transcriptional modules consisting of hundreds of genes, new drugs might be developed to target the upstream signal-transducing molecules that are responsible for the expression of pathological transcriptional programs.

Similar findings have also been accomplished in solid tumor malignancies. A previously unrecognized taxonomy based on molecular profiling has been proposed by Bittner et al.[14] for discrimination of various types of melanomas. Through cluster analysis, they discovered a distinct subset of melanomas whose characteristic genes were differentially regulated in invasive melanomas that form primitive tubular networks in vitro, a feature of some of the most highly aggressive melanomas. Notably, no statistically significant association was found between the cluster groups and any clinical or histological variable, such as age, sex, biopsy site, or in vitro pigmentation. In their analysis, Bittner et al. generated a ranked list of individual genes (e.g., WNT5A, MART-1, pirin, HDHB) with the most power to define the clusters of the 19 samples studied, providing a sound molecular basis for the discovery of other clinically relevant melanoma subtypes and for greater understanding of the more aggressive forms of this cancer.

Molecular Classifiers and Predictors

Analysis of gene expression data with respect to cancer classification is divided into two broad tasks: class discovery and class prediction. Class discovery refers to the identification of previously unknown cancer subtypes and can be achieved through the use of unsupervised machine learning, such as hierarchical clustering. Class prediction refers to the assignment of unknown tumor samples to previously defined classes. Classification methods such as the supervised methods ANN and SVM discussed previously are generally used to predict the classes of unknown samples.[15] Using these methods, research work on breast, lung, colon, skin, kidney, soft tissue, parathyroid, prostate, and other conditions has led to many significant findings, demonstrating that molecular profiling can not only improve the accuracy of diagnosis but can also be used to predict therapeutic response and clinical outcome.

A prognostic system based on gene expression profiling can be constructed by identifying distinct molecular profiles with particular clinical behaviors and outcomes. The utilization of gene profiling improves the predictive power of clinical prognosis by correlating molecular fingerprinting to clinical data. Evidence of the potential and progress of this approach is illustrated by the clustering of breast cancer patients by Perou et al.[16] into two major subdivisions: an estrogen receptor-positive group, characterized by the relatively high expression of many genes expressed by breast luminal cells, and an estrogen receptor-negative group. It was discovered that the estrogen-positive group could be further subdivided into two groups, each with a distinctive expression profile and significantly different survival outcomes.

Further gene expression-based research into the clinical behavior of breast cancer was performed by van't Veer et al.[17] Using supervised clustering on microarray data taken from 117 breast cancer patients, van't Veer et al. identified a gene expression signature predictive of a short interval to distant metastases ("poor prognosis" signature) in patients without tumor cells in local lymph nodes at diagnosis. This breast cancer prognosis classifier consisting of 70 genes predicted to 83% accuracy the actual outcome of disease. Using the same 70-gene prognosis profile, van de Vijver et al.[18] classified a series of 295 consecutive patients with primary breast carcinomas as having a gene expression signature associated with either a poor prognosis or a good prognosis. The study evaluated the predictive power of the gene prognosis profile and found it to be a more powerful predictor of outcome than the traditional system based on clinical and histological criteria.

Similar success has also been found with other solid organ malignancies. Tomida et al.[19] created a prediction classifier based on the expression profiling of 50 patients with non-small cell carcinoma of the lung. The resultant classifier yielded 82% accuracy for forecasting survival or death 5 years after surgery. Furthermore, unsupervised hierarchical clustering analysis revealed for the first time the existence of clinically and biologically relevant subclasses of squamous cell carcinomas of the lung with marked differences in invasive growth and prognosis.

For the third most common cancer worldwide, prostate cancer, three previously unknown subclasses were discovered, with high-grade and advanced-stage tumors disproportionately represented among two of the subclasses. Expression levels of MUC1, highly expressed in the more aggressive tumor subgroups, and AZGP1, highly expressed in the non-advanced subgroup, were found to be strong predictors of tumor recurrence independent of tumor grade, stage, and preoperative prostate-specific antigen levels. The discovery of such differentially expressed genes as well as distinct molecular subtypes has great potential not only in uncovering new cancer subtypes but also in identifying potential biomarkers and therapeutic targets.[20]

Novel biomarkers and molecular targets identified by gene profiling can also be used to predict survival. For example, vascular cell adhesion molecule 1 (VCAM-1) was found to be the gene most predictive for patients with kidney cancer, whose clinical course can be highly variable, with many patients dying within 1 year of diagnosis and others living for years with slowly progressive disease. Survival for patients with metastatic renal cancer has been correlated with the expression of various genes based solely on the molecular profile of the primary kidney tumor.[21] More recently, Dave et al.[22] used gene expression profiling to construct a molecular predictor of survival length for the second most common form of non-Hodgkin's lymphoma, follicular lymphoma. The gene expression signatures used to construct the survival predictor, which included genes that encode T-cell markers (e.g., CD7 and STAT4) and genes highly expressed in macrophages (e.g., ACTN1 and TNFSF13B), allowed patients to be divided into four quartiles with widely disparate median lengths of survival (ranging from 13.6 to 3.9 years), independently of any clinical prognostic variables. Surprisingly, these signatures were derived from nonmalignant cells in the tumors, revealing the important role of the host immune system in the development of this type of malignancy and pointing the way to possible new targets for therapy.

Perhaps the most exciting demonstration of the potential for molecular signatures is the development of multitissue tumor classifiers. Recently, Bloom et al. demonstrated that an artificial neural network could be trained with microarray data to classify more than 500 specimens from 21 different types of cancer into their respective diagnostic categories with extremely high accuracy, indicating that a microarray-based tumor classifier can objectively complement existing histomorphological techniques in the accurate diagnosis of cancer origin. In fact, such a classifier might be the most promising method in solving the vexing problem, cancer of unknown primary (CUP).[23]

The utility of a molecular-based prognostic system can also be enhanced using epidemiological databases. Variables such as ethnicity, gender, age, social, economic, environmental, and behavioral factors can be integrated into the analysis and modeling to identify risk factors that will assist in devising new prevention strategies. Bhattacharjee et al.[24] have proposed a gene expression-based taxonomy of lung cancer. Using oligonucleotide microarrays, mRNA expression levels in 186 lung tumor samples were analyzed, including 139 adenocarcinomas resected from the lung. Clustering of expression data defined distinct subclasses of lung adenocarcinoma. One subclass, characterized by several neuroendocrine markers such as dopa decarboxylase and achaete-scute homologl, showed a significantly less favorable survival outcome than all other groups, whereas another subclass, characterized by the highest expression of type II alveolar pneumocyte markers, was associated with a more favorable clinical outcome. Interestingly, two adenocarcinoma subclasses were associated with lower tobacco smoking histories.

Novel Therapeutic Targets

A primary challenge of cancer treatment has been to create specific therapies that differentiate among cancer types which are genetically and clinically distinct, although similar in their histological and morphological manifestations. As patients diagnosed with the same type of cancer may differ in their genetic pathology, therapies that target specific cancer subtypes could minimize adverse side effects while maximizing efficacy. A natural dividend of gene profiling in cancer is the identification of genes and pathways involved in carcinogenesis and metastasis. For example, in the van't Veer et al.[17] study on breast cancer, genes significantly overexpressed in the poor prognosis signature include those involved in cell cycle, invasion, and metastasis, angiogenesis, and signal transduction (e.g., cyclin E2, MCM6, MMp9, PK428, and the VEGF receptor FLT1) and represent potential targets for the rational development of new cancer drugs. Furthermore, many biological variations in growth rate, in the activity of signaling pathways, and in the cellular composition of the tumors were all reflected in the corresponding differences in the gene expressions. Again, in the Perou et al. study on breast cancer, the expression of a large cluster of genes regulated by the interferon pathway (including STAT1) varied widely among the tumor samples. Such variation in biological activity also can be exploited as therapeutic targets.[16]

Personalized Medicine

The diagnosis and treatment of malignancies using gene expression profiling could achieve the ultimate promise of the practice of medicine—treating our patients as individuals. Rather than offering patients "one size fits all" therapy, wherein many patients are treated to benefit an unknown few, the molecular fingerprints of each patient can be used to identify cancer and guide clinicians to customize therapy based on predicted therapeutic response.[25] This approach begins with the collection of a patient's biological specimen for gene expression profiling. This molecular fingerprint will then be used to generate an objective diagnosis that can be paired with the clinical diagnosis for accuracy. Medications will be tailored according to how the patient is predicted to respond based on his or her gene expression profile. Potential adverse reactions toward particular therapy can also be avoided using the same one-patient, one-gene-chip approach.[1] This concept of personalized genomic medicine will lead to a more evidence-based, outcome-driven, and cost-effective cancer care.

References

1. Yeatman TJ. The future of cancer management: translating the genome, transcriptome, and proteome. Ann Surg Oncol 2003; 10(1):7–14.
2. Lander ES, Linton LM, Birren B, et al. Intitial sequencing and analysis of the human genome. Nature (Lond) 2001;409:860–921.
3. Venter JC, Adams MD, Myers EW, et al. The sequence of the human genome. Science 2001;291:1304–1351.
4. Schena M, Shalon D, Heller R, Chai A, Brown PO. Quantitative monitoring of gene expression patterns with a complementary DNA microarray. Science 1995;270:467–470.
5. Aebersold R, Mann, M. Mass spectrometry-based proteomics. Nature (Lond) 2003;422:198–207.
6. Steen H, Mann M. The ABC's (and XYZ's) of peptide sequencing. Nat Rev Mol Cell Biol 2004;5:699–711.
7. Kononen J, Bubendorf L, Kallioniemi A, et al. Tissue microarrays for high-throughput molecular profiling of tumor specimens. Nat Med. 1998;4(7):844–847.
8. Torhorst J, Bucher C, Kononen J, et al. Tissue microarrays for rapid linking of molecular changes to clinical endpoints. Am J Pathol 2001;159(6):2249–2256.
9. Eschrich S, Yeatman TJ. DNA microarrays and data analysis: an overview. Surgery (St. Louis) 2004;136(3):500–503.
10. Shimkets RA, LaRochelle WJ. The Oncogenomics Handbook: Understanding and Treating Cancer in the 21st Century. Totowa, NJ: Humana Press, 2004.
11. Quackenbush J. Computational analysis of microarray data. Nat Rev Genet 2001;6(2):418–427.
12. Golub TR, Slonim DK, Tamayo P, et al. Molecular classification of cancer: class discovery and class prediction by gene expression monitoring. Science 1999;286(5439):531–537.
13. Alizadeh AA, Eisen MB, Davis RE, et al. Distinct types of diffuse large B-cell lymphoma identified by gene expression profiling. Nature (Lond) 2000;403(6769):503–511.
14. Bittner M, Meltzer P, Chen Y, et al. Molecular classification of cutaneous malignant melanoma by gene expression profiling. Nature (Lond) 2000;406(6795):536–540.
15. Golub TR, Slonim DK, Tamayo P, et al. Molecular classification of cancer: class discovery and class prediction by gene expression monitoring. Science 1999;286:531–537.
16. Perou CM, Sorlie T, Eisen MB, et al. Molecular portraits of human breast tumours. Nature (Lond) 2000;406(6797):747–752.
17. van't Veer LJ, Dai H, van de Vijver MJ, et al. Gene expression profiling predicts clinical outcome of breast cancer. Nature (Lond) 2002;415:530–535.
18. van de Vijver MJ, He YD, van't Veer LJ, et al. A gene-expression signature as a predictor of survival. N Engl J Med 2002;347(25):1999–2009.
19. Tomida S, Koshikawa K, Yatabe Y, et al. Gene expression-based, individualized outcome prediction for surgically treated lung cancer patients. Oncogene 2004;23(31):5360–5370.
20. Lapointe J, Li C, Higgins JP, et al. Gene expression profiling identifies clinically relevant subtypes of prostate cancer. Proc Natl Acad Sci U S A 2004;101(3):811–816.
21. Vasselli JR, Shih JH, Iyengar SR, et al. Predicting survival in patients with metastatic kidney cancer by gene-expression profiling in the primary tumor. Proc Natl Acad Sci USA 2003; 100(12):6958–6963.
22. Dave S, Wright G, Tan B, et al. Prediction of survival in follicular lymphoma based on molecular features of tumor-infiltrating immune cells. *N Engl J Med* 2004;351:2159–2169.
23. Bloom G, Yang IV, Boulware D, et al. Multi-platform, multi-site, microarray-based human tumor classification. Am J Pathol 2004;164(1):9–16.
24. Bhattacharjee A, Richards WG, Staunton J, et al. Classification of human lung carcinomas by mRNA expression profiling reveals distinct adenocarcinoma subclasses. Proc Natl Acad Sci U S A 2001;98(24):13790–13795.
25. Evans W, Relling M. Moving towards individualized medicine with pharmacogenomics. Nature (Lond) 2004;429(6990):464–468.

92

Fundamentals of Cancer Cell Biology and Molecular Targeting

Steven N. Hochwald, David Bloom, Vita Golubovskaya, and William G. Cance

Despite recent advances in surgery, chemotherapy, and radiation treatment, survival of patients with advanced malignancy remains suboptimal. Fortunately, our understanding of the origins of cancer has changed dramatically during the past 25 years, owing in large part to the revolution in molecular biology that has changed all biomedical research. Powerful experimental tools are available to cancer biologists and have made it possible to uncover and dissect the complex molecular machinery operating inside normal and malignant cells. In addition, these tools have allowed researchers to pinpoint the defects that cause cancer cells to signal and proliferate abnormally.

Cancer cells acquire aberrations that favor their growth in the complex environments of living tissues; this includes their ability to recruit blood vessels into tumor masses, that is, the process of angiogenesis, their ability to invade and metastasize, and their ability to grow and divide indefinitely. Thanks to an increased understanding of the biological basis of cancer, investigators are turning to molecularly targeted therapy to further improve patient outcomes. Recent years have seen the advent of a new generation of agents that directly target alterations in the malignant cell itself or the cells supporting tumor growth. This specific targeted therapy should avoid the nonspecific toxicities that limit dosages that can be given with standard chemotherapy. Targeted therapies are changing the scope of anticancer care and challenging healthcare professionals to understand cancer at a cellular level. In this chapter, common molecular alterations that have been uncovered in cancer cells and recent advances in the development and clinical use of molecular targeted agents are discussed.

Signal Transduction

Loss of regulation of cell growth is the defining feature of benign and malignant neoplasms.[1] Both proliferation and suppression of cell growth are associated with overexpression of a family of proteins called tyrosine kinases. Signal transduction is the chemistry that allows communication at the cellular level, frequently through tyrosine kinases which phosphorylate other proteins on tyrosine residues, generally activating the target protein or providing binding sites for protein–protein interactions. These kinases are important regulators of intracellular signaling pathways. Perturbation and changes of protein–kinase signaling by mutations or other genetic alterations result in loss of regulation of kinase activity and malignant transformation.[1,2]

Approximately 90 tyrosine kinases have been identified, of which 58 are the transmembrane receptor type and 32 the cytoplasmic nonreceptor type. Tyrosine kinases transduce signals from both outside and inside the cell and play a central role in message transduction, acting as relay points for a complex network of interdependent signaling molecules that ultimately affect gene transcription within the nucleus. Strict regulation of tyrosine kinase activity controls the most fundamental processes of cells, such as the cell cycle, proliferation, differentiation, motility, and cell death or survival.

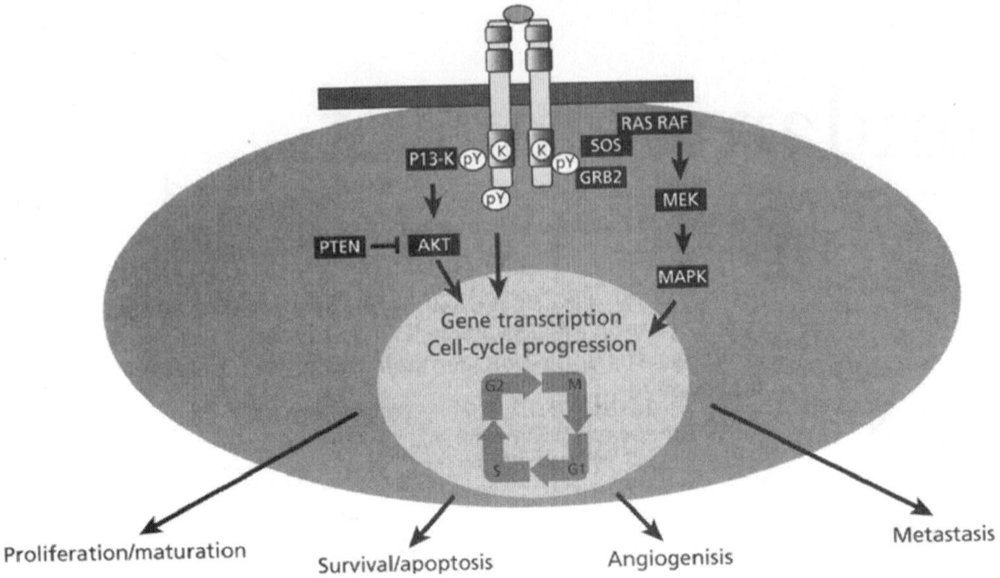

FIGURE 92.1. Epidermal growth factor receptor (EGFR) signal transduction and its effects on tumor cell growth and survival. EGFR signal transduction affects a variety of pathways involved in tumor cell survival. Binding of ligands activates EGFR dimerization and autophosphorylation on tyrosine residues, producing docking sites for signal transducers and adapter molecules. These factors then initiate signaling pathways that result in cell proliferation, differentiation, migration, adhesion, and transformation and inhibition of apoptosis. (Adapted from Baselga J. Eur J Cancer 2001;37:S16–S22.)

In tumor cells, it is common that key tyrosine kinases are no longer adequately controlled, and excessive phosphorylation sustains signal transduction pathways in an activated state.[1]

Growth Factors and Receptors

Usually, signaling pathways begin with binding of a ligand to a receptor, which results in stimulation of intrinsic activity of the receptor or of associated proteins. Receptors can have intrinsic enzymatic activity or can associate with protein kinases, guanine nucleotide exchange factors, and transcription factors. An example of a family of receptor tyrosine kinases are the EGF (epidermal growth factor) group, which consists of four related receptors: the EGFR (Erb I/HER1), Erb2 (HER2/*neu*), Erb3 (HER3), and ErbB4 (HER4). ErbB receptors are composed of an extracellular ligand-binding domain, a transmembrane domain, and intracellular tyrosine kinase domain with a regulatory carboxyl-terminal segment. A variety of EGFR family ligands drive the formation of homo- or heterodimeric complexes. Receptor activation by dimerization leads to its autophosphorylation and phosphorylation of several downstream intracellular substrates and activation of downstream signaling (Fig. 92.1).

The EGF receptor family are abnormally activated in a variety of tumor types. For example, both EGFR and HER-2/*neu* are overexpressed in breast tumors. The forced overexpression of either EGFR and HER-2/*neu* can transform murine fibroblasts into a deregulated, tumorigenic cell type. EGFR and HER-2/*neu* activation leads to elevated MAP kinase and phosphatidylinositol 3-kinase (PI3-K) recruitment. PI3-K suppresses apoptosis by activating the Akt antiapoptotic protein kinase. Through phosphorylation of a variety of kinases and transcription factors, the ERK kinases disable regulation of the cell cycle. Signaling through MAP kinases and PI3-kinases is a common feature of many tyrosine kinases[2] (see Fig. 92.1).

Activation of other growth factor receptors, such as platelet-derived growth factor receptor (PDGFR), fibroblast growth factor receptor (FGFR), vascular endothelial growth factor receptor (VEGFR), and insulin-like growth factor receptor (IGF-1R), is also important for intracellular signaling pathways involved in cell proliferation, migration, angiogenesis, and invasion.

Regulators of Cell Signaling

Ras-Raf-MAP Kinase

A major downstream signaling of the Erb family is the Ras-Raf-MAP kinase pathway. Activation of Ras and Raf initiates a multistep phosphorylation cascade leading to activation of mitogen-activated protein kinases (MAPKs) and ERK1/2 kinases. ERK1 and ERK2 regulate transcription of genes, associated with cell proliferation, survival, and transformation. As previously mentioned, another target of EGFR signaling is PI3-K and the downstream serine-threonine kinase, Akt. Another downstream pathway from EGFR is the PKC-Jak/Stat pathway. Activation of these pathways mediates cell proliferation, survival (apoptosis), motility, invasion, adhesion, and metastasis.

Phosphatidylinositol 3-Kinase

Phosphatidylinositol 3-Kinase (PI3-K) belongs to a family of lipid kinases defined by their ability to phosphorylate the 3′-OH group of the inositol ring in inositol phospholipids.[1] Classical PI3-K is a heterodimer consisting of a 85-kDa regulatory subunit and a 110-kDa catalytic subunit, containing two SH2 domains and an SH3 domain.[3] Activation of PI3-K and production of phosphoinotide-3 lipids stimulates a number of plekstrin homology-containing serine kinases. These activated serine kinases activate the Akt/PKB class of serine kinase, leading to antiapoptotic signaling.

Akt/PKB

A serine/threonine protein kinase B (PKB; also known as Akt) mediates many downstream events under the control of PI3-K. PKB/Akt is the cellular homologue of the transforming viral oncogene v-Akt and bears a significant homology to the cyclic AMP-dependent protein kinase A (PKA) and the protein kinase C (PKC). Akt contains a N-terminal PH domain, a central kinase domain with an activation loop Thr 308 phosphorylation site, and a conserved regulatory serine phosphorylation site, Ser473, near the C-terminus.[1] Numerous substrates of Akt fall into two main classes: regulators of apoptosis and cell cycle regulators. The Akt substrates involved in apoptosis include the Bcl-2 family member, Bad, Forkhead transcription factors, and the cyclic AMP response binding protein, CREB.[1,4] The antiapoptotic effects of Akt are mediated also by blocking glycogen synthase kinase-3 (GSK-3), cyclin D, and p21WAF1 pathways.

Focal Adhesion Kinase

Attachment to the underlying extracellular matrix provides cells both with a means of anchorage needed for traction during migration via a link to the actin cytoskeleton and also with intracellular structures that house membrane-associated signaling proteins. This action leads to the transmission of biochemical signals into the cell interior to induce multiple biological responses. Loss of regulation of the process of adhesion formation or turnover, or of downstream signaling, is likely to contribute to primary tumor development and/or tumor dissemination. Signaling via adhesion-associated kinases controls the changes that are necessary for cell migration, including regulation of cell–matrix adhesion turnover and coordination of remodeling of the actin cytoskeleton network.[5]

Focal adhesion kinase (FAK) is an adhesion-associated nonreceptor protein tyrosine kinase that plays key roles in regulation of the migratory process and has been implicated in key aspects of malignant cell behavior and in tumor development. FAK was discovered as a 125-kDa tyrosine-phosphorylated protein on Src-transformed cells. FAK is localized in the focal adhesions, sites of cell attachment to the underlying extracellular matrix. FAK contains a N-amino-terminal domain, central catalytic domain, and a carboxy-terminal domain. The carboxy-terminal region of FAK contains the focal adhesion targeting (FAT) domain, responsible for its localization to the focal adhesions. Alternative splicing of FAK results in autonomous expression of a carboxy-terminal part of FAK, called FRNK (FAK related non-kinase protein). An autophosphorylation (Y397) site is located in the N-terminal domain of FAK, and the kinase domain has Y576/577 tyrosines important for the catalytic activity of FAK. The C-terminal part of FAK has Y861 and Y925 tyrosines. A model has been proposed for FAK activation: integrins bind the N-terminal part of FAK and induce its autophosphorylation at Y397, which creates a high-affinity binding for the Src family kinases via a SH2 Src domain and for the regulatory p85 subunit of PI3-kinase. Src-FAK binding activates Src and enhances FAK phosphorylation at Y576/577 on carboxy-terminal sites. FAK tyrosine phosphorylation creates additional binding sites for other proteins, Grb2, Cas, and paxillin, that links integrin engagement to the Ras/MAP kinase pathway and causes downstream transcriptional and cytoskeletal changes.[2,5]

Abnormal Survival Signaling in Cancer

In tumor cells, EGFR overexpression or inappropriate activation can cause ligand-independent receptor dimerization and receptor activation. In some tumors, such as glioblastoma, mutant forms of the EGFR can result in activation of downstream signaling. EGFR was proposed as a target for cancer therapy about 20 years ago.[6] There are several drugs that inhibit EGFR signaling which have been studied in humans and are discussed next.

Mutations in PI3-K/Akt signaling pathways are causally involved in a high percentage of human malignancies. Akt is constitutively activated in a significant number of different types of cancer. Akt plays a role in cancer by stimulating cell proliferation and inhibiting apoptosis. Deregulation of PI3-K/Akt signaling can contribute to the malignant phenotype.

FAK is a point of convergence of a number of signaling pathways associated with cell adhesion, invasion, motility, mitogenesis, angiogenesis, and oncogenic transformation. FAK was found to be overexpressed in a number of tumors.[3] Introduction of antisense oligonucleotides or the dominant-negative C-terminal part of FAK leads to cell detachment and apoptosis. Thus, deregulated FAK could affect the ability of cancer cells to die in response to cytotoxic drugs.

Invasion and Metastases

Cancer cell invasion and metastasis are both hallmarks of tumor malignancy. Invasion and metastasis depend on the "cross talk" between the invaders and host cells.[7] The molecular analysis of invasion and metastases cellular activities include cell–cell adhesion, cell–extracellular interactions, migration, and signal transduction pathways.

Invasive Phenotype

The term *invasion* means penetration of cells into neighboring tissues and their occupation.[7] The acquisition of invasive phenotype requires changes in cell–cell and cell–extracellular matrix contacts. The transition from a benign (noninvasive) to an invasive, malignant phenotype requires reprogramming of cells, known as epithelial-mesenchymal transition (EMT).[8] To trigger EMT, cells need to activate different signal transduction pathways (Src, Ras/MAPK, PI3K, Rho).[8] Activation of major signaling pathways leads to transcriptional changes in the nucleus, changes in cellular adhesion, and cytoskeletal remodeling. Among important transcription factors that control EMT are the Jun/Fos transcription complex and Snail, Slug, and Ets transcription factors downstream of the Ras pathway (Fig. 92.2).

Cells must progress through a multistep process of invasion to metastasize. This process includes (1) invasion of cells from the tissue where the cancer has originated, into the surrounding tissues; (2) entry into the blood or lymph system; 3) transport through circulation; (4) exit from circulation at the

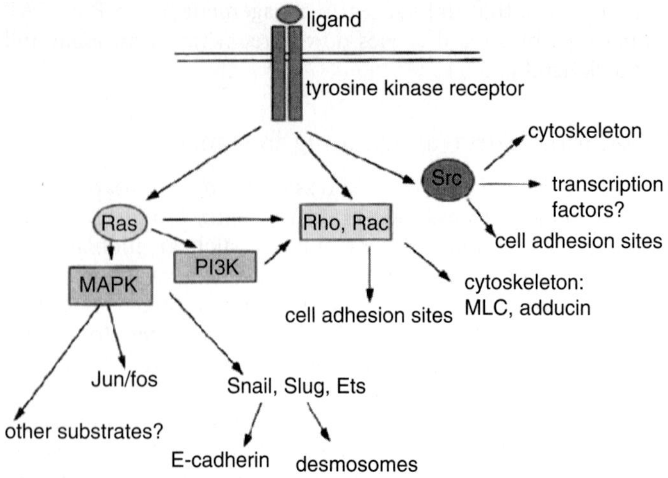

FIGURE 92.2. Signaling induced during epithelial-mesenchymal transition. Ligand-induced dimerization of tyrosine kinase receptor induces activation of several signaling pathways, causing changes in cell adhesion, cytoskeleton and gene induction. MLC, myosin light chain. (Adapted from Boyer B, Valles AM, Edme N. Induction and regulation of epithelial-mesenchymal transitions. Biochem Pharmacol 2000;60:1091–1099.)

potential metastasis site; and (5) invasion into the tissues of the occupied organ.[7]

Cell–Cell Adhesion and Invasion

Epithelial cells interact with each other via four types of junctions: adherens junctions, tight junctions, desmosomes, and gap junctions.[7] Adherens junction and desmosomes junctions are the main adhesive junctions that give the cells mechanical strength.[8] The main adhesion receptors of these junctions are cadherins (predominantly E-cadherin), and they link epithelial cells to the actin and intermediate filament cytoskeleton. Expression of E-cadherin is downregulated in most epithelial cancers. Tight junctions constitute morphological and functional boundaries between the apical and basolateral cell-surface domains, maintaining cell-surface polarity. The tight junctions restrict intermixing of apical and basolateral plasma membrane components. Tight junctions contain different membrane proteins, such as claudins and occludins. However, gap junctions are communicating junctions between cells and are formed of connexins. Connexins assemble into connexons (hemichannels that link cytoplasm of neighboring cells by forming intercellular channels).

All adhesion complexes have the same structure: different transmembrane components that interact with ligands outside of the cells (extracellular matrix components, such as fibronectin, collagen, or components of neighboring cells by homotypic and heterotypic interactions) and inside in the cytoplasm with large multiprotein complexes, signal transduction proteins, cytoskeletal proteins, and regulatory proteins.[9]

Adherens junctions and desmosomes have main adhesion receptors, cadherins, and also secondary types of receptors, nectins linked to the actin cytoskeleton. The predominant cadherin, E-cadherin, recruits β-catenin dimers and p120 catenin. The catenins belong to the family of armadillo proteins that have a similar structural domain, armadillo repeats, and are named after the *Drosophila* gene armadillo. β-Catenin is a multifunctional protein that regulates gene expression. One of the regulators of β-catenin is the Wnt/Wingless growth factor signaling pathway.[9]

In many cases, investigators have found a direct correlation between increased in vitro cell–cell adhesion and lack of invasion. Downregulation of adhesion proteins has been shown to correlate with invasion and metastasis in some human cancers. In prostate, head, and neck cancer, migration of epithelial cells was correlated with the loss of E-cadherin.[7]

Cell–Extracellular Interactions and Invasion

Integrins are the main mediators of signal transduction from the extracellular matrix to the cell. Integrins control many cellular activities, such as adhesion, migration, proliferation, differentiation, and survival. Integrins are composed of two membrane-spanning polypeptides, α- and β-subunits. The particular α/β pairing specifies the ligand-binding ability of integrins. Several extracellular molecules are recognized by more than one integrin. Epithelial cancer cells tend to express fewer integrins. Invasive cells leave their natural extracellular environment above the basement membrane and arrive in a completely different extracellular environment in the stroma. When these cells fail to turn on survival pathways, they undergo a detachment-induced apoptosis called anoikis.[10,11]

One important pathway initiated by integrins involves activation of focal adhesion kinase (FAK). Cell–substrate attachment, mediated by binding of integrin extracellular domains with the extracellular matrix, causes clustering of integrins, recruitment to the focal adhesion complexes, and phosphorylation of FAK, which is essential for downstream signaling from the extracellular matrix to the actin cytoskeleton. Activation of FAK involves its autophosphorylation at Tyr 397, which is recognized by the SH2 domain of Src-family tyrosine kinase members.[12] Src members phosphorylate other tyrosine residues of FAK, creating binding sites for other focal adhesion proteins. FAK is a nonreceptor tyrosine kinase, and signaling through FAK is important in regulation of several cellular functions, such as cell spreading, migration, invasion, and survival.

Apoptosis

During the development of multicellular organisms, excess cells are produced that must be removed. Similarly, cells that have sustained irreparable damage must be eliminated. To this end, a tightly controlled and evolutionarily conserved process of programmed cell death, apoptosis, has been established.

Apoptosis is distinct from necrosis. When cells die a necrotic death they rupture, releasing their contents into the extracellular space, which can adversely affect neighboring cells. Apoptosis, on the other hand, results in an orderly disassembly of the cell. During apoptosis, the nuclear chromatin is condensed and the nucleus is fragmented. The entire cell is then divided into membrane-bound bodies that are phagocytized. This process leaves no trace of the apoptotic cell.

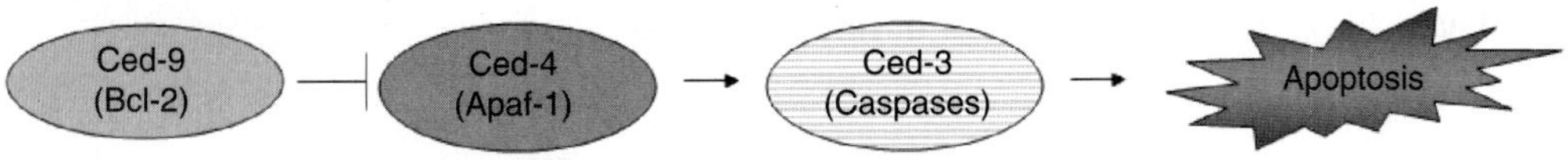

FIGURE 92.3. Regulation of apoptosis in *Caenorhabditis elegans*. Ced-4 activates the protease Ced-3, leading to cell death. Cell death can be inhibited by Ced-9. The mammalian homologues of the *C. elegans* genes are shown in *parentheses*.

Genetics of Cell Death

The study of *Caenorhabditis elegans* was instrumental in defining the genetic pathways that participate in programmed cell death. *C. elegans* was a very attractive model system because the fate of all 1090 cells generated during development has been determined. Of the 1090 cells, 131 die. Two genes, *ced* (cell death abnormal)-*3* and *ced-4*, were shown to be necessary for the death of all 131 cells.[13] Inactivation of either gene results in the survival of all 131 cells that would normally die.

Both *ced-3* and *ced-4* have mammalian counterparts. *ced-3* is a cysteine protease homologous to caspase 1.[14,15] *ced-4* is homologous to apoptotic protease-activating factor-1 (Apaf-1), which activates caspases in a cytochrome *c*-dependent manner.

Another gene, *ced-9*, represses cell death by inhibiting *ced-4*. Loss of *ced-9* function results in rampant cell death, whereas overexpression represses cell death. *ced-9* is a homologue of the mammalian antiapoptotic gene Bcl-2.[16–18] The structure and function of these genes have been so well conserved evolutionarily that expressing Bcl-2 in *C. elegans*, lacking *ced-9* activity, rescues them from cell death.

The pathway leading to cell death in *C. elegans* is very simple. Apoptosis is carried out by a *ced-3*. *ced-3* activity is regulated by *ced-4*, which is inhibited by *ced-9* (Fig. 92.3).

Extrinsic and Intrinsic Pathways of Caspase Activation

Caspases are the main effector molecules of apoptosis, although it should be noted that several caspase-independent cell death mechanisms have been reported.[19] Caspases comprise a family of cysteine proteases that cleave specific substrates after aspartic acid residues.[20–22] They are produced as proenzymes that contain three domains separated by aspartic acid residues: N-terminal prodomain, large subunit, and small subunit (Fig. 92.4). Caspase activation requires proteolytic cleavage of the domains, followed by formation of a heterotetramer of two identical large subunits and two identical small subunits. Caspases can cleave themselves and other caspases, resulting in an amplification of the apoptotic signal.

Apoptotic signaling leads to the activation of caspases through two pathways: an extrinsic pathway activated by death receptors, and an intrinsic pathway activated when cytochrome *c* is released from the mitochondrial membrane. Death receptors are activated when bound by their ligands, such as tumor necrosis factor-α (TNF-α), Fas, or TNF-related apoptosis-inducing ligand (TRAIL). Once activated, the receptors recruit adaptor proteins such as TNF receptor-associated death domain protein (TRADD), Fas-associated death domain protein (FADD), and receptor interacting protein (RIP).[23–26] These adaptor proteins then bind the death effector domain (DED) of caspase-8, leading to the activation of caspase-8, an initiator caspase (Fig. 92.5). Caspase-8 then activates the effector caspases, resulting in apoptosis.

The intrinsic pathway is activated by stress signals such as oxidative-stress, DNA damage, and changes in cell homeostasis. The mediators of these signals are the Bcl-2 family of proteins. The Bcl-2 family members regulate the permeability of the mitochondrial membrane and release of cytochrome *c*. It is a change in the ratio of the antiapoptotic family members, such as Bcl-2 and Bcl-xl, to the proapoptotic family members, such as Bax, Bak, Bid, and Bad, that results in release of cytochrome *c*.[27,28] Once in the cytoplasm, cytochrome *c* binds to the adaptor protein Apaf-1. This complex, known as the apop-

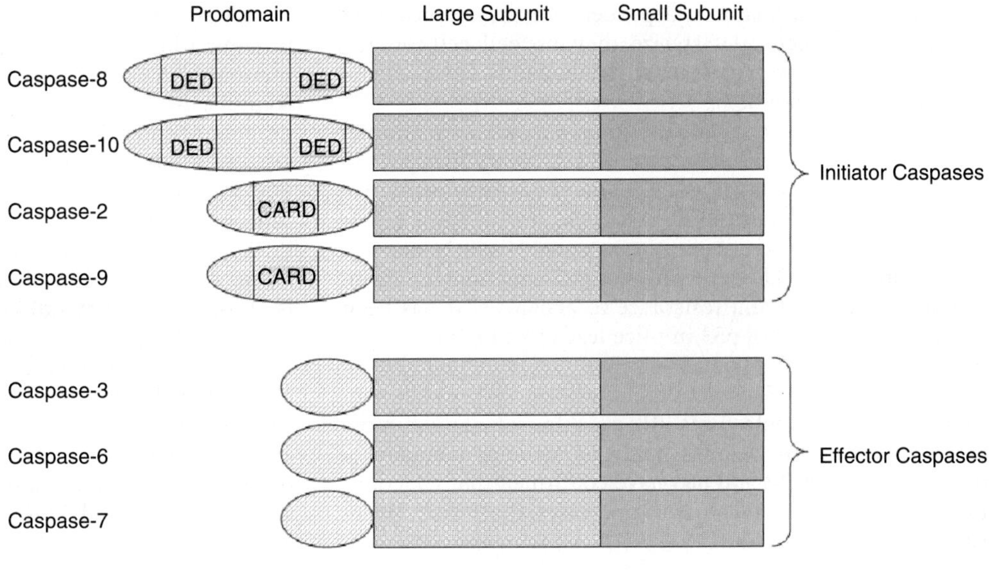

FIGURE 92.4. Caspase family of cysteine proteases. The caspases are synthesized as inactive pro-caspases that must be processed to be active. They are cleaved into three domains: the pro domain, large subunit, and small subunit. The initiator caspases contain death effector domains (*DED*) or the caspase activation and recruitment domain (*CARD*), which aid in transduction and activation of the apoptotic signal.

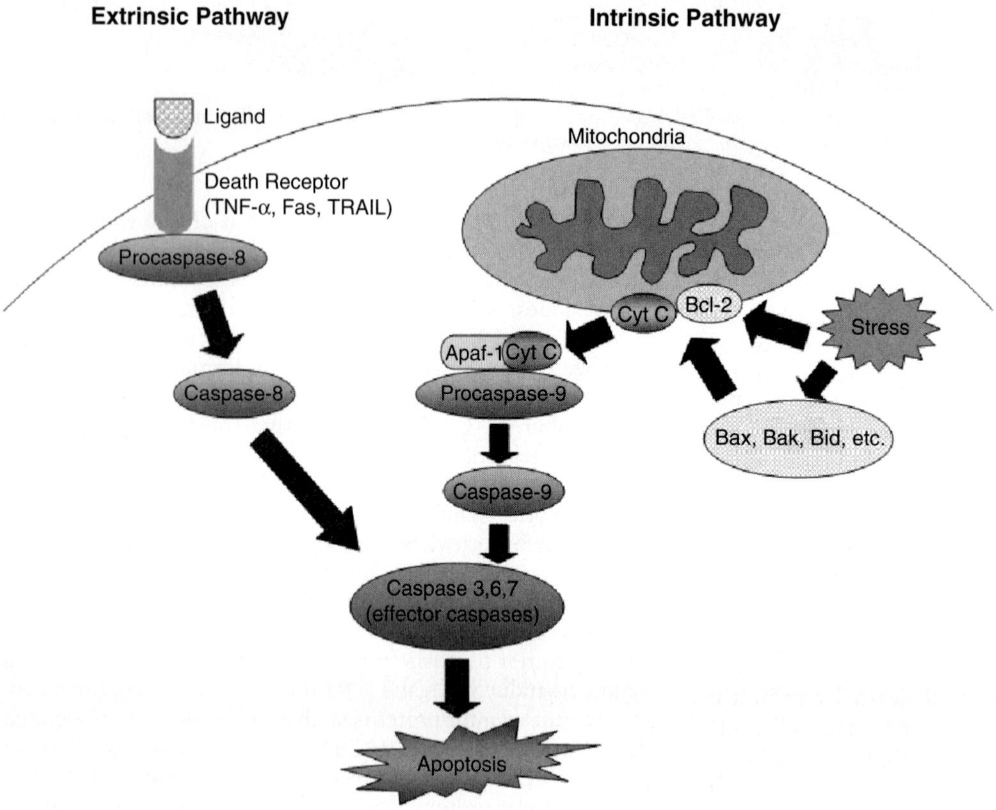

FIGURE 92.5 Extrinsic and intrinsic pathways of caspase activation. The extrinsic pathway is activated when a death receptor binds its ligand. Pro-caspase-8 is recruited to the receptor by interaction with its death effector domain (DED) and is cleaved into its subunits and activated. Caspase-8 then activates the effector caspases initiating apoptosis. The intrinsic pathway is activated when a stress signal results in cytochrome *c* release from the mitochondria; this leads to the formation of a complex containing cytochrome *c*, Apaf-1, and pro-caspase-9 (the apoptosome). The apoptosome activates caspase-9, which in turn activates caspase-3, initiating apoptosis.

tosome, activates procaspase-9. Caspase-9 then activates the effector caspases, resulting in apoptosis (see Fig. 92.5).

Loss of Normal Apoptosis in Cancer

Tumorigenesis requires several genetic alterations that lead to both an increase in cell proliferation and a decrease in apoptosis. The inhibition of apoptosis is critical for the survival of tumor cells because tumors grow quickly and can outpace the ability of the existing vasculature to provide nutrients. These cells would undergo apoptosis if the apoptotic machinery were not inhibited. Furthermore, the ability of tumors to metastasize is dependent on the inhibition of apoptosis. When cells metastasize, they lose cell–cell contact, a condition that normally leads to detachment-induced apoptosis, known as anoikis.

One of the most frequently mutated genes in human cancers is the tumor suppressor gene, p53. Wild-type p53 serves as a "guardian of the genome" by detecting DNA damage and either halting the cell cycle and allowing repair of the damaged DNA, or by initiating apoptosis if the damage is too extensive.[29] Therefore, loss of p53 function results in genomic instability and resistance to apoptosis. It has been shown that deletion of p53 in mice leads to a high incidence of spontaneous tumors at a young age.[30]

Another tumor suppressor that is often mutated in human cancers is the retinoblastoma (RB) gene. In fact, many tumors carry mutations in both RB and p53. Studies using mice deficient for both RB and p53 have confirmed that concomitant loss of these two proteins increases the formation of tumors.[31]

The Bcl-2 family is also implicated in the resistance of tumor cells to apoptosis. Cells lacking both proapoptotic Bcl-2 family members Bak and Bax are resistant to many apoptotic stimuli including staurosporine, ultraviolet radiation, and growth factor deprivation.[32] The importance of Bax in preventing tumors has been supported by the finding that it is inactivated in more than half of microsatellite mutator phenotype class of colon tumors.[33]

Upregulation of Antiapoptotic Signals: NF-κB and Bcl-2

NF-κB is a transcription factor involved in immunity and inflammation[34,35] as well as in cell proliferation and transformation.[36,37] More recently, the importance of NF-κB in tumorigenesis, by inhibition of apoptosis, has been realized.[38–41] Because of the role of NF-κB in cell proliferation and apoptosis, and the fact that many human cancers express constitutively activated NF-κB,[42] it could be an important target for cancer therapy.

Under normal conditions, NF-κB is retained in the cytoplasm by the inhibitor of NF-κB (IκB). Upon stimulation, IκB is phosphorylated by IκB kinase (IKK); this results in the degradation of IκB by the proteasome. NF-κB then translocates to the nucleus and induces the expression of genes that inhibit both intrinsic and extrinsic apoptotic pathways (Fig. 92.6). These genes include the cellular inhibitors of apoptosis (cIAPs), which bind to and inhibit caspases 3 and 7 and prevent the activation of procaspases 6 and 9; TNF receptor-associated factor 1 (Traf1) and Traf2, which are involved in recruiting cIAPs; and caspase 8-FADD-like IL-1β-converting enzyme

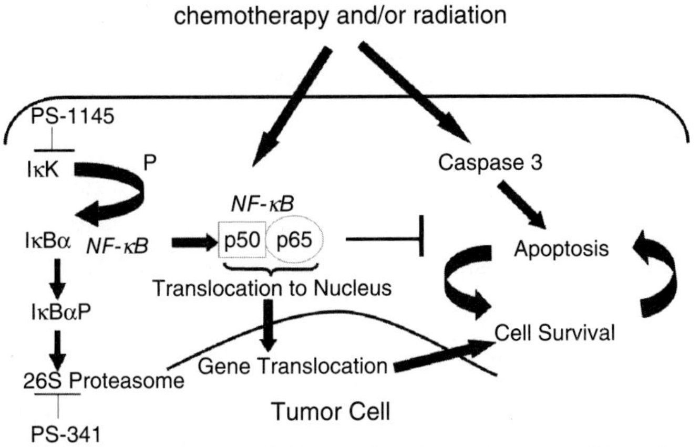

FIGURE 92.6. Activation of NF-κB by chemotherapy and/or radiation. Translocation of NF-κB subunits to the nucleus results in gene transcription leading to enhanced activation of antiapoptotic pathways. Inhibition of proteasome activity (via PS-1145 or PS-341) leads to increased stabilization of the IκBα–NF-κB complex and reduced activation of NF-κB.

inhibitory protein (cFLIP). This explanation is a very simplified view, and NF-κB biology and interactions are detailed elsewhere.[43]

Another target of NF-κB may be the Bcl-2 family. As stated before, the balance of pro- and antiapoptotic Bcl-2 family members is critical for cell survival or entry into apoptosis. Elevated levels of Bcl-X_L and Bcl-2, as well as other antiapoptotic family members, have been found in many human tumors.[37] It is known that inducers of NF-κB increase the expression of the antiapoptotic family member Bcl-X_L.[44,45] Although direct regulation of Bcl-2 by NF-κB has not been shown, B cells deficient in certain NF-κB family members have aberrant Bcl-2 expression.[46] It is clear that in some instances constitutive activation of NF-κB might lead to dysregulation of the Bcl-2 family. However, the Bcl-2 family can be dysregulated by other mechanisms such as increased copy of number of genes, gene deletions, or aberrant regulation by other signal transduction pathways.[27,28]

Angiogenesis

In 1971, Judah Folkman first published the hypothesis that a solid tumor and capillary endothelial cells might have a reciprocal growth relationship.[47] His hypothesis was correct. It is now known that a developing solid tumor will not grow to more than a few cubic millimeters without the formation of new vessels to supply the tumor with blood.[48] Folkman also hypothesized that drugs that could prevent angiogenesis in tumors might be effective in the treatment of cancer. He coined the term "antiangiogenesis" to define this type of effect.

Angiogenesis requires multiple steps. It starts with the degradation of the basement membrane surrounding the capillaries and is followed by migration of endothelial cells into the surrounding stroma. Finally, the cells proliferate and reorganize into vessels that join with the existing vasculature.[49] Preventing angiogenesis as a treatment for disease might appear to be risky, because a person, as much as a tumor, needs blood vessels for survival. However, endothelial cells in normal individuals are quiescent and divide only once every couple of years. Furthermore, endothelial cells that are stimulated to divide by a tumor act very differently from endothelial cells stimulated to divide by other processes such as wound healing. Tumor-induced neovascularization is disordered and lacks many of the features of normal vessels that provide structure and support, resulting in vasculature that is weak and "leaky."[50] These properties make tumor vasculature an attractive target for therapy. Drugs that either block the formation of these vessels or attack newly formed tumor vasculature are currently in clinical trials and have little effect on existing vessels.

Mediators of Angiogenesis

The process of angiogenesis is quite complex. In normal endothelial cells, there is a balance of positive and negative regulators of angiogenesis. Activators of angiogenesis include acidic and basic fibroblast growth factors (aFGF and bFGF), angiogenin, estrogen, and vascular endothelial growth factor (VEGF). Inhibitors of angiogenesis include thrombospondin-1, 16-kDa prolactin, interferon-α/β, platelet factor-4, endostatin, and angiostatin.[51] The angiogenic "switch" seen in tumor vasculature is a result of a change in the balance of these regulatory factors; it may be caused by a downregulation of angiogenesis inhibitors, or an upregulation of endothelial growth factors/angiogenesis activators, or both.[52] Once the endothelial cells are stimulated to proliferate, they begin production of proteases that subsequently degrade the endothelial basement membrane and allow the infiltration of the new vessels into the stroma.[48] These proteases include urokinase, collagenase, and the matrix metalloproteinases (MMPs).[53]

Endogenous Inhibitors of Angiogenesis

Endostatin and angiostatin are naturally occurring angiogenesis inhibitors. Angiostatin is a 38-kDa fragment of plasminogen.[54] Endostatin is a 20-kDa fragment of collagen XVIII. It had been observed that a growing tumor could suppress the growth of its metastases. Folkman's group implanted a Lewis lung carcinoma subcutaneously in the rat, and it was able to inhibit the growth of distant metastases. They then removed the primary tumor, and the metastases grew. When samples of the animals' urine were tested, the inhibitory activity copurified with a 38-kDa protein, angiostatin.[55]

There are many other endogenous inhibitors of angiogenesis, including interferon-α/β, interleukin 1, interleukin 6, interleukin 12, platelet factor 4, prolactin fragment, thrombospondin 1, -2, and tissue inhibitors of metalloproteinases (TIMPs). Many of these, as well as inhibitors of many proangiogenic factors, are being exploited as potential cancer therapies.[56]

Prognostic Significance of Angiogenesis in Tumors

Highly vascularized tumors usually grow quickly whereas benign neoplasms tend to be poorly vascularized and grow slowly.[57] Highly vascularized tumors also have a higher propensity to become metastatic,[58] which could result from the "leaky" nature of the tumor neovasculature.

Many studies have measured the microvessel density of surgically resected tumors. These studies have shown an inverse relationship between microvessel density (angiogenesis) and patient prognosis.[59–62] Other studies have tested the relevance of using secreted angiogenic factors such as VEGF or MMPs as prognostic factors.[63,64] Although the results are not always consistent, it appears that the presence of these factors may have negative prognostic value in predicting survival.

TABLE 92.1. HER1/EGFR Overexpression in Human Solid Tumors.

Tumor type	*HER1/EGFR expression rate*	*Reference*
NSCLC	40%–80%	66–68
Colon	25%–77%	69, 70
Ovarian	35%–70%	69, 71, 72
Breast	14%–91%	73–75
Pancreatic	30%–50%	69, 76

Molecular Targets for Cancer Therapy

A new understanding of genetics and tumor biology has allowed for the development of novel approaches for the targeted treatment of cancer. These innovative strategies herald a promising era of hope for oncologists and their patients, particularly in the treatment of solid tumors, which traditionally have a poor prognosis and are refractory to conventional therapy.

Agents that Target Egfr

The human epidermal growth factor receptor (EGFR), HER, family of receptor proteins play an important role in tumorigenesis and progression of disease.[65] HER1/EGFR and HER2 are the most widely studied HERs. In many cancers, HER1/EGFR expression is abnormal or upregulated, indicative of a possible role in tumorigenesis (Table 92.1).[66–76] These proteins have formed the basis of extensive and growing drug development programs in both public and private research companies.

A range of potential therapeutic targets exists within the HER signaling system, both inside and outside the cell. Monoclonal antibodies and tyrosine kinase inhibitors, acting extracellularly and intracellularly, respectively, comprise two classes of agents most advanced in clinical development. Monoclonal antibodies were the earliest approach to targeting HERs, binding to the extracellular portion of the HER molecule and preventing activation. Mouse monoclonal antibodies that inhibited these receptors were genetically engineered to contain human antibody motifs. Two examples are cetuximab (Erbitux), a HER1/EGFR-targeted monoclonal antibody (mAb) now in the late stages of clinical development in many cancers and approved for use in metastatic colorectal carcinoma, and the HER2-specific trastuzumab (Herceptin), already established in the care of breast cancer patients (Fig. 92.7).

Trastuzumab is the first HER-directed therapy to gain approval from the U.S. Food and Drug Administration (FDA) for the treatment of patients with metastatic breast cancer. In preclinical studies, trastuzumab has been demonstrated to downregulate HER2, lead to G_1 growth arrest and apoptosis, act as an angiogenic inhibitor, and have synergistic effect with doxorubicin, taxanes, vinorelbine, and flavopiridol in breast cancer cells.[77–80] Response rates to trastuzumab given as a single agent ranged from 12% to 40%, in part depending on the method used to determine HER2 status and prior treatment received.[79–81] In an important study, Slamon et al. showed that combining trastuzumab with either doxorubicin plus cyclophosphamide (AC) or single-agent paclitaxel produced higher response rates and survival times than chemotherapy alone.[82] However, severe cardiac dysfunction was seen with combinations of AC and trastuzumab; this led to the development of trastuzumab-based combinations that do not contain doxorubicin. Perhaps the most promising applications of trastuzumab mAb therapy will be in the adjuvant setting. Large randomized trials are being performed by the cancer cooperative groups in node-positive HER2 breast cancer patients. In these studies, trastuzumab is being added

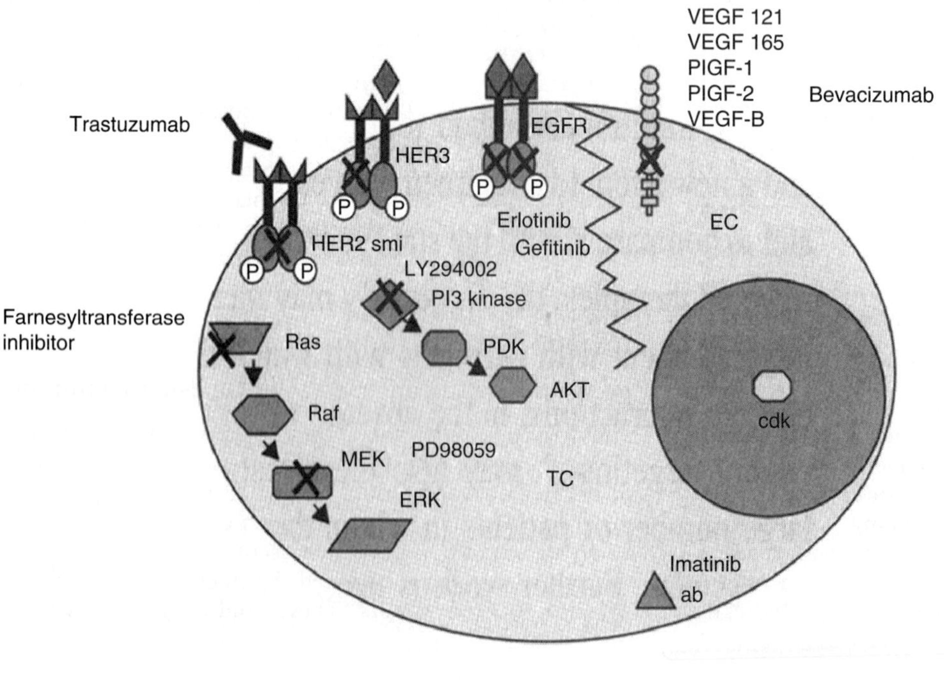

FIGURE 92.7. Schematic of tumor cell (*TC*) and endothelial cell (*EC*) signaling pathways targeted by select molecular-targeted therapies. *VEGF*, vascular endothelial growth factor; *PIGF*, placental growth factor. (Adapted from Slamon DJ. The future of ErbB-1 and ErbB-2 pathway inhibition in breast cancer: targeting multiple receptors. Oncologist 2004;9:1–3.)

TABLE 92.2. HER Tyrosine Kinase Inhibitors.

Inhibitor	*Binding*	*Specificity*	*Tumor types*	*Development phase*
Gefitinib (Astra Zeneca; Wilmington, DE)	Reversible	ErbB-1 TK	Locally advanced or metastatic NSCLC, head and neck, breast, ovarian, prostate, glioma, pancreatic, colorectal	Approved
Erlotinib (Genentech, Inc.; San Francisco, CA)	Reversible	ErbB-1 TK	NSCLC, head and neck, breast ovarian, prostate, pancreatic, colorectal, glioma	III
EKB-569 (Wyeth-Ayerst Labs, Inc.; St. Davids, PA)	Irreversible	ErbB-1/2 TK	NSCLC, breast, other ErbB-dysregulated solid tumors	I/II
CI-1033 (Pfizer Inc.; Groton, CT)	Irreversible	ErbB-1 to 4 TK	NSCLC, breast, other ErbB-dysregulated solid tumors	I/II
Lapatinib (GlaxoSmithKline; Research Triangle Park, NC)	Reversible	ErbB-1/2 TK	ErbB-dysregulated solid tumors	II

NSCLC, non–small cell lung cancer; TK, tyrosine kinase.

to the current chemotherapeutic regimen standard of care in an effort to improve response and survival.

On February 12, 2004, the FDA approved cetuximab (Erbitux; Imclone Systems, Inc.) for use in combination with irinotecan for the treatment of EGFR-expressing, metastatic colorectal carcinoma in patients who are refractory to irinotecan-based chemotherapy. This antibody was also approved for use as a single agent for the treatment of EGFR-expressing, recurrent metastatic colorectal carcinoma in patients who are intolerant of irinotecan-based chemotherapy. Cetuximab binds specifically to the EGFR on both normal and tumor cells and competitively inhibits the binding of EGF and other ligands, such as transforming growth factor-alpha. Binding of cetuximab blocks phosphorylation and activation of receptor-associated kinases, resulting in inhibition of cell growth, induction of apoptosis, and decreased matrix metalloproteinase and vascular endothelial growth factor production.

The data establishing the efficacy and safety of cetuximab were derived mainly from the results of a multicenter, randomized, controlled clinical trial conducted in 329 patients. These patients were randomized to received either cetuximab plus irinotecan (218 patients) or cetuximab monotherapy (111 patients). All patients had EGFR-expressing, recurrent, metastatic colorectal cancer. The overall response rate was 23% with a median duration of response of 5.7 months in the cetuximab plus irinotecan arm. The overall response rate was 12% with a median duration of response of 4.1 months in the cetuximab monotherapy arm. The median time to progression was significantly longer for patients receiving combination therapy (4.1 versus 1.5 months). The most common adverse events seen in patients receiving cetuximab plus irinotecan were acneform rash (88%), asthenia/malaise (73%), diarrhea (72%), nausea (55%), abdominal pain (45%), and vomiting (41%).[83]

Small molecule tyrosine kinase inhibitors (TKIs) are given orally and may be the most promising class of targeted agents currently in development. They block downstream signaling by inhibiting the intracellular portion of the target HER. Examples include gefitinib (Iressa) and erlotinib (Tarceva), which are both HER1/EGFR-targeted reversible TKIs (see Figure 92.7). Other TKIs can be irreversible and can have single, dual, or pan-HER specificity. TKIs are in varying stages of development, and several clinical trials studying their toxicity and efficacy are underway or have been completed (Table 92.2).

In phase II trials, gefitinib monotherapy has shown promising results in solid malignancies. In patients with non-small cell lung cancer (NSCLC), response rates (complete, partial, and stable disease) were 54% and 42% in those who had received prior chemotherapy (Table 92.3).[84–88] Despite these encouraging findings, two phase III trials involving a total of 2130 patients with untreated, advanced NSCLC, evaluating

TABLE 92.3.
Phase II Studies Evaluating Tyrosine Kinase Inhibitors in Solid Malignancies.

Drug	*Gefitinib*	*Gefitinib*	*Erlotinib*	*Erlotinib*	*Erlotinib*
Reference	84	85	86	87	88
Design	Double-blind, Randomized	Double-blind, Randomized	Open-label	Open-label	Open-label
No. of patients	209	216	124	34	57
Cancer type	Advanced NSCLC	Advanced NSCLC	HNSCC-refractory	Advanced ovarian cancer	Advanced NSCLC
Adverse events	Rash, GI	Rash, GI	Rash, diarrhea	Rash, diarrhea	Rash, diarrhea
Response and survival	CR/PR, 18%; CR/PR/SD, 54%;OS 7.6 months at 250mg/day	CR/PR, 12%; CR/PR/SD, 42%; OS 6.5 months at 250mg/day	PR, 6%; PR/SD, 46%	PR, 6%; PR/SD, 51%	CR/PR, 12%; CR/PR/SD, 51%; OS 8.4 months

CR, complete response; GI, gastrointestinal; HNSCC, head and neck squamous cell cancer; NSCLE, non-small cell lung cancer; OS, overall survival; PR, partial response; SD, stable disease.

gefitinib in combination with one of two standard chemotherapeutic regimens found no significantly greater survival associated with the addition of this TKI to chemotherapy, compared with chemotherapy plus placebo.[89,90] Of note, these phase III trial results also differ dramatically from data obtained from preclinical studies in murine models.[91] The cause for the lack of concordance between preclinical and clinical studies is not clear but could be different drug administration schedules or the inability to identify appropriate patient populations, that is, those with molecular target alterations that are important for the expression of the disease being treated. These failures emphasize the need for a better understanding of patient and disease characteristics that increase the likelihood of therapeutic response. In addition, a better understanding of how the targeted signaling pathways act individually and with one another in the pathogenesis of the disease being treated is necessary.

Agents that Target Bcr/Abl and c-Kit

Perhaps the most dramatic example demonstrating the potential of kinase-targeted therapy comes from chronic myeloid leukemia (CML). CML is characterized by constitutive activity of the Abl (Abelson) tyrosine kinase as a result of chromosomal translocation that produces the Bcr-Abl fusion protein. Because unrestricted tyrosine kinase activity was known to be the principal pathogenetic defect in CML, investigators tested the hypothesis that a small molecule signal transduction inhibitor (STI571) would target the neoplastic cells selectively in this disease. STI571 was discovered at Novartis Pharmaceuticals during a search for inhibitors of platelet-derived growth factor receptor. STI571 selectively inhibits specific tyrosine kinases, including Abl, Bcr-Abl, kit, and platelet-derived growth factor receptor.[92] STI571 induces growth arrest or apoptosis specifically in Bcr-Abl expressing hematopoietic cells with no obvious effects on normal cells or in cells transformed by other tyrosine kinase oncogenes.[93] Initial studies were done in patients with CML and demonstrated that STI571 treatment resulted in a complete response rate of approximately 90% in the chronic phase. Additionally, only a small percentage of patients had to discontinue therapy because of adverse events as toxicity from STI571 treatment was relatively uncommon.

Because of its ability to also inhibit the c-Kit receptor tyrosine kinase, STI571 has been shown to be an effective treatment for gastrointestinal stromal tumor (GIST), the most common mesenchymal neoplasm of the intestinal tract (see Chapter 99). GISTs have a gain-of-function mutation in the kit proto-oncogene. Normally, kit protein is activated only when its ligand binds to it and induces receptor dimerization, resulting in intracellular signaling and cell growth and survival. However, c-Kit is activated in GIST in the absence of its natural ligand, resulting in unopposed neoplastic proliferation.

The standard of care for patients with primary GIST without metastasis is surgical resection. However, even after complete resection of a primary GIST, most patients experience recurrence and eventually die of the disease. The 5-year survival rate after complete gross resection is approximately 50% and the median time to recurrence after resection of a primary GIST is 2 years. The site of first recurrence typically involves the liver, peritoneum, or both.[94] Before the development of STI571, recurrent GIST was treated with very limited success. GIST is refractory to chemotherapy, and in a phase II study, only 1 (5%) of 21 patients with metastatic GIST treated with doxorubicin, dacarbazine, mitomycin, cisplatin, and granulocyte-macrophage colony-stimulating factor had a therapeutic response.[95]

In February 2000, the first patient with metastatic GIST was treated with STI571. The patient's tumor rapidly responded with partial regression and a dramatic reduction in tumor uptake of [^{18}F]fluorodeoxyglucose on positron emission tomography.[96] Following this, two clinical trials in the United States and Europe were initiated. In a phase II trial of 36 patients with unresectable or metastatic GIST, STI571 demonstrated minimal toxicity and substantial activity, with a partial response rate of approximately 60%. The trial size was then expanded, and a total of 147 patients were randomly assigned to receive 400mg or 600mg STI571 daily. Overall, 79 patients (53.7%) had a partial response and 41 patients (27.9%) had stable disease. No patient had a complete response to the treatment. The median duration of response had not been reached after a median follow-up of 24 weeks after the onset of response. Early resistance to imatinib was noted in 20 patients (13.6%).[97] Of note, toxicity with STI571 was generally acceptable. There were a few patients who developed bleeding as a result of rapid tumor necrosis induced by the agent. The common side effects were diarrhea, periorbital edema, and fatigue. In the other trial performed by the EORTC, there was a 69% response (major and minor) in 36 patients (Table 92.4). Again, progression was observed in only a small percentage of patients.[97]

As experience with STI571 treatment of patients with metastatic GIST has grown, kinase mutations and response to treatment have been correlated. In one study, activating mutations of kit or platelet-derived growth factor receptor-alpha (PDGFRA) were found in 112 (88.2%) and 6 (4.7%) GISTs, respectively. Most mutations involved exon 9 ($n = 23$) or exon 11 ($n = 85$). In patients with GISTs harboring exon 11 kit mutations, the partial response was 83.5%, whereas patients with tumors containing an exon 9 kit mutation or no detectable mutation of kit or PDGFRA had partial response rates of 47.8% ($P = 0.0006$) and 0.0% ($P < 0.0001$), respectively. Patients whose tumors contained exon 11 kit mutations had a longer event-free and overall survival than those whose tumors expressed either exon 9 KIT mutations or had no detectable kinase mutation.[98] For those patients with tumors that are refractory to STI571 therapy, multitargeted tyrosine kinase inhibitors may prove beneficial. SU11248 is a pleiotrophic inhibitor with antitumor and antiangiogenic activity through targeting platelet-derived growth factor receptor, vascular endothelial growth factor receptor, kit, and FLT3. Preliminary results have shown clinical responses with the use

TABLE 92.4. Imatinib Response Rate in Metastatic Gastrointestinal Stromal Tumor (GIST) (400-mg Dose).

	U.S.-Finland	*EORTC*
N	147	36
Partial response (%)	54	69
Stable disease (%)	28	19
Progression (%)	14	11

EORTC, European Organization for Research and Treatment of Cancer.

of SU11248 in patients with GISTs that are resistant to STI571 therapy.[99]

In addition to its role in metastatic GIST, STI571 is being evaluated as an adjuvant therapy after complete resection of primary GIST because (1) the risk of recurrence after surgical resection alone is high, (2) conventional chemotherapy is ineffective in preventing or treating recurrent disease, and (3) STI571 has demonstrated considerable activity in metastatic GIST. It is possible that STI571 may have its greatest effect on survival when there is minimal disease, as is the case after complete gross tumor resection when only residual microscopic disease may exist. Because STI571 treatment in the setting of metastatic disease has not produced any complete responses, avoidance of recurrent disease is important. It is hoped that STI571 may prevent, or at least delay, recurrence and consequently prolong survival.[100]

Agents that Target VEGF

Virtually all existing anticancer drugs, and those in development, are designed to directly attack cancer cells by exploiting some property of the cancer cells that distinguishes them from normal cells. Antiangiogenic therapy is based on a fundamentally different approach: attacking a tumor's lifelines—its growing blood vessel supply—upon which tumor cells depend for oxygen and nutrients. Currently there is a large and diverse group of drugs being developed and tested as angiogenesis inhibitors, for example, monoclonal antibodies to VEGF, small molecule inhibitors of VEGF receptor-2 (which is expressed by activated endothelial cells of growing blood vessels and conveys proangiogenic signals into such cells after binding VEGF), or small peptide fragments of thrombospondin-1 (endogenous inhibitor of angiogenesis) (see Figure 92.7). In addition to specifically designed antiangiogenic drugs, evidence suggests that many other anticancer drugs that were not developed as angiogenesis inhibitors can actually express this activity. This group of antiangiogenic drugs include radiation, many chemotherapeutic agents, thalidomide, COX-2 inhibitors, and signal transduction inhibitors (Herceptin and STI571).

Bevacizumab is a recombinant humanized monoclonal antibody directed against vascular endothelial growth factor that has been recently studied in a variety of solid malignancies. When VEGF is targeted and bound to bevacizumab, it cannot stimulate the growth of blood vessels, thus denying tumors blood, oxygen, and other nutrients needed for growth (see Figure 92.7). Angiogenesis inhibitors such as bevacizumab have been studied in the laboratory for three decades, with the hope they might prevent the growth of cancer. A recent phase III randomized double blind study in 925 patients has demonstrated efficacy and safety when bevacizumab was added to irinotecan/5-fluorouracil/leucovorin chemotherapy as first-line therapy for metastatic colorectal cancer.[101] In this study, the addition of bevacizumab, compared to placebo, resulted in an improved response rate, survival benefit and time to progression. Median survival was increased by 4.5 months ($P = 0.00003$) and overall response increased by 10% ($P < 0.003$) in the bevacizumab arm. Relatively few side effects were demonstrated with the administration of bevacizumab, and most were related to mild increases in blood pressure that were easily controlled with oral antihypertensives. Of note, this is the first molecular targeted antiangiogenic product that has been proven to delay tumor growth and, more importantly, significantly extend the lives of patients. As a result, bevacizumab has been approved by the FDA as first-line treatment for metastatic colorectal cancer. However, other studies, including some in patients with breast cancer, have not demonstrated a beneficial effect with the addition of bevacizumab. At present, the role of antiangiogenic-targeted therapy in other solid malignancies is not known.

The application of targeted agents represents a new era in cancer therapeutics and is a major change in philosophy from the use of conventional chemotherapy and radiation treatment. The development of these novel compounds stems directly from our increasing understanding of the biological and molecular pathways of cancer. STI571 serves as a paradigm of targeted molecular therapy and represents a landmark in cancer therapeutics. The efficacy of this drug is the result of the inhibition of the single molecular defect at the center of the pathogenesis of CML and GIST. Other cancers are more complex and contain multiple genetic aberrations. Strategies designed to interfere with multiple molecular abnormalities will be necessary to impact on survival and are under development.

References

1. Blume-Jensen P, Hunter T. Oncogenic kinase signalling. Nature (Lond) 2001;411:355–365.
2. Craven RJ, Lightfoot H, Cance WG. A decade of tyrosine kinases: from gene discovery to therapeutics. Surg Oncol 2003;12:39–50.
3. Jones RJ, Brunton VG, Frame MC. Adhesion-linked kinases in cancer: emphasis on src, focal adhesion kinase and PI 3-kinase. Eur J Cancer 2000;36:1595–1606.
4. Lawlor MA, Alessi DR. PKB/Akt: a key mediator of cell proliferation, survival and insulin responses? J Cell Sci 2001;114:2903–2910.
5. McLean G, Avizienyte E, Frame MC. Focal adhesion kinase as a potential target in oncology. Expert Opin Pharmacother 2003;4:227–234.
6. Mendelsohn J, Baselga J. Status of epidermal growth factor receptor antagonists in the biology and treatment of cancer. J Clin Oncol 2003;21:2787–2799.
7. Mareel M, Leroy A. Clinical, cellular, and molecular aspects of cancer invasion. Physiol Rev 2003;83:337–376.
8. Boyer B, Valles AM, Edme N. Induction and regulation of epithelial-mesenchymal transitions. Biochem Pharmacol 2000;60:1091–1099.
9. Balda MS, Matter K. Epithelial cell adhesion and the regulation of gene expression. Trends Cell Biol 2003;13:310–318.
10. Frisch SM, Vuori K, Ruoslahti E, Chan-Hui PY. Control of adhesion-dependent cell survival by focal adhesion kinase. J Cell Biol 1996;134:793–799.
11. Ruoslahti E, Reed JC. Anchorage dependence, integrins and apoptosis. Cell 1994;77:477–478.
12. Rodriguez-Fernandez JL. Why do so many stimuli induce tyrosine phosphorylation of FAK? Bioessays 1999;21:1069–1075.
13. Sulston JE, Schierenberg E, White JG, et al. The embryonic cell lineage of the nematode *Caenorhabditis elegans*. Dev Biol 1983;100:64.
14. Cerretti DP, Kozlosky CJ, Mosley B, et al. Molecular cloning of the interleukin-1 beta converting enzyme. Science 1992;256:97–100.
15. Thornberry NA, Bull HG, Calaycay JR, et al. A novel heterodimeric cysteine protease is required for interleukin-1 beta processing in monocytes. Nature (Lond) 1992;356:768–774.

16. Yuan J, Shaham S, Ledoux S, et al. The *C. elegans* cell death gene ced-3 encodes a protein similar to mammalian interleukin-1 beta-converting enzyme. Cell 1993;75:641–652.
17. Hengartner MO, Horvitz HR. *C. elegans* cell survival gene ced-9 encodes a functional homolog of the mammalian proto-oncogene bcl-2. Cell 1994;76:665–676.
18. Vaux DL, Weissman IL, Kim SK. Prevention of programmed cell death in *Caenorhabditis elegans* by human bcl-2. Science 1992;258:1955–1957.
19. Leist M, Jäättelä M. Four deaths and a funeral: from caspases to alternative mechanisms. Nat Rev Mol Cell Biol 2001;2:589–598.
20. Thornberry NA, Lazebnik Y. Caspases: enemies within. Science 1998;281:1312–1316.
21. Earnshaw WC, Martins LM, Kaufmann SH. Mammalian caspases: structure, activation, substrates and functions during apoptosis. Annu Rev Biochem 1999;68:383–424.
22. Strasser A, O'Connor L, Dixit VM. Apoptosis signaling. Annu Rev Biochem 2000;69:217–245.
23. Chinnaiyan AM, O'Rourke K, Tewari M, Dixit VM. FADD, a novel death domain-containing protein, interacts with the death domain of Fas and initiates apoptosis. Cell 1995;81:505–512.
24. Chinnaiyan AM, Tepper CG, Seldin MF, et al. FADD/MORT1 is a common mediator of CD95 (Fas/APO-1) and tumor necrosis factor receptor-induced apoptosis. J Biol Chem 1996;271:4961–4965.
25. Hsu H, Xiong J, Goeddel DV. The TNF receptor 1-associated protein TRADD signals cell death and NF-kappa B activation. Cell 1995;81:495–504.
26. Stanger BZ, Leder P, Lee TH, et al. RIP: a novel protein containing a death domain that interacts with Fas/APO-1 (CD95) in yeast and causes cell death. Cell 1995;81:513–523.
27. Cory S, Adams J. The Bcl2 family: regulators of the cellular life-or-death switch. Nat Rev Cancer 2002;2:647–656.
28. Kirkin V, Joos S, Zornig M. The role of Bcl-2 family members in tumorigenesis. Biochim Biophys Acta 2004;1644:229–249.
29. Lane DP. p53, guardian of the genome. Nature (Lond) 1992; 358:15–16.
30. Donehower LA, Harvey M, Slagle BL, et al. Mice deficient for p53 are developmentally normal but susceptible to spontaneous tumors. Nature (Lond) 1992;356:215–221.
31. Williams BO, Remington L, Albert DM, et al. Mice deficient in both p53 and Rb develop tumors primarily of endocrine origin. Cancer Res 1995;55:1146–1151.
32. Wei MC, Zong WX, Cheng EG, et al. Proapoptotic BAX and BAK: a requisite gateway to mitochondrial dysfunction and death. Science 2001;292:727–730.
33. Ionov Y, Yamamoto H, Krajewski S. Mutational inactivation of the proapoptotic gene BAX confers selective advantage during tumor clonal evolution. Proc Natl Acad Sci U S A 2000;97:10872–10877.
34. Karin M, Ben-Neriah Y. Phosphorylation meets ubiquitination: the control of NF-κB activity. Annu Rev Immunol 2000;18:621–663.
35. Ghosh S, Karin M. Missing pieces in the NF-κB puzzle. Cell 2002;109(suppl):S81–S96.
36. Baldwin AS. Control of oncogenesis and cancer therapy resistance by the transcription factor NF-κB. J Clin Invest 2001;107: 241–246.
37. Karin M, Cao Y, Greten FR, et al. NF-κB in cancer: from innocent bystander to major culprit. Nat Rev Cancer 2002;2:301–310.
38. Beg AA, Baltimore D. An essential role for NF-κB in preventing TNF-α-induced cell death. Science 1996;274:782–784.
39. Wang C-Y, Mayo MW, Baldwin AS Jr. TNF- and cancer therapy-induced apoptosis: potentiation by inhibition of NF-κB. Science 1996;274:784–787.
40. Van Antwerp DJ, Martin SJ, Kafri T, et al. Suppression of TNF-α-induced apoptosis by NF-κB. Science 1996;274:787–789.
41. Liu Z-G, Hu H, Goeddel DV, et al. Dissection of TNF receptor 1 effector functions: JNK activation is not linked to apoptosis, while NF-κB activation prevents cell death. Cell 1996;87:565–576.
42. Rayet B, Gelinas C. Aberrant rel/nfkb genes and activity in human cancer. Oncogene 1999;18:6938–6947.
43. Lin A, Karin M. NF-kappaB in cancer: a marked target. Semin Cancer Biol 2003;13:107–114.
44. Lee HH, Dadgostar H, Cheng Q, et al. NF-κB-mediated up-regulation of Bcl-x and Bfl-1/A1 is required for CD40 survival signaling in B lymphocytes. Proc Natl Acad Sci USA 1999; 96:9136–9141.
45. Chen C, Edelstein LC, Gelinas C. The Rel/NF-κB family directly activates expression of the apoptosis inhibitor Bcl-x(L). Mol Cell Biol 2000;20:2687–2695.
46. Grossmann M, O'Reilly LA, Gugasyan R, et al. The anti-apoptotic activities of Rel and RelA required during B-cell maturation involve the regulation of Bcl-2 expression. EMBO J 2000;19:6351–6360.
47. Folkman J. Tumor angiogenesis: therapeutic implications. N Engl J Med 1971;285:1182–1186.
48. Folkman J, Shing Y. Angiogenesis. J Biol Chem 1992;267:10931–10934.
49. Folkman J, Watson K, Ingber D, et al. Induction of angiogenesis during the transition from hyperplasia to neoplasia. Nature (Lond) 1989;339:58–61.
50. Eckhardt G. Angiogenesis inhibitors as cancer therapy. Hosp Pract 1999;34(1):63–68, 77–79, 83–84.
51. Folkman J. Fundamental concepts of the angiogenic process. Curr Mol Med 2003;3:643–651.
52. Hanahan D, Folkman J. Patterns of emerging mechanisms of the angiogenic switch during tumorigenesis. Cell 1996;86:353–364.
53. Hojilla CV, Mohammed FF, Khokha R. Matrix metalloproteinases and their tissue inhibitors direct cell fate during cancer development. Br J Cancer 2003;89:1817–1821.
54. O'Reilly MS, Holmgren L, Shing Y, et al. Angiostatin: a novel angiogenesis inhibitor that mediates the suppression of metastases by a Lewis lung carcinoma. Cell 1994;79:315–328.
55. O'Reilly MS, Boehm T, Shing Y, et al. Endostatin: an endogenous inhibitor of angiogenesis and tumor growth. Cell 1997; 88:277–285.
56. Sridhar SS, Shepherd FA. Targeting angiogenesis: a review of angiogenesis inhibitors in the treatment of lung cancer. Lung Cancer 2003;Suppl 1:S81–S91.
57. Fidler IJ, Ellis LM. The implications of angiogenesis to the biology and therapy of cancer metastasis. Cell 1994;79:185–188.
58. Liotta LA, Steeg PS, Settler-Stevenson WG. Cancer metastasis and angiogenesis: an imbalance of positive and negative regulation. Cell 1991;64:327–336.
59. Meert AP, Paesmans M, Martin B, et al. The role of microvessel density on the survival of patients with lung cancer: a systematic review of the literature with meta-analysis. Br J Cancer 2002;87:694–701.
60. Sauer G, Deissler H. Angiogenesis: prognostic and therapeutic implications in gynecologic and breast malignancies. Curr Opin Obstet Gynecol 2003;15:45–49.
61. Poon RT, Fan ST, Wong J. Clinical significance of angiogenesis in gastrointestinal cancers: a target for novel prognostic and therapeutic approaches. Ann Surg 2003;238:9–28.
62. Shirabe K, Shimada M, Tsujita E, et al. Prognostic factors in node-negative intrahepatic cholangiocarcinoma with special reference to angiogenesis. Am J Surg 2004;1 87:538–542.
63. Delmotte P, Martin B, Paesmans M, et al. VEGF and survival of patients with lung cancer: a systematic literature review and meta-analysis. Rev Mal Respir 2002;19:577–584.
64. Vihinen P, Kahari VM. Matrix metalloproteinases in cancer: prognostic markers and therapeutic targets. Int J Cancer 2002; 99:157–166.

65. Yarden Y, Sliwkowski MX. Untangling the ErbB signalling network. Nat Rev Mol Cell Biol 2001;2:127–137.
66. Fujino S, Enokibori T, Tezuka N, et al. A comparison of epidermal growth factor receptor levels and other prognostic parameters in non-small cell lung cancer. Eur J Cancer 1996;32A: 2070–2074.
67. Rusch V, Klimstra D, Venkatraman E, et al. Overexpression of the epidermal growth factor receptor and its ligand transforming growth factor is frequent in resectable non-small cell lung cancer but does not predict tumor progression. Clin Cancer Res 1997;3:515–522.
68. Fontanini G, De Laurentiis M, Vignati S, et al. Evaluation of epidermal growth factor-related growth factors and receptors and of neoangiogenesis in completely resected stage I-IIIA non-small cell lung cancer: amphiregulin and microvessel count are independent prognostic indicators of survival. Clin Cancer Res 1998;4:241–249.
69. Salomon DS, Brandt R, Ciardiello F, et al. Epidermal growth factor-related peptides and their receptors in human malignancies. Crit Rev Oncol Hematol 1995;53:167–176.
70. Messa C, Russo F, Caruso MG, et al. EGF, TGF-α, and EGF-R in human colorectal adenocarcinoma. Acta Oncol 1998;37:285–289.
71. Fischer-Colbrie J, Witt A, Heinzl H, et al. EGFR and steroid receptors in ovarian carcinoma: comparison with prognostic parameters and outcome of patients. Anticancer Res 1997;17:613–619.
72. Bartlett JM, Langdon SP, Simpson BJ, et al. The prognostic value of epidermal growth factor receptor mRNA expression in primary ovarian cancer. Br J Cancer 1996;73:301–306.
73. Walker RA, Dearing SJ. Expression of epidermal growth factor receptor mRNA and protein in primary breast carcinomas. Breast Cancer Res Treat 1999;53:167–176.
74. Beckmann MW, Niederacher D, Massenkeil G, et al. Expression analyses of epidermal growth factor receptor and HER-2/neu: no advantage of prediction of recurrence or survival in breast cancer patients. Oncology 1996;53:441–447.
75. Bucci B, D'Agnano I, Botti C, et al. EGF-R expression in ductal breast cancer: proliferation and prognostic implications. Anticancer Res 1997;17:769–774.
76. Uegaki K, Nio Y, Inoue Y, et al. Clinicopathological significance of epidermal growth factor and its receptor in human pancreatic cancer. Anticancer Res 1997;17:3841–3847.
77. Xu F, Lupu R, Rodriguez GC, et al. Antibody-induced growth inhibition is mediated through immunochemically and functionally distinct epitopes on the extracellular domain of the c-erb-2 (HER-2/neu) gene product p185. Int J Cancer 1993;53: 401–408.
78. Baselga J, Tripathy D, Mendelsohn J, et al. Phase II study of weekly intravenous recombinant humanized anti-p185HER2 monoclonal antibody in patients with HER2/neu-overexpressing metastatic breast cancer. J Clin Oncol 1996;14:737–744.
79. Cobleigh MA, Vogel CL, Tripathy D, et al. Multinational study of the efficacy and safety of humanized anti-HER2-overexpressing metastatic breast cancer that has progressed after chemotherapy for metastatic disease. J Clin Oncol 1999;17:2639–2648.
80. Nahta R, Iglehart JD, Kempkes B, et al. Rate-limiting effects of cyclin D1 in transformation by ErbB2 predicts synergy between herceptin and flavopiridol. Cancer Res 2002;62:2267–2271.
81. Vogel CL, Cobleigh MA, Tripathy D, et al. Efficacy and safety of trastuzumab as a single agent in first-line treatment of HER2-overexpressing metastatic breast cancer. J Clin Oncol 2002; 20:719–726.
82. Slamon DJ, Leyland-Jones B, Shak S, et al. Use of chemotherapy plus a monoclonal antibody against HER2 for metastatic breast cancer that overexpresses HER2. N Engl J Med 2001;344:783–792.
83. Cunningham D, Humblet Y, Siena S, et al. Cetuximab (C225) alone or in combination with irinotecan (CPT-11) in patients with epidermal growth factor receptor (EGFR)-positive, irinotecan-refractory metastatic colorectal cancer (MCRC). Proc Am Soc Clin Oncol 2003;22:1012.
84. Fukuoka M, Yano S, Giaccone G, et al. Multi-institutional randomized phase II trial of gefitinib for previously treated patients with advanced non-small-cell lung cancer. J Clin Oncol 2003;21: 2237–2246.
85. Kris MG, Natale RB, Herbst RS, et al. A phase II trial of ZD1839 (Iressa) in advanced non-small cell lung cancer (NSCLC) patients who had failed platinum- and docetaxel-based regimens (IDEAL 2). Proc Am Soc Clin Oncol 2002;21:292a.
86. Senzer NN, Soulieres D, Siu L, et al. Phase 2 evaluation of OSI-774, a potent oral antagonist of the EGFR-TK in patients with advanced squamous cell carcinoma of the head and neck. Proc Am Soc Clin Oncol 2001;20:2a.
87. Finkler N, Gordon A, Crozier M, et al. Phase 2 evaluation of OSI-774, a potent oral antagonist of the EGFR-TK in patients with advanced ovarian carcinoma. Proc Am Soc Clin Oncol 2001;20:208a.
88. Perez-Soler R, Chachoua A, Huberman M, et al. Final results from a phase II study of erlotinib (Tarceva) monotherapy in patients with advanced non-small cell lung cancer following failure of platinum-based chemotherapy. Lung Cancer 2003; 41(suppl 2):S246.
89. Giaccone G, Johnson DH, Manegold C, et al. A phase III clinical trial of ZD1839 (Iressa) in combination with gemcitabine and cisplatin in chemotherapy-naïve patients with advanced non-small-cell lung cancer (INTACT 1). Ann Oncol 2002;13(suppl 5):2.
90. Johnson DH, Herbst R, Giaccone G, et al. ZD1839 (Iressa) in combination with paclitaxel and carboplatin in chemotherapy-naïve patients with advanced non-small-cell lung cancer (NSCLC): results from a phase III clinical trial (INTACT 2). Ann Oncol 2002;13 (suppl 5):127.
91. Sirotnak FM. Studies with ZD1839 in preclinical models. Semin Oncol 2003;30(suppl 1):12–20.
92. Mellinghoff IK, Sawyers CL. Kinase inhibitor therapy in cancer. Princ Pract Oncol 2000;14:1–11.
93. Druker BJ, Lydon NB. Lessons learned from the development of an Abl tyrosine kinase inhibitor for chronic myelogenous leukemia. J Clin Invest 2000;105:3–7.
94. DeMatteo RP, Lewis JL, Leung D, et al. Two hundred gastrointestinal stromal tumors: recurrence patterns and prognostic factors for survival. Ann Surg 2000;231:51–58.
95. Edmondson J, Marks R, Buckner J, et al. Contrast of response to D-MAP + sargramostim between patients with advanced malignant gastrointestinal stromal tumors and patients with other advanced leiomyosarcomas. Proc Am Soc Clin Oncol 1999; 18:541.
96. Joensuu H, Roberts PJ, Sarlomo-Rikala M, et al. Effect of the tyrosine kinase inhibitor STI571 in a patient with a metastatic gastrointestinal stromal tumor. N Engl J Med 2001;344:1052–1056.
97. Demetri GD, von Mehren M, Blanke CD, et al. Efficacy and safety of imatinib mesylate in advanced gastrointestinal stromal tumors. N Engl J Med 2002;347:472–480.
98. Heinrich MC, Corless CL, Demetri GD, et al. Kinase mutations and imatinib response in patients with metastatic gastrointestinal stromal tumor. J Clin Oncol 2003;21:4342–4349.
99. Smith JK, Mamoon NM, Duhe RJ. Emerging roles of targeted small molecule protein-tyrosine kinase inhibitors in cancer therapy. Oncol Res 2004;14:175–225.
100. DeMatteo RP. The GIST of targeted cancer therapy: a tumor (gastrointestinal stromal tumor), a mutated gene (c-kit), and a molecular inhibitor (STI571). Ann Surg Oncol 2002;9:831–839.
101. Hurwitz H, Fehrenbacher L, Novotny W, et al. Bevacizumab plus irinotecan, fluorouracil, and leucovorin for metastatic colorectal cancer. N Engl J Med 2004;350:2335–2342.

93

Immunology of Cancer

Craig L. Slingluff, Jr.

A central principle of tumor immunology is that cancer can be prevented or controlled by a host immune response. Thus, a significant corollary is that the progression of cancer represents, in some measure, a failure of the host immune system to control cancer growth. In the lay community, it is commonly accepted that immunological control of cancer is possible, but the medical community has traditionally been more skeptical. Increasingly, however, host–tumor interactions that affect the progression of cancer are being defined, and clinical trials are providing evidence for the benefit of immunological therapies.

The concept of immune surveillance was formally described as a hypothesis in 1970 by Burnet,[1] and it arose out of earlier descriptions by Ehrlich.[2] This hypothesis states that the immune system normally detects and destroys malignant cells as they arise, preventing the outgrowth of clinically apparent cancers in most individuals. Thus, this hypothesis of immune surveillance states that the presentation of a patient with cancer would represent a failure of immune protection.

As the molecular genetic basis for oncogenesis has become elucidated, however, the complexity of oncogenesis and cancer progression has become apparent. The malignant phenotype of individual cancers can be explained by many factors, including the loss of tumor suppressor gene function, alterations in the expression of integrins and other adhesion molecules, autocrine production of growth factors, and the stimulation of angiogenesis. Certainly, alterations in the host immune responses to cancer are not the only cause of cancer. However, failures of the host immune response certainly contribute to cancer progression. Thus, modulation of immune function can control or cure cancers, and immune therapy has emerged as an effective form of therapy for some cancer patients. Many of the exciting novel forms of immune therapy remain to be optimized; investigations in these areas represent exciting opportunities for laboratory and clinical investigation for the next decade. This chapter summarizes some of the basic and clinical science that defines the current status of tumor immunology and the prospects for advances in immunotherapy of cancer. This review addresses multiple antibody, cytokine, and cellular aspects of tumor immunology.

Antibody Responses to Tumor Antigens

Antibodies are polymorphic molecules produced by B lymphocytes, which contain a hypervariable region with an extraordinary repertoire for recognizing a multitude of proteins and other complex molecules. Antibody responses to human tumor antigens have been described for many tumors, and the antigens they recognize have been characterized. Many of the antigens are expressed on both normal cells and malignant cells but are overexpressed on malignant cells. Efforts have been made to target tumor cells with antibodies, both for diagnostic purposes and for therapy of cancer. Some antigens for which antibodies have been developed for clinical use are listed in Table 93.1.

Diagnostic Uses of Antibodies

In vivo, diagnostic uses of antibody have involved labeling antibodies with radionuclides such as indium-111, iodine-123, iodine-131, yttrium-90, and technetium-99 and injecting them systemically, with the expectation that they will bind specifically to tumor cells, allowing scintigraphic imaging of tumor deposits. This approach results in images that, in the more ideal situations, permit identification of tumor deposits over background radioactivity. However, nonspecific binding of antibodies and failure of clearance from the bloodstream

TABLE 93.1. Examples of Major Tumor-Associated Antigens Targeted by Monoclonal Antibodies in Clinical Trials or in Clinical Use.

Categories	*Examples of antigen*	*Tumor types*
Lymphomas/leukemias	CD5	T cell leukemia/lymphoma
Differentiation antigens	CD19, CD20, CD21, CD22, CD37	B cell lymphoma
	CD30	Hodgkin's lymphoma
	CD33, CD45	AML
	CAMPATH-1 (CDw52)	Lymphoid malignancies (T and B cell)
	HLA-DR	B cell lymphoma
	Anti-idiotype	B cell lymphoma
Solid tumors	CEA, TAG-72, Ep-CAM, MUC1	Epithelial tumors (breast, colon, lung)
Cell-surface antigens	Folate-binding protein	Ovarian tumors
Glycoproteins	GA733-2 (17-1A antigen)	Gastrointestinal neoplasms[196]
	A33	Colorectal carcinoma
	G250	Renal carcinoma
Glycolipids	Gangliosides (e.g., GD2, GD3)	Neuroectodermal tumors, melanoma
Carbohydrates	Le^y	Epithelial tumors (breast, colon, lung)
	CA-125	Ovarian carcinoma
Intracellular antigens	Ferritin	Hodgkin's disease, hepatoma
Growth factor receptors	EGF-R	Lung, breast, head and neck tumors
	$P185^{HER2}$	Breast, ovarian tumors
	IL-2 receptor	T and B cell neoplasms
Stromal/extracellular antigens	FAP-α	Epithelial tumors (breast, colon, lung)
	Tenascin	Glioblastoma multiforme
	Metalloproteinases	Epithelial tumors
	VEGF	Colorectal cancers and others

Source: Modified with permission from Scott AM, Welt S. Antibody-based immunological therapies. Current Opinion in Immunology 1997;9(5):718.[197] [Current Biology Ltd]. References for each of these antigens/antibodies are available from that source.

usually result in background radioactivity in many tissues, and this limits the sensitivity for detection of small tumor deposits. Often the sensitivity of these scans is not better than the sensitivity of more anatomic imaging approaches such as computed tomography (CT), or approaches that identify tumors by neovascularity such as positron emission tomography (PET) scanning and gadolinium-enhanced magnetic resonance imaging (MRI).[3] However, some antibodies tagged with radionuclides have been FDA-approved for tumor imaging in humans and have been promoted, in particular, for identification of occult metastases in patients with elevated serum tumor markers (e.g., carcinoembryonic antigen, CEA).[4] Overall accuracy has been reported in the range of 85% to 90% for CEA scans in patients with elevated serum CEA levels.[5]

A more surgical application is radioimmunoguided surgery (RIGS), in which the goal is to use a gamma probe intraoperatively to identify "hot spots" directly in the operating room. In two recent studies, RIGS approaches resulted in identification of occult metastases, especially in lymph nodes, in up to 50% of patients studied at the time of laparotomy.[6,7] Whether this will impact on patient outcomes remains to be determined.

Major limitations of antibody approaches to diagnostic whole-body imaging are the nonspecific or cross-reactive binding to nontargeted tissues and binding to soluble antigen shed into the circulation.[8] In cytological preparations and histological sections, however, this limitation can be controlled significantly, because cellular morphology and the subcellular localization of staining can be correlated with the antibody findings. Thus, antibodies are very useful for pathologists to aid in characterizing and in diagnosing tumors. A clinical setting in which this is very useful is the characterization of poorly differentiated tumors, especially those of unknown primary. Antibodies commonly used in such settings are antibodies to leukocyte common antigen (LCA, a pan-leukocyte antigen), which can be helpful in ruling in or out a lymphoma, and cytokeratin antibodies, which can identify carcinomas. Antibodies to melanoma that are used clinically include S100, HMB45 (reactive to gp100/Pmel17), T311 (reactive to tyrosinase), and A103 (reactive to MART-1/Melan-A). Antibodies to prostate-specific antigen (PSA) are useful in ruling in or out prostatic carcinoma.[9] Many other antibodies are commercially available and well characterized for use in these settings and can also help to distinguish cancer cells from reactive epithelial cells in cytological preparations.[10]

Therapeutic Uses of Antibodies

Antibodies, by targeting tumor antigens, have value as therapeutic tools. Murine studies, especially in tumor xenograft models, have revealed significant therapeutic effects. The approaches have included either attaching toxins or radioactive particles to the antibodies or simply administering the antibodies directly. In the latter case, tumor cell death may be mediated by complement. However, early clinical application of antibody therapy was disappointing.

Several reasons for those results have been cited[8] and include the following:

1. Less than 0.1% of the injected antibody dose actually reaches the tumor.
2. The total dose of radiation exposure to the tumor is usually less than 2 Gy, whereas doses of 30–60 Gy have been obtained in optimized animal models.
3. Bone marrow is the dose-limiting organ.
4. Human antimouse antibodies (HAMA) form readily after administration of murine monoclonal antibody prepara-

TABLE 93.2. FDA-Approved Monoclonal Antibodies (MAb) for Human Cancer Therapy.

MAb name (trade name)	*Epitope specificity*	*Used to treat:*	*Conjugate*	*Approved in:*
Rituximab (Rituxan)	B-cell surface antigen CD20	Relapsed non-Hodgkin B-cell lymphoma		1997
Trastuzumab (Herceptin)	Her-2/neu	Breast cancer		1998
Gemtuzumab ozogamicin[a] (Mylotarg)	CD33, present on most leukemia cells	Acute myelogenous leukemia (AML)	Calicheamycin	2000
Alemtuzumab (Campath)	CD52 (on T and B cells)	B-cell chronic lymphocytic leukemia (CLL), after prior chemotherapy		2001
Ibritumomab tiuxetan[b] (Zevalin)	CD20	B-cell non-Hodgkin lymphoma, after failing standard therapy	^{90}Y or ^{111}I	2002
Tositumomab[b] (Bexxar)	CD20	Non-Hodgkin lymphoma	^{131}I	2003
Cetuximab (Erbitux)	EGF-R	Colorectal cancer, with irinotecan		2004
Bevacizumab (Avastin)	VEGF	Colorectal cancer, with chemotherapy		2004

[a]Monoclonal antibody conjugated to immunotoxin.

[b]Monoclonal antibodies conjugated to radiolabel.

Source: Data from reference 198 and from American Cancer Society web site: http://www.cancer.org/docroot/ETO/content/ETO_1_4X_Monoclonal_Antibody_Therapy_Passive_Immunotherapy.asp?sitearea=ETO).

tions, and these HAMA responses usually result in clearance of the murine antibodies such that repeated administration of the antibodies is not effective.

However, subsequent technological advances have made it possible to create humanized antibodies as a means of permitting repeat administration, and this has breathed new life into the field of antibody-based immunotherapy of cancer. In the past few years, numerous monoclonal antibodies have been approved for use in therapy of various cancer. Those with formal FDA approval for cancer therapy (as of 2005) are listed in Table 93.2. Commonly, these antibody therapies have been approved for use in conjunction with cytotoxic chemotherapy, and the combination therapy is found to be more effective than either therapy alone. These new therapies are changing our strategies for management of advanced cancer. Those antibodies useful in treatment of advanced solid tumors should be investigated for their role in adjuvant therapy or neoadjuvant therapy, where they are likely to have particular relevance to surgeons.

SEREX (Serological Analysis of Recombinant cDNA Expression Libraries)

Because in vivo tumor destruction by antibodies depends on antibody recognition of viable cells, the target molecules for most antibodies are at the cell surface. However, it is also clear that apoptotic or necrotic tumor cells release intracellular proteins, against which antibodies are generated in vivo. These antibodies to intracellular proteins are not likely to have clinically significant antitumor effects, but the fact that they exist is evidence of immune recognition of these tumor proteins. B-cell responses, similar to cytotoxic T-lymphocyte (CTL) responses, depend on T-helper responses, so it has been proposed that proteins recognized by antibodies must also be recognized by T-helper cells and thus may also be recognized by cytotoxic T cells.

This concept has resulted in development of an approach for identifying new tumor antigens that may have relevance both to T-cell recognition and to B-cell (antibody) recognition. This approach, called SEREX (serological analysis of recombinant cDNA expression libraries) has been described in detail.[11] The technology has resulted in the identification of hundreds of proteins that are immunogenic in humans, some of which were previously known, some of which have since been confirmed to induce T-cell responses as well, and many of which remain to be characterized. Current summaries of the known antigenic profile for human cancers, by SEREX, are available on the Cancer Immunity web site.[12]

One of the antigens identified by SEREX is the NY-ESO-1 antigen,[13] which is a member of the C-T (cancer-testis) class of antigens whose expression is limited to cancer cells and to testis, with occasional expression in ovary or placenta. Members of this class of antigens (MAGE, BAGE, GAGE) are expressed in only a subset of cancers from different individuals and in major histocompatibility complex (MHC)-negative cells in the testis,[14] so preexisting tolerance to this antigen is not likely to exist. In a patient with an ESO+ tumor, antibody reactivity to NY-ESO-1 was detected at a 1:1,000,000 titer, and a CTL response has been identified as well.[15] Thus, there is proof of principle that the SEREX approach can identify new antigens relevant to both the humoral and the cellular arms of the immune system.

Another antigen defined by SEREX is HOM-MEL-40, encoded by the SSX-2 gene, which is involved in a genetic translocation in synovial cell sarcomas. This antigen is also expressed in 50% of melanomas, 25% of colon cancers, and some hepatomas and breast cancers, but not in normal tissues other than testis.[16] The fact that this antigen is associated with a translocation suggests that it may be part of the malignant transformation process.

Thus, in addition to the established therapeutic value of monoclonal antibodies in cancer therapy, antibodies also have defining tumor antigens recognized by the cellular arm of the immune system, which will lead to new therapeutic approaches directed at tumor antigens.

Natural Killer Immunity: LAK

Innate immunity to cancer has often been attributed to natural killer cells. These cells are capable of lysing target cells in an antigen-independent manner, and the mechanism of this recognition is now being elucidated. Storkus et al.

TABLE 93.3.
Responses to High-Dose IL-2 Therapy in Human Trials.

Cancer treated	*Author*	*Year*	*Number evaluable patients*	*% PR*	*% CR*	*Total response rate*	*Median duration of CR*
Renal cell cancer (RCC)	Yang[36]	2003	156	14	7	21%	More than 100 months
Melanoma	Atkins[199]	2000	270	10	6	16%	More than 59 months
Melanoma, RCC	Rosenberg[34]	1994	283	12	7	19%	More than 91 months

PR, partial response; CR, complete response.

demonstrated that the ability of NK cells to lyse a target cell was inversely correlated with the expression of MHC molecules by the target cell.[17] Some viruses induce downregulation of host cell MHC expression, so NK cells may be able to recognize those virally infected cells; that may be one teleological explanation for the evolution of NK cells in animals. A similar observation has been made about cancers; downregulation of HLA-A2 expression has been observed in 21% of primary melanomas and 44% of metastatic melanomas,[18] and downregulation of MHC molecules has been observed generally in as many as 16% to 50% of many cancers.[19,20]

During the past decade, a family of cell-surface receptors has been identified that explains, in part, the reactivity profile of NK cells. This family of receptors is called killer inhibitor receptors (KIRs), which are members of the immunoglobulin superfamily.[21] Although the effector functions of T cells, NK cells, and B cells had been well described, the inhibitory mechanisms that promote homeostasis and prevent indiscriminant target cell lysis had not been previously defined. This family of KIRs contains dozens of different receptors with specificities that are quite varied.[22,23] Although the trigger for activating NK cells remains incompletely defined, the inhibitory signal relayed by these KIRs is partially understood and may involve SHP-1.[24] When an NK cell encounters another normal host cell, a KIR on the cell surface will bind to a normal MHC molecule on that cell, which in turn transmits an intracellular signal that blocks activation pathways which otherwise would result in initiation of a cytotoxic event. On the other hand, if the target cell lacks a certain normal MHC molecule, then some NK cells in that patient will express KIRs that will be unable to bind their ligand; thus, the NK cells will lyse those target cells. In addition to their expression on NK cells, these receptors have been described on a subset of cytotoxic T cells.[25,26] At least one case is described in which a T-cell response to a ubiquitous antigen, in a patient with melanoma, permitted recognition and lysis of a tumor cell that had lost expression of several MHC molecules[27]; this was possible because the T cell expressed a KIR reactive to one of the lost MHC molecules. Thus, the expression of KIR molecules by T cells permits the immune system to adapt to the loss of MHC molecules by tumors.

Lymphokine-Activated Killer Cells and Interleukin 2

In 1976, interleukin 2 (IL-2) was described as T-cell growth factor.[28] This cytokine is produced by activated T-helper cells and provides help in expanding T cells responding to defined antigens. It was further described that IL-2 activated peripheral blood lymphocytes in vitro and turned them into very active killer cells, with specificity similar to that of NK cells, but substantially more active.[29] These lymphokine-activated killer (LAK) cells can lyse many different types of cancer cells in vitro, but they have little activity against normal cells of various histological types.

Studies in murine tumor models showed that IL-2 therapy or LAK cell therapy was capable of destroying micrometastatic disease, such that treated mice had dramatic reductions in lung metastases of each of several different experimental tumors.[30] In addition, high-dose IL-2 therapy of established metastases caused tumor regressions in murine models.[30,31] Thus, there was great enthusiasm in the 1980s for therapy with adoptive transfer of LAK cells or systemic administration of high-dose IL-2 for several cancers, and clinical trials in humans were performed in the mid-1980s, mostly with melanoma, renal cell cancer, and breast cancer. Some dramatic responses were seen in a minority of patients, but the overall response was less than that predicted from the animal models. The most convincing responses were observed in melanoma and in renal cell cancer. Some examples of those results are listed in Table 93.3. In general, response rates [complete response (CR) + partial response (PR)] for IL-2 therapy were approximately 15% to 20% in melanoma and renal cell cancer.[32–34] Although these response rates are low, they approximate the response to single-agent chemotherapy. However, for melanoma, the cure rate for cytotoxic chemotherapy is estimated to be less than 1%. On the other hand, a significant minority of patients receiving IL-2 therapy for metastatic melanoma have durable CRs.[34,35] This subset of patients includes those who have remained clinically free of disease (NED) for beyond 10 years. Whether these will translate into cures requires a longer follow-up, but it appears that approximately 5% to 7% of patients receiving high-dose IL-2 therapy will experience durable CRs. On this basis, IL-2 is approved for use in metastatic renal cell cancer and in metastatic (stage IV) melanoma at 600,000 IU/kg per dose IV q 8 h. The toxicity of high-dose IL-2 is substantial and limits its applicability to patients with comorbidities. However, a randomized trial of low-dose IL-2 versus high-dose IL-2 in renal cell cancer supported the superiority of high-dose over low-dose IL-2.[36] There are some clinical features that may predict response to IL-2 therapy; in particular, patients with disease limited to skin and lymph node sites have response rates approaching 50%.[37,38]

Antigen-Specific Tumor Cell Recognition by Human T Cells

In animal models, it is possible to generate tumor-specific immunity by vaccinating naïve animals against syngeneic tumors, and those vaccinated animals subsequently reject a challenge with those same tumor cells. This immunity can be transferred by transferring lymphocytes to a naïve animal. Thus, it appeared that tumor immunity in these models is mediated by cellular elements.[39] Furthermore, work by Greenberg in a murine leukemia virus tumor system, in the early 1980s, revealed that adoptive transfer of tumor-specific T cells (helper and cytotoxic) was capable of mediating leukemia rejections,[40] and a number of studies have shown that immune-mediated tumor rejection can be blocked by depleting CD8+ T cells or CD4+ T cells. Thus, there has been an increasing interest in identifying T-cell responses to tumors.

In 1982, Vose and Bonnard showed that cytotoxic T-cell lines could be generated in vitro against autologous tumors by stimulation of peripheral blood lymphocyte (PBL) blasts with autologous tumor cells in the presence of IL-2.[41] This work was done with cancers of several different histologies, including lung, breast, and melanoma. Subsequent studies have demonstrated that CTL lines can be generated reliably in a substantial proportion of cases.[42] A clinical application of this work was the use of these ex vivo generated CTL in adoptive therapy of humans with cancer, which has been done initially using tumor-infiltrating lymphocytes (TILs) expanded ex vivo in high-dose IL-2. The resultant CTL lines were not restimulated with tumor over time but were simply exposed initially to the tumor cells naturally present in the metastatic deposit. When melanoma patients have been treated with these TILs, plus high-dose systemic IL-2, a response rate of about 30% to 35% has been reported.[43] Some of that response may be caused by nonspecific antitumor effects of IL-2. However, the response rate is higher than that observed with IL-2 alone, and responses were seen even in patients who had previously failed IL-2 therapy. Thus, some of that response is believed to be the result of specific antitumor effector cells.

Adoptive T-Cell Therapy

Recent studies have combined adoptive T-cell therapy with nonmyeloablative chemotherapy, with excellent response rates in patients with melanoma. Cyclophosphamide and fludarabine were administered to patients with advanced melanoma to create peripheral lymphopenia before administration of tumor-reactive lymphocytes and IL-2. This combination therapy results in high percentages of circulating lymphocytes with melanoma antigen reactivity. Of 35 patients who received that therapy, major clinical responses have been observed in 51% (18 patients), including 3 complete responses and 15 partial responses, with a mean response duration of 11.5 months.[44] This continues to be an aggressive and toxic therapy, and one that has not been developed widely at other centers yet, but it provides strong proof of principle for the effectiveness of T-cell therapy for advanced metastatic melanoma.

Identification of Tumor Antigens Recognized by T Cells

Adoptive T-cell therapy currently is available only for patients with metastatic disease to sites that are resectable and which contain substantial amounts of tumor. In the interest of being able to generate tumor-reactive T cells from patients with minimal disease, there has been heightened interest in understanding the nature of the antigens, on melanoma and other cancers, that are recognized by T cells. A goal has been to use these antigens directly to stimulate T-cell responses even in the absence of available autologous tumor cells.

An observation that was critical to the current and future direction of tumor immunology research was the observation of shared antigens on melanoma and other tumors. It was observed that, although CTL lines reactive to autologous tumor failed to lyse most allogeneic tumor cells or autologous normal cells, they did lyse HLA-matched allogeneic cancers of the same histological type (sarcomas, melanoma).[45,46] All that was required was matching of a single Class I MHC molecule, and because HLA-A2 is the most common serologically defined allele in humans, many studies have focused on that molecule as a restricting element. Using cellular assays, it was possible to confirm that shared antigens, restricted by HLA-A2, were being recognized on melanoma cells by CTL, and this led to work on characterizing these shared antigens.[45]

T cells recognize target cells through a T-cell receptor, which interacts with cell-surface antigens. The form of antigen recognized by T cells consists of a short peptide bound in a special peptide-binding groove on the exposed surface of an MHC molecule.[47–49] These MHC-associated peptides represent degradation products of cellular proteins that are processed through one of several intracellular pathways.

Thus, substantial effort has been directed toward identifying the peptides, presented by human cancer cells, that are recognized by tumor-reactive cytotoxic T cells and T-helper cells. Using several different approaches, many of these immunogenic peptides have been identified, and it is likely that many more will be identified, not only for melanoma but also for many of the common human cancers. A list of categories of antigenic proteins is provided in Table 93.4. As identification of these epitopes is proceeding very rapidly, the list

TABLE 93.4. Proteins Encoding Peptide Epitopes for Human Tumor-Specific CTL.

Category of antigenic protein	*Example(s) for which specific epitopes have been described or postulated*
Nonmutated tissue differentiation proteins	Melanoma: Tyrosinase, gp100/Pmel17, MART-1/Melan-A, gp75/TRP-1, trp2; Prostate cancer: PSA, PMSA; Colon cancer: CEA
Cancer-testis antigens	MAGE-A1, MAGE-A3, BAGE, GAGE-1 and –2, NY-ESO-1, SSX-2, TAG
Other nonmutated cancer-associated antigens upregulated in cancer cells and often integral to cancer cell phenotype	EphA2 (tyrosine kinase), survivin, telomerase, mesothelin
Oncogenes or tumor suppressor genes (mutated and/or overexpressed)	HER-2/neu, mutated ras, p53
Commonly mutated cellular proteins other than known oncogenes or tumor suppressor genes	B-raf kinase
Viral proteins	E6, E7 of human papilloma virus (HPV)
Unique antigens caused by patient-specific mutations	Beta-catenin, elongation factor 2, CASP-8, MUM-1

may be expected to grow as well. A recent updated summary listing of defined antigens is available.[50] There are at least seven categories of antigenic proteins (see Table 93.4): (i) nonmutated tissue differentiation protein (TDP); (ii) cancer-testis antigens; (iii) other nonmutated cancer-associated antigens upregulated in cancer cells, and often integral to cancer cell phenotype; (iv) oncogenes or tumor suppressor genes; (v) commonly mutated cellular proteins other than known oncogenes or tumor suppressor genes; (vi) viral proteins; and (vii) unique antigens resulting from patient-specific mutations. The shared antigens include those in groups i–vi.

The TDPs have been described in detail for melanoma, where immune-mediated destruction of melanoma cells is possible by targeting peptides from the melanocytic tissue proteins gp100, tyrosinase, MART-1/Melan-A, and gp75.[50] Interestingly, the regression of melanoma, either after systemic therapy or by spontaneous remission, has occasionally been associated with loss of skin melanocytes (vitiligo).[51,52] Although the etiology of vitiligo in those patients has not been proven to be associated with the immune response, there are strong circumstantial data implicating cross-reactive immunity. In particular, with IL-2 therapy, vitiligo was observed in 15% (11/74) of melanoma patients but in 0% (0/104) of patients with renal cell cancer receiving the same therapy.[52] More striking is the fact that vitiligo was seen in 26% (11/43) of melanoma patients responding to IL-2 therapy but was not seen in nonresponders.[52] These data are consistent with prior reports of an association between vitiligo and an improved prognosis in patients with melanoma.[51,53]

A risk of immune therapy directed at TDPs is the possibility of inducing autoimmune destruction of normal tissues that express those proteins. However, the morbidity of loss of melanocytes is quite trivial, and except for theoretical risks of associated injury to retinal pigment epithelium, should be well tolerated. Thus, targeting these antigens, even though they are not strictly tumor-specific, is a reasonable goal for immunotherapy. Meanwhile, it has not been possible to assess with confidence, for technical reasons, primarily, whether these peptides are presented on melanocytes at the same level that they are on melanomas. One report by Wagner suggests in fact that one of these antigens, gp100, is expressed at much lower levels in melanocytes than in melanoma.[54] Certainly if any TDP-derived peptides are upregulated on melanoma as a result of differences in gene expression, in antigen processing, or in MHC expression, then they may be more appropriately considered tumor-specific antigens.

Similarly, there has been an effort to identify cancers other than melanoma in which TDPs can be targeted. The knowledge of prostate-specific antigen as a prostatic protein has led to clinical trials of immunotherapy for prostate cancer, directed at PSA and prostate-specific membrane antigen (PSMA).[55] Results with a five-arm trial of two PSMA peptides were associated with partial responses in seven patients, five of whom were in the groups receiving dendritic cells pulsed with peptide.[55] Other related trials are ongoing and, again, they are based on the premise that loss of the entire normal prostate would not be associated with significant morbidity and would be acceptable if the prostate cancer also is destroyed. It has been proposed, similarly, that immune targeting of TDPs of breast epithelium, ovary, or thyroid also are reasonable therapeutic targets.

MHC-associated peptides are transported to the MHC molecules in the endoplasmic reticulum by a series of steps, and it has been proposed that heat shock proteins function in that process as molecular chaperones.[56] Thus, heat shock proteins isolated from whole tumor cells may be expected to contain the full repertoire of potentially immunogenic peptides from those cells. Srivastava has demonstrated that vaccination of animals with tumor-derived heat shock proteins can produce tumor-specific protective immunity.[57] A few human clinical trials of vaccines with heat shock proteins are underway; so it will be possible in the next few years to determine if these promising findings in preclinical models can be translated to the human system.[58]

Cytokine Modulation of Immune Responses to Cancer

Cytokines are molecules that are produced by cells and which have local effects on other cells; many cytokines have specific and critical functions in the immune system. In particular, they have dramatic effects on tumor immunity. A detailed explanation of the diverse effects of cytokines is beyond the scope of this chapter but is available in numerous immunology texts. Several salient facts about some of these cytokines, however, are worth mentioning as key aspects of our current understanding of tumor immunology.

The cytokine most commonly linked to tumor immunity is interleukin 2 (IL-2), originally described as T-cell growth factor, which was outlined briefly earlier. It is secreted by activated T-helper cells and is a critical signal to cytotoxic T lymphocytes (CTLs) responding to antigen.[59] When CTLs recognize their cognate antigen through the T-cell receptor (TCR), they upregulate expression of the IL-2 receptor (IL-2R), and if IL-2 is available in the microenvironment, expansion/proliferation of the activated CTL occurs. Thus, the presence of activated T-helper cells or of exogenous IL-2 is critical to the maximal expansion of an immune response.[60] The therapeutic use of IL-2 has already been described in the generation of LAK cells, and that occurs both in vitro and in vivo in the presence of IL-2. IL-2 therapy has been approved for use in advanced renal cell cancer and melanoma. Still under investigation is its use in treatment of other cancers and its use in conjunction with experimental vaccine therapies and/or chemotherapy. An interesting new discovery is that regulatory T cells (detailed below) are commonly characterized by the surface expression of CD25, the high affinity IL-2 receptor, and these regulatory cells are stimulated by IL-2. The molecular signaling pathways in these regulatory T cells differ from those in activated CD8 T cells, but IL-2 appears to increase cell survival signals.[61] Thus, IL-2 has both immunostimulatory and immunoregulatory properties, depending on the status of other elements of the immune system locally and systemically.[62,63]

The interferons are a set of molecules that have diverse effects, acting through two receptors (type I and type II). The type I interferons include interferons-α and -β, and type II interferons include interferon-γ.[64–66] IFN-α has direct antitumor properties and complex immunomodulatory effects. It has been approved for use in some leukemias and in melanoma; however, the mechanisms of its antitumor effects remain to be fully elucidated. The effects may be caused by the immunological function of IFN-α or other more direct effects on tumor cells.

IFN-γ induces upregulation of class I MHC, class II MHC, antigen-processing pathways, and costimulatory molecule expression (e.g., ICAM-1), and it also induces upregulation of expression of numerous other cellular proteins. Thus, the effects on immune responses in vitro can be dramatic. Because of the effects seen experimentally, IFN-γ has been administered systemically in hopes of increasing tumor immunity in vivo. However, these trials have not been associated with any significant therapeutic responses.[67–71]

IFN-γ is, however, a key cytokine at a cellular level, being one of three major cytokines released by CTL upon activation by antigen recognition [IFN-γ, tumor necrosis factor-alpha (TNF-α), and granulocyte-macrophage colony-stimulating factor (GM-CSF)]. It also is secreted by T-helper cells in the T_H1 pathway. Thus, induction of expression of IFN-γ in tumor cells in tumor vaccines has been attempted as an approach to augment tumor immunity, with some encouraging results in a murine B16 melanoma model.[72] Also, a human clinical trial of vaccination with autologous melanoma cells modified to express IFN-γ led to some evidence of antibody responses to melanoma antigens.[73]

The cytokine most strongly associated with improved immune responses to a cellular tumor vaccine is GM-CSF, which has been approved for human use in patients recovering from bone marrow transplant, as a means of speeding the recovery of transplanted bone marrow cells. In a study using a murine B16 melanoma model, tumor cells were transfected with retroviral vectors, each expressing 1 of 12 different cytokines, and these cytokine-expressing tumor cells were used to vaccinate syngeneic mice. Protective immunity was dramatically improved by the expression of GM-CSF in tumor cell vaccines, compared to the expression of other cytokines, and compared to vaccination with unmodified tumor cells alone.[74] The effect was dose-dependent, as low expressors of GM-CSF were much less effective immunogens than high expressors of GM-CSF. Phase II human studies of GM-CSF as monotherapy for melanoma have been associated with good clinical outcomes,[75] and a definitive trial of GM-CSF versus placebo is underway through the Eastern Cooperative Oncology Group (E4697).

TNF-α also is a critical effector molecule in T-cell responses. Similar to IFN-γ and GM-CSF, it is secreted by activated CTL after recognition of their cognate antigens. It can effect target cell lysis directly.[76,77] It has been investigated as a therapeutic agent in cancer patients, especially in isolated limb perfusion studies, where response rates of melanoma and sarcomas have exceeded 90%.[78] It has effects on neovasculature, which may well mediate some of its therapeutic effects. However, TNF is a mediator of septic shock in humans, and this toxicity has limited its role in systemic therapy of cancer.[79,80]

In addition to cytokines that have a role in T-cell immune responses, other cytokines with a significant impact on tumor immune responses are those with immunosuppressive function. It is likely that they have a role in suppressing effective tumor immunity and may be key effectors responsible for immune escape mechanisms expressed by tumors. Many tumors secrete transforming growth factor (TGF)-β, IL-10, and/or prostaglandin (PG)E-2 in vitro and in vivo.[81] TGF-β is a growth factor for many epithelial tissues and can be expressed by many cells. In some settings, it may also have growth regulatory functions, but advanced breast and ovarian cancers, among others, often are resistant to these growth regulator effects while they also produce substantial quantities of TGF-β constitutively.[82–86] This cytokine has strong immunosuppressive qualities, blocking generation of CTL and LAK cells. In vivo studies in murine models show that coadministration of IL-2 and anti-TGF-β monoclonal antibodies (MoAbs) is associated with significantly better control of syngeneic tumors than administration of IL-2 alone.[87] Also, antisense DNA for TGF-β, administered at sites of rat brain tumors, or intraperitoneally for murine ovarian cancer, was associated with increased tumor control.[88,89] Thus, there is significant evidence that TGF-β secreted by tumor cells can downmodulate immune responses that otherwise may be protective. TGF-β also may be secreted by regulatory T cells or by other cells in the tumor microenvironment and may have negative regulatory effects.[90]

Similarly, IL-10 and PGE-2 are also secreted by many tumor cells.[81,91] IL-10 has potent immunosuppressive effects and may render tumor cells resistant to lysis by T cells.[92,93] Serum levels have been reported to be elevated in patients with melanoma and in patients with adenocarcinomas of the stomach and pancreas.[94] Although less well studied to date than TGF-β, both IL-10 and PGE-2 may well have clinically significant effects in blocking tumor immunity. New approaches to interfere with these immunosuppressive cytokines will likely be added to immune therapy trials in the future.

Regulatory T Cells

The human immune system is a highly regulated and complex system. Its numerous effector functions as already detailed are regulated at several levels. A critical regulatory element is a T-cell subset known as regulatory T cells. These cells are classically identified as CD4+ CD25+ cells and also express FoxP3.[95] They are capable of inhibiting proliferation of antigen-specific T cells in response to antigen or mitogen and have been found in high proportions among tumor-infiltrating lymphocytes. Their function is not fully elucidated, but TGF-β and IL-10 have been implicated in their regulatory function. Because they express CD25, an IL-2 receptor, they appear to be regulated in part by IL-2.[63,95] In addition to what was originally described as a monomorphic population of regulatory T cells, there is increasing evidence that there may be multiple populations of regulatory T cells. Collectively, they may well be a critical obstacle to immune control of cancer, and mechanisms to downregulate or to deplete them may be helpful as tools for effective immune therapy of cancer.

Autoimmunity and Antigen-Loss Variants: Evidence of Immune Responses In Vivo

A major goal in tumor immunology has long been to identify truly tumor-specific antigens; so targeting of the immune response to tissue differentiation antigens, which are not strictly tumor-specific, is not entirely satisfying from an immunological standpoint. On the other hand, it is a reasonable clinical goal to target immune therapy against tissue differentiation antigens when the normal tissue expressing those antigens is not required for life. Certainly this is true for melanoma, where loss of skin melanocytes is little more than a cosmetic complication. One potential difficulty of targeting cells with melanocytic tissue differentiation, however, is the possible cross-reactivity on retinal pigment epithelium and on the pigmented tissues in the brain, locus ceruleus, and substantia nigra. Such tissues, however, may be protected by the blood–brain barrier, by downregulation of MHC expression in those tissues, and by some differences in the melanin pathways compared to normal melanocytes.

More dramatic autoimmunity, however, does occur in association with anticancer immune responses, in rare cases. These cases include a number of paraneoplastic syndromes, the best described of which are caused by antibody responses to tumor antigens that cross-react with normal tissue antigens.[96] One example of a dramatic presentation is the anti-Yo antibody, which occurs usually as a result of antibodies to ovarian or breast cancers. The anti-Yo antibodies cross-react with an antigen naturally present on cerebellar Purkinje cells.[97] The result can be the total destruction of Purkinje cells and very severe ataxia and loss of coordination; this leads to physical incapacitation even though the cancer may be controlled. Thus, it is clear that immune responses to cancer cells can occur naturally, can be very dramatic, and can be capable of target cell destruction; however, these antibody responses do not predictably cause destruction of the tumor. Thus, there may be mechanisms by which the tumor cells, although stimulating an immune response, ultimately evade destruction by that immune response. Possible mechanisms for immune escape are discussed next.

Furthermore, the expression of tumor-associated antigens in normal tissues can be predicted to induce some tolerance to these antigens in the normal host and may present an obstacle to tumor immunity.[98] Elucidation of mechanisms for overcoming tolerance will be important in future immunotherapy trial design. Regardless, the fact that antitumor responses, such as those evident in the case of anti-Yo antibodies, can arise in the presence of those antigens on normal cells is evidence that tolerance to normal tissue antigens can be overwhelmed. Similarly, the finding of immune responses to melanocyte tissue differentiation antigens is evidence that tolerance is not absolute and may be subject to therapeutic intervention.

Toleragenic Presentation by Tumors

For most cancers, it has been very well demonstrated that in vitro stimulation of patient lymphocytes with autologous tumor results in generation of autologous tumor-specific CTLs.[46,99–105] These CTLs may also cross-react on HLA-matched allogeneic tumors, where shared antigens are being targeted. Presumably, their targets include both shared and unique antigens. Regardless, the fact that those CTLs can be generated ex vivo simply by coculture with autologous tumor and IL-2 is evidence that the host repertoire includes tumor-reactive CTLs. The fact that the patient's tumor progresses in vivo despite the presence of antigens that can be targeted by these CTLs is one of the central paradoxes in tumor immunology. It suggests that the in vivo setting protects the tumor from immune eradication. It is important to characterize the mechanisms by which tumors escape immune recognition in vivo. Hopefully, such an understanding will lead to new approaches to counteract those immune escape mechanisms.

One feature of tumor cells, which can explain their failure to stimulate T-cell responses directly, is their lack of the costimulatory molecules B7-1 and B7-2.[106] These molecules are ligands for CD28 on T cells. As such, these molecules provide the second signal required for T-cell activation.[107,108] They appear on antigen-presenting cells such as dendritic cells, macrophages, and B cells.[109] When a T-cell receptor binds its cognate antigen on a professional antigen-presenting cell (APC), CD28 on the T cell binds to B7-1 or B7-2 molecules on the APC, providing a second signal required for activation. Without that second signal, ligation of the TcR results in tolerance to that antigen. Many different tumors fail to express either of these costimulatory molecules, a fact that is a partial explanation for the relative failure of T-cell immunity to tumor antigens in vivo.

Other mechanisms for immune escape include failure to express tumor antigens as a result of heterogeneity or immune selection,[110–113] downregulation of MHC expression,[114–119] failure of antigen-processing pathways,[120–124] expression of Fas ligand,[125] or secretion of immunosuppressive cytokines.[81] Tumors are well described as heterogeneous, with expression of some tumor-associated antigens often downregulated or lost as they become more metastatic.[126] In particular, the tissue differentiation antigens in melanoma are commonly downregulated in advanced melanoma, and nonpigmented metastases are commonly observed. On one hand, the loss of expression of these antigens may be the result of selective immune pressure. On the other hand, it is a mechanism of immune escape that may complicate immune therapy with these antigens.

Other recent studies have identified two enzymes that may be critical mediators of immune dysfunction at sites of tumor: arginase and indoleamine 2,3-dioxygenase (IDO). Arginase degrades arginine[127] and IDO degrades tryptophan.[128,129] The effects of these enzymes on immune function in the tumor microenvironment can be dramatic. Gene microarray studies on metastatic melanoma suggest a high prevalence of these mechanisms.[130] Targeted inhibition of the function of these enzymes is a rational strategy to augment immune therapy of cancer.[131]

MHC class II molecules are not expressed on most normal somatic cells but are expressed by activated T cells and by professional APCs. Class I MHC molecules, however, are widely expressed on almost all normal somatic cells. Tumor cells usually fail to express Class II MHC molecules, but Class I MHC molecules are often expressed. On the other hand, downregulation of Class I MHC molecules has been observed on tumors. In an interesting example, a patient with metastatic melanoma had circulating T cells reactive to antigens restricted by three different MHC molecules, and she was vaccinated repeatedly with an autologous tumor cell vaccine. A subsequent metastasis was resected and contained tumor cells that had lost expression of all three of those MHC molecules. However, reactivity to an antigen presented by a fourth MHC molecule was observed, and the patient has done well after resection of that metastasis plus repeated vaccination with the autologous tumor cells.[27] This example illustrates immunoselection in vivo, presumably caused by loss of MHC molecule expression.

In another detailed study of immune escape, multiple mechanisms of immune escape were identified in the patient's metastatic melanoma, but the patient's immune response spontaneously developed reactivity to a previously cryptic antigenic target, resulting in a broader antitumor immune repertoire. This adaptive immune response was associated with long-term survival after surgery.[132] This observation supports the hypothesis that surgery can cure patients with metastatic cancer in cases where there is also induction of protective antitumor immunity, either spontaneously or induced by immune therapy.

Downregulation of antigen-processing pathways has also been described in several tumor cell lines in vitro.[120–124] Although its role in tumor escape from immune recognition in vivo has not been defined, it is likely is a factor in vivo. IFN-γ can reverse the antigen-processing defects that have been described.[120,122] Another mechanism of possible tumor-induced immune escape may be related to tumor-induced apoptosis of tumor-reactive T cells. Activated CTLs express the apoptotic signaling protein Fas, and some tumors have been reported to express FasL.[125] There have been conflicting reports on this subject, but it remains an intriguing possibility.[133]

Costimulation as a Regulatory Mechanism

As explained earlier, costimulatory signals mediated by interaction between CD28 and B7-1/B7-2 are critical to the effective stimulation of T-cell immunity. In addition to CD28, another T-cell surface molecule is a ligand for B7-1 and B7-2. This molecule, CTLA4, is expressed after T-cell stimulation occurs, and when it binds to B7-1 or B7-2, it mediates a negative signal that limits the T-cell proliferative response.[134–136] The importance of this interaction is evidenced by the fact that CTLA4-knockout mice experience rapid and dramatic proliferation of lymphocytes in lymph nodes, such that the animals become overwhelmed and deformed by this expansion of nodal tissue.[137] Thus, it appears that CTLA4/B7 interactions limit T-cell responses once an adequate response occurs. However, if the initial response is weak, CTLA4 may prevent expansion of that initial response and may lead to failure of the response. Thus, it has been postulated that blocking CTLA4/B7 interactions with antibody to CTLA4 may augment antitumor responses. Initial animal studies support this hypothesis, as vaccination against syngeneic tumors is markedly more effective when administered with anti-CTLA4 antibodies.[135]

Recent clinical trials with humanized antibodies against CTLA4 have led to provocative results. Patients with advanced melanoma treated with that antibody have experienced major objective tumor regressions in 10% to 20% of cases and have also experienced dramatic autoimmune-like toxicities including a severe colitis and hypophysitis.[138] The autoimmune toxicities are typically reversible with steroids. These findings provide dramatic evidence for the role of immune dysregulation in cancer therapy, but also highlight the complexities of such interventions. Larger studies with these CTLA4 antibodies are being initiated. Similarly, new therapies targeting other costimulatory interactions (e.g., PD-1) are in the pipeline for cancer immunotherapy.[139]

Prognostic Implications of Immune Responses to Cancer Cells

Numerous studies have shown that humoral and cellular immunity to cancer cells is strongly associated with the prognosis of patients with cancer. Several nonrandomized clinical trials of tumor vaccines have been performed in which patients with demonstrated immune responses to the vaccine have prolonged survival compared to nonresponders.[140] Furthermore, there is strong evidence now that the finding of a "brisk" infiltrate of lymphocytes in tumor deposits correlates with a good prognosis.[141–144] Thus, there is evidence that immune responses to tumor may be associated with an improved clinical outcome, and the challenge remains to induce an effective immune response in patients where one does not exist naturally.

Clinical Trials of Cancer Vaccines

Nonspecific Active Immunotherapy

The concept that the immune system may effect some control over tumor progression is not new. Immune therapy has been investigated for the treatment of cancer in an increasingly systematic way over the past hundred years or so. Even before the twentieth century, some clinical studies provided intriguing evidence for the power of immune responses to affect cancer progression. Clinical studies of bacterial toxins in the eighteenth and nineteenth centuries associated exposure to bacterial toxins with tumor regressions.[145–147] These were anecdotal observations that suggested an association between nonspecific immune stimulation and augmentation of antitumor immune responses.

Following from those studies and other observations, a surgeon named William B. Coley initiated investigations with injection of several different toxins in patients with advanced cancer. In particular, he administered *Cryptospiridium parvum* and BCG (Bacille Calmette–Guerin) to patients with advanced cancer. Although he reported responses in only a few percent of patients, these were more significant than what was possible with other existing therapy.[148,149] Use of bacterial toxins as therapy in patients with cancer continued sporadically throughout the twentieth century. Intravesical BCG therapy is still used for treatment of superficial bladder cancer and is FDA approved for that indication. However, the precise mechanism by which BCG exerts its therapeutic effects is unknown.[150]

For adjuvant therapy of patients, after resection of solid tumors, cutaneous injections of bacterial toxins have been studied extensively. However, randomized trials of BCG and/or *C. parvum* "vaccines" have shown no survival benefit in a large number of studies. The use of BCG as direct injection in tumor deposits is associated with ulcerative local inflammatory reactions and local tumor destruction. BCG has also been used as an adjuvant for whole cell vaccines, where it is believed to augment T-cell responses to vaccinating antigens.

Cancer Vaccines Based on Whole Tumor Cells

Coley, Morton, and others reported that direct injection of metastatic deposits with bacterial toxins such as BCG usually resulted in destruction of the tumor deposits and, in a minority of cases, destruction of other metastatic sites not injected with BCG.[148,151,152] The suggestion was that the BCG injection turned the tumor deposits into tumor vaccines, with tumor cells serving as the antigen source. BCG continues to be used as an adjuvant in whole cell vaccines. A randomized prospective trial of autologous tumor cell vaccines plus BCG versus no therapy was performed in colon cancer patients, after surgical resection, and revealed a 50% to 60% reduction in recurrence among stage II patients, which correlated well with DTH responses to the autologous tumor cells.[153] However, a subsequent multicenter trial by the Eastern Cooperative Oncology Group failed to show a survival advantage with an autologous whole cell vaccine for colon cancer.[154]

Few other randomized prospective trials of tumor cell-derived vaccines have been completed to date, even though the approach is not a new one. Several investigators have administered whole cell vaccines, with clinical results suggestive of therapeutic benefit. T-cell responses and antibody responses have correlated with good clinical outcomes in these patients as well. Mastrangelo and Berd reported improved survival rates in melanoma patients, compared to institutional controls, after vaccination with autologous whole cell vaccines coupled with the hapten dinitrophenol (DNP) in patients.[155] The only large randomized trial of a melanoma cell vaccine was the vaccinia melanoma oncolysate (VMO) trial, where patients with high-risk resected melanoma were randomized to receive a lysate of allogeneic whole cells infected with vaccinia virus. There was no significant survival advantage for the treatment group.[156] Morton has reported cellular and humoral immune responses to melanoma antigens in patients with advanced melanoma treated with surgical resection and postoperative adjuvant immunotherapy using Canvaxin, a mixture of three allogeneic whole cell lines, plus BCG.[140,157] The survival results in these patients significantly exceed the survival of patients with stage IV disease previously treated at that institution.[158] Two phase III randomized placebo-controlled trials were initiated using this vaccine preparation in patients with resected stage III or stage IV melanoma. The trial in stage IV patients was closed early from failure to show improved outcomes with vaccination. However, the final results of that trial have not been reported formally. The trial in stage III patients has completed accrual, but clinical results are pending.

Instead of using whole cells or lysates of whole cells, Bystryn has administered a vaccine composed of cultured whole cell supernatants, excluding small molecules. He has demonstrated that melanoma antigens such as MART-1 and MAGE-A3 are represented as intact proteins in these shed antigens in the supernatant,[159] and he has shown that antibodies to some of the vaccine components are induced in serum of vaccinated patients.[160] In addition, vaccination with this crude preparation is associated with increased T-cell responses to defined epitopes from these proteins.[159] In a small randomized trial, patients receiving this vaccine had improved disease-free survival over controls.[161]

Another approach to whole cell vaccines has been to vaccinate with allogeneic whole tumor cells transfected with a gene for human GM-CSF. Murine studies demonstrated the value of this approach,[74] and human studies in melanoma, lung cancer, renal cell cancer, and pancreatic cancer are underway and are promising.[162–165]

A vaccine approach for melanoma specifically targeted to stimulation of antibody responses used the ganglioside GM2, coupled to KLH, administered in the adjuvant QS-21.[166] This approach, led by Phil Livingston, does induce specific IgG and IgM responses[167] and was associated with some evidence of clinical efficacy in phase I and phase II trials.[168,169] However, in a phase III trial, where patients were randomized to receive the vaccine or interferon-α, survival of patients receiving the ganglioside vaccine did not exceed that of patients receiving interferon.[170]

Another approach that has promise in patients with B-cell lymphomas is the use of antiidiotype antibodies.[171] In this approach, the aim is to induce antibodies that mimic the idiotype recognized by the membrane-bound immunoglobulin on clonal B-cell lymphoma cells, thus leading to antibody-mediated clearance of the malignant cells expressing that immunoglobulin. Early results with this approach in clinical trials are promising.[171–173]

Vaccines with Defined Antigen Vaccines

Since the early 1990s, many antigens have been identified that function as targets for T-cell responses as categorized in Table 93.4. Not only are the genes and proteins characterized, by many peptides from those proteins have also been defined that function as MHC-associated epitopes for cancer-reactive T cells. Clinical trials using defined antigens have been performed in the past decade, and more are underway; these involve multiple different strategies, including viral vaccines encoding defined antigens and direct peptide injections, among others (Table 93.5). Each of these usually is administered with some form of adjuvant, designed to induce inflammation and to augment antigen-specific immunity (Table 93.6). All these various approaches have led to promising immunological responses, and objective clinical responses have been observed in patients on various trials. However, the large majority of immune responses are of low magnitude and are not associated with clinical responses. The goals of future vaccine development are to augment immunological and clinical responses.

Results of many vaccine trials using defined antigens are summarized and referenced in a recent report.[174] Overall, clinical response rates with such vaccines are in the range of 3% to 6% for melanoma. Approaches to augment clinical responses should involve rational approaches to augment

TABLE 93.5. Forms of Defined Cancer Antigens in Vaccines.

Intact or modified proteins
Gangliosides or other molecules
DNA encoding whole proteins
DNA encoding protein subunits
DNA encoding MHC-associated peptides
RNA encoding whole proteins or peptides
Viral constructs encoding antigenic proteins or peptides
MHC-associated peptides

TABLE 93.6. Antigen-Delivery Systems and Adjuvants.

Bacille Calmette–Guerin (BCG)
Incomplete Freund's adjuvant (e.g., Montanide ISA-51)
Alum
Saponins (e.g., QS-21)
Toll-like receptor (TLR) agonists TLR7 agonist (e.g., imiquimod) TLR9 agonist (CPGs)
Viral vectors
Viral vectors encoding costimulatory molecules (TRICOM)
Cytokines (IL-2, GM-CSF, IL-12) or genes encoding them
Dendritic cells Immature Mature Other

immune responses and/or to modulate immunoregulation systemically or at sites of tumor. Some of these are listed in Table 93.7 and were described.

One approach has been to vaccinate with dendritic cells pulsed with antigen. Dendritic cells (DCs) are particularly effective antigen-presenting cells (APCs), and a current understanding of their role in the generation of immune responses to cutaneous antigens is that dendritic cells in the skin (Langerhans cells) take up antigens, then migrate to draining lymph nodes, where they encounter T cells and stimulate T-cell responses to the antigens presented by the DC.[175] Thus, it has been suggested that optimal vaccination strategies must involve use of dendritic cells, either by induction of them in vivo, or by adoptive transfer of them after ex vivo culture. In animal studies, pulsing dendritic cells with tumor-derived peptides, or with tumor lysates, resulted in dramatic protective immunity.[176–181] In some of these murine studies, dendritic cell vaccines induced regression of palpable tumors. As a result, there has been enthusiasm for evaluating similar approaches in human clinical trials. Numerous vaccine approaches using dendritic cells have been initiated, and promising clinical results have been reported.[182,183] On the other hand, some of these promising results have been difficult to replicate to the same degree in other centers.[174,184] Also, there is a growing body of evidence that some dendritic cells can be powerful mediators of tolerance, rather than immunity.[185–189] It is increasingly clear that dendritic cells are critical in controlling or directing immune responses, that they can be either immunostimulatory or immunoregulatory, and that the factors controlling their function remain incompletely understood. A randomized prospective clinical trial was performed in Europe through the EORTC, comparing clinical response to (a) DTIC chemotherapy versus (b) vaccination with dendritic cells pulsed with defined peptides. These DC were generated in a rigorously defined manner based on good laboratory science; the trial was halted early because of lower clinical response rates in the DC vaccine arm.[190] This result, along with awareness of the complexity of DC regulation, has introduced greater caution into current studies of DC vaccines.

An alternative approach is to vaccinate with defined antigens directly into the skin or subcutaneous tissues, combined with local adjuvants to induce innate immune responses and inflammation. Examples of adjuvants that appear to augment T-cell responses are IL-12,[191] Montanide-ISA 51 (a form of incomplete Freund's adjuvant) with or without GM-CSF,[192,193] combinations of KLH and GM-CSF,[194] and CpG molecules.[195] There is new enthusiasm for using defined agonists for toll-like receptors such as imiquimod and CpG molecules as vaccine adjuvants. However, there is a great deal of work to do toward identifying optimal adjuvants and in understanding the cellular and molecular effects of vaccine adjuvants.

The next decade will be marked by the development of more robust cancer vaccines that target both CD8 and CD4 T cells while also upregulating innate immunity and downregulating regulatory T cells and other immune regulation. Furthermore, combination immunotherapies for human cancers are already in development; these will include the combination of vaccines with therapies that interfere with immunoregulatory processes (e.g., CTLA4 antibody, cyclophosphamide), that modulate the Th1/Th2 balance of immune responses (cytokines or cytokine modulators, e.g., IL-12), those that deplete circulating or tumor-infiltrating regulatory T cells (e.g., Ontak, CD25 antibodies), and those that synergize for tumor cell destruction (small molecule inhibitors of critical cell signaling pathways, e.g., B-raf kinase inhibitors, mTOR), or for destruction of tumor vasculature (bevacizumab, VEGF signaling inhibitors). It is appears that the new work with adoptive T-cell transfer, after lymphodepletion, is likely to become part of the future of immune therapy for cancer and that innovations in this area will contribute to new approaches for management of advanced cancer. Some of these areas for ongoing and future investigation are listed in Table 93.7.

TABLE 93.7. Opportunities for Basic and Translational Research to Improve Cancer Vaccines.

Antigen identification • Identification of the complete "immunome" of shared defined antigens • Technology for rapid identification of relevant patient-specific tumor-rejection antigens
Induction of T-cell responses • Characterization of the optimal antigen-presenting cell and how to induce its activation and function in vivo and ex vivo • Identification of optimal vaccine adjuvants (TLR agonists, cytokines) • Strategies for reliable induction of T-cell responses to multiple antigens • Optimizing adoptive T-cell therapy
Controlling the T-cell response to vaccination in multiple compartments • Understanding factors that control regional versus systemic immunity • Understanding factors that control organ- or tissue-specific immunity • Technology to direct responding immune cells to sites of tumor • Regulatory T cells and what controls them
Immune monitoring • Technology for monitoring T-cell responses in real time • Characterization of the quality of the T-cell response
Overcoming immune escape • Patient-specific characterization of immune escape phenotypes • Tailoring vaccines to overcome patient-specific/tumor-specific immune escape • Combination therapies (chemotherapy, antibodies to CTLA4, others)

TABLE 93.8. FDA-Approved Immunological Treatments.

Type of therapy	*Specific approved treatments*
Nonspecific immune stimulants	• Bacille Calmette–Guerin (BCG)
Cytokines	• Interleukin 2 (IL-2) • Interferon-α (IFN-α) • TNF-α (Europe)
Antibodies	• Herceptin (humanized anti-Her-2/neu) • Rituximab (humanized anti-CD20) • Avastin (anti-VEGF)

Summary

There is substantial evidence now that immune responses to human tumor antigens occur in vivo, and that such immune responses may be associated with improved prognosis. Clinical trials completed within the past few years now provide evidence that some manipulations of that immune response can be therapeutic, and may even lead to durable complete responses. These observations offer promise that antibody therapy, cytokine therapy, adoptive immunotherapy, and tumor vaccines all may have a role in the therapy of human cancers in the near future. In fact, several immunological treatments have been approved by the FDA for use in cancer therapy (Table 93.8).

On the other hand, it is clear that the immune response to cancer is complicated by mechanisms tumor cells use to evade immune recognition, and that successful immune therapy will likely require new approaches to overcome such immune escape mechanisms. It will also be necessary to develop more robust immune therapies that simultaneously or sequentially target multiple effector arms of the immune responses. Advances in this field have been significant over the past few years, with a new understanding of the antigens targeted by cytotoxic T cells, and with an awareness of the role of immune regulation mediated both by the host and by the tumor cells. It is expected that continued advancement in these areas will lead to significant changes in the treatment of human cancer in the next decade.

References

1. Burnet FM. The concept of immunologic surveillance. Prog Exp Tumor Res 1970;13:1–27.
2. Ehrlich P. Uber den jetzigen Stand der Karzinomforschung. Ned Tijdschr Geneesk 1909;5:273–290.
3. Delaloye AB, Delaloye B. Radiolabelled monoclonal antibodies in tumour imaging and therapy: out of fashion? Eur J Nucl Med 1995;22:571–580.
4. Zuckier LS, DeNardo GL. Trials and tribulations: oncological antibody imaging comes to the fore. Semin Nucl Med 1997;27:10–29.
5. Sirisriro R, Podoloff DA, Patt YZ, et al. 99Tcm-IMMU4 imaging in recurrent colorectal cancer: efficacy and impact on surgical management. Nucl Med Commun 1996;17:568–576.
6. LaValle GJ, Martinez DA, Sobel D, et al. Assessment of disseminated pancreatic cancer: a comparison of traditional exploratory laparotomy and radioimmunoguided surgery. Surgery (St. Louis) 1997;122:867–871.
7. Schneebaum S, Papo J, Graif M, et al. Radioimmunoguided surgery benefits for recurrent colorectal cancer. Ann Surg Oncol 1997;4:371–376.
8. Stigbrand T, Ullen A, Sandstrom P, et al. Twenty years with monoclonal antibodies: state of the art—where do we go? Acta Oncol 1996;35:259–265.
9. Gamble AR, Bell JA, Ronan JE, et al. Use of tumour marker immunoreactivity to identify primary site of metastatic cancer. Br Med J 1993;306:295–298.
10. Mottolese M, Venturo I, Donnorso RP, et al. Use of selected combinations of monoclonal antibodies to tumor associated antigens in the diagnosis of neoplastic effusions of unknown origin. Eur J Cancer Clin Oncol 1998;28:1277–1284.
11. Tureci O, Usener D, Schneider S, Sahin U. Identification of tumor-associated autoantigens with SEREX. Methods Mol Med 2005;109:137–154.
12. Chen YT. Identification of human tumor antigens by serological expression cloning: an online review on SEREX. Cancer Immun 2004;[updated 2004 Mar 10; cited 2004 Apr 1]. http://www.cancerimmunity.org/SEREX/.
13. Chen YT, Scanlan MJ, Sahin U, et al. A testicular antigen aberrantly expressed in human cancers detected by autologous antibody screening. Proc Natl Acad Sci U S A 1997;94:1914–1918.
14. Van den Eynde BJ, van der Bruggen P. T cell defined tumor antigens. Curr Opin Immunol 1997;9:684–693.
15. Jager E, Chen YT, Drijfhout JW, et al. Simultaneous humoral and cellular immune response against cancer-testis antigen NY-ESO-1: definition of human histocompatibility leukocyte antigen (HLA)-A2-binding peptide epitopes. J Exp Med 1998;187:265–270.
16. Tureci O, Sahin U, Schobert I, et al. The SSX-2 gene, which is involved in the t(X;18) translocation of synovial sarcomas, codes for the human tumor antigen HOM-MEL-40. Cancer Res 1996;56:4766–5772.
17. Storkus WJ, Howell DN, Salter RD, et al. NK susceptibility varies inversely with target cell class I HLA antigen expression. J Immunol 1987;138:1657–1659.
18. Kageshita T, Wang Z, Calorini L, et al. Selective loss of human leukocyte class I allospecificities and staining of melanoma cells by monoclonal antibodies recognizing monomorphic determinants of class I human leukocyte antigens. Cancer Res 1993;53:3349–3354.
19. Khanna R. Tumour surveillance: missing peptides and MHC molecules. Immunol Cell Biol 1998;76:20–26.
20. Chang CC, Campoli M, Ferrone S. HLA class I antigen expression in malignant cells: why does it not always correlate with CTL-mediated lysis? Curr Opin Immunol 2005;16:644–650.
21. Chouaib S, Thiery J, Gati A, et al. Tumor escape from killing: role of killer inhibitory receptors and acquisition of tumor resistance to cell death. Tissue Antigens 2002;60(4):273.
22. Steffens U, Vyas Y, Dupont B, et al. Nucleotide and amino acid sequence alignment for human killer cell inhibitory receptors (KIR). Tissue Antigens 1998;51:398–413.
23. Uhrberg M, Valiante NM, Shum BP, et al. Human diversity in killer cell inhibitory receptor genes. Immunity 1997;7:753–763.
24. Christensen MD, Geisler C. Recruitment of SHP-1 protein tyrosine phosphatase and signalling by a chimeric T cell receptor-killer inhibitory receptor. Scand J Immunol 2000;51:557–564.
25. Bakker AB, Phillips JH, Figdor CG, et al. Killer cell inhibitory receptors for MHC class I molecules regulate lysis of melanoma cells mediated by NK cells, gamma delta T cells, and antigen-specific CTL. J Immunol 1998;160:5239–5245.
26. Mingari MC, Moretta A, Moretta L. Regulation of KIR expression in human T cells: a safety mechanism that may impair protective T-cell responses. Immunol Today 1998;19:153–157.
27. Ikeda H, Lethe B, Lehmann F, et al. Characterization of an antigen that is recognized on a melanoma showing partial HLA loss by CTL expressing an NK inhibitory receptor. Immunity 1997;6:199–208.

28. Morgan DA, Ruscetti FW, Gallo R. Selective in vitro growth of T lymphocytes from normal human bone marrow. Science 1976;193:1007–1008.
29. Kedar E, Ikejiri BL, Gorelik E, et al. Natural cell-mediated cytotoxicity in vitro and inhibition of tumor growth in vivo by murine lymphoid cells cultured with T cell growth factor (TCGF). Cancer Immunol Immunother 1982;13:14–23.
30. Rosenberg SA, Mule JJ, Spiess PJ, et al. Regression of established pulmonary metastases and subcutaneous tumor mediated by the systemic administration of high-dose recombinant interleukin 2. J Exp Med 1985;161:1169–1188.
31. Eberlein TJ, Rosenstein M, Rosenberg SA. Regression of a disseminated syngeneic solid tumor by systemic transfer of lymphoid cells expanded in interleukin 2. J Exp Med 1982;156: 385–397.
32. Fisher RI, Coltman CA Jr, Doroshow JH, et al. Metastatic renal cell cancer treated with interleukin-2 and lymphokine-activated killer cells. A phase II clinical trial. Ann Intern Med 1998;108:518–523.
33. Dutcher JP, Creekmore S, Weiss GR, et al. A phase II study of interleukin-2 and lymphokine-activated killer cells in patients with metastatic malignant melanoma. J Clin Oncol 1989;7:477–485.
34. Rosenberg SA, Yang JC, Topalian SL, et al. Treatment of 283 consecutive patients with metastatic melanoma or renal cell cancer using high-dose bolus interleukin 2 [see comments]. Comment in JAMA 1994;271(12):945–946; comment in JAMA 1994;272(17):1327. JAMA 1994;271:907–913.
35. Fisher RI, Rosenberg SA, Fyfe G. Long-term survival update for high-dose recombinant interleukin-2 in patients with renal cell carcinoma. Cancer J Sci Am 2000;6(suppl 1):S55–S57.
36. Yang JC, Sherry RM, Steinberg SM, et al. Randomized study of high-dose and low-dose interleukin-2 in patients with metastatic renal cancer. J Clin Oncol 2003;21:3127–3132.
37. Phan GQ, Attia P, Steinberg SM, et al. Factors associated with response to high-dose interleukin-2 in patients with metastatic melanoma. J Clin Oncol 2001;19:3477–3482.
38. Chang E, Rosenberg SA. Patients with melanoma metastases at cutaneous and subcutaneous sites are highly susceptible to interleukin-2-based therapy. J Immunother 2001;24:88–90.
39. Gross L. Intradermal immunization of C3H mice against a sarcoma that originated in an animal of the same line. Cancer Res 1943;3:326–333.
40. Klarnet JP, Matis LA, Kern DE, et al. Antigen-driven T cell clones can proliferate in vivo, eradicate disseminated leukemia, and provide specific immunologic memory. J Immunol 1987; 138:4012–4017.
41. Vose BM, Bonnard GD. Human tumor antigens defined by cytotoxicity and proliferative responses of cultured lymphoid cells. Nature (Lond) 1982;296:359–361.
42. Slingluff CL Jr, Darrow T, Vervaert C, et al. Human cytotoxic T cells specific for autologous melanoma cells: successful generation from lymph node cells in seven consecutive cases. J Natl Cancer Inst 1988;80:1016–1026.
43. Rosenberg SA, Yannelli JR, Yang JC, et al. Treatment of patients with metastatic melanoma with autologous tumor-infiltrating lymphocytes and interleukin 2 [see comments]. J Natl Cancer Inst 1994;86:1159–1166.
44. Dudley ME, Wunderlich JR, Yang JC, et al. Adoptive cell transfer therapy following non-myeloablative but lymphodepleting chemotherapy for the treatment of patients with refractory metastatic melanoma. J Clin Oncol 2005;23:2346–2357.
45. Darrow TL, Slingluff CLJ, Seigler HF. The role of HLA class I antigens in recognition of melanoma cells by tumor-specific cytotoxic T lymphocytes. Evidence for shared tumor antigens. J Immunol 1989;142:3329–3335.
46. Slovin SF, Lackman RD, Ferrone S, et al. Cellular immune response to human sarcomas: cytotoxic T cell clones reactivity with autologous sarcomas. I. Development, phenotype, and specificity. J Immunol 1986;137:3042–3048.
47. Van Bleek GM, Nathenson SG. Isolation of endogenously processed immunodominant viral peptides form the class I H-$2K^b$ molecule. Nature (Lond) 1990;348:213.
48. Falk K, Rotzschke O, Deres K, et al. Identification of naturally processed viral nonapeptides allow their quantification in infected cells and suggests an allele-specific T cell epitope forecast. J Exp Med 1991;174:425–434.
49. Udaka K, Tsomides TJ, Eisen HN. A naturally occurring peptide recognized by alloreactive CD8+ cytotoxic T lymphocytes in associateion with a class I MHC protein. Cell 1992;69:989.
50. Novellino L, Castelli C, Parmiani G. A listing of human tumor antigens recognized by T cells: March 2004 update. Cancer Immunol Immunother 2005;54:187–207.
51. Bystryn JC, Rigel D, Friedman RJ, et al. Prognostic significance of hypopigmentation in malignant melanoma. Arch Dermatol 1987;123:1053–1055.
52. Rosenberg SA, White DE. Vitiligo in patients with melanoma: normal tissue antigens can be targets for cancer immunotherapy. J Immunother Emphasis Tumor Immunol 1996;19:81–84.
53. Gregor RT. Vitiligo and malignant melanoma: a significant association? S Afr Med J 1976;50:1447–1449.
54. Wagner SN, Wagner C, Schultewolter T, et al. Analysis of Pmel17/gp100 expression in primary human tissue specimens: implications for melanoma immuno- and gene-therapy. Cancer Immunol Immunother 1997;44:239–247.
55. Tjoa BA, Erickson SJ, Bowes VA, et al. Follow-up evaluation of prostate cancer patients infused with autologous dendritic cells pulsed with PSMA peptides. Prostate 1997;32:272–278.
56. Multhoff G, Botzler C. Heat-shock proteins and the immune response. Ann N Y Acad Sci 1998;851:86–93.
57. Tamura Y, Peng P, Liu K, et al. Immunotherapy of tumors with autologous tumor-derived heat shock protein preparations. Science 1997;278:117–120.
58. Castelli C, Rivoltini L, Rini F, et al. Heat shock proteins: biological functions and clinical application as personalized vaccines for human cancer. Cancer Immunol Immunother 2004;53:227–233.
59. Cantrell DA, Smith KA. Transient expression of interleukin 2 receptors. Consequences for T cell growth. J Exp Med 1983;158: 1895–1911.
60. Hefeneider SH, Conlon PJ, Henney CS, et al. In vivo interleukin 2 administration augments the generation of alloreactive cytolytic T lymphocytes and resident natural killer cells. J Immunol 1983;130:222–227.
61. Bensinger SJ, Walsh PT, Zhang J, et al. Distinct IL-2 receptor signaling pattern in CD4+CD25+ regulatory T cells. J Immunol 2004;172:5287–5296.
62. Setoguchi R, Hori S, Takahashi T, et al. Homeostatic maintenance of natural Foxp3(+) CD25(+) CD4(+) regulatory T cells by interleukin (IL)-2 and induction of autoimmune disease by IL-2 neutralization. J Exp Med 2005;201:723–735.
63. Scheffold A, Huhn J, Hofer T. Regulation of CD4+ CD25+ regulatory T cell activity: it takes (IL-)two to tango. Eur J Immunol 2005;35:1336–1341.
64. Muller U, Steinhoff U, Reis LF, et al. Functional role of type I and type II interferons in antiviral defense. Science 1994;264: 1918–1921.
65. Colamonici OR, Porterfield B, Domanski P, et al. Ligand-independent anti-oncogenic activity of the alpha subunit of the type I interferon receptor. J Biol Chem 1994;269:27275–27279.
66. Platanias LC, Uddin S, Domanski P, et al. Differences in interferon alpha and beta signaling. Interferon beta selectively induces the interaction of the alpha and betaL subunits of the type I interferon receptor. J Biol Chem 1996;271:23630–23633.
67. Kowalzick L, Weyer U, Lange P, et al. Systemic therapy of advanced metastatic malignant melanoma with a combination

of fibroblast interferon-beta and recombinant interferon-gamma. Dermatologica 1990;181:298–303.
68. Creagan ET, Loprinzi CL, Ahmann DL, et al. A phase I-II trial of the combination of recombinant leukocyte A interferon and recombinant human interferon-gamma in patients with metastatic malignant melanoma. Cancer (Phila) 1988;62:2472–2474.
69. Creagan ET, Schaid DJ, Ahmann DL, et al. Recombinant interferons in the management of advanced malignant melanoma. Updated review of five prospective clinical trials and long-term responders. Am J Clin Oncol 1988;11:652–659.
70. Gleave ME, Elhilali M, Fradet Y, et al. Interferon gamma-1b compared with placebo in metastatic renal-cell carcinoma. Canadian Urologic Oncology Group. N Engl J Med 1988;38:1265–1271.
71. Brown TD, Goodman PJ, Fleming T, et al. Phase II trial of recombinant DNA gamma-interferon in advanced colorectal cancer: a Southwest Oncology Group study. J Immunother 1991;10:379–382.
72. Abdel-Wahab Z, Dar M, Osanto S, et al. Eradication of melanoma pulmonary metastases by immunotherapy with tumor cells engineered to secrete interleukin-2 or gamma interferon. Cancer Gene Ther 1997;4:33–41.
73. Abdel-Wahab Z, Weltz C, Hester D, et al. A phase I clinical trial of immunotherapy with interferon-gamma gene-modified autologous melanoma cells: monitoring the humoral immune response. Cancer (Phila) 1997;80:401–412.
74. Dranoff G, Jaffee E, Lazenby A, et al. Vaccination with irradiated tumor cells engineered to secrete murine granulocyte-macrophage colony-stimulating factor stimulates potent, specific, and long-lasting anti-tumor immunity. Proc Natl Acad Sci U S A 1993;90:3539–3543.
75. Spitler LE, Grossbard ML, Ernstoff MS, et al. Adjuvant therapy of stage III and IV malignant melanoma using granulocyte-macrophage colony-stimulating factor [see comments]. J Clin Oncol 2000;18:1614–1621.
76. Ando K, Hiroishi K, Kaneko T, et al. Perforin, Fas/Fas ligand, and TNF-alpha pathways as specific and bystander killing mechanisms of hepatitis C virus-specific human CTL. J Immunol 1997;158:5283–5291.
77. Lee RK, Spielman J, Zhao DY, et al. Perforin, Fas ligand, and tumor necrosis factor are the major cytotoxic molecules used by lymphokine-activated killer cells. J Immunol 1996;157:1919–1925.
78. Bartlett DL, Ma G, Alexander HR, et al. Isolated limb reperfusion with tumor necrosis factor and melphalan in patients with extremity melanoma after failure of isolated limb perfusion with chemotherapeutics. Cancer (Phila) 1997;80:2084–2090.
79. Tracey KJ, Fong Y, Hesse DG, et al. Anti-cachectin/TNF monoclonal antibodies prevent septic shock during lethal bacteraemia. Nature (Lond) 1987;330:662–664.
80. Jones AL, Selby P. Tumour necrosis factor: clinical relevance. Cancer Surv 1989;8:817–836.
81. Wojtowicz-Praga S. Reversal of tumor-induced immunosuppression: a new approach to cancer therapy. J Immunother 1997;20:165–177.
82. Vanky F, Nagy N, Hising C, et al. Human ex vivo carcinoma cells produce transforming growth factor beta and thereby can inhibit lymphocyte functions in vitro. Cancer Immunol Immunother 1997;43:317.
83. Hirte H, Clark DA. Generation of lymphokine-activated killer cells in human ovarian carcinoma ascitic fluid: identification of transforming growth factor-beta as a suppressive factor. Cancer Immunol Immunother 1991;32:296.
84. Dalal BI, Keown PA, Greenberg AH. Immunocytochemical localization of secreted transforming growth factor-beta 1 to the advancing edges of primary tumors and to lymph node metastases of human mammary carcinoma. Am J Pathol 1993;143:381.
85. McCune BK, Mullin BR, Flanders KC, et al. Localization of transforming growth factor-beta isotypes in lesions of the human breast. Hum Pathol 1992;23:13.
86. Walker RA, Dearing SJ. Transforming growth factor beta 1 in ductal carcinoma in situ and invasive carcinomas of the breast. Eur J Cancer 1992;28:641.
87. Wojtowicz-Praga S, Verma UN, Wakefield L, et al. Modulation of B16 melanoma growth and metastasis by anti-transforming growth factor beta antibody and interleukin-2. J Immunother Emphasis Tumor Immunol 1996;19:169.
88. Fakhrai H, Dorigo O, Shawler DL, et al. Eradication of established intracranial rat gliomas by transforming growth factor beta antisense gene therapy. Proc Natl Acad Sci U S A 1996;93:2909–2914.
89. Dorigo O, Shawler DL, Royston I, et al. Combination of transforming growth factor beta antisense and interleukin-2 gene therapy in the murine ovarian teratoma model. Gynecol Oncol 1998;71:204–210.
90. Hussain SF, Paterson Y. CD4+ CD25+ regulatory T cells that secrete TGF-beta and IL-10 are preferentially induced by a vaccine vector. J Immunother 2004;27:339–346.
91. Nakagomi H, Pisa P, Pisa EK, et al. Lack of interleukin-2 (IL-2) expression and selective expression of IL-10 mRNA in human renal cell carcinoma. Int J Cancer 1995;63:366–371.
92. Tanchot C, Guillaume S, Delon J, et al. Modifications of CD8+ T cell function during in vivo memory or tolerance induction. Immunity 1998;8:581–590.
93. Petersson M, Charo J, Salazar-Onfray F, et al. Constitutive IL-10 production accounts for the high NK sensitivity, low MHC class I expression, and poor transporter associated with antigen processing (TAP)-1/2 function in the prototype NK target YAC-1. J Immunol 1998;161:2099–2105.
94. Fortis C, Foppoli M, Gianotti L, et al. Increased interleukin-10 serum levels in patients with solid tumours. Cancer Lett 1996;104:1–5.
95. Sakaguchi S. Naturally arising Foxp3-expressing CD25+CD4+ regulatory T cells in immunological tolerance to self and non-self. Nat Immunol 2005;6:345–352.
96. Tomer Y, Sherer Y, Shoenfeld Y. Autoantibodies, autoimmunity and cancer. Oncol Rep 1998;5:753–761.
97. Peterson K, Rosenblum MK, Kotanides H, et al. Paraneoplastic cerebellar degeneration. I. A clinical analysis of 55 anti-Yo antibody-positive patients. Neurology 1992;42:1931–1937.
98. Golumbek P, Levitsky H, Jaffee L, et al. The antitumor immune response as a problem of self-nonself discrimination: implications for immunotherapy. Immunol Res 1993;12:183–192.
99. Schendel DJ, Gansbacher B, Oberneder R, et al. Tumor-specific lysis of human renal cell carcinomas by tumor-infiltrating lymphocytes. I. HLA-A2 restricted recognition of autologous and allogeneic tumor lines. J Immunol 1993;151:4209–4220.
100. Slingluff CLJ, Cox AL, Stover JMJ, et al. Cytotoxic T-lymphocyte response to autologous human squamous cell cancer of the lung: epitope reconstitution with peptides extracted from HLA-Aw68. Cancer Res 1994;54:2731–2737.
101. Ioannides CG, Fisk B, Pollack MS, et al. Cytotoxic T-cell clones isolated from ovarian tumor-infiltrating lymphocytes recognize common determinants to non-ovarian tumour clones. Scand J Immunol 1993;37:413–424.
102. Yasumura S, Hirabayashi H, Schwartz DR, et al. Human cytotoxic T-cell lines with restricted specificity for squamous cell carcinoma of the head and neck. Cancer Res 1993;53:1461–1468.
103. Peoples GE, Goedegebuure PS, Andrews JV, et al. HLA-A2 presents shared tumor-associated antigens derived from endogenous proteins in ovarian cancer. J Immunol 1993;151:5481–5491.

104. Schwartzentruber DJ, Solomon D, Rosenberg SA, et al. Characterization of lymphocytes infiltrating human breast cancer: specific immune reactivity detected by measuring cytokine secretion. J Immunother 1992;12:1–12.
105. Wolfel T, Herr W, Coulie P, et al. Lysis of human pancreatic adenocarcinoma cells by autologous HLA-class I-restricted cytolytic T-lymphocyte (CTL) clones. Int J Cancer 1993;54:636–644.
106. Dessureault S, Graham F, Gallinger S. B7-1 gene transfer into human cancer cells by infection with an adenovirus-B7 (Ad-B7) expression vector. Ann Surg Oncol 1996;3:317–324.
107. Turka LA, Ledbetter JA, Lee K, et al. CD28 is an inducible T cell surface antigen that transduces a proliferative signal in CD3+ mature thymocytes. J Immunol 1990;144:1646–1653.
108. Koulova L, Clark EA, Shu G, et al. The CD28 ligand B7/BB1 provides costimulatory signal for alloactivation of CD4+ T cells. J Exp Med 1991;173:759–762.
109. Hathcock KS, Laszlo G, Pucillo C, et al. Comparative analysis of B7-1 and B7-2 costimulatory ligands: expression and function. J Exp Med 1994;180:631–640.
110. deVries TJ, Fourkour A, Wobbes T, et al. Heterogeneous expression of immunotherapy candidate proteins gp100, MART-1, and tyrosinase in human melanoma cell lines and in human melanocytic lesions. Cancer Res 1997;57:3223.
111. Kawakami Y, Zakut R, Topalian SL, et al. Shared human melanoma antigens. Recognition by tumor-infiltrating lymphocytes in HLA-A2.1-transfected melanomas. J Immunol 1992;148:638–643.
112. Hom SS, Topalian SL, Simonis T, et al. Common expression of melanoma tumor-associated antigens recognized by human tumor infiltrating lymphocytes: analysis by human lymphocyte antigen restriction. J Immunother 1991;10:153–164.
113. Bakker AB, Schreurs MW, de Boer AJ, et al. Melanocyte lineage-specific antigen gp100 is recognized by melanoma-derived tumor-infiltrating lymphocytes. J Exp Med 1994;179:1005–1009.
114. Elliott BE, Carlow DA, Rodricks AM, et al. Perspectives on the role of MHC antigens in normal and malignant cell development. Adv Cancer Res 1989;53:181–245.
115. Doyle A, Martin WJ, Funa K, et al. Markedly decreased expression of class I histocompatibility antigens, protein, and mRNA in human small-cell lung cancer. J Exp Med 1985;161:1135–1151.
116. Lassam N, Jay G. Suppression of MHC class I RNA in highly oncogenic cells occurs at the level of transcription initiation. J Immunol 1989;143:3792–3797.
117. Lehmann F, Marchand M, Hainaut P, et al. Differences in the antigens recognized by cytolytic T cells on two successive metastases of a melanoma patient are consistent with immune selection. Eur J Immunol 1995;25:340–347.
118. Jager E, Ringhoffer M, Altmannsberger M, et al. Immunoselection in vivo: independent loss of MHC class I and melanocyte differentiation antigen expression in metastatic melanoma. Int J Cancer 1997;71:142–147.
119. Rivoltini L, Barracchini KC, Viggiano V, et al. Quantitative correlation between HLA class I allele expression and recognition of melanoma cells by antigen-specific cytotoxic T lymphocytes. Cancer Res 1995;55:3149–3157.
120. Restifo NP, Esquivel F, Kawakami Y, et al. Identification of human cancers deficient in antigen processing. J Exp Med 1993;177:265–272.
121. Restifo NP, Esquivel F, Asher AL, et al. Defective presentation of endogenous antigens by a murine sarcoma. Implications for the failure of an anti-tumor immune response. J Immunol 1991;147:1453–1459.
122. Sanda MG, Restifo NP, Walsh JC, et al. Molecular characterization of defective antigen processing in human prostate cancer. J Natl Cancer Inst 1995;87:280–285.
123. Sibille C, Gould KG, Willard-Gallo K, et al. LMP2+ proteasomes are required for the presentation of specific antigens to cytotoxic T lymphocytes. Curr Biol 1995;5:923–930.
124. Maeurer MJ, Gollin SM, Martin D, et al. Tumor escape from immune recognition: lethal recurrent melanoma in a patient associated with downregulation of the peptide transporter protein TAP-1 and loss of expression of the immunodominant MART-1/Melan-A antigen. J Clin Invest 1996;98: 1633–1641.
125. Hahne M, Rimoldi D, Schroter M, et al. Melanoma cell expression of Fas(Apo-1/CD95) ligand: implications for tumor immune escape [see comment]. Science 1996;274:1363–1366.
126. Jager E, Ringhoffer M, Karbach J, et al. Inverse relationship of melanocyte differentiation antigen expression in melanoma tissues and CD8+ cytotoxic-T-cell responses: evidence for immunoselection of antigen-loss variants in vivo. Int J Cancer 1996;66:470–476.
127. Bansal V, Ochoa JB. Arginine availability, arginase, and the immune response. Curr Opin Clin Nutr Metab Care 2003;6:223–228.
128. Munn DH, Mellor AL. IDO and tolerance to tumors. Trends Mol Med 2004;10:15–18.
129. Munn DH, Sharma MD, Lee JR, et al. Potential regulatory function of human dendritic cells expressing indoleamine 2,3-dioxygenase. Science 2002;297:1867–1870.
130. Gajewski TF, Peterson AC, Slingluff C, McKee M, Harlin H. Reciprocal expression of indoleamine-2,3-dioxygenase (IDO) and arginase-I in metastatic melanoma tumors. J Clin Oncol 2005; ASCO abstract 7523.
131. Gajewski TF. Overcoming immune resistance in the tumor microenvironment by blockade of indoleamine 2,3-dioxygenase and programmed death ligand 1. Curr Opin Invest Drugs 2004; 5:1279–1283.
132. Yamshchikov GV, Mullins DW, Chang CC, et al. Sequential immune escape and shifting of T cell responses in a long-term survivor of melanoma. J Immunol 2005;174:6863–6871.
133. Chappell DB, Restifo NP. T cell-tumor cell: a fatal interaction? Cancer Immunol Immunother 1998;47:65–71.
134. Perkins D, Wang Z, Donovan C, et al. Regulation of CTLA-4 expression during T cell activation. J Immunol 1996;156:4154–4159.
135. Hurwitz AA, Yu TF, Leach DR, et al. CTLA-4 blockade synergizes with tumor-derived granulocyte-macrophage colony-stimulating factor for treatment of an experimental mammary carcinoma. Proc Natl Acad Sci U S A 1998;95:10067–10071.
136. Krummel MF, Allison JP. CD28 and CTLA-4 have opposing effects on the response of T cells to stimulation. J Exp Med 1995;182:459–465.
137. Chambers CA, Sullivan TJ, Allison JP. Lymphoproliferation in CTLA-4-deficient mice is mediated by costimulation-dependent activation of CD4+ T cells. Immunity 1997;7:885–895.
138. Attia P, Phan GQ, Maker AV, et al. Autoimmunity correlates with tumor regression in patients with metastatic melanoma treated with anti-cytotoxic T-lymphocyte antigen-4 [see comment]. J Clin Oncol 2005;23:6043–6053.
139. Blank C, Gajewski TF, Mackensen A. Interaction of PD-L1 on tumor cells with PD-1 on tumor-specific T cells as a mechanism of immune evasion: implications for tumor immunotherapy. Cancer Immunol Immunother 2005;54:307–314.
140. Hsueh EC, Gupta RK, Qi K, et al. Correlation of specific immune responses with survival in melanoma patients with distant metastases receiving polyvalent melanoma cell vaccine. J Clin Oncol 1998;16:2913–2920.
141. Clemente CG, Mihm MC Jr, Bufalino R, et al. Prognostic value of tumor infiltrating lymphocytes in the vertical growth phase of primary cutaneous melanoma. Cancer (Phila) 1996;77:1303–1310.

142. Aaltomaa S, Lipponen P, Eskelinen M, et al. Lymphocyte infiltrates as a prognostic variable in female breast cancer. Eur J Cancer 1992;28A:859–864.
143. Clark WH Jr, Elder DE, Guerry D, et al. Model predicting survival in stage I melanoma based on tumor progression. J Natl Cancer Inst 1989;81:1893–1904.
144. Naito Y, Saito K, Shiiba K, et al. CD8+ T cells infiltrated within cancer cell nests as a prognostic factor in human colorectal cancer. Cancer Res 1998;58:3491–3494.
145. DeLisle D. Traite du Vice Cancereux. Paris: Couturier Fils, 1774.
146. Fehleisen F. Uber die Zuchtung der Erysipel-Kokken auf Kunstlichen Nahrboden und die Ubertragbarkeit auf den Menschen. Deutsch Med Wochenschr 1882;8:533.
147. Bruns P. Die Heilwirkung des Erysipels auf Geschwulste. Beitr Klin Chir 1887;3:443.
148. Coley WB. The mixed toxins of erysipelas and *Bacillus prodigiosus* in the treatment of sarcoma. JAMA 1900;34:906–908.
149. Coley WB. The treatment of inoperable sarcoma by bacterial toxins (the mixed toxins of the *Streptococcus erysipelatis* and the *Bacillus prodigiousis*. Proc R Soc Med Surg Sect 1909;3:1.
150. Patard JJ, Saint F, Velotti F, et al. Immune response following intravesical bacillus Calmette-Guerin instillations in superficial bladder cancer: a review. Urol Res 1998;26:155–159.
151. Morton DL, Eilber FR, Malgrem RA, et al. Immunological factors which influence response to immunotherapy in malignant melanoma. Surgery (St. Louis) 1970;68:158–164.
152. Lieberman R, Wybran J, Epstein W. The immunologic and histopathologic changes of BCG-mediated tumor regression in patients with malignant melanoma. Cancer (Phila) 1975;35:756–777.
153. Vermorken JB. Active specific immunotherapy for stage II and stage III human colon cancer: a randomised trial. Lancet 1999; 353:345–350.
154. Harris JE, Ryan L, Hoover HC Jr, et al. Adjuvant active specific immunotherapy for stage II and III colon cancer with an autologous tumor cell vaccine: Eastern Cooperative Oncology Group Study E5283. J Clin Oncol 2000;18:148–157.
155. Berd D, Maguire HC Jr, Schuchter LM, et al. Autologous hapten-modified melanoma vaccine as postsurgical adjuvant treatment after resection of nodal metastases. J Clin Oncol 1997;15:2359–2370.
156. Wallack MK, Sivanandham M, Balch CM, et al. Surgical adjuvant active specific immunotherapy for patients with stage III melanoma: the final analysis of data from a phase III, randomized, double-blind, multicenter vaccinia melanoma oncolysate trial. J Am Coll Surg 1998;187:69–77.
157. Tafra L, Dale PS, Wanek LA, et al. Resection and adjuvant immunotherapy for melanoma metastatic to the lung and thorax. J Thorac Cardiovasc Surg 1995;110:119–129.
158. Morton DL, Foshag LJ, Hoon DS, et al. Prolongation of survival in metastatic melanoma after active specific immunotherapy with a new polyvalent melanoma vaccine. Ann Surg 1992;216: 463–482.
159. Reynolds SR, Oratz R, Shapiro RL, et al. Stimulation of CD8+ T cell responses to MAGE-3 and Melan A/MART-1 by immunization to a polyvalent melanoma vaccine. Int J Cancer 1997;72: 972–976.
160. Applebaum J, Reynolds S, Knispel J, et al. Identification of melanoma antigens that are immunogenic in humans and expressed in vivo. J Natl Cancer Inst 1998;90:146–149.
161. Bystryn JC, Zeleniuch-Jacquotte A, Oratz R, et al. Double-blind trial of a polyvalent, shed-antigen, melanoma vaccine [see comment]. Clin Cancer Res 2001;7:1882–1887.
162. Zhou X, Jun dY, Thomas AM, et al. Diverse CD8+ T-cell responses to renal cell carcinoma antigens in patients treated with an autologous granulocyte-macrophage colony-stimulating factor gene-transduced renal tumor cell vaccine. Cancer Res 2005;65:1079–1088.
163. Soiffer R, Hodi FS, Haluska F, et al. Vaccination with irradiated, autologous melanoma cells engineered to secrete granulocyte-macrophage colony-stimulating factor by adenoviral-mediated gene transfer augments antitumor immunity in patients with metastatic melanoma. J Clin Oncol 2003;21:3343–3350.
164. Salgia R, Lynch T, Skarin A, et al. Vaccination with irradiated autologous tumor cells engineered to secrete granulocyte-macrophage colony-stimulating factor augments antitumor immunity in some patients with metastatic non-small-cell lung carcinoma [see comment]. J Clin Oncol 2003;21:624–630.
165. Jaffee EM, Hruban RH, Biedrzycki B, et al. Novel allogeneic granulocyte-macrophage colony-stimulating factor-secreting tumor vaccine for pancreatic cancer: a phase I trial of safety and immune activation. J Clin Oncol 2001;19:145–156.
166. Helling F, Zhang S, Shang A, et al. GM2-KLH conjugate vaccine: increased immunogenicity in melanoma patients after administration with immunological adjuvant QS-21. Cancer Res 1995;55:2783–2788.
167. Livingston P, Zhang S, Adluri S, et al. Tumor cell reactivity mediated by IgM antibodies in sera from melanoma patients vaccinated with GM2 ganglioside covalently linked to KLH is increased by IgG antibodies. Cancer Immunol Immunother 1997;43:324–330.
168. Livingston PO, Adluri S, Helling F, et al. Phase 1 trial of immunological adjuvant QS-21 with a GM2 ganglioside-keyhole limpet haemocyanin conjugate vaccine in patients with malignant melanoma. Vaccine 1994;12:1275–1280.
169. Livingston PO, Wong GY, Adluri S, et al. Improved survival in stage III melanoma patients with GM2 antibodies: a randomized trial of adjuvant vaccination with GM2 ganglioside. J Clin Oncol 1994;12:1036–1044.
170. Kirkwood JM, Ibrahim JG, Sosman JA, et al. High-dose interferon alfa-2b significantly prolongs relapse-free and overall survival compared with the GM2-KLH/QS-21 vaccine in patients with resected stage IIB-III melanoma: results of intergroup trial E1694/S9512/C509801. J Clin Oncol 2001;19:2370–2380.
171. Davis TA, Maloney DG, Czerwinski DK, et al. Anti-idiotype antibodies can induce long-term complete remissions in non-Hodgkin's lymphoma without eradicating the malignant clone. Blood 1998;92:1184–1190.
172. Weng WK, Czerwinski D, Timmerman J, et al. Clinical outcome of lymphoma patients after idiotype vaccination is correlated with humoral immune response and immunoglobulin G Fc receptor genotype. [Erratum appears in J Clin Oncol 2005; 23(1):248.] J Clin Oncol 2004;22:4717–4724.
173. Timmerman JM, Czerwinski DK, Davis TA, et al. Idiotype-pulsed dendritic cell vaccination for B-cell lymphoma: clinical and immune responses in 35 patients. Blood 2002;99:1517–1526.
174. Rosenberg SA, Yang JC, Restifo NP. Cancer immunotherapy: moving beyond current vaccines. Nat Med 2004;10:909–915.
175. Huang AYC, Golumbek P, Ahmadzadeh M, et al. Role of bone marrow-derived cells in presenting MHC class I-restricted tumor antigens. Science 1994;264:961–965.
176. Tuting T, DeLeo AB, Lotze MT, et al. Genetically modified bone marrow-derived dendritic cells expressing tumor-associated viral or "self" antigens induce antitumor immunity in vivo. Eur J Immunol 1997;27:2702–2707.
177. Mayordomo JI, Zorina T, Storkus WJ, et al. Bone marrow-derived dendritic cells serve as potent adjuvants for peptide-based antitumor vaccines. Stem Cells 1997;15:94–103.
178. Dematos P, Abdel-Wahab Z, Vervaert C, et al. Vaccination with dendritic cells inhibits the growth of hepatic metastases in B6 mice. Cell Immunol 1998;185:65–74.

179. Gilboa E, Nair SK, Lyerly HK. Immunotherapy of cancer with dendritic-cell-based vaccines. Cancer Immunol Immunother 1998;46:82–87.
180. Morse MA, Lyerly HK, Gilboa E, et al. Optimization of the sequence of antigen loading and CD40-ligand-induced maturation of dendritic cells. Cancer Res 1998;58:2965–2968.
181. Nair SK, Snyder D, Rouse BT, et al. Regression of tumors in mice vaccinated with professional antigen-presenting cells pulsed with tumor extracts. Int J Cancer 1997;70:706–715.
182. Nestle FO, Alijagic S, Gilliet M, et al. Vaccination of melanoma patients with peptide- or tumor lysate-pulsed dendritic cells. Nat Med 1998;4:328–332.
183. Banchereau J, Palucka AK, Dhodapkar M, et al. Immune and clinical responses in patients with metastatic melanoma to CD34(+) progenitor-derived dendritic cell vaccine. Cancer Res 2001;61:6451–6458.
184. Hersey P, Menzies SW, Halliday GM, et al. Phase I/II study of treatment with dendritic cell vaccines in patients with disseminated melanoma. Cancer Immunol Immunother 2004;53:125–134.
185. Munn DH, Sharma MD, Hou D, et al. Expression of indoleamine 2,3-dioxygenase by plasmacytoid dendritic cells in tumor-draining lymph nodes. [Erratum appears in J Clin Invest 2004;114(4):599.] J Clin Invest 2004;114:280–290.
186. Dhodapkar MV, Steinman RM, Krasovsky J, et al. Antigen-specific inhibition of effector T cell function in humans after injection of immature dendritic cells. J Exp Med 2001;193:233–238.
187. Bhardwaj N. Interactions of viruses with dendritic cells: a double-edged sword. J Exp Med 1997;186:795–799.
188. Chakraborty A, Li L, Chakraborty NG, et al. Stimulatory and inhibitory differentiation of human myeloid dendritic cells. Clin Immunol 2000;94:88–98.
189. Starzl TE, Demetris AJ, Rao AS, et al. Migratory nonparenchymal cells after organ allotransplantation: with particular reference to chimerism and the liver. Prog Liver Dis 1994;12:191–213.
190. Schadendorf D, Nestle FO, Broecker E-B, et al. Dacarbacine (DTIC) versus vaccination with autologous peptide-pulsed dendritic cells (DC) as first-line treatment of patients with metastatic melanoma: results of a prospective-randomized phase III study. J Clin Oncol 2004;22:7508 (abstr 7508).
191. Lee P, Wang F, Kuniyoshi J, et al. Effects of interleukin-12 on the immune response to a multipeptide vaccine for resected metastatic melanoma. J Clin Oncol 2001;19:3836–3847.
192. Slingluff CL Jr, Petroni GR, Yamshchikov GV, et al. Clinical and immunologic results of a randomized phase II trial of vaccination using four melanoma peptides either administered in granulocyte-macrophage colony-stimulating factor in adjuvant or pulsed on dendritic cells. J Clin Oncol 2003;21:4016–4026.
193. Weber J, Sondak VK, Scotland R, et al. Granulocyte-macrophage-colony-stimulating factor added to a multipeptide vaccine for resected stage II melanoma. Cancer (Phila) 2003;97:186–200.
194. Scheibenbogen C, Schadendorf D, Bechrakis NE, et al. Effects of granulocyte-macrophage colony-stimulating factor and foreign helper protein as immunologic adjuvants on the T-cell response to vaccination with tyrosinase peptides. Int J Cancer 2003;104:188–194.
195. Speiser DE, Lienard D, Rufer N, et al. Rapid and strong human CD8+ T cell responses to vaccination with peptide, IFA, and CpG oligodeoxynucleotide 7909. J Clin Invest 2005;115:739–746.
196. Fagerberg J, Ragnhammar P, Liljefors M, et al. Humoral anti-idiotypic and anti-anti-idiotypic immune response in cancer patients treated with monoclonal antibody 17-1A. Cancer Immunol Immunother 1996;42:81–87.
197. Scott AM, Welt S. Antibody-based immunological therapies. Curr Opin Immunol 1997;9:718.
198. Stern P, Herrmann R. Overview of monoclonal antibodies in cancer therapy: present and promise. Crit Rev Oncol-Hematol 2005;54:11–29.
199. Atkins MB, Kunkel L, Sznol M, et al. High-dose recombinant interleukin-2 therapy in patients with metastatic melanoma: long-term survival update. Cancer J Sci Am 2000;6(suppl 1):S11–S14.

94

Principles of Cancer Surgery

John H. Donohue

Surgery remains the single most effective modality for treating most malignancies. Solid tumors must be localized to allow complete resection that offers a patient the potential for curative treatment. Although adjuvant therapies have improved disease-free and overall survivals, most notably in breast[1] and colorectal[2] cancers, these treatments are effective in only a minority of patients.

A team of specialists including surgeons, medical oncologists, radiation oncologists, rehabilitation personnel, and, in inherited forms of cancer, medical geneticists needs to be involved in the management of most cancer patients to assure the longest and highest quality of life. Given the central role of surgical treatment, the surgical oncologist needs to take a leading role in therapeutic planning. With the explosion of molecular biology and minimally invasive and noninvasive methods of tissue ablation, the surgeon caring for oncology patients must be aware of new methods of tumor prevention, detection, staging, and treatment that will improve patient care and outcome. This chapter outlines the basic principles of the surgical management of cancer, including its use in prevention, diagnosis, staging, debulking, palliation, rehabilitation, and cure.

Tumor Biology

Cancer is an aberration of cell growth. Malignant cells (1) grow without the orderly histology of the primary organ; (2) do not function as normal cells; (3) impinge upon and destroy neighboring normal tissue; (4) invade adjacent, distinct structures if given sufficient time; and (5) often spread and grow at distant sites as metastases. The isolated or combined effects of loss of primary organ function, impingement on vital structures, loss of distant vital organ function, and cachexia cause the afflicted person's death.

Much remains to be learned about the actual mechanisms of the biological transformation of malignant cells. Recent developments in molecular biology have shown mutations in specific oncogenes and tumor suppressor genes to be critical in the development of neoplastic cells. Fearon and Vogelstein[3] have outlined the sequential molecular process that results in a histological progression from normal colonic epithelium to hyperplastic polyp, epithelial dysplasia, carcinoma in situ, and finally invasive carcinoma of the colon (Fig. 94.1). Although not all cancers of the large bowel follow this sequence of molecular events, this schema nicely outlines the cumulative effect of multiple mutations on the growth pattern and biology of the transformed cells.

Once a malignant transformation has occurred, the invasion of the normal surrounding tissue structures, both cellular and stromal, occurs. For a cancer to progress beyond microscopic size, new blood vessels must be formed to provide oxygen and nutrients and dispose of metabolic by-products. Recent developments in tumor biology have included the recognition of potent angiogenesis factors that abet the growth of malignancies. Inhibitors of tumor blood vessel growth offer a potentially valuable method of tumor control.

Until a tumor has spread from its primary site, local treatments such as surgery are potentially curative. Cancers most commonly spread by vascular or lymphatic routes. Tumors that grow to reach a free body surface, such as the visceral peritoneum, can also metastasize by exfoliation of viable cells. Most patients die of their malignancy because the disease has metastasized before diagnosis, and systemic treatments cannot eradicate all tumor cells. The process of metastasis formation is a complex one involving adhesion, stromal and tissue invasion, new tumor growth, and vascular recruitment steps. Without completing all these processes, a metastasis will not develop. Fortunately, the metastatic efficiency, that is, the percent of tumor cells entering a cancer's lymphatic or vascular drainage systems that successfully form metastases, is very low. Most malignancies have been growing for years before detection, and circulating tumor cells are commonly found in the circulation. If most cancer cells shed from the primary tumor were able to grow at distant sites, no patient with invasive cancer would have localized disease at diagnosis.

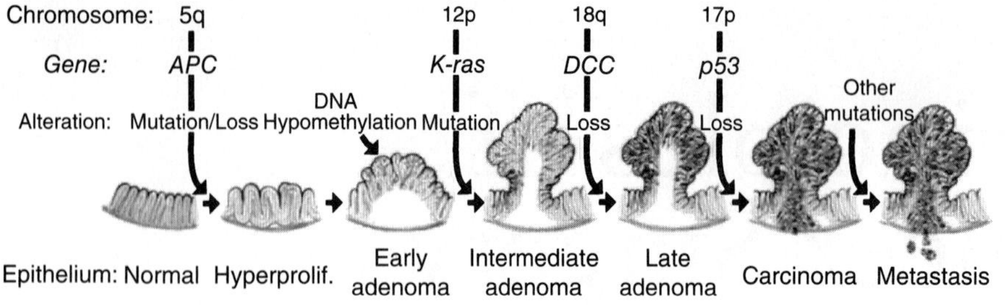

FIGURE 94.1. A Genetic model for colorectal tumorigenesis. (Revised from Fearon E, Vogelstein B. Cell 1990;61:759–767,[3] with permission.)

The patterns of metastasis formation are well established for individual cancer types. Most sarcomas spread to distant sites only by vascular routes, with lymphatic involvement being uncommon. Most carcinomas, such as adenocarcinomas of the breast and colon, readily metastasize via both the lymphatics and blood. The actual mechanisms for site-specific metastasis, including surface–molecule interactions, are still incompletely understood. The probable sites of tumor spread determine the preoperative evaluation, operative management, and postoperative follow-up tests for cancer patients. Although some tumor characteristics such as type of malignancy, histological grade, and molecular markers including oncogene mutations are known to increase the risk of metastatic disease, the precise prediction of which patients harbor established but clinically occult metastases is not possible at present. Clinically apparent distant metastases almost always eliminate the chance of curative treatment in solid tumors. In some instances, limited distant metastatic disease can be successfully resected with a chance of cure (see "Curative Surgical Therapy"). Many patients with apparently localized cancers harbor occult metastatic disease, meaning that surgical therapy alone will not be curative.

Prognosis and Tumor Staging

Because the biology of cancer is still poorly understood, no biological marker of cancer prognosis is currently in routine clinical use. Because of the inability to predict individual tumor behavior, the extent of tumor spread remains the most powerful predictor of patient outcome, assuming appropriate treatment is delivered. The American Joint Commission on Cancer (AJCC)[4] has formulated staging systems for most common cancers. These staging schemata categorize tumor involvement using both clinical and pathological data into T (primary tumor), N (regional lymph node), and M (distant metastasis) classifications. Except for soft tissue sarcomas, histological grade (G) has no role in tumor staging. By combining the information of known TNM extent, the tumor stage is determined. The stage of disease predicts the probability of patient survival. The current AJCC staging system and survival curves by stage for colorectal cancer are shown in Table 94.1[4] and Figure 94.2,[5] respectively. It is imperative for the surgeon to be familiar with standardized staging systems to adequately treat and counsel their cancer patients. Accurate staging using AJCC guidelines is critical when comparing results between different therapies and institutions. The use of standardized staging criteria should be required in all publications reporting cancer outcomes. Regular revisions of the staging systems have been made, and the addition of molecular prognostic markers will likely occur in the future.

Preoperative Assessment

Physiological Preparation

Preoperatively, the surgeon must assess a patient's ability to tolerate the appropriate anesthetic and surgical procedure. Correction of acute physiological decompensations and evaluation of chronic medical conditions are undertaken preoperatively. A patient's overall state of health, as reflected by their performance status, is commonly used in cancer research protocols as an inclusion (or exclusion) criterion. The Eastern Cooperative Oncology Group (ECOG) and Karnofsky[6] performance status scales are depicted in Table 94.2. These measurements of patient well-being also help in considering the prudence of a major surgical treatment for a cancer patient. Care must be paid to situations where an acute and reversible decline in performance status has occurred. If preoperative medical or surgical intervention can significantly improve a patient's functioning, a poor performance status may be overlooked, although patients with poor performance statuses (ECOG more than 2 or Karnofsky less than 60) are at higher risk for perioperative complications. The risk of perioperative mortality can be assessed, as with any o'perative candidate, using the risk classification of the American Society of Anesthesia (ASA).[7] If partial resection of a vital organ such as the lung or liver is scheduled, the postoperative physiological reserve must be calculated before proceeding with an operation.

Cachexia and malnutrition frequently occur with metastatic malignancies and certain *clinically* localized cancers (i.e., ductal adenocarcinoma of the pancreas). Tumors cause a depletion of lean body mass with shunting of nutrients to support tumor growth. Unfortunately, supplemental nutrition neither totally reverses the wasting of normal tissue nor limits the caloric consumption of the cancer. Multiple randomized trials[8–10] have evaluated the effects of nutritional supplementation in cancer patients (see Chapter 102). These studies have not shown objective benefit of perioperative parenteral[8,9] or enteral[10] feedings. Enteral nutrition is preferred whenever possible because it is more physiological, less costly, and has fewer complications. Although the entire population of patients *may* not enjoy improved outcomes, occasional severely debilitated individuals appear to benefit from a preoperative course of medical therapy including alimentation.[9] A minimum of 10 to 14 days of nutritional support is necessary to have any real benefit in the preoperative preparation of a patient. Isolated nutritional deficits that significantly affect the surgical procedure must also be reversed. For example, in patients with obstructive jaundice whose fat-soluble vitamin absorption is inhibited, a vitamin K deficiency must be anticipated and corrected preoperatively. Failure to do so may result in major intraoperative hemorrhage.

TABLE 94.1. Definition of TMN, Stage Grouping, Histopathologic Type, Histologic Grade, and Residual Tumor for Colorectal Carcinoma.

Definition of TMN
The same classification is used for both clinical and pathological staging.

Primary Tumor (T)

TX	Primary tumor cannot be assessed
T0	No evidence of primary tumor
Tis	Carcinoma *in situ:* intraepithelial or invasion of lamina propria[1–3]
T1	Tumor invades submucosa
T2	Tumor invades muscularis propria
T3	Tumor invades through the muscularis propria into the subserosa, or into non-peritonealized pericolic or perirectal tissues
T4	Tumor directly invades other organs or structures, and/or perforates visceral peritoneum[2,3]

Notes: [1]Tis includes cancer cells confined within the glandular basement membrane (intraepithelial) or lamina propria (intramucosal) with no extension through the muscularis mucosae into the submucosa.

[2]Direct invasion in T4 includes invasion of other segments of the colorectum by way of the serosa; for example, invasion of the sigmoid colon by a carcinoma of the cecum.

[3]Tumor that is adherent to other organs or structures, macroscopically, is classified T4. However, if no tumor is present in the adhesion, microscopically, the classification should be pT3. The V and L substaging should be used to identify the presence or absence of vascular or lymphatic invasion.

Regional Lymph Nodes (N)

NX	Regional lymph nodes cannot be assessed[4]
N0	No regional lymph node metastasis
N1	Metastasis in 1 to 3 regional lymph nodes
N2	Metastasis in 4 or more regional lymph nodes
	Total nodes examined = ____

[4]A tumor nodule in the pericolorectal adipose tissue of a primary carcinoma without histologic evidence of residual lymph node in the nodule is classified in the pN category as a regional lymph node metastasis if the nodule has the form and smooth contour of a lymph node. If the nodule has an irregular contour, it should be classified in the T category and also coded as V1 (microscopic venous invasion) or as V2 (if it was grossly evident), because there is a strong likelihood that it represents venous invasion.

Distant Metastasis (M)

MX	Distant metastasis cannot be assessed
M0	No distant metastasis
M1	Distant metastasis
	Biopsy of metastatic site performed . . . ☐Y . . . ☐N
	Source of pathologic metastatic specimen ___

Stage Grouping

Stage	*T*	*N*	*M*	*Dukes*	*MAC*
0	Tis	N0	M0	—	—
I	T1	N0	M0	A	A
	T2	N0	M0	A	B1
IIA	T3	N0	M0	B	B2
IIB	T4	N0	M0	B	B3
IIIA	T1-T2	N1	M0	C	C1
IIIB	T3-T4	N1	M0	C	C2/C3
IIIC	Any T	N2	M0	C	C1/C2/C3
IV	Any T	Any N	M1	—	D

Histologic Grade (G)

GX	Grade cannot be assessed
G1	Well differentiated
G2	Moderately differentiated
G3	Poorly differentiated
G4	Undifferentiated

Residual Tumor (R)

R0	Complete resection, margins histologically negative, no residual tumor left after resection
R1	Incomplete resection, margins histogically involved, microscopic tumor remains after resection of gross disease
R2	Incomplete resection, margins involved or gross disease remains after subtotal resection

Additional Descriptors
For identification of special cases of TNM or pTNM classifications, the "m" suffix and "y", "r", and "a" prefixes are used. Although they do not affect the stage grouping, they indicate cases needing separate analysis.

m suffix indicates the presence of multiple primary tumors in a single site and is recorded in parentheses: pT(m)NM

y prefix indicated those cases in which classification is performed during or following initial multimodality therapy. The cTNM or pTNM category is identified by a "y" prefix. The ycTNM or ypTNM categorizes the extent of tumor actually present at the time of that examination. The "y" categorization is not an estimate of tumor prior to multimodality therapy.

r prefix indicates a recurrent tumor when staged after a disease-free interval, and is identified by the "r" prefix: rTNM.

a prefix designates the stage determined at autopsy: aTNM

Prognostic Indicators
For CRC
CEA level: __________ ng/ml

Notes
Additional Descriptors

Lymphatic Vessel Invasion (L)

LX	Lymphatic vessel invasion cannot be assessed
L0	No lymphatic vessel invasion
L1	Lymphatic vessel invasion

Venous Invasion (V)

VX	Venous invasion cannot be assessed
V0	No venous invasion
V1	Microscopic venous invasion
V2	Macroscopic venous invasion

Source: Used with the permission of the American Joint Committee on Cancer (AJCC), Chicago, Illinois. The original source for this material is the *AJCC Cancer Staging Manual, Sixth Edition* (2002) published by Springer Science and Business Media LLC, www.springerlink.com.

Hematological abnormalities frequently are present in the cancer patient. Many patients with malignancy have anemia as a consequence of chronic or acute hemorrhage, impaired hematopoiesis, or a combination of causes. Adequate erythrocyte replacement to ensure sufficient tissue oxygenation and offset anticipated operative blood losses is an essential component of perioperative care. Neutropenic patients present a difficult scenario because transfusions will have little effect in raising white blood cell counts, and patients with an absolute neutropenia ($<500 \times 10^9$/L) are at substantial risk of perioperative infection and death. Delaying an elective operation until the white blood cell count rises, as occurs following systemic chemotherapy, is the best approach whenever possible.

Some patients with hematological neoplasms may have profound thrombocytopenia. Platelet transfusions should be given as close to the start of the surgical procedure as possible.

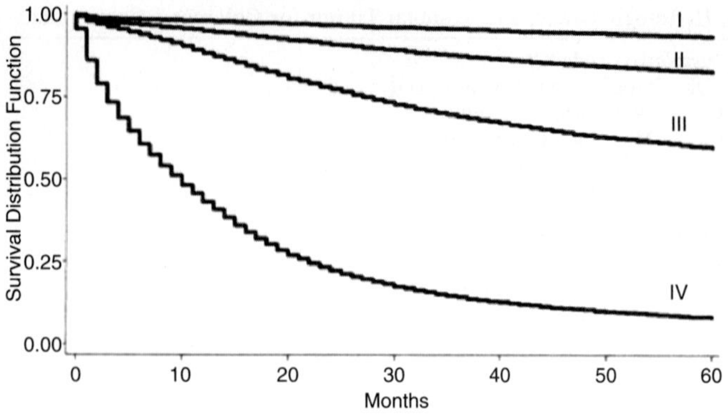

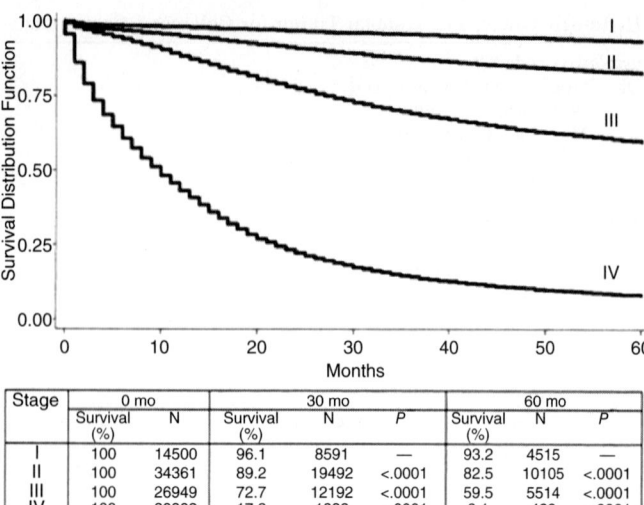

Stage	0 mo		30 mo			60 mo		
	Survival (%)	N	Survival (%)	N	*P*	Survival (%)	N	*P*
I	100	14500	96.1	8591	—	93.2	4515	—
II	100	34361	89.2	19492	<.0001	82.5	10105	<.0001
III	100	26949	72.7	12192	<.0001	59.5	5514	<.0001
IV	100	20802	17.3	1832	<.0001	8.1	432	<.0001

FIGURE 94.2. Five-year survival for colorectal cancer by the American Joint Committee on Cancer (6th edition) system, stages I–IV. *P* value determined by the log-rank test refers to the corresponding stage and the stage in the row above, unless otherwise indicated. All statistical tests were two-sided. *mo*, months. (Used with permission of the American Joint Committee on Cancer (AJCC), Chicago, IL. The original source for this material is O'Connell JB, Maggard MA, Ko CY. J Natl Cancer Inst 2004;96:1420–1425, by Oxford University Press.)

Early administration provides little benefit because of the short half-life of transfused platelets. In thrombocytopenic patients having a splenectomy, delaying platelet transfusions until after control of the vascular hilum will prevent the transfused platelets from being sequestered in the spleen. Aminosalicylic acid-containing drugs cause irreversible dysfunctions of platelets. Stopping these drugs 7 to 10 days before a major cancer operation allows the replacement of affected platelets with normal functioning platelets. This precaution should be routine practice in any major cancer operation, especially when postoperative coagulopathy is expected (i.e., major hepatectomy). Platelet transfusions may be necessary for patients preoperatively taking aspirin who are operated on in an emergency situation.

Coagulopathies can be corrected acutely with fresh-frozen plasma, cryoprecipitate, or both blood products. Common causes of abnormal hemostasis in the cancer patient are (1) a prolonged prothrombin time because of malabsorption of fat-soluble vitamins including vitamin K or (2) chronic anticoagulation therapy with coumadin, both of which result in depressed levels of Factors II, VII, IX, and X. Parenteral vitamin K will correct these protein deficiencies in 24 to 48 h if normal hepatic function is present. For an emergency procedure or if coumadin anticoagulation is to be reinstituted postoperatively, transfusions of fresh-frozen plasma should be used. Plasma treatment is preferable in the latter situation because of problems offsetting the effect of exogenous vitamin K with postoperative coumadin. After initial treatment of the coagulopathy, a repeat prothrombin time should be drawn to ensure adequate correction of the defect.

Informed Consent

An important component of preoperative preparation is a frank discussion with the patient of the goals, risks, and alternatives of the surgical procedure. Patients must be aware whether an operation is merely for palliative purposes or possibly curative. The potential for intraoperative findings to change the scope and effect of surgical therapy must be outlined as fully as possible. Significant changes in bodily function or quality of life (i.e., tracheostomy, mastectomy, bowel stoma, infertility, impotence, and amputation) must be included in the informed consent discussion. Preoperative consultation with medical support personnel or volunteer groups may be valuable for patient education and adaptation to their postoperative status. Potential life-threatening (i.e., death, myocardial infarction, pulmonary embolism, etc.) and lesser major (i.e., hemorrhage, infection) complications should also be enumerated, as with any operative procedure. Patients should also be asked about whether they have advance directives; that is, a living will, and should be offered help in completing such a document preoperatively, if desired. Adequate preoperative physical and mental preparation of the cancer patient reduces the incidence of both medical and legal complications.

TABLE 94.2. Eastern Cooperative Oncology Group (ECOG) and Karnofsky Performance Status Criteria.

Grade	*ECOG*	*Karnofsky*
0	Fully active, able to carry on all predisease performance without restriction.	100—Normal, no complaints; no evidence of disease 90—Able to carry on normal activity; minor signs or symptoms of disease
1	Restricted in physically strenuous activity but ambulatory and able to carry out work of a light or sedentary nature, e.g., light housework, office work.	80—Normal activity with an effort, some signs or symptoms of disease 70—Cares for self but unable to carry on normal activity or to do active work
2	Ambulatory and capable of all self-care but unable to carry out any work activities. Up and about more than 50% of waking hours.	60—Requires occasional assistance but is able to care for most of personal needs 50—Requires considerable assistance and frequent medical care
3	Capable of only limited self-care, confined to bed or chair more than 50% of waking hours.	40—Disabled; requires special care and assistance 30—Severely disabled; hospiptalization is indicated, although death not imminent
4	Completely disabled. Cannot carry on any self-care. Totally confined to bed or chair.	20—Very ill; hospitalization and active supportive care necessary 10—Moribund
5	Dead	0—Dead

Source: Reprinted from Oken M, Creech R, Tormey D, et al. Toxicity and response criteria of the Eastern Cooperative Oncology Group. Am J Clin Oncol (CCT) 1982;5:649–655, with permission.

Neoadjuvant Therapy

Some adult cancers are best treated first with nonsurgical therapies. This strategy is most often undertaken because (1) nonoperative therapy is preferable for a cancer and surgery best reserved for removal of residual nonresponsive tumor, or (2) a malignancy is locally advanced, preventing the complete excision of the neoplasm with standard or even extended radical surgical procedures.

Nowhere is the successful application of nonsurgical treatment to replace radical operations better demonstrated than in advanced-stage testicular carcinomas. Physicians at the University of Indiana[11] were instrumental in developing the modern management of bulky testicular cancer. Radical surgical procedures, including retroperitoneal lymphadenectomy, formerly were a routine part of the therapy for patients with this disease. Currently, after histological confirmation of malignancy, usually by orchiectomy, multiple cycles of cisplatin-based combination chemotherapy are delivered. Operative therapy for advanced-stage disease is limited to those patients in whom residual tumor is noted on follow-up imaging. Many of these lesions are found to be necrotic tumor or benign mature teratoma, rather than unresponsive malignancy. With the traditional treatment approach for nonseminomatous testicular cancers, there was a 5-year survival rate of 5% or 10%. Despite the relegation of surgery to a secondary role in carcinomas of the testes, 70% to 80% of men with bulky metastatic testicular carcinoma are presently cured of their disease.[12]

Another striking example of improved solid tumor management with nonoperative therapy is squamous cell carcinoma of the anus. At one time, abdominoperineal resection was considered the only effective therapy. Radiation therapy and chemotherapy were given in advanced disease cases and to patients with disease relapse. Nigro and colleagues at Wayne State University[13] spearheaded efforts to alter the management of this disease. With a combination of mitomycin C and fluorouracil-based chemotherapy plus external-beam radiation therapy, most patients are now spared major surgical resections. Only those patients having local failure after primary chemoirradiation and salvage chemotherapy undergo abdominoperineal resection. Rectal sphincter function is now preserved in 75% to 85% of patients, and overall 5-year survival for patients with squamous cell cancer of the anus is 75% to 90%.[14] These rates compare favorably to the results of radical surgical treatment where abdominoperineal resection was the rule and only 40% to 50% of patients survived 5 years.[14]

Unfortunately, most malignancies do not manifest a sufficient response to available nonsurgical treatments to allow the abandonment of extirpative procedures. Neoadjuvant therapy has been utilized increasingly in several forms of cancer to allow complete removal of locally advanced disease with less extensive operations. Patients treated in this fashion do not necessarily have improved survival because occult metastases are frequently present; however, the resectability rates and incidence of local tumor control are usually improved, often with less radical procedures than needed at the time of disease presentation.

Locally advanced rectal cancers can involve the pelvic side walls, sacrum, and anterior pelvic organs, resulting in a fixed tumor. Primary surgical management of these malignancies leaves microscopic disease at the lateral pelvic margins. The application of external-beam radiation therapy plus fluorouracil-based chemotherapy as a radiosensitizer provides sufficient tumor regression in 60% to 70% of patients to allow gross resection of disease.[15] Because the radial margins are still often microscopically involved with cancer, intraoperative[16] or postoperative[17] radiation boosts are utilized in an effort to enhance local disease control by sterilizing residual cancer cells. Anal sphincter preservation is possible with proximal rectal tumors, whereas abdominoperineal resection is still advised for low rectal cancers, even with major tumor regression. Recent trials[18,19] have shown improved disease-free and overall survival rates with preoperative chemoirradiation compared to surgery alone; patients presenting with resectable rectal cancer may also have a curative operation followed by adjuvant chemotherapy and radiation therapy.[20]

Surgical Treatment Goals

There are six major objectives of the surgical management for malignancy: prevention of cancer, diagnosis and staging of disease, disease cure, tumor debulking, symptom palliation, and patient rehabilitation. With the development of genetic markers for inherited forms of cancer and the clear recognition of acquired premalignant disease conditions, preventative operations have become feasible for tumors of nonvital organs. Indications for prophylactic surgical management of genetic or acquired conditions predisposing a patient to cancer will likely continue to increase as more genetic mutations are identified (see Chapter 90). Ultimately, however, effective chemoprevention, gene therapy, or other means of treatment will become the preferred methods of management. Because of donor organ shortages and the high costs, low efficacy, and substantial morbidity of transplantation in cancer patients, prophylactic transplantation is not routinely practiced for premalignant conditions.

Many surgical procedures are merely for diagnosis, usually to document disease histology or to determine the extent of spread (staging) to best plan the type and timing of therapy. Although complete resection for cure is the desired goal of many oncological operations, this result is not feasible in the majority of cancer patients because metastatic disease exists at diagnosis. In a limited number of tumors, debulking tumor enhances the effect of postoperative therapy. In most patients with metastatic or locally advanced incurable cancer, debulking the tumor does not prolong survival or significantly impact the quality of life. In selected noncurable cancer patients, surgical palliation of symptoms should be undertaken for emergent or progressive conditions. Palliative surgical therapy should not be offered in instances in which the patient is moribund with advanced disease or has no meaningful remaining quality of life. Months, or even years, of unimpaired and productive life may result from prudent palliative surgical procedures in carefully selected patients.

Last among the roles of operative therapy for cancer are the reconstruction of normal structures and rehabilitation of normal function. These procedures have no effect on tumor control, but will markedly improve quality of life for the patient. This component of surgery therapy can be simultaneous to a resectional procedure or delayed. Illustrative examples of each goal of surgery are provided in the following sections.

Cancer Prevention

Both inherited genetic mutations and acquired diseases may predispose a patient to malignant transformation. With the decoding of the entire human genome, more genes responsible for specific cancers are being identified regularly. Theoretically, once the causative gene has been isolated, genetic screening for relevant mutations can be initiated and cancer preventative treatment implemented. In most instances, preventive therapy presently means the surgical removal of the organ at risk. As the mechanisms of genetic causes of cancer become better understood, nonsurgical treatment should replace extirpative surgery. In patients with certain chronic inflammatory processes, a significantly increased risk of cancer is present. In many of these situations, patients can be routinely screened and surgical resection undertaken when atypical, but ideally not malignant, histological changes are found with screening biopsies.

Diseases of the large intestine best demonstrate the role of preventative surgery for both genetic and acquired causes of malignancy. The familial adenomatous polyposis coli (FAP) syndrome has been long recognized because of the diffuse involvement of the colon and rectum with adenomatous polyps, which usually develop in the second or third decade of life. FAP has a high penetrance, and colorectal cancer nearly always develops if the large intestine is left in situ. The gene responsible for this condition, the adenomatous polyposis coli (APC) gene, has been isolated on the long arm of chromosome 5 (5q21). Most FAP patients have a missense mutation of the APC gene, usually a nonsense or termination codon that results in nonexpression or truncation of the 300-kDa protein encoded by this gene.[21] Loss of the APC gene sequence is also a common occurrence in sporadic colorectal cancers.[22] In families in which a germline APC gene mutation has been identified, children at risk can have genetic screening before polyps become apparent. The age that polyps appear and time of progression to cancer differs between FAP families and may correlate with specific APC mutations.[23] Once polyps are present, the large bowel should be removed, usually in the late teens or early twenties for FAP patients. Although preservation of the distal rectum improves bowel function, risk of cancer in the rectal stump is as high as 59% with a median follow-up of 23 years.[24] Recent studies[25,26] have shown that the APC genotype predicts rectal stump cancers and allows some FAP patients to have an ileorectostomy without undue risk. Although the functional results are not perfect, when the rectal stump needs to be removed for a rectal cancer, a total abdominal colectomy, mucosal protectomy, and ileoanal pouch anastomosis is the best operation.[27] This surgical procedure was developed to preserve anal continence while removing the entire large bowel mucosa. In most patients, continence is good to excellent, although stool frequency increases and soilage occurs occasionally in many patients. In some FAP patients, such as those having an invasive rectal cancer or poor anal sphincter tone, a total proctocolectomy with standard or continent ileostomy is performed.

Chronic ulcerative colitis (CUC) is a disease of unknown etiology, variable severity, and unpredictable clinical course. Patients with involvement of the entire large bowel mucosa, onset of disease at a young age, and long duration of CUC are most at risk for developing colorectal cancer.[28] More than 10% of patients with pancolitis will develop colorectal cancer within 25 years of the onset of this disease. Routine screening colonoscopies are recommended for all CUC patients. Any morphological abnormalities should be biopsied in addition to multiple, random, mucosal samplings. The diagnosis of carcinoma or high-grade dysplasia is an indication for removal of the entire large bowel mucosa with ileostomy or ileal pouch anal anastomosis reconstruction.[29] At some centers, low-grade dysplasia is also used as an indicator for proctocolectomy. Unfortunately, unrecognized cancers are already present in some patients with dysplasia. Some carcinomas in CUC patients are not visible and can be missed with random sampling. Improved surveillance techniques or predictors of those CUC patients who will develop cancer are needed. For now, routine colonoscopy and surgical resection based on histological findings provide the most reasonable opportunity to prevent cancer development and provide cancer detection at an early stage.

The multiple endocrine neoplasia (MEN) type 2 syndromes provide a preview of the future interaction of genetic testing and preventative treatment. MEN-2A (patients develop medullary thyroid cancer, pheochromocytoma, and hyperparathyroidism) and MEN-2B (affected family members have medullary thyroid cancer, pheochromocytoma, hyperparathyroidism, mucosal neuromata, intestinal ganglioneuromatosis, and skeletal deformities) are both autosomal dominant diseases. The gene responsible for both conditions and for familial medullary thyroid cancer (FMTC) has been mapped to the region near the centromere of chromosome 10.[30] Mutations of the RET proto-oncogene have been shown to be the cause for MEN-2A, MEN-2B, and FMTC. The protein encoded by the RET proto-oncogene is a transmembrane receptor tyrosine kinase; 95% of MEN-2A patients have a missense mutation in one of five codons, which results in the substitution of another amino acid for a highly conserved cystine residue.[31] These mutations cause configuration changes in the protein. All patients with MEN-2B have the same point mutation.[32]

Before the discovery of these specific genetic mutations, family members at risk for MEN-2A would undergo annual screening for elevated calcitonin levels to detect medullary thyroid cancer (MTC). Now a total thyroidectomy can be performed at a young age in patients with known germline RET mutations, before the development of an MTC. Wells and colleagues[33] first reported a series of 13 patients ranging from 6 to 20 years old whose total thyroidectomy was recommended solely on DNA testing showing a RET mutation. None had metastatic disease, but all had C-cell hyperplasia or localized MTC. Postoperatively, the stimulated plasma calcitonin levels were normal in each patient.

The imperfections of surgery for cancer prevention are clearly seen in the case of familial breast cancer syndromes. The discovery of the genes BRCA-1 and BRCA-2, which are responsible for many familiar breast and ovarian cancer pedigrees, allows identification of some patients at very high risk for these malignancies. Prophylactic bilateral mastectomies have been suggested for cancer prevention, but even in high-risk patients (not proven gene carriers), this surgery has only been 90% effective.[34]

In a large, controlled trial in the United States,[35] tamoxifen reduced breast cancer incidence in a similar patient population by 45%. Two smaller European studies[36,37] did not show a significant reduction in cancer risk with tamoxifen.

Tamoxifen appears to have an effect in reducing the risk of breast cancer in women with BRCA2 mutations but not women with BRCA1 mutations.[38] Preventative mastectomies are not widely recommended because of (1) the relative rarity of familial breast cancer patients; (2) the current inability to detect a genetic defect in most patients with a family history of breast cancer; (3) the imperfect results with bilateral simple mastectomies; and (4) the presence of other reasonable alternatives, including tamoxifen and close clinical monitoring. Prophylactic oophorectomies suffer from similar problems with respect to a small population at risk, inability to confirm all patients at risk with DNA analysis, the occurrence of primary peritoneal adenocarcinoma despite bilateral oophorectomy, and the alternative strategy of screening women with serum CA125 levels and pelvic ultrasonography.

Surgical Diagnosis of Malignancy

When a biopsy is needed to diagnosis a malignancy, the surgeon must remember several principles of management: these are (1) obtain sufficient tissue for a definitive diagnosis; (2) specimen handling to maximize tumor information including stage, microscopic margins (when indicated), and special pathological evaluations; and (3) the biopsy process must not interfere with future treatment or adversely impact on patient outcome. Not all tumors need to be biopsied preoperatively. If the findings are consistent with cancer and a benign biopsy result would not change the operative approach, tumor sampling should not be pursued. An example of this is a patient with painless jaundice and a mass in the head of the pancreas. If resectable for potential cure, a pancreaticoduodenotomy should be performed, regardless of preoperative or intraoperative primary tumor biopsy results. All biopsy procedures should be performed under sterile conditions, with more extensive procedures being undertaken in an operating room. Local anesthetic is sufficient for needle biopsies and superficial procedures, whereas regional or general anesthesia should be used for larger biopsy specimens or biopsies of deep-seated tumors. There are four types of biopsy used for tumor diagnosis: fine-needle aspirate (FNA), core needle biopsy, incisional biopsy, and excisional biopsy.

Fine-needle aspirate involves the removal of a cytology specimen from the tumor using a fine-caliber hollow needle (often 22-gauge) and suction (usually a pistol grip aspiration system with a small syringe) (Fig. 94.3). Superficial palpable masses, such as a thyroid nodule, cervical or other superficial adenopathies, and breast masses, can be sampled by fixing the palpable target between the physician's fingers and passing the needle through the tumor mass several times while applying suction on the syringe. Smears are made of the aspirate on microscopic slides, which are immediately fixed in alcohol, then stained. Deeper situated or nonpalpable abnormalities can be biopsied with ultrasound or computed tomography guidance. Because only a cytological diagnosis is made with FNA, care should be taken before performing a radical surgical procedure based on cytological information. Ideally, a histological diagnosis is obtained before mastectomy or other extensive procedures. Rare, but well-documented, false-positive FNA results have been reported.[39] If curative surgery is undertaken, the FNA tract is ideally included in the dissection, although tumor seeding with small-needle FNA biopsies is uncommon. Because of the limitations of FNA biopsy, its use should be limited to the following situations: (1) confirmation of recurrent metastatic disease, (2) proof of a primary or metastatic cancer before initiating nonoperative therapy, and (3) obtaining a diagnosis of malignancy preoperatively when this information affects surgical treatment. A common use of an FNA biopsy is for an abnormal cervical lymph node to rule out metastatic squamous cell cancer. If an excisional lymph node biopsy were done and metastatic head and neck cancer diagnosed, the efficacy of subsequent surgical therapy could be compromised by an open node biopsy.

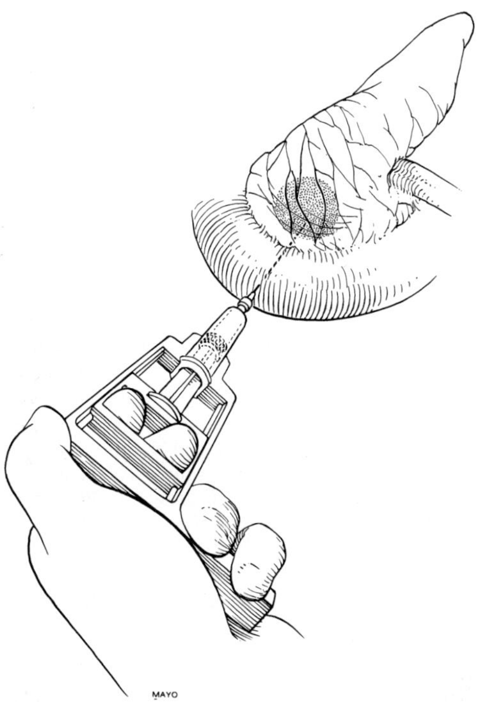

FIGURE 94.3. Intraoperative fine-needle aspirate (FNA) biopsy of unresectable pancreatic carcinoma. (Reprinted from McIlrath D, van Heerden J. Subtotal pancreatectomy: the Whipple procedure. In: Donohue J, van Heerden J, Monson J, eds. Atlas of Surgical Oncology. Cambridge: Blackwell Science, 1995:172, with permission.)

Core needle biopsies provide a cylinder of tissue for examination by the pathologist and allow a histological diagnosis of cancer. Larger needle diameters increase the risk of complications such as hemorrhage and tumor seeding along the biopsy tract. Core needle biopsies of mammographic abnormalities have become commonplace. The use of stereotactic core needle biopsies has reduced the number of open diagnostic biopsies and treatment costs for indeterminate mammographic abnormalities.[40,41] False-negative results may occur in as many as 5% of patients because of technical error or insufficient sampling. Patients with a negative biopsy result must have close follow-up (6 months or less) to avoid an excessive delay in diagnosis.

Incisional biopsies are used mostly in preparation for a more definitive procedure (confirm diagnosis of sarcoma before neoadjuvant chemotherapy or definitive surgical resection) or to obtain a larger amount of tissue than core biopsy in a nonoperable malignancy; for example, an incisional biopsy including a skin ellipse for a suspected inflammatory carcinoma of the breast allows documentation of dermal lymphatic involvement, plus confirming the diagnosis of breast cancer and assessing tumor hormone receptor status. Immu-

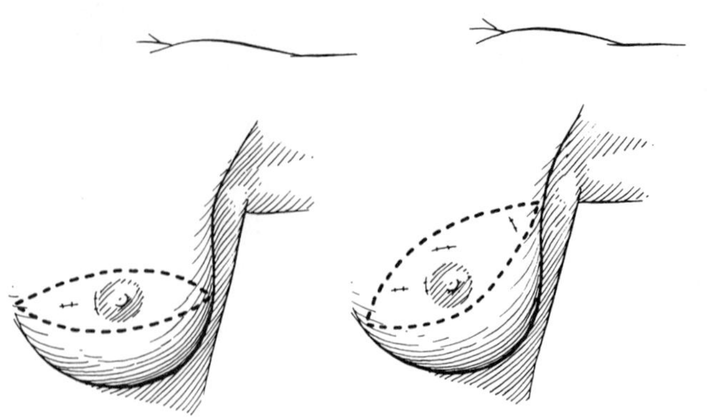

FIGURE 94.4. Placement of a diagnostic biopsy incision of the breast where it may be encompassed by a subsequent mastectomy if indicated. (Reprinted from Donohue J, Meland N. Breast excision, axillary dissection, and reconstruction. In: Donohue J, van Heerden J, Monson J, eds. Atlas of Surgical Oncology. Cambridge: Blackwell Science, 1995:100, with permission.)

nohistochemical techniques for hormone receptor [estrogen (ER) and progesterone (PR)] assays using tissue from needle biopsies are sufficient for ER and PR determination in breast cancer patients.

Because a larger operation often follows an incisional biopsy, the placement and orientation of the incision are critical. On the extremities, longitudinal incisions should be used because they are more readily encompassed during wide local excision. The scar should overlie the tumor and avoid subcutaneous tunneling because the entire biopsy cavity should be removed with the definitive resection (Fig. 94.4). It is imperative to achieve hemostasis at the time of incisional biopsy because large hematomas and ecchymosis may impair subsequent surgical management and result in local tumor spread. If an incisional biopsy is performed for a suspected cutaneous melanoma, the procedure should take a full-thickness sample of the pigmented lesion (Fig. 94.5). Tangential shave biopsies are not acceptable because the primary staging of a melanoma requires an accurate measurement of tumor thickness.

Small tumor masses, particularly superficial tumors and peripheral adenopathy suspected to be lymphoma, are best managed by excisional biopsy. For primary tumors, a rim of grossly uninvolved tissue should be included if excisional biopsy provides adequate local therapy. In the example of a breast mass believed to be cancerous, a 1-cm margin of normal breast tissue is included with the specimen. To enable the pathologists to assess microscopic involvement of margins, the specimen must be marked with ink, sutures, or clips to allow orientation (Fig. 94.6). Alternatively, additional normal tissue specimens from the periphery of the biopsy cavity can be sent separately to document adequate microscopic clearance around the cancer. Complete evaluation of a lymphoma requires special tissue handling with both fixed and fresh-frozen tissue. The surgeon must be certain to notify the pathology laboratory and ensure rapid transportation and handling of the specimen.

Diagnostic exploratory operations represent a key element of the surgical management of cancer. Because stage I and some stage II Hodgkin's disease patients did not traditionally receive chemotherapy, staging laparotomy with splenectomy, liver biopsies, and sampling of the intraabdominal nodal groups was commonly performed to prevent undertreatment of occult stage III and IV patients. The indicators for staging laparotomy have dwindled as chemotherapy is usually given for most early-stage Hodgkin's disease patients. Laparoscopic staging for Hodgkin's disease is feasible[42] but rarely performed. Laparoscopic exploration has proven to be of great benefit in assessing gastrointestinal cancer patients for occult metastasis. In patients with gastric cancer[43] and carcinoma of the head of the pancreas[44] not requiring palliative surgical procedures, diagnostic laparoscopy avoids nontherapeutic laparotomy in 21% and 27% of patients, respectively. Diagnostic laparoscopy is even more beneficial in adenocarcinomas of

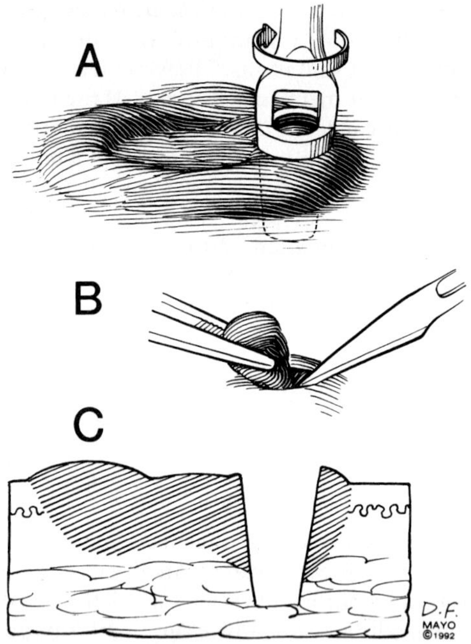

FIGURE 94.5. A. Punch biopsy. B. The base of the biopsy specimen is being transected. C. Cross section of the biopsy site with a full-thickness sampling of the pigmented skin lesion. (Reprinted from Bland K, Dudrick P, Copeland E. Surgical management of primary cutaneous melanoma. In: Donohue J, van Heerden J, Monson J, eds. Atlas of Surgical Oncology. Cambridge: Blackwell Science, 1995:10, with permission.)

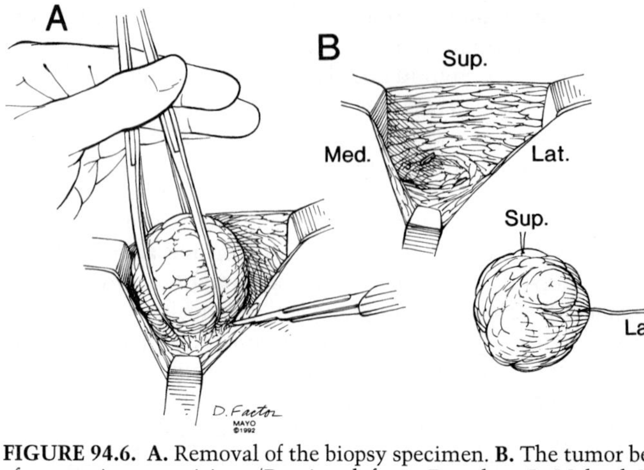

FIGURE 94.6. A. Removal of the biopsy specimen. B. The tumor bed after specimen excision. (Reprinted from Donohue J, Meland N. Breast excision, axillary dissection, and reconstruction. In: Donohue J, van Heerden J, Monson J, eds. Atlas of Surgical Oncology. Cambridge: Blackwell Science, 1995:97, with permission.)

the pancreatic body and tail. Laparoscopy can detect metastases in 65% of these patients.[44] Diagnostic laparoscopy is most sensitive in detecting small hepatic and peritoneal metastases not visible with noninvasive imaging modalities. Positive peritoneal cytology obtained at laparoscopy indicates incurable disease in pancreatic cancer[45] and can further reduce the incidence of nontherapeutic celiotomies.

Curative Surgical Therapy

Primary Tumor

Whenever possible, the primary cancers should not be violated during surgical manipulation. En bloc surgical resection of cancer is a well-established principle of oncological surgery. Any violation of the cancer has the potential for tumor spillage and wound implantation. If adjacent structures are adherent or fixed to the tumor, the attachment is assumed to be malignant in nature (this is often not demonstrable histologically) and the involved tissue is removed together with the neoplasm. Figure 94.7 shows a colon cancer with loop of adherent small bowel. A small part of the intestine is removed along with an adequate length of colon and mesocolon. Retroperitoneal sarcoma resections not uncommonly involve en bloc removal of several adjacent normal organs including a kidney and a segment of colon. Figure 94.8 demonstrates en bloc resection of the left kidney, left colon, spleen, and distal pancreas with a large left upper quadrant liposarcoma. If tumor abuts on structures not amenable to en bloc resection, metallic surgical clips are placed to mark the site at risk for microscopic residual tumor. Postoperative radiation therapy can be more accurately delivered with the placement of these radiopaque markers.

The treatment of breast cancer is the best example of equivalent outcomes with different surgical operations. A radical mastectomy was once the only acceptable therapy for this disease. Multiple large prospective trials[46–50] (Table 94.3) have shown wide local excision plus radiation therapy to be as effective as mastectomy in treating breast cancer (see Chapter 96). Breast conservation therapy has become the preferred method of treatment for breast cancer because of the improved cosmesis.[51]

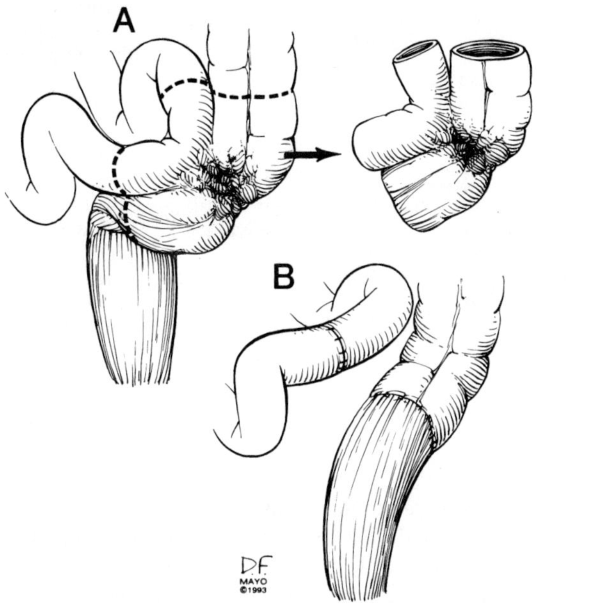

FIGURE 94.7. **A.** Sigmoid colon cancer with a loop-adherent small bowel. **B.** Colonic and small bowel intestinal anastomoses completed after en bloc tumor resection. (Reprinted from Donohue J. Principles of surgical oncology. In: Donohue J, van Heerden J, Monson J, eds. Atlas of Surgical Oncology. Cambridge: Blackwell Science, 1995:5, with permission.)

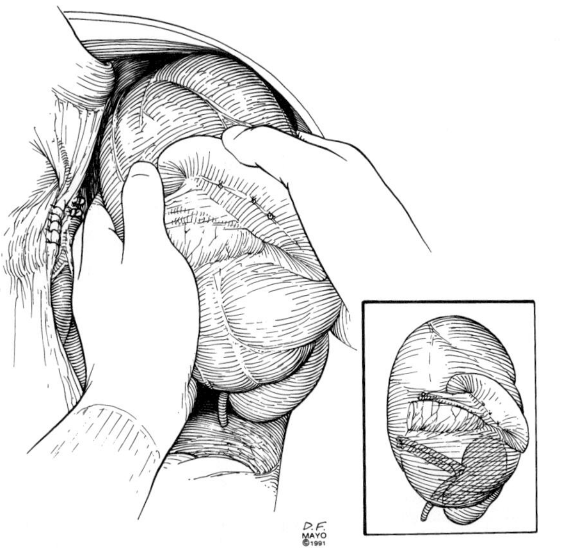

FIGURE 94.8. En bloc resection of left upper quadrant retroperitoneal liposarcoma with involved viscera (kidney, pancreas, spleen, and colon). (Reprinted from Donohue J, Mucha P. Retroperitoneal sarcoma excision. In: Donohue J, van Heerden J, Monson J, eds. Atlas of Surgical Oncology. Cambridge: Blackwell Science, 1995:262, with permission.)

Adequate margins of clearance for a curative resection vary depending on the tumor site and extent of the disease. Randomized, prospective studies have shown that 1-cm[52] or 2-cm[53] skin margins are adequate for cutaneous melanoma (see Chapter 97). The latter degree of tumor clearance is preferred for melanomas thicker than 1 mm. For other tumor sites, only uncontrolled data exist regarding the optimal surgical margin. Although a 5-cm distal margin was once considered necessary for adequate treatment of rectal adenocarcinoma, retrospective review has shown that a 2-cm margin would include all microscopic tumor in curative cases.[54] Ironically, the radial margins of rectal resections were not evaluated routinely until Quirke and associates[55] noted the frequent microscopic involvement (27%) of the lateral resection margins in patients believed to have had curative rectal operations. Wider tumor margins should be obtained in cancer types with diffuse infiltrative growth patterns. At least 5-cm proximal and distal longitudinal margins are recommended for gastric cancers. Although some authors prefer a 10-cm gastric margin, which would necessitate a total gastrectomy for nearly all tumors, total gastrectomy has proven no more curative than subtotal gastrectomy in a controlled trial.[56]

Regional Lymph Nodes

The curative impact of surgical resection of regional lymph nodes remains controversial in most solid tumors. There is little dispute that part of the en bloc resection of the primary

TABLE 94.3.
Comparison of Mastectomy and Breast Conservation Therapy for Early-Stage Breast Carcinoma: Prospective Trials.

Trial	*Year*	*Level of evidence*	*Randomized groups (n)*	*Intervention/design*	*Median follow-up (years)*	*Minor endpoint*	*Major endpoint*	*Interpretations/ comments*
NCI Milan	2002	I			20	Local recurrence (%)	Overall survival (%)	No survival difference despite more local recurrences with quandrantectomy. Only T1 cancers included and both operations more radical than current practice.
			Mastectomy (349)	Radical mastectomy		2.3	58.8	
						$P < 0.001$	$P = 1.0$	
			Breast conservation (352)	Quandrantectomy, axillary dissection, radiation therapy		8.8	58.3	
NSABP	2002	I			20.7	In breast failure (%)	Overall survival (%)	Significantly higher risk of breast failure with lumpectomy without radiation therapy. Disease-free and overall survival the same for all treatments. Both stage I and II cancer patients treated.
			Mastectomy (589)	Modified radical mastectomy			47	
			Lumpectomy (634)	Lumpectomy, axillary dissection		39.2	46	
						$P = 0.001$	$P = 0.57$	
			Lumpectectomy + radiation (628)	Lumpectomy, axillary dissection, radiation therapy		14.3	46	
NCI Bethesda	2003	I			18.4	Disease-free survival (%)	Overall survival (%)	Small study but no difference in disease-free or overall survival. Included stage I and II breast cancer patients.
			Mastectomy (116)	Modified radical mastectomy		67	58	
						$P = 0.64$	$P = 0.67$	
			Lumpectomy (121)	Lumpectomy, axillary dissection, radiation therapy		63	54	
EORTC	2000	I			13.4	Locoregional recurrence (%)	Overall survival (%)	Despite significantly more locoregional recurrences with lumpectomy, no difference in distant failure or overall survival; 80% of patients had T2 cancers (stage II disease).
			Mastectomy (420)	Modified radical mastectomy		12	66	
						$P = 0.01$	$P = 0.11$	
			Lumpectomy (448)	Lumpectomy, axillary dissection, radiation therapy		20	65	
Danish Breast Cancer Group	1992	I			3.3	Recurrence-free survival (%)	6-year overall survival (%)	Only short-term follow-up published, but comparable disease control and patient survival for both operations.
			Mastectomy (429)	Modified radical mastectomy		66	82	
						$P = 0.74$	$P = 0.81$	
			Lumpectomy (430)	Lumpectomy, axillary dissection, radiation therapy		70	79	

carcinoma should include adjacent draining lymph nodes. However, the benefit of extended lymphadenectomy in cancers where nodal removal may be more of a staging procedure rather than a therapeutic maneuver is debatable (Table 94.4).

For cutaneous malignant melanomas, there is a close correlation between the primary tumor thickness and the risk of metastasis. Balch and colleagues[57] demonstrated that melanomas less than 0.76 mm in thickness have a very small risk of metastasis, whereas melanomas 4.0 mm or more in diameter have a high probability of distant metastases. For patients with intermediate thickness tumors, namely 0.76 to 3.99 mm, an empiric regional lymph node dissection was recommended by a retrospective analysis that demonstrated improved survival for patients undergoing elective lymphadenectomy (no clinical evidence of regional nodal involvement) compared to patients treated with primary melanoma excision alone.[57] The results of this publication differed from two randomized

TABLE 94.4.
Effect of Regional Lymph Node Dissection: Prospective Trials.

Trial	*Disease*	*Year*	*Level of evidence*	*Randomized groups (n)*	*Median follow-up (years)*	*Minor endpoint*	*Major endpoint*	*Interpretations/ comments*
WHO	Melanoma	1982	I		8.2	Lymph node metastases (%)	20-year survival (%)	No benefit of immediate lymph node dissection. Many patients with unknown T stage and/or low risk of metastases.
				Wide local excision (286)		22.3	~60	
				Wide local excision and lymph node dissection (267)		20.2	~60	
Mayo	Melanoma	1986	I		4.5	Recurrent melanoma (%)		No benefit of immediate or delayed lymph node dissection. Small sample size limits statistical power of study.
				Wide local excision (62)		26	Survival ($P = 0.9$) and distant disease-free survival ($P = 0.8$) equivalent	
				Wide local excision, immediate lymph node dissection (54)		17 $P = 0.26$		
				Wide local excision, delayed lymph node dissection (55)		15		
Intergroup Melanoma Surgical Program	Melanoma	1996	I		7.4	—	5-year survival (%)	No benefit of elective lymph node dissection seen for whole group. Subsets did better, but the analysis was retrospective.
				Wide local excision (361)			72 $P = 0.25$	
				Wide local excision, elective lymph node dissection (379)			86	
Dutch Gastric Cancer Group	Gastric cancer	2004	I		11	Postoperative complications	11-year overall survival (%)	D2 nodal dissection caused more morbidity with no survival benefit compared to standard D1 gastrectomy.
				Curative gastrectomy (D1) (380)		25% $P < 0.001$	30 $P = 0.53$	
				Curative gastrectomy with extended lymphadenectomy (D2) (331)		43%	35	
Medical Research Committee	Gastric cancer	1999	I		6.5	Significantly worse outcome with splenectomy and pancreatectomy ($P = 0.01$)	5-year survival (%)	No benefit of D2 dissection for patient survival, having significantly more mortality.
				Curative gastrectomy (D1) (200)			35 NS	
				Curative gastrectomy with extended lymphadenectomy (D2) (200)			33	
NSABP B04	Breast cancer	2002	I		More than 25 years (mean)	25-year disease-free survival (%)	25-year overall survival (%)	Type of axillary treatment did not significantly affect long-term disease-free or overall survival for either women with involved or uninvolved lymph nodes.
				Lymph node– Radical mastectomy (362)		19	25	
				Total mastectomy + irradiation (352)		13 $P = 0.65$	19 $P = 0.49$	
				Total mastectomy (365)		19	26	
				Lymph node + Radical mastectomy (292)		11 $P = 0.20$	14 $P = 0.49$	
				Total mastectomy + irradiation (294)		10	14	

prospective trials,[58,59] both of which showed no benefit of routine regional lymphadenectomy for cutaneous melanoma. However, these trials were both initiated before the prognostic importance of melanoma thickness was recognized.

Patient entry criteria did not exclude patients not expected to benefit from elective nodal dissection based on Balch and coworkers' retrospective analysis.[57] Because a real benefit of nodal dissection may have been missed, another randomized prospective trial comparing local surgery alone and wide local excision and elective regional nodal dissection was initiated. This study by the Intergroup Melanoma Surgical Program entered 740 melanoma patients. With a median follow-up of 7.4 years, there was no overall survival benefit for patients undergoing an elective lymph node dissection.[60] Although patients 60 years old or younger with nonulcerated tumors 1 to 2mm thick had significantly better survival with lymphadenectomy compared to observation of the nodes, the dangers of such subset analysis were discussed at the time these data were presented.[60]

Part of the problem with the elective lymph node trials in melanoma is that most patients with indeterminate-thickness melanomas will not have regional nodal metastases; the incidences of nodal disease ranged from 17% in 1- to 2-mm melanomas to 37% in the 3- to 4-mm-thickness group in the Intergroup Melanoma study.[60] Because of this, the majority of patients are not at risk for disease failure if the regional lymph nodes are observed. A better evaluation of the efficacy of elective nodal dissection would be a comparison of treatments in the subset of patients with documented microscopic nodal metastases.

Morton and colleagues[61] first reported the mapping of lymphatic drainage to regional lymph nodes for primary melanomas using a vital dye. Krag and associates at the University of Vermont[62] subsequently used radiolabeled colloid to localize the first node draining the tumor site, the so-called sentinel lymph node. Standardized techniques have been proposed.[63] Multiple studies[64,65] have demonstrated that the sentinel node can be identified in more than 95% of cutaneous melanomas using radioactive colloid injections, with or without lymphangiogram dye. If nodal metastases are present, the sentinel node is an excellent predictor of their existence when carefully examined histologically using standard hematoxylin and eosin plus immunohistochemical stains. A negative sentinel lymph node is also an excellent indicator that no regional melanoma metastases are present; however, false-negative sentinel lymph node results occur.[64,65]

Because of an approximately 5% incidence of nodal recurrence after negative sentinel lymph node biopsy, more thorough pathological examination of the sentinel nodes, including multiple sections and immunohistochemical stains, has been recommended.[63,66] Completed trials using sentinel lymph node biopsy for selective application of nodal dissection should provide objective data comparing delayed versus immediate lymphadenectomy but still do not provide a definitive answer to whether elective lymph node dissection in cutaneous melanoma patients with microscopic nodal metastases improves patient survival.

Another malignancy for which the therapeutic effect of lymphadenectomy is hotly debated is gastric adenocarcinoma. In standard Occidental gastrectomy specimens, only the perigastric nodes along the lesser and greater curvatures of the stomach (N1) are excised (a D1 dissection). Many surgeons, particularly the Japanese,[67] have advocated an extended lymphadenectomy that includes nodal groups along the branches of the celiac axis (N2 nodes; a D2 dissection when these are excised) or even more distant nodal basins (N3 nodes, a D3 dissection). The survival data for gastric cancer in Japan are far superior to most from the Western world. Pathological stage migration, based on the tissues available and the thoroughness of evaluation,[67,68] differences in tumor biology between Japan and the West, and other hypotheses have been proposed as alternative explanations for the improved survival of Japanese gastric cancer patients. Small randomized prospective trials from Cape Town[69] and Hong Kong[70] attempted to compare a D1 operation with a D2 or D3 procedure, respectively. Both were discontinued before a sufficient number of patients were accrued.

The protocol of Robertson and colleagues noted significantly more complications following the extended resection.[70] A large multicenter, prospective, but not randomized, trial from Germany[71] reported significant improvement in outcome for some patients following extended (D2) lymphadenectomy. Only D1 resections were performed at some centers, and the extent of the lymph node dissection was based on the number of nodes examined histologically, rather than by the operative procedure. Randomized prospective trials comparing D1 and D2 resections in adenocarcinoma of the stomach have recently been reported from both the Netherlands and the United Kingdom. Analyses of patient outcome for both studies[72,73] reported significantly higher postoperative morbidity and mortality for the more extensive operation without any improvement in patient survival. No objective data exist supporting an extended lymphadenectomy for improved survival in gastric cancer. Unfortunately many patients with gastric cancer in the Western world present with peritoneal or distant metastases. These patients would not benefit from more extensive surgery, even if a D2 resection was proven better for less extensive cancers of the stomach.

The en bloc removal of regional lymph nodes along with the breast in radical and ultraradical mastectomies was thought to be critical in enhancing the cure rate for carcinoma of the breast. With the realization that nodal metastases in breast cancer were usually an indicator of distant metastatic risk, rather than the cause of further tumor dissemination,[74] the rationale for axillary node dissection in breast cancer patients changed to accurate staging of the disease and, to a lesser degree, improved regional control. The National Adjuvant Breast and Bowel Project (NSABP) B-04 study[75] considered the effect of axillary nodal treatment in a controlled fashion. Women with clinically negative axillae were randomized to radical mastectomy (removal of the axillary nodes), simple mastectomy followed by axillary radiation, or simple mastectomy alone. Although 40% of the women in the radical mastectomy arm had nodal metastases, only half that many women in the simple mastectomy cohort developed their first clinical relapse in the axilla. There was no difference in patient survival among the three groups.[75] Surgical removal had no impact on patient survival but did lower the incidence of regional tumor failure.

Improved public education and screening have resulted in more early-stage breast cancers being diagnosed. Because women with tumors 1cm in diameter or less are usually not given systemic therapy unless lymph node metastases are present, axillary staging is key to therapeutic decision making in a growing number of breast cancer patients. Even tumors 0.5 cm or smaller have a 4% to 12% incidence of axillary metastases.[76,77] A combination of prognostic factors for small breast cancers do not accurately predict the absence of nodal metastasis.[78] Axillary lymphadenectomy is no longer standard therapy for most women with invasive adenocarcinoma. Sentinel lymph node biopsy has gained favor as an accurate and less morbid method of staging breast cancer.[79–81] Similar techniques for melanoma sentinel lymph node biopsy using a vital dye, radiolabeled colloid, or both techniques, are utilized. Sentinel lymph node excision has become the surgical procedure of choice to determine axillary nodal involvement in breast cancer. Formal lymphadenectomy is usually limited to patients with clinically apparent metastases or patients at high risk for residual disease based on the sentinel node biopsy findings.

Metastatic Tumor

For most patients with distant metastases, surgery is of no benefit as a curative treatment. Although no prospective controlled trials have been performed, there are several clinical situations in which an aggressive surgical approach can result in the long-term survival and cure of patients with metastatic cancer. Before embarking on surgical excision of metastatic disease, several conditions must be fulfilled. The patient must be able to tolerate the proposed operation. There must be no evidence of locoregional recurrence, or with the discovery of synchronous metastases, the primary cancer must be amenable to curative resection. A full evaluation of all sites of metastasis must be undertaken. Metastasis to more than one distant site is usually a contraindication to resection. Resectable metastases are usually in a vital organ, most commonly the lungs or the liver. All metastases must be ablated and sufficient functional normal parenchyma left to be compatible with an acceptable lifestyle. Hepatic resections can be more extensive (as much as 75% of a healthy liver) because of the liver's ability to regenerate. No absolute number of metastases should be used to deny a healthy patient an aggressive treatment plan for metastatic disease; however, the larger the number of preoperatively detected metastases, the more likely additional disease will be found at exploration or be present occultly.

The most extensive experience with surgical treatment for metastatic disease is in hepatic colorectal cancer metastases. Multiple single-institution[82,83] and collaborative[84,85] reports have shown 25% to 40% 5-year survival for patients undergoing complete resection of their intrahepatic disease. Uncontrolled comparisons of resected patients to patients not undergoing hepatic surgery show a significant difference in survival.[86] Although no prospective, randomized trial has been performed, it is well established that patients with untreated metastatic colorectal carcinoma rarely survive more than 5 years. At least a quarter of the hepatectomy patients reach this endpoint. Long-term studies[87,88] have shown that disease-free survival to 5 years following hepatectomy for colorectal metastases is usually indicative of disease cure. The most common site for disease failure following hepatectomy is in the liver remnant. Multiple reports[89–91] have demonstrated comparable patient survival curves after repeat hepatectomy compared to the results following initial liver resection for colorectal metastases.

Unfortunately, most patients with recurrent colorectal cancer are not candidates for hepatic resection because of multiple sites of disease recurrence, extensive liver involvement, underlying health problems, or other contraindications. Hepatic tumors can be destroyed in situ using a number of techniques, including radiofrequency ablation, cryotherapy, high-intensity focused ultrasonography, and ethanol ablation. Ablation is only used in place of resection for patients not suited for or unwilling to have an operation.[92] Combining resection and ablation allows more patients to have potentially curative procedures, however, recurrence rates are higher and survival lower than with resection alone.[93] Bismuth and colleagues[94] were the first to show that neoadjuvant chemotherapy with an oxaliplatin-containing regimen can cause sufficient tumor regression to render some (13%) patients resectable with curative intent. At 5 years, these patients had a 35% survival,[95] comparable to or perhaps improved[96] when compared to patients resectable without neoadjuvant chemotherapy.

Patients with colorectal metastases to the lungs amenable to complete resection should also be treated surgically. Several institutions[97,98] have reported 30% to 40% 5-year survivals for these patients. Both soft tissue and osteogenic sarcomas show a propensity to metastasize to the lungs. Five-year survival of approximately 30%[99–101] can be achieved following complete resection of metastatic sarcoma. Repeat pulmonary resections for metastatic colorectal and sarcoma patients can salvage some patients and should be considered.

For most other metastatic cancers, there are limited data or poor results for curative metastasis resections. Many common malignancies, such as breast, lung, and pancreatic carcinomas, regularly metastasize to multiple sites making the removal of limited single-organ metastases unlikely to be curative. Why some patients with adenocarcinoma of the large bowel and sarcomas have limited tumor spread to a single organ that allows curative operative therapy remains unknown. Improvements in adjuvant therapy are needed to increase the rate of success in the select tumors where metastasis resection is an accepted treatment and also to expand this approach to other cancers.

Tumor Debulking

There are no controlled data indicating incomplete tumor removal or debulking increases patient survival. Patients and their families frequently ask why the surgeon will not remove as much disease as possible during an operation. Despite the intuitive notion that such therapy would prolong survival, the increased mortality from an extensive operation and the unchanged natural history of the underlying cancer are both reasons to not perform routine debulking procedures. In select instances, there is evidence that subtotal resection of disease improves patient outcome.

Epithelial ovarian carcinomas normally present with extensive intraperitoneal metastases. Because of the usually diffuse nature of the intraabdominal involvement, often with carcinomatosis and ascites, curative resections are generally not feasible. No randomized prospective trial comparing aggressive cytoreductive resection and less extensive ovarian cancer surgery has been completed. Griffiths[102] first reported the benefit of maximal debulking surgery in women who received postoperative chemotherapy. The median survival was 39 months for women in whom all gross disease was removed. The median survival decreased with larger residual tumor masses. The least successful cytoreduction group (residual tumors > 1.5 cm) had a median survival of only 11 months.[102] Multiple other reports[103–105] have shown similar results. In each study, optimal cytoreductive procedures (minimal residual tumor diameter either <1 cm or <2 cm) resulted in at least a 40-month median survival when postoperative combination chemotherapy (a variety of regimens, all containing cisplatin) was given. In contrast, patients less completely debulked had median survivals less than half as long (16–21 months).[103–105]

The benefits of this combination of surgical debulking and chemotherapy treatment are thought to be a result of improved chemotherapy sensitization, reduced probability of drug resistance, or simply the several log diminishment of tumor mass in optimally debulked patients (as much as a 99.9% reduction in tumor mass in some ovarian cancer patients, in contrast to most other solid tumors, in whom a much larger percentage of tumor is left in situ). Hoskins and colleagues[106] showed several nonsurgical factors, including patient age, tumor grade, and the number of residual tumor masses, to be independent prognostic factors. A large cooperative study organized by the Gynecologic Oncology Group[107] demonstrated that all tumors larger than 2 cm need to be removed to gain a significant survival benefit. Another report[108] demonstrated the efficacy of optimal cytoreductive surgery even in stage IV ovarian cancer patients in whom hepatic and extraabdominal metastases are present. The rates of successful optimal cytoreduction vary between institutions based on the aggressiveness of the surgeon plus patient and tumor characteristics. Maximum ovarian cancer debulking can be achieved in approximately 35% of patients.[109] The use of second-look laparotomy with repeat cytoreduction and further chemotherapy based on intraoperative findings attempt to further prolong patient survival. The data for these treatments are uncontrolled, limited in extent, and do not show as distinct an advantage as primary cytoreductive surgery. Despite such an aggressive treatment approach, the vast majority of women with advanced-stage ovarian carcinoma eventually succumb to their disease, even when a complete response is achieved with combination therapy.

Neuroendocrine tumors of the gastrointestinal tract should also be considered for cytoreductive surgery. These neoplasms, which include metastatic carcinoid tumors and islet cell cancers, are generally indolent in nature. In contrast to the typical epithelial cancers of the gut, patients with neuroendocrine malignancies may live for years, even with distant metastases.[110] Midgut carcinoid tumors are most likely to cause the carcinoid syndrome when they metastasize to the liver. Most of these cancers present with extensive bilobar metastases, not amenable to total surgical removal. In these patients, hepatic devascularization (embolization or surgical arterial ligation) will result in short-term relief from carcinoid syndrome symptoms.[110] Hepatic transplantation has been performed in small numbers of patients in the United States[111] and Europe.[112,113] Although the duration of symptomatic relief and patient survival are excellent (up to an actuarial 5-year survival of 69%),[113] most transplantation surgeons will not treat these patients because of the scarcity of donor organs and better long-term recipient survival with benign diseases.

In a selected group of patients (approximately 10%) in whom the metastases are clustered sufficiently to allow debulking of 90% to 95% of the hepatic disease, conventional hepatic resection can result in improved or even complete response of symptoms. Unfortunately, the duration and degree of response are quite variable.[110,114] The rare patient with metastatic neuroendocrine malignancy may undergo complete resection of all known disease and potentially be cured.[114,115] Functioning islet cell cancers that are resistant to medical therapy may also benefit from cytoreductive surgery, but the benefit of surgical intervention is frequently uncertain and patients need to be carefully chosen. The best results follow near-complete or total tumor excision in a malignancy that has limited sites of disease involvement.

Palliative Surgery

In many patients with advanced primary or recurrent cancer, the growth of the malignancy causes symptoms related to luminal obstruction, tissue infiltration, or perforation of a hollow viscus. Medical treatment, radiation therapy, or increasingly minimally invasive procedures are utilized to relieve tumor-induced symptoms. Surgical palliation often has the advantage of a longer duration of efficacy. Before treating a patient with incurable cancer surgically, it is imperative to consider the patient's status, in particular their ability to tolerate the operation, their functional limitations, the anticipated duration of survival, and the expected quality of their remaining life. Although difficult for the patient and family to accept, nonintervention is the best surgical approach when there is no realistic possibility of providing an acceptable lifestyle for a reasonable period of time. Loss of normal body function, such as intestinal stoma formation, is often necessary for malignant bowel obstruction and should be clearly explained to the patient beforehand. The surgeon must also mention that no or limited therapeutic benefit may result from the surgical procedure because of intraoperative findings, postoperative complications, or further progression of the cancer.

The most common type of palliative surgery is for the obstruction of a hollow viscus. Bowel obstructions may be resected when limited disease is present and healthy bowel is present on either side of the anastomosis. Bypass or proximal diversion with an enterostomy is indicated when locally advanced or multifocal tumors are present. In the case of extensive carcinomatosis where safe dissection of the intestine is not possible, no bypass or diversion may be technically feasible or safe. If a gastrostomy tube can be placed, this may provide some relief in lieu of a nasogastric tube. When a procedure to relieve an intestinal obstruction is complicated by extensive carcinomatosis and a future celiotomy is unlikely to be therapeutic, the surgeon should comment on these findings in the operative dictation to aid other clinicians in subsequent patient management.

Obstructive jaundice commonly occurs with a number of primary upper gastrointestinal malignancies and less commonly from distant metastatic disease. Biliary drainage can be achieved by surgical, endoscopic, or percutaneous routes. For patients with limited life expectancy, the least invasive procedure, usually endoscopic stent placement, is preferred (Table 94.5). A randomized trial of endoscopic and percutaneous drainage[116] showed endoscopic biliary decompression to

TABLE 94.5.
Comparison of Biliary Decompression Techniques in Cancer Patients.

Trial	Year	Level of evidence	Randomized groups (n)	Intervention/ design	Median follow-up (months)	Minor endpoint	Major endpoint	Interpretations/ comments
King's College	1987	I		Randomized to percutaneous or endoscopic biliary stenting	4	Successful stenting (%)	30-day mortality (%)	Endoscopic stenting more successful and less morbid in elderly, debilitated patients with biliary obstruction
			Percutaneous (36)			61	33	
						$P = 0.017$	$P = 0.016$	
			Endoscopic (39)			81	15	
Southhampton	1988	I		Randomized to endoscopic or surgical biliary decompression	4.5	Relief of jaundice (%)	Median survival (days)	Significantly shorter hospital stay with endoscopic stenting but greater need for additional treatment (stent change)
			Endoscopic stent (23)			92	152	
						ns	ns	
			Surgical bypass (25)			91	124.5	
Middlesex	1994	I		Randomized endoscopic stent or surgical bypass	5.5	Relief of jaundice (%)	Median survival (months)	Less hospital morbidity and mortality and shorter stay with stents but more likely to need stent replacement and gastric bypass than surgical group
			Endoscopic stent (101)			95	21	
						ns	$P = 0.065$	
			Surgical bypass (103)			94	26	
Amsterdam	1992	I		Randomized to plastic or expandable metal endoscopic stent	4.0	Median stent patency (days)	Median survival (days)	Longer patency of self-expanding metal stents,but no improvement in survival
			Plastic stent (56)			126	147	
						$P = 0.006$	$P = 0.45$	
			Expandable metal stent (49)			273	175	

ns, not significant.

be significantly less morbid and more likely to successfully decompress the obstructed biliary tree. Prospective controlled trials[117,118] of endoscopic decompression versus surgical biliary bypass procedures have shown comparable success rates with significantly reduced cost, earlier hospital dismissal, and less morbidity in the endoscopic stent group. Self-expanding metal stents provide longer relief of jaundice than plastic stents.[119] Unfortunately, this advantage is lessened for patients who survive longer, requiring repeated stent changes resulting in an increased rate of complications.[120,121] If intestinal obstruction develops, as occurs in 15% to 20% of periampullary malignancies, this needs to be treated. As a rule, the longer the life expectancy of the patient with malignant biliary obstruction, the more a surgical bypass procedure needs to be performed. Gastrojejunostomy can be performed as an open or laparoscopic procedure. Expandable metal stents have been successfully used for bowel obstructions. A small study[122] found stent use to have significant advantages to either form of surgical bypass.

Urinary obstruction must be treated if a patient is to maintain maximum renal function; this is of special importance in allowing continued chemotherapy. Cystoscopically placed internal ureteral stents are the preferred method of renal decompression, whenever possible. Regular stent changes are required. If stents cannot be placed or the bladder outflow is compromised, percutaneously placed nephrostomy or cystostomy catheters provide alternative methods of urinary drainage.

Hemorrhage from a malignancy that requires transfusion or causes hemodynamic instability must be localized and treated expeditiously. Tumor bleeding is generally not amenable to long-term control by nonsurgical means. The hemorrhagic tumor usually must be resected to stop blood loss. Endoscopic methods of temporary control include cauterization, laser ablation, or vasoconstrictor injection. Devascularization by either radiologic embolization or surgical ligation are usually only efficacious transiently. These techniques should be employed to stabilize the patient or when surgical resection is not feasible.

The perforation of a hollow viscus may occur at the site of necrotic tumor or proximal to the malignancy. Acute perforation in this setting is a surgical emergency and requires urgent stabilization of the patient and expeditious operative therapy. In addition to controlling the site of perforation, resection of the causative tumor should be undertaken when the patient status and tumor extent allow it. Stoma formation is often required because of intraperitoneal soilage in the patients with intestinal or colonic perforations. Reestablishment of intestinal continuity can be achieved at a later date in appropriate patients.

Pain caused by a solid tumor is often secondary to infiltration of adjacent nerves. Severe back pain complicates the management of the majority of patients with advanced pancreatic carcinoma. This symptom results from involvement of the retroperitoneal splanchnic nerves. Lillimoe and colleagues,[123] in a controlled trial, demonstrated that intraoperative chemical splanchnicectomy, using 50% alcohol solution injected on either side of the aorta at the celiac axis, significantly improves preexistent pain and significantly delays the development of this problem postoperatively. Most malignant pain is best managed by oral or parenteral narcotics, percutaneous nerve blocks, and, in some patients, localized radiation therapy. In patients with osseous metastases, it is important to evaluate for impending pathological fractures, particularly in weight-bearing bones. Patient morbidity is markedly reduced by prophylactic orthopedic management of these situations, rather than urgent treatment of a pathological fracture.

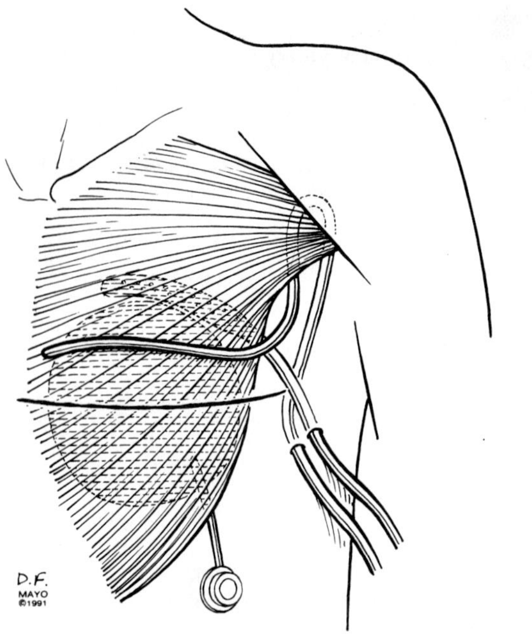

FIGURE 94.9. Immediate reconstruction with breast prosthesis. (Reprinted from Donohue J, Meland N. Breast excision, axillary dissection, and reconstruction. In: Donohue J, van Heerden J, Monson J, editors. Atlas of Surgical Oncology. Cambridge: Blackwell Science, 1995:110, with permission.)

Rehabilitative/Reconstructive Surgery

As our understanding of tumor biology and the increased application of adjuvant therapies have developed, less radical surgical procedures have replaced older more extensive extirpative procedures for many types of cancer. Two clear-cut examples are extremity sarcomas and breast cancer. In the past, most larger or proximal extremity sarcomas were treated with a major amputation. Because prospective data showed no difference in patient outcome when treated with amputation or wide local excision with postoperative radiation therapy[124] and temporal changes in institutional practice,[125] most extremity sarcoma patients now undergo limb salvage procedures. For carcinoma of the breast, multiple, long-term, controlled trials[46–49] have conclusively demonstrated that breast conservation surgery plus postoperative chemotherapy have similar rates of disease control and overall patient survival. Experiences with both sarcoma[126,127] and breast cancer[128,129] patients have shown that preoperative treatment can reduce tumor size, allowing even more patients to undergo organ-sparing curative operations.

Some women still require mastectomy to achieve total removal of disease. There is extensive experience with breast reconstruction using prosthetics (Fig. 94.9) and autologous tissue transfers (Fig. 94.10). These reconstructive procedures

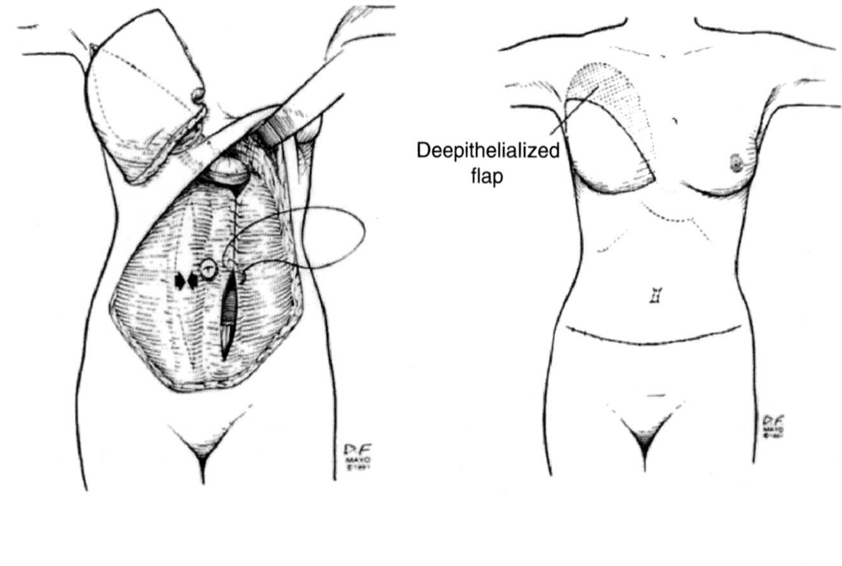

FIGURE 94.10. Pedicled transverse rectus abdominis myocutaneous (TRAM) flap breast reconstruction. (Reprinted from Donohue J, Meland N. Breast excision, axillary dissection, and reconstruction. In: Donohue J, van Heerden J, Monson J, eds. Atlas of Surgical Oncology. Cambridge: Blackwell Science, 1995:112, with permission.)

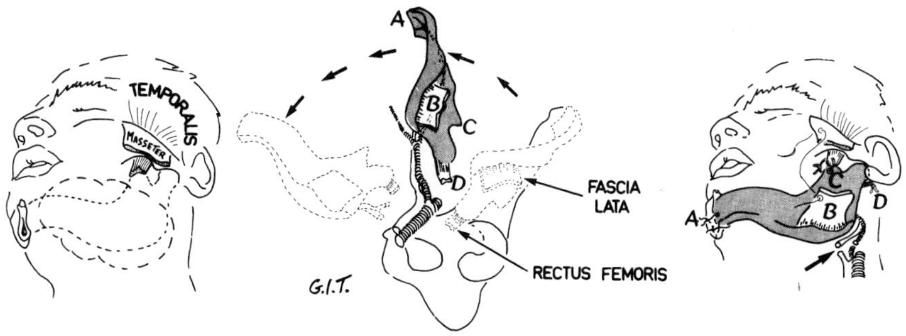

FIGURE 94.11. Composite tissue flap using iliac crest and muscle based on deep circumflex iliac vessels for reconstruction of oral cavity defect. (Reprinted from Taylor G, Townsend P, Corlett R. Superiority of the deep circumflex iliac vessels as the supply for free groin flaps. Clinical work. Plast Reconstr Surg 1979;64:745, with permission.)

can be performed immediately or subsequent to mastectomy in most women. Despite concern about impairing tumor control or affecting postoperative detection of recurrent disease, no data have suggested an adverse effect on tumor control by appropriately performed breast reconstruction.[130–132] Breast reconstruction has a marked impact on improving a woman's psychosocial adjustment to mastectomy.

Composite resections of head and neck cancers involve removal of soft tissue, bone, and regional lymph nodes. These procedures result in substantial deficits in patient function, including speech, nutrition, and respiration, and cause a significant cosmetic defect. A large variety of reconstructive procedures, including composite free flaps including bone to bridge a skeletal defect, have been developed to reduce the cosmetic and functional defects after these radical excisions (Fig. 94.11). These operations improve the physiological and psychological results after surgery.

Large wounds caused by the resection of irradiated tissue are notoriously difficult to manage. These wounds heal slowly and result in substantial morbidity and mortality. Pedicled and free tissue transfer flaps provide healthy, well-vascularized tissue bulk to fill the surgical defect (eliminate dead space) and provide coverage for the wound that will heal spontaneously in a shorter period of time with fewer complications. Because radiation therapy is commonly used in cervical and rectal adenocarcinomas, patients undergoing resections of local tumor recurrence are left with high-risk wounds in their perineum. A number of myocutaneous tissue transfers, including gracilis and rectus abdominis flaps, can be used to repair perineal defects caused by radical rectal or gynecological resection.

Conclusion

Surgery continues to play a pivotal role in the treatment of the cancer patient, primarily for diagnosis, eradication of disease, and treatment of symptoms. Although the role of surgery is no longer a primary one in some malignancies, it remains the single most effective form of management in most adult solid tumors. Although new advances in molecular biology and nonsurgical therapies will diminish the role of the surgeon in treating cancer, surgery will continue as a prominent component of therapy for the foreseeable future. Because of the rapid developments in oncological treatments, it behooves the surgical oncologist to keep abreast of changes in therapy and utilize them once they have objectively proven superior to conventional treatments.

References

1. NIH Consensus Development Panel. National Institute of Health consensus development conference statement: adjuvant therapy for breast cancer, November 1–3, 2000. J Natl Cancer Inst 2001;93:979–989.
2. MacDonald JS. Adjuvant therapy of colon cancer. CA Cancer J Clin 1999;49:202–219.
3. Fearon ER, Vogelstein B. A genetic model for colorectal tumorigenesis. Cell 1990;61:759–767.
4. Greene FL, Page DL, Fleming ID, et al., eds. AJCC Cancer Staging Manual, 6th ed. New York: Springer-Verlag, 2002.
5. O'Connell JB, Maggard MA, Ko KY. Colon cancer survival rates with the new American Joint Committee on Cancer, 6th ed. Staging. J Natl Cancer Inst 2004;96:1420–1425.
6. Oken M, Creech R, Tormey D, et al. Toxicity and response criteria of the Eastern Cooperative Oncology Group. Am J Clin Oncol 1982;5:649–655.
7. Dripps R, Lamont A, Eckenhoff J. The role of anesthesia in surgical mortality. JAMA 1961;178:261–266.
8. The Veterans Affairs Total Parenteral Nutrition Cooperative Study Group. Preoperative total parenteral nutrition in surgical patients. N Engl J Med 1991;325:525–531.
9. von Meyenfeldt M, Meyerink W, Soeters P, et al. Perioperative nutritional support results in a reduction of major postoperative complications, especially in high risk patients. Gastroenterology 1991;100:A5553.
10. Heslin M, Latkany L, Leung D, et al. A prospective randomized trial of early enteral feeding after resection of upper gastrointestinal malignancy. Ann Surg 1997;226:567–580.
11. Einhorn L. Testicular cancer as a model for a curable neoplasm: the Richard and Hinda Rosenthal Foundation Award Lecture. Cancer Res 1981;41:3275–3280.
12. Willilams S, Birch R, Einhorn L, et al. Treatment of disseminated term-cell tumors with cisplatin, bleomycin, and either vinblastine or etoposide. N Engl J Med 1987;316:1435–1440.
13. Nigro N, Vaitkevicius V, Considine B. Combined therapy for cancer of the anal canal: a preliminary report. Dis Colon Rectum 1974;17:354–356.
14. Fuchshuber P, Rodriquez-Bigas M, Weber T, et al. Anal canal and perianal epidermoid cancers. J Am Coll Surg 1997;185:494–505.
15. Minsky B, Cohen A, Kemeny N, et al. Enhancement of radiation-induced downstaging of rectal cancer by fluorouracil and high-dose leucovorin chemotherapy. J Clin Oncol 1992;10:79–84.
16. Gunderson LL, Nelson H, Martenson JA, et al. Locally advanced primary colorectal cancer: intraoperative electron and external beam irradiation ± 5FU. Int J Radiat Oncol Biol Phys 1997; 137:601–614.
17. Allee P, Tepper J, Gunderson L, et al. Postoperative radiation therapy for incompletely resected colorectal carcinoma. Int J Radiat Oncol Biol Phys 1989;17:1171–1176.

18. Oates G, Stenning S, Harcastle J, et al. Randomised trial of surgery alone versus radiotherapy followed by surgery for potentially operable locally advanced rectal cancer: Medical Research Council Rectal Cancer Working Party. Lancet 1996;348:1605–1610.
19. Pahlman L, Glimelius B. Improved survival with preoperative radiotherapy in resectable rectal cancer: Swedish Rectal Cancer Trial. N Engl J Med 1997;336:980–987.
20. Krook J, Moertel C, Gunderson L, et al. Effective surgical adjuvant therapy for high-risk rectal carcinoma. N Engl J Med 1991;324:709–715.
21. Miyoshi Y, Nagase H, Ando H, et al. Somatic mutations of the APC gene in colorectal tumors: mutation cluster region in the APC gene. Hum Mol Genet 1992;1:229–233.
22. Solomon E, Voss R, Hall V, et al. Chromosome 5 allele loss in human colorectal carcinomas. Nature (Lond) 1987;328:616–619.
23. Nagase H, Miyoshi Y, Horii A, et al. Correlation between the location of germ-line mutations in the APC gene and the number of colorectal polyps in familial adenomatous polyposis patients. Cancer Res 1992;52:4055–4057.
24. Moertel C, Hill J, Adson M. Surgical management of multiple polyposis. The problem of cancer in the retained bowel segment. Arch Surg 1970;100;521–526.
25. Wu JS, Paul P, McGannon EA, Church JM. APC genotype, polyp number, and surgical options in familial adenomatous polyposis. Ann Surg 1998;227:57–62.
26. Bertario L, Russo A, Radice P, et al. Genotype and phenotype factors as determinants for rectal stump cancer in patients with familial adenomatous polyposis. Ann Surg 2000;231:438–443.
27. Ambroze W Jr, Dozois R, Pemberton J, et al. Familial adenomatous polyposis: results following ileal pouch-anal anastomosis and ileorectostomy. Dis Colon Rectum 1992;35:12–15.
28. Ekborn A, Helmick C, Zack M, et al. Ulcerative colitis and colorectal cancer: a population-based study. N Engl J Med 1990;323:1228–1233.
29. Taylor B, Pemberton J, Carpenter H, et al. Dysplasia in chronic ulcerative colitis: implications for colonoscopic surveillance. Dis Col Rectum 1992;35:950–956.
30. Lairmore T, Howe J, Korte J, et al. Familial medullary thyroid carcinoma and multiple endocrine neoplasia type 2B map to the same region of chromosome 10 as multiple endocrine neoplasia type 2A. Genomics 1991;9:181–192.
31. Mulligan L, Ponder B. Genetic basis of endocrine disease: multiple endocrine neoplasia type 2. J Clin Endocrinol Metab 1995; 80:1989–1995.
32. Carlson K, Dou S, Chi D, et al. Single missense mutation in the tyrosine kinase catalytic domain of the RET protooncogene is associated with multiple endocrine neoplasia type 2B. Proc Natl Acad Sci U S A 1994;91:1579–1583.
33. Wells S Jr, Chi D, Toshima K, et al. Predictive DNA testing and prophylactic thyroidectomy in patients at risk for multiple endocrine neoplasia type 2A. Ann Surg 1994;220:237–247.
34. Hartmann LC, Sellers SA, Schaid DJ, et al. Efficacy of bilateral prophylactic mastectomy in BRCA1 and BRCA2 gene mutation carriers. J Natl Cancer Inst 2001;93:1633–1637.
35. Fisher B, Costantino JP, Wickerham DL, et al. Tamoxifen for prevention of breast cancer: report of the National Surgical Adjuvant Breast and Bowel Project P-1 Study. J Natl Cancer Inst 1998;90:1371–1388.
36. Veronesi U, Maisonneuve P, Costa A, et al. Prevention of breast cancer with tamoxifen: preliminary findings from Italian randomized trial among hysterectomised women. Lancet 1998;352: 93–97.
37. Powles T, Eeles R, Ashley S, et al. Interim analysis of the incidence of breast cancer in the Royal Marsden Hospital tamoxifen randomised chemoprevention trial. Lancet 1998;352:98–101.
38. King M-C, Wieand S, Hale K, et al. Tamoxifen and breast cancer incidence among women with inherited mutations in BRCA1 and BRCA2: National Surgical Adjuvant Breast and Bowel Project (NSABP-P1) Breast Cancer Prevention Trial. JAMA 2001;286:2251–2256.
39. Kline T, Joshi L, Neal H. Fine-needle aspiration of the breast: diagnosis and pitfalls—a review of 3545 cases. Cancer (Phila) 1979;44:1458–1464.
40. Jackman R, Nowels K, Shepard M, et al. Stereotaxic large-core needle biopsy of 450 nonpalpable breast lesions with surgical correlation in lesions with cancer or atypical hyperplasia. Radiology 1994;193:91–95.
41. Parker S, Burbank F, Jackman R, et al. Percutaneous large-core breast biopsy: a multi-institutional study. Radiology 1994;193: 359–364.
42. Baccarani U, Carroll B, Hiatt J, et al. Comparison of laparoscopic and open staging in Hodgkin disease. Arch Surg 1998;133:517–522.
43. Burke E, Karpeh M, Conlon K, et al. Laparoscopy in the management of gastric adenocarcinoma. Ann Surg 1997;225:262–267.
44. Fernandez-del Castillo C, Warshaw A. Laparoscopy for staging in pancreatic carcinoma. Surg Oncol 1993;2(suppl 1):25–29.
45. Makary M, Warshaw A, Centeno B, et al. Implications of peritoneal cytology for pancreatic cancer management. Arch Surg 1998;133:361–365.
46. Veronesi U, Cascinelli N, Mariani L, et al. Twenty-year follow-up of a randomized study comparing breast-conserving surgery with radical mastectomy for early breast cancer. N Engl J Med 2002;2347:1227–1232.
47. Fisher B, Anderson S, Bryant J, et al. Twenty-year follow-up of a randomized trial comparing total mastectomy, lumpectomy, and lumpectomy plus irradiation for the treatment of invasive breast cancer. N Engl J Med 2002;347:1233–1241.
48. Poggi MM, Danforth DN, Sciuto LC, et al. Eighteen-year results in the treatment of early breast carcinoma with mastectomy versus breast conservation therapy. The National Cancer Institute randomized trial. Cancer (Phila) 2003;98:697–702.
49. van Dongen JA, Voogd AC, Fentiman IS, et al. Long-term results of a randomized trial comparing breast-conserving therapy with mastectomy: European Organization for Research and Treatment of Cancer 10801 trial. J Natl Cancer Inst 2000;92:1143–1150.
50. Blichert-Toft M, Rose C, Andersen JA, et al. Danish randomized trial comparing breast conservation therapy with mastectomy: six years of life-table analysis. J Natl Cancer Inst Monogr 1992;11:19–25.
51. Consensus statement: treatment of early-stage breast cancer. NIH Consensus Development Conference, June 18–21, 1990, vol 8, no. 6. Bethesda, MD: National Institutes of Health, 1990:1–19.
52. Veronesi U, Cascinelli N, Adamus J, et al. This stage I primary cutaenous malignant melanoma: comparison of excision with margins of 1 or 3 cm. N Engl J Med 1988;318:1159–1162.
53. Balch C, Urist M, Karakousis C, et al. Efficacy of 2-cm surgical margins for intermediate-thickness melanomas (1 to 4): results of a multi-institutional randomized surgical trial. Ann Surg 1993;218:262–269.
54. Williams N, Dixon M, Johnston D. Reappraisal of the 5 centimeter rule of distal excision for carcinoma of the rectum: a study of distal intramural spread and a patients' survival. Br J Surg 1983;70:150–154.
55. Quirke P, Durdey P, Dixon M, et al. Local recurrence of rectal adenocarcinoma due to inadequate surgical resection. Histopathological study of lateral tumour spread and surgical excision. Lancet 1986;2:996–999.
56. Bozzetti F, Marubini E, Bonfanti G, et al. Subtotal versus total gastrectomy for gastric cancer: five-year survival rates in a multicenter randomized Italian trial. Ann Surg 1999;230:170–178.

57. Balch C, Soong S, Milton G. A comparison of prognostic factors and surgical results in 1,786 patients with localized (stage I) melanoma treated in Alabama, USA, and New South Wales, Australia. Ann Surg 1982;196:677–684.
58. Veronesi U, Adamus J, Bandiera D, et al. Delayed regional lymph node dissection in Stage I melanoma of the skin of the lower extremities. Cancer (Phila) 1982;49:2420–2430.
59. Sim F, Taylor W, Pritchard D, et al. Lymphadenectomy in the management of Stage I malignant melanoma: a prospective randomized study. Mayo Clin Proc 1986;61:697–705.
60. Balch C, Soong S, Bartolucci A, et al. Efficacy of an elective regional lymph node dissection of 1 to 4 mm thick melanomas for patients 60 years of age and younger. Ann Surg 1996;224:225–266.
61. Morton D, Wen D, Wong J, et al. Technical details of intraoperative lymphatic mapping for early stage melanoma. Arch Surg 1992;127:392–399.
62. Krag D, Meijer S, Weaver D, et al. Minimal-access surgery for staging of malignant melanoma. Arch Surg 1995;130:654–660.
63. Cochran AJ, Balda B-R, Starz H, et al. The Augsburg Consensus. Techniques of lymphatic mapping, sentinel lymphadenectomy, and completion lymphadenectomy in cutaneous malignancies. Cancer (Phila) 2000;89:236–241.
64. Cascinelli N, Belli F, Santinami M, et al. Sentinel lymph node biopsy in cutaneous melanoma: the WHO Melanoma Program experience. Ann Surg Oncol 2000;7:469–474.
65. Morton DL, Hoon SDB, Cochran AJ, et al. Lymphatic mapping and sentinel lymphadenectomy for early-stage melanoma: therapeutic utility and implications of nodal microanatomy and molecular staging for improving the accuracy of detection of nodal micrometastases. Ann Surg 2003;238:538–550.
66. Gershenwald J, Colome M, Lee J, et al. Patterns of recurrence following a negative sentinel lymph node biopsy in 243 patients with Stage I or II melanoma. J Clin Oncol 1998;16:2253–2260.
67. Noguchi Y, Imada T, Matsumoto A, et al. Radical surgery for gastric cancer: a review of the Japanese experience. Cancer (Phila) 1989;64:2053–2062.
68. Noda N, Sasako M, Yamaguchi N, et al. Ignoring small lymph nodes can be a major cause of staging error in gastric cancer. Br J Surg 1998;85:831–834.
69. Dent D, Madden M, Price S. Randomized comparison of R1 and R2 gastrectomy for gastric carcinoma. Br J Surg 1988;75:110–112.
70. Robertson C, Chung S, Woods S, et al. A prospective randomized trial comparing R1 subtotal gsatrectomy with R3 total gastrectomy for antral cancer. Ann Surg 1994;220:176–182.
71. Siewert JR, Bottcher K, Stein HJ, et al. Relevant prognostic factors in gastric cancer: ten-year results of the German Gastric Cancer Study. Ann Surg 1998;228:449–461.
72. Hartgrink HH, van de Velde CJH, Putter H, et al. Extended lymph node dissection for gastric cancer: who may benefit? Final results of the randomized Dutch Gastric Cancer Group Trial. J Clin Oncol 2004;22:2069–2077.
73. Cuschieri A, Weeden S, Fielding J, et al. Patient survival after D1 and D2 resections for gastric cancer: long-term results of the MRC randomized surgical trial. Br J Cancer 1999;79:1522–1530.
74. Fisher B. Laboratory and clinical research in breast cancer—a personal adventure: the David A. Karnofsky Memorial Lecture. Cancer Res 1980;40:3863–3874.
75. Fischer B, Jeong J-H, Anderson S, et al. Twenty-five year follow-up of a randomized trial comparing radical mastectomy, total mastectomy, and total mastectomy followed by irradiation. N Engl J Med 2002;347:567–575.
76. Chontos A, Maher D, Ratzer E, et al. Axillary lymph node dissection: is it required in T1a breast cancer? Am J Surg 1996;172:501–505.
77. McGee Y, Youmans R, Clingan F, et al. The value of axillary dissection in T1a breast cancer. Am J Surg 1996;172:501–505.
78. Barth A, Craig P, Silverstein M. Predictors of axillary lymph node metastases in patients with T1 breast carcinoma. Cancer (Phila) 1997;79:1918–1922.
79. Giuliano A, Jones R, Brennan M, et al. Sentinel lymphadenectomy in breast cancer. J Clin Oncol 1997;15:2345–2350.
80. Veronesi U, Paganelli G, Balimberti V, et al. Sentinel-node biopsy to avoid axillary dissection in breast cancer with clinically negative lymph nodes. Lancet 1997;349:1864–1867.
81. Ollila D, Brennan M, Giuliano A. Therapeutic effect of sentinel lymphadenectomy in T1 breast cancer. Arch Surg 1998;133:647–651.
82. Scheele J, Stang R, Altendorf-Hofmann A, et al. Resection of colorectal liver metastases. World J Surg 1995;19:59–71.
83. Fong Y, Cohen A, Fortner J, et al. Liver resection for colorectal metstases. J Clin Oncol 1997;15:938–946.
84. Hughes KS, Simon R, Songhorabodi S, et al. Resection of the liver for colorectal carcinoma metastases: a multi-institutional study of indications for resection. Surgery (St. Louis) 1988;103:278–288.
85. Nordlinger B, Jaeck D, Guiguet M, et al. Multicentric retrospective study by the French Surgical Association. In: Nordlinger B, Jaeck D, eds. Treatment of Hepatic Metastases of Colorectal Cancer. Paris: Springer-Verlag, 1992, pp 129–146.
86. Wilson S, Adson M. Surgical treatment of hepatic metastases from colorectal cancers. Arch Surg 1976;111:330–334.
87. Jamison R, Donohue J, Nagorney D, et al. Hepatic resection for metastatic colorectal cancer results in cure for some patients. Arch Surg 1997;132:505–511.
88. Scheele J, Rudroff C, Altendorf-Hofmann A. Resection of colorectal liver metastases revisited. J Gastrointest Surg 1997;1:408–422.
89. Fernandez-Trigo V, Shamsa F, Sugarbaker P, et al. Repeat liver resections from colorectal metastasis. Surgery (St. Louis) 1995;117:296–304.
90. Neeleman N, Andersson R. Repeated liver resection for recurrent liver cancer. Br J Surg 1996;83:893–901.
91. Adam R, Bismuth H, Castaing D, et al. Repeat hepatectomy for colorectal liver metastases. Ann Surg 1997;225:51–62.
92. Erce C, Parks RW. Interstitial ablative techniques for hepatic tumors. Br J Surg 2003;90:272–289.
93. Abdalla EK, Vauthey J-N, Ellis LM, et al. Recurrence and outcomes following hepatic resection, radiofrequency ablation, and combined resection/ablation for colorectal liver metastases. Ann Surg 2004;239:818–827.
94. Bismuth H, Adam R, Levi F, et al. Resection of nonresectable liver metastases from colorectal cancer after neoadjuvant chemotherpay. Ann Surg 1996;224:509–522.
95. Adam R, Avisar E, Ariche A, et al. Five-year survival following hepatic resection after neoadjuvant therapy for nonresectable colorectal [liver] metastases. Ann Surg Oncol 2001;8:347–353.
96. Tanaka K, Adam R, Shimada H, et al. Role of neoadjuvant chemotherapy in the treatment of multiple colorectal metastases to the liver. Br J Surg 2003;90:963–969.
97. McCormack P, Burg M, Bains M, et al. Lung resection for colorectal metastases: 10-year results. Arch Surg 1992;127:1403–1406.
98. McAfee M, Allen M, Trastek V, et al. Colorectal lung metastases: results of surgical excision. Ann Thorac Surg 1992;53:780–786.
99. Martini N, McCormack P, Bains M, et al. Surgery for solitary and multiple pulmonary metastases. N Y State J Med 1978;78:1711–1714.
100. Creagan E, Fleming T, Edmonson J, et al. Pulmonary resection for metastatic nonosteogenic sarcoma. Cancer (Phila) 1979;44:1908–1912.
101. Putnam J, Roth J, Wesley M, et al. Analysis of prognostic factors in patients undergoing resection of pulmonary metastases from soft tissue sarcomas. J Thorac Cardiovasc Surg 1984;87:260–268.

102. Griffiths C. Surgical resection of tumor bulk in the primary treatment of ovarian carcinoma. Natl Cancer Inst Monogr 1975;42:101–104.
103. Vogl S, Pagano M, Kaplan B, et al. Cisplatin based combination chemotherapy for advanced ovarian cancer: high overall response rate with curative potential only in women with small tumor burdens. Cancer (Phila) 1983;51:2024–2030.
104. Pohl R, Dallenbach-Hellweg G, Plugge T, et al. Prognostic parameters in patients with advanced ovarian malignant tumors. Eur J Gynaecol Oncol 1984;3:160–169.
105. Omura G, Bundy B, Berek J, et al. Randomized trial of cyclophosphamide plus cisplatin with or without doxorubicin in ovarian carcinoma: a gynecologic oncology study group. J Clin Oncol 1989;7:457–465.
107. Hoskins W, Bundy B, Thigpen J, et al. The influence of cytoreductive surgery on recurrence-free interval and survival in small-volume stage III epithelial ovarian cancer: a gynecologic oncology group study. Gynecol Oncol 1992;47:159–166.
107. Hoskins W, McGuire W, Brady M, et al. The effect of diameter of largest residual disease on survival after primary cytoreductive surgery in patients with suboptimal residual epithelial ovarian carcinoma. Am J Obstet Gynecol 1994;170:974–980.
108. Curtin J, Malik R, Venkatraman E, et al. Stage IV ovarian cancer: impact on surgical debulking. Gynecol Oncol 1997;64:9–12.
109. Boente M, Chi D, Hoskins W. The role of surgery in the management of ovarian cancer: primary and interval cytoreductive surgery. Semin Oncol 1998;25:326–334.
110. Moertel C. An odyssey in the land of small tumors (Karnofsky Memorial Lecture). J Clin Oncol 1987;5:1502–1522.
111. Iwatsuki S, Tzakis A, Todo S, et al. Liver transplantation for metastatic hepatic malignancy. Hepatology 1993;18:723.
112. Lang H, Oldhafer K, Weinmann A, et al. Liver transplantation for metastatic neuroendocrine tumors. Ann Surg 1997;225:355–364.
113. Le Treut Y, Delpero J, Dousset B, et al. Results of liver transplantation in the treatment of metastatic neuroendocrine tumors: a 31-case French multicentric report. Ann Surg 1997;225:355–364.
114. Sarmiento JM, Heywood G, Rubin J, et al. Surgical treatment of neuroendocrine metastases to the liver: a plea for resection to increase survival. J Am Coll Surg 2003;197:29–37.
115. Chen H, Hardacre J, Uzar A, et al. Isolated liver metastases from neuroendocrine tumors: does resection prolong survival? J Am Coll Surg 1998;198:88–93.
116. Speer A, Cotton P, Russell R, et al. Randomized trial of endoscopic versus percutaneous stent insertion in malignant obstructive jaundice. Lancet 1978;2:57–62.
117. Shepherd H, Royle G, Ross A, et al. Endoscopic biliary endoprostheses in the palliation of malignant obstruction of the distal common bile duct: a randomized trial. Br J Surg 1988;75:1166–1168.
118. Smith A, Dowsett J, Russell R, et al. Randomized trial of endoscopic stenting versus surgical bypass in malignant low bile duct obstruction. Lancet 1994;334:1655–1660.
119. Davids PHP, Groen AK, Rauws EAJ, et al. Randomised trial of self-expanding metal stents versus polyethylene stents for distal malignant biliary obstruction. Lancet 1992;340:1488–1492.
120. Gilbert D, DiMarino A, Jensen D, et al. Status evaluation: biliary stents. Gastrointest Endosc 1992;38:750–752.
121. Deviere J, Baize M, de Toeuf J, et al. Long-term follow-up of patients with hilar malignant stricture treated by endoscopic internal biliary drainage. Gastrointest Endosc 1988;34:95–101.
122. Mittal A, Windsor J, Woodfield J, et al. Matched study of three methods for palliation of malignant pyloroduodenal obstruction. Br J Surg 2004;91:205–209.
123. Lillemoe K, Cameron J, Kaufman H, et al. Chemical splanchnicectomy in patients with unresectable pancreatic cancer: a prospective, randomized trial. Ann Surg 1993;217;447–457.
124. Rosenberg S, Kent H, Costa J, et al. Prospective, randomized evaluation of the role of limb-sparing surgery, radiation therapy, and adjuvant chemoimmunotherapy in the treatment of adult soft-tissue sarcomas. Surgery (St. Louis) 1978;84:62–69.
125. Brennan M, Shiu M, Collin C, et al. Extremity soft tissue sarcomas. Cancer Treat Symp 1985;3:71–81.
126. Eilber F, Guiliano A, Huth J, et al. Limb salvage for high grade soft tissue sarcomas of the extremity: experience at the University of California, Los Angeles. Cancer Treat Symp 1985;3:49–57.
127. Denton J, Dunham W, Salter M, et al. Preoperative regional chemotherapy and rapid-fraction irradiation for sarcomas of the soft tissue and bone. Surg Gynecol Obstet 1984;158:545–551.
128. Veronesi U, Bonadonna G, Zurrida S, et al. Conservation surgery after primary chemotherapy in large carcinomas of the breast. Ann Surg 1995;222:612–618.
129. Fisher B, Brown A, Mamounas E, et al. Effect of preoperative chemotherapy on local-regional disease in women with operable breast cancer: findings from National Surgical Adjuvant Breast and Bowel Project B-18. J Clin Oncol 1997;15:2483–2493.
130. Johnson C, van Heerden J, Donohue J, et al. Oncological aspects of immediate breast reconstruction following mastectomy for malignancy. Arch Surg 1989;124:819–824.
131. Noone R, Frazier T, Noone G, et al. Recurrence of breast carcinoma following immediate reconstruction: a 13-year review. Plast Reconstr Surg 1994;93:96–108.
132. Carlson G, Bostwick J, Styblo T, et al. Skin-sparing mastectomy: oncologic and reconstructive considerations. Ann Surg 1997;225: 570–578.

95

Radiation as an Adjunct to Surgery

Barbara-Ann Millar and Laura A. Dawson

Almost one-half of all cancer patients are treated with radiation at some time during the duration of their illness. This chapter focuses on the role of radiotherapy as an adjunct to surgery, both as adjuvant treatment to standard surgery (e.g., in rectal cancer) and as adjuvant therapy to organ-preserving surgery, as a substitute to more radical surgery (e.g., lumpectomy and radiation rather than mastectomy for breast cancer). We begin by briefly reviewing the biological and physical basis for using radiotherapy and the rationale for combining surgery and radiation for the treatment of cancer. It should be noted that radiation is a primary curative modality for several cancer subtypes (e.g., seminoma, lymphoma, head and neck cancer) and has a critical role in the palliation of patients with locally advanced or metastatic disease. The role of radiation in these settings is well addressed in other textbooks.[1,2]

Physical Basis of Radiation

Radiation therapy refers to the use of radiation (defined as the emission and propagation of energy through space or material) for clinical use. X-rays, gamma rays, and particulate radiation are all used in the treatment of cancer. X-rays and gamma rays constitute part of the continuous electromagnetic radiation spectrum. X-rays are man made, whereas gamma rays refer to radiation produced naturally (e.g., produced during decay of cobalt-60). Particulate radiation refers to radiation propagated by traveling corpuscles within a resting mass. Particulate radiation causes direct ionization of atoms via interactions with electrons or protons. X-rays and gamma rays are also ionizing radiation because individual photons can lead to the complete displacement of an electron from its orbit around the nucleus of an atom. When photons interact with tissue, they give up energy by one of three main processes: the photoelectric effect, the Compton effect, or electron–positron "pair" production. The most important interaction in clinical radiotherapy is the Compton effect, in which a photon interacts with a loosely bound electron. The incident photon transfers energy to the electron and is deflected with a lower energy. The energy dissipated by ionizing events leads to the disruption of chemical bonds, including those in DNA, leading to biological effects. The unit for an absorbed dose from radiation is a gray (Gy), which is equal to one joule absorbed per kilogram of tissue.

The photon energies used in clinical radiotherapy range from kiloelectron volts (keV) to more than 20 million electron volts (MeV). As the energy increases, the penetration of the radiation in tissue increases, and the skin is spared a dose by the production of higher-energy electrons that travel forward and achieve full intensity at a depth below the skin's surface (Figure 95.1). Low-energy radiation (50–500 keV) is useful for the treatment of superficial skin cancers, and megavoltage radiation is generally used for the treatment of deeper tumors.

Electrons, protons, and neutrons are the types of particulate radiation used most often clinically. Electrons are commonly used to treat superficial targets. As a function of energy, they demonstrate a sharp falloff in penetration at a particular depth (see Figure 95.1). Other charged particles (e.g., protons) have the unusual but useful characteristic of delivering radiation at a depth while sparing the superficial areas. Neutrons produce a distribution of energy in tissue similar to that produced with photons, although with more ionizations per unit path. Neither charged-particle therapy nor neutron therapy is available in most centers across North America.

Brachytherapy refers to radiation delivered from a short distance to the target, typically by placing radioactive sources within or adjacent to the tumor. The radioactive sources come in sealed containers such as thin wires or seeds. Sources placed permanently are referred to as implants.

Sources placed temporarily in the body are removed after the prescribed dose of radiation has been delivered. An advantage of brachytherapy is that as the source to target distance decreases, the penetration of radiation falls off quickly. This characteristic offers a potential advantage compared with external-beam radiation to deliver a high dose of radiation to the volume adjacent to the brachytherapy source while sparing the normal tissue at a distance from the source. A potential disadvantage of brachytherapy compared with external-beam radiation is the difficulty in obtaining a homogeneous dose distribution across the tumor volume. Very high dose radiation in some sites may result in a high risk of necrosis, whereas too little dose in other sites could lead to tumor persistence.

External-beam radiation, delivered at a distance from the patient (usually 100 cm), usually from a *linear accelerator* that produces high-energy X-rays or electrons, is most commonly used in the adjuvant setting. The radiation dosimetry is optimized by using shaped radiation fields, varying the number of beams, the beam weighting, and the beam orientation, and using beam-modifying devices.

Before planning radiation therapy, the target volume is chosen based on physical examination, imaging, operative findings, and pathology. To ensure that the tumor is treated with the prescribed radiation dose, a margin of normal tissue around the target must be treated to account for potential variations in patient setup and organ motion. Patient positioning, immobilization, and tumor localization tools can help patients to be treated in as reproducible a position as possible. Immobilization devices include custom-made face masks and body casts (Figure 95.2). Localization methods involve the use of external reference marks (e.g., skin tattoos and stereotactic frames), IV contrast, radiopaque dyes, surgical clips, and applicators to outline hollow organs. Target volumes and relevant normal tissues are delineated using computed tomography (CT), magnetic resonance imaging (MRI), and/or positron emission tomography (PET) scans incorporated into the radiation planning system. *Conformal radiation therapy* (CRT) refers to the use of three-dimensional imaging to facilitate precise targeting of the tumor and avoidance of radiation dose to adjacent normal tissues. Another method of conforming radiation to unusually shaped target volumes is by using beams with variable intensities of photons across the beam cross section (*intensity modulated radiation therapy*, IMRT). The intensity patterns are generally obtained with the aid of computer optimization algorithms.

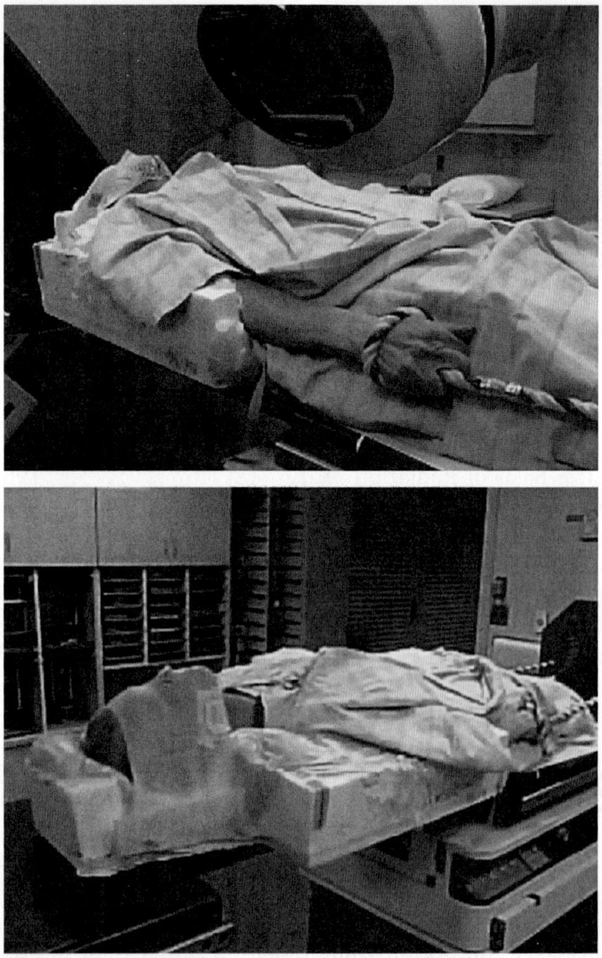

FIGURE 95.2. **A.** A patient with a head and neck cancer is seen in the treatment position, with a mask and body cast used for immobilization. **B.** Arm pulls are used to keep the shoulders as low as possible. (Courtesy of Dr. Eisbruch, University of Michigan.)

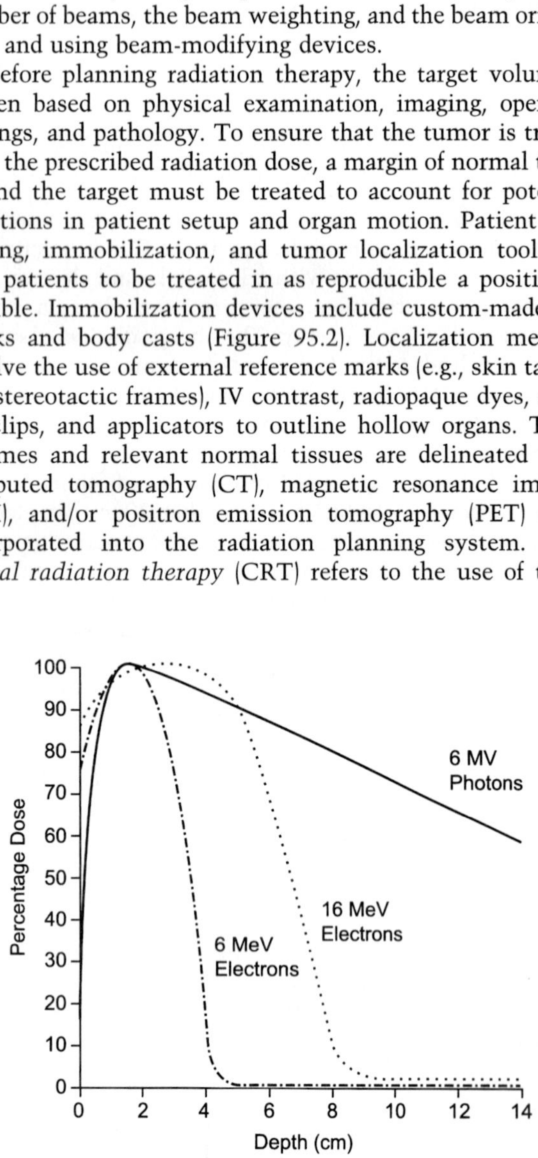

FIGURE 95.1. Percentage depth dose distribution is displayed for a 6-MV photon beam, which is compared to the sharp falloff that occurs at depth for two electron beams of different energies (6 MeV and 18 MeV).

Stereotactic radiotherapy is a form of conformal radiation in which sophisticated immobilization, setup, and image guidance systems are so accurate that very little normal tissue surrounding the tumor needs to be treated to the prescription dose. *Radiosurgery* generally refers to stereotactic radiotherapy delivered in a single fraction. The most common type of radiosurgery is for the treatment of brain tumors, in which the tumors are localized using a stereotactic frame that is fixed to the patient's skull.

Biological Basis for Radiation

The primary target of radiation is DNA that is affected directly or indirectly by ionizing radiation. Most radiation-induced cell death results from reproductive death, which manifests

TABLE 95.1. Preoperative Radiotherapy Versus Postoperative Radiotherapy.

Preoperative radiation	*Postoperative radiation*
Advantage	
Downstaging, which leads to:	Surgical and pathological staging
Potential for organ preservation	Patient selection for radiation
Potential for an increase in resectibility	Patient selection for chemotherapy
Less chance of a positive margin	No delay in definitive therapy
Potential for less toxicity, e.g., in abdomen less small bowel irradiated, fewed adhesions, smaller adhesions, smaller volume possible	Opportunity to help optimize radiation delivery by: Localization of high-risk areas with clips; Moving normal tissues away from target
Less risk of seeding during surgery	
Less hypoxia leading to more effective radiation	
Disadvantage	
Delays definitive treatment (surgery)	Increase in toxicity, due to:
No pathological staging, leading to:	Larger volume radiated
Overtreatment of some patients (with radiation)	More small bowel irradiated
Undertreatment of some patients (with chemotherapy) who would normally be offered therapy	More adhesions irradiated
	Less chance for organ preservation
Increased wound complications	Hypoxic tumor leading to less effective radiation
Psychological impact of waiting for surgery	Potential for tumor seeding at surgery

itself after several cell divisions. An alternate type of cell death, apoptosis, occurs as a direct consequence of radiation in some cell types (e.g., lymphocytes and oocytes). Apoptosis is an energy-dependent process that occurs hours to days after radiation treatment and involves the activation of a cell death program. In addition to DNA damage, radiation produces a variety of cellular perturbances in signal transduction pathways and alterations in cell cycle progression.

Radiosensitivity is an intrinsic measure of the susceptibility of cells to injury by radiation. Radiosensitivity does not necessarily translate into clinical radioresponsiveness because many other factors are important in determining whether all clonogens are eradicated. These factors include the tumor growth kinetics, the rate of clearance of dead cells, the rate of clonogen proliferation, the rate of repair of radiation-induced damage, the hypoxic fraction of cells, and the number of malignant clonogens. Proliferating cells are more radiosensitive than nonproliferating cells, with mitosis being the most sensitive phase of the cell cycle. Some tumors, such as meningiomas, can be cured without "responding" because much of the tumor may be noncellular material.

Both sensitive and resistant cells sustain approximately the same amount of DNA damage after radiation. In contrast, the level of repair of radiation-induced double-strand DNA breaks varies between cell lines and may be partially responsible for the different cell survival curves seen after radiation to different cell lines. In general, tumors have a decreased capacity for sublethal damage repair compared to late-reacting tissues. This difference between tumors and normal tissues may be responsible for the increase in therapeutic gain that is produced by fractionating radiation treatments. The fact that normal cells outside the radiation portal can migrate in and out may also play a role.

Oxygen must be present at the time of radiation for maximal cell killing. Oxygen "fixes" the free radicals produced by photons in tissue, causing nonrepairable DNA damage. In vitro, hypoxia may reduce cellular radiosensitivity by as much as threefold. Although the hypoxic fraction of cells has been found to be a prognostic factor in sarcoma, cervical, and head and neck cancer,[3,4] the role of hypoxia in clinical radiation responsiveness remains controversial.

In addition to the total dose of radiation being important for tumor cell kill, the biological effectiveness of dose is modified by dose per fraction, dose rate, interfraction interval, time, volume irradiated, and host factors. Chemotherapy can also modify radiation sensitivity.

As an in-depth discussion of the biological basis for radiation is beyond the scope of this chapter, the interested reader is referred to more detailed radiobiology references.[5]

Combining Surgery and Radiation

One rationale for combining surgery and radiation in the treatment of cancer relates to the ability of radiation to treat potential microscopic disease in the structures surrounding the surgical bed, while preserving the structure and function of the surrounding tissues. The goal of adjuvant radiation is to decrease the probability of cancer recurrence. Radiation may be delivered preoperatively or postoperatively. Advantages and disadvantages of preoperative radiation compared with postoperative radiation are outlined in Table 95.1. Some advantages of preoperative radiation include the potential for an increase in resectability, organ preservation, and less toxicity. Disadvantages include the lack of surgical and pathological staging, which may lead to unnecessary irradiation of some patients. Conversely, the lack of pathological staging with preoperative radiation may lead to avoidance of adjuvant chemotherapy that may have otherwise been offered. When postoperative radiation is used, radiopaque markers placed at the time of surgery to delineate the tumor bed can facilitate radiation planning, especially when the high-risk volume is to be treated to higher radiation doses, as with sarcoma. Surgical maneuvers may also be used to reduce normal tissue irradiation. Small bowel toxicity from pelvic radiation can be reduced with tissue expanders, with absorbable meshes, or by retroperitonealizing the pelvic floor, retroverting the uterus, or constructing an omental sling.

When preoperative radiation is used with the goal of improving resectability, a 4- to 6-week break between the completion of radiation and surgery is usually required for substantial tumor shrinkage. Postoperative radiation is generally not recommended until 3 to 4 weeks following surgery when healing of surgical scars is complete. Shorter intervals between surgery and radiation are well tolerated for some tumors, such as Wilms tumor, where postoperative radiation is delivered 10 days following surgery. When delivering postoperative radiation to grafted skin, late complications are rare so long as chemotherapy is not given in conjunction with radiation and the graft is allowed to heal adequately before initiating therapy (usually by 6 weeks).[6] Longer delays between surgery and radiation may allow tumor proliferation and be associated with a reduction in the efficacy of radiation.

The collaboration of surgical, medical, and radiation oncologists will help to ensure optimal treatment for the patient. For example, at the time of surgery for a soft tissue sarcoma, the surgeon may define the high-risk operative bed, and the radiation oncologist may place catheters in an arrangement that will ensure radiation delivery to that area, using afterloaded radioactive sources. With a multidisciplinary approach, improvements in survival, local control, and quality of life are increasingly possible.

Clinical Evidence-Based Guidelines

The following section is a site-based review of the role of radiotherapy in organ-preserving treatment and as adjuvant treatment to surgery in the most common clinical sites and the sites where the evidence supporting the use of radiotherapy is strongest. This overview is not all inclusive. The interested reader is referred to one of the major oncology textbooks.[1,2,7]

Breast Cancer

Breast Radiotherapy Following Lumpectomy

Breast cancer provides a classic example of how the use of radiation has led to organ-conserving therapy. Multiple randomized studies have shown that breast-conserving surgery and breast radiotherapy produce the same ultimate local control and survival rates as mastectomy[8–13] (Table 95.2). Other randomized trials of patients treated with breast-conserving surgery have demonstrated that postoperative breast radiation improves local control compared to conservative surgery alone[9,14–18] (Table 95.3). The results of two meta-analyses from the Early Breast Cancer Trialists confirmed these results, demonstrating a 75% reduction in the risk of local recurrence with radiotherapy, with no significant difference in survival.[19,20] Given the strong evidence supporting breast-conserving surgery and radiation, the National Cancer Institute's Consensus Development Conference in 1990 recommended that lumpectomy and radiation are preferable to mastectomy in the treatment of T1 and T2 breast cancer.[21] Reduction in local recurrence has also been demonstrated by the European Organization for Research and Treatment of Cancer (EORTC) in the setting of ductal carcinoma in situ (DCIS) where the addition of radiation following local excision gave a local recurrence-free rate of 85% compared to 74% for local excision alone.[22] Regional nodal irradiation in the context of breast-conserving surgery is under review in the management of women with one to three positive axillary nodes or high-risk node-negative disease in the ongoing NCIC CTG MA-20 study.

Whether a group of breast cancer patients with a good prognosis may not require adjuvant radiotherapy following lumpectomy has been investigated. Three randomized trials of low-risk patients found that radiation improved local control, but not survival, compared to adjuvant tamoxifen alone.[23–25] The National Surgical Adjuvant Bowel and Breast Project (NSABP) B-21 study[23] randomized 1851 women with tumors 1 cm or less to tamoxifen alone, radiotherapy and placebo, or tamoxifen and radiotherapy, with a cumulative

TABLE 95.2.
Randomized Trials of Mastectomy Compared to Breast-Conserving Surgery and Radiotherapy (Level I Evidence).

Trial	*Reference*	*Median follow-up (years)*	*No. of patients*	*Stage*	*Study arm*	*Local recurrence (%)*	*Significance*	*Survival (%)*
Gustave–Roussy	13	15	179	I	L+RT	13[a]		73[a]
					MRM	18	NS	65
Milan	11	20	701	I	Q+RT	4		71
					RM	2		69
NSABP B-06	9	20	2163	I-II	L	39[b]	$P < 0.001$	46[b]
					L+RT	14		46
			MRM	NR		47		
NCI	10	10	237	I-II	L+RT	5[c]		77[c]
					MRM	10	NS	75
EORTC	12	13.5	868	I-II	L+RT	20[d]	$P = 0.01$	65[d] NS
					MRM	12		66
Danish	8	8	904	I-III	Q/L+RT	3	NS	79
					MRM	4		82

L, lumpectomy; MRM, modified radical mastectomy; RM, radical mastectomy; Q, quandrentectomy; Q/L, quadrentectomy or lumpectomy; NS, nonsignificant (P = 0.0.05); NSABP, National Surgical Adjuvant Bowel and Breast Project; NCI, National Cancer Institute; EORTC, European Organization for Research and Treatment of Cancer; LRR, local recurrence rate.

[a]15-year results.

[b]20-year results.

[c]10-year results.

[d]13.5 year results.

TABLE 95.3.
Randomized Trials of Breast-Conserving Surgery Compared to Breast-Conserving Therapy and Radiotherapy (Level I Evidence).

Trial	*Reference*	*Median follow-up (years)*	*No. of patients*	*Size of tumor (cm)*	*Study arm*	*Five-year local recurrence (%)*	*Significance*	*Five-year survival*	*Significance*
NSABP B-06	9	20	2163	4	L+RT	14[a]	$P > 0.001$	46[a]	NS
					L	39		46	
Swedish	14	7–8	381	2	Q+RT	8.5	$P < 0.0001$	77.5	NS
					Q	24		78	
Candian	16	5.5	837	4	L+RT	18[b]	$P < 0.0001$	87[b]	NS
					L	40		85	
Milan III	15	9	579	2.5	Q+RT	5.8	$P = 0.001$	82.4	Node +ve OS $P = 0.04$ for RT group
					Q	23.5		76.9	
Scottish	17	5.7	585	4	L+RT	5.8	$P = 0.05$	88	NS
					L	24.5		85	
British	18	5[c]	399	5	L+RT	13	$P < 0.05$	NR	NR
					L	35			
<u>**Low-risk patients**</u>									
Canadian	23	5.6	769	5	L+T+RT	0.6	$P < 0.001$	93	NS
					L+T	7.7		93	
CALGB	24	5	636	2	L+RT+T	1	$P < 0.01$	87	NS
					L+T	5		86	

L, lumpectomy; Q, quadrantectomy; RT, breast radiation; NS, nonsignificant ($P = 0.0.05$); NR, not reported; NSABP, National Surgical Adjuvant Breast Project, T, tamoxifen.

[a]20-year follow-up.

[b]10-year follow-up.

[c]Minimum follow-up.

incidence of ipsilateral breast tumor recurrence at 8 years of 16.5%, 9.3%, and 2.8% for each treatment group. A Canadian study randomized 769 women of 50 years of age or older with T1/T2 N0 breast cancer to breast radiation plus tamoxifen or tamoxifen alone. At 5 and 8 years, the local relapse rate with tamoxifen alone was 7.7% and 15.2% compared to 0.6% and 3.6% with tamoxifen plus radiation ($P < 0.001$).[24] A third study investigated the role of radiotherapy in a very low-risk subset of patients, those over 70 years, with T1, estrogen receptor-positive tumors. Radiotherapy reduced the local relapse rate from 4% to 1% at 5 years ($P < 0.001$).[25] Given the small absolute benefit, the authors recommend an individualized treatment approach in such patients, with lumpectomy and tamoxifen and no radiotherapy being an option in highly selected low-risk patients. Longer follow-up may demonstrate more substantial differences in outcome, as seen in the NSABP and Canadian trials.

Factors that increase the rate of local recurrence in breast cancer, but do not preclude the use of breast-conserving surgery and radiotherapy, include extensive intraductal component (EIC), young age, and positive margins. In the latter situation, local control is improved if reexcision is carried out before radiotherapy. Contraindications to breast-conserving surgery and radiotherapy include pregnancy, gross tumor in separate quadrants of the breast, diffuse microcalcifications (absolute), previous breast radiotherapy, large tumor/breast ratio, and history of scleroderma or systemic lupus erythematosus (relative).[26,27]

Postmastectomy Locoregional Radiotherapy

All randomized trials of mastectomy and postoperative locoregional radiotherapy compared to mastectomy alone have demonstrated an improvement in locoregional control with radiation.[28–35] However, the majority of the studies have not shown an improvement in overall survival. The statistical power of many of these studies to detect a survival difference was low because of small patient numbers, the inclusion of some patients who may not benefit from regional radiation (e.g., node-negative patients), and limited follow-up. In addition, cardiac mortality secondary to outdated radiation techniques may have masked improvements in cancer-specific mortality. The introduction of effective chemotherapy offered a new opportunity to evaluate the role of postmastectomy radiation. Two studies in premenopausal women treated with CMF chemotherapy demonstrated an improvement in survival with locoregional radiotherapy.[36,37] An increase in 10-year survival from 45% to 54% was seen in a Danish study of 1708 patients ($P < 0.001$),[36] and an increase in 20-year survival from 37% to 47% was seen in a study from Canada of 318 patients ($P = 0.03$).[37]

Because of concerns regarding the potential late toxicities from anthracycline-based chemotherapy and radiation, controversy remains over which patients should be offered locoregional radiation and what are the optimal radiation volumes and techniques. One might hypothesize that with more effective systemic agents controlling occult distant metastasis locoregional radiation may lead to more significant gains in survival. We recommend locoregional radiotherapy to patients with T3 and T4 tumors and to patients with four or more positive lymph node metastases based on the results from Denmark and British Columbia.

Soft Tissue Sarcoma

Another example of the effectiveness of radiation in organ preservation is in the management of patients with extremity soft tissue sarcomas (Figure 95.3). The National Cancer Institute (NCI) performed a randomized trial of limb-sparing surgery (wide local excision) plus radiotherapy versus amputation in 43 patients with high-grade sarcomas. Local control and survival were equivalent with either approach, with less morbidity in the limb-preserving arm.[38] Another trial from Memorial Sloan-Kettering Cancer Center randomized 164 patients with wide local excision to postoperative brachytherapy or no further therapy.[39] In patients who received brachytherapy, a statistically significant increase in 5-year local control was seen (69% to 82%, $P = 0.04$). The local control advantage was limited to patients with high-grade lesions, with local control rates of 89% versus 66% ($P = 0.003$) with and without brachytherapy, respectively. The 5-year local control rate of low-grade lesions was 70% with brachytherapy and 80% without brachytherapy ($P = 0.49$). The NCI is currently conducting a randomized trial in patients with low-grade sarcomas. A preliminary analysis of 50 patients demonstrated a significant reduction in local recurrences in patients treated with radiation.[40] Low-grade local recurrences in some sites can be salvaged with organ conservation, whereas high-grade recurrences require amputation more frequently. Thus, the benefit of radiotherapy in resected low-grade soft tissue sarcomas is not well defined.

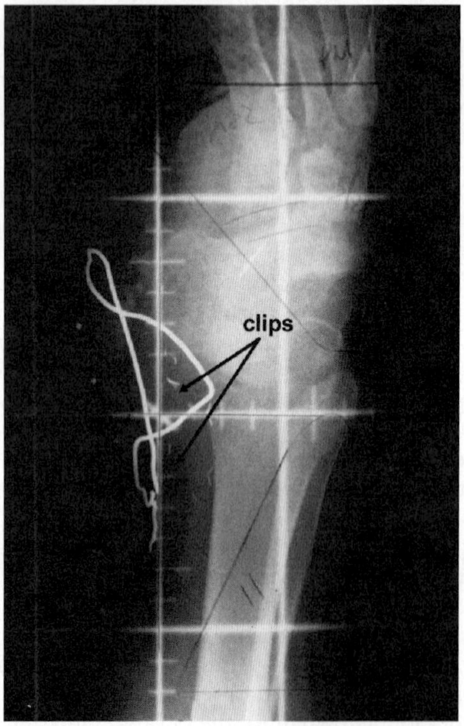

FIGURE 95.3. Clips placed at the high-risk areas during surgery for an ankle soft tissue sarcoma may be used to guide the position and shape of oblique radiation fields. (Courtesy of Dr. Lawrence, University of Michigan.)

The National Cancer Institute of Canada (NCIC) Clinical Trials Group conducted a randomized trial of preoperative radiotherapy versus postoperative radiotherapy in 190 patients with extremity soft tissue sarcoma treated with wide local excision.[41] The trial was closed early because of a significant increase in postoperative wound complications with preoperative radiation compared to postoperative radiation (35% versus 17%). With a median follow-up of 3.3 years, overall survival was slightly improved in patients who had preoperative radiotherapy compared to postoperative treatment ($P = 0.048$).

Retroperitoneal sarcomas are a major challenge to treat. They often present at an advanced stage, making it difficult to obtain adequate margins of resection. They are also adjacent to radiosensitive normal tissues such as small bowel, kidney, and liver, which make delivery of radiation challenging. A randomized trial conducted at the NCI compared adjuvant intraoperative radiation (IORT) (20Gy) followed by low-dose external-beam radiation (35–40Gy) to external-beam radiation alone (50–55Gy) in 35 patients with retroperitoneal sarcoma. A significant improvement in local control was seen in patients treated with IORT, although there was no difference in survival.[42,43] Because of the numerous dose-limiting normal tissues that are often present within the radiation fields following surgery, retroperitoneal sarcomas are especially well suited for preoperative radiation. An Intergroup randomized trial of preoperative versus postoperative radiotherapy for retroperitoneal sarcomas is ongoing.

Lung Cancer

Non-Small Cell Lung Cancer

The optimal therapy for non-small cell lung cancer (NSCLC) is complete resection. Unfortunately, most patients present with unresectable lesions, metastases, or medical contraindications to surgery and are treated with primary radiation therapy or chemoradiation. The role of pre- and postoperative adjuvant radiation (with or without chemotherapy) is described next.

Postoperative Radiation

Randomized trials have demonstrated that postoperative radiation therapy in stage I and II NSCLC is associated with no improvement in survival and little improvement in local control.[44–47] In patients with stage III NSCLC, postoperative radiation has been shown to significantly improve local control.[48–53] The Lung Cancer Study Group (LCST) randomized 210 patients with completely resected stage II and IIIA squamous cell carcinoma to postoperative radiation (50Gy) or no further therapy. The locoregional failure rate (as first site of failure) was reduced from 41% to 3% with radiation, and a trend toward improved survival was observed in patients with N2 disease.[48] The Medical Research Council (MRC) conducted a randomized trial in 308 patients with stage II and III NSCLC of postoperative radiation (40 Gy) versus no further treatment.[53] Again, a trend toward improved survival was seen in the T2N2 subgroup. An individual-based meta-analysis of nine randomized trials of 2128 patients with stage I, II, and III NSCLC treated with excision and postoperative radiation demonstrated that overall survival is not improved with postoperative radiation. On subgroup analysis, there was a trend toward improved survival in patients with stage III, N2 disease. Problems with this meta-analysis include the inclusion of patients with stage I disease, who would not be expected to benefit from postoperative radiation, the long time frame over which the studies were conducted (1965 to 1995), and the variable, now outmoded treatment techniques used in some of the studies (including large fields, high doses per fraction, and shielding over disease).[54] One of the studies included in the meta-analysis was a study of 728 patients who were randomized to postoperative radiotherapy (60 Gy) or observation alone following complete surgical resection.[55] The 5-year overall survival was reduced in the radiotherapy group compared to observation only (43% versus 30%, $P = 0.002$). This result was believed to be related to an excess of intercurrent deaths in the radiation group compared to the observation only group (31% versus 8%, $P = 0.0001$). In summary, postoperative radiation is only indicated in patients with N2 disease to improve local control.

Postoperative Radiation and Chemotherapy

Surgery (with or without radiation) and postoperative chemotherapy have been compared to surgery and no further therapy in several trials.[56,57] No trial has compared postoperative chemoradiation to no further therapy. A trial of patients treated with surgery and postoperative radiation found that the addition of chemotherapy was not associated with improved survival.[56] Another trial in patients with a high risk of residual disease following surgery (positive margin, or tumor present in the highest lymph node removed) demonstrated an increase in recurrence-free survival with adjuvant treatment.[57]

Preoperative Radiation

Randomized and nonrandomized trials have found that preoperative radiation therapy alone for stage I and II NSCLC did not improve survival.[58] However, single institutional experiences have suggested that preoperative radiation has a role in the treatment of superior sulcus tumors.[59] Despite the locally advanced nature of these tumors, they often have no mediastinal lymph node metastases. The goal of preoperative radiation therapy is to improve the chance of complete resection. Preoperative chemoradiation and chemoradiation alone have also been used to treat superior sulcus tumors.

Preoperative Radiation and Chemotherapy

As the outcomes of stage IIIA and IIIB NSCLC treated with chemoradiation are poor (15% and 5% 5-year survival rates, respectively), induction chemoradiation followed by surgery has been carried out in several phase I/II studies. A large phase III trial of induction chemoradiation followed by surgery compared to chemoradiation alone has been initiated in patients with stage IIIA (N2) disease.

Small Cell Lung Cancer (SCLC)

The main role of surgery in the treatment of small cell lung cancer (SCLC) is to obtain a tissue diagnosis. The standard treatment for limited-stage SCLC is chemotherapy and thoracic radiation. The addition of thoracic radiotherapy to chemotherapy has been shown to improve local control and prolong survival in patients with limited-stage SCLC.[60] The use of prophylactic cranial irradiation also improves overall and disease-free survival in this group of patients.[61]

Gastrointestinal Cancer

Rectal Cancer

Postoperative Radiation

As local recurrence following rectal cancer treatment is associated with substantial morbidity, radiation has been used in the adjuvant setting to improve local control. No randomized trials comparing surgery and postoperative radiation to surgery alone in rectal cancer have detected a difference in overall survival.[62–69] The Medical Research Council (MRC) trial detected a significant decrease in local recurrence with postoperative radiation alone from 33% to 20%,[67] and a trend to decreased local recurrence was seen in the NSABP trial.[63]

Postoperative Radiation and Chemotherapy

Three large randomized trials of postoperative chemoradiation have been conducted (Table 95.4).[63,69,70] One trial, by the Gastrointestinal Tumor Study Group, compared observation alone with combined radiation and chemotherapy following surgery in 227 patients. There was a significant improvement in overall survival favoring chemoradiation compared with observation alone (56% versus 36%, $P = 0.04$) and a trend toward a reduction in local failure (11% versus 24%, $P = 0.08$). There was no significant difference in survival between adjuvant radiation or chemotherapy compared to surgery alone.[70] The North Central Cancer Trial Group (NCCTG) compared surgery plus radiation to surgery plus radiation and chemotherapy in 204 patients. There was no surgery-alone arm. A significant improvement in overall survival and a reduction in local recurrence were seen for the chemotherapy and radiation compared with radiation alone (53% versus 43%, $P = 0.025$, and 13.5% versus 25%, $P = 0.036$, respectively).[69] The NSABP RO1 trial of 528 patients demonstrated a significant increase in 5-year survival (53% versus 43%, $P = 0.05$) in patients who received chemotherapy compared with surgery alone. There was no significant difference in survival in patients who received radiation alone compared with surgery.[63] The NSABP RO2 trial showed no difference in survival between postoperative chemoradiation and chemotherapy. Local control was, however, significantly improved with chemoradiation compared to chemotherapy alone (local relapse, 11.3% versus 6.7%, $P = 0.05$).[71]

Preoperative Radiation

Advantages of preoperative radiation in rectal cancer include reduced small bowel toxicity, primarily because a lesser volume of small bowel was irradiated, the potential for

TABLE 95.4.
Randomized Trials of Postoperative Adjuvant Radiation and Chemotherapy for Rectal Cancer (Level I Evidence).

Trial	*Reference*	*No. of patients*	*Treatment arm*	*Chemo-therapy*	*Five-year local failure overall (%)*	*Significance*	*Five-year survival (%)*	*Significance*	*Eight-year survival*	*Significance*
NSABP-RO1	62	185	OR	FSV	25	$P = 0.06$	43		NR	
		184	OR-RT		16	NS	41	NS		
		187	OR-CT		21		53	$P = 0.05$		
GITSG	69	58	OR		24	NS	44		28%	NS
		50	OR-RT		20		52	NS	43%	
		48	OR-CT	FS	27	NS	56	NS	43%	NS
		46	OR-RT-CT	FS	11		59	$P = 0.07$	57%	$P = 0.05$
NCCTG	68	100	OR-RT		25	$P = 0.08$	47	$P = 0.04$	NR	
		104	OR-RT-CT	FS	14	$P = 0.04$	58			
NSABP-RO2	70	348	OR-CT	MOF or FLv	14		58	NS		
		346	OR-RT-CT		8	$P = 0.02$	58			

RT, pelvic radiation; OR, radical surgery (low anterior resection or abdominal perineal resection); NS, nonsignificant ($P = 0.05$); NR, not reported; F, 5-FU; S, semustine; V, vincristine; NSABP, National Surgical Adjuvant Bowel and Breast Project; GITSG, Gastrointestinal Tumor Study Group; NCCTG, North Central Cancer Trial Group.

increased organ preservation, and increased resectability. There are more than 10 randomized trials of preoperative radiation and surgery versus surgery alone (Table 95.5).[72–85] The time from completion of radiation to the time of surgery was short in most of the trials, and there were significant variations in radiation schedules. In general, lower doses than used in other settings were used, with large fraction sizes (up to 500cGy) and large treatment portals, both of which contribute to increased late toxicity. The incidence of postoperative complications with preoperative radiation in the first Stockholm trial was increased from 19% to 26% ($P < 0.01$) with preoperative radiation, and postoperative wound infections were increased from 29% to 48% ($P < 0.001$).[80] Despite the unconventional methods of radiation delivery, these trials demonstrated a significant decrease in the rate of local recurrence with preoperative radiation (see Table 95.5). The Swedish group has demonstrated an improvement in 5-year survival rates with 58% in the radiotherapy plus surgery group compared to 48% in the surgery only group ($P = 0.004$).[76] Two meta-analyses confirmed a significant benefit in local control with preoperative radiation for rectal cancer.[86,87] Camma et al.[86] also found a reduced overall mortality rate ($P = 0.03$), and cancer related mortality ($P < 0.001$) from preoperative radiation compared to the surgery-alone group. The Colorectal Cancer Collaborative Group[87] failed to demonstrate a survival advantage. The development of total mesorectal excision (TME) and the increased recognition of the requirement of specialist colorectal cancer units have contributed to lower local failure rates. One study from the Dutch Colorectal Cancer Group compared preoperative radiotherapy (25Gy in five fractions) followed by TME to TME alone. The local recurrence rate at 2 years for TME alone versus preoperative radiotherapy and TME was 8.2% and 2.4%, respectively ($P < 0.001$).[88]

A clear situation in which preoperative radiation should be recommended is for rectal cancers that are tethered and fixed, that is, in tumors which are borderline resectable. The adverse prognosis of a cut-through may be prevented if preoperative radiation can downstage the tumor so that it may be resected with negative margins. In addition, with preoperative radiation some unresectable tumors may become resectable. In one randomized trial of preoperative radiation in 284 patients with tethered or fixed tumors, a highly significant reduction in local recurrences was seen in the irradiated group (12.8% versus 36.5%, $P = 0.0001$). In addition, there was a survival benefit for the subset of patients who underwent curative resections.[81]

Preoperative Radiation and Chemotherapy

The EORTC, in a randomized trial of 247 patients, compared surgery and preoperative radiation (34.5Gy, 2.3Gy per fraction) to the same preoperative radiation with concurrent 5-fluorouracil (5FU) (375 mg/m^2 day 1–4).[89] There was no difference in local control between the two groups. However, the addition of chemotherapy had a negative effect on overall survival (46% versus 59%, $P = 0.06$). This difference in survival was caused mainly by an increase in perioperative and intercurrent deaths. Criticisms of this study include the use of large radiation fields, high doses per fraction, and nonstandard chemotherapy that may have contributed to increased toxicity and decreased efficacy of the chemoradiation arm.

A more recent French study evaluated T3 and T4 resectable rectal tumors treated with radiation to 45Gy in 25 fractions with or without concurrent 5FU on days 1 to 5 in weeks 1 and 5, followed by surgery 3 to 10 weeks after radiation therapy. The overall survival rates were similar, but local control in the preoperative chemoradiation arm was improved (5-year local recurrence rate of 8.1% compared to 16.5% for radiation therapy alone).[90]

Preoperative Radiation Versus Postoperative Radiation

Preoperative radiation and surgery were compared to surgery and postoperative radiation in a Swedish trial of 471 patients.[91] The preoperative radiation consisted of 25.5Gy in five fractions 1 week before surgery. The postoperative radiation consisted of 60Gy in 2-Gy fractions with a week break after

TABLE 95.5.
Randomized Trials of Preoperative Adjuvant Radiation for Resectable Rectal Cancer (Level I Evidence).

Study	*Reference*	*No. of patients*	*Treatment arm*	*Dose RT (Gy)*	*Fraction size (Gy)*	*Local recurrence (%)*	*Significance*	*Five-year survival (%)*	*Significance*
PMH	74	60	RT-OR	5	5	NR		35%	NS
		65	OR						
VASOG I	81	302	RT-OR	20–25	2–2.5	29%	NS	43%	$P < 0.02$
		311	OR			40%		32%	
VASOG II	72	180	RT-OR	31.5	1.75	NR		50%	NS
		181	OR					50%	
Stockholm I[a]	78	424	RT-OR	25	5	14% (16%[b])	$P < 0.01$	30% (37%[b])	NS
		425	OR			28% (30%[b])		31% (37%[b])	
Stockholm II[c]	77	272	RT-OR	25	5	10%	$P < 0.01$	50%	NS
		285	OR			21%		45%	
MRC I[d]	82	277	RT-OR	5	5	45%	NS	55%	NS
		272	RT-OR	20	2	47%		53%	NS
		275	OR			43%		57%	
MRC II[d]	76	139	RT-OR	40	2	HR 0.68 [0.47–0.98]	$P = 0.04$	HR 0.79 [0.60–1.04]	$P = 0.10$
		140	OR						
Norway	83	159	RT-OR	31.5	1.75	15%	NS	58%	NS
		150	OR			21%		57%	
EORTC[e]	84	231	RT-OR	34.5	2.3	22% (15%[b])	$P = 0.02$	60% (69%[b])	$P = 0.08$
		228	OR			34% (30%[b])		60% (59%[b])	
San Paulo	73	34	RT-OR	40	2	3%	NR	71%	NR
		34	OR			24%		30%	
BRCG	71	228	RT-OR	15	5	17%	$P < 0.05$	39%	NS
		239	OR			24%		40%	
Swedish[c]	75	583	RT-OR	25	5	11%	$P < 0.001$	58%	$P = 0.004$
		585	OR			27%		48%	
Dutch TME	87	924	RT-TME	25	5	2.4% (2 years)	$P < 0.001$	8.2% (2 years)	$P = 0.84$
		937	TME			82% (2 years)		81.8% (2 years)	

RT, pelvic radiation; OR, radial surgery (low anterior resection or abdominal perineal resection); NS, nonsignificant ($P = 0.05$); NR, not reported; HR, hazards ratio; [ ], 95% confidence interval; PMH, Princess Margaret Hospital, Toronto; MRC, Medical Research Council; VASOG, Veterans Administration Surgical Oncology Group; EORTC, European Organization Research Treatment of Cancer; BRCG, British Rectal Cancer Group.TME, Total Mesorectal Excision.

[a]Includes 165 patients with noncurative resections.

[b]Survival for patients treated with curative resection only.

[c]A subset of patients was included in both trials.

[d]Includes some partially fixed tumors.

[e]Includes 108 patients with noncurative resections.

40 Gy. Five-year local recurrence rate was decreased with preoperative radiation compared with postoperative radiation (13% versus 22%, $P = 0.02$), with no significant difference in overall survival (42% versus 38%). Operative morbidity was similar in the two treatment arms, with the exception of wound infection (33% and 18% in preoperative and postoperative patients respectively; $P < 0.01$). Late small bowel toxicity was increased in the postoperative patients (11% compared to 5% for surgery alone and 6% for preoperative radiation; $P < 0.01$).

More recently, the German Rectal Cancer Study Group reported a study of 823 patients randomized to preoperative chemoradiation (50.4 Gy with 5FU) or postoperative chemoradiation (50.4 Gy with 5FU, with possible boost of 5.4 Gy).[92] The 5-year local recurrence rate was significantly reduced in the preoperative arm (6% versus 13%, $P = 0.006$), with no change in overall survival. Acute and long-term complications were also reduced, providing a rationale for the preoperative approach.

Anal Canal Cancer

The standard treatment of anal canal cancer is combined radiation and chemotherapy, with surgery reserved for residual and recurrent cancer. Radiation and chemotherapy allows anorectal preservation with good sphincter control in the majority of patients. Although preoperative chemoradiation and radical surgery were used to treat many patients before the use of primary chemoradiation for this malignancy, there is no evidence that surgery improves the outcome of patients treated with chemoradiation. For patients with bulky groin metastasis at presentation, local excision may improve the regional control.

A series of protocols at the Princess Margaret Hospital (PMH) established that a combination of 5FU and mitomycin C and radiation is more effective than radiation alone in the treatment of anal canal carcinoma.[93] A split-course radiation regimen was found to be the most tolerable method of delivering radiation and chemotherapy and is now considered the new standard for the EORTC, based upon their phase 2 study of a shortened irradiation scheme with mitomycin C in each radiotherapy sequence and continuous-infusion 5FU.[94] However, others have successfully treated patients with continuous chemoradiation and radiation alone.[95,96] Good outcomes have also been reported using radiation and cisplatin-based chemotherapy.

Three randomized trials have studied the benefit of chemotherapy in addition to radiation.[97–99] The UK Co-ordinating Committee on Cancer Research (UKCCCR) compared radiation alone to radiation and 5FU and mitomycin C in 585 patients. The colostomy-free local control was significantly improved with radiation (61% compared to 39%), but survival was not statistically different [3-year survival, 58% (radiation) and 65% (chemoradiation); $P = 0.25$].[97] The Netherlands Cancer Institute randomized study of 110 patients similarly demonstrated increased local control and colostomy-free survival with chemotherapy, with no survival benefit.[98] The Radiation Therapy Oncology Group (RTOG) and Eastern Cooperative Oncology Group (ECOG) studied the benefit of mitomycin C over radiation and 5FU in 310 patients. The local control, disease-free survival, and colostomy-free survival were all significantly increased with mitomycin C, demonstrating the requirement of this drug in anal canal treatment. Survival was not significantly improved at a follow-up of 4 years.[99] Salvage surgery was required in 10% to 40% of patients treated radically, either for local failure or treatment toxicity necessitating an abdominoperineal resection (APR).

Esophageal Cancer

Treatment strategies for esophageal cancer include surgery, radiation therapy, chemotherapy, or a combination of these modalities. There remains controversy over the optimal treatment strategy for esophageal cancer. Selection bias makes results from pathologically staged surgery series difficult to compare to clinically staged radiation therapy series. In addition, the outcomes of palliative patients are often pooled with those of patients treated with radical radiation. Despite these adverse factors, the poor local control and survival rates with nonsurgical approaches are not very different from those with surgery. One randomized trial comparing chemoradiation to radiation alone demonstrated an improved 3-year survival from 0% to 30% with chemoradiation, which remains the standard treatment in patients who are not surgical candidates.[100,101] There are no randomized trials comparing surgery to primary chemoradiation for esophageal cancer, nor has preoperative chemoradiation and surgery been compared to primary chemoradiation. Studies of preoperative and postoperative radiation, with and without chemotherapy, as adjuvant treatment to surgery are reviewed here.

Postoperative Radiation

Randomized trials of surgery compared to surgery and radiation suggest that radiation does not improve survival.[102–104] In addition, significant toxicity (e.g., gastritis and hemorrhage) has been associated with radiation to the esophageal substitute.[103] Only one randomized trial demonstrated an improvement in recurrence-free survival and local control in lymph node-negative patients but not in lymph node-positive patients.[102] Given the high probability of local failure in patients with positive margins, it is not unreasonable to offer postoperative radiation to improve local control, although there is no evidence that this improves survival. Postoperative chemoradiation has not been studied in randomized trials.

Preoperative Radiation

Six randomized studies have compared preoperative radiation (in variable dose regimens) and surgery to surgery alone in patients with resectable esophageal cancer, with no survival benefit from preoperative radiation.[105–110] An EORTC study[107] demonstrated improved local control with preoperative radiation (33 Gy over 2 weeks) compared to surgery alone, whereas Wang et al. found no difference in local control with preoperative radiation.[110] In a randomized study by Nygaard et al. there was a significant difference in 5-year survival from 5% to 18% ($P < 0.01$) when preoperative radiation and preoperative chemoradiation were compared to surgery alone. There was, however, no significant difference in survival between preoperative radiation and surgery.[108] A recent patient-based meta-analysis of 1147 patients also failed to find a survival benefit with preoperative radiation.[111]

Preoperative Radiation and Chemotherapy

Several randomized trials of preoperative radiation and chemotherapy have been reported with variable outcomes[112–114] (Table 95.6). In a randomized study of 100 patients with adenocarcinoma (75%) and squamous cell carcinoma (25%), Urba et al.[115] reported a nonstatistically significant increase in 3-year survival from 16% to 30% ($P = 0.14$) with preoperative radiation and 5FU, vinblastine, and cisplatin chemotherapy compared to surgery alone. Another randomized trial compared preoperative radiation (40 Gy) with 5FU and cisplatin to surgery alone in patients with adenocarcinoma of the esophagus.[112] Median survival was improved from 11 months to 16 months ($P = 0.001$), and the 3-year survival was improved from 6% to 32% ($P = 0.01$) with preoperative chemoradiation and surgery. These positive results are in contrast to other randomized studies of primarily squamous cell carcinoma, which have not found significant survival differences.[113,114] Thus, it appears that adenocarcinoma and squamous cell carcinoma may respond differently to therapy.

Improved local control has been demonstrated in most studies of preoperative chemoradiation, at the expense of increased operative mortality (12% compared to 4%). One randomized trial was stopped early because of increased postoperative morbidity and mortality.[116] A meta-analysis of nine randomized trials of neoadjuvant chemoradiation versus surgery alone for esophageal cancer found an odds ratio (OR) of 0.66 for 3-year survival ($P = 0.016$) and reduced local recurrence (OR, 0.88) in favor of chemoradiation and surgery.[117] A nonsignificant trend to increased treatment mortality was also noted. The variability in reported complications suggests that the success of the preoperative approach depends on the type of radiation and surgical techniques utilized.

TABLE 95.6.
Preoperative Radiation and Chemotherapy for Resectable Esophageal Cancer Randomized Trials (Level I Evidence).

Trial	*Reference*	*No. of patients*	*%SCC (SCC1adeno)*	*Treatment arm*	*Pathological CR*	*Local control*	*Significance*	*Median survival*	*Three-year survival (%)*	*Significance*
Walsh	112	58	0	CMT-E	25%	NR		16 months	32	$P = 0.01$
		55		E				11 months		
Urba	115	50	24	CMT-E	28%	NR		16.9 months	30	$P = 0.15$
		50		E				17.6 months	16	
Le Prise	113	45	100	CMT-E	NR	NR		10 months	19.2	NS
		41		E					13.8	
Bosset	114	139	100	CMT-E	26%	RR = 0.6[a]	$P = 0.01$	18.6 months	36	NS
		143		E				18.6 months	34	

CMT, combined chemotherapy and radiation; E, esophagectomy; NR, not reported; NS, nonsignificant ($P = 0.05$).
[a]Risk reduction (RR) 50.6 (0.4–0.9) for time free of local recurrence.

Pancreatic Cancer

Postoperative Radiation and Chemotherapy

The Gastrointestinal Tumor Study Group (GITSG) conducted a small randomized study of postoperative radiation and chemotherapy in 42 patients treated with pancreatoduodenectomy for pancreatic cancer.[118] Adjuvant radiation and 5FU was associated with an improvement in median survival from 11 to 21 months ($P = 0.03$), and an improvement in 2-year survival from 15% [95% confidence interval (CI), 6%–33%] to 49% (95% CI, 29%–68%). Thirty additional patients treated by the GITSG with the same adjuvant therapy had a median survival of 18 months and a 2-year survival of 46%.[119] However, the overall 5-year survival with chemoradiation was only 14%. A small randomized study of 30 patients, presented in abstract form, also demonstrated an increase in median survival with postoperative chemoradiation (from 11 to 23 months).120 However, two European large randomized trials have subsequently failed to show a statistical survival benefit from adjuvant radiation.[121,122] The EORTC study of 218 patients randomized to adjuvant radiotherapy and 5FU or observation following surgery demonstrated a small nonsignificant benefit for adjuvant therapy (median survival, 19 versus 24.5 months, $P = 0.208$).[121] The European Study Group for Pancreatic Cancer Trial of 289 patients (ESPAC-1) demonstrated a survival advantage from adjuvant chemotherapy but decreased survival with adjuvant chemoradiation compared to adjuvant chemotherapy alone (5-year survival, 20% with no adjuvant chemotherapy, 10% with adjuvant chemoradiation, 21% with adjuvant chemotherapy, and 8% with no further therapy).[122] The latter trial has been criticized because of the high local recurrence rate and suboptimal radiation dose and schedule, with the use of outdated large radiation fields that may have contributed to late toxicity. Thus, adjuvant radiation should continue to be investigated in clinical trials, using modern radiation techniques and modern systemic therapy.[123]

Preoperative Radiation and Chemotherapy

Preoperative chemoradiation has been used in several phase 2 studies, with encouraging outcomes.[124,125] The rationale for preoperative radiation includes the benefits of preoperative radiation outlined in Table 95.1, as well as the fact that more patients may be able to complete radiation before surgery. Preoperative treatment for pancreatic cancer should be done in a study setting where the toxicity and benefits can be prospectively evaluated. Ideally, preoperative chemoradiation for pancreatic cancer will be investigated in randomized trials.

Gastric Cancer

The only potentially curative modality for localized gastric cancer is surgery. Even in patients with lymph node-negative disease, locoregional failure occurs in up to 40% of patients and 5-year survival is 50% at best.

Postoperative Radiation

The British Stomach Cancer Group randomized patients with gastric cancer to postoperative radiation, postoperative chemotherapy, or surgery alone. No difference in 3-year survival was seen between the treatment arms, but the local failure rate was decreased from 54% in the surgery arm to 32% in the radiation arm ($P < 0.01$).[126,127]

Hallissey et al. randomized patients with locally advanced resected gastric cancer to surgery alone, postoperative chemotherapy, or postoperative radiation (45 Gy in 25 fractions). At 5-year follow-up, there was no significant difference in survival.[127]

Postoperative Radiation and Chemotherapy

Three randomized studies compared patients treated with surgery followed by concurrent chemoradiation to no further therapy.[128,129] Dent and colleagues randomized 142 patients with completely and incompletely resected tumors to no further therapy or 20 Gy in eight fractions with 5FU given for 4 days before radiation and 4 weeks later. In 67 patients with no gross residual disease following surgery, there was no difference in survival.[128] Another study from the Mayo Clinic randomized 62 patients treated with gastrectomy for advanced gastric cancer to radiation (37.5 Gy in 24 fractions) and 5FU or no further treatment.[129] The treated patients had a 5-year survival of 20% compared to 4% in controls ($P < 0.05$).

More recently, the Intergroup 0116 study[130] of observation or adjuvant therapy with 5FU/FA and 45 Gy following curative resection reported improved 3-year survival (52% versus 41%, $P = 0.03$) and 3-year disease-free survival (49% versus 32%, $P = 0.001$) for adjuvant treatment. Adjuvant radiation for gastric cancer is now the standard of care based on this landmark study.

Genitourinary Cancer

Bladder Cancer

Traditional treatment for bladder cancer has been cystectomy. As in breast cancer and soft tissue sarcoma, preservation of a functional organ is possible in the treatment of bladder cancer. Radiotherapy may be used alone or with chemotherapy for bladder preservation, reserving cystectomy for salvage treatment. With transurethral resection of the bladder tumor (TURBT) plus concurrent chemotherapy and radiation, long-term survival is comparable to treatment with immediate cystectomy, although no direct comparisons have been made.

A randomized trial from the National Cancer Institute of Canada (NCIC) demonstrated that in stage T2 to T4b bladder cancer patients, concurrent cisplatin with radiation therapy improved local control from 29% to 52% compared to radiation alone ($P = 0.04$).[131] Using this approach, the chance of bladder preservation was 70% with radiation and cisplatin compared to 36% with radiation alone ($P = 0.16$). An alternative regimen for bladder preservation has been described by Shipley et al.[132,133] In patients treated with maximal TURBT, two cycles of neoadjuvant MCV chemotherapy were followed by radiation and concurrent cisplatin. Patients were examined after receiving 39.6 Gy, and only patients with complete responses were treated with the remaining course of radiation (to 64.8 Gy); the others were treated with immediate cystectomy. The bladder preservation rate in patients treated with a full course of radiation was 80%.[133,134]

Several randomized trials comparing preoperative radiation and cystectomy to cystectomy alone in bladder cancer patients demonstrated no difference in survival with preoperative radiation therapy.[135,136]

Prostate Cancer

Two randomized studies have been conducted to identify the role of postoperative radiation therapy in the setting of prostate cancer.[137,138] Bolla et al., in EORTC 22911, randomized 1005 men postradical retropubic prostatectomy (with pT3 prostate cancer or positive surgical margins) to immediate postoperative radiation (60 Gy in 30 fractions) or observation.[137] At a median follow-up of 5 years, in the irradiated group there was improvement in biochemical progression-free survival (74% versus 52.6%, $P < 0.0001$), clinical progression-free survival ($P = 0.0009$), and locoregional control ($P < 0.0001$). This finding was confirmed by a North American multiinstitutional study of 425 patients with pathologically advanced stage prostate cancer (defined as one or more of extraprostatic extension, positive surgical margins, or seminal vesicle invasion) who were randomly assigned to postoperative radiation therapy (60–64 Gy) versus observation.[138] With a median follow-up of 10.6 years, no statistically significant difference was seen in either group for overall or metastasis-free survival. However, the time to prostate-specific antigen (PSA) relapse (10.3 years for radiation therapy versus 3.1 years for observation) and the time to disease recurrence (13.8 years versus 9.9 years,) were both significantly reduced with radiation therapy.

Head and Neck Cancer

Radiotherapy plays a key role in the management of head and neck cancer. Radiation (with or without chemotherapy) is the primary treatment for some malignancies such as nasopharyngeal cancers. Radiation may be used as an alternative to surgery for organ preservation (e.g., larynx cancer). Unresectable disease in sites usually managed by surgery can also be treated with radiation. In addition to these definitive applications, in patients with a high risk of local or regional relapse, postoperative or preoperative radiation can decrease the risk of relapse. However, few prospective studies have addressed the role of radiation therapy as an adjunct to surgery.

Three completed trials of organ-preserving treatment versus surgery have been conducted in larynx and hypopharynx cancer.[139–141] The Veterans Administration (VA) randomized trial compared three cycles of induction chemotherapy plus radiotherapy with surgery plus radiotherapy in 332 patients with stage III and IV larynx cancer.[139] The initial EORTC study had a similar design for 202 patients with stage II, III, or V squamous cell carcinoma of the hypopharynx.[140] In these two studies, radiation therapy was only offered to patients who had responses to chemotherapy (partial response, VA; complete response, EORTC); patients who did not respond to chemotherapy were treated with surgery. In these trials, the 3- and 5-year survival rates were no different for the organ-preserving treatment approaches. In the organ preservation treatment arms, a functional larynx was preserved in 64% and 52% of patients in the VA and the EORTC trials, respectively. The RTOG 91-11 Intergroup study[141] investigated three radiation-based treatment options for larynx cancer; induction chemotherapy (cisplatin plus fluorouracil) followed by radiation, radiotherapy with concurrent chemotherapy (cisplatin alone), and radiation alone. A significant increase in the proportion of patients with an intact larynx was seen in the radiation and concurrent cisplatin group (88%) versus induction chemotherapy and radiation (75%, $P = 0.005$) and radiation alone (70%, $P = 0.001$). Locoregional control was also improved with concurrent chemoradiation [78% versus 61% and 56% for induction and radiation therapy (RT) and RT alone], although no significant difference was seen in survival. There was a substantial increase in the adverse effects in the combined therapy groups (77% grade 3 or greater acute adverse effects; $P < 0.001$) (Table 95.7).

In another trial of 320 patients, patients with advanced operable supraglottic laryngeal or hypopharyngeal cancers were randomly allocated to receive either preoperative radiation therapy (50 Gy) or postoperative radiation therapy (60 Gy), and patients with oral cavity or oropharyngeal lesions were randomly assigned either preoperative radiation, postoperative radiation, or definitive radiation therapy (65–70 Gy), with

TABLE 95.7.
Randomized Trials for Organ Preservation in Head and Neck Cancer.

Trial	Reference	No. of patients	Treatment arm	Chemotherapy	Site	Stage	Criteria for organ preservation with RT	PC/CR rate	Three-Year larynx preservation rate	Three-year survival with preserved larynx	Three-year local regional failure rates	Significance	Three-year survival	Significance	Five-year survival		Median survival (months)
VA	134	166	CFR RT	CF33[a]	Glottis/ supraglottis	III (57%), IV (43%), (excluding T1N1)	PR after CF×2	85% 31% CR 54% PR	64%	31%	12% (L), 8% (R)	$P = 0.04$	53%	NS	42%	NS	42
		166	ORR RT						0%	0%	2% (L), 5% (R)		56%		45%		53
EORTC	135	100	CFR RT	CF33[a]	Hypopharynx/ aryepiglottic fold	II (7%), III (57%), IV (37%)	CR after Cx3	88% 54% CR 32% PR	52%	28%	12% (L), 19% (R)	NS	57%	NS	30%	NS	44 $P = 0.006$
		94	ORR RT						0%	0%	17% (L), 23% (R)		43%		35%		25
RTOG 91-11	136	173 172 173	Ind Ch+RT ConCh+RT RT		Glottis/ Supraglottis	III /IV	PR after Cx2	21%CR 64% PR	84% 72% 67%	61% 35% 72%		$P = 0.004$ $P < 0.001$	76%[b] 74%[b] 75%[b]	NS	55% 54% 56%	NR NS NR	NR

C, cisplatin; F, 5-fluorouracil; OR, radical surgery (not larynx preserving); RT, radiotherapy; PR, partial response: greater than 50% reduction in tumor at examination under anesthesia; CR, complete response: at examination under anesthesia; NR, not reported; NS, nonsignificant ($P = 0.05$); L, local; R, regional; VC, vocal cord; VA, Veterans Administration; EORTC, European Organization for Research and Treatment of Cancer; RTOG, Radiation Therapy Oncology Group; Ind Ch + RT, induction cisplatin and fluorouracil (cisplatin 100 mg/m^2 day 1, fluorouracil 1000 mg/m^2 continous every 24 h for 120 h, every 3 weeks for 3 courses) and radiotherapy; ConCh + RT, concurrent chemotherapy (cisplatin 100 mg/m^2 day1, 22, 43) and radiotherapy.

[a]Cisplatin 100 mg/m^2 IV day 1 and 5FU 1 g/m^2 day 1–5 every 4 weeks.

[b]Two-year estimates of survival.

surgery reserved for salvage.[142] At a median follow-up of 60 months, locoregional control was significantly better for patients assigned to postoperative radiation therapy (65%) compared with preoperative radiation therapy (48%, $P = 0.04$). There was also a trend for improved survival (38% versus 33%, $P = 0.10$). In 43 evaluable patients with oral cavity or oropharyngeal lesions, there were no statistically significant differences in overall survival (4-year survival: 30% preoperative, 36% postoperative, 33% definitive radiation therapy) or locoregional control (43% preoperative, 52% postoperative, 38% definitive radiation therapy) (Figure 95.4).

Regarding the role of postoperative radiation, a randomized trial by Peters et al. in patients with American Joint Commission (AJC) stage III or IV oral cavity, oropharyngeal, hypopharyngeal, or laryngeal cancer compared three doses of postoperative radiation, delivered in 1.8Gy per fraction.[143] Patients treated with low doses (54Gy or less) had a significantly higher primary failure rate than those receiving higher doses (57.6Gy or more). In patients with extracapsular nodal disease, the regional control rate was best in patients who received the highest dose of radiation (63Gy or greater). The only independent prognostic factor for locoregional relapse was extracapsular extension of disease; however, other factors associated with an increased risk of recurrence included two or more of the following: oral cavity primary, close or positive margins, perineural invasion, more than two nodal metastases, node size greater than 3cm, treatment delay greater than 6 weeks, and poor performance status. Other prognostic factors for local failure include stage, primary tumor size, and lymphatic space invasion. With respect to neck node metastasis, in addition to extracapsular spread, the size, number, and bilaterality of node metastasis are prognostic factors for regional recurrence.[144] A combined modality approach for treatment of neck metastasis with adverse factors has been recommended to improve the regional control rates in these patients.

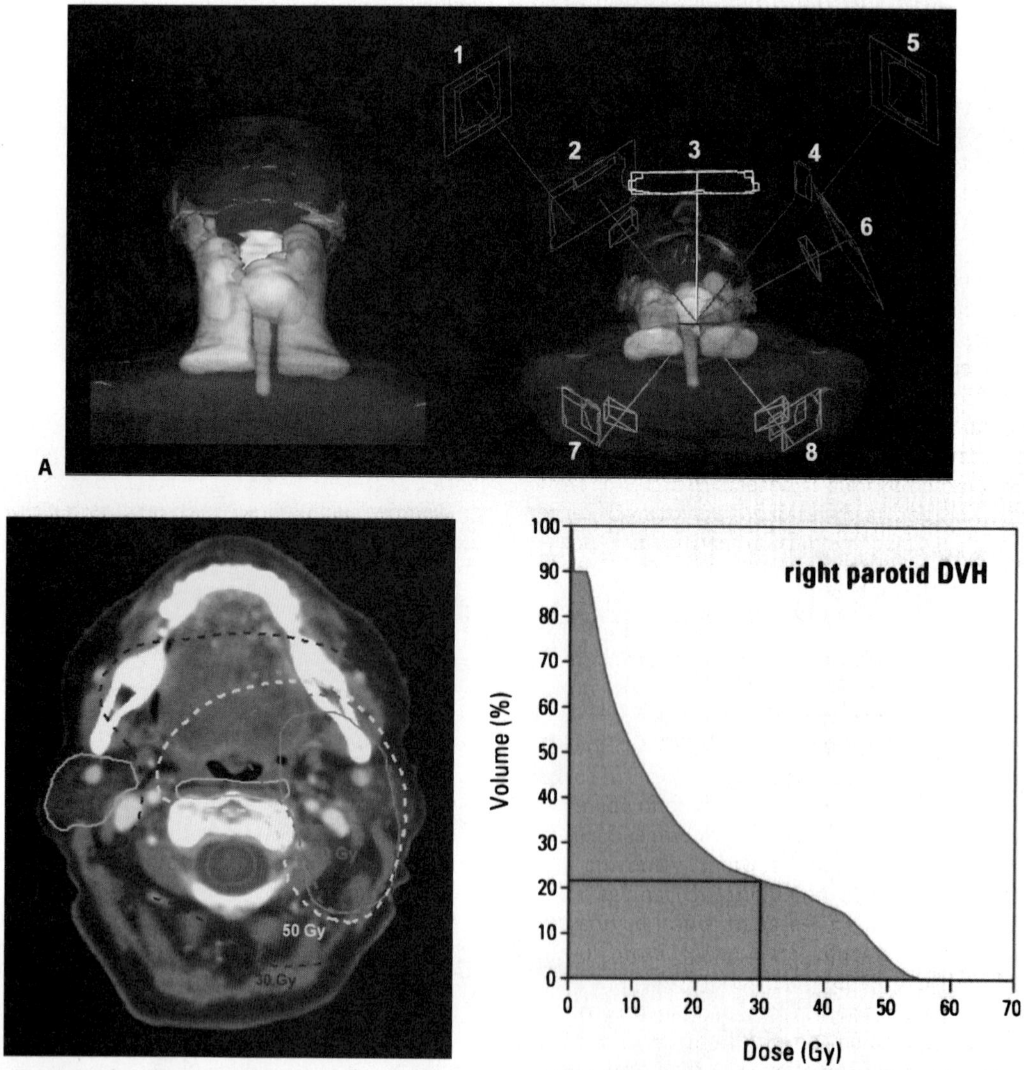

FIGURE 95.4. A, B. Example of a three-dimensional radiotherapy plan to treat a supraglottic cancer while sparing part of the right parotid gland. Each field is composed of multiple segments that produce a uniform dose distribution in the target volumes: 70Gy will be delivered to the gross tumor, 60Gy will be delivered to the left neck and retropharyngeal nodes, and 50Gy will be delivered to the right neck. As shown in the dose–volume histogram (DVH) of the right parotid gland (C), only 20% of the gland receives a dose greater than 30Gy; this allows some saliva flow to be preserved. (Courtesy of Dr. Eisbruch, University of Michigan.)

Two recent randomized trials (EORTC 22931 and RTOG 9501/Intergroup) have reported their results of adjuvant radiation (60–66 Gy) with or without concomitant cisplatin following surgical resection of head and neck tumors. Both recruited patients with high-risk disease following curative resection. In the EORTC study[145] of 334 patients with a median follow-up of 60 months, overall survival was 53% for the combined therapy group and 40% for the radiation alone group ($P = 0.02$), with reduced local and regional relapses (18% combined therapy and 31% radiation alone; $P = 0.007$). The RTOG study[146] randomized 459 patients with pathological features of high-risk disease and with a median follow-up of 45.9 months also demonstrated an improvement in local and regional control for the combination therapy group (82% versus 72% for radiation alone at 2 years). Disease-free survival was significantly better in the combined therapy group ($P = 0.04$), but there was no significant impact on overall survival. Based on these two studies, adjuvant chemoradiation should be considered in high-risk patients.

Central Nervous System Cancers

Primary brain tumors are a heterogeneous group of tumors, with outcomes ranging from commonly curable with surgery alone to never curable despite multimodality therapy. Postoperative radiation has been used to improve local control (e.g., incompletely resected meningioma) and to improve survival (e.g., medulloblastoma). This section reviews only the role of radiation in the treatment of the most common primary brain tumors in adults, astrocytomas.

High-Grade Astrocytoma

High-grade astrocytomas include Kernohan grade III (anaplastic astrocytoma) and grade IV (glioblastoma multiforme) tumors. The median survival, despite optimal therapy, is 18 months for grade III tumors and 12 months for grade IV tumors. These outcomes are highly dependent on prognostic factors such as performance status and age. In contrast with other malignancies, a surgical excision of an astrocytoma with clear margins is unusual. Postoperative radiation has been found to double the median survival of patients with malignant gliomas.[147,148] A randomized trial from the 1970s compared postoperative supportive care, radiation (50–60 Gy), chemotherapy (BCNU), and radiation and BCNU in 222 patients with high-grade astrocytomas. The 1-year survival rates were 3% with surgery alone, 12% with BCNU, 24% with radiation, and 32% with radiation and BCNU ($P = 0.001$ for radiation versus no radiation). The median survival rates were 14 weeks for supportive care, 19 weeks for BCNU, and 36 weeks for radiotherapy (alone and with BCNU).[147]

Several studies have compared escalated dose radiotherapy to standard radiotherapy. An MRC randomized trial of 474 patients demonstrated a 3-month improvement in median survival with higher-dose radiation.[149] A retrospective comparison of 621 patients entered on three different Brain Tumor Cooperative Group (BTCG) trials found that 60 Gy was associated with an improvement in median survival compared to 55 and 50 Gy.[150] However, a RTOG/ECOG randomized study of 626 patients demonstrated that survival was the same with 60 Gy and 70 Gy.[151] A trial of 140 patients who received 50 Gy postoperatively randomized patients to more radiation (60 Gy using brachytherapy) versus no further therapy.[152] Although brachytherapy was associated with improved survival on multivariate analysis (relative risk 0.7, $P = 0.07$) and two long-term survivors were seen at 6 and 9 years from surgery, the median survival was not significantly different with brachytherapy (13.8 months) compared to no brachytherapy (13.2 months) ($P = 0.49$).

As age is a significant prognostic factor for glioblastoma multiforme, shortened course radiation (40 Gy in 15 fractions) was compared to standard radiation (60 Gy) in patients 60 years or older following surgery.[153] Overall survival times were similar for both groups (5.1 months for standard RT versus 5.6 months for shortened RT), and there was a decreased requirement for increase in steroid in the shortened treatment group.

The addition of chemotherapy to radiation for glioblastoma multiforme has recently been shown to improve survival. A recent EORTC/NCIC randomized control study of 573 patients randomized to radiotherapy (60 Gy) versus radiotherapy plus concomitant temozolamide followed by adjuvant temozolamide for 6 months demonstrated a significant improvement in progression-free (7.2 versus 5 months, $P < 0.0001$) and median survival (15 versus 12 months) with chemoradiation.[154]

Low-Grade Astrocytoma

The median survival of patients with low-grade astrocytomas is 5 to 7 years. The main goal of radiation is to delay local recurrences, although randomized studies have not addressed this question. It is unclear when the optimal time for radiation is in patients who present with no neurological symptoms or mass effect. Advantages of using radiotherapy at the time of diagnosis include the theoretical benefit of using radiation when the number of clonogens is low, whereas delaying radiation until tumor progression postpones potential radiation-induced toxicities. A randomized trial of 311 patients found that immediate radiation improved the progression-free survival but not overall survival.[155] In patients with neurological symptoms, mass effect or recurrence following excision of a low-grade astrocytoma, radiation therapy should be offered. In young patients (less than 45 years) who present with seizures alone, radiation may be delayed until tumor progression occurs. These patients must be followed carefully with regular imaging studies so that tumor progression may be detected before the development of neurological compromise.

Conclusion

Radiation therapy is an important adjunct treatment to surgery for many cancers. Potential benefits of radiotherapy include an improvement in local control, overall survival, and organ functional preservation. The evidence supporting the use of radiation therapy in addition to surgery is very strong in some sites (e.g., breast cancer), but less strong in others (e.g., low-grade astrocytoma). The optimal timing of radiation, chemotherapy, and surgery is best determined in a multidisciplinary setting before the initiation of any treatment. Future studies should determine the optimal strategy of combining surgery, radiation therapy, and chemotherapy. Endpoints for such studies should include organ function as well as tumor control and cure.

References

1. Halperin EC, Perez CA, Brady LW, Wazer DE, Freeman C. Perez and Brady's Principles and Practic of Radiation Oncology. Philadelphia: Lippincott Williams and Wilkins, 2007.
2. DeVita VT, Hellman S, Rosenberg SA. Cancer: Principles and Practice of Oncology. Philadelphia: Lippincott Williams & Wilkins, 2004.
3. Hockel M, Knoop C, Schlenger K, et al. Intratumoral pO_2 predicts survival in advanced cancer of the uterine cervix. Radiother Oncol 1993;26(1):45–50.
4. Hockel M, Schlenger K, Hockel S, Aral B, Schaffer U, Vaupel P. Tumor hypoxia in pelvic recurrences of cervical cancer. Int J Cancer 1998;79(4):365–369.
5. Vaupel P, Kelleher DK, Hockel M. Oxygen status of malignant tumors: pathogenesis of hypoxia and significance for tumor therapy. Semin Oncol 2001;28(2 suppl 8):29–35.
6. Lawrence WT, Zabell A, McDonald HD. The tolerance of skin grafts to postoperative radiation therapy in patients with soft-tissue sarcoma. Ann Plast Surg 1986;16(3):204–210.
7. Abeloff MAJ, Lichter A, Niederhuber J. Clinical Oncology. New York: Churchill Livingston, 1995.
8. Blichert-Toft M, Rose C, Andersen JA, et al. Danish randomized trial comparing breast conservation therapy with mastectomy: six years of life-table analysis. Danish Breast Cancer Cooperative Group. J Natl Cancer Inst Monogr 1992(11):19–25.
9. Fisher B, Anderson S, Bryant J, et al. Twenty-year follow-up of a randomized trial comparing total mastectomy, lumpectomy, and lumpectomy plus irradiation for the treatment of invasive breast cancer. N Engl J Med 2002;347(16):1233–1241.
10. Jacobson JA, Danforth DN, Cowan KH, et al. Ten-year results of a comparison of conservation with mastectomy in the treatment of stage I and II breast cancer. N Engl J Med 1995;332(14):907–911.
11. Veronesi U, Banfi A, Salvadori B, et al. Breast conservation is the treatment of choice in small breast cancer: long-term results of a randomized trial. Eur J Cancer 1990;26(6):668–670.
12. van Dongen JA, Voogd AC, Fentiman IS, et al. Long-term results of a randomized trial comparing breast-conserving therapy with mastectomy: European Organization for Research and Treatment of Cancer 10801 trial. J Natl Cancer Inst 2000;92(14):1143–1150.
13. Arriagada R, Le MG, Rochard F, Contesso G. Conservative treatment versus mastectomy in early breast cancer: patterns of failure with 15 years of follow-up data. Institut Gustave-Roussy Breast Cancer Group. J Clin Oncol 1996;14(5):1558–1564.
14. Liljegren G, Holmberg L, Bergh J, et al. 10-Year results after sector resection with or without postoperative radiotherapy for stage I breast cancer: a randomized trial. J Clin Oncol 1999;17(8):2326–2333.
15. Veronesi U, Marubini E, Mariani L, et al. Radiotherapy after breast-conserving surgery in small breast carcinoma: long-term results of a randomized trial. Ann Oncol 2001;12(7):997–1003.
16. Clark RM, Whelan T, Levine M, et al. Randomized clinical trial of breast irradiation following lumpectomy and axillary dissection for node-negative breast cancer: an update. Ontario Clinical Oncology Group. J Natl Cancer Inst 1996;88(22):1659–1664.
17. Forrest AP, Stewart HJ, Everington D, et al. Randomised controlled trial of conservation therapy for breast cancer: 6-year analysis of the Scottish trial. Scottish Cancer Trials Breast Group. Lancet 1996;348(9029):708–713.
18. Renton SC, Gazet JC, Ford HT, Corbishley C, Sutcliffe R. The importance of the resection margin in conservative surgery for breast cancer. Eur J Surg Oncol 1996;22(1):17–22.
19. Anonymous. Effects of radiotherapy and surgery in early breast cancer. An overview of the randomized trials. Early Breast Cancer Trialists Collaborative Group. N Engl J Med 1995; 333(22):1444–1455.
20. Anonymous. Favourable and unfavourable effects on long-term survival of radiotherapy for early breast cancer: an overview of the randomised trials. Early Breast Cancer Trialists Collaborative Group. Lancet 2000;355(9217):1757–1770.
21. Carlson RW, Goldstein LJ, Gradishar WJ, et al. NCCN Breast Cancer Practice Guidelines. The National Comprehensive Cancer Network. Oncology (Huntingt) 1996;10(11 suppl):47–75.
22. Bijker N, Meijnen P, Peterese J, et al. Breast-conserving treatment with or without radiotherapy in ductal carcinoma in situ: ten year results of European Organisation for research and treatment of cancer randomised phase III trial 10853. A study by the EORTC breast cancer cooperative group and EORTC radiotherapy group. J Clin Oncol Vol 2006;24:3381–3387.
23. Fisher B, Bryant J, Dignam JJ, et al. Tamoxifen, radiation therapy, or both for prevention of ipsilateral breast tumor recurrence after lumpectomy in women with invasive breast cancers of one centimeter or less. J Clin Oncol 2002;20(20):4141–4149.
24. Fyles AW, McCready DR, Manchul LA, et al. Tamoxifen with or without breast irradiation in women 50 years of age or older with early breast cancer. N Engl J Med 2004;351(10):963–970.
25. Hughes KS, Schnaper LA, Berry D, et al. Lumpectomy plus tamoxifen with or without irradiation in women 70 years of age or older with early breast cancer. N Engl J Med 2004;351(10):971–977.
26. Robertson JM, Clarke DH, Pevzner MM, Matter RC. Breast conservation therapy. Severe breast fibrosis after radiation therapy in patients with collagen vascular disease. Cancer (Phila) 1991;68(3):502–508.
27. Ross JG, Hussey DH, Mayr NA, Davis CS. Acute and late reactions to radiation therapy in patients with collagen vascular diseases. Cancer (Phila) 1993;71(11):3744–3752.
28. Griem KL, Henderson IC, Gelman R, et al. The 5-year results of a randomized trial of adjuvant radiation therapy after chemotherapy in breast cancer patients treated with mastectomy. J Clin Oncol 1987;5(10):1546–1555.
29. Velez-Garcia E, Carpenter JT Jr, Moore M, et al. Postsurgical adjuvant chemotherapy with or without radiotherapy in women with breast cancer and positive axillary nodes: a South-Eastern Cancer Study Group (SEG) Trial. Eur J Cancer 1992;28A(11):1833–1837.
30. Rutqvist LE, Pettersson D, Johansson H. Adjuvant radiation therapy versus surgery alone in operable breast cancer: long-term follow-up of a randomized clinical trial. Radiother Oncol 1993;26(2):104–110.
31. Jones JM, Ribeiro GG. Mortality patterns over 34 years of breast cancer patients in a clinical trial of post-operative radiotherapy. Clin Radiol 1989;40(2):204–208.
32. Host H, Brennhovd IO, Loeb M. Postoperative radiotherapy in breast cancer: long-term results from the Oslo study. Int J Radiat Oncol Biol Phys 1986;12(5):727–732.
33. Early Breast Cancer Trialists' Collaborative Group. Treatment of Early Breast Cancer, vol 1. Worldwide Evidence, 1985–1990. Oxford: Oxford University Press, 1990.
34. Muss HB, Cooper MR, Brockschmidt JK, et al. A randomized trial of chemotherapy (L-PAM vs. CMF) and irradiation for node positive breast cancer. Eleven year follow-up of a Piedmont Oncology Association trial. Breast Cancer Res Treat 1991; 19(2):77–84.
35. Buzdar AU, Blumenschein GR, Smith TL, et al. Adjuvant chemotherapy with fluorouracil, doxorubicin, and cyclophospha-

mide, with or without Bacillus Calmette-Guerin and with or without irradiation in operable breast cancer. A prospective randomized trial. Cancer (Phila) 1984;53(3):384–389.
36. Overgaard M, Hansen PS, Overgaard J, et al. Postoperative radiotherapy in high-risk premenopausal women with breast cancer who receive adjuvant chemotherapy. Danish Breast Cancer Cooperative Group 82b Trial. N Engl J Med 1997;337(14):949–955.
37. Ragaz J, Olivotto I, Spinelli J, et al. Locoregional radiation therapy in patients with high risk breast cancer receiving adjuvant chemotherapy: 20 year results of the British Columbia randomised trial. J Natl Cancer Inst 2005;97,2:116–126.
38. Rosenberg SA, Tepper J, Glatstein E, et al. The treatment of soft-tissue sarcomas of the extremities: prospective randomized evaluations of (1) limb-sparing surgery plus radiation therapy compared with amputation and (2) the role of adjuvant chemotherapy. Ann Surg 1982;196(3):305–315.
39. Pisters PW, Harrison LB, Leung DH, Woodruff JM, Casper ES, Brennan MF. Long-term results of a prospective randomized trial of adjuvant brachytherapy in soft tissue sarcoma. J Clin Oncol 1996;14(3):859–868.
40. Yang JC, Chang AE, Baker AR, et al. Randomized prospective study of the benefit of adjuvant radiation therapy in the treatment of soft tissue sarcomas of the extremity. J Clin Oncol 1998;16(1):197–203.
41. O'Sullivan B, Davis AM, Turcotte R, et al. Preoperative versus postoperative radiotherapy in soft-tissue sarcoma of the limbs: a randomised trial. Lancet 2002;359(9325):2235–2241.
42. Sindelar WF, Kinsella TJ, Chen PW, et al. Intraoperative radiotherapy in retroperitoneal sarcomas. Final results of a prospective, randomized, clinical trial. Arch Surg 1993;128(4):402–410.
43. Chang AE, Kinsella T, Glatstein E, et al. Adjuvant chemotherapy for patients with high-grade soft-tissue sarcomas of the extremity. J Clin Oncol 1988;6(9):1491–1500.
44. Van Houtte P, Rocmans P, Smets P, et al. Postoperative radiation therapy in lung cancer: a controlled trial after resection of curative design. Int J Radiat Oncol Biol Phys 1980;6(8):983–986.
45. Bangma PJ. Postoperative radiotherapy. In: Deeley TJ (ed) Carcinoma of the Bronchus: Modern Radiotherapy. New York: Appleton-Century-Crofts, 1972:163–170.
46. Paterson R, Russell MH. Clinical trial in malignant disease. IV. Lung cancer. Value of postoperative radiotherapy. Clin Radiol 1962;13:141–144.
47. Smolle-Juettner FM, Mayer R, Pinter H, et al. "Adjuvant" external radiation of the mediastinum in radically resected non-small cell lung cancer. Eur J Cardiothorac Surg 1996;10(11):947–950.
48. Anonymous. Effects of postoperative mediastinal radiation on completely resected stage II and stage III epidermoid cancer of the lung. The Lung Cancer Study Group. N Engl J Med 1986;315(22):1377–1381.
49. Choi NC, Carey RW, Daly W, et al. Potential impact on survival of improved tumor downstaging and resection rate by preoperative twice-daily radiation and concurrent chemotherapy in stage IIIA non-small-cell lung cancer. J Clin Oncol 1997;15(2):712–722.
50. Astudillo J, Conill C. Role of postoperative radiation therapy in stage IIIa non-small cell lung cancer. Ann Thorac Surg 1990;50(4):618–623.
51. Chung CK, Stryker JA, O'Neill M Jr, DeMuth WE Jr. Evaluation of adjuvant postoperative radiotherapy for lung cancer. Int J Radiat Oncol Biol Phys 1982;8(11):1877–1880.
52. Israel L Bonadonna G, Sylvester R. Controlled study with adjuvant radiotherapy, chemotherapy, immunotherapy, and chemoimmunotherapy in operable squamous cell carcinoma of the lung. In: Muggia FM, Rozencweig M, eds. Lung Cancer: Progress in Therapeutic Research. New York: Raven Press, 1979:443–452.
53. Stephens RJ, Girling DJ, Bleehen NM, Moghissi K, Yosef HM, Machin D. The role of post-operative radiotherapy in non-small-cell lung cancer: a multicentre randomised trial in patients with pathologically staged T1–2, N1–2, M0 disease. Medical Research Council Lung Cancer Working Party. Br J Cancer 1996;74(4):632–639.
54. Anonymous. Postoperative radiotherapy in non-small-cell lung cancer: systematic review and meta-analysis of individual patient data from nine randomised controlled trials. PORT Meta-analysis Trialists Group. Lancet 1998;352(9124):257–263.
55. Dautzenberg B, Arriagada R, Chammard AB, et al. A controlled study of postoperative radiotherapy for patients with completely resected nonsmall cell lung carcinoma. Groupe d'Etude et de Traitement des Cancers Bronchiques. Cancer (Phila) 1999; 86(2):265–273.
56. Dautzenberg B, Chastang C, Arriagada R, et al. Adjuvant radiotherapy versus combined sequential chemotherapy followed by radiotherapy in the treatment of resected nonsmall cell lung carcinoma. A randomized trial of 267 patients. GETCB (Groupe d'Etude et de Traitement des Cancers Bronchiques). Cancer (Phila) 1995;76(5):779–786.
57. Anonymous. The benefit of adjuvant treatment for resected locally advanced non-small-cell lung cancer. The Lung Cancer Study Group. J Clin Oncol 1988;6(1):9–17.
58. Trakhtenberg A, Kiseleva ES, Pitskhelauri VG, et al. Preoperative radiotherapy in the combined treatment of lung cancer patients. Neoplasma 1988;35(4):459–465.
59. Okubo K, Wada H, Fukuse T, et al. Treatment of Pancoast tumors. Combined irradiation and radical resection. Thorac Cardiovasc Surg 1995;43(5):284–286.
60. Perry MC, Herndon JE III, Eaton WL, Green MR. Thoracic radiation therapy added to chemotherapy for small-cell lung cancer: an update of Cancer and Leukemia Group B Study 8083. J Clin Oncol 1998;16(7):2466–2467.
61. Auperin A, Arriagada R, Pignon JP, et al. Prophylactic cranial irradiation for patients with small-cell lung cancer in complete remission. Prophylactic Cranial Irradiation Overview Collaborative Group. N Engl J Med 1999;341(7):476–484.
62. Anonymous. Prolongation of the disease-free interval in surgically treated rectal carcinoma. Gastrointestinal Tumor Study Group. N Engl J Med 1985;312(23):1465–1472.
63. Fisher B, Wolmark N, Rockette H, et al. Postoperative adjuvant chemotherapy or radiation therapy for rectal cancer: results from NSABP protocol R-01. J Natl Cancer Inst 1988;80(1):21–29.
64. Bentzen SM, Balslev I, Pedersen M, et al. Time to loco-regional recurrence after resection of Dukes' B and C colorectal cancer with or without adjuvant postoperative radiotherapy. A multivariate regression analysis. Br J Cancer 1992;65(1):102–107.
65. Balslev I, Pedersen M, Teglbjaerg PS, et al. Postoperative radiotherapy in Dukes' B and C carcinoma of the rectum and rectosigmoid. A randomized multicenter study. Cancer (Phila) 1986;58(1):22–28.
66. Arnaud JP, Nordlinger B, Bosset JF, et al. Radical surgery and postoperative radiotherapy as combined treatment in rectal cancer. Final results of a phase III study of the European Organization for Research and Treatment of Cancer. Br J Surg 1997;84(3):352–357.
67. Anonymous. Randomised trial of surgery alone versus surgery followed by radiotherapy for mobile cancer of the rectum. Medical Research Council Rectal Cancer Working Party. Lancet 1996;348(9042):1610–1614.
68. Treurniet-Donker AD, van Putten WL, Wereldsma JC, et al. Postoperative radiation therapy for rectal cancer. An interim analysis of a prospective, randomized multicenter trial in The Netherlands. Cancer (Phila) 1991;67(8):2042–2048.
69. Krook JE, Moertel CG, Gunderson LL, et al. Effective surgical adjuvant therapy for high-risk rectal carcinoma. N Engl J Med 1991;324(11):709–715.

70. Thomas PR, Lindblad AS. Adjuvant postoperative radiotherapy and chemotherapy in rectal carcinoma: a review of the Gastrointestinal Tumor Study Group experience. Radiother Oncol 1988;13(4):245–252.
71. Wolmark N, Wieand HS, Hyams DM, et al. Randomized trial of postoperative adjuvant chemotherapy with or without radiotherapy for carcinoma of the rectum: National Surgical Adjuvant Breast and Bowel Project Protocol R-02. J Natl Cancer Inst 2000;92(5):388–396.
72. Goldberg PA, Nicholls RJ, Porter NH, Love S, Grimsey JE. Long-term results of a randomised trial of short-course low-dose adjuvant pre-operative radiotherapy for rectal cancer: reduction in local treatment failure. Eur J Cancer 1994;30A(11):1602–1606.
73. Higgins GA, Humphrey EW, Dwight RW, Roswit B, Lee LE Jr, Keehn RJ. Preoperative radiation and surgery for cancer of the rectum. Veterans Administration Surgical Oncology Group Trial II. Cancer (Phila) 1986;58(2):352–359.
74. Reis Neto JA, Quilici FA, Reis JA Jr. A comparison of nonoperative vs. preoperative radiotherapy in rectal carcinoma. A 10-year randomized trial. Dis Colon Rectum 1989;32(8):702–710.
75. Rider WD, Palmer JA, Mahoney LJ, Robertson CT. Preoperative irradiation in operable cancer of the rectum: report of the Toronto trial. Can J Surg 1977;20(4):335–338.
76. Anonymous. Improved survival with preoperative radiotherapy in resectable rectal cancer. Swedish Rectal Cancer Trial. N Engl J Med 1997;336(14):980–987.
77. Anonymous. Randomised trial of surgery alone versus radiotherapy followed by surgery for potentially operable locally advanced rectal cancer. Medical Research Council Rectal Cancer Working Party. Lancet 1996;348(9042):1605–1610.
78. Anonymous. Randomized study on preoperative radiotherapy in rectal carcinoma. Stockholm Colorectal Cancer Study Group. Ann Surg Oncol 1996;3(5):423–430.
79. Cedermark B, Johansson H, Rutqvist LE, Wilking N. The Stockholm I trial of preoperative short term radiotherapy in operable rectal carcinoma. A prospective randomized trial. Stockholm Colorectal Cancer Study Group. Cancer (Phila) 1995;75(9):2269–2275.
80. Anonymous. Preoperative short-term radiation therapy in operable rectal carcinoma. A prospective randomized trial. Stockholm Rectal Cancer Study Group. Cancer (Phila) 1990;66(1): 49–55.
81. Marsh PJ, James RD, Schofield PF. Adjuvant preoperative radiotherapy for locally advanced rectal carcinoma. Results of a prospective, randomized trial. Dis Colon Rectum 1994;37(12): 1205–1214.
82. Roswit B, Higgins GA, Keehn RJ. Preoperative irradiation for carcinoma of the rectum and rectosigmoid colon: report of a National Veterans Administration randomized study. Cancer (Phila) 1975;35(6):1597–1602.
83. Duncan W. Adjuvant radiotherapy in rectal cancer: the MRC trials. Br J Surg 1985;72(suppl):S59–S62.
84. Dahl O, Horn A, Morild I, et al. Low-dose preoperative radiation postpones recurrences in operable rectal cancer. Results of a randomized multicenter trial in western Norway. Cancer (Phila) 1990;66(11):2286–2294.
85. Gerard A, Buyse M, Nordlinger B, et al. Preoperative radiotherapy as adjuvant treatment in rectal cancer. Final results of a randomized study of the European Organization for Research and Treatment of Cancer (EORTC). Ann Surg 1988;208(5):606–614.
86. Camma C, Giunta M, Fiorica F, Pagliaro L, Craxi A, Cottone M. Preoperative radiotherapy for resectable rectal cancer: a meta-analysis. JAMA 2000;284(8):1008–1015.
87. Anonymous. Adjuvant radiotherapy for rectal cancer: a systematic overview of 8,507 patients from 22 randomised trials. Lancet 2001;358(9290):1291–1304.
88. Kapiteijn E, Marijnen CA, Nagtegaal ID, et al. Preoperative radiotherapy combined with total mesorectal excision for resectable rectal cancer. N Engl J Med 2001;345(9):638–646.
89. Boulis-Wassif S, Gerard A, Loygue J, Camelot D, Buyse M, Duez N. Final results of a randomized trial on the treatment of rectal cancer with preoperative radiotherapy alone or in combination with 5-fluorouracil, followed by radical surgery. Trial of the European Organization on Research and Treatment of Cancer Gastrointestinal Tract Cancer Cooperative Group. Cancer (Phila) 1984;53(9):1811–1818.
90. Gerard JP, Conroy T, Bonnetain F, et al. Preoperative radiotherapy with or without concurrent fluorouracil and leucovorin in T3–4 rectal cancers:results of FFCD 9203.J Clin Oncol 2006;24(28):4620–4625
91. Pahlman L, Glimelius B. Pre- or postoperative radiotherapy in rectal and rectosigmoid carcinoma. Report from a randomized multicenter trial. Ann Surg 1990;211(2):187–195.
92. Sauer Rolf BH, Hohenberger W, Rodel C, et al. Preoperative versus postoperative chemoradiotherapy for rectal cancer. N Engl J Med 2004;351:1731–1740.
93. Cummings BJ, Keane TJ, O'Sullivan B, Wong CS, Catton CN. Epidermoid anal cancer: treatment by radiation alone or by radiation and 5-fluorouracil with and without mitomycin C. Int J Radiat Oncol Biol Phys 1991;21(5):1115–1125.
94. Bosset JF, Roelofsen F, Morgan DA, et al. Shortened irradiation scheme, continuous infusion of 5-fluorouracil and fractionation of mitomycin C in locally advanced anal carcinomas. Results of a phase II study of the European Organization for Research and Treatment of Cancer. Radiotherapy and Gastrointestinal Cooperative Groups. Eur J Cancer 2003;39(1):45–51.
95. Peiffert D, Bey P, Pernot M, et al. Conservative treatment by irradiation of epidermoid cancers of the anal canal: prognostic factors of tumoral control and complications. Int J Radiat Oncol Biol Phys 1997;37(2):313–324.
96. Gerard JP, Ayzac L, Hun D, et al. Treatment of anal canal carcinoma with high dose radiation therapy and concomitant fluorouracil-cisplatinum. Long-term results in 95 patients. Radiother Oncol 1998;46(3):249–256.
97. Anonymous. Epidermoid anal cancer: results from the UKCCCR randomised trial of radiotherapy alone versus radiotherapy, 5-fluorouracil, and mitomycin. UKCCCR Anal Cancer Trial Working Party. UK Co-ordinating Committee on Cancer Research. Lancet 1996;348(9034):1049–1054.
98. Bartelink H, Roelofsen F, Eschwege F, et al. Concomitant radiotherapy and chemotherapy is superior to radiotherapy alone in the treatment of locally advanced anal cancer: results of a phase III randomized trial of the European Organization for Research and Treatment of Cancer Radiotherapy and Gastrointestinal Cooperative Groups. J Clin Oncol 1997;15(5):2040–2049.
99. Flam M, John M, Pajak TF, et al. Role of mitomycin in combination with fluorouracil and radiotherapy, and of salvage chemoradiation in the definitive nonsurgical treatment of epidermoid carcinoma of the anal canal: results of a phase III randomized intergroup study. J Clin Oncol 1996;14(9):2527–2539.
100. al-Sarraf M, Martz K, Herskovic A, et al. Progress report of combined chemoradiotherapy versus radiotherapy alone in patients with esophageal cancer: an intergroup study. J Clin Oncol 1997;15(1):277–284.
101. Herskovic A, Martz K, al-Sarraf M, et al. Combined chemotherapy and radiotherapy compared with radiotherapy alone in patients with cancer of the esophagus. N Engl J Med 1992; 326(24):1593–1598.
102. Teniere P, Hay JM, Fingerhut A, Fagniez PL. Postoperative radiation therapy does not increase survival after curative resection for squamous cell carcinoma of the middle and lower esophagus as shown by a multicenter controlled trial. French University Association for Surgical Research. Surg Gynecol Obstet 1991;173(2):123–130.

103. Fok M, Sham JS, Choy D, Cheng SW, Wong J. Postoperative radiotherapy for carcinoma of the esophagus: a prospective, randomized controlled study. Surgery (St. Louis) 1993;113(2):138–147.
104. Zieren HU, Muller JM, Jacobi CA, Pichlmaier H, Muller RP, Staar S. Adjuvant postoperative radiation therapy after curative resection of squamous cell carcinoma of the thoracic esophagus: a prospective randomized study. World J Surg 1995;19(3):444–449.
105. Huang G. Combined Irradiation and Surgery for Esophageal Carcinoma. St. Louis: Mosby, 1988.
106. Arnott SJ, Duncan W, Kerr GR, et al. Low dose preoperative radiotherapy for carcinoma of the oesophagus: results of a randomized clinical trial. Radiother Oncol 1992;24(2):108–113.
107. Gignoux M, Roussel A, Paillot B, et al. The value of preoperative radiotherapy in esophageal cancer: results of a study of the E. O.R.T.C. World J Surg 1987;11(4):426–432.
108. Nygaard K, Hagen S, Hansen HS, et al. Pre-operative radiotherapy prolongs survival in operable esophageal carcinoma: a randomized, multicenter study of pre-operative radiotherapy and chemotherapy. The second Scandinavian trial in esophageal cancer. World J Surg 1992;16(6):1104–1109; discussion 1110.
109. Launois B, Delarue D, Campion JP, Kerbaol M. Preoperative radiotherapy for carcinoma of the esophagus. Surg Gynecol Obstet 1981;153(5):690–692.
110. Wang M, Gu XZ, Yin WB, Huang GJ, Wang LJ, Zhang DW. Randomized clinical trial on the combination of preoperative irradiation and surgery in the treatment of esophageal carcinoma: report on 206 patients. Int J Radiat Oncol Biol Phys 1989;16(2):325–327.
111. Arnott SJ, Duncan W, Gignoux M, et al. Preoperative radiotherapy in esophageal carcinoma: a meta-analysis using individual patient data (Oesophageal Cancer Collaborative Group). Int J Radiat Oncol Biol Phys 1998;41(3):579–583.
112. Walsh TN, Noonan N, Hollywood D, Kelly A, Keeling N, Hennessy TP. A comparison of multimodal therapy and surgery for esophageal adenocarcinoma. N Engl J Med 1996;335(7):462–467.
113. Le Prise E, Etienne PL, Meunier B, et al. A randomized study of chemotherapy, radiation therapy, and surgery versus surgery for localized squamous cell carcinoma of the esophagus. Cancer (Phila) 1994;73(7):1779–1784.
114. Bosset JF, Gignoux M, Triboulet JP, et al. Chemoradiotherapy followed by surgery compared with surgery alone in squamous-cell cancer of the esophagus. N Engl J Med 1997;337(3):161–167.
115. Urba SG, Orringer MB, Turrisi A, Iannettoni M, Forastiere A, Strawderman M. Randomized trial of preoperative chemoradiation versus surgery alone in patients with locoregional esophageal carcinoma. J Clin Oncol 2001;19(2):305–313.
116. Schlag PM. Randomized trial of preoperative chemotherapy for squamous cell cancer of the esophagus. The Chirurgische Arbeitsgemeinschaft Fuer Onkologie der Deutschen Gesellschaft Fuer Chirurgie Study Group. Arch Surg 1992;127(12):1446–1450.
117. Urschel JD, Vasan H. A meta-analysis of randomized controlled trials that compared neoadjuvant chemoradiation and surgery to surgery alone for resectable esophageal cancer. Am J Surg 2003;185(6):538–543.
118. Kalser MH, Ellenberg SS. Pancreatic cancer. Adjuvant combined radiation and chemotherapy following curative resection. Arch Surg 1985;120(8):899–903.
119. Anonymous. Further evidence of adjuvant combined radiation and chemotherapy following curative resection of pancreatic cancer. Cancer (Phila) 1987;59:2006–2010.
120. Bakkevold KE, Arnesjo B, Dahl O, Kambestad B. Adjuvant combination chemotherapy (AMF) following radical resection of carcinoma of the pancreas and papilla of Vater—results of a controlled, prospective, randomised multicentre study. Eur J Cancer 1993;29A(5):698–703.
121. Klinkenbijl JH, Jeekel J, Sahmoud T, et al. Adjuvant radiotherapy and 5-fluorouracil after curative resection of cancer of the pancreas and periampullary region: phase III trial of the EORTC gastrointestinal tract cancer cooperative group. Ann Surg 1999;230(6):776–782; discussion 82–84.
122. Neoptolemos JP, Stocken DD, Friess H, et al. A randomized trial of chemoradiotherapy and chemotherapy after resection of pancreatic cancer. N Engl J Med 2004;350(12):1200–1210.
123. Knaebel HP, Marten A, Schmidt J et al. Phase III trial of postoperative cisplatin, interferon alpha 2b, and 5FU combined with external radiation treatment versus 5FU alone for patients with resected pancreatic adenocarcinoma: CapRI study protocol. BMC Cancer 2005,5:37
124. Hoffman JP, Weese JL, Solin LJ, et al. A pilot study of preoperative chemoradiation for patients with localized adenocarcinoma of the pancreas. Am J Surg 1995;169(1):71–77; discussion 77–78.
125. Allum WH, Hallissey MT, Ward LC, Hockey MS. A controlled, prospective, randomised trial of adjuvant chemotherapy or radiotherapy in resectable gastric cancer: interim report. British Stomach Cancer Group. Br J Cancer 1989;60(5):739–744.
126. Fielding JW, Fagg SL, Jones BG, et al. An interim report of a prospective, randomized, controlled study of adjuvant chemotherapy in operable gastric cancer: British Stomach Cancer Group. World J Surg 1983;7(3):390–399.
127. Hallissey MT, Dunn JA, Ward LC, Allum WH. The second British Stomach Cancer Group trial of adjuvant radiotherapy or chemotherapy in resectable gastric cancer: five-year follow-up. Lancet 1994;343(8909):1309–1312.
128. Dent DM, Werner ID, Novis B, Cheverton P, Brice P. Prospective randomized trial of combined oncological therapy for gastric carcinoma. Cancer (Phila) 1979;44(2):385–391.
129. Moertel CG, Childs DS, O'Fallon JR, Holbrook MA, Schutt AJ, Reitemeier RJ. Combined 5-fluorouracil and radiation therapy as a surgical adjuvant for poor prognosis gastric carcinoma. J Clin Oncol 1984;2(11):1249–1254.
130. Macdonald JS, Smalley SR, Benedetti J, et al. Chemoradiotherapy after surgery compared with surgery alone for adenocarcinoma of the stomach or gastroesophageal junction. N Engl J Med 2001;345(10):725–730.
131. Coppin CM, Gospodarowicz MK, James K, et al. Improved local control of invasive bladder cancer by concurrent cisplatin and preoperative or definitive radiation. The National Cancer Institute of Canada Clinical Trials Group. J Clin Oncol 1996;14(11):2901–2907.
132. Kachnic LA, Kaufman DS, Heney NM, et al. Bladder preservation by combined modality therapy for invasive bladder cancer. J Clin Oncol 1997;15(3):1022–1029.
133. Shipley WU, Winter KA, Kaufman DS, et al. Phase III trial of neoadjuvant chemotherapy in patients with invasive bladder cancer treated with selective bladder preservation by combined radiation therapy and chemotherapy: initial results of Radiation Therapy Oncology Group 89–03. J Clin Oncol 1998;16(11):3576–3583.
134. Shahab N. Bladder preservation trial: Radiation Therapy Oncology Group 89–03. J Clin Oncol 1999;17(4):1327–1328.
135. Sell A, Jakobsen A, Nerstrom B, Sorensen BL, Steven K, Barlebo H. Treatment of advanced bladder cancer category T2 T3 and T4a. A randomized multicenter study of preoperative irradiation and cystectomy versus radical irradiation and early salvage cystectomy for residual tumor. DAVECA protocol 8201. Danish Vesical Cancer Group. Scand J Urol Nephrol Suppl 1991;138:193–201.
136. Bloom HJ, Hendry WF, Wallace DM, Skeet RG. Treatment of T3 bladder cancer: controlled trial of pre-operative radiotherapy and radical cystectomy versus radical radiotherapy. Br J Urol 1982;54(2):136–151.

137. Bolla M, van Poppel H, Collette L, et al. Postoperative radiotherapy after radical prostatectomy: a randomised controlled trial (EORTC trial 22911). Lancet 2005;366(9485):572–578.
138. Thompson IM, Tangen CM, Paradelo J, et al. Adjuvant radiotherapy for pathologically advanced prostate cancer. A randomised clinical trial. JAMA 2006;296(19):2329–2335.
139. Anonymous. Induction chemotherapy plus radiation compared with surgery plus radiation in patients with advanced laryngeal cancer. The Department of Veterans Affairs Laryngeal Cancer Study Group. N Engl J Med 1991;324(24):1685–1690.
140. Lefebvre JL, Chevalier D, Luboinski B, Kirkpatrick A, Collette L, Sahmoud T. Larynx preservation in pyriform sinus cancer: preliminary results of a European Organization for Research and Treatment of Cancer phase III trial. EORTC Head and Neck Cancer Cooperative Group. J Natl Cancer Inst 1996;88(13):890–899.
141. Forastiere AA, Goepfert H, Maor M, et al. Concurrent chemotherapy and radiotherapy for organ preservation in advanced laryngeal cancer. N Engl J Med 2003;349(22):2091–2098.
142. Kramer S, Gelber RD, Snow JB, et al. Combined radiation therapy and surgery in the management of advanced head and neck cancer: final report of study 73–03 of the Radiation Therapy Oncology Group. Head Neck Surg 1987;10(1):19–30.
143. Peters LJ, Goepfert H, Ang KK, et al. Evaluation of the dose for postoperative radiation therapy of head and neck cancer: first report of a prospective randomized trial. Int J Radiat Oncol Biol Phys 1993;26(1):3–11.
144. Lavertu P, Adelstein DJ, Saxton JP, et al. Management of the neck in a randomized trial comparing concurrent chemotherapy and radiotherapy with radiotherapy alone in resectable stage III and IV squamous cell head and neck cancer. Head Neck 1997;19(7):559–566.
145. Bernier J, Domenge C, Ozsahin M, et al. Postoperative irradiation with or without concomitant chemotherapy for locally advanced head and neck cancer. N Engl J Med 2004;350(19):1945–1952.
146. Cooper JS, Pajak TF, Forastiere AA, et al. Postoperative concurrent radiotherapy and chemotherapy for high-risk squamous-cell carcinoma of the head and neck. N Engl J Med 2004;350(19):1937–1944.
147. Kristiansen K, Hagen S, Kollevold T, et al. Combined modality therapy of operated astrocytomas grade III and IV. Confirmation of the value of postoperative irradiation and lack of potentiation of bleomycin on survival time: a prospective multicenter trial of the Scandinavian Glioblastoma Study Group. Cancer (Phila) 1981;47(4):649–652.
148. Walker MD, Alexander E Jr, Hunt WE, et al. Evaluation of BCNU and/or radiotherapy in the treatment of anaplastic gliomas. A cooperative clinical trial. J Neurosurg 1978;49(3):333–343.
149. Bleehen NM, Stenning SP. A Medical Research Council trial of two radiotherapy doses in the treatment of grades 3 and 4 astrocytoma. The Medical Research Council Brain Tumour Working Party. Br J Cancer 1991;64(4):769–774.
150. Walker MD, Strike TA, Sheline GE. An analysis of dose-effect relationship in the radiotherapy of malignant gliomas. Int J Radiat Oncol Biol Phys 1979;5(10):1725–1731.
151. Chang CH, Horton J, Schoenfeld D, et al. Comparison of postoperative radiotherapy and combined postoperative radiotherapy and chemotherapy in the multidisciplinary management of malignant gliomas. A joint Radiation Therapy Oncology Group and Eastern Cooperative Oncology Group study. Cancer (Phila) 1983;52(6):997–1007.
152. Laperriere NJ, Leung PM, McKenzie S, et al. Randomized study of brachytherapy in the initial management of patients with malignant astrocytoma. Int J Radiat Oncol Biol Phys 1998;41(5):1005–1011.
153. Roa W, Brasher PM, Bauman G, et al. Abbreviated course of radiation therapy in older patients with glioblastoma multiforme: a prospective randomized clinical trial. J Clin Oncol 2004;22(9):1583–1588.
154. Stupp R, Mason WP, Van Den Bent MJ, et al. Concomitant and adjuvant temozolamide (TMZ) and radiotherapy (RT) for newly diagnosed glioblastoma multiforme (GBM). Proc Am Soc Clin Oncol 2004;23:1.
155. Karim AB, Afra D, Cornu P, et al. Randomized trial on the efficacy of radiotherapy for cerebral low-grade glioma in the adult: European Organization for Research and Treatment of Cancer Study 22845 with the Medical Research Council study BRO4: an interim analysis. Int J Radiat Oncol Biol Phys 2002;52(2):316–324.

96

Benign and Malignant Diseases of the Breast

Helen A. Pass

Embryology

Appreciation of the embryological development, anatomy, and physiology of the breast is critical for the rational evaluation and treatment of both benign and malignant breast disease. The breast develops from the ectodermally derived milk streak. Early in fetal life, the milk streak extends from the axilla to the pubis (Fig. 96.1). At the end of the first trimester, all but the pectoral portion of the milk streak atrophies, leaving the nipple bud. The ducts and lobules form from ingrowth of the ectoderm from the nipple surface. Breast development continues in puberty because of an interplay of mammotrophic hormones. By the age of 20, the breast has reached its greatest development. By 40, it begins to undergo atrophic change.

Anatomy

The breast parenchyma lies between the subcutaneous fat and the fascia of the pectoralis major and serratus anterior muscles (Fig. 96.2). Small branching lymphatics and blood vessels course through the retromammary space between the posterior surface of the breast parenchyma and the fascia of the pectoralis major muscle. Spanning from the dermis to the deep fascia are the suspensory ligaments of Cooper, the supporting framework of the breast. Because of this, even small tumors that involve Cooper's ligaments may cause skin dimpling and skin retraction. In women, breast tissue extends from the level of the clavicle to the sixth rib on the anterior chest wall. The medial margin is the sternocostal junction. The lateral is the midaxillary line. The areola is the circular, darkly pigmented area surrounding the nipple. At the periphery there are Montgomery tubercles, small, raised glands that lubricate the nipple–areolar complex during lactation. Beneath the epithelium of the areola, and extending throughout the entire ductal system, is a specialized myoepithelial cell with contractile properties under the regulation of oxytocin. This cell facilitates expulsion of milk during lactation.

Deep to the pectoralis major muscle lies the pectoralis minor muscle. The pectoralis minor muscle is invested by the clavipectoral fascia that fuses with the axillary fascia. Division of this fascia allows entry into the axillary space. The axillary lymph nodes are separated into three levels based upon their location relative to the pectoralis minor muscle (Fig. 96.3). Level I lymph nodes are lateral to the border of the pectoralis minor muscle. Level II nodes are found beneath the muscle. Level III nodes are medial to the edge of the muscle. To access level III nodes surgically, often the pectoralis minor muscle must be detached from the coracoid process. Rotter's nodes, or the interpectoral lymph nodes, are anterior to the axillary space located between the pectoralis major and minor muscles. Intramammary nodes are found within or along the lateral edge of the breast and axillary tail. Although the majority of the lymphatic flow is laterally to the axillary lymph nodes, as much as 30% courses medially to the internal mammary lymph nodes. Distal spread to the sub- and supraclavicular nodes can occur in advanced breast cancer.

Paralleling the lymphatic pathways of the breast, the venous drainage is to the axillary, internal mammary, and intercostal veins. The arterial supply to the breast is rich. The medial and central breast is supplied from perforating branches of the internal mammary artery. Branches from the long

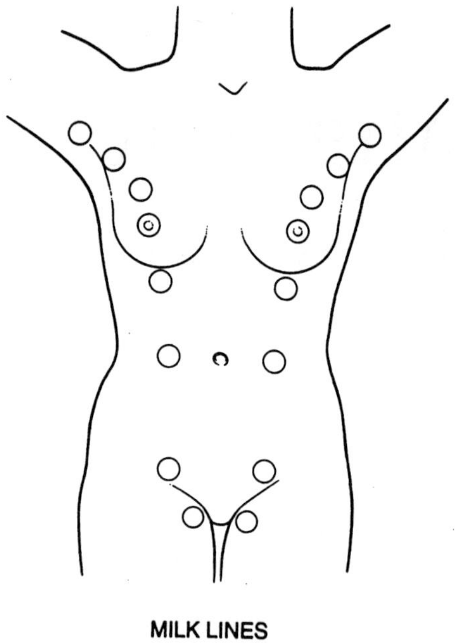

FIGURE 96.1. Extent of embryological milk streak. The mammary milk line atrophies by week 9 of gestation and only the nipple bud remains. Supernumerary nipples and accessory breast tissue may be found anywhere along the milk streak. (From Hindle WH, ed. Breast Care: A Clinical Guidebook for Women's Primary Healthcare Providers. ©1999 by permission of Springer-Verlag, New York.)

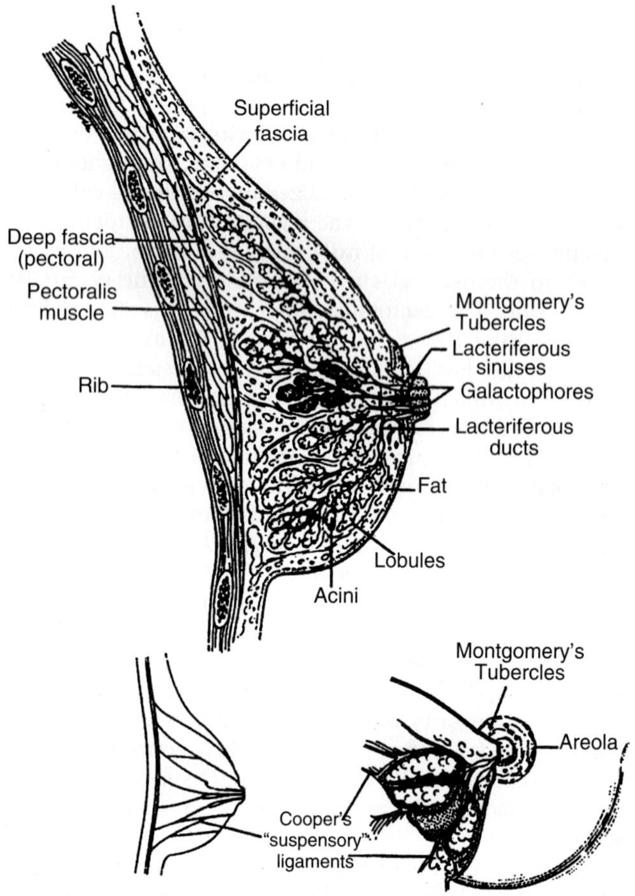

FIGURE 96.2. Tangential view of breast and chest wall. (From Hindle WH, ed. Breast Care: A Clinical Guidebook for Women's Primary Healthcare Providers. ©1999 by permission of Springer-Verlag, New York.)

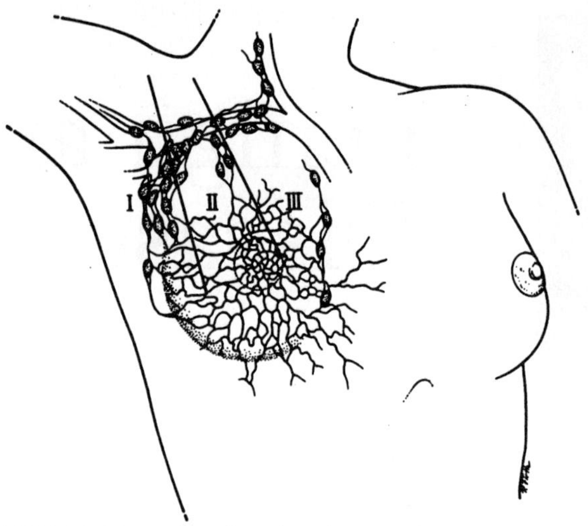

FIGURE 96.3. The axillary lymph nodes are defined by their relationship to the pectoralis minor muscle. Level I nodes are lateral to the border of the pectoralis minor muscle and include the inframammary, axillary vein, and scapular lymph nodes. Level II nodes are deep to the pectoralis minor muscle and encompass the central and some subclavicular lymph nodes. Level III nodes are medial to the border of the pectoralis minor muscle and involve the remainder of the subclavicular lymph nodes. (From Hindle WH, ed. Breast Care: A Clinical Guidebook for Women's Primary Healthcare Providers. ©1999 by permission of Springer-Verlag, New York.)

thoracic, thoracodorsal, and subscapular arteries provide the remainder of the blood supply to the lateral breast.

Knowledge of the location of the major neural structures in the axilla is necessary for the performance of a complication-free axillary dissection (Fig. 96.4). The long thoracic nerve of Bell courses along the chest wall at the medial edge of the axilla. It innervates the serratus anterior muscle and

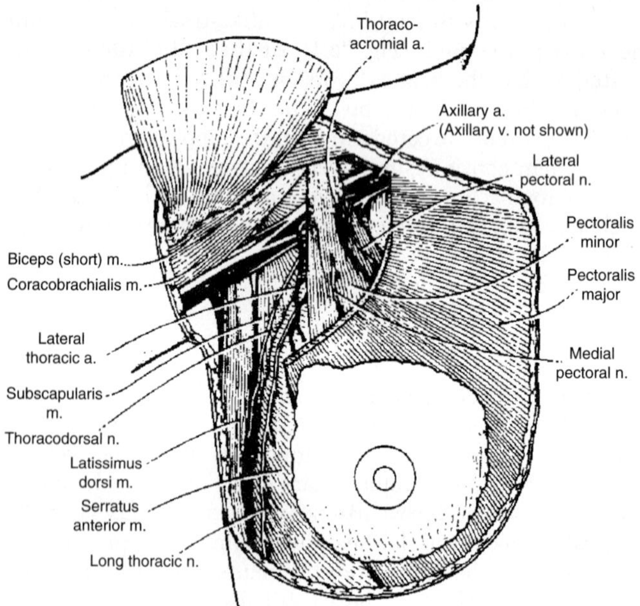

FIGURE 96.4. Topography of the axilla. (From Skandalakis JE, Gray SW, Rowe JR. Anatomical Complications in General Surgery. New York: McGraw-Hill, 1983:103, with permission.)

provides fixation of the scapula to the chest wall during arm extension. Injury to the long thoracic nerve results in a winged scapula deformity. The thoracodorsal nerve innervates the latissimus dorsi muscle. Transection of this nerve causes weakness in abduction and external rotation of the arm. Spanning the axillary space are the large sensory intercostal brachial (brachial cutaneous) nerves. Sacrifice results in numbness or dysesthesia along the posterior and medial surface of the forearm and skin of the axilla along the chest wall. The medial pectoral nerve is encountered upon division of the clavipectoral fascia, traveling around the lateral border of the pectoralis minor muscle to innervate the lower one-third of the pectoralis major muscle. Inadvertent injury results in atrophy of the muscle with less tissue coverage in patients who are treated with mastectomy. Although preservation of each of these named neural structures is preferred, sacrifice may become necessary in case of direct tumor involvement.

Developmental Disorders

Mastitis Neonatorum

As a result of the natural maternal hormonal influences, transient stimulation of the newborn's breast bud may occur. In 10% of infants, palpation of a breast disk is possible and may be associated with the secretion of a milk-like substance (witch's milk). As the maternal circulating hormone levels in the newborn fall after delivery, the production of witch's milk ceases after 2 to 3 weeks.

Amastia, Athelia, and Amazia

Difficulties during the first 6 to 12 weeks of fetal life may interfere with normal breast development. Absence of the breast (amastia) or nipple (athelia) is very rare. In 90% of patients, amastia is associated with Poland's syndrome. Poland's syndrome is characterized by hypoplasia of the breast, chest wall, and pectoral muscles along with multiple deformities of digits.

Amazia occurs in the rare instance when the nipple is present but the glandular tissue is absent. It is usually iatrogenic in origin, either as the result of a breast biopsy or drainage of an abscess. Chest wall radiation therapy before puberty may also cause amazia. Prepubertal gynecomastia may be unilateral and present as enlargement of the breast bud before other changes of puberty. Biopsy in this circumstance results in amazia.

Polythelia and Polymastia

Supranumerary nipples (polythelia) and accessory breast tissue (polymastia) are both more common. Accessory nipples may form anywhere along the milk streak from axilla to pubis, may occur in both males and females, and usually are only of cosmetic concern. Polythelia specifically refers to the very unusual instance when more than one nipple drains a breast.

Polymastia may also occur anywhere along the milk line. Complete breast development is possible, especially in the axilla. During pregnancy, the patient may present with an expanding axillary mass, pain, or mastitis. Removal may be necessary for palliation of symptoms, improvement of cosmesis, or in the rare instances when primary breast cancer arises within the accessory breast.

Clinical Evaluation of the Breast Patient: History and Risk Assessment

There are a variety of items specific to the evaluation of patients with benign and malignant breast diseases. When obtaining the history of a patient with a breast mass, one needs to evaluate when and how it was found, if it has changed since its discovery, timing relative to menstrual cycle, and if it is painful. Similarly, complaints of breast pain need to be correlated with timing of menstrual cycles and aggravating factors identified. Nipple discharge should be classified as unilateral versus bilateral, spontaneous versus induced, and characterized by color and consistency (bloody, milky, yellow, or clear). Concern regarding the possibility of cancer should prompt inquiry of constitutional symptoms such as fatigue, weight loss, or bone pain.

Risk Assessment

As with other malignancies, an assessment for the development of breast cancer is important to define populations that may benefit from early and more aggressive screening programs or preventive interventions. The average American female's lifetime risk of developing breast cancer is 11% and her risk of death from breast cancer is 3% to 4%. Numerous factors have been implicated including reproductive or hormonal history, dietary fat and alcohol use, a personal or family history of breast cancer, a past history of benign proliferative breast disease (especially if associated with atypia), and a history of radiation exposure. Nevertheless, more than two-thirds of women diagnosed with breast cancer have no identifiable risk factor (Table 96.1).

A personal history of cancer in one breast increases that individual's risk of a second, contralateral breast primary. In general, the actual risk is cited as 1% per year; however, this risk varies with age at diagnosis. For women less than 45 years at the diagnosis of the first breast cancer, the relative risk is fivefold the normal population, whereas for older patients it is twofold or less. Fortunately, women who have estrogen receptor-positive tumors and receive adjuvant tamoxifen therapy for 5 years reduce their incidence of contralateral breast cancer by almost 50%.[1]

Much attention has been focused on the influence of family history on the risk of developing breast cancer. It is first important to remember that because breast cancer is a common disease, the presence of one relative with unilateral breast cancer, especially if postmenopausal, does not seem to markedly increase risk.[2] The risk of developing breast cancer is two- to threefold greater in first-degree relatives (mother, sisters, daughters) of breast cancer patients.[2,3] The excess risk is much greater (up to ninefold) if the relative was affected by bilateral, premenopausal breast cancer.[1,4] Number of affected relatives has inconsistently been positively correlated with increased risk. Only 5% of women have true hereditary breast cancer.

Exposure to ionizing radiation has been demonstrated to increase breast cancer risk. There is a long latency period, and

TABLE 96.1. Epidemiological Risk Factors for Breast Cancer.

Factors of proven significance	*Strength of the association*	*Size of the effect*	*Evidence from prospective, randomized studies*	*Evidence from case-control or observational studies*
Factors that increase risk				
Age	+++	++	X	X
Early age at menarche (less than 12 years)	++	+	X	X
Late age at first live birth (more than 30 years)	++	+	X	X
Genetic mutations	+++	+++	X	X
Benign breast disease (proliferation ± atypia)	+++	++	X	X
Elevated levels of endogenous sex hormones	+++	+	X	X
Estrogen metabolism	+	+		X
Hormone replacement therapy	+++	++	X	X
Environmental factors				
Alcohol	++			X
Smoking	+?			X
Ionizing radiation	+++			X
Large body size (height and weight)	+	+		X
Factors that decrease risk or cause no change				
Lactation	++	–		X
Oral contraceptives	No effect	0		X
Induced abortion	No effect	0		X
Weight loss	+?	–		X
Exercise	+?	–		X
Dietary factors				X
Fat	No effect	0	X	X
Red meat	No effect	0		X
Dietary fiber	No effect	0		X
Caffeine	No effect	0		X
Micronutrients				
Vitamin A	No effect	0		X
Vitamin C	No effect	0		X
Vitamin E	No effect	0		X
Selenium	No effect	0		X
Organochlorines	No effect	0		X
Phytoestrogens	+?	–		X

Source: From Bland KI, Copeland EM. The Breast: Comprehensive Management of Benign and Malignant Disorders, 3rd ed, vols 1, 2. Philadelphia: Saunders, 2004:342, with permission.

age at exposure is correlated to risk.[5,6] Exposure during adolescence causes the highest risk whereas radiation after the age of 40 only minimally increases risk. Common scenarios of radiation exposure include mantle radiation for Hodgkin's disease, thymic radiation during infancy for thymic enlargement, breast radiation for mastitis, and exposure to ionizing radiation from nuclear war. Newer, high-risk screening guidelines recommend that women 25 years or older begin annual mammographic screening and biannual clinical breast evaluation 10 years after their radiation exposure. Because of the limited usefulness of mammography in dense breasts, current guidelines recommend that women younger than 25 should be evaluated yearly by physical examination only. There is increasing evidence that magnetic resonance imaging (MRI) may be beneficial in screening high-risk, young women with dense breasts.[7]

A personal history of a benign breast biopsy has previously been linked to an increased risk of breast cancer; however, as demonstrated by Dupont and Page, the histopathological classification of the benign lesion was critical in assessing risk.[8] Seventy percent of palpable lesions are nonproliferative and thus are not associated with an increased risk of cancer. Examples of nonproliferative lesions include adenosis, fibrosis, mild hyperplasia, squamous or apocrine metaplasia, duct ectasia, mastitis, cysts, and fibroadenomas. Women with proliferative fibrocystic disease (moderate or florid hyperplasia, sclerosing adenosis, or papilloma with fibrovascular core) have a 1.5- to 2-fold increased risk. The most substantial increased risk was seen in patients with atypical ductal or lobular hyperplasia. These women with proliferative disease with atypia have a 4.4-fold increased cancer risk, which increases to 9-fold if combined with a positive family history. It must be realized that these women are at increased risk not because of the biopsy itself but as a result of what prompted, and was found on, the biopsy.

Patients may desire an individualized estimate of invasive breast cancer risk over a 5-year period or over a lifetime. Lifetime risk is best interpreted in the context of age. For example, an American women's lifetime breast cancer risk is 11%, but more than half of that risk is manifest after age 65. Furthermore, the risk of death is one-third the risk of developing breast cancer. The Gail Model of risk assessment is a useful tool.[9] The National Cancer Institute has made a breast cancer risk assessment tool available based upon the Gail Multivariate Logistic Regression Model as a computer program (the "Risk Disk").[9,10] The risk factors included are those for which the evidence is conclusive and a relative weight can be assigned. Several factors are used to estimate risk: age, race, age at menarche, age at first live birth, a personal history of ductal carcinoma in situ (DCIS) or lobular carcinoma in situ (LCIS), personal history of a breast biopsy revealing proliferative changes with atypia, and a family history of breast cancer among first-degree relatives. Other risk factors, while viewed as important, were believed to be more difficult to quantify and therefore were not included. It is acknowledged that the Gail Model underestimates risk in patients with numerous second-degree relatives with breast or ovarian cancer. These factors should therefore be used to modify the Gail recommendations.

Management of High-Risk Patients

Screening Guidelines

Risk factor assessment is imprecise at best, but certain high-risk populations can be identified. As previously mentioned, women with a personal history of atypia, radiation exposure, or family history of breast and/or ovarian cancer or are a known BRCA1 or BRCA2 kindred are at increased risk for the development of breast cancer. Additionally, a personal history of breast cancer or lobular carcinoma in situ increases risk and thereby influences screening recommendations.

Screening guidelines are most specific for women with a personal history of breast cancer, lobular carcinoma in situ, and true hereditary breast cancer syndromes. For women with less strong family histories or a history of atypia on breast biopsy, the recommendations are still evolving. To date, there is no evidence that the additive radiation from the frequent mammograms increases breast cancer risk in these high-risk women. Nevertheless, it is important to note that, currently, there are also no data demonstrating that increased surveillance reduces breast cancer mortality in high-risk patients; however, an indirect benefit may be derived from the reassurance these women feel from participating in a prescribed regimen of close surveillance.

For women with a personal history of breast cancer, follow-up is determined by time from diagnosis. Physical examination should be performed every 3 to 4 months within the first 2 years from diagnosis, biannually from 2 until 5 years, and annually thereafter. Mammography should be obtained annually. Other laboratory and radiologic evaluation should be determined by stage at presentation. Women with lobular carcinoma in situ have twice-yearly clinical breast examinations and annual mammography. Those with atypia may be followed annually with both clinical breast examination and mammography.

Women with a significant radiation exposure or family history may benefit from earlier screening, as proposed by Lynch.[11] Patients with an autosomal dominant pattern of transmission of breast cancer, including those with a BRCA mutation, should have twice-yearly physical examination (see Familial/Hereditary Breast Cancer section).[12,13] Screening mammograms should be obtained annually or semiannually beginning 10 years younger than the youngest affected relative but not younger than 30 to 35 years old. There is increasing evidence that MRI may be used as an effective screening tool in this subset of young patients.[7,14] The lifetime risk for the development of breast cancer in a known BRCA1 or BRCA2 carrier has been estimated at between 60% and 80%.[15,16] BRCA1 mutations are linked to the development of breast, ovarian, and prostate cancers whereas BRCA2 families have an increased incidence of male and female breast cancers.[17–19] Undoubtedly, practice recommendations will change as more is learned about the natural history of these patients.

Chemoprevention

The only drug that is currently approved for reducing the risk of breast cancer in high-risk women is tamoxifen. The National Surgical Adjuvant Breast and Bowel Project P-1 Study (NSABP-P1) demonstrated a 49% reduced risk of invasive breast cancer in high-risk women randomized to tamoxifen versus placebo.[20] High-risk women were defined as those with a history of lobular carcinoma in situ, a 5-year predicted risk for breast cancer of at least 1.66% as defined by the Gail Model, or 60 years of age or older. The findings of the NSABP-P1 study are consistent with tamoxifen's demonstrated benefit in lowering the incidence of contralateral breast cancer in women with a previous history of breast cancer, prolonging survival when used as a postoperative adjuvant in women with stage I or II disease, and efficacy with or without chemotherapy in the treatment of advanced breast cancer.[21–23] The authors were careful to point out that even though tamoxifen prevented the occurrence of breast cancer in a substantial number of patients over the duration of the study, there was no evidence to support the assumption that carcinogenesis was inhibited or that tumors were permanently prevented.

Women considering tamoxifen chemoprevention need to be counseled about the increased risk of serious side effects in women over 50. The most common mild side effects reported were hot flashes and vaginal discharge. Furthermore, women over 50 had an increased incidence of endometrial cancer, deep venous thrombosis, and pulmonary embolism. This risk of developing endometrial cancer was similar to that for postmenopausal women on hormone replacement therapy. Women on tamoxifen must receive annual gynecological examinations, and any abnormal vaginal bleeding must be rigorously evaluated. With this approach, all women who developed endometrial cancer in the NSABP-P1 trial were stage I at the time of diagnosis.[20]

Women at risk for or with a previous history of deep venous thrombosis should not take tamoxifen for chemoprevention. Pulmonary embolism occurred in almost three times as many women on tamoxifen as in the placebo group. Nevertheless, this increased risk is similar to that observed in women taking oral contraceptives or hormone replacement therapy, which are routinely widely prescribed.

Two European trials, with different eligibility criteria, have failed to demonstrate that tamoxifen was an effective prophylactic agent.[24,25] Significant differences in the European trials include a potentially lower risk for eligibility, a higher rate of noncompliance, and, most importantly, an allowance of the concomitant use of hormone replacement therapy.

These differences, combined with the smaller study sizes, do not permit direct comparison of the trials and therefore do not invalidate the results of NSABP-P1.

The current NSABP chemoprevention trial, P-2 (STAR), is comparing the benefits and side effects of tamoxifen versus raloxifene in a prospective randomized fashion. Raloxifene is a selective estrogen receptor modulator (SERM) that had been used primarily to treat osteoporosis. Trials that have evaluated the effectiveness of raloxifene with respect to treating osteoporosis have shown a decrease in breast cancer by 54% without the increased incidence of endometrial cancer.[26] The Multiple Outcomes of Raloxifene Evaluation (MORE) is a multicenter trial that randomized women to raloxifene versus placebo. At a median follow-up of 40 months, the risk of developing invasive breast cancer was decreased by 76% with 3 years of treatment with raloxifene. It is clear that, as newer agents with fewer detrimental effects become available, more women will become candidates for chemoprevention.[27]

Prophylactic Mastectomy

It is likely that the indications for prophylactic mastectomy will continue to evolve as the long-term outcomes of both chemoprevention and genetic testing become better defined. There are currently no absolute indications for prophylactic mastectomy, and decisions are best made on a case-by-case basis. The most common indications include hereditary breast cancer (i.e., BRCA1 or -2 carriers), strong family history of breast cancer, a personal history of lobular carcinoma in situ, or a personal history of atypia combined with a family history of breast cancer. Softer criteria include women with unduly high anxiety about cancer development (after appropriate psychiatric counseling and screening), women in whom clinical or radiographic surveillance is difficult, and patients with contralateral breast cancer.

To date there are no prospective, randomized trials. The best study regarding the efficacy of bilateral prophylactic mastectomy is a retrospective study by Hartman. She evaluated the outcomes of 639 women with a family history of breast cancer who underwent the procedure.[28] After a median follow-up of 14 years, prophylactic mastectomy was associated with a 90% reduction in the incidence and risk of death from breast cancer as compared to untreated sisters. This finding may be more significant because a significant proportion of patients (90%) received bilateral subcutaneous mastectomies, which is no longer considered optimal for prophylaxis. However, the benefit may have also been overestimated because the risk of death was extrapolated from the Surveillance, Epidemiology and End Results (SEER) Program, was not stage specific, and therefore may have been too high. Nevertheless, when adjustments were made for high- and moderate-risk groups, as well as other potential sources of bias, the risk reduction remained unchanged. Thus, for select women, bilateral prophylactic mastectomy remains a valid treatment option.

All women considering prophylactic mastectomy benefit from extensive preoperative education and counseling. Ideally, they should receive an individualized risk assessment; psychiatric evaluation with psychosocial support; evaluation for plastic surgical reconstruction; and frank, honest dialogue with peer counselors who have been gratified by their decisions to undergo prophylactic mastectomies, as well as with those who have been disappointed with their decisions. With this structured approach, selection is optimized and patient satisfaction is maximized.

Screening Recommendations

Breast cancer screening relies upon the triad of self-breast examination (SBE), clinical breast examination (CBE) by a trained examiner, and screening mammography. Screening refers to the evaluation of an asymptomatic patient in an effort to identify disease at a stage before the onset of symptoms. Controversy exists regarding all three modalities, although intuitively all have appeal.

Self-Breast Examination

All major medical organizations endorsed self-breast examination (SBE) until the U.S. Preventive Health Service Task Force in 1995 and the National Comprehensive Cancer Network (NCCN) Breast Cancer Screening Guidelines Committee in 1998 categorized SBE as optional. This modification was made once the results of the St. Petersburg and Shanghai studies became available.[29,30] Both panels of experts asserted that, currently, there is insufficient evidence to recommend for or against the inclusion of SBE in screening guidelines. Unresolved issues in assessing the utility of SBE include the cost of provider time for education and evaluation of false positives. It is important to remember that, because there are insufficient data to recommend for or against SBE, current practice patterns should not be changed until additional and longer-term data are available.

Clinical Breast Examination

Accurate interpretation of the clinical breast examination (CBE) can be difficult. In a study of 15 patients with lesions proven malignant at surgery were evaluated preoperatively by four experienced surgeons. The diagnostic accuracy of concordance for the need for biopsy was only 73%.[30a] Nevertheless, CBE should be viewed as a complementary modality to mammography because up to 10% of breast cancers are mammographically occult.

There has never been a trial of CBE versus an unexamined control group. The Canadian National Breast Screening Study (NBSS2) has been the only trial designed to evaluate the additive impact of mammography over CBE only.[31] In this study, 39,405 women volunteers between 50 and 59 years old were randomized to annual mammography plus CBE versus CBE alone. Compliance was 85% after the first screening, and both groups were taught SBE. This trial has been criticized for lack of sensitivity of the mammographic units, the quality of the interpretation of the films, and the inclusion of some symptomatic patients. Nevertheless, these criticisms, some of which have not stood up over time, do not account for the lack of significance demonstrated in this trial. In NBSS2, although mammography detected smaller tumors, there was no difference in breast cancer mortality between the two groups. Additionally, 10% to 15% of cancers were mammographically occult.[32] It has been suggested that CBE may have been so effective in the NBSS2 because of the expertise of the nurse examiners, again highlighting the importance of adequate training and attention to detail in the performance of CBE.

Mammography: The Screening Trials and Surveillance Recommendations

Mammography remains the cornerstone of early detection programs for breast cancer. Multiple trials have demonstrated a reduction in breast cancer mortality as a result of mammographic screening of women over 50, and more recent analyses have now shown a statistically significant benefit for women 40 to 49 years old. Although the benefit of earlier mammogram is substantial and the risks from screening are relatively small, screening recommendations still vary slightly among organizations.[33] The American Cancer Society, however, is the most current in its recommendations and most organizations now follow their recommendations. This includes a monthly SBE and annual CBE, as well as annual mammography for all women 40 years or older.

Although there have been persuasive data for many years supporting annual screening mammography for women 50 to 69 years, and more recent data favoring screening in women 40 to 49 years, little evidence exists for or against screening in the elderly. An upper age limit for screening has not been defined. Several studies have found that screening mammography in older patients is underutilized.[34,35] In a retrospective review of women 75 years and older, Wilson et al. found that women who participated in annual screening mammography presented with statistically smaller tumors than women who were not screened (1.1 versus 2.1 cm, respectively; $P = 0.005$).[36] Given that the annual incidence of breast cancer increases with age, and the density of breast tissue decreases with age, the sensitivity and specificity of mammography are greatest

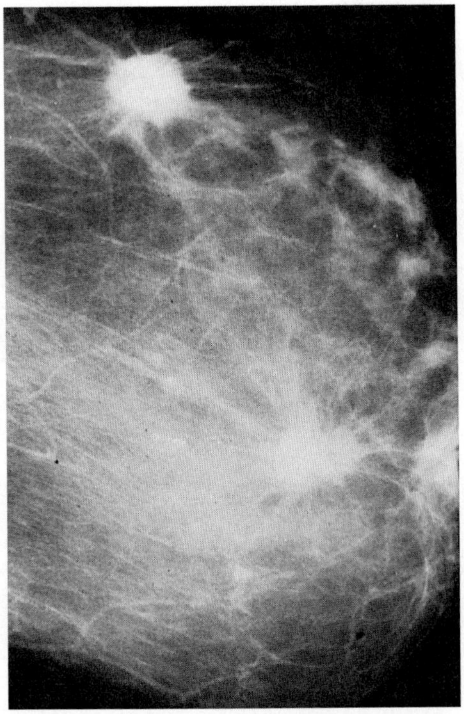

FIGURE 96.5. Mammogram demonstrating two spiculated masses characteristic of breast cancer. (Courtesy of M. Helvie, M.D.)

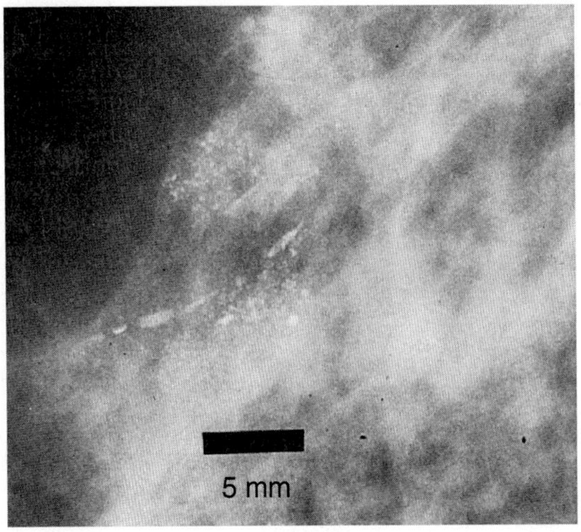

FIGURE 96.6. Mammogram demonstrating linear branching microcalcifications suspicious for cancer. (Courtesy of M. Helvie, M.D.)

in the elderly. Therefore, unless the patient has a significant comorbidity, annual screening mammography should be continued in the elderly.

To summarize, the data support that annual screening mammography can reduce breast cancer mortality and therefore should be incorporated into an overall strategy of SBE, CBE, and radiologic screening. Because 10% of palpable cancers are mammographically occult, all modalities must be incorporated into a comprehensive screening policy. Nevertheless, mammography remains the cornerstone because the 10-year survival for cancers detectable only by mammography nears 95%. The most common reason identified for failure to undergo annual mammography has been failure of the women's physician to recommend screening. All healthcare professionals should incorporate SBE instructions, CBE annually at the time of health maintenance examination, and recommendation for annual screening mammography in women of the appropriate age.

Diagnostic Mammography

Although screening mammography is performed in an asymptomatic woman, diagnostic mammography is obtained in a woman with a palpable abnormality, breast complaints, or lesion identified on screening. Mammographic abnormalities include densities, calcifications, or both. The most worrisome radiologic features include spiculated masses (Fig. 96.5), mass with associated microcalcifications, and linear branching calcifications (Fig. 96.6). Overall, about one-third of nonpalpable lesions discovered on mammography prove to be malignant. In abnormalities for which no biopsy is recommended, short-term mammographic follow-up must be obtained. The American College of Radiology has adopted standard definitions and established six mammographic categories (Table 96.2).[37] These definitions assist patients and their physicians in treatment planning.

Digital Mammography

Digital mammography is a newer technique of performing mammograms whereby images that are acquired are collected electronically and are stored on a computer in a digital format

TABLE 96.2. Ameican College of Radiology BIRADS Classification.

BIRADS classification	*Interpretation*	*Follow-up*
0: Assessment is incomplete	Finding on screening evaluation; more workup is needed	Complete the radiologic evaluation
1: Negative	Normal	Annual mammography after 40
2: Benign finding	No evidence of malignancy, but a characteristic benign lesion found (i.e., implant, cyst, intramammary lymph node)	Annual mammography after 40
3: Probably benign finding	Risk of malignancy 1%–2%	Short-term (4–6 month) mammographic follow-up
4: Suspicious abnormality	Lesion does not have absolute malignant characteristics, but a definite probability of cancer exists	Biopsy recommended
5: Highly suggestive of malignancy	High probability of breast cancer	Biopsy required

BIRADS, Breast Imaging Reporting and Data System.

analogous to a digital camera. These images can then be transferred to a monitor or to film. Radiologists are then able to easily manipulate the images by either enhancing or magnifying certain areas. A computer-assisted image checker can also be used. The Digital Mammographic Imaging Screening Trial (DMIST) prospectively evaluated 49,528 asymptomatic women with both digital and film screen mammography. Overall, both modalities were equivalent for screening, but digital was superior for women under fifty or premenopausal, or with dense breasts.[37a]

Other Imaging Modalities

Ultrasound is not a useful modality for screening but has a pivotal role in the evaluation of a palpable mass. It is increasingly being utilized because state-of-the-art, high-frequency, linear array, handheld transducers can interrogate lesions as small as 2 mm. Sonography is operator dependent and, if used for screening, irregularities in the normal glandular composition of the breast may be mistaken for masses. Additionally, cancers that are manifest as microcalcifications cannot be detected by ultrasound. Once a lesion is located, however, ultrasound is the only modality to reliably delineate solid from cystic structures. By ultrasound, a simple cyst is seen as a round, well-circumscribed, smooth-walled, hypoechoic structure, devoid of internal echoes with enhanced through transmission (Fig. 96.7). If the lesion is solid, ultrasound will accurately define size and contour. Ultrasound is also very useful to radiographically guide biopsies.

Breast magnetic resonance imaging (MRI) provides complementary information to the conventional modalities of mammography and ultrasound. In some studies, MRI has a sensitivity of 94% to 100% for invasive cancer but a specificity of only 37% to 97%.[38] Unfortunately, MRI has a sensitivity of only 17% in detecting DCIS.[39] Currently, MRI is the most sensitive method for determining the capsular integrity of the implants. It is especially sensitive for the detection of recurrent breast cancer, identification of multifocal cancers, evaluation of surgical scars, and assessment of brachial plexus involvement by tumor. Because dedicated breast coils are expensive, and construction of images labor intensive, MRI is reserved for those special circumstances where it has demonstrated utility.

Computed tomography (CT) may require contrast, results in higher radiation exposure, and is less able to identify small abnormalities. Its role, currently, is limited to evaluation of the internal mammary lymph nodes, as well as the chest wall and axilla postmastectomy. Furthermore, it is routinely used to detect symptomatic sites of metastatic disease.

Positron emission tomography (PET) is still under investigation. Because of uptake of radiolabeled tracer by the heart, evaluation of left-sided lesions can sometimes be compromised. Nevertheless, it holds promise for the detection of multicentric breast lesions, as well as evaluation of the nodal basins. Although CT can only identify lymph nodes that are abnormally enlarged, PET can localize normal-size nodes with increased tracer uptake. In a prospective study that evaluated the accuracy of PET in axillary nodal staging in 360 women with newly diagnosed breast cancer, PET had a 61% sensitivity and 80% specificity. PET was the least accurate in patients with small nodal metastases and with only a few lymph nodes involved. Based on these data, PET is believed not to be accurate enough to replace the sentinel lymph node mapping.[40]

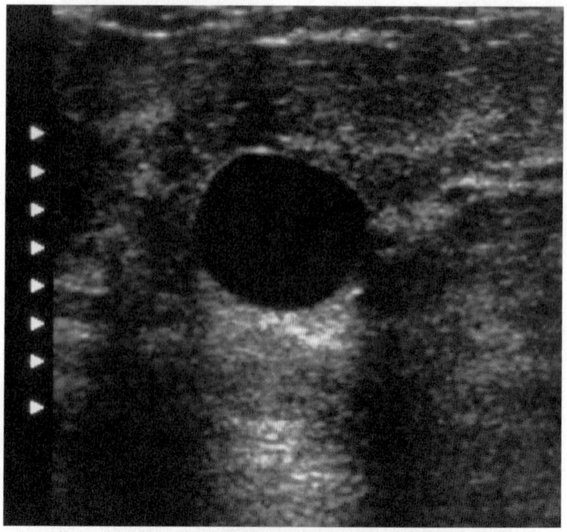

FIGURE 96.7. Ultrasound with characteristic findings of a simple cyst: a round, well-circumscribed, smooth-walled hypoechoic structure, devoid of internal echoes with enhanced through transmission. (Courtesy of M. Helvie, M.D.)

Ductoscopy and Ductal Lavage

Recently ductoscopy and ductal lavage have gained in popularity in screening women at high risk or those that have a nipple discharge. It is believed that by using these techniques it may be possible to detect hyperplastic noncancerous lesions early. Because these patients are at higher risk for breast cancer, they may benefit from chemoprevention. Ductal lavage uses microcatheters to obtain and identify malignant cells from small ducts. Ductoscopy is a technique that allows direct visualization of the ductal system, thereby detecting small abnormalities which may not be seen on mammogram or ultrasound. The first experiences were reported from Japan where their experience was limited by the scope size, inability to distend the duct, and the fragility of the fiberoptic scopes. American manufacturers have solved some of these problems, but clinical questions still exist of how best to apply these techniques in clinical practice.

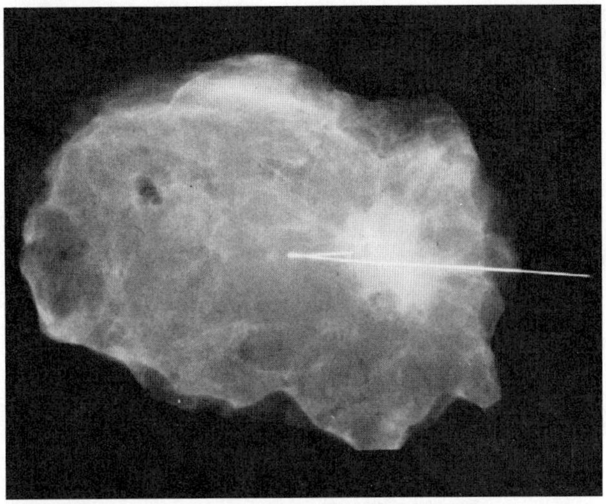

FIGURE 96.9. Specimen mammogram demonstrates removal of area with microcalcifications. (Courtesy of M. Helvie, M.D.)

Management of Nonpalpable Abnormalities

The widespread use of screening mammography has resulted in the increased detection of clinically occult breast lesions. Mammographic evaluation is best performed by an experienced radiologist, and some studies have shown that reading by two independent radiologists ("double reading") may improve sensitivity. Approximately 5% to 10% of all screened women require additional radiologic evaluation after a screening study. Most will have a normal diagnostic evaluation; however, for the subset of women classified as Breast Imaging Reporting and Data System (BIRADS) 4 or 5, biopsy is recommended.

Wire localization excisional breast biopsy historically has been the routine method for the diagnosis of the nonpalpable, mammographically detected, breast lesion (Fig. 96.8). The needle localization procedure begins with mammographically or sonographically guided needle placement into the site of radiologic abnormality. A wire is threaded through the needle, its location radiographically confirmed, and then the hook deployed. In the operating room, open surgical biopsy is performed with excision of tissue around the hook wire. A specimen radiograph must be performed to confirm the adequacy of excision (Fig. 96.9). Although still effective, it has been largely replaced by the less invasive percutaneous needle biopsy.

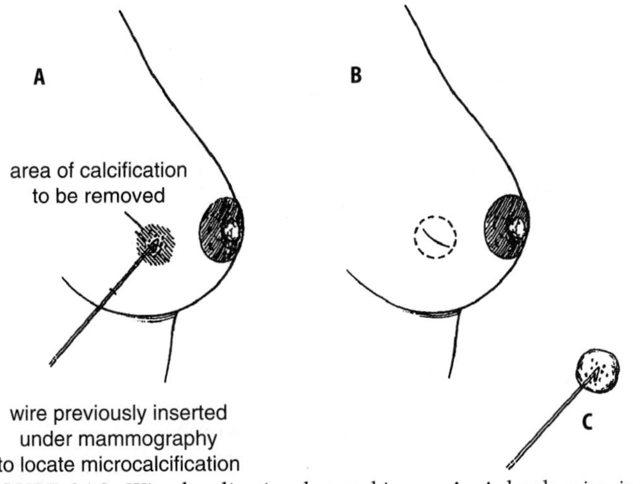

FIGURE 96.8. Wire localization breast biopsy. A. A hook wire is placed under mammographic guidance. B. Abnormal area is encompassed by excisional biopsy using the wire as a guide. C. Specimen and wire are sent for confirmatory mammogram and pathological examination. (From Hindle WH, ed. Breast Care: A Clinical Guidebook for Women's Primary Healthcare Providers. ©1999 by permission of Springer-Verlag, New York.)

Mammogram-guided percutaneous stereotactic core biopsy has several advantages over open wire localization biopsy (Fig. 96.10). It is faster, produces less scarring and breast deformity by limiting tissue removal, requires shorter convalescence, and is less costly. Diagnostic costs can be reduced at least 50% by performing stereotactic core versus open surgical biopsies.[41] Core biopsy is performed with a 9- to 14-gauge vacuum-assisted automated biopsy gun. The lesion to be biopsied is imaged in two projections, the position of the mammographic abnormality triangulated, and the three-dimensional location determined within the breast. With computer assistance, the *x*-, *y*-, and *z*-coordinates are calculated and relayed to the biopsy apparatus. Through a puncture site in the breast, successive samples are obtained. Specimen radiographs and postbiopsy images are obtained.

Many patients are ideally suited for core biopsy. In patients who do not desire breast conservation or are not candidates for it, core biopsy documentation of malignancy can eliminate premastectomy open biopsy. For a probably benign lesion, a definitive benign diagnosis by core biopsy obviates the need for excisional biopsy. In patients who have suspicious lesions and desire breast conservation, core biopsy is favored by some surgeons. For patients with a malignant diagnosis by core, a one-stage definitive surgical procedure can be performed with a large lumpectomy with greater likelihood of negative margins by this technique.[42] Some surgeons, however, prefer to proceed directly to wire localization biopsy for suspicious lesions. Benefits to this approach include a more thorough histological analysis, the ability to reexcise if margins are positive or close at the time of axillary dissection, and an early assessment by the patient of the acceptability of cosmesis of the lumpectomy, which may aid in decision making.

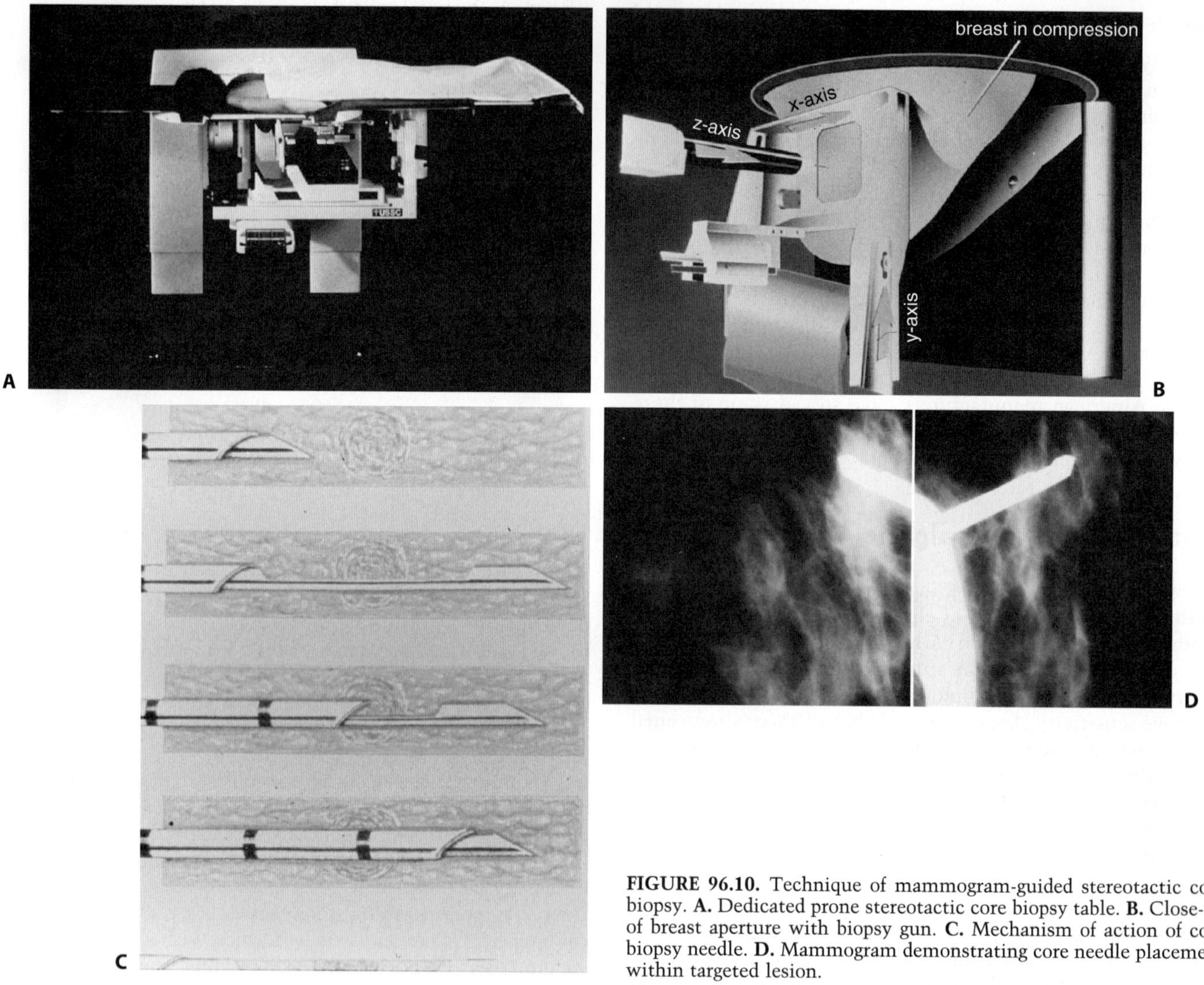

FIGURE 96.10. Technique of mammogram-guided stereotactic core biopsy. **A.** Dedicated prone stereotactic core biopsy table. **B.** Close-up of breast aperture with biopsy gun. **C.** Mechanism of action of core biopsy needle. **D.** Mammogram demonstrating core needle placement within targeted lesion.

Contraindications to stereotactic core biopsy include both patient-related and technical considerations. The patient must be able to lie unmoving in the prone position for as long as 45 min. Patients with significant anxiety, clinical arthritis, chronic cough, or severe kyphosis may not be able to meet this restriction. Technically, lesions located close to the chest wall, in the axillary tail, very superficial, or in small breasts that compress to less than 2.5 cm may not be amenable to core biopsy.

If pathological concordance with image characteristics is obtained, the specificity and sensitivity of core biopsy is greater than 90%.[43,44] If concordance is not established, rebiopsy must be undertaken. Cases of atypical ductal hyperplasia (ADH) or atypical lobular hyperplasic (ALH) diagnosed by core biopsy should undergo reexcision with wire localization because approximately 30% of lesions diagnosed as ADH/ALH by core will be found to have carcinoma at excisional biopsy.[45,46] A complete excision is also necessary to confirm the diagnosis of radial scar. In two of six radial scars, carcinoma was found at definitive surgical excision after core biopsy.[47] Similarly, as core biopsy is a sampling procedure, Jackman et al. observed that 8 of 43 (19%) cases of ductal carcinoma in situ diagnosed by core biopsy were found to contain areas of invasion after excision.[45] The multicenter trial by Parker and colleagues similarly demonstrated incomplete classification in 57 of 173 (33%) lesions initially classified as in situ or atypical hyperplasia.[48] Clinicians need to incorporate these data when counseling patients and determining treatment strategies.

Benign Breast Disease

It is estimated that one of every two women will see a physician for a breast complaint during her life.[49] Although breast cancer is the most common malignancy of American women, 80% to 90% of clinical evaluations for breast disorders are for benign conditions. Thus, the goal in the evaluation of a patient with an abnormal clinical breast examination is to avoid missing the diagnosis of a malignancy while providing reassurance for benign conditions.

Abnormal Clinical Breast Examination

An initial determination should be made whether the abnormality represents a true dominant mass versus a vague area of thickening or nodularity (Fig. 96.11). Normal breast texture, especially in premenopausal women, is heterogeneous and therefore vague thickening and nodularity is a common finding. The initial step in evaluating these areas is to compare that site with the mirror image area of the opposite breast. Symmetrical areas, especially in the upper outer quadrant, are seldom pathological. Reassurance with repeat clinical evaluation in 6 weeks [ideally on day 5–7 (follicular phase) for premenstrual women] is appropriate initial management. If the area remains stable on reexamination, no further intervention is necessary. If the area seems to progress, further workup with mammogram or breast ultrasound, depending on the patient's age, should be obtained. A radiographic abnormality with a subtle or vague palpable abnormality is best managed with a stereotactic core biopsy of the imaged lesion. Asymmetrical thickening and nodularity should be imaged initially. If radiologic evaluation is negative, 6-week clinical reevaluation is indicated. Stable areas at short-term follow-up can continue to be managed conservatively, whereas biopsy is warranted for any progressive abnormality. If a radiologic abnormality is identified, image-guided biopsy should be obtained.

The initial step in the evaluation of a dominant mass is to determine degree of suspicion (Fig. 96.12). Breast cancer generally presents as a hard, nontender, irregular mass; however, it is impossible to rule out cancer by clinical evaluation alone. Low-suspicion lesions in premenopausal women may be observed through one cycle. Complete resolution implies that the mass was a cyst.

A dominant mass that occurs in a postmenopausal woman, persists for one or more cycles in a premenopausal woman, or is suspicious requires additional evaluation and definitive histological diagnosis. Fine-needle aspiration (FNA), core needle biopsy, or urgent radiologic evaluation within 1 week is appropriate; however, there are some advantages in obtaining imaging studies first. Biopsy results in tissue disruption and even when performed by experienced physicians may result in hematoma formation significant enough to interfere with radiographic imaging. Additionally, mammography will ultimately be required to evaluate the remainder of the ipsilateral breast parenchyma and contralateral breast if a malignancy is diagnosed. In the ideal setting, same-day imaging followed by biopsy would be performed. If, however, there is a delay in radiologic evaluation, consider performing the biopsy first. Importantly, a negative mammogram in the setting of a clinically dominant mass should not delay biopsy because 10% of cancers are radiologically occult.

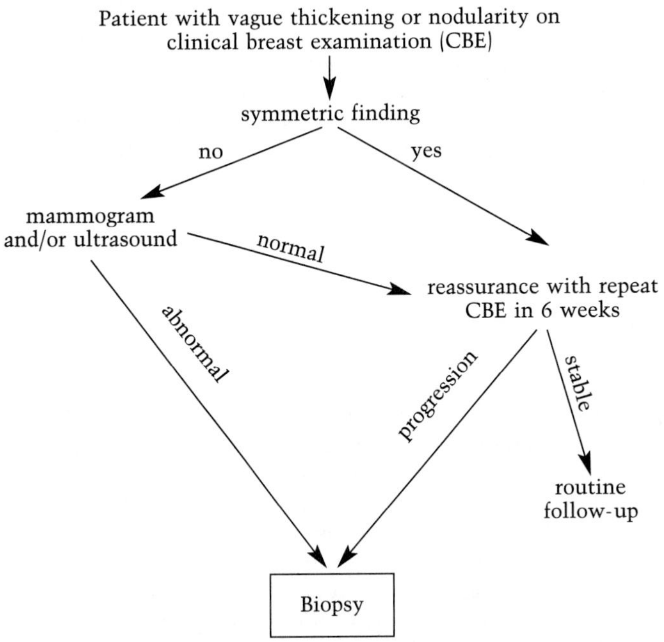

FIGURE 96.11. Algorithm for the management of vague thickening or nodularity.

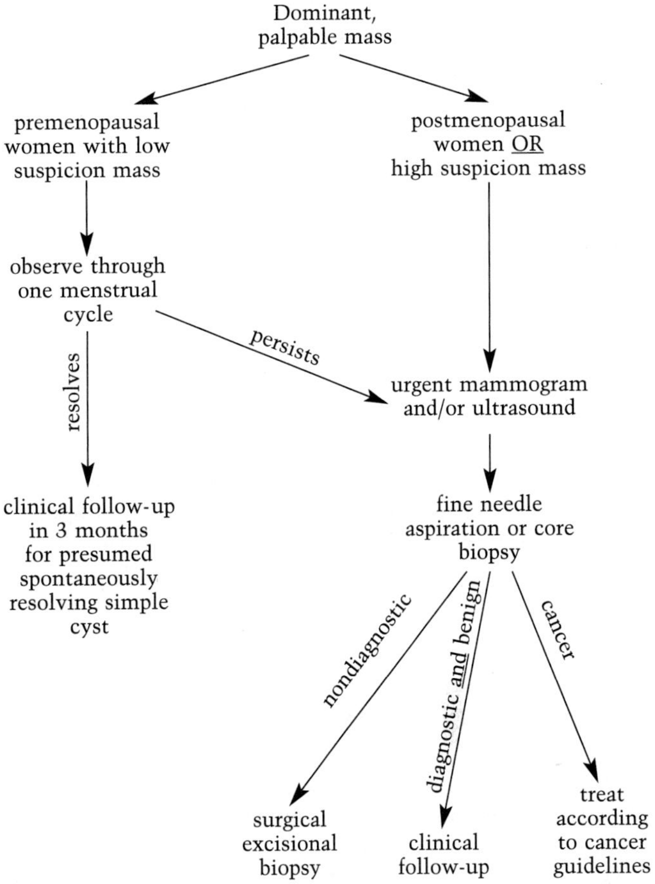

FIGURE 96.12. Algorithm for the management of a dominant palpable mass.

Specific Entities

Cyst

If a cyst is suspected clinically or documented sonographically, an FNA can be both diagnostic and therapeutic. Determination that a palpable mass is a cyst is impossible by physical examination alone, but sonography can confirm the diagnosis. Cysts may be classified as simple or complex based upon their appearance on ultrasound. A simple cyst is a round, well-circumscribed, smooth-walled structure that is anechoic and has enhanced through transmission. A complex cyst has central septations, indistinct margins, or internal echoes. An asymptomatic, simple cyst found incidentally on screening evaluation may be observed. Simple cysts that are large, painful, or interfere with radiologic evaluation should be aspirated. Complex cysts should be aspirated to confirm the diagnosis. Indications for excisional biopsy after cyst aspiration include grossly bloody fluid, residual mass postaspiration, or cyst reaccumulation in the same location two or three times postaspiration. Therefore, a follow-up physical examination should be performed 4 to 6 weeks postaspiration. Cytological analysis of clear, straw-colored fluid is not necessary or helpful; however, if the character of the fluid is atypical, cytological analysis must be obtained.

The pathogenesis of cyst formation is not well understood; however, cyst formation is undoubtedly influenced by ovarian hormones. Cysts often suddenly appear in midmenstrual cycle then spontaneously regress with the onset of menses. Cysts most commonly occur after age 35. The incidence of cystic disease increases steadily until menopause, when cysts are rare except in women on hormone replacement therapy. Therefore, any lesion presumed to be a cyst in a postmenopausal woman not on hormone replacement therapy must be proven to be fluid filled by needle aspiration. Intracystic carcinoma, however, is very rare.

Fibrocystic Breast Disease

Fibrocystic breast disease is a generalized process of microscopic cyst formation, often accompanied by breast nodularity, with stromal proliferation. Ovarian hormones are again implicated, and fibrocystic changes seem to represent an exaggerated response of the breast epithelium. Because these alterations represent variation in normal physiology some clinicians prefer to term the process a fibrocystic condition, reserving "disease" for patients with symptoms significant enough to require intervention. Clinical evaluation of women with fibrocystic changes reveal firm nodular breast tissue with multiple palpable abnormalities corresponding to macrocysts. These women often have significant tenderness with examination and may have clear, greenish, or brown nipple discharge. Although pain is not an indication for surgical therapy, a dominant mass, even in the setting of fibrocystic changes, requires confirmation by aspiration or biopsy. Cancer risk varies with histological type. As demonstrated by Dupont and Page, the greatest risk occurs in women with proliferative disease with atypia.[8] Women with biopsy-proven atypical ductal or lobular hyperplasia have a 4.4-fold increased cancer risk. If this is combined with a positive family history, the risk increases to 9-fold. A more mild risk elevation, 1.5- to 2-fold, is found in women with proliferative changes without atypia such as sclerosing adenosis, moderate or florid hyperplasia, and papilloma with fibrovascular core. Women with nonproliferative fibrocystic breast disease do not have a demonstrable increased breast cancer risk.

Mastalgia

Breast pain (mastalgia or mastodynia) is one of the most common breast symptoms. Evaluation should include a thorough history of the character, chronicity, and aggravating factors for the pain. Mastalgia should be characterized as cyclic or noncyclic. Cyclical mastalgia varies in intensity throughout the menstrual cycle. It is most severe immediately before menstruation, then resolves with the onset of menses. It is the most frequent type, and may occur unilaterally or bilaterally. Noncyclic mastalgia bears no relationship to the menstrual cycle. It may be continuous or intermittent, is more commonly unilateral and sharp in character, and often occurs in the fourth decade. Chest wall musculoskeletal abnormalities (i.e., costochondritis) may mimic noncyclic mastalgia.

Breast examination should determine the presence of fibrocystic changes (diffuse tender nodularity), whether a dominant mass distinct from the background nodularity is present, and if skin changes or nipple discharge are present. Women over 35 years should have a mammogram or ultrasound. In the absence of findings on physical examination and mammography, treatment of mastalgia should consist of reassurance and conservative measures. Eighty-five percent of patients will have some relief of their symptoms after having been reassured.[50] Breast pain in the absence of palpable or mammographic abnormality rarely represents carcinoma.

Of the 15% of patients who require further treatment, one-half to one-third of women achieve significant improvement in their symptoms with conservative measures such as caffeine elimination and nicotine and alcohol reduction, as well as change to a better-fitting or more supportive brassiere. Also patients who decrease their fat content to less than 15% have a significant improvement in their tenderness.[51] If symptoms persist, medications may be indicated. In one of the only positive prospective randomized trials of intervention for mastalgia, oral administration of evening primrose oil reduced or eliminated breast pain in 50% of women with cyclic mastalgia.[52] For women with disabling pain, and a negative physical and mammographic evaluation, danazol (an androgenic agent) or bromocriptine (a prolactin antagonist) may be effective therapy.[53,54] The significant side effects including weight gain, hirsutism, acne, irregular menses, and headache often limit patient acceptance and compliance with therapy, reducing the overall response rate. For most patients, reassurance and nonsteroidal analgesics are the only necessary therapy. Cyclic mastalgia is more responsive to therapy and usually spontaneously resolves with menopause. Nevertheless, several studies have failed to demonstrate a difference in circulating estrogen levels in women with mastalgia and pain-free controls. Follow-up is required to evaluate symptom management with intervention as well as to document the absence of an evolving abnormality on physical examination.

Nipple Discharge

Evaluation of a patient with nipple discharge should begin with an attempt to classify it as physiological, pathological, or galactorrhea. Although frightening for the patient, nipple discharge usually has a benign etiology. Only 6% to 12% of patients with nipple discharge have carcinoma.[55,56] The likelihood of carcinoma is increased if the discharge is bloody (however, 10% of cancers have serous discharge), there is an associated mass, or the patient is postmenopausal.

Physiological discharge is usually bilateral, nonspontaneous, and from multiple ducts. It is clear, yellow, green, or brown. The drainage may be evoked by mammography, sexual stimulation, or multiple medications. Many drugs, especially phenothiazines, tricyclic antidepressants, reserpine, butyrophenones, cimetidine, verapamil, metoclopramide, thiazide

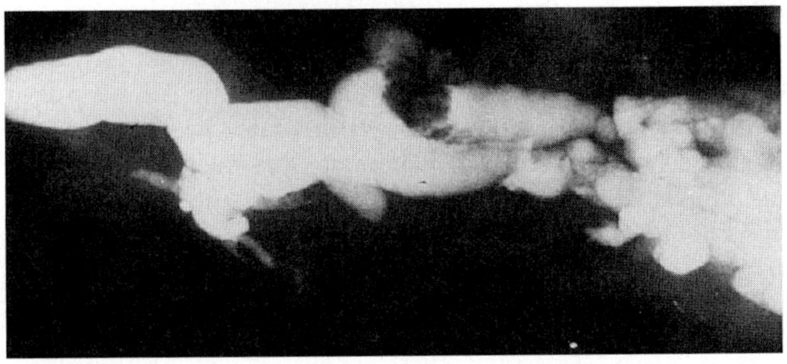

FIGURE 96.13. Ductogram demonstrating multiple intraluminal filling defects. (Courtesy of M. Helvie, MD.)

diuretics, or hormone replacement can be associated with nipple discharge. If physical examination, mammography, and hemoccult testing for blood are all negative, no additional treatment or testing is necessary, and the patient may be reassured the discharge is benign.

Pathological nipple discharge is unilateral, spontaneously arising from one duct. The drainage may be clear, brownish, or bloody. Benign intraductal papilloma is the most common cause of bloody nipple discharge. The specific location of the draining duct may be elicited by manually expressing the drainage, working circumferentially around the areolar complex. Hemoccult testing of the drainage should be performed. Cytological evaluation is rarely useful. As with the evaluation of any breast complaint, a thorough breast examination, and mammogram in women over 35 years of age, must be performed and any abnormality further investigated. In the absence of another lesion, ductogram may be pursued (Fig. 96.13). Galactography may provide a surgical road map by identifying an intraluminal filling defect consistent with an intraductal papilloma. An approximate distance from the nipple, and in cases of diffuse papillomatosis extent of ductal involvement, can be determined by ductogram, and this information may alter surgical treatment. Additionally, a ductogram may identify diffusely dilated subareolar ducts consistent with duct ectasia. In women who still desire preservation of the ability to breastfeed, solitary duct excision may be performed for an isolated abnormality; this is greatly facilitated by insertion of a small lacrimal probe into the discharging duct. For other women, excision of all the central ducts is the procedure of choice.

Not all whitish discharge is galactorrhea. True galactorrhea contains fat, lactose, and milk-specific proteins. The discharge is bilateral, and arises from multiple ducts. Lactation is the most common cause of galactorrhea; however, medications, chest wall trauma, and hypothyroidism are also implicated. In one-third of women with galactorrhea, especially if associated with amenorrhea, an elevated serum prolactin will confirm a pituitary origin. If the prolactin level is elevated, an MRI scan of the sella turcica should be obtained.

Gynecomastia

Gynecomastia is hypertrophy of male breast tissue. Pubertal hypertrophy occurs during adolescence, whereas senescent hypertrophy occurs in the elderly. Imbalance in the testosterone to estrogen ratio has been implicated in both forms. In puberty, estrogen levels may rise before testosterone production, and in the elderly testosterone levels may fall with maintenance of physiological estrogen levels. This relative hormonal imbalance accounts for the bimodal prevalence of gynecomastia. Gynecomastia can also be seen in any condition that alters hormonal production or clearance, such as Klinefelter's syndrome, testicular feminization, testicular failure, testicular tumors, ectopic estrogen secretion, hepatic failure, renal failure, or drug related. Several commonly used medications can exacerbate senescent gynecomastia including cimetidine, thiazides, digoxin, theophylline, phenothiazines, androgens or estrogens, and marijuana. Discontinuation of the implicated drug may not result in regression; however, it may halt further hypertrophy.

Clinical evaluation must begin with a thorough history of prescribed and illicit drug use, evaluation for signs of kidney or liver dysfunction, and testicular examination to rule out the existence of a tumor. Breast examination is critical. Gynecomastia presents as a smooth, firm, symmetrical, discoid lesion immediately beneath the nipple–areolar complex. This must be differentiated from generalized fat deposition in the obese and the often eccentric, hard, irregular mass of male breast cancer. Gynecomastia can often be unilateral. Mammography can accurately differentiate these clinical scenarios. If a testicular tumor is suspected, testicular sonogram can be confirmatory. Laboratory evaluation of liver and renal function can confirm other suspected etiologies.

Management of gynecomastia involves identification and correction of the underlying cause. If any question exists regarding the benignity of the condition, biopsy may be required. For patients with aesthetic concerns, chest wall sculpting with liposuction is now replacing subcutaneous mastectomy as the treatment of choice for optimal cosmesis.

Breast Infection and Abscess

Breast infections are broadly categorized as lactational versus nonpuerperal, and mastitis versus abscess. Puerperal mastitis is thought to originate from the reflux of bacteria into the milk-containing breast by the nursing infant. It is especially prevalent during periods of increased engorgement such as weaning. Duct obstruction, inspissation of milk, and incomplete emptying have been implicated as factors facilitating bacterial growth. Treatment involves oral antibiotics to cover gram-positive cocci, local heat or ice packs, and frequent nursing or pumping to prevent engorgement. Women do not need to discontinue breast feeding as there is no risk of transmission of the bacterial infections to the infant; however, antibiotics approved for use by nursing mothers should be selected.

Nonlactational mastitis is often a complication of duct ectasia, an irregular dilatation of the subareolar ducts. The ducts fill with secretions, debris, and keratin, and chronic inflammation results. Manifestations of this periductal mastitis include nipple discharge, recurrent subareolar abscesses, mammary fistula (Zuska's disease), and nipple retraction. These infections are more likely to be polymicrobial with a mix of gram-positive cocci and skin anaerobes. Treatment involves broad-spectrum oral antibiotics, analgesics, and local comfort measures.

Once abscess formation occurs, therapy must include surgical incision and drainage. Breast abscesses in lactating women rarely present with a fluctuant mass because of the dense fibrous septa. Clinically, these women present with fever, leukocytosis, and point tenderness. Ultrasonography can be confirmatory. Incision and drainage should be performed under general anesthesia because it is too painful to adequately break up the loculations under local anesthesia. Breastfeeding must be discontinued because the cavity should be left open and packed. The wall of the abscess cavity should be biopsied to rule out necrotic cancer as an etiology of the infections, especially for spontaneous abscesses in nonlactating women. Subareolar abscesses can be especially difficult to eradicate, are often recurrent, and may require excision of the entire subareolar duct complex.

All patients with mastitis or abscess should be followed until complete resolution is documented. Inflammatory carcinoma may mimic mastitis with erythema and skin edema; however, it will not improve with a trial of antibiotic therapy. Failure to respond to an initial cycle of antibiotics should not prompt a change to another antibiotic until mammography and punch biopsy of the skin rule out malignancy.

Mondor's Disease

Mondor's disease, thrombophlebitis of the superficial breast veins (lateral thoracic or cutaneous superior thoracoepigastric), is another benign condition that may mimic carcinoma. Clinically, this may cause breast retraction associated with a palpable cord usually leading to the axilla, or coursing inferomedially onto the anterior abdominal wall. Mammography must be performed to rule out associated malignancy, and duplex ultrasound often can document the presence of the thrombosis. Antiinflammatory analgesics and local measures can improve patient comfort. Rarely, excision of residual bands may be necessary for cosmetic reasons.

Fibroadenoma

Fibroadenoma is a benign, solid lesion composed of both stromal and epithelial elements. Clinically, they are the most common mass in women under 30 years of age, with a peak incidence of 21 to 25 years. They present as rubbery, lobulated, well-circumscribed, highly mobile masses on physical examination. Although usually single, multiple fibroadenomas occur in 15% of affected patients. Radiographically, they may have a lobulated appearance suggestive of a fibroadenoma. In postmenopausal women, fibroadenomas may involute, hyalinize, or calcify and on mammography have dense calcifications or a popcorn-like appearance. As with any solid mass, malignancy cannot be excluded on clinical or radiographic criteria alone and tissue confirmation must be obtained. Fine-needle aspiration or core needle biopsy can be confirmatory and obviate the need for open biopsy in select patients. Cryoablation is a newer technique that has been used to treat both benign and malignant breast disease. A noninsulated probe is positioned in the area by ultrasound guidance and liquid nitrogen or argon is used to create a freezing effect. Multiple freeze-thaw cycles are used to create maximum local tissue destruction. This technique has been shown to eliminate the need of excision as the majority of lesions regress over time. Percutaneous large-core needle vacuum-assisted excision has also been used successfully as a minimally invasive strategy for the treatment of patients with fibroadenomas. Most women, however, choose to undergo excisional biopsy to establish the diagnosis, obviate the need for long-term follow-up, and prevent the possibility of growth during pregnancy when biopsy is slightly more complicated. Fibroadenoma growth has not been found to be influenced by oral contraceptive use; however, premenstrual tenderness, and growth with pregnancy and lactation, are common features. Although fibroadenomas themselves are not thought to have malignant potential, the epithelial elements, as all breast epithelium, are at risk. More than 160 cases of carcinomas arising in fibroadenomas appear in the literature.[57,58] Of these cases, 20% to 50% were clinically misdiagnosed. Nevertheless, the risk of carcinoma in a young woman with fibroadenoma is exceedingly rare and should not influence therapy.

Juvenile Fibroadenoma

Juvenile or giant fibroadenomas are fibroadenomas that attain unusually large size (greater than 5 cm) and commonly occur in adolescence. These lesions may display rapid growth, but are benign, and excisional surgery is curative. Histologically, these lesions tend to be more cellular than typical fibroadenomas and must be differentiated from cystosarcoma phyllodes. At least one author has proposed that these lesions can be managed nonoperatively if physical examination, ultrasound, and fine-needle aspiration are concordant.[58]

Hamartoma

Hamartoma of the breast is a benign lesion best characterized as an adenofibrolipoma. It is an exceptionally soft lesion and may be difficult to appreciate on physical examination even when very sizable. On mammography, it is an easily visualized, well-circumscribed lesion impossible to differentiate from the more common fibroadenoma. Because of the fatty composition of the mass, it is often difficult to obtain an adequate specimen for cytological evaluation by fine-needle aspiration. Therefore, if hamartoma is clinically suspected, surgical excision is preferable as well as curative.

Adenoma

Tubular and lactational adenomas are also histologically benign lesions related to fibroadenomas. They are characterized by glandular structures with minimal to absent supporting stromal structures. Clinically and radiographically, they resemble fibroadenomas as well. Lactational adenomas occur during pregnancy and lactation, may increase in size under the influence of gestational hormones, and have secretory differentiation on histological analysis. Again, excisional biopsy is diagnostic and curative.

Papillary Lesions

Solitary intraductal papilloma is the most common papillary breast lesion. They most frequently occur in women 35 to 55 years of age, usually arise as a single lesion, in a subareolar duct, and are manifest by bloody nipple discharge. Intraductal papillomas occurring in peripheral ducts present as mammographic or palpable masses. Ductography may be helpful, and solitary or central duct excision is the treatment of choice.

Multiple papillomas are usually located grouped together in the periphery of the breast and thus rarely present as nipple discharge. More than 98% of multiple papillomas are palpable, and clinically they mimic fibroadenomas. They are bilateral in 15% of patients, and after excision almost one-third will recur. They are frequently associated with atypical ductal hyperplasia, and up to 30% of women with multiple papillomas will develop breast cancer, which is believed to arise in the altered adjacent epithelium.

Juvenile papillomatosis is a lesion characterized by epithelial hyperplasia and not true papillary growth. Two-thirds of the cases occur in women under 20, the remainder in women under 30. Seventy percent of affected females have a family history of breast carcinoma; however, evidence does not support an increased risk of cancer development in these women. The degree of subsequent cancer risk appears more directly related to the presence of atypia in the lesion and the positive family history. Treatment is surgical excision of the involved tissue.

Sclerosing Adenosis

Sclerosing adenosis is the benign proliferation of both stromal tissue (sclerosis) associated with an increase in the small terminal ductules (adenosis). It is usually a component of fibrocystic disease and is manifest as microcalcifications found on screening mammogram. Stereotactic core or wire localization biopsy is diagnostic. No further therapy is necessary if this lesion is found as the etiology of microcalcifications on biopsy.

Fat Necrosis

Fat necrosis is another sclerosing lesion. Because it is not an epithelial abnormality, it has no malignant potential. Lipid-laden macrophages against a background of chronic inflammation and scar tissue establishes the diagnosis. Fat necrosis may present as a mass, or mammographic density with distortion of the surrounding tissue secondary to the chronic inflammation, thereby simulating cancer. It may follow an episode of recognized or occult trauma, prior surgical intervention, or in large pendulous breasts. It is usually biopsied to differentiate it from cancer.

Breast Cancer Staging

Even though pathological evaluation of the primary breast tumor and axillary lymph node status are the most important determinants of survival, accurate clinical staging is important. Preoperative diagnostic and therapeutic interventions are based on careful assessment of the clinical extent of disease. Many staging classifications exist; however, the TNM system of the American Joint Committee on Cancer (AJCC) and the International Union Against Cancer (UICC) is the one most widely used for breast cancer.[59] The three significant events in the natural history of tumorigenesis are included in the TNM classification: local tumor growth (T), spread to regional lymph nodes (N), and distant metastatic spread (M).

At presentation, a patient's TNM status should be determined (Table 96.3). On staging physical examination primary tumor size and degree of axillary nodal involvement should be estimated. It is recognized that clinical staging of the axilla has a false negative rate of 30%.[60] Furthermore, breast cancer is currently believed to have systemic micrometastases at the time of diagnosis. Nevertheless, some general treatment guidelines can be based on clinical tumor staging.

All patients with invasive breast cancer should have a thorough history and physical examination, chest X-ray, complete blood count, and chemical profile. Asymptomatic stage I or II patients with normal findings on these studies do not require further metastatic evaluation because the likelihood of finding occult metastatic disease has been estimated to be 2% to 3%. Patients with stage IIIA or B disease, however, should undergo screening bone scan and computed tomography because of the increased possibility of distant metastases. Additionally, as discussed earlier, neoadjuvant chemotherapy may be appropriate for patients with stage III breast cancer. Metastatic, stage IV disease occurs most frequently in the bone, lung, or liver; however, any nodal or visceral site may become involved.

Ductal Carcinoma In Situ

Ductal carcinoma in situ (DCIS), noninvasive ductal carcinoma, and intraductal carcinoma are the same entities. Before the widespread use of screening mammography, DCIS presented as a palpable mass, nipple discharge, or an incidental finding on biopsy and accounted for 2% of diagnosed malignancies. Today, in some series it represents 30% of all malignancies found by screening.[61] DCIS is thought to be a precursor of invasive carcinoma, and therefore once recognized, treatment is indicated. Data supporting this position are multiple. First, if left untreated DCIS will progress to invasive carcinoma in up to 50% of women; moreover, the cancers that develop are ductal in origin and occur at the site of the original biopsy. These data are from instances in which the in situ lesion was initially misclassified as benign then found on further review of the pathology to be DCIS; thus, these women were treated with biopsy alone. Page et al. found progression to invasive carcinoma in 7 of 25 patients, and in a similar study Rosen et al. documented subsequent invasive cancer in 8 of 15 patients.[62,63]

The second piece of evidence that DCIS is a precursor lesion is from recurrence data after breast-conserving therapy. In patients with DCIS treated with lumpectomy, 87% of treatment failures occur at or close to the lumpectomy bed rather than at distant sites.[64] Left untreated, DCIS will progress to invasive ductal carcinoma 30% of the time over 10 years.[62,65] Invasive ductal carcinoma is found in 50% of treatment failures from DCIS, and one-third of women with invasive cancer develop metastatic disease. Further, assessment of the natural history of DCIS may be possible by determining the incidence of DCIS on autopsy studies of women who expired of nonbreast causes. Because the breasts are not generally examined in the routine performance of an autopsy, several investigators specifically addressed this question. Alpers et al. found a 6% incidence of DCIS and Bartow et al. a 0.2% incidence in a younger population.[66,67] These data imply that the identification of this lesion is significant and that therapy is warranted.

For many years, simple mastectomy was the treatment of choice for DCIS. Survival approached 99%.[68,69] The 1% to 4%

TABLE 96.3. Definition of TMN, Stage Grouping, Histopathologic Type, and Histologic Grade for Breast Carcinoma.

Definition of TMN

Primary Tumor (T)

Definitions for classifying the primary tumor (T) are the same for clinical and for pathologic classification. If the measurement is made by physical examination, the examiner will use the major headings (T1, T2, or T3). If other measurements, such as mammographic or pathologic measurements, are used, the subsets of T1 can be used. Tumors should be measured to the nearest 0.1 cm increment.

TX	Primary tumor cannot be assessed
T0	No evidence of primary tumor
Tis	Carcinoma *in situ*
Tis (DCIS)	Ductal carcinoma *in situ*
Tis (LCIS)	Lobular carcinoma *in situ*
Tis (Paget's)	Paget's disease of the nipple with no tumor

Note: Paget's disease associated with a tumor is classified according to the size of the tumor.

T1	Tumor 2 cm or less in greatest dimension
T1mic	Microinvasion 0.1 cm or less in greatest dimension
T1a	Tumor more than 0.1 cm but not more than 0.5 cm in greatest dimension
T1b	Tumor more than 0.5 cm but not more than 1 cm in greatest dimension
T1c	Tumor more than 1 cm but not more than 2 cm in greatest dimension
T2	Tumor more than 2 cm but not more than 5 cm in greatest dimension
T3	Tumor more than 5 cm in greatest dimension
T4	Tumor of any size with direct extension to (a) chest wall or (b) skin, only as described below
T4a	Extension to chest wall, not including pectoralis muscle
T4b	Edema (including peau d'orange) or ulceration of the skin of the breast, or satellite skin nodules confined to the same breast
T4c	Both T4a and T4b
T4d	Inflammatory carcinoma

Regional Lymph Nodes (N)

Clinical

NX	Regional lymph nodes cannot be assessed (e.g., previously removed)
N0	No regional lymph node metastasis
N1	Metastasis to movable ipsilateral lymph node(s)
N2	Metastasis to ipsilateral axillary lymph nodes fixed or matted, or clinically apparent* ipsilateral internal mammary nodes in the *absence* of clinically evident axillary lymph node metastasis
N2a	Metastasis to ipsilateral axillary lymph nodes fixed to one another (matted) or to other structures
N2b	Metastasis only in clinically apparent* ipsilateral internal mammary nodes and in the *absence* of clinically evident axillary lymph node metastasis
N3	Metastasis in ipsilateral infraclavicular lymph node(s) with or without axillary lymph node involvement, or in clinically apparent* ipsilateral internal mammary node(s) and in the *presence* of clinically evident axillary lymph node metastasis; or metastasis in ipsilateral supraclavicular lymph node(s) with or without axillary or internal mammary lymph node involvement
N3a	Metastasis in ipsilateral infraclavicular lymph node(s)
N3b	Metastasis in ipsilateral internal mammary node(s) and axillary lymph node(s)
N3c	Metastasis in ipsilateral supraclavicular lymph node(s)

**Clinically apparent* is defined as detected by imaging studies (excluding lymphoscintigraphy) or by clinical examination or grossly visible pathologically.

Pathologic (pN)[a]

pNX	Regional lymph nodes cannot be assessed (e.g., previously removed, or not removed for pathologic study)
pN0	No regional lymph node metastasis histologically, no additional examination for isolated tumor cells (ITC)

Note: Isolated tumor cells (ITC) are defined as single tumor cells or small cell clusters not greater than 0.2 mm, usually detected only by immunohistochemical (IHC) or molecular methods but which may be verified on H&E stains. ITCs do not usually show evidence of malignant activity, e.g., proliferation or stromal reaction.

pN0(i–)	No regional lymph node metastasis histologically, negative IHC
pN0(i+)	No regional lymph node metastasis histologically, positive IHC, no IHC cluster greater than 0.2 mm
pN0(mol–)	No regional lymph node metastasis histologically, negative molecular findings (RT-PCR)[b]
pN0(mol+)	No regional lymph node metastasis histologically, positive molecular findings (RT-PCR)[b]

[a]Classification is based on axillary lymph node dissection with or without sentinel lymph node dissection. Classification based solely on sentinel lymph node dissection without subsequent axillary lymph node dissection is designated (sn) for "sentinel node," e.g., pN0(i+) (sn).

[b]RT-PRC: reverse transcriptase/polymerase chain reaction.

pN1	Metastasis in 1 to 3 axillary lymph nodes and/or in internal mammary nodes with microscopic disease detected by sentinel lymph node dissection but not clinically apparent**
pN1mi	Micrometastasis (greater than 0.2 mm, none greater than 2.0 mm)
pN1a	Metastasis in 1 to 3 axillary lymph nodes
pN1b	Metastasis in internal mammary nodes microscopic disease detected by sentinel lymph node dissection but not clinically apparent**
pN1c	Metastasis in 1 to 3 axillary lymph nodes and in internal mammary lymph nodes with microscopic disease detected by sentinel lymph node dissection but not clinically apparent.** (If associated with greater than 3 positive axillary lymph nodes, the internal mammary nodes are classified as pN3b to reflect increased tumor burden)
pN2	Metastasis in 4 to 9 axillary lymph nodes, or in clinically apparent* internal mammary lymph nodes in the *absence* of axillary lymph node metastasis
pN2a	Metastasis in 4 to 9 axillary lymph nodes (at least one tumor deposit greater 2.0 mm)
pN2b	Metastasis in clinically apparent* internal mammary lymph nodes in the *absence* of axillary lymph node metastasis
pN3	Metastasis in 10 or more axillary lymph nodes, or in infraclavicular lymph nodes, or in clinically apparent* ipsilateral internal mammary lymph nodes in the *presence* of 1 or more positive axillary lymph nodes; or in more than 3 axillary lymph nodes with clinically negative microscopic metastasis in internal mammary lymph nodes; or in ipsilateral supraclavicular lymph nodes
pN3a	Metastasis in 10 or more axillary lymph nodes (at least one tumor deposit greater than 2.0 mm), or metastasis to the infraclavicular lymph nodes
pN3b	Metastasis in clinically apparent* ipsilateral internal mammary lymph nodes in the *presence* of 1 or more positive axillary lymph nodes; or in more than 3 axillary lymph nodes and in internal mammary lymph nodes with microscopic disease detected by sentinel lymph node dissection but not clinically apparent**
pN3c	Metastasis in ipsilateral supraclavicular lymph nodes

**Clinically apparent* is defined as detected by imaging studies (excluding lymphoscintigraphy) or by clinical examination.

***Not clinically apparent* is defined as not detected by imaging studies (excluding lymphoscintigraphy) or by clinical examination.

TABLE 96.3. *Continued*

Distant Metastasis (M)			
MX	Distant metastasis cannot be assessed		
M0	No distant metastasis		
M1	Distant metastasis		
Stage Grouping			
Stage 0	Tis	N0	M0
Stage I	T1*	N0	M0
Stage IIA	T0	N1	M0
	T1*	N1	M0
	T2	N0	M0
Stage IIB	T2	N1	M0
	T3	N0	M0
Stage IIIA	T0	N2	M0
	T1*	N2	M0
	T2	N2	M0
	T3	N1	M0
	T3	N2	M0
Stage IIIB	T4	N0	M0
	T4	N1	M0
	T4	N2	M0
Stage IIIC	Any T	N3	M0
Stage IV	Any T	Any N	M1

*T1 includes T1mic.

Note: Stage designation may be changed if post-surgical imaging studies reveal the presence of distant metastases, provided that the studies are carried out within 4 months of diagnosis in the absence of disease progression and provided that the patient has not received neoadjuvant therapy.

Source: Used with the permission of the American Joint Committee on Cancer (AJCC), Chicago, Illinois. The original source for this material is the *AJCC Cancer Staging Manual, Sixth Edition* (2002) published by Springer Science and Business Media LLC, www.springerlink.com

incidence of lymph node metastasis as well as 1% mortality has often been attributed to unrecognized foci of microinvasion.[70] Currently, breast conservation is deemed an acceptable alternative in select patients. Lumpectomy must be to negative margins, and radiation therapy is routinely advocated. The NSABP B-17 study compared wide excision alone to excision plus radiation therapy in patients with localized DCIS and clinically negative axillary lymph nodes. Preliminary results indicate that radiation decreased recurrence rates by 50% from 16.4% to 7%, decreased ipsilateral invasive cancer from 8.2% to 2%, and improved 5-year event-free survival from 74% to 84%. Eight-year follow-up confirmed these preliminary results.[71]

Survival with breast conservation is believed to be equivalent to that with mastectomy. Patient choice is one factor in deciding between breast conservation and mastectomy. The patient must weigh the small but real risk of a local recurrence, possibly as invasive cancer, versus the cosmetic implications of mastectomy. Careful mammographic and pathological assessment can often determine which patients are not candidates for lumpectomy. Patients better treated by mastectomy include those with multicentric disease, disease not able to be encompassed in a cosmetically acceptable lumpectomy, and those with persistently positive margins after reexcision lumpectomy.

Because of the low (2%) risk of axillary involvement, routine axillary lymph node dissection is not performed. Certain patients, however, may benefit from one or more sampling procedures. Patients undergoing mastectomy for diffuse DCIS have up to a 20% incidence of invasive carcinoma being found on final pathology when the DCIS as manifest by microcalcifications covered more than a 2.5-cm mammographic area[72]; this is especially true when the DCIS was diagnosed by stereotactic core biopsy and thus only a pathological sampling was performed. If indicated, sentinel lymph node biopsy may provide a more precise surgical staging of DCIS. Currently, there are no trials evaluating routine addition of sentinel lymph node biopsy to standard surgery for DCIS; however, Albertini and co-workers found a 4% incidence of sentinel lymph nodal positivity in patients undergoing mastectomy for diffuse DCIS.[73]

Another controversial issue is the omission of radiation therapy in a select subset of well-informed patients with favorable presentations of DCIS. Many classification schemes have been devised to further characterize DCIS. The most popular is the Van Nuys Prognostic Index for DCIS.[73a] Patients are stratified into three groups based upon primary tumor characteristics (Table 96.4). Comedo-type DCIS has prominent intraductal necrosis and is believed to represent a more aggressive form of DCIS. Tumor grade is also of prognostic significance. In 2001, the University of California found that age was an independent prognostic factor for local recurrence. The index was thus modified to reflect a patient's age. Local recurrence in 238 patients with DCIS was 3.8% in group 1, 11.1% in group 2, and 26.5% in group 3[73a]; this translated into a difference in 8-year survival as well. Although data are limited, some advocate that women with non-comedo DCIS less than 1 cm in size and excised to widely negative margins (approximately 1 cm) may forego radiation. These patients often have had the DCIS found incidentally on biopsy performed for another indication, or with a very small cluster of microcalcifications. Women who opt to not undergo radiation must understand that this is currently not the standard of care and that long-term data are unavailable.

Management of the contralateral breast in patients with DCIS continues to evolve. Surgical procedures on the opposite breast are hard to support in absence of data documenting an increased contralateral risk. Tamoxifen is now given as an adjuvant therapy in those patients with estrogen receptor-positive DCIS. The NSABP B-24 trial randomized 1804 patients with DCIS treated by lumpectomy plus radiation therapy to placebo versus tamoxifen. After a mean follow-up of 64 months, the addition of tamoxifen was associated with a decrease in all breast cancer events. Invasive ipsilateral breast cancers had a 3.4% cumulative incidence at 5 years in the control group versus 2.1% in the tamoxifen-treated patients. In the contralateral breast, the risk was reduced from 3.4% with placebo to 2.0% with tamoxifen. A similar decrease in noninvasive carcinomas was also identified. Interestingly, 15% of patients in each arm had histologically

TABLE 96.4. The University of Southern California/Van Nuys Prognostic Index Scoring System.

Score	*1*	*2*	*3*
Size (mm)	<15	16–40	>41
Margin (mm)	>10	1–9	<1
Pathological classification	Non-high grade without necrosis	Non-high grade with necrosis	High grade with or without necrosis
Age (years)	≥61	40–60	≤39

One to three points are awarded for each of four different predictors of local breast recurrence (size, margin, width, pathological classification, and age). Scores for each of the predicators are totaled to yield a USC/VNPI score ranging from a low of 4 to a high of 12.

positive margins that did not appear to affect the benefit of tamoxifen.[74] Based on the only study available, it appears that addition of tamoxifen to standard therapy for DCIS may be warranted in patients without a contradiction to the drug. Extrapolation of these data to women with DCIS treated by mastectomy because of the reduction in contralateral breast cancer risk is tempting, but further studies are necessary to validate the original finding and to specifically address this population. The NSABP B35 trial is currently comparing anastrozole to tamoxifen in the treatment of postmenopausal patients with DCIS.

Lobular Carcinoma In Situ

Lobular carcinoma in situ (LCIS) is a poorly understood disease of the ductal and glandular system. There are some theories that LCIS is a precursor to breast cancer and others that suggest that LCIS is merely a risk factor. Multiple molecular studies have been performed to try to evaluate these theories. From the data, one might suggest that LCIS may actually represent more than one entity. At this time, further molecular studies are indicated.

Currently, LCIS is believed to represent a predictor of increased risk of the development of breast cancer rather than a precursor of invasive disease. As seen in Table 96.5, LCIS differs markedly from DCIS. Because it is found incidentally during biopsy for another cause, its true incidence is unknown. However, in a variety of series, LCIS was found in 0.8% to 8.0% of benign breast biopsies.[75,76] It occurs in asymptomatic premenopausal women, and is not manifest by a palpable mass, mammographic microcalcifications, or architectural distortion.

Because the paradigm has shifted from viewing LCIS as a premalignant lesion to a precursor lesion, treatment recommendations have changed. It was previously believed that LCIS was a premalignant lesion, based on the work initially by McDivitt et al. and updated by Rosen et al. from Memorial Sloan-Kettering Cancer Center.[77,78] Their data found an increasing risk of breast cancer with increasing time from biopsy. At 15 years, the risk of ipsilateral cancer was 30% and that of contralateral cancer 15%. For this reason, Rosen recommended ipsilateral simple mastectomy with contralateral mirror image biopsy. It is now more widely believed that LCIS is a risk factor for the development of breast cancer rather than a precursor lesion.[61,79]

TABLE 96.5. Comparison of LCIS and DCIS.

	LCIS	*DCIS*
Age at presentation	Premenopausal	Postmenopausal
Physical examination	Negative	Occasionally palpable mass
Mammogram	Negative	Microcalcifications
Diagnosis	Incidental	Workup of abnormality
Risk	In all breast tissue	At site of diagnosis
Treatment	Observation vs. chemoprevention vs. bilateral prophylactic mastectomy	Lumpectomy plus radiation vs. ipsilateral simple mastectomy Consider tamoxifen

LCIS, lobular carcinoma in situ; DCIS, ductal carcinoma in situ.

Importantly, the histological type of carcinomas that develop in women with a personal history of LCIS parallels the incidence in women without a history of LCIS and are of a ductal type.[80,81] Although some studies such as Rosen's demonstrate a greater risk in the ipsilateral breast, others, most notably Haagensen's, found the subsequent cancer risk equal in both breasts.[65] The actual probability of developing carcinoma was 21% at 35 years. Forty percent of new carcinomas were in situ lesions; half occurred in the contralateral breast, and the rest were scattered throughout the remainder of the ipsilateral breast.

Treatment recommendations for women with LCIS have been modified to align with this change in philosophy. Because the area in which LCIS was found is at no higher risk than the rest of the breast parenchyma, surgery to negative margins is not indicated. Similarly, contralateral mirror image or blind biopsy does not make sense because all breast tissue is at equal risk. Thus, the treatment options include careful observation as for any high-risk patient, chemoprevention with tamoxifen as per the NSABP-P1 trial, or bilateral prophylactic mastectomies as discussed in previous sections. These recommendations may change if further studies can show that a subset of LCIS is indeed a precursor lesion.

Familial Hereditary Breast Cancer: Molecular Genetics and Syndromes

Families that are characterized by having hereditary breast cancer are distinguished by the following characteristics: (1) early onset of breast cancer, classically less than 45 years of age; (2) an excess of bilateral breast cancer; (3) autonomic dominant inheritance for the cancer; and (4) greater frequency of multiple primary cancers. Individuals with hereditary breast cancer are really a subset of the larger group of individuals with familial breast cancer who have one or more first- or second-degree relatives with breast cancer but who do not fulfill the other criteria. It is estimated that individuals in families having familial breast cancer have a threefold increased risk of breast cancer than sporadic breast cancer cases. Any individual with a history of familial breast cancer should be referred for genetic counseling.

Paul Broca in 1866 was the first person to note the importance of a family history of breast cancer.[82] He did this when he described four generations of breast cancer and occurrences of cancer of the gastrointestinal tract in his wife's family. Lynch is credited with the first description of the hereditary breast ovarian cancer syndrome, by reporting families with two or more first-degree relatives with breast cancer and a variety of other cancer sites.[83]

Breast Cancer Susceptibility Genes

BRCA1

In 1990, Marie-Clare King reported mapping, by segregation analysis, the first breast cancer susceptibility gene (BRCA1) to chromosome 17q21. This gene was determined to have linkage with the hereditary breast and ovarian cancer syndrome.[84] BRCA1 encompasses 22 coding exons over 100 kb, and hereditary breast cancer is associated with mutations in the coding regions for BRCA1. The majority of these mutations result in a decreased or truncated BRCA1 protein. Overall, the BRCA1 gene confers an 80% to 85% risk of breast and 40% to 60% risk of ovarian cancer by the age of 70.[85] BRCA1 hereditary breast cancers are characterized pathologically as having a high grade and cell proliferation with a significantly higher occurrence of medullary and atypical medullary carcinomas.[86] Moreover, in situ carcinomas are seen less often in BRCA1-associated breast cancer than in the general breast cancer population.[86]

A second breast cancer susceptibility gene, BRCA2, was mapped to chromosome 13q12 in 1995.[87] In contrast to BRCA1, BRCA2 is associated with male breast cancer and confers only a 15% risk of ovarian cancer. Similar to BRCA1, mutations of the gene have been found in BRCA2-associated breast cancers.[87] The pathology of BRCA2-associated breast cancers is weighted toward tubular-lobular invasive carcinomas and invasive cribriform carcinomas, which tend to be lower-grade tumors with less proliferation.[86]

The most optimal treatment for BRCA-associated breast cancers has yet to be defined. There are multiple studies evaluating the risk and benefits of both bilateral mastectomies versus breast conservation, the role of bilateral salpingo-oophorectomy (BSO), and the administration of tamoxifen as chemoprevention. Hafftey et al. in 2002 showed that patients with the BRCA gene have almost double the rate of local recurrence after breast conservation as well as four times the rate of developing a contralateral tumor. There have also been some data to suggest that a prophylactic BSO not only reduces the risk of developing ovarian cancer but also decreases the risk of breast cancer in BRCA patients.[88] Unfortunately, the data regarding the implications of BRCA1 and BRCA2 on prognosis of patients are limited and paradoxical. Indeed, despite the aggressive-appearing pathological manifestations of BRCA1-associated tumors, they are associated with fewer recurrences in node-negative patients, and survival may be better for hereditary breast cancer cases in general and BRCA1-related tumors in particular.[86]

Hereditary Breast Cancer Syndromes and High-Risk Groups

Hereditary Breast/Ovarian Cancer Syndromes

These families have predominantly breast and ovarian cancers, with a lifetime risk of 85% for breast cancer in BRCA1 and BRCA2 carriers and of 40% to 60% for ovarian cancer in BRCA1 carriers.[84] The majority of the hereditary breast/ovarian cancer (HBOC) families have mutations of the BRCA1 gene. The risk of colon cancer and prostate cancer is also elevated in carriers of the gene by a factor of 3 to 4 compared to national incidence rates.[84]

Li–Fraumeni Syndrome

This syndrome is characterized by families with p53 germline mutations, causing a higher than expected occurrence of sarcomas, breast cancers, brain tumors, lung and laryngeal cancers, leukemias, and adrenal cortical carcinomas.[89] There is an autosomal dominant pattern of transmission, and 30% of the tumors occur before 15 years of age; 77% of the women who develop breast cancer with Li–Fraumeni syndrome are between 22 and 45 years old, and 25% have bilateral disease. Overall, the prevalence of germline p53 mutations in women diagnosed with breast cancer younger than 40 years is 1%, thus limiting the widespread application of p53 for screening breast cancer.[90]

Cowden Syndrome

Multiple benign keratoses located at mucocutaneous sites on the face as well as on the front and back of feet, hands, and forearms are characteristic of the Cowden syndrome.[91] Other manifestations include goiter, adenomas, polyps, uterine leiomyomas, and lipomas. Thirty percent of women with this syndrome develop infiltrating ductal carcinoma of the breast, and a significant proportion (close to 30%) will have bilateral breast cancer.[92] As yet, there are no biological markers for the syndrome.

Muir Syndrome

Germline mutations of the genes responsible for autosomal dominant inherited forms of colon cancer (MSH2, MLH1) are associated with a syndrome of multiple skin tumors and multiple benign and malignant tumors of the gastrointestinal and the genitourinary tract.[3] These individuals have an increased tendency for breast cancer, but the magnitude of risk remains uncharacterized.

Ataxia Telangiectasia

Ataxia telangiectasia is a syndrome characterized by progressive neuromotor and cerebellar deterioration, multiple telangiectasia, immune dysfunction, and hypersensitivity to ionizing radiation. It is caused by chromosomal fragility. The gene responsible for this disorder is located on chromosome 11q, and as many as 1% of the general population are homozygous mutated gene carriers.[93,94] Heterozygotic individuals with the mutated gene have a fivefold greater risk of developing breast cancer than the general population, and it is estimated that 7% of the general population is heterozygotic for the gene.[94] The implications for screening mammography with its ionizing radiation effects in the ataxia telangiectasia population remain controversial.

Ashkenazi Jews

There is an increased incidence of BRCA1 mutations in Ashkenazi Jews, which might explain the increased risk of breast cancer among Jewish women.[95] It is estimated that 1% of women of Ashkenazi descent are at increased risk for breast and ovarian cancer.[96]

Treatment of Stage I or II Breast Cancer

Primary Surgical Therapy

Once malignant cells invade the basement membrane of the breast ducts or lobules, the lesion is classified as an invasive or infiltrating cancer. Because of the current belief that inva-

TABLE 96.6. Tissues Resected in Various Types of Mastectomies.

Lymph	*Skin of entire chest wall (skin grafting internal mammary required)*	*Nipple–areolar complex*	*Breast mound*	*Pectoralis minor and major muscles*	*Axillary nodes*	*Lymph nodes*
Urban extended radical mastectomy	X	X	X	X	X	X
Halstead radical mastectomy	X	X	X	X	X	
Patey modified radical mastectomy		X	X	Pectoralis minor only	X	
Auchincloss modified radical mastectomy		X	X		X	
Simple mastectomy		X	X			
Subcutaneous mastectomy			X			

sive cancer is a micrometastatic disease at diagnosis, local therapies are no longer believed to influence long-term survival. Nevertheless, the Halstedian theory of orderly tumor progression dramatically influenced early breast cancer therapies.

The Halsted radical mastectomy (Table 96.6) was first described in 1894 with a report of the first 50 patients treated.[97] For 75 years after the introduction of the radical mastectomy, it remained the standard of care for women with breast cancer. Its popularity stemmed from the fact that most tumors could be resected via this approach, and afterward local recurrences were rare. This aggressive surgical approach, however, can be quite morbid. Removal of the pectoralis major muscle and skin results in significant aesthetic chest wall deformity that is difficult to reconstruct except with myocutaneous flaps. Impaired range of motion and chronic lymphedema occur in 25% to 53% of women after a radical mastectomy and significantly impair quality of life.[98,99] The radical mastectomy is no longer performed, and its failure began the challenge to the idea that more radical surgery would result in improved survival. The lack of survival advantage combined with the superior functional and cosmetic results of modified radical mastectomy (MRM) has made MRM a viable and standard treatment option for all women with operable breast cancer.

The migration toward less radical surgery prompted the evaluation of breast conservation as an option in women with breast cancer. Several trials have confirmed that lumpectomy with axillary lymph node dissection plus radiation is as effective as modified radical mastectomy for patients with early-stage breast cancer (Table 96.7) The rationale for breast conservation is the present belief that breast cancer is a systemic disease from the time of diagnosis. Therefore, local treatment options have little impact on survival and are performed only to achieve local disease control. Several additional important conclusions have resulted from the seven randomized trials comparing breast conservation treatment (BCT) and mastectomy. The NCI-Milan trial demonstrated that BCT can be successfully performed in lymph node-positive patients if they receive adjuvant chemotherapy.[100,101] NSABP-B06 further confirmed that local recurrence does not alter survival.[102] Additionally, in 10% of patients randomized to BCT, negative margins could not be achieved. NSABP-B06 also convincingly demonstrated the importance of adequate radiation therapy (XRT) in patients treated with BCT. At 8 years, breast recurrence occurred in 10% of patients treated with BCT plus XRT versus 39% of patients with lumpectomy alone ($P < 0.001$).[102]

Several factors influence the success of BCT. The goal of BCT is to minimize the risk of local recurrence while optimizing cosmetic results. Several criteria can accurately predict the optimal candidates for BCT (Table 96.8). It is important to note that patient age, nodal status, and anticipated need for adjuvant therapy are factors irrelevant to the choice of surgical procedure. The extent of tissue that should be removed remains a controversial matter. Initially, it was feared that removal of less than the entire breast would result in unacceptably high rates of local relapse because of the multicentricity of breast cancer. It is important to accurately distinguish between multifocal (multiple foci in the vicinity of the primary tumor) and multicentric (multiple independent foci of cancer not within the same quadrant as the primary tumor) cancers. The frequency of multicentricity has been variously estimated to range from 9% to 75%.[103] However, using strict definitions, Holland et al. demonstrated that breast cancer is commonly multifocal but rarely multicentric.[104]

Local recurrence after BCT is also influenced by the presence of an extensive intraductal component (EIC). EIC occurs when DCIS comprises greater than 25% of the infiltrating tumor and is present in grossly normal adjacent breast tissue. The Joint Center for Radiation Therapy (JCRT) series found a 27% local recurrence in EIC-positive tumors versus 8% in EIC-negative tumors treated with BCT.[105] The effect of EIC on local recurrence can be overcome by increasing the amount of tissue excised.[106] Additionally, the increased risk of local failure in BCT patients less than 40 years old can be explained in part by the increased incidence of EIC-positive tumors in young women.[107]

Based on the findings from these trials as well as the availability of mature results, the National Institutes of Health Consensus Development Conference on the Treatment of Early Breast Cancer issued a consensus statement in 1990.[108] They stated that BCT provided equivalent survival to mastectomy and, because it spared the breast, it is the preferable choice in women with stage I or II tumors.

Surgical Management of the Axilla

Axillary lymph node status remains the most powerful predictor of recurrence and survival in breast cancer. Axillary lymph node dissection had been an integral part of surgery

TABLE 96.7.
Randomized Trial of Mastectomy Versus Breast Conservation (Level I Evidence).

Trial	*Reference*	*Year*	*n*	*Randomized*	*Stage*	*Median Design*	*Follow-up*	*Results*
Guy's Hospital	147	1961–1970	376	Yes	T1N_0 or T1N_1	WLE1XRT vs. radical mastectomy	11 years	(1) Treatment deemed inadequate (omission of ALND and low-dose XRT)
		1971–1976	250	Yes	T1N_0	1XRT Radical Mastectomy1 XRT vs. WLE 1XRT		(2) Higher regional recurrence and lower survival in WLE1XRT group, especially in stage II patients
Gustave-Roussay	148	1972–1979	179	Yes	T1N_0 or T1N_1	Tumorectomy 1 XRT vs. MRM	10 years	No difference in overall survival, local control, distant metastasis, or contralateral breast cancer rate
NCI Milan	100	1973–1980	701	Yes	T1N_0	Quadrentectomy, ALND, and XRT vs. radical mastectomy	10 years	(1) No difference in local recurrence or survival (2) BCT can be performed in lymph node-positive patients if there is adjuvant chemotherapy
NSABP-B06	102	1976–1984	1843	Yes	T, 4 cm N_0	Lumpectomy, ALND, and XRT vs. Lumpectomy/ ALND, vs. MRM	8 years	(1) 10% of patients assigned to BCT-negative margins could not be achieved (2) XRT critically important for local control as breast recurrence occurred in 10% of lumpectomy/ XRT vs. 39% of lump alone (*p*,0.001) (3) No difference in survival thus local recurrence does not predict survival
NCI Bethesda	149	1979–1987	247	Yes		Lumpectomy/ ALND1XRT vs. MRM	8 years	No difference in survival or local control
EORTC	150	1980–1986	148 755	Yes Yes	I II	Lumpectomy/ ALND1XRT vs. MRM	8 years	No difference in survival, local control, or distant recurrence
Danish Breast Cancer Group	151	1983–1989	905	Yes	I or II	Quadrantectomy/ ALND1 XRT vs. MRM	6 years	(1) Identical overall survival (2) Fewer local/regional recurrences in BCT group (NS)

NCI, National Cancer Institute; EORTC, European Organization for Research and Treatment of Cancer; ALND, axillary lymph node dissection; XRT, radiation therapy; MRM, modified radical mastectomy; WLE, wide local excision; BCT, breast conservation treatment; NS, not significant.

TABLE 96.8. Breast Conservation.

A: Indications for breast conservation
- Ability to achieve negative margins
- Favorable tumor to breast size ratio to achieve good aesthetic result
- Unifocal malignancy
- Minimal changes in residual breast tissue allowing adequate follow-up by physical examination and mammography

B: Contraindications to breast conservation
- Patient preference for mastectomy
- Primary tumor greater than 5 cm
- Any size primary tumor unable to be resected without major deformity
- Multicentric disease
- Persistently positive margins on reexcision lumpectomy
- Diffuse mammographic changes that impair follow-up
- Lack of access to radiation facility
- Noncompliant patient
- First- or second-trimester pregnancy in whom delay of radiation therapy to the postpartum period is contraindicated
- Patients with significant collagen vascular disease (i.e., scleroderma or lupus)
- Patients who have previously received radiotherapy encompassing the chest wall (i.e., mantle for Hodgkin's disease)

for the past 100 years. Although major complications from axillary lymph node dissection are rare, minor complications are not infrequent and may cause significant morbidity.

In an effort to eliminate routine axillary lymph node dissection without losing the prognostic information obtained, sentinel lymph node dissection (SLND) was developed. The sentinel lymph node (SLN) is defined as the first lymph node to receive lymphatic drainage from the tumor. Injecting vital blue dye, radiolabeled colloid, or both in the vicinity of the primary tumor site identifies the SLN. SLND is much more challenging for breast cancer than melanoma because the breast parenchymal lymphatics are not as rich as the dermal lymphatics. Also, the upper outer quadrant location of most breast cancers can make identification of the SLN with radiocolloid mapping difficult because of the high background activity at the primary tumor site. Variation still exists among techniques at different experienced centers. Some rely on blue dye alone, other solely on radioisotope, and yet others on the dual technique. Injections can be performed peritumorally, retroareolarly, subdermally, or intradermally. When radioisotope is used, the timing, dose, type of colloid employed, and use of lymphoscintigraphy vary. Nevertheless, in all mappings the SLN is located by injecting a vital blue dye or radioisotope at the location of choice. The blue dye is visually identified leaving the periphery of the breast and the afferent lymphatic channel is traced to the blue stained lymph node (Fig. 96.14). When radiocolloid is used, the SLN can be identified by preoperative lymphoscintigraphy (Fig. 96.15), or intraoperatively with a hand-held gamma detector. There is no significant difference in success based on protocol implemented. At all major institutions the SLN can be identified in 95% of patients and is accurate in up to 100% of cases (Table 96.9). A significant learning curve exists as evidenced by the improved success by Giuliano from 66% to 94% with maturation of the techniques.

Patient selection is also critical. SLND is contraindicated in patients with palpably enlarged suspicious axillary lymph nodes or inflammatory cancers. Historically, it was thought initially that patients receiving neoadjuvant chemotherapy, patients with multicentric tumors, patients with extensive prior breast biopsy or axillary surgeries, or patients with large excisional biopsy cavities also were not to be candidates for SLN mapping. With increased experience, these are now believed at best to be relative contraindications to SLN biopsy.

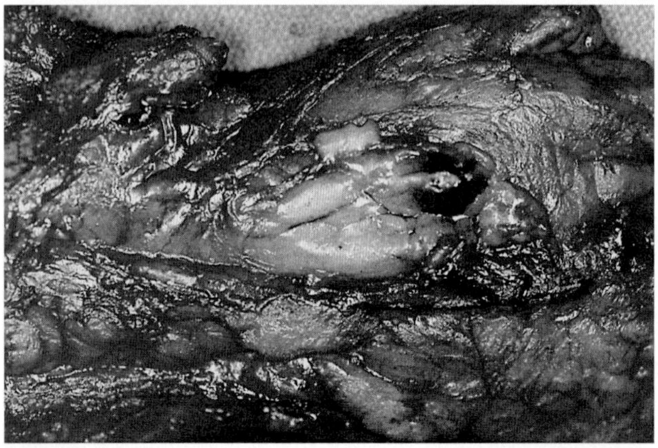

FIGURE 96.14. Lymphatic mapping with vital blue dye. Dissected specimen clearly demonstrates blue afferent lymphatic leading into blue stained sentinel lymph node. (Courtesy of A.E. Chang, MD.)

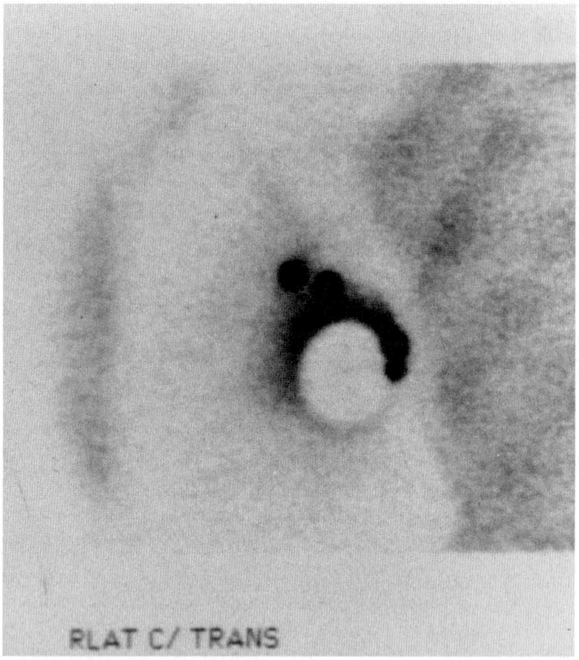

FIGURE 96.15. Unfiltered sulfur colloid lymphoscintogram demonstrating uptake in two axillary lymph nodes. A lead shield is placed over the breast to minimize interference from the injection site.

An additional important issue is that SLN mapping, by providing the pathologist with the lymph node most likely to contain disease, may be more sensitive for the detection of metastatic disease. With only one or two lymph nodes to process, a more detailed examination with thin serial sectioning, immunohistochemical staining, or potentially reverse transcriptase-polymerase chain reaction (RT-PCR) analysis is possible. In a trial of SLND followed by complete axillary lymph node dissection in 103 patients, the SLN was positive in 42% of the patients by thin serial sectioning and immunohistochemical staining; only 29% of the remainder of the axillary lymph nodes were positive by conventional processing ($P < 0.03$).[109] In a similar study, routine hematoxylin and eosin (H&E) staining of SLN identified metastatic foci in 32% of the patients; however, with immunohistochemical staining, 42% of patients were node positive.[110] Thus, 10% of patients were upstaged.

The prognostic importance of micrometastases has historically been questioned, and as our pathological evaluation improves so does the ability to detect smaller micrometastasis. In 2002, the TMN staging was modified to differentiate isolated tumor clusters from micrometastasis. The new AJCC staging classification also denotes whether the micrometastasis of the sentinel lymph node was found by H&E or only with the use of immunohistochemistry. Currently, the discovery of micrometastases has been proved clinically relevant with poorer survival for patients with micrometastases detected by serial staining, anticytokeratin immunohistochemical staining, and RT-PCR.[111–113] It is currently recommended that any SLN-positive patients undergo formal level I and II lymph node dissection whether the metastasis was found by H&E or by immunohistochemical staining. Even though the probability of detecting additional positive lymph

TABLE 96.9.
Sentinel Lymph Node (SLN) Mapping Trials.

Source	*Year*	*False-negative rate (%)*	*n*	*Technique*	*Injection site*	*SLN identified %*	*Accuracy[a] %*
Krag[152]	1993	0	22	Radiocolloid	Peritumoral	82	100
Giuliano[109]	1994	12	174	Dye	Peritumoral	66	96
Albertini[73]	1996	0	62	Both	Peritumoral	92	100
Krag[153]	1996	0	70	Radiocolloid	Peritumoral	71	100
Borgstein[154]	1997	0	33	Dye plus Radiocolloid	Intradermal Peritumoral	100	100
Giuliano[155]	1997	0	107	Dye	Peritumoral	94	100
Guenther[156]	1997	10	145	Dye	Peritumoral	71	97
Veronesi[157]	1997	5	163	Radiocolloid	Subdermal	98	98
Barnwell[158]	1998	0	42	Both	Peritumoral	90	100
Borgstein[159]	1998	2	130	Radiocolloid	Peritumoral	94	99
Krag[160]	1998	11	443	Radiocolloid	Peritumoral	93	97
O'Hea[161]	1998	15	59	Both	Peritumoral	93	95

[a]Accuracy equals total number of the positive SLN plus the negative SLN divided by the total number of patients in whom the SLN was identified.

nodes may be small, as suggested by the nomogram by Zee at Memorial Sloan-Kettering, additional nodal metastases have been detected in a significant proportion of patients.[114] Until further information from recently completed randomized trials is available, management should be decided on a case-by-case basis.

Adjuvant Chemotherapy or Hormonal Therapy for Lymph Node-Negative Breast Carcinoma

The current paradigm for breast cancer asserts that it is a systemic disease from the time of diagnosis. In patients with lymph node-negative disease, tumor size is the most important prognostic factor for relapse.[115] Patients with tumors less than 1 cm have a favorable prognosis, with greater than 90% 10-year disease-free survival.[115] The National Institutes of Health 1990 Breast Cancer Conference recommended that these patients rarely receive adjuvant chemotherapy.[108] This remains an area of controversy in patients that have less favorable tumor characteristics. A retrospective analysis of the NSABP trial has shown that a small number of patients have a decrease in their risk of recurrence with the use of adjuvant chemotherapy. Women who were estrogen receptor negative had a disease-free survival of 87% without chemotherapy. When adjuvant chemotherapy was added, this increased to 90%. This decrease in recurrence rates also holds true for those patients who were estrogen receptor positive. Some question the validity of this study because of possible selection bias. The NCCN guidelines still state that patients who have tumors less than 1 cm and favorable prognosis do not require chemotherapy; however, in patients with unfavorable prognostic factors, chemotherapy can be considered on an individual basis.

It is also recommended that all invasive tumors now be tested for the level of Her 2-neu expression. Overexpression is not only thought to be a predictor of poorer prognosis, but it is also being used as a way to determine the need for an anthracycline-based chemotherapy regimen. Patients with Her 2-neu-overexpressing tumors should preferentially receive anthracycline-based chemotherapy because data have demonstrated that there is significantly longer disease-free survival and overall survival.[116]

Patients with node-negative tumors larger than 1 cm, however, have a sufficiently significant risk of relapse that adjuvant systemic therapy is warranted. Almost 25% of stage I and 33% to 44% of stage II node-negative patients will develop recurrent disease.[115]

Several trials have documented an improvement in disease-free or overall survival in node-negative women treated with adjuvant chemotherapy. The NSABP B-13 trial randomized 760 node-negative, estrogen- and progesterone receptor-negative tumors to chemotherapy (methotrexate plus 5-fluorouracil with leucovorin times 12 versus observation).[117] At 4 years, an improvement in disease-free survival could be demonstrated in the chemotherapy-treated group

(74% versus 59%; $P < 0.001$). With longer than 8-year follow-up, a survival advantage was also observed (89% versus 80%; $P = 0.03$).[118] These benefits were noted in both pre- and postmenopausal women. In a follow-up study, NSABP B-19, the identical patient cohort was randomized to methotrexate/5-fluorouracil (M/F) versus cyclophosphamide/methotrexate/5-fluorouracil (CMF). At 5 years, CMF demonstrated an improved disease-free survival (88% versus 73%; $P < 0.001$) and overall survival (88% versus 85%; $P = 0.06$).

In a parallel trial, NSABP B-14, 2644 node-negative, estrogen receptor-positive patients were randomized to receive tamoxifen or no postsurgical therapy.[119] Treatment with tamoxifen increased disease-free survival at 4 years from 77% to 83% ($P < 0.001$). No improvement in overall survival was noted. At 10-year follow-up, tamoxifen-treated patients had an improved disease-free survival ($P < 0.001$) and overall survival ($P = 0.02$).[120]

Two multidrug regimens are currently used to treat node-negative women with tumors greater than 1 cm, doxorubicin (adriamycin)/cyclophosphamide (AC) and cyclophosphamide, methotrexate and 5-flurouracil (CMF). Although neither regimen has been proven superior, recently there has been a trend toward AC, especially for HER2/neu-expressing tumors. The Early Breast Cancer Trialists' Collaborative Group (EBCTG) has conducted meta-analyses of data from all the randomized trials comparing chemotherapies. In 1998, they published their results. These data showed that polychemotherapy reduced recurrence risk by 35% in women under 50 and 20% for women between 50 and 69. Polychemotherapy was also shown to reduce the mortality rates. There was no added benefit if the chemotherapy was given for more than 6 months. Compared with CMF, anthracycline-containing regimens produced a greater reduction in both recurrence and mortality rates.[121] In estrogen- or progesterone receptor-positive patients, systemic chemotherapy should be followed by tamoxifen.

Additional data from NSABP-B14 revealed that the benefit from 5 years of tamoxifen therapy persisted at 10 years of follow-up, with no additional advantage to more than 5 years of therapy. These conclusions resulted from a secondary randomization. After 5 years on tamoxifen, patients in NSABP-B14 underwent rerandomization to tamoxifen versus placebo. Similarly, comparison of many trials with different tamoxifen regimens suggest that more than 2 years of therapy is superior to less than 2 years of tamoxifen.[122] A randomized trial of 4742 patients was also performed in women who had been taking tamoxifen for at least 2 years. These women were either randomized to continue their tamoxifen for the remaining 3 years or to switch to exemestane for the remaining years. Patients who were switched to exemestane had an improved 3-year disease-free survival versus those who completed their tamoxifen (92% versus 87%). There was no difference in overall survival.[123]

Several side effects of tamoxifen have been described. Statistically significant increases in hot flashes (57% versus 41%) and vaginal discharge (24% versus 12%) were found in tamoxifen versus placebo patients in NSABP-B14. Other reported toxicities include thromboembolic events, endometrial cancer, retinopathy, liver cancer, and benign ovarian cysts. Balancing the known survival advantage with incidence of therapy-related complications, the current recommendation is to treat women with estrogen- or progesterone receptor-positive tumors greater than 1 cm with tamoxifen (20 mg daily) for 5 years.

There are also newer data to suggest that the aromatase inhibitor, anastrazole, provides a superior disease-free survival and a more favorable toxicity profile than tamoxifen for the treatment of estrogen receptor-positive postmenopausal women. These studies do not suggest that women on tamoxifen should switch to anastrazole. Anastrazole should not be used in premenopausal women.

Adjuvant Chemotherapy for Lymph Node-Positive Breast Carcinoma

As previously stated, lymph node status is the most important prognostic factor. Multiple studies have demonstrated that adjuvant systemic chemotherapy can prolong disease-free and overall survival in node-positive patients.[124] Meta-analysis of 11,000 women randomized to adjuvant chemotherapy versus no treatment revealed a 30% reduction in recurrence rate odds and 18% reduction in death odds for node-positive patients.[124] Premenopausal women had an even larger benefit with adjuvant therapy. The most frequent regimens used include AC, CMF, and AC followed by taxol.

Newer dosing techniques which shorten the interval between doses (dose-dense regimens) have also been evaluated. Cancer and Leukemia Group B (CALGB) compared dose-dense schedule paclitaxel to conventional dosing. There was a 26% improvement in disease-free survival and a 31% improvement in overall survival when the dose-dense regimen was used. There was no difference in the incidence of treatment-related leukemias in the two dosing schedules. Patients receiving dose-dense therapy did, however, require the administration of growth factors more often than those who received conventional dosing. At this time there are no further data to suggest that dose-dense therapy should be applied to other regimens. Further randomized studies are ongoing.

In patients who have metastatic cancer and an overexpression of their HER 2-neu genes, a newer agent, trastuzumab (Herceptin), is indicated. Multiple studies have shown efficacy when used as a single-agent chemotherapy for those patients who have recurrent disease and had undergone prior adjuvant therapy. It also has efficacy when used in patients with metastatic disease. Slamon et al. in 2001 showed that the addition of trastuzumab to standard regimens was associated with a longer time to disease progression, a higher rate of objective response, a longer duration of response, a longer survival, and a 20% reduction in the risk of death. In early studies, there was a greater risk of cardiotoxicity, especially when added to the anthracycline-based regimens. More studies are awaiting this association. Symptoms were generally improved with medical therapy.[125] Trastuzumab should be considered in all patients who overexpress the Her 2-neu gene.

Adjuvant Radiation Therapy

As demonstrated in previous sections (NSABP-B06), the need for postlumpectomy radiation therapy is absolute. The current controversy centers on the sequencing of adjuvant chemotherapy and radiation after breast conservation. In a study by Recht et al., 244 women were randomized to receive a 12-week course of systemic chemotherapy (cyclophosphamide/

methotrexate/5-fluorouracil, prednisone, and doxorubicin) either before or after radiation therapy.[126] All patients had breast-conserving surgery. The difference in overall survival between the chemotherapy-first group versus the radiotherapy-first group was 81% versus 73% ($P = 0.11$), and local recurrence was 14% versus 5% ($P = 0.07$). These data implied that delaying radiation for several months to allow systemic therapy first might be preferable in women at risk for systemic relapse. Two additional studies confirmed these results but failed to demonstrate a higher local relapse rate with chemotherapy first.[127] Currently, treatment is frequently individualized on the basis of risk assessment. Sequencing is based on the greatest perceived risk. For patients with a high risk of systemic relapse, chemotherapy precedes radiation; for patients with local control issues (see postmastectomy chest wall radiation, next), radiation may be given first.

Because 85% of local recurrences after lumpectomy occur in the tumor bed, and only 3% of breast recurrences occur elsewhere, there have been some that question the benefit of whole-breast radiation. Some investigators have shown that accelerated partial breast irradiation may achieve adequate local control. Added benefits of partial breast radiation include shorter treatment time, less breast tissue radiated, and potentially less damage to surrounding structures. It also seems that the cosmetic outcomes are the same. The past use of brachytherapy has given us some data to suggest that a certain subgroup of patients may be good candidates for partial breast irradiation. In the initial trials, these highly selected patients are those over 50, have tumors less than 2 cm, have widely clear margins, and no residual calcifications on mammograms, and have primarily an invasive ductal histology without an extensive in situ component. In addition to needle-based brachytherapy, other technology that allows us to deliver accelerated radiation includes the use of an implantable brachytherapy balloon (the MammoSite device) and external-beam accelerated partial breast radiation with three-dimensional or CT guidance. Currently a randomized trial is under way to determine the effectiveness of partial breast irradiation.[128]

Indications for postmastectomy radiation are still evolving. As with other variables, the risk of postoperative chest wall recurrence is influenced by nodal status. Local relapse occurs in 25% of node-positive patients versus 5% of node-negative women.[129] Total number of positive nodes also correlates with risk of local recurrence. Stefanik et al., in a study of patients treated with CMF, reported local recurrences in 9% of patients with one to three positive nodes versus 36% for those with four or more involved nodes.[130] Similarly, the Eastern Cooperative Oncology Group (ECOG) had a 7% versus 15% local recurrence rate in patients with one to three versus four or more positive nodes, respectively. For this reason, most patients with four or more positive nodes, or those with large primaries (T3), receive chest wall radiation. This position is further strengthened by the realization that only 50% of local recurrences respond to treatment.[131] It may therefore be easier to prevent local relapses then to treat them when they occur.

Despite the documented improvement in local control, until 1997 no trial demonstrated a survival benefit to postmastectomy chest wall radiation.[131] Two very similar studies were reported in 1997. The Danish Breast Cancer Group randomized 1708 high-risk patients to receive radiotherapy versus observation; all patients received CMF. Local regional recurrence was 9% in the radiotherapy plus CMF group versus 32% in the CMF-alone group ($P < 0.001$).[132] Overall 10-year survival was 54% versus 45%, respectively ($P < 0.001$). Similarly, at 15 years follow-up, Ragaz et al. completed a randomized study that demonstrated a 33% reduction in recurrence and a 29% reduction in mortality in the women who received postmastectomy radiation and chemotherapy versus women treated with chemotherapy alone.[133] Analysis of these trials, however, reveals an unusually high rate of axillary failure and a correspondingly low mean number of nodes resected. It has been suggested that if a more complete surgical procedure had been performed the results might have been negative, and thus the benefit of radiation was in compensating for inadequate surgery. Unfortunately, as a consequence of treating physician and patient bias, planned prospective randomized controlled trials failed to accrue adequate patient numbers to better delineate the role of postmastectomy radiation.

Currently, postmastectomy radiation should be performed for women with T3 or T4 primary tumors, four or more positive nodes, or positive margins, and should be considered in premenopausal women who have one to three positive nodes based on these studies.

Treatment of Locally Advanced (Stage III) Breast Cancer

Locally advanced breast cancers (LABC) include patients with tumors greater than 5 cm (T3 lesions), fixed to the chest wall or skin (T4 tumors), and/or those with bulky fixed axillary lymph nodes (N2 disease). Inflammatory cancer is a distinct entity and is discussed separately. For both these situations, neoadjuvant chemotherapy has become the treatment of choice.[134,135]

Although rare, management of patients with LABC has altered the role of neoadjuvant chemotherapy in patients with stage I or II disease. Historically, 5-year survival of LABC patients was less than 5% for women treated by surgery alone. Primary radiotherapy produced 5-year survival of 12% to 38%.[135] The addition of radiation therapy to surgery improved 5-year survival to 58% in T3 N-positive patients and 49% for T4 patients.[136]

Numerous studies have demonstrated an improvement in survival with multimodal sequential therapy. Treatment is initiated with neoadjuvant chemotherapy. Response rates of 60% to 80% have been demonstrated, with 10% to 15% being complete responses.[136,137] As demonstrated by Hortobagyi et al., with aggressive multimodal therapy the 5-year disease-free survival was 64% in patients with IIIA disease and 33% for IIIB disease, with an overall survival of 84% and 94%, respectively.[136]

Patients with inflammatory cancer present with brawny induration of the skin, often with peau d'orange (skin edema) and erythema (Fig. 96.16). These changes are caused by tumor embolization of dermal lymphatics. Historically, when treated with surgery alone, survival was infrequent and local recurrence occurred in nearly three-quarters of patients. Neoadjuvant chemotherapy produces similar response rates (up to 80%) as in LABC patients. Most patients can then be resected by mastectomy with clear margins. Local control rates up to

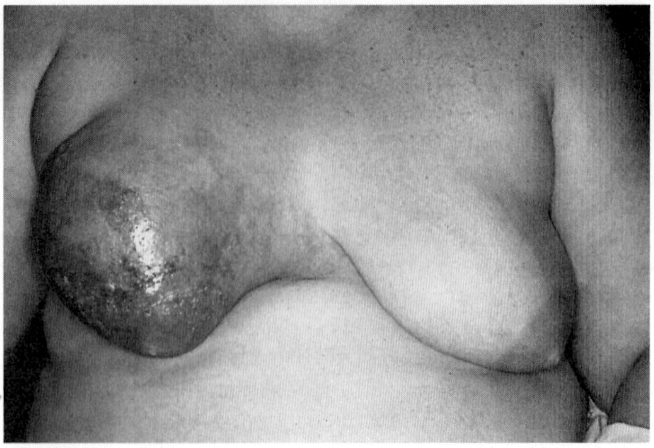

FIGURE 96.16. Patient with inflammatory breast cancer. Note the diffuse erythema, peau d'orange, and near tumor ulceration. (Courtesy of A.E. Chang, MD.)

70% can now be achieved with a 50% 5-year survival.[138,139] To achieve these results, surgery must be followed by radiation and chemotherapy.

Because of the dramatic response rates to neoadjuvant chemotherapy, some patients who might otherwise not be candidates for breast-conserving surgery because of large tumor to breast size can be salvaged. To be eligible for lumpectomy, a patient should be evaluated with a postchemotherapy mammogram that must demonstrate limited disease. Negative margins must be achieved, and an acceptable cosmetic outcome should be anticipated. Newman prospectively studied 100 consecutive patients who were given neoadjuvant chemotherapy with paclitaxel followed by adriamycin. The median tumor size was decreased from 2.4 to 1 cm, and there was an increase in breast conservation eligibility by 34%; 28 patients had a complete pathological response.[139a] Although neoadjuvant chemotherapy has been demonstrated in numerous trials to improve breast conservation rates, no study to date has shown improved survival with neoadjuvant versus adjuvant chemotherapy.

Treatment of Metastatic (Stage IV) Breast Cancer

Metastatic breast cancer is rarely cured. The median survival of women with stage IV disease is 2 years. Therefore, palliation and prolongation of life are the goals of treatment. Thus, when two therapeutic choices are equally efficacious, the least toxic should be selected.

The bone is the most common site of disease, followed in order by lung, pleura, and soft tissue. Isolated locoregional recurrence occurs in 15% of patients, distant disease only in 60%, and combined failure in 25%. Specific treatment of bony metastasis may include bisphosphonates. When added to chemotherapy or hormonal treatments, they reduce pain and prolong survival free of bone-related events.[140] For patients with disease in nonthreatening locations such as bone or soft tissue whose tumors are known to be hormone sensitive, or for older or poor performance status patients, endocrine manipulation can be tried first. In patients with life-threatening metastases or hormone-negative tumors, multiagent chemotherapy is the treatment of choice.

Treatment of Unusual Presentations of Breast Cancer

Paget's Disease

Paget's disease of the breast is a rare form of in situ carcinoma involving the nipple and is often associated with an underlying invasive or intraductal carcinoma.[141] Clinically it is manifest as eczematoid changes of the nipple with accompanying edema, erythema, pruritus, and nipple discharge. Punch biopsy of the nipple is diagnostic and reveals large cells with prominent nucleoli and pale cytoplasm (Paget's cells). Because of its unusual presentation, there is often a delay in making the diagnosis. The majority of women with Paget's disease have an underlying cancer within their breast at the time of diagnosis; therefore, a careful physical examination coupled with a mammogram must be performed. For patients with an associated lesion, mastectomy is the preferred treatment unless the associated cancer can be resected en bloc with the nipple–areolar complex. Axillary lymph node dissection should be performed only if the associated cancer has an invasive component. For patients without palpable breast masses or mammographic densities, breast conservation may be considered. Recent data demonstrate that complete resection of the nipple–areola complex followed by definitive radiotherapy has an acceptable disease-free and overall survival.[142] The prognosis of Paget's disease is that of the underlying cancer and approaches 100% for patients without an associated invasive cancer.

Occult Breast Cancer Presenting as Axillary Metastases

Although breast cancer presenting with axillary lymphadenopathy without an identifiable primary represents less than 1% of breast cancers, this entity has been recognized since the time of Halstead. Evaluation should include a thorough physical examination. Radiologic workup should include a mammography. If no primary is discovered, a high-quality dedicated breast MRI should be obtained.

Women with axillary metastasis from an occult breast primary historically have been treated with mastectomy. The likelihood of identifying an occult primary have decreased as high-resolution mammography and MRI have become widely available. Summation data by Harris et al. reported a 64% incidence of identification of a primary tumor in 228 mastectomies for occult breast cancer, with a range of 93% to 8%.[143]

As with other breast cancers, there has been a trend toward breast conservation. Some groups advocate axillary lymph node dissection followed by radiation therapy. The limitation of this approach is the inability to deliver a boost dose of radiation therapy to the whole breast. Even though the reported local recurrence rates of 17% to 37% are higher than for standard breast-conserving therapy, there is no reported difference in survival for women treated with breast preservation versus mastectomy.[144]

Overall survival is the same as for women with stage II cancer in whom a breast primary was identified, reinforcing the prognostic importance of axillary staging. Because of the nodal involvement, adjuvant systemic therapy is recommended for these women.

Breast Cancer During Pregnancy

It used to be believed that breast cancer arising during pregnancy was especially aggressive; however, when stratified by stage, survival is similar to that of nonpregnant women. Delay in diagnosis and treatment along with the increased incidence in inflammatory cancers detected in pregnant women resulting in presentation at a later stage is now implicated in the poorer prognosis overall for pregnant women with breast cancer.

Clearly, the management of breast cancer in pregnancy poses a difficult dilemma. Termination of pregnancy has not been demonstrated to affect survival; therefore, local therapy decisions are usually influenced by gestational age. Because of the unknown effects of radiation on fetal development it has been recommended that a mastectomy is the procedure of choice in the first two trimesters. Lumpectomy may be considered in the third trimester in a select group of patients who can delay their radiation therapy until after delivery. Patients who opt for surgery should be aware of the increased risk of spontaneous abortion, especially early in development. There also has been an increased risk of infant death within 1 week of delivery.[145] Reconstruction is usually delayed because the increased operative time increases fetal risk. Additionally, it would be difficult to achieve symmetry with the postpartum breast.

The use and timing of adjuvant chemotherapy also remains problematic. Fetal malformations have been reported with first-trimester administration and low fetal birth weight with later treatments. For cancers diagnosed later in pregnancy, delay until after delivery is induced would seem prudent. As with all treatment decisions, the risk versus benefit must be determined on an individual basis.

Nonepithelial Tumors

Phyllodes Tumor (Cystosarcoma Phyllodes)

Phyllodes tumors are the most common nonepithelial tumors of the breast. Despite the older designation of cystosarcoma, the majority of these lesions are benign. Therefore, "malignant" or "benign" should qualify the diagnosis of "phyllodes tumor the breast."

These tumors exclusively occur in the female breast. They present as large, mobile, well-circumscribed masses that are mammographically indistinguishable from fibroadenomas. They occasionally can grow rapidly. For benign tumors, local excision to widely negative margins is appropriate. Some advocate mastectomy for malignant phyllodes tumors, especially if they are of large size. Because the risk of axillary metastasis is less than 1%, axillary lymph node dissection is not indicated. Most recurrences tend to be local; however, metastasis to the lung and bones may be seen. The role of radiation therapy is limited to the treatment of symptomatic metastatic disease. Currently there is no effective chemotherapy regimen. Additionally, hormonal therapy is of no value.

Even though mesenchymal tumors arising in the breast are rare, it is important to correctly recognize this entity as the treatment of sarcoma varies markedly from breast carcinoma. These soft tissue sarcomas may arise anywhere within the breast. Treatment generally is by mastectomy, especially because these tumors tend to be of large size. The usual route of spread is hematogenous, and therefore axillary dissection is not indicated.

The role of radiation and chemotherapy can only be extrapolated from treatment of sarcomas in other sites. At least for high-grade lesions, adjuvant therapies may be warranted. An academically interesting subset of patients are those with radiation-induced sarcomas. Angiosarcoma is the most common histological type. In a population-based, case-controlled cohort study, it was demonstrated that there was a twofold relative risk (overall risk less than 1%) of a soft tissue sarcoma developing in women treated with surgery plus radiation for breast cancer.[146] Most sarcomas occurred within the vicinity of the primary breast cancer or within the lymph-edematous ipsilateral extremity. Treatment can be difficult and follows the foregoing principles.

Male Breast Cancer

Male breast cancer typically presents as a hard, irregular, nontender, eccentric mass often fixed to the chest wall. It must be distinguished from gynecomastia, which is more commonly bilateral, symmetrical, and retroareolar. Mammography is extremely helpful in differentiating between the two entities. If any question persists, tissue diagnosis via fine-needle aspiration, core, or surgical biopsy should be undertaken. Almost all male breast cancers are ductal in origin because of the paucity of lobular elements in the male breast. Both ductal carcinoma in situ and Paget's disease have been described.

Traditionally, male breast cancer presented at a later stage, often because of delay either in the patient seeking medical care or in diagnosis. Treatment depends on extent of involvement. If there is invasion of the pectoralis major muscle, either saucerization of a portion of pectoralis muscle or a radical mastectomy will be necessary. For earlier tumors, simple mastectomy with sentinel lymph node biopsy is the preferred procedure. For close or positive margins, postmastectomy radiation should be added. Breast conservation, although theoretically acceptable, is often not feasible because of the limited amount of tissue of the male breast. If all criteria for breast conservation are met, however, there is no absolute contraindication to its use.

The value of systemic adjuvant chemotherapy has been extrapolated from the large trials on women, and should be considered at least for patients with stage II or greater disease. The majority of patients (80%) are estrogen receptor positive, and treatment with tamoxifen should be considered in these male patients. Stage for stage, survival curves parallel those of female epithelial breast cancers.

References

1. Early Breast Cancer Trialists' Collaborative Group. Tamoxifen for early breast cancer: an overview of the randomised trials. Lancet 1998;351:1451–1467.
2. Ottman R, King M, Pike M, Henderson B. Practical guide for estimating risk for familial breast cancer. Lancet 1983;2:556–558.
3. Anderson D. Genetic study of breast cancer: identification of a high risk group. Cancer (Phila) 1974;34:1090–1097.

4. Anderson D, Badzioch M. Bilaterality in familial breast cancer patients. Cancer (Phila) 1985;56:2092–2098.
5. Tokunaga M, Land C, Yamamoto T, et al. Incidence of female breast cancer among atomic bomb survivors, Hiroshima and Nagasaki, 1950–1980. Radiat Res 1987;112:243–272.
6. Hildreth N, Shore L, Dvoretsky P. The risk of breast cancer after irradiation of the thymus in infancy. N Engl J Med 1989;321:146–151.
7. Morris EA. Breast cancer imaging with MRI. Radiol Clin N Am 2002:40:443–66.
8. Dupont W, Page D. Risk factors for breast cancer in women with proliferative breast disease. N Engl J Med 1985;312:146–151.
9. Gail M, Brinton L, Byar D, et al. Projecting individualized probabilities of developing breast cancer for white females who are being examined annually. J Natl Cancer Inst 1989;81:1879–1886.
10. National Cancer Institute. http://cancertrials.nci.nih.gov/ 1998.
11. Lynch HT. Introduction to breast cancer genetics. In: Lynch HT, ed. Genetics and Breast Cancer. New York: Van Nostrand Reinhold, 1992:1–13.
12. Miki Y, Swensen J, Shattuck-Eiden D, et al. A strong candidate gene for the breast and ovarian cancer susceptibility gene BRCA1. Science 1994;266:66.
13. Wooster R, Bignell G, Lancaster J, et al. Identification of the breast cancer susceptibility gene BRCA2. Nature (Lond) 1995; 378:789–792.
14. Kriege MS, Brekelmans C, Boetes C, et al. Efficacy of MRI and mammography for breast cancer screening in women with a familial or genetic predisposition. N Engl J Med 7/2004;351:427–437.
15. Claus EB, Schildkraut J, Iversen ES Jr, et al. Effect of BRCA1 and BRCA2 on the association between breast cancer risk and family history. J Natl Cancer Inst 1998;90:1824–1829.
16. Brody LC, Biesecker BB. Breast cancer susceptibility genes: BRCA1 and BRCA2. Rev Mol Med 1998;77:208–226.
17. Narod SA, Reuteun J, Lynch HT, et al. Familial breast-ovarian cancer locus on chromosome 17q12-q23. Lancet 1991;338:82–83.
18. Akashi-Tanaka S, Fukutomi T, Tukami A, et al. Male breast cancer in patients with a familial history of breast cancer. Surg Today 1996;26:975–979.
19. Stratton MR, Ford D, Neuhasen S, et al. Familial male breast cancer is not linked to the BRCA1 locus on chromosome 17q. Nat Genet 1994;7:103–107.
20. Fisher B, Costantino JP, Wickerham L, et al. Tamoxifen for the prevention of breast cancer: report of the National Surgical Adjuvant Breast and Bowel Project P1 study. J Natl Cancer Inst 1998;90:1371–1388.
21. Fisher B, Costantino JP, Redmond C, et al. A randomized clinical trial evaluating Tamoxifen in the treatment of patients with node negative breast cancer who have estrogen receptor positive tumors. N Engl J Med 1989;320:479–484.
22. Fisher B, Redmond C, Brown A, et al. Adjuvant chemotherapy with and without Tamoxifen in the treatment of primary breast cancer: 5 year results from the National Surgical Adjuvant Breast and Bowel Project Trial. J Clin Oncol 1986;4:459–471.
23. Mouridsen H, Palshof T, Patterson J, et al. Tamoxifen in advanced breast cancer. Cancer Treat Rev 1978;5:137–141.
24. Veronesi U, Maisonneuve P, Costa A, et al. Prevention of breast cancer with Tamoxifen: preliminary findings from the Italian Tamoxifen Prevention Study. Lancet 1998;352:93–97.
25. Powles T, Eeles R, Ashley S, et al. Interim analysis of the incidence of breast cancer in the Royal Marsden Hospital Tamoxifen randomised chemoprevention trial. Lancet 1998;352:98.
26. Jolly EE, Bjarnason NH, Neven P, et al. Prevention of osteporosis and uterine effects in postmenopausal women taking raloxifene for 5 years. Menopause 2003;10(4):337–344.
27. Cummings SR, Eckert S, Krueger KA, et al. The effect of raloxifene on risk of breast cancer in postmenopausal women results from MORE. JAMA 1999;281:2189–2197.
28. Hartmann LC, Schaid DJ, Woods JE, et al. Efficacy of bilateral prophylactic mastectomy in women with a family history of breast cancer. N Engl J Med 1999;340:77–84.
29. Thomas DB, Gao DL, Self SG, et al. Randomized trial of breast self examination in Shanghai: methodology and preliminary results. J Natl Cancer Inst 1997;89:355–365.
30. Boyd NF, Sutherland HF, Fish EB, et al. Prospective evaluation of physical examination of the breast. Am J Surg 1981;142: 331.
30a. Boyd NF, Sutherland HF, Fish EB, et al. Prospective evaluation of physical examination of the breast. Am J Surg 1981;142: 1477.
31. Miller AB, Baines CJ, To T, et al. Canadian National Breast Screening Study 2: breast cancer detection and death rates among women 50 to 59 years. Can Med Assoc J 1992;147:1477.
32. Ciatto J, Catalion L, Distante V. Nonpalpable breast lesions detected with mammography: review of 512 consecutive cases. Radiology 1987;165:99–102.
33. Feig SA, Kopans DB, Sickles EA, et al. Rationale for annual screening mammography for women ages 40–49. Breast Dis 1998;10(3–4):13–21.
34. Morrow M. Surgery in the elderly patient, I: breast disease in elderly women. Surg Clin N Am 1994;74:145.
35. Rimer BK, Ross E, Cristinzio S. Older women's participation in breast screening. J Gerontol 1992;47:85.
36. Wilson TE, Helvie MA, August DA. Breast imaging: breast cancer in elderly patients, early detection with mammography. Radiology 1994;190:203.
37. American College of Radiology. Breast Imaging Reporting and Data System (BI-RADS). Reston, VA: American College of Radiology, 1993.
37a. Pisano ED, Gatsonis C, Hendrick E, et al. Diagnostic performance of digital versus film mammography for breast-cancer screening. NEJM 2005;252:1773–1783.
38. Liberman L, Morris E, Joo-Young Lee M et al. Breast lesions detected on MR imaging: features and positive predictive value. Am J Roentgenol 2002;179:171–178.
39. Liberman L. Breast cancer screening with MRI: what are the data for patients at high risk? N Engl J Med 7/2004;351:497–500.
40. Clinical diagnosis, breast cancer [session 36]. Proceedings of the Society of Nuclear Medicine, 50th Annual Meeting, June 21–25, 2003, New Orleans, LA.
41. Schmidt RA. Stereotactic breast biopsy. CA Cancer J Clin 1994;44:172–191.
42. Al-Sobhi S, Helvie MA, Pass HA, Chang AE. Extent of lumpectomy for breast cancer after diagnosis by stereotactic core versus wire localization biopsy. Ann Surg Oncol 1999;6:330–335.
43. Dronkers DJ. Stereotaxic core biopsy of breast lesions. Radiology 1992;183:631–634.
44. Parker SH, Lovin JD, Jobe WE, et al. Nonpalpable breast lesions: stereotactic automated large-core biopsies. Radiology 1991;180: 403–407.
45. Jackman RJ, Nowels KW, Shepard MJ, et al. Stereotaxic large-core needle biopsy of 450 nonpalpable breast lesions with surgical correlation in lesions with cancer or atypical hyperplasia. Radiology 1994;193:91–95.
46. Liberman L, Cohen MA, Dershaw DD, et al. Atypical ductal hyperplasia diagnosed at stereotaxic core biopsy of breast lesions: an indication for surgical biopsy. Am J Roentgenol 1995;164:1111–1113.
47. Jackman RJ, Finkelstein SI, Marzoni FA. Stereotaxic large-core needle biopsy of histologically benign, nonpalpable breast lesions: false-negative results and failed follow up. Radiology 1995;193:91–95.

48. Parker S, Burbank F, Jackman RJ, et al. Percutaneous large-core breast biopsy: a multi-institutional study. Radiology 1994; 193:359–364.
49. Smith BL, Souba WW. Algorithm and explanation: assessment and management of breast complaints. Common Clin Prob 1995:1–17.
50. Gately CA, Mottola J, Ruiz CA et al. Reassurance in the treatment of mastalgia. Br J Hosp Med 1990;43(5):330–332.
51. Boyd NF, McGuire V, Shannon P, et al. Effect of a low fat high carbohydrate diet on symptoms of cyclic mastopathy. Lancet 1998;2(8603):128–132.
52. Pashby NL, Mansel RE, Hughes LE, et al. A clinical trial of evening primrose oil in mastalgia. Br J Surg 1981;68:801.
53. Baker H, Snedecor P. Clinical trial of danazol for benign breast disease. Am Surg 1979;45:727.
54. Mansel R, Preece P, Hughes L. A double blind trial of the prolactin inhibitor bromocriptine in painful benign breast disease. Br J Surg 1978;65:724.
55. Devitt JE. Management of nipple discharge by clinical findings. Am J Surg 1985;149:789.
56. Leis HP Jr, Greene FL, Cammarata A, et al. Nipple discharge: surgical significance. South Med J 1988;81:20.
57. Page DL, Anderson TJ, eds. Diagnostic Histopathology of the Breast. Edinburgh: Churchill-Livingstone, 1987.
58. Dixon JM, Dobie V, Laub J, et al. Assessment of the acceptability of conservative management of fibroadenoma of the breast. Br J Surg 1996;83:264–265.
59. Fleming ID, Cooper JS, Henson DE, et al. Cancer Staging Manual, 5th ed. Philadelphia: Lippincott-Raven, 1997:171–178.
60. Van Lancker M, Goor C, Sacre R, et al. Patterns of axillary lymph node metastasis in breast cancer. Am J Clin Oncol 1995;18:267–272.
61. Frykberg ER, Bland KI. Management of in situ and minimally invasive breast carcinoma. World J Surg 1994;18:45.
62. Page DL, Dupont W, Rogers L, Landenberger M. Intraductal carcinoma of the breast: follow-up after biopsy only. Cancer (Phila) 1982;49:751–758.
63. Rosen P, Brown D, Kinne D. The clinical significance of preinvasive breast carcinoma. Cancer (Phila) 1980;46:919–925.
64. Fisher B, Costantino JP, Redmond C, et al. Lumpectomy compared with lumpectomy and radiation therapy for the treatment of intraductal breast cancer. N Engl J Med 1993;328:1581–1586.
65. Haagensen CD, Lane N, Lattes R, et al. Lobular neoplasia (so-called lobular carcinoma in situ) of the breast. Cancer (Phila) 1978;42:737–769.
66. Alpers C, Wellings S. The prevalence of carcinoma in situ in normal and cancer-associated breast. Hum Pathol 1985;16:796–807.
67. Bartow S, Pathak D, Black W, Key C, Teaf S. Prevalence of benign, atypical, and malignant breast lesions in populations at different risk for breast cancer. Cancer (Phila) 1987;60:2751–2760.
68. Silverstein MJ, Waisman JR, Gierson ED, Colburn W, Gamagami P, Lewinsky B. Radiation therapy for intraductal carcinoma: is it an equal alternative? Arch Surg 1991;126:424–427.
69. Kinne D, Petrek J, Osborne M, Fracchia A, De Palo A, Rosen PP. Breast carcinoma in situ. Arch Surg 1989;124:33–36.
70. Silverstein MJ, Gierson ED, Waisman JR, et al. Axillary lymph node dissection for T1a breast carcinoma: is it indicated? Cancer (Phila) 1994;73:664–667.
71. Fisher B, Dignam J, Wolmark N, et al. Lumpectomy and radiation therapy for the treatment of intraductal breast cancer: findings from National Surgical Breast and Bowel Project B-17. J Clin Oncol 1998;16:441–452.
72. Lagios MD, Margolin FR, Westdahl PR, et al. Mammographically detected duct carcinoma in situ: frequency of local recurrence following tylectomy and prognostic effect of nuclear grade on local recurrence. Cancer (Phila) 1989;63:618.
73. Albertini JJ, Lyman GH, Cox C, et al. Lymphatic mapping and sentinel node biopsy in the patient with breast cancer. JAMA 1996;276:1818–1822.
73a. Silverstein MJ. The University of Southern California/Van Nuys Prognostic Index in Ductal Carcinoma in Situ of the Breast Second Edition Silverstein MJ, Recht, A, and Lagios MD. Editors, Chapter 45, Lippincott, Williams & Wilkins, Philadelphia 2002.
74. Wolmark N, Dignam J, Fisher B. The addition of tamoxifen to lumpectomy and radiotherapy in the treatment of ductal carcinoma in situ (DCIS): preliminary results of NSABP protocol B-24 [abstract]. Br Cancer Res Treat 1998;50:227.
75. Schwartz G, Feig S, Rosenberg A. Staging and treatment of clinically occult breast cancer. Cancer (Phila) 1984;53:1379.
76. Frykberg E, Santiago F, Betsill W, O'Brien P. Lobular carcinoma in situ of the breast. Surg Gynecol Obstet 1987;164:285–301.
77. McDivitt R, Hutter R, Foote F, Stewart F. In situ lobular carcinoma. A prospective follow-up study indicating cumulative patient risks. JAMA 1967;201:82–86.
78. Rosen P, Lieberman P, Braun D. Lobular carcinoma in situ of the breast. Am J Surg 1978;2:225–251.
79. Page DL, Jensen RA. Evaluation and management of high risk and premalignant lesions of the breast. World J Surg 1994;18:32.
80. Rosen PP, Kosloff C, Lieberman P, et al. Lobular carcinoma in situ of the breast: detailed analysis of 99 patients with average follow-up of 24 years. Am J Pathol 1978;2:225.
81. Fisher ER, Fisher B. Lobular carcinoma of the breast: an overview. Ann Surg 1977;185:377.
82. Broca PP. Traite des Tumeurs. Paris: Asselin, 1866.
83. Lynch HT, Krush AJ, Lemon HM, Kaplan AR, Condit PT, Bottomley RH. Tumor variation in families with breast cancer. JAMA 1972;222:1631–1635.
84. Easton DF, Ford D, Bishop DT. Breast and ovarian cancer incidence in BRCA1-mutation carriers: Breast Cancer Linkage Consortium. Am J Hum Genet 1995;56:265–271.
85. Easton DF, Bishop DT, Ford D, et al. Genetic linkage analysis in familial breast and ovarian cancer: results from 214 families. Am J Hum Genet 1993;52:678.
86. Marcus JN, Watson P, Page DL, et al. Hereditary breast cancer: pathobiology, prognosis, and BRCA1 and BRCA2 gene linkage [see comments]. Cancer (Phila) 1996;77:697–709.
87. Stratton MR, Ford D, Neuhasen S, et al. Familial male breast cancer is not linked to the BRCA1 locus on chromosome 17q. Nat Genet 1994;7:103–107.
88. Kauff ND, Sutagopan JM, Robson ME, et al. Risk reducing salpingooophorectomy in women with a BRCA 1 or BRCA 2 mutation. N Engl J Med 2002;346:1609–1615.
89. Li FP, Fraumeni JF Jr. Soft-tissue sarcomas, breast cancer, and other neoplasms: a familial syndrome? Ann Intern Med 1969;71:747–752.
90. Sidransky D, Tokino T, Helzlsouer K, et al. Inherited p53 gene mutations in breast cancer. Cancer Res 1992;52:2984–2986.
91. Brownstein MH, Wolf M, Bikowski JB. Cowden's disease: a cutaneous marker of breast cancer. Cancer (Phila) 1978;41:2393–2398.
92. Williard W, Borgen P, Bol R, Tiwari R, Osborne M. Cowden's disease: a case report with analyses at the molecular level. Cancer (Phila) 1992;69:2969–2974.
93. Gatti RA, Berkel I, Boder E, et al. Localization of an ataxia-telangiectasia gene to chromosome 11q22*23. Nature (Lond) 1988;336: 577–580.
94. Swift M, Morrell D, Cromartie E, Chamberlin AR, Skolnick MH, Bishop DT. The incidence and gene frequency of ataxia-telangiectasia in the United States. Am J Hum Genet 1986;39:573–583.

95. Roa BB, Boyd AA, Volcik K, Richards CS. Ashkenazi Jewish population frequencies for common mutations in BRCA1 and BRCA2. Nat Genet 1996;14:185–187.
96. Struewing JP, Brody LC, Erdos MR, et al. Detection of eight BRCA1 mutations in 10 breast/ovarian cancer families, including 1 family with male breast cancer. Am J Hum Genet 1995;57:1–7.
97. Halsted W. The results of operations cure of cancer of the breast performed at Johns Hopkins Hospital. Johns Hopkins Hosp Bull 1894;4:497–555.
98. Say C, Donegan WL. A biostatistical evaluation of complications from mastectomy. Surg Gynecol Obstet 1974;138:370–376.
99. Forrest A, Roberts M, Cant E. Simple mastectomy and pectoral node biopsy: the Cardiff-St. Mary's Trial. World J Surg 1977;1:320–323.
100. Veronesi U, Saccozzi R, Del Vecchio M, et al. Comparing radical mastectomy with quadrantectomy, axillary dissection, and radiotherapy in patients with small cancers of the breast. N Engl J Med 1981;305:6.
101. Veronesi U, Banfi A, Salvadori B, et al. Breast conservation is the treatment of choice in small breast cancer: long-term results of a randomized clinical trial. Eur J Cancer 1990;26:668.
102. Fisher B, Redmond C, Poisson R, et al. Eight-year results of a randomized clinical trial comparing total mastectomy and lumpectomy with or without irradiation in the treatment of breast cancer. N Engl J Med 1989;320:822.
103. Lagios MD, Westdahl PR, Rose M. The concept and implications of multicentricity in breast carcinoma. Pathol Annu 1981;16:83–102.
104. Holland R, Velig S, Mravunac M, Hendricks J. Histologic multifocality of Tis, T1–2 breast carcinomas: implications for clinical trials of breast-conserving surgery. Cancer (Phila) 1985;56:979–990.
105. Harris J, Recht A. Conservative surgery and radiotherapy. In: Harris J, Hellman S, Henderson IC, Kinne D, eds. Breast Diseases. Philadelphia: Lippincott, 1991:399–404.
106. Vicini F, Eberlein T, Connolly J, et al. The optimal extent of resection for patients with stages I or II breast cancer treated with conservative surgery and radiotherapy. Ann Surg 1991;214:200–205.
107. Kurtz J, Jacquemier J, Amalric R, et al. Why are local recurrences after breast-conserving therapy more frequent in younger patients? J Clin Oncol 1990;8:591–598.
108. NIH Consensus Development Conference Treatment of early-stage breast cancer. NIH Consensus Statement 1990;8:1–19.
109. Giuliano AE, Kirgan DM, Guenther JM, Morton DL. Lymphatic mapping and sentinel lymphadenectomy for breast cancer. Ann Surg 1994;220:391–401.
110. Turner RR, Ollila DW, Krasne DL, Giuliano AE. Histopathologic validation of the sentinel lymph node hypothesis for breast carcinoma. Ann Surg 1997;226:271–276.
111. Prognostic importance of occult axillary lymph node micrometastases from breast cancers. International (Ludwig) Breast Cancer Study Group [see comments]. Lancet 1990;335:1565–1568.
112. Trojani M, de Mascarel I, Bonichon F, Coindre JM, Delsol G. Micrometastases to axillary lymph nodes from carcinoma of breast: detection by immunohistochemistry and prognostic significance. Br J Cancer 1987;55:303–306.
113. Noguchi S, Aihara T, Motomura K, Inaji H, Imaoka S, Koyama H. Detection of breast cancer micrometastases in axillary lymph nodes by means of reverse transcriptase-polymerase chain reaction: comparison between MUC1 and mRNA and keratin 19 mRNA amplification. Am J Pathol 1996;148:649–656.
114. Menes TS, Tartter PI, Mizrachi H et al. Breast cancer patients with pN0 and pN1 sentinel nodes have high rate of nonsentinel node metastases. J Am Coll Surg 3/2005;(3):323–327.
115. Rosen PP, Groshen S, Kinne DW, Norton L. Factors influencing prognosis in node-negative breast carcinoma: analysis of 767 T1N0M0/T2N0M0 patients with long-term follow-up. J Clin Oncol 1993;11:2090–2100.
116. Thor AD, Berry DA, Budman DR, et al. Erb-2, p53, and efficacy of adjuvant therapy in lymph node-positive breast cancer. J Natl Cancer Inst 1998;90(18):1346–1360.
117. Fisher B, Redmond C, Dimitrov NV, et al. A randomized clinical trial evaluating sequential methotrexate and fluorouracil in the treatment of patients with node-negative breast cancer who have estrogen-receptor-negative tumors. N Engl J Med 1989;320:473–478.
118. Fisher B, Dignam J, Mamounas EP, et al. Sequential methotrexate and fluorouracil for the treatment of node-negative breast cancer patients with estrogen receptor-negative tumors: eight-year results from National Surgical Adjuvant Breast and Bowel Project (NSABP) B-13 and first report of findings from NSABP B-19 comparing methotrexate and fluorouracil with conventional cyclophosphamide, methotrexate, and fluorouracil [see comments]. J Clin Oncol 1996;14:1982–1992.
119. Fisher B, Costantino J, Redmond C, et al. A randomized clinical trial evaluating tamoxifen in the treatment of patients with node-negative breast cancer who have estrogen-receptor-positive tumors. N Engl J Med 1989;320:479–484.
120. Fisher B, Dignam J, Bryant J, et al. Five versus more than five years of tamoxifen therapy for breast cancer patients with negative lymph nodes and estrogen receptor-positive tumors [see comments]. J Natl Cancer Inst 1996;88:1529–1542.
121. Polychemotherapy for early breast cancer: an overview of the randomized trials. Early Breast Cancer Trialists' Collaborative Group. Lancet 1998;352(9132):930–942.
122. Early Breast Cancer Trialists' Collaborative Group. Systemic treatment of early breast cancer by hormonal, cytotoxic, or immune therapy: 133 randomised trials involving 31,000 recurrences and 24,000 deaths among 75,000 women [see comments]. Lancet 1992;339:71–85.
123. Coombes RC, Hall E, Gibson LJ, et al. A randomized trial of exemestane after two to three years of tamoxifen therapy in postmenopausal women with primary breast cancer. N Engl J Med 2004;350(11):1081–1092.
124. Jones SE, Moon TE, Bonadonna G, et al. Comparison of different trials of adjuvant chemotherapy in stage II breast cancer using a natural history data base. Am J Clin Oncol 1987;10:387–395.
125. Slamon DJ, Leyland-Jones B, Shaks S, et al. Use of chemotherapy plus a monoclonal antibody against Her 2 for metastatic breast cancer that overexpresses Her 2. N Engl J Med 2001;344(11):783–792.
126. Recht A, Come SE, Henderson IC, et al. The sequencing of chemotherapy and radiation therapy after conservative surgery for early-stage breast cancer [see comments]. N Engl J Med 1996;334:1356–1361.
127. Fisher B, Brown AM, Dimitrov NV, et al. Two months of doxorubicin-cyclophosphamide with and without interval reinduction therapy compared with 6 months of cyclophosphamide, methotrexate, and fluorouracil in positive-node breast cancer patients with tamoxifen-nonresponsive tumors: results from the National Surgical Adjuvant Breast and Bowel Project B-15. J Clin Oncol 1990;8:1483–1496.
128. Arthur DW, Morris MM, Vicini FA. Breast cancer: new radiation treatment options. Oncology 2004(13):1621–1629.
129. Bedwinek JM, Lee J, Fineberg B, Ocwieza M. Prognostic indicators in patients with isolated local-regional recurrence of breast cancer. Cancer (Phila) 1981;47:2232–2235.
130. Stefanik D, Goldberg R, Byrne P, et al. Local-regional failure in patients treated with adjuvant chemotherapy for breast cancer. J Clin Oncol 1985;3:660–665.

131. Jones JM, Ribeiro GG. Mortality patterns over 34 years of breast cancer patients in a clinical trial of post-operative radiotherapy [see comments]. Clin Radiol 1989;40:204–208.
132. Overgaard M, Hansen PS, Overgaard J, et al. Postoperative radiotherapy in high-risk premenopausal women with breast cancer who receive adjuvant chemotherapy: Danish Breast Cancer Cooperative Group 82b Trial [see comments]. N Engl J Med 1997;337:949–955.
133. Ragaz J, Jackson SM, Le N, et al. Adjuvant radiotherapy and chemotherapy in node-positive premenopausal women with breast cancer [see comments]. N Engl J Med 1997;337:956–962.
134. Swain SM, Sorace RA, Bagley CS, et al. Neoadjuvant chemotherapy in the combined modality approach of locally advanced nonmetastatic breast cancer. Cancer Res 1987;47:3889–3894.
135. Booser DJ, Hortobagyi GN. Treatment of locally advanced breast cancer. Semin Oncol 1992;19:278–285.
136. Hortobagyi GN, Ames FC, Buzdar AU, et al. Managements of stage III primary breast cancer with primary chemotherapy, surgery, and radiation therapy. Cancer (Phila) 1988;62:2507–2516.
137. Lippman ME, Sorace RA, Bagley CS, Danforth DW Jr, Lichter A, Wesley MN. Treatment of locally advanced breast cancer using primary induction chemotherapy with hormonal synchronization followed by radiation therapy with or without debulking surgery. Monogr Natl Cancer Inst 1986:1:153–159.
138. Rouesse J, Friedman S, Sarrazin D, et al. Primary chemotherapy in the treatment of inflammatory breast carcinoma: a study of 230 cases from the Institut Gustave-Roussy. J Clin Oncol 1986;4:1765–1771.
139. Perez CA, Fields JN, Fracasso PM, et al. Management of locally advanced carcinoma of the breast, II: Inflammatory carcinoma. Cancer (Phila) 1994;74(suppl 1):466–476.
139a. Newman LA, Buzdar AU, Singletary SE, et al. A prospective trial of preoperative chemotherapy in resectable breast cancer: predictors of breast-conservation therapy feasibility. Annals of Surgical Oncology 2002;9:217–219.
140. Hortobagyi GN, Theriault RL, Porter L, et al. Efficacy of pamidronate in reducing skeletal complications in patients with breast cancer and lytic bone metastases: protocol 19 Aredia Breast Cancer Study Group [see comments]. N Engl J Med 1996;335:1785–1791.
141. Paget J. Disease of the mammary areola preceding cancer of the mammary gland. St Bart Hosp Rep 1874;10:79–89.
142. Pierce LJ, Haffty BG, Solin LJ, et al. The conservative management of Paget's disease of the breast with radiotherapy. Cancer (Phila) 1997;80:1065–1072.
143. Harris J, Morrow M, Bonadonna G. Cancer of the breast. In: Harris J, Lippman M, Morrow M, eds. Diseases of the Breast. Philadelphia: Lippincott-Raven, 1996:129.
144. Campana F, Forquet A, Ashby M. Presentation of axillary lymphadenopathy without detectable breast primary: experience at Institut Curie. Radiol Oncol 1989;15:321–325.
145. Mazze RI, Kallean B. Reproductive outcome after anaesthesia and operation during pregnancy: a registry study of 5405 cases. Am J Obstet Gynecol 1980;138:1165.
146. Karlsson P, Holmberg E, Johansson KA, Kindblom LG, Carstensen J, Wallgren A. Soft tissue sarcoma after treatment for breast cancer. Radiother Oncol 1996;38:25–31.
147. Hayward J. The Guy's trials on "early" breast cancer. World J Surg 1977;1:314.
148. Sarrazin D, Le M, Arriagada R, et al. Ten-year results of a randomized trial comparing a conservative treatment to mastectomy in early breast cancer. Radiother Oncol 1989;14:177.
149. Lichter A, Lippman M, Danforth D, et al. Mastectomy versus breast-conserving therapy in the treatment of stage I and II carcinoma of the breast: a randomized trial at the National Cancer Institute. J Clin Oncol 1992;10:976.
150. Van Dongen J, Bartelink K, Fentimen I, et al. Randomized clinical trial to assess the value of breast conserving therapy in Stage I and II breast cancer: EORTC 10801 trial. Monogr J Natl Cancer Inst 1992;11:15.
151. Blichert-Toft M, Rose C, Andersen J, et al. Danish randomized trial comparing breast conservation therapy with mastectomy: six years of life-table analysis. Monogr J Natl Cancer Inst 1992;11:19.
152. Krag D, Harlow S, Weaver D, Ashikaga T. Technique of sentinel node resection in melanoma and breast cancer: probe-guided surgery and lymphatic mapping. Eur J Surg Oncol 1998;24:89–93.
153. Krag DN, Weaver DL, Alex JC, Fairbank JT. Surgical resection and radiolocalization of the sentinel lymph node in breast cancer using a gamma probe. Surg Oncol 1993;2:335–339.
154. Borgstein PJ, Meijer S, Pijpers R. Intradermal blue dye to identify sentinel lymph-node in breast cancer [letter] [see comments]. Lancet 1997;349:1668–1669.
155. Giuliano AE. Intradermal blue dye to identify sentinel lymph node in breast cancer (letter; comment), Lancet 1997;350:958.
156. Guenther JM, Krishnamoorthy M, Tan LR. Sentinel lymphadenectomy for breast cancer in a community managed care setting. Cancer J Sci Am 1997;3:336–340.
157. Veronesi U, Paganelli G, Galimberti V, et al. Sentinel-node biopsy to avoid axillary dissection in breast cancer with clinically negative lymph-nodes. Lancet 1997;349:1864–1867.
158. Barnwell JM, Arredondo MA, Kollmorgen D, et al. Sentinel node biopsy in breast cancer. Ann Surg Onc 1998;126–130.
159. Borgstein PJ, Pijpers R, Comans EF, Van Diest PJ, Boom RP, Meijer S. Sentinel lymph node biopsy in breast cancer: guidelines and pitfalls of lymphoscintigraphy and gamma probe detection. J Am Coll Surg 1998;186:275–283.
160. Krag D, Weaver D, Ashikaga T, et al. The sentinel node in breast cancer—a multicenter validation study (see comments). N Engl J Med 1998;339:941–946.
161. O'Hea BJ, Hill ADK, El-Shirbiny AM, et al. Sentinel lymph node biopsy in breast cancer: initial experience at Memorial Sloan-Kettering Cancer Center. J Am Coll Surg 1998;186:423–427.

97

Melanoma and Other Cutaneous Malignancies

Vernon K. Sondak, Eric H. Jensen, and Kim A. Margolin

Cancers of the skin constituted nearly one-half of all cancers diagnosed in 2006, at least 1,000,000 new cases in the United States alone. In fact, the skin is by far the most common primary site for human cancer development. Although skin cancer is often thought of as causing relatively little morbidity and mortality, more than 10,000 deaths were attributed to cutaneous malignancies in the United States in 2005, most (7,770) from malignant melanoma.[1] Moreover, both the incidence and mortality of skin cancers are increasing in the United States and throughout most of the world.[2,3] Although this chapter focuses primarily on melanoma, a discussion of other cutaneous malignancies is included.

Melanoma

The incidence of melanoma has climbed steadily since 1930; the rate of this increase is higher than that for any other type of cancer.[4] Because of its relatively young age of onset, melanoma is second only to leukemia in terms of the years of potential life lost per death among all types of malignancy in the United States.[5] Melanoma was expected to be diagnosed in more than 60,000 U.S. individuals in 2006.

Demographics and Epidemiology

The major etiological factor in the development of melanoma is exposure to ultraviolet (UV) radiation. In particular, intermittent, high-intensity exposure (e.g., blistering sunburns) contributes most dramatically to the development of melanoma. Fair-skinned individuals who lack the protective effect of melanin are at highest risk, whereas dark-skinned individuals are much less likely to develop melanoma. Even in individuals with a genetic predisposition, exposure to UV radiation is the primary factor determining whether an at-risk person actually develops melanoma.[6,7]

Disease Sites

Most melanomas (more than 90%) are cutaneous lesions; however, melanomas also occur in the pigmented cells of the retina and on mucous membranes of the nasopharynx, vulva, and anal canal. These noncutaneous primary sites frequently go unnoticed until they reach an advanced stage, at which point they are rarely curable. Little is known about the epidemiology or biological differences of noncutaneous melanomas from cutaneous melanomas. The risk factors and demographic data related here apply to cutaneous melanomas, unless specified otherwise. About 2% of melanoma cases present as metastatic disease to regional lymph nodes or distant sites without a known primary.[8,9]

Age

Melanoma affects a broad age range, with an average age of onset of 55 years. Three-quarters of all cases occur before age 70. More than 20% of cutaneous melanomas occur in individuals under 40 years of age.[8]

Gender

Melanoma is slightly more common in men than in women, with a male-to-female ratio of approximately 1.2:1. The most common site of melanoma development in males is the trunk, whereas the extremities are most frequently affected in females. Melanoma is now the most common malignancy in women 25 to 29 years of age and is exceeded only by breast cancer in women aged 30 to 35. It appears that women have a slightly better prognosis, stage for stage, compared to men.[8]

Race

Skin cancer is uncommon in people of African descent, with an annual age-adjusted incidence of only 0.9% compared to that of Caucasians. Asian and Latino individuals are also at low risk.[10] It is important to recognize, however, that melanoma and other skin cancers do occur in these groups, and suspicious lesions should be evaluated appropriately. The presentation of melanoma is different in more deeply pigmented races, with most melanomas occurring on the relatively nonpigmented skin of the palms and soles.[11,12]

Geography

Incidence rates of melanoma are highest in areas of the world where fair-skinned peoples live in a very sunny climate near the equator.[3] Thus, Australia and Israel have among the highest melanoma rates in the world (more than 40 cases per 100,000 Caucasian individuals per year) followed by the southwestern United States and Hawaii (about 20–30 cases per 100,000 Caucasian individuals annually). The incidence of melanoma in the United States decreases with increasing latitude (i.e., more northerly regions). Overall, about 12 cases of melanoma are seen per 100,000 U.S. whites.

Specific Risk Factors

Ultraviolet Light

Most dangerous is UVB radiation (wavelength, 290–320nm), but UVA (320–400nm) probably also has carcinogenic potential.[13] There are two likely explanations for the increasing incidence of melanoma and nonmelanoma skin cancers: people spend more time in the sunlight, and the atmosphere's ability to screen out UV radiation is impaired as the result of depletion of the ozone layer. Different types of skin cancer are associated with different patterns of sun exposure: intermittent exposure appears to be more important in most cases of melanoma, with a number of studies implicating blistering sunburns during childhood as a major risk factor for later melanoma development.[13,14] It has recently been observed that chronic sun exposure, as evidenced by the presence of solar elastosis, is associated with a more favorable melanoma biology.[15] Melanoma is more common in indoor workers than outdoor laborers and occurs most often on parts of the body that are only occasionally exposed to the sun. The one exception is lentigo maligna melanoma, which occurs most frequently on the head and neck of older individuals with a long history of chronic sun exposure and evidence of severe actinic skin damage, as is the case for nonmelanoma skin cancer. Melanoma is quite rare on skin surfaces that are never exposed to the sun (the "bathing suit" or doubly covered areas).

Typical and Atypical Moles

Melanoma occurs most frequently in fair-skinned, light-haired individuals who sunburn easily and rarely or never tan. The size, number, and appearance of moles on an individual's skin also affect the risk of melanoma development.

Typical moles or benign moles, also called melanocytic nevi, are small (less than 6mm), round, uniformly tan or brown, and symmetrical (Fig. 97.1). They are generally raised above the skin surface, as opposed to freckles, which are flat. Patients with many (25 or more) melanocytic nevi are at increased risk for melanoma development[16,17]; most of these patients are also fair-skinned, light-haired individuals who burn easily and rarely tan.

Atypical moles, also called clinically atypical nevi or dysplastic nevi, are larger (generally 6mm or more), asymmetrical, and often raised with a pebbly surface (Fig. 97.2). Although atypical moles are frequently referred to as dysplastic nevi, pathological analysis does not always demonstrate the presence of dysplasia. Hence, the term clinically atypical nevi is preferred. Atypical nevi are usually tan or brown but may have various shades of coloration within them. At least 5% of the white population of the United States has one or more clinically atypical nevus. Otherwise normal individuals with at least one clinically atypical nevus have a 6% lifetime risk of developing melanoma. This risk rises to as high as 80% or more in individuals who have a family history of melanoma in addition to one or more atypical nevi.[18] Some clinically atypical nevi eventually develop into melanoma. Even if every atypical mole is surgically removed, however, the patient remains at increased risk for melanoma development in the remaining normal skin. Until such time, if any, that genetic testing identifies those individuals with atypical moles who are at greatest risk of melanoma development, all individuals with clinically atypical nevi should be carefully followed.[19,20] Close follow-up is particularly important in those with a family history of melanoma.

Dysplastic nevus syndrome is a familial tendency to develop atypical moles and also melanoma. Approximately

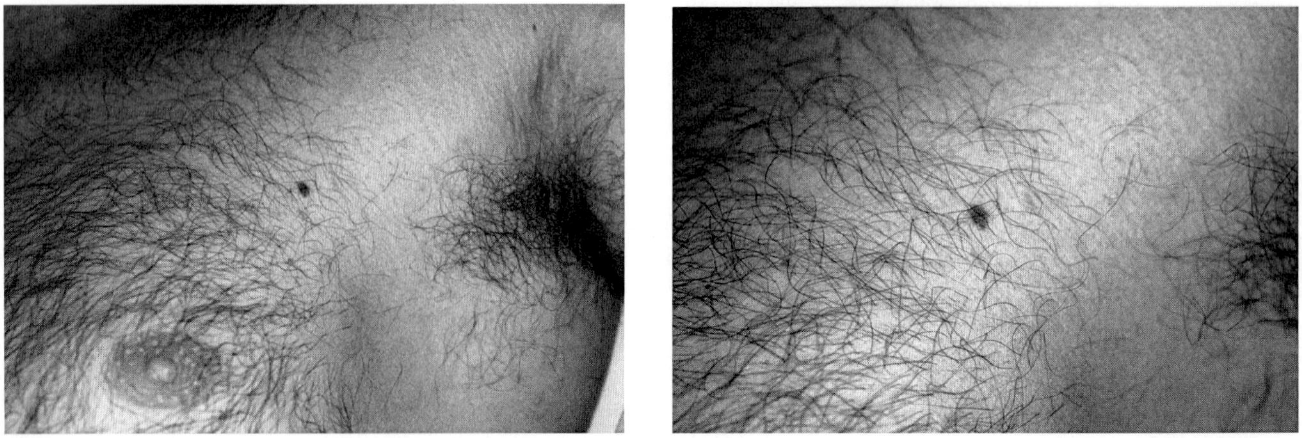

A B

FIGURE 97.1. A, B. Typical moles, also called melanocytic nevi, are small (less than 6mm), round symmetrical, and uniformly tan or brown.

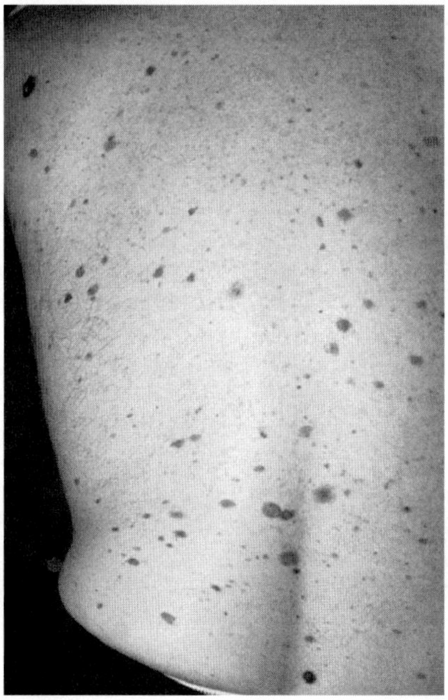

FIGURE 97.2. Clinically atypical moles, also called dysplastic nevi, are large (generally greater than 6 mm), asymmetrical, and have a pebbly surface. They may have various shades of coloration.

10% of melanomas occur in patients with a family history, most often in association with multiple clinically atypical nevi. The dysplastic nevus syndrome was initially named the B-K mole syndrome (after the initials of the last names of the two families in which it was recognized).[21] The name familial atypical multiple mole melanoma (FAMMM) syndrome has also been proposed as an alternative.[22] Familial patients tend to be diagnosed at a younger age and often develop multiple primaries. Studies in several kindreds suggest an autosomal-dominant pattern of inheritance, with some cases being linked to markers on either chromosomes 1p or 9p.[23,24]

Giant congenital nevi are pigmented lesions actually present at birth, as opposed to developing months or years later. (Most typical and atypical nevi are not present at birth, and many develop after puberty.) Among congenital nevi, only the giant congenital nevus (defined as greater than 20 cm in maximum diameter), a very rare lesion, is a documented precursor to melanoma.[25] Most melanomas that occur in children under 10 years of age arise within these lesions. Whenever the cosmetic result permits, giant congenital nevi should be excised in early childhood. If complete excision is impossible, even with staged procedures, close follow-up is indicated.

Genetic Predisposition

Multiple genes have been implicated in the development and progression of melanoma. CDKN2A (which codes for the proteins p16 and p14^{ARF}) and CDK4 are susceptibility genes located on chromosomes 9p21 and 12q14, respectively. These genes encode cyclin-dependent kinases (CDK) that are integral to cell cycle regulation.[19] p16 in particular plays a vital inhibitory role in maintaining cells at the G_1/S interface through interactions with CDK4 and CDK6, which control phosphorylation of the retinoblastoma family of proteins. Inactivating mutations of p16 lead to uninhibited phosphorylation of RB-1 protein, causing transcription factor E2F-1 to be released, thereby inducing S-phase genes and resulting in uninhibited progression through the cell cycle.[20]

Although CDKN2A has been implicated in the development of melanoma, there are clearly multiple other factors involved, including environmental exposure and other, as yet undiscovered susceptibility genes. Germline mutations in CDKN2A have been identified in only 40% of familial melanoma pedigrees. The penetrance of these mutations has been shown to be highly dependent on geographic location. Comparison of European, American, and Australian pedigrees reveals mutation penetrance by age 80 of 0.57, 0.70, and 0.91 respectively, indicating the importance of environmental factors in addition to genetic predisposition.[26] Polymorphisms in the melanocortin-1 receptor gene may contribute further to this environmental influence,[6] as may inherited variations in the capacity to handle oxidative stress, which results when UV radiation interacts with intracellular melanin pigment.[27]

Genetics

No single genetic change is found in all melanomas. In addition to inherited or sporadic loss of p16 or CDK4 function, mutations in the mitogen-activated protein kinase (MAPK) pathway are extremely common in melanoma. Proteins in this pathway act as mediators of intracellular signaling, with particular importance in the regulation of cell growth and response to UV radiation. It has been noted that 60% to 90% of melanomas contain a mutation in the B-*raf* gene; encoding a serine/threonine kinase involved in the MAPK pathway. A single transversion (T1799A) in exon 15 results in a missense mutation (V600E), resulting in constitutive activation of the kinase, which accounts for 80% or more of B-*raf* mutations.[28] The Ras family of genes is upstream of B-*raf* in the MAPK pathway. Mutations in either *Ras* (N-*ras* in particular) or *Raf* are common in melanomas, but mutations in both are extremely rare.[20,29,30] Thus, it is likely that the pathway need only be perturbed at one level for melanomagenesis to occur. The observation that B-*raf*-activating mutations can be found in a significant percentage of benign nevi as well as melanoma cell lines[31,32] highlights the fact that much remains to be learned about the key molecular events in the process of melanoma development.[33]

Diagnosis and Prognosis

The prognosis for melanoma is directly related to the stage at initial diagnosis. The most commonly used staging system is the TNM system (Tables 97.1, 97.2). If detected early (stage I or II), most cutaneous melanomas can be cured with surgical excision. The prognosis of patients with lymphatic dissemination decreases significantly, and only a minority of patients who develop metastatic disease survive beyond 5 years (Fig. 97.3).

Early Diagnosis of Melanoma

Because melanoma is situated on the skin, early detection of melanoma should be the goal in every case. This aim requires that melanomas be differentiated from typical and atypical benign moles, and that amelanotic melanomas be recognized as well.

TABLE 97.1. American Joint Committee on Cancer (AJCC) Melanoma T Classification by Thickness and Ulceration Status.

T classification	*Thickness*	*Ulceration status*
T1	1.0mm or less	a: without ulceration and level II/III b: with ulceration or level IV/V
T2	1.01–2.0mm	a: without ulceration b: with ulceration
T3	2.01–4.0mm	a: without ulceration b: with ulceration
T4	More than 4.0mm	a: without ulceration b: with ulceration
N classification	No. of metastatic nodes	Nodal metastatic mass
N1	1 node	a: micrometastasis* b: macrometastasis†
N2	2–3 nodes	a: micrometastasis* b: macrometastasis† c: in transit met(s)/ satellite(s) without metastatic nodes
N3	4 or more metastatic nodes, or matted nodes, or in transit met(s)/ satellite(s) with metastatic node(s)	
M classification	Site	Serum lactate dehydrogenase
M1a	Distant skin, subcutaneous, or nodal metastases	Normal
M1b	Lung metastases	Normal
M1c	All other visceral metastases	Normal
	Any distant metastasis	Elevated

*Micrometastases are diagnosed after sentinel or elective lymphadenectomy.

†Macrometastases are defined as clinically detectable nodal metastases confirmed by therapeutic lymphadenectomy or when nodal metastasis exhibits gross extracapsular extension.

Source: With permission from Balch CM, Buzaid AC, Soong SJ, et al. Final version of the American Joint Committee on Cancer staging system for cutaneous melanoma. J Clin Oncol 2001;19:3635–3648.

TABLE 97.2. AJCC Stage Groupings for Cutaneous Melanoma.

	*Clinical staging**			*Pathological staging*†		
	T	*N*	*M*	*T*	*N*	*M*
0	Tis	N0	M0	Tis	N0	M0
IA	T1a	N0	M0	T1a	N0	M0
IB	T1b T2a	N0 N0	M0 M0	T1b T2a	N0 N0	M0 M0
IIA	T2b T3a	N0 N0	M0 M0	T2b T3a	N0 N0	M0 M0
IIB	T3b T4a	N0 N0	M0 M0	T3b T4a	N0 N0	M0 M0
IIC	T4b	N0	M0	T4b	N0	M0
III‡	Any T	N1 N2 N3	M0			
IIIA				T1-4a T1-4a	N1a N2a	M0 M0
IIIB				T1-4b T1-4b T1-4a T1-4a T1-4a/b	N1a N2a N1b N2b N2c	M0 M0 M0 M0 M0
IIIC				T1-4b T1-4b Any T	N1b N2b N3	M0 M0 M0
IV	Any T	Any N	Any M1	Any T	Any N	Any M1

*Clinical staging includes microstaging of the primary melanoma and clinical/radiologic evaluation for metastases. By convention, it should be used after complete excision of the primary melanoma with clinical assessment for regional and distant metastases.

†Pathological staging includes microstaging of the primary melanoma and pathological information about the regional lymph nodes after partial or complete lymphadenectomy. Pathological stage 0 or stage 1A patients are the exception; they do not require pathological evaluation of their lymph nodes.

‡There are no stage III subgroups for clinical staging.

Source: With permission from Balch CM, Buzaid AC, Soong SJ, et al. Final version of the American Joint Committee on Cancer staging system for cutaneous melanoma. J Clin Oncol 2001;19:3635–3648.

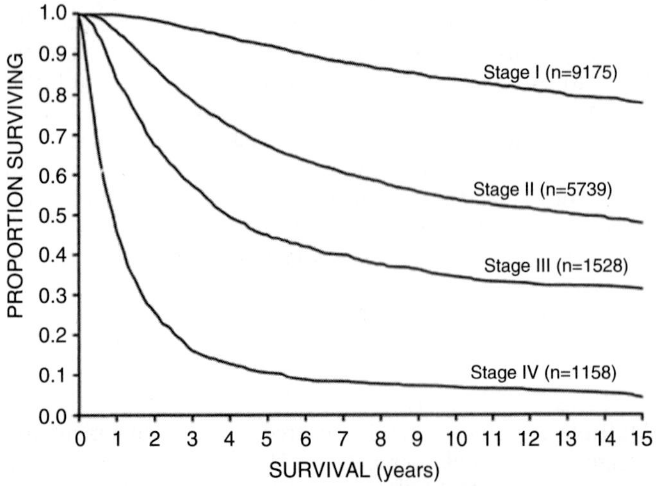

FIGURE 97.3. Fifteen-year survival curves comparing localized melanoma (stages II and I), regional metastases (stage III), and distant metastases (stage IV). The *numbers in parentheses* are patients from the AJCC melanoma staging database used to calculate the survival rates. The differences between the curves are significant ($P < 0.0001$). (With permission from Balch CM, Buzaid AC, Soong SJ, et al. Final version of the American Joint Committee on Cancer staging system for cutaneous melanoma. J Clin Oncol 2001;19:3635–3648.)

Differentiation from Benign Moles

Early melanomas (Fig. 97.4) may be differentiated from typical benign moles (see Figure 97.1) by assessing for asymmetry, border irregularity, color (variable or very dark), and diameter greater than 6mm (the so-called ABCDs; Table 97.3). Recently, an "E" has been added, representing enlargement of the lesion over time, which is another sign associated with malignancy. Other signs of melanoma include itching, bleeding, ulceration, or changes in a preexisting mole.

Clinically Atypical Nevi

Clinically atypical nevi have some, but not all, the features of melanoma: They are generally larger than 6mm, asymmetrical, and often show border irregularity (see Fig. 97.2). Significantly raised areas or regions of dark brown or black pigmentation in an atypical nevus suggest the development of melanoma. Biopsy of any suspicious skin lesion should be carried out. Patients with too many atypical nevi to excise require careful follow-up. Periodic total-body skin examinations combined with photographs of any atypical nevi and, most importantly, thorough patient education on the need to watch for changes in existing moles or the development of

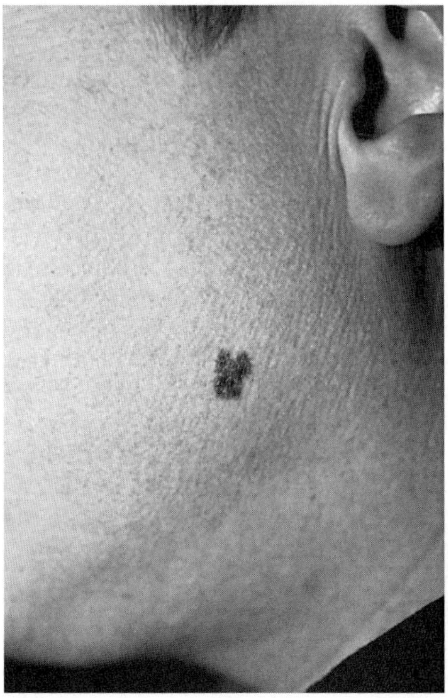

FIGURE 97.4. Early melanomas generally demonstrate asymmetry, border irregularity, dark or variable coloration, and diameter greater than 6 mm.

new lesions are essential components of the management of patients with atypical moles.[21]

AMELANOTIC MELANOMA

Most (but not all) melanomas are pigmented. Nonpigmented melanomas are referred to as "amelanotic" melanomas. These are among the hardest types of melanoma to diagnose, and they are often mistaken for basal and squamous cell cancers or benign lesions such as pyogenic granuloma. A high index of suspicion and a low threshold for conducting biopsies of persistent or suspicious nonpigmented lesions is the only way amelanotic melanomas can be diagnosed at a relatively early stage. Even then, they are characteristically diagnosed at a more advanced stage than the average pigmented melanoma.

SKIN AND REGIONAL LYMPH NODE EXAMINATION

Total-body skin examination is a critical part of the initial evaluation and subsequent follow-up of patients with melanoma, nonmelanoma skin cancer, or clinically atypical nevi. Because of the common denominator of solar exposure in the causation of most skin cancers, patients with one skin cancer are at significant risk of harboring or developing a second or even multiple skin cancers, often of a different histological type. A complete skin examination is essential for patients with clinically atypical nevi, because they are at increased risk for the development of melanoma on their entire skin surface, not just within recognized moles. A thorough skin examination requires a well-lit room, a completely disrobed patient, and a relaxed and unhurried approach. Useful adjuncts in selected cases include serial skin photography and special techniques such as dermoscopy, also called epiluminescence microscopy (direct application of a magnifying lens to an area of the skin with oil applied to minimize reflectance).[34] Wood's lamp ("black light") illumination can be helpful in the evaluation of the rare patient who presents without a known primary; areas of depigmentation stand out clearly under the Wood's lamp and can be biopsied to look for histological evidence of a regressed melanocytic lesion.

All accessible lymph nodes groups (cervical, supraclavicular, axillary, and inguinal regions) should be carefully examined in melanoma patients at the time of presentation and at each follow-up visit. Lymphatic metastasis is the most frequently encountered type of dissemination in melanoma.

BIOPSY TECHNIQUES

When the decision is made to biopsy a suspicious pigmented or nonpigmented skin lesion, several factors must be taken into consideration. First and foremost, the pathologist must receive adequate tissue to permit assessment of all relevant histological features. Also, the initial biopsy should be planned so as not to complicate subsequent surgical treatment.[35]

TECHNIQUES TO AVOID

Partial-thickness shave biopsies, cryosurgery, or electrodesiccation do not allow for pathological analysis of margins and depth of invasion and should be avoided.

COMPLETE EXCISION

Ideally, most clinically suspicious skin lesions should be biopsied by complete excision using local anesthesia, taking a 1- to 2-mm margin of normal skin and including some subcutaneous fat. Unusually large lesions or those situated in cosmetically sensitive areas, such as the face, may be approached by incisional or punch biopsy. In these cases, sampling the most elevated portion of the lesion provides the best estimate of tumor thickness. Frozen-section analysis is not routinely employed for the diagnosis of skin lesions.

BIOPSY OF LYMPH NODES

Lymph node basins are predominantly evaluated by physical examination, although the potential role of ultrasonography is receiving increasing attention.[36,37] Enlarged lymph nodes suspected of representing melanoma metastasis are initially evaluated by fine-needle aspiration cytology.[38] A positive cytology is grounds for performing a full lymph node dissection. If the cytology is nondiagnostic or negative, or if the node is in a location that precludes aspiration, an open biopsy is appropriate. Only the enlarged node should be removed, with minimal dissection of the surrounding tissue. In this setting, frozen-section analysis may be conducted and, if indicative of melanoma, a lymph node dissection carried out during the same procedure in an appropriately informed and consenting patient.

TABLE 97.3. Differentiating Melanoma from Typical Benign Moles: the ABCDs.

	Characteristic	*Melanoma*	*Benign moles*
A:	Asymmetry	Asymmetrical	Symmetrical
B:	Border irregularity	Irregular, notched	Regular, round
C:	Color	Very dark or variable	Uniform, brown or tan
D:	Diameter	Usually more than 6 mm	Always less than 6 mm

Sentinel Lymph Node Biopsy. Clinically normal lymph nodes harbor microscopic or even macroscopic deposits of melanoma in up to 30% of patients. A technique for identifying those lymph nodes most likely to be involved by melanoma, called the "sentinel" nodes, is described in detail later in this chapter.

Histological Types of Melanoma

Melanomas are classified into four major histological categories: superficial spreading melanoma, nodular melanoma, lentigo maligna melanoma, and acral-lentiginous melanoma. *Superficial spreading melanomas* constitute up to 70% of cutaneous melanomas. They often arise within a preexisting nevus and are surrounded by a zone of atypical melanocytes that may extend beyond the visible borders of the lesion. *Nodular melanomas* represent about 8% to 10% of cutaneous melanomas. They are generally dark blue-black and are more symmetrical and uniform in color than other melanomas. *Lentigo maligna melanomas* also account for about 10% of cutaneous melanomas. They typically occur on the sun-exposed areas of the head and neck and the hands. Clinically, they are large (often >3 cm), flat, tan lesions with areas of dark brown or black coloration. These lesions arise from a precursor lesion known as lentigo maligna, or Hutchinson's melanotic freckle. *Acral-lentiginous melanomas* occur on the palms, soles, and beneath the nails (subungual melanoma), and make up only 1% of melanoma cases.[8] Subungual melanomas can easily be confused with subungual hematomas, and delays in diagnosis and proper treatment are common with these sites; the presence of pigmentation in the paronychial skin is generally indicative of melanoma.

Acral-lentiginous melanoma is a distinct variant of melanoma that occurs in equal frequency among light- and darker-pigmented races. Because of their higher incidence of other types of cutaneous melanoma, acral-lentiginous melanomas account for only 1% of melanomas in Caucasians, as opposed to about 40% of melanomas in Africans, Latinos, and Asians.[10–12]

Growth Phases of Melanoma

The local growth of melanoma has been characterized as occurring in two distinct phases: a radial and a vertical phase.[39] *Radial growth phase* is characterized by melanoma tumor cells extending laterally ("radially") within the epidermis and papillary dermis. Although pure radial growth phase melanomas may be fully invasive lesions, they are extremely unlikely to metastasize to the regional nodes or beyond, and have a prognosis nearly as good as melanoma in situ. *Vertical growth phase*, defined as the presence of either one or more dermal mitoses or a dermal nest of melanoma cells larger than the largest epidermal nest, is associated with a much greater potential for metastasis. As discussed next, the depth of dermal invasion correlates directly with prognosis. This correlation is valid only for lesions in the vertical growth phase because radial growth phase lesions have an excellent prognosis regardless of depth.

Pathological Staging of Melanoma

In the absence of distant metastatic disease, the single most important prognostic factor in melanoma is the status of the regional lymph nodes. Currently, 85% of melanoma patients present with clinically normal lymph nodes. In clinically node-negative patients, most investigators have found the microscopic degree of invasion of the melanoma, or *microstage*, to be of critical importance in predicting outcome. Two methods have been described for microscopic staging of primary cutaneous melanomas.

Clark's levels were devised by Wallace Clark and associates to classify melanomas according to the level of invasion relative to histologically defined landmarks in the skin. Clark's five levels are depicted in Figure 97.5. Clark's levels correlate with prognosis: lesions with deeper levels of invasion have a greater risk of recurrence. The biggest drawback to Clark's system is that the thickness of the skin, and hence the distance between the various dermal layers, varies widely in different areas of the body. Except for Clark's level I (melanoma in situ), there is no scientific rationale for considering these dermal layers to be biological barriers to tumor growth. For example, there is no compelling evidence to suggest that a lesion that reaches but does not invade the reticular dermis is inherently less aggressive than an equivalent melanoma that penetrates into the reticular dermis because it is situated in an area where the skin is thinner. Current American Joint Committee on Cancer (AJCC) staging criteria incorporate Clark's level as a prognostic factor for stage I tumors only (i.e., those 1.0 mm or less), but even this association has been the subject of debate.

Breslow's thickness, an alternative microstaging method described by Alexander Breslow, addresses some of the problems associated with Clark's levels. In this method, the thickness of the primary tumor is measured from the top of the granular layer of the epidermis to the deepest contiguous tumor cell at the base of the lesion using a micrometer in the microscope eyepiece. Many investigators have documented an inverse correlation between the maximum measured tumor thickness and survival. More importantly, several studies have demonstrated that tumor thickness conveys more prognostic information than does Clark's level of invasion. In addition, the measurement of tumor thickness is generally more reproducible and less subjective than is the determination of Clark's level. For these reasons, Breslow's thickness is preferred for clinical decision making and staging classification. Occasionally, usually because of technical factors related to the nature of the biopsy or the preparation of the pathology specimen, Breslow's thickness is impossible

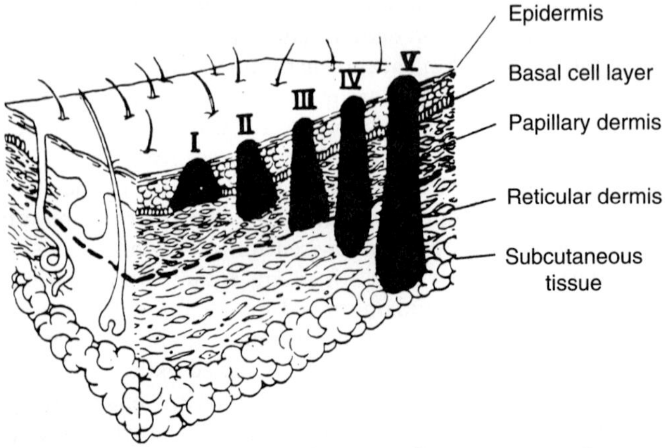

FIGURE 97.5. Clark's levels of invasion for cutaneous melanoma.

to determine and only the Clark's level is available for microstaging. These situations, which inevitably result in the loss of important prognostic information, can usually be avoided by performing full-thickness (not partial-thickness shave) biopsies and by careful attention to detail when preparing histology specimens.

Regional Lymph Node Involvement

There is a direct relationship between the thickness of a primary melanoma and the likelihood of metastatic involvement of the regional lymph nodes. The presence of regional lymph node metastases is a poor prognostic sign regardless of the microstage of the primary lesion. As in other cancers, the number of involved lymph nodes has an inverse correlation with survival. In general, patients with palpable nodes fare worse than those with only microscopic involvement. Extranodal invasion (also called extracapsular extension) of melanoma into the soft tissue of the node basin increases the chance of regional recurrence after lymphadenectomy and is associated with a poorer overall prognosis. The survival rate for patients with nodal metastases varies over a broad range: patients with one to three nodes involved with microscopic metastases have a 5-year survival of 50% to 69%, whereas patients with multiple (four or more) grossly positive nodes have a 5-year survival of 13% to 27%.[40]

TNM Staging System

The AJCC staging system for melanoma incorporates prognostic factors that were validated on a multiinstitutional sample of more than 17,000 patients (see Table 97.1). The tumor (T) classification is based on Breslow's thickness of the primary tumor (T1, 1 mm or less; T2, 1.1–2.0 mm; T3, 2.1–4.0 mm; T4, more than 4 mm), and is modified by the absence (a) or presence (b) of ulceration (and for T1 melanomas only, the presence of Clark's level IV or V).[40] The presence of ulceration in a primary melanoma has been recognized as one of the strongest negative predictive factors for long-term survival. Ulceration is defined as the lack of a complete epidermal layer overlying the melanocytic lesion. The presence of ulceration "upstages" patients to the next highest T level. In other words, patients with 1.1- to 2.0-mm melanomas that are ulcerated carry the same long-term prognosis as those with 2.1- to 4.0-mm nonulcerated melanomas. The risk of ulceration is directly related to tumor depth; patients with melanomas 1.0 mm or less have a very low rate of ulceration (6% or less), whereas those with 4-mm melanomas have a rate as high as 63%.[40]

The node (N) classification is based on the number of nodes (N1 = 1, N2 = 2–3, N3 = 4 or more or matted nodes) and is modified by the size of the nodal metastasis (a = microscopic, b = macroscopic). The metastasis (M) classification is based on the site of distant metastasis and the serum lactate dehyrogenase (LDH) level (M1a = skin, soft tissue, or distant nodes with normal LDH level, M1b = lung metastases with normal LDH level, M1c = visceral metastases or elevated LDH level). Figure 97.3 shows the 5-year survival rates associated with each stage. Although this system does not take into account all known prognostic factors, it does provide a useful classification relevant to clinical decision making, and its use should be encouraged in all cases.[40]

Other Prognostic Factors

Histological Type

In general, nodular and acral-lentiginous melanomas are significantly thicker at the time of diagnosis than superficial spreading or lentigo maligna melanomas. Even when TNM stage was taken into account, however, nodular and acral-lentiginous melanomas had a significantly worse prognosis in a recent review of more than 84,000 melanoma cases.[8]

Site of the Primary

Several studies have shown that patients with melanomas of the extremities have a better survival rate than patients with lesions arising on the trunk or head and neck. In particular, the subset of melanomas occurring on the back, back of the upper arms, neck, and scalp—the so-called BANS area—have been reported to have a worse prognosis.[41] What these parts of the body have in common is that they are relatively hidden from a person's view, and hence melanomas in these locations tend to present as thicker lesions. Some studies suggest, however, that when lesions of equivalent thickness are compared, overall survival for BANS melanomas is similar to that for other sites. Thus, whether primary site can be considered an independent prognostic factor for survival in cutaneous melanoma remains a matter of debate. It is likely that molecular genetic differences in the pathogenesis of these melanoma subtypes contribute to these differences in their clinical behavior.

Other Pathological Features

Angiolymphatic invasion is defined as invasion of tumor cells into the wall and/or lumen of vessels or lymphatics of the dermis or deeper structures and is uncommon in melanoma. When present, this finding is clearly associated with more aggressive tumors: multiple studies have shown higher rates of lymph node involvement and worsened long-term survival in patients with angioinvasive melanomas. In fact, risk of lymphatic involvement increases as much as threefold whereas 5-year survival is reduced by as much as 50% when comparing matched patients with and without angiolymphatic invasion.

Angiogenesis is the development of new blood vessels in and around a tumor and differs from angiolymphatic invasion. Angiogenesis appears to be a marker of invasive potential and is found more frequently in thicker lesions. Multiple studies have suggested that angiogenesis may be an independent factor affecting long-term survival as well as local recurrence.[42]

Mitotic rate is typically measured as the number of mitotic figures/mm^2 in the most mitotically active region of the primary tumor. High mitotic rates have been found to be predictive of increased metastatic potential and decreased long-term survival in numerous studies.[43,44]

Regression is a histological finding indicative of a host immune response to invasive melanoma. Areas where melanoma cells once existed are replaced by inflammatory reaction and fibrosis; this may make it impossible to determine the maximum thickness attained by the primary lesion. There is continuing debate regarding the prognostic importance of regression; however, it is clear that even lesions with extensive or total regression can develop lymph node metastases.

Tumor-infiltrating lymphocytes (TIL) are found in variable numbers in primary melanomas. Brisk TIL are associated with an improved prognosis, likely representing an active host response to the tumor.[45,46]

Desmoplastic melanomas represent an uncommon spindle cell variant of melanoma with dense fibrosis and frequent neurotropism, a tendency to grow along nerves and nerve sheaths. Clinically, they are raised, firm nodules that are amelanotic in up to 40% of cases, frequently resulting in delayed diagnosis. Likely because of their neurotropism, these tumors have reported local recurrence rates as high as 40%, which has led many to advocate local radiation therapy following excision of these lesions. Whether pure desmoplastic melanomas, those without neurotropism, have a significantly greater risk of local recurrence than other melanomas remains a subject of considerable debate. Although many desmoplastic melanomas are deeply invasive at the time of diagnosis, overall they are less likely to metastasize to regional lymph nodes and may be more likely to develop distant metastases without lymph node involvement than nondesmoplastic melanomas.[47]

Gender and Age

Female gender and age less than 60 years have been found to be independent favorable prognostic factors in many but not all studies.[8,39,48] Older males seem to be particularly at risk of presenting with a locally advanced primary lesion. The prognosis for melanoma occurring in childhood has not been extensively studied, but appears to be similar or slightly improved compared to adults. Anecdotal experience suggests that young children (under 10) have a better prognosis than adolescents or adults with melanoma.[49,50]

Surgical Treatment of Cutaneous Melanoma

Surgery remains the mainstay of treatment for local/regional cutaneous melanoma (stages I–III) and occasionally plays a role in selected patients with stage IV disease as well. Initial surgical management of the patient with clinically localized melanoma involves adequate excision of the primary lesion and, in many cases, staging of the regional lymph nodes.

Excision of the Primary Lesion

It was recognized more than a century ago that tumor cells could extend within the skin for several centimeters beyond the visible borders of a melanoma, so that the risk of local recurrence is reduced if an area of normal skin is excised around the primary. Initially, a "one size fits all" approach of taking a 5-cm margin around all cutaneous melanomas was adopted. With such wide margins, skin grafts were required in all but a few cases. More recently, it was recognized that the thickness of the primary tumor influenced the likelihood of local recurrence and not all melanomas require the same excision margin. For instance, retrospective reviews indicated that melanomas less than 1 mm thick had very low recurrence rates even when less than the full 5-cm margin was excised. This realization prompted a number of randomized trials to determine the optimal excision margins for melanomas based on Breslow's thickness.

One randomized trial found that when a 1-cm margin of normal skin was taken around a melanoma less than 1 mm thick, the local recurrence rate was exceedingly low (<1%) and patient survival was just as good as if 3-cm margins were taken. For melanomas 1 to 2 mm in thickness, patient survival was the same for both margins of excision, but the local recurrence rate was slightly higher with the 1-cm margin (about 2%).[51,52] Another randomized trial compared 2-cm to 4-cm margins for all cutaneous melanomas between 1 and 4 mm in thickness. In this trial, both local recurrence and survival were the same whether 2- or 4-cm margins were taken. Skin grafts were less frequent and hospital stays shorter with the narrower margin, however.[53,54] Recently, a randomized trial conducted in patients with melanomas 2 mm in thickness compared 1-cm to 3-cm margins. The combined frequency of local and regional recurrences was higher in the patients who had a 1-cm margin, mostly because of an increased rate of nodal relapses. This finding raises the possibility that a narrow margin for thicker lesions could be associated with unrecognized persistent disease leading to subsequent nodal metastasis, but it may be nothing more than an imbalance in the preexisting incidence of nodal disease, because no surgical staging of the lymph nodes was done in this trial.[55,56]

Current Recommendations

The current recommendations for excision margins of cutaneous melanomas are summarized in Table 97.4. Based on randomized trial data, for lesions less than 1 mm in thickness, the recommended excision margin is 1 cm. Lesions 1 to 2 mm in thickness are treated with a 2-cm margin if they are situated in an area that permits such an excision to be closed primarily, but may be excised with a 1-cm margin if doing so would avoid the need for a skin graft. Tumors between 2 mm and 4 mm in thickness are treated with a 2-cm margin wherever possible. The optimal excision margins for thicker lesions and tumors with satellitosis have not been addressed in prospective, randomized trials. Based on retrospective data, at least a 2-cm margin should be taken for these high-risk primary melanomas.[57]

Several facts should be borne in mind regarding these recommendations. Regardless of the recommended width of excision, a histologically negative margin is necessary. Thus, if a 2-cm margin is taken and the pathology report reveals melanoma cells or atypical melanocytic hyperplasia at the margins, further excision is indicated. When the anatomic location of the primary precludes excision of the desired margin (e.g., on the hands and feet or the face), excision with at least 1 cm of normal tissue is appropriate so long as the margins are histologically negative. If a minor compromise in excision margin can allow primary closure without a skin graft, this may be worthwhile, particularly for lesions between 1 and 2 mm in thickness.

Although the current recommendations for excision margins are narrower than what was once the norm, the importance of an adequately wide excision cannot be overstressed. When excessively narrow margins are taken, local recurrence rates inevitably rise, and local recurrence of melanoma is associated with as much as an 85% chance of eventual death from the disease. The critical role of Breslow's thickness in determining excision margins also highlights

TABLE 97.4.
Current Recommendations for Excision Margins for Cutaneous Melanomas.

Location	*Tumor thickness*	*Recommended margin evidence*	*Reference*
Trunk and proximal extremity	<1 mm 51,52	1 cm	Randomized trial[a]
	1–2 mm 51,52,53,54	2 cm if able to be closed primarily, otherwise 1 cm	Randomized trials[a]
	2–4 mm 53,54	2 cm	Randomized trial[a]
	>4 mm or with satellitosis 57	At least 2 cm	Nonrandomized clinical series[b] Accepted surgical practice[c]
Head and neck and distal extremity	<1 mm 51, 52	1 cm	Randomized trial[a]
	≥1 mm	At least 1 cm	Accepted surgical practice[c]

[a]Level I evidence. Level I evidence is defined as prospective, randomized clinical trials.
[b]Level II evidence. Level II evidence is defined as clinical trials without randomization or case-controlled retrospective studies.
[c]Level III evidence. Level III evidence is defined as retrospective analyses without case controls, accepted clinical practice, or anecdotal case reports.

the importance of careful biopsy technique and pathological analysis in the treatment of localized melanoma.

Mohs surgery is a technique in which a cutaneous lesion is completely excised with a narrow margin of normal skin and the periphery is evaluated microscopically at the time of surgery to determine whether wider excision of specific areas is required. This technique has only limited applicability to melanoma, and significant limitations should be recognized. The artifacts in cellular morphology that are inherent in frozen sections, even those of the best technical quality, make it very difficult to distinguish melanoma from normal melanocytes at the excision margin. Although immunohistochemical stains can help, these have been performed mostly in research settings and are not part of the routine evaluation of Mohs specimens. Mohs surgery is not recommended for the treatment of invasive melanomas, and should play only a very limited role in the treatment of melanoma in situ in cosmetically sensitive areas such as the face.

Management of Regional Lymph Nodes

Melanoma patients with clinical evidence of lymph node involvement but no evidence of distant disease (AJCC clinical stage III) should undergo a fine-needle aspiration cytology or, when necessary, an open biopsy to document the presence of metastatic melanoma. If the cytology or biopsy confirms the presence of nodal involvement, complete regional lymph node dissection should be carried out. Depending on the number of lymph nodes found to contain melanoma, the prognosis for long-term survival is approximately 20% to 50% for these patients.

For decades, the management of melanoma patients with clinically normal lymph nodes has been controversial. It is clear that the likelihood of occult nodal involvement rises with increasing thickness of the primary tumor. Thus, patients with very thin lesions would be less likely to harbor metastases—and to benefit from any nodal surgery—than patients with thicker lesions. Recommendations regarding surgical management of patients with clinically negative regional nodes are therefore best made in the context of the thickness of the primary tumor.

Thin Melanomas

Patients with thin melanomas (1 mm or less in thickness) have a very low likelihood of nodal involvement (less than 5%) and generally require only wide excision of the primary with a 1-cm margin. These patients should undergo periodic physical examinations to detect the rare cases of nodal recurrence, as well as annual or more frequent total-body skin examinations to detect second primary melanomas and nonmelanoma skin cancers. There may be a subset of patients with thin melanomas who have a higher risk of nodal metastases, and for whom surgical staging of the regional nodes should be considered, but this subset remains poorly defined.[58–60]

Intermediate-Thickness Melanomas

Melanomas 1 to 4 mm in thickness are associated with a 20% to 25% chance of occult nodal involvement. Intermediate-thickness lesions are generally treated with a 2-cm excision margin, which can be performed as an outpatient procedure. To evaluate for nodal disease, selective lymphadenectomy (described later) is generally performed; this is followed by complete lymphadenectomy in patients found to have metastatic nodal disease.

Randomized Trials of Elective Versus Therapeutic Lymph Node Dissection in Intermediate-Thickness Melanoma

Retrospective data suggested that there was, indeed, a survival benefit for immediate (elective) lymph node dissection at the time of excision of the primary in patients with intermediate-thickness melanoma.[61] These data led to a number of randomized trials in the United States and around the world (Table 97.5). The largest study was a United States intergroup trial in which 786 patients with melanomas between 1 and 4 mm thick and clinically negative nodes were randomized to either observation or elective node dissection. Overall, there was no significant difference in survival between patients randomized to (or actually treated with) node dissection and those in the observation group. Subset analysis did suggest the existence of some subgroups of

TABLE 97.5.
Randomized Trials of Elective Node Dissection in Clinically Localized Cutaneous Melanoma (Level I Evidence).

Trial	*Eligible patients*	*No. of patients*	*Outcome versus observation with therapeutic LND if necessary*	*Reference*
WHO Trial 1	Extremity primary, all thicknesses	533	No advantage for ELND in OS, DFS	64
Mayo Clinic	Extremity primary, all thicknesses	171	No advantage for immediate ELND or ELND delayed 30–60 days in OS, DFS	63
Intergroup Surgical Trial	All sites, 1–4 mm thick	786	No advantage for ELND in OS, DFS; some subsets appeared to benefit from ELND	62
WHO Trial 14	Trunk primary, ≥1.5 mm thick	252	No advantage for ELND in OS, DFS; subset with 1.5- to 4-mm-thick primary appeared to benefit from ELND	65

DFS, disease-free survival; ELND, elective lymph node dissection; LND, lymph node dissection; OS, overall survival; WHO, World Health Organization.

patients who may have benefited from elective node dissection [notably, patients with thinner (1–2 mm) tumors who were 60 years of age or younger].[62] The other randomized studies have not indicated a benefit for elective node dissection in any specific subset of patients.[63–65] These results argue strongly against the routine use of elective dissection in patients who have intermediate-thickness melanomas and clinically negative lymph nodes. Nonetheless, as indicated next, sentinel node biopsy-guided *staging* of the regional nodes (selective lymphadenectomy) may be of benefit in selecting patients for adjuvant therapy, and perhaps even improve the outcome for patients with involved lymph nodes.

Thick Melanomas

Patients with thick melanomas (4 mm or more) have a high likelihood of nodal involvement but also have a high incidence of occult systemic metastasis at the time of diagnosis. For this reason, even strong proponents of elective node dissection agree that patients with thick primaries do not benefit from elective removal of clinically negative lymph nodes.[61] Wide excision of the primary with at least a 2-cm margin is appropriate in these patients,[57] with surgical treatment of the nodes reserved for those who develop clinical evidence of nodal recurrence without signs of metastatic disease. Because of the high likelihood of microscopic nodal involvement in patients with thick primaries, sentinel node biopsy with selective lymphadenectomy is an attractive alternative to observation of the nodes.

Selective Lymphadenectomy

In pioneering studies, Morton and associates showed that the lymphatics from any given spot on the skin drain to a single or at most two or three specific lymph nodes within a regional basin. The node or nodes that are the initial drainage site can be identified in nearly all patients with cutaneous melanoma. These nodes, which Morton called the "sentinel" nodes, are almost always the first site of nodal involvement when melanoma spreads to the regional nodes. If the sentinel nodes are negative for melanoma, the remaining nodes are also free of involvement in at least 96% of cases.[66] A number of other investigators have confirmed Morton's original observations,[67] and the technique of selective lymphadenectomy has been adopted as an alternative to "watch and wait" or routine elective node dissection strategies. Patients with melanoma involving the sentinel node often have other nonsentinel nodes involved, and hence complete node dissection is indicated in sentinel node-positive patients.

Techniques of Sentinel Node Biopsy

Two techniques are available for identifying the sentinel node draining a cutaneous melanoma. Morton originally described the use of a blue lymphangiogram dye [either isosulfan blue (Lymphazurin) or patent blue] injected intradermally at the site of the primary or adjacent to the biopsy scar if the primary has been excised (Fig. 97.6). About 5 min later, an incision is made over the lymph node basin, and the blue lymphatic channel or channels coursing to the sentinel node are identified and traced until a blue-stained node is identified and removed (Fig. 97.7). This technique allows for identification of the sentinel node at least 80% of the time. The alternative technique involves injection of a radiolabeled colloid solu-

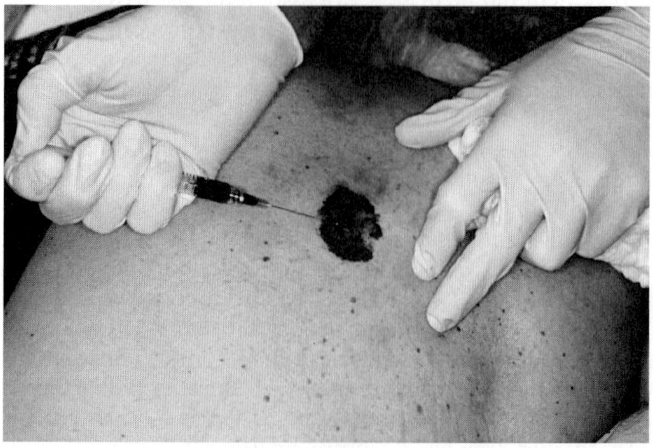

FIGURE 97.6. Intradermal injection of 1% isosulfan blue dye at the site of a primary melanoma, performed as part of intraoperative lymphatic mapping for sentinel lymph node identification. (See *color insert.*)

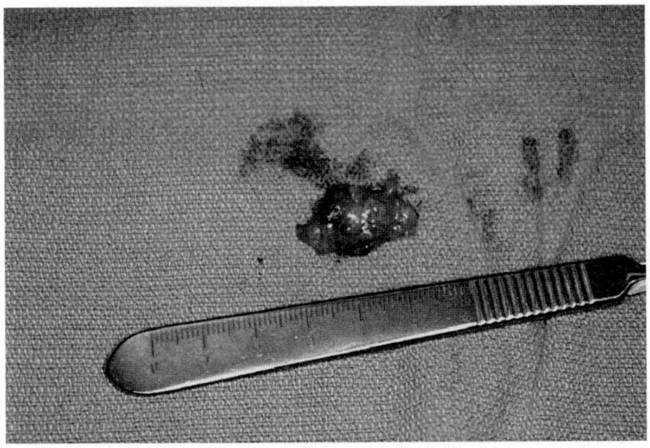

FIGURE 97.7. Following intradermal injection of 1% isosulfan blue dye and technetium 99m-labeled sulfur colloid, the sentinel lymph node is readily identified by finding a blue-stained lymphatic channel leading to a blue lymph node. A hand-held gamma detector confirms that the blue node is also radioactive.

tion, which can be done up to 4h before surgery, combined with intraoperative identification of the sentinel node using a hand-held gamma detector. Because the radiolabeled technique provides no visual clues to the sentinel node's location, most surgeons combine the two techniques. The combined use of blue lymphangiogram dye plus radiolabeled colloid enables the detection of the sentinel node in more than 98% of cases.[67,68] The use of the radiolabeled colloid is combined with preoperative lymphoscintigraphy; imaging of the drainage pathways can identify sentinel nodes outside the traditional nodal basins (Fig. 97.8). Wide excision of the primary melanoma can alter the lymphatic drainage patterns sufficiently to make identification of the sentinel node unreliable. Patients who have had more than 1 cm of skin excised around their primary melanoma can still undergo successful sentinel node biopsy in carefully selected cases, however.[69]

Pathological Evaluation of the Sentinel Node

Reliable prediction of the status of the nodal basin requires careful examination of the sentinel nodes. Generally, this examination involves techniques not routinely applied to full node dissection specimens, such as serial sectioning and immunohistochemical staining with anti-S100 and anti-MART1 antibodies. There have been several reports of regional failures in patients whose sentinel node was considered to be tumor free by standard examination but was subsequently shown to contain melanoma cells by more sophisticated evaluation.[70]

Results of a Randomized Trial of Sentinel Node Biopsy

Morton et al. conducted a randomized trial comparing wide excision alone to wide excision plus sentinel node biopsy in 2001 patients with clinically node-negative cutaneous melanoma.[71] Detailed results have been published for a subset of 1347 patients with primary melanomas between 1.2 and 3.6mm in thickness.[72] In this subset of patients, one or more sentinel nodes was microscopically positive in 16%. Among the patients with a negative sentinel node, 3.4% have developed a nodal recurrence to date, a so-called "false-negative" sentinel node biopsy. In the wide excision alone arm, 15.6% have had a nodal recurrence to date, with a projected cumulative incidence of nodal recurrence at 8 years of 18.5%. Thus, the rate of nodal involvement in both arms is very similar, suggesting that most if not all sentinel node metastases eventually develop into clinically detectable regional disease. The average time to nodal recurrence in the wide excision alone arm was only 1.33 years, indicating that many of these regional failures will occur relatively soon after initial treatment. The status of the sentinel node was confirmed to be the strongest predictor of melanoma recurrence and overall survival: 5 years after study entry, 83.2% of patients with a negative sentinel node were disease free, with a melanoma-specific survival of 90.2%, compared to 53.4% disease-free survival and 72.3% melanoma-specific survival if the sentinel node was positive.

When all patients on the sentinel node arm were compared to those on the wide excision alone arm, the 5-year recurrence-free survival was statistically significantly better for those randomized to sentinel node biopsy (78.3% versus 73.1%, $P = 0.009$). This difference resulted almost entirely from the lower likelihood of regional relapse; melanoma-specific survival was not significantly different between the two study arms. When patients with a positive sentinel node were compared to those who developed clinical evidence of nodal recurrence on the wide excision arm, however, the differences in recurrence-free survival and melanoma-specific survival strongly favored the sentinel node-positive patients. After a median follow-up of 48 months, the 5-year melanoma-specific survival among sentinel node biopsy-positive patients was 72.3% compared to 52.4% for patients developing nodal recurrence on the wide excision arm. The strong implication of these results is that early treatment of sentinel node-positive patients decreases the likelihood of disease recurrence and potentially results in improved survival compared to observation of the nodes with node dissection at the time of clinically detectable relapse. Until long-term results of the entire study population are available, the data thus far strongly support the continued use of sentinel node biopsy in properly selected patients with cutaneous melanoma.

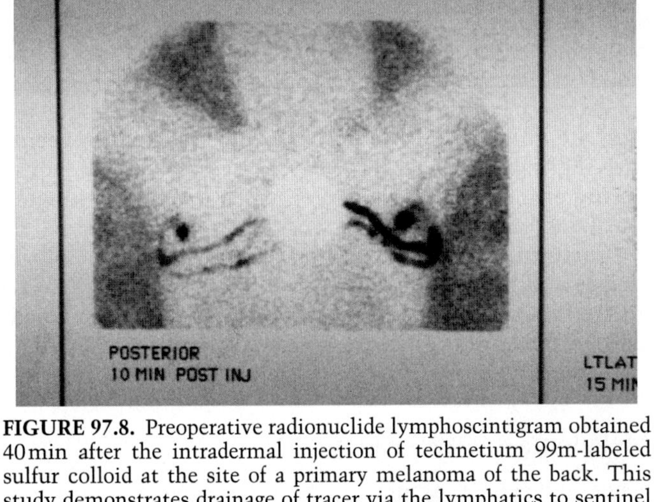

FIGURE 97.8. Preoperative radionuclide lymphoscintigram obtained 40min after the intradermal injection of technetium 99m-labeled sulfur colloid at the site of a primary melanoma of the back. This study demonstrates drainage of tracer via the lymphatics to sentinel nodes in the axilla and also in the soft tissues of the back.

Ultrastaging of the Sentinel Nodes

Immunohistochemical examination of sentinel nodes clearly identifies more foci of metastatic disease than routine staining techniques, yet even more sensitive techniques for detecting melanoma cells are now available. The reverse transcriptase-polymerase chain reaction (RT-PCR) can be used to detect minute quantities of messenger RNA that are expressed by tumor cells but not the normal cells of the lymph node. RT-PCR for the detection of tyrosinase messenger RNA has been reported to detect a single melanoma cell in 1 million normal cells.[73] Using this technique, patients whose sentinel node was histologically negative but RT-PCR positive were determined to have a significantly worse outcome than those whose node was histologically and RT-PCR negative for melanoma.[74] Patients with thicker tumors were more likely to have RT-PCR-positive nodes. The Sunbelt Melanoma Trial is an ongoing study in which patients with a sentinel node that is positive only by RT-PCR will be randomized to no further treatment, a full lymph node dissection, or a full lymph node dissection plus adjuvant interferon. Results to date, however, fail to substantiate a role for RT-PCR analysis of the sentinel node: the recurrence-free and overall survival rates for PCR-positive and -negative patients were basically identical.[75]

Postoperative Follow-Up of the Melanoma Patient

The main goals of postoperative follow-up are to detect treatable (i.e., locoregional) recurrences and new primary tumors in an expeditious fashion. Hence, physical examination plays a more important role than laboratory or radiologic examination. Patients with thin melanomas are often at greater risk of developing a second primary tumor than they are of developing recurrence of their original lesion. Patients with melanomas of all thicknesses are at increased risk of both second primary melanomas and second primary nonmelanoma skin cancers. A thorough skin examination is therefore a routine part of the follow-up physical examination. The primary site and regional nodes are both common sites of recurrence for patients with cutaneous melanoma, and distant nodes are a frequent site of metastatic disease as well. The primary site and all accessible lymph node basins should also be examined at each follow-up visit. The exact frequency of follow-up visits varies with the stage of the original tumor (patients with thick tumors being seen somewhat more often), the length of time since surgery (the most intensive follow-up is conducted in the first 3 to 5 postoperative years), and the presence or absence of atypical moles (melanoma patients with multiple atypical moles, especially those with a family history of melanoma requiring the most frequent follow-up schedules).

Intensive surveillance with laboratory and radiologic studies adds little to the follow-up of melanoma patients. The overwhelming majority of recurrences (and almost all surgically treatable recurrences) are detected by the patient or by a routine history and physical examination.[76]

Melanoma and Pregnancy

When melanoma occurs during pregnancy, a number of unique considerations arise. Hormones, in particular estrogen, stimulate the proliferation of normal melanocytes, and there is abundant evidence to suggest they affect melanoma cells as well. Furthermore, melanoma is one of the few malignancies that have been recognized to metastasize to the placenta and even cross the placenta to involve the fetus.[77] Although these facts merit careful consideration, the bulk of the available evidence suggests that, stage for stage, the outcome of a pregnant patient with stage I or II melanoma is not different from a nonpregnant patient.[78] Subsequent pregnancy also does not seem to be associated with an adverse outcome, although patients are frequently advised to refrain from childbearing for at least 2 years after diagnosis of a melanoma. This restriction represents a prudent recommendation in most cases, as it allows those patients whose melanoma is destined for rapid recurrence to be identified before they become pregnant and complicate the management of their recurrence. Oral contraceptives and postmenopausal replacement estrogens are frequently avoided in patients who have been treated for melanoma, although evidence demonstrating a survival disadvantage for such treatment is lacking.[78]

Surgical Treatment of Noncutaneous Melanomas

Noncutaneous melanomas generally present at a more advanced stage than cutaneous lesions. The site of the lesion greatly affects the approach to the primary tumor and regional lymph nodes.

Ocular Melanoma

Prognostic factors for ocular melanoma are not nearly as well characterized as for cutaneous melanomas. Ocular melanomas generally do not have access to lymphatic channels, so regional spread is rarely seen. Ocular primaries metastasize hematogenously (most commonly to the liver), often many years after initial diagnosis. For an ocular melanoma without evidence of distant disease, size of the primary is the main determinant of treatment and prognosis. Small ocular melanomas, defined as tumors 1.0 to 3.0mm in apical height and between 5.0 and 16.0mm in diameter, comprised 28% of cases in a recent collaborative series.[79] Only 6 of the 204 cases died of melanoma, and 4 of these died more than 5 years after initial diagnosis. Twenty-seven patients (13%) ultimately required enucleation (total removal) of the eye. For medium-sized lesions, treatment options are enucleation or implanted radiotherapy with a radioactive gold plaque fitted to the back of the eyeball immediately behind the tumor. A multiinstitution randomized trial indicated that implanted radiotherapy is equivalent to enucleation in terms of disease control and overall survival.[80] Large ocular melanomas have traditionally been treated with enucleation, often with preoperative radiation, which on the basis of retrospective data was thought to decrease the likelihood of distant metastases. A randomized trial involving more than 1000 patients, however, demonstrated no significant survival advantage for preoperative radiation. Disease-specific 5-year survival was 72% for enucleation alone versus 74% for enucleation plus radiation.[81]

Anal and Vulvar Melanoma

Melanomas of the anus and vulva pose challenges in the treatment of both the primary lesion and regional nodes. They usually present at an advanced stage, with thick primary tumors and a high likelihood of clinically occult regional and distant metastases at the time of diagnosis. Excision of primary tumors in these areas should not be overly radical: abdominoperineal resection or radical vulvectomy are unnecessarily deforming and are not associated with improved survival compared to wide local excision. Abdominoperineal resection, with its attendant permanent colostomy, is indicated only for very large primary melanomas, locally recurrent melanomas after prior sphincter-conserving excision, or melanomas with radiographic evidence of mesorectal node involvement. Anal and vulvar melanomas often present with inguinal lymph node metastases; if no evidence of distant disease is present, both the primary site and regional nodes should be removed. Elective dissection of clinically normal inguinal nodes has never been demonstrated to be of any survival value in either anal or vulvar melanoma; sentinel node biopsy may have a role and is the preferred approach if surgical staging of the nodes is to be conducted. In the National Cancer Data Base melanoma study, 5-year survival for anal melanoma was 19.8% and for vulvar melanoma was 11.4%.[8]

Nasal or Nasopharyngeal Melanoma

Melanomas arising in the nasal or nasopharyngeal mucosa should be conservatively excised, with node dissection reserved for patients who have proven nodal involvement. Because of the difficulty achieving wide, tumor-free margins around the primary site, postoperative radiation is often employed.[82] Five-year survival for these tumors in the National Cancer Data Base melanoma study was 31.7%.[8]

Adjuvant Therapy of Cutaneous Melanoma

Although the prognosis for patients with early-stage cutaneous melanoma is quite good, far fewer patients with deep primaries (4mm or more) or regional lymph node involvement will be cured by surgery alone. The development of effective adjuvant therapy capable of increasing postsurgical survival has been a long-standing goal of melanoma researchers.

Chemotherapy and Nonspecific Immunostimulants

The use of DTIC (dacarbazine) chemotherapy in the adjuvant treatment of high-risk melanoma is ineffective. This result is not surprising considering the limited effectiveness of dacarbazine chemotherapy in metastatic melanoma. In contrast, a large body of evidence from animal models shows that immunostimulatory interventions could be highly active for animals with very low tumor burdens but not for animals with extensive tumor. As research efforts shifted to the investigation of adjuvant immunotherapy for human melanoma, the first agent to undergo widespread testing was bacillus Calmette–Guérin (BCG), a live mycobacteria that had been shown to induce regression when directly injected into cutaneous melanoma metastases. Although nonrandomized, historically controlled trials suggested a role for BCG following surgery, subsequent randomized trials failed to show any benefit for BCG in the adjuvant therapy of high-risk melanoma.[83,84]

Other nonspecific agents that have undergone evaluation in at least two randomized trials are levamisole, an anthelminthic drug predominantly affecting macrophages, and *Corynebacterium parvum*. No clear evidence of benefit has emerged for either agent, although levamisole is still occasionally used in Canada.[83,85]

Interferons

The availability of recombinant interferons (α, β "leukocyte" interferon, type 1, derived predominantly from phagocytic leukocytes, and γ type 2, "immune" interferon, derived from lymphocytes) facilitated the application of immunotherapy in human cancers. Melanoma was a particularly promising target, in view of its poor responsiveness to chemotherapy, as well as observations of immune phenomena such as vitiligo that appeared to be associated with more favorable outcomes. In many patients with melanoma, an additional advantage has been an accessible source of tumor (subcutaneous metastases) for locoregional therapies and tissue for correlative studies.

Clinical trials of interferon (IFN) -β and -γ proved to be disappointing (despite the large body of preclinical work suggesting a promising role for IFN-γ in immunotherapy) for advanced melanoma and, in the case of IFN-γ, in the adjuvant setting for high-risk patients as well. IFN-α, however, showed sufficient activity in patients with advanced disease to justify its investigation in the adjuvant setting, using high-dose IFN-α regimens that were tested in a series of randomized cooperative group trials for patients with deep primary and/or nodal disease. These trials, which began in the 1980s, demonstrated that high-dose IFN-α, administered as a daily (5 days per week) intravenous dose for 4 weeks followed by a thrice-weekly subcutaneous dose for 11 months, could prolong relapse-free survival and probably overall survival as well (Table 97.6).[86,87] Lower doses of IFN-α were clearly less active, although several trials with suggested prolongation of relapse-free but not overall survival.[87–89] Updates of the data from high-dose IFN trials have indicated that the survival benefit appears to diminish over long follow-up times, although the impact on relapse-free survival has been durable.[90] Given the significant morbidity of high-dose IFN-α, there is a clear need for investigation of innovative and promising alternative approaches, such as vaccines.[91]

Adjuvant Vaccine Therapy

The adjuvant therapy of melanoma provides an ideal setting for the study of other innovative strategies, and many randomized trials have been conducted with vaccines and other agents. To date, other than high-dose IFN-α, all other interventions tested have not proven sufficiently effective to support their widespread adoption. Most disappointingly, two large randomized trials testing an allogeneic whole cell vaccine called Canvaxin in patients with resected stage III or IV melanoma showed no advantage for the vaccine arm compared to placebo.[92] Recent observations suggested the immunomodulatory properties of granulocyte-macrophage colony-stimulating factor (GM-CSF), and historical data suggested its potential benefit in the adjuvant setting for high-risk melanoma following resection.[93] Peptide fragments from

TABLE 97.6.
Published Randomized Trials of Adjuvant Interferon Therapy in Resected Cutaneous Melanoma (Level I Evidence).

Trial	*Disease stage*	*Intervention*	*Results*	*Reference*
SWOG-8642	Stage II, III	IFN-g 0.1 mg/day ×1 year vs. observation	No benefit for OS or DFS (treatment arm slightly worse)	128,129
NCCTG-83–70–52	Stage II (≥1.67 mm), III	IFN-α2a 20 MU/m^2 IM 3 days/week ×3 months vs. observation	No overall benefit for OS or DFS; DFS benefit for stage III patients	88
ECOG-1684	Stage IIB (≥4 mm), III	IFN-α2b 20 MU/m^2 IV 5 days/week ×1 month, then 10 MU/m^2 SC 3 days/week 311 months vs. observation	**Significant improvement in OS and DFS**	86
ECOG-1690	Stage IIB (≥4 mm), III	IFN-α2b 20 MU/m^2 IV 5 days/week31 month, then 10 MU/m^2 SC. 3 days/week ×11 months vs. IFN-α a2b 3 MU SC × 2 years vs. observation	Significant improvement in DFS for high-dose IFN arm; no OS benefit	87
WHO-16	Stage III	IFN-α2a 3 MU SC 3 days/week ×3 years vs. observation	No benefit in OS or DFS	89
Italian multicenter	Stage I, II	IFN- α2b 3 MU SC ×3 years vs. observation	Significant improvement in DFS, no OS benefit	130
Austrian multicenter	Stage II	IFN-α2a 3 MU SC daily × 3 weeks then 3 days/week × 1 year vs. observation	Significant improvement in DFS, no OS benefit	131
French multicenter	Stage II	IFN-α2a 3 MU SC 3 18 months vs. observation	Significant improvement in DFS, no OS benefit	132

DFS, disease-free survival; ECOG, Eastern Cooperative Oncology Group; IFN, interferon; MU, million international units; NCCTG, North Central Cancer Treatment Group; OS, overall survival; SWOG, Southwest Oncology Group; WHO, World Health Organization.

melanoma differentiation antigens may also stimulate melanoma immunity when administered with nonspecific immunostimulatory adjuvants potentially superior to BCG (for example, CpG oligonucleotides and Montanide ISA).[94] A recently completed trial for patients with metastatic melanoma who have undergone complete resection of all metastatic lesions will assess the value of GM-CSF as an adjuvant therapy. In selected patients with histocompatibility type that can respond to the available melanoma peptides (HLA-A*0201), the value of peptides with and without GM-CSF will also be tested in this trial (ECOG 4697).

Radiation Therapy

Radiation therapy is rarely employed after surgical therapy for primary or nodal melanoma, although recent reports have demonstrated that the pessimistic impression that melanoma is a "nonradioresponsive" tumor is simply not justified. Nonrandomized studies suggest that postoperative radiation to the neck or axilla after radical lymph node dissections decreases regional recurrence rates in node-positive patients.[95–97] A small randomized trial addressing the issue was inconclusive,[98] but until larger randomized trials are conducted, it seems reasonable to consider the use of postoperative radiation therapy in patients with multiple (4 to 10 or more) involved lymph nodes or with gross extracapsular extension, because these patients are at very high risk of regional recurrence despite an adequate lymph node dissection. As these patients are also candidates for IFN-α2b adjuvant therapy, the optimal schedule for integrating radiation with IFN needs to be determined. In the absence of definitive data, we defer the start of radiation until after the completion of the initial month of intravenous interferon and administer it during the subcutaneous phase of treatment.

Treatment of Metastatic Melanoma

Stage IV melanoma is associated with a very poor overall prognosis, yet some patients are long-term survivors with aggressive treatment (see Figure 97.3). Surgery, radiation therapy, and systemic treatments all have a role to play. In general, solitary metastases in any location should be considered for resection. It is important to recognize that melanoma metastases to certain sites call for specific treatments before discussing systemic therapies that can be used for widely disseminated disease.

Management of Metastatic Disease in Selected Sites

In-Transit Skin Metastases

In-transit metastases, that is, cutaneous or subcutaneous nodules arising between the primary site and the regional lymph node basin, are a well-recognized but fairly uncommon site of failure in cutaneous melanoma. A surgical technique developed to treat in-transit metastases, isolation limb perfusion, involves cannulating the artery and vein to an extremity and connecting the cannulas to a cardiopulmonary bypass machine. This procedure effectively isolates the blood flow to that extremity and allows for prolonged perfusion with cytotoxic or biological agents. Most commonly, the chemotherapeutic agent melphalan (L-phenylalanine mustard, Alkeran) has been used for isolation limb perfusion; this drug is generally heated to an elevated temperature (up to 41.5°C) and perfused for 60 to 90 min.[99] Major complications, such as neutropenia from systemic absorption of the cytotoxic agent, amputation of the limb, and death, each occur in less than 1% of cases.[100] Hyperthermic isolation perfusion with melphalan alone or combined with tumor necrosis factor-α (TNF-α) results in the regression of more than 90% of cutaneous in-transit metastases.[99,101,102] The addition of TNF-α increases response rates but also toxicity, and is currently available only in Europe. Isolation limb infusion has recently been advocated as a less invasive way to deliver chemotherapy to the limb.[103] Adjuvant use of hyperthermic isolation limb perfusion after resection of high-risk primary melanomas demonstrated no significant benefit in a large, international intergroup trial and cannot be recommended.[104]

Central Nervous System

The brain and central nervous system (CNS) are the initial site of metastasis in 12% to 20% of patients with metastatic melanoma, but CNS metastasis is diagnosed more commonly in association with one or more extracranial sites of metastatic disease. Because the frequency of this devastating complication appears to increase with the duration of disease, and because of its resistance to the improving therapies for systemic disease, the brain can be considered a "sanctuary" site in many patients with advanced melanoma. Although CNS metastasis is frequently discovered at an asymptomatic stage when the patient undergoes brain imaging for staging purposes, it sometimes presents as an acute intracranial event occurring as a result of sudden hemorrhage into a highly vascular metastasis. The best outcomes are in patients with minimal or no extracranial metastatic disease whose CNS metastases are limited in size and number and who can undergo surgical resection or stereotactic radiosurgery. Surgery is particularly valuable in this situation, where metastases are often hemorrhagic, requiring prompt evacuation to limit the neurological deficit. This approach can also minimize the use of glucocorticoids, which are generally excluded in patients being considered for immunotherapy trials. The value of whole-brain radiotherapy alone or in addition to surgery or stereotactic radiotherapy has not been adequately defined, and the sobering results of two recent trials of temozolomide-based chemotherapy (chosen for its similarity to dacarbazine and its high penetration across the blood–brain barrier) plus whole-brain radiotherapy in patients with good performance status and no prior chemotherapy (less than 10% objective response in the pooled 75-patient experience of the two trials) are a grim reminder that this disease is indeed relatively radioresistant and that CNS metastatic disease is the major cause of morbidity and mortality in a substantial fraction of patients with metastatic melanoma.[105,106]

When radiation therapy is used for patients with multiple or unresectable brain metastases, the majority of treated patients show some improvement in tumor size, symptomatology, or performance status.[107] Corticosteroids should be given concomitantly with brain irradiation to minimize intracranial swelling, then tapered off rapidly after the completion of therapy. Although anticonvulsants are not routinely given to patients with brain metastases from most solid tumors in the absence of frank seizures, melanoma is associated with a higher-than-average incidence of seizures for which prophylactic anticonvulsant therapy may be warranted.

Gastrointestinal Tract and Abdominal Viscera

Melanoma has a propensity for metastases involving the gastrointestinal tract, otherwise a decidedly unusual site of tumor spread. The highly vascular nature of melanoma metastases accounts for the high rate of gastrointestinal hemorrhage as a complication of this site of involvement. Other manifestations that mandate surgical intervention include obstruction, intussusception, and even perforation. Surgical resection is indicated whenever feasible, even if extraintestinal spread is present that cannot be removed. Other intraabdominal sites of involvement include liver, spleen, and adrenal metastases, which are occasionally amenable to resection when there is no known extraabdominal spread.

Systemic Therapy of Metastatic Melanoma

The systemic therapy of melanoma is one of the most frustrating tasks for the medical oncologist. Despite great strides in the understanding of tumor biology, immunology, and pharmacology, the treatment of advanced melanoma yields few durable remissions and minimal impact on survival at the cost of considerable toxicity.

Cytotoxic Chemotherapy and Targeted Therapy

Among the numerous available chemotherapeutic agents, only dacarbazine (DTIC), which has been reported to have a 15% to 20% objective response rate as a single agent, is currently approved for treatment of advanced melanoma. More recent studies have shown that the response rate to this drug is probably no higher than 8% to 12%. Responses to chemotherapy are nearly always of brief duration (less than 6 months), are rarely complete, and occur most often in asymptomatic, good performance status patients with small-volume metastases in soft tissue, skin, lymph nodes, or lung.

Combination Regimens

Most combination regimens in current use or under investigation include DTIC or its orally administered analogue, temozolomide. Temozolomide is commonly used because of its ease of administration and relatively mild toxicity compared to DTIC, as well as its CNS penetration. Other drugs with demonstrated single-agent activity that are frequently included in combination regimens are vinca alkaloids and cisplatin. The use of chemotherapy combinations in first-line therapy for metastatic melanoma, while associated with a higher rate of response in pilot studies, has been disappointing when evaluated in larger, cooperative group trials.

Recent studies of the biology of melanoma led to the discovery of genes, such as Ras and Raf in the mitogen-activated kinase pathway and AKT in the PTEN/PI3/AKT/mTOR pathway, that are mutated or deleted in many melanomas and hence could provide relatively tumor-specific targets for therapy.[20,108,109] New drugs such as sorafenib (commercial name, Nexavar), a potent inhibitor of the B-Raf kinase and other important cellular kinases are entering clinical trials. Sorafenib, while known to affect B-Raf, also inhibits several other cellular kinases associated with membrane signaling, including the platelet-derived growth factor (PDGF) and vascular endothelial growth factor (VEGF) receptors. Sorafenib showed relatively minimal activity in initial single-agent trials in previously treated melanoma patients, but it may have significant value when combined with cytotoxic chemotherapy.[109] Clinical trials are now under way to determine if this combination approach represents a major advance. Similar investigations and drug development strategies are ongoing with other agents that inhibit enzymes in the other pathways or target the tumor vasculature itself (angiogenesis inhibitors).

Immunological Therapies for Advanced Melanoma

IFN-α

When used as a single agent, interferon-α produces objective responses in 15% or less of patients with metastatic melanoma.[110] As with chemotherapy, the best responses occur in patients with small-volume, nonvisceral metastatic disease and a good performance status. The toxicities of interferon are predominantly constitutional, consisting of fever and chills (which subside in most patients after the first few doses), nausea and anorexia, myalgias, and arthralgias. Fatigue, which may be progressive as therapy continues, is generally the most troublesome side effect and is often dose limiting. The most common laboratory abnormalities consist of asymptomatic elevations of serum transaminases and mild myelosuppression, as well as occasional nephrotoxicity. Virtually all these effects are reversible and occur in a dose- and schedule-dependent pattern. Currently, interferon-α is widely used in the adjuvant therapy of high-risk melanoma, but its use as a single agent in the advanced disease setting is largely limited to patients with major comorbidities that preclude using more toxic therapies.

Interleukin 2

Interleukin 2 (IL-2) (Proleukin), a potent stimulator of T-cell growth and function, is the only other immune therapy with demonstrated antitumor activity in melanoma. The majority of published data are from trials of high doses of IL-2 given at toxicity levels requiring inpatient management. At these dose-intensity levels, objective response rates of approximately 15% to 20% have been achieved with substantial but generally reveresible multiorgan toxicity,[111,112] with a small fraction of patients experiencing durable complete remissions lasting in excess of 5 years. Based on these favorable results, high-dose IL-2 was approved by the FDA in 1998 for treatment of metastatic melanoma.

Although the frequency of durable complete responses to IL-2 therapy appears to be higher than that reported for other single agents and combination regimens, it is important to consider that patients selected for their ability to tolerate the serious toxicities of high-dose IL-2 may represent a more favorable group with a higher a priori likelihood of tumor response. Only limited data are available on the activity of outpatient low-dose IL-2 regimens in melanoma, and this form of therapy is not recommended outside a clinical trial. The therapeutic potential of other interleukins (such as IL-4, IL-6, and IL-12) remains under investigation.

The potential for enhanced activity of combinations containing the most active chemotherapeutic agents (generally, cisplatin, dacarbazine and vinblastine) and both IL-2 and IFN-α has been studied in several large, randomized trials, the results of which have failed to confirm earlier promise of this form of "biochemotherapy."[113] Although biochemotherapy combinations are still considered appropriate for young, otherwise fit individuals who have symptomatic metastatic disease that would benefit from even a brief remission, less aggressive therapy (or, preferably, enrollment in a clinical trial) is recommended for the majority of patients.

Melanoma Vaccines

Vaccines produced from allogeneic melanoma cell lines administered with one of several available nonspecific immunostimulants (which stimulate antigen-presenting cells and enhance other aspects of immune recognition of antigens) have shown limited antitumor activity in patients with metastatic disease (generally less than 10% objective response rates in patients with limited metastatic disease).[114–116] The specific tumor antigens most critical to mediating an antimelanoma immune response are under intense investigation. Ganglioside (glycoprotein) vaccines that represent surface molecules relatively specific to melanoma cells have undergone extensive testing. However, the results of a large phase III adjuvant trial comparing a promising ganglioside vaccine with high-dose IFN-α showed that patients receiving the vaccine had inferior survival.[90,117]

Peptide antigens are small fragments of processed proteins that interact with HLA molecules and the T-cell receptor to initiate the cell-mediated immune response. Peptide vaccines for melanoma have been extensively studied, including clinical trials that use either naturally occurring antigen peptides or chemically altered peptides that have been optimized for their interaction with specific HLA molecules. Many imaginative strategies for delivering and enhancing peptide-based immunotherapies in advanced and adjuvant settings for melanoma patients are under active investigation, and the details of some of the most promising current strategies are included in Table 97.7. Both immune responses and clinical activity have been observed in a fraction of patients, although the expected correlation between these outcomes has not generally occurred. Many of these studies have contributed to our understanding of mechanisms for resistance to immune destruction, which will be important information for the design of future clinical trials.

A full description of the vast number of vaccine-related approaches is beyond the scope of this chapter, but they have been reviewed recently.[118,119] Selected aspects of some of the most important vaccine strategies are provided in Table 97.7.

Encouraging results have emerged from recent studies directed at blocking negative regulatory signals mediated by the cytolytic T-cell antigen CTLA4 on T lymphocytes. A human antibody to this receptor recently has been shown to have immunological and clinical activity in patients with advanced melanoma. Interestingly, an important toxicity has been the development of so-called autoimmune breakthrough events, including uveitis, hypophysitis, hepatitis, dermatitis, and colitis. This finding suggests that successfully breaking tolerance to tumor antigens will be accompanied by a loss of

TABLE 97.7. Melanoma Vaccine Strategies.

Target	*Antigen used to immunize*	*Route/site of administration*	*Immune-asjuvant*	*Preclinical status*	*Clincal status*	*Reference*
Melanoma cell	Allogeneic line	Subcutaneous	BCG	Induces cellular and humoral responses	In Phase III investigation	133
Melanoma cell	Allogeneic cell lysate	Subcutaneous	DETOX	Induces mainly cellular responses	Approved for metastatic melanoma in Canada; adjuvant benefit limited to selected HLA types	114–116
Melanoma cell	DNP-modified cells	Intradermal	DNP	Induces mainly cellular responses; hallmark is strong delayed-type hypersensitiviy reaction	In Phase II evaluation	134
Surface glycoprotein	Gangliosides GM2, GD2, GD3 conjugated to KLH	Subcutaneous	QS-21	Induces mainly humoral responses	Phase III adjuvant trials begun with GM2; others in earlier phase of investigation	117, 135
Melanoma differentiation proteins	Peptides of Melan-A/ MART-1, tyrosinase, gp-100, others	Intravenous, subcutaneous	IFA, with IL-2, other cytokine	Induces cellular responses, HLA-restricted	In Phase II/ laboratory investigations; most promising is following lymphodepletion	136, 137
Gene mutation-defined antigens	Peptides of MAGE, NY-ESO-1, others	Intravenous, subcutaneous	Recombinant viral fusion protein	Induces mainly cellular responses	In Phase I/ laboratory investigations	138
Various proteins	Peptides, tumor-cell RNA with dendritic cells	Intravenous, intradermal, intranodal	DC is own adjuvant	Induces mainly cellular responses depending on conditions of preparation	In Phase I-III/ laboratory investigations	139
Melanoma cell	Endogenous tumor antigen, added melanoma peptides	Subcutaneous	CpG oligodeoxynucleotides	Induces B- and T-cell responses	In Phase III investigation with peptide	140

BCG, Bacille Calmette–Guerin; DC, dendritic cells; DNP, dinitrophenol; IFA, incomplete Freund's adjuvant; KLH, keyhole limpet hemocyanin; QS-21, Quilla saponari 21.

tolerance to certain normal tissue determinants. The overall risk:benefit of this and related approaches remains under active investigation.[120]

Nonmelanoma Skin Cancer

With more than 1 million cases annually in the United States alone, nonmelanoma skin cancer is by far the most common form of human malignancy.[1] Most are basal and squamous cell cancers. For these two tumor types, chronic solar exposure is the predominant etiological factor, with fair-skinned individuals who have had a long history of sun exposure at highest risk. Little is known about the etiologies of other histological types of cutaneous malignancy, but at least some of them (for example, angiosarcomas of the scalp in elderly patients) appear to be related to chronic sun exposure as well. In addition to chronic sun damage, there are some other risk factors that are associated with nonmelanoma skin cancer development.[121,122]

Risk Factors for Nonmelanoma Skin Cancer Development

Actinic Keratoses

Actinic keratoses are scaly, rough, erythematous patches that occur in chronically sun-exposed areas. They are both markers for and precursors to nonmelanoma skin cancer development. These lesions may progress to squamous cell cancers or, in some cases, regress spontaneously in response to prolonged avoidance of sun exposure. Actinic keratoses can be removed or destroyed with liquid nitrogen, if few in number. For multiple lesions, topical 5-fluorouracil (5-FU) and more recently, imiquimod cream has been used successfully.

Burns

Squamous cell cancers occasionally arise in burns or other scars. Burn scar cancers (so-called Marjolin's ulcers) often have a more aggressive clinical course than the usual nonmelanoma skin cancer.

Xeroderma Pigmentosum

Xeroderma pigmentosum, a rare congenital disorder in which patients lack the capacity to repair UV-induced DNA damage, is associated with the development of innumerable nonmelanoma skin cancers at a very early age and also with an increased risk of developing melanoma.[122]

Immunosuppression or Prior Hematological Malignancy

Nonmelanoma skin cancers and, to a much lesser degree, melanomas are increased in patients who are immunosuppressed or who have had previous hematological malignancies. Furthermore, the aggressiveness of the skin tumors can be significantly greater in these patients.

Histological Types of Nonmelanoma Skin Cancer

Basal Cell and Squamous Cell Carcinomas

The two most common types of nonmelanoma skin cancer are basal cell carcinoma and squamous cell carcinoma. Bowen's disease is the name given to squamous cell carcinoma in situ involving the skin. A rarer, more aggressive skin cancer, presumably arising from the neuroendocrine cells of the skin, is Merkel's cell cancer. Nonmelanoma skin cancers can occur on any part of the skin surface but are largely found on the head and neck, hands, and forearms.

Cancers Arising in the Skin Appendages

The skin appendages (e.g., hair follicles and sweat glands) can be the site of origin of adenocarcinomas or apocrine cancers; these are exceedingly rare.

Sarcomas

The most common primary sarcoma affecting the skin is dermatofibrosarcoma protuberans; leiomyosarcoma, angiosarcoma, and malignant fibrous histiocytoma can also arise entirely within the skin. Generally speaking, cutaneous and subcutaneous sarcomas have a better prognosis than lesions that involve or are deep to the muscular fascia.[123] Angiosarcomas, however, tend to have a poor prognosis even when confined to the skin.

Differentiating Nonmelanoma Skin Cancers

Nonmelanoma skin cancers usually are not confused with melanomas because most melanomas are pigmented and most nonmelanoma skin cancers are not. Basal and squamous cell cancers may be harder to distinguish from one another, but certain features are more characteristic of one type than the other. Basal cell cancers often have a pearly, translucent appearance with a rolled border, whereas squamous cell cancers are often keratinized or ulcerated. Dermatofibrosarcoma protuberans and angiosarcomas present as raised nodules or plaques and are frequently multifocal. Both often have a purplish or violaceous hue. Merkel's cell cancers present as a raised, ulcerated lesion that can achieve very large size (Fig. 97.9).

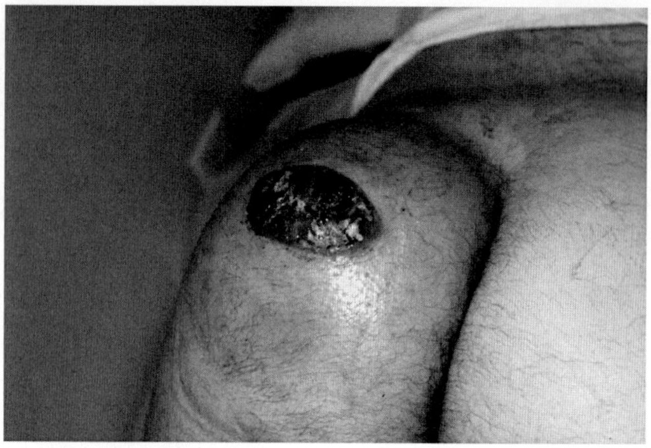

FIGURE 97.9. Large, ulcerated tumor involving the skin, subcutaneous tissue, and muscle of the buttock. Biopsy revealed Merkel's cell carcinoma (neuroendocrine carcinoma) of the skin.

Nonmelanoma Skin Cancers in African Americans

The presentations of nonmelanoma skin cancer differ in more deeply pigmented races. Basal cell cancers, which are usually nonpigmented in whites, are almost always pigmented in black patients. Most cases of squamous cell cancer of the skin occur on the sun-exposed skin of the head and neck or arms, but in blacks the majority of cases develop on less exposed areas, such as the legs, often in association with burns.[10]

Surgical Treatment of Nonmelanoma Skin Cancers

Surgery is the mainstay of treatment for nonmelanoma skin cancers, just as for melanoma. Less radical resections than required for melanoma are generally adequate. Because so many nonmelanoma skin cancers occur on cosmetically critical areas, a number of special techniques are used in their removal.

Margins of Excision

Most nonmelanoma skin cancers can be conservatively excised with much narrower margins than are required for cutaneous melanomas. Excision margins of 0.5 to 1.0cm are adequate for most nonrecurrent basal and squamous cell cancers and yield local recurrence rates under 5% provided that histologically negative margins are achieved. For most tumors in most anatomic sites, these excision margins can be achieved using standard surgical techniques with local anesthesia and primary closure.

Recurrent Cancers and Lesions in Difficult Sites

More sophisticated techniques are required for recurrent skin cancers or those in cosmetically difficult areas, such as the tip of the nose or the eyelid. For these lesions, a variation of Mohs micrographic surgery is frequently employed. This type of surgery is simply a very controlled surgical excision in which the removed tissue is precisely oriented and carefully examined histologically, and serial reexcisions are performed wherever residual disease is noted.[124] Although this technique may take quite a bit longer than routine surgical excision, the extra precision can be helpful for identifying the often asymmetrical extensions of skin cancers, thus minimizing the amount of normal tissue resected. After Mohs surgery has achieved complete excision, reconstruction is done by whatever means is appropriate, but often involves skin grafts or local flaps rather than primary closure.

More aggressive histological types of skin cancers, particularly Merkel's cell cancers and sarcomas, generally require wider excision than the more common basal and squamous cell cancers. Margins of 2 to 3 cm are usually taken, similar to a thick melanoma. Dermatofibrosarcoma protuberans in particular, however, may spread in a very eccentric fashion, with little extension in one direction but many centimeters of subclinical tumor growth in another. Careful examination of the histological status of the margins is a must. Mohs surgery may be useful in some cases.[125]

Radiation Therapy

Radiation therapy is a potential treatment for skin cancers located in critical sites where surgical excision would be disfiguring. Primary basal and squamous cell cancers treated with radiation have nearly identical cure rates (about 95%) as those treated with surgical excision. Radiation is also employed postoperatively to reduce local recurrence rates after excision of high-grade or recurrent sarcomas of the skin.

Topical and Intralesional Therapy

Occasionally, patients present with numerous skin cancers that would be impossible to resect completely; this is particularly common in the immunosuppressed patient who is predisposed to skin cancer development. For these patients, topical therapy with 5-fluorouracil or imiquimod cream can dramatically reduce the number of excisions required. Direct intralesional injections of IFN-α have been reported to successfully treat basal cell cancers. This technique may be particularly helpful for locally recurrent lesions after surgery or radiation.

Management of Recurrent Disease

Locoregional Recurrence

The vast majority of nonmelanoma skin cancers are successfully treated with surgery or primary radiation, with fewer than 5% recurring locally. Of those that do recur locally, at least 80% are cured by further local treatment. Regional lymph node metastases develop in up to 5% of squamous cell cancers and less than 2% of basal cell cancers. Nodal metastasis is more common in Merkel's cell cancers but is very unusual in sarcomas of the skin. Regardless of the histological type, whenever clinically obvious nodal enlargement occurs, a needle biopsy should be performed and a therapeutic lymph node dissection carried out if regional spread is documented. There is essentially no role for elective dissections of clinically normal nodes in any form of nonmelanoma skin cancer, but there may be a role for sentinel node biopsy in Merkel cell cancers.[126]

Distant Metastasis

Distant spread occurs in about 2% of squamous cell cancers and 0.1% of basal cell cancers, most frequently after nodal recurrence. No effective therapy exists for metastatic nonmelanoma skin cancer, although there have been a few reports of responses to chemotherapy or the combination of IFN-α and 13-*cis*-retinoic acid (isotretinoin, Accutane).[127]

References

1. Jemal A, Murray T, Ward E, et al. Cancer statistics, 2005. CA Cancer J Clin 2005;55:10–30.
2. Rigel DS. Malignant melanoma: incidence issues and their effect on diagnosis and treatment in the 1990s. Mayo Clin Proc 1997;72:367–371.
3. Weinstock MA. Issues in the epidemiology of melanoma. Hematol Oncol Clin N Am 1998;12:681–698.
4. Wingo PA, Ries LAG, Rosenberg HM, Miller DS, Edwards BK. Cancer incidence and mortality. Cancer (Phila) 1998;82:1197–1207.
5. Albert VA, Koh HK, Geller AC, Miller DR, Prout MN, Lew RA. Years of potential life lost: another indicator of the impact of cutaneous malignant melanoma on society. J Am Acad Dermatol 1990;23:308–310.
6. Chaudru V, Chompret A, Bressac-de Paillerets B, Spatz A, Avril M-F, Demenais F. Influence of genes, nevi, and sun sensitivity on melanoma risk in a family sample unselected by family history and in melanoma-prone families. J Natl Cancer Inst 2004;96:785–795.
7. Rouzaud F, Kadekaro AL, Abdel-Malek ZA, Hearing VJ. MC1R and the response of melanocytes to ultraviolet radiation. Mutat Res 2005;571:133–152.
8. Chang AE, Karnell LH, Menck HR. The National Cancer Data Base report on cutaneous and non-cutaneous melanoma: a summary of 84,836 cases from the past decade. Cancer (Phila) 1998;83:1664–1678.
9. Katz KA, Jonasch E, Hodi FS, et al. Melanoma of unknown primary: experience at Massachusetts General Hospital and Dana-Farber Cancer Institute. Melanoma Res 2005;15:77–82.
10. Cress RD, Holly EA. Incidence of cutaneous melanoma among non-Hispanic whites, Hispanics, Asians, and blacks: an analysis of California cancer registry data, 1988-93. Cancer Causes Control 1997;8:246–252.
11. Byrd KM, Wilson DC, Hoyler SS, Peck GL. Advanced presentation of melanoma in African Americans. J Am Acad Dermatol 2004;50:21–24.
12. Halder RM, Bridgeman-Shah S. Skin cancer in African Americans. Cancer (Phila) 1995;75:667–673.
13. Elwood JM, Jopson J. Melanoma and sun exposure: an overview of published studies. Int J Cancer 1997;73:198–203.
14. Langley RGB, Sober AJ. A clinical review of the evidence for the role of ultraviolet radiation in the etiology of cutaneous melanoma. Cancer Invest 1997;15:561–567.
15. Berwick M, Armstrong BK, Ben-Porat L, et al. Sun exposure and mortality from melanoma. J Natl Cancer Inst 2005;97:195–199.
16. Tsao H, Sober A. Acquired precursor lesions and markers of increased risk for cutaneous melanoma. In: Balch C, Houghton A, Sober A, Soong S, eds. Cutaneous Melanoma, 4th ed. St. Louis: Quality Medical, 2003:121–134.
17. Tsao H, Bevona C, Goggins W, Quinn T. The transformation rate of moles (melanocytic nevi) into cutaneous melanoma: a population-based estimate. Arch Dermatol 2003;139:282–288.
18. Tucker MA, Halpern A, Holly EA, et al. Clinically recognized dysplastic nevi. A central risk factor for cutaneous melanoma. JAMA 1997;277:1439–1444.
19. Chin L. The genetics of malignant melanoma: lessons from mouse and man. Nat Rev Cancer 2003;3:559–570.

20. Chudnovsky Y, Khavari PA, Adams AE: Melanoma genetics and the development of rational therapeutics. J Clin Invest 2005;115:813–824.
21. Greene MH, Clark WH Jr, Tucker MA, et al. Acquired precursors of cutaneous malignant melanoma: the familial dysplastic nevus syndrome. N Engl J Med 1985;312:91–97.
22. Lynch HT, Fusaro RM, Pester J, Lynch JF. Familial atypical multiple mole melanoma (FAMMM) syndrome: genetic heterogeneity and malignant melanoma. Br J Cancer 1980;42:58–70.
23. Bale SJ, Dracopoli NC, Tucker MA, et al. Mapping the gene for hereditary cutaneous malignant melanoma: dysplastic nevus to chromosome 1p. N Engl J Med 1989;320:1367–1372.
24. Nancarrow DJ, Mann GJ, Holland EA, et al. Confirmation of chromosome 9p linkage in familial melanoma. Am J Hum Genet 1993;53:936–942.
25. Marghoob AA, Schoenbach SP, Kopf AW, Orlow SJ, Nossa R, Bart RS. Large congenital melanocytic nevi and the risk for the development of malignant melanoma: a prospective study. Arch Dermatol 1996;132:170–175.
26. Nancarrow D, Platz A, Tucker MA for the Melanoma Genetics Consortium. Geographical variation in the penetrance of CDKN2A mutations for melanoma. J Natl Cancer Inst 2002; 94:894–903.
27. Meyskens FL, Farmer PJ, Anton-Culver H. Etiologic pathogenesis of melanoma: a unifying hypothesis for the missing attributable risk. Clin Cancer Res 2004;10:2581–2583.
28. Wellbrock C, Ogilvie L, Hedley D, Karasarides M, et al. ^{V599E}B-RAF is an oncogene in melanocytes. Cancer Res 2004;64:2338–2342.
29. Tsao H, Zhang X, Fowlkes K, Haluska FG. Relative reciprocity of NRAS and PTEN/MMAC1 alterations in cutaneous melanoma cell lines. Cancer Res 2000;60:1800–1804.
30. Tsao H, Goel V, Wu H, Yang G, Haluska FG. Genetic interaction between NRAS and BRAF mutations and PTEN/MMAC1 inactivation in melanoma. J Invest Dermatol 2004;122:337–341.
31. Uribe P, Wistuba II, Gonzalez S. BRAF mutation: a frequent event in benign, atypical, and malignant melanocytic lesions of the skin. Am J Dermatopathol 2003;25:365–370.
32. Pollock PM, Harper UL, Hansen KS, et al. High frequency of BRAF mutations in nevi. Nat Genet 2003;33:19–20.
33. Dong J, Phelps RG, Qiao R, Yao S, Benard O, Ronai Z, Aaronson SA. BRAF oncogenic mutations correlate with progression rather than initiation of human melanoma. Cancer Res 2003;63:3883–3885.
34. Argenziano G, Soyer HP. Dermoscopy of pigmented skin lesions: a valuable tool for early diagnosis of melanoma. Lancet Oncol 2001;2:443–449.
35. Riker AI, Glass F, Perez I, Cruse CW, Messina J, Sondak VK. Cutaneous melanoma: methods of biopsy and definitive surgical excision. Dermatol Ther 2005;18:387–393.
36. Saiag P, Bernard M, Beauchet A, Bafounta ML, Bourgault-Villada I, Chagnon S. Ultrasonography using simple diagnostic criteria vs palpation for the detection of regional lymph node metastases of melanoma. Arch Dermatol 2005;141:183–189.
37. Starritt EC, Uren RF, Scolyer RA, Quinn MJ, Thompson JF. Ultrasound examination of sentinel nodes in the initial assessment of patients with primary cutaneous melanoma. Ann Surg Oncol 2005;12:18–23.
38. Basler GC, Fader DJ, Yahanda A, Sondak VK, Johnson TM. The utility of fine needle aspiration in the diagnosis of melanoma metastatic to lymph nodes. J Am Acad Dermatol 1997;36:403–408.
39. Clark WH, Elder DE, Guerry D, et al. Model predicting survival in stage I melanoma based on tumor progression. J Natl Cancer Inst 1989;81:1893–1904.
40. Balch CM, Soong S-J, Gershenwald JE, et al. Prognostic factor analysis of 17,600 melanoma patients: validation of the American Joint Committee on Cancer Melanoma Staging System. J Clin Oncol 2001;19:3622–3234.
41. Weinstock MA, Morris BT, Lederman JS, Bleicher P, Fitzpatrick TB, Sober AJ. Effect of BANS location on the prognosis of clinical stage I melanoma: new data and meta-analysis. Br J Dermatol 1988;119:559–565.
42. Fidler IJ, Ellis LM. Neoplastic angiogenesis. Not all blood vessels are created equal. N Engl J Med 2004;351:215-216.
43. Sondak VK, Taylor JM, Sabel MS, et al. Mitotic rate and younger age are predictors of sentinel lymph node positivity: lessons learned from the generation of a probabilistic model. Ann Surg Oncol 2004;11:247–258.
44. Barnhill RL, Katzen J, Spatz A, Fine J, Berwick M. The importance of mitotic rate as a prognostic factor for localized cutaneous melanoma. J Cutan Pathol 2005;32:268–273.
45. Clemente CG, Mihm MC Jr, Bufalino R, Zurrida S, Collini P, Cascinelli N. Prognostic value of tumor infiltrating lymphocytes in the vertical growth phase of primary cutaneous melanoma. Cancer (Phila) 1996;77:1303–1310.
46. Tuthill RJ, Unger JM, Liu PY, Flaherty LE, Sondak VK, for the Southwest Oncology Group. Risk assessment in localized primary cutaneous melanoma: a Southwest Oncology Group study evaluating nine factors and a test of the Clark logistic regression prediction model. Am J Clin Pathol 2002;118:504–511.
47. Hawkins WG, Busam KJ, Ben-Porat L, et al. Desmoplastic melanoma: a pathologically and clinically distinct form of cutaneous melanoma. Ann Surg Oncol 2005;12:207–213.
48. Balch CM, Soong S, Shaw HM, Urist MM, McCarthy WH. An analysis of prognostic factors in 8500 patients with cutaneous melanoma. In: Balch CM, Houghton AN, Milton GW, Sober AJ, Soong S, ed. Cutaneous Melanoma, 2nd ed. Philadelphia: Lippincott, 1992:165–187.
49. Ferrari A, Bono A, Baldi M, et al. Does melanoma behave differently in younger children than in adults? A retrospective study of 33 cases of childhood melanoma from a single institution. Pediatrics 2005;115:649–654.
50. Chao MM, Schwartz JL, Wechsler DS, Thornburg CD, Griffith KA, Williams JA. High-risk surgically resected pediatric melanoma and adjuvant interferon therapy. Pediatr Blood Cancer 2004;43:1–8.
51. Veronesi U, Cascinelli N, Adamus J, et al. Thin stage I primary cutaneous malignant melanoma. Comparison of excision with margins of 1 or 3 cm. N Engl J Med 1988;318:1159–1162.
52. Veronesi U, Cascinelli N. Narrow excision (1-cm margin): a safe procedure for thin cutaneous melanoma. Arch Surg 1991;126:438–441.
53. Karakousis CP, Balch CM, Urist MM, Ross MM, Smith TJ, Bartolucci AA. Local recurrence in malignant melanoma: long-term results of the multiinstitutional randomized surgical trial. Ann Surg Oncol 1996;3:446–452.
54. Balch CM, Urist MM, Karakousis CP, et al. Efficacy of 2-cm surgical margins for intermediate-thickness melanomas (1–4 mm): results of a multi-institutional randomized surgical trial. Ann Surg 1993;218:262–269.
55. Thomas JM, Newton-Bishop J, Ahern R, et al. Excision margins in high-risk malignant melanoma. N Engl J Med 2004;350:757–766.
56. Johnson TM, Sondak VK. Melanoma margins: the importance and need for more evidence-based trials. Arch Dermatol 2004;140:1148–1150.
57. Heaton KM, Sussman JJ, Gershenwald JE, et al. Surgical margins and prognostic factors in patients with thick (0.4 mm) primary melanoma. Ann Surg Oncol 1998;5:322–328.
58. Kesmodel SB, Karakousis GC, Botbyl JD, et al. Mitotic rate as a predictor of sentinel lymph node positivity in patients with thin melanomas. Ann Surg Oncol 2005;12:1–10.

59. Gimotty PA, Van Belle P, Elder DE, et al. Biologic and prognostic significance of dermal Ki67 expression, mitoses, and tumorigenicity in thin invasive cutaneous melanoma. J Clin Oncol 2005;23:8048–8056.
60. Puleo CA, Messina JL, Riker AI, et al. Sentinel node biopsy for thin melanomas: which patients should be considered? Cancer Control 2005;12:230–235.
61. Balch CM. The role of elective lymph node dissection in melanoma: rationale, results, and controversies. J Clin Oncol 1988;6:163–172.
62. Balch CM, Soong SJ, Bartolucci AA, et al. Efficacy of an elective regional lymph node dissection of 1 to 4mm thick melanomas for patients 60 years of age and younger. Ann Surg 1996;224:255–263.
63. Sim FH, Taylor WF, Ivins JC, et al. A prospective randomized study of the efficacy of routine elective lymphadenectomy in management of malignant melanoma: preliminary results. Cancer (Phila) 1978;41:948–956.
64. Veronesi U, Adamus J, Bandiera DC, et al. Delayed regional node dissection in stage I melanoma of the skin of the lower extremities. Cancer (Phila) 1982;49:2420–2430.
65. Cascinelli N, Morabito A, Santinami M, MacKie RM, Belli F. Immediate or delayed dissection of regional nodes in patients with melanoma of the trunk: a randomised trial. WHO Melanoma Programme. Lancet 1998;351:793–796.
66. Morton DL, Wen D-R, Wong JH, et al. Technical details of intraoperative lymphatic mapping for early stage melanoma. Arch Surg 1992;127:392–399.
67. Reintgen DS, Brobeil A. Lymphatic mapping and selective lymphadenectomy as an alternative to elective lymph node dissection in patients with malignant melanoma. Hematol Oncol Clin N Am 1998;12:807–821.
68. Bostick P, Essner R, Glass E, et al. Comparison of blue dye and probe-assisted intraoperative lymphatic mapping in melanoma to identify sentinel nodes in 100 lymphatic basins. Arch Surg 1999;134:43–49.
69. Evans HL, Krag DN, Teates CD, et al. Lymphoscintigraphy and sentinel node biospy accurately stage melanoma in patients presenting after wide local excision. Ann Surg Oncol 2003;10:416–425.
70. Gershenwald JE, Colome MI, Lee JE, et al. Patterns of recurrence following a negative sentinel lymph node biopsy in 243 patients with stage I or II melanoma. J Clin Oncol 1998;16:2253–2260.
71. Morton DL, Thompson JF, Cochran AJ, et al. Interim results of the Multicenter Selective Lymphadenectomy Trial (MSLT-1) in clinical stage I melanoma. J Clin Oncol 2005;23:abstract 7500.
72. Morton DL, Thompson JF, Cochran AJ, et al. Sentinel-node biopsy or nodal observation for melanoma. N Engl J Med 2006;355:1307–1317.
73. Wang X, Heller R, VanVoorhis N, et al. Detection of submicroscopic lymph node metastases with polymerase chain reaction in patients with malignant melanoma. Ann Surg 1994;220:768–774.
74. Shivers SC, Wang X, Li W, et al. Molecular staging of malignant melanoma: correlation with clinical outcome. JAMA 1998; 280:1410–1415.
75. Scoggins CR, Ross MI, Reintgen DS, et al. Prospective multi-institutional study of reverse transcriptase polymerase chain reaction for molecular staging of melanoma. J Clin Oncol 2006;24:2849–2857.
76. Poo-Hwu WJ, Ariyan S, Lamb L, et al. Follow-up recommendations for patients with American Joint Commission on Cancer stages I–III malignant melanoma. Cancer (Phila) 1999;86:2252–2258.
77. Baergen RN, Johnson D, Moore T, Benirschke K. Maternal melanoma metastatic to the placenta. Arch Pathol Lab Med 1997;121:508–511.
78. Mackie RM. Pregnancy and exogenous hormones in patients with cutaneous malignant melanoma. Curr Opin Oncol 1999;11:129–131.
79. Collaborative Ocular Melanoma Study Group. Mortality in patients with small choroidal melanoma. COMS report no. 4. Arch Ophthalmol 1997;115(7):886–893.
80. Jampol LM, Moy CS, Murray TG, et al. The COMS randomized trial of iodine 125 bryachytherapy for choroidal melanoma: IV. Local treatment failure and enucleation in the first 5 years after brachytherapy. COMS report no. 19. Ophthalmology 2002;109: 2197–2206.
81. Collaborative Ocular Melanoma Study Group. The Collaborative Ocular Melanoma Study (COMS) randomized trial of pre-enucleation radiation of large choroidal melanoma II: initial mortality findings. COMS report no. 10. Am J Ophthalmol 1998;125:779–796.
82. Cooper JS. The evolution of the role of radiation therapy in the management of mucocutaneous malignant melanoma. Hematol Oncol Clin N Am 1998;12:849–862.
83. Sondak VK, Wolfe JA. Adjuvant therapy for melanoma. Curr Opin Oncol 1997;9:189–204.
84. Veronesi U, Adamus J, Aubert C, et al. A randomized trial of adjuvant chemotherapy and immunotherapy in cutaneous melanoma. N Engl J Med 1982;307:913–916.
85. Quirt IC, Shelley WE, Pater JL, et al. Improved survival in patients with poor-prognosis malignant melanoma treated with adjuvant levamisole: a phase III study by the National Cancer Institute of Canada Clinical Trials Group. J Clin Oncol 1991;9:729–735.
86. Kirkwood JM, Strawderman MH, Ernstoff MS, Smith TJ, Borden EC, Blum RH. Interferon alfa-2b adjuvant therapy of high-risk resected cutaneous melanoma: the Eastern Cooperative Oncology Group trial EST 1684. J Clin Oncol 1996;14:7–17.
87. Kirkwood JM, Ibrahim JG, Sondak VK, et al. High- and low-dose interferon alfa-2b in high-risk melanoma: first analysis of intergroup trial E1690/S9111/C9190. J Clin Oncol 2000;18:2444–2458.
88. Creagan ET, Dalton RJ, Ahmann DL, et al. Randomized, surgical adjuvant clinical trial of recombinant interferon alfa-2a in selected patients with malignant melanoma. J Clin Oncol 1995;13:2776–2783.
89. Cascinelli N, Bufalino R, Morabito A, MacKie RM. Results of adjuvant interferon study in WHO melanoma programme. Lancet 1994;343:913–914.
90. Kirkwood JM, Manola J, Ibrahim J, Sondak V, Ernstoff MS, Rao M. A pooled analysis of Eastern Cooperative Group and Intergroup trials of adjuvant high-dose interferon for melanoma. Clin Cancer Res 2004:10:1670–1677.
91. Schuchter LM. Adjuvant interferon therapy for melanoma: high-dose, low-dose, no dose, which dose? J Clin Oncol 2004;22:7–10.
92. Morton DL, Mozzillo N, Thompson JF, et al. An international randomized double blind, phase 3 study of the specific active immunotherapy agent, onamelatucel-L (Canvaxin), compared to placebo as a post-surgical adjuvant in AJCC stage IV melanoma. Ann Surg Oncol 2006;13:5(abstract).
93. Spitler LE, Grossbard ML, Ernstoff MS, et al. Adjuvant therapy of stage III and IV malignant melanoma using granulocyte-macrophage colony-stimulating factor. J Clin Oncol 2000;18:1614–1621.
94. Speiser DE, Lienard D, Rufer N, et al. Rapid and strong human CD8+ T cell responses to vaccination with peptide, IFA, and CpG oligodeoxynucleotide 7909. J Clin Invest 2005;115:739–746.
95. Ang KK, Peters LJ, Weber RS, et al. Postoperative radiotherapy for cutaneous melanoma of the head and neck region. Int J Radiat Oncol Biol Phys 1994;30:795–798.

96. Strom EA, Ross MI. Adjuvant radiation therapy after axillary lymphadenectomy for metastatic melanoma: toxicity and local control. Ann Surg Oncol 1995;2:445–449.
97. O'Brien CJ, Petersen-Schaefer K, Stevens GN, et al. Adjuvant radiotherapy following neck dissection and parotidectomy for metastatic malignant melanoma. Head Neck 1997;19:589–594.
98. Creagan ET, Cupps RE, Ivins JC, et al. Adjuvant radiation therapy for regional nodal metastases from malignant melanoma: a randomized, prospective study. Cancer (Phila) 1978;42:2206–2210.
99. Eggermont AM, Brunstein F, Grunhagen D, ten Hagen TL. Regional treatment of metastasis: role of regional perfusion. State of the art isolated limb perfusion for limb salvage. Ann Oncol 2004;15(suppl 4):iv-107–iv-112.
100. Taber SW, Polk HC Jr. Mortality, major amputation rates, and leukopenia after isolated limb perfusion with phenylalanine mustard for the treatment of melanoma. J Surg Oncol 1997;4:440–445.
101. Lienard D, Ewalenko P, Delmotte J-J, Renard N, Lejeune FJ. High-dose recombinant tumor necrosis factor alpha in combination with interferon gamma and melphalan in isolation perfusion of the limbs for melanoma and sarcoma. J Clin Oncol 1992;10:52–60.
102. Fraker DL, Alexander HR, Andrich M, Rosenberg SA. Treatment of patients with melanoma of the extremity using hyperthermic isolated limb perfusion with melphalan, tumor necrosis factor, and interferon gamma: results of a tumor necrosis factor dose-escalation study. J Clin Oncol 1996;14:479–489.
103. Thompson JF, Kam PC. Isolated limb infusion for melanoma: a simple but effective alternative to isolated limb perfusion. J Surg Oncol 2004;88(1):1–3.
104. Schraffordt Koops H, Vaglini M, Suciu S, et al. Prophylactic isolated limb perfusion for localized, high-risk limb melanoma: results of a multicenter randomized phase III trial. J Clin Oncol 1998;16:2906–2912.
105. Margolin K, Atkins MB, Thompson JA, et al. Temozolomide and whole brain irradiation in melanoma metastatic to the brain: a phase II trial of the Cytokine Working Group. J Cancer Res Clin Oncol 2002;128:214–218.
106. Atkins MB, Sosman J, Agarwala S, et al. A Cytokine Working Group phase II study of temozolomide (TMZ), thalidomide (THAL) and whole brain radiation therapy (WBRT) for patients with brain metastases from melanoma. Proc Am Soc Clin Oncol 2005;23:723S.
107. Ang KK, Geara FB, Byers RM, Peters LJ. Radiotherapy of melanoma. In: Balch CM, Houghton AN, Sober AJ, Soong S, eds. Cutaneous Melanoma, 3rd ed. St. Louis: Quality Medical, 1998:389–403.
108. Wu H, Goel V, Haluska FG. PTEN signaling pathways in melanoma. Oncogene 2003;22:3113–3122.
109. Flaherty KT. New molecular targets in melanoma. Curr Opin Oncol 2004;16:150–154.
110. Legha SS. The role of interferon alfa in the treatment of metastatic melanoma. Semin Oncol 1997;24(1 suppl 4):S24–S31.
111. Atkins MB. Immunotherapy and experimental approaches for metastatic melanoma. Hematol Oncol Clin N Am 1998;12:877–902.
112. Atkins MB, Lotze MT, Dutcher JP, et al. High-dose recombinant interleukin 2 therapy for patients with metastatic melanoma: analysis of 270 patients treated between 1985 and 1993. J Clin Oncol 1999;17:2105–2116.
113. Margolin K. Biochemotherapy for melanoma: rational therapeutics in the search for weapons of melanoma destruction. Cancer (Phila) 2004;101:435–438.
114. Sondak VK, Sosman JA. Results of clinical trials with an allogeneic melanoma tumor cell lysate vaccine: Melacine®. Semin Cancer Biol 2003;13:409–415.
115. Mitchell MS, Harel W, Kempf RA, et al. Active-specific immunotherapy for melanoma. J Clin Oncol 1990;8:856–869.
116. Demierre M-F, Swetter SM, Sondak VK. Vaccine therapy of melanoma: an update. Curr Cancer Ther Rev 2005;1:115–125.
117. Kirkwood JM, Ibrahim JG, Sosman JA, et al. High-dose interferon alfa-2b significantly prolongs relapse-free and overall survival compared with the GM2-KLH/QS-21 vaccine in patients with resected stage IIB-III melanoma: results of intergroup trial E1694/S9512/C509801. J Clin Oncol 2001;19:2370–2380.
118. Panelli MC, Wang E, Monsurro VV, et al. Overview of melanoma vaccines and promising approaches. Curr Oncol Rep 2004;6:414–420.
119. Perales MA, Wolchok JD. Melanoma vaccines. Cancer Invest 2002;20:1012–1026.
120. Antonia S, Mule JJ, Weber JS. Current developments of immunotherapy in the clinic. Curr Opin Immunol 2004;16:130–136.
121. Preston DS, Stern RS. Nonmelanoma cancers of the skin. N Engl J Med 1992;327:1649–1662.
122. Halpern AC, Altman JF. Genetic predisposition to skin cancer. Curr Opin Oncol 1999;11:132–138.
123. Brooks AD, Heslin MJ, Leung DH, Lewis JJ, Brennan MF. Superficial extremity soft tissue sarcoma: an analysis of prognostic factors. Ann Surg Oncol 1998;5:41–47.
124. Swanson NA. Mohs surgery: technique, indications, applications, and the future. Arch Dermatol 1983;119:761–773.
125. Ratner D, Thomas CO, Johnson TM, et al. Mohs micrographic surgery for the treatment of dermatofibrosarcoma protuberans: results of a multi-institutional series with an analysis of the extent of microscopic spread. J Am Acad Dermatol 1997;37:600–613.
126. Messina JL, Reintgen DS, Cruse CW, et al. Selective lymphadenectomy in patients with Merkel cell (cutaneous neuroendocrine) carcinoma. Ann Surg Oncol 1997;4:389–395.
127. Lippman SM, Parkinson DR, Itri LM, et al. 13-*cis*-Retinoic acid and interferon alpha-2a: effective combination therapy for advanced squamous cell carcinoma of the skin. J Natl Cancer Inst 1992;84:235–241.
128. Meyskens FL Jr, Kopecky K, Taylor CW, et al. Randomized trial of adjuvant human interferon gamma versus observation in high-risk cutaneous melanoma. J Natl Cancer Inst 1995;87:1710–1713.
129. Sondak VK, Kopecky KJ, Smith JW II, et al. Is interferon-α detrimental? Results of a Southwest Oncology Group randomized trial of adjuvant human interferon-α versus observation in malignant melanoma. In: Salmon SE, ed. Adjuvant Therapy of Cancer, vol VIII. Philadelphia: Lippincott-Raven, 1997:259–272.
130. Rusciani L, Petraglia S, Alotto M, et al. Postsurgical adjuvant therapy of melanoma: evaluation of a 3-year randomized trial with recombinant interferon-α after 3 and 5 years of follow-up. Cancer (Phila) 1997;79:2354–2360.
131. Pehamberger H, Soyer HP, Steiner A, et al. Adjuvant interferon alfa-2a treatment in resected primary stage II cutaneous melanoma. J Clin Oncol 1998;16:1425–1429.
132. Grob JJ, Dreno B, de la Salmonière P, et al. Randomised trial of interferon α-2a as adjuvant therapy in resected primary melanoma thicker than 1.5 mm without clinically detectable node metastases. Lancet 1998;351:1905–1910.
133. Berd D, Sato T, Maguire HC Jr, Kairys J, Mastrangelo MJ. Immunopharmacologic analysis of an autologous, hapten-modified human melanoma vaccine. J Clin Oncol 2004;22:403–415.
134. Hsueh EC, Morton DL. Antigen-based immunotherapy of melanoma: Canvaxin therapeutic polyvalent cancer vaccine. Semin Cancer Biol 2003;13:401–417.
135. Livingston PO, Wong GYC, Adluri S, et al. Improved survival in stage III melanoma patients with GM2 antibodies: a randomized trial of adjuvant vaccination with GM2 ganglioside. J Clin Oncol 1994;12:1036–1044.

136. Rosenberg SJ, Yang JC, Restifo NP. Cancer immunotherapy: moving beyond current vaccines. Nat Med 2004;10:909–915.
137. Dudley ME, Wunderlich JR, Yang JC, et al. Adoptive cell transfer therapy following non-myeloablative but lymphodepleting chemotherapy for the treatment of patients with refractory metastatic melanoma J Clin Oncol 23:2346–2357.
138. Lonchay C, van der Bruggen P, Connerotte T, et al. Correlation between tumor regression and T cell responses in melanoma patients vaccinated with a MAGE antigen. Proc Natl Acad Sci U S A 2004;101(suppl 2):14631–14638.
139. Slingluff CL Jr, Petroni GR, Yamshchikov GV, et al. Immunologic and clinical outcomes of vaccination with a multiepitope melanoma peptide vaccine plus low-dose interleukin-2 administered either concurrently or on a delayed schedule. J Clin Oncol 2004;22:4474–4485.
140. Klinman D. Immunotherapeutic uses of CpG oligodeoxynucleotides. Nat Rev Immunol 2004;4:249–258.

98

Soft Tissue Sarcoma

Peter W.T. Pisters

Soft tissue sarcomas comprise a group of relatively rare, anatomically and histologically diverse neoplasms. These tumors share a common embryological origin, arising primarily from tissues derived from the mesoderm. The notable exceptions are neurosarcomas, primitive neuroectodermal tumors, and possibly Ewing's sarcomas, which are believed to arise from tissues of ectodermal origin.

Despite the fact that the somatic soft tissues account for as much as 75% of total body weight, neoplasms of the soft tissues are comparatively rare, accounting for 1% of adult malignancies and 15% of pediatric malignancies. The annual incidence of soft tissue sarcomas in the United States is about 7800 new cases with 4400 deaths annually.[1] This chapter reviews current concepts in the diagnosis, staging, and management of patients with soft tissue sarcoma. Extremity sarcoma, which accounts for approximately 50% of all sarcomas (and is therefore the anatomic site with the largest literature base), is the focus of the first section of the chapter. Retroperitoneal sarcomas are covered in a separate subsection at the end of the chapter.

Etiology and Epidemiology

In the United States, the race and sex distribution of adult soft tissue sarcomas approximates that of the U.S. population.[2] No specific etiological agent is identified in the majority of patients with soft tissue sarcoma. There are, however, a number of recognized associations between specific environmental factors and the subsequent development of sarcoma: these include a history of previous exposure to ionizing radiation or alkylating chemotherapeutic agents; occupational exposure to phenoxy acetic acids, chlorophenols, vinyl chloride, or arsenic; or exposure to the previously employed intravenous contrast agent Thorotrast. In addition, chronic lymphedema of congenital origin, infectious etiology (filariasis), or posttreatment (postsurgical or postirradiation) etiology have been implicated in the subsequent development of lymphangiosarcoma.

In clinical practice, the most commonly observed nongenetic predisposing factors are previous irradiation and chronic lymphedema. By definition, radiation-induced sarcomas arise no sooner than 3 years after completion of therapeutic radiation and often arise decades later.[3,4] Most of these sarcomas are high grade (87%), and the predominant histology of radiation-induced sarcomas is osteosarcoma,[3] possibly because of the greater absorption of radiation by bone than by other tissues. Chronic lymphedema is seen as a contributing factor in the development in lymphangiosarcoma arising in the chronically lymphedematous arms of women treated for breast cancer with radical mastectomy (Stewart–Treves syndrome).

A number of genetic conditions are also associated with an increased risk for the development of soft tissue sarcoma. These conditions include neurofibromatosis, Li–Fraumeni syndrome, familial retinoblastoma, and Gardner's syndrome. The most commonly encountered genetically related soft tissue sarcomas occur in patients with neurofibromatosis or Gardner's syndrome. Patients with neurofibromatosis have a 7% to 10% lifetime risk of developing a malignant neurofibroma or fibrosarcoma.[5,6] Gardner's syndrome is characterized by colonic polyposis associated with various benign and malignant extracolonic manifestations. Desmoid tumors occur in 8% to 12% of patients with the Gardner's variant of familial polyposis.[7]

In summary, a small fraction of patients with soft tissue sarcoma present with a sarcoma that could be related to one of these environmental or genetic factors, but the majority of patients have spontaneous development of soft tissue sarcoma without any known etiological agent. The precise etiology of an individual sarcoma is of little clinical significance because this does not affect on therapeutic decision making beyond the obvious fact that patients who have sarcomas arising in a previously irradiated field usually cannot receive further external-beam radiotherapy (EBRT).

Pathology

Anatomic Site Distribution

Soft tissue sarcomas have been described at virtually all anatomic sites. The anatomic sites and site-specific histological subtypes of 1182 sarcomas treated at a single referral institution are outlined in Figure 98.1. Approximately one-third to one-half of all soft tissue sarcomas occur in the lower extremities, where the most common histopathological subtypes are malignant fibrous histiocytoma and liposarcoma. Retroperitoneal sarcomas comprise 15% to 20% of all soft tissue sarcomas, with liposarcoma and leiomyosarcoma being the predominant histological subtypes. The visceral sarcomas make up an additional 24%, and head and neck sarcomas comprise approximately 4% of all sarcomas seen at a tertiary care cancer center (see Fig. 98.1).

Histological Classification

In broad terms, sarcomas can be classified into neoplasms arising in bone and those arising from the periosseous soft tissue. Sarcomas of the soft tissues can be further grouped into those that arise from viscera (gastrointestinal, genitourinary, and gynecological organs) and those that originate in nonvisceral soft tissues such as muscle, tendon, adipose tissue, pleura, synovium, and connective tissue.

The most universally applied classification scheme for soft tissue sarcoma is based on histogenesis, as outlined in the recent World Health Organization (WHO) classification system for sarcomas.[8] This classification system is reproducible for the better-differentiated tumors. However, as the degree of histological differentiation declines, the determination of cellular origin becomes increasingly difficult. In particular, despite advanced immunohistochemical techniques and electron microscopy, determining the cellular origin for many spindle cell and round cell soft tissue tumors is difficult, occasionally arbitrary, and sometimes impossible. This difficulty leads to significant disparity in diagnosis among pathologists. A discrepancy between the original histological assessment and that of a subsequent expert review has been noted in as many as 25% of cases.[9,10]

Difficulties in establishing the specific cellular origin have limited clinical importance because the histological subtype is not generally directly related to biological behavior. Important exceptions to this generalization include epithelioid sarcoma, clear cell sarcoma, angiosarcoma, and embryonal rhabdomyosarcoma, all of which have a greater risk of regional lymph node metastasis.[11,12] In one single-institution study, the overall rate of nodal metastasis at the time of presentation was only 2.7%; however, the rate was much higher for the histological subtypes angiosarcoma (13.5%), embryonal rhabdomyosarcoma (13.6%), and epithelioid sarcoma (16.7%).[11] Thus, treatment strategies may differ for these histological subtypes. For the remaining histological

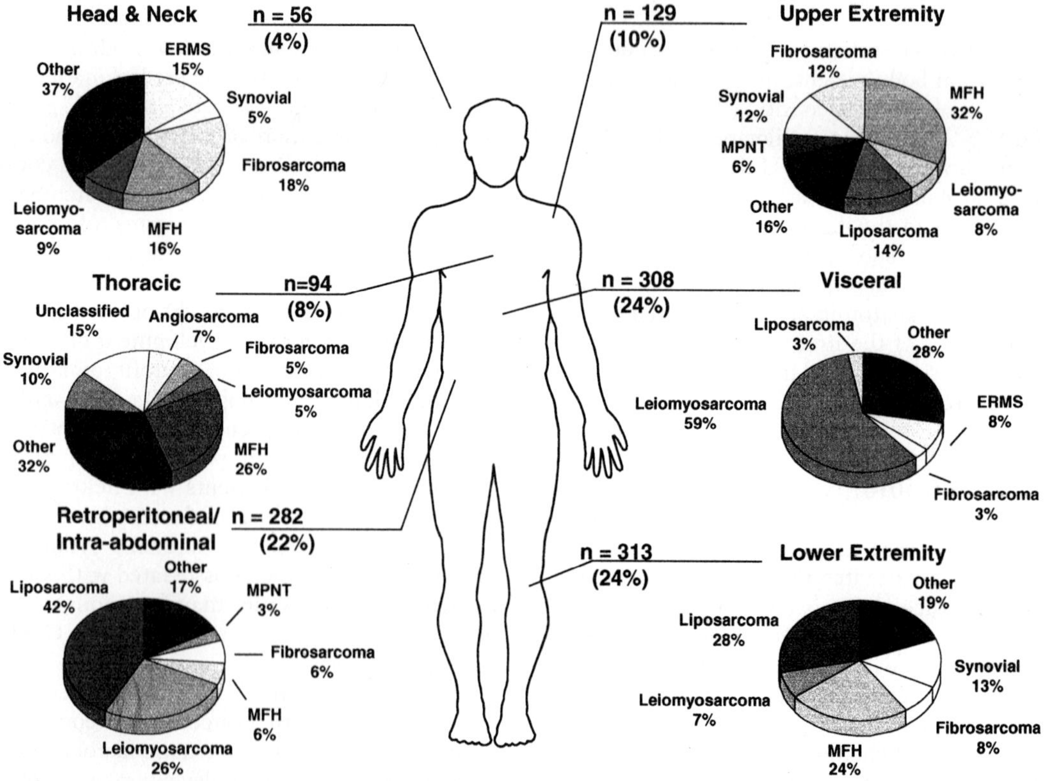

FIGURE 98.1. Anatomic distribution and site-specific histological subtypes of 1182 consecutive patients with soft tissue sarcomas seen at The University of Texas M.D. Anderson Cancer Center (University of Texas M.D. Anderson Cancer Center Sarcoma Database, June 1996–December 1998). *MFH*, malignant fibrous histiocytoma; *ERMS*, embryonal rhabdomyasarcoma; *MPNT*, malignant peripheral nerve sheath tumor.

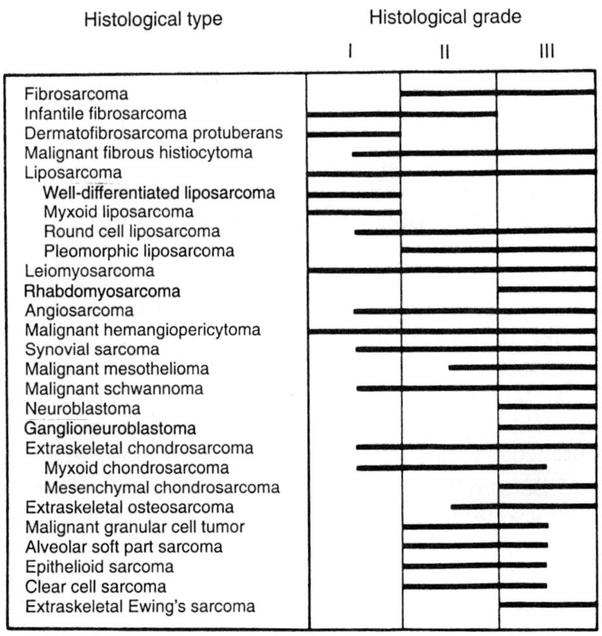

FIGURE 98.2. The spectrum of grades (*right*) observed among histological subtypes (*left*) of soft tissue sarcoma. (From Enzinger FN, Weiss SW, eds. Soft Tissue Tumors, 3rd ed. St. Louis: Mosby-Year Book, 1995, with permission.)

subtypes, biological behavior is more determined by histological grade than histological subtype.[13]

Histological Grading

Biological aggressiveness can be best predicted on the basis of histological grade.[13,14] The spectrum of grades varies among specific histological subtypes (Fig. 98.2). In careful comparative multivariate analyses, histological grade has been the most important prognostic factor in assessing the risk for distant metastasis and tumor-related mortality.[13,14] Several grading systems have been proposed, but there is no consensus regarding the specific morphological criteria that should be employed in the grading of soft tissue sarcomas.

Two of the most commonly employed grading systems are the U.S. National Cancer Institute (NCI) system developed by Costa and colleagues[15] and the FNCLCC system (Federation Nationale des Centres de Lutte Contre le Cancer) developed by the French Federation of Cancer Centers Sarcoma Group.[16] The NCI system is based on tumor histological subtype, location, and amount of tumor necrosis, but cellularity, nuclear pleomorphism, and mitosis count are also to be considered in certain situations. The FNCLCC system employs a score generated by the evaluation of three parameters: tumor differentiation, mitotic rate, and amount of tumor necrosis. The prognostic values of these two grading systems were retrospectively compared in a population of 410 adult patients with nonmetastatic soft tissue sarcoma.[17] Univariate and multivariate analyses suggested that the FNCLCC system has a slightly better ability to predict distant metastasis development and tumor-related mortality. Significant discrepancies were observed in one-third of cases. An increased number of grade 3 tumors, a reduced number of grade 2 tumors, and better correlation with overall and metastasis-free survival were observed in favor of the FNCLCC system.[17] Thus, in the absence of other comparative data, the FNCLCC system may be the best presently available grading system.

Clinical Presentation and Diagnosis

The majority of patients present with a painless mass, although pain is noted at presentation in up to a third of cases.[2] Delay in diagnosis or sarcomas is common, with the most common incorrect diagnosis for extremity and trunk lesions being hematoma or "pulled muscle."

Physical examination should include an assessment of the size and mobility of the mass. Its relationship to the fascia (superficial versus deep) and nearby neurovascular and bony structures should be noted. A site-specific neurovascular examination and assessment of regional lymph nodes should also be performed.

Imaging

Optimal imaging of the primary tumor is dependent on the anatomic site. For soft tissue masses of the extremities, magnetic resonance imaging (MRI) has been regarded as the imaging modality of choice (Figs. 98.3, 98.4) because MRI enhances the contrast between tumor and muscle and between tumor and adjacent blood vessels and provides multiplanar

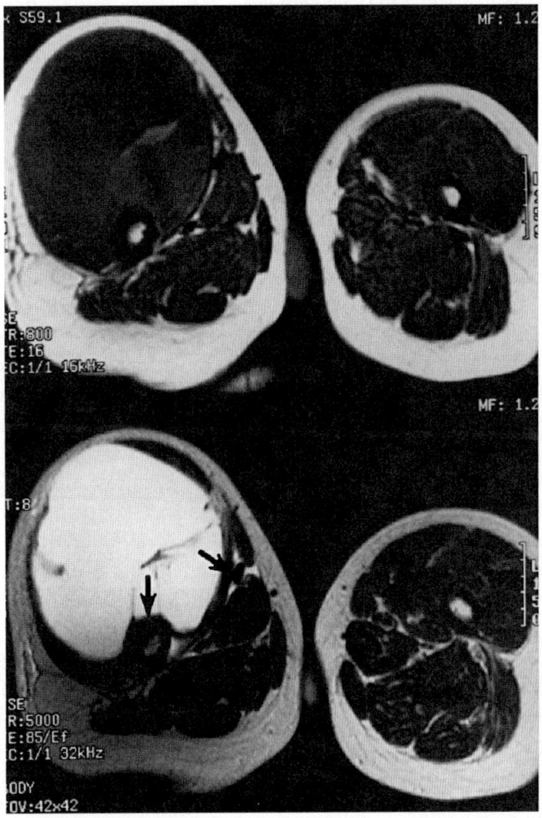

FIGURE 98.3. A 37-year-old man with T2 right proximal thigh malignant fibrous histiocytoma. *Top*: Axial T_1-weighted magnetic resonance (MR) image. Note abutment of femoral cortex and plane between mass and superficial femoral and profunda femoris vessels (*arrows*). *Bottom*: Axial T_2-weighted fast-spin-echo MR image reveals high-intensity necrotic nature of the tumor mass.

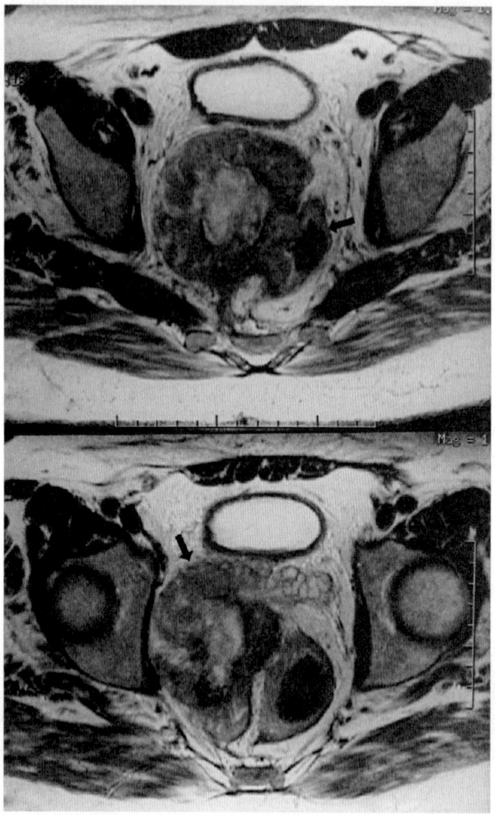

FIGURE 98.4. A 57-year-old man with T2 pelvic leiomyosarcoma. *Top*: Axial T_2-weighted fast-spin-echo MR image reveals heterogenous mass involving the rectum (note air in rectal lumen, *arrow*). *Bottom*: Note abutment of mass to right seminal vesicle (*arrow*).

definition of the lesion.[18,19] However, a recent study by the Radiation Diagnostic Oncology Group that compared MRI and computed tomography (CT) in patients with malignant bone (n = 183) and soft tissue (n = 133) tumors showed no specific advantage of MRI over CT.[20] For pelvic lesions, the multiplanar capability of MRI may provide superior single-modality imaging (see Figure 98.4). In the retroperitoneum and abdomen, CT usually provides satisfactory anatomic definition of the lesion. Occasionally, MRI with gradient sequence imaging can better delineate the relationship of the tumor with midline vascular structures, particularly the inferior vena cava and aorta. More invasive studies such as angiography or cavography are almost never required for the evaluation of soft tissue sarcomas.

Cost-effective imaging to exclude the possibility of distant metastatic disease is dependent on the size, grade, and anatomic location of the primary tumor. In general, patients with low- and intermediate-grade tumors or high-grade tumors less than 5 cm in diameter require only a chest X-ray for satisfactory staging of the chest; this directly reflects the comparatively low risk for presentation with pulmonary metastases in these patients.[21] In contrast, patients with high-grade tumors 5 cm or larger in size should undergo more thorough staging of the chest by CT. Patients with retroperitoneal and intrabdominal visceral sarcomas should undergo single-modality imaging of the liver to exclude the possibility of synchronous hepatic metastases; the liver is a more common site for first metastasis for these lesions.

Biopsy

Biopsy of the primary tumor is essential for most patients presenting with soft tissue masses. In general, any soft tissue mass in an adult that is asymptomatic or enlarging, is larger than 5 cm, or persists beyond 4 to 6 weeks should be biopsied. The preferred biopsy approach is generally the least invasive technique required to allow a definitive histological diagnosis and assessment of grade. In most centers, core needle biopsy provides satisfactory tissue for diagnosis[22–24] and has been demonstrated to result in substantial cost savings compared to open surgical biopsy.[24] Direct palpation can be used to guide needle biopsy of most superficial lesions, but less accessible sarcomas often require imaging-guided biopsy for accurate percutaneous sampling of the most heterogeneous component of the mass. Needle tract tumor recurrences after percutaneous biopsy are rare but have been reported,[25] leading some surgeons to advocate tattooing the biopsy site for subsequent excision. In some centers, fine-needle aspiration may be an acceptable biopsy technique for primary soft tissue masses provided that an experienced sarcoma cytopathologist is available.[26–29] However, because of the frequent difficulty in accurately diagnosing these lesions even when adequate tissue is available, the major utility of fine-needle aspiration in most centers is in the diagnosis of suspected recurrences of sarcoma.

Incisional or excisional biopsy is rarely required but may be performed when a definitive diagnosis cannot be achieved by less invasive means. Several technical points merit comment. Relatively small, superficial masses that can easily be removed should be biopsied by complete excision with microscopic assessment of surgical margins. Incisional and excisional biopsies should be performed with the incision oriented to facilitate subsequent wide local excision (i.e., longitudinal orientation for extremity soft tissue masses). The incision should be centered over the mass at its most superficial point. Care should be taken not to raise tissue flaps. Meticulous hemostasis should be ensured to prevent dissemination of tumor cells into adjacent tissue planes by hematoma. All excisional biopsy specimens should be sent fresh, sterile, and anatomically oriented for pathological analysis. At definitive resection of a previously biopsied sarcoma, the previous surgical biopsy scar should be excised en bloc with the tumor.

A practical approach for biopsy and staging of the patient who presents with a primary extremity soft tissue mass is outlined in Figure 98.5. Small superficial lesions in locations on the extremity where the morbidity of excisional biopsy is minimal (i.e., remote from joints, tendons, and neurovascular structures that would compromise the surgical margin) are easily biopsied by excisional biopsy with assessment of microscopic surgical margins. T2 lesions, T1 lesions located deep to the investing fascia of the extremity, or superficial T1 lesions situated in proximity to joints, tendons, or neurovascular structures are best biopsied by percutaneous core needle biopsy.

Staging

The relative rarity of soft tissue sarcomas, the anatomic heterogeneity of these lesions, and the presence of more than 30 recognized histological subtypes of variable grade have made it difficult to establish a functional system that can accurately stage all forms of this disease. The revised staging system (sixth edition) of the American Joint Committee on Cancer (AJCC) and the International Union Against Cancer (UICC) is the most widely employed staging system for soft tissue sarcomas.[30] This staging system incorporates histological grade into the conventional TNM system (Table 98.1). All soft tissue sarcoma subtypes are included except dermatofibrosarcoma protuberans, a condition considered to have only borderline malignant potential. Four distinct histological grades are recognized, ranging from well differentiated to undifferentiated. Histological grade and tumor size are the primary determinants of clinical stage (see Table 98.1). Tumor size is further substaged as "a" (a superficial tumor that arises outside the investing fascia) or "b" (a deep tumor that arises beneath the fascia or invades the fascia). The system is designed to optimally stage extremity tumors but is also applicable to torso, head and neck, and retroperitoneal lesions; it should not be used for sarcomas of the gastrointestinal tract.

A major limitation of the present staging system is that it does not take into account the anatomic site of soft tissue sarcomas. Anatomic site, however, is an important determinant of outcome. Patients with retroperitoneal and visceral sarcomas have a worse overall prognosis than do patients with extremity tumors. Although site is not incorporated as a specific component of any present staging system, outcome data should be reported on a site-specific basis.

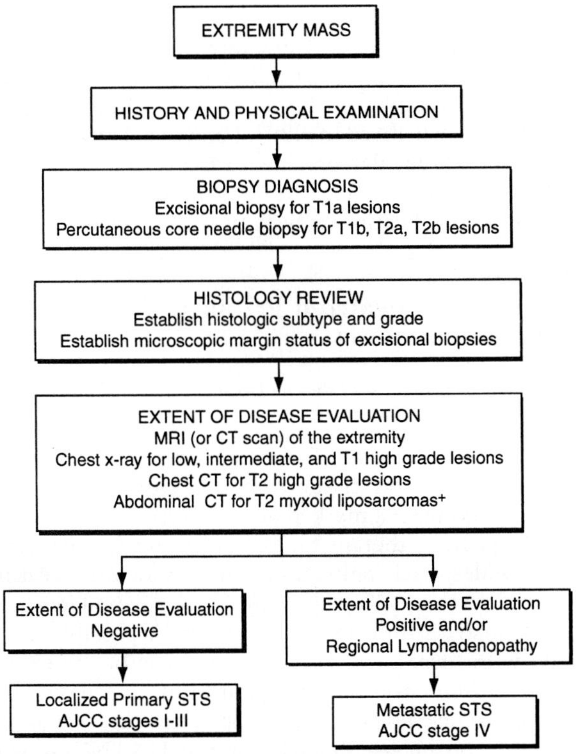

FIGURE 98.5. Approach for pretreatment evaluation and staging of the patient with a primary extremity soft tissue mass. *AJCC*, American Joint Commission on Cancer. (From Pisters PWT. Ann Surg Oncol 1998;5:464–472, with permission.)

TABLE 98.1. Definition of TMN, Stage Grouping, Histopathologic Type, and Histologic Grade for Soft Tissue Sarcomas.

Definition of TMN

Primary Tumor (T)

TX	Primary tumor cannot be assessed
T0	No evidence of primary tumor
T1	Tumor 5 cm or less in greatest dimension
	T1a superficial tumor
	T1b deep tumor
T2	Tumor more than 5 cm in greatest dimension
	T2a superficial tumor
	T2b deep tumor

Note: Superficial tumor is located exclusively above the superficial fascia without invasion of the fascia; deep tumor is located either exclusively beneath the superficial fascia, superficial to the fascia with invasion of or through the fascia, or both superficial yet beneath the fascia. Retroperitoneal, mediastinal, and pelvic sarcomas are classified as deep tumors.

Regional Lymph Nodes (N)

NX	Regional lymph nodes cannot be assessed
N0	No regional lymph node metastasis
N1*	Regional lymph node metastasis

**Note:* Presence of positive nodes (N1) is considered Stage IV.

Distant Metastasis (M)

MX	Distant metastasis cannot be assessed
M0	No distant metastasis
M1	Distant metastasis

Stage Grouping

Stage I	T1a, 1b, 2a, 2b	N0	M0	G1-2	G1	Low
Stage II	T1a, 1b, 2a	N0	M0	G3-4	G2-3	High
Stage III	T2b	N0	M0	G3-4	G2-3	High
Stage IV	Any T	N1	M0	Any G	Any G	High or Low
	Any T	N0	M1	Any G	Any G	High or Low

Source: Used with the permission of the American Joint Committee on Cancer (AJCC), Chicago, Illinois. The original source for this material is the *AJCC Cancer Staging Manual, Sixth Edition* (2002) published by Springer Science and Business Media LLC, www.springerlink.com

Prognostic Factors

Conventional Clinicopathological Factors

Thorough understanding of the clinicopathological factors known to impact outcome is essential in formulating a treatment plan for the patient with soft tissue sarcoma. Over the past decade, more than a dozen multivariate analyses of prognostic factors for patients with localized sarcoma have been reported.[16,31–45] With few exceptions,[13,14,31,37] most studies have analyzed fewer than 300 patients (range, 82–297 patients).

Three detailed analyses of prognostic factors in soft tissue sarcoma merit discussion.[13,14,31] The initial study of prognostic factors in extremity sarcoma from Memorial Sloan-Kettering Cancer Center evaluated clinicopathological prognostic factors in a series of 423 patients with localized extremity soft tissue sarcoma seen from 1968 to 1978.[31] This analysis, among the first to discriminate between specific clinical endpoints, clearly established the clinical profile of what is now accepted as the high-risk patient with extremity soft tissue sarcoma: the patient with a large (5cm or larger), high-grade, deep lesion. The adverse prognostic significance of a high tumor grade, deep tumor location, and tumor size 5cm or larger were also noted in the recent report of the French Federation of Cancer Centers study of 546 patients with sarcomas of the extremities, head and neck, trunk wall, retroperitoneum, and pelvis.[14] A follow-up report from Memorial Sloan-Kettering

TABLE 98.2. Multivariate Analysis of Prognostic Factors in Patients with Extremity Soft Tissue Sarcoma.

Endpoint	*Adverse prognostic factor*	*Relative risk*
Local recurrence	Fibrosarcoma	2.5
	Local recurrence at presentation	2.0
	Microscopically positive surgical margin	1.8
	Malignant peripheral nerve sheath tumor	1.8
	Age more than 50 years	1.6
Distant recurrence	High grade	4.3
	Deep location	2.5
	Size 5.0–9.9 cm	1.9
	Leiomyosarcoma	1.7
	Nonliposarcoma histology	1.6
	Local recurrence at presentation	1.5
	Size 10.0 cm or more	1.5
Disease-specific survival	High grade	4.0
	Deep location	2.8
	Size 10.0 cm or more	2.1
	Malignant peripheral nerve sheath tumor	1.9
	Leiomyosarcoma	1.9
	Microscopically positive surgical margin	1.7
	Lower extremity site	1.6
	Local recurrence at presentation	1.5

Adverse prognostic factors identified are independent by Cox regression analysis.

Source: From Pisters et al.,[13] by permission of Journal of Clinical Oncology.

evaluated clinicopathological prognostic factors that had been documented prospectively in a population of 1041 patients with extremity soft tissue sarcoma.[13] The endpoints for the multivariate analyses were local recurrence, distant recurrence (metastasis), and disease-specific survival. Results of the regression analyses for each of these endpoints are summarized in Table 98.2. These results, using prospectively acquired data, confirm the initial observations made at that institution.[31] In addition, the previously unappreciated prognostic significance of certain specific histological subtypes and the increased risk for adverse outcome associated with a microscopically positive surgical margin or presentation with locally recurrent disease were noted.

In contrast to those for other solid tumors, the adverse prognostic factors for local recurrence of a soft tissue sarcoma are different from those that predict distant metastasis and tumor-related mortality (see Table 98.2).[13] In other words, patients with a constellation of adverse prognostic factors for local recurrence are not necessarily at increased risk for distant metastasis or tumor-related death. Therefore, staging systems that are designed to stratify patients for risk of distant metastasis and tumor-related mortality using these prognostic factors (such as the AJCC/UICC system) will not stratify patients for risk of local recurrence.

Potential Molecular Prognostic Factors

Attention has recently been focused on the evaluation of molecular pathological prognostic factors. Specific molecular parameters evaluated for prognostic significance have included p53,[46] mdm2,[46] Ki-67,[46] altered expression of the retinoblastoma gene product (pRb)[47,48] in high-grade sarcomas, and the presence of SYT-SSX fusion transcripts in synovial sarcoma[49] or EWS-FL11 fusion transcripts in Ewing's sarcoma.[50,51] Complete discussion of the extensive literature on molecular prognostic factors in sarcoma is beyond the scope of this chapter. Readers are referred to recent detailed reviews.[52,53] Data evaluating the prognostic significance of the most widely studied molecular factor, Ki-67, are summarized next.

Ki-67, an antigen expressed throughout the majority of the cell cycle, is utilized as a measure of the fraction of cells undergoing division.[54] Preliminary reports of series of heterogeneous sarcomas in adults suggested that the proliferation index as measured by Ki-67 nuclear staining correlated with histological grade but was not of independent prognostic significance when histological grade was taken into account.[55,56] However, additional studies in larger numbers of patients have demonstrated that Ki-67 status is an independent prognostic factor.[46,57,58] An initial immunohistochemical analysis of a cohort of 65 soft tissue sarcomas and a subsequent analysis of 132 soft tissue sarcomas from the French Federation of Cancer Centers Sarcoma Group demonstrated the adverse prognostic significance of increased Ki-67 activity.[57,58]

Heslin and colleagues evaluated the potential prognostic significance of pRb, p53, mdm2, and Ki-67 by immunohistochemical techniques in a population of 121 patients with primary, high-grade extremity sarcomas and compared these factors to conventional clinicopathological prognostic factors (median follow-up, 64 months).[46] Clinicopathological and molecular factors found to be statistically significant adverse prognostic factors in both univariate and multivariate analyses for the separate endpoints of distant metastasis and tumor-related mortality included T2 tumor size, microscopically positive surgical margin, and a Ki-67 score greater than 20 (more than 20% nuclear staining). Overexpression of p53 or mdm2 or deletion of pRb did not correlate with an increased risk of distant metastasis or tumor-related mortality.

Although specific cellular and molecular parameters have been identified as having independent prognostic significance, there is presently no consensus on how these prognostic factors should be utilized in clinical practice. Until more data are available, molecular prognostic factors proven to be of prognostic significance (e.g., Ki-67) should be considered for inclusion as stratification criteria in clinical trials.

Treatment of Localized Primary Soft Tissue Sarcoma

Surgery

Surgical resection remains the cornerstone of therapy for localized primary soft tissue sarcoma. During the past 20 years, there has been a marked decline in the rate of amputation as the primary therapy for extremity soft tissue sarcoma. With the widespread application of multimodality treatment strategies, less than 10% of patients presently undergo amputation.[59,60] Instead, limb-sparing treatment is possible in most patients with localized soft tissue sarcomas of the extremities. The current use of limb-sparing multimodality treatment approaches for patients with extremity sarcoma is largely based on a phase III trial from the (U.S.) NCI in which patients with extremity sarcomas amenable to limb-sparing surgery were randomly assigned to receive amputation or limb-sparing surgery with postoperative radiotherapy.[61,62]

Both arms of this trial included postoperative chemotherapy with doxorubicin, cyclophosphamide, and methotrexate. With more than 9 years of follow-up evaluation, 5 (19%) of 27 patients randomly assigned to receive limb-sparing surgery and postoperative radiation with chemotherapy had local recurrences, as compared to 1 (6%) of 17 patients in the amputation plus chemotherapy arm ($P = 0.22$).[62] The overall survival rate was 63% for limb-sparing surgery versus 71% for amputation ($P = 0.52$), and the overall survival rate was 70% for limb-sparing surgery versus 71% for amputation ($P = 0.97$). This study established that, for patients for whom limb-sparing surgery is an option, a multimodality approach employing limb-sparing surgery combined with postoperative radiotherapy yields disease-related survival rates comparable to those for amputation while simultaneously preserving a functional extremity.

Currently, at least 90% of patients with localized extremity sarcomas can undergo limb-sparing procedures.[59,63] Most surgeons consider definite major vascular, bony, or nerve involvement as relative indications for amputation. Complex en bloc bone, vascular, and nerve resections with interposition grafting can be undertaken, but the associated morbidity is high. Therefore, for a few patients with critical involvement of major bony or neurovascular structures, amputation remains the only surgical option but offers the prospect of prompt rehabilitation with excellent local control and survival.[62]

Satisfactory local resection involves resection of the primary tumor with a margin of normal tissue around the lesion. It is clear that dissection along the tumor pseudocapsule (enucleation) is associated with local recurrence rates ranging between 33% and 63%.[64–66] In contrast, wide local excision with a margin of normal tissue around the lesion is associated with local recurrence rates in the range of 10% to 31%, as noted in the control arms (surgery alone) of the randomized trials evaluating postoperative radiotherapy[67,68] and in single-institution reports.[69] In contrast to malignant melanoma, a disease for which there are randomized data to address adequate margin size, there are no comparable data available to define what constitutes a satisfactory gross resection margin for a sarcoma. In general, every effort should be made to achieve a wide margin (2cm is often an arbitrary choice) around the tumor mass, except in the immediate vicinity of functionally important neurovascular structures, where, in the absence of frank neoplastic involvement, dissection is performed in the immediate perineural or perivascular tissue planes. Technical details of the surgical approach to extremity sarcomas are beyond the scope of this chapter but are reviewed in a recent surgical atlas.[70]

Given the low (2%–3%) prevalence of lymph node metastasis in adults with sarcomas,[11,12] there is no role for routine regional lymph node dissection. Patients with angiosarcoma, embryonal rhabdomyosarcoma, and epithelioid histiotypes have an increased incidence of lymph node metastasis and should be carefully examined for lymphadenopathy. Therapeutic lymph node dissection results in a 34% actuarial survival rate,[11] and thus the rare patients with regional nodal involvement who have no evidence of extranodal disease should undergo therapeutic lymphadenectomy.

Surgery Alone

Although the majority of patients with extremity soft tissue sarcoma should receive pre- or postoperative radiotherapy (see following section), recent reports suggest that radiotherapy may not be required for selected patients with completely resected, small, primary soft tissue sarcomas (Table 98.3).[69,71–74]

Rydholm and colleagues have reported their experience with 70 patients with subcutaneous or intramuscular extremity sarcomas treated with wide surgical resection and microscopic assessment of surgical margins.[72] Negative histological margins were obtained for 32 of 40 subcutaneous and 24 of 30 intramuscular tumors. The 56 patients with microscopically negative margins received no postoperative radiotherapy, yet only 4 (7%) developed local recurrence. A study from Brigham and Women's Hospital reported similar results for 54 patients with small (T1) soft tissue sarcomas [AJCC (fourth edition) stages IA and IIB] treated with surgical resection without radiotherapy.[73] Resection margins were microscopically clear for all but 1 patient. Only 4 (7%) of 54 patients developed local recurrence, and distant metastases were observed in only 4 patients (7%), all with intermediate- or high-grade lesions. Karakousis and colleagues have reported results of 152 patients with extremity sarcoma, 116 of whom were managed by surgical resection without radiotherapy (with or without chemotherapy).[69] Twelve local recurrences (10%) were observed. The favorable local recurrence rates reported in these series are comparable to local recurrence rates observed with conventional multimodality therapy

TABLE 98.3.
Results of Surgery Alone for Selected Patients with Soft Tissue Sarcoma.

First author	*Institution*	*No. of patients*	*Selection criteria*	*No. with adjuvant radiation*	*Local recurrence, %*	*Distant recurrence, %*
Geer[71]	MSKCC	174	T1 size, primary tumor	117	10	5
Rydholm[72]	Lund, Sweden	56	G/M margin negative	0	7	NR
Healey[73]	BWH	54	T1 size, G/M margin negative	0	4	4
Karakousis[69]	RPCI	116	2-cm G margin	0	10	NR
Respondek[74]	MDACC	40	T1 size, primary tumor, G/M margin negative	4	8	NR

MSKCC, Memorial Sloan-Kettering Cancer Center; G/M, gross/microscopic; NR, not reported; BWH, Brigham and Women's Hospital; RPCI, Roswell Park Cancer Institute; MDACC, The University of Texas M.D. Anderson Cancer Center.

TABLE 98.4.
Local Control with Surgery and Radiotherapy for Localized Soft Tissue Sarcoma: Randomized Phase III Trials and Selected Nonrandomized Retrospective Reviews (Level I and Level III Evidence).

Radiotherapy approach	*First author*	*Institution*	*Radiation dose, Gy*	*Study design*	*No. of patients*	*Local failure, %*
Preoperative EBRT	Suit[75]	MGH	50–56	Retrospective	89	17
	Barkley[76]	MDACC	50	Retrospective	110	10
	Brant[77]	U. FL.	50.4	Retrospective	58	9
Brachytherapy	Pisters[68]	MSKCC	42–45	Prospective (RCT)	119	9 (high grade)
					45	23 (low grade)
Postoperative EBRT	Lindberg[82]	MDACC	60–75	Retrospective	300	22
	Karakousis[80]	RPMI	45–60	Retrospective	53	14
	Suit[85]	MGH	60–68	Retrospective	131	12
	Yang[67]	NCI	45 + 18 (boost)	Prospective (RCT)	91	0 (high grade)
					50	5 (low grade)

EBRT, external-beam radiotherapy; RCT, randomized controlled trial; MGH, Massachusetts General Hospital; MDACC, M.D. Anderson Cancer Center; U.FL., University of Florida; MSKCC, Memorial Sloan-Kettering Cancer Center; RPMI, Roswell Park Memorial Institute; NCI, National Cancer Institute.

incorporating pre- or postoperative radiotherapy (Table 98.4).[67,68,75–81] These data support the hypothesis that selected patients with small, primary soft tissue sarcomas can be treated with surgical resection alone without pre- or postoperative radiotherapy.

It is difficult to provide a precise estimation of what, if any, size or gross margin restriction should be used to identify patients with primary sarcoma who can safely undergo surgery without radiotherapy. In the study by Rydholm and colleagues, the median tumor size of the deep lesions treated with wide surgical resection was 7 cm.[72] Other studies, however, utilized a smaller tumor size as a criterion for surgery without radiotherapy (see Table 98.3). In contrast, Karakousis and colleagues did not consider absolute tumor size but instead reserved surgical resection alone for patients in whom a minimum intracompartmental margin of 2 cm could be maintained circumferentially, irrespective of tumor size.[69] The most conservative recommendation that can be made at this time would be to use 5 cm as an approximate size cutoff. Treatment of patients with large (5 cm or more) primary lesions by surgery alone should not be done outside the confines of a clinical trial.

Preoperative or Postoperative Radiotherapy

Radiotherapy has been combined with conservative (limb-sparing) surgery to optimize local control for patients with localized soft tissue sarcoma. Concomitant radiotherapy can be administered preoperatively,[75–77,82,83] postoperatively,[79,84,85] or by interstitial techniques (brachytherapy).[68,78,86–90]

Data from two phase III trials[67,68] have confirmed several retrospective reports suggesting that surgery combined with radiotherapy results in superior local control compared to surgery alone (Table 98.5).[76,79,81] Yang and colleagues from the NCI recently reported on a randomized prospective trial of postoperative EBRT[67] in which 141 patients with localized extremity soft tissue sarcomas amenable to limb-sparing resection were randomly assigned to receive postoperative EBRT or no radiotherapy (Figs. 98.6, 98.7). All 91 patients with high-grade lesions also received postoperative chemotherapy. No local recurrences have been noted in the 44 patients with high-grade lesions who received postoperative radiotherapy (with chemotherapy) versus 9 local recurrences (19%) in the 47 patients who received postoperative chemotherapy alone ($P = 0.0003$). In the 50 patients with low-grade sarcomas, 1 (4%) of 26 patients who received adjuvant radiotherapy has had a local recurrence versus 8 (33%) of 24 patients treated by surgical resection alone ($P = 0.016$). However, there was no improvement in survival noted with adjuvant radiotherapy in the entire cohort of patients or in any subgroup (see Fig. 98.7).

The second randomized trial of postoperative radiotherapy was conducted at Memorial Sloan-Kettering Cancer

TABLE 98.5.
Phase III Trials of Adjuvant Radiotherapy for Localized Extremity and Trunk Sarcomas Stratified by Grade (Level I Evidence).

Histological grade	*First author/institution*	*Treatment group*	*Radiation dose, Gy*	*No. of patients*	*No. with local failure*	*LRFS*	*OS*
High grade	Pisters/MSKCC[68]	Surgery + BRT	42–45	56	5 (9%)	89%	27%
	—	Surgery	—	63	19 (30%)	66%	67%
	Yang/NCI[67]	Surgery + XRT	45 + 18 (boost)	47	0 (0%)	100%	75%
	—	Surgery	—	44	9 (20%)	78%	74%
Low grade	Pisters/MSKCC[68]	Surgery + BRT	42–45	22	8 (36%)	73%	96%
	—	Surgery	—	23	6 (26%)	73%	95%
	Yang/NCI[67]	Surgery + XRT	45 + 18 (boost)	26	1 (4%)	96%	NR
		Surgery	—	24	8 (33%)	63%	NR

LRFS, local recurrence-free survival; OS, overall survival; MSKCC, Memorial Sloan-Kettering Cancer Center; BRT, brachytherapy; NCI, National Cancer Institute; XRT, external-beam radiation therapy.

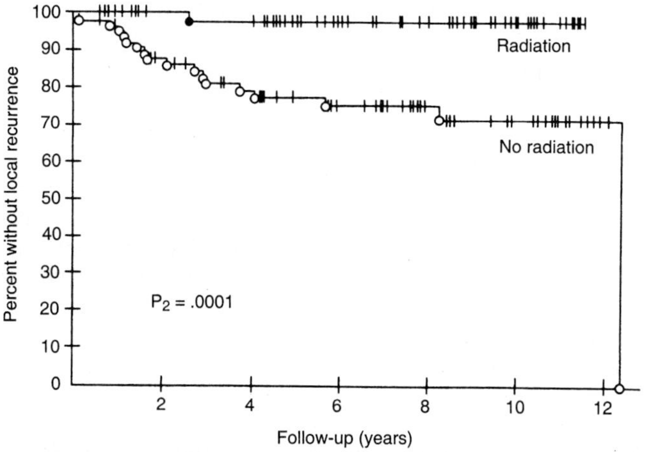

FIGURE 98.6. Local recurrence-free survival for all patients with extremity sarcoma treated in the U.S. National Cancer Institute phase III trial of surgery plus postoperative external-beam radiotherapy versus surgery alone. The median follow-up was 9.6 years. (From Yang et al.,[67] by permission of Journal of Clinical Oncology.)

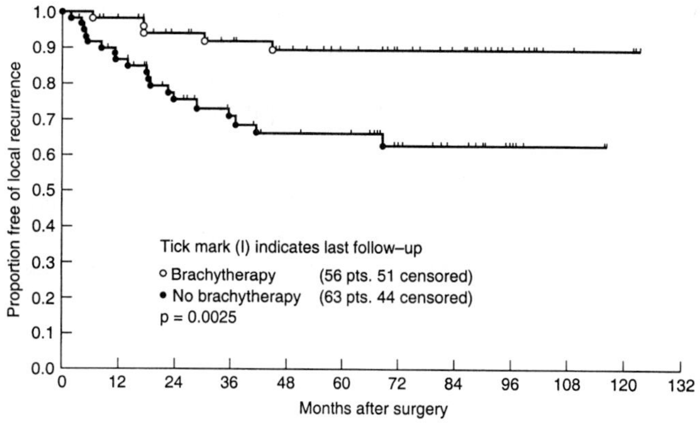

FIGURE 98.8. Local recurrence-free survival in patients with high-grade soft tissue sarcoma treated in the Memorial Sloan-Kettering Cancer Center randomized trial of surgery plus perioperative brachytherapy versus surgery alone. A statistically significant difference was noted in local recurrence-free survival with perioperative brachytherapy ($P = 0.0025$). (From Pisters et al.,[68] by permission of Journal of Clinical Oncology.)

Center, where investigators studied adjuvant brachytherapy for patients with extremity and superficial trunk soft tissue sarcomas[68]; 164 patients with extremity or superficial trunk soft tissue sarcomas were randomly assigned to receive adjuvant brachytherapy (42–45 Gy with an iridium-192 implant) or no postoperative radiotherapy following complete resection of their sarcomas. Sixty-eight of 119 patients with high-grade tumors also received chemotherapy. With a median follow-up of 76 months, 5-year actuarial local control rates were significantly better in the group treated with adjuvant brachytherapy (82%) than in those who received surgery alone (69%). Subset analysis demonstrated that the local control advantage of brachytherapy was confined to patients with high-grade lesions for whom the 5-year local control rate was 89% (versus 66% in the surgery-only group) (Fig. 98.8). Patients with low-grade soft tissue sarcomas did not appear to experience the same local control benefit with adjuvant brachytherapy.[68,90] As noted in the NCI randomized trial,[67] the improvement in local control did not translate into any detectable survival difference between the brachytherapy and no-brachytherapy arms of the trial.

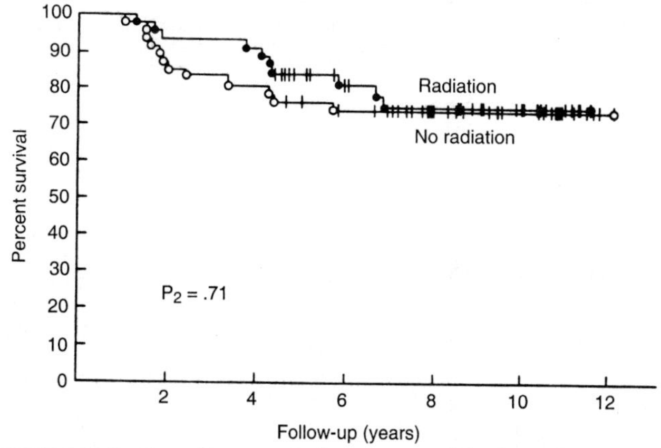

FIGURE 98.7. Overall survival of patients with high-grade extremity soft tissue sarcoma treated in the U.S. National Cancer Institute phase III trial of surgery plus postoperative external-beam radiotherapy versus surgery alone. The median follow-up was 9.6 years. (From Yang et al.,[67] by permission of Journal of Clinical Oncology.)

Local failure rates with combined-modality regimens incorporating surgery and radiotherapy are generally less than 15% (see Table 98.4). Despite theoretical advantages that may favor preoperative radiation, brachytherapy, or postoperative radiation, there does not appear to be a major difference in local control rates among these radiation techniques, although no presently available phase III trial data allow for direct comparison of the techniques. Single-institution retrospective series suggest that preoperative radiation, particularly in the setting of gross palpable or radiographically definable disease, provides superior local control as compared to postoperative treatment.[81,91] A phase III trial of preoperative EBRT compared to postoperative EBRT for patients with localized extremity soft tissue sarcoma is presently nearing completion under the direction of the National Cancer Institute of Canada Clinical Trials Group/Canadian Sarcoma Group. The results of this important study may provide insight into the comparative efficacy, functional outcome, economic costs, and complication rates of these two options for EBRT.

In the absence of a clear local control advantage to any specific radiation technique, clinicians have considered other factors in formulating standards of care. Such factors have included wound complication rates, financial costs, and patient convenience. It is clear that although field size and radiation dose may be minimized with preoperative radiotherapy,[92] major wound complications following preoperative radiotherapy and surgery have been reported to be in the 20% to 30% range.[93,94] This range is at least double the anticipated major wound complication rate when surgical resection and primary wound closure are accomplished in a nonirradiated field. This fact alone has caused some groups to favor postoperative radiotherapy. On the other hand, with brachytherapy, the patient's entire local treatment (surgery plus radiation) can be completed within 10 to 14 days, which has significant cost advantages[95] and also has significant implications in terms of overall patient convenience. In the absence of comparative data addressing the efficacy of these techniques in achieving local control, these additional considerations assume increased importance. Until data from the Canadian Sarcoma Group phase III comparative study are available, it appears reasonable to treat most patients with postoperative EBRT because local control rates are comparable to preoperative techniques but major wound complication rates are significantly lower. Where the necessary expertise is available for brachytherapy, this technique provided an excellent, cost-effective alternative for patients with high-grade lesions. Brachytherapy should not be used for patients with low-grade sarcomas.[90]

Postoperative Chemotherapy

Efficacy of Postoperative Chemotherapy

Despite two decades of randomized trials, the role of postoperative chemotherapy in the management of localized soft tissue sarcoma remains controversial. Table 98.6 outlines 12 published randomized trials evaluating postoperative chemotherapy in patients with localized soft tissue sarcoma.[96–109] Each of these trials had a control arm that received surgery (± radiotherapy) without postoperative chemotherapy and a group that received surgery plus postoperative systemic therapy with doxorubicin alone or doxorubicin-based combination chemotherapy. Four of the trials reported significantly improved relapse-free survival rates with postoperative chemotherapy, but only 2 of 12 trials found a statistically significant improvement in overall survival rates (see Table 98.6). In the trial from the Instituto Ortopedico Rizzoli (Bologna),[104] improved disease-free and overall survival rates were seen in the patients receiving adjuvant doxorubicin therapy after amputation for high-grade extremity sarcomas. This difference was not seen in the patients undergoing limb-sparing surgery, although all limb-salvage patients received preoperative doxorubicin before randomization.[104] In the other trial demonstrating an overall survival advantage, investigators from the Fondation Bergonie (Bordeaux) reported results for 59 patients with stage IIB–IVA (AJCC staging, fourth edition) high-grade sarcomas randomly assigned to observation or adjuvant chemotherapy with doxorubicin, cyclophosphamide, vincristine, and dacarbazine following surgery.[96] With a relatively short 40-month median follow-up, statistically significant increases in disease-free (65% versus 37%) and overall (83% versus 43%) survival rates were seen in patients who received postoperative chemotherapy. Initial data from the NCI randomized trial demonstrated an overall survival advantage to adjuvant chemotherapy[110,111]; however, with longer follow-up, an overall survival advantage is no longer evident.[112] Two other groups have also reported an improvement in disease-free survival without a significant impact on overall survival.[100,101,113] Thus, with the exception of the small trial from the Fondation Bergonie and a subset of patients from the Instituto Ortopedico Rizzoli trial, none of the studies comparing single-agent or multidrug adjuvant chemotherapy to observation have found a durable, statistically significant overall survival advantage for patients who received chemotherapy, although the majority show a trend in favor of the chemotherapy group over the control group.

All the randomized trials of adjuvant chemotherapy published thus far contain recognized deficiencies in design and conduct. The most commonly cited deficiencies of these trials as a group relate to the relatively small sample size and to the fact that small differences in survival require relatively large numbers of patients to detect with sufficient statistical power. The statistical tool of meta-analysis is designed to address these deficiencies by examining a group of similarly designed clinical trials. Recently, the Sarcoma Meta-Analysis Collaboration (SMAC) group reported on a comprehensive meta-analysis of the published randomized trials evaluating local therapy plus adjuvant doxorubicin-based chemotherapy versus local therapy alone.[114] This meta-analysis demon-

TABLE 98.6.
Randomized Trials of Adjuvant Chemotherapy Versus Observation in Soft Tissue Sarcoma (Level I Evidence).

Group[a]	Regimen[b]	No. of patients	Median follow-up, months	Disease-free survival, %			Overall survival, %		
				Chemotherapy	Observation	P value	Chemotherapy	Observation	P value
Bergonie[96]	ACVD	59	40	65	37	0.003	83	43	0.002
EORTC[97]	ACVD	332	44	61	62	NS	74	68	NS
MDACC[113]	ACVAD	43	120	60	35	0.05	75	61	NS
NCI[98,99,112]	ACM	67	85	75	54	0.037	83	60	NS
Mayo[100,101]	AVDAd	61	64	65	68	NS	70	70	NS
UCLA[102]	A	119	28	58	54	NS	84	80	NS
Scand[103]	A	154	40	62	56	NS	75	70	NS
RIZZOLI[104]	A	77	.28	73	45	<0.02	91	70	<0.05
MGH/DFC[105–107]	A	46	46	67	62	NS	71	72	NS
ISTSS[108]	A	86	20	73	55	NS	67	49	NS
ECOG[105,106]	A	36	59	66	55	NS	65	52	NS
GOG[109]	A	156	60	60	45	NS	60	47	NS

[a]Bergonie, Fondation Bergonie; EORTC, European Organization for The Research and Treatment of Cancer; MDACC, M.D. Anderson Cancer Center; NCI, National Cancer Institute; Mayo, Mayo Clinic; UCLA, University of California, Los Angeles; Scand, Scandinavian Sarcoma Group; RIZZOLI, Instituto Ortopedico Oncology Group; MGH/DFC, Massachusetts General Hospital/Dana Farber Cancer Center; GOG, Gynecologic Oncology Group.

[b]A, doxorubicin (Adriamycin); C, cyclosphosphamide; V, vincristine, D, dacarbazine; Ad, dactinomycin; M, methotrexate.

TABLE 98.7.
Sarcoma Meta-Analysis Collaboration Group Meta-Analysis of Randomized Doxorubicin-Based Postoperative Chemotherapy in Soft Tissue Sarcoma.

Endpoint	*Hazard ratio*	*Absolute benefit*	P *value*
Local recurrence-free interval	0.74	6% (75%→81%)	0.024
Distant recurrence-free interval	0.69	10% (60%→70%)	0.0003
Overall recurrence-free interval	0.69	13% (45%→58%)	0.000008
Overall recurrence-free survival	0.74	11% (40%→51%)	0.00008
Overall survival	0.87	5% (50%→55%)	0.087

Source: Tierney et al.,[114] by permission of Lancet.

strated statistically significantly improved local and distant recurrence-free survival and disease-free survival rates in patients who received doxorubicin-containing postoperative chemotherapy (Table 98.7). However, there was no statistically significant improvement in overall survival rates in this meta-analysis of individual patient data. As a significant improvement in survival with postoperative chemotherapy has not been detected with these advanced statistical techniques, it appears reasonable to conclude that if such a benefit exists, it must be quite small. Indeed, the meta-analysis suggests that if a survival benefit exists, it may be 4% or less (see Table 98.7).

Recent investigations have focused on the possible benefits of newer agents in the postoperative treatment of localized soft tissue sarcomas. A recently reported randomized trial of five cycles of epirubicin (120 mg/m^2) and ifosfamide (9 g/m^2) following definitive local therapy versus local therapy alone showed preliminary evidence of a survival advantage in favor of the group receiving postoperative chemotherapy.[115] This study initially reported with a short 21-month median follow-up and longer follow-up of this trial reveals no statistically signficant differences between treatment and control groups.

At this time, given the overall results of the SMAC meta-analysis and negative second-generation (post-meta-analysis) randomized trials, postoperative chemotherapy cannot be considered standard therapy for patients with localized soft tissue sarcoma. Most investigators agree that postoperative chemotherapy should not be given to patients with low-grade sarcomas because of their inherently low rates of systemic disease spread. Other subsets of patients, such as patients with small (AJCC stage IIB) extremity sarcomas, have excellent overall survival rates (more than 90%) and are not appropriate candidates for clinical trials evaluating the efficacy of postoperative chemotherapy.[71]

Postoperative Chemotherapy Dosing and Delivery

Doxorubicin, the agent most commonly employed against sarcoma, is associated with a significant risk of cardiotoxicity. Doxorubicin cardiotoxicity is dose dependent, with the incidence of clinically significant cardiomyopathy in excess of 18% when the cumulative dose of doxorubicin administered exceeds 550 mg/m^2 body surface area.[116–118] Two randomized studies have addressed adjuvant drug combinations, dosage, and delivery in an effort to minimize cardiotoxicity.[112,119] The NCI group has demonstrated comparable overall and disease-free survival rates in 88 patients with localized soft tissue sarcoma randomly assigned to receive high-dose doxorubicin, cyclophosphamide, and methotrexate or lower-dose doxorubicin and cyclophosphamide without methotrexate.[112] No patient in the lower-dose chemotherapy group developed congestive heart failure. Investigators from Memorial Sloan-Kettering Cancer Center demonstrated that the rate of cardiotoxicity (defined as a 10% or greater decrease in left ventricular ejection fraction as assessed by radionuclide cineangiography) as a function of the cumulative dose of doxorubicin was significantly reduced in a randomized study when the drug was given by 72-h continuous infusion rather then bolus infusion ($P = 0.0017$) in a randomized study of 82 patients with high-grade extremity or trunk sarcomas.[119] However, there was a significantly lower rate of disease-related mortality in the group that received bolus chemotherapy ($P = 0.036$), and an equal number of patients in each group experienced clinical congestive heart failure or died of cardiac causes.

Preoperative Chemotherapy

Preoperative chemotherapy has specific theoretical advantages over postoperative treatment. First, preoperative chemotherapy provides an in vivo test of chemosensitivity. Patients whose tumors show objective evidence of response are presumed to be the subset who will benefit most from further postoperative systemic treatment. In contrast, it is assumed that the population of nonresponding patients defined by this in vivo assessment will derive minimal or no benefit from further chemopostoperative therapy and can therefore be spared its toxicity. A second theoretical advantage of preoperative chemotherapy is that it treats occult micrometastatic disease as soon after the cancer diagnosis as possible. This may prevent the development of chemoresistance by isolated clones of metastatic cells or prevent the postoperative growth of micrometastases. Finally, chemotherapy-induced cytoreduction may permit a less radical and consequently less morbid surgical resection than would have been required initially. In patients with large soft tissue sarcomas of the extremities, cytoreduction may reduce the morbidity of limb-salvage surgical procedures and possibly even allow patients who might otherwise have required an amputation to undergo limb-salvage surgery.

Investigators from The University of Texas M.D. Anderson Cancer Center have reported long-term results with doxorubicin-based preoperative chemotherapy for AJCC/UICC stages IIC and III (formerly AJCC stage IIIB) extremity soft tissue sarcomas.[120] In a series of 76 patients treated with doxorubicin-based preoperative chemotherapy, radiologic response rates were complete response, 9%; partial response, 19%; minor response, 13% stable disease, 30%; and disease progression, 30%. The overall objective major response rate (complete plus partial responses) was 27%. At a median follow-up of 85 months, 5-year actuarial rates of local recurrence-free survival, distant metastasis-free survival, disease-free survival, and overall survival were 83%, 52%, 46%, and

59%, respectively. The event-free outcomes reported from M.D. Anderson are comparable to those observed with chemotherapy in the phase III postoperative chemotherapy trials. Furthermore, comparison of responding patients (complete and partial responses) and nonresponding patients did not reveal any significant differences in event-free outcome.[120]

In a prospective study from Memorial Sloan-Kettering, 29 patients with AJCC stage IIIB (AJCC, fourth edition) soft tissue sarcomas larger than 10cm were treated with two cycles of a doxorubicin-based regimen before local therapy.[121] Subjective changes in the degree of primary tumor firmness and in imaging characteristics of the tumor (intratumoral necrosis and hemorrhage) were observed in many patients but were not quantifiable. Only one patient met the standard criteria for a partial response. Survival results in this population of high-risk patients were similar to those in historical controls treated with postoperative doxorubicin or patients treated with local therapy alone. The reasons for the apparent discrepancy in response rates between the reports from M.D. Anderson and Memorial Sloan-Kettering remain unclear. Possible explanations include the fact that the population treated at Memorial Sloan-Kettering appears to be a higher-risk population, with all patients having high-grade lesions larger than 10cm. Moreover, the patients treated at Memorial Sloan-Kettering received a lower doxorubicin dose (60mg/m^2) for a fewer number of cycles (two). This fact may be important given the known dose–response relationship for doxorubicin.[122]

Recently, ifosfamide-containing combinations have been used in the preoperative setting. Selected patients treated with aggressive doxorubicin- and ifosfamide-based regimens have had major responses, and preliminary results suggest that response rates may be higher than in historical controls treated with non-ifosfamide-containing regimens.[123] A randomized trial of preoperative chemotherapy (50mg/m^2 doxorubicin and 5mg/m^2 ifosfamide) versus local therapy alone has recently been completed by the European Organization for the Research and Treatment of Cancer Bone and Soft Tissue Sarcoma Group (EORTC protocol 62874). Toxicity results of this trial have been presented,[124] but event-free outcome has not yet been formally reported.

Combined Preoperative Chemotherapy and Radiotherapy

With the advances made with combined modality treatment of other solid tumors, there has been interest in combined modality preoperative treatment (concurrent or sequential chemotherapy and radiation) for patients with localized soft tissue sarcomas. Concurrent doxorubicin-based chemoradiation has been employed extensively by Eilber and colleagues at the University of California, Los Angeles.[125,126] This treatment protocol involved intraarterial doxorubicin with unusually high dose per fraction radiotherapy (35Gy external-beam radiation delivered in 10 daily fractions, which was reduced to 17.5Gy in 5 daily fractions to minimize local toxicity). A subsequent prospective randomized trial compared preoperative intraarterial doxorubicin to intravenous doxorubicin, both followed by 28Gy of radiation delivered over 8 days followed by surgical resection.[127] No differences in local recurrence or survival were noted.

The combination of regional chemotherapy and concurrent radiotherapy originally pioneered by Eilber et al. has been modified and utilized by other groups.[128–130] Investigators from the University of Illinois treated 55 patients with a 10-day preoperative regimen of intraarterial doxorubicin (10mg/m^2/day) and concomitant radiotherapy (25Gy; 2.5Gy/fraction × 10 fractions).[130] With a mean follow-up of 94 months, the local control rate was 85%. Complications related to the therapy occurred in 26% of patients and required operative management in 7% of patients. Temple and colleagues treated a group of 42 patients with a similar regimen of 60 to 90mg doxorubicin infused intraarterially or intravenously over a 3-day period followed by sequential radiotherapy (30Gy; 3Gy/fraction × 10 fractions).[129] Resection of the residual posttreatment mass was performed 4 to 6 weeks later. At a median follow-up of 6 years, local control was achieved in 39 (98%) of 40 patients; 2 patients were excluded from this analysis because clear margins were not obtained at the time of surgery. Intraarterial infusion-related complications occurred in 4 (11%) of 35 patients. Objective radiologic and pathological response rates were not reported, and thus the efficacy of concurrent chemoradiation therapy in achieving cytoreduction to an extent sufficient to convert lesions resectable only by amputation to lesions amenable to a limb-sparing approach remains largely anecdotal. Moreover, whether preoperative chemoradiation approaches offer local control advantages over conventional treatment approaches employing surgery with pre- or postoperative radiotherapy is also unknown.

Alternative chemoradiation sequencing has been employed by investigators from the Massachusetts General Hospital, who have investigated a novel sequential chemoradiation strategy in the treatment of patients with localized, high-grade large (more than 8cm) extremity soft tissue sarcomas.[131] This treatment protocol involved alternating courses of chemotherapy and radiotherapy: three courses of doxorubicin, ifosfamide, mesna, and dacarbazine (MAID); and two 22-Gy courses of radiation (11 fractions each) for a total preoperative radiation dose of 44Gy. This step was followed by surgical resection with careful microscopic assessment of surgical margins. An additional 16-Gy (8 fractions) boost dose was delivered for microscopically positive surgical margins. The outcomes of 47 patients treated with this regimen have been compared to those of matched historical controls (Fig. 98.9). With a median follow-up of 36 months, 5-year actuarial local control, distant metastasis-free survival, and overall survival rates for the sequential chemoradiation group are 94%, 73%, and 95%, respectively. For the matched historical controls, these rates are 87%, 46%, and 57%, respectively (I. Spiro, personal communication). These encouraging results will require longer follow-up, and additional studies are needed for confirmation. An ongoing phase II trial from the Radiation Therapy Oncology Group and Eastern Cooperative Oncology Group (RTOG, ECOG protocol 95-14) is further investigating sequential chemoradiation for patients with localized sarcomas. The results of this phase II study will help to better define the efficacy of sequential chemoradiation. Until more data are available, sequential chemoradiation should not be given outside the context of a clinical trial.

Hyperthermic Isolated Limb Perfusion

Hyperthermic isolated limb perfusion (HILP) is an investigational technique that has received considerable recent

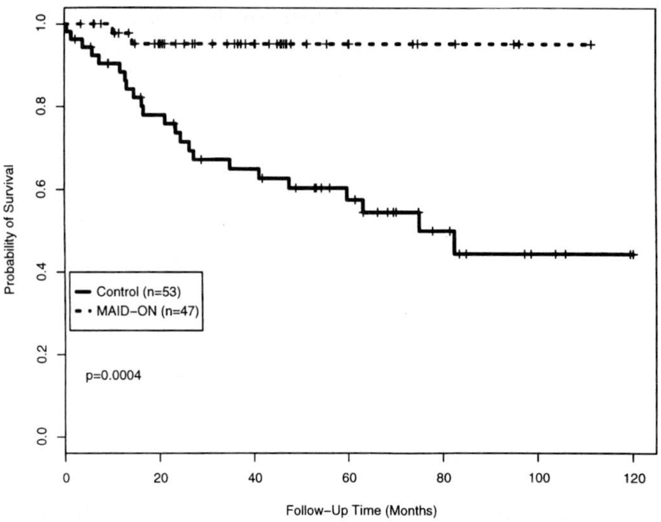

FIGURE 98.9. Overall survival for 47 patients treated at the Massachusetts General Hospital with sequential mesna, doxorubicin, ifosfamide, dacarbazine (MAID)-based chemoradiation followed by surgical resection as compared to a historical control group of 53 similar-stage patients treated by surgery and radiotherapy alone ($P = 0.0004$). (From Spiro I, personal communication; with permission.) The median follow-up in the MAID-based chemoradiation group is 36 months. This treatment strategy is currently being evaluated in a multicenter phase II trial (Radiation Therapy Oncology Group/Eastern Cooperative Oncology Group 95-14).

attention in the treatment of soft tissue sarcomas. HILP is an experimental technique that has been evaluated for the treatment of extremity soft tissue sarcomas in the setting of (1) locally advanced extremity lesions amenable only to amputation used in an attempt to preserve the limb, and (2) locally advanced extremity lesions with synchronous pulmonary metastases, for which HILP is employed in an effort to preserve a functional extremity for the short survival anticipated in the setting of stage IV disease. A multicenter phase II trial has evaluated a series of 55 patients with radiologically unresectable extremity soft tissue sarcomas treated with HILP using high-dose tumor necrosis factor-α, interferon-γ, and melphalan.[132] A major tumor response was seen in 87% of patients: complete responses in 20 (36%) and partial responses in 28 (51%). Limb salvage was achieved in 84% of patients. Regional toxicity was limited, and systemic toxicity was minimal to moderate. There were no treatment-related deaths. This approach is presently being further evaluated in ongoing trials in Europe.

Treatment of Sarcoma Patients at Specialty Centers

Recent data on other tumor types have demonstrated improved outcomes for patients requiring complex treatment who are treated at specialty centers.[133,134] Similar data confirm the same phenomenon in soft tissue sarcoma.[135,136] Given the rarity of soft tissue sarcoma and the complexity of multimodality treatment for this disease, soft tissue sarcoma patients should be referred to a specialty center with a multidisciplinary sarcoma group to facilitate optimal treatment, for participation in clinical trials, and to provide the best chance for a favorable outcome.

Gustafson and colleagues analyzed the quality of treatment in a population-based series of 375 patients with primary soft tissue sarcomas arising in the extremities ($n = 329$) or the trunk ($n = 46$).[136] Comparison was made between patients referred to a specialty soft tissue tumor center before surgery ($n = 195$), those referred to a specialty center after surgery ($n = 102$), and those not referred to a specialty center for treatment of the primary tumor ($n = 78$). The total number of operations for the primary tumor was 1.4 times higher in patients not referred and 1.7 times higher in patients referred after surgery than in patients referred before surgery. Of greatest significance, however, was the finding that the local recurrence rate was 2.4 times higher in patients not referred and 1.3 times higher in patients referred after surgery than in patients referred to a specialty soft tissue tumor center before any manipulation of their tumors. These findings support the principle of centralizing treatment of these rare tumors, which frequently require complex multimodality therapy. Similar observations were noted in a recent population-based study from the South-East Thames Region in the United Kingdom,[135] reaffirming the recommendation of Gustafson and colleagues that all sarcoma patients be treated in a referral center with a multidisciplinary group.

Treatment of Locally Recurrent Soft Tissue Sarcoma

Incidence of Local Recurrence

Despite optimal multimodality therapy, at least 20% to 30% of soft tissue sarcoma patients will develop locally recurrent disease, with a median disease-free interval of 18 months.[13,137] Not surprisingly, local recurrence rates are a function of the primary site and are highest for retroperitoneal and head and neck sarcomas, partly because adequate surgical margins are technically more difficult to attain in these locations. Indeed, by multivariate analysis, a positive surgical margin and operation for recurrent disease are adverse prognostic factors associated with local recurrence.[13,14] In addition, employment of standard-dose postoperative radiotherapy (60–65 Gy) is often limited in these sites by the relative radiosensitivity of surrounding structures. These factors result in local recurrence rates of 38% for high-grade retroperitoneal sarcomas[138] and 48% for high-grade head and neck sarcomas,[139] compared to 5% to 23% for extremity lesions (see Table 98.4).

Surgery and Radiotherapy

Locally recurrent disease generally presents as a nodular mass or series of nodules arising in the surgical scar or radiation port. Treatment approaches for patients with locally recurrent soft tissue sarcoma need to be individualized based on local anatomic constraints and the limitations on present treatment options imposed by prior therapies. Whenever possible, such patients should be referred to a specialized sarcoma center with a multidisciplinary sarcoma group. In general, all patients with locally recurrent sarcoma should be evaluated for reresection of their local recurrence. The results of such "salvage surgery" are good, with two-thirds of patients experiencing long-term survival.[140,141]

If no prior radiotherapy was employed, adjuvant radiation should be utilized after surgery for locally recurrent disease. If subtherapeutic or low-dose radiation was previously employed, patients may be candidates for additional adjuvant radiation by external-beam or brachytherapy approaches. Patients who have had a full course of prior radiation should be managed on an individual basis. Several centers have reported experience with reirradiation of such patients by brachytherapy[142,143] or external-beam[144] approaches. In a series of 40 such patients with recurrent extremity sarcoma treated at Memorial Sloan-Kettering Cancer Center, the 5-year actuarial local control rate was 68%, with satisfactory limb preservation.[142] The recently reported experience with reirradiation by brachytherapy from M.D. Anderson also emphasizes the importance of wound closure by rotational or free tissue transfer because major wound complications are frequent when reirradiation by brachytherapy is employed with primary wound closure.[143] It is important to note that brachytherapy should be used with caution in patients with locally recurrent low-grade sarcomas as it appears to be ineffective against low-grade sarcomas.[68,90]

Notwithstanding these encouraging results for selected patients with locally recurrent sarcoma arising in an irradiated field, for many such patients the best option for local control may be amputation or protocol-based HILP.

Relationship Between Local Control and Survival

Whether local control affects overall survival for patients with soft tissue sarcoma remains unclear and highly controversial.[44,145–148] Only a prospective randomized trial can assess the precise nature of any relationship between local control and overall survival. Three major phase III trials have evaluated local control and survival in the context of defining treatment approaches for soft tissue sarcoma. In a randomized trial of amputation versus conservative surgery plus radiation from the NCI, local recurrence rates were 19% in the limb-sparing arm versus 6% in the amputation arm ($P = 0.022$).[61,62] Despite this, overall survival rates were equal, at 70% for limb-sparing surgery versus 71% for amputation ($P = 0.97$). In addition, in the randomized trials of postoperative radiotherapy,[67,68] the improvement in local control noted in patients treated with surgery plus radiotherapy did not translate into any detectable survival advantage. Thus, none of the currently available prospective randomized data support the hypothesis that better local control enhances survival in patients with sarcoma. Furthermore, data from nonrandomized studies support the concept that there is little, if any, relationship between local control and survival. In a recent series from Sweden, the outcome of patients treated with an inadequate excision was compared with the outcome of those who had an adequate operation.[147] Local recurrence was 3.5 times more common after inadequate excision, but there was no difference in the incidence or timing of distant metastases.

The power of the reported randomized trials to detect a difference in survival is relatively small, and a large number of patients may be required to demonstrate that prevention of local recurrence impacts survival.[145] Stotter et al. have argued that local recurrence is a time-dependent variable and should be considered as such in multivariate studies.[44] Analysis of nonrandomized data in this fashion demonstrates a statistically significant relationship between local control and survival. Other retrospective analyses have yielded similar conclusions.[36,43]

It is clearly important to distinguish between the well-defined adverse prognostic impact of subsequent local recurrence on survival[13,148] and the unproven positive effect of improved local control (i.e., prevention of local recurrence with improved local therapy) on survival. The former phenomenon may be a manifestation of more aggressive tumor biology; that is, biologically more aggressive lesions may recur locally and metastasize more frequently.

Treatment of Metastatic Soft Tissue Sarcoma

The most common site of metastasis from soft tissue sarcoma of the extremity is the lungs. Indeed, the lungs are the only site of recurrence in approximately 80% of all patients with metastases from primary extremity and trunk soft tissue sarcomas.[137,149] Primary visceral and gastrointestinal sarcomas also commonly metastasize to the liver. Extrapulmonary metastases are uncommon forms of first metastasis and usually occur as a late manifestation of widely disseminated disease.[137] The median survival after development of distant metastases is 11.6 months (Figure 98.10).[150] Optimal treatment of patients with metastatic soft tissue sarcoma requires an understanding of the natural history of the disease and individualized selection of treatment options based on specific patient factors, disease factors, and limitations imposed by prior treatment.

Surgical Resection

Multiple investigators have reported their experience with pulmonary metastasectomy for metastatic soft tissue sarcoma in adults.[151–160] Three-year survival rates following thoracotomy for pulmonary metastasectomy range from 23% to 54%, as outlined in the selected series summarized in Table 98.8.[151–153,160–163] Because the ability to achieve complete resection of all metastatic disease is an important determinant of outcome,[150,153,162] the interinstitution variability reported in

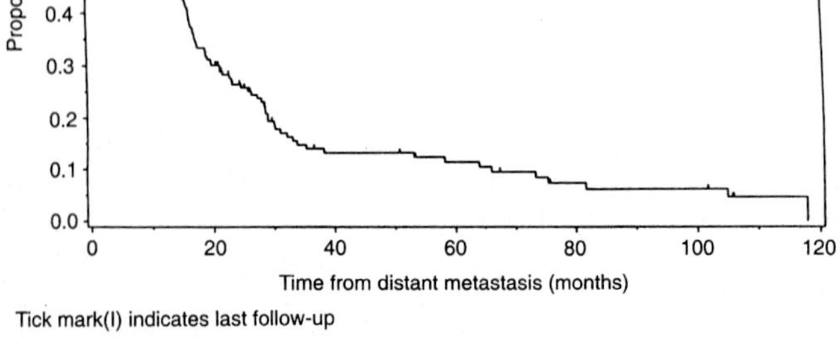

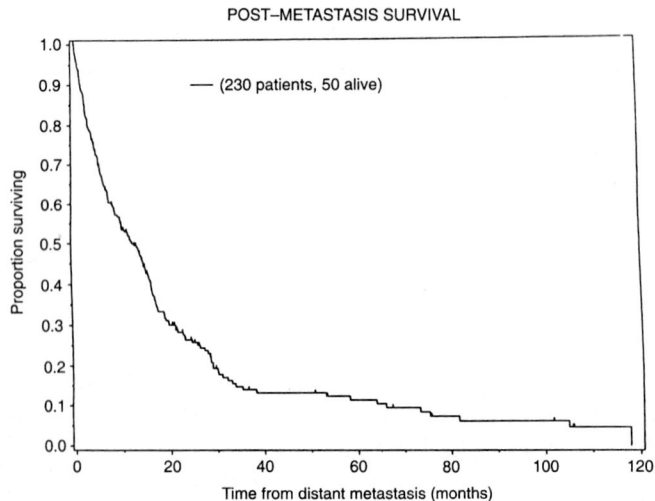

FIGURE 98.10. Postmetastasis survival (from time of diagnosis of M1 disease) in a cohort of 230 patients with primary soft tissue sarcomas of the extremities. The median postmetastasis survival was 11.6 months (From Billingsley et al.,[150] by permission of Cancer.)

TABLE 98.8.
Survival Following Complete Resection of Pulmonary Metastases from Soft Tissue Sarcoma in Adults.

	No. of patients					
First author/institution	*Total*	*Pulmonary metastases*	*Surgical treatment*	*Complete resection, %*	*Median survival, months*	*Three-year survival, %*
Creagan/Mayo[151]	112	112	112	64 (57)	18	29
Putnam/NCI[161,167]	487	93	68	51 (75)	23	32
Jablons/NCI[162]	74	57	57	49 (86)	27	35
Casson/MDACC[165]	68	68	68	58 (85)	25	42
Verazin/Roswell[171]	78	78	78	61 (78)	21	21.5 (5 years)
Gadd/MSKCC[153]	716	135	78	65 (83)	19	23
van Geel/EORTC[160]	255	255	255	255 (100)	NR	54

Mayo, Mayo Clinic; NCI, U.S. National Cancer Institute; MDACC, The University of Texas M.D. Anderson Cancer Center; Roswell, Roswell Park Cancer Institute; MSKCC, Memorial Sloan-Kettering Cancer Center; EORTC, European Organization for The Research and Treatment of Cancer; NR, not reported.

postmetastesectomy survival rates is partially a function of whether survival was reported among all patients who underwent thoracotomy or among the subset who underwent complete resection.

Many investigators believe that repeat thoracotomy to render patients free of disease from pulmonary soft tissue sarcoma metastases is justified in the absence of effective systemic therapy. Several series of reoperative pulmonary metastasectomy have been published.[164,165] In a series of 43 such patients treated at the NCI, 72% of patients could be rendered free of disease at the second thoracotomy, with a median survival duration from the time of second thoracotomy of 25 months.[164] In a report from M.D. Anderson Cancer Center of a series of 39 patients undergoing reoperation for a second pulmonary metastasis after successful initial metastasectomy, factors predicting long-term survival included the presence of a solitary metastasis and the ability to perform a complete resection.[165] This study also illustrates the significant survival duration many of these patients enjoy; the median survival in the 19 patients who had complete resection of unifocal recurrent metastatic disease was 65 months as compared to 14 months in the 15 patients with complete resection of two or more sites of recurrent disease.

It remains difficult to predict which patients with pulmonary metastases will benefit from pulmonary resection. A number of different clinical criteria have been evaluated by univariate analysis in this regard, including the disease-free interval,[151,161,163,166] number of metastatic nodules,[163,166–169] and tumor doubling time.[163,169,170] Multivariate analyses from both the NCI and Roswell Park Cancer Institute confirm that a short disease-free interval and incomplete pulmonary resection are adverse prognostic factors for survival for patients with pulmonary metastases.[162,171] A multivariate analysis from M.D. Anderson Cancer Center suggested that, in addition, the presence of more than three metastatic pulmonary nodules on preoperative chest CT is an adverse prognostic sign.[152] Perhaps the most important prognostic factor impacting survival, however, is the ability to completely resect all disease.[150,153,162] In the review of postmetastasis outcome by Billingsley and colleagues from Memorial Sloan-Kettering, the median survival among patients who were able to undergo complete resection of metastases was 20 months as compared to 10 months among patients who did not have complete resection (Figure 98.11).[150] In summary, the clinical criteria (disease-free interval, tumor doubling time, and number of nodules) serve as general prognostic indicators, and no single criterion should be used to exclude patients from surgery. Postoperatively, the ability to achieve complete resection and the number of pulmonary nodules present appear to best define the prognosis for these patients.

Unfortunately, metastasectomy benefits only a small (less than 15%) fraction of patients who develop pulmonary metastases. This situation is best illustrated by data from Memorial Sloan-Kettering, where a population of 716 patients who presented with primary extremity sarcoma were followed for the subsequent development and treatment of pulmonary metastases (Fig. 98.12).[149] Of the initial cohort of 716 patients, 148 patients (21%) developed pulmonary metastases. Isolated pulmonary metastases occurred in 135 (91%) of these 148 patients. Of the 135 patients with pulmonary-only metasta-

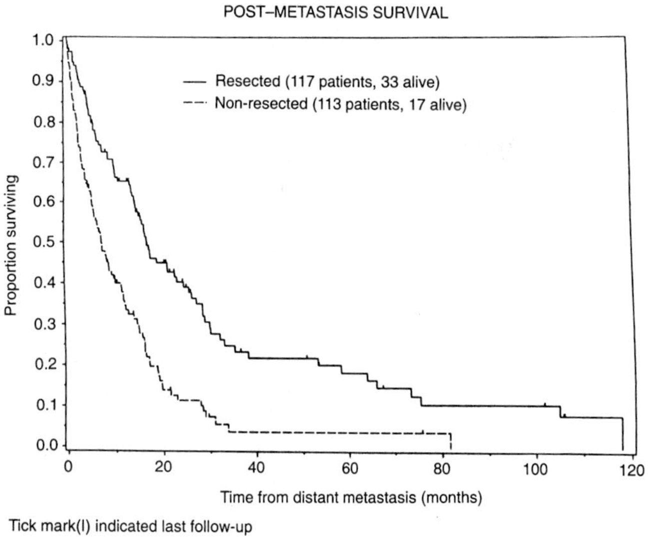

FIGURE 98.11. Postmetastasis survival stratified by resection of pulmonary metastatic disease. The median survival among patients undergoing complete resection of metastatic disease was 20 months. (From Billingsley et al.,[150] by permission of Cancer.)

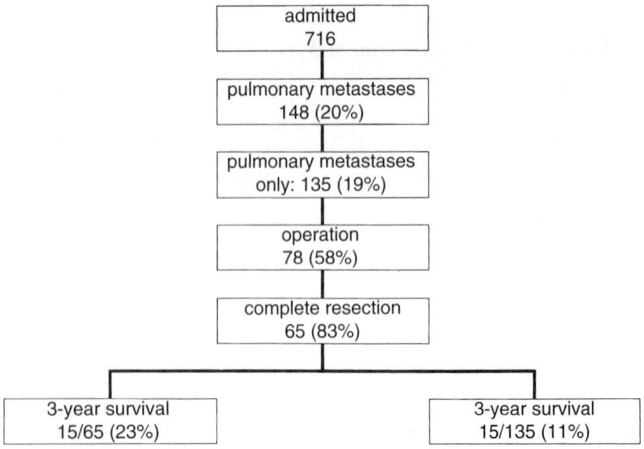

FIGURE 98.12. Risk for and subsequent management of pulmonary metastases in 716 patients with primary or locally recurrent extremity soft tissue sarcoma. (From Brennan,[149] by permission of Journal of the American College of Surgeons.)

ses, 78 (58%) were considered to have operable disease, and 65 (83%) of those taken to thoracotomy were able to undergo complete resection of all their pulmonary metastatic disease. Thus, 44% of all patients with pulmonary metastases were able to undergo complete metastasectomy. The median survival from the time of complete resection was 19 months, and the 3-year survival rate was 23%. All patients who did not undergo thoracotomy died within 3 years. For the entire cohort of 135 patients developing pulmonary-only metastases, the 3-year survival rate was only 11% (see Fig. 98.12).

The rather disappointing overall results of treatment for metastatic disease underscore the importance of careful patient selection for resection of pulmonary metastases. The following criteria are generally agreed: (1) the primary tumor is controlled or is controllable, (2) there is no extrathoracic disease, (3) the patient is a medical candidate for thoracotomy and pulmonary resection, and (4) complete resection of all disease appears possible.[172] With careful patient selection, the morbidity of thoracotomy can be limited to the subset of patients who are most likely to benefit from this aggressive treatment approach.

Chemotherapy

Soft tissue sarcoma patients with unresectable pulmonary metastases or extrapulmonary metastatic disease have a generally poor prognosis and usually are best treated with systemic chemotherapy or supportive care. A number of agents including cyclophosphamide, dactinomycin, and vincristine have been studied and have produced response rates between 5% and 10%.[173,174] Doxorubicin was the first and remains the most active single chemotherapeutic agent in soft tissue sarcoma.[122,175–178] A variety of schedules and doses have been employed,[175,176,179] with objective overall response rates of approximately 25% in the advanced disease setting.[180] Unfortunately, however, there is little difference in survival rates between responders and nonresponders to chemotherapy.

Several studies have established that there is a dose–response relationship for doxorubicin in soft tissue sarcomas,[122,175,179] and doses greater than 50 mg/m^2 are required to achieve response rates exceeding 20%. Combining doxorubicin with a number of agents including dacarbazine, vincristine, and ifosfamide has improved response rates; these investigations are outlined next. However, randomized comparisons evaluating the addition of cyclophosphamide[181,182] and vincristine[183] to doxorubicin-based regimens have not demonstrated any survival benefit in patients with advanced sarcoma.

Dacarbazine has been found to have activity against soft tissue sarcomas.[184] When dacarbazine is used as a single agent for advanced sarcoma, response rates are of the order of 17%,[184,185] but when it is used in combination with doxorubicin (ADIC), investigators from both the Eastern Cooperative Oncology Group[179] and the Gynecologic Oncology Group[186] have observed higher response rates (significantly in the Eastern Cooperative Oncology Group study), approaching 30%.[179] However, these improved response rates have been associated with significant bone marrow and gastrointestinal toxicity and have not translated into enhanced objective complete response or overall survival rates. In the largest study of ADIC, from the Southwest Oncology Group, an overall response rate of 42% was observed in 218 evaluable patients.[180] This result included an 11% complete response rate, and the disease-free survival rate was significantly improved compared to that of patients treated with doxorubicin alone.[184] Giving the combination by 96-h continuous infusion (versus bolus therapy) reduces cardiotoxicity and improves patient tolerance without compromising therapeutic effect.[187] Thus, despite substantial toxicity, with response rates in the 30% to 40% range, considerable interest remains in combination therapies based on ADIC.

A phase III randomized comparative trial from the Southwest Oncology Group has evaluated the addition of a third drug (cyclophosphamide or dactinomycin) to ADIC.[181] There was no statistically significant difference in response rates for the ADIC (33% of 104 patients), cyclophosphamide/ADIC (34% of 112 patients), and dactinomycin/ADIC (24% of 119 patients) regimens ($P = 0.22$). Toxicities were substantial and equivalent in the three treatments arms.

Vincristine has modest activity against advanced sarcomas, with a single-agent response rate of 5% to 10%.[188,189] In an effort to further improve response rates without increasing myelosuppression, vincristine was added to ADIC in a series of 107 patients with advanced sarcoma, with a resulting objective response rate of 42%.[180] This result was not different from that of historical controls treated with ADIC only. The addition of cyclophosphamide (which has a single-agent activity of 9%) to produce the CyVADIC regimen (subsequently utilized in a number of postoperative adjuvant chemotherapy studies)[96,190,191] resulted in a 50% major response rate in a multiinstitutional series of 125 patients.[192] These favorable response rates for CyVADIC confirmed previous findings from the Southwest Oncology Group, which had reported a 45% overall response rate for CyVADIC in a series of 229 patients with advanced sarcoma in 1976.[184] However, a randomized trial comparing CyVADIC to doxorubicin alone revealed no significant difference in response rates or survival.[193]

Ifosfamide has been found to have significant activity against sarcoma, with response rates ranging from 24% to

TABLE 98.9.
Randomized Phase III Trials with Ifosfamide-Containing Treatment Arms in Advanced Soft Tissue Sarcoma (Level I Evidence).

Group	*Treatment arm*[a] *(dose in mg/m^2)*	*No. of patients*	*Response rate, %*[b]	*Median survival, months*
SWOG/CALGB[205]	A (60), D (1000)	170	17	12
	A (60), D (1000), I (7.5)	170	32[b]	13[b]
ECOG[204]	A (80)	90	20	9
	M (8), A (40), P (60)	88	34[b]	12
EORTC[193]	A (75)	263	23	13
	A (50), I (5)	258	25	12.8
	Cy (500), V (1.5), A (50), D (750)	142	18	13.8

SWOG, Southwest Oncology Group; CALGB, Cancer and Leukemia Study Group B; ECOG, Eastern Cooperative Oncology Group; EORTC, European Organization for The Research and Treatment of Cancer.

[a]A, doxorubicin (Adriamycin); D, dacarbazine; I, ifosfamide; M, mitomycin C; P, cisplatin; Cy, cyclophosphamide; V, vincristine.

[b]Complete responses plus partial responses.

38% in patients with advanced sarcoma who have failed to respond to doxorubicin-based treatment.[194–196] Ifosfamide is a cyclophosphamide analogue that does not have cross-resistance with cyclophosphamide.[195,197,198] Similar to cyclophosphamide, the major toxicity of ifosfamide is hemorrhagic cystitis. However, uroprotection with mesna prevents cystitis by inactivating toxic metabolites and thereby allows administration of larger doses of ifosfamide.[199] In a randomized comparison of cyclophosphamide and ifosfamide in 171 patients with advanced sarcoma, higher response rates were seen in the ifosfamide treatment arm (18% versus 8%) with less myelosuppression.[197] Combinations of ifosfamide and doxorubicin have resulted in response rates of 35% and 36% in two separate studies.[200,201] Dose-limiting myelosuppression (grade 4) was seen in 34% of patients.[201] Investigators from the Dana-Farber Cancer Institute have evaluated the combination of mesna, ifosfamide, doxorubicin, and dacarbazine (MAID) and have found a 47% response rate with 10% complete responses.[202] Median survival in this series of 108 patients was 16 months, with life-threatening myelosuppression occurring in 12% of patients.[202] Twenty-five percent of patients treated with the MAID regimen required hospitalization and antibiotics for neutropenic fever.[203]

The evaluable phase III trials with ifosfamide-containing treatment arms are summarized in Table 98.9.[193,204,205] The most comprehensive comparative study performed to date was reported by the EORTC.[193] In that study, 663 eligible patients were randomly assigned to receive doxorubicin (75 mg/m^2) (arm A), CyVADIC (arm B), or ifosfamide (5 g/m^2) plus doxorubicin (50 mg/m^2) (arm C). There was no statistically significant difference detected among the three study arms in terms of response rate (arm A, 23.3%; arm B, 24.4%; arm C, 28.1%), remission duration, or overall survival (median, 52 weeks for arm A, 51 weeks for arm B, and 55 weeks for arm C). The degree of myelosuppression was significantly greater for the combination of ifosfamide and doxorubicin than for the other two regimens. Cardiotoxicity was also more frequent in arm C. This study and the aggregate data suggest that single-agent doxorubicin is still the standard against which more intensive or new drug treatments should be compared.

Treatment of Retroperitoneal Sarcomas

Presentation and Pretreatment Evaluation

Retroperitoneal sarcomas are relatively uncommon, accounting for approximately 15% of all sarcomas (see Figure 98.1). The most common histological subtypes are liposarcoma and leiomyosarcoma (Figure 98.1). Nearly 80% of patients present with an abdominal mass, and 50% of patients report pain at the time of presentation.[206] Patients commonly describe nonspecific gastrointestinal symptoms. Other commonly noted symptoms include neurological symptoms (primarily sensory) in 27% and weight loss in 7%.[206,207] These tumors often grow to substantial size before the patient's nonspecific complaints are evaluated or an abdominal mass is noted on physical examination.

The differential diagnosis for a retroperitoneal mass is relatively limited when soft tissue neoplasms are considered as a group. Physical examination should include a testicular examination in men to evaluate the possibility of a primary testicular neoplasm. Laboratory tests should include the common serum markers for germ cell tumors, beta-human chorionic gonadotropin, and alpha-fetoprotein. If physical examination is suggestive of malignancy or biochemical markers are elevated, testicular ultrasonography should be performed. This modality may obviate laparotomy for patients with metastatic testicular tumors and allow for identification of primary retroperitoneal germ cell tumors.

CT and MRI are the primary methods used to image retroperitoneal tumors.[208–210] These modalities allow for assessment of the consistency of the mass (cystic or solid components, associated necrosis), precise anatomic location of the mass, and the extent of any regional disease and for confirmation of function of the kidneys. CT of the abdomen and pelvis usually provides images satisfactory for treatment planning. Occasionally, MRI with flow-sensitive gradient sequence imaging may be helpful in defining vascular anatomy for surgical planning. For patients with an abnormal chest radiograph, chest CT should be performed to exclude the possibility of metastatic disease.

In general, preoperative biopsy is not necessary when surgical resection is planned for a resectable primary retroperitoneal mass. Fine-needle or core biopsy of presumed *primary* retroperitoneal (extravisceral) masses that appear resectable based on radiologic studies is not indicated; this is because the overall therapeutic plan is rarely altered by preoperative attempts to ascertain a histological diagnosis and because the histologically heterogeneous nature of individual lesions precludes a plan of "observation" for biopsies that are read as "benign" or indeterminate. Preoperative imaging-directed biopsy is invasive and expensive and rarely modifies treatment for patients in whom surgical exploration is planned. However, there are specific circumstances in which biopsy of primary retroperitoneal masses should be performed: these include (1) clinical suspicion of lymphoma or germ cell tumor, (2) tissue diagnosis for preoperative treatment, (3) tissue diagnosis of radiologic unresectable disease, and (4) suspected retroperitoneal or intraabdominal metastasis from another primary tumor. In the main, however, for patients for whom exploratory laparotomy is planned, surgical resection of intraoperative incisional biopsy (for unresectable lesions) is the best means of establishing a tissue diagnosis of a potentially resectable retroperitoneal mass.

Surgical Resection

Surgical resection with negative margins remains the standard primary treatment for patients with localized retroperitoneal sarcoma. Because en bloc multiorgan resection may be required to achieve negative margins, all patients should have preoperative bowel preparation and assessment of bilateral renal function by CT. Resectability rates in recent series combining patients with primary and recurrent retroperitoneal sarcomas range from 25% to 95% (Table 98.10).[98,206,207,211–215] Resectability rates at different institutions are difficult to compare and interpret because the reported rates are a function of whether the series included primary and recurrent lesions, the referral pattern of the reporting institution, the criteria used for determining which patients underwent surgical exploration, and the skill and experience of the surgeons.[214,216,217] The ability to achieve complete surgical resection (resection of all gross tumor) is also a function of presentation—primary lesions are more likely to be completely resected than are locally recurrent retroperitoneal sarcomas, and the ability to achieve complete resection declines as the number of local recurrences increases (Fig. 98.13).

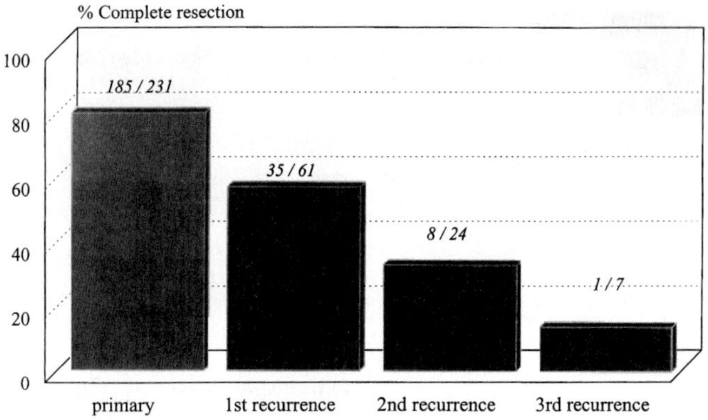

FIGURE 98.13. Rate of initial complete resection for 231 patients presenting with primary retroperitoneal sarcoma and rates of complete resection for subsequent local recurrences stratified by recurrence number. The number of patients who underwent complete resection divided by those undergoing attempted resection is indicated *above each bar*. The ability to achieve complete tumor resection declined as the number of recurrences increased. (From Lewis et al.,[218] by permission of Annals of Surgery.)

For patients with primary lesions, grossly complete resection is possible in up to 78% of cases.[138,214,218] The most common reasons for unresectability are the presence of major vascular involvement (aorta or vena cava), peritoneal implants, or distant metastases.[206] Resection of adjacent retroperitoneal or intraabdominal organs, frequently the kidney, colon, or pancreas, is required in the majority (50%–80%) of cases to permit complete resection.[206,212,219] Partial resections or debulking procedures have been performed, but there is no evidence that partial resection improves survival.[206,219] In general, until effective adjuvant therapy is available for gross residual disease, deliberate partial resection outside the confines of a clinical trial should be reserved for relief of bowel obstruction or palliation of other symptoms of advanced disease.

The survival of patients with retroperitoneal sarcoma is largely related to clinical presentation: the median disease-specific survivals of patients with primary disease, locally recurrent disease, and metastatic disease are 72 months, 28 months, and 10 months, respectively (Figure 98.14). Results from recent series demonstrate 5-year actuarial survival rates

TABLE 98.10.
Resectability Rates for Retroperitoneal Sarcomas in Selected Series.

First author	*Institution*	*Accrual period, years*	*Total no. of patients*	*No. completely resected*	*Resectability rate, %*
Glenn[98]	NCI	19	50	37	74
Karakousis[214]	Roswell Park	24	68	27	40
Dalton[212]	Mayo Clinic	19	116	63	54
Jaques[206]	MSKCC	5	114	67	59
Alvarenga[207]	Royal Marsden	20	110	28	25
Karakousis[217]	Roswell Park	17	87	83	96
Kilkenny[215]	University of Florida	25	63	49	78

NCI, National Cancer Institute; MSKCC, Memorial Sloan-Kettering Cancer Center.

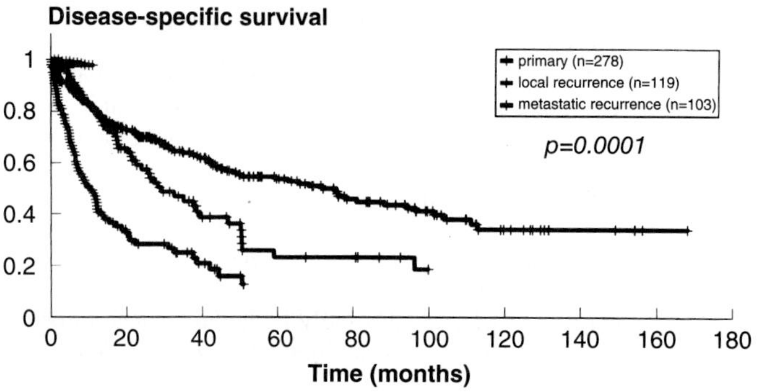

FIGURE 98.14. Disease-specific survival of a cohort of 500 patients presenting with retroperitoneal sarcoma stratified by presentation status: primary (n = 5278) versus locally recurrent (n = 119) versus metastatic (n = 103). Median survival was 72 months for those with primary disease, 28 months for those with locally recurrent disease, and 10 months for those with metastases at presentation. (From Lewis et al.,[218] by permission of Annals of Surgery.)

in the range of 54% to 64% for patients with completely resected retroperitoneal sarcomas.[138,206,211,212,214,215,218] The median survival of patients with incompletely resected retroperitoneal sarcomas is 18 months and is comparable to that of patients who do not undergo resection.[218]

Adequate margins are often difficult to obtain in retroperitoneal sarcoma surgery because of the proximity of critical organs, vascular structures, and the spine. Consequently, local recurrence remains a significant problem (Fig. 98.15). With short-term follow-up, local recurrence rates approximate 40% to 50%.[206,212,214,218,220] However, with longer follow-up, it appears that patients continue to have local recurrences, even well beyond 5 years after complete surgical resection, such that true local recurrence rates may be well in excess of 50%.[221] Thus, improving local control for patients with retroperitoneal sarcoma remains one of the most clinically significant challenges.

Postoperative follow-up strategies are based on the continuing risk for local failure and the difficulties inherent in detecting recurrent disease by clinical criteria alone. Serial CT or MRI should be utilized for follow-up as detection of recurrent retroperitoneal sarcoma by physical examination of identification of symptoms is unreliable. There are no published data to make specific follow-up recommendations, but because many patients develop late (more than 5 years) recurrence, it is clear that follow-up should continue at least 10 years after initial treatment.[220,221] Any sign of recurrent disease should be investigated promptly because complete resection of recurrent disease is often possible and is associated with 5-year survival rates of 50% or greater.[206,214]

A number of recent studies have evaluated prognostic factors for retroperitoneal sarcomas by univariate[206] and multivariate analysis.[138,207,212,218,220,221] For patients presenting without metastatic disease, complete surgical resection and histological grade were primary determinants of survival in several multivariate analyses.[138,207,212,215,221] Some investigators have also found that large tumor size (more than 10cm) and fixation to adjacent retroperitoneal structures other than neurovascular bundles or bone were significant adverse prognostic factors for survival by multivariate analysis.[212] In a comprehensive analysis of 500 patients with retroperitoneal sarcoma treated at Memorial Sloan-Kettering Cancer Center, unresectable disease [relative risk (RR) = 4.7], incomplete resection (RR = 4.0), and high histological grade (RR = 3.2) were predictive of sarcoma-related mortality.[218]

Postoperative Radiation Therapy and Chemotherapy

Postoperative EBRT has been shown to reduce local recurrence rates for extremity and superficial trunk sarcomas. However, gastrointestinal or neural toxicities often limit the delivery of sufficient radiation doses to the retroperitoneum. Several retrospective studies have suggested that postoperative EBRT improves local control after grossly complete resection.[221–226] However, these series are difficult to compare and interpret because they include small numbers of patients (fewer than 30–40), no standard treatment protocol, and variable details on histopathology, extent of resection, and margin status. Other investigators have found no benefit to adjuvant radiation for retroperitoneal sarcomas.[89,206,211] Thus, there is no current consensus on the role of postoperative EBRT following complete resection of retroperitoneal sarcomas.

Preoperative EBRT offers certain theoretical and practical advantages: (1) high-dose treatment may minimize the risk of tumor implantation in the peritoneal cavity after resection by sterilizing a large number of tumor cells; (2) tumor reponse to preoperative treatment may facilitate grossly complete resection; and (3) the tumor displaces critical radiosensitive organs away from the preoperative radiation field, thereby reducing toxicity and improving tolerance. At the Massachusetts General Hospital, the combination of preoperative high-dose EBRT (40–50Gy) with intraoperative radiation therapy (10–20Gy) has been employed.[227] The small number of patients in this preliminary study and short follow-up preclude definitive conclusions, but preliminary results were encouraging, with local control achieved in 9 of 12 patients. Given the theoretical advantages associated with preoperative treatment, additional studies of preoperative radiotherapy for retroperitoneal sarcomas are certainly warranted.

Given the relatively high complication rates of high-dose external-beam radiation to the retroperitoneum and the lack of phase III data demonstrating clinical benefit, routine pre- or postoperative EBRT cannot be recommended for retroperito-

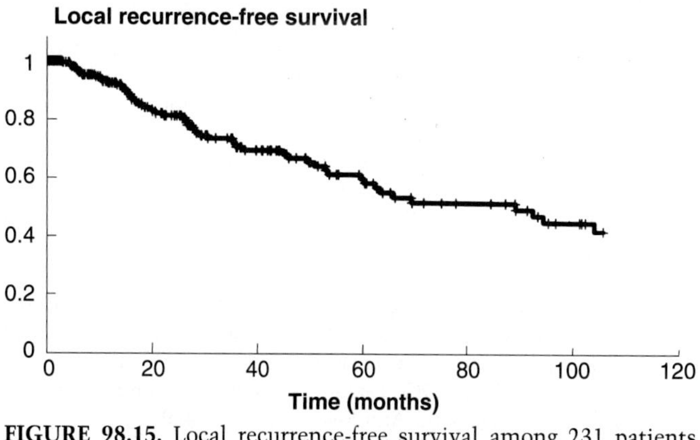

FIGURE 98.15. Local recurrence-free survival among 231 patients with primary retroperitoneal sarcoma. With a median follow-up of 28 months, 61 patients had experienced local recurrence. The local recurrence-free survival rate was 81% (confidence interval, 76%–86%) at 2 years and 59% (95% confidence interval, 55%–63%) at 5 years. (From Lewis et al.,[218] by permission of Annals of Surgery.)

neal sarcomas outside the setting of a clinical trial. In selected patients with advanced disease, some disabling symptoms may be palliated by EBRT.

Intraoperative radiotherapy (IORT) offers the advantage of a direct boost dose to the tumor bed, thereby allowing a reduction in the dose of relatively toxic external-beam radiation. The efficacy of combined adjuvant IORT and EBRT have been evaluated in two recent series.[227–229] In a randomized prospective trial from the NCI, 30 patients with completely resected retroperitoneal sarcomas were randomly assigned to receive IORT (11–15 MeV electron beam to a dose of 20 Gy) with low-dose postoperative EBRT (35–40 Gy) or high-dose postoperative EBRT (50–55 Gy) alone.[228,229] IORT with low-dose EBRT was associated with a significantly lower rate of gastrointestinal toxicity (7% versus 60%), but no differences were noted in local control, disease-free survival, or overall survival. The rates of 5-year disease-free and overall survival reported in this study are comparable to those observed with surgery alone.[89,212] At the Massachusetts General Hospital, the combination of preoperative high-dose EBRT (40–50 Gy) with IORT (9–15 MeV electron beam to a dose of 10–20 Gy) had been employed.[227] The small number of patients in this preliminary study and short follow-up preclude definitive conclusions, but preliminary results are encouraging, with local control seen in 9 of 12 patients overall and 9 of 10 patients treated for microscopic residual disease. However, larger studies are needed before conclusions can be reached.

Retrospective studies have not demonstrated any benefit to preoperative[230] or postoperative[138,206,211] doxorubicin-based chemotherapy for retroperitoneal sarcomas. The role of adjuvant chemotherapy (doxorubicin, cyclophosphamide, and methotrexate) following complete resection of retroperitoneal sarcomas has been investigated in a small phase III trial at the NCI.[98] Only 15 patients were randomized, and the 2-year actuarial survival rate was lower in the chemotherapy arm than in the surgery-only arm (47% versus 100%; $P = 0.06$). Thus, as for extremity sarcomas, presently there are no data available to support the use of routine postoperative chemotherapy for patients with retroperitoneal sarcoma.

References

1. Landis SH, Murray T, Bolden S, et al. Cancer statistics, 1999. CA J Clin 1999;49:8–31.
2. Lawrence W Jr, Donegan WL, Natarajan N, et al. Adult soft tissue sarcomas. a pattern of care survey of the American College of Surgeons. Ann Surg 1987;205:349–359.
3. Feigen M. Should cancer survivors fear radiation-induced sarcomas? Sarcoma 1997;1:5–15.
4. Brady MS, Gaynor JJ, Brennan MF. Radiation-associated sarcoma of bone and soft tissue. Arch Surg 1992;127:1379–1385.
5. Sorensen SA, Mulvihill JJ, Nielsen A. Long-term follow-up of von Recklinghausen neurofibromatosis: survival and malignant neoplasms. N Engl J Med 1986;314:1010–1015.
6. Zoller MET, Rembeck B, Oden A, et al. Malignant and benign tumors in patients with neurofibromatosis type 1 in a defined Swedish population. Cancer (Phila) 1997;79:2125–2131.
7. Jones IT, Jagelman DG, Fazio VW, et al. Desmoid tumors in familial polyposis coli. Ann Surg 1986;204:94–97.
8. Weiss SW, Sobin LH. Histologic Typing of Soft Tissue Tumors, 2nd ed. Berlin: Springer-Verlag, 1994.
9. Presant CA, Russell WO, Alexander RW, et al. Soft-tissue and bone sarcoma histopathology peer review: the frequency of disagreement in diagnosis and the need for second pathology opinions: the Southeastern Cancer Study Group experience. J Clin Oncol 1986;4:1658–1661.
10. Shiraki M, Enterline HT, Brooks JJ, et al. Pathologic analysis of advanced adult soft tissue sarcomas, bone sarcomas, and mesotheliomas: the Eastern Cooperative Oncology Group (ECOG) experience. Cancer (Phila) 1989;64:484–490.
11. Fong Y, Coit DG, Woodruff JM, et al. Lymph node metastasis from soft tissue sarcoma in adults: analysis of data from a prospective database of 1772 sarcoma patients. Ann Surg 1993; 217:72–77.
12. Weingrad DN, Rosenberg SA. Early lymphatic spread of osteogenic and soft-tissue sarcomas. Surgery (St. Louis) 978;84:231–240.
13. Pisters PWT, Leung DHY, Woodruff J, et al. Analysis of prognostic factors in 1041 patients with localized soft tissue sarcomas of the extremities. J Clin Oncol 1996;14:1679–1689.
14. Coindre JM, Terrier P, Bui NB, et al. Prognostic factors in adult patients with locally controlled soft tissue sarcoma. A study of 546 patients from the French Federation of Cancer Centers Sarcoma Group. J Clin Oncol 1996;14:869–877.
15. Costa J, Wesley RA, Glatstein E, et al. The grading of soft tissue sarcomas. Results of a clinicohistopathologic correlation in a series of 163 cases. Cancer (Phila) 1984;53:530–541.
16. Trojani M, Contesso G, Coindre JM, et al. Soft-tissue sarcomas of adults: study of pathological prognostic variables and definition of a histopathological grading system. Int J Cancer 1984;33:37–42.
17. Guillou L, Coindre JM, Bonichon F, et al. Comparative study of the National Cancer Institute and French Federation of Cancer Centers Sarcoma Group grading systems in a population of 410 adult patients with soft tissue sarcoma. J Clin Oncol 1997;15:350–362.
18. Chang AE, Matory YL, Dwyer AJ, et al. Magnetic resonance imaging versus computed tomography in the evaluation of soft tissue tumors of the extremities. Ann Surg 1987;205:340–348.
19. Hanna SL, Fletcher BD. MR imaging of malignant soft-tissue tumors. Magn Reson Imaging Clin N Am 1995;3:629–650.
20. Panicek DM, Gatsonis C, Rosenthal DI, et al. CT and MR imaging in the local staging of primary malignant musculoskeletal neoplasms: report of the Radiology Diagnostic Oncology Group. Radiology 1997;202:237–246.
21. Fleming JB, Holtz D, Cantor SB, et al. The utility and cost-effectiveness of computerized tomography (CT) to screen for pulmonary metastases in patients presenting with T1 extremity soft tissue sarcomas (STS) [abstract]. Proc Am Soc Clin Oncol 1998;17:1989.
22. Heslin MJ, Lewis JJ, Woodruff JM, et al. Core needle biopsy for diagnosis of extremity soft tissue sarcoma. Ann Surg Oncol 1997;4:425–431.
23. Ball AB, Fisher C, Pittam M, et al. Diagnosis of soft tissue tumours by Tru-Cut biopsy. Br J Surg 1990;77:756–758.
24. Skrzynski MC, Biermann JS, Montag A, et al. Diagnostic accuracy and charge-savings of outpatient core needle biopsy compared with open biopsy of musculoskeletal tumors. J Bone Joint Surg [Am] 1996;78:644–649.
25. Schwartz HS, Spengler DM. Needle tract recurrences after closed biopsy for sarcoma: three cases and review of the literature. Ann Surg Oncol 1997;4:228–236.
26. Akerman M. Fine-needle aspiration cytology of soft tissue sarcoma: benefits and limitations. Sarcoma 1998;2:155–161.
27. Akerman M, Idvall I, Rydholm A. Cytodiagnosis of soft tissue tumors and tumor-like conditions by means of fine needle aspiration biopsy. Arch Orthop Trauma Surg 1980;96:61–67.
28. Kissin MW, Fisher C, Webb AJ, et al. Value of fine needle aspiration cytology in the diagnosis of soft tissue tumours: a preliminary study on the excised specimen. Br J Surg 1987;74: 479–480.

29. Layfield LJ, Anders, KH, Glasgow BJ, et al. Fine-needle aspiration of primary soft-tissue lesions. Arch Pathol Lab Med 1986;110:420–424.
30. Soft tissue sarcoma. In: Fleming ID, Cooper JS, Henson DE, et al., eds. American Joint Committee on Cancer (AJCC) Staging Manual, 5th ed. Philadelphia: Lippincott-Raven, 1997:149–156.
31. Gaynor JJ, Tan CC, Casper ES, et al. Refinement of clinicopathologic staging for localized soft tissue sarcoma of the extremity: a study of 423 adults. J Clin Oncol 1992;10:1317–1329.
32. Markhede G, Angervall L, Stener B. A multivariate analysis of the prognosis after surgical treatment of malignant soft-tissue tumors. Cancer (Phila) 1982;49:1721–1733.
33. Sears HF, Hopson R, Inouye W, et al. Analysis of staging and management of patients with sarcoma: a ten-year experience. Ann Surg 1980;191:488–493.
34. Rydholm A, Berg NO, Gullberg B, et al. Prognosis for soft-tissue sarcoma in the locomotor system: a retrospective population-based follow-up study of 237 patients. APMIS 1984;92:375–386.
35. Heise HW, Myers MH, Russell WO, et al. Recurrence-free survival time for surgically treated soft tissue sarcoma patients: multivariate analysis of five prognostic factors. Cancer (Phila) 1986;57:172–177.
36. Rooser B, Attewell R, Berg NO, et al. Survival in soft tissue sarcoma: prognostic variables identified by multivariate analysis. Acta Orthop Scand 1987;58:516–522.
37. Collin CF, Godbold J, Hajdu S, et al. Localized extremity soft tissue sarcoma: an analysis of factors affecting survival. J Clin Oncol 1987;5:601–612.
38. Tsujimoto M, Aozasa K, Ueda T, et al. Multivariate analysis for histologic prognostic factors in soft tissue sarcomas. Cancer (Phila) 1988;62:994–998.
39. Ueda T, Aozasa K, Tsujimoto M, et al. Multivariate analysis for clinical prognostic factors in 163 patients. Cancer (Phila) 1988;62:1444–1450.
40. Rooser B, Attewell R, Berg NO, et al. Prognostication in soft tissue sarcoma: a model with four risk factors. Cancer (Phila) 1988;61:817–823.
41. Mandard AM, Petiot JF, Marnay J, et al. Prognostic factors in soft tissue sarcomas: a multivariate analysis of 109 cases. Cancer (Phila) 1989;63:1437–1451.
42. Bell RS, O'Sullivan B, Liu FF, et al. The surgical margin in soft-tissue sarcoma. J Bone Joint Surg [Am] 1989;71:370–375.
43. Emrich LJ, Ruka W, Driscoll DL, et al. The effect of local recurrence on survival time in adult high-grade soft tissue sarcomas. J Clin Epidemiol 1989;42:105–110.
44. Stotter AT, Ahern RP, Fisher C, et al. The influence of local recurrence of extremity soft tissue sarcoma on metastasis and survival. Cancer (Phila) 1990;65:1119–1129.
45. Alvegard TA, Berg NO, Baldetorp B, et al. Cellular DNA content and prognosis of high-grade soft tissue sarcoma: the Scandinavian Sarcoma Group experience. J Clin Oncol 1990;8:538–547.
46. Heslin MJ, Cordon-Cardo C, Lewis JJ, et al. Ki-67 detected by MIB-1 predicts distant metastasis and tumor mortality in primary, high grade extremity soft tissue sarcoma. Cancer (Phila) 1998;83:490–497.
47. Cance WG, Brennan MF, Dudas ME, et al. Altered expression of the retinoblastoma gene product in human sarcomas. N Engl J Med 1990;323:1457–1462.
48. Karpeh MS, Brennan MF, Cance WG, et al. Altered patterns of retinoblastoma gene product expression in adult soft-tissue sarcomas. Br J Cancer 1995;72:986–991.
49. Kawai A, Woodruff J, Healey JH, et al. SYT-SSX gene fusion as a determinant of morphology and prognosis in synovial sarcoma. N Engl J Med 1998;338:153–160.
50. Zoubek A, Dockhorn-Dworniczak B, Delattre O, et al. Does expression of different EWS chimeric transcripts define clinically distinct risk groups of Ewing tumor patients? J Clin Oncol 1996;14:1245–1251.
51. de Alava E, Kawai A, Healey JH, et al. EWS-FLII fusion transcript structure is an independent determinant of prognosis in Ewing's sarcoma. J Clin Oncol 1998;16:1248–1255.
52. Pisters PWT, Brennan MF. Sarcomas of soft tissue. In: Abeloff M, Armitage J, Lichter A, et al, eds. Clinical Oncology, 1st ed. New York: Churchill Livingstone, 1995:1799–1832.
53. Pisters PWT, Pollock RE. Staging and prognostic factors in soft tissue sarcoma. Semin Radiat Oncol 1999:307–314.
54. Gerdes J. Ki-67 and other proliferation markers useful for immunohistological diagnostic and prognostic evaluations in human malignancies. Semin Cancer Biol 1990;1:199–206.
55. Drobnjak M, Latres E, Pollack D, et al. Prognostic implications of p53 nuclear overexpression and high proliferation index of Ki-67 in adult soft-tissue sarcomas. J Natl Cancer Inst 1994;86:549–554.
56. Yang P, Hirose T, Hasegawa T, et al. Prognostic implication of the p53 protein and Ki-67 antigen immunohistochemistry in malignant fibrous histiocytoma. Cancer (Phila) 1995;76:618–625.
57. Levine EA, Holzmayer T, Bacus S, et al. Evaluation of newer prognostic markers for adult soft tissue sarcomas. J Clin Oncol 1997;15:3249–3257.
58. Rudolph P, Kellner U, Chassevent A, et al. Prognostic relevance of a novel proliferation marker, ki-s11, for soft-tissue sarcoma: a multivariate study. Am J Pathol 1997;150:1997–2007.
59. Williard WC, Collin CF, Casper ES, et al. The changing role of amputation for soft tissue sarcoma of the extremity in adults. Surg Gynecol Obstet 1992;175:389–396.
60. Williard WC, Hajdu SI, Casper ES, et al. Comparison of amputation with limb-sparing operations for adult soft tissue sarcoma of the extremity. Ann Surg 1992;215:269–275.
61. Rosenberg SA, Tepper J, Glatstein E, et al. The treatment of soft-tissue sarcomas of the extremities: prospective randomized evaluations of (1) limb-sparing surgery plus radiation therapy compared with amputation and (2) the role of adjuvant chemotherapy. Ann Surg 1982;196:305–315.
62. Yang JC, Rosenberg SA. Surgery for adult patients with soft tissue sarcomas. Semin Oncol 1989;16:289–296.
63. Brennan MF, Casper ES, Harrison LB, et al. The role of multimodality therapy in soft-tissue sarcoma. Ann Surg 1991;214:328–337.
64. Bowden L, Booher RJ. The principles and techniques of resection of soft parts for sarcomas. Surgery (St. Louis) 1958;44:963–977.
65. Cantin J, McNeer GP, Chu FC, et al. The problem of local recurrence after treatment of soft tissue sarcoma. Ann Surg 1968;168:47–53.
66. Gerner RD, Moore GE, Pickren JW. Soft tissue sarcomas. Ann Surg 1975;181:803–808.
67. Yang JC, Chang AE, Baker AR, et al. A randomized prospective study of the benefit of adjuvant radiation therapy in the treatment of soft tissue sarcomas of the extremity. J Clin Oncol 1998;16:197–203.
68. Pisters PWT, Harrison LB, Leung DHY, et al. Long-term results of a prospective randomized trial of adjuvant brachytherapy in soft tissue sarcoma. J Clin Oncol 1996;14:859–868.
69. Karakousis CP, Proimakis C, Walsh DL. Primary soft tissue sarcoma of the extremities in adults. Br J Surg 1995;82:1208–1212.
70. Karakousis CP. Surgery for soft tissue sarcomas. In: Bland KI, Karakousis CP, Copeland EM, eds. In: Atlas of Surgical Oncology, 1st ed. Philadelphia: Saunders, 1995:283–400.
71. Geer RJ, Woodruff J, Casper ES, et al. Management of small soft-tissue sarcoma of the extremity in adults. Arch Surg 1992;127:1285–1289.

72. Rydholm A, Gustafson P, Rooser B, et al. Limb-sparing surgery without radiotherapy based on anatomic location of soft tissue sarcoma. J Clin Oncol 1991;9:1757–1765.
73. Healey B, Corson JM, Demetri GD, et al. Surgery alone may be adequate treatment for select stage IA–IIIA soft tissue sarcomas [abstract]. Proc Am Soc Clin Oncol 1995;14:517.
74. Respondek P, Pollack A, Feig BW, et al. Prospective trial of conservative surgery and selective use of radiotherapy for AJCC T1 extremity and trunk soft tissue sarcomas [abstract]. Sarcoma 1997;1:219.
75. Suit HD, Mankin HJ, Schiller AL. Results of treatment of sarcoma of soft tissue by radiation and surgery at Massachusetts General Hospital. Cancer Treat Symp 1985;3:33–47.
76. Barkley HT Jr, Martin RG, Romsdahl MM, et al. Treatment of soft tissue sarcomas by preoperative irradiation and conservative surgical resection. Int J Radiat Oncol Biol Phys 1988;14:693–699.
77. Brant TA, Parsons JT, Marcus RB Jr, et al. Preoperative irradiation for soft tissue sarcomas of the trunk and extremities in adults. Int J Radiat Oncol Biol Phys 1990;19:899–906.
78. Harrison LB, Franzese F, Gaynor JJ, et al. Long term results of a prospective trial of adjuvant brachytherapy in the management of completely resected soft tissue sarcomas of the extremity and superficial trunk. Int J Radiat Oncol Biol Phys 1993;27:259–265.
79. Lindberg RD, Martin RG, Romsdahl MM, et al. Conservative surgery and postoperative radiotherapy in 300 adults with soft-tissue sarcomas. Cancer (Phila) 1981;47:2391–2397.
80. Karakousis CP, Emrich LJ, Rao U, et al. Feasibililty of limb salvage and survival in soft tissue sarcomas. Cancer (Phila) 1986;57:484–491.
81. Suit HD, Mankin HJ, Wood WC, et al. Treatment of the patient with stage M0 soft tissue sarcoma. J Clin Oncol 1988;6:854–862.
82. Lindberg R. Treatment of localized soft tissue sarcomas in adults at MD Anderson Hospital and Tumor Institute (1960–1981). Cancer Treat Symp 1985;3:59–65.
83. Enneking WF, McAuliffe JA. Adjunctive preoperative radiation therapy in treatment of soft tissue sarcomas: a preliminary report. Cancer Treat Symp 1985;3:37–42.
84. Leibel SA, Tranbaugh RF, Wara WM, et al. Soft tissue sarcomas of the extremities: survival and patterns of failure with conservative surgery and postoperative irradiation compared to surgery alone. Cancer (Phila) 1982;50:1076–1083.
85. Suit HD, Mankin HJ, Wood W, et al. Preoperative, intraoperative, and postoperative radiation in the treatment of primary soft tissue sarcoma. Cancer (Phila) 1985;55:2659–2667.
86. Shiu MH, Hilaris BS, Harrison LB, et al. Brachytherapy and function-saving resection of soft tissue sarcoma arising in the limb. Int J Radiat Oncol Biol Phys 1991;21:1485–1492.
87. Willett CG, Suit HD. Limited surgery and external beam irradiation in soft tissue sarcoma. Adv Oncol 1989;5:26–29.
88. Habrand JL, Gerbaulet A, Pejovic MH, et al. Twenty years experience of interstitial iridium brachytherapy in the management of soft tissue sarcomas. Int J Radiat Oncol Biol Phys 1991;20:405–411.
89. Brennan MF, Hilaris B, Shiu MH, et al. Local recurrence in adult soft-tissue sarcoma: a randomized trial of brachytherapy. Arch Surg 1987;122:1289–1293.
90. Pisters PWT, Harrison LB, Woodruff JM, et al. A prospective randomized trial of adjuvant brachytherapy in the management of low grade soft tissue sarcomas of the extremity and superficial trunk. J Clin Oncol 1994;12:1150–1155.
91. Pollack A, Zagars GK, Goswitz MS, et al. Preoperative vs. postoperative radiotherapy in the treatment of soft tissue sarcomas: a matter of presentation. Int J Radiat Oncol Biol Phys 1998;42:563–572.
92. Nielsen OS, Cummings B, O'Sullivan B, et al. Preoperative and postoperative irradiation of soft tissue sarcomas: effect of radiation field size. Int J Radiat Oncol Biol Phys 1991;21:1595–1599.
93. Bujko K, Suit HD, Springfield DS, et al. Wound healing after preoperative radiation for sarcoma of soft tissues. Surg Gynecol Obstet 1993;176:124–134.
94. Peat BG, Bell RS, Davis A, et al. Wound-healing complications after soft-tissue sarcoma surgery. Plast Reconstr Surg 1994;93:980–987.
95. Janjan NA, Yasko AW, Reece GP, et al. Comparison of charges related to radiotherapy for soft tissue sarcomas treated by preoperative external beam irradiation versus interstitial implantation. Ann Surg Oncol 1994;1:415–422.
96. Bui NB, Maree D, Coindre JM, et al. First results of a prospective randomized study of CYVADIC adjuvant chemotherapy in adults with operable high risk soft tissue sarcoma [abstract]. Proc Am Soc Clin Oncol 1989;8:318.
97. Bramwell VHC, Rouesse J, Steward W, et al. Adjuvant CYVADIC chemotherapy for adult soft tissue sarcoma—reduced local recurrence but no improvement in survival: a study of the European Organization for Research and Treatment of Cancer Soft Tissue and Bone Sarcoma Group. J Clin Oncol 1994;12:1137–1149.
98. Glenn J, Sindelar WF, Kinsella T, et al. Results of multimodality therapy of resectable soft-tissue sarcomas of the retroperitoneum. Surgery (St. Louis) 1985;97:316–325.
99. Glenn J, Kinsella T, Glatstein E, et al. A randomized, prospective trial of adjuvant chemotherapy in adults with soft tissue sarcomas of the head and neck, breast, and trunk. Cancer (Phila) 1985;55:1206–1214.
100. Edmonson JH, Fleming TR, Ivins JC, et al. Randomized study of systemic chemotherapy following complete excision of nonosseous sarcomas. J Clin Oncol 1984;2:1390–1396.
101. Edmonson JH. Role of adjuvant chemotherapy in the management of patients with soft tissue sarcomas. Cancer Treat Rep 1984;68:1063–1066.
102. Eiber FR, Giuliano AE, Huth JF, et al. A randomized prospective trial using postoperative adjuvant chemotherapy (Adriamycin) in high-grade extremity soft-tissue sarcoma. Am J Clin Oncol 1988;11:39–45.
103. Alvegard TA, Sigurdsson H, Mouridsen H, et al. Adjuvant chemotherapy with doxorubicin in high-grade soft tissue sarcoma: a randomized trial of the Scandinavian Sarcoma Group. J Clin Oncol 1989;7:1504–1513.
104. Picci P, Bacci G, Gherlinzoni F, et al. Results of a randomized trial for the treatment of localized soft tissue tumors (STS) of the extremities in adult patients. In: Ryan JR, Baker LO, eds. Recent Concepts in Sarcoma Treatment. Dordrecht: Kluwer, 1988:144–148.
105. Antman K, Amato D, Lerner H. Eastern Cooperative Oncology Group and Dana-Farber Cancer Institute/Massachusetts General Hospital study. In: Jones S, Salmon S, eds. Adjuvant Therapy of Cancer, 4th ed. Orlando: Grune & Stratton, 1984:611–620.
106. Antman K, Anato D, Lerner H, et al. Adjuvant doxorubicin for sarcoma: data from the Eastern Cooperative Oncology Group and Dana-Farber Cancer Institute/Massachusetts General Hospital studies. Cancer Treat Symp 1985;3:109–115.
107. Antman K, Suit H, Amato D, et al. Preliminary results of a randomized trial of adjuvant doxorubicin for sarcomas: lack of apparent difference between treatment groups. J Clin Oncol 1984;2:601–608.
108. Antman K, Amato D, Pilepich M, et al. A preliminary analysis of a randomized Intergroup (SWOG, ECOG, CALBG, NCOG) trial of adjuvant doxorubicin for soft tissue sarcomas. In: Salmon S, ed. Adjuvant Therapy of Cancer, 5th ed. Orlando: Grune & Stratton, 1987:725–734.
109. Omura GA, Blessing JA, Major F, et al. A randomized clinical trial of adjuvant Adriamycin uterine sarcomas: a Gynecologic Oncology Group study. J Clin Oncol 1985;3:1240–1245.

110. Rosenberg SA, Tepper J, Glatstein E, et al. Prospective randomized evaluation of adjuvant chemotherapy in adults with soft tissue sarcomas of the extremities. Cancer (Phila) 1983;52:424–434.
111. Rosenberg SA. Prospective randomized trials demonstrating the efficacy of adjuvant chemotherapy in adult patients with soft tissue sarcomas. Cancer Treat Rep 1984;68:1067–1078.
112. Chang AE, Kinsella T, Glatstein E, et al. Adjuvant chemotherapy for patients with high-grade soft-tissue sarcomas of the extremity. J Clin Oncol 1988;6:1491–1500.
113. Benjamin RS, Terjanian TO, Fenoglio CJ, et al. The importance of combination chemotherapy for adjuvant treatment of high risk patients with soft-tissue sarcomas of the extremities. In: Salmon S, ed. Adjuvant Therapy of Cancer, 5th ed. Orlando: Grune & Stratton, 1987:735–744.
114. Tierney JF. Adjuvant chemotherapy for localised resectable soft-tissue sarcoma of adults: meta-analysis of individual data. Lancet 1997;350:1647–1654.
115. Frustaci S, Gherlinzoni F, De Paoli A, et al. Preliminary results of an adjuvant randomized trial on high risk extremity soft tissue sarcomas (STS): the interim analysis [abstract]. Proc Am Soc Clin Oncol 1997;16:1785.
116. Dresdale A, Bonow RO, Wesley R, et al. Prospective evaluation of doxorubicin-induced cardiomyopathy resulting from postsurgical adjuvant treatment of patients with soft tissue sarcomas. Cancer (Phila) 1983;52:51–60.
117. Singal PK, Iliskovic N. Doxorubicin-induced cardiomyopathy. N Engl J Med 1998;339:900–905.
118. Singal PK, Iliskovic N, Li T, et al. Adriamycin cardiomyopathy: pathophysiology and prevention. FASEB J 1997;11:931–936.
119. Casper ES, Gaynor JJ, Hajdu SI, et al. A prospective randomized trial of adjuvant chemotherapy with bolus versus continuous infusion of doxorubicin in patients with high-grade extremity soft tissue sarcoma and an analysis of prognostic factors. Cancer (Phila) 1991;68:1221–1229.
120. Pisters PWT, Patel SR, Varma DGK, et al. Preoperative chemotherapy for stage IIIB extremity soft tissue sarcoma: long-term results from a single institution. J Clin Oncol 1997;15:3481–3487.
121. Casper ES, Gaynor JJ, Harrison LB, et al. Preoperative and postoperative adjuvant combination chemotherapy for adults with high grade soft tissue sarcoma. Cancer (Phila) 1994;73:1644–1651.
122. O'Bryan RM, Baker LH, Gottlieb JE, et al. Dose response evaluation of adriamycin in human neoplasia. Cancer (Phila) 1977;39:1940–1948.
123. Patel SR, Vadhan-Raj S, Papadopolous N, et al. High-dose ifosfamide in bone and soft tissue sarcomas: results of phase II and pilot studies—dose-response and schedule dependence. J Clin Oncol 1997;15:2378–2384.
124. Gortzak E, Rouesse J, Verwey J, et al. Randomised phase II study of neoadjuvant chemotherapy in soft tissue sarcomas in adults: protocol 62874. Eur J Cancer 1993;29A(suppl 6):S183.
125. Eilber FR, Giuliano A, Huth JH, et al. Neoadjuvant chemotherapy, radiation, and limited surgery for high grade soft tissue sarcoma of the extremity. In: Ryan JR, Baker LO, eds. Recent Concepts in Sarcoma Treatment. Dordrecht: Kluwer, 1988:115–122.
126. Eilber FR, Giuliano AE, Huth JF, et al. Postoperative adjuvant chemotherapy (Adriamycin) in high grade extremity soft tissue sarcoma: a randomized prospective trial. In: Salmon SE, ed. Adjuvant Therapy of Cancer, 5th ed. Orlando: Grune & Stratton, 1987:719–723.
127. Eilber FR, Giuliano AE, Huth JF, et al. Intravenous (IV) vs. intra-arterial (IA) Adriamycin, 2800r radiation and surgical excision for extremity soft tissue sarcomas: a randomized prospective trial [abstract]. Proc Am Soc Clin Oncol 1990;9:309.
128. Wanebo HJ, Temple WJ, Popp MB, et al. Preoperative regional therapy for extremity sarcoma: a tricenter update. Cancer (Phila) 1995;75:2299–2306.
129. Temple WJ, Temple CLF, Arthur K, et al. Prospective cohort study of neoadjuvant treatment in conservative surgery of soft tissue sarcomas. Ann Surg Oncol 1997;4:586–590.
130. Levine EA, Trippon M, DasGupta TK. Preoperative multimodality treatment for soft tissue sarcomas. Cancer (Phila) 1993;71:3685–3689.
131. Spiro IJ, Suit H, Gebhardt MC, et al. Neoadjuvant chemotherapy and radiotherapy for large soft tissue sarcomas [abstract]. Proc Am Soc Clin Oncol 1996;15:524.
132. Eggermont AMM, Shraffordt Koops H, Lienard D, et al. Isolated limb perfusion with high-dose tumor necrosis factor-α in combination with interferon-g and melphalan for nonresectable extremity soft tissue sarcomas: a multicenter trial. J Clin Oncol 1996;14:2653–2665.
133. Begg CB, Cramer LD, Hoskins WJ, et al. Impact of hospital volume on operative mortality for major cancer surgery. JAMA 1998;280:1747–1751.
134. Birkmeyer JD, Finlayson SR, Tosteson AN, et al. Effect of hospital volume on in-hospital mortality with pancreaticoduodenectomy. Surgery (St. Louis) 1999;125:250–256.
135. Clasby R, Tilling K, Smith MA, et al. Variable management of soft tissue sarcoma: regional audit with implications for specialist care. Br J Surg 1997;84:1692–1696.
136. Gustafson P, Dreinhofer KE, Rydholm A. Soft tissue sarcoma should be treated at a tumor center: a comparison of quality of surgery in 375 patients. Acta Orthop Scand 1994;65:47–50.
137. Potter DA, Glenn J, Kinsella T, et al. Patterns of recurrence in patients with high-grade soft-tissue sarcomas. J Clin Oncol 1985;3:353–366.
138. Bevilacqua RG, Rogatko A, Hajdu SI, et al. Prognostic factors in primary retroperitoneal soft-tissue sarcomas. Arch Surg 1991;126:328–334.
139. Farhood AI, Hajdu SI, Shiu MH, et al. Soft tissue sarcomas of the head and neck in adults. Am J Surg 1990;160:365–369.
140. Singer S, Antman K, Corson JM, et al. Long-term salvageability for patients with locally recurrent soft-tissue sarcomas. Arch Surg 1992;127:548–553.
141. Midis GP, Pollock RE, Chen NP, et al. Locally recurrent soft tissue sarcoma of the extremities. Surgery (St. Louis) 1998;123:666–671.
142. Nori D, Schupak K, Shiu MH, et al. Role of brachytherapy in recurrent extremity sarcoma in patients treated with prior surgery and irradiation. Int J Radiat Oncol Biol Phys 1991;20:1229–1233.
143. Pearlstone D, Janjan NA, Feig BW, et al. Re-resection with brachytherapy for locally recurrent soft tissue sarcoma arising in a previously radiated field. Cancer J Sci Am 1999;5:26–33.
144. Catton CN, Davis A, Bell RS, et al. Soft tissue sarcoma of the extremity: limb salvage after failure of combined conservative therapy. Radiother Oncol 1996;41:209–214.
145. Barr LC, Stotter AT, A'Hern RP. Influence of local recurrence on survival: a controversy reviewed from the perspective of soft tissue sarcoma. Br J Surg 1991;78:648–650.
146. Rooser B, Gustafson P, Rydholm A. Is there no influence of local control on the rate of metastases in high-grade soft tissue sarcoma? Cancer (Phila) 1990;65:1727–1729.
147. Gustafson P, Rooser B, Rydholm A. Is local recurrence of minor importance for metastases in soft tissue sarcoma? Cancer (Phila) 1991;67:2083–2086.
148. Lewis JJ, Leung D, Heslin M, et al. Association of local recurrence with subsequent survival in extremity soft tissue sarcoma. J Clin Oncol 1997;15:646–652.
149. Brennan MF. The surgeon as a leader in cancer care: lessons learned from the study of soft tissue sarcoma. J Am Coll Surg 1996;182:520–529.

150. Billingsley KG, Lewis JJ, Leung DH, et al. Multifactorial analysis of the survival of patients with distant metastasis arising from primary extremity sarcoma. Cancer (Phila) 1999;85:389–395.
151. Creagan ET, Fleming TR, Edmonson JH, et al. Pulmonary resection for metastatic nonosteogenic sarcoma. Cancer (Phila) 1979;44:1908–1912.
152. Casson AG, Putnam JB, Natarajan G, et al. Five-year survival after pulmonary metastasectomy for adult soft tissue sarcoma. Cancer (Phila) 1992;69:662–668.
153. Gadd MA, Casper ES, Woodruff JM, et al. Development and treatment of pulmonary metastases in adult patients with extremity soft-tissue sarcoma. Ann Surg 1993;218:705–712.
154. Huth JF, Holmes EC, Vernon SE, et al. Pulmonary resection for metastatic sarcoma. Am J Surg 1980;140:9–16.
155. McCormack PM, Martini N. The changing role of surgery for pulmonary metastases. Ann Thorac Surg 1979;28:139–145.
156. Morrow CE, Vassilopoulos PP, Grage TB. Surgical resection for metastatic neoplasms of the lung: experience at the University of Minnesota Hospitals. Cancer (Phila) 1980;45:2981–2985.
157. Mountain CF, McMurtney MJ, Hermes KE. Surgery for pulmonary metastasis: a 20-year experience. Ann Thorac Surg 1984; 38:323–330.
158. Pastorino U, Valente M, Gasparini M, et al. Lung resection for metastatic sarcomas: total survival from primary treatment. J Surg Oncol 1989;4:275–280.
159. Rizzoni WE, Pass HI, Wesley MN, et al. Resection of recurrent pulmonary metastases in patients with soft-tissue sarcomas. Arch Surg 1986;121:1248–1252.
160. van Geel AN, Pastorino U, Jauch KW, et al. Surgical treatment of lung metastases: the European Organization for Research and Treatment of Cancer-Soft Tissue and Bone Sarcoma Group study of 255 patients. Cancer (Phila) 1996;77:675–682.
161. Putnam JB Jr, Roth JA, Wesley MN, et al. Analysis of prognostic factors in patients undergoing resection of pulmonary metastases from soft tissue sarcomas. J Thorac Cardiovasc Surg 1984;87:260–268.
162. Jablons D, Steinberg SM, Roth J, et al. Metastasectomy for soft tissue sarcoma: further evidence for efficacy and prognostic indicators. J Thorac Cardiovasc Surg 1989;97:695–705.
163. Roth JA, Putnam JB Jr, Wesley MN, et al. Differing determinants of prognosis following resection of pulmonary metastases from osteogenic and soft tissue sarcoma patients. Cancer (Phila) 1985;55:1361–1366.
164. Pogrebniak HW, Roth JA, Steinberg SM, et al. Reoperative pulmonary resection in patients with metastatic soft tissue sarcoma. Ann Thorac Surg 1991;52:197–203.
165. Casson AG, Putnam JB, Natarajan G, et al. Efficacy of pulmonary metastasectomy for recurrent soft tissue sarcoma. J Surg Oncol 1991;47:1–4.
166. Takita H, Edgerton F, Karakousis C, et al. Surgical management of metastases to the lung. Surg Gynecol Obstet 1981;152:191–194.
167. Putnam JB Jr, Roth JA, Wesley MN, et al. Survival following aggressive resection of pulmonary metastases from osteogenic sarcoma: analysis of prognostic factors. Ann Thorac Surg 1983;36:516–523.
168. Regnard JF, Cerrina J, Silbert D. Curative surgical treatment of pulmonary metastases. In: Proceedings of 3rd European Conference on Clinical Oncology, Stockholm, Sweden, 1985:58.
169. Ramming KP. Surgery for pulmonary metastases. Surg Clin N Am 1980;60:815–824.
170. Joseph WL, Morton DL, Adkins PC. Prognostic significance of tumor doubling time in evaluating operability in pulmonary metastatic disease. J Thorac Cardiovasc Surg 1971;61:23–32.
171. Verazin GT, Warneke JA, Driscoll DL, et al. Resection of lung metastases from soft-tissue sarcomas: a multivariate analysis. Arch Surg 1992;127:1407–1411.
172. McCormack P. Surgical resection of pulmonary metastases. Semin Surg Oncol 1990;6:297–302.
173. Jacobs EM. Combination chemotherapy of metastatic testicular germinal cell tumors and soft part sarcomas. Cancer (Phila) 1970;25:324–332.
174. Greenhall MJ, Magill GB, DeCosse JJ, et al. Chemotherapy for soft tissue sarcoma. Surg Gynecol Obstet 1986;162:193–198.
175. Schoenfeld DA, Rosenbaum C, Horton J, et al. A comparison of Adriamycin versus vincristine and Adriamycin, and cyclophosphamide versus vincristine, actinomycin-D, and cyclophosphamide for advanced sarcoma. Cancer (Phila) 1982;50: 2757–2762.
176. O'Bryan RM, Luce JK, Talley R, et al. Phase II evaluation of Adriamycin in human neoplasia. Cancer (Phila) 1973;32:1–8.
177. Cruz AB Jr, Thames EA Jr, Aust JB, et al. Combination chemotherapy for soft-tissue sarcomas: a phase III study. J Surg Oncol 1979;11:313–323.
178. Creagan ET, Hahn RG, Ahmann DL, et al. A clinical trial of Adriamycin (NSC 123127) in advanced sarcomas. Oncology 1977;34:90–91.
179. Borden EC, Amato DA, Rosenbaum C, et al. Randomized comparison of three Adriamycin regimens for metastatic soft tissue sarcomas. J Clin Oncol 1987;5:840–850.
180. Gottlieb JA, Baker LH, O'Bryan RM, et al. Adriamycin (NSC-123127) used alone and in combination for soft tissue and bony sarcoma. Cancer Chemother Rep 1975;6(part 3):271–282.
181. Baker LH, Frank JA, Fine G, et al. Combination chemotherapy using Adriamycin, DTIC, cyclophosphamide, and actinomycin D for advanced soft tissue sarcomas: a randomized comparative trial (a phase III, Southwest Oncology Group Study (7613)). J Clin Oncol 1987;5:851–861.
182. Muss HB, Bundy B, DiSaia PJ, et al. Treatment of recurrent or advanced uterine sarcoma: a randomized trial of doxorubicin versus doxorubicin and cyclophosphamide (a phase III trial of the Gynecologic Oncology Group). Cancer (Phila) 1985;55:1648–1653.
183. Borden EC, Amato DA, Edmonson JH, et al. Randomized comparison of doxorubicin and vindesine to doxorubicin for patients with metastatic soft-tissue sarcomas. Cancer (Phila) 1990;66:862–867.
184. Gottlieb JA, Benjamin RS, Baker LH, et al. Role of DTIC (NSC-45388) in the chemotherapy of sarcomas. Cancer Treat Rep 1976;60:199–203.
185. Luce JK, Thurman WG, Isaacs BL, et al. Clinical trials with the antitumor agent 5-(3,3-dimethyl-1-triazeno)imidazole-4-carboxamide(NSC-45388). Cancer Chemother Rep 1970;54:119–124.
186. Omura GA, Major FJ, Blessing JA, et al. A randomized study of Adriamycin with and without dimethyl triazenoimidazole carboxamide in advanced uterine sarcomas. Cancer (Phila) 1983;52:626–632.
187. Zalupski M, Metch B, Balcerzak SP, et al. Phase III comparison of doxorubicin and dacarbazine given by bolus versus infusion in patients with soft-tissue sarcomas: a Southwest Oncology Group study. J Natl Cancer Inst 1991;83:926–932.
188. Selawry OS, Holland JF, Wolman IJ. Effect of vincristine (NSC-67574) on malignant solid tumors in children. Cancer Chemother Rep 1968;52:497–500.
189. Korbitz BC, Davis HL Jr, Ramirez G, et al. Low doses of vincristine (NSC-67574) for malignant disease. Cancer Chemother Rep 1969;53:249–253.
190. Ravaud A, Nguyen BB, Coindre JM, et al. Adjuvant chemotherapy with CyVADIC in high-grade soft tissue sarcoma: a randomized prospective trial. In: Salmon S, ed. Adjuvant Therapy of Cancer, 6th ed. Philadelphia: Saunders, 1990:556–566.
191. Bramwell VHC, Rouesse J, Steward W, et al. European experience of adjuvant chemotherapy for soft tissue sarcoma: interim report of a randomized trial of CYVADIC versus control. In:

Ryan JR, Baker LO, eds. Recent Concepts in Sarcoma Treatment. Dordrecht: Kluwer, 1988:157–159.
192. Yap BS, Baker LH, Sinkovics JG, et al. Cyclophosphamide, vincristine, Adriamycin, and DTIC (CYVADIC) combination chemotherapy for the treatment of advanced sarcomas. Cancer Treat Rep 1980;64:93–98.
193. Santoro A, Tursz T, Mouridsen H, et al. Doxorubicin versus CYVADIC versus doxorubicin plus ifosfamide in first-line treatment of advanced soft tissue sarcomas: a randomized study of the European Organization for Research and Treatment of Cancer Soft Tissue and Bone Sarcoma Group. J Clin Oncol 1995;13:1537–1545.
194. Antman KH, Ryan L, Elias AD, et al. Response to ifosfamide and mesna: 124 previously treated patients with metastatic or unresectable sarcoma. J Clin Oncol 1989;7:126–131.
195. Antman KH, Montella D, Rosenbaum C, et al. Phase II trial of ifosfamide with mesna in previously treated metastatic sarcoma. Cancer Treat Rep 1985;69:499–504.
196. Stuart-Harris R, Harper PG, Kaye SB, et al. High-dose ifosfamide by infusion with mesna in advanced soft tissue sarcoma. Cancer Treat Rev 1983;10(suppl A):163–164.
197. Bramwell VHC, Mouridsen HT, Santoro A, et al. Cyclophosphamide versus ifosfamide: final report of a randomized phase II trial in adult soft tissue sarcomas. Eur J Cancer Clin Oncol 1987;23:311–321.
198. Morgan LR, Posey LE, Rainey J, et al. Ifosfamide: a weekly dose fractionated schedule in bronchogenic carcinoma. Cancer Treat Rep 1981;65:693–695.
199. Brock N, Pohl J. The development of mesna for regional detoxification. Cancer Treat Rev 1983;10(suppl A):33–43.
200. Wiltshaw E, Westbury G, Harmer C, et al. Ifosfamide plus mesna with and without Adriamycin in soft tissue sarcoma. Cancer Chemother Pharmacol 1986;18(suppl 2):S10–S12.
201. Schutte J, Mouridsen HT, Stewart W, et al. Ifosfamide plus doxorubicin in previously untreated patients with advanced soft tissue sarcoma: the EORTC Soft Tissue and Bone Sarcoma Group. Eur J Cancer 1990;26:558–561.
202. Elias AD, Ryan L, Sulkes A, et al. Response to mesna, doxorubicin, ifosfamide, and dacarbazine in 108 patients with metastatic or unresectable sarcoma and no prior chemotherapy. J Clin Oncol 1989;7:1208–1216.
203. Elias AD, Ryan L, Aisner J, et al. Mesna, doxorubicin, ifosfamide, dacarbazine (MAID) regimen for adults with advanced sarcoma. Semin Oncol 1990;17:41–49.
204. Edmonson JH, Ryan LM, Blum RH, et al. Randomized comparison of doxorubicin alone versus ifosfamide plus doxorubicin or mitomycin, doxorubicin, and cisplatin against advanced soft tissue sarcomas. J Clin Oncol 1993;11:1269–1275.
205. Antman K, Crowley J, Balcerzak SP, et al. An Intergroup phase III randomized study of doxorubicin and dacarbazine with or without ifosfamide and mesna in advanced soft tissue and bone sarcomas. J Clin Oncol 1993;11:1276–1285.
206. Jaques DP, Coit DG, Hajdu SI, et al. Management of primary and recurrent soft-tissue sarcoma of the retroperitoneum. Ann Surg 1990;212:51–59.
207. Alvarenga JC, Ball AB, Fisher C, et al. Limitations of surgery in the treatment of retroperitoneal sarcoma. Br J Surg 1991;78:912–916.
208. Neifeld JP, Walsh JW, Lawrence W Jr. Computed tomography in the management of soft tissue tumors. Surg Gynecol Obstet 1982;155:535–540.
209. Sundaram M, McLeod RA. MR imaging of tumor and tumor like lesions of bone and soft tissue. AJR Am J Roentgenol 1990; 155:817–824.
210. Manaser BJ, Ensign MF. Imaging of musculoskeletal tumors. Semin Oncol 1991;18:140–149.
211. Karakousis CP, Velez AF, Emrich LJ. Management of retroperitoneal sarcomas and patient survival. Am J Surg 1985;150:376–380.
212. Dalton RR, Donohue JH, Mucha P Jr, et al. Management of retroperitoneal sarcomas. Surgery (St. Louis) 1989;106:725–733.
213. Storm FK, Mahvi DM. Diagnosis and management of retroperitoneal soft-tissue sarcoma. Ann Surg 1991;214:2–10.
214. Karakousis CP, Velez AF, Gerstenbluth R, et al. Resectability and survival in retroperitoneal sarcomas. Ann Surg Oncol 1996;3:150–158.
215. Kilkenny JW III, Bland KI, Copeland EM III. Retroperitoneal sarcoma: the University of Florida experience. J Am Coll Surg 1996;182:329–339.
216. Karakousis CP, Kontzoglou K, Driscoll DL. Resectability of retroperitoneal sarcomas: a matter of surgical technique? Eur J Surg Oncol 1995;21:617–622.
217. Karakousis CP, Gerstenbluth R, Kontzoglou K, et al. Retroperitoneal sarcomas and their management. Arch Surg 1995;130:1104–1109.
218. Lewis JJ, Leung D, Woodruff JM, et al. Retroperitoneal soft-tissue sarcoma: analysis of 500 patients treated and followed at a single institution. Ann Surg 1998;228:355–365.
219. McGrath PC, Neifeld JP, Lawrence W Jr, et al. Improved survival following complete excision of retroperitoneal sarcomas. Ann Surg 1984;200:200–204.
220. Heslin MJ, Lewis JJ, Nadler E, et al. Prognostic factors associated with long-term survival for retroperitoneal sarcoma: implications for management. J Clin Oncol 1997;15:2832–2839.
221. Catton CN, O'Sullivan B, Kotwall C, et al. Outcome and prognosis in retroperitoneal soft tissue sarcoma. Int J Radiat Oncol Biol Phys 1994;29:1005–1010.
222. Bose B. Primary malignant retroperitoneal tumours: analysis of 30 cases. Can J Surg 1979;22:215–220.
223. Cody HSI, Turnbull AD, Fortner JG, et al. The continuing challenge of retroperitoneal sarcomas. Cancer (Phila) 1981;47:2147–2152.
224. Harrison LB, Gutierrez E, Fischer JJ. Retroperitoneal sarcomas: the Yale experience and a review of the literature. J Surg Oncol 1986;32:159–164.
225. Wist E, Solheim OP, Jacobsen AB, et al. Primary retroperitoneal sarcomas: a review of 36 cases. Acta Radiol Oncol 1985;24:305–310.
226. Tepper JE, Suit HD, Wood WC, et al. Radiation therapy of retroperitoneal soft tissue sarcomas. Int J Radiat Oncol Biol Phys 1984;10:825–830.
227. Willett CG, Suit HD, Tepper JE, et al. Intraoperative electron beam radiation therapy for retroperitoneal soft tissue sarcoma. Cancer (Phila) 1991;68:278–283.
228. Kinsella TJ, Sindelar WF, Lack E, et al. Preliminary results of a randomized study of adjuvant radiation therapy in resectable adult retroperitoneal soft tissue sarcomas. J Clin Oncol 1988; 6:18–25.
229. Sindelar WF, Kinsella TJ, Chen PW, et al. Intraoperative radiotherapy in retroperitoneal sarcomas. Final results of a prospective, randomized, clinical trial. Arch Surg 1993;128:402–410.
230. Storm FK, Eilber FR, Mirra J, et al. Retroperitoneal sarcomas: a reappraisal of treatment. J Surg Oncol 1981;17:1–7.

99

Gastrointestinal Stromal Tumors

Jason S. Gold and Ronald P. DeMatteo

Despite its relative rarity as a clinical entity, gastrointestinal stromal tumor (GIST) has garnered much interest in the past several years. The recognition of KIT activation as essential in the tumorigenesis of GIST and the subsequent treatment of GISTs with a molecular inhibitor of KIT signaling, imatinib mesylate (STI 571, Gleevec; Novartis Pharmaceuticals, Basel, Switzerland), represent landmark achievements in solid tumor oncology. The use of imatinib in the management of GIST most likely signals the beginning of the application of specific molecular and genetic approaches to cancer therapy. Thus, the integration of surgery and targeted therapy in the treatment of GIST, which is currently the subject of much investigation, may serve as a paradigm for the multimodality management of other solid malignancies.

Background

GIST is the most common mesenchymal tumor of the gastrointestinal tract. However, until recently, GISTs were generally regarded as smooth muscle neoplasms and thus were often misclassified as leiomyomas or leiomyosarcomas. Electron microscopy and immunohistochemistry revealed that few of these tumors show ultrastructural or immunophenotypic features of smooth muscle differentiation, and this led to the introduction of the term stromal tumor (Fig. 99.1). The widespread utilization of KIT (CD 117) immunostaining, which is positive in at least 95% of GISTs, and the increased recognition of the histopathological appearance of this tumor in recent years has revealed that true leiomyomas and leiomyosarcomas of the gastrointestinal (GI) tract are rare. It is believed that GISTs are derived from or share a common lineage with the interstitial cell of Cajal, an intestinal pacemaker cell.

Epidemiology

As a consequence of previous inconsistencies in the classification of GIST, its true incidence has been difficult to determine. A recent population-based study from Sweden suggests an incidence of about 13 cases per million persons per year.[1] Older Surveillance, Epidemiology, and End Results (SEER) data from the National Cancer Institute (NCI) suggested 500 to 600 new cases per year in the United States.[2] The rapid accrual of patients in clinical trials has led to the upward revision of previous incidence estimates. Although there are no data on the true incidence in the United States, it may be as high as a few thousand cases per year.

GIST affects men slightly more often than women. Most patients are between 40 and 80 years old, with a median age of approximately 60 at the time of diagnosis.[3–7] GIST is nearly always sporadic, although it has been identified in a few families and has been associated with von Recklinghausen's disease and Carney's triad (gastric GIST, paraganglioma, and pulmonary chondroma).

GIST can occur anywhere along the GI tract. The most common site of origin is the stomach, accounting for about 65% of cases. The small intestine accounts for about 25% of cases. Approximately 5% to 10% of cases arise in the colon and rectum and about 5% arise in the esophagus.[1,3,8] In fact, most esophageal mesenchymal tumors are leiomyomas. Occasionally GIST can occur in the omentum, mesentery, or retroperitoneum. Rarely have GISTs been reported in unusual sites such as the urinary bladder or gallbladder.

Clinical Presentation

There is wide variation in the presentation of GIST. Some are asymptomatic and found incidentally on physical examination, radiologic imaging, endoscopy, or laparotomy.

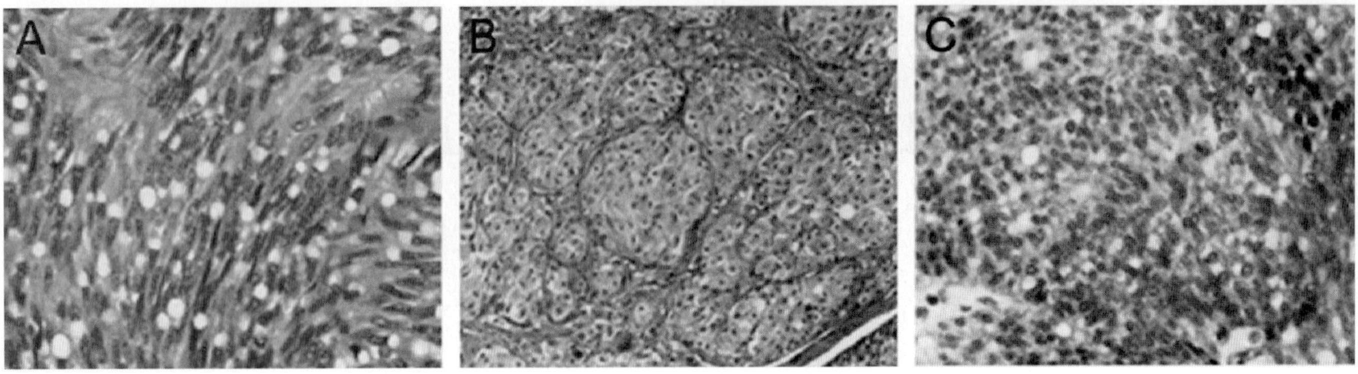

FIGURE 99.1. **A–C.** Histology of gastrointestinal stromal tumors (GIST).

Figure 99.2 shows the appearance of a GIST at laparotomy. Symptoms typically result from mass effect or bleeding. Similar to other sarcomas, GISTs tend to displace adjacent structures without invasion. Thus, they can grow quite large before becoming symptomatic. In this manner, GISTs can cause vague abdominal discomfort, pain, bloating, early satiety, or increased abdominal girth. GISTs can also exert symptoms particular to their site of origin, such as dysphagia for esophageal tumors, biliary obstruction for periampullary tumors, and intussusception or rarely, intestinal obstruction for small bowel tumors.[9]

GISTs can erode into the lumen of the GI tract, causing clinically significant bleeding or occult bleeding resulting in symptoms caused by anemia. Furthermore, they can cause life-threatening hemorrhage from intraperitoneal rupture. Overall, in a recent population-based study, about 70% of GISTs were symptomatic, 20% were asymptomatic, and 10% were detected at autopsy. Symptomatic GISTs tended to be larger, with an average size of 6cm versus 2cm for asymptomatic GISTs and 1.5cm for GISTs detected at autopsy.[1]

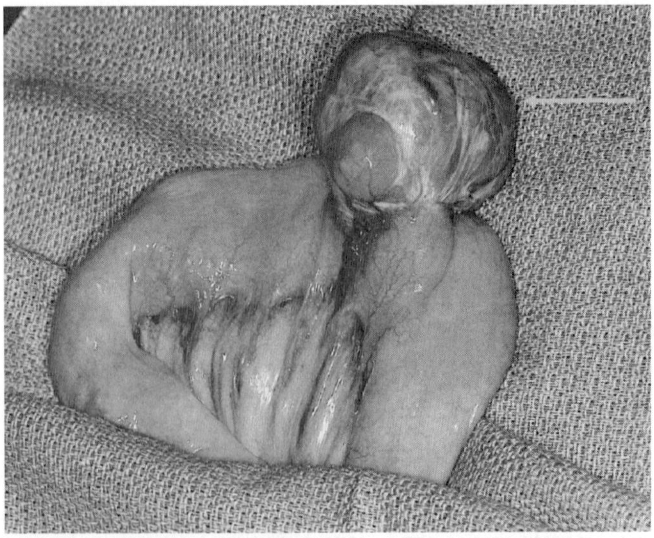

FIGURE 99.2. Gastrointestinal stromal tumor (GIST) of the small intestine. GISTs typically present as well-demarcated masses that arise within the submucosa or muscularis propria.

Diagnosis

Clinical Diagnosis

GIST is often not diagnosed before formal pathological examination after resection as it is an uncommon tumor and not familiar to many clinicians. The preoperative diagnosis of GIST requires a high degree of suspicion. GIST is often detected on cross-sectional imaging, usually contrast-enhanced computed tomography (CT) and, less commonly, magnetic resonance imaging (MRI), as these studies are commonly employed to evaluate abdominal symptoms. Cross-sectional imaging is useful to evaluate the primary tumor as well as detect metastases to the liver or peritoneum. Primary GIST usually appears as a well-circumscribed, often well-vascularized mass closely associated with the stomach or intestine. Larger GISTs often show necrosis or intratumoral hemorrhage. On CT, GIST typically appears as a hyperdense-enhancing mass.

GIST can also be detected by endoscopy where it appears as a submucosal mass. Endoscopic ultrasound is often useful to characterize the tumor or determine extramural extent. For masses diagnosed endoscopically, contrast-enhanced CT is advocated to assess for metastases. A chest radiograph is satisfactory to assess the thorax, as GIST seldom initially metastasizes to the chest. Bone scans are necessary only to evaluate symptoms. ^{18}Fluorodeoxyglucose (FDG) positron emission tomography (PET) is highly sensitive but less specific for the diagnosis of GIST. ^{18}FDG-PET can detect small tumors or metastases missed by CT as well as provide functional information about the tumor that may be useful in treatment. However, its limited availability and high cost make it less commonly employed.

Pathological Diagnosis

The majority of GISTs fall into one of three categories based on histological appearance: spindle-cell type (70%), epithelioid type (20%), or, rarely, mixed type where both features are present.[10] Spindle cell GIST is characterized by uniform fusiform cells in intersecting fascicles or whorls. Epithelioid GIST has rounded cells typically in a nested pattern. GIST usually has uniform cytology with fibrillary eosinophilic cytoplasm and nuclei containing fine chromatin and inconspicuous nucleoli. There is also usually scant stroma.

GISTs have a characteristic immunohistochemical profile that has proven very helpful in diagnosis. Most importantly, they show immunopositivity for KIT with rare exceptions. Furthermore, 60% to 70% are positive for CD34, 30% to 40% are positive for smooth-muscle actin (SMA), and approximately 5% are positive for the S-100 protein. GISTs very rarely express desmin, which is characteristic of smooth muscle tumors, and when they do, it is invariably focal with only a small number of immunopositive cells.[10]

The use of percutaneous biopsy for a resectable primary tumor is controversial. Biopsy can theoretically precipitate tumor rupture and lead to tumor dissemination or hemorrhage. Furthermore, GIST is often difficult to reliably diagnose from a percutaneous biopsy, especially from a fine-needle aspirate when only a few cells are obtained, or from a core biopsy when a necrotic or hemorrhagic area of the tumor may be sampled. Percutaneous biopsy may be more appropriate if it will change the clinical management, such as when the diagnosis of lymphoma is in question or if a mass is marginally resectable and neoadjuvant imatinib may be considered.

Treatment Modalities

Small Molecule Tyrosine Kinase Inhibitors

Since Gustav Lindskog, a surgeon at Yale University, first used nitrogen mustard to treat a patient with sarcoma in 1942, the chemotherapy of cancer has traditionally employed cytotoxic agents. These nonspecific therapies have essentially functioned by interfering with cellular machinery shared by neoplastic and normal cells. Thus, chemotherapy has usually induced toxicity and had a narrow therapeutic index. Imatinib mesylate, in contrast, is a selective potent inhibitor of structurally related tyrosine kinase signaling molecules including KIT, which is known to be important in the pathogenesis of GIST.

In 1998, Hirota and colleagues found that there were mutations in the KIT gene in five of six GISTs they examined, causing transcription of a protein that is constitutively active and results in ligand-independent signaling.[11] KIT was originally discovered as the oncogene in a feline sarcoma retrovirus. The cellular homologue of the KIT oncogene encodes for a transmembrane receptor tyrosine kinase signaling molecule. Binding of KIT to its ligand (known as KIT ligand, stem-cell factor, steel factor, or mast-cell growth factor) causes dimerization of KIT molecules on the cell surface; this results in activation of the KIT tyrosine kinase moiety. The subsequent autophosphorylation and phosphorylation of downstream signaling molecules results in inhibition of apoptosis and in increased cell proliferation. Activating KIT mutations are present in approximately 80% of GISTs.[12,13]

Although it was known that the oncogenesis of chronic myeloid leukemia (CML) entails a chromosomal translocation generating a chimeric fusion protein BCR-ABL that functions via uncontrolled tyrosine kinase activity, the development of an inhibitor of BCR-ABL was initially hampered by philosophical and logistical concerns. It was argued that since the ATP-binding pocket of most kinases is highly conserved, an inhibitor would not be selective to BCR-ABL. Also, because CML is a rare disease, it was argued that developing such an inhibitor would not be economically feasible. After overcoming these barriers, the development of an orally administered selective tyrosine kinase inhibitor, imatinib mesylate, was quite rapid. In vitro studies identifying imatinib and demonstrating its activity against CML cells were published in 1996.[14] Preliminary human data were presented in 1999. Phase I human trials were published in early 2001,[15,16] and the U.S. Food and Drug Administration (FDA) approved imatinib for use in CML the next month. Imatinib subsequently has been shown to have a more than 90% complete response rate in the chronic phase of CML.

Because imatinib is not completely specific to BCR-ABL and was soon found to inhibit signaling of KIT, this opened the door for the experimental use of imatinib in GIST. Preclinical studies demonstrated that imatinib causes growth arrest and apoptosis of GIST cells in vitro.[17] The first patient with metastatic GIST began treatment with imatinib in 2000 after failing other treatments. Within a few weeks, the patient exhibited a major objective clinical response as evaluated by MRI, ^{18}FDG-PET, and histopathological examination of serial biopsies.[18] The dramatic response of this first patient led to the rapid implementation of clinical trials formally testing the efficacy of imatinib in metastatic GIST (Table 99.1).

TABLE 99.1.
Trials of Imatinib Mesylate in Metastatic Gastrointestinal Stromal Tumor (GIST).

					Best response			
Trial	*Phase*	*Year*	*Imatinib mesylate dose (n)*	*Follow-up*	*PR*	*SD*	*PD*	*Comments*
EORTC[31,33]	I	2001, 2002	400, 600, 800, or 1000 mg/day (35)	8–12 months	51%	31%	8%	TTR = 1 week MTD = 800 mg/day
U.S. multicenter[36,37]	II	2002, 2004	400 mg/day (73) 600 mg/day (74)	34 months	67%	16%	17%	No difference between groups
EORTC[35]	III	2003	400 mg/day (470) 800 mg/day (472)	2 years	50% 54%	32% 32%	13% 9%	32% Grade III-IV toxicity 50% Grade III-IV toxicity Improved PFS for 800 mg/d ($P = 0.03$)
Intergroup[34]	III	2003	400 mg/day (350) 800 mg/day (352)	12 months	49% 48%	22% 22%		36% Grade III-IV toxicity 52% Grade III-IV toxicity No difference in PFS

PR, partial response; SD, stable disease; PD, progressive disease; TTR, time to recurrence; MTD, maximal tolerated dose; CR, complete response; PFS, progression-free survival.[36,37]

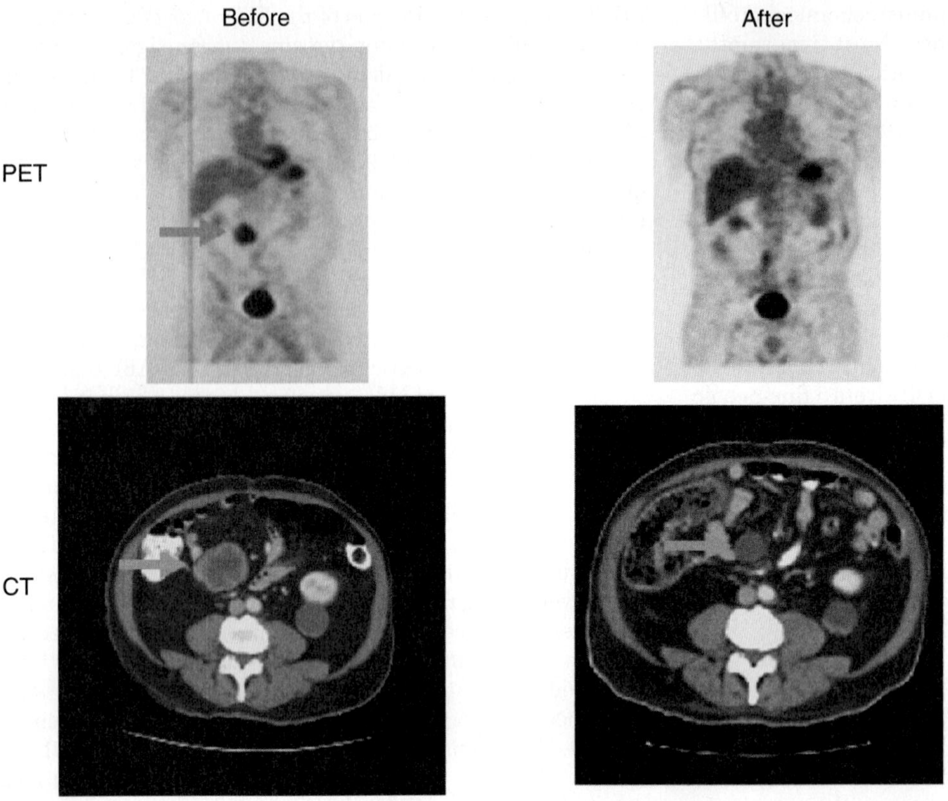

FIGURE 99.3. Response to imatinib mesylate in a patient with recurrent gastrointestinal stromal tumor (GIST). The patient presented with a large peritoneal mass seen in the computed tomography (*CT*) scan in the *lower left* with corresponding activity on ^{18}fluorodeoxyglucose (^{18}FDG) positron emission tomography (*PET*) seen in the *upper left*. After several weeks of therapy with imatinib mesylate, the patient experienced a partial response with reduction of tumor size (*lower right*) and loss of ^{18}FDG activity (*upper right*). (Reproduced with permission from DeMatteo RP. The GIST of targeted cancer therapy: a tumor (gastrointestinal stromal tumor), a mutated gene (c-kit), and a molecular inhibitor (STI571). Ann Surg Oncol 2002;9:831–839.)

Figures 99.3 and 99.4 show response to imatinib treatment. The current treatment of metastatic GIST is further delineated next.

Lessons learned from clinical use of imatinib include that, although the progression of disease is halted in the majority of patients, complete responses are rare. It appears that imatinib works as more of an oncostatic agent, suppressing disease that can reemerge after withdrawal of the agent. Major toxicities of imatinib therapy are usually manageable and include mild fatigue, periorbital edema, diarrhea, muscle cramps, nausea, abdominal pain, and rash.

The reasons for variation in the response of GIST to imatinib are beginning to be understood. It appears that advanced GISTs with exon 11 mutations (which occur in 70% of cases) are more responsive to imatinib than GISTs with exon 9 mutations.[13] A subgroup of GISTs without KIT mutations have been shown to have mutations in the homologous tyrosine kinase platelet-derived growth factor receptor (PDGFR)-α (5-7%).[19] GISTs with PDGFR-α mutations also have a favorable response to imatinib, except those with D842V mutations. Furthermore, the 10% to 15% of GISTs without a known tyrosine kinase mutation have an unfavorable response to imatinib.[13] Mechanisms of acquired resistance to imatinib are beginning to be understood and include the acquisition of additional KIT mutations, KIT amplification, or additional oncogene mutations.[20]

The development of other small molecule tyrosine kinase inhibitors and their application to GIST is under way. SU11248 (Sugen) is another agent with activity against KIT and PDGFR. In Phase I/II trials, of patients with metastatic GIST who are intolerant of or resistant to imatinib, 8% to 15% have a

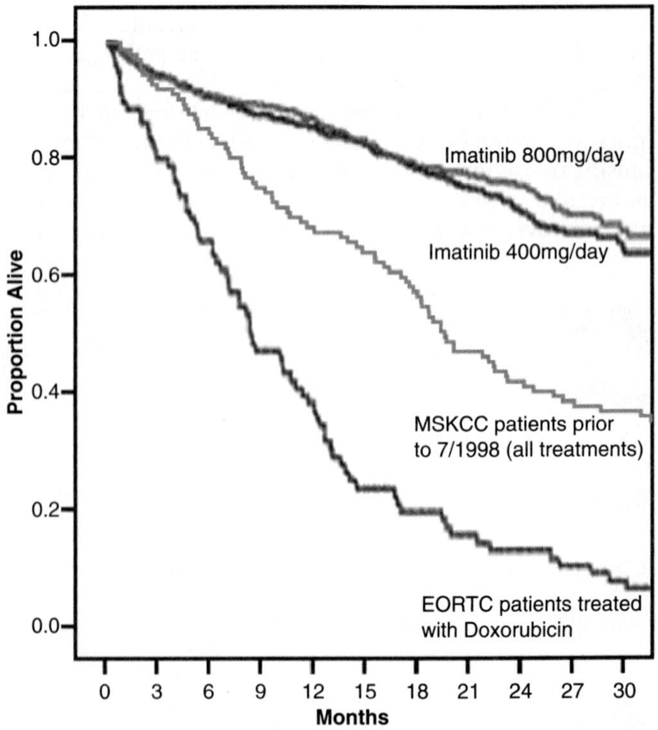

FIGURE 99.4. Response to imatimib: Memorial Sloan Kettering Cancer Center (MSKCC) patients before July 1998, and European Organization for Research and Treatment of Cancer (EORTC) patients treated with doxorubicin.

response to SU11248 and 39% to 58% have stable disease.[21,22]

Surgery

Surgery represents the cornerstone of treatment for localized GIST and can also be an integral part of the treatment of recurrent and metastatic disease. Before the advent of imatinib, surgery was the only effective therapy available. Today, surgery still represents the best chance of cure for primary disease that has not metastasized. Nevertheless, many resected GISTs will eventually recur. The role of surgery in the multidisciplinary treatment of advanced disease is evolving.

Conventional Chemotherapy

Although the historical confusion between GIST and leiomyosarcoma makes it difficult (if not impossible) to discern the response of GIST to chemotherapy in older trials, it appears to be minimal (less than 10%) (Table 99.2). In fact, it is now apparent that leiomyosarcoma is more sensitive to conventional chemotherapeutic agents than GIST. Several agents have been employed for GIST without success. Agents that are commonly used for sarcoma (such as doxorubicin and ifosfamide) have negligible activity. The mechanisms of resistance of GIST to chemotherapy are unknown but may include increased expression of *p*-glycoprotein and multidrug resistance protein, or the activation of antiapoptotic signaling through KIT.[23]

Intraperitoneal chemotherapy has been used after resection or debulking of peritoneal recurrences, but only data from nonrandomized phase I and II trials support its use. Topical chemotherapy is attractive in the treatment of recurrent GIST because of its superficial pattern of spread. Sugarbaker et al. pioneered this strategy in the late 1980s by using doxorubicin with or without cisplatin.[24] Eilber et al. extended this work by employing intraperitoneal mitoxantrone, a derivative of doxorubicin. This approach proved to be both technically feasible and safe. Furthermore, in the 27 patients who were treated, the median time to recurrence was increased from 8 months to 21 months, although the overall survival was not changed.[25,26] The role of intraperitoneal chemotherapy in the era of imatinib is not known. A small trial at Memorial Sloan-Kettering Cancer Center employing intraperitoneal chemotherapy for metastatic GIST did not confirm its benefit (DeMatteo and Brennan, unpublished data).

TABLE 99.2.
Response Rates to Chemotherapy in Patients with Metastatic GIST (Level III Evidence).

Regimen	*No. of patients*	*Partial response n (%)*
DOX + DTIC	43	3 (7%)
DOX + DTIC +/- IF	60	10 (15%)
DOX + DTIC+ IF	11	3 (27%)
IF + VP-16	10	0 (0%)
Paclitaxel	15	1 (7%)
Gemcitabine	17	0 (0%)
Liposomal DOX	15	0 (0%)
DOX	12	0 (0%)
DOX or Docetaxel	9	0 (0%)
High-dose IF	26	NR (0%–8%)
EPI + IF	13	0 (0%)
Various (e.g., DOX, Gemcitabine, CT2584)	40	4 (10%)
DTIC + MMC + DOX + CDDP + GM-CSF	21	1 (5%)
TOTAL	**266**	**22 (8.3%)**

DOX, doxorubin; DTIC, dacarbazine; IF, ifosfamide; CDDP, cisplatin; VP16, etoposide; EPI, epirubicin; NR, not reported.

Source: Adapted from DeMatteo RP, Heinrich MC, El-Rifai Wa'el M, Demetri G. Clinical management of gastrointestinal stromal tumors: before and after STI-571. Hum Pathol 2002;33:466–477.

Radiation Therapy

Radiation is rarely valuable in the treatment of GIST. Delivery of radiation to the peritoneal cavity is mired in complications related to exposure of the small intestine. Furthermore, the diffuse nature of recurrent GIST makes radiation not feasible. Anecdotal evidence supports the use of radiation for the palliation of GI bleeding or pain from liver, pelvic, or bone metastases.

Treatment of Primary Disease

Surgery represents the only chance for cure in patients with localized primary GIST. Unfortunately, about 20% to 30% of GISTs are metastatic at initial diagnosis. In tumors that are confined to the stomach or intestine, resection can usually be accomplished without significant morbidity. The role of adjuvant treatment with imatinib and its timing in relationship to surgery for primary resectable disease is currently unknown. When resection would require the risk of severe organ dysfunction or where negative margins would be difficult to achieve because of the size and location of the tumor, it may be best to consider the use of neoadjuvant imatinib (see algorithm in Fig. 99.5). The role of imatinib in the neoadjuvant treatment of GIST is currently being evaluated in a prospective nonrandomized fashion by the Radiation Therapy Oncology Group (RTOG) trial 0132.

There are several noteworthy surgical principles. A thorough abdominal exploration should be performed to evaluate for early metastases to the liver or peritoneum. GISTs are soft and friable, so special care should be taken to avoid rupture, which increases the risk of recurrence. GIST tends to be contained within a pseudocapsule, and infiltration of surrounding tissues is not common. GIST should be removed with an intact pseudocapsule, which can usually be accomplished with a wedge resection of the stomach or a segmental resection of the intestine. Every effort should be taken to ensure negative margins; wider margins have not been shown to be beneficial. Surgical staplers can be used, although removal of the staples from wedge resections of the stomach during pathological processing may obscure the true margin. Therefore, we often prefer to open the stomach to ensure a 1- to 2-cm margin of uninvolved tissue. GISTs can usually be lifted away from surrounding structures, but when GIST is densely adherent to adjacent tissues, en bloc resection

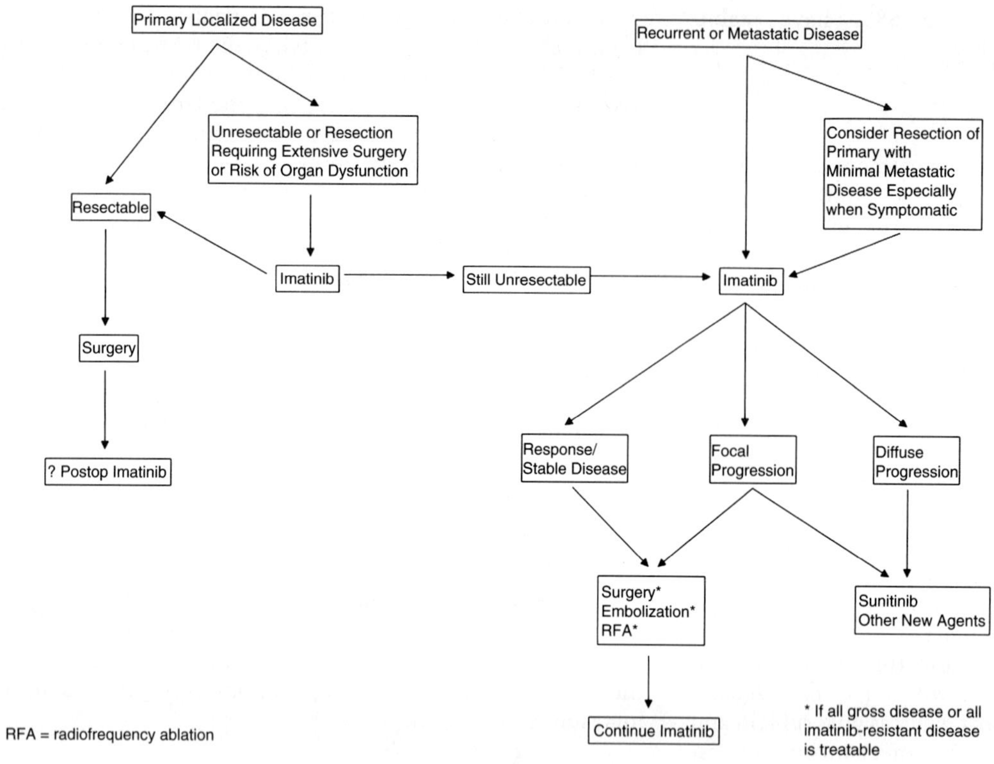

FIGURE 99.5. Algorithm for the management of gastrointestinal stromal tumor (GIST). RFA, radiofrequency ablation.

should be performed. Lymphadenectomy is not indicated as GIST rarely metastasizes to lymph nodes. Although laparoscopic resection of small GISTs may be technically possible, laparoscopic resection of GIST is generally not advocated for larger tumors for reasons of the possibility of tumor rupture.

Although the goal of surgical resection is negative margins, the role of negative margins on the resected organ is uncertain for GISTs larger than 10cm, which may shed tumor cells into the peritoneum from anywhere along their surface. The management of a positive microscopic margin on final pathological review depends on whether the surgeon thinks the margin is truly positive as well as whether the area of positive margin could be reidentified on exploration and whether further resection is technically feasible.

In patients with localized disease, complete gross resection is possible about 85% of the time.[3,5,7,27] Negative microscopic margins are achieved in 70% to 95% of these completely resected cases.[3–5,7,27] Unfortunately, recurrence is common (almost 50%), even after complete resection of localized GISTs. Five-year survival after complete resection of localized GISTs is usually about 50%.[3,4,27] Results of published series reporting outcome for completely resected localized primary GIST are shown in Table 99.3.

The two most important prognostic features of GISTs are their size and mitotic index.[28] Anatomic site of origin has also been identified as a prognostic factor.[8] Gastric GISTs tend to behave more favorably than small intestinal GISTs. Colonic GISTs are malignant at least as often as those from the small bowel. Esophageal GISTs are often diagnosed late and have a poor outcome.

Despite these prognostic features, it is difficult to predict the clinical behavior of any particular GIST. It is now accepted that all GISTs can exhibit malignant behavior and none, except perhaps 1-cm tumors, can be labeled as definitely benign based on clinicopathological features. A commonly accepted system for predicting the malignant behavior of GISTs is shown in Table 99.4.[8]

As GIST is refractory to conventional chemotherapeutic agents and radiotherapy, the standard of care after complete resection historically has been observation. Because of the significant risk of recurrence with surgery alone, the use of imatinib in the adjuvant setting is currently under investigation. The American College of Surgeons Oncology Group (ACOSOG) is conducting two prospective trials for completely resected GIST. The Z9000 trial met accrual in September 2003; 110 patients underwent complete resection of a high-risk GIST (10cm or larger, intraperitoneal rupture or bleeding, or multifocal tumors) and then were treated for 1 year with imatinib 400mg/day. The patients are being followed for recurrence and survival. The Z9001 trial is a randomized, double-blind trial of adjuvant imatinib following the complete resection of GIST of 3cm or larger. Patients are randomized to either imatinib 400mg/day or placebo for 1 year, and there is a crossover in the event of recurrence. In April, 2007 the ACOSOG Data Monitoring Committee recommended early closure of the study because the trial had statistically demonstrated improved recurrence-free survival with imatinib.

There is no standard of care regarding the proper follow-up of patients with completely resected GIST. There is no proof that earlier detection of recurrent GIST improves survival. Nevertheless, because there is therapy that can halt the progression of disease in most patients, it appears reasonable to perform routine surveillance. Most recurrences occur within the first 3 to 5 years, so the recent National Comprehensive Cancer Network (NCCN) consensus guidelines advocate CT scans of the abdomen and pelvis with intravenous con-

TABLE 99.3.
Outcome of Complete Surgical Resection of Primary Localized GIST.

Author	*Year*	*Level of evidence*	*No. of patients*	*Number with completely resected primary localized disease*	*Median follow-up (months)*	*Number with recurrence (%)*	*5-year survival*	*Comments*
DeMatteo[3]	2000	III	200	80	24	32 (40%)	54% DSS	Tumor size prognostic variable
Crosby[27]	2001	III	50	34	24	15 (43%)[a]	42% OS[a]	All cases small bowel in location
Pierie[4]	2001	III	69	39	38[b]	16 (41%)[c]	42% OS[c]	Tumor size, grade prognostic variables
Fujimoto[6]	2003	III	140	129		14 (11%)	93% OS	All cases gastric in location
Langer[7]	2003	III	39	37	26	10 (27%)		

DSS, disease-specific survival; OS, overall survival.
[a]One patient with completely resected metastatic disease included in analysis.
[b]Follow-up of surviving patients.
[c]Two patients with completely resected metastatic disease included in analysis.

trast every 3 to 6 months during this interval and yearly afterward.[29]

Treatment of Recurrent and Metastatic Disease

The median time to recurrence after surgery is about 19 to 25 months.[3,4,7,27] The site of first recurrence is typically within the abdomen. Metastases to lung and bone may develop subsequently. Approximately two-thirds of patients have recurrence in the liver, about half have recurrence on peritoneal surfaces, and about one-fifth have recurrence at both sites.[3,27] Surgery is usually not effective treatment for recurrent GIST. Complete resection can be achieved in less than 50% of patients with locally recurrent disease. Although peritoneal disease usually rests on top of tissues without deeper invasion, making removal possible with limited resection, this is tempered by the fact that the extent of disease is usually greater than evidenced on cross-sectional imaging and subsequent recurrence after resection is very common. Liver metastases from GIST are usually multifocal and diffuse and thus not amenable to resection. In patients who have resectable liver lesions, resection is usually complicated by recurrence and the 5-year survival was reported as 30% before imatinib.[30]

TABLE 99.4. Estimation of Malignant Potential of GIST.

	Gastric		*Intestinal*	
	Size (cm)	*Mitoses per 50 HPF*	*Size (cm)*	*Mitoses per 50 HPF*
Likely benign	5 or less	5 or fewer	2 or less	5 or fewer
Intermediate	5–10	5 or fewer	2–5	5 or fewer
Probably malignant	More than 10	More than 5	More than 5	More than 5

Source: Adapted from Miettinen M, El-Rifai WE, Leslie HS, Lasota J. Evaluation of malignancy and prognosis of gastrointestinal stromal tumors: a review. Hum Pathol 2002;33:478–483.

Because of the multifocal nature of recurrent GIST and its predilection for further recurrence after resection, recurrent and metastatic GIST should be managed similarly. Imatinib is considered first-line treatment, with further intervention employed after maximal response or lack of response when elimination of all gross disease or unresponsive clones is possible. Results of trials of imatinib in the setting of metastatic GIST are shown in Table 99.1. Approximately 50% of patients will have a response and about 75% to 85% at least will have stable disease.[31–36] Approximately 70% of patients with metastatic disease will be alive 2 years after starting imatinib mesylate and about 50% will be free of progression.

Initial response to imatinib treatment can be followed by CT or ^{18}FDG-PET. On CT, lesions that are responsive to imatinib may regress or change in appearance from hypervascular to hypoattenuating and homogeneous. On ^{18}FDG-PET, responsive lesions become "cold." CT is the preferred modality for serial monitoring as it provides more anatomic information. Although imatinib can keep metastatic GIST from progressing and complete responses are rare, lifelong treatment is recommended and withdrawal is not advocated unless toxicities are not manageable. In patients who do not respond to imatinib at 400 mg/day or who become refractory to that dose, dose escalation to 800 mg/day may be of benefit.

In patients who respond to imatinib, surgery should be considered if all gross disease can be resected, as resistance to imatinib may be encountered as treatment is continued. Similarly, in patients who exhibit a variable response with some tumors progressing through imatinib and others remaining dormant, surgery can be considered for the progressive disease. In addition to formal hepatic resection, radiofrequency ablation (RFA) and hepatic artery embolization may be used to control liver metastases (Fig. 99.6). The benefit of cytoreduction in combination with imatinib is currently unknown.

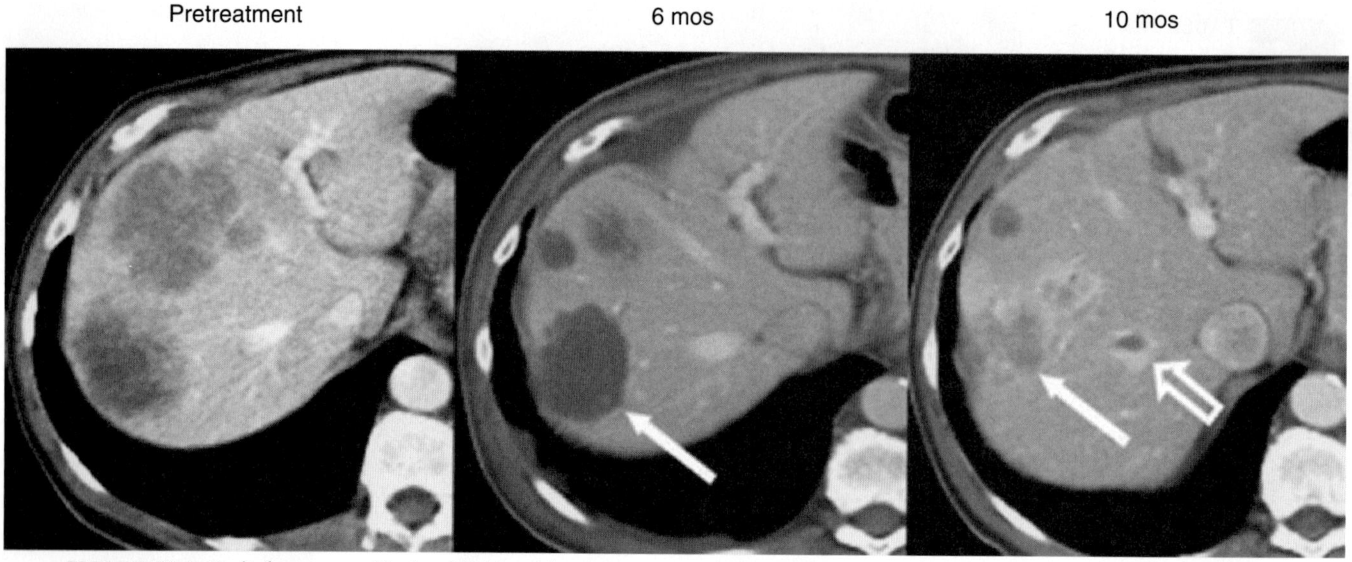

FIGURE 99.6. Radiofrequency ablation (RFA) and hepatic artery embolization may be used to control liver metastases (*arrows*).

Summary

Although it is a rare tumor, GIST has garnered much attention for its response to a novel targeted anticancer agent. Although the treatment for localized primary disease is still primarily surgical, recurrence is unfortunately a frequent event. The role of imatinib in the adjuvant and neoadjuvant setting is under investigation. Evolving questions about the optimal management of GIST will need to be addressed in a multidisciplinary fashion. The integration of surgery and targeted therapy in GIST will likely be a prototype for the management of other solid tumors as new targeted agents become available.

References

1. Kindblom LG. Gastrointestinal stromal tumors: diagnosis, epidemiology, prognosis. Presented at ASCO Annual Meeting, Chicago, IL, 2003.
2. Thomas RM, Sobin LH. Gastrointestinal cancer. Cancer (Phila) 1995;75:154–170.
3. DeMatteo RP, Lewis JJ, Leung D, et al. Two hundred gastrointestinal stromal tumors: recurrence patterns and prognostic factors for survival. Ann Surg 2000;231:51–58.
4. Pierie J-PEN, Choudry U, Muzikansky A, et al. The effect of surgery and grade on outcome of gastrointestinal stromal tumors. Arch Surg 2001;136:383–389.
5. Singer S, Rubin BP, Lux ML, et al. Prognostic value of KIT mutation type, mitotic activity, and histologic subtype in gastrointestinal stromal tumors. J Clin Oncol 2002;20:3898–3905.
6. Fujimoto Y, Nakanishi Y, Yoshimura K, Shimoda T. Clinicopathologic study of primary malignant gastrointestinal stromal tumor of the stomach, with special reference to prognostic factors: analysis of results in 140 surgically resected patients. Gastric Cancer 2003;6:39–48.
7. Langer C, Gunawan B, Schuler P, et al. Prognostic factors influencing surgical management and outcome of gastrointestinal stromal tumours. Br J Surg 2003;90:332–339.
8. Emory TS, Sobin LH, Lukes L, et al. Prognosis of gastrointestinal smooth-muscle (stromal) tumors: dependence on anatomic site. Am J Surg Pathol 1999;23:82–87.
9. DeMatteo RP, Maki RG, Antonescu CC, Brennan MF. Targeted molecular therapy for cancer: the application of STI571 to gastrointestinal stromal tumor. Curr Probl Surg 2003;40:144–193.
10. Fletcher CDM, Berman JJ, Corless C, et al. Diagnosis of gastrointestinal stromal tumors: a consensus approach. Hum Pathol 2002;33:459–465.
11. Hirota S, Isozaki K, Moriyama Y, et al. Gain-of-function mutations of c-KIT in human gastrointestinal stromal tumors. Science 1998;279:577–580.
12. Antonescu CR, Viale A, Sarran L, et al. Gene expression in gastrointestinal stromal tumors is distinguished by KIT genotype and anatomic site. Clin Cancer Res 2004;10:3282–3290.
13. Heinrich MC, Corless CL, Demetri GD, et al. Kinase mutations and imatinib response in patients with metastatic gastrointestinal stromal tumor. J Clin Oncol 2003;21:4342–4349.
14. Druker BJ, Tamura S, Buchdunger E, et al. Effects of a selective inhibitor of the ABL tyrosine kinase on the growth of BCR-ABL positive cells. Nat Med 1996;2:561–566.
15. Druker BJ, Sawyers CL, Kantarjian H, et al. Activity of a specific inhibitor of the BCR-ABL tyrosine kinase in the blast crisis of chronic myeloid leukemia and acute lymphoblastic leukemia with the Philadelphia chromosome. N Engl J Med 2001;344:1038–1042.
16. Druker BJ, Talpaz M, Resta DJ, et al. Efficacy and safety of a specific inhibitor of the BCR-ABL tyrosine kinase in chronic myeloid leukemia. N Engl J Med 2001;344:1031–1037.
17. Tuveson DA, Willis NA, Jacks T, et al. STI571 inactivation of the gastrointestinal stromal tumor c-KIT oncoprotein: biological and clinical implications. Oncogene 2001;20:5054–5058.
18. Joensuu H, Roberts PJ, Sarlomo-Rikala M, et al. Effect of the tyrosine kinase inhibitor STI571 in a patient with a metastatic gastrointestinal stromal tumor. N Engl J Med 2001;344:1052–1056.
19. Heinrich MC, Corless CL, Duensing A, et al. PDGFRA activating mutations in gastrointestinal stromal tumors. Science 2003;299:708–710.
20. Fletcher JA, Corless CL, Dimitrijevic S, et al. Mechanisms of resistance to imatinib mesylate (IM) in advanced gastrointestinal stromal tumor (GIST). Proc Am Soc Clin Oncol 2003;22:815.
21. Demetri GD, Desai J, Fletcher JA, et al. SU11248, a multitargeted tryosine kinase inhibitor, can overcome imatinib (IM)

resistance caused by diverse genomic mechanisms in patients (pts) with metastatic gastrointestinal stromal tumor (GIST). J Clin Oncol 2004;22(14S):3001.
22. Desai J, Maki R, Heinrich MC, et al. Activity and tolerability of the multitargeted tyrosine kinase inhibitor SU11248 in patients (pts) with metastatic gastrointestinal stromal tumor (GIST) refractory to imatinib mesylate. Presented at 2004 Gastrointestinal Cancers Symposium, San Francisco, CA, 2004.
23. DeMatteo RP, Heinrich MC, El-Rifai WeM, Demetri G. Clinical management of gastrointestinal stromal tumors. Hum Pathol 2002;33:466–477.
24. Berthet B, Sugarbaker TA, Chang D, Sugarbaker PH. Quantitative methodologies for selection of patients with recurrent abdominopelvic sarcoma for treatment. Eur J Cancer 1999;35:413–419.
25. Eilber FC, Rosen G, Forscher C, et al. Recurrent gastrointestinal stromal sarcomas. Surg Oncol 2000;9:71–75.
26. Eilber FC, Rosen G, Forscher C, et al. Surgical resection and intraperitoneal chemotherapy for recurrent abdominal sarcomas. Ann Surg Oncol 1999;6:645–650.
27. Crosby JA, Catton CN, Davis A, et al. Malignant gastrointestinal stromal tumors of the small intestine: a review of 50 cases from a prospective database. Ann Surg Oncol 2001;8:50–59.
28. Miettinen M, El-Rifai WeM, Leslie HS, Lasota J. Evaluation of malignancy and prognosis of gastrointestinal stromal tumors: a review. Hum Pathol 2002;33:478–483.
29. Demetri GD, Benjamin R, Blanke CD, et al. Optimal management of patients with gastrointestinal stromal tumors (GIST): expansion and update of NCCN Clinical Practice Guidelines. J Comprehensive Cancer Network 2004;(in press).
30. DeMatteo RP, Shah A, Fong Y, et al. Results of hepatic resection for sarcoma metastatic to liver. Ann Surg 2001;234:540–547; discussion 547–548.
31. van Oosterom AT, Judson I, Verweij J, et al. Safety and efficacy of imatinib (STI571) in metastatic gastrointestinal stromal tumours: a phase I study. Lancet 2001;358:1421–1423.
32. Heinrich MC, Rubin BP, Longley BJ, Fletcher JA. Biology and genetic aspects of gastrointestinal stromal tumors: KIT activation and cytogenetic alterations. Hum Pathol 2002;33:484–495.
33. van Oosterom AT, Judson IR, Verweij J, et al. Update of phase I study of imatinib (STI571) in advanced soft tissue sarcomas and gastrointestinal stromal tumors: a report of the EORTC Soft Tissue and Bone Sarcoma Group. Eur J Cancer 2002;38:S83–S87.
34. Benjamin RS, Rankin C, Fletcher C, et al. Phase III dose-randomized study of imatinib mesylate (STI571) for GIST: Intergroup S0033 early results. Proc Am Soc Clin Oncol 2003;22:814.
35. Verweij PJ, Casali PG, Zalcberg PJ, et al. Progression-free survival in gastrointestinal stromal tumours with high-dose imatinib: randomized trial. Lancet 2004;364:1127–1134.
36. Blanke C, Joensuu H, Demetri G, et al. Long-term follow-up of advanced gastrointestinal stromal tumor (GIST) patients treated with imatinib mesylate. Presented at 2004 Gastrointestinal Cancers Symposium, San Francisco, CA, 2004.
37. Demetri GD, von Mehren M, Blanke CD, et al. Efficacy and safety of imatinib mesylate in advanced gastrointestinal stromal tumors. N Engl J Med 2002;347:472–480.

100

Head and Neck Malignancies

Jeffrey S. Moyer and Carol R. Bradford

Head and neck cancer accounts for 4% of all new cancer cases and 2% of all cancer deaths in the United States annually. This statement translates into 40,000 new diagnoses of head and neck cancer (30,300 with oral cavity and pharyngeal cancer and 12,500 with laryngeal cancer).[1] Head and neck cancer has a much greater incidence in certain parts of the world, particularly in India, and is a leading cause of cancer mortality worldwide.[2]

Survival rates in head and neck cancer have not significantly improved over the past three decades despite improvements in diagnosis and local management. Development of second primary tumors remains a major threat to long-term survival in patients initially cured of head and neck squamous cell carcinoma (HNSCC).[3] In addition to the problem of long-term survival in the face of a second primary risk, HNSCC patients also face tremendous quality-of-life effects following definitive treatment. Occurring in several distinct sites and linked only by common squamous histology, HNSCC may be the most diverse class of malignancies lumped together under one diagnostic heading. Squamous cell carcinoma of the vocal cord and pyriform sinus illustrate the diversity of HNSCC. Although the anatomic sites are only a small distance apart, cancer of the vocal cord has a low metastatic potential and high curability whereas cancer of the pyriform sinus metastasizes early and has a grim prognosis, despite matching for tumor stage. The difference in survival is explained not only by anatomic factors but also by major differences in tumor biology across sites.

New strategies for the management of HNSCC are desperately needed. A team approach is essential and should include head and neck surgeons, radiation oncologists, medical oncologists, plastic and reconstructive surgeons, specialized radiologists and pathologists, speech pathologists, dentists, maxillofacial prosthedontists, nurses, social workers, nutritionists, and physical therapists. The clinical manifestations of disease are varied and may impact the cosmetic and functional integrity of the head and neck region. The associated morbidities of tumor and/or treatment impact all the special senses to a great or lesser degree, most notably speech, swallowing, breathing, and mastication. Advances in organ preservation utilizing chemoradiation approaches are beginning to offer realistic hopes for improvements in HNSCC patient survival and quality of life.

Etiology and Epidemiology

Tobacco and Alcohol Exposure

Approximately 90% of head and neck cancers occur after exposure to known carcinogens, specifically tobacco and alcohol. Tobacco is a carcinogen that initiates a linear dose–response carcinogenic effect in which duration is more important than intensity of exposure.[4] In heavy smokers, roughly 15 years must pass before the risk approximates the level of nonsmokers. Smokeless tobacco and betel nut significantly elevate the risk of oral cavity cancers. For example, squamous cell carcinoma (SCC) of the oral cavity and hypopharynx account for only 3% of all cancers in the United States, where smokers outnumber chewers. In contrast, 50% of all cancers in Bombay, where chewing betel nut is endemic, are SCCs of the oral cavity and hypopharynx.[5] Marijuana use appears to confer an even greater risk for HNSCC than does cigarette smoking.[6]

Alcohol is an equally important promoter of carcinogenesis and is a contributing factor in at least 75% of HNSCC.[7] The major clinical significance is that it potentiates the carcinogenic effect of tobacco at every level of tobacco use. The causative effect is most striking at the highest exposure levels to both. The magnitude of the effect is synergistic rather than simply additive.

Viruses

Viral agents have been implicated in the pathogenesis of oral, laryngeal, and nasopharyngeal carcinomas. Increasing data have emerged supporting a role for human papilloma virus (HPV) in the development of head and neck neoplasms. HPVs comprise a heterogeneous group of more than 70 viral types, each of which induces the proliferation of epithelium at various body sites. Although the role is less clear in head and neck cancer than for cervical cancer, HPV DNA has been identified in primary tumors of the tonsil,[8,9] larynx,[10] hypopharynx,[10] oral cavity,[11] tongue,[12] nasopharynx,[13] in cell lines derived from a variety of head and neck carcinomas,[14] and in inverted papillomas that have progressed to SCC.[15] Precancerous lesions[16] and metastatic lymph nodes[8,17] have also been shown to contain DNA of the same HPV type as the primary tumor, supporting the involvement of HPV in the development of SCC. The detection of HPV DNA varies widely, from 0% to 100%, depending on the site examined and methods used.[18] The overwhelming majority of these studies have primarily focused on detection of HPV genomic material in upper aerodigestive tract tissues. Consequently, the actual mechanisms by which HPV functions in malignant transformation remain ill defined. A study using polymerase chain reaction (PCR) techniques and antibodies to HPV type 16 capsid in a population-based case-control study supports a role for HPV type 16 in development of a small proportion of oral cancers, most likely in combination with cigarette smoking.[19]

There is a strong epidemiological link between Epstein–Barr virus and nasopharyngeal carcinoma (NPC). Regardless of the histopathological subtype [World Health Organization (WHO) I–III], ethnicity, or epidemiological pattern, NPC is an EBV-associated malignancy. Epstein–Barr nuclear antigen, DNA, and transmissible virus have been identified in WHO types II and III, and EBV DNA has been identified in well-differentiated NPC (WHO type I).[20,21] Of note, NPC is 20 times more common in the Far East than in North America, particularly in the southern areas of mainland China, and is typically WHO type II or III.[22]

Diet and Chemoprevention

Considerable preclinical evidence suggests that vitamin A, vitamin E, and β-carotene play a protective role in epithelial neoplasia.[23–25] Several large clinical chemoprevention studies, however, have not demonstrated a significant survival benefit of the use of vitamin A or vitamin E analogues for oral premalignant lesions or second primary tumors of the upper aerodigestive tract.[26] In fact, some studies have shown that vitamin E actually increases the risk for recurrence and second primaries.[27] Significant toxicity has been associated with some vitamin A regimens.

Radiation

There is no strong association between exposure to ionizing radiation and development of squamous carcinoma of the head and neck. Gamma irradiation, however, is associated with thyroid cancers, sarcomas of the head and neck, and malignancies of the salivary glands and paranasal sinuses. Lip cancer is associated with ultraviolet B exposure. Paranasal sinus cancers are related to radium dial painting.[28]

Occupation

Exposure to nickel refining, woodworking, and leather working are risk factors for adenocarcinomas of the sinonasal region.[29,30]

Anatomy

The term "cancer of the head and neck" describes a diverse collection of cancers arising from a variety of anatomic sites in the upper aerodigestive tract with a varied histopathology. Most commonly this terminology has applied to those cancers arising from the mucosal surfaces of the upper aerodigestive tract and are typically squamous cell carcinomas. Other relevant sites include the nose and paranasal sinuses as well as the salivary glands (major and minor).

Oral Cavity

The oral cavity includes the lips, buccal mucosa, anterior or oral tongue (two-thirds), floor of mouth, hard palate, as well as the upper and lower alveolar ridges and retromolar trigone (Fig. 100.1).

Pharynx

The pharynx is a musculomembranous tube extending from the skull base to the cervical esophagus. The muscular support is from the superior, middle, and inferior constrictor muscles as well as other muscles arising from the styloid process and skull base. The pharynx can be subdivided into three distinct

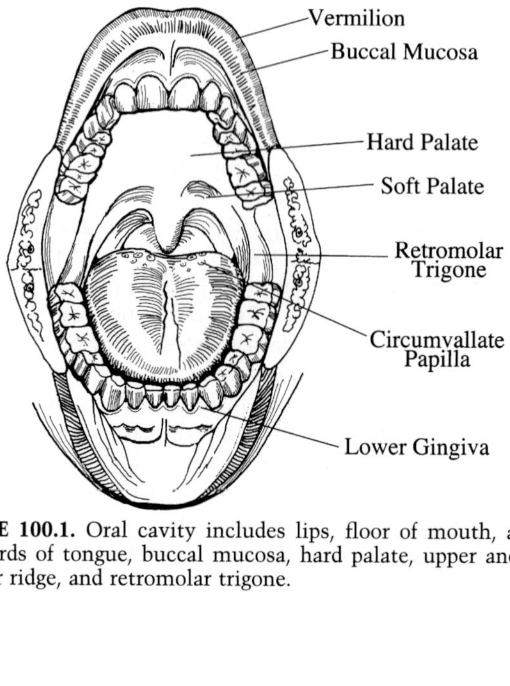

FIGURE 100.1. Oral cavity includes lips, floor of mouth, anterior two-thirds of tongue, buccal mucosa, hard palate, upper and lower alveolar ridge, and retromolar trigone.

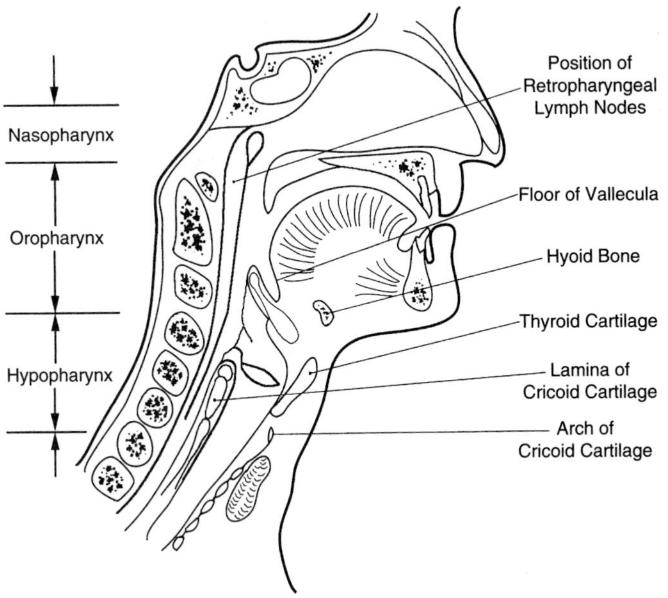

FIGURE 100.2. Sagittal view of the face and neck depicting the subdivisions of the pharynx as described in the text.

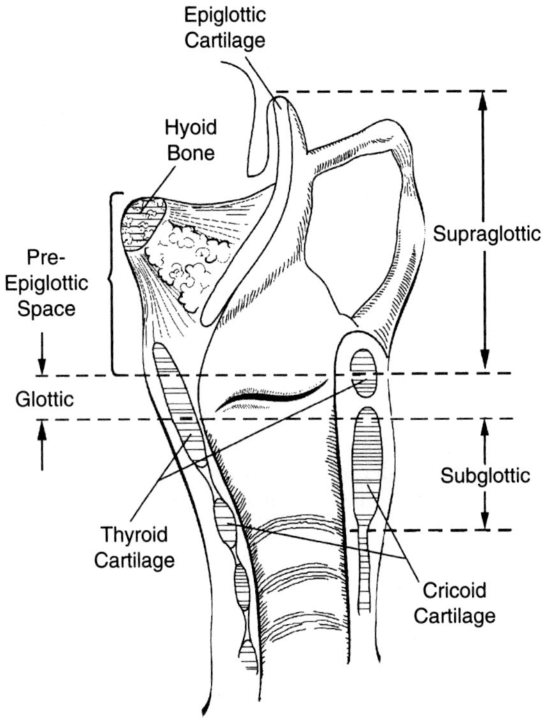

FIGURE 100.3. Sagittal view of the larynx depicting the subdivisions of the larynx. The preepiglottic space is that area anterior to the epiglottis bordered by the hyoid bone superiorly and the thyrohyoid membrane and superior rim of the thyroid cartilage anteriorly.

sites: the nasopharynx, oropharynx, and hypopharynx (Fig. 100.2). The level of the free border of the soft palate separates the nasopharynx from the oropharynx and the level of the hyoid bone separates the oropharynx from the hypopharynx.[31] The nasopharynx begins anteriorly at the posterior nasal choana and extends along the plane of the airway to the free border of the soft palate (Fig. 100.2). It includes the vault, lateral walls, and posterior wall. The oropharynx includes the tonsillar area (tonsillar fossa, anterior and posterior pillars), the tongue base, the inferior surface of the soft palate and uvula, and the lateral and posterior pharyngeal walls. The hypopharynx extends from the plane of the hyoid bone to the plane of the cricoid cartilage. The hypopharynx is divided into three subsites for staging purposes: the pyriform sinuses, the postcricoid mucosa, and the posterior and lateral hypopharyngeal walls.

Larynx

The larynx is composed of a mucosally covered cartilaginous framework (the thyroid and cricoid cartilages). The larynx is divided into three anatomically distinct regions: the supraglottis, the glottis, and the subglottis (Fig. 100.3). The supraglottic larynx includes the laryngeal and lingual surfaces of the epiglottis, aryepiglottic folds, arytenoids, and false vocal folds (Fig. 100.4). The glottic larynx includes the true vocal cords and the anterior and posterior commissures. The glottic larynx occupies a horizontal plane 1 cm in thickness that extends inferiorly from the lateral margin of the ventricle. The subglottic larynx extends from the lower boundary of the glottis to the inferior border of the cricoid cartilage. The supraglottic lymphatics drain to the cervical lymph nodes through the thyrohyoid membrane; the subglottic lymphatics drain through the cricothyroid membrane. The level of the glottic larynx is a relative watershed for lymphatic drainage.

Neck

Anatomic considerations in the treatment of cancers of the head and neck must include a thorough understanding of the neural, vascular, and lymphatic structures of the neck. There are 10 major groups of lymph nodes in the head and neck: these include the occipital, mastoid, parotid, submandibular, facial, submental, sublingual, retropharyngeal, anterior

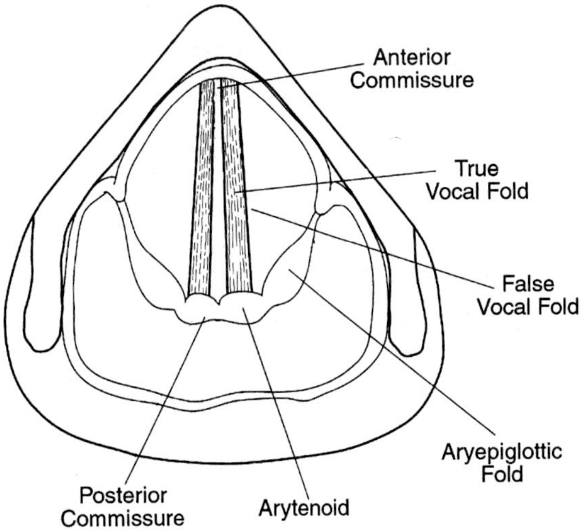

FIGURE 100.4. Laryngoscopic view of endolarynx. Relevant structures are identified.

cervical, and lateral cervical lymph node groups. Primary and secondary echelon lymph node drainage has been determined for each major site in the head and neck (Fig. 100.5). For the purposes of regional treatment, the various lymph node groups have been divided into six levels (Fig. 100.6). Level I includes the submental and submandibular nodal groups. Level II consists of the upper jugular or jugulodigastric lymph nodes (from the skull base to the carotid bifurcation). Level III includes the middle jugular nodes (from the carotid bifurcation to the omohyoid muscle). Level IV includes the lower jugular group (from the omohyoid muscle to the clavicle). The anterior border of the jugular nodal stations is the anterior border of the sternocleidomastoid muscle, and the posterior border is the posterior border of the sternocleidomastoid muscle. Level V nodes include the posterior accessory chain and transverse cervical nodes. Level V is bounded anteriorly by the posterior border of the sternocleidomastoid muscle and posteriorly by the anterior border of the trapezius muscle. Level VI contains the lymph nodes of the anterior compartment from the hyoid bone superiorly to the suprasternal notch inferiorly. The medial border of the carotid sheath forms the lateral border of level VI.[31]

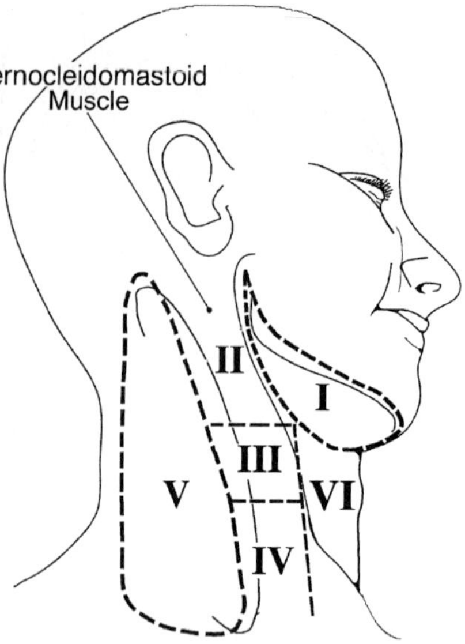

FIGURE 100.6. Division of cervical lymph nodes by levels. The level system for describing location of cervical lymph nodes is demonstrated. Refer to the text for a description of nodal stations I–VI.

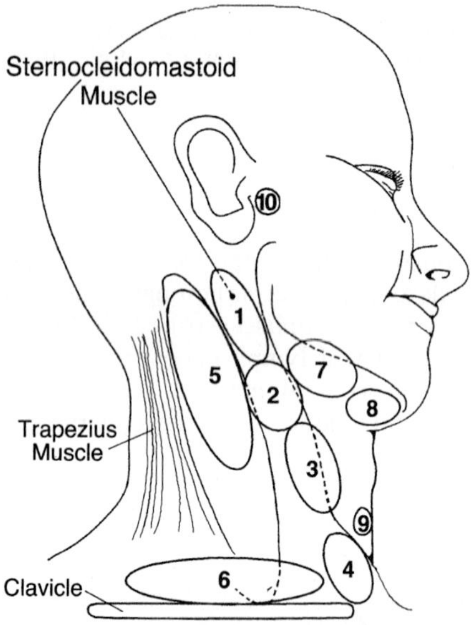

FIGURE 100.5. Depicted is a guide to usual lymphatic drainage patterns for head and neck malignancies as it pertains to usual patterns of early metastases. The primary lesions are listed under each level. (*1*) Superior jugular nodes: (a) nasopharynx, (b) base of tongue, (c) palatine tonsil, (d) parotid gland, and (e) larynx. (*2*) Subdigastric lymph nodes: (a) palatine tonsil, (b) tongue and other intraoral structures, (c) larynx, (d) oro- and hypopharynx, and (e) paranasal sinuses. (*3*) Middle jugular nodes: (a) larynx, (b) cervical esophagus, (c) hypopharynx, and (d) thyroid. (*4*) Inferior jugular nodes: (a) thyroid, (b) larynx, and (c) cervical esophagus. (*5*) Posterior cervical triangle (spinal accessory): (a) nasopharynx, (b) thyroid, and (c) posterior wall of hypopharynx (occasionally). (*6*) Supraclavicular: (a) lung, (b) breast, (c) virtually any head and neck primary, and (d) other locations below clavicles. (*7*) Submandibular: (a) intraoral primary (floor of mouth, buccal mucosa) and (b) submandibular salivary gland. (*8*) Submental: (a) lip, (b) anterior floor of mouth and alveolar ridge, (c) buccal mucosa and (d) breast. (*9*) Cricothyroid (delphian): (a) larynx and (b) thyroid. (*10*) Preauricular: (a) parotid salivary gland, (b) external auditory canal, (c) skin of lateral face, temple region, and scalp, and (d) genitourinary tract.

Pathology

More than 90% of head and neck cancers are squamous cell carcinomas. The comprehensive histological evaluation of head and neck squamous cell carcinomas includes characteristics of tumor–host interactions. Jakobsson and colleagues[32] incorporated degree of keratinization, nuclear grade, mitotic rate, inflammatory response, vascular-stromal response, vascular invasion, and pattern of invasion into the comprehensive histological evaluation. These characteristics have variably correlated with biological behavior. For example, tumors that invade the stroma with thin cords or single disassociated cells behave more aggressively than tumors which invade with a pushing border or thick cords. Other features reflecting aggressive behavior include presence of lymphatic invasion, perineural invasion, lymph node metastasis, and extracapsular spread (penetration of tumor through the capsule of the involved lymph node).[33] The presence of extracapsular spread in cervical lymph node metastasis has been associated with decreased disease-free and overall survival.[34]

Diagnosis

Early identification and treatment of squamous cell carcinomas of the upper aerodigestive tract is the most important component in reducing mortality from this devastating disease. Physicians and dentists must harbor a high index of suspicion and a low threshold for biopsy of any mucosal abnormality such as leukoplakia (a white patch) or erythroplasia (a red patch).[35] In addition, symptoms such as hoarseness, chronic sore throat, referred otalgia, or dysphagia warrant a careful examination of the larynx, oropharynx, and hypopharynx.

Dysphagia, odynophagia, referred otalgia, hoarseness, mucosal abnormalities, weight loss, and neck mass are the most common presenting complaints of HNSCC.[36] Unilateral serous otitis media is a sign of nasopharyngeal carcinoma. Nasal cavity or paranasal sinus neoplasms commonly present with unilateral nasal polyps, nasal obstruction, or epistaxis. A firm unilateral neck mass is cancer until proven otherwise. In an adult, 80% of firm neck masses represent cancer and most are cervical metastasis from HNSCC.

Most commonly, occult or unknown primaries responsible for cervical metastasis arise in the nasopharynx, tongue base, tonsil, or hypopharynx. Close visual inspection in the operating room and random biopsies from these sites are recommended in the setting of unknown primary with cervical metastasis. The use of positron emission tomography has also increased the likihood of identifying the location of an unknown primary. Fine-needle aspiration cytology of suspicious neck masses has greatly reduced the necessity of open cervical node biopsy for diagnosis of squamous cell carcinoma.

Staging

Staging criteria for cancers arising in the upper aerodigestive tract, paranasal sinuses, and salivary glands have been developed by the American Joint Council on Cancer (AJCC). The stage groupings for head and neck cancer are based upon T (primary tumor) stage, N (regional nodal status) stage, and M (distant metastasis). The regional lymph node staging for nasopharyngeal carcinoma varies slightly and the reader is encouraged to review the 2002 American Joint Committee on Cancer Staging Manual for this information[31] (Table 100.1).

TABLE 100.1. Definition of Regional Lymph Node and Metastasis for Head and Neck Cancer.

Regional Lymph Node (N)	
NX	Regional lymph nodes cannot be assessed
N0	No regional lymph node metastasis
*N1	Metastasis in a single ipsilateral lymph node, 3 cm or less in greatest dimension
*N2	Metastasis in a single ipsilateral lymph node, more than 3 cm but not more than 6 cm in greatest dimension; or in multiple ipsilateral lymph nodes, none more than 6 cm in greatest dimension; or in bilateral or contralateral lymph nodes, none more than 6 cm in greatest dimension
*N2a	Metastasis in a single ipsilateral lymph node more than 3 cm but not more than 6 cm in greatest dimension
*N2b	Metastasis in multiple ipsilateral lymph nodes, none more than 6 cm in greatest dimension
*N2c	Metastasis in bilateral or contralateral lymph nodes, none more than 6 cm in greatest dimension
*N3	Metastasis in a lymph node more than 6 cm in greatest dimension

**Note:* A designation of "U" or "L" may be used to indicate metastasis above the lower border of the cricoid (U) or below the lower border of the cricoid (L).

Distant Metastasis (M)	
MX	Distant metastasis cannot be assessed
M0	No distant metastasis
M1	Distant metastasis

Source: Used with the permission of the American Joint Committee on Cancer (AJCC), Chicago, Illinois. The original source for this material is the *AJCC Cancer Staging Manual, Sixth Edition* (2002) published by Springer Science and Business Media LLC, www.springerlink.com

Treatment

General Principles

Surgery, with or without radiation therapy, has traditionally been the mainstay of treatment for most head and neck cancers. Stage I and II tumors (T1N0M0 or T2N0M0) are typically treated with a single modality, either radiation therapy or surgery.[37] Stage III and IV tumors require a combined modality approach, typically surgery plus chemotherapy and/or radiation therapy. To preserve function at the primary site as well as to potentially improve survival, chemotherapy plus radiation therapy as a primary treatment modality may be offered to patients with advanced cancers of the oropharynx, larynx, or hypopharynx as an alternative to surgery plus radiation. Surgical salvage of nonresponders or persistent/recurrent tumors is essential in patients treated with chemoradiation strategies.

The workup of a newly diagnosed head and neck cancer patient should include a complete history and physical examination, including a comprehensive head and neck examination. Biopsy should be performed of the primary and/or neck mass either in the office setting or in the operative room at the time of formal endoscopy. Triple or panendoscopy has traditionally been defined as direct laryngoscopy, full-length esophagoscopy, and bronchoscopy. As both bronchoscopy and full-length esophagoscopy are directed at the identification of synchronous primary lesions and are of moderately low yield, many head and neck surgeons perform only direct laryngoscopy and cervical esophagoscopy as part of the staging workup. A preoperative chest X-ray or chest computed tomography (CT) scan is routinely indicated. Chest CT for advanced disease is probably preferable to routine chest X-ray given the greater incidence of lung metastasis in this population and the greater sensitivity of this screening modality.[38,39] A barium esophagram may be helpful if rigid esophagoscopy is planned. Further radiologic studies such as panorex and neck CT are ordered as indicated for primary tumor evaluation and/or extent of cervical adenopathy.[37] Positron emission tomography with or without CT is being used increasingly for intial tumor staging, the evaluation of unknown primary tumors, the assessment of recurrent disease, and the monitoring of treatment response.

Surgical Principles

Wide surgical resection for primary squamous cell carcinoma of the head and neck generally can be interpreted as resection of tumor with 1- to 2-cm margins, often with frozen-section control of surgical margins. In conservation laryngeal surgery, much narrower surgical margins are acceptable. There is a body of literature to support the benefit of clear surgical margins in terms of overall patient outcome in HNSCC.[40–43] When tumor is adherent to mandibular periosteum without bony erosion, a cortical or rim mandibulectomy is advisable. When the mandible is invaded, segmental mandibular resection is recommended.

Surgical management of the neck is an evolving science. In general terms, when the risk of occult nodal metastasis exceeds 25% to 30%, selective nodal dissection is recommended, particularly when postoperative radiation therapy is not planned. Selective neck dissection refers to any type of cervical lymphadenectomy where there is preservation of one or more lymph node groups removed by radical neck dissection (levels I–V).[44] In addition, if the surgeon must enter the neck to resect the primary tumor, a selective neck dissection is recommended. Staging of the neck for primary tumors of the oral cavity and oropharynx can be accomplished with a supraomohyoid neck dissection that encompasses the submental and submandibular triangles (level I), the upper jugular nodes (level II), and the midjugular lymph nodes (level III). Many surgeons also dissect level IV in this instance because of the occasional isolated level IV metastasis in tumors of the oral cavity and oropharynx and the limited additional effort and morbidity required with this dissection. Similarly, staging of the neck for primary tumors of the larynx or hypopharynx can be accomplished with a lateral neck dissection, which includes the upper, mid-, and lower jugular nodes (levels II, III, IV).

Surgical management of the N1 neck is controversial. Some surgeons perform selective neck dissection and others perform modified neck dissection. Modified radical neck dissection refers to the excision of all lymph node stations routinely removed by radical neck dissection (levels I–V) with preservation of one or more nonlymphatic structures; that is, spinal accessory nerve, internal jugular vein, and sternocleidomastoid muscle.[44] Modified or radical neck dissection is indicated for N2 or N3 nodal disease.

Radiation Therapy Principles

Radiation therapy is an effective modality in treating local/regional disease. For early lesions (stage I/II), radiation therapy offers comparable cure rates to surgical excision. Local tumor control rates are generally better with primary surgical resection, but local recurrences after primary radiation can be managed successfully with salvage surgery. Surgical complication rates are increased following radiation therapy. The choice between radiation therapy and surgery as definitive primary treatment depends upon a consideration of treatment morbidity and functional outcome.

For stage III/IV disease (extensive primary tumors or regional metastases), planned combined modality treatment offers improved local/regional control rates. Although radiotherapy can be given either preoperatively or postoperatively, postoperative radiation therapy had improved local/regional control rates (65% versus 48%, $P = 0.04$) in a randomized clinical trial of 277 patients with cancers of the oral cavity, oropharynx, larynx, or hypopharynx.[45] Optimally, postoperative radiation therapy should be initiated within 6 weeks of extirpative surgery.[46] During the past 20 years in the United States, a regimen of 1.8 to 2.0 Gy once a day for 5 days a week has become standard for most head and neck cancer patients. Microscopic or subclinical disease requires 50 to 60 Gy delivered over 5 to 6 weeks; macroscopic tumors require 70 Gy over 7 weeks or more. Doses exceeding 70 Gy are associated with high rates of normal tissue complications. A typical head and neck regimen involves shrinking field techniques in which the various regions at risk receive dosages commensurate with the tumor mass they are thought to contain. The acute effects of radiation include mucositis and skin erythema. The late sequelae include fibrosis, xerostomia, and altered taste.

Three major developments have evolved in recent years in the practice of radiation for head and neck tumors. First is the change in the number and frequency of radiation fractions. Hyperfractionated radiation schemes (involving twice-daily treatments, each delivering a relatively small dose of 1.15–1.25 Gy) allow an increase of the total radiation dose to 80 Gy without increasing complications. Four randomized studies comparing hyperfractionated to standard radiation for advanced head and neck tumors have been conducted to date.[47] All four studies reported improved locoregional control, and three of four studies reported improved survival using hyperfractionation compared with standard radiation. The second major development is the addition of concurrent chemotherapy to hyperfractionated radiation schemes. A recent randomized study compared hyperfractionated irradiation with or without chemotherapy (concomitant cisplatin and 5-fluorouracil) in patients with locally advanced head and neck cancer.[48] This study, which included patients with unresectable disease, demonstrated an improvement in locoregional control, disease-free survival, and overall survival in the combined therapy arm ($P = 0.01$, 0.08, and 0.07, respectively).[48] The third recent development has been the increased use of intensity-modulated radiation therapy (IMRT). This technique utilizes three-dimensional CT imaging and radiation dose–tumor volume histograms to visually assess the risk to surrounding normal tissue and refine delivery of radiation to the tumor. A recent study conducted at the University of Michigan demonstrated that parotid gland salivary flow could be preserved utilizing this technique.[49] Improvement in subjective xerostomia has been demonstrated as well.

Table 100.2 shows representative local control rates and survival data for patients with HNSCC of various sites treated with definitive radiation therapy.

Chemotherapy Principles

Data from many different trials do not demonstrate a survival advantage for use of chemotherapy ALONE for HNSCC compared to standard surgery and/or radiation therapy. Chemotherapy does play a role in the palliation of recurrent or unresectable disease and has proven effective when combined with radiation for organ preservation in trials of the oropharynx, larynx, and hypopharynx.[52–55] The most active agents in head and neck squamous cell carcinoma are cisplatin or carboplatin and 5-fluorouracil. The role of taxanes in head and neck squamous cell carcinoma continues to evolve. Several other agents, including bleomycin, hydroxyurea, and methotrexate, have a high activity in squamous cell carcinoma of the head and neck. Aside from utilization of chemotherapy for these specific indications, chemotherapy must be considered investigational in previously untreated, advanced, resectable HNSCC. Single-arm trials utilizing chemotherapy in primary HNSCC (previously untreated) should be limited to feasibility testing and innovative treatment design.

Large-scale multicenter randomized trials of specific HNSCC sites are critical to establish the benefit of chemotherapy or other novel treatments in this disease. The need for more effective treatments for HNSCC, however, is clear. Although the combination of optimal surgery and radiation therapy has improved locoregional control, it has not improved survival, mainly because of distant metastasis and second

TABLE 100.2. Local Control and Survival Rates for Patients with Head and Neck Squamous Cell Carcinoma (HNSCC) Treated with Definitive Radiation Therapy.

T stage by site	*Local control (%)*[a]	*Five-year survival (%)*[a]
Oral Cavity		
Oral tongue		
T1	80–90	75–80
T2	60–85	40–60
T3	30–50	20–30
T4	25–45	10–15
Floor of mouth		
T1	75–85	70–85
T2	60–80	50–60
T3	30–50	15–40
T4	5–30	5–20
Oropharynx		
Base of tongue		
T1	80–95	65–85
T2	60–75	40–55
T3	40–65	15–20
T4	30–50	5–20
Tonsil		
T1	75–95	65–85
T2	60–80	55–60
T3	40–65	20–40
T4	30–50	10–15
Soft Palate		
T1	90–100	90–95
T2	75–85	65–75
T3	60–70	30–40
T4	25–35	10–15
Nasopharynx		
T1	70–85	60–75
T2	50–60	50–65
T3	20–45	25–50
T4	15–35	5–30
Hypopharynx		
Pyriform sinus		
T1	60–70	30–50
T2	40–50	20–45
T3	30–40	15–25
T4	10–25	5–20
Larynx		
Supraglottis		
T1	80–90	65–90
T2	60–80	50–65
T3	35–70	35–55
T4	30–60	15–40
Glottis		
T1	85–95	80–95
T2	65–75	60–85
T3	20–35	35–60
T4	15–30	10–30

[a]Survival data include surgical salvage for radiation failures.

Source: Adapted from Laramore.[50,51]

primaries. Two years after standard treatment, less than 40% of advanced HNSCC patients will be disease free: local recurrence accounts for 40% of treatment failures, regional recurrence accounts for 15%, and distant metastasis for 50%.[54] Several studies have suggested that chemotherapy may have some activity in reduction of distant metastatic rate.[52,56,57]

Chemotherapy approaches for HNSCC fall into three main categories: (1) neoadjuvant (primary or induction) chemotherapy (before standard surgery and/or radiation therapy), (2) maintenance (adjuvant) chemotherapy (following definitive standard primary therapy), and (3) concomitant chemotherapy (in combination with radiation therapy). The principal goals of primary chemotherapy in HNSCC are to enhance locoregional control, to decrease distant metastases, and to improve overall survival. "Organ preservation" is a term that means preservation of organ function and typically refers to efforts to avoid surgery at the primary site with the use of chemoradiation protocols. A handful of well-designed, multicenter randomized trials have been conducted in head and neck cancer that have added to the standard treatment options available to patients with advanced HNSCC of the oropharynx, larynx, and hypopharynx.[52–55,58] Although none of these trials has shown a survival advantage to date, they have clearly demonstrated the role of chemotherapy and radiation in achieving organ preservation in HNSCC without negatively impacting survival rates.

Three of these studies are summarized here. The completed multiinstitutional clinical trial (VA Cooperative Study 268) showed that induction chemotherapy (cisplatin and 5-FU) combined with radiation therapy is an effective alternative to traditional laryngectomy plus radiation therapy for patients with advanced laryngeal squamous carcinoma.[52] Analysis of the results in 332 patients with 60 months median follow-up revealed that the larynx was preserved in 66% of surviving patients receiving induction chemotherapy plus radiation therapy without a decrease in survival rates.[52] Estimated 3-year survival in both groups of patients was 53% to 56%. Patterns of failure are shown in Table 100.3. Ten-year follow-up on this study revealed no significant difference in overall survival rate, with 30% alive in the surgery arm and 25% of patients alive in the chemotherapy arm.

A second well-designed trial was conducted by the European Organization for Research and Treatment of Cancer (EORTC).[53] This study compared a larynx-preserving treatment (induction chemotherapy plus definitive radiation therapy in complete responders) to conventional treatment (total laryngectomy with partial pharyngectomy, radical neck dissection, and postoperative radiation therapy) in patients with stage II–IV cancers of the pyriform sinus or aryepiglottic fold. Analysis of results in 194 patients with 51 months median follow-up revealed equivalent survival in the two groups (39% in the surgery arm and 41% in the chemotherapy arm). The 3- and 5-year estimates of retaining a functional larynx were 42% and 35%, respectively. Interestingly, there were fewer failures at distant sites in the induction chemotherapy arm than in the immediate surgery arm (25% versus 36%, respectively; $P = 0.041$).

Recently, the National Cancer Center Institute Cooperative Trials Head and Neck Intergroup (R91-11)[58] examined the exact role of chemotherapy in advanced laryngeal cancer with

TABLE 100.3.
Patterns of Failure in the Department of Veterans Affairs Laryngeal Cancer Group Trial (Level I Evidence).

Site of failure	*Surgery arm*	*Chemotherapy arm*
Local	4	20
Regional	9	14
Distant	29	18
Second Primary	10	3
Total	52 (31%)	55 (33%)

Source: Data from Wolf et al.[52]

a randomized, three-arm trial examining whether radiation alone with surgical salvage was superior to either induction chemoradiation (VA larynx protocol) or concurrent chemoradiation. With a median follow-up of 36 months in 497 evaluable patients, there were no differences in survival among the groups studied, but laryngectomy-free survival was greater in the concurrent chemoradiation arm (66%) compared with either the induction chemotherapy arm (58%) or the radiation-alone arm (52%). Distant metastatic failure rates and disease-free survival were both statistically better with concurrent and induction chemoradiation compared with radiation alone.

The postoperative use of chemotherapy and radiation in high-risk patients has also been shown to be highly effective in both the United States and Europe. Two recent studies have demonstrated that postoperative chemotherapy and radiation in high-risk patients (histological evidence of invasion of two or more regional lymph nodes, extracapsular extension of nodal disease, microscopically positive margins, perineural or perivascular invasion) improves locoregional control and probably improves overall survival.[59,60]

Recently, a meta-analysis was performed on three randomized trials comparing surgery plus radiation therapy to chemotherapy followed by radiation therapy in responders in patients with laryngeal and hypopharyngeal cancer.[61] Nonresponders received surgery plus radiation therapy. The two studies summarized earlier are included in this analysis. As before, no significant differences in overall survival or disease-free survival were observed between the chemotherapy and control arms of the studies. Overall survival results are shown in Table 100.4. In the chemotherapy arm, the proportion of patients with an intact larynx was 67% and 58% among patients alive at 3 and 5 years, respectively.

Another large meta-analysis of chemotherapy in head and neck cancer was performed.[62] This study compared the results of locoregional treatment versus the same treatment plus chemotherapy in patients with locally advanced HNSCC. The overall pooled relative risk of death was 0.91, corresponding to an absolute benefit of 4% for chemotherapy (32%–36% 5-year survival rate; Table 100.5). There was a significant interaction between chemotherapy timing and treatment result, with concomitant treatment showing the greatest advantage. Browman et al.[63] confirmed these findings in another meta-analysis of 18 randomized controlled trials of 3192 patients. This study found an 11% relative risk reduction for patients with locally advanced head and neck cancer treated with concurrent chemoradiation compared with radiation alone.

TABLE 100.5.
Meta-Analysis of Chemotherapy (CT) According to Timing of Chemotherapy.

Trials timing	*Patients*		*Survival*		
CT	(n)	(n)	*RR*	P	*Benefit (%)*
Adjuvant	8	1,854	0.98	NS	1
Neoadjuvant	31	5,245	0.95	NS	2
Concomitant	26	3,727	0.81	<0.0001	8
Total	65	10,826	0.91	<0.0001	4

Source: Data from Pignon et al.[62]

An active area of head and neck oncology research continues to be concomitant chemoradiation for advanced HNSCC with the goal of improving survival as well as development of novel, molecularly targeted therapies.

Natural History and Treatment by Site

Oral Cavity

Tumor growth and treatment affect speech and swallowing, particularly for patients with oral cavity cancers. The current T staging of oral cavity carcinoma is shown in Table 100.6.[31] The principles of treatment of oral cavity cancers are stage dependent. For early lesions (T1N0, T2N0), excision of the primary tumor with or without a unilateral or bilateral selective (supraomohyoid) neck dissection is usually the treatment of choice.[37] Pathological assessment of the primary and neck contents at risk can be carried out. Chemotherapy and/or postoperative radiation therapy is indicated for close surgical margins, perineural/lymphatic/vascular invasion, multiple positive lymph nodes, and/or extracapsular extension. Adjuvant radiation therapy is optional for a single positive lymph node without extracapsular extension. An alternative treatment approach is radiation therapy to the primary (70 Gy) and to the neck at risk (50 Gy).

For resectable advanced oral cavity tumors, combined surgery and postoperative radiation therapy is the standard treatment approach.[37] Although many phase I/II trials have demonstrated the feasibility of chemotherapy and radiation for advanced oral cavity cancers, to date no randomized trial has been conducted for this site.[64] As such, this author would strongly advise that chemotherapy plus radiation remain an

TABLE 100.4.
Survival Rates for Larynx Preservation Trials Using Neoadjuvant Chemotherapy (Level I Evidence).

Study	n	*Site*	*Overall survival Chemotherapy arm (n)*	*Surgery arm (n)*	*(chemotherapy/surgery arm)*
Wolf	332	Larynx	166	166	39%/48%
Lefebvre	202	Hypopharynx or AE Fold	103	99	29%/33%
Richard	68	Larynx	36	32	31%/66%
Meta-analysis	602	Larynx/Hypopharynx	305	297	39%/45% ($p = 0.1$)

Source: Data from Lefebvre et al.[61]

TABLE 100.6. Definition of TMN, Stage Grouping, Histopathologic Type, Characteristics of Tumor, and Histologic Grade for Lip and Oral Cavity Carcinoma.

Definition of TMN

Primary Tumor (T)

TX	Primary tumor cannot be assessed
T0	No evidence of primary tumor
Tis	Carcinoma *in situ*
T1	Tumor 2 cm or less in greatest dimension
T2	Tumor more than 2 cm but not more than 4 cm in greatest dimension
T3	Tumor more than 4 cm in greatest dimension
T4 (lip)	Tumor invades through cortical bone, inferior alveolar nerve, floor of mouth, or skin of face, i.e., chin or nose
T4a	(oral cavity) Tumor invades adjacent structures (e.g., through cortical bone, into deep [extrinsic] muscle of tongue [genioglossus, hyoglossus, palatoglossus, and styloglossus], maxillary sinus, skin of face)
T4b	Tumor invades masticator space, pterygoid plates, or skull base and/or encases internal carotid artery

Note: Superficial erosion alone of bone/tooth socket by gingival primary is not sufficient to classify a tumor as T4.

Regional Lymph Nodes (N)

NX	Regional lymph nodes cannot be assessed
N0	No regional lymph node metastasis
N1	Metastasis in a single ipsilateral lymph node, 3 cm or less in greatest dimension
N2	Metastasis in a single ipsilateral lymph node, more than 3 cm but not more than 6 cm in greatest dimension; or in multiple ipsilateral lymph nodes, none more than 6 cm in greatest dimension; or in bilateral or contralateral lymph nodes, none more than 6 cm in greatest dimension
N2a	Metastasis in single ipsilateral lymph node more than 3 cm but not more than 6 cm in greatest dimension
N2b	Metastasis in multiple ipsilateral lymph nodes, none more than 6 cm in greatest dimension
N2c	Metastasis in bilateral or contralateral lymph nodes, none more than 6 cm in greatest dimension
N3	Metastasis in a lymph node more than 6 cm in greatest dimension

Distant Metastasis (M)

MX	Distant metastasis cannot be assessed
M0	No distant metastasis
M1	Distant metastasis

Stage Grouping

Stage 0	Tis	N0	M0
Stage I	T1	N0	M0
Stage II	T2	N0	M0
Stage III	T3	N0	M0
	T1	N1	M0
	T2	N1	M0
	T3	N1	M0
Stage IVA	T4a	N0	M0
	T4a	N1	M0
	T1	N2	M0
	T2	N2	M0
	T3	N2	M0
	T4a	N2	M0
Stage IVB	Any T	N3	M0
	T4b	Any N	M0
Stage IVC	Any T	Any N	M1

Source: Used with the permission of the American Joint Committee on Cancer (AJCC), Chicago, Illinois. The original source for this material is the *AJCC Cancer Staging Manual, Sixth Edition* (2002) published by Springer Science and Business Media LLC, www.springerlink.com

experimental treatment for advanced oral cavity tumors and should be limited to patients enrolled in experimental protocols or those refusing standard therapy. Early results of a protocol conducted at the University of Michigan suggest that the oral cavity is a poor site for the use of chemoradiation strategies.[65]

Lip

Squamous cell carcinoma of the lip is the most common oral cavity cancer. Most occur on the lower lip (90%). Early lesions without neck metastasis can be treated most efficiently with wide excision and closure. Neck dissection is indicated for nodal metastasis. Radiation therapy can be utilized as first-echelon treatment in patients with increased surgical risk or as adjuvant treatment in high-risk tumors. The indications for adjuvant radiation in lip cancers are close or positive margins, perineural/vascular/lymphatic invasion, and recurrent and/or large primary tumors (more than 3 cm).

Tongue

Occult nodal metastasis is present in 30% to 40% of early oral tongue cancers.[66] Therefore, selective neck dissection for all early tongue cancers except the most superficial lesions is advisable. Tumors that are minimally invasive (2mm thick or less) probably do not require neck dissection because of the low risk of regional metastasis.[67] Adequate surgical margins are required for tongue carcinomas, and most early lesions require hemiglossectomy. For radiation therapy to control cancer of the mobile (anterior) tongue, interstitial brachytherapy should be utilized along with external-beam irradiation. For more advanced tongue carcinomas, surgical management often includes subtotal glossectomy, neck dissection, and often mandibulectomy. The pull-through or lip split/paramedian mandibulotomy approaches are most commonly utilized for advanced tongue tumors. When tumors extend across the midline or involve the base of tongue, subtotal or total glossectomy may be required. Modern reconstructive techniques, particularly free tissue transfer, have greatly improved the functional outcome in these patients.[68] In spite of these improvements, total glossectomy patients often require permanent feeding gastrostomy.

Floor of Mouth

Surgery is the treatment of choice for most patients with floor of mouth cancer. Because of the occult metastatic rate of 40% (T2) to 70% (T3), patients with lesions greater than 2 cm in diameter should have either selective (supraomohyoid) neck dissection or irradiation of the cervical nodes.[69] This strategy appears to offer a survival advantage for T2–T4 tumors.[70] For lesions approaching the midline, bilateral supraomohyoid neck dissection versus radiation is recommended. The rates of mandibular invasion increase with T stage (7% of T1, 55% of T2, and 63% of T3).[71] Involvement of periosteum dictates partial-thickness mandibular resection. Exploration by elevation of the periosteum at the time of surgery is recommended when partial-thickness mandibular resection is planned. Depending upon the site of mandibular attachment, one can perform a rim (superior edge) or lingual cortical plate mandibulectomy. When there is radiologic or clinical evidence of bony invasion, a segmental mandibulectomy (full thickness) should be performed.

Several reconstructive options are available for floor-of-mouth defects, ranging from primary closure, allowing to granulate, skin grafting, to local, regional, or free flaps. Small T1 lesions can be treated with wide excision (2-cm margins should be obtained when possible). These defects are best treated with either skin grafting or allowing to granulate when neck dissection is not planned. When the neck is entered, an attractive alternative in nonirradiated patients that provides pliable, thin tissue is the plastyma myocutaneous flap.[72] State-of-the-art reconstruction for larger defects is the radial forearm free fasciocutaneous flap. This flap provides well-vascularized tissue with the capacity for sensory reinnervation that is not as bulky as the traditional pectoralis major myocutaneous flap.[68] Advanced tumors with involvement of the anterior mandibular arch require reconstruction with free osteocutaneous flaps (fibula, iliac crest, or scapula).[68]

Buccal Mucosa

Buccal carcinoma is an uncommon form of oral cavity carcinoma. Buccal cancers often arise in areas of leukoplakia. Early-stage squamous cell carcinoma of the buccal mucosa without bony involvement is best treated with primary radiation therapy based upon a report by Strome et al.[73] Because of the poor anatomic confines of the buccal space it is often difficult to obtain an adequate surgical margin. Surgery plus postoperative radiation therapy is the preferred mode of treatment of stage III/IV buccal cancer. Advanced buccal cancers are challenging to reconstruct because of the creation of a through-and-through facial defect and the risk to the facial nerve. However, modern reconstructive techniques utilizing free tissue transfer allow internal and external resurfacing.

Retromolar Trigone/Alveolar Ridge

Most early tumors of the retromolar trigone or alveolar ridge can be treated effectively with transoral resection including rim mandibulectomy. Advanced lesions require segmental mandibulectomy plus neck dissection (composite resection) and postoperative radiation therapy. Many options are available for reconstruction of lateral mandibular defects including primary closure (permitting the mandible to "swing"), reconstruction bar and regional flap, or osseocutaneos free tissue transfer (i.e., fibular flap).

Oropharynx

The most common presenting symptom of oropharyngeal cancers is chronic sore throat and referred otalgia. Change in voice, dysphagia, and trismus are later signs. The clinical staging of oropharynx cancers is shown in Table 100.7. Survival rates for advanced primary lesions are less than 50%. The presence of lymph node metastasis drops survival rates to the 25% range. Generally, T1 or T2 primary tumors of the oropharynx can be treated equally well with surgery or radiation therapy. Because lymphatic drainage of the oropharynx can be bilateral in all sites except lateralized tonsillar primaries, radiation is often an attractive first-treatment approach. An added benefit is treatment of the retropharyngeal lymph nodes, which are not typically addressed in neck dissection. Advanced oropharyngeal tumors can be treated with surgery followed by radiation or with an organ preservation strategy utilizing concurrent chemotherapy and radiation.[55,74] In this site, an advantage of primary chemotherapy and radiation is the opportunity to spare the patient surgical treatment of the primary. Surgical management of advanced oropharyngeal tumors historically has resulted in significant functional morbidity. Larngectomy may also be required for larger lesions involving functionally important portions of the larynx. Persistent disease at the primary site after chemotherapy and/or radiation, however, dictates surgical salvage. Persistent disease in the neck requires comprehensive neck dissection.

Tonsil

Early-stage tonsil cancers can be treated equally well with surgery or radiation. An advantage of primary radiation therapy is irradiation of the retropharyngeal and cervical lymph nodes. The treatment of advanced tonsillar carcinoma is more controversial.[75] The advantage of surgery and postoperative radiation therapy for advanced tonsillar cancer is that both the primary site and neck receive combined modality treatment. Historically, tonsillar fossa lesions have been treated with radiation therapy primarily, with surgery reserved for salvage. However, several reports indicate that such an approach may decrease locoregional control.[76,77] More recently, the findings of several large randomized trials have shown that the addition of chemotherapy to either radiation alone[55] or surgery and radiation[78] has improved survival relative to control arms. In addition, overall survival with concurrent chemoradiation at this subsite compares favorably to historical surgical controls with improved functional outcomes. Advanced tonsillar cancers encroaching on the mandible require composite resection. Tumors that do not invade the medial pterygoid muscle can be approached with lip-split and paramedian mandibulotomy (preserving the mandible, mental nerve, and chin sensation) and wide local excision with neck dissection. The radial forearm free flap is an ideal flap for recontouring the oropharynx and has significantly improved functional outcomes when surgery is performed for either primary or salvage treatment.

Base of Tongue

Base of tongue cancers present a more challenging management problem. These tumors are often diagnosed late, metastases are more common, and treatment morbidity is greater. Early tumors, especially superficial ones, are best treated with external-beam irradiation because of the functional morbidity of surgical resection of the base of tongue, but some smaller, localized tumors can be resected with the CO_2 laser or electrocautery. Advanced tumors are probably best treated with concurrent chemotherapy and radiation with surgery reserved for persistant disease or recurrence. Patients undergoing surgical resection of base of tongue tumors can have significant problems with swallowing and aspiration that are probably less frequent and severe after successful organ preservation approaches.

TABLE 100.7. Definition of TMN, Stage Grouping, Histopathologic Type, and Histologic Grade for Nasopharynx, Oropharynx, and Hypopharynx Carcinoma.

Definition of TMN

Primary Tumor (T)

TX	Primary tumor cannot be assessed
T0	No evidence of primary tumor
Tis	Carcinoma *in situ*

Nasopharynx

T1	Tumor confined to the nasopharynx
T2	Tumor extends to soft tissues
T2a	Tumor extends to oropharynx and/or nasal cavity without parapharyngeal extension*
T2b	Any tumor with parapharyngeal extension*
T3	Tumor involves bony structures and/or paranasal sinuses
T4	Tumor with intracranial extension and/or involvement of cranial nerves, infratemporal fossa, hypopharynx, orbit, or masticator space

**Note:* Parapharyngeal extension denotes posterolateral infiltration of tumor beyond the pharyngobasilar fascia.

Oropharynx

T1	Tumor 2 cm or less in greatest dimension
T2	Tumor more than 2 cm but not more than 4 cm in greatest dimension
T3	Tumor more than 4 cm in greatest dimension
T4a	Tumor invades the larynx, deep/extrinsic muscle of tongue, medial pterygoid, hard palate, or mandible
T4b	Tumor invades the lateral pterygoid muscle, pterygoid plates, lateral nasopharynx, or skull bases or encases carotid artery

Hypopharynx

T1	Tumor limited to one subsite of hypopharynx and 2 cm or less in greatest dimension
T2	Tumor invades more than one subsite of hypopharynx or an adjacent site, or measures more than 2 cm but not more than 4 cm in greatest diameter without fixation of hemilarynx
T3	Tumor more than 4 cm in greatest dimension or with fixation of hemilarynx
T4a	Tumor invades thyroid/cricoid cartilage, hyoid bone, thyroid gland, esophagus, or central compartment soft tissue*
T4b	Tumor invades prevertebral fascia, encases carotid artery, or involves mediastinal structures

**Note*: Central compartment soft tissue includes prelaryngeal strap muscles and subcutaneous fat.

Regional Lymph Nodes (N)

Nasopharynx

The distribution and the prognostic impact of regional lymph node spread from nasopharynx cancer, particularly of the undifferentiated type, are different from those of other head and neck mucosal cancers and justify the use of a different N classification scheme.

NX	Regional lymph nodes cannot be assessed
N0	No regional lymph node metastasis
N1	Unilateral metastasis in lymph node(s), 6 cm or less in greatest dimension, above the supraclavicular fossa*
N2	Bilateral metastasis in lymph node(s), 6 cm or less in greatest dimension, above the supraclavicular fossa*
N3	Metastasis in a lymph node(s)* >6 cm and/or to supraclavicular fossa
N3a	Greater than 6 cm in dimension
N3b	Extension to the supraclavicular fossa**

*Note: Midline nodes are considered ipsilateral nodes.

**Supraclavicular zone or fossa is relevant to the staging of nasopharyngeal carcinoma and is the triangular region originally described by Ho. It is defined by three points: (1) the superior margin of the sternal end of the clavicle, (2) the superior margin of the lateral end of the clavicle, (3) the point where the neck meets the shoulder. Note that this would include caudal portions of Levels IV and V. All cases with lymph nodes (whole or part) in the fossa are considered N3b.

Oropharynx and Hypopharynx

NX	Regional lymph nodes cannot be assessed
N0	No regional lymph node metastasis
N1	Metastasis in a single ipsilateral lymph node, 3 cm or less in greatest dimension
N2	Metastasis in a single ipsilateral lymph node, more than 3 cm but not more than 6 cm in greatest dimension, or in multiple ipsilateral lymph nodes, none more than 6 cm in greatest dimension, or in bilateral or contralateral lymph nodes, none more than 6 cm in greatest dimension
N2a	Metastasis in a single ipsilateral lymph node more than 3 cm but not more than 6 cm in greatest dimension
N2b	Metastasis in multiple ipsilateral lymph nodes, none more than 6 cm in greatest dimension
N2c	Metastasis in bilateral or contralateral lymph nodes, none more than 6 cm in greatest dimension
N3	Metastasis in a lymph node more than 6 cm in greatest dimension

Distant Metastasis (M)

MX	Distant metastasis cannot be assessed
M0	No distant metastasis
M1	Distant metastasis

Stage Grouping

Nasopharynx

Stage 0	Tis	N0	M0
Stage I	T1	N0	M0
Stage IIA	T2a	N0	M0
Stage IIB	T1	N1	M0
	T2	N1	M0
	T2a	N1	M0
	T2b	N0	M0
	T2b	N1	M0
Stage III	T1	N2	M0
	T2a	N2	M0
	T2b	N2	M0
	T3	N0	M0
	T3	N1	M0
	T3	N2	M0
Stage IVA	T4	N0	M0
	T4	N1	M0
	T4	N2	M0
Stage IVB	Any T	N3	M0
Stage IVC	Any T	Any N	M1

Oropharynx, Hypopharynx

Stage 0	Tis	N0	M0
Stage I	T1	N0	M0
Stage II	T2	N0	M0
Stage III	T3	N0	M0
	T1	N1	M0
	T2	N1	M0
	T3	N1	M0
Stage IVA	T4a	N0	M0
	T4a	N1	M0
	T1	N2	M0
	T2	N2	M0
	T3	N2	M0
	T4a	N2	M0
Stage IVB	T4b	Any N	M0
	Any T	N3	M0
Stage IVC	Any T	Any N	M1

Source: Used with the permission of the American Joint Committee on Cancer (AJCC), Chicago, Illinois. The original source for this material is the *AJCC Cancer Staging Manual, Sixth Edition* (2002) published by Springer Science and Business Media LLC, www.springerlink.com

There are several ways to surgically approach the base of tongue, including mandibulotomy, lateral pharyngotomy, suprahyoid, and median glossotomy.[79–81] Tumors encroaching upon the supraglottic larynx require supraglottic or total laryngectomy. Advanced tumors of the base of tongue frequently require total glossectomy, and the rate of persistant G-tube dependance postoperatively is typically greater than 50%. Reconstruction of this region is frequently performed with larger-volume flaps such as the rectus abdominis myocutaneous flap. This particular site continues to be an area of active investigation for organ preservation utilizing chemotherapy plus radiation therapy approaches.

Soft Palate and Posterior Pharyngeal Wall

Both these tumor sites have bilateral lymphatic drainage. Radiation therapy alone is preferred for most T1 and T2 lesions with the addition of chemotherapy for stage 3 and 4 tumors. The addition of chemotherapy concurrent with radiation for advanced tumors has shown promise in both phase 2 and phase 3 studies. Resection of all but the smallest soft palate tumors is associated with significant functional disability as it pertains to velopharyngeal incompetence. Soft palate reconstruction utilizing free tissue transfer is an evolving art and may offer improved functional results in the future. Small tumors of the posterior pharyngeal wall can be treated surgically and reconstructed with a skin graft. The benefit of radiation therapy over surgery, however, is the management of occult nodal disease in the retropharyngeal region.

Hypopharynx

Squamous cell carcinoma of the hypopharynx is an aggressive disease with a poor prognosis irrespective of the therapeutic regimen instituted.[82] Stage III and IV squamous cell carcinoma of the hypopharynx has 5-year survival rates of 25% and 5%, respectively.[83] The staging of hypopharynx cancer is based primarily upon the subsite of pharynx involved, the presence of vocal cord fixation, and the extent of lymph node metastasis (Table 100.7). Because of the necessity of removing the larynx as part of the surgical management of most hypopharyngeal cancers, chemotherapy plus radiation therapy approaches have been investigated. Lefebvre and colleagues published the results of a European cooperative group study which indicated that induction chemotherapy followed by radiation can be offered as an alternative standard treatment modality for stage II–IV hypopharyngeal cancers.[53] In this study, complete response of the primary tumors to three cycles of chemotherapy was required to proceed with radiation. If a complete response was not achieved, patients received early surgical salvage.

Larynx

The cardinal symptom of laryngeal cancer is hoarseness. Other symptoms include airway obstruction, hemoptysis, odynophagia, otalgia (referred), dysphagia, neck mass, and weight loss. Because of the prominent role the larynx plays in speech, swallowing, and airway, treatment decisions about cancer of the larynx involve significant quality-of-life issues. Anatomic studies have defined the basis for natural anatomic barriers to cancer spread within the larynx and have contributed to the development of precise surgical techniques for partial conservation procedures in early-stage disease. The true vocal cords present an effective boundary between supraglottic and subglottic lymphatic spread. Modern clinical evaluation of laryngeal cancers includes indirect mirror-assisted or fiberoptic laryngoscopy, direct laryngoscopy, computerized tomography, and magnetic resonance imaging (MRI) scanning. The radiologic studies permit assessment for direct extension of tumor into the preepiglottic or paraglottic spaces of the larynx and for detection of cartilage invasion.

In general, stage I and II disease can be managed with radiation therapy or conservation surgery. Stage III and IV disease often requires laryngectomy with or without neck dissection plus postoperative radiation therapy or concurrent chemoradiation with or without induction chemotherapy with surgical salvage for patients who do not respond to the induction chemotherapy.[52] For salvage surgery following radiation therapy, one can perform hemilaryngectomy after radiation therapy whereas supraglottic laryngectomy after radiation therapy is fraught with complications.[84] Laryngectomy after chemoradiation has a high fistula rate (75%), which may require free tissue transfer.[85]

Another alternative is supracricoid laryngectomy with cricohyoidoepiglottopexy.[86] This procedure is a useful alternative to radiotherapy, partial vertical laryngectomy, and total laryngectomy in selected cases of glottic carcinoma, specifically glottic cancers with extension beyond the confines of the membranous true vocal cord or limited vocal cord mobility. Some authors advocate laser CO_2 resection for advanced laryngeal tumors, but this technique appears to be highly dependent on surgical exposure and the surgeon's skill with endoscopic techniques.

Supraglottis

Supraglottic primary tumors account for 25% to 50% of all laryngeal cancers. The staging of supraglottic cancers is based upon the number of subsites involved, vocal cord fixation, and tumor invasion of cartilage or extension beyond larynx (Table 100.8). Supraglottic tumors commonly invade the preepiglottic space. Supraglottic cancers (T2 or greater) have a high rate of lymph node metastasis. T1–2N0 tumors of the supraglottic larynx can be treated with endoscopic laser resection,[87] open supraglottic laryngectomy (Fig. 100.7) with or without selective neck dissection, or primary radiation therapy. As supraglottic laryngectomy is contraindicated after radiation, primary surgery is likely the best way to preserve the larynx in patients who are candidates for supraglottic laryngectomy. In clinically N0 patients undergoing supraglottic laryngectomy, bilateral neck dissection is advocated.[88] Pathological node-negative patients are able to avoid postoperative radiation, which has significant sequelae in patients who have had supraglottic laryngectomy (prolonged dysphagia and airway edema, usually requiring tracheostomy and gastrostomy). Contraindications to supraglottic laryngectomy include transglottic tumors, vocal cord fixation, and anterior or posterior commissure extension as well as patients with pulmonary or other significant medical problems.[89] Supraglottic tumors with preepiglottic space involvement are amenable to supraglottic laryngectomy. T3–T4 tumors requiring total laryngectomy can be treated surgically with

TABLE 100.8. Definition of TMN, Stage Grouping, Histopathologic Type, and Histologic Grade for Larynx Carcinoma.

Definition of TMN

Primary Tumor (T)

TX	Primary tumor cannot be assessed
T0	No evidence of primary tumor
Tis	Carcinoma *in situ*
Supraglottis	
T1	Tumor limited to one subsite of supraglottis with normal vocal cord mobility
T2	Tumor invades mucosa of more than one adjacent subsite of supraglottis or glottis or region outside the supraglottis (e.g., mucosa of base of tongue, vallecula, medial wall of pyriform sinus) without fixation of the larynx
T3	Tumor limited to larynx with vocal cord fixation and/or invades any of the following: postcricoid area, pre-epiglottic tissues, paraglottic space, and/or minor thyroid cartilage erosion (e.g., inner cortex)
T4a	Tumor invades through the thyroid cartilage and/or invades tissues beyond the larynx (e.g., trachea, soft tissues of neck including deep extrinsic muscle of the tongue, strap muscles, thyroid, or esophagus)
T4b	Tumor invades prevertebral space, encases carotid artery, or invades mediastinal structures
Glottis	
T1	Tumor limited to vocal cord(s) (may involve anterior or posterior commissure) with normal mobility
T1a	Tumor limited to one vocal cord
T1b	Tumor involves both vocal cords
T2	Tumor extends to supraglottis and/or subglottis and/or with impaired vocal cord mobility
T3	Tumor limited to the larynx with vocal cord fixation and/or invades paraglottic space, and/or minor thyroid cartilage erosion (e.g., inner cortex)
T4a	Tumor invades through the thyroid cartilage and/or invades tissues beyond the larynx (e.g., trachea, soft tissues of neck including deep extrinsic muscle of the tongue, strap muscles, thyroid, or esophagus)
T4b	Tumor invades prevertebral space, encases carotid artery, or invades mediastinal structures
Subglottis	
T1	Tumor limited to subglottis
T2	Tumor extends to vocal cord(s) with normal or impaired motility
T3	Tumor limited to larynx with vocal cord fixation
T4a	Tumor invades cricoid or thyroid cartilage and/or invades tissues beyond the larynx (e.g., trachea, soft tissues of neck including deep extrinsic muscles of the tongue, strap muscles, thyroid, or esophagus)
T4b	Tumor invades prevertebral space, encases carotid artery, or invades mediastinal structures

Regional Lymph Nodes (N)

NX	Regional lymph nodes cannot be assessed
N0	No regional lymph node metastasis
N1	Metastasis in a single ipsilateral lymph node, 3 cm or less in greatest dimension
N2	Metastasis in a single ipsilateral lymph node, more than 3 cm but not more than 6 cm in greatest dimension, or in multiple ipsilateral lymph nodes, none more than 6 cm in greatest dimension, or in bilateral or contralateral lymph nodes, none more than 6 cm in greatest dimension
N2a	Metastasis in a single ipsilateral lymph node, more than 3 cm but not more than 6 cm in greatest dimension
N2b	Metastasis in multiple ipsilateral lymph nodes, none more than 6 cm in greatest dimension
N2c	Metastasis in bilateral or contralateral lymph nodes, none more than 6 cm in greatest dimension
N3	Metastasis in a lymph node, more than 6 cm in greatest dimension

Distant Metastasis (M)

MX	Distant metastasis cannot be assessed
M0	No distant metastasis
M1	Distant metastasis

Stage Grouping

Stage 0	Tis	N0	M0
Stage I	T1	N0	M0
Stage II	T2	N0	M0
Stage III	T3	N0	M0
	T1	N1	M0
	T2	N1	M0
	T3	N1	M0
Stage IVA	T4a	N0	M0
	T4a	N1	M0
	T1	N2	M0
	T2	N2	M0
	T3	N2	M0
	T4a	N2	M0
Stage IVB	T4b	Any N	M0
	Any T	N3	M0
Stage IVC	Any T	Any N	M1

Source: Used with the permission of the American Joint Committee on Cancer (AJCC), Chicago, Illinois. The original source for this material is the *AJCC Cancer Staging Manual, Sixth Edition* (2002) published by Springer Science and Business Media LLC, www.springerlink.com

laryngectomy plus neck dissection or with concurrent chemoradiation.[52] A third alternative is definitive radiation therapy alone, but this has a lower rate of local control than combined modality treatment.[58] A fourth alternative is the recently described supracricoid partial laryngectomy (SCPL) procedure for selected T1–T3 supraglottic and transglottic cancers.[90] Contraindications for SCPL include tumor extension to the cricoid cartilage, arytenoid fixation, and extralaryngeal spread of tumor. Careful evaluation of quality of life and functional measures will be necessary to determine which treatment approach yields the best outcome. Indications for postoperative radiation therapy for supraglottic cancer include T4 tumors, close surgical margins, and positive lymph nodes.[91]

Glottis

Early glottic cancers are amenable to radiation therapy or microsurgical resection. Vocal results are typically better with radiation therapy, but is dependant on tumor location and surgeon experience. T1/T2 glottic cancers are also amenable to laser resection or hemilaryngectomy (Fig. 100.8). Contraindications to hemilaryngectomy include posterior commissure involvement, transglottic tumor spread, and cricoarytenoid joint involvement. More advanced tumors that would require laryngectomy can be alternatively treated with concurrent chemoradiation, with or without induction chemotherapy.

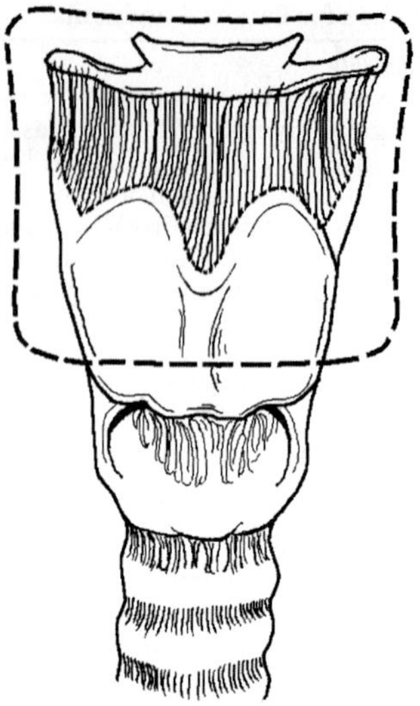

FIGURE 100.7. Supraglottic laryngectomy. The mucosa and cartilage cuts are shown. Resection will include the hyoid bone, the upper half of the thyroid cartilage, and the supraglottic larynx from the ventricle to the vallecula.

Subglottis

Primary subglottic cancers account for less than 5% of all laryngeal cancers. Limited data do support the role of radiation therapy in early-stage disease. More advanced tumors require total laryngectomy combined with resection of adjacent soft tissue. Neck dissection is recommended, as histologically positive lymph nodes are present in roughly 65% of cases. The risk of stomal recurrence is increased in subglottic tumors.

Nasopharynx

Nasopharyngeal carcinoma (NPC) accounts for 2% of all HNSCCs in the United States. One-third of patients initially present with a neck mass, and 70% to 75% have enlarged neck nodes at time of presentation. Presenting symptoms may also include epistaxis, nasal obstruction, headache, or unilateral hearing loss. Unilateral serous otitis media is an indication for evaluation of the nasopharynx. CT and/or MRI are critical for evaluation of base of skull involvement and/or presence of occult lymph nodes.

The World Health Organization (WHO) has defined three histopathological types of NPC: type 1, differentiated squamous cell carcinoma; type 2, nonkeratinizing carcinoma; and type 3, undifferentiated or lymphoepithelial carcinoma.[92] The staging of nasopharyngeal carcinoma is shown in Table 100.7.

The treatment of stage I/II nasopharyngeal cancer is definitive radiotherapy to the nasopharynx. Surgical resection even of early-stage disease is difficult because of proximity to the base of skull. Stage III/IV NPC (M0) is treated with concomitant chemotherapy plus radiation according to the Intergroup Trial, which showed a survival benefit in patients treated this way rather than with radiation therapy alone.[93] Surgery, utilizing various approaches to the skull base, is reserved for very selected patients with recurrent tumors and for some tumors of unusual histology (chondrosarcoma, adenocarcinoma).[37] Patients with metastatic disease can be treated with platinum-based combination chemotherapy regimens. If a complete response occurs, definitive radiation therapy may be added.

Paranasal Sinus and Nasal Cavity

Cancers arising in the paranasal sinuses and nasal cavity are relatively rare, accounting for only 0.2% of all human cancers. Approximately two-thirds arise in the maxillary sinus, and one-third arise in the ethmoid sinus. Malignant tumors arising in the frontal or sphenoid sinuses are exceedingly rare. Sinus cancers are associated with woodworking, nickel refining, and inhalation of noxious fumes (nitrosamines, dioxanes), as well as tobacco exposure. Eighty percent are squamous cell carcinomas but other cell types exist: these include adenocarcinoma, esthesioneuroblastoma, sinonasal undifferentiated carcinoma (SNUC), malignant melanoma, lymphoma, and inverting papilloma. Inverting papilloma is an HPV-associated tumor that characteristically arises from the lateral nasal wall. Inverting papilloma has a propensity for local recurrence and can progress to squamous cell carcinoma, particularly when associated with high-risk HPV types.[94] Malignant melanoma of the nasal cavity/paranasal sinus region has historically been associated with a dismal prognosis. Modern skull base and reconstructive techniques, which have permitted wide local excision, have improved the bleak outlook for this neoplasm.[95] Adjuvant radiation therapy appears to be beneficial for mucosal malignant melanoma.

Malignant tumors of the paranasal sinuses often present at a late stage. Most have bony involvement at the time of presentation. Symptoms are often vague and mimic more benign conditions such as sinusitis. Ohngren's line is a line joining the medial canthus of the eye with the angle of the mandible. This line separates the maxillary antrum into an anteroinferior portion (infrastructure) and a superoposterior portion (suprastructure; Fig. 100.9). The location as well as

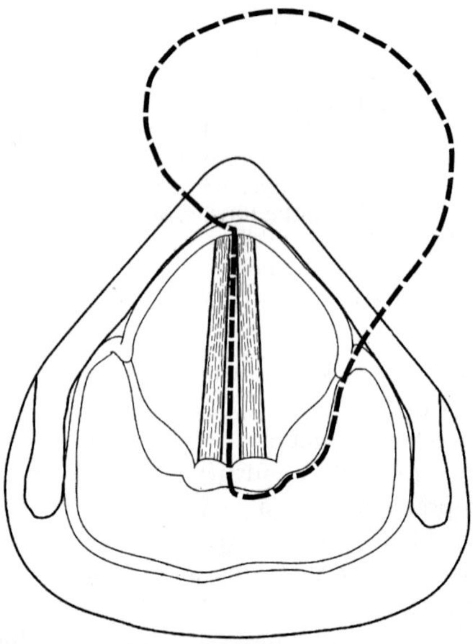

FIGURE 100.8. Vertical hemilaryngectomy involves resection of most of the ipsilateral thyroid cartilage with the underlying vocal cord and thyroarytenoid muscle. The arytenoid can be included in the resection (as shown) or excluded if the tumor does not extend to the arytenoid.

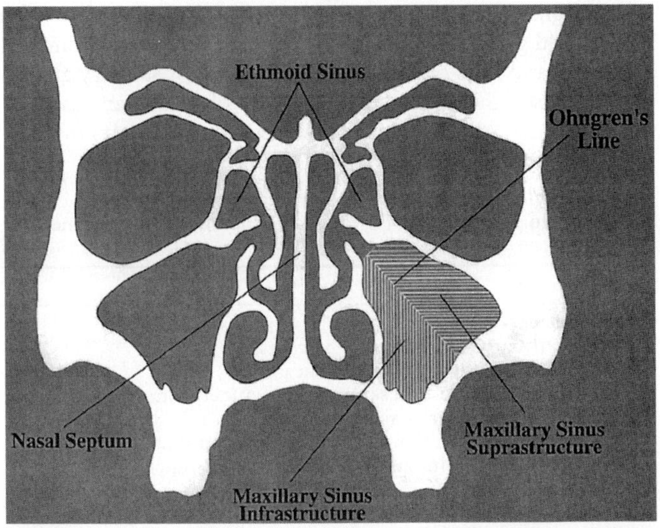

FIGURE 100.9. Anatomy of ethmoid and maxillary sinuses. Ohngren's line divides the maxillary sinus into two components: suprastructure (superolateral) and infrastructure (inferomedial).

extent of tumor has prognostic significance. Tumors involving the suprastructure of the maxillary antrum have a worse prognosis than those involving the infrastructure. Cross-sectional imaging with MRI or CT is mandatory for accurate pretreatment staging of malignant tumors of the sinuses. Primary tumor staging for maxillary and ethmoid sinus cancers is shown in Table 100.9.

Advancement in the treatment of tumors of the paranasal sinuses and nasal cavity is linked to the development of approaches to the skull base and adequate surgical extirpation. Modern techniques include lateral rhinotomy, midface degloving, and subcranial approaches.[96–98] Microvascular free tissue transfer of skin, soft tissue, and/or bone as well as maxillofacial prosthedontics have allowed functional and esthetic rehabilitation of defects arising from resection of sinus and nasal cavity tumors.[95]

Surgical therapy with curative intent is considered in patients without evidence of distant disease who have no medical contraindications, if consistent with a reasonable functional outcome.[37] Maxillary sinus cancers can be managed with medial maxillectomy (preserving hard palate), total maxillectomy, and radical maxillectomy with or without orbital

TABLE 100.9. Definition of TMN, Stage Grouping, Histopathologic Type, and Histologic Grade for Maxillary Sinus, Nasal Cavity, and Ethmoid Sinus Carcinoma.

Definition of TMN

Primary Tumor (T)

TX	Primary tumor cannot be assessed
T0	No evidence of primary tumor
Tis	Carcinoma *in situ*

Maxillary Sinus

T1	Tumor limited to maxillary sinus mucosa with no erosion or destruction of bone
T2	Tumor causing bone erosion or destruction including extension into the hard palate and/or middle nasal meatus, except extension to posterior wall of maxillary sinus and pterygoid plates
T3	Tumor invades any of the following: bone of the posterior wall of maxillary sinus, subcutaneous tissues, floor or medial wall of orbit, pterygoid fossa, ethmoid sinuses
T4a	Tumor invades anterior orbital contents, skin of the cheek, pterygoid plates, infratemporal fossa, cribriform plate, sphenoid or frontal sinuses
T4b	Tumor invades any of the following: orbital apex, dura, brain, middle cranial fossa, cranial nerves other than maxillary division of trigeminal nerve (V_2), nasopharynx, or clivus

Nasal Cavity and Ethmoid Sinus

T1	Tumor restricted to any one subsite, with or without bony invasion
T2	Tumor invading two subsites in a single region or extending to involve an adjacent region within the nasoethmoidal complex, with or without bony invasion.
T3	Tumor extends to invade the medial wall or floor of the orbit, maxillary sinus, palate, or cribriform plate
T4a	Tumor invades any of the following: anterior orbital contents, skin of the nose or cheek, minimal extension to anterior cranial fossa, pterygoid plates, sphenoid or frontal sinuses
T4b	Tumor invades any of the following: orbital apex, dura, brain, middle cranial fossa, cranial nerves other than V_2, nasopharynx, or clivus

Regional Lymph Nodes (N)

NX	Regional lymph nodes cannot be assessed
N0	No regional lymph node metastasis
N1	Metastasis in a single ipsilateral lymph node, 3 cm or less in greatest dimension
N2	Metastasis in a single ipsilateral lymph node, more than 3 cm but not more than 6 cm in greatest dimension, or in multiple ipsilateral lymph nodes, none more than 6 cm in greatest dimension, or in bilateral or contralateral lymph nodes, none more than 6 cm in greatest dimension
N2a	Metastasis in a single ipsilateral lymph node, more than 3 cm but not more than 6 cm in greatest dimension
N2b	Metastasis in multiple ipsilateral lymph nodes, none more than 6 cm in greatest dimension
N2c	Metastasis in bilateral or contralateral lymph nodes, none more than 6 cm in greatest dimension
N3	Metastasis in a lymph node, more than 6 cm in greatest dimension

Distant Metastasis (M)

MX	Distant metastasis cannot be assessed
M0	No distant metastasis
M1	Distant metastasis

Stage Grouping

Stage 0	Tis	N0	M0
Stage I	T1	N0	M0
Stage II	T2	N0	M0
Stage III	T3	N0	M0
	T1	N1	M0
	T2	N1	M0
	T3	N1	M0
Stage IVA	T4a	N0	M0
	T4a	N1	M0
	T1	N2	M0
	T2	N2	M0
	T3	N2	M0
	T4a	N2	M0
Stage IVB	T4b	Any N	M0
	Any T	N3	M0
Stage IVC	Any T	Any N	M1

Source: Used with the permission of the American Joint Committee on Cancer (AJCC), Chicago, Illinois. The original source for this material is the *AJCC Cancer Staging Manual, Sixth Edition* (2002) published by Springer Science and Business Media LLC, www.springerlink.com.

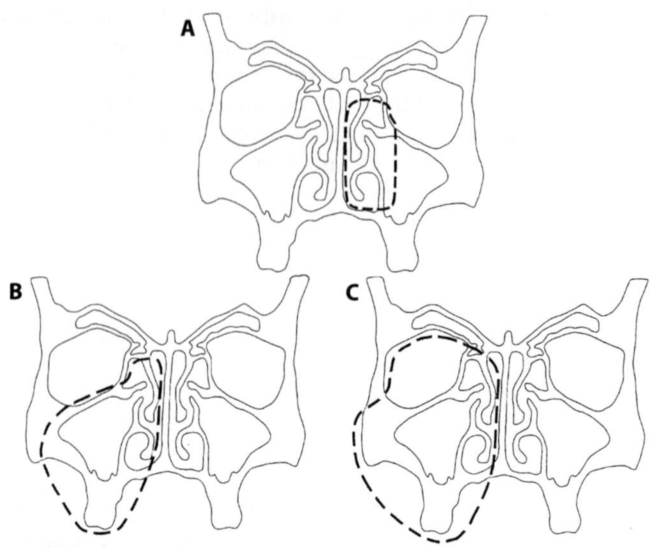

FIGURE 100.10. A. Medial maxillectomy for tumors of the lateral nasal wall (usually inverted papilloma). Medial maxillectomy can be approached via midface degloving or lateral rhinotomy. **B.** Subtotal maxillectomy with preservation of the orbit for carcinoma of the maxillary antrum. **C.** Radical maxillectomy with orbital exenteration for tumors which penetrate the orbital periosteum and/or involve the orbital apex.

exenteration (Fig. 100.10). Orbital exenteration is indicated for tumors involving the periorbita and/or orbital apex. Early cancers of the ethmoid sinus can be treated with external ethmoidectomy. More advanced tumors involving the roof of the ethmoid or cribriform plate require craniofacial resection. Tumors that involve the skull base can be resected via a subcranial approach and reconstructed with pericranial flaps, split calvarial bone grafts, and/or microvascular free flaps.[95] Survival rates appear to be better in patients treated with surgery plus postoperative radiation therapy.[99] For patients in whom adequate surgical resection is not consistent with a reasonable functional outcome (i.e., bilateral orbital involvement, extensive intracranial extension), chemotherapy and/or radiation therapy may be employed. In patients with advanced squamous cell carcinoma, esthesioneuroblastoma, and SNUC, an appropriate chemotherapy regimen may be utilized in combination with radiation therapy, surgery, or both. Advanced tumors in this location have a poor prognosis, and response rates of 50% to 70% have been documented in esthesioneuroblastoma utilizing a regimen of cyclophosphamide and vincristine (with or without doxyrubicin). A retrospective series reported survival benefit with multimodality therapy (including primary chemotherapy) for advanced-stage esthesioneuroblastoma.[100]

Salivary Gland Malignancies

Tumors can arise in major or minor salivary glands. The major salivary glands include the parotid gland and submandibular and sublingual glands. Minor salivary glands are distributed throughout the hard palate, base of tongue, and buccal mucosa. Staging of primary salivary gland tumors is based upon size and extraparenchymal extension (Table 100.10).

Malignant tumors account for 20% of tumors arising in the parotid gland, 50% of tumors arising in the submandibular gland, and 75% of tumors arising in minor salivary glands. Table 100.11 shows the various types of malignant salivary gland tumors. Mucoepidermoid carcinoma accounts for 26%

TABLE 100.10. Definition of TMN, Stage Grouping, Histopathologic Type, and Histologic Grade for Salivary Gland Carcinoma.

Definition of TMN

Primary Tumor (T)

TX	Primary tumor cannot be assessed
T0	No evidence of primary tumor
T1	Tumor 2 cm or less in greatest dimension without extraparenchymal extension*
T2	Tumor more than 2 cm but not more than 4 cm in greatest dimension without extraparenchymal extension*
T3	Tumor more than 4 cm and/or tumor having extraparenchymal extension*
T4a	Tumor invades skin, mandible, ear canal, and/or facial nerve
T4b	Tumor invades skull base and/or pterygoid plates and/or encases carotid artery

**Note:* Extraparenchymal extension is clinical or macroscopic evidence of invasion of soft tissues. Microscopic evidence alone does not constitute extraparenchymal extension for classification purposes.

Regional Lymph Nodes (N)

NX	Regional lymph nodes cannot be assessed
N0	No regional lymph node metastasis
N1	Metastasis in a single ipsilateral lymph node, 3 cm or less in greatest dimension
N2	Metastasis in a single ipsilateral lymph node, more than 3 cm but not more than 6 cm in greatest dimension, or in multiple ipsilateral lymph nodes, none more than 6 cm in greatest dimension, or in bilateral or contralateral lymph nodes, none more than 6 cm in greatest dimension
N2a	Metastasis in a single ipsilateral lymph node, more than 3 cm but not more than 6 cm in greatest dimension
N2b	Metastasis in multiple ipsilateral lymph nodes, none more than 6 cm in greatest dimension
N2c	Metastasis in bilateral or contralateral lymph nodes, none more than 6 cm in greatest dimension
N3	Metastasis in a lymph node, more than 6 cm in greatest dimension

Distant Metastasis (M)

MX	Distant metastasis cannot be assessed
M0	No distant metastasis
M1	Distant metastasis

Stage Grouping

Stage I	T1	N0	M0
Stage II	T2	N0	M0
Stage III	T3	N0	M0
	T1	N1	M0
	T2	N1	M0
	T3	N1	M0
Stage IVA	T4a	N0	M0
	T4a	N1	M0
	T1	N2	M0
	T2	N2	M0
	T3	N2	M0
	T4a	N2	M0
Stage IVB	T4b	Any N	M0
	Any T	N3	M0
Stage IVC	Any T	Any N	M1

Source: Used with the permission of the American Joint Committee on Cancer (AJCC), Chicago, Illinois. The original source for this material is the *AJCC Cancer Staging Manual, Sixth Edition* (2002) published by Springer Science and Business Media LLC, www.springerlink.com

TABLE 100.11. Malignant Tumors of the Salivary Glands.

Classification	*Five-year survival*
Mucoepidermoid carcinoma	97% (low grade) 56% (high grade)
Acinic cell carcinoma	95% (low grade) 58% (high grade)
Adenoid cystic carcinoma	75%
Adenocarcinoma	75%
Carcinoma expleomorphic adenoma	50%
Squamous cell carcinoma	47%

Source: Eneroth and Hamberger (1974)[101]; Johns and Coulthard (1977).[102]

of minor salivary gland tumors and 21% of parotid tumors. In fact, mucoepidermoid carcinoma is the most common malignant tumor of the parotid gland. Low-grade tumors are characterized by slow growth and low recurrence rates following complete surgical excision. High-grade mucoepidermoid cancers are highly aggressive tumors with a local recurrence rate of 60%, a regional metastatic rate of 50%, and a distant metastatic rate of 30%. These high-grade tumors are best treated with radical surgery, including neck dissection, and postoperative radiation therapy.

Adenoid cystic carcinomas account for 58% of malignant submandibular and minor salivary gland tumors and 12% of malignant parotid tumors. This tumor has a propensity for perineural invasion and spread. Although many tumors follow an indolent course, as many as 40% develop regional or distant metastasis over a 10- or 20-year horizon. Surgical management includes radical resection (sacrificing nerves only for direct tumor extension) and postoperative radiation therapy.

Carcinoma ex-pleomorphic adenoma arises from a preexisting pleomorphic adenoma. The risk of malignant transformation increases with duration of presence of pleomorphic adenoma. Adenomas present for more than 15 years have a 9.4% incidence of malignant transformation.[103] True malignant mixed tumors of the salivary gland are exceedingly rare, constituting 2% to 5% of all malignant salivary gland tumors. Acinic cell carcinomas account for 13% of malignant parotid tumors. These tumors have a spectrum of behavior from very indolent to very aggressive. Adenocarcinomas account for 12% of parotid gland malignancies and a high percentage of minor salivary gland tumors. Most are high grade, with a propensity for regional and distant metastasis. Primary squamous cell carcinoma of the salivary gland is rare, if it exists. Batsakis contended that all squamous cell carcinomas of the salivary glands were, in fact, metastases rather than primary tumors.[104] Squamous cell carcinomas in the salivary glands require a search for the primary tumor (including facial skin and scalp) and aggressive treatment including neck dissection.

Surgery is the mainstay of treatment in patients with resectable salivary gland cancer. All malignant tumors of the parotid gland typically warrant total parotidectomy, although in many cases the facial nerve is actually the closest tumor margin. The facial nerve should be sacrificed only for direct tumor invasion. The goal of parotid surgery for malignant tumors is complete tumor removal with the widest possible margins with facial nerve preservation unless the tumor invades and/or encases the nerve. Patients with high-grade tumors prone to metastasis (high-grade mucoepidermoid carcinoma, adenocarcinoma) should also undergo selective neck dissection (N0/N1) or modified or radical neck dissection (N2/N3). Postoperative radiotherapy is indicated for all high-grade tumors (any histology except low-grade mucoepidermoid and acinic cell less than 3 cm), close surgical margins, recurrent disease, skin, bone, nerve, or extraparotid involvement, positive nodes, and for gross residual or unresectable disease.[37] Fast-neutron radiation therapy has a role in patients with large, inoperable salivary gland cancers.[105]

References

1. Boring CC, Squires TS, Tong T, et al. Cancer Statistics 1992; 42:19.
2. Decker J, Goldstein JD. Risk factors in head and neck cancer. N Engl J Med 1982;306:1151.
3. Lippman SM, Hong WK. Second malignant tumors in head and neck squamous cell carcinoma: the overshadowing threat for patients with early-stage disease [editorial]. Int J Radiat Oncol Biol Phys 1989;17:691.
4. Wynder EL, Hoffman D. Tobacco. In: Schottenfield D, Fraumeri JF Jr, eds. Cancer Epidemiology and Prevention. Philadelphia: Saunders, 1982:277–292.
5. Boyle P, Macfarlane GJ, McGinn R, et al. International epidemiology of head and neck cancer. In: de Vries N, Gluckman JL, eds. Primary Tumors in the Head and Neck. Stuttgart: Thieme, 1990:80–138.
6. Caplan GA, Brigham BA. Marijuana smoking and carcinoma of the tongue: is there an association? Cancer (Phila) 1990; 66:1005.
7. Blot WJ, McLaughlin JK, Winn DM, et al. Smoking and drinking in relation to oral and pharyngeal cancer. Cancer Res 1998; 48:3282.
8. Paz B, Cook N, Odom-Maryon T, et al. Human papillomavirus (HPV) in head and neck cancer. Cancer (Phila) 1997;79:595–604.
9. Snijders PJF, Cromme FV, Van Den Brule AJC, et al. Prevalence and expression of human papillomavirus in tonsillar carcinomas, indicating a possible viral etiology. Int J Cancer 1992;51:845–850.
10. Clayman GL, Stewart MG, Weber RS, et al. Human papillomavirus in laryngeal and hypopharyngeal carcinomas. Arch Otolaryngol Head Neck Surg 1994;120:743–748.
11. Kashima HK, Kutcher M, Kessis T, et al. Human papillomavirus in squamous cell carcinoma, leukoplakia, lichen planus, and clinically normal epithelium of the oral cavity. Ann Otol Rhinol Laryngol 1990;99:55–61.
12. De Villers EM, Weidauer H, Otto H, et al. Papillomavirus DNA in human tongue carcinomas. Int J Cancer 1985;36:575–578.
13. Hording U, Nielsen HW, Daugaard S, et al. Human papillomavirus types 11 and 16 detected in nasopharyngeal carcinomas by the polymerase chain reaction. Laryngoscope 1994;104:99–102.
14. Bradford CR, Zacks SE, Androphy EJ, et al. Human papillomavirus DNA sequences in cell lines derived from head and neck squamous cell carcinomas. Otolaryngol Head Neck Surg 1991;104:303–310.
15. Beck JC, McClatchey KD, Lesperance MM, et al. Human papillomavirus types important in progression of inverted papilloma. Otolaryngol Head Neck Surg 1995;113:558–563.
16. Fouret P, Martin F, Flahault A, et al. Human papillomavirus infection in the malignant and premalignant head and neck epithelium. Diagn Mol Pathol 1995;4:122–127.
17. Miller CS, White DK. Human papillomavirus expression in oral mucosa, premalignant conditions, and squamous cell carcinoma. Oral Surg Oral Med Oral Pathol 1996;82:58–68.

18. Steinberg BM, DiLorenzi TP. A possible role for human papilloma virus in head and neck cancer. Cancer Metastasis Rev 1996;15:91–112.
19. Schwartz SM, Daling JR, Doody DR, et al. Oral cancer risk in relation to sexual history and evidence of human papillomavirus infection. J Natl Cancer Inst 1998;90:1626–1636.
20. Connors JM, Jacobs C. Nasopharyngeal carcinoma: relationship to Epstein–Barr virus and treatment with interferon. In: Jacob CJ, ed. Cancers of the Head and Neck. Boston: Martinus Nijhoff, 1987:167–175.
21. Raab-Traub N, Flynn K, Pearson G, et al. The differentiated form of nasopharyngeal carcinoma contains Epstein–Barr virus DNA. Int J Cancer 1987;39:25.
22. Henderson BE, Louis E, SooHoo Jing J, et al. Risk factors associated with nasopharyngeal carcinoma. N Engl J Med 1997; 295:1101.
23. Graham S. Epidemiology of retinoids and cancer. J Natl Cancer Inst 1984;73:1423.
24. Lippman SM, Meyskens FL. Retinoids for the prevention of cancer. In: Moon TE, Micozzi M, eds. Nutrition and Cancer Prevention: The Role of Micronutrients. New York: Dekker, 1989:243–272.
25. McLaughlin JK, Gridley G, Block G, et al. Dietary factors in oral and pharyngeal cancer. J Natl Cancer Inst 1988;80: 1237.
26. Jain S, Khuri FR, Shin DM. Prevention of head and neck cancer: current status and future prospects. *Curr Probl* Cancer 2004;28(5):265.
27. Bairati I, Meyer F, Gelinas M, et al. A randomized trial of antioxidant vitamins to prevent second primary cancers in head and neck cancer patients. J Natl Cancer Inst 2005;97(7):481.
28. Goolden AWG. Radiation cancer: a review with special reference to radiation tumors in the pharynx, larynx, and thyroid. Br J Radiol 1957;30:626.
29. Barton RT, Hogetveit AC. Nickel-related cancers of the respiratory tract. Cancer (Phila) 1980;45:3061.
30. Cann CI, Fried MP, Rotman KJ. Epidemiology of squamous cell cancer of the head and neck. Otolaryngol Clin N Am 1985; 18:367.
31. American Joint Committee on Cancer. AJCC Cancer Staging Handbook, 6th ed. New York: Springer, 2002.
32. Jakobsson PA, Erneroth DM, Killander D, et al. Histologic classification and grading of malignancy in carcinoma of the larynx. Acta Radiol Ther Phys Biol 1973;12:1.
33. Cooper JS, Pajak TF, Forastiere A. Precisely defining high-risk operable head and neck tumors based on RTOG:85093 and RTOG:88–24: targets for postoperative radiochemotherapy? Head Neck 1998;20:588–594.
34. Bradford CR, Wolf GT, Carey TE, et al. Predictive markers for response to chemotherapy, organ preservation, and survival in patients with advanced laryngeal carcinoma. Otolaryngol Head Neck Surg, 1999;121:534–538.
35. Mashberg AL. Erythoplasia vs. leukoplakia in the diagnosis of early asymptomatic oral squamous carcinoma. N Engl J Med 1977;297:109.
36. Jacobs C. The internist in the management of head and neck cancer. Ann Intern Med 1990;113:771.
37. American Society for Head and Neck Surgery and the Society of Head and Neck Surgeons. Cancer of the Head and Neck: Clinical Practice Guidelines. 1996. Available at: www.ahns.info/
38. Arunachalam PS, Putnam G, Jennings P, et al. Role of computerized tomography (CT) scan of the chest in patients with newly diagnosed head and neck cancers. Clin Otolaryngol 2002; 27(5):409.
39. Warner GC, Cox GJ. Evaluation of chest radiography versus chest computed tomography in screening for pulmonary malignancy in advanced head and neck cancer. J Otolaryngol 2003;32(2):107.
40. Byers RM, Bland KI, Borlase B, et al. The prognostic and therapeutic value of frozen section determinations in the surgical treatment of squamous carcinoma of the head and neck. Am J Surg 1978;136:525–528.
41. Bauer WC, Lesinski SG, Ogura JH. The significance of positive margins in hemilaryngectomy specimens. Laryngoscope 1975;85:1–13.
42. Batsakis JG. Surgical margins in squamous cell carcinomas. Ann Otol Rhinol Laryngol 1988;97:213–214.
43. Looser KG, Shah JP, Strong EW. The significance of "positive" margins in surgically resected epidermoid carcinomas. Head Neck Surg 1978;1:107–111.
44. Robbins KT, Clayman G, Levine PA, et al. Neck dissection classification update: revisions proposed by the American Head and Neck Society and the American Academy of Otolaryngology-Head and Neck Surgery. Arch Otolaryngol–Head Neck Surg 2002;128(7):751–758.
45. Kramer S, Gelber RD, Snow JB, et al. Combined radiation therapy and surgery in the management of advanced head and neck cancer: final report of the study 73-03 of the Radiation Therapy Oncology Group. Head Neck Surg 1987;10:19.
46. Vikram B, Strong EW, Shah J, et al. Elective postoperative irradiation in stages III and IV epidermioid carcinoma of the head and neck. Am J Surg 1980;140:580.
47. Stuscke M, Thames HD. Hyperfractionated radiotherapy of human tumors: overview of the randomized clinical trials. Int J Radiat Oncol Biol Phys 1997;37:259.
48. Brizel DM, Albers ME, Fisher SR, et al. Hyperfractionated irradiation with or without concurrent chemotherapy for locally advanced head and neck cancer. N Engl J Med 1998;338:1798–1804.
49. Eisbruch A, Kim HM, Terrell JE, et al. Xerostomia and its predictors following parotid-sparing irradiation of head-and-neck cancer. Int J Radiat Oncol Biol Phys 2001;50:695.
50. Laramore GE. Radiation Therapy of Head and Neck Cancer. Berlin: Springer-Verlag, 1988.
51. Wolf GT, Lippman SM, Laramore GE, Hong WK. Head and neck cancer. In: Holland JF, Frei E, eds. Cancer Medicine. Philadelphia: Lea & Febieger, 1993:1211–1274.
52. Wolf GT, Hong WK, Fisher SG, et al. Induction chemotherapy plus radiation compared with surgery plus radiation in patients with advanced laryngeal cancer. N Engl J Med 1991;324:1685–1690.
53. Lefebvre J-L, Chevalier D, Luboinski B, et al. Larynx preservation in pyriform sinus cancer: preliminary results of a European Organization for Research and Treatment of Cancer phase III trial. J Natl Cancer Inst 1996;88:890–899.
54. Richard JM, Sancho-Garnier H, Pessey JJ, et al. Randomized trial of induction chemotherapy in larynx carcinoma. Oral Oncol 1998;34:224–228.
55. Calais G, Alfonsi M, Bardet E, et al.: Randomized trial of radiation therapy versus concomitant chemotherapy and radiation therapy for advanced-staged oropharynx carcinoma. J Natl Cancer Inst 1999; 91:2081.
56. Schuller DE, Stein DW, Metch B. Analysis of treatment failure patterns: a Southwest Oncology Group study. Arch Otolaryngol Head Neck Surg 1989;115:834–836.
57. Laramore GE, Scott CB, al-Sarraf M, et al. Adjuvant chemotherapy for resectable squamous cell carcinomas of the head and neck: report on Intergroup 0035. Int J Radiat Oncol Biol Phys 1992;23:885–886.
58. Forastiere AA, Goepfert H, Maor M, et al. Concurrent chemotherapy and radiotherapy for organ preservation in advanced laryngeal cancer. N Engl J Med 2003;349:2091.
59. Cooper JS, Pajak TF, Forastiere AA, et al. Postoperative concurrent radiotherapy and chemotherapy in high-risk squamous-cell carcinoma of the head and neck. N Engl J Med 2004;350: 1937.

60. Bernier J, Domenge C, Ozsahin M, et al. Postoperative irradiation with or without concomitant chemotherapy for locally advanced head and neck cancer. N Engl J Med 2004;350: 1945.
61. Lefebvre JL, Wolf GT, Luboinski B, et al. Meta-analysis of chemotherapy in head and neck cancer (MACH-NC): (2) larynx preservation using neoadjuvant chemotherapy in laryngeal and hypopharyngeal carcinoma [abstract]. 1998. Proc Am Soc Clin Oncol 1998;17:382a.
62. Pignon JP, Bourhis J, Domenge C, et al. Chemotherapy added to locoregional treatment for head and neck squamous-cell carcinoma: three meta-analyses of updated individual data. Lancet 2000, 355:949-955.
63. Browman GP, Hodson DI, Mackenzie RJ, et al. Choosing a concomitant chemotherapy and radiotherapy regimen for squamous cell head and neck cancer: a systematic review of the published literature with subgroup analysis. Head Neck 2001;23:579.
64. Urba SG, Wolf GT, Bradford CR, et al. Neoadjuvant therapy for organ preservation in head and neck cancer. Laryngoscope 2000;110(12):2074.
65. Urba S, Worden F, Carey T, et al. One cycle of induction chemotherapy to select for organ preservation for patients with advanced squamous carcinoma of the oral cavity [abstract]. J Clin Oncol 2005;23 (suppl):61s (abstract 5555).
66. Spiro RH, Alfonso AE, Farr HW, et al. Cervical node metastases from epidermoid carcinoma of the oral cavity and oropharynx: a critical assessment of current staging. Am J Surg 1974;128: 562.
67. Spiro RH, Huvos AG, Wong GY, et al. Predictive value of tumor thickness in squamous carcinoma confined to the tongue and floor of the mouth. Am J Surg 1986;152(4):345.
68. Bradford CR, Chepeha DB. Microvascular free flaps in head and neck reconstruction. In: Bailey BJ, Calhoun KH, eds. Head and Neck Surgery—Otolaryngology, 2nd ed. Philadelphia: Lippincott-Raven 1998:2389–2410.
69. DiTroia JF. Nodal metastases and prognosis in carcinoma of the oral cavity. Otolaryngol Clin N Am 1972;5:333.
70. Baker SR. Malignant neoplasms of the oral cavity. In: Cummings CW, Frederickson JM, Harker LA, et al, eds. Otolaryngology—Head and Neck Surgery, 1st ed. St. Louis: Mosby, 1986:1281–1344.
71. Bradford CR, Krause CJ. Floor of mouth cancer. In: Gates G, ed. Current Therapy of Head and Neck Cancer, 5th ed. St. Louis: Mosby 1994:266–267.
72. Esclamado RM, Burkey BB, Carroll WR, et al. The platysma myocutaneous flap: indications and caveats. Arch Otolaryngol Head Neck Surg 1994;120:32–35.
73. Strome SE, To Waiyat, Strawderman M, Gerstin K, Bradford CR, Esclamado RM. Squamous cell carcinoma of the buccal mucosa. Otolaryngol Head Neck Surg 1999;120(3):375–379.
74. Worden FP, Urba S, Bradford C, et al. One cycle of induction chemotherpay in advanced oropharyngeal cancer to select patients for organ preservation [abstract]. J Clin Oncol 2005; 23(suppl):61s (abstract 5512).
75. Bradford CR, Futran N, Peters G. Controversies: management of tonsil cancer. Head Neck 1999;21:657–662.
76. O'Brien CJ, Castle GK, Steven GN, et al. Limitations of radiotherapy in the definitive treatment of squamous carcinoma of the tonsillar fossa. Aust N Z J Surg 1992;62:709–713.
77. Hicks WL, Kuriakose A, Loree TR, et al. Surgery versus radiation therapy as a single-modality treatment of tonsillar fossa carcinoma: the Roswell Park Cancer Institute experience. Laryngoscope 1998;108:1014–1019.
78. Domenge C, Hill C, Lefebvre JL, et al. Randomized trial of neoadjuvant chemotherapy in oropharyngeal carcinoma. Br J Cancer 2000; 83:1594.
79. Stern SJ. Anatomy of the lateral pharyngotomy approach. Head Neck 1992;14:153–156.
80. Zeitels SM, Vaughan CW, Toomey JM. A precision technique for suprahyoid pharyngotomy. Laryngoscope 1991;101:565–566.
81. Sessions DG, Cummings CW, Weymuller EA, et al. Oropharynx. In: Atlas of Access & Reconstruction in Head and Neck Surgery. St. Louis: Mosby Year Book 1992:71–106.
82. Bradford CR, Esclamado RM, Carroll WR, et al. Analysis of recurrence, complications, and functional results with free jejunal flaps. Head Neck 1994:150–154.
83. Razack M, Sako K, Marchetta F, et al. Carcinoma of the hypopharynx: success and failure. Am J Surg 1977;134:489.
84. DelGaudio JM, Fleming DJ, Esclamado RM, et al. Hemilaryngectomy for glottic carcinoma after radiation therapy failure. Arch Otolaryngol Head Neck Surg 1994;120:959–963.
85. Sassler AM, Esclamado RM, Wolf GT. Surgery after organ preservation therapy: analysis of wound complications. Arch Otolaryngol 1995;121:162–165.
86. Laccourreye H, Laccourreye O, Weinstein G. Supracricoid laryngectomy with cricohyoidoepiglottopexy: a partial laryngeal procedure for glottic carcinoma. Ann Otol Rhinol Laryngol 1990;99:421–426.
87. Zeitels SM, Koufman JA, Davis RK, et al. Endoscopic treatment of supraglottic and hypopharynx cancer. Laryngoscope 1994; 104:71–78.
88. Lutz CK, Wagner RL, Johnson JT, Myers EN. Supraglottic carcinoma: patterns of recurrence. Ann Otol Rhinol Laryngol 1990;99:12–17.
89. Silver C. The Larynx and Hypopharynx. In: Silver CE, ed. Atlas of Head and Neck Surgery. New York: Churchill Livingstone 1986:167–251.
90. Laccourreye H, Laccourreye O, Weinstein G, et al. Supracricoid laryngectomy with cricohyoidopexy: a partial laryngeal procedure for selected supraglottic and transglottic carcinomas. Laryngoscope 1990;100:735–741.
91. Bradford CR, Wolf GT, Fisher SG, et al. Prognostic importance of surgical margins in advanced laryngeal squamous cell carcinoma. Head Neck 1996;18:11–16.
92. Shanmugaratnam K, Path FRC, Sobin LH. The World Health Organization histological classification of tumors of the upper respiratory tract and ear: a commentary on the second edition. Cancer (Phila) 1993;71:2689–2697.
93. Al-Sarraf M, LeBlanc M, Giri PG, et al. Chemoradiotherapy versus radiotherapy in patients with advanced nasopharyngeal cancer. J Clin Oncol 1998;16:1310–1317.
94. Beck JC, McClatchey KD, Bradford CR, et al. Human papillomavirus types important in progression of inverted papilloma. Otolaryngol Head Neck Surg 1995;113:558–563.
95. Moyer JS, Chepeha DB, Teknos TN. Contemporary skull base reconstruction. Curr Opin Otolaryngol Head Neck Surg 2004;12:294–299.
96. Sessions D, Cummings C, Weymuller E, et al., eds. Nasal cavity, paranasal sinuses, and anterior cranial fossa. In: Atlas of Access & Reconstruction in Head and Neck Surgery. St. Louis: Mosby Year Book 1992:107–162.
97. Price J, Holiday M, Johns M, et al. The versatile midfacial degloving approach. Laryngoscope 1988;98:291–295.
98. Moore CE, Marentette LJ, Ross D, et al. Subcranial approach to tumors of the anterior cranial base: analysis of current and traditional surgical techniques. Otolaryngol Head Neck Surg 1999;120:387–390.
99. Isaacs J, Mooney S, Mendenhall W, et al. Cancer of the maxillary sinus treated with surgery and/or radiation therapy. Am Surg 1990;56:327.
100. Spaulding CA, Kranyak MS, Constable WC, et al. Esthesioneuroblastoma: a comparison of two treatment eras. Int J Radiat Oncol Biol Phys 1988;15:581.
101. Eneroth C, Hamberger C. Principles of treatment of different types of parotid tumors. Laryngoscope 1974;84:1732.

102. Johns M, Coulthard S. Survival and follow-up in malignant tumors of the salivary glands. Otolaryngol Clin N Am 1977;10:455.
103. Bjorkland A, Eneroth C. Management of parotid gland neoplasms. Am J Otolaryngol 1980;1:155.
104. Batsakis JG. Tumors of the head and neck. In: Batsakis JG, ed. Clinical and Pathological Considerations. Baltimore: Williams & Wilkins, 1974.
105. Griffin T, Pajak T, Laramore G, et al. Neutron vs. photon irradiation of inoperable salivary gland tumors: results of an RTOG-MRC Cooperative Randomized Study. Int J Radiat Oncol Biol Phys 1988;15:1085.

101

Surgical Emergencies in the Cancer Patient

Jeffrey J. Sussman

Emergency care is needed in cancer patients under a variety of circumstances. These interventions can be divided into medical and surgical emergencies, and further subdivided into those related to the cancer diagnosis or cancer therapy and those unrelated to the cancer and only occurring incidentally in the cancer patient. Although it is tempting to always connect the new surgical problem to a cancer recurrence, in many instances the new problem is unrelated and the cancer diagnosis is of no consequence. Those surgical emergencies not related to a cancer diagnosis are not discussed in detail within this chapter and are covered elsewhere in this volume. Nongeneral surgical emergencies in the cancer patient are listed in Table 101.1.

Basic general surgical principles are generally still used to handle general surgical emergencies in the cancer patient. The main difference is that these techniques and strategies are used with an eye toward the overall status of the patient, their cancer-related prognosis, and their need for ongoing cancer treatment including chemotherapy, radiation, and/or additional surgery. Thus, as much information as possible relating to the patient's cancer diagnosis and current cancer stage should be sought. Of particular importance is an assessment of the patient's individual tumor's biological aggressiveness. The preemergency performance status of the patient is critically important, and, ideally, frank conversations with the patient and his/her family in a nonemergency setting about the patient's wishes regarding aggressive medical and surgical interventions in case of deterioration or an unexpected emergency should have already occurred. How aggressive an intervention should be undertaken in a particular patient varies from patient to patient and from tumor to tumor, even given exactly the same complication. Living wills, power of attorney documents, and prior discussions with the patient all are useful in helping to determine the most appropriate intervention. Balancing the risks of surgical intervention with the risks, both short term and long term, of more minimally invasive interventions and the potential benefits of these interventions with regard to the patient's cancer prognosis all need to be taken into account. Sound judgment and good communication skills are critical.

Table 101.2 lists common general surgical emergencies in cancer patients and serves as an outline for this chapter. Some are more cancer type specific, others are more general in nature, but each is covered in a specific following section. Treatments are evolving to minimize surgical interventions and speed recovery, particularly when palliation only is the goal. Randomized trials are lacking as a consequence of the great variability of clinical situations and the difficulty involved in randomizing patients to surgical interventions in an emergency setting, but applicable trials are referenced when available.

Obstruction

Obstructive problems in the cancer patient require emergent attention but often do not require emergent surgery. A third of obstructions are benign in nature and unrelated to the cancer diagnosis. Gastrointestinal obstructions can often be decompressed with nasogastric suction, the patient can be rehydrated, staging studies are performed to evaluate the extent of cancer involvement, and therefore the best approach to the treatment and/or palliation of the patient as a whole can be undertaken. Biliary obstructive complications accompanied by sepsis also requires emergent decompression but in the setting of sepsis is best performed minimally invasively through endoscopic and/or percutaneous transhepatic drainage.

Esophageal Obstruction

Locally advanced esophageal cancer can present initially with obstruction, or obstruction can occur as a result of recurrent disease. One needs to assess the degree of obstruction and determine if the patient can handle his or her own salivary secretions. A nasogastric tube can be placed above the level of the obstruction to clear secretions and prevent aspiration

TABLE 101.1. Nongeneral Surgical Emergencies in the Cancer Patient.

Metabolic/Paraneoplastic Syndromes
SIADH (syndrome of inappropriate antidiurectic hormone)
Hypoglycemia
Hypercalcemia
Hyperuricemia
Adrenal insufficiency
Lambert–Eaton syndrome
Polymyositis/dematomyositis
Tumor lysis syndrome
Brain edema/cord compression
Intracranial hemorrhage
Status epilecticus
Deep venous thrombosis/pulmonary embolus
Superior vena caval syndrome
Cardiac complications
Pericardial tamponade
Nonbacterial thrombotic endocarditis
Urological complications
Bleeding
Ureteral obstruction
Infectious
Priapism
Orthopedic/fractures
Airway compromise

in the completely obstructed patient as a short-term solution. Most commonly, however, patients can manage their own secretions but are unable to adequately receive oral nutrition. Liquid dietary supplements can be used while obtaining staging imaging studies to determine the extent of disease both locally and distantly as well as assessing the patient's performance status and comorbidities. If judged to be a potential surgical candidate, the patient then can be properly prepared for surgery. If nutritionally depleted, the patient may benefit from either a feeding tube placed past the obstruction if possible or a laparoscopically or radiologically placed percutaneous jejunostomy tube. Alternatively intravenous nutrition can be instituted. A gastrostomy tube can be placed; however, if surgery is anticipated a jejunostomy tube may be preferred to avoid repairing the usual conduit.

If primary or neoadjuvant chemotherapy/radiation therapy is planned, one should be prepared for treatment-related edema and initial worsening of the obstructive symptoms before improvement in esophageal patency. This situation may also require feeding tube placement to help with nutritional support as a result of both tumor obstruction and treatment-related mucosal erosions.

For patients with a complete obstruction, advanced disease, or recurrent cancer after failed initial treatment, endoscopically placed self-expanding metal wire stents have been successfully utilized. Prospective trial evidence demonstrates wire stents to be an improvement upon previously placed plastic prostheses, which had significant problems with erosion and migration[1–3] and laser ablation.[4] Stents may be combined with endoscopic ablative techniques such as laser, photodynamic therapy, bipolar cautery, or injection of sclerosing agents. These ablative techniques, however, do risk perforation, and even if successful, the patient's esophageal motility may still be decreased in the area of tumor treatment, requiring careful patient instructions for thorough mastication with plenty of liquids to prevent clogging of the newly formed passage. Rarely subtotal palliative resection or substernal surgical bypass may be necessary because of the typical aggressive biology of locally advanced esophageal cancers.

Gastric Obstruction

Because of the size of the body of the stomach, mechanical obstruction is uncommon in this location. Functional obstruction can, however, occur with tumor infiltration of the wall of the stomach or neural structures, making it noncompliant and dysmotile. Physical obstruction can occur more commonly at the gastroesophageal (GE) junction (which can be treated similar to esophageal cancer) or in the antrum where the stomach is narrower.

Analogous to esophageal cancer, nasogastric decompression can be used for complete or near-complete obstructions to relieve the acute distension and patient emesis. The patient should be rehydrated, electrolytes corrected as necessary, and proton pump inhibitors used to decrease gastric fluid output; this provides time to properly stage the cancer patient and discuss an overall treatment plan. Operative candidates can more electively undergo resection with consideration of neoadjuvant treatment. Some patients with good performance status may be candidates for a palliative resection, even in the setting of early metastatic disease, to relieve gastric obstruction but consideration to systemic chemotherapy may help define the tumor biological aggressiveness before submitting a patient to surgery and prolonged recovery if life expectancy is short.

Patients unresectable for cure may be palliated with endoscopic stent placement. Migration and long-term durability of the stents is still problematical, however, and a surgical gastrojejunostomy bypass for distal obstructing lesions or proximal resection and either antral- or jejunoesophagostomy for proximal lesions should be considered for patients with a life expectancy greater than several months. Often this is combined with a jejunostomy tube and/or gastrostomy tube placement to help speed nutritional recovery, particularly if the stomach fails to empty promptly through the new anastomosis or becomes reobstructed.

Small Bowel Obstruction

If small bowel obstruction is caused by the primary tumor, resection is recommended as the primary treatment option. Nasogastric decompression may also allow time to optimize the patient's hydration, correct electrolytes, and stage the cancer for appropriate treatment planning. More commonly, small bowel obstruction, if tumor related, is caused by a carcinomatosis. Again, performance status, extent of metastatic

TABLE 101.2. General Surgical Emergencies.

Obstruction
Perforation
Fistulas
Bleeding
Pain
Neutropenic Enterocolitis

tumor burden, and aggressiveness of tumor biology need to be considered in this situation. No randomized trial evidence exists to help select the most appropriate therapy, and sound surgical judgment is required.[5] Some patients are best served by hospice care without operative intervention. A percutaneous endoscopic gastrostomy (PEG) tube can be placed for palliation in such situations to eliminate the need for nasogastric intubation. Intravenous nutrition decisions are left for patient–physician discussion, with the realization that once started such feedings are sometimes emotionally difficult for the patient and/or the family to stop.

Carcinomatosis rarely leads to bowel ischemia, except in cases of closed loop obstruction. Therefore, time is often available for nasogastric decompression, prolonged observation, full cancer staging, and detailed patient–family discussions. Computed tomography (CT) scan imaging can often delineate the extent of tumor involvement and level of obstruction. Many times nasogastric decompression alone allows a partial small bowel obstruction to resolve after a few days of supportive care. Once resolved, however, an outpatient elective contrast study may be helpful to define the level and degree of a partial obstruction for either elective repair or further expectant observation.

Nonresolving small bowel obstructions in a patient with an otherwise good performance status should be operatively explored. Even with carcinomatosis, patients can often be best palliated for the longest period of time by surgical intervention. If a localized implant of tumor is causing the obstruction, resection of the small bowel segment is preferred. In many instances, an adhesive band is the source of the obstruction and not tumor at all. If resection cannot be performed safely, bypass to a distal small bowel loop or to the colon may be preferred. If extensive bowel involvement by cancer is noted, proximal decompression with an intestinal stoma or gastrostomy tube may be in order. Care needs to be taken to prevent inadvertent enterotomies and fistula formation, which may be difficult to heal and treat. Attention to additional, more distant obstructive lesions or impending obstructions should be noted. Additional bypass or resections may be necessary. Creation of mucous fistulas to decompress closed loops no longer in intestinal continuity may also be in order. One should define in the operative report the extent of disease, and, if a reobstruction were to occur, if the patient would likely benefit from an additional operation.

In selected patients, aggressive cytoreduction may be indicated, and ongoing trials appear to support this in appendiceal and colorectal cancer, sarcoma, mesothelioma, and ovarian cancers where the spread is primarily peritoneally based.[6,7] This intervention is often combined with hyperthermic chemotherapy perfusion. Ideally, the patient should not be acutely obstructed when undergoing this procedure, however, and may require an initial decompressive procedure before undergoing definitive cytoreduction. Complete or near-complete gross cytoreduction should be anticipated for this procedure to have any hope of effectiveness.

To prevent future bowel obstructions, there is randomized trial evidence that if one is operating on a patient who is found to have unresectable periampullary cancer, prophylactic gastrojejunostomy bypass is indicated.[8] This intervention can be done without incurring additional morbidity or mortality and prevents reoperation for obstruction in approximately 20% of patients.

Colorectal Obstruction

Obstructing colorectal lesions are an emergency as an intact ileocecal valve leads to a closed-loop situation with the risk of colonic perforation. In addition, pseudoobstruction or an "Ogilvie's syndrome" may simulate a mechanical obstruction. CT or water-soluble contrast enema studies may differentiate the two conditions. Nonmechanical obstruction should be initially treated nonoperatively if possible by addressing the underlying cause of the colonic ileus with electrolyte correction, sepsis control, ambulation, and narcotic medication minimization. Neostigmine and/or endoscopic decompression may be necessary.[9]

Mechanical obstruction may be amenable to decompression with endoscopy with or without stent placement or ablative techniques to allow bowel preparation and elective resection in non-end-stage patients.[10] If relief cannot be achieved expeditiously, then operative intervention for resection and/or diversion is mandated.

Biliary Obstruction

As mentioned previously, endoscopic or transhepatic percutaneous drainage is often well tolerated when the obstruction is associated with sepsis. Initial decompression and stenting can be converted to a covered wire stent without the need for frequent plastic stent exchanges if definitive resectional therapy is not possible. If a long prognosis is anticipated or if surgical intervention is contemplated for other reasons, then a surgical biliary-enteric anastomosis provides good long-term durability although with higher initial morbidity than endoscopic techniques.[11] In poor performance status patients, decompression and external drainage of bile flow via PTC (percutaneous transhepatic cholangiogram) tube placement is palliative. Similarly, gallbladder outlet obstruction can be treated with cholecystectomy, enteric bypass, or percutaneous external drainage. Biliary obstruction without cholangitis does not mandate immediate decompression, and patients can be fully staged and evaluated for definitive resection and treatment.

Perforation

Perforation of the gastrointestinal (GI) tract and concomitant infectious complications are life-threatening events that can occur in cancer patients. Perforation may present after prolonged obstruction that has led to distention and ischemia. Perforation may also result from localized tumor replacement of the bowel wall with subsequent tumor necrosis or from a lack of normal mucosal integrity. Occasionally, perforation may result from treatment such as steroids or from complications of chemotherapy, for example, severe dehydration and decreased bowel perfusion. The antiangiogenesis drug bevacizumab has also been associated with bowel perforation in approximately 2% of treated patients.

If an abscess develops from a walled-off, contained perforation, then image-guided percutaneous drainage may be preferred to control the infection and convert the situation into a controlled enteric-cutaneous fistula, particularly in a palliative setting. The drain tract in this circumstance may now be seeded with tumor. In situations involving a primary tumor perforation where a formal resection can remove both the primary and the entire perforated space, then this would be preferred.

If an uncontrolled perforation exists into the chest or abdomen, surgery is usually necessary for the patient's survival. Surgical considerations are detailed below. Occasionally, in a poor performance status patient with end-stage disease, palliative pain control is all that may be appropriate.

If perforation occurs during chemotherapy treatment and the patient is neutropenic, mortality is high. Treatment should include broad-spectrum antibiotics/antifungals and colony-stimulating factors to reverse the immunosuppression. Treatment responses in full-thickness bowel wall tumor deposits do not typically lead to perforation; however, this may occur with very chemoradiation sensitive tumors such as lymphoma. The rapid necrosis of the malignant lymphocytes that have replaced the bowel wall in certain areas can lead to a perforation. However, this scenario is not so common that prophylactic surgery is required in high-risk patients or that the chemotherapy regimens should be changed to be those less efficacious.

Principles of treatment include drainage and control of the perforation. If resection of the tumor involved area is possible, this is preferable, but the risk of prolonged surgery, the patient's hemodynamic status, and degree of intestinal spillage need to be assessed. Decreased performance status and possible immunosuppression should also be taken into account. In many cases, drainage and proximal diversion or tube drainage is more appropriate to control sepsis and salvage the patient. Surgeons should keep in mind the potential need for subsequent chemotherapy and/or radiation therapy, as well as the need for a speedy recovery in a patient with a limited life expectancy in assessing the extent of surgical intervention.

The perforation of a primary cancer is associated with a high risk of peritoneal spread of cancer cells in addition to the infectious complications. Colorectal cancer, in particular, may present in this manner. If the perforation is contained in the retroperitoneum or into the abdomen side wall, the affected area can be marked with radiopaque clips for adjuvant postoperative radiation therapy. If the perforation is subsequent to a biopsy of prepped bowel, a formal resection in an otherwise stable patient would be most appropriate. If a large amount of spillage of unprepped bowel or delayed presentation has occurred, proximal diversion with limited resection may be appropriate, allowing a more elective formal resection and reanastomosis to be performed at a later date. These patients may also be candidates for an adjuvant hyperthermic intraperitoneal perfusion because of the risk of peritoneal spread. There is a decrease in survival and increase in morbidity when patients undergo emergent colorectal cancer operations secondary to perforation as compared to elective resections.[12,13] This survival decrement is also seen in acutely obstructed colorectal cancer patients.

Perforation of esophageal tumors is also poorly tolerated; however, the same general surgical principles apply. As drainage alone is often not sufficient because the cancerous tissue will not heal and a persistent fistula may develop, resection is usually necessary; this may be performed transhiatally or transthoracically depending on tumor location, local extension, and extent of inflammation. Reconstruction can be safely performed in stable patients; however, cervical esophagostomy, gastrostomy tube placement, and mediastinal drainage with or without primary tumor resection may be necessary, with elective anastomosis at a later date.

Fistulas

As in other general surgery patients, fistulas can develop for a number of reasons in cancer patients (Table 101.3). Fistulas can be postoperative from anastomotic leaks or bowel injury, or they can be the end result of percutaneous drainage for a perforation. In addition, fistulas can result from tumor involvement and invasion between hollow viscous, such as small bowel loop to small bowel loop, bowel to bladder, or bowel to vagina or skin or other organ. General principles of drainage and sepsis control are followed. Some fistulas may heal with time only, but distal obstruction, irradiation, malnutrition, and the presence of tumor at the fistula site all may contribute to the nonhealing of a fistula in a cancer patient.

As with other emergent conditions already discussed, medical treatment initially with proximal nasogastric decompression, skin care, antibiotics if associated with infection/sepsis, rehydration, electrolyte correction, and associated abscess drainage may be necessary to allow time for full cancer staging, appropriate discussions with the patient and their families, formation of an overall treatment plan for the patient's cancer, and how the fistula repair can be managed within that plan. Treatment may involve resection of the fistula's tract and involved organs, bypass, or diversion of intestinal flow away from the fistula, hyperbaric oxygen therapy, prolonged nutritional support, and possibly chemotherapy to treat the cancer if it is the underlying cause. In some patients, simply palliation of any fistula-related symptoms and skin care is all that is necessary as the treatment may be worse than leaving the fistula alone. Fistulograms/bowel contrast studies/CT scans all can be particularly helpful in treatment planning.

Tracheal esophageal fistulas usually result from esophageal cancer penetration and perforation into the respiratory tract. Overall prognosis is usually poor as a result of the locally advanced nature of these cancers; however, short-term palliation is achievable with covered metal stents placed in both trachea and esophagus.

TABLE 101.3. Gastrointestinal (GI) Fistulas: Reasons for Failure to Heal.

Significant bowel integrity disruption
Cancer
Irradiation
Foreign body
Distal obstruction
Inflammatory bowel disease
Malnutrition
Immunosuppression
Abscess/sepsis
Epithelization

Bleeding

Bleeding can be a particularly emergent situation occurring in the cancer patient. In the majority of instances, bleeding is from non-cancer-related causes, such as gastritis or diverticulosis. It may be exacerbated, however, by cancer-related treatments, for example, as with chemotherapy-induced thrombocytopenia or anticoagulation instituted for other cancer-related conditions. Non-cancer-related causes are typically treated as in the noncancer patient with consideration of the overall prognosis of the patient. A specific source of the bleeding should be determined so that treatment can be effected to prevent recurrent bleeding with additional cancer treatments. Occasionally, bleeding can be the sole manifestation of recurrent cancer such as colon cancer, a local recurrence, or a melanoma small bowel metastasis.

Portal hypertensive bleeding can be particularly difficult to manage when induced by cancer-related portal vein thrombosis. Therapy is directed at the bleeding source with variceal banding or sclerosis and pharmacological control of portal hypertension. Bleeding gastric and esophageal varicies caused by splenic vein thrombosis can be treated if symptomatic with splenectomy when portal hypertension is not present.

Bleeding can also occur directly from the tumor bed, either the primary or a distant metastasis; this can be immediately life threatening, if in the brain, or can be asymptomatic, if very slow into the GI tract, or in the case of tamponade, for example, in the retroperitoneum. Supportive care is necessary with correction of underlying coagulopathies and quantitative or qualitative platelet defects. Operative resection may be in order for resectable lesions in the stomach or bowel. Selected patients may benefit from angiographic embolization with or without eventual elective resection, particularly if the source is a liver metastasis bleeding into a biliary system. Radiation therapy is also effective for slowly bleeding lesions, but several days to weeks are required for the therapy to take effect.

Pain

Pain control, although not typically emergent, deserves mention. Acute cancer-related fractures require orthopedic attention and fixation; radiation therapy can be helpful for pain control. Most sources of pain can be relieved through a combination of oral and/or transdermal routes of narcotics and nonnarcotic pain medications. Excess sedation and other narcotic side effects can become particularly problematical. Surgical or percutaneous celiac plexus blockade, as well as other regional blocks, can also be helpful to control abdominal pain.[14–17] Thoracic sympathetectomy can also be useful and can be performed minimally invasively. Implantable epidural pumps or subcutaneous continuous infusion devices are also useful in selective circumstances. Acute pain service consultation can often be very helpful. Other adjuvant treatments such as nonsteroidal antiinflammatory medications, visual imaging, exercise, massage, biofeedback, acupuncture, and other alternative medicine practices may be extremely useful. In selected patients, resection of the tumor in an otherwise noncurative fashion can sometimes result in pain relief. For example, decompression of distended bowel loops that could cause extreme pain may be helpful even if noncurative. However, as a rule, the part of the tumor that can be resected is not usually the area of the tumor which is invading the nerves and causing the pain.

Neutropenic Enterocolitis

Neutropenic enterocolitis, which goes by many other names, including typhlitis from the Greek word for cecum, agranulocytic colitis, neutropenic enteropathy, and ileocecal syndrome, all refer to an inflammatory condition of the right colon and particularly the cecum in a setting of neutropenia.[18] Presentation is often characterized by fever, right lower quadrant pain, decreased neutrophil count, abdominal distension, diarrhea, nausea, vomiting, and bloody stools. Mortality is as high as 20%. Differential diagnosis includes other causes of inflammation including *Clostridia difficile* colitis, diverticulitis, inflammatory bowel disease, appendicitis, intussusception, bowel ischemia, cholecystitis, diffuse peritonitis, mesenteric adenitis, and constipation. Physical examination is usually consistent with localized peritonitis, and a CT scan of the abdomen is often characterized by right colonic and cecal bowel wall thickening with occasional air within the bowel wall and pericecal fat stranding. The absolute neutrophil count is usually less than 500/μL. Barium enema is usually contraindicated in this situation. The pathophysiology is not completely understood. However, as the cecum is often the most dilated portion of the large colon, as per Laplace's law, it is often this area that becomes most distended with increased intraluminal pressure within the colon, leading to localized ischemia, increased stasis, low-grade sepsis, and bacterial translocation. Concomitant steroid medication use, dehydration, decreased blood supply, malnutrition, and change in bowel flora may also contribute. Susceptibility of the right colon may also relate to a decrease in normal lymphoid tissue in this region with chemotherapy.

Treatment involves broad-spectrum antibiotic use and bowel rest, colony-stimulating factors to increase neutrophil count, and supportive care. In the majority of instances medical management is sufficient. Surgical intervention (Table 101.4) is reserved for cases in which there is a lack of improvement or suspected perforation, bleeding, or uncontrolled sepsis. CT imaging is often helpful. Most often surgical intervention requires resection of the right colon with diversion. Some authors have recommended surgical intervention even after a medically successfully treated episode of neutropenic enterocolitis to prevent recurrences with subsequent chemotherapy cycles.[19,20] This method is not,

TABLE 101.4. Surgical Indications in Neutropenic Enterocolitis.

1. Evidence of free entraperitoneal perforation
2. Ongoing sepsis/acidosis despite initial resuscitative therapy
3. Ongoing bleeding after correction of platelet and coagulation defects
4. Failure to improve after reversal of neutropenia
5. Uncertainty in diagnosis
6. Selectively to prevent future episodes with additionally planned chemotherapy

however, widely practiced because of the delays incurred in chemotherapy administration by the intervening surgery and recovery.

Summary

In summary, management of general surgical complications in the cancer patient is not that dissimilar to management of complications in the noncancer patient. However, not only the particular complication, but how that particular complication fits into the overall treatment plan and prognosis for the patient, needs to be considered. Risks and benefits to the patient need to be addressed in the context of the potential need for subsequent radiation and/or chemotherapy or additional surgical interventions related to the cancer diagnosis. Treatment must consider the nonhealing and progressive nature of any residual cancer remaining after surgical intervention and overall patient prognosis. Although very challenging, there is great opportunity for helping cancer patients with surgical interventions and personal satisfaction in working with cancer patients and their families at this particularly stressful time in their lives.

References

1. Segalin A, Bonavina L, Carazzone A, et al. Improving results of esophageal stenting: a study on 160 consecutive unselected patients. Endoscopy 1997;29:701–709.
2. Siersema PD, Hop WC, Dees J, et al. Coated self-expanding metal stents versus latex prostheses for esophagogastric cancer with special reference to prior radiation and chemotherapy: a controlled, prospective study. Gastrointest Endosc 1998;47:113–120.
3. De Palma GD, di Matteo E, Romano G, et al. Plastic prosthesis versus expandable metal stents for palliation of inoperable esophageal thoracic carcinoma: a controlled prospective study. Gastrointest Endosc 1996;43:478–482.
4. Adam A, Ellul J, Watkinson AF, et al. Palliation of inoper-able esophageal carcinoma: a prospective randomized trial of laser therapy and stent placement. Radiology 1997;202:344–348.
5. Feuer DJ, Broadley KE, Shepherd JH, et al. Systematic review of surgery in malignant bowel obstruction in advanced gynecological and gastrointestinal cancer. The Systematic Review Steering Committee. Gynecol Oncol 1999;75:313–322.
6. Verwaal VJ, van Ruth S, de Bree E, et al. Randomized trial of cytoreduction and hyperthermic intraperitoneal chemotherapy versus systemic chemotherapy and palliative surgery in patients with peritoneal carcinomatosis of colorectal cancer. J Clin Oncol 2003;21:3737–3743.
7. Glehen O, Kwiatkowski F, Sugarbaker PH, et al. Cytoreductive surgery combined with perioperative intraperitoneal chemotherapy for the management of peritoneal carcinomatosis from colorectal cancer: a multi-institutional study. J Clin Oncol 2004;22:3284–3292.
8. Lillemoe KD, Cameron JL, Hardacre JM, et al. Is prophylactic gastrojejunostomy indicated for unresectable periampullary cancer? A prospective randomized trial. Ann Surg 1999;230:322–328; discussion 328–330.
9. Ponec RJ, Saunders MD, Kimmey MB. Neostigmine for the treatment of acute colonic pseudo-obstruction. N Engl J Med 1999;341:137–141.
10. Tamim WZ, Ghellai A, Counihan TC, et al. Experience with endoluminal colonic wall stents for the management of large bowel obstruction for benign and malignant disease. Arch Surg 2000;135:434–438.
11. Gouma DJ, van Geenen R, van Gulik T, et al. Surgical palliative treatment in bilio-pancreatic malignancy. Ann Oncol 1999;10(suppl 4):269–272.
12. Chen HS, Sheen-Chen SM. Obstruction and perforation in colorectal adenocarcinoma: an analysis of prognosis and current trends. Surgery (St. Louis) 2000;127:370–376.
13. Smothers L, Hynan L, Fleming J, et al. Emergency surgery for colon carcinoma. Dis Colon Rectum 2003;46:24–30.
14. Lillemoe KD, Cameron JL, Kaufman HS, et al. Chemical splanchnicectomy in patients with unresectable pancreatic cancer. A prospective randomized trial. Ann Surg 1993;217:447–455; discussion 456–457.
15. Mercadante S. Celiac plexus block versus analgesics in pancreatic cancer pain. Pain 1993;52:187–192.
16. Kawamata M, Ishitani K, Ishikawa K, et al. Comparison between celiac plexus block and morphine treatment on quality of life in patients with pancreatic cancer pain. Pain 1996;64:597–602.
17. Polati E, Finco G, Gottin L, et al. Prospective randomized double-blind trial of neurolytic coeliac plexus block in patients with pancreatic cancer. Br J Surg 1998;85:199–201.
18. Bavaro MF. Neutropenic enterocolitis. Curr Gastroenterol Rep 2002;4:297–301.
19. Moir CR, Scudamore CH, Benny WB. Typhlitis: selective surgical management. Am J Surg 1986;151:563–566.
20. Keidan RD, Fanning J, Gatenby RA, et al. Recurrent typhlitis. A disease resulting from aggressive chemotherapy. Dis Colon Rectum 1989;32:206–209.

102

Nutritional Care of Cancer Patients

David A. August and Maureen B. Huhmann

The lay press and professional journals are replete with articles concerning the use of various nutrition interventions to treat, palliate, and support cancer patients.

Three major issues need to be addressed when considering the role of nutrition in cancer:

1. Cancer cachexia and the metabolic consequences of cancer.
2. Nutrition care of cancer patients.
3. The relationship of diet to carcinogenesis and cancer prevention.

Historical Overview

More than 60 years ago, it was observed that malnutrition and weight loss often contribute to the death of cancer patients.[1,2] In 1936 it was noted that patients with a greater than 20% preoperative loss of their usual body weight were at eightfold increased risk of dying following a surgical procedure.[3] Little could be done about these devastating consequences of malnutrition until techniques of effective nutrition support were developed. The modern era of nutrition intervention began in 1968 with the description by Dudrick and colleagues of the support of growth and development in a newborn solely using parenteral nutrition.[4] Because of the prominent role of malnutrition in malignancy, it was natural that the use of parenteral nutrition be studied in humans with cancer. By 1974, the initial reports of such investigations had been published.[5,6] Since that time, despite the performance of numerous studies investigating the role of specialized nutrition support (SNS; administration of nonoral enteral or parenteral nutrition products to supplement or replace oral nutrient intake) in cancer patients, the role of nutrition support in malignancy remains to be defined.[7] This lack in large measure results from the effects of the presence of a malignancy on the metabolic milieu of the cancer-bearing host. Simple provision of nutrients does not ensure that they can be effectively utilized by the host to overcome the metabolic impact of the malignancy. Recognition of this fact has spurred research into the metabolic consequences of cancer and methods to alter host metabolism and host–tumor interactions to the benefit of the patient. These clinical and research issues may be grouped under the heading of cancer cachexia.

Cancer Cachexia and the Metabolic Consequences of Cancer

Cancer cachexia is a syndrome characterized by progressive, involuntary weight loss. The term cachexia is derived from two Greek words, *kakos* (bad) and *hexis* (condition). Indeed, weight loss in a cancer patient is indicative of a "bad condition" and carries with it adverse prognostic implications. Clinical features of cancer cachexia include host tissue wasting, anorexia, skeletal muscle atrophy, anergy, fatigue, anemia, and hypoalbuminemia (Table 102.1). If diminished intake resulting from anorexia were the only problem, aggressive SNS would successfully treat the syndrome. This, however, is not the case. The cancer cachexia syndrome (CCS) involves a heterogeneous medley of physiological and

TABLE 102.1. Clinical and Laboratory Features of Cancer Cachexia.

Clinical	*Laboratory*
Tissue wasting	Microcytic anemia
Anorexia	Hypoalbuminemia
Weight loss	Hyperlipidemia
Muscle atrophy	Skin test anergy
Weakness	
Lethargy	
Myalgia	

metabolic derangements resulting in potentially life-threatening malnutrition.[8,9] Although often seen in patients with advanced malignancies, CCS may be present in the early stages of tumor growth and may even be the iatrotropic stimulus.[10]

Incidence

Anorexia and weight loss are frequent findings in cancer patients. Between 15% and 40% of patients present with weight loss[11,12]; as many as 80% with advanced malignancies will evidence CCS. The extent of weight loss is related to tumor type and is of prognostic significance. The lowest frequency of weight loss is observed in patients with favorable prognosis lymphomas, leukemias, breast cancers, and soft tissue sarcomas. More aggressive lymphomas, and colon, prostate, and lung cancers, are associated with an approximate 50% incidence of weight loss. The highest incidence and severity are seen in pancreatic and gastric cancer (approximately 85%) (Table 102.2).[12]

The importance of CCS is highlighted by the prognostic significance of weight loss. For any given tumor type, survival is shorter in patients who experience pretreatment weight loss (see Table 102.2).[12] Furthermore, CCS is a problematical cause of symptom distress in cancer patients. Anorexia, weight loss and the associated fatigue, and changes in body image can contribute to depression and decreased social interactions.[13,14] Early recognition and intervention to prevent worsening of CCS may afford the best opportunity to prevent its debilitating consequences.[13,15]

TABLE 102.3. Causes of Cancer Cachexia.

Anorexia
Mechanical factors
Side effects of therapy
Altered energy metabolism
Changes in cytokine and hormonal milieu

Causes of Cancer Cachexia

Multiple factors contribute to the development of CCS (Table 102.3). The interplay of these factors varies from patient to patient.

Anorexia

Anorexia is a prominent component of CCS. The anorexia of malignancy is characterized by a spontaneous decrease in food intake.[8] The causes are unknown but likely relate to an altered cytokine milieu in the host (see following).[16,17] It is unlikely that anorexia is a primary event in CCS; it is more likely a secondary effect. A number of lines of evidence support this contention. First, SNS may be used to meet the nutrient requirements of cachectic cancer patients, but often this does not reverse either the weight loss or the other clinical stigmata of CCS. Second, in animal models, pair-feeding of nontumor-bearing animals with food intake of matched tumor-bearing animals does not reproduce the metabolic or clinical changes seen in tumor-bearing hosts. In animals and humans, the consequences of starvation differ markedly from those seen in tumor-bearing hosts.[18] Third, CCS may be present early in the pathogenesis of cancer despite the fact that food intake is normal.[19,20] Fourth, in some situations, the apparent anorexia may not be real; it is an adaptive decrease in food intake in response to cancer-induced weight loss.[21]

TABLE 102.2. Weight Loss and Life Expectancy in Cancer Patients.

				Median survival (weeks)	
Tumor type	*No weight loss*	*1%–10% weight loss*	*More than 10% weight loss*	*No weight loss*	*Weight loss*
Lymphoma, favorable prognosis	69	22	10	—[a]	138
Lymphoma, unfavorable prognosis	52	33	15	107	55
Acute leukemia	61	35	4	8	4
Sarcoma	60	33	7	46	25
Breast	64	30	6	70	45
Colon	46	40	14	43	21
Prostate	44	46	10	46	24
Lung, small cell	43	43	14	34	27
Lung, non-small cell	39	46	15	20	14
Pancreas	17	57	26	14	12
Stomach, early	17	53	30	41	27
Stomach , advanced	13	49	38	18	16

[a]Fewer than 50% of patients had died.

Source: Adapted from Dewys WD, Begg C, Lavin PT, et al. Prognostic effect of weight loss prior to chemotherapy in cancer patients. Eastern Cooperative Oncology Group. Am J Med 1980;69(4):491–497.[12]

Mechanical Factors

Mechanical factors related to tumor or complications of therapy may compromise gastrointestinal tract continuity and normal motility. This effect occurs most commonly as a result of malignant obstruction of the esophagus, stomach, small intestine, colon, or biliary tract, or secondary to tumor-induced changes in gastric wall compliance. Cancer is the most common cause of gastrointestinal fistulae.[22] Symptoms related to mechanical factors may include alterations in taste sensation, early satiety, pain, cramps, vomiting, diarrhea, and constipation.[23]

Cancer Therapy

Cancer treatments may induce anorexia and weight loss. Surgery invariably leads to a temporary catabolic state and decreased nutrient intake, which may be exacerbated when surgical complications occur. Chemotherapy often induces transient nausea and vomiting or injury to gastrointestinal mucosa with resultant stomatitis, mucositis, diarrhea, and/or typhlitis. These side effects may be particularly severe in profoundly neutropenic patients, such as those receiving chemotherapy for leukemias and lymphomas and those undergoing high-dose chemotherapy with either autologous or allogeneic bone marrow reconstitution. Radiation therapy may cause acute gastrointestinal injury similar to that seen with some chemotherapy; it may also cause chronic radiation enteritis with malabsorption and stricture formation. These changes may induce anorexia, malabsorption, or mechanical obstruction.

Altered Energy Metabolism

The hallmark of the energetics of the metabolic response to cancer is its variability. In comparison with control groups, cancer patients may have reduced, normal, or increased energy expenditure (Fig. 102.1).[24–27] The variability is in part caused by the inherent heterogeneity of "cancer," but is also likely the result of variability in host responses to tumor such as infection, elaboration of an acute-phase reaction, and organ-specific reactions.[24,28] This variability in host energetics in response to cancer makes prediction of the nutritional requirements of cancer patients problematical.

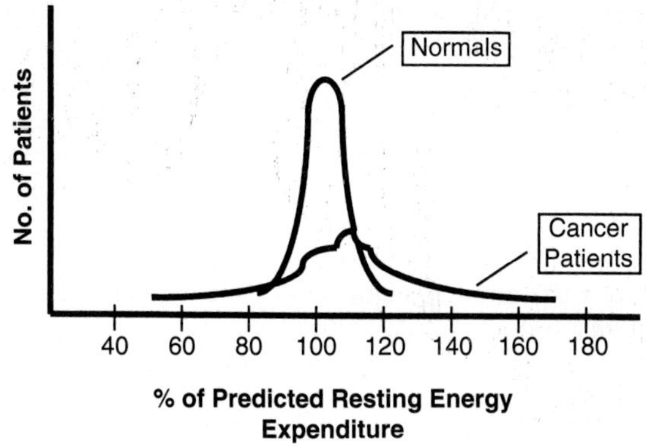

Figure 102.1. Resting energy expenditure in cancer patients is unpredictable. In comparison with normal subjects, the measured resting energy expenditure in cancer patients has a wider standard deviation and more extreme maxima and minima. This variability in host energetics in response to cancer makes prediction of nutritional requirements difficult.

TABLE 102.4. Putative Mediators of Cancer Cachexia Syndrome (CCS).

Major factors:
Tumor necrosis factor
Interferon-γ
Interleukin-1
Interleukin-6
Other factors:
Proteolysis-inducing factor
Lipid-mobilizing factor
Uncoupling proteins 1, 2, 3

Changes in the Cytokine and Hormonal Milieu

Information from parabiotic[29] and serum transfer experiments[30] in tumor-bearing and normal animals implicates circulating factors as primary mediators of CCS. Recent research has focused interest on the proinflammatory cytokines tumor necrosis factor (TNF), interferon-γ (IFN-γ), and interleukins 1 and 6 (IL-1 and IL-6) as the most important effectors in the pathogenesis of CCS (Table 102.4). Other catabolic molecules implicated in CCS include proteolysis-inducing factor (PIF), lipid-mobilizing factor (LMF), and mitochondria-uncoupling proteins (UCP) 1, -2, and -3. These products, in contrast to the cytokines, do not affect appetite. There is a strong correlation between high levels of these factors and the presence of cachexia.[31] It must be noted, however, that there is no currently accepted model that adequately explains the etiology of CCS in most patients.[32]

Tumor necrosis factor was first described as a metabolically active circulating factor in septic rabbits.[33] The substance was subsequently found to cause hemorrhagic necrosis of tumors and to mediate severe cachexia.[34] Animal experiments show that intermittent administration of TNF causes acute anorexia and transient weight loss, but tachyphylaxis rapidly develops.[35] When similar experiments were performed using tumor cell lines constitutively producing TNF, tachyphylaxis did not develop, and 80% of animals developed progressive weight loss and died. Autopsy revealed features similar to cancer cachexia.[36] Interestingly, the site of TNF production in animals inoculated with TNF-producing tumors alters the metabolic profile of CCS. Brain inoculation induces anorexia, whereas muscle implantation causes chronic cachexia with severe loss of carcass mass.[37]

These site-specific findings may explain some of the heterogeneity that characterizes CCS. Paracrine, organ-specific effects of TNF may be more important than distant, hormone-like circulating effects. In animal models, TNF administration in an episodic fashion does not induce CCS but can induce cachexia-like symptoms. These effects include increased energy expenditure and lipolysis and decreased protein synthesis.[34,37–39] In contrast to CCS, repeated doses of TNF over a longer period of time seem to generate tolerance and the CCS symptoms are overcome.[40] To demonstrate a role for TNF in human cancer cachexia, investigators have attempted to measure TNF levels in the plasma of cancer patients. Levels of TNF are consistently elevated in patients experiencing CCS[41,42]; however, these values may also be elevated in noncachectic patients.[43] This inconsistency may be a result of the variable nature of CCS and the possibility that undetectable or bound concentrations of TNF may be biologically active.[34] It is likely that TNF does play a significant role in many instances of CCS, but its effects are heterogeneous and likely modulated or overshadowed by other mediators in many situations.

Interferon-γ mimics some of the metabolic effects of TNF on fat metabolism and protein synthesis. In an animal model, implantation of tumors constitutively producing IFN-γ transiently induced a CCS-like syndrome.[44] Passive immunization against IFN-γ can eliminate this response.[45,46] Similar to TNF, IFN-γ levels have not been consistently found to be elevated in cachectic cancer patients.

Recent interest has focused on IL-1 and IL-6 as mediators of CCS. Both TNF and IL-1 can induce the production and release of IL-6,[47,48] and IL-6 can be detected in the blood of tumor-bearing animals.[49] IL-1 activity may be more paracrine in nature, similar to TNF. IL-1 seems to act centrally[40] and causes early satiety, possibly via serotonergic activity, and enhances intracellular lipolysis.[20] IL-6 has a paradoxical effect in that it inhibits tumor growth and promotes CCS.[40] Interleukins 1 and 6 independently recreate many of the metabolic changes seen in CCS. Acting in concert, IL-1, IL-6, and TNF can increase protein turnover and prevent utilization of stored and circulating lipids.[50]

The proteolytic pathway has been identified as extremely important in the muscle atrophy seen in cancer.[31] PIF is a secretory protein isolated from the urine of cachectic patients that appears to be produced exclusively by primary and metastatic tumor. PIF transcripts are absent in all normal human tissue except brain and skin. Transcripts for PIF have been found in breast, prostate, and colon tumors.[51] It is hypothesized that PIF induces an upregulation of the ubiquitin proteosome proteolytic pathway, causing an increase in skeletal muscle degredation.[52] PIF also depresses plasma amino acid levels, which in turn leads to a decrease in protein synthesis.[31] In cell culture, PIF has been shown to increase production of IL-6, IL-8, and C-reactive protein (CRP).[53]

Recent data suggest an important role for cytokine-mediated inhibition of the synthesis of myosin heavy chain relative to that of other myofibrillar proteins such as actin and tropomyosin in the pathogenesis of CCS.[54] TNF, IFN-γ, and IL-6 effects mediated by the nuclear transcription factor Myo-D and ubiquitin lipase-dependent proteosome pathway can lead to the functional loss of contractile units with resultant muscle atrophy and wasting.[55–57]

CCS is also associated with a loss of fat mass. LMF causes an increase in the UCPs and subsequently induces lipolysis in adipocytes.[31] This action appears to be mediated through the beta-3 adrenoreceptors.[52] UCP 1, -2, and -3 are involved in thermogenesis in brown adipose tissue and possibly skeletal muscle. Increased thermogenesis causes an increase in energy expenditure and contributes to tissue wasting.[53]

Changes in hormone regulation and sensitivity may also play a role in the pathogenesis of CCS. Weight loss in cancer patients is often associated with insulin resistance.[58] Infusion of insulin sufficient to induce hypoglycemia can reverse some of the nutritional and biochemical abnormalities of CCS in tumor-bearing rats.[59–61] Other hormonal factors may also play a role.[14]

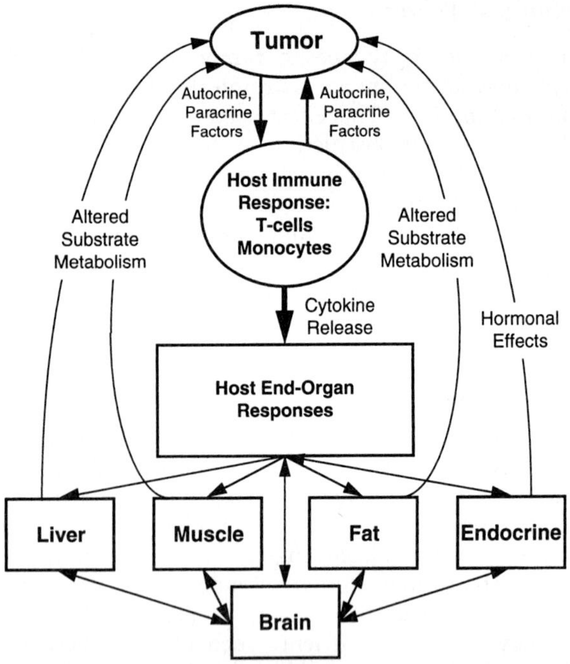

Figure 102.2. Interleukin-1, interleukin-6, interferon-γ, and tumor necrosis factor, as well as other cytokines, are important mediators of cancer cachexia syndrome (CCS). The host response to the tumor releases cytokines that have direct effects upon the tumor and its milieu and which have broad-ranging effects on host end organs. These end-organ effects, in turn, may cause release of hormones, alterations in intermediary metabolism, and central nervous system responses that further change the host milieu and affect tumor growth and metastasis. The host response may cause even seemingly localized cancers to produce systemic effects.

It is likely that IL-1, IL-6, TNF, and PIF, as well as other cytokines and growth factors,[18] are important mediators of CCS. They create a milieu in which the host may be unable to effectively utilize enterally or parenterally administered nutrients (Fig. 102.2). Interventions targeted at altering this tumor-mediated environment to favor host anabolism are actively being investigated. The complex interplay of host, tumor, and mediators makes this a challenging endeavor.[50]

Metabolic Consequences of the Cancer Cachexia Syndrome

The metabolic changes seen in CCS are multiple and variable (Table 102.5). They are generally characterized by decoupling of supply and demand, resulting in excessive substrate cycling and turnover. These changes emphasize that CCS is more than a failure to meet nutritional requirements with substrate intake. The metabolic derangements must be corrected or co-opted if the clinical sequelae of cancer cachexia are to be remediated and prevented.

Energetics

As noted, it is unlikely that energy demands created by tumor physiology or the host response to the tumor are etiological in cancer cachexia. The energy requirements of cancer patients, in contrast to those of nontumor-bearing hosts, do not follow a normal, Gaussian distribution. They vary between

TABLE 102.5. Metabolic Alterations Observed in Patients with Cancer Cachexia Syndrome.[8]

Carbohydrate metabolism
Glucose intolerance
Insulin resistance
Increased glucose production
Increased glucose turnover
Increased gluconeogenesis
Increased Cori cycle activity
Protein metabolism
Increased protein turnover
Increased hepatic protein synthesis
Decreased muscle protein synthesis
Increased muscle protein catabolism
Decreased plasma concentrations of branched-chain amino acids
Lipid metabolism
Depletion of fat stores
Increased lipolysis
Decreased lipogenesis
Hyperlipidemia
Increased free fatty acid and glycerol turnover
Decreased serum lipoprotein lipase activity

Source: From Kern KA, Norton JA. Cancer cachexia. JPEN J Parenter Enteral Nutr 1988;12(3):286–298.[8]

individuals and among tumor types. What is constant, however, is the failure of tumor-bearing hosts to adjust food intake to changes in metabolic rate. Whether metabolic rate is increased, decreased, or unchanged, food intake in patients with CCS is chronically below energy expenditure, inevitably resulting in weight loss.[8]

Carbohydrate Metabolism

Multiple derangements in carbohydrate metabolism have been observed in cancer patients. Weight loss in CCS is often associated with glucose intolerance and abnormal insulin responsiveness[62]; this may be a result of insulin resistance or decreased pancreatic function.[58] Gluconeogenesis may be increased as a result of upregulated Cori cycle activity in response to tumor production of lactic acid.[63,64] Additional upregulation of hepatic gluconeogenesis may be caused by increased release of other glucose precursors, especially alanine and glycerol, from the periphery.[65,66] Cancer cachexia mediators may also induce gluconeogenic enzymes in the liver, further driving glucose synthesis. One net effect of increased hepatic gluconeogenesis may be host energy depletion. Recycling of precursors to produce glucose is an energy-consuming process. The magnitude of this effect may be clinically significant in some patients.[8,19]

Triglyceride and Fat Metabolism

Depletion of fat stores is one of the characteristic features of CCS. This phenomenon accounts for the wasted, "skin-and-bones" appearance of many cancer patients. It is often accompanied by hyperlipidemia.[67,68] As with carbohydrates, increased turnover of glycerol and fatty acids compared with normal subjects is observed. Glucose infusion fails to suppress lipolysis in cancer patients.[69] Lipoprotein lipase levels are decreased in many cancer patients, resulting in a type IV hyperlipidemia type picture.[70] Alterations in lipid metabolism and serum lipid profiles may have profound effects upon the tumor-bearing host. Increased lipid levels in the blood may help the host by fueling the increased substrate turnover characteristic of CCS. Unfortunately, the same lipids may also be utilized by the tumor to meet essential requirements for polyunsaturated fats such as linoleic and arachidonic acids.[19,71] Furthermore, plasma from hyperlipidemic patients is immunosuppressive and may impair monocyte and macrophage function.[8] A variety of "lipid-mobilizing factors" have been described that may mediate some of the abnormalities of lipid metabolism seen in cancer patients.[19,31,52,53]

Protein Metabolism

Muscle wasting is a prominent finding in patients with CCS. It contributes to the fatigue, weakness, asthenia, and respiratory complications observed in patients with advanced cancer. It is heralded by signs including muscle atrophy and myopathy and the accompanying loss of visceral mass and hypoalbuminemia. Increased host nitrogen turnover is a prominent metabolic correlate.

There is an apparent failure in cancer patients of the normal mechanisms of protein metabolism adaptation seen during simple starvation.[8] Despite protein depletion, protein turnover remains normal or is even increased; this change is unaffected by administration of exogenous nitrogen.[72,73] The peripheral depletion is primarily caused by decreased muscle protein synthesis.[74,75] Simultaneously, hepatic protein synthesis appears preserved or even supranormal[76,77]; this includes albumin, despite the consistent observation of hypoalbuminemia, suggesting an important effect of increased albumin degradation.[78] The mediators of altered protein metabolism are not known. In addition to TNF, interleukins, and other cytokines, a protein-mobilizing factor has been described.[19]

Treatment of Cancer Cachexia

The clinical use of SNS to ameliorate the effects of CCS is discussed in detail next. As is evident from the previous discussion, however, SNS alone would not be expected to have a major impact on the clinical consequences of CCS. Simple administration of substrate does not address the fundamental metabolic derangements associated with cancer wasting. An obvious approach is the use of antibodies or other agents to block the putative mediators of CCS. The results of this approach in animal models have been summarized by others.[14,79–81] To date, there have been no trials in humans utilizing TNF-directed antibodies or other similar interventions. Design of such trials is difficult because (a) the multifactorial etiology of CCS makes it unlikely that an intervention directed at a single mediator will be consistently effective; (b) there are few agents appropriate and available for clinical testing; and (c) the prolonged treatment likely to be necessary would be both impractical and prohibitively expensive.

Pharmacological Treatments

A variety of pharmacological agents (Table 102.6) have been tested for use to treat or provide symptomatic relief for patients with CCS.[14,82–110] Most agents are directed at improving appetite and sense of well-being. These agents can be placed in three categories: agents with demonstrated

TABLE 102.6.
Pharmacological Treatments for Weight Loss.

Agent	*Drug class (mechanism of action)*	*Level of evidence*	*Clinical outcomes*	*Adverse outcomes*	*Comments*
Agents with demonstrated effectiveness:					
Megestrol acetate (Megace)	Progestational (appetite stimulant)	3	Increased appetite Enhanced food intake Weight gain Improved sense of well-being[14,82] Inhibition of cytokine activity[82,83]	Weight gain primarily fat[84] Risk of thrombosis[85] Edema[82,83]	No increase in benefit if combined with dronabinol[86]
Medroxyprogesterone acetate (MPA)	Progestational (appetite stimulant)	3	Increased appetite Enhanced food intake[87,88]	No change in body composition No change in quality of life[87,88] Weight gain primarily fat[88]	
Agents with possible effectiveness:					
Growth hormone	Hormone (promotes nitrogen balance)	3	Reduced nitrogen loss[89]	Improvements not seen with severe weight loss[89]	
Oxandrolone	Anabolic steroid (promotes increase in lean body mass)	3	Weight gain Increased lean body mass Improved performance scores Improved QOL[90]	Increases in liver function tests[90]	
Dronabinol (Marinol)	Cannabinoid (antiemetic, appetite stimulant)	3	Improved mood Improved appetite[91,92]	Improvement in appetite slow (up to 4 weeks) Tumor cell proliferation in cell culture[93]	Not as effective as megestrol acetate[86]
Melatonin	Hormone (inhibition of TNF production)	3	Weight loss slowed[94,95]	No increase in food intake[94]	
Thalidomide	Immunomodulatory (inhibition of TNF production)	3	Weight gain Increased lean body mass[96] Decreased GI side effects[97]	Reduced clearance in the elderly[97]	
Eicosapentanoic acid (EPA)	Essential fatty acid/ nutraceutical (immunomodulatory[98])	3	Weight stabilization or gain[99]	No change in body composition[99]	Dose-dependent effect
Agents without proven effectiveness:					
Hydrazine sulfate	(gluconeogenic enzyme inhibitor)	3		No effect on weight loss No effect on nutritional indices Decreased QOL[100–102]	
Pentoxifylline	Inhibition of TNF production[103–105]	3	Protection against radiation-induced skin and tissue changes[106,107]	No improvement in appetite[108]	
Cyproheptadine hydrochloride	(histamine/serotonin antagonist)	3	Mild increase in appetite Decrease in nausea and vomiting[109]	No effect on weight loss[109]	
Prednisolone	Corticosteroid (appetite stimulant)	3	Increased appetite[82]	No weight gain	
Methylprednisolone	Corticosteroid (appetite stimulant)	3	Increased appetite[82]	Short duration Progressive muscle wasting Muscle weakness Hyperglycemia Osteoporosis Immunosuppression No weight gain[82] Improved QOL[110]	Recommended for palliative care only

QOL, quality of life; TNF, tumor necrosis factor.

TABLE 102.7. Prognostic Nutrition Assessment Formulae.

	History/uses	*Formula*
Prognostic nutritional index (PNI)[117]	Validated prospectively Calculates percentage risk of an operative complication occurring in an individual Can distinguish patients at low risk for nutrition related complications (<10%) from those at high risk (>50%)	Percentage risk of complication = 158 – 16.6(s. albumin; g/dl) – 0.78(TSF; mm) – 0.20(s. transferrin; g/dl) – 5.8 (delayed-type hypersensitivity reaction)
Nutrition risk index (NRI)[118,119]	Used to stratify nutrition risk in the Veterans Affairs Total Parenteral Nutrition Cooperative Study Group trial of perioperative PN Classifies individuals as either well nourished or malnourished	NRI = 1.519(s. albumin; g/dl) + 41.7(current weight/usual weight)
Hospital prognostic index (HPI)[120]	Identifies high-risk patients and evaluates the efficacy of hospital therapy	HPI = 0.91(s. albumin; g/dl) – 1.0(delayed hypersensitivity reaction) – 1.44(sepsis rating) + 0.98(diagnosis rating) – 1.09

TSF, triceps skin fold; delayed-type hypersensitivity reaction: 0 = nonreactive, 1 = <5 mm induration, 2 = >5 mm induration; PN, total parenteral nutrition; sepsis rating: 1 = present, 2 = absent; diagnosis rating: 1 = cancer present, 2 = cancer not present.

effectiveness, agents with possible effectiveness, and agents without proven effectiveness.

Megestrol acetate (MA) and medroxyprogesterone acetate (MPA) have some demonstrated effectiveness in slowing tumor-induced weight loss.[87,111] Multiple studies have demonstrated that MA can enhance food intake, weight gain, and sense of well-being in patients with advanced cancer.[14,82] Much of the associated weight gain, however, is fat rather than lean body mass.[84] MPA also stimulates appetite and food intake in cancer patients; however, it is not clear if sense of well-being or quality of life are improved.[87,111]

Growth hormone has been suggested for use as an anabolic agent in patients with CCS. In animal models, growth hormone preferentially supports lean body mass over tumor growth.[112] This effect has also been observed in humans.[113] Oxandrolone, an anabolic steroid, has been associated with increases in weight, lean body mass, performance status, and quality of life in preliminary studies.[90] Tetrahydrocannabinol derivatives (THCs; Dronabinol) have been observed to stimulate appetite and food intake. In practice, uncertainty regarding optimum dose and delayed onset of effect limit the use of these agents.[91,92] Melatonin and thalidomide have been proposed to treat cancer-induced weight loss. The theorized mechanism of action of these drugs is inhibition of TNF production. Preliminary studies of melatonin suggest reduction in weight loss.[94,95] Thalidomide can induce weight gain and increased lean body mass.[96,97]

Corticosteroids,[82] hydrazine sulfate,[100–102] pentoxifylline,[108] and cyproheptadine[109] have failed to demonstrate sustained benefit, and long-term use can be associated with unacceptable side effects.

Nutrition Care of Cancer Patients

The process of nutrition care may be broken down into a series of steps with feedback loops; these include nutrition screening, formal nutrition assessment, formulation of a nutrition care plan, implementation of the plan, patient monitoring, reassessment of the care plan, and then either reformulation of the care plan or termination of therapy.[114] Because all cancer patients are either malnourished or at risk for becoming malnourished, nutrition screening is unnecessary; the presence of cancer in and of itself defines an at-risk population and mandates formal nutrition assessment.

Significance of Malnutrition in Surgical Patients

The existence of a correlation between degree of malnutrition and increased risk of perioperative complications is undeniable. Since the first description of this relationship by Studley, in 1936,[3] numerous investigators have demonstrated the value of a variety of nutrition status parameters for predicting risk of surgical complications.[115–118] Particularly useful parameters include weight loss, serum protein levels (especially albumin), anthropometric indices (especially triceps skinfold thickness), and immunocompetence (as assessed by total lymphocyte count and delayed-type cutaneous hypersensitivity). Combinations of these indicators can stratify patients into low-, moderate-, and high-risk categories for nutrition-related surgical complications[117–120] (Table 102.7). More sophisticated measurement techniques involving isotope methods and electrical impedance may be used to assess specific body compartments, but they are not generally used in clinical practice and have not been validated for prediction of surgical risk.[121]

Given the relationship between nutrition status and operative risk, it seems obvious that nutrition support of perioperative, malnourished patients should improve clinical outcomes. Unfortunately, beneficial effects of SNS in perioperative patients have been difficult to demonstrate consistently.[7] This difficulty may be caused, in part, by methodological problems with trials performed in this setting, including the use of suboptimal feeding regimens and the inclusion of well-nourished patients unlikely to benefit from SNS. As detailed here, the issues are even more clouded in cancer patients.

Approaches to Nutrition Assessment in Cancer Patients

Nutrition assessment in perioperative patients may be performed using multivariate risk equations (Table 102.7). In clinical practice, such "objective" criteria, however, may not be necessary. The Patient Generated Subjective Global

TABLE 102.8. Elements of Patient-Generated Subjective Global Assessment, a Validated Tool for Determination of Nutrition Status and Nutrition-Related Risk.[125]

History	
	Weight change
	Change in dietary intake
	Gastrointestinal tract-related symptoms
	Change in functional capacity
	Diagnosis
Physical examination	
	Loss of subcutaneous fat
	Muscle wasting
	Ankle edema
	Sacral edema
	Ascites

Source: Blackburn GL, Bistrian BR, Maini BS, Schlamm HT, Smith MF. Nutritional and metabolic assessment of the hospitalized patient. JPEN J Parenter Enteral Nutr 1977;1:11–22.

Assessment (PG-SGA)[122] is based on a tool developed by Baker and colleagues, the Subjective Global Assessment (SGA).[122–124] Both the SGA and PG-SGA combine known prognostic indicators such as weight loss, performance status, and nutrition-related symptoms.[122] The PG-SGA uses criteria obtained from a history and physical examination performed by an experienced clinician to classify nutrition status (Table 102.8). Historical features assessed include weight change, change in dietary intake, presence of gastrointestinal symptoms, functional capacity (performance status), and primary diagnosis. The physical examination concentrates on loss of subcutaneous fat and presence of muscle wasting, ankle edema, sacral edema, and ascites. These factors are combined into a global assessment of nutrition status (A, well nourished; B, moderately malnourished; C, severely malnourished).[125] The "scored PG-SGA" additionally incorporates a numerical score in addition to the global rating.[122,125] The Oncology Dietetics Practice Group of the American Dietetics Association uses scored PG-SGA as the standard nutrition assessment for oncology patients.

In general, nutrition assessment of cancer patients is easily accomplished by taking a nutrition history and conducting a complete physical examination guided by the SGA and the PG-SGA. Diagnosis, stage of cancer, weight loss history, and changes in diet are especially informative. Serum albumin may also be helpful, as it has been shown to be of prognostic significance.[126,127] Perhaps most important is a commitment to thorough nutritional evaluation of all cancer patients serially. Despite the important role of malnutrition in the pathogenesis of cancer, nutrition assessment and nutrition care are often overlooked in this patient population.[128]

The Metabolic Effects of Specialized Nutrition Support in Cancer Patients

Nutrition care of cancer patients should focus on improvement of substrate delivery and alteration of the host metabolic milieu to improve nutrient utilization. Pharmacologic interventions, to date, play only a limited role in overcoming cancer-associated anorexia. Nutrient intake by spontaneous oral feeding is not sufficiently improved by drugs such as megestrol acetate; additional measures must be used to increase nutrient delivery to meet metabolic demands. Clinical research has focused on the use of SNS to overcome CCS-related anorexia, bypassing oral intake as the primary mode for nutrition support. To understand whether SNS is indeed helpful in cancer patients, the effect of SNS on the host and upon the tumor must be understood.

The Effects of Specialized Nutrition Support on the Host

For SNS to achieve its ultimate goal of improving outcomes in cancer patients, it must first be able to effect demonstrable changes in "intermediate endpoints" related to the nutrition status of the cancer-bearing host. Numerous studies have looked at the effect of SNS on nutritional parameters in cancer patients.

In 2002, Bozzetti authored a comprehensive overview of the effects of enteral (EN) and parenteral (PN) SNS on the nutrition status of cancer patients.[129] Citing more than 100 relevant studies, he reviewed the effect of EN and PN on body composition, protein and carbohydrate metabolism, and immune function (Table 102.9). Parenteral nutrition consistently causes weight gain, increases body fat, and improves nitrogen balance. The effects of EN on body composition are less consistent; EN usually causes weight gain and improves nitrogen balance. Despite achievement of an anabolic state as evidenced by positive nitrogen balance, neither EN nor PN, when administered for 7 to 49 days, have demonstrably beneficial effects on either serum proteins or whole-body protein kinetics. Specialized nutrition support has less of an effect on nutritional indices in cancer patients than in noncancer patients.[129,130]

The relevance of immune parameters to clinical immunocompetence and outcomes is uncertain. Patients receiving preoperative PN versus oral nutrition undergoing colorectal cancer surgery had exaggerated inflammatory responses as assessed by plasma interleukin-6 and interleukin-8 responses in the immediate postoperative period.[131] The clinical significance of these findings is unclear, but the immunosuppressive effects of these inflammatory cytokines may partially explain the apparent increase in septic complications seen in many studies of perioperative PN in cancer patients.[118]

These data demonstrate that SNS interventions can measurably affect nutrition status parameters in cancer patients, but the effects are not consistent or dramatic. The data,

TABLE 102.9. Effects of Specialized Nutrition Support on Nutrition Status and Metabolic Parameters in Cancer Patients.[129]

Parameter	*Total parenteral nutrition*	*Enteral nutrition*
Weight	⇑	⇑
Body fat	⇑	⇑
Lean body mass	⇔	⇔
Nitrogen balance	⇑	⇑
Albumin	⇔	⇔ ⇓
Plasma glucose, insulin[130]	⇑	⇔ ⇑
Humoral immunity	⇔	⇔
Cellular immunity	⇔	⇔ ⇑

⇑ Increased; ⇓ decreased; ⇔ unchanged; two symbols, data conflicted.

Source: From Bozzetti F. Rationale and indications for preoperative feeding of malnourished surgical cancer patients. Nutrition 2002;18(11-12):953–959.[129]

however, do not shed light on the impact of SNS on patient outcomes. Only clinical trials, as summarized below, can answer this most relevant question.

The Effects of Specialized Nutrition Support on the Tumor

Enthusiasm for the use of SNS in cancer patients has historically been tempered by concern that provision of nutrients may stimulate tumor growth and metastasis. Investigators have studied these issues in animal models.[132,133] Popp et al. demonstrated a dose–response relationship between PN caloric intake and growth of methylcholanthrene-induced sarcomas in Fischer-344 rats (Fig. 102.3). Tumor weight increased more than 3.5 times faster in animals receiving 167% of normal caloric intake than in those receiving 33% of normal caloric requirements. Tumor growth occurred to a greater extent than host lean body mass growth, especially at the highest caloric intakes.[134]

Composition of the SNS has been shown to have an effect on tumor growth and metastasis in rats. Torosian and Donoway compared the effect of three PN solutions (carbohydrate alone; carbohydrate plus amino acid; and carbohydrate plus amino acid plus lipid) and two oral diets (standard; and protein depleted) on primary tumor growth and lung metastasis in Lobund rats with prostate adenocarcinoma implants.[135] Tumor growth and metastasis was decreased in animals receiving an oral, protein-depleted diet. Growth and metastasis were greatest in animals receiving the complete PN diet.

These and numerous other provocative animal studies lend urgency to the question of possible deleterious stimulatory effects of SNS on tumor growth and metastasis in humans. There are few relevant clinical studies. Baron et al. studied the effect of 3 to 17 days of PN on tumor ploidy in head and neck cancer patients.[136] The percentage of hyperdiploid cells almost doubled following PN administration, whereas no such change occurred in normal mucosa or in control patients not receiving PN. Frank et al. found increased cellular proliferation in tumor tissue from all studied head and neck cancer patients after 7 days of PN.[137] The effect of PN on tumor cell kinetics was studied by Franchi et al. in 44 patients with gastrointestinal malignancies.[138] Cellular proliferation decreased 24% in patients receiving lipid-based PN (80% of total calories as fat), increased 32% in patients receiving isocaloric, fat-free PN, and increased 25% in control patients receiving oral diets. These results suggest that high parenteral lipid intakes may actually suppress tumor cell proliferation. Heys and colleagues gave nine patients with colorectal cancer PN for 24h before tumor resection and compared protein synthesis in the removed tumors with tumor protein synthesis in nine patients undergoing resection following a 24-h fast.[139] Tumor protein synthesis rates were 89% higher in patients receiving PN than in fasting patients. A commonly cited potential harm of PN is the possibility of stimulating tumor growth. Given that glucose is the preferred fuel for tumor cells, the concern that PN may "feed the tumor" has been posed. Recently, Bozzetti et al. showed that glucose-based PN does not increase glucose uptake by human tumors when compared to lipid-based PN. The patients receiving lipid-based PN did not experience a suppression of glucose uptake by tumors.[140]

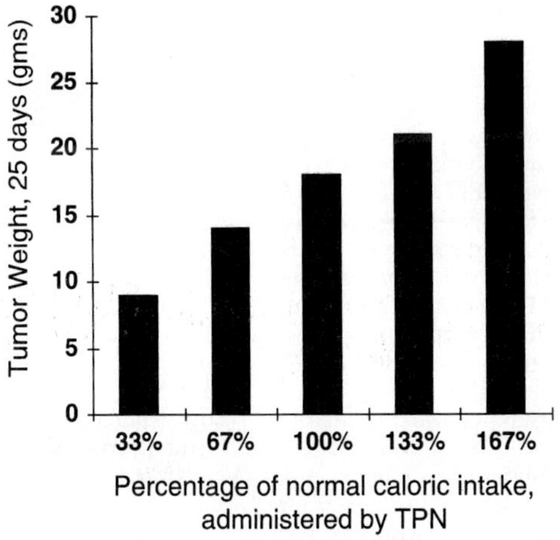

Figure 102.3. Animal data suggest that provision of nutrients to the host may stimulate tumor growth and metastasis. Popp et al. demonstrated a dose–response relationship between parenteral nutrition (PN) caloric intake and growth of methylcholanthrene-induced sarcomas in Fischer-344 rats.[134] Twenty-five days after tumor implantation, tumor weight was more than 3.5 times greater in animals receiving 167% of normal caloric intake than in those receiving 33% of normal caloric requirements via PN.

Clearly, nutritional intake may affect tumor biology in humans as well as animals. The relevance of these studies to the clinical effects of SNS in cancer patients is not known. To date, no human studies have demonstrated deleterious, clinically evident effects of SNS on tumor growth or metastasis. Absent any overt effects, it is reasonable to ignore these theoretical considerations when contemplating the use of SNS in patients. These studies even raise the intriguing possibility that SNS may be used to modulate tumor cell kinetics to increase sensitivity to chemotherapy and radiation therapy. Clinical trials are needed to investigate these concepts.

Clinical Trials of Specialized Nutrition Support in Cancer Patients

The data discussed so far may be interpreted to show that:

1. The cancer cachexia syndrome occurs commonly in cancer patients.
2. Cancer patients with CCS have poorer surgical outcomes and poorer overall survival.
3. Because current understanding of the etiology of CCS is limited, it is not yet possible to reverse the underlying metabolic, hormonal, and cytokine abnormalities associated with CCS.
4. Specialized nutrition support, either enteral or parenteral, is nutritionally effective in cancer patients as assessed by markers of nutrition status.
5. There are no obvious deleterious effects of SNS on tumor growth or metastasis in humans.

These conclusions emphasize the importance of CCS in cancer patients, and suggest that SNS may be used to counteract the nutritional sequelae of CCS. Given the complexity of SNS interventions, and potential associated complications, beneficial effects of SNS in cancer patients cannot be assumed. Clinical trial data must be reviewed to answer the question,

TABLE 102.10.

Prospective, Randomized Trials Involving 20 or More Subjects of Perioperative Specialized Nutrition Support in Cancer Patients (Level 1 Evidence).

First author	*Year*	*Level of evidence*	*Study design/eligibility criteria*	*n*	*Results*	*Comments*
PN versus standard oral diet (SOD):						
Holter[142]	1977	I	Pre- and postoperative PN vs. SOD: GI cancer; weight loss >10 lb	56	No difference in morbidity or mortality	
Sako[143]	1981	I	Post- ± preoperative PN vs. SOD; poor prognosis head and neck cancer	69	No difference in morbidity, 2 early deaths in PN group; 18-month survival better in SOD group	PN also not beneficial in patients stratified as malnourished
Muller[144]	1982	I	Preoperative PN vs. SOD; GI cancer	125	Reduced major morbidity and mortality in PN group	Well-nourished patients included
Yamada[145]	1983	I	Postoperative PN vs. SOD; gastric cancer	34	Reduced morbidity and longer disease-free survival in PN group	Randomization scheme not clearly reported
Muller[146]	1986	I	Preoperative PN vs. SOD; esophageal and gastric cancer	113	Reduced major morbidity in PN group	Various operative techniques used in different groups
Askanazi[147]	1986	I	Postoperative PN vs. D5W; cystectomy for bladder cancer	35	No difference in morbidity, 2 deaths in D5W group; LOS 17 days in PN group vs. 24 days in D5W group	Post hoc LOS analysis
Brennan[148]	1994	I	Postoperative PN vs. SOD; major pancreatic resection for cancer	117	Fewer major complications in SOD group; trend to fewer minor complications and deaths in SOD group	Well-nourished patients included
Fan[149]	1994	I	Pre- and postoperative PN vs. SOD; hepatocellular carcinoma	124	Fewer septic complications in PN group; no differences in mortality	Differences seen in patients with and without cirrhosis
Bozzetti[162]	2000	I	Preoperative and postoperative PN vs. SOD + postoperative hypocaloric PN; gastrointestinal cancer, 10% weight loss	90	Fewer complications and lower mortality in perioperative group; longer LOS in perioperative group	Malnourished patients only; hypocaloric PN included 960 Kcal, 85 g protein
Hyltander[163]	2005	I	Postoperative PN/EN vs. SOD; upper gastrointestinal malignancies	126	No difference in mortality, nutritional indices or hospital LOS; more complications in EN/PN group	Ten noncancer patients included
Wu[164]	2006	I	Preoperative and postoperative PN/EN vs. SOD + postoperative hypocaloric PN; gastrointestinal cancer, moderately to severely malnourished by SGA	468	Fewer complications, lower mortality, shorter LOS in perioperative group	Malnourished patients only; hypocaloric PN included 600 Kcal, 60 g protein
EN versus PN:						
Meijerink[150]	1992	I	Preoperative PN vs. EN vs. SOD; gastric or colorectal cancer	151	No differences in mortality; reduced intraabdominal abscess with severe malnutrition in PN and EN groups; no differences between EN and PN groups	Malnourished patients only
Gianotti[151]	1997	I	Postoperative PN vs. EN vs. isEN; gastric or pancreatic cancer	260	No differences in mortality or surgical morbidity; trend to fewer septic complications in isEN group; LOS shorter in isEN group	
Sand[152]	1997	I	Postoperative PN vs. EN; gastric cancer	29	No differences in morbidity or mortality	
Braga[153]	2001	I	Postoperative PN vs. EN; gastric, pancreatic, or esophageal cancer	257	No difference in complication rates, LOS, or mortality; higher incidence of hyperglycemia in PN group; improved intestinal oxygen tension in EN group	Lower percentage reached nutrition goals in EN group
Bozzetti[154]	2001	I	Postoperative PN vs. EN; malnourished gastrointestinal cancer	317	Decreased overall incidence of complications, incidence of minor complications, and incidence of infectious complications, and LOS in EN group; increased incidence of GI side effects in EN group	Nine percent of patients in EN group switched to PN because of complications; nutrient provision similar between groups

TABLE 102.10. (continued)

First author	*Year*	*Level of evidence*	*Study design/eligibility criteria*	*n*	*Results*	*Comments*
Aiko[155]	2001	I	Postoperative PN vs. EN; esophageal cancer	24	No difference in nutrition indices or morbidity	
Papapietro[156]	2002	I	Postoperative PN plus EN vs. early EN alone; gastric cancer	28	Nutritional indices improved and less hyperglycemia in early EN group	EN initiated in PN group after resolution of postop ileus
Jiang[157]	2003	I	Postoperative PN vs. EN; gastric or colon cancer	40	Decreased intestinal permeability in EN group	SNS started POD 3
Aiko[165]	2003	I	Postoperative PN vs. EN; esophageal cancer (± thoracic duct ligation)	39	Increase in lymphocyte count and decrease in CRP in EN group with preserved thoracic duct; total bilirubin decreased in EN groups	Small numbers when stratified by thoracic ligation
Wu[164]	2003	I	Postoperative PN vs. EN vs. SOD; chronic liver damage	135	EN group reached positive nitrogen balance first and lowest loss of body weight; increase in gut barrier permeability in PN group	Included noncancer patients (n = 98); 32 in EN group complained of abdominal distension, relieved with rate change
EN versus SOD:						
Sagar[158]	1979	I	Postoperative EN vs. SOD; "major intestinal surgery"	30	No differences in morbidity or mortality; LOS shorter in EN group	Cancer status of patients not clearly reported
Smith[159]	1985	I	Postoperative EN vs. SOD; GI cancer	50	No differences in morbidity or mortality	Only 56% of EN patients successfully fed
Foschi[160]	1986	I	Preoperative EN vs. SOD; patients with percutaneous biliary drains undergoing operation	60	Reduced in morbidity and mortality in EN group	Cancer status of patients not clearly reported; 4 EN patients also received PN
Heslin[161]	1997	I	Postoperative isEN vs. SOD	195	No differences in morbidity or mortality	
Seven[167]	2003	I	EN vs. SOD; laryngectomy	67	No differences in morbidity or mortality	

PN, parenteral nutrition; EN, enteral nutrition; isEN, immune-supplemented enteral nutrition; SOD, standard oral diet; LOS, length of hospital stay.

"Nutrition support in patients with cancer: what do the data really show?"[141] Fortunately, hundreds of studies have been conducted that address this issue. Even limiting review to prospective, randomized studies of sufficient size, many questions concerning the appropriateness and effectiveness of SNS in cancer patients may be answered with confidence.

Perioperative Nutrition Support in Cancer Patients

Table 102.10 summarizes the results of 26 prospective, randomized clinical trials that investigated the use of perioperative SNS in cancer patients.[142–167] Consideration was limited to studies published in the English language of at least 20 or more subjects, all of whom had cancer (or in which the outcomes in the subset of cancer patients were separately reported). Only studies reporting clinical outcomes (morbidity, mortality, or length of stay) were analyzed. In all these studies, SNS was initiated some time during the period starting 14 days preoperatively to 3 days postoperatively.

Before drawing conclusions from the studies in Table 102.10, a number of points must be emphasized: (1) the studies involved heterogeneous populations with different tumor types and stages undergoing different operations; (2) some studies excluded severely malnourished patients (for fear of denying them SNS), thus excluding those who might be expected to benefit most from SNS; (3) the SNS composition and route of administration varied widely between studies, and in many studies the SNS regimen would today be considered suboptimal because of overfeeding and inappropriate substrate composition; and (4) there are no studies that report functional status and quality-of-life endpoints, outcomes that are perhaps most likely to be affected by SNS.[7,168]

The studies authored by Muller et al.[144,146] are the only large studies that showed improved outcomes in patients receiving perioperative SNS (PN for 10 days before operation). The authors themselves suggest that the failure to see a difference in mortality in their second study may be attributable to improved surgical technique. In both studies, the mortality rate in the control, standard oral diet (SOD) group was quite high (approximately 20%). Discounting these two studies, the data summarized in Table 102.10 are quite consistent. There is little evidence that routine perioperative SNS improves surgical outcomes in cancer patients. This conclusion is bolstered by the results of two well-designed, prospective randomized trials of postoperative PN versus SOD[148] and of postoperative EN versus SOD.[161] Neither study showed a benefit to routine use of SNS, true for both EN and PN. The results of the comparisons of EN versus PN are inconsistent. More recent studies indicate EN may have a beneficial effect on intestinal permeability and incidence of hyperglycemia in comparison to the PN group.

Not included in the summary table is the Veterans Affairs Cooperative Study Group trial of perioperative PN in surgical patients. The report of this study did not separate outcomes in cancer patients (who comprised approximately two-thirds of the subjects) from those in subjects with benign diagnoses.[118] This randomized study of 395 patients undergoing major abdominal or thoracic procedures failed to demonstrate any benefit to PN given 7 to 15 days preoperatively and for at least 3 days postoperatively. Furthermore, PN actually increased the risk of perioperative infectious complications (primarily pneumonia and bacteremia) in mildly and moderately malnourished patients.

Forty-six trials of the use of specialized nutrition support were reviewed in narrative to assess the clinical efficacy of enteral and parenteral nutrition in cancer patients. This analysis suggested that at least 7 days of preoperative PN were required to decrease the rate of major perioperative complications in surgical patients. The majority of the trials suggested that there was no improvement in length of hospital stay.[141]

The data are conclusive. Routine use of SNS in patients undergoing major cancer operations does not improve surgical outcomes when either morbidity or mortality is used as endpoint. Preoperative SNS may be beneficial in moderately or severely malnourished patients if administered for 7 to 14 days preoperatively. In this situation, the potential benefits of nutrition support must be weighed against the potential risks of the SNS itself, and of delaying the operation.

Nutrition Support in Patients Receiving Stem Cell Transplants

PN may be beneficial in stem cell transplant (SCT) patients. Table 102.11 summarizes prospective, randomized trials of 30 subjects or more receiving SNS after stem cell transplant.[169–172] Although SNS does not appear to reduce toxicity, it may reduce length of stay.[169,173–175] Furthermore, one study demonstrated a long-term survival advantage in patients who received PN compared with SOD controls.[169] This significant benefit (21 months versus 7 months) is hard to interpret, however, because it was not evident until 6 months after transplantation. More recent studies seem to indicate that PN may prevent weight loss in SCT patients.[172]

Nutrition Support in Patients Receiving Chemotherapy

Table 102.12 summarizes the results of 14 prospective, randomized clinical trials that investigated the use of adjunctive SNS in cancer patients receiving chemotherapy.[176–189] Consideration was limited to studies published in the English language of at least 30 or more subjects. Only studies reporting clinical outcomes (morbidity, mortality, and/or functional status and quality of life) were analyzed. In these studies, SNS was generally given for 3 to 6 weeks before and/or during chemotherapy administration. The limitations of these studies are similar to those enumerated for studies of perioperative SNS. Study design and inclusion criteria heterogeneity, exclusion of malnourished patients, and use of suboptimal SNS regimens limits the application of these studies to current patient care.

Despite these limitations, the data are once again clear. Except in the study of Tandon et al.[182] (the interpretation of which is limited by the lack of any statistical analysis), there was no benefit to the routine use of SNS as an adjunct to chemotherapy. Toxicity (defined by severity of bone marrow suppression) was not reduced, and tumor responses and patient survival were not improved. Because of an increased risk of infection associated with the use of PN (approximately fourfold), routine adjunctive use was actually deleterious. These findings are bolstered by the results of three meta-analyses, which all reached similar conclusions.[190–192]

From these data, it can be firmly recommended that SNS not be used routinely as an adjunctive therapy in cancer

TABLE 102.11.
Prospective, Randomized Trials Involving 30 or More Subjects of Specialized Nutrition Support in Stem Cell Transplantation.

First author	*Year*	*Level of evidence*	*Study design/eligibility criteria*	*n*	*Results*	*Comments*
Weisdorf[169]	1987	I	PN vs. IVF + vitamins and minerals; SCT in patients with hematological and solid malignancies	137	Improved survival and time to relapse in PN group; no effect on GVHD or infection	
Charuhas[170]	1997	I	PN vs. IVF; post-SCT in outpatients with hematologic and solid malignancies	258	Resumption of oral intake earlier in IVF group; less weight loss in PN group	
Muscaritoli[171]	1998	I	Glucose-based PN vs. lipid-based PN; allogenic SCT in patients with hematological malignancies	60	Increased incidence of acute GVHD and hyperglycemia in glucose group; trend toward better survival in lipid group	Glucose-based PN – 100% NPC from glucose; lipid based PN – 20% NPC from glucose
Roberts[172]	2003	I	PN vs. SOD; autologous SCT in breast cancer patients	55	Improved nutrition status and increased preservation of LBM in PN group; trend to improved QOL in PN group	PN started 1 day prior to HCT; 50% of SOD group received PN due to poor intake

GVHD, graft-versus-host disease; NPC, nonprotein calories; SCT, stem cell transplant; SOD, standard oral diet; QOL, quality of life.

TABLE 102.12.

Prospective, Randomized Trials Involving 30 or More Subjects of Specialized Nutrition Support in Cancer Patients Undergoing Chemotherapy.

First author	*Year*	*Level of evidence*	*Study design*	*n*	*Results*	*Comments*
Jordan[176]	1981	I	PN vs. SOD; advanced lung cancer	65	No differences in toxicity or response rate; reduced survival in PN group	Randomization scheme not strictly followed
Nixon[177]	1981	I	PN vs. SOD; advanced colorectal cancer	50	No differences in toxicity or response rate; reduced survival in PN group	
Popp[178]	1981	I	PN vs. SOD; advanced diffuse lymphoma	42	No differences in toxicity, response rate, or survival	High rate of catheter-related thrombosis
Samuels[179]	1981	I	PN vs. SOD; stage III testicular cancer	30	No differences in toxicity, response rate, or survival; septicemia more frequent in PN group	Randomization scheme not strictly followed
Serrou[180]	1982	I	PN vs. SOD; small cell lung cancer	39	No differences in toxicity, response rate, or survival	
Shamberger[181]	1984	I	PN vs. SOD; adjuvant therapy in sarcoma patients	32	No differences in toxicity, response rate, or survival; disease-free survival reduced in PN group; treatment deaths more common in SOD group	
Tandon[182]	1984	I	EN vs. SOD; advanced GI cancer	70	Decreased toxicity, improved response rate in EN group	No formal statistical analysis
Clamon[183]	1985	I	PN vs. SOD; small cell lung cancer	119	No differences in toxicity, response rate, or survival	No benefit to PN seen even in malnourished patients
Valdivieso[184]	1987	I	PN vs. SOD; small cell lung cancer	65	No differences in toxicity or survival; trend to improved complete response rate in SOD group	
Evans[185]	1987	I	SOD vs. SOD + nutrition counseling vs. SOD + oral supplementation; metastatic lung and colorectal cancer		No differences in toxicity, response rate, or survival	Oral supplementation brought intake to 25% of calories as protein, 150 mg/day Zn and 266 mg/day Mg; patients counseled to maintain weight as determined by Harris Benedict equation; crossover of patients with poor intake to EN or PN
Hyltander[188]	1991	I	PN + SOD vs. SOD	33	Higher percentage patients in positive energy balance, weight gain in PN group; weight gain attributed to fat gain; nitrogen loss similar between groups	PN group provided with 150% caloric needs
De Cicco[186]	1993	I	Crossover study, one of two consecutive chemotherapy cycles with PN and one without; bladder cancer, small cell lung cancer, and Hodgkin's disease	43	No differences in toxicity	
Bozzetti[187]	1998	I	EN vs. SOD; esophageal cancer	50	Decreased body weight, total protein, and serum albumin in SOD group; no effect on chemotherapy tolerance, response, or survival	EN group more malnourished before treatment
Jin[189]	1999	I	PN vs. PN + chemotherapy vs. SOD + chemotherapy vs. SOD; gastrointestinal cancer patients with severe to moderate malnutrition	92	Proliferation of tumor cells in PN only group; improved prealbumin, transferrin, nitrogen balance in PN groups; no difference in weight	Ten-day PN intervention

Year, year of publication; *n*, number of patients; PN, total parenteral nutrition; SOD, standard oral diet; Zn, zinc; Mg, magnesium.

patients receiving chemotherapy. Specialized nutrition support is clearly appropriate in patients receiving active anticancer treatment who are malnourished and who are anticipated to be unable to absorb adequate nutrients for a prolonged period of time.[114]

Nutrition Support in Patients Receiving Radiation Therapy

There are few prospective, randomized clinical trials investigating the routine use of SNS as an adjunct to radiation therapy in cancer patients, which may in part be explained by the relatively milder acute physiological impact of radiation therapy in comparison with either surgery or chemotherapy. A number of reviews have tried to summarize the role of SNS in this setting.[7,141,193] As might be expected, there is no clearly defined role for routine EN, PN, or oral supplements during head and neck, abdominal, or pelvic irradiation. A recent retrospective study of 45 patients by Sikora et al. considered the impact of PN on outcomes in patients receiving preoperative chemoirradiation for esophageal cancer.[194] Although patients receiving PN were able to receive a greater proportion of their planned chemotherapy, there were no differences observed in chemotherapy- or radiation therapy-related complication rates, in tumor response rates, or in surgical morbidity or mortality.

Nutritional Pharmacology in Cancer Patients

Some nutrients have specific biologic effects on tumor and host tissues and cells. These effects extend beyond the nutritional value of these substrates. Some nutrients are claimed to enhance host immunocompetence or to alter host or tumor metabolism. Use of specific substances for effects beyond their nutritional role may be referred to as nutritional pharmacology. Four nutrients have been the subject of recent research: glutamine, arginine, nucleic acids, and essential fatty acids (Table 102.13).

Glutamine

Glutamine (GLN), the most abundant amino acid in the human body, is considered nonessential. It is an important substrate for rapidly proliferating cells such as lymphocytes, macrophages, enterocytes, fibroblasts, and renal epithelium.[195] It acts as a nitrogen shuttle between tissues and is a precursor for the synthesis of purines, pyrimidines, and amino acids.[196] It is also a major respiratory fuel for tumor cells. Alterations in glutamine metabolism in the tumor-bearing host suggest that in cancer patients glutamine may be conditionally essential. Peripheral muscle stores of GLN are reduced in cancer patients.[197] It is hypothesized that glutamine supplementation in cancer patients may restore immunocompetence and gut barrier function by providing substrate to glutamine-requiring tissues that are made conditionally deficient by the presence of a tumor.

GLN has been supplemented in both enteral nutrition and parenteral nutrition.[198–202] GLN-supplemented enteral formulas commonly contain other immunonutrients, such as arginine and omega-3 fatty acids (*n*-3FA). Therefore, there are limited data on the effectiveness of enteral GLN alone as an immunonutrient. However, there is some research utilizing GLN powder indicating glutamine may play a role in the prevention of chemotherapy- and radiation-induced toxicity. A meta-analysis of human and animal studies suggests it may be effective in decreasing the incidence and severity of chemotherapy-induced mucositis, irinotecan-induced diarrhea,

TABLE 102.13. Substrates with Potential Beneficial Effects for Use as Nutritional Pharmacological Agents in Cancer Patients.

Substrate	*Metabolic activities*	*Clinical use*
Glutamine	Most abundant amino acid in the human body, nonessential Important substrate for rapidly proliferating cells such as lymphocytes,macrophages, enterocytes, fibroblasts, and renal epithelium Nitrogen shuttle between tissues Precursor for the synthesis of purines, pyrimidines, and amino acids Major respiratory fuel for tumor cells May be conditionally essential in tumor-bearing hosts	Potentially beneficial as a supplement to PN in bone marrow transplant patients Currently being evaluated for prevention of chemotherapy and radiation toxicity
Arginine	Nonessential amino acid, may become conditionally essential during periods of physiological stress Substrate in the urea cycle, roles in protein, creatinine, and polyamine synthesis Effects nitrogen metabolism, wound healing, immunocompetence, and tumor metabolism Immune-enhancing effects include inhibition of tumor growth by improving natural killer, lymphokine-activated killer, and macrophage cytotoxicity, and by stimulating host (but not tumor) protein synthesis	May improve immunological indices postoperatively
Nucleic acids	Stimulatory effects on nonspecific parameters of immune function Mechanism of action not understood	No clinical studies performed
Essential fatty acids	*n*-3 polyunsaturated fatty acids (PUFAs) favor production of 3-series prostaglandins (PGE_3) and 5-series leukotrienes (immune-enhancing and antiinflammatory) *n*-3 PUFAs reduce production of 2-series prostaglandins (PGE_2) and 4-series leukotrienes (immunosuppressive and proinflammatory)	Possibly beneficial in cachexic patients

paclitaxel-induced neuropathy, and hepatic venoocclusive disease.[195]

Standard PN does not contain GLN because it is unstable in its free form. Common GLN dipeptides that are stable in an aqueous solution are alanyl-glutamine and glycyl-glutamine.[203] One prospective, randomized study of perioperative parenteral GLN in colorectal cancer patients indicated improved nitrogen balance with glutamine supplementation.[199] A recent study of acute myeloid leukemia patients receiving high-dose chemotherapy without SCT indicated quicker return of neutrophil count with GLN-supplemented PN.[203]

GLN supplementation has been studied in patients receiving stem cell transplant. Enteral GLN has been associated with decreased length of stay and decreased need for PN.[200,201] It is hypothesized that GLN provides a gut protective effect when it is supplemented enterally, although parenteral GLN is metabolized similarly.[195] One study of GLN-supplemented PN in SCT indicates improved lymphocyte recovery but worse mucositis.[202] The significance of these results is unclear.

Arginine

Arginine (ARG) has been demonstrated in animal models to have effects on nitrogen metabolism, wound healing, immunocompetence, and tumor metabolism. It is a nonessential amino acid that may become conditionally essential during periods of physiological stress. It is a substrate in the urea cycle and plays a role in protein, creatinine, and polyamine synthesis.[196] The immune-enhancing effects of arginine have been reported to inhibit tumor growth in animals by improving natural killer, lymphokine-activated killer, and macrophage cytotoxicity and by stimulating host (but not tumor) protein synthesis. Similar effects have been demonstrated in humans.[196]

Similar to glutamine, ARG is commonly supplemented enterally in conjunction with other immunonutrients. Table 102.14 includes studies of arginine alone and in combination with *n*-3 FA, GLN, and RNA.[161,198,204–212] Studies of ARG in combination with other immunonutrients indicate improved immune parameters and decreased incidence of infection. Enterally supplemented ARG alone had little impact on morbidity and mortality in two studies; however, both studies were flawed.[211,212] Perioperative parenteral ARG supplementation was studied by Song et al. in colorectal cancer patients. Patients receiving ARG-supplemented PN experienced enhanced immune responsiveness when compared to controls.[213]

Nucleic Acids

Nucleotides, administered in the form of nucleic acids, have stimulatory effects on nonspecific parameters of immune function.[196] The mechanism of action is not understood. The effects of nucleotide supplementation in cancer patients is not well characterized because nucleotides have not been administered as the single experimental agent in controlled clinical trials. A series of studies by Lacour et al. in breast cancer patients raises the possibility of a beneficial effect on disease-free and overall survival, but it is not clear that the polyadenylic-polyuridylic acid supplement administered in these studies was the active agent.[214,215] There was no effect on survival with nucleotide supplementation in colorectal cancer patients.[216]

Essential Fatty Acids

Certain polyunsaturated fatty acids (PUFAs) cannot be synthesized by humans and are therefore required in the diet. The essential fatty acids fall into two main categories, the *n*-6 series derived from linoleic acid and the *n*-3 series derived from linolenic acid (fish oils). The *n*-3 fatty acids favor production of prostaglandins in the 3-series (PGE_3) and leukotrienes in the 5-series (which are associated with improved immunocompetence and reduced inflammatory responses) and reduce levels of the PGE_2 and leukotrienes in the 4-series (immunosuppressive and proinflammatory).[217,218] *n*-3 fatty acids have been supplemented enterally in pill form and in liquid nutrition supplements, as well as parenterally. They have also been supplemented in combination with other immunonutrients. In addition to the effects of *n*-3 fatty acids on prostaglandin synthesis and cyclooxygenase (COX)-2 inhibition, they also seem to be effective in reducing proinflammatory cytokines in CCS.[217] Early studies of *n*-3 fatty acid were performed in pancreatic cancer patients; more recent studies have looked at other cancer types. Enteral *n*-3 fatty acids appear to stabilize weight in cancer patients (see Table 102.14).[219–221] Currently, additional studies are underway to assess the effectiveness of liquid nutritional supplements containing *n*-3 fatty acids. Wachtler et al. studied parenteral *n*-3 fatty acid supplementation in colorectal cancer patients. The patients who received *n*-3 fatty acids had improved LT5 levels and decreased TNF levels.[222]

In summary, the role of supplementation with these nutrients (GLN, ARG, nucleic acids, and PUFAs) individually is not known. Interpretation of studies performed to date is confounded by uncertainties in dose and route of administration and by failure of investigators to study the nutrients in isolation.

Combinations of Specific Nutrients

The largest clinical trials that have investigated nutritional pharmacological interventions in perioperative cancer patients have all used a commercially available enteral formula (Impact; Novartis Nutrition) containing supplemental arginine, RNA, and *n*-3 fatty acids (isEN). Eight studies evaluated the effect of isEN on nonspecific parameters of immunocompetence such as immunoglobulin levels, cytokine profiles, T-cell profiles, and macrophage function. Table 102.14 summarizes the results of these studies, all prospective, randomized clinical trials published in the English language of at least 20 or more subjects, all of whom had cancer.[161,204–210,223–227] In all these studies, SNS was initiated at some time during the period from 7 days preoperatively to 3 days postoperatively.

Nutrition parameters were improved in three studies.[204,205,207] Six of the studies indicated an improvement in immune parameters or incidence of infections.[204–206,208–210] Given the difficulties in assessing immune status in a fashion that is clinically meaningful, these results are interesting but of questionable significance.

TABLE 102.14.
Prospective, Randomized Trials Involving 20 or More Subjects of Immune-Supplemented Enteral Nutrition Support in Cancer Patients (Level 1 Evidence).

First author	*Year*	*Level of evidence*	*Study design*	*n*	*Results*	*Comments*
Arginine, RNA, and omega-3 fatty acids:						
Daly[204]	1992	I	EN vs. isEN	85	Improved nutrition and immune parameters, clinical outcomes in isEN group	Criticized because of post hoc grouping of endpoints exclusions
Senkal[205]	1995	I	EN vs. isEN; upper GI cancer	42	Improved nutrition and immune parameters in isEN group	No clinical endpoints
Daly[206]	1995	I	EN vs. isEN; upper GI cancer	60	Improved immune parameters, clinical outcomes in isEN group	
Braga[207]	1996	I	Preoperative, oral EN vs. isEN; colorectal and stomach cancer	40	Improved nutrition and gut function parameters in isEN group	No clinical endpoints
Heslin[161]	1997	I	Intravenous crystalloid vs. isEN; upper GI cancer surgery	195	Trend toward increased morbidity, mortality in isEN group	isEN outcomes not attributable to jejunostomy-related complications. Mean volume of isEN 300 ml/day
Braga[208]	1998	I	PN vs. EN vs. isEN; gastric and pancreatic cancer	166	Increased incidence of cardio-pulmonary complications in PN group. Lower severity of postoperative infections and shorter LOS in malnourished isEN group compared to PN group. Earlier return of bowel function in EN groups	78% of subjects classified as malnourished pre-op
Di Carlo[209]	1999	I	PN vs. EN vs. isEN; pancreatic cancer	100	Decreased morbidity, infections, LOS in the isEN group. Earlier return of bowel function in EN groups	EN not tolerated in 16% of patients
Senkal[223]	1999	I	Pre- and postoperative isEN vs. Pre- and postoperative EN; upper gastrointestinal cancer	154	Decreased infection complications and decreased cost of complications in isEN group	
Braga[224]	2002	I	Preoperative and postoperative isEN vs. pre-op isEN and postoperative EN vs. postoperative EN; cancer of the gastrointestinal tract, weight loss >10%	150	Decreased morbidity and LOS in preoperative and postoperative isEN group	Malnourished patients only
Gianotti[210]	2002	I	Preoperative isEN + SOD vs. pre and postoperative isEN + SOD vs. SOD alone; cancer of the gastrointestinal tract	305	Decreased postoperative infections and shorter LOS in isEN groups	Malnourished patients excluded
Farreras[225]	2005	I	Postoperative isEN vs. EN; gastric cancer	66	Higher markers of healing and lower incidence of wound healing complication in isEN group	
Arginine, glutamine, and n-3 fatty acids:						
Wu[198]	2001	I	Postoperative EN vs. postoperative supplemented EN; gastrointestinal cancers	48	Improved immune parameters, decreased pro-inflammatory cytokines in immune supplemented EN group	
Chen[226]	2005	I	Postoperative EN vs. postoperative supplemented EN; gastric cancers	40	Increased prealb, transferrin (day 9), increased IG, CD4, IL-2 in isEN group; decreased IL-6 and TNF in isEN group	
Arginine and n-3 fatty acids:						
Braga[227]	2002	I	Preoperative enriched EN vs. pre- and postoperative enriched EN vs. preoperative EN vs. SOD alone; colorectal cancer	200	Improved immune response, gut oxygenation, microprofusion in enriched EN group; decreased infection rate in enriched EN group	

TABLE 102.14. (continued)

First author	*Year*	*Level of evidence*	*Study design*	*n*	*Results*	*Comments*
Arginine						
van Bokhorst-De Van Der Schueren[211]	2001	I	Postoperative EN vs. pre & postoperative EN vs. pre-op EN with arginine; malnourished head and neck cancer	49	Trend toward better survival in arginine group. No effect on morbidity	
de Luis[212]	2004	I	Post op EN vs. EN with arginine; head and neck cancer	90	Decreased incidence of fistula and LOS in arginine group; increased gastrointestinal intolerance in arginine group	Severely malnourished (weight loss > 10%) patients excluded
Omega-3 fatty acids:						
Fearon[220]	2001	I	SOD + standard oral supplement vs. SOD + *n*-3 FA enriched liquid supplement; pancreatic cancer	200	Gain of weight and LBM in n-3 fatty acid group	
Jatoi[219]	2004	I	*n*-3 FA enriched oral supplement vs. megestrol acetate vs. *n*-3 FA enriched oral supplement + megestrol acetate; incurable malignancies	421	Weight stabilization and improved appetite in both groups; No effect on mortality or QOL	
Moses[221]	2004	I	SOD + standard oral supplement vs. SOD + *n*-3 FA enriched oral supplement; pancreatic cancer	24	Increased physical activity and total energy expenditure in *n*-3 fatty acid group	Patients with BMI >30 excluded

Year, year of publication; n, number of subjects; EN, enteral nutrition; isEN, enteral nutrition supplemented with arginine, RNA, and *n*-3 fatty acids; LOS, length of hospital stay; SOD, standard oral diet; LBM, lean body mass; BMI, body mass index.

Daly and colleagues conducted two trials comparing isEN to unsupplemented EN in cancer patients undergoing major upper gastrointestinal surgery. Their first study reported a significant reduction in infectious/healing complications and length of stay in the isEN group; there was no difference in mortality between the groups.[204] This study of 85 patients has been criticized because of apparent post hoc grouping of various categories of complications, and because of exclusion of patients from the supplemented group who were apparently more ill than those excluded from the control group.[228] Their second study of 60 patients randomized to either isEN or unsupplemented EN also demonstrated a reduction in perioperative morbidity and length of stay, but no difference in mortality.[206] A well-designed study by Heslin et al. randomized patients undergoing major gastrointestinal resection for malignancy to receive either isEN or intravenous fluids for 10 days postoperatively (or until the initiation of oral intake, whichever came first).[161] No statistically significant differences in morbidity or mortality were noted between the groups.

Subsequently, five prospective randomized trials of isEN in cancer patients have been performed.[161,207–210] A meta-analysis that summarizes these studies demonstrates a lower incidence of infectious complications with the use of isEN, especially with those formulas that were high in arginine. This benefit was more significant in surgical patients as opposed to critically ill patients.[229]

From the foregoing discussion, it is evident that supplementation with nutritional pharmaceuticals holds promise for cancer patients. Biomarkers such as immune status and nitrogen balance may be favorably affected by specific nutrients. The information regarding specific nutrients is mounting. For some of the nutrients, such as glutamine and *n*-3FA, more information is needed on dosing and administration. Combinations of immunonutrients need to be studied in larger populations of cancer patients, but currently available data suggest a role for isEN in malnourished cancer patients undergoing major thoracic or abdominal procedures.[210,227,230,231] Forethought in the operating room to establish reliable enteral access can facilitate administration of isEN.

Specialized Nutrition Support in Terminally Ill Cancer Patients

Despite published guidelines that state that the palliative use of SNS is rarely appropriate,[114] this issue remains controversial. As has recently been asked, "Is parenteral nutrition ever appropriate in palliative care?"[232] This question is unlikely to ever be the subject of a prospective, randomized trial because of the emotionally charged circumstances under which these clinical decisions are made. However, given the increasing frequency of the use of home PN in patients with a cancer diagnosis, it is important to address this issue; patients' quality of life and significant health care resources are at stake.[233]

In general, PN is only indicated when incurable patients are receiving active anticancer therapy, are malnourished, and are unable to take in adequate oral or enteral nutrients for a significant period of time.[114] Some investigators have identified a small subset of terminally ill cancer patients with dysfunctional gastrointestinal tracts in whom long-term

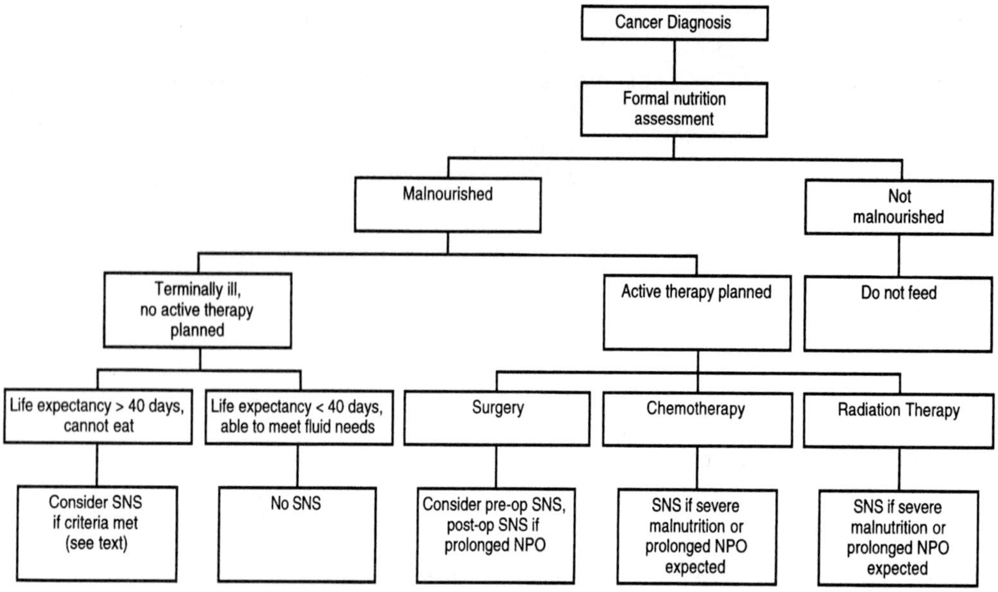

Figure 102.4. An evidence-based algorithm for decisions regarding the appropriate use of specialized nutrition support (*SNS*) in cancer patients.

home PN may provide palliative benefits.[234–237] In carefully selected patients, home PN can lengthen survival and improve quality of life. There is general consensus that, if patients are to benefit from this complex, intrusive, and expensive therapy, they (1) must be very strongly motivated and physically capable of participating in the their own care; (2) should have an estimated life expectancy of greater than 40 to 60 days; and (3) require strong social and financial support at home, including a dedicated in-home lay care provider. Furthermore, they must fail trials of less invasive therapies, including aggressive medical management with antiemetics, narcotics, anticholinergics, and antidepressants.[235,238] Those patients with a life expectancy of less than 40 days are often well palliated with home intravenous fluid therapy. Most patients evaluated for palliative care with home PN do not meet these criteria. Frank, compassionate discussions with these patients, their families, and their referring physicians are crucial if optimal decisions are to be made and accepted by all involved.

Clinical Algorithm

These data allow evidence-based decisions to be made regarding the appropriate use of SNS in many situations involving cancer patients (Figs. 102.4, 102.5). Foremost, a diagnosis of cancer in and of itself identifies the patient as nutritionally at risk. All hospitalized cancer patients, and many outpatients, should undergo a formal nutrition status assessment. The goal of this assessment is to identify those patients who are indeed malnourished and to counsel patients concerning the nutritional impact of cancer and potential dietary changes to ameliorate the effects of the disease and its treatment.

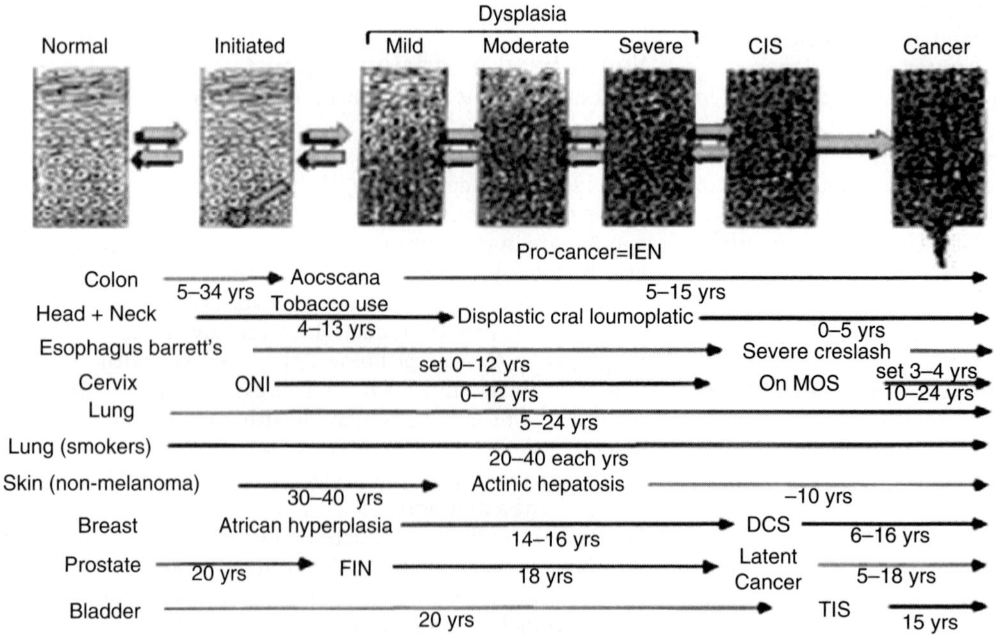

Figure 102.5. Human tumors evolve over decades. The estimate of time for the progression through initiation, dysplasia, and carcinoma in situ (CIS) to cancer varies among tumor types. (From O'Shaughnessy et al., with permission of Clinical Cancer Research 2002;8(2):314.)

There is no indication for the *routine* use of SNS in cancer patients. Adequately nourished patients do not benefit from "adjuvant" nutrition support, and this may actually harm some patients.

For patients undergoing surgery, preoperative SNS should be considered in those who are moderately or severely malnourished. Oral supplements may occasionally be adequate; most often, either EN or PN is required to meet nutritional needs and initiate nutritional repletion. To be effective, preoperative support should be initiated at least 7 days before surgery, and preferably 10 to 14 days preoperatively. For malnourished patients in whom surgery cannot be delayed, or who are recognized postoperatively as unlikely to be able to meet nutritional needs orally within 7 days, SNS is indicated. Forethought to establish enteral feeding access (a gastrostomy or jejunostomy tube) during an abdominal surgical procedure can simplify the decision to initiate SNS by providing an efficient, secure route for EN. In those patients without enteral access or in whom the gastrointestinal tract is nonfunctional, PN should be used. Because of the variable nutrient requirements in cancer patients, and because perioperative needs are most often dictated by the physiological status of the patient, protein and calorie requirements must be measured or estimated for each patient. Currently, there is no proven role for nutritional pharmacological supplements.

In patients receiving chemotherapy or radiation therapy, SNS should be reserved for those patients who are moderately to severely malnourished and in whom oral intake is expected to be inadequate for a prolonged period of time (14 days or longer).

Patients who are terminally ill and who are not receiving active anticancer treatment rarely benefit from SNS. The risk, inconvenience, and discomfort outweigh the potential palliative benefit. Patients who are unable to meet their fluid requirements orally because of malignant bowel obstruction or treatment-related side effects may benefit from intravenous fluid therapy administered intermittently in an ambulatory care setting or at home. On rare occasions, a terminally ill patient not receiving active therapy may derive benefit from home parenteral nutrition if life expectancy is greater than 40 to 60 days, functional status is good, there is a dedicated and capable care provider living with the patient, and the costs of the therapy do not place a prohibitive burden upon the patients or their heirs.

Given the general physiological and nutritional equivalence of EN and PN in cancer patients, EN is the preferred method of SNS whenever possible. EN is simpler, cheaper, and safer if the gastrointestinal tract is functional and secure enteral access can be established.

The Role of Diet in Carcinogenesis and Cancer Prevention

In 1981, Doll and Peto published a widely quoted estimate that 35% of all cancer deaths may be avoidable by changes in diet.[239] This estimate was updated by Willett in 1995.[240] Although arriving at a similar estimate (32%), use of more recent data allowed a narrowing of the likely upper and lower bounds of that number to 20% to 42%. These estimates identify a crucial opportunity for the safe reduction of cancer morbidity and mortality through dietary interventions. They also raise a series of questions: What is the quality of the evidence upon which such estimates are made? What are the mechanisms by which diet affects cancer risk? Are there appropriate recommendations that can be made when counseling patients? What about "alternative/complementary therapies?"

The Nature of the Evidence Relating Diet and Cancer

A range of evidence is available relating cancer risk and dietary intake. The nature of the problem, unfortunately, limits the availability of controlled clinical trials.[241]

Epidemiological studies are the primary source of information regarding the effects of specific diets on cancer risk. Population studies have been particularly informative. However, these studies cannot control for all confounding factors. Exposures to exogenous and endogenous carcinogens including radiation, physical agents, bacteria, and viruses impact carcinogenesis and therefore further confound studies.[242]

Case-control studies can control for confounding factors that cannot be accounted for in population studies. Although more powerful, these types of studies are more expensive, and by their nature require retrospective assessment of exposure (i.e., dietary intake). There are numerous methodological difficulties with retrospective determination of dietary intake and nutrient exposure.[243] Cohort studies, because they are prospective, overcome many of these methodological limitations. Unfortunately, cohort studies are complex and expensive because they involve collecting detailed data in large populations over an extended period of time.

In vitro and animal studies are very useful to generate hypotheses and to test mechanisms of carcinogenesis and of cancer prevention. These systems permit the use of strictly defined interventions under tightly controlled circumstances. Species differences, however, make it impossible to reliably extrapolate these data to humans.

Human dietary intervention studies are the strongest source of information concerning the diet–cancer relationship. They may be used to actually investigate the effect of dietary interventions on intermediate endpoints (for example, regression of preneoplastic lesions, or change in a proliferation marker associated with cancer risk). Dietary intervention studies are very complex and expensive. Large numbers of subjects must be included, as even in high-risk populations the number of cases is small. Subjects must be followed over a long period of time because of the latency of cancer development. Dietary compliance in intervention groups and dietary changes in control groups stimulated by greater diet awareness may blunt the observable effect of interventions.[244] It is also unknown if the effectiveness of individual nutrients relies on a critical exposure period or is tumor specific.[245]

In light of these methodological difficulties, pronouncements concerning dietary effects on cancer risk must be regarded with caution. Absent data from controlled clinical trials, interpretation of epidemiological data should be performed only with knowledge of mechanistic and biological observations that make the epidemiological associations observed biologically plausible. In general, claims about overall dietary influences (e.g., caloric intake, food groups such as fresh fruits and vegetables) are more reliable than those concerning specific foods or nutrients. Putative protective individual nutrients identified in epidemiological studies may be ineffective when administered alone outside the context of associated nutrients that may be required for activation or as cofactors. Furthermore, such putative nutrients may in fact only be measurable "passengers," accompanying unidentified trace compounds that are the true active agents.

How Does Diet Affect Cancer Risk?

Multiple mechanisms have been proposed whereby dietary intake may influence carcinogenesis.[243,246,247] It is likely that all these mechanisms play a role to some extent.

Procarcinogenic factors in the diet include sedentary lifestyle, energy intake, and specific substances. The correlation of dietary fat intake to cancer incidence is somewhat controversial. Although initial studies indicated a link between high dietary fat intake and cancer, more recently several epidemiological studies have indicated a weak or no association.[241] Energy intake is also positively correlated with cancer risk and mortality.[166] Specific dietary substances associated with increased cancer risk include smoked, broiled, and charred foods and those rich in nitrites (both of which contain procarcinogens and carcinogens), and pickled and other salty foods (salt is a cocarcinogen in the stomach, increasing oxidative stress and thereby inducing lipid peroxidation and cellular proliferation).

Dietary elements may protect against carcinogens by altering components of the cytochrome P-450 system. Specific nutrients and foods may induce detoxifying pathways that metabolize individual carcinogens or may block precarcinogen access to activating enzymes. For example, smokers who are active metabolizers of the antihypertensive agent debrisoquine appear to be at higher risk for development of lung and bladder cancer.[248] A dietary constituent that competitively blocks this pathway could potentially reduce lung and bladder cancer incidence in some smokers who are poor metabolizers.

The antioxidant hypothesis has received much attention in both scientific and lay publications.[249–251] The proposed anticarcinogenic properties of substances such as vitamin E, vitamin C, selenium, carotenoids, and bioflavonoids are thought to result from their antioxidant function. It is postulated that oxidative damage to DNA caused by normal metabolism, aging, and various environmental and dietary exposures results in DNA damage. Antioxidant nutrients may scavenge free oxygen radicals before they cause mutagenic changes to DNA.[252]

There may also be a relationship between dietary intake and in vivo apoptosis. Nutrients that increase mitogenesis in target tissues are often implicated in tissue-specific carcinogenesis; they may increase the risk for mutations and chance development of malignant genotypes. Apoptosis, the process of programmed cell death, may protect against the development of cancer by eliminating unrepairable, potentially mutagenic changes in chromosomal DNA.[253]

Interestingly, caloric restriction may be very effective in both reducing oxidative damage and stimulating apoptosis (the latter particularly in preneoplastic cells). Especially intriguing is the role that dietary caloric restriction may play in the reduction of cancer incidence.[251,253–255] Human studies provide evidence of a link between cancer incidence and mortality and caloric intake.[166] There are also nutrient-specific mechanisms by which dietary constituents may reduce cancer risk. Fiber may reduce colorectal carcinogenesis by decreasing stool transit time and altering mucosal exposure to bile constituents and metabolites.[256] Calcium ameliorates proliferative changes in colorectal epithelium in rodents and humans. Vitamin D appears to have similar effects.[257] Folate's role in DNA synthesis and repair as well as possible effects on DNA methylation indicates a paradoxical role for folate in both colorectal cancer prevention and possibly in carcinogenesis.[258] Pseudoestrogenic effects of genistein and other phytoestrogens (which are found in high concentrations, relatively, in soybeans) may exert cancer-preventive effects as estrogen antagonists.[259] Polyphenols found in tea, curcumin, and in some fruits and vegetables have a variety of antiproliferative, antioxidant, and cytochrome P-450-inducing effects, all of which may be anticarcinogenic.[245,260,261]

What Recommendations Can Be Made to Patients?

Patients diagnosed with cancer often ask what they can do with their lifestyle and diet to improve their odds of being cured. The simple answer is "Nothing." There are no controlled trials that demonstrate any specific or general dietary interventions that can influence the clinical behavior of any type of cancer or responses to therapy. This lack must be emphasized, given the multitude of alternative diets (macrobiotic, coffee enemas, etc.) that purport to help cure cancer (and at a steep price!).

There are, however, general recommendations that can be made that common sense and clinical data strongly suggest can prevent the development of new cancers. To be effective, these must be adhered to lifelong. The guidelines suggested by the American Cancer Society include the following[262]:

1. Eat a variety of healthful foods, with an emphasis on plant sources.
   a. Eat five or more servings daily of a variety of fruits and vegetables.
   b. Choose whole grains in preference to processed grains.
   c. Limit consumption of red meats, especially those high in fat and that are processed.
   d. Choose foods that help maintain a healthful weight.
2. Adopt a physically active lifestyle.
   a. Adults: engage in moderate activity for 30 minutes or more, 5 or more days per week.
   b. Children and adolescents: moderate-vigorous activity for 45 minutes or more, 5 or more days per week.
3. Maintain a healthful weight throughout life.
   a. Balance caloric intake with physical activity.
   b. Lose weight if you are currently overweight or obese.
4. Limit alcohol intake.
5. Do not use tobacco in any form.

Is There a Role for "Complementary/Alternative Therapies"?

Patients often ask questions about the use of "complementary/alternative therapies" (CAM) to prevent or treat cancer. CAM use is more common in cancer patients than in patients with any other disease state. Among cancer patients, women appear to utilize CAM approaches more frequently than men.[263] The use of CAM in cancer is highest in breast cancer patients, with estimates of 20% to 66% utilizing some type of alternative therapy.[264–266] Unfortunately, only a small percentage of these patients actually communicate this use with their oncologist or healthcare provider.[267,268]

These data must be interpreted carefully, however, because the meanings of the terms alternative and complementary are not well defined.[269] In fact, the most sensible approach may be to insist that such therapies do not exist. Treatment alternatives that pass the rigorous testing of well-designed clinical trials should be considered "proven," whatever their nature. Conversely, no therapeutic modality, whether mainstream or complementary, should be accepted unless it is demonstrably safe and effective in clinical trials.[270] The pernicious effects of unproven therapies should not be underestimated. They may produce unwanted and dangerous side effects, interfere with the activity of proven therapies, and confound interpretation of responses to proven therapies.[271] Use of unproven therapies by patients may also diminish their commitment and ability to pursue proven therapies and impose potentially staggering financial burdens on patients and their families. Cancer physicians should be familiar with commonly used complementary/alternative techniques to communicate effectively and persuasively with patients and to be able to recognize side effects and confounding treatment responses that may harm them.[269]

References

1. Warren S. The immediate cause of death in cancer. Am J Med Sci 1932;185:610–615.
2. Inagaki J, Rodriguez V, Bodey GP. Proceedings: Causes of death in cancer patients. Cancer (Phila) 1974;33(2):568–573.
3. Studley H. Percentage of weight loss. JAMA 1936;106:458–460.
4. Dudrick SJ, Wilmore DW, Vars HM, Rhoads JE. Long-term total parenteral nutrition with growth, development, and positive nitrogen balance. Surgery (St. Louis) 1968;64(1):134–142.
5. Copeland EM III, Jonathan E. Rhoads lecture. Intravenous hyperalimentation and cancer. A historical perspective. JPEN J Parenter Enteral Nutr 1986;10(4):337–342.
6. Copeland EM, Macfayden BV Jr, Dudrick SJ. Intravenous hyperalimentation in cancer patients. J Surg Res 1974;16(3):241–247.
7. Klein S, Kinney J, Jeejeebhoy K, et al. Nutrition support in clinical practice: review of published data and recommendations for future research directions. National Institutes of Health, American Society for Parenteral and Enteral Nutrition, and American Society for Clinical Nutrition. JPEN J Parenter Enteral Nutr 1997;21(3):133–156.
8. Kern KA, Norton JA. Cancer cachexia. JPEN J Parenter Enteral Nutr 1988;12(3):286–298.
9. Brennan MF. Total parenteral nutrition in the cancer patient. N Engl J Med 1981;305(7):375–382.
10. Kritchevsky SB, Wilcosky TC, Morris DL, Truong KN, Tyroler HA. Changes in plasma lipid and lipoprotein cholesterol and weight prior to the diagnosis of cancer. Cancer Res 1991;51(12):3198–3203.
11. DeWys WD. Anorexia as a general effect of cancer. Cancer (Phila) 1979;43(5 suppl):2013–2019.
12. Dewys WD, Begg C, Lavin PT, et al. Prognostic effect of weight loss prior to chemotherapy in cancer patients. Eastern Cooperative Oncology Group. Am J Med 1980;69(4):491–497.
13. Ottery FD. Supportive nutrition to prevent cachexia and improve quality of life. Semin Oncol 1995;22(2 suppl 3):98–111.
14. Puccio M, Nathanson L. The cancer cachexia syndrome. Semin Oncol 1997;24(3):277–287.
15. MacDonald N. Is there evidence for earlier intervention in cancer-associated weight loss? J Support Oncol 2003;1(4):279–286.
16. Laviano A, Meguid MM, Rossi-Fanelli F. Cancer anorexia: clinical implications, pathogenesis, and therapeutic strategies. Lancet Oncol 2003;4(11):686–694.
17. Tisdale MJ. Pathogenesis of cancer cachexia. J Support Oncol 2003;1(3):159–168.
18. Lowry SF. Cancer cachexia revisited: old problems and new perspectives. Eur J Cancer 1991;27(1):1–3.
19. Costa G, Bewley P, Aragon M, Siebold J. Anorexia and weight loss in cancer patients. Cancer Treat Rep 1981;65(suppl 5):3–7.
20. Tisdale MJ. Cancer cachexia: metabolic alterations and clinical manifestations. Nutrition 1997;13(1):1–7.
21. Grosvenor M, Bulcavage L, Chlebowski RT. Symptoms potentially influencing weight loss in a cancer population. Correlations with primary site, nutritional status, and chemotherapy administration. Cancer (Phila) 1989;63(2):330–334.
22. Chang A, August D. Acute abdomen, bowel obstruction, and fistula. In: Abeloff M, Armitage J, Lichter A, Niederhuber J, eds. Clinical Oncology. New York: Churchill Livingstone, 1995:583–597.
23. Nelson KA, Walsh D, Sheehan FA. The cancer anorexia-cachexia syndrome. J Clin Oncol 1994;12(1):213–225.
24. Falconer JS, Fearon KC, Plester CE, Ross JA, Carter DC. Cytokines, the acute-phase response, and resting energy expenditure in cachectic patients with pancreatic cancer. Ann Surg 1994;219(4):325–331.
25. Hansell DT, Davies JW, Burns HJ. The relationship between resting energy expenditure and weight loss in benign and malignant disease. Ann Surg 1986;203(3):240–245.
26. Arbeit JM, Lees DE, Corsey R, Brennan MF. Resting energy expenditure in controls and cancer patients with localized and diffuse disease. Ann Surg 1984;199(3):292–298.
27. Knox LS, Crosby LO, Feurer ID, Buzby GP, Miller CL, Mullen JL. Energy expenditure in malnourished cancer patients. Ann Surg 1983;197(2):152–162.
28. Hyltander A, Drott C, Korner U, Sandstrom R, Lundholm K. Elevated energy expenditure in cancer patients with solid tumours. Eur J Cancer 1991;27(1):9–15.
29. Norton JA, Moley JF, Green MV, Carson RE, Morrison SD. Parabiotic transfer of cancer anorexia/cachexia in male rats. Cancer Res 1985;45(11 pt 1):5547–5552.
30. Stovroff MC, Fraker DL, Norton JA. Cachectin activity in the serum of cachectic, tumor-bearing rats. Arch Surg 1989;124(1):94–99.
31. Tisdale MJ. Tumor–host interactions. J Cell Biochem 2004;93(5):871–877.
32. Lind D, Souba W, Copeland E. Weight loss and cachexia. In: Abeloff M, Armitage J, Lichter A, Niederhuber J, eds. Clinical Oncology. New York: Churchill Livingstone, 1995:393–407.
33. Beutler B, Mahoney J, Le Trang N, Pekala P, Cerami A. Purification of cachectin, a lipoprotein lipase-suppressing hormone secreted by endotoxin-induced RAW 264.7 cells. J Exp Med 1985;161(5):984–995.
34. Garcia-Martinez C, Costelli P, Lopez-Soriano FJ, Argiles JM. Is TNF really involved in cachexia? Cancer Invest 1997;15(1):47–54.
35. Tracey KJ, Wei H, Manogue KR, et al. Cachectin/tumor necrosis factor induces cachexia, anemia, and inflammation. J Exp Med 1988;167(3):1211–1227.
36. Oliff A, Defeo-Jones D, Boyer M, et al. Tumors secreting human TNF/cachectin induce cachexia in mice. Cell 1987;50(4):555–563.
37. Tracey KJ, Morgello S, Koplin B, et al. Metabolic effects of cachectin/tumor necrosis factor are modified by site of

production. Cachectin/tumor necrosis factor-secreting tumor in skeletal muscle induces chronic cachexia, while implantation in brain induces predominantly acute anorexia. J Clin Invest 1990;86(6):2014–2024.
38. Tracey KJ, Vlassara H, Cerami A. Cachectin/tumour necrosis factor. Lancet 1989;1(8647):1122–1126.
39. Toomey D, Redmond HP, Bouchier-Hayes D. Mechanisms mediating cancer cachexia. Cancer (Phila) 1995;76(12):2418–2426.
40. Ramos EJ, Suzuki S, Marks D, Inui A, Asakawa A, Meguid MM. Cancer anorexia-cachexia syndrome: cytokines and neuropeptides. Curr Opin Clin Nutr Metab Care 2004;7(4):427–434.
41. Wang YY, Lo GH, Lai KH, Cheng JS, Lin CK, Hsu PI. Increased serum concentrations of tumor necrosis factor-alpha are associated with disease progression and malnutrition in hepatocellular carcinoma. J Chin Med Assoc 2003;66(10):593–598.
42. Mantovani G, Maccio A, Mura L, et al. Serum levels of leptin and proinflammatory cytokines in patients with advanced-stage cancer at different sites. J Mol Med 2000;78(10):554–561.
43. Dulger H, Alici S, Sekeroglu MR, et al. Serum levels of leptin and proinflammatory cytokines in patients with gastrointestinal cancer. Int J Clin Pract 2004;58(6):545–549.
44. Matthys P, Dijkmans R, Proost P, et al. Severe cachexia in mice inoculated with interferon-gamma-producing tumor cells. Int J Cancer 1991;49(1):77–82.
45. Matthys P, Heremans H, Opdenakker G, Billiau A. Anti-interferon-gamma antibody treatment, growth of Lewis lung tumours in mice and tumour-associated cachexia. Eur J Cancer 1991;27(2):182–187.
46. Langstein HN, Doherty GM, Fraker DL, Buresh CM, Norton JA. The roles of gamma-interferon and tumor necrosis factor alpha in an experimental rat model of cancer cachexia. Cancer Res 1991;51(9):2302–2306.
47. Fischer E, Marano MA, Barber AE, et al. Comparison between effects of interleukin-1 alpha administration and sublethal endotoxemia in primates. Am J Physiol 1991;261(2 pt 2):R442–R452.
48. Fong Y, Tracey KJ, Moldawer LL, et al. Antibodies to cachectin/tumor necrosis factor reduce interleukin 1 beta and interleukin 6 appearance during lethal bacteremia. J Exp Med 1989;170(5):1627–1633.
49. Gelin J, Moldawer LL, Lonnroth C, et al. Appearance of hybridoma growth factor/interleukin-6 in the serum of mice bearing a methylcholanthrene-induced sarcoma. Biochem Biophys Res Commun 1988;157(2):575–579.
50. Espat NJ, Moldawer LL, Copeland EM III. Cytokine-mediated alterations in host metabolism prevent nutritional repletion in cachectic cancer patients. J Surg Oncol 1995;58(2):77–82.
51. Monitto CL, Dong SM, Jen J, Sidransky D. Characterization of a human homologue of proteolysis-inducing factor and its role in cancer cachexia. Clin Cancer Res 2004;10(17):5862–5869.
52. Martignoni ME, Kunze P, Friess H. Cancer cachexia. Mol Cancer 2003;2(1):36.
53. Tisdale MJ. Cachexia in cancer patients. Nat Rev Cancer 2002;2(11):862–871.
54. Chamberlain JS. Cachexia in cancer–zeroing in on myosin. N Engl J Med 2004;351(20):2124–2125.
55. Acharyya S, Ladner KJ, Nelsen LL, et al. Cancer cachexia is regulated by selective targeting of skeletal muscle gene products. J Clin Invest 2004;114(3):370–378.
56. Sandri M, Sandri C, Gilbert A, et al. Foxo transcription factors induce the atrophy-related ubiquitin ligase atrogin-1 and cause skeletal muscle atrophy. Cell 2004;117(3):399–412.
57. Bergstrom DA, Penn BH, Strand A, Perry RL, Rudnicki MA, Tapscott SJ. Promoter-specific regulation of MyoD binding and signal transduction cooperate to pattern gene expression. Mol Cell 2002;9(3):587–600.
58. Rofe AM, Bourgeois CS, Coyle P, Taylor A, Abdi EA. Altered insulin response to glucose in weight-losing cancer patients. Anticancer Res 1994;14(2B):647–650.
59. Moley J, Peacock J, Morrison S. Insulin reversal in cancer induced protein loss. Surg Forum 1985;36:416–419.
60. Moley JF, Morrison SD, Norton JA. Insulin reversal of cancer cachexia in rats. Cancer Res 1985;45(10):4925–4931.
61. Morrison SD. Feeding response of tumor-bearing rats to insulin and insulin withdrawal and the contribution of autonomous tumor drain to cachectic depletion. Cancer Res 1982;42(9):3642–3647.
62. Lundholm K, Holm G, Schersten T. Insulin resistance in patients with cancer. Cancer Res 1978;38(12):4665–4670.
63. Holroyde CP, Gabuzda TG, Putnam RC, Paul P, Reichard GA. Altered glucose metabolism in metastatic carcinoma. Cancer Res 1975;35(12):3710–3714.
64. Waterhouse C. Lactate metabolism in patients with cancer. Cancer (Phila) 1974;33(1):66–71.
65. Waterhouse C, Jeanpretre N, Keilson J. Gluconeogenesis from alanine in patients with progressive malignant disease. Cancer Res 1979;39(6 pt 1):1968–1972.
66. Lundholm K, Edstrom S, Karlberg I, Ekman L, Schersten T. Glucose turnover, gluconeogenesis from glycerol, and estimation of net glucose cycling in cancer patients. Cancer (Phila) 1982;50(6):1142–1150.
67. Kralovic RC, Zepp FA, Cenedella RJ. Studies of the mechanism of carcass fat depletion in experimental cancer. Eur J Cancer 1977;13(10):1071–1079.
68. Mueller PS, Watkin DM. Plasma unesterfiled fatty acid concentrations in neoplastic disease. J Lab Clin Med 1961;57:95–108.
69. Shaw JH, Wolfe RR. Fatty acid and glycerol kinetics in septic patients and in patients with gastrointestinal cancer. The response to glucose infusion and parenteral feeding. Ann Surg 1987;205(4):368–376.
70. Dilman VM, Berstein LM, Ostroumova MN, Tsyrlina YV, Golubev AG. Peculiarities of hyperlipidaemia in tumour patients. Br J Cancer 1981;43(5):637–643.
71. Hussey HJ, Tisdale MJ. Effect of polyunsaturated fatty acids on the growth of murine colon adenocarcinomas in vitro and in vivo. Br J Cancer 1994;70(1):6–10.
72. Jeevanandam M, Legaspi A, Lowry SF, Horowitz GD, Brennan MF. Effect of total parenteral nutrition on whole body protein kinetics in cachectic patients with benign or malignant disease. JPEN J Parenter Enteral Nutr 1988;12(3):229–236.
73. Norton JA, Stein TP, Brennan MF. Whole body protein synthesis and turnover in normal man and malnourished patients with and without known cancer. Ann Surg 1981;194(2):123–128.
74. Lundholm K, Bylund AC, Holm J, Schersten T. Skeletal muscle metabolism in patients with malignant tumor. Eur J Cancer 1976;12(6):465–473.
75. Lundholm K, Bennegard K, Eden E, Svaninger G, Emery PW, Rennie MJ. Efflux of 3-methylhistidine from the leg in cancer patients who experience weight loss. Cancer Res 1982;42(11):4807–4811.
76. Warren RS, Jeevanandam M, Brennan MF. Comparison of hepatic protein synthesis in vivo versus in vitro in the tumor-bearing rat. J Surg Res 1987;42(1):43–50.
77. Fearon KC, McMillan DC, Preston T, Winstanley FP, Cruickshank AM, Shenkin A. Elevated circulating interleukin-6 is associated with an acute-phase response but reduced fixed hepatic protein synthesis in patients with cancer. Ann Surg 1991;213(1):26–31.
78. Moldawer L, Andersson C, Lonnroth C. Mechanisms of hypoalbuminemia in experimental cancer. J Parenter Enteral Nutr 1987;11:3S.
79. Moldawer LL, Rogy MA, Lowry SF. The role of cytokines in cancer cachexia. JPEN J Parenter Enteral Nutr 1992;16(6 suppl):43S–49S.

80. McNamara MJ, Alexander HR, Norton JA. Cytokines and their role in the pathophysiology of cancer cachexia. JPEN J Parenter Enteral Nutr 1992;16(6 suppl):50S–55S.
81. Argiles JM, Alvarez B, Lopez-Soriano FJ. The metabolic basis of cancer cachexia. Med Res Rev 1997;17(5):477–498.
82. Langer CJ, Hoffman JP, Ottery FD. Clinical significance of weight loss in cancer patients: rationale for the use of anabolic agents in the treatment of cancer-related cachexia. Nutrition 2001;17(1 suppl):S1–S20.
83. Yeh S, Wu SY, Levine DM, et al. Quality of life and stimulation of weight gain after treatment with megestrol acetate: correlation between cytokine levels and nutritional status, appetite in geriatric patients with wasting syndrome. J Nutr Health Aging 2000;4(4):246–251.
84. Loprinzi CL, Schaid DJ, Dose AM, Burnham NL, Jensen MD. Body-composition changes in patients who gain weight while receiving megestrol acetate. J Clin Oncol 1993;11(1):152–154.
85. Bolen JC, Andersen RE, Bennett RG. Deep vein thrombosis as a complication of megestrol acetate therapy among nursing home residents. J Am Med Dir Assoc 2000;1(6):248–252.
86. Jatoi A, Windschitl HE, Loprinzi CL, et al. Dronabinol versus megestrol acetate versus combination therapy for cancer-associated anorexia: a North Central Cancer Treatment Group study. J Clin Oncol 15 2002;20(2):567–573.
87. Anonymous. More on megestrol for prevention and treatment of cancer-associatied cachexia. Cancer Oncol Alerts 1998;13:21–22.
88. Simons JP, Schols AM, Hoefnagels JM, Westerterp KR, ten Velde GP, Wouters EF. Effects of medroxyprogesterone acetate on food intake, body composition, and resting energy expenditure in patients with advanced, nonhormone-sensitive cancer: a randomized, placebo-controlled trial. Cancer (Phila) 1998;82(3):553–560.
89. Tayek JA, Brasel JA. Failure of anabolism in malnourished cancer patients receiving growth hormone: a clinical research center study. J Clin Endocrinol Metab 1995;80(7):2082–2087.
90. Von Roenn JH, Tchekmedyian S, Hoffman RM, Chang C-Y, Ottery FD. Oxandrolone in cancer-related weight loss: improvement in weight, body cell mass (BCM), performance status, and quality of life (QOL). Paper presented at: 38th Annual ASCO Meeting; May 15–22, 2002, Orlando, FL.
91. Nelson K, Walsh D, Deeter P, Sheehan F. A phase II study of delta-9-tetrahydrocannabinol for appetite stimulation in cancer-associated anorexia. J Palliat Care 1994;10(1):14–18.
92. Wadleigh R, Spaulding M, Lembersky B, et al. Dronabinol enhancement of appetite in cancer patients (abstract). Proc Am Soc Clin Oncol 1990;9:1280.
93. Hart S, Fischer OM, Ullrich A. Cannabinoids induce cancer cell proliferation via tumor necrosis factor alpha-converting enzyme (TACE/ADAM17)-mediated transactivation of the epidermal growth factor receptor. Cancer Res 2004;64(6):1943–1950.
94. Lissoni P, Paolorossi F, Tancini G, et al. Is there a role for melatonin in the treatment of neoplastic cachexia? Eur J Cancer 1996;32A(8):1340–1343.
95. Lissoni P, Barni S, Tancini G, et al. Role of the pineal gland in the control of macrophage functions and its possible implication in cancer: a study of interactions between tumor necrosis factor-alpha and the pineal hormone melatonin. J Biol Regul Homeost Agents 1994;8(4):126–129.
96. Khan ZH, Simpson EJ, Cole AT, et al. Oesophageal cancer and cachexia: the effect of short-term treatment with thalidomide on weight loss and lean body mass. Aliment Pharmacol Ther 2003;17(5):677–682.
97. Zhou S, Kestell P, Tingle MD, Paxton JW. Thalidomide in cancer treatment: a potential role in the elderly? Drugs Aging 2002;19(2):85–100.
98. Gogos CA, Ginopoulos P, Salsa B, Apostolidou E, Zoumbos NC, Kalfarentzos F. Dietary omega-3 polyunsaturated fatty acids plus vitamin E restore immunodeficiency and prolong survival for severely ill patients with generalized malignancy: a randomized control trial. Cancer (Phila) 1998;82(2):395–402.
99. Wigmore SJ, Barber MD, Ross JA, Tisdale MJ, Fearon KC. Effect of oral eicosapentaenoic acid on weight loss in patients with pancreatic cancer. Nutr Cancer 2000;36(2):177–184.
100. Kosty MP, Fleishman SB, Herndon JE II, et al. Cisplatin, vinblastine, and hydrazine sulfate in advanced, non-small-cell lung cancer: a randomized placebo-controlled, double-blind phase III study of the Cancer and Leukemia Group B. J Clin Oncol 1994;12(6):1113–1120.
101. Loprinzi CL, Goldberg RM, Su JQ, et al. Placebo-controlled trial of hydrazine sulfate in patients with newly diagnosed non-small-cell lung cancer. J Clin Oncol 1994;12(6):1126–1129.
102. Loprinzi CL, Kuross SA, O'Fallon JR, et al. Randomized placebo-controlled evaluation of hydrazine sulfate in patients with advanced colorectal cancer. J Clin Oncol 1994;12(6):1121–1125.
103. Lissoni P, Ardizzoia A, Perego MS, et al. Inhibition of tumor necrosis factor-alpha secretion by pentoxifylline in advanced cancer patients with abnormally high blood levels of tumor necrosis factor-alpha. J Biol Regul Homeost Agents 1993;7(2):73–75.
104. Laviano A, Renvyle T, Yang ZJ. From laboratory to bedside: new strategies in the treatment of malnutrition in cancer patients. Nutrition 1996;12(2):112–122.
105. Dezube BJ, Sherman ML, Fridovich-Keil JL, Allen-Ryan J, Pardee AB. Down-regulation of tumor necrosis factor expression by pentoxifylline in cancer patients: a pilot study. Cancer Immunol Immunother 1993;36(1):57–60.
106. Aygenc E, Celikkanat S, Kaymakci M, Aksaray F, Ozdem C. Prophylactic effect of pentoxifylline on radiotherapy complications: a clinical study. Otolaryngol Head Neck Surg 2004;130(3):351–356.
107. Ozturk B, Egehan I, Atavci S, Kitapci M. Pentoxifylline in prevention of radiation-induced lung toxicity in patients with breast and lung cancer: a double-blind randomized trial. Int J Radiat Oncol Biol Phys 2004;58(1):213–219.
108. Goldberg RM, Loprinzi CL, Mailliard JA, et al. Pentoxifylline for treatment of cancer anorexia and cachexia? A randomized, double-blind, placebo-controlled trial. J Clin Oncol 1995;13(11):2856–2859.
109. Kardinal CG, Loprinzi CL, Schaid DJ, et al. A controlled trial of cyproheptadine in cancer patients with anorexia and/or cachexia. Cancer (Phila) 1990;65(12):2657–2662.
110. Popiela T, Lucchi R, Giongo F. Methylprednisolone as palliative therapy for female terminal cancer patients. The Methylprednisolone Female Preterminal Cancer Study Group. Eur J Cancer Clin Oncol 1989;25(12):1823–1829.
111. Simons JP, Aaronson NK, Vansteenkiste JF, et al. Effects of medroxyprogesterone acetate on appetite, weight, and quality of life in advanced-stage non-hormone-sensitive cancer: a placebo-controlled multicenter study. J Clin Oncol 1996;14(4):1077–1084.
112. Bartlett DL, Stein TP, Torosian MH. Effect of growth hormone and protein intake on tumor growth and host cachexia. Surgery (St. Louis) 1995;117(3):260–267.
113. Wolf RF, Pearlstone DB, Newman E, et al. Growth hormone and insulin reverse net whole body and skeletal muscle protein catabolism in cancer patients. Ann Surg 1992;216(3):280–288; discussion 288–290.
114. Directors AASfPaENBo. Guidelines for the use of parenteral and enteral nutrition in adult and pediatric patients. JPEN J Parenter Enteral Nutr 2002;26(1 suppl):1SA–138SA.
115. Hill G. The perioperative patient. In: Kinney J, Jeejeebhoy K, Hill G, Owen O, eds. Nutrition and Metabolism in Patient Care. Philadelphia: Saunders, 1988:643–655.

116. Smale BF, Mullen JL, Buzby GP, Rosato EF. The efficacy of nutritional assessment and support in cancer surgery. Cancer (Phila) 1981;47(10):2375–2381.
117. Buzby GP, Mullen JL, Matthews DC, Hobbs CL, Rosato EF. Prognostic nutritional index in gastrointestinal surgery. Am J Surg 1980;139(1):160–167.
118. Perioperative total parenteral nutrition in surgical patients. The Veterans Affairs Total Parenteral Nutrition Cooperative Study Group. N Engl J Med 1991;325(8):525–532.
119. Franch-Arcas G. The meaning of hypoalbuminaemia in clinical practice. Clin Nutr 2001;20(3):265–269.
120. Harvey KB, Moldawer LL, Bistrian BR, Blackburn GL. Biological measures for the formulation of a hospital prognostic index. Am J Clin Nutr 1981;34(10):2013–2022.
121. Kirby D, DeLegge M. Nutritional assessment in the high tech and low tech tour. In: Kirby D, Dudrick S, eds. Practical Handbook of Nutrition in Clinical Practice. Boca Raton: CRC Press, 1994:1–18.
122. Ottery FD. Definition of standardized nutritional assessment and interventional pathways in oncology. Nutrition 1996;12(1 suppl):S15–S19.
123. Detsky AS, McLaughlin JR, Baker JP, et al. What is subjective global assessment of nutritional status? JPEN J Parenter Enteral Nutr 1987;11(1):8–13.
124. Isenring E, Bauer J, Capra S. The scored Patient-generated Subjective Global Assessment (PG-SGA) and its association with quality of life in ambulatory patients receiving radiotherapy. Eur J Clin Nutr 2003;57(2):305–309.
125. Ottery FD. Instruments of proactive assessment and intervention in the context of outcomes-based research and clinical care. In: Improving Clinical Practice with Nutrition in a Managed Care Environment. Columbus: Ross Products Division, Abbott Laboratories, 1997:29–36.
126. Falconer JS, Fearon KC, Ross JA, et al. Acute-phase protein response and survival duration of patients with pancreatic cancer. Cancer (Phila) 1995;75(8):2077–2082.
127. Deehan D, Heys S, Walker L, et al. Serum albumin an indepedent progonostic factor in patients with colorectal cancer. Br J Surg 1995;82:691.
128. Delmore G. Assessment of nutritional status in cancer patients: widely neglected? Support Care Cancer 1997;5(5):376–380.
129. Bozzetti F. Rationale and indications for preoperative feeding of malnourished surgical cancer patients. Nutrition 2002;18(11–12):953–959.
130. Bozzetti F. Effects of artificial nutrition on the nutritional status of cancer patients. JPEN J Parenter Enteral Nutr 1989;13(4):406–420.
131. Lin MT, Saito H, Fukushima R, et al. Preoperative total parenteral nutrition influences postoperative systemic cytokine responses after colorectal surgery. Nutrition 1997;13(1):8–12.
132. Daly J, Thorn A. Neoplastic diseases. In: Kinney J, Jeejeebhoy K, Hill G, Owen O, eds. Nutrition and Metabolism in Patient Care. Philadelphia: Saunders, 1988:567–587.
133. Torosian MH. Stimulation of tumor growth by nutrition support. JPEN J Parenter Enteral Nutr 1992;16(6 suppl):72S–75S.
134. Popp MB, Wagner SC, Brito OJ. Host and tumor responses to increasing levels of intravenous nutritional support. Surgery (St. Louis) 1983;94(2):300–308.
135. Torosian MH, Donoway RB. Total parenteral nutrition and tumor metastasis. Surgery (St. Louis) 1991;109(5):597–601.
136. Baron PL, Lawrence W Jr, Chan WM, White FK, Banks WL Jr. Effects of parenteral nutrition on cell cycle kinetics of head and neck cancer. Arch Surg 1986;121(11):1282–1286.
137. Frank JL, Lawrence W Jr, Banks WL Jr, McKinnon JG, Chan WM, Collins JM. Modulation of cell cycle kinetics in human cancer with total parenteral nutrition. Cancer (Phila) 1992;69(7):1858–1864.
138. Franchi F, Rossi-Fanelli F, Seminara P, Cascino A, Barone C, Scucchi L. Cell kinetics of gastrointestinal tumors after different nutritional regimens. A preliminary report. J Clin Gastroenterol 1991;13(3):313–315.
139. Heys SD, Park KG, McNurlan MA, et al. Stimulation of protein synthesis in human tumours by parenteral nutrition: evidence for modulation of tumour growth. Br J Surg 1991;78(4):483–487.
140. Bozzetti F, Gavazzi C, Mariani L, Crippa F. Glucose-based total parenteral nutrition does not stimulate glucose uptake by humans tumours. Clin Nutr 2004;23(3):417–421.
141. Klein S, Koretz RL. Nutrition support in patients with cancer: what do the data really show? Nutr Clin Pract 1994;9(3):91–100.
142. Holter AR, Fischer JE. The effects of perioperative hyperalimentation on complications in patients with carcinoma and weight loss. J Surg Res 1977;23(1):31–34.
143. Sako K, Lore JM, Kaufman S, Razack MS, Bakamjian V, Reese P. Parenteral hyperalimentation in surgical patients with head and neck cancer: a randomized study. J Surg Oncol 1981;16(4):391–402.
144. Muller JM, Brenner U, Dienst C, Pichlmaier H. Preoperative parenteral feeding in patients with gastrointestinal carcinoma. Lancet 1982;1(8263):68–71.
145. Yamada N, Koyama H, Hioki K, Yamada T, Yamamoto M. Effect of postoperative total parenteral nutrition (TPN) as an adjunct to gastrectomy for advanced gastric carcinoma. Br J Surg 1983;70(5):267–274.
146. Muller JM, Keller HW, Brenner U, Walter M, Holzmuller W. Indications and effects of preoperative parenteral nutrition. World J Surg 1986;10(1):53–63.
147. Askanazi J, Hensle TW, Starker PM, et al. Effect of immediate postoperative nutritional support on length of hospitalization. Ann Surg 1986;203(3):236–239.
148. Brennan MF, Pisters PW, Posner M, Quesada O, Shike M. A prospective randomized trial of total parenteral nutrition after major pancreatic resection for malignancy. Ann Surg 1994;220(4):436–441; discussion 441–444.
149. Fan ST, Lo CM, Lai EC, Chu KM, Liu CL, Wong J. Perioperative nutritional support in patients undergoing hepatectomy for hepatocellular carcinoma. N Engl J Med 1994;331(23):1547–1552.
150. Meijerink WJ, von Meyenfeldt MF, Rouflart MM, Soeters PB. Efficacy of perioperative nutritional support. Lancet 1992; 340(8812):187–188.
151. Gianotti L, Braga M, Vignali A, et al. Effect of route of delivery and formulation of postoperative nutritional support in patients undergoing major operations for malignant neoplasms. Arch Surg 1997;132(11):1222–1229; discussion 1229–1230.
152. Sand J, Luostarinen M, Matikainen M. Enteral or parenteral feeding after total gastrectomy: prospective randomised pilot study. Eur J Surg 1997;163(10):761–766.
153. Braga M, Gianotti L, Gentilini O, Parisi V, Salis C, Di Carlo V. Early postoperative enteral nutrition improves gut oxygenation and reduces costs compared with total parenteral nutrition. Crit Care Med 2001;29(2):242–248.
154. Bozzetti F, Braga M, Gianotti L, Gavazzi C, Mariani L. Postoperative enteral versus parenteral nutrition in malnourished patients with gastrointestinal cancer: a randomised multicentre trial. Lancet 2001;358(9292):1487–1492.
155. Aiko S, Yoshizumi Y, Sugiura Y, et al. Beneficial effects of immediate enteral nutrition after esophageal cancer surgery. Surg Today 2001;31(11):971–978.
156. Papapietro K, Diaz E, Csendes A, et al. Early enteral nutrition in cancer patients subjected to a total gastrectomy. Rev Med Chil 2002;130(10):1125–1130.
157. Jiang XH, Li N, Li JS. Intestinal permeability in patients after surgical trauma and effect of enteral nutrition versus parenteral nutrition. World J Gastroenterol 2003;9(8):1878–1880.

158. Sagar S, Harland P, Shields R. Early postoperative feeding with elemental diet. Br Med J 1979;1(6159):293–295.
159. Smith RC, Hartemink RJ, Hollinshead JW, Gillett DJ. Fine bore jejunostomy feeding following major abdominal surgery: a controlled randomized clinical trial. Br J Surg 1985;72(6):458–461.
160. Foschi D, Cavagna G, Callioni F, Morandi E, Rovati V. Hyperalimentation of jaundiced patients on percutaneous transhepatic biliary drainage. Br J Surg 1986;73(9):716–719.
161. Heslin MJ, Latkany L, Leung D, et al. A prospective, randomized trial of early enteral feeding after resection of upper gastrointestinal malignancy. Ann Surg 1997;226(4):567–577; discussion 577–580.
162. Bozzetti F, Gavazzi C, Miceli R, et al. Perioperative total parenteral nutrition in malnourished, gastrointestinal cancer patients: a randomized, clinical trial. JPEN J Parenter Enteral Nutr 2000; 24(1):7–14.
163. Hyltander A, Bosaeus I, Svedlund J, et al. Supportive nutrition on recovery of metabolism, nutritional state, health-related quality of life, and exercise capacity after major surgery: a randomized study. Clin Gastroenterol Hepatol 2005;3(5):466–474.
164. Wu GH, Liu ZH, Wu ZH, Wu ZG. Perioperative artificial nutrition in malnourished gastrointestinal cancer patients. World J Gastroenterol 2006;12(15):2441–2444.
165. Aiko S, Yoshizumi Y, Matsuyama T, Sugiura Y, Maehara T. Influences of thoracic duct blockage on early enteral nutrition for patients who underwent esophageal cancer surgery. Jpn J Thorac Cardiovasc Surg 2003;51(7):263–271.
166. Calle EE, Rodriguez C, Walker-Thurmond K, Thun MJ. Overweight, obesity, and mortality from cancer in a prospectively studied cohort of U.S. adults. N Engl J Med 2003;348(17):1625–1638.
167. Seven H, Calis AB, Turgut S. A randomized controlled trial of early oral feeding in laryngectomized patients. Laryngoscope 2003;113(6):1076–1079.
168. August DA. Creation of a specialized nutrition support outcomes research consortium: if not now, when? JPEN J Parenter Enteral Nutr 1996;20(6):394–400.
169. Weisdorf SA, Lysne J, Wind D, et al. Positive effect of prophylactic total parenteral nutrition on long-term outcome of bone marrow transplantation. Transplantation 1987;43(6):833–838.
170. Charuhas PM, Fosberg KL, Bruemmer B, et al. A double-blind randomized trial comparing outpatient parenteral nutrition with intravenous hydration: effect on resumption of oral intake after marrow transplantation. JPEN J Parenter Enteral Nutr 1997; 21(3):157–161.
171. Muscaritoli M, Conversano L, Torelli GF, et al. Clinical and metabolic effects of different parenteral nutrition regimens in patients undergoing allogeneic bone marrow transplantation. Transplantation 1998;66(5):610–616.
172. Roberts S, Miller J, Pineiro L, Jennings L. Total parenteral nutrition vs oral diet in autologous hematopoietic cell transplant recipients. Bone Marrow Transplant 2003;32(7):715–721.
173. Szeluga DJ, Stuart RK, Brookmeyer R, Utermohlen V, Santos GW. Nutritional support of bone marrow transplant recipients: a prospective, randomized clinical trial comparing total parenteral nutrition to an enteral feeding program. Cancer Res 1987;47(12):3309–3316.
174. Ziegler TR, Young LS, Benfell K, et al. Clinical and metabolic efficacy of glutamine-supplemented parenteral nutrition after bone marrow transplantation. A randomized, double-blind, controlled study. Ann Intern Med 1992;116(10):821–828.
175. Schloerb PR, Amare M. Total parenteral nutrition with glutamine in bone marrow transplantation and other clinical applications (a randomized, double-blind study). JPEN J Parenter Enteral Nutr 1993;17(5):407–413.
176. Jordan WM, Valdivieso M, Frankmann C, et al. Treatment of advanced adenocarcinoma of the lung with ftorafur, doxorubicin, cyclophosphamide, and cisplatin (FACP) and intensive iv hyperalimentation. Cancer Treat Rep 1981;65(3–4):197–205.
177. Nixon D, Moffitt S, Lawson D, et al. Total parenteral nutrition as an adjunct to chemotherapy for metastatic colorectal cancer. Cancer Treat Rep 1981;65(suppl 5):123–128.
178. Popp MB, Fisher RI, Wesley R, Aamodt R, Brennan MF. A prospective randomized study of adjuvant parenteral nutrition in the treatment of advanced diffuse lymphoma: influence on survival. Surgery (St. Louis) 1981;90(2):195–203.
179. Samuels ML, Selig DE, Ogden S, Grant C, Brown B. IV hyperalimentation and chemotherapy for stage III testicular cancer: a randomized study. Cancer Treat Rep 1981;65(7–8):615–627.
180. Serrou B, Cupissol D, Plagne R, et al. Follow-up of a randomized trial for oat cell carcinoma evaluating the efficacy of peripheral intravenous nutrition (PIVN) as adjunct treatment. Recent Results Cancer Res 1982;80:246–253.
181. Shamberger RC, Brennan MF, Goodgame JT Jr, et al. A prospective, randomized study of adjuvant parenteral nutrition in the treatment of sarcomas: results of metabolic and survival studies. Surgery (St. Louis) 1984;96(1):1–13.
182. Tandon SP, Gupta SC, Sinha SN, Naithani YP. Nutritional support as an adjunct therapy of advanced cancer patients. Indian J Med Res 1984;80:180–188.
183. Clamon GH, Feld R, Evans WK, et al. Effect of adjuvant central iv hyperalimentation on the survival and response to treatment of patients with small cell lung cancer: a randomized trial. Cancer Treat Rep 1985;69(2):167–177.
184. Valdivieso M, Frankmann C, Murphy WK, et al. Long-term effects of intravenous hyperalimentation administered during intensive chemotherapy for small cell bronchogenic carcinoma. Cancer (Phila) 1987;59(2):362–369.
185. Evans WK, Nixon DW, Daly JM, et al. A randomized study of oral nutritional support versus ad lib nutritional intake during chemotherapy for advanced colorectal and non-small-cell lung cancer. J Clin Oncol 1987;5(1):113–124.
186. De Cicco M, Panarello G, Fantin D, et al. Parenteral nutrition in cancer patients receiving chemotherapy: effects on toxicity and nutritional status. JPEN J Parenter Enteral Nutr 1993; 17(6):513–518.
187. Bozzetti F, Cozzaglio L, Gavazzi C, et al. Nutritional support in patients with cancer of the esophagus: impact on nutritional status, patient compliance to therapy, and survival. Tumori 1998;84(6):681–686.
188. Hyltander A, Drott C, Unsgaard B, et al. The effect on body composition and exercise performance of home parenteral nutrition when given as adjunct to chemotherapy of testicular carcinoma. Eur J Clin Invest 1991;21(4):413–420.
189. Jin D, Phillips M, Byles JE. Effects of parenteral nutrition support and chemotherapy on the phasic composition of tumor cells in gastrointestinal cancer. JPEN J Parenter Enteral Nutr 1999; 23(4):237–241.
190. Klein S, Simes J, Blackburn GL. Total parenteral nutrition and cancer clinical trials. Cancer (Phila) 1986;58(6):1378–1386.
191. McGeer AJ, Detsky AS, O'Rourke K. Parenteral nutrition in cancer patients undergoing chemotherapy: a meta-analysis. Nutrition 1990;6(3):233–240.
192. Parenteral nutrition in patients receiving cancer chemotherapy. American College of Physicians. Ann Intern Med 1989;110(9): 734–736.
193. Donaldson SS. Nutritional support as an adjunct to radiation therapy. JPEN J Parenter Enteral Nutr 1984;8(3):302–310.
194. Sikora SS, Ribeiro U, Kane JM III, Landreneau RJ, Lembersky B, Posner MC. Role of nutrition support during induction chemoradiation therapy in esophageal cancer. JPEN J Parenter Enteral Nutr 1998;22(1):18–21.
195. Savarese DM, Savy G, Vahdat L, Wischmeyer PE, Corey B. Prevention of chemotherapy and radiation toxicity with glutamine. Cancer Treat Rev 2003;29(6):501–513.

196. Heys SD, Gough DB, Khan L, Eremin O. Nutritional pharmacology and malignant disease: a therapeutic modality in patients with cancer. Br J Surg 1996;83(5):608–619.
197. O'Riordain MG, Fearon KC, Ross JA, et al. Glutamine-supplemented total parenteral nutrition enhances T-lymphocyte response in surgical patients undergoing colorectal resection. Ann Surg 1994;220(2):212–221.
198. Wu GH, Zhang YW, Wu ZH. Modulation of postoperative immune and inflammatory response by immune-enhancing enteral diet in gastrointestinal cancer patients. World J Gastroenterol 2001;7(3):357–362.
199. Morlion BJ, Stehle P, Wachtler P, et al. Total parenteral nutrition with glutamine dipeptide after major abdominal surgery: a randomized, double-blind, controlled study. Ann Surg 1998; 227(2):302–308.
200. Schloerb PR, Skikne BS. Oral and parenteral glutamine in bone marrow transplantation: a randomized, double-blind study. JPEN J Parenter Enteral Nutr 1999;23(3):117–122.
201. Coghlin Dickson TM, Wong RM, Offrin RS, et al. Effect of oral glutamine supplementation during bone marrow transplantation. JPEN J Parenter Enteral Nutr 2000;24(2):61–66.
202. Piccirillo N, De Matteis S, Laurenti L, et al. Glutamine-enriched parenteral nutrition after autologous peripheral blood stem cell transplantation: effects on immune reconstitution and mucositis. Haematologica 2003;88(2):192–200.
203. Scheid C, Hermann K, Kremer G, et al. Randomized, double-blind, controlled study of glycyl-glutamine-dipeptide in the parenteral nutrition of patients with acute leukemia undergoing intensive chemotherapy. Nutrition 2004;20(3):249–254.
204. Daly JM, Lieberman MD, Goldfine J, et al. Enteral nutrition with supplemental arginine, RNA, and omega-3 fatty acids in patients after operation: immunologic, metabolic, and clinical outcome. Surgery (St. Louis) 1992;112(1):56–67.
205. Senkal M, Kemen M, Homann HH, Eickhoff U, Baier J, Zumtobel V. Modulation of postoperative immune response by enteral nutrition with a diet enriched with arginine, RNA, and omega-3 fatty acids in patients with upper gastrointestinal cancer. Eur J Surg 1995;161(2):115–122.
206. Daly JM, Weintraub FN, Shou J, Rosato EF, Lucia M. Enteral nutrition during multimodality therapy in upper gastrointestinal cancer patients. Ann Surg 1995;221(4):327–338.
207. Braga M, Gianotti L, Cestari A, et al. Gut function and immune and inflammatory responses in patients perioperatively fed with supplemented enteral formulas. Arch Surg 1996;131(12):1257–1264; discussion 1264–1265.
208. Braga M, Gianotti L, Vignali A, Cestari A, Bisagni P, Di Carlo V. Artificial nutrition after major abdominal surgery: impact of route of administration and composition of the diet. Crit Care Med 1998;26(1):24–30.
209. Di Carlo V, Gianotti L, Balzano G, Zerbi A, Braga M. Complications of pancreatic surgery and the role of perioperative nutrition. Dig Surg 1999;16(4):320–326.
210. Gianotti L, Braga M, Nespoli L, Radaelli G, Beneduce A, Di Carlo V. A randomized controlled trial of preoperative oral supplementation with a specialized diet in patients with gastrointestinal cancer. Gastroenterology 2002;122(7):1763–1770.
211. van Bokhorst-De Van Der Schueren MA, Quak JJ, von Blomberg-van der Flier BM, et al. Effect of perioperative nutrition, with and without arginine supplementation, on nutritional status, immune function, postoperative morbidity, and survival in severely malnourished head and neck cancer patients. Am J Clin Nutr 2001;73(2):323–332.
212. de Luis DA, Izaola O, Cuellar L, Terroba MC, Aller R. Randomized clinical trial with an enteral arginine-enhanced formula in early postsurgical head and neck cancer patients. Eur J Clin Nutr 2004;58(11):1505–1508.
213. Song JX, Qing SH, Huang XC, Qi DL. Effect of parenteral nutrition with L-arginine supplementation on postoperative immune function in patients with colorectal cancer. Di Yi Jun Yi Da Xue Xue Bao 2002;22(6):545–547.
214. Lacour J, Lacour F, Spira A, et al. Adjuvant treatment with polyadenylic-polyuridylic acid in operable breast cancer: updated results of a randomised trial. Br Med J (Clin Res Ed) 1984; 288(6417):589–592.
215. Lacour J, Laplanche A, Delozier T, et al. Polyadenylic-polyuridylic acid plus locoregional and pelvic radiotherapy versus chemotherapy with CMF as adjuvants in operable breast cancer. A $6^1/_2$ year follow-up analysis of a randomized trial of the French Federation of Cancer Centers (F.F.C.C.). Breast Cancer Res Treat 1991;19(1):15–21.
216. Lacour J, Laplanche A, Malafosse M, et al. Polyadenylic-polyuridylic acid as an adjuvant in resectable colorectal carcinoma: a $6^1/_2$ year follow-up analysis of a multicentric double blind randomized trial. Eur J Surg Oncol 1992;18(6):599–604.
217. Jho DH, Cole SM, Lee EM, Espat NJ. Role of omega-3 fatty acid supplementation in inflammation and malignancy. Integr Cancer Ther 2004;3(2):98–111.
218. Hardman WE. Omega-3 fatty acids to augment cancer therapy. J Nutr 2002;132(11 suppl):3508S–3512S.
219. Jatoi A, Rowland K, Loprinzi CL, et al. An eicosapentaenoic acid supplement versus megestrol acetate versus both for patients with cancer-associated wasting: a North Central Cancer Treatment Group and National Cancer Institute of Canada collaborative effort. J Clin Oncol 2004;22(12):2469–2476.
220. Fearon K, von Meyenfeldt MF, Moses A, et al. An energy and protein dense, high n-3 fatty acid oral supplement promotes weight gain in cancer cachexia. Eur J Cancer 2001;37(suppl 6): S27–S28.
221. Moses AW, Slater C, Preston T, Barber MD, Fearon KC. Reduced total energy expenditure and physical activity in cachectic patients with pancreatic cancer can be modulated by an energy and protein dense oral supplement enriched with n-3 fatty acids. Br J Cancer 2004;90(5):996–1002.
222. Wachtler P, Konig W, Senkal M, Kemen M, Koller M. Influence of a total parenteral nutrition enriched with omega-3 fatty acids on leukotriene synthesis of peripheral leukocytes and systemic cytokine levels in patients with major surgery. J Trauma 1997;42(2):191–198.
223. Senkal M, Zumtobel V, Bauer KH, et al. Outcome and cost-effectiveness of perioperative enteral immunonutrition in patients undergoing elective upper gastrointestinal tract surgery: a prospective randomized study. Arch Surg 1999;134(12):1309–1316.
224. Braga M, Gianotti L, Nespoli L, Radaelli G, Di Carlo V. Nutritional approach in malnourished surgical patients: a prospective randomized study. Arch Surg 2002;137(2):174–180.
225. Farreras N, Artigas V, Cardona D, Rius X, Trias M, Gonzalez JA. Effect of early postoperative enteral immunonutrition on wound healing in patients undergoing surgery for gastric cancer. Clin Nutr 2005;24(1):55–65.
226. Chen DW, Wei Fei Z, Zhang YC, Ou JM, Xu J. Role of enteral immunonutrition in patients with gastric carcinoma undergoing major surgery. Asian J Surg 2005;28(2):121–124.
227. Braga M, Gianotti L, Vignali A, Carlo VD. Preoperative oral arginine and n-3 fatty acid supplementation improves the immunometabolic host response and outcome after colorectal resection for cancer. Surgery (St. Louis) 2002;132(5):805–814.
228. Koretz RL. Immunonutrition. Surgery (St. Louis) 1993;114(3):631–632.
229. Heyland DK, Novak F, Drover JW, Jain M, Su X, Suchner U. Should immunonutrition become routine in critically ill patients? A systematic review of the evidence. JAMA 2001; 286(8):944–953.
230. Tepaske R, Velthuis H, Oudemans-van Straaten HM, et al. Effect of preoperative oral immune-enhancing nutritional supplement on patients at high risk of infection after cardiac surgery: a ran-

domised placebo-controlled trial. Lancet 2001;358(9283):696–701.
231. Bistrian BR. Practical recommendations for immune-enhancing diets. J Nutr 2004;134(10 suppl):2868S–2872S; discussion 2895S.
232. Fainsinger RL, Gramlich LM. How often can we justify parenteral nutrition in terminally ill cancer patients? J Palliat Care 1997;13(1):48–51.
233. Howard L. Home parenteral nutrition in patients with a cancer diagnosis. JPEN J Parenter Enteral Nutr 1992;16(6 suppl):93S–99S.
234. Bozzetti F. Home total parenteral nutrition in incurable cancer patients: a therapy, a basic humane care or something in between? Clin Nutr 2003;22(2):109–111.
235. August DA, Thorn D, Fisher RL, Welchek CM. Home parenteral nutrition for patients with inoperable malignant bowel obstruction. JPEN J Parenter Enteral Nutr 1991;15(3):323–327.
236. King LA, Carson LF, Konstantinides N, et al. Outcome assessment of home parenteral nutrition in patients with gynecologic malignancies: what have we learned in a decade of experience? Gynecol Oncol 1993;51(3):377–382.
237. Cozzaglio L, Balzola F, Cosentino F, et al. Outcome of cancer patients receiving home parenteral nutrition. Italian Society of Parenteral and Enteral Nutrition (S.I.N.P.E.). JPEN J Parenter Enteral Nutr 1997;21(6):339–342.
238. Baines M, Oliver DJ, Carter RL. Medical management of intestinal obstruction in patients with advanced malignant disease. A clinical and pathological study. Lancet 1985;2(8462):990–993.
239. Doll R, Peto R. The causes of cancer: quantitative estimates of avoidable risks of cancer in the United States today. J Natl Cancer Inst 1981;66(6):1191–1308.
240. Willett WC. Diet, nutrition, and avoidable cancer. Environ Health Perspect 1995;103(suppl 8):165–170.
241. Willett WC. Diet and cancer: one view at the start of the millennium. Cancer Epidemiol Biomarkers Prev 2001;10(1):3–8.
242. Forman MR, Hursting SD, Umar A, Barrett JC. Nutrition and cancer prevention: a multidisciplinary perspective on human trials. Annu Rev Nutr 2004;24:223–254.
243. Schatzkin A. Dietary change as a strategy for preventing cancer. Cancer Metastasis Rev 1997;16(3–4):377–392.
244. Hill MJ. Diet and cancer: a review of scientific evidence. Eur J Cancer Prev 1995;4(suppl 2):3–42.
245. McCullough ML, Giovannucci EL. Diet and cancer prevention. Oncogene 2004;23(38):6349–6364.
246. Ames BN. Dietary carcinogens and anticarcinogens. Oxygen radicals and degenerative diseases. Science 1983;221(4617):1256–1264.
247. Chesson A, Collins A. Assessment of the role of diet in cancer prevention. Cancer Lett 1997;114(1-2):237–245.
248. Caporaso NE, Tucker MA, Hoover RN, et al. Lung cancer and the debrisoquine metabolic phenotype. J Natl Cancer Inst 1990;82(15):1264–1272.
249. Greenwald P. Chemoprevention of cancer. Sci Am 1996;275(3):96–99.
250. Trichopoulos D, Li FP, Hunter DJ. What causes cancer? Sci Am 1996;275(3):80–87.
251. Weindruch R. Caloric restriction and aging. Sci Am 1996;274(1):46–52.
252. Bjelakovic G, Nikolova D, Simonetti RG, Gluud C. Antioxidant supplements for prevention of gastrointestinal cancers: a systematic review and meta-analysis. Lancet 2004;364(9441):1219–1228.
253. Albright CD, Liu R, Mar MH, et al. Diet, apoptosis, and carcinogenesis. Adv Exp Med Biol 1997;422:97–107.
254. Weindruch R, Albanes D, Kritchevsky D. The role of calories and caloric restriction in carcinogenesis. Hematol Oncol Clin N Am 1991;5(1):79–89.
255. Wachsman JT. The beneficial effects of dietary restriction: reduced oxidative damage and enhanced apoptosis. Mutat Res 1996;350(1):25–34.
256. Bostick R. Diet and nutrition in the etiology and primary prevention of colon cancer. In: Bendich A, Deckelbaum R, eds. The Comprehensive Guide for Health Professionals. Totowa: Humana Press, 1997:57–95.
257. Slattery ML, Neuhausen SL, Hoffman M, et al. Dietary calcium, vitamin D, VDR genotypes and colorectal cancer. Int J Cancer 2004;111(5):750–756.
258. Kim YI. Folate, colorectal carcinogenesis, and DNA methylation: lessons from animal studies. Environ Mol Mutagen 2004;44(1):10–25.
259. Pike MC, Pearce CL, Wu AH. Prevention of cancers of the breast, endometrium and ovary. Oncogene 2004;23(38):6379–6391.
260. Moyers SB, Kumar NB. Green tea polyphenols and cancer chemoprevention: multiple mechanisms and endpoints for phase II trials. Nutr Rev 2004;62(5):204–211.
261. Aggarwal K, Pahuja S, Chadha R. Botryoid rhabdomyosarcoma of common bile duct. Indian J Pediatr 2004;71(4):363–364.
262. Byers T, Nestle M, McTiernan A, et al. American Cancer Society guidelines on nutrition and physical activity for cancer prevention: reducing the risk of cancer with healthy food choices and physical activity. CA Cancer J Clin 2002;52(2):92–119.
263. Spiegel W, Zidek T, Vutuc C, Maier M, Isak K, Micksche M. Complementary therapies in cancer patients: prevalence and patients' motives. Wien Klin Wochenschr 2003;115(19–20):705–709.
264. Gray RE, Fitch M, Goel V, Franssen E, Labrecque M. Utilization of complementary/alternative services by women with breast cancer. J Health Soc Policy 2003;16(4):75–84.
265. Malik IA, Gopalan S. Use of CAM results in delay in seeking medical advice for breast cancer. Eur J Epidemiol 2003;18(8):817–822.
266. Henderson JW, Donatelle RJ. Complementary and alternative medicine use by women after completion of allopathic treatment for breast cancer. Altern Ther Health Med 2004;10(1):52–57.
267. Navo MA, Phan J, Vaughan C, et al. An assessment of the utilization of complementary and alternative medication in women with gynecologic or breast malignancies. J Clin Oncol 2004;22(4):671–677.
268. Eng J, Ramsum D, Verhoef M, Guns E, Davison J, Gallagher R. A population-based survey of complementary and alternative medicine use in men recently diagnosed with prostate cancer. Integr Cancer Ther 2003;2(3):212–216.
269. Cassileth BR, Chapman CC. Alternative cancer medicine: a ten-year update. Cancer Invest 1996;14(4):396–404.
270. Angell M, Kassirer JP. Alternative medicine: the risks of untested and unregulated remedies. N Engl J Med 1998;339(12):839–841.
271. DiPaola RS, Zhang H, Lambert GH, et al. Clinical and biologic activity of an estrogenic herbal combination (PC-SPES) in prostate cancer. N Engl J Med 1998;339(12):785–791.

103

Regional Therapy of Cancer

Douglas L. Fraker

Surgical resection is the primary treatment and typically the only curative therapy for most solid malignancies. Throughout this surgical textbook, virtually all chapters dealing with individual organs have some portion of that chapter devoted to the surgical treatment of primary cancer at that site. For example, Chapter 96 on breast disease primarily discusses the treatment of cancer because this is by far the predominant surgical disease in that organ. On the other hand, Chapter 49 on the small intestine has a much smaller proportion dealing with cancer as primary malignancies comprise a smaller fraction of the surgical diseases involving the small intestine. A specialized type or category of surgical treatment for cancer can be categorized as regional therapy. As opposed to straightforward surgical resection, in this type of therapy a specific region or area of the body is treated. Regional therapy is primarily applicable to metastatic disease limited to one site or area of the body. There are two broad categories of regional therapy of cancer: (1) vascular-based treatments and (2) intracavitary treatments. The most successfully treated areas of the body by vascular means are the extremities and the liver. There is also potential to treat other sites such as the lung or pelvis. The peritoneal cavity and the pleural cavity are areas amenable to intracavitary treatments.

The theoretical advantage of regional therapy lies in the ability to have either a significant dose escalation of an antineoplastic agent to increase the therapeutic index or a specific targeting of treatment to one region (Table 103.1). The majority of regional treatment strategies use standard chemotherapeutic agents. For most antineoplastic drugs, dose escalation to the maximally tolerated level leads to the optimal response rate for that agent. Dose-limiting toxicities vary among different antineoplastic agents, but specific side effects most commonly seen are bone marrow suppression, gastrointestinal toxicity, or neurotoxicity, which provide well-defined limits beyond which it is unsafe to administer any more systemic treatments. If a patient has tumor that is only in one region of the body, such as an extremity, or in one organ, such as the liver, delivery of drug only to that site may allow dose escalation to achieve tissue levels well beyond what can be achieved with maximal systemic drug delivery. When the location of the metastatic cancer differs from the target organ of drug toxicity, the therapeutic index is improved if technical means exist to allow the successful delivery of regional therapy.

Although a large proportion of regional therapies of cancer deliver standard chemotherapeutic agents that have well-characterized responses and toxicities via systemic administration, regional approaches facilitate the use of other potential tools against cancer which cannot be readily achieved systemically (Table 103.2). Examples of alternative agents or techniques to treat cancer that can be used in conjunction with regional treatment include hyperthermia, photodynamic light therapy, and cancer gene therapy. Malignant cells are known to be more sensitive to hyperthermia than nontransformed cells.[1–3] The ability of the entire body to withstand temperatures that are in the range that would have a significant effect against cancer may produce unacceptable systemic toxicity. By applying hyperthermia regionally, this therapy can be tolerated with fewer untoward effects.[2] Also, hyperthermia has been shown to act synergistically with both standard chemotherapeutic agents as well as biological agents.[3] Photodynamic therapy, such as external-beam radiation therapy, is a local treatment as the therapy is only delivered to the sites where laser light of a defined wavelength is directed; this is discussed in detail in the section on intracavitary treatments.[4–6] Gene therapy of cancer is a topic of intense investigation with multiple strategies that can be employed to target genetic mutations in tumor suppressor genes and proto-oncogenes, deliver suicide genes, deliver anti-angiogenic therapies, or utilize virus that cause lysis selectively in tumor cells.[7,8] However, this type of treatment,

TABLE 103.1. Advantages and Disadvantages of Regional Therapy.

Advantages
- Dose escalation at treatment site
- Limited toxicity
- Ability to add hyperthermia

Disadvantages
- Regional treatment for a potentially systemic disease
- Complicated procedure to deliver therapy
- Other single treatment possible

which has been shown to be effective in vitro to reverse malignant phenotypes, often cannot be translated into in vivo therapies because the vector cannot be delivered successfully to the sites of cancer. Regional delivery techniques may provide an opportunity to ameliorate the current deficiencies of systemic genetic vector administration.[7,9]

The two categories of regional therapy, intravascular therapy and intracavitary therapy, are discussed generally, and then specific clinical experience for each treatment is discussed (Table 103.3). New techniques or treatments that are in development are also described.

Intravascular Regional Treatment

Intravascular regional therapy of cancer is based on delivering antineoplastic treatments via the bloodstream, targeting a specific organ such as the liver or a specific region of the body such as an extremity. Within the category of regional vascular treatment are two general categories differentiated by the mechanism of drug delivery: (1) regional vascular infusion and (2) isolated vascular perfusion. Regional infusion is technically more straightforward than isolation perfusion and is often performed by an interventional radiologist working in conjunction with medical oncologists. However, the degree of advantage gained in improving the therapeutic index based on regional infusion compared to systemic intravascular delivery is much less than can be achieved by isolated perfusion. By far the most important site of treatment for regional intravascular infusion is the liver. The ability of infusion to be effective in this location is predominantly because of the role the liver plays in drug metabolism. This ability to metabolize drug allows the liver to clear certain agents on the first pass through the liver parenchyma, which is not applicable

TABLE 103.2. Agents/Modulation Utilized in Regional Cancer Therapies.

Agents/modalities	*Examples*
Chemotherapeutics	Melphalan in isolated limb perfusion. FUDR in hepatic artery infusion, cisplatin/mitomycin in peritoneal perfusion
Biological agents	Tumor necrosis factor in isolated limb perfusion and isolated liver perfusion
Hyperthermia	Isolated limb perfusion, isolated liver perfusion, continuous hyperthermic peritoneal perfusion
Photodynamic therapy	Photofrin in peritoneal cavity and pleural cavity, Foscan in pleural cavity
Gene therapy	Wild-type p53 gene into hepatic artery, TK suicide gene in intrapleural treatment

TABLE 103.3. Categories of Regional Treatment of Cancer.

Area of treatment	*Procedure*	*Target disease*
Limb	Isolated limb perfusion	In-transit melanoma
	Isolated limb infusion	Extremity sarcoma
Liver	Hepatic artery infusion pump	Colorectal metastases, other metastatic tumors
	Isolated hepatic perfusion	
	Percutaneous hepatic perfusion with hemofiltration	Hepatomas
	Gene therapy	
Lung	Isolated lung perfusion	Metastatic lung cancer (sarcoma, renal cell cancer), primary lung tumor
	Isolated lung infusion	
Pelvis	Isolated pelvic infusion	Recurrent rectal cancer
Kidney	Isolated renal perfusion	Multifocal renal cancer
Intracavitary treatment:		
Peritoneal cavity	Continuous hyperthermic peritoneal perfusion	Carcinomatosis from gastric, colorectal, appendiceal, pancreas and ovarian
	Photodynamic therapy	
	Gene therapy	Sarcomatosis
Pleural cavity	Photodynamic therapy	Mesothelioma
	Gene therapy	Lung cancer
		Metastatic cancer

to other areas or regions of the body.[10,11] A variation of regional intravascular infusion that has been applied to other areas besides the liver is a stop-flow technique in which an antineoplastic drug is infused into an organ or region with a balloon devise applied to temporarily decrease the normal vascular inflow to that site.[12,13] By blocking the normal inflow at the time of infusion, the level of drug exposure is improved as there is less rapid drug washout. Also, tissue ischemia is generally produced to some degree by blocking normal arterial inflow, and this may augment the response. This technique has been applied to situations such as tumors of the pancreas[13] as well as regions to the body such as an extremity.[14] Thompson and colleagues have promoted isolated limb infusion (ILI) as a similar and less costly procedure than isolated limb perfusion (ILP) for advanced extremity melanoma.

The second type of vascular regional treatment is isolation perfusion. Isolation perfusion is a surgical procedure in which control of the inflow and outflow vessels to and from an organ or region of the body is achieved by operative dissection. That area of the body is then perfused using an extracorporeal bypass circuit which allows continuous recirculation of antineoplastic agent into that area of the body. This technique is advantageous as it not only eliminates the target organ of toxicity for a particular drug, but also may eliminate the organ of metabolism for that drug such that the area under the curve of drug exposure during the time of isolation perfusion is markedly increased. The ability to perform isolation perfusion was dependent upon the technological advance of extracorporeal bypass that was designed primarily to facilitate cardiac operations. With the development of this technology in the midpart of the twentieth century, surgical oncologists recognized the ability to apply extracorporeal bypass to regional vascular perfusion.[15] In this initial experience, many areas of the body were attempted to be treated with isolation perfusion.[16–18] Only treatment of the extremities primarily for in-transit melanoma produced results with positive objective antitumor responses and acceptable toxicity such that the operation became accepted as a standard procedure. Recently, partly because of improved technical aspects of complex surgical procedures as well as the availability of alternative treatment agents, isolation perfusion has been applied to other organs that were abandoned by the earlier investigators 30 to 40 years ago (see Table 103.3). Specifically, isolation perfusion procedures of the liver[19,20] and lung,[21,22] which had been reported as failures as a result of technical difficulties and low response rates, are being actively studied once again. Additional work has been performed on isolation perfusion procedures of the pelvis[23,24] as well as the kidney.[25] Because of the multiple areas of vascular inflow and areas of vascular outflow in the pelvis, this has not been as successful as isolation perfusion of the limb or liver. Isolation perfusion of the kidney is technically easier but is limited by the lack of clinical situations in which isolation perfusion would be an optimal outcome as compared to unilateral nephrectomy or renal wedge resection. The application of intravascular regional therapy to the extremities and liver is discussed here in great detail, and experience with isolated perfusion of other areas is also mentioned.

Intracavitary Treatment

The second broad category of regional therapy is intracavitary treatments. The two sites that are potentially treatable are the peritoneal cavity and the pleural cavity (Table 103.3). The bladder also provides an area for potential intracavitary treatment, but this is different in that it is typically applied to superficial bladder cancer as a primary neoplasm in an organ that has a contained accessible lumen. Regional therapies for the peritoneal cavity and the pleural cavity primarily target metastatic disease or diffuse primary malignancies such as mesothelioma of the pleura or peritoneum.

Many tumors have a natural history in which there is widespread disease in the peritoneal cavity without any evidence of hematogenous or even lymphatic spread.[26,27] Carcinomatosis from either primary ovarian tumors[28,29] or gastrointestinal tumors, including colorectal, appendiceal, gastric, and pancreatic cancers, constitute adenocarcinomas that spread in this manner.[30–32] Sarcomatosis from either primary gastrointestinal stromal tumors[33] or retroperitoneal sarcoma[34] comprise the second major group of tumors that spread in this way. There is no effective standard treatment available for peritoneal carcinomatosis and sarcomatosis, and tumor progression in these patients inevitably leads to considerable morbidity and eventual death.[35] Peritoneal carcinomatosis represents direct extension into a contained cavity with a complex surface where malignant cells may implant on any available surface and form nodules or plaques as well as causing ascites.[27,28] Ovarian tumors gain access to the peritoneal cavity as they represent free organs within the peritoneum, and this is the most common pattern of spread for that histology. Similarly, the pancreas, although retroperitoneal in location, may have direct seeding of the peritoneal cavity from tumors on the surface of the pancreas. Cancers of the colon, appendix, stomach, bile duct, and gallbladder uniformly start on the inner surface or mucosal layer but can have transmural invasion such that cells are seeded into the peritoneal cavity.

Standard oncological therapies including surgical resection, radiation therapy, and systemic chemotherapy uniformly fail in patients afflicted with this pattern of disease. Although all grossly visible surgical implants may be technically resected, recurrent disease always develops as a consequence of microscopic seeding throughout other surfaces that cannot be appreciated at the time of surgery. To attempt to improve these results, more aggressive surgical procedures called peritonectomy procedures have been advocated, as the peritoneal lining is often a barrier against this disease because tumor implants spread on the surface but do not invade through the peritoneum.[33] Although peritonectomy including stripping of the lining of the diaphragms, pericolic gutter, anterior abdominal wall, and pelvis is technically possible, the extensive operation removes less than half the potential surfaces available for contamination with intraperitoneal spread.[36] Specifically, the capsule of the liver and the capsule of the spleen cannot be completely stripped without leading to life-threatening blood loss. Similarly, the serosa of the stomach, small bowel, and colon cannot be excised, and these are frequently sites where tumor implants will grow. Finally, the mesenteric peritoneum for the small intestine and the transverse mesocolon, although it can be removed in small areas, cannot be completely removed without considerable blood loss and potential ischemic injury to the intestine by damaging mesenteric vessels. Therefore, an effective adjuvant therapy to add to peritonectomy or tumor debulking is needed.

Radiation therapy of the entire peritoneal cavity has been utilized as an adjunct in certain situations, including treatment of ovarian tumors.[37,38] However, the dose of radiation that can be administered to the entire abdominal cavity is limited by normal tissue toxicity to a level that is not generally cytotoxic. Finally, standard systemic chemotherapy is generally ineffectual against intraperitoneal disease caused by gastrointestinal tumors. Ovarian cancers are more chemoresponsive, but once gross peritoneal carcinomatosis is present (i.e., stage 3 disease), this tumor is almost never cured. This lack of efficacy stems from the general failure of available antineoplastic agents against solid malignancies at any location and is compounded by the inability of intravascular drug delivery to reach peritoneal disease that may be poorly vascularized. Intraperitoneal chemotherapy given via one or even more catheters placed at the time of an operative procedure has been attempted as regional infusional therapy.[39] However, after any surgical procedure, particularly when malignancy is involved, the contents of the abdominal cavity become densely adherent to one another, creating multiple isolated areas of peritoneal surfaces. Therefore, intraperitoneal drug delivery even when multiple catheters are used does not allow distribution of the treatment to all surfaces of the peritoneum that are at risk for tumor.

Two types of surgical peritoneal treatments are discussed: hyperthermic peritoneal perfusion and photodynamic therapy of the peritoneal cavity. Intraperitoneal gene therapy is also in initial clinical trials as an innovative approach using a different treatment agent against this pattern of disease.

The second area of the body in which intracavitary treatment may be applied for extensive disease is the pleural cavity. Intrapleural treatments are primarily directed against mesothelioma and locally advanced lung cancers. Pleural mesothelioma, as is peritoneal carcinomatosis, is typically considered incurable but often is a relatively isolated disease at the time of diagnosis.[40] There is no currently available surgical and chemotherapy treatment to obtain a complete response. Primary lung carcinomas often may have intrapleural effusions and recurrences; however, application of intracavitary treatments to that histology is limited by the fact that the majority of patients develop both lymphatic and hematogenous metastases simultaneously with intrapleural recurrences. In other words, as opposed to patients with carcinomatosis and sarcomatosis, patients with widespread intrapleural lung cancer generally do not have disease limited only to that site. Similar intracavitary approaches have been applied to the pleural space (photodynamic therapy, gene therapy) in certain patients with metastatic disease, and these are also discussed.

Extremity Procedures

Although the number of patients with diffuse in-transit melanoma of the extremity who are eligible for isolated limb perfusion is relatively small, the technical ease of the procedure and the early success rates of this procedure for extremity melanoma made this the most accepted and widely applied isolation perfusion procedure. Recent clinical trials have evaluated the addition of tumor necrosis factor and extended this application from in-transit melanoma to unresectable extremity sarcomas and other soft tissue neoplasms of the limb.[41,42] An additional procedure that has recently been reported with favorable objective response rates is isolated limb infusion, which is a nonsurgical intervention for in-transit melanoma. The technique of ILP, the results in melanoma both for adjuvant and therapeutic perfusion, and the results for soft tissue sarcoma are discussed.

Technique of Isolated Limb Perfusion

Anatomically the extremities are excellent areas for isolation perfusion procedures because of the straightforward vascular anatomy. For both the upper and lower extremity, there is essentially one artery into the extremity and one vein out of the extremity. The exception is the upper extremity where there may be multiple axillary veins, but typically these run in parallel and there is one dominant vessel. Isolated limb perfusion involves cannulating an artery leading to the extremity and a vein leading from the extremity, ligating collateral vascular branches, placing a tourniquet at the root of the extremity, and by these maneuvers there is control over the circulation to that portion of the body. This cannulation can be performed at multiple sites in both the upper and lower extremities. The potential levels for cannulation in the lower extremity are the external iliac vessels via a retroperitoneal approach, the common femoral vessels, and the popliteal vessels. Options for cannulation of the upper extremities are the axillary vessels and the brachial vessels just above the elbow. The level of cannulation is dictated by the disease that is being treated and other factors such as previous surgical dissection, body habitus, or anatomic variations. For in-transit melanoma in which the entire extremity is at risk for disease, the most proximal technically possible cannulation site is utilized. This site is always the axillary vessels for the upper extremity and typically the external iliac vessels for the lower extremity. For soft tissue tumors such as single large extremity sarcomas, the most distal site that can perfuse the entire tumor is utilized as this histology tends not to spread via intradermal lymphatics. An exception to this rule is multifocal sarcomas which act as melanoma such as epithelioid sarcomas and angiosarcomas in which proximal perfusion is indicated.

One of the most important technical aspects of isolated limb perfusion is gaining vascular control to prevent leak of the perfusate with the antineoplastic agents to the systemic circulation. With the use of high-dose tumor necrosis factor at several times the lethal systemic dose level, this problem has been magnified. There is much greater potential for leak from the extremity to the rest of the body in isolated limb perfusion compared to isolated organ perfusions including the liver, lung, and kidney in which the dissection can completely isolate that organ and obviate any significant leak. The cross-sectional area of the lower extremity at the pelvis is quite large, and significant potential collaterals exist posteriorly in the gluteal and pudendal vessels and centrally in the obturator vessels. An upper extremity perfusion is more easily controlled as the cross-sectional area of the arm at the shoulder is much smaller and more complete control can be obtained. The maneuvers utilized to achieve vascular isolation of the lower extremity at the external iliac vessels are complete skeletonization of the external iliac artery and vein down into the proximal common femoral vessels, ligating all branches circumferentially. The internal iliac artery is dissected and clamped and the obturator artery is tied. Either the main internal iliac vein or branches of that vein which appear to be going inferiorly to the leg can also be encircled and either tied or clamped. Finally, a tourniquet is placed around the root of the extremity, typically using an Esmarch tape placed in the medial groin crease and controlled laterally with a Steinmann pin in the anterior superior iliac spine. Approaching the lower extremity via the common femoral vessels utilizes a similar application of a tourniquet but does not control the branches above the inguinal ligament and therefore has a greater potential for leak of the perfusate to the systemic circulation. Cannulation via the popliteal vessels utilizes a pneumatic cuff tourniquet in the proximal thigh at 300 mmHg, which leads to virtual total isolation of that lower portion of the extremity. For upper extremity perfusions, dissection of all the axillary artery and vein branches and placement of an Esmarch tourniquet around the axilla secured with a small Steinmann pin in the head of the humerus lead to almost complete control of perfusate leak. In fact, the greatest problem with upper extremity ILP is to avoid causing brachial plexus trauma with excessive tightness in the tourniquet.

An essential component of ILP is monitoring the perfusate leak to the systemic circulation and making adjustments during treatment to reduce that leak.[41] Techniques such as injecting fluorescein into the perfusate have been utilized but are highly imprecise and nonquantitative. Virtually all ILP circuits use a gravity return venous line to a reservoir such that a visible assessment of the volume in the reservoir is possible. If the reservoir is decreasing in volume, it would indicate that perfusate is being lost into the systemic circulation. If the reservoir volume is rising, it would indicate that blood is leaking from the systemic circulation into the perfusion circuit. However, if there is a two-way leak of similar magnitude there would be no change in the reservoir yet considerable perfusate exposure. The standard of care, particularly in operations with high-dose tumor necrosis factor (TNF), uses a gamma counter over the precordium with radionuclide in the perfusion circuit that allows continuous readings and estimations of the leak of the perfusion solution into the systemic circulation.[43] This assessment is both quantitative and continuous, allowing the surgeon to react to changes almost immediately to control a perfusate leak.

TABLE 103.4. Incidence of In-Transit Melanoma of the Extremity.

Group	*n*	*Incidence of in-transit disease (%)*
Total population	3832	171 (4.46%)
Incidence based on Breslow levels		
<1.0mm	1891	30 (1.59%)
1.01–2.0mm	1074	41 (3.82%)
2.01–4.0mm	610	55 (9.02%)
>4.0mm	257	23 (8.95%)
Incidence based on surgery of lymph nodes		
Wide local excision only	2771	93 (3.36%)
Sentinel lymph node biopsy	1061	37 (3.64%)
Elective lymph node dissection	625	41 (6.56%)

Source: Adapted from Kang JC, Wanek LA, Essner R, Faries MB, Foshag LJ, Morton DL. Sentinel lymphadenectomy does not increase the incidence of in-transit metastases in primary melanoma. J Clin Oncol 2005;23:4764–4770.[48]

Natural History of In-Transit Melanoma

Isolated limb perfusion (ILP) has been applied most successfully against a pattern of disease spread called in-transit melanoma metastases. This pattern of recurrence represents lymphatic spread in the dermal and subcutaneous tissue with multiple nodules appearing throughout the extremity.[44] The entire limb is at risk for this pattern of spread, including areas distal to the site of the primary (Fig. 103.1). Because this represents intralymphatic spread, it is considered stage III disease, with in-transit nodules being N3 disease (AJCC stage 3C). The incidence of in-transit melanoma metastases from primary melanomas of the extremity is best demonstrated by clinical trials of adjuvant limb perfusion after resection of an intermediate and high-risk primary melanoma (>1.5mm) (Table 103.4). Patients in the control arm of these trials who do not receive ILP therapy have an incidence of 9.9% in-transit melanoma or local recurrence by satellite lesions.[45] The incidence of in-transit melanoma for stage I primary lesions (<1.5mm thick) is not as clearly known but would certainly be expected to be much less than the incidence for thicker melanoma. Local resection of in-transit melanoma nodules is almost uniformly destined to fail as the entire extremity is at risk.[46] Because in-transit melanoma nodules are often quite some distance from the primary location, all the intervening tissue is at risk as well as any other area in the dermal and subcutaneous tissue of that extremity. Therefore, simple excision with narrow margins with primary closure is the most appropriate procedure for resection of in-transit melanoma lesions instead of wide excision with split-thickness skin graft. Patients may develop very bulky disease in the extremity without evidence of systemic spread. Literature from a series of major limb amputations for extensive extremity melanoma report 25% to 30% 5-year disease-free survival rates, indicating that even with regional disease remarkable enough to mandate an amputation, systemic spread may not have occurred.[47] Therefore, an effective therapy to treat the entire limb may be beneficial for this patient population. Some investigators have postulated an increase in in-transit melanoma in the past 10 years since the practice of sentinel lymph node biopsy has been widely used.[48,49] Theoretically, the specific ligation of the primary draining lymphatic vessels may cause more in-transit disease. However, analysis of a large series of cases at John Wayne Cancer Institute showed no increase with sentinel lymph node biopsy, and it was an excellent demonstration of the expanded incidence of in-transit disease.

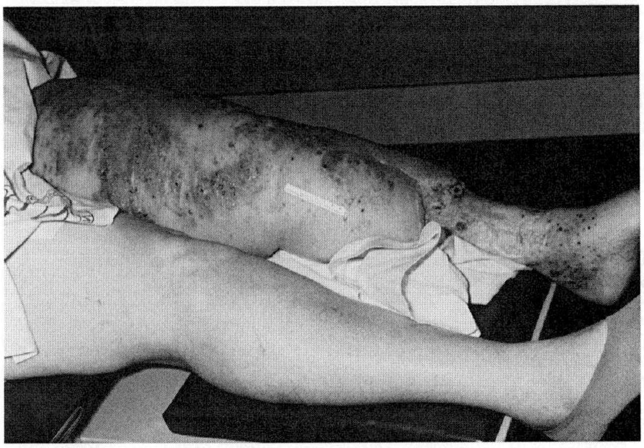

FIGURE 103.1. Patient with extensive in-transit melanoma from a calf primary. Note the extent of surgical resection of the distal calf, yet recurrent melanoma both distally and extensive disease proximal to that resection site. At the time of this photograph, the patient had no evidence by radiologic studies or physical examination of any extraextremity disease.

Adjuvant Isolated Limb Perfusion for Extremity Melanoma

An adjuvant ILP is one in which all gross disease has been resected from an extremity but there is a high risk of local recurrence. Historically, the largest number of ILP procedures have been performed in the adjuvant setting, most commonly after resection of high-risk primary melanoma but also for resection of limited satellite or in-transit metastases.[50] Although individual investigators who believe in the benefit of ILP applied this regional technique after resection of high-risk primary lesions (typically primary melanomas more than 1 or 1.5mm thick), both retrospective case-controlled studies and prospective randomized studies have failed to verify a benefit for this use of ILP.[51,52] A small study from Germany published in the 1980s reported a significant improvement in survival after adjuvant ILP. However, the numbers of patients treated were small, and the outcome in the control group was

TABLE 103.5.
Prospective Randomized Trials of Adjuvant Isolated Limb Perfusion (ILP) for Resected High-Risk Primary or In-Transit Melanoma.

Stage II primary melanoma (45):		
	Excision alone	***Excision + ILP***
No. of patients	412	420
Incidence of recurrent disease (%)		
— Local	3.3	2
— In transit	6.6	1.5
— Lymph nodes	16.7	12.6
— Distant metastases	6	8
— Overall survival	No difference	No difference
Resected in-transit melanoma (53):		
	Excision Alone	***Excision + ILP***
n	36	33
Disease-free survival		
— Overall (%)	17	33
— Median (months)	10	17
Survival		
— Overall (%)	44	55
— Median (months)	39	57
Regional recurrence	53%	36%
Distal recurrence	16%	18%

so much worse than expected compared to historical controls that this trial is not to be utilized in arguing for adjuvant ILP. The best information regarding adjuvant ILP for resected high-risk primary extremity melanoma comes from a recently published very large prospective randomized study[45] (Table 103.5). With almost 400 patients in a wide local excision-alone group or a wide local excision plus isolated limb perfusion with melphalan group, there was a decrease in the regional recurrence rate but no increase in the systemic recurrence rate and no change in survival. With the publication of this study as a negative trial, no adjuvant ILP should ever be performed after resection of primary melanoma.

A second setting for adjuvant ILP perfusion is for patients who have developed in-transit metastases that have been excisionally biopsied. These patients are clearly at much greater risk for additional recurrences in the limb than patients with high-risk primary cutaneous melanoma who have not had a regional recurrence. One could argue that an adjuvant regional treatment would be beneficial in this setting.[53] Again, there was a positive study reported from Germany, but the success rate with an adjuvant ILP with melphalan in that study was much greater than any other study reported in the medical literature with a small number of patients, and this study should not be trusted.[51,52] The best adjuvant isolated limb perfusion trial for resected in-transit disease comes from Sweden; there was a significant improvement in local control in the perfusion field, but this did not translate into improvement in overall survival[53] (see Table 103.5). Again, only small numbers of patients (fewer than 40 per arm) were studied, and with larger numbers there may have been a significant benefit. At the present time, adjuvant ILP should never be used for high-risk primary disease that has been resected and should be utilized for resected in-transit metastases only in the setting of a clinical trial.

Therapeutic Isolated Limb Perfusion for Extremity Melanoma

Therapeutic ILP is defined as procedures that treat measurable disease in the extremity. The response rates that are obtained with ILP are considerably higher than any other systemic therapy for this type of tumor. Although melphalan has very limited activity given systemically against melanoma, it is the optimal chemotherapeutic drug for ILP.[41,45,54] Objective response rates with melphalan ILP under either normothermic (37°C) conditions or with mild hyperthermia (38.5°–40°C) have been reported as high as 90% to 100%. These response rates should be placed in context of the responses seen with systemic chemotherapy. The best combination systemic chemotherapy gives a 25% to 40% response rate and a 0% to 5% complete response[44] (Table 103.6). Interleukin 2 treatment results in an 18% to 25% overall response rate and a 7% complete response.[44] There have never been any randomized clinical trials comparing melphalan ILP to systemic treatments because of this clear difference in response.[55,56] What is not known is whether this difference in regional response translates into any improvement in survival. The optimal dose of melphalan is calculated based on limb volume, because basing melphalan dose on patient weight may undertreat or overtreat an individual dependent on body habitus.[57] Limb volume measurements either with water displacement or sequential circumferential measurements can be obtained with lower extremities treated with 10 mg melphalan/L limb volume and upper extremities treated with 13 mg melphalan/L limb volume. Even with melphalan dosing based on limb volume, recent studies have shown highly variable perfusate in tissue drug levels, possibly contributing to variable response rates.[58]

The two best current studies of the objective response rates that can be achieved with melphalan ILP come from northern Europe. One is a multiinstitutional study of more than 100 patients reporting a complete response rate of 54% and an overall response rate of 85%.[59] The median duration of response was slightly more than 9 months. A more updated study from two centers in the Netherlands reported a complete response rate of 45% with melphalan ILP and time to complete response of 3 months. Median limb recurrence-free survival was 14 months, limb salvage rate was 96%, and overall 5-year survival was 29%.[60]

Other standard chemotherapeutic agents used in therapeutic ILP for melanoma have yielded either much lower subjective response rates or, if responses are seen, the toxicity is much greater. The most successful alternative would be cisplatin, but the response rates are somewhat lower, in the

TABLE 103.6. Objective Treatment Response for Metastatic Melanoma.

	Complete response rate	*Overall response rate*
DTIC	0%–2%	20%
Combination chemotherapy	5%–15%	13%–55%
IL-2	8%	20%–30%
ILP-melphalan	54%–65%	79%–95%
ILP-melphalan + TNF	78%–90%	95%–100%

TNF, tumor necrosis factor; DTIC, dacarbazine.
Source: Data from references 44, 54, 56, 59, 60.

range of 50% to 60% objective response rates, and this agent when used in ILP is complicated by peripheral neuropathy.[54] The most successful systemic treatment agent for melanoma is DTIC but used in regional perfusion this agent leads to minimal responses.[61]

Tumor Necrosis Factor in Isolated Limb Perfusion

Tumor necrosis factor (TNF) is a protein derived from multiple cellular sources believed to be a mediator of the inflammatory cascade in acute sepsis as well as in chronic autoimmune diseases; this protein causes complete necrosis of established 1-cm subcutaneous sarcomas in mice with a single treatment.[62] Systemic use of recombinant TNF in patients did not translate into the responses seen in the preclinical murine models. In fact, virtually no patients responded to TNF in multiple phase I and phase II clinical trials of advanced cancer.[63] The dose-limiting toxicity is universally hypotension, and serum levels of TNF at maximal doses in patients are 100 fold lower than levels achieved in mice. Because the preclinical evidence that TNF is an effective antineoplastic drug is overwhelming and because the doses that led to responses in mice could not be achieved with systemic administration, TNF was utilized in regional perfusion.[64] In this setting, the equivalent intravascular levels that led to responses in mice (1–3 μg/ml) could be achieved in the perfusate. TNF alone in ILP for melanoma led to minimal antineoplastic effects that were not sustained.[65] However, high-dose TNF combined with a standard dose of melphalan seemed to augment the response, with the initial phase II trial reporting a 90% complete response rate and a 100% overall response rate[66,67] (Table 103.7). There was also a suggestion that the duration of response was improved.[66] These initial trials of TNF also incorporated low-dose preoperative subcutaneous interferon-γ and low-dose interferon-γ in the perfusion. A phase III trial in Europe comparing melphalan plus TNF with or without interferon-γ demonstrated that the addition of interferon resulted in marginal benefit.[68] Also, in the setting of a multiinstitutional study, the initial phase II results were not reproduced, with complete response rates with melphalan, TNF, and interferon seen at 78% instead of 90%.[68]

TABLE 103.7.
Results of ILP Trials Using TNF to Treat In-Transit Melanoma of the Extremity.

Reference	*Type of trial*	*Treatment regimen*	*n*	*Percent CR*
67	II	Melp/TNF/IFN	29	90%
70	II	Melp/TNF/IFN	26	76%
69	III	Melphalan	23	61%
		Melp/TNF/IFN	20	80%
68	III	Melphalan + TNF	33	69%
		Melp/TNF/IFN	31	78%

CR, complete response; Melp, melphalan; IFN, interferon-γ.

A North American trial comparing melphalan alone to melphalan, TNF, and interferon-γ demonstrated some benefit with TNF for patients with high tumor burden but showed equivalent results when patients with low tumor burden or small tumors were treated with either of these two regimens.[69] Patients with low tumor burden had equivalent complete response rates with melphalan alone (81%) and melphalan, TNF, and interferon-γ (87%) (see Table 103.7). However, in patients with high tumor burden, the addition of TNF and interferon increased response rates from 17% to 67%.[69] Figure 103.2 shows a patient with high tumor burden who had a sustained complete response after melphalan and TNF ILP. A follow-up randomized trial in North America compared melphalan alone to melphalan plus TNF. Preliminary results indicated no significant improvement in the experimental arm, and the trial was halted by the data safety

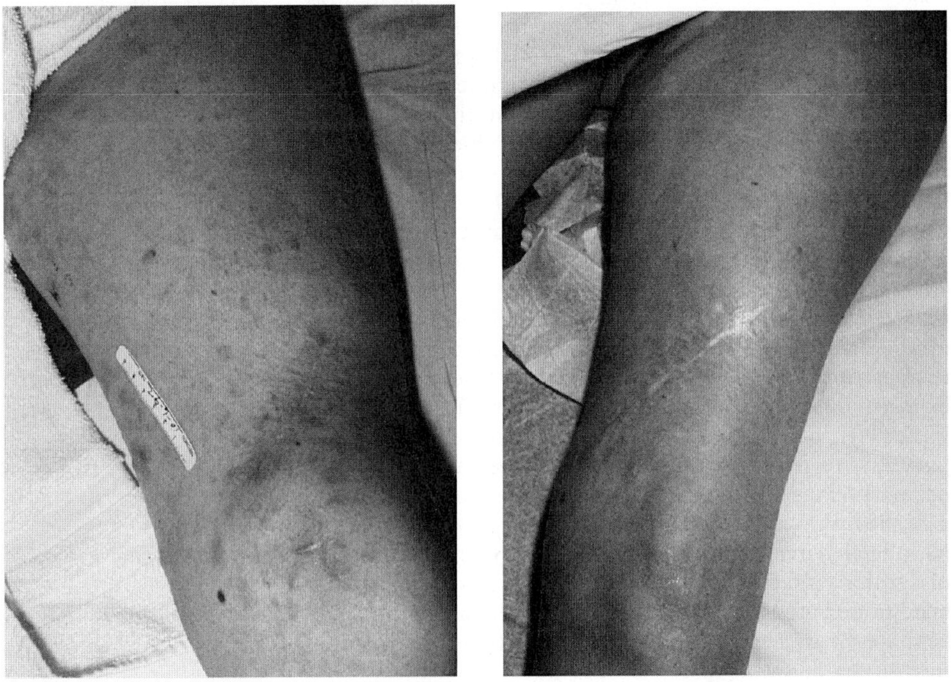

A B

FIGURE 103.2. Patient with in-transit melanoma of the thigh. **A.** Preoperative photograph with multiple dermal and subcutaneous melanoma nodules. **B.** Same leg 1 year after an isolated limb perfusion with melphalan, tumor necrosis factor, and interferon-γ demonstrating a complete clinical response. This patient had a sustained complete response for more than 3 years, until she had systemic recurrence and succumbed to the disease.

and monitoring committee. The final results of this study have yet to be reported. In Europe, as TNF is an approved agent for ILP for unresectable extremity sarcoma, investigators use TNF selectively in melanoma for reperfusion after melphalan failure or for bulky disease. A phase I/II dose escalation study demonstrated no benefit for increased TNF levels but increased systemic and regional toxicity.[70]

In summary, all subsequent reports show that the response rate achieved with TNF and melphalan for melanoma are not as good as the initial complete response rates of 90%. However, there is value in the use of TNF in patients with bulky disease and in patients who have failed prior melphalan-alone ILP.[71] One study showed that the overall response rate achieved with melphalan plus TNF was 59%, and in a nonrandomized trial compared to their melphalan-alone perfusions there was no difference in recurrence rate or median limb recurrence-free survival. Another study of patients with very bulky disease and symptoms within the extremity[72] showed that TNF and melphalan achieved a complete response rate of only 13% but an overall response rate of 88%. Palliation of symptoms within the extremity occurred in 75% of the patients.[72,73] Evidence for the TNF effect includes enhanced response rates in bulky disease as well as responses in patients who have failed melphalan-alone isolated limb perfusion. As randomized studies have failed to demonstrate any significant improvement in duration of response or survival, TNF is unavailable in North America.

Toxicity of Isolated Limb Perfusion

Toxicity after ILP procedures can be categorized as side effects from systemic exposure of the drugs and side effects caused by the regional effects of high-dose exposure. The systemic exposure depends on the adequacy of the isolation in the perfusion circuit. Perfusate leak with melphalan at the doses utilized in limb perfusion can be tolerated up to a 10% to 20% leak in which patients receive what would be a typical systemic bolus dose of melphalan; this dose leads to early postoperative nausea and vomiting and a delayed bone marrow suppressive effect that is transient. The use of high-dose TNF at levels 10 times the maximally tolerated systemic intravenous bolus dose limits the acceptable leak rate to 10% in ILP use with TNF.[63,74] The side effects seen are those seen with systemic administration of TNF, including high fever, hypotension, and potentially acute respiratory distress syndrome (ARDS) and renal failure.[63] All these side effects are transient and are managed with appropriate resuscitative techniques.

The most important toxicities in ILP are the regional effects in the extremity.[41,59] All tissues of the extremity including skin, muscle, bone, and peripheral nerve are exposed to the same additions of chemotherapy concentration and temperatures to which the tumors within the extremities are exposed. The toxicities seen with melphalan are skin erythema, with areas of blistering and subcutaneous edema in virtually all patients.[75–77] The skin changes as well as this edema universally return to baseline after several months. The most important toxicities are the effects on muscle and peripheral nerve. Myopathy can be seen with mild muscle discomfort and in the worst situation causes compartment syndrome with potential muscle necrosis and subsequent limb loss. Peripheral neuropathies lead to transient electrical shock sensations in more than half the patients treated, which typically resolve. Approximately 5% to 10% of the patients have significant long-term discomfort in their extremity after ILP. The addition of TNF to melphalan appears to add virtually nothing to the regional side effects.

Use of Isolated Limb Perfusion in Nonmelanoma Tumors

Although by far the most widespread use of ILP is for extremity melanoma, this procedure was also applied to other tumors in the extremity, most commonly, soft tissue sarcomas, in the 1960s and 1970s. The early experience with treatment of soft tissue sarcomas showed minimal objective responses, and this application was not generally utilized by most investigators after the initial disappointing results.[78] Also, it was more acceptable to undergo an extremity amputation for a soft tissue tumor than for diffuse in-transit melanoma. Recently, alternative strategies for limb preservation by compartmental excisions with preoperative or postoperative radiation therapy were able to provide adequate local control for most extremity sarcoma, which is different than from the outcome in in-transit melanoma.[79]

When the benefit of TNF when added to melphalan in ILP for bulky melanoma was seen, this same regimen was applied to sarcoma.[66] The results were much more positive with this combination compared to melphalan alone, and several series have been published demonstrating limb preservation in patients deemed to have unresectable tumors with amputation as the only surgical option[80–82] (Table 103.8). The overall approach with large extremity sarcomas that have no local resection options because of relationship to neurovascular and bony structures is to conduct an isolated limb perfusion with TNF and melphalan. This treatment generally results in significant tumor shrinkage by 8 to 12 weeks. At that time, a second procedure is undertaken to resect this smaller tumor. Objective response rates by size criteria in a large European trial of 186 patients were 17% complete response rates and 54% partial response rate.[81] When patients do not undergo the secondary resection, there is a high incidence of local recurrence.[66] Other groups have similar although not quite so dramatic response rates. A group from Amsterdam of 48 evaluable patients had a complete response rate of 2% and partial response rate of 47% based on standard size criteria. When they incorporated pathological responses, this increased to

TABLE 103.8.
Response Rates and Limb Salvage in Phase II Trials of ILP to Treat Unresectable Soft Tissue Sarcomas of the Extremity.

Reference	*No. of patients*	*CR (%)*	*PR (%)*	*Overall response (%)*	*Limb salvage*
81	186	18%	57%	75%	82%
87	43	27%	32%	59%	58%
82	35	37%	54%	91%	85%
85	53	42%	46%	88%	82%
86	30	20%	50%	70%	65%

CR, complete response; PR, partial response.

8% complete response rate and 57% partial response rate.[83] However, because high-grade sarcomas often have a large degree of necrosis without any treatment, it is hard to differentiate tumor necrosis resulting from rapid growth from that induced by the regional therapy. A study from France has questioned whether the dose of tumor necrosis factor used in perfusion for sarcoma is too high. They performed a clinical trial with four doses of TNF (0.5, 1, 2, and 3 or 4 mg).[84] The response rates of extremity sarcoma in these four dose groups were 68%, 56%, 72%, and 64%, respectively, showing absolutely no dose effect, and none was significantly different from another. The long-term overall survival and disease-free survival were no different. The authors did comment that the systemic toxicity seen in this patient population was always higher in the higher TNF groups and questioned whether a lower dose may be equally effective but safer.

A separate group of sarcoma patients are those in which multifocal disease behaves more as in-transit melanoma metastasis than a single bulky sarcoma; examples include angiosarcoma, epithelioid sarcoma, and multifocal malignant fibrous histiocytoma. In a series published from Europe, 64 isolated limb perfusions were performed on 53 patients with multifocal disease.[85] The overall response rate was 88% with 42% complete response rate and a 46% partial response rate. In this same group of patients, single large lesions had an overall response rate of 69% (see Table 103.8). Just as for melanoma, this perfusion strategy seems to achieve better results when administered for smaller volume, but multifocal, disease. A second clinical situation that often rises in extremity sarcoma is local recurrence after initial resection with maximal radiation therapy. In these situations, the local recurrence often grows in a way in which repeat excision is not possible and, as there is no way to deliver additional radiation therapy, amputation may be the only option. A group of 30 isolated limb perfusions were performed for this indication, with a response rate of 70% with 20% complete responses and 50% partial responses.[86] The overall limb salvage was 65%. There was no increased toxicity seen in this patient group compared to the patients who have not had radiation therapy.

These studies on bulky extremity sarcomas have demonstrated that the tumor necrosis factor is acting by targeting the tumor vasculature with fairly rapid elimination of tumor blood flow within days of the treatment to these tumors.[64] The success rate has varied from an 80% to 85% limb salvage rate in European studies to a 65% limb salvage rate in North American trials[87] (see Table 103.8). As opposed to melanoma, the addition of TNF to a melphalan ILP has demonstrated a clear improvement in tumor response and benefit in terms of limb salvage. For these reasons, TNF is approved and available for ILP for extremity sarcoma in Europe.

In addition to treatment of melanoma and sarcoma, other more unusual tumors of the extremity such as Merkel cell carcinoma, which often spreads by in-transit metastases within the limb, as well as eccrine adenocarcinoma and basal and squamous cell skin carcinoma have been reported to respond to ILP with melphalan plus tumor necrosis factor.[88] Again, as this treatment acts via an apparent antiangiogenic mechanism, it may be applicable against all solid malignancies with a target tissue of the tumor endothelium that is similar across several histologies.

Isolated Limb Infusion

Although the success rate with isolated limb perfusion (ILP) is significant, this treatment requires a surgical procedure, one that generally lasts 4 to 5 h and has the disadvantage that it is quite difficult to administer a second treatment in a reoperative setting. Reperfusions using the ILP technique have been reported, but again this is more technically challenging and also there is some cumulative toxicity within the extremity.[71] An alternative regional treatment for extremity melanoma that has been proposed by Thompson from Australia isolated limb infusion (ILI).[14,89] In this setting, a radiologic procedure in which balloon cannulas are utilized is essentially a stop-flow infusion into an extremity with a tourniquet, which allows a relatively acceptable dose of melphalan to be present within the extremity for 15 to 20 min. The objective response rates seen in gross disease in melanoma are significant, considering the ease and dose of agent utilized in this technique. Complete response rates of 30% to 40% and overall response rates of 70% have been reported, and this technique has the advantage of being much easier for reperfusion.[14] The Sydney Melanoma Group has furthered this field of isolated limb infusion by developing a salvage regimen. They treated patients who have failed one or more ILIs with melphalan in whom amputation was the only other treatment option with ILI with fotemustine after systemic chemosensitization with DTIC.[90] They treated 13 of these patients; 4 had a complete response and 8 had a partial response. However, the median duration of the response was only 3 months, resulting in limb salvage in 5 of 12 assessable patients; this is a very good response rate in a heavily pretreated patient population.

Isolated limb infusion is just now being investigated at select centers in the United States, and the ability to achieve similar response rates as seen in the Australian experiments has yet to be reported. This is a less expensive technique than isolated limb perfusion, but the early reports of toxicity are no different. If there are not equal or improved response rates, then this technique would be inferior to isolated limb perfusion. Furthermore, the conduct of this treatment does not allow regional therapy to the proximal one-third to one-half of the thigh and, because of the pattern of spread of the in-transit melanoma, there will be a patient population that will be not eligible as a consequence of proximal disease spread. Ongoing trials will determine the role of this procedure in the regional treatment of extremity melanoma.

Regional Treatment of Liver Malignancies

The liver is the archetypal organ for regional treatment of cancer for several reasons. First, it is commonly the sole site of metastatic disease for a variety of malignancies such as colorectal cancer, gastrointestinal stromal tumors, gastrointestinal/pancreatic neuroendocrine tumors, and ocular melanoma. Also, as an essential organ as opposed to the extremity, liver failure is often the cause of death in patients with metastatic cancer from these primary lesions, so that an effective regional therapy may improve survival. Second, the liver is able to be dissected such that there is essentially no vascular connection to the remainder of the body except via bile duct collaterals. Third, the vascular anatomy favors regional intravascular therapy. Although the dual vascular supply of the hepatic arterial system and the portal vein would appear to complicate regional treatment of the liver to some extent, it offers advantages as well. The branching vasculature in and around the liver offers a straightforward cannulation site via cutdown on the gastroduodenal artery in most patients to allow simple access to the hepatic arterial system for both infusion or isolated hepatic perfusion. Also, studies have demonstrated that the majority of the blood supply from metastatic tumors growing in the hepatic parenchyma is parasitized from the hepatic arterial system, as opposed to the portal venous system, which allows better drug delivery via the hepatic artery.[91,92] The final reason why the liver is an excellent organ for regional perfusion is that, as a central component of the body's system to metabolize drugs, extensive clearance of infused agents often occurs after a first pass through the hepatic vasculature, limiting systemic exposure with hepatic infusion.[10,11]

The regional vascular treatments of liver metastases can be categorized as hepatic arterial infusion therapy, chemoembolization, isolated hepatic perfusion, and percutaneous hepatic perfusion with hemofiltration (see Table 103.3). Although isolated hepatic infusion can be delivered via radiologic catheters, the ability to have an indwelling pump with continuous flow has made this primarily a surgical procedure. The procedure of chemoembolization is clearly an interventional radiology procedure.[93] Isolated hepatic perfusion is a very extensive and complex surgical operation,[17,18] and isolated hepatic perfusion with hemofiltration is a percutaneous operation that has been primarily developed by surgical oncologists.

Colorectal Metastasis to the Liver and Regional Infusion Therapy

The most important metastatic tumor in the liver that is treated by regional therapy is metastases from colon or rectal primary adenocarcinomas. The incidence of adenocarcinoma of the colon/rectum has decreased recently in the United States but there were still an estimated 139,000 cases in 1999. There will be an estimated 42,000 patients with metastases to the liver, and in approximately half these cases the liver will initially be the sole site of metastatic disease. It is estimated that only 10% of these patients would be eligible for complete resection, meaning there are approximately 37,000 new patients per year with colorectal metastases to the liver who are not resectable.[94] Historically, the first line of systemic therapy for metastatic colon cancer was fluorouracil (5-FU) plus leucovorin, with response rates in the range of 12% to 20% and duration of response less than 1 year. There has been tremendous progress in the treatment regimens available for colon cancer, with several new agents and several new treatment combinations reported over the past 5 to 10 years (Table 103.9). New standard antineoplastic agents such as irinotecan and oxaliplatin as well as targeted therapy such as an antivascular epithelial growth factor (anti-VEGF) antibody (Bevacizimab) and antiepidermal growth factor (anti-EGF antibodies) (Erbitux) have greatly improved the response rate and duration of response for metastatic colorectal cancer in the liver as well as elsewhere.[95] With this greatly improved systemic therapy, the role of regional treatment with intraarterial infusion therapy has greatly diminished in the past 5 years. The theory and results of hepatic arterial infusion therapy are reviewed briefly, and how this regional treatment may be incorporated into current protocols is discussed.

TABLE 103.9. Response Rates and Duration of Response for Metastatic Colon Cancer.

	Response rate	*Duration*
Systemic therapies:		
5-FU/leucovorin	11%–23%	3–5 months
IFL (irinotecan/5-FU/leucovorin)	31%–35%	6.9 months
FOLFIRI (irinotecan/5-FU)	56%	8.5 months
FOLFOX (oxaliplatin/5-FU/leucovorin)	54%	8.1 months
IFL + bevacizumab	45%	10.6 months
Intraarterial therapies:		
FUDR	42%–68%	8–10 months
FUDR + systemic oxaliplatin	90%	9.8 months
FUDR + systemic irinotecan	74%	8.1 months

5-FU, 5-fluorouracil; FUDR, fluorodeoxyuridine.

The initial regimen used for continuous intraarterial infusion therapy was floxuridine (FUDR). The reason for use of FUDR as opposed to 5-FU is that the extraction in the first pass through the liver with FUDR is in the range of 98% to 99% whereas with 5-FU it is 65% to 70%.[10,11] More than 20 years ago, a device was developed that would serve as a subcutaneous pump which at body temperatures would infuse a small quantity of medication such as intraarterial FUDR on a daily basis continually, and these pumps replaced catheters placed percutaneously by radiologists.[96]

The initial phase II trials of hepatic arterial infusion therapy were FUDR at 0.3mg/kg/day given as 2 weeks of treatment and 2 weeks off with reported response rates between 50% and 70%.[10,11] It became clear with this initial experience that there was toxicity to the normal liver, to the gallbladder via the cystic artery from the right hepatic artery, and to the lesser curvature of the stomach and duodenum via collateral branches.[97] The complications of gastritis or duodenitis are prevented by a complete intraoperative dissection including cholecystectomy. During placement of an intraarterial infusion catheter, fluorescein is injected via the pump, and under Wood's lamp evaluation the stomach and duodenum are inspected to see if there is any direct infusion from the pump into those areas. If a collateral vessel develops or a small vessel is missed at the time of the surgical dissection, this vessel can normally be occluded by coil embolization in radiology.

The most important side effect of hepatic arterial infusion therapy is chemical hepatitis, and in many cases this toxicity limits treatment more than progressive disease.[98] This inflammation of the normal liver can lead to biliary sclerosis that in advanced cases causes liver failure with intrahepatic bile duct obstruction leading to overwhelming jaundice. Two advances have occurred in the past decade to circumvent this complication.[99] First, it was noted that addition of dexamethasone to the infusate limits this complication. A phase II trial reported improved response rates with the combination of dexamethasone plus FUDR and leucovorin with a much lower rate of biliary sclerosis at 3% incidence. Second, biliary sclerosis has been prevented by understanding and awareness of this side effect and using elevations of alkaline phosphatase as indicators to decrease the infused dose of drug or even hold therapy.

The response rates achieved by infusional FUDR were in the range of 50% to 78%.[99,100] At the time initial phase II trials were performed of hepatic arterial infusion therapy, the standard systemic therapy was 5-FU and leucovorin with response rates between 12% and 20%. This clinical situation was appropriately evaluated by several prospective randomized clinical trials in both the United States and Europe[98,101–105] (Table 103.10). In all these trials, the overall response rate achieved by infusional therapy was much higher than that with systemic therapy, but in the majority of trials this was not translated into improved survival. Reasons why the response rates were superior without survival benefit included crossover of patients from systemic therapy to infusional therapy, significant hepatotoxicity in the infusional therapy group, and systemic extrahepatic recurrences in the perfusion group. The response rates achieved with current combination systemic therapy regimens (also shown in Table 103.9) have improved so they are similar to those achieved with intraarterial infusion therapy.[95] Furthermore, these treatment regimens are systemic and would treat not only known hepatic disease but also any extrahepatic disease that is either present or in the microscopic stage. Finally, these therapies of course do not require any major abdominal procedure to administer and, for all these reasons, the utilization of intraarterial infusion pump treatment as an early-line treatment for metastatic colon cancer, even if liver-only disease, has diminished markedly.

New protocols are utilizing a combination of intraarterial FUDR with systemic agents that act by a different mechanism (see Table 103.9). The primary impetus from this comes from Memorial Sloan-Kettering Cancer Center where they have reported phase I/II trials combining hepatic artery FUDR plus systemic irinotecan and infusional FUDR plus systemic oxaliplatin. The maximally tolerated dose of irinotecan was 100mg/m^2 weekly with concurrent FUDR at 0.16mg/kg/day with dose-limiting toxicities of diarrhea and neutropenia. The response rate in evaluable patients was 76%.[106]

A subsequent trial combined FUDR intraarterially with systemic irinotecan for patients who had undergone complete resection of liver metastases from colorectal cancer (1072A). They were treated with six monthly cycles of FUDR and escalating doses of systemic irinotecan. The maximally tolerated dose levels were FUDR at 0.12mg/kg/day for 14 days and irinotecan at 200mg/m^2 every other week. Dose-limiting toxicities were diarrhea and neutropenia. With a follow-up time of 26 months, at 2 years the survival rate was 89%, and all 27 patients treated at the maximal dose level were alive.[107] The second phase I/II trial treated patients with established disease.[108] Two treatment groups were designed: one was given concurrent hepatic arterial therapy with FUDR plus systemic oxaliplatin plus irinotecan, and a second group received intraarterial FUDR plus systemic oxaliplatin and 5-FU and leucovorin. The overall response rate for the group receiving oxaliplatin plus irinotecan was 90%, and the complete overall response rate for the group receiving oxaliplatin plus systemic 5-FU was 87%.[108] These response rates compared to current systemic regimens incorporating oxaliplatin in the range of 35% to 45%, indicating that the addition of intraarterial FUDR may be beneficial in combination with these current systemic therapies (see Table 103.9).

A second regional therapy is as an adjuvant treatment after resection of hepatic disease or more recently in trials in which tumor debulking of gross tumors are treated by combination of resection plus ablative techniques. For patients who have metastatic disease to their colon who are eligible for resection, approximately half the recurrences will be in the remaining liver. In other words, microscopic disease will be present at the time of the resection that cannot be appreciated by palpation or preoperative imaging or intraoperative ultrasound. Two randomized trials evaluated patients who had complete resection and were randomized either to intraarterial FUDR or either systemic therapy or observation[109,110] (Table 103.11). Both these trials suggest improvement in local recurrences within the liver in the hepatic arterial infusion arm, but neither trial utilized currently available systemic agents in the control arm. Again, the progress in response rates with systemic requests has limited the use of intraarterial pump treatment in an adjuvant setting after liver resection. Also, other institutions have utilized intraarterial therapy in combination with ablative techniques.[111,112] Usage of radiofrequency ablation initially for primary hepatomas but also for metastatic colorectal cancer has been greatly increased. Ablative treatments can be done either alone or in combination with major lobar liver resections or wedge resections. In fact, the criteria for trying to eliminate gross disease in colorectal cancer has changed from a maximum of 3 or 4 separate nodules to sometimes up to 10 or more nodules that can be treated with this technique. Because these surgical resection and ablation procedures are open techniques, it is possible to place an hepatic arterial infusion pump. The protocols combining these two technologies show that it is safe but that the disease-free survival may be no different from that of patients who have adjuvant systemic therapy.

TABLE 103.10.
Randomized Trials of Intraarterial Chemotherapy for Colorectal Metastases to the Liver.

Reference	No. of patients	Objective Response (%) IA vs. systemic	Survival (median) IA vs. systemic
98	110	42% vs. 10% ($P < 0.0001$)	NA–crossover
101	64	68% vs. 17% ($P < 0.003$)	22% vs. 15% (2-year survival)
102	99	50% vs. 20% ($P < 0.001$)	NA–crossover
103	69	48% vs. 21% ($P < 0.05$)	13 vs. 11 months
104	163	43% vs. 9%	15 vs. 11 months
105	100	NA	13.5 vs. 7.5 ($P < 0.05$)

Isolated Hepatic Perfusion

Although there are many advantages to the liver both anatomically and by its drug metabolism for hepatic arterial infusion, the technique of isolated hepatic perfusion (IHP) is complicated by the vascular activity of the liver. At the time when isolated limb perfusion was performed initially in the

TABLE 103.11.
Phase II and III Trials of Adjuvant Intraarterial Chemotherapy After Resection of Colorectal Metastases.

	MSKCC (109)		*SWOG/ECOG (110)*		*MSKCC*
	HAI + SYS + 5-FU	*SYS alone*	*HAI + SYS + 5-FU*	*No treatment*	*HAI + SYS + irinotecan*
n	74	82	53	56	46%
Two-year survival	85%	69%	80%	79%	89%
Phase	III		III		II
Hepatic DFS	89%	57%	85%	57%	88%
Overall DFS	55%	41%	58%	34%	47%
Overall 5-year survival	—	—	63%	32%	—

HAI, hepatic arterial therapy; SYS, systemic therapy; DFS, disease-free survival; MSKCC, Memorial Sloan Kettering Cancer Center; SWOG, Southwest Oncology Group; ECOG, Eastern Cooperative Oncology Group.

1950s, isolated hepatic perfusion was also attempted but, as stated by Dr. Chung, "the technique for complete isolation of the liver is a relatively complicated procedure because of its anatomic peculiarity."[16] Specifically, the dual blood supply as well as the reality that the inferior vena cava essentially passes through the posterior liver, with the hepatic veins being broad short structures, make this a much more complex situation than isolated limb perfusion. One recent strategy attempted in performing an isolated hepatic perfusion was a double-lumen cannula that allowed inferior vena cava blood returning from the lower extremities and kidney to pass behind the liver at the same time that hepatic venous return was collected in a recirculating system. A major advance for IHP was the application of a venovenous bypass extracorporeal circuit to shunt both the portal venous flow and the inferior vena cava flow below the level of the liver back to the axillary vein.[20,113] This circuit is utilized in liver transplantation when patients are anhepatic, and while the liver is completely isolated it can be used to shunt blood flow peripherally. The hepatic artery can be cannulated via the gastroduodenal artery as in hepatic infusional therapy. The retrohepatic vena cava can be cannulated directly for venous return and with a complete dissection including ligation of phrenic veins and the right adrenal vein, the entire liver is completely isolated.[17,20] The only connection that does not allow complete vascular control is the bile duct, and the amount of blood flow there is minimal.

The initial trials of isolated hepatic perfusion reported recently used mitomycin C, which led to significant objective responses but were complicated by life-threatening venoocclusive disease, and this dose-limiting toxicity made this treatment impractical.[114] Even though melphalan is not an active agent against colorectal adenocarcinoma given systemically, because it is an excellent perfusion drug with outstanding tissue levels as seen with isolated limb perfusion it was utilized in isolated hepatic perfusion. A series of studies have evaluated isolated hepatic perfusion with melphalan either in combination with tumor necrosis factor,[115] alone, or with additional intraarterial hepatic infusion with FUDR and leucovorin. The initial study was a mixed group of tumors treated with melphalan and tumor necrosis factor with a 72% partial response rate and a 3% complete response rate occurring in an ocular melanoma patient. Subsequent follow-up studies have shown the response rates are between 71% and 77% for colorectal cancer; however, the median duration of response is 10 months[116] (Table 103.12). The addition of post-isolated hepatic perfusion intraarterial FUDR did not appear to augment the response rate. Another tumor type that may be very appropriate for treatment with isolated hepatic perfusion is metastatic ocular melanoma. For unknown reasons, approximately 70% of patients with this tumor when it metastasizes have liver disease only. Furthermore, this tumor has been very resistant to treatment with standard agents that show benefit for cutaneous melanoma. A trial of melphalan isolated liver perfusion for ocular melanoma, showing a 10% complete response rate and a 52% partial response rate (see Table 103.12). For patients who had lactate dehydrogenase (LDH) in the mid- to low normal range, there was prolonged survival, but the overall duration of response was 9 months; this seemed to be greatly improved with the addition of tumor necrosis factor in the perfusate. Trials in Europe have generally reproduced these results in small series in the Netherlands and Germany. Typically, the response rates are in the range of 60% to 80% for melanoma, but the duration of response tends to be between 9 and 11 months.[116] In a recent report from the National Cancer Institute (NCI) of nine patients with primary hepatoma, a partial response rate of 67% (six of nine) was reported with a median time to progres-

TABLE 103.12.
Results of Clinical Trials with Isolated Hepatic Perfusion for Metastatic Cancers.

n	*Histology*	*Drug*	*Response rate*
29	Colorectal	Melphalan	17.2% (3%–4% CR, 13.8% PR)
22	Ocular melanoma	Melphalan ± TNF	62% (9.5% CR, 52% PR)
32	Colorectal	Melphalan + TNF	77% (0% CR, 77% PR)
19	Colorectal	Melphalan + ia FUDR	74% (0% CR, 79% PR)
29	Ocular melanoma	Melphalan	62% (10% CR, 52% PR)
9	Primary hepatic	Melphalan	67% (0% CR, 67% PR)
28	Colorectal + ocular melanoma	Melphalan (percutaneous perfusion with hemofiltration)	30% (7.1% CR, 23% PR)

CR, complete response; PR, partial response.
Source: Grover and Alexander,[116] Feldman et al.,[117] and Pingpank et al.[119]

sion of 7.7 months. Because of the complexity of this procedure, it has not been widely accepted, and efforts to streamline the operation by use of percutaneous catheter techniques are being studied.[117]

Percutaneous Perfusion with Hemofiltration

A variation on isolated hepatic perfusion that is much less invasive is percutaneous hepatic perfusion with hemofiltration. This technique uses a percutaneous arterial catheter into the common hepatic artery.[118] A double-balloon inferior vena cava catheter collects the hepatic venous effluent, and then this collected blood is recirculated externally into a large-bore cannula into the subclavian vein. Two significant problems exist with this percutaneous technique compared to the open isolated hepatic perfusion technique. First, the portal venous flow is not controlled, and therefore the majority of the blood coming through the liver does not contain chemotherapeutic drug and a large outflow from the hepatic veins is from this portal system. Second, the type of drug in the dose escalation is limited by the ability of the extracorporeal charcoal filter system to remove the agent before reinfusion into the subclavian vein. Technological limitations on this clearance at rapid flow rates limit the ability to significantly escalate the drug as can occur in isolated hepatic perfusion. Third, the isolated hepatic perfusion uses hyperthermia by heating the perfusate. Again, in this closed technique it would be technically impossible to successfully utilize hyperthermia to augment chemotherapy response. The initial use of this technique treated patients with 5-FU, adriamycin, or melphalan.[118] Although the procedure was technically possible, there were only limited objective responses of very short duration following this treatment.

A recent phase I trial was reported using this type of technique from the group at the Surgery Branch at the NCI. A total of 74 percutaneous treatments were administered to 28 patients.[119] The drug used was melphalan initially at a dose of 2.0mg/kg, escalating up to 3.5mg/kg, with a treatment time of 30min. The dose-limiting toxicity, seen at 3.5mg/kg, was neutropenia and thrombocytopenia. The radiographic response rate overall was 30%, and in 10 patients with ocular melanoma a 50% overall response rate was seen with 20% (2 patients) having complete responses.[119] These results are much more promising than the earlier studies on this technique using other agents. This percutaneous technique is much less involved in terms of the technical aspects of the procedure than an open isolated hepatic perfusion performed surgically and allows retreatment. Further studies are needed to define the response rates in the patient population that will benefit from this regional treatment in light of the improved systemic therapies and alternative treatments for colorectal cancer. Perhaps this treatment may become a standard for the patient population with ocular melanoma who have limited alternative options.

Isolated Lung Perfusion

If the extremities are straightforward in terms of anatomic considerations to perform isolation perfusion and the liver is a challenge, isolation perfusion of the lung provides another level of technical difficulty. The pulmonary artery and vein have an extremely high flow rate as each lung receives approximately half the total cardiac output at any one time. These are large short vessels that may be fragile in terms of cannulation, and to perform perfusion in an isolated way is a technical challenge. The other considerations that limit the use of this technique are the bronchial vessels, which provide a second source of blood flow that is difficult to control. Another limitation is that of a clinical indication for this treatment and whether this induction justifies the complexity of the procedure. Although the lung is often the sole site of metastatic disease in patients with soft tissue sarcomas, as well as renal cell carcinomas and occasionally melanoma, the metastatic spread is typically to both the right and left lung. Therefore, not only is it a complex procedure needed to perfuse the one lung, but a second procedure is necessary to provide the patient with a complete therapy for their metastatic disease in this clinical situation. Also, although for the histologies listed here the primary set of metastasis is often the lung, it is more likely than with other malignancies to have extrapulmonary spread as well. A series of publications were reported from Pass from the National Cancer Institute[21] on the preclinical models of isolated lung perfusion and a subsequent clinical trial. This trial utilized escalating high-dose tumor necrosis factor (0.3–6.0mg) and lower-dose interferon-γ. Although this study showed isolated lung perfusion was technically possible by a skilled thoracic surgeon, there were only 3 partial responses in 16 patients treated, and all these responses were of short duration.[21]

A different strategy was employed by investigators at Memorial Sloan-Kettering Cancer Center in which an isolated lung infusion was performed.[120] In this preclinical model, direct infusion into the pulmonary artery was performed with infusion of a catheter without a recirculation perfusion. This technique, applied in a preclinical model of a rat with sarcoma metastasis, led to improved response rates but has yet to be utilized to any large extent in clinical trials.

Intracavitary Treatments

As already described, several types of malignancies spread within the generalized body cavity in which they originate. Two surgical techniques have been applied to the problem of diffuse peritoneal disease, and one of these techniques has also been applied to advanced disease of the pleural cavity. The first procedure is tumor debulking from the peritoneum with hyperthermic peritoneal perfusion at the time of operation with high-dose chemotherapy. The second procedure is photodynamic therapy for intraperitoneal disease, and this has also been evaluated in clinical trials for the pleural cavity. The rationale behind these experimental approaches, the technical considerations, and the results of these regional therapies are discussed.

Continuous Hyperthermic Peritoneal Perfusion of the Abdominal Cavity

The concept of continuous hyperthermic peritoneal perfusion (CHPP) was developed as an intraoperative technique to circumvent the problem of poor drug distribution with postoperative intraperitoneal therapy. This treatment may be given to patients who have demonstrated advanced intraperitoneal disease or as an adjuvant treatment based on the natural history of a specific tumor (e.g., ovarian cancer, gastric cancer). This approach provides excellent drug distribution as the treatment is done at the conclusion of a tumor resection/debulking operation.[121] Another advantage of this approach is that there is a significant decrease in the tumor burden immediately before the treatment. The initial application of this technique was done in Japan in conjunction with gastrectomy for advanced disease.[122–124] A follow-up prospective randomized trial treated 60 patients undergoing gastric resection with curative intent who were then treated in an adjuvant manner with either mitomycin C at 8 to 10mg/L perfusate with significant hyperthermia versus no further treatment.[125] In the 47 patients in this study who had evidence of serosal invasion, the survival rate was improved in the CHPP group, with 83% 3-year survival compared to the control group with 67% 3-year survival.

Two recent studies from Japan have been reported randomizing patients to receive hyperthermic peritoneal perfusion after resection of primary gastric cancer for T2 through T4 primary lesions. The results are variable, as one study reported a positive benefit and the other did not. The negative trial was not randomized, but included patients of younger age and better performance status who received the hyperthermic perfusion and patients who were older or had decreased performance status or major organ function who received surgery alone. A total of 124 patients were treated, 45 patients in the peritoneal perfusion group and 79 in the nonperfusion group.[126] The tumor characteristics including depth of penetration and nodal status were no different between the two groups. Patients received a combination of mitomycin C, cisplatin, and etoposide hyperthermic peritoneal perfusion following resective surgery. The 5-year survival rate for the perfusion group was 49% and for the nonperfusion group was 56%.[126] Again, this was not a randomized study, but the tumor characteristics were similar, and because the performance status was better in the perfusion group, one could argue that they would be expected to have an improved outcome. This trial would then argue against any benefit from prophylactic CHPP. A second study recently reported was a true randomized trial for patients with T2 through T4 primary gastric cancers but no evidence of peritoneal carcinomatosis.[127] One hundred and thirty-nine patients were randomized to either surgery alone, surgery plus a normothermic peritoneal perfusion with mitomycin C, or surgery plus a hyperthermic peritoneal perfusion with mitomycin C. In this trial, a positive result with 5-year survival rates for surgery alone were 42%, surgery plus normothermic peritoneal perfusion 43%, and surgery plus hyperthermic perfusion were 61%.[127] This trial achieved statistical significance, and the authors conclude that this is beneficial only when given as a hyperthermic peritoneal perfusion in this patient population. They did notice increased toxicity with peritoneal perfusion of either type, not dependent on temperature.

The North American experience with CHPP has been almost exclusively treating advanced disease as opposed to adjuvant treatment after resection of high-risk primary lesions[128,129] (Table 103.13). Investigators at Bowman Gray University[120] as well as M.D. Anderson have utilized mitomycin C as the primary chemotherapeutic agent with this technique. At the Surgery Branch of the National Cancer Institute,[130] cisplatin has been primarily studied as the chemotherapeutic agent. Both these drugs are alkylating agents and are much more suitable for a short-term high-dose treatment such as CHPP than drugs that are antimetabolites such as 5-FU. These trials varied in terms of the perfusate inflow temperature and the target intraperitoneal temperature. The study from Bowman Gray utilizes an inflow temperature of 42°C with a target intraperitoneal temperature between 40° and 40.5°C. The inflow perfusion temperature at MD Anderson is 44.5°C, also seeking a target temperature between 40° and 41°C in the peritoneum. The NCI studies utilize a higher inflow temperature of 48°C with a target temperature between 41.5° and 43°C intraperitoneally.[128]

The results of the initial phase I studies of CHPP report toxicity and pharmacokinetics.[121] Partly because the initial reports are phase I trials and partly because the intraperitoneal disease after debulking is generally not detectable by any standard imaging study, it is very difficult to ascertain the response rates or benefit from this regional treatment. In a recent report of the NCI phase I trial of cisplatin with or without tumor necrosis factor with a median follow-up time of 12.3 months, the 1-year survival rate was 49%.[130] Patients with colorectal carcinoma recurred at a median time interval of 3 months. Patients with sarcoma recurred at a median time of almost 3 months as well. Patients with low-grade pseudomyxoma-type lesions such as appendiceal carcinoma include 1 patient who recurred at 20 months and 1 who is free of disease 42 months after treatment. Also, benefit was seen in

TABLE 103.13.
Phase I/II Trial of Continuous Hyperthermic Peritoneal Perfusion for Advanced Peritoneal Disease.

	NCI, Surgery Branch (130)	*Bowman Gray (120)*	*NCI (128)*
n	27	34	49
Agents	Cisplatin 100–350 mg/m^2 TNF 0–3μg/L	Mitomycin C 30mg initial + 10 at later time	Cisplatin + 5-FU trial
Inflow temperature	48°C	42°C	42°C
Peritoneal temperature	41.5°–43°C	40°–40.5°C	41.5°–43°C
Duration of treatment	90min	120min	90min
Tumor type	Mixed	Gastric	Mesothelioma
Outcome	1-year survival 49%	1-year survival 75% 2-year survival 48% 75% ascites controlled	17 months progression-free survival; 92 months median overall survival

patients with primary peritoneal mesothelioma with recurrence at 3, 5, 24, and 31 months.[130] The field has matured enough that individual investigators are now accumulating significant follow-up for specific types of cancer. The group at Wake Forest has reported studies evaluating experience with gastric cancer as well as colorectal cancer.[131] In 34 patients with gastric cancer treated with hyperthermic peritoneal perfusion with mitomycin C for carcinomatosis and compared to a historical population, the overall survival rate was 11.2% versus 3.3%, with a 2-year survival rate of 45% versus 8%.[131] Again, this was not a randomized trial but a historical comparison against patients who have a very poor prognosis. This same group reported on 77 patients with colorectal cancer and peritoneal carcinomatosis.[132] In this patient group, the 2-year survival rate after tumor debulking and hyperthermic peritoneal perfusion was 25% and the 5-year survival rate was 17%. Bowel obstruction, malignant ascites, and incomplete debulking were all correlated with poor outcomes. The Loggie group has reported using hyperthermic peritoneal perfusion with mitomycin in 109 patients with carcinomatosis. For patients who could have complete debulking of all gross tumor, the median survival was 15.5 months with a 5-year survival of 13%. For patients who did not achieve complete debulking, the median survival was 7.9 months with a 2% 5-year survival. Conclusions from these studies would be that in select patient populations that have fairly minimal disease, this strategy may have some benefit in achieving long-term survival in a subset of the population.[133] Patients who had more bulky disease in which gross disease is being treated with hyperthermic peritoneal perfusion do not do as well. However, one could also interpret that the patients who achieved complete debulking had fairly nonaggressive tumors and may benefit from the surgical procedure alone as there has been no randomized trial comparing surgery alone in this patient population to surgery plus hyperthermic peritoneal perfusion.

A disease type that has no other reasonable treatment options is peritoneal mesothelioma. The group at the NCI[134] has reported remarkable results for this patient population with cisplatin hyperthermic peritoneal perfusion with or without a postperfusion treatment with Taxol plus 5-FU. In 49 patients with peritoneal mesothelioma treated in this study, there was a 17-month median disease-free survival and a remarkable 92-month overall median survival in patients who historically did not have good results even with surgery alone or surgery plus systemic therapy[134] (see Table 103.13).

The technique of continuous hyperthermic peritoneal perfusion involves a laparotomy with the lysis of all adhesions to the anterior abdominal wall as well as between bowel loops. Tumor is debulked to the maximum possible degree and then two large-bore catheters are placed, one in the upper abdomen and one in the pelvis.[128] The abdomen is filled with perfusate and the abdominal incision is closed. Multiple thermal probes are placed at various locations throughout the abdomen to monitor the temperature at those sites to ensure good distribution of treatment. The abdomen then is perfused with a volume of 2 and 6L perfusate that is recirculated with an extracorporeal circuit with a pump and heater. The setpoint of the inflow temperature of the perfusate will define the maximally achieved temperature as read by the thermisters. During the perfusion, the abdomen is gently manipulated and the table is turned side to side to ensure even distribution. At the conclusion of the treatment interval, generally either 90 or 120min, the perfusate is washed out of the abdomen into a waste container. The abdomen is then reopened with removal of the thermisters and formal closure of the incision. Another key component in perfusing CHPP is to place ice around the extremities, chest, and head to prevent core body temperature arising to above 40°C.[135] This technique allows exposure to small-volume disease or microscopic disease on peritoneal surfaces to high concentrations of chemotherapeutic agent that may be augmented by hyperthermia. The major disadvantage of CHPP, as for all other surgical regional therapies, is that this is limited to a single treatment. Some investigators leave intraperitoneal catheters behind at the time of surgery for additional postoperative treatment. However, shortly after an operation the formation of adhesions limits the utility of the indwelling cannulae.

Photodynamic Therapy

A second technique to address to the problem of surface malignancies throughout the peritoneum is photodynamic therapy (PDT).[4,5] As in CHPP, PDT combines a surgical debulking procedure with an additional procedure as treatment of surface malignancies. Instead of using chemotherapeutic agents augmented by hyperthermia, PDT uses a laser light treatment of all surface areas. The three components of photodynamic therapy that are essential for cytotoxicity are light and specific wavelength, a photosensitizer retained by tumor cells, and oxygen.[4] When the photosensitizer is stimulated with the appropriate wavelength light, then the energy absorbed is transferred to oxygen, and oxygen-free radicals are generated that lead to cell death. One potential limitation of this treatment is the depth of penetration of the light, which is variable depending on the wavelength of light used for a given sensitizer, typically in the range of 3 to 5mm. Although this is a disadvantage because larger nodules of disease cannot be treated, it has an advantage as it protects normal tissues from toxic effects. The theoretical selectivity of the antitumor effect with PDT after systemic photosensitizer administration is in selective uptake and retention of the photosensitizer within malignant cells to a greater degree than normal cells; this has been shown to be true for a variety of these porphyrin-derivative sensitizers that are retained in tumor and skin primaries for reasons that are not clear.[4,5] The time interval between administration of photosensitizers and light delivery varies depending on the pharmacokinetics of the specific photosensitizer that is used. For trials with the initial clinically sensitized hematoporphyrin derivative, the time interval is 48h.

Initial preclinical data from a murine ovarian carcinomatosis model demonstrated benefit from treatment with intraperitoneal hematoporphyrin derivative and laser light therapy.[136,137] On the basis of these preclinical data, a phase I study was performed at the NCI alternating escalations of the dose of light energy and the dose of photosensitizer. The results of this phase I trial were published[138] and recently updated in abstract form.[139] In an initial report, 56 patients were entered and received photosensitizer. Two patients had no evidence of disease at operation and 15 patients had tumors that could not be debulked below 5mm as required by the protocol. Therefore, only 39 patients were treated, including

21 with ovarian cancer, 12 with sarcomatosis, and 6 with gastrointestinal (GI) carcinomatosis. Nine of 39 patients remained disease free between 3 and 27 months later; 9 patients died of progressive tumor, and 21 were alive with disease with follow-up of approximately 1 year. Three patients with ovarian tumors were free of disease at 3, 4, 15, and 27 months after treatment. Three patients with GI tumors that were low-grade pseudomyxomas were free of disease at 8, 9, and 18 months, and 1 patient with sarcomatosis was free of disease at 20 months.[138,139]

A phase II trial was designed based on these data utilizing photofrin given at a dose of 2.5 mg/kg 48 h before debulking surgery. The inclusion criteria of this trial were disease confined to the peritoneal cavity with no evidence of hematogenous spread. To receive light treatments, the patient had to have tumors debulked down to 5 mm or smaller. Patients were divided into ovarian carcinomatosis, carcinomatosis from gastrointestinal tumors including stomach, pancreas, colon, and appendix, and sarcomatosis from gastrointestinal stromal tumors or retroperitoneal sarcomas. One hundred patients were entered in this trial, although only 71 could be debulked to a degree where light therapy was administered. All patients showed signs of recurrent disease typically within 3 to 4 months, but the median overall survival for this heavily pretreated population was 22.0 months for the ovarian carcinoma group, 13.2 months for the gastrointestinal group, and 21.9 months for the sarcoma group.[140] Tissue analysis suggested that, particularly for gastrointestinal tumors and sarcomas, there was no detected retention of the photosensitizer within the tumor compared to normal tissue contributing to the early recurrences. However, the fairly prolonged median survival in the patient population that at entry was very heavily pretreated indicates some essential benefit for this difficult disease.

New trials with second- and third-generation photosensitizers with either better optical properties or better tumor retention are being conducted.[141] Also, the way the light is administered and distributed in the complex peritoneal surface is being studied with measurements of light distribution at various locations within the peritoneum. Photodynamic therapy for endobronchial and esophageal lesions has been approved, but treatment for the peritoneal cavity is certainly considered investigational at present.

Intrapleural Treatments

Two types of regional therapy have been applied to the pleural cavity, primarily for mesothelioma. One is analogous to the PDT that has been utilized and described for intraperitoneal diseases.[6,142,143] A second treatment for pleural mesothelioma is with intracavitary gene therapy.[8,144] Mesothelioma is a tumor of the lining of the pleural cavity, and it often encases the lung at the time of presentation but has not spread outside of a single pleural cavity.[40] Surgery alone generally does not result in cure, and the tumor is relatively chemotherapy resistant, which provides an ideal setting for attempts at regional intracavitary therapy.

In many ways, the pleural spaces are better suited for photodynamic therapy than the peritoneum,[6,143] because of the relatively simple geometry of the surfaces in which there are no hidden areas between bowel loops and in the pelvis. An initial phase I trial of intraperitoneal PDT with photofrin II was conducted treating mesothelioma with escalating intraoperative light doses between 15 and 35 J/cm^2 48 h after receiving photosensitizer.[145] Forty-two patients were treated, and it established that the maximal tolerated light dose was 30 J/cm^2. This phase I trial was then followed by a phase II trial comparing maximally debulking of mesothelioma with postoperative cisplatin, interferon-α, and tamoxifen with or without PDT.[145] Forty-eight patients were randomized to receive PDT or not, and there was no difference in median survival, median disease-free survival, and sites of first recurrence.[142] The conclusions from this study were with the first-generation sensitizers available, and although the treatment could be technically delivered, there was no benefit over surgery plus chemotherapy. Again, second-generation sensitizers with more selective uptake into tumor tissue as well as depth of penetration may provide benefit with this adjunctive regional therapy.

A phase II trial using Foscan, a second-generation sensitizer, has been recently reported from the group at Penn.[146] Four dose levels of Foscan were utilized in this study, and the maximal tolerated dose was 0.1 mg/kg injected 6 days before debulking surgery. The next higher dose level led to multisystem organ failure and capillary leak syndrome, and two of three patients at that dose level expired. As this was a phase I study, the clinical response results were not reported, but it was thought that this treatment deserved further study.

A recent clinical trial has been reported treating non-small cell lung cancer with pleural spread using intrapleural PDT.[147] The median survival rate for this patient population has historically been quite dismal, with most series reporting 6- to 9-month survival. This trial treated 22 patients with non-small cell lung cancer and, of the 22 enrolled, 17 were able to undergo complete debulking and photodynamic therapy. Fifteen of these 17 were available for response assessment. The local control of pleural disease at 6 months was achieved in 11 of 15 patients (73%).[147] Medial survival for the entire patient population entered on this trial was 21.7 months. For this disease, there were measurements of the tissue levels of photofrin and the ratio between tumor to normal tissue ranged between 1.19 and 22.4. These response rates, although not in a randomized trial, would argue strongly that there is significant benefit from photodynamic therapy for this difficult clinical problem compared to historical results. However, because very aggressive surgery is being performed that would otherwise not be indicated outside a clinical trial, one cannot at this time differentiate between the benefit achieved from the surgical intervention and the additional benefit from light treatment.

Regional Gene Therapy

This same patient population with regional advanced pleural mesothelioma has also been studied in a gene therapy trial. A phase I trial used adenovirus to deliver herpes simplex virus thymidine kinase gene with follow-up treatment with ganciclovir.[144] Twenty-one patients were treated with viral doses ranging from 1×10^9 up to 1×10^{12} by forming units. Dose-limiting toxicity was not reached in this trial. Patients underwent thoracoscopic pleural biopsies, which demonstrated strong gene transfer and expression as well as an intratumor immune response with this adenoviral vector. These studies of gene therapy into the pleural cavity are in their infancy and may serve as a proof of principle concerning the ability to administer viral vectors to an intracavitary space. No data regarding response or regression of tumor are available with current studies.

As the molecular genetics of malignancies have been defined as well as development of molecular techniques to alter gene expression with gene therapy, much preclinical work as well as clinical trials has been performed utilizing gene therapy for treatment of malignancy. The most commonly used transgene is a thymidine kinase gene or suicide gene that, if expressed in malignant tissues, make these susceptible to subsequent drug treatment. Other strategies include replacement of mutated tumor suppressor genes such as adenovirus vectors expressing wild-type p53 genes.[8]

One of the major obstacles in gene therapy, even if an effective agent were available, would be a systemic distribution to all sites of malignant disease. In the application of this technology, often the regional treatment is the most optimal mode of effective delivery. For example, intrapleural administration of adenoviral vectors expression suicide genes has been studied for treatment of mesothelioma.[144] Similarly, intraperitoneal administration of wild-type p53 adenovirus vectors has been evaluated for ovarian carcinoma. In addition to the intracavitary treatments, intraarterial treatments are under investigation, primarily to the liver.[7] In many cases, surgical oncologists are either the principal investigators or important coinvestigators as these early trials of gene therapy generally rely on regional delivery systems.[9] Many of the clinical scenarios mentioned here may provide suitable clinical models for either intracavitary or intravascular gene therapy in the next decade.

In summary, surgical oncologists have played a major role in designing treatment strategies that target regions or specific areas of the body primarily to treat metastatic disease. Again, the opportunity to employ these treatments depends on the natural history of a particular malignancy in terms of having locally advanced disease with limited or no systemic spread. The surgical strategies combining debulking operations in some cases or vascular isolation in other cases may, it is hoped, provide meaningful improvements in disease-free survival for patients for whom there are no other effective therapies.

References

1. Cavaliere R, Ciogatto EC, Giovanelli BC, et al. Selective heat sensitivity of cancer cells. Cancer (PHila) 1967;20:1351–1381.
2. DiFilippo F, Anza M, Rossi CR, et al. The application of hyperthermia in regional chemotherapy. Semin Surg Oncol 1998; 14(3):215–223.
3. Christophi C, Winkworth A, Muralihdaran V, Evans P. The treatment of malignancy by hyperthermia. Surg Oncol 1998; 7(1-2):83–90.
4. Dougherty TJ, Gomer CJ, Henderson BW, et al. Photodynamic therapy. J Natl Cancer Inst 1998;90(12):889–905.
5. Kessel D. Photodynamic therapy. Sci Med 1998:46–55.
6. Rodriguez E, Baas P, Friedberg JS. Innovative therapies: photodynamic therapy. Thorac Surg Clin 2004;14(4):557–566.
7. Van der Eb MM, Hoeben RC, van de Velde CJ. Towards gene therapy for colorectal liver metastases. Recent Results Cancer Res 1998;147:173–186.
8. Albelda SM, Wiewrodt R, Sterman DH. Gene therapy for lung neoplasms. Clin Chest Med 2002;23(1):265–277.
9. Milas M, Feig B, Yu D, et al. Isolated limb perfusion in the sarcoma-bearing rat: a novel preclinical gene delivery system. Clin Cancer Res 1997;3:2197–2203.
10. Collins JM. Pharmacologic rationale for hepatic arterial therapy. Recent Results Cancer Res 1986;100:140–147.
11. Sigurdson ER, Ridge JA, Kemeny N, Daly JM. Tumor and liver drug uptake following hepatic artery and portal vein infusion in man. J Clin Oncol 1987;5:1836–1840.
12. Guadagni S, Aigner KR, Palumbo G, et al. Pharmacokinetics of mitomycin C in pelvic stop flow infusion and hypoxic pelvic perfusion with and without hemofiltration: a pilot study of patients with recurrent unresectable rectal cancer. J Clin Pharmacol 1998;38(10):936–944.
13. Lorenz M, Petrowsky H, Heinrich S, et al. Isolated hypoxic perfusion with mitomycin C in patients with advanced pancreatic cancer. Eur J Surg Oncol 1998;24(6):542–547.
14. Thompson JF, Kam PC, Waugh RC, Harman CR. Isolated limb perfusion with cytotoxic agents: a simple alternative to isolated limb perfusion. Semin Surg Oncol 1998;14(3):238–247.
15. Creech O, Krementz ET, Ryan RF, Winblad JN. Chemotherapy of cancer: regional perfusion utilizing an extracorporeal circuit. Ann Surg 1958;148:616–632.
16. Chung WB, Moore JR, Mersereau W. A technique of isolated perfusion of the liver. Surgery (St. Louis) 1962;51:508–511.
17. Shingleton WW, Parker RT, Mahaley S. Abdominal perfusion for cancer: regional perfusion utilizing an extracorporeal circuit. Ann Surg 1969;152:583–593.
18. Mulcare RJ, Solis A, Fortner JG. Isolation and perfusion of the liver for cancer chemotherapy. J Surg Res 1973;15:87–95.
19. Alexander HR, Bartlett DL, Libutti SK, Fraker DL, Moser T, Rosenberg SA. Isolated hepatic perfusion with tumor necrosis factor and melphalan for unresectable cancers confined to the liver. J Clin Oncol 1998;16(4):1479–1489.
20. Oldhafer KJ, Lang H, Frerker M, et al. First experience and technical aspects of isolated liver perfusion for extensive liver metastasis. Surgery (St. Louis) 1998;126(6):622–631.
21. Pass HI, Mew DJ, Kranda KC, Temeck BK, Donington JS, Rosenberg SA. Isolated lung perfusion with tumor necrosis factor for pulmonary metastases. Ann Thorac Surg 1996;61(6):1609–1617.
22. Hendriks JM, Van Schil PE. Isolated lung perfusion for the treatment of pulmonary metastases. Surg Oncol 1998;7(1–2): 59–63.
23. Turk PS, Belleveau JF, Dranowski JW, Weinberg MC, Leenen L, Wanebo HJ. Isolated pelvic perfusion for unresectable cancer using a balloon occlusion technique. Arch Surg 1993;128(5):533–538, discussion 538–539.
24. Wanebo HJ, Chung MA, Levy AI, Turk PS, Vezeridis MP, Belliveau JF. Preoperative therapy for advanced pelvic malignancy by isolated pelvic perfusion with the balloon-occlusion technique. Ann Surg Oncol 1996;3(3):295–303.
25. Walther MM, Jennings SB, Choyke PL, et al. Isolated perfusion of the kidney with tumor necrosis factor for localized renal-cell carcinoma. World J Urol 1996;14:S2–S7.
26. Deraco M, Santoro N, Carraro O, et al. Peritoneal carcinomatosis: feature of dissemination. A review. Tumori 1999;85(1): 1–5.
27. Sugarbaker PH. Observations concerning cancer spread within the peritoneal cavity and concepts supporting an ordered pathophysiology. In: Sugerbaker PH (ed) Peritoneal Carcinomatosis, Diagnosis, and Treatment. Boston: Kluwer, 1995.
28. Berek JS, Bertelsen K, duBois A, et al. Advanced epithelial ovarian cancer: 1998 consensus statements. Ann Oncol 1999; 10(1):87–92.
29. Eltabbakh GH, Piver MS, Natarajan N, Mettline CJ. Epidemiologic differences between women with extraovarian primary peritoneal carcinoma and women with epithelial ovarian cancer. Obstet Gynecol 1998;91(2):254–259.
30. Jacquet P, Vidal-Jove J, Zhu B, Sugarbaker PH. Peritoneal carcinomatosis from gastrointestinal malignancy. Natural history and new prospects for management. Acta Belg Chir 1994;94:191–197.

31. Sugarbaker PH, Schillinx MET, Chang D, Koslowe P, Meyenfeldt MV van. Peritoneal carcinomatosis from adenocarcinoma of the colon. World J Surg 1996;20:585–592.
32. Vasseur B, Cadiot G, Zins M, et al. Peritoneal carcinomatosis in patients with digestive endocrine tumors. Cancer (Phila) 1996;78(8):1686–1692.
33. Ng EH, Pollock RE, Munsell MF, Atkinson ENM, Romsdahl MM. Prognostic factors influencing survival in gastrointestinal leiomyosarcomas. Implications for surgical management and staging. Ann Surg 1992;215:68–77.
34. Jaques DP, Coit DG, Hajdu SI, Brennan MF. Management of primary and recurrent soft-tissue sarcoma of the retroperitoneum Ann Surg 1990;212(12):511–518.
35. Shen P, Levine EA, Loggie BW. Peritoneal carcinomatosis: what can we do about it? J Clin Oncol 2004;22(1):202.
36. Sugarbaker PH. Perionectomy procedures. Ann Surg 1995; 221(1):29–42.
37. Wong CS, Harwood AR, Cummings BJ, Keane TJ, Thomas GM, Rider WD. Total abdominal irradiation for cancer of the colon. Radiother Oncol 1984;2(3):209–214.
38. Fabian C, Giri S, Estes N, et al. Adjuvant continuous infusion 5-FU, whole-abdominal radiation, and tumor bed boost in high-risk stage III colon carcinoma: a Southwest Oncology Group Pilot study. Int J Radiat Oncol Biol Phys 1995;32(2):457–464.
39. Markmann M. Intraperitoneal therapy of ovarian cancer. Oncologist 1996;1:18–21.
40. Price B. Analysis of current trends in United Stated mesothelioma incidence. Am J Epidemiol 1997;145(3):211–218.
41. Fraker DL. Hyperthermic regional perfusion for melanoma and sarcoma of the limbs. Curr Probl Surg 1999;36(11):841–908.
42. Eggermont AM, Brunstein F, Grunhagen D, ten Hagen TL. Regional treatment of metastasis: role of regional perfusion. State of the art isolated limb perfusion for limb salvage. Ann Oncol 2004;15(4):107–112.
43. Barker WC, Andrich MP, Alexander HR, Fraker DL. Continuous intraoperative external monitoring of perfusate leak using iodine-131 human serum albumin during isolated perfusion of the liver and limbs. Eur J Nucl Med 1995;22:1242–1248.
44. Balch CM, Houghton AN, Peters LJ. Cutaneous melanoma. In: DeVita VT, Hellman S, Rosenberg SA, eds. Cancer: Principles and Practice of Oncology, 4th ed. Philadelphia: Lippincott, 1997:1947–1997.
45. Koops HS, Vaglini M, Cuciu S, et al. Prophylactic isolated limb perfusion for localized, high risk limb melanoma: results of a multicenter randomized phase III trial. European Organization for Research and Treatment of Cancer Malignant Melanoma Cooperative Group Protocol 18832, the World Health Organization Melanoma Program Trial 15, and the North American Perfusion Group Southwest Oncology Group-8593. J Clin Oncol 1998;16:2906–2912.
46. Hayes AJ, Clark MA, Harries M, Thomas JM. Management of in transit metastases from cutaneous malignant melanoma. Br J Surg 2004;91(6):673–682.
47. Jaques DP, Coit DG, Brennan MF. Major amputation for advanced malignant melanoma. Surg Gynecol Obstet 1989;169:1–6.
48. Kang JC, Wanek LA, Essner R, Faries MB, Foshag LJ, Morton DL. Sentinel lymphadenectomy does not increase the incidence of in-transit metastases in primary melanoma. J Clin Oncol 2005;23:4764–4770.
49. Pawlik TM, Ross MI, Thompson JF, Eggermont AMM, Gershenwald JE. The risk of in-transit melanoma metastasis depends on tumor biology and not the surgical approach to regional lymph nodes. J Clin Oncol 2005;23:4588–4590.
50. Krementz ET, Carter RD, Sutherland CM, Muchmore JH, Ryan RF, Creech O Jr. Regional chemotherapy for melanoma: a 35 year experience. Ann Surg 1994;220:520–535.
51. Ghussen F, Nagel K, Groth W, Muller JM, Stutzer H. A prospective randomized study of regional extremity perfusion in patients with malignant melanoma. Ann Surg 1984;200:764–768.
52. Ghussen F, Kruger I, Groth W, Stutzer H. The role of regional hyperthermic cytostatic perfusion in the treatment of extremity melanoma. Cancer (Phila) 1988;61:654–659.
53. Hafstrom L, Rudenstam CM, Blomquist E, et al. Regional hyperthermic perfusion with melphalan after surgery for recurrent malignant melanoma of the extremities. J Clin Oncol 1991;9:209–214.
54. Thompson JF, Giantoutsos MP. Isolated limb perfusion for melanoma: effectiveness and toxicity of cisplatin compared with that of melphalan and other drugs. World J Surg 1992;16:227–233.
55. Noorda EM, Vrouenraets BC, Nieweg OE, Van Coevorden F, Kroon BB. Isolated limb perfusion: what is the evidence for its use? Ann Surg Oncol 2004;11(9):837–845.
56. Lens MB, Dawes M. Isolated limb perfusion with melphalan in the treatment of malignant melanoma of the extremities: a systematic review of randomized controlled trials. Lancet Oncol 2003;4(6):359–364.
57. Wieberdink J, Benckhuysen C, Braat RP, van Slooten EA, Olthuis GAA. Dosimetry in isolation perfusion of the limbs by assessment of perfused tissue volume and grading of toxic tissue reactions. Eur J Cancer Clin Oncol 1982;18:905–910.
58. Cheng TY, Grubbs E, Abdul-Wahab O, et al. Marked variability of melphalan plasma drug levels during regional hyperthermic isolated limb perfusion. Am J Surg 2003;186(5):460–467.
59. Klaase JM, Kroon BBR, van Geel AN, Eggermont AMM, Franklin HR, Hart AAM. Prognostic factors for tumor response and limb recurrence-free interval in patients with advanced melanoma of the limbs treated with regional isolated perfusion with melphalan. Surgery (St. Louis) 1994;115:39–45.
60. Noorda EM, Vrouenraets BC, Nieweg OE, vanGeel BN, Eggermont AM, Kroon BB. Isolated limb perfusion for unresectable melanoma of the extremities. Arch Surg 2004;139(11):1237–1242.
61. Vaglini M, Belli F, Marolda R, Prada A, Santinami M, Cascinelli N. Hyperthermic antiblastic perfusion with DTIC in stage IIIA-IIIB melanoma of the extremities. Eur J Surg Oncol 1987;13: 127–129.
62. Carswell EA, Old LJ, Kassel R, Green S, Fiore N, Williamson B. An endotoxin-induced serum factor that causes necrosis of tumors. Proc Natl Acad Sci U S A 1975;72:3666–3670.
63. Fraker DL, Alexander HR, Pass HI. Biologic therapy of tumor necrosis factor: clinical applications by systemic and regional administration. In: DeVita V, Hellman S, Rosenberg SA, eds. Biologic Therapy of Cancer, 2nd ed. Philadelphia: Lippincott, 1995:329–346.
64. Lejeune FI. High dose recombinant tumour necrosis factor (rTNFi-1) administered by isolation perfusion for advanced tumours of the limbs: a model for biochemotherapy of cancer. Eur J Cancer 1995;31:1009–1016.
65. Posner MC, Lienard D, Lejeune FJ, Rosenfelder D, Kirkwood J. Hyperthermic isolated limb perfusion with tumor necrosis factor alone for melanoma. Cancer J Sci Am 1995;1:274–280.
66. Leinard D, Lejeune F, Delmotte J, et al. High doses of rTNF in combination with IFN-gamma and melphalan in isolation perfusion of the limbs for melanoma and sarcoma. J Clin Oncol 1992;10:52–60.
67. Lienard D, Lejeune F, Ewalenko I. In transit metastases of malignant melanoma treated by high dose rTNF in combination with interferon-gamma and melphalan in isolation perfusion. World J Surg 1992;16:234–240.
68. Lienard D, Eggermont AM, Kroon B, Schraffordt Koops H, Lejeune FJ. Isolated limb perfusion in primary and recurrent melanoma: indications and results. Semin Surg Oncol 1998; 14:202–209.

69. Fraker DL, Alexander HR, Bartlett DL, Rosenberg SA. A prospective randomized trial of therapeutic isolated limb perfusion (ILP) comparing melphalan (M) versus melphalan, tumor necrosis factor (TNF) and interferon: an initial report [abstract]. Proc Soc Surg Oncol 1996;49:6.
70. Fraker DL, Alexander HR, Andrich M, Rosenberg SA. Treatment of patients with melanoma of the extremity using hyperthermic isolated limb perfusion with melphalan, tumor necrosis factor, and interferon-gamma: results of a TNF dose escalation study. J Clin Oncol 1996;14:479–489.
71. Bartlett DL, Ma G, Alexander HR, Libutti SK, Fraker DL. Isolated limb reperfusion with tumor necrosis factor and melphalan in patients with extremity melanoma after failure of isolated limb perfusion with chemotherapeutics. Cancer (Phila) 1997; 80:2084–2090.
72. Takkenberg RB, Vrouenraets BC, vanGeel AN, et al. Palliative isolated limb perfusion for advanced limb disease in stage IV melanoma patients. J Surg Oncol 2005;91(2):107–111.
73. Fraker DL, Alexander HR, Andrich M, Rosenberg SA. Palliation of regional symptoms of advanced extremity melanoma by isolated limb perfusion with melphalan and high-dose tumor necrosis factor. Cancer J Sci Am 1995;1:122–130.
74. Thom AK, Alexander HR, Andrich MP, Barker WC, Rosenberg SA, Fraker DL. Cytokine levels and systemic toxicity in patients undergoing isolated limb perfusion with high dose tumor necrosis factor, interferon-gamma and melphalan. J Clin Oncol 1995;13:264–273.
75. Van Geel AN, van Wijk J, Weieberdink J. Functional morbidity after regional isolated perfusion of the limb for melanoma. Cancer (Phila) 1989;63:1092–1096.
76. Olieman AFT, Koops HS, Geertzen JHB, Kingma H, Hoekstra HU, Oldhoff J. Functional morbidity of hyperthermic isolated regional perfusion of the extremities. Ann Surg Oncol 1994;3:382–388.
77. Vrouenraets BC, Klaase JM, Nieweg OE, Kroon BB. Toxicity and morbidity of isolated limb perfusion. Semin Surg Oncol 1998;14:224–231.
78. Krementz ET, Carter RD, Sutherland CM, Hutton I. Chemotherapy of sarcomas of the limbs by regional perfusion. Ann Surg 1977;195:555–564.
79. Williard WC, Hajdu SI, Casper ES, Brennan MF. Comparison of amputation with limb-sparing operations for adult soft tissue sarcoma of the extremity. Ann Surg 1992;215:269–75.
80. Eggermont AM, Koops HS, Lienard D, et al. Isolated limb perfusion with high dose tumor necrosis factor-α in combination with interferon-γ and melphalan for nonresectable extremity soft tissue sarcomas: a multicenter trial. J Clin Oncol 1996;14:2653–2665.
81. Eggermont AMM, Koops HS, Lkausner JM, et al. Isolated limb perfusion with tumor necrosis factor and melphalan for limb salvage in 186 patients with locally advanced soft tissue extremity sarcomas. Ann Surg 1996;244:756–765.
82. Gutman M, Inbar M, Lev-Shluch D, et al. High dose tumor necrosis factor-alpha and melphalan administered via limb perfusion for advanced limb soft tissue sarcoma results in a ≥90% response rate and limb preservation. Cancer (Phila) 1997;79:1129–1137.
83. Noorda EM, Vrouenraets BC, Nieweg OE, van Coevorden F, van Slooten GW, Kroon BB. Isolated limb perfusion with tumor necrosis factor-alpha and melphalan for patients with unresectable soft tissue sarcoma of the extremities. Cancer (Phila) 2003;98(7):1483–1490.
84. Bonvalot S, Laplanche A, Lejeune F, et al. Limb salvage with isolated limb perfusion for soft tissue sarcoma: could less TNF-alpha be better? Ann Oncol 2005;16(7):1061–1068.
85. Grunhagen DJ, Brunstein F, Graveland WJ, van Geel AN, deWilt JH, Eggermont AM. Isolated limb perfusion with tumor necrosis factor and melphalan prevents amputation in patients with multiple sarcomas in arm or leg. Ann Surg Oncol 2005;12(6):473–479.
86. Lans TE, Grunhagen DJ, deWilt JH, vanGeel AN, Eggermont AM. Isolated limb perfusion with tumor necrosis factor and melphalan for locally recurrent soft tissue sarcoma in previously irradiated limbs. Ann Surg Oncol 2005;12(5):4-6–4-11.
87. Fraker DL, Alexander HR, Ross M, Tyler D, Bartlett D, Bauer T. A phase II trial of isolated limb perfusion with high dose tumor necrosis factor and melphalan for unresectable extremity sarcomas (abstract). Soc Surg Oncol Cancer Symp 1999;52:22.
88. Olieman AF, Lienard D, Eggermont AM, et al. Hyperthermic isolated limb perfusion with tumor necrosis factor alpha, interferon gamma, and melphalan for locally advanced nonmelanoma skin tumors of the extremities: a multicenter study. Arch Surg 1999;134(3):303–307.
89. Thompson JF, Kam PC. Isolated limb infusion for melanoma: a simple but effective alternative to isolated limb perfusion. J Surg Oncol 2004;88(1):1–3.
90. Bonenkamp JJ, Thompson JF, deWitt JH, Doubrovsky A, deFarla Lima R, Kam PC. Isolated limb perfusion with fotemustine after dacarbazine chemosensitisation for inoperative loco-regional melanoma recurrence. Eur J Surg Oncol 2004;30(10):1107–1112.
91. Lin G, Lunderquist A, Hagerstrand I, Boijsen E. Postmortem examination of the blood supply and vascular pattern of small liver metastases in man. Surgery (St. Louis) 1984;96:517–526.
92. Ridge JA, Bading JR, Gelbard AS, et al. Perfusion of colorectal hepatic metastases: relative distribution of flow from the hepatic artery and portal vein. Cancer (Phila) 1987;59:1547–1553.
93. Soulen MC. Chemoembolization of hepatic malignancies. Oncology 1994;8:77–93.
94. Cohen AM, Minsky BD, Schilsky RL. Cancer of the Colon. In: *Cancer: Principles and Practice of Oncology*, 5th ed. Philadephia: Lippincott-Raven, 1997:1144–1197.
95. Diaz-Rubio E. New chemotherapeutic advances in pancreatic, colorectal, and gastric cancers. Oncologist 2004;9(3):282–294.
96. Neiderhuber JE, Ensminger W, Gyves J, Thrall J, Walker S, Cozzi E. Regional chemotherapy of colorectal cancer metastatic to the liver. Cancer (Phila) 1984;53:1336–1343.
97. Allen PJ, Nissan A, Picon AI, et al. Technical complications and durability of hepatic artery infusion pumps for unresectable colorectal liver metastases: an institutional experience of 544 consecutive cases. J Am Coll Surg 2005;201:57–65.
98. Hohn DC, Stagg RJ, Friedman MA, et al. A randomized trial of continuous intravenous versus hepatic intra-arterial floxuridine in patients with colorectal cancer metastatic to the liver: the Northern California Oncology Group Trial. J Clin Oncol 1989;7:1646–1654.
99. Kemeny N, Conti J, Cohen A, et al. A phase II study of hepatic arterial FUDR, leucovorin, and dexamethasone for unresectable liver metastases from colorectal carcinoma. J Clin Oncol 1994;12:2288–2295.
100. Stagg R, Venook A, Chase J, et al. Alternating hepatic intra-arterial floxuridine and fluorouracil: a less toxic regimen for treatment of liver metastases from colorectal cancer. J Natl Cancer Inst 1991;83:423–428.
101. Chang A, Schneider PD, Sugarbaker PH, et al. A prospective randomized trial of regional versus systemic continuous 5-fluorodeoxyuridine chemotherapy in the treatment of colorectal metastases. Ann Surg 1987;206:685–693.
102. Kemeny N, Daly J, Reichman B, Geller N, Botet J, Oderman P. Intrahepatic or systemic infusion of fluorodeoxyuridine in patients with liver metastases from colorectal carcinoma. Ann Intern Med 1987;107:459–465.
103. Martin J, O'Connell M, Wieand H, et al. Intra-arterial floxuridine versus systemic fluorouracil for hepatic metastases from colorectal cancer: a randomized trial. Arch Surg 1990;125:1022–1027.

104. Rougier PH, Laplanche A, Huguier M, et al. Hepatic arterial infusion of floxuridine in patients with liver metastases from colorectal carcinoma: long term results of a prospective randomized trial. J Clin Oncol 1992;10:1112–1118.
105. Allen-Mersh TG, Earlam S, Fordy C. Quality of life and survival with continuous hepatic artery infusion for colorectal liver metastases. Lancet 1994;344:1255–1260.
106. Kemeny N, Gonen M, Sullivan D, et al. Phase I study of hepatic arterial infusion of floxuridine and dexamethasone with systemic irinotecan for unresectable hepatic metastases from colorectal cancer. J Clin Oncol 2001;19(10):2687–2695.
107. Kemeny N, Narnagin W, Gonen M, et al. Phase I/II Study of hepatic arterial therapy with floxuridine and dexamethasone in combination with intravenous irinotecan as adjuvant treatment after resection of hepatic metastases from colorectal cancer. J Clin Oncol 2003;21(17):3303–3309.
108. Kemeny N, Jarnagin W, Paty P, et al. Phase I trial of systemic oxaliplatin combination chemotherapy with hepatic arterial infusion in patients with unresectable liver metastases from colorectal cancer. J Clin Oncol 2005;23:4888–4896.
109. Kemeny N, Cohen A, Huang Y, et al. Randomized study of hepatic arterial infusion (HAI) and systemic chemotherapy (SYS) versus SYS alone as adjuvant therapy after resection of hepatic metastases from colorectal cancer. Proc Am Soc Clin Oncol 1999;18:1011.
110. Kemeny M, Adak S, Lipsitz S, Gray B, MacDonald J, Benson AB. Results of the Intergroup Eastern Cooperative Oncology Group (ECOG) and Southwest Oncology Group (SWOG) prospective randomized study of surgery alone versus continuous hepatic artery infusion of FUDR and continuous systemic infusion of 5FU after hepatic resection for colorectal liver metastases. Proc Am Soc Clin Oncol 1999;18:1012.
111. Scaife CL, Curley SA, Izzo F, et al. Feasibility of adjuvant hepatic arterial infusion of chemotherapy after radiofrequency ablation with or without resection in patients with hepatic metastases from colorectal cancer. J Surg Oncol 2003;10(4):348–354.
112. Fraker DL. Combination of radiofrequency ablation and intraarterial chemotherapy for metastatic cancer in the liver. In: Ellis LM, Curley SA, Tanabe KK, eds. Radiofrequency Ablation for Cancer. New York: Springer, 2004:47–66.
113. Shaw BW, Martin DJ, Marquez JM, et al. Venous bypass in clinical liver transplantation. Ann Surg 1984;200:524–533.
114. Walther H, Link KH. Isolated liver perfusion with MMC/5-FU: surgical technique, pharmacokinetics, clinical results. In: Aigner KR, Patt YZ, Lind KH Kreidler J, eds. Regional Cancer Treatment. Basel: Karger, 1988:229–246.
115. Fraker DL, Alexander HR, Thom AK. Use of tumor necrosis factor in isolated hepatic perfusion. Circ Shock 1994;44:45–50.
116. Grover A, Alexander HR. The past decade of experience with isolated hepatic perfusion. Oncologist 2004;9:653–664.
117. Feldman ED, Wu PC, Beresneva T, et al. Treatment of patients with unresectable primary hepatic malignancies using hyperthermic isolated hepatic perfusion. J Gastrointest Surg 2004; 8(2):200–207.
118. Ravikumar TS, Pizzorno G, Bodden W, et al. Percutaneous hepatic vein isolation and high-dose hepatic arterial infusion chemotherapy for unresectable liver tumors. J Clin Oncol 1994;12:2723–2736.
119. Pingpank JF, Libutti SK, Chang R, et al. Phase I study of hepatic arterial melphalan infusion and hepatic venous hemofiltration using percutaneously placed catheters in patients with unresectable hepatic malignancies. J Clin Oncol 2005;23(15):3465–3474.
120. Furrer M, Lardinois D, Thormann W, et al. Cytostatic lung perfusion by use of an endovascular blood flow occlusion technique. Ann Thorac Surg 1998;65(6):1523–1528.
121. Panteix G, Beaujard A, Garbit F, et al. Population pharmacokinetics of cisplatin in patients with advanced ovarian cancer during intraperitoneal hyperthermia chemotherapy. Anticancer Res 2002;22(2B):1329–1336.
122. Fujimoto S, Shrestha RD, Kokubun M, et al. Intraperitoneal hyperthermic perfusion combined with surgery effective for gastric cancer patients with peritoneal seeding. Ann Surg 1988; 208(1):36–41.
123. Fujimoto S, Takahashi M, Kobayashi K, et al. Cytohistologic assessment of antitumor effects of intraperitoneal hyperthermic perfusion with mitomycin C for patients with gastric cancer with peritoneal metastasis. Cancer (Phila) 1992;70(12):2754–2760.
124. Yonemura Y, Kawamura T, Bandou E, Takahashi S, Sawa T, Matsuki N. Treatment of peritoneal dissemination from gastric cancer by peritonectomy and chemohyperthermic peritoneal perfusion. Br J Surg 2005;92(3):370–375.
125. Koga S, Hamazoe R, Maeta M, et al. Prophylactic therapy for peritoneal recurrence of gastric cancer by continuous hyperthermic peritoneal perfusion with mitomycin C. Cancer (Phila) 1988;61:232.
126. Kunisaki C, Shimada H, Nomura M, Akiyama H, Takahashi M, Matsuda G. Lack of efficacy of prophylactic continuous hyperthermic peritoneal perfusion on subsequent peritoneal recurrence and survival in patients with advanced gastric cancer. Surgery (St. Louis) 2002;131(5):521–528.
127. Yonemura Y, de Aretxabala X, Fujimura T, et al. Intraoperative chemohyperthermic peritoneal perfusion as an adjuvant to gastric cancer: Final results of a randomized controlled study. Hepato-Gastroenterology 2001;48(42):1776–1782.
128. Alexander HR, Buell JF, Fraker DL. Rationale and clinical status of continuous hyperthermic peritoneal perfusion for the treatment of peritoneal carcinomatosis. In: Devita VT, Hellman S, Rosenberg SA, eds. Principles and Practice of Oncology. Philadelphia: Lippincott, 1995:9:1–9.
129. Loggie BW, Perini M, Fleming RA, Russell GB, Geisinger K. Treatment and prevention of malignant ascites associated with disseminated intraperitoneal malignancies by aggressive combined-modality therapy. Am Surg 1997;63(2):137–143.
130. Bartlett DL, Buell JF, Libutti SK, et al. A phase I trial of continuous hyperthermic peritoneal perfusion with tumor necrosis factor and cisplatin in the treatment of peritoneal carcinomatosis. Cancer (Phila) 1998;83(6):1251–1261.
131. Hall JJ, Loggie BW, Shen P, et al. Cytoreductive surgery with intraperitoneal hyperthermic chemotherapy for advanced gastric cancer. J Gastrointest Surg 2004;8(4):454–463.
132. Shen P, Hawksworth J, Lovato J, et al. Cytoreductive surgery and intraperitoneal hyperthermic chemotherapy with mitomycin C for peritoneal carcinomatosis from nonappendiceal colorectal carcinoma. Ann Surg Oncol 2004;11(2):178–186.
133. McQuellon RP, Loggie BW, Lehman AB, et al. Long-term survivorship and quality of life after cytoreductive surgery plus intraperitoneal hyperthermic chemotherapy for peritoneal carcinomatosis. Ann Surg Oncol 2003;10(2):155–162.
134. Feldman AL, Libutti SK, Pingpank JF, et al. Analysis of factors associated with outcome in patients with malignant peritoneal mesothelioma undergoing surgical debulking and intraperitoneal chemotherapy. J Clin Oncol 2003;21(24):4560–4567.
135. Shido A, Ohmura S, Yamamoto K, Kobayashi T, Fujimura T, Yonemura Y. Does hyperthermia induce peritoneal damage in continuous hyperthermic peritoneal perfusion? World J Surg 2000;24(5):507–511.
136. Tochner Z, Mitchell JB, Harrington FS, Smith P, Russo DT, Russo A. Treatment of murine intraperitoneal ovarian ascitic tumor with hematoporphyrin derivative and laser light. Cancer Res 1985;45:2983–2987.
137. Tochner Z, Mitchell JB, Smith P, et al. Photodynamic therapy of ascites tumours within the peritoneal cavity. Br J Cancer 1986;53:733–736.

138. Delaney TF, Sindelar WF, Tochner Z, et al. Phase I study of debulking and photodynamic therapy for disseminated intraperitoneal tumors. J Radiat Oncol 1993;25(3):445–447.
139. Sindelar WF, Sullivan FJ, Abraham E, et al. Intraperitoneal photodynamic therapy shows efficacy in phase I trial. Proc Am Soc Clin Oncol 1995;14:447.
140. Hahn SM, Fraker DL, Mick R, et al. A phase II trial of intraperitoneal photodynamic therapy for patients with peritoneal carcinomatosis and sarcomatosis. Clin Cancer Res 2006;12(8): 2517–2525.
141. Young SW, Woodburn KW, Wright M, et al. Lutetium texaphyrin (PCI-0123): a near-infrared, water-soluble photosensitizer. Photochem Photobiol 1997;63(6):892–897.
142. Pass HI, Temeck BK, Kranda K, et al. Phase III randomized trial of surgery with or without intraoperative photodynamic therapy and postoperative immunochemotherapy for malignant pleural mesothelioma. Ann Surg Oncol 1997;4(8):628–633.
143. Pass HI. Photodynamic therapy in thoracic surgery. Ann Thorac Surg 2002;73(6):2012–2013.
144. Sterman DH, Treat J, Litzky LA, et al. Adenovirus-mediated herpes simplex virus thymidine kinase/ganciclovir gene therapy in patients with localized malignancy: results of a phase I clinical trial in malignant mesothelioma. Hum Gene Ther 1992;9(7):1083–1092.
145. Pass HI, DeLaney TF, Tochner Z, et al. Intrapleural photodynamic therapy: results of a phase I trial. Ann Surg Oncol 1994;1(1):28–37.
146. Friedberg JS, Mick R, Stevenson J, et al. A phase I study of Foxcan-mediated photodynamic therapy and surgery in patients with mesothelioma. Ann Thorac Surg 2003;75(3):952–959.
147. Friedberg JS, Mick R, Stevenson JP, et al. Phase II trial of pleural photodynamic therapy and surgery for patients with non-small cell lung cancer with pleural spread. J Clin Oncol 2004;22(11): 2192–2201.

SECTION TEN

Associated Disciplines

104

Urology

Joseph C. Presti, Jr.

This chapter is designed to cover some of the common situations in which the nonurological surgeon might be required to perform surgery on the urinary tract. It focuses primarily on surgery involving the kidney, ureter, and bladder. The end of each section addresses injuries of each organ as a result of external trauma, including the evaluation and management. The last part of this chapter provides a brief overview of urological oncology.

Kidney

Kidney Anatomy

The kidneys are paired structures residing deep within the retroperitoneum, obliquely oriented on the psoas muscle with the lower poles lying more lateral than the upper poles. The right kidney usually lies lower than the left as a result of the position of the liver. Both kidneys are surrounded by perirenal fat, which is contained within Gerota's fascia. Outside of Gerota's fascia is the pararenal, or retroperitoneal fat. Gerota's fascia has both anterior and posterior leaves, which course anteriorly and posteriorly, respectively, around the kidney. These two leaves fuse superiorly, medially, and laterally but remain open inferiorly, allowing the ureter and gonadal vessels to exit. A separate envelope of Gerota's fascia encloses each adrenal gland. Gerota's fascia acts as an important barrier in preventing most renal malignancies from directly invading adjacent structures. It also prevents the spread of perinephric fluid (urine, pus, or blood) from crossing the midline; however, extension into the bony pelvis can occur as the inferior leaves are not fused.

The right kidney lies behind the liver and is separated from it by a reflection of the peritoneum. However, a small portion of Gerota's fascia overlying the upper pole of the right kidney does contact the retroperitoneal bare spot of the liver. The hepatorenal ligament is a condensation of the parietal layer of the peritoneum, attaching the anterior leaf of Gerota's fascia over the upper pole of the right kidney with the posterior portion of the liver. Excessive traction on this ligament may result in a capsular tear of the liver. In mobilizing the kidney in preparation for nephrectomy, this avascular ligament should be divided sharply. The second portion of the duodenum lies over the medial aspect of the right kidney and renal hilum. The hepatic flexure of the colon crosses the lower pole of the right kidney.

The upper and midpole of the left kidney is crossed anteriorly by the tail of the pancreas and splenic vessels. More superiorly, the left kidney is related to the posterior wall of the stomach. The lower pole of the left kidney is crossed by the splenic flexure of the colon. The splenorenal ligament is a condensation of the parietal peritoneum attaching Gerota's fascia overlying the lateral aspect of the upper pole of the left kidney to the inferior aspect of the spleen. Excessive traction on this ligament may result in a capsular tear of the spleen. In mobilizing the kidney in preparation for nephrectomy, this avascular ligament should be divided sharply.

Typically, a single artery and vein enter the renal hilum. The vein lies anterior to the artery, which in turn lies anterior to the renal pelvis (Fig. 104.1). The renal arteries leave the aorta just below the superior mesenteric artery at the level of the second lumbar vertebra. The right renal artery usually courses underneath (posterior) the inferior vena cava on its way to the right kidney. Both arteries usually branch into anterior and posterior divisions before entering the renal hilum. The anterior division usually gives four segmental branches after entering the renal parenchyma. All renal arteries are "end arteries" without collateral circulation, and occlusion of any branch results in ischemia and infarction of its corresponding segment. Supernumerary or "accessory" renal arteries are common, occurring in up to one-fourth of patients. These anomalous vessels are also "end arteries," and thus inadvertent ligation or injury results in segmental renal infarction. More common on the left than the right, these arteries usually arise from the lateral aspect of the aorta and may either enter the kidney via the hilum or directly enter the upper or lower poles. Lower pole supernumerary arteries on the right tend to cross anterior, rather than posterior, to the inferior vena cava. The right renal vein is short and usually enters the inferior vena cava without receiving any branches.

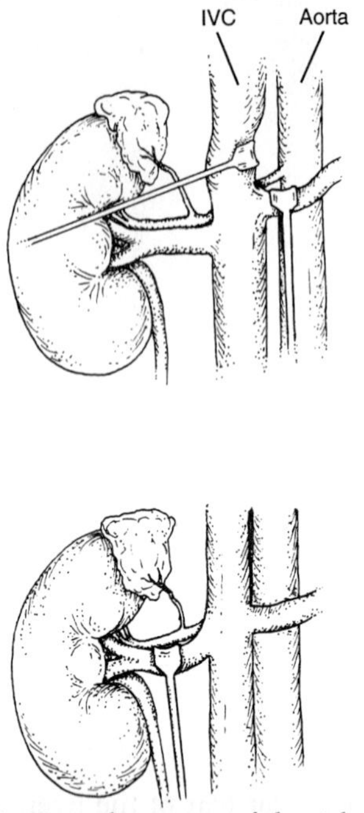

FIGURE 104.1. Normal anatomy of the right renal hilum.

The left renal vein usually crosses anterior to the aorta and receives three branches: (1) the left adrenal vein enters superiorly; (2) the left gonadal vein enters inferiorly; (3) the left lumbar vein enters posteriorly. In contrast to the arterial system, the venous drainage system has extensive collateral circulation, thus making venous occlusion more tolerable. Variations in venous drainage anatomy, although possible, are much less common than variations in arterial anatomy.

Nephrectomy

Preoperative Considerations

The general surgeon may be faced with the possible need for nephrectomy under various circumstances, perhaps most commonly relating to oncological surgery such as retroperitoneal sarcoma or colorectal carcinoma resections. Such tumors might be directly adjacent to or invading into the kidney or renal hilum, necessitating a nephrectomy to attain adequate margins. Other possible indications might result from extensive ureteral involvement requiring a wide resection of a large ureteral segment; however, ureteral reconstruction as described (following) can often spare the patient a nephrectomy. Before deciding on nephrectomy, the surgeon should address several key points.

Foremost, the need for a nephrectomy should be critically assessed. With respect to surgical margins, if a nephrectomy is needed to attain negative margins in one area of the resection, ideally all other areas of resection should also result in negative margins. Often extensive en bloc resections including adjacent bowel and kidney are performed for retroperitoneal tumors solely to leave positive surgical margins along the aorta, vena cava, or iliac vessels. This is a mistake and should be avoided.

Second, an important consideration is maintenance of renal function. Current global renal function should be assessed by serum creatinine. The status of the contralateral kidney should be assessed. Any pathology that might be present should be noted, such as obstruction, kidney stones, or masses. Systemic problems that might impact upon future renal function such as diabetes or hypertension or a history of urinary stone disease should be noted. In addressing global renal function, if the kidney under consideration for removal has obstruction, its relative contribution to global renal function can be assessed preoperatively by isotope renography. In dealing with extrinsic malignant obstruction, such processes tend to be chronic in nature, resulting in less return of function when the obstruction is relieved. Relative function less than 15% to 20% may warrant nephrectomy rather than preservation; however, if additional systemic therapy is planned that is renal toxic, attempts at renal preservation are indicated.

Surgical Technique of Nephrectomy

Urologists utilize several surgical approaches to the kidney including the flank, dorsal lumbotomy, transabdominal, or thoracoabdominal approaches. This discussion addresses only the transabdominal approach as this would be the most typical approach for the general surgeon who is performing a nephrectomy as a secondary procedure in association with another procedure. A simple nephrectomy refers to removal of the kidney within Gerota's fascia and is commonly utilized by the urologist for removal of a nonfunctioning kidney. A radical nephrectomy is the usual treatment of choice for patients with renal cell carcinoma and is often the procedure needed by the general surgeon when performing a nephrectomy in association with resection of an adjacent malignancy. A radical nephrectomy removes the kidney outside of Gerota's fascia. As classically described for renal cell carcinoma, it also implies early ligation of the renal artery and vein with en bloc removal of the kidney and adrenal gland outside of Gerota's fascia. Unless needed for adequate surgical margins, as when performing this procedure for a nonrenal or adrenal malignancy, this procedure can be easily performed while preserving the adrenal gland, which resides within its own separate envelope of Gerota's fascia.

In a transperitoneal approach, on the left side the colon is reflected medially and the splenocolic ligament is divided to expose the aorta (Fig. 104.2A). On the right side, the colon and duodenum are reflected medially to expose the inferior vena cava (Fig. 104.2B). In addressing the renal hilum, the renal artery should be ligated before the renal vein to avoid congestion of the kidney. The artery resides posterior to the vein (see Fig. 104.1). It can be approached either anteriorly or, if the kidney is first mobilized, posteriorly. On the right side, the renal artery is usually ligated lateral to the inferior vena cava; however, if difficulty is encountered in this area, it can also be identified and ligated in the interaortocaval area. On the left, the three branches of the renal vein (adrenal, lumbar, gonadal) can be divided first, facilitating retraction on the left renal vein to identify the artery anteriorly. The artery is usually ligated with 2-0 silk sutures, and an additional 2-0 silk suture ligature is placed on the aortic side distal to the first ligature. The renal vein is divided and ligated in a similar manner. The kidney is then mobilized outside of Gerota's fascia, with care being taken to preserve the adrenal gland, and the ureter is ligated and divided to complete the nephrectomy.

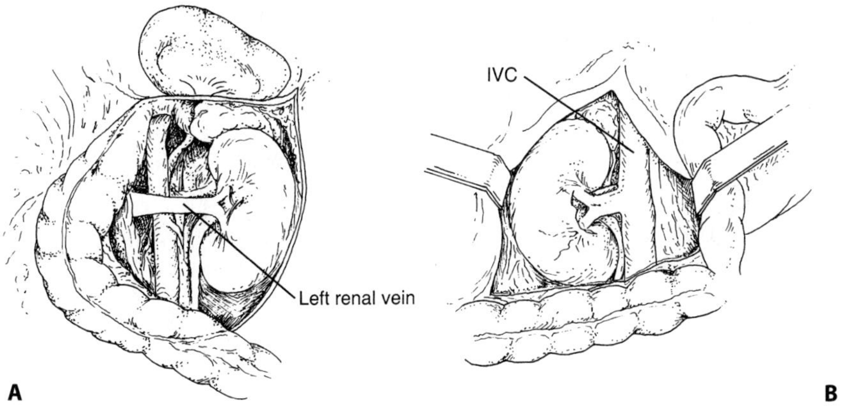

FIGURE 104.2. A. Transperitoneal approach to the left kidney with descending colon reflected medially. **B.** Transperitoneal approach to the right kidney with ascending colon reflected medially. *IVC*, inferior vena cava.

During the performance of a nephrectomy, troublesome bleeding can occur from the inferior vena cava or some of its tributaries. Several of the most common sites are discussed with some surgical tips to assist in their management. Lumbar veins enter the posterolateral aspect of the inferior vena cava at each vertebral level. Avulsion can occur if undue traction is applied to the vena cava without first identifying, dissecting, and ligating these branches. Ligatures of 3-0 or 4-0 silk are used to divide these vessels. If avulsion does occur, bleeding on the vena cava can be controlled with digital compression above and below the site of the avulsion. By rolling the vena cava medially, the posterolateral site of entry of the lumbar vein can be identified, and an Allis clamp can be used to grasp both sides of the vena cava at the site of injury to enable oversewing. Bleeding from the proximal end of the lumbar vein can also be problematic. The vein may retract into the psoas muscle. If the vein is visible, it can be grasped end-on with a hemostat, which is then twisted, resulting in occlusion of the vein and elevation for suture ligation. Alternatively, a figure-of-eight suture ligature in the psoas muscle overlying the vein can control the proximal end. Failure to identify and ligate lumbar veins entering the posterior aspect of the left renal vein can also result in problematical bleeding.

Another problematical site for venous bleeding occurs at the insertion of the right gonadal vein into the anterior wall of the inferior vena cava. Excessive traction can result in an avulsion at this site; however, this is usually easily controlled with a figure-of-eight suture ligature.

The insertion of the right adrenal vein into the lateral wall of the vena cava can also be avulsed if excessive traction is applied. Careful identification and dissection of the adrenal vein from adjacent structures will prevent this injury. If it is incurred, however, use of an Allis clamp to grasp both sides of the vena cava at the site of injury facilitates oversewing.

Renal Injuries from External Trauma

Classification of Renal Injuries

The American Association for the Surgery of Trauma has established the following categories for renal injuries: grade I, contusions, bruises, or subcapsular hematomas with an intact renal capsule; grade II, minor lacerations of the parenchyma extending into the superficial renal cortex, not involving the medulla or collecting system; grade III, major renal parenchymal lacerations extending through the renal cortex into the medulla, but not involving the collecting system; grade IV, major parenchymal laceration extending through the cortex and medulla and into the collecting system as well as any vascular injury to main or segmental vessels with locally contained hemorrhage; grade V, multiple deep parenchymal lacerations extending into the cortex, medulla, and collecting system as well as any major vascular injury causing extensive hemorrhage or main vessel thrombosis (Fig. 104.3).[1]

Evaluation of Renal Traumas: Indications and Methods

The following criteria should be used to identify the need for assessment of renal trauma in adults: (1) penetrating trauma to the flank or abdomen regardless of the degree of hematuria; (2) blunt trauma in adults with either gross hematuria or microscopic hematuria and shock (systolic blood pressure

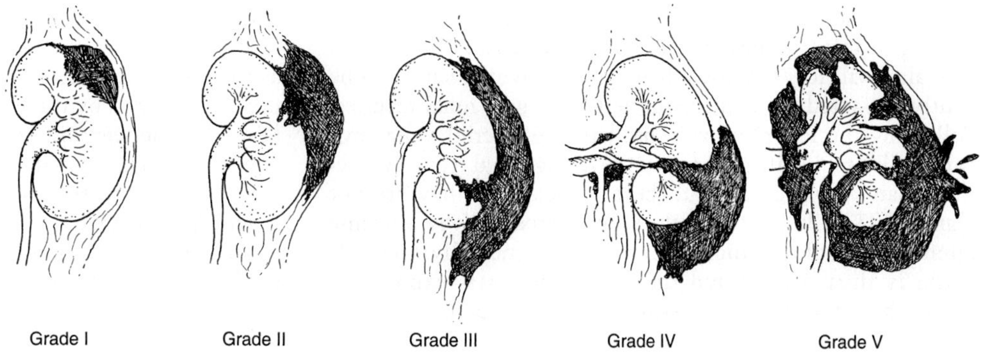

FIGURE 104.3. Renal trauma grading classification.

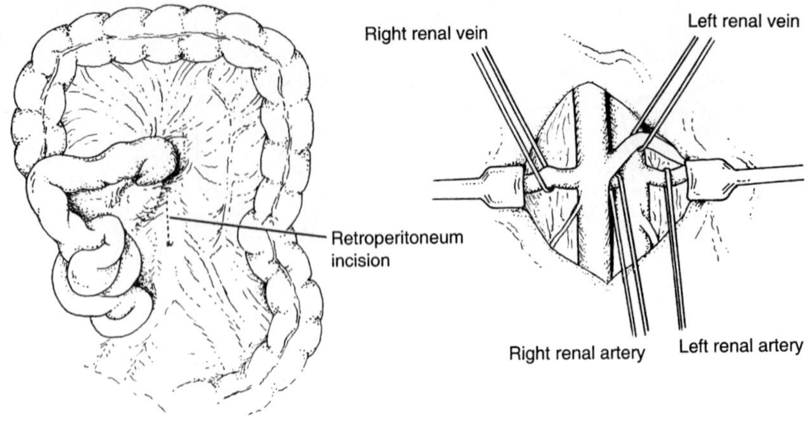

FIGURE 104.4. Transperitoneal approach to the renal vasculature. The posterior peritoneum is incised over the aorta, medial to the inferior mesenteric vein and superior to the inferior mesenteric artery.

<90 mmHg); (3) deceleration injuries; and (4) major associated intraabdominal injuries and microhematuria.[2]

In hemodynamically stable patients in whom renal injury alone is suspected, intravenous urography with tomography is considered adequate renal staging. If this study is equivocal or multiple injuries are suspected, a computed tomography (CT) scan should be performed. Arteriography is reserved only for patients with suspected renovascular injuries in whom CT scan findings are inconclusive. Surgical exploration to completely stage suspected renal injuries is required if radiologic staging is incomplete or not feasible because of hemodynamic instability. If the patient is subsequently stabilized on the operating room table, an intravenous urogram should be performed intraoperatively to assess the status of the potentially injured kidney and establish the presence of a normal contralateral kidney. If this study is indeterminate or abnormal, or if an expanding or pulsatile retroperitoneal hematoma is encountered, exploration is warranted.

Renal Exploration: Indications and Technique

Blunt traumatic renal injuries rarely require exploration. Accurate clinical staging can be achieved with appropriate imaging, and currently less than 10% require intervention.[3,4] Injuries that require repair include all grade V and some grade IV injuries (see Fig. 104.3). Penetrating injuries often require exploration; however, if accurate staging is achieved and no associated injuries are identified or suspected, observation is warranted in grades I to III and possibly some grade IV injuries.

Early isolation and control of the renal artery and vein have been suggested to decrease the risk of nephrectomy at time of renal exploration for trauma.[5,6] If desired, vascular control can be obtained by lifting the small bowel cephalad and then incising the posterior peritoneum over the aorta above the inferior mesenteric artery (Fig. 104.4). Dissection cephalad will identify the left renal vein, which can then be gently retracted to identify the left and right renal arteries. Following the left renal vein back to the inferior vena cava can facilitate identification of the right renal vein. Vessel loops can be placed around these vessels, but they are not clamped. The kidney can then be approached by incising lateral to the colon, which is then reflected medially. Gerota's fascia is then opened and the entire kidney is exposed to assess the extent of the injury. If excessive bleeding is identified, the renal artery can be clamped; however, warm ischemia times in excess of 20 to 30 min must be avoided.

Principles of repair included the following. (1) Debride nonviable tissue: margins of the injury are sharply incised until active bleeding is observed. Care is taken to preserve as much of the renal capsule as possible for subsequent closure. (2) Obtain hemostasis: figure-of-eight sutures of 4-0 chromic are used to obtain hemostasis. Suture ligation of veins does not result in any sequelae; however, ligation of major renal artery branches will result in distal parenchymal infarction. (3) Close the collecting system: a watertight closure can be accomplished using a running 4-0 chromic suture. (4) Cover the defect: the capsule is approximated using interrupted 2-0 chromic sutures over bolsters of absorbable gelatin sponge (Gelfoam). Large defects can be covered with omental flaps if the margins of the repair cannot be approximated.

Ureter

Ureteral Anatomy

The ureter lies entirely within the retroperitoneum and is fixed to other structures at three sites: the ureteropelvic junction (connection with the renal pelvis), the ureterovesical junction (connection with the urinary bladder), and, to a lesser extent, at the pelvic brim as it crosses the iliac vessels. Anatomically, the ureter is often divided into three segments—the upper, middle, and lower segments—but from a functional standpoint it can be divided into two segments of approximately equal length, the abdominal ureter and the pelvic ureter. The abdominal ureter originates from the renal pelvis and courses inferiorly on the anterior surface of the psoas muscle. On the right side, the cranial 5 cm of ureter lies behind the second portion of the duodenum, and as it descends it lies posterior to the right colic and ileocolic vessels as well as the root of the small bowel mesentery. On the left side the ureter is crossed by the left colic vessels and at the rim of the pelvis by the sigmoid vessels. As the ureters enter the false pelvis, they are crossed anteriorly by the gonadal vessels. The pelvic ureter crosses anteriorly over the iliac vessels at the junction of the external and internal iliac vessels. In the male, it courses anteromedial to the obturator vessels. It then turns medially at the level of the ischial spine and just before entering the bladder is crossed anteriorly by the superior vesical

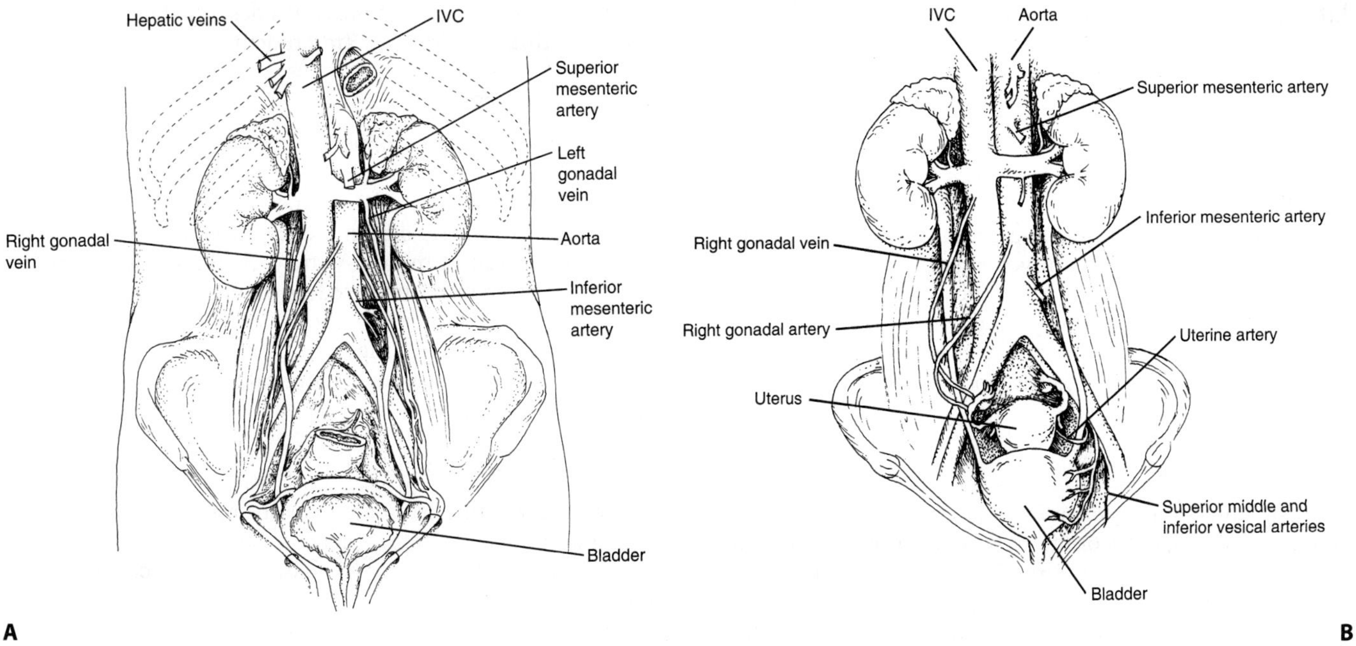

FIGURE 104.5. **A.** Normal ureteral anatomy in the male. **B.** Normal ureteral anatomy in the female.

artery and ductus deferens (Fig. 104.5A). In the female, the ureter travels posterior to the ovary as it turns medially in the base of the broad ligament and is crossed anteriorly by the uterine artery just before its entry into the bladder (Fig. 104.5B).

Histologically, the ureter is composed of three layers: an inner mucosal layer lined by transitional epithelium; a middle, helically oriented, smooth muscular layer; and an outer adventitial layer (Fig. 104.6). The ureteral blood supply travels through the adventitial layer and is quite variable. In up to 80% of cases, a single artery runs through its entire length and is supplied by multiple collateral arteries. In the remaining 20% of cases, multiple noncollateralizing arteries are seen. Sources of blood supply include the aorta, and the renal, gonadal, iliac, uterine, middle hemorrhoidal, vaginal, and superior vesical arteries (Fig. 104.7). Because the blood supply is not predictable, the surgeon must exercise great care in ureteral mobilization so as to avoid devascularization. In general, dissection should be lateral to the ureter above the pelvic brim and anterior and medial below the pelvic brim. Care must be taken to avoid skeletonizing the ureter during dissection.

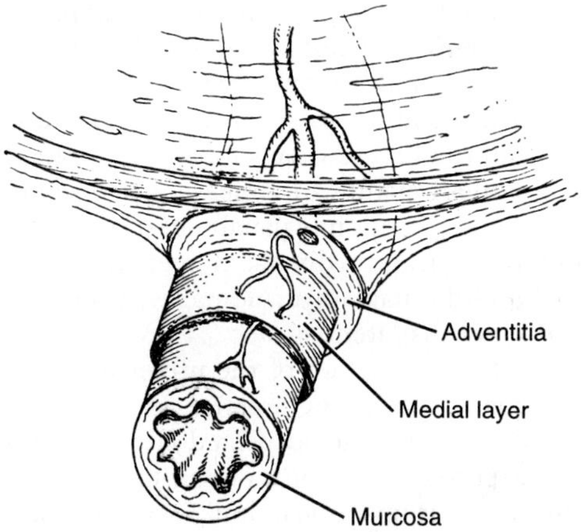

FIGURE 104.6. Cross-section view of normal ureteral histology.

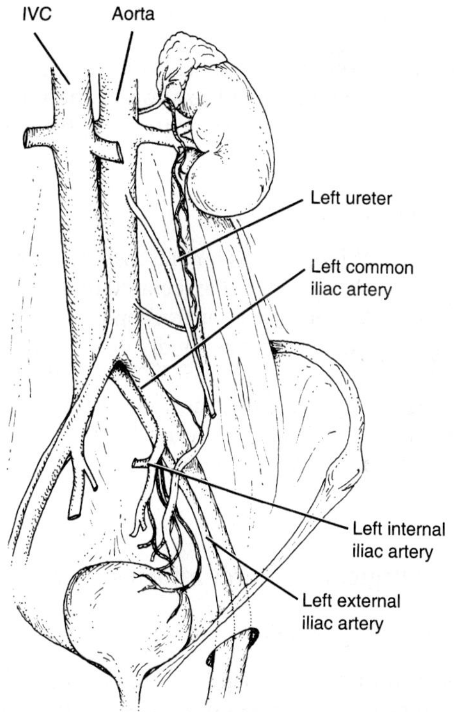

FIGURE 104.7. Ureteral blood supply. Note that above the pelvic brim most blood supply comes medially whereas below the pelvic brim most blood supply comes laterally.

Iatrogenic Intraoperative Ureteral Injury

Gynecological Surgery

Most intraoperative ureteral injuries result from gynecological surgery and occur at the pelvic brim or at the level of the broad ligament where the ureter passes beneath the uterine vessels.[7] The highest rates of injury are associated with hysterectomy, cesarean section, and laparotomy for pelvic inflammatory disease. Tumorous involvement of the parametrium represents a significant risk for subsequent ureteral injury during attempted debulking procedures. Preoperative identification of hydronephrosis should heighten one's awareness of ureteral involvement and the close proximity of the ureter to the neoplastic process.

General Surgery

Rectosigmoid surgery for inflammatory or malignant disease comprises the most common general surgical procedures associated with ureteral injury. The four areas identified that may result in ureteral injury during these procedures are (1) during ligation of the inferior mesenteric artery; (2) near the cul-de-sac where the ureter crosses under the vas deferens at the sacral promontory; (3) during division of the lateral pedicles of the rectum; and (4) during reperitonealization when the ureter may be included in ligatures.[8]

Vascular Surgery

Vascular reconstructive surgery may result in ureteral injury in the region of the iliac artery or in the abdominal segment of the ureter if aneurysm is present.[9] Risk of injury seems to be increased when perianeurysmal inflammation is present.

Orthopedic Surgery

Anterior and posterior approaches to lumbar spinal surgery, as well as open reduction and fixation of the sacroiliac joint associated with an unstable pelvic fracture, have been associated with ureteral injury.[10]

Laparoscopy

As the number of indications for laparoscopic surgery continues to increase, the number of associated ureteral injuries has also increased. As with most laparoscopic-associated complications, this incidence most assuredly will decline with operator experience. Laparoscopic-assisted vaginal hysterectomy and laser-assisted endometriosis ablative procedures have been associated with ureteral injuries.[11,12] Laparoscopic pelvic lymphadenectomy has also been associated with ureteral injury.

Types of Surgical Ureteral Injuries

Sutures and Ligatures

The most common intraoperative ureteral injury is ligation of the ureter during division of a major vessel, such as the uterine artery during hysterectomy or the inferior mesenteric artery during colorectal surgery. If recognized acutely, simple deligation is often all that is necessary. If ureteral integrity is in question following the measures described next, then ureteral stenting and drainage are prudent.

Crush Injuries

Crush injuries most commonly occur during blind clamping of bleeding vessels in an attempt to obtain hemostasis. The most common site is the uterine artery during abdominal hysterectomy. Clamp size and duration of clamping contribute to the extent of injury. A small clamp applied for only a few minutes may be removed without long-term sequelae; however, all such injuries should at least be stented and drained. Many crush injuries require resection of the involved segment with appropriate surgical repair, as described (following).

Laceration and Excision

Sharp division of the ureter usually results in little or no ischemic injury, and repair depends upon the level of injury. Partial transections caused by sharp dissection can usually be closed with fine interrupted absorbable sutures. When partial transections approach 50% of the ureteral circumference, usually complete transections with a spatulated anastomosis are advised to avoid stricture. If complete transection is encountered or a segment of ureter is excised, the level of the injury is the most important factor in determining the type of repair. Upper ureteral injuries that enable adequate mobilization of both proximal and distal segments are usually managed by ureteroureterostomy. Complete transections of the distal ureter are usually managed by reimplantation.

Devascularization

If a segment of ureter is obviously identified as nonviable in the operating room, it should be excised with appropriate repair being performed depending on the level and extent of injury. If a ureteral segment is of questionable viability, stenting and drainage should be performed.

Identification of Ureteral Injury and Timing of Repair

Surgically induced ureteral injury may be identified intraoperatively, in the early postoperative period, or in the delayed postoperative period. The timing of presentation or identification of a ureteral injury has significant impact upon the timing of repair. Intraoperative recognition is optimal, and immediate repair should be undertaken, resulting in minimal morbidity. Identification in the early postoperative setting (usually within the first few days following surgery) warrants early repair unless significant infection or inflammation is present. Late identification is usually best handled with temporary proximal urinary diversion (percutaneous nephrostomy tube) and drainage of urinoma, with delayed elective repair 2 to 3 months later.

Intraoperative inspection of the ureter remains the most reliable means of assessing ureteral integrity. Hemostasis must be obtained, and the suspected site of injury must be adequately exposed. Inspection of the ureter may be facilitated by intravenous injection of indigo carmine or methylene blue, but this may be unreliable in the face of hypotension. Alternatively, the dye may be directly injected into the ureter with a 25-gauge needle to assess ureteral integrity. Ureteral integrity may be present despite a significant vascular injury, and careful inspection of the ureteral wall is important, noting discoloration of the wall or absence of capillary refill as a prelude to impending ischemia.

Early postoperative identification of ureteral injury may occur by identification of a ureteral segment in a pathological specimen. Clinical presentation may include urine drainage from the surgical wound, unexplained fever, flank pain, or more subtle signs including prolonged ileus or nausea and vomiting.

Delayed identification of a ureteral injury may present with hydronephrosis and flank pain. If from an ischemic injury, symptoms and signs described above for early postoperative identification may be observed as the ischemic segment sloughs in a delayed setting.

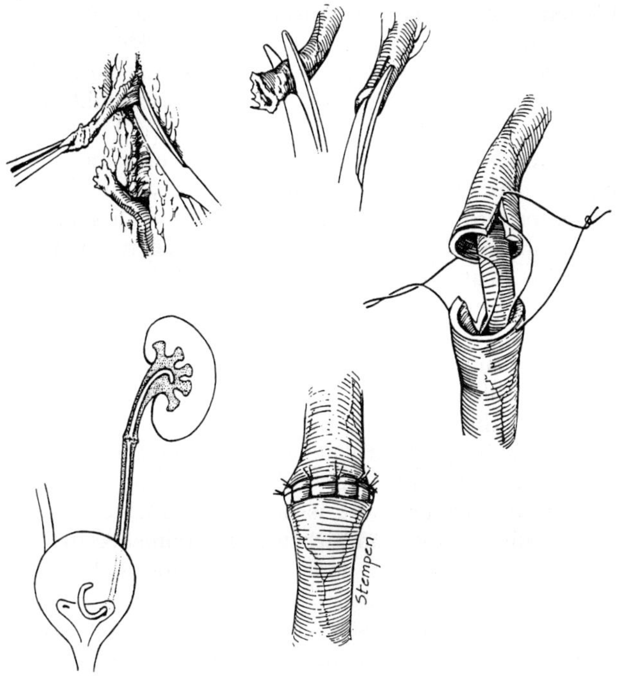

FIGURE 104.8. Ureteroureterostomy showing proximal and distal ureteral segment mobilization, debridement, spatulation, and anastomosis over a double-J stent. (Reprinted with permission from Presti JC, PR Caroll PR. Intraoperative management of the injured ureter. In: Perspectives in Colon and Rectal Surgery, vol 1, no. 2. © 1998 Thieme Medical Publishers.)

Surgical Repair of Ureteral Injuries

General principles of ureteral repair include (1) debridement of nonviable tissue; (2) a tension-free anastomosis; (3) precise mucosal approximation and watertight closure; (4) internal ureteral stents, in most cases; (5) isolation of repair with omentum or fat in patients at high risk for infection (simultaneous bowel, vascular, or pancreatic surgery); and (6) retroperitoneal drainage.

Primary Closure of Partial Transection of the Ureter

If a partial transection of the ureter resulting from a scalpel or scissors is encountered, then often primary closure can be accomplished. Mobilization of proximal and distal ureteral segments is necessary to avoid any tension on the repair. Closure can be accomplished with interrupted 4-0 or 5-0 absorbable sutures. Stenting is not mandatory, yet we typically use stents if the degree of transection approaches 50% of the ureteral circumference. Stent placement is facilitated by placing the guidewire through a side hole of the double-J stent and directing one end of the stent upward to the renal pelvis. The wire is then withdrawn, reinserted in a side hole, and directed toward the opposite end of the stent, which is then directed downward to the bladder. Retroperitoneal drainage of the repair is mandatory, and in selected cases one should employ omental flaps for further isolation of the repair (see following). Stenting is usually maintained for 6 weeks.

Primary Ureteroureterostomy

Any complete transection can often be repaired by primary ureteroureterostomy. Such a repair should be undertaken only if a tension-free anastomosis can be accomplished. Careful mobilization of the proximal and distal ureteral segments should be performed, with care being taken to avoid devascularization.

Debridement of nonviable tissue from both proximal and distal ureteral segments should be performed back to tissue that readily bleeds; this will delineate the length of the defect. Both segments should be mobilized and ends spatulated on contralateral sides to allow for an anastomosis of wide caliber. Interrupted 4-0 or 5-0 absorbable sutures are then placed at the apex of each spatulation and brought through the opposite segment of ureter in appropriate positions to allow knot placement on the outside. These two sutures can be tagged with clamps and provide stabilization while serving to minimize direct handling of the ureter. A double-J stent may now be inserted, as previously described, and interrupted sutures placed in the anterior surface of the repair. The ureter can now be rotated by use of the two tagged apical sutures, and the posterior wall closure is now performed (Fig. 104.8). Retroperitoneal drainage of the repair is mandatory, and in selected cases one should employ omental flaps for further isolation of the repair (see following). Stenting is usually maintained for 6 weeks.

Ureteral Reimplantation and Psoas Hitch

Injuries of the pelvic ureter in which the distal ureteral segment is of poor quality or of insufficient length are best managed by ureteral reimplantation, the modified submucosal tunnel technique.

The proximal ureteral segment is first debrided, and a traction suture is then placed to facilitate handling of the ureter. The ureter is mobilized proximally to avoid tension on the repair. A site is selected in the posterior bladder wall, superior and medial to the original ureteral hiatus. A tonsil clamp is then passed from within the bladder to the outside, creating a new ureteral hiatus. The ureter is then brought through the bladder via the traction suture. Placement in the more mobile lateral wall should be avoided as this may result in kinking of the ureter with bladder filling and subsequent obstruction. A submucosal tunnel is then developed with tenotomy scissors, directed toward the bladder neck, with a ratio of length to diameter of 3:1 to avoid reflux. The ureter is then passed through the submucosal tunnel with aid of the traction suture. It is now spatulated on its anterior surface with Potts scissors and sutured to the bladder with interrupted 4-0 or 5-0 absorbable sutures. The initial suture should be placed in the posterior ureteral wall and should incorporate detrusor muscle as well as mucosa to avoid retraction of the ureter. The remainder of the sutures may include only mucosa. The mucosal defect at the initial point of entry of the ureter into the bladder is then closed with some interrupted absorbable sutures (Fig. 104.9). The ureter may be stented with an internal double-J stent or a pediatric feeding tube, which may be brought out via a separate stab wound. The cystotomy may be closed in two layers: a running 4-0 absorbable suture in the mucosal layer and an interrupted 2-0 absorbable suture in the seromuscular layer. Drains are placed near the cystotomy and the site of the ureteral hiatus. Catheter drainage of the bladder is maintained for 7 days, and if pediatric feeding tubes are utilized, these may be removed at 7 to 10 days. Drainage is monitored after catheter and feeding tube removal, and when it is diminished the drains are removed. If internal double-J stents are used, these are removed at 4 to 6 weeks.

Occasionally, extensive injury to the distal ureter is encountered that prevents the proximal ureter from reaching the bladder without tension. Under these circumstances, a psoas hitch may allow for a tension-free reimplantation. Before performing the reimplantation, the bladder is mobilized by stripping the peritoneum from the bladder dome. The ipsilateral obliterated umbilical vessels and, in more difficult cases, the contralateral superior vesical vessels are divided and ligated to provide greater bladder mobilization. The bladder is anchored to the tendon of the psoas minor muscle with 2-0 absorbable sutures. This maneuver may be facilitated by placement of the index finger through the cystotomy. Care must be taken to avoid incorporation of the genitofemoral nerve into these sutures. In the 10% of patients with congenital absence of the psoas minor tendon, the bladder may be sutured directly to the psoas major muscle belly. The anchoring sutures are not tied until after the submucosal tunnel has been created. The ureter enters the bladder medial to the anchoring sutures and travels a straight course along the posterior bladder wall. Fixation of the bladder in this fashion should prevent kinking of the ureter with bladder filling (Fig. 104.10).

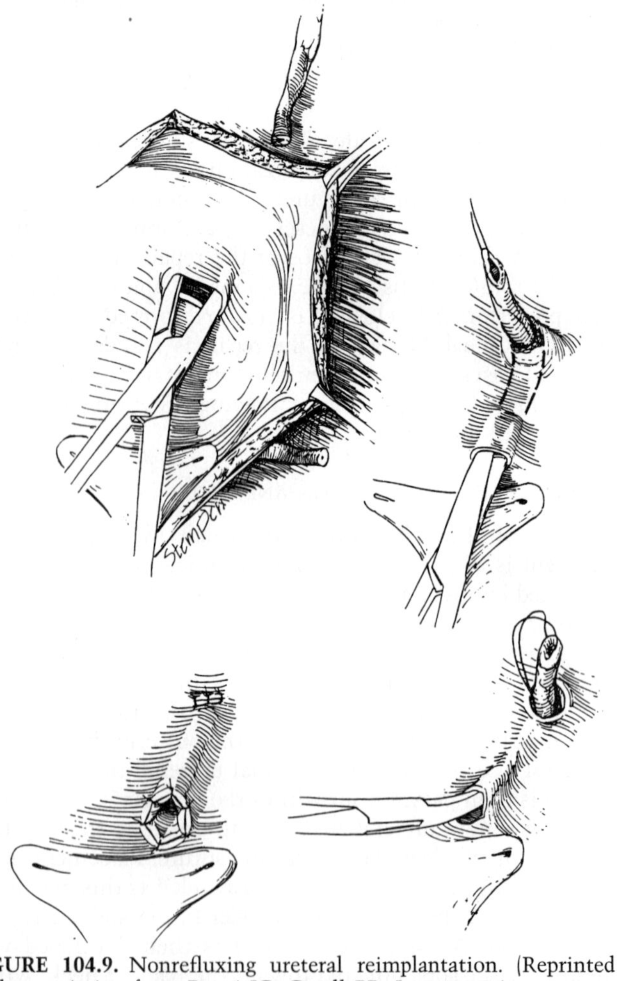

FIGURE 104.9. Nonrefluxing ureteral reimplantation. (Reprinted with permission from Presti JC, Caroll PR. Intraoperative management of the injured ureter. In: Perspectives in Colon and Rectal Surgery, vol 1, no. 2. © 1998 Thieme Medical Publishers.)

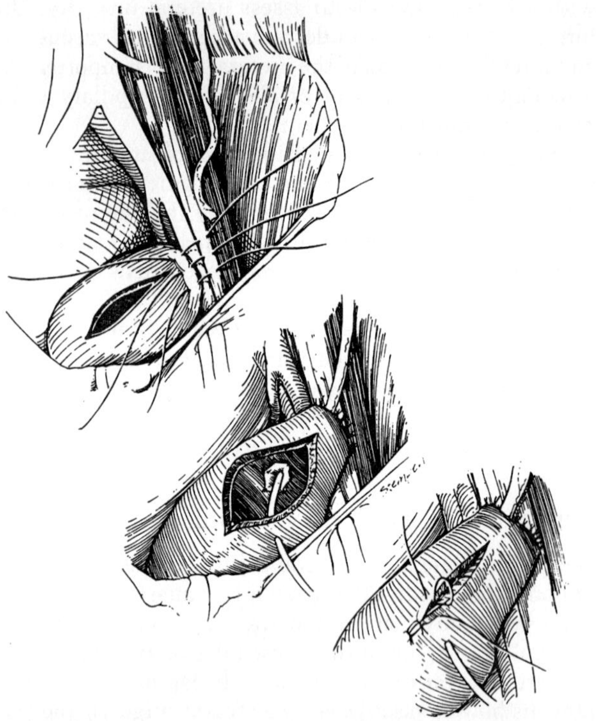

FIGURE 104.10. Psoas hitch maneuver. (Reprinted with permission from Presti JC, Caroll PR. Intraoperative management of the injured ureter. In: Perspectives in Colon and Rectal Surgery, vol 1, no. 2. © 1998 Thieme Medical Publishers.)

Boari Flap

If a psoas hitch does not provide adequate length for a tension-free vesicoureteral anastomosis, then a Boari flap may be considered. However, such considerations must be made before performing the cytostomy because the bladder incision will become one side of the flap. The peritoneum is swept off the bladder dome, and a posteriorly based flap is created. The flap should be at least 4 cm wide and be of sufficient length to allow for a tension-free ureteral anastomosis (at least 3 cm longer than the measured deficit). The flap is folded back, a submucosal tunnel is developed in the flap as described earlier, and the ureteral reimplantation is completed. The flap is tubularized and closed in two layers as described for cystotomy. Drainage and stenting should be performed as described previously.

Transureteroureterostomy

In cases of extensive pelvic ureteral loss where remaining proximal ureteral length is inadequate to allow reimplantation into the bladder, or concomitant significant ipsilateral pathology is present, a transureteroureterostomy (TUU) may be considered. The recipient ureter is mobilized as little as possible to avoid any devascularization, and the injured ureter is brought under the mesentery above or below the inferior mesenteric artery, depending upon the degree of ureteral loss as well as the site selected for anastomosis. The injured ureter must follow a smooth course under the mesentery, avoiding any acute angulation. The injured ureter is then debrided and spatulated. A 2-cm longitudinal ureterotomy is made in the recipient ureter, and the anastomosis is performed with interrupted 4-0 or 5-0 absorbable sutures. Initially, sutures are placed in the superior and inferior aspects of the ureterotomy and brought through the corresponding points on the spatulated ureter. These are tied on the outside, and may be tagged for further aid in stabilizing the anastomosis. An internal double-J stent should be inserted and retroperitoneal drainage utilized (Fig. 104.11).

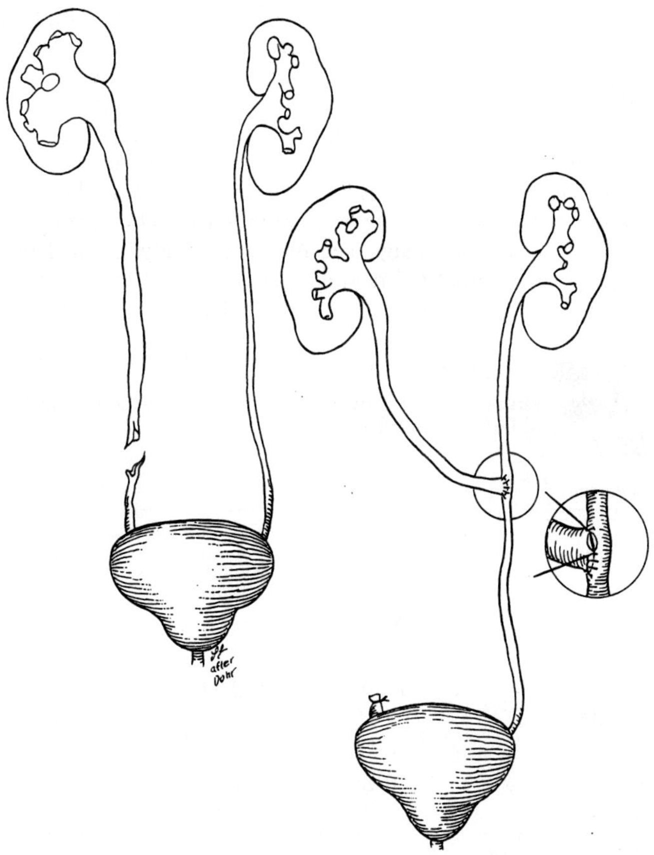

FIGURE 104.11. Transureteroureterostomy. (Reprinted with permission from Presti JC, Caroll PR. Uretal and renal pelvic trauma. In: McAninch JW, ed. Traumatic and Reconstructive Urology. © 1996 WB Saunders.)

Isolation and Drainage

Depending upon the side of injury, omental flaps can be based upon either the right or the left gastroepiploic vessels along the greater curvature of the stomach. The short gastric vessels are divided as they enter the gastroepiploic vessels, and the flap can be swung into the retroperitoneum either by going through the mesentery of the colon or by going around the lateral gutters adjacent to the colon. Once in the retroperitoneum, the omentum can be wrapped around the ureteral repair, providing physical isolation from adjacent pathology.

Drains should be placed in the retro- or extraperitoneal space. Closed drainage systems are preferable to decrease the likelihood of infection.

Ureteral Injuries from External Trauma

Ureteral and renal pelvic injuries resulting from external trauma are rare, accounting for less than 1% of all urological trauma. The ureter, because of its location in the retroperitoneum surrounded by fat and muscle, is well protected from external trauma. Patients with ureteral injuries tend to be severely injured and often have multiple associated injuries. Penetrating rather than blunt trauma is the more common cause for ureteral injury, and early diagnosis and reconstruction are paramount for a favorable outcome. The importance of immediate recognition of ureteral injury has been demonstrated previously, as one series reported a 32% incidence of nephrectomy in cases of delayed recognition compared with a 4.5% incidence when the injury was recognized immediately.[13]

Mechanisms of Injury

Penetrating trauma is by far the most common etiology of ureteral injury resulting from external trauma, with gunshot wounds being more common than stab wounds. The incidence of ureteral injuries following gunshot wounds to the abdomen has been estimated to range from 2% to 3%.[14,15] In addition to directly causing an acute injury, gunshots may also result in delayed injuries from blast effect.[16] Any segment of the ureter may be injured from penetrating trauma. Injuries to the renal pelvis and upper ureter have been reported more frequently than mid- or lower ureteral injuries (Table 104.1). Blunt trauma is a rare cause of ureteral injury and is more commonly associated with ureteral injuries in the pediatric age group. Deceleration-type injuries (falls or motor vehicle accidents) account for the majority of ureteral injuries resulting from blunt trauma, and the region of the ureteropelvic junction seems to be the most vulnerable.[17]

Patients sustaining ureteral injuries represent a high-risk group because they tend to have multiple associated injuries. In our series at San Francisco General Hospital, 53% of patients presented in shock, the mean transfusion requirement was 2483 mL per patient, and 94% of patients had major associated organ injuries with the mean number of organs injured per patient being 3.7.[18] It has been suggested that the observed incidence of ureteral injuries may be increasing as trauma evacuation and resuscitative measures continue to expand and improve; larger numbers of seriously injured patients now survive and get in-depth evaluations at trauma centers.[19]

TABLE 104.1.
Mechanism and Site of Ureteral Injuries.

Reference	*n*[a]	*GSW*[b]	*SW*[c]	*Blunt*[d]	*Upper*[e]	*Mid*[f]	*Lower*[g]	*Data class*
Peterson[20]	18	17	1	0	5	7	6	III
Liroff[21]	20	N/A	N/A	N/A	5	11	4	III
Stutzman[47]	22	22	0	0	6	3	13	III
Holden[14]	63	63	0	0	20	27	16	III
Lankford[24]	10	10	0	0	6	3	1	III
Carlton[22]	39	36	1	2	N/A	N/A	N/A	III
Eickenberg[23]	17	17	0	0	6	2	9	III
Presti[18]	18	10	6	2	15	1	2	III
Steers[48]	18	17	0	1	12	4	2	III
Rober[49]	16	16	0	0	8	4	4	III
Campbell[19]	15	12	0	3	7	4	4	III
Totals	256	219	8	8	90 (42%)	66 (30%)	61 (28%)	

N/A, not available.
[a]Number of patients in study.
[b]Gunshot wound.
[c]Stab wound.
[d]Blunt trauma.
[e]Upper one-third of ureter or renal pelvis.
[f]Middle one-third of ureter.
[g]Lower one-third of ureter.

Evaluation

The physical findings associated with ureteral injuries are nonspecific. Unless the surgeon maintains a high index of suspicion, the diagnosis may go unnoticed with serious consequences. Any patient who sustains a penetrating wound to the flank or to the abdomen is at risk for ureteral injury. Patients sustaining blunt trauma associated with rapid deceleration or hyperextension of the lower thoracic and upper lumbar regions should also be evaluated for ureteral injuries.

The presence of gross or microscopic hematuria is not a reliable indicator of ureteral injury. Our experience demonstrated a false-negative rate of 31%, similar to that reported in other series (23%–31%).[20,21] Thus, the absence of hematuria on the initial urinalysis does not exclude an ureteral injury (Table 104.2).

The sensitivity of intravenous urography (IVU) in detecting ureteral injuries in many series ranges from 78% to 100%.[22–24] It must be emphasized, however, that these series typically utilized complete studies (see Table 104.2). Patients sustaining severe abdominal trauma are often evaluated with "limited studies" because the extent of associated injuries requires prompt surgical intervention. Such studies are performed by giving a 150-mL bolus of intravenous contrast, and a single flat-plate film of the abdomen is then performed approximately 10 min later. Although such limited studies may be useful for the initial evaluation of the injured kidney and for establishing the presence of a contralateral kidney, they are unreliable in assessing injuries to the ureter. Although extravasation of contrast on IVU may be diagnostic of ureteral injury, other findings such as delayed excretion, nonvisualization, deviation, or dilation of the ureter are commonly identified. Retrograde pyelography is probably the most sensitive radiographic tool in detecting ureteral injuries, but because of the need for prompt surgical intervention for associated injuries in these patients it is performed rarely in such cases. The exact sensitivity of CT scanning in detecting ureteral injuries is not known. As with IVU, the urinary excretion of contrast may be delayed secondary to hypotension or concomitant renal injury, and the injured ureter may be incompletely opacified. In the setting of large amounts of urinary extravasation, the exact site of injury may also be obscured.

Intraoperative inspection of the ureter remains the most reliable means of assessing ureteral integrity. The majority of ureteral injuries are diagnosed intraoperatively. Even if preoperative radiographic imaging does not reveal injury to the ureter, if one has a high index of suspicion for injury then

TABLE 104.2.
Urinalysis and Intravenous Urography in the Diagnosis of Ureteral Injuries.

Reference	*n*[a]	*Urinalysis*[b]	*IVU*[c]	*Data class*
Peterson[20]	18	10/13	7/11	III
Liroff[21]	20	9/13	N/A	III
Lankford[24]	10	9/9	8/8	III
Carlton[22]	39	N/A	17/21	III
Eickenberg[23]	17	N/A	7/9	III
Presti[18]	18	11/16	3/11	III
Steers[47]	18	14/16	7/8	III
Rober[49]	16	8/11	8/8	III
Campbell[19]	15	10/13	4/12	III
Totals	171	71/91 (78%)	61/88 (69%)	

N/A, not available.
[a]Number of patients in study.
[b]Microscopic (more than 5 red cells/high-power field) or gross hematuria on initial urinalysis.
[c]Intravenous urography demonstrating ureteral injury.

exploration is warranted. Inspection of the ureter may be facilitated by the use of indigo carmine or methylene blue, as described. One must exercise greater caution when assessing for ureteral injury following a gunshot wound, especially if a high-velocity weapon is involved (muzzle velocity greater than 2500 feet/s). Under these circumstances, a ureteral injury may have occurred even in the absence of urine, contrast, or dye extravasation. The kinetic energy of a projectile is directly proportional to the mass of the projectile and the square of its velocity. Military assault rifles such as the M-16 and the AK-47 have muzzle velocities of 3300 and 2625 feet per second, respectively, and upon entering the body projectiles fired from these weapons produce a cavity 30 to 40 times their size because of their high energy, which is transferred to surrounding tissues. Ureteral contusions may occur from the projectile passing in proximity to the ureter, causing damage to the intima of the blood vessels within the ureteral wall and resulting in a bruised appearance of the ureter from thrombosis or hemorrhage. If unrecognized, this may result in ischemia with delayed necrosis and urinary leakage.

Considerations Regarding Repair of Ureteral Injuries from External Trauma

Penetrating injuries to the ureter often require debridement of nonviable tissue, which is particularly important in the management of gunshot injuries to the ureter. Tissue should be resected both proximally and distally to a point that bleeds freely. All complete transections and partial transections of the abdominal ureter resulting from gunshot wounds should be completely transected and debrided to viable tissue before formation of a ureteroureterostomy. All complete transections and partial transections of the pelvic ureter resulting from gunshot wounds should be completely transected and debrided to viable tissue. Then, if sufficient length is available, a primary ureteroureterostomy may be performed. If the distal ureteral segment is inadequate or insufficient length is available, then a ureteral reimplantation should be performed. If significant distal ureteral length is lost, then a psoas hitch may be performed to provide a tension-free anastomosis. Occasionally, a Boari flap may be required in addition to a psoas hitch if there has been extensive loss of the distal ureteral segment. If concomitant injuries within the pelvis do not allow for an ipsilateral repair, then a transureteroureterostomy may be performed. Rarely in the trauma setting would autotransplantation or an ileal ureteral substitution be attempted in cases of extensive ureteral loss.

Partial transections of the abdominal or pelvic ureter resulting from stab wounds or blunt trauma can often be closed primarily with little or no debridement.

Urinary Bladder

Bladder Anatomy

The urinary bladder resides within the extraperitoneal space of the pelvis. The dome of the bladder is covered by a reflection of the peritoneal envelope. The urachus (median umbilical ligament) extends from the bladder dome to the umbilicus. The mucosal lining of the bladder is composed of transitional cell epithelium. The submucosa, or lamina propria, is composed of blood vessels, connective tissue, and thin wisps of smooth muscle, the muscularis mucosa. The muscularis propria layer is composed of large fascicles of detrusor muscle bundles, which are randomly oriented except at the bladder neck where they form three distinct layers: an inner longitudinal, a middle circular, and an outer longitudinal layer. The serosa is the thin outer membranous layer separating the bladder from the perivesical fat. Blood supply to the bladder comes from the anterior trunk of the internal iliac vessels: the superior, middle, and inferior vesical branches. Of note, the obliterated umbilical vessels (medial umbilical ligament) are the first branch of the anterior trunk of the internal iliac, and the ureter courses under this branch as well as the superior vesical branches before entering the bladder at the ureteral hiatus.

Enterovesical Fistulas

Etiology and Diagnosis

Enterovesical fistulas are more common in men than women. Colovesical fistulas are the most common of the enterovesical fistulas, and almost two-thirds of these result from diverticular disease. Colon cancer accounts for about 20% of colovesical fistulas. Other etiologies of enterovesical fistulas include Crohn's disease, radiation exposure, bladder cancer, appendicitis, gynecological tumors, and some infections (tuberculosis, actinomycosis).

Pneumaturia and fecaluria are reported in 63% and 43% of patients, respectively. Urinary tract infections are present in 95% of patients, and therefore irritable voiding complaints are common. Infections with multiple organisms are only seen in one-third of patients.

The most accurate diagnostic test for making the diagnosis of an enterovesical fistula is computer tomography (CT).[25] Typical CT findings include air within the bladder, focal bladder wall and bowel wall thickening in apposition with one another, extravesical soft tissue mass, and presence of contrast within the bladder before administration of intravenous contrast. Conventional cystograms are diagnostic in only one-third of cases. Cystoscopy, although diagnostic in less than one-half of patients, should be performed in all patients to exclude a bladder malignancy as the primary etiology.[26] Colonoscopy or sigmoidoscopy is diagnostic in only 10% of patients, but this is also mandatory to exclude a colonic malignancy as the underlying etiology. Biopsy of the fistula tract either endoscopically or cystoscopically is usually recommended to exclude a malignant etiology.

Surgical Treatment

A midline transperitoneal approach is used to expose the segment of bowel communicating with the bladder. The fistula tract is identified and is circumferentially dissected as close to the bladder as possible. The bladder is then opened around the fistula site with adequate margins for a malignant fistula or until healthy mucosa and bladder musculature are seen for an inflammatory fistula. Once adequate margins are obtained, the bladder is inspected for hemostasis and closed in two layers using absorbable sutures. The inner layer is a running stitch including the mucosa and portion of the muscularis, while the outer layer is a running seromuscular stitch. The segment of bowel is then resected. If the underlying etiology is a colonic malignancy, the appropriate colectomy is performed. If secondary to inflammation, the involved bowel segment is resected. An omental interposition between bladder and bowel segment should be performed. Catheter drainage of the bladder is maintained for approximately 2 weeks.

Intraoperative Bladder Injury

Any pelvic surgery may result in an injury to the bladder. The most common is hysterectomy, both abdominal and vaginal. However, injury may also occur in general surgical procedures including colorectal surgery for both benign and malignant disease, other pelvic surgery for malignancy, hernia repairs, and laparoscopic surgery. Prompt intraoperative identification is critical to decrease morbidity.

If in question, identification of bladder injury can be facilitated by the instillation of a diluted methylene blue solution into the Foley catheter. If an injury is identified, successful repair can usually be obtained by adherence to a few basic principles: (1) evaluating the site and extent of the bladder injury; (2) obtaining adequate exposure of the area of perforation and adjacent structures; (3) debriding edges as needed and closing in two layers; (4) interposition of omental flap if a second suture line is in proximity of the bladder closure (e.g., vaginal cuff following hysterectomy, bowel anastomosis following bowel resection); (5) extraperitoneal drainage of repair; and (6) prolonged catheter drainage of the bladder. Some of these points are now further expanded.

The site and extent of injury affect the surgical approach employed. A small injury in the anterior or lateral bladder wall might be closed primarily without opening the remainder of the bladder. A large injury or one extending toward the posterior wall and trigone (region where ureteral orifices are located) usually warrants the performance of an anterior cystotomy to enable direct inspection of the ureteral orifices. Ureteral integrity can be established by the administration of intravenous indigo carmine or methylene blue. Closure is then performed while keeping the ureteral orifices under direct vision. Internal stenting or externalized ureteral catheters can be used if needed to avoid injury during closure.

Adequate exposure is important to completely visualize the entire injury, and it also facilitates separation of the bladder closure from other suture lines to decrease fistula formation. Interposition of an omental flap should always be used when dealing with prior radiated tissue or if a second suture line might overlap the bladder closure. Catheter drainage is usually maintained for at least 2 weeks, and should be extended if radiated or infected tissue is involved.

Bladder Injuries from External Trauma

Classification and Mechanisms of Injury

Bladder injury from external trauma can be classified into either extraperitoneal rupture, intraperitoneal rupture, or combined intra- and extraperitoneal rupture. Almost all bladder injuries resulting from external trauma are associated with a pelvic fracture. It is most likely the shearing force of the pelvic ring, as it becomes distorted by the external trauma, that results in a tear in the bladder wall. Less than one-third of bladder injuries result from a bony spicule actually penetrating the bladder wall. Approximately one-third of bladder injuries are intraperitoneal whereas two-thirds are extraperitoneal in the adult.

Evaluation

Blunt trauma patients who present with gross hematuria or a pelvic fracture with microscopic hematuria and shock need imaging of the urinary bladder to exclude an injury. Before passing a urethral catheter, the urethral meatus and perineum should be inspected, because if blood is present at the meatus or a perineal hematoma is observed, then a retrograde urethrogram is required to exclude urethral injury before urethral catheterization. Conventional CT scans or IVU can frequently miss significant bladder injuries.[27] A cystogram, either conventional or CT, is performed by instilling at least 300 mL contrast under gravity. Images are taken before filling, after the bladder is full, and after drainage. Extravasation is indicative of bladder rupture. If using plain films, extraperitoneal rupture demonstrates a characteristic "flame" appearance of contrast, whereas intraperitoneal rupture shows contrast surrounding loops of bowel or in the pericolic gutters.

Management of Traumatic Bladder Rupture

Patients sustaining a bladder injury, both intra- and extraperitoneal, resulting from penetrating trauma warrant surgical exploration. Associated injuries to other major organs are common. As the course of projectiles may be quite erratic, often ureteral integrity must be assessed as well.

Isolated extraperitoneal bladder rupture can be adequately managed with catheter drainage alone. A follow-up cystogram is recommended at 2 weeks to ensure complete healing before catheter removal. If patients with extraperitoneal bladder ruptures are undergoing exploration for other reasons, and the patient is not critically ill, the bladder rupture is usually repaired transvesically. However, if a larger pelvic hematoma is present, care must be taken to avoid entry into it as massive hemorrhage may ensue.

Intraperitoneal bladder ruptures should always be repaired. Although sterile, urinary leakage into the peritoneum results in a chemical peritonitis and electrolyte abnormalities. Conservative management can also result in problems resulting from persistent hematuria and bowel or omentum prolapse into the bladder injury.

Urological Oncology

Prostate Cancer

Epidemiology and Risk Factors

Prostate cancer (CaP) is the most common cancer diagnosed and is the second leading cause of cancer death in American men. In the United States, approximately 218,890 cases will be diagnosed and 27,050 deaths will result from CaP in 2007. Of all cancers, the prevalence of CaP increases the most rapidly with age. However, in contrast to most cancers, which have a peak age of incidence, the incidence of CaP continues to increase with advancing age. The lifetime risk of a 50-year-old man for latent CaP (detected as an incidental finding at autopsy, not related to the cause of death) is 40%, that for clinically apparent CaP is 9.5%, and for death from CaP it is 2.9%. Thus, many prostate cancers are indolent and inconsequential to the patient, whereas others are virulent and, if detected too late or left untreated, result in a patient's demise.

This broad spectrum of biological activity can make decision making for individual patients difficult.

Several risk factors have been identified for prostate cancer. As discussed, increasing age increases one's risk of developing CaP. What factors associated with the aging process responsible for this observation are unknown. The probability of developing CaP in a man under the age of 40 is 1 in 10,000; for men ages 40 to 59 it is 1 in 103, and for men ages 60 to 79 it is 1 in 8. African-Americans are at a higher risk of developing CaP than Caucasians. In addition, African-American men tend to present at a later stage of disease than Caucasians. Controversial data have been reported suggesting that mortality may also be greater for African-Americans.[28,29] A positive family history of CaP also increases one's relative risk of developing CaP. The age of onset of the relative diagnosed with CaP impacts a patient's relative risk. If the age of onset is at age 70, the relative risk is fourfold increased; if the age of onset is 60, the relative risk is fivefold increased; and if the age of onset is 50, the relative risk is sevenfold increased. High dietary fat intake also increases one's relative risk of developing CaP by almost a factor of 2.

Histopathology and Clinical Staging

The Gleason grading system is the most commonly employed grading system in the United States. It is truly a system that relies upon the "low-power" appearance of the glandular architecture under the microscope. In assigning a grade to a given tumor, pathologists assign a primary grade to that pattern of cancer which is most commonly observed and a secondary grade to the pattern of cancer that is the second most commonly observed grade in the specimen. Grades range from one to five. If the entire specimen has only one pattern present, then both the primary and secondary grade are reported as the same grade. The Gleason score or Gleason sum is obtained by adding the primary and secondary grades together. As Gleason grades range from 1 to 5, Gleason scores or Gleason sums thus range from 2 to 10. Well-differentiated tumors have a Gleason sum of 2 to 4, moderately differentiated tumors have a Gleason sum of 5 to 7, and poorly differentiated tumors have a Gleason sum of 8 to 10. The TNM staging system of the American Joint Cancer Committee (AJCC) for CaP is presented in Table 104.3.

TABLE 104.3. Definition of TMN, Stage Grouping, Histopathologic Type, and Histologic Grade for Prostate Carcinoma.

Definition of TMN

Primary Tumor (T)

Clinical

TX	Primary tumor cannot be assessed
T0	No evidence of primary tumor
T1	Clinically inapparent tumor neither palpable nor visible by imaging
T1a	Tumor incidental histologic finding in 5% of less of tissue resected
T1b	Tumor incidental histologic finding in more than 5% of tissue resected
T1c	Tumor identified by needle biopsy (e.g., because of elevated PSA)
T2	Tumor confined within the prostate*
T2a	Tumor involves one-half of one lobe or less
T2b	Tumor involves more than one-half of one lobe but not both lobes
T2c	Tumor involves both lobes
T3	Tumor extends through the prostate capsule**
T3a	Extracapsular extension (unilateral or bilateral)
T3b	Tumor invades seminal vesicle(s)
T4	Tumor is fixed or invades adjacent structures other than seminal vesicles: bladder neck, external sphincter, rectum, levator muscles, and/or pelvic wall

*Note: Tumor found in one or both lobes by needle biopsy, but not palpable or reliably visible by imaging, is classified as T1c.

**Note: Invasion into the prostatic apex or into (but not beyond) the prostatic capsule is classified not as T3 but as T2.

Pathologic (pT)

pT2*	Organ confined
pT2a	Unilateral, involving one-half of one lobe or less
pT2b	Unilateral involving more than one-half of one lobe but not both lobes
pT2c	Bilateral disease
pT3	Extraprostatic extension
pT3a	Extraprostatic extension**
pT3b	Seminal vesicle invasion
pT4	Invasion of bladder, rectum

*Note: There is no pathologic T1 classification.

**Note: Positive surgical margin should be indicated by an R1 descriptor (residual microscopic disease).

Regional Lymph Nodes (N)

Clinical

NX	Regional lymph nodes were not assessed
N0	No regional lymph node metastasis
N1	Metastasis in regional lymph node(s)

Pathologic

pNX	Regional nodes not sampled
pN0	No positive regional nodes
pN1	Metastases in regional node(s)

Distant Metastasis (M)*

MX	Distant metastasis cannot be assessed (not evaluated by any modality)
M0	No distant metastasis
M1	Distant metastasis
M1a	Non-regional lymph node(s)
M1b	Bone(s)
M1c	Other site(s) with or without bone disease

*Note: When more than one site of metastasis is present, the most advanced category is used. pM1c is most advanced.

Stage Grouping

Stage I	T1a	N0	M0	G1
Stage II	T1a	N0	M0	G2, 3-4
	T1b	N0	M0	Any G
	T1c	N0	M0	Any G
	T1	N0	M0	Any G
	T2	N0	M0	Any G
Stage III	T3	N0	M0	Any G
Stage IV	T4	N0	M0	Any G
	Any T	N1	M0	Any G
	Any T	Any N	M1	Any G

Source: Used with the permission of the American Joint Committee on Cancer (AJCC), Chicago, Illinois. The original source for this material is the *AJCC Cancer Staging Manual, Sixth Edition* (2002) published by Springer Science and Business Media LLC, www.springerlink.com.

Clinical Presentation

The majority of patients with early stage CaP are asymptomatic. The presence of symptoms often suggest locally advanced or metastatic disease. Obstructive or irritative voiding complaints can result from local growth of the tumor into the urethra or bladder neck or as a result of direct extension into the trigone of the bladder. Metastatic disease to the bones may result in bone pain. Metastatic disease to the vertebral column with impingement on the spinal cord may be associated with symptoms of cord compression, including paresthesias and weakness of the lower extremities and urinary or fecal incontinence.

A physical examination including a digital rectal examination (DRE) is needed. Induration, if detected, must alert the physician to the possibility of cancer and further evaluation is needed (biopsy). Locally advanced disease with bulky regional lymphadenopathy may result in lymphedema of the lower extremities.

Prostate-specific antigen (PSA) is a glycoprotein produced only in the cytoplasm of benign and malignant prostate cells. The serum level of PSA correlates with the volume of both benign and malignant prostatic tissue. With regard to prostatic carcinoma, measurement of PSA may be useful in detecting and staging prostatic cancer, monitoring response to treatment, and detecting recurrence well before it becomes obvious clinically. As a first-line screening test, PSA is elevated in approximately 8% to 15% of men self-referred for screening. Approximately 30% to 40% of men with intermediate degrees of elevation (4.1–10ng/mL; normal, <4ng/mL) will be found to have prostate cancer, and almost two-thirds of those with elevations greater than 10ng/mL have prostate cancer. Patients with intermediate levels of PSA usually have localized, and therefore potentially curable, cancers.

Transrectal ultrasound (TRUS)-guided biopsy seems to be a superior method to detect prostatic cancer compared to finger-guided biopsy. The use of a spring-loaded, 18-gauge biopsy needle has allowed transrectal biopsy to be performed with little patient discomfort and low attendant morbidity. Systematic prostate biopsy most commonly involves the taking of 10 to 12 needle cores from the apex, midsection, and base of each side of the prostate at the midsagittal line as well as the more lateral aspect of the gland. These extended systematic biopsy schemes have demonstrated an improved cancer detection rate over standard sextant biopsies. Transrectal ultrasound is useful for both performing prostatic biopsies as well as providing some useful local staging information if cancer is detected. TRUS provides more accurate local staging than DRE.[30]

When prostate cancer metastasizes, it does so most commonly to the bone. Soft tissue metastases (i.e., lung and liver) are rare at the time of initial presentation. Although a bone scan has been considered a standard part of the initial evaluation of men with newly diagnosed prostate cancer, good evidence has been accumulated that it can be excluded in the majority of such men on the basis of serum PSA. Oesterling and colleagues have conducted studies to assess the ability of serum PSA to predict bone scan findings.[31] On the basis of their results, bone scans can be omitted in patients with newly diagnosed, untreated prostate cancer who are asymptomatic and have serum PSA concentrations less than 10ng/mL.

Differential Diagnosis

Not all patients with an elevated PSA have CaP. Other factors that elevate serum PSA include benign prostatic hypertrophy (BPH), urethral instrumentation, infection, prostatic infarction, or vigorous prostate massage. Induration of the prostate can also be seen in chronic granulomatous prostatitis, prior transurethral resection of the prostate gland (TURP) or needle biopsy, or prostatic calculi.

Treatment and Prognosis

Localized Disease

General Considerations. The optimal form of treatment for all stages of CaP remains a subject of great debate. Well-designed, randomized trials comparing various treatment modalities for localized disease are lacking. Treatment dilemmas persist in the management of localized disease (T1 and T2) because of the uncertainty surrounding the relative efficacy of various treatment modalities including radical prostatectomy, radiation therapy, and surveillance. Presently, treatment decisions are based on the grade and stage of the tumor, life expectancy of the patient, the ability of each treatment to ensure disease-free survival, the morbidity of treatment, and patient and physician preferences.

Watchful Waiting. Small well-differentiated prostate cancers are often associated with very slow growth rates. Several recent publications have shown that surveillance alone may be an appropriate form of management for highly selected patients with prostate cancer (Table 104.4). However,

TABLE 104.4.
Results of Watchful Waiting Series for Prostate Cancer.

	Follow-up					
Author	*n*	*(years)*	*Overall mortality (%)*	*Disease-specific mortality (%)*	*CaP progression (%)*	*Level of evidence*
Johansson[50]	223	10.2	56	8	34	III
Whitmore[51]	75	9.5	39	15	69	III
Hanash[52]	179	15	55	45	NA	III
George[53]	120	7	44	4	83	III
Madsen[54]	50	10	52	6	18	III

most patients in such series are older and have very small, well-differentiated cancers. Even in such a selected population, cancer death rates approach 10%. In addition, endpoints for intervention in patients on surveillance regimens have not been defined. Therefore, in general, watch waiting is not recommended unless the patient has significant comorbid conditions that relatively contraindicate treatment. A recent randomized trial between watchful waiting and radical prostatectomy has demonstrated a survival advantage in patients undergoing surgery.[32]

Radical Prostatectomy. Radical prostatectomy can either be performed through a lower midline incision (radical retropubic prostatectomy) or through a perineal incision (radical perineal prostatectomy). The seminal vesicles, entire prostate, and ampullae of the vas deferens are removed. The technique has gained considerable popularity because of refinements in technique that allow for maintenance of urinary continence in almost all patients (93%) and erectile function in many patients. More recently laparoscopic and robotic prostatectomy have gained in popularity, yet comparative outcome data relative to experienced open surgeons are lacking.

The prognosis of patients treated by radical prostatectomy correlates with the pathological stage of the specimen. Patients with positive lymph nodes or seminal vesical involvement at radical prostatectomy are destined to distant failure. Fortunately, the number of these patients with these adverse prognostic factors coming to surgery are decreasing, because enhanced surgical selection has occurred as a result of appropriate use of preoperative clinical parameters as described previously. Patients with organ-confined cancer have 10-year disease-free survival ranging from 70% to 85% in several series.[33–35] Patients with focal extracapsular extension demonstrate 85% and 75% disease-free survival at 5 and 10 years, respectively. Patients with more extensive extracapsular extension demonstrate 70% and 40% disease-free survival at 5 and 10 years, respectively.[36] High-grade tumors (Gleason sum 7–10) have a higher risk of progression than low-grade tumors. Disease-free survival at 10 years for Gleason sum 2 to 6 tumors is in excess of 70%, for Gleason sum 7 it is 50%, and for Gleason sum of 8 or more it is 15%. Positive surgical margins significantly impact only upon tumors with extensive extracapsular extension.

Radiation Therapy. Radiation can be delivered by a variety of techniques, including use of external-beam radiotherapy (XRT) and transperineal implantation of radioisotopes. Morbidity is limited, and the survival of patients with localized cancers (T1, T2, and selected T3) approaches 65% at 10 years. As with surgery, the likelihood of local failure correlates with technique and tumor stage. The likelihood of a positive, prostatic biopsy more than 18 months after surgery varies between 19% and 61% in selected series. Patients with local recurrence are at an increased risk of cancer progression and cancer death compared to those with negative biopsies. Inadequate target definitions and radiation doses, and understaging of patients, may be responsible for the failure noted in some series. Newer techniques of radiation (implantation, conformal therapy using three-dimensional reconstruction of CT-based tumor volumes, heavy-particle, charged-particle, and heavy charged-particle) may improve local control rates.

Locally Advanced Disease

Radiation Therapy. The majority of patients with T3 CaP are currently treated with neoadjuvant hormonal therapy followed by external-beam radiotherapy (XRT). This approach has been proven to be superior to external-beam therapy alone in several randomized trials. One study reported on 456 evaluable patients with high-volume T2, T3, and T4 patients randomized to receive 4 months of neoadjuvant complete androgen blockade with XRT (2 months before and 2 months during XRT) compared to XRT alone and demonstrated an improvement in local control and disease-free survival in the patients treated with neoadjuvant therapy.[37] Another study reported on 401 evaluable patients with locally advanced CaP (predominantly T3) randomized to receive 3 years of androgen ablation therapy and XRT versus XRT alone and demonstrated an improved survival in patients treated with combination therapy.[38]

Metastatic Disease

Because death from CaP is almost invariably a result of failure to control metastatic disease, a great deal of research has concentrated on efforts to improve control of distant disease. It is well known that most prostatic carcinomas are hormone dependent and that approximately 70% to 80% of men with metastatic CaP respond to various forms of androgen deprivation. Testosterone, the major circulating androgen, is produced by the Leydig cells in the testes (95%), with a smaller amount being produced by peripheral conversion of other steroids. Use of a class of drugs delivered as depot injections, either monthly or, more recently, at 3-month intervals, luteinizing hormone-releasing hormone (LHRH) agonists, has allowed induction of androgen deprivation without orchiectomy or administration of diethylstilbestrol (DES). Presently, administration of LHRH agonists or orchiectomy are the most common forms of primary androgen blockade used.

Although androgen deprivation is effective, most patients with advanced disease so treated experience disease relapse, usually within 3 years. Once relapse has been identified, survival is limited. Palliative care including adequate pain control and focal irradiation of symptomatic or unstable bone disease should be instituted in patients who have failed standard hormonal therapy. Secondary therapy with chemotherapeutic agents has had limited results but should be considered in patients with a reasonable performance status. A modest survival advantage has recently been reported with the use of taxanes in hormone-refractory prostate cancer.

Kidney Cancer

Epidemiology and Risk Factors

Renal cell carcinoma (RCC) accounts for 2.3% of all adult cancers. In the United States, approximately 51,190 cases will be diagnosed and 12,890 deaths will result from RCC in 2007. RCC has a peak incidence in the sixth decade of life and has a male-to-female ratio of 2:1.

The etiology of RCC is unknown. Cigarette smoking is the only significant environmental risk factor that has been identified. Familial settings for RCC have been identified (von Hippel–Lindau syndrome), as well as an association with acquired cystic disease of renal failure, yet sporadic tumors are far more common.

Histopathology and Clinical Staging

RCC originates from the proximal tubule cells. Histological subtypes include clear cell, papillary, chromophobe, and collecting duct carcinomas. However, histological subtype does not affect treatment. The TNM classification of the AJCC for kidney cancer is shown in Table 104.5.

TABLE 104.5. Definition of TMN, Stage Grouping, Histopathologic Type, and Histologic Grade for Kidney Carcinoma.

Definition of TMN

Primary Tumor (T)

TX	Primary tumor cannot be assessed
T0	No evidence of primary tumor
T1	Tumor 7 cm or less in greatest dimension, limited to the kidney
T1a	Tumor 4 cm or less in greatest dimension, limited to the kidney
T1b	Tumor more than 4 cm but not more than 7 cm in greatest dimension, limited to the kidney
T2	Tumor more than 7 cm in greatest dimension, limited to the kidney
T3	Tumor extends into major veins or invades adrenal gland or perinephric tissues but not beyond Gerota's fascia
T3a	Tumor directly invades adrenal gland or perirenal and/or renal sinus fat but not beyond Gerota's fascia
T3b	Tumor grossly extends into the renal vein or its segmental (muscle-containing) branches, or vena cava below the diaphragm
T3c	Tumor grossly extends into vena cava above diaphragm or invades the wall of the vena cava
T4	Tumor invades beyond Gerota's fascia

Regional Lymph Nodes (N)*

NX	Regional lymph nodes cannot be assessed
N0	No regional lymph node metastasis
N1	Metastases in a single regional lymph node
N2	Metastasis in more than one regional lymph node

*Laterality does not affect the N classification.

Note: If a lymph node dissection is performed, then pathologic evaluation would ordinarily include at least eight nodes.

Distant Metastasis (M)

MX	Distant metastasis cannot be assessed
M0	No distant metastasis
M1	Distant metastasis

Stage Grouping

Stage I	T1	N0	M0
Stage II	T2	N0	M0
Stage III	T1	N1	M0
	T2	N1	M0
	T3	N0	M0
	T3	N1	M0
	T3a	N0	M0
	T3a	N1	M0
	T3b	N0	M0
	T3b	N1	M0
	T3c	N0	M0
	T3c	N1	M0
Stage IV	T4	N0	M0
	T4	N1	M0
	Any T	N2	M0
	Any T	Any N	M1

Source: Used with the permission of the American Joint Committee on Cancer (AJCC), Chicago, Illinois. The original source for this material is the *AJCC Cancer Staging Manual, Sixth Edition* (2002) published by Springer Science and Business Media LLC, www.springerlink.com.

Clinical Presentation

Historically, 60% of patients presented with gross or microscopic hematuria. Flank pain or an abdominal mass was detected in approximately 30% of cases. The triad of flank pain, hematuria, and mass was found in only 10% to 15% of patients and is often a sign of advanced disease. Symptoms of metastatic disease (cough, bone pain) occurred in 20% to 30% of patients at presentation. Of note, because of the more widespread use of ultrasound and CT scanning, more incidentally found renal tumors are detected and thus a stage migration is occurring toward lower-stage tumors.

Hematuria is seen in 60% of patients. Paraneoplastic syndromes are common in patients with RCC. Erythrocytosis occurs in 3% to 10%, hypercalcemia in 3% to 13%, and hypertension in 40% of patients. Stauffer's syndrome is a reversible syndrome of hepatic dysfunction in the absence of metastatic disease.

Renal masses are often first detected by IVP. Further evaluation requires an ultrasound to determine whether the mass is solid or cystic. CT scanning is perhaps the most valuable imaging test for RCC. It enables the determination of whether the mass is solid as well as further staging the lesion with respect to regional lymph nodes, renal vein, or hepatic involvement. It also gives valuable information on the contralateral kidney (function, bilaterality of neoplasm). Chest radiographs are necessary to exclude pulmonary metastases, and bone scans should be performed for large tumors and patients with bone pain or elevated serum levels of alkaline phosphatase. Magnetic resonance imaging (MRI) is an excellent means of assessing for the presence and extent of tumor thrombus within the renal vein or vena cava in selected patients.

Differential Diagnosis

The differential diagnosis of a renal mass starts by the determination of whether it is solid or cystic. Solid lesions of the kidney are RCC until proven otherwise. Other solid lesions involving the kidney include angiomyolipomas (fat density usually visible by CT); renal abscesses (fever, flank pain, pyuria); transitional cell cancers of the renal pelvis (more centrally located, involvement of the collecting system, positive urinary cytologies); adrenal tumors (superoanterior to kidney); and oncocytomas (indistinguishable from RCC preoperatively).

Treatment and Prognosis

Radical nephrectomy is the primary treatment for localized RCC. Tumors confined to the renal capsule (T1–T2) demonstrate 5-year disease-free survival rates of 88% to 100%. Tumors extending beyond the renal capsule (T3 or T4) and node-positive tumors have 50% to 60% and 0% to 15% 5-year disease-free survival rates, respectively.

No effective chemotherapy is available for metastatic RCC. Biological response modifiers, including alpha interferon (α-IFN) and interleukin 2 (IL-2), have received much attention. Partial response rates of 15% to 20% and 16% to 35%, respectively, have been reported. Responders tended to have lower tumor burdens (primary tumor removed), lung metastases only, and a high performance status. Multicenter trials with these agents are ongoing. In patients with metastatic disease and a good performance status, nephrectomy results in improved response rates and survival to biological response modifiers.[39]

Of note, one subgroup of metastatic patients has demonstrated long-term survival, namely, those with solitary resectable metastases. In this setting, radical nephrectomy with resection of the metastasis has resulted in 5-year disease-free survival rates of 15% to 30%.

Bladder Cancer

Epidemiology and Risk Factors

Bladder cancer is the second most common urological cancer. It occurs more commonly in men than women (2.7:1), and the mean age at diagnosis is 65 years. In the United States, approximately 67,160 cases will be diagnosed and 13,750 deaths will result from bladder cancer in 2007. Cigarette smoking and exposure to industrial dyes or solvents are risk factors for the disease and account for approximately 60% and 15% of new cases, respectively.

Pathology

Ninety-eight percent of primary bladder cancers are epithelial malignancies, with the majority being transitional cell carcinomas (90%). These latter cancers most often appear as papillary growths, but higher-grade lesions are often sessile and ulcerated. Grading is based on histological architecture: size, pleomorphism, mitotic rate, and hyperchromatism. The frequency of recurrence and progression is strongly correlated with grade. Although progression may be noted in few grade I cancers (19%–37%), it is common with poorly differentiated lesions (33%–67%). Carcinoma in situ is recognizable as a flat, nonpapillary, anaplastic epithelium and may occur focally or diffusely but is most often found in association with papillary bladder cancers. Its presence identifies a patient at an increased risk of recurrence and progression.

Adenocarcinomas and squamous cell cancers account for approximately 2% and 7% of all bladder cancers detected in the United States. The latter is often associated with bilharzias infection, vesical calculi, or chronic catheter use.

Bladder cancer staging is based on the extent of bladder wall penetration and the presence of either regional or distant metastases. The TNM classification of the AJCC for bladder cancer is shown in Table 104.6.

TABLE 104.6. Definition of TMN, Stage Grouping, Histopathologic Type, and Histologic Grade for Bladder Carcinoma.

Definition of TMN

Primary Tumor (T)

TX	Primary tumor cannot be assessed
T0	No evidence of primary tumor
Ta	Noninvasive papillary carcinoma
Tis	Carcinoma *in situ*: "flat tumor"
T1	Tumor invades subepithelial connective tissue
T2	Tumor invades muscle
pT2a	Tumor invades superficial muscle (inner half)
pT2b	Tumor invades deep muscle (outer half)
T3	Tumor invades perivesical tissue
pT3a	Microscopically
pT3b	Macroscopically (extravesical mass)
T4	Tumor invades any of the following: prostate, uterus, vagina, pelvic wall, abdominal wall
T4a	Tumor invades prostate, uterus, vagina
T4b	Tumor invades pelvic wall, abdominal wall

Regional Lymph Nodes (N)

Regional lymph nodes are those within the true pelvis; all others are distant lymph nodes.

NX	Regional lymph nodes cannot be assessed
N0	No regional lymph node metastasis
N1	Metastasis in a single lymph node, 2 cm or less in greatest dimension
N2	Metastasis in a single lymph node, more than 2 cm but not more than 5 cm in greatest dimension; or multiple lymph nodes, none more than 5 cm in greatest dimension
N3	Metastasis in a lymph node, more than 5 cm in greatest dimension

Distant Metastasis (M)

MX	Distant metastasis cannot be assessed
M0	No distant metastasis
M1	Distant metastasis

Stage Grouping

Stage 0a	Ta	N0	M0
Stage 0is	Tis	N0	M0
Stage I	T1	N0	M0
Stage II	T2a	N0	M0
	T2b	N0	M0
Stage III	T3a	N0	M0
	T3b	N0	M0
	T4a	N0	M0
Stage IV	T4b	N0	M0
	Any T	N1	M0
	Any T	N2	M0
	Any T	N3	M0
	Any T	Any N	M1

Source: Used with the permission of the American Joint Committee on Cancer (AJCC), Chicago, Illinois. The original source for this material is the *AJCC Cancer Staging Manual, Sixth Edition* (2002) published by Springer Science and Business Media LLC, www.springerlink.com.

The natural history of bladder cancer is based on two separate but related processes: tumor recurrence and progression to higher-stage disease. Both are related to tumor grade and stage. At initial presentation, approximately 50% to 80% of bladder cancers are superficial: Ta, Tis, T1. Lymph node metastases and progression are uncommon in such patients when they are properly treated, and survival is excellent at 81%. Patients with superficial cancers (Ta, T1) are treated with complete transurethral resection and the selective use of intravesical chemotherapy; the latter is used to prevent or delay recurrence. Patients who present with large, high-grade, recurrent Ta lesions, T1 cancers, and those with CIS are good candidates for intravesical chemotherapy. Patients with more invasive (T2, T3) but still localized cancers are at risk of both nodal metastases and progression, and they require more aggressive surgery, irradiation, or the combination of chemotherapy and selective surgery or irradiation because of the much higher risk of progression compared to patients with lower-stage lesions. Patients with evidence of lymph node or distant metastases should undergo systemic chemotherapy initially.

Clinical Presentation

Hematuria, gross or microscopic, chronic or intermittent, is the presenting symptom in 85% to 90% of patients with bladder cancer. Irritative voiding symptoms (urinary frequency and urgency) will occur in a small percentage of the patients because of the location or size of the cancer. Most patients with bladder cancer fail to have signs of the disease because of its superficial nature. Masses detected on bimanual exam may be present in patients with large-volume or deeply infiltrating cancers. Hepatomegaly or supraclavicular lymphadenopathy may be present in patients with metastatic disease and, rarely, lymphedema of the lower extremities may be present as the result of locally advanced cancers or metastases to pelvic lymph nodes.

A urinalysis reveals hematuria in the majority of cases. On occasion, it may be accompanied by pyuria. Azotemia may be present in a small number of cases associated with ureteral obstruction. Anemia may be the result of chronic blood loss, which is unusual, or of replacement of the bone marrow with metastatic disease. Exfoliated cells from normal and abnormal urothelium can readily be detected in voided urine specimens. Cytology may be useful in detecting the disease at the time of initial presentation or to detect recurrence. Cytology is very sensitive in detecting higher-grade and higher-stage cancers (82%–90%) but is less sensitive in detecting superficial or well-differentiated lesions (50%). Sensitivity of detection using exfoliated cells may be enhanced by flow cytometry.

Bladder cancers may be detected using intravenous urography, ultrasound, CT, or MRI where filling defects within the bladder are noted. However, the presence of cancer is confirmed by cystoscopy and biopsy, so imaging is useful primarily for evaluating the upper urinary tracts and in staging the more advanced lesions.

Treatment and Prognosis

Cystourethroscopy and Biopsy

The diagnosis and staging of bladder cancers is made by cystoscopy and transurethral resection. If cystoscopy, usually performed under local anesthesia, confirms the presence of bladder cancer, the patient is scheduled for transurethral resection under general or regional anesthesia. A careful bimanual exam is performed initially and at the end of the procedure, noting the size, position, and degree of fixation of a mass, if present. Any suspicious lesions are resected using electrocautery. Resection is carried down to the muscular elements of the bladder wall so as to allow complete staging. Random bladder and, on occasion, prostatic urethral biopsies are performed to detect occult disease elsewhere in the bladder and therefore identify patients at high risk of recurrence and progression.

Intravesical Chemotherapy

Immuno- or chemotherapeutic agents can be delivered directly into the bladder by a urethral catheter. They can be used to eradicate existing disease or to reduce the likelihood of recurrence in those who have undergone complete transurethral resection. They seem to be more effective in the latter situation. Most agents are administered weekly for 6 to 12 weeks. The use of maintenance therapy after the initial induction regimen may be beneficial. Efficacy may be increased by prolonging contact time to 2 h. Common agents include thiotepa, mitomycin C, doxorubicin, and bacillus Calmette–Guerin (BCG); the latter seems to be the most effective agent when compared to mitomycin C or doxorubicin. Side effects of intravesical chemotherapy include irritative voiding symptoms and hemorrhagic cystitis. Systemic effects are rare. Those patients who develop symptoms as a result of BCG may require antituberculous therapy.

Surgery

Although transurethral resection is the initial form of treatment for all bladder cancers because it is diagnostic, allows for proper staging, and controls superficial cancers, muscle-infiltrating cancers require more aggressive treatment. Partial cystectomy may be indicated in patients with solitary lesions and those with cancers in a bladder diverticulum. Radical cystectomy entails removal of the bladder, prostate, seminal vesicles, and surrounding fat and peritoneal attachments in men and inclusion of the uterus, cervix, urethra, anterior vaginal vault, and usually the ovaries, in addition to the bladder, in women. A bilateral pelvic lymph node dissection is performed simultaneously.

Urinary diversion can be performed using a conduit of small or large bowel. However, continent forms of diversion have been developed that avoid the necessity of an external appliance. Continent orthotopic bladder replacement may be performed in select men and women. Such diversions utilize segments of small bowel, which are detubularized and reconfigured into a sphere and are then anastomosed to the urethra.

Radiotherapy

External-beam radiotherapy delivered in fractions over a 6- to 8-week period is generally well tolerated, but approximately 10% to 15% of patients will develop bladder, bowel, or rectal complications. Unfortunately, local recurrence is common after radiotherapy (33%–68%). Increasingly, radiotherapy is being combined with systemic chemotherapy in an effort to improve local and distant relapse rates.

Chemotherapy

Fifteen percent of patients with newly diagnosed bladder cancer present with metastatic disease, and 40% of those thought to have localized disease at the time of cystectomy or definitive radiotherapy develop metastases, usually within 2 years of treatment. Cisplatin-based, combination chemotherapy will result in partial or complete response in 13% to 37% and 17% to 47% of patients, respectively. The most active regimens tested to date include MVAC (methotrexate, velban, doxorubicin, cisplatin) and CMV (cisplatin, methotrexate, velban). The median response in those who achieve a complete response is approximately 14 to 38 months. More recently, less toxic regimens consisting of carboplatinum and the taxanes or cisplatin and gemcitabine have been investigated in phase II clinical trials.

Combination chemotherapy has been integrated into trials of surgery and radiotherapy. It has been used before each (neoadjuvant) in an attempt to preserve the bladder and decrease recurrence rates. Alternatively, it has been used postoperatively (adjuvant) in patients who have undergone cystectomy and have been found to be at high risk of recurrence (P3 or N1). Both approaches seem to have merit and are the subject of ongoing clinical trials.

Testicular Cancer

Epidemiology and Risk Factors

Malignant tumors of the testis are rare, with approximately 9 new cases per 100,000 males being reported in the United

States each year. Ninety percent to 95% of all primary testicular tumors are germ cell tumors (seminoma and nonseminoma) while the remainder are nongerminal neoplasms (Leydig cell, Sertoli cell, gonadoblastoma). For the purposes of this review, we only consider germ cell tumors. The lifetime probability of developing testicular cancer is 0.2% for an American white male. Survival in testis cancer has improved dramatically in recent years as a result of the development and application of effective combination chemotherapy. Overall 5-year survival rates have increased from 78% in 1974–1976 to 91% in 1980–1985 ($P < 0.05$).

Testis cancer is slightly more common on the right than on the left, which parallels the increased incidence of cryptorchidism on the right side. One percent to 2% of primary testis tumors are bilateral and up to 50% of these men have a history of uni- or bilateral cryptorchidism. Primary bilateral testis tumors may occur synchronously or asynchronously but tend to be of the same histology. Seminoma is the most common histology in bilateral *primary* testis tumors whereas malignant lymphoma is the most common bilateral testis tumor.

Although the etiology of testis cancer is unknown, both congenital and acquired factors have been associated with tumor development. Approximately 6% of testis tumors develop in a patient with a history of cryptorchidism, with seminoma being the most common.[40] However, 5% to 10% of these tumors occur in the contralateral, normally descended testis. The relative risk of development of malignancy is highest for the intraabdominal testis (1 in 20) and is lower for the inguinal testis (1 in 80). Placement of the cryptorchid testis into the scrotum (orchiopexy) does not alter the malignant potential of the cryptorchid testis; however, it does facilitate examination and tumor detection.

Exogenous estrogen administration during pregnancy has been associated with an increased relative risk for testis tumors, ranging from 2.8 to 5.3.[41,42] Other acquired factors such as trauma and infection-related testicular atrophy have been associated with testicular tumors; however, a causal relationship has not been established.

Pathology

From a treatment standpoint, testicular carcinoma can be divided into two major categories: (1) nonseminomas, which include embryonal cell carcinomas (20%), teratomas (5%), choriocarcinomas (<1%), and mixed-cell types (40%); and (2) seminomas (35%). Many clinical staging systems have been proposed for nonseminoma testis cancer; however, most are variations of the original system proposed by Boden and Gibb in 1951.[43] In this system, a stage A lesion was confined to the testis, stage B demonstrated regional lymph node spread to the retroperitoneum, and stage C was spread beyond retroperitoneal lymph nodes. For seminoma, the M.D. Anderson system is commonly used. In this system a stage I lesion is confined to the testis, a stage II lesion has spread to the retroperitoneal lymph nodes, and a stage III lesion has supradiaphragmatic nodal or visceral involvement. The TNM classification of the AJCC for testis cancer is shown in Table 104.7.

Patterns of Spread

With the exception of choriocarcinoma, which demonstrates early hematogenous spread, germ cell tumors of the testis typically spread via lymphatics in a stepwise fashion. Lymph nodes of the testis extend from T1 to L4 but are concentrated at the level of the renal hilum as a consequence of their common embryological origin with the kidney. The primary landing site for the right testis is the interaortocaval area at the level of the right renal hilum. Stepwise spread, in order, is to the precaval, preaortic, paracaval, right common iliac, and right external iliac lymph nodes. The primary landing site for the left testis is the periaortic area at the level of the left renal hilum. Stepwise spread, in order, is to the preaortic, left common iliac, and left external iliac lymph nodes. In the absence of disease on the left side, no crossover metastases to the right side have ever been identified. However, right-to-left crossover metastases are common.[44,45] These observations have resulted in modified surgical dissections to preserve ejaculation in select patients (see following).

Certain factors may alter the primary drainage of a testis neoplasm. Invasion of the epididymis or spermatic cord may allow spread to the distal external iliac and obturator lymph nodes. Scrotal violation or invasion of the tunica albuginea may result in inguinal metastases.

The retroperitoneum is the site most commonly involved in metastatic disease; however, visceral metastases may be seen in advanced disease. The sites involved in decreasing frequency include lung, liver, brain, bone, kidney, adrenal, gastrointestinal tract, and spleen.[46]

As mentioned, choriocarcinoma is the exception to the rule and is characterized by early hematogenous spread, especially to the lung. Choriocarcinoma also has a predilection for unusual sites of metastasis such as the spleen.

Clinical Presentation

The most common symptom of testis cancer is a painless enlargement of the testis. Sensations of heaviness are not unusual. Patients are usually the first to recognize an abnormality, yet the typical delay in seeking medical attention ranges from 3 to 6 months. Acute testicular pain resulting from intratesticular hemorrhage occurs in approximately 10% of cases. Ten percent of patients are asymptomatic at presentation, and 10% manifest symptoms relating to metastatic disease such as back pain (retroperitoneal metastases), cough (pulmonary metastases), or lower extremity edema (vena cava obstruction).

A testicular mass or diffuse enlargement of the testis is found in the majority of cases on physical examination. Secondary hydroceles may be present in 5% to 10% of cases. In advanced disease, supraclavicular adenopathy may be detected, and abdominal examination may palpate a retroperitoneal mass. Gynecomastia is seen in 5% of germ cell tumors.

Several biochemical markers are important in the diagnosis and treatment of testicular carcinoma, including human chorionic gonadotropin (hCG), alpha-fetoprotein (AFP), and lactic acid dehydrogenase (LDH). AFP is never elevated in seminomas and, although hCG is occasionally elevated in seminomas, levels tend to be lower than those seen in nonseminomas. LDH may be elevated in either type of tumor. Liver function tests may be elevated in the presence of hepatic metastases, and anemia may be present in advanced disease. In patients with advanced disease who will receive chemotherapy, renal function is assessed with a 24-h creatinine clearance urine collection.

TABLE 104.7. Definition of TMN, Serum Tumor Markers, Stage Grouping, and Histopathologic Type for Testis Carcinoma.

Definition of TMN

Primary Tumor (T)

The extent of primary tumor is usually classified after radical orchiectomy, and for this reason, a *pathologic* stage is assigned.

*pTX	Primary tumor cannot be assessed
pT0	No evidence of primary tumor (e.g., histologic scar in testis)
pTis	Intratubular germ cell neoplasia (carcinoma *in situ*)
pT1	Tumor limited to the testis and epididymis without vascular/lymphatic invasion; tumor may invade into the tunica albuginea but not the tunica vaginalis
pT2	Tumor limited to the testis and epididymis with vascular/lymphatic invasion, or tumor extending through the tunica albuginea with involvement of the tunica vaginalis
pT3	Tumor invades the spermatic cord with or without vascular/lymphatic invasion
pT4	Tumor invades the scrotum with or without vascular/lymphatic invasion

*Note: Except for pTis and pT4, extent of primary tumor is classified by radical orchiectomy. TX may be used for other categories in the absence of radical orchiectomy.

Regional Lymph Nodes (N)

Clinical

NX	Regional lymph nodes cannot be assessed
N0	No regional lymph node metastasis
N1	Metastasis with a lymph node mass 2 cm or less in greatest dimension; or multiple lymph nodes, none more than 2 cm in greatest dimension
N2	Metastasis in a lymph node mass more than 2 cm but not more than 5 cm in greatest dimension; or multiple lymph nodes, any one mass greater than 2 cm but not more than 5 cm in greatest dimension
N3	Metastasis with a lymph node mass more than 5 cm in greatest dimension

Pathologic (pN)

pNX	Regional lymph nodes cannot be assessed
pN0	No regional lymph node metastasis
pN1	Metastasis with a lymph node mass 2 cm or less in greatest dimension and less than or equal to 5 nodes positive, none more than 2 cm in greatest dimension
pN2	Metastasis with a lymph node mass more than 2 cm but not more than 5 cm in greatest dimension; or more than 5 nodes positive, none more than 5 cm; or evidence of extranodal extension of tumor
pN3	Metastasis with a lymph node mass more than 5 cm in greatest dimension

Distant Metastasis (M)

MX	Distant metastasis cannot be assessed
M0	No distant metastasis
M1	Distant metastasis
M1a	Non-regional nodal or pulmonary metastasis
M1b	Distant metastasis other than to non-regional lymph nodes and lungs

Serum Tumor Markers (S)

SX	Marker studies not available or not performed
S0	Marker study levels within normal limits
S1	LDH < 1.5 × N* **AND** hCG (mIu/ml) < 5000 **AND** AFP (ng/ml) < 1000
S2	LDH 1.5–10 × N **OR** hCG (mIu/ml) 5000–50,000 **OR** AFP (ng/ml) 1000–10,000
S3	LDH > 10 × N **OR** hCG (mIu/ml) > 50,000 **OR** AFP (ng/ml) > 10,000

*N indicates the upper limit of normal for the LDH assay.

Stage Grouping

Stage 0	pTis	N0	M0	S0
Stage I	pT1-4	N0	M0	SX
Stage IA	pT1	N0	M0	S0
Stage IB	pT2	N0	M0	S0
	pT3	N0	M0	S0
	pT4	N0	M0	S0
Stage IS	Any pT/Tx	N0	M0	S1-3
Stage II	Any pT/Tx	N1-3	M0	SX
Stage IIA	Any pT/Tx	N1	M0	S0
	Any pT/Tx	N1	M0	S1
Stage IIB	Any pT/Tx	N2	M0	S0
	Any pT/Tx	N2	M0	S1
Stage IIC	Any pT/Tx	N3	M0	S0
	Any pT/Tx	N3	M0	S1
Stage III	Any pT/Tx	Any N	M1	SX
Stage IIIA	Any pT/Tx	Any N	M1a	S0
	Any pT/Tx	Any N	M1a	S1
Stage IIIB	Any pT/Tx	N1-3	M0	S2
	Any pT/Tx	Any N	M1a	S2
Stage IIIC	Any pT/Tx	N1-3	M0	S3
	Any pT/Tx	Any N	M1a	S3
	Any pT/Tx	Any N	M1b	Any S

Source: Used with the permission of the American Joint Committee on Cancer (AJCC), Chicago, Illinois. The original source for this material is the *AJCC Cancer Staging Manual, Sixth Edition* (2002) published by Springer Science and Business Media LLC, www.springerlink.com.

Scrotal ultrasound can readily determine whether the mass is intra- or extratesticular in origin. Once the diagnosis of testicular cancer has been established by inguinal orchiectomy, clinical staging of the disease is accomplished by chest radiography (CXR) and abdominal and pelvic CT.

Differential Diagnosis

An incorrect diagnosis is made at the initial examination in up to 25% of patients with testicular tumors. The differential diagnosis of scrotal masses includes epididymitis, spermatoceles, hydroceles, varicoceles, and hernias. Scrotal ultrasonography should be performed if any uncertainty exists with respect to the diagnosis. Although most intratesticular masses are malignant, one benign lesion, an epidermoid cyst, may rarely been seen. Usually these are very small benign nodules located just underneath the tunica albuginea, but on occasion they can be large.

Treatment and Prognosis

Inguinal exploration with early vascular control of the spermatic cord structures is the initial intervention to exclude neoplasm. If cancer cannot be excluded by examination of the testis, then radical orchiectomy is warranted. Scrotal approaches and open testicular biopsies should be avoided. Further therapy is dependent upon the histology of the tumor as well as the clinical stage.

Five-year disease-free survival rates for stage I seminomas treated by radical orchiectomy and retroperitoneal irradiation (2500–3000 cGy). Higher-stage seminomas involving the retroperitoneum and stage III receive primary chemotherapy (etoposide and cisplatin or cisplatin, etoposide and bleomycin); 95% of patients with stage III disease attain a complete response following orchiectomy and chemotherapy. Surgical resection of residual retroperitoneal masses is only warranted if the mass is larger than 3 cm in diameter, under which circumstances 40% will harbor residual carcinoma.

Up to 75% of stage A nonseminomas are cured by orchiectomy alone. Currently such patients may be treated by modified retroperitoneal lymph node dissections designed to preserve the sympathetic innervation for seminal fluid emission. Select patients who meet specific criteria may be offered surveillance. These criteria are (1) tumor is confined within the tunica albuginea, (2) tumor does not demonstrate vascular invasion, (3) tumor markers normalize after orchiectomy, (4) radiographic imaging shows no evidence of disease (CXR and CT), and (5) the patient is considered reliable. Surveillance should be considered an active process on the part of both the physician and the patient. Patients are followed monthly for the first 2 years and bimonthly in the third year. Tumor markers are obtained at each visit, and CXR and CT scans are obtained every 3 to 4 months. Follow-up continues beyond the initial 3 years; however, the majority of relapses occur within the first 8 to 10 months. With rare exception, patients who relapse can be cured by chemotherapy and/or surgery. The 5-year disease-free survival for patients with stage A disease ranges from 96% to 100%. For low-volume stage B disease, a 90% 5-year disease-free survival rate is attainable.

Patients with bulky retroperitoneal disease (>3-cm nodes) or metastatic nonseminoma are treated with primary platinum-based combination chemotherapy following orchiectomy (etoposide and cisplatin or cisplatin, etoposide and bleomycin). If tumor markers normalize and a residual mass is apparent on imaging studies, then resection of that mass is mandatory because 20% of the time it will harbor residual cancer, 40% of the time it will be teratoma, and 40% of the time it will be necrosis. Even if patients have a complete response to chemotherapy, a recent study suggests that retroperitoneal lymphadenectomy is warranted in some patients as 10% of patients may harbor residual carcinoma and 10% may have teratoma in the retroperitoneum. If tumor markers fail to normalize following primary chemotherapy, then salvage or high-dose chemotherapy is required (cisplatin, etoposide, bleomycin, ifosfamide). Patients with bulky retroperitoneal or disseminated disease treated with primary chemotherapy followed by surgery have a 5-year disease-free survival rate of 55% to 80%.

References

1. Moore EE, Shackford SR, Pachter HL, et al. Organ injury scaling: spleen, liver and kidney. J Trauma 1989;29:1664–1666.
2. Miller KS, McAninch JW. Radiographic assessment of renal trauma: our 15-year experience. J Urol 1995;154:352–355.
3. Wein AJ, Murphy JJ, Mulholland SG, et al. A conservative approach to the management of blunt renal trauma. J Urol 1977;117:425–427.
4. Nash PA, Bruce JE, McAninch JW. Nephrectomy for traumatic renal injuries. J Urol 1995;153:609–611.
5. Carroll PR, Klosterman P, McAninch JW. Early vascular control for renal trauma: a critical review. J Urol 1989;141:826–829.
6. McAninch JW, Carroll PR, Armenakas NA, et al. Renal gunshot wounds: methods of salvage and reconstruction. J Trauma 1993;35:279–283.
7. Daly JW, Higgins KA. Injury to the ureter during gynecologic procedures. Surg Gynecol Obstet 1988;167:19–22.
8. Higgins CC. Ureteral injuries during surgery. JAMA 1967; 199:82.
9. Blasco FJ, Saladie JM. Ureteral obstruction and ureteral fistula after aortofemoral or aortoiliac bypass surgery. J Urol 1991; 145:237–242.
10. Bec A. Ureteric injury during laminectomy for a prolapsed disc. Br J Urol 1989;63:552–553.
11. Woodland MB. Ureter injury during laparoscopy-assisted vaginal hysterectomy with the endoscopic lineal stapler. Am J Obstet Gynecol 1992;167:756–757.
12. Saidi MH, Sadler RK, Vancaillie TG, et al. Diagnosis and management of serious urinary complications after major operative laparoscopy. Obstet Gynecol 1996;87:272–276.
13. McGinty DM, Mendez R. Traumatic ureteral injuries with delayed recognition. Urology 1977;10:115–117.
14. Holden S, Hicks CC, O'Brien DP, et al. Gunshot wounds of the ureter: a 15-year review of 63 consecutive cases. J Urol 1976;116:562–564.
15. Walker JA. Injuries of the ureter due to external violence. J Urol 1969;102:410–413.
16. Cass AS. Ureteral contusion with gunshot wounds. J Trauma 1984;24:59–60.
17. Reznichek RC, Brosman SA, Rhodes DB. Ureteral avulsion from blunt trauma. J Urol 1973;109:812–816.
18. Presti JC Jr, Carroll PR, McAninch JW. Ureteral and renal pelvic injuries from external trauma: diagnosis and management. J Trauma 1989;29:370–374.
19. Campbell EW, Filderman PS, Jacobs SC. Ureteral injury due to blunt and penetrating trauma. Urology 1992;40:216–220.
20. Peterson NE, Pitts JC. Penetrating injuries of the ureter. J Urol 1981;126:587–590.
21. Liroff SA, Pontes JES, Pierce JM Jr. Gunshot wounds of the ureter: 5 years of experience. J Urol 1977;118:551–553.
22. Carlton CE Jr, Scott R Jr, Guthrie AG. The initial management of ureteral injuries: a report of 78 cases. J Urol 1971;105:335–341.
23. Eickenberg H, Amin M. Gunshot wounds to the ureter. J Trauma 1976;16:562–565.
24. Lankford R, Block NL, Politano VA. Gunshot wounds of the ureter: a review of ten cases. J Trauma 1974;14:848–852.
25. Goldman SM, Fishman EK, Gatewood OMD, et al. CT in the diagnosis of enterovesical fistula. Am J Radiol 1985;144:1229–1233.
26. Karamchandani MC, West CF. Vesicoenteric fistulas. Am J Surg 1984;147:681–683.
27. Mee SL, McAninch JW, Federle MP. Computerized tomography in bladder rupture—diagnostic limitations. J Urol 1987;137:207–209.
28. Morton RA Jr. Racial differences in adenocarcinoma of the prostate in North American men. Urology 1994;44:637–645.
29. Fowler JE Jr, Terrell F. Survival in blacks and whites after treatment for localized prostate cancer. J Urol 1996;156:133–136.
30. Perrapato SD, Carothers GG, Maatman TJ, et al. Comparing clinical staging plus transrectal ultrasound with surgical-pathological staging of prostate cancer. Urology 1989;33:103–105.

31. Oesterling J, Martin SK, Bergstralh EJ, et al. The use of prostate-specific antigen in staging patients with newly diagnosed prostate cancer. JAMA 1993;269:57–60.
32. Walsh PC, Partin AW, Epstein JI. Cancer control and quality of life following anatomical radical retropubic prostatectomy: results at 10 years. J Urol 1994;152:1831–1836.
33. Holmberg L, Bill-Axelson A, Helgesen F, et al. A randomized trial comparing radical prostatectomy with watchful waiting in early prostate cancer. N Engl J Med 2002;347:781–789.
34. Paulson DF. Impact of radical prostatectomy in the management of clinically localized disease. J Urol 1994;152:1826–1830.
35. Trapasso JG, deKernion JB, Smith RB, et al. The incidence and significance of detectable levels of serum prostate specific antigen after radical prostatectomy. J Urol 1994;152:1821–1825.
36. Epstein JI, Carmichael MJ, Pizov G, et al. Influence of capsular penetration on progression following radical prostatectomy: a study of 196 cases with long term follow-up. J Urol 1993;150:135–141.
37. Pilepich MV, Krall JM, al-Sarraf M, et al. Androgen deprivation with radiation therapy compared with radiation therapy alone for locally advanced prostatic carcinoma: a randomized comparative trial of the Radiation Therapy Oncology Group. Urology 1995;45:616–623.
38. Bolla M, Gonzalez D, Warde P, et al. Improved survival in patients with locally advanced prostate cancer treated with radiotherapy and goserelin. N Engl J Med 1997;337:295–300.
39. Flanigan RC, Salmon SE, Blumenstein BA, et al. Nephrectomy followed by interferon alpha 2b compared with interferon alpha 2b alone for metastatic renal cell cancer. N Engl J Med 2001;345:1655–1659.
40. Batata MA, Chu FCH, Hilaris BS, et al. Testicular cancer in cryptorchids. Cancer (Phila) 1982;49:1023–1030.
41. Henderson BE, Ross RK, Pike MC. Epidemiology of testicular cancer. In: Skinner DG, Lieskovsky G, eds. Diagnosis and Management of Genitourinary Cancer. Philadelphia: Saunders, 1988.
42. Schottenfeld D, Warshauer ME, Sherlock S, et al. The epidemiology of testicular cancer in young adults. Am J Epidemiol 1980;112:232–246.
43. Boden G, Gibb R. Radiotherapy and testicular neoplasms. Lancet 1951;2:1195–1202.
44. Donahue JP, Zachary JM, Magnard BR. Distribution of nodal metastases in nonseminomatous testis cancer. J Urol 1982; 128:315–320.
45. Biswamay R, Hajdu SI, Whitmore WF Jr. Distribution of retroperitoneal lymph node metastases in testicular germinal tumors. Cancer (Phila) 1974;33:340–348.
46. Bredael JJ, Vugrin D, Whitmore WF Jr. Autopsy findings in 154 patients with germ cell tumors of the testis. Cancer (Phila) 1982;50:548–551.
47. Stutzman RE. Ballistics and the management of ureteral injuries from high velocity missiles. J Urol 1977;118:947–949.
48. Steers WD, Corriere JN Jr, Benson GS, et al. The use of indwelling ureteral stents in managing ureteral injuries due to external violence. J Trauma 1985;25:1001–1003.
49. Rober PE, Smith JB, Pierce JM. Gunshot injuries of the ureter. J Trauma 1990;30:83–86.
50. Johansson J-E, Adami H-O, Andersson S-O, et al. High 10-year survival rate in patients with early, untreated prostatic cancer. JAMA 1992;267:2191–2196.
51. Whitmore WF, Warner JA, Thompson IM. Expectant management of localized prostatic cancer. Cancer (Phila) 1991;67:1091–1096.
52. Hanash KA, Utz DC, Cook EN, et al. Carcinoma of the prostate: a 15 year follow-up. J Urol 1972;107:450–453.
53. George NJR. Natural history of localized prostatic cancer managed by conservative therapy alone. Lancet 1988;1:494–497.
54. Madsen PO, Graverson PH, Gasser TC, et al. Treatment of localized prostatic cancer: radical prostatectomy versus placebo: a 15 year follow-up. Scand J Urol Nephrol Suppl 1988;110: 95–100.

105

Gynecology

Hillary B. Boswell, Janet S. Rader, and David E. Cohn

Given the anatomic proximity of the female reproductive system to other abdominal and pelvic structures, surgeons commonly find themselves faced with a decision regarding these organs. Similarly, the overlap of signs and symptoms in gynecological and surgical diseases commonly leads to the inclusion of a gynecological disease in a differential diagnosis.[1] Thus, it is imperative that the surgeon has a general understanding of operative and nonoperative gynecology.

Reproductive Anatomy

The organs of the female reproductive system develop embryologically with the gastrointestinal and urinary systems, and their anatomic relationships account for the overlap in signs and symptoms of gynecological disease and other surgical disorders. The vulva, labia, clitoris, and urethra are visible on the perineum and are thus designated the external genitalia (Fig. 105.1). Bartholin's glands are small, paired glands located at the 4 and 8 o'clock positions of the vulva, whose ducts are approximately 2 cm in length. Infection arising in these glands or ducts leads to vulvovaginal pain, erythema, and swelling (Fig. 105.2). Treatment is generally conservative in mild cases, employing hot compresses and analgesics, but incision and drainage may be necessary in severe, recurrent, or persistent cases. This intervention may be accomplished by making a small incision along the vaginal margin of the enlarged gland and inserting a Word catheter for continuous drainage over a 4- to 6-week period. The gland may also be marsupialized, where the edges are sewn to the surrounding vaginal mucosa. Definitive surgery involves resection of the duct and gland. There exists small risk of malignancy in an enlarged Bartholin's gland after the age of 40; however, there are no data to support the routine excision of enlarged glands to obtain a histological diagnosis.[2]

The vagina extends from the vulva to the uterine cervix; it is a collapsed fibromuscular tube composed of stratified, nonkeratinizing squamous epithelium, which, similar to the cervix, can harbor a preinvasive or invasive neoplasm. Given the anatomic proximity of the vagina and uterus to the bladder and rectum (Fig. 105.3), infection in one organ may lead to symptoms referred to the other. The cervix is the fibrous opening to the uterus. It is covered by stratified squamous epithelium (ectocervix) and columnar epithelium (endocervix). The Papanicolaou smear, which is used as a screening tool for preinvasive and invasive cervical neoplasia, evaluates cells sampled from both ectocervix and endocervix. The arterial supply of the cervix arises from the descending branch of the uterine artery, with rich anastomoses with the vaginal and middle hemorrhoidal systems. The ureter, which is approximately 1.5 cm lateral to the internal os of the uterine cervix, is most commonly injured at this anatomic location during hysterectomy (Fig. 105.4).

The uterus continues from the cervix cephalad and is composed of a visceral peritoneum, a middle layer of smooth muscle (the myometrium), and an inner lining (the endometrium). The vascular supply of the uterus is derived from the uterine arteries, a branch of the internal iliac artery, as well as the ovarian arteries from the aorta. Clinically, this is important as the lymphatic drainage from the uterus is through the pelvic as well as paraaortic lymph nodes, and metastatic disease may be present in both these regions. The uterine artery crosses over the ureter near the cervix within the broad ligament (Fig. 105.4). The fallopian tubes arise from the superolateral aspects of the uterus. The mesosalpinx is the anastomosis of the termination of the uterine and ovarian arteries, which supply the fallopian tubes. A ruptured ectopic pregnancy may cause significant bleeding because of the rich vascularization. The ovaries are suspended laterally from the uterus by the uteroovarian ligament. The lateral pole of the ovary is suspended by the suspensory ligament of the ovary,

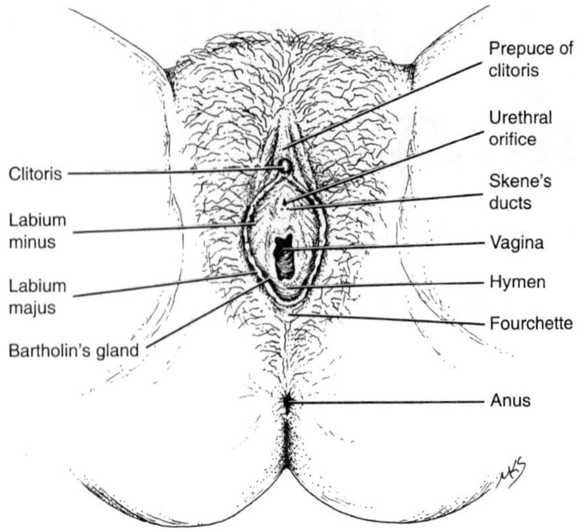

FIGURE 105.1. Diagram of female external genitalia.

also known as the infundibulopelvic ligament. Within it run the ovarian vessels, branching from the aorta below the renal arteries. During laparotomy for certain gynecological cancers, the lymph nodes are sampled in the pelvis, along the aorta, and to the level of the renal arteries.

Physiology of the Reproductive System

The physiology of the reproductive system involves endocrine organs acting in concert to secrete hormones that act interdependently (Fig. 105.5).[3] These organs include the hypothalamus (gonadotropin-releasing hormone, GnRH), pituitary gland (luteinizing hormone, LH, and follicle-stimulating hormone, FSH), ovaries (androgens, estrogens, and progesterone), and the uterus. The hypothalamus is the major regulatory organ for the hormones involved in reproductive endocrinology. The pulsatile release of GnRH has been demonstrated to be critical for proper function of the reproductive apparatus, in that some women with altered GnRH pulse frequency or amplitude develop anovulation. GnRH analogues have demonstrated utility in inducing a "chemical menopause" through the saturation of pituitary GnRH receptors and subsequent downregulation of the hormonal cascade. Thus, GnRH analogues are useful in treating hormonally sensitive conditions such as uterine leiomyomata (fibroids) and endometriosis.

The pulsatile stimulation of GnRH on the gonadotrope cells of the anterior pituitary leads to the release of the gonadotropins LH and FSH. LH and FSH share the same alpha-subunit, which is similar to the alpha-subunit of both thyroid-stimulating hormone (TSH) and human chorionic

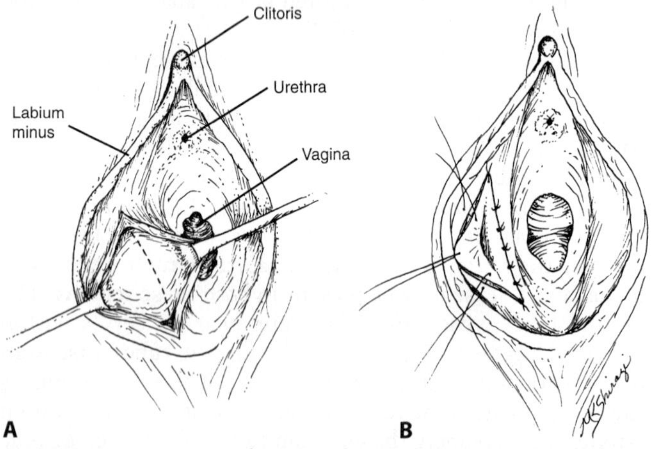

FIGURE 105.2. Marsupialization of a Bartholin's gland abscess. **A.** When the duct of Bartholin's gland becomes blocked, a small incision through the vaginal epithelium into Bartholin's gland can be made to relieve pressure. **B.** The cyst wall is then sutured to the vaginal epithelium to allow for continued drainage.

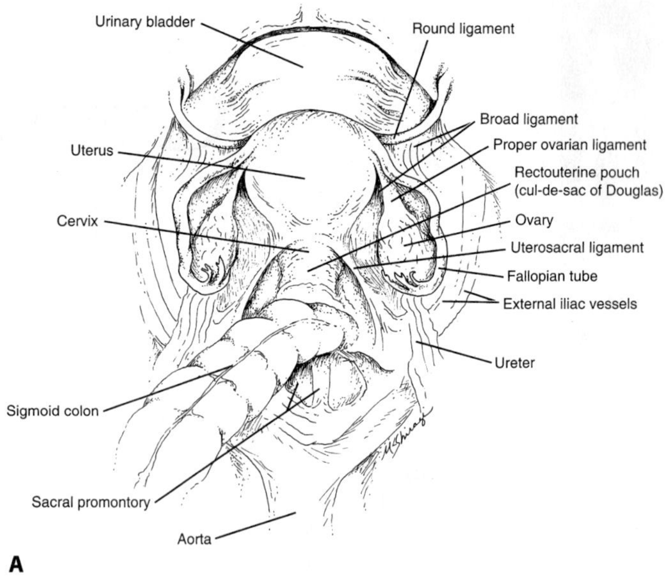

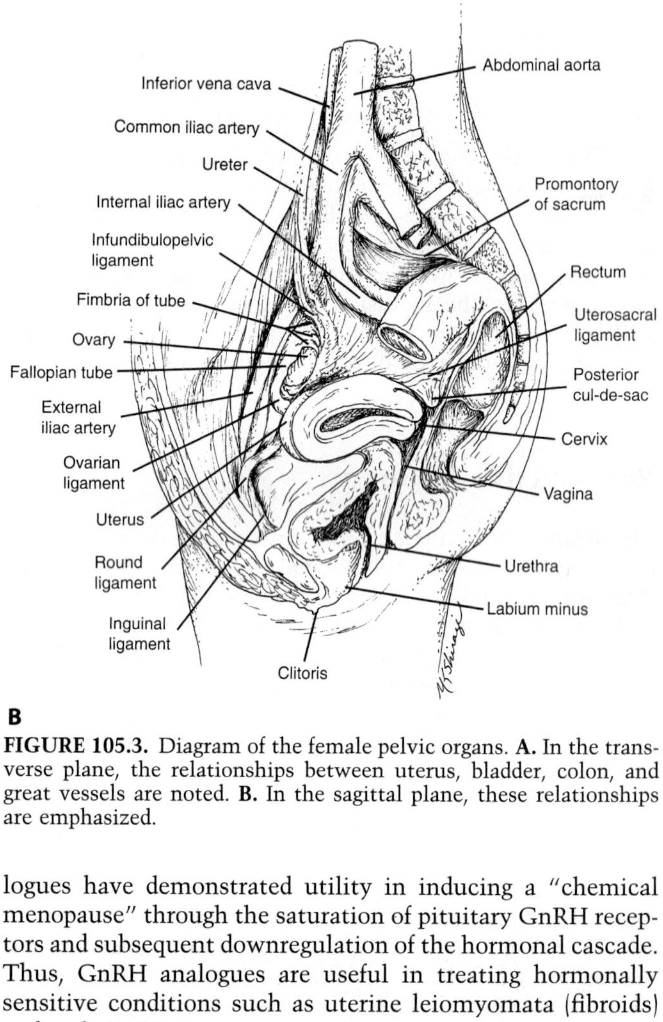

FIGURE 105.3. Diagram of the female pelvic organs. **A.** In the transverse plane, the relationships between uterus, bladder, colon, and great vessels are noted. **B.** In the sagittal plane, these relationships are emphasized.

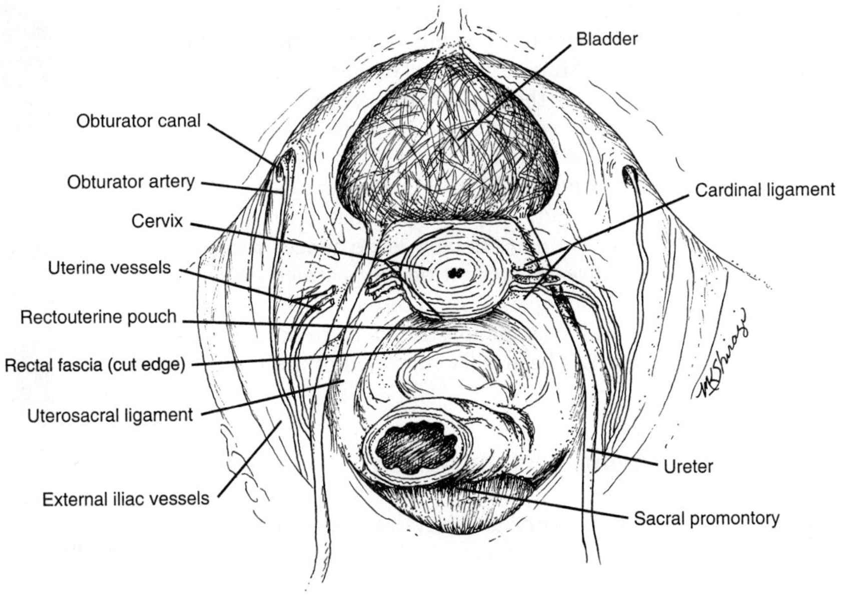

FIGURE 105.4. Relationship between ureter, cervix, and uterine artery. With the body of the uterus removed at the level of the uterine blood vessels (at the endocervix), the ureter runs below the uterine artery, approximately 1.5 cm lateral to the cervix.

gonadotropin (hCG). LH acts primarily on the theca cells of the ovary to induce steroidogenesis, whereas FSH acts on the granulosa cells of the ovary to stimulate follicle growth. Under the influence of LH on the theca cells, the ovary synthesizes androgens (androstenedione and testosterone), which are converted to estrogens (estrone and estradiol) in the granulosa cells by the enzyme aromatase under the influence of FSH. Estrogen is then utilized by target organs, such as the uterus. Fine control of estrogen, progesterone, FSH, and LH is required for the appropriate timing of the menstrual cycle (see Fig. 105.5). During the first half of the menstrual cycle (days 1–14), FSH increases during this follicular phase of the cycle, with a sharp peak at midcycle (day 14) and a subsequent decline during the luteal phase (days 15–28). This rise in FSH stimulates the ovarian follicles, leading to an estrogen-dominated cycle before ovulation (day 14). LH levels are generally low during both the follicular and luteal phases but increase sharply before ovulation. This precipitous rise in LH acting on an FSH-primed follicle leads to ovulation. During the luteal phase of the menstrual cycle, LH and FSH levels decline, and the corpus luteum of the ovary begins producing progesterone, which dominates this half of the menstrual cycle. If no embryo is implanted into the endometrium, menstruation occurs because progesterone levels decline as a result of the regression of the corpus luteum.

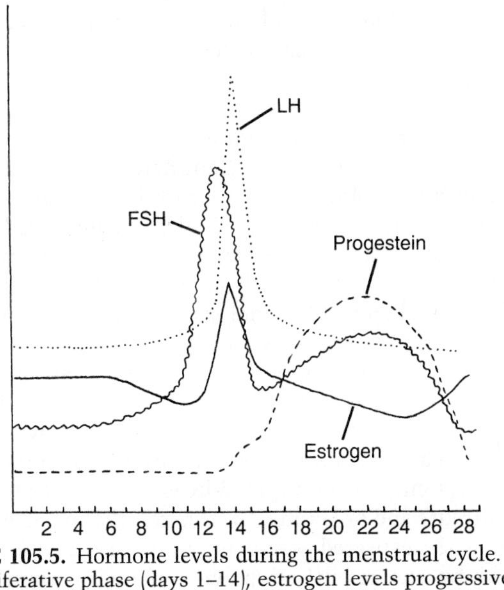

FIGURE 105.5. Hormone levels during the menstrual cycle. During the proliferative phase (days 1–14), estrogen levels progressively rise. Ovulation (day 14) is preceded by an increase in the gonadotropins, and is signaled by a sharp rise in luteinizing hormone (*LH*). During the secretory phase (days 15–28), the corpus luteum produces increasing levels of progesterone. In the absence of fertilization, menstruation (days 1–5) occurs as the endometrium is shed. *FSH*, follicle-stimulating hormone.

During menopause, FSH levels rise in an effort to continue ovarian production of estrogen. Given the lack of ovarian estrogen production, no negative feedback to FSH production exists, resulting in the elevated FSH levels that indicate menopause. Signs and symptoms of menopause include abnormal bleeding (increased or decreased, irregular intervals), infertility, vasomotor instability (hot flashes), psychological symptoms (anxiety, irritability, or depression), and atrophy of the vaginal epithelium. Before the findings of the Women's Health Initiative randomized controlled primary prevention trial, hormone replacement therapy was routinely used for symptom management as well as prevention of osteoporosis and heart disease. The study was stopped early when the risks of estrogen plus progesterone therapy were determined to outweigh the benefits (Table 105.1).[4] Coronary

TABLE 105.1. Risks Versus Benefits of Estrogen Plus Progesterone Therapy.

Excess risks per 10,000 person-years	*Risk reductions per 10,000 person-years*
+7 more cardiac events	–6 fewer colorectal cancers
+8 more strokes	–5 fewer hip fractures
+8 more pulmonary emboli	
+8 more invasive breast cancers	

Source: Writing Group for Women's Health Initiative Investigators. Rossouw JE, et al. Risks and benefits of estrogen plus progestin in healthy postmenopausal women: principal results from the Women's Health Initiative randomized controlled trial. JAMA 2002;288(3):321–333.[4]

heart disease, stroke, and venous thromboembolic disease were all increased in women assigned to treatment with estrogen plus progestin. Similar findings were associated with the estrogen alone arm of the study,[5] and review of studies using different preparations or methods of investigation also suggested that the risk–benefit analysis reported by the Women's Health Initiative study could be generalized to all hormone replacement therapy products.[6] Based on these studies, hormone replacement therapy is no longer recommended for chronic disease prevention in postmenopausal women, but rather for menopausal symptom management for as short a time as possible at the lowest tolerated dose, once the individual patient has been fully informed of the risks.

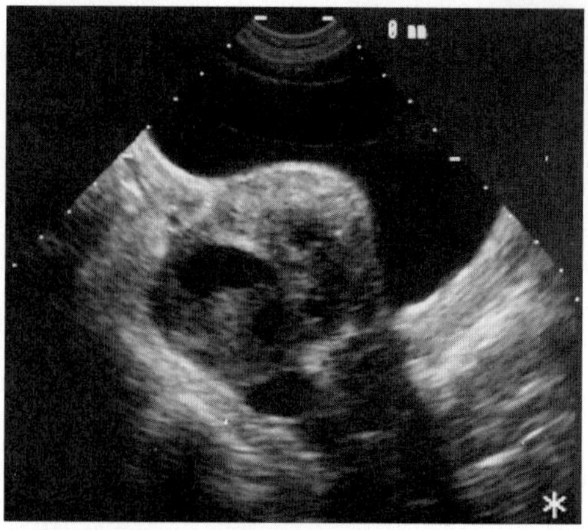

FIGURE 105.6. Ultrasound of a tuboovarian abscess (TOA) by transvaginal ultrasound of the left adnexa. A complex, cystic, and solid mass is seen in the left tube, representing a tuboovarian abscess. (Courtesy of Diana Gray, M.D., Washington University School of Medicine.)

History and Physical Examination

Obtaining a thorough history and physical examination is imperative in the evaluation of a gynecological patient. This information should include a history regarding gravity and parity, menses (age of onset and menopause, frequency, duration, flow, date of last menstrual period, intermenstrual bleeding, postcoital bleeding), contraceptive use, vaginal discharge (amount, color, odor, associated symptoms, history of previous infection), review of systems with emphasis on gastrointestinal and genitourinary symptoms, and results of the most recent Pap smears and sexually transmitted disease testing. Along with the general physical examination, specific components of a gynecological examination include these findings:

- External genitalia: pubic hair, clitoris, labia, urethra, vulva, vaginal introitus
- Speculum: evaluate the vagina (including the anterior and posterior vagina upon withdrawal of the speculum) and cervix; perform wet preparation and obtain cervical or vaginal cytology for Papanicolaou smear
- Bimanual: uterus (consistency, shape, size, position, mobility), adnexa (shape, size, tenderness with movement; i.e., cervical motion tenderness)
- Rectovaginal: uterosacral ligaments, posterior uterus, parametrium, stool guaiac

Pelvic Inflammatory Disease

Pelvic inflammatory disease (PID) is an infection of the upper female reproductive tract, including the uterus (endometritis/myometritis), fallopian tubes (salpingitis), ovary (oophoritis), adnexa (tuboovarian abscesses; Fig. 105.6), and peritoneum. It is an acute polymicrobial inflammatory condition caused by microorganisms ascending from the vagina. The sexually transmitted organisms *Neisseria gonorrhoeae* and *Chlamydia trachomatis* are often implicated, but PID may also be caused by other pathogens found in the vaginal flora, including *Gardnerella vaginalis*, *Haemophilus influenzae*, enteric gram-negative rods, and *Streptococcus agalactiae* as well as mycoplasmas and in some cases herpes simplex and cytomegalovirus.[7] PID affects as many as 1.5 million women annually in the United States, and the direct medical expenditures for PID and its three major sequelae (chronic pelvic pain, ectopic pregnancy, and infertility) have been estimated to be at least $2,150 per person.[8]

An accurate diagnosis of PID is often difficult, because signs and symptoms of the disease are varied and there exists no single historical, physical, laboratory, or diagnostic entity that is both sensitive and specific for the disease. Guidelines have been established to assist in the diagnosis of PID as well as to determine the appropriate timing of the initiation of therapy (Table 105.2).[9] In general, any patient presenting with the minimal criteria for the diagnosis of PID and a clinical suspicion for the disease should be treated to prevent complications. Epidemiological factors should also be considered when evaluating a patient with possible PID. The frequency of exposure to sexually transmitted disease has been correlated with the age of first intercourse, marital status, and the number of sexual partners. The use of certain types of contraceptives, including condoms, diaphragms, spermicides, and oral contraceptives, has been demonstrated to reduce the risk of PID. Alternatively, the risk of PID increases in the first 20 days following the insertion of an intrauterine device (IUD)[10] and with vaginal douching.[11]

Most diagnoses of pelvic inflammatory disease are based on clinical history and physical examination. Patients often complain of acute lower abdominal pain; increased vaginal discharge, fevers, and urinary frequency.[12] On examination, adnexal tenderness is frequently elicited, and an adnexal mass may be palpated on rectovaginal examination. Patients generally experience tenderness when the cervix is moved during examination (cervical motion tenderness), although this symptom is commonly present with any disease causing peritoneal irritation. All reproductive-age women with pelvic pain should have a determination of the beta-subunit of serum human chorionic gonadotropin (β-hCG) to exclude pregnancy, either intrauterine or ectopic. In general, the management of patients with suspected pelvic inflammatory disease is rarely modified by the results of pelvic, including transvaginal, ultrasonography.[13–15] If examination is not possible because of tenderness, ultrasound may be useful in assessing the adnexa for a tuboovarian abscess. Pelvic laparoscopy serves as the most sensitive and specific method of diagnosing pelvic inflammatory disease. During the procedure, cultures of the

TABLE 105.2.
Studies Evaluating Ultrasonography in Pelvic Inflammatory Disease (Level II Evidence).

Outcome measure	*Level of evidence*	*References*	*Comments/recommendations*
Correlating US with laparoscopy	Class II	10	Prospective trial evaluating 16 cases of PID confirmed by laparoscopy. US findings were correlated with laparoscopy. The authors determined that prospectively transvaginal sonography is a sensitive and specific tool in diagnosing PID.
Correlating US with endometrial biopsy-proven PID	Class II	11	Prospective trial of 51 patients with suspected PID, 13 of whom were confirmed with an EMB; 11/13 had thickened tubes by ultrasound. In 34 patients with a negative EMB, none had thickened tubes by ultrasound, leading to a sensitivity of 85%, and a specificity 100%.
Utility of US in diagnosing PID	Class II	12	Evaluation of 55 patients with suspected PID with abdominal and endovaginal US. Specificity of ultrasound in diagnosing abnormal tubes was 97%, but the sensitivity was only 32%.

US, ultrasound; PID, pelvic inflammatory disease; EMB, endometrial biopsy.

Conclusion: Transvaginal pelvic sonography may be a useful adjunct in confirming the diagnosis of an adnexal mass. However, it infrequently modifies the diagnosis of pelvic inflammatory disease or its treatment.

Source: From Centers for Disease Control and Prevention. 2002. Guidelines for treatment of sexually transmitted diseases. MMWR (Morb Mortal Wkly Rep) 2002;51(RR-6):48–51.[9]

peritoneum as well as any abscess should be obtained to individualize antimicrobial coverage.

Although it is imperative to rule out other common causes of lower abdominal pain such as ectopic pregnancy, acute appendicitis, and functional pain, initiating empiric antimicrobial therapy for PID as soon as it is suspected is unlikely to hinder diagnosis and management of these other conditions. Table 105.3 reviews the current Centers for Disease Control and Prevention guidelines for treatment of acute PID.[9] In all patients with a suspected diagnosis of PID, antibiotic treatment should be initiated following examination and culture of the endocervix for *N. gonorrhoeae* and *C. trachomatis*. All treatment regimens need to be effective against these two pathogens, because negative endocervical screening does not eliminate the possibility of upper genital tract infection. Anaerobic coverage must also be included, as these bacteria have been isolated from the upper reproductive tract of women with PID. When selecting a treatment regimen the clinician must consider patient compliance, cost, availability, and antimicrobial susceptibility.

Results from the pelvic inflammatory disease evaluation and clinical health (PEACH) randomized trial demonstrated no difference in reproductive outcomes between women with mild to moderate PID who were treated with cefoxitin and doxycycline as inpatients versus those treated as outpatients.[16] It is uncertain if this reflects a true parity of enteral versus parenteral antibiotics in terms of treatment, or if the damage resulting in sequelae tends to occur before presentation. In any case, the decision of whether hospitalization is necessary is at the discretion of the healthcare provider. Guidelines for inpatient treatment are listed in Table 105.4. For those patients requiring parenteral antibiotics, treatment should be

TABLE 105.3. Guidelines for Treatment of Acute Pelvic Inflammatory Disease (PID).

Parenteral regimen A:
Cefotetan 2g IV every 12h
Or
Cefoxitin 2g IV every 6h
Plus
Doxycycline 100mg orally or IV every 12h

Parenteral regimen B:
Clindamycin 900mg IV every 8h
Plus
Gentamicin loading dose IV or IM (2mg/kg body weight) followed by a maintenance dose (1.5mg/kg) every 8h
Single daily dosing may be substituted

Alternative parenteral regimens:
Ofloxacin 400mg IV every 12h
Or
Levofloxacin 500mg IV once daily
With or without
Metronidazole 500mg IV every 8h
Or
Ampicillin/Sulbactam 3g IV every 6h
Plus
Doxycycline 100mg orally or IV every 12h

Oral regimen A:
Ofloxacin 400mg orally twice a day for 14 days
Or
Levofloxacin 500mg orally once daily for 14 days
With or without
Metronidazole 500mg orally twice a day for 14 days

Oral and intramuscular/parenteral regimen B:
Ceftriaxone 250mg IM in a single dose
Or
Cefoxitin 2g IM in a single dose and **Probenecid** 1g orally administered concurrently in a single dose
Or
Other parenteral third-generation **cephalosporin** (e.g., **ceftizoxime** or **ceftaxime**)
Plus
Doxycycline 100mg orally twice a day for 14 days
With or without
Metronidazole 500mg orally twice a day for 14 days

Source: From Centers for Disease Control and Prevention. 2002 Guidelines for treatment of sexually transmitted diseases. MMWR (Morb Mortal Wkly Rep) 2002;51(RR-6):48–51.[9]

TABLE 105.4. Indications for Hospitalization for Patients with Suspected Pelvic Inflammatory Disease (PID).

- A surgical emergency (e.g., appendicitis, ovarian torsion) cannot be excluded
- The patient is pregnant
- The patient does not respond clinically to oral antimicrobial therapy for PID
- The patient is unable to follow or tolerate an outpatient oral regimen for PID
- The patient has severe illness, nausea and vomiting, or high fever
- The patient has a tuboovarian abscess (TOA) on imaging studies or examination

Source: From Centers for Disease Control and Prevention. 2002 Guidelines for treatment of sexually transmitted diseases. MMWR (Morb Mortal Wkly Rep) 2002;51(RR-6):48–51.[9]

continued for at least 24h following clinical improvement. At that time, enteral treatment can be initiated. Patients should be evaluated 48 to 72h following initiation of outpatient treatment. In the absence of a clinical response, the patient should be hospitalized for parenteral therapy.

Given the limited effectiveness of antibiotic treatment in patients with a tuboovarian abscess (TOA), consideration must be given to surgical therapy in patients who do not respond to broad-spectrum intravenous antibiotics. In general, surgery for PID should be limited to patients with symptomatic pelvic masses, ruptured TOAs, and drainage of abscesses in patients failing antibiotic therapy. In an effort to minimize surgery and preserve reproductive function, there has been increasing interest in radiologically guided aspiration of pelvic abscesses in patients not responding to antibiotic treatment. Modalities described include percutaneous computed tomography (CT)-guided drainage, and transabdominal, transvaginal, and transrectal ultrasonographically guided drainage. Investigation of these therapeutic modalities has generally been reported as case series[17–21]; randomized studies are needed.

Ectopic Pregnancy

A common and potentially life-threatening cause of abdominal pain in women is ectopic pregnancy. An ectopic pregnancy is defined as a gestation in which implantation has taken place in a site other than the endometrium, 97% of which occurs in the fallopian tubes.[22] Ectopic pregnancies are responsible for approximately 9% of all pregnancy-related deaths and account for the most common cause of maternal death in the first trimester of pregnancy.[23] It has become difficult to assess the incidence of ectopic pregnancies because surveillance has relied on inpatient discharge records, but as a result of changing medical practices in the late 1980s, an increasing proportion of women with this condition are treated as outpatients. Centers for Disease Control and Prevention reported approximately 64,000 hospitalizations for ectopic pregnancy in 1990; this rate has been climbing since ectopic pregnancy surveillance began in 1970.[24] Reviewing the available data from 1992 to 1999, consisting mostly of provider-based surveys, yearly averages of ectopic pregnancy range between 10,221 and 67,234.[25]

Risk factors for ectopic pregnancy include prior pelvic inflammatory disease, especially that caused by *Chlamydia trachomatis*, prior ectopic pregnancy, increasing age, smoking, and prior tubal surgery.[26] Approximately one-third of all pregnancies in women who have previously undergone tubal sterilization are ectopic.[27] Although the overall risk of ectopic pregnancy is decreased in users of intrauterine devices (IUD) compared to women who do not use contraception, ectopic pregnancy risk is 5% if pregnancy occurs in the presence of an IUD.[28] The use of assisted reproductive technologies for patients with infertility has also a significant risk factor; in vitro fertilization and embryo transfer is associated with a 2.1% to 9.4% risk of ectopic pregnancy.[29]

Abdominal pain and irregular vaginal bleeding (especially the lack of menses with spotting) are the most common complaints of women with ectopic pregnancies. In early (unruptured) ectopic pregnancies, pain may be perceived as vague and colicky; it may be unilateral or bilateral. Upon rupture, the pain often becomes intense. Patients may feel pain radiating to the shoulder as a result of diaphragmatic irritation. If intraperitoneal bleeding ensues, patients may feel dizzy or experience syncope. Patients may report having passed tissue vaginally; however, this never excludes ectopic pregnancy from a differential, as 10% of women with ectopic pregnancies pass a cast of decidualized endometrium. On examination, patients experience tenderness in the adnexa, and often a mass can be appreciated. The uterus should be smaller than expected for the appropriate gestational age of the fetus by menstrual dating. Following rupture, hypotension and tachycardia may be apparent. Temperature usually does not change with ectopic pregnancy. With the increased use of transvaginal ultrasound and sensitive tests for β-hCG, many ectopic pregnancies are diagnosed before they become symptomatic. Any woman of reproductive age with abdominal or pelvic complaints should be tested for pregnancy with a urine or serum β-hCG.

As the technology of transvaginal sonography has evolved, the diagnosis of ectopic pregnancies has been made at earlier gestations and with more accuracy (Fig. 105.7). With transvaginal sonography, it is possible to identify a gestational sac in the uterus when the β-hCG level reaches 1,500mIU/mL. At a β-hCG level of 2,500mIU/mL, absence of an intrauterine gestational sac indicates either a nonviable intrauterine preg-

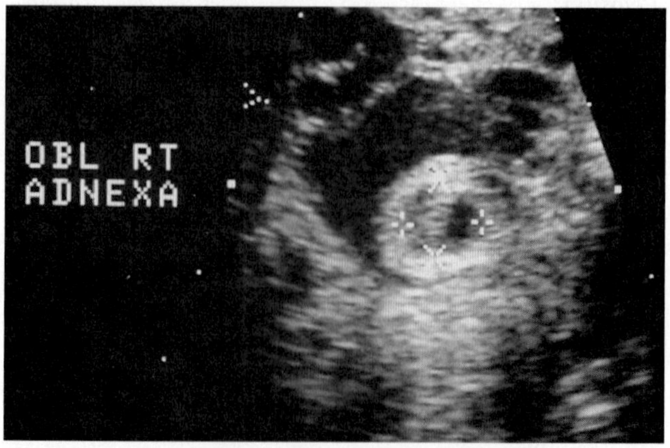

FIGURE 105.7. Ectopic pregnancy seen by transvaginal ultrasound of the right fallopian tube. A gestational sac is identified and marked on this image. The pregnancy is seen within the sac. (Courtesy of Diana Gray, M.D., Washington University School of Medicine.)

TABLE 105.5.
Studies Evaluating the Surgical Approach to Hemodynamically Stable Ectopic Pregnancy (Level I Evidence).

Outcome measure	*Level of evidence*	*References*	*Comments*
Safety and efficacy of laparotomy vs. laparoscopy	Class I	33	63 patients with suspected EP were randomized to either laparoscopy (26) or laparotomy (37). There was shorter hospital stay, less blood loss, and less narcotic requirement with laparoscopy.
Safety and efficacy of laparotomy vs. laparoscopic salpingostomy	Class I	34	60 patients underwent diagnostic laparoscopy to confirm EP, and were then randomized to either laparoscopic salpingostomy (30) or laparotomy with salpingostomy (30); 2 patients in the laparoscopy group required laparotomy for control of bleeding. There was equivalent fertility and decline of β-hCG with both treatments.
Effect on fertility of laparotomy vs. laparoscopic salpingostomy	Class I	35	105 patients with EP randomized to laparotomy with salpingostomy vs. laparoscopic salpingostomy. Fertility was reported to be equivalent in both groups for those women who desired to become pregnant.

EP, ectopic pregnancy; β-hCG, β-subunit of human chorionic gonadotropin.

Conclusion: Laparoscopy is superior to laparotomy in the treatment of hemodynamically stable ectopic pregnancy. There appears to be decreased morbidity with equivalent postprocedure fertility rates in those patients treated with laparoscopic salpingostomy compared with those patients treated by laparotomy.

nancy or an ectopic pregnancy. This level of β-hCG is usually reached at 5 to 6 weeks after the last normal menstrual period, or a gestational age of 38 days.[30] If the β-hCG value falls below the discriminatory zone for vaginal ultrasound (1,500 mIU/mL), serial determinations of β-hCG should be obtained. β-hCG concentrations increase 67% over 48 h,[31] but recent studies suggest that even a 53% increase in 2 days can represent a viable intrauterine pregnancy.[32] In the absence of an appropriate doubling time, an abnormal pregnancy (either intrauterine or ectopic) is likely, and further diagnostic procedures, such as dilatation and curettage (D&C) or laparoscopy, are indicated. If the β-hCG is more than 100,000 mIU/mL, the likelihood of an ectopic or abnormal intrauterine pregnancy is low and an alternative explanation for the patient's symptoms should be sought. Consideration must be given to appendicitis, nephrolithiasis, degenerating uterine leiomyomata (fibroids), and adnexal torsion arising in conjunction with an intrauterine pregnancy. Transvaginal ultrasound is used to determine whether the pregnancy is intrauterine or ectopic at β-hCG levels between 1,500 and 100,000 mIU/mL.

If the patient is hemodynamically stable, conservative surgical or medical management can be considered. If surgery is to be performed, the laparoscopic management of ectopic pregnancy has consistently been shown to be superior to laparotomy (Table 105.5).[33–35] Data suggest that rates of intrauterine pregnancy following conservative surgical treatment of ectopic pregnancy (i.e., linear salpingostomy) is equivalent if not superior to the rate following radical surgery (i.e., salpingectomy). However, there may be an increased risk of recurrent ectopic pregnancy following linear salpingostomy when compared to salpingectomy (Table 105.6).[36–39]

TABLE 105.6.
Studies Evaluating Radical Versus Conservative Surgical Management of Ectopic Pregnancy (Level II Evidence).

Outcome measure	*Level of evidence*	*References*	*Comments*
Rate of intrauterine and ectopic pregnancy following salpingostomy with or without tubal suturing	Class II	36	34 patients with EP were randomized to salpingostomy with or without suturing of the tubal incision. This group was compared to a historical control group of 24 patients treated with salpingectomy. Intrauterine pregnancy rate was higher following salpingostomy than salpingectomy, and occurred earlier in the group without suturing. Recurrent EP was more common following salpingostomy with and without suturing compared with salpingectomy.
Fertility following conservative vs. radical surgery for EP	Class II	37	1025 patients with EP were treated initially with either conservative (salpingostomy) or radical (wedge resection) surgery, and followed prospectively with questionnaires. The pregnancy rates were similar following surgery, as were EP recurrence rates (16%).
Fertility following laparoscopy	Class II	38	143 patients with EP were followed prospectively following laparoscopic treatment for EP. Pregnancy rates following salpingostomy were similar to those following salpingectomy.
Fertility following conservative vs. radical surgery for EP	Class II	39	90 patients with EP (56 treated with salpingectomy, 34 treated with conservative, tube-sparing surgery) were followed for at least 3 years. The rates of pregnancy were similar in both groups, as were the recurrence rates for EP.

EP, ectopic pregnancy.

Comment: Conservative surgical management is an appropriate treatment for hemodynamically stable ectopic pregnancy. Fertility is at least equivalent in patients treated with salpingostomy, although the recurrence rate for EP may be higher than in patients treated with salpingectomy.

Laparoscopic salpingostomy is generally performed with a fine-tip electrocautery unit. The pregnancy is removed through the tubal incision, and the base of the ectopic is irrigated. Hemostasis is obtained with electrocautery. To exclude persistence of trophoblastic tissue following salpingostomy, a repeat β-hCG level should be obtained 1 week postoperatively or if the patient develops increasing abdominal pain. If β-hCG levels continue to rise during follow-up, treatment for persistent ectopic pregnancy must be initiated.

Many patients with hemodynamically stable ectopic pregnancies are candidates for either medical or surgical therapy. The decision of which modality is used is generally based on the characteristics of the ectopic pregnancy, the patient's medical status, and her ability to comply with strict follow-up. Recommendations regarding the use of methotrexate for ectopic pregnancy are largely based on retrospective reviews of the experience of individual institutions. Nonetheless, most studies have found that methotrexate is a feasible alternative to radical or conservative surgical treatment for ectopic pregnancy, with reported success rates ranging from 67% to 100% with a median of 84% for the single-dose methotrexate regimen.[40–45] Criteria and contraindications to medical management are listed in Table 105.7.[46] Methotrexate is most often administered as a single intramuscular dose of 50 mg/m^2. Potential problems associated with medical management include drug-related side effects, treatment-related complications, and treatment failure. Although drug side effects such as myelosuppression, nephrotoxicity, and hepatitis are rare and can be monitored with laboratory studies, treatment effects such as increase in abdominal pain occur in as many as two-thirds of patients. Significantly worsening abdominal pain, hemodynamic instability, or levels of β-hCG that do not decline by at least 15% between day 4 and 7 postinjection suggest treatment failure and require subsequent appropriate medical or surgical intervention.

Ectopic pregnancy, similar to other first- and second-trimester clinical events associated with fetomaternal hemorrhage, may lead to alloimmunization in susceptible women. Therefore, whether treatment is medical or surgical, the patient's blood type should be obtained to evaluate the need for anti-D immunoglobulin. Women who are RhD antigen negative should receive a dose of 50 μg anti-D globulin within 72 h following surgery or initial methotrexate injection. Although this dose is sufficient to protect against 2.5 mL fetal red blood cells and is more than adequate to cover first-trimester fetal loss, second-trimester events, such as abortion, should be covered with the standard 300 μg dose.[47]

TABLE 105.7. Criteria and Contraindications for Use of Methotrexate for Management of Ectopic Pregnancy.

Criteria for receiving methotrexate
Absolute indications:
Hemodynamically stable without active bleeding or signs of hemoperitoneum
Patient desires future fertility
General anesthesia poses a significant risk
Patient is able to return for follow-up care
Patient has no contraindications to methotrexate
Relative indications:
Unruptured mass <3.5 cm at its greatest dimension
No fetal cardiac motion detected
Contraindications to medical therapy with methotrexate
Absolute contraindications:
Breastfeeding
Overt or laboratory evidence of immunodeficiency
Alcoholism, alcoholic liver disease, or other chronic liver disease
Preexisting blood dyscrasias
Known sensitivity to methotrexate
Active pulmonary disease
Peptic ulcer disease
Hepatic, renal, or hematological dysfunction
Relative contraindications:
Gestational sac >3.5 cm
Embryonic cardiac motion

Source: From ACOG Practice Bulletin. Medical Management of Tubal Pregnancy. Number 3, December 1998. Obstet Gynecol 1998;92(6):510–511.[46]

Adnexal Torsion

Adnexal torsion occurs when the ovary and/or fallopian tube becomes twisted and its vascular supply becomes compromised. Adnexal torsion is generally a disease of reproductive-age women. Torsion is commonly related to ovarian or tubal enlargement, including benign neoplasms (benign cystic teratoma, paraovarian cyst, cystadenoma, fibroma), pregnancy-related changes (corpus luteum cyst, ovarian enlargement from ovulation induction as infertility treatment), or rarely an ovarian malignancy.[48,49] The differentiation between appendicitis and adnexal torsion is made more difficult by the fact that ovarian torsion occurs 1.5 times more commonly on the right than the left side.

Patients with adnexal torsion often present with the acute onset of severe, intermittent lateralizing pain. Frequently, patients have complained of this type of pain in the preceding days or weeks, likely from previous episodes of partial and resolved torsion of the adnexa. Patients often complain of nausea and vomiting, and may also attribute signs to urinary tract infection. Often a unilateral adnexal enlargement is palpable on physical examination. There are no reliable laboratory tests to diagnose adnexal torsion. The use of Doppler ultrasound has been evaluated in the diagnosis and management of adnexal torsion (Table 105.8).[50–52] From these data, it appears that Doppler ultrasound has moderate sensitivity and specificity in the diagnosis of adnexal torsion. The demonstration of vascular flow to the adnexa may support conservative management of the torsion. Clearly, prospective clinical studies are needed to further elucidate the role of Doppler ultrasound in adnexal torsion.

The management of patients with adnexal torsion is aimed at preserving the health of the patient without compromising her reproductive capabilities. Thus, untwisting of twisted adnexa is the recommended surgical procedure for adnexal torsion, with ovarian or tubal cystectomy where appropriate[53]; this may be performed via laparoscopy or laparotomy.[54] If there is evidence of necrosis of the adnexa, adnexectomy is the most appropriate procedure. To further select patients in whom conservative therapy may be undertaken in the presence of adnexal torsion, authors have used intravenous fluorescein in an attempt to determine whether the untwisted adnexa demonstrates fluorescence under ultraviolet light, suggesting viable tissue.[55]

TABLE 105.8.
Studies Evaluating the Use of Color Doppler Sonography in the Diagnosis and Management of Ovarian Torsion (Level II Evidence).

Outcome Measure	*Level of Evidence*	*References*	*Comments*
Vascular flow and adnexal viability	Class II	50	24/27 patients with adnexal torsion were identified preoperatively by color Doppler sonography. In 10/10 patients with arterial and venous flow, no ovarian necrosis was noted at surgery. In 9/9 adnexa demonstrating only arterial flow, all had evidence of hemorrhagic necrosis of the adnexa.
Vascular flow and adnexal viability	Class II	51	28/32 patients with adnexal torsion were identified preoperatively by color Doppler sonography. In 10/11 patients who underwent adnexectomy with normal arterial and venous flow, no necrosis was noted. In 12/12 patients with no flow, necrosis was noted. In 5/5 patients with flow who were treated with untwisting of the adnexa without resection, all had normal postoperative ovarian follicular development.
Correlation of venous flow with ovarian viability	Class II	52	13 patients with surgically documented adnexal torsion had preoperative color flow Doppler sonography; 10/13 ovaries were considered nonviable at surgery, 6/10 of which lacked preoperative evidence of venous flow. All ovaries considered viable at surgery had evidence of central venous flow documented preoperatively.

Conclusion: Doppler sonography has moderate sensitivity and specificity in the diagnosis of ovarian torsion. The preoperative lack of vascular flow may aid in assessing the risk of adnexal necrosis and thus improve preoperative patient counseling regarding the likely surgical outcome. Randomized clinical trials of Doppler sonography are needed to further evaluate this radiographic technique. The long-term effects of conservative management of adnexal torsion on fertility are unknown.

Adnexal Masses

Surgeons frequently find themselves faced with the discovery of an adnexal mass, either on pelvic examination or during the intraoperative assessment of pelvic organs. With the increasing use of transvaginal sonography, many of these masses are being detected and evaluated preoperatively. To guide the surgeon in the management of an adnexal mass, it is of critical importance to determine the risk that the mass is malignant. Criteria have been developed to aid in assessing the potential of an adnexal mass to be malignant so that proper preoperative management or referral to a specialist can be arranged (Table 105.9). Unfortunately, these criteria are neither completely sensitive nor specific, and thus cancer will be discovered in masses believed to be benign. When an adnexal mass is considered to have a significant risk of being malignant, surgery to obtain a histological diagnosis is imperative. In patients who have an adnexal mass greater than 10 cm, the risk of malignancy or other complications such as adnexal torsion is high enough to justify laparotomy. If a pelvic mass is diagnosed in a premenopausal woman, a period of observation may be appropriate in the absence of other factors that make malignancy likely. If after 6 to 8 weeks the mass is stable or has grown, surgery is indicated.

TABLE 105.9. Indications for Operative Intervention of Adnexal Masses.

Mass >10 cm
Ascites
Solid and fixed
Persistence following 8 weeks of observation
Size increase, following observation
Symptomatic, large (>5 cm), or complex mass in postmenopausal women
Family history of ovarian, breast, or colon carcinoma

Controversy exists in the management of postmenopausal women with small, asymptomatic adnexal masses. Laparotomy had been recommended for all pelvic masses in women older than 50. Recent data, however, have suggested that some older women with asymptomatic, small, unilocular ovarian cysts may be observed rather than explored.[56,57] However, the overall risk of an ovarian malignancy in the presence of a palpable postmenopausal ovary is not insignificant. In general, if a malignancy is suspected, laparotomy with an opportunity for complete surgical staging of an ovarian cancer is the appropriate technique. Laparoscopy may be appropriate in certain circumstances, such as those in which there is a lower suspicion for malignancy. A prospective randomized trial of laparoscopy versus laparotomy in women with benign ovarian masses randomized 102 women with masses less than 10 cm to either operative laparoscopy or laparotomy. The authors demonstrated a significant reduction in operative morbidity, postoperative pain, hospitalization time, and recovery time in those patients treated laparoscopically. They also noted an equal rate of inadvertent cyst rupture in both groups.[58] The authors concluded that operative laparoscopy should replace laparotomy in the management of ovarian masses thought to be benign. If an ovarian neoplasm suspicious for cancer is discovered incidentally during laparoscopy, all peritoneal surfaces (i.e. pelvis, pouch of Douglas, diaphragm, paracolic gutters, omentum, bowel surfaces) should be examined, peritoneal washings should be obtained, and, if possible, the mass should be removed without spilling cyst contents into the peritoneal cavity. Biopsy, puncture, and partial resection are not appropriate. Frozen section should be performed when available. If the plan is to abort the procedure in favor of laparotomy at a later date, this should be scheduled within the week if possible.

Other recent retrospective series and case reports have examined the use of laparoscopy for the management of adnexal masses suspicious for malignancy (Table 105.10).[59–62] In these studies, frozen section was used to direct surgical

TABLE 105.10.
Laparoscopic Management of Suspicious Adnexal Masses (Level II Evidence).

Outcome measure	*Level of evidence*	*Reference*	*Comments*
Appropriate management of malignant adnexal masses initially evaluated via laparoscopy	II	59	Of 757 patients with 819 masses who were evaluated laparoscopically, 6% were suspicious, and 41% of these masses were found to be malignant or low malignant potential. No malignant masses missed at time of exploration; 7 of 15 malignant tumors ruptured during laparoscopy.
Morbidity and hospital length of stay associated with appropriate management of suspicious adnexal masses	II	60	Of 138 patients with suspicious adnexal masses based on US criteria and CA-125 values who underwent laparoscopy, 14% (19/138) were found to have malignancies and 8% were converted to laparotomy. Overall, 95% of benign and 74% of malignant masses were managed laparoscopically. Mean stay was 1.5 days, and 3 major surgical complications were noted. Two patients with apparent stage I disease had recurrence diagnosed at 6 and 38 months after laparoscopy.
Appropriate management of malignant adnexal masses initially evaluated via laparoscopy	II	61	Of 230 patients with suspicious adnexal masses who were evaluated with laparoscopy, 204/230 (82.6%) were successfully treated with laparoscopy, including 7/37 with malignant tumors and 197/210 benign tumors. One case of tumor dissemination occurred following morcellation of an ovarian tumor; 3 cases were thought to be benign at the time of frozen section and were subsequently found to be malignant.
Safety and feasibility of laparoscopic adnexal mass removal without exclusion of suspicious masses	II	62	Of 160 patients who underwent laparoscopic evaluation for adnexal masses, 87% were found to have benign pathology and 88% were managed laparoscopically. Frozen-section diagnosis was discordant with final pathology in 5 patients, which did not result in delay of treatment.

management, with the histological results leading to either conservative treatment or complete staging via laparotomy or continued laparoscopy. Laparoscopic management is first and foremost tailored to the individual patient, and factors such as tumor size and consistency, age and weight of the patient, her past medical and surgical history, and the skill of the surgeon all need to be taken into account before proceeding. It is also imperative that a plan is in place for management of cancer if it is discovered, before proceeding with a laparoscopic approach, and the patient must be consented for the possibility of laparotomy, cytoreduction, etc. Some of the special concerns associated with laparoscopic management of ovarian cancer include the risk of port site metastasis, risk of rupture and tumor spillage, and the difficulty of performing adequate staging with this approach.

Ovarian masses that are encountered most commonly by the surgeon can be divided into those that are functional and those which are neoplastic (Table 105.11). Follicular cysts are the most common physiological ovarian cysts in premenopausal women. They may enlarge and become symptomatic, undergo torsion along the blood supply, or they may rupture and cause irritation of the peritoneum, leading to symptoms requiring emergent evaluation. Following ovulation, the ovary develops a corpus luteum, which secretes progesterone to support a fertilized ovum. Most cysts arising from an enlarged corpus luteum are asymptomatic, but some may cause unilateral abdominal or pelvic pain. Patients may complain of a delay in their menses, likely from the high progesterone levels supplied by the functioning corpus luteum. Given the similar signs and symptoms of a corpus luteum cyst and ectopic pregnancy (menstrual irregularity, pain, and an adnexal mass), a urine or serum β-hCG must be obtained. If a corpus luteum cyst ruptures, intraperitoneal bleeding may ensue, which can be significant. If operative intervention is

TABLE 105.11. Functional and Neoplastic Ovarian Masses.

Functional ovarian masses:		
	Tissue of origin	*Comments*
Follicular cysts	Graafian follicle	Most common physiological cyst in premenopausal women.
Corpus luteum cysts	Corpus luteum, which develops after ovulation	Called a cyst when more than 3 cm in diameter. May lead to delay in menses. May lead to significant hemorrhage if ruptures.
Theca lutein cysts	Luteinized ovarian follicle	Associated with high levels of circulating gonadotropins such as pregnancy, molar pregnancies, and choriocarcinoma.
Benign ovarian neoplasms:		
	Tissue of origin	*Comments*
Mature cystic teratomas	Arise from autofertilization of germ cells	Accounts for one-fourth of all ovarian tumors. All three germ cell layers present.
Cystadenomas	Ovarian epithelium	Serous type more common than mucinous and often bilateral. Mucinous cysts can be extremely large.
Thecoma and fibroma	Gonadal stroma	Fibromas are most common ovarian stromal tumors. Thecomas are hormonally active and produce androgens or estrogens.

necessary, ovarian cystectomy is generally recommended, with oophorectomy or salpingo-oophorectomy if the ovary is not salvageable or bleeding cannot be controlled by more conservative measures. If a patient with a hemorrhagic corpus luteum cyst is explored during the first 12 weeks of pregnancy, an attempt at preserving the cyst should be made, as it provides the hormonal support to the pregnancy. Theca lutein cysts develop under the stimulation of endogenous or exogenous gonadotrophins, especially during infertility treatment or in pregnancies with high β-hCG levels (twins or gestational trophoblastic disease). Theca lutein cysts are generally asymptomatic, but approximately 3% undergo complications such as torsion or hemorrhage.[63]

Benign cystic teratomas (dermoid cysts) are a common ovarian neoplasm (Fig. 105.8). Because elements from all three germ cell layers may be present, it is not uncommon to find gross evidence of teeth, hair, and sebum, as well as microscopic evidence of neural or respiratory tissue, in these neoplasms. They generally cause no symptoms, but may twist or rupture, leading to a reactive peritonitis from the spill of sebaceous material. Management is generally with ovarian cystectomy, but oophorectomy or salpingo-oophorectomy is occasionally necessary. As these neoplasms are bilateral in 10% to 15% of cases, the contralateral ovary must be inspected and managed appropriately. In rare instances, the squamous component of dermoids may undergo malignant degeneration. Immature teratomas are the malignant counterparts to benign cystic teratomas. They demonstrate elements of immature embryonic tissue, are almost exclusively unilateral, and are managed with unilateral salpingo-oophorectomy and biopsies of suspicious peritoneal surfaces.

Cystadenomas are the benign counterpart of epithelial ovarian cancers and may be either serous or mucinous in histology. Serous are more common than mucinous cystadenomas and are much more likely to be bilateral. Mucinous cystadenomas may grow extremely large, and there are reports of mucinous tumors weighing more than 100 pounds. Mucinous tumors may rupture, spilling mucin in the peritoneal cavity. In rare instances, the peritoneal mesothelium may undergo mucinification under the influence of the cystadenoma, resulting in pseudomyxoma peritoneii.[64] If this situation is encountered, it is important to evaluate the appendix as well as the ovaries because an appendiceal mucocele or carcinoma may also lead to pseudomyxoma peritoneii. Surgical management of ovarian cystadenomas should be identical to that for other benign ovarian masses. Other benign ovarian masses, including Brenner tumors, ovarian fibromas, and thecomas, may be encountered during surgical exploration.

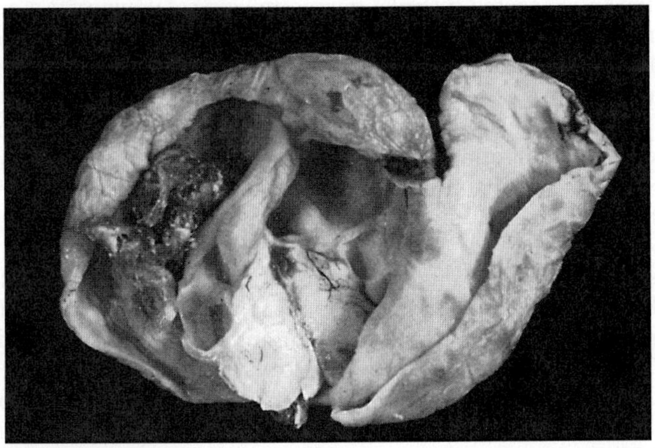

FIGURE 105.8. Dermoid cyst (benign cystic teratoma). This left ovary was removed from a 16-year-old girl with an enlarged (14-cm) adnexa. Grossly, the surface is white, glistening, and without excrescences. The cut surface reveals sebum and hair, consistent with a teratoma. Microscopically, this mass was determined to be a benign cystic (mature) teratoma. (Courtesy of Phyllis Huettner, M.D., Washington University School of Medicine.)

Endometriosis

Endometriosis is defined by ectopic implants of tissue resembling functioning endometrial glands and stoma, located outside the uterine cavity. These lesions can be found throughout the pelvic cavity, commonly in the rectovaginal septum, uterine ligaments, ovaries, parietal peritoneum of the uterus and bladder, as well as the appendix and intestinal serosa. Less common sites include the umbilicus or hernia sacs, laparotomy and episiotomy scars, and the pleural and pericardial cavities. Endometriosis occurs in 7% to 10% of women in general, with a prevalence of 38% in infertile women and 71% to 87% of women with chronic pelvic pain.[65] It is important to note, however, that many women with the incidental finding of endometriosis have no symptoms. Although endometriosis has been extensively studied, it is as yet poorly understood. Endometriosis is understood to be an estrogen-dependent condition, and medical or surgical castration is capable of alleviating symptoms.

The classic presenting symptoms for endometriosis are dysmenorrhea, dysperunia, and infertility. Often presenting symptoms reflect implantation sites. For example, pain with defecation can result from rectal or sigmoid endometriosis and can even be associated with cyclical rectal bleeding. Rarely a patient will present with recurrent pneumothorax as a result of diaphragmatic involvement or with azotemia as a result of complete ureteral obstruction. On physical examination, tender nodules on the uterosacral ligaments, cul-de-sac nodularity, induration of the rectovaginal septum, a fixed and retroverted uterus, adnexal masses, and pelvic tenderness are all possible findings. An enigmatic aspect of the disease is the lack of association between severity of endometriosis, as defined by the American Society for Reproductive Medicine classification system (stage I–IV, based on size, location, and extent of lesions), and patient symptoms or infertility.[66] Studies have shown, however, that the depth of infiltration correlates well with pain severity.[67,68]

The mechanisms whereby endometriosis causes infertility and pain are a subject of considerable debate. Individual inflammatory response may play a key role in the local peritoneal response to the endometrial lesion, leading to an abundance of prostaglandins and cytokines that could interfere with reproduction and stimulate pain receptors. Although it is clear that anatomic distortion as a result of extensive, invasive endometriosis and adhesions can lead to infertility, a cause-and-effect relationship between mild to moderate endometriosis and infertility has not been proven. Clinically, however, surgical treatment of endometriosis has been shown to be beneficial in the management of infertility. In general, a pregnancy rate of approximately 65% can be reached within 1 to 2 years following surgical treatment of endometriosis.[69]

In a meta-analysis of studies comparing surgery with medical treatments for endometriosis-associated infertility, the surgical approach was superior, with pregnancy rates up to 38% higher than for nonsurgical approaches.[69]

The standard for diagnosing endometriosis remains direct visualization confirmed by histological examination. Identification of endometriosis can be difficult, even for experienced surgeons, because of the subtle and varied appearance of lesions. Small, darkly pigmented adherent masses, often attached to the posterior cul-de-sac and posterior surface of the uterus, are characteristic. However, lesions can appear as clear vesicles, flat plaques, raised or polypoid lesions, areas of fibrosis, adhesion formation, or peritoneal defects. Hemosiderin deposition determines the extent of yellow, brown, blue, or black discoloration. Histologically, presence of two or more of the following features is diagnostic: endometrial epithelium, glands, and/or stroma, as well as hemosiderin-laden macrophages. These ectopic foci respond to estrogen by proliferating and to progesterone by showing secretory change, but these functional changes are less uniform than for the uterine mucosa. Although rare, up to 1% of patients with endometriosis have lesions that undergo malignant transformation, with the majority being ovarian endometrioid adenocarcinomas. The use of CA-125 measurement has not been shown to be useful in screening patients for endometriosis or determining response to medical therapy, although there is correlation between elevated CA-125 and the presence of moderate to severe disease.[70,71]

Imaging studies for patients with suspected endometriosis are useful only in the assessment of pelvic or adnexal masses. The mass resulting from a cystic enlargement of an implant of endometriosis on the ovary is termed an endometrioma. Many patients with endometriomas do not have the classic symptoms of endometriosis. Endometriomas are usually resistant to medical management, and thus surgery via laparotomy or laparoscopy is usually employed to remove the endometrioma without sacrificing reproductive function. Endometriomas are usually less than 10cm and usually develop over several months as a result of intracystic hemorrhage. They are also known as "chocolate cysts" because of the dark brown, thick fluid contained within the endometrial cyst.

Although a persistent pelvic mass is certainly an indication for surgery, and the standard for diagnosis is direct visualization, not everyone with pelvic pain and/or infertility associated with endometriosis needs to go to the operating room. When a patient presents with pelvic pain, and a thorough diagnostic evaluation fails to reveal any other gynecological or nongynecological cause, medical treatment can be empirically initiated. Progestins, danazol, oral contraceptives, nonsteroidal antiinflammatory drugs (NSAIDs), and gonadotropin-releasing hormone (GnRH) agonists have all been used to treat the pain associated with endometriosis. Based on a prospective, randomized, controlled, double-blind clinical trial, a patient with suspected endometriosis who has failed initial treatment with oral contraceptives and NSAIDs can be tried on a 3-month course of a GnRH agonist.[72] This course of treatment is associated with improvement in dysmenorrhea, pelvic pain, and tenderness.

When laparoscopy is employed, a methodical and complete survey of the pelvis needs to be performed, requiring at least two ports for adequate manipulation and visualization. One prospective, double-blind, randomized, controlled trial has demonstrated the effectiveness of laparoscopic surgery for women with pelvic pain.[73] Of the women in the study who underwent laparoscopic evaluation with laser ablation and uterosacral nerve ablation, 62% experienced pain relief after surgery compared to 22% who underwent inspection of the pelvis alone. With continued follow-up, however, 44% of women experienced recurrence of symptoms within 1 year postoperatively.[74] Debate continues over the best means of surgical therapy as no one method has been shown to be superior, and options include excision, coagulation, electrocautery, and vaporization. Operative success rate correlates with meticulous surgical techniques directed toward removal of all endometrial implants in an atraumatic, hemostatic fashion.[69] When appropriate, a laparotomy is performed, especially in instances of excessive adhesions (which need to be removed rather than lysed as endometriosis can be present within them) or a large endometrioma. In situations where a woman has completed her childbearing and medical management has failed, definitive surgery of hysterectomy and salpingo-oophorectomy is very effective, providing pain relief in up to 90% of patients.[75]

Ovarian Cancer

A woman's lifetime risk of being diagnosed with ovarian cancer is 1 in 75 (15%).[76] It is estimated that 22,430 new cases of ovarian cancer will be diagnosed in the United States in 2007.[77] Ovarian cancer ranks eighth and accounts for 3% of all cancers among women, ranking second, behind endometrial cancer, among gynecological malignancies.[77] It is estimated that 15,280 patients with ovarian cancer will die of their disease in 2007, more deaths than from any other cancers of the female reproductive system.[77] The peak incidence of invasive ovarian cancer is 62 years, with more than two-thirds of cancers being diagnosed in postmenopausal women. Because most women with ovarian cancer have very few symptoms with early-stage disease, two-thirds of the cases of ovarian cancer are diagnosed in the later stages. Cancer may be either diagnosed preoperatively through physical examination or suspected by radiographic imaging. Likewise, a diagnosis may be made upon discovering an ovarian mass or intraperitoneal disease during surgical exploration for other reasons.

In later stages, women with ovarian cancer may complain of vague abdominal pain or pressure, nausea, early satiety, constipation, abdominal swelling, loss of weight, urinary frequency, and occasionally abnormal vaginal bleeding. If a pelvic mass is felt on examination, transvaginal sonography is an effective tool for determining the etiology of the mass (Fig. 105.9). Preoperatively, if malignancy is suspected, determination of serum CA-125 tumor antigen is recommended, as in many patients with ovarian cancer it serves as a marker for disease status. Furthermore, the American College of Obstetricians and Gynecologists (ACOG), in combination with the Society of Gynecologic Oncologists (SGO), has recommended that in postmenopausal women with a pelvic mass the CA-125 measurement can stratify the risk for malignancy preoperatively so that consultation or referral can be made before the patient is taken to the operating room. Unfortunately, CA-125 lacks the sensitivity and specificity to be

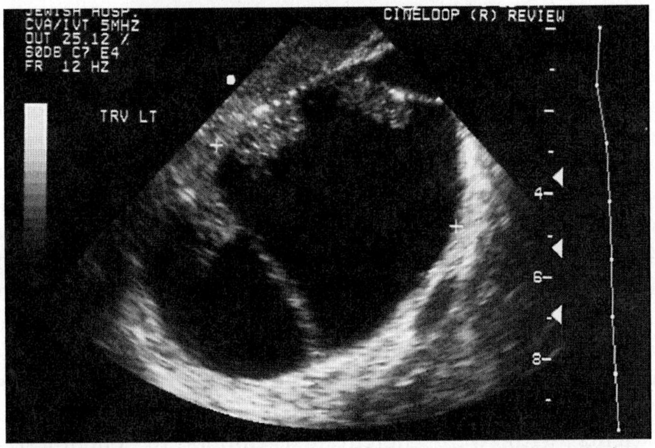

FIGURE 105.9. Invasive ovarian carcinoma by transvaginal ultrasound of the left ovary. A large cystic mass with a septum comprises the majority of this mass. Solid areas are seen on the upper surface of this cyst. Histologically, a papillary serous adenocarcinoma of the ovary was diagnosed. (Courtesy of Diana Gray, M.D., Washington University School of Medicine.)

useful in screening for ovarian cancer, especially in patients with early-stage disease.[78] Similarly, the combination of CA-125 and routine transvaginal sonography in an asymptomatic population has been shown to be neither sensitive nor specific for the early diagnosis of ovarian cancer. The diagnosis of ovarian cancer is thus made surgically.

Based on the recommendations of ACOG and the SGO, referral to a gynecological oncologist should be considered in situations in which an ovarian cancer is more likely; these include (1) a postmenopausal woman with a suspicious pelvic mass (elevated CA-125, ascites, fixed on examination, evidence of extrapelvic disease, or a family history of a first-degree relative with breast or ovarian cancer) and (2) a premenopausal woman with a suspicious mass as defined above with the exception that the CA-125 is extremely high (>200 U/mL).

In general, the intraoperative evaluation of a patient with ovarian cancer involves complete surgical staging to determine precisely the extent of the disease and thus determine whether adjuvant postoperative treatment is necessary (Table 105.12). In patients with advanced or bulky disease, cytoreduction is performed to reduce the tumor burden and improve response to adjuvant therapy and thus survival. Because it is necessary to thoroughly sample all peritoneal surfaces of the abdomen and pelvis, a vertical midline incision gives the surgeon the best exposure during laparotomy. If an ovarian cancer is discovered incidentally in a patient who has undergone a transverse incision, a Maylard or Cherney incision can be used to improve exposure. Upon entering the peritoneum, any ascites should be collected and sent for cytological evaluation. If no ascites is present, 50 mL saline should be introduced into the peritoneal cavity and collected for cytology. A thorough assessment of all abdominal and pelvic contents should then be performed, with biopsies of any suspicious nodules or adhesions. The ovarian mass should be resected and evaluated by frozen section to confirm malignancy.

If inspection of the abdomen and pelvis demonstrates an ovarian malignancy apparently confined to the pelvis, random biopsies of the peritoneum overlying the pelvis, bladder, rectosigmoid, abdominal gutters, and diaphragm should be taken. An infracolic omentectomy should then be performed, as the omentum often harbors metastasis (Fig. 105.10). The retroperitoneal spaces should be evaluated, with pathological assessment of the pelvic and paraaortic lymph nodes. In a woman with an apparently localized ovarian malignancy who desires to retain her fertility, a unilateral oophorectomy, peritoneal biopsies, and unilateral lymphadenectomy may be performed, with hysterectomy and contralateral oophorectomy delayed until after completion of childbearing.[79] In all other situations, a total abdominal hysterectomy with bilateral salpingo-oophorectomy is recommended. Although few randomized clinical trials have evaluated the concept of "debulking surgery" to reduce the volume of ovarian cancer to a microscopic residual, it is generally accepted that patients with smaller volumes of tumor following staging laparotomy ("optimal debulking," <1 cm maximum residual tumor diameter) have an improved survival when compared to patients in whom cytoreduction is unable to be performed ("suboptimal debulking," >1 cm maximum residual tumor diameter). Thus, it is often necessary to perform extensive surgery, including intestinal resection with reanastamosis or colostomy, if the procedure renders the patient with minimal residual disease. With appropriate experience, colostomy is rarely necessary for ovarian cancer debulking surgeries.

TABLE 105.12. Surgical Technique for Staging of Epithelial Ovarian Cancer.

Vertical midline incision
Peritoneal cytology
Exploration of abdomen and pelvis
Biopsy of any nodules or adhesions
Removal of ovarian tumor for frozen section
Hysterectomy and salpingo-oophorectomy
Biopsy of peritoneal surfaces (pelvis, bladder, rectosigmoid, abdominal gutters, and diaphragm)
Omentectomy
Retroperitoneal lymphadenectomy (pelvic and paraaortic)
Cytoreduction where appropriate

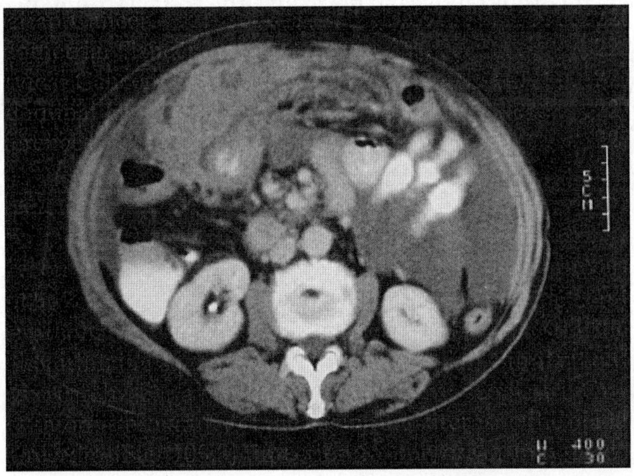

FIGURE 105.10. Advanced ovarian cancer with omental metastasis, shown by computed tomography (CT) of the abdomen of a patient with a stage IIIC papillary serous adenocarcinoma of the ovary. Ascites is seen in the right upper quadrant. The omentum has been infiltrated by tumor, leading to an "omental cake." (Courtesy of Vamsi Narra, M.D., Washington University School of Medicine.)

The goal of cytoreduction is to minimize the diameter of the remaining disease, as survival is directly proportional to the tumor volume following cytoreduction.[80,81] Following completion of initial staging and cytoreduction, patients with disease outside the ovary are treated with six cycles of paclitaxel and platinum-based chemotherapy.[82] In certain research settings, a reassessment surgery ("second-look" laparotomy or laparoscopy) is performed after appropriate chemotherapeutic management to gather precise histological data and evaluate response to therapy. In the presence of macroscopic disease, interval cytoreduction may also be performed. Outside the research setting, there exist few data to support routine reassessment surgery in ovarian cancer.

Endometrial Cancer

Endometrial cancer is the most common gynecological malignancy in the United States, with 39,080 new cases expected to be diagnosed in 2007.[77] Overall, it is expected that 7,400 women will die in 2007 as a result of endometrial cancer.[77] Endometrial cancer is generally a disease of more affluent Caucasian women, many of whom are obese. Any factor that increases exposure to estrogen increases the risk of developing endometrial cancer. Thus, early menarche, late menopause, nulliparity, unopposed estrogen for hormone replacement, anovulatory menstrual cycles, and estrogen-secreting tumors are implicated in the pathogenesis of this malignancy. Factors that decrease endogenous estrogen, such as oral contraceptives and smoking, decrease the risk of developing endometrial cancer. Endometrial hyperplasia with nuclear atypia has been identified as a precursor to some cases of endometrial cancer. Patients with untreated atypical endometrial hyperplasia have a 23% risk of progression to cancer, whereas patients with simple or complex hyperplasia without atypia have a 1% to 3% risk, respectively.[83] Similarly, women with endometrial hyperplasia who respond to a trial of progestin therapy have a lower risk for progression to cancer than patients whose hyperplasia persists following treatment.[84]

Patients with endometrial hyperplasia without atypia are treated with hormones to normalize the endometrium, using medroxyprogesterone acetate, combination estrogen/progestin oral contraceptives, or clomiphene citrate (to induce ovulation in patients who desire to become pregnant). Extrafascial hysterectomy is appropriate if the hyperplasia persists or if other indications for hysterectomy exist. Treatment for patients who desire to retain their reproductive function with atypical hyperplasia is initially with progestins, using escalating doses in an effort to normalize the endometrium. If repeat endometrial sampling demonstrates persistent atypical hyperplasia, hysterectomy is appropriate.

The median age of diagnosis of patients with endometrial cancer is 61 years, and three-fourths are postmenopausal. Approximately three-fourths of patients with endometrial cancer are diagnosed with early or stage I disease, as most patients experience abnormal vaginal bleeding and thus seek medical attention. On examination, evidence of hyperestrogenism may be appreciated. The uterus may be enlarged but is usually of a normal size. In advanced cases, an omental cake or ascites may be appreciated. Any peri- or postmenopausal patients who are at risk for endometrial cancer, experience abnormal bleeding, or demonstrate abnormal glandular cells on Papanicolaou smear should be evaluated with an endometrial biopsy or curettage. Transvaginal sonography may be useful in determining whether any intrauterine abnormalities exist.

Once a diagnosis of endometrial cancer is made, the extent of disease should be determined surgically. Surgical staging of endometrial cancer was established in 1988 in an effort to gain more accurate prognostic information. Despite this, not all centers or physicians follow the recommendations for complete surgical staging, and thus prognostic information is not uniform. In general, surgery for endometrial cancer should include obtaining peritoneal fluid for cytology, extrafascial hysterectomy, and bilateral salpingo-oophorectomy.[85] In patients with well-differentiated tumors by endometrial biopsy and comorbid conditions making laparotomy dangerous, vaginal hysterectomy may be the appropriate treatment.[86] Laparoscopically assisted surgical staging of endometrial cancer has also been employed with success; aspiration of pelvic fluid for cytology and salpingo-oophorectomy (with or without lymphadenectomy) are performed laparoscopically, followed by vaginal hysterectomy. Otherwise, a vertical midline incision affords adequate visualization in most patients for an abdominal hysterectomy. In morbidly obese patients, a transverse (Pfannenstiel, Maylard, or Cherney) incision may be superior. Other incision techniques, such as a supraumbilical midline incision, may also be appropriate in morbidly obese patients undergoing pelvic surgery.[87]

On entering the peritoneal cavity, any fluid should be aspirated and sent for cytology. If no ascites exists, 50 mL saline should be instilled, aspirated, and sent for cytological evaluation. A comprehensive evaluation of the abdomen and pelvis should then be undertaken, with biopsies of any suspicious areas. An extrafascial hysterectomy and bilateral salpingo-oophorectomy should be performed next. On completion of the hysterectomy, the uterus should be bivalved in the sagittal plane to evaluate the depth of tumor penetration into the myometrium, as this is one factor that predicts the risk of lymph node metastasis in endometrial cancer. Studies have shown that there is good correlation between gross and microscopic estimation of tumor permeation into the myometrium in patients with well-differentiated tumors.[88] The decision whether to pursue pelvic and paraaortic lymph node sampling following completion of hysterectomy is controversial. As more data are collected, it appears that no preoperative or intraoperative factors (such as tumor grade, spread, and depth of myometrial invasion) are adequately sensitive in predicting retroperitoneal lymph node metastasis. As such, a lymphadenectomy should be strongly considered in all cases in which it is technically feasible. Other factors that predict lymph node metastasis include lymph–vascular space invasion,[89] adnexal metastasis, and clear cell[90] or papillary serous[91] histology.

The decision to recommend adjuvant radiation following surgical staging of endometrial cancer depends on the risk of disease recurrence. Thus, the extent of disease at staging, tumor grade, and depth of invasion are important prognostic factors in determining which patients will benefit from adjuvant therapy.[92] Patients with well- and moderately differentiated tumors localized to the endometrium or with superficial myometrial invasion have a 5-year survival of 98% following surgical treatment alone, compared with a 94% survival following surgery and adjuvant radiation.[93] Thus, most patients in this low-risk group do not receive adjuvant radiation. Patients with poorly differentiated tumors have a significant risk of pelvic recurrence and thus are candidates for adjuvant external-beam pelvic radiation.[94] In patients with disease spread outside the uterus, the response to chemotherapy has been poor, with a Gynecologic Oncology Group trial demonstrating a 66% response rate to doxorubicin and cisplatin, a progression-free interval of 6.2 months, and a median survival of 9 months.[95] Response to other chemotherapeutic agents has also been poor.[96,97] In patients who are not candidates for surgical therapy, clinical staging is applied according to the International Federation of Gynecology and Obstetrics (FIGO) guidelines of 1971, which include evaluation of the length of the endometrial canal, tumor grade, endocervical curettage, and radiographic assessment of distant metastasis. In these patients, primary radiation therapy may be appropriate.

Cervical Cancer

Worldwide, cervical cancer is a major health concern, with a yearly incidence of 371,000 cases and an annual death rate of 190,000.[98] Since the development of the Papanicolaou (Pap) smear in 1943, however, and its acceptance in the role of screening for cervical cancer, a significant decrease in both the incidence and mortality of this disease has been possible. Currently, cervical cancer is the third most common gynecological malignancy in the United States, with 10,520 new cases and 3,900 deaths expected in 2004.[76] The reason for the dramatic decrease in the incidence of cervical cancer in the United States lies in the ability of the Pap smear to detect a premalignant precursor of cervical cancer, cervical intraepithelial neoplasia (CIN). CIN progresses slowly to carcinoma, allowing intervention before the development of malignancy. Algorithms have been developed for the management of an abnormal Pap smear. Recommendations for the initiation and frequency of cervical cytological screenings have recently changed from the traditional annual Pap smear and are still evolving as more epidemiological data accrue. Based on a review of the studies to date, the American College of Obstetricians and Gynecologists (ACOG) recommends that annual cervical cytology screening to detect CIN should begin 3 years after initiation of sexual intercourse but no later than age 21 years. Annual screening is recommended for women younger than 30 years, but for those over age 30 who have had three consecutive negative cervical cytology screening test results, have no history of CIN 2 or -3, are not immunocompromised or infected with human immunodeficiency virus (HIV), and are without in utero diethylstilbestrol (DES) exposure, the interval between Pap smears may be extended to every 2 to 3 years. Results from a recently reported randomized trial (Atypical squamous cells of undetermined significance [ASC-US]/Low-grade squamous intraepithelial lesions [LSIL] Triage Study for cervical cancer [ALTS]) evaluating the role of testing for the human papillomavirus (HPV) for the detection of cervical dysplasia suggests that in women with minimally abnormal cervical cytology, the absence of oncogenic strains of HPV predicts an extremely low risk for developing cervical cancer; in this situation, repeat annual cytology rather than further evaluation is acceptable.[99]

Signs and symptoms of cervical cancer vary considerably. Many patients are asymptomatic at the time of their diagnosis. Pelvic examination with a speculum may demonstrate a lesion on the cervix, or bimanual rectovaginal examination may reveal a palpable nodule on the cervix. Cervical cancer spreads from cervix to vagina to the paracervical and parametrial tissues as a result of direct extension. Thus, symptoms may be related to the tumor location. Both ulcerating and exophytic cervical lesions can cause abnormal bleeding, a thin serosanguineous discharge, or bleeding after intercourse. As the tumor necroses, a malodorous discharge may become noticeable. As the tumor progresses from the cervix to other pelvic tissues, bimanual rectovaginal pelvic examination may reveal tumor extension. With advanced primary or recurrent cervical cancer, ureteral obstruction, hydronephrosis or hydroureter, and azotemia may result, as well as lower extremity edema, neurological deficits, or pain as a result of tumor infiltration around the pelvic lymphatics, vasculature, and nerves.

Staging of cervical cancer is based on physical examination (bimanual rectovaginal examination, cystoscopy, proctoscopy) and appropriate adjuvant radiographs [chest radiography, barium enema, intravenous pyelogram (IVP)]. The stage of a cervical cancer is never changed by information gained at the time of surgical exploration. Stage at diagnosis has been shown to be the most important prognostic factor in cervical cancer. In general, the 5-year survival in stage I (cancer confined to the cervix) disease is 88%, compared with 63% for stage II (invasion beyond the uterus but not the pelvic wall) and 38% for stage III (pelvic wall involvement).[100] The presence of metastasis in pelvic or paraaortic lymph nodes (as determined by either lymphangiography or retroperitoneal lymphadenectomy) has also been shown to be a significant negative prognostic factor.

Treatment of primary cervical cancer is dependent on stage and lymph node status. Microinvasive cervical cancer is adequately treated with either a cervical conization or extrafascial hysterectomy. Early-stage cancers are candidates for either radical hysterectomy or irradiation. The decision to pursue one treatment option over another is generally guided by the patient's age, general health, and other complicating factors. Radiotherapy is applicable to any patient with early-stage cervical cancer, but radical hysterectomy is appropriate for only a subset of these patients. The goals of radical hysterectomy are to remove the uterus, parametrial tissue, upper one-third of the vagina, and pelvic lymph nodes, with or without the paraaortic lymph nodes. In the hands of an experienced gynecologic oncologist, the morbidity of radical hysterectomy is 1% to 5%. Bladder dysfunction is the most common postoperative complication as a result of transection of the nerves supplying the bladder. Ureteral fistulae occur rarely (0%–3%), as do pelvic infection, hemorrhage, and lymphocyst formation. Pulmonary embolism is the most common fatal complication of radical pelvic surgery.

Radiotherapy is the appropriate treatment for locally advanced cancers as well as for early-stage disease. The prescription of radiation is generally based on the stage, lesion size, and lymph node status, with the use of both external-beam irradiation (teletherapy) and intracavitary radiation (brachytherapy) in various combinations. Complications from radiation therapy are related to treatment dose, volume, and the tolerance of the tissues included in the radiated field. Diarrhea and nausea are common acute complications, but these are generally transient and resolve on completion of therapy. Early complications occur within 6 months of therapy, and include skin ulceration, cystitis, and proctitis. Late complications, occurring more than 6 months following therapy, may include intestinal obstruction, fistulization, and chronic proctosigmoiditis. Recent studies have demonstrated improved survival when cisplatin is added to radiation for patients with locally advanced disease as well as early-stage, high-risk disease (pelvic lymph node metastasis, parametrial metastasis, positive surgical margins) following radical hysterectomy. Together, these studies indicate that concurrent chemoradiation decreases the risk of death from cervical cancer by 30% to 50% when compared with radiation alone.[101–105]

Following treatment for invasive cervical cancer, patients are followed closely with bimanual rectovaginal examination and cytological assessment of the upper vagina every 3 to 4 months for the first 2 years after therapy. Death resulting from cervical cancer occurs most commonly during the first year of observation (50%), decreasing to 25% by the second year. The prognosis of a patient with a recurrence of cervical cancer depends on the location of the disease. Patients with a pelvic recurrence who were initially treated with radical hysterectomy are frequently treated with radiation. Following primary radiation therapy, patients with a central (cervical or upper vaginal) recurrence may be candidates for a pelvic exenteration, which involves removal of the uterus, tubes, ovaries, bladder, and rectosigmoid with urinary diversion and creation of a colostomy. Five-year survival rates following pelvic exenteration range between 20% and 62%, with the operative death rate approaching 10%. Careful patient selection will lead to the most favorable survival rates while minimizing operative morbidity and mortality. Unfortunately, the response to chemotherapy for recurrent cervical cancer is generally poor.

Abdominal Hysterectomy

Abdominal hysterectomy is second to cesarean section as the most common major gynecological operation performed in the United States, with approximately 645,000 cases completed in 1998.[106] This procedure is the treatment for many gynecological conditions, including benign and malignant tumors, bleeding, and infection. As in any surgical procedure, thorough preoperative evaluation, proper intraoperative technique, and appropriate postoperative care are required to minimize morbidity and mortality. Although general surgeons are occasionally involved in the primary management of a gynecological condition requiring hysterectomy, this procedure is most commonly performed either as an adjunct to colon cancer surgery (infiltration of the uterus or adnexa, or prophylaxis against ovarian metastasis) or because of the incidental discovery of gynecological pathology during surgery for an unrelated condition.

The indications for hysterectomy are not reviewed here. In many circumstances, hysterectomy can be accomplished by either a vaginal or abdominal approach. The decision to pursue one over the other depends on the condition to be treated as well as the patient's medical condition. The technique of vaginal hysterectomy is beyond the scope of this chapter. It is important to note that recent advancements in minimally invasive surgery and interventional radiology are providing effective alternatives to hysterectomy for benign disease. Along with medical management, issues of menorrhagia are now routinely treated with a variety of hysteroscopic approaches to endometrial ablation. Symptomatic uterine fibroids are the largest single indication for hysterectomy.[107] In addition to abdominal or laparoscopic myomectomy for those wishing to preserve fertility, hysteroscopic resection can also be attempted. A recent study has demonstrated that uterine artery embolization, a technique barely a decade old, is a cost-effective alternative to hysterectomy for the treatment of fibroids.[108] Treatment modalities currently under investigation include high-intensity focused ultrasound, which may provide a completely noninvasive approach to the treatment of uterine fibroids.[109]

Before hysterectomy, one dose of prophylactic antibiotic is recommended to reduce the risk of infectious morbidity. A first- or second-generation cephalosporin is usually administered 30 min before the incision. In general, most abdominal hysterectomies are performed through a transverse incision in the lower abdomen. The Pfannenstiel incision provides excellent exposure of the pelvic organs and is used most commonly. A Maylard or Cherney incision can be made if more exposure is necessary. For malignant conditions or cases in which visualization of the upper abdomen is necessary, a vertical midline incision is used. A heavy (O or OO) absorbable suture such as polyglycolic acid or chromic gut is generally used in an abdominal hysterectomy.

On opening the abdomen, a thorough visual inspection and palpation of the upper abdomen and pelvic organs and surfaces is imperative. The bowels are then packed in the upper abdomen, and a retractor is placed. Heavy clamps are then placed across the uterine cornua (including the utero-ovarian ligament and fallopian tube) for retraction. The round ligament is then divided, and the broad ligament is entered (Fig. 105.11). The peritoneum overlying the broad ligament is then divided parallel to the infundibulopelvic ligament, which contains the ovarian blood vessels. The ureter is identified on the medial leaf of the broad ligament to avoid injury during the procedure (Fig. 105.12). If the ovaries are to be removed,

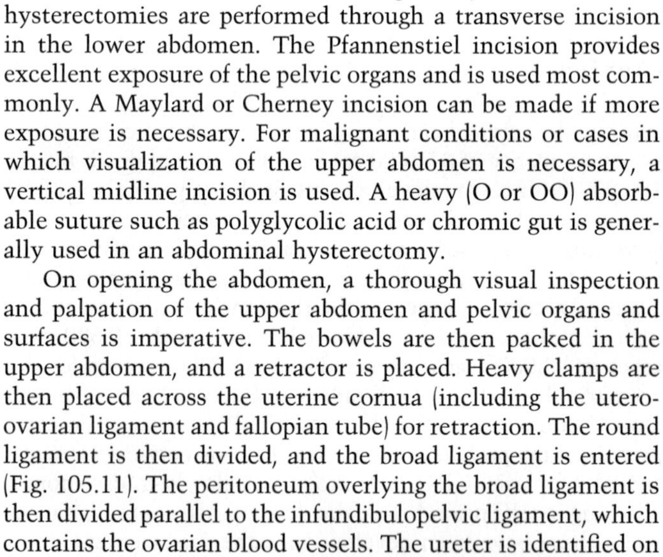

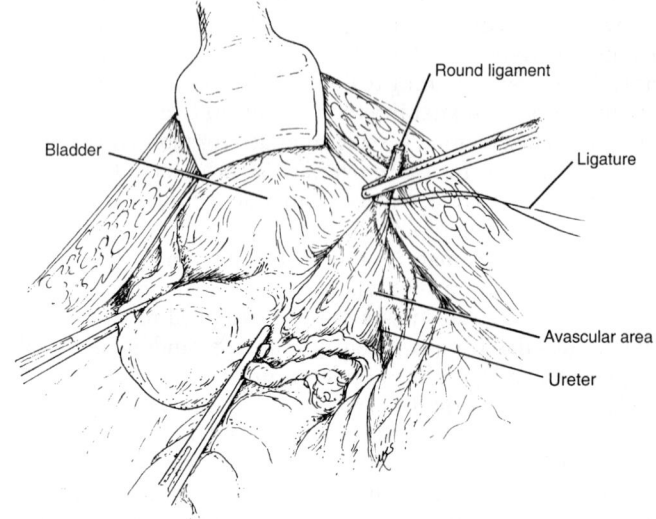

FIGURE 105.11. Entering the retroperitoneal space. The round ligaments are clamped and divided. The posterior leaf of the broad ligament is then divided parallel to the infundibulopelvic ligament, and the ureter is identified in the retroperitoneal space.

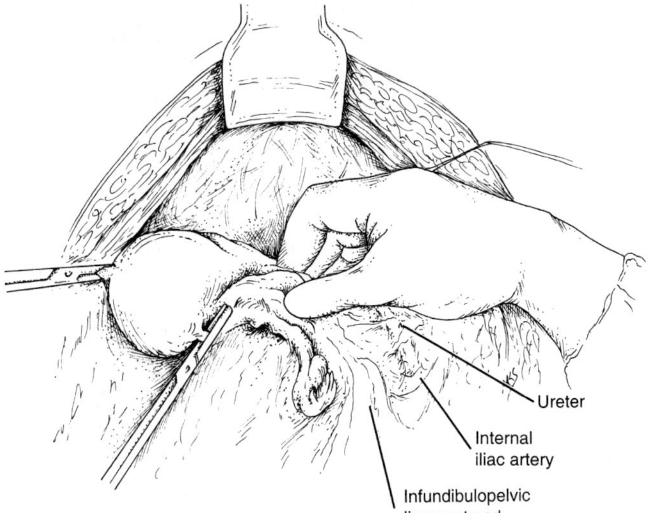

FIGURE 105.12. Dividing the infundibulopelvic ligament. Once the ureter has been identified along the medial leaf of the broad ligament, a window in the peritoneum is created above the ureter and below the infundibulopelvic ligament. The ovarian blood vessels are then clamped, divided, and ligated.

a window in the broad ligament between the ureter and the infundibulopelvic ligament is developed, doubly clamped, divided, and ligated. If the ovaries are to be preserved, transection of the infundibulopelvic ligament is not performed. In this situation, a window in the peritoneum below the utero-ovarian ligament medial to the adnexa is created sharply, clamped, divided, and ligated. The uterovesical peritoneum is then divided, and the plane between the bladder and cervix is developed sharply (Fig. 105.13). The bladder is then advanced below the level of the cervix and upper vagina. The uterine blood vessels are then clamped at the level of the endocervix. A second clamp can be placed above the first to control bleeding from within the uterus. This pedicle is then cut and suture-ligated. The remaining portion of the cardinal and uterosacral ligaments are clamped, cut, and suture-ligated in a similar fashion. Once these ligaments have been divided down to the ectocervix, clamps are placed from both corners across the upper vagina, and the hysterectomy specimen is divided above the clamps. These pedicles are then suture ligated. The remainder of the vaginal cuff is then closed. Once hemostasis is confirmed, the fascia and skin incisions are closed.

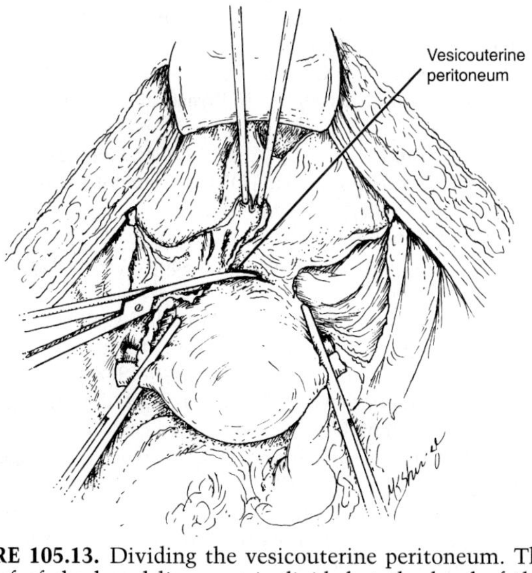

FIGURE 105.13. Dividing the vesicouterine peritoneum. The anterior leaf of the broad ligament is divided at the level of the lower uterine segment. The bladder is then advanced from the uterus until it is below the level of the cervix. This step is important in avoiding injury to the bladder when the upper vagina is divided below the cervix.

References

1. Curtis KM, Hillis SD, Kieke BA Jr, Brett KM, Marchbanks PA, Peterson HB. Visits to emergency departments for gynecologic disorders in the United States, 1992–1994. Obstet Gynecol 1998; 91:1007–1012.
2. Visco AG, Del Priore G. Postmenopausal Bartholin gland enlargement: a hospital-based cancer risk assessment. Obstet Gynecol 1996;87:286–290.
3. Speroff L, Glass RH, Kase NG. Clinical Gynecologic Endocrinology and Infertility, 5th ed. Baltimore: Williams & Wilkins, 1994.
4. Rossouw JE, Anderson GL, Prentice RL, et al. Risks and benefits of estrogen plus progestin in healthy postmenopausal women: principal results From the Women's Health Initiative randomized controlled trial. JAMA 2002;288(3):321–333.
5. Anderson GL, Limacher M, Assaf AR, et al. Effects of conjugated equine estrogen in postmenopausal women with hysterectomy: the Women's Health Initiative randomized controlled trial. JAMA 2004;291(14):1701–1712.
6. Warren MP. A comparative review of the risks and benefits of hormone replacement therapy regimens. Am J Obstet Gynecol 2004;190(4):1141–1167.
7. Beigi RH, Wiesenfeld HC. Pelvic inflammatory disease: new diagnostic criteria and treatment. Obstet Gynecol Clin N Am 2003;30(4):777–793.
8. Yeh JM, Hook EW 3rd, Goldie SJ. A refined estimate of the average lifetime cost of pelvic inflammatory disease. Sex Transm Dis 2003;30(5):369–378.
9. Centers for Disease Control and Prevention. 2002 Guidelines for treatment of sexually transmitted diseases. MMWR (Morb Mortal Wkly Rep) 2002;51(RR-6):48–51.
10. Farley TM, Rosenberg MJ, Rowe PJ, Chen JH, Meirik O. Intrauterine devices and pelvic inflammatory disease: an international perspective. Lancet 1992;339:785–788.
11. Scholes D, Stergachis A, Ichikawa LE, Heidrich FE, Holmes KK, Stamm WE. Vaginal douching as a risk factor for cervical *Chlamydia trachomatis* infection. Obstet Gynecol 1998;91:993–997.
12. Jacobson L. Differential diagnosis of acute pelvic inflammatory disease. Am J Obstet Gynecol 1980;138:1006–1011.
13. Patten RM, Vincent LM, Wolner-Hanssen P, Thorpe E Jr. Pelvic inflammatory disease. Endovaginal sonography with laparoscopic correlation. J Ultrasound Med 1990;9:681–689.
14. Cacciatore B, Leminen A, Ingman-Friberg S, Ylostalo P, Paavonen J. Transvaginal sonographic findings in ambulatory patients with suspected pelvic inflammatory disease. Obstet Gynecol 1992;80:912–916.
15. Boardman LA, Peipert JF, Brody JM, Cooper AS, Sung J. Endovaginal sonography for the diagnosis of upper genital tract infection. Obstet Gynecol 1997;90:54–57.
16. Ness RB, Soper DE, Holley RL, et al. Effectiveness of inpatient and outpatient treatment strategies for women with pelvic inflammatory disease: results from the Pelvic Inflammatory Disease Evaluation and Clinical Health (PEACH) Randomized Trial. Am J Obstet Gynecol. 2003;188(2):598–600.

17. Perez-Medina T, Huertas MA, Bajo JM. Early ultrasound-guided transvaginal drainage of tubo-ovarian abscesses: a randomized study. Ultrasound Obstet Gynecol 1996;7:435–438.
18. Aboulghar MA, Mansour RT, Serour GI. Ultrasonographically guided transvaginal aspiration of tuboovarian abscesses and pyosalpinges: an optional treatment for acute pelvic inflammatory disease. Am J Obstet Gynecol 1995;172:1501–1503.
19. Nelson AL, Sinow RM, Renslo R, Renslo J, Atamdede F. Endovaginal ultrasonographically guided transvaginal drainage for treatment of pelvic abscesses. Am J Obstet Gynecol 1995; 172:1926–1932.
20. Feld R, Eschelman DJ, Sagerman JE, Segal S, Hovsepian DM, Sullivan KL. Treatment of pelvic abscesses and other fluid collections: efficacy of transvaginal sonographically guided aspiration and drainage. AJR Am J Roentgenol 1994;163:1141–1145.
21. vanSonnenberg E, D'Agostino HB, Casola G, Goodacre BW, Sanchez RB, Taylor B. US-guided transvaginal drainage of pelvic abscesses and fluid collections. Radiology 1991;181:53–56.
22. Breen JL. A 21 year survey of 654 ectopic pregnancies. Am J Obstet Gynecol 1970;106:1004–1019.
23. Centers for Disease Control and Prevention. Advanced report of final mortality statistics. Mon Vital Stat Rep 1995;43:11–13.
24. Centers for Disease Control and Prevention. Ectopic pregnancy—United States 1990–1992. MMWR (Morb Mortal Wkly Rep) 1995;44:46–48.
25. Zane SB, Kieke BA Jr, Kendrick JS, Bruce C. Surveillance in a time of changing health care practices: estimating ectopic pregnancy incidence in the United States. Matern Child Health J 2002;6(4):227–236.
26. Chow WH, Daling JR, Cates W Jr, Greenberg RS. Epidemiology of ectopic pregnancy. Epidemiol Rev 1987;9:70–94.
27. Peterson HB, Xia Z, Hughes JM, Wilcox LS, Tylor LR, Trussell J. The risk of ectopic pregnancy after tubal sterilization. U.S. Collaborative Review of Sterilization Working Group. N Engl J Med 1997;336:762–767.
28. Sulak, PJ. Intrauterine device practice guidelines: patient types. Contraception 1998;58(3 suppl):55S–58S.
29. American Society for Reproductive Medicine. Assisted Reproductive Technology in the United States: 2000 results generated from the ASRM/SART Registry. Fertil Steril 2004;81(5):1207–1215.
30. Kadar N, Bohrer M, Kemmann E, Shelden R. The discriminatory human chorionic gonadotropin zone for endovaginal sonography: a prospective, randomized study. Fertil Steril 1994;61:1016–1020.
31. Kadar N, Caldwell BV, Romero R. A method of screening for ectopic pregnancy and its indications. Obstet Gynecol 1981; 58:162–166.
32. Barnhart KT, Sammel MD, Rinaudo PF, Zhou L, Hummel AC, Guo W. Symptomatic patients with an early viable intrauterine pregnancy: HCG curves redefined. Obstet Gynecol 2004;104(1):50–55.
33. Murphy AA, Nager CW, Wujek JJ, Kettel LM, Torp VA, Chin HG. Operative laparoscopy versus laparotomy for the management of ectopic pregnancy: a prospective trial. Fertil Steril 1992;57:1180–1185.
34. Vermesh M, Silva PD, Rosen GF, Stein AL, Fossum GT, Sauer MV. Management of unruptured ectopic gestation by linear salpingostomy: a prospective, randomized clinical trial of laparoscopy versus laparotomy. Obstet Gynecol 1989;73:400–404.
35. Lundorff P, Thorburn J, Lindblom B. Fertility outcome after conservative surgical treatment of ectopic pregnancy evaluated in a randomized trial. Fertil Steril 1992;57:998–1002.
36. Tulandi T, Guralnick M. Treatment of tubal ectopic pregnancy by salpingotomy with or without tubal suturing and salpingectomy. Fertil Steril 1991;55:53–55.
37. Korell M, Albrich W, Hepp H. Fertility after organ-preserving surgery of ectopic pregnancy: results of a multicenter study. Fertil Steril 1997;68:220–223.
38. Silva PD, Schaper AM, Rooney B. Reproductive outcome after 143 laparoscopic procedures for ectopic pregnancy. Obstet Gynecol 1993;81:710–715.
39. de la Cruz A, Cumming DC. Factors determining fertility after conservative or radical surgical treatment for ectopic pregnancy. Fertil Steril 1997;68:871–874.
40. Hajenius PJ, Engelsbel S, Mol BW, et al. Randomised trial of systemic methotrexate versus laparoscopic salpingostomy in tubal pregnancy. Lancet 1997;350:774–779.
41. Stovall TG, Ling FW. Single-dose methotrexate: an expanded clinical trial. Am J Obstet Gynecol 1993;168:1759–1762.
42. Lipscomb GH, Bran D, McCord ML, Portera JC, Ling FW. Analysis of three hundred fifteen ectopic pregnancies treated with single-dose methotrexate. Am J Obstet Gynecol 1998;178:1354–1358.
43. Stika CS, Anderson L, Frederiksen MC. Single-dose methotrexate for the treatment of ectopic pregnancy: Northwestern Memorial Hospital three-year experience. Am J Obstet Gynecol 1996;174:1840–1846.
44. Glock JL, Johnson JV, Brumsted JR. Efficacy and safety of single-dose systemic methotrexate in the treatment of ectopic pregnancy. Fertil Steril 1994;62:716–721.
45. Alexander JM, Rouse DJ, Varner E, Austin JM Jr. Treatment of the small unruptured ectopic pregnancy: a cost analysis of methotrexate versus laparoscopy. Obstet Gynecol 1996;88:123–127.
46. ACOG Practice Bulletin. Medical Management of Tubal Pregnancy. Number 3, December 1998. Obstet Gynecol 1998; 92(6):510–511.
47. ACOG Practice Bulletin. Prevention of Rh D Alloimmunization. Number 4, May 1999. Obstet Gynecol 1999;93(5):627–633.
48. Sommerville M, Grimes DA, Koonings PP, Campbell K. Ovarian neoplasms and the risk of adnexal torsion. Am J Obstet Gynecol 1991;164:577–578.
49. Merritt DF. Torsion of the uterine adnexa: a review. Adolesc Pediatr Gynecol 1991;4:3–13.
50. Chang KH, Hwang KJ, Kwon HC, et al. Conservative therapy of adnexal torsion employing color Doppler sonography. J Am Assoc Gynecol Laparosc 1998;5:13–17.
51. Lee EJ, Kwon HC, Joo HJ, Suh JH, Fleischer AC. Diagnosis of ovarian torsion with color Doppler sonography: depiction of twisted vascular pedicle. J Ultrasound Med 1998;17:83–89.
52. Fleischer AC, Stein SM, Cullinan JA, Warner MA. Color Doppler sonography of adnexal torsion. J Ultrasound Med 1995;14:523–528.
53. Zweizig S, Perron J, Grubb D, Mishell DR Jr. Conservative management of adnexal torsion. Am J Obstet Gynecol 1993;168:1791–1795.
54. Chapron C, Capella-Allouc S, Dubuisson JB. Treatment of adnexal torsion using operative laparoscopy. Hum Reprod (Oxf) 1996;11:998–1103.
55. McHutchinson LL, Koonings PP, Ballard CA, d'Ablaing G III. Preservation of ovarian tissue in adnexal torsion with fluorescein. Am J Obstet Gynecol 1993;168:1386–1388.
56. Goldstein SR, Subramanyam B, Snyder JR, Beller U, Raghavendra BN, Beckman EM. The postmenopausal cystic adnexal mass: the potential role of ultrasound in conservative management. Obstet Gynecol 1989;73:8–10.
57. Bailey CL, Ueland FR, Land GL, et al. The malignant potential of small cystic ovarian tumors in women over 50 years of age. Gynecol Oncol 1998;69:3–7.
58. Yuen PM, Yu KM, Yip SK, Lau WC, Rogers MS, Chang A. A randomized prospective study of laparoscopy and laparotomy in the management of benign ovarian masses. Am J Obstet Gynecol 1997;177:109–114.

59. Canis M, Mage G, Pouly JL, Wattiez A, Manhes H, Bruhat MA. Laparoscopic diagnosis of adnexal cystic masses: a 12-year experience with long-term follow-up. Obstet Gynecol 1994;83(5 Pt 1):707–712.
60. Childers JM, Nasseri A, Surwit EA. Laparoscopic management of suspicious adnexal masses. Am J Obstet Gynecol 1996;175(6):1451–1457; discussion 1457–1459.
61. Canis M, Pouly JL, Wattiez A, Mage G, Manhes H, Bruhat MA. Laparoscopic management of adnexal masses suspicious at ultrasound. Obstet Gynecol 1997;89(5 Pt 1):679–683.
62. Dottino PR, Levine DA, Ripley DL, Cohen CJ. Laparoscopic management of adnexal masses in premenopausal and postmenopausal women. Obstet Gynecol 1999;93(2):223–228.
63. Montz FJ, Schlareth JB, Morrow CP. The natural history of theca lutein cysts. Obstet Gynecol 1988;72:247–251.
64. Sandenbergh HA, Woodruff JD. Histogenesis of pseudomyxoma peritonei. Review of 9 cases. Obstet Gynecol 1977;49:339–345.
65. Wheeler JM. Epidemiology of endometriosis-associated infertility. J Reprod Med 1989;34(1):41–46.
66. American Society for Reproductive Medicine. Revised classification of endometriosis: 1996. Fertil Steril 1997;67(5):817–821.
67. Koninckx PR, Martin DC. Deep endometriosis: a consequence of infiltration or retraction or possibly adenomyosis externa? Fertil Steril 1992;58(5):924–928.
68. Koninckx PR, Oosterlynck D, D'Hooghe T, Meuleman C. Deeply infiltrating endometriosis is a disease whereas mild endometriosis could be considered a non-disease. Ann N Y Acad Sci 1994;734:333–341.
69. Adamson D. Surgical management of endometriosis. Semin Reprod Med 2003;21(2):223–234.
70. Mol BW, Bayram N, Lijmer JG, et al. The performance of CA-125 measurement in the detection of endometriosis: a meta-analysis. Fertil Steril 1998;70(6):1101–1108.
71. Colacurci N, Fortunato N, De Franciscis P, et al. Serum and peritoneal CA-125 levels as diagnostic test for endometriosis. Eur J Obstet Gynecol Reprod Biol 1996;66(1):41–43.
72. Ling FW. Randomized controlled trial of depot leuprolide in patients with chronic pelvic pain and clinically suspected endometriosis. Pelvic Pain Study Group. Obstet Gynecol 1999; 93(1):51–58.
73. Sutton CJG, Ewen SP, Whitelaw N, Haines P. Prospective, randomized, double-blind controls: trial of laser laparoscopy in the treatment of pelvic pain associated with minimal, mild and moderate endometriosis. Fertile Steril 1994;62:696–700.
74. Jones KD, Haines P, Sutton CJG. Long-term follow-up of a controlled trial of laser laparoscopy in the treatment of pelvic pain associated with minimal, mild and moderate endometriosis. J Surg Laparosc Surg 2002;5:111–115.
75. Olive DL, Shwartz LB. Endometriosis. N Engl J Med 1993; 328:1759–1769.
76. Ries LAG, Eisner MP, Kosary CL, et al., eds. SEER Cancer Statistics Review, 1975–2001. National Cancer Institute, Bethesda, MD: http://seer.cancer.gov/csr/1975_2001/, 2004.
77. Jemal A, Siegel R, Ward E, Murray T, Xu J, Thun MJ. Cancer statistics, 2007. CA Cancer J Clin 2007;57(1):43–66.
78. Einhorn N, Sjovall K, Knapp RC, et al. Prospective evaluation of serum CA 125 levels for early detection of ovarian cancer. Obstet Gynecol 1992;80:14–18.
79. Colombo N, Chiari S, Maggioni A, Bocciolone L, Torri V, Mangioni C. Controversial issues in the management of early epithelial ovarian cancer: conservative surgery and role of adjuvant therapy. Gynecol Oncol 1994;55:S47–S51.
80. Griffiths CT. Surgical resection of tumor bulk in the primary treatment of ovarian carcinoma. Natl Cancer Inst Monogr 1975;42:101–104.
81. Hoskins WJ, McGuire WP, Brady MF, et al. The effect of diameter of largest residual disease on survival after primary cytoreductive surgery in patients with suboptimal residual epithelial ovarian carcinoma. Am J Obstet Gynecol 1994;170:974–979.
82. NIH Consensus Development Panel on Ovarian Cancer. Ovarian cancer: screening, treatment, and follow-up. JAMA 1995;273:491–497.
83. Kurman RJ, Kaminski PF, Norris HJ. The behavior of endometrial hyperplasia. A long-term study of "untreated" hyperplasia in 170 patients. Cancer (Phila) 1985;56:403–412.
84. Ferenczy A, Gelfand M. The biologic significance of cytologic atypia in progestogen-treated endometrial hyperplasia. Am J Obstet Gynecol 1989;160:126–131.
85. Maggino T, Romagnolo C, Landoni F, Sartori E, Zola P, Gadducci A. An analysis of approaches to the management of endometrial cancer in North America: a CTF study. Gynecol Oncol 1998;68:274–279.
86. Peters WA III, Anderson WA, Thornton WN Jr, Morley GW. The selective use of vaginal hysterectomy in the management of adenocarcinoma of the endometrium. Am J Obstet Gynecol 1983;146:285–289.
87. Greer BE, Cain JM, Figge DC, Shy KK, Tamimi HK. Supraumbilical upper abdominal midline incision for pelvic surgery in the morbidly obese patient. Obstet Gynecol 1990;76:471–473.
88. Goff BA, Rice LW. Assessment of depth of myometrial invasion in endometrial adenocarcinoma. Gynecol Oncol 1990;38:46–48.
89. Creasman WT, Morrow CP, Bundy BN, Homesley HD, Graham JE, Heller PB. Surgical pathologic spread patterns of endometrial cancer: a Gynecologic Oncology Group study. Cancer (Phila) 1987;60:2035–2041.
90. Wilson TO, Podratz KC, Gaffey TA, Malkasian GD Jr, O'Brien PC, Naessens JM. Evaluation of unfavorable histologic subtypes in endometrial adenocarcinoma. Am J Obstet Gynecol 1990; 162:418–423.
91. Sherman ME, Bitterman P, Rosenshein NB, Delgado G, Kurman RJ. Uterine serous carcinoma. A morphologically diverse neoplasm with unifying clinicopathologic features. Am J Surg Pathol 1992;16:600–610.
92. Society of Gynecologic Oncologists. Clinical practice guidelines: uterine corpus—endometrial cancer. Oncology 1998;12:122–126.
93. Fanning J, Evans MC, Peters AJ, Samuel M, Harmon ER, Bates JS. Adjuvant radiotherapy for stage I, grade 2 endometrial adenocarcinoma and adenoacanthoma with limited myometrial invasion. Obstet Gynecol 1987;70:920–922.
94. Keys HM, Roberts JA, Brunetto VL, et al; Gynecologic Oncology Group. A phase III trial of surgery with or without adjunctive external pelvic radiation therapy in intermediate risk endometrial adenocarcinoma: a Gynecologic Oncology Group study. Gynecol Oncol 2004;92:744–751.
95. Thigpen JT, Blessing J, Holmsley HD, Lia S. Phase III trial of doxorubicin versus doxorubicin plus cisplatin in advanced or recurrent endometrial carcinoma. Proc Am Soc Clin Oncol 1993;12:261.
96. Ball HG, Blessing JA, Lentz SS, Mutch DG. A phase II trial of paclitaxel in patients with advanced or recurrent adenocarcinoma of the endometrium: a Gynecologic Oncology Group study. Gynecol Oncol 1996;62:278–281.
97. Fleming GF, Fowler JM, Waggoner SE, et al. Phase I trial of escalating doses of paclitaxel combined with fixed doses of cisplatin and doxorubicin in advanced endometrial cancer and other gynecologic malignancies: a Gynecologic Oncology Group study. J Clin Oncol 2001;19:1021–1029.
98. Parkin DM, Pisani P, Ferlay J. Global cancer statistics. CA Cancer J Clin 1999;49(1):33–64.
99. Solomon D, Schiffman M, Tarone R; ALTS Study Group. Comparison of three management strategies for patients with atypical squamous cells of undetermined significance: baseline results from a randomized trial. J Natl Cancer Inst 2001;93:293–299.

100. Benedet J, Odicono F, Maisonneuve P, et al. FIGO annual report on the results of treatment in gynaecological cancer: carcinoma of the cervix uteri. J Epidemiol Biostat 1998;3:5–34.
101. Whitney CW, Sause W, Bundy BN, et al. Randomized comparison of fluorouracil plus cisplatin versus hydroxyurea as an adjunct to radiation therapy in stage IIB–IVA carcinoma of the cervix with negative para-aortic lymph nodes: a Gynecologic Oncology Group and Southwest Oncology Group study. J Clin Oncol 1999;17:1339–1348.
102. Morris M, Eifel PJ, Lu J, et al. Pelvic radiation with concurrent chemotherapy compared with pelvic and para-aortic radiation for high-risk cervical cancer. N Engl J Med 1999;340:1137–1143.
103. Rose PG, Bundy BN, Watkins EB, et al. Concurrent cisplatin-based radiotherapy and chemotherapy for locally advanced cervical cancer. N Engl J Med 1999;340:1144–1153.
104. Peters WA III, Liu PY, Barrett RJ II, et al. Concurrent chemotherapy and pelvic radiation therapy compared with pelvic radiation therapy alone as adjuvant therapy after radical surgery in high-risk early-stage cancer of the cervix. J Clin Oncol 2000; 18:1606–1613.
105. Keys HM, Bundy BN, Stehman FB, et al. Cisplatin, radiation, and adjuvant hysterectomy compared with radiation and adjuvant hysterectomy for bulky stage IB cervical carcinoma. N Engl J Med 1999;340:1154–1161.
106. Kozak LJ, Owings MF, Hall MJ. National Hospital Discharge Survey: 2002 annual summary with detailed diagnosis and procedure data. Vital Health Stat 13 2005;(158):1–199.
107. Wilcox LS, Koonin LM, Pokras R, Strauss LT, Xia Z, Peterson HB. Hysterectomy in the United States, 1988–1990. Obstet Gynecol 1994;83:549–555.
108. Beinfeld MT, Bosch JL, Isaacson KB, Gazelle GS. Cost-effectiveness of uterine artery embolization and hysterectomy for uterine fibroids. Radiology 2004;230(1):207–213.
109. Stewart EA, Gedroyc WM, Tempany CM, et al. Focused ultrasound treatment of uterine fibroid tumors: safety and feasibility of a noninvasive thermoablative technique. Am J Obstet Gynecol 2003;189(1):48–54.

106

Neurosurgery

Philip Starr

Overview of Neurosurgery

Brain Anatomy and Physiology

The brain and spinal cord are bathed in 150 mL cerebrospinal fluid (CSF), covered by three layers of connective tissue, the meninges, and encased in bone. The meninges, from innermost to outermost layers, consist of the pia mater, the arachnoid mater, and the dura mater. CSF is secreted mainly by the choroid plexus within the cerebral ventricles, flows through the ventricular system, and exits from the fourth ventricle into the subarachnoid space. Approximately 500 mL CSF is produced per day. CSF is absorbed into the venous system at the arachnoid granulations, which are specialized villi of the arachnoid membrane invaginating into the superior sagittal sinus.

Brain parenchyma is categorized as gray matter or white matter. Gray matter consists of groups of neuronal cell bodies and white matter consists of thickly myelinated axons. In the brain, gray matter exists primarily in the surface cortical mantle, and in a few large "nuclei" or clusters of neuronal cells that are deep to cortex. The largest subcortical nuclei are the basal ganglia and thalamus. Each cerebral hemisphere is divided into four lobes on the basis of surface anatomy: frontal, parietal, occipital, and temporal lobes.

The brain's blood supply is derived primarily from the internal carotid arteries and the vertebral arteries, which anastomose at the base of the brain to form the circle of Willis. Cerebral arteries travel in the subarachnoid space, within which they may dive into brain sulci, and divide into much smaller "perforating" vessels before entering brain parenchyma. Cerebral veins also travel in the subarachnoid space but ultimately empty into the venous sinuses, which run between the inner and outer leaves of the dura mater.

Nerve cells communicate with one another mainly by action potentials, which are transient changes in transmembrane voltage. Although generated at or near the cell body, the action potentials can propagate long distances down axons as they course through white matter pathways. For example, within the axons of the corticospinal tract, action potentials propagate as much as 1 m from their origin in motor cortex to their termination on the anterior horn cells of the spinal cord. During surgery of the basal ganglia, neuronal action potentials are recorded because their discharge rate and pattern are helpful for precise surgical navigation (Fig. 106.1).

Proper function of brain tissue is exquisitely dependent on adequate perfusion with oxygenated blood. When perfusion is compromised, brain tissue may be irreversibly damaged within minutes. Cerebral perfusion is compromised by globally increased pressure, or by locally increased pressure that causes a shift (herniation) of brain tissue from one intracranial compartment to another.

For the purpose of clinical treatment of neurological disease, cortical areas are divided into "eloquent" and "noneloquent" areas. Although all the cortex probably has some function, the eloquent cortex consists of those regions where function is highly localized and specific, such that small lesions can produce dramatic and consistent neurological deficits. Such regions include the motor cortex at the posterior margin of the frontal lobes, speech cortex in the perisylvian area, and primary visual cortex at the occipital pole. Noneloquent cortex, representing the majority of the cortical mantle, are regions of "delocalized" function such that damage to a noneloquent area produces little or no evident clinical syndrome unless the damage is very extensive or occurs in a bilateral, symmetrical manner. A fundamental principal of brain surgery is that surgical approaches to subcortical targets are designed to transgress only noneloquent cortical regions.

Along with eloquent cortical areas, several subcortical areas are unforgiving with respect to surgical manipulation or trauma. The brainstem and hypothalamus are the primary examples. The hypothalamus controls many endocrine functions, vegetative behavior, and emotional state. The brainstem consists of the midbrain, pons, and medulla. Bounded by the tentorial notch superiorly and the foramen magnum inferiorly, it connects the forebrain with the spinal cord. Most of the major motor and sensory pathways of the central nervous system traverse the brainstem. Although small in size, the brainstem is critically important for nearly all neurological functions and is thus frequently the focus of clinical

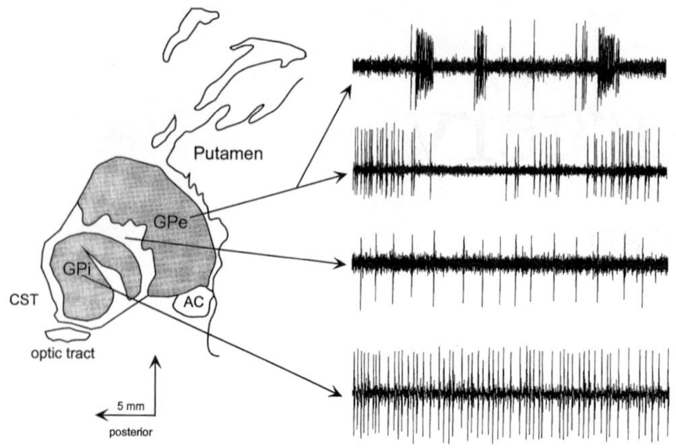

FIGURE 106.1. Action potential discharges recorded from the basal ganglia during surgery for Parkinson's disease. A drawing of basal ganglia nuclei in a parasagittal plane, 20mm for the midline, is shown with characteristic action potential discharges (1-s traces) from different nuclear regions. *GPe*, globus pallidus, external segment; *GPi*, globus pallidus, internal segment; *CST*, corticospinal tract.

examination. Consciousness requires function of the midbrain along with function of one of the two cerebral hemispheres. Most of the cranial nerves (nerves 3–10, 12, and part of 11) have their origin at various levels of the brainstem. Thus, detailed clinical examination of cranial nerve function may provide important, precise localizing information in evaluating brainstem dysfunction.

Conditions Treated by Neurosurgeons

Neurosurgeons manage diseases of the brain, cranial cavity, cerebral blood vessels, spinal cord, and spinal column that are amenable to surgical treatment. In addition, neurosurgeons manage most cases of trauma to the brain and spinal canal whether the case requires surgical treatment or not. The most common neurosurgical disease processes may be categorized as follows:

Hydrocephalus
Trauma to the head or spine
Degenerative spine diseases, including disk herniations, spondylotic disease, and spinal instability
Neurovascular disease: aneurysms and arteriovenous malformations of the brain and spinal cord, carotid stenosis, and intracranial hemorrhage of any etiology
Neurooncology: tumors of the brain and meninges, pituitary gland, spine, and spinal column
Medically intractable disorders of brain physiology, including movement disorders, epilepsy, and chronic pain
Infections of the brain and spinal canal, including brain abscess and spinal epidural abscess
Peripheral nerve injury or entrapment
Congenital malformations involving the neuraxis, such as spinal dysraphism and craniosynostosis

Some neurosurgical procedures may also be performed by other surgical specialties. Examples include carotid endarterectomy (also performed by vascular surgery), spinal instrumentation for instability (also performed by orthopedic surgery), and traumatic injury or entrapment of peripheral nerves (also managed by plastic or orthopedic surgery).

The Neurological Exam for Neurosurgery: What Is Important?

The neurological examination as performed by medical neurologists tends to be detailed. In contrast, the neurological examination for neurosurgery is more concise. Rapid examination of the neurosurgery patient with known or suspected brain pathology is summarized in Table 106.1. The critical parts of the examination are level of consciousness, cranial nerve examination, presence of a lateralizing (e.g., unilateral) motor deficit, and speech. Although hemiplegia or severe hemiparesis are obvious and important lateralizing motor deficits, subtle lateralizing motor deficits, manifested only by pronator drift or flattening of a nasolabial fold, may be important early signs of a mass lesion.

The clinical syndrome of temporal (or uncal) herniation is important to recognize immediately because it often heralds an emergent but surgically treatable problem. It is caused by mass lesions or edema forcing the medial temporal lobe below the tentorial edge, where the herniated tissue compresses the midbrain and third nerve. Clinically, the temporal herniation syndrome consists of the triad of a depressed state of consciousness, pupillary dilatation (ipsilateral to the side of the brain lesion), and lateralized motor deficit (usually, but not always, contralateral to the brain lesion).

For patients with spinal problems, the focus of the neurological exam is on the identification of myelopathy (dysfunction of the spinal cord) or radiculopathy (dysfunction of a spinal nerve root). The exam focuses on deep tendon reflexes, motor strength in relevant muscle groups, sphincter function, and presence or absence of a sensory level. Myelopathy is clinically diagnosed by one or several of the following findings: (1) motor weakness, usually bilateral but not always symmetrical, below a specific spinal level, (2) hyperreflexia, (3) presence of a sensory level (a dermatomal level below which sensation to any modality is objectively or subjectively different), and (4) sphincter dysfunction (urinary retention, lax anal sphincter). Radiculopathy is diagnosed by numbness, weakness, or diminished reflexes in a specific nerve root (that is, dermatomal or myotomal) distribution.

Diagnostic Imaging in Neurosurgery

The introduction of computed tomography (CT) in the 1970s and magnetic resonance (MR) imaging in the 1980s radically altered the practice of neurosurgery. These tools allow rapid and accurate preoperative localization and diagnosis of most

TABLE 106.1. Rapid Neurological Examination for Important Brain Pathology.

Examination category	*What to look for*
State of consciousness	Awake, drowsy, stuporous, or unresponsive
Cranial nerves	Pupillary asymmetry, visual fields, conjugate eye movements, facial muscle asymmetry, gag or cough
Motor examination	Lateralizing motor deficit: hemiplegia, hemiparesis, pronator drift, facial asymmetry
Speech	Fluency of speech production, speech comprehension, Repetition

brain and spinal disorders and precise postoperative evaluation of the results of surgery.

The choice of CT versus MR depends on the type of pathology that is clinically suspected. In general, MR scanning provides superior resolution of soft tissues. CT is superior for examination of bone and acute hemorrhage, especially subarachnoid hemorrhage. Both are excellent for visualizing the ventricles. In the evaluation of most intracranial emergencies (such as head trauma or suspected spontaneous hemorrhage), CT is the exam of choice. In most other situations, MR is the exam of choice. Some situations call for both studies, such as spinal fracture with myelopathy. In this case, CT is used to delineate bony structures whereas MR is used for disk herniation and spinal cord parenchyma. The use of intravenous contrast for a cranial CT or MR study is primarily for imaging tumors or infection. Tumors cause a breakdown in the blood–brain barrier that permits the entry of contrast, thus delineating the tumor margins on the image.

General Care of the Neurosurgical Inpatient

Intracranial Pressure Control

After closure of the fontanelles in infancy, the cranium is a closed cavity. Thus, hydrocephalus, brain edema, or intracranial mass lesions can cause increased intracranial pressure (ICP). Normal ICP, in a supine person who is relaxed, is 0 to 10 mm Hg. Intracranial pressure should be treated aggressively when more than 20 mm Hg and very aggressively when over 25 mm Hg.[1] Elevated ICP interferes with cerebral perfusion and, if not quickly controlled, can lead to a downward spiral in which ischemia further increases the ICP, which exacerbates ischemia, leading to brain death.

The difference between the mean arterial pressure and the ICP is the cerebral perfusion pressure (CPP). The CPP must be above 60 mm Hg for adequate cerebral perfusion.[1,2] Thus, hypotension is particularly dangerous in the setting of elevated ICP. There is debate as to whether maintenance of CPP greater than 70 confers additional protection.[3]

Intracranial pressure may be monitored in several ways. The most common methods are hydrostatic measurement via a catheter placed in the ventricular system, or with a fiberoptic transducer ("ICP bolt") placed in the subarachnoid space or inserted slightly into brain parenchyma. A ventricular catheter has the advantage of allowing CSF drainage to treat ICP in addition to measuring it but may be difficult to place in a patient with very small ventricles. The most common indication for ICP monitoring is severe head trauma. ICP monitoring is recommended in head trauma patients with a Glascow Coma Score of 3–8 (described later) who also have abnormal CT scans, although this is considered a practice guideline, not a practice standard.[1]

Additional options for monitoring brain physiology in the setting of severe trauma include direct measurement of brain tissue oxygenation with an intraparenchymal probe, or of brain oxygen extraction using an oxygen sensor in the jugular bulb and an arterial oxygen saturation monitor. Titration of therapeutic maneuvers to optimize brain oxygenation and oxygen extraction can improve outcomes in severe head trauma, but there is insufficient evidence for these measures at this time to support them as guidelines.[4,5]

If elevated ICP is caused by a surgically accessible mass lesion, such as hematoma, the mass lesion should be removed. The other measures used for controlling elevated ICP, in roughly the order in which they are instituted, are listed in Table 106.2.[1] The interventions listed represent practice guidelines, not practice standards, as there exists little Class I outcomes evidence to support most measures commonly used to treat elevated intracranial pressure.[6]

Other medical measures can reduce secondary injury in the setting of high ICP. Fever and hyperglycemia increase neuronal metabolism and thus can exacerbate ischemic damage to the brain. Acetaminophen or ibuprofen, with or without a cooling blanket, may be used for fever. Hyperglycemia should be controlled with subcutaneous insulin injections or, in difficult cases, by an insulin drip.

The Use of Corticosteroids in Neurosurgery

Corticosteroids were introduced into neurosurgery in the 1960s and have radically improved the acute management of brain tumors. By stabilizing the blood–brain barrier, corticosteroids effectively reduce vasogenic edema in the brain or spinal cord associated with tumors. Steroids are also used to treat edema caused by recent surgical manipulation. They are of no proven use in treating the cytotoxic edema associated with hemorrhagic stroke[7] or head trauma.[8] Decadron (dexamethasone) is the most commonly used corticosteroid in neurosurgery because it is a pure glucocorticoid with no mineralocorticoid effect (unlike prednisone or hydrocortisone) and can be given intravenously or enterally. The relative glucocorticoid potency of decadron, for equivalent milligram doses, is 25 fold greater than hydrocortisone, 5 fold greater than prednisone, and 4 fold greater than methylprednisolone. Following surgery, decadron is usually tapered over a period ranging from 24 h to many weeks. Steroids should be tapered slowly (over weeks to months) in a patient who has been on steroids for more than 1 month because the patient's production of endogenous cortisol is suppressed after long-term therapy. Steroid therapy can be withdrawn only after a positive adrenocorticotropic hormone (ACTH) stimulation test.

Common side effects of steroid use are gastrointestinal (GI) bleeding, hyperglycemia, immunosuppression, poor wound healing, and psychosis. Long-term steroid use may produce osteoporosis, fat redistribution, or myopathy.

Seizures

Seizures are caused by synchronous paroxysmal discharge from the cerebral cortex. Frequently, a seizure is the first presentation of an intracranial lesion, especially with brain tumors. Infratentorial lesions do not produce seizures. Patients with an intracranial lesion that affects the cerebral cortex are at risk for seizures and are usually placed on an anticonvulsant for prophylaxis before surgical treatment. Most of the major anticonvulsants are titrated according to blood levels as well as seizure control.

Dilantin is the most commonly used first-line anticonvulsant for a patient with a new presentation of generalized or focal seizures. It may be loaded enterally or intravenously and rarely causes drowsiness. Dilantin allergies are common and may present as a red macular rash, unexplained fever, or

TABLE 106.2.
Techniques for Controlling Elevated Intracranial Pressure (ICP) (Level II and Level III Evidence).

Technique	*Description*	*Level of evidence*
Surgical evacuation of mass lesions	When a mass lesion is greater than 30 mL and is surgically accessible, craniotomy for removal will contribute to ICP control	III
Head elevation	The head should be elevated to 30° or greater, slightly extended, and not rotated.	III
Optimize venous drainage	Loosen devices that constrict venous return in the neck, such as a cervical collar or an excessively tight tie, for the endotracheal tube	III
Intravenous mannitol	Osmotic diuretics such as mannitol may be given to keep serum osmolarity at 290–310 mOsm/dL; diuresis beyond 320 mOsm/dL is counterproductive as it diminishes cerebral perfusion and may cause renal failure	I[64]
CSF drainage	Drainage performed by ventriculostomy, NOT by spinal tap or spinal drain; may be impractical when ventricles are very small; increasingly performed, but not yet convincingly supported by class I evidence	II[6]
Sedation	Indicated for patients with elevated ICP who are agitated and straining against mechanical ventilation; may use 2% propofol infusion; shown to lower ICP (day 3) in comparison with controls; increasingly performed, but not yet convincingly supported by class I evidence	II[6]
Mild temporary hyperventilation	For temporary control of elevated ICP, mild reduction of P_{CO_2} to 30–35 may be useful. However, randomized studies have shown that long-term or aggressive hyperventilation is harmful because it lowers cerebral perfusion, and efficacy of mild temporary hyperventilation for improved outcomes has not been demonstrated	III[65]
Pentobarbital coma	Load 10 mg/kg over 30 min, then 5 mg/kg q 1 h for 3 doses, then 1 mg/kg/h; titrate to keep serum pentobarbital level 3–4 mg/dl, or to maintain a "burst suppression pattern" on a portable EEG (only some randomized studies have supported the effectiveness of pentobarbital coma for lowering ICP)	II[6,66,67]
Mild hypothermia	Now under study for severely elevated ICP in head trauma; preliminary class II evidence suggests efficacy	II[68]

CSF, cerebrospinal fluid.

altered liver function. Signs of dilantin overdose include arrhythmias, hyperreflexia, dysarthria, confusion, ataxia, and nystagmus. For a patient with allergies or side effects to dilantin who require rapid control of partial or generalized seizures, phenobarbital may be used. Phenobarbital is used only if the patient requires intravenous administration or needs to rapidly achieve a therapeutic level as it tends to be sedating.

An acute generalized seizure requires urgent pharmacological treatment with a benzodiazepine if it does not stop spontaneously within 30 to 60 s because ventilation may be compromised. Ativan (1–2 mg IV) or versed (1–2 mg IV) is frequently used. Intubation is rarely necessary if the seizure lasts less than 2 min. Focal seizures rarely result in airway compromise. Benzodiazepines only halt a seizure acutely and are not useful long-term anticonvulsants. Electrolyte abnormalities predispose the patient to acute seizures. After an unexpected seizure, the serum sodium, magnesium, calcium, and glucose, and anticonvulsant drug level (if applicable), should be checked and corrected.

Blood Pressure Control

During and after intracranial surgery, control of hypertension is critical for the prevention of brain hemorrhage. In the intensive care unit (ICU) postoperatively, blood pressure is kept equal to or slightly less than what it was intraoperatively when brain hemostasis was achieved (usually 120–140 mm Hg systolic). For short-term control of blood pressure in the ICU, a continuous drip such as nipride or trinitroglycerine (TNT) is used. The new onset of hypertension in a neurosurgical patient may signify rising ICP, so intracranial causes should be considered and evaluated by ICP measurement (if an ICP monitor is present) and by changes in the neurological examination.

Fluid and Electrolyte Management

Volume Status

For intracranial pathology, fluid and electrolyte management is specific for the type of pathology. In the setting of large brain tumors, major head trauma, extensive posterior fossa surgery, or intractable postoperative cerebral edema, patients are kept normo- to hypovolumic and normo- to hyperosmolar. This status may be achieved with a fluid restriction of 1000 to 1500 mL/day, or more aggressively with osmotic diuretics such as mannitol. A patient on a diuretic regimen should be monitored for rising creatinine, metabolic alkalosis, and hypokalemia. Following aneurysmal subarachnoid hemorrhage, fluid management is quite different: patients are kept *hyper*volemic because of the risk of stroke from cerebral vasospasm.

Hyponatremia

Hyponatremia should be avoided in neurosurgery patients because it exacerbates brain edema and lowers seizure threshold. The usual treatment for a sodium less than 133 is fluid restriction, ranging from 1500 to 800 mL/day, depending on the degree of hyponatremia. For a patient with fairly acute (less than 48 h) hyponatremia with a sodium below 126 who is not hypervolemic, it is reasonable to give a brief course of 3% saline, usually 50 mL/h over 6 h; this will raise an adult's serum sodium by 2 to 3 mEq/dL, which may be enough to prevent generalized seizures. As overcorrection of hyponatremia may cause pontine myelinolysis,[9] it is not appropriate to give 3% saline as a continuous intravenous infusion or for a patient with long-standing hyponatremia.

Disorders of ADH Regulation

Antidiuretic hormone (ADH, or vasopressin) is synthesized in the hypothalamus, transported through the pituitary stalk, and secreted by the posterior pituitary. Disordered regulation of ADH arises commonly in neurosurgery. Diabetes insipidus (DI) is caused by diminished or absent secretion of ADH; it may arise because of lesions of the sella, suprasellar region, or hypothalamus, or following surgical intervention in these regions. If untreated it leads to excessive water loss, hypernatremia, and hypovolemia. The syndrome of inappropriate ADH secretion (SIADH) may occur transiently following pituitary surgery. It causes hyponatremia with normo- or hypervolemia.

Roughly 30% of patients who undergo transphenoidal surgery of the pituitary develop temporary DI, usually between 12 and 36 h after surgery. Rarely, the DI is permanent. Sometimes it can be preceded by a period of SIADH as traumatized cells of the posterior pituitary rupture and release excess ADH. Patients are written for strict intake and output monitoring, frequent checks of urine specific gravity, and frequent measurement of serum electrolytes. The patient is allowed fluids PO ad lib, with a pitcher of water kept at the bedside.

Following transphenoidal surgery, DI is strongly suspected if urine output is consistently greater than 300/h with urine specific gravity less than 1.003, in the setting of normal or elevated serum sodium. Initial treatment consists of fluid replacement alone, without ADH replacement. In awake patients with DI, the thirst mechanism is intact. Often the patient is able to compensate adequately for DI just by drinking water ad lib. However, if the patient's serum sodium rises above 148, treatment with desmopressin (DDAVP) is appropriate. If DDAVP is given, it is important to stop any IV fluids to avoid severe iatrogenic SIADH. If the serum sodium drops below 140 on DDAVP, fluid restriction is initiated and DDAVP is stopped.

Severe DI arises in brain death (as a result of primary hypothalamic failure) or following transection of the pituitary stalk. Pituitary stalk transection may occur following severe head trauma or because of surgical removal of a craniopharyngioma or other large suprasellar tumor. Management may initially require a pitressin drip, titrated to keep urine output below 100 mL/h. Brain-dead organ donors almost always require a pitressin drip to maintain intravascular volume until organ harvest.

Activity Orders

Head elevation decreases intracranial CSF pressure but increases spinal CSF pressure. Because of this, there are a number of specific conditions in neurosurgery in which the postoperative head position is important for management. Raised intracranial pressure or cranial CSF leak are treated by raising the head of the bed (HOB). Following placement of a new ventriculoperitoneal shunt, overdrainage of CSF can cause severe headache or result in subdural hygromas or hematomas, especially in the elderly. Thus, the HOB should be kept flat for several days and then slowly elevated. During catheter drainage of chronic subdural hematoma, a HOB flat position encourages further fluid drainage and helps the brain to reexpand. Following intradural thoracic or lumbar spinal surgery, there is a risk of CSF leak, so the HOB is initially flat to decrease pressure on the dural closure.

Postoperative Intracranial Hemorrhage

One of the most serious and frequent perioperative complications is intracranial hemorrhage. Although most common in the first 24 h following surgery, it can also occur a few days after surgery. Attention to blood pressure control is critical to avoid this. Any new, unexpected neurological deficit in a postoperative patient warrants an emergent noncontrast head CT to look for evidence of acute bleeding. Bleeding following a posterior fossa operation can cause extremely rapid life-threatening deterioration.

The best preventive measure for perioperative hemorrhage is attention to coagulopathy in the preoperative workup.[10] Coagulation abnormalities are more important to neurosurgery than in other surgical fields because the consequences of intraoperative or postoperative hemorrhage are devastating. Patients on chronic aspirin therapy must stop this medication at least 1 week before surgery. If a preoperative patient has *any* abnormality (however small) of coagulation times or bleeding time, the test should be immediately repeated and the cause determined. Coagulation studies must be completely normal for an elective case.

Common Medical Complications

Certain types of medical complications arise frequently in neurosurgical inpatients: pneumonia, meningitis, and deep venous thrombosis. Major risk factors for pneumonia include immobility, depressed alertness, and lower cranial nerve palsies, all of which are common in neurosurgical patients. Patients who are not awake and ambulatory with a good cough reflex should have chest physical therapy and bronchodilator therapy as prophylaxis. Any postoperative craniotomy patient is at risk for meningitis. There is a very high risk of meningitis following penetrating head injury, after a craniotomy that has violated the frontal sinus, or in a patient with an ongoing CSF leak. In these settings, fever, nuchal rigidity, or change in mental status should prompt a lumbar puncture for CSF culture, if not contraindicated by a large intracranial mass or severe brain edema. Two major risk factors for deep venous thromboses (DVT) and pulmonary emboli are hypercoaguability and immobility, which are especially prevalent in brain tumor patients. Brain tumors are associated with a hypercoagulable state, and associated neurological deficits may immobilize an extremity. All brain tumor patients who are not ambulatory should be treated with sequential compression devices or compressive stockings and should start subcutaneous heparin on postoperative day 1.[10] Sudden tachypnea, hypoxia, or pleuritic chest pain, especially in a bedridden patient, may indicate a pulmonary embolus.

Management of Common Neurosurgical Problems

Hydrocephalus

Hydrocephalus refers to dilation of the cerebral ventricles in which ventricular CSF is, or has been, under elevated pressure. Blockage of CSF circulation may occur within the ventricular system or within the subarachnoid space. Acute hydrocephalus in adults is usually the result of tumors, hemorrhage, or infection; in children, it is usually caused by congenital malformation. Acute hydrocephalus is a common and easily treated neurosurgical emergency.

CSF Diversion Procedures

Acute, life-threatening hydrocephalus may be rapidly treated by placing a catheter within the ventricular system and draining CSF externally (ventriculostomy). External drains may be left in place for as long as several weeks. If the cause of the hydrocephalus resolves (for example, by removal of a tumor obstructing CSF flow), temporary drainage is the only treatment needed. However, if permanent CSF drainage will be required, a totally internal CSF drainage device must be placed. The most common is the ventriculoperitoneal shunt, in which the ventricular catheter drains CSF through a one-way valve into a catheter placed in the intraperitoneal space. CSF shunts may also drain into the pleural space (ventriculopleural shunt) or into the venous system (ventriculoatrial shunt).

In cases of adult hydrocephalus that are caused by obstruction of the Sylvian aqueduct, endoscopic techniques may be used to create a hole in the base of the third ventricle ("third ventriculostomy"), allowing egress of CSF directly into the interpeduncular cistern; this bypasses the obstruction and obviates the need for a shunting procedure.[11]

Management of External Ventricular Drains

Ventriculostomies are prone to infection. For patients on continuous ventricular drainage, antibiotic prophylaxis has been shown to reduce infection risk.[12] Regular changes of the ventriculostomy catheter does not reduce the risk of infection.[13] Patients should have CSF cultured for fever, using sterile technique to handle all components. Intraventricular antibiotics may be administered in the case of a ventriculitis or meningitis.[14] To regulate the amount of drainage and the intracranial pressure, the drainage bag is kept at a certain height above the patient's head, usually 100 to 200 mm above the external auditory canal.

Shunt Complications

Complications of long-term CSF shunting are common.[15] Shunt blockage requires urgent revision. Shunt infection requires shunt removal and temporary external drainage.[16] Shunts may produce excessive CSF drainage, which can lead to the formation of subdural hygromas or hematomas, low-pressure headaches, or the slit ventricle syndrome.[15]

Neurotrauma

Head Trauma: Types of Pathology

Head trauma may produce a variety of intracranial pathologies (Table 106.3). Any of the pathologies listed may be associated with brain edema. Skull fractures are classified by the specific cranial bones involved. Basilar skull fractures are fractures involving the petrous or sphenoid bones, often traverse an air-filled sinus, and may be associated with CSF rinorrhea or otorrhea.

Spine Trauma: Types of Pathology

Traumatic myelopathy is classified by severity (complete or incomplete) and by the spinal level of injury. The incidence of complete myelopathy associated with spinal fractures is decreasing, probably because of improved immobilization and transport. Incomplete myelopathy, even if the degree of residual function is small, has a much better prognosis than complete myelopathy.[17,18]

Spinal fractures are classified into stable and unstable injuries. Spinal instability is defined as "excessive deformation of the spine under physiological loading." There are several schemes for classifying spinal instability; one of the most useful is the three-column model of Denis.[19] In this model, the vertebral column is divided into anterior, middle, and posterior columns; disruption of two or more of the columns predicts spinal instability. Any spine fracture that is associated with acute neurological deficit is presumed to be unstable.

Physical Examination of the Neurotrauma Patient

Following is a suggested initial assessment and management sequence for the neurosurgical consultant asked to see a

TABLE 106.3. Types of Intracranial Pathology Caused by Head Trauma.

Pathology	*Comments*
Epidural hematoma	Usually caused by arterial bleeding associated with a skull fracture; appears biconvex on computed tomography (CT) scan; delimited by bony sutures
Subdural hematoma	Usually caused by venous bleeding and often associated with underlying brain contusion
Subarachnoid	Traumatic subarachnoid hemorrhage (SAH) is more common than aneurysmal SAH but is rarely associated with delayed vasospasm hemorrhage (SAH)
Intraventricular	May be associated with acute hydrocephalus hemorrhage
Brain contusion	Contusions are foci of intraparenchymal hemorrhages or edema, most frequently in the frontal and temporal lobes; "coup" injuries are at the site of the impact; "contrecoup" injuries are opposite to the site of impact
Diffuse axonal injury	A diffuse white matter injury caused by a rapid deceleration of the head; tends to affect the cortical gray–white interface, the corpus callosum, and midbrain; may not be visible on CT

newly arrived *major* trauma victim that is based on the principles of advanced trauma life support. The following assumes that someone else (usually the emergency medicine physician or trauma surgeon) is attending to the nonneurological aspects of initial trauma care.

Initial Assessment

1. Obtain initial history from the emergency medical technicians who transported the patient. Key elements are the mechanism of injury, time of injury, and the patient's neurological examination and vitals at the scene.

2. Confirm appropriate immobiliation of the patient's cervical spine with a hard cervical collar *and* a rigid backboard to which the patient's body and head are fixed by straps or tape.

3. Check the pupils for size and reactivity. A difference of more than 1 mm between the pupils is considered abnormal.

Note: A victim of severe head trauma may arrive brain dead—if both pupils are dilated more than 6 mm and unreactive, check corneal reflexes and cough reflex (by gently tugging on the endotracheal tube) to see if other signs of brainstem function are present.

4. Determine the patient's level of consciousness by the three categories of the Glasgow Coma Scale (GCS).[13] The GCS is summarized in Table 106.4. It assigns a point value to the level of consciousness (from 3 to 15) based on evaluation of three functions: motor response, eye opening, and verbal response.

When describing the patient to a colleague, it is best to give the patient's actual responses (e.g., "moving purposefully with eyes opening to pain") rather than just a cumulative point score. The patient often is intubated, making the verbal response subscale of the GCS inapplicable.

Secondary Assessment

5. Inspect and palpate the head and neck for scalp contusions, lacerations, and fractures. Palpate any head lacerations for underlying open skull fractures. To inspect the neck and palpate the cervical spine to elicit tenderness, it is all right to temporarily remove the cervical collar with a colleague holding the head in gentle traction. Palpate the thoracic and lumbar vertebrae for deformity or tenderness.

6. Perform otoscopy for hemotympanum, blood in the external canal, or CSF otorrhea. Look for CSF draining from the nares. The ophthalmoscopic exam is not very useful in acute trauma because *acute* changes in ICP do not produce papilledema. The exception is the evaluation of children with a question of child abuse. In this case, the fundoscopic exam may show retinal hemorrhages.

7. Determine if the patient is able to move all extremities. If the patient is not following commands, do this by looking for movement to painful stimuli. If able to follow commands, check the strength and symmetry of hand grip, elbow flexion and extension, straight leg lifting, and plantar- and dorsiflexion.

If the patient is weak or paralyzed below a certain level, the sensory exam is very important. March down the neck, thorax, and thighs with a pin or needle to see if there is a level below which sensation is diminished or absent. If the patient is not cooperative, sensation may be confirmed by facial grimacing or purposeful avoidance caused by a painful stimulus applied to successively lower dermatoses.

8. Rectal examination: check for sphincter tone. In a comatose patient, absent anal tone may be the only objective sign of spinal cord trauma. If the preceding motor examination suggested spinal cord injury, check for a bulbocavernosus reflex by feeling for anal sphincter contraction in response to tugging on the Foley catheter. Absence of this reflex in the setting of spinal cord injury indicates "spinal shock," a temporary loss of intrinsic spinal reflexes in acute myelopathy.[20]

9. Reflexes: check the biceps, patellar, and achilles tendon reflexes, and the plantar response. Absent reflexes below a certain level is suggestive of acute spinal cord injury. Diffuse hyperreflexia in an acute trauma patient is suggestive of diffuse axonal injury to the brainstem.

TABLE 106.4. The Glasgow Coma Scale (GCS).

Category	*Level of function*	*Point value*
Motor response	Following commands	6
	Spontaneous purposeful movements	5
	Withdraws to pain	4
	Decorticate posturing	3
	Decerebrate posturing	2
	No motor response with stimuli	1
Eye opening	Spontaneous	4
	To voice command	3
	To pain only	2
	No eye opening	1
Verbal response	Speaks coherently	5
	Uses sentences but disoriented	4
	Uses only isolated words	3
	Vocalizes but does not verbalize	**2**
	No vocalization	1

Source: Teasdale and Jennett (1974).[69]

Radiologic Evaluation of Neurotrauma

CT (without contrast) is the examination of choice for the evaluation of head trauma because it images bone and blood better than MRI. The only type of traumatic intracranial pathology that is better imaged by MRI is diffuse axonal injury[21]; there is no specific treatment for this, however, so emergent diagnosis is not necessary. If the initial physical examination assessment reveals a GCS less than 15 or any lateralizing motor deficit, emergency CT is indicated. In addition, CT is indicated for anyone with a normal GCS who has a suspicious mechanism of injury (for example, fall from a height of 12 feet with extensive scalp lacerations), or any person who is systemically anticoagulated and suffers even minor head trauma.[21] A CT scan of a patient with a large acute traumatic subdural hematoma is shown in Figure 106.2.

Plain spine films are indicated in any awake patient with traumatic myelopathy, focal spine pain or tenderness following trauma, or in any person who is comatose following trauma. Discovery of a spinal fracture at one level warrants careful plain films of the rest of the spine, as up to 15% of spinal fractures are associated with a second fracture at a different level.[22] Any fracture seen on plain films must be further evaluated with a spinal CT. Traumatic myelopathy with or

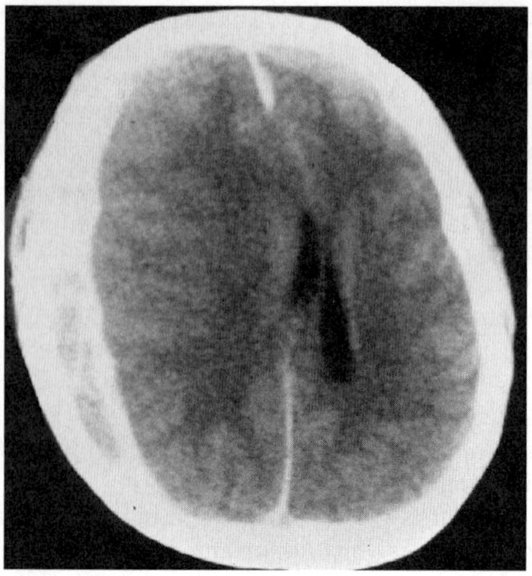

FIGURE 106.2. Axial noncontrast head computed tomography (CT) scan showing large subdural hematoma with shift of the midline structures. This patient had temporal herniation syndrome at the time of this CT.

without fracture should be evaluated by spinal MR to assess soft tissue elements (disk or blood) that may be compressing the spinal cord.

To "clear" the cervical spine in the setting of major head trauma, the patient must not only have a normal cervical spine *series* including lateral, anteroposterior (AP), and odontoid views and both obliques, but the patient must also have grossly normal neurological function below the cervical level and be awake enough to determine that there is no neck tenderness. In the setting of major trauma, a cervical spine CT with coronal and sagittal reconstruction is often obtained in addition to or instead of plain films of the cervical spine because the former has greater sensitivity and specificity for cervical fractures.[23]

Initial Management of Head Trauma

Because brain injury is so heterogeneous, it is very difficult to conduct rigorous, controlled clinical studies of medical or surgical interventions for head trauma. The best guidelines for the management of head trauma are contained in a 1996 publication of the American Association of Neurological Surgeons, *Guidelines for the Management of Severe Head Trauma*.[1] Updates to these guidelines appear periodically on the Brain Trauma foundation website, http://www2.braintrauma.org/guidelines/.

Some medications may be indicated in the emergency room before a CT diagnosis of type and extent of trauma. Immediate (before head CT) treatment with osmotic diuretics (mannitol) is considered a treatment option in a patient with a GCS less than 9 who has unequal pupils or lateralized motor deficit (hemiparesis).[1] A recent prospective trial indicated that early mannitol administration improves brainstem function and clinical outcome in severe head trauma (GCS = 3).[24] Mannitol is contraindicated in hypotension or hypovolemic shock. Corticosteroids are not indicated for head trauma.[8] Although antibiotic prophylaxis is frequently used for deep lacerations with exposed bone, its use for traumatic CSF fistulae is still debated.[25] Seizure prophylaxis in head trauma is controversial, but one study has suggested that phenytoin is protective against posttraumatic seizures for 1 week in patients who present with GCS less than 9.[26]

Craniotomy for drainage of an intracranial hematoma is indicated if the hematoma is surgically accessible, large enough to produce mass effect, and is believed to be causing neurological symptoms because of its mass effect.[27] A large, acute hematoma, particularly one causing temporal lobe herniation, is a neurosurgical emergency. Figures 106.2 and 106.3 illustrate the consequence of a delay in surgical treatment. The hematoma in Figure 106.2 was evacuated about 1 h after the temporal lobe herniation syndrome was evident. The follow-up CT scan 2 days after evacuation (see Figure 106.3) was performed because the patient remained comatose with decerebrate posturing. Infarction of the basal ganglia and brainstem occurred because of ischemic insult from the hematoma before its removal.

Depressed fractures of the convexity should be elevated for cosmesis and to repair any dural tears that may be present.[28] Indications for ICP monitoring in head trauma are GCS of 8 or less, or any patient with an abnormal head CT who will be under prolonged general anesthesia and therefore inaccessible for neurological examination.[1] Treatment of elevated ICP was discussed previously and summarized in Table 106.2.

Initial Management of Spine Trauma

For acute myelopathy (complete or partial), with or without spinal fracture, high-dose methylprednisolone infusion has been shown in randomized trials to improve outcome if initiated within 8 h of injury.[29,30] It should be given immediately and *must* be given within 8 h of the injury. This is the first agent proven in a prospective, randomized study to be efficacious in decreasing secondary injury following trauma to the central nervous system.

In unstable cervical spine fractures in which the spine is misaligned, reduction is performed emergently, by either closed (with cervical traction under X-ray control) or open

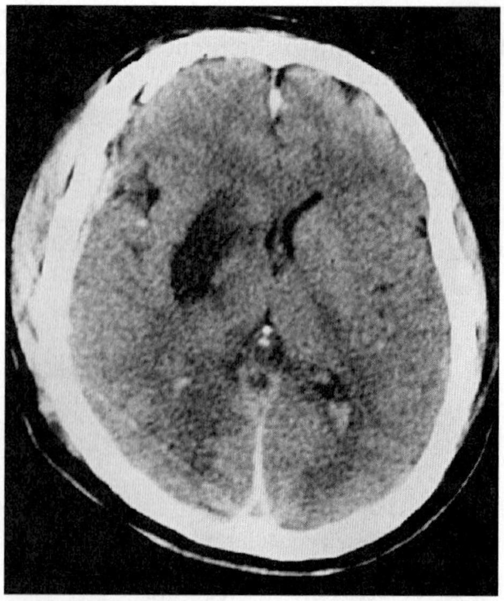

FIGURE 106.3. Same case as shown in Figure 106.2, 2 days following surgical evacuation of the subdural hematoma. The herniation syndrome was not reversed rapidly enough, resulting in a large infarction of the basal ganglia and internal capsule.

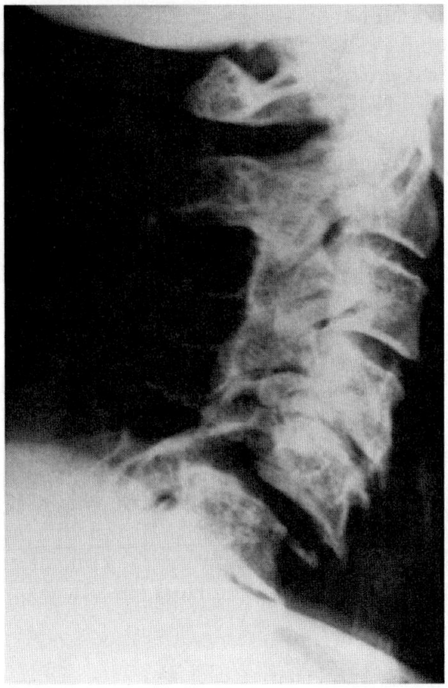

FIGURE 106.4. Lateral radiograph of the cervical spine following traumatic fracture-dislocation between C5 and C6, associated with severe quadriparesis.

surgical reduction. Figures 106.4 and 106.5 show pre- and postoperative lateral spine films for a patient with traumatic dislocation of C4–C5. If available, MR should be performed before closed reduction to rule out anterior disk herniation because, rarely, closed reduction in the setting of a large traumatic disk herniation may exacerbate neurological deficit.[18] If an unstable thoracolumbar fracture is found, the patient must be kept flat and turned by log-rolling (that is, the spine cannot be twisted or flexed). The patient cannot be kept indefinitely on the hard backboard used for transport, even if an unstable fracture is present, because backboards may cause skin breakdown in about 6h.

Surgical treatment of posttraumatic spinal instability is a topic that is complex and evolving. Some general principles, however, are as follows. Compression of neural elements requires surgical decompression. Ligamentous injuries must be surgically fused and internally fixed (see Figure 106.5).[31] Pure bony injuries with good spinal alignment and no neurological deficit can often be treated with external immobilization, such as a halo vest. In these cases, however, the option of early internal (surgical) fixation may avoid a prolonged period of wearing a bulky, uncomfortable external fixator.

Degenerative Spine Disease

Disk Disease

One of the most common problems in neurosurgery is compression of the spinal cord or nerve roots caused by disease of the intervertebral disk. Normally, the central disk material (nucleus pulposus) is contained by a firm band of connective tissue (annulus fibrosis). The major types of disk pathology are diffuse bulging of the annulus without actual herniation, herniation of the disk through a rupture in the annulus, and

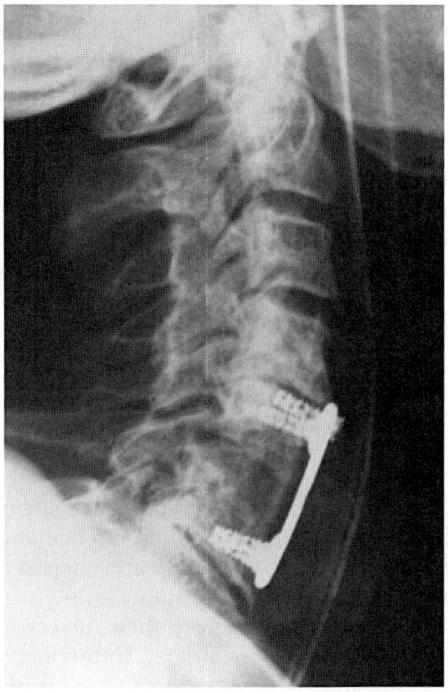

FIGURE 106.5. Lateral radiograph of the cervical spine, same case as in Figure 106.2, following closed reduction, anterior fusion of the C5–C6 disk space with autologous iliac crest bone graft, and placement of spinal instrumentation for internal fixation.

migration of a "free fragment" of disk within the spinal canal. Disk pathology can produce radiculopathy by pressing on nerve roots or myelopathy by pressing on the spinal cord. Disk herniations are most common at the mid- and low cervical and low lumbar levels (Fig. 106.6).

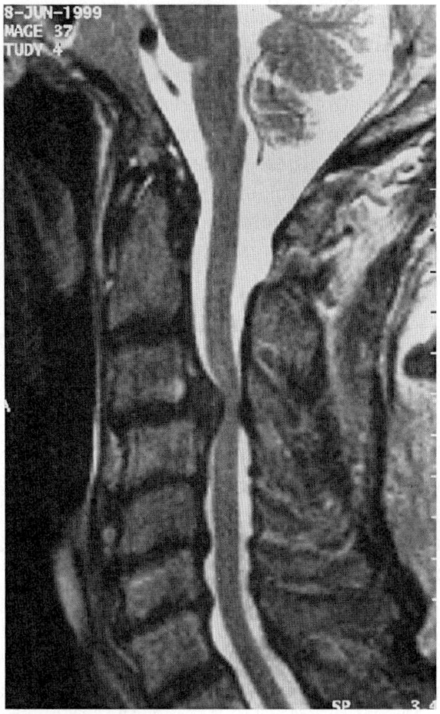

FIGURE 106.6. Large cervical disk herniation at C3–C4, producing cord compression and clinical signs of myelopathy. This patient underwent urgent diskectomy from an anterior approach.

Usually, painful radiculopathy from intervertebral disk herniation resolves without specific treatment. A new presentation of painful radiculopathy (without motor deficit) should be treated with nonsteroidal antiinflammatory drugs (NSAIDs) for at least 6 weeks. For lumbar disk herniations, a period of bed rest of 1 to 2 weeks often provides relief.

The indications for surgical removal of a disk herniation are (1) painful radiculopathy for a minimum of 6 weeks unresponsive to conservative therapy, (2) radiculopathy (of any duration) with significant motor deficit, and (3) myelopathy or cauda equina syndrome (of any duration). MRI must show focal disk disease that correlates anatomically with the neurological symptoms.

Spondylosis

Spinal spondylosis refers to a common pathological process in which bony overgrowth at the intervertebral endplate produces osteophytes (bone spurs). The initial step in this pathological process is desiccation and volume loss of intervertebral disks. Vertebral body endplates are then subjected to excessive stress and respond by new bone formation, leading to bony spurs. This process is most pronounced in the cervical spine because of its mobility. Osteophytes may produce stenosis of the central spinal canal, leading to myelopathy, and/or impinge on exiting nerve roots, producing radiculopathy.

Surgical decision making in multilevel cervical spondylotic disease can be complex. Detailed preoperative evaluation may require both CT and MR to adequately visualize both bony and neural elements. Neurological examination must document exactly which roots are symptomatic and whether myelopathy is present. For myelopathy, associated with motor weakness, radiculopathy, or persistent (greater than 6 weeks) painful radiculopathy, surgical decompression is indicated in the regions where symptoms clearly correlate with CT or MR evidence of neural compression. Abnormalities on imaging that are not symptomatic need not be included in the decompression. When the indication and precise anatomic location for surgical decompression are established, the type of procedure must be determined. Choices for cervical spondylosis include anterior versus posterior approaches, with or without bony fusion, and with or without spinal instrumentation. Fusion across an intervertebral segment is a useful adjunct to decompression because it arrests the pathological process (excessive joint stress) that originally resulted in osteophyte formation.

Degeneration of one or more lumbar intervertebral disks is commonly associated with chronic low back pain, in the absence of a specific neural compression syndrome. Although lumbar fusion is frequently performed for this condition, very few good clinical trials of this procedure have been performed. In carefully selected cases, Fritzell et al.[32,33] recently showed that surgical fusion resulted in decreased long-term pain and a higher rate of return to gainful employment than conservative treatment.

Ruptured Intracranial Aneurysms

Autopsy studies show that about 5% of the population harbors at least one intracranial aneurysm.[34] These aneurysms are usually associated with the circle of Willis and its immediate branches, which are located in the subarachnoid space at the base of the brain. Rupture of a brain aneurysm is a common neurosurgical emergency. It usually produces subarachnoid hemorrhage (SAH), but may also produce intraparenchymal or intraventricular hemorrhage, depending on which way the aneurysm dome points.

Initial Evaluation of Suspected SAH

The most important point on the history is the timing and character of the headache. Ruptured aneurysms typically produce a sudden, massive headache ("worst headache of my life"). Aneurysms often rupture during activities that alter blood pressure or intracranial pressure, such as having an argument, sexual intercourse, or defecation. The most important points on physical examination: (1) look for cranial nerve palsies, which may help localize an aneurysm; a third nerve palsy suggests a posterior communicating artery aneurysm; a monocular field cut or monocular visual loss suggests an ophthalmic aneurysm; (2) determine the clinical grade of the SAH according to the Hunt and Hess classification[35] given in Table 106.5.

Radiologic Evaluation

Emergent head CT (without contrast) is indicated for anyone with a history or physical suggestive of SAH. CT examination is useful not only for diagnosing the type and location of hemorrhage but also for diagnosing SAH-associated hydrocephalus (Fig. 106.7). Aneurysmal SAH is usually in the basal cisterns and/or Sylvian fissures. There may be intraventricular blood as well. If the blood is only over the convexities or is purely intraventricular, a nonaneurysmal etiology is more likely. Look for asymmetries in the subarachnoid clot. The largest clot in the Sylvian fissure suggests a middle cerebral artery aneurysm; clot in the inferior frontal lobe or interhemispheric fissure anteriorly suggests an anterior communicating artery aneurysm; clot in the prepontine/interpeduncular cistern suggests a basilar aneurysm. Clot thickness is graded according to the Fischer scale, which predicts the likelihood of symptomatic delayed vasospasm based on clot thickness.[36] A large aneurysm (>1 cm) may itself be visible as a mass on CT, but aneurysms less than 1 cm usually are not.

If CT confirms SAH, a four-vessel angiogram or CT angiogram should be obtained. All cranial vessels must be examined because 15% of intracranial aneurysms are multiple.

TABLE 106.5. The Hunt and Hess Classification of the Clinical Presentation of Ruptured Cerebral Aneurysms.

Grade	*Description*
I	Asymptomatic or minimal headache
II	Moderate to severe headache, and/or nuchal rigidity; no deficit other than CN palsy
III	Drowsiness, confusion, or mild focal deficit
IV	Stupor, moderate to severe hemiparesis
V	Deep coma, decerebrate rigidity

CN, central nervous system.

Source: Hunt and Hess (1968).[35]

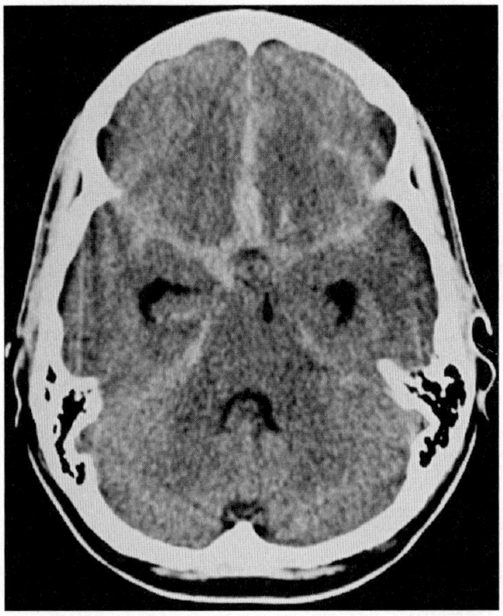

FIGURE 106.7. Axial noncontrast CT scan showing acute subarachnoid hemorrhage from rupture of an anterior communicating artery aneurysm. Acute hydrocephalus, manifested by dilatation of the temporal horns, is also evident.

Treatment

The goals in treating a patient with aneurysmal SAH are to treat hydrocephalus, repair the aneurysm to prevent rerupture, and prevent or treat delayed cerebral vasospasm.

Hydrocephalus. If the CT scan shows hydrocephalus and if the patient's state of consciousness is impaired, a ventriculostomy should be placed. Weaning from external ventricular drainage may be attempted over 1 to 4 days, with weaning failures requiring permanent internalized ventricular shunt placement.[37]

Aneurysm repair. After an initial aneurysm rupture, the incidence of early rerupture is about 4% in the first 24h, then 1% per day.[38] Thus, the aneurysm must be repaired emergently. Many aneurysms are amenable to either surgical clipping or endovascular occlusion (coiling). A large randomized multicenter trial of clipping versus coiling showed improved survival-free disability with coiling, but the difference between groups was small.[39] Aneurysms with a wide-based neck usually cannot be coiled. Most middle cerebral artery aneurysms fit this description. Some types of aneurysms, especially fusiform dilatation of a vessel, may be impossible to clip or to coil. The only option in this case may be to trap and bypass the involved segment.[40] Patients who remain Hunt and Hess grade V after ventriculostomy have a poor prognosis and are not always treated.[41]

Vasospasm. Most (60%) of patients with aneurysmal SAH develop vasospasm 4 to 7 days after the SAH,[42] which is seen on angiography as narrowing of the arteries at the circle of Willis or its proximal branches. The exact cause of this is unknown. It may be diagnosed and followed by transcranial Doppler ultrasonography.

From the initial presentation, SAH patients are kept well hydrated (IV at 100–125mL/h) to maintain cerebral perfusion as spasm commences. Hypervolemic therapy should not be stopped suddenly (except in the case of cardiopulmonary decompensation), but is weaned over 2 to 4 days as the period of vasospasm risk passes. While on hypervolemic therapy, the patient should be monitored for desaturation (heralding pulmonary edema) and myocardial ischemia.

Some patients develop cerebral ischemia as the result of severe vasospasm. It is diagnosed clinically by new neurological deficits not caused by hydrocephalus or aneurysm rerupture and may be confirmed by Doppler or angiography. If not rapidly treated, symptomatic vasospasm may lead to infarction with devastating consequences. Symptomatic vasospasm is treated by induced hypertension and increased cardiac output, in addition to hypervolemia. Pressors and inotropes are given, usually to keep systolic pressure at 170 to 200mmHg and cardiac index above 5. Although numerous retrospective or nonrandomized studies have described the effectiveness of hypervolemic hypertensive therapy for vasospasm, its efficacy has not been proven in randomized trials.[43] Endovascular techniques, such as balloon dilatation of the involved arterial segments, are additional treatment options in severe symptomatic vasospasm.[44,45]

Unruptured Intracranial Aneurysms

Unruptured intracranial aneurysms are often discovered incidentally during neuroimaging studies for other suspected pathologies. Treament recommendations were recently formulated by the International Study of Unruptured Intracranial Aneurysms (ISUIA), a longitudinal study risk of rupture and risk of surgical treatment of intracranial aneurysms.[46] For unruptured aneurysms less than 10mm in diameter, the risk of rupture was 0.05% per year. For lesions in this size group, the risk of prophylactic surgical treatment was found to be greater than the risk of nontreatment.

Brain Tumors

Brain tumors typically present with seizure, focal neurological deficit, or headache. Headaches caused by brain tumor are characteristically worse upon awakening and improve during the day as intracranial pressure lowers with upright posture. MR with and without gadolinium contrast is an excellent study for delineating the presence and detailed anatomy of brain tumors. An MR image and operative photograph of an exophytic brainstem glioma are shown in Figures 106.8 and 106.9.

Brain tumors may be primary or metastatic. The malignancies with the greatest tendency to metastasize to brain are lung, breast, renal, and thyroid cancers. MR allows early diagnosis and treatment of small, asymptomatic brain metastasis during initial workup of malignancy in other organs.

Primary brain tumors may be benign or malignant, and may arise from glial cells, neuronal cells, or the meninges. Primary malignant brain tumors rarely metastasize, but are locally invasive of surrounding parenchyma, whereas benign tumors are encapsulated. Grade IV astrocytoma (glioblastoma) is the most common primary brain tumor of adults.

Treatment

Corticosteroids result in a rapid decrease in tumor-associated edema and may allow remarkable resolution of neurological

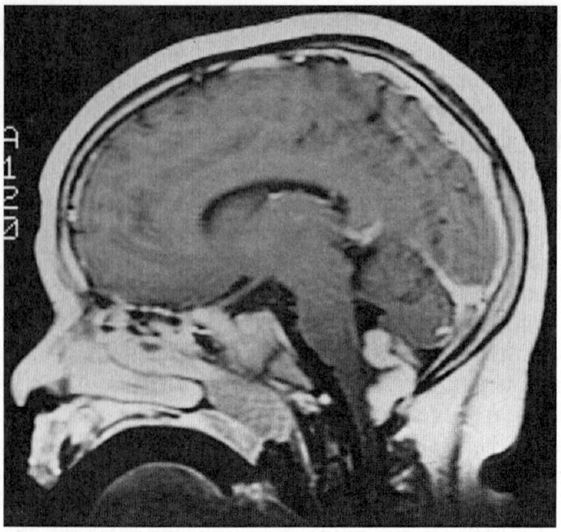

FIGURE 106.8. Contrast-enhanced T_1-weighted magnetic resonance (MR) scan in the sagittal plane, showing an exophytic glioma growing from the cervicomedullary junction.

deficits. However, steroids treat only edema, not the tumor itself. The definitive management of brain tumors may include surgery, radiation, chemotherapy, or all of these. Unfortunately, surgical or radiation treatment for brain tumors have rarely been subjected to prospective, randomized trials.

The mainstay of treatment of most primary tumors and large (>3 cm) solitary metastases is surgical excision. For low-grade gliomas, extent of resection correlates with survival[47]; this is probably true for higher-grade lesions also, but the data are less clear and the degree of benefit is small.[48,49]

Surgery of intraparenchymal tumors has become more precise with the advent of image-guided surgery.[50] This technique is based on the fact that the borders of a tumor are much better defined on preoperative MR than by direct visual or tactile cues at craniotomy. Once the patient's head is fixed in position for surgery, preoperative images are coregistered on a computer monitor with fiducial markers or surface landmarks visible on the patient's scalp. An infrared light detector can then track the position of surgical instruments in the operative field and display the precise position of instruments with respect to the tumor boundaries on the monitor. Some centers are now performing tumor resections within a specially adapted intraoperative MRI unit, for real-time imaging of the brain as the resection progresses, but the utility and necessity of this in relationship to standard image-guided techniques are unclear.[51]

Most malignant brain tumors cannot be completely excised because of extensive invasion of surrounding parenchyma. Some benign tumors, such as skull-based meningiomas, may be so intimately associated with cranial nerves that total excision is impossible without unacceptable morbidity. Standard fractionated radiation therapy is a useful adjunct for most malignant brain tumors but has long-term side effects on neurological function in survivors. Stereotactic radiosurgery is an emerging therapy in brain tumor treatment that allows high dosage to the treatment area, sparing normal brain. Small (<3 cm) brain metastases are as well controlled by stereotactic radiosurgery as by standard surgical excision with whole-brain radiation.[52] Length of survival is then determined by systemic disease outside the central nervous system. Radiosurgery as a boost to standard open surgery may add survival benefit for malignant glioma.[53] Radiosurgery is increasingly used as the sole technique for control of benign intracranial neoplasms, such as acoustic schwannoma[54] and meningioma,[55] but has not been proven superior in randomized trials.[56]

Chemotherapy, following surgical debulking, is of proven benefit in only a few types of malignancies such as medulloblastoma and germinoma. In most of the common adult brain tumors, such as glioblastoma, its use remains experimental. For malignant gliomas, limited benefit of interstitial chemotherapy with implanted carmustine or BCNU "wafers" has recently been shown.[57,58] Trials of antiangiogenic agents for malignant glioma are now underway.[59]

Pituitary Tumors

Pituitary tumors may be "functional" (hormone-producing) or "nonfunctional." If larger than 1 cm in diameter, they are classified as macroadenomas. They may produce symptoms by excessive hormone production or, in the case of macroadenomas, by compression of the optic chiasm. Classically, chiasmatic compression produces bitemporal hemianopsia. Prolactin-secreting adenomas may be treated medically with bromocriptine, but withdrawal of bromocriptine results in regrowth of the tumor. Most other functional adenomas, and most macroadenomas producing visual symptoms, are best treated by surgical excision.

For pituitary tumors that do not transgress the diaphragm sellae, the surgical approach is through the sphenoid sinus to the base of the sella turcica. Postoperatively, it is important to monitor the patient for new ocular motor palsies or visual field loss as these may herald "cavernous sinus syndrome" (palsy of nerve III, V-1, and VI) or chiasmal compression, which usually mandates a return to the operating room for exploration of the sella and sphenoid sinus. During and after transphenoidal pituitary surgery, the patient is assumed to be

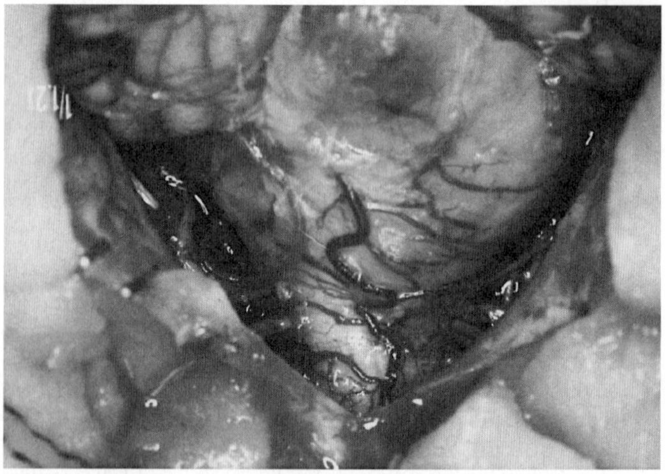

FIGURE 106.9. Intraoperative photograph of the exophytic glioma shown in Figure 106.8. The inferior occipital bone and the posterior arch of C1 have been removed, and the dura has been opened over the cervicomedullary junction. The cervical spinal cord with exiting nerve roots is seen inferiorly, and the cerebellar tonsils are superior. The exophytic mass, before surgical resection, is shown in the center.

deficient in cortisol. Steroid coverage is continued until a fasting serum cortisol or an ACTH stimulation test is documented to be adequate.

Brain Death

Each hospital may set its own policy for diagnosis of brain death, but most policies are based on the recommendations of a presidential commission on death.[60] Several reasonable formulas are as follows:

A. Two clinical examinations showing no brainstem function, and two positive apnea tests, separated by at least 6h; OR
B. A clinical examination showing no brainstem function, a positive apnea test, AND a cerebral blood flow study (done in nuclear medicine) showing no cerebral blood flow.

The brainstem examination consists of pupillary light reaction, corneal reflex, oculovestibular reflex (icewater calorics), cough, and gag.

When a brain death workup is beginning, the local organ bank should be notified. It is a law in many states that a brain-dead patient's family must be asked about donating organs. The neurosurgeon is not personally required to discuss organ donation with the family so long as the organ bank is involved, as their representative will discuss it. It is important to keep the patient's organs in good condition for donation. Regional organ banks can provide a set of standard "brain death orders," designed to keep all organs in optimal condition. A key concern is adequate hydration so that the systolic blood pressure remains greater than 100mmHg and the urine output greater than 100mL/h. Eventually, the brain-dead patient develops severe diabetes insipidus as a result of hypothalamic failure, usually necessitating a pitressin drip.

Peripheral Nerve Compression Syndromes

Decompression of a peripheral nerve is a frequent neurosurgical procedure. The most common nerve compression syndromes amenable to surgical treatment are compression of the median nerve at the carpal tunnel ("carpal tunnel syndrome") and compression of the ulnar nerve in the ulnar groove at the medial epicondyle of the elbow joint.

Carpal tunnel syndrome usually presents with painful numbness in the region of the hand innervated by the distal median nerve: the palmar aspect of the thumb, index finger, middle finger, and radial half of the fourth finger. There may be weakness of grip strength as a result of weakness of the thenar musculature. Two clinical signs are useful in its diagnosis: Phalen's sign (30–60s of complete wrist flexion reproduces or exacerbates pain) and Tinnel's sign (percussing over the carpal tunnel reproduces or exacerbates pain). In equivocal cases, nerve conduction studies are useful for diagnosis; these show reduced conduction velocity in the median nerve through the carpal tunnel in 80% of cases. When conservative therapy (splinting) fails, microsurgical sectioning of the transverse carpal ligament is usually effective.

Ulnar neuropathy presents with painful numbness in the ulnar sensory distribution, which includes the palmar aspect of the fifth finger and ulnar half of the fourth finger. Motor signs include wasting of the interosseus muscles, abduction of the little finger because of weakness of the third dorsal interosseus muscle (Wartenburg's sign), and, in advanced cases, a claw deformity of the hand. Nerve conduction studies usually show decreased velocity in the ulnar nerve as it crosses the elbow. Surgical options include simple decompression of the nerve in the ulnar groove, versus transposition of the nerve out of its groove to a position where it is protected by forearm musculature.

Movement Disorders, Epilepsy, and Pain

Functional neurosurgery is the area of neurosurgery that deals with altering the function of the nervous system rather than removing or repairing a lesion. This subspecialty includes the surgical treatment movement disorders, epilepsy, and pain. Table 106.6 describes recent randomized clinical trials in functional neurosurgery. There is now Class I evidence for the surgical treatment of medically intractable temporal lobe epilepsy using temporal lobectomy and for the treatment of "failed back syndrome" (chronic severe low back pain following previous lumbar spine surgery) with implantation of dorsal column stimulators.

The surgical treatment of Parkinson's disease (PD) has been the subject of intense study. Several trials have focused on lesioning surgery (pallidotomy) or chronic deep brain stimulation (DBS) of the globus pallidus or subthalamic nucleus (see Table 106.6). The rationale for these surgeries was developed during study of a nonhuman primate model of PD, based on the discovery that the neurotoxin 1-methyl-4-phenyl-1,2,3,6-tetrahydropyridine (MPTP), a by-product of illicit narcotic synthesis, causes parkinsonism in man and in nonhuman primates. In PD, loss of dopaminergic neurons of the substantia nigra compacta (SNc) results in excessive and abnormally patterned activity in the subthalamic nucleus (STN) and in its major target nuclei, the internal segment of the globus pallidus (GPI) and the substantia nigra, pars reticulata (SNr). Because GPi and SNr have inhibitory projections to motor regions of the thalamus, thalamocortical activity is suppressed; this is thought to be the basis for many of the motor abnormalities in PD. As predicted by this model, lesioning or inactivation of brain tissue in STN or GPi—effectively decreasing the inhibitory influence on the motor thalamus and, thus, "normalizing" thalamocortical activity—has been found to be effective in treating parkinsonism in animal models.[61] The use of pallidotomy and deep brain stimulation of the subthalamic nucleus for PD is now supported by Class I evidence.

Lesioning surgery and DBS surgery compensate for the electrical abnormalities present in the parkinsonian brain but do not treat the underlying dopamine deficiency and do not arrest progression of the disease. Attempts are underway to treat PD by intrastriatal transplantation of dopamine-producing fetal cells or by intrastriatal infusion of dopaminergic growth factors (see Table 106.6). Efficacy of these therapies has not yet been demonstrated. Trials of fetal cell transplantation in PD, however, have pioneered the use of sham surgery controls for the study of major surgical procedures.[62,63]

Techniques for Stereotactic Treatment of Parkinson's Disease

Because the basal ganglia are deep structures, they are approached through small skull openings without direct

TABLE 106.6.
Class I Evidence in Functional Neurosurgery (Epilepsy, Pain, and Movement Disorders).

Reference	*Disease*	*Year*	*n*	*Intervention/design*	*Median follow-up*	*Major endpoint*	*Interpretations/comments*
Wiebe et al.[70]	Epilepsy	2001	80	Temporal lobectomy for temporal lobe epilepsy	1 year	Freedom from seizures	Fifty-eight percent of surgical patients were seizure free versus 8% of medical patients
North et al.[71]	Back pain	1995	27	Reoperation versus spinal cord stimulation in failed back syndrome	6 months	Relief of low back pain	Showed SCS provides superior pain relief compared with reoperation for "failed back"
Vitek et al.[72]	PD	2003	36	Pallidotomy versus best medical therapy for Parkinson's disease	6 months	Motor improvement by the Unified Parkinson's Disease Rating Scale	Pallidotomy showed a 32% improvement compared to an 5% decline in medical treatment alone
De Bie et al.[73]	PD	1999	37	Pallidotomy versus best medical therapy for Parkinson's disease	6 months	Motor improvement by the Unified Parkinson's Disease Rating Scale	Pallidotomy showed a 31% improvement compared to an 8% decline in medical treatment alone
Schuurman et al.[74]	PD	2000	68	DBS of the thalamus versus thalamotomy for tremor	6 months	Change in functional ability by the Frenchay activities index	Thalamic DBS and thalamotomy have similar efficacy but DBS has fewer complications
Esselink et al.[75]	PD	2004	34	Pallidotomy versus bilateral DBS of the STN	6 months	Motor improvement by the Unified Parkinson's Disease Rating Scale	Bilateral subthalamic DBS is superior to unilateral pallidotomy for relief of PD signs at 6 months
Nutt et al[76]	PD	2003	50	Intraventricular injection of GDNF for PD	8 months	Motor improvement by the Unified Parkinson's Disease Rating Scale	GDNF delivered intraventricularly does not improve motor signs of Parkinson's disease
Olanow et al.[63]	PD	2003	34	Intrastriatal grafting of fetal ventral mesencephalon for PD	2 years	Motor improvement by the Unified Parkinson's Disease Rating Scale	Intrastriatal grafting of fetal mesencephalon does not improve motor signs of Parkinsons' disease
Freed et al.[62]	PD	2001	40	Intrastriatal grafting of fetal ventral mesencephalon for PD	1 year	Subjective global rating of change in disease severity	Intrastriatal grafting of fetal mesencephalon produced some improvement in PD motor signs in younger patients only

PD, Parkinson's disease; DBS, deep brain stimulation; GDNF, glial-derived neurotrophic factor.

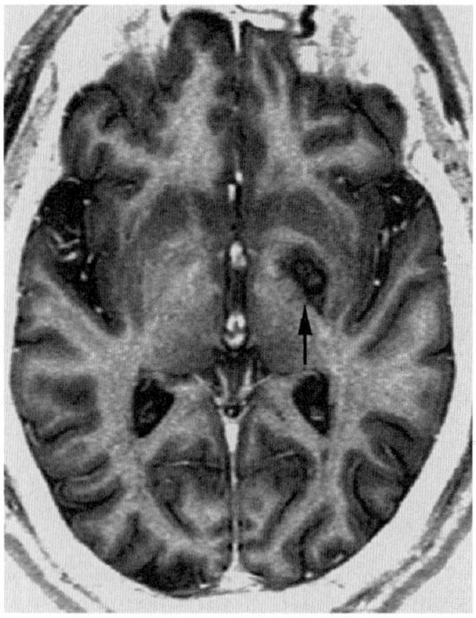

FIGURE 106.10. Postoperative axial MR scan 24h following stereotactic pallidotomy for Parkinson's disease. Two thermolytic lesions and surrounding edema (indicated by *black arrow*) are located in the posterior part of the internal segment of the globus pallidus.

visualization of the target structures, rather than by open craniotomy. Target localization is performed by the method of *stereotaxis*. In stereotactic neurosurgery, a stereotactic frame is fixed to the patient's head to provide both an external coordinate system and a mechanical platform on which to mount instruments and direct them to known coordinates in the patient's brain. A brain image, such as CT or MR, is then obtained to visualize both the frame and the target within the patient's brain. The coordinates of the brain target, in the coordinate system defined by the frame, are calculated. In the operating room, instruments are mounted on the frame and directed toward the image-defined stereotactic target. Correct identification of the target is confirmed by intraoperative physiological studies, such as neuronal recording with microelectrodes (see Fig. 106.1). The neurological status of the patient (such as strength, vision, and improvement of motor function) must be monitored frequently during the procedure.

Pallidotomy, or lesioning of the internal segment of the globus pallidus, is now a commonly performed stereotactic procedure for Parkinson's disease. A postoperative MR showing a pallidotomy lesion is shown in Figure 106.10.

References

1. Guidelines for the management of severe head injury. Brain Trauma Foundation, American Association of Neurological Surgeons, Joint Section on Neurotrauma and Critical Care. J Neurotrauma 1996;13:641–734.
2. Robertson CS, Valadka AB, Hannay HJ, et al. Prevention of secondary ischemic insults after severe head injury. Crit Care Med 1999;27:2086–2095.
3. Juul N, Morris GF, Marshall SB, Marshall LF. Intracranial hypertension and cerebral perfusion pressure: influence on neurological deterioration and outcome in severe head injury. The Executive Committee of the International Selfotel Trial. J Neurosurg 2000;92:1–6.
4. Cruz J. The first decade of continuous monitoring of jugular bulb oxyhemoglobinsaturation: management strategies and clinical outcome. Crit Care Med 1998;26:344–351.
5. Manley GT, Pitts LH, Morabito D, et al. Brain tissue oxygenation during hemorrhagic shock, resuscitation, and alterations in ventilation. J Trauma 1999;46:261–267.
6. Allen CH, Ward JD. An evidence-based approach to management of increased intracranial pressure. Crit Care Clin 1998;14:485–495.
7. Poungvarin N, Boopat W, Viriyavejakul A, et al. Effects of dexamethasone in primary supratentorial intracerebral hemmorhage. N Engl J Med 1987;316:1229–1233.
8. Braakman R, Schouten HJA, Dishoeck MB. Megadose steroids in severe head injury. J Neurosurg 1983;58:326–330.
9. Ayus JC, Krothapalli RK, Arieff A. Treatment of symptomatic hyponatremia and its relation to brain damage. N Engl J Med 1987;317:1190–1195.
10. Lazio BE, Simard JM. Anticoagulation in neurosurgical patients. Neurosurgery 1999;45:838–847; discussion 847–848.
11. Hopf NJ, Grunert P, Fries G, Resch KD, Perneczcky A. Endoscopic third ventriculostomy: outcome analysis of 100 consecutive procedures. Neurosurgery 1999;44:795–804.
12. Poon WS, Ng S, Wai S. CSF antibiotic prophylaxis for neurosurgical patients with ventriculostomy: a randomised study. Acta Neurochir Suppl (Wien) 1998;71:146–148.
13. Wong GK, Poon WS, Wai S, Yu LM, Lyon D, Lam JM. Failure of regular external ventricular drain exchange to reduce cerebrospinal fluid infection: result of a randomised controlled trial. J Neurol Neurosurg Psychiatry 2002;73:759–761.
14. Pfausler B, Spiss H, Beer R, et al. Treatment of staphylococcal ventriculitis associated with external cerebrospinal fluid drains: a prospective randomized trial of intravenous compared with intraventricular vancomycin therapy. J Neurosurg 2003;98:1040–1044.
15. Kestle JR. Pediatric hydrocephalus: current management. Neurol Clin 2003;21:883–895, vii.
16. Schreffler RT, Schreffler AJ, Wittler RR. Treatment of cerebrospinal fluid shunt infections: a decision analysis. Pediatr Infect Dis J 2002;21:632–636.
17. Ikata T, Iwasa K, Morimoto K, Tonai T, Taoka Y. Clinical considerations and biochemical basis of prognosis of cervical spinal cord injury. Spine 1989;14:1096–1101.
18. Selden N, Quint D, Patel N, d'Arcy H, Papadopoulos S. Emergency magnetic resonance imaging of cervical spinal cord injuries: clinical correlation and prognosis. Neurosurgery 1999;44:785–792.
19. Denis F. The three column spine and its significance in the classification of acute thoracolumbar injuries. Spine 1983;8:817–831.
20. Atkinson P, Atkinson J. Spinal shock. Mayo Clin Proc 1996;71:384–389.
21. Takaoka M, Tabuse H, Kumura E, et al. Semiquantitative analysis of corpus callosum injury using magnetic resonance imaging indicates clinical severity in patients with diffuse axonal injury. J Neurol Neurosurg Psychiatry 2002;73:289–293.
22. Keenan TL, Anthony J, Benson DR. Non-contiguous spinal fractures. J Trauma 1990;30:489–491.
23. Widder S, Doig C, Burrowes P, Larsen G, Hurlbert RJ, Kortbeek JB. Prospective evaluation of computed tomographic scanning for the spinal clearance of obtunded trauma patients: preliminary results. J Trauma 2004;56:1179–1184.
24. Cruz J, Minoja G, Okuchi K, Facco E. Successful use of the new high-dose mannitol treatment in patients with Glasgow Coma Scale scores of 3 and bilateral abnormal pupillary widening: a randomized trial. J Neurosurg 2004;100:376–383.
25. Friedman JA, Ebersold MJ, Quast LM. Post-traumatic cerebrospinal fluid leakage. World J Surg 2001;25:1062–1066.
26. Temkin NR. A randomized, double-blind study of phenytoin for the prevention of post-traumatic seizures. N Engl J Med 1990;323:497–502.
27. Meyer SH, Chestnut RM. Post-trauamatic extra-axial mass lesions: subdural and extradural hematoma. In: Tindall GT, Cooper PR, Barrow DL, eds. The Practice of Neurosurgery, vol 2. Baltimore: Williams & Wilkins, 1996:1443–1460.
28. Weiner HL, Cooper PR. Significance and management of cranial vault fractures. In: Tindall GT, Cooper PR, Barrow DL, eds. The Practice of Neurosurgery, vol 2. Baltimore: Williams & Wilkins, 1996:1541–1552.
29. Bracken MB, Shepard MJ, Collins WF. A randomized, controlled trial of methylprednisolone or nalozone in the treatment of acute spinal-cord injury. Results of the second national Acute Spinal Cord Injury Study. N Engl J Med 1990;322:1405–1411.
30. Bracken MB, Shepard MJ, Holford TR, et al. Administration of methylprednisolone for 24 or 48 hours or tirilazad mesylate for 48 hours in the treatment of acute spinal cord injury. Results of the Third National Acute Spinal Cord Injury Randomized Controlled Trial. National Acute Spinal Cord Injury Study. JAMA 1997;277:1597–1604.
31. Bucholz RD, Cheung KC. Halo vest versus spinal fusion for cervical injury: evidence from an outcome study. J Neurosurg 1989;70:884–892.
32. Fritzell P, Hagg O, Jonsson D, Nordwall A. Cost-effectiveness of lumbar fusion and nonsurgical treatment for chronic low back pain in the Swedish Lumbar Spine Study: a multicenter, randomized, controlled trial from the Swedish Lumbar Spine Study Group. Spine 2004;29:421–434; discussion Z423.
33. Fritzell P, Hagg O, Wessberg P, Nordwall A. 2001 Volvo Award Winner in Clinical Studies. Lumbar fusion versus nonsurgical treatment for chronic low back pain: a multicenter randomized controlled trial from the Swedish Lumbar Spine Study Group. Spine 2001;26:2521–2532; discussion 2532–2534.
34. Wiebers DO, Whisnant JP, Sundt TM. The significance of unruptured intracranial saccular aneurysms. J Neurosurg 1987;66:23–29.
35. Hunt WE, Hess RM. Surgical risk as related to timing of intervention in the repair of intracranial aneurysms. J Neurosurg 1968;28:14–20.
36. Fisher CM, Kistler JP, Davis JM. Relation of cerebral vasospasm to subarachnoid hemmorhage visualized by CT scanning. Neurosurgery 1980;6:1–9.
37. Klopfenstein JD, Kim LJ, Feiz-Erfan I, et al. Comparison of rapid and gradual weaning from external ventricular drainage in

patients with aneurysmal subarachnoid hemorrhage: a prospective randomized trial. J Neurosurg 2004;100:225–229.
38. Inagawa T, Kamiya K, Ogasawara H. Rebleeding of ruptured intracranial aneurysms in the acute stage. Surg Neurol 1987; 28:93–99.
39. Molyneux A, Kerr R, Stratton I, et al. International Subarachnoid Aneurysm Trial (ISAT) of neurosurgical clipping versus endovascular coiling in 2143 patients with ruptured intracranial aneurysms: a randomised trial. Lancet 2002;360:1267–1274.
40. Wanebo JE, Zabramski JM, Spetzler RF. Superficial temporal artery-to-middle cerebral artery bypass grafting for cerebral revascularization. Neurosurgery 2004;55:395–398; discussion 398–399.
41. Laidlaw JD, Siu KH. Ultra-early surgery for aneurysmal subarachnoid hemorrhage: outcomes for a consecutive series of 391 patients not selected by grade or age. J Neurosurg 2002;97:250–258; discussion 247–259.
42. Macdonald RL, Rosengart A, Huo D, Karrison T. Factors associated with the development of vasospasm after planned surgical treatment of aneurysmal subarachnoid hemorrhage. J Neurosurg 2003;99:644–652.
43. Treggiari MM, Walder B, Suter PM, Romand JA. Systematic review of the prevention of delayed ischemic neurological deficits with hypertension, hypervolemia, and hemodilution therapy following subarachnoid hemorrhage. J Neurosurg 2003;98:978–984.
44. Andaluz N, Tomsick TA, Tew JM Jr, van Loveren HR, Yeh HS, Zuccarello M. Indications for endovascular therapy for refractory vasospasm after aneurysmal subarachnoid hemorrhage: experience at the University of Cincinnati. Surg Neurol 2002;58:131–138; discussion 138.
45. Newell DW, Elliott JP, Eskridge JM, Winn HR. Endovascular therapy for aneurysmal vasospasm. Crit Care Clin 1999;15:685–699, v.
46. Wiebers DO, Whisnant JP, Huston J III, et al. Unruptured intracranial aneurysms: natural history, clinical outcome, and risks of surgical and endovascular treatment. Lancet 2003;362:103–110.
47. Berger MS, Deliganis AV, Dobbins J, Keles GE. The effect of extent of resection on recurrence in patients with log grade hemisphere gliomas. Cancer (Phila) 1994;74:1784–1791.
48. Albert FK, Forsting M, Sartor K, Adams HP, Kunze S. Early postoperative magnetic resonance imaging after resection of malignant glioma: objective evaluation of residual tumor and its influence on regrowth and prognosis. Neurosurgery 1994; 34:45–60.
49. Vuorinen V, Hinkka S, Farkkila M, Jaaskelainen J. Debulking or biopsy of malignant glioma in elderly people: a randomised study. Acta Neurochir (Wien) 2003;145:5–10.
50. Barnett GH, Kormos DW, Steiner CP, Weisenberger J. Intraoperative localization using an armless, frameless stereotactic wand. J Neurosurg 1993;78:510–514.
51. Black PM, Alexander E, Martin C, et al. Craniotomy for tumor treatment in an intraoperative magnetic resonance imaging unit. Neurosurgery 1999;45:423–433.
52. Muacevic A, Kreth F, Horstmann GSE, et al. Surgery and radiotherapy compared with gamma knife radiosurgery in the treatment of solitary cerebral metastases of small diameter. J Neurosurg 1999;91:35–43.
53. Shrieve D, Alexander ER, Black P, et al. Treatment of patients with primary glioblastoma multiforme with standard postoperative radiotherapy and radiosurgical boost: prognostic factors and long-term outcome. J Neurosurg 1999;90:72–77.
54. Kondziolka D, Lunsford LD, McLaughlin MR, Flickinger JC. Long-term outcomes after radiosurgery for acoustic neuromas. N Engl J Med 1998;339:1426–1433.
55. Kondziolka D, Levy E, Niranjan A, Flickinger J, Lunsford L. Long-term outcomes after meningioma radiosurgery: physician and patient perspectives. J Neurosurg 1999;91:44–50.
56. Nikolopoulos TP, O'Donoghue GM. Acoustic neuroma management: an evidence-based medicine approach. Otol Neurotol 2002;23:534–541.
57. Valtonen S, Timonen U, Toivanen P, et al. Interstitial chemotherapy with carmustine-loaded polymers for high-grade gliomas: a randomized double blind study. Neurosurgery 1997;41:44–48.
58. Westphal M, Hilt DC, Bortey E, et al. A phase 3 trial of local chemotherapy with biodegradable carmustine (BCNU) wafers (Gliadel wafers) in patients with primary malignant glioma. Neuro-Oncology 2003;5:79–88.
59. Van Meir EG, Bellail A, Phuphanich S. Emerging molecular therapies for brain tumors. Semin Oncol 2004;31:38–46.
60. Cohen LM, Germain MJ, Poppel DM. Practical considerations in dialysis withdrawal. JAMA 2003;289:2113–2119.
61. Bergman H, Wichmann T, DeLong MR. Reversal of experimental parkinsonism by lesions of the subthalamic nucleus. Science 1990;249:1436–1438.
62. Freed CR, Greene PE, Breeze RE, et al. Transplantation of embryonic dopamine neurons for severe Parkinson's disease. N Engl J Med 2001;344:710–719.
63. Olanow CW, Goetz CG, Kordower JH, et al. A double-blind controlled trial of bilateral fetal nigral transplantation in Parkinson's disease. Ann Neurol 2003;54:403–414.
64. Smith HP, McWhorter JM, Armstrong D, Johnson R, Transou C, Howard G. Comparision of mannitol regimens in patients with severe head injury undergoing intracranial pressure monitoring. J Neurosurg 1986;65:820–824.
65. Muizelaar JP, Marmarou A, Ward JD, et al. Adverse effects of prolonged hyperventilation in patients with severe head injury. J Neurosurg 1991;75:731–739.
66. Ward JD, Becker DP, Miller JD, et al. Failure of prophylactic barbiturate coma in the treatment of severe head injury. J Neurosurg 1985;62:383–388.
67. Eisenberg HM, Frankowski RF, Constant CF, et al. High-dose barbiturate control of elevated intracranial pressure in patients with severe head injury. J Neurosurg 1988;69:15–23.
68. Clifton GL, Allen S, Barrodale P, et al. A phase II study of moderate hypothermia in severe brain injury. J Neurotrauma 1993;10:263–271; discussion 273.
69. Teasdale G, Jennett B. Assessment of coma and impaired consciousness: a practical scale. Lancet 1974;2:81–84.
70. Wiebe S, Blume WT, Girvin JP, Eliasziw M. A randomized, controlled trial of surgery for temporal-lobe epilepsy. N Engl J Med 2001;345:311–318.
71. North RB, Kidd DH, Piantadosi S. Spinal cord stimulation versus reoperation for failed back surgery syndrome: a prospective, randomized study design. Acta Neurochir Suppl (Wien) 1995;64:106–108.
72. Vitek JL, Bakay RA, Freeman A, et al. Randomized trial of pallidotomy versus medical therapy for Parkinson's disease. Ann Neurol 2003;53:558–569.
73. de Bie RM, de Haan RJ, Nijssen PC, et al. Unilateral pallidotomy in Parkinson's disease: a randomised, single-blind, multicentre trial. Lancet 1999;354:1665–1669.
74. Schuurman PR, Bosch DA, Bossuyt PM, et al. A comparison of continuous thalamic stimulation and thalamotomy for suppression of severe tremor. N Engl J Med 2000;342:461–468.
75. Esselink RA, de Bie RM, de Haan RJ, et al. Unilateral pallidotomy versus bilateral subthalamic nucleus stimulation in PD: a randomized trial. Neurology 2004;62:201–207.
76. Nutt JG, Burchiel KJ, Comella CL, et al. Randomized, double-blind trial of glial cell line-derived neurotrophic factor (GDNF) in PD. Neurology 2003;60:69–73.

107

Orthopaedic Surgery

David W. Lowenberg and Andrew Fang

The field of orthopedic surgery involves caring for patients with injuries and afflictions to the musculoskeletal system. It involves treating the widest array of anatomic structures of any surgical subspecialty and requires a detailed knowledge of the anatomy of the muscles, bones, and vital structures of both the extremities and axial skeleton. The field is also unique as a surgical subspecialty in that nonoperative treatment often represents the preferred method of care for many musculoskeletal conditions. In fact, one would dare say that the majority of musculoskeletal afflictions are at least initially treated with nonoperative intervention. This statement means that the astute physician must often be as knowledgeable in medical management as surgical technique.

Bone Physiology

The skeleton provides a framework for human function. The bones represent a system in constant homeostatic remodeling. This remodeling process is carried out primarily by three cell lines. These cells are responsible for the continual turnover of cortical and cancellous bone so as to maintain its tensile and compressive strength and thereby prevent it from becoming brittle. Just as all materials (i.e., metals, wood, plastic, rope) fail with time after being put through enough cyclic loads, the same would be true of bone if it were not going through this continual remodeling process.

Osteoblasts are the body's bone-forming cells. They require a collagen scaffold matrix in which to work and form bone on the scaffold of the periosteum, endosteum, or haversian canal network inside the cortical bone. The osteoblasts synthesize osteoid. Osteoid is the predominant organic component of bone, and 95% of the osteoid is composed of mainly type 1 collagen. The osteoid is the precursor of mature bone. Once calcification of this matrix occurs, mature bone is now formed.

Once osteoblasts mature and become encased in the mineralized bone matrix, they then grow in size and become osteocytes. Within the bone matrix, these osteocytes reside in small openings called lacunae. The osteocyte cells themselves have tentacle-like extensions that travel along canals, or canaliculi, and provide a means of communication between osteocytes. This communication network plays a role in the process of calcium and phosphate ion homeostasis in the body's extracellular fluid.

Osteoclasts are the largest of the three major cell lines involved in bone formation and remodeling. They are from the hematopoietic lineage and function to resorb mature bone. Osteoclasts reside in the lacunar regions of the bone where resorption is occurring. On a trabecula, this is classically at the opposite end of the region where the osteoblasts are functioning and laying down new osteoid. Thus, in a steady state, the osteoblasts are working laying down new bone at the same rate that the osteoclasts are working to resorb bone.

Osteoblasts, osteocytes, and osteoclasts represent only 2% of the entire organic composition of bone.[1] The primary organic component is the osteoid. Ninety-five percent of osteoid is composed of type 1 collagen.[1] The inorganic component of bone is primarily in the form of a hydroxyapatite matrix, which constitutes roughly 70% of the dry weight of bone.[1]

In the developing skeleton, bone is formed by two similar but distinctly different pathways. The long bones of the body grow in length by a process called *enchondral ossification*.

This process involves the orderly conversion of a cartilage precursor into mature bone. In the flat bones of the body, bone is formed independently of the structured cartilage precursor in a process called *intramembranous ossification*. These two processes create the initial "modeling" of bone that occurs early in life.[2] Actual growth of the long bones and vertebrae involves a combination of these two growth processes in that lengthening occurs via endochondral ossification at the physes, while widening of the bone occurs by intramembranous ossification at the periosteal lining of the bone.

"Remodeling" of bone[2] occurs throughout the rest of skeletal life. The process of remodeling of bone is integral to maintaining the strength and durability of the skeleton. Just as all materials, including the strongest metals, fail after a certain number of cyclic loads, so also would bone fatigue and fracture with normal use if it were not continually being remodeled.

To treat the basic afflictions of the musculoskeletal system, it is important to understand the basic principles of bone homeostasis and remodeling. One must also remember that the skeleton represents the body's primary "mineral bank" for calcium and phosphorus (as phosphate ions). Less than 1% of the body's calcium stores exist in extracellular fluid, and it is this fraction that represents the metabolically active form. Bone represents the site of rapid mobilization and storage of the body's calcium supplies.

Two hormones represent the primary systemic modulators of calcium homeostasis, parathyroid hormone (PTH) and 1,25-dihydroxy vitamin D. PTH stimulates bone resorption with resultant mobilization of calcium into the systemic circulation. New work suggests that prolonged intermittent administration of PTH actually has a biphasic effect and causes an increase in bone formation.[3] It also stimulates conversion of 25-hydroxy vitamin D to 1,25-dihydroxy vitamin D in the kidney. Its net effect is an increase in serum calcium with a decrease in serum phosphate. 1,25-Dihydroxy vitamin D stimulates calcium and phosphate absorption from the intestine. It also stimulates osteoclastic activity. Its net effect is an increase in both serum calcium and phosphate.

Besides the stimulatory effects on bone mass development of activity and weight-bearing, several hormones promote the formation of bone: these include estrogen, testosterone, thyroid hormone, and growth hormone. Decreasing circulatory estrogen levels in postmenopausal women seem to be the primary cause of osteoporosis in this population group.[4]

Joint Physiology

Two types of joints exist in the human skeleton. Symphyseal joints, typified by the intervertebral disk articulations of the spine, consist of a central portion of fibrocartilage serving as an articulation between two vertebrae, with hyaline cartilage present on the appositional ends of the vertebrae. Limited motion is possible across these joints, but no true gliding occurs. The symphysis pubis is the only symphyseal joint in the appendicular skeleton.[1] Symphyseal joints represent a phylogenetic intermediary in the development of the more common synovial joints.

Synovial joints are the kind that one commonly pictures. Also known as diarthrodial joints, they are composed of two hyaline-covered appositional bone ends encased in a synovial lining and bathed with synovial fluid, which is a transudate. The synovial capsule or lining is composed on the innermost side by a several-cell-thick synovial membrane and on the outermost side by a thick, fibrous capsule. Two distinct cell lines have been identified in the thin synovial membrane. Type B cells secrete the hyaluronic acid, which gives the synovial fluid its viscosity. They also secrete prostaglandins and other proteinacious elements of synovial fluid. Type A cells are phagocytic and originate from monocytes. A fine capillary network lies just under the synovial membrane, allowing for a transudate to cross into the joint as a component of the joint fluid.

The synovial fluid is what provides the chondrocytes with nourishment, as articular (hyaline) cartilage is avascular. Motion is therefore critical to the well-being of diarthrodial joints, as this is how the synovial fluid is pumped around and transported to the chondrocytes. The act of cyclic loading of the joint also serves as a means of enhancing exchange of waste products and nutrients between the cartilage matrix and synovial fluid.

Hyaline cartilage is the bearing surface of the joint. It is composed of collagen, proteoglycan, and water. It is able to tolerate large compressile loads without injury to the cartilage or chondrocytes, which is possible because of the viscoelastic behavior of articular cartilage. This viscoelastic characteristic exists because of interstitial fluid flow with compressive load in the cartilage matrix and is known as the flow-dependent viscoelastic behavior of cartilage.[5–7] It is the interstitial fluid pressurization within the collagen–proteoglycan matrix that allows for the biphasic nature of articular cartilage and provides its primary load-carrying mechanism.[5] Under normal conditions, the opposing articular cartilage surfaces function in a nearly frictionless manner, with a very low coefficient of friction. Ideally, there is no wear of these surfaces throughout life; however, the failure in these bearing surfaces is what results in the arthritic process.

Synovial joints differ widely in their motion planes and actual architecture throughout the body. Some are uniaxial (i.e., interphalangeal joints), some are multiaxial (i.e., wrist joint), and others, such as the hip, are "ball-and-socket" type joints. The thickness of the articular cartilage differs widely among the various joints of the body. The ankle and elbow joints are covered by a thin layer of articular cartilage whereas the knee is covered by a thick layer of articular cartilage (approximately 5 mm in young adults). It has been shown that congruent joints have a thinner layer of articular cartilage and incongruent joints have a resultant thicker layer of articular cartilage.[8] This understanding has led to the concept that the thickness of articular cartilage in a joint is inversely proportional, in a linear fashion, to the congruence of the joint surfaces (Fig. 107.1). It is important that this relationship exists, as this allows for equalization of the forces across congruent and incongruent joints in the same extremity.[8] It has been postulated that the loss of this relationship of congruence to joint thickness secondary to trauma is one cause of resultant degenerative joint disease (arthritis).

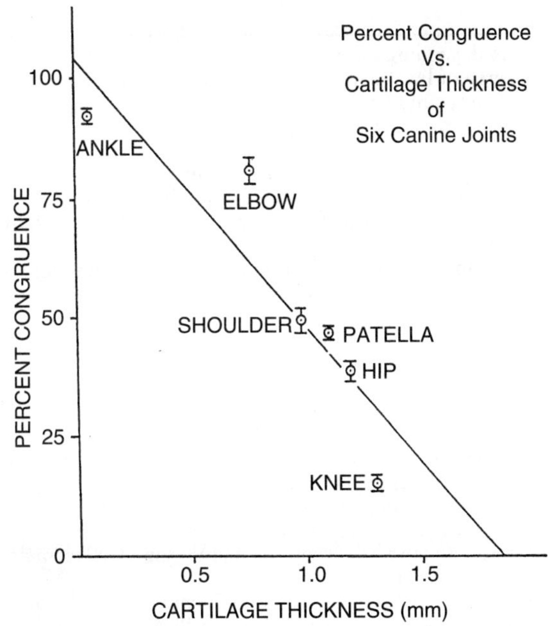

FIGURE 107.1. Graph of percent congruence versus cartilage thickness of canine joints demonstrating a straight-line, inverse relationship. The *r* value for the simple linear regression line is 0.9049. (From Simon WH, Friedenberg S, Richardson S. Joint congruence. J Bone Joint Surg 1973;55A(8):1614–1620.[8])

Fracture Healing

Although the skeleton has evolved to withstand high loads and trauma, fractures still represent one of the most common types of injury seen in the body. A basic knowledge of fractures and their care is essential to the surgeon involved in any aspect of trauma care. Hip fractures in the elderly alone accounted for 3.5 million hospital days with a cost of 8.7 billion dollars in the United States in 1988.[9]

Fractures can be categorized according to the anatomic location in the bone, cause of the fracture, geometry of the fracture, and whether the injury is open (bone exposed to the outside environment) or closed (Table 107.1). To think of fractures in terms of these categorization parameters helps one communicate the nature of the injury to others.

The degree of soft tissue involvement associated with a fracture has classically been described according to the Gustilo and Anderson classification of open fractures[10] (Table 107.2). This fracture classification aids the surgeon in the appropriate treatment for open fractures. In general, open fractures should be treated with an immediate irrigation and debridement of the wound and exposed bone ends. Any devascularized segments of bone should generally be removed to prevent chronic infection and osteomyelitis. Depending on the extent of contamination and the original injury, the patient should then be taken back to the operating room at 48 to 72h either for redebridement, if necrotic tissue remains, or for a delayed primary closure.

Certain open fractures may be primarily closed if, at the time of the original irrigation and debridement, the wound is clean. Type 2 and 3 wounds may need several further visits to the operating room until definitive debridement is achieved. Ideally, soft tissue coverage should be obtained with the appropriate soft tissue procedures (i.e., split-thickness skin grafting, rotational flap, or free vascularized muscle flap) within the first week after the injury.

TABLE 107.1. Fracture Categorization.

Category	*Description*
Anatomic location	Intraarticular Periarticular Proximal, middle, or distal shaft Physeal fractures
Cause	Traumatic Stress fracture Pathological (tumor/metastatic, osteoportic, osteomalacia, etc.)
Fracture geometry	Transverse fracture Spiral fracture Oblique fracture Linear pattern Comminuted pattern Segmental pattern Impacted pattern Greenstick pattern (in children)
Soft tissue	Closed fracture Open fracture

Fracture healing can occur by one of two pathways: primary osteonal healing, or callus formation. Primary osteonal healing occurs only when a fracture is rigidly fixed via plate and screw fixation utilizing interfragmentary compression with either an interfragmentary screw or dynamic compression plate. These principles were first established in a cohesive and experimentally proven form by the Acta Orthopedica (AO) group of surgeons from Switzerland. In 1963, Schenk published work on a dog model confirming primary healing of bone via *primary vascular bone formation*.[11] He confirmed that when such rigid fixation of bone is achieved, the bone ends heal without any callus formation, and instead unite via direct (appositional) bone formation. He later documented the same results in human studies.[12] The hallmark finding in this mode of healing is the absence of fibrous or cartilaginous tissue at the healing site. Radiographically, the bones heal without any periosteal reaction, and bone appositionally grows directly between the two fracture ends.

TABLE 107.2. Gustilo and Anderson Classification of Open Fractures.

Open fracture grade	*Description*
Type 1	Low-energy injury Wound <1 cm in length
Type 2	Moderate-energy injury Wound 1–10 cm in length
Type 3A	High-energy injury Wound <10 cm in length; requires no major soft tissue procedure for wound closure
Type 3B	As above, but more extensive soft tissue injury with wound requiring major soft tissue procedure for closure
Type 3C	Similar to grade 3B injury, but in addition with major arterial injury requiring revascularization for limb salvage

Source: Gustilo and Anderson.[10]

TABLE 107.3. Factors Influencing Fracture Healing.

I. Systemic factors
- A. Age
- B. Activity level including
  - 1. General immobilization
  - 2. Space flight
- C. Nutritional status
- D. Hormonal factors
  - 1. Growth hormone
  - 2. Corticosteroids [microvascular avascular necrosis (AVN)]
  - 3. Others [thyroid, estrogen, androgen, calcitonin, parathyroid hormone (PTH), prostaglandins]
- E. Diseases: diabetes, anemia, neuropathies, tabes
- F. Vitamin deficiencies: A, C, D, K
- G. Drugs: nonsteroidal antiinflammatory drugs (NSAIDs), anticoagulants, factor XIII, calcium channel blockers [verapamil, cytotoxins, diphosphonates, phenytoin (Dilantin), sodium fluoride, tetracycline]
- H. Other substances (nicotine, alcohol)
- I. Hyperoxia
- J. Systemic growth factors
- K. Environmental temperature
- L. Central nervous system trauma

II. Local factors
- A. Factors independent of injury, treatment, or complications
  - 1. Type of bone
  - 2. Abnormal bone
    - a. Radiation necrosis
    - b. Infection
    - c. Tumors and other pathological conditions
  - 3. Denervation
- B. Factors depending on injury
  - 1. Degree of local damage
    - a. Compound fracture
    - b. Comminution of fracture
    - c. Velocity of injury
    - d. Low circulatory levels of vitamin K_1
  - 2. Extent of disruption of vascular supply to bone, its fragments (macrovascular AVN), or soft tissues; severity of injury
  - 3. Type and location of fracture (one or two bones, e.g., tibia and fibula or tibia alone)
  - 4. Loss of bone
  - 5. Soft tissue interposition
  - 6. Local growth factors
- C. Factors depending on treatment
  - 1. Extent of surgical trauma (blood supply, heat)
  - 2. Implant-induced altered blood flow
  - 3. Degree and kind of rigidity of internal or external fixation and the influence of timing
  - 4. Degree, duration, and direction of load-induced deformation of bone and soft tissues
  - 5. Extent of contact beween fragments (gap, displacement, overdistraction)
  - 6. Factors stimulating posttraumatic osteogenesis [bone grafts, bone morphogenetic protein (BMP), electrical stimulation, surgical technique, intermittent venous stasis (Bier)]
- D. Factors associated with complications
  - 1. Infection
  - 2. Venous stasis
  - 3. Metal allergy

Source: Uhthoff HK. Fracture healing. In: Gustilo RB, Kyle RF, Templeman DC, eds. Fractures and Dislocations. St. Louis: Mosby, 1993.[14]

All other methods of achieving healing of fractures rely on the callus formation pathway. Brighton has described the six stages of natural bone repair in which callus is formed. These stages are (1) *impact* [the bone absorbs energy until structural failure occurs]; (2) *induction* [a change in the microenvironment, possibly hypoxia or an acidic pH, which induces periosteal and endosteal osteoblast formation as well as differentiation of mesenchymal cells]; (3) *inflammation* [fibrovascular tissue invades the fracture gap and lays down collagen and matrix]; (4) *soft callus* [osteoid is formed in the fracture gap and an intermediary cartilaginous matrix is formed, which causes the fracture ends to begin to "stick" together]; (5) *hard callus* [enchondral bone formation proceeds on to full bony union with accompanying development of an endosteal blood supply spanning the fracture site]; and (6) *remodeling* [osteoclastic remodeling of the callus with accompanying simultaneous osteoblastic bone formation to convert the woven bone to lamellar bone with reconstitution of the medullary canal].[13]

Fractures heal at different rates. Many factors contribute to the rate and success of fracture healing. Uhthoff has characterized those endogenous and environmental factors that act to either promote or inhibit fracture healing[14] (Table 107.3).

Spinal Injuries

Epidemiology

The overall incidence of spinal injuries is more than 1 million cases per year. Approximately 50,000 of these injuries involve fractures of the spine. Actual spinal cord injury with neurological deficit affects approximately 10,000 patients per year.[15] These devastating injuries most commonly affect young male adults through high-energy blunt and penetrating trauma. One recent study from a Level I trauma center found that 75% of patients with cervical spine injuries were less than 50 years old. Furthermore, 30% of the injured patients were from the third decade alone.[16] The cost to our society of treating spinal cord injuries is enormous. The lifetime cost of treating a 25-year-old patient with quadriplegia is estimated to be 1.3 million dollars.[17]

Initial Management

The initial management of spinal injuries is crucial because inappropriate management in the early phases can exacerbate an existing injury. Stabilization of the spine should begin at the site of the injury by placing the patient on a rigid full-length backboard with additional cervical stabilization through a cervical orthosis. Sandbags and tape immobilizing the head to the backboard provide additional stability.[18] This method limits flexion and extension, which are the major causes of additional cervical injury. The patient should be moved in log-roll fashion with the cervical spine stabilized in a neutral position.

Initial trauma resuscitation should begin with the basic tenets of airway, breathing, and circulation. The physicians performing the resuscitation should always keep in mind the possibility of a head or spinal injury. The patient should be kept immobilized pending a thorough evaluation of the patient's injuries through physical examination and appropriate radiographs. If the patient is awake, all subjective complaints of pain should be investigated. Evaluation of the injured patient's spine should include an understanding of the patient's mechanism of injury. High-speed motor vehicle accidents, falls from height, or penetrating injuries are all mechanisms commonly associated with spinal column injury. The trauma surgeon should look for signs of injury to the patient's face, neck, shoulders, or scalp. These types of injuries are associated with cervical trauma. The presence of thoracic or intraabdominal injuries should clue the investigator to look more closely at the patient's thoracolumbar spine.

Examination of the spine should be undertaken by log-rolling the patient onto their side. Note should be made of any deformity, swelling, lacerations, or abrasions. Palpation of the entire spine should be performed with the patient's cervical spine stabilized in a neutral position. The physician who coordinates the movement of the patient should stabilize the head. Any areas of tenderness, swelling, or stepoff should be identified; these may represent areas of injury secondary to fractures, dislocations, or ligamentous disruptions. The mental status of the patient is crucial in the subjective portion of the exam. Unconscious or impaired patients are not able to appropriately protect themselves and should be kept in a cervical orthosis until they are better able to relate any symptomatology.

Imaging

During the initial assessment, trauma radiographs of the cervical spine should include three separate views of the cervical spine: anteroposterior, lateral, and open mouth odontoid views. The lateral view is the most important view and should include the occiput to T1; 77% of cervical fractures can be identified on the lateral cervical film.[19] X-rays should also be obtained for any portion of the thoracolumbar spine for which the patient complains of pain or for which there are obvious signs of injury. Imaging of thoracolumbar injuries requires two views of the affected region (anteroposterior and lateral).

In some cases, a patient's body habitus, pain, or muscle spasm make it difficult to obtain adequate views of the lateral cervical spine. In these cases, a "swimmer's view" can be ordered. This view requires the patient to abduct one arm above the head with downward traction on the resting arm. The X-ray beam is then angled at approximately 60° across the patient's cervical spine (c-spine). This view allows for better visualization of the cervicothoracic junction to the level of T1. To further assess cervical stability, flexion/extension views can be ordered; these should be done only in the neurologically intact and awake patient. Flexion/extension views can demonstrate instability or subluxation that was not apparent on the standard trauma series.

Computed tomography (CT) scans provide excellent resolution of bony detail in spinal fractures. In cases in which injury to the posterior elements (lamina, pars, and pedicles) or the posterior vertebral body is suspected, a CT scan should be obtained; this allows for more accurate assessment of canal compromise by any bony fragments. The CT is also useful in providing additional information about cervical injuries that are often difficult to visualize on plain radiographs. A study of the value of thin-cut CT scans found that they identified 70% of fractures that were not evident on plain radiographs.[19]

Magnetic resonance imaging (MRI) allows for the best evaluation of the neural elements and the intervertebral disks. An MRI should be obtained in all cases of neurological injury to further define the damage to the neural elements. MRI imaging can help differentiate between spinal cord edema, hematoma, and transection.

Neurological Examination

A complete neurological examination should be performed in all cases of spinal injury. Respiratory function is dependent on cervicothoracic innervation and can be severely compromised as a result of spinal cord injury. C3 and C4 provide innervation to the diaphragm, and injury at these levels can cause the loss of respiratory function. The lower cervical roots and the thoracic roots provide innervation to the intercostal muscles. Loss of the intercostal muscles causes paradoxical breathing. The diaphragm displaces inferiorly, causing abdominal distension rather than retraction during inspiration.

Strength testing should be performed for all major upper- and lower extremity muscle groups. Muscle function should be graded on a 0 to 5 scale.

0. No muscle contraction
1. Flicker of muscle contraction
2. Active movement of the muscle with gravity removed
3. Active movement against gravity
4. Active movement against gravity and mild resistance
5. Normal muscle strength, active movement against full resistance

A dermatomal sensory examination should be done to identify any areas of sensory loss. Pinprick, light touch, and temperature should be tested to localize the area of the lesion within the spinal cord.

The physician should also perform a complete check of all reflexes. Pathological reflexes such as a positive Babinski sign and clonus are pathognomonic of upper motor neuron lesions. The rectal exam serves to identify the status of sacral nerve root function. The presence of rectal sphincter tone and sensation demonstrates sacral sparing if there is an injury at the levels above. The presence of sacral sparing is important as it is used to define a complete versus incomplete neurological lesion. A test of the bulbocavernosus reflex alludes to the presence of spinal shock if it is absent. A patient's rectal sphincter should contract when the glans penis is squeezed in a male; in a female patient, the bulbocavernosus reflex can be elicited by tugging on the Foley catheter.

Neurological Injury

Patients with spinal column injuries may present with associated neurological compromise, which may manifest initially as neurogenic shock. In the initial minutes after a spinal cord injury, a patient may exhibit hypertension and tachycardia. Subsequently, the patient becomes bradycardic and hypotensive; this results from what is essentially a traumatic sympathectomy. The patient exhibits what is unopposed vagal tone from the parasympathetic nervous system.

Neurogenic shock can last from several hours to several days. The bulbocavernosus reflex is important in heralding the end of neurogenic shock. Testing the bulbocavernosus reflex involves squeezing the glans penis while performing a rectal exam. The rectal sphincter should contract when the glans penis is stimulated. In a female, the reflex may be elicited by tugging on the Foley catheter. This reflex is a sensorimotor pathway independent of white matter long-tract axons. It is the lowest spinal cord-mediated reflex and is the first one to return following spinal shock. The bulbocavernosus reflex will function regardless of whether the more cephalad cord is intact.

Careful neurological examination should be performed on patients in whom spinal injury has been demonstrated or is suspected. Careful documentation of the neurological deficits should be made to facilitate further treatment. Motor weakness, dermatomal sensory deficits, and the reflex exam allow for characterization of the level of injury. It is essential to know if a neurological deficit is stable or progressive. Serial neurological exams must be performed because a progressive neurological deficit often warrants prompt surgical intervention.When determination of a spinal cord injury is made, steroids should be administered. The following recommendations have been made as a result of the National Acute Spinal Cord Injury Study (NASCIS-III). In the first 8 h following the injury, methylprednisolone should be given. If the patient is receiving methylprednisolone within 3 h after the injury, a bolus of 30 mg/kg should be followed by an infusion of 5.4 mg/kg/h for 23 h. If the patient starts receiving steroids 3 to 8 h after the injury, the same infusion should be continued for a total of 47 h.[20]

Classification of neurological injury should then be made as to the level of the injury and also as to whether the injury is complete or incomplete. An incomplete injury refers to the presence of some neurological function beyond the level of the injury. This function may be either motor, or sensory, or both. Patients with complete injuries show absolutely no neurological function beyond the site of injury. The prognosis of complete injuries is dismal. In a study of 142 patients with complete paraplegia 1 month following their injury, only 5% regained enough function to ambulate independently with assistive devices.[21]

The Frankel classification is a commonly used measure of function after spinal injury.[22] Another newer system in use is the International Standards for classifying spinal injury. These standards are based upon the level of the lesion and whether a lesion is complete or incomplete.

Incomplete Spinal Cord Injury Syndromes

The common types of incomplete injury in the spinal cord are discussed next.

Central Cord Syndrome

This injury commonly occurs in older patients with preexisting degenerative changes in their cervical spine. It is the most common incomplete spinal cord injury. The patient presents with decreased motor function that is more profound in the upper extremities than the lower extremities. There is generally sacral sparing, although patients can develop urological difficulties. These injuries frequently occur as a result of a blow to the anterior head that causes the cervical spine to hyperextend. This hyperextension mechanism causes the spinal cord to become pinched between the posterior elements and any preexisting degenerative osteophytes or disks anteriorly. Prognosis is fair, with approximately 50% of patients regaining functional recovery.[23]

Anterior Cord Syndrome

Injury to the anterior spinal cord is generally attributed to compression or flexion injuries. The damage can be related to a vascular insult secondary to the compression or direct impingement on the spinal cord. Patients generally have no motor function below the level of injury as a result of damage to the anterior corticospinal tracts. Preservation of proprioception and vibratory sense is maintained through preservation of the dorsal columns. The prognosis of this type of injury is exceedingly poor. It is estimated that only 10% of patients obtain a useful recovery.[23]

Posterior Cord Syndromes

Injury to the posterior aspect of the cord only is rare and results in a profound proprioceptive and vibratory deficit. These neurological functions are mediated by the posterior columns of the spinal cord. The patient retains motor function and often sensation because the anterior aspect of the cord is spared. These patients will develop a slapping gait secondary to their lack of proprioception.

Brown–Sequard Syndrome

This incomplete spinal cord injury is often caused by penetrating trauma. An asymmetrical neurological deficit develops below the level of the lesion. The loss of motor function is greatest on the ipsilateral side of the injury. Damage to the ascending dorsal columns cause proprioceptive and vibratory deficits on the ipsilateral side of the injury. A contralateral pain and temperature sensory loss develops one to two levels below the injury because of damage to the crossing spinothalamic tracts. The prognosis for the Brown–Sequard injury is very good, with up to 75% of patients developing functional recovery.[24]

Cauda Equina Syndrome

The cauda equina is composed of lumbosacral nerve roots below the level of the spinal cord. The etiology of cauda equina syndrome is nerve root impingement secondary to trauma, tumors, or disk herniation, or is iatrogenic secondary to surgery. The term cauda equina syndrome refers to a constellation of symptoms relating to lumbosacral nerve root dysfunction. Bowel and bladder function is usually impaired, with decreased sphincter tone and elevated postvoiding residuals. The patient may also have radiculopathy and back pain related to nerve impingement. Bilateral radiculopathy should increase the suspicion for a central caudal nerve root impingement.

The onset of a cauda equina syndrome can be subtle, and the findings just mentioned may manifest themselves slowly. Treatment depends on the etiology, but rapid decompression is required. The prognosis for recovery is dependent on the time between onset of the lesion and decompression. Overall, return of motor and sensory function is more reliable than bowel and bladder function.

Common Cervical Fractures

Upper Cervical Spine Injuries

Anatomy of the Craniovertebral Junction

The craniovertebral junction (occipitoatlantoaxial complex) is composed of the occiput, the atlas (C1), and the axis (C2). This region is characterized by specific fracture patterns that differ from those of the lower cervical spine. The occiput articulates with the cervical spine through the occipital condyles. The foramen magnum allows the spinal cord to pass into the skull. The atlas supports the occiput through the lateral masses upon which the occipital condyles rest. The axis contains the dens around which the atlas rotates.

Trauma and surgery at these levels can severely impair both rotation and flexion of the head and cervical spine. The occipitoatlantoaxial complex allows the majority of head motion. The occipitoatlantal articulation allows approximately 50% of normal cervical flexion. The atlantoaxial articulation allows 50% of normal cervical rotation.

Ligamentous integrity is crucial to maintaining stability in the upper cervical spine. At the level of the occiput, the tectorial membrane forms the primary ligamentous restraint against flexion and extension. The alar ligaments extending from the lateral portion of the foramen magnum to the posterolateral odontoid are the primary rotational stabilizers of the craniovertebral junction. The transverse ligament provides support to the lateral masses by inserting on their medial side.

Occipitoatlantal Dislocation

This devastating injury is usually fatal. The mechanism of injury involves distraction or translation of the head on the cervical spine. If the patient survives the initial trauma, this injury is often missed because of the difficulty in imaging this region. Clues to the injury include vertebral artery injuries and cranial nerve palsies. Cranial nerve palsy can be associated with this injury. An example is involvement of the abducens (CN VI) nerve. This injury can be diagnosed on the lateral radiograph by using Power's ratio.

Traction should be avoided because this will cause overdistraction and most likely the patient's death. Treatment involves stabilizing the patient in a halo vest and then performing an occiput to C2 fusion.

C1 Burst Fracture (Jefferson Fracture)

A fracture of the atlas (C1) occurs primarily through axial loading. The addition of rotational and flexion/extension moments result in different fracture patterns. It is frequently associated with other cervical fractures. The majority of associated fractures occur in the C2 vertebrae. Craniofacial trauma is associated with 25% of atlas fractures.[25] Neurological injury with this type of injury is rare. Axial loading causes the C1 vertebrae to fracture outward, thus creating an increase in the space available for the spinal cord.

On the lateral view of the cervical spine, there may be an abnormal atlanto–dens interval or increased soft tissue swelling. This fracture is most readily diagnosed on plain radiographs through the open mouth odontoid view. Using this view it is possible to measure the atlantoaxial offset (AAO). The AAO allows diagnosis of the stability of a C1 fracture. An AAO less than 5.7 mm predicts that the transverse longitudinal ligament (TLL) is intact and that the fracture is stable. However, an AAO greater than 6.9 mm predicts rupture of the TLL and thus represents an unstable injury.[25]

Treatment of these injuries is generally nonsurgical. There exists debate about whether halo vest or traction is the best method of treatment. If surgery is required, then transarticular screws or occipitocervical fusion should be performed.

C2 Odontoid Fracture

The odontoid can be fractured by a mechanism involving flexion, extension, or a combination of both. Odontoid fractures make up approximately 10% to 15% of all cervical fractures.[26] Most fractures are caused by motor vehicles and falls. A significant number of patients have associated skull, mandible, and other cervical fractures.[27]

Anderson and D'Alonzo classified odontoid fractures into categories based upon the location of the fracture.[28] A type I fracture is an oblique fracture through the apex of the dens where the alar ligaments attach. The type II fracture occurs at the junction of the vertebral body and dens. The type III fracture occurs through the body of the axis.

Odontoid fractures can be very difficult to diagnose on plain radiographs. The fracture is often best visualized on the open mouth odontoid radiograph. Sagittal and coronal reconstructions on the CT scan are often useful to better define fracture morphology. Axial CT scan cuts must be interpreted with caution as the fracture is in the plane of the CT and can be missed by the plane of imaging.

One of the major complications of this type of injury is nonunion. The type II odontoid fracture is at the greatest risk for nonunion. Patient characteristics including age greater than 65 years and a history of smoking increase the risk of nonunion. Similarly, if the fracture fragment is more than 5 mm displaced or the angular deformity is greater than 10°, the rate of nonunion is increased.[29] The risk for nonunion is exacerbated by the tenuous blood supply to the odontoid and presence of synovial fluid that bathes it.

Treatment must take into account the risk factors for nonunion. If the fracture is nondisplaced, the patient can be placed into halo immobilization for 12 weeks. However, if the patient is older and/or a smoker, they must be counseled about the possibility of nonunion. If the fragment is significantly displaced (more than 5 mm), then posterior fusion from C1–C2 can be performed with the understanding that this treatment will cause the patient to lose 50% of the rotation of his or her head. Another approach that helps avoid this loss of rotation is the placement of an odontoid screw. Preoperative planning and intraoperative imaging is crucial to avoid damage to the neurovascular structures that lie in close proximity to the odontoid.

C2 Pedicle Fracture (Hangman's Fracture)

Fracture of the pedicles of the axis can occur through hyperextension and axial loading. This type of mechanism can be seen when a patient falls or their face strikes the windshield during a motor vehicle accident. These particular fractures have the eponym "hangman's fractures." These fractures are best demonstrated on the lateral cervical film. These fractures show a high association with other types of cervical fractures.[30] Close examination of the entire cervical spine must be undertaken.

Treatment is dependent on the displacement and angulation of the fracture fragments. The most commonly used classification is the one proposed by Levine.[30] A type I hangman's fracture is minimally or nondisplaced. There is no significant angulation or translation of the C2 body on C3. These fractures can be treated with the use of a rigid cervical collar for a period of 12 weeks.

A type II hangman's fracture shows displacement, translation, or angulation. Initially, a closed reduction of these injuries may be undertaken. The patient should then be treated with a halo vest. If the displacement is significant (more than 6 mm), the patient should be placed into halo immobilization with 6 to 9 pounds of traction applied for as long as 5 days.[30] Lateral X-rays are then obtained to look at the reduction. If an acceptable reduction is maintained, then the patient should be kept in halo immobilization for 12 weeks. If the reduction is unsuccessful, the patient should be continued in traction for 4 to 6 weeks, followed by halo immobilization for 6 more weeks.

The rare type III fracture occurs concomitantly with a unilateral or bilateral facet dislocation. Closed reduction is rarely successful, and open reduction is usually required. Surgical stabilization should be performed.

Lower Cervical Spine Injuries

Cervical Sprains and Strains

Sprains refer to ligamentous injuries without evidence of bony injury. The patient typically presents with cervical pain and an inability to fully range their neck. These injuries can be classified into four categories on the basis of the grade of injury.

C3–C7 Facet Dislocation (Jumped Facet)

Dislocation of the cervical facets can occur through flexion-distraction and rotation of the cervical spine. These injuries can involve unilateral or bilateral facets, and they can often be identified on both the anteroposterior and lateral views. On the anteroposterior view, the spinous processes are rotated toward the side of injury above the level of injury. On the lateral view, the vertebral body is displaced. The degree of displacement is helpful in determining whether the facet dislocation is unilateral or bilateral. A unilateral dislocation usually involves less than 25% displacement of the body, whereas a bilateral facet dislocation usually involves 25% to 50% displacement of the body. The "bow-tie" sign may also be visible on the lateral view. This "bow-tie" is created secondary to rotation and is actually caused by overlapping of the lateral masses of the vertebral body above the dislocation.

MRI should be obtained in the presence of a unilateral or bilateral facet dislocation. Disk herniation can occur at the time of injury, and this can cause further neurological impingement during reduction of a dislocation. If a disk is present, surgery is indicated to remove the disk before reduction and stabilization of the spine.[31]

Dislocations may be reduced by either open or closed techniques. Closed reduction is typically attempted before open treatment. Reduction can be performed using Gardner–Wells tongs; usually, 5 to 10 pounds is added as the starting weight. An additional 5 pounds is then added at 15-min intervals for each level above the dislocation. X-rays should be obtained after the addition of any weight. The attempted reduction should be stopped if the facets reduce, if distraction greater than 1 cm occurs at any level, or if there is any change in neurological status.[32] Open reduction and posterior fusion is required if the closed reduction fails or remains unstable.

Compression Fractures of the Lower Cervical Spine (C3–C7)

Compression fractures occur during axial compression and flexion injuries. Examination of the lateral cervical film helps to determine stability of these fractures. Stability of these fractures is dependent on the degree of angulation and translation. If a vertebral level is greater than 3.5 mm translated or 11° angulated, the current management is to proceed with fusion.[33] In terms of compression, the vertebral body should be evaluated. If there is less than 25% loss of body height and the body has an intact posterior wall, the patient can be treated nonoperatively. The presence of neurological injury or impairment and the need for decompression will modify these guidelines. If the fracture is unstable or if cord compression is present, then anterior decompression with strut grafting should be performed.

C3–C7 Spinous Process Fractures

Spinous process fractures represent avulsions of the paraspinal muscles. The eponym associated with these fractures is "clayshoveler's fractures." If these are symptomatic, the patient should be immobilized in a hard cervical collar for approximately 1 to 2 weeks and then weaned to a soft collar.

Thoracolumbar Spine Injuries

Anatomy of the Thoracolumbar Spine

The thoracic spine contains 12 vertebral bodies, which increase gradually in size toward the lumbar spine. Each of the vertebrae has costal articulations where the ribs attach. The thoracic spine has characteristic spinous processes that are long and oriented caudally. Their facets are different from the cervical and lumbar spine and paired such that the superior articular facet faces posterolaterally and the inferior facets face anteromedially. This orientation helps provide for rotation of the thorax.

The lumbar spine is made up of five vertebral bodies. The lumbar vertebrae have short thick spinous processes that face directly posteriorly. The orientation of the facets changes toward the inferior vertebral bodies. They start out, at the first lumbar vertebra, oriented medial to lateral and end up facing anterior to posterior. This arrangement resists rotation but provides a considerable degree of flexion (60°). The most common location of thoracic and lumbar fractures is at their junction (T12–L1), where relatively stiff thoracic segments transition to more relatively more mobile lumbar segments.

Spinal stability in the lumbar spine is currently based upon the three-column system as described by Denis in 1983. The posterior column includes the spinous processes, laminae, facets, and the pedicles. The middle column includes the posterior half of the vertebral bodies, the posterior annulus fibrosis, and the posterior longitudinal ligament. The anterior column includes the anterior longitudinal ligament, the anterior annulus fibrosis, and the anterior half of the vertebral body.[34]

In Denis' review of 482 patients, he identified stable versus unstable injuries. Stable fractures are those fractures with minimal and moderate compression fractures and an intact posterior column. He defined three types of instability. The first type of instability is mechanical instability, which includes severe compression fractures and seatbelt-type injuries. In these cases, the anterior and posterior columns are disrupted and the vertebrae can hinge around the middle column. The second type of instability is neurological instability. In these cases, the middle column is disrupted, such as in a burst fracture. These patients may develop late neurological sequelae to their injury secondary to compression from the middle column. The last type of instability is mechanical and neurological instability. Examples of this type of injury include fracture-dislocations and severe burst fractures with neurological deficits. Fracture displacement and further neurological injury can occur with this category of instability.[34]

Common Thoracolumbar Spine Injuries

Compression Fractures

Compression fractures involve disruption of the anterior column with an intact middle column and posterior column. Compression fractures are common in elderly persons with osteoporotic bone and may be the result of relatively minor trauma. The mechanism of injury is anterior flexion or lateral flexion. In evaluating these fractures, anteroposterior and lateral films of the spine should be obtained. Most commonly there is collapse of the superior endplate with wedging of the vertebral body. These injuries are graded according to the amount of body height lost and the degree of kyphosis. A loss of body height greater than 40% to 50% is indicative of posterior column compromise.[35] A correlation was also found between continued back pain at 2 years when the degree of kyphosis was greater than 30°.[36]

In cases where the loss of body height is less than 40% to 50% and there is less than 30° of kyphosis, conservative management is recommended. Management of these fractures includes a short period of rest and then a hyperextension brace or thoracolumbosacral orthosis (TLSO). Surgery may be recommended in cases in which the criteria for instability is met. Surgery will help to prevent any further deformity caused by collapse into kyphosis. The current approach to these fractures is posterior with fixation through a distraction rodding construct.

Burst Fractures

Burst fractures involve the anterior and middle columns of the spine. The mechanism of injury is axial loading as well as some degree of flexion. The treatment of burst fractures is dependent on the amount of spinal canal compromise, the percentage of body height lost, the degree of kyphosis, and whether neurological injury is present. On plain radiographs, widening of the pedicles is a sign of disruption of the posterior elements. A CT scan can then further define the bony pathology and determine the amount of canal compromise.

If the degree of canal compromise is less than 50%, the patient is neurologically intact, and there is not a significant degree of vertebral body collapse (<40%) and kyphosis (30°), then the patient can generally be treated conservatively.[37] This treatment should consist of a short period of rest and then mobilization while supported in an orthosis. The type of orthosis is dependent on the level at which the fracture occurs.

In cases in which there is more than 50% canal compromise or there is concern about late instability, fixation of the fracture can be recommended. Burst fractures can be approached either anteriorly or posteriorly. Decompression and fusion of the affected levels are performed.

Flexion-Distraction Injuries

These spinal injuries are flexion injuries where the center of rotation lies anterior to the spinal column. The eponym associated with these fractures is "seatbelt injuries." The injury may involve bone, ligaments, or both. If the injury is purely bony in nature, then the prognosis is better than for a mixed or pure soft tissue injury. A purely bony flexion-distraction injury is known as a "Chance fracture." These purely bony injuries tend to heal well, often without any operative intervention. Again, treatment should consist of a short period of bed rest and then mobilization with a TLSO or extension cast. The stability of these fractures should be assessed routinely with radiographs. However, if the injury involves the ligaments and/or the disk, then these are considered unstable injuries that should be stabilized with the use of instrumentation, usually performed through a posterior approach.

Fracture-Dislocations

Fracture-dislocations are very high energy injuries that disrupt all three columns of the spine. The mechanism of injury may be flexion-rotation, shear, or a continuation of the flexion-distraction injury. The majority of fractures are the flexion-rotation type[34] and are often accompanied by neurological injury. Surgical intervention is usually necessary in these injuries to decompress the neural elements and provide stability. If the patient is neurologically intact at the time of injury, surgery helps prevent future instability or neurological injury. The most common surgical approach to the fractures is posterior. Instrumentation is indicated to provide rigid fixation of the fracture.

Sacral Fractures

Five sacral vertebrae fuse to form the sacrum. There are no true spinous processes. However, there exists a median sacral crest formed from fused spinous processes. Sacral fractures are often the result of high-energy trauma and can occur in conjunction with pelvic fractures. Fractures through the sacrum may compromise the stability of the pelvic ring. The mechanism of these fractures is often axial loading and vertical shear or lateral compression.

Neurological examination is critical, and strict observation of bowel and bladder function is required. A rectal exam should be performed and perianal sensation documented. Sacral fractures are sometimes visible on standard trauma series anteroposterior pelvic X-rays. Additional views are helpful to define the fracture pattern. Pelvic inlet and outlet view and lateral views of the sacrum may help define the pathology. If there is no clear documentation of the fracture and one is suspected, then a CT scan should be ordered.

The classification of sacral fractures is based upon dividing the sacrum into three zones[38]:

Zone I: alar fractures (lateral to the sacral foramina)
Zone II: foraminal fractures (fractures passing through the foramina)
Zone III: central sacral fractures (fractures medial to the foramina)

The treatment of sacral fractures is dependent on the neurological status of the patient. If there is neurological impingement, then decompression may be required. Additionally, if the fracture compromises the stability of the pelvic ring, stabilization with instrumentation may be required.

Common Shoulder Fractures

Anatomy of the Shoulder

The shoulder consists of the clavicle, scapula, and the humeral head. The humeral head articulates with the glenoid portion of the scapula at the glenohumeral joint. The clavicle connects to the scapula at the acromioclavicular joint. The glenohumeral joint is the most mobile joint in the body. It is a ball-and-socket joint that allows for flexion/extension, abduction/adduction, and rotation. The shallow nature of the glenoid helps give the shoulder its mobility but also renders it prone to instability. An array of ligaments including the glenohumeral, coracoclavicular, and coracoacromial ligaments help support the joint. Dynamic stability of the shoulder joint is provided by the rotator cuff muscles, which include the subscapularis, supraspinatus, infraspinatus, and teres minor.

Proximal Humerus Fracture

Proximal humeral fractures involve the humeral head, the greater and lesser tuberosities, and extend to the region of the surgical neck of the humerus. These fractures show a bimodal incidence with younger patients suffering high-energy trauma and older osteoporotic patients who may sustain the fracture through relatively minor trauma. The most common mechanisms are a fall onto an outstretched arm or direct trauma to the shoulder region.

Physical examination reveals swelling and ecchymosis over the shoulder region. The patient has pain with glenohumeral motion. It is important to perform a complete neurovascular assessment of the patient. Distal pulses in the extremity should be palpated to ensure that circulation to the extremity is not impaired. The most common neurological deficit is that of an axillary nerve deficiency.[39] This deficit may be difficult to detect at the time of the acute trauma. One way to assess axillary nerve function is to question that patient about sensation over the deltoid muscle. It is generally difficult to accurately assess the motor function of the deltoid muscle in a patient with pain secondary to a fracture.

When shoulder trauma is suspected, radiographs must include anteroposterior and axillary views. These two views constitute the standard trauma series for the shoulder. The axillary view is important in determining whether the humeral head is concentrically located within the glenoid. It provides information about fracture configuration and may help demonstrate any fractures of the glenoid. It is often difficult to visualize posterior shoulder dislocations or glenoid fractures solely on the anteroposterior view. CT scan can be a useful complement to plain radiographs. It allows for better assessment of fracture pattern and assessment of the joint surface.[40]

Proximal humerus fractures are most commonly described by the Neer classification.[41] This system divides the proximal humerus into four parts: (1) articular segment or humeral head, (2) greater tuberosity, (3) lesser tuberosity, and (4) shaft. A part is defined by a fragment that is displaced 1 cm or greater and/or angulated more than 45°. If the fragment does not meet these criteria, it does not qualify as a "part." For example, a proximal humerus fracture that has a greater tuberosity fragment that is 1 cm displaced is classified as a "two-part" proximal humerus fracture. A nondisplaced fracture line through the lesser tuberosity does not change the classification of the fracture. Each of these fragments is affected by the muscle insertions acting on them. The greater and lesser tuberosities are affected by the insertion of the rotator cuff muscles. The humeral shaft fragment is displaced by the action of the pectoralis major and deltoid muscles.

Proximal humerus fractures can be very difficult to treat given the frequent poor nature of the bone stock in many elderly patients. The fracture fragments can be small and difficult to reduce. Fortunately, 80% of proximal humerus fractures are nondisplaced or minimally displaced.[42] These fractures can be treated with a sling and then with early range of motion to prevent shoulder stiffness.

There exist a myriad of ways to treat more comminuted or displaced humeral head fractures. An attempted closed reduction can be performed with a well-relaxed patient. Reduction is more successful in two-part fractures versus three- and four-part fractures. After reduction, the patient can be immobilized in a sling and swathe or a velpeaux sling. Unsuccessful attempts at stable reduction require percutaneous pinning or open reduction and internal fixation.

In three-part and four-part fractures (Fig. 107.2), it is extremely difficult to achieve and maintain a reduction. Closed reduction can be attempted and stabilized with percutaneous pinning if possible. Otherwise, open reduction and internal fixation are necessary. Various plate/screw, tension band, suture, and intramedullary devices have been reported in fixation of the proximal humerus. In four-part fractures, prosthetic replacement is often used. The comminuted nature of these fractures makes successful reduction and fixation very difficult. Furthermore, given the high degree of damage to the bone, these patients often develop avascular necrosis of the head fragment, thus compromising the results of any stable fixation.[43]

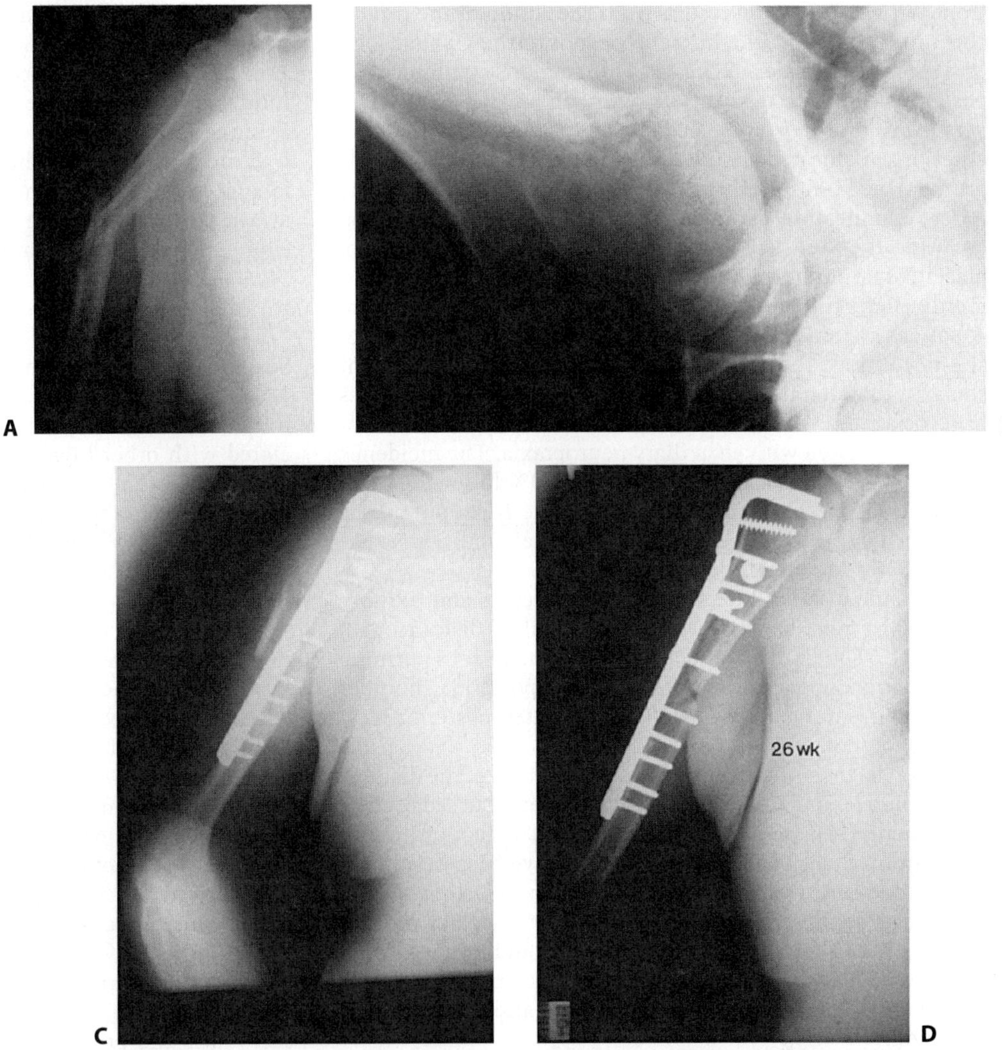

FIGURE 107.2. A. Proximal humerus fracture dislocation with humeral shaft fracture in a 41-year-old patient. Anteroposterior view. **B.** Axillary lateral view. **C.** Anteroposterior view of humerus with blade plate fixation postoperatively. **D.** Anteroposterior view of fracture 26 weeks later.

Clavicle Fractures

Clavicle fractures occur commonly as the result of a direct blow or a fall onto an outstretched hand. The majority of clavicle fractures involve the middle third of the bone (85%). Medial-third and lateral-third fractures make up 5% and 10% of clavicle fractures, respectively.[44]

Physical examination reveals tenderness and ecchymosis over the clavicle. Displaced fractures commonly present with superior displacement of the medial portion secondary to the muscular pull of the sternocleidomastoid muscle. The weight of the humerus on the lateral portion causes it to be displaced inferiorly. It is important to examine the skin over the fracture carefully. The skin overlying the clavicle is thin and can be punctured by the sharp edges of the fracture. Documentation of the patient's neurovascular status must be undertaken during evaluation. The subclavian artery and vein as well as the brachial plexus lie in close proximity under the clavicle.

The majority of middle-third clavicle fractures do not require operative intervention. The patient should be placed into a sling to help support the weight of the arm. Fracture healing is generally swift, and nonunion is rare.[45] The healing of the fracture commonly results in some shortening of the clavicle and often some mild loss of abduction at the shoulder.

Surgical intervention is required in cases of open fracture and may be necessary in cases where the fracture fragments threaten to penetrate the skin. Neurological or vascular injuries are also an indication to explore the fracture and stabilize it. The proximity of the brachial plexus and the subclavian artery and vein place them at risk during a fracture.

Shoulder Dislocation

The shoulder is the most commonly dislocated joint in the body. It is inherently less stable than other joints in the body secondary to its wide range of mobility. This mobility is related to the shallow glenohumeral joint. Stability of the shoulder is achieved through muscular and ligamentous restraints as well as the biomechanical properties of the shoulder itself. The rotator cuff muscles combine with the glenoid labrum and the glenohumeral ligaments to help provide stability. Biomechanically, concavity compression has also been proposed as an important shoulder stabilizer.

Concavity compression results from the action of the rotator cuff muscles forcing the humeral head into the glenoid.

Anterior shoulder dislocation is far more common than posterior shoulder dislocation, with an incidence of 95% versus 5% for posterior dislocation.[42] Examination of an anteriorly dislocated shoulder often demonstrates a palpable humeral head anteriorly. A sulcus sign is also commonly noted, manifesting as an indentation below the acromion denoting the void left from the humeral head being out of place. Palpation of the posterior aspect of the shoulder commonly elicits the presence of a hollow beneath the acromion. A patient with a locked dislocated shoulder shows a lack of ability to move the affected arm. Neurovascular assessment should be undertaken to ensure that no associated injuries have occurred. Anterior shoulder dislocation is most commonly associated with an axillary neuropraxia. The incidence of axillary neuropraxia is approximately 10% following anterior dislocation.[46] Testing of axillary nerve function can be performed by questioning patients about their ability to sense stimuli over the lateral deltoid muscle.

A trauma series including anteroposterior and axillary radiographs must be obtained when a shoulder dislocation is suspected. The axillary lateral view is crucial to determine the direction of the dislocation. Often a posterior shoulder dislocation is not readily apparent on an anteroposterior view of the shoulder.

After diagnosis of the dislocation, reduction of the dislocation should be undertaken. Muscle relaxation and sedation of the patient are paramount to a successful reduction. Many different methods of shoulder reduction have been described. After reduction, a period of immobilization in a sling up to 3 weeks can be prescribed. Therapy to regain range of motion and strengthen the dynamic stability of shoulder should then be started. It is important to assess for the possibility of a rotator cuff tear as early diagnosis can allow for prompt treatment.[46]

Posterior dislocations can result from seizures or electrical shock injuries. A strong posteriorly directed force may also result in a posterior dislocation. The patient has severe pain over the affected shoulder. Motion at the glenohumeral joint is severely impeded, and the patient lacks external rotation. There is often a void anteriorly over the shoulder combined with a palpable fullness posteriorly. A prominent coracoid can also be a sign of a posterior dislocation.

Fractures of the humeral head or glenoid are often associated with posterior dislocations. There is frequently a compression fracture of the anteromedial humeral head caused by impaction against the posterior cortical rim of the glenoid. This fracture is often called a "reverse Hill–Sachs lesion." The posterior cortical rim of the glenoid can also be fractured during a posterior shoulder dislocation.

Treatment of a posterior shoulder dislocation should begin with an attempted closed reduction. Success is highly dependent upon a relaxed patient with adequate analgesia. Conscious sedation may be inadequate to allow for sufficient relaxation to reduce the shoulder. General anesthesia may be necessary if the sedation and analgesia available in the emergency room are inadequate. Occasionally, the humeral head may become locked on the glenoid. In these cases, an open reduction is required.[47]

The reduction maneuver should be performed with the patient supine. Longitudinal traction should be applied to the adducted arm and pressure should be applied from posteriorly to the humeral to reduce it and bring it back into the glenoid. A laterally directed force may be necessary to unlock the humeral head from the posterior glenoid. Force involving external rotation should be avoided because it can result in a fracture of the head or shaft of the humerus. If the reduction is successful, the patient should be placed into a sling and swath position with the shoulder adducted across the body. The patient should be immobilized for 3 to 4 weeks.

Scapula Fractures

Scapular fractures are relatively infrequent, making up only 1% of all fractures and 5% of all shoulder fractures. Scapular fractures are often the result of high-energy trauma and associated with other high-energy thoracic injuries. The mechanism of fracture is generally a direct blow. Fractures of the body represent approximately 50% of scapular fractures, glenoid fractures make up approximately 35%, and fractures of the coracoid and acromion represent approximately 7% each.[42]

Diagnosis of scapular fractures is often difficult, and any injuries of the thorax should make the physician suspicious for a scapular fracture. Furthermore, patients usually present with pain and ecchymosis in the region of the scapula or shoulder joint. If a scapular fracture is suspected, several radiographs should be obtained. A "trauma series" of the shoulder including anteroposterior and axillary view of the shoulder should be ordered. In addition, an anteroposterior and lateral view of the scapula should be obtained. Given the difficulty in visualizing many scapular fractures, a CT scan is a useful adjunct in determining fracture morphology.

Scapular body fractures can usually be treated nonoperatively. The majority of scapular body fractures are minimally or nondisplaced. There is a thick soft tissue envelope that surrounds and protects the bone. The affected limb can be placed into a sling and, after the initial swelling and pain have resolved, early motion can be started. The fractures heal rapidly, and generally by 6 weeks no further immobilization or support is needed.

The portion of the scapula that articulates with the humeral head is the glenoid. Glenoid fractures occur from the humeral impacting into the glenoid. It is important to distinguish whether glenoid fractures are extra- or intraarticular. Extraarticular fractures generally do not need any type of reduction. The humeral head usually remains concentric within the glenoid. After a period of immobilization in a sling, range-of-motion exercises can be started to prevent shoulder stiffness.

Exceptions include glenoid neck fractures that are significantly displaced or angulated. Only about 10% of glenoid fractures are severely displaced. Intraarticular glenoid fractures have been classified by Ideberg.[48] Type I fractures involve the glenoid rim: these are further subdivided into IA, anterior rim, and IB, posterior rim. A type II fracture is a fracture through the glenoid fossa. The type III fracture is an oblique fracture through the middle and superior border of the scapula; it can be associated with acromion fractures and AC separations. The type IV glenoid fracture is a horizontal fracture that exits the medial border of the blade of the glenoid. The type V fracture is a type IV fracture with the additional component of an inferior glenoid fragment. The type VI fracture was described by Goss and refers to severely comminuted fractures of the articular surface.[49]

Operative indications have arisen from several small series of fractures. Some authors recommend fixation of fractures that are more than 40° angulated or with more than 5 mm of articular stepoff.[50] Angulation greater than 40° can later compromise glenohumeral motion. Late correction of these deformities can be exceedingly difficult. Other operative indications include fracture that result in subluxation of the humeral head and also severely displaced fragments (larger than 1 cm) where nonunion might result.

Fractures of the Humerus

Fractures of the Humeral Shaft

Fractures of the humeral shaft involve the diaphyseal region of the humerus from below the surgical neck of the humerus and extending to the area above the humeral condyles. Humeral shaft fractures most often occur as a result of a direct blow to the arm. Mast, in a review of 240 humeral shaft fractures, found that the majority of the fractures occurred in the middiaphyseal region of the humerus (69%).[51]

The patient with a humeral shaft fracture may present with angulation or deformity over the upper arm. There may be signs of direct trauma such as abrasions or lacerations in the region of the fracture. Care should be taken to ensure that the fracture did not penetrate the skin, thus rendering it an open fracture. Examination of the neurovascular status should include attention to the radial nerve, which is the nerve most frequently damaged with this type of injury.[52] Sensation in the doral first web space, as well as wrist and finger extension, should be checked. When a humerus fracture is suspected, radiographs should include anteroposterior and lateral views of the humerus. Classification of humerus fractures is based upon the radiographic appearance of the fracture. They are described by location (proximal third, middle third, and distal third) and fracture morphology (transverse, spiral, segmental, or oblique).

Fractures of the humeral shaft tend to heal well without surgical intervention. Given the wide range of mobility at the shoulder, up to 30° of varus and 20° of anterior angulation has been reported as well tolerated.[53] The treatment of these fractures is varied, but coaptation splints, hanging arm casts, and velpeaux slings have all been utilized with success. Functional bracing has also become more common, and excellent results have been achieved using this method.[54,55] Bracing may be undertaken 1 to 2 weeks after pain and swelling have subsided. The soft tissue compression afforded by the fracture brace has led to improved results regarding fracture angulation and displacement. Furthermore, the patient can participate in shoulder and elbow range-of-motion exercises during the healing period.

Surgery for humeral shaft fractures should be undertaken for open fractures, poorly aligned fractures despite closed reduction, vascular injury, multiple trauma patients to facilitate mobilization, and floating elbows (ipsilateral humerus fracture with a concomitant both-bones forearm fracture).[56,57] Humerus fractures can be stabilized in a variety of manners, most commonly by plating or intramedullary nailing.

Surgical intervention is not strictly indicated in the case of radial nerve injury. The path of the radial nerve crosses the posterior aspect of the humerus from medial to lateral. Near the middiaphyseal portion, it lies in direct contact with the humerus. The incidence of radial nerve injury varies in the literature from 1.8% to 24% of fractures.[58] The most common fracture type associated with a radial nerve palsy is a spiral distal third fracture, also known as a Holstein–Lewis fracture. Most nerve injuries are neuropraxias and resolve spontaneously with time.[51] These injuries will generally resolve after 3 to 4 months. If after a waiting period of 3 to 4 months the palsy remains, then electrodiagnostic studies are indicated. At this time, it is recommended to pursue surgical exploration if a radial nerve palsy develops during a closed reduction. However, this remains a controversial subject, with a large number of secondary nerve palsies also resolving with time.

Distal Humerus Fractures

The distal humerus articulates with the radius and the ulna to form the elbow joint. The humeroulnar joint is composed of the trochlea of the humerus and the trochlear notch of the ulna. This articulation allows for flexion/extension at the elbow. The humeroradial joint is formed by the humeral capitellum and the radial head. The distal humerus is also the origin of the wrist flexors and extensors. The medial epicondyle serves as the origin of the flexor mass, and the lateral epicondyle is the origin of the extensor wad. Distal humeral fractures are rare, making up only about 2% of adult fractures. They generally occur during high-energy trauma and can be intra- or extraarticular. These difficult-to-treat fractures include supracondylar and intercondylar fracture types.

Supracondylar Fractures

Supracondylar fractures are by definition extraarticular and involve the region of bone just above the humeral condyles. Supracondylar fractures occur primarily as the result of an extension injury. In this form of injury, the humeral condyles are displaced posterior to the humeral shaft. The mechanism is often a fall onto an outstretched hand with the elbow extended. Less common are flexion-type fractures of the supracondylar region. In flexion-type fractures, the condyles are displaced anterior to the humeral shaft. Flexion-type injuries are caused by a force directed against the posterior aspect of the elbow while it is held in a flexed position. Supracondylar fractures are more common in skeletally immature individuals. In adults, the more common fracture pattern involves the intercondylar region of the humerus.

Physical examination of the patient usually reveals extensive swelling around the elbow joint. Open fractures occur not infrequently, and the wound is usually caused by the humeral shaft penetrating the skin anteriorly. Careful examination of the neurovascular status of the extremity should be undertaken. Injury to the brachial artery can occur as well as injury to the radial, ulnar, and/or the median nerves. The radial nerve is the most frequently injured nerve in supracondylar fractures. Imaging including anteroposterior and lateral X-rays of the elbow should be obtained. If there is a diminished or absent pulse, some authors recommend immediate angiography.[59]

Treatment of supracondylar fractures is dependent upon the degree of displacement and factors including the neurovascular status of the patient, the degree of swelling, and whether it is open or closed. If the fracture is nondisplaced or minimally displaced, it can be treated with splinting or casting for approximately 2 weeks. After 2 weeks, range-of-motion exercise is started at the elbow. The elbow is particularly prone to stiffness during extended periods of immobilization.

If the fracture is unstable or displaced, then it is best treated through open reduction and internal fixation. The fracture should be reduced as anatomically as possible. Stable fixation allows for early range of motion and helps prevent future elbow stiffness. Because supracondylar fractures are extraarticular, any remaining incongruity of the fracture fragments is better tolerated than in the case of intraarticular intercondylar fractures.

Intercondylar Fractures

If a humerus fracture extends into the humeral condyles, it is classified as an intercondylar fracture. The fracture usually separates the medial and lateral condyles into separate fragments. The fracture patterns observed are thought to be caused by the impact of the ulna in the trochlear groove. This impact acts as a wedge to split apart the condyles. These fractures can occur with the elbow in flexion or in extension.

Patients present with severe pain and swelling around the elbow joint. Landmarks including the medial and lateral epicondyles, and the olecranon are often distorted secondary to their displacement. Anteroposterior and lateral X-rays of the affected elbow should be obtained. It is also important to obtain radiographs that include the entire humerus, as the fracture can extend to the supracondylar region and the shaft. Often comminution is present on the films, and it may be difficult to ascertain the full extent of the fracture. Given the importance of restoring articular congruity, some surgeons recommend CT scans to further define the fracture pattern.[60] Assessment of neurovascular status is crucial, and angiography should be performed if there are absent or severely diminished distal pulses.[59]

Intercondylar fractures are most commonly classified by Riseborough and Radin.[54] There are four fracture patterns based upon radiographic appearance:

Type I: Nondisplaced fracture between the capitellum and trochlea
Type II: Separation of the capitellum and the trochlea without appreciable rotation of the fragments in the frontal plane
Type III: Separation of the fragments with rotational deformity
Type IV: Severe comminution of the articular surface with wide separation of the humeral condyles

Treatment of intercondylar fractures is currently primarily operative given the need to restore articular congruity to the joint surface. Cast immobilization has been described in the past but there have been no recent studies of its efficacy. Traction can be utilized for intercondylar fractures if necessary. Placement of an olecranon pin allows the arm to be suspended and help correct some of the shortening that occurs with these fractures. Treatment with traction alone can lead to less than optimal results. Utilizing traction does not allow for correction of any rotational deformity that may be present.

Restoration of the articular congruity should be the major goal of any surgery. Stiffness of the elbow joint occurs quickly and any operative intervention should be rigid enough to allow the patient early range of motion. The distal humerus should be considered to have a medial and a lateral column. Stable fixation should seek to restore the integrity of both these columns. Fixation using dual plates in perpendicular planes is termed 90–90 plating and is recommended. Generally one plate is placed medially along the medial condyle and a second plate is placed posterolaterally along the distal humerus. This construct orients the plates at approximately 90° to each other and has been found to be the most biomechanically stable during testing.[56]

Elbow and Forearm Fractures

Radial Head Fractures

The radial head is the proximal portion of the radius that articulates with the capitellum of the distal humerus. This humeroradial joint allows two planes of movement; it allows for supination/pronation as well as flexion and extension through the neighboring humeroulnar joint. The radial head is an important valgus stabilizer of the elbow. Significant fractures or loss/excision of the radial head can result in elbow instability. The most common mechanism of injury in radial head fractures is a fall onto an outstretched hand that is held in a pronated position. Radial head fractures can also be seen with elbow dislocations.

Physical examination reveals tenderness on the lateral aspect of the proximal forearm. There may or may not be mild swelling present at the elbow. The patient commonly has pain with flexion/extension of the elbow joint as well as in supination/pronation. Examination of the forearm and wrist should also be undertaken when a radial head fracture is suspected. Radial head fractures can be associated with injury to the distal radioulnar joint and disruption of the interosseous membrane. This associated injury is known by the eponym Essex–Lopresti lesion.

Anteroposterior and lateral X-rays of the elbow should be taken. If there is any question of forearm or wrist pathology, then additional anteroposterior and lateral X-rays of the forearm and wrist should be obtained. In cases where open reduction and fixation of the radial head may be considered, some authors have recommended CT scans to provide better information regarding fracture displacement and angulation.[61]

Radial head fractures are most commonly classified according to the system proposed by Mason in 1954.[62] Several authors have made modifications to this system but retain the three types of fractures. The severity of the fractures increases from type I to type III.

Type I: nondisplaced or minimally displaced fractures
Type II: marginal fractures of the radial head that are displaced
Type III: comminuted fracture of the radial head

A type I fracture can be treated nonoperatively with a short period of splinting or a sling. Once the patient's pain and swelling subside, early range of motion should be started. Aspiration of the associated effusion and injection of a local anesthetic can be performed to help with pain after the initial injury. Regular follow-up radiographs should be obtained to ensure that the fracture does not displace.

A type II fracture typically involves displaced fractures to margin of the radial head. Most commonly these fractures occur on the anterolateral aspect of the radial head. The displaced fragment can lead to a mechanical blockage of motion at the elbow. If this occurs, surgical intervention is usually necessary.[63] The bias has changed from early excision of these fractures to open reduction and fixation. Attempts should be made to restore the radial head as anatomically as possible. Fixation of this fracture is typically performed through an anterolateral elbow incision. Fixation should be stable enough to allow for early range of motion at the elbow. Reduction and fixation of the fracture is commonly accomplished with plates, screws, or k-wires.

In cases of comminuted radial head fractures (Mason type III), it is critical to assess for the presence of an Essex–Lopresti lesion. In type III fractures, the radial head fracture is comminuted. If possible, reconstruction of the radial head should be performed.[61] When it cannot be reconstructed, excision may be required. If excision is required, it is critical to assess for the presence of an Essex–Lopresti lesion. This injury involves the rupture of the interosseous membrane and the triangular fibrocartilage complex at the wrist. Patients may demonstrate wrist and forearm pain in addition to pain at the elbow. Forearm and wrist radiographs may or may not reveal any abnormality. There may be some subtle widening of the distal radioulnar joint when compared to radiographs of the contralateral side.

An Essex–Lopresti lesion leads to proximal migration of the radius if radial head excision is performed. The interosseous membrane serves to provide stability between the radius and ulna. The loss of the interosseous membrane allows the radius to migrate proximally independent of the ulna, leading to disruption of the proper anatomic relationship at the distal radioulnar joint. In these cases, a radial head spacer is necessary to maintain proper radial length. Currently, metal implants have shown the best results, and silicone implants have fallen into disfavor.[64]

Olecranon Fractures

The olecranon is the most proximal portion of the ulna that articulates with the trochlea of the distal humerus. Fractures to the olecranon usually occur through direct trauma and generally result in transverse or oblique fracture patterns. Separation of the fracture fragments is caused by the pull of the triceps insertion on the proximal fragment.

Patients usually complain of pain directly over the olecranon. Pain is elicited with range of motion. Anteroposterior and lateral views of the elbow should be ordered. The fracture will be most visible on the lateral view, and assessment should be made of its displacement. It is important to assess the articular congruency at the site of the fracture.

Most olecranon fractures, unless they are nondisplaced, benefit from operative reduction and fixation. Only nondisplaced fractures should be treated with a short period of immobilization and then started on a range-of-motion protocol. These fractures should be watched carefully to ensure that range of motion does not cause any displacement secondary to the muscle pull of the triceps.

If there is any articular stepoff noted at the fracture site, open reduction and internal fixation should be done to restore articular congruency. A persistent articular stepoff can predispose the patient to posttraumatic arthritis. Fixation of olecranon fractures can be done with tension-band wire constructs as well as with plating.[65] Prominence of the hardware remains an issue because hardware impingement can occur when patients rest their elbows on hard surfaces. In cases of severely comminuted or segmental fractures with bone loss, excision of the fragment may be undertaken. As much as 60% of the olecranon can be excised without destabilizing the elbow.[66] Care must be taken to reattach the triceps insertion to the remaining distal ulna after resection.

Anatomy of the Forearm

The bones of the forearm are composed of the ulna and the radius. They are joined together by the interosseous membrane and articulate with each other at the distal radioulnar joint and also proximally at the elbow. At this level, their articulation is stabilized by the elbow joint capsule and the annular ligament. At the wrist, the radioulnar joint is supported by the triangular fibrocartilage and the wrist capsule. The volar side of the forearm contains the wrist flexor musculature and the dorsal side contains the extensor muscles.

Isolated Ulnar Shaft Fracture

Isolated ulnar shaft fractures are also known by the eponym nightstick fracture. The most common mechanism of injury is a direct blow. Often the affected arm was raised in an attempt to deflect a blow. These fractures are often minimally or nondisplaced and can be treated conservatively. Functional bracing and cast immobilization are two frequent methods of treatment.[67] Nonunion of these fractures is rare.

Operative indications include open fractures, fractures with neurovascular deficits, and fractures that are significantly angulated or displaced. Angulation greater than 10° or displacement greater than 50% of the diaphysis should be treated with operative intervention.[67] Plate fixation is the preferred method of fixation for most authors.

Monteggia Fractures

A Monteggia fracture is defined as a fracture of the proximal ulna that results in dislocation of the proximal radioulnar joint. This type of fracture was first described by Giovanni Battista Monteggia in 1814. Later, Bado further defined four types of Monteggia fractures.[68] The mechanism of injury varies in each of the four different types of injuries.

The patient with a Monteggia fracture commonly complains of severe pain around the elbow. Severe swelling and deformity over the elbow and forearm often accompany these injuries. Radiographs of both the elbow and forearm should be obtained to fully define the extent of the injury. Evaluation of the neurovascular status of the patient is important, as these fractures can be associated with neurological deficits. Most commonly, the radial nerve (posterior interosseous branch) is injured.[69] The posterior interosseous nerve lies in close contact with the radial neck and is a purely motor nerve. Injury to the posterior interosseous nerve causes a weakness in wrist extension as it innervates the extensor musculature.

Treatment of this injury in adults requires open reduction and internal fixation of the ulna as well as reduction of the radial head. The key to successful treatment lies in a stable and anatomic reduction of the ulna. Without first stabilizing the ulna, it is nearly impossible to obtain a congruent reduction of the radial head. Direct repair of the ligamentous structures stabilizing the radiocapitellar joint is rarely necessary once congruent reduction has been obtained.

Isolated Radial Shaft Fracture

A radial shaft fracture in the proximal two-thirds is rare. If a radius fracture occurs in the distal third, it is usually associated with a disruption of the distal radioulnar joint and is known by the eponym Galleazi fracture. (Galleazi fractures are described separately.) Evaluation of radial shaft fractures is identical to other forearm fractures. Two views (anteroposterior and lateral) should be obtained of the entire forearm. Serial neurovascular checks and assessment of the forearm compartments are needed.

If the fracture is nondisplaced, it can be treated with cast immobilization. The patient should be casted in some degree of supination to offset the pull of the biceps and supinator muscles. If the fracture involves the proximal portion of the radius before the insertion of pronator teres, the distal fragment will be pronated. In this case, the patient should be placed in full supination to help neutralize the pull of the pronator teres and prevent displacement. If the fracture occurs distal to the insertion of pronator teres, then mild supination should be used to bring the distal fragment into contact with the proximal one.

In the case of displaced fractures, open reduction and internal fixation are recommended. The standard approach to the radius is volar. Care should be taken to maintain the radial bow because this can affect forearm rotation if it is not reproduced.

Galleazzi Fracture

"Galleazzi fracture" is an eponym that refers to a fracture of the distal third of the radius with disruption of the distal radioulnar joint. The mechanism of this fracture is thought to be a fall on an outstretched hand held in pronation. Another mechanism is a direct blow to the distal radius.

Patients often demonstrate deformity related to the radius fracture. There also will be pain related to the disruption of the distal radioulnar joint. The disruption of the distal radioulnar joint is not always immediately evident. The gradual widening of the joint can occur later during the healing phase. The entire forearm should be imaged in two planes to evaluate the fracture and the distal radioulnar joint.

Closed reduction of this fracture has shown poor results. The fracture tends to displace with time even with cast immobilization; this is secondary to the deforming forces on the fracture fragments. If anatomic alignment is not maintained, the disruption of the distal radioulnar joint will progress, leading to posttraumatic degenerative changes at the level of the wrist.

The fracture should be reduced in open fashion and stabilized. The most common method of fixing the radius involves using a plate.[70] In addition to fixation of the radius, the distal radioulnar joint must be congruently reduced. In most cases this joint will reduce after anatomic fixation of the radius fracture. Positioning of the forearm in supination may be necessary to allow for a stable reduction. If this position does not allow for stable reduction, then the joint should be pinned to secure it. This pin is generally removed after 3 weeks. Radiographs must be taken to follow all Galleazi fractures very closely; this is to ensure that there is no further loss of reduction despite fixation.

Both-Bones Forearm Fractures

A both-bones forearm fracture refers to a simultaneous radius and ulna fracture. The most common mechanism of injury is direct violence such as a motor vehicle accident or a direct blow. The majority of these fractures are displaced, and this is obvious on examination. Anteroposterior and lateral radiographs of the forearm should be obtained. The classification of these fractures is based upon location (proximal, middle, distal third) and fracture pattern. Note should be made as to whether the fracture is comminuted or segmental and whether it is open or closed. The neurovascular status of the patient should be established and recorded. The amount of forearm swelling should also be evaluated. It is critical to assess whether the patient is developing a compartment syndrome, which can happen given the discrete nature of the forearm compartments. If the forearm is tense and the patient demonstrates pain with passive motion, compartment pressures should be measured.

Treatment of these fractures usually requires open reduction and internal fixation if there is any displacement of the fracture fragments. Only nondisplaced fractures or those patients who are unable to undergo surgery should be treated with cast immobilization. For each degree of angulation of the fracture fragments, the patient typically loses 1° of rotation. Thus, an attempt should be made to reduce the fragments as anatomically as possible. Common methods of fixation include compression plating of the radius and ulna, typically through a two-incision approach.[71] Intramedullary fixation can also be used to stabilize these fractures.

Distal Radius Fractures

Anatomy of the Wrist

The distal radius is the main foundation to support the carpus. It has three separate articulations, including the scaphoid and lunate fossas, which articulate with the carpus, and the sigmoid notch that articulates with the distal ulna. The distal radius has a specific alignment that is important to note when treating fractures. The articular surface of the radius is aligned at 14° of volar tilt and 22° of ulnar inclination. The bones of the wrist are supported by the triangular fibrocartilage, the wrist capsule, and the dorsal and palmar ligaments.

Distal Radius Fractures

Distal radius fractures are very common. The most frequent mechanism of injury is a fall onto an outstretched hand. The patient generally presents with pain and swelling over the distal radius. Deformity may be present if the fracture fragment is displaced. Examination should include the condition of the skin and neurovascular status. Assessment of the elbow and more proximal forearm are important, as pathology may be masked by the more painful wrist fracture.

There are many eponyms for the various types of distal radius fractures. Furthermore, there exist a multitude of classification schemes for distal radius fractures. Several eponyms are used to describe the most common types of fractures. The most frequent type fracture is the Colles' fracture, a fracture of the distal radius metaphysis. The distal fracture fragment is dorsally angulated and displays what is known as a "dinner-fork deformity." This type of fracture occurs when a patient attempts to catch themselves with their hand and wrist outstretched. The counterpart to the Colles' fracture is the Smith fracture, which is a volarly angulated fracture. A common system used to classify the range of distal radius fractures is the Frykman classification.[72]

Treatment depends heavily on whether the fracture is intraarticular or extraarticular. The age, handedness, occupation, and activity level of the patient should be taken into account. Intraarticular fractures run the risk of posttraumatic arthritis if they are not satisfactorily reduced. Some authors have found that even 2 mm of stepoff will predispose the patient to the development of arthritis.[73]

If the fracture is nondisplaced then the patient can be immobilized in a cast, typically for 4 to 6 weeks. After removal of the cast, active range of motion should be started to prevent wrist stiffness. The patient should be encouraged to move their fingers and elbow during the healing phase to maintain suppleness at these joints.

If the fracture is displaced, closed reduction should be attempted and then assessed again radiographically. The patient should be anesthetized with local anesthetic in the form of a hematoma block. Additional sedation may be required, as the hematoma block is often insufficient to block all the patient's pain. Fingertraps may be used to help align the fracture site through traction and ligamentotaxis. The reduction maneuver involves initially recreating the deformity and then providing traction and a counterforce to relocate the fracture. For a Colles' fracture, the distal fragment should be hyperextended first to unlock the fragment. Next, traction and pressure dorsally on the distal fragment should be applied. Ulnar deviation is often necessary to help return radial length. A well-molded cast should be applied. A three-point mold helps to hold the fracture in place.

In cases of intraarticular fractures, there are several methods of closed versus open reduction. Percutaneous pinning of fractures allows fixation after reduction of the fracture fragments; this may be combined with external fixator placement. An external fixator bridges the wrist joint and is secured percutaneously to the radius and usually the second metacarpal; this helps to maintain traction on the fracture while it is healing and allows ligamentotaxis to align the fracture fragments. Using this method, it is usually not necessary to directly violate the fracture site.

In cases where percutaneous fixation methods are insufficient to hold the fracture fragments, open reduction and plate fixation can be used; this is particularly useful in cases such as volar rim fractures where closed reduction is usually unsuccessful in providing satisfactory reduction of the fragments.

Hip Fractures

Roughly 300,000 hip fractures occur each year in the United States. It is by far the most common fracture-related cause for admission to a hospital. Ninety percent of these fractures occur in those over 60 years of age. Hip fractures in the elderly are distinctly different from those in younger individuals. In people under 60, fractures about the hip are usually caused by a higher mechanism of injury (i.e., motor vehicle versus pedestrian accident, fall from a height, etc.). There are henceforth often other associated injuries. In the elderly, hip fractures occur secondary to a low-energy injury, most commonly from a simple fall, and associated injuries are rare. Also of importance is that in the elderly population that sustains a hip fracture there are usually concomitant medical illnesses, with the most common being hypertension, coronary artery disease, chronic obstructive pulmonary disease (COPD), cardiac arrhythmia, diabetes mellitus, and cancer.[74] The mortality rate in this population within the first year following fracture ranges from 13% to 30%.[75]

Many classification systems have emerged to help categorize hip fractures from both an anatomic and a treatment-related perspective. The anatomic location, degree of displacement, and characterization of the major fracture fragments are the three most important factors in describing a hip fracture and deciding on optimal treatment. The three general types of proximal femur fractures are (1) femoral neck fractures, (2) intertrochanteric fractures, and (3) subtrochanteric fractures. Most authors concur that, in the elderly, 95% of hip fractures are either femoral neck or intertrochanteric fractures, with a roughly equal distribution of each.[74] Subtrochanteric fractures are more common in a younger age group and usually represent a higher-energy type of fracture.

Femoral neck fractures occur from the base of the femoral neck to the subcapital region, just distal to the femoral head. These fractures are therefore subdivided into subcapital fractures, transcervical fractures, and basilar neck fractures. Subcapital and transcervical fractures are treated by either screw fixation of the fracture or replacement hemiarthroplasty. In younger patients it is uniformly agreed that every effort should be made to save the hip and perform an anatomic reduction (either opened or closed) with screw fixation of these fractures; this is the case because prosthetic replacement has a limited lifespan and invariably fails with time because of loosening or osteolysis of the bone. In the elderly population, this is a different story.

The debate over whether to repair versus primarily replace (hemiarthroplasty) a subcapital or transcervical hip fracture in the elderly has now continued for several decades.[76–79] In general, most orthopedic surgeons would agree that for non-displaced or impacted type fractures the treatment of choice is generally screw fixation, best accomplished with cannulated screws placed over a guidewire. Ideally, three such screws are placed in a parallel fashion with proximal purchase in the subchondral bone of the femoral head (Figure 107.3). Optimally, these screws should provide enough fixation that the patient can begin weight-bearing early in the postoperative period because the elderly are not able to partially weight-bear on a limb. Hemiarthroplasty is the treatment of choice for the displaced fractures, because the displaced fractures have a much higher incidence of avascular necrosis of the femoral head as a consequence of disruption of the blood supply. Garden[80] has described a useful classification system commonly referred to for femoral neck fractures. He was able to equate the degree of displacement with the risk of developing avascular necrosis. Replacement hemiarthroplasty offers the patient to immediately return to a full weight-bearing status. In general, the longevity of the implant will far outlast the lifespan of the patient in this age group (see Fig. 107.3).

Basilar neck fractures, by definition, are extracapsular. They are best treated with open reduction and internal fixation with the same type of implants used for intertrochanteric fractures. In certain instances in the very elderly population, an argument can be made to proceed with a hemiarthroplasty instead of repair, as this does generally allow for more immediate unprotected weight-bearing by the patient.

Intertrochanteric fractures are located from an area just distal to the base of the neck to the inferior border of the lesser trochanter. The primary fracture line invariably traverses through a zone between the greater and lesser trochanter. The categorization scheme used most commonly involves

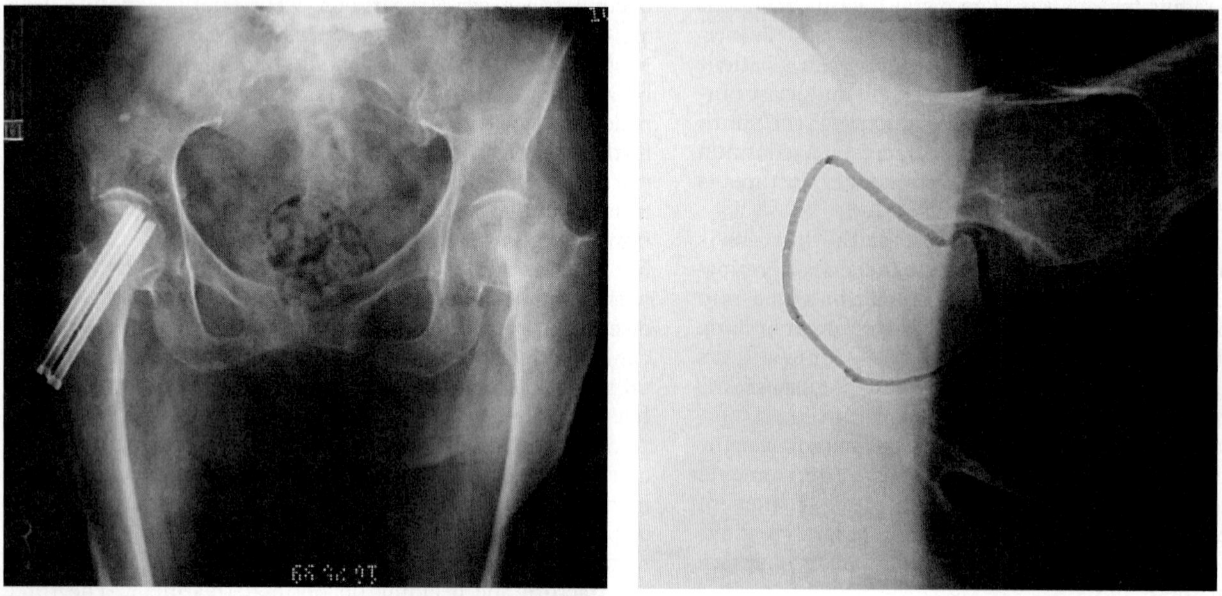

A B

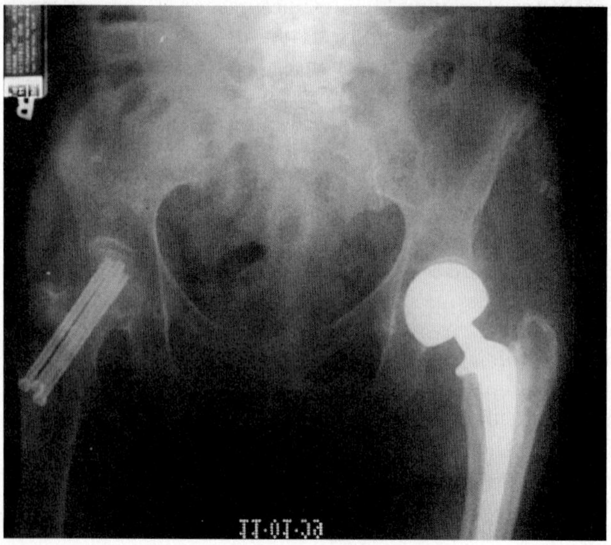

C

FIGURE 107.3. Radiographs of a 95-year-old woman who suffered an impacted and nondisplaced right subcapital femur fracture 5 years in the past that was successfully treated with screw fixation; this allowed for healing of the fracture, and the patient returned to her preambulatory status. The patient then fell again and presented at this time with a displaced left subcapital femur fracture. **A.** Anterior-to-posterior radiograph showing new displaced left subcapital femur fracture with old, healed right hip fracture. **B.** Lateral radiograph of the left hip showing the posterior displacement of the head of the femur (femoral head fragment *outlined in black*). **C.** Anterior-to-posterior radiograph of the pelvis showing cemented hemiarthroplasty of the left hip.

determining how many major fracture fragments exist. Two-part fractures are those in which an isolated fracture line exists at the intertrochanteric line, thereby separating the proximal femur from the shaft; these are inherently more stable fractures. Three-part fractures again have the primary fracture line through the intertrochanteric zone; however, the lesser trochanter is now broken off and represents the third major fragment. Four-part fractures are three-part fractures with a displaced and separate fracture of the greater trochanter as well. Four-part fractures are far more unstable and represent a greater challenge for fixation.

Intertrochanteric fractures are generally treated with open reduction and internal fixation utilizing a hip screw and side plate. The barrel of the side plate allows for telescoping of the hip screw so as to prevent distraction of the fracture site and to promote compression, to allow for a more rapid union. This method revolutionized the fixation of these fractures, as fixation devices previously did not allow for telescoping and compression of the proximal segment on the distal segment. Without this ability for axial compression of the fragments, the incidence of nonunion and hardware failure was previously unacceptably high, but with this simple modification excellent results have been achieved.[81,82]

Another fixation device gaining greater popularity is the intramedullary hip screw. This device achieves fixation of the proximal segment (femoral head and neck) with the same type of screw used in the screw and side plate device. The screw can telescope within a barrel portal of an intramedullary rod. This device is particularly well suited for treatment of the more unstable three- and four-part fractures. It is more load sharing, and the rod also acts as an internal buttress to limit the amount of medial displacement of the distal fragment, as this leads to further overall shortening of the limb. Excellent results have been achieved with this device; however, it has been found to have a higher learning curve for proper utilization as compared to the hip screw and side plate.[83]

Subtrochanteric fractures extend from a region just distal to the lesser trochanter and involve the proximal several inches of the femoral shaft. They are often a higher-energy injury than standard hip fractures. In general, they are best treated with the new generation ("second-generation") intramedullary nails. These rods allow for screw fixation into the femoral head and neck as well as fixation distally along the entire shaft of the femur (Fig. 107.4). Hip screw and long side plate devices have also been used with success in the past. However, this requires a much greater surgical dissection with resultant blood loss.

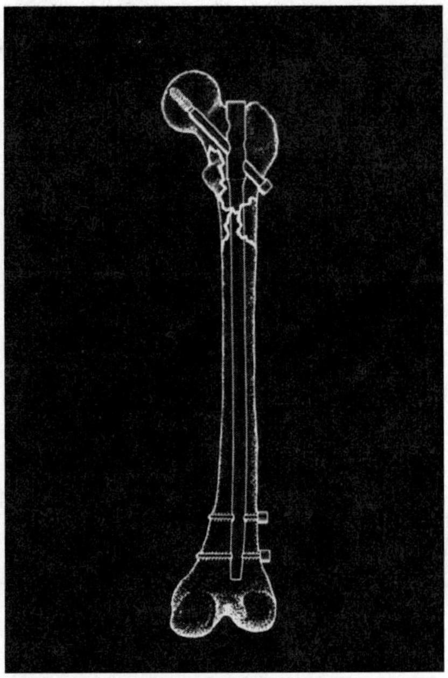

FIGURE 107.4. Schematic diagram of a "second-generation" design femoral rod. The proximal interlocking screw allows for fixation of femoral fractures as far proximal as the subcapital region (if augmented by at least a second screw). Stabilization distally is the same as for any other femoral rod (to the distal femoral metaphysis). This rod design allows for stabilization of segmental or combined fracture patterns to span nearly the entire femur.

Femoral Shaft Fractures

Femoral shaft fractures are usually the result of a high-energy type of injury. They are commonly seen in motor vehicle-related accidents, and associated injuries are common. In a large series of such fractures treated at a major Level I trauma center,[84] 78% of the fractures involved a motor vehicle or motorcycle. In this series of 520 consecutive femoral shaft fractures, there was a 29% incidence of associated head, chest, or abdominal injuries, and many had multiple fractures.

Blood loss from a femoral shaft fracture can be significant, with 3 to 4 units of blood loss occurring into the thigh even with a closed fracture. Immediate placement of the affected limb into skeletal traction is of great value to the patient because the traction restores a cylindrical shape to the thigh. This restoration is important as it helps decrease blood loss, because for a mass with the same surface area, the volume of a cylinder is less than the volume of a sphere.

Following appropriate resuscitation and treatment of life-threatening associated injuries, the femoral fracture should be stabilized as soon as possible to allow for mobilization of the patient. Early mobilization is quite important as it helps reduce the incidence of pulmonary complications, including adult respiratory distress syndrome (ARDS).

The current standard of care for the treatment of these injuries is placement of a locked intramedullary nail, allowing for restitution of limb length, control of rotation, prevention of shortening of the fracture, mobilization of the patient, and early weight-bearing. This technique, when performed properly, leads to a very high rate of union with low associated morbidity and complications[85–87] (Fig. 107.5). It can also be safely performed in most open fractures.[88,89] In treating closed fractures, the technique involves the use of a fracture table to apply traction with accompanying closed manipulation of the fracture so that a guidewire can be placed proximally to distally across the fracture fragments from an entrance point at the piriformis fossa. Under certain circumstances, retrograde statically locked intramedullary nails have also been used. The entrance site is through the knee joint at the intercondylar notch of the femur.

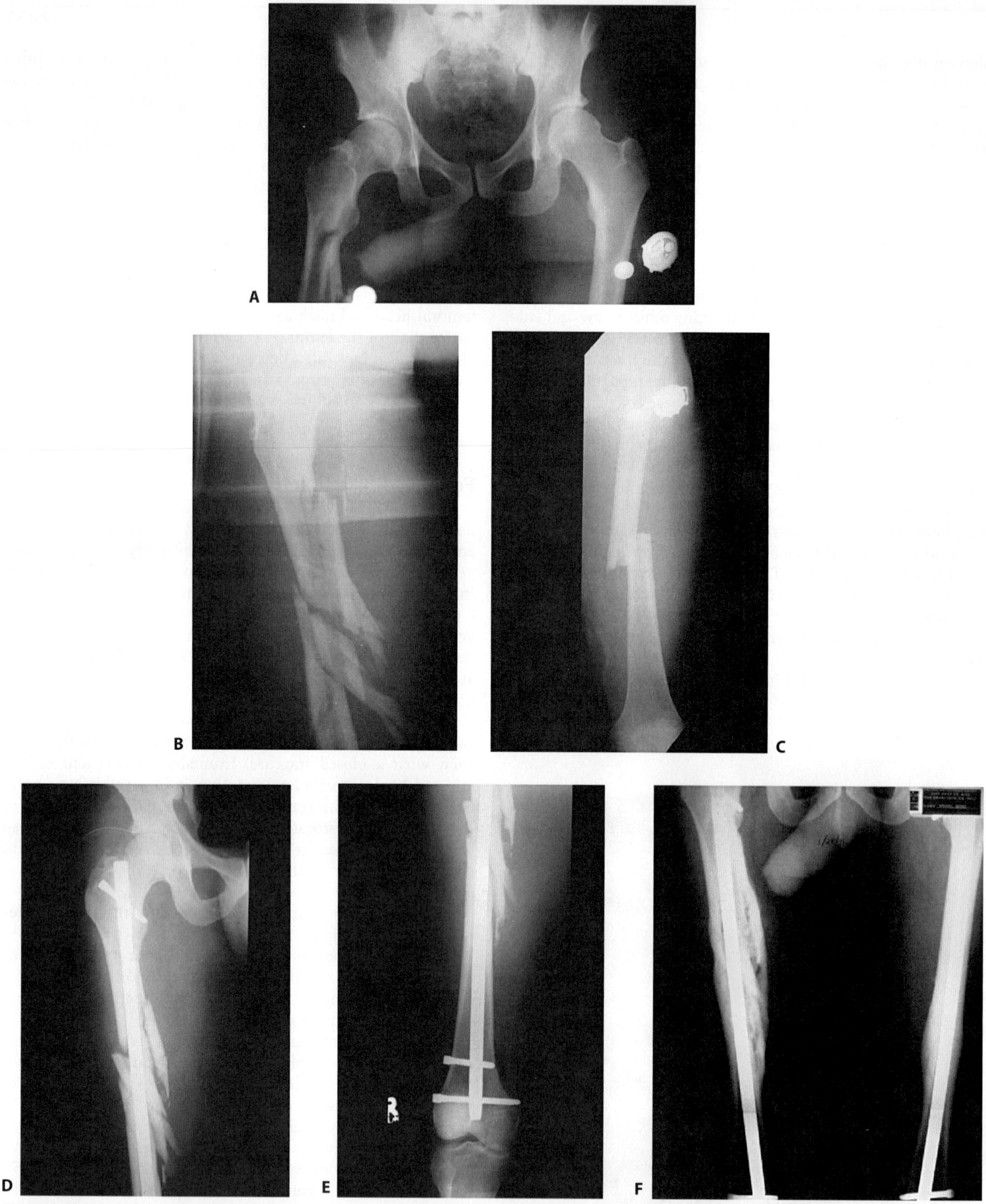

FIGURE 107.5. Radiographs of a 30-year-old man involved in a high-speed motor vehicle accident in which the engine block of his car was driven off its mountings and landed on the driver"s lap, with resultant bilateral femur fractures. **A.** Anterior-to-posterior radiograph of the pelvis showing comminuted segmental left femur fracture extending proximally to a level just below the lesser trochanter. **B.** Lateral radiograph of the comminuted right femoral shaft fracture. **C.** Anterior-to-posterior radiograph of the left femur showing the midshaft fracture. The patient was taken to the operating room where he underwent bilateral closed femoral interlocked roddings. He had an uneventful postoperative course and required no blood transfusion. He was rapidly mobilized with weight-bearing. **D, E.** Anterior-to-posterior radiographs of the right femur showing successful stabilization of the right femur with restoration of alignment. **F.** Anterior-to-posterior radiograph of both femora taken 13 months postoperatively. The femora are healed with the patient having equal limb lengths. He returned to work as an automobile mechanic.

Tibia Fractures

Tibial shaft fractures represent the most common site of long bone fracture in the body. They have posed a great challenge in treatment over the years because there is a relatively high incidence of nonunion with these fractures; this is partly because there is a poor soft tissue envelope surrounding the tibia, as the entire anteromedial cortex is covered only by subcutaneous fat and skin. With the increase in higher-velocity injuries associated with the use of motorcycles, there is also a higher incidence of open fractures of the tibia than of other bones.

Treatment modalities for this fracture depend on fracture pattern, location of the fracture, opened or closed fracture, degree of soft tissue injury, functionality and age of the patient, and whether the fracture is the result of a high- or low-energy injury. The classic treatment method for closed tibial fractures has been closed reduction with long leg cast immobilization. Overall good results have been achieved with this treatment method.[90,91] Sarmiento et al. popularized the use of prefabricated cast bracing of these fractures[92] and reported good results with this treatment method, although others have not had as great a result.

However, with the advent of improved intramedullary nailing techniques, many surgeons prefer intramedullary stabilization of displaced shaft fractures as this allows for more rapid mobilization of the knee and ankle with resultant decreased morbidity from cast immobilization to these joints. Bone et al.[93] performed an age-matched retrospective study of patients with an isolated closed and displaced tibial diaphyseal fracture treated with either cast immobilization or closed intramedullary nailing of the fractures. The time to bony union was shorter in those patients managed with a nail as compared to those managed with a cast. There was also a 10% incidence of nonunion in those managed with a cast as compared to 2% in those treated with an intramedullary nail. Also of importance was that 4 years after the fracture, those patients treated with intramedullary nailing had statistically significant better knee and ankle function than those patients treated with cast immobilization. These authors concluded that intramedullary nailing of displaced closed tibial diaphyseal fractures provided a better long-term result than conventional cast immobilization. In fact, intramedullary nailing has now become the "gold standard" for treatment of displaced tibial shaft fractures in the United States.

Open fractures present a bit of a different problem. They are fraught with a higher incidence of infection and nonunion. Recent studies have documented good results for the treatment of grade 1, 2, and 3A open tibial shaft fractures with placement of the newer unreamed smaller-diameter tibial nails.[94,95] The infection rate in these studies was comparable to other treatment methods (Fig. 107.6). The classic treatment method for these injuries is placement of the tibia in external fixation. With the advent of the newer circular external fixators, excellent results have also now been achieved with this treatment method.

Regardless of the type of hardware used in the treatment of open tibial fractures, it is imperative to adhere to certain basic principles. It is imperative that all nonviable and necrotic soft tissue and bone be debrided. It is also necessary to obtain early delayed primary closure or closure following subsequent debridements with a muscle flap. These principles help reduce the incidence of deep infection and chronic osteomyelitis.

Treatment of tibial plateau (proximal tibial epiphysis and metaphysis) and tibial plafond (distal tibial epiphysis and metaphysis) fractures is usually with plate and screw fixation. An exception to this is in high-energy fractures with significant soft tissue injury or severely comminuted fractures. In these instances better results are being reported with external fixation using fine wire external fixators at the plafond or plateau segments.[96–98] This approach allows for less soft tissue stripping and has a significantly lower instance of deep wound infection in these two subsets of fractures. The fine wire external fixators have a high learning curve and can be plagued with complications if careful attention to detail is not followed.

Ankle Fractures

Fractures of the ankle represent the most common fracture around a joint in the lower extremity, just as wrist fractures represent the most common fracture around a joint in the upper extremity. Although initially one would think that the ankle moves in several different planes, in fact it only moves in one plane. The ankle joint has the ability to plantar and dorsiflex the foot in the sagittal plane. The motions of inversion and eversion occur through the subtalar joint. These two joints function in unison to allow for the complex arc of motion of the foot on the leg.

The ankle mortise functions as a "roof" (in French, *plafond*) over the talus. The lateral and medial malleoli support the ankle to allow for the constained plantar and dorsiflexion of the joint. This geometry, combined with the supporting ligamentous structures, resists rotation of the talus within the ankle mortise.

Ankle fractures are generally described according to the malleoli involved. Therefore, one can have an isolated lateral malleolar, or medial malleolar fracture, a bimalleolar fracture (both the lateral and medial malleolus), a trimalleolar fracture (the lateral and medial malleoli along with the posterior lip of the tibial plafond, which is referred to as the posterior malleolus), Dupuytren's fracture (fracture of the lateral malleolus with complete rupture of the deltoid ligament), and Maisonneuve's fracture (medial malleolar fracture with rupture of the syndesmotic ligament and proximal fibular fracture).

Numerous classification systems have been developed to describe ankle fractures. The most commonly utilized classification system was described by Lauge-Hansen in 1950 and is based on the mechanism of injury (Table 107.4).[99] It is able to accurately describe 95% of those ankle fractures seen. He stressed freshly amputated limbs to failure in combinations of supination, pronation, adduction, abduction, and eversion. These movements refer to the position of the patient's foot at the instance of injury. By doing this he was able to describe four major mechanisms of injury corroborated with real-life situations: (1) supination adduction, (2) supination eversion, (3) pronation abduction, and (4) pronation eversion. He then added a pronation dorsiflexion mechanism of injury so as to include certain tibial plafond fractures because this is more a compression-type injury.

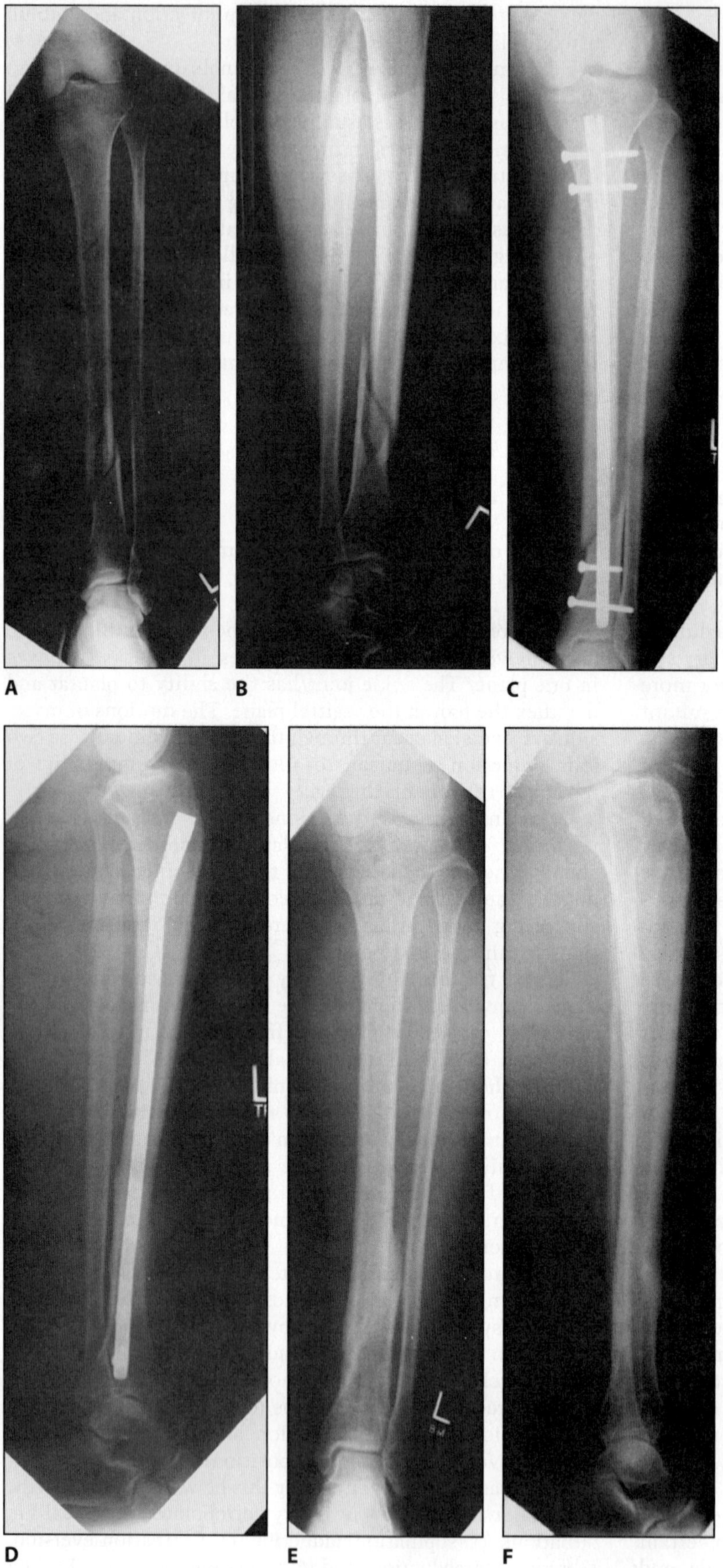

FIGURE 107.6. Radiographs of a 32-year-old woman who suffered a spiral left distal tibial shaft and proximal fibular fracture following a fall while skiing. **A, B.** Anterior-to-posterior and lateral views of the tibia and fibula fractures. The patient was taken to the operating room where she underwent reduction and stabilization with a closed interlocked left tibial rodding. **C, D.** Anterior-to-posterior and lateral radiographs following placement of the interlocked tibial rod. The patient healed uneventfully and returned to full activities. **E, F.** Anterior-to-posterior and lateral radiographs taken following rod removal 18 months after sustaining the fracture.

TABLE 107.4. Lauge-Hansen Classification System for Ankle Fractures.

Foot position and direction of force	*Stage*	*Description of injury*
Pronation and abduction	I	Tear of deltoid ligament or fracture of medial malleolus
	II	Stage I plus fracture of posterior lip of tibia and rupture of anterior and posterior syndesmosis ligaments
	III	Stage II plus oblique fracture of fibula above ankle mortise
Pronation and eversion	I	Tear of deltoid ligament or fracture of medial malleolus
	II	Stage I plus tear of interosseous ligament and anterior inferior tibiofibular
	III	Stage II plus spiral fracture of fibula, 5–6 cm above tibial plafond, and tear of interosseous membrane
	IV	Stage III plus avulsion fracture of posterior tibial lip
Supination and abduction	I	Tear of lateral collateral ligaments or transverse fracture of lateral malleolus
	II	Stage I plus fracture of medial malleolus
Supination and eversion	I	Rupture or avulsion fracture of anterior inferior tibiofibular ligament
	II	Stage I plus oblique or spiral fracture of lateral malleolus
	III	Stage II plus fracture of posterior tibial lip
	IV	Stage III plus tear of deltoid ligament or fracture of medial malleolus

Source: Adapted from Lauge-Hansen N. Fractures of the ankle. II. Combined experimental-surgical and experimental-roentgenologic investigations. Arch Surg 1950;60:957.[99]

Chapman[100] outlined the four criteria that must be met to optimize treatment of ankle fractures. These are (1) fractures and dislocations should be close reduced as soon as possible, (2) the joint surfaces must be precisely and anatomically restored, (3) the fracture fragments must be held and maintained in a reduced position during fracture healing, and (4) early joint motion should be initiated.

As mentioned, at the time of presentation the ankle fracture or fracture-dislocation should initially be close reduced and splinted. The isolated nondisplaced lateral malleolar fracture (supination eversion stage 2) can then be successfully treated with simple cast or splint immobilization. The other fracture patterns are best treated with formal open reduction and internal fixation; this allows one to then achieve the other three criteria as listed. Screw and plate systems have been specially developed for the surgical repair of ankle fractures.

Care must be taken to gently handle the soft tissues about the ankle, as further injury to them can cause devastating wound healing problems. With careful attention to detail an anatomic stable reduction can usually be achieved. It is important to initially keep these patients non-weight-bearing for at least 6 weeks after open reduction and internal fixation of these fractures to allow the bone as well as the articular cartilage to heal.

Nonunions, Malunions, and Osteomyelitis

As a rule, most fractures heal. The evolutionary process builds certain safeguards into the living system for functions essential to its survival. The healing of fractures has evolved in just such a manner. Different external forces, be they chemical, mechanical, or electrical, can work alone or in conjunction with one another to lead to a final common pathway for bony healing. Despite the fact that several pathways exist to stimulate fracture healing, sometimes these inductive forces still fail to achieve healing of the bone.

The treatment of nonunited fractures has developed into a subspecialty of orthopedic surgery. Newer methods of treatment have led to improved clinical results in even those fractures most difficult to heal. Currently, the U.S. Food and Drug Administration defines a nonunion as a fracture that has failed to show progressive evidence of healing during a 4- to 6-month time period. Delayed unions are defined as those fractures that have failed to fully unite after 6 months. These are rather arbitrary definitions, however, as a fracture with a 5-cm bony deficit clearly is a nonunion (or a nonunion waiting to happen) from the instant of the time of injury.

Many variables play a role on why some fractures go on to nonunion. Rosen[101] has previously outlined many of the known factors that can impair fracture healing (Table 107.5). By far the two most common reasons for nonunion are lack of adequate vascular supply at the fracture site and suboptimal stabilization of the fracture. It should also be mentioned that the use of nicotine has been shown to be the one major exogenous factor contributing to impaired fracture healing. As would be expected, certain specific sites have a higher incidence of nonunion. Three of the more common sites in the body are the distal tibial diaphysis, the carpal navicular, and the proximal diaphyseal region of the fifth metatarsal.

Presently, the "gold standard" in nonunion treatment remains rigid fixation with supplemental iliac crest bone grafting. In the hands of the experienced nonunion surgeon, this can lead to a success rate greater than 90% for achieving union in long bones. To date, the bone graft substitutes have

TABLE 107.5. Causes of Nonunion.

1. Excess motion: inadequate immobilization
2. Diastasis of fracture fragments
   a. Soft tissue interposition
   b. Distraction from traction or internal fixation
   c. Malposition
   d. Loss of bone
3. Compromised blood supply
   a. Damage to nutrient vessels
   b. Stripping or injury to periosteum and muscle
   c. Free fragments; severe comminution
   d. Avascularity due to internal fixation devices
4. Infection
   a. Bone death (sequestrum)
   b. Osteolysis (GAP)
   c. Loosening of implants (motion)
5. General: age, nutrition, steroids, anticoagulants, radiation, burns, predisposure to nonunion.
6. Distraction from traction or internal fixation

Source: Adapted from Rosen H. Treatment of nonunions: General principles. In: Chapman MW, ed. Operative Orthopedics, 2nd ed. Philadelphia: Lippincott, 1988.[101]

not yet proved as effective as cancellous bone grafting from the ilium. It has been demonstrated that mesenchymal stem cells from the bone marrow from the iliac crest graft have great osteoinductive properties.

With the explosion in genetic engineering techniques and molecular genetics, it is conceivable that in the future nonunions will successfully be treated with the delivery of the proper combination of osteoinductive hormones directly to the nonunion site. Information to date suggests that this will not be one single agent, such as one of the bone morphogenic proteins (BMPs), but rather several different hormones either delivered at once or sequentially over time.

A technique that has revolutionized the treatment of nonunions is the Ilizarov method. This treatment method relies on the use of a ring external fixator with fixation to bone achieved via fine wires under tension. It was developed by a surgeon in Siberia in 1948 as a technique to treat post-World War II-related injuries.[102] The first cases utilizing this technique in the United States were performed in the mid-1980s. It allows for regeneration of segmental defects of bone as well as limb lengthening with relatively low morbidity and high predictability. Its use in the treatment of nonunions and malunions has markedly improved treatment results, for atrophic or devascularized segments of bone can now be resected, and new healthy bone regenerated in their place.

Results with the Ilizarov method for treatment of nonunions have been quite good.[103,104] The technique not only allows for the healing of nonunions, but also allows for elimination of deformity and restitution of limb length. When incorporated with free tissue transfers,[105] even the worst nonunions, infected nonunions, and limb deformities can be predictably corrected with a success rate greater than 90%, whereas previously many of these limbs would have been amputated.

Malunions, as the name implies, are fractures that heal in a nonanatomic position with resultant deformity or functional limb shortening. As expected, limb length inequality is much better tolerated in the upper extremity than unilaterally in the lower extremity. Most orthopedic surgeons agree that lower limb inequality as great as 2 cm can be successfully corrected with a shoe lift. Inequalities greater than 2 cm in the young healthy individual are probably best treated with limb lengthening. Deformity correction secondary to malunion is less well defined. If the malunion causes significant enough malalignment of the limb, particularly in the lower extremity, then higher than tolerated forces across the knee or ankle occur, resulting in posttraumatic arthritis of these joints. In this situation the malunion should be surgically corrected.

Osteomyelitis is the infection of bone. It can either occur secondary to hematogenous spread (*hematogenous osteomyelitis*) or via direct inoculation of the bone, usually secondary to trauma. The infection can either be acute (*acute osteomyelitis*) or chronic (*chronic osteomyelitis*). Chronic osteomyelitis refers to a long-standing infection of the bone that has never been treated or has failed treatment regimens.

Acute osteomyelitis of the spine can often be successfully treated with a long course of intravenous antibiotics. In the pediatric population, acute hematogenous osteomyelitis can also usually be successfully treated with intravenous antibiotics alone, provided there is no joint involvement. However, in adults, in any site other than the spine, antibiotics alone rarely eradicate the infection, as is generally true in all bones of the body when chronic osteomyelitis exists.

The hallmark of chronic osteomyelitis is a chronic draining sinus tract. The infection persists because of a necrotic nidus of bone, the *sequestrum*. Often an *involucrum* of reactive, viable bone forms around this necrotic nidus. Infection cannot be permanently eradicated without complete removal of the sequestrum. Good long-term results have been obtained with thorough debridement and sequestrectomy followed by free flap placement to fill the resultant dead space in the bone and increase blood supply locally.[106] In some instances, however, the amount of infected bone is so great that an entire diaphyseal or metaphyseal segment must be excised to fully debride all infected tissue. In such cases excellent results have been documented with a wide debridement of all infected bone and soft tissue followed by combined Ilizarov frame placement (to restore bone) and application of a free muscle (to provide immediate soft tissue coverage).[105] With experience in this armamentarium of techniques, most cases of osteomyelitis can now be eradicated.

Joint Pathology: Osteoarthritis

Epidemiology

Osteoarthritis or degenerative joint disease is the most common musculoskeletal disease. It is a significant source of pain and disability, especially in the older population.[107] Osteoarthritis is a degenerative condition that leads to the destruction of articular cartilage and formation of new bone at the weight-bearing surface. Osteoarthritis can be found in both males and females and is present in all races. The incidence increases with age, and it is estimated that more than 50% of individuals older than 50 years have some degree of degenerative joint disease.[108]

Degenerative joint disease affects certain joints preferentially. It is found more commonly in the fingers, hip, knee, and spine.[109] Women seem to have a wider range of joints affected, although it appears that they are equally susceptible to the disease. Marked differences have been found in the rates of degenerative joint disease in various ethnic populations.[110–112]

There are two different categories of osteoarthritis. The first is primary osteoarthritis, which is the classic form that presents in predisposed individuals without a specific etiology. Although still not clearly elucidated, the cause is multifactorial. Secondary osteoarthritis is a result of a preceding injury or stress to the joint; examples are posttraumatic arthritis or a dysplastic condition affecting the joint.

Predisposing factors to arthritis include occupation, previous trauma, congenital or developmental joint dysplasia, and family history. Those individuals who are engaged in manual labor show an increased incidence of osteoarthritis,[108] likely secondary to repetitive trauma or loading of the joints. Families often present with a strong history of degenerative joint disease. Although still unclear, several genetic mechanisms have been proposed. Joint damage secondary to intraarticular fractures can lead to degeneration of the joint. Fracture fixation is often predicated upon achieving anatomic articular congruency to prevent this sequela. Last, the presence of dysplastic joint conditions can lead to joint damage and degeneration. Developmental dysplasia of the hip and Perthes' disease are examples of conditions that, if left untreated, can lead to osteoarthritis.

Pathophysiology

Much of the pathology that occurs in osteoarthritis is a result of changes within the articular cartilage that surfaces the joint. Articular cartilage provides the necessary gliding motion of the joints. It serves to redistribute the high body loads that the joints must accommodate. Articular cartilage is compressible, elastic, and lubricated, allowing it to protect the underlying subchondral bone.

Normal articular cartilage is composed of chondrocytes and a large percentage of hyaline extracellular matrix. Within this extracellular matrix are collagen, protein, and proteoglycans. The primary type of collagen in articular cartilage is type II collagen. Healthy articular cartilage contains a high percentage of water, up to 80% of its weight. This water content increases in osteoarthritic cartilage. Much of this shift is caused by changes in the makeup of the proteoglycans. The proteoglycans decrease and change in composition as the disease worsens. As the extracellular matrix changes, it is less able to provide support and lubrication to the joint and advances the cascade of degenerative changes.

In addition to changes in the composition of the articular cartilage, enzymes play an important role in the advancement of osteoarthritis. Matrix-destroying enzymes have been found to be greatly increased during the disease process. These enzymes include collagenase, stromelysin, and gelatinase.[112] After they are activated they can act to break down the extracellular cartilage matrix. Cytokines such as interleukin 1 (IL-1) are also found in high concentrations in osteoarthritis. They may play an important role in activating the enzymes that slowly destroy the joint.

The bone within an arthritic joint also demonstrates changes with osteoarthritis. One of the clinical hallmarks of degenerative joint disease is osteophyte formation. Several theories have been advanced to explain the development of this new bone. Some authors believe that it may be secondary to penetration of blood vessels into the bottom layers of damaged cartilage.[113] It may also result from the healing of multiple stress fractures that occur as the shock-absorbing properties of the cartilage are lost.[114]

Clinical Presentation

Pain is the most common presentation of osteoarthritis. The patient may complain of pain within a particular joint that has been slowly progressive over time. Often, the pain is exacerbated by activity and improved by rest. Capsular fibrosis may lead to contractures of the joint and decreased motion. Swelling and grinding within the joint may also be present. More advanced arthritis often presents with bony deformity, and changes in the alignment of an extremity may become evident. For example, the knee joint may fall into a varus or valgus alignment.

Radiographs of the affected joint will show characteristic changes as the disease advances. The normal joint space becomes narrowed and osteophytes become visible. There will be changes within the subchondral bone, including sclerosis and subchondral cysts.

Laboratory test results from patients with osteoarthritis are generally normal. Visual examination of the synovial fluid shows that it is generally clear. Cell count demonstrates low noninflammatory white cell counts (150–1500/mm^3). Calcium pyrophosphate crystals can be found on occasion within the fluid.

Treatment

Treatments of osteoarthritis can be grouped into nonsurgical and surgical management. Nonsurgical etiologies include drugs, dietary changes, physical therapy, and activity modification. Surgery entails total joint replacements, various open and arthroscopic debridement procedures, and techniques to realign deformities.

Nonsteroidal Antiinflammatories

Nonsteroidal antiinflammatory medications (NSAIDs) form the mainstay of osteoarthritis therapy. Along with their antiinflammatory properties, they provide some degree of analgesia that can help to relieve symptoms. Often there is an inflammatory component to the arthritis that benefits from pharmacological management. For example, in the knee, there is often an element of synovial inflammation.

It is important to note that NSAIDs have significant gastrointestinal (GI) side effects. They inhibit prostaglandin secretion in the GI tract, which can lead to ulceration and bleeding. In a study of older patients, 16 of 1000 patients per year required hospitalization for peptic ulcer disease; this was four times higher than the control group, which was not placed on NSAIDs.[115] A newer class of NSAIDs is the COX-2 inhibitor group. This class of medication is thought to prevent GI side effects by preferentialy inhibiting the inducible inflammatory cascade over the constitutive cyclooxygenase (COX) pathway responsible for protecting the gastric mucosa. These newer medications may lead to a decrease in the gastrointestinal complications seen with older antiinflammatories. However, several COX-2 inhibitors have been pulled from sale because of concerns about drug safety.

Physical Therapy and Activity Modification

A structured physical therapy program can be of significant benefit to the patient with osteoarthritis. Patients can lose mobility and strength as a result of degenerative changes. Range-of-motion exercises can help to combat flexion contractures and improve overall mobility. Strengthening various muscle groups has a protective effect on the joint as it helps to provide increased shock absorption and reduce the stresses across the joint.[116] Regular exercise can also play a role in weight reduction. Obesity is a recognized etiology in osteoarthritis.[117] Diet modification should also be recommended for the same reason. Weight loss has been correlated with a decrease in patient symptoms.

Total Joint Replacement

The use of total joint replacement in the United States continues to accelerate yearly. The majority of patients who undergo joint replacements are older (more than 65 years of age), and as the population ages, the number of procedures will likely continue to increase. More than 120,000 total hip arthroplasties are performed each year. The cost of these procedures has been estimated to be $2.5 billion dollars per year.[118] Studies have shown the benefits of joint replacement in terms of pain relief, mobility, and other psychosocial factors. In one study of patients 3 months postoperatively, patients who underwent a primary total hip arthroplasty showed improvements in overall health, physical function, and even social interaction.[119]

Total joint arthroplasty involves surgically resecting the degenerated joint and replacing it through implantation of a prosthesis. The two most commonly replaced joints are the hip and the knee. Joint replacements have been in use for several decades, and overall survivorship of the components has been excellent. Various studies quote a greater than 85% survival of total hip arthroplasty components at 15 to 20 years.[120]

The decision to implant a total joint should be made only after the patient has failed conservative treatments. Younger patients should be counseled to wait as long as possible before undergoing procedures as the lifespan of the components does remain limited. The results of revision arthroplasty surgery are not as impressive as those of primary replacement. Furthermore, arthroplasty is not a benign surgery, and a myriad of complications can occur, including bleeding, infection, deep vein thrombosis, and component failure.

Arthroscopy

The technique of arthroscopy has revolutionized the field of orthopedic surgery. It involves the placement of a small-caliber fiberoptic lens into joints and defined spaces (i.e., bursae) of the musculoskeletal system. The lens instrument is attached to a small camera, and visualization is achieved on a video monitor. The current arthroscopes range in diameter from the conventional 4-mm diameter (used for most major large joints of the body, i.e., hip, knee, shoulder, elbow) down to the 1.8-mm-diameter miniscopes. Small hand-operated and motorized instruments complement the arthroscope so that surgical procedures can be performed in the joints.

Arthroscopic surgery was developed in Japan in the mid-1970s as a diagnostic tool for disorders of the knee. It has evolved since then to the point where many procedures that were previously done in an open fashion can now successfully be performed arthroscopically. This development has dramatically reduced the need for hospitalization as well as the associated morbidity of a more extensive open procedure. Presently, the most widely performed orthopedic surgical procedure performed in the United States is arthroscopy. The most common joint that is arthroscoped is the knee, followed by the shoulder.

In general, arthroscopic surgery of a joint is performed in a fluid environment (usually sterile lactated Ringer's solution or saline). Because of improvements in the field of video electronics, the resolution of structures that can be seen far exceeds the detail seen in conventional treatment methods. The knee has become the paradigm as a model for arthroscopic procedures. Most ligamentous, meniscal, and articular cartilage-related problems can now be addressed via arthroscopic surgical procedures. The posterior regions of the knee, which previously could only be adequately visualized through massive surgical dissections, can now be well visualized through as few as two 6-mm-length incisions.

Arthroscopic surgery has been of paramount importance in the evolution of the subspecialty of sports medicine. With the continued improvement in microelectronics and fiberoptics, it is almost certain that more and more orthopedic surgical procedures will be performed in a video-assisted manner.

References

1. Netter FH. The Ciba Collection of Medical Illustrations, vol 8. Musculoskeletal System. Summit, NJ: Ciba-Geigy, 1987.
2. Raisz LG. Physiology and pathophysiology of bone remodeling. Clin Chem 1999;45(8B):1353–1358.
3. Dempster DW, Cosman F, Parisien M, Shen V. Anabolic actions of parathyroid hormone on bone. Endocr Rev 1993;14:690–709.
4. Riggs BL, Khosla S, Melton LJ. A unitary model for involutional osteoporosis: estrogen deficiency causes both type 1 and type 2 osteoporosis in postmenopausal women and contributes to bone loss in aging men. J Bone Miner Res 1998;13:763–773.
5. Mow VC, Ratcliffe A, Poole AR. Cartilage and diarthrodial joints as paradigms for hierarchical materials and structures. Biomaterials 1992;13(2):67–97.
6. Mow VC, Ratcliffe A, Woo SL-Y, eds. Biomechanics of Diarthrodial Joints, vols I, II. New York: Springer-Verlag, 1990.
7. Mow VC, Holmes MH, Lai WM. Fluid transport and mechanical properties of articular cartilage. J Biomech 1984;17:377–394.
8. Simon WH, Friedenberg S, Richardson S. Joint congruence. J Bone Joint Surg 1973;55:8(A):1614–1620.
9. Praemer A, Furner S, Rice DP. Musculoskeletal Conditions in the United States. Rosemont: American Academy of Orthopaedic Surgeons, 1992.
10. Gustilo RB, Anderson JT. Prevention of infection in the treatment of 1025 open fractures of long bones. J Bone Joint Surg 1976;58(A):453.
11. Schenk RK, Willenegger H. Zum Histologischen Bild der Sogenannten Primarheilung der Knochenkompakta nach Experimentellen Osteotomien am Hund. Experientia (Basel) 1963;19: 593–595.
12. Schenk RK, Willenegger H. Morphological findings in primary fracture healing. Symp Biol Hung 1967;7:75–86.
13. Brighton CT. Principles of fracture healing. 1. The biology of fracture repair. AAOS Instr Course Lect 1984;32:60.
14. Uhthoff HK. Fracture healing. In: Gustilo RB, Kyle RF, Templeman DC, eds. Fractures and Dislocations. St. Louis: Mosby, 1993.
15. Delamarter RB, Coyle J. Acute management of spinal cord injury. J Am Assoc Orthop Surg 1999;7:166–175.
16. Prasad VS, Schwartz A, Bhutani R, et al. Characteristics of injuries to the cervical spine and spinal cord in polytrauma patient population: experience from a regional trauma unit. Spinal Cord 1999;37(8):560–568.
17. Factsheet. Spinal Cord Injury Statistics. Birmingham, AL: National Spinal Cord Injury Statistical Center, 1999.
18. Podolsky S, Baraff LJ, Simon RR, et al. Efficacy of cervical spine immobilization methods. J Trauma 1983;3:471–493.
19. Streitwisen DR, Knopp R, Wales LR, et al. Accuracy of standard radiographic views detecting cervical spine fractures. Ann Emerg Med 1983;12:538–542.
20. Bracken MB, Shepard MJ, Holford TR, et al. Administration of methylprednisolone for 24 to 48 hours or tirilazad meysylate for 48 hours in the treatment of acute spinal cord injury: results of the Third National Acute Spinal Cord Injury Randomized Controlled Trial–National Acute Spinal Cord Injury Study. JAMA 1997;1597–1604.
21. Waters RL, Yakura JS, Adkins RH, et al. Recovery following complete paraplegia. Arch Phys Med Rehabil 1992;73:784–789.

22. Frankel HL, Hancock DO, Hyslop G, et al. The value of postural reduction in the initial management of closed injuries of the spine with paraplegia and tetraplegia. Paraplegia 1969;7:179–192.
23. Stauffer ES, MacMillan M. Fractures and dislocations of the cervical spine. In: Rockwood C, Green DP, Bucholz RW, Heckman JD, eds. Rockwood and Green's Fractures in Adults. Philadelphia: Lippincott-Raven, 1996.
24. Roth EJ, Park T, Pang T, et al. Traumatic cervical Brown–Sequard and Brown–Sequard plus syndromes: the spectrum of presentations and outcomes. Paraplegia 1991;29:582–589.
25. Heller JG. The atlas vertebra: fractures and ligamentous injuries. In: Levine AM, ed. Orthopaedic Knowledge Update: Trauma. Rosemont: American Academy of Orthopedic Surgeons, 1996.
26. Southwick WO. Current concepts review: Management of fractures of the dens (odontoid process). J Bone Joint Surg 1980; 62A:482–486.
27. Bucholz RW, Burkhead WZ. The pathological anatomy of fatal atlanto-occipital dislocations. J Bone Joint Surg 1979;61A:248–250.
28. Anderson LD, D'Alonzo RT. Fractures of the odontoid processes of the axis. J Bone Joint Surg 1974;56A:1663–1674.
29. Clark CR, White AA. Fractures of the dens: a multicenter study. J Bone Joint Surg 1985;67A:1340–1348.
30. Levine AM, Edwards CC. The management of traumatic spondylolisthesis of the axis. J Bone Joint Surg 1985;67A:217–226.
31. Eismont FJ, Arena MJ, Green BA. Extrusion of an intervertebral disc associated with traumatic subluxation or dislocation of cervical facets: case report. J Bone Joint Surg 1991;73A:1555–1560.
32. Delamarter RB. Lower cervical injuries: classification and initial management. In: Levine AM, ed. Orthopaedic Knowledge Update: Trauma. Rosemont: American Academy of Orthopedic Surgeons, 1996.
33. White AW, Southwick WO, Panjabi MM. Clinical instability of the lower cervical spine. Spine 1976;1(1):15–27.
34. Denis F. The three column spine and its significance in the classification of acute thoracolumbar spinal injuries. Spine 1983;8(8):817–831.
35. Spivak JM, Vaccaro AR, Cotler JM. Thoracolumbar spine trauma. I. Evaluation and classification. J Am Assoc Orthop Surg 1995; 3(6):345–352.
36. Gertzbein SD. Scoliosis Research Society Multicenter Spine Fracture Study. Spine 1992;17:528–540.
37. McAfee PC, Yuan HA, Frederickson BE, et al. The value of computed tomography in thoracolumbar fractures: an analysis of 100 consecutive cases and a new classification. J Bone Joint Surg 1983;65A:461–473.
38. Denis F, Davis S, Comfort T. Sacral fractures: an important problem. Retrospective analysis of 236 cases. Clin Orthop 1988;227:67–81.
39. Bigliani LU, Flatow EL, Pollock RG. Fractures of the proximal humerus. In: Rockwood C, Green DP, Bucholz RW, Heckman JD, eds. Rockwood and Green's Fractures in Adults. Philadelphia: Lippincott-Raven, 1996:1059.
40. Kilcoyne RF, Shuman WP, Matsen FA III, et al. The Neer classification of displaced proximal humeral fractures: spectrum of findings on plain radiographs and CT scans. Am J Radiol 1990;154:1029–1033.
41. Neer CS II. Displaced proximal humerus fractures: part I. Classification and evaluation. J Bone Joint Surg 1970;52A:1077–1089.
42. Cornell C. Fractures of the proximal humerus and dislocation of the glenohumeral joint. In: Levine AM, ed. Orthopaedic Knowledge Update: Trauma. Rosemont: American Academy of Orthopedic Surgeons, 1996:18, 17, 222.
43. Neer CS II. Displaced proximal humerus fractures: part II. Treatment of three-part and four-part displacement. J Bone Joint Surg 1970;52A:1090–1103.
44. Kasser J, ed. Shoulder Trauma: Bone, Orthopaedic Knowledge Update 5. Rosemont: American Academy of Orthopaedic Surgeons, 1996:224.
45. Zeni EJ Jr, Krieg JK, Rosen MJ. Open reduction and internal fixation of clavicular fractures. J Bone Joint Surg 1981;63A:147–151.
46. Neviaser RJ, Neviaser TJ, Neviaser JS. Concurrent rupture of the rotator cuff and anterior dislocation of the shoulder in the older patient. J Bone Joint Surg 1988;70A:1308–1311.
47. Stableforth PG, Sarangi PP. Posterior fracture-dislocation of the shoulder: a superior subacromial approach for open reduction. J Bone Joint Surg 1992;74B:579–584.
48. Ideberg R. Fractures of the scapula involving the glenoid fossa. In: Bateman JE, Welsh RP, eds. Surgery of the Shoulder. Toronto: Decker, 1984:63–66.
49. Goss TP. Scapular fractures and dislocations: diagnosis and treatment. J Am Assoc Orthop Surg 1995;3:22–33.
50. Ada JR, Miller ME. Scapular fractures: analysis of 113 cases. Clin Orthop Relat Res 1991;269:174–180.
51. Mast JW, Spiegel PG, Harvey JP Jr, Harrison C. Fractures of the humeral shaft: a retrospective study of 240 adult fractures. Clin Orthop Relat Res 1975;112:254–262.
52. Lange RH, Foster RJ. Skeletal management of humeral shaft fractures associated with forearm fractures. Clin Orthop Relat Res 1985;195:173–177.
53. Helfet DL, Hotchkiss RN. Internal fixation of the humerus: a biomechanical comparison of methods. J Orthop Trauma 1990;4:260–264.
54. Riseborough EJ, Radin EL. Intercondylar T-fractures of the humerus in the adult: a comparison of operative and non-operative treatment in twenty-nine cases. J Bone Joint Surg 1969;51A:130–141.
55. Webb LX. Distal humerus fractures in adults. J Am Assoc Orthop Surg 1996;4:336–344.
56. Gainor BJ, Metzler M. Humeral shaft fracture with brachial artery injury. Clin Orthop Relat Res 1986;204:154–161.
57. Lange RH. Fractures of the humeral shaft. In: Levine AM, ed. Orthopaedic Knowledge Update: Trauma. Rosemont: American Academy of Orthopedic Surgeons, 1996:29.
58. Klenerman L. Fractures of the shaft of the humerus. J Bone Joint Surg 1966;48B:105–111.
59. Sarmiento A, Kinman PB, Galvin EG, Schmitt RH, Phillips JG. Functional bracing of the shaft of the humerus. J Bone Joint Surg 1977;59A(5):596–601.
60. Aspirnio D, Helfet DL. Fractures of the distal humerus. In: Levine AM, ed. Orthopaedic Knowledge Update: Trauma. Rosemont: American Academy of Orthopedic Surgeons, 1996:40.
61. Hotchkiss RN. Displaced fractures of the radial head: internal fixation or excision? J Am Assoc Orthop Surg 1997;5:1–10.
62. Mason ML. Some observations on fractures of the head of the radius with a review of one hundred cases. Br J Surg 1954;42:123–132.
63. Khalfayan EE, Culp RW, Alexander AH. Mason type II radial head fractures: operative versus non-operative treatment. J Orthop Trauma 1992;6:283–289.
64. Knight, DJ, Rymaszewski LA, Amis AA, et al. Primary replacement of the fractured radial head with a metal prosthesis. J Bone Joint Surg 1993;75:845–850.
65. Wolfgang G, Burke F, Bush D, et al. Surgical treatment of displaced olecranon fractures by tension band wiring technique. Clin Orthop Relat Res 1987;224:192–204.
66. Gartsman GM, Sculco TP, Otis JC. Operative treatment of olecranon fractures: excision or open reduction with internal fixation. J Bone Joint Surg 1981;63A:718–721.
67. Zych GA, Latta LL, Zagorski JB. Treatment of isolated ulnar shaft fractures with prefabricated functional fracture braces. Clin Orthop Relat Res 1987;219:194–200.

68. Bado JL. The Monteggia lesion. Clin Orthop Relat Res 1967;50:71–76.
69. Boyd HB, Boals JC. The Monteggia lesion: a review of 159 cases. Clin Orthop Relat Res 1969;94–100.
70. Strehle J, Gerber C. Distal radioulnar joint function after Galeazzi fracture-dislocations treated by open reduction and internal plate fixation. Clin Orthop Relat Res 1993;293:240–245.
71. Schemitsch EH, Richards RR. The effect of malunion on functional oucome after plate fixation of fractures of both bones of the forearm in adults. J Bone Joint Surg 1992;74A:1068–1078.
72. Frykman G. Fracture of the distal radius including sequelae—shoulder-hand-finger syndrome, disturbance in the distal radio-ulnar joint, and impairment of nerve function: a clinical and experimental study. Acta Orthop Scand 1967;108(suppl):1–153.
73. Bradway JK, Amadio PC, Cooney WP. Open reduction and internal fixation of displaced, comminuted intra-articular fractures of the distal end of the radius. J Bone Joint Surg 1989;71A:839–847.
74. Feldman D, Zuckerman JD, Frankel VH. Geriatric hip fractures: preoperative decision making. J Musculoskel Med 1990;Sept:69–78.
75. Kenzora JE, McCarthy RE, Lowell JD, et al. Hip fracture mortality: relation to age, treatment, preoperative illnesses, time of surgery, and complications. Clin Orthop 1984;186:45–56.
76. Hunter GA. Should we abandon primary prosthetic replacement for fresh displaced fractures of the neck of the femur? Clin Orthop 1980;152:158–161.
77. Sikorski JM, Barrington R. Internal fixation versus hemiarthroplasty for the displaced subcapital fracture of the femur. J Bone Joint Surg 1981;63:3(B):357–361.
78. Bochner RM, Pellicci PM, Lyden JP. Bipolar hemiarthroplasty for fracture of the femoral neck. J Bone Joint Surg 1988;70:7(A):1001–1010.
79. Bray TJ, Smith-Hoefer E, Hooper A, Timmerman L. The displaced femoral neck fracture. Clin Orthop 1988;230:127–140.
80. Garden RS. Stability and union in subcapital fractures of the femur. J Bone Joint Surg 1964;46(B):630–647.
81. Rao JR, Banzon MT, Weiss AB, Rayhack J. Treatment of unstable intertrochanteric fractures with anatomic reduction and compression hip screw fixation. Clin Orthop 1983;175:65–71.
82. Kyle RF, Gustilo RB, Premer RF. Analysis of 622 intertro-chanteric hip fractures. J Bone Joint Surg 1979;61A(2):216–221.
83. Hardy DCR, Descamps PY, Krallis P, et al. Use of an intramedullary hip-screw compared with a compression hip-screw with a plate for intertrochanteric femoral fractures. J Bone Joint Surg 1998;80A(5):618–630.
84. Winquist RA, Hansen ST, Clawson DK. Closed intramedullary nailing of femoral fractures. J Bone Joint Surg 1984;66A(4):529–534.
85. Brumback RJ, Reilly JP, Poka A, et al. Intramedullary nailing of femoral shaft fractures. Part 1: Decision-making errors with interlocking fixation. J Bone Joint Surg 1988;70A(10):1441–1452.
86. Brumback RJ, Uwagie-Ero S, Lakatos R, et al. Intramedullary nailing of femoral shaft fractures. Part II: Fracture-healing with static interlocking femoral fixation. J Bone Joint Surg 1988;70A(10):1453–1462.
87. Brumback RJ, Ellison TS, Poka A, et al. Intramedullary nailing of femoral shaft fractures. Part III: Long-term effects of static interlocking fixation. J Bone Joint Surg 1992;74A(1):106–112.
88. Lhowe DW, Hansen ST. Immediate nailing of open fractures of the femoral shaft. J Bone Joint Surg 1988;70A(6):812–820.
89. Brumback RJ, Ellison TS, Poka A, et al. Intramedullary nailing of open fractures of the femoral shaft. J Bone Joint Surg 1989;71A(9):1324–1331.
90. Bostman OM. Spiral fractures of the shaft of the tibia: initial displacement and stability of reduction. J Bone Joint Surg 1986;68B:462–466.
91. Nicoll EA. Fractures of the tibial shaft: a survey of 705 cases. J Bone Joint Surg 1964;46B:373–387.
92. Sarmiento A, Sobol PA, Sew Hoy AL, et al. Prefabricated functional braces for the treatment of fractures of the tibial diaphysis. J Bone Joint Surg 1984;66A:1328–1339.
93. Bone LB, Sucato D, Stegemann PM, Rohrbacher BJ. Displaced isolated fractures of the tibial shaft treated with either a cast or intramedullary nailing. J Bone Joint Surg 1997;79A(9):1336–1341.
94. Sanders R, Jersinovich I, Anglen J, Dipasquale T, Herscovici D. The treatment of open tibial shaft fractures using an interocked intramedullary nail without reaming. J Orthop Trauma 1994;8(6):504–510.
95. Bonatus T, Olson SA, Lee S, Chapman MW. Nonreamed locking intramedullary nailing for open fractures of the tibia. Clin Orthop 1997;339:58–64.
96. Stamer DT, Schenk R, Staggers B, Aurori K, Aurori B, Behrens FF. Bicondylar tibial plateau fractures treated with a hybrid ring external fixator: a preliminary study. J Orthop Trauma 1994:8(6):455–461.
97. Mikulak SA, Gold SM, Zinar DM. Small wire external fixation of high energy tibial plateau fractures. Clin Orthop 1998;356:230–238.
98. Barbieri R, Schenk R, Koval K, Aurori K, Aurori B. Hybrid external fixation in the treatment of tibial plafond fractures. Clin Orthop 1996;332:16–22.
99. Lauge-Hansen N. Fractures of the ankle. II. Combined experimental-surgical and experimental-roentgenologic investigations. Arch Surg 1950;60:957–985.
100. Chapman MW. Fractures and fracture-dislocations of the ankle. In: Mann RA, ed. Surgery of the Foot, 5th ed. St. Louis: Mosby, 1986.
101. Rosen H. Treatment of Nonunions. In: Chapman MW, ed. Operative Orthopaedics. Philadelphia: Lippincott, 1988.
102. Ilizarov GA, Ledyaev VI. The replacement of long tubular bone defects by lengthening distraction osteotomy of one of the fragments. Vestnik Khururgii 1979;6:78. (Clin Orthrop 1992;280:7. Transl. Vladimir Schwartzman and abridged.)
103. Cattaneo R, Catagni M, Johnson EE. The treatment of infected nonunions and segmental defects of the tibia by the methods of Ilizarov. Clin Orthop 1992;280:143–152.
104. Dipasquale D, Ochsner MG, Kelly AM, Maloney DM. The Ilizarov method for complex fracture nonunions. J Trauma 1994;37(4):629–634.
105. Lowenberg DW, Feibel RJ, Louie KW, Eshima I. Combined muscle flap and Ilizarov reconstruction for bone and soft tissue defects. Clin Orthop 1996;332:37–51.
106. Anthony JP, Mathes SJ, Alpert BSL. The muscle flap in the treatment of chronic lower extremity osteomyelitis: results in patients over 5 years after treatment. Plast Reconstr Surg 1991;88:311–318.
107. Peyron JG, Altman RD. The epidemiology of osteoarthritis. In: Moskowitz RW, Howell DS, Goldberg VM, Mankin HJ, eds. Osteoarthritis: Diagnosis and Management. Philadelphia: Saunders, 1992:15–38.
108. Lawrence JS. Rheumatism in Populations. London: William Heinemann, 1977.
109. Cushnaghan J, Dieppe P. Study of 500 patients with limb joint osteoarthritis: I. Analysis by age, sex and distribution of symptomatic joint sites. Ann Rheum Dis 1991;50:8.
110. Hoagland FT, Yau ACMC, Wong WL. Osteoarthritis of the hip and other joints in southern Chinese in Hong Kong. J Bone Joint Surg 1973;55A:545.
111. Solomon L, Beighton P, Lawrence JS. Osteoarthritis in a rural South African Negro population. Ann Rheum Dis 1976;45:274.
112. Richards AJ, Hamilton EBD. Destructive arthropathy in chondrocalcinosis articularis. Ann Rheum Dis 1986;45:272.

113. Trueta J. Studies of the Development and Decay of the Human Frame. Philadelphia: Saunders, 1968.
114. Swanson SAV, Freeman MAR. The mechanics of synovial joints. In: Simpson DC, ed. Modern Trends in Biomechanics, vol 1. London: Butterworths, 1970.
115. Griffin MR, Ray WA, Schaffner W. Nonsteroidal anti-inflammatory drug use and death from peptic ulcer in elderly persons. Ann Intern Med 1988;109:359.
116. Radin EL, Yang KH, Riegger C, et al. Relationship between lower limb dynamics and knee joint pain. J Orthop Res 1991;9:398.
117. Felson DT, Anderson JJ, Naimack A, et al. Obesity and symptomatic knee osteoarthritis: results of the Framingham Study. Arthritis Rheum 1987;30:S130.
118. Kasser J, ed. Shoulder Trauma: Bone. Orthopaedic Knowledge Update 5. Rosemont: American Academy of Orthopaedic Surgeons, 1996:397.
119. Laupacis A, Bourne R, Rorabeck C, et al. The effect of elective total hip replacement on health-related quality of life. J Bone Joint Surg 1993;75A:1619–1626.
120. Joshi AB, Porter ML, Trail IA, et al. Long-term results of Charnley low-friction arthroplasty in young patients. J Bone Joint Surg 1993;75B:616–623.

108

Plastic Surgery

W. Thomas Lawrence and Adam Lowenstein

Plastic surgery has been defined as a field that involves the study of the skin and its contents (E.E. Peacock, Jr., personal communication). Although this description may seem overly broad, it accurately reflects the variety of patients and problems managed by plastic surgeons. In contrast to pediatrics or orthopedics, plastic surgery is not a field defined by patient age or anatomy. Instead, it is a field characterized by a method of managing problems. The name of the specialty, plastic surgery, derives from the Greek word *plastikos*, which means "to change or mold." The theme of changing or molding is the common thread that binds the often diverse problems managed by plastic surgeons. The defects and abnormalities treated by plastic surgeons include congenital problems, traumatic injuries, skin cancers, defects created in the management of oncological problems, hand abnormalities, chronic wounds, and problems caused by aging. In managing all these problems, the purpose of plastic surgery is to change or mold to restore form and function.

Much of this work is optimally done as part of a team including other specialists. Craniofacial teams, for example, involve neurosurgeons, dentists, oral surgeons, speech pathologists, and other healthcare professionals to provide optimal care for patients with cleft and craniofacial abnormalities. The management of chronic wounds also involves a variety of medical specialists including vascular surgeons, dermatologists, and rheumatologists. Combining the differing expertises of individuals from a variety of medical and surgical specialties frequently optimizes patient outcomes.

This chapter considers many of the types of problems managed by plastic surgeons. Some are components of plastic surgery such as hand surgery, burns, cutaneous malignancies, malignancies of the head and neck, and wound healing that are discussed in other chapters and are not considered here.

Wound Management

Much of plastic surgery involves the management of wounds. Some of the wounds are acute, and some are chronic. Some are caused by trauma, some are congenital, and some result from medical disorders and their treatment. Common principles of wound management apply to all wounds, regardless of etiology and duration.

The treatment of any wound must be prioritized in relation to coexistent injuries or problems. Wounds are generally obvious and easily diagnosed, but they are not life threatening. Their treatment is only undertaken after all more urgent problems have been addressed.

Wounds are first examined to determine whether the wounded tissues are clean and viable and to determine whether foreign bodies are present. Knowledge of local anatomy dictates whether the possibility of injuries to adjacent nerves, ducts, muscle, or bone must also be considered, and appropriate evaluations are obtained if needed (Fig. 108.1).

The first decision that the treating (Fig. 108.2) physician must make in terms of wound management relates to the timing of wound closure (see "wound decision tree"). Primary wound closure refers to closing a wound at the time of presentation. This approach is preferred unless coexisting factors preclude it. Factors that prevent primary closure include uncontrollable bleeding, necrotic tissue and/or foreign material that cannot be completely removed from the wound by irrigation or debridement, and excessive bacterial contamination.

Wounds with bacterial concentrations greater than 10^5 organisms/gram of tissue[1] are defined as infected and should not be closed. Beta-hemolytic streptococci are an exception to this rule in that they can produce clinical infections at lower concentrations.[2] It is difficult to assess the degree of

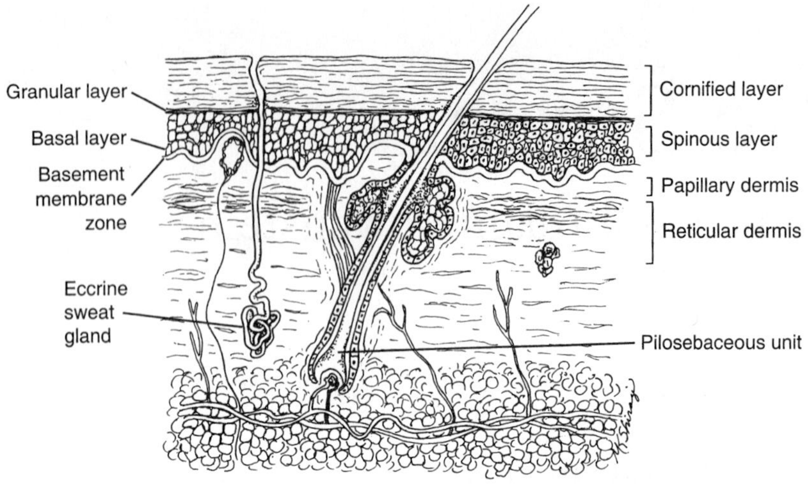

FIGURE 108.1. Normal skin and subcutaneous tissue.

bacterial contamination of a wound solely by visual inspection, and levels of bacterial contamination are optimally determined by quantitative bacteriology. This assessment requires biopsy of the wound, which is not always available, however.

The degree of bacterial contamination is suggested by several clinical features of the wound. The age of acute wounds is one factor correlated with the degree of bacterial contamination. The early postwounding time frame has been called the golden period because closure can usually be accomplished safely during this period. The exact length of the golden period has been variably defined as lasting between 6 and 15h. The mechanism of injury is another factor associated with the degree of bacterial contamination. Saliva contains large quantities of bacteria, and human bites are therefore considered infected from their inception and should rarely if ever be closed. Farm injuries are associated with intermediate levels of bacterial contamination and may or may not be safely closed depending on coexistent factors. The location of injury also affects the decision as to when wounds can be safely closed. The head and neck are better vascularized than the lower extremity, and one can close slightly older wounds that have a less favorable mechanism of injury in the head and neck than the foot. The patient's overall health status also impacts the decision as to when primary wound closure is safe. Malnourished or steroid-treated patients have less competent systems and may not be able to tolerate levels of bacteria acceptable for more healthy patients. For chronic wounds, excessive bacterial contamination may be suggested by excessive wound exudate, limited healing progress, and/or signs of cellulitis in the surrounding tissues.

Another variable in considering whether to close a wound is how aggressively the wound can be treated before closure. If a wound can be completely excised back to fresh tissue, primary closure can be successfully carried out even in wounds with some unfavorable characteristics. Aggressive debridement may be contraindicated by a lack of excess tissue or because structures adjacent to the wound such as nerve, blood vessels, or bone must be preserved.

If primary closure is not feasible, a period of wound management is initiated. Wounds with uncontrollable bleeding are generally packed or wrapped tightly. Surgical debridement is the most definitive method of removing quesitonable tissue from a wound. This process is often facilitated by the use of the Versajet device. Dressing change regimens can also be utilized for wounds with excessive bacterial contamination or necrotic tissue. Wet to dry dressings are effective at debriding necrotic tissue from wounds. Collagenolytic ointments may also facilitate wound debridement.[3] Bacterial counts are most effectively lowered by dressing changes with antibacterial agents such as silver sulfadiazine.[4] The vacuum assisted closure (VAC) device applies negative pressure to wounds improving their blood supply and thereby accelerating their healing and limiting bacterial counts. The VAC has been commonly used recently in the treatment of wound before definitive closure. Wounds may be closed in a tertiary fashion once the problem preventing primary closure has been corrected.

Wounds not closed primarily or in a tertiary fashion may be allowed to heal secondarily. Secondary healing is healing through wound contraction and epithelialization. This method of healing is often preferred for infected wounds, superficial wounds, small wounds, and puncture wounds. Allowing infected wounds to heal secondarily limits the likelihood of recurrent infection. The functional and aesthetic results of secondary healing for small and superficial wounds are generally as good as or better than those obtained by closing them. Small wounds on concave surfaces such as the medial canthal and nasolabial regions heal secondarily with particularly excellent aesthetic results as well.[5] For puncture wounds, secondary healing is preferred because it diminishes the likelihood of infection and produces an aesthetically acceptable scar.

Wound Closure

The "reconstructive ladder" defines the options available for the closure of any wound (Table 108.1). In general, the simplest method of wound closure that can be used is preferred. Wound closure by direct wound approximation is appropriate for most lacerations as well as wounds that involve limited tissue loss. This method generally allows wound closure with the least scarring and deformity. For more extensive wounds, skin grafts may be required. Skin grafts require a wound bed that can revascularize the graft and permit it to survive. Skin grafts cannot be used for wounds exposing bone denuded of periosteum, cartilage denuded of perichondrium, nerve

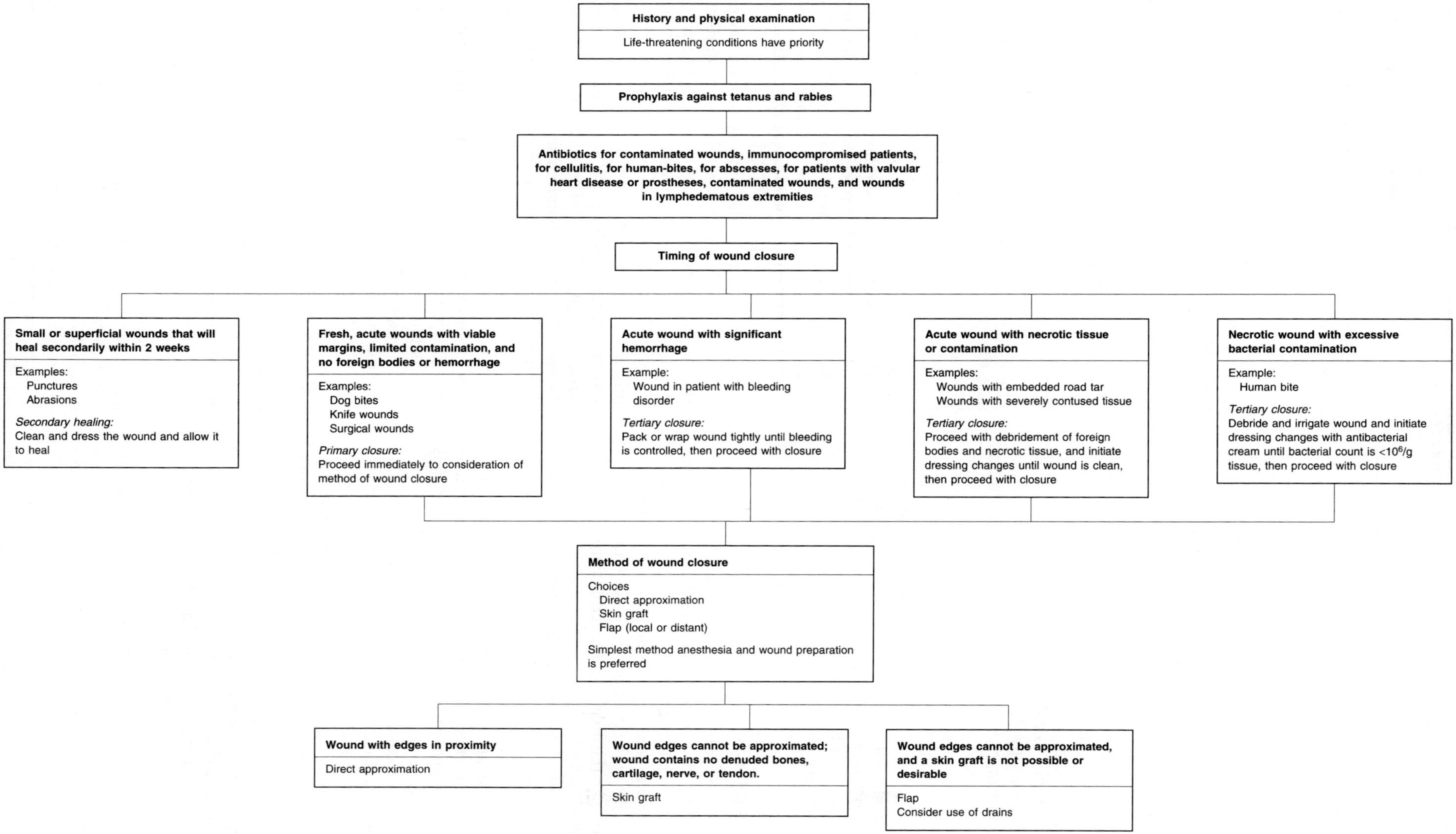
History and physical examination
Life-threatening conditions have priority
Prophylaxis against tetanus and rabies
Antibiotics for contaminated wounds, immunocompromised patients, for cellulitis, for human-bites, for abscesses, for patients with valvular heart disease or prostheses, contaminated wounds, and wounds in lymphedematous extremities
Timing of wound closure
Small or superficial wounds that will heal secondarily within 2 weeks
Examples:
Punctures
Abrasions
Secondary healing:
Clean and dress the wound and allow it to heal
Fresh, acute wounds with viable margins, limited contamination, and no foreign bodies or hemorrhage
Examples:
Dog bites
Knife wounds
Surgical wounds
Primary closure:
Proceed immediately to consideration of method of wound closure
Acute wound with significant hemorrhage
Example:
Wound in patient with bleeding disorder
Tertiary closure:
Pack or wrap wound tightly until bleeding is controlled, then proceed with closure
Acute wound with necrotic tissue or contamination
Examples:
Wounds with embedded road tar
Wounds with severely contused tissue
Tertiary closure:
Proceed with debridement of foreign bodies and necrotic tissue, and initiate dressing changes until wound is clean, then proceed with closure
Necrotic wound with excessive bacterial contamination
Example:
Human bite
Tertiary closure:
Debride and irrigate wound and initiate dressing changes with antibacterial cream until bacterial count is <10^6/g tissue, then proceed with closure
Method of wound closure
Choices
Direct approximation
Skin graft
Flap (local or distant)
Simplest method anesthesia and wound preparation is preferred
Wound with edges in proximity
Direct approximation
Wound edges cannot be approximated; wound contains no denuded bones, cartilage, nerve, or tendon.
Skin graft
Wound edges cannot be approximated, and a skin graft is not possible or desirable
Flap
Consider use of drains

FIGURE 108.2. Approach to acute wound management.

TABLE 108.1. Reconstructive Ladder.

Direct wound approximation
Skin graft
Local flap
Distant flap

denuded of perineurium, or tendon denuded of peritendon. All these structures have a limited blood supply and are not capable of revascularizing a skin graft. Skin grafts also have certain limitations that must be accepted if they are to be utilized. Skin grafts do not provide bulk, and they cannot be elevated secondarily to allow subsequent surgery to be performed underneath them. In addition, their appearance differs from that of intact skin. Local flaps are often used for wounds that cannot be closed by direct wound approximation and where a skin graft cannot be used or has unacceptable limitations. A variety of flaps are available that vary in size, bulk, and tissue characteristics. In general, a flap that includes tissue as similar as possible to the tissue lost is preferred. At times, local tissue is either unavailable or has limitations in volume or other characteristics. For wounds such as these, distant tissue transferred by microvascular methods may be desirable. In all cases, the benefits of closure must be balanced against the morbidity related to the method of closure chosen.

Direct Wound Approximation

Wound closure by direct wound approximation generally involves five steps: (1) induction of anesthesia, (2) wound irrigation, (3) shave and prepping of the wounded area, (4) wound debridement, and (5) wound closure. Anesthesia should virtually always be induced first and wound closure is always last, although the order of the intermediate three steps sometimes varies.

For small wounds, local anesthesia is generally utilized. Most commonly, the local anesthetic is injected into the wound edge. In some locations, such as digits, a regional block is simple and appropriate. Extensive injuries to an extremity may make an axillary block or spinal anesthetic more desirable. Coexistent problems or extensive wounds may necessitate a general anesthetic.

A large variety of local anesthetics are available. Lidocaine is commonly used in that it has the advantages of relatively rapid onset, a duration of action of 2 to 3h, which is adequate for most wound closures, and a low incidence of allergic reactions. It is commonly used with epinephrine except in locations where vasospasm in axial vessels could lead to tissue loss, such as on the digits. Epinephrine contributes to hemostasis and increases the maximum dose of lidocaine that can be safely utilized. The classic maximum dosages for lidocaine are 4mg/kg without epinephrine and 7mg/kg with epinephrine, respectively, although the validity of these maximal doses has been questioned recently.

Topical local anesthetics have also been gaining popularity as an altenative or adjunct to injectable local anesthetics in accute wound management. TAC, a solution of 0.5% tetracaine, 1:2000 adrenaline, and 11.8% cocaine, effectively induces local anesthesia when applied topically to an open wound, especially in the face and scalp.[6] A variety of other topical combinations of agents have also been succussfully used to induce topical anesthesia in wounds with success. EMLA, an eutectic mixture of lidocaine and prilocaine, is effective at inducing anesthesia in intact skin, although it must be in contact with skin for 1 to 2h to be effective.[7]

Wound irrigation is carried out to decrease the number of bacteria in the wound and wash out foreign material. High-pressure irrigation (>8p.s.i.) is more effective at diminishing bacterial concentrations than low-pressure irrigation or scrubbing with a saline-soaked sponge.[8–10] Pulsatile irrigation is the best mechanism for cleansing fragments of foreign debris from soft tissue. Acceptable agents for irrigation include Ringer's lactate, 0.9% saline, and Pluronic F-68.[11–13] There is some evidence that antibiotic supplements decrease bacterial counts in contaminated wounds more effectively than saline solution.[14]

In hair-bearing areas, hair can get in the wound and make wound closure more difficult. Hair may be clipped to eliminate this problem. Shaving displaces bacteria from hair follicles, potentiating wound infections, and should be avoided if possible, however. Preparation of the skin surrounding the wound is carried out to limit contamination of the wound by bacteria residing on the skin surface.

The goals of wound debridement differ depending on the nature of the wound. Debridement may be required to remove devitalized tissue, to excise tissue heavily contaminated by bacteria or foreign bodies, or to create perpendicular wound edges. Perpendicular wound edges are desirable in that they make a fine line scar more likely.

The final step in the process is actual wound closure, accomplished with sutures, staples, tapes, or tissue adhesives. An optimal method of wound closure is to precisely align the wound edges, support the wound for at least 6 weeks until it has gained adequate strength, not cause any ischemia or inflammation, and not penetrate the adjacent epidermis and possibly generate additional scars. No method of wound closure accomplishes all these goals, so any method of wound closure represents a compromise.

Sutures are probably used most frequently for wound closure. Sutures allow precise alignment of wound edges and can be left in for varying lengths of time for wound support. Skin sutures have the disadvantage of penetrating the epidermis. An epithelialized tract develops around a suture left in skin for longer than 7 to 10 days, and the tract will be replaced by an unwanted scar after stitch removal.[15] If sutures are tied too tightly, they can cause ischemia, slowing healing and contributing to additional scarring. They are also foreign bodies that can contribute to inflammation. The suture utilized should be the one with the smallest diameter that still has the strength to maintain wound edge approximation to limit the quantity of foreign material placed in the wound. In general, monofilament suture material is less reactive than braided sutures and is preferable for skin closure. Braided sutures are more pliable and generally tie more easily, providing advantages in some locations.

Suture-induced epidermal scarring can be alleviated by placing sutures in the dermis and not penetrating the epidermis; this can be accomplished either with absorbable sutures or nonabsorbable sutures that are removed secondarily. If absorbable materials are to be utilized, synthetic material such as polyglactin 910 (Vicryl), polyglycolic acid (Dexon), poliglecaprone 25 (monocryl), polyglyconate (Maxon), or polydioxanone (PDS) are preferable to chromic or plain catgut. The former are absorbed by simple hydrolysis with little inflammatory response, whereas the latter materials provoke an active cellular inflammatory response that slows the healing process (see Table 108.2 for absorption characteristics). There is some evidence that protracted wound support with a dermal permanent suture may maximally limit scar spreading. Dermal sutures can be supplemented with tapes such as Steri-Strips or fine epidermal sutures if epidermal alignment is not adequate with subcuticular sutures alone.

Staples may be somewhat less precise than sutures, although they are quicker to place and are elevated from the wound surface, limiting the possibility of ischemic tissue damage as can be created by a tightly tied suture. Similar to sutures, staples penetrate the epidermis and are foreign bodies, thus having similar disadvantages in this regard.

Tapes avoid the problems that can result from epidermal penetration and foreign bodies, and in addition are comfortable for patients.[16] Tapes avoid the inflammation and ischemia sutures or staples can produce as well. Tapes alone may not lead to accurate approximation of the deeper dermis, however, and wound edema may cause inversion of taped wound edges. In addition, tapes may inadvertently come off prematurely and are difficult to use in hair-bearing areas.

The decision as to when to remove sutures or staples from a particular wound necessitates developing a compromise between factors that favor prolonged wound support and those which favor early removal. Optimal cosmesis demands early removal of sutures or staples before inflammation can develop and before epithelialization can occur along the suture tracts. On the other hand, it takes a number of weeks for the wound to gain significant tensile strength, and early removal of sutures or staples can result in scar widening or even wound disruption. Skin wounds in most anatomic locations are generally not subjected to significant tension and can maintain satisfactory closure with 15% or less of the tensile strength of normal skin. Facial wounds are subjected to very little stress and may heal faster than wounds in other locations because of the excellent blood supply, allowing especially early suture removal in this anatomic location. Facial skin sutures are generally removed at 3 to 5 days. Abdominal skin sutures are generally left in slightly longer and are removed at 7 to 10 days. Sutures on the lower extremity are left in place 10 to 14 days because injured lower extremities are more frequently edematous, producing more stress on the wound, and because the blood supply to the lower extremity is often not so good as that in other locations.[17] Wounds subjected to excessive tension, such as those overlying joints, often require 3 or more weeks of suture support to avoid disruption as well. Wounds in individuals with impaired healing because of diabetes, steroids, or other factors may also require protracted suture support. Less aesthetic consequences must be accepted in these cases.

Fibrin glues approximate wounds with a natural molecule that is eventually broken down enzymatically. Fibrin has been utilized clinically to improve the adherence of skin grafts[18] and to limit seroma formation under flaps.[19] Fibrin has been used together with a limited number of sutures for the closure of wounds subjected to minimal tension such as blepharoplasty incisions.[20] Although helpful in these clinical settings, fibrin glue is not strong enough to allow its independent use for the closure of wounds subjected to even limited tension.

Cyanoacrylate tissue adhesives have been used by surgeons for more than 30 years. They are strong, reasonably flexible, and biocompatible. When they first became available, isobutyl cyanoacrylate and trifluoropropyl cyanoacrylate were placed directly in wounds to approximate the wound edges. Adhesives used in this manner created a mechanical barrier to healing and increased wound inflammation and infection rates, so their use was abandoned relatively quickly. More recently, cyanoacrylates have been applied topically to intact skin at the edge of wounds to hold injured surfaces together. Contact with the open wound itself is carefully avoided to limit wound toxicity. Dermabond (octylcyanoacrylate) has been compared to sutures as a wound closure method in a prospective, randomized trial in Canada.[21] Few wound dehiscences were seen, and aesthetic results of wounds assessed 3 months after closure were similar to those obtained with sutures. As would be expected, octylcyanoacrylate clo-

TABLE 108.2. Characteristics of Absorbable Suture Materials.[a]

	Time to 50% breaking strength	*Time to complete absorption*	*Breaking strength at 2 weeks (%)*	*Breaking strength at 3 weeks (%)*
Natural				
Gut	6 days	70 days	5	0
Chromic gut	10 days	90 days	30	0
Synthetic				
Braided				
Dexon S (polyglycolic acid)	18 days	60–90 days	65	35
Polysorb (lactomer)	14 days	60–90 days	57	21
Vicryl (polyglactin 910)	21 days	56–70 days	75	50
Vicryl Rapide (polyglactin 910)	5 days	42 days	0	0
Monofilament				
Biosyn (glycomer)	15 days	90–110 days	54	29
Maxon (polyglyconate)	28 days	6 months	75	65
Monocryl (polyglecaprone 25)	7 days	91–119 days	20–30	5
PDS II (polydiaxone)	28 days	6 months	70	60

[a]Data derived from package inserts and company-provided information.

sures were faster and less painful. Octylcyanoacrylate was not used in deep wounds that penetrated fascia. It is also not recommended for use on the hands and over joints where either washing or repetitive motion might lead to premature removal of the adhesive.

Deep wounds that involve structural and functional units such as muscle and fascia require multiple layers of closure. Closure of these deeper layers almost invariably involves sutures. The question of how many layers to close arises with deeper wounds. Both laboratory animal and human studies have demonstrated that closure of the subcutaneous fat contributes to an increased incidence of infection,[22] so sutures should only be placed in more structural tissues such as fascia (including Scarpa's fascia). If concern exists regarding the possibility of fluid collecting in an unclosed subcutaneous space, drains are a suitable alternative to subcutaneous stitches. In addition to preventing the accumulation of blood or serum, suction drains also aid in the approximation of tissues. They are particularly useful in aiding tissue approximation under flaps. Removal of drains can usually be safely accomplished when drainage reaches levels of 25 to 50 mL/day. All drains have the potential for bacterial infections and should be removed from a wound as soon as possible.[23]

Skin Grafts

As mentioned, skin grafts are generally utilized for well-vascularized wounds that are too large to allow direct wound approximation. Skin is 5% epidermis and 95% dermis. Skin grafts transfer epidermis and a variable amount of dermis from the donor area to the wound to close it. Any reconstructive method has some cost associated with it. For skin grafts, the primary cost is the second wound at the donor site. Split-thickness skin grafts (STSGs) that include only a portion of the dermis are more commonly utilized because the epidermal appendages (hair follicles, sweat glands, and sebaceous glands) left in the remaining dermis of the donor site allow spontaneous reepithelialization of the donor wound. If a full thickness of skin is harvested as a graft, additional techniques need to be utilized for closure of the donor wound; this limits the size of full-thickness skin grafts (FTSGs) that can practically be used.

Skin varies in thickness with age and among various parts of the body. Children less than 10 years of age have relatively thin skin. The skin thickens with age until the fourth decade when it subsequently begins to thin again. Eyelid skin and other facial skin to a lesser degree is relatively thin, whereas skin from the back is extremely thick. Full-thickness grafts need to be harvested from areas where the skin is thinner to achieve reliable graft survival.

Split-thickness grafts can also be designed to include greater or lesser portions of dermis. Thin and thick grafts have different advantages and disadvantages (Table 108.3). Thin grafts take more readily and allow quicker secondary healing of the donor wound. They also allow the recipient wound to secondarily contract to a greater degree than grafts that include greater amounts of dermis and especially full-thickness skin grafts.[24] Although more effective at limiting secondary contraction, thick grafts contract more immediately after harvest in that they contain more elastin fibers within the dermis. This process is referred to as primary graft contraction and can shrink the size of a full-thickness graft 40%.

TABLE 108.3. Types of Skin Grafts.

Split-thickness skin grafts:
- Advantages
  1. Grafts "take" more readily
  2. Donor site heals more readily, allowing secondary harvesting at an earlier date (particularly important in large burns)
  3. Recipient site contracts to a greater degree, limiting the size of the graft (advantageous if the graft does not overlie a joint but disadvantageous if it does)
- Disadvantages
  1. Color and texture of grafted skin are not well maintained
  2. Grafts are less likely to have normal sebaceous activity and sweating
  3. Hair is not transferred with the graft (advantageous if hair-bearing donor site to be used for non-hair-bearing recipient site)
  4. Grafts in children will not grow as the child grows

Full-thickness skin grafts:
- Advantages
  1. Color and texture of grafted skin are optimally maintained
  2. More normal sweating and sebaceous activity maintained
  3. Contraction at recipient site is limited (important when the graft overlies a joint)
  4. Hair is transferred with the graft
  5. Grafts in children will grow as the child grows
- Disadvantages
  1. Grafts require careful attention to ensure "take"
  2. Donor sites will not heal secondarily and require separate closure

Meshed grafts (generally split-thickness grafts although full-thickness grafts can be meshed):
- Advantages
  1. Grafts can be expanded to cover larger areas
  2. Interstices prevent blood and serum from accumulating under the graft and limiting "take"
  3. Grafts may contour better to irregular recipient sites
- Disadvantages
  1. Graft appearance is "cobblestoned" and less aesthetic
  2. Recipient site may contract to a greater degree (can contribute to contractures over joints)

Thick grafts and full-thickness grafts in particular are more likely to maintain a more natural appearance and to allow the functional transfer of epithelial appendages. The successful transfer of these appendages allows the graft to grow hair, sweat, and maintain normal sebaceous activity. Full-thickness grafts are more likely to maintain their color than split-thickness grafts, which generally darken after transfer. Independent of thickness, grafts taken from below the clavicle are more likely to darken after transfer whereas those taken from the head and neck area are more likely to retain a pinker hue. Full-thickness grafts also maintain the ability to grow, in contrast to split-thickness grafts. The ability of full-thickness grafts to limit contracture of the recipient site is particularly helpful when grafts are placed over joints.[24] Sensitivity similar to that of the recipient site gradually returns in all grafts.[25] Wounds closed with both STSG and FTSG are very durable once the graft has healed.

The ideal graft donor site from the point of view of color and texture match is tissue from the contralateral structure in that humans are relatively symmetrical. It is also desirable, however, for donor sites to be relatively inconspicuous. Donor sites for skin grafts are chosen after balancing the desire for optimal color and texture match with the desire for a minimally visible donor location.

As mentioned, skin harvested from the supraclavicular area and above more closely resembles facial skin than skin from the buttocks. For that reason, head and neck donor sites are preferred for grafts in the facial region. Commonly used donor sites include the postauricular area, the supraclavicular area, and the scalp. The postauricular area is commonly utilized for smaller full-thickness grafts. Larger full- or split-thickness grafts can be harvested from the supraclavicular area, although this donor site has limitations in women who prefer low-cut tops. The scalp is an excellent donor site for both split-thickness grafts and full-thickness grafts. The donor area is hidden after hair regrowth. Split-thickness scalp grafts generally do not grow hair. The head must be shaved to take the graft, however, and this may be unacceptable to some patients. Full-thickness scalp grafts are used to transfer hair-bearing tissue, although the amount of scalp skin that can be transferred is limited. The buttocks and upper thighs are covered by clothes and are the most commonly used donor sites for wounds below the clavicles in that the color match is reasonable and the sites are inconspicuous.

Skin grafts are often meshed before placing them on a wound. Meshing involves cutting multiple slits into the graft, which allow it to expand before transplantation. Meshing has advantages and disadvantages. It allows the graft to cover a wider area and allows better contouring of the graft to irregular recipients beds. It also allows blood and exudate to flow through the graft interstices instead of collecting under the graft, potentially limiting graft take. The disadvantages of meshing are that the aesthetic appearance of the graft is frequently less satisfactory and the interstices heal secondarily partly by wound contraction, which may increase secondary contraction of the recipient site.

Flaps

Flaps differ from grafts in that flaps maintain their own blood supply when transferred for closure of a wound. The decision to use a flap for wound closure is based on the nature of the wound and the desired aesthetic and functional result. Skin grafts require a well-vascularized wound bed and, as mentioned, flaps are indicated for the closure of wounds exposing relatively avascular tissue such as bone, cartilage, nerve, or tendon. Flaps are also preferred for wounds including tissue rendered relatively avascular by radiation or chronic scarring.

Flaps may sometimes be used where grafts might be an alternative to provide either an improved aesthetic result or improved functionality. In general, local flaps are used if a flap of the appropriate dimensions and type is available, whereas distant or free flaps are used when local tissue of the desired type is not available. Ideally, flaps are taken from areas where there is adequate tissue laxity to allow direct approximation of the donor wound. The aesthetic and functional cost of any flap must be considered carefully before flap transfer to ensure that the gain is worth the cost.

The size and components transferred with any flap depend on the blood supply of the tissues. A variety of descriptive classification schemes exist for flaps, relating to the type of blood supply, the technique of flap transfer, or the tissues incorporated in the flap (Table 108.4). Many of the transfer methods are shown diagrammatically in Figure 108.3. The schemes can be somewhat confusing in that they overlap significantly, and any one flap can often be described in several ways. Perhaps the most meaningful classification relates to blood supply. Random flaps survive on perforating blood vessels extending from underlying blood vessels into the dermal–subdermal plexus proximal to the flap base. The tissue of the flap itself depends on flow in this dermal–subdermal plexus for survival. Such flaps are limited in length with various length to width ratios between 5:1 for the face and 1:1 for the lower extremity, sometimes cited as defining the limits of dependable flap survival. Axial flaps, in contrast, receive their blood supply from specific, defined blood vessels. The size and tissue composition of axial flaps are dependent on the volume and type of tissue nourished by the axial vessel. In many parts of the body, these vessels run underneath and within muscles that need to be included in the flap, for example, a latissimus dorsi flap. In other anatomic locations, axial vessels run adjacent to fascia overlying muscle, allowing transfer of axial fasciocutaneous units. In some areas, axial vessels course within the subcutaneous layer and allow transfer of flaps containing only the skin and subcutaneous layers, for example, a groin flap. In still other locations, axial flaps are based on small septal vessels that extend from deeper axial vessels directly to the overlying skin, such as a radial forearm flap.

TABLE 108.4. Classification of Flaps.

Blood supply:
Random flap
Axial flap
Tissue composition:
Cutaneous flap
Fasciocutaneous flap
Musculocutaneous flap
Muscle flap
Osteocutaneous flap
Osseous flap
Transfer method:
Advancement flap
Single pedicle advancement flap
V–Y, Y–V flap
Bipedicle flap
Pivot flap
Rotation flap
Transposition flap
Simple transposition flap
Bilobed flap
Rhomoboid flap
Z-plasty
Interpolation/island flap
Distant
Direct flap, e.g., crossleg flap
Tubed pedicle
Free flap

Essentially any axial flap has the possibility of being completely detached and transferred as a free flap using microvascular techniques. As mentioned, the utilization of free flaps is generally reserved for clinical situations where inadequate local tissue exists for transfer or a particular tissue characteristic is required that is unavailable locally. Examples include extensive defects of the head and neck created by extirpation of oropharyngeal cancers, where bone is often required for mandibular reconstruction in conjunction with large volumes of soft tissue.

The ability to transfer tissue with specific characteristics is currently being expanded by flap "prefabrication."[26] Prefab-

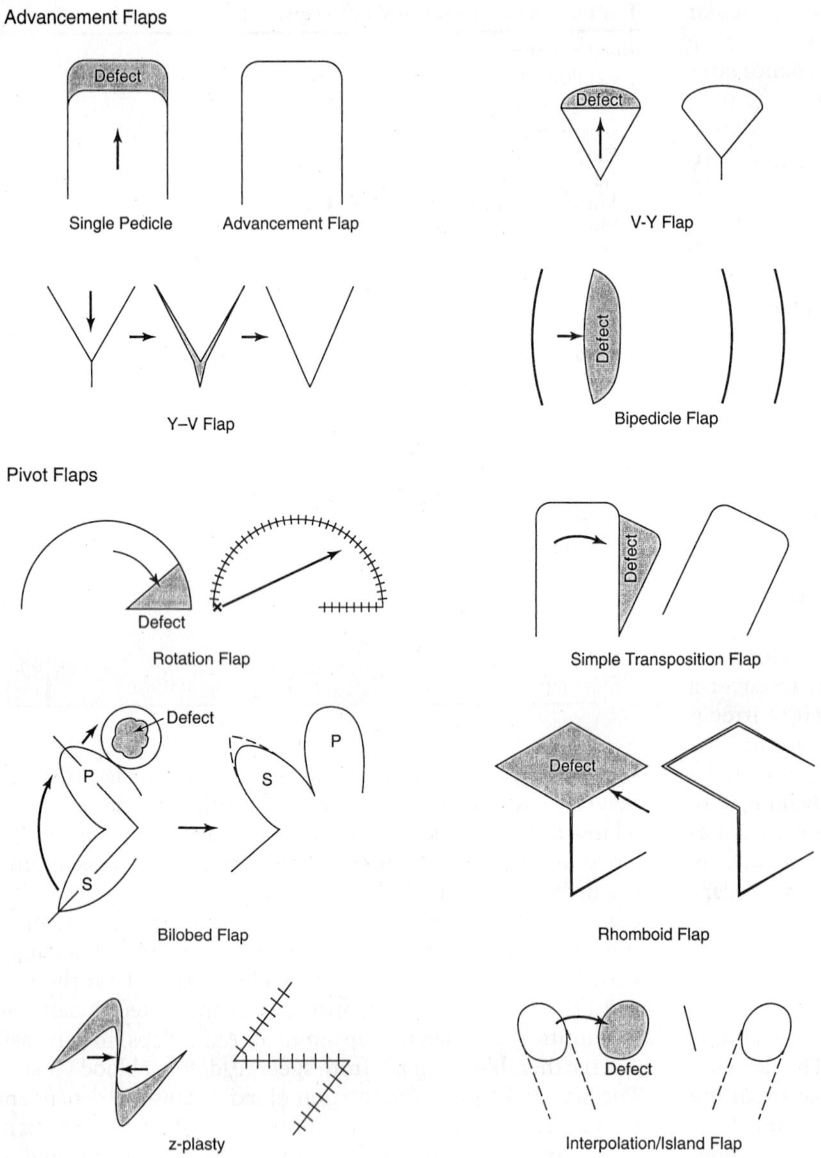

FIGURE 108.3. Flap transfer methods.

rication involves manipulation and refinement of the tissue characteristics of an existing flap before transfer of that flap, which might involve placement of grafts of skin and cartilage on the undersurface of the flap and/or preliminary repositioning of the tissues before secondary transfer to the defect requiring closure. This technique has been used with success for nasal reconstruction.

Flaps transfer tissue that is unchanged in color, texture, thickness, hair-bearing characteristics, and sebaceous activity by the transfer process. Flaps will grow with the patient. Sensation and sweating will be maintained if a nerve supply is transferred with the flap. When a nerve supply is not maintained, some sensation usually returns to the flap in time. Flaps can be designed that allow the transfer of viable bone or specialized structures such as jejunum when such tissue is required for complex restorations.

Tissue Expansion

In situations where the local tissue has desired characteristics but is inadequate in volume, tissue expansion is a clinical option. The first step in tissue expansion is the placement of an empty synthetic bag under the tissue for which expansion is desired. The bag includes a valve either incorporated within it or attached to it by a tube. Most tissue expanders used at this time are made of silastic material. The valve is accessed percutaneously with a needle in the outpatient clinic setting, generally beginning 2 to 3 weeks after tissue expander placement. During each expansion, the expander is inflated until the overlying tissue is taut; the tissue subsequently stretches and relaxes, allowing additional expansion. Although further expansion can sometimes be carried out within days, an interval of 1 to 2 weeks between expansion episodes is more commonly used clinically. Expansion is continued until the desired degree of expansion of the donor area has been achieved. Overexpansion is often carried out in that expanded skin will retract to some degree after the expander is removed during flap transfer. Two or more expanders may be concurrently placed to allow expansion circumferentially around a wound or defect to recruit skin from several different anatomic locations. Although tissue expansion has great clinical utility, it does require that the patient accept an obvious deformity during the period of expansion and two operations to achieve eventual wound closure.

Scar Characteristics

No matter what wound approximation techniques are utilized, it is critical that one adhere to basic surgical principles regarding the meticulous handling of tissues to optimize chances for an aesthetic scar. When sutures or staples are used, care should be taken to ensure that wound edges are gently approximated but that the tissue is not strangulated. Excessive tension on the wound should be avoided whenever possible. Wounded tissues should not be exposed to potentially harmful materials such as hexachlorophene or povidone-iodine.[27]

Regardless of how the wound is managed, inherent characteristics of the wound and patient have a major influence on the ultimate appearance of the scar. Wounds with two perpendicular, well-vascularized wound edges that are approximated in a tension-free manner are more likely to result in aesthetic scars. Wounds designed to parallel relaxed skin tension lines, which generally follow wrinkle lines, generally result in a more favorable scar as well. Wounds on the deltoid or sternal area, wounds in dark-skinned individuals, and wounds in patients between the ages of 2 and 40 are more likely to result in less favorable scars. No individual or combination of factors allows a surgeon to predict with assurance how any wound will heal in any given patient, however, given the multiplicity of variables involved.

Because wounds almost invariably improve in appearance with time, scar revisions for any wound are generally postponed for at least 6 months after any injury. This time period allows wounds closed by direct approximation or flaps to become metabolically stable.

Reconstructive Surgery

Reconstructive surgery involves the utilization of one of the wound closure methods previously discussed to close wounds or restore deformities created by trauma, infection, ablative surgery, or congenital defects. The principles of reconstructive surgery were summarized by Millard, who emphasized the need to "Know the ideal beautiful normal. Diagnose what is present, what is diseased, destroyed, displaced, or distorted, and what is in excess. Then, guided by the normal in your mind's eye, utilize what you have to make what you want and when possible go for even better than would have been."[28] Although some of these statements seem intuitive, their importance is often better appreciated in their application in that defects that seem simple are sometimes more complex than they initially appear. Detailed discussions of all the reconstructive methods available for specific parts of the body are beyond the scope of this chapter, but special concerns and common reconstruction options for different anatomic areas are highlighted.

Head and Neck

Because of their prominent location, restoration of form and function is particularly important in the head and neck. Reconstructing deformities of the head and neck can be especially challenging, however, because of the specialized structures in the area including the scalp, eyelids, ears, nose, and mouth. In most areas of the head and neck, one needs to consider aesthetic units. Aesthetic units are areas of the face whose borders are at the natural junctures of facial structure.[29] Reconstructive methods ideally place scars at the juncture of the aesthetic units (Fig. 108.4).

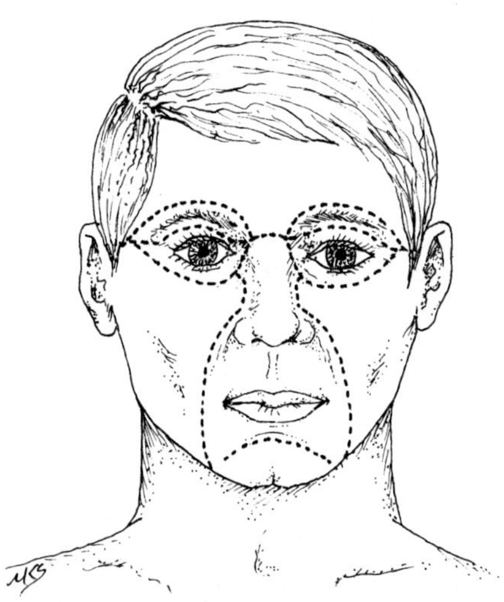

FIGURE 108.4. Aesthetic units of the face.

Scalp

Scalp defects are ideally reconstructed with hair-bearing skin in a manner that restores the original pattern of hair growth. The skin of the scalp is normally stretched tightly across the cranium, limiting the degree of skin edge mobilization that can be achieved for closure of scalp defects. Although direct wound approximation of small scalp defects is sometimes possible, larger defects are ideally closed by rotation of flaps of adjacent hair-bearing tissue. The flaps must be large and broad based becuase of the limited ability of scalp skin to stretch. Orticochea[30,31] developed three- and four-flap methods that include mobilization of essentially all the skin of the scalp for closure of moderate-sized scalp defects. Scoring of the underlying galea extends the area a scalp flap can span. Alternatively, skin expansion can be utilized to increase the inventory of hair-bearing skin available for reconstruction of hair-bearing areas. Still larger defects force compromise of ideal reconstructive goals to accept non-hair-bearing skin. In these cases, skin grafts can be utilized if the wound does not extend through periosteum. For more extensive defects, free tissue transfer may be required. Unfortunately, no other part of the body provides hair-bearing skin similar to that of the scalp.

Eyelids

Eyelids are extremely specialized structures that provide significant reconstructive challenges. The lids include an outer layer of thin skin and an inner conjunctival component. The intermediate portion of the lid includes a tarsus at the lid margin and the orbicularis oculi muscle, which serves to close the eye. Additionally, in the upper eyelid, the levator palpebrae superioris and aponeurosis and Muller's muscle contribute to lid opening. The more mobile upper eyelid is responsible for 90% of the eye-opening action. The periorbital area also includes the medial and lateral canthi, which help define eye shape and position, and the lacrimal system, which is responsible for tear production, distribution, and drainage.

Limited effects that do not involve the full thickness of the eyelid can often be reconstructed with grafts. Mucosa of the cheek or nose can be used to replace significant conjunctival defects, and cartilage from the nasal septum or ear can be used to replace the tarsal plate. Full-thickness defects involving 25% to 30% of the eyelid can frequently be directly approximated.[32] Slightly larger defects can be approximated if the lateral canthus is divided. More extensive defects provide a greater reconstructive challenge. The lower lid is somewhat easier to restore because it is relatively static, and flaps from the cheek or upper eyelid combined with grafts of mucosa and cartilage for lining have often been successful.[33] The upper eyelid must remain mobile, however. Transfer of tissue from the lower lid to the upper lid by one of several methods is often carried out to correct such defects in that no other part of the body mimics the complex anatomy of the eyelid.[33]

Nose

The nose includes nasal lining and overlying skin with bone and cartilage as structural elements between them. One has to consider which elements are missing when developing a reconstructive plan. In addition, the skin of the more cephalad aspect of the nose is thinner whereas the skin of the tip tends to be thicker and more oily. The nasal bone in the proximal nose is rigid, and the cartilage in the distal nose is more flexible. These anatomic characteristics influence decisions regarding reconstruction.

For simpler defects requiring only overlying skin, skin grafts and local flaps are generally used for wound closure. When grafts are used, postauricular skin is the most commonly used donor site, although the supraclavicular area can also be used successfully. Full-thickness skin grafts can replace the thinner skin of the cephalad aspect of the nose with aesthetic results, but grafts on the caudal nose are often less attractive. Composite grafts containing cartilage and two layers of skin can be harvested from the ear for closure of complex defects of the nostril rim. The upper limit of predictable composite graft survival is generally 1.5 cm, however. Local flaps replace like with like and often heal with a more satisfactory aesthetic result than grafts, especially on the nasal tip. Smaller flaps can be created on the nose itself, and a larger number of such flaps have been described. More extensive defects generally require a regional donor site such as the forehead or cheek. The nasolabial area of the cheek is an excellent donor site for lateral nasal defects[34] (Fig. 108.5). Nasolabial flaps as well as other local flaps can also be used as turnover flaps for nasal lining. Alternatively, skin grafts or hinged septal tissue can be used for lining restoration. Forehead flaps are the workhorse for reconstruction of significant defects involving nasal skin. These flaps are generally rotated to the nose from the paramedian area of the forehead based on the supratrochlear vessels. Alternatively, lateral forehead skin can be transposed to the nose using the scalp as a pedicle.[35] Another option is to transfer postauricular skin to the nose, again using the scalp as a pedicle, as described by Washio.[36] These three methods all require secondary division of the scalp pedicle. If replacement of skeletal support is required, it should be done at the same time that the soft tissue is replaced to prevent skin contraction and maintain nasal structure.[37] Depending on the size and nature of the defect, either bone or cartilage may be successfully used. Total nasal defects often require either a cantilevered bone graft rigidly fixed to the frontal bone or an L-shaped strut of bone or cartilage affixed to the frontal area and the nasal spine. Hinged septal cartilage can also be used to provide skeletal support for less extensive defects. Free tissue transfers have also been utilized for the reconstruction of all or part of the nose when local tissues are inadequate.

Lip

The lip provides the challenge of reconstructing a mobile, multilaminated, sensate structure that maintains oral competence, facilitates speech and alimentation, and allows facial expression when necessary. Defects involving only the skin or mucosa can be closed in a relatively straightforward fashion with local flaps or grafts. Grafts or flaps from the tongue and cheek can provide mucosa, whereas skin is often transferred from the adjacent cheek or submental area if local tissue is inadequate. Care must be taken to align the vermilion border as naturally as possible to maximize result quality. As in the eyelid, limited defects that involve all three layers of the lip can be closed by direct wound approximation. Defects involving one-quarter of the upper lip and one-third of the lower lip

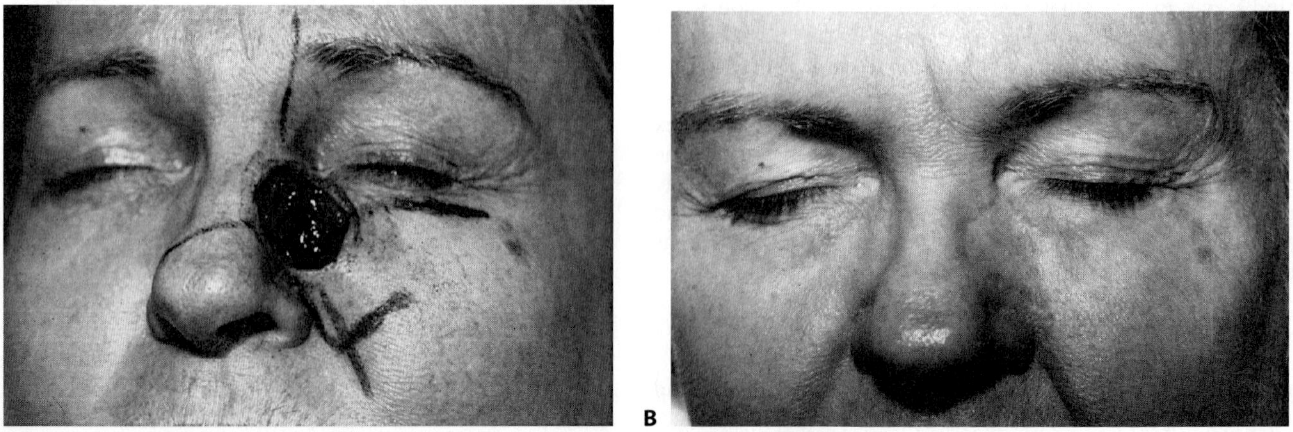
A B

FIGURE 108.5. Lateral nasal reconstruction with nasolabial rhomboid flap. **A.** Preoperative view. **B.** Postoperative view.

may be closed in this manner. Larger full-thickness defects may require transfer of a cross lip flap. Although probably not the originator of the concept, Abbe described the procedure in 1898, and cross lip flaps are commonly known as Abbe flaps.[38] Such flaps involve two stages. The initial stage involves the transfer of a full-thickness lip segment from one lip to the opposite lip to fill a defect while maintaining a vascular connection to the lip of origin. The second procedure, performed 2 to 3 weeks after the initial procedure, involves division of the vascular pedicle. There are a number of variations of Abbe flaps, including the Estlander flap, which involves transfer of lip tissue around the commissure from one lip to the other.[39] More extensive lip defects may require more complex transfers of tissue from one lip to the other. Karapandzic[40] described one technique that maximally preserves orbicularis oris muscle function, although even more extensive defects require the transfer of distant tissue, often including a tendinous, muscle, or fascia component to provide lip support. Lips reconstructed from distant tissue sources are generally deficient in sensory and muscular function and are functionally less satisfactory.

Ear

Reconstruction of ear defects is also extremely challenging. The ear includes anterior and posterior layers of thin skin with a delicately contoured cartilaginous framework between them. Limited defects involving only skin are relatively easily closed, either with skin grafts or by direct wound approximation after ear cartilage reduction. More limited, marginal defects may be closed by advancement of helical rim flaps.[41] Defects that do not involve the full thickness of the ear but are ungraftable because of exposed cartilage are often well managed by flaps of preauricular or postauricular skin, often in multistaged procedures. More extensive defects of the upper and middle portions of the ear can be managed by rotation of conchal tissue to take the place of lost tissue from the helix.[42] Defects that leave little or no auricular tissue remaining require transfer of a new auricular framework in a similar manner to that utilized for the reconstruction of congenital auricular aplasia.[43] The auricular cartilage framework is most commonly carved from rib cartilage. The framework is placed under the postauricular skin and is secondarily elevated with placement of a postauricular skin graft. If there is no remaining skin of good quality, a temporoparietal fascia flap or free flap may be necessary to provide coverage for the cartilaginous framework.

Forehead, Cheek, and Neck

Reconstruction of defects of the forehead, cheek, and neck is more straightforward in that skin cover alone is all that is generally required. The principles previously discussed regarding wound management remain applicable in these settings. Only a limited array of flaps is available for extensive forehead defects because of the lack of skin laxity in this area. Grafts are commonly used if periosteum is intact. Tissue expansion is also frequently utilized. Cheek tissue lends itself more effectively to the utilization of local flaps for wound closure. Extensive flaps involving both cheek and neck skin are sometimes used. Tissue expansion can be a valuable reconstructive tool for cheek defects, as well. When possible, flap margins are hidden in the natural folds and boundaries of the face as defined by aesthetic units (see Figure 108.4). Musculocutaneous flaps available from the neck include the sternocleidomastoid flap, the platysma flap and the submental flap. The sternocleidomastoid flap can provide limited amounts of skin and muscle for the closure of local complex wounds, and the platysma myocutaneous flap and submental flap have utility in cheek reconstruction.

Oropharyngeal Reconstruction

The surgical treatment of complex oropharyngeal tumors frequently involves extensive excisions of facial and oropharyngeal tissue, in addition, on occasion, to portions of the mandible or cervical esophagus. Regional flaps such as the pectoralis major myocutaneous flap, the trapezius myocutaneous flap, and the deltopectoral flap are commonly used for soft tissue coverage. Free tissue transfers often involving the thin pliable radial forearm flap are also commonly used. Mandibular reconstruction requires bone that can survive the radiation therapy these patients frequently require as adjuvant treatment. Free fibular flaps[44] have been used most commonly for these defects, although free scapular flaps, iliac crest grafts, and radial artery flaps including bone have also been used. Reconstruction of the cervical esophagus frequently involves the microvascular transfer of jejunum, especially when the defects are circumferential.[45] Defects that are not circumferential can be closed by local flaps such as the pectoralis major myocutaneous flap. Some prefer this flap even for circumferential defects.[46]

Back

Reconstruction of back wounds includes the usual options of direct wound approximation, skin grafts, and local flaps. More extensive or complex wounds may require use of the latissimus dorsi myocutaneous flap or latissimus dorsi muscle flap with a skin graft applied for cutaneous coverage. These flaps can be based laterally on the primary thoracodorsal blood supply or medially on the secondary paraspinal perforators. The trapezius muscle or myocutaneous flap has utility in the upper back, and the transverse back flap is an option for lower back defects. More extensive defects may require free tissue transfer or sometimes tissue expansion.

Chest (Not Including the Breast)

The normal chest wall has properties of elasticity, compliance, and structural support to facilitate ventilation. The rib cage also protects the underlying heart and lungs. These normal anatomic and functional characteristics must be considered in reestablishing form and function in chest defects. For most defects involving only skin and soft tissue, wound closure can be accomplished in a relatively straightforward manner either by direct wound approximation or with skin grafts or local flaps.

Extensive wounds that involve ribs or sternum sometimes require reestablishment of structural support. At least two adjacent ribs can be removed without reestablishing structural support, although the critical size of defects requiring reconstruction of structural elements remains undefined. Sternal defects that include the manubrium and upper sternal body with adjacent ribs produce severe physiological deficits if not reconstructed and generally require reconstruction. Defects confined to the sternal body and adjacent ribs produce moderate physiological deficits. Wounds limited to the upper sternal body and adjacent ribs alone produce minimal physiological deficit. The decision regarding the need for reconstruction of structural elements is based on evaluation of whether the patient can tolerate the functional impairment created by the loss of these elements. Wounds where there is significant scarring from radiation or infection generally remain stable with soft tissue reconstruction alone. When structural reconstruction is required, alloplastic materials such as polytetrafluoroethylene (PTFE, Gore-Tex)[47] or polypropylene mesh (Marlex) are commonly used. Marlex has also been used in a sandwich technique in conjunction with methylmethacrylate to provide a more rigid and stable construct.[48] Autogenous materials such as split ribs or fascia lata have been used as well. Flaps are required to cover these more extensive chest wall defects, with or without structural reconstruction. Latissimus dorsi or rectus abdominis myocutaneous flaps are used most commonly, although pectoralis major myocutaneous flaps, external oblique myocutaneous flaps, random pattern flaps, and deltopectoral flaps may at times be of value.

Dehisced, infected postsurgical median sternotomy wounds represent one of the most common indications for reconstructive surgery of the chest. All infected sternum and adjacent costal cartilage must be resected. Secondary healing of such wounds is prolonged, so the wounds are generally closed using local flaps. There is generally enough skin for wound closure, but the flaps are needed to fill the defect created by the sternal debridement. Unilateral or bilateral pectoralis major muscles are often used. The rectus abdominis muscle or omentum can also be used. The use of the internal mammary artery for coronary revascularization may preclude the use of the rectus abdominis flap or medially based pectoralis flap on the side utilized in that the artery represents the primary blood source for both flaps.

Intrathoracic postpneumonectomy empyema defects may require rotation of flaps into the thoracic cavity to facilitate wound closure and healing of the frequently coexistent bronchopleural fistulae. This is accomplished through a defect created by a double rib resection 4 to 5 cm long. Latissimus dorsi, serratus anterior, rectus abdominis, and omental flaps have all been used for this purpose.

Abdomen

As in the chest, simple wounds involving skin and soft tissues can be closed either by direct wound approximation or with skin grafts or local flaps, sometimes augmented by tissue expansion. Defects involving structural elements of the abdominal wall represent more substantial reconstructive challenges. For fistulae patients with multiple coexistent problems, wound closure of complex abdominal wounds should generally be accomplished in stages from the underlying viscera, which may require concurrent treatment as well and add to the complexity of wound management. As a general rule, the more complex the coexistent intraabdominal pathology requiring treatment, such as fistulae or an obstruction, the less involved the acute abdominal reconstruction should be. The treatment of complex abdominal problems generally requires a team approach involving a general surgeon and a plastic surgeon as a minimum. In these cases, simple reconstructive methods are generally used initially with the understanding that definitive reconstruction will be carried out at a later date.

One simple alternative for the initial stage of closure in very ill patients is to use bipedicle flaps of skin and subcutaneous tissue, leaving a persistent fascial defect. Another alternative is to close the fascial defect with an absorbable mesh and allow it to dissolve. A skin graft can then be applied to the underlying bowel, which at that point is covered by granulation tissue. Alloderm, a dermal construct, can also be used to fill an abdominal fascial defect and has the advantage of becoming vacularized and incorporated as a neostructural element to the abdomen. With all these methods, a secondary, more definitive reconstructive procedure is required secondarily when the the acute pathology has been treated and edema has subsided.

After providing such a time interval, fascial defects that could not initially be closed can often be approximated by direct wound approximation. When this is not possible, the technique of "component separation" is sometimes of value[49] (Fig. 108.6). With this technique, the rectus muscle is separated from the external oblique muscle to allow advancement of the rectus abdominis, internal oblique, and transversus abdominis muscles for up to 10 cm on each side of the abdomen.

For wounds involving a more extensive fascial deficit, autogenous fascia can be transferred either as a graft or as a component of a flap. Tensor fascia lata is a commonly used fascial graft donor site,[50] and it can also be used as a component of a tensor fascia lata myocutaneous flap for lower abdominal defects or as a component of a mutton chop rectus femoris flap for upper abdominal defects.[51] Alternative flaps for abdominal wall reconstruction include the rectus abdominis flap, latissimus dorsi flap, and the gracilis flap. The rectus abdominis flap can be utilized as a superiorly based, inferiorly based, or bipedicled flap. The use of these tissue rearrangements may be restricted by the size and location of the

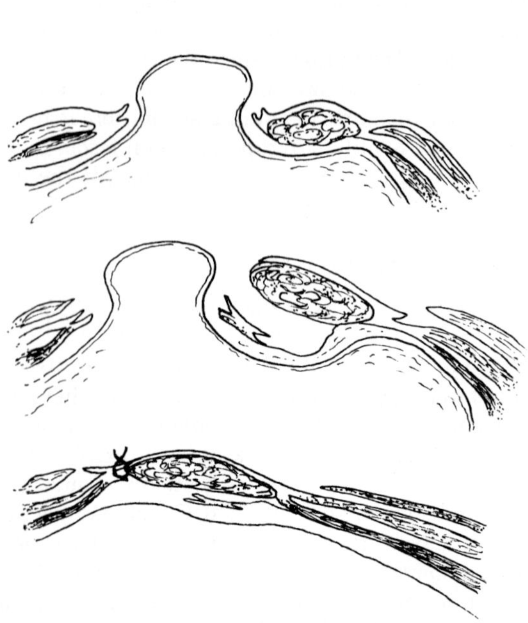

FIGURE 108.6. Abdominal wall bipartition for the closure of difficult abdominal wounds.

abdominal defect. The tensor fascia lata flap, for example, will rarely reach the medial upper abdomen, which is the most difficult area of the abdomen to reconstruct. If the patient's own adjacent tissues cannot be utilized, synthetic materials such as polypropylene, polyester, and PTFE may be used to provide structural support to the abdomen.[52] PTFE may have advantages when applied over viscera in that fewer adhesions that may predispose to fistulae are seen. There are newer constructs that include more than one material to allow exposure of a nonadherent material intraabdominally and a more adhering material subcutaneously. All synthetic materials share the disadvantage of being susceptible to infection and extrusion. In addition, they require adequate soft tissue to be present for skin closure over them.

Perineum: Including Pressure Sores

The most commonly seen defects in the perineal region are pressure-induced ulcerations, although trauma, infectious disease, congenital problems, and surgery or radiation performed to treat oncological problems can also produce substantial wounds. Pressure sores are seen primarily in chronically debilitated or acutely ill individuals who are unable to move themselves adequately and in spinal cord-injured patients who are unable to sense pressure-induced tissue ischemia. Areas particularly prone to pressure sores include the soft tissues overlying the sacrum, ischial tuberosities, and greater trochanters. Friction and shearing forces are significant cofactors that contribute with pressure to the development of these wounds.

Direct wound closure and skin grafts have a limited role in the management of small defects, but flap closure is almost always required for more substantial wounds.[53] Complete wound excision involving the underlying bony prominence is required before flap rotation. In pressure sore patients, patient factors other than those considered in the management of most wounds weigh heavily in the decision-making process as when to operate on a patient. One must be certain that the patient is physically able and psychologically motivated to prevent the development of recurrent pressure sores. The underlying pathology that renders the patients susceptible to pressure sores generally cannot be corrected. In spite of teaching regarding frequent repositioning and the utilization of pressure-relieving cushions and mattresses, recurrence rates up to 61%[54] are often seen after pressure sore closure.

Sacral wounds develop in patients lying supine for prolonged periods. Closure of sacral wounds can be accomplished with fasciocutaneous rotation flaps, gluteus maximus myocutaneous flaps in a variety of configurations, and lumbosacral flaps.

Pressure is placed on the ischii when sitting, and patients develop ischial sores from sitting for prolonged periods without changing position. Posterior thigh rotation flaps, gluteal thigh flaps, gluteus maximus myocutaneous flaps, gracilis myocutaneous flaps, biceps femoris or hamstring myocutaneous flaps, and tensor fascia lata myocutaneous flaps are available for the closure of ischial wounds.

Trochanteric defects arise when patients lie on their sides without moving for protracted periods. The tensor fascia lata (TFL) flap is the workhorse for coverage of trochanteric defects, although the gluteal thigh flap and myocutaneous flaps involving the vastus lateralis and rectus femoris muscles are also useful. In considering surgical treatment for any pressure sore, flaps should be chosen realizing that recurrence is likely and alternative flap donor sites need to be preserved.

Intrapelvic defects resulting from oncological extirpations can be filled with gracilis myocutaneous flaps or gluteal thigh flaps from the legs or rectus abdominis flaps rotated intraabdominally. Cutaneous paddles associated with any of these flaps can be used for vaginal reconstructions. Local fasciocutaneous flaps such as the Singapore flap are excellent alternatives for less extensive defects of the vagina and perineal area.[55,56]

Muscle flaps have also been used to restore anal continence. The gracilis was initially wrapped around the distal anus to restore this function.[57] More recently, gluteus muscle flaps have been used for this purpose.[58] Electrical stimulation can provide preconditioning, which increases the utility of muscular neosphincters.[59] Urinary sphincters have been reconstructed in experimental models with electrically stimulated free gracilis flaps as well.[60]

Penile reconstruction represents a particular challenge. Although local flaps are available, free radical forearm flaps provide the best reconstructions available at this time.[61]

Upper Extremity

Reconstruction of hand deformities involves multiple considerations in relationship to reestablishing form and function, and these are addressed in a separate chapter. Defects of the proximal arm are generally closed in a straightforward fashion with skin grafts or local flaps. Flaps derived from the area such as the deltoid flap and the lateral arm flap are more commonly used as free tissue transfers at distant sites than as local flaps. At the elbow, there is little soft tissue naturally covering the olecranon, which predisposes the area to bone exposure. Skin grafts applied in this area do not provide adequate padding and frequently break down. Flaps are therefore generally preferred for wound closure over the elbow. The reverse lateral arm flap based on the anterior or posterior radial recurrent vessel is most commonly used,[62] although the ulnar recurrent upper arm flap[63] is another local option. Other approaches include the utilization of random flaps transferred from the chest wall that are secondarily divided, brachioradialis muscle flaps, and local fasciocutaneous flaps. The distal forearm can also provide challenges in that the underlying tissues are primarily tendinous. Wounds that expose tendons are not amenable to grafts. Reversed flow flaps based on the radial, ulnar, or posterior interosseous vessels are often utilized for wound closure in this area.

Lower Extremity

Lower extremity defects are common and generally result from trauma, complications of diabetes, or arterial or venous vascular disease. Smaller wounds will often heal secondarily with an appropriate wound care regimen. Somewhat larger defects are amenable to closure with skin grafts or local flaps, including transposition and bipedicle flaps. Significant defects require more involved techniques for wound closure, however. In the upper leg, flaps previously discussed for perineal and abdominal reconstruction including the tensor fascia lata, rectus femoris, gracilis, and gluteal thigh flaps are often of use. The inferiorly based epigastric flap can also be used.[64]

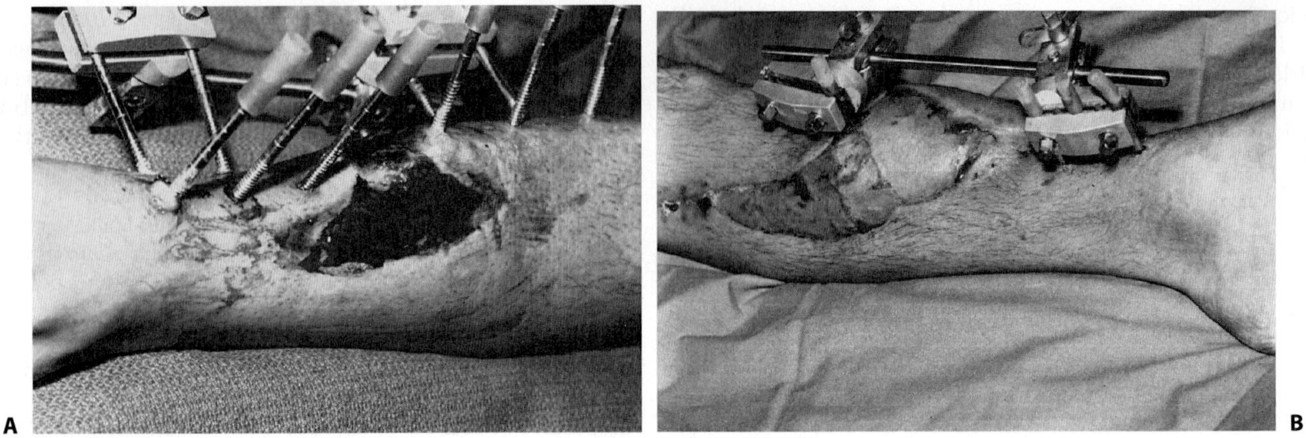

FIGURE 108.7. Free latissimus dorsi flap covered with skin graft for closure of distal leg wound. A. Preoperative view. B. Postoperative view.

The sartorius muscle can be transposed to cover small defects. In the area around the knee, local flaps based distally on the lateral[65] or medial[66] genicular artery can be used, as can gastrocnemius muscle or myocutaneous flaps. The vastus medialis musculocutaneous flap has also been utilized.

The lower leg is anatomically divided into thirds when evaluating reconstructive options. Muscles used for coverage of the upper third include the medial and lateral heads of the gastrocnemius and the soleus. The larger medial gastrocnemius muscle is the workhorse in this area. The middle third of the leg can often be reached by the soleus muscle as well. Other muscles of the leg have been used as local flaps for closure of defects in the middle third of the lower leg in addition to the soleus; these include the tibialis anterior, flexor digitorum longus, extensor digitorum longus, extensor hallucis longus, peroneus brevis, and peroneus longus. Distal defects often require free tissue transfers because of the paucity of sizeable local flaps (Fig. 108.7). Some local flaps are available, however. Reversed flow fasciocutaneous flaps based on perforators from the posterior tibial artery[67] and flaps based on the dorsalis pedis[68] can be used for defects in the ankle area. V-Y flaps,[69] medial[70] and lateral[71] plantar flaps, the flexor digitorum longus flap,[72] and other local flaps are available for smaller defects of the foot.

Breast

Breast cancer is currently the most common malignancy in American women. Although breast-conserving surgery is increasingly utilized for the treatment of smaller breast cancers, mastectomy is still indicated for more extensive lesions and for cancers that recur after breast-conserving treatment. In addition, prophylactic mastectomies are sometimes indicated in patients at high risk for the development of cancer because of a strong family history, genetic predisposition, or previously noted atypia. Women undergoing mastectomy for any of these reasons are potential candidates for reconstruction. Concerns previously expressed regarding the possibility of breast reconstruction limiting the detection of recurrent cancers have not been substantiated.[73] In addition, no increased risk of recurrent cancer has been seen in women undergoing breast reconstruction.[74]

The benefits of reconstruction in terms of improvement in self-image are well documented.[75] Not all women eligible for reconstruction choose it in that they cope with the deformity in other ways. The most commonly cited reasons for undergoing reconstruction include the improved ability to utilize a wider variety of clothing styles. Reconstruction is more commonly of importance to younger women than older women, although age is not a contraindication to undergoing breast reconstruction.

Reconstruction can be carried out at the time of mastectomy or in a delayed fashion. Immediate reconstruction is more commonly associated with a lower amount of perioperative stress and is often preferred.[76] The previously popular idea that women undergoing delayed reconstruction would appreciate the result more after actually seeing the mastectomy defect has not been substantiated. Delayed reconstruction is preferable to some women, and is sometimes recommended to optimize aesthetic results if aggressive radiation is planned in the postoperative period.

There are a large number of reconstructive methods available for breast reconstruction, and all have advantages and disadvantages. The simplest methods involve breast implants similar to those used in breast augmentation. The implants that are generally available at this time are saline-filled implants with a silicone outer shell. They require adequate skin and ideally muscle coverage to assure an adequate result that matches the contralateral breast; this is frequently not the case unless a skin-sparing mastectomy is utilized.[77] If inadequate skin cover exists, the chest skin can be preliminarily expanded using a tissue expander before placement of a permanent breast implant in a second operative procedure. No additional incisions are required, and only limited additional surgery is necessary to reconstruct a breast in this manner. This method has the disadvantage of requiring a minimum of 3 to 4 months to complete, however. The patient must return to the outpatient office approximately weekly for 4 to 8 weeks until the expander is fully expanded. The expander is ideally overexpanded 1.5- to 2 fold to generate surplus skin to provide a more natural ptotic contour to the ultimate reconstructive result. After expansion is completed, the skin is generally allowed to relax for approximately 4 to 6 weeks before replacement of the expander with a permanent prosthesis. Although reconstructive results are often adequate, especially for smaller, nonptotic breasts, the accuracy of reconstruction is often less precise when implants are utilized as opposed to when autogenous tissue is utilized.[78] In

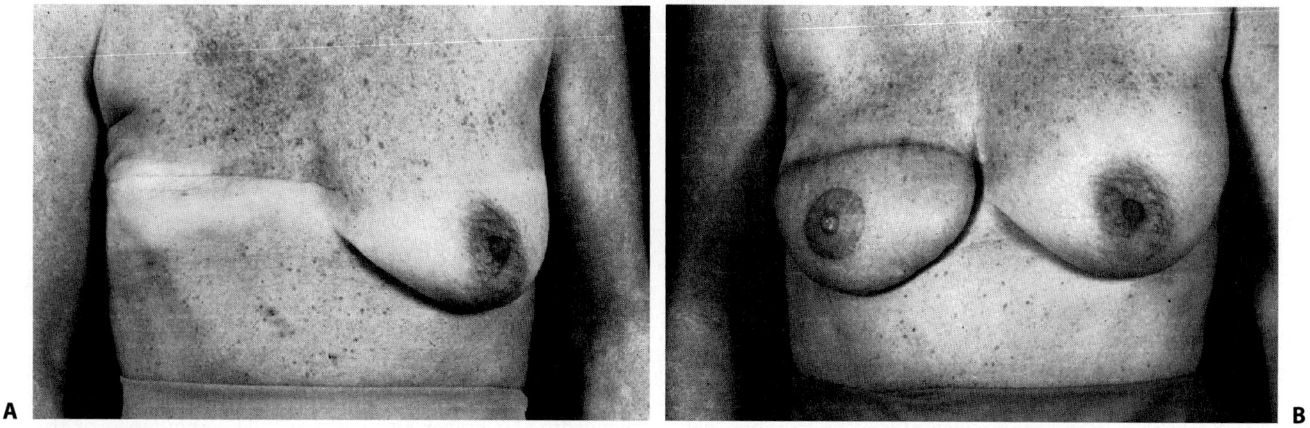

FIGURE 108.8. Breast reconstruction with transverse rectus myocutaneous (TRAM) flap. A. Preoperative view. B. Postoperative view.

addition, possible complications specifically related to the implant make this method of reconstruction less desirable to some. These complications include capsular contracture, which can produce an unnatural firmness, wrinkling of the implant that is visible through the skin, and the rare implant deflation that requires implant replacement.

More involved methods of reconstruction utilize flaps of different sorts. Local flaps and breast-sharing procedures have been utilized, and the microvascular transfer of gluteal or other tissue is preferred by some.[79] The most commonly utilized flaps, however, are the transverse rectus myocutaneous (TRAM) flap[80] and, to a lesser degree, the latissimus dorsi flap.[81] The TRAM flap involves the transfer of skin and subcutaneous fat from the lower abdomen to the chest for reconstruction of the breast mound (Fig. 108.8). This flap can be transferred while maintaining its myocutaneous pedicle or by free transfer, anastamosing the inferior epigastric vessels to either the thoracodorsal vessels or internal mammary vessels in the chest area. The advantage of microvascular transfer is primarily improved tissue reliability because of dependence on the primary blood supply to the lower abdominal area (deep inferior epigastric vessels) as opposed to the secondary blood supply (deep superior epigastric vessels) that is relied upon when the flap is transferred while maintaining its muscular pedicle. Improved postoperative abdominal muscle function as the result of more limited muscle harvest with the free flap has not been substantiated.[82] More recently, the utilization of perforator flaps based on the deep inferior epeigastric artery, which preserve nearly the entire muscle, have been popularized. Somewhat less tissue can be reliably transferred with these perforator flaps than the more traditional free TRAM flaps. Disadvantages of microvascular transfer are increased technical complexity, which may lengthen operative time, and an increased, although limited, likelihood of complete as opposed to marginal flap loss.

Most commonly, women must basically choose between methods of reconstruction involving an expander and/or implant and methods involving myocutaneous flaps. The ultimate decision is generally made by the patient based on her individual assessment of the different advantages of the two approaches (Table 108.5).

TABLE 108.5. Decision Making in Breast Reconstruction.

Reasons for choosing an expander/implant:
1. No additional scars
2. Less additional time in surgery
3. Lower risk of complications and no risk of problems such as abdominal hernia or other donor site wound complications
4. No additional time in hospital
5. No functional loss from muscle transfer

Reasons for choosing a myocutaneous flap:
1. Better aesthetic result on average
2. Avoid concern regarding long-term problems with implant such as rupture, capsular contracture
3. With transverse rectus myocutaneous (TRAM) flap, get concomitant abdominoplasty
4. Result nearly complete after one stage; prolonged period of expansion requiring 4–8 clinic visits over several months followed by second procedure for implant placement is avoided

Other Breast Surgery and Congenital Chest Wall Deformities

Plastic surgeons are often involved in the correction of other breast deformities. Congenital abnormalities include breast aplasia and Poland's syndrome. Poland's syndrome involves congenital absence of the sternal head of the pectoralis major and sometimes other muscles in conjunction with chest wall deformities, breast hypoplasia or aplasia, and hand deformities. Surgical treatment involves reconstruction of the muscle contour with a latissimus dorsi muscle flap[83] or prosthetic device and reconstruction of the breast mound by one of the previously discussed methods. Chest wall reconstruction may be required in individuals with severe deformities.[84]

Reduction mammoplasty is performed for correction of macromastia. Macromastia can lead to back pain, neck pain, shoulder pain and grooving from bra straps, generalized breast discomfort, and intertriginous irritation in the skin underneath the breast. In addition, physical activities can be substantially limited by the weight and discomfort of excessively large breasts. Breast reduction is carried out to improve these symptoms and is considered a functional procedure more than an aesthetic one. There are a variety of methods available for breast reduction but all involve excision of excess skin and glandular tissue and reshaping of the remaining tissue in a near-anatomic manner. All methods have the disadvantages of creating significant scarring and possibly interfering with normal nipple sensation and glandular function. In spite of these limitations, patient satisfaction with reduction mammoplasty is high. Outcome studies evaluating the results of reduction mammoplasty have demonstrated improvement in symptoms in more than 90% of patients.[85]

Individuals without excess breast tissue but with a ptotic breast form as the result of age or pregnancy sometimes desire a mastopexy to lift the breast to a more youthful position. Breast shape can be improved, but incisions somewhat similar to those used in reduction mammoplasties are often required, resulting in significant scarring.

Breast augmentation is indicated for the correction of mammary hypoplasia. In breast augmentation, a breast implant is placed behind the breast mound, and often the underlying pectoralis muscle to increase breast projection. Most currently used implants are saline-filled silicone implants because a moratorium was placed on silicone gel-filled implants in April 1992. Silicone implants are generally well tolerated, regardless of the fill material, and have proved superior to other prosthetic materials used in the past. Although patient satisfaction with implants is high, women with implants must be counseled that special techniques need to be utilized for mammography[86] and that the quality of mammograms is somewhat impaired by the presence of implants.[87] Implants are not associated with any increase in the development of carcinoma, however,[88] and have not been associated with a delay in the diagnosis of cancer.[89] Concerns have been expressed about a possible association of silicone implants with autoimmune disease, but evidence accumulated to date has not supported such an association.[90]

Capsular contracture is a possible complication of augmentation mammoplasty and is related to the foreign-body reaction generated by the implant.[91] The foreign-body response results in the formation of a capsule of scar tissue surrounding the implant that can contract and make the breast feel abnormally firm. The variables that determine whether the scar capsule which forms around the implants becomes firm or remains soft have not been fully elucidated, although low-grade infection, blood collections, submammary (as opposed to subpectoral) implant positioning, and silicone gel implants have all been implicated as potentially contributing to increasing degrees of firmness.

Gynecomastia is enlargement of the male breast. The condition is common during puberty because of proliferation of breast parenchyma. Most commonly, the breast tissue involutes in 3 to 18 months, although in some individuals it persists. Gynecomastia can have a number of alternative etiologies that must be considered, including endocrine imbalances, testicular or endocrine tumors, a variety of drugs, liver disease, and marijuana and anabolic steroid use. Nonresolving gynecomastia may require surgical treatment, either by direct excision, suction-assisted lipectomy, or a combination of the two modalities.

Congenital Defects

One of the major categories of problems treated by plastic surgeons is defects of a congenital nature. All parts of the body are susceptible to congenital deformities, and plastic surgeons are involved in the treatment of many of them, either independently or as members of a multidisciplinary team. For some deformities, rehabilitation of function is the primary goal, while for others restoration of form may be more critical. Several of the more commonly treated congenital deformities are discussed.

Cleft Lip and Palate

Clefts of the lip and palate are one of the most common congenital defects of the head and neck. The cause of the deformities is unknown, although genetic as well as environmental factors most likely play a role. The lip and palate normally develop through migration of neural crest cells in the developing embryo between the 3rd and 12th week of gestation. Defects in this cellular migration generate the cleft deformities. The ratio of isolated cleft lips to combined clefts of the lip and palate to isolated cleft palate is 21:46:33, according to Fraser and Calnan.[92] The incidence of the cleft lip and palate deformity varies among individuals of different racial backgrounds from 2.1 in 1000 live births in Asians to 1 in 1000 live births in Caucasians to 0.41 in 1000 in African Americans, although such a racial predilection is not seen for cleft palate alone.[93–95] Cleft lip and palate may be a component of a number of other syndromes such as Stickler syndrome.

Repair of clefts of the lip and palate are generally carried out at different times. Neither problem is life threatening, and repairs can be electively planned. The classic timing for repair of cleft lips follows the rule of tens: 10 weeks of age, 10g of hemoglobin, and 10 pounds in weight. Surgery is postponed for this interval to allow the neonate to develop immunocompetence and limit the risk of anesthesia. The delay also allows the baby to grow, and the larger structures facilitate the surgery. Although the traditional time frame has been modified in some centers, it remains a good general guideline.

Cleft palates have traditionally been repaired in the 12- to 24-month time frame. Cleft palate repair is delayed to allow further growth and development to minimize bleeding or airway difficulties. It is undesirable to postpone cleft palate repair indefinitely, however, in that an intact palate is required for normal speech development. Formal speech does not usually develop until 18 to 24 months, and it was therefore thought for some time that surgery could be safely postponed until that time point.[96] More recent information suggests that rudiments of speech begin to develop at 3 to 9 months, and many now perform cleft palate repairs in this earlier time interval. There is some evidence that operating at 3 to 9 months improves speech results.[97]

An additional consideration in the timing of surgical repairs of cleft structures is the effect of surgical intervention on subsequent facial development. Both lip and palate repairs most likely interfere with subsequent facial growth, although opinions differ as to whether lip or palate repair has the greatest effect. There is little evidence that limited delays in repair of the cleft lip or palate during the first 2 years of life make a significant difference in facial growth in that growth normally continues until the teen years.

Numerous methods of cleft lip repair have been described, but the two most commonly used methods are the rotation advancement method described by Ralph Millard[98] and the triangular flap method described by Tennison and modified by Randall[99] (Fig. 108.9). These techniques utilize a variant of a Z-plasty to provide lip lengthening on the cleft side. The Millard method involves a Z-plasty at the superior portion of the lip under the nostril sill whereas the Randall–

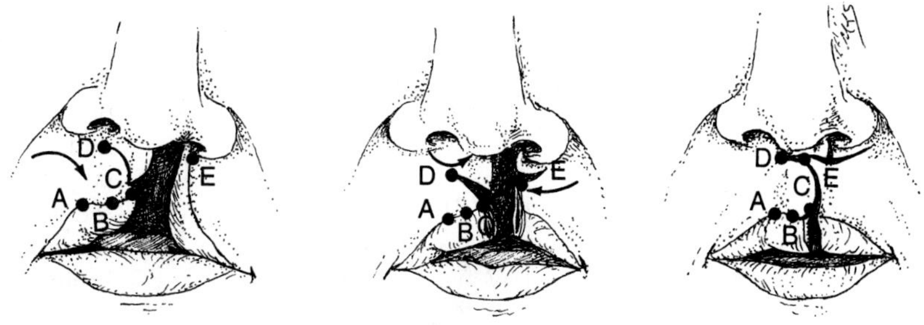

FIGURE 108.9. Cleft lip repair using Millard's rotation advancement technique.

Tennison technique utilizes a Z-plasty variant in the lower portion of the lip. Reported advantages of Millard's method include tightness in the upper lip where it more normally occurs, a scar that better mimics a normal philtrum, and greater flexibility in its application. Some believe the Millard method creates more nasal distortion of the cleft side, however, particularly in wide clefts. The Randall–Tennison method is less likely to distort the nose but it generates a less anatomic scar and is more difficult to modify secondarily. Holtmann and Wray compared the two techniques in unilateral clefts and could not demonstrate a statistically significant difference between the two.[100] All current techniques involve repair of the upper and lower components of the orbicularis muscle.

The bilateral cleft lip deformity repair generally has less satisfactory long-term results because of the greater severity of the deformity. As for unilateral cleft lip repairs, a large number of methods of repair have been described. Some involve more of a straight line repair while others involve slight lengthening of the medial lip segment (the prolabium) with Z-plasty, such as tissue rearrangements either in the upper or lower portion of the lips. There is less unanimity concerning which method of repair is optimal.

With wide clefts and particularly with wide bilateral clefts, preliminary lip adhesions are sometimes done. A lip adhesion is a preliminary straight line closure that provides tension to realign widely separated lip and palatal segments before a secondary, more definitive repair. Another technique gaining more popularity is the utilization of presurgical maxillary orthopedics to apply tension on displaced bones to better align them before surgical intervention. This method limits the amount of surgical dissection that is sometimes required and may improve ultimate aesthetic and functional results.

Many methods of palatoplasty have been described, although none is uniformly associated with normal speech. The oldest method of repair is the von Langenbeck palatoplasty, which involves elevating bilateral bipedicled flaps of mucoperiosteum from the palate through incisions at the cleft margin and on the lingual side of the alveolus.[101] Although still used by some, the von Langenbeck method has been supplanted for the most part by methods that provide additional palatal lengthening. Variations on the Veau–Wardill–Kilner method, which involves transposing flaps of mucoperiosteum posteriorly in a V–Y fashion, are used by many.[102] Alternatively, double-opposing Z-plasties as described by Furlow[103] are also commonly used. Intravelar veloplasty involving repair of the levator palati within the hemipalates can be performed as a component of any of the repairs, and it is often carried out in hopes of improving speech result.[104] The critical measure of success for palate repairs is normal speech, which may be achieved in 85% to 90% of patients with palatoplasty combined with postoperative speech therapy. In patients in whom speech inadequacy from velopharyngeal incompetence persists after palatoplasty, a secondary procedure is often required. Most commonly, this involves a pharyngeal flap. Pharyngeal flaps are elevated from the posterior pharyngeal wall and affixed to the palate to facilitate velopharyngeal closure.[105] Alternatively, a pharyngoplasty involving transfer of lateral pharyngeal tissue to the posterior pharyngeal wall has been used.[106] More recently, some have used Furlow's double opposing Z-plasty as a secondary procedure in patients with velopharyngeal incompetence after an alternative primary technique has been utilized. These secondary procedures are successful at establishing normal speech in 50% to 95% of patients.

Other components of the cleft lip and palate deformity are the cleft of the dental alveolus and the cleft lip nasal deformity, which differs in unilateral and bilateral clefts. Although more is being done for the nasal deformity at the time of lip repair,[107] additional nasal procedures are often performed before school age, and definitive nasal repair is often delayed until nasal growth is complete in the teens. Alveolar repair often involves bone grafts and is commonly carried out before the eruption of the canine teeth at the age of 9 to 10.[108]

Craniofacial Surgery

The field of craniofacial surgery is concerned with the correction of congenital abnormalities of the skull and facial structures. Clefts of the lip and palate, the most common craniofacial anomalies, have already been discussed. A variety of additional deformities can occur; similar to clefts of the lip and palate, these deformities result from defects in embryological development, primarily during the first 12 weeks of gestation (Fig. 108.10). The etiology of these additional craniofacial deformities is unknown, although they also most likely result from a combination of genetic and environmental factors. The list of potential environmental contributors is extensive, including radiation, infections of various sorts, drugs including diphenylhydantoin (Dilantin) and isotretinoin (Accutane), and chemical exposure. In most cases, a specific etiological factor cannot be identified. Recent advances in molecular biology have provided greater insight into the role of genetic factors in the etiology of several craniofacial syndromes. Crouzon's syndrome has been mapped to a defect on the long arm of chromosome 10 in the gene for fibroblast growth factor 2.[109] Other syndromes, including Apert's and Pfeiffer's syndromes, have been related to a mutation in the same gene.[110,111]

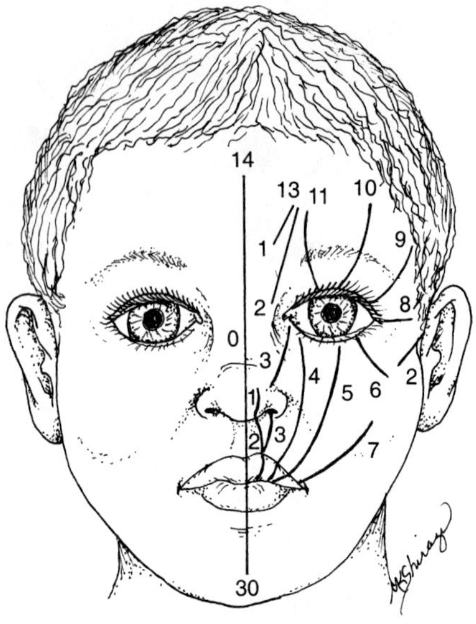

FIGURE 108.10. Tessier's classification of facial clefts.

The evaluation of a child with craniofacial anomalies almost always involves both computed tomography (CT) scans and cephalometric X-rays,[112–114] and often photometric or computerized imaging information as well. Cephalometric X-rays involve standardized radiographs taken so as to allow precise evaluation of the relationships of the various craniofacial structures. These films assist in planning the amount of surgical movement required to create normal anatomic harmony. Limited deformities may require only orthognathic surgery in which the maxilla, mandible, or both jaws are surgically repositioned. More extensive craniofacial deformities may require extensive reconstruction involving the entire skull.

Facial Trauma

Soft tissue injuries to the face can result from blunt or sharp trauma. In most cases, repair involves reapproximating tissues as anatomically as possible. Special attention needs to be given to more specialized anatomic structures such as the eyelid, ear, nose, and mouth to ensure that proper anatomic alignment is achieved.

Facial fractures are most commonly a result of either a motor vehicle accident or an assault by another individual. The nature of the injury produced is determined by the mechanism of injury and the anatomic location involved. The bones of the face vary in their susceptibility to fractures; their resistance to injury is demonstrated in Figure 108.11.[115] Greater force is required to break the stronger bones of the face, such as the supraorbital portion of the frontal bone, as compared to weaker bones such as the nose. The fracture pattern gives insight into the severity of the traumatic insult that occurred and the likelihood of coexistent injuries. For example, nasal fractures are often isolated injuries resulting from relatively minor trauma. A fracture of the supraorbital rim requires a significant traumatic insult and is frequently associated with other major injuries.

Most fractures can be diagnosed on physical examination. Inspection often demonstrates ecchymoses surrounding fracture sites and asymmetries in injured facial structures. Intraoral examination may demonstrate malocclusion when there are mandibular fractures, maxillary fractures, or both. Careful palpation of the bony structures of the face both externally and intraorally identifies fractures as points where there are stepoffs in the normally smooth bony contours. Fracture sites are generally also noted to be extremely tender to palpation in the awake patient. Midfacial mobility can be strongly indicative of a maxillary fracture.

The management of facial fractures has become more sophisticated in recent years. Diagnosis has been improved by the routine use of CT scans, sometimes with three-dimensional reconstructions. CT scans provide extremely detailed information regarding the nature of the injury and are particularly useful for areas that are difficult to visualize, such as the orbital floor. The surgical approach to these injuries includes direct anatomic exposure of as many fracture sites as possible, precise anatomic reduction of these fractures, rigid internal fixation of the damaged bones, and primary bone grafting when needed to accurately reconstruct skeletal deficiencies. Bony repair is supplemented by periosteal suspension of the soft tissues after fracture fixation.

Fractures of the zygoma frequently involve condurrent fractures at or near the points of articulation of the zygoma with the surrounding bones, producing what is known as a zygomatic complex fracture. Zygomatic complex fractures involve fractures to the zygomaticofrontal region along the lateral orbital rim, the zygomaticotemporal region in the vicinity of the zygomatic arch, the zygomaticomaxillary region along the infraorbital rim and lateral buttress of the maxilla, and in the zygomaticopterygoid region deep within the fascial skeleton. The masseter muscle provides the primary deforming force on the zygoma after such injuries. The signs and symptoms that may be present when a zygoma is fractured, in addition to localized stepoffs and tenderness, include cheek and eyelid edema, circumorbital ecchymosis, subconjunctival ecchymosis, unilateral epistaxis, anesthesia or hypoesthesia of the cheek, upper lip, and gingiva (infraorbital nerve), and diplopia or displacement of the globe. Occasionally the zygomatic arch may be fractured in an isolated

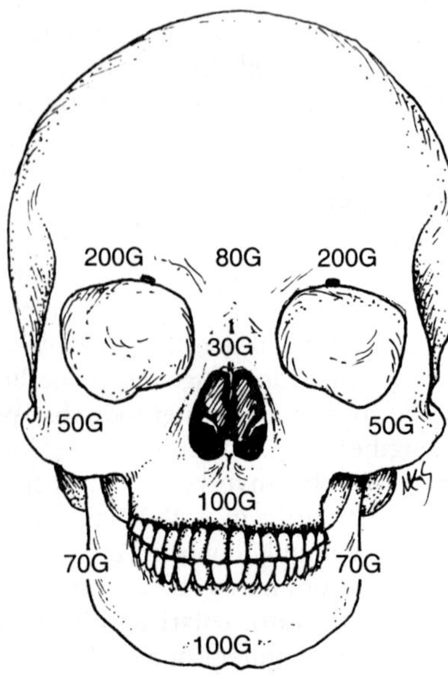

FIGURE 108.11. Resistance to fracture of facial bones.

fashion, resulting in depression on the involved side of the face.

Nondisplaced fractures require no specific treatment other than a soft diet and a follow-up evaluation to ensure that no bony displacement develops with time. Isolated zygomatic arch fractures can generally be treated by reduction without internal fixation through incisions in the temporal scalp or mouth. Displaced quadrapod fractures almost always require open reduction and fixation, however.

Zygomatic fractures by definition involve the floor of the orbit in that the zygomatic bone makes up the lateral and anterior portions of the orbital wall. Orbital floor fractures that occur as a component of zygomatic complex fracture are considered impure blowout fractures. Orbital fractures that occur without involving the bones of the orbital rim are considered pure blowout fractures. Isolated orbital floor fractures most commonly involve the inferior wall of the orbit where the bone is thin and concave. The infraorbital nerve runs through the bone in this location, creating additional bony weakness.

In addition to facial deformities related to bony displacement, the main problems resulting from orbital floor fractures are diplopia and enophthalmus. Diplopia most commonly occurs as the result of restricted upward gaze, which is most commonly caused by entrapment of the inferior rectus or inferior oblique muscle in the fracture line. Other periorbital structures such as periorbital fat or Lockwood's ligament, which supports the eye, can less commonly become incarcerated in fracture lines and restrict eye movement. Diplopia resulting from entrapment must be differentiated from diplopia caused by damage to the extraocular muscles or the nerves that innervate them. The etiology of diplopia can often be determined by a forced duction test in which the inferior rectus muscle is held with a forcep and the eye is mechanically rotated within the orbit. The inability to rotate the eye on a forced duction test is diagnostic of mechanical entrapment. The indications for surgical exploration of an orbital floor fracture in a patient with diplopia include a positive forced duction test, radiographic evidence of extraocular muscle entrapment, or no symptomatic improvement within 7 to 10 days after an injury.

Enophthalmus after orbital floor injuries results from either enlargement of the bony orbital cavity, escape of orbital fat into the maxillary sinus, orbital fat necrosis, or muscle entrapment in the fracture line with scarring and contracture pulling the globe backward and downward. Early enophthalmus, a large orbital floor defect likely to result in late enophthalmus, and dystopia are indications for surgical exploration of orbital floor fractures.

Surgical correction of orbital floor fractures involves reduction of fracture fragments in as anatomical a manner as possible and often includes placement of either a bone graft or alloplastic implant to provide additional support. Titanium or vitallium implants made of materials similar to those used for facial plates are commonly used for correction of orbital floor defects.

Nasal fractures occur relatively commonly in that the nasal bones are among the weakest in the facial skeleton and the nose is a prominent anatomic structure. Simple displaced nasal fractures can generally be managed by closed reduction and external stabilization with a splint. More complex fractures, and especially those that include the nasoorbitoethmoid complex with resulting telecanthus, generally require open reduction and fixation, combined often with bone grafting and reestablishment of normal medial canthal positioning.

Frontal bone injuries involving the frontal sinus require open treatment when there is significant displacement of the anterior wall creating a contour irregularity, significant displacement of the posterior wall of the sinus with sinus disruption, and a persistent cerebrospinal fluid leak and/or injury or obstruction to the nasofrontal duct that drains the sinus into the nasal cavity. For simple fractures of the anterior sinus wall, that are not associated with significant disruption of the sinus or the nasofrontal ducts, simple fracture reduction and fixation are adequate. When the nasofrontal ducts are severely damaged and drainage from the sinus is questionable, the sinus must be obliterated. To accomplish this, the walls of the sinus are first stripped of mucosa and then burred to remove any mucosal remnants. The ducts are then plugged, and the sinus is obliterated with bone, muscle, or fat. The sinus may also be allowed to spontaneously ossify.[116] Alternatively, the posterior wall of the sinus can be removed, allowing the sinus cavity to fill with cranial matter.[117] This latter approach, known as cranialization, is also of use in severe injuries to the posterior sinus wall.

LeFort described the three lines of weakness through which maxillary fractures generally occur.[118,119] The fracture patterns are shown in Figure 108.12. Signs and symptoms of maxillary fractures include bilateral circumorbital and subconjunctival ecchymosis and edema, facial lengthening, and malocclusion. Maxillary movement can often be detected when anterior traction is applied to the upper alveolus while stabilizing the head in the region of the nasal root. Although a soft diet may be adequate for nondisplaced fractures, particularly in edentulous patients, most maxillary fractures require open reduction and fixation. Whenever possible, stabilization based on occlusion to a normal mandible provides the best assurance of a good result.

Mandibular fractures are relatively common as a result of the prominence of the jaw in the facial contour. The curved anatomy of the mandible predisposes to concurrent fractures

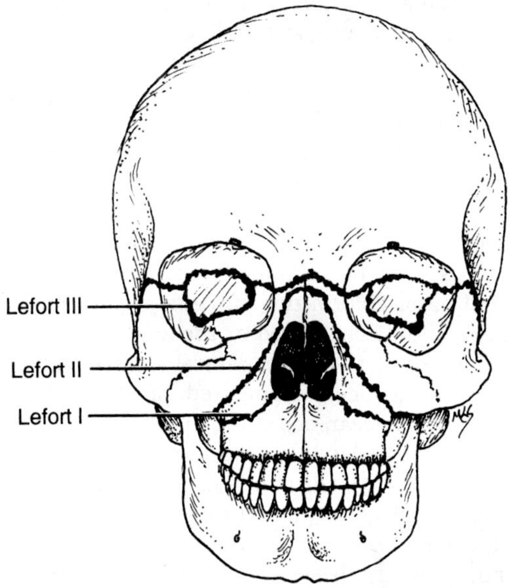

FIGURE 108.12. LeFort fracture patterns.

in more than one location. The mental foramen and the long roots of the canine teeth as well as impacted third molars create points of weakness that are particularly prone to fracture. The subcondylar area is the weakest part of the bone and is also a common fracture site. In addition to localized pain and palpable fracture edges, mandibular fractures may also lead to malocclusion, trismus caused by injury to the masseter, and lip anesthesia or paraesthesias caused by damage to the inferior alveolar nerve that runs through the body of the mandible. The goals of treatment for mandibular fractures are to achieve anatomical reduction and stabilization of the fractured segments. Such treatment reestablishes pretraumatic occlusion and restores facial contour, height, and symmetry. Although nondisplaced, immobile fractures may be treated with a soft diet alone, most mandibular fractures require surgical treatment. Stabilization alone in maxillomandibular fixation may be adequate for simple, relatively stable fractures. This is accomplished by fixation of arch bars to the upper and lower teeth and immobilizing the jaws by fixing them together with either wires or elastics. The period for which maxillomandibular fixation is required for nonfixed fractures is not clear. Chuong suggested clinical union by 4 weeks in 79% of patients and by 5 weeks in 90%,[120] and a 4- to 6-week period of immobilization is often used. Immobilization for as little as 10 to 14 days is often recommended for intracapsular condylar fractures to limit late ankylosis of the temporomandibular joint, however.

Comminuted fractures and less stable fractures such as those involving the parasymphyseal area require more stabilization than maxillomandibular fixation alone can provide and generally require open reduction and internal fixation; this is carried out after initially reestablishing normal occlusion by maxillomandibular fixation. Sometimes internal fixation is utilized to limit the period of jaw immobilization required when it is not otherwise absolutely required.

Aesthetic Surgery

Aesthetic surgery is that component of plastic surgery which involves enhancing or modifying anatomic features that are otherwise normal to improve their appearance. Some procedures are done to modify anatomic characteristics that were never believed to be attractive. Breast augmentation, which was discussed earlier, falls into this category, as do liposuction and rhinoplasty. Other aesthetic procedures are done to rejuvenate features that were previously felt to be attractive but which have become less so because of the effects of pregnancy and/or aging. Rhytidectomy, abdominoplasty, brachioplasty, thigh lifts, and mastopexy fall into this category.

Rhinoplasty can be performed to correct either congenital or acquired nasal deformities. In rhinoplasty, the structural components of the nose including the lower lateral cartilages, the dorsal septum, the upper lateral cartilages, and/or the nasal bones are reduced, augmented, or otherwise modified so as to alter the appearance of the nose. This intervention is ideally accomplished while maintaining or improving the nasal functions of facilitating air flow and humidifying inspired air. Ideal nasal proportions have been described,[121] but the ultimate decisions regarding the optimal appearance of any nose and the best methods for achieving it remain largely subjective.

Liposuction is currently the most commonly performed aesthetic surgical procedure. Liposuction is carried out to remove excess fat that does not respond to diet and exercise from specific anatomic areas. Although adipocytes multiply during early childhood and puberty, no new adipocytes are formed after adolescence under normal circumstances. In adults, moderate weight gain is accompanied by an increase in the amount of lipid stored by individual adipocytes and not an increase in the number of adipocytes. New adipocytes are formed only if weight gain exceeds approximately 40 kg.[122] The number of adipocytes and their distribution vary from individual to individual in a manner determined by their genetic background. All individuals have specific anatomic locations that harbor more fatty tissue than others. Women characteristically have greater amounts of fat in the lower trunk, upper thighs, and buttocks, a gynoid pattern. In contrast, men accumulate extra fat in the trunk and flank areas, an android pattern.

Ideal liposuction candidates are not overweight and have good skin tone to allow skin redraping in a natural fashion. Although the indications for liposuction have broadened to include somewhat overweight individuals, liposuction is clearly not a treatment for obesity, and it does not treat skin irregularities caused by cellulite. Liposuction involves removal of fat by negative pressure applied by means of subcutaneously placed cannulae. Negative pressure of 1 atm and cannulae with a maximal diameter of 4 to 5 mm are currently used most commonly. Suction is ideally carried out using at least two incisions for each anatomic area treated to create a crisscross pattern in the subcutaneous layers (Fig. 108.13); this is done to diminish the likelihood of contour irregularities. Klein made a major contribution to liposuction when he described the "tumescent" anesthetic technique;[123] this involves infusing the areas to be treated with large volumes of saline including a dilute solution of lidocaine (0.1% or 0.05%) and epinephrine (1:1,000,000). Classically, the endpoint of the infusion is tumescence, although many prefer somewhat smaller volumes of infusate, using what is known as the superwet technique. In addition to sometimes allowing procedures to be performed without general anesthesia, the

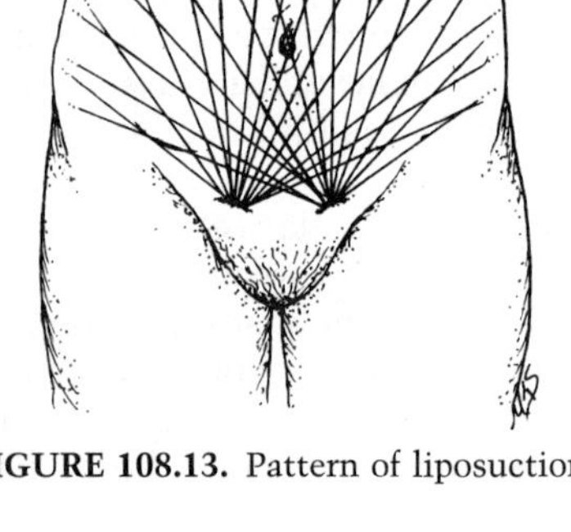

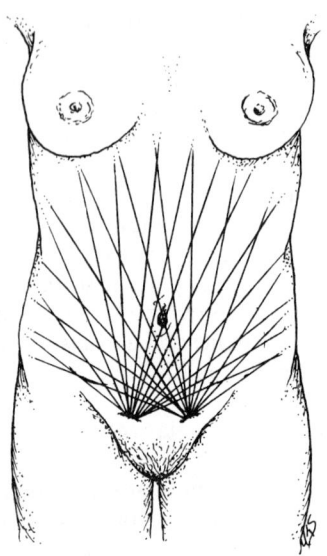

FIGURE 108.13. Pattern of liposuction.

tumescent technique also limits blood loss. Up to 35 mg/kg lidocaine has been successfully administered without causing lidocaine toxicity.[124] When general anesthesia is utilized for liposuction, tumescence is frequently generated with fluid containing epinephrine alone without the lidocaine to minimize blood loss and eliminate any concern regarding lidocaine toxicity. Recent additions to the liposuction armamentarium are power assistance and ultrasonic energy. Using the ultrasonic technique, an ultrasonic probe is advanced through the subcutaneous fat to emulsify the fat before aspiration. This technique allows easier and perhaps improved treatment of more fibrous areas such as the back and male chest. It is also believed by some to improve skin remodeling.

Abdominoplasty is often preferred as an alternative or adjunctive procedure to liposuction in individuals with excess, lax skin, and musculofascial laxity or diastasis in the abdominal area. These conditions most commonly result from massive weight loss or pregnancy. The technique utilized for abdominoplasty varies depending on the specific anatomic abnormality as well as surgeon preference. In individuals of near-normal weight whose primary deformity results from past pregnancies, techniques using transversely oriented suprapubic incisions and undermining of the abdominal skin are most commonly utilized. After skin flap mobilization, the abdominal fascia is plicated, and excess skin, often including a significant number of stretch marks, is excised. The abdominal skin is then repositioned, creating a smooth, taut contour. The umbilicus is circumscribed and left in situ during elevation of the abdominal skin flap, and it is later translocated through the abdominal flap after the flap repositioning. Alternatively, a miniabdominoplasty is sometimes performed when the skin excess is less pronounced and isolated to the infraumbilical area.[125] With this technique, a smaller incision is utilized, skin mobilization is less extensive, less skin is removed, and the umbilicus is not circumscribed. At times the umbilicus is freed and translocated up to 2 cm inferiorly. This procedure is frequently combined with liposuction.

Different abdominoplasty techniques are required in patients who were formerly morbidly obese and whose weight loss has left them with significant amounts of excess skin.[126] In these patients, extensive skin undermining is likely to result in skin necrosis in that the vascularity of the skin is much less dependable than in patients with skin excess from pregnancy. Also, the location of skin excess is less localized, and more extensive incisions are frequently required. These patients are generally less concerned about the extensive scarring generated by these incisions in that their body habitus is often not conducive to clothing and swimwear that bare the abdomen. A commonly used technique in these patients includes both transverse and vertical skin excisions, which result in an inverted-T incision line. The transverse incision at times extends circumferentially around the body. Abdominoplasty frequently facilitates the correction of coexistent ventral hernias that are common in these patients.

In the extremities, the effects of aging are seen as sagging of tissues. These effects can be exacerbated in individuals who have experienced significant weight fluctuations. Correction of skin excess in the upper extremities necessitates a brachioplasty; in the lower extremity, it requires a thigh lift. A brachioplasty involves excision of redundant tissue from the posterior upper arm, and a thigh lift involves excision of excess tissue in the region of the groin crease.

Other aesthetic procedures are performed to reverse the effects of aging. As the body ages, skin thins and becomes less elastic, subcutaneous tissues droop, and even the bony structure of the face changes to a limited degree. These changes are manifested in different ways in different parts of the face (Fig. 108.14). In the upper face, the brow droops, transverse and glabellar skin creases become more prominent, the nasal tip droops, and the eyelids become redundant and lax. In the lower face, drooping subcutaneous fat and thinning of the skin results in a prominent nasolabial fold, jowls, and a poorly defined jawline, often with prominent bands produced by the underlying platysma muscle. Brow lifts address drooping brows and prominent glabellar and transverse skin creases. Traditionally this procedure was performed through a bicoronal incision, but more recently the endoscopic approach through limited incisions has become more popular. Blepharoplasty addresses skin laxity and contour irregularities that develop in the eyelids. It includes excision of excess eyelid

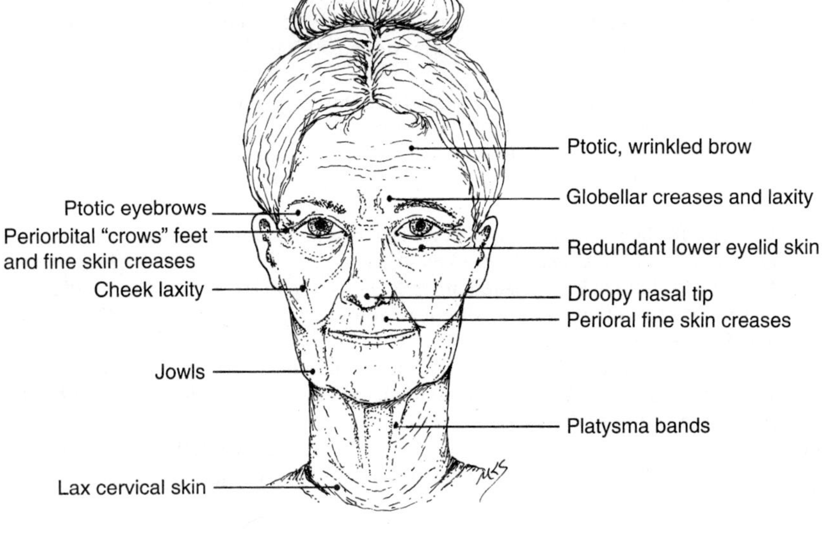

FIGURE 108.14. Stigmata of facial aging.

skin along with fat bulging through the often attenuated orbital septum. The cheek, jowl, and neck areas are best addressed by rhytidectomy. Excess skin is excised, deeper structures of the face are often tightened, and the facial skin is repositioned in a more youthful, taut manner during a rhytidectomy.

Although each of these procedures can be performed individually, they are frequently performed together in that the effects of aging are often manifest throughout the face. Fine wrinkling resulting from age and often excessive actinic exposure may require chemical peels, dermabrasion, or CO_2 laser treatment either independently or as an adjunct to the aforementioned procedures. In spite of all these treatment modalities, some effects of aging remain relatively resistant to surgical correction. Deep nasolabial folds, for example, are rarely eradicated by any currently existing surgical manipulation.

Conclusion

Plastic surgeons are dedicated to the restoration of form and function lost as the result of congenital defects, trauma, infectious diseases, neoplasia, or previous surgery. This chapter highlights the management of some of the major problems treated by plastic surgeons. The chapter should be viewed more as a sampler than an encyclopedic treatise in that the space available does not permit a comprehensive discussion of all problems managed by plastic surgeons. The key element that defines plastic surgery, however, is the approach to treating these problems, and this sampler has, hopefully, conveyed the essence of this thought process.

References

1. Teplitz C, Davis D, Mason AD, et al. Pseudomonas burn wound sepsis: I. Pathogenesis of experimental burn wound sepsis. J Surg Res 1964;5:200–216.
2. Robson MC, Heggers JP. Surgical infection, II: the beta-hemolytic streptococcus. J Surg Res 1969;9:289–292.
3. Kucan JO, Robson MC, Heggers JP, et al. Comparison of silver sulfadiazine, povidone-iodine and physiological saline in the treatment of chronic pressure ulcers. J Am Geriatr Soc 1981; 29:232–235.
4. Hebda PA, Flynn KJ, Dohar JE. Evaluation of the efficacy of enzymatic debriding agents for removal of necrotic tissue and promotion of healing in porcine skin wounds. Wounds 1988; 10:83–96.
5. Zitelli JA. Wound healing by secondary intention: a cosmetic appraisal. J Am Acad Dermatol 1983;9:407–415.
6. Anderson AB, Colecchi C, Baronoski R, et al. Local anesthesia in pediatric patients: topical TAC versus lidocaine. Ann Emerg Med 1990;19:519–522.
7. Lander J, Hodgins M, Nazarali S, et al. Determinants of success and failure of EMLA. Pain 1996;64:89–97.
8. Madden H, Edlich RF, Schauerhamer R, et al. Application of principles of fluid dynamics to surgical wound irrigation. Curr Top Surg Res 1971;3:85–93.
9. Gross A, Cutright DE, Bhaskar SN. Effectiveness of pulsating water jet lavage in treatment of contaminated crushed wounds. Am J Surg 1972;124:373–377.
10. Hamer ML, Robson MC, Krizek TJ, et al. Quantitative bacterial analysis of comparative wound irrigations. Ann Surg 1975;181: 819–822.
11. Schauerhamer RA, Edlich RF, Panek P, et al. Studies in the management of contaminated wounds, VII: susceptibility of surgical wounds to postoperative surface contamination. Am J Surg 1971;122:74–77.
12. Branemark PI, Albrektsson B, Lindstrom J, et al. Local tissue effects of wound disinfectants. Eur J Surg Suppl 1966; 357(suppl):166–176.
13. Rodeheaver GT, Smith SL, Thacker JG, et al. Mechanical cleansing of contaminated wounds with a surfactant. Am J Surg 1975;129:241–245.
14. Dirschl DR, Wilson FC. Topical antibiotic irrigation in the prophylaxis of operative wound infections in orthopedic surgery. Orthop Clin N Am 1991;22:419–426.
15. Ordman LJ, Gillman T. Studies in the healing of cutaneous wounds. II. The healing of epidermal, appendageal, and dermal injuries inflicted by suture needles and by suture material in the skin of pigs. Arch Surg 1966;93:883–910.
16. Conolly WB, Hun TK, Zederfeldt B, et al. Clinical comparison of surgical wounds closed by suture and adhesive tapes. Am J Surg 1969;117:318–322.
17. VanWinkle N, Hastings JC. Considerations in the choice of suture material for various tissues. Surg Gynecol Obstet 1972;135:113–126.
18. Jabs AD, Wider TM, DeBellis J, et al. The effect of fibrin glue on skin grafts in infected sites. Plast Reconstr Surg 1992;89:268–271.
19. Ersek RA, Schade K. Subcutaneous pseudobursa secondary to suction and surgery. Plast Reconstr Surg 1991;85:442–444.
20. Mandel MA. Minimal suture blepharoplasty: closure of incisions with autologous fibrin glue. Aesth Plast Surg 1992;16:269–272.
21. Quinn J, Wells G, Sutcliffe T, et al. A randomized trial comparing octylcyanoacrylate tissue adhesive and sutures in the management of lacerations. JAMA 1997;277:1527–1530.
22. deHoll D, Rodeheaver G, Edgerton MT, et al. Potentiation of infection by suture closure of dead space. Am J Surg 1974;127:716–720.
23. Magee C, Rodeheaver GT, Golden GT, et al. Potentiation of wound infection by surgical drains. Am J Surg 1976;131:547–549.
24. Rudolph R. The effect of skin graft preparation on wound contraction. Surg Gynecol Obstet 1976;142:49–56.
25. Ponten B. Grafted skin. Observations on innervation and other qualities. Eur J Surg Suppl 1960;267(suppl):1–78.
26. Pribaz JJ, Fine NA. Prelamination: defining a prefabricated flap—a case report and review. Microsurgery 1994;15:618–623.
27. Custer J, Edlich RF, Prusak M, et al. Studies in the management of the contaminated wound. V. An assessment of the effectiveness of pHisoHex and betadine surgical scrub solutions. Am J Surg 1971;121:572–575.
28. Millard DR Jr. Principlization of Plastic Surgery. Boston: Little, Brown, 1986.
29. Gonzlez-Ulloa M. Restoration of the face covering by means of selected skin in regional aesthetic units. Br J Plast Surg 1956;9:212–221.
30. Orticochea M. Four flap reconstruction technique. Br J Plast Surg 1967;20:159–171.
31. Orticochea M. New three-flap reconstruction technique. Br J Plast Surg 1971;24:184–188.
32. Ross JJ, Pham R. Closure of eyelid defects. J Dermatol Surg Oncol 1992;18:1061–1064.
33. Mustarde JC. Reconstruction of eyelids. Ann Plast Surg 1983;11:149–169.
34. Lawrence WT. The nasolabial rhomboid flap. Ann Plast Surg 1992;29:269–273.
35. Converse JM. New forehead flap for nasal reconstruction. Proc R Soc Med 1942;35:811–812.

36. Washio H. Retroauricular-temporal flap. Plast Reconstr Surg 1969;43:162–166.
37. Millard DR Jr. Total reconstructive rhinoplasty and a missing link. Plast Reconstr Surg 1966;37:167–183.
38. Abbe R. A new plastic operation for the relief of deformity due to double harelip [reprinted in Plast Reconstr Surg 1968;42:480–482]. Med Rec 1898;53:477.
39. Estlander JA. A method of reconstructing loss of substance in one lip from the other lip [reprinted in Plast Reconstr Surg 1968;42:361–366]. Arch Klin Chir 1872;14:622.
40. Karapandzic M. Reconstruction of lip defects by local arterial flaps. Br J Plast Surg 1974;27:93–97.
41. Antia NH, Buch VI. Chondrocutaneous advancement flap for the marginal defect of the ear. Plast Reconstr Surg 1967;39:472–477.
42. Orticochea M. Reconstruction of partial losses of the auricle. Plast Reconstr Surg 1970;46:403–405.
43. Brent B. Auricular repair with autogenous rib cartilage: two decades of experience with 600 cases. Plast Reconstr Surg 1992;90:355–374.
44. Hidalgo DA. Free fibula flap: a new method of mandibular reconstruction. Plast Reconstr Surg 1989;84:71–79.
45. Coleman JJ III, Tan KC, Searles JM, et al. Jejuanal free autograft: analysis of complications and their resolution. Plast Reconstr Surg 1989;84:589–595.
46. Cusumano RJ, Silver CE, Brauer RJ, et al. Pectoralis myocutaneous flap for replacement of the cervical esophagus. Head Neck 1989;11:450–456.
47. Hyans P, Moore JH Jr, Sinha L. Reconstruction of the chest wall with e-PTFE following major resection. Ann Plast Surg 1992;29:321–327.
48. McCormack PM. Use of prosthetic materials in chest wall reconstruction. Assets and liabilities. Surg Clin North Am 1989;69:965–976.
49. Ramirez OM, Ruas E, Dellon AL. Components separation method for closure of abdominal wall defects: an anatomic and clinical study. Plast Reconstr Surg 1990;86:519–526.
50. Hamilton JE. The repair of large or difficult hernias with mattress onlay grafts of fascia lata: a 21 year experience. Ann Surg 1968;167:85–90.
51. Dibbell DG Jr, Mixter RC, Dibbell DG Sr. Abdominal wall reconstruction (the mutton chop flap). Plast Reconstr Surg 1991;87:60–65.
52. Brown GL, Richardson JD, Malangoni MA. Comparison of prosthetic materials for abdominal wall reconstruction in the presence of contamination and infection. Ann Surg 1985;201: 705–711.
53. Griffith BH, Schultz RC. The prevention and surgical treatment of recurrent decubitus ulcers in patients with paraplegia. Plast Reconstr Surg 1961;27:248–260.
54. Disa JJ, Carlton JM Jr, Goldberg NH. Efficacy of operative cure of pressure sores. Plast Reconstr Surg 1992;89:272–278.
55. Wee JT, Joseph VT. A new technique of vaginal reconstruction using neurovascular pudendal-thigh flaps: a preliminary report. Plast Reconst Surg 1989;83:701–709.
56. Woods JE, Alter G, Meland B, et al. Experience with vaginal reconstruction utilizing the modified Singapore flap. Plast Reconstr Surg 1992;90:270–274.
57. Pickrell KS, Masterrn F, Georgiade N, et al. Rectal sphincter reconstruction using gracilis muscle technique. Plast Reconstr Surg 1954;13:46–55.
58. Orgell MG, Kucan JO. A double-split gluteus maximus muscle flap for the reconstruction of the rectal sphincter. Plast Reconstr Surg 1985;75:62–67.
59. Wexner SD, Gonzalez-Padron A, Teoh TA, et al. The stimulated gracilis neosphincter for fecal incontinence: a new use of an old concept. Plast Reconstr Surg 1996;98:693–699.
60. van Aalst VC, Werker PM, Stremel RW, et al. Electrically stimulated free-flap graciloplasty for urinary sphincter reconstruction: a new surgical procedure. Plast Reconstr Surg 1998; 102:84–91.
61. Byun JS, Cho BC, Baik BS. Results of a one stage penile reconstruction using an innervated radial osteocutaneous flap. J Reconstr Microsurg 1994;10:321–331.
62. Maruyama Y, Takeuchi S. The radial recurrent fasciocutaneous flap: reverse upper arm flap. Br J Plast Surg 1986;39:458–461.
63. Maruyama Y, Onishi K, Iwahira Y. The ulnar recurrent fasciocutaneous flap: reverse medial arm flap. Plast Reconstr Surg 1987;79:381–388.
64. Taylor GI, Corlett RJ, Boyd JB. The extended deep inferior epigastric flap: a clinical technique. Plast Reconstr Surg 1983;72:751–765.
65. Hayashi A, Maruyama Y. The lateral genicular artery flap. Ann Plast Surg 1990;24:310–317.
66. Hayashi A, Maruyama Y. The medial genicular artery flap. Ann Plast Surg 1990;25:174–180.
67. Hong G, Steffens K, Wang FG. Reconstruction of the lower leg with the reverse pedicled posterior tibial fasciocutaneous flap. Br J Plast Surg 1989;42:512–516.
68. McCraw JB, Furlow LT Jr. The dorsalis pedis arterialized flap. Plast Reconstr Surg 1975;55:177–185.
69. Colen LB, Replogle SL, Mathes SV. The V-Y plantar flap for reconstruction of the forefoot. Plast Reconstr Surg 1988;81:220–228.
70. Shanahan RE, Gingrass RP. Medial plantar sensory flap for the coverage of heel defects. Plast Reconstr Surg 1979;64:295–298.
71. Shaw WW, Hidalgo DA. Anatomic basis of plantar flap design: clinical applications. Plast Reconstr Surg 1986;78:637–649.
72. Hartrampf CR Jr, Scheflan M, Bostwick J III. The flexor digitorum brevis muscle island pedicle flap: a new dimension in heel reconstruction. Plast Reconstr Surg 1980;66:264–270.
73. Noone RB, Frazier TG, Noone GC, et al. Recurrence of breast carcinoma following immediate reconstruction: a 13-year review. Plast Reconstr Surg 1994;93:96–106.
74. Patel RJ, Webster DJ, Mansel RE, et al. Is immediate postmastectomy reconstruction safe in the long term? Eur J Surg Oncol 1993;19:372–375.
75. Rowland JH, Holland JC, Chaglassian T, et al. Psychological response to breast reconstruction: expectations for and impact on postmastectomy functioning. Psychosomatics 1993;34:241–250.
76. Wellisch DK, Schain WS, Noone RB, et al. Psychosocial correlates of immediate versus delayed reconstruction of the breast. Plast Reconstr Surg 1985;76:713–718.
77. Carlson GW, Bostwick J III, Stylbo TM, et al. Skin-sparing mastectomy: oncologic and reconstructive considerations. Ann Surg 1997;225:570–578.
78. Kroll SS, Baldwin B. A comparison of outcomes using three different methods of breast reconstruction. Plast Reconstr Surg 1992;90:455–462.
79. Schusterman MA, Kroll SS, Weldon ME. Immediate breast reconstruction: why the free TRAM over the conventional TRAM flap? Plast Reconstr Surg 1992;90:255–261.
80. Hartrampf CR, Scheflan M, Black PW. Breast reconstruction with transverse abdominal island flap. Plast Reconstr Surg 1982;69:216–225.
81. McCraw JB, Papp C, Edwards A, et al. The autogenous latissimus breast reconstruction. Clin Plast Surg 1994;21:279–288.
82. Kind GM, Rademaker AW, Mustoe TA. Abdominal-wall recovery following TRAM flap: a functional outcome study. Plast Reconstr Surg 1997;99:417–428.
83. Hester TR, Bostwick J III. Poland's syndrome: correction with latissimus muscle transposition. Plast Reconstr Surg 1982;69:226–233.
84. Shamberger RC, Welch KJ, Upton J III. Surgical treatment of thoracic deformity in Poland's syndrome. J Pediatr Surg 1989;24:760–765.

85. Boshert MT, Barone CM, Puckett CL. Outcome analysis of reduction mammoplasty. Plast Reconstr Surg 1996;98:451–454.
86. Eklund GW, Busby RC, Miller SH, et al. Improved imaging of the augmented breast. AJR Am J Roentgenol 1988;151:469–473.
87. Hayes H Jr, Vandergrift J, Diner WC. Mammography and breast implants. Plast Reconstr Surg 1988;82:1–8.
88. Bryant H, Brasher P. Breast implants and breast cancer—reanalysis of a linkage study. N Engl J Med 1995;332:1535–1539.
89. Cahan AC, Ashikari R, Pressman P, et al. Breast cancer after breast augmentation with silicone implants. Ann Surg Oncol 1995;2:121–125.
90. Blackburn WD Jr, Everson MP. Silicone-associated rheumatic disease: an unsupported myth. Plast Reconstr Surg 1997;99:1362–1367.
91. McGrath MH, Burkhardt BR. The safety and efficacy of breast implants for breast augmentation. Plast Reconstr Surg 1984;74:550–560.
92. Fraser GR, Calnan JS. Cleft lip and palate: seasonal incidence, birth weight, birth rank, sex, site, associated malformations and parenteral age. Arch Dis Child 1961;36:420–423.
93. Fraser FC. The genetics of cleft lip and palate. Am J Hum Genet 1970;22:336–352.
94. Neel JV. A study of major congenital defects in Japanese infants. Am J Hum Genet 1958;10:398–445.
95. Chung CS, Myrianthopolous NC. Racial and prenatal factors in major congenital malformations. Am J Hum Genet 1968;20:44–60.
96. Slaughter WB, Pruznasky S. The rationale for velar closure as a primary procedure in the repair of cleft palate defects. Plast Reconstr Surg 1954;13:341–357.
97. Randall P, LaRossa DD, Fakhree SM, et al. Cleft palate closure at 3 to 7 months of age: a preliminary report. Plast Reconstr Surg 1983;71:624–628.
98. Millard DR. Complete unilateral clefts of the lip. Plast Reconstr Surg 1960;25:595–605.
99. Randall P. A triangular flap operation for the primary repair of unilateral clefts of the lip. Plast Reconstr Surg 1959;23:331–347.
100. Holtmann B, Wray RC. A randomized comparison of triangular and rotation-advancement unilateral cleft lip repairs. Plast Reconstr Surg 1983;71:172–179.
101. Trier WC, Dreyer TM. Primary von Langenbeck palatoplasty with levator reconstruction: rationale and technique. Cleft Palate J 1984;21:254–262.
102. Krause CJ, Tharp RF, Morris HG. A comparative study of results of the von Langenbeck and the V-Y pushback palatoplasties. Cleft Palate J 1976;13:11–19.
103. Furlow LT Jr. Cleft palate repair by double opposing Z-plasty. Plast Reconstr Surg 1986;78:724–738.
104. Dryer TM, Trier WC. A comparison of palatoplasty techniques. Cleft Palate Cranofac J 1984;21:251–253.
105. Seyfer AE, Prohazka D, Leahy E. The effectiveness of the superiorly based pharyngeal flap in relation to the type of palatal defect and the timing of operation. Plast Reconstr Surg 1988;82:760–764.
106. Witt PD, D'Antonio LL, Zimmerman GJ, et al. Sphincter pharyngoplasty: a preoperative and postoperative analysis of perceptual speech characteristics and endoscopic studies of velopharyngeal function. Plast Reconstr Surg 1994;93:1154–1168.
107. LaRossa D, Donath G. Primary nasoplasty in unilateral and bilateral cleft nasal deformity. Clin Plast Surg 1993;20:781–791.
108. El Deeb M, Messer LB, Lehnert MW, et al. Canine eruption into grafted bone in maxillary alveolar defects. Cleft Palate J 1982; 19:9–16.
109. Reardon W, Winter R, Rutland P, et al. Mutations in the fibroblast growth factor receptor 2 gene cause Crouzon syndrome. Nat Genet 1994;8:98–103.
110. Wilkie A, Slaney S, Oldridge M, et al. Apert syndrome results from localized mutations of FGFR2 and is allelic with Crouzon syndrome. Nat Genet 1995;9:165–172.
111. Rutland P, Pulleyn L, Reardon W, et al. Identical mutations in the FGFR2 gene cause both Pfeiffer and Crouzon syndrome phenotypes. Nat Genet 1995;9:173–176.
112. Zide B, Grayson B, McCarthy JG. Cephalometric analysis: part I. Plast Reconstr Surg 1981;68:816–823.
113. Zide B, Grayson B, McCarthy JG. Cephalometric analysis for upper and lower midface surgery. Part II. Plast Reconstr Surg 1981;68:961–968.
114. Zide B, Grayson B, McCarthy JG. Cephalometric analysis for mandibular surgery. Part III. Plast Reconstr Surg 1982;69:155–164.
115. Luce EA, Tubb TD, Moore AM. Resistance of various parts of the facial skeleton to fracture-producing forces. Plast Reconstr Surg 1979;63:26–30.
116. Mickel TJ, Rohrich RJ, Robinson JB Jr. Frontal sinus obliteration: a comparison of fat, muscle, bone, and spontaneous osteogenesis in the cat model. Plast Reconstr Surg 1995;95:586–592.
117. Donald PJ. Frontal sinus ablation by cranialization: report of 21 cases. Arch Otolaryngol 1982;108:142–146.
118. LeFort R. Experimental study of fractures of the upper jaw, parts I and II [reprinted in Plast Reconstr Surg 1972;50:497–506]. Rev Chir Paris 1901;23:208–227; 360–379.
119. LeFort R. Experimental study of fractures of the upper jaw, part III. [reprinted in Plast Reconstr Surg 1972;50:600–607]. Rev Chir Paris 1901;23:479–507.
120. Chuong R, Donoff RB, Guralnick WC. A retrospective analysis of 327 mandibular fractures. J Oral Maxillofac Surg 1983;41:305–309.
121. Byrd HS, Hobar PC. Rhinoplasty: a practical guide for surgical planning. Plast Reconstr Surg 1992;91:642–654.
122. Hirsch J, Knittle JL. Cellularity of obese and nonobese human adipose tissue. Fed Proc 1970;29:1516–1521.
123. Klein JA. Tumescent technique for local anesthesia improves safety in large-volume liposuction. Plast Reconstr Surg 1993;92:1085–1089.
124. Samdal F, Amland PF, Bugge JF. Plasma lidocaine levels during suction-assisted lipectomy using large doses of dilute lidocaine with epinephrine. Plast Reconstr Surg 1994;93:1217–1223.
125. Greminger RF. The mini-abdominoplasty. Plast Reconstr Surg 1987;79:356–364.
126. Petty P, Manson PN, Black R, et al. Panniculus morbidus. Ann Surg 1992;28:442–452.

SECTION ELEVEN

Modern Practice of Surgery

Technology, the Surgeon, and Surgical Innovation: An Introduction

Michael E. Gertner and Thomas Krummel

The daily work of the surgeon relies heavily on technology for both efficiency and enablement. Outside the operating room, surgeons rely on technology to make diagnoses with sophisticated imaging equipment, to quickly transmit patient information, and to monitor patients. In the operating room, the use of technology is obvious: the Bovie, the videoscopic equipment used in laparoscopy and endoscopy, staplers, and, most recently, robots.

For the most part, these innovations were not developed in isolation. They were developed through close collaboration between physicians and "technology enablers." These enablers include engineers, managers, and suppliers of capital (e.g., NIH, DARPA, and private investment). The technology *vision* typically originates with the physician and/or any of the technology enablers. For the most part, however, the technology would not have been developed were it not for close collaboration, and equal contribution, among these groups.

There is often a tendency for physicians to trivialize technology; for example, the answer to a medical student's question of how the newest electrocautery device works, "It's magic!" Similarly, it is common for surgeons to "fit" a technological solution into a clinical problem because it is the only technology known (have a tool, find a nail) and the one with which they feel most comfortable. For example, a new wound closure technology has to be a mechanical device because "I don't know chemistry."

Going forward, it will be ever more crucial that surgeons collaborate with the technology enablers. Technology is advancing at a rapid pace, becoming more complex and specialized. At the same time, clinical practice is demanding increased specialization and focus. Therefore it is increasingly difficult for surgeons to do it all—to maintain a clinical practice, to stay abreast of advances in fundamental technologies, to innovate, and to maintain close collaboration with the enablers.

Surgeons also have an ethical responsibility to understand the technology they are working with on a daily basis. It can be argued that it is as important that surgeons understand the energy sources that they are applying to their patients or the material they are permanently placing in their patients as it is to make the decision to operate in the first place. Surgeons must understand the limitations of the technology and the principles behind the limitations so that the appropriate applications and assumptions are made and the next-generation devices developed. Unknowing use of a technology is as unconscionable as the unknowing use of a drug.

We believe that it is time for a formal educational process that teaches surgeons how to identify clinical needs, work with technology enablers, and realize a relevant solution. Such an educational process would facilitate innovation by emphasizing the critical components of the innovation process and the critical components involved in bringing an innovation to the patient bedside. It would also emphasize breaking down old paradigms and thinking "outside the box." The Surgical Innovation Program at Stanford (*surgery.stanford.edu/innovation* for more information) is designed to achieve these ends.

The ensuing chapters represent the beginnings of such educational programs; indeed, two of the chapters are directly written by surgeons and engineers in the inaugural classes of the innovation program at Stanford. The chapters describe the most common surgical technology in use today and the data to support their use. Chapters 109, 110, and 111 outline the development of hernia biomaterials from their beginnings to the future, Chapter 112 discusses the wide range of injectable biomaterials and their "magic," Chapter 113 discusses energy transfer in the practice of surgery, and Chapter 114 describes the evolution and evolving uses of robotics in surgery.

The chapters are organized such that the technology is discussed in the clinical context and the specifics of the technology are discussed in somewhat greater detail. Where possible, Class I clinical data are presented.

109

Biomaterials and the Evolution of Hernia Repair I: The History of Biomaterials and the Permanent Meshes

Raul A. Cortes, Edward Miranda, Hanmin Lee, and Michael E. Gertner

Increasingly, bioprosthetic materials are being used for a variety of surgical applications. In general surgery, for example, surgical techniques for hernia repair have been influenced directly by the development of different prosthetic meshes. As the field of biomaterial science advances, new insight into the physiological response to materials guides the development of newer classes of biomaterials including synthetic, partially synthetic, and natural tissue derivatives. This chapter, the first of three parts on materials for hernia repair, outlines historical aspects of bioprosthetic materials, details experimental (often animal) and clinical evidence for use of current materials, and establishes a framework for understanding the principles used for development of new prostheses. Although hernias serve as the model disease, the fundamentals of bio–prostheses interactions are applicable to many different genres in medicine.

History of Biomaterials in Hernia Repair

A hernia is defined as a "protrusion or projection of an organ or part of an organ through the wall of the cavity that normally contains it."[1] Inherent to this interpretation is the concept of tissue *failure* and implied in it is the need for tissue *augmentation*. This need has been long recognized as necessary for proper management of hernias; in fact, Billroth is known to have pondered the development of a material that could "artificially produce tissue of the density and toughness of fascia and tendon . . . (so as to provide) . . . the radical cure of hernia(s)."[2] During the past two centuries, this need for a fascial reinforcement has fueled surgical innovation into the development of multiple varied prostheses.

The development of reinforcements or abdominal wall replacements has been traced back in the English literature to 1894 when Phelps introduced the concept of silver wire coils on the floor of the inguinal canal.[3] This concept progressed to the use of silver filigrees, or wire arrangements, that were known to incite an inflammatory process that promoted scar formation and reinforcement. Successful in providing a strong reinforcing scar, these and other early efforts were limited, however, by patient discomfort, resultant sinus tracts, and material failure secondary to metal corrosion.

These failures guided early twentieth-century efforts to utilize less corrosive substances such as annealed stainless steel formed into wire-ring meshes. Ultimately abandoned, these meshes had an extensive history of use; in fact, relatively recently (1986), one series reported a relatively low 9.5% recurrence frequency, a low complication rate, and "good clinical results" in 95% of patients followed to 4 years.[4] Despite this favorable review, overall utilization of these metallic derivatives soon declined. Accounts of critical device failure manifest by mesh fragmentation and material erosion into intraabdominal structures abruptly curbed initial enthusiasm.[5]

With advances in polymer science early in the second half of the twentieth century providing a backdrop for biotechnological innovation, clinicians implemented use of nonmetallic prostheses as the newest class for abdominal wall defect replacements. A wide variety of materials were created and evaluated, including regenerated cellulose (Fortisan), polyvinyl alcohol (Ivalon), nylon, acrylic cloth (Orlon), fiberglass, polyester sheeting (Mylar), polytetrafluoroethylene (Teflon), and, carbon fiber.[2,3] These substances were advantageous in providing increased flexibility compared to their less rigid predecessors (increasing patient comfort) and in minimizing the detrimental risks of erosive fragmentation. With increased clinical use, however, it quickly became apparent that these materials deteriorated with time leading to rejection and extrusion. In addition, in the presence of infection, these materials consistently disintegrated and necessitated removal.

Despite these failures, the experience gained from use of these materials led to new understanding of the physiological responses to implanted foreign materials. These observations guided the design and development of yet another generation of *plastic* biomaterials. These newer modern meshes showed improved mechanical stress resistance, withstood physical modifications, and maintained both immunological inertness and noncarcinogenicity. These improved properties, along with a capacity for material sterilization, fulfilled the principles of "the ideal prosthetic" as suggested originally by Cumberland and Scales in 1950 in their guidelines for biomaterial development.[6]

Arguably, the modern era of mesh hernia repair can be documented as beginning in 1958 when Francis Cowgill Usher published his landmark experiences with the use of biomaterials as fascial reinforcements and replacements.[7] An extremely resourceful surgeon, Usher worked with engineers and chemists to develop "optimal" hernia repair materials. He introduced the use of Marlex mesh, originally composed of polyethylene but then changed to polypropylene, for repair/reinforcement of experimentally created canine abdominal, chest, and diaphragmatic defects (Fig. 109.1).

These early animal successes led to clinical applications of Marlex for subcutaneous reinforcement of primarily closed incisional hernias. This role quickly expanded from tissue reinforcement to tissue replacement when Usher reported success with intraperitoneal Marlex for use in ventral defects not otherwise amenable to primary closure. Reported recurrence rates were quite low; in fact, Usher et al. documented a 4% recurrence rate for subcutaneous reinforcement and a 0% recurrence rate for intraperitoneal replacement.[8] Of interest, Usher also advocated for mesh reinforcements of inguinal hernias and advocated for subfascial reinforcement by "fixing mesh to the overlying fascia and the conjoined tendon."[8] In yet another foretelling example, Usher emphasized a "technique . . . of reconstruction without tension" and endorsed Marlex as quite utile given its "biological inertness in the presence of infection."[8]

Usher's introduction of Marlex mesh heralded the arrival of the three major modern meshes: derivatives of *polypropylene* (Marlex, Atrium, Surgipro, Prolene, and, Trelex), *polyester* (Dacron, Mersilene, Parietex), *expanded polytetrafluoroethylene* ("Gore-Tex meshes": Soft Tissue Patch, DualMesh), and the two newer types, *absorbable* (e.g., Vicryl) and *composite* (e.g., ePTFE/polypropylene composite: Composix) meshes.

Introduction of polyester meshes, interestingly, actually preceded Usher's introduction of Marlex mesh by 2 years. In 1956, Walstenholme reported on the use of a new biomaterial, Dacron (a polyester made of polymers of polyethylene terephthalate), as an adjunct for abdominal and groin hernia repair (Fig. 109.2).[9] For reasons explained in the section on polyester meshes, widespread clinical acceptance of Dacron or Mersilene, however, did not occur until popularization by French surgeons (Rives and Stoppa) 13 years later.[3,10] During the interim, Dacron did gain favor for use as a biomaterial construct for vascular and cardiac surgery prostheses.

Similarly to polyester, expanded polytetrafluoroethylene (ePTFE), the third of the three major groups of modern mesh material bases, served initially as a biomaterial for vascular and cardiac surgery applications (Fig. 109.3). ePTFE mesh did differ, however, from the previous two meshes in that it was derived from a modification of a previously known material, polytetrafluoroethylene (Teflon). This softer, microporous material proved to be more flexible and stronger than

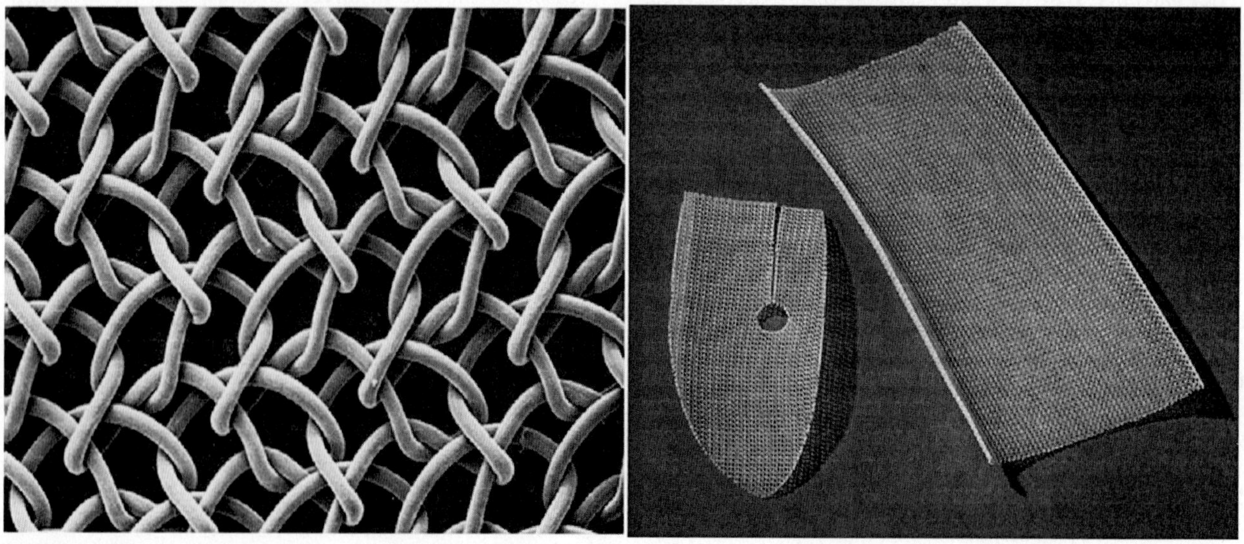

FIGURE 109.1. Scanning electron micrograph (SEM) (*left*) and product view (*right*) of "modern day" Marlex mesh, Bard Mesh. (Images obtained by permission from Davol, Inc.)

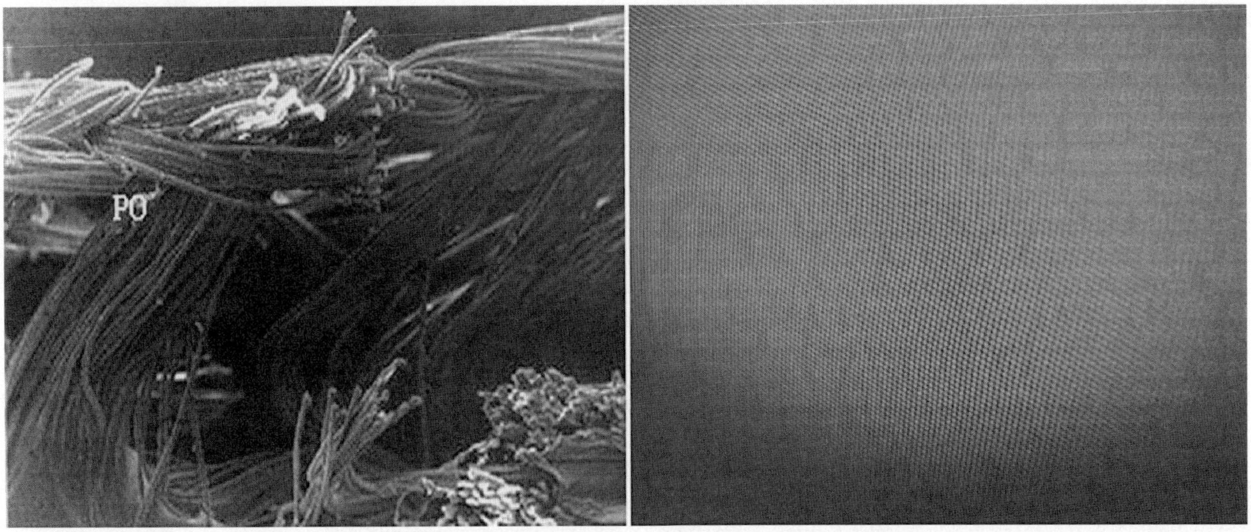

FIGURE 109.2. SEM (*left*) and product view (*right*) of Mersilene mesh. *PO*, polyester fibers. (SEM image provided by Dr. Juan Bellon; product image by Ethicon, Inc.)

Teflon, which had previously been shown to have poor incorporation, intolerance to infection, and excessive wound complications.[3]

Elliot and Juler were the first authors to generate experimental evidence for the utility of ePTFE and showed preferable qualities compared to Marlex when used as a fascial buttress in rabbit inguinal defects.[11] Histological investigation into why significantly fewer adhesions formed with intraperitoneal ePTFE revealed an organized tissue reaction with minimal peritoneal involvement compared to the chaotic dense inflammatory response noted for Marlex. This characteristic drove initial clinical interest for hernia repair application in 1985; in fact, this property continues to serves as an impetus for the development of ePTFE mesh combinations that, theoretically, provide adhesion prevention surfaces.[12–15]

Many of these "modern" meshes currently remain in clinical practice despite disagreement (sometimes significant) over the reporting of favorable or unfavorable characteristics (Tables 109.1–109.3). More recent derivations represent newer versions developed on modifications intended to capitalize and minimize good and bad properties, respectively. For example, modern-day ePTFE derivatives include second-generation products that have had surface qualities modified to enhance tissue ingrowth. The meshes described in this chapter are all derived from synthetic materials and are thus nonabsorbable. However, the most recent material classes, the absorbable meshes (e.g., Vicryl) and the biologically derived meshes (Surgisis, AlloDerm, and Permacol), represent the latest advances in implantable biomaterial technology and are discussed in separate chapters.

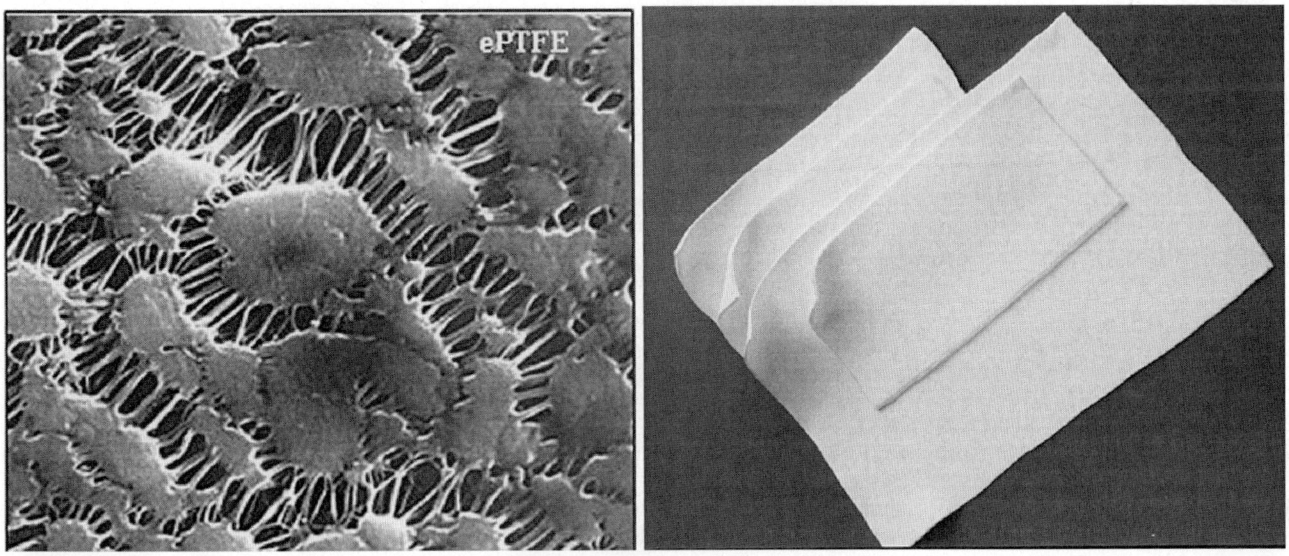

FIGURE 109.3. SEM (*left*) and product view (*right*) of Soft Tissue Patch mesh, the expanded polytetrafluoroethylene (ePTFE) prototype. (SEM image provided by Dr. Juan Bellon; product images obtained by permission from W.L. Gore Associates, Inc.)

TABLE 109.1.
Seminal Studies and Reports Describing the Use of Polypropylene Mesh.

Animal studies	*Animal*	*Primary study mesh*	*Comparison mesh*	*Mesh placement location*
Usher[8]	Dogs	Marlex (polyethylene)	Teflon	Intraperitoneal (IP)
Law et al.[44]	Rats	Marlex®	ePTFE	IP
Bleichrodt et al.[47]	Rats	Marlex®	ePTFE	IP
Beets et al.[19]	Pigs	Surgipro®	Prolene®	Preperitoneal (PP)
Bellon et al.[13]	Rabbits	Marlex®	Prolene®; Trelex®	PP, IP
Baykal et al.[74]	Mice	Prolene®	Vicryl®; Tutoplast®[a]	IP
Baptista et al.[24]	Rats	Polypropylene (not specified)	None	IP
Greca et al. (Hernia 5, 59 June 2001)	Dogs	Prolene®	T mesh®[b]	PP, SC
Ferrando et al.[75]	Rats	Marlex®	None	IP
Human studies	*Hernia type*	*Primary study mesh*	*Comparison mesh*	*Mesh placement location*
Stone et al.[21]	Abdominal	Marlex®	Prolene®	IP
Kaufman et al.[36]	Abdominal	Marlex®	None	IP
Voyles et al.[76]	Abdominal	Marlex®	None	IP
Jones et al. (Am Surg 55, 73 Jan 1989)	Abdominal	Marlex®	None	IP
Lichtenstein et al.[77]	Inguinal	Marlex®	None	PP
Lichtenstein et al.[78]	Inguinal	Marlex®	None	PP
Molloy et al.[79]	Abdominal	Marlex®	None	IP, PP
Shulman et al.[29]	Inguinal	Marlex®	None	PP
Amid et al.[40]	Abdominal	Marlex®	None	PP
DeGuzman et al.[37]	Abdominal	Polypropylene (not specified)	None	IP
Brandt et al.[80]	Abdominal	Marlex®	None	IP
Friis et al.[31]	Inguinal	Prolene®	None	PP
Sugerman et al.[35]	Abdominal	Marlex®	Prolene®	SC
McGillicuddy[30]	Inguinal	Marlex®	Trelex®	PP
Chuback et al.[38]	Inguinal	Polypropylene (not specified)	None	PP
Luijendijk et al.[34]	Abdominal	Marlex®	None	IPb
Vrijland et al.[32]	Inguinal	Marlex®	Prolene®	PP
Amid[81]	Inguinal	Bard LHI preshaped®	None	PP

ePTFE, expanded polytetrafluoroethylene.

[a]Tutoplast is cadaveric dura mater.

[b]T mesh is an experimental polypropylene mesh with pore size 4 × 3 mm.

TABLE 109.2.
Seminal Articles Describing the Use of Polyester and Polyester-Derived Meshes.

Human studies[a]	*Hernia type*	*Primary study mesh*	*Comparison mesh*	*Mesh placement location*
Wolstenholme[9]	Both	Dacron®	Heavier Dacron fabric	IP
Stoppa et al.[10]	Inguinal	Dacron®	None	PP
Wantz[62]	Abdominal	Mersilene®	None	PP or IP
Thill et al.[69]	Inguinal	Mersilene®	None	IP
Taizo et al. (Surg Lap End Percut Tech Aug 1998)	Inguinal	Polyester/Bard®	None	Lap PP
Gilbert et al.[73]	Abdominal	Mersilene®	Prolene®	PP
Stoppa[71]	Abdominal	Mersilene®	None	PP
Wantz[72]	Both	Mersilene®	None	PP
Moreno-Egea et al.[82]	Abdominal	Parietex®	None	IP
Lepere et al.[83]	Inguinal	Parietex®	None	IP and PP
Ramshaw et al.[68]	Inguinal	Parietex®	None	Lap PP
Moreno-Egea et al.[84]	Abdominal	Parietex®	None	Lap PP
Arnaud et al.[85]	Abdominal	Parietex®	Mersilene®	IP
Ammaturo et al.[86]	Abdominal	Parietex®	None	IP

LAP, laparoscopy.

[a]Data in the English literature examining the use of Dacron and Parietex mesh in animal experiments have primarily been focused in multiple mesh comparison studies; see Table 109.3.

TABLE 109.3.
Seminal Articles Describing the Use of ePTFE and ePTFE-Derived Meshes.

Animal studies	*Animal*	*Study mesh*	*Comparison mesh*	*Mesh placement location*
Elliot et al.[11]	Rabbits	ePTFE	Marlex®	PP
Lamb et al.[49]	Rabbits	ePTFE	Marlex®; Vicryl®	IP
Brown et al.[42]	Guinea pig	ePTFE	Marlex®	IP
Murphy et al.[87]	Rats	ePTFE	Marlex®	IP
Simmermacher et al.[88]	Rats	ePTFE + Perforations	ePTFE + Alcohol Rx	SC
Naim et al.[89]	Rats	ePTFE + Marlex®	Marlex® + Interceed or Poloxamer	IP
Bellon et al.[13]	Rabbits	DualMesh®	None	IP
Bellon et al.[12]	Rabbits	MycroMesh®	Marlex®	IP
Bellon et al.[18]	In vitro	MycroMesh®	Surgilene®	In vitro
Bellon et al.[48]	Rabbits	Soft Tissue Patch®/ePTFE	None	IP
Zieren et al.[90]	Rats	DualMesh®	Polyur Dacron/Polyester Composite	IP
Bellon et al.[50]	Rabbits	DualMesh®	CV-4 Gore-Tex Suture Mesh	IP
LeBlanc et al.[91]	Rabbits	DualMesh®	DualMesh with Corduroy Surface®	IP
Ferrando et al.[92]	Rats	Composix®	None	IP
Kapan et al.[93]	Rats	DualMesh®	Tutopatch®[a]; Tutoplast®[a]	PP, IP
Bellon et al.[94]	Rabbits	CV-4 Composite ePTFE	DualMesh®	IP
Human studies	***Hernia type***	***Study mesh***	***Comparison mesh***	***Mesh placement location***
Bauer et al.[59]	Abdominal	Soft Tissue Patch®/ePTFE	None	IP
van der Lei et al.[60]	Abdominal	Soft Tissue Patch®/ePTFE	None	IP
Toy et al.[57]	Abdominal	Soft Tissue Patch®/ePTFE	None	Lap IP
Deysine[58]	Both	Soft Tissue Patch®/ePTFE	None	IP
Vogt et al.[95]	Inguinal	Soft Tissue Patch® "Modified"	None	Lap IP
Toy et al.[96]	Abdominal	Soft Tissue Patch® or DualMesh®	None	Lap IP
Tsimoyiannis et al.[97]	Abdominal	Soft Tissue Patch®	None	Lap IP
LeBlanc et al.[55]	Abdominal	DualMesh®	None	Lap IP
Lau et al.[98]	Abdominal	DualMesh®	None	Lap IP
Berger et al.[99]	Abdominal	DualMesh®	None	Lap IP
LeBlanc[100]	Abdominal	DualMesh®	None	Lap IP
Lau et al.[101]	Abdominal	DualMesh®	None	Lap, open IP
Araki et al.[102]	Abdominal	Composix®	None	Lap IP
Gillian et al.[103]	Abdominal	Composix®	None	Lap IP
LeBlanc et al.[104]	Abdominal	Composix®	DualMesh®	IP
Cobb et al.[105]	Abdominal	Composix®	None	IP

[a]Tutoplast is cadaveric dura mater.

The Coming of Age of Biomaterials: The Permanent Meshes

For the most part in hernia practice today, there are three common groups of nonabsorbable, or permanent, hernia meshes: polypropylene and its derivatives, polyester and its derivatives, and ePTFE and its derivatives. Combinations of these materials, that is, "composites" are becoming quite popular and are discussed in a separate chapter. Physical properties, experimental findings, and clinical experiences with each mesh are described.

Of note, given potential confusion that may occur with purely biochemical descriptions, one common descriptor, woven versus knitted, refers to a categorization based on the textile manufacturing processes. Woven refers to a weave created without the use of a needle and generally results in a less porous, less flexible material. Figure 109.4 depicts a woven braid, the simplest of all braids. Knitted materials are created by looping of a thread; products created this way are generally more porous and flexible materials (Fig. 109.5). Furthermore, some meshes are made from individual strands that may be woven; that is, braided strands are used as individual strands in a higher-order knitted mesh.

Polypropylene Meshes

Physical Properties

Polypropylene is the most widely used mesh material.[6] Monofilament polypropylene is commonly used as a suture material that resists biodegradation (i.e., permanent).[16] Meshes derived from polypropylene are typically knitted from monofilaments of polypropylene (Marlex, see Fig. 109.1; Atrium; Trelex), double filaments of polypropylene (Prolene, see Fig.

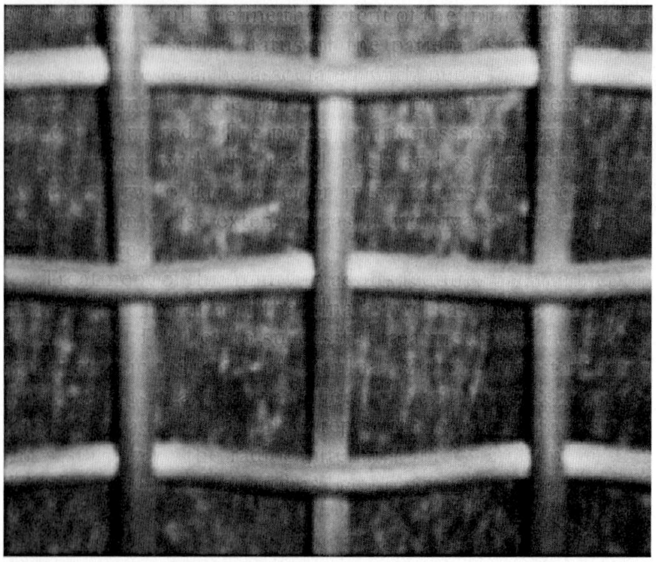

FIGURE 109.4. An example of a woven pattern. As exhibited at the Museum of Technology and Science in Berlin, woven patterns were the simplest to mass produce with the early machines of the industrial revolution.

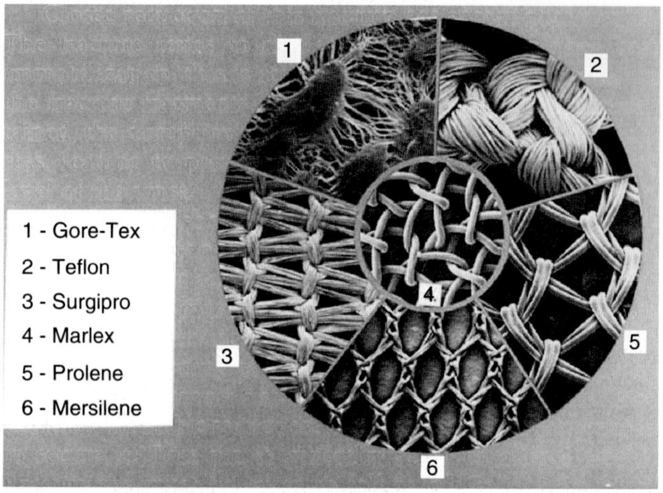

FIGURE 109.6. SEMs of several different mesh types. *4* (Marlex), *5* (Prolene), and *3* (Surgipro) are produced from knits of single, double, or multiple polypropylene strands, respectively. (Reproduced with permission from P.K. Amid, M.D.)

109.7), or more than two filaments (i.e., braided) of polypropylene (Surgipro, Fig. 109.6). The addition of multiple strands decreases the stiffness of the mesh (the knit can be looser) while maintaining excellent strength. The additional strands increase the surface area at overlapping junctions, which, in turn, helps to prevent unraveling and increases the mesh–tissue interface. This property aids incorporation into the existing fascia and thus facilitates postoperative healing.[16] Unfortunately, as surface area increases, so do interstices available for microorganism invasion.

Animal/Experimental Data

Experimental observations with polypropylene meshes, in general, have demonstrated that they induce favorable fibrous

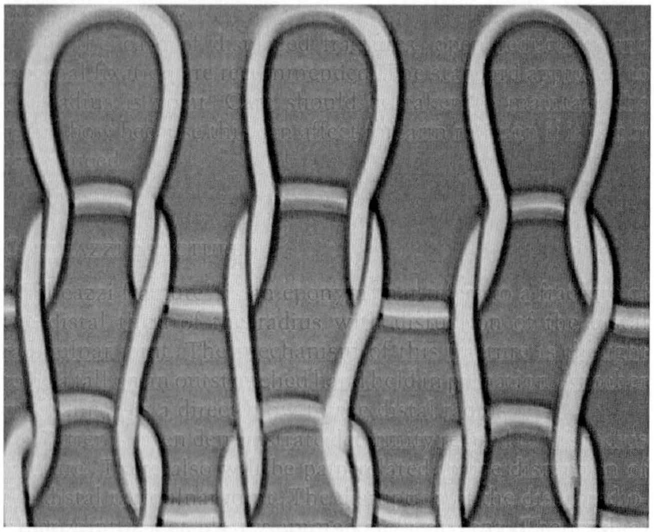

FIGURE 109.5. An example of a knitted pattern, also from a historical fabric display at the Berlin Museum of Technology and Science. The loop-within-loop pattern results in a more form-fitting material with greater open area than the woven pattern shown in Figure 109.4.

ingrowth, that they are relatively strong with excellent tensile properties, and that they are relatively resistant to infection. However, these typically favorable qualities are counterbalanced by increased inflammatory reactions and subsequently higher adhesion formation rates. The degree of these reactions is not uniform across all polypropylene based meshes, however. Single- and double-filament polypropylene meshes induce different peritoneal inflammatory reactions compared to multifilament polypropylene meshes. This variability (despite biochemical similarity) has led to a distinct classification method based on experimentally observed pore/interstice sizes (see Figure 109.6).[2] Amid et al. chose to emphasize the importance of pore size based on prior demonstrations that optimal fibrous tissue infiltration occurred at pore sizes of 90 μm or greater.[17] Using this system, polypropylene *monofilament* meshes (single- or double-stranded) are considered type I biomaterials, having an average pore size greater than 75 μm (Table 109.4). These "totally macroporous" meshes allow for dense cellular infiltration and lead to intense fibrotic and brisk immune responses.[2] Braided *multifilament* meshes, on the other hand, are considered type III [along with Teflon, polyester, and perforated ePTFE (MycroMesh)] and are characterized as "macroporous with multifilament or microporous components."[2]

In comparison to the other type III biomaterials, Surgipro differs in that it elicits an intense inflammatory reaction. Similarly to the other type III meshes, on the other hand, Surgipro contains microporous interstices (a product of overlapping multifilaments) that allow microbial colonization and increased infectious potential. In fact, one recent in vitro investigation into the interaction of meshes with bacteria showed that although microcolonies of bacteria formed on both type I and type III polypropylene pores, immune cells were allowed "passage" into the former but not into the latter.[18] Immune cell restriction from type III micropores isolates bacteria from immune clearance. One other limitation of type III polypropylene meshes is an increased inflammatory reaction attributed to the braided versus monofilament composition.[19]

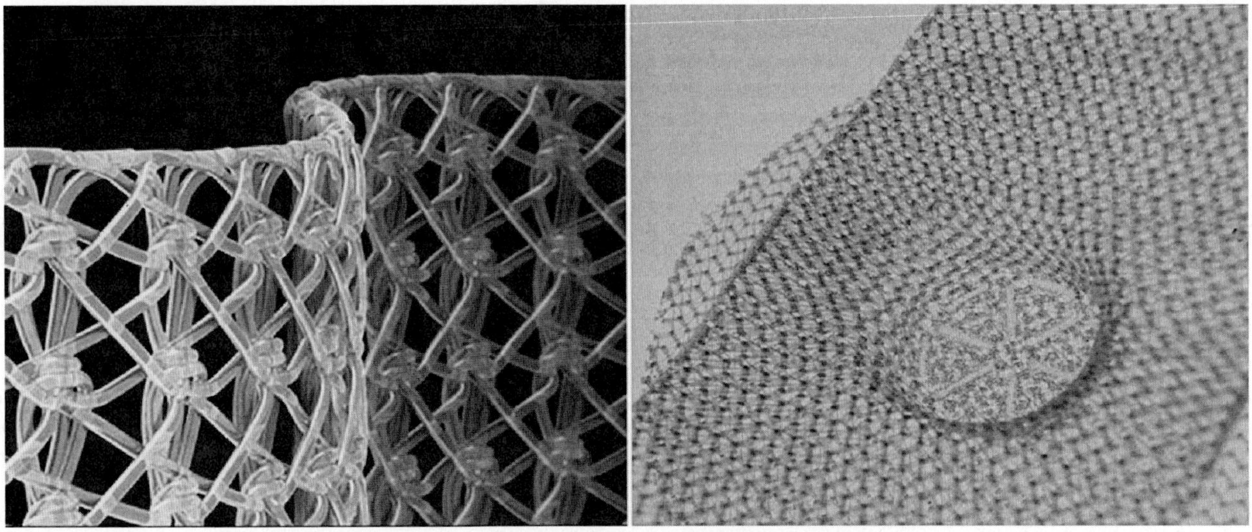

FIGURE 109.7. SEM (*left*) and product view (*right*) of Prolene mesh. Prolene differs from other polypropylene meshes by its double-stranded polypropylene pattern (see Figure 109.6). (Images obtained by permission from Ethicon, Inc.)

TABLE 109.4. Amid Classification of Biomaterials Used for Hernia Repair.

Type	*Description*	*Mesh types*
Nonabsorbable:		
Type I	Totally *macroporous* meshes containing pores larger 75 μm required for admission of macrophages, fibroblasts, blood vessels, and collagen fibers	Atrium, Marlex, Prolene, Trelex
Type II	Totally *microporous* prostheses containing pores smaller than 10 μm in at least one of their two surface dimensions	Soft Tissue Patch, DualMesh
Type III	*Macroporous* prostheses with multifilament or *microporous* components	Teflon, Mersilene (braided polyester), Surgipro (braided polypropylene), MycroMesh (perforated ePTFE)
Type IV	Biomaterials with *submicronic* pore size not suitable alone as bioprostheses but can be used in combination with Type I as barriers between mesh and viscera to form adhesion-free composites	Silastic, polypropylene films, Preclude Pericardial Membrane, Preclude Dura-Substitute
Absorbable:		
	Claimed to be replaced by host tissue and recommended for contaminated cases (but no evidence for new replacement tissue having collagen type I/III ratio to withstand intraabdominal pressure)	a: Synthetic: Dexon, Vicryl b: Biological: Surgisis, AlloDerm, Permacol

Considerable data exist confirming the adequate (i.e., supraphysiological) in vitro strength and tensile properties of nearly all modern nonabsorbable meshes. In vivo, the biomechanical profiles of these prostheses are less well defined because tensiometric measurements, such as mesh–fascial tensile strength and abdominal burst pressures, prove unreliably reproducible from study to study.[20] Morris-Stiff et al. undertook an extensive comparative review of the experimental literature and drew broad categorical conclusions on the strength and tensile properties of the three major types of meshes (excluding newer composite and absorbable derivatives.) They affirmed that tensile strength and incorporation of both polypropylene and polyester meshes were equivalent and that both performed favorably compared to ePTFE meshes in clean and contaminated environments.[6] Differences aside, all the meshes were supraphysiological in strength.

As already noted, a propensity for adhesion formation is yet another variable by which to compare the different meshes. For polypropylene meshes, significant adhesion formation is known to occur if placed intraperitoneally.[15,21] This reaction, however, differs among the polypropylene meshes, and the mechanism that accounts for this difference is poorly understood. Initially thought to be a product of reactivity to the material composition, recent experimentation has implicated other factors such as material weight and mass as more relevant. For example, some authors attribute differences between inflammatory reactions generated by double-stranded polypropylene meshes versus single-stranded meshes as functions of material "weight." In fact, newer composite polypropylene meshes such as Vypro and Ti-Mesh have been specifically designed with the concept of reducing mesh mass (see Chapter 110).

An alternative factor thought to account for the development of peritoneal adhesions is a configurational change that occurs with polypropylene mesh "shrinkage" after implantation (disproportionate to wound contracture.) A resulting decrease in mesh area (usually by 20%) creates sharp edges that potentially irritate underlying peritoneum and intestinal serosa, leading to adhesion formation.[2,22,23] The importance of a propensity for shrinkage has driven the development of yet other "modified" polypropylene meshes and justified the use of composite combinations.[14,15,22,24–28]

Clinical Data

Extensive clinical experience has been compiled with the use of polypropylene mesh in inguinal and ventral/incisional hernia repair. The use of polypropylene for inguinal hernias was initially advocated based on the premise that the mesh permits a tension-free repair and prevents late-appearing direct hernias that result from progressive physiological deterioration of the inguinal floor (after primary repair).[29] As expected, the concept of utilizing a prosthetic garnered a large amount of reservation; however, the data ultimately proved overwhelming. Shulman et al. retrospectively reviewed the combined results of 3019 groin hernias repaired with a tension-free mesh-reinforced technique (using Prolene or Marlex), noting a 0.2% recurrence rate and 0.03% infection rate at an average follow-up of 7.5 years.[29] Three more recent "prospectively randomized" trials have confirmed superiority of mesh compared to traditional primary non-mesh repair in regards to postoperative hernia recurrence rates (Prolene, Marlex, and Trelex) (see Table 109.1).[30–32]

Extensive reported experience with the use of polypropylene mesh in elective *incisional* hernia repair has reaffirmed its safety characteristics and underscored its compelling low recurrence statistics. Starting with the initial reports by Usher, lower frequency of recurrences favored use of polypropylene mesh over primary closure under tension (0%–10% versus 30%–50%).[33] One recent, prospectively randomized multicenter 6-year trial by Luijendijk et al. confirmed the statistically significant superiority of mesh repair (using Marlex or Prolene) compared to primary suture repair for incisional hernia repair.[34] Although overall recurrence rates were higher than historically reported (primary repair, 43%; mesh repair, 24%), the study authors were quick to point out that historical rates were based on retrospective (rather than prospective) case studies.[34] Another investigation of the rates of hernia development after elective surgery in a group of high-risk patients (gastric bypass or colectomy patients, most of whom were on chronic steroids), demonstrated only a 4% recurrence rate after using prefascial polypropylene (Marlex or Prolene). Compared to their own recurrence rates for primarily closed defects, 31%, they concluded that tension-free mesh closure proved more beneficial in these high-risk patient populations.[35]

In examining the complications associated with the use of either pre- or intraperitoneal placed polypropylene, clinical experience has verified experimental observations of the mesh's propensity for extensive adhesion formation. In addition, numerous other complications have been attributed to intraperitoneal mesh placement such as late fistulization and mechanical obstruction as a consequence of mesh migration.[36–38] These more deleterious complications, however, are thought by some to represent exceedingly rare circumstances.[39] In a recent retrospective evaluation, Vrijland et al. demonstrated a 0% fistula formation rate for mesh placed subfascially (with or without intact underlying peritoneum) in more than 130 patients undergoing incisional hernia repairs followed at 3 years.[39] In addition, the authors performed a meta-analysis of literature ascribing to polypropylene use for incisional hernia repair and showed a combined 0.5% enterocutaneous fistula rate. In fact, the authors concluded that "polypropylene mesh can be placed safely intraperitoneal" and that "enterocutaneous fistula formation need not be feared in elective incisional hernia repair with polypropylene mesh, (although), this should be performed under antibiotic cover." Most others, however, do not advocate for placement of traditional polypropylene mesh directly in contact with bowel serosa (intraperitoneal) and alternatively advocate for use of composites when confronted with this scenario (see Chapter 110).[2,23,40] Notwithstanding the debate over intraperitoneal placement, when possible, subfascial placement or intraperitoneal composite mesh use is preferable. However, when these alternatives are impossible, intraperitoneal placement can be done with the small but real risk of subsequent fistulization and related complications.

The primary use of polypropylene mesh for complex abdominal wall reconstruction such as "loss of abdominal domain" has not gained universal acceptance because of concern with direct mesh–bowel contact. In fact, concern for mesh-induced erosion of bowel serosa and consequent fistulization led to the application of nonabsorbable/absorbable mesh sandwiches for closure of "open abdominal cases." Fabian et al. further modified this technique by implementing a two-stage approach. After placement of a presumably "low adhesion risk" absorbable mesh (see section on absorbable meshes), the subsequent incisional hernia is repaired with polypropylene mesh after 6 to 12 months.[41]

Other approaches to the open abdomen involve the use of polypropylene, specifically in cases that require repeated peritoneal lavage. Placement of a stronger, better incorporated mesh is justified as facilitating gradual closure of the abdominal cavity.[23] Other favorable characteristics include easily draining nature of the open pores, documented ability of the mesh to allow for infectious clearance, and a similar adhesion and fistula formation rate found for absorbable meshes.[23] Alternative points of view argue for ePTFE or ePTFE derivatives (in the form of composites) use based on in vitro evidence for lower organism adherence to ePTFE compared to polypropylene.[42] One retrospective review pointed to less morbidity (0% versus 75% fistula formation) and mortality outcomes with Soft Tissue Patch (ePTFE) compared to Marlex in acute "loss of domain" scenarios.[43] The superior results were attributed to decreased adhesion formation with ePTFE as well as "ease of removal" of the mesh at the time of definitive repair, less risk of fistula development, and decreased inflammatory reaction. Despite this view, however, most authors recommend against ePTFE placement under infectious circumstances, based on experimental demonstration of impaired microorganism clearance of bacteria-colonized ePTFE mesh.[42,44]

Overall, polypropylene has been used extensively, and support remains very high for its application in most clinical scenarios. Although still often debated, a consensus appears to be developing in recommending against intraperitoneal placement of polypropylene mesh under elective circumstances. With infection, avoidance of any inert prosthesis seems preferable. However, when needed, polypropylene appears to serve as an acceptable (although not ideal) fascial surrogate.

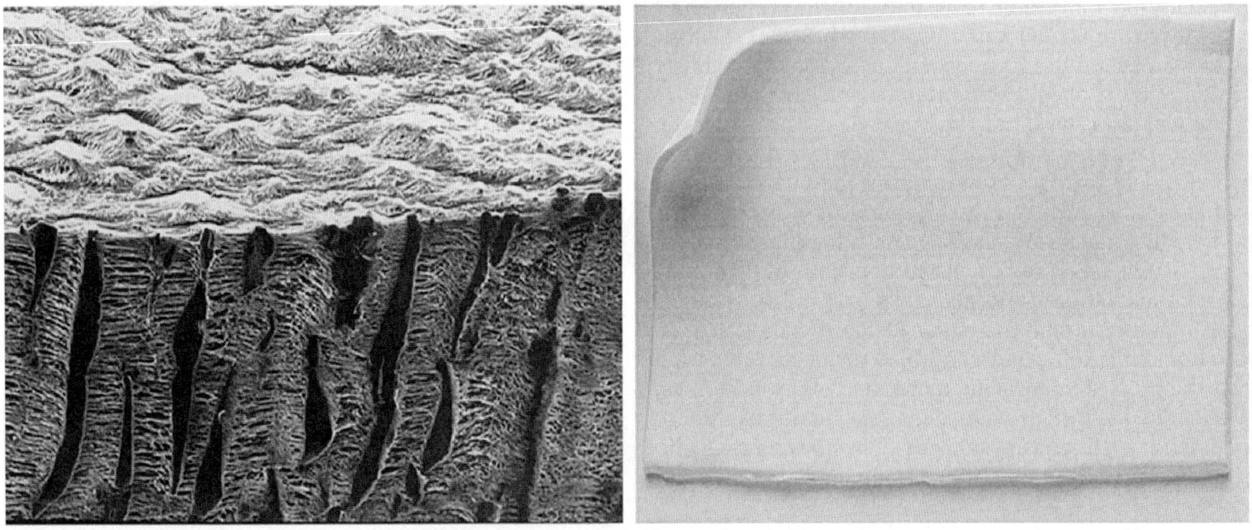

FIGURE 109.8. SEM (*left*) and product view (*right*) of Soft Tissue Patch mesh, the ePTFE prototype. This view shows the smooth laminar mesh surface. (Images provided by W.L. Gore Associates, Inc.)

Expanded Polytetrafluoroethylene Meshes

Physical Properties

Expanded polytetrafluoroethylene (Gore-Tex, ePTFE) mesh is the expanded version of Teflon, a material derived from a powdered polymer form of the gas tetrafluoroethylene.[16] The expanded mesh is a woven microporous sheet that is composed of "compact nodules of polytetrafluoroethylene interconnected by fine fibers of the same material" (Fig. 109.8).[45] These "internodal" areas are equivalent to the pores of the other meshes and are located approximately 17 to 41 μm apart. The material is inherently hydrophobic (and negatively charged) and, with pore sizes of 17 to 41 μm, can be considered impervious to water. ePTFE is classified as an Amid type II biomaterial (totally microporous) in contrast to its unexpanded predecessor, Teflon, which is characterized as a type III biomaterial.[2] Similar to the other meshes, its superior tensile strength has been well documented both ex vivo and in vitro. In vivo, some evidence has pointed to greater suture retention strength for ePTFE compared to that of Marlex, Prolene, or Mersilene likely because of its multidirectional fibrillary arrangement.[3,16,46] Fibrous ingrowth and correspondingly, abdominal integration of ePTFE, however, is considered to be inferior to these other meshes. ePTFE is commercially available as Soft Tissue Patch, although recent modifications with varied pore sizes have been introduced to enhance fibrous ingrowth (MycroMesh, DualMesh.) These variations are discussed in the composite mesh chapter (Chapter 110).

Animal/Experimental Data

Expanded polytetrafluoroethylene was utilized primarily for vascular prostheses before introduction by Elliot and Juler in 1979 as a fascial replacement in animal experiments.[11] In contrast to polypropylene and polyester meshes, the distinct biophysical properties of ePTFE have led to its incorporation into a greater range of clinical applications. Many modified forms of ePTFE exist, however; also, biological properties attributed to ePTFE mesh vary and conflicting studies exist.

Experimental consensus does exist, however, with regard to the degree of mesh–tissue incorporation. Histological evaluations of ePTFE meshes explanted from animal models have revealed *decreased* fibrous fixation and *weaker* tensiometric properties compared to polypropylene explants.[46,47] Ultrastructural evaluation of implanted mesh show tissue incorporation by way of fine collagen fibrils versus dense and disorganized large collagen fibers associated with polypropylene tissue reactions. Amid et al. suggest that inferior tissue integration occurs as a result of poor fibroblast infiltration through ePTFE "micropores."[2]

The behavioral properties of ePTFE mesh placed under infectious experimental conditions remain unclear. Brown et al. used an animal peritonitis model to demonstrate a statistically significant decrease in the adherence of bacteria to ePTFE compared to polypropylene mesh.[42] Additionally, a significant decrease in the rate of adhesion formation was found in ePTFE-treated animals compared to those with polypropylene. Bleichrodt et al., on the other hand, demonstrated contrasting properties of ePTFE placed in contaminated fields.[47] The authors showed diminished mesh–fascial tensile strength for ePTFE compared to polypropylene when placed in contaminated environments. Corroborative histological evaluation showed poorer collagen fiber penetration into the ePTFE mesh–tissue interface. The authors used these experimental findings to explain the mechanism by which "ePTFE disintegration" occurred in their patient population who had ePTFE placed under infectious conditions.

Additional animal work has substantiated unfavorable ePTFE properties when placed in infectious scenarios.[46,47] Law et al. reported that higher recurrence rates observed with ePTFE occurred because of pore-size limitation of immune cell trafficking. Unopposed colonization of bacteria induced deformation of prosthetic filaments and subsequent mesh weakening and consequent failure. Based on these experimental observations, most investigators avoid placement of ePTFE into infected operative fields and recommend either prompt removal or debridement of infected portions.[2,18,46,48]

Low adhesion formation tendencies, on the other hand, account for the most favorable aspects of ePTFE. Consistently, numerous studies have documented a lower quantity and/or structurally weaker/finer adhesions attributable to ePTFE when compared to polypropylene or polyester meshes.[13,46,49] Bellon et al. specifically investigated the mechanisms of these properties by examining the relative importance of mesh structure versus biochemical composition.[50] The authors hypothesized that the smooth laminar surface of Soft Tissue Patch prevented extensive adhesions by "guiding" ordered and layered neoperitoneum deposition. By showing differential properties of the same ePTFE mesh based on structural modifications, they confirmed that structure rather than biochemical composition modulated peritoneal reaction. Reticulated ePTFE (patterned into a structure similar to polypropylene mesh) caused as many adhesions as that normally noted for intraperitoneal polypropylene mesh.

Clinical Data

Direct clinical comparisons of Soft Tissue Patch to other meshes for use in incisional or inguinal hernia repairs are limited. A multitude of retrospective reviews describe outcomes with ePTFE mesh; however, recurrence statistics are difficult to compare with other meshes because many studies evaluate different hernia techniques. Overall, studies have focused on using ePTFE for elective application intraperitoneal in laparoscopic hernia repair.[51–55] In one favorable semi-comparative review, DeMaria et al. showed improved rehospitalization rates, postoperative pain scores, and decreased disability with use of ePTFE in laparoscopic hernia repair compared to traditional open Prolene mesh repair (follow-up at 2 years).[56]

Other studies examining specific etiologies for ePTFE hernia recurrences have found that surgical technique rather than material failure predisposes to unsuccessful repair.[57–59] Authors investigating the mechanisms of mesh/hernia repair failure concluded by recommending a wide overlap of the mesh-to-abdominal-wall interface (by way of a two-layer suture fixation) to maximize graft incorporation and prevent development of "button-hole" hernia lead points.

As noted earlier, considerable debate has prevented a uniform consensus on the appropriateness of clinical usage of ePTFE in contaminated settings. Many authors do agree, however, that mesh that has become infected usually requires excision based on the possibility of material deterioration.[58–60] Clinical rates of other more serious mesh-related complications such as mesh-induced fistula formation have also been inconsistent. Some authors suggest that implanted ePTFE has low to no fistula formation rates whereas others indicate that the ePTFE mesh has significant potential for erosion.[2,46]

In summary, the data regarding ePTFE mesh primarily focuses on its use for intraperitoneal placement, given a low propensity for adhesion formation. Accurate reherniation rates as well as ePTFE properties when placed in contaminated settings are difficult to determine because of conflicting retrospective reports. As with most of the other biomaterials, prospectively randomized comparative studies are still needed.

Polyester Meshes

Physical Properties

Polyester meshes derive from a polymer of ethylene glycol and terphthalic acid, polyethylene terephthalate. As noted in the historical review, its use as a bioprosthesis preceded polypropylene mesh. Nevertheless, widespread implementation of polyester materials was initially limited to cardiac and vascular surgery forums. It did not gain favor until French surgeons pioneering newer hernia surgical techniques advocated for its use as an adjunct to groin and incisional hernia repairs. Rives and Stoppa noted that polyester meshes contained inherent qualities that were ideal for use as an unsutured adjunct in their novel inguinal hernias repair technique.[10]

Polyester meshes are typically knitted (Dacron is composed of monofilaments and Mersilene is composed of multifilaments) and interlocked with pore sizes of $120 \times 85\,\mu m$ (see Fig. 109.9). They are characterized as a type III biomaterial, macroporous with multifilament components (see Table 109.4).[2] Physical "handling" is consistently described as light, elastic, and highly pliable "with little fraying upon cutting."[3,10,16,61,62] Biomechanical testing, however, has not held so favorably. In comprehensive ex vivo and in vivo assessments of bursting pressure and tensile wound strength, studies have demonstrated inferior polyester properties compared to polypropylene.[14,63] As well, newer evidence has sur-

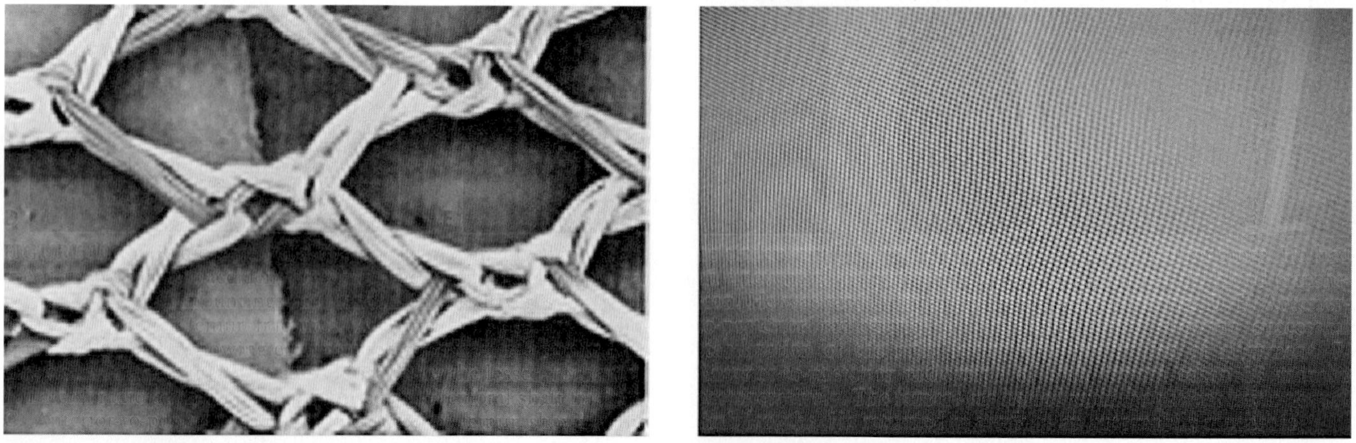

FIGURE 109.9. SEM (*left*) and product view (*right*) of Mersilene mesh. (Images obtained by permission from Ethicon, Inc.)

faced that Dacron-based vascular graphs show in vivo degradation.[16] In light of this and other reported cases of polyester mechanical failures, the question is raised as to whether polyester is durable over decades of implantation.[16,64]

Animal/Experimental Data

Many of the data regarding polyester meshes have been extrapolated from clinical experience rather than animal/experimental data. Of the few animal studies published in the English literature, most have examined polyester performance within the context of comparisons to polypropylene or ePTFE meshes.

Initial animal experimentation with polyester meshes revealed the importance of an open structured mesh form of polyester rather than an impervious cloth form for use in repair of fascial defects.[65] Subsequent evaluations of its use for reinforcement of large defects showed superiority of polyester mesh over primary suture closure with tension.[66] Despite these initial favorable reviews, however, trends in clinical application favored polypropylene meshes based on superior incorporation and fibrous fixation.[61] Histological evaluation of the polyester-induced inflammatory response have varied; some have described "a rapid fibroblastic response" whereas others emphasize "little acute inflammatory reaction compared with Prolene."[14,62]

Use of this mesh under infectious circumstances is neither advocated nor supported by evidence derived from animal experimentation.[33,61,67] As a type III biomaterial, polyester meshes are equated to braided suture, containing interstices that can harbor bacteria but prevent immune cell passage.[2] Assessments of adhesion formation elicited by intraperitoneally placed polyester have been found to be similar to those for polypropylene mesh.[15,68]

Clinical Data

Much of the push for the clinical application of polyester-based meshes can be attributed to the reported successes of Rives and Stoppa with their novel hernia repair adaptation, giant prosthetic reinforcement of the visceral sac (GPRVS).[61,62,69] In his initial descriptive study of the French technique, Wantz described favorable outcomes of 30 complex patients treated with Mersilene GPRVS repair.[62] Held in place solely by intraabdominal pressure (suture-less placement far beyond the hernia defect), Mersilene "grips" the abdominal wall as a product of its "elastic and supple" material properties.[62] Other studies have since corroborated both the ease of use and the favorable low recurrence rates obtained with use of Mersilene mesh for inguinal and femoral hernias, as well as for use in laparoscopic hernia repairs.[69,70] These studies, however, never compared this mesh directly to the other more commonly used meshes.

In a more recent, large review of clinical experience with use of the three modern types of synthetic meshes for ventral hernia repairs, Morris-Stiff et al. demonstrated that polyester meshes had lower rates of seroma formation (0.8% versus 5.5%), greater incidences of infection (8.3% versus 4.7%), and lower incidences of sinus formation (1.2% versus 1.6%) compared to polypropylene.[6] An additional review of the French collective experience (the Association of French Surgeons, AFS) demonstrated equivalent rates of hematoma and infectious complications for polyester meshes compared to traditional nonmesh primary repairs of groin and incisional hernias.[61] Of note, in his reporting of the AFS results, Soler also commented that the AFS reached a consensus recommending against the placement of polyester mesh in infected fields. Interestingly, he noted that they did *not* recommend complete removal of the mesh if it became infected.[6,61]

In contrast to the conflicting clinical data for ePTFE and polypropylene mesh, clinical experience with polyester meshes has shown more consistency in regard to adhesion rates and its associated complications. Leber et al., in a landmark article that likely influenced American surgical practice patterns, showed a significantly higher number of overall complications per patient with Mersilene mesh compared to Marlex, Prolene, or ePFTE (Soft Tissue Patch) (4.7 versus 1.4–2.3).[33] Furthermore, they described a 15.6% incidence of fistula formation in 30 patients treated with Mersilene mesh (6.7 years follow-up) and increased rates of infection (16% versus 0%–6%) and recurrence (34% versus 10%–14%).

In addition to the described limitations of intraperitoneal placed Mersilene mesh, other studies evaluating mesh incorporation have documented inferior polyester mesh tissue integration and cases of actual material failure.[33,61] Heeding the described limitations of polyester mesh, Soler and Stoppa, proponents for Mersilene placement in GPRVS, recommended only select usage of polyester and recommended "the use of polypropylene [and not polyester] when the abdominal wall is very fragile." The authors also discouraged the intraperitoneal use of both polypropylene or polyester meshes based on known visceral migration and fistula formation.[61]

Despite the growing French experience with successful application of polyester meshes, the majority of American surgical opinion of polyester prosthetics remains negative. Interestingly, responses to Leber's review have revealed more favorable long-term outcomes with use of Mersilene mesh. Stoppa reported a much more favorable 5.93% recurrence rate for 751 patients treated with Mersilene mesh followed up between 2 and 12 years. Wantz described an even lower 1.5% recurrence rate for 184 treated patients (no follow-up time point reported.) Finally, Gilbert relayed a 0% recurrence rate for 27 treated patients (followed up for 3 years) and reported successful experience with nonoperative management of three patients with mesh infection.[71–73] In summary, the preponderance of conflicting evidence suggests that the in vivo response to the permanent biomaterials may actually be indistinguishable; indeed, one author has convincingly suggested that because of this, possibly, "cost should be the deciding factor."[6]

Conclusion

Although this is far from an in-depth overview of the surgical innovations that led to current biomaterials used in surgery as it is practiced today, this chapter provides a glimpse of what is possible as well as what can be expected in the future for biomaterials.

References

1. Thomas CL, ed. Taber's Cyclopedic Medical Dictionary, 17th ed. Philadephia: Davis, 1993.

2. Amid PK. Complications of the use of prostheses: Part I. In: Bendavid MR, ed. Abdominal Wall Hernias: Principles and Management. New York: Springer, 2001:707–713.
3. Debord J. Prostheses in hernia surgery: a century of evolution. In: Bendavid MR, ed. Abdominal Wall Hernias: Principles and Management. New York: Springer, 2001:16–32.
4. Validire JIP, Dutet D, Duron JJ. Large abdomnial incliscional hernias: repair by fascial approximation reinforced with a stainless steel mesh. Br J Surg 1986;73(1):8–10.
5. Majeski J. Migration of wire mesh into the intestinal lumen causing an intestinal obstruction 30 years after repair of a central hernia. South Med J 1998;91(5):496–498.
6. Morris-Stiff GJ. The outcomes of nonabsorbable mesh placed within the abdominal cavity: literature review and clinical experience. J Am Coll Surg 1997;186(3):352–367.
7. Usher FC. Marlex mesh, a new plastic mesh for replacing tissue defects. Arch Surg 1959;78:131–137.
8. Usher FC, Ochsner JL. Hernia repair with Marlex mesh. A comparison of techniques. Surgery (St. Louis) 1959;46(1):718–724.
9. Wolstenholme JT. Use of commercial dacron fabric in the repair of inguinal hernias and abdominal wall defects. Arch Surg 1956;73:1004–1008.
10. Stoppa RE, Henry X. Unsutured dacron prosthesis in groin hernias. Int Surg 1975;60:411–412.
11. Elliot MP. Comparison of marlex mesh and microporous teflon sheets when used for hernia repair in the experimental animal. Am J Surg 1979;137(3):342–344.
12. Bellon JM, Contreras LA, Carrera-San Martin A, Jurado F. Comparison of a new type of PTFE patch (mycro mesh) and polypropylene prostheses (marlex) for repair of abdominal wall defects. J Am Coll Surg 1996;183:11–18.
13. Bellon JM, Carrera-San Martin A. Experimental assay of a dual mesh PTFE (non-porous on one side) in the repair of abdominal wall defects. Biomaterials 1996;17:2367–2372.
14. Klinge U, Conze J, Limberg W, et al. Modified mesh for hernia repair that is adapted to the physiology of the abdominal wall. Eur J Surg 1998;164:951–960.
15. Amid PK, Lichtenstein IL, Sostrin S, Young J, Hakakkha M. Experimental evaluation of a new composite mesh with the selective property of incorporation to the abdominal wall without adhering to the intestines. J Biomed Mater Res 1994; 28:373–375.
16. Kossovsky NFC, Horwath D. Biomaterials pathology. In: Bendavid MR, ed. Abdominal Wall Hernias: Principles and Management. New York: Springer, 2001:221–234.
17. Bobyn JD, Wilson GJ, MacGregor DC, Pilliar RM, Weatherly GC. Effect of pore size on the peel strength of attachment of fibrous tissue to porous-surfaced implants. J Biomed Mater Res 1982;16(5):571–584.
18. Bellón JM, G-Honduvilla N, Jurado F, Carranza A, Buján J. In vitro interaction of bacteria with polypropylene/ePTFE prostheses. Biomaterials 2001;22(14):2021–2024.
19. Beets GL, Go PM, van Mameren H. Foreign body reactions to monofilament and braided polypropylene mesh used as preperitoneal implants in pigs. Eur J Surg 1996;162(10):823–825.
20. Jenkins SD, Klamer TW, Parteka JJ, Condon RE. A comparison of prosthetic materials used to repair abdominal wall defects. Surgery (St. Louis) 1983;94(2):392–398.
21. Stone HH, Fabian TC, Turkleson ML, Jurkiewicz MJ. Management of acute full-thickness losses of the abdominal wall. Ann Surg 1981;193(5):612–618.
22. Junge K, Klinge U, Rosch R, Klosterhalfen B, Schumpelick V. Functional and morphologic properties of a modified mesh for inguinal hernia repair. World J Surg 2002;26(12):1472–1480.
23. Simmermacher R. Intraperitoneal prostheses. In: Bendavid MR, ed. Abdominal Wall Hernias: Principles and Management. New York: Springer, 2001:299–305.
24. Baptista ML, Bonsack ME, Delaney JP. Seprafilm reduces adhesions to polypropylene mesh. Surgery (St. Louis) 2000;128(1):86–92.
25. Bellón JM, García-Carranza A, Jurado F, García-Honduvilla N, Carrera-San Martín A, Buján J. Peritoneal regeneration after implant of a composite prosthesis in the abdominal wall. World J Surg 2001;25(2):147–152.
26. Bellón JM, García-Carranza A, Jurado F, García-Honduvilla N, Carrera-San Martín A, Buján J. Evaluation of a new composite prosthesis (PL-PU99) for the repair of abdominal wall defects in terms of behavior at the peritoneal interface. World J Surg 2002;26(6):661–666.
27. Altuntas I, Tarhan O, Delibas N. Seprafilm reduces adhesions to polypropylene mesh and increases peritoneal hydroxyproline. Am Surg 2002;68(9):759–761.
28. van 't Riet M, de Vos van Steenwijk PJ, Bonthuis F, et al. Prevention of adhesion to prosthetic mesh: comparison of different barriers using an incisional hernia model. Ann Surg 2003;237(1): 123–128.
29. Shulman AG, Amid PK, Lichtenstein LL. The safety of mesh repair for primary inguinal hernias: results of 3,019 operations from five diverse surgical sources. Am Surg 1992;58(4):255–257.
30. McGillicuddy JE. Prospective randomized comparison of the Shouldice and Lichtenstein hernia repair procedures. Arch Surg 1998;133(9):974–978.
31. Friis E, Lindahl F. The tension-free hernioplasty in a randomized trial. Am J Surg 1996;172(4):315–319.
32. Vrijland WW, van den Tol MP, Luijendijk RW, et al. Randomized clinical trial of non-mesh versus mesh repair of primary inguinal hernia. Br J Surg 2002;89(3):293–297.
33. Leber GE, Garb JL, Alexander AI, Reed WP. Long-term complications associated with prosthetic repair of incisional hernias. Arch Surg 1998;133(4):378–382.
34. Luijendijk RW, Hop WC, van den Tol MP, et al. A comparison of suture repair with mesh repair for incisional hernia. N Engl J Med 2000;343(6):392–398.
35. Sugerman HJ, Kellum JM Jr, Reines HD, DeMaria EJ, Newsome HH, Lowry JW. Greater risk of incisional hernia with morbidly obese than steroid-dependent patients and low recurrence with prefascial polypropylene mesh. Am J Surg 1996;171(1):80–84.
36. Kaufman Z, Engelberg M, Zager M. Fecal fistula: a late complication of Marlex mesh repair. Dis Colon Rectum 1981;24(7):543–544.
37. DeGuzman LJ, Nyhus LM, Yared G, Schlesinger PK. Colocutaneous fistula formation following polypropylene mesh placement for repair of a ventral hernia: diagnosis by colonoscopy. Endoscopy 1995;27(6):459–461.
38. Chuback JA, Singh RS, Sills C, Dick LS. Small bowel obstruction resulting from mesh plug migration after open inguinal hernia repair. Surgery (St. Louis) 2000;127(4):475–476.
39. Vrijland WW, Jeekel J, Steyerberg EW, Den Hoed PT, Bonjer HJ. Intraperitoneal polypropylene mesh repair of incisional hernia is not associated with enterocutaneous fistula. Br J Surg 2000;87(3):348–352.
40. Amid PK. Intraperitoneal polypropylene mesh repair of incisional hernia is not associated with enterocutaneous fistula. Br J Surg 2000;87(10):1436–1437.
41. Fabian TC, Croce MA, Pritchard FE, et al. Planned ventral hernia. Staged management for acute abdominal wall defects. Ann Surg 1994;219(6):643–650; discussion 651–653.
42. Brown GL, Richardson JD, Malangoni MA, Tobin GR, Ackerman D, Polk HC Jr. Comparison of prosthetic materials for abdominal wall reconstruction in the presence of contamination and infection. Ann Surg 1985;201(6):705–711.
43. Nagy KK, Fildes JJ, Mahr C, et al. Experience with three prosthetic materials in temporary abdominal wall closure. Am Surg 1996;62(5):331–335.

44. Law NW, Ellis H. A comparison of polypropylene mesh and expanded polytetrafluoroethylene patch for the repair of contaminated abdominal wall defects: an experimental study. Surgery (St. Louis) 1991;109(5):652–655.
45. Matthews BD, Pratt BL, Pollinger HS, et al. Assessment of adhesion formation to intra-abdominal polypropylene mesh and polytetrafluoroethylene mesh. J Surg Res 2003;114(2):126–132.
46. Law N. Expanded polytetrafluoroethylene. In: Bendavid MR, ed. Abdominal Wall Hernias: Principles and Management. New York: Springer, 2001:279–285.
47. Bleichrodt RP, Simmermacher RK, van der Lei B, Schakenraad JM. Expanded polytetrafluoroethylene patch versus polypropylene mesh for the repair of contaminated defects of the abdominal wall. Surg Gynecol Obstet 1993;176(1):18–24.
48. Bellon JM, Contreras LA, Bujan J. Ultrastructural alterations of polytetrafluoroethylene prostheses implanted in abdominal wall provoked by infection: clinical and experimental study. World J Surg 2000;24(5):528–531; discussion 532.
49. Lamb JP, Vitale T, Kaminski DL. Comparative evaluation of synthetic meshes used for abdominal wall replacement. Surgery (St. Louis) 1983;93(5):643–648.
50. Bellón JM, Jurado F, García-Honduvilla N, López R, Carrera-San Martín A, Buján J. The structure of a biomaterial rather than its chemical composition modulates the repair process at the peritoneal level. Am J Surg 2002;184(2):154–159.
51. Gillion JF, Bégin GF, Marecos C, Fourtanier G. Expanded polytetrafluoroethylene patches used in the intraperitoneal or extraperitoneal position for repair of incisional hernias of the anterolateral abdominal wall. Am J Surg 1997;174(1):16–19.
52. Heniford BT, Park A, Ramshaw BJ, Voeller G. Laparoscopic repair of ventral hernias: nine years' experience with 850 consecutive hernias. Ann Surg 2003;238(3):391–399; discussion 399–400.
53. Koller R, Miholic J, Jakl RJ. Repair of incisional hernias with expanded polytetrafluoroethylene. Eur J Surg 1997;163(4):261–266.
54. LeBlanc KA, Booth WV. Laparoscopic repair of incisional abdominal hernias using expanded polytetrafluoroethylene: preliminary findings. Surg Laparosc Endosc 1993;3(1):39–41.
55. LeBlanc KA, Booth WV, Whitaker JM, Bellanger DE. Laparoscopic incisional and ventral herniorrhaphy: our initial 100 patients. Hernia 2001;5(1):41–45.
56. DeMaria EJ, Moss JM, Sugerman HJ. Laparoscopic intraperitoneal polytetrafluoroethylene (PTFE) prosthetic patch repair of ventral hernia. Prospective comparison to open prefascial polypropylene mesh repair. Surg Endosc 2000;14(4):326–329.
57. Toy FK, Smoot RT Jr. Laparoscopic hernioplasty update. J Laparoendosc Surg 1992;2(5):197–205.
58. Deysine M. Hernia repair with expanded polytetrafluoroethylene. Am J Surg 1992;163(4):422–424.
59. Bauer JJ, Salky BA, Gelernt IM, Kreel I. Repair of large abdominal wall defects with expanded polytetrafluoroethylene (PTFE). Ann Surg 1987;206(6):765–769.
60. van der Lei B, Bleichrodt RP, Simmermacher RK, van Schilfgaarde R. Expanded polytetrafluoroethylene patch for the repair of large abdominal wall defects. Br J Surg 1989;76(8):803–805.
61. Soler M, Stoppa R. Polyester (dacron) mesh. In: Bendavid MR, ed. Abdominal Wall Hernias: Principles and Management. New York: Springer, 2001:266–271.
62. Wantz GE. Incisional hernioplasty with Mersilene. Surg Gynecol Obstet 1991;172(2):129–137.
63. Chu CC, Welch L. Characterization of morphologic and mechanical properties of surgical mesh fabrics. J Biomed Mater Res 1985;19(8):903–916.
64. Schumpelick V, Klinge U, Kloseterhalfen B. Biomaterials for the repair of abdominal wall hernia: structural and compositional considerations. In: Greenberg FA, ed. Nyhus and Condon's Hernia. Philadelphia: Lippincott Williams & Wilkins, 2002:551–565.
65. Arnaud JP, Eloy R, Adloff M, Grenier JF. Critical evaluation of prosthetic materials in repair of abdominal wall hernias: new criteria of tolerance and resistance. Am J Surg 1977;133(3):338–345.
66. Cerise EJ, Busuttil RW, Craighead CC, Ogden WW 2nd. The use of Mersilene mesh in repair of abdominal wall hernias: a clinical and experimental study. Ann Surg 1975;181(5):728–734.
67. Francioni G. Complications of the use of prostheses: part II. In: Bendavid MR, ed. Abdominal Wall Hernias: Principles and Management. New York: Springer, 2001:714–720.
68. Ramshaw B, Abiad F, Voeller G, Wilson R, Mason E. Polyester (Parietex) mesh for total extraperitoneal laparoscopic inguinal hernia repair: initial experience in the United States. Surg Endosc 2003;17(3):498–501.
69. Thill RH, Hopkins WM. The use of Mersilene mesh in adult inguinal and femoral hernia repairs: a comparison with classic techniques. Am Surg 1994;60(8):553–556; discussion 556–557.
70. Kimura T, Wada H, Yoshida M, et al. Laparoscopic inguinal hernia repair using fine-caliber instruments and polyester mesh. Surg Laparosc Endosc 1998;8(4):300–303.
71. Stoppa R. Long-term complications of prosthetic incisional hernioplasty. Arch Surg 1998;133(11):1254–1255.
72. Wantz GE. Incisional hernioplasty with polyester mesh. Arch Surg 1998;133(10):1137.
73. Gilbert AI, Graham MF. Problems associated with prosthetic repair of incisional hernias. Arch Surg 1998;133(10):1137.
74. Baykal A, Bagci M, Aran O, et al. Experimental study of the effect of different meshes on bacterial translocation. World J Surg 1999;23(7):625–628; discussion 629.
75. Ferrando JM, Vidal J, Armengol M, et al. Experimental evaluation of a new layered prosthesis exhibiting a low tensile modulus of elasticity: long-term integration response within the rat abdominal wall. World J Surg 2002;26(4):409–415.
76. Voyles CR, Richardson JD, Bland KI, et al. Emergency abdominal wall reconstruction with polypropylene mesh: short-term benefits versus long-term complications. Ann Surg 1981;194:219–223.
77. Lichtenstein L, Shulman AG, Amid PK. Use of mesh to prevent recurrence of hernias. Postgrad Med 1990;87:155–158.
78. Lichtenstein IL, Shulman AG, Amid PK, Willis PA. Hernia repair with polypropylene mesh. An improved method. AORN J 1990;52(3):559–565.
79. Molloy RG, Moran KT, Waldron RP, Brady MP, Kirwan WO. Massive incisional hernia: abdominal wall replacement with Marlex mesh. Br J Surg 1991;78(2):242–244.
80. Brandt CP, McHenry CR, Jacobs DG, et al. Polypropylene mesh closure after emergency laparotomy: morbidity and outcome. Surgery (St. Louis) 1995;118(4):736–740.
81. Amid PK. Lichtenstein tension-free hernioplasty: its inception, evolution, and principles. Hernia 2004;8(1):1–7.
82. Moreno-Egea A, Liron R, Girela E, Aguayo JL. Laparoscopic repair of ventral and incisional hernias using a new composite mesh (Parietex): initial experience. Surg Laparosc Endosc Percutan Tech 2001;11(2):103–106.
83. Lepere M, Benchetrit S, Debaert M, et al. A multicentric comparison of transabdominal versus totally extraperitoneal laparoscopic hernia repair using PARIETEX meshes. J Surg Laparosc Surg 2000;4(2):147–153.
84. Moreno-Egea A, Castillo JA, Girela E, Canteras M, Aguayo JL. Outpatient laparoscopic incisional/ventral hernioplasty: our experience in 55 cases. Surg Laparosc Endosc Percutan Tech 2002;12(3):171–174.
85. Arnaud JP, Hennekinne-Mucci S, Pessaux P, et al. Ultrasound detection of visceral adhesion after intraperitoneal ventral hernia treatment: a comparative study of protected versus unprotected meshes. Hernia 2003;7(2):85–88.

86. Ammaturo C, Bassi G. Surgical treatment of large incisional hernias with an intraperitoneal Parietex composite mesh: our preliminary experience on 26 cases. Hernia 2004;8(3):242–246.
87. Murphy JL, Freeman JB, Dionne PG. Comparison of Marlex and Gore-Tex to repair abdominal wall defects in the rat. Can J Surg 1989;32(4):244–247.
88. Simmermacher RK, van der Lei B, Schakenraad JM, et al. Improved tissue ingrowth and anchorage of expanded polytetrafluoroethylene by perforation: an experimental study in the rat. Biomaterials. 1991;12(1):22–24.
89. Naim JO, Pulley D, Scanlan K, et al. Reduction of postoperative adhesions to Marlex mesh using experimental adhesion barriers in rats. J Laparoendosc Surg. 1993 Apr;3(2):187–90.
90. Zieren J, Paul M, Osei-Agyemang T, et al. Polyurethane-covered dacron mesh versus polytetrafluoroethylene DualMesh for intraperitoneal hernia repair in rats. Surg Today 2002;32(10):884–886.
91. LeBlanc KA, Bellanger D, Rhynes KV 5th, et al. Tissue attachment strength of prosthetic meshes used in ventral and incisional hernia repair. A study in the New Zealand White rabbit adhesion model. Surg Endosc 2002;16(11):1542–1546.
92. Ferrando JM, Vidal J, Armengol M, et al. Experimental evaluation of a new layered prosthesis exhibiting a low tensile modulus of elasticity: long-term integration response within the rat abdominal wall. World J Surg 2002;26(4):409–415.
93. Kapan S, Kapan M, Goksoy E, Karabicak I, Oktar H. Comparison of PTFE, pericardium bovine and fascia lata for repair of incisional hernia in rat model, experimental study. Hernia 2003; 7(1):39–43.
94. Bellon JM, Rodrigues M, Serrano N, et al. Improved biomechanical resistance using an expanded polytetrafluoroethylene composite-structure prosthesis. World J Surg 2004;28(5):461–465.
95. Vogt DM, Curet MJ, Pitcher DE, Martin DT, Zucker KA. Preliminary results of a prospective randomized trial of laparoscopic onlay versus conventional inguinal herniorrhaphy. Am J Surg 1995;169(1):84–89.
96. Toy FK, Bailey RW, Carey S, et al. Prospective, multicenter study of laparoscopic ventral hernioplasty. Preliminary results. Surg Endosc 1998;12(7):955–959.
97. Tsimoyiannis EC, Tassis A, Glantzounis G, et al. Laparoscopic intraperitoneal onlay mesh repair of incisional hernia. Surg Laparosc Endosc 1998;8(5):360–362.
98. Lau H, Lee F, Patil NG. Laparoscopic repair of incisional hernia. Hong Kong Med J 2001;7(3):319–321.
99. Berger D, Bientzle M, Muller A. Postoperative complications after laparoscopic incisional hernia repair. Incidence and treatment. Surg Endosc 2002;16(12):1720–1723.
100. LeBlanc KA. Outpatient laparoscopic incisional/ventral hernioplasty: our experience in 55 cases by Moreno-Egea et al. Surg Laparosc Endosc Percutan Tech 2002;12(3):171–174.
101. Lau H, Patil NG, Yuen WK, Lee F. Laparoscopic incisional hernioplasty utilising on-lay expanded polytetrafluoroethylene DualMesh: prospective study. Hong Kong Med J 2002;8(6):413–417.
102. Araki Y, Ishibashi N, Kanazawa M, et al. Laparoscopic intraperitoneal repair of postoperative ventral incisional hernia using Composix mesh. Kurume Med J 2002;49(4):167–170.
103. Gillian GK, Geis WP, Grover G. Laparoscopic incisional and ventral hernia repair (LIVH): an evolving outpatient technique. J Surg Laparosc Surg 2002;6(4):315–322.
104. LeBlanc KA, Whitaker JM. Management of chronic postoperative pain following incisional hernia repair with Composix mesh: a report of two cases. Hernia 2002;6(4):194–197.
105. Cobb WS, Harris JB, Lokey JS, McGill ES, Klove KL. Incisional herniorrhaphy with intraperitoneal composite mesh: a report of 95 cases. Am Surg 2003;69(9):784–787.

110

Biomaterials and the Evolution of Hernia Repair II: Composite Meshes

Raul A. Cortes, Edward Miranda, Hanmin Lee, and Michael E. Gertner

The term composite is used in a number of different ways in the literature and, depending on the background of the author, the definition is interpreted differently. In its broadest and simplest meaning, it refers to a structure composed of two or more different materials, independent of the manufacturing method. Methods used to combine materials vary from simple techniques such as sutured or glued meshes to more complex processing such as thermopressing and vapor deposition. Central to all these techniques is a desire to obtain favorable properties and minimize negative characteristics of respective components.

Composite meshes developed as a consequence of better understanding of the physiological response to the traditional biomaterials. Various combinations and modifications of the three major synthetic mesh types have been created to optimize prosthesis engraftment, minimize peritoneal reaction, increase durability under infection, and improve patient comfort. Given their recent development, however, the majority of data about these meshes derive from animal experimentation, and, as such, clinical consideration should be weighed appropriately. Composite descriptions in this chapter are grouped based on the associated nonabsorbable mesh.

Polypropylene Derivatives

Polypropylene composites have been designed to ameliorate the dense inflammatory reactions elicited by the single component polypropylene meshes previously described. In particular, these derivatives have been designed to allow intraperitoneal placement for both open and (more commonly) laparoscopic surgical repair. Early composites, simple in design, were created by adding an additional absorbable mesh layer to the polypropylene layer to theoretically provide time for mesothelialization over the absorbed surface. J.C. Porter described one of the more influential clinical series with the use of a Vicryl/Marlex composite for closure of emergent "open abdomen" cases.[1] Treated patients were ascribed to having "good results," that is, no fistula formations, hernia recurrences, or mesh extrusions. These results echoed earlier reports by Naim and Dayton in experimental and clinical investigations, respectively.[1–3]

The concept that adhesions could be prevented by adding an absorbable mesh to polypropylene was somewhat refuted, however, by Amid et al. in a series of formal animal experiments.[4] Using a full-thickness abdominal defect in rabbits, they showed that *nonabsorbable* composites (impervious) prevented adhesion formation whereas absorbable composites (porous) caused adhesion formation. Contrary to expectations, adhesions occurred with all the absorbable combinations. Addition of polyglactin, polyglycolic acid, or a fibrin layer proved to be unsuccessful. On the other hand, use of a nonabsorbable silastic layer or modified polypropylene sheet (impervious) led to a zero percent adhesion rate. Although results were derived from a limited sample size, the study was the first to show experimental evidence for the failure of absorbable meshes to prevent adhesion formation.

These described failures of the absorbable/polypropylene mesh combinations fueled the biomaterial industry's development of an entire new class of "modified" polypropylene derivatives. These new varieties are notable for surfaces that theoretically induce formation of an organized "neoperitoneum" and thus reduce the intraabdominal inflammatory reaction. The derivatives discussed in this section,

Sepramesh, Vypro, TiMesh, and PLPU99, have been selected for review on the basis of the availability of published clinical and animal experimental evidence. Composix mesh, a polypropylene/expanded polytetrafluoroethylene (ePTFE) combination, is discussed under the ePTFE derivatives.

Sepramesh is a recently developed composite that is composed of a co-knitted polypropylene and polyglycolic acid mesh coated with an absorbable adhesion barrier (composed of carboxymethylcellulose, polyethylene glycol, and hyalurante) on the polyglycolic acid surface (Fig. 110.1). These layers are considered to be hydrophilic, nonimmunogenic, and viscoelastic. These properties "allow for coating and lubrication of serosal surfaces, thus, preventing or reducing serosal trauma—a predisposing factor for adhesion development" (Genzyme website).

Although few clinical series describing the use of Sepramesh exist, experimental evaluations of intraabdominally placed Sepramesh show varied reports of effective antiadhesive properties. One favorable study demonstrated a smaller percentage of mesh covered with adhesions for Sepramesh-treated animals compared to those treated with either polypropylene alone or polypropylene placed with different liquid antiadhesive barriers. At 7 days, 55% of Sepramesh surfaces were covered with adhesions compared to 81% for Prolene (68%–90% for the other composites). At 30 days, percent of adhesion-covered surface areas dropped to 25% compared to 48% for Prolene mesh.[5] Another comparative study evaluating Sepramesh, Composix, and polypropylene mesh (Bard Mesh) showed that adhesion prevention was "better" (animals without adhesions, 8/10 versus 3/10) and that tissue incorporation was "comparable" for implanted Sepramesh (compared to both other meshes, measured using a tensiometer that measured disruption-force).[6] When comparing Sepramesh to other composites, van Reit and Gonzalez et al., in separate studies, found that Sepramesh had superior incorporation compared to the ePTFE dual-layer composite DualMesh, based on histological assessments and gross observation, respectively.[5,7]

Other comparisons demonstrated contrary, negative qualities of Sepramesh. One well-designed recent article tested the properties of five composite meshes placed in infected scenarios. Using a cecal serosal injury model, the authors examined adhesion formation and tensile strength of incorporation for meshes placed over denuded bowel. Sepramesh not only showed greater adhesion formation tendencies but also inferior incorporation (tensiometer data) compared to the other meshes (see below for more detail on this study).[8] Matthews et al. also showed the inferiority of Sepramesh placed over "naked bowel" compared to DualMesh in an experimental laparoscopic ventral hernia repair model.[9] Of note, critical review of the experimental literature on Sepramesh must be distinguished from experiences with nonbound polypropylene/Seprafilm combinations.

Utilizing a different approach for polypropylene modification, Klinge et al. focused attention on the concept of reducing material *mass* or *weight* to minimize tissue reaction.[10] This modification stemmed from the theory that mesh weight accounted for "shrinkage" that caused abdominal wall restriction and subsequent pain in patients treated with traditional polypropylene mesh (found in up to 25% of patients in their series). They developed a lighter and more porous mesh, Soft Hernia Mesh (later renamed Vypro II), that was composed of a *braided* polypropylene (<30% of the weight of Prolene mesh) stiffened by addition of a polyglactin 910 coating "to optimize intraoperative handling"[11] (Fig. 110.2). To assure that tissue incorporation remained adequate, they compared tensile strength of implanted mesh to Prolene mesh and showed that textile analysis after 90 days did not demonstrate significant differences. However, when they evaluated abdominal wall mobility (using a novel three-dimensional "photogrammetry" technique) and inflammatory response [histological and cellular response (apoptosis, heat shock protein analysis)], Vypro II showed significantly improved characteristics. Junge concluded that less mass, an increased pore size, and the addition of the polyglactin coating diminished side effects while retaining favorable tissue infiltration properties.[11] Which polypropylene alteration (i.e., lower weight, absorbable coating, or increased pore size) accounted for the effect was not determined.

Not all experimental data have affirmed the benefits of mass-reduced polypropylene. Recent animal experimentation with open intraperitoneal placement of Vypro (an earlier formulation of Vypro II) by Zieren et al. pointed to adhesion formation rates similar to that noted with intra-peritoneal placed Prolene.[12] They graded adhesions by subjective qualification of dissection "effort" needed to take down adhesions.

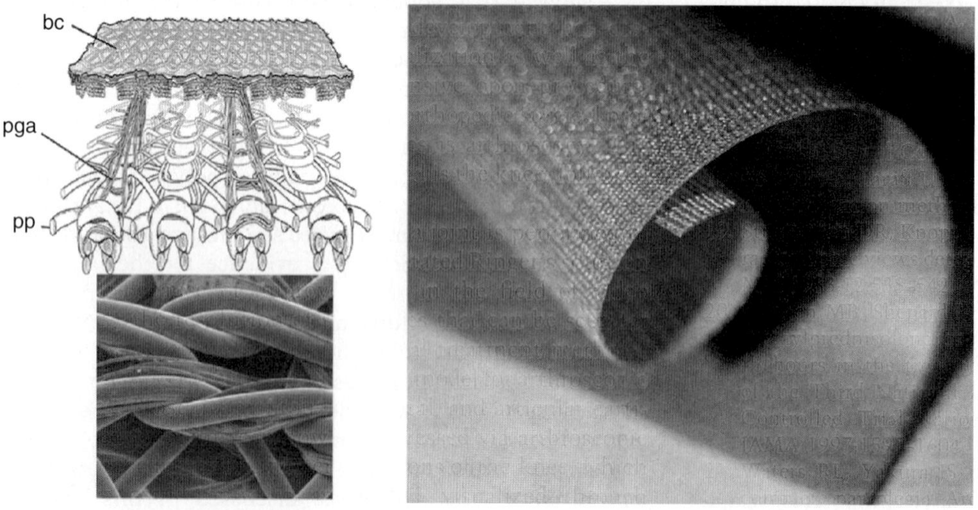

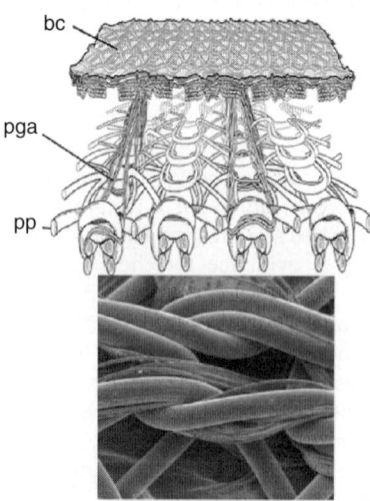

FIGURE 110.1. Schematic (*upper left*), scanning electron micrograph (SEM; *lower left*), and product view (*right*) of Sepramesh. Polyglycolic acid is shown as strands on the SEM view. *Bc*, bioresorbable coating; *pga*, polyglycolic acid; *pp*, polypropylene. (Images provided by Genzyme, Inc.)

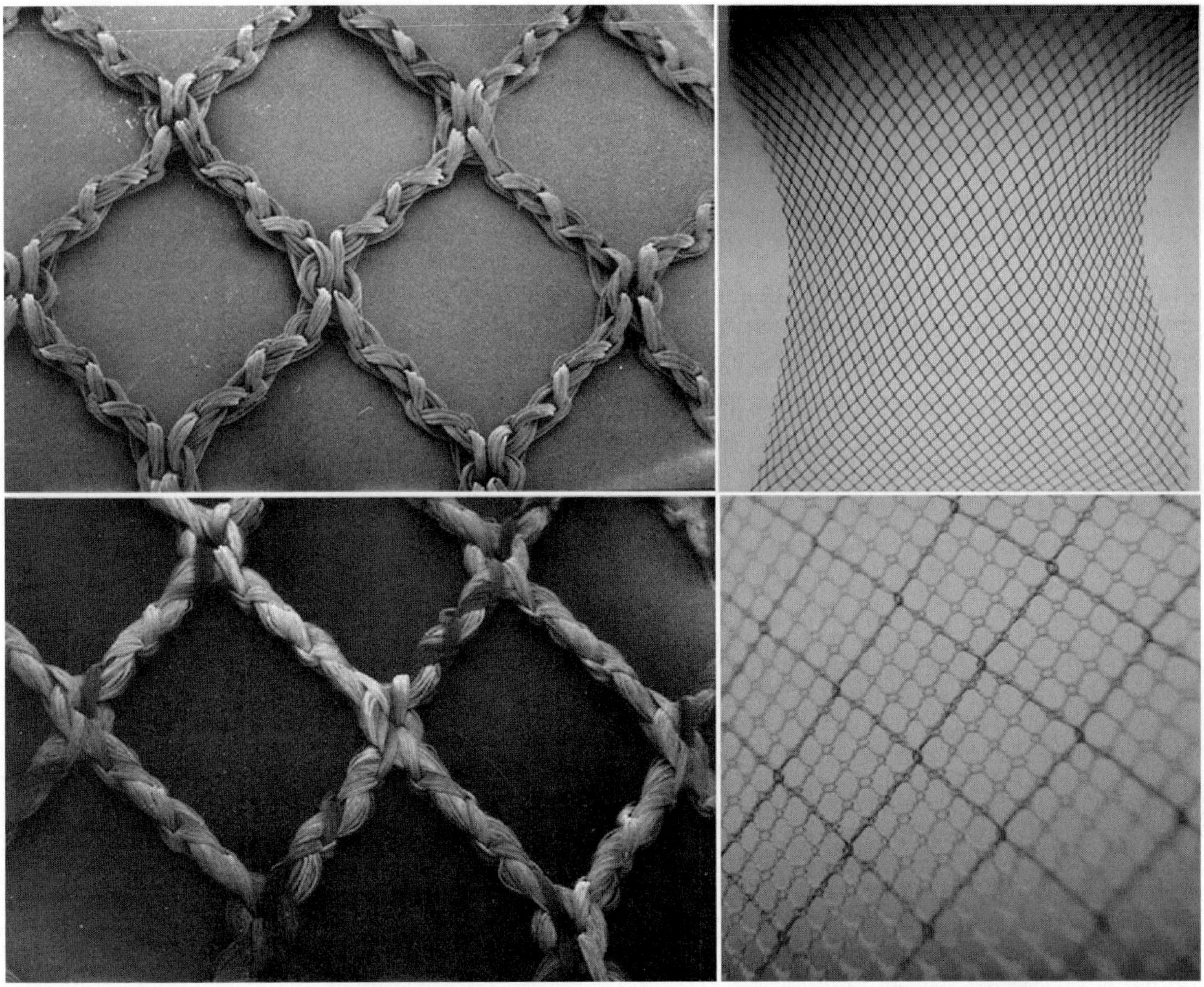

FIGURE 110.2. SEMs (*left*) and corresponding product views (*right*) of Vypro (*top*) and Vypro II (*bottom*) meshes. (SEMs provided by Drs. Joachim Conze and Volker Schumpelick; product images obtained by permission from Ethicon, Inc.).

Despite finding lower-grade adhesions with Vypro, they still recommended against intraperitoneal placement given concern that adhesion presence indicated a potential for subsequent clinical problems.

Clinical experience with Vypro or Vypro II has only recently been published and, similarly to the experimental data, reports range from positive to negative. Schmidbauer et al. reviewed 69 patients with either Prolene or Vypro preperitoneal open incisional hernia repair. They found that chronic pain (determined subjectively at 14 months follow-up) and minor perioperative complications were higher for heavier polypropylene meshes compared to lower-weight meshes. Recurrence rates and major complications, however, were similar between groups.[13] In contrast, one other prospectively randomized study showed *no* difference between Vypro II and Prolene in regard to chronic pain (measured by a validated pain assessment questionnaire) or recurrence rate in more than 500 patients followed up for 13 months.[14] Yet another review of Vypro II found no experimental or clinical evidence for advantage with the lighter mesh. Histological and biochemical analyses of Vypro II [partial volume of the inflammatory infiltrate and quantification of proliferation of apoptosis (MMP1, TGF-β, uPA, type 1 collagen)] were noted to be comparable to that obtained with "heavy" polypropylene, Atrium (corresponding mass for Atrium and Vypro II were measured at 90 versus 35 g/m^2).[15] Both clinically and experimentally, they also noted difficult "endoscopic handling" of Vypro II when used for laparoscopic total extraperitoneal repair (TEP) and advocated for use of another, even "lighter" weight polypropylene, titanium-coated mesh, Ti-Mesh Extralight[15] (Fig. 110.3).

Hypothetical advantages of lighter or less rigid forms of polypropylene mesh led to the development of other *monofilament* polypropylene modifications. One mesh, Ti-Mesh Extralight, is a newly introduced titanium mesh derivative composed of thin polypropylene monofilaments (16 g/m^2) that allow "sustained support of cell growth" as a function of the hydrophilic coating.[16] Other derivatives include lighter monofilament polypropylene mesh such as Serapren Mesh and polypropylene monofilament meshes coated with polyurethane, PL-PU99.

Langenbach et al. conducted a prospectively randomized double-blinded study of the intraperitoneal reactions of "thinner" polypropylene meshes by comparing outcomes of 40 patients undergoing laparoscopic transabdominal preperitoneal repair with either thicker or thinner polypropylene

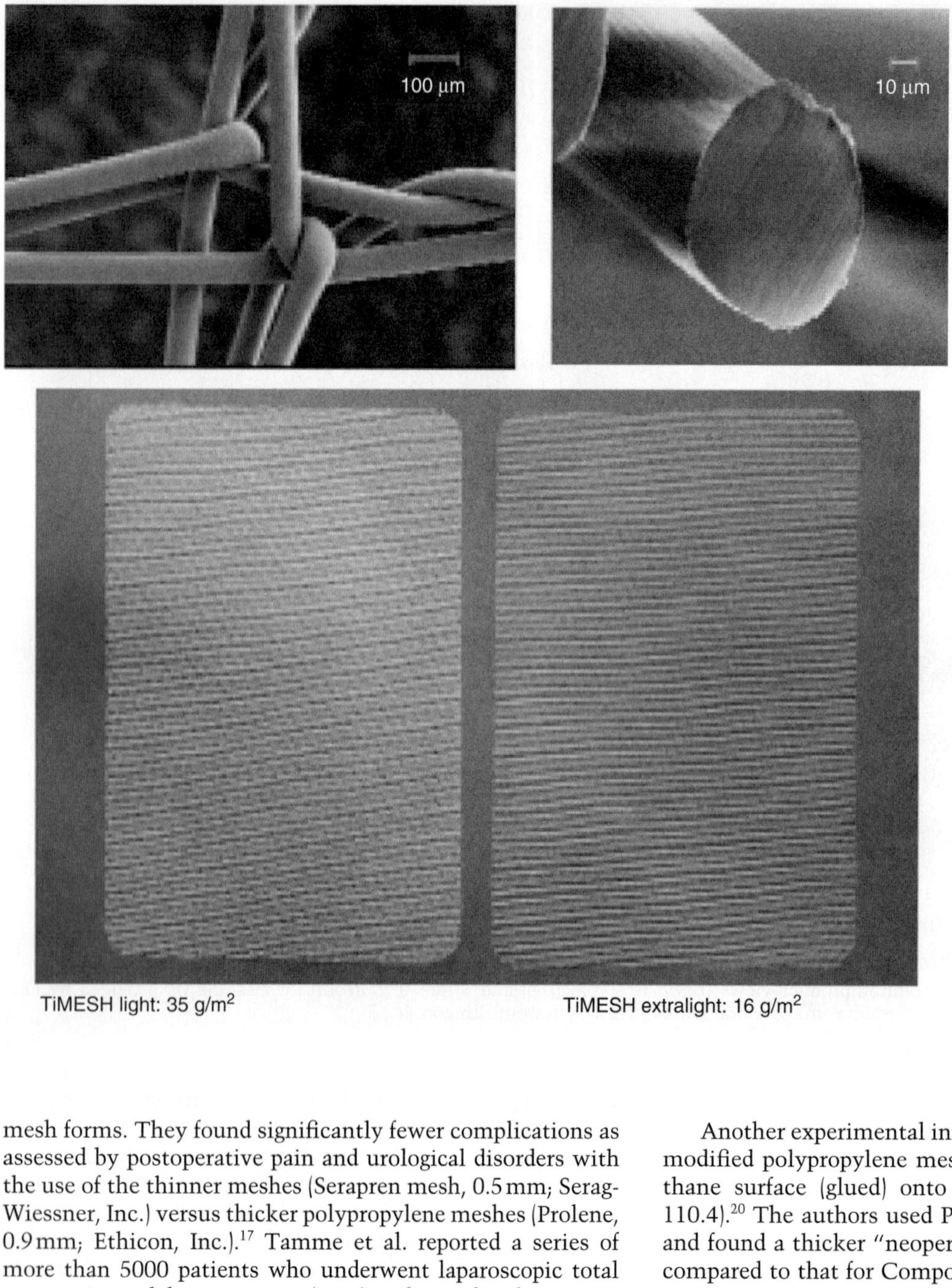

FIGURE 110.3. SEMs (*top*) and product views (*bottom*) of Ti-Mesh Light (*left*) and Extralight (*right*). Titanium is embedded on the polypropylene surface. (SEMs and product images obtained by permission from Gesellschaft fur Elektrometallurgie, Inc.)

mesh forms. They found significantly fewer complications as assessed by postoperative pain and urological disorders with the use of the thinner meshes (Serapren mesh, 0.5 mm; Serag-Wiessner, Inc.) versus thicker polypropylene meshes (Prolene, 0.9 mm; Ethicon, Inc.).[17] Tamme et al. reported a series of more than 5000 patients who underwent laparoscopic total extraperitoneal hernia repair (TEP) and noted only a 0.6% complication rate (recurrence, infection) with use of a "material reduced" polypropylene mesh (40 g/m^2) compared to a traditional polypropylene mesh (82 g/m^2).[18] Although the actual mesh was not identified, the reported weight resembles the weight noted for Ti-Mesh Light (35 g/m^2). In a follow-up study, these authors attested to the safety of the most recent Ti-Mesh derivation, the "lighter" Ti-Mesh Extralight (16 g/m^2). Used in TEP repair, they reported a 0.2% early recurrence rate, a 0.5% complication rate, and .03% bleeding rate in 400 patients followed up to 6 weeks. Despite the observed low recurrence rates and corresponding lower morbidity, they reserved comment on the long-term efficacy of this mesh to reduce chronic pain (as it was intentionally designed to prevent) until future reevaluation of this patient group at 12 months follow-up.[19]

Another experimental innovation reported by Bellon et al. modified polypropylene mesh by adding a laminar, polyurethane surface (glued) onto the peritoneal mesh side (Fig. 110.4).[20] The authors used PL-PU99 in full-thickness defects and found a thicker "neoperitoneum" formed with PL-PU99 compared to that for Composix or Parietex (a polyester composite). As well, a significantly smaller percentage of mesh area covered by adhesions and "less firm" adhesions (ease with which the prosthesis and visceral surfaces could be separated) formed with PL-PU99 and Parietex meshes compared to untreated polypropylene meshes.[20]

In summary, a great number of polypropylene composites exist. None, however, completely prevents adhesion formation, although a clinically significant reduction is attributed to each of these modifications. All composites should be considered within the context of their structural and biochemical composition, given that these factors most likely determine in vivo human inflammatory response. Given the very recent development of these and other composite meshes, application of these bioprosthetics requires judicious selection considering the wide disparity in experimental reports.

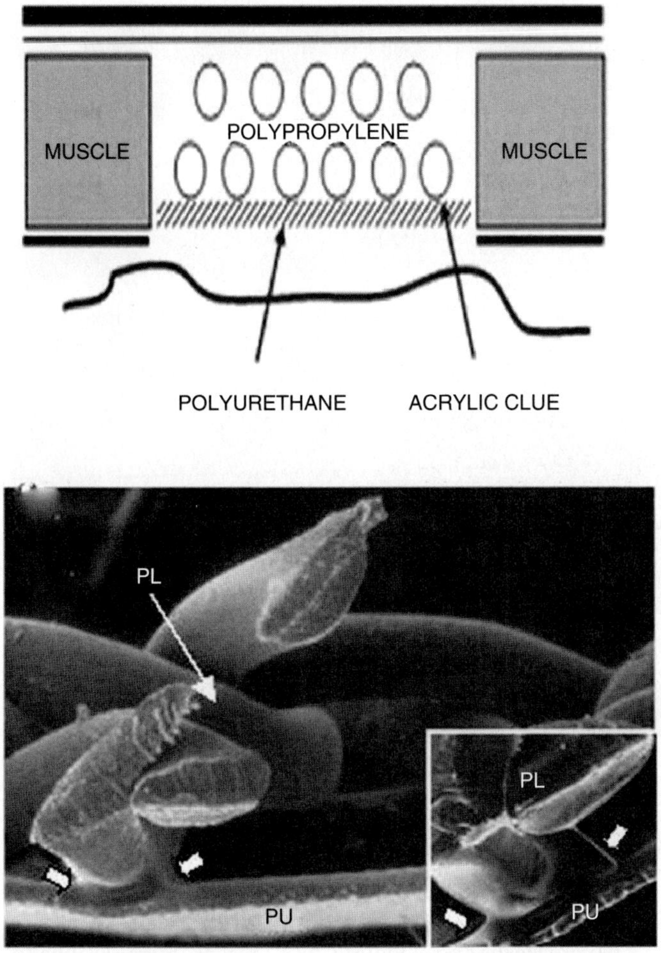

FIGURE 110.4. SEMs (*bottom*) and schematic (*top*) of PL-PU99. Polyurethane coating is shown on peritoneal side. *PL*, polypropylene; *PU*, polyurethane; *thick arrows*, acrylic glue used to attach the polyurethane layer to the polypropylene. (SEMs and product images obtained by permission from Dr. Juan Bellon.)

Polyester Derivatives

Polyester composites have been developed primarily to take advantage of the pliability and "ease of use" aspects of the material while minimizing the peritoneal inflammatory reaction. Similarly to some of the polypropylene derivatives, polyester composites have been modeled on creation of a dual interface with one face serving as the tissue integration side and the other as the adhesion barrier. The most common polyester composite is Parietex, a "double layer mesh with a three-dimensional multifiber polyester . . . on one side and a hydrophilic absorbable nonstick collagen membrane [on the other side] . . . containing a mixture of oxidized atelcollagen type I, polyethylene glycol, and glycerol"[21] (Fig. 110.5). Other polyester composites include Fluoropassiv, composed of polyester fibers treated with a fluorinated polymer and gelatin interface, and a compound (sutured) prosthesis that combines polyglactin-910 and polyester meshes (available in France; reports in the French literature).[22,23] The majority of experience has been with implementation of Parietex mesh, as reviewed next.

Published reports of animal experimentation with Parietex have yielded mostly favorable reviews. Bellon et al. investigated the potential antiadhesive properties of Parietex by comparing it to polypropylene and to a sutured polypropylene/ePTFE "sandwich" (polypropylene + ePTFE–Preclude dura substitute). They found that the two composites minimized adhesion formation while maintaining comparable abdominal wall integration as evaluated by tensiometer testing.[24] A follow-up study specifically designed to compare Parietex to the commercially available polypropylene/ePTFE composite, Composix (processed by heat rather than suture), found that both Parietex and PL-PU99 showed better adhesion prevention.[5,25]

Another comparison evaluating liquid antiadhesive barriers also showed favorable antiadhesive properties with Parietex.[5] Both Sepramesh and Parietex completely prevented adhesion formation in "clean" experimentally created wounds.[5] On histological analysis, however, Parietex, was found to be associated with greater infection rates (57% vs. 14%).[5] A more recent infected wound model (cecal injury) comparing the incidence of adhesion formation for five meshes [Parietex, Composix, Sepramesh, Parietene (polypropylene coated with a "collagen oxidized film"), and DualMesh] showed that Parietex demonstrated superior adhesion prevention compared to control (no mesh) or compared to monofilament polypropylene mesh.[8] Of note, all meshes maintained comparable strength of incorporation. The only difference found among the composites was a significantly inferior adhesion prevention rate found with Sepramesh.

Clinical usage of Parietex has primarily focused on use in laparoscopic ventral hernia repair (intraperitoneal placement). Lepere et al. and Moreno-Egea et al. recently described their experience with use of the mesh for laparoscopic transabdominal and total extraperitoneal hernia repair in a combined 1992 patients.[21,26] The former review comprised a 4-year experience with Parietex and documented a less than 1% recurrence rate and only 1 infectious complication ($n = 1972$ patients). The latter review ($n = 20$ patients) reported no documentation of infections, rejections, or recurrences in their patient population at up to 10 months. Notably, however, one author commented on the preliminary nature of these results given the inadequate follow-up period for detecting complications with intraperitoneal placement.[27,28] Leber's report on poor outcomes with intraperitoneally placed polyester noted an average follow-up of 6.7 years before any demonstration of severe polyester mesh-related complications (fistulas or erosions).[28,29] Others have since supported use of Parietex for laparoscopic total extraperitoneal hernia repair with reported complication rates of only 6% ($n = 400$ patients) at 11 month average follow-up [complications were genitourinary, pain, recurrence ($n = 1$), seromas, hematomas].[30]

Some recent studies, favorable for intraperitoneal Parietex, nevertheless bring into light the *potential* morbidity of intraperitoneal placement. Ammaturo and Arnaud, in separate studies of Parietex, showed proof of ultrasound-detected adhesions with intraperitoneal Parietex mesh.[31,32] Ammaturo et al. reported their experience with their first 26 patients treated with intraperitoneal Parietex for use in complicated ventral hernias [large defects, history of multiple prior recurrences, associated gastrointestinal (GI) pathology, and hernias located at flank borders]. Arnaud et al. directly compared rates of ultrasound-detected adhesions in patients treated with Parietex versus Mersilene mesh. Both found comparable rates of adhesion formation (12% and 18% patients, respectively,

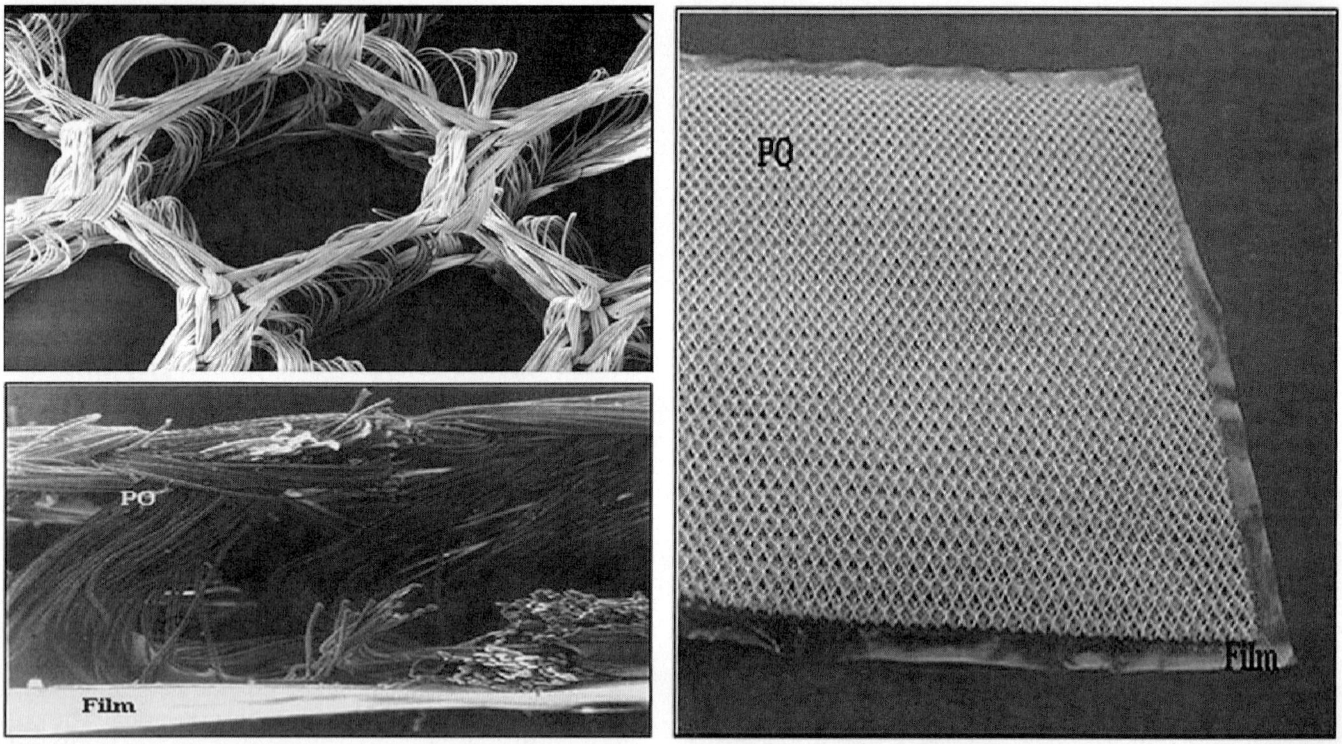

FIGURE 110.5. SEMs (*left*) and product view (*right*) of Parietex Mesh. Polyester multifibers and three-dimensional structures are shown. *PO*, polyester; *Film*, film attached to mesh, see text. (Lower SEM obtained by permission from Dr. Juan Bellon, remaining images obtained by permission from Sofradim, Inc.)

versus 77% for Mersilene) without any associated major complications (i.e., intestinal obstruction or fistulae) by 2-year and 1-year follow-up, respectively. Without knowing the clinical significance of ultrasound-detected adhesions, however, the potential morbidity of those 12% to 18% of patients remains unknown.

In summary, accumulating evidence favors many of the characteristics of Parietex mesh. It retains the pliability and integrative aspects of the traditional polyester mesh while protecting against adhesion formation on the membranous side. As noted for the other composites, long-term follow-up for this and all the others remain limited.

Expanded Polytetrafluoroethylene Derivatives

Modifications of ePTFE have been derived to overcome the observed limitations of the initial proprietary formulation of ePTFE, Soft Tissue Patch. As noted previously, the ePTFE formulation used for Soft Tissue Patch is unique in that its structure is microporous and in that it elicits less of an inflammatory response (and correspondingly fewer associated adhesions) compared to polyester or polypropylene meshes.[33] One concern weighed against the benefits of *potential* fewer intraabdominal complications is the reality of inferior tissue incorporation attributed to the muted inflammatory response. All modifications of ePTFE meshes, therefore, have been directed toward maximizing fibrous tissue ingrowth by manipulating surface characteristics of the original ePTFE form or by including a novel "separate" additional mesh surface. Last, brief mention is made of a very recent development that employs the addition of silver/clorhexidine coating to ePTFE and its derivations (PLUS meshes) designed to withstand infectious potential.

MycroMesh and DualMesh represent formulations of ePTFE devised with the intent of optimizing tissue ingrowth while maintaining reduced visceral reactions (Fig. 110.6). Simmermacher et al. were one of the first groups to show in animal models that resurfacing ePTFE by adding perforations (thus making it macroporous) created better tissue ingrowth. In fact, in their original study of ePTFE meshes, the only histological ingrowth occurred for perforated ePTFE meshes.[34] Interestingly, however, they found that this better incorporation came at the cost of decreased mechanical/tensile strength (diminished by 25%). W.L. Gore & Associates, Inc., capitalized on this experimentally demonstrated concept and developed MycroMesh by creating through-and-through perforations and stampings to the smooth laminar face of microporous Soft Tissue Patch (Fig. 110.7),[35] which created a theoretically simultaneous microporous and macroporous mesh.[36] Of the few published experimental evaluations of MycroMesh, one comparison to Marlex mesh showed improved histological tissue integration and significantly fewer and looser adhesions.[35] However, one other direct comparison with polypropylene *explants* showed significantly diminished tensile strength with MycroMesh.[35]

DualMesh offers another variation of Soft Tissue Patch that has two mesh faces, one that remains true to the Soft Tissue Patch surface and the other that enhances incorporative strength.[36] A nonporous surface retains the propensity for little adhesion formation while a newly developed, *macroporous* surface allows for better tissue integration.[36] Experiments with DualMesh have shown lower or comparable adhesion rates to those observed for both MycroMesh and Soft

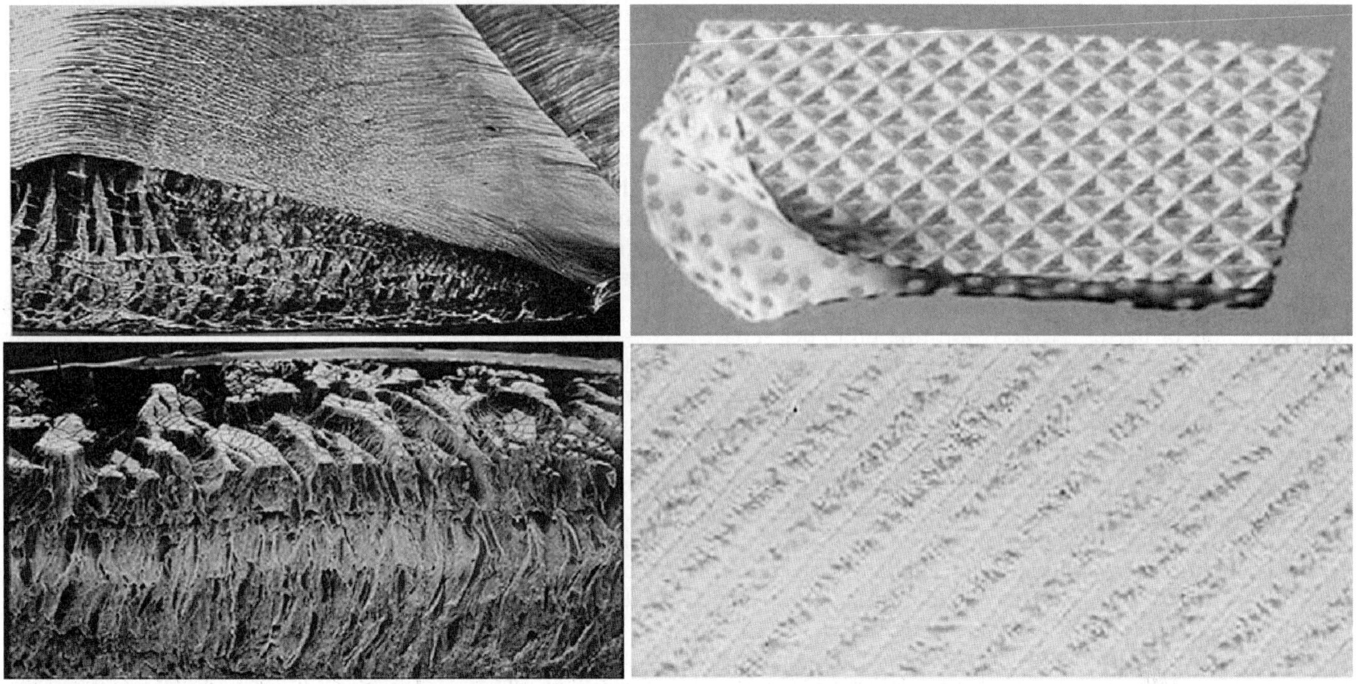

FIGURE 110.6. SEMs (*left*) and product views (*right*) of MycroMesh (*top*) and DualMesh (*bottom*). Note that textural differences shown in the micrographs account for the different mesh characteristics. Corduroy modification also shown in inset of Figure 110.7. (Images obtained by permission from W.L. Gore & Associates, Inc.)

Tissue Patch.[37–39] Integration, however, has not been as thoroughly evaluated against other meshes as had been for Soft Tissue Patch. Of those few studies that performed vigorous assessments of DualMesh incorporation, most comparisons show improved or equivalent integration of DualMesh compared to other mesh derivatives (a polyurethane-covered Dacron mesh) or other types of mesh not commonly used (bovine pericardium).[39,40] Of interest, one group showed that DualMesh was unique in its integration in that explants showed an increasing tensile strength incorporation over time in contrast to those properties observed for Soft Hernia Mesh or MycroMesh (no direct comparison was made to polypropylene or polyester mesh).[37]

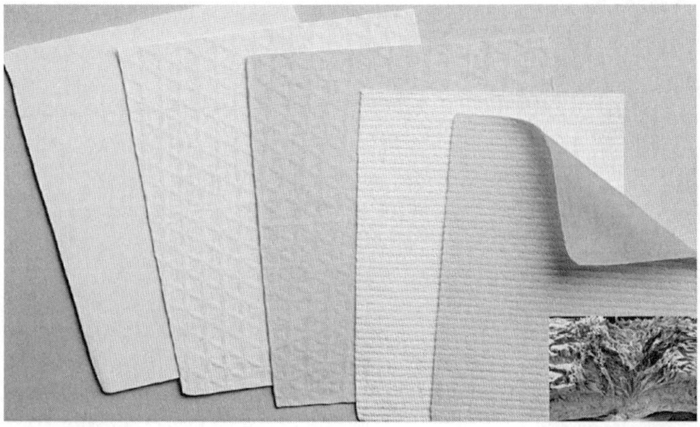

FIGURE 110.7. Product views from *left to right*: Soft Tissue Patch, MycroMesh, MycroMesh Plus, DualMesh (with corduroy surface), and DualMesh Plus. *Inset* shows the "Corduroy" modification on magnification of DualMesh. (Images obtained by permission from W.L. Gore & Associates, Inc.)

A more recent direct comparison study examining yet a newer derivative of DualMesh, DualMesh Biomaterial with Corduroy (DMBC), by Leblanc et al. specifically compared the tensiometric properties of polypropylene, DualMesh, and DMBC.[41] They noted similar tensile strengths of attachments for the former two meshes but noted superior integration with DMBC. This observation has led W.L. Gore & Associates, Inc., to modify the manufacturing process for both commercially available MycroMesh and DualMesh so that all current meshes produced under those trade names have this corduroy surface (personal communication, Jared Parker, Ph. D., product specialist, W.L. Gore & Associates, Inc.). Interestingly, some authors have remarked that the observed differences in bioincorporation of ePTFE-derived meshes underscores the importance of pattern structure (reticular versus smooth/laminar) over biochemical composition of materials as the true determinant of visceral/adhesion reactions.[34,42,43]

Clinical reports of DualMesh have primarily focused on its application in laparoscopic ventral and inguinal hernia repair. As noted in the other derivative sections, it is difficult to compare reherniation or complication rates between meshes used in these studies because the experiments were designed primarily for evaluating different surgical techniques. DeMaria et al. compared patient outcomes between laparoscopically placed intraperitoneal DualMesh compared to open prefascially placed polypropylene.[44] Less pain during recovery, a shorter hospital stay, and less total expense was found with DualMesh. The study results have been scrutinized, however, because of concerns of potential selection bias ("easier" cases) in the laparoscopic repair group. Other case reports and larger clinical experiences have affirmed, at a minimum, safety with use of this mesh, and, as well, have attested to low recurrence and low complication rates with use of DualMesh.[45–49]

The most recent modifications of the ePTFE derivatives already listed (those produced by W.L Gore & Associates, Inc) include the recently described PLUS line. These meshes have an antiinfectious coating impregnated onto the ePTFE materials placed for the purpose of withstanding/preventing of infections. Developed after reports showed lower infection rates with implanted catheters coated with antibacterial surfaces, the PLUS line has a silver and chlorhexidine combination impregnated onto the meshes. Although only one preliminary experimental reports exists at the time of this review, this comparative evaluation showed significantly lower numbers of bacteria (colony-forming units per square centimeter of mesh) for washes of and cultures of (broths) DualMesh PLUS mesh inoculated with bacteria compared to nontreated DualMesh, AlloDerm, Sepramesh, an ePTFE/polypropylene combination, and polypropylene. The authors conclude by hypothesizing that "silver/chlorhexidine impregnated meshes may be the prosthetics of choice to prevent the occurrence of mesh infection."[50]

Bard Composix mesh represents another derivative of ePTFE, consisting of a bonded ePTFE/polypropylene combination (Fig. 110.8). Rather than modifying the ePTFE mesh surface (as in MycroMesh), or adding an extra "macroporous" side (as in DualMesh), Composix maximizes tissue integration, theoretically, by utilizing two polypropylene layers added onto an ePTFE mesh.[51] Historical reports of success with the use of manually sutured combinations of polypropylene and ePTFE meshes served as the initial impetus for developing Composix mesh. Walker et al. were the first to formally experiment with a double-layer technique for combining ePTFE (Soft Tissue Patch) and polypropylene mesh (Bard Marlex mesh).[52] ePTFE/polypropylene "composites" showed lower adhesion scores (defined by the force/dissection required to free the bowel from the mesh) compared to polypropylene mesh. Bellon et al. later tested a slightly different sutured ePTFE/polypropylene combination (Preclude Dura Substitute and Prolene mesh) and similarly showed superior adhesion scores compared to polypropylene alone. Scanning electron micrographs demonstrated formation of smooth neoperitoneal layers at the intraabdominal/ePTFE interface.[24]

Experience with the commercial form, Composix, is slightly more varied. In a follow-up evaluation of the available bonded (Composix) commercial form, Bellon et al. showed surprisingly inferior intraperitoneal adhesion qualities.[20] They found dense adhesions associated with Composix mesh, in particular at points where the material had been "heat sealed." The authors utilized scanning electron microscope analysis to show less laminar surface area and hypothesized this to be a consequence of the polypropylene/ePTFE bonding process.[25] In a favorable Composix study, both Besim et al. and Greenawalt et al. reviewed the "adhesiogenic potential" of untreated polypropylene, Composix and polypropylene with added sodium hyalurontae/carboxmethylcellulose film (Seprafilm). The authors found reduced adhesion-covered mesh areas, better tissue integration, and a more optimal formation of neoperitoneum with both Composix and the polypropylene/Seprafilm composite.[6,53] Ferrando et al. specifically evaluated Composix-caused mesh shrinkage, degradation, abdominal wall inflexibility, and tissue reactivity. Favorable histological/morphometric assessments, scanning

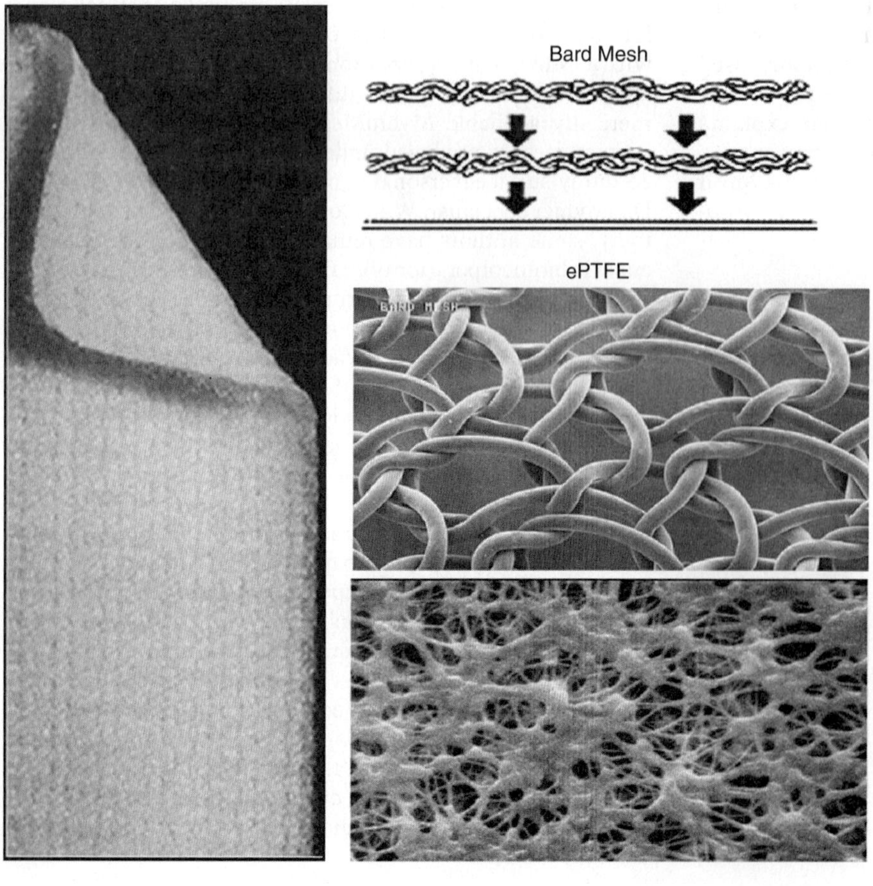

FIGURE 110.8. Product view (*left*) and schematic/SEMs (*right*) of Composix surfaces. *Upper right inset* shows the dual polypropylene layer of Composix, *middle right inset* shows a polypropylene mesh (Bard Mesh), and *lower right inset* shows expanded polytetrafluoroethylene (ePTFE). (Images obtained by permission from Davol, Inc.)

electron micrograph analyses of integration, and tensile load tests, led the authors to conclude that Composix was "a potentially optimal bio-implant for the surgical management of abdominal wall defects."[54] Winslow and Matthews, in separate studies, evaluated adhesion scores for Composix placed in an experimental laparoscopic repair model.[9,55] They both found lower adhesion scores for Composix when compared to that for intraperitoneal polypropylene mesh. Similarly, Alimoglu et al. also found low adhesion scores with Composix compared to polypropylene mesh but observed even lower adhesion scores for implanted DualMesh.[56] Despite these lower adhesion scores, however, mean histological scores for inflammation and mesothelialization did not differ between groups (possibly a less biased assessment compared to adhesion grading.) Given these wide disparities it is therefore not surprising that one recent, well-designed "multi-composite mesh" comparative study showed did not find differences adhesion prevention amongst a number of different composite meshes. Compared to untreated polypropylene, Dacron, or ePTFE, however, all composites demonstrated superior adhesion prevention.[8]

Clinical reports of use with Composix parallel DualMesh in that the studies were predominantly designed to evaluate the safety of laparoscopic intraperitoneal ventral hernia repair rather than to compare different mesh types.[57–59] The few case reports and retrospective reviews vary in complication reporting and, therefore preclude definitive conclusions with use of Composix mesh. One favorable review of 100 patients followed from 12 to 27 months postoperatively documented a 1% recurrence rate and minimal morbidity (wound infections and seromas) for laparoscopically placed Composix (ventral and inguinal hernia repair).[59–61] Another less favorable review of 95 patients followed up to 54 months, however, documented bowel fistulization in one patient and an 8% mesh infection rate for Composix-treated patients (recurrence remained low at 2%).[58] Despite these and additional case series attributing to the safety of Composix, other critics point to anecdotal observations of an associated Composix chronic pain syndrome speculated to be a consequence of mesh shrinkage.[62]

In summary, as has been to shown to be the case for the other recently developed composites, the true efficacy of Composix in preventing adhesions and thus abdominal complications remains unknown despite favorable experimental observations. The lack of consistency in complication reporting, a paucity of prospectively randomized studies, and the lack of comparative evaluations should alert the modern-day surgeon to balance carefully the potential benefits of these biomaterials against their potential for disastrous consequences, especially when considering intraperitoneal placement.

Conclusion

The composite meshes described in this section were developed as a consequence of improved insight into the prosthetic–host tissue interaction. Despite extensive experience with usage of the permanent meshes, however, data regarding the safety and clinical efficacy of these composites remain limited and should be weighed appropriately. We caution clinicians to consider the context of industrial claims of composite mesh performance, especially, when considering application of composites for high-risk complex abdominal hernia repairs.

References

1. Porter JM. A combination of Vicryl and Marlex mesh: a technique for abdominal wall closure in difficult cases. J Trauma 1995;39(6):1178–1180.
2. Naim JO, Pulley D, Scanlan K, Hinshaw JR, Lanzafame RJ. Reduction of postoperative adhesions to Marlex mesh using experimental adhesion barriers in rats. J Laparoendosc Surg 1993;3(2):187–190.
3. Dayton MT, Buchele BA, Shirazi SS, Hunt LB. Use of an absorbable mesh to repair contaminated abdominal-wall defects. Arch Surg 1986;121(8):954–960.
4. Amid PK, Lichtenstein IL, Sostrin S, Young J, Hakakkha M. Experimental evaluation of a new composite mesh with the selective property of incorporation to the abdominal wall without adhering to the intestines. J Biomed Mater Res 1994; 28:373–375.
5. van 't Riet M, de Vos van Steenwijk PJ, Bonthuis F, et al. Prevention of adhesion to prosthetic mesh: comparison of different barriers using an incisional hernia model. Ann Surg 2003;237(1): 123–128.
6. Greenawalt KE, Butler TJ, Rowe EA, Finneral AC, Garlick DS, Burns JW. Evaluation of sepramesh biosurgical composite in a rabbit hernia repair model. J Surg Res 2000;94(2):92–98.
7. Young RM, Gustafson R, Dinsmore RC. Sepramesh vs. Dualmesh for abdominal wall hernia repairs in a rabbit model. Curr Surg 2004;61(1):77–79.
8. Gonzalez R, Rodeheaver GT, Moody DL, Foresman PA, Ramshaw BJ. Resistance to adhesion formation: a comparative study of treated and untreated mesh products placed in the abdominal cavity. Hernia 2004;8:213–219.
9. Matthews BD, Mostafa G, Carbonell AM, et al. Evaluation of adhesion formation and host tissue response to intra-abdominal polytetrafluoroethylene mesh and composite prosthetic mesh. J Surg Res 2005;123(2):227–234.
10. Klinge U, Conze J, Limberg W, Obolenski B, Ottinger AP, Schumpelick V. Modified mesh for hernia repair that is adapted to the physiology of the abdominal wall. Eur J Surg 1998;164:951–960.
11. Junge K, Klinge U, Rosch R, Klosterhalfen B, Schumpelick V. Functional and morphologic properties of a modified mesh for inguinal hernia repair. World J Surg 2002;26(12):1472–1480.
12. Zieren J, Neuss H, Ablassmaier B, Müller JM. Adhesions after intraperitoneal mesh repair in pigs: Prolene vs. Vypro. J Laparoendosc Adv Surg Tech A 2002;12(4):249–252.
13. Schmidbauer S, Ladurner R, Hallfeldt KK, Mussack T. Heavy-weight versus low-weight polypropylene meshes for open sublay mesh repair of incisional hernia. Eur J Med Res 2005;10(6):247–253.
14. Bringman S, Wollert S, Osterberg J, et al. One year results of a randomised controlled multi-centre study comparing Prolene and Vypro II-mesh in Lichtenstein hernioplasty. Hernia 2005;9:223–227.
15. Scheidbach H, Tamme C, Tannapfel A, Lippert H, Köckerling F. In vivo studies comparing the biocompatibility of various polypropylene meshes and their handling properties during endoscopic total extraperitoneal (TEP) patchplasty: an experimental study in pigs. Surg Endosc 2004;18(2):211–220.
16. Heinlein M. Effectiveness of titanium containing coatings.GFE website: www.gfe.com., 2005.
17. Langenbach MR, Schmidt J, Zirngibl H. Comparison of biomaterials in the early postoperative period. Surg Endosc 2003;17:1105–1109.

18. Tamme C, Scheidbach H, Hampe C, Schneider C, Köckerling F. Totally extraperitoneal endoscopic inguinal hernia repair (TEP). Surg Endosc 2003;17(2):190–195.
19. Tamme C, Garde N, Klingler A, Hampe C, Wunder R, Köckerling F. Totally extraperitoneal inguinal hernioplasty with titanium-coated lightweight polypropylene mesh: early results. Surg Endosc 2005;19:1125–1129.
20. Bellón JM, García-Carranza A, Jurado F, García-Honduvilla N, Carrera-San Martín A, Buján J. Evaluation of a new composite prosthesis (PL-PU99) for the repair of abdominal wall defects in terms of behavior at the peritoneal interface. World J Surg 2002;26(6):661–666.
21. Moreno-Egea A, Lirón R, Girela E, Aguayo JL. Laparoscopic repair of ventral and incisional hernias using a new composite mesh (Parietex): initial experience. Surg Laparosc Endosc Percutan Tech 2001;11(2):103–106.
22. Soler M, Stoppa R. Polyester (Dacron) mesh. In: Bendavid MR, ed. Abdominal Wall Hernias: Principles and Management. New York: Springer, 2001:266–271.
23. Soares BM, King MW, Marois Y. In vitro characterization of a fluoropassivated gelatin-impregnated polyester mesh for hernia repair. J Biomed Mater Res 1996;32(2):259–270.
24. Bellón JM, García-Carranza A, Jurado F, García-Honduvilla N, Carrera-San Martín A, Buján J. Peritoneal regeneration after implant of a composite prosthesis in the abdominal wall. World J Surg 2001;25(2):147–152.
25. Bellón JM, Jurado F, García-Moreno F, Corrales C, Carrera-San Martín A, Buján J. Healing process induced by three composite prostheses in the repair of abdominal wall defects. J Biomed Mater Res 2002;63(2):182–190.
26. Lepere M, Benchetrit S, Debaert M, et al. A multicentric comparison of transabdominal versus totally extraperitoneal laparoscopic hernia repair using PARIETEX meshes. J Surg Laparasc Surg 2000;4(2):147–153.
27. Moreno-Egea A, Castillo JA, Girela E, Canteras M, Aguayo JL. Outpatient laparoscopic incisional/ventral hernioplasty: our experience in 55 cases. Surg Laparosc Endosc Percutan Tech 2002;12(3):171–174.
28. LeBlanc KA. Outpatient laparoscopic incisional/ventral hernioplasty: our experience in 55 cases by Moreno-Egea et al. Surg Laparosc Endosc Percutan Tech 2002;12(6):451–452; author reply 452.
29. Leber GE, Garb JL, Alexander AI, Reed WP. Long-term complications associated with prosthetic repair of incisional hernias. Arch Surg 1998;133(4):378–382.
30. Ramshaw B, Abiad F, Voeller G, Wilson R, Mason E. Polyester (Parietex) mesh for total extraperitoneal laparoscopic inguinal hernia repair: initial experience in the United States. Surg Endosc 2003;17(3):498–501.
31. Arnaud JP, Hennekinne-Mucci S, Pessaux P, Tuech JJ, Aube C. Ultrasound detection of visceral adhesion after intraperitoneal ventral hernia treatment: a comparative study of protected versus unprotected meshes. Hernia 2003;7(2):85–88.
32. Ammaturo C, Bassi G. Surgical treatment of large incisional hernias with an intraperitoneal Parietex Composite mesh: our preliminary experience on 26 cases. Hernia 2004;8:242–246.
33. Kossovsky N, Horwath D. Biomaterials pathology, In: Bendavid MR, ed. Abdominal Wall Hernias: Principles and Management. New York: Springer, 2001:221–234.
34. Simmermacher RK, van der Lei B, Schakenraad JM, Bleichrodt RP. Improved tissue ingrowth and anchorage of expanded polytetrafluoroethylene by perforation: an experimental study in the rat. Biomaterials 1991;12(1):22–24.
35. Bellon JM, Contreras LA, Carrera-San Martin A, Jurado F. Comparison of a new type of PTFE patch (Mycro mesh) and polypropylene prostheses (Marlex) for repair of abdominal wall defects. J Am Coll Surg 1996;183:11–18.
36. Website http://www.goremedical.com/English/Products/GeneralSurgery.htm.
37. Bellon JM, Carrera-San Martin A. Experimental assay of a dual mesh PTFE (non-porous on one side) in the repair of abdominal wall defects. Biomaterials 1996;17:2367–2372.
38. Matthews BD, Pratt BL, Pollinger HS, et al. Assessment of adhesion formation to intra-abdominal polypropylene mesh and polytetrafluoroethylene mesh. J Surg Res 2003;114(2):126–132.
39. Zieren J, Paul M, Osei-Agyemang T, Maecker F, Müller JM. Polyurethane-covered dacron mesh versus polytetrafluoroethylene DualMesh for intraperitoneal hernia repair in rats. Surg Today, 2002;32(10):884–886.
40. Kapan S, Kapan M, Goksoy E, Karabicak I, Oktar H. Comparison of PTFE, pericardium bovine and fascia lata for repair of incisional hernia in rat model, experimental study. Hernia 2003;7(1):39–43.
41. LeBlanc KA, Bellanger D, Rhynes KV 5th, Baker DG, Stout RW. Tissue attachment strength of prosthetic meshes used in ventral and incisional hernia repair. A study in the New Zealand White rabbit adhesion model. Surg Endosc 2002;16(11):1542–1546.
42. Bellón JM, Jurado F, García-Honduvilla N, López R, Carrera-San Martín A, Buján J. The structure of a biomaterial rather than its chemical composition modulates the repair process at the peritoneal level. Am J Surg 2002;184(2):154–159.
43. Simmermacher R. Intraperitoneal prostheses. In: Bendavid MR, ed. Abdominal Wall Hernias: Principles and Management. New York: Springer, 2001:299–305.
44. DeMaria EJ, Moss JM, Sugerman HJ. Laparoscopic intraperitoneal polytetrafluoroethylene (PTFE) prosthetic patch repair of ventral hernia. Prospective comparison to open prefascial polypropylene mesh repair. Surg Endosc 2000;14(4):326–329.
45. Tsimoyiannis EC, Tassis A, Glantzounis G, Jabarin M, Siakas P, Tzourou H. Laparoscopic intraperitoneal onlay mesh repair of incisional hernia. Surg Laparosc Endosc 1998;8(5):360–362.
46. Lau H, Patil NG, Yuen WK, Lee F. Laparoscopic incisional hernioplasty utilising on-lay expanded polytetrafluoroethylene DualMesh: prospective study. Hong Kong Med J 2002;8(6):413–417.
47. Lau H, Lee F, Patil NG. Laparoscopic repair of incisional hernia. Hong Kong Med J 2001;7(3):319–321.
48. LeBlanc KA, Booth WV, Whitaker JM, Bellanger DE. Laparoscopic incisional and ventral herniorraphy: our initial 100 patients. Hernia 2001;5(1):41–45.
49. Berger D, Bientzle M, Muller A. Postoperative complications after laparoscopic incisional hernia repair. Incidence and treatment. Surg Endosc 2002;16(12):1720–1723.
50. Carbonell AM, Matthews BD, Dréau D, et al. The susceptibility of prosthetic biomaterials to infection. Surg Endosc 2005;19(3):430–435.
51. Website http://www.perfixplug.com/compos.htm.
52. Walker AP, Henderson J, Condon RE. Double-layer prostheses for repair of abdominal wall defects in a rabbit model. J Surg Res 1993;55(1):32–37.
53. Besim H, Yalçin Y, Hamamcí O, et al. Prevention of intraabdominal adhesions produced by polypropylene mesh. Eur Surg Res 2002;34(3):239–243.
54. Ferrando JM, Vidal J, Armengol M, et al. Experimental evaluation of a new layered prosthesis exhibiting a low tensile modulus of elasticity: long-term integration response within the rat abdominal wall. World J Surg 2002;26(4):409–415.
55. Winslow ER, Diaz S, Desai K, Meininger T, Soper NJ, Klingensmith ME. Laparoscopic incisional hernia repair in a porcine model: what do transfixion sutures add? Surg Endosc 2004;18(3):529–535.
56. Alimoglu O, Akcakaya A, Sahin M, et al. Prevention of adhesion formations following repair of abdominal wall defects with prosthetic materials (an experimental study). Hepatogastroenterology 2003;50(51):725–728.

57. Araki Y, Ishibashi N, Kanazawa M, et al. Laparoscopic intraperitoneal repair of postoperative ventral incisional hernia using Composix mesh. Kurume Med J 2002;49(4):167–170.
58. Cobb WS, Harris JB, Lokey JS, McGill ES, Klove KL. Incisional herniorrhaphy with intraperitoneal composite mesh: a report of 95 cases. Am Surg 2003;69(9):784–787.
59. Gillian GK, Geis WP, Grover G. Laparoscopic incisional and ventral hernia repair (LIVH): an evolving outpatient technique. J Surg Laparosc Surg 2002;6(4):315–322.
60. Furukawa K, Taniai N, Suzuki H, et al. Abdominal incisional hernia repair using the Composix Kugel Patch: two case reports. J Nippon Med School 2005;72(3):182–186.
61. Settembre A, Cuccurullo D, Pisaniello D, Capasso P, Miranda L, Corcione F. Laparoscopic repair of congenital diaphragmatic hernia with prosthesis: a case report. Hernia 2003;7(1):52–54.
62. LeBlanc KA, Whitaker JM. Management of chronic postoperative pain following incisional hernia repair with Composix mesh: a report of two cases. Hernia 2002;6(4):194–197.

111

Biomaterials and the Evolution of Hernia Repair III: Biologically Derived Prosthetic Meshes

Raul A. Cortes, Edward Miranda, Hanmin Lee, and Michael E. Gertner

The concept of using biologically based tissues as constructs is not new. For example, tissue-based heart valves have been used in cardiac surgery for more than three decades with excellent clinical success. Using protein fixation techniques, long-term host recognition of cadaveric or porcine antigens have been successfully repressed.

In addition to the field of cardiac surgery, biological constructs have been increasingly implemented in a wide array of other clinical settings. One particular expanding niche has been for application in hernia repair. Greater understanding of the biology behind the tissue fixation process, more advanced protein purification techniques, and better substrate attachment have allowed for greater biomaterial application. As well, limitations in the function of traditional meshes for use in complicated abdominal wall defects have driven the field of mesh biocomposites.

The list of biologically derived meshes and their indications for use seem to be expanding daily. Novel materials continue to be developed as advances are made in other branches of materials science (e.g., nanotechnology). Described below are the most advanced hernia meshes (Surgisis, AlloDerm, and Permacol) (Table 111.1). The science behind biocomposite manufacture/production as well as supporting animal and clinical data are reviewed. The reader must note, however, that most current animal data are limited and that clinical data are relegated to retrospective or small case series. Irregardless, investigations and examinations into the in vivo response to these biomaterials continue to evolve, especially as trends in innovative clinical applications expand experimental efforts.

Biologically derived composite meshes, biocomposites, have been developed to overcome the limits of traditional synthetic prostheses. These materials were initially designed to overcome the challenges of complex hernia repair such as repair with unstable skin coverage, extensive loss of abdominal fascia, intraabdominal contamination, or after removal of infected mesh. Interestingly, use of biocomposites has been increasingly applied to more standard hernia repairs. This change has been driven by the outstanding safety profiles of tissue-based meshes and by the opportunity to avoid using traditional meshes fraught with high recurrence rates and fistulous/infections complications.[1]

Repair with *autologous* tissues marked initial efforts to find mesh alternatives to the traditional mesh materials. This approach developed from well-documented evidence of the resilience of autologous tissues placed within infected operative fields. Donor site morbidity and factors such as the location of the defect, however, quickly became constraints for this type of repair.[2,3] Newer efforts, based on this biological design, led to productions of the current biocomposites. Porcine small intestinal submucosa (Surgisis), human cadaveric acellular dermal matrix (AlloDerm), and porcine dermis (Permacol) represent these newer biological derivatives.

In general, the principles of creating these materials include separation of tissue layers (the submucosa from the small intestine or the dermis from epidermis), removal of cellular components (typically with detergents), and tissue strengthening by cross-linking collagen (Fig. 111. 1). In fact, these strengthening and immunomodulatory steps likely con-

TABLE 111.1. Overview of Current Biocomposite Formulations.

Current bioprosthetic materials	*Composition*
Surgisis	Porcine intestine submucosa: antigens removed, sterilized
AlloDerm	Human dermis: antigens removed, sterilized and cross-linked
Permacol	Porcine dermis: antigens removed, sterilized and cross-linked

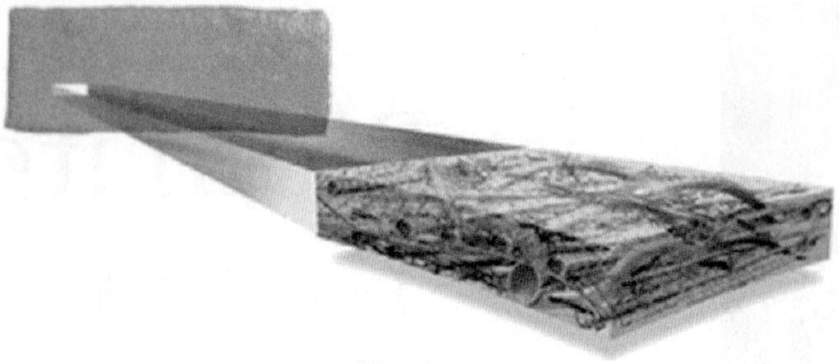

FIGURE 111.1. Schematic view of AlloDerm. The matrix retains native dermis architecture but is processed to destroy antigenicity and maximize mesh strength (Courtesy of LifeCell.)

tribute to increased mesh effectiveness more so than the mesh tissue-specific origin. Indeed, in vitro studies have underscored that importance of adding fixatives such as formaldehyde and glutaraldehyde to biological tissue replacements to ameliorate the deleterious effects of native or nonnative collagenases.[4]

Porcine Small Intestinal Submucosa

Physical Properties

Mesh derived from porcine small intestinal submucosa is commercially available as small intestinal submucosa (SIS) by Cook Corporation. The submucosa, the strongest layer of the intestinal wall, is resected from the small intestines of slaughtered pigs. After dissection and removal of the mesentery, the small intestine is opened longitudinally and the mucosal and muscular layers removed mechanically. The remaining layer is composed of submucosa, extracellular matrix, and a cellular portion that includes fibroblasts and leukocytes. Using detergent-based chemical lysis, the cellular layer is then removed to produce the final product, an acellular submucosal matrix (Fig. 111.2).

Animal/Experimental Data

Animal studies of SIS have focused on graft xenogenicity, graft–host integration, and strength of graft–host tissue interfaces. Allman et al. used a murine model to investigate histological and cytokine patterns of the xenograft–host immune response. SIS, a negative syngeneic control (mouse abdominal muscle), urinary bladder submucosa, and a positive xenogeneic control (rat abdominal muscle) were placed in a subcutaneous pocket and then harvested for examination at different postsurgical time points.[5] Examination of the immune reactions to SIS implants were noteworthy for an initial acute inflammatory response *not* characterized by hyperacute rejection (as expected to occur with the xenogeneic material) but rather characterized by a *muted* response similar to that elicited by syngeneic tissue. Serum and graft site cytokine profiles corroborated histological findings and showed increased interleukin (IL)-4 and IgG-1 but not interferon (IFN)-γ or IL-12. The authors concluded that the T_H2-restricted immune cell response represented immunogenic tolerance. Indeed, by 28 days, SIS was histologically indistinguishable from syngeneic implants, thereby signifying graft tolerance and complete incorporation.[6] Further investigations into the mechanisms of this immune tolerance have suggested that it is mediated, in part, by porcine transforming growth factor (TGF)-β activity inherent to the implanted xenografts.[7] Despite this inherent immunomodulation, however, Allman et al. showed that host responses to foreign materials remained intact.[6]

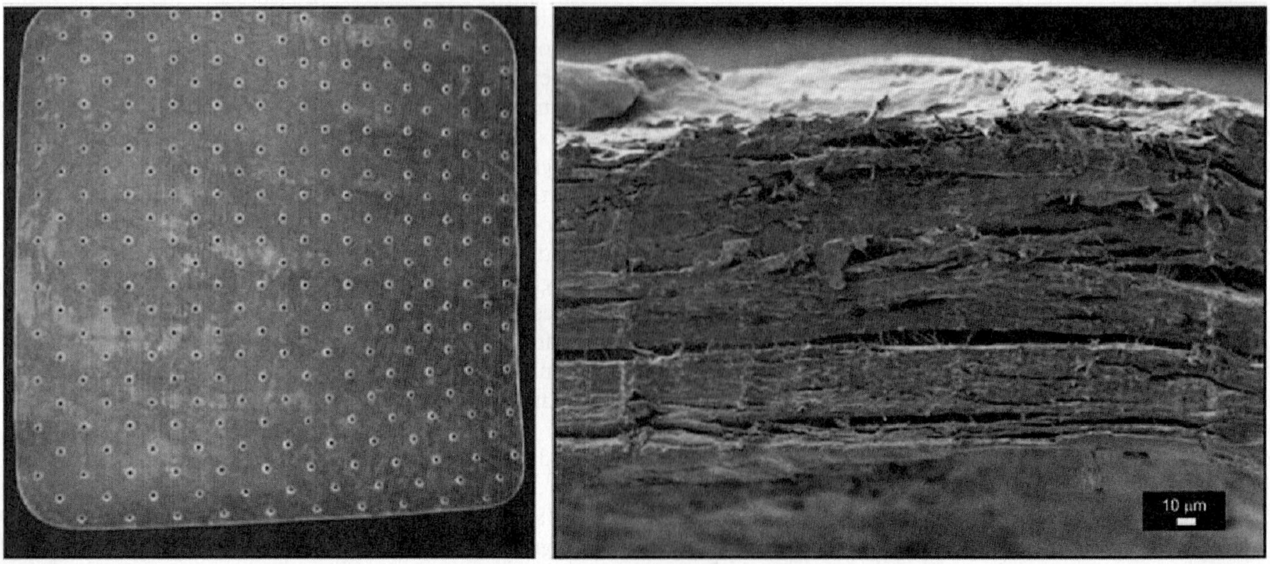

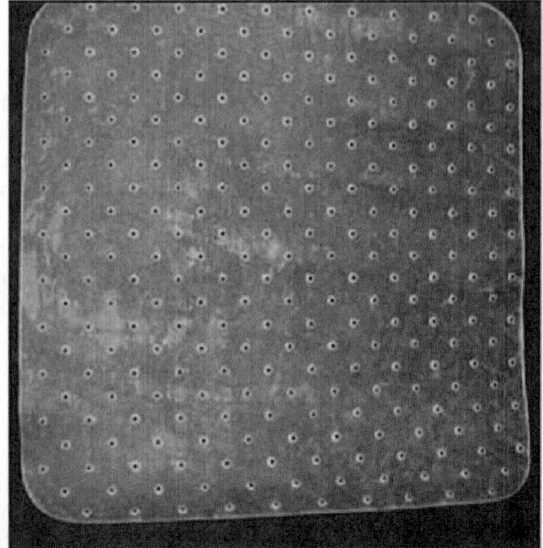

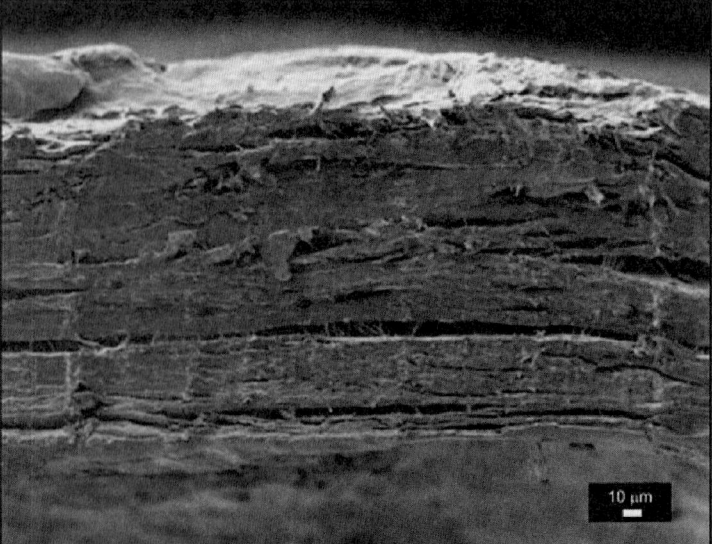

FIGURE 111.2. Product view (*left*) and scanning electron micrograph (SEM) (*right*) of porcine small intestinal submucosa (SIS) mesh. (Images obtained by permission from Cook Corporation.)

Host integration of SIS has been shown to occur through production of a histological structure characteristic of local connective tissue. In recently described rodent and canine abdominal defect models, SIS was shown to result in production of "neoconnective tissue" more typical of native fascia rather than the typical scar produced by nonabsorbable mesh materials.[8,9] In fact, in a separate examination, Dejardin et al. showed that cellular ingrowth and angiogenesis (at 12 weeks) of integrated SIS resembled native architecture of central and peripheral fascia lata.[10]

The biomechanical strength of incorporated SIS was measured by Badylak et al. and found to be within a supraphysiological range after implantation.[11] Using a canine "body wall repair" model, the authors collected and analyzed abdominal explants of incorporated SIS and determined graft–tissue burst strengths using a ball-constant compression device at numerous time points of sacrifice. At early time points (10 days), strength diminished progressively until a nadir of approximately 55% of the initial device strength; however, beyond this, strength increased progressively to approximately 200% of the preimplantation level by 2 years follow-up.

Clinical Data

Reports of clinical experience with SIS include application in laparoscopic inguinal and ventral hernia repair, application in infected inguinal/ventral hernias, and use in laparoscopic paraesophageal hernia repair. As has been the case with many of the newer synthetic meshes to date, few prospectively randomized direct comparisons of SIS to other meshes exist. The predominant focus of investigations, rather, has been on mesh performance in high-risk patients and in complicated hernia repairs. Available data are presented in Table 111.2.

In a recent prospectively nonrandomized comparison, Edelman et al. reported on the outcomes of 12 patients who underwent laparoscopic total extraperitoneal (TEP) inguinal

TABLE 111.2.
Summary of Major Clinical Studies of Porcine Small Intestinal Submucosa (SIS) Used in Herniorrhaphy.

Study	*Reference*	*Year*	*Type*	*n*	*Follow-up*	*Outcomes*	*Class*	*Notes*
Lap inguinal/ ventral	Franklin[13]	2004	Consecutive patients	53	1–30 months (median, 19)	0% recurrence; 0% complications	3	20 (34% clean-contaminated), 13 (22% contaminated)
Inguinal/ ventral	Ueno[14]	2004	Prospective nonrandomized, uncontrolled	20 (18 ventral, 2 inguinal)	—	1 (5%) mortality from fasciitis with breakdown of mesh, 8 (40%) wound infections, 6 (30%) recurrence by CT	—	50% clean contaminated, 50% contaminated/ infected; 5/6 recurrences occurred in patients operated on for a grossly infected wound or mesh
Lap para-esophageal	Oelschlage[16]	2003	Retrospective case series	9	3–16 months (median, 8)	1/9 recurrence, 1/9 mortality (CVA); no prosthetic complications	3	The 9 study patients were selected from 18 total who were intraoperatively judged that tension-free closure was not possible.
TEP	Edelman[12]	2002	Prospective non-randomized, Prolene controls	24	—	No differences	2	15 inguinal herniae in 12 test patients were compared with 12 patients who underwent repair with Prolene mesh
Lap Stoppa–Rives with lap gastric bypass	Eid	2003	Retrospective non-randomized case series	85	7–53 months (mean, 26)	0% recurrence in SIS vs. 22% recurrence in primary repair	3	59 primary repairs, 12 SIS via Stoppa-rives technique, 14 deferred repair. SIS only had mean follow-up of 13 (7–18) months vs. 30 (18–53) months in primary repair; 3/12 wound infections in SIS, 4/12 seromas in SIS

Lap, laparoscopy; TEP total extraperitoneal, total extraperitoneal.

hernia repair with SIS and compared their outcomes to historical outcomes for 12 others who had undergone repair with polypropylene mesh.[12] Fewer complications were noted compared to the historical controls, and those that did occur were limited to 3 postoperative seromas (25%) and 1 case of postoperative dysuria (phone interviews at 1 year).

Other retrospective/observational studies have specifically examined differences in treated patient-outcomes for SIS placed in clean-contaminated and contaminated operative fields. Franklin et al. followed 53 patients in a prospectively nonrandomized fashion who underwent complicated laparoscopic ventral or inguinal hernia repairs in clean (n = 20), clean-contaminated (e.g., concurrent laparoscopic colectomy/cholecystectomy or exploratory laparoscopy for incarcerated or strangulated bowel; n = 20), or grossly contaminated environments (gross pus or fecal spillage; n = 13). At 19 months follow-up, no recurrences had occurred, and only 1 wound infection was observed for a patient who had been intraoperatively noted to have nonviable bowel.[13] Ueno et al. also evaluated outcomes for patients (n = 20) who had SIS placed in clean-contaminated or grossly infected circumstances (most commonly after removal of infected mesh). Fifty percent of patients sustained early postoperative complications including 7 wound infections (6 in grossly infected scenarios), 2 postoperative seromas, and 1 death from fascial infection. At mean follow-up of 16 months, recurrences were present in 30% of patients (5 of these 6 patients had had mesh placed in grossly infected wounds). In spite of their higher complication rates, the authors still advocated use of SIS in the management of grossly contaminated hernias. They suggested that SIS offered relatively low recurrence rates without evidence for chronic infection or risk of early evisceration when compared to the poor outcomes with the available alternatives: closure under tension, component separation, polypropylene mesh, polyglactin mesh, or simple skin closure.[14]

Helton et al. performed a more recent retrospective review of 53 patients who underwent SIS ventral hernia repair (median follow-up, 14 months) and stratified outcomes based on both wound classifications (clean, clean-contaminated, and dirty) and clinical status (i.e., critically ill, elective, etc.).[15] In what now appears to be a growing pattern in the clinical data, 66% of patients who had the mesh placed into dirty wounds required reoperations and 39% sustained recurrences. In the "clean" and "clean-contaminated" cohorts, the recurrence rates were 4% and 9%, respectively. Although overall these rates represented significant improvement over the typically quoted incisional hernia recurrence rates of 30% to 50%, the authors acknowledged that larger comparative studies were still needed.

Another unique application for SIS has been for use in paraesophageal or primary diaphragmatic repairs. Oelschlager et al. reported on nine SIS repairs with a median follow-up of 8 months and noted only one recurrence (one death from an unrelated cause [stroke] did occur).[16] No other additional prosthetic-related complications were reported.

To conclude, the use of SIS remains in its early stages. The available studies suggest that it may be useful as a fascial replacement in both routine and complicated abdominal hernias. In particular, many studies have focused on its role as a prosthetic for infected or contaminated operative fields. Although SIS appears to have utility for use in all situations, Level I data are still needed.

Acellular Human Dermal Matrix

Physical Properties

Acellular human dermis is commercially available as AlloDerm by LifeCell Corporation. It is prepared from cadaveric human dermis by a proprietary method and then cryopreserved in a manner that avoids the structural damage that normally occurs with ice crystal formation (Fig. 111.3). Although this matrix preparation method is proprietary, an initial "pilot" harvest method has been previously described in a porcine model.[17] In this model, harvested split thickness skin (0.025 inches) is separated from the epidermis via overnight incubation in 1 M NaCl. Dermal cells (fibroblasts and endothelial cells) are removed by digestion with 0.5% sodium dodecyl sulfate, after which the absence of cellular organelles is affirmed by electron microscopy. The remaining matrix is cryoprotected in a solution of 6% sucrose, 7% dextran, 6% raffinose/1 mM ethylenediaminetetraacetic acid (EDTA), and freeze-dried at −23°C. Rewarmed product (20°C) is then stored for later rehydration at room temperature just prior to use. On immunohistochemical analysis, the remaining dermal matrix is composed of undamaged collagen, elastin, and laminin.

Animal/Experimental Data

Allograft dermal matrices have had vast applications in other fields outside of fascial/hernia surgery including use as replacements for skin (burns), gingiva, dura mater, and soft tissue (augmentation).[18–23] Similarly to the other biocomposite meshes, initial AlloDerm investigations focused on evaluating its immunogenic potential in vivo.

Knowing that the epidermis and skin cellular components accounted for the source of rejection of allografts used in full-thickness burns, Livesey et al. hypothesized that a "de-epidermized" porcine dermal allograft could achieve tolerance in a rat (xenotransplant) model.[17] Prepared as described above, dermal matrices were implanted into full-thickness wounds and subsequently removed and analyzed histologically. By 21 days postimplantation, explants revealed minimal inflammation (no lymphocytes) and a thin scar capsule (few cell layers thick). Grafts were integrated into host tissues as evidenced by fibroblast infiltration/neovascularization and matrices maintained structural integrity as confirmed by ultrastructural analysis (transmission electron microscopy). Wainwright et al. similarly showed neovascularization and neoepithelization of dermal grafts applied clinically for coverage of full-thickness burn wounds.[18]

Menon et al. specifically evaluated the efficacy of AlloDerm for use as a fascial replacement in a rabbit hernia model.[24] Full-thickness abdominal wall resections were repaired by either primary closure, expanded polytetrafluoroethylene (ePTFE; MycroMesh), or acellular human dermal matrix. After 28 days, no recurrences were noted; however, all MycroMesh animals developed visceral adhesions whereas none formed in those treated with AlloDerm. Furthermore, fluorescein injections showed revascularization of acellular matrices without evidence of rejection.

Acellular dermal matrices have also been evaluated for use as prosthetic replacements in the context of peritoneal

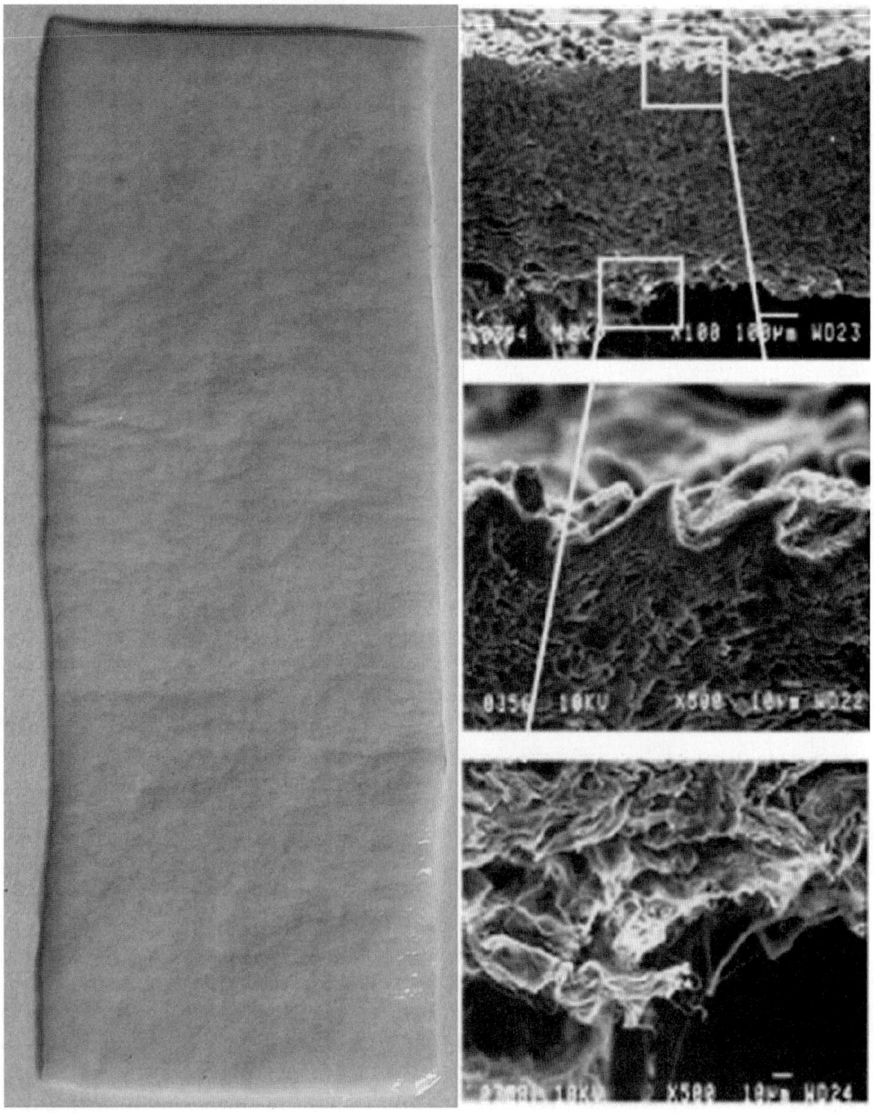

FIGURE 111.3. Product view (*left*) and SEM images (*right*) of AlloDerm mesh. *Upper right*, 100×; *middle right*, 500× reticular surface view; *lower right inset*, 500× basement surface view. (Images obtained by permission from LifeCell, Inc.)

infection and loss of skin coverage. An et al. used rat stool slurry to "contaminate" wounds during repair of full-thickness abdominal defects with either an acellular rat dermal matrix or ePTFE (Soft Tissue Patch)(25). They observed a lower mortality with the acellular dermal matrix compared to ePTFE and noted faster epithelialization and overall wound healing in the matrix group. Of interest, however, both groups were noted to have equivalent evisceration/fistulalization rates as well as visceral adhesion formation (graded as moderate) by 21 days postimplantation.

Tensiometric analyses of integrated AlloDerm explants have also been shown to be either comparable or superior to other synthetic meshes. Menon et al. found no differences in patch–fascial interface breaking strengths between integrated MycroMesh and AlloDerm meshes (of note, primarily closed defects had significantly higher breaking strengths). Additionally, there was no incidence of reherniation or contraction of the matrix; in fact, 2 of 10 matrix grafts were noted to have expanded approximately 1 cm (not significant).[24] Interestingly, Silverman et al. found that AlloDerm patch–fascial interfaces had *higher* breaking strengths than ePTFE mesh interfaces and *comparable* breaking strengths compared to primarily closed defects.[20]

Clinical Data

Few clinical studies describe the role of AlloDerm for application in human herniorraphy. Of those reported, experience has been with its use for complex abdominal wall reconstruction, for repair of enterocutaneous fistulae, and for fascial repair after transverse rectus abdominis musculocutaneous (TRAM) flap harvest (for breast reconstruction).[26–29] Clinical experience is summarized in Table 111.3.

Guy et al. described use of AlloDerm for an early one-stage closure in patients with abdominal compartment syndrome.[27] In their study, they describe outcomes of patients who had AlloDerm implanted as a fascial substitute during decompressive celiotomies. Before discharge from the trauma unit, three patients (33%) demonstrated complications including one flap hematoma, wound infection, and hernia recurrence.[27]

TABLE 111.3.
Summary of Major Clinical Studies of AlloDerm (Acellular Dermal Matrix) Used in Herniorrhaphy.

Study	*Reference*	*Year*	*Type*	*n*	*Follow-up*	*Outcomes*	*Class*	*Notes*
Primary TRAM or complex abdominal wall reconstructions	Buinewicz[28]	2004	Retrospective case series, no controls	44	8–31 months (mean, 20)	0/18 TRAM hernias; 2/26 recurrences; 3 SS infections, 2 dehiscences, 2 seromas, 0 reoperations, 0 removal of prosthesis	3	18 TRAMs and 26 abdominal wall reconstructions; double-layer interpositions were used for complex abdominal wall reconstructions after the 2 recurrences were detected
Fascial replacement after abdominal compartment syndrome	Guy[27]	2003	Retrospective case series, no controls	9	—	1/9 recurrence, 1 hematoma, 1 wound infection	3	Average closure on POD #9
Abdominal wall reconstructions	Silverman[20]	2004	Retrospective case series, no controls, nonrandom ("highly selected")	13	3–12 months (mean, 6)	0 recurrences, 0 removals of dermal matrix allografts	4	Non-peer-reviewed (preliminary comment)

TRAM, transverse rectus abdominis musculocutaneous flap.

Buinewicz et al. described AlloDerm use for both prophylactic rectus fascial reinforcement after TRAM procedures and ventral/incisional hernia repair.[28] Of 44 patients evaluated at an average 20-month follow-up, 9 (21%) had surgically related complications. Although none required reoperation, 3 patients experienced postoperative infection (7%), 2 underwent dehiscences (5%), 2 had recurrences (5%) and 2 developed postoperative seromas (5%). The authors report that recurrences subsequently dropped to 0% after a modification of their mesh implantation technique (a multilayer repair.) The significance of these results are unclear, however, as similarly low hernias and infection rates have been shown to occur with other prosthetic meshes (1.5%).[30] Finally, Girard et al. reported on a novel application of AlloDerm for sealing deserosalized bowel and treating intestinal fistulae in complicated abdominal wounds.[29] The authors applied AlloDerm to open abdomens either directly over deserosalized bowel (2 patients) or as a barrier over an enterocutaneous fistula (one patient). No fistulae developed after "patching" bowel, and the treated fistula eventually closed. The authors concluded by cautiously recommending further investigation into their new "patching" technique.

In conclusion, AlloDerm is a relatively new bioprosthetic similar to SIS in its utility as a fascial substitute for contaminated settings. Although preliminary clinical data appear favorable, further animal evaluations are needed in light of reported variability in AlloDerm outcomes.

Acellular Porcine Dermis (Permacol)

A new arrival to the bioartificial material market is the porcine dermal mesh, Permacol (Tissue Science Laboratories, Aldershot, UK). Similarly to its human counterpart, AlloDerm, Permacol is harvested from porcine skin from which cellular elements are removed (trypsin digestion and solvent extraction) that is then gamma irradiated to extract all genetic material (Fig. 111.4). The remaining extracellular matrix is cross-linked with an isocyanate derivative so as to "stabilize the structure in order to resist degradation by native and foreign (bacterial) collagenases" (Permacol website). With the foreign-body response minimized, the diminished inflammatory response is presumed to prevent formation of adhesions.[31]

Animal Studies

Macleod et al. were one of the first groups to describe the in vivo response to implanted Permacol. Permacol, SIS, and glycerol-treated/ethylene oxide porcine dermis were implanted subcutaneously and subsequently excised to evaluate the degree of inflammation and ingrowth vascularity.[32] Excised specimens were graded based on severity of acute and chronic inflammation (mild, moderate, severe) and degree of fibrosis/stromal reaction (Fig. 111.5). Glycerol-treated implants showed the severest acute and chronic inflammatory scores whereas Permacol showed the least severe *acute* inflammatory scores. Interestingly, SIS and Permacol *chronic* inflammatory scores did not differ. Coinciding with the inflammatory response, early harvest date (4 weeks) collagen content and vascular ingrowth assessments were lower for Permacol explants. By 10 and 20 weeks, however, vascular ingrowth did not differ between the different meshes. The authors concluded by attesting to Permacol's likely biocompatibility but questioned the clinical implications of Permacol's initial decreased in vivo vascularization.

In a comparative evaluation of Permacol versus polypropylene mesh, Kaleya used a bilateral rat incisional hernia

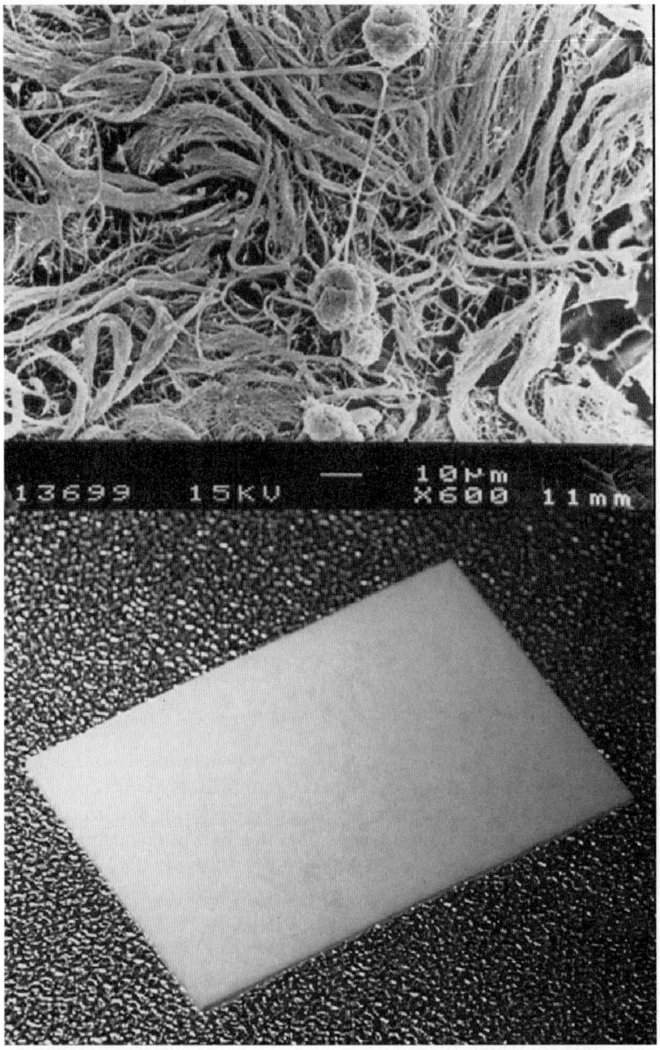

FIGURE 111.4. Product view (*bottom*) and SEM (*top*) of Permacol mesh. (Images obtained by permission from Aldershot, UK.)

model (different meshes on opposite sides of the same animal) to compare adhesion formation rates at 4 and 12 weeks.[31] Surprisingly, striking differences were found between different mesh sides within the same animal. Polypropylene sides demonstrated uniform dense adhesions by 12 weeks whereas none were found on the Permacol side. Furthermore, Permacol treated sides underwent neoperitonization by 12 weeks, compared to the relative absence of mesothelium formed on the polypropylene sides.

In a follow-up to their initial evaluation, Macleod et al. manipulated Permacol mesh porosity by perforating the mesh with a CO_2 laser.[33] Perforations resulted in improved fibrovascular ingrowth into "neopores" but not surrounding (untreated/nonperforated) matrix. They hypothesized that increased porosity likely promoted improved ingrowth and, therefore, promoted improved mesh integration.

Clinical Studies

Unfortunately, to date, clinical evaluations of Permacol are limited to one retrospective review and a few case reports. Of interest, one older study published in 1984 by Sarmah et al. reported long-term clinical results with use of a Permacol-like implant.[34] Cross-linked collagen derived from pig dermis was implanted into 11 patients undergoing incisional hernia repair. Within a median follow-up of 4.8 years, no complications or recurrences were reported.

In their review of Permacol implanted for use in complicated fascial defects, Parker et al. described outcomes for nine patients followed up at a median of 18.2 months.[35] Overall, five patients (56%) remained complication-free at follow-up. Of the remaining group, one had expired secondary to unrelated causes, another developed an abdominal wall abscess that required mesh removal, and two others required local mesh debridement secondary to either a developed abscess (after a missed enterotomy) or skin separation. The authors concluded that Permacol was a safe and acceptable alternative to prosthetic meshes in the repair of complicated abdominal wall defects. Other recent reports of Permacol comment on its implementation as a fascial adjunct in pediatric renal transplant recipients (0% recurrence at 18 months follow-up) to use in repair of parastomal herniae (0% recurrence rate at 12 months follow-up).[36,37]

Conclusion

Currently, a variety of biocomposites are available for clinical use. It is tempting to speculate that biocomposites will replace current artificial materials as additional data appear and costs decrease. Prospectively randomized trials may be needed to further delineate the most appropriate mesh for a given clinical scenario; however, these are very difficult to perform well in surgical series. Nonetheless, early trends are evolving with these materials. In patients with infected open abdomens, a 50% or lower hernia recurrence rate compares superiorly to the 100% hernia rate attributed to use of absorbable meshes (the standard of care in infected surgical fields). Furthermore, there appears to be an excellent safety and low recurrence profile emerging for bioprosthetic use in elective incisional

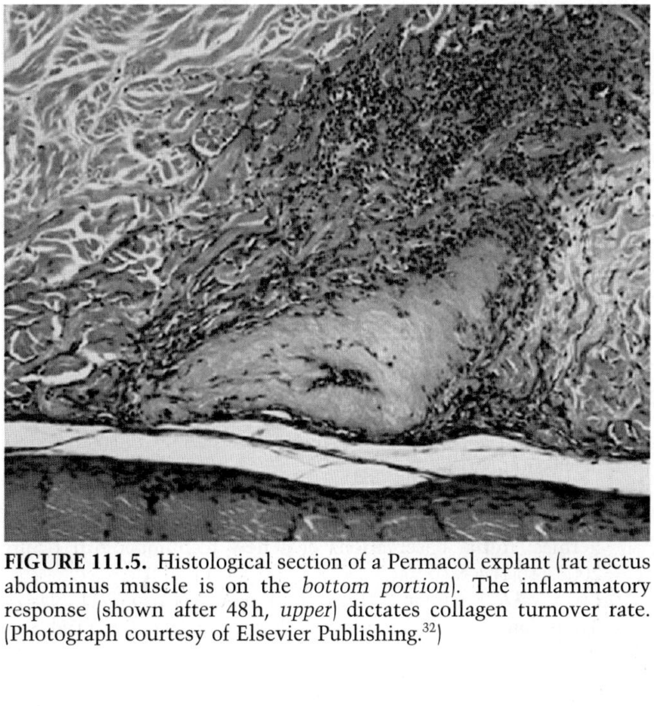

FIGURE 111.5. Histological section of a Permacol explant (rat rectus abdominus muscle is on the *bottom portion*). The inflammatory response (shown after 48h, *upper*) dictates collagen turnover rate. (Photograph courtesy of Elsevier Publishing.[32])

hernia repair. With evolving insight into the principle of tissue engineering, better understanding of the parameters that affect mesh incorporation and/or host response (immune tolerance) will likely lead to further application of these meshes in clinical practice.

References

1. Mathes SJ, Steinwald PM, Foster RD, Hoffman WY, Anthony JP. Complex abdominal wall reconstruction: a comparison of flap and mesh closure. Ann Surg 2000;232(4):586–596.
2. Disa JJ, Klein MH, Goldberg NH. Advantages of autologous fascia versus synthetic patch abdominal reconstruction in experimental animal defects. Plast Reconstr Surg 1996;97(4):801–806.
3. Disa JJ, Goldberg NH, Carlton JM, Robertson BC, Slezak S. Restoring abdominal wall integrity in contaminated tissue-deficient wounds using autologous fascia grafts. Plast Reconstr Surg 1998;101(4):979–986.
4. Oliver RF, Barker H, Cooke A, Grant RA. Dermal collagen implants. Biomaterials 1982;3(1):38–40.
5. Allman AJ, McPherson TB, Badylak SF, et al. Xenogeneic extracellular matrix grafts elicit a TH2-restricted immune response. Transplantation 2001;71(11):1631–1640.
6. Allman AJ, McPherson TB, Merrill LC, Badylak SF, Metzger DW. The Th2-restricted immune response to xenogeneic small intestinal submucosa does not influence systemic protective immunity to viral and bacterial pathogens. Tissue Eng 2002;8(1):53–62.
7. Palmer EM, Beilfuss BA, Nagai T, Semnani RT, Badylak SF, van Seventer GA. Human helper T cell activation and differentiation is suppressed by porcine small intestinal submucosa. Tissue Eng 2002;8(5):893–900.
8. Clarke KM, Lantz GC, Salisbury SK, Badylak SF, Hiles MC, Voytik SL. Intestine submucosa and polypropylene mesh for abdominal wall repair in dogs. J Surg Res 1996;60(1):107–114.
9. Prevel CD, Eppley BL, Summerlin DJ, Jackson JR, McCarty M, Badylak SF. Small intestinal submucosa: utilization for repair of rodent abdominal wall defects. Ann Plast Surg 1995;35(4):374–380.
10. Dejardin LM, Arnoczky SP, Clarke RB. Use of small intestinal submucosal implants for regeneration of large fascial defects: an experimental study in dogs. J Biomed Mater Res 1999;46(2):203–211.
11. Badylak S, Kokini K, Tullius B, Whitson B. Strength over time of a resorbable bioscaffold for body wall repair in a dog model. J Surg Res 2001;99(2):282–287.
12. Edelman DS. Laparoscopic herniorrhaphy with porcine small intestinal submucosa: a preliminary study. J Surg Laparosc Surg 2002;6(3):203–205.
13. Franklin ME Jr, Gonzalez JJ Jr, Glass JL. Use of porcine small intestinal submucosa as a prosthetic device for laparoscopic repair of hernias in contaminated fields: 2-year follow-up. Hernia 2004;8(3):186–189.
14. Ueno T, Pickett LC, de la Fuente SG, Lawson DC, Pappas TN. Clinical application of porcine small intestinal submucosa in the management of infected or potentially contaminated abdominal defects. J Gastrointest Surg 2004;8(1):109–112.
15. Helton WS, Fisichella PM, Berger R, Horgan S, Espat NJ, Abcarian H. Short-term outcomes with small intestinal submucosa for ventral abdominal hernia. Arch Surg 2005;140(6):549–560; discussion 560–562.
16. Oelschlager BK, Barreca M, Chang L, Pellegrini CA. The use of small intestine submucosa in the repair of paraesophageal hernias: initial observations of a new technique. Am J Surg 2003;186(1):4–8.
17. Livesey SA, Herndon DN, Hollyoak MA, Atkinson YH, Nag A. Transplanted acellular allograft dermal matrix. Potential as a template for the reconstruction of viable dermis. Transplantation 1995;60(1):1–9.
18. Wainwright D, Madden M, Luterman A, et al. Clinical evaluation of an acellular allograft dermal matrix in full-thickness burns. J Burn Care Rehabil 1996;17(2):124–136.
19. Harris RJ. A comparative study of root coverage obtained with an acellular dermal matrix versus a connective tissue graft: results of 107 recession defects in 50 consecutively treated patients. Int J Periodont Restor Dent 2000;20(1):51–59.
20. Silverman RP, Li EN, Holton LH 3rd, Sawan KT, Goldberg NH. Ventral hernia repair using allogenic acellular dermal matrix in a swine model. Hernia 2004;8(4):336–342.
21. Chaplin JM, Costantino PD, Wolpoe ME, Bederson JB, Griffey ES, Zhang WX. Use of an acellular dermal allograft for dural replacement: an experimental study. Neurosurgery 1999;45(2):320–327.
22. Sclafani AP, Romo T 3rd, Jacono AA, McCormick S, Cocker R, Parker A. Evaluation of acellular dermal graft in sheet (AlloDerm) and injectable (micronized AlloDerm) forms for soft tissue augmentation. Clinical observations and histological analysis. Arch Facial Plast Surg 2000;2(2):130–136.
23. DeSagun EZ, Botts JL, Srivastava A, Hanumadass M, Walter RJ. Long-term outcome of xenogenic dermal matrix implantation in immunocompetent rats. J Surg Res 2001;96(1):96–106.
24. Menon NG, Rodriguez ED, Byrnes CK, Girotto JA, Goldberg NH, Silverman RP. Revascularization of human acellular dermis in full-thickness abdominal wall reconstruction in the rabbit model. Ann Plast Surg 2003;50(5):523–527.
25. An G, Walter RJ, Nagy K. Closure of abdominal wall defects using acellular dermal matrix. J Trauma 2004;56(6):1266–1275.
26. Silverman RP, Singh NK, Li EN, et al. Restoring abdominal wall integrity in contaminated tissue-deficient wounds using autologous fascia grafts. Plast Reconstr Surg 2004;113(2):673–675.
27. Guy JS, Miller R, Morris JA Jr, Diaz J, May A. Early one-stage closure in patients with abdominal compartment syndrome: fascial replacement with human acellular dermis and bipedicle flaps. Am Surg 2003;69(12):1025–1028; discussion 1028–1029.
28. Buinewicz B, Rosen B. Acellular cadaveric dermis (AlloDerm): a new alternative for abdominal hernia repair. Ann Plast Surg 2004;52(2):188–194.
29. Girard S, Sideman M, Spain DA. A novel approach to the problem of intestinal fistulization arising in patients managed with open peritoneal cavities. Am J Surg 2002;184(2):166–167.
30. Bucky LP, May JW Jr. Synthetic mesh. Its use in abdominal wall reconstruction after the TRAM. Clin Plast Surg 1994;21(2):273–277.
31. Kaleya RN. Evaluation of implant/host tissue interactions following intraperitoneal implantation of porcine dermal collagen prosthesis in the rat. Hernia 2005;9(3):269–276.
32. Macleod TM, Williams G, Sanders R, Green CJ. Histological evaluation of Permacol as a subcutaneous implant over a 20-week period in the rat model. Br J Plast Surg 2005;58(4):518–532.
33. Macleod TM, Sarathchandra P, Williams G, Sanders R, Green CJ. The diamond CO_2 laser as a method of improving the vascularisation of a permanent collagen implant. Burns 2004;30(7):704–712.
34. Sarmah BD, Holl-Allen RT. Porcine dermal collagen repair of incisional herniae. Br J Surg 1984;71(7):524–525.
35. Parker DM, Armstrong PJ, Frizzi JD, North JH Jr. Porcine dermal collagen (Permacol) for abdominal wall reconstruction. Curr Surg 2006;63(4):255–258.
36. Liyanage SH, Purohit GS, Frye JN, Giordano P. Anterior abdominal wall reconstruction with a Permacol implant. Br J Plast Surg 2006;59:553–555.
37. Richards SK, Lear PA, Huskisson L, Saleem MA, Morgan JD. Porcine dermal collagen graft in pediatric renal transplantation. Pediatr Transplant 2005;9(5):627–629.

112

Injectable Biomaterials in Surgery

Bilal Shafi, Carlos Mery, Gary Binyamin, Joseph Knight, and Michael E. Gertner

Biomaterials in clinical practice encompass an enormous breadth of different materials, performing varied functions and taking different forms. Injected biomaterials are a unique subset within the biomaterial field, really entering the mainstream in recent years with the proliferation of minimally invasive technologies. Undoubtedly, as the breadth and depth of minimally invasive technology continues to grow, there will be a continued and even growing emphasis on newer materials or in some cases adaptation of older materials for novel applications.

This chapter relates evidence to support the clinical use of injectable biomaterials. For many of the materials in use today, data to support their clinical indications (either approved or off-label) are sparse at best and therefore further studies need to be performed to justify many of the newest biomaterial applications. Furthermore, currently used materials have been developed for disparate applications and in many case are used "off label" by physicians. For example, fibrin sealant was originally developed to aid in hemostasis and now is applied to wound closure, albeit with limited success. Future biomaterials will likely build upon the fundamental mechanisms of processes such as wound healing as well as the underlying biophysical principles of materials and will likely be more specifically effective for the problem at hand (e.g., wound healing).

This chapter highlights the creative uses of injectable biomaterials to treat a variety of diseases in a variety of fields (Table 112.1). In many cases, these materials enable new procedures and techniques to treat disease both in and out of general surgery. The materials in this chapter are ordered somewhat chronologically in terms of dates of first use and widespread acceptance.

Cements

Cements have been used for decades in dentistry and orthopedics to fill osseous defects and to allow stable fixation of metallic and plastic prostheses. Recent advances in synthetic and analytical biomaterials science have allowed the development of new cements as well as their use in novel applications.

Cements, and in general, all biomaterials applied to bone, can be described as osteogenic, osteoconductive, or osteoinductive. *Osteogenic* materials are those that contain living cells capable of differentiating into bone (e.g., bone autograft). *Osteoconductive* materials promote bone apposition onto its surface, serving as a receptive scaffold to facilitate bone formation (e.g., hydroxyapatite). *Osteoinductive* materials provide a biologic stimulus to actively induce cells to differentiate into osteoblasts and create bone (e.g., demineralized bone matrix).[1]

Polymethylmethacrylate

Polymethylmethacrylate (PMMA) is a very common biomaterial in the clinic today. It was first described in 1960 by Charnley as a self-curing material for anchoring femoral head prostheses in place.[2] Since then, PMMA cement (also known as acrylic cement) has been widely used in the fixation of implants and artificial joints by filling the space between the prosthesis and bone.

Numerous formulations of PMMA cement have been developed by a host of companies but they all have similar characteristics. The cements are packaged in two components, a powder and a liquid, which are combined to produce the cement. The powder contains some previously polymerized PMMA, an initiator required for curing of the cement (dibenzoyl peroxide), and a radiopacifier (either barium sulfate or zirconium oxide) to allow visibility of the cement in radiographs. The liquid contains methylmethacrylate (MMA) monomer to be polymerized, an activator (usually dimethyl-para-toluidine), and a stabilizer (hydroquinone) to prevent polymerization during storage of the product. Some cements may also contain a dye or an antibiotic. Differences in powder composition between different brands are responsible for the variations in their properties.

When the powder and liquid are mixed, a viscous fluid or dough is formed. The initiator in the powder and the activator

TABLE 112.1. Selected Injectable Biomaterials: Overview of Commercially Available Biomaterials on the Market or that Have Been on the Market.

Biomaterial	*Selected commercial names*	*Examples of applications*
Cements:		
Polymethylmethacrylate (PMMA)	C-ment 1–3, CMW1–3, Endurance, Osteobond, Palacos R, Simplex P, Versabond	Cementing of prostheses and fixation devices; cranioplasty; intertrocantheric, calcaneus, distal radius fractures; vertebroplasty / kyphoplasty
Calcium phosphate cements	Biobone™, Bonesource™, α-BSM, Cementek™, Mimix™, Norian™ CRS/SRS	Cementing of prostheses and fixation devices; cranioplasty; intertrochanteric, femoral neck, calcaneus, distal radius fractures
Demineralized bone matrix	Allomatrix™ Injectable Putty	Benign bone lesions; ankle and hindfoot fusions
Calcium sulfate	Osteoset™	Distraction osteogenesis; tibial plateau and pilon fractures
Bisphenol-*a*-glycidyl dimethacrylate (Bis-GMA)	Cortoss™	Cementing of fixation devices; vertebroplasty
Sealants:		
Cyanoacrylates	Dermabond™	Skin closure
Albumin-based compounds	Bioglue™	Sealing vascular anastomosis at suture holes, aortic dissection repair to glue the dissection flaps together, patch placement in cardiac defects
Hydrogels	FocalSeal™, CoSeal™, DuraSeal™	Sealing air leaks after lung resection, suture hole bleeding at vascular anastomosis sites, CSF leak after craniotomy or spinal surgery
Fibrin glue	Tisseal™, Hemaseel™	Sealing suture hole bleeding at vascular anastomosis sites, sealing air leaks after lung resection, sealing bleeding after liver resection, sealing the pancreas to prevent pancreatic leak, seal bleeding peptic ulcer
Miscellaneous Biomaterials:		
Silicone oil	Silikon™ 1000, Adato Sil-ol 5000	Prolonged retinal tamponade for select cases of retinal detachments
n-Butyl cyanoacrylate	Trufill™ n-BCA Liquid Embolic System	Embolization of cerebral arteriovenous malformations when devascularization is desired
Hyaluronic acid	Hyalgan™, Synvisc™, Orthovisc™, Supartz™	Intrajoint viscosupplementation of knee fluid for the treatment of osteoarthritis
Polytetrafluoroethylene paste (PTFE)		Reported use in vesicoureteral reflux and vocal fold augmentation
Protein emulsion	Ethibloc™	Not approved for use in the USA; reported for vascular embolization
Ethylene vinyl alcohol	Onyx™ Liquid Emobolization System, Enteryx Procedure	Embolization of cerebral arteriovenous malformations when presurgical devascularization is desired; bulking agent to narrow the esophageal sphincter

in the liquid interact to produce free radicals that in turn start the polymerization process of MMA into PMMA. The process ends when all reactive sites have been incorporated into polymers. The process of polymerization of MMA is an exothermic reaction with in vivo temperatures reaching approximately 104°–115°F during curing. By converting a large number of monomers into a smaller number of polymers, there is volume shrinkage of approximately 6% to 7% during the process, which is accompanied by inclusion of small air bubbles and the absorption of water within the hardened cement.[3]

The compressive strength of PMMA cements (75–105 MPa) is higher than their flexural (bending) strength (60–75 MPa), which in turn is higher than their tensile strength (50–60 MPa).[4] Strength is determined by the particular composition of each cement but can be altered by the inadvertent incorporation of air during mixing, therefore increasing porosity and decreasing strength. The viscosity of the cement is determined by both the chemical composition and the powder-to-monomer ratio. High-viscosity cements are injectable almost directly after mixing and have a longer application phase; however, because of their viscosity, these may entrap air more easily during mixing.[3]

In addition to implant fixation, PMMA cement has been widely used as an adjunct to fracture fixation. Several decades ago, it was recognized that the injection of acrylic cement into the femoral neck and the femoral shaft in intertrochanteric fractures improved the stability of internal fixation devices and allowed for immediate weight-bearing.[5] The application of PMMA cement can improve the union rates in unstable fractures, but in some studies it has been suggested that PMMA may hinder long-term functional outcomes.[6] In another series of randomized studies and in patients with Colles' fractures that had redisplaced after two closed reductions, Schmalholz showed that the application of cement into the dorsal bone defect improves outcomes when compared with either reduction/immobilization[7] or reduction/external fixation of the fractures.[8] Rehabilitation was faster and the treatment was more comfortable with the application of cement.

As it turns out (and not surprisingly), the type of cement used in arthroplasties (implant fixation) has a significant impact on the stability of long-term prosthetics. In a Norwegian retrospective study of 17,323 total hip replacements, lower failure rates were observed in implants fixed with Palacos (Schering-Plough International, Kenilworth, NJ, USA) or Simplex (Howmedica, London, UK) cements compared to CMW1 or CMW3 (DePuy, Leeds, UK).[9] Low-viscosity cements (e.g., CMW3) fared the worst. Although no clear explanation exists as to why low-viscosity cements may be associated with higher failure rates, the authors suggested that it could be the result of differences in stress-related fatigue.

Antibiotic-containing cements versus nonantibiotic-containing cements showed no difference in long-term outcomes. However, more recent studies have shown that the use of antibiotic-containing cements in addition to systemic antibiotics on the day of surgery decreases the long-term risk of failure.[10]

Some of the most interesting advances and novel applications of cements during the past two decades are the vertebroplasty and kyphoplasty procedures. These procedures are mainly intended for the treatment of osteoporotic vertebral collapse and fractures. In percutaneous vertebroplasty, a transpedicular puncture of the vertebral body is performed under fluoroscopy and PMMA cement is instilled under pressure directly into the vertebral body.[11] In balloon kyphoplasty (Fig. 112.1), an inflatable tamp is percutaneously inserted into the vertebral body to restore vertebral height and create an intravertebral cavity before injection of the cement, therefore decreasing the amount of pressure needed for instillation of the cement.[12] These techniques represent innovative applications of old materials (PMMA cement) to treat unsolved clinical needs. The results of selected clinical studies on vertebroplasty and kyphoplasty are summarized in Table 112.2; as can be seen immediately in the table, the clinical results of vertebroplasty and kyphoplasty are stellar.[12–21]

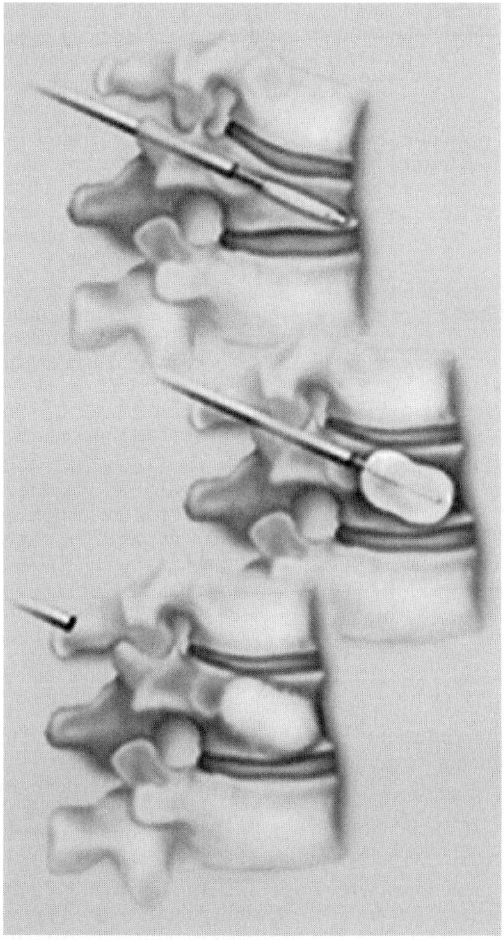

FIGURE 112.1. Depiction of the balloon kyphoplasty procedure. A balloon is inserted through the pedicle of a spinous process, the balloon is expanded, and cement is then injected into the fracture space. (Courtesy of Kyphon, Inc.)

PMMA cement has also been used in the repair of craniofacial defects (i.e. cranioplasty)[22] as well as injection of cement into calcaneus fractures, allowing for early weight-bearing in these patients.[23]

Calcium Phosphate Cements

The high exothermic setting phase of PMMA, its tendency to encapsulate, and its lack of osseointegration prompted the search for more biocompatible and osteoconductive cements. Because of their similarity to bone, hydroxyapatite and tricalcium phosphate have been used for several decades as ceramic implants. In the 1980s, liquid calcium phosphate cements (CPCs) that harden in situ (i.e., they could be used as injectable biomaterials) were developed. As discussed next, however, the injectability of CPCs is limited by some of their mechanical properties.

Calcium phosphate cements are produced by the reaction of a calcium phosphate powder with a wetting medium such as deionized water or a calcium- or phosphate-containing solution. On mixing, the calcium phosphate dissolves and precipitates into an apatite, brushite, or amorphous calcium phosphate. The latter material is further transformed into apatite after several weeks in the body.[24] The resultant apatite has a composition similar to bone and is therefore highly biocompatible and osteoconductive.[25]

Overall, calcium phosphate cements have mechanical properties inferior to PMMA. Because of the nature of calcium phosphates, their compressive strength (10–100 MPa) is much greater than their tensile strength (1–10 MPa). Furthermore, to maintain cohesion, CPCs need to be more viscous than PMMA, ultimately rendering them less injectable.[24]

CPCs have been used to augment internal fixation in the treatment of complex calcaneal fractures. By injecting CPCs into the fracture space after the internal fixation of 36 calcaneal fractures, Schildhauer et al. were able to allow their patients to bear full weight as soon as 3 weeks after the procedure, compared to the usual recommended period of more than 12 weeks.[26] Similar results were obtained in a second study where 26 patients with intraarticular tibial plateau fractures underwent reduction, internal fixation, and injection of CPCs in the subchondral bone defect.[27] Two cases required early revisions because of sterile drainage and two other patients had partial loss of the fracture reduction. The application of cement did allow for a shorter postoperative period before the initiation of partial weight-bearing and overall functional improvement.

Calcium phosphate cements have also been used in the treatment of fractures of the distal radius. Cassidy et al. reported the results of a randomized controlled trial where 323 patients with fractures of the distal radius were randomized to either conventional treatment (closed reduction and application of a cast or external fixator for 6–8 weeks) or treatment with CPC (open or percutaneous application of cement into the fracture site followed by a cast for 2 weeks).[28] Patients with CPC treatment had a faster recovery of wrist and forearm motion and a decreased incidence of complications when compared to the control group. Similar results were found in another randomized control study of 110 patients.[29]

TABLE 112.2.
Selected Clinical Studies of Vertebroplasty and Balloon Kyphoplasty.

Authors	*Level of evidence*	*Procedure*	*Cement*	*Study population*	*Results*
Berlemann et al. 2004[13]	III	Kyphoplasty	PMMA	24 patients (27 procedures) with osteoporotic vertebral fractures	All but one patient had pain relief after procedure; after 1 year, two patients had recurrence of pain; cement leaks in 33% of procedures with no clinical sequelae; no other complications
Diamond et al. 2003[14]	II	Vertebroplasty	PMMA	55 patients (71 procedures) with osteoporotic fractures compared with 15 patients that refused vertebroplasty (controls)	Treated patients reported 53% reduction in pain and 29% improvement in physical functioning compared with no changes in controls; complications: fractured transverse processes (n = 2), psoas hemorrhage (n = 1)
Han et al. 2005[15]	III	Vertebroplasty	PMMA	27 patients (34 procedures) with vertebral compression fractures	Pain relief and mobility improved immediately after the procedure; leakage of PMMA in one vertebral treatment; no other complications
Komemushi et al. 2005[16]	III	Vertebroplasty	PMMA	49 patients (104 procedures) with vertebral compression fractures from osteoporosis (n = 41), trauma (n = 7), metastasis (n = 1)	Significant improvement in visual analogue pain score (from 7.4 ± 2.2 to 2.5 ± 2.7); no correlation between change in pain score and vertebral body volume or amount of bone cement injected
Lee et al. 2004[17]	III	Vertebroplasty	PMMA	200 patients with painful single-level osteoporotic vertebral fractures	Regain of anterior, middle, and posterior vertebral body height in 81%, 76%, and 26% of patients, respectively; PMMA leakage in 14% of patients; no clinical consequences
Lieberman et al. 2001[12]	III	Kyphoplasty	PMMA	30 patients (70 procedures) with painful vertebral fractures from osteoporosis (n = 24) or multiple myeloma (n = 5)	Immediate relief of fracture pain; some height restored in 70% of patients; improvement in quality of life scores in all patients; cement extravasation in 9% of procedures; no other complications
Martin et al. 1999[18]	III	Vertebroplasty	PMMA	40 patients (67 procedures) for osteoporotic collapse (n = 11), hemangioma (n = 7), metastases (n = 19), primary tumors (n = 3)	Pain relief within 3 days; cement leak "frequently" found; one patient required infiltration of the area to treat consequent radicular pain; complications: DVT (n = 1), aspiration pneumonia (n =), and death 3 days after procedure (n = 1)
Palussière et al. 2005[19]	III	Vertebroplasty	Bis-GMA	53 patients (83 procedures) with vertebral compression fractures from osteoporosis (n = 48), angioma (n = 2), postradiotherapy necrosis (n = 4), myeloma (n = 2)	44% decrease in visual analogue pain scale; 9/11 patients evaluated at 6 months had pain reduction and improvement in quality of life; leakage of cement in 70% of procedures; 6 patients with mild clinical symptoms and one required corticosteroid injection for pain; other complications included vertebral body fractures (n = 2) and pneumonia (n = 1)
Phillips et al. 2003[20]	III	Kyphoplasty	PMMA	29 patients (61 procedures) with osteoporotic vertebral fractures	29/30 patients had decrease in discomfort; 96% patients satisfied; extravertebral cement leaks in 10% of procedures with no clinical consequences; complications: MI (n = 1), AF (n = 1)
Winking et al. 2004[21]	III	Vertebroplasty	PMMA	38 patients (43 procedures) with osteoporotic vertebral fractures	Significant improvement in pain and disability that persisted over a year; extravasation of PMMA in 26% of patients with one patient developing transient sciatica; no other complications

Classification into a table reveals the dramatic clinical results of these procedures.

AF, atrial fibrillation; Bis-GMA, bisphenol-*a*-glycidyl dimethacrylate; DVT, deep venous thrombosis; MI, myocardial infarction; PMMA, polymethylmethacrylate.

Other instances in which CPCs have been used include the correction of skull defects[30] and internal fixation of femoral neck and intertrochanteric fractures.[31] It has also been suggested that CPCs may be better than PMMA for vertebroplasty because of their remodeling profile and the nonexothermic reaction (which in theory could injure the neural elements). In a study conducted in cadaveric thoracolumbar vertebrae, no differences were observed in the height, fracture strength, or stiffness after application of CPC versus PMMA.[32] Clinical studies are the next step in the assessment of the use of CPCs compared to PMMA in vertebroplasty and/or kyphoplasty.

Other Cements

Calcium sulfate (a.k.a. plaster of paris) is a biocompatible, osteoconductive, and inexpensive material that has been used in its solid form in orthopedics because of its faster reabsorption and substitution by bone when compared to apatites. Cho et al. have used grounded pellets of calcium sulfate and combined them with carboxymethylcellulose to produce an injectable material. They have successfully used this material for early bone consolidation in distraction osteogenesis for treatment of craniofacial microsomia.[33]

More recently, an injectable calcium sulfate paste was developed (Minimally Invasive Injectable Graft; Wright Medical Technology, Arlington, TN, USA). The clinical results of injecting this paste into compression defects in tibial fractures are encouraging. In a small study, eight patients with comminuted tibial plateau or pilon fractures underwent injection of calcium sulfate paste followed by internal fixation and temporary external fixation or functional bracing.[34] Bone regrowth was observed in all patients, and seven of the eight patients had complete osteointegration of the graft within 12 weeks postoperatively. This material has also been used in combination with demineralized bone matrix for treatment of benign bone lesions.[35]

Demineralized bone matrix (DBM) is an osteoinductive material prepared by acid extraction of cadaveric allograft bone, resulting in loss of most of the mineralized component but retention of collagen and noncollagenous proteins (e.g., bone morphogenic proteins).[36] DBM is combined with substances such as glycerol, sodium hyaluronate, carboxymethylcellulose, or poloxamer 407 to create a putty that can be manipulated by the surgeon. DBM has been used for treatment of benign bone lesions[35] and ankle and hindfoot fusion.[37] Percutaneous injection of autologous bone marrow[38] and bone marrow–DBM composites[39] have also been described for treatment of nonunion and bone defects. The experience with DBM is remains limited, but because of its excellent osteoinductivity it will likely play an increasing role in the management of difficult fractures.

Another family of cements is based on the bisphenol-*a*-glycidyl dimethacrylate (Bis-GMA) resin. Similar to PMMA, Bis-GMA is a member of the methacrylate class of resins. Bis-GMA has a rigid bisphenol aromatic core, several double bonds that participate in the process of polymerization, and two hydroxyl groups positioned diametrically across the aromatic core structure which participate in the intermolecular hydrogen bonding that leads to the high viscosity of the material.[40] Therefore, bioactive glass–ceramic composites based on Bis-GMA have a three-dimensional cross-linked polymerized structure that provides tight physical binding and are therefore stronger than PMMA, with mechanical properties approaching that of human cortical bone.[41] One of these composites, Cortoss (Orthovita, Malvern, PA, USA) is a matrix mainly composed of Bis-GMA, bisphenol-*a*-ethoxy dimethacrylate (Bis-EMA), and silica particles. This material is provided in an automatic mixing gun and hardens within 5 to 8 min of mixing in an exothermic reaction. A recent study described the use of Cortoss in 53 patients undergoing percutaneous vertebroplasty.[19] Vertebroplasty provided adequate pain control but there was leakage of cement in 70% of augmented vertebrae; other complications included two vertebral body fractures and one case of back pain from leakage of cement into surrounding soft tissue.

Sealants

Hemostasis, wound healing, and closure of tissue defects have challenged surgeons for centuries. In recent decades, a number of devices and methods have been developed including suturing, stapling, and cauterization that address these challenges. Although many of these have been successful, there still exists a need to rapidly and effectively address the constant ooze of blood from a vascular anastomosis, the closure of a tissue defect without causing more damage to the tissue, or to assist in rapid wound healing. In response to this need, many soft tissue adhesives, sealants, and hemostatic agents have been developed.

A sealant is defined as a substance capable of holding materials together by surface attachment.[42] This substance can consist of one or more organic or inorganic compounds that start as a liquid and form a thin solid impervious layer on the targeted tissue. Ideally, a tissue sealant should aid in hemostasis, promote wound healing, allow easy and accurate application, work in bloody or a wet environment, and be biocompatible and biodegradable. There is no one sealant that satisfies all these requirements. Currently the tissue sealants and adhesives utilized in the operating room include cyanoacrylate esters, albumin-based sealants, and hydrogel sealants. In contrast to the tissue sealants, hemostatic agents take advantage of the clotting cascade to achieve hemostasis. Fibrin glue was the first injectable biomaterial used as a hemostatic agent.

Cyanoacrylates Esters

Cyanoacrylates were discovered in the 1940s as a very strong adhesive. Cyanoacrylate esters are liquid monomers whose chain can be altered by adding to or altering the alkoxycarbonyl (–COOR) group.[43] Upon contact with a weak base, water, or NH_2, the monomer rapidly polymerizes via hydroxylation to form a very strong bond to proteinaceous tissue. The polymer film that is created is brittle, especially with the shorter chain monomers. The cyanoacrylates degrade into their components, yielding formaldehyde and cyanoacetate. The longer-chain cyanoacrylates spread more rapidly on surfaces, polymerize more quickly, degrade more slowly, and allow the film more flexibility.[42,43]

Many attempts were made to find internal applications for cyanoacrylates. The rapid polymerization in blood allowed for rapid hemostasis as well as a strong bond to the tissue, but the early lower molecular weight forms of cyanoacrylate were not biocompatible. The degradation product, formaldehyde, causes severe acute or chronic inflammatory response in humans and is carcinogenic in laboratory animals.[44] This response was found to be dose dependent. During the past couple of years longer-chain cyanoacrylates have been developed that degrade less rapidly, releasing a lower concentration of formaldehyde and therefore causing less toxicity and opening the possibility for more clinical applications (Fig. 112.2).

"Krazy Glue," ethylcyanoacrylate, is the most popular cyanoacrylate on the commercial market because of its ability to rapidly and effectively bond materials. Clinical applications of cyanoacrylates are limited because of their toxicity to internal tissues. The U.S. Food and Drug Administration (FDA) has approved a long-chain polymer, Dermabond (2-octylcyanoacrylate), for topical medical applications to approximate skin wounds. Dermabond allows for faster skin closure while having the added benefit of eliminating the suture as a source of infection and forming a mechanical barrier to bacteria.[45] Currently, efforts are underway to expand the use of long-chain cyanoacrylates (e.g., vascular and/or intestinal anastamoses) because of their improved biocompatibility. Indeed, 2-octylcyanoacrylate was shown to be highly effective in sealing vascular anastomoses without significant inflammation, thereby opening the possibility for numerous internal applications.[44,46,47]

Albumin-Based Sealants

In response to the (now previous) toxicity of cyanoacrylate esters, Falb et al. developed an albumin based glue. This glue

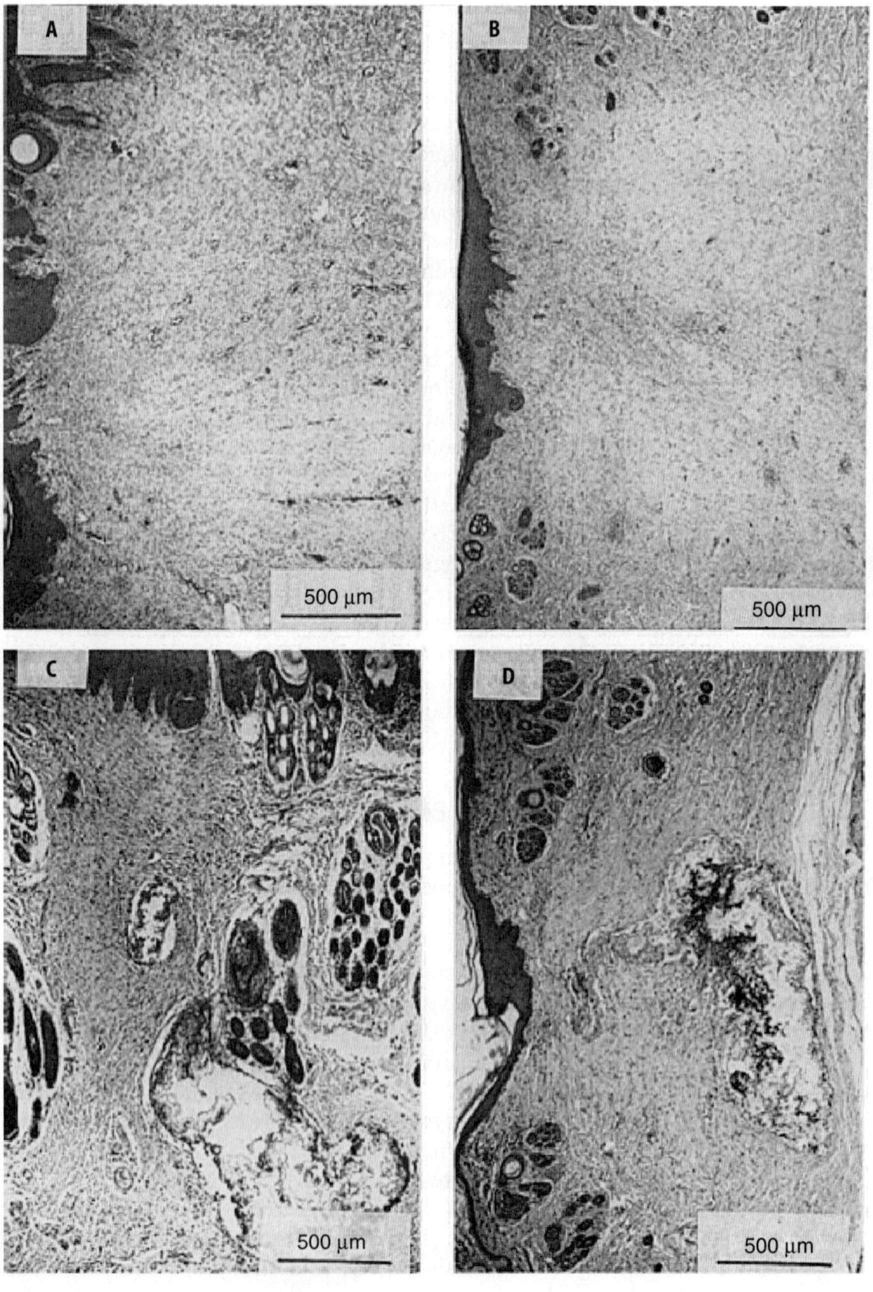

FIGURE 112.2. Cyanoacylate was used in this experiment of primary wound healing. **A, B.** Methyl-2-cyanoacrylate and ethoxyethyl-cyanoacrylate, respectively: effect of the fastest degrading cyanoacrylates on wound healing after 15 days. Note that by 15 days the fastest degrading cyanoacrylates show excellent tissue apposition with minimal inflammatory response; however, at 2–5 days, these cyanoacrylates show an intense inflammatory response because of the rapidly degrading material. The toxicity in the slower dissolving cyanoacrylates in the bottom two figures (**C, D**) (ethyl-2-cyanoacrylate and isobutyl-2-cyanolacrylate) is more drawn out and less intense over a longer period of time. (From Tseng et al.,[47] by permission of Journal of Applied Biomaterials.)

contained gelatin, resorcinol, formaldehyde, and glutaraldehyde (GRF glue).[48] GRF glue has proven its efficacy over many years in Europe for the treatment of acute type A aortic dissections. The glue was never approved by the FDA and was eventually abandoned by the European market because of (presumed) carcinogenic, inflammatory, and mutagenic effects of formaldehyde (at least in mice). Recognizing the effectiveness of this sealant in the treatment of aortic dissections, Cryolife (Atlanta, GA, USA) offered an alternative, Bioglue.

Bioglue is composed of 10% glutaraldehyde and 45% albumin. These components are mixed using a double-barrel syringe delivery system at the time of application. When glutaraldehyde contacts the amines of the albumin, the extracellular matrix, and the cell surface, the adhesive covalently binds to both the adhesive and the tissue. The glue bonds within 30 s and obtains maximum strength within 2 min.[49,50] This glue forms a firm cohesive sealant that is not brittle. Although long-term data are not currently available, initial animal studies have shown minimal inflammation in sheep at 3 months following thoracic aortic operations.[51] Because of the relative biocompatibility of Bioglue, it has obtained FDA approval and found many clinical applications.

Bioglue obtained FDA approval as a tissue sealant to aid in hemostasis at anastomotic sites in cardiac and vascular procedures. Bioglue effectively achieves hemostasis at suture lines, reinforces and provides stability to fragile tissues, and glues tissues together. Gundry et al. showed that Bioglue provided leak-free and suture-less coronary artery anastomoses at high pressures in pigs.[52] Furthermore, Hewitt et al. showed that the volume and rate of postsurgical bleeding were significantly reduced in coagulopathic sheep undergoing thoracic aortic operations.[51]

Clinically, Bioglue effectively added support to friable dissected tissue and approximated tissue flaps in acute aortic dissections. Bioglue also achieved hemostasis at suture lines in coagulopathic patients, allowing for quicker and more thorough anastomoses, which allowed surgeons to decrease periods of circulatory arrest, cardiopulmonary bypass times, and operating room (OR) times, improving the morbidity and mortality associated with this operation.[49,50,53] In a multicenter, randomized controlled trial comparing Bioglue with standard repair, patients treated with Bioglue showed a significant reduction in anastomotic bleeding over the use of pledgets[54] (Table 112.3). More recently, Bioglue has been shown to aid in the repair of intracardiac structural defects caused by infection or infarction. It seals the patch at suture lines and provides support to friable cardiac tissue, preventing leaks and/or formation of pseudoaneurysms.[55]

TABLE 112.3.
Selected Clinical Trials for Bioglue™.

Authors	*Level of evidence*	*Procedure*	*Material*	*Study population*	*Results*
Bavaria et al. 2002[53]	III	Aortic root replacement	Bioglue™	58 patients with type A aortic dissections	Significant reduction in circulatory arrest times, cardiopulmonary bypass times, and operative times with 2/58 late distal aortic reoperations
Chao et al. 2003[50]	II	Aortic root replacement	Bioglue™	25 patients with type A aortic dissections; 13 treated with Bioglue™	Hypothermic arrest time, blood transfusions, and hospital stays were all decreased in the treatment group; 4/12 in the conventional group had to be taken back for bleeding compared to 0/13 for the Bioglue™
Fink et al. 2004[55]	IV	Repair of intracardiac structural defects with patch	Bioglue™	2 patients with mitral annular defect, 1 patient with aortic annular defect, 1 patient with ventricular septal rupture, and 1 with atrioventricular groove after MVR	All patients underwent patch repair without any early or late evidence of leak, embolization; all patients remained in NYHA class I–II after 6–29 months postoperatively
Passage et al. 2002[49]	II	Valve repair/replacement (12), aortic root replacement (36), aorta repair/replacement (39), other (23)	Bioglue™	115 patients with aortic dissection (30), aortic aneurysm (49), aortic valvular disease (17), CAD (6), left ventricular aneurysm (6), other (17)	14/115 (12%) patients were taken back to the operating room, of whom only 1 was bleeding from a site where Bioglue™ had been applied; overall mortality was 11/115 (10%), of which none was attributed to the use of Bioglue™
Coselli et al. 2003[54]	II	Cardiac (49), aortic (105), peripheral vascular (48)	Bioglue™	105 patients randomized to Bioglue™ or control (75) with a variety of cardiac, aortic, and peripheral vascular diseases	Immediate hemostasis was achieved in 60.5% of patients treated with Bioglue™ compared to 39.2% of the control group; pledget use was reduced in the Bioglue group (26.2%) compared to control (35.9%); there was no difference in any other factors including use of blood products, morbidity, or mortality except for a threefold reduction in neurological events in the Bioglue™ group

Despite the many clinical applications of Bioglue, there are limitations. Bioglue must be applied to a dry surface to form an effective bond to the tissue and itself. In addition, because of the strong cohesive properties and slow biodegradation (more than 2 years) of Bioglue, it is relatively contraindicated in children because the glue will not grow with the child.[49] Furthermore, the adhesive must be applied sparingly and in a controlled fashion so as to prevent circumferential application, scarring, and subsequent stricture. There are reported cases of strictures in the superior vena cava (SVC) because of spillage.[56]

Hydrogels

In an effort to find more biocompatible and functional surgical sealants, hydrogels were offered as an alternative. Hydrogels have innate elastic and biocompatible properties that offer intrinsic advantages over other sealants, which is particularly important when the size of the tissue changes under normal physiological conditions.

Hydrogels were introduced as injectables in a two-component system that used a blue-green xenon light to induce photopolymerization. The two-component hydrogel system consists of an eosin-based polyethylene glycol (PEG) primer with acrylate end caps and a second polyethylene glycol in combination with polylactic acid. The first primer is brushed onto the target tissue, bonding to itself and to the tissue. Next, the sealant is laid down and a xenon light is used to photopolymerize the components, resulting in a highly cross-linked hydrogel. Photo polymerization takes about 40 s.[57,58]

Because of the complicated process of applying the photopolymerized sealant, it never made commercial inroads. The next-generation PEG hydrogel sealant did not require photopolymerization. This sealant consisted of two PEG solutions, one containing a sodium phosphate buffer and the other a sodium carbonate buffer. These two solutions are mixed using a double-barrel syringe, producing a semisolid sealant that bonds to the tissue, cross-linking in 60 s.[59–61]

Hydrogels offer many advantages over previously introduced tissue sealants and hemostatic agents. Because hydrogels are completely synthetic and highly diverse, they can be made to be relatively inert and biodegradable, posing little threat of antigenicity or risk of viral transmission, making them more biocompatible. Furthermore, the sealant polymerizes without significant tissue damage because a mechanical bond is formed with the irregular tissue surface without generating a large amount of heat. The resulting mechanical barrier provides homeostasis without relying on the clotting cascade, forming a barrier against infection and reinstating the integrity of organs to which it is applied. The polymer can be made to ultimately degrade by hydrolysis with a minimal inflammatory response after 10 months.[58] The target tissue surface does not need to be dry as the hydrogel absorbs water (for up to 24 h after its application, and growing to 300% of its original size). Furthermore, the highly cross-linked structure allows for strength to withstand tensile stress but has a component of elasticity allowing stretch without compromising the sealant.[59]

Currently, the FDA has approved the following hydrogels for clinical use: FocalSeal–L (Genzyme Biosurgery, Cambridge, MA), the photopolymerizable tissue sealant mentioned above, and, more recently, CoSeal (Baxter Healthcare, Fremont, CA) as one of the nonphotopolymerizable hemostatic agents, and just recently DuraSeal (Confluent Surgical, Waltham, MA), also a nonphotopolymerizable tissue sealant (Table 112.4).

Hydrogels have shown efficacy in a number of clinical scenarios. FocalSeal–L is FDA approved as a tissue sealant to control air leaks by sealing lung tissue following pulmonary resection, allowing for earlier removal of chest tubes and earlier discharge from the hospital.[54] The relative elasticity allows for the sealant to stretch upon lung expansion, making it ideal for sealing lung tissue.[57,62]

Although not approved as such, FocalSeal–L also demonstrated efficacy as a hemostatic agent to prevent anastomotic bleeding. Torchiana was able to seal openings as large as 2.5 mm in canine arteries so long as there was no active bleeding at the time of application.[58] Furthermore, given the relative strength and elasticity of hydrogels, it was found that application to vein grafts prevented graft injury and intimal hyperplasia by providing external support; this allowed for perivenous support, reducing wall tension and increasing shear stress, ultimately promoting long-term patency.[58,60]

CoSeal has been approved as a mechanical hemostatic agent to aid vascular anastomoses. A randomized, controlled trial comparing CoSeal with Gelfoam (oxidized regenerated cellulose, and gelatin sponges that initiate the clotting cascade) showed equivalent suture hole hemostasis on polytetrafluoroethylene (PTFE) grafts placed for infrainguinal revascularization after observation for a specified period of time.[63] CoSeal also showed equivalent efficacy in a randomized-controlled trial for suture hole bleeding during aortic reconstructions where immediate hemostasis occurred in 81% of subjects compared to 37% in the Gelfoam group.[64]

DuraSeal has been approved by the FDA to aid in repair of dural leaks. DuraSeal was shown to effectively allow for dural healing without adhesions or inflammatory reactions in canines after durotomy.[65] Furthermore, initial data (unpublished) from a prospective, nonrandomized trial showed 100% efficacy in sealing dural cerebrospinal fluid leaks following application of Duraseal and simulation of a valsalva maneuver to test the seal.[66]

As already discussed, hydrogels have shown efficacy in a wide range of areas as both a tissue sealant and a hemostatic agent. These effects are mainly achieved by forming a mechanical bond with the surrounding tissue and subsequently a barrier. The strength of the barrier as well as its degradation kinetics and ability (or inability) to induce wound healing leads to its efficacy (or nonefficacy) in specific scenarios. Spraygel (Confluent Surgical, Waltham, MA), which is currently under review by the FDA for approval, is taking advantage of a mechanical barrier with speedy degradation kinetics for use as a spray to prevent postoperative adhesions. Initial animal studies have shown that adhesions were significantly reduced following pelvic surgery in pigs and pericardial abrasion in rabbits.[67]

Fibrin Glue

Fibrin glues capitalize on the human body's coagulation cascade for hemostasis. They have been used for many years to allow surgeons to achieve adequate hemostasis. These glues provide the components needed for coagulation to

TABLE 112.4.
Selected Clinical Trials for Hydrogels.

Authors	*Level of evidence*	*Indication*	*Material*	*Study population*	*Results*
Wain et al. 2001[62]	II	Air leak after lung resection	Photopolymerizable polyethylene glycol (FocalSeal™)	172 patients undergoing lung resection randomized to sealant group (117) and control (39)	Application of a sealant resulted in 92% of patients without an air leak on closure compared to 29% of controls; significantly more patients in the sealant group remained free of air leaks (39% vs. 11%) with earlier removal of the chest tube and discharge than the control group; no difference in mortality or morbidity was observed
Porte et al. 2001[57]	II	Air leak after lung resection	Photopolymerizable polyethylene glycol (FocalSeal™)	124 patients undergoing lung resection randomized to sealant group (62) or control group (62)	Patients treated with sealants had smaller volumes of intraoperative air leaks and time to last observable air leak was shorter postoperatively; however, there was no difference in hospital stay or occurrence of incomplete lung expansion; 4/62 patients developed a localized empyema requiring a chest tube
Glickman et al. 2002[63]	II	Suture hole bleeding at vascular anastomosis with PTFE	Polyethylene glycol (CoSeal™)	148 patients undergoing revascularization procedures or dialysis access randomized to sealant (74) or Gelfoam™/Thrombin (74)	CoSeal (16.5 s) achieved more rapid sealing than the Gelfoam (189.0 s) treated group; aAt 10 min both groups had equal efficacy in sealing the anastomosis
Hagberg et al. 2004[64]	II	Suture hole bleeding after aortic reconstruction with Dacron	Polyethylene glycol (CoSeal™)	54 patients undergoing repair of aortic aneurysm randomized to sealant (37) or Gelfoam™/Thrombin (17)	81% of the sealant group compared to 37% of Gelfoam™ group achieved immediate hemostasis; this significance was maintained at 5 min with 85% of the sealant group and 52% of the control group achieving hemostasis
Grotenhuis et al. 2005[66]	III	CSF leak via dural defect	Polyethylene glycol (Duraseal™)	47 patients undergoing cranial or spinal intradural surgery with dural leaks	94% of patients had an intradural leak that stopped 100% with the sealant and valsalva; postoperatively, 3/47 patients had overt leak

proceed adequately, which became especially effective at bleeding surfaces.

Most formulations of fibrin glue consist of two components which when mixed together mimic the final step in the coagulation cascade. The first component is a combination of fibrinogen and Factor XIII and the second component is a combination of thrombin and calcium chloride. When these two components are mixed together using a double-barrel syringe, the thrombin and calcium convert the fibrinogen into fibrin monomers that polymerize into long fibrin strands. These strands are stabilized by Factor XIII, forming a physiological fibrin clot independently of the coagulation cascade that binds to surrounding tissue and allows for hemostasis. Depending on the formulation of the fibrin glue, it may or may not contain aprotinin. The aprotinin inhibits fibrinolysis to achieve better hemostasis, especially in the presence of heparin. Following the formation of the fibrin clot, fibroblasts and granulocytes form granulation tissue and eventually proliferation of collagen fibers, allowing for improved hemostasis and wound healing.[42,68]

Fibrin glues have many advantages over the various synthetic tissue sealants and hemostatic agents available on the market. Fibrin glues are inherently biocompatible because of their natural origin, but they are not necessarily safe. All the components of fibrin glues are derived from either human or bovine sources. They are not associated with inflammatory reactions, tissue necrosis, or foreign-body reactions as are many of the other sealants. Furthermore, the clot is reabsorbed by the body within days to weeks during the normal process of wound healing.[69] The thrombin and fibrinogen provide almost immediate hemostasis, while the concentration of the fibrinogen determines its tensile strength. This tensile strength is not as high as the other synthetic tissue sealants such as Bioglue or hydrogels.[70]

Despite the various advantages of fibrin glues, they do have their shortcomings. The FDA initially did not approve fibrin glues for use in the United States because of the risk of viral transmission. Fibrinogen is obtained from autologous or homologous pooled human plasma. These homologous preparations may be contaminated with a number of viruses including hepatitis, human immunodeficiency virus (HIV), herpes simplex virus (HSV), or cytomegalovirus (CMV).[69] In response to these concerns, multiple methods have been introduced to reduce the viral load and risk of viral transmission, including treating the pooled fibrinogen via precipitation, chromatography, pH treatment, filtration, pasteurization, vapor heating, and solvent detergent treatment.[68,71] Furthermore, thrombin is obtained from bovine or human sources. The bovine thrombin added the additional (theoretical) risk of contamination with bovine spongiform encephalopathy (BSE) and immunomediated coagulopathy because of antibodies to bovine Factor V reacting with human Factor V.[42,68] Minimizing the risk of viral transmission facilitated approval from the FDA; to date, there have been no documented cases of viral transmission.

The FDA initially approved fibrin glues as a hemostatic agent (Table 112.5). Tisseel (Baxter Immuno, Vienna, Austria), the first commercially approved fibrin glue, ultimately found a place in cardiac and vascular surgery applications as an adjunct to hemostasis. In a multicenter randomized control trial, Tisseel achieved complete hemostasis in 92.6% of patients compared to 12.4% in the control group at 5 min before sternotomy closure[72]; this resulted in shorter hospital stays and improved patient outcomes. Furthermore, Tisseel was shown to reduce postoperative blood loss in patients undergoing various cardiac procedures, including coronary artery bypass graft surgery (CABG) and valvular procedures, as measured by chest tube output.[73]

Tisseel also found efficacy in achieving hemostasis in traumatic liver injury, elective liver resection, and bleeding gastroduodenal ulcers. In a prospective, randomized trial, Crosseal (Johnson & Johnson, Sommerville, NJ), which contains no animal products, was shown to significantly reduce the time to hemostasis as compared to other accepted hemostatic agents in elective liver resections with fewer complications.[74] Furthermore, repeated injections of fibrin glue in the treatment of bleeding gastroduodenal ulcers during endoscopy was shown to be more effective than polidocanol injection in a randomized controlled trial of 854 patients.[75] Finally, fibrin glue was effective in controlling bleeding in patients who had coagulation disorders or who were on anticoagulant therapy as it did not rely on the body's coagulation cascade.

After its efficacy as a hemostatic agent was shown, the FDA expanded the use of fibrin glue as a tissue sealant. Figure 112.3 depicts the time course of wound healing induced by fibrin sealant in the epicardium of a rat. The lasting effect of Tisseel appears to be on collagen synthesis.[76]

In the clinical setting, the rate of postoperative air leak following thoracic surgery was significantly lower in patients treated with fibrin sealants undergoing thoracic procedures including lobectomy, pneumonectomy, or decortication.[77] Tisseel has also shown efficacy in reducing the rate of anastomotic leak and abscess formation following a gastrojejunostomy in laparoscopic gastric bypass surgery of swine.[78] Fibrin glue was also shown to prevent pancreatic leak and subsequent fistula formation by 25% in patients undergoing a Whipple procedure.[79] Finally, fibrin glue has found applications in neurosurgery to prevent cerebrospinal fluid (CSF) leak, in orthopedics to achieve hemostasis during total knee arthroplasty, and in plastic surgery to achieve skin graft survival.[69]

Floseal was introduced as an alternative to fibrin sealants to address the lack of tensile strength seen in fibrin glues. Floseal is a formulation containing human thrombin in combination with cross-linked gelatin granules composed of collagen to allow for hemostasis. Floseal relies on active bleeding to work effectively. The gelatin granules occupy irregular surfaces to tamponade bleeding surfaces by absorbing the blood and swelling further to create hemostatic pressure. The thrombin converts the fibrinogen in the blood to fibrin to form a clot that incorporates the gelatin granules, allowing for a sealing effect on the bleeding site.[80] Floseal was shown to be a more effective hemostatic agent at 3 min than Gelfoam in a multicenter, multispecialty, prospective randomized trial. The sealant is more effective than conventional fibrin glues with higher tensile strengths.

Soft Tissue (Dermal) Fillers

During the past few decades, a significant increase in the number of plastic surgery procedures has resulted in an increase in the number of available injectable soft tissue fillers. These tissue fillers are most often used in facial procedures that add or reconstruct contours and/or the shapes of facial features, such as wrinkle removal and nasolabial reconstruction. In a natural transition, many fillers are now being placed internally (e.g., lower esophageal sphincter), within body lumens, or within the walls of solid organs, which will make further inroads into various surgical fields. Consequently, these materials are discussed in some depth and should be of interest to all surgeons.

The materials that make up the fillers can be divided into three broad categories based upon composition: natural polymers, synthetic polymers, and combinations of these two. Most synthetic tissue fillers are produced from poly-L-lactic acid (Sculptra), polyacrylamide gel (PAAG) (Aquamid), calcium hydroxyapatite, or polysaccharide gel (Radiesse).

The natural polymer and combination category of materials can be divided into several groups: (1) acrylic hydrogels in combination with hyaluronic acid (DermaLive & DermaDeep, Restylane and Perlane, Hylaform); (2) autologous collagen from fat; (3) human collagen (CosmoDerm and CosmoPlast, Dermalogen, Autologen); (4) bovine collagen (Zyderm I, Zyderm II, and Zyplast); and (5) a natural polymer/synthetic combination consisting of PMMA and collagen (Artecoll). Zyplast was one of the first collagen soft tissue fillers, and many of the newer formulations are therefore compared to Zyplast in clinical studies.

Bovine Collagen

Zyderm I, Zyderm II, and Zyplast are each composed of different combinations of bovine-derived collagen that have been cross-linked with glutaraldehyde. These products have been used for more than 20 years and serve as a benchmark for new implantable fillers. Zyderm and Zyplast are both injected into the dermal layer of the skin (mid- to deep tissue for Zyplast). The implant then undergoes syneresis, and, as the saline is lost, the suspended collagen condenses into a soft

TABLE 112.5.
Selected Clinical Trials for Fibrin Glues.

Authors	*Level of evidence*	*Indication*	*Material*	*Study population*	*Results*
Johnson et al. 2005[140]	II	Prevention of seroma formation after breast surgery	Hemaseel™	82 patients undergoing breast surgery and/or axillary lymph node dissection with placement of drain (42) or sealant (38)	Sealant group had a seroma in 36% of patients compared to 45.5% for the drain group; at 10 days the seroma was much higher in the sealant group; authors suggested that sealant was a good option but because of the cost may not be worth it (Sealant $440 vs. Drain $67)
Sentovich 2003[141]	II	Fistula-in-ano	Fibrin Glue	48 patients with anal fistula because of cryptoglandular disease, Crohn's disease, or other	33/48 (69%) had closure of the fistula after 1 or 2 treatments at 22 months; remaining patients required fistulotomy; 3/33 patients had recurrence of which 2 were retreated with the sealant; no incidences of incontinence or obstruction
Suc et al. 2003[142]	II	Pancreatic leak after pancreatic resection	Fibrin glue	182 patients undergoing distal pancreatectomy or Whipple randomized to duct occlusion with fibrin glue (102) or no occlusion (80)	No difference between the two groups in the incidence or severity of intraabdominal complications (25%) or pancreatic fistula (16%); this was comparable to previous studies
Lau 2005[143]	II	Extraperitoneal hernioraplasty	Tisseel™	93 patients undergoing endoscopic extraperitoneal hernioplasty with either a fibrin glue (46) or mechanical stapling (47) for fixation	Fibrin sealant group required less analgesic (4.5 vs. 7 tablets) but the subjective reporting of pain at rest or on coughing and return to normal activity was equivalent; 17% of the fibrin glue patients had a seroma vs. 5% for the stapled group; at median follow-up time of 1.2 years, incidence of chronic pain was higher in the staple group (20% vs. 13%)
Fabian et al. 2003[144]	II	Air leaks after pulmonary resection	Hemaseel™	100 patients undergoing lung resection for cancer randomized to sealant (50) or no sealant (50)	There was a significant reduction in immediate postoperative air leak (34% vs. 68%), time to remove chest tube (3.5 vs. 5.0 days), and prolonged air leak (2% vs. 16%); no difference in volume of drainage or complications
Schenk et al. 2003[145]	II	Vascular anastomosis	Fibrin glue	48 patients undergoing dialysis access with an AV graft randomized to fibrin sealant (24), Surgicel™ (14), or pressure (10)	Time to hemostasis was significantly less for the fibrin glue (56.3 s) compared to Surgicel™ (772.9 s) and pressure (1269.6 s); complete hemostasis was 54% in the fibrin group compared to 0% for the others; adverse events were comparable
Levy et al. 1999[146]	II	Bleeding after total knee replacement (TKA)	Fibrin glue	58 patients undergoing TKA for arthritis randomized to sealant (29) and no sealant (29)	Average blood loss was significantly less in the sealant group (360 mL) vs. control (878 mL); 83% patients in the control group required blood transfusion compared to 3% in the sealant group; no adverse events were reported

cohesive network of fibers. This network is responsible for restoring skin contour.[81] Zyderm and Zyoplast have stood the test of time as far as safety and reproducibility of results, but their stability in tissue and their clinical effects are short lived, and thus they require frequent reimplantation.[82]

Hyaluronic Acid-Based Biomaterials

DermaLive and DermaDeep are composed of a combination of hyaluronic acid produced by cell culture and acrylic hydrogel particles, the acrylic material rendering the materials

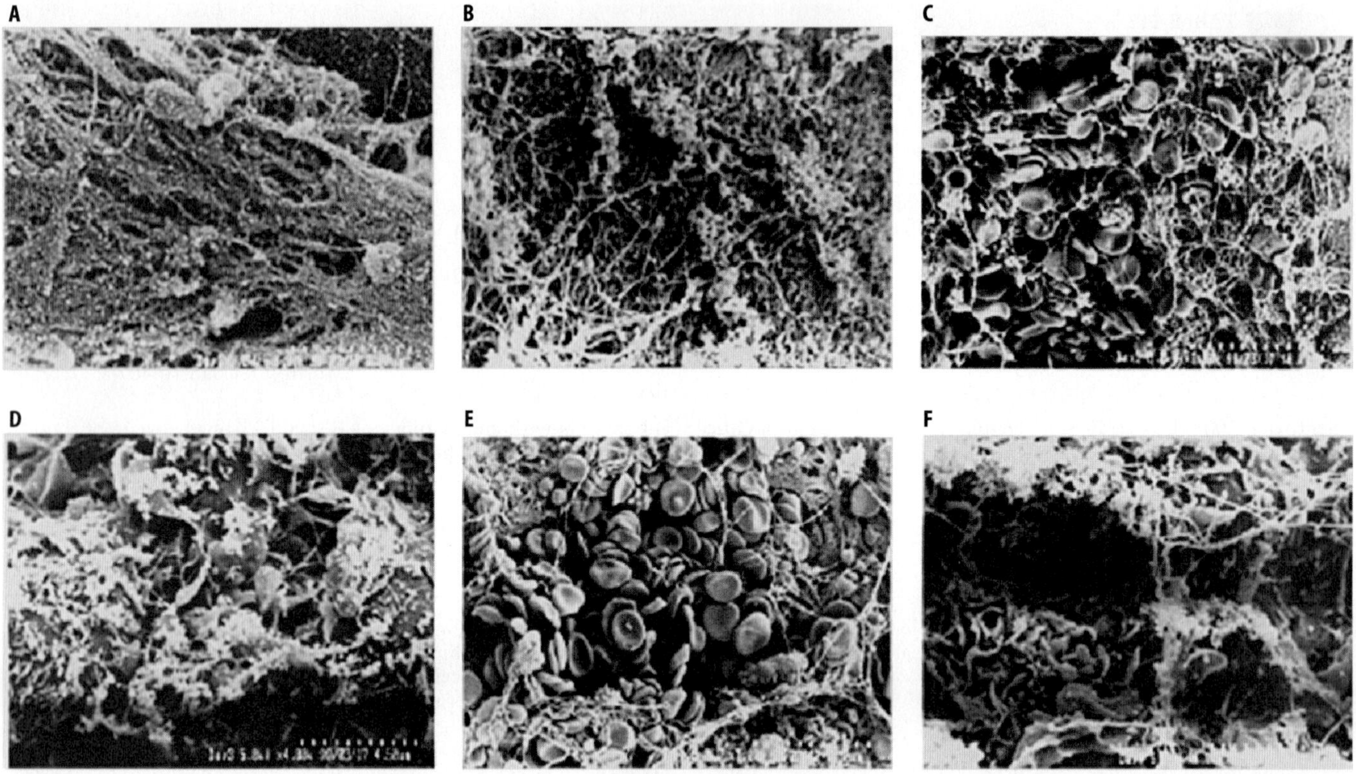

FIGURE 112.3. Time course of the healing response induced by fibrin sealant in a rat model. An incision was made in the eipcardium, sewn with suture, and then buttressed with glue. On day 1 (**A**), a thick fibrin network can be seen. On day 3, a dense fibrin network remained (**B**). **C, D.** A network of fibroblasts are observed and depicted by the *dashed bars* (18.0µm). By postoperative day 7 (**E, F**), the fibrin network had dissipated and was thinner. (From Hattori et al.,[76] by permission of Annals of Thoracic Surgery.)

semipermanent in nature. Hyaluronic acid is naturally found as an interstitial substance within the dermal layer of skin.[83] Both DermaLive and DermaDeep are injectable mixtures of 40% hydroethylmethacrylate (HEMA) and ethylmethacrylate (EMA) (HEMA and EMA are part of the acrylate family) suspended in 60% hyaluronic acid. The acrylic hydrogel particles are intentionally irregularly shaped with smooth walls, which prevents concentric fibrosis and promotes a smoother integration of the product into the body through the formation of an extremely loose network of collagen fibers around the particles. To evaluate the biocompatibility of DermaLive, the University of Technology of Compiegne in France performed an implant study in the dermis of a rat. The study results showed that there was an excellent integration of DermaLive into the dermis and that DermaLive had a long-lasting clinical effect. DermaLive and DermaDeep have been used extensively overseas but have not yet been approved by the FDA for use within the United States.

Restylane and Perlane are pure formulations of hyaluronic acid. Restylane is produced thorough the use of *Streptococcus equi* bacteria in saline and is used for more superficial wrinkling whereas Perlane is meant for use on deeper wrinkles (Table 112.6). The difference between the two products lies in their particle size, 250µm for Restylane and 1000µm for Perlane; it is generally accepted that the larger the particle size, the deeper the implantation should be. The biocompatibility and durability of Restylane (along with nine other substances) were tested on the forearms of authors in a study by Lemperle et al. which showed that Restylane was phagocytosed slowly (9 months) and with a minimal histological reaction.[84] A randomized, double-blind, multicenter comparison of the efficacy and tolerability of Perlane versus Zyplast (see following, or Table 112.6) in the correction of nasolabial folds was performed on 68 patients. The study found (by investigator-based and patient-based ratings) that Perlane was more effective than Zyplast in maintaining cosmetic correction. Also, reactions at the injection site (such as redness and swelling) were less frequent with Perlane than with Zyplast.[85]

Hylaform (hylan B gel) is composed of cross-linked molecules of hyaluronan derived from avian (bird) sources. A prospective, double-blind, multicenter clinical study conducted to evaluate the safety and effectiveness of Hylaform gel when used as a dermal filler in the nasolabial folds found Hylaform to be equivalent to the control material, Zyplast.[86]

Human Collagen

CosmoDerm and CosmoPlast are composed of human-derived collagen and are considered safer than bovine-derived collagen because they are human derived and do not require a skin test as do bovine injectables. CosmoDerm and CosmoPlast are the first FDA-approved dermal fillers not requiring a skin test and, as such, are an advance in the field. CosmoDerm is typically used for minor defects whereas CosmoPlast is used for more serious defects. In a study to determine immunological response, 428 patients were injected in the forearm

TABLE 112.6.
Selected Clinical Trials for Dermal Fillers.

Authors	*Level of evidence*	*Indication*	*Material*	*Study population*	*Results*
Lindqvist et al. 2005[85]	I	Intradermal nasolabial fold correction	Perlane	68	Randomized, evaluator-blind, multicenter comparison of the efficacy and tolerability of Perlane versus Zyplast in the correction of nasolabial folds; investigator-based and patient-based ratings indicated that Perlane was more effective than Zyplast in maintaining cosmetic correction; reactions at the injection site (such as redness and swelling) were less frequent with Perlane than with Zyplast
Kanchwala 2005[97]	I	Treatment of nasolabial folds and glabella, and lips	Radiesse	976	Study involving 976 patients using four common injectable fillers (autologous fat, Hylaform, Restylane, and Radiesse) concluded a preference for the use of Radiesse for the isolated treatment of nasolabial folds and glabella, but also recommended that Radiesse not be used in the lips because of the increased risk of complications
Cassidy et al. 2003[28]	I	Treatment of wrinkles of the glabella, nasolabial fold, radial upper lip lines, and corner-of-the-mouth lines	Artecoll	251	Multicenter clinical trail of 251 subjects comparing safety and efficacy of Artecoll to Zyoderm and Zyplast showed a definite improved efficacy of Artecoll over the others; Artecoll was also shown to be highly safe and biocompatible

with CosmosDerm and followed for 2 months. The most common side effect was cold symptoms (4.1%), with other adverse events, including flu-like symptoms, urinary tract infection, bronchitis, strep throat, and sinus infection, being 8.6%.[87]

Dermalogen is an injectable human tissue matrix (HTM) implant that is composed of collagen procured from donor tissue which has gone through a patented process to neutralize antigen and remove cellular components. It is used for treating facial contour folds, most commonly nasolabial folds, perioral lines, the vermillion ridge, glabellar frown lines, oral commissures, and depressed scars. Similar to CosmoDerm and CosmoPlast, Dermalogen does not require pretesting because it is human derived.

Autologen is unique in that it is derived from collagen harvested and processed from a patient's own skin and therefore required minimal FDA oversight. After processing, the formulation is adequate on the shelf for 6 months. Five patients of the Facial Plastic Surgery Clinic at The New York Eye and Ear Infirmary were injected with Autologen in one postauricular area and Zyplast on the contralateral side. The study showed that all implants were well tolerated and suggested that autologous collagen (Autologen) dispersion may represent a viable alternative to bovine collagen. The study also found the persistence and histological behavior of Autologen to be at least as good as those of Zyoplast.[88] As Autologen does not require any allergy testing and as it is harvested from the patient, eliminating the threat of disease transmission, it may provide a better overall option than the older Zyplast.

Polymethylmethacrylate/Collagen

Artecoll is composed of PMMA in uniformly smooth microspheres of diameter of 32 to 40 μm, blended with partly denatured 3.5% bovine collagen (which serves as a vehicle for deep dermal implantation) and 0.3% lidocaine (which aids in post-treatment discomfort). The smooth surface of the microspheres cause each individual microsphere to become encapsulated by the patient's own collagen fibers, thus preventing dislocation.[28] Indications for Artecoll are facial folds, lip and philtrum augmentation, chin and malar augmentation, dark-shadowed eyelids, enopthalmos, bony defects in face and hands, nipple reconstruction and augmentation, and urinary incontinence.[89] Not including the United States (it is not approved by the FDA), worldwide usage of Artecoll is estimated at 200,000 patients since 1994 with a low complication rate.[84] A multicenter clinical trial of 251 subjects that compared the safety and efficacy of Artecoll to Zyoderm and Zyplast showed a definitive improved efficacy of Artecoll over the others. Artecoll was also shown to be highly safe and biocompatible.[28] Artecoll is currently pending FDA approval for cosmetic usage.

Poly-L-Lactic Acid

Sculptra is a synthetic, biodegradable polymer composed of poly-L-lactic acid, sodium carboxymethylcellulose, nonpyrogenic mannitol, and sterile water for injection. This polymer has been used successfully in the correction of nasolabial folds, mid- and lower facial volume loss, jawline laxity, and other signs of aging. Sculptra is popular in Europe for the correction of lipoatrophy. Once Sculptra has been injected, over time the microparticles in the site will degrade as the tissue in the area responds to the compound. The poly-L-lactic acid portion of the compound will be broken down into carbon dioxide and water, but the collagen production that occurs in response to the injected implant remains and provides the source of the long-term correction. Sculptra is FDA approved for the treatment of lipoatrophy in people with HIV but is not approved as a cosmetic facial filler in the United States. It has been used in 30 other countries as a dermal filler for many years.

Polyacrylamide Gel

Aquamid is composed of 97.5% water and 2.5% cross-linked polyacrylamide. Because of its unique characteristics, the gel is highly biocompatible. The main toxicological concern with polyacrylamide is the content of monomer in the acrylamide. However, the content of acrylamide in Aquamid is lower than the exposure to drinking water in 1 or 2 days and therefore is largely not a concern.[90]

Several studies have been performed to determine the tolerability of a polyacrylamide hydrogel for soft tissue augmentation. Multicenter studies have been performed in Europe (228 patients),[91] France (68 patients),[92] Brazil (123 patients),[93] and studies of lipodystrophy in Brazil (patients included 18 HIV patients),[94] Italy (50 patients),[95] and Spain (about 100 patients).[96] In the majority of these studies patients were at least satisfied with the results.

Calcium Hydroxyapatite and Polysaccharide Gel

Radiesse (formerly known as Radiance) is the first calcium hydroxyapatite injectable filler used for soft tissue augmentation. Radiesse is composed of calcium hydroxyapatite microspheres, with diameter range 25 to 45 μm, suspended in a biocompatible carboxymethylcellulose gel. Radiesse has FDA approval for certain bone applications, oral/maxillofacial defects, vocal fold augmentation, and radiographic tissue marking, but not for cosmetic usage. A study involving 976 patients was performed using four common injectable fillers: autologous fat, Hylaform, Restylane, and Radiesse. The study concluded a preference for the use of Radiesse for the isolated treatment of nasolabial folds and glabella, but also recommends that Radiesse not be used in the lips because of the increased risk of complications.[97] Radiesse has also been studied for the treatment of lipoatrophy in the cheeks of HIV patients because of the severe psychosocial consequences involved with lipoatrophy as an identifying marker of HIV infection. One such study of 3 patients showed that although there was some loss of improvement over time, there was significant persistence for up to 9 months, and that Radiesse could be a potentially valuable tool for treating facial lipoatrophy.[98]

Unique Applications and Unique Biomaterials

In the previous sections of this chapter, the direct application of materials has been described within general material categories; in this section, various materials are described with specific clinical applications. In some cases, completely new materials are introduced. In many cases, these new materials/applications have only one or two unique applications and the materials are not even fully characterized because they were introduced into the clinic before the medical device act of the Food and Drug Administration.

Silicone Oil

Silicone oil is a sterile, nonpyrogenic liquid material that is clear and colorless. Chemically described as polydimethylsiloxane, this synthetic polymer is immiscible in an aqueous environment and varies in viscosity depending on chain length. It is indicated to prolong retinal tamponade in select cases of complicated retinal detachments and for detachments because of viral infections resulting from acquired immunodeficiency syndrome (AIDS) and cytomegalovirus retinitis. The oil is introduced after vitrectomy (removal of the aqueous humor of the posterior chamber of the eye) by transconjunctival or transcleral injection into the vitreous cavity. Overfilling or underfilling should be avoided to prevent inadequate tamponade and high intraocular pressures, respectively. Care should be taken because of the inherent property of the oil being less dense than the aqueous fluid of the aqueous humor, which could lead to papillary block or glaucoma.[99–103]

Prospective, multicenter U.S.-based trials have been performed to demonstrate the safety and effectiveness of silicone oil for the described indications[99–103] (Table 112.7). One such trial examined the efficacy, defined as complete reattachment, preservation of visual acuity, and safety, as measured by the number of complications. The results of patients with retinal detachments secondary to necrotizing retinitis because of HIV infection showed that the macula was completely attached in 94% ($n = 393$) of eyes, with visual acuity preserved in 56% ($n = 388$) of eyes. Complications were observed in less than 7% of eyes studied; only 1 eye had elevated intraocular pressure.[99] Commercially, silicon oil is available under the trade names of Silikon 1000 (Alcon Laboratories, Fort Worth, TX) and ADATO SIL-OL 5000 (Bausch & Lomb Surgical, San Dimas, CA).[104,105]

Silicone oil had been previously used as a dermal filler for soft tissue augmentation but was found to cause foreign-body reaction and chronic inflammation.[84,106–108] Although it continues to be used around the world for these applications, it is no longer available in the United States for corrective cosmetic applications.

n-Butyl Cyanoacrylate

The cyanoacrylate class has been previously described in the tissue sealant section of this chapter. This "super glue" analogue is also used as an embolization agent in cerebrovascular applications. *n*-Butyl cyanoacrylate is a small molecule that rapidly polymerizes in the presence of nucleophilic media such as water or alkali vapor. It is indicated for the embolization of cerebral arteriovenous malformations (AVM) when presurgical devascularization is desired. Typically, this liquid adhesive is combined with a polymerization regulating agent and a visualization agent. Application of the mixture through an appropriate delivery catheter is performed under real-time visual guidance; upon contact with fluids, there is instant

TABLE 112.7.
Selected Clinical Studies of "Miscellaneous Biomaterials."

Authors	*Level of evidence*	*Indication*	*Material*	*Study population*	*Results*
Davis et al. 1995[99]	II	Retinal tamponade	Silicone (PDMS)	350 patients with human immunodeficiency (HIV) infection (407 eyes with retinal detachment secondary to necrotizing retinitis)	Efficacy described anatomically as macula attachment in 94% of eyes and complete retinal attachment in 73% of eyes; complications including increased intraocular pressure (<1%), emulsification (1%), hypotony (2%), and corneal opacification (4%)
Tomsick et al. 2002[110]	I	Preoperative devascularization of cerebral arteriovenous malformations (AVM)	*n*-Butyl cyanoacrylate (n-BCA)	104 patients randomized to *n*-butyl cyanoacrylate or polyvinyl alcohol (PVA) (control)	AVM dimensional reduction per patient was 86.9% with PVA and 79.4% with n-BCA; 106 total complications reported; 54 were associated with n-BCA, resulting in only one device-related, adverse clinical event
Altman et al. 1998[120]	I	Knee osteoarthritis	Hyaluronic acid (HA)	495 patients with idiopathic osteoarthritis of the knee having moderate to severe pain, equally randomized to placebo, NSAIDs, or HA	At 26 weeks, analysis of visual analogue scale (VAS) for pain during a 50-foot walk test for HA group showed a statistically significant difference (1/3 SD) compared to placebo group; patient assessment of reduced pain was 73% with HA, 63% with placebo, and 67% with NSAIDs; adverse events across groups were comparable
Adamsbaum et al. 2003[130]	III	Aneurysmal bone cyst (ABC)	Protein emulsions	17 patients (children) injected for ABC located in the femur ($n = 6$), humerus ($n = 3$), pelvis ($n = 2$), fibula ($n = 2$), clavicle ($n = 2$), ulna ($n = 1$), and metacarpal ($n = 1$) with zein alcohol emulsion	Healing including normal cortex thickening and bone diameter observed in 82% of patients; most patients exhibited inflammatory response to injection; surgical excision was needed for 3 patients (18%); no major complications were reported
Dubois et al. 2003[133]	III	Aneurysmal bone cyst (ABC)	Protein emulsions	17 patients (children) injected for ABC with either zein alcohol emulsion ($n = 14$) or histoacryl glue ($n = 3$) located in metatarsal ($n = 2$), fibula ($n = 1$), humerus ($n = 3$), mandible ($n = 5$), pelvis ($n = 2$), spine ($n = 2$), rib ($n = 1$), and sphenoid bone ($n = 1$)	Excellent results (<20% of initial cyst involvement) seen in 94% of patients; remaining patient showed satisfactory results (30%–50% of initial cyst involvement); no major adverse clinical events noted and recurrence was not observed
Molyneux et al. 2004[139]	II	Intracranial aneurysm	Ethylene vinyl alcohol	Results for 71 aneurysms presented	Complete occlusion of 79% of patients was observed at 1 year with incomplete occlusion in 8%; adverse clinical events resulting in neurological deficit attributed to device or procedure failure observed in 8% of patients with a 2% procedural mortality
Johnson et al. 2003[138]	II	Gastroesophageal reflux disease (GERD)	Ethylene vinyl alcohol	81 patients with >3 months history of daily proton pump inhibitor (PPI) therapy	80.3% ($n = 65$) of patients decreased PPI dosage by more than half at 1-year follow-up including 57 patients (70.4%) without further PPI treatment; need for reimplantation in >23% of all patients; no adverse clinical events reported

HA, hyaluronic acid; NSAID, nonsteroidal antiinflammatory drug; PDMS, polydimethylsiloxane.

polymerization and adhesion to tissue, reducing or occluding the blood flow. Premature polymerization and adhesion of the delivery device to tissue must be avoided during the procedure. There are no data regarding the long-term implantation of these materials.[109]

A prospective, randomized, single-blind, multicenter trial in the United States has been performed to demonstrate safety and efficacy of an embolization mixture that contains *n*-butyl cyanoacrylate.[109,110] In a study of 104 patients equally randomized to *n*-butyl cyanoacrylate or polyvinyl alcohol treatment, efficacy and safety were evaluated. The primary efficacy endpoints were defined as AVM reduction and mean number of vessels embolized per patient, and secondary efficacy endpoints were surgical time and fluid replacement. The primary endpoints were comparable for both groups, 79.4% reduction in the *n*-butyl acrylate group and 86.9% in the polyvinyl alcohol group with a similar number of occluded vessels. Mean surgical time and volume of fluid replacement for both procedures were equivalent. Similarly, there was no difference detected in the incidence of adverse events between the two groups.[110] Cordis Neurocascular (Miami Lakes, FL) offers the TRUFILL n-BCA Liquid Embolic System[111]; this kit contains *n*-butyl acrylate, tantalum powder (radiopaque additive), and ethiodized oil (polymerizing retardant).

Hyaluronic Acid

Earlier in this chapter hyaluronic acid and sodium hyaluronate, the salt form of the acid, were described for application as a dermal filler. This polymer, naturally found in synovial fluid, can also be used as a viscosupplement of intrajoint fluid in the treatment of knee osteoarthritis.[61,112,113] Hyaluronic acid is a natural glycosaminoglycan polymer consisting of repeating disaccharides of glucuronic acid and *N*-acetylglucosamine. It is described as not provoking humoral or cell-mediated immune responses and is not species specific,[114] although there have been rare reports of allergic reaction to this polymer when derived from nonhuman sources.[115] Aspiration of the joint before hyaluronic acid injection is recommended if a joint effusion is present. Select commercial sources of hyaluronic acid include Hyalgan (Sanofi-Synthelabo, NewYork, NY), Synvisc (Genzyme Biosurgery, Ridgefield, NJ), Orthovisc (Ortho Biotech, Bridgewater, NJ), and Supartz (Smith & Nephew, Memphis, TN).[116–119]

Several prospective, multicenter, randomized, double-blind clinical trials of hyaluronic acid injection for the treatment of osteoarthritis have been performed.[61,120,121] Altman et al. in a study of 495 patients found that hyaluronic acid either exceeded or was comparable to the placebo in both primary and secondary efficacy categories. Safety studies showed that adverse effects were equivalent across groups.[120] Dahlberg reported overall improvements in efficacy endpoints in a study of 52 patients, although no differences were observed between placebo and hyaluronic acid groups. Some of the primary endpoints measured in these studies included range of motion, evaluation of knee pain and knee function, and activity level.[121]

Meta-analysis of the various hyaluronic acid studies for osteoarthritis has examined these for efficacy,[113,122] and again contradictory data are presented. Lo et al. in an analysis of 22 trials that met inclusion criteria found that there was modest efficacy of hyaluronic acid injection with a trend toward higher molecular weight being more efficacious.[113] In another meta-analysis of 8 trials, George et al. reported that there was a statistically significant effect of hyaluronic acid compared to placebo.[122]

Polytetrafluoroethylene Paste

Polytetrafluoroethylene paste (PTFE) as a solid material has been used successfully for several decades as a biomaterial and possesses many attractive characteristics for use as an implantable; see, for example, the preceding chapters on hernia biomaterials. A paste composed of PTFE particles can be injected as a filler and has been extensively used in cases for the treatment of vesicoureteral reflux[123–126] and vocal fold augmentation.[114] However, there are reports suggesting that the particles have an inadequate safety profile, including complications such as granuloma formation[127] and migration to distant organ systems.[128,129] Future improvements should address these safety concerns.

Protein Emulsions

Ethibloc (Ethicon, Norderstedt, Germany) is an emulsion in ethanol containing zein (an agriculturally derived protein), papaverin, oleum (for consistency), propylene glycol for sterility, and a contrast agent. Although not currently available in the United States, there have been observational reports and retrospective studies performed worldwide, mainly in Europe and Canada.[130–133] Ethibloc is applied as a single solution and acts as a fibrosing agent, the zein precipitating on contact with aqueous solution. Subsequently, the zein natural peptide polymer degrades over time because of enzymatic cleavage. It has been used for vascular embolization, including venous malformations (AVM) and aneurysmal bone cysts (ABC). Injection of Ethibloc is performed under direct visualization or with imaging; both CT and fluoroscopy have been advocated.[134,135]

Adamsbaum et al. reported on the percutaneous treatment of aneurysmal bone cysts in 17 pediatric patients[130] who were followed for an average of 5 years. In 14 (82%) of the patients, healing was observed, with the remainder requiring surgical excision. All but 1 patient exhibited an inflammatory response to the Ethibloc, and repeat injections were required in a third of the patients. In a retrospective study of 17 aneurysmal bone cysts in pediatric patients, Dubois et al. described sclerotherapy with Ethibloc (14 patients) and arterial embolization (3 patients).[133] The average follow-up time was almost 5 years, with all patients exhibiting a similar outcome. Less than 20% of residual cyst was seen in 16 patients (94%), which were classified as excellent results, and the remaining patient had a satisfactory result of 30% to 50% remaining cyst. The authors do caution that Ethibloc must be carefully considered around the brain because of risk of leakage or misapplication to surrounding tissue, causing damage to the central nervous system.

Kramer et al. performed a retrospective study composed of 32 patients having gastrointestinal hemorrhage.[132] Embolization was performed using metal coils (14 patients), Ethibloc (12 patients), gelfoam and tissue adhesive (2 patients), Ethibloc and tissue adhesive (1 patient), metal coils and Ethibloc (2 patients), or gelfoam with coils (1 patient). Bleeding was stopped in 83% of the cases, which included both upper and lower gastrointestinal cases. A 14% ischemic complication rate related to the intestine and spleen was attributed to the use of Ethibloc during the interventions.

Ethylene Vinyl Alcohol

Ethylene vinyl alcohol copolymer is a water-insoluble, biocompatible, nonresorbable material that becomes a spongy precipitate upon contact with aqueous solution. When dissolved in dimethyl sulfoxide (DMSO) and with the addition of a radiopaque contrast agent, the three components are delivered as a single solution for use in multiple applications. The Onyx Liquid Embolization System (MicroTherapeutics, Irvine, California) is intended for the embolization of cerebral arteriovenous malformations (AVM) when presurgical devascularization is desired. The solution is delivered through an appropriate catheter under real-time visualization for the reduction or occlusion of blood flow. Premature polymerization and adhesion of the delivery device to tissue must be avoided during the Onyx procedure.[136] In the Enteryx Procedure (Boston Scientific, Natick, MA), the mixture is delivered within and along the muscle layer of the lower esophageal sphincter under real-time visualization. The solid polymer acts as a bulking agent to narrow the sphincter and reduce symptoms of gastroesophogeal reflux disease (GERD).[137,138]

A prospective, multicenter European trial has been performed to demonstrate the safety and efficacy of an embolization mixture resembling the Onyx formulation. The clinical groups were patients with difficult aneurysms versus those who failed previous treatment ($n = 71$); 79% exhibited complete occlusion with 13% having subtotal occlusion and the remainder having incomplete occlusion at 1 year.[139] Of the 97 patients studied, there was an 8% permanent neurological morbidity and 2% mortality rate related to the device or procedure. Recurrence was observed in 10% of the aneurysms, related to the technical difficulty of the procedure. The authors concluded that the Onyx system can provide occlusion in patients with large and wide-neck aneurysms for whom there is minimal chance of success using other methods and that occlusion rates with the Onyx method are deemed to be better than those following coil techniques.

The safety and efficacy of using Enteryx as a bulking agent to narrow the gastroesophageal sphincter was performed in a prospective, multicenter, international trial.[138] The study consisted of 81 patients with gastroesophageal reflux disease, all of whom were receiving the standard medical treatment, proton pump inhibitor (PPIs). The primary endpoint was a decrease in PPI use, and the secondary endpoints were physiological parameters, symptoms, and quality of life scores. The results of the study showed that 70.4% of patients completely discontinued PPIs and 9.9% reduced their dosage by more than half; the remaining 19.7% of patients were not treatment responders after 1 year. It should be noted that 22.4% of the study participants required reimplantation of Enteryx between months 1 and 3 of the study and that 68.4% of these patients became treatment responders. Secondary endpoints similarly demonstrated improvements in most categories, including a statistically significant reduction in the median percent of time of esophageal exposure with pH less than 4 and a mean decease of 29.1% in the number of episodes at pH less than 4 at 12 months. No clinically serious adverse complications were recorded during the study.

Conclusion

In summary, the future for injectable biomaterials is very bright. Intervention-minded physicians need to know and appreciate all types of injectable materials in use in the clinical arena, regardless of the field of current application. Indeed, as evidenced here, an understanding of more traditional biomaterials can further the appreciation of injectables. With such knowledge and integration, it is likely that there will be many new disease-driven procedures involving injectable biomaterials.

References

1. Bauer TW, Muschler GF. Bone graft materials. An overview of the basic science. Clin Orthop Relat Res 2000;371:10–27.
2. Charnley J. Anchorage of the femoral head prosthesis to the shaft of the femur. J Bone Joint Surg Br 1960;42B:28–30.
3. Kuehn KD, Ege W, Gopp U. Acrylic bone cements: composition and properties. Orthop Clin N Am 2005;36(1):17–28, v.
4. Kuehn KD, Ege W, Gopp U. Acrylic bone cements: mechanical and physical properties. Orthop Clin N Am 2005;36(1):29–39, v–vi.
5. Muhr G, Tscherne H, Thomas R. Comminuted trochanteric femoral fractures in geriatric patients: the results of 231 cases treated with internal fixation and acrylic cement. Clin Orthop Relat Res 1979;138:41–44.
6. Bartucci EJ, Gonzalez MH, Cooperman DR, Freedberg HI, Barmada R, Laros GS. The effect of adjunctive methylmethacrylate on failures of fixation and function in patients with intertrochanteric fractures and osteoporosis. J Bone Joint Surg Am 1985;67(7):1094–1107.
7. Schmalholz A. Bone cement for redislocated Colles' fracture. A prospective comparison with closed treatment. Acta Orthop Scand 1989;60(2):212–217.
8. Schmalholz A. External skeletal fixation versus cement fixation in the treatment of redislocated Colles' fracture. Clin Orthop Relat Res 1990;254:236–241.
9. Espehaug B, Furnes O, Havelin LI, Engesaeter LB, Vollset SE. The type of cement and failure of total hip replacements. J Bone Joint Surg Br 2002;84(6):832–838.
10. Engesaeter LB, Lie SA, Espehaug B, Furnes O, Vollset SE, Havelin LI. Antibiotic prophylaxis in total hip arthroplasty: effects of antibiotic prophylaxis systemically and in bone cement on the revision rate of 22,170 primary hip replacements followed 0–14 years in the Norwegian Arthroplasty Register. Acta Orthop Scand 2003;74(6):644–651.
11. Deramond H, Depriester C, Galibert P, Le Gars D. Percutaneous vertebroplasty with polymethylmethacrylate. Technique, indications, and results. Radiol Clin N Am 1998;36(3):533–546.
12. Lieberman IH, Dudeney S, Reinhardt MK, Bell G. Initial outcome and efficacy of "kyphoplasty" in the treatment of painful osteoporotic vertebral compression fractures. Spine 2001;26(14):1631–1638.
13. Berlemann U, Franz T, Orler R, Heini PF. Kyphoplasty for treatment of osteoporotic vertebral fractures: a prospective non-randomized study. Eur Spine J 2004;13(6):496–501.
14. Diamond TH, Champion B, Clark WA. Management of acute osteoporotic vertebral fractures: a nonrandomized trial comparing percutaneous vertebroplasty with conservative therapy. Am J Med 2003;114(4):257–265.
15. Han KR, Kim C, Eun JS, Chung YS. Extrapedicular approach of percutaneous vertebroplasty in the treatment of upper and midthoracic vertebral compression fracture. Acta Radiol 2005; 46(3):280–287.

16. Komemushi A, Tanigawa N, Kariya S, Kojima H, Shomura Y, Sawada S. Percutaneous vertebroplasty for compression fracture: analysis of vertebral body volume by CT volumetry. Acta Radiol 2005;46(3):276–279.
17. Lee ST, Chen JF. Closed reduction vertebroplasty for the treatment of osteoporotic vertebral compression fractures. Technical note. J Neurosurg 2004;100(4 suppl spine):392–396.
18. Martin JB, Jean B, Sugiu K, et al. Vertebroplasty: clinical experience and follow-up results. Bone (NY) 1999;25(2 suppl):11S–15S.
19. Palussière J, Berge J, Gangi A, et al. Clinical results of an open prospective study of a bis-GMA composite in percutaneous vertebral augmentation. Eur Spine J 2005;14:982–991.
20. Phillips FM, Ho E, Campbell-Hupp M, McNally T, Todd Wetzel F, Gupta P. Early radiographic and clinical results of balloon kyphoplasty for the treatment of osteoporotic vertebral compression fractures. Spine 2003;28(19):2260–2265; discussion 2265–2267.
21. Winking M, Stahl JP, Oertel M, Schnettler R, Böker DK. Treatment of pain from osteoporotic vertebral collapse by percutaneous PMMA vertebroplasty. Acta Neurochir (Wien) 2004;146(5): 469–476.
22. Moreira-Gonzalez A, Jackson IT, Miyawaki T, Barakat K, DiNick V. Clinical outcome in cranioplasty: critical review in long-term follow-up. J Craniofac Surg 2003;14(2):144–153.
23. Kiyoshige Y, Takagi M, Hamasaki M. Bone-cement fixation for calcaneus fracture: a report on 2 elderly patients. Acta Orthop Scand 1997;68(4):408–409.
24. Bohner M. Physical and chemical aspects of calcium phosphates used in spinal surgery. Eur Spine J 2001;10(suppl 2):S114–S121.
25. Ooms EM, Wolke JG, van der Waerden JP, Jansen JA. Trabecular bone response to injectable calcium phosphate (Ca-P) cement. J Biomed Mater Res 2002;61(1):9–18.
26. Schildhauer TA, Bauer TW, Josten C, Muhr G. Open reduction and augmentation of internal fixation with an injectable skeletal cement for the treatment of complex calcaneal fractures. J Orthop Trauma 2000;14(5):309–317.
27. Lobenhoffer P, Gerich T, Witte F, Tscherne H. Use of an injectable calcium phosphate bone cement in the treatment of tibial plateau fractures: a prospective study of twenty-six cases with twenty-month mean follow-up. J Orthop Trauma 2002;16(3):143–149.
28. Cassidy C, Jupiter JB, Cohen M, et al. Norian SRS cement compared with conventional fixation in distal radial fractures. A randomized study. J Bone Joint Surg Am 2003;85A(11):2127–2137.
29. Sanchez-Sotelo J, Munuera L, Madero R. Treatment of fractures of the distal radius with a remodellable bone cement: a prospective, randomised study using Norian SRS. J Bone Joint Surg Br 2000;82(6):856–863.
30. Verheggen R, Merten HA. Correction of skull defects using hydroxyapatite cement (HAC): evidence derived from animal experiments and clinical experience. Acta Neurochir (Wien) 2001;143(9):919–926.
31. Goodman SB, Bauer TW, Carter D, et al. Norian SRS cement augmentation in hip fracture treatment. Laboratory and initial clinical results. Clin Orthop Relat Res 1998;348:42–50.
32. Bai B, Jazrawi LM, Kummer FJ, Spivak JM. The use of an injectable, biodegradable calcium phosphate bone substitute for the prophylactic augmentation of osteoporotic vertebrae and the management of vertebral compression fractures. Spine 1999; 24(15):1521–1526.
33. Cho BC, Park JW, Baik BS, Kim IS. Clinical application of injectable calcium sulfate on early bony consolidation in distraction osteogenesis for the treatment of craniofacial microsomia. J Craniofac Surg 2002;13(3):465–475; discussion 475–477.
34. Watson JT. The use of an injectable bone graft substitute in tibial metaphyseal fractures. Orthopedics 2004;27(1 suppl):s103–s107.
35. Kelly CM, Wilkins RM. Treatment of benign bone lesions with an injectable calcium sulfate-based bone graft substitute. Orthopedics 2004;27(1 suppl):s131–s135.
36. Peterson B, Whang PG, Iglesias R, Wang JC, Lieberman JR. Osteoinductivity of commercially available demineralized bone matrix. Preparations in a spine fusion model. J Bone Joint Surg Am 2004;86A(10):2243–2250.
37. Thordarson DB, Kuehn S. Use of demineralized bone matrix in ankle/hindfoot fusion. Foot Ankle Int 2003;24(7):557–560.
38. Matsuda Y, Sakayama K, Okumura H, Kawatani Y, Mashima N, Shibata T. Percutaneous autologous bone marrow transplantation for nonunion of the femur. Nippon Geka Hokan 1998;67(1):10–17.
39. Connolly JF. Injectable bone marrow preparations to stimulate osteogenic repair. Clin Orthop Relat Res 1995;313:8–18.
40. Sideridou I, Tserki V, Papanastasiou G. Effect of chemical structure on degree of conversion in light-cured dimethacrylate-based dental resins. Biomaterials 2002;23(8):1819–1829.
41. Pomrink GJ, DiCicco MP, Clineff TD, Erbe EM. Evaluation of the reaction kinetics of CORTOSS, a thermoset cortical bone void filler. Biomaterials 2003;24(6):1023–1031.
42. Bauer TW, Smith ST. Bioactive materials in orthopaedic surgery: overview and regulatory considerations. Clin Orthop Relat Res 2002(395):11–22.
43. Schwade ND. Wound adhesives, 2-octyl cyanoacrylate. 2005 (cited; available from: http://www.emedicine.com/ent/topic375.htm).
44. Ellman PI, Maxey PS, Tache-Leon C, et al. Evaluation of an absorbable cyanoacrylate adhesive as a suture line sealant. J Surg Res 2005;125:161–167.
45. Axel Nitsch AP, Franz Honig J, Verheggen R, Merton H-A. Cellular, histomorphologic, and clinical characteristics of a new octyl-2-cyanoacrylate skin adhesive. Aesth Plastic Surg 2005; 29:53–58.
46. Hallock GG. Expanded applications for octyl-2-cyanoacrylate as a tissue adhesive. Ann Plast Surg 2001;46(2):185–189.
47. Tseng YC, Hyon SH, Ikada Y, Shimizu Y, Tamura K, Hitomi S. In vivo evaluation of 2-cyanoacrylates as surgical adhesives. J Appl Biomater 1990;1(111):111–119.
48. Falb RD. Adhesives in surgery. New Sci 1966:308–309.
49. Passage J, Tam RK, Harrocks S, O'Brien MF. Bioglue surgical adhesive: an appraisal of its indications in cardiac surgery. Ann Thorac Surg 2002;74:432–437.
50. Chao HH. BioGlue: albumin/glutaraldehyde sealant in cardiac surgery. J Cardiac Surg 2003;18:500–503.
51. Hewitt CW, Kann BR, Tran HS, et al. Bioglue surgical adhesive for thoracic aortic repair during coagulopathy: efficacy and histopathology. Ann Thorac Surg 2001;71:1609–1612.
52. Gundry SR, Izutani H. Sutureless coronary artery bypass with biologic glued anastomoses: preliminary in vivo and in vitro results. J Thorac Cardiovasc Surg 2000;120(3):473–477.
53. Bavaria JE, Gorman RC, Woo YJ, Gleason T, Pochettino A. Advances in the treatment of acute type A dissection: an integrated approach. Ann Thorac Surg 2002;74(5):S1848–S1852; discussion S1857–S1863.
54. Coselli JS, Fehrebacher J, Stowe CL, Macheers SK, Gundry SR. Prospective randomized study of a protein-based tissue adhesive used as a hemostatic and structural adjunct in cardiac and vascular anastomotic repair procedures. J Am Coll Surg 2003; 197(2):243–252.
55. Fink D, Kang H, Ergin MA. Application of biological glue in repair of intracradiac structural defects. Ann Thorac Surg 2004;77:506–511.
56. Economopoulos GC, Brountzos E, Kelekis DA. Superior vena cava stenosis: a delayed Bioglue complication. J Thorac Cardiovasc Surg 2004;127(6):1819–1821.
57. Porte HL, Akkad R, Conti M, Gillet PA, Guidat A, Wurtz AJ. Randomized controlled trial of a synthetic sealant for preventing

alveolar air leaks after lobectomy. Ann Thorac Surg 2001;71: 1618–1622.

58. Torchiana DF. Polyethylene glycol based synthetic sealants: potential uses in cardiac surgery. J Cardiac Surg 2003;18:504–506.
59. Wallace DG, Rhee WM, Schroeder JA, et al. A tissue sealant based on reactive multifunctional polyethylene glycol. J Biomed Mater Res 2001;58:545–555.
60. Stooker W, Jansen EK, Fritz J, et al. Surgical sealant in the prevention of early vein graft injury in an ex vivo model. Cardiovasc Pathol 2003;12:202–206.
61. Wen DY. Intra-articular hyaluronic acid injections for knee osteoarthritis. Am Fam Physician 2000;62(3):565–570, 572.
62. Wain JC, Johnstone DW, Yang SC, et al. Trial of a novel synthetic sealant in preventing air leaks after lung resection. Ann Thorac Surg 2001;71:1623–1629.
63. Glickman M, Money S, Martin J, Ballard JL. A polymeric sealant inhibits anastomotic suture hole bleeding more rapidly than gelfoam/thrombin: results of a randomized controlled trial. Arch Surg 2002;137(3):326–331; discussion 332.
64. Hagberg RC, Sabik J, Conte J, Block JE. Improved intraoperative management of anastomotic bleeding during aortic reconstruction: results of a randomized controlled trial. Am Surg 2004; 70(4):307–311.
65. Preul MC, Muench TR, Spetzler RF. Toward optimal tissue sealants for neurosurgery: use of a novel hydrogel sealant in a canine durotomy repair model. Neurosurgery 2003;53(5):1189–1198; discussion 1198–1199.
66. Grotenhuis JA, Bartels RHMA, Beems T. A novel absorbable hydrogel for dural repair: results of a pilot clinical study. Department of Neurosurgery, University Medical Center, Nijmegen, St. Radboud Canisus Wilhelmina Hospital, Nijmegen Netherlands: 2005.
67. Ferland R, Campbell PK. Evaluation of a sprayable polyethylene glycol adhesion barrier in a porcine efficacy model. Hum Reprod 2001;16(12):2718–2723.
68. Spotnitz WD. Commercial fibrin sealants in surgical care. Am J Surg 2001;182:8S–14S.
69. Jackson MR. Fibrin sealants in surgical practice: an overview. Am J Surg 2001;182:1S–7S.
70. Saltz R, Sierra D, Feldman D, Saltz MB, Dimick A, Vasconez LO. Experimental and clinical applications of fibrin glue. Plastic Reconst Surg 1991;88:1005–1015.
71. Sidentop KH, Shah AN, Bhattacharyya TK, O'Grady KM. Safety and efficacy of currently available fibrin tissue adhesives. Am J Otolaryngol 2001;22(4):230–235.
72. Rousou J, Levitsky S, Gonzalez-Lavin L, et al. Randomized clinical trial of fibrin sealant in patients undergoing resternotomy or reoperation after cardiac operations. J Thorac Cardiac Surg 1989;97:194–203.
73. Matthew TL, Spotnitz WD, Kron IL, Daniel TM, Tribble CG, Nolan SP. Four years' experience with fibrin sealant in thoracic and cardiovascular surgery. Ann Thorac Surg 1990;50:40–44.
74. Schwartz M, Hirose R, Shaver TR, et al. Comparison of a new fibrin sealant with standard topical hemostatic agents. Arch Surg 2004;139:1148–1154.
75. Rutgeerts P, Wara P, Swain P, et al. Randomised trial of single and repeated fibrin glue compared with injection of poidocaol in treatment of bleeding peptic ulcer. Lancet 1997;350:692–696.
76. Hattori R, Otani H, Omiya H, et al. Fate of fibrin sealant in pericardial space. Ann Thorac Surg 2000;70:2132–2136.
77. Mouritzen C, Keinecke HO. The effect of fibrin glueing to seal bronchial and alveolar leakages after pulmonary resections and decortications. Eur J Cardiothorac Surg 1993;7:75–80.
78. Nguyen NT, Stevens M, Steward E, Paya M. The efficacy of fibrin sealant in prevention of anastomotic leak after laparoscopic gastric bypass. J Surg Res 2004;122:218–224.
79. Suzuki Y, Kuroda Y, Morita A, et al. Fibrin glue sealing for the prevention of pancreatic fistulas following distal pancreatectomy. Arch Surg 1995;130:152–155.
80. Oz MC, Shargill NS. Floseal matrix: new generation topical hemostatic sealant. J Cardiac Surg 2003;18:486–493.
81. MM Corporation. Zyderm Collagen Implant Physician Package Implant. 2000.
82. Alster TS, West TB. Fagien: human-derived and new synthetic injectable materials for soft-tissue augmentation: current status and role in cosmetic surgery. Plastic Reconst Surg 2000; 105(7):2526–2528.
83. Hotta TT. Dermal fillers. The next generation. Plastic Surg Nurs 2004;24(1):14–19.
84. Lemperle G, Morhenn V, Charrier U. Human histology and persistence of various injectable filler substances for soft tissue augmentation. Aesthet Plast Surg 2003;27(5):354–366; discussion 367.
85. Lindqvist C, Tveten S, Bondevik BE, Fagrell D. A randomized, evaluator-blind, multicenter comparison of the efficacy and tolerability of Perlane versus Zyplast in the correction of nasolabial folds. Plast Reconst Surg 2005;115(1):282–289.
86. Carruthers A, Carey W, De Lorenzi C, Remington K, Schachter D, Sapra S. Randomized, double-blind comparison of the efficacy of two hyaluronic acid derivatives, Restylane Perlane and Hylaform, in the treatment of nasolabial folds. Dermatol Surg 2005;31(11 pt 2):1591–1598.
87. I Corporation. CosmoDerm Human-Based Collagen Implant. 2003.
88. Sclafani AP, Romo T 3rd, Parker A, McCormick SA, Cocker R, Jacono A. Autologous collagen dispersion (Autologen) as a dermal filler: clinical observations and histologic findings. Arch Facial Plast Surg 2000;2(1):48–52.
89. Kessels RR, Santanchè PP, Bonarrigo CC. Re: PMMA-microspheres (Artecoll) for long-lasting correction of wrinkles: refinements and statistical results. Aesthet Plastic Surg 2000; 24(1):73–75.
90. Breiting V, Aasted A, Jørgensen A, Opitz P, Rosetzsky A. A study on patients treated with polyacrylamide hydrogel injection for facial corrections. Aesthet Plastic Surg 2004;28(1):45–53.
91. Aasted, A. A prospective European multi-center study on 228 patients followed one year after facial correction with Aquamid. 2003.
92. Trevidic P. Prospective French multi-center study. 2003.
93. Freitas F. Prospective Brazilian multi-center study.
94. Tariki V. Lipodystrophy study, Brazil. 2003.
95. Santis D. Lipodystrophy study, Italy.
96. Clotet B. Lipodystrophy study, Spain.
97. Kanchwala. Reliable soft tissue augmentation: a clinical comparison of injectable soft-tissue fillers for facial-volume augmentation. Ann Plast Surg 2005;55(1):30–35.
98. Comite SL, Liu JF, Balasubramanian S, Christian MA. Treatment of HIV-associated facial lipoatrophy with Radiance FN (Radiesse). Dermatology Online J 2004;10(2):2.
99. Davis JL, Serfass MS, Lai MY, Trask DK, Azen SP. Silicone oil in repair of retinal detachments caused by necrotizing retinitis in HIV infection. Arch Ophthalmol 1995;113(11):1401–1409.
100. Brourman ND, Blumenkranz MS, Cox MS, Trese MT. Silicone oil for the treatment of severe proliferative diabetic retinopathy. Ophthalmology 1989;96(6):759–764.
101. Aylward GW, Cooling RJ, Leaver PK. Trauma-induced retinal detachment associated with giant retinal tears. Retina 1993;13(2):136–141.
102. Sell CH, McCuen BW 2nd, Landers MB 3rd, Machemer R. Long-term results of successful vitrectomy with silicone oil for advanced proliferative vitreoretinopathy. Am J Ophthalmol 1987;103(1):24–28.

103. Brinton GS, Aaberg TM, Reeser FH, Topping TM, Abrams GW. Surgical results in ocular trauma involving the posterior segment. Am J Ophthalmol 1982;93(3):271–278.
104. Silikon 1000 website. (cited: available from: www.silikon1000.com.)
105. Bausch & Lomb website. (cited: available from: http://www.bausch.com/us/resource/surgical/vitreo/adatostatement.jsp.)
106. Bernal-Sprekelsen M, Caballero M, Farrè X, Calvo C, Alòs L. Particulate silicone for vocal fold augmentation: morphometric evaluation in a rabbit model. Ann Otol Rhinol Laryngol 2004;113(3 pt 1):234–241.
107. Maas CS, Papel ID, Greene D, Stoker DA. Complications of injectable synthetic polymers in facial augmentation. Dermatol Surg 1997;23(10):871–877.
108. Pollack SV. Silicone, fibrel, and collagen implantation for facial lines and wrinkles. J Dermatol Surg Oncol 1990;16(10):957–961.
109. Summary of Safety and Effectiveness Data for TRUFILL. FDA Review Application 2000;1–22.
110. N-Butyl cyanoacrylate embolization of cerebral arteriovenous malformations: results of a prospective, randomized, multicenter trial. AJNR Am J Neuroradiol 2002;23(5):748–755.
111. TRUFILL n-BCA Liquid Embolic System website. (cited: available from: http://www.jnjgateway.com/public/USENG/EndoNeuroOct2003ProductCatalog.pdf).
112. Bayramoglu M, Karatas M, Cetin N, Akman N, Sözay S, Dilek A. Comparison of two different viscosupplements in knee osteoarthritis: a pilot study. Clin Rheumatol 2003;22(2):118–122.
113. Lo GH, LaValley M, McAlindon T, Felson DT. Intra-articular hyaluronic acid in treatment of knee osteoarthritis: a meta-analysis. JAMA 2003;290(23):3115–3121.
114. Kwon TK, Buckmire R. Injection laryngoplasty for management of unilateral vocal fold paralysis. Curr Opin Otolaryngol Head Neck Surg 2004;12(6):538–542.
115. Fernandez-Acenero MJ, Zamora E, Borbujo J. Granulomatous foreign body reaction against hyaluronic acid: report of a case after lip augmentation. Dermatol Surg 2003;29(12):1225–1226.
116. Hyalgan. (cited: Available from: www.hyalgan.com.)
117. Synvisc. (cited: Available from: www.synvisc.com.)
118. Orthovisc. (cited: Available from: www.orthovisc.com.)
119. Supartz (cited: Available from: http://www.smithnephew.com/US/Standard.asp?NodeId=3242.)
120. Altman RD, Moskowitz R. Intraarticular sodium hyaluronate (Hyalgan) in the treatment of patients with osteoarthritis of the knee: a randomized clinical trial. Hyalgan Study Group. J Rheumatol 1998;25(11):2203–2212.
121. Dahlberg L, Lohmander LS, Ryd L. Intraarticular injections of hyaluronan in patients with cartilage abnormalities and knee pain. A one-year double-blind, placebo-controlled study. Arthritis Rheum 1994;37(4):521–528.
122. George E. Intra-articular hyaluronan treatment for osteoarthritis. Ann Rheum Dis 1998;57(11):637–640.
123. Sugiyama T, Hanai T, Hashimoto K, Umekawa T, Kurita T. Long-term outcome of the endoscopic correction of vesicoureteric reflux: a comparison of injected substances. BJU Int 2004;94(3):381–383.
124. Kumon H, Tsugawa M, Ozawa H, Monden K, Ohmori H. Endoscopic correction of vesicoureteral reflux by subureteric Teflon (polytetrafluoroethylene) injection: review of 6-year experience. Int J Urol 1997;4(6):541–545.
125. Puri, Granata C. Multicenter survey of endoscopic treatment of vesicoureteral reflux using polytetrafluoroethylene. J Urol 1998;160(3 pt 2):1007–1011; discussion 1038.
126. Engel JD, Palmer LS, Cheng EY, Kaplan WE. Surgical versus endoscopic correction of vesicoureteral reflux in children with neurogenic bladder dysfunction. J Urol 1997;157(6):2291–2294.
127. Malizia AA Jr, Reiman HM, Myers RP, et al. Migration and granulomatous reaction after periurethral injection of polytef (Teflon). JAMA 1984;251(24):3277–3281.
128. Frey P, Lutz N, Jenny P, Herzog B. Endoscopic subureteral collagen injection for the treatment of vesicoureteral reflux in infants and children. J Urol 1995;154(2 pt 2):804–807.
129. Steyaert H, Sattonnet C, Bloch C, Jaubert F, Galle P, Valla JS. Migration of PTFE paste particles to the kidney after treatment for vesico-ureteric reflux. BJU Int 2000;85(1):168–169.
130. Adamsbaum C, Mascard E, Guinebretière JM, Kalifa G, Dubousset J. Intralesional Ethibloc injections in primary aneurysmal bone cysts: an efficient and safe treatment. Skeletal Radiol 2003;32(10):559–566.
131. Cottalorda J, Kohler R, Chotel F. Recurrence of aneurysmal bone cysts in young children: a multicentre study. J Pediatr Orthop B 2005;14(3):212–218.
132. Krämer SC, Görich J, Rilinger N, et al. Embolization for gastrointestinal hemorrhages. Eur Radiol 2000;10(5):802–805.
133. Dubois J, Chigot V, Grimard G, Isler M, Garel L. Sclerotherapy in aneurysmal bone cysts in children: a review of 17 cases. Pediatr Radiol 2003;33(6):365–372.
134. Guibaud L, Herbreteau D, Dubois J, et al. Aneurysmal bone cysts: percutaneous embolization with an alcoholic solution of zein: series of 18 cases. Radiology 1998;208(2):369–373.
135. Garg NK, Carty H, Walsh HP, Dorgan JC, Bruce CE. Percutaneous Ethibloc injection in aneurysmal bone cysts. Skeletal Radiol 2000;29(4):211–216.
136. Summary of Safety and Effectiveness Data for Onyx. FDA Review Application 2003;1–39.
137. Louis H, Closset J, Deviere J. Enteryx. Best Pract Res Clin Gastroenterol 2004;18(1):49–59.
138. Johnson DA, Ganz R, Aisenberg J, et al. Endoscopic implantation of enteryx for treatment of GERD: 12-month results of a prospective, multicenter trial. Am J Gastroenterol 2003;98(9): 1921–1930.
139. Molyneux AJ, Cekirge S, Saatci I, Gál G. Cerebral Aneurysm Multicenter European Onyx (CAMEO) trial: results of a prospective observational study in 20 European centers. AJNR Am J Neuroradiol 2004;25(1):39–51.
140. Johnson L, Helmer SD, Osland JS. Influence of fibrin glue on seroma formation after breast surgery. Am J Surg 2005;189:319–323.
141. Sentovich SM. Fibrin glue for anal fistulas: long-term results. Dis Colon Rectum 2003;46(4):498–502.
142. Suc B, Fingerhut A, Fourtanier G, et al. Temporary fibrin glue occlusion of the main pancreatic duct in the prevention of intra-abdominal complications after pancreatic resection. Ann Surg 2003;237(1):5765.
143. Lau H. Fibrin sealant versus mechanical stapling for mesh fixation during endoscopic extraperitoneal inguinal hernioplasty: a randomized prospective trial. Ann Surg 2005;242:670–675.
144. Fabian T, Ponn RB. Fibrin glue in pulmonary resection: a prospective randomized, blinded study. Ann Thorac Surg 2003;75: 1587–1592.
145. Schenk WG, Gagne PJ, Kagan SA, Lawson JH, Spotnitz WD. Fibrin sealant improves hemostasis in peripheral vascular surgery: a randomized prospective trial. Ann Surg 2003;237(6): 871–876.
146. Levy BO, Martinowitz U, Oran A, Hashomer T, Tauber C, Horoszowski H. The use of fibrin tissue adhesive to reduce blood loss and the need for blood transfusion after total knee arthroplasty: a prospective randomized multicenter study. J Bone Joint Surg 1999;81:1580–1588.

113

Energy Transfer in the Practice of Surgery

James Wall and Michael E. Gertner

Energy is a fundamental tool of the modern surgeon. Transduction of energy can take many forms, including the oldest, which is basically manual energy transduction, to effect a change. Modern surgical instruments use electrons, photons, and sound waves to transfer energy to human tissue. Surgeons expect specific and repeatable results from these tools. An understanding of the basic underpinnings of energy transfer and its effects on biological tissue is necessary to adapt current technologies to specific surgical situations.

Safety and effectiveness are studied in accordance with U.S. Food and Drug Administration (FDA) requirements on the basis of device classification. Once approved for use, devices are evaluated by individual physicians. High-level clinical evidence is often lacking in the field of surgical devices. Devices that offer significant and/or perceived advantages in the operating room are often widely adopted often without being studied in a randomized controlled fashion.

This chapter briefly discusses the most commonly used energy transduction devices in use by today's surgeons. Many of these are indispensable but are nonetheless imperfect. In particular, spatial control of energy distribution is a very difficult variable to predict and control. Data, albeit limited, are outlined where appropriate in this chapter. The purpose of this chapter is to place energy transfer devices into the proper perspective, stimulate thought and study of the clinical use of these devices, and catalyze innovation in the field.

History

The most primitive use of energy transfer in surgery dates back hundreds of year to the use of heat for coagulation. The house of a surgeon was frozen in the year 79 AD by the eruption of Mount Vesuvius in the Roman city of Pompeii. More than 100 instruments have been identified in the house including blades, needles, speculums, and cautery rods (Fig. 113.1).[1–3] These tools were conceived centuries before the eruption of Mount Vesuvius by the likes of Hippocrates but saw no significant innovation until the twentieth century.

The 1920s saw a major advance for surgical technology with the advent of electrosurgery. Neurosurgeon Harvey Cushing teamed with physicist William T. Bovie to develop a device that delivered high-frequency electrical current for the purpose of hemostasis. This device, commonly referred to as the "Bovie," allowed Cushing to call back patients he had previously deemed inoperable because of a high risk of hemorrhage.[4] The Bovie has become a cornerstone of modern surgical technique.

Over the near century since the introduction of electrosurgery, there have been many advances in the "bovie" (Fig. 113.2A). Electrosurgical generators have evolved from bulky unreliable units to modern and compact devices run by sophisticated and computer-controlled generators (Fig. 113.2B). Furthermore, the delivery of radiofrequency energy has undergone many refinements and now takes many forms. Devices including endovascular catheters, percutaneous instruments, and laparoscopic tools have been developed to reach every part of the body. Modern conductive pathways, including argon plasma and saline, have also been developed to control and modulate the delivery of energy in new, practical ways. Recently, feedback controls have been developed to optimize electrosurgical vessel sealing and minimize surrounding tissue damage.

The twentieth century has also seen the development of ultrasound as a diagnostic and therapeutic modality in medicine. The piezoelectric effect was described by the Curie brothers in 1880,[5] who received a Nobel Prize in 1901. Ultrasonic energy was subsequently noted to have a variety of effects on biological tissue including heat and cavitation (a vacuum-induced destruction of tissue). In 1968, American surgeon Charles Kelman adapted the technology for the removal of cataracts and called it phacoemulsification.[6] More recently, surgeons have adopted ultrasonic tools for the purpose of dissection and vessel sealing.

LASER stands for light amplification by stimulated emission of radiation. The first laser was discovered at the Hughes Aircraft Corporation in 1960, but the theoretical basis dates back to work by Einstein in the early part of the century. To date, lasers have been used sparingly in general surgery while

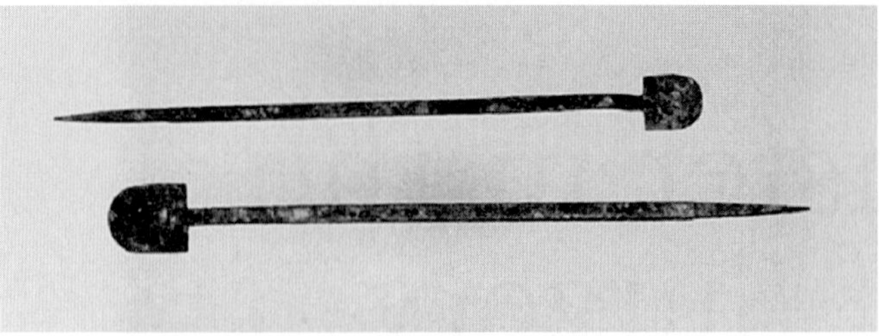

FIGURE 113.1. Iron cautery rods from Pompeii.

having been used extensively in other fields such as dermatology, ophthalmology, and otolaryngology. Laser light has many advantages over other forms of radiation. Photons emitted from a laser travel in a straight line after emission and form a tight coherent line of light. This light can be directed to a region of tissue and be rapidly absorbed by the tissues, creating heat; in some cases, enough heat is generated so that the tissue vaporizes, or is "ablated."

Early lasers were considered bulky, difficult to use, and expensive (Fig. 113.3). However, current lasers are produced from semiconductor technologies and their delivery tips are made from optical fibers. These laser systems are smaller, less expensive, and require less maintenance than their ancestors. These newer lasers are used extensively to cut and coagulate tissue in ophthalmology, plastic surgery, and dermatology. It is likely that many applications in general surgery will surface with the "next generation."

Electrosurgery

Electrosurgery is a form of energy transfer via electrons from the instrument to the tissues. All matter is composed of atoms with a nucleus, composed of positively charged protons and neutral neutrons, all orbited by negatively charged electrons. Atoms may become ionized by losing or gaining electrons, creating a charged state. When positive and negative ions are placed in opposition, a gradient or voltage is created. A conductor provides a path so that electrons may flow along the gradient, creating a current. The current is proportional to the voltage and inversely proportional to the resistance of the conductor. Current will always follow the path of least resistance and will always seek an electron reservoir (typically called the "ground" in a circuit). Living tissue is a good conductor of electrical current because of its high electrolyte content.

Electricity can be delivered as direct current in which a fixed voltage drives a unidirectional current. Handheld electrocautery devices are an example of a direct current system. They employ battery power through a high-resistance wire loop. The wire loop heats up and is capable of coagulation. Use of this device is limited to ophthalmic surgery and minor procedures as it is unable to cut tissue or control significant hemorrhage.

Electricity is most commonly delivered as an alternating current in the operating room. Typical alternating currents, that is, household current, operate at a frequency of 60 hertz (Hz). Electrical current traveling through muscle and other tissues at 60 Hz causes polarization and depolarization of the neuromuscular junction, which manifests clinically as twitching; high amounts of energy delivered at this frequency lead to electrocution. At 100,000 (100 kHz), passage of current results in tetanic contraction. At levels greater than 200 kHz and up to 5 MHz (5 million hertz), the muscle does not have a chance to depolarize but the molecular oscillations produce heat instead. At the high end of this range, the energy is not contained within the tissues and heat is not generated. Therefore, the frequency at which there is a compromise between electrocution and no effect is typically 500 kHz. The radiofrequency portion of the electromagnetic spectrum ranges from 300 to 10 MHz. Hence, the high-frequency current used in electrosurgery is often referred to as "radiofrequency."

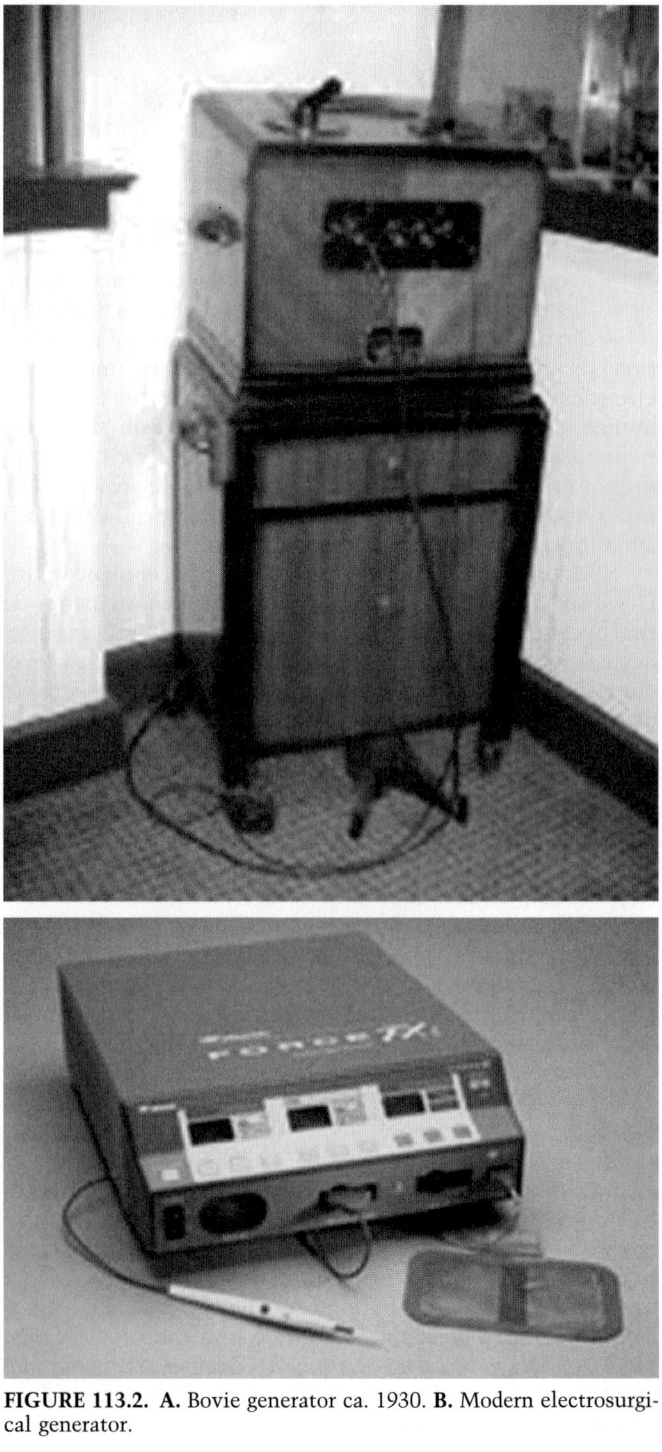

A

B

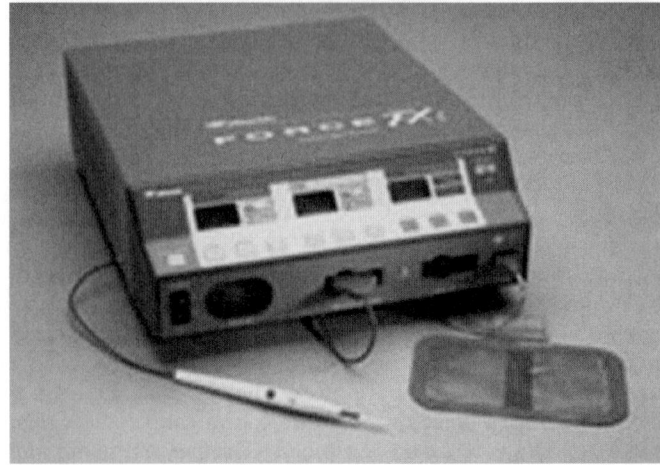

FIGURE 113.2. **A.** Bovie generator ca. 1930. **B.** Modern electrosurgical generator.

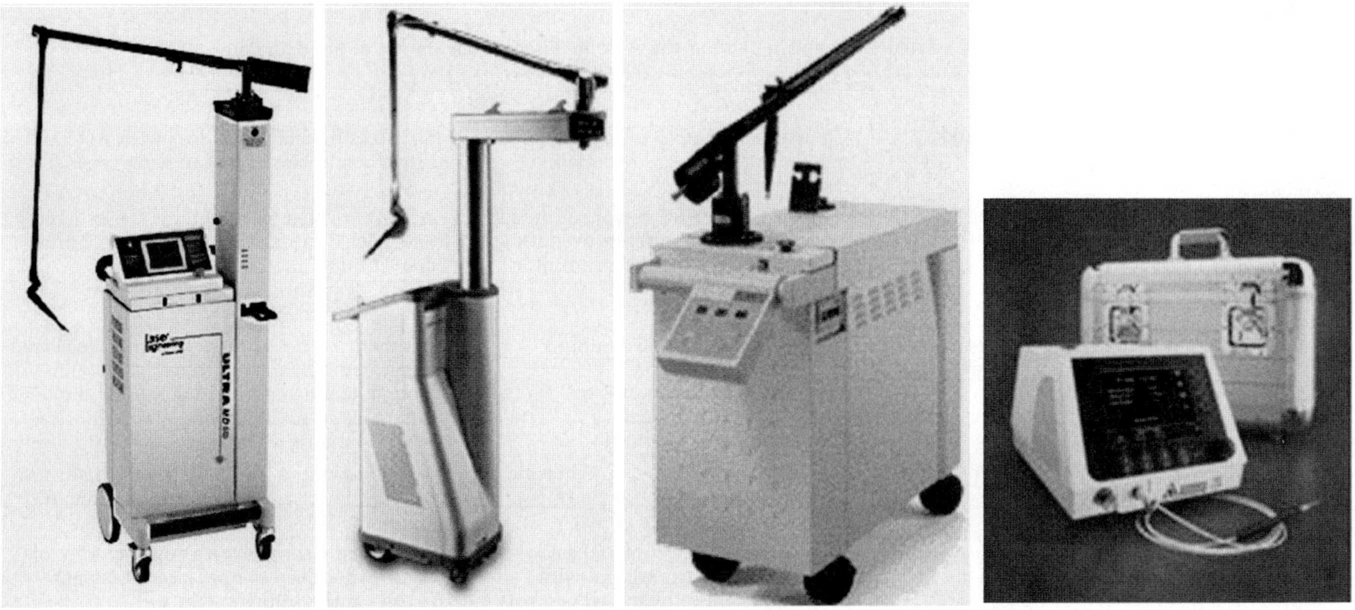

A B C D

FIGURE 113.3. A–D. Modern lasers.

Monopolar

Electrosurgery is most commonly delivered in the operating room via a monopolar circuit. This circuit incorporates the entire patient as a resistor. A generator produces radiofrequency current that is delivered to the tissue by an active electrode, known to the surgeon as the "bovie tip." The current then passes through the patient to a return electrode to complete the circuit. The desired effect occurs at the tip of the active electrode as a result of the high concentration of current at that location; the current quickly disperses from the higher concentration, en route to the broad return electrode. Because of the dispersion of current though the patient, a given amount of lateral damage must always be considered by the surgeon close to the bovie tip. The amount of lateral tissue damage varies based on the tissue and amount of current delivered; however it can be significantly higher than other electrosurgical methods.[7]

Monopolar surgical generators have two basic modes, cut and coagulate. These modes are differentiated by their voltage and duty cycle (the percentage of time current is delivered). The cut mode uses a continuous duty cycle, providing a stream of electrical current that vaporizes and cleanly divides tissue when the electrode is held just above the tissue. When placed in direct contact with tissue, the cut mode tends to desiccate tissue. Because of its continuous nature, it relies on a relatively low voltage to produce current. The coagulation mode uses an interrupted duty cycle, providing energy 6% of the time. The limited duty (time on versus off) time relies on high voltage to create energy spikes and heat tissue. The 94% off-time allows tissue to cool and coagulate between energy spikes. When activated just above the tissue, the coagulation mode has the effect of fulguration, which describes the combination of coagulation and tissue charring. Many generators also offer a blend mode, which provides a mix of cutting and coagulation. The mix varies among manufacturers; however, in general a higher blend means a larger component of coagulation.

Argon Plasma-Enhanced Electrosurgery

An argon plasma is basically current delivered through a fluid of ionized particles, where the ionized gas conducts the electrocautery current rather than the tissues. Energy is delivered much as in the bovie but because the gas is heavy, surfaces can easily be covered. Inert gases contain a stable number of electrons and are chemically unreactive and not combustible. Argon is the most abundant and widely accessible of the inert gases. It is heavier than air and therefore can sit on the surface of tissue and displace the air; it also ionizes easily. Argon's chemical properties make it ideal for delivering monopolar current in a controlled fashion.

Argon beam coagulators deliver a stream of ionized argon from their tip, creating a homogeneous current bridge to the target tissue. Electricity ionizes the argon, allowing a smooth conduction of current without electrode contact. Being heavier than air, the ionized gas settles uniformly on the tissue, creating a consistent and malleable eschar. As an added benefit, the stream of gas also disperses blood and oxygen, increasing visibility and decreasing smoke production.[8,9]

The argon beam coagulator (ABC) has found success in the control of significant diffuse visceral hemorrhage.[10] It has proven an effective method for hemostasis in hepatic resection, contributing to decreased transfusion requirements.[11,12] Studies have also found an advantage to use of the ABC in splenic salvage.[13–16] Table 113.1 summarizes the uses and clinical trials that involve the argon beam coagulator.

The surgical team should always consider the possibility of gas embolus with use of the ABC. Although rare, reports of clinically significant embolus exist.[17–19] With the natural extension of the ABC to laparoscopic procedures, there are additional considerations. For example, intraabdominal pressure may be elevated by extended use of the device, which can further increase the probability of significant gas embolus.[20,21] Limited use of the ABC has also been described in the thoracic, gynecological, and ENT (ear, nose, and throat) literature.

TABLE 113.1.
Argon Beam Coagulator (ABC): Studies Supporting Use of the ABC in Tissue Coagulation of Solid Organs.

Postema et al.[11]	Level I animal study	Comparison of ABC to conventional methods of hemostasis in pig liver resections	80% less median blood loss with ABC and significantly faster time to hemostasis
Go et al.[10]	Level I animal study	Comparison of ABC to conventional methods of hemostasis in liver and spleen lacerations of heparinized dogs	ABC controlled bleeding in 100% of liver and splenic lacerations in less than 3 min; conventional methods failed in 14/15 attempts at 3 min, all of which were salvaged by the ABC
Glover et al.[9]	Level I animal study	Comparison of wound healing measures between ABC, electrocautery, laser, and steel scalpel in mouse model	All thermal knives showed similar localized tissue damage, with 3- to 6-day delay in wound healing compared to scalpel; no difference in final breaking strength of the wounds among all modalities
Rees et al.[12]	Level IV human study	Retrospective review of 150 hepatic resections with ABC, no controls (not even historical control?)	Mean blood loss, 814 mL; mean transfusion rate, 0.5 units; mean hemoglobin drop, 0.7
Dunham et al.[14]	Level III human study	Retrospective review of 160 cases of blunt splenic injury treated with ABC compared to historical controls	85% splenic salvage with ABC vs. 47% of controls for deep splenic lacerations not involving the hilum

Radiofrequency Ablation

Radiofrequency ablation (RFA) uses a monopolar circuit for the purpose of ablation; that is, to devitalize tissue without having to surgically remove it. An active electrode is inserted into the tissue with return electrodes placed on the surface of the patient. In this respect, RFA is very similar to bovie electrocautery. Typically, the active electrode takes a shape that spreads current over a larger area than the bovie, which gives the device the ability to define an ablative volume.

It should be noted that ablation as used in RFA refers to controlled temperature thermal denaturation. The collagen macromolecules are denatured by heat generated by RF inside the tissue, destroying blood vessels and cell membranes in the process. As discussed below, "ablation" in the context of laser has a very different physical basis.

In RFA, the active electrode delivers a current that heats the surrounding tissue. At temperatures above 60°C, proteinis denatured and cells are destroyed. The denatured collagen can be pressed together under pressure; when the collagen cools, the newer bonds will result in a greater tensile strength than in the previous bonds. The extent of ablation can be extended by shape variations of the active electrode including coaxial umbrellas, internally cooled probes, and multiple probes.[22]

The RFA electrical generators require a feedback system that monitors tissue impedance to deliver optimal energy. Energy delivered too quickly results in charred tissue adjacent to the electrode, which impedes further local tissue destruction. By relating the output of the active electrode to the measured impedance, charring can be avoided to some degree. After being first described in cardiac electrophysiology, ablation technology has been adapted to several uses in surgery.[23] The most common application is the destruction of tumors, particularly involving the liver.[24]

Although resection continues to be the gold standard in both primary and metastatic liver tumors, many patients present with unresectable lesions.[25] RFA can play an effective role in regional control of these lesions as well as other solid tumors.[26–31] RFA, whether done via percutaneous, laparoscopic, or open means, carries a morbidity of 7% to 10% and a mortality of 0.1% to 0.5%.[32] Table 113.2 summarizes some of the clinical data available today to support RFA.

Bipolar Electrocautery

Bipolar circuits deliver current between two closely opposed electrodes, one of which is the ground and the other is the active electrode. Forceps tines are the most commonly used electrodes, but other delivery methods such as scissor blades and clamps are available. The circuit incorporates the tissue between the oppositely charged electrodes. A return electrode (i.e., the bovie pad) is not necessary because one of the tines serves as the ground.

Bipolar generators historically have used a lower voltage than monopolar circuits and offer only a coagulation mode. However, some of the newer generators offer a high voltage cut mode. The bipolar circuit has the advantage of precise delivery; however, it is not as effective as the monopolar circuit at both cutting and large vessel hemostasis.[33] Bipolar electrosurgery has found extensive use in microvascular surgery where precise coagulation of individual vessels is warranted.[34–38]

Bipolar Electrocautery with Pressure and Current Control

Several specialized bipolar devices (e.g., the Ligasure) have been developed to enhance vessel sealing while minimizing damage to surrounding tissue. The basic bipolar coagulator delivers current between pressure-generating jaws. The current denatures collagen and elastin within the blood vessel walls and connective tissue. The compression serves two purposes: (1) pressure applied by the instrument allows the denatured, pliable tissue to remodel, creating a vessel seal;

TABLE 113.2.

Radiofrequency Ablation (RFA) Can Treat Disease as Well as Assisting in Surgical Procedures: Clinical Outcomes Can Be Measured as Shown Here.

Lencioni et al. 2003[27]	Level I human study	Prospective randomized comparison in 102 patients between RFA and percutaneous ethanol injection (PEI) for hepatocellular carcinoma	Local recurrence-free survival at 1 and 2 years were 98% and 96% for RFA vs. 83% and 62% for PEI; trend toward survival benefit in RFA patients
Abdalla et al.[25]	Level II human study	Prospective nonrandomized comparison in 418 patients of resection vs. RFA vs. both vs. chemotherapy only for colorectal liver metastases	Resection when anatomically possible conferred the highest survival: 4-year survival after resection, resection + RFA, and RFA only was 65%, 36%, and 22% respectively; unresectable patients treated with RFA or resection + RFA had better survival than chemotherapy alone
Miao et al.[29–31]	Level I animal studies	Multiple animal studies evaluating RFA ablation of carcinoma tumor model vs. controls	High rate of complete tumor eradication, from 22% to 83%, proven by animal survival and pathology
Mulier et al.[32]	Level IV human study	Metanalysis of RFA complications reported in the world literature	Complication rates of 7.2%, 9.5%, and 9.9% for percutaneous, laparoscopic, and open RFA, respectively; complication rate of 31.8% for patients undergoing combined RFA + additional treatment such as resection, cryotherapy, or debulking; complications included bleeding, hepatic abscess, peritoneal infection, and biliary tract damage

and (2) the initial compression forces blood out of the vessels and water out of the interstitium, both of which allow for quicker and more uniform heating.

Further development of bipolar coagulation technology led to feedback mechanisms by which the active electrodes can sense tissue impedance and adjust voltage to maintain a constant current.[39] The impedance setpoint is reached at the moment of coagulation and the current is shut off; this minimizes charring, lateral thermal damage, and sticking of tissue to the electrodes. The Ligasure (Valleylab, Boulder, CO) and PlasmaKinetic (Gyrus, Maple Grove, MN) have been shown to seal vessels up to 7mm in diameter with similar burst strength as surgical clips.[40–44]

The EnSeal (SurgRx, Palo Alto, CA) is able to adjust energy delivery to each area of tissue within the instrument using a proprietary nanomaterial that replaces computer-controlled feedback. The material changes its resistance instantaneously as a result of material property changes related to temperature.[45]

Use of bipolar vessel sealing has decreased operative time in open bowel resections[46]; however, the same is not true for thyroid resection.[47] Although effective in transecting the mesentery and other vascular beds, the devices have shown mixed results in sealing other luminal structures, such as the cystic duct[48,49] (Table 113.3). Bipolar vessel sealers have been shown to cause lateral thermal damage up to 4mm.[50]

Saline-Modulated Electrosurgery

Saline modulation of monopolar and bipolar current is yet another strategy aimed at refining the delivery of electrical current. It is similar to the argon beam coagulator in that it provides a current bridge from the instrument to the tissue and spreads the ionization across a surface. The TissueLink (TissueLink Medical, Dover, NH) focuses energy through continuous low-volume saline irrigation (Table 113.4). The saline facilitates energy transfer between the device–tissue interface and provides temperature uniformity as the saline will not heat above 100°C until vaporized. Once the current ceases, the saline solution provides surface cooling to maximize eschar formation.[51] The device seals vascular and biliary structures up to 3mm in diameter and 5 to 10mm deep by the fusion of collagen.[52]

The surgeon must always consider the ability of this device to heat tissue without charring (that is, there may not be a clinical indicator of damage). When left in one area for an extended period, it may cause steam formation and tissue destruction to 20mm below the surface.[53] In the case of the tissue link, the thermal spread of the instrument can be advantageous, offering surgeons the ability to coagulate deeply (beneath the cutting surface), so that when the tissue below the surface is reached, it will not bleed (Fig. 113.4).

Ultrasonic Surgery

Sound waves are longitudinal mechanical pressure waves. The human ear can detect sound in the range of 20 to 20,000 cycles per second. Above that range, pressure waves are termed ultrasonic. Ultrasonic waves are created by transducers that convert electrical energy into mechanical vibration. The most common ultrasonic transducers are ceramic piezo-

TABLE 113.3.
Majority of Bipolar Sealing Data Are from Animal Studies: Similar Results Seen Across Various Platforms.

Kennedy et al.[42]	Level I animal data	Reports initial use of feedback-controlled bipolar vessel sealer in porcine vessels and compares its burst strength measurements to ultrasonic coagulator, regular bipolar, clip, and ligature	Bipolar sealer an average burst strength of 738 mmHg ± 237 in 1–7 mm arteries with the only failures coming in the 5- to 7-mm group (38%); burst strength declined in larger vessels but was comparable to clips and suture ligation up to 7 mm; ultrasonic coagulator and regular bipolar showed considerable variability in burst strengths, often falling below 400 mmHg in small vessels
Heniford et al.[46]	Level IV human data plus animal data	Case series using Ligasure™ and animal model of bowel resection comparing Ligasure™ to clamp and tie technique	Safe and effective use of Ligasure™ with rare need (0.3%) for additional hemostatic techniques; Ligasure™ was faster than classic technique for open bowel resection in an animal model (252 s vs. 702 s)
Carbonell et al.[40]	Level I animal data	Comparison of burst pressure and lateral thermal spread between Ligasure™ and PlasmKinetic™ using porcine vessels of 2–3 mm, 4–5 mm, and 6–7 mm	Ligasure™ had average bursting pressures of 326, 573, and 585 mmHg in the three groups; PlasmaKinetic™ had average burst pressures of 397, 389, and 317 mmHg; although comparable in the 2–3 mm group, Ligasure™ produced significantly higher burst pressures in the 4–5 mm and 6–7 mm group; thermal spread was similar between instruments and increased with increasing vessel size up to 3.2 mm in the 6- to 7-mm vessels

electric crystals, which convert electricity into high-frequency pressure waves.

Depending on the frequency and directionality of the ultrasonic transducers, sound waves can be used in a variety of different ways by the surgeon. For example, in the case of lithotripsy, sound waves can be focused to destroy kidney stones. HIFU is the acronym for high intensity focused ultrasound, which is essentially the same concept of lithotripsy except that it is performed over a smaller area to create heat and ablate tissue. In general surgery, a favored instrument is the Ethicon Harmonic Scalpel, which locally cuts and heats tissue to dissect through the tissue. Other devices utilize the cavitation effect (generation of high local pressure waves) to very locally rip through tissue.

Phacoemulsification

Ultrasonic surgery has met with huge success in the treatment of cataracts. Phacoemulsification employs a small ultrasonic probe that is inserted into the lens capsule. The mechanism of action is likely different from that seen in surgical procedures. There are likely two mechanisms at work in this technology: (1) direct mechanical destruction of the tissue with the vibrating probe; and (2) cavitating waves that emanate from the probe and liquefy the cataractous lens without damaging the surrounding tissues. The emulsified fragments of the lens are then removed with suction.

A folded intraocular lens is inserted through the small incision. The difference between phacoemulsification and the

TABLE 113.4.
Tissue Link: Limited Clinical Studies: In Animals, the Saline-Modulated Electrosurgical Device (SMED) Appears Efficacious in Controlling Vessels Below Organ Surface.

Topp et al.[53]	Level I animal data	180 lesions were created in pig livers using saline-modulated electrosurgical device SMED and effect of several variables on depth of injury and steam popping were studied	Steam popping can be avoided with appropriate choice of power for a given size lesion; depth of liver injury is to 20 mm and is directly related to power, lesion size, inflow occlusion
Di Carlo et al.[51]	Level IV human data	Case series of 9 patients undergoing liver resection; SMED used to achieve hemostasis at the cut liver surface	Average liver resection performed in 20 min with 150 mL (50–300 mL) blood loss; Pringle maneuver required in 1 case
Sundaram et al.[52]	Level IV human data	Case series of 3 patients undergoing laparoscopic partial nephrectomy; SMED used to control bleeding from cut parenchyma	Feasible system for local renal vascular control

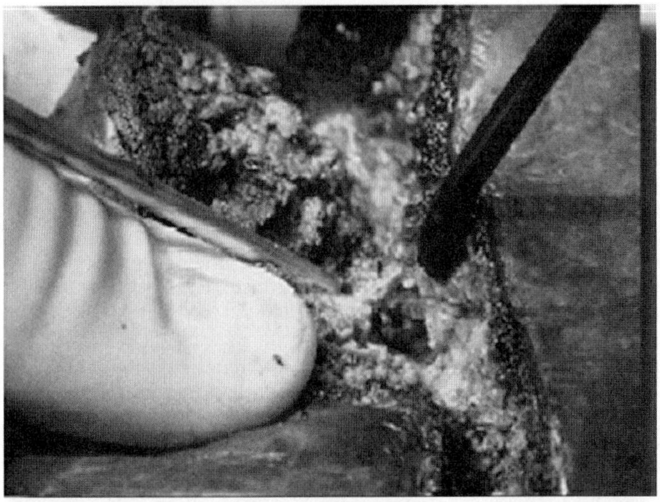

FIGURE 113.4. Gross pathology of a liver section after coagulation with a TissueLink™ floating ball device. A 5- to 10-mm rind of coagulation can be seen at the surface of the liver, which allows surgeons to "coagulate prior to cutting." (From TissueLink Medical, with permission.)

harmonic scalpel (see below) likely lies in the geometry of the tip. In phacomemulsification, the tip is the size of an 18-gauge needle, which results in a very intense field around the tip. In the case of the harmonic scalpel, the pressure waves emanate from a larger surface area and do not necessary create cavitatation.[54]

Harmonic Scalpel

Harmonic scalpel systems deliver ultrasonic waves at a frequency of about 55,500 vibrations per second (55.5 kHz). The ultrasonic energy can be delivered by a variety of instruments including scissors, blades, and ball tips. The high-frequency vibrations of the instrument create both a saw effect and coagulation effect but not a cavitation effect. When using a blade, the saw effect tends to cut tissue at the center of the instrument, while coagulation of the tissue edges occurs by vibration-induced heat. The heat causes protein denaturation that forms a coagulum to seal small vessels. When the effect is prolonged, secondary heat is produced that seals larger vessels.[55] The UltraCision (Ethicon Endo-Surgery, Cincinnati, OH) is approved to seal vessels as large as 5 mm.

In contrast to the bipolar/pressure vessel sealing devices, the harmonic scalpel does not have a defined endpoint for optimal vessel sealing, but relies on the judgment of the surgeon. Ultrasound dissection is associated with minimal lateral thermal spread. However, in one study, a comparison between UltraCision and Ligusure did not reveal a significant difference in lateral tissue damage during ureteral dissection, with both damaging tissue up to 4 mm[50] (Table 113.5).[56–61]

Laser Surgery

The detailed science behind stimulated emission and the extensive clinical results in fields outside general surgery is outside the scope of this chapter but is covered briefly to introduce general surgeons to the technology to stimulate innovation in the field.

Briefly, the two forms of photon emission (light) are spontaneous and stimulated emission. Spontaneous emission of light is the process encountered every day in our world. Atoms (specifically electrons) are electrically excited and then spontaneously return to a resting state, emitting photons (visible light) in the process. Importantly, this light is not in phase and typically consists of many different wavelengths in a process that is difficult to control.

Stimulated emission, on the other hand, is the process whereby a photon is emitted after an electron that is already in a stimulated state is hit with a photon. The exiting photon continues on to hit a second and a third photon, etc. This process, photon-stimulated photon emission, leads to emission of "quanta" of light, which are monochromatic and in phase, or "coherent."[62,63] The utility of a laser for a given application is the result of a complex, non-linear interaction between the wavelength of the laser, the power intensity, and energy content of the laser and the properties of the tissue with which it interacts. The tissue properties include absorption by the biologic molecules, tissue water content, scattering (reflection), thermal conductivity, and blood flow in the region.

There are three essential categories of laser–tissue interactions, depending on the aforementioned tissue parameters. Photochemical effects typically occur at the milliwatt to watt per square centimeter power density. A photochemical effect is a chemical reaction induced directly by the light (e.g., photosynthesis, curing of adhesives). Photothermal effects occur at the $1–10^6\,W/cm^2$ power level. Photothermal effects include heating interactions such as ablation and coagulation. Photomechanical and photoionizing effects occur at 10^8 to $10^{12}\,W/cm^2$ and include effects such as direct destruction of cell membrane lipid bilayers, proteins, and DNA.[64]

Of note, the "ablation" described above in the context of radiofrequency ablation is different from that used in laser "photoablation." In laser photoablation molecular bonds are directly disrupted whereas ablation in the radiofrequency world refers to tissue destruction from heating and denaturation of proteins; these are "photothermal effects" and not "photoablative" effects in the laser realm.

Another concept in laser phototherapy is that of photodynamic therapy. In this case, an exogenous chromophore (light-absorbing molecule) is introduced into the tissue. The light is then absorbed by the chromophore and converted to (e.g.) heat or a cytotoxic oxygen radical.[65,66] Clinical use of phototherapy is discussed with respect to regional therapy of cancer.

Conclusion

This chapter presents a brief overview of devices that modulate energy to produce reliable tissue effects. Modern surgeons depend on these tools to increase the effectiveness and efficiency of their art. Understanding the conceptual basis of each tool allows the surgeon to apply the correct device to the correct situation. To reiterate the quote of Dr. Andrew Brill (University of Illinois at Chicago), "It's not the wand, but the magician." Further understanding of the limitations of these devices will continue to force new innovations.

TABLE 113.5.
Results with Harmonic Scalpel Show Equivalence and Superior Results in Some Cases to Electrocautery.

Sugo et al.[56]	Level III human data	Case-control series comparing hepatic resection using ultrasonic scalpel (n = 18) vs. conventional crush and clamp technique (n = 34)	No difference in morbidity and mortality, with no specific morbidity attributed to the ultrasonic scalpel; operating time significantly longer in the ultrasonic scalpel group, average 281 vs. 223 min; in subset of patients undergoing minor hepatectomy, ultrasonic scalpel had lower average blood loss, 657 ± 588 vs. 1447 ± 984 mL
Takayama et al.[57]	Level II human data	Randomized comparison comparing hepatic resection using ultrasonic scalpel (n = 66) and conventional crush and clamp technique (n = 66)	No significant difference in blood loss (515 vs. 452 min) or transection time (61 vs. 54 min) between ultrasonic scalpel and conventional technique, respectively; ultrasonic scalpel caused more histological tumor exposure at the surgical margin, with no difference in morbidity
Schmidbauer et al.[58]	Level IV human data	Case series of 41 patients undergoing 64 open liver resections and 2 laparoscopic liver resections using ultrasonic scalpel	Average blood loss 820 mL in open resections and 50 mL in laparoscopic resections; 1 death from postoperative liver failure; no major complications; author reports advantage of limited heat and smoke production
Takao et al.[59]	Level IV human data plus animal data	Comparison between ultrasonic scalpel, steel scalpel, and electrocautery in 5 canine pancreatic resections; case series of 50 pancreatic resections using ultrasonic scalpel	Ultrasonic scalpel showed significantly less bleeding volume in the canine model then the other modalities, with less local tissue damage (up to 0.5 mm) than electrocautery; case series showed feasibility of instrument for pancreatic surgery with minimal bleeding and no postoperative pancreatic fistula
Sugo et al.[60]	Level III human data	Retrospective case-control series comparing ultrasonic scalpel (n = 11) to conventional technique (n = 20) in transecting the parenchyma during distal pancreatectomy	Significantly higher rate of pancreatic fistula (6 vs. 0, $P = 0.04$) in the conventional technique group, as well as a higher level of postoperative serum amylase, $P < 0.01$; no difference in hemorrhage or abscess formation found; no additional methods of hemostasis were required in the ultrasound group
Janssen et al.[61]	Level I human data	Prospective randomized controlled trial comparing UltraCision™ to electrocautery dissection during laparoscopic cholecystectomy; primary endpoint was gallbladder perforation; secondary endpoints were operative time, optical lens cleaning, and use of electrocautery for hemostasis in the ultrasound group	Groups were matched for age, sex, body mass index (BMI), and operating surgeon experience; less gallbladder perforation seen using UltraCision™ (19 vs. 69, $P < 0.001$); no overall difference in operative time and optical lens cleaning; in the subset of complicated operations, UltraCision™ showed less operative time (60 vs. 80 min, $P = 0.049$) and less optical lens cleaning (2 vs. 4, $P = 0.035$); electrocautery used in 41% of ultrasound cases for purpose of hemostasis

References

1. Ciarallo A, De Carolis E. Pompeii: Life in a Roman Town. Milan: Electra, 1999.
2. Sigurdsson HEA. The eruption of Vesuvius in A.D. 79. Am J Archaeol 1982;86.
3. Wallace-Hadrill A. Houses and Society in Pompeii and Herculaneum. Princeton: Princeton University Press, 1994.
4. Cushing H. Electro-surgery as an aid to the removal of intracranial tumors. With a preliminary note on a new surgical-current generator by W.T. Bovie. Surg Gynecol Obstet 1928;47:751–784.
5. Curie J, Curie P. Bulletin de la Societe Mineralogique de France 1880;3:90.
6. Kelman CD Symposium: Phacoemulsification. History of emulsification and aspiration of senile cataracts. Trans Am Acad Ophthalmol Otolaryngol 1974;78(1):OP5–OP13.
7. Lantis JC II, Durville FM, Connolly R, Schwaitzberg SD. Comparison of coagulation modalities in surgery. J Laparoendosc Adv Surg Tech A 1998;8(6):381–394.
8. Link WJ, Incropera FP, Glover JL. A plasma scalpel: comparison of tissue damage and wound healing with electrosurgical and steel scalpels. Arch Surg 1976;111(4):392–397.
9. Glover JL, Bendick PJ, Link WJ, Plunkett RJ. The plasma scalpel: a new thermal knife. Lasers Surg Med 1982;2(1):101–106.

10. Go PM, Goodman GR, Bruhn EW, Hunter JG. The argon beam coagulator provides rapid hemostasis of experimental hepatic and splenic hemorrhage in anticoagulated dogs. J Trauma 1991;31(9):1294–1300.
11. Postema RR, Plaisier PW, ten Kate FJ, Terpstra OT. Haemostasis after partial hepatectomy using argon beam coagulation. Br J Surg 1993;80(12):1563–1565.
12. Rees M, Plant G, Wells J, Bygrave S. One hundred and fifty hepatic resections: evolution of technique towards bloodless surgery. Br J Surg 1996;83(11):1526–1529.
13. Dowling RD, Ochoa J, Yousem SA, Peitzman A, Udekwu AO. Argon beam coagulation is superior to conventional techniques in repair of experimental splenic injury. J Trauma 1991;31(5):717–720; discussion 720–721.
14. Dunham CM, Cornwell EE III, Militello P. The role of the argon beam coagulator in splenic salvage. Surg Gynecol Obstet 1991;173(3):179–182.
15. Kwon AH, Inui H, Kamiyama Y. Successful laparoscopic haemostasis using an argon beam coagulator for blunt traumatic splenic injury. Eur J Surg 2001;167(4):316–318.
16. Stylianos S, Hoffman MA, Jacir NN, Harris BH. Sutureless hemisplenectomy. J Pediatr Surg 1991;26(1):87–89.
17. Palmer M, Miller CW, van Way CW 3rd, Orton EC. Venous gas embolism associated with argon-enhanced coagulation of the liver. J Invest Surg 1993;6(5):391–399.
18. Stojeba N, Mahoudeau G, Segura P, Meyer C, Steib A. Possible venous argon gas embolism complicating argon gas enhanced coagulation during liver surgery. Acta Anaesthesiol Scand 1999;43(8):866–867.
19. Veyckemans F, Michel I. Venous gas embolism from an argon coagulator. Anesthesiology 1996;85(2):443–444.
20. Fatal gas embolism caused by overpressurization during laparoscopic use of argon enhanced coagulation. Health Devices 1994;23(6):257–259.
21. Daniell J, Fisher B, Alexander W. Laparoscopic evaluation of the argon beam coagulator. Initial report. J Reprod Med 1993;38(2):121–125.
22. Choi D, Lim HK, Kim MJ, et al. Overlapping ablation using a coaxial radiofrequency electrode and multiple cannulae system: experimental study in ex-vivo bovine liver. Korean J Radiol 2003;4(2):117–123.
23. McGahan JP, Brock JM, Tesluk H, Gu WZ, Schneider P, Browning PD. Hepatic ablation with use of radio-frequency electrocautery in the animal model. J Vasc Intervent Radiol 1992;3(2):291–297.
24. Gillams AR. The use of radiofrequency in cancer. Br J Cancer 2005;92(10):1825–1829.
25. Abdalla EK, Vauthey JN, Ellis LM, et al. Recurrence and outcomes following hepatic resection, radiofrequency ablation, and combined resection/ablation for colorectal liver metastases. Ann Surg 2004;239(6):818–825; discussion 825–827.
26. Lencioni R, Cioni D, Crocetti L, et al. Early-stage hepatocellular carcinoma in patients with cirrhosis: long-term results of percutaneous image-guided radiofrequency ablation. Radiology 2005;234(3):961–967.
27. Lencioni RA, Allgaier HP, Cioni D, et al. Small hepatocellular carcinoma in cirrhosis: randomized comparison of radio-frequency thermal ablation versus percutaneous ethanol injection. Radiology 2003;228(1):235–240.
28. Lee JM, Jin GY, Li CA, et al. Percutaneous radiofrequency thermal ablation of lung VX2 tumors in a rabbit model using a cooled tip-electrode: feasibility, safety, and effectiveness. Invest Radiol 2003;38(2):129–139.
29. Miao Y, Ni Y, Bosmans H, et al. Radiofrequency ablation for eradication of pulmonary tumor in rabbits. J Surg Res 2001; 99(2):265–271.
30. Miao Y, Ni Y, Bosmans H, et al. Radiofrequency ablation for eradication of renal tumor in a rabbit model by using a cooled-tip electrode technique. Ann Surg Oncol 2001;8(8):651–657.
31. Miao Y, Ni Y, Mulier S, et al. Treatment of VX2 liver tumor in rabbits with "wet" electrode mediated radio-frequency ablation. Eur Radiol 2000;10(1):188–194.
32. Mulier S, Mulier P, Ni Y, et al. Complications of radiofrequency coagulation of liver tumours. Br J Surg 2002;89(10):1206–1222.
33. Chehrazi B, Collins WF Jr. A comparison of effects of bipolar and monopolar electrocoagulation in brain. J Neurosurg 1981; 54(2):197–203.
34. Caffee HH, Ward D. Bipolar coagulation in microvascular surgery. Plast Reconstr Surg 1986;78(3):374–377.
35. DeLong WB, Fox JL. Automatic cycling bipolar coagulator. Surg Neurol 1977;8(1):15–16.
36. Dujovny M, Dujovny N, Gundamraj NR, Misra M. Bipolar coagulation in neurosurgery. Surg Neurol 1998;49(3):328–332.
37. Jacques S, Bullara LA, Pudenz RH. Microvascular bipolar coagulator. Technical note. J Neurosurg 1976;44(4):523–524.
38. Sugita K, Tsugane R. Bipolar coagulator with automatic thermocontrol. Technical note. J Neurosurg 1974;41(6):777–779.
39. Bergdahl B, Vallfors B. Studies on coagulation and the development of an automatic computerized bipolar coagulator. Technical note. J Neurosurg 1991;75(1):148–151.
40. Carbonell AM, Joels CS, Kercher KW, Matthews BD, Sing RF, Heniford BT. A comparison of laparoscopic bipolar vessel sealing devices in the hemostasis of small-, medium-, and large-sized arteries. J Laparoendosc Adv Surg Tech A 2003;13(6):377–380.
41. Harold KL, Pollinger H, Matthews BD, Kercher KW, Sing RF, Heniford BT. Comparison of ultrasonic energy, bipolar thermal energy, and vascular clips for the hemostasis of small-, medium-, and large-sized arteries. Surg Endosc 2003;17(8):1228–1230.
42. Kennedy JS, Stranahan PL, Taylor KD, Chandler JG. High-burst-strength, feedback-controlled bipolar vessel sealing. Surg Endosc 1998;12(6):876–878.
43. Landman J, Kerbl K, Rehman J, et al. Evaluation of a vessel sealing system, bipolar electrosurgery, harmonic scalpel, titanium clips, endoscopic gastrointestinal anastomosis vascular staples and sutures for arterial and venous ligation in a porcine model. J Urol 2003;169(2):697–700.
44. Presthus JB, Brooks PG, Kirchhof N. Vessel sealing using a pulsed bipolar system and open forceps. J Am Assoc Gynecol Laparosc 2003;10(4):528–533.
45. Brill A. Mapping the thermal gradient of a new radiofrequency bipolar vessel sealing device, EnSeal, using real-time thermography. J Am Assoc Gynecol Laparosc 2004;11(suppl 3):S7, S19.
46. Heniford BT, Matthews BD, Sing RF, Backus C, Pratt B, Greene FL. Initial results with an electrothermal bipolar vessel sealer. Surg Endosc 2001;15(8):799–801.
47. Kiriakopoulos A, Dimitrios T, Dimitrios L. Use of a diathermy system in thyroid surgery. Arch Surg 2004;139(9):997–1000.
48. Matthews BD, Pratt BL, Backus CL, et al. Effectiveness of the ultrasonic coagulating shears, LigaSure vessel sealer, and surgical clip application in biliary surgery: a comparative analysis. Am Surg 2001;67(9):901–906.
49. Schulze S, Krisitiansen VB, Fischer Hansen B, Rosenberg J. Sealing of cystic duct with bipolar electrocoagulation. Surg Endosc 2002;16(2):342–344.
50. Goldstein SL, Harold KL, Lentzner A, et al. Comparison of thermal spread after ureteral ligation with the Laparo-Sonic ultrasonic shears and the Ligasure system. J Laparoendosc Adv Surg Tech A 2002;12(1):61–63.
51. Di Carlo I, Barbagallo F, Toro A, Sofia M, Guastella T, Latteri F. Hepatic resections using a water-cooled, high-density, monopolar device: a new technology for safer surgery. J Gastrointest Surg 2004;8(5):596–600.
52. Sundaram CP, Rehman J, Venkatesh R, et al. Hemostatic laparoscopic partial nephrectomy assisted by a water-cooled, high-density, monopolar device without renal vascular control. Urology 2003;61(5):906–909.

53. Topp SA, McClurken M, Lipson D, et al. Saline-linked surface radiofrequency ablation: factors affecting steam popping and depth of injury in the pig liver. Ann Surg 2004;239(4):518–527.
54. Packer M, Fishkind WJ, Fine IH, Seibel BS, Hoffman RS. The physics of phaco: a review. J Cataract Refract Surg 2005;31(2):424–431.
55. Lee SJ, Park KH. Ultrasonic energy in endoscopic surgery. Yonsei Med J 1999;40(6):545–549.
56. Sugo H, Matsumoto K, Kojima K, Fukasawa M, Beppu T. Role of ultrasonically activated scalpel in hepatic resection: a comparison with conventional blunt dissection. Hepatogastroenterology 2005;52(61):173–175.
57. Takayama T, Makuuchi M, Kubota K, et al. Randomized comparison of ultrasonic vs clamp transection of the liver. Arch Surg 2001;136(8):922–928.
58. Schmidbauer S, Hallfeldt KK, Sitzmann G, Kantelhardt T, Trupka A. Experience with ultrasound scissors and blades (UltraCision) in open and laparoscopic liver resection. Ann Surg 2002;235(1):27–30.
59. Takao S, Shinchi H, Maemura K, Aikou T. Ultrasonically activated scalpel is an effective tool for cutting the pancreas in biliary-pancreatic surgery: experimental and clinical studies. J Hepatobiliary Pancreat Surg 2000;7(1):58–62.
60. Sugo H, Mikami Y, Matsumoto F, Tsumura H, Watanabe Y, Futagawa S. Comparison of ultrasonically activated scalpel versus conventional division for the pancreas in distal pancreatectomy. J Hepatobiliary Pancreat Surg 2001;8(4):349–352.
61. Janssen IM, Swank DJ, Boonstra O, Knipscheer BC, Klinkenbijl JH, van Goor H. Randomized clinical trial of ultrasonic versus electrocautery dissection of the gallbladder in laparoscopic cholecystectomy. Br J Surg 2003;90(7):799–803.
62. Sulieman M. An overview of the use of lasers in general dental practice: 1. Laser physics and tissue interactions. Dent Update 2005;32(4):228–230, 233–234, 236.
63. Sulieman M. An overview of the use of lasers in general dental practice: 2. Laser wavelengths, soft and hard tissue clinical applications. Dent Update 2005;32(5):286–288, 291–294, 296.
64. Knappe V, Frank F, Rohde E. Principles of lasers and biophotonic effects. Photomed Laser Surg 2004;22(5):411–417.
65. Dougherty TJ, Gomer CJ, Henderson BW, et al. Photodynamic therapy. J Natl Cancer Inst 1998;90(12):889–905.
66. Kessel D. Photodynamic therapy and neoplastic disease. Oncol Res 1992;4(6):219–225.

114

Robot-Assisted Surgery: Technology and Current Clinical Status

Russell K. Woo, David A. Peterson, David Le, Michael E. Gertner, and Thomas Krummel

Since their commercial introduction in the early 1990s, robotic telemanipulator surgical systems have been increasingly used to facilitate complex minimal access surgical procedures. In the field of general surgery, such systems have been used to perform a wide variety of operations including foregut procedures, colon resections, and bariatric operations. In addition, these systems have seen significant use in several surgical subspecialties including urology, cardiothoracic surgery, and pediatric surgery. With improvements in robotic instrumentation and technology, interest and experience with robotic surgery has grown. This chapter reviews the current experience with robotic surgical systems in general surgery, highlighting the origins, current state, and future directions of robotic surgery.

Historical Background

Although robotics is generally viewed as a young and developing field, the fundamental concept of automation is actually centuries old. As far back as the fourth century BC, Aristotle wrote "if every instrument could accomplish its own work, obeying or anticipating the will of others . . . if the shuttle could weave, and the pick touch the lyre, without a hand to guide them, chief workmen would not need servants."[1] Stemming from this concept, the earliest generation of robots consisted of self-moving machines designed to imitate the actions of humans or animals. These "automatons" often utilized clock-derived mechanisms and included examples such as an automated rooster that flapped its wings and crowed as well as a mechanical armored knight designed by Leonardo da Vinci to amuse royalty.[1,2]

Although the original automatons were often ornamental in nature, later versions were designed to serve more practical purposes. In 1801, Joseph Jacquard invented an automated loom.[2] This was followed by the development of the first industrial robot—a motorized crane used to remove ingots from a furnace—in 1892 by Seward Babbit.[1] Although examples of automatons had existed for centuries, the first reference to the word "robot" is thought to have appeared in the play "Rossum's Universal Robots" by the Czechoslovakian playwright, Karel Capek, which debuted in London in 1921. The word robot was derived from the Czech word *robota*, which refers to a serf or a person whose role is to perform "forced labor." In the play, Capek describes a society where menial labor is performed by robots, allowing humans to pursue more enlightened activities. However, as the play progresses, the robots begin to be used for destructive purposes. As the robots develop, they gain more and more intelligence and eventually decide that they no longer need their human masters and begin to exterminate the population.[3]

Since Capek's original play, the concept of robots as artificially intelligent, independent anthropomorphic machines has been perpetuated in many famous works of science fiction. However, to date, this image has had little grounding in modern, practical technology. Originally developed in the 1940s, modern robotic technology has generally been focused around the production of reprogrammable, nonanthropomorphic industrial manipulators designed to reproducibly perform specific tasks. In accordance, modern robots may be more appropriately described using a broader definition: a robot is a reprogrammable, computer-controlled mechanical device equipped with sensors and actuators.[3]

For several decades now, robots have served in numerous and varied applications such as high-volume manufacturing, deep-sea exploration, detonation of munitions, military surveillance, and entertainment.[2] In contrast, the use of robotic technology in medicine and surgery is still a relatively young field. Surgical procedures have advanced rapidly in the past two decades because of the large technology base that has been developed in robotics research. Improvements in mechanical design, kinematics, and control algorithms that were originally created for industrial robots have been directly applied toward the development of surgical robotic systems. Conversely, the unique characteristics inherent to human surgical applications have required the development of specific technological features that have advanced and will continue to advance the field of robotics in new directions.

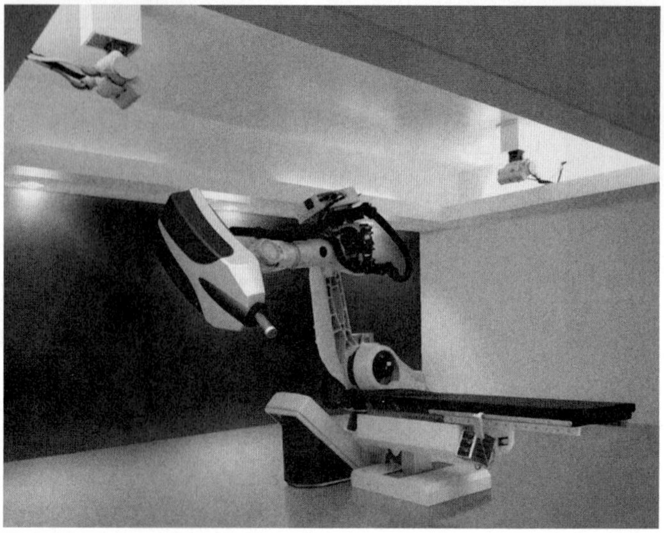

FIGURE 114.1. CyberKnife radiosurgery OR image guided robotic radiosurgery system components. (Courtesy of Accuray, Sunnyvale, CA.)

Robots in Medicine and Surgery

The application of robotic technology in the medical field has been a recent occurrence. In the healthcare system, robots have been used for supportive roles, laboratory assistance, rehabilitation, and surgery. In hospitals and clinics, systems such as the Help-Mate (Pyxis Corporation, San Diego, CA) are used as delivery systems transporting radiographs, records, and medications.[4] In the field of rehabilitation medicine, robotic systems such as the Robbie (Adaptive Abilities, Kelowno, BC, Canada) and the Assistive Robotic Manipulator (ARM) (Exact Dynamics, s-Heerenberg, The Netherlands) have been developed to aid physically disabled patients gain independence and mobility.[4]

Robots were first utilized in surgery in the mid-1980s.[4] Used to assist with neurosurgical and orthopedic procedures, these early surgical devices were designed to aid with predefined tasks that required a high degree of accuracy and reproducibility. Examples of these include the Neuromate System (Integrated Surgical Systems, Sacramento, CA) designed to facilitate stereotactic neurosurgical procedures and the Robodoc System (Integrated Surgical Systems, Sacramento, CA) used in orthopedic surgery to accurately mill out the femoral canal for hip implants.

TABLE 114.1. Classification of Robotic Surgical Systems.

Type of system	*Definition*	*Example*
Autonomous	System carries out treatment without immediate input from the surgeon	Cyberknife® Robodoc®
Surgical assist	Surgeon and robot share control	Aesop®
Teleoperators	Input from the surgeon directs movement of instruments	da Vinci® System Zeus® System

Since the introduction of robots to the operating room in the 1980s, technological advancements have led to the development of several different types of robotic systems. These systems vary significantly in complexity and function. One method of classifying surgical robots is by their level of autonomy. Under this classification, there are currently three types of robots used in surgery: autonomous robots, surgical assist devices, and teleoperators (Table 114.1).

An autonomously operating robot carries out a preoperative plan without any immediate control from the surgeon. The tasks performed are typically focused or repetitive but require a degree of precision not attainable by human hands. The early surgical robots such as the Neuromate and Robodoc fit into this category. Another more recent example is the CYBERKNIFE system (Accuray, Sunnyvale, CA), which consists of a linear accelerator mounted on a robotic arm that is used to precisely deliver radiotherapy to treat intracranial and spinal tumors[5,6] (Fig. 114.1).

The second class of robots is the surgical assist devices, where the surgeon and robot share control. The best known example of this group is the AESOP (Automatic Endoscopic System for Optimal Positioning; formerly Computer Motion, Inc., Goleta, CA, now Intuitive Surgical, Sunnyvale, CA). This system allows a surgeon to attach an endoscope to a robotic arm that provides a steady image by eliminating the natural movements inherent in a live camera holder. The surgeon is then able to reposition the camera by voice commands. To date, the AESOP has been used in many different surgical disciplines including general surgery,[7,8] gynecological surgery,[9] cardiothoracic surgery,[10] and urology.[11]

The final class consists of robots whose every function is explicitly controlled by the surgeon. The hand motions of the surgeon at a control console are tracked by the electronic controller and then relayed to the slave robot in such a manner that the instrument tips perfectly mirror every movement of the surgeon. Because the control console is physically separated from the slave robot, these systems are referred to as teleoperators. All the recent advances in robot-assisted surgery have involved this class of machines.

Teleoperator Systems

The foundations of teleoperator surgical system can be traced back to the 1970s, when the U.S. National Aeronautics and Space Administration (NASA) began the development of telepresence surgical systems to provide surgical care for astronauts in space.[3] This effort subsequently took a major step forward in the late 1980s and early 1990s. At that time, a U.S. government organization known as DARPA (Defense Advanced Research Project Administration) funded telepresence surgery projects at a number of centers in the United States. Spearheaded by Dr. Richard Satava, the goal of these projects was to investigate and develop battlefield surgical systems through which military surgeons would be able to remotely operate on injured soldiers using robots installed on armored vehicles. The soldiers could thereby be stabilized in the battlefield until they could be evacuated to a military hospital. The sites involved in these projects included the Stanford Research Institute (SRI), the Massachusetts Institute of Technology (MIT), IBM's Watson Laboratory, NASA's Jet Propulsion Laboratory (JPL), and Computer Motion Inc.[12]

As envisioned by Dr. Satava and DARPA, these battlefield surgical systems represented a form of telemanipulator robot, where the motions of a human operator are remotely translated into movements of mechanical arms. Also described as "master–slave" systems, telemanipulator devices have been used for many years in other industries to assist in the safe handling of hazardous materials. In fact, the first mechanical master–slave system was developed in 1948 by Raymond Goertz at Argonne National Laboratories. This robot, named the M1, used mechanical linkages and cables to connect an operator-controlled "master" manipulator to an identical "slave" manipulator on the other side of a protective barrier.[12]

Funded by the NIH and DARPA, SRI International developed the first robotic telemanipulator system capable of performing remote surgical tasks. This system, known as the SRI system, consisted of a surgeon's workstation and a remote surgical unit.[3] It featured remote articulating robotic arms capable of basic force feedback, stereoscopic imaging, and an ergonomic design. Although the SRI system was never commercialized, the technological foundations achieved during its development, combined with technology developed at other institutions, have formed the basis for the commercial systems in use today.[12]

State of the Art

From a clinical standpoint, there previously were two systems commercially available: the da Vinci Surgical System by Intuitive Surgical, Inc. (Sunnyvale, CA) and the Zeus system by the former Computer Motion (Goleta, CA). Recently, the two companies have merged, and the da Vinci system has become the predominant robotic operative platform. However, at the current time, both systems are in active clinical use and are therefore described in detail. From a clinical evidence standpoint, the majority of the literature reviewed in this chapter focuses on the worldwide experience with the da Vinci Surgical System as it is the only commercially available system at this current time.

Reported Advantages of Robotic Surgical Systems

The integration of computer technology into both the da Vinci and Zeus helps to resolve many of the limitations of standard laparoscopic surgery. By scanning the surgeon's hand motions, information is relayed to the instruments to move them in the corresponding direction and orientation. Intuitive nonreversed instrument control is therefore restored, while preserving the minimal access nature of the approach.

The presence of a computer control system allows one to filter out inherent hand tremor, thus making the motion of the endoscope and the instrument tips steadier than with the unassisted hand. In addition, the system allows for variable motion scaling from the surgeon's hand to the instrument tips. For instance, a 3 : 1 scale factor maps 3 cm of movement of the surgeon's hand into 1 cm of motion at the instrument tip. In combination with image magnification from the video endoscope, motion scaling makes delicate motions easier and more precise to perform.[13]

In both systems, the instruments are also engineered with articulations at the "wrist" distally that increases their dexterity compared to simpler MAS tools. The da Vinci system alone possesses instruments capable of the full 6° of freedom of motion of the human wrist. Finally, both systems have the option to utilize stereo endoscopes, restoring true three-dimensional (3-D) visualization for the operating surgeon.

The Zeus System

The Zeus system (formerly Computer Motion, Goleta, CA, USA; now Intuitive Surgical, Sunnyvale, CA, USA) is a telemanipulator system that consists of a surgeon's console and three robotic arms (Figs. 114.2, 114.3). The surgeon operates from a console several feet away from the operating table. There, handheld manipulators are used to control the two robotic arms and surgical instruments, a foot pedal activates the computer-driven system, and voice commands direct a camera controlled by an AESOP arm.[14] Similar to the da Vinci

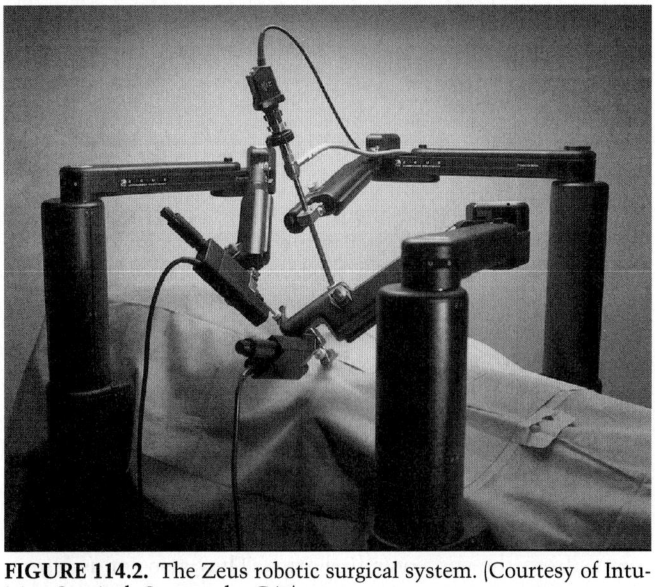

FIGURE 114.2. The Zeus robotic surgical system. (Courtesy of Intuitive Surgical, Sunnyvale, CA.)

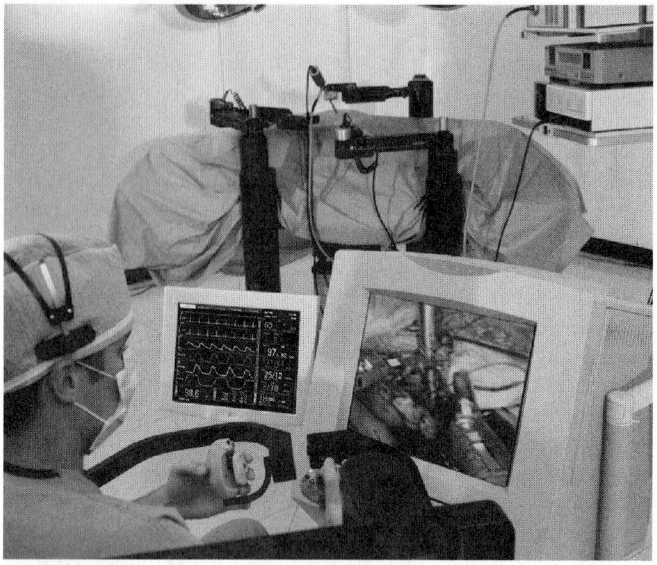

FIGURE 114.3. The Zeus surgeon's console with its video display and master controls. (Courtesy of Intuitive Surgical, Sunnyvale, CA.)

system, the Zeus system offers tremor reduction and motion scaling.

The Zeus system consists of three modular, free-standing robotic arms that are attached to the operating table. This design allows the system to be oriented to many different configurations. The Zeus system also features 3.5- to 5-mm instruments, several of which are capable of increased articulation through the Zeus Microwrist. This joint provides the instrument with an additional degree of freedom at the wrist, giving a total of 5° of freedom. The Zeus system also features the ability to accommodate a variety of visualization options (3-D and 2-D) and telescope sizes.

The Zeus system has received generalized clearance for surgery under Conformité Européenne (CE) guidelines. In the United States, the Zeus system received U.S. Food and Drug Administration (FDA) clearance for general laparoscopy and has been used for thoracic and cardiac procedures as well. To date, the Zeus system has been used to perform multiple operations in adults in different surgical specialties throughout the world.

The da Vinci System

The da Vinci system is made up of two major components (Figs. 114.4–114.7). The first is the surgeon's console, which houses the visual display system, the surgeon's control handles, the user interface buttons, and the electronic controller. The second component is the patient-side cart, which consists of two arms that control the operative instruments and a third arm which controls the video endoscope.

The operative surgeon is seated at the surgeon's console, which can be located up to 10 m away from the operating table. Within the console are located the surgeon's control handles, or masters, which act as high-resolution input devices that read the position, orientation, and grip commands from the surgeon's fingertips. They also act as haptic displays that transmit forces and torques back to the surgeon's hand in response to various measured and synthetic

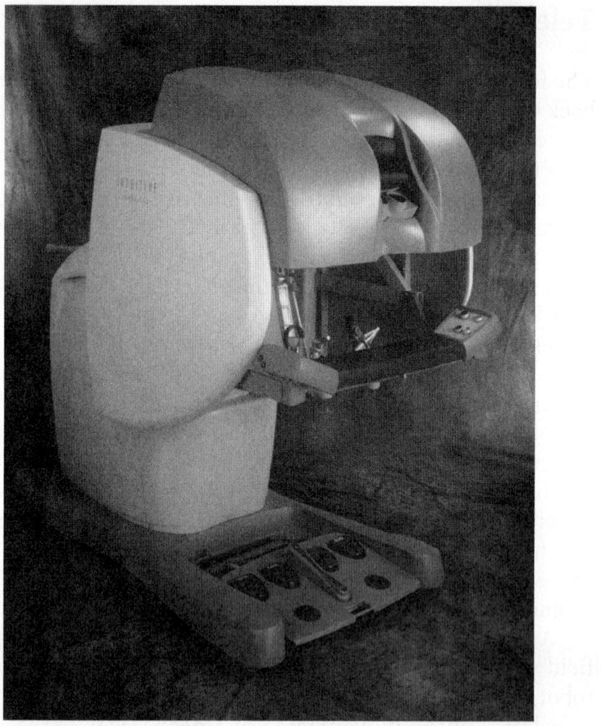

FIGURE 114.4. The Intuitive Surgical da Vinci robotic surgical system: surgeon's console. (Courtesy of Intuitive Surgical, Sunnyvale, CA.)

force cues. This control system also allows for computer enhancement of functions such as motion scaling and tremor reduction.

The image of the operative site is projected to the surgeon through a high-resolution stereo display system that uses two

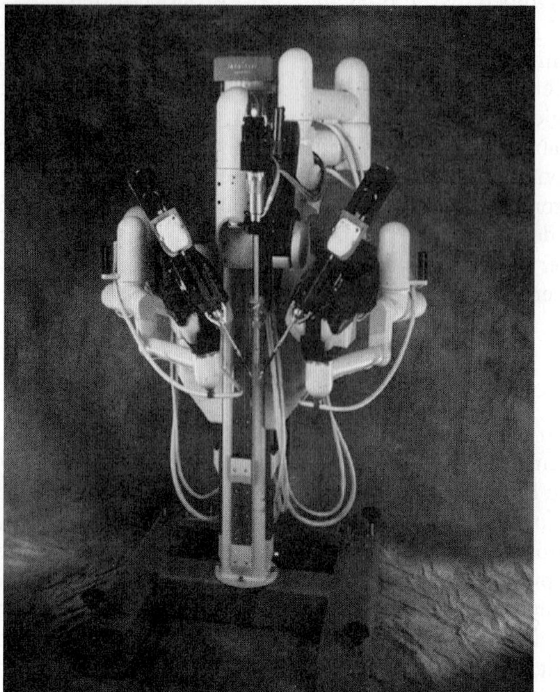

FIGURE 114.5. The Intuitive Surgical da Vinci robotic surgical system: patient-side cart. (Courtesy of Intuitive Surgical, Sunnyvale, CA.)

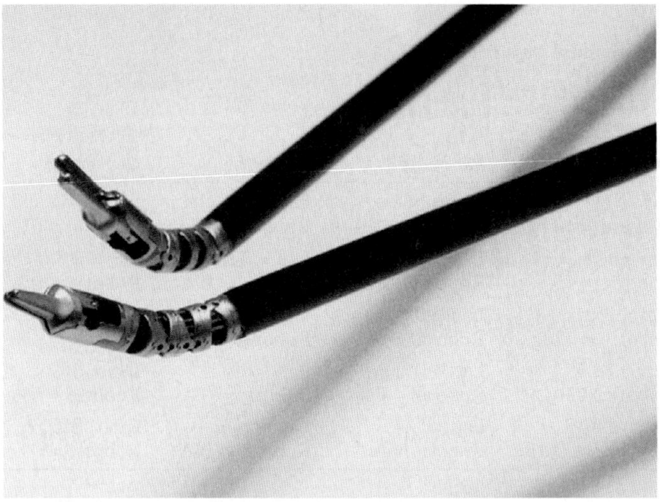

FIGURE 114.6. Articulated 5-mm robotic instrument. (Courtesy of Intuitive Surgical, Sunnyvale, CA.)

medical-grade cathode ray tube (CRT) monitors to display a separate image to each of the surgeon's eyes. The surgeon's brain then fuses the two separate images into a virtual three-dimensional construct. The image plane of the stereo viewer is superimposed over the range of motion of the masters, which restores visual alignment and hand–eye coordination. In addition, because the image of the endoscopic instrument tips is overlaid on top of where the surgeon senses his or her hands, the end effect is that the surgeon feels that his or her hands are virtually inside the patient's body.

Since its introduction in 1995, the da Vinci system has received generalized clearance under European CE guidelines for all surgical procedures; in the United States it has received clearance for general surgery, thoracic surgery, and urological procedures. In addition, the da Vinci system recently received FDA clearance for cardiac procedures involving a cardiotomy. To date, thousands of surgical procedures in multiple disciplines have been performed using the da Vinci system.

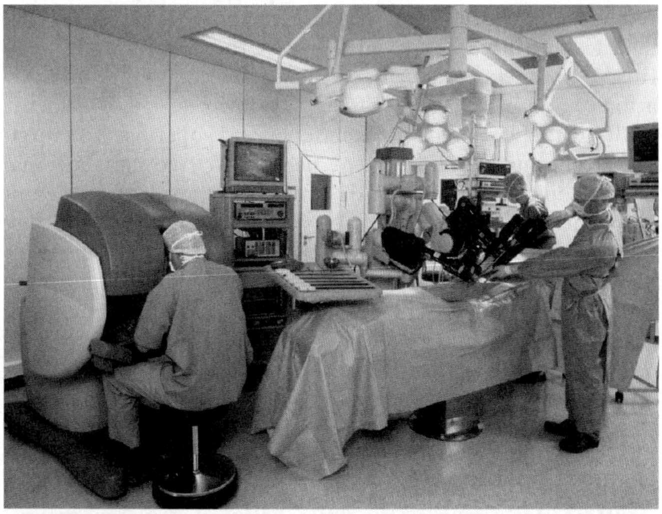

FIGURE 114.7. The Intuitive Surgical da Vinci robotic surgical system OR simulation. (Courtesy of Intuitive Surgical, Sunnyvale, CA.)

Current Clinical Experience with Robot-Assisted Surgery

Introduced in the 1990s, robotic surgical systems are currently used to facilitate operations in multiple fields of surgery including general surgery, urology, pediatric surgery, vascular surgery, and cardiothoracic surgery. This section highlights the published experience with robot-assisted surgery in these fields with particular attention paid to the developing experience in general surgery.

Robot-Assisted General Surgery

To date, robotic surgical systems have been used to perform a variety of general surgical procedures. Beginning with cholecystectomy in 1998, robotic systems have now been used to facilitate complex laparoscopic operations such as colon resections, esophageal myotomies, and gastric bypass procedures. Currently, the worldwide experience with robot-assisted general surgery is entering a second phase. Multiple case reports have demonstrated safety and feasibility, but more recent clinical trials are seeking to elucidate demonstrable clinical benefits compared to standard operations.

Cholecystectomy

Himpens et al. published the first case of robot-assisted laparoscopic cholecystectomy in a human patient in 1998 using a protoype of the da Vinci Surgical System.[15] Since then, multiple authors have published their experience with robot-assisted cholecystectomy using both the Zeus and da Vinci systems. To date, more than 900 robot-assisted cholecystectomies have been reported in the published literature, although it is estimated that the number actually performed worldwide is much larger.[16,17] The authors of these case series report that robot-assisted cholecystectomy can be performed safely and reproducibly with conversion, complication, and mortality rates similar to standard laparoscopic cholecystectomy. Operating times ranged from 62 to 152 min with a described learning curve of approximately 10 to 20 operations.[17] A unique complication reported in several series has been the conversion to an open procedure through a mini-laparotomy to recover a lost robotic instrument part.[16]

Although the published experience with robot-assisted cholecystectomy is primarily retrospective case series, five authors have compared the robot-assisted procedure to standard laparoscopy in prospective trials (Table 114.2). Two sets of authors utilized the da Vinci Surgical System and three sets utilized the Zeus Surgical System.

Ruurda et al. prospectively studied 20 consecutive patients requiring elective cholecystectomy for symptomatic cholelithiasis with gallstones confirmed by ultrasound evaluation. These patients were randomly assigned to receive either robot-assisted laparoscopic cholecystectomy ($n = 10$) or standard laparoscopic cholecystectomy ($n = 10$). For the robot-assisted procedure, the authors utilized the da Vinci Surgical System. The robot-assisted procedures were performed by one of three experienced surgeons with an assistant crew that had performed at least 15 robotic procedures. The conventional laparoscopic procedures were performed by one of five

TABLE 114.2.
Clinical Trials Comparing Robot-Assisted Cholecystectomy to Standard Laparoscopy.

Reference	*System*	*No. of patients*	*Study design*	*Total operating room time (min)*[a]	*Morbidity*	*Mortality*	*Conversion*
Ruurda et al.[77]	da Vinci®	Lap = 10 Robotic = 10	Prospective, randomized	Lap = 119 Robotic = 144	Lap = NA Robotic = NA	Lap = NA Robotic = NA	Lap = 0% Robotic = 0%
Hourmont et al.[19]	da Vinci®	Lap = 25 Robotic = 25	Prospective, nonrandomized	Lap = 138 Robotic = 152	Lap = 12% Robotic = 12%	Lap = 0% Robotic = 0%	Lap = 0% Robotic = 0%
Nio et al.[20]	Zeus®	Lap = 10 Robotic = 10	Prospective, nonrandomized	Lap = 95.4 Robotic = 123.5	Lap = 0% Robotic = 0%	Lap = 0% Robotic = 0%	Lap = 0% Robotic = 0%
Zhou et al.[21]	Zeus®	Lap = 20 Robotic = 20	Prospective, randomized	Lap = 78.6[b] Robotic = 104.9[b]	Lap = 0% Robotic = 0%	Lap = 0% Robotic = 0%	Lap = 5% Robotic = 5%
Kornprat et al.[22]	Zeus®	Lap = 26 Robotic = 20	Prospective, nonrandomized	Lap = 141.5 Robotic = 222.5	Lap = NA Robotic = NA	Lap = NA Robotic = NA	Lap = 0% Robotic = 0%

LAP, laparoscopy.
[a]Represents total time in operating room.
[b]Represents time from disinfection of operative field to skin closure; total operating room time not available.

surgical residents, supervised and assisted by an experienced surgeon. The authors divided total operating room time into preoperative, operative, and postoperative phases. These three phases were further divided into smaller, task-specific time frames. Upon completion of the study, the authors reported a total mean operating room time for the robot-assisted procedure of 144 min versus 119 min for the conventional laparoscopic procedure. This difference did not reach statistical significance ($P = 0.131$). When the smaller time frames were analyzed, the robot-assisted procedure was found to take longer than conventional laparoscopy for all three phases. However, only the difference in the preoperative phase reached statistical significance with a mean preoperative phase time of 47 min for the robot-assisted procedure compared to a mean time of 27 min for standard laparoscopy ($n < 0.001$). The authors concluded that robot-assisted cholecystectomy led to time loss compared to conventional laparoscopic cholecystectomy for routine, elective cases. This time loss was attributed to increased time spent on the preoperative steps of the procedure because of the need for additional robotic equipment and the novelty of the technology. Based on this analysis, they recommended dedicated, robotic surgical workplaces, improvements in the robotic technology, and improved time management by the surgical team as methods to decrease the time loss associated with the robot-assisted procedure.[18]

Hourmont et al. prospectively studied 50 consecutive patients undergoing laparoscopic cholecystectomy at a single institution over a period of approximately 1 year.[19] No patients were excluded, and the report included all the patients who underwent laparoscopic cholecystectomy by the senior author for the period of the study. Patients were assigned in a nonrandomized fashion to either a robot-assisted procedure using the da Vinci Surgical System ($n = 25$) or a standard laparoscopic cholecystectomy using an Aesop (voice-activated) camera holder ($n = 25$) based on robot availability and patient preference. Patient characteristics were similar between the two groups. There was a tendency to assign patients who had had previous abdominal operations to the laparoscopic group and patients with higher body mass indexes to the robotic group. All operations were completed by the intended method with no conversions. The mean surgical time for the laparoscopic group (99 min) was shorter than the robotic group (110 min), although this did not reach statistical significance ($P > 0.05$) The total operating room time for the laparoscopic group (138 min) was also shorter than for the robotic group (152 min). This difference did reach statistical significance by *t* test. Furthermore, the setup times, surgical times, and total operating room times did not differ through the course of the study, indicating no overall significant learning curve effect. Outcomes with respect to blood loss, morbidity, mortality, and length of stay were similar between the two groups. The authors concluded that robot-assisted cholecystectomy achieved similar clinical outcomes compared to standard laparoscopic cholecystectomy with slightly longer total operating room times.[19]

Nio et al. prospectively studied 20 consecutive patients undergoing elective laparoscopic cholecystectomy at a single institution. Similar to Hourmont's report, the patients were assigned to receive either conventional laparoscopic cholecystectomy or robot-assisted cholecystectomy in a nonrandomized fashion based on availability of the robotic system. In this case, the authors utilized the Zeus system and the operations were performed primarily by two surgical residents with limited laparoscopic experience and supervised by surgical attendings. Each resident performed five conventional laparoscopic and five robotic cholecystectomies after completing specific training courses. Clinical outcomes, operating times, and number of actions (grasping, dissection) were evaluated prospectively. All operations were completed by the intended method with no conversions. Setup time and dissection time was significantly longer for the robotic group compared to the conventional laparoscopy group. Total operating room time was also longer for the robotic group (123.5 min) compared to the laparoscopic group (95.4 min) although this difference did not reach statistical significance ($P = 0.056$). Number of actions and patient outcomes (morbidity, hospital stay) did not significantly differ between the two groups. Overall, the authors concluded that robot-assisted laparoscopic cholecystectomy was feasible but required longer operating times compared to conventional laparoscopic cholecystectomy.[20]

Also utilizing the Zeus system, Zhou et al. randomly assigned 40 patients undergoing elective cholecystectomy to receive either a robot-assisted procedure ($n = 20$) or a conventional laparoscopic procedure ($n = 20$). Patient characteristics were similar between the two groups. Procedure times, conversion rates, postoperative complication rates, and length of hospital stay were tracked. In addition, the authors tracked several operative parameters including the number of camera clearing events, the time spent adjusting the operative field, the number of grasping actions, the number of dissecting actions, and the rate of operative errors such as gallbladder perforation or liver laceration. All procedures were completed using the intended technique with one conversion to an open procedure in both groups because of "tight adherence in the triangle of Calot." Blood loss, complication rates, and hospital stay were similar between the two groups. The mean total operative time (time from skin disinfection to skin closure) was significantly longer for the robot-assisted group compared to the conventional laparoscopic group (104.9 versus 78.6 min). The number of camera clearing events and the time spent adjusting the operative field was statistically greater in the conventional laparoscopic group compared to the robot-assisted group. The number of operative actions and operative errors was generally less in the robot-assisted group although these differences were not statistically significant. Overall, the authors reported that robot-assisted laparoscopic cholecystectomy was safe and feasible using the Zeus system. Although the robot-assisted procedure required longer operative times, the authors believed that robotic assistance provided a better ability to control the operative field and enabled more precise and stable operative manipulations.[21]

Similar to Ruurda's group, Kornprat et al. in Austria performed a time analysis comparing robot-assisted laparoscopic cholecystectomy using the Zeus system (Z group) to standard laparoscopic cholecystectomy (S group). They enrolled 46 consecutive patients scheduled for elective cholecystectomy for symptomatic cholelithiasis, with 26 patients assigned to the S group and 20 patients assigned to the Z group. There were no significant differences in patient characteristics between the two groups. All procedures were completed using the intended method with no conversions to conventional laparoscopy or open in the robot-assisted group and no conversions to open in the conventional laparoscopic group. Total procedure mean time was significantly longer for group Z compared to group S (222.5 versus 141.5 min). This difference was highly significant. Upon subdivision analysis, the authors reported longer times for the robotic group for the preoperative, operative, and postoperative phases of the procedure. In particular, the authors cited the setup and deinstallation times associated with the robot-assisted procedure as contributing to the overall longer procedure times. Interestingly, the net dissection time for the cystic duct, cystic artery, and gallbladder was not statistically different between the two groups. In conclusion, the authors reported that the robot-assisted procedure was safe and effective, but required longer operating room times and offered no further benefit compared to the standard laparoscopic procedure.[22]

Overall, these five prospective randomized and nonrandomized studies consistently demonstrated the safety and feasibility of robot-assisted cholecystectomy using either the da Vinci Surgical System or the Zeus Surgical System. Compared to conventional laparoscopic cholecystectomy, conversion rates, hospital stay, and morbidity and mortality rates were not statistically different. However, procedure times were significantly longer for the robot-assisted operations in all five studies. Furthermore, only one of the studies demonstrated any significant benefit from robotic assistance in the form of decreased camera clearing events and decreased time spent positioning the operative field.[21] Because of this, several authors have advocated the use of robot-assisted cholecystectomy only for robotic training.

Fundoplication

Fundoplications for the treatment of gastroesophageal reflux disease have been one of the most common general surgical procedures to utilize robotic surgical systems. To date, multiple authors have published case reports and series highlighting the safety and feasibility of a robot-assisted operation. In 2004, Gutt et al. estimated that more than 500 robot-assisted fundoplications had been performed worldwide. At that time, a review of the published literature demonstrated nine case series encompassing 243 total operations. The majority of these procedures were Nissen fundoplications. Intraoperative complication rates ranged from 0% to 5.1%; postoperative complication rates ranged from 0% to 2.4%.[16] Surgical technique including the extent of robotic system use varied. Conversion rates to either traditional laparoscopy or to an open procedure ranged from 0% to 5%. The reasons for conversion were not specifically delineated. Although no specific advantages have been reported, several authors have suggested the robotic system provides enhanced dexterity, which may facilitate delicate dissection and suturing, especially in the case of patients with paraesophageal hernias.[23] In addition, authors have advocated robotic fundoplication as a high-volume, "stepping stone" operation that provides robotic surgeons with the experience needed to perform more complex robot-assisted operations.[17]

At this time, three prospective, randomized clinical trials have been published comparing traditional, laparoscopic Nissen fundoplication to robot-assisted Nissen fundoplication (Table 114.3) The earliest study, published in 2001 by Cadiere et al., utilized the Mona, an early version of the Intuitive Surgical da Vinci Surgical System.[24] Twenty-one patients undergoing laparoscopic Nissen fundoplication for treatment of gastroesophageal reflux disease (GERD) were randomized to have their operation performed either using standard laparoscopy or with robot assistance. Mean total operating times were statistically longer in the robotic group compared to the standard laparoscopy group (76 versus 52 min; $P < 0.01$). The authors also divided the procedure into several steps or tasks. Operating times for each step were also longer for the robot-assisted procedure. Blood loss, hospital stay, and complication rates were similar between the two groups. As an early study, the authors only concluded that robot-assisted Nissen fundoplication was feasible.[24]

The next two studies were both published in 2006, after wider spread adoption of robotic surgical systems throughout the world. The first of these, published by Nakadi et al. from Erasme Hospital in Brussels, was a prospective, randomized clinical trial evaluating 20 patients assigned to either a laparoscopic ($n = 11$) or robotic ($n = 9$) procedure using the da Vinci

TABLE 114.3.
Clinical Trials Comparing Robot-Assisted Nissen Fundoplication to Standard Laparoscopy.

Reference	*System*	*No. of patients*	*Study design*	*Total operating time (min)*	*Morbidity*	*Mortality*	*Conversion*
Cadiere et al.[78]	da Vinci®	Lap = 11 Robotic = 10	Prospective, randomized	Lap = 52 Robotic = 76	Lap = 9% Robotic = 10%	Lap = 0% Robotic = 0%	Lap = 0% Robotic = 0%
Nakadi et al.[25]	da Vinci®	Lap = 11 Robotic = 9	Prospective, randomized	Lap = 96 Robotic = 137	Lap = 0% Robotic = 11%	Lap = 0% Robotic = 0%	Lap = 0% Robotic = 11%
Draaisma et al.[26]	da Vinci®	Lap = 25 Robotic = 25	Prospective, randomized	Lap = 95 Robotic = 120	Lap = 16% Robotic = 4%	Lap = 0% Robotic = 0%	Lap = 8% Robotic = 0%

Surgical System.[25] Studied variables included procedure times, the efficacy of the instrumentation, intraoperative events, postoperative morbidity, and cost. Patient characteristics were similar between the two groups. Fundoplication was completed in all 20 patients. There was one conversion from a robotic procedure to a laparoscopic procedure secondary to instrument length in an obese patient. The patients were followed up to 12 months postoperatively. Postoperative complication rates, return to oral intake, and length of stay were similar between the two groups. Total procedure time was significantly longer for the robotic group (137 ± 12 min.) compared to the laparoscopic group (96 ± 5 min.) Operative costs were also significantly higher for the robotic group. The authors concluded that robot-assisted procedure was safe and feasible but offered no clear advantages over the standard laparoscopy. Furthermore, they found that procedure times and cost were higher with the robotic procedure.[25]

Similarly, Draaisma et al. published a prospective, randomized trial evaluating 50 patients assigned to either laparoscopic Nissen fundoplication (n = 25) or robot-assisted Nissen fundoplication (n = 25) using the da Vinci Surgical System.[26] Subjective assessment of dysphagia, regurgitation, heartburn, and general well-being was performed before and 6 months after surgery. Objective studies obtained 6 months postoperation included esophageal manometry, 24-h pH monitoring, barium esophagram series, and upper endoscopy. Perioperative measures including operating time, blood loss, postoperative pain scores, hospital stay, and complication rates were not statistically different between the two groups. Qualitative measures including postoperative self-rated change in GERD symptoms and quality of life were similarly improved in both groups. Results of the objectives studies were also similar between the two groups. The authors therefore concluded that the robot-assisted procedure added no additional benefit over standard laparoscopic Nissen fundoplication over a follow-up period of 6 months.[26]

Overall, these three prospective, randomized clinical trials represent the best evidence to date comparing robot-assisted Nissen fundoplication to standard, laparoscopic Nissen fundoplication. Although all three studies demonstrate the safety and feasibility of the robot-asssisted procedure, all the studies also demonstrated that there was no statistically significant benefit attained through the use of the robot. Furthermore, all three studies demonstrated significantly longer operating times with the robot-assisted procedure. Table 114.3 summarizes the design and results of these trials.

Colon Resection

Weber et al. reported the first two robot-assisted laparoscopic colon resections in 2002.[27] Using the da Vinci Surgical System to mobilize the bowel, Weber and group performed both a sigmoid colectomy and right hemicolectomy for diverticular disease. For both procedures, the mesenteric dissection, bowel transaction, and anastomosis were completed using conventional laparoscopy. Overall, the authors concluded that robot-assisted laparoscopic colon resections were safe and feasible but required longer operative times compared to their standard laparoscopic techniques.[27]

Since this initial report, multiple authors have published case reports and case series reiterating the safety and feasibility of robot-assisted colon resections. However, these reports have varied significantly with regard to the type of procedures performed and the parameters studied. Because of this, morbidity, mortality, and oncological parameters are difficult to analyze. In general, these reports demonstrate feasibility, but also longer operative times.[28]

Although no prospective randomized studies have been completed, three case-control studies have recently been published highlighting more extensive experience with robot-assisted colorectal surgery (Table 114.4). In 2003, Delaney and group compared six robot-assisted laparoscopic colon operations (two right hemicolectomies, three sigmoid colectomies, and one rectompexy) to case-matched controls from a prospective conventional laparoscopic colorectal surgery database.[29] The da Vinci Surgical System was used to perform the mobilization of the colon and the vascular ligation for all cases. All procedures were completed, and there were no complications or conversions. Upon comparison, the robot-assisted procedures were found to require significantly longer times with a mean operative time of 165 min compared to 108 min for conventional laparoscopy (P = 0.313); this was primarily attributed to additional setup time. Other variables such as blood loss, length of hospital stay, and hospital cost were not significantly different. A mean additional equipment cost of $350 was observed for each robot-assisted operation. This figure included limited use items such as the robot drapes and instruments and did not include the capital costs of the robotic system. Overall the authors found robot-assisted colorectal operations to be safe and feasible. However, they thought that the use of the robotic system resulted in longer mean operative times and overall additional expense.[29]

Also using the da Vinci Surgical System, D'Annibale et al. in Padua, Italy, compared their first 53 robot-assisted

TABLE 114.4.
Clinical Trials Comparing Robot-Assisted Colon Resection to Standard Laparoscopy.

Reference	*System*	*No. of patients*	*Study design*	*Total operating room time (min)*[a]	*Morbidity*	*Mortality*	*Conversion*
Delaney et al.[29]	da Vinci®	Lap = 6 Robotic = 6	Case control	Lap = 165 Robotic = 108	Lap = NA Robotic = NA	Lap = NA Robotic = NA	Lap = 0% Robotic = 0%
D'Annibale et al.[30]	da Vinci®	Lap = 53 Robotic = 53	Case control	Lap = NA Robotic = NA	Lap = 15% Robotic = 7%	Lap = 0% Robotic = 0%	Lap = 5.6% Robotic = 6.7%
Anvari et al.[31]	Zeus®	Lap = 10 Robotic = 10	Case control	Lap = 94 Robotic = 155	Lap = 0% Robotic = 0%	Lap = 0% Robotic = 0%	Lap = 0% Robotic = 0%

[a]Represents total time in operating room.

colorectal resections to their last 53 conventional laparoscopic colorectal resections.[30] Before performing these cases, their group was noted to have performed more than 300 laparoscopic colorectal resections and more than 70 robot-assisted noncolorectal surgical procedures. A variety of colorectal operations were performed including segmental colon resections, low anterior resection, abdominal perineal resection, and total colectomy. There were no significant differences in patient characteristics between the two groups. All procedures were completed, with 3 conversions to open laparotomy in the conventional laparoscopy group and 1 conversion to standard laparoscopy and 3 conversions to hand-assistance in the robot-assisted group. Upon analysis, no significant differences were found between the two groups with respect to operating time, intraoperative blood loss, specimen length, and number of lymph nodes resected. There were no mortalities in either group, and 1 patient in each group required reoperation. Complications were varied including surgical and medical complications. Overall morbidity was 7% in the robot-assisted group and 15% in the conventional laparoscopy group. The robot-assisted group did require a longer mean setup time, defined as the time between inducing anesthesia and starting the surgical procedure compared to the conventional laparoscopic group (24 versus 18 min). In addition, the robot-assisted group generally required more ports compared to the conventional laparoscopy group. Of note, a hand-sewn intracorporeal anastomosis was performed in one robot-assisted operation. All other anastomoses were performed either extracorporeally or with a surgical stapling device. In conclusion, the authors found the robot-assisted procedures to be comparable with conventional laparoscopy with regard to surgical accuracy, oncological radicality, and postoperative outcomes. They also highlight the usefulness of robotic assistance for specific stages of operations such as splenic flexure takedown, dissection of the inferior mesenteric artery with identification of the nervous plexus, and dissection of a narrow pelvis. They also highlight the fact that robotic assistance enabled the completion of an intracorporeal hand-sewn anastomosis, allowing movement of the minilaparotomy site required to remove the specimen to a cosmetically dictated location.[30]

Last, Anvari et al. prospectively followed 10 patients undergoing robot-assisted laparoscopic colon resections using the Zeus Surgical System.[31] The postoperative outcomes of these patients were then compared to 10 case-matched consecutive conventional laparoscopic controls. The procedures performed included right hemicolectomy, left hemicolectomy, low anterior resection, subtotal colectomy, and sigmoid colectomy. Six of the 10 patients underwent operation for malignant disease. Study outcomes included operative time, blood loss, length of hospital stay, complications, time to passing of flatus, and time to initiation of oral diet. All operations were completed using the robotic system. There were no intraoperative complications, conversions, or mortalities, and the estimated blood loss was less than 150 mL for all cases. There were no significant differences in any of the outcome measures between the two groups except for operative time. Specifically, the mean operative time for the robot-assisted group was significantly longer compared to the conventional laparoscopy group (155.3 versus 94.4 min; $P = 0.0009$). In conclusion, the authors stated that robot-assisted laparoscopic colon resection was safe and feasible for both benign and malignant disease. Although the operative times were longer for the robot-assisted procedures, they thought that robotic assistance may confer significant benefit to novice surgeons.[31]

Based on these three studies, robotic colon resection appears to be safe and feasible with similar postoperative and oncologic outcomes compared to conventional laparoscopy. In all three studies, the robot-assisted procedures required longer operative times with no documented additional benefit. Early concerns over the ability of robotic systems to work in multiple abdominal quadrants were not addressed in detail in these reports, likely because of significant variations in the actual procedures performed, with most operations being performed as hybrid procedures with both open and conventional laproscopic components. Furthermore, the inability to move the operating table while the da Vinci system is docked was not thoroughly addressed in the literature. Despite these unanswered concerns, most authors agreed that with technological improvements, operative times for robot-assisted colon resections may decrease and additional benefits may arise.

Heller Myotomy

Robot-assisted laparoscopic Heller myotomy is one of the best studied robot-assisted general surgical procedures to date. First reported by Melvin et al. in 2001, multiple authors have since published case reports and case series demonstrating the safety and feasibility of the operation.[32] Although the laparoscopic approach has become increasingly common, a reported rate of perforation of 5% to 10% has been well described even among experienced surgical teams.[33] With the features of improved visualization and instrument articulation, many surgeons have hypothesized that robot-assistance may facilitate more accurate myotomy, decreasing the perforation rate. In a review in 2007, Ballantyne summarized the published experience with robot-assisted Heller myotomy for the treatment of esophageal achalasia.[17] At that time, eight case series had been reported with a total of 244 patients. Mucosal perforation was reported in only 2 of the 244 cases, resulting in a perforation rate of less than 1%; this is significantly different from the 5% to 10% perforation rates reported for conventional laparoscopic Heller myotomy. In addition, general morbidity and mortality rates for robot-assisted myotomy appeared to be similar to those reported for conventional laparoscopy.

Although the pooled data from these case series are promising, to date only one study has directly compared robot-assisted myotomy to conventional laparoscopic myotomy. Published by a multiinstitutional group of academic surgeons, the report retrospectively reviewed prospectively collected data on all the robot-assisted and conventional laparoscopic myotomies performed at three separate institutions. A total of 121 patients were included in the study, with 59 patients in the robot-assisted group and 62 patients in the conventional laparoscopy group. Patient characteristics were similar between the two groups. All procedures were completed using the intended techniques. Mean operative time was significantly longer in the robot-assisted group (141 versus 129 min; $P < 0.05$). However, this difference disappeared during the last 30 cases. Esophageal perforation rates were significantly higher in the conventional laparoscopic group compared to the robot-assisted group (16% versus 0%). Postoperative relief of dysphagia was comparably achieved in both groups, with 90% to 92% relief rates at 18 to 22 months of follow-up. Overall, the authors thought that robot-assisted myotomy resulted in decreased esophageal perforation rates compared to conventional laparoscopy and was therefore a safer operation.[33]

Bariatric Surgery

Over the past several decades, morbid obesity has become an increasingly prevalent healthcare problem. In response to this, the field of bariatric surgery has grown rapidly. Recently, laparoscopic approaches to bariatric surgical procedures have become the standard of care given the benefits of decreased pain, length of hospital stay, and wound complications. However, laparoscopic bariatric surgical procedures are often technically challenging given the complex reconstructive nature of the procedures and the size of the patients. Because of this, several authors have investigated the use of robotic assistance to facilitate both laparoscopic adjustable gastric banding procedures and laparoscopic Roux-en-Y gastric bypass procedures. Specifically, Moser et al.[34] and Cadiere et al.[35] both reported the safety and feasibility of robot-assisted adjustable gastric band placement. Operative times and outcomes appeared comparable to conventional laparoscopy. In addition, the authors thought that robotic assistance was particularly useful in superobese patients in whom the thickness of the abdominal wall limits instrument mobility and affects surgeon ergonomics. Ballantyne also reported the use of the four-arm da Vinci system to facilitate solo surgery, enabling gastric band placement without an operative assistant.[17]

Robot-assisted laparoscopic Roux-en-Y gastric bypass has also been described. Most authors have used robotic surgical systems to perform the hand-sewn gastrojejunal anastomosis. In this situation, the features of intuitive movement, articulated instrumentation, tremor filtration, and improved visualization facilitate intracorporeal suturing. Ballantyne states that "clearly, suturing of gastrointestinal anastomoses with the wristed instruments, tremor filtration, and 3-D imaging is substantially easier than attempting this with traditional laparoscopic instruments and 2-D imaging."[17]

In a series of publications, the bariatric surgical group at Stanford University investigated the efficacy of a totally robotic Roux-en-Y laparoscopic gastric bypass procedure using the da Vinci Surgical System. Requiring an active surgical assistant as well as intraoperative repositioning and redocking of the surgical system to work in different abdominal quadrants, this procedure utilizes the robot to facilitate all aspects of the operation including a hand-sewn, double-layer gastrojejunal anastomosis. In their first publication, Mohr et al. compared the group's first 10 conventional laparoscopic Roux-en-Y gastric bypass procedures completed in 2002 to their first 10 robotic Roux-en-Y gastric bypass procedures. Morbidity (20%) and mortality (0%) rates were comparable in both groups. The robot-assisted procedures demonstrated significantly shorter mean operating times compared to traditional laparoscopy (169 versus 208 min). Furthermore, this difference was magnified for larger patients.[36] In a separate report, the group randomized a new laparoscopic fellow's first 50 patients to receive either a totally robotic Roux-en-Y laparoscopic gastric bypass or a conventional laparoscopic Roux-en-Y laparoscopic gastric bypass. Patient characteristics were similar between the two groups. Mean operating times were significantly shorter for the robot-assisted procedures compared to the conventional laparoscopic procedures (130.8 versus 149.4 min; $P = 0.02$). Once again, this difference was magnified for larger patients, with the most significant difference in mean operative times occurring in patients with a body mass index greater than 43 kg/m^2. The authors concluded that totally robotic Roux-en-Y gastric bypass was safe and feasible and required shorter operative times compared to convenional laparoscopy during a surgeon's learning curve. Based on this, they thought that the robot-assisted procedure may be superior to conventional laparoscopy when a hand-sewn gastrojejunal anastomosis is performed.[37]

Conclusion

Since their introduction in the 1990s, robotic surgical systems have been increasingly used to facilitate general surgical procedures. Review of the published literature demonstrates multiple case reports and case series, with a few prospective clinical trials. Early use was focused on common laparoscopic procedures such as cholecystectomy and Nissen fundoplication. For these procedures, robot assistance appears to be both safe and feasible. However, prospective trials comparing robot-assisted procedures to conventional laparoscopy demonstrate significantly longer operative times and higher cost with no additional benefit. Recently, more complex robot-assisted procedures have been reported, such as esophageal myotomy and bariatric operations. Once again, robot-assisted procedures appear to be safe and feasible. However, the features of the robotic systems such as intuitive movement, articulated instrumentation, and three-dimensional visualization may provide additional benefits leading to improved outcomes compared to conventional laparoscopy. In the case of esophageal myotomy, Horgan et al. reported a 0% mucosal perforation rate with robot-assisted Heller myotomy compared to a 16% rate with conventional laparoscopic Heller myotomy. In the case of Roux-en-Y gastric bypass for morbid obesity, Mohr and Sanchez reported shorter operating times and more rapid learning curves with robot assistance. Furthermore, this benefit appeared to magnify in larger patients.

Overall, published data suggest that robotic surgical systems show no benefit when routine laparoscopic procedures are performed but may be advantageous when performing complex, reconstructive procedures. Issues particular to general surgery such as multiquadrant abdominal surgery, and the ability to reposition the table during an operation were not clearly addressed, although authors believe that these concerns may be resolved with experience and technological improvements.

Robot-Assisted Urology

To date, multiple urological procedures have been performed using robotic surgical systems. Compared to other surgical fields, robot-assisted urological surgery has seen relatively rapid adoption. Procedures such as radical prostatectomy, cystectomy, and pyeloplasty have all been reported in the surgical literature and appear to be well suited to robotic assistance. In particular, robot-assisted radical prostatectomy—a procedure that involves complex dissection and reconstruction in a single, difficult-to-access anatomic area—seems to take advantage of the strengths of robotic technology while minimizing the drawbacks. Because of this, robot-assisted radical prostatectomy has become one of the most commonly performed robot-assisted procedures in the United States.

Similar to general surgical procedures, the published experience with robotic prostatectomy primarily consists of case reports and case series. No prospective randomized clinical trials have been performed comparing robot-assisted prostatectomy to conventional laparoscopy or even open procedures. However, several large, prospective clinical series and nonrandomized clinical studies have been published.

In the case of robot-assisted radical prostatectomy, the group at Henry Ford Hospital in Detroit, Michigan, has published the largest experience. Since the year 2000, this group has performed more than 2600 transperitoneal robot-assisted radical prostatectomies using the da Vinci Surgical System. In a recent publication, data on 1142 patients with at least 12-month follow-up were obtained evaluating both oncological and functional outcomes. On review, their actuarial 5-year biochemical recurrence rate was 8.4%. By 12 months, only 0.8% patients had total incontinence, and in men with no preoperative erectile dysfunction who underwent nerve-sparing surgery, the intercourse rate was 93%.[38] In an earlier review of their first 1100 cases, the group reported mean operative times of 70 to 160 min with a mean operative blood loss of 50 to 150 mL. Furthermore, 95% of their patients were discharged within 24 h of the operation.[39]

In another report, Menon and colleagues compared their robot-assisted prostatectomy (RAP) experience to their own experience with open, radical retropubic prostatectomy (RRP). In a single-institution, nonrandomized prospective study, this group compared 100 patients undergoing RRP with 200 patients undergoing RAP.[40] Patient characteristics including cancer stage were similar between the two groups. Mean operative times were also comparable (163 min for RRP versus 160 min for RAP). Intraoperative blood loss was significantly greater for the RRP group (910 mL for RRP versus 150 mL for RAP), and 67% of the RRP group received a blood transfusion compared to 0% of the RAP group. Hospital stay, duration of catheterization, time to resumption of urinary continence, and time to achievement of erections were also significantly longer for the RRP group compared to the RAP group. Last, positive margins on pathological review were more frequent in the RRP group versus the RAP group (23% versus 9% respectively; $P < 0.05$).[40]

In similar nonrandomized studies, both Ahlering et al.[41] and Farnham et al.[42] demonstrated significantly lower mean intraoperative blood loss with robot-assisted prostatectomy compared to open prostatectomy. Specifically, mean blood loss was 191 mL[41] and 103 mL[42] for the robot-assisted procedures and 418 mL[41] and 664 mL[42] for the open procedures. Furthermore, Ahlering and colleagues demonstrated similar operative times for the two techniques but a positive margin rate of 20% for the open prostatectomy versus 16% for the robot-assisted prostatectomy.[41]

Overall, the use of robotic surgical systems in urology appears to be growing. In particular, robot-assisted radical prostatectomy has seen increased adoption since its introduction. In fact, it is estimated that in the year 2005, more than 10% of all prostatectomies performed in the United States were performed using the da Vinci Surgical System.[43] This number appears to be increasing. Currently, large case series and nonrandomized clinical trials suggest that robot-assisted radical prostatectomy may result in decreased blood loss, shorter hospital stay, improved continence and potency rates, and lower positive margin rates compared to open retropubic radical prostatectomy. However, prospective randomized trials have yet to be reported. Furthermore, no high-quality studies have been published comparing robot-assisted prostatectomy to conventional laparoscopic prostatectomy.

Robot-Assisted Cardiac Surgery

Both the da Vinci and Zeus robotic surgical systems were initially conceived in large part to enable cardiac surgery to be performed via a minimally invasive endoscopic approach. Although the techniques of abdominal laparoscopy and thoracoscopy have grown and developed over the past two decades, their application toward cardiac procedures has been slow. The constraints imposed by operating within a closed, minimally expandable chest, the technical requirements of cardiopulmonary bypass, and the technical difficulties of operating on a beating heart have made the development of minimally invasive cardiac surgical approaches challenging. In many ways, the current robotic surgical systems were designed to overcome these challenges. Features of intuitive control of the instrument tips, articulated instrumentation, tremor reduction, and motion scaling further were intended to enhance control and precision to enable technically demanding tasks such as suturing a coronary anastomosis and repairing a mitral valve. To date, multiple cardiac surgical procedures have been performed using both the da Vinci and Zeus robotic surgical systems. Worldwide experience has been limited to a few centers in Europe and North America, although this number is growing. Compared to general surgery and urology, robot-assisted cardiac surgery requires additional, complimentary technologies to allow for femoral cannulation during arrested heart procedures or cardiac stabilization for beating heart procedures.

Mohr et al. reported the first robot-assisted harvest of an internal mammary artery to be used for coronary artery bypass grafting in 1998[44]; this was quickly followed by the first reported use of a robotic surgical system to sew a coronary anastomosis through a small left anterior thoracotomy by Falk et al.[45] Loulmet et al. from Paris reported the first totally endoscopic coronary artery bypass (TECAB) on an arrested heart in 1999 using a prototype of the da Vinci surgical system.[46] Kappert et al.[47], Falk et al.[48], and Mohr et al.[49] subsequently described early success in performing closed chest coronary bypass on the arrested heart. Cardiac arrest was achieved using femoral cannulation by modification of the Port-Access technique (Heartport, Redwood City, CA). Although shown to be technically feasible, the full benefits of MIS cardiac surgery were yet to be realized given the need for cardiac bypass, with all its attendant risks and physiological sequelae.

Beating heart totally endoscopic coronary artery bypass (TECAB) was realized with the creation of a novel endoscopic cardiac stabilizer (Intuitive Surgical, Sunnyvale, CA). Kappert et al. described a series of 37 patients who underwent this procedure, which involves three 1-cm incisions in the left thorax and an additional 1-cm incision in the subxyphoid position for the cardiac stabilizer.[50,51] The da Vinci Surgical System was utilized to harvest the internal mammary artery (IMA) and perform the anastomosis to the left anterior descending (LAD) artery. Average times for the IMA harvest was 35 min, anastomosis time was 30 min, and total operating time was 174 min. Of the initial group of 56 patients intended to undergo TECAB, 34% required conversion to a minithoracotomy. Challenges encountered include difficulties with endoscopic stabilization of the beating heart, exposure of intramural coronary target vessels, and occlusion of the LAD during the anastomosis. Similarly, Mohr et al. describe a subseries of beating heart TECAB procedures using the da Vinci Surgical System. Four of eight attempted procedures were completed with anastomosis times ranging from 24 to 48 min and coronary artery occlusion times ranging from 38 to 65 min.[49]

Mitral valve repair has also been demonstrated using the da Vinci Surgical System. Carpentier et al. reported the first successful robot-assisted mitral valve repair using a prototype of the da Vinci Surgical System in 1998.[52] In 2000, Chitwood et al. reported the first robot-assisted mitral valve repair in North America requiring a trapezoidal resection as well as placement of an annuloplasty band.[53] Since these initial reports, Nifong et al.[54] and Mohr et al.[49] have described their experience with quadrangular resections and sliding plasties, as well as chordal transfers and replacements. These procedures still necessitate cardiac arrest using the Port Access technique as well as a minithoracotomy to provide retraction and surgical assistance.

Recently, the results of several large clinical trials evaluating robot-assisted mitral valve surgery have been reported. In a multicenter, phase II FDA trial, 112 patients at 10 U.S. centers underwent robot-assisted mitral valve repairs using the da Vinci Surgical System.[55] The types of procedures included quadrangular resections, sliding plasties, edge-to-edge approximations, chordal transfers, and chordal replacements. Overall, few differences were seen between the different centers with respect to operating times. Specifically, mean leaflet repair time was 37 min and mean annuloplasty time was 39 min. Mean aortic cross-clamp time was 2.1 h, and mean cardiopulmonary bypass time was 2.8 h. Transthoracic echocardiography performed at 1 month postoperative demonstrated significant mitral regurgitation (grade 2) in 9 patients (8%), 6 of whom underwent reoperation.[56]

Recently, other innovative minimally invasive cardiac procedures have been reported using the da Vinci Surgical System: these include implantation of biventricular epicardial pacing wires for advanced heart failure,[57] repair of atrial septal defects,[58–60] and epicardial ablation for atrial fibrillation.[61]

Robotic-Assisted Vascular Surgery

Open aortic surgery for aneurysmal and occlusive disease is hindered by significant morbidity and mortality. First performed in the late 1990s, laparoscopic aortobifemoral bypass attempted to mitigate the trauma of aortic surgery.[62] Reported advantages of laparoscopic aortic surgery include decreased ileus, hospital stay, and narcotic use.[63] Laparoscopic aortic surgery is limited by a steep learning curve and resultant long operative times. Robotic approaches to aortic pathology were proposed to address these deficiencies of totally laparoscopic techniques, primarily by decreasing anastomotic times. Robotic aortic surgery is currently nascent and requires laparoscopic exposure of the aorta, meaning these procedures are most aptly described as "robotic-assisted." Table 114.5 presents the two largest published experiences with robotic-assisted aortic surgery.[64,65]

As outlined by Stadler et al., robotic-assisted aortic surgery requires placing the patient on his or her right side in slight Trendelenburg position. Six 11- or 12-mm ports are introduced in the left flank. Conventional laparoscopy is used to mobilize the descending colon through a transperitoneal approach. The posterior and parietal peritoneum are sewn together to maintain exposure of the aorta. In the case of an aortobifemoral bypass, clamps are passed from the groin into the abdomen under laparoscopic visualization. The robot is introduced into the field and is used for all suturing. The patient is heparinized, and aortic cross-clamps are applied. The aorta is opened, and lumbar arteries are oversewn with 4-0 polytetrafluoroethylene sutures. Proximal and distal anastomoses are created using 3-0 or 4-0 Gore-Tex (W.L. Gore and Associates, Flagstaff, AZ) sutures.[64]

Stadler's published experience with robotic-assisted aortic surgery involved 30 procedures over an 8 month period. Results included a median operating time of 236 (range, 180–

TABLE 114.5.
Published Experience with Robot-Assisted Aortic Surgery.

Reference	*System*	*No. of patients*	*Study design*	*Total operating room time (min)*[a]	*Morbidity*	*Mortality*	*Conversion*
Stadler et al.[64]	da Vinci®	Robotic = 30	Case series	236	2	1	0
Diks et al.[65]	da Vinci®	Robotic = 17	Case series	365	1	1	3

[a]Represents total time in operating room.

360) min, an aortic clamp time of 54 min, an anastomotic time of 27 min, and blood loss of 320 mL. Median intensive care unit (ICU) time and length of stay were 1.8 and 5.4 days, respectively. Perioperative morbidity included one episode of atrial fibrillation and a transient elevation of liver function tests. There were no mortalities or conversions to an open approach. The primary advantage of the robot in this experience was a decreased aortic cross-clamp time.[64]

A subsequent report by Diks et al. evaluated the effects of experience on outcomes of robotic-assisted aortic surgery, dividing their series into early (group 1, $n = 8$) and late (group 2, $n = 9$) cohorts. Median cross-clamp and anastomotic times were statistically significantly shorter in the second group, 111 min (range, 85–205 min) versus 57.5 min (range, 25–130 min), and 74 min (range, 40–110 min) versus 36 min (range, 22–69 min), respectively. Although the data reveal clear trends in favor of the latter group, differences in total operative time 405 min (range, 260–589 min) versus 339 min (range, 225–465 min), blood loss, and hospital stay were not statistically significant. The authors concluded that their longer operative times were explained by the fact that they remained on the steep part of the learning curve.[65]

In sum, current data suggest that a robotic approach to aortic pathology decreases aortic cross-clamp and anastomotic times in comparison to those achieved using laparoscopy alone. Equipment costs, reliance on laparoscopy for exposure, a compromised ability to address bleeding, and the absence of tactile feedback presently limit the utility of robotics in vascular surgery. Moreover, intense competition from endovascular approaches along with minimal or absent laparoscopic and robotic capabilities among many vascular surgeons have curtailed rapid adoption of robotic assistance in the treatment of aortic pathology. Refinements in techniques and technology, including aortic stapling devices, are next steps in the progression toward robotic vascular procedures. Ultimately, comparisons to the surgical standard of care are necessary to define the advantages of robotics in the care of the patient with vascular disease.

Robotic-Assisted Pediatric Surgery

To date there is only a small body of literature regarding the application of robotic technology for pediatric surgical procedures. Hollands et al.[14,66,67] and Lorincz et al.[68] have both described the application of the Zeus robotic system in a porcine model. Technically challenging procedures such as enteroenterostomy, hepaticojejunostomy, portoenterostomy, and esophagoesophagostomy were all demonstrated to be technically feasible. Similarly, Malhotra et al.,[69] Aaronson et al.,[70] and Olsen et al.[71] have described the application of the da Vinci system in animal models to perform complex pediatric cardiovascular, neurosurgical, and urological procedures.

Several authors have reported a small but assorted variety of human pediatric cases performed with both the Zeus and da Vinci systems (Table 114.6). On average, setup and operative times were longer with the robotic cases when compared to standard laparoscopy. The rate of complications or conversion to open surgery has been low. Significant long-term follow-up for any differences in clinical outcome have yet to be reported. Specialized training of the surgical teams and the expense of the equipment remain substantial obstacles to widespread adoption. However, the authors in common have applauded the introduction of high-quality three-dimensional vision, articulated instrument tips, and intuitive instrument control which all seem to enhance surgical precision. To fully evaluate the potential benefits and application to pediatric surgery, further studies are warranted.

Discussion

During the past decade, robotic surgical systems have emerged as unique, somewhat controversial, and increasingly utilized tools in today's operating rooms. Originally driven by the U.S. government's interest in battlefield surgical systems, followed by technological capability and market forces, these systems have been utilized in multiple surgical disciplines. To date, these systems have generally been used to facilitate complex minimal access operations, given their unique features of three-dimensional visualization, articulated intuitive instrumentation, motion scaling, and tremor reduction. However, their clinical value to the patient and to the surgeon is still being determined. Early reports demonstrated the safety and feasibility of robot-assisted procedures. More recently, prospective studies have compared robot-assisted procedures to conventional laparoscopic procedures. Overall, the literature indicates that robotic assistance adds little to no benefit to more routine laparoscopic procedures such as cholecystectomy and Nissen fundoplication with longer mean operating times and additional cost. However, early studies suggest improved outcomes with robot assistance for more complex procedures such as Heller myotomy, Roux-en-Y gastric bypass, and prostatectomy. In addition, robotic assistance has enabled a minimal access approach to procedures that were largely performed via open incisions, such as coronary artery bypass grafting and mitral valve repair. The widespread applicability and clinical value of these procedures have yet to be fully determined.

TABLE 114.6.
Pediatric Clinical Experience with the Zeus® and da Vinci® Robotic Systems.

Reference	*System*	*No. of patients*	*Operative procedure*	*Results*	*Comments*
Le Bret et al.[79]	Zeus®	56	Patent ductus arteriosus ligation (28 thoracoscopic, 28 robotic)	Operating room time: thoracoscopic = 83 min; robotic = 162 min Surgical procedure time: thoracoscopic = 24 min; robotic = 50 min	Longer operative time for robotic group; 1 conversion to videothoracoscopic; no significant difference in complications or outcome
Lorincz et al.[68]	Zeus®	7	5 Nissen fundoplication; 1 cholecystectomy; 1 Heller myotomy	Operative time for fundoplication reduced from 4.5 h to 1.5 h	Rapid improvement in case times as team progressed along learning curve
Gutt et al.[80] and Heller et al.[81]	Da Vinci®	14	11 fundoplication; 2 cholecystectomy; 1 bilateral salpingo-oophorectomy	Operative times: fundoplication = 146 min (mean); cholecystectomy 105, 150 min; salpingo-oophorectomy 95 min	No complications or conversion to laparotomy
Luebbe et al.[82]	Da Vinci®	20	10 fundoplication; 3 cholecystectomy; 2 splenectomy; 1 urachus resection; 1 Morgagni diaphragmatic hernia; 3 biopsies; 1 lymphadenectomy	Mean times: OR setup = 45 min; patient preparation = 17 min; console operating time = 93 min (range, 10–299 min)	15% complications (2 conversions to laparotomy for bleeding, 1 pneumothorax)
Mihaljevic et al.[83]	Da Vinci®	2	Vascular ring dissection	Total operative times: 172.5 min (mean) Robotic procedure times: 106.5 min (mean)	Total operative time longer than usually required for standard thoracoscopic procedure due to setup; dissection time slightly shorter in robotic cases

From a technological standpoint, today's robotic surgical systems represent a significant advance in surgical instrumentation. Despite these improvements, there remain significant obstacles to the widespread adoption of these robotic systems. Chief among these is cost for both the robotic systems and their array of instruments. Robotic procedure times are predictably longer when compared to the conventional laparoscopic approach, at least for the initial series of cases until the surgical team becomes facile with the use of the new technology. The robotic systems themselves are somewhat large and obtrusive, at times impeding access by the anesthesiologist or patient-side surgeon. In addition, the current da Vinci system does not allow for repositioning of the patient without undocking the system. Until recently, the robotic instruments were significantly larger than their laparoscopic equivalents. For instance, the da Vinci instruments required 8-mm ports; the 3-D endoscope required a 12-mm port. Currently, 5-mm instruments and 5-mm 2-D endoscopes are available. Finally, the lack of significant haptic feedback continues to be a major drawback to precise surgical dissection. Undoubtedly, many of these issues will need to be addressed in the next generation of equipment as the technology continues to improve.

Future Directions

Although the current robotic systems represent significant strides in technology, possibilities for innovation remain. The use of a video image that is processed through a computer system, rather than direct vision, allows for the overlay of any number of images or information. With this type of "augmented reality" display, vital signs, preoperative imaging studies, and other patient information may be projected directly in front of the surgeon's eyes throughout the course of an operation. Incorporating preoperative image registration techniques, computer systems may be made aware of both the patient's anatomy as well as the position of the operative instruments. Using these data, a virtual "safety envelope" may be defined and used to warn a surgeon away from inadvertent damage to collateral tissues.

Currently, research and development of haptic feedback systems is occurring around the world at the university and industry levels. Current robotic surgical systems only provide extremely gross force reflection. However, accurate tactile sensation is often an important element of surgery. If developed, haptic feedback-enabled instrument tips would represent a significant new advance for minimal access surgery. In addition to tensile feedback, other biological data could be relayed back to the surgeon including temperature, oxygen tension, and tissue density. The NASA Smartprobe project is already developing these types of sensors.[72]

From a surgeon's ergonomic standpoint, advances in robotic technology may focus in minimizing the size and space requirements of the robotic systems. Improved robotic arm articulations will better facilitate multiquadrant surgery, and changes in the way that surgical robots interface with intracorporeal instruments will allow the robots to adjust while a patient is repositioned.

Improvements in robotic surgical systems may also be used to enhance ergonomics in the operating room. For instance, the operative instruments can be programmed to align with the axis of view of the endoscope. Thus, wherever the endoscope is angled, it would appear to the surgeon that he or she is positioned at the end of the endoscope. For example, an angled endoscope inserted into the mouth and directed back toward the nasopharynx could establish a vantage point for the operative instruments such that one would seem to operate through the back of the patient's head.

From a training standpoint, robotic surgical systems may be used to track and record a surgeon's hand movements in relation to real-time patient data. Using this information, a surgeon in training may be able to first mimic, and then perform, an operation as it was performed by an experienced surgeon. This "player piano" model may be valuable to surgical education and may help in the development of more accurate and realistic surgical simulators.

A much-popularized idea is the concept of telesurgery, whereby a surgeon can perform an operation from a distance by means of a remote interface. This concept, first conceived for military applications, would allow for the delivery of surgical care to remote or inhospitable areas. It also allows a surgical authority to perform operations far beyond his immediate geographic vicinity. Recently, the world's first trans-Atlantic laparoscopic cholecystectomy was performed remotely, in which a surgeon located in New York operated on a patient in Strasbourg, France.[73] However, this concept is still severely restricted by the cost and capacity of current bandwidth technology, as well as the inviolate limit of the speed of light. A less ambitious application is telementoring, whereby an experienced specialist can observe and advise a surgical team operating in a remote location. Already, a growing number of procedures have been accomplished using this technology.[74–76]

Conclusion

Currently, robotic surgical systems represent novel and technologically advanced surgical tools that have the potential to facilitate complex minimal access procedures. Since their introduction in the late 1990s, worldwide experience has demonstrated the safety and feasibility of robot-assisted procedures across multiple surgical disciplines. However, the true clinical value of these systems has yet to be fully determined. As the technology continues to be refined, the ultimate acceptance or robotic surgical systems as valuable surgical tools will demand that the issues of cost, training, safety, efficacy, and clinical utility all must be addressed.

References

1. Diodato MD Jr, Prosad SM, Klingensmith ME, Damiano RJ Jr. Robotics in surgery. Curr Probl Surg 2004;41(9):752–810.
2. Dharia SP, Falcone T. Robotics in reproductive medicine. Fertil Steril 2005;84(1):1–11.
3. Camarillo DB, Krummel TM, Salisbury JK Jr. Robotic technology in surgery: past, present, and future. Am J Surg 2004;188(4A suppl):2S–15S.
4. Allaf M, Patriciu A, Mazilu D, Kavoussi L, Stoianovici D. Overview and fundamentals of urologic robot-integrated systems. Urol Clin N Am 2004;31(4):671–682, vii.
5. Adler JR Jr, Chang SD, Murphy MJ, Doty J, Geis P, Hancock SL. The Cyberknife: a frameless robotic system for radiosurgery. Stereotact Funct Neurosurg 1997;69(1–4):124–128.
6. Kuo JS, Yu C, Petrovich Z, Apuzzo ML. The CyberKnife stereotactic radiosurgery system: description, installation, and an initial evaluation of use and functionality. Neurosurgery 2003; 53(5):1235–1239; discussion 1239.
7. Kasalicky MA, Svab J, Fried M, Melechovsky D. AESOP 3000—computer-assisted surgery, personal experience. Rozhl Chir 2002;81(7):346–349.
8. Arezzo A, Testa T, Ulmer F, Schurr MO, Degregori M, Buess GF. Positioning systems for endoscopic solo surgery. Minerva Chir 2000;55(9):635–641.
9. Mettler L, Ibrahim M, Jonat W. One year of experience working with the aid of a robotic assistant (the voice-controlled optic holder AESOP) in gynaecological endoscopic surgery. Hum Reprod 1998;13(10):2748–2750.
10. Okada S, Tanaba Y, Yaegashi S, et al. Initial use of the newly developed voice-controlled robot system for a solitary pulmonary arterio-venous malformation. Kyobu Geka 2002;55(10):871–875.
11. Lee BR, Chow GK, Ratner LE, Kavoussi LR. Laparoscopic live donor nephrectomy: outcomes equivalent to open surgery. J Endourol 2000;14(10):811–819; discussion 819–820.
12. Luebbe B, Woo R, Wolf S, Irish M. Robotically assisted minimally invasive surgery in a pediatric population: initial experience, technical considerations, and description of the da Vinci Surgical System. Pediatr Endosurg Innov Tech 2003;7(4):385–402.
13. Falk V, Diegeler A, Walther T, et al. Endoscopic coronary artery bypass grafting on the beating heart using a computer enhanced telemanipulation system. Heart Surg Forum 1999;2(3):199–205.
14. Hollands CM, Dixey LN. Applications of robotic surgery in pediatric patients. Surg Laparosc Endosc Percutan Tech 2002; 12(1):71–76.
15. Himpens J, Leman G, Cadiere GB. Telesurgical laparoscopic cholecystectomy. Surg Endosc 1998;12(8):1091.
16. Gutt CN, Oniu T, Mehrabi A, Kashfi A, Schemmer P, Buchler MW. Robot-assisted abdominal surgery. Br J Surg 2004; 91(11):1390–1397.
17. Ballantyne GH. Telerobotic gastrointestinal surgery: phase 2—safety and efficacy. Surg Endosc 2007;21:1054–1062.
18. Ruurda JP, Visser PL, Broeders IA. Analysis of procedure time in robot-assisted surgery: comparative study in laparoscopic cholecystectomy. Comput Aided Surg 2003;8(1):24–29.
19. Hourmont K, Chung W, Pereira S, Wasielewski A, Davies R, Ballantyne GH. Robotic versus telerobotic laparoscopic cholecystectomy: duration of surgery and outcomes. Surg Clin N Am 2003;83(6):1445–1462.
20. Nio D, Bemelman WA, Busch OR, Vrouenraets BC, Gouma DJ. Robot-assisted laparoscopic cholecystectomy versus conventional laparoscopic cholecystectomy: a comparative study. Surg Endosc 2004;18(3):379–382.
21. Zhou HX, Guo YH, Yu XF, et al. Clinical characteristics of remote Zeus robot-assisted laparoscopic cholecystectomy: a report of 40 cases. World J Gastroenterol 2006;12(16):2606–2609.
22. Kornprat P, Werkgartner G, Cerwenka H, et al. Prospective study comparing standard and robotically assisted laparoscopic cholecystectomy. Langenbecks Arch Surg 2006;391(3):216–221.
23. Ruurda JP, Draaisma WA, van Hillegersberg R, et al. Robot-assisted endoscopic surgery: a four-year single-center experience. Dig Surg 2005;22(5):313–320.
24. Cadiere GB, Himpens J, Vertruyen M, et al. Evaluation of telesurgical (robotic) NISSEN fundoplication. Surg Endosc 2001;15(9):918–923.

25. Nakadi IE, Melot C, Closset J, et al. Evaluation of da Vinci Nissen fundoplication clinical results and cost minimization. World J Surg 2006;30(6):1050–1054.
26. Draaisma WA, Ruurda JP, Scheffer RC, et al. Randomized clinical trial of standard laparoscopic versus robot-assisted laparoscopic Nissen fundoplication for gastro-oesophageal reflux disease. Br J Surg. Nov 2006;93(11):1351–1359.
27. Weber PA, Merola S, Wasielewski A, Ballantyne GH. Telerobotic-assisted laparoscopic right and sigmoid colectomies for benign disease. Dis Colon Rectum 2002;45(12):1689–1694; discussion 1695–1686.
28. Ballantyne GH, Ewing D, Pigazzi A, Wasielewski A. Telerobotic-assisted laparoscopic right hemicolectomy: lateral to medial or medial to lateral dissection? Surg Laparosc Endosc Percutan Tech 2006;16(6):406–410.
29. Delaney CP, Lynch AC, Senagore AJ, Fazio VW. Comparison of robotically performed and traditional laparoscopic colorectal surgery. Dis Colon Rectum. 2003;46(12):1633–1639.
30. D'Annibale A, Morpurgo E, Fiscon V, et al. Robotic and laparoscopic surgery for treatment of colorectal diseases. Dis Colon Rectum 2004;47(12):2162–2168.
31. Anvari M, Birch DW, Bamehriz F, Gryfe R, Chapman T. Robotic-assisted laparoscopic colorectal surgery. Surg Laparosc Endosc Percutan Tech 2004;14(6):311–315.
32. Melvin WS, Needleman BJ, Krause KR, Wolf RK, Michler RE, Ellison EC. Computer-assisted robotic Heller myotomy: initial case report. J Laparoendosc Adv Surg Tech A 2001;11(4):251–253.
33. Horgan S, Galvani C, Gorodner MV, et al. Robotic-assisted Heller myotomy versus laparoscopic Heller myotomy for the treatment of esophageal achalasia: multicenter study. J Gastrointest Surg 2005;9(8):1020–1029; discussion 1029–1030.
34. Moser F, Horgan S. Robotically assisted bariatric surgery. Am J Surg 2004;188(4A suppl):38S–44S.
35. Cadiere GB, Himpens J, Vertruyen M, Favretti F. The world's first obesity surgery performed by a surgeon at a distance. Obes Surg 1999;9(2):206–209.
36. Mohr CJ, Nadzam GS, Curet MJ. Totally robotic Roux-en-Y gastric bypass. Arch Surg 2005;140(8):779–786.
37. Sanchez BR, Mohr CJ, Morton JM, Safadi BY, Alami RS, Curet MJ. Comparison of totally robotic laparoscopic Roux-en-Y gastric bypass and traditional laparoscopic Roux-en-Y gastric bypass. Surg Obes Relat Dis 2005;1(6):549–554.
38. Menon M, Shrivastava A, Kaul S, et al. Vattikuti Institute prostatectomy: contemporary technique and analysis of results. Eur Urol 2007;51(3):648–657; discussion 657–658.
39. Menon M, Tewari A, Peabody JO, et al. Vattikuti Institute prostatectomy, a technique of robotic radical prostatectomy for management of localized carcinoma of the prostate: experience of over 1100 cases. Urol Clin N Am 2004;31(4):701–717.
40. Tewari A, Srivasatava A, Menon M. A prospective comparison of radical retropubic and robot-assisted prostatectomy: experience in one institution. BJU Int 2003;92(3):205–210.
41. Ahlering TE, Woo D, Eichel L, Lee DI, Edwards R, Skarecky DW. Robot-assisted versus open radical prostatectomy: a comparison of one surgeon's outcomes. Urology 2004;63(5):819–822.
42. Farnham SB, Webster TM, Herrell SD, Smith JA Jr. Intraoperative blood loss and transfusion requirements for robotic-assisted radical prostatectomy versus radical retropubic prostatectomy. Urology 2006;67(2):360–363.
43. Rocco B, Djavan B. Robotic prostatectomy: facts or fiction? Lancet 2007;369(9563):723–724.
44. Mohr FW, Falk V, Diegeler A, Autschback R. Computer-enhanced coronary artery bypass surgery. J Thorac Cardiovasc Surg 1999;117(6):1212–1214.
45. Falk V, Fann JI, Grunenfelder J, Daunt D, Burdon TA. Endoscopic computer-enhanced beating heart coronary artery bypass grafting. Ann Thorac Surg 2000;70(6):2029–2033.
46. Loulmet D, Carpentier A, d'Attellis N, et al. Endoscopic coronary artery bypass grafting with the aid of robotic assisted instruments. J Thorac Cardiovasc Surg 1999;118(1):4–10.
47. Kappert U, Cichon R, Gulielmos V, et al. Robotic-enhanced Dresden technique for minimally invasive bilateral internal mammary artery grafting. Heart Surg Forum 2000;3(4):319–321.
48. Falk V, Diegeler A, Walther T, et al. Total endoscopic computer enhanced coronary artery bypass grafting. Eur J Cardiothorac Surg 2000;17(1):38–45.
49. Mohr FW, Falk V, Diegeler A, et al. Computer-enhanced "robotic" cardiac surgery: experience in 148 patients. J Thorac Cardiovasc Surg 2001;121(5):842–853.
50. Kappert U, Cichon R, Schneider J, et al. Technique of closed chest coronary artery surgery on the beating heart. Eur J Cardiothorac Surg. 2001;20(4):765–769.
51. Kappert U, Schneider J, Cichon R, et al. Development of robotic enhanced endoscopic surgery for the treatment of coronary artery disease. Circulation 2001;104(12 suppl 1):I102–I107.
52. Carpentier A, Loulmet D, Aupecle B, et al. Computer assisted open heart surgery. First case operated on with success. C R Acad Sci III 1998;321(5):437–442.
53. Chitwood WR Jr, Nifong LW, Elbeery JE, et al. Robotic mitral valve repair: trapezoidal resection and prosthetic annuloplasty with the da Vinci surgical system. J Thorac Cardiovasc Surg 2000;120(6):1171–1172.
54. Nifong LW, Chu VF, Bailey BM, et al. Robotic mitral valve repair: experience with the da Vinci system. Ann Thorac Surg 2003;75(2):438–442; discussion 443.
55. Nifong LW, Chitwood WR, Pappas PS, et al. Robotic mitral valve surgery: a United States multicenter trial. J Thorac Cardiovasc Surg 2005;129(6):1395–1404.
56. Kypson AP. Recent trends in minimally invasive cardiac surgery. Cardiology 2007;107(3):147–158.
57. Mair H, Jansens JL, Lattouf OM, Reichart B, Dabritz S. Epicardial lead implantation techniques for biventricular pacing via left lateral mini-thoracotomy, video-assisted thoracoscopy, and robotic approach. Heart Surg Forum 2003;6(5):412–417.
58. Argenziano M, Oz MC, DeRose JJ Jr, et al. Totally endoscopic atrial septal defect repair with robotic assistance. Heart Surg Forum 2002;5(3):294–300.
59. Argenziano M, Oz MC, Kohmoto T, et al. Totally endoscopic atrial septal defect repair with robotic assistance. Circulation 2003;108(suppl 1):II191–II194.
60. Argenziano M, Williams MR. Robotic atrial septal defect repair and endoscopic treatment of atrial fibrillation. Semin Thorac Cardiovasc Surg 2003;15(2):130–140.
61. van Brakel TJ, Bolotin G, Nifong LW, et al. Robot-assisted epicardial ablation of the pulmonary veins: is a completed isolation necessary? Eur Heart J 2005;26(13):1321–1326.
62. Dion YM, Gracia CR, Estakhri M, et al. Totally laparoscopic aortobifemoral bypass: a review of 10 patients. Surg Laparosc Endosc 1998;8(3):165–170.
63. Coggia M, Di Centa I, Javerliat I, Alfonsi P, Kitzis M, Goeau-Brissonniere OA. Total laparoscopic abdominal aortic aneurysms repair. J Cardiovasc Surg (Torino) 2005;46(4):407–414.
64. Stadler P, Matous P, Vitasek P, Spacek M. Robot-assisted aortoiliac reconstruction: a review of 30 cases. J Vasc Surg 2006; 44(5):915–919.
65. Diks J, Nio D, Jongkind V, Cuesta MA, Rauwerda JA, Wisselink W. Robot-assisted laparoscopic surgery of the infrarenal aorta: the early learning curve. Surg Endosc 2007;21:1760–1763.
66. Hollands CM, Dixey LN. Robotic-assisted esophagoesophagostomy. J Pediatr Surg 2002;37(7):983–985; discussion 983–985.
67. Hollands CM, Dixey LN, Torma MJ. Technical assessment of porcine enteroenterostomy performed with ZEUS robotic technology. J Pediatr Surg 2001;36(8):1231–1233.

68. Lorincz A, Langenburg S, Klein M. Robotics and the pediatric surgeon. Curr Opin Pediatr 2003;15(3):262–266.
69. Malhotra SP, Le D, Thelitz S, et al. Robotic-assisted endoscopic thoracic aortic anastomosis in juvenile lambs. Heart Surg Forum 2002;6(1):38–42.
70. Aaronson OS, Tulipan NB, Cywes R, et al. Robot-assisted endoscopic intrauterine myelomeningocele repair: a feasibility study. Pediatr Neurosurg 2002;36(2):85–89.
71. Olsen LH, Deding D, Yeung CK, Jorgensen TM. Computer assisted laparoscopic pneumovesical ureter reimplantation a.m. Cohen: initial experience in a pig model. APMIS Suppl 2003;109:23–25.
72. Andrews RJ, Mah RW. The NASA Smart Probe Project for real-time multiple microsensor tissue recognition. Stereotact Funct Neurosurg 2003;80(1–4):114–119.
73. Marescaux J, Leroy J, Rubino F, et al. Transcontinental robot-assisted remote telesurgery: feasibility and potential applications. Ann Surg 2002;235(4):487–492.
74. Marescaux J, Mutter D, Soler L, Vix M, Leroy J. The Virtual University applied to telesurgery: from tele-education to tele-manipulation. Bull Acad Natl Med 1999;183(3):509–521.
75. Marescaux J, Rubino F. Telesurgery, telementoring, virtual surgery, and telerobotics. Curr Urol Rep 2003;4(2):109–113.
76. Marescaux J, Soler L, Mutter D, et al. Virtual university applied to telesurgery: from teleeducation to telemanipulation. Stud Health Technol Inform 2000;70:195–201.
77. Ruurda JP, Visser PL, Broeders IA. Analysis of procedure time in robot-assisted surgery: comparative study in laparoscopic cholecystectomy. Comput Aided Surg 2003;8(1):24–29.
78. Cadiere GB, Himpens J, Vertruyen M, et al. Evaluation of telesurgical (robotic) NISSEN fundoplication. Surg Endosc 2001;15(9):918–923.
79. Le Bret E, Papadatos S, Folliguet T, et al. Interruption of patent ductus arteriosus in children: robotically assisted versus videothoracoscopic surgery. J Thorac Cardiovasc Surg 2002;123(5):973–976.
80. Gutt CN, Markus B, Kim ZG, Meininger D, Brinkmann L, Heller K. Early experiences of robotic surgery in children. Surg Endosc 2002;16(7):1083–1086.
81. Heller K, Gutt C, Schaeff B, Beyer PA, Markus B. Use of the robot system da Vinci for laparoscopic repair of gastrooesophageal reflux in children. Eur J Pediatr Surg 2002;12(4):239–242.
82. Luebbe B, Wolf SA, Irish MS. Robotically assisted minimally invasive surgery in a pediatric population: initial experience, technical considerations, and description of the da Vinci® Surgical System. Pediatr Endosurg Innov Tech. 2003;7(4):385–402.
83. Mihaljevic T, Cannon JW, del Nido PJ. Robotically assisted division of a vascular ring in children. J Thorac Cardiovasc Surg 2003;125(5):1163–1164.

Index

Index

D

F

J

K

P

W